Medical and Health Information Directory

Volume 1:

Organizations, Agencies, and Institutions

ISSN 0749-9973

SIXTEENTH EDITION
(In Three Volumes)

Medical and Health Information Directory

A Guide to Organizations, Agencies, Institutions, Programs, Publications, Services, and Other Resources Concerned with Clinical Medicine, Basic Biomedical Sciences, and the Technological and Socioeconomic Aspects of Health Care

Volume 1:

Organizations, Agencies, and Institutions

Amanda C. Quick
Project Editor

GALE®

THOMSON
GALE™

Detroit • New York • San Diego • San Francisco • Cleveland • New Haven, Conn. • Waterville, Maine • London • Munich

THOMSON
GALE

Medical and Health Information Directory, 16th Edition
Volume 1

Project Editor
Amanda C. Quick

Editorial
Jaime E. Noce

Editorial Support Services
Scott Flaugher

Product Design
Cynthia Baldwin, Kate Scheible

Composition and Electronic Prepress
Evi Seoud

Manufacturing
Rita Wimberley

For more information, contact
The Gale Group, Inc.
27500 Drake Rd.
Farmington Hills, MI 48331-3535
Or you can visit our Internet site at
http://www.gale.com

ISBN 0-7876-6910-5 (Volume 1)
ISBN 0-7876-6911-3 (Volume 2)
ISBN 0-7876-6912-1 (Volume 3)
ISBN 0-7876-6909-1 (Set)
ISSN 0749-9973

Printed in the United States of America
10 9 8 7 6 5 4 3 2 1

Contents

Volume 1 of the *Medical and Health Information Directory (MHID)*, now in its sixteenth edition, is a convenient one-stop source of contact and descriptive information on medical and health-related organizations, agencies, and institutions. It directs health care professionals and the public alike to a wide variety of organizations, including:

- National & International Organizations
- State & Regional Organizations
- Foundations & Funding Organizations
- Consultants & Consulting Organizations
- Peer Review Organizations
- Medical Ethics Organizations
- Hospital Management Companies
- Pharmaceutical Companies
- Federal Government Agencies
- Federal Domestic Assistance Programs
- State Government Agencies
- University-Related & Other Nonprofit Research Centers
- Federal Government Research Agencies, Facilities & Programs
- Medical & Allied Health Schools Comprehensive Coverage

Volume 1 profiles nearly 30,000 organizations, agencies, and institutions, primarily in the United States, that are involved in some aspect of the medical or health care fields. Entries represent a wide range of subject matter within the following broad areas:

- basic biomedical sciences
- clinical medicine
- technological and socioeconomic aspects of health care

Content and Arrangement

Volume 1 consists of Descriptive Listings and an Alphabetical Name and Keyword Index.

Descriptive Listings are organized within 18 separate chapters, according to type of organization, agency, or institution, as outlined on the "Contents" pages.

Alphabetical Name and Keyword Index speeds access to Volume 1 entries through a consolidated listing of all organizations, agencies, and institutions included in the book, as well as to significant keywords appearing in organization names.

For additional information on the content, arrangement, and indexing of Volume 1, consult the "User's Guide" following this introduction.

Method of Compilation

The sixteenth edition of Volume 1 represents a complete revision and updating of all material presented in the previous edition, incorporating thousands of changes to addresses, telephone numbers, personnel, and other key details.

Many sources were used to update this edition. Entries relevant to the medical and allied health fields were carefully selected from Gale directories, federal government documents, state government publications, and lists and directories supplied by numerous national organizations. Telephone inquiries were also employed to gather data and/or verify information.

Companion Volumes Profile Information Resources and Health Services

The companion volumes in this set complement volume 1's coverage of health and medical organizations, agencies, and institutions:

- **Volume 2** covers over 13,000 publications, libraries, and other information resources
- **Volume 3** lists over 33,000 health services, including clinics, treatment centers, care programs, and counseling/diagnostic services

Together, these volumes provide complete coverage of the medical and health care information and delivery system.

Comments Welcome

We encourage users to bring new or unlisted resources to our attention. Every effort will be made to include them in subsequent editions of *MHID.* Comments and suggestions for improving the directory are also welcome. Please contact:

Medical and Health Information Directory
The Gale Group, Inc.
27500 Drake Rd.
Farmington Hills, MI 48331-3535
Telephone: (248)699-GALE
Toll-Free: (800)347-GALE
Fax: (248)699-8070
E-mail: BusinessProducts@gale.com

Volume 1 of the *Medical and Health Information Directory (MHID)* consists of a main body of Descriptive Listings grouped within separate chapters by organization type, and an Alphabetical Name and Keyword Index, which provides a convenient alphabetical listing of all organizations, agencies, and institutions included in Volume 1. Each part is described below.

Listings are numbered sequentially within 18 separate chapters, as outlined on the "Contents" pages. Details on the content, arrangement, indexing, and sources for each chapter are provided in the following descriptions.

National & International Organizations

- Scope: Primarily nonprofit membership groups, including national organizations of the United States, as well as organizations that are international in scope, membership, or interest and are headquartered outside the United States.
- Entries Include: Organization name, address, telephone number, toll-free and fax numbers, e-mail address, web site, name and title of the chief official, and a brief description, including former/alternate names, founding date, number of members, purpose, and publications. In non-U.S. entries, the principal foreign-language name is listed in parentheses following the English-language version of the organization name.
- Arrangement: Alphabetical by organization names.
- Indexed by: Organization names, both English- and foreign-language; former/alternate names; and significant keywords within names.
- Source: *Encyclopedia of Associations, Volume 1: National Organizations of the U.S.* and *Encyclopedia of Associations: International Organizations* (published by Gale).

State & Regional Organizations

- Scope: State and regional affiliates of 46 national organizations.
- Entries Include: Organization name, address, telephone number, fax number, e-mail address, and web site.
- Arrangement: Geographical by states, then alphabetical by organization names within subject category.

Foundations & Funding Organizations

- Scope: U.S. funding organizations, including major private and corporate foundations that provide charitable support to nonprofit organizations, as well as professional associations and special interest groups that administer scholarship, fellowship, and grant programs, and provide other financial assistance for a variety of medical and health-related interests.
- Entries Include: Organization name, address, telephone number, toll-free and fax numbers, e-mail address, web site, and basic descriptive information on the funding program, including foundation philosophy, giving priorities, typical health-related recipients, and geographic distribution of funds.
- Arrangement: Alphabetical by organization names within three sections: 1) Private Foundations, 2) Corporate Foundations, and 3) Other Funding Organizations.
- Indexed by: Organization names and significant keywords within names.
- Source: *Foundation Reporter* and *Corporate Giving Directory* (both published by the Taft Group); and *Encyclopedia of Associations, Volume 1: National Organizations of the U.S.* (published by Gale).

Consultants & Consulting Organizations

- Scope: Individuals and firms that provide consulting services to the health care industry.
- Entries Include: Consultant or consulting organization name, address, telephone number, toll-free and fax numbers, e-mail address, web site, founding date, and a brief description of consulting activities.

- Arrangement: Geographical by states and cities, then alphabetical by consultant/organization names within cities.
- Indexed by: Consultant or consulting organization names and significant keywords within names.
- Source: *Consultants & Consulting Organizations Directory* (published by Gale).

Peer Review Organizations

- Scope: Local peer review organizations contracted by the U.S. Health Care Financing Administration to monitor the hospital care of Medicare beneficiaries.
- Entries Include: Organization name, address, telephone number, and toll-free and fax numbers.
- Arrangement: Geographical by states.
- Indexed by: Organization names.
- Source: *Directory of Peer Review Organizations* (provided by the Health Care Financing Administration, U.S. Department of Health and Human Services).

Medical Ethics and History Organizations

- Scope: Organizations and institutions interested in medical ethics and its history.
- Entries Include: Organization name, address, telephone number, fax number, e-mail address, web site, and contact person.
- Arrangement: Alphabetical by organization names.
- Indexed by: Organization names.
- Source: Original research by the editorial staff.

Hospital Management Companies

- Scope: Hospital management companies.
- Entries Include: Organization name, address, telephone number, toll-free and fax numbers, e-mail address, web site, and total number of hospitals and beds, both domestic and foreign, that are owned and/or managed by the company listed.
- Arrangement: Alphabetical by organization names.
- Indexed by: Organization names.
- Source: *Directory of Privately-Owned Community Hospitals, Hospital Management Companies and Health-Systems, and Residential Treatment Facilities and Centers* (published for the Federation of American Health Systems by FAHS, 1405 N Pierce, Ste. 311, Little Rock, AR 72207).

Pharmaceutical Companies

- Scope: Pharmaceutical and related healthcare companies that manufacture a variety of human and veterinary prescription or over-the-counter drugs and diagnostic products.
- Entries Include: Organization name, address, telephone number, toll-free and fax numbers, e-mail address, and web site.
- Arrangement: Alphabetical by organization names.
- Indexed by: Organization names.
- Source: Original research by the editorial staff.

Dental Care Plans

- Scope: Dental service corporations that are active members of Delta Dental Plans Association. These dental service plans provide prepaid dental care coverage to the public on a group basis.
- Entries Include: Organization name, address, telephone number, and toll-free and fax numbers.
- Arrangement: Geographical by states.
- Indexed by: Organization names.
- Source: List provided by Delta Dental Plans Association (1515 W 22nd St., Ste. 1200, Oak Brook, IL 60521).

Blue Cross & Blue Shield Plans

- Scope: Blue Cross and Blue Shield Plans.
- Entries Include: Organization name, address, telephone number, toll-free and fax numbers, e-mail address, and web site.
- Arrangement: Geographical by states, then alphabetical by organization names within states.
- Indexed by: Organization names.
- Source: Original research by the editorial staff.

Commercial Insurance Companies

- Scope: Companies that offer various types of individual or group indemnity health insurance plans.
- Entries Include: Organization name, address, telephone number, toll-free and fax numbers, e-mail address, and web-site.
- Arrangement: Alphabetical by organization names.
- Indexed by: Organization names.
- Source: Original research by the editorial staff.

Managed Health Care Organizations

- Scope: Health Maintenance Organizations (HMOs), Preferred Provider Organizations (PPOs), and Point-of-Service (POS) Plans. HMOs are health delivery systems that offer plan enrollees comprehensive health coverage for hospital and physician services for a prepaid, fixed fee. HMOs contract with or directly employ participating health care providers, which HMO members are required to choose from for all health care services. A PPO is a health care benefit arrangement between a panel of providers (physicians, hospitals, and other health care professionals) and the purchasers of care (employers, insurance companies, or others) to provide health care services to its enrollees on a discounted fee-for-service basis. Patients may receive care from non-PPO physicians or hospitals, but are given financial incentives to select those providers affiliated with the PPO. POS Plans are similar to PPOs in that they provide in-network health services to enrollees at a lower cost than the services of non-network providers. The primary difference is that PPO enrollees are free to contact network specialists at their discretion, while POS participants must first receive authorization from a primary care physician in order to receive full benefits.

- Entries Include: Organization name, address, telephone number, toll-free and fax numbers, e-mail address, and web site.
- Arrangement: Geographical by states, then alphabetical by organization names within three sections: 1) Health Maintenance Organizations (HMOs), 2) Preferred Provider Organizations (PPOs), and 3) Point-of-Service (POS) Plans.
- Indexed by: Organization names.
- Source: Original research by the editorial staff.

Federal Government Agencies

- Scope: Units of the federal government concerned with medicine and health.
- Entries Include: Agency name, address, telephone number, and, in many cases, a brief description of agency programs and purposes.
- Arrangement: Alphabetical by agency names.
- Indexed by: Parent agency and specific unit names, as well as significant intermediate agency names and keywords within names.
- Source: *United States Government Manual* (published by the U.S. National Archives and Records Administration and available from the U.S. Government Printing Office) and original research by the editorial staff.

Federal Domestic Assistance Programs

- Scope: Federally-funded programs, projects, services, and activities that provide assistance or benefits (financial and non-financial) to the American public in areas relating to medicine and health.
- Entries Include: Parent agency name, program name, address, telephone number, and a brief program description. *Catalog of Federal Domestic Assistance* numbers are also included for easy cross-reference to complete Catalog listings.
- Arrangement: Alphabetical by agency and program names.
- Indexed by: Parent agency name, program name, and significant keywords within names.
- Source: *Catalog of Federal Domestic Assistance* (published by the U.S. General Services Administration and available from the U.S. Government Printing Office).

State Government Agencies

- Scope: Agencies that function in 27 areas relating to medicine and health.
- Entries Include: Agency name, address, telephone number, fax number, e-mail address, and web site.
- Arrangement: Geographical by states within subject category.
- Indexed by: State designations in agency names; for example: Michigan Department of Public Health, Alabama State Board of Pharmacy, etc.
- Source: Individual state government directories, lists provided by organizations and federal government agencies, and original research by the editorial staff.

University-Related & Other Nonprofit Research Centers

- Scope: Nonprofit university research centers and independent, nonprofit research organizations engaged in medical and health-related research on a continuing basis. Research is broadly interpreted to include fundamental, applied, and developmental studies, as well as data gathering, analysis, and synthesis activities. It does not, for the most part, include research supporting or research coordinating activities.
- Entries Include: Parent institution or organization name, research unit name, address, telephone number, toll-free and fax numbers, e-mail address, web site, director name, a brief description of principal activities and fields of research, and a listing of publications issued by the research unit.
- Arrangement: Alphabetical by institution or organization names.
- Indexed by: Parent institution or organization names, research unit names, and significant keywords within names.
- Source: *Research Centers Directory* (published by Gale).

Federal Government Research Agencies, Facilities & Programs

- Scope: U.S. government research centers and programs, including federal agencies and bureaus that are themselves research organizations, research facilities owned and operated by the federal government, government-owned/contractor-operated facilities, test centers and facilities, cooperative research programs, data collection and analysis activities, and offices that support research by awarding grants and/or contracts.

- Entries Include: Agency name, address, telephone number, fax number, e-mail address, web site, director name, a brief description of principal activities and fields of research, and a listing of serial or periodical publications issued by the research unit.

- Arrangement: Alphabetical by agency names.

- Indexed by: Parent agency names, research unit names, significant intermediate agency names, and significant keywords within names.

- Source: *Government Research Directory* (published by Gale).

Medical & Allied Health Schools

- Scope: Educational institutions and training programs in 29 occupational categories. Coverage is limited primarily to baccalaureate and advanced degree programs. To obtain information on related educational programs at other levels, consult the section description referred to under the "Arrangement" heading below. For other occupational categories not covered, consult the last section of the chapter, "Other Allied Health Educational Programs." It provides names, addresses, and telephone numbers of professional organizations to contact for information on careers and programs in the fields indicated. Information on schools and programs is also available from the American Medical Association (515 N State St., Chicago, IL 60610, (312)464-4635).

- Entries Include: Institution name, address, telephone number, fax number, e-mail address, web site.

- Arrangement: Geographical by state, then alphabetical by institution names within subject category. Each section of schools is accompanied by a description of the programs listed there, along with references to professional organizations that may be contacted for general information concerning accreditation or careers in that field.

- Indexed by: Institution names.

- Source: Lists provided by national organizations and original research by the editorial staff.

Alphabetical Name and Keyword Index

The Alphabetical Name and Keyword Index provides access to all entries included in Volume 1, as well as to former or alternate names that appear within the text of entries. Each organization, agency, and institution is indexed by the name listed and by significant keywords that are a part of that name. Index references are to book entry numbers rather than page numbers. Entry numbers appear in the index in boldface type if the reference is to a main entry, and in lightface type if the reference is to a former or alternate name included within the text of the cited entry.

Many of the entries in Volume 1 use a hierarchical organization name structure, with a parent organization and often intermediate sub-units preceding the specific unit name. The Alphabetical Name and Keyword Index offers access to all multiple-part organization names via the parent organization name. Some entries are also referenced under the specific unit name and some under a significant intermediate unit name. Multiple parts of names are separated in index citations by a bullet (•). If several entries have the same parent organization, as is the case with many of the government and university groups listed in Volume 1, the related units appear as a group under the name of the parent organization. The parent agencies of most federal government organizations are indexed under "U.S." (e.g., U.S. House of Representatives, U.S. Department of Health and Human Services, etc.).

Alphabetizing Rules

In both the descriptive listings chapters and the index, organization names are sorted on a word-by-word basis, so that "New York Easter Seal Society" comes before "Newark Beth Israel Medical Center." Initial articles ("A," "An," or "The") are ignored for sorting purposes. Conjunctions, articles, and most prepositions elsewhere in the names are also not considered in alphabetizing. In addition:

- Numbers are sorted as if spelled-out and interfiled alphabetically with other non-number words.

- Abbreviations such as "U.S.," "St.," "Mt.," "Ft.," and "Dr.," are sorted as if spelled-out and interfiled with names in which the full version of those words are used.

- Personal names are sorted under the first name, or initial, within the descriptive listings chapters. In the index, they can be accessed under both the first and last names.

Act.	Acting
Adj.	Adjutant
Admin.	Administrator
AFB	Air Force Base
AK	Alaska
AKA	Also Known As
AL	Alabama
Alt. Contact	Alternate Contact
Apt.	Apartment
AR	Arkansas
Assoc.	Associate
Asst.	Assistant
Ave.	Avenue
AZ	Arizona
Bldg.	Building
Blvd.	Boulevard
Br.	Branch
CA	California
Cat. No.	Catalogue Number
CEO	Chief Executive Officer
Chf.	Chief
Chm.	Chairman
Cir.	Circle
Clghse.	Clearinghouse
c/o	Care of
CO	Colorado
Co.	Company
Coll.	Collection
Comdr.	Commander
Commun.	Communication
Coord.	Coordinator
Corp.	Corporation
Couns.	Counselor
CT	Connecticut
Ct.	Court
Ctr.	Center
DC	District of Columbia
DE	Delaware
Dept.	Department
Desc	Description
Dir.	Director
Dr.	Drive
E.	East
Educ.	Education
Exec.	Executive
Expy.	Expressway
Ext.	Extension
First Pub	First Published
FL	Florida
Flr.	Floor
Fnded	Founded
Freq	Frequency
Frmly	Formerly
Ft.	Fort
Fwy.	Freeway
GA	Georgia
Gen.	General
Geo. Dist.	Geographical Distribution
GU	Guam
Hd.	Head
HI	Hawaii
Hwy.	Highway
IA	Iowa
ID	Idaho
IL	Illinois
IN	Indiana
Inc.	Incorporated
Info.	Information
KS	Kansas
KY	Kentucky
LA	Louisiana
Lang	Language
Lib.	Library
Libn.	Librarian
Ln.	Lane
MA	Massachusetts
MD	Maryland
ME	Maine
Med.	Medical
Mem	Members
Mgr.	Manager
MI	Michigan
MN	Minnesota
MO	Missouri
MS	Mississippi
MT	Montana
Mt.	Mount
N.	North
Natl.	National
NC	North Carolina
ND	North Dakota
NE	Nebraska, Northeast
NH	New Hampshire
NJ	New Jersey
No.	Number
NV	Nevada
NW	Northwest
NY	New York
Off.	Officer
OH	Ohio
OK	Oklahoma
OR	Oregon
PA	Pennsylvania
Pgs	Pages
Pkwy.	Parkway
Pl.	Place
Plz.	Plaza
PO Box	Post Office Box
PR	Puerto Rico
Pres.	President
Prog.	Program
Pub	Publication
RD	Rural Delivery
Rd.	Road
Ref.	Reference
Reg.	Regional
Res.	Research
RFD	Rural Free Delivery
RI	Rhode Island
Rm.	Room
RR	Rural Route
Rte.	Route
S.	South
SC	South Carolina
Sci.	Science
SD	South Dakota
SE	Southeast
Sec.	Secretary
Sect.	Section
Serv.	Service
Soc.	Social
Spec.	Specialist
Sq.	Square
Sr.	Senior
St.	Saint, Street

Sta.	Station
Ste.	Suite, Sainte
Subscript	Subscription(s)
Supv.	Supervisor
SW	Southwest
Telecom	Telecommunications
Ter.	Terrace
TN	Tennessee
Tpke.	Turnpike
Trl.	Trail
TX	Texas
Univ.	University
U.S.	United States
U.S. Dist	U.S. Distributor
UT	Utah
VA	Virginia
VI	Virgin Islands
VP	Vice President
VT	Vermont
W.	West
WA	Washington
WV	West Virginia
WY	Wyoming

Chapter 1
National & International Organizations

Entries in this chapter are arranged alphabetically by organization names. See the "User's Guide" at the front of this directory for additional information.

★ 1 ★ A-T Medical Research Foundation
c/o Pam Smith
5241 Round Meadow Rd.
Hidden Hills, CA 91302
Phone: (818)703-0151 **Fax:** (818)703-0176
Email: Becca4435@aol.com
Website: http://www.gspartners.com/at
George Smith, Chm.

Fnded: 1989. **Desc:** Works to fund medical research to find a cure for Ataxia-Telangiectasia (A-T), a degenerative genetic disease of the nervous system. Sponsors pioneering research as well as advanced work. **Pub:** Newsletter, annual.

★ 2 ★ Aboriginal Nurses Association of Canada (ANAC)
56 Sparks St., Ste. 502
Ottawa, ON, Canada K1P 5A9
Phone: (613)724-4677 **Fax:** (613)724-4718
Email: info@anac.on.ca
Website: http://www.anac.on.ca/

Fnded: 1975. **Desc:** Promotes Aboriginal nursing in Canada in order to meet and better understand the health needs of Aboriginal people; maintains a registry of Aboriginal Registered Nurses.

★ 3 ★ Abortion Access Project (AAP)
552 Massachusetts Ave., Ste. 215
Cambridge, MA 02139
Phone: (617)661-1161 **Fax:** (617)492-1915
Email: info@abortionaccess.org
Website: http://www.abortionaccess.org

Fnded: 1992. **Desc:** Works to ensure access to abortion for all women by increasing abortion services, training new abortion providers, raising awareness. **Pub:** Newsletter, quarterly. • Report.

★ 4 ★ AboutFace International (AF)
123 Edward St., Ste. 1003
Toronto, ON, Canada M5G 1E2
Phone: (416)597-2229 **Free:** 800-665-3223
Fax: (416)597-8494
Email: info@aboutfaceinternational.org
Website: http://www.aboutfaceinternational.org

Fnded: 1985. **Mem:** 6,000. **State Groups:** 30. **Lang(s):** Portuguese, Spanish. **Desc:** Individuals with facial difference resulting from birth conditions, surgery, or accidents; family members and health care providers. Serves as a network for mutual support and information exchange on coping skills and resources for recovery. Offers continuing education program to medical, nursing, and allied health professionals concerned with facial difference. Provides phone consultation services. Booklets of information/resources on specific conditions, a quarterly newsletter; hospital visits, school programs and local chapter across North America. **Pub:** *About Face Pamphlet.* Pamphlet. Provides general overview of programs, services, and mission. • *Apert, Crouzon and Other Craniosynostosis.* Booklet. Provides detailed look at Apert, Crouzon and other craniosynostosis in layman terms. • *Face Values: Women, Body Image and Facial Differences.* Pamphlet. Written for everyone concerned with body image, diversity and violence prevention issues. • *My Newborn Has a Facial Difference.* Pamphlet. Provides basic overview for parents of newborns with facial differences. • *You, Your Child and The Craniofacial Team.* Outlines the craniofacial team.

★ 5 ★ Absorbent Hygiene Products Manufacturers Association
46 Bridge St.
Godalming GU7 1HL, United Kingdom
Phone: 44 1483 418221

★ 6 ★ Abstinence Clearinghouse
801 E 41st St.
Sioux Falls, SD 57105
Website: http://www.abstinence.net/AboutUs.cfm

Desc: Promotes the practice of sexual abstinence through age-appropriate, factual and medically-accurate materials. **Pub:** *Abstinence Clearinghouse Directory of Abstinence Resources.* Directory. Contains abstinence-until-marriage resources. • *The Abstinence Network*, quarterly. Newsletter. Assists those working with young people to abstain from premarital sexual intercourse.

★ 7 ★ Academia Nacional de Agronomia y Veterinaria
Av Alvear 1711
1014 Buenos Aires, Argentina
Phone: 54 1 8124168 **Fax:** 54 1 8124168
Fnded: 1909.

★ 8 ★ Academia Nacional de Medicina
Bolsa a San Francisco
Caracas 1010, Venezuela
Phone: 58 212 421868
Fnded: 1904.

★ 9 ★ Academic Orthopaedic Society (AOS)
6300 N River Rd., Ste. 505
Rosemont, IL 60018-4226
Phone: (847)318-7330 **Fax:** (847)318-7339
Email: aos@aoassn.org
Website: http://www.a-o-s.org
John D. Lubahn, Pres.

Fnded: 1971. **Desc:** Chairpersons and faculty members of orthopedic departments and divisions of medical schools; directors of orthopedic residency programs; fellowship directors. Provides forum for discussion of administrative and departmental problems concerning undergraduate and graduate orthopedics education in medical schools. Coordinates and plans activities requiring cooperation between orthopedic departments and residencies. Acts as liaison between orthopedic organizations and organizations interested in medical education. **Pub:** *Presidential Newsletter*, semiannual. Newsletter. • Directory, annual. **Frmly:** (1989) Association of Orthopaedic Chairmen; (1991) American Orthopaedic Society.

★ 10 ★ Academy of Ambulatory Foot and Ankle Surgery (AAFS)
1601 Walnut, Ste. 1005
Philadelphia, PA 19102
Phone: (215)569-3303 **Free:** 800-433-4892
Dr. Harriet Waloss, Program Coordinator

Fnded: 1972. **Mem:** 1,500. **Desc:** Podiatric physicians who advocate performing foot surgery in their offices or on an outpatient basis, thereby keeping patients ambulatory and able to function normally, and lowering the patients' medical costs. Promotes the advancement of podiatric surgical procedures that can eliminate the necessity of hospital admission. Sponsors national and regional continuing medical education seminars and semiannual research program. Compiles statistics. **Pub:** *Action Letter*, bimonthly. Newsletter. • *Journal of the Academy of Ambulatory Foot Surgery*, periodic. Journal. • Directory, periodic.

★ 11 ★ Academy of Aphasia (AA)
c/o Luci Varian
East Bay Institute for Research and Education
150 Muir Rd. 126-S
Martinez, CA 94553
Fax: (925)372-2553
Email: contact@academyofaphasia.org
Website: http://www.academyofaphasia.org

Fnded: 1962. **Mem:** 189. **Desc:** Neurologists, psychologists, linguists, speech pathologists, and others specializing in aphasia (impairment of language caused by focal brain damage). Seeks to encourage research and promote communication among the scientific disciplines that can contribute to the understanding of aphasia.

★ 12 ★ Academy of Behaviorial Medicine Research (ABMR)
3600 Forbes Ave., Ste. 405
Pittsburgh, PA 15213
Phone: (412)624-4800 **Fax:** (412)647-1936
Email: haywardmc@msx.upmc.edu
Lori McBurney, Contact

Fnded: 1979. **Mem:** 275. **Desc:** Individuals actively involved in research in more than one aspect of biobehavioral science, and who have been published in refereed journals relevant to the field. Seeks to foster the integration of research in biomedical and behavioral science; identify current and future areas of research in the field; provide a multidisciplinary forum for review of research findings and assessment of applicability of such findings to prevention, diagnosis, and treatment of and rehabilitation from illness; serve as a technical and educational resource for academic, governmental, and public bodies. Promotes research and professional standards within the field. Assists in developing guidelines for research training in behavioral medicine. **Pub:** *AMBR Membership Directory*, periodic. Directory. • *Experimental Foundations of Behavioral Medicine*, annual. • *Perspectives on Behavioral Medicine*, annual.

★ 13 ★ Academy of Canadian Executive Nurses
(Academie des infirmieres et infirmiers du Canada)
c/o Providence Health Care
St. Paul's Hospital, No. 548
1081 Burrard St.
Vancouver, BC, Canada V6Z 1Y6
Phone: (604)806-8088
Website: http://www.acen-cjonl.org

State Groups: mie de. **Local Groups:** irmier. **Desc:** Promotes the interests of executive nurses in Canada.

★ 14 ★ Academy of Clinical Laboratory Physicians and Scientists (ACLPS)
c/o William L. Roberts
500 Chipeta Way
Salt Lake City, UT 84108
Phone: (801)583-2787 **Fax:** (801)584-5207
Email: william.roberts@aruplab.com
Website: http://www.aclps.org
William L. Roberts, MD, Ph, Sec. -Treas.

Fnded: 1966. **Mem:** 500. **Desc:** Physicians, Scientists, and Educators. Encourages and promotes the highest standards of education, service and research in clinical pathology at universities and medical schools. Sponsors journal. **Pub:** *ACLPS Newsletter*, periodic. Newsletter. *Price:* Included with membership. • *The American Journal of Clinical Pathology*. Journal. Publication sponsored by ACLPS and the American Society for clinical pathology.

★ 15 ★ Academy of Counseling Psychology (ACoP)
514 E Capitol Ave.
Jefferson City, MO 65101
Phone: (573)634-7157 **Fax:** (573)634-7157
Website: http://academyofabpps.org/
W. James Cosse, PhD, Pres.

Fnded: 1992. **Desc:** Counseling psychologists. Promotes standards of professional practice and conduct within the specialization of Counseling Psychology; seeks to protect the well-being of the public, the profession, and the Academy. Provides education and training. **Pub:** *ACoP*. Newsletter.

★ 16 ★ Academy of Dental Materials (ADM)
WVU School of Dentistry
HSC North
Morgantown, WV 26506-9403
Phone: (304)293-3370 **Fax:** (304)293-2859
Email: mbagby@hsc.wvu.edu
Website: http://www.academydentalmaterials.org
Mike Bagby, Treas.

Fnded: 1940. **Mem:** 300. **Desc:** Active members are licensed dentists, members of academic institutions, industrial employees, and individuals active or interested in dental materials. Coordinates activities relating to the use of dental materials. **Pub:** *ADM Newsletter*, 3/year. Newsletter. • *Dental Materials*, bimonthly. Journal. Covers scientific research. *Price:* Included in membership dues; $195 for nonmembers. • *Transactions of the Academy of Dental Materials*. • Directory, periodic. **Frmly:** (1983) American Academy for Plastics Research in Dentistry.

★ 17 ★ Academy of Dental Sleep Medicine
Westbrooke Corporate Center, Ste. 920
Westchester, IL 60154
Phone: (708)273-9335 **Fax:** (708)492-0943
Email: info@dentalsleepmed.org
Website: http://www.dentalsleepmed.org

Fnded: 1991. **Mem:** 500. **Desc:** Dentists, physicians, and PhD's active in sleep disorder medicine. Seeks to improve the treatment of patients with sleep disorders through the involvement of dental practicioners and use of oral appliances in overall therapy and to enhance the lives of people suffering form sleep disorders. Supports research in application of dental appliances in the treatment of sleep disorders, such as snoring and sleep apnea; conducts educational and certification programs; establishes dental treatment protocol; disseminates information on sleep disorder treatment; facilitates the exchange of information; operates the SDDS Resource Center. **Pub:** *ADSM Dialogue*, quarterly. Newsletter.

★ 18 ★ Academy of Dentistry International (ADI)
3813 Gordon Creek Dr.
PO Box 307
Hicksville, OH 43526
Phone: (419)542-0101
Website: http://www.adint.org
Robert L. Ramus, DDS, Exec. Dir.

Fnded: 1974. **Mem:** 2,400. **Nat'l Groups:** 55. **Reg. Groups:** 10. **State Groups:** 4. **Desc:** Dentists; membership by invitation only. Works to further dentistry and the prevention of dental diseases worldwide. Disseminates and promotes the exchange of scientific information and fosters research. **Pub:** *International Communicator*, semiannual. Newsletter. *Price:* Included in membership dues. • *Roster of ADI*, periodic.

★ 19 ★ Academy of Dispensing Audiologists (ADA)
3008 Millwood Ave.
Columbia, SC 29205
Phone: (803)252-5646 **Free:** 800-445-8629
Fax: (803)765-0860
Email: info@audiologist.org
Website: http://www.audiologist.org
Robert D. Manning, Pres.

Fnded: 1977. **Mem:** 525. **Desc:** Individuals with graduate degrees in audiology who dispense hearing aids as part of a rehabilitative practice. Fosters and supports professional dispensing of hearing aids by qualified audiologists; encourages audiology training programs to include pertinent aspects of hearing aid dispensing in their curriculums; conducts seminars on the business aspects of the hearing aid industry. **Pub:** *ADA Feedback*, quarterly. Newsletter. Includes book reviews and new members listing. *Price:* Free. • *ADA Membership Directory*, annual. Membership Directory. Arranged alphabetically and geographically. *Price:* Included in membership dues.

★ 20 ★ Academy for Eating Disorders (AED)
6728 Old McLean Village Dr.
Mc Lean, VA 22101
Phone: (703)556-9222 **Fax:** (703)556-8729
Email: aed@degnon.org
Website: http://www.aedweb.org/

Fnded: 1993. **Desc:** Eating disorders research and treatment, particularly anorexia nervosa, bulimia nervosa, binge eating disorder, and related disorders; promotes effective treatment and care to patients; develops and advances primary and secondary preventions; disseminates information; advocates on behalf of patients, the public and eating disorder professionals; assists in developing guidelines for training, practice and professionals within the field. **Pub:** Newsletter.

★ 21 ★ Academy of General Dentistry (AGD)
211 E Chicago Ave., Ste. 900
Chicago, IL 60611
Phone: (312)440-4300 **Free:** 888-243-3368
Fax: (312)440-0559
Email: agddented@agd.org
Website: http://www.agd.org
Harold E. Donnell, Jr., Exec. Dir.

Fnded: 1952. **Mem:** 37,000. **Nat'l Groups:** 1. **Reg. Groups:** 20. **State Groups:** 62. **Local Groups:** 35. **Desc:** Seeks to serve the needs and represent the interest of general dentists. Fosters their dentists' continued proficiency through quality continuing dental education to better serve the public. **Pub:** *AGD Impact*, 11/year. Magazine. Covers issues, legislation, and trends that affect the practice and role of dentistry in the health care community. *Price:* Included in membership dues; $25/year for nonmembers. • *Dentalnotes*, quarterly. Newsletter. Provides information on the latest dental issues and trends; intended for the national media and to be displayed in dentists' reception areas. *Price:* $20 /year for members; $40 /year for nonmembers. • *General Dentistry*, bimonthly. Journal. Provides research and clinical reports for the continuing education of general dentists. Contains advertisers' index, book reviews, and quizzes. *Price:* Included in membership dues; $30/year for nonmembers.

★ 22 ★ Academy Health Sciences
2578 Broadway, Ste. 112
New York, NY 10025
Phone: (212)932-2381
Email: naturaltherapy@verizon.net
Website: http://www.naturaltherapy.com
Dr. Shoshana Margolin, Coord.

Fnded: 1996. **Mem:** 120. **Desc:** Arranges conferences where researchers and practitioners share innovative ideas on upgrading the skills of healthcare professionals. Conducts research and educational programs.

★ 23 ★ Academy for Health Services Research and Health Policy
1801 K St. NW, Ste. 701-L
Washington, DC 20006-1301
Phone: (202)292-6700 **Fax:** (202)292-6800
Email: info@ahsrhp.org
Website: http://www.academyhealth.org
David Helms, Pres.

Fnded: 1981. **Mem:** 2,800. **Desc:** Individuals and organizations concerned with health services research. Objectives are to educate the public concerning the need for and contribution of health services research in improving health care in the U.S.; to foster productive cooperation among researchers, public and private funding agencies, health professionals, policymakers, and the public; to represent the views of members in the development and implementation of national legislative and administrative policies concerning health services research. Disseminates research findings to public and private sector officials. **Pub:** *HSR Reports*, quarterly. Newsletter. Covers legislative news and association activities. Includes conference calendar, employment listings, and training opportunities. *Price:* Free with membership. **Frmly:** (2002) Association for Health Services Research.

★ 24 ★ Academy of Hospice and Palliative Medicine (AAHPM)
4700 W Lake Ave.
Glenview, IL 60025-1485
Phone: (847)375-4712 **Free:** 877-734-8671
Website: http://www.aahpm.org
Carla Alexander, MD, Pres.

Fnded: 1988. **Desc:** Physicians. Committed to improvement of care of the dying.

★ 25 ★ Academy for Implants and Transplants (AIT)
PO Box 223
Springfield, VA 22150
Phone: (703)451-0001 **Fax:** (703)451-0004
Anthony J. Viscido, D.D.S., Sec. -Treas.

Fnded: 1972. **Mem:** 180. **Reg. Groups:** 15. **Desc:** Dentists united to: motivate and assist men and women in the general practice of dentistry in the field of implants and transplants; encourage and promote the art and science of implant and transplant dentistry; assist in research in this and allied fields. Conducts seminars; teaches implantology. **Pub:** *Implant Update*, quarterly. Newsletter. Discusses developments in the field of implant and transplant dentistry. *Price:* Included in membership dues. • Journal, periodic.

★ 26 ★ Academy for International Health Studies (AIHS)
621 Georgetown Pl.
Davis, CA 95616
Phone: (530)758-8600 **Fax:** (916)313-3410
Email: jlewis@aihs.com
Website: http://www.aihs.com
Jonathan C. Lewis, Pres.

Fnded: 1993. **Desc:** Senior health care executives from multinational health industries including health plans, health care providers, medical device manufacturers, pharmaceutical companies, and information technology vendors. Seeks to improve understanding of the international health care market and the American health system. Brings together members for the discussion of matters of mutual concern; serves as a clearinghouse on the health care industries; organizes trade and study missions. Operates Mexico-U.S.A. CrossBorder Health Insurance Initiative, which assists in the development of commercially viable health insurance for Mexican nationals living in the United States. Maintains speakers' bureau; functions as the North American Office of the International Federation of Health Funds. **Pub:** *Modern Healthcare International*, weekly. Magazine.

★ 27 ★ Academy of Laser Dentistry
PO Box 8667
Coral Springs, FL 33075
Phone: (954)346-3776 **Fax:** (954)757-2598
Email: memberservices@laserdentistry.org
Website: http://www.laserdentistry.org
Gail S. Siminovsky, Exec. Dir.

Fnded: 1993. **Mem:** 600. **Nat'l Groups:** 3. **Desc:** Dentists, hygienists, dental academicians and researchers, and corporate laser and laser accessory dental vendors. Promotes clinical education, research, and development of standards and guidelines for the safe and ethical use of dental laser technology. Conducts educational programs. Provides certification. **Pub:** *Wavelengths*, quarterly. Journal. Clinical case studies, industry and academy news. *Price:* Included in membership.

★ 28 ★ Academy of Managed Care Pharmacy (AMCP)
100 N Pitt St., Ste. 400
Alexandria, VA 22314-2747
Phone: (703)683-8416 **Free:** 800-827-2627
Fax: (703)683-8417
Email: amcp@amcp.org
Website: http://www.amcp.org
Judith A. Cahill, Exec. Dir.

Fnded: 1989. **Mem:** 4,800. **Desc:** Dedicated to the concept and practice of pharmaceutical care in managed health care environments. Promotes the development and application of pharmaceutical care in order to ensure appropriate health care outcomes for all individuals. Represents the views and interest of managed care pharmacy. **Pub:** *AMCP News*, monthly. Newsletter. • *Concept Series in Managed Care Pharmacy*, periodic. Paper. • *JMCP*, bimonthly. Journal. • *Who's Who*, annual. Directory.

★ 29 ★ Academy of Managed Care Providers (AMCP)
1945 Palo Verde Ave. Ste. 202
Long Beach, CA 90815-3445
Phone: (562)682-3559 **Free:** 800-297-2627
Fax: (562)799-3355
Email: members@academymcp.org
Website: http://www.academymcp.org
Dr. John Russell, Pres.

Fnded: 1993. **Mem:** 2,500. **Desc:** Clinicians and Managed Care Industry executives. Provides a mulititude of services to members. Awards diplomate status to qualified members who meet criteria and pass written exam. **Pub:** *Managed Care Times*, monthly. Newsletter. Contains update on all aspects of the healthcare industry. *Price:* Included in membership dues.

★ 30 ★ Academy of Medical Surgical Nurses (AMSN)
East Holly Ave.
PO Box 56
Pitman, NJ 08071-0056
Phone: (856)256-2323 **Fax:** (856)589-7463
Email: amsn@ajj.com
Website: http://www.medsurgnurse.org/cover.htm

Desc: Adult/health, medical-surgical nurses. Promotes standards of nursing. Collaborates with other nursing organizations to provide educational programs, practice guidelines and new ideas for its members. **Pub:** *Certification Review Course Manual*. Manual. Available to educators providing continuing nursing education.

★ 31 ★ Academy of Medicine, Singapore
College of Medicine Bldg., 16 College Rd.
Singapore 0316, Singapore
Phone: 65 2238968 **Fax:** 65 2255155

Fnded: 1957.

★ 32 ★ Academy of Molecular Imaging (AMI)
PO Box 951735
Los Angeles, CA 90095-1735
Email: kpierce@mednet.ucla.edu
Website: http://www.ami-imaging.org/
Kim Pierce, Exec. Dir.

Desc: Promotes molecular diagnostics and molecular therapies. **Pub:** *Molecular Imaging and Biology*, bimonthly. Journal. Contains information about various technologies of molecular imaging. • Newsletter, quarterly.

★ 33 ★ Academy of Operative Dentistry (AOD)
PO Box 991
Midway, UT 84049
Dr. Ebb A. Berry, III, Pres.

Fnded: 1972. **Mem:** 1,000. **Desc:** Dentists and persons in allied industries. Seeks to ensure quality in all of operative dentistry, teaching, service, research. **Pub:** *Membership Roster*, periodic. • *Operative Dentistry*, 6/year.

★ 34 ★ Academy of Oral Dynamics (AOD)
8919 Sudley Rd.
Manassas, VA 20110
Phone: (703)368-8527 **Fax:** (703)331-0356
Dr. E. Paul Byrne, Sec.

Fnded: 1950. **Mem:** 75. **Desc:** Professional society of dentists. Promotes the study of oral dynamics, especially as it applies to the use of natural teeth in restoring and maintaining a healthy, functioning mouth; disseminates information gained through research. Conducts educational programs. **Frmly:** (1950) International Academy of Oral Dynamics.

★ 35 ★ Academy of Organizational and Occupational Psychiatry (AOOP)
717 Princess St.
Alexandria, VA 22314
Free: 877-789-2667 **Fax:** 877-789-6050
Email: staff@aoop.com
Website: http://www.aoop.org
Carol Montoya, Contact

Fnded: 1990. **Mem:** 160. **Desc:** Strives to provide a forum for exchanging ideas between psychiatry and the world of work. The association is dedicated to the advancement of psychiatric solutions to the problems of organizations, workers, and leaders. **Pub:** *The Bulletin of Organizational and Occupational Psychiatry*, quarterly. Bulletin. Contains scholarly articles regarding occupational and organizational psychiatry for publication. *Price:* included in membership dues. • Membership Directory.

★ 36 ★ Academy of Osseointegration (AO)
85 W Algonquin Rd., Ste. 550
Arlington Heights, IL 60005-4460
Phone: (847)439-1919 **Free:** 800-656-7736
Fax: (847)439-1569
Email: academy@osseo.org
Website: http://www.osseo.org
Kevin P. Smith, Exec. Dir.

Fnded: 1987. **Mem:** 4,500. **Desc:** Works for the advancement of osseointegration among dentists, physicians and related professionals. Conducts research and educational programs; disseminates information to the public and medical agencies; provides a forum for interdisciplinary discussions. **Pub:** *Academy News*, bimonthly. Newsletter. • *International Journal of Oral & Maxillofacial Implants*, bimonthly. Journal. Includes current information related to the management of patients utilizing implant modalities. *Price:* $118 in U.S.; $158 outside U.S.

★ 37 ★ Academy of Pharmaceutical Research and Science (APRS)
American Pharmaceutical Association
2215 Constitution Ave. NW
Washington, DC 20037-2985
Phone: (202)628-4410 **Free:** 800-237-2742
Fax: (202)783-2351
Email: apha-aprs@mail.aphanet.org
Website: http://www.aphanet.org/about/aprs.html
Arthur H. Kibbe, Pres.

Fnded: 1965. **Mem:** 3,000. **Desc:** A part of American Pharmaceutical Association. Pharmaceutical scientists from industry and academia. Objective is to serve the profession of pharmacy by developing knowledge and integrating the process of science into the profession. Sponsors national meetings to provide a forum for presentation and discussion of original research, controversial topics, and continuing communication. Provides consultation and advice to: pharmacists on scientific matters as they relate to policy; congressional committees on bills of interest to pharmaceutical scientists; governmental agencies. **Pub:** *Abstracts of Papers*, annual. Published in Journal of the American Pharmaceutical Ass'n. • *Journal of Pharmaceutical Sciences*, monthly. Journal. • Manuals. • Monographs. **Frmly:** (1987) Academy of Pharmaceutical Sciences.

★ 38 ★ Academy of Psychosomatic Medicine (APM)
5824 N Magnolia
Chicago, IL 60660
Phone: (773)784-2025 **Fax:** (773)784-1304
Email: apsychmed@aol.com
Website: http://www.apm.org
Evelyne A. Hallberg, Exec. Dir.

Fnded: 1954. **Mem:** 1,000. **Desc:** Interdisciplinary organization of health care professionals dedicated to the concept of total health care of the physical and emotional needs of the patient. Objectives are: to advance scientific knowledge and the practice of medicine relating to the interaction of mind, body, and environment through study and research; to cooperate with other workers in these and related disciplines; to provide a forum for the presentation and discussion of these problems; to publish the results of research; to facilitate total and comprehensive care. **Pub:** *Academy of Psychosomatic Medicine–Directory*, annual. Directory. • *Psychosomatics*, bimonthly. Journal. Includes book reviews and calendar of events. *Price:* Included in membership dues; $99/year for nonmembers.

★ 39 ★ Academy of Rehabilitative Audiology (ARA)
c/o Frances Laven
PO Box 26532
Minneapolis, MN 55426
Phone: (952)920-0484 **Fax:** (952)920-6098
Email: ara@incnet.com
Website: http://www.audrehab.org
Jodell Newman Ryan, PhD, Pres.

Fnded: 1966. **Mem:** 400. **Nat'l Groups:** 1. **Desc:** Individuals who hold graduate degrees in audiology, language, or speech pathology, education of the deaf, or allied fields, and who have at least two years of post-degree involvement in rehabilitative or educational programs for the hearing impaired. Provides a forum for exchange of ideas in audiology; fosters professional education, research, and interest in programs for hearing handicapped persons. Maintains speakers' bureau. **Pub:** *ARA Membership Directory*, annual. Membership Directory. • *Journal of the Academy of Rehabilitative Audiology*, annual. Journal. *Price:* $25/year. • *Monograph of Academy of Rehabilitative Audiology*, quinquennial. *Price:* $20.

★ 40 ★ Academy of Scientific Hypnotherapy (ASH)

PO Box 12041
San Diego, CA 92112
Phone: (619)427-6225 **Fax:** (619)427-5650
Email: docbill@e-machines.net
Website: http://www.health.gov/nhic/NHICScripts/Entry.cfm?HRCode=HR0670
William E. Kemery, PhD, Pres.

Fnded: 1977. **Mem:** 250. **Desc:** Professionals in the healing arts who have been properly trained in hypnosis, and who are known to the academy to be ethical and of good professional reputation. The academy plans to fill the need for training programs, continuing education, and certification throughout the U.S. Maintains placement and referral service; compiles statistics. **Pub:** *Hypnotherapy in Review*, periodic. Newsletter. Reports on medical and psychological research in hypnotherapy. Includes book reviews. *Price:* Included in membership dues. • Bulletin, periodic. • Monograph, periodic. *Price:* Included in membership dues.

★ 41 ★ Academy of Surgical Research (ASR)

13355 10th Ave. N, Ste. 108
Minneapolis, MN 55441-5510
Phone: (763)765-2300 **Fax:** (763)765-2329
Email: director@surgicalresearch.org
Website: http://www.surgicalresearch.org
Patricia Nolt, Exec. Dir.

Fnded: 1982. **Mem:** 425. **Desc:** Individuals, organizations, and corporations with an interest in surgical research. Seeks to advance surgical techniques and equipment through improved research. Facilitates cooperation and exchange of information among members; fosters interdisciplinary transfer of ideas to advance surgical research. **Pub:** *Journal of Investigative Surgery*, periodic. Journal. Discusses advances in surgical research techniques and education. *Price:* $29.95.

★ 42 ★ Academy of Upper Cervical Chiropractic Organizations (AUCCO)

1637 Westbridge Dr., Unit H4
Fort Collins, CO 80526
Website: http://www.aucco.org/

Fnded: NNst. **Mem:** udent (,Chi.) **Reg. Groups:** nd doc. **State Groups:** withi. **Local Groups:** ileges. **Desc:** Chiropractors and chiropractic organizations. Fosters and promotes information about atlas subluxation complex; disseminates information in order to preserve the science of upper cervical adjustment; provides resources and health tips **Pub:** Newsletter.Contains information of interest to members.

★ 43 ★ Academy of Veterinary Allergy and Clinical Immunology (AVA)

c/o Richard Rossman, Treas.
330 Waukegan Rd.
Glenview, IL 60025
Phone: (847)729-5200 **Fax:** (847)729-5214
Email: richlge@aol.com
Website: http://www.avaci.org
Dr. Richard Rossman, DVM, Treas.

Fnded: 1960. **Mem:** 300. **Desc:** Veterinarians, research M.D.s, and allergy extract firms. Promotes education and research in veterinary and comparative allergy and immunology. **Pub:** *Membership List*, periodic. • *Veterinary Allergist*, quarterly.

★ 44 ★ Academy of Veterinary Cardiology (AVC)

48 Notch Rd.
Little Falls, NJ 07424
Fax: (973)890-5617
Andrew Beardow, Exec. VP

Fnded: 1967. **Mem:** 600. **Desc:** Persons with an interest in veterinary or comparative cardiology. Purpose is to disseminate literature, reviews, and materials of interest to veterinary practitioners. Maintains specialized education program. **Pub:** Membership Directory, biennial. • Newsletter, periodic. • Also publishes abstracts and bibliography.

★ 45 ★ Academy of Veterinary Homeopathy (AVH)

PO Box 9280
Wilmington, DE 19809
Free: (866)652-1590
Email: webmaster@theavh.org
Website: http://www.theavh.org/
Susan H. Pitcaim, Off. Mgr.

Fnded: 1996. **Desc:** Works to promote education and research in veterinary homeopathy. Offers an accreditation training program for veterinarians; provides referrals to the public; sponsors continuing education conferences; supports practical and clinical research.

★ 46 ★ Academy of Zoology

Church Rd. 2/95, Civil Lines
Agra 282 002, India
Fnded: 1954.

★ 47 ★ Access Technology Association

3612 Bent Branch Ct.
Falls Church, VA 22041
Phone: (703)941-4329 **Fax:** (703)941-4329
Dr. William J. Tobin, Exec. Dir.

Fnded: 1990. **Desc:** Provides forum and national clearinghouse on a variety of issues related to the disabled. Represents manufacturers and suppliers of assistive devices for the disabled.

★ 48 ★ Accessibility Equipment Manufacturers Association (AEMA)

PO Box 380
Metamora, IL 61548-0380
Free: 800-514-1100 **Fax:** (309)923-7964
Email: host@aema.com
Website: http://www.aema.com/

Fnded: 1990. **Desc:** Promotes awareness of accessibility equipment, including the design, installation and servicing of vertical, inclined and horizontal conveying systems that are used to provide access and/or egress for physically challenged people in public and residential areas. Accessibility products are platform lifts, wheelchair lifts, access elevators, residence elevators, stairway chairlifts, and similar products.

★ 49 ★ Accreditation Association for Ambulatory Health Care (AAAHC)

3201 Old Glenview Rd., Ste. 300
Wilmette, IL 60091
Phone: (847)853-6060 **Fax:** (847)853-9028
Email: info@aaahc.org
Website: http://www.aaahc.org
John E. Burke, PhD, Exec. Dir.

Fnded: 1979. **Mem:** 16. **Desc:** Operates a voluntary, peer-based accreditation and consulting program for ambulatory health care organizations as a means of assisting them in efficiently providing a high level of care for patients. Distributes free lists of accredited organizations. **Pub:** *Accreditation Handbook for Ambulatory Health Care*, biennial. Standards for accreditation of ambulatory health care centers. Includes subject index. *Price:* $120/copy prepaid. • Also publishes related survey materials.

★ 50 ★ Accreditation Commission for Acupuncture and Oriental Medicine (ACAOM)

7501 Greenway Ctr. Dr., Ste. 820
Greenbelt, MD 20770
Phone: (301)313-0580 **Fax:** (301)313-0912
Email: 73352.2467@compuserve.com
Website: http://www.acaom.org
Dort Bigg, Exec. Dir.

Fnded: 1982. **Mem:** 51. **Desc:** Acts as an independent body to evaluate first professional master's degree and first professional master's level certificate and diploma programs in acupuncture and first professional master's degree and first professional master's level certificate and diploma programs in Oriental medicine with concentrations in both acupuncture and herbal therapy for a level of performance, integrity and quality that entitles them to the confidence of the educational community and the public they serve. Also acts to evaluate doctoral programs in oriental medicine. Establishes accreditation criteria, arranges site visits, evaluates those programs that desire accredited status and publicly designates those programs that meet the criteria. **Pub:** *Accreditation Handbook*. Handbook. *Price:* $25. • *Acupuncture and Oriental Medicine Accreditation*, semiannual. Newsletter. *Price:* Free. • Brochure. • Manuals. **Frmly:** (1998) National Accreditation Commission for Schools and Colleges of Acupuncture and Oriental Medicine.

★ 51 ★ Accreditation Council for Continuing Medical Education (ACCME)

515 N State St., Ste. 2150
Chicago, IL 60610
Phone: (312)464-2500 **Fax:** (312)464-2586
Email: postmaster@accme.org
Website: http://www.accme.org
Murray Kopelow, MD, Exec. Dir.

Fnded: 1981. **Desc:** Acts as an accrediting agency for sponsors of continuing medical education for physicians. Sponsoring participants are: American Board of Medical Specialties; American Hospital Association; American Medical Association; Association of American Medical Colleges; Association for Hospital Medical Education; Council of Medical Specialty Societies; Federation of State Medical Boards of the United States. **Frmly:** Liaison Committee on Continuing Medical Education.

★ 52 ★ Accreditation Council on Optometric Education (ACOE)

243 N Lindbergh Blvd.
Saint Louis, MO 63141
Phone: (314)991-4100 **Fax:** (314)991-4101
Email: acoe@aoa.org
Website: http://www.aoa.org/students/accreditation.asp
Joyce L. Urbeck, Admin. Dir.

Fnded: 1934. **Mem:** 11. **Desc:** Accrediting body for professional optometric degree (O.D.) programs (examination, diagnosis, and treatment and management of diseases and disorders of the vision system, the eyes and associated structures as well as diagnosis of related systemic conditions), paraoptometric educational programs, and optometric residency programs. Members are appointed by the president of the American Optometric Association. Works to ensure the quality of optometric education by establishing and applying valid educational standards and announces list of accredited programs. **Frmly:** (2002) Council on Optometric Education.

★ 53 ★ Accreditation Review Commission on Education for Physician Assistants (ARC-PA)

1000 N Oak Ave.
Marshfield, WI 54449-5788
Phone: (715)389-3785 **Fax:** (715)387-5163
Email: mccartyj@mfldclin.edu
Website: http://www.arc-pa.org
John E. McCarty, Exec. Dir.

Fnded: 1971. **Mem:** 16. **Desc:** Serves as an accrediting body for physician assistant education nationwide. **Frmly:** (1972) Joint Review Committee on Educational Programs for Physician's Assistants; (1987) Joint Review on Educational Programs for Physician Assistants; (1989) Accreditation Committee on Education for Physicians Assistants; (2000) Accreditation Review Committee on Education for Physician Assistants.

★ 54 ★ Accreditation Review Committee on Education in Surgical Technology (ARC-ST)

c/o Paul Price, CST/CFA, MBA
7108-C S Alton Way
Centennial, CO 80112-2106
Phone: (303)694-9262 **Fax:** (303)741-3655
Email: acollinsworth@ast.org
Website: http://www.arcst.org
Paul Price, Exec. Dir.

Fnded: 1974. **Mem:** 317. **Desc:** Reviews accreditation applications of surgical techology programs in hospitals, community colleges, technical schools, and universities and makes recommendations to the Commission on Accreditation of Allied Health Education Programs. Collaborates with American College of Surgeons, American Hospital Association, and the Association of Surgical Technologists. **Pub:** *Surgical Technology: A Growing Career*. Brochure. Contains information on careers in surgical technology, educational requirements, and a list of accredited programs. *Price:* Free (first copy); $1/each additional copy. **Frmly:** (1987) Joint Review Committee on Education for the Surgical Technologist; (1990) Accreditation Review Committee for Educational Programs in Surgical Technology.

★ 55 ★ Accrediting Bureau of Health Education Schools (ABHES)

7777 Leesburg Pke., Ste. 730
Falls Church, VA 22043-2403
Phone: (703)917-9503
Email: info@abhes.org
Website: http://www.abhes.org
Carol A. Moneymaker, Exec. Dir.

Fnded: 1964. **Mem:** 180. **Desc:** Serves as a nationally recognized accrediting agency of health education institutions and schools conducting medical laboratory technician and medical assistant education programs. Establishes criteria and standards for the administration and operation of health education institutions. Seeks to enhance the profession through the improvement of schools, courses, and the competence of graduates. Schools must apply voluntarily for accreditation; once accredited, they must report to the bureau annually and be reexamined at least every 6 years. Has accredited 15 programs for medical laboratory technicians, 124 medical assistants, and 80 institutions of allied health. **Pub:** *Accrediting Bureau of Health Education Schools–Directory of Accredited Schools and Programs*, annual. Directory. Lists education institutions and programs accredited by the com missioners of the ABHES. • *Advantage*, quarterly. Newsletter. Includes calendar of events, news, lists personnel and comissioners. **Frmly:** Accrediting Bureau of Medical Laboratory Schools.

★ 56 ★ Accrediting Commission on Education for Health Services Administration (ACEHSA)

730 11th St. NW, No. 400
Washington, DC 20001
Phone: (202)638-5131 **Fax:** (202)638-3429
Email: acehsa@aupha.org
Website: http://www.acehsa.org
Jeptha W. Dalton, PhD, Pres. & CEO

Fnded: 1968. **Mem:** 67. **Desc:** Accredits graduate degree programs in health services administration, health planning, and health policy. Goal is the improvement of professional education. **Pub:** *Official List of Accredited Programs*, semiannual. *Price:* Free. **Frmly:** (1976) Accrediting Commission on Graduate Education for Hospital Administration.

★ 57 ★ Achilles Track Club (ATC)

42 W 38th St., 4th Fl.
New York, NY 10018-6210
Phone: (212)354-0300 **Fax:** (212)354-3978
Email: achillesclub@aol.com
Website: http://www.achillestrackclub.org/
James M. Benson, Pres.

Fnded: 1982. **Mem:** 3,400. **Nat'l Groups:** 43. **Local Groups:** 40. **Desc:** Disabled runners; volunteer coaches. (Membership, though drawn primarily from New York City, also includes international members who are coached by mail.) Purpose is to encourage people with all types of disabilities to participate in running, and to improve the self-image of the disabled and demonstrate that they are energetic and capable people. Encourages the disabled to be aerobically fit and to run in competitions beside the able-bodied. Stresses that no previous athletic experience is necessary, just a desire to improve fitness with regular training. Conducts childrens' programs. Maintains speakers' bureau. Group is named for the mythical Greek hero whose disability was a vulnerable heel on an otherwise invincible body. **Pub:** *The Achilles Heel and Kid's Bits*, 3/year. Newsletter.

★ 58 ★ Achromatopsia Network

PO Box 214
Berkeley, CA 94701-0214
Phone: (510)540-4700 **Fax:** (510)540-4767
Email: publications@acromat.org
Website: http://www.achromat.org/
Frances Futterman, Contact

Fnded: 1994. **Desc:** Provides information and support for individuals and families concerned with the vision disorder achromatopsia, including both rod monochromacy and blue cone monochromacy.

★ 59 ★ Acid Maltase Deficiency Association (AMDA)

PO Box 700248
San Antonio, TX 78270-0248
Phone: (210)494-6144 **Fax:** (210)497-3810
Email: tianrama@aol.com
Website: http://www.amda-pompe.org/
Marylyn House, Contact

Fnded: 1995. **Mem:** 500. **Desc:** Promotes awareness of Acid Maltase Deficiency, also known as Pompe's Disease; assists in funding research.

★ 60 ★ Acoustic Neuroma Association (ANA)

600 Peachtree Pkwy., No. 108
Cumming, GA 30041
Phone: (770)205-8211 **Fax:** (770)205-0239
Email: anausa@aol.com
Website: http://www.anausa.org
Lois White, Exec. Dir.

Fnded: 1981. **Mem:** 5,000. **Local Groups:** 43. **Desc:** Provides information and support to patients who have been diagnosed with or experienced an acoustic neuroma or other benign problem affecting the cranial nerves. The association also furnishes information on patient rehabilitation to physicians and health care personnel, promotes research on acoustic neuroma, thus promoting early diagnosis and successful treatment. **Pub:** *A Glimpse of the Brain*. Booklet. • *Acoustic Neuroma, Basic Overview*. Booklet. • *The Acoustic Neuroma Experience 1988/Member Survey*. Booklet. • *ANA Notes*, quarterly. Newsletter. • *Diagnosis Acoustic Neuroma: What Next?*. Booklet. • *Eye Care after Acoustic Neuroma Surgery*. Booklet. • *Facial Nerve and Acoustic Neuroma: Possible Damage and Rehabilitation*. Booklet. • *Headache Following Acoustic Neuroma*. Booklet. • *Improving Balance Following Treatment for AN*. Booklet. • Newsletter, quarterly. Newsletter covering advances in the treatment of acoustic neuroma, patient letters, support group information. *Price:* Included in membership dues. • Booklets.*Price:* included in membership dues.

★ 61 ★ Acoustic Neuroma Association of Canada (ANAC)

PO Box 369
Edmonton, AB, Canada T5J 2J6
Phone: (780)428-3384 **Free:** 800-561-2622
Fax: (780)438-4837
Email: anac@compusmart.ab.ca
Website: http://www.anac.ca

Fnded: 1983. **Mem:** 451. **Lang(s):** English, French. **Desc:** For people with acoustic neuroma, Bell's Palsy, and other neuromuscular disorders, their families, health care professionals, and other interested individuals. Seeks to improve the quality of life of people with neuromuscular diseases; promotes research into the causes and treatment of acoustic neuroma. Conducts charitable programs; provides support and services to people with neuromuscular disorders; maintains speakers' bureau. **Pub:** *Connection*, quarterly. Newsletter.

★ 62 ★ ACROD

PO Box 60
Curtin, ACT 2605, Australia
Phone: 61 2 62833200 **Fax:** 61 2 62813488
Email: acrodnat@acrod.org.au
Website: http://www.acrod.org.au

Fnded: 1962. **Mem:** 550. **State Groups:** 8. **Desc:** National industry association for disability services. Seeks to promote the development of quality services and life opportunities for Australians with disabilities. **Pub:** *ACROD Newsletter*, bimonthly. Newsletter. • *Discussion Papers*. Papers.

★ 63 ★ ACT UP

332 Bleecker St., No. G5
New York, NY 10014-2980
Phone: (212)966-4873 **Fax:** (212)966-4873
Email: actupny@panix.com
Website: http://www.actupny.org

Fnded: 1987. **Desc:** Individuals "united in anger and committed to direct action to end the AIDS crisis." Seeks to increase public awareness and government involvement in the fight against AIDS. Conducts rallies and demonstrations aimed at public figures or institutions that the group feels should be doing more to combat AIDS. Lobbies for quicker availability of experimental AIDS drugs. **Pub:** *Act Up Americans*. Catalog. • *AIDS, Act Up and Activism*. Handbook. • *Merchandise Catalog*. *Price:* Free upon request. • *Women and AIDS Handbook*. Handbook. **AKA:** AIDS Coalition to Unleash Power.

★ 64 ★ Action Against Allergy (AAA)

PO Box 278
Twickenham
Middlesex
Twickenham TW1 4QQ, United Kingdom
Phone: 44 20 8922711 **Fax:** 44 20 8924950
Email: aaa@freeserve.co.uk

Fnded: 1978. **Mem:** 1,200. **Lang(s):** English, French, German, Italian. **Desc:** Campaigns for diagnosis and treatment of allergies through the British national health service institutions and physicians. Provides information to chronic allergy sufferers. Coordinates medical reference center. **Pub:** *Allergy Newsletter*, 3/year. Newsletter. • Brochures, periodic. • Directory, periodic. Information on suppliers of additive-free and non-allergenic foods and materials.

★ 65 ★ Action for Blind People

14-16 Verney Rd.
London SE16 3DZ, United Kingdom
Phone: 44 207 6354800 **Fax:** 44 207 6354900
Email: info@afbp.org
Website: http://www.afbp.org

Fnded: 1857. **Desc:** Provides services for visually impaired people in the UK, including employment services, hotels and holidays, accommodation and residential care, and information and welfare rights advice.

★ 66 ★ Action Cancer
1 Marlborough Park
Belfast BT9 6XS, United Kingdom
Phone: 44 2890 803344 **Fax:** 44 2890 803356
Email: info@actioncancer.org
Website: http://www.actioncancer.org

Fnded: 1973. **Local Groups:** 40. **Desc:** Works to heighten awareness of the importance of early cancer detection. Offers breast and cervical cancer screening services for women, and testicular and prostatic screening services for men. Provides counselling for cancer patients, families, and friends. Maintains research lab. Disseminates information. **Pub:** *Action Cancer News Update*, quarterly. Magazine. • Annual Report. Selection of Cancer information leaflets.

★ 67 ★ Action on Disability and Development (ADD)
Vallis House
57 Vallis Rd.
Somerset
Frome BA11 3EG, United Kingdom
Phone: 44 1373 473064 **Fax:** 44 1373 452075
Email: add@add.org.uk
Website: http://www.add.org.uk

Fnded: 1985. **Lang(s):** English. **Desc:** Development organizations. Seeks to increase participation by people with disabilities in the development process. Conducts educational and training courses to enhance the income-generation potential of people with disabilities; supports inclusion of people with disabilities in community rehabilitation initiatives.

★ 68 ★ Action Health - Nigeria (AHI)
PO Box 803
Yaba Post Office
Lagos, Lagos, Nigeria
Phone: 234 1 7743745 **Fax:** 234 1 863198
Email: ahi@linkserve.com.ng
Website: http://www.actionhealthinc.org

Fnded: 1989. **Lang(s):** English. **Desc:** Individuals interested in the health and well-being of Nigerian youth. Promotes increased availability of health and social services for youth; works to improve public understanding of reproductive health and related issues. Conducts educational programs for youth; sponsors reproductive health clinics. **Pub:** *Growing Up*, periodic. Newsletter. Addresses sexual and reproductive health of young people.

★ 69 ★ Action in International Medicine (AIM)
125 High Holborn
London WC1V 6QA, United Kingdom
Phone: 44 171 4053090 **Fax:** 44 171 4053093
Email: actintmed@aol.com

Fnded: 1988. **Mem:** 100. **Lang(s):** English. **Desc:** Health care institutions and health services. Promotes adoption of of "CCI," a self-help health improvement program which empowers local communities to address their health and poverty issues. Works to establish health care infrastructure in developing areas; provides support and assistance to grass roots health services. **Pub:** *AIM Bulletin*, quarterly. Newsletter.

★ 70 ★ Action on Smoking and Health (ASH)
2013 H St. NW
Washington, DC 20006
Phone: (202)659-4310 **Fax:** (202)833-3921
Email: webmaster@ash.org
Website: http://www.ash.org
John F. Banzhaf, III, Exec. Dir.

Fnded: 1967. **Desc:** Works for the rights of nonsmokers against the problems of smoking. Provides scientific, educational, legal, and advocacy services. Accomplishments include: ban of tobacco ads from radio and television; establishment of no-smoking sections on airplanes, trains, and interstate buses; persuading the National Association of Insurance Commissioners to adopt a resolution urging insurance companies to force smokers to pay their fair share of health insurance costs by charging them higher rates than non smokers; sued the Occupational Safety and Health Administration (OSHA) to ban smoking in all workplaces. **Pub:** *ASH Smoking and Health Review*, bimonthly. Newsletter. Covers medical, legal, regulatory, commercial, institutional, and humorous news related to smoking. *Price:* $25/year. • Also publishes informational handouts on addiction to nicotine, effects of passive smoking, workplace smoking costs, workplace nonsmokers' rights, filing for workers' compensation, and other materials.

★ 71 ★ Action on Smoking and Health - England (ASH)
102 Clifton St.
London EC2A 4HW, United Kingdom
Phone: 44 207 7395902 **Fax:** 44 207 6130531
Email: enquiries@ash.org.uk
Website: http://www.ash.org.uk

Fnded: 1971. **Mem:** 1,000. **Reg. Groups:** 13. **Lang(s):** English. **Desc:** Publicizes the dangers of smoking. Campaigns for smoke-free public areas and for tobacco control legislation. Liaises with medical charities, health promotion organizations, and private groups. Disseminates information; monitors media, scientific, and trade publications. **Pub:** *Burning Views*, bimonthly. Bulletin. Digest of news on smoking and health.

★ 72 ★ Action on Smoking and Health - Ireland (ASH-NI)
5 Northumberland Rd.
Dublin BT9 6DX, Ireland
Phone: 353 1 2310500 **Fax:** 353 1 2310555
Email: admin@irishcancer.ie
Website: http://www.ash.ie

Fnded: 1970. **Desc:** Supports cancer research/prevention and care. Individuals united to disseminate information on the dangers of smoking. Seeks to establish smoke-free public areas and help those addicted to smoking. Works with medical and health groups in support of its aims. Support groups for cancer patients and families, nurses in cancer centres and units, patient advocacy.

★ 73 ★ Action on Smoking and Health - Scotland
8 Frederick St.
Edinburgh EH2 2HB, United Kingdom
Phone: 44 131 2254725 **Fax:** 44 131 2206604
Email: ashscotland@ashscotland.org.uk
Website: http://www.ashscotland.org.uk

Fnded: 1973. **Nat'l Groups:** 1. **Lang(s):** English. **Desc:** National organisation dedicated to campaigning for a tobacco-free Scotland. Aims to: keep the tobacco issue on the public agenda; promote non-smoking as the norm; contribute to the reduction in the uptake of smoking; support stop smoking initiatives. **Pub:** *Unfiltered News*, semiannual. Newsletter. **Frmly:** (1992) Scottish Committee Action on Smoking and Health.

★ 74 ★ Action for Victims of Medical Accidents
44 High St.
Croydon CR0 1YB, United Kingdom
Phone: 44 208 6868333

Desc: Provides independent advice and support to anyone who has suffered a medical accident.

★ 75 ★ Acupuncture Foundation of Canada Institute (AFCI)
2131 Lawarence Ave. E, Ste. 204
Scarborough, ON, Canada M1R 5G4
Phone: (416)752-3988 **Fax:** (416)752-4398
Email: info@afcinstitute.com
Website: http://www.afcinstitute.com

Fnded: 1995. **Mem:** 1,200. **Reg. Groups:** 10. **Desc:** Promotes acupuncture's legitimate place in health care by initiating and supporting research in acupuncture. **Pub:** Newsletter, periodic.

★ 76 ★ Acupuncture and Oriental Medicine Alliance
6405 43rd Ave. Ct. NW, Ste. B
Gig Harbor, WA 98335
Phone: (253)851-6896 **Fax:** (253)851-6883
Website: http://www.aomalliance.org
Tierney Tully, Exec. Dir.

Fnded: 1994. **Mem:** 1,600. **Desc:** Dedicated to the advancement of acupuncture and Oriental medicine. **Pub:** *The Forum*, quarterly. Newsletter. **AKA:** AOMAlliance.

★ 77 ★ Ad Hoc Group for Medical Research Funding (AHGMRF)
c/o Association of American Medical Colleges
2450 N St. NW
Washington, DC 20037-1126
Phone: (202)828-0525 **Fax:** (202)862-6218
Email: adhoc@aamc.org
Website: http://www.aamc.org/research/adhocgp/start.htm
Richard M. Knapp, PhD, Chmn.

Fnded: 1982. **Mem:** 300. **Desc:** Organizations engaged in or supporting biomedical and behavioral research. Goals are to assess federal funding for biomedical and behavioral research and advocate appropriate funding for the National Institutes of Health. **Pub:** *Annual Funding Proposal*, annual. Brochure. • *NIH Resource Guide*, biennial. Directory. • Annual Report.*Price:* Free.

★ 78 ★ Adaptive Sports Association
PO Box 1884
Durango, CO 81302
Phone: (970)259-0374 **Fax:** (970)259-2175
Email: asa@frontier.net
Website: http://www.asadurango.org
Timothy S. Kroes, Exec. Dir.

Fnded: 1983. **Mem:** 420. **Desc:** Provides ski lessons to people with disabilities. Also offers summer sports opportunities to individuals with disabilities including river rafting, kayaking, canoeing, hiking, and fishing. **Pub:** *Membership Newsletter*, quarterly. Newsletter. • Newsletter, quarterly. *Price:* $30. **Frmly:** (1995) Durango/Purgatory Adaptive Sports Association.

★ 79 ★ ADARA: Professionals Networking for Excellence in Service Delivery with Individuals Who are Deaf or Hard of Hearing
PO Box 727
Lusby, MD 20657
Phone: (410)495-8440 **Fax:** (410)495-8442
Email: adaraorgn@aol.com
Website: http://www.adara.org
Sherri Gallagher, Natl. Off. Coord.

Fnded: 1966. **Mem:** 600. **State Groups:** 12. **Desc:** Psychiatrists, mental health counselors, students, teachers, researchers, rehabilitation facility personnel, interpreters, speech therapists, social workers, doctors, and rehabilitation counselors who serve deaf and deaf-blind persons. Promotes the development and expansion of quality services to deaf and hard-of-hearing persons. Strives to bring about a better understanding of deaf, hard-of-hearing, and deaf-blind people as a whole by encouraging students, professionals, and laymen to develop more than a superficial understanding of the needs and problems of this group, especially the problems related to communication techniques needed to work effectively with deaf, hard-of-hearing, and deaf-blind persons in human services or a rehabilitation setting. Encourages scientific research of the needs and problems engendered by deafness. Promotes and develops recruitment and training of professional workers with deaf, hard-of-hearing, and deaf-blind persons. Sponsors a professional publication for the promotion of inter- and intradisciplinary communication among professionals concerned with deaf adults and others interested in such activities. Cooperates with other organizations in promoting and encouraging legislation pertinent to the development of professional services and facilities for deaf, hard-of-hearing, and deaf-blind persons. **Pub:**

ADARA Update, quarterly. Newsletter. Includes membership activities information, research reports, and list of employment opportunities. *Price:* Included in membership dues. • *JADARA: A Journal for Professionals Networking for Excellence in Service Delivery with Individuals who are Deaf or Hard of Hearing*, 3/year. Journal. Provides research findings and information on new ideas within the field. Includes reviews of current literature. *Price:* Included in membership dues; $55/year for nonmembers in U.S.; $65/year for nonmembers outside U.S. • Monographs. **Frmly:** American Deafness and Rehabilitation Association; (2003) ADARA.

★ 80 ★ Addiction Research and Treatment Corp. (ARTC)

22 Chapel St.
Brooklyn, NY 11201
Phone: (718)260-2900 **Fax:** (718)260-8276
Email: rsage@artcny.org
Website: http://www.Artcny.org
Dr. Beny J. Primm, Pres.

Fnded: 1969. **Mem:** 250. **Desc:** Operates a multimodality drug treatment program with nine ambulatory treatment clinics and a Vocational Evaluation Center. Funded by the state of New York Substance Abuse Services and Medicaid reimbursements. Treatments employed are primarily detoxification, methadone maintenance, and drug-free services. Other services include: individual counseling, group therapy, job development, vocational counseling, mental health care, and recreation. Participates in national research programs. Sponsors substance abuse and AIDS research projects. Maintains speakers' bureau. Publishes abstracts.

★ 81 ★ Adelaide Hospital Society

c/o Adelaide and Meath Hospital
Tallaght
Dublin 24, Ireland
Phone: 353 1 4142072 **Fax:** 353 1 4142070
Email: info@adelaide.ie
Website: http://www.adelaide.ie

Fnded: 1839. **Mem:** 1,000. **Desc:** Promotes the participation of the Protestant community in the Irish health system. Makes available financial support to Adelaide and Meath Hospital. Conducts fundraising activities; sponsors charitable programs.

★ 82 ★ ADHD-foreningen (MBD-foreningen)

Alexandragarden
Arnstein Arnebergsv 30
N-1366 Lysaker, Norway
Phone: 47 67583757 **Fax:** 47 67583747
Email: post@adhd-foreningen.no
Website: http://www.mbd.no

Fnded: 1979. **Mem:** 5,000. **Reg. Groups:** 18. **Local Groups:** 18. **Lang(s):** English, Norwegian. **Desc:** Parents of children with ADHD - Attention Deficit/Hyperactivity Disorder; health personnel. Acts as support group. **Pub:** *Artikkelsamling om MBD*. Book. • *Ett Oyeblikk, Noe Barm / Volksne Med ADHD*, quarterly, always March, June, July, and December. Brochure. • *Sta Pa*, quarterly, always March, June, September, and December. Magazine. • *Sta Pa Temanummer om ADHD 1998*.

★ 83 ★ Advanced Medical Technology Association (AdvaMed)

1200 G St. NW, Ste. 400
Washington, DC 20005-3814
Phone: (202)783-8700 **Fax:** (202)783-8750
Email: info@advamed.org
Website: http://www.advamed.org
Mary Plock, VP Pub. Affairs

Fnded: 1974. **Mem:** 800. **Desc:** Represents domestic (including U.S. territories and possessions) manufacturers of medical devices, diagnostic products, and healthcare information systems. Develops programs and activities on economic, technical, medical, and scientific matters affecting the industry. Gathers and disseminates information concerning the United States and international developments in legislative, regulatory, scientific or standards-making areas. Conducts scientific and educational seminars and programs. **Pub:** *Health Industry Manufacturers Association–Directory*, annual. Directory. Covers issues facing the health industry. *Price:* Free. For members only. • *In Brief*, monthly. *Price:* Free. For members only. • Manuals. • Proceedings. • Reports. • Also publishes a catalogue. **Frmly:** (2001) Health Industry Manufacturers Association.

★ 84 ★ Adventures in Movement for the Handicapped (AIM)

945 Danbury Rd.
Dayton, OH 45420
Phone: (937)294-4611 **Free:** 800-332-8210
Fax: (937)294-3783
Email: aimkids@siscom.net
Dr. Jo A. Geiger, Exec. Dir.

Fnded: 1958. **Mem:** 4,000. **Desc:** Organizes activities for people with physical challenges. **Pub:** *Adventures in Movement*. Book. • Brochure. **Frmly:** (1969) DANCE, Inc.

★ 85 ★ Advisory Council for Children with Impaired Hearing

137 Blackburn Rd.
Blackburn, VIC 3130, Australia
Phone: 61 3 98771300 **Fax:** 61 3 98771922
Email: moreinfo@edumail.vic.gov.au

Fnded: 1968. **Lang(s):** English. **Desc:** Individuals with a specific interest in the field of hearing impairment, and/or early childhood development. Seeks to maximize the opportunity for deaf children to develop oral skills. Maintains an early intervention center and unit within a school setting.

★ 86 ★ Advocate Health Care (AHC)

25455 Martin Luther King Dr.
Chicago, IL 60616
Phone: (312)808-5573 **Free:** 800-323-8622
Fax: (630)572-9139
Website: http://www.advocatehealth.com/
Richard Risk, Pres.

Fnded: 1995. **Mem:** 10. **Desc:** Health care corporations. Promotes the philosophy that good health care involves an understanding of human ecology and must meet the emotional and spiritual as well as the physical needs of patients. (Human ecology is the "understanding and care of human beings as whole persons in light of their relationships to God, themselves, their families, and the society in which they live.") Supports the concept of holistic health care. Sponsors teaching programs at hospitals; maintains support groups. Sponsors the Park Ridge Center, an institute for the study of health, faith, and ethics; and Parkside Alcoholic Research Foundation, which studies the cause and course of alcoholism and substance abuse. Maintains speakers' bureau. **Pub:** *Human Ecology Booklet*, semiannual. Booklet. • *Ounce of Prevention*, quarterly. • *Second Opinion: Health, Faith, and Ethics*, 3/year. Journal. *Price:* $35/year. • Annual Report. • Bulletin, bimonthly.

★ 87 ★ Advocates for Youth

1025 Vermont Ave. NW, Ste. 200
Washington, DC 20005
Phone: (202)347-5700 **Fax:** (202)347-2263
Email: info@advocatesforyouth.org
Website: http://www.advocatesforyouth.org
James Wagoner, Pres.

Fnded: 1980. **Desc:** Mission is to create programs and promote policies that help young people make informed and responsible decisions about their sexual and reproductive health. Provides information, training and advocacy to youth-serving Organizations, youth leaders, policymakers, and the media in the US and developing countries. Implements numerous programs and promotes evidence-based policies on effective pregnancy and HIV/STI prevention for youth; sexuality education; gay, lesbian, bisexual and transgender youth issues, in addition to forming online communities for sexual health activists. The Resource Center online offers journal databases of information on youth sexual health, as well as model programs in developing countries. **Pub:** *Linkx*, quarterly. Newsletter. Details school-based health care. • *Options*, quarterly. Newsletter. • *Passages*, quarterly. • Reports. • Also publishes fact sheets, resource guides, and life planning education curricula. **Frmly:** Center for Population Options.

★ 88 ★ Advocates for Youth's Media Project

10999 Riverside Dr., Ste. 300
North Hollywood, CA 91602-2239
Phone: (818)762-9668 **Fax:** (818)762-9769
Email: healthytv@aol.com
Website: http://www.themediaproject.com
Robin Smalley, Dir.

Fnded: 1983. **Desc:** A project of Advocates for Youth and the Kaiser Family Foundation. Serves as an advisory and information resource for the entertainment industry to encourage positive and relevant messages about family planning, sexuality, and reproductive health, especially in programming directed toward adolescents. Operates speakers' bureau. **Frmly:** Center for Population Options' Media Project.

★ 89 ★ Aerobics and Fitness Association of America (AFAA)

15250 Ventura Blvd., Ste. 200
Sherman Oaks, CA 91403
Phone: 800-446-2322 **Free:** 877-968-7263
Fax: (818)788-6301
Email: contactafaa@afaa.com
Website: http://www.afaa.com
Linda D. Pfeffer, R.N., Pres.

Fnded: 1983. **Mem:** 145,000. **Desc:** Promotes safety and excellence in exercise instruction. World's largest fitness educator offering certifications in Aerobics, Personal Training, Weightroom, Step, KickBoxing, Emergency Response and the AFAA Fitness Practioner. **Pub:** *American Fitness*, bimonthly. Magazine. Features exercise trends, research, interviews, products, health, and nutrition. *Price:* included in membership dues; $27 /year for nonmembers. • *Fitness Theory and Practice*. Book.

★ 90 ★ Aerospace Medical Association (AsMA)

320 S Henry St.
Alexandria, VA 22314-3579
Phone: (703)739-2240 **Fax:** (703)739-9652
Email: rrayman@asma.org
Website: http://www.asma.org
Russell B. Rayman, MD, Exec. Dir.

Fnded: 1929. **Mem:** 3,300. **Desc:** Medical and scientific personnel engaged in clinical, operational, and research activities in aviation, space, and environmental medicine. Sponsors continuing professional education programs. **Pub:** *Aviation, Space, and Environmental Medicine*, monthly. Journal. Covers the medical aspects of survival in aviation, space, and undersea exploration. Includes annual index; book reviews; meetings calendar. *Price:* Included in membership dues; $140/year for nonmembers; $173/year foreign (agency discount available). • *Aviation, Space and Environmental Medicine*, annual. Membership Directory. • *Scientific Abstracts*, annual. **Frmly:** (1959) Aero Medical Association.

★ 91 ★ Aesculapian Club (AC)

c/o Dr. Sam Kim
25 Shattuck St., Bldg. A Rm. 206
Boston, MA 02115
Phone: (617)726-8858
Dr. Sam Kim, Contact

Desc: Social organization of graduates of Harvard Medical School or physicians who have held teaching appointments there for three years.

★ 92 ★ Aestheticians International Association (AIA)

2611 N Belt Line, Ste. 140
Sunnyvale, TX 75182
Phone: (972)203-8530 **Free:** 877-968-7539
Fax: (972)226-2339
Email: aiathekey@aol.com
Douglas Preston, Pres.

Fnded: 1975. **Mem:** 600. **Desc:** Committed to raise standard of aesthetics with advancement of education and public awareness through legislation, educational institutes, certification, instructors, continuing education and to create a national standard for education.

★ 93 ★ AFAPAC Foundation

Daalwijk 29
NL-1102 AA Amsterdam, Netherlands
Phone: 31 20 6003454 **Fax:** 31 20 6006269
Email: 1.afapac@wxs.nl

Fnded: 1993. **Desc:** Seeks to prevent the spread of the AIDS virus. Provides counseling services.

★ 94 ★ AFASIC - Overcoming Speech Impairments

50 - 52 Great Sutton St.
London EC1V 0DJ, United Kingdom
Phone: 44 20 74909410 **Fax:** 44 20 72512834
Email: info@afasic.org.uk
Website: http://www.afasic.org.uk/

Fnded: 1968. **Mem:** 2,300. **Local Groups:** 30. **Lang(s):** English. **Desc:** Promotes the interests of young people with speech and/or language difficulties. Seeks to enhance understanding of speech and language disorders and improve educational and employment opportunities for young adults with such disorders. Offers advice and support for parents of individuals with speech and language disorders. Conducts research on children's language development. Organizes international symposia, national seminars, and workshops. Maintains speakers' bureau; compiles statistics. **Pub:** *Annual Review*, annual. • *Newsletter*, 3/year, always January, May, and September. Newsletter.

★ 95 ★ African American Breast Cancer Alliance (AABCA)

PO Box 8981
Minneapolis, MN 55408-0981
Phone: (612)825-3675 **Fax:** (612)825-3675
Email: aabcainc@yahoo.com
Website: http://www.geocities.com/aabcainc/

Fnded: 1990. **Desc:** Committed to helping Black women, people of color, families and communities cope with breast cancer. Sponsors a breast cancer support group for patients and survivors at various stages of their experiences; addresses the specific needs of Black women diagnosed with breast cancer; also sponsors celebrations and health events for survivors, families, friends and communities. **Pub:** *Being There*. Brochure. Contains advice to empower women to take charge of their health and care of their lives by becoming more informed about breast cancer.

★ 96 ★ African Association for the Study of Liver Diseases

Dept. of Medicine, Liver Research Centre, University of Cape
Cape Town, Republic of South Africa
Phone: 27 21 471250 **Fax:** 27 4486815

★ 97 ★ African Council of AIDS Service Organizations

c/o ENDA Tiers Monde
54 rue Cannot
Boite Postale 3370
Dakar, Senegal
Phone: 221 8231935 **Fax:** 221 8236615
Email: icaso@endadak.gn.apc.org

Lang(s): English, French. **Desc:** Organizations providing services to people with AIDS. Seeks to improve the quality of life of people with aids; promotes increased availability of AIDS services; works to stop the spread of AIDS. Serves as a forum for communication among members; coordinates members' activities; functions as a clearinghouse on AIDS and AIDS services.

★ 98 ★ African Gerontological Society (AGS)

c/o Dr. Nana Apt, PRes.
Department of Sociology
University of Ghana
Accra, Ghana
Phone: 233 21 556382 **Fax:** 233 21 228397

Lang(s): English. **Desc:** Health care professionals with an interest in gerontology. Seeks to advance the study, teaching, and practice of gerontology. Serves as a forum for the exchange of information among members; sponsors continuing professional development courses.

★ 99 ★ African Medical and Research Foundation (AMREF USA)

19 W 44th St., Ste. 710
New York, NY 10036
Phone: (212)768-2440 **Fax:** (212)768-4230
Email: amrefusa@amrefusa.org
Website: http://www.amref.org
Lisa Meadowcroft, Exec. Dir.

Fnded: 1957. **Reg. Groups:** 11. **Desc:** U.S. branch of the African Medical & Research Foundation. Voluntary organization providing medical services to aid and augment health programs in developing nations and in rural areas of East Africa. Attempts to reach isolated peoples and outlying medical facilities through a network of 100 two-way radios, clinic-equipped mobile units, and a "Flying Doctor Service." Undertakes research programs in the field of medicine and general health surveys. Designs and implements primary health care projects. Provides health education courses through its training center to train health educators and is implementing a program of continuing education for health workers. health workers. **Pub:** *AFYA*, bimonthly. Journal. • *Defender: Health Journal for Africa*, bimonthly. Journal. • *Rural Health Series*, periodic. **Frmly:** African Research Foundation; (1973) African Medical and Research Foundation; (1981) International Medical and Research Foundation.

★ 100 ★ African Medical and Research Foundation - Canada (AMREF Cana)

489 College St., Ste. 407
Toronto, ON, Canada M5G 1A5
Phone: (416)961-6981 **Fax:** (416)961-6984
Email: amref@web.ca
Website: http://www.amref.org/no.htm

Fnded: 1973. **Lang(s):** English, French. **Desc:** Medical and public health professionals in Africa. Seeks to identify and address health needs in rural areas of Africa. Develops, implements, and evaluates public health programs and services; encourages enhancement of local administrative capabilities through training, education, and community participation; facilitates increased participation by women in community development. Conducts outreach and fundraising activities. **Pub:** Newsletter, 3/year. • Brochure, periodic.

★ 101 ★ African Medical and Research Foundation - France (AMRFF)

c/o Mrs. Zarina de Bagneux, Dir.
21 rue Cassette
F-75006 Paris, France
Phone: 33 1 662579458
Email: tzarina@club-internet.fr
Website: http://www.amref.org

Lang(s): English, French. **Desc:** Medical and public health professionals. Seeks to identify and address health needs in rural Africa. Develops, implements, and evaluates public health programs; encourages enhancement of local administrative capacities through training.

★ 102 ★ African Medical and Research Foundation - Italy (AMREF - It) (Fondazione Africana per la Medicina e la Ricerca)

Via Settembrini, 30
I-00195 Rome, Italy
Phone: 39 06 3202222 **Fax:** 39 06 3202227
Email: info@amref.it
Website: http://www.amref.it

Fnded: 1988. **Mem:** 30,000. **Lang(s):** French, German, Italian, Spanish. **Desc:** Provides health care services to people in eastern Africa. Identifies health needs and evaluates and implements methods and programs to meet those needs. Maintains projects which emphasize affordable health care for people in underdeveloped, rural areas. Operates mobile health service facilities, airborn support for health centers in remote areas, and radio communication services with over 100 two-way radio stations. Conducts training programs for rural health care workers and research into the control of hydatid disease, malaria, and sleeping sickness. Applies knowledge from the behavioral and social sciences to health care improvement initiatives. Writes articles and information for training manuals, health education materials, and medical journals. Disseminates information. Offers consultancy services. **Pub:** *Amref News*, every four months. Newsletter. Eight pages of information about our projects and general conditions and problems of the Horn of Africa Where AMREF works.

★ 103 ★ African Medical and Research Foundation - Kenya (AMREF)

PO Box 00506-27691
Langata Rd.
Nairobi, Kenya
Phone: 254 20 605220 **Fax:** 254 20 609518
Email: fundraising@amrefhq.org
Website: http://www.amref.org

Fnded: 1957. **Nat'l Groups:** 5. **Lang(s):** English, Kiswahili. **Desc:** Purpose is to improve the health of people living in 9 east and south African countries. Focuses efforts on developing low-cost healthcare for people in rural areas. Program includes: training of community health workers; planning and evaluation of health projects; consulting services; primary healthcare education; operation of a medical radio communication network within the region; ground mobile health services for nomadic and pastoral peoples; the Flying Doctor Service (funded by the Flying Doctors' Society of Africa), which provides airborne support for remote medical, surgical, and public health facilities. Conducts medical research, particularly into the control of malaria, and hydatid disease; applies behavioral and social sciences in health improvement. Offers computerized services. Produces health manuals and promotes research and advocacy. Promotes capacity building. **Pub:** *Afya*, quarterly. Journal. Covers developments in medical education. • *AMREF Annual Report*, annual. Annual Report. **Frmly:** Flying Doctors Service.

★ 104 ★ African Medical and Research Foundation - Sweden (AMREF - Sw)

Djurgårdsvagen 230
S-115 21 Stockholm, Sweden
Phone: 46 8 6620910 **Fax:** 46 8 6674494
Email: amref@telia.com
Website: http://www.amref.org

Desc: Aims to improve the health of people in eastern Africa. Seeks to indentify health needs and develop, implement, and evaluate methods and programmes to meet those needs through service, training and research. Programmes include: primary health care; training of community health workers; training of rural health staff through continuing education, teacher training and correspondence courses; development, printing, and distribution of training manuals, medical journals, and health education materials; application of behavioral and social sciences to health improvement; airborne support for remote health facilities, including surgical, medical, and public health services; grounds mobile health services for nomadic pastoralists; medical research into the control of hydatid disease, and malaria.

★ 105 ★ African Medical and Research Foundation - Tanzania (AMREF)
PO Box 2773
Upanga Rd.
Dar es Salaam, United Republic of Tanzania
Phone: 255 51 116610 **Fax:** 255 51 115823
Email: info@amreftz.org
Website: http://www.amref.org

Fnded: 1957. **Desc:** Works to develop health programs among communities in Africa. Conducts research; compiles and disseminates information on health issues. Networks with other organizatins with similar objectives, providing a forum for information exchange and cooperation in projects and research.

★ 106 ★ African Medical and Research Foundation - Uganda (AMREF)
PO Box 10663
Kampala, Uganda
Phone: 256 41 250319 **Fax:** 256 41 344565
Email: info@amrefug.org
Website: http://www.amref.org

Fnded: 1957. **Desc:** Purpose is to improve the health of people living in Uganda. Focus is on public heath education, sanitation, medical auxilaries, preventive medicine, health care teams, and clinics.

★ 107 ★ African Network on HIV/AIDS - Europe
Focus Consultancy
32B Warwick Sq.
London SW1 V2AQ, United Kingdom
Phone: 44 171 9320072 **Fax:** 44 171 9320074
Email: london@fcwsq.demon.co.uk

Lang(s): English. **Desc:** National European AIDS organizations with an interest in the AIDS epidemic in Africa. Seeks to slow the spread of AIDS and increase the availability of AIDS treatment services in African countries. Makes available educational and consulting services.

★ 108 ★ African Regional Council for Mental Health
PO Box 50209
Lusaka, Zambia
Phone: 260 1 2812880 **Fax:** 260 1 282880
Email: arcofwfmh@zamtel.zm

Fnded: 1992. **Mem:** 2. **Lang(s):** English. **Desc:** Mental health professionals and organizations. Seeks to advance the diagnosis and treatment of mental illness. Facilitates exchange of information among members; provides assistance and consulting services to mental health care programs.

★ 109 ★ African Society for Traumatic Stress Studies (AFSTSS)
Senderwood, 28 Spencer Ave
Bedfordview 2007, Republic of South Africa
Phone: 27 11 4533489 **Fax:** 27 4533489
Email: merle@icon.co.za

★ 110 ★ African Union of the Blind - Kenya (AUB)
North Airport Rd.
PO Box 72872
Embakasi
Nairobi, Kenya
Phone: 254 20 823989 **Fax:** 254 20 823776
Email: afub@kenyaweb.com
Website: http://www.afub.net

Fnded: 1987. **Mem:** 42. **Nat'l Groups:** 44. **Reg. Groups:** 6. **State Groups:** 44. **Lang(s):** English, French. **Desc:** Works to improve the quality of life of the blind and people with visual impairments in Africa. Represents the interests of people with visual impairments before government agencies, international organizations, and the public. **Pub:** *AFUB Newsletter*, semiannual. Newsletter. Contains exchange of information between national organizations.

★ 111 ★ Africans in Partnership Against AIDS
517 College St., Ste. 338
Toronto, ON, Canada M8G 4A2
Phone: (416)924-5256 **Fax:** (416)924-6575
Email: apaa@on.aibn.com

Fnded: 1993. **Mem:** 150. **Lang(s):** English, French. **Desc:** Individuals of African descent. Seeks to stop the spread of AIDS and HIV among Africans. Conducts educational programs on AIDS prevention. Provides a supportive environment for those infected or affected by HIV/AIDS, their partners, friends, and families. **Pub:** *Kibaru*, monthly. Newsletter.

★ 112 ★ Africans United to Control AIDS
c/o African Community Health Services
219-339 Bloor St. W
Toronto, ON, Canada M5S 1W7
Phone: (416)519-7600 **Fax:** (416)519-7317
Email: aches@globalserve.net

Lang(s): English, French. **Desc:** Individuals of African descent. Seeks to stop the spread of AIDS and HIV among Africans. Conducts educational programs on AIDS prevention.

★ 113 ★ Afro-Asia-Oceania Association of Anatomists (AAOAA)
Room No 1025 PC Block, Ansari Nagar
New Delhi 110 029, India

Fnded: 1985.

★ 114 ★ Agape Center
c/o Japan Church World Service
2-10-14 Komatsubara
Zama-shi
Kanagawa 228-0002, Japan
Phone: 81 46 2547111 **Fax:** 81 46 2552915
Email: agape@mb.infoweb.ne.jp

Fnded: 1980. **Lang(s):** English, Japanese. **Desc:** Works to improve the living conditions of people with disabilities throughout Asia. Conducts social work, rehabilitation, and vocational training programs. Sends Japanese social workers to assist in programs for people with disabilities overseas; distributes equipment to facilities for people with disabilities. **Frmly:** (1998) Agape Workshop for the Disabled.

★ 115 ★ Age Action Ireland
30/31 Lower Camden St.
Dublin 2, Ireland
Phone: 353 1 4756989 **Fax:** 353 1 4756011
Email: info@ageaction.ie
Website: http://www.ageaction.ie

Fnded: 1992. **Mem:** 970. **Nat'l Groups:** 32. **Reg. Groups:** 1. **State Groups:** 18. **Local Groups:** 84. **Desc:** Works to improve the quality of life of all older people, especially those who are most disadvantaged and vulnerable, by enabling them to live full, independent and satisfying lives for as long as they wish in their own homes. Membership is open to all organizations and individuals concerned with aging and older people. Main activities include information and publishing, library, education and training, U3A, Carer Support Programme, innovative projects, research, policy development and campaigning. **Pub:** *Bulletin*, monthly.

★ 116 ★ Age Concern England (ACE)
Astral House
1268 London Rd.
London SW16 4ER, United Kingdom
Phone: 44 20 87657200 **Fax:** 44 20 87657240
Email: ace@ace.org.uk
Website: http://www.ageconcern.org.uk

Fnded: 1940. **Mem:** 98. **Local Groups:** 1100. **Lang(s):** Dutch, English, French, German, Spanish. **Desc:** Involved in campaigning, parliamentary work, policy analysis, research, specialist information and advice provision and publishing. Raises funds. Member of the federation of over 400 Age Concern organizations operating in England. Provides both financial and development support to assist the other members in their provision of vital local services. **Pub:** *Information Bulletin*, monthly. Journal. • Books, periodic. • Pamphlets, periodic. • Papers, periodic.

★ 117 ★ Age Concern Institute of Gerontology
Franklin-Wilkins Bldg.
150 Stamford St.
London SE1 9NN, United Kingdom
Phone: 44 40 78483035 **Fax:** 44 20 78483235
Email: aciog@kcl.ac.uk
Website: http://www.kcl.ac.uk/kis/schools/life_sciences/health/gerontology/top.html

Lang(s): English. **Desc:** Health care professionals treating the elderly; scientists and clinicians with an interest in the aging process and diseases of the aged. Works to insure high standards of research and practice in gerontology, and to maximize availability of gerontological services. Conducts research and educational activities. **Frmly:** (1997) British Society of Gerontology.

★ 118 ★ Age Concern Scotland (ACS)
113 Rose St.
Edinburgh EH2 3DT, United Kingdom
Phone: 44 131 2203345 **Fax:** 44 131 2202779
Email: enquiries@acscot.org.uk
Website: http://www.ageconcernscotland.org.uk

Fnded: 1943. **Mem:** 500. **Nat'l Groups:** 1. **Local Groups:** 240. **Lang(s):** English. **Desc:** Works to make the lives of older people in Scotland more secure, comfortable, dignified and enjoyable. **Pub:** *Adage*, bimonthly. Newsletter. • Brochures, periodic.

★ 119 ★ Age - The European Older People's Platform
111 rue Froissart
B-1040 Brussels, Belgium
Phone: 32 2 2801470 **Fax:** 32 2 2801522
Email: info@age-platform.org
Website: http://www.age-platform.org

Fnded: 2000. **Mem:** 103. **Lang(s):** Dutch, English, French, German, Italian, Portuguese, Spanish. **Desc:** Works to improve the quality of life of older people. Gathers and disseminates information on issues including social issues, pensions, and employment, focusing on European Union's policy. **Pub:** *Rapport AGE*, MON. Newsletter. Conference reports, fact sheets, and policy papers.

★ 120 ★ Aggressive Aids Prevention
Federal PO Box 26227
San Francisco, CA 94126-6227
Phone: (415)255-6022
Email: bod@aggressive.org
Website: http://www.aggressive.org
Devin Kordt-Thomas, Media

Fnded: 1998. **Desc:** Promotes HIV/AIDS awareness. Provides information, materials and education.

★ 121 ★ Aging in America (AIA)
1500 Pelham Pky. S
Bronx, NY 10461
Phone: (718)824-4004 **Fax:** (718)409-8781
William Smith, CEO

Fnded: 1979. **Desc:** Research and service organization for professionals in gerontology. Objectives are: to produce, implement, and share effective and affordable programs and services that improve the quality of life for the elderly community; to better prepare professionals and students interested in, or currently involved with, aging and the aged. Conducts research projects, educational and training seminars, and inservice curricula for long-term and acute care facilities. Operates: Education and Training Program to educate professionals and para-professionals; Projects With Industry Program to help both able-bodied and disabled elderly individuals enter into the work force. Conducts local programs in New York City including: In-Home Services, which provides Meals-on-Wheels, transportation, and housekeeping; Alzheimer's Day Care; Respite and Long-Term Residence; Self-Governing Senior Centers. Provides social services, including case management, information, referral, and advocacy; Research. Maintains speakers' bureau; compiles statistics. **Pub:** *Sharing Newsletter*, quarterly. Newsletter. • Brochure.Outlines various programs. **Frmly:** (1952) Morningside House.

★ 122 ★ Aicardi Syndrome Newsletter
c/o Denise Parsons
1510 Polo Fields Ct.
Louisville, KY 40245
Phone: (502)244-9152
Email: aicnews@aol.com
Website: http://www.aicardi.org
Denise Parsons, Trustee

Fnded: 1983. **Mem:** 200. **Nat'l Groups:** 5. **Desc:** Families with daughters affected by Aicardi Syndrome (Aicardi Syndrom is a rare genetic disorder affecting females only; and characterized by absence of the corpus callosum, and retinal lesions, seizures, and mental retardation.) Provides information, research opportunities, networking, and communication. Acts as a reference and resource contact for medical, educational, and professional organizations. Conducts research programs. **Pub:** *Aicardi Syndrome Newsletter*, 2-3/year. Newsletter. • *ASN Brief*, bimonthly. Newsletter. • Brochure. • Directory.

★ 123 ★ Aid for International Medicine (AIM)
PO Box 119
Rockland, DE 19732
Phone: (302)655-8290 **Fax:** (302)655-0487
Dr. John Levinson, Pres.

Fnded: 1965. **Mem:** 25. **Reg. Groups:** 2. **Desc:** To extend medical help through areas where one or more members of the board have personally served and documented a need. Funding and/or materials have been provided for hospitals, medical schools, and orphanages in Asia, Africa, and the U.S. Has established medical textbook program which makes available new books to medical schools and hospitals.

★ 124 ★ AIDS Action
1906 Sunderland Place NW
Washington, DC 20036
Phone: (202)530-8030 **Fax:** (202)530-8031
Email: aidsaction@aidsaction.org
Website: http://www.aidsaction.org

Fnded: 1984. **Mem:** 3,200. **Desc:** National AIDS service organizations. Dedicated to responsible federal policy for improved HIV/AIDS care and services, vigorous medical research and effective prevention. Operates the Pedro Zamora Center national AIDS youth advocacy program.

★ 125 ★ AIDS Care Education and Training (ACET)
The Oasis Centre
115 Southwark Bridge Rd.
London SE1 0AX, United Kingdom
Phone: 44 207 4509082 **Fax:** 44 207 4509001
Email: acet@acetuk.org
Website: http://www.oasistrust.org

Fnded: 1988. **Nat'l Groups:** 7. **Reg. Groups:** 6. **Lang(s):** English. **Desc:** Promotes effective and unconditional care for people with HIV and AIDS worldwide. Conducts educational and training programs for AIDS care providers; works with national and international AIDS care organizations to improve the quality and availability of AIDS care. **Pub:** *ACET Newsletter*, 3/year. Newsletter. • *HIV - Facts for Life*. Booklet.

★ 126 ★ AIDS Evaluation
Swiss Federal Office of Public Health
Evaluation Management & Resource Centre
CH-3003 Bern, Switzerland
Phone: 41 31 3238761 **Fax:** 41 31 3229900
Email: evaluation@bag.admin.ch
Website: http://www.health-evaluation.admin.ch
Lang(s): English, French, German, Italian.

★ 127 ★ AIDS Foundation of Canada
885 Dunsmuir St., Ste. 1000
Vancouver, BC, Canada V6C 1N5
Phone: (604)688-7294 **Fax:** (604)689-4888
Email: ganapath@axionet.com

Fnded: 1986. **Mem:** 6. **Lang(s):** English, French. **Desc:** Individuals and corporations with an interest in the prevention and treatment of AIDS and HIV. Promotes an improved quality of life for people with HIV and AIDS; seeks to advance AIDS and HIV treatment and prevention techniques. Conducts public awareness programs to slow the spread of AIDS; provdies financial and other assistance to innovative programs assisting people with HIV and AIDS. Sponsors charitable programs.

★ 128 ★ AIDS Helpline Northern Ireland
7 James St. S
Belfast BT2 8DN, United Kingdom
Phone: 44 28 90249268 **Fax:** 44 28 90329845
Email: admin@aidshelpline.org.uk
Website: http://www.aidshelpline.org.uk

Fnded: 1985. **Mem:** 48. **Desc:** Makes available counselors to offer advice to those affected by AIDS. Offers home support. Conducts preventative education and a outreach programs. Promotes fundraising. Provides a range of complementary therapies freephone helpline, health enquiries, advice line.

★ 129 ★ AIDS Resource Foundation for Children (ARFC)
St. Clare's Home for Children
182 Roseville Ave.
Newark, NJ 07107
Phone: (973)483-4250 **Fax:** (973)483-1998
Email: info@aidsresource.org
Website: http://www.aidsresource.org/
Terrence P. Zealand, Exec. Dir.

Fnded: 1985. **Desc:** Operates homes for children ages birth thru 12 years of age with HIV, AIDS, or AIDS-Related Complex (ARC) medically fragile (ie: cerebral palsy, menigitis, mentally retarded, etc.) who are well enough to be released from the hospital but are in need of foster care placement or respite care; provides support services to families coping with AIDS or related diseases. Operates foster parent recruitment, training, and support programs; collects and distributes toys and clothing. Sponsors summer camp for families. Conducts HIV training workshops, community outreach programs, and agency networking; maintains speakers' bureau. Provides referrals, bereavement counseling, and emergency assistance. Acts as a model program for transitional foster homes nationwide; although all homes are currently operating in the New Jersey area, any child with AIDS or a related disease is eligible for assistance. **Pub:** Newsletter, periodic. **AKA:** St. Clare's Home for Children; St. Clare's Home Properties.

★ 130 ★ AIDS School Education Resource Centre
c/o Programme of Education for the Prevention of AIDS
UNESCO
Section de l'Education Preventive
Division de la Renovation de l'Enseignement Secondaire et Pr
7 Place de Fontenoy
F-75352 Paris, France
Phone: 33 1 45681622 **Fax:** 33 1 45685621
Email: s.bahri@unesco.org

Lang(s): English, French. **Desc:** AIDS education programs and institutions. Seeks to slow the spread of AIDS through increasing public awareness of the disease. Sponsors educational programs and produces and distributes curricular materials.

★ 131 ★ AIDS Secretariat - Antigua-Barbuda
Ministry of Health and Civil Service Affairs
AIDS Secretariat
AFLAK Bldg.
Friar's Hill Rd.
Saint Johns, Antigua-Barbuda
Phone: (268)462-5039 **Fax:** (268)462-5039
Email: aidssec@candw.ag

Fnded: 1989. **Lang(s):** English. **Desc:** Individuals in Antigua-Barbuda interested in fighting the spread of HIV/AIDS. Conducts public awareness and health programs.

★ 132 ★ AIDS Society for Asia and the Pacific
Edmund Blacket Bldg., 1st Fl. S Wing
Prince of Wales Hospital
Randwick, NSW 2031, Australia
Phone: 61 2 93822775 **Fax:** 61 2 93822787
Email: j.dwyer@unsw.edu.au

Fnded: 1990. **Mem:** 3,600. **Nat'l Groups:** 3. **Reg. Groups:** 3. **Lang(s):** English. **Desc:** AIDS organizations and agencies. Seeks to prevent the spread of AIDS through increased public awareness of the disease and its prevention; promotes improved treatment of AIDS and HIV. Sponsors educational programs; conducts research.

★ 133 ★ AIDS Trust of Australia (ATA)
PO Box 1030
Darlinghurst, NSW 1300, Australia
Phone: 61 2 93610610 **Fax:** 61 2 93610665
Email: info@aidstrust.com.au
Website: http://www.aidstrust.com.au

Fnded: 1987. **Reg. Groups:** 1. **State Groups:** 1. **Local Groups:** 1. **Lang(s):** English. **Desc:** Works to raise funds which are then employed in the continuing struggle against HIV/AIDS in Australia.

★ 134 ★ Air Medical Physician Association (AMPA)
c/o Pat Petersen
383 F St.
Salt Lake City, UT 84103
Phone: (801)534-0829 **Fax:** (801)534-0434
Email: patp@ampa.org
Website: http://www.ampa.org
Pat Petersen, Exec. Dir.

Fnded: 1992. **Mem:** 400. **Desc:** Physicians and professionals involved in medical transport. Promotes safe and effective patient transportation through medical direction, research, education, leadership and collaboration. **Pub:** *Air Medical Journal*, quarterly. Journal. Peer-reviewed journal. • *Air Medical Physician Handbook*. Handbook. *Price:* included in membership dues; $65 for nonmembers; $50 additional copies for members.

★ 135 ★ Air and Surface Transport Nurses Association (ASTNA)
9101 E Kenyon Ave., Ste. 3000
Denver, CO 80237
Free: 800-897-6362 **Fax:** (303)770-1812
Email: astna@gwami.com
Website: http://www.astna.org
Karen Wojdyla, CAE, Exec. Dir.

Fnded: 1981. **Mem:** 1,700. **Reg. Groups:** 10. **Desc:** Transport nurses. Seeks to promote the quality of transport nursing by developing standards for the profession and exploring educational opportunities. Seeks optimum working conditions for members. Provides assistance to hospitals for developing air medical services programs. Maintains speakers' bureau. **Pub:** *Across the Board*, bimonthly. Newsletter. • *Journal of Air Medical Transport*, monthly. Journal. • Also produces educational learning module. **AKA:** (1999) National Flight Nurses Association.

★ 136 ★ AirLifeLine (ALL)
50 Fullerton Ct., Ste. 200
Sacramento, CA 95825
Phone: (916)641-7800 **Free:** 877-AIR-LIFE
Fax: (916)641-0600
Email: staff@airlifeline.org
Website: http://www.airlifeline.org
Randall R. Quast, CEO

Fnded: 1978. **Mem:** 1,120. **Nat'l Groups:** 1. **Desc:** Voluntary association of pilots who donate their time, skills, fuel, and aircraft to fly medical missions. Provides free air transportation for financially needy patients who require specialized treatment at medical facilities far from their homes. **Pub:** *Pilot and Patient*, quarterly. Newsletter. Includes Victory Roll, a list of volunteer pilots who have flown medical missions and stories of patients. *Price:* Free. • *Skylines*, 3/year. Newsletter. Provides information on the program and on aviation in general. • Membership Directory, 3/year.

★ 137 ★ Airlines Medical Directors Association (AMDA)
c/o Ralph G. Fennell, M.D.
United Airlines Medical
Denver International Airport
Denver, CO 80249-6363
Phone: (303)348-4300 **Fax:** (303)348-4338
Ralph G. Fennell, MD, Sec. Dir.

Fnded: 1946. **Mem:** 130. **Desc:** Physicians employed by, or consulting to, commerical airlines.

★ 138 ★ Airspace Action on Smoking and Health (ASASH)
6200 McKay Ave.
Box 141-831
Burnaby, BC, Canada V5H 4M9
Phone: (604)444-8016 **Free:** 888-621-7233
Fax: (604)276-3247
Email: airspace@airspace.bc.ca
Website: http://airspace.bc.ca/

Lang(s): English, French. **Desc:** Individuals and organizations. Seeks to eliminate tobacco smoking. Lobbies for more stringent laws banning smoking in public places; provides assistance to individuals wishing to quit smoking.

★ 139 ★ Al-Anon/Alateen/Alcoholics Anonymous
Box 1672
Yellowknife, NT, Canada X1A 2N1
Phone: (867)873-5096

Lang(s): English, French. **Desc:** Alcoholics and their families. Promotes abstinence from liquor. Assists individuals wishing to abstain from drinking using a twelve-step program facilitated by participation in support groups; provides assistance to families of alcoholics. **Pub:** Report, periodic.

★ 140 ★ Al-Anon Family Group Headquarters, World Service Office (AFG)
1600 Corporate Landing Pkwy.
Virginia Beach, VA 23454-5617
Phone: (757)563-1600 **Free:** 888-4AL-ANON
Fax: (757)563-1655
Email: wso@al-anon.org
Website: http://www.al-anon.alateen.org

Fnded: 1951. **Reg. Groups:** 26000. **Desc:** Relatives and friends of individuals with an alcohol problem. Operates Alateen for members 12-20 years of age whose lives have been adversely affected by someone else's drinking problem, usually a parent's. **Pub:** *Al-Anon Family Group Headquarters–The Forum: A Meeting in My Pocket*, monthly. Magazine. Written by Al-Anon members. Includes calendar of events. *Price:* $10/year. • *Al-Anon Speaks Out*, semiannual. For the professional community regarding alcohol abuse. *Price:* Free. • *Alateen Talk*, bimonthly. Newsletter. Contains written and artistic contributions from Alateen members. Includes articles written by adult Alateen sponsors and coordinators. *Price:* Included in Alateen Group Registration; $2.50/year for individuals; $.15/copy. • *Loner's Letter Box*, bimonthly. Newsletter. *Price:* available to members only. • Also publishes leaflets, pamphlets, and books.

★ 141 ★ Al-Anon Family Groups - United Kingdom and Eire
61 Great Dover St.
London SE1 4YF, United Kingdom
Phone: 44 20 74030888 **Fax:** 44 20 73789910
Email: alanonuk@aol.com
Website: http://www.hexnet.co.uk/alanon/

Fnded: 1951. **Nat'l Groups:** 900. **Lang(s):** English, Irish. **Desc:** Offers understanding and support for families and friends of problem drinkers, whether alcoholic is still drinking or not. **Pub:** *Al-Anon - A Community Resource*. Brochure. • *Facts About Al-Anon and Alateen*. Brochure.

★ 142 ★ Alagille Syndrome Alliance (ASA)
c/o Cindy L. Hahn
10630 SW Garden Park Pl.
Tigard, OR 97223
Phone: (503)639-6217
Email: alagille@earthlink.net
Website: http://www.alagille.org
Cindy L. Hahn, Pres.

Fnded: 1993. **Desc:** Works to provide a support network for family, friends and healthcare providers as well as children and adults with Alagille Syndrome, a liver disorder affecting the bile ducts and/or the pulmonary arteries, heart and lungs, spinal column, eyes, facial features and less frequently, the pancreas, renal system and arteries in the brain. **Pub:** *Fact Sheet*. • *LiverLink*, bimonthly. Newsletter. Back issues are available. • Brochure.Available for schools.

★ 143 ★ Alan Guttmacher Institute (AGI)
120 Wall St., 21st Fl.
New York, NY 10005
Phone: (212)248-1111 **Fax:** (212)248-1951
Email: info@agi-usa.org
Website: http://www.guttmacher.org
Sara Seims, Pres.

Fnded: 1968. **Desc:** The Alan Guttmacher Institute (AGI) is a non-profit organization focused on reproductive health research, policy analysis and public education. The Institute's mission is to protect the reproductive choices of all women and men in the United States and throughout the world. It is to support their ability to obtain the information and services needed to achieve their full human rights, safeguard their health and exercise their individual responsibilities in regard to sexual behavior, reproduction and family information. **Pub:** *Fulfilling the Promise: Public Policy and U.S. Family Planning Clinics*. Report. • *The Guttmacher Report on Public Policy*, bimonthly. Journal. • *In Their Own Right: Addressing the Sexual and Reproductive Health Needs of American Men*. Report. • *International Family Planning Perspectives*, quarterly. Journal. • *Perspectives on Sexual and Reproductive Health*, bimonthly. Journal. **Frmly:** (1975) Center for Family Planning Program Development; (1977) Research and Development Division of Planned Parenthood Federation of America.

★ 144 ★ Alateen
1600 Corporate Landing Pkwy.
Virginia Beach, VA 23454-5617
Phone: (757)563-1600 **Free:** 888-425-2666
Fax: (757)563-1655
Email: wso@al-anon.org
Website: http://www.alateen.org

Fnded: 1957. **Nat'l Groups:** 3000. **Local Groups:** 1826. **Desc:** Individuals ages 12-19 who have been adversely affected by a relative or friend with an alcohol problem. **Pub:** *Alateen Talk*, quarterly. Newsletter.

★ 145 ★ Alateen
1771 Ave. Rd.
Box 54533
North York, ON, Canada M5M 4N5
Phone: (905)770-1060

Lang(s): English, French. **Desc:** Alcoholic teens. Promotes abstinence from alcohol among members. Facilitates recovery among members using a 12step program utilizing support groups. **Pub:** *SDSA News*, quarterly. Newsletter. • *You See Down's Syndrome. We See Potential*. Brochure.

★ 146 ★ Albanian Association of Gerontology and Geriatrics
University Hospital Centre "Mother Teresa"
Tirana, Albania
Phone: 355 42 23883 **Fax:** 355 43 62627
Email: drspit@sanx.net

Fnded: 1996. **Lang(s):** Albanian, English. **Desc:** Provides services to the aged.

★ 147 ★ Albanian Association in Support of Asthma and Allergy Patients
c/o Aristo Uruci
Rr. Anastas Kullorioti 8/1
Tirana, Albania
Phone: 355 42 69200 **Fax:** 355 42 69200
Email: aasap@icc-al.org

Desc: Protects the interests of asthma and allergy patients. Conducts educational programs; offers medical advice to patients. **Pub:** Booklet.

★ 148 ★ Albanian Dental Association
Rrugo Dibres
Pallaati 375, Shk. 2, Ap. 8
Tirana, Albania
Phone: 355 43 63241 **Fax:** 355 43 63241
Email: rqafmolla@yahoo.com
Website: http://www.asa.org.al

Fnded: 1993. **Mem:** 400. **Nat'l Groups:** 18. **Reg. Groups:** 12. **State Groups:** 6. **Lang(s):** Albanian, English, German. **Desc:** Promotes dentistry in Albania. **Pub:** *Albanian Stomatological Journal*, every semester. Journal.

★ 149 ★ Albanian Society for Cardiology
c/o University Hospital Centre
Rruga e Dibres 370
Tirana, Albania
Phone: 355 4 274294 **Fax:** 355 4 374294
Email: drspit@sanx.net
Website: http://www.escardio.org/society/natsoc/albania.htm

Fnded: 1994. **Mem:** 134. **Nat'l Groups:** 11. **Desc:** Cardiologists in Albania. Fosters research of cardiac diseases.

★ 150 ★ Albert Ellis Institute
45 E 65th St.
New York, NY 10021
Phone: (212)535-0822 **Free:** 800-323-4738
Fax: (212)249-3582
Email: info@rebt.org
Website: http://www.rebt.org
Dominic J. DiMattia, Ed.D, Exec. Dir.

Fnded: 1968. **Desc:** Provides professional training; moderate-cost treatment services, including individual and group psychotherapy, marriage and family counseling, and crisis intervention; consultative services for mental health professionals, corporations, and community agencies; research programs in applied psychology. Operates speakers' bureau. Rational emotive behavior therapy, the institute's chief treatment approach, is a psychological theory and technique devised in 1955 based on the assumption that human beings become disturbed through acquiring irrational thoughts, beliefs, philosophies, or attitudes. REBT asserts that people can be taught to change their negative and disturbed feelings and behaviors by consciously correcting the false beliefs and inaccurate perceptions that underlie and accompany these feelings. **Frmly:** (1978) Institute for Advanced Study in Rational Psychotherapy; (1996) Institute for Rational-Emotive Therapy.

★ 151 ★ Albinism World Alliance (AWA)
PO Box 959
East Hampstead, NH 03826-0959
Free: 800-473-2310 **Fax:** (603)887-6049
Email: awa@albinism.org
Website: http://www.albinism.org/awa.html
Janice L. Knuth, Co-Chair

Fnded: 1992. **Desc:** Albinism support groups in 15 countries. (Albinism is an inherited metabolic disorder that results in reduced pigment in the hair, eyes, and/or skin of those it affects; people with albinism also have impaired eye function including decreased visual acuity, involuntary eye movements, and increased sensitivity to light.) Fosters communication among albinism support groups, and promotes development of albinism support groups worldwide. Disseminates information.

★ 152 ★ Alcohol and Drug Concerns (ADC)
112-4500 Sheppard Ave. E
Toronto, ON, Canada M1S 3R6
Phone: (416)293-3400 **Fax:** (416)293-1142
Email: info@concerns.ca
Website: http://www.concerns.ca

Fnded: 1876. **Mem:** 1,200. **Reg. Groups:** 1. **Lang(s):** English, French. **Desc:** Individuals and organizations. Seeks to eliminate the harm associated with substance abuse among youth. Serves as a clearinghouse on substance abuse and related social problems; makes available support and services to teens, their families, and schools. **Pub:** *Concerns*, quarterly. Newsletter. Contains information for those interested in helping youth learn responsible drug use.

★ 153 ★ Alcohol and Drug Free Traffic - International (ADFTI)
Gammelgardsvagen 38
S-112 64 Stockholm, Sweden
Phone: 46 8 6726165 **Fax:** 46 8 6726167
Email: landsradet@sobernet.org

Lang(s): English, Swedish. **Desc:** Individuals and organizations. Seeks to eliminate driving while under the influence of alcohol or other substances. Lobbies for heavier penalties for individuals convicted of driving under the influence; conducts educational programs to raise public awareness of the dangers of drinking and driving.

★ 154 ★ Alcohol and Drug Problems Association of North America (ADPA)
307 N Main
Saint Charles, MO 63301
Phone: (314)589-6702 **Fax:** (314)940-2358
Email: blefilm@juno.com
Website: http://www.adpana.com
Barbara Eisenstadt, EdD, Contact

Fnded: 1949. **Mem:** 1,325. **Desc:** Individuals (1100), official state or provincial alcoholism program members (75), and other alcoholism and/or drug agencies and institutions (150). Seeks to facilitate governmental and professional activities in the fields of alcoholism, alcohol-related problems, and drug abuse by exchange of information, promotion of legislation and standards which will contribute to the care and control of alcoholism, and research and cooperation. Maintains continuing education program and placement service. **Pub:** *ADPA Professional*, bimonthly. Newsletter. On public policy concerning drug and alcohol abuse. Includes book reviews; calendar of events; educational opportunities. *Price:* Included in membership dues. • *Special Reports*, periodic. **Frmly:** (1956) National States Conference on Alcoholism; (1972) North American Association of Alcoholism Programs.

★ 155 ★ Alcohol Focus Scotland
166 Buchanan St.
Glasgow G1 2LW, United Kingdom
Phone: 44 141 3339677 **Fax:** 44 141 3331606
Email: jacklaw@alcohol-focus-scotland.org.uk
Website: http://www.alcohol-focus-scotland.org.uk

Fnded: 1973. **Lang(s):** English. **Desc:** Seeks to reduce the level of alcohol abuse in Scotland. Conducts educational and training programs for health care professionals and therapists working with people who abuse alcohol; serves as a clearinghouse on alcohol abuse programs and services. Participates in charitable activities; compiles statistics. **Pub:** *Alcohol Focus Annual Report*, annual. Annual Report. • *Alcohol Update*, quarterly. Newsletter. • Books. • Reports. **Frmly:** (2002) Scottish Council on Alcohol.

★ 156 ★ Alcohol and Other Drugs Council of Australia (ADCA)
PO Box 269
Woden, ACT 2606, Australia
Phone: 61 2 62810686 **Fax:** 61 2 62810995
Email: pennys@adca.org.au
Website: http://www.adca.org.au

Fnded: 1967. **Mem:** 400. **Desc:** Develops and promotes national policies and advises on all issues concerning alcohol and other drugs. Conducts research. Runs media campaigns on alcohol and drug use. **Pub:** *ADCA Annual Report*, annual. • *ADCA Update*, monthly. Newsletter. • *AIM*. • *Drug Contents.*

★ 157 ★ Alcohol Research Information Service (ARIS)
430 Lathrop St.
Lansing, MI 48912
Phone: (517)485-9900 **Fax:** (517)485-1928
Email: alcoholresearch@ameritech.net
Robert Hammond, Exec. Dir.

Fnded: 1931. **Desc:** Individual and corporate contributors. Collects, correlates, and disseminates information regarding alcohol and alcoholic products, their manufacture, sale, and use for beverage, industrial, or other purposes, and their relation to the health and well-being of the people of the United States. Operates clearinghouse for information on alcohol, drugs, and compulsive and problem gambling. Compiles statistics. **Pub:** *Monday Morning Report*, bimonthly. Newsletter. Contains six pages. *Price:* $100 first class mail. • Also provides teaching materials for elementary and secondary school levels, and adults. **Frmly:** (1984) American Business Men's Research Foundation.

★ 158 ★ Alcoholics Anonymous Australia
National Office
48 Firth St.
Arncliffe, NSW 2205, Australia
Phone: 61 2 95998866 **Fax:** 61 2 95998844
Email: national.office@aa.org.au
Website: http://www.alcoholicsanonymous.org.au

Lang(s): English. **Desc:** Individuals recovering from alcoholism in Australia. Members believe that they can free themselves from alcohol abuse by following a 12-step program that includes sharing of experiences, strength, and hope with fellow members. Refuses alliance with any sect, denomination, political organization, or institution and does not endorse or oppose any cause.

★ 159 ★ Alcoholics Anonymous - Brazil (Junaab-Junta de Servicos Gerais de A.A. do Brasil)
Av. Senador Queiros 101, 2 andar, cj 205
Caixa Postal 3180
01060-970 Sao Paulo, SP, Brazil
Phone: 55 11 2293611 **Fax:** 55 11 2293611
Email: aa@alcoolicosanonimos.org.br
Website: http://www.alcoolicosanonimos.org.br

Fnded: 1947. **Mem:** 120,000. **Nat'l Groups:** 5300. **Reg. Groups:** 130. **State Groups:** 420. **Lang(s):** Dutch, English, Portuguese. **Desc:** Individuals recovering from alcoholism in Brazil. Members believe that they can free themselves from alcohol by following a 12-step program that includes sharing of experiences, strength, and hope with fellow members. Refuses alliance with any sect, denomination, political organization, or institution and does not endorse or oppose any cause. **Pub:** *Bob Mural*, bimonthly. Newsletter. • *Revista Vivencia*, bimonthly. Magazine. • Books. • Pamphlets.

★ 160 ★ Alcoholics Anonymous - England
PO Box 1
Stonebow House
Stonebow
York YO1 7NJ, United Kingdom
Phone: 44 1904 644026 **Fax:** 44 1904 629091
Website: http://www.alcoholics-anonymous.org.uk

Lang(s): English. **Desc:** Individuals recovering from alcoholism in the United Kingdom and the Republic of Ireland. Members believe that they can free themselves from alcohol abuse by following a 12step program that includes sharing of experiences, strength, and hope with fellow members. Refuses alliance with any sect, denomination, political organization, or institution and does not endorse or oppose any cause. **Frmly:** Alcoholics Anonymous World Services - United Kingdom and Eire General Services Office.

★ 161 ★ Alcoholics Anonymous - French General Services Office
21, rue Trousseau
F-75011 Paris, France
Phone: 33 1 48064368 **Fax:** 33 1 40210535
Email: aaf2@club-internet.fr
Website: http://perso.club-internet.fr/aafr/

Fnded: 1960. **Mem:** 11,000. **Reg. Groups:** 23. **Local Groups:** 580. **Lang(s):** French. **Desc:** Individuals recovering from alcoholism in France. Members believe that they can free themselves from alcohol abuse by following a 12-step program that includes sharing of experiences, strength, and hope with fellow members. Refuses alliance with any sect, denomination, political organization, or institution and does not endorse or oppose any cause. **Frmly:** (1997) Alcoholics Anonymous World Services - French General Services Office; (1997) Services Generaux Al-Anon.

★ 162 ★ Alcoholics Anonymous World Services (AA)
Box 459
Grand Central Sta.
475 Riverside Dr., 11th Fl.
New York, NY 10163
Phone: (212)870-3400 **Fax:** (212)870-3003
Website: http://www.aa.org
Greg Muth, Gen. Service Mgr.

Fnded: 1935. **Desc:** Individuals recovering from alcoholism. AA maintains that members can solve their common problem and help others achieve sobriety through a twelve step program that includes sharing their experience, strength, and hope with each other. Self-supported through members' contributions, AA is not allied with any sect, denomination, political organization, or institution and does not endorse nor oppose any cause. **Pub:** *AA Comes of Age.* • *Alcoholics Anonymous.* • *As Bill Sees It.* • *Dr. Bob and the Good Oldtimers.* • *Pass it On.* • *Twelve Steps and Twelve Traditions.*

★ 163 ★ Alcoholics Anonymous World Services - General Service Board for French-Speaking Belgium
Boulevard Clovis, 81
B-1000 Brussels, Belgium
Phone: 32 2 5114030 **Fax:** 32 1 1844658
Email: bsg@alcooliquesanonymes.be
Website: http://www.alcooliquesanonymes.be

Fnded: 1953. **Nat'l Groups:** 230. **Reg. Groups:** 8. **Lang(s):** French. **Desc:** French-speaking individuals recovering from alcoholism in Belgium. Members believe that they can free themselves from alcohol abuse by following a 12-step program that includes sharing of experiences, strength, and hope with fellow members. Refuses alliance with any sect, denomination, political organization, or institution and does not endorse or oppose any cause.

★ 164 ★ Alcoholics Anonymous World Services - New Zealand General Services Office

PO Box 6458, level 2, Unit 4
The Harbour City Centre
Panana, New Zealand
Phone: 64 9 47924250

Lang(s): English. **Desc:** Individuals recovering from alcoholism in New Zealand. Members believe that they can free themselves from alcohol abuse by following a 12-step program that includes sharing of experiences, strength, and hope with fellow members. Refuses alliance with any sect, denomination, political organization, or institution and does not endorse or oppose any cause.

★ 165 ★ Alcoholics Anonymous World Services - Swedish General Services Office
(Al-Anon Familjegrupper i Sverige)

Erstagatan 1
S-116 28 Stockholm, Sweden
Phone: 46 8 6431393 **Fax:** 46 8 641193
Email: afg@al-anon.a.se
Website: http://www.al-anon.a.se

Lang(s): Swedish. **Desc:** Individuals recovering from alcoholism in Sweden. Members believe that they can free themselves from alcohol abuse by following a 12-step program that includes sharing of experiences, strength, and hope with fellow members. Refuses alliance with any sect, denomination, political organization, or institution and does not endorse or oppose any cause.

★ 166 ★ Alcor Life Extension Foundation (ALEF)

7895 E Acoma Dr., Ste. 110
Scottsdale, AZ 85260-6916
Phone: (480)905-1906 **Free:** 877-462-5267
Fax: (480)922-9027
Email: jennifer@alcor.org
Website: http://www.alcor.org
Jerry B. Lemler, Pres.

Fnded: 1972. **Mem:** 555. **Reg. Groups:** 10. **Desc:** Individuals who have made anatomical donation for purpose of being cryonically suspended. Seeks to extend lives of Alcor members; currently 47 members in suspension. **Pub:** *ALCOR: Reaching for Tomorrow*, quarterly. Magazine. Covers cryonics, life extension, and immortality. *Price:* $35/year; $25/year in Canada and Mexico; $30/year in all other countries. • *Cryonics: Reaching for Tomorrow*, biennial. Booklet. Covers cryonics, life extension, and immortality. *Price:* $8.95/year in the U.S.; $20/year in Canada and Mexico; $25/year overseas. • Brochures. **AKA:** Alcor Foundation.

★ 167 ★ Alexander Graham Bell Association for the Deaf and Hard of Hearing (AGBELL)

3417 Volta Pl. NW
Washington, DC 20007
Phone: (202)337-5220 **Fax:** (202)337-8314
Email: info@agbell.org
Website: http://www.agbell.org
K. Todd Houston, PhD, Exec. Dir.

Fnded: 1890. **Mem:** 5,000. **State Groups:** 17. **Local Groups:** 110. **Desc:** An international membership organization and resource center on hearing loss and spoken language approaches and related issues. Founded in 1890 by Alexander Graham Bell, the association offers members a wide range of programs and services and provides to all inquirers information on a vast array of issues pertaining to hearing loss. Members include parents of children with hearing loss, educators, adults with hearing loss, and hearing health professionals. Publishes books and provides financial aid to qualifying applicants for mainstreamed, auditory-based education at pre-school, school-age and university levels. Provides governmental and education advocacy services through its national office and state chapters, children's rights coordinators and international affiliates. **Pub:** *Alexander Graham Bell Association for the Deaf–Our Kids Magazine*, 2-3/year. Newsletter. For parents of hearing impaired children. *Price:* Included in membership dues. • *Children's Corner*. • *Newsounds*, 10/year. Membership activities newsletter. Includes chapter news and calendar of events. *Price:* Included in membership dues. • *OK Kids*. • *Volta Review*, bimonthly. Professional journal covering issues related to hearing impairment for teachers of the hearing impaired. *Price:* Included in membership dues; $35/year for institutions. • *Volta Voices*, bimonthly. Magazine. • Also publishes bibliographies, teachers' and clinicians' textbooks, lipreading books, and references; produces audiovisuals. **Frmly:** (1948) American Association to Promote the Teaching of Speech to the Deaf; (1953) Volta Speech Association for the Deaf; (2003) Alexander Graham Bell Association for the Deaf.

★ 168 ★ Alexander Technique International (ATI)

c/o Jan Baty, Corr.Sec.
1692 Massachusetts Ave., 3rd Fl.
Cambridge, MA 02138
Phone: (617)497-2242 **Free:** 888-668-8996
Fax: (617)497-2615
Email: usa@ati-net.com
Website: http://www.ati-net.com/
Jan Baty, Corr. Sec.

Mem: 320. **Nat'l Groups:** 13. **Desc:** Worldwide organization of Alexander technique teachers, students and supporters of the technique, created to promote and advance the work discovered by F.M. Alexander. Alexander technique is a bodywork described as a preventative technique which can improve health and overcome present harmful habits that cause unnecessary stress and restrict physical and mental capabilities. **Pub:** Books. • Videos.

★ 169 ★ Alfred Adler Institute (AAI)

594 Broadway, Ste. 1213
New York, NY 10012
Phone: (212)254-1048 **Fax:** (212)254-8271
Website: http://www.alfredadler-ny.org/
Dr. Robert Ellenbogen, PhD, Exec. Dir.

Fnded: 1948. **Mem:** 220. **Desc:** Offers training in psychotherapy, analytic psychotherapy, and analysis to psychiatrists, psychologists, social workers, teachers, clergymen, lawyers, counselors and other related professional persons. Conducts part-time, evening three-year-plus program to provide an understanding of the dynamics of personality and interpersonal relationships and to teach therapeutic methods and techniques. Presents the theory of Individual Psychology as formulated by the Austrian psychiatrist Alfred Adler (1870-1937). Maintains the Alfred Adler Consultation Center. **Pub:** *Journal of Individual Psychology*, quarterly. Journal. • Bulletin, annual. • Newsletter, quarterly. **Frmly:** Alfred Adler Institute for Individual Psychology.

★ 170 ★ Algerian Ostomy Association

c/o Rachid Rezgui, Pres.
Clinique Mohamed Boudiaf
12, rue Kesri Amar
Tizi-Ouzou, Algeria
Phone: 213 3 211521 **Fax:** 213 3 217960
Email: aoa@djaznir-connect.com
Website: http://www.ostomyinternational.org/regioneurope.htm

Fnded: 1988. **Mem:** 600. **Nat'l Groups:** 1. **State Groups:** 1. **Local Groups:** 2. **Lang(s):** English, French. **Desc:** Works to put into the disposition of ostomates in Algeria the different medical apparatus they need and to provide information on therapies and medical assistance in our clinics.

★ 171 ★ All Africa Leprosy, Tuberculosis and Rehabilitation Training Centre (ALERT)

PO Box 165
Addis Ababa, Ethiopia
Phone: 251 1 711524 **Fax:** 251 1 711199
Email: leprosytb@telecom.net.et
Website: http://www.telecom.net.et/~tdalert

Fnded: 1965. **Lang(s):** English. **Desc:** Health care services working with people with leprosy. Seeks to advance the diagnosis, prevention, and treatment of leprosy. Makes available medical services; conducts training programs for health care personnel. Main emphasis is on international training related to leprosy and tuberculosis.

★ 172 ★ All-India Ophthalmological Society

Kotla Rd.
New Delhi 110 002, India
Phone: 91 11 23318813
Fnded: 1937.

★ 173 ★ All Russia Association of the Blind
(Vserossiiskoe Obschestvo Slepykn — VOS)

Novaya ploschad' 14
101999 Moscow, Russia
Phone: 7 95 9253730 **Fax:** 7 95 9239149
Email: info@vos.org.ru
Website: http://www.vos.org.ru

Fnded: 1925. **Mem:** 274,341. **Nat'l Groups:** 147. **Reg. Groups:** 74. **Local Groups:** 932. **Lang(s):** Russian. **Desc:** People with visual impairments, health care professionals, and others with an interest in the situation of people with visual impairments. Promotes the rights of people with visual impairments; represents members' interests. **Pub:** *Dialogue*, bimonthly. Audiotape. • *Literary Reading*, monthly. Magazine. Arts digest. Provides the readers with the most recent literary publications. • *Modern Prose, Modern Poetry, In the World of Music, Culture and Health, The Knowledge, Computer Technologies*, quarterly. Magazine. Covers the life of the association and international relations. • *Our Life*, monthly. Covers the life of the association and international relations. **Frmly:** (1999) All Russian Association of the Blind.

★ 174 ★ All-Russian Society of the Deaf (ARFD)
(Vserossiiskoe Obshchestvo Glukhikh — VOG)

ulitsa 1905-goda 10A
123022 Moscow, Russia
Phone: 7 95 2556704 **Fax:** 7 95 2522381
Email: centrvog@umail.ru

Fnded: 1926. **Mem:** 107,062. **Reg. Groups:** 74. **Local Groups:** 74. **Lang(s):** Russian. **Desc:** Assists in the decision-making process regarding education, vocational training, and job placement for the hearing impaired; organizes cultural and leisure activities for hearing-impaired individuals, including creative work and physical training. **Pub:** *Tikhiye vesti*. Newsletter. • *V yedinom stroyu*, monthly. Magazine. **Frmly:** (1991) All-Union Society of the Deaf; (1993) All-Russian Society of the Deaf.

★ 175 ★ All-Russian Society for Disabled

Udaltzova 11
117415 Moscow, Russia
Phone: 7 95 9350064 **Fax:** 7 95 9350064
Email: id.voi@relcom.ru

Fnded: 1988. **Mem:** 2500,000. **Reg. Groups:** 80. **Lang(s):** Russian. **Desc:** Promotes the interests of disabled people. **Pub:** *Nadedgda*, monthly. Newspaper. Also publishes 23 other magazines and newspapers all over the Russia.

★ 176 ★ Allergy/Asthma Information Association (AAIA)
PO Box 100
Etobicoke, ON, Canada M9W 5K9
Phone: (416)679-9521 **Free:** 800-611-7011
Fax: (416)679-9524
Email: national@aaia.ca
Website: http://www.aaia.ca/aaia/index.htm

Fnded: 1964. **Mem:** 6,000. **Reg. Groups:** 5. **Local Groups:** 85. **Lang(s):** English, French. **Desc:** Seeks to develop societal awareness of the seriousness of allergic disease, including asthma, and to enable allergic individuals, their families, and caregivers to increase control over allergy symptoms. Provides leadership in information, education, and advocacy through partnership with healthcare professionals, businesses, industry, and government. Maintains speakers' bureau. **Pub:** *Awareness and Info Allergie*, quarterly. Newsletter. Provides the latest medical finding and coping tips. Also publishes info-letters on allergies, asthma and oraphylaxis.

★ 177 ★ Allergy and Asthma Network/ Mothers of Asthmatics (AAN/MA)
2751 Prosperity Ave., Ste. 150
Fairfax, VA 22031
Phone: (703)641-9595 **Free:** 800-878-4403
Fax: (703)573-7794
Email: aanma@aol.com
Website: http://www.aanma.org
Nancy Sander, Pres.

Fnded: 1985. **Mem:** 6,000. **Desc:** Professional associations, physicians, patients, parents, and educators. Dedicated to the education and support of people with allergies and asthma. Nonprofit patient education organization dedicated to people with allergies and asthma. Members include individuals, parents, physicians, patients, educators and professional associations. Resources include monthly newsletter books, quarterly magazines, videos, pamphlets on asthma and allergies. **Pub:** *Allergy & Asthma Health*, quarterly. Magazine. Provides in-depth coverage of allergy and asthma issues from leading medical and consumer experts. Includes a mini-magazine for kids. *Price:* $15. • *Breathing Easy with Day Care*. • *Consumer Update on Asthma*. • *I'm a Meter Reader*. Video. • *MA Report*, monthly. Newsletter. Provides patients and families of children with asthma and allergies with coping strategies, medical information, product reviews & how to articles. *Price:* $25/year. • *So You Have Asthma Too!*. Book. **Frmly:** (1991) Mothers of Asthmatics; (1993) National Allergy and Asthma Network.

★ 178 ★ Allergy Society of South Africa (ALLSA)
PO Box 88
Observatory 7935
Cape Town, Republic of South Africa
Phone: 27 21 44790919 **Fax:** 27 21 4480846
Website: http://allergysa.org

Desc: Works to advance the practice of allergy and immunology. Fosters education and research.

★ 179 ★ Alliance for Aging Research (AAR)
2021 K St. NW, Ste. 305
Washington, DC 20006-1003
Phone: (202)293-2856 **Free:** 800-497-0360
Fax: (202)785-8574
Email: info@agingresearch.org
Website: http://www.agingresearch.org
Daniel Perry, Exec. Dir.

Fnded: 1986. **Desc:** Gerontologists and other medical professionals, executives, and members of Congress are participants. Works to increase private and public research into aging. Supports policies concerning: productive aging; independence for older Americans; successful aging; human genome initiative. **Pub:** *Age-Related Macular Degeneration*. Report. • *Aging Research on the Threshold of Discovery*. • *Alliance Reports*. Reports. • *Americans' View on Aging*. • *Health Care Options under MEDICARE: The Choice is Yours*. Report. • *Independence for Older Americans: Task Force for Aging Research Funding*. • *Investing in Older Women's Health*. • *Is it Time for a Heart to Heart?*. An educational kit for CHF. • *Issue Reports*, periodic. • *Last Year of Life: Exposing Seven Deadly Myths About the High Costs of Dying in America*. Report. • *Meeting the Medical Needs of the Senior Boom: The National Shortage of Geriatricians*. • *Putting Aging on Hold–Delaying the Diseases of Old Age*. • *Report on Public Opinion*. Report. • *The Research Gap*. • *Will You Still Treat Me When I'm 65?*. Report.

★ 180 ★ Alliance for Alternatives in Healthcare (AAH)
PO Box 6279
Thousand Oaks, CA 91359-6279
Phone: (818)226-9829 **Fax:** (818)226-9820
Email: althlthins@aol.com
Website: http://www.alternativeinsurance.com
Steve Gorman, Pres.

Fnded: 1983. **Mem:** 1,500. **Desc:** Holistic physicians; employers; interested individuals. Seeks to enhance public recognition of holistic, homeopathic, naturopathic, chiropractic, and acupuncture treatments. (Holistic medicine focuses on the treatment of the entire body, rather than on any one organ or system; homeopathic medicine treats diseases by administering minute quantities of a substance that would produce the disease's symptoms in a healthy person; naturopathic medicine avoids the use of surgery and drugs, focusing instead on natural agents, such as sunshine and fresh air, or on physical means, such as manipulation or acupuncture.) Encourages health insurance systems to cover holistic, homeopathic, and naturopathic treatments in their policies. Attends exhibitions to disseminate information on holistic, homeopathic, and naturopathic medicine to health care providers and the public. Offers group medical, dental, and vision plans to members. Manages network of holistic and natural providers who offer discounts to subscribers of the Holistic Health Network. **Pub:** *Natural Marketing News*, periodic. • *Press Releases*, periodic. **Frmly:** Alternative Health Insurance Services; (1989) Natural Marketing Association.

★ 181 ★ Alliance of the American Dental Association (AADA)
211 E Chicago Ave., Ste. 730
Chicago, IL 60611
Phone: (312)440-2865 **Free:** 800-621-8099
Fax: (312)440-2587
Email: allianceada@mindspring.com
Website: http://www.allianceADA.org
Sheila Duda, Exec. Dir.

Fnded: 1955. **Mem:** 12,000. **Nat'l Groups:** 1. **State Groups:** 32. **Local Groups:** 160. **Desc:** Spouses of dentists. Promotes public dental health and creates public awareness of dentistry. Conducts preventive dental health education programs and assists organized dentistry in encouraging state and national legislation that benefits the public and dentistry. Maintains legislative projects and leadership skill development. **Pub:** *Key*, quarterly. Newsletter. **Frmly:** Auxiliary to the American Dental Association; (1982) Women's Auxiliary to the American Dental Association.

★ 182 ★ Alliance of Cardiovascular Professionals
4456 Corporation Ln., No. 120
Virginia Beach, VA 23462
Phone: (757)497-1225 **Fax:** (757)497-0010
Email: seanmce@aol.com
Peggy McElgunn, Exec. Dir.

Fnded: 1967. **Mem:** 3,200. **Desc:** Dedicated to meeting educational needs, developing programs to meet those needs, and providing a structure to offer the cardiovascular and pulmonary technology professional a key to the future as a valuable member of the medical team. Seeks advancement for members through communication and education. Provides coordinated programs to orient the newer professional to his field and continuing educational opportunities for technologist personnel. Has established guidelines for educational programs in the hospital and university setting. Works with educators and physicians to provide basic, advanced, and in-service programs for technologists. Sponsors registration and certification programs which provide technology professionals with further opportunity to clarify their level of expertise. Compiles statistics. **Pub:** *ACP Membership Directory*, annual. Membership Directory. Arranged alphabetically; includes field specialty, geographical location, and chapter affiliation. *Price:* Included in membership dues; $25/year for nonmembers. • *Beat Goes On*. • *CP Digest*, bimonthly. Newsletter. Includes employment opportunity listings, legislative reports, and new member information. *Price:* Included in membership dues; $35/year for nonmembers. • *Heart to Heart*. • *Pulmonary News*, quarterly. • *Strategies*. • Books. • Monographs. **Frmly:** (1980) National Society of Cardiopulmonary Technologists; (1986) National Society for Cardiopulmonary Technology; (1988) National Alliance of Cardiovascular Technologists; (1989) American Cardiology Technologists Association; (1998) American Society of Cardiovascular Professionals/Society for Cardiovascular Management.

★ 183 ★ Alliance of Community Health Plans (ACHP)
2000 M St., NW, Ste. 201
Washington, DC 20036-3307
Phone: (202)785-2247 **Fax:** (202)785-4060
Email: jebeler@achp.org
Website: http://www.achp.org
Jack C. Ebeler, Pres.

Fnded: 1984. **Desc:** Members are twenty-two not-for-profit and provider-based health plans, non-investor owned and provider-based, that serve more than 12 million Americans in 18 states and the District of Columbia. These plans have distinguished themselves through the National Committee for Quality Assurance accreditation, and with superior scores in both the Health Plan Data and Information Set and the Consumer Assessment of Health Plan Survey. The Alliance provides aid to contributing plans to enhance the wellbeing of their members and their communities and promotes the improvement in health care services of member plans by supporting activities which focus on the achievement of the highest standards of health care delivery. **Frmly:** The HMO Group.

★ 184 ★ Alliance for Continuing Medical Education (ACME)
1025 Montgomery Hwy., Ste. 105
Birmingham, AL 35216
Phone: (205)824-1355 **Fax:** (205)824-1357
Email: acme@acme-assn.org
Website: http://www.acme-assn.org
Bruce J. Bellande, PhD, Contact

Fnded: 1978. **Mem:** 2,500. **Desc:** Professionals engaged in continuing medical educational programs. Seeks to "educate and support continuing medical education professionals and to promote leadership in the development of continuing medical education to improve health care outcomes and the performance of health care providers." Facilitates exchange of information among members; makes available educational and continuing professional development opportunities; works to "shape and influence policy in the field of continuing medical education." Makes available discounts on product and services to members. **Pub:** *Almanac*, monthly. Newsletter. *Price:* included in membership dues. • *Journal of Continuing Education in the Health Professions*, quarterly. Journal.

★ 185 ★ Alliance for Health Reform (AHR)
1900 L St. NW, Ste. 512
Washington, DC 20036
Phone: (202)466-5626 **Fax:** (202)466-6525
Email: edhoward@allhealth.org
Website: http://www.allhealth.org
Edward F. Howard, Exec. V. Pres.

Fnded: 1991. **Desc:** Individuals and organizations with an interest in health care. Promotes increased public awareness of health care issues and proposals for health care reform in the United States. Serves as a clearinghouse on health care reform.

★ 186 ★ Alliance of Independent Academic Medical Centers (AIAMC)
c/o Glenn Craig Davis
233 E Erie St., Ste. 306
Chicago, IL 60611
Phone: (313)874-2181 **Fax:** (313)874-2180
Email: nancie@aiamc.org
Website: http://www.aiamc.org
Dr. Glenn Craig Davis, Pres.

Fnded: 1989. **Desc:** Independent academic medical center that sponsor four or more accredited residency programs, supports an institutional research program, and serves as a major affiliate for a significant number of medical school student clerkships. Promotes the roles and contributions of independent academic medical centers, fosters professional collegiality among their leaders, and works with other professional organizations to achieve mutual goals.

★ 187 ★ Alliance for Lung Cancer Advocacy, Support and Education (ALCASE)
PO Box 849
500 W 8th St., Ste. 240
Vancouver, WA 98666
Phone: (360)696-2436 **Free:** 800-298-2436
Fax: (360)735-1305
Email: info@alcase.org
Website: http://www.alcase.org
Cynthia M. Langhorne, Exec. Dir.

Fnded: 1995. **Mem:** 35,000. **Desc:** Dedicated to helping people living with or at risk of lung cancer on a worldwide basis. **Pub:** *Information for the Asking.* Booklet. Designed to increase communication between survivors and their healthcare team. *Price:* Free. • *The Lung Cancer Manual.* Manual. Contains information on lung cancer treatments, diagnosis and staging , complementary medicine, financial issues, and end-of-life issues. *Price:* Free. • *Lung Cancer Resource Guide.* Booklet. Includes list of organizations, programs, and other services for people living with lung cancer. *Price:* Free. • *Spirit and Breath,* quarterly. Newsletter. Provides information on new treatments, patient profiles, symptom management and advocacy issues. *Price:* Free. **Frmly:** (1998) Spirit and Breath.

★ 188 ★ Alliance for the Prudent Use of Antibiotics (APUA)
75 Kneeland St.
Boston, MA 02111-1901
Phone: (617)636-0966 **Fax:** (617)636-3999
Email: apua@tufts.edu
Website: http://www.healthsci.tufts.edu/apua/
Kathleen T. Young, Exec. Dir.

Fnded: 1981. **Mem:** 1,000. **Nat'l Groups:** 24. **Desc:** International membership of physicians, scientists, and medical and public health personnel; other individuals supporting prudent use of antibiotics. (Believes that extensive use of antibiotics leads to development of resistant strains of pathogenic and common, nonpathogenic bacteria with resistance traits transferable from one bacterium to others. These resistant strains are no longer susceptible to antibiotics and therefore can undermine treatment of infectious bacterial diseases.) Advocates and defines "good usage" of antibiotics; informs and educates the public about the dangers of misusing and overusing antibiotics and other antimicrobial agents; provides data to individuals and organizations interested in preventing antibiotic misuse and overuse. Informs and educates medical and paramedical personnel worldwide about the defined and specific action of antibiotics and the necessity of controlling their dispensation and prescription. Supports research projects. Maintains speakers' bureau. **Pub:** *APUA Newsletter*, quarterly. Newsletter. Includes pharmacology reviews. *Price:* Included in membership dues.

★ 189 ★ Alliance for South Asian AIDS Prevention (ASAAP)
20 Carlton St., Ste. 126, Fl. M
Toronto, ON, Canada M5B 2H5
Phone: (416)599-2727 **Fax:** (416)599-6011
Email: asaap@asaap.ca
Website: http://www.asaap.ca

Fnded: 1989. **Mem:** 120. **Lang(s):** Bengali, English, Gujarati, Hindi, Punjabi, Tamil, Urdu. **Desc:** Seeks to stop the spread of HIV and AIDS in Toronto's South Asian communities. Provides support and services to South Asian individuals affected by HIV/AIDS. Conducts AIDS and HIV advocacy, networking, prevention, and education programs. **Pub:** *WASPNews*, periodic. Newsletter.

★ 190 ★ Almshouse Association
Billingbear Lodge
Wokingham RG40 5RU, United Kingdom
Phone: 44 1344 452922 **Fax:** 44 1344 862062
Email: naa@almshouses.org
Website: http://www.almshouses.org

Fnded: 1946. **Mem:** 1,850. **Desc:** Members are almshouse foundations which provide accommodation for the elderly. Advises members on any matters, concerning almshouses and the welfare of the elderly; promotes improvements in almshouses; promotes study and research into all matters affecting almshouses; makes grants or loans to members. **Pub:** *The Almshouses Gazette*, quarterly.

★ 191 ★ Alpha Omega Alpha Honor Medical Society
525 Middlefield Rd., Ste. 130
Menlo Park, CA 94025
Phone: (650)329-0291 **Fax:** (650)329-1618
Email: eharris@alphaomegaalpha.org
Website: http://www.alphaomegaalpha.org
Edward D. Harris, Jr., Exec. Sec.

Fnded: 1902. **Mem:** 72,000. **Reg. Groups:** 124. **Desc:** Honor society for men and women studying medicine at graduate and postgraduate levels. Sponsors "Leaders in American Medicine" videotape series; underwrites visiting professorships. Also sponsors student research, student essay, and medical student service project awards. **Pub:** *The Pharos*, quarterly. Journal. Contains nontechnical articles of medical interest. **Frmly:** Alpha Omega Alpha.

★ 192 ★ Alpha Omega International Dental Fraternity
500 Commonwealth Dr.
Warrendale, PA 15086
Phone: (724)778-3419 **Free:** 800-677-8468
Fax: (724)772-8349
Email: headquarters@ao.org
Website: http://www.ao.org/
Susan Branscum, Ch. Staff Off.

Fnded: 1907. **Mem:** 15,000. **Local Groups:** 125. **Desc:** Professional fraternity - dentistry. Encourages fraternalism and monitors discrimination in dental schools. Maintains the Alpha Omega Foundation, which sends funds to dental schools in Israel and the U.S. Holds continuing education seminars. **Pub:** *Alpha Omegan*, quarterly. • *AO Today*, quarterly. Newsletter. Provides information on dental education in the United States and Israel. *Price:* Included in membership dues.

★ 193 ★ The Alpha 1 Foundation
2937 SW 27th Ave., Ste. 302
Miami, FL 33133
Phone: (305)567-9888 **Free:** 877-228-7321
Fax: (305)567-1317
Website: http://www.alphaone.org
John W. Walsh, Pres. /CEO

Fnded: 1995. **Desc:** Strives to provide leadership and resources that will result in increased research, improved health, worldwide detection and a cure for Alpha1-Antitrypsin Deficiency (Alpha-1). Devoted solely to research and a cure through grant award programs, research registry, DNA and tissue bank and various programs.

★ 194 ★ Alpha 1 National Association
815 Connecticut Ave. NW, Ste. 1200
Washington, DC 20006-4004
Phone: (202)887-1900 **Free:** 800-521-3025
Fax: (202)887-1964
Email: info@alpha1.org
Website: http://www.alpha1.org
Richard Sharp, Contact

Fnded: 1989. **Mem:** 1,239. **Nat'l Groups:** 81. **State Groups:** 35. **Local Groups:** 2. **Desc:** Individuals with Alpha 1 Antitrypsin deficiency emphysema. Provides advocacy and educational programs. **Pub:** *Alpha 1 Quarterly Review*, quarterly. Newsletter. *Price:* For members only. **Frmly:** (1991) Alpha 1 Antitrypsin Support Group.

★ 195 ★ Alpha Tau Delta (ATD)
150 Cruickshank Dr.
Folsom, CA 95630
Phone: (916)984-9150
Email: kerrik@atdnursing.org
Website: http://www.atdnursing.org
Kerri L. Kaye, Pres.

Fnded: 1921. **Mem:** 6,000. **Nat'l Groups:** 1. **Reg. Groups:** 2. **State Groups:** 12. **Desc:** Professional fraternity - nursing. Seeks to further educational standards for the nursing profession. Maintains scholarship program for members only. **Pub:** *President's Letter*, quarterly. • *The Pulse...A publication of Alpha Tau Delta*, quarterly. Newsletter. Contains reports, member and chapter news, and calendar of events, CEU, interview and nursing news. *Price:* Included in membership dues. • Brochure.

★ 196 ★ ALS Diagnostic Support Group (Vereniging Spierziekten Nederland — VSN)
van Heutszlaan 6
NL-3743 JN Baarn, Netherlands
Phone: 31 33 5480480
Email: vsn@vsn.nl
Website: http://www.vsn.nl

Fnded: 1967. **Reg. Groups:** 10. **Desc:** Individuals in The Netherlands affected by Amyotrophic Lateral Sclerosis (ALS), a muscle wasting condition. Provides a forum for support and exchange of information.

★ 197 ★ ALS March of Faces
984 Hathaway Dr.
Trenton, OH 45067-9214
Phone: (513)988-0796 **Fax:** (513)988-0796
Email: als@march-of-faces.org
Website: http://www.march-of-faces.org/

Desc: Promotes public awareness of Amyotrophic Lateral Sclerosis (ALS), or Lou Gehrig's Disease. Hosts fundraisers.

★ 198 ★ ALS Research Fund (Stichting ALS Onderzoekfonds)
Joos van Clevelaan 8
NL-3723 PG Bilthoven, Netherlands
Phone: 31 30 2533591 **Fax:** 31 30 2533665
Email: etrietsch@ktu.ruu.nl
Website: http://www.alsmndalliance.org/directory/netherlands.html

Fnded: 1981. **Desc:** Individuals interested in amyotropic lateral sclerosis or ALS (also known as Lou Gehrig's Disease). Works to: heighten public awareness and understanding of the disease; encourage research among medical and scientific communities. Sponsors researchers.

★ 199 ★ ALS Support Group - Belgium (ALS Zelfhulpgroep Belgie)
Klein Broekstraat 38
B-3350 Linter, Belgium
Phone: 32 16 789954 **Fax:** 32 16 781175
Email: alssecretariaat@pi.be
Website: http://www.als-mnd.be

Fnded: 1994. **Desc:** Individuals in Belgium affected by Amyotrophic Lateral Sclerosis (ALS), a muscle wasting condition. Provides a forum for support and exchange of information. **Pub:** Newsletter, periodic.

★ 200 ★ ALSAC/St. Jude Children's Research Hospital
501 St. Jude Pl.
Memphis, TN 38105
Phone: (901)578-2000 **Free:** 800-877-5833
Fax: (901)578-2200
Email: joe.hanna@stjude.org
Website: http://www.stjude.org/
Joe Hanna, Senior Information Specialist

Fnded: 1957. **Mem:** 2,000. **Reg. Groups:** 8. **Local Groups:** 60. **Desc:** Fundraising organization maintaining St. Jude Children's Research Hospital and laboratories in Memphis, TN. Conducts research and children's services and provides patient care in children's catastrophic diseases. Incorporated as American Lebanese Syrian Associated Charities, ALSAC was organized through the auspices of Danny Thomas, television and theatre personality. **Pub:** *ALSAC News*, quarterly. Tabloid informing members of St. Jude Hospital activities and ALSAC fundraising programs. Covers regional news. *Price:* Included in membership dues. • *Partners in Hope*, quarterly. Tabloid providing human interest stories and news of St. Jude Hospital activities. *Price:* Available to donors only. **Frmly:** (1972) Aiding Leukemia Stricken American Children.

★ 201 ★ Alstrom Syndrome - Canada
RR No. 2, Box 204
Finch, ON, Canada K0C 1K0
Phone: (613)346-2604
Email: randy.douglas@nbpcd.com
Website: http://www.jax.org/alstrom/documents/sasf.html

Fnded: 1995. **Desc:** Provides support to those affected by Alstrom Syndrome and their families, friends, and professionals.

★ 202 ★ Alstrom Syndrome International
49 Southfield Ave.
Paignton TQ3 1LH, United Kingdom
Email: alstrom@syndromeuk.freeserve.co.uk
Website: http://www.jax.org/alstrom/documents/sasf.html

Fnded: 1995. **Desc:** Provides support to those affected by Alstrom Syndrome and their families, friends, and professionals worldwide.

★ 203 ★ Alstrom Syndrome International
14 Whitney Farm Rd.
Mount Desert, ME 04660
Phone: (207)288-6385 **Free:** 800-371-3628
Fax: (207)288-6078
Email: jdm@jax.org
Website: http://www.jax.org/alstrom
Jan D. Marshall, Ch.

Fnded: 1995. **Nat'l Groups:** 3. **Desc:** Individuals with Alstrom's syndrome (a genetic disorder resulting in multiple organ failures) and their families; health care professionals with an interest in the syndrome and its diagnosis and treatment. Seeks to improve the quality of life of people with Alstrom's syndrome. Serves as a clearinghouse on the syndrome and its treatment; functions as a support group for people with Alstrom's syndrome and their families. Encourages and fosters genetic and clinical research on Alstion Syndrome. **Pub:** *The Alstrom Syndrome Handbook*. Book. • *The Alstrom Syndrome Newsletter*, 3/year. Newsletter. **Frmly:** (2002) International Society for Alstrom Syndrome Families.

★ 204 ★ Alzheimer Angehorige Austria (AAA)
Obere Augartenstrasse 26-28
A-1020 Vienna, Austria
Phone: 43 1 3325166 **Fax:** 43 1 3342141
Website: http://www.alzheimer-selbsthilfe.at/

Lang(s): English, German. **Desc:** Individuals and organizations. Seeks to improve the quality of life of people with Alzheimer's disease and their families. Makes available support and services; facilitates research on Alzheimer's disease and related disorders; conducts educational programs.

★ 205 ★ Alzheimer Europe (AE)
Alzheimer Society of Ireland
Alzheimer House
43 Northumberland Ave.
Dun Laoghaire, Dublin, Ireland
Phone: 353 1 2846616 **Fax:** 353 1 2846030
Email: moconnell@alzheimer.ie
Website: http://www.alzheimer-europe.org

Fnded: 1990. **Mem:** 27. **Lang(s):** English, French, German. **Desc:** Health care providers and other individuals and organizations with an interest in Alzheimer's disease. Promotes improvement in the diagnosis, prevention, and treatment of Alzheimer's disease; seeks to improve the quality of life of people with Alzheimer's disease and their families. Makes available health care and nursing services; sponsors research and educational programs.

★ 206 ★ Alzheimer Keskuslitto (AK)
Luotsikatu 4E
SF-00160 Helsinki, Finland
Phone: 358 9 6226200 **Fax:** 358 9 62262020
Email: varpu.kettunen@alzheimer.fi
Website: http://www.alzheimer.fi

Lang(s): English, Finnish. **Desc:** Individuals and organizations. Seeks to improve the quality of life of people with Alzheimer's disease and their families. Makes available support and services; facilitates research on Alzheimer's disease and related disorders; conducts educational programs.

★ 207 ★ Alzheimer Nederland
Postbus 183
NL-3980 CD Bunnik, Netherlands
Phone: 31 30 6596900 **Fax:** 31 30 6596901
Email: info@alzheimer-nederland.nl
Website: http://www.alzheimer-nederland.nl

Fnded: 1984. **Mem:** 200. **Lang(s):** Dutch, English. **Desc:** Individuals and organizations. Seeks to improve the quality of life of people with Alzheimer's disease and their families. Makes available support and services; facilitates research on Alzheimer's disease and related disorders; conducts educational programs.

★ 208 ★ Alzheimer Scotland-Action on Dementia (ASAD)
22 Drumsheugh Gardens
Edinburgh EH3 7RN, United Kingdom
Phone: 44 131 2431453 **Fax:** 44 131 2431450
Email: alzheimer@alzscot.org
Website: http://www.alzscot.org

Fnded: 1994. **Mem:** 2,100. **Reg. Groups:** 60. **Lang(s):** Scottish. **Desc:** Works to help individuals with dementia and their carers in Scotland. **Pub:** *Dementia in Scotland*, quarterly. Newsletter.

★ 209 ★ Alzheimer Society of Canada (ASC)
20 Eglington Ave. W, Ste. 1200
Toronto, ON, Canada M4R 1K8
Phone: (416)488-8772 **Free:** 800-616-8816
Fax: (416)488-3778
Email: info@alzheimer.ca
Website: http://www.alzheimer.ca

Fnded: 1978. **Mem:** 10. **Nat'l Groups:** 1. **State Groups:** 10. **Local Groups:** 145. **Lang(s):** English, French. **Desc:** Volunteers with an interest in helping individuals with Alzheimer's disease. Promotes an improved quality of life for people with Alzheimer's disease and their families. Supports research and educational programs; undertakes fundraising; creates awareness of Alzheimer's disease.

★ 210 ★ Alzheimer Society of Ireland (ASI)
Alzheimer House
43 Northumberland Ave.
Dublin, Ireland
Phone: 353 1 2846616 **Fax:** 353 1 2846030
Email: info@alzheimer.ie
Website: http://www.alzheimer.ie

Fnded: 1982. **Mem:** 5,000. **Reg. Groups:** 8. **Local Groups:** 30. **Lang(s):** English, Irish. **Desc:** Individuals and organizations. Seeks to improve the quality of life of people with Alzheimer's disease and their families; promotes advancement in the diagnosis and treatment of Alzheimer's disease. Makes available home support and day care service to people with Alzheimer's disease and their families; maintains respite home; serves as a clearinghouse on Alzheimer's disease and services available to people with the disease. **Pub:** *Alheimer Society of Ireland Newsletter*, quarterly. Newsletter.

★ 211 ★ Alzheimer Society Romania (SA) (Societatea Alzheimer)
Bd. Mihail Kogalniceanu 49
Sc. A et. 1 ap. 8 sector 5
70603 Bucharest, Romania
Phone: 40 21 3113411 **Fax:** 40 21 3348940
Email: alzsocro@fx.ro

Fnded: 1992. **Mem:** 900. **Nat'l Groups:** 6. **Lang(s):** English, Romanian. **Desc:** Individuals and organizations. Seeks to improve the quality of life of people with Alzheimer's disease and their families. Makes available support and services; facilitates research on Alzheimer's disease and related disorders; conducts educational programs. **Pub:** Newsletter, quarterly.

★ 212 ★ Alzheimerforeningen
Skt. Lukas Vej 6
DK-2900 Hellerup, Denmark
Phone: 45 39400488 **Fax:** 45 39616669
Email: post@alzheimer.dk
Website: http://www.alzheimer.dk

Fnded: 1969. **Mem:** 3,000. **Nat'l Groups:** 1. **Local Groups:** 16. **Lang(s):** Danish, English. **Desc:** Individuals and organizations. Seeks to improve the quality of life of people with Alzheimer's disease and their families. Makes available support and services; facilitates research on Alzheimer's disease and related disorders; conducts educational programs.

★ 213 ★ Alzheimerforeningen I Sverige (AIS)
PO Box 4109
S-227 22 Lund, Sweden
Phone: 46 46 147318 **Fax:** 46 46 188976
Email: info@alzheimerforeningen.nu
Website: http://www.alzheimerforeningen.nu

Fnded: 1986. **Mem:** 4,000. **Lang(s):** English, Swedish. **Desc:** Individuals and organizations. Seeks to improve the quality of life of people with Alzheimer's disease and their families. Makes available support and services; facilitates research on Alzheimer's disease and related disorders; conducts educational programs. **Pub:** *Alzheimer Foreningen*. Newsletter.

★ 214 ★ Alzheimer's Association (ADRDA)
919 N Michigan Ave., Ste. 1100
Chicago, IL 60611-1676
Phone: (312)335-8700 **Free:** 800-272-3900
Fax: (312)335-1110
Email: info@alz.org
Website: http://www.alz.org
Patricia Pinkowski, Dir. Library

Fnded: 1980. **Local Groups:** 83. **Desc:** Alzheimer's disease is a progressive, degenerative brain disease in which changes occur in the central nervous system and regions of the brain causing memory loss and other changes in thought, personality, and behavior. Promotes research to find the cause, treatment, and cure for the disease; provides educational programs for the public, media, and health care and medical professionals; represents the continuing care needs of the affected population before government and social service agencies. Seeks to destroy the myth that what were once called "senile behaviors" are a natural part of aging. Works to develop family support systems for relatives of persons with the disease. Sponsors educational forums; operates speakers' bureau. Compiles statistics. Library available. **Pub:** *Advances*, quarterly. Newsletter. Covers stories and developments of interest to patients with Alzheimer's disease and related disorders, and their families and friends. *Price:* Free. • Brochures. • Also publishes a variety of fact sheets, video kits, and patient care publications. **Frmly:** (1989) Alzheimer's Disease and Related Disorders Association.

★ 215 ★ Alzheimer's Association of Australia
PO Box 108
Higgins, ACT 2615, Australia
Phone: 61 2 62544233 **Fax:** 61 2 62787225
Email: secretariat@alzheimers.org.au
Website: http://www.alzheimers.org.au

Lang(s): English. **Desc:** Represents member interests on all matters relating to dementia and caregiver issues.

★ 216 ★ Alzheimer's Association Japan
Kyoto Social Welfare Hall
Horikawa-Marutamachi
Kamigyo
Kyoto 602-8143, Japan
Phone: 81 75 8118195 **Fax:** 81 75 8118188
Email: office@alzheimer.or.jp
Website: http://www.alzheimer.or.jp

Fnded: 1980. **Mem:** 7,000. **Reg. Groups:** 39. **Lang(s):** English, Japanese. **Desc:** Family caregivers, medical professionals, and volunteers involved with and concerned for people affected with dementia, including Alzheimer's disease. Seeks to raise awareness of Alzheimer's Disease and other forms of dementia in Japan, and to help dementia patients and their families. Provides public education and professional training; appeals to the Ministry of Health and Welfare and local governments. **Pub:** *Caring for the Elderly*, monthly. Newsletter.

★ 217 ★ Alzheimer's Australia NSW
PO Box 6042
North Ryde, NSW 1670, Australia
Phone: 61 2 98050100 **Fax:** 61 2 98051665
Email: admin@alznsw.asn.au
Website: http://www.alzheimers.org.au

Fnded: 1982. **Lang(s):** English. **Desc:** Provides support to people with dementia and their families and works to raise community awareness in New South Wales about Alzheimer's disease and other dementias. **Pub:** Handbooks. HelpNotes covering dementia.

★ 218 ★ Alzheimer's Disease Association of Nigeria
c/o Department of Psychiatry
Nnamdi Azikiwe University Teaching Hospital
Nnewi, Nigeria
Phone: 234 46 4636613 **Fax:** 234 46 460124
Email: tfine@infoweb.abs.net

Fnded: 1998. **Mem:** 320. **Desc:** Seeks to improve health and welfare of people with Alzheimer's disease in Nigeria. Seeks to raise public awareness of dementia.

★ 219 ★ Alzheimer's Disease Foundation Malaysia (ADFM)
14, Lorong Utara A
PO Box 28
46700 Petaling Jaya, Selangor, Malaysia
Phone: 60 3 79581522 **Fax:** 60 3 79581507
Email: alzheimers@pd.jaring.my
Website: http://www.adfm.org.my

Fnded: 1997. **Mem:** 18. **State Groups:** 3. **Lang(s):** English. **Desc:** Seeks to raise awareness of Alzheimer's Disease and other forms of dementia in Malaysia, and to help dementia patients and their families. **Pub:** *Sharing*, quarterly. Newsletter. Includes information on past and future activities, caregiver stories, and tips.

★ 220 ★ Alzheimer's Disease International (ADI)
45/46 Lower Marsh
London SE1 7RG, United Kingdom
Phone: 44 207 6203011 **Fax:** 44 207 4017351
Email: info@alz.co.uk
Website: http://www.alz.co.uk

Fnded: 1984. **Mem:** 60. **Lang(s):** English. **Desc:** Umbrella organization of 60 national Alzheimer associations worldwide. Main goal is to build and strengthen these associations so that they are better able to meet the needs of people with dementia and their carers. **Pub:** *Global Perspective*, quarterly. Newsletter. Booklets

★ 221 ★ Alzheimers NZ
71 Armagh St.
PO Box 2808
Christchurch, New Zealand
Phone: 64 3 3651590 **Fax:** 64 3 3798744
Email: alzheimers@alzheimers.org.nz
Website: http://www.alzheimers.org.nz

Fnded: 1983. **Mem:** 22. **Desc:** Seeks to improve health and welfare of people with dementia. Seeks to raise public awareness of dementia. **Pub:** *Alzheimers News*, quarterly. Newsletter.

★ 222 ★ Alzheimer's and Related Dementias Association (ARDA)
PO Box 81183
Parkhurst
Johannesburg 2120, Republic of South Africa
Phone: 27 11 4782234 **Fax:** 27 11 4782251
Email: alzheimerssa@icon.co.za

Fnded: 1985. **Mem:** 2,000. **Reg. Groups:** 5. **Lang(s):** Afrikaans. **Desc:** Works to create awareness about Alzheimer's disease and other dementias; provides support network for persons with dementia and their caregivers. **Pub:** *Alzheimer's News/Nuus*. Newsletter. • Annual Report.

★ 223 ★ Alzheimer's and Related Disorders Society of India (ARDSI)
PO Box 53
Kunnamkulam 680 503, Kerala, India
Phone: 91 488 2522939 **Fax:** 91 488 523801
Email: alzheimr@md2.vsnl.net.in
Website: http://www.alzheimerindia.org

Fnded: 1984. **Lang(s):** English. **Desc:** Seeks to raise awareness of Alzheimer's Disease and other forms of dementia in India, and to help dementia patients and their families.

★ 224 ★ Alzheimer's Society (AS)
Gordon House
10 Greencoat Pl.
London SW1P 1PH, United Kingdom
Phone: 44 20 73060606 **Fax:** 44 20 73060808
Email: info@alzheimers.org.uk
Website: http://www.alzheimers.org.uk

Fnded: 1979. **Mem:** 25,000. **Reg. Groups:** 12. **Lang(s):** English. **Desc:** Provides care and research charity for people with Alzheimer's disease and other forms of dementia, their families and carers. **Pub:** Booklets. • Newsletter, monthly. **Frmly:** (1999) Alzheimer's Disease Society.

★ 225 ★ Ambucs Resource Center
3315 North Main St.
High Point, NC 27265
Phone: (336)869-2166 **Fax:** (336)887-8451
Email: ambucs@ambucs.com
Website: http://www.ambucs.com

Fnded: 1922. **Mem:** 5,600. **Desc:** Dedicated to creating independence and opportunities for people with disabilities. Conducts service projects designed to give children with disabilities their first set of wheels. **Pub:** *AMBUC Magazine*, quarterly. Magazine.

★ 226 ★ Ambulance Service Association
Friars House, 2nd Fl.
157-168 Blackfriars Rd.
London SE1 8EU, United Kingdom
Phone: 44 20 79289620 **Fax:** 44 20 79289502
Email: richard@bizuk.com
Website: http://www.the-asa.org

Fnded: 1948. **Reg. Groups:** 6. **Desc:** Ambulance services in the United Kingdom. Promotes members' interests. Fosters collaboration and sharing of best practices among members. **Pub:** *ASA News*, bimonthly. Magazine. **Frmly:** Association of Chief Ambulance Officers.

★ 227 ★ Ambulatory Pediatric Association (APA)
6728 Old McLean Village Dr.
Mc Lean, VA 22101
Phone: (703)556-9222 **Fax:** (703)556-8729
Email: info@ambpeds.org
Website: http://www.ambpeds.org
Marge Degnon, Exec. Dir.

Fnded: 1960. **Mem:** 2,000. **Reg. Groups:** 10. **Desc:** Health care providers interested in the care of children in ambulatory care facilities, particularly directors of outpatient departments in private, university, and other teaching hospitals and those engaged in public health work or private practice. Aims to improve methods of care of children. Studies methods of research and the teaching of outpatient care. Conducts collaborative research; compiles statistics; presents annual scientific program. **Pub:** *Ambulatory Pediatric Association–Membership Directory*, biennial. Membership Directory. *Price:* included in membership dues. • *Ambulatory Pediatric Association–Newsletter*, 3/year. Newsletter. Includes book reviews, calendar of events, listing of employment opportunities, research reports, and statistics. *Price:* included in membership dues. • *Ambulatory Pediatrics, (The Journal of the Ambulatory Pediatric Assn.)*, 6/year. • Also publishes abstracts of scientific papers. **Frmly:** (1967) Association for Ambulatory Pediatric Services.

★ 228 ★ America Association for Homecare
625 Slaters Ln., Ste. 200
Alexandria, VA 22314-1171
Phone: (703)836-6263 **Fax:** (703)836-6730
Email: info@aahomecare.org
Website: http://www.aahomecare.org

Mem: 1,000. **Desc:** Home care providers. Advocate for quality medical care at home to the extent technically feasible. **Pub:** *HME Answer Book*, quarterly. Manual. Provides information and guidance on Medicare coverage, billing and payment rules for DMEPOS claims processing under DMERCs.

★ 229 ★ America Association of Integrative Medicine
2750 E Sunshine
Springfield, MO 65804
Phone: (417)881-9995 **Free:** 877-718-3053
Fax: (417)881-6414
Email: info@aaimedicine.com
Website: http://www.aaimedicine.com
Jennifer Leimkuehler, Ch. Assn. Off.

Fnded: 2000. **Mem:** 600. **Desc:** Seeks to bring together health care providers of both traditional and nontraditional medicine, from varied backgrounds such as acupuncture, massage therapy, herbology, pain management, pastoral counseling. **Pub:** Newsletter, monthly.

★ 230 ★ America Medical Billing Association (AMBA)
4297 Forrest Dr.
Sulphur, OK 73086

Phone: (580)622-2624
Website: http://www.ambanet.net/ambajoin.htm

Fnded: 1998. **Desc:** Promotes the medical billing profession; assists small and home medical billing professionals.

★ 231 ★ America Society of Plastic Surgeons (ASPS)

444 E Algonquin Rd.
Arlington Heights, IL 60005
Phone: (847)228-9900 **Free:** 888-4-PLASTIC
Fax: (847)228-9131
Website: http://www.plasticsurgery.org
James Wells, MD, Pres.

Fnded: 1931. **Mem:** 5,000. **Reg. Groups:** 29. **State Groups:** 35. **Desc:** Plastic surgeons. Dedicated to quality patient care and to maintain professional and ethical standards through education, research, and advocacy of socioeconomic and other professional activities. **Pub:** *Plastic and Reconstructive Surgery*, monthly. Journal. Includes research reports and book reviews. *Price:* included in membership dues; $420 for non-members. **Frmly:** ASPRS - American Society of Plastic and Reconstructive Surgery.

★ 232 ★ American Academy of Acupuncture and Oriental Medicine (AAAOM)

1925 County Rd., B2 W
Saint Paul, MN 55113-2703
Website: http://www.acuall.org/

Desc: Seeks to advance acupuncture and oriental medicine.

★ 233 ★ American Academy of Addiction Psychiatry (AAAP)

7301 Mission Rd., Ste. 252
Prairie Village, KS 66208
Phone: (913)262-6161 **Fax:** (913)262-4311
Email: info@aaap.org
Website: http://www.aaap.org
Becky Stein, Exec. Dir.

Fnded: 1985. **Mem:** 1,000. **Reg. Groups:** 9. **Desc:** Psychiatrists and other health care and mental health professionals treating people with addictive behaviors. Promotes accessibility to highest quality treatment for all who need it; promotes excellence in clinical practice in addiction psychiatry; educates the public to influence public policy regarding addictive illness; provides continuing education for addiction professionals; disseminates new information in the field of addiction psychiatry; and encourages research on the etiology, prevention, identification, and treatment of the addictions. **Pub:** *AAAP News*, 3/year. Journal. • *American Journal on Addictions*, 5/year. Journal.

★ 234 ★ American Academy of Allergy, Asthma and Immunology (AAAAI)

611 E Wells St.
Milwaukee, WI 53202
Phone: (414)272-6071 **Fax:** (414)272-6070
Email: membership@aaaai.org
Website: http://www.aaaai.org
Audrey Mudek, Membership Service Mgr.

Fnded: 1943. **Mem:** 6,200. **Desc:** Professional society of physicians specializing in allergy and allergic diseases. Sponsors annual two-day postgraduate course and three-day scientific session. Conducts research and educational programs. Maintains speakers' bureau; operates placement service; compiles statistics. **Pub:** *American Academy of Allergy Asthma and Immunology–Abstract Book*, annual. Journal. Contains abstracts of papers presented at annual meeting. *Price:* $30/copy. • *American Academy of Allergy, Asthma and Immunology–Academy News*, bimonthly. Newspaper. *Price:* Included in membership dues. • *American Academy of Allergy, Asthma and Immunology–Membership Directory*, biennial. Membership Directory. *Price:* Included in membership dues; $200/copy for nonmembers. • *Journal of Allergy and Clinical Immunology*, monthly. Journal. *Price:* Included in membership dues. **Frmly:** (1982) American Academy of Allergy.

★ 235 ★ American Academy of Alternative Medicine (AAAM)

c/o Dr. Alex Cougar
16126 E Warren, Box 24224
Detroit, MI 48224-0224
Phone: (313)882-0641 **Fax:** (313)882-0979
Dr. Alex Cougar, Contact

Fnded: 1984. **Mem:** 800. **Nat'l Groups:** 2. **Desc:** Advocates of alternative medicine. Promotes increased reliance on alternative treatments by professionals. Conducts research; sponsors training programs for health care professionals wishing to make use of alternative therapies. Conducts continuing education leading to American Board of Alternative Medicine Certification for members. **Pub:** *Restricted*, periodic. Newsletter. *Price:* Free for members.

★ 236 ★ American Academy of Ambulatory Care

2813 S Hiawassee Rd., Ste. 206
Orlando, FL 32835
Phone: (407)521-5789 **Fax:** (407)521-5790
Email: info@ambulatorymedicine.org
Website: http://www.ambulatorymedicine.org
Franz Ritucci, Jr.,MD, Dir.

Fnded: 1997. **Desc:** Licensed practitioners advancing the profession of Ambulatory Care/Acute Care Medicine by elevating standards through education, basic and advanced training, and board certification. Contributes to the field in the areas of professional growth, scientific and medical research, and medical education, to improve the overall quality of medical care. **Pub:** *Ambulatory Medicine Today*, quarterly. Newsletter. Features current issues and relevant reviews on ambulatory medicine. *Price:* included in membership dues.

★ 237 ★ American Academy of Ambulatory Care Nursing (AAACN)

East Holly Ave., Box 56
Pitman, NJ 08071-0056
Phone: (856)256-2350 **Free:** 800-262-6877
Fax: (856)589-7463
Email: aaacn@ajj.com
Website: http://www.aaacn.org
Cynthia R. Nowicki, EdD,RN, Contact

Fnded: 1978. **Mem:** 1,900. **Local Groups:** 17. **Desc:** AAACN is the association of professional nurses who identify ambulatory care nursing as essential to the continuum of high quality, cost-effective patient care. The mission of the Academy is to advance the art and science of ambulatory care nursing. The goals of the Academy are to be the voice of ambulatory care nursing, promote professional practices, stimulate innovative thinking, build collaborating relationships, and strengthen the AAACN resource base. **Pub:** *Ambulatory Care Nursing Administration and Practice Standards*, periodic. Manual. Reference manual. *Price:* $15 for members; $25 for nonmembers. • *American Academy of Ambulatory Care Nursing Administration Membership Directory*, annual. Directory. Arranged alphabetically and geographically. *Price:* Included in membership dues. • *Dermatology Nursing*. Journal. • *MedSurg Nursing*. Journal. • *Nursing Economics*, bimonthly. Journal. • *Pediatric Nursing*. Journal. • *Viewpoint*, bimonthly. Newsletter. Includes legislative updates and synopses of articles in current journals. *Price:* Included in membership dues; $80 institutional. **Frmly:** American Academy of Ambulatory Nursing Administration.

★ 238 ★ American Academy of Anesthesiologist Assistants (AAAA)

PO Box 13978
Tallahassee, FL 32317
Phone: (850)656-8848 **Free:** (866)328-5858
Fax: (850)656-3038
Email: susan@anesthetist.org
Website: http://www.anesthetist.org
Susan Cabrera, Exec. Dir.

Fnded: 1975. **Mem:** 412. **Desc:** Active anesthesiologist assistants who have graduated from an accredited training program and full-time students currently enrolled in an accredited program. Establishes and maintains the standards of the profession. Fosters and encourages continuing education and research. Sponsors educational meetings for graduates and student anesthesiologist assistants. **Pub:** *The Anesthesia Record*, 5/year. Newsletter. *Price:* included in membership dues. • *Membership Directory*. Membership Directory.

★ 239 ★ American Academy of Anti-Aging Medicine (A4M)

c/o Dr. Ronald Klatz
2415 North Greenview Ave.
Chicago, IL 60614
Phone: (773)528-4333 **Fax:** (773)528-5390
Email: media@worldhealth.net
Website: http://www.worldhealth.net
Dr. Ronald Klatz, Pres.

Fnded: 1993. **Mem:** 10,000. **Desc:** Dedicated to the advancement of technology to detect, prevent, and treat aging related disease and to promote research into methods to retard and optimize the human aging process. Also educates physicians, scientists and members of the public on anti-aging issues. Seeks to disseminate information concerning innovative science and research as well as treatment modalities designed to prolong human lifespan. **Pub:** *Anti-Aging Medical News*, quarterly. Newsletter. • *Report of the Medical Committee on Aging Research & Education*, quarterly. Newsletter.

★ 240 ★ American Academy of Audiology (AAA)

11730 Plaza America Dr., Ste. 300
Reston, VA 20190
Phone: (703)790-8466 **Free:** 800-AAA-2336
Fax: (703)790-8631
Email: mail@audiology.org
Website: http://www.audiology.org
Brad Stach, PhD, Pres.

Fnded: 1988. **Mem:** 8,300. **Nat'l Groups:** 1. **Desc:** Professionals in the field of audiology. Seeks to "enhance the ability of our members to achieve career and practice objectives through professional development." Conducts research and educational programs; sponsors public education campaigns to raise awareness of hearing disorders and audiological services. **Pub:** *Audiology Today*, bimonthly. Magazine. • *Journal of the American Academy of Audiology*, 10/year. Journal.

★ 241 ★ American Academy for Cerebral Palsy and Developmental Medicine (AACPDM)

6300 N River Rd., Ste. 727
Rosemont, IL 60018
Phone: (847)698-1635 **Fax:** (847)823-0536
Email: king@aaos.org
Website: http://www.aacpdm.org
Sheril King, Exec. Dir.

Fnded: 1947. **Mem:** 1,600. **Desc:** Professional organization of physicians, Ph.D.s, and allied health care individuals concerned with dignosis, care, treatment, and research of cerebral palsy and developmental disorders. **Pub:** *AACPDM News*, biennial. Newsletter. Includes academy news. *Price:* Included in membership dues. • *Journal of Developmental Medicine and Child Neurology*, monthly. • *Membership Roster*, annual. **Frmly:** (1976) American Academy for Cerebral Palsy.

★ 242 ★ American Academy of Child and Adolescent Psychiatry (AACAP)

3615 Wisconsin Ave. NW
Washington, DC 20016-3007
Phone: (202)966-7300 **Free:** 800-333-7636
Fax: (202)966-2891

Email: executive@aacap.org
Website: http://www.aacap.org
Marilyn Benoit, MD, Pres.

Fnded: 1953. **Mem:** 6,500. **Reg. Groups:** 57. **Desc:** Professional society of degreed physicians who have completed an additional five years of residency in child and adolescent psychiatry. Seeks to stimulate and advance medical contributions to the knowledge and treatment of psychiatric illnesses of children and adolescents. **Pub:** *AACAP News*, bimonthly. Newsletter. Includes listing of employment opportunities, research updates, and statistics. *Price:* Included in membership dues. • *Journal of the AACAP*, monthly. Journal. • Bulletin, periodic. • Catalog. • Manuals. • Membership Directory, periodic. **Frmly:** (1986) American Academy of Child Psychiatry.

★ 243 ★ American Academy of Clinical Neurophysiology

100 E San Francisco
Santa Fe, NM 87501
Phone: (505)982-5511 **Free:** 800-523-5002
Email: asumnel@lsumc.edu
Website: http://www.pressenter.com/~dtjorneh/
Austin J. Summer, Pres.

Fnded: 1985. **Mem:** 800. **Desc:** Clinical neurophysiologists. Fosters an understanding of the function of the nervous system among health professionals, scientists, and the public by serving as a forum for interaction and the communication of new developments. Offers educational programs.

★ 244 ★ American Academy of Clinical Psychiatrists (AACP)

PO Box 458
Glastonbury, CT 06033
Phone: (860)633-5045 **Fax:** (860)633-6023
Email: info@aacp.com
Website: http://www.aacp.com
Gregory Teas, MD, Pres.

Fnded: 1975. **Mem:** 600. **Desc:** Practicing board-eligible or board-certified psychiatrists. Promotes the scientific practice of psychiatric medicine. Conducts educational and teaching research. **Pub:** *Annals of Clinical Psychiatry*, quarterly. Journal. *Price:* Included in membership dues.

★ 245 ★ American Academy of Clinical Toxicology (AACT)

777 E Park Dr.
PO Box 8820
Harrisburg, PA 17105-8820
Phone: (717)558-7750 **Free:** 888-633-5784
Fax: (717)558-7845
Email: jreisinger@pamedsoc.org
Website: http://www.clintox.org
Jan Reisinger, Interim

Fnded: 1968. **Mem:** 600. **Desc:** Physicians, veterinarians, pharmacists, nurses research scientists, and analytical chemists. Objectives are to: unite medical scientists and facilitate the exchange of information; encourage the development of therapeutic methods and technology; Conducts professional training in poison information and emergency service personnel. **Pub:** *Journal of Toxicology-Clinical Toxicology*, 7/year. Journal. *Price:* Included in membership dues. • Current Awareness-Publication of Contemporary References in clinical toxicology and AACTion-organization newsletter.

★ 246 ★ American Academy of Cosmetic Dentistry (AACD)

5401 World Dairy Dr.
Madison, WI 53718
Phone: (608)222-8583 **Free:** 800-543-9220
Fax: (608)222-9540
Email: info@aacd.com
Website: http://www.aacd.com
Robert A. Hall, Exec. Dir.

Fnded: 1984. **Mem:** 4,300. **Desc:** Cosmetic dentists. Seeks to advance the study, teaching, and practice of cosmetic dentistry. Facilitates exchange of information among members; conducts educational programs.

★ 247 ★ American Academy of Cosmetic Surgery (AACS)

737 N Michigan Ave., Ste. 820
Chicago, IL 60611
Phone: (312)981-6760
Website: http://www.cosmeticsurgery.org
Jeffrey P. Knezovich, Exec. VP

Fnded: 1985. **Mem:** 1,400. **Desc:** Licensed cosmetic surgeons. Seeks to encourage high-quality cosmetic medical and dental care; provides continuing education for cosmetic surgeons; promotes research. Compiles statistics. Maintains hall of fame and speakers' bureau. **Pub:** *American Journal of Cosmetic Surgery*, quarterly. Journal. *Price:* $110 in U.S.; $130 outside U.S. • *Membership Roster*, annual. Membership Directory. • *Newsline*, bimonthly. Newsletter.

★ 248 ★ American Academy of Craniofacial Pain (AACP)

516 W Pipeline Rd.
Hurst, TX 76053-4924
Phone: (817)282-1501 **Free:** 800-322-8651
Fax: (817)282-8012
Email: central@aacfp.org
Website: http://www.aacfp.org
Cordelia Mason, Exec. Sec.

Fnded: 1985. **Mem:** 525. **Desc:** Health Care Practitioners who treat head, facial, and neck pain. Functions as a referral service for patients suffering from head, facial, and neck pain worldwide. Plans to establish computerized medical procedures and insurance database. **Pub:** *Membership List*, periodic.

★ 249 ★ American Academy of Dental Group Practice (AADGP)

2525 E Arizona Biltmore Cir., Ste. 127
Phoenix, AZ 85016
Phone: (602)381-1185 **Fax:** (602)381-1093
Email: info@aadgp.org
Website: http://www.aadgp.org
Dr. Hugh Norsted, Pres.

Fnded: 1973. **Mem:** 2,000. **Nat'l Groups:** 1. **Desc:** Active dentists and dental group practices. Purpose is to improve the level of dental service provided by members through exchanging and expanding of ideas and techniques for patient treatment and practice administration. Promotes group practice and research; accumulates and disseminates information; seeks to achieve the proper recognition for the aims and goals of group practice. Helps support an accreditation program as a system of voluntary peer review. **Pub:** *AADGP Contact*, quarterly. Newsletter. *Price:* included in membership dues. • Membership Directory, annual.

★ 250 ★ American Academy of Dental Practice Administration (AADPA)

c/o Kathleen Uebel
1063 Whippoorwill Ln.
Palatine, IL 60067-7064
Phone: (847)934-4404 **Fax:** (847)934-4410
Email: aadpa@aol.com
Website: http://www.aadpa.org
Kathleen S. Uebel, Exec. Dir.

Fnded: 1956. **Mem:** 250. **Desc:** Professional society of dentists interested in efficient administration of dental practice. Offers educational programs. **Pub:** *American Academy of Dental Practice Administration–Communicator*, 3/year. Newsletter. *Price:* Free. For members only. • *American Academy of Dental Practice Administration–Roster*, annual. *Price:* For members only. • *Essay Tapes*, annual.

★ 251 ★ American Academy of Dermatology (AAD)

PO Box 4014
Schaumburg, IL 60168-4014
Phone: (847)330-0230 **Free:** 888-462-DERM
Fax: (847)330-0050
Email: memsrv@aad.org
Website: http://www.aad.org
Thomas P. Conway, Exec. Dir.

Fnded: 1938. **Mem:** 14,000. **Desc:** Professional society of medical doctors specializing in skin diseases. Provides educational opportunities through meetings and publications. Provides support to members' practices. Promotes dermatologists as experts in treating skin, hair, and nail conditions. Maintains liaison with Congress, Federal agencies, State legislatures and State agencies. **Pub:** *Derm Coding Consult*, quarterly. • *Dermatology Insights*, quarterly. Magazine. • *Dermatology World*, monthly. Magazine. • *Dialogues in Dermatology*, monthly. Audiotapes. • *Journal of the American Academy of Dermatology*, monthly. Journal. Scientific journal. **Frmly:** American Academy of Dermatology and Syphilology.

★ 252 ★ American Academy of Disability Evaluating Physicians (AADEP)

150 N Wacker Dr., Ste. 1420
Chicago, IL 60606-1605
Phone: (312)658-1171 **Free:** 800-456-6095
Fax: (312)658-1175
Website: http://www.aadep.org
Sandra L. Yost, Exec. Dir.

Fnded: 1987. **Mem:** 1,300. **Desc:** Physicians. Seeks to provide graduate and continuing medical education programs to qualify doctors of medicine and doctors of osteopathy to meet the needs of the public in the practice of the medical science of disability evaluation as well as disability consultation. Works to develop educational programs and training programs in disability evaluation and disability consultation for health care professionals. Fosters and develops the medical science of disability evaluation. Sponsors research programs. Establishes standards for physicians in the practice of disability evaluation and disability consultation. **Pub:** *AADEP Membership Directory*, annual. Directory. *Price:* $100. • *AADEP News*, quarterly. Newsletter. • *Disability*, quarterly. Journal. Papers pertaining to information useful to physicians' disability arena. *Price:* Free. For members only; $100 /year for nonmembers.

★ 253 ★ American Academy of Emergency Medicine (AAEM)

c/o Kay Whalen
611 E Wells St.
Milwaukee, WI 53202-3816
Phone: (414)276-7390 **Free:** 800-884-AAEM
Fax: (414)276-3349
Email: info@aaem.org
Website: http://www.aaem.org
Kay Whalen, Dir.

Fnded: 1993. **Mem:** 3,500. **State Groups:** 6. **Desc:** Board certified physicians specializing in emergency medicine or pediatric emergency medicine; medical students and residents. Promotes "unencumbered access to quality emergency care provided by a specialist in emergency medicine" for every individual. Seeks to advance the study and profession of emergency medicine. Represents members economic and professional interests; supports growth of medical residency and graduate medical education programs; works to create a professional and legal environment conducive to the delivery of quality emergency medical care. **Pub:** *Common Sense*, bimonthly. Newsletter. • *Official Journal: Journal of Emergency Medicine*. Journal.

★ 254 ★ American Academy of Environmental Medicine (AAEM)

7701 E Kellogg Dr. Ste. 625
Wichita, KS 67207-1705
Phone: (316)684-5500 **Fax:** (316)684-5709
Email: aaem@swbell.net
Website: http://www.aaem.com
Bobbie Hinshaw, Exec. Dir.

Fnded: 1965. **Mem:** 400. **Desc:** Physicians, and others interested in the clinical aspect of environmental medicine. Supports physicians and other professionals in serving the public through education about the interactions between humans and their environment. **Pub:** *AAEM Directory*, annual. Directory. *Price:* $50/copy for nonmembers. • *Environmental Physician*, quarterly. Newsletter. • *Journal of Nutritional and Environmental Medicine*, quarterly. Journal. **Frmly:** (1984) Society for Clinical Ecology.

★ 255 ★ American Academy of Esthetic Dentistry (AAED)

401 N Michigan Ave.
Chicago, IL 60611
Phone: (312)321-5121 **Fax:** (312)673-6952
Email: aaed@sba.com
Website: http://www.estheticacademy.org/
Ronald I. Maitland, DMD, Pres.

Fnded: 1975. **Mem:** 138. **Desc:** Dentists seeking to advance the art and science of esthetic dentistry (dentistry concerned with restorative procedures of natural teeth). **Pub:** *Journal of Esthetic and Restorative Dentistry*, quarterly. Journal.

★ 256 ★ American Academy of Experts in Traumatic Stress

368 Veterans Memorial Hwy.
Commack, NY 11725
Phone: (631)543-2217 **Fax:** (631)543-6977
Website: http://www.aaets.org/abtaaets.htm

Mem: 200. **Nat'l Groups:** 41. **Desc:** Committed to the advancement of intervention for survivors of trauma. **Pub:** *The Academy Update.* • *Trauma Response.*

★ 257 ★ American Academy of Facial Plastic and Reconstructive Surgery (AAFPRS)

310 S Henry St.
Alexandria, VA 22314
Phone: (703)299-9291 **Free:** 800-332-FACE
Fax: (703)299-8898
Email: info@aafprs.org
Website: http://www.facemd.org
Stephen C. Duffy, Exec. VP

Fnded: 1964. **Mem:** 2,600. **Desc:** Physicians specializing in facial plastic surgery. Promotes research and study in the field. Maintains speakers' bureau. Conducts educational and charitable programs; compiles statistics. **Pub:** *The Face Book: The Pros and Cons of Facial Plastic Surgery.* • *Face Facts*, quarterly. • *Facial Plastic Surgery Today*, quarterly. • *Facial Plastic Times*, monthly. Newsletter. Includes calendar of events and book reviews. *Price:* available to members only. • Brochures. • Membership Directory, annual. Includes buyers' guide. *Price:* $35/copy for members; $75/copy for nonmember physicians; $300/copy for others. • Monographs. • Videos.

★ 258 ★ American Academy of Family Physicians (AAFP)

11400 Tomahawk Creek Pkwy.
Leawood, KS 66211-2672
Phone: (913)906-6000 **Free:** 800-274-2237
Fax: (913)906-6077
Email: fp@aafp.org
Website: http://www.aafp.org
Douglas E. Henley, MD, Exec. VP

Fnded: 1947. **Mem:** 93,500. **State Groups:** 55. **Local Groups:** 200. **Desc:** Professional society of family physicians who provide continuing comprehensive care to patients. **Pub:** *AAFP Reporter*, monthly. Newsletter. Covers socioeconomic issues and legislative news affecting medicine; includes member news. Available to selected media. • *American Family Physician*, 16/year. Journal. Includes book reviews, newsletter, calendar of events, and therapeutic, product, and subject indexes. *Price:* Free to qualified recipients; $50/year for nonmembers. • *Family Practice Management*, 10/year. Covers practice management and socioeconomic issues. • Annual Report. **Frmly:** (1971) American Academy of General Practice.

★ 259 ★ American Academy of Fixed Prosthodontics (AAFP)

PO Box 1409
Bodega Bay, CA 94923-1409
Phone: (707)875-3040 **Free:** 800-785-9188
Fax: (707)875-2927
Email: secaafp@monitor.net
Website: http://www.prosthodontics.org/aafp
Dr. Robert S. Staffanou, Sec.

Fnded: 1951. **Mem:** 606. **Desc:** Dentists. Provides 2-day professional continuing education course in the specialty of fixed prosthodontics. **Pub:** *American Academy of Fixed Prosthodontics Newsletter*, semiannual. Newsletter. *Price:* Included in membership dues. • *Journal of Prosthetic Dentistry*, monthly. Journal. *Price:* included in membership dues. • *Meeting Program/Directory*, annual. Directory. **Frmly:** (1991) American Academy of Crown and Bridge Prosthodontics.

★ 260 ★ American Academy of Gnathologic Orthopedics (AAGO)

2651 Oak Grove Rd.
Walnut Creek, CA 94598
Free: 800-510-AAGO **Fax:** (925)676-7678
Website: http://www.aago.com
John Rothchild, D.D.S., Exec. Dir.

Fnded: 1970. **Mem:** 700. **Nat'l Groups:** 1. **Reg. Groups:** 9. **State Groups:** 16. **Desc:** Dentists dealing with the prevention or correction of malocclusion and bony misformation of the jaw and face. Conducts activities in the fields of maxillofacial orthopedics/orthodontics and preventative and corrective orthodontics. **Pub:** *American Academy of Gnathologic Orthopedics–Journal*, quarterly. Journal. Includes scientific articles and case reports on orthodontic treatment. *Price:* $80 plus postage in U.S.; $85 Canada; $100 foreign. • *American Academy of Gnathologic Orthopedics–Membership Roster*, annual. Membership Directory. *Price:* Included in membership dues. • Articles.On the Crozat Method.

★ 261 ★ American Academy of Gold Foil Operators (AAGFO)

17922 Tallgrass Ct.
Noblesville, IN 46060
Phone: (317)867-3011 **Fax:** (317)867-3011
Email: piperon@earthlink.net
Website: http://www.goldfoil.org
Dr. Ronald K. Harris, Sec. -Treas.

Fnded: 1952. **Mem:** 285. **Desc:** Dentists who perform restorative procedures utilizing gold foil, cast gold, and the rubber dam. Formulates and applies new ideas for research on gold restorations and the rubber dam; encourages members of the dental profession and research institutions in the armed forces, government, dental schools, and private enterprise to study gold restorations and rubber dam procedures. Presents chair demonstrations at dental schools. **Pub:** *Gold Leaf*, semiannual. • *Journal of Operative Dentistry*, bimonthly. Journal. • *Roster*, biennial. • Also prepares slides, charts, models, and written materials.

★ 262 ★ American Academy of Health Care Providers

314 W Superior St., Ste. 702
Duluth, MN 55802
Phone: (218)727-3940 **Free:** 888-429-3701
Fax: (218)722-0347
Email: info@americanacademy.org
Website: http://www.americanacademy.org
Lorraine D. Grymala, Exec. Dir.

Fnded: 1989. **Desc:** Nurses, doctors, psychologists, psychiatrists, social workers, and counselors. Established and maintains Certified Addiction Specialist (CAS) credentials. Strives to create a national unity of standards. **Pub:** *Academy E-News*, bimonthly. Newsletter. *Price:* Free. • *Academy News*, semiannual. Newsletter. *Price:* Free for members.

★ 263 ★ American Academy of Health Care Providers in the Addictive Disorders (AAHCPAD)

314 West Superior St., Ste. 702
Duluth, MN 55802
Phone: (218)727-3940 **Fax:** (218)722-0346
Email: info@americanacademy.org
Website: http://www.americanacademy.org
Lorraine D. Grymala, Exec. Dir.

Fnded: 1989. **Desc:** Health care professionals, mental health care providers, and social workers treating individuals with addictive disorders. Promotes excellence in the care of people with addictions. Develops and enforces standards of ethics and practice for addiction medicine; facilitates exchange of information among members; holds examination and confers certification to qualified addiction care providers. **Frmly:** (2003) American Academy of Health Care Providers.

★ 264 ★ American Academy of Health Physics (AAHP)

1313 Dolley Madison Blvd., Ste. 402
Mc Lean, VA 22101
Phone: (703)790-1745 **Fax:** (703)790-2672
Email: aahp@burkinc.com
Website: http://www.hps1.org/aahp

Desc: Certified Health Physicists. Works to promote the profession. Actively participates in the certification program.

★ 265 ★ American Academy of the History of Dentistry (AAHD)

c/o Aletha A. Kowitz
100 S Vail Ave.
Arlington Heights, IL 60005-1866
Phone: (847)670-7561
Aletha A. Kowitz, Sec. -Treas.

Fnded: 1951. **Mem:** 450. **Desc:** Seeks to stimulate interest, study, and research in the history of dentistry and promote the teaching of dental history. **Pub:** *Journal of the History of Dentistry*, 3/year. Journal. Includes articles on the history of dentistry, book reviews, and 5yr cumulative index. *Price:* $55/year.

★ 266 ★ American Academy of Home Care Physicians (AAHCP)

PO Box 1037
Edgewood, MD 21040-0337
Phone: (410)676-7966 **Fax:** (410)676-7980
Email: aahcp@mindspring.com
Website: http://www.aahcp.org
Constance F. Row, Exec. Dir.

Desc: Physicians, home care professionals and agencies, and student affiliates and corporate sponsors-members. Patient referral services.

★ 267 ★ American Academy of Hospice and Palliative Medicine (AAHPM)

4700 W Lake Ave.
Glenview, IL 60025-1485
Phone: (847)375-4712 **Fax:** 877-734-8671
Email: aahpm@aahpm.org
Website: http://www.aahpm.org

Fnded: 1988. **Desc:** Physicians and other medical professionals dedicated to excellence in palliative medicine and prevention and relief of suffering; fosters research; provides public advocacy. training programs in hospice and palliative care. Educates the public regarding the rights of the dying and other issues affecting hospice and palliative medicine. **Pub:** *Hospice and Palliative Medicine Core Curriculum and Review Syllabus.* • *Position Statements*, periodic. Reports. • *UNIPACs: Hospice/Palliative Care Training for Physicians and other Medical Professionals.* **Frmly:** Academy of Hospice Physicians.

★ 268 ★ American Academy of Husband-Coached Childbirth (AAHCC)
PO Box 5224
Sherman Oaks, CA 91413-5224
Phone: (818)788-6662 **Free:** 800-4-A-BIRTH
Fax: (818)788-1580
Website: http://www.bradleybirth.com
Marjie Hathaway, Exec. Dir.

Fnded: 1970. **Mem:** 1,200. **Desc:** Trains instructors in the Bradley method of natural childbirth. Provides referals to Bradley teachers. **Pub:** *Directory of Instructors*, 2-3/year. *Price:* Free. • *Fetal Advocate*, periodic.

★ 269 ★ American Academy of Implant Dentistry (AAID)
211 E Chicago Ave., Ste. 750
Chicago, IL 60611
Phone: (312)335-1550 **Free:** 877-335-2243
Fax: (312)335-9090
Email: aaid@aaid-implant.org
Website: http://www.aaid-implant.org
J. Vincent Shuck, Exec. Dir.

Fnded: 1952. **Mem:** 2,200. **Reg. Groups:** 4. **Desc:** Dedicated to furthering scientific research and development in the field of implantology. **Pub:** *AAIDNEWS*, quarterly. Newsletter. Includes news and calendar updates of Academy events. *Price:* Free to members. • *American Academy of Implant Dentistry*, annual. Directory. Arranged geographically and alphabetically. *Price:* Free to members. • *Journal of Oral Implantology*, bimonthly. Journal. Contains original manuscripts, clinical presentations, research annotations, and educational reports pertinent to dental studies. *Price:* Included in membership dues; $75/year for nonmembers; $100/year for libraries, corporations, and institutes. **Frmly:** American Academy of Implant Dentures.

★ 270 ★ American Academy of Implant Prosthodontics (AAIP)
709 Haddonfield-Berlin Rd.
Voorhees, NJ 08043
Phone: (856)782-3990 **Fax:** (856)782-3775
Website: http://perso.wanadoo.fr/piezoklein
Sheldon Winkler, Exec. Dir.

Fnded: 1982. **Mem:** 1,400. **Nat'l Groups:** 1. **Desc:** Experts in dental implantology; dental school professors, clinicians, and researchers. Encourages continuing education, advancement, and research in implant dentistry; believes that prosthodontics and implantology education and research should take place in academic institutions. Promotes the surgical insertion of dental implants and the design and insertion of prosthodontic devices to replace missing teeth. Emphasizes research on the construction and maintenance of fixed and removable prostheses. Conducts continuing education courses in conjunction with dental schools. Maintains speakers' bureau and small library. **Pub:** *The Dental Implant - Clinical and Biological Response of Oral Tissues*. • *Implant Prosthodontics - Surgical and Prosthetic Techniques for Dental Implants*, periodic. Membership Directory. • *Journal of Oral Implantology*, bimonthly. Journal. • Membership Directory, periodic. • Newsletter, 3/year.

★ 271 ★ American Academy of Insurance Medicine (AAIM)
c/o Robert W. Watson, MD
Allianz Life Insurance Co. of North America
5701 Golden Hills Dr.
Minneapolis, MN 55416-1297
Phone: (612)721-7061 **Fax:** (612)721-3581
Email: ellyn@unconventionalplanning.com
Website: http://www.aaimedicine.org
Ellyn Holzman, Exec. Sec.

Fnded: 1889. **Mem:** 500. **Desc:** Professional society of medical directors of life insurance companies. **Pub:** *Journal of Insurance Medicine*, quarterly. Journal. *Price:* Included in membership dues; $65/year for nonmembers. **Frmly:** (1992) Association of Life Insurance Medical Directors of America.

★ 272 ★ American Academy of Maxillofacial Prosthetics (AAMP)
c/o Rhonda Jacob, M.D.
Anderson Cancer Center
1515 Holcomb Blvd.
PO Box 441
Houston, TX 77030
Phone: (713)792-6917 **Fax:** (713)794-4662
Email: rjacob@mail.mdanderson.org
Website: http://www.maxillofacialprosth.org/maxillofacial/
Dr. Rhonda Jacobs, Pres.

Fnded: 1953. **Mem:** 148. **Desc:** Dentists specializing in maxillofacial prosthetics. **Pub:** *Journal of Prosthetic Dentistry*, monthly. Journal.

★ 273 ★ American Academy of Medical Acupuncture
4929 Wilshire Blvd., Ste. 428
Los Angeles, CA 90010
Phone: (323)937-5514 **Fax:** (323)937-0959
Email: jdowden@prodigy.net
Website: http://www.medicalacupuncture.org
C. James Dowden, Exec. Admin.

Fnded: 1987. **Mem:** 1,710. **State Groups:** 8. **Desc:** Professional society of physicians and osteopaths who utilize acupuncture in their practices. Provides ongoing training and information related to the Chinese practice of puncturing the body at specific points to cure disease or relieve pain. Offers educational and research programs. **Pub:** *Medical Acupuncture*, semiannual. Journal.

★ 274 ★ American Academy of Medical Administrators (AAMA)
701 Lee St., Ste. 600
Des Plaines, IL 60016
Phone: (847)759-8601 **Fax:** (847)759-8602
Email: info@aameda.org
Website: http://www.aameda.org
Renee S. Schleicher, CAE, Pres. /CEO

Fnded: 1957. **Mem:** 2,800. **Reg. Groups:** 8. **State Groups:** 50. **Desc:** Individuals involved in healthcare management at all levels. Promotes healthcare administration through educational courses and research. **Pub:** *American Academy of Medical Administrators–Executive*, quarterly. Newsletter. Covers membership activities. Includes triennial membership directory;also contains calendar of events, book reviews, and lists of new members. *Price:* Included in membership dues; $60/year for nonmembers. • *Journal of Cardiovascular Management*, bimonthly. Journal. • *Journal of Oncology Management*, bimonthly. Journal.

★ 275 ★ American Academy of Medical Administrators Research and Educational Foundation (AAMA)
701 Lee St., Ste. 600
Des Plaines, IL 60016
Phone: (847)759-8601 **Fax:** (847)759-8602
Email: info@aameda.org
Website: http://www.aameda.org/AboutAAMA/aboutfoundation.html
Renee S. Schleicher, CAE, Pres.

Fnded: 1957. **Mem:** 3,800. **Reg. Groups:** 7. **State Groups:** 50. **Desc:** Individuals with health care backgrounds. Conducts research in the health care field and seminars geared toward professional development. Maintains placement services. **Pub:** *AAMA Executive*, bimonthly. Newsletter. Covers management topics, industry trends, current developments in health care administration, and association news. Includes book reviews. *Price:* Included in membership dues; $110/year for nonmembers.

★ 276 ★ American Academy of Medical Hypnoanalysts (AAMH)
5628 Murray Rd., Ste. 4
Memphis, TN 38119-3876
Phone: 888-454-9766 **Free:** 888-454-9766
Fax: (901)683-1224
Website: http://www.aamh.com
John Scott, Jr., Admin.

Fnded: 1974. **Mem:** 125. **Reg. Groups:** 8. **Desc:** Medical doctors, doctors of osteopathy, psychologists, social workers, and professional counselors. Provides training in and promotes the use of medical hypnoanalysis. (Medical hypnoanalysis employs an analytic approach to resolving emotional disorders that is applied while the subject is hypnotized.) Conducts 3-month residency training programs. **Pub:** Membership Directory, annual.

★ 277 ★ American Academy of Medical Management
Crossville Commons
560 West Crossville Rd., Ste. 103
Roswell, GA 30075
Phone: (770)649-7150 **Fax:** (770)649-7552
Email: webmaster@epracticemanagement.com
Website: http://www.epracticemanagement.com
Roger G. Bonds, Exec. Dir.

Fnded: 1990. **Mem:** 400. **Desc:** Health care administrators with an interest in continuing professional development; continuing medical education programs. Seeks to increase the quality and availability of continuing medical education courses. Serves as a clearinghouse on continuing medical education; formulates model practice management and recruitment and physician employment contracts; sponsors fellowship and certification programs for continuing medical educators. **Pub:** *Medical Staff Development Professional*, periodic. Journal. **Frmly:** (2000) American College of Medical Staff Development; (2003) American College of Medical Practice Management.

★ 278 ★ American Academy on Mental Retardation (AAMR)
c/o Linda Hickon, PhD
Center for Opportunities and Outcome
Teachers College
Columbia University
New York, NY 10027
Email: mseltzer@waisman.wisc.edu
Website: http://www.academyonmr.org/
Dr. Linda Hickson, Sec.

Fnded: 1960. **Mem:** 250. **Desc:** Scientists actively engaged in research in any discipline relating to mental retardation; active membership is limited to scientists possessing a doctorate degree. Encourages and promotes investigative work in the clinical and experimental field of mental retardation; provides a forum for research workers in this field. Facilitates relations between various disciplines and stimulates cooperative research. Cooperates with national and international organizations and cosponsors colloquia, symposia, and other meetings. **Pub:** Newsletter, semiannual.

★ 279 ★ American Academy of Neurological and Orthopaedic Surgeons (AANOS)
2300 S Rancho Dr., Ste. 202
Las Vegas, NV 89102-4508
Phone: (702)388-7390 **Fax:** (702)388-7395
Email: aanos@lasvegas.net
Website: http://www.aanos.org
Dr. Kazem Fathie, MD, Chair

Fnded: 1977. **Mem:** 280. **Desc:** Neurological and orthopaedic surgeons, neurologists, physiatrists, and professionals in allied medical or surgical specialties. Provides and encourages information about and understanding of neurological and orthopaedic medicine and surgery, a branch of medicine that deals with diseases and injuries to the human neuromusculoskeletal system; seeks to improve patient care. Maintains American Board of Neurological and Orthopaedic Medicine and Surgery and American Board of Spinal Surgery. Sponsors charitable program. Maintains a complete collection of recordings of scientific meetings since 1977. Operates 40 colleges of experts in individual disciplines related to neurological and orthopaedic medicine and surgery. Acronym stands for Fellowship of the American Academy of Neurological and Orthopaedic Surgeons. **Pub:** *Journal of Neurological and Orthopaedic Medicine and Surgery (JONOMS)*, quarterly. Journal. *Price:* $125/year in U.S.; $135/year outside U.S.

★ 280 ★ American Academy of Neurology (AAN)
1080 Montreal Ave.
Saint Paul, MN 55116-2325
Phone: (651)695-2717 **Free:** 800-879-1960
Fax: (651)695-2791
Email: memberservices@aan.com
Website: http://www.aan.com
Catherine M. Rydell, Exec. Dir.

Fnded: 1948. **Mem:** 17,200. **Desc:** Professional society of medical doctors specializing in brain and nervous system diseases. Maintains placement service. Sponsors research and educational programs. Compiles statistics. Publishes scientific journal. **Pub:** *AAN Governmental Report*, bimonthly. Newsletter. Includes news on legislative affairs. • *AANews*, monthly. Newsletter. General information and placement publication. • *American Academy of Neurology Membership Directory*, annual. Membership Directory. • *ICD-9-CM for Neurologists*. Booklet. To aid users of ICD-9 diagnostic codes. • *Medical Specialty of Neurology*. Brochure. Discusses neurology as a career. • *Neurologist*. Brochure. For patients. • *Neurology*, monthly. Journal. Includes research reports. • *Patient Information Guide for Neurology*. Handbook for patients to find educational information about disorders.

★ 281 ★ American Academy of Nurse Practitioners (AANP)
National Administrative Office
PO Box 12846
Austin, TX 78711
Phone: (512)442-4262 **Fax:** (512)442-6469
Email: admin@aanp.org
Website: http://www.aanp.org
Zo DeMarchi, Dir. of Association Services

Fnded: 1985. **Mem:** 13,000. **Desc:** Promotes high standards of health care delivered by nurse practitioners. Acts as a forum to enhance the identity and continuity of nurse practitioners. Addresses national and state legislative issues that affect members; acts as a resource center on legislative activity. Supports continuing education programs. Encourages research in the field. Compiles statistics. **Pub:** *Academy Update*, monthly. Newsletter. • *Journal of the American Academy of Nurse Practitioners*, monthly. Journal. Focuses on clinical practice, management, and education. • Brochures.

★ 282 ★ American Academy of Nursing (AAN)
600 Maryland Ave., NW, Ste. 100 West
Washington, DC 20024-2571
Phone: (202)651-7238 **Fax:** (202)554-2641
Email: tgaffney@ana.org
Website: http://www.nursingworld.org/aan
Terri Gaffney, Dir.

Fnded: 1973. **Mem:** 800. **Desc:** Purposes are to: advance new concepts in nursing and health care; identify and explore issues in health, the professions, and society that concern nursing; examine interrelationships among the segments within nursing and the interaction among nurses as these affect the development of the nursing profession; identify and propose resolutions to issues and problems confronting nursing and health, including alternative plans for implementation. Sponsors symposia. **Pub:** *American Academy of Nursing Directory*, biennial. Directory. *Price:* Included in membership dues. • *Differentiating Nursing Practice: Into the 21st Century*. • *Knowledge About Care and Caring: State of the Art and Future Directions*. • *Nursing Outlook*, bimonthly. Journal. Includes calendar of events, obituaries, and research reports. *Price:* Included in membership dues; $25/year for nonmembers. • *Practice and Inquiry for Nursing Administration: Intra- and Interdisciplinary Perspectives*.

★ 283 ★ American Academy of Ophthalmology (AAO)
PO Box 7424
San Francisco, CA 94120-7424
Phone: (415)561-8500 **Fax:** (415)561-8533
Email: customer_service@aao.org
Website: http://www.aao.org
H. Dunbar Hoskins Jr.,, MD, Exec. VP

Fnded: 1896. **Mem:** 26,000. **Desc:** Works to achieve accessible, appropriate and affordable eye care for the public by serving the educational and professional needs of the ophthalmologist. Provides clinical education, ophthalmic practice, federal and state advocacy, patient information, and other services to its members. Provides accurate, appropriate and timely information to the public through its media and public information programs. Current activities of the foundation include National Eye Care Project; Oral Histories Program. **Pub:** *Basic and Clinical Science Course*. • *Eye Net*, monthly. Magazine. *Price:* Free to members; $128/year US non-members. • *Member Directory*, biennial. Directory. • *Ophthalmology*, monthly. Journal. • Manuals. • Videos. • Also publishes slide script packages and study guides, special interest newsletters, modules, procedures assessments, issue briefs, brochures.

★ 284 ★ American Academy of Optometry (AAO)
6110 Executive Blvd., Ste. 506
Rockville, MD 20852
Phone: (301)984-1441 **Fax:** (301)984-4737
Email: loiss@aaoptom.org
Website: http://www.aaopt.org
Lois Schoenbrun, Exec. Dir.

Fnded: 1921. **Mem:** 5,000. **Local Groups:** 20. **Desc:** Optometrists, educators, and scientists interested in optometric education, and standards of care in visual problems. Conducts continuing education for optometrists and visual scientists. Sponsors 5-day annual meeting. **Pub:** *Geographic Directory of Members*, biennial. Membership Directory. Complete geographical/alphabetical listing of academy fellows. *Price:* $15. • *Optometry and Vision Science*, monthly. Includes academy news, book reviews, and periodic index. *Price:* Included in membership dues; $55/year for nonmembers; $70/year for institutions; $30/year for students. • Newsletter, bimonthly.

★ 285 ★ American Academy of Optometry - British Chapter (ACABC)
Andrew Field
2 Doric Pl.
Woodbridge IP12 1BT, United Kingdom
Phone: 44 1394 380139 **Fax:** 44 7967 446413
Email: academy@debenlogic.co.uk
Website: http://www.academy.org.uk

Fnded: 1952. **Mem:** 110. **Lang(s):** English. **Desc:** Optometrists. Seeks to advance the study, teaching, and practice of optometry. Maintains standards of training, ethics, and practice for members; conducts continuing professional development courses for optometrists.

★ 286 ★ American Academy of Oral and Maxillofacial Pathology (AAOMP)
710 E Ogden Ave, Ste. 600
Naperville, IL 60563-8614
Phone: (630)579-3252 **Free:** 888-552-2667
Fax: (630)369-2488
Email: aaomp@b-online.com
Website: http://www.aaomp.org
Carl M. Allen, Pres. Elect

Fnded: 1946. **Mem:** 700. **Desc:** Professional society of oral pathologists. **Pub:** *Oral Surgery, Oral Medicine, Oral Pathology*, monthly. **Frmly:** (1994) American Academy Oral Pathology.

★ 287 ★ American Academy of Oral and Maxillofacial Radiology (AAOMR)
PO Box 55722
Jackson, MS 39296
Phone: (601)984-6060 **Fax:** (601)984-6086
Email: mocarroll@sod.umsmed.edu
Website: http://www.aaomr.org
Dr. M. Kevin O Carroll, Exec. Dir.

Fnded: 1949. **Mem:** 400. **Nat'l Groups:** 1. **Desc:** Dentists and other professionals who specialize in oral and maxillofacial rediology in clinical practice, teaching or research. Serves as authoritative body on radiation hygiene and hazards for the American Dental Association. **Pub:** *AAOMR Newsletter*, quarterly. Newsletter. Features news, president's messages, & announcements. *Price:* Free. • *Oral and Maxillofacial Radiology Section of Oral Surgery, Oral Medicine, Oral Pathology, Oral Radiology, and Endodontics*, monthly. Journal. *Price:* Included in active membership dues; $52 corporate, associate, affiliate, student, life. • *Roster of Membership*, annual. **Frmly:** (1951) American Academy of Oral Roentgenology; (1967) American Academy of Dental Radiology.

★ 288 ★ American Academy of Oral Medicine (AAOM)
2910 Lightfoot Dr.
Baltimore, MD 21209
Phone: (410)602-8585
Email: info@AAOM.com
Website: http://www.aaom.com
Joyce Caplan, Exec. Sec.

Fnded: 1945. **Mem:** 800. **Reg. Groups:** 4. **Desc:** Dental educators, specialists, general dentists, and physicians interested in the study of the oral health care of medically compromised patients and the nonsurgical management of medically related diseases and disorders affecting the maxillofacial region. Promotes an improved quality of life for people with oral and maxillofacial diseases and disorders; fosters better scientific understanding between the fields of dentistry and medicine. Maintains speakers' bureau; offers continuing education lectures and seminars. **Pub:** *AAOM News*, semiannual. Newsletter. *Price:* for members only. • *The Clinician's Guide to Oral Health in Geriatric Patients*. Monograph. *Price:* $21. • *The Clinician's Guide to the Treatment of the Medically-Complex Dental Patient*. Monograph. *Price:* $21. • *The Clinician's Guide to Treatment of Common Oral Conditions*, every 3-5 years. Monograph. *Price:* $21. • *The Clinician's Guide to Treatment of HIV-infected Patients*, periodic. Monograph. *Price:* included in membership dues; $15/year for nonmembers. • *Diagnosis and Treatment of Chronic Orofacial Pain*. Monograph. *Price:* $21. • *Oral Surgery, Oral Medicine, Oral Pathology, Oral Radiology and Endodontics*. Journal.

★ 289 ★ American Academy of Orofacial Pain (AAOP)
19 Mantua Rd.
Mount Royal, NJ 08061
Phone: (856)423-3629 **Fax:** (856)423-3420
Email: aaopco@talley.com
Website: http://www.aaop.org
Robert Rosenbaum, Pres.

Fnded: 1975. **Mem:** 330. **Desc:** Medical and dental doctors. Seeks to further knowledge of Orofacial Pain and Temporomandibular Disorders. Maintains patient referral program. **Pub:** *Journal of Orofacial Pain*, quarterly. Journal. *Price:* included in membership dues. • *Orofacial Pain: Guidelines for Classification, Assessment, and Management*. • *Temporomandibular Disorders: Guidelines for Classificiation, Assessment, and Management*. **Frmly:** (1979) American Academy of Craniomandibular Orthopedics; (1992) American Academy of Craniomandibular Disorders.

★ 290 ★ American Academy of Orthodontics for the General Practitioner (AAOGP)
9701 Wesley St., Ste. 202
Greenville, TX 75402
Free: 800-634-2027 **Fax:** 888-634-2028
Email: cborde9321@aol.com
Website: http://www.academygportho.com/
Cynthia Bordelon, Dir.

Fnded: 1959. **Mem:** 250. **Reg. Groups:** 2. **State Groups:** 5. **Desc:** Licensed dentists. Provides dentists in general practice with an organization through which they can augment their basic knowledge and training in orthodontics. Offers continuing education courses for dentists and auxiliary personnel; sponsors seminars. Provides facilities and audiovisual material for its affiliated study clubs. **Pub:** *American Academy of Orthodontics for the General Practitioner–Continuing Education*, annual. Brochure. Lists AAOGP-sponsored continuing education courses, seminars, and meetings for the coming year. *Price:* Free. • *International Journal of Orthodontics*, semiannual. Journal.

★ 291 ★ American Academy of Orthopaedic Surgeons (AAOS)

6300 N River Rd.
Rosemont, IL 60018-4262
Phone: (847)823-7186 **Free:** 800-346-AAOS
Fax: (847)823-8125
Email: custserv@aaos.org
Website: http://www.aaos.org
Dr. William Tipton, Exec. VP

Fnded: 1933. **Mem:** 24,000. **Reg. Groups:** 6. **State Groups:** 30. **Desc:** Professional society of orthopedic surgeons certified by the American Board of Orthopedic Surgery to practice orthopedic (bone and joint) surgery. Promotes physician education and skills enhancement by offering textbooks, clinical videotapes, courses and self-assessment exams. **Pub:** *Journal of the American Academy of Orthopaedic Surgeons: A Comprehensive Review.* • Bulletin, bimonthly.

★ 292 ★ American Academy of Orthotists and Prosthetists (AAOP)

526 King St., Ste. 201
Alexandria, VA 22314
Phone: (703)836-0788 **Fax:** (703)836-0737
Email: academy@oandp.com
Website: http://www.oandp.org
Thomas Gorski, CAE, Exec. Dir.

Fnded: 1970. **Mem:** 2,100. **Reg. Groups:** 15. **Desc:** Professional practitioners certified by the American Board for Certification in Orthotics and Prosthetics. Dedicated to the advancement of the profession and the improvement of patient care. Provides continuing education designed to increase professional competence of the individual practitioner. **Pub:** *Academician*, monthly. Newsletter. *Price:* included in membership dues. • *Journal of Prosthetics and Orthotics*, quarterly. Journal. Scientific, research articles on latest products, fitting techniques and patient care regimens. • *JPO Selected Readings.* • Handbooks. • Manuals. • Also publishes home study videos.

★ 293 ★ American Academy of Osteopathy (AAO)

3500 DePauw Blvd., Ste. 1080
Indianapolis, IN 46268
Phone: (317)879-1881 **Fax:** (317)879-0563
Email: snoone@academyofosteopathy.org
Website: http://www.academyofosteopathy.org
Stephen J. Noone, CAE, Exec. Dir.

Fnded: 1937. **Mem:** 6,000. **Reg. Groups:** 14. **Desc:** Doctors of osteopathy. Seeks to develop and teach the science and art of osteopathic manipulative treatment and encourage greater proficiency in the use of osteopathic structural diagnostic and therapeutic procedures. Conducts graduate courses and seminars; offers structural consultation and treatment service at meetings. Conducts research. **Pub:** *AAO Yearbooks.* Yearbooks. A collection of 52 yearbooks on one CD-ROM, over 9,000 pages of osteopathic literature. • *American Academy of Osteopathy–Quarterly Journal*, quarterly. Journal. *Price:* $60/year. • *Membership Directory*, annual. Directory. • *Millennial Edition of AAO Yearbook (2001).* Yearbook. • Videos. **Frmly:** (1944) Osteopathic Manipulative Therapeutic and Clinical Research Association; (1970) Academy of Applied Osteopathy.

★ 294 ★ American Academy of Otolaryngic Allergy Foundation (AAOA)

1990 M St. NW, Ste. 680
Washington, DC 20036
Phone: (202)955-5010 **Fax:** (202)955-5016
Email: aaoa@aaoaf.org
Jami Lucas, Exec. Dir.

Fnded: 1941. **Mem:** 2,300. **Desc:** Otolaryngologists who are interested in the study, research, and practice of otolaryngic allergy. Offers research fellowship in allergy related to the head and neck. Sponsors scientific meetings and continuing medical education programs. **Pub:** *AAOA News*, quarterly. Newsletter. *Price:* Free. • Directory, annual. **Frmly:** American Society of Ophthalmologic and Otolaryngologic Allergy.

★ 295 ★ American Academy of Otolaryngology - Head and Neck Surgery (AAO-HNS)

1 Prince St.
Alexandria, VA 22314-3357
Phone: (703)836-4444 **Fax:** (703)683-5100
Email: webmaster@entnet.org
Website: http://www.entnet.org
David R. Nielsen, MD, Exec. VP

Fnded: 1896. **Mem:** 11,000. **Desc:** Professional society of medical doctors specializing in otolaryngology (diseases of the ear, nose, and throat) and head and neck surgery. Represents otolaryngology in governmental and socioeconomic areas and provides high-quality medical education for otolaryngologists. Coordinates Combined Otolaryngological Spring Meetings for ten national otolaryngological societies. Operates job information exchange service and museum. **Pub:** *American Academy of Otolaryngology-Head and Neck Surgery–Bulletin*, monthly. Magazine. Includes academy news, calendar of events, employment opportunity listings, legislative news, and research updates. *Price:* Included in membership dues; $55/year for nonmembers. • *Conjoint Directory of the American Academy of Otolaryngology - Head and Neck Surgery*, semiannual. Directory. • *Otolaryngology - Head and Neck Surgery*, monthly. Journal. *Price:* Included in membership dues; $205/year for domestic nonmembers; $365/year for domestic institutions. • Monographs. • Videos.

★ 296 ★ American Academy of Pain Management

13947 Mono Way, No. A
Sonora, CA 95370
Phone: (209)533-9744 **Fax:** (209)533-9750
Email: aapm@aapainmanage.org
Website: http://www.aapainmanage.org
Kathryn A. Weiner, PhD, Exec. Dir.

Fnded: 1988. **Mem:** 6,000. **Desc:** To establish the core body of knowledge necessary to become a pain management professional. Provides educational and research programs and a speakers bureau. **Pub:** *American Journal of Pain Management*, quarterly. Journal. • *Pain Management A Practical Guide for Clinicians.* Textbook. • *The Pain Practitioner*, quarterly. Newsletter.

★ 297 ★ American Academy of Pain Medicine (AAPM)

4700 W Lake Ave.
Glenview, IL 60025
Phone: (847)375-4731 **Fax:** 877-734-8750
Email: aapm@amctec.com
Website: http://www.painmed.org
Kathryn M. Checea, Dir. of Professional Relations

Fnded: 1983. **Mem:** 1,200. **Desc:** Anesthesiologists, internists, neurologists, neurosurgeons, orthopedic surgeons, physiatrists, and psychiatrists. Promotes a socioeconomic and political climate conducive to the effective and efficient practice of pain medicine. Ensures quality medical care by physicians specializing in pain medicine. Participates in networking and liaison activities with other organizations dealing in pain medicine. Conducts educational programs. Holds a seat in the American Medical Association House of Delegates. **Pub:** *A Guide to Pain Medicine.* Brochure. • *AAPM Membership Directory*, annual. Membership Directory. Lists primary care and specialty physicians with an interest in pain medicine. • *Pain Medicine*, quarterly. Journal. Contains clinical articles, research information, articles concerning socioeconomic issues, and news. *Price:* Included in membership dues. • *Pain Medicine Network*, quarterly. Newsletter. Covers news about the academy and its members. **Frmly:** American Academy of Algology.

★ 298 ★ American Academy of Pediatric Dentistry (AAPD)

211 E Chicago Ave., Ste. 700
Chicago, IL 60611-2663
Phone: (312)337-2169 **Fax:** (312)337-6329
Email: aapdinfo@aapd.org
Website: http://www.aapd.org
Dr. John Rutkauskas, Exec. Dir.

Fnded: 1947. **Mem:** 5,600. **Reg. Groups:** 6. **Desc:** Professional society of dentists whose practice is limited to children; teachers and researchers in pediatric dentistry. Seeks to advance the specialty of pediatric dentistry through practice, education, and research. Sponsors graduate student pediatric dentistry award program. **Pub:** *American Academy of Pediatric Dentistry–Membership Roster*, annual. Membership Directory. • *American Academy of Pediatric Dentistry–Today*, bimonthly. Newsletter. Includes employment listings, meetings calendar, research updates, and obituaries. *Price:* Included in membership dues. • *Pediatric Dentistry*, bimonthly. Journal. Includes employment listings and conference proceedings. *Price:* Included in membership dues; $50/year for nonmembers; $65/year for institutions. • Pamphlets. **Frmly:** (1984) American Academy of Pedodontics.

★ 299 ★ American Academy of Pediatrics (AAP)

141 Northwest Point Blvd.
Elk Grove Village, IL 60007-1098
Phone: (847)434-4000 **Fax:** (847)434-8000
Email: kidsdocs@aap.org
Website: http://www.aap.org
E. Stephen Edwards, MD, Pres.

Fnded: 1930. **Mem:** 55,000. **State Groups:** 66. **Desc:** Professional medical society of pediatricians and pediatric subspecialists. Operates small member library of books and journals on pediatric medicine, office practice, and child health care policy. Maintains 42 committees, councils, and tasks forces including: Accident and Poison Prevention; Early Childhood, Adoption and Dependent Care; Infectious Diseases. Operates 47 sections. Sponsors Pediatrics Review and Education Program (PREP), a self-assessment, continuing education program for practicing pediatricians. **Pub:** *AAP News*, monthly. Newspaper. Covers the social, economic, and professional aspects of pediatric care. Includes association news and chapter news. *Price:* Included in membership dues; $40/year for nonmembers. • *Fellowship List*, annual. • *Pediatrics*, monthly. Journal. Includes employment listings. *Price:* $110/year for individuals; $180/year for institutions; $70/year for students; $70/nurses. • *Pediatrics in Review*, monthly. Journal. Contains review articles and abstracts. Subscribers are eligible for Category/Continuing Medical Education credit. *Price:* $130/year for members; $165/year for nonmembers and institutions. • Also publishes professional manuals and patient education materials.

★ 300 ★ American Academy of Periodontology (AAP)

737 N Michigan Ave., Ste. 800
Chicago, IL 60611-2615
Phone: (312)787-5518 **Fax:** (312)787-3670
Email: aapsite@perio.org
Website: http://www.perio.org
Alice DeForest, Exec. Dir.

Fnded: 1914. **Mem:** 7,500. **Desc:** Professional society of dentists specializing in the prevention, diagnosis, and treatment of diseases affecting the gums and supporting structures of the teeth and in the placement and maintenance of dental implants. **Pub:** *AAP News*, bimonthly. Newsletter. • *Annals of Periodontology*, annual. Journal. • *Directory of Members*, annual. • *Journal of Periodontology*, monthly. Journal.

★ 301 ★ American Academy of Pharmaceutical Physicians Education Foundation
c/o Anne G. Arella, Executive Director
1031 Pemberton Hill Rd., Ste. 101
Apex, NC 27502
Phone: (919)355-1000 **Fax:** (919)355-1010
Email: office@aapp.org
Website: http://www.aapp.org
Anne G. Arella, Exec. Dir.

Fnded: 1993. **Mem:** 1,200. **Reg. Groups:** 9. **Desc:** Physicians dedicated to pharmaceutical medicine, research, education and practice who spend 50% of their professional time practicing pharmaceutical medicine. **Pub:** *AAPP...Rx*, quarterly. Newsletter. *Price:* included in membership dues.

★ 302 ★ American Academy of Physical Medicine and Rehabilitation (AAPM&R)
1 IBM Plz., Ste. 2500
Chicago, IL 60611-3604
Phone: (312)464-9700 **Fax:** (312)464-0227
Email: info@aapmr.org
Website: http://www.aapmr.org
Ronald A. Henrichs, CAE, Exec. Dir.

Fnded: 1938. **Mem:** 6,700. **Desc:** National medical specialty society of physical medicine and rehabilitation physicians whose patients include people with physical disabilities and chronic, disabling illnesses. Mission is to maximize quality of life, minimize the incidence and prevalence of impairments, disability, and handicaps, promote societal health, and enhance the understanding and development of psychiatry. Offers educational opportunities and advocacy support to members and provides information, referrals, and patient education materials. **Pub:** *AAPM&R Membership Directory*, annual. Membership Directory. Arranged alphabetically, geographically, and by special interest group. *Price:* Included in membership dues. • *Archives of Physical Medicine and Rehabilitation*, monthly. Journal. Provides original research and clinical reports to health professionals who work with the disabled, elderly, and handicapped. *Price:* Included in membership dues; $159/year for nonmembers; $200/year for institutions; $72/year for students. • *The Physiatrist*, 10/year. Newsletter. Provides information on organizational activities, legislative and practice issues. Includes research updates, calendar, and quarterly inserts. *Price:* Included in membership dues. • *Study Guide*. Published part of Self-Directed Medical Knowledge Program. **Frmly:** (1956) American Society of Physical Medicine and Rehabilitation.

★ 303 ★ American Academy of Physician Assistants (AAPA)
950 N Washington St.
Alexandria, VA 22314-1552
Phone: (703)836-2272 **Fax:** (703)684-1924
Email: aapa@aapa.org
Website: http://www.aapa.org
Timi Agar-Barwick, Exec. Dir.

Fnded: 1968. **Mem:** 36,000. **Reg. Groups:** 5. **State Groups:** 57. **Local Groups:** 59. **Desc:** Physician assistants and other interested parties. Seeks to promote quality, cost-effective, and accessible healthcare, and the professional and personal development of PAs. Provide services for members. Organizes annual National PA Day. Develops research and education programs; compiles statistics. **Pub:** *AAPA News*, biweekly. Newsletter. News on physician assistant programs, AAPA's activities, and employment information and opportunities. *Price:* included in membership dues. • *Journal of the American Academy of Physician Assistants*, monthly, 12/year. Journal. Covers clinical and scholarly research. Includes book reviews. *Price:* Included in membership dues; $50/year for nonmembers; $75/year for institutions. • *Legislative Watch*, monthly. • Membership Directory, annual.

★ 304 ★ American Academy of Physician Assistants in Occupational Medicine (AAPA-OM)
950 N Washington St.
Alexandria, VA 22314-1552
Free: 800-596-4398 **Fax:** (703)684-1924
Email: aapaom@aapa.org
Website: http://www.aapa.org/paom.html
Tom Moreno, Membership Mgr.

Fnded: 1981. **Mem:** 200. **Nat'l Groups:** 1. **Desc:** Physicians, physician assistants, students and graduates of PA programs. Designed for an exchange of information and ideas within occupational health field. Endorses the code of ethical conduct established by the American College of Occupational Medicine. **Pub:** *AAPA-OM Membership Directory*. Directory. • *AAPA-OM Newsletter*, quarterly. Newsletter.

★ 305 ★ American Academy on Physician and Patient
6728 Old McLean Village Dr.
Mc Lean, VA 22101
Phone: (703)556-9222 **Fax:** (703)556-8729
Email: aappatient@degnon.org
Website: http://www.physicianpatient.org

Desc: Research and education professionals. Dedicated to research, education and improving professional standards in doctor-patient communication. Sponsors scholarships and grants.

★ 306 ★ American Academy of Podiatric Practice Management
707 Turnpike St.
North Andover, MA 01845
Phone: (978)686-6185 **Fax:** (978)685-9410
Email: aappmexecdir@aappm.com
Website: http://www.aappm.com
Hal Ornstein, D.P.M., Pres.

Fnded: 1961. **Mem:** 200. **Desc:** Doctors of podiatric medicine interested in practice administration. Works to standardize office management procedures to create more efficient podiatry practices; conducts research on the administration and function of podiatry offices; develops formalized procedures for obtaining and training podiatry office assistants. Disseminates pedal information and material on practice management. Investigates methods of delivering improved podiatric care to an increasing number of patients; seeks effective participation in the public health team. Maintains collection of newsletters and position papers; sponsors seminars and workshops. Compiles statistics. **Pub:** *AAPA Newsletter*, quarterly. Newsletter. • *Directory of Membership*, annual. Directory. **Frmly:** (1969) American Academy of Practice Management in Podiatry; (1970) American Academy of Podiatric Management; (1993) American Academy Podiatric Administration.

★ 307 ★ American Academy of Podiatric Sports Medicine (AAPSM)
PO Box 723
Rockville, MD 20848-0723
Phone: (301)845-9888 **Free:** 888-854-3338
Email: info@aapsm.org
Website: http://www.aapsm.org
Rita J. Yates, Exec. Dir.

Fnded: 1970. **Mem:** 600. **Desc:** Podiatrists, medical doctors, and athletic trainers interested in promoting professional participation and research in sports medicine. Directs 12 committees that deal with individual sports. Compiles statistics. **Pub:** *AAPSM Newsletter*, quarterly. Newsletter. Features articles on the treatment of sports injuries in the field of podiatry. Includes calendar of events and research updates. *Price:* included in membership dues.

★ 308 ★ American Academy of Professional Coders (AAPC)
309 West 700 South
Salt Lake City, UT 84101-2608
Free: 800-626-2633 **Fax:** (801)236-2258
Email: info@aapc.com
Website: http://www.aapc.org
Lan C. England, Exec. Dir.

Fnded: 1988. **Mem:** 24,000. **State Groups:** 50. **Local Groups:** 250. **Desc:** Certified professional coders. Promotes high standards of physician and outpatient facility coding through education and cerification. **Pub:** *AAPC Coding Edge*, monthly. Newsletter. *Price:* included in membership dues. **Frmly:** (2001) American Academy of Procedural Coders.

★ 309 ★ American Academy of Psychoanalysis and Dynamic Psychiatry (AAPDP)
PO Box 30
1 Regency Dr.
Bloomfield, CT 06002-0030
Phone: (860)243-0437 **Free:** 888-691-8281
Fax: (860)286-0787
Email: info@aapsa.org
Website: http://aapsa.org
Jacquelyn Coleman, Exec. Dir.

Fnded: 1956. **Mem:** 750. **Desc:** Psychoanalysts are fellows of the academy; psychiatric members are psychiatrists who meet specific requirements; associates are psychiatrists, scientists, or educators; candidates. Seeks to develop communication among psychoanalysts and persons in other disciplines in science and the humanities; provides a forum for inquiry into the phenomena of individual motivation and social behavior; encourages and supports research in psychoanalysis; fosters acceptance of psychoanalysis. Sponsors seminars and symposia. **Pub:** *Academy Forum*, biennial. Magazine. Contains articles on psychoanalysis and related topics and book reviews. *Price:* $20. • *Academy News*. Newsletter. • *Journal of the American Academy of Psychoanalysis*, quarterly. Journal. *Price:* $35. **Frmly:** (1966) Academy of Psychoanalysis; (2001) American Foundation for Psychoanalysis and Psychoanalysis in Groups; (2003) American Academy of Psychoanalysis.

★ 310 ★ American Academy of Psychotherapists (AAP)
PO Box 1611
New Bern, NC 28563
Phone: (252)634-3066 **Fax:** (252)634-3067
Email: aapoffice@coastalnet.com
Website: http://www.coe.iup.edu/aap/
Nancy R. Hunt, Dir.

Fnded: 1955. **Mem:** 725. **Reg. Groups:** 4. **Desc:** Professional society of psychologists, psychiatrists, clergy, and social workers engaged in the practice of psychotherapy. Provides meeting ground for psychotherapists of differing backgrounds and orientations. Facilitates cross-discipline thinking, planning, and research in psychotherapy. Sponsors workshops. **Pub:** *AAP Newsletter*, monthly. Newsletter. • *VOICES*, quarterly. Journal. *Price:* $30/year. • Directory, biennial.

★ 311 ★ American Academy of Restorative Dentistry (AARD)
985 Fuller Rd.
Colorado Springs, CO 80920
Phone: (719)633-1060 **Fax:** (719)593-7926
Email: rbrianullmann@restorativedentistry.com
Website: http://www.aard-dental-video.org/
Ned Van Roekel, D.D.S., Pres.

Fnded: 1928. **Mem:** 285. **Desc:** Professional society of dentists practicing restorative dentistry, and educators interested in dentistry as it applies to treatment of the natural teeth to restore and maintain a healthy functioning mouth as part of a healthy body. **Pub:** *Journal of Prosthetic Dentistry*, periodic. Journal. • *Roster*, annual. **Frmly:** (1928) American Society of Dental Ceramics.

★ 312 ★ American Academy of Sanitarians (AAS)
c/o Gary Noonan
720 S Colorado Blvd., Ste. 960-S
Denver, CO 80246

Phone: (303)758-5667 **Fax:** (303)691-9490
Website: http://Sanitarians.org
Gary Noonan, contact

Fnded: 1966. **Mem:** 400. **Desc:** Legally registered sanitarians who possess at least a master's degree in public health, environmental health sciences, or environmental management. Purpose is to improve the environmental health status of humanity through certification of those sanitarians who have helped or who are helping to achieve this long-range goal. **Pub:** *Register of Professional Sanitarians*, quinquennial. • *Roster of Diplomates*, annual. • Newsletter, semiannual. **Frmly:** American Intersociety Academy for Certification of Sanitarians.

★ 313 ★ American Academy of Sleep Medicine (AASM)

One Westbrook Corp. Ctr., Ste. 920
Westchester, IL 60154
Phone: (708)492-0930 **Fax:** (708)492-0943
Email: info@aasmet.org
Website: http://www.aasmnet.org/
Jerry Barrett, Exec. Dir.

Fnded: 1975. **Mem:** 2,900. **Desc:** Sleep disorders centers and individuals united to provide full diagnostic and treatment services and to improve the quality of care for patients with all types of sleep disorders. Fosters educational activities at medical schools and in continuing medical education programs; conducts site visits to assure minimum standards at member centers; trains and evaluates the competence of individuals who care for patients with sleep disorders. Conducts research programs, including a cooperative case study series on all patients seen by sleep disorders centers throughout the country. **Pub:** *ASDA News*, quarterly. Newsletter. • *SLEEP*, 9/year. Journal. *Price:* $129 individual; $185 institutional. • Also publishes a roster of centers. **Frmly:** American Association of Sleep Disorders Centers; (1987) Association of Sleep Disorders Centers; (2000) American Association of Sleep Disorders.

★ 314 ★ American Academy of Somnology (AAS)

PO Box 27077
Las Vegas, NV 89126
Phone: (702)222-6463
Email: somnology@aol.com
Website: http://www.hopperinstitute.com/aas_intro.html
Dr. David L. Hopper, PhD, Founder & Pres.

Fnded: 1986. **Mem:** 75. **Desc:** Clinicians, researchers, and students in the field of somnology; interested individuals. Promotes advancement of somnology as a health care specialty. (Somnology is the study of sleep and sleep disorders.) Advocates standardization of university programs in somnology and a multidisciplinary approach to the study and treatment of sleep disorders; conducts continuing education program. Sponsors American Board of Somnology to evaluate qualifications of applicants, administer examinations, and confer diplomate status on qualified individuals. Provides a forum for somnology clinicians and researchers to present findings and exchange ideas. Maintains speakers' bureau. **Pub:** *AAS Membership Directory*, annual. Membership Directory. • *Certification Handbook*, periodic. • *Journal of Somnology*, annual. Journal. • *The Somnologist*, quarterly. • Also publishes constitution, ethical standards, and bylaws.

★ 315 ★ American Academy of Sports Physicians (AASP)

17445 Oak Creek Court
Encino, CA 91316
Phone: (818)501-4433 **Fax:** (818)501-8855
Janie Zimmer, Coord.

Fnded: 1979. **Mem:** 150. **Desc:** Clinical physicians engaged in the practice of sports medicine who have made contributions in research, academics, or related fields. Objectives are to educate and inform physicians whose practices comprise mainly sports medicine and to register and recognize physicians who have expertise in sports medicine. Sponsors seminars. **Pub:** Newsletter, quarterly.

★ 316 ★ American Academy of Tropical Medicine (AATM)

16126 E Warren
PO Box 24224
Detroit, MI 48224
Phone: (313)882-0641 **Fax:** (313)882-0979
Ben Allie, MD, Pres.

Fnded: 1984. **Mem:** 2,600. **Nat'l Groups:** 10. **Reg. Groups:** 10. **Desc:** Physicians and allied health professionals interested in tropical medicine. Provides postgraduate continuing medical education; confers certificates and diplomas. Maintains speakers' bureau; provides placement service. Conducts research and compiles statistics. Conducts educational programs; offers children's services. **Pub:** *Journal of the American Academy of Tropical Medicine*, semiannual. Journal. Includes book reviews, employment opportunities, and information on new diagnostic equipment. *Price:* $125/year. • Monographs. • Newsletter, periodic. • Also publishes case studies and plans to publish directory of physicians and hospitals in tropical countries.

★ 317 ★ American Academy of Veterinary and Comparative Toxicology (AAVCT)

c/o Dr. Ramesh Gupta
Murray State University in Kentucky
Breathitt Veterinary Center
715 North Dr.
PO Box 2000
Hopkinsville, KY 42240
Phone: (270)886-3959 **Fax:** (270)886-4295
Email: ramesh.gupta@murraystate.edu
Dr. Ramesh Gupta, Contact

Fnded: 1957. **Mem:** 178. **Desc:** Veterinarians specializing in toxicology and others interested in veterinary comparative toxicology. Sponsors and encourages scientific and technical meetings and promotes discussion and interchange of information in the following fields of veterinary comparative toxicology: teaching, research and development, diagnosis, nomenclature, public health, and other problems of common interest. Reviews manuscripts and literature pertaining to toxicology and keeps a file of such literature for use by its members. Encourages the use of uniform toxicologic nomenclature. Facilitates and implements the exchange of proven methods among veterinary comparative toxicologists. **Pub:** *Veterinary and Human Toxicology*, quarterly. Journal. Contains annual directory. **Frmly:** American College of Veterinary Toxicologists.

★ 318 ★ American Academy of Veterinary Nutrition (AAVN)

1080 North Cobb Pky.
Marietta, GA 30062
Email: s.wynn@mindspring.com
Susan G. Wynn, DVM, Sec. -Treas.

Fnded: 1956. **Mem:** 475. **Desc:** Veterinarians and nutritional scientists interested in animal nutrition and health. Works to promote research and discussion in fields where health of animals may be influenced by nutrition. Sponsors programs on animal nutrition. Maintains speakers' bureau. **Pub:** Membership Directory, annual. **Frmly:** (1978) American Association of Veterinary Nutritionists.

★ 319 ★ American Academy of Veterinary Pharmacology and Therapeutics (AAVPT)

c/o Dr. Carol A. Davis
621 W Hill St.
Champaign, IL 61820
Phone: (217)359-0661
Email: cdavis@short.net
Website: http://www.aavpt.org/
Carol A. Davis, PhD, Sec. -Treas.

Fnded: 1977. **Mem:** 187. **Desc:** Veterinary pharmacologists and clinicians interested in clinical therapeutics; representatives of academia, industry, and government; private practitioners. Supports and promotes education and research in comparative pharmacology, clinical veterinary pharmacology, and other aspects of pharmacology of interest to the veterinary profession; aims to enhance the exchange of educational materials and ideas among veterinary pharmacologists. Organizes committees of experts to research and make recommendations to the profession on current problems in veterinary therapeutics. Sponsors and conducts workshops and other scientific and educational meetings. **Pub:** *Journal of Veterinary Pharmacology and Therapeutics*, bimonthly. Journal. • Directory, periodic. • Newsletter, quarterly.

★ 320 ★ American Academy of Wound Management (AAWM)

1255 23rd St., NW, No. 200
Washington, DC 20037-1174
Phone: (202)521-0368 **Fax:** (202)833-3636
Email: woundnet@aawm.org
Website: http://www.aawm.org
Melissa T. Forburger, Exec. Dir.

Fnded: 1995. **Mem:** 2,000. **Nat'l Groups:** 1. **Desc:** Medical practitioners, representing numerous professional specialties, with an interest in wound management. Seeks to advance the study and practice of wound treatment. Formulates standards of wound management practice; sponsors examinations and confers certification. Conducts continuing professional education programs. **Pub:** *AAWM Quarterly News Briefing*, quarterly. Journal. • *National Registry of Board Certified Wound Specialists*, annual. • Brochure.

★ 321 ★ American Accreditation Healthcare Commission (URAC)

1275 K St. NW, Ste. 1100
Washington, DC 20005
Phone: (202)216-9010 **Fax:** (202)216-9006
Email: gcarneal@urac.org
Website: http://www.urac.org
Garry Carneal, Pres. /CEO

Fnded: 1990. **Mem:** 300. **Desc:** Accreditation body for the managed health care industry. Seeks to establish and enforce standards for the managed care industry. Examines managed health care providers and bestows accreditation upon qualifying case management, health utilization management, health network, health plan, practitioner credentialling, credentials verification, workers' compensation utilization management, workers' compensation network, and health call center programs. **Pub:** *Directory of Accredited Organizations*, annual. Directory. *Price:* $39/copy. • *Models of Care: Case Studies of Healthcare Delivery Innovation*. Book. *Price:* $195/copy.

★ 322 ★ American Action Fund for Blind Children and Adults (AAFBCA)

1800 Johnson St., Ste. 100
Baltimore, MD 21230
Phone: (410)659-9315 **Fax:** (410)685-5653
Email: acc@roudley.com
Website: http://www.actionfund.org

Fnded: 1919. **Desc:** Works to assist blind persons in securing reading material, to educate the public about blindness, to give aid to the deaf-blind and to improve the quality of life for blind persons. Provides information and referral services on Social Security Disability Insurance, employment, civil rights, products and aids, education of blind children and public rehabilitation agencies; disseminates information on Braille and sign language; distributes publications free of charge to libraries and schools. **Pub:** *Great Documents Series*. Books. Features Braille copies of Great American documents. • *Twin Vision*. Books. Children's books containing Braille and print side by side. • Also publishes Braille calendars. **Frmly:** (1990) American Brotherhood for the Blind.

★ 323 ★ American Acupuncture Association (AAA)
4262 Kissena Blvd.
Flushing, NY 11355
Phone: (718)886-4431 **Fax:** (718)463-0808
Dr. David P. J. Hung, Chm.

Fnded: 1972. **Mem:** 400. **Desc:** Physicians, nurses, acupuncturists, physical therapists, and herbologists. Promotes acceptance of acupuncture as a viable medical method. Works to legalize acupuncture on the state level. Offers continuing education course. Maintains speakers' bureau. Conducts lectures to educate public on acupuncture. **Pub:** *Journal of Chinese Acupuncture*, annual. Journal.

★ 324 ★ American Aging Association (AGE)
c/o The Sally Balin Medical Center
110 Chesley Dr.
Media, PA 19063
Phone: (610)627-2626 **Fax:** (610)565-9747
Email: ameraging@aol.com
Website: http://www.americanaging.org
Arthur K. Balin, MD, Exec. Dir.

Fnded: 1970. **Mem:** 500. **Desc:** Laymen and scientists primarily in the biomedical field. Dedicated to "helping people live better, longer" by promoting biomedical aging studies directed toward slowing down the aging process, informing the public of the progress of aging research and of practical means of achieving a long and healthy life, and increasing knowledge of gerontology among physicians and other health workers. **Pub:** *Age News*, quarterly. Newsletter. *Price:* included in membership dues. • *Journal of the American Aging Association*, quarterly. Journal. Covers biomedical aging research. *Price:* $221/year for individuals.

★ 325 ★ American Ambulance Association (AAA)
8201 Greensboro Dr., Ste. 300
Mc Lean, VA 22102
Phone: (703)610-9018 **Free:** 800-523-4447
Fax: (703)610-9005
Email: questions@the-aaa.org
Website: http://www.the-aaa.org
Lori Green, Contact

Fnded: 1977. **Mem:** 830. **Desc:** Private suppliers of ambulance service. Purposes are: to aid in developing private enterprise pre-hospital emergency medical treatment and medical transportation services as a viable cost-effective alternative to publicly-operated services; to promote improved patient care; to develop efficient medical transportation at a reasonable cost; to improve personnel and equipment standards; to work with organizations offering medical transportation; to encourage high standards of ethics and conduct. Acts as an information clearinghouse; informs members of developments in the industry. Offers advice on federal statutes and regulations related to the medical transportation industry, such as insurance and antitrust regulations. Holds four regional seminars per year on topics such as training requirements, insurance systems, medicare reimbursement, and local, state, and federal legislation and regulations. Conducts quarterly emergency medical services management seminar. **Pub:** *Ambulance Industry Journal*, quarterly. Journal. Includes book reviews and legislative reports. *Price:* Free to members; $25 for nonmembers. **Frmly:** (1978) Ambulance and Medical Service Association of America.

★ 326 ★ American Amputee Foundation (AAF)
Box 250218, Hillcrest Sta.
Little Rock, AR 72225
Phone: (501)666-2523 **Fax:** (501)666-8367
Email: cjwaiden@hotmail.com
C.J. Waiden, Exec. Dir. /CEO

Fnded: 1975. **Nat'l Groups:** 1. **State Groups:** 13. **Local Groups:** 2. **Desc:** Provides information and referral service to new amputees and their families to aid them in their adjustment to amputation. Sponsors programs and resources on state-of-the-art prosthetics, coalition building, and self-help life care planning services to those with catastrophic injury. on a very limited basis, aid in buying the first limb for amputees who qualify. Sponsors programs on state-of-the-art prosthetics, coalition building, and selfhelp. **Pub:** *National Resource Directory*, biennial. Directory. • Books.Provides information on self-help methods.

★ 327 ★ American Animal Hospital Association (AAHA)
12575 West Bayaud Ave.
Lakewood, CO 80228
Phone: (303)986-2800 **Free:** 800-252-2242
Fax: (303)986-1700
Email: info@aahanet.org
Website: http://www.aahanet.org
John W. Albers, D.V.M., Exec. Dir.

Fnded: 1933. **Mem:** 17,000. **Desc:** Veterinarians engaged in small animal practice who own or staff small animal hospitals. Works for the promotion of excellence in small animal medicine and improvement of hospital facilities. Operates AAHA Foundation, which gives grants for small animal medical research. Compiles statistics. **Pub:** *American Animal Hospital Association Scientific Proceedings*, annual. Proceedings. Includes manuscripts of papers delivered at AAHA meeting. Contains authors index. *Price:* Included in membership dues; $55 for nonmembers plus shipping and handling. • *Journal of the American Animal Hospital Association*, bimonthly. Journal. Includes advertisers' index. *Price:* Included in membership dues; $107/year U.S. & Canada; $127/year Foreign Countries. • *TRENDS Magazine*, bimonthly. Magazine. Covers management trends, social issues, paraprofessional topics in veterinary medicine; includes association news, and CE calendar. *Price:* Included in membership dues; $60/year for nonmembers. • Membership Directory, annual. • Has also published atlases for ophthalmology, behavior, oncology, dermatology, cytology, and cardiology and a manual of standards.

★ 328 ★ American Apitherapy Society (AAS)
1209 Post Rd.
Scarsdale, NY 10583
Phone: (914)725-7944 **Fax:** (914)723-0920
Email: aas.office@apitherapy.org
Website: http://www.apitherapy.org/
Sara Cornwell, Exec. Dir.

Fnded: 1989. **Mem:** 800. **Reg. Groups:** 9. **Desc:** Beekeepers, physicians, scientists, and others interested in apitherapy, the therapeutic use of honey bee products. Purpose is to collect and disseminate information in the field and to provide a forum for researchers to present the results of their work. Encourages investigation of hive products in order to provide a scientific foundation for their curative properties and use in human medicine. Seeks to prove the effectiveness of bee venom in treating inflammatory diseases such as arthritis and rheumatism. Gains funding for clinical laboratory studies through contributions. Supports selected research and fundraising projects for the investigation of apiotherapeutic agents. Compiles statistics. **Pub:** *Journal of the American Apitherapy Society*, quarterly. Journal. *Price:* Free with membership. • Brochures.Contains information on bee venom, honey, pollen, and beeswax. • Journal, annual. **Frmly:** (1989) North American Apio-Therapy Society.

★ 329 ★ American Art Therapy Association (AATA)
1202 Allanson Rd.
Mundelein, IL 60060-3808
Phone: (847)949-6064 **Free:** 888-290-0878
Fax: (847)566-4580
Email: info@arttherapy.org
Website: http://www.arttherapy.org
Shaun McNiff, Pres.

Fnded: 1969. **Mem:** 4,300. **Local Groups:** 30. **Desc:** Art therapists, students, and individuals in related fields. Supports the progressive development of therapeutic uses of art, the advancement of research, and improvements in the standards of practice. Has established specific professional criteria for training art therapists. Facilitates the exchange of information and experience. Compiles statistics. **Pub:** *American Art Therapy Association–Newsletter*, quarterly. Newsletter. Provides information on related organizations and available resources; includes calendar of events, legislative news, and member news. *Price:* Included in membership dues; $16/year for nonmembers. • *Art Therapy*, quarterly. Journal. Includes referred articles and illustrations, news and summaries of national conferences, books reviews, media, and commentaries. *Price:* Included in membership dues; $40/year for nonmembers; $57/year for institutions; $64/year for nonmembers outside the U.S. • *Proceedings of Annual Conference*. Proceedings.

★ 330 ★ American Assembly for Men in Nursing (AAMN)
c/o NYSNA
11 Cornell Rd.
Latham, NY 12110-1499
Phone: (518)782-9400 **Fax:** (518)782-9530
Email: aamn@aamn.org
Website: http://aamn.org
Russell G. Tranbarger, RN, Pres.

Fnded: 1971. **Mem:** 200. **Reg. Groups:** 5. **State Groups:** 4. **Desc:** Registered nurses. Works to: help eliminate prejudice in nursing; interest men in the nursing profession; provide opportunities for the discussion of common problems; encourage education and promote further professional growth; advise and assist in areas of professional inequity; help develop sensitivities to various social needs; promote the principles and practices of positive health care. Acts as a clearinghouse for information on men in nursing. Conducts educational programs. Promotes education and research about men's health issues. **Pub:** *Interaction*, quarterly. Newsletter. Contains statement of objectives and information on officers, events, and activities. *Price:* Included in membership dues. **Frmly:** (1982) National Male Nurse Association.

★ 331 ★ American Association for Accreditation of Ambulatory Surgery Facilities (AAAASF)
1202 Allanson Rd.
Mundelein, IL 60060
Phone: (847)949-6058 **Free:** 888-545-5222
Fax: (847)566-4580
Email: info@aaaasf.org
Website: http://www.aaaasf.org
Michael McGuire, MD, Pres.

Fnded: 1981. **Desc:** Board-certified surgeon-operated ambulatory surgical facilities. To maintain high standards through adherence to a voluntary program of inspection and accreditation of ambulatory surgery facilities. **Pub:** Newsletter, semiannual. **Frmly:** (1994) American Association for Accreditation of Ambulatory Plastic Surgery Facilities.

★ 332 ★ American Association of Ambulatory Surgery Centers (AAASC)
PO Box 23220
San Diego, CA 92193
Phone: (858)490-8085 **Free:** 800-237-3768
Fax: (858)490-9016
Email: aaasc@mtgsunlimited.com
Website: http://www.aaasc.org
Michelle Freeland, Admin. Dir.

Fnded: 1978. **Mem:** 500. **Desc:** Assists physicians, corporations, healthcare administrators to provide excellence in ambulatory care; provides information to build free-standing surgery center by addressing legal, accreditation and leadership issues. **Pub:** *Monitor*, quarterly. Newsletter. • Membership Directory, annual. For members only on website. *Price:* Free to members. **Frmly:** (1986) Society for Office-Based Surgery; (1996) American Society of Outpatient Surgeons.

★ 333 ★ American Association of Anatomists (AAA)
9650 Rockville Pike
Bethesda, MD 20814
Phone: (301)634-7910 **Fax:** (301)634-7965
Email: exec@anatomy.org
Website: http://www.anatomy.org
John Fallon, Pres.

Fnded: 1888. **Mem:** 2,500. **Desc:** Professional society of anatomists and scientists in related fields. **Pub:** *Anatomical News*, quarterly. Newsletter. Includes list of employment opportunities. *Price:* Included in membership dues. • *Anatomical Record*, monthly. • *Developmental Dynamics*, monthly. • *Directory, Departments of Anatomy, U.S. and Canada*, triennial. Directory. • *New Anatomist*, bimonthly.

★ 334 ★ American Association of Avian Pathologists (AAAP)
382 West St. Rd.
New Bolton Center
Kennett Square, PA 19348
Phone: (610)444-4282 **Fax:** (610)925-8106
Email: aaap@vet.upenn.edu
Website: http://www.aaap.info/
Dr. Robert J. Eckroade, Sec. -Treas.

Fnded: 1957. **Mem:** 1,100. **Desc:** Membership limited to graduates of recognized veterinary colleges. Associate members are not veterinarians but are engaged in some form of avian medicine. Maintains 29 committees. **Pub:** *Avian Diseases*, quarterly. Journal. Contains case reports. *Price:* Included in membership dues; $110/year for nonmembers in U.S.; $120/year for nonmembers outside U.S. • Manuals. • Videos.

★ 335 ★ American Association of Bioanalysts (AAB)
917 Locust St., Ste. 1100
Saint Louis, MO 63101-1419
Phone: (314)241-1445 **Fax:** (314)241-1449
Email: aab@aab.org
Website: http://www.aab.org
Mark S. Birenbaum, PhD, Admin.

Fnded: 1956. **Mem:** 1,000. **Desc:** Professional organization of directors, owners, managers, supervisors, technologists and technicians of bioanalytical clinical laboratories devoting their efforts to clinical laboratory procedure and testing. Sponsors Proficiency Testing Service open to individuals engaged in the clinical laboratory field. Provides specialized education and representation before federal and state legislatures and regulatory agencies. **Pub:** *AAB Bulletin*, bimonthly. Bulletin. • *AAB Update*, periodic.

★ 336 ★ American Association of Bioanalysts Board of Registry (ABOR)
917 Locust St., Ste. 1100
Saint Louis, MO 63101-1419
Phone: (314)241-1445 **Fax:** (314)241-1449
Email: aab@aab.org
Website: http://www.aab.org
Mark S. Birenbaum, PhD, Admin.

Fnded: 1962. **Desc:** Autonomous certifying agency for medical technologists, laboratory technicians, and physician office laboratory technicians. Maintains Continuing Education for Professional Advancement (CEPA) program to approve and record continuing education unit credits. **Frmly:** Accrediting Commission; (2000) Credentialing Commission.

★ 337 ★ American Association of Blood Banks (AABB)
8101 Glenbrook Rd.
Bethesda, MD 20814-2749
Phone: (301)907-6977 **Fax:** (301)907-6895
Email: aabb@aabb.org
Website: http://www.aabb.org
Sara Foer, Contact

Fnded: 1947. **Mem:** 11,500. **Desc:** Community and hospital blood centers and transfusion and transplantation services, physicians, nurses, technologists, administrators, blood donor recruiters, scientists, and individuals involved in related activities. Encourages the voluntary donation of blood and other tissues and organs through education, public information, and research. Operates the National Blood Exchange; inspects and accredits blood banks and parentage testing laboratories; sponsors the National Blood Foundation; maintains a rare donor file and reference laboratory system. Maintains over 40 scientific, technical, and administrative committees and three councils. **Pub:** *AABB News Briefs*, 11/year. Newsletter. Includes calendar of events, employment listings, and government affairs update. *Price:* Included in membership dues. • *American Association of Blood Banks–Membership Directory*, biennial. Directory. Lists institutional and individual members in alphabetical and geographic order. *Price:* Included in membership dues; $50 for nonmembers. • *Blood Bank Week*. Newsletter. Covers scientific, legislative, and regulatory events affecting blood banking and transfusion medicine. *Price:* $98/year for members; $128/year for nonmembers. • *Directory of Community Blood Centers*, biennial. Directory. *Price:* $25 for participating members; $50 for nonmembers. • *Standards for Blood Banks and Transfusion Services*, every 18 months. *Price:* $20 for members; $35 for nonmembers. • *Technical Manual*, triennial. Manual. *Price:* $48 for members; $60 for nonmembers; $45 for students. • *Transfusion*, monthly. Journal. Presents scientific, technical, and administrative papers relating to the field of blood banking. Includes advertisers index and convention abstract. *Price:* Included in membership dues; $135/year for nonmember individuals; $195/year for institutions. • Books. • Monographs.

★ 338 ★ American Association of Bovine Practitioners (AABP)
Box 1755
Rome, GA 30162
Phone: (706)232-2220 **Fax:** (706)232-2232
Email: aabphq@aabp.org
Website: http://www.aabp.org
James A Jarrett, Exec. Dir.

Fnded: 1965. **Mem:** 5,800. **Desc:** Veterinarians who practice bovine medicine. Aims to elevate standards in the field; cooperates with veterinary and agricultural organizations and regulatory agencies. **Pub:** *AABP Newsletter*, monthly. Newsletter. Contains meetings calendar. *Price:* Included in membership dues. • *American Association of Bovine Practitioners Directory*, annual. Directory. Includes annual supplements. *Price:* Included in membership dues; $25/copy for select others. • *American Association of Bovine Practitioners Proceedings of Annual Meeting*. *Price:* Included in membership dues; $40/copy for nonmembers. • *Bovine Practitioner*, annual. Covers new developments in bovine practice. *Price:* Included in membership dues; $20/copy for nonmembers.

★ 339 ★ American Association for Cancer Research (AACR)
615 Chestnut St., 17th Fl.
Philadelphia, PA 19106
Phone: (215)440-9300 **Fax:** (215)440-9313
Email: membership@aacr.org
Website: http://www.aacr.org
Margaret Foti, PhD, CEO

Fnded: 1907. **Mem:** 19,000. **Local Groups:** 3. **Desc:** Works to facilitate communication and dissemination of information among scientists and others dedicated to cancer research; seeks to advance understanding of cancer etiology, prevention, diagnosis and treatment throughout the world. Fosters research on cancer, public and science education and training. **Pub:** *Cancer Epidemiology, Biomarkers & Prevention*, monthly. Journal. Contains original research on causes and prevention of cancer. *Price:* $165/year for individual nonmembers. • *Cancer Research*, semimonthly. Journal. Contains reports in subfields of cancer research: biochemistry, biophysics, carcinogenesis, endocrinology, immunology, and molecular biology. *Price:* Included in membership; $640/year for individual nonmembers. • *Clinical Cancer Research*, monthly. Journal. Features articles on clinical and translational cancer research. *Price:* $225/year for individual nonmembers. • *Molecular Cancer Research*, monthly. Journal. Peer-reviewed research on the molecular and cellular biology of cancer (formerly Cell Growth & Differentiation). *Price:* $145/year for nonmembers. • *Molecular Cancer Therapeutics*, monthly. Journal. Contains research on emerging disciplines with implications for cancer therapeutics. *Price:* $100/year for nonmembers. • *Supplement to Journal*, periodic. Journal. • Directory, annual. • Proceedings, annual.

★ 340 ★ American Association of Cardiovascular and Pulmonary Rehabilitation (AACVPR)
401 N Michigan Ave., Ste. 2200
Chicago, IL 60611-4267
Phone: (312)321-5146 **Fax:** (312)527-6635
Email: aacvpr@tmahq.com
Website: http://www.aacvpr.org
John Porcari, Pres.

Fnded: 1985. **Mem:** 3,000. **Desc:** Allied health professionals involved in the field of cardiovascular and pulmonary rehabilitation. Fosters the improvement of clinical practice in CVPR; promotes scientific CVPR research; seeks the advancement of CVPR education for health care professionals and the public. **Pub:** *AACVPR Directory*, annual. Directory. • *Directory of Cardiovascular and Pulmonary Rehabilitation Programs*, annual. Directory. • *Journal of Cardiopulmonary Rehabilitation*, bimonthly. Journal. Provides theoretical and practical information on cardiovascular and pulmonary rehabilitation. Includes reviews and calendar of events. *Price:* Included in membership dues; $120/year for nonmembers. • *News and Views of AACVPR*, monthly. Newsletter.

★ 341 ★ American Association of Certified Allergists (AACA)
85 W Algonquin Rd. Ste. 550
Arlington Heights, IL 60005
Phone: (847)427-8111 **Fax:** (847)427-1294
Richard Slawny, Exec. Dir.

Fnded: 1968. **Mem:** 510. **Desc:** Physicians specializing in allergy and clinical immunology. Objectives are to: improve expertise in allergy treatment; disseminate information pertaining to undergraduate and graduate education in allergology; promote improved standards for the practice and teaching of allergy; exchange information between physicians facing similar problems under different circumstances. **Pub:** Newsletter, 3/year. *Price:* Included in membership dues.

★ 342 ★ American Association of Certified Orthoptists (AACO)
c/o UIHC-Ophthalmology
200 Hawkins Dr.
Iowa City, IA 52242
Phone: (319)356-3863 **Fax:** (319)384-9831
Email: Pamela-kutschke@uiowa.edu
Website: http://www.orthoptics.org
Pamela Kutschke, Pres.

Fnded: 1940. **Mem:** 250. **Reg. Groups:** 4. **Desc:** Orthoptists certified by the American Orthoptic Council, after completing a minimum of 24 months' special training, to treat defects in binocular function. Assists in postgraduate instruction courses; conducts programs and courses at international, national, and regional meetings; helps individual orthoptists with special or unusual problem cases; trains new orthoptists. Operates a placement listing. **Pub:** *American Association of Certified Orthoptists–Directory*, annual. Directory. *Price:* Included in membership dues. • *American Orthoptic Journal*, annual. Journal. Presents new material in the fields of amblyopia and strabismus. Includes book reviews and abstracts of current English and French literature. *Price:* $25/copy for individuals; $56/copy for institutions. • *The Prism*, quadrennial. Newsletter. **Frmly:** (1963) American Association of Orthopic Technicians.

★ 343 ★ American Association of Chairs of Departments of Psychiatry (AACDP)

AACDP
UCHC-Dept Psychiatry, MC 1935
263 Farmington Ave.
Farmington, CT 06030-1935
Phone: (860)679-8113 **Fax:** (860)679-1246
Email: info@aacdp.org
Website: http://www.aacdp.org
Daniel K. Winstead, MD, Pres.

Fnded: 1967. **Mem:** 136. **Desc:** Chairmen of departments of psychiatry in colleges of medicine. Purposes are: to promote medical education, research, and patient care, particularly as these concern psychiatry; to promote the growth and continuing development of psychiatry; to provide a forum for discussion and exchange of ideas among the chairmen of departments of psychiatry in medical schools; to provide appropriate liaison between chairmen and individuals and organizations whose activities bear on the objectives of the association. Membership list.

★ 344 ★ American Association for Chronic Fatigue Syndrome (AACFS)

34693 Bookhammer Landing Rd.
Lewes, DE 19958
Phone: (302)947-9634
Email: info@aacfs.org
Website: http://www.aacfs.org
Dharam V. Ablashi, DVM, Pres.

Fnded: 1992. **Mem:** 500. **Nat'l Groups:** 1. **Desc:** Research scientists, physicians and other health care professionals, and institutions with and interest in chronic fatigue syndrome (CFS). Seeks to advance the diagnosis and treatment of CFS. Facilitates exchange of information among members; sponsors research; serves as a clearinghouse on CFS diagnosis and patient care. Maintains speakers' bureau. **Pub:** *AACF'S Newsletter*, quarterly. Newsletter. • Position papers and conference proceedings.

★ 345 ★ American Association of Clinical Anatomists (AACA)

c/o R. Benton Adkins, Jr.
Vanderbilt University Medical Center
D5220 Medical Center N
1161 21st Ave. S
Nashville, TN 37232-2577
Phone: (713)500-6169 **Fax:** (713)500-0621
Email: benton.adkins@mcmail.vanderbilt.edu
Website: http://www.clinicalanatomy.org/
Dr. Lawrence M. Ross, Sec.

Desc: Dedicated to the advancement of science and art of clinical anatomy; encourages research and publication in the field and maintaining high standards in teaching of anatomy. **Pub:** *Clinical Anatomy*. Journal. Provides a medium for the exchange of current information between anatomists and clinicians.

★ 346 ★ American Association for Clinical Chemistry (AACC)

2101 L St. NW, Ste. 202
Washington, DC 20037-1558
Phone: (202)857-0717 **Free:** 800-892-1400
Fax: (202)887-5093
Email: info@aacc.org
Website: http://www.aacc.org
Richard Flaherty, Exec. VP

Fnded: 1948. **Mem:** 10,000. **Local Groups:** 22. **Desc:** Clinical laboratory scientists and others engaged in the practice of clinical laboratory science in independent laboratories, hospitals, and allied institutions. Sponsors education programs; publishes books. **Pub:** *Clinical Chemistry Journal*, monthly. Journal. • *Clinical Laboratory News*, monthly. • *Clinical Laboratory Strategies*, monthly. • Annual Report, annual. • Books. • Membership Directory.*Price:* for members only. **Frmly:** (1976) American Association of Clinical Chemists.

★ 347 ★ American Association of Clinical Endocrinologists (AACE)

1000 Riverside Ave., Ste. 205
Jacksonville, FL 32204
Phone: (904)353-7878 **Fax:** (904)353-8185
Email: djones@aace.com
Website: http://www.aace.com
Donald C. Jones, CEO

Fnded: 1991. **Mem:** 4,000. **Desc:** Clinical endocrinologists and physicians with special education in diabetes, osteoporosis, thyroid illness, lipid-cholesterol problems, reproductive disorders, obesity and nutrition. Seeks to enhance the practice of clinical endocrinology. **Pub:** *Endocrine Practice*, bimonthly. Journal. Features peer reviewed scientific articles on clinical endocrinology. • *The First Messenger*, bimonthly. Newsletter.

★ 348 ★ American Association of Clinical Urologists (AACU)

1111 N Plaza Dr., No. 550
Schaumburg, IL 60173-6021
Phone: (847)517-1050 **Fax:** (847)517-7229
Email: aacu@wjweiser.com
Website: http://aacuweb.org
Wendy J. Weiser, Exec. Dir.

Fnded: 1970. **Mem:** 5,600. **Desc:** Clinical urologists who are members of the American Urological Association or its sections and the American Medical Association. Purposes are to stimulate interest in the science and practice of urology and to promote understanding of socioeconomic and political affairs affecting medical practice. Does not abstract statistical information or function as a referral service for people with urological/ medical problems. **Pub:** *AACU Fax*, 3-4/year. Newsletter. • *AACU News*. • *Membership Roster*, annual. • Journal, bimonthly.

★ 349 ★ American Association of Colleges of Nursing (AACN)

1 Dupont Cir. NW, Ste. 530
Washington, DC 20036
Phone: (202)463-6930 **Fax:** (202)785-8320
Email: webmaster@aacn.nche.edu
Website: http://www.aacn.nche.edu
Polly Bednash, Exec. Dir.

Fnded: 1969. **Mem:** 570. **Desc:** Institutions offering baccalaureate and/or graduate degrees in nursing. Seeks to advance the practice of professional nursing by improving the quality of baccalaureate and graduate programs, promoting research, and developing academic leaders. Works with other professional nursing organizations and organizations in other health professions to evaluate and improve health care. Conducts educational programs on masters and doctoral nursing education and faculty practice; sponsors executive development series for new and aspiring deans of nursing. **Pub:** *A Guide to Grassroots Activism. Price:* $5. • *A Model for Differentiated Nursing Practice. Price:* $10. • *Annual State of the Schools*. Annual Report. • *Enrollment and Graduations in Baccalaureate and Graduate Programs in Nursing*, annual. Report. • *Essential Clinical Resources for Nursing's Academic Mission. Price:* $7 for members; $10 for nonmembers. • *Essentials of Baccalaureate Education for Professional Nursing Practice. Price:* $7 for members; $10 for nonmembers. • *Essentials of Master's Education for APN. Price:* $7 for members; $10 for nonmembers. • *Faculty Salaries in Baccalaureate and Graduate Programs in Nursing*, annual. Report. • *Issue Bulletin*, 3/year. Bulletin. Examines issues in nursing education and research. • *Journal of Professional Nursing*, bimonthly. Journal. • *Meet the Press. . .and Succeed: A Handbook for Nurse Educators. Price:* $4.75 for members; $5.75 for nonmembers. • *Position Statement on Nursing Research. Price:* $3. • *Salaries of Administrative Nursing Faculty in Baccalaureate and Graduate Programs in Nursing*, biennial. Report. • *Salaries of Deans in Baccalaureate and Graduate Programs in Nursing*, annual. Report. *Price:* $28. • *Syllabus*, bimonthly. Newsletter.

★ 350 ★ American Association of Colleges of Osteopathic Medicine (AACOM)

5550 Friendship Blvd., Ste. 310
Chevy Chase, MD 20815-7231
Phone: (301)968-4100 **Fax:** (301)968-1554
Email: ckearns@aacom.org
Website: http://www.aacom.org
Douglas L. Wood, PhD,DO, Pres.

Fnded: 1898. **Mem:** 20. **Desc:** Osteopathic medical colleges. Operates centralized application service; monitors and works with Congress and other government agencies in the planning of health care programs. Gathers statistics on osteopathic medical students, on innovations in medical education, faculty, administers federal contract, develops national communication programs on behalf of member colleges. **Pub:** *American Association of Colleges of Osteopathic Medicine–Annual Statistical Report*. Covers activities of the colleges of osteopathic medicine; provides information on enrollment , student costs, and scholarships and loans. *Price:* $18/copy. • *College Information*, annual. Book. • *Debts and Career Plans of Osteopathic Medical Students*, annual. Report describing financial debt and career plans of freshmen and seniors in osteopathic colleges. Contains statistics on debts. *Price:* $16/copy. **Frmly:** (1970) American Association of Osteopathic Colleges.

★ 351 ★ American Association of Colleges of Pharmacy (AACP)

1426 Prince St.
Alexandria, VA 22314
Phone: (703)739-2330 **Fax:** (703)836-8982
Email: aconnelly@aacp.org
Website: http://www.aacp.org
Amy B. Connelly, Mgr.

Fnded: 1900. **Mem:** 3,000. **Desc:** College of pharmacy programs accredited by American Council on Pharmaceutical Education; corporations and individuals. Compiles statistics. **Pub:** *AACP News*, monthly. Newsletter. Includes information on association activities, employment opportunities, and new members. *Price:* Included in membership dues; $100/year for nonmembers. • *American Association of Colleges of Pharmacy–Graduate Programs in the Pharmaceutical Sciences*, annual. Directory. Lists graduate programs in pharmacy; provides comparative analysis of pharmacy schools and admissions criteria for graduate programs. *Price:* $25/copy. • *American Journal of Pharmaceutical Education*, quarterly. Journal. Includes book reviews, listing of recent publications, and statistics. *Price:* Included in membership dues; $40/ year for nonmembers in the U.S. and Canada; $65/ year for nonmembers outside the U.S. and Canada; $100/year for libraries. • *Pharmacy School Admission Requirements*, annual. Directory. Lists pharmacy schools arranged by state; provides comparative analysis of pharmacy schools and admissions criteria for professional programs. *Price:* $25/copy. • *Roster of Teaching Personnel in Colleges of Pharmacy*, annual. Includes calendar of events. *Price:* Included in membership dues; $100/copy for nonmembers. **Frmly:** (1925) American Conference of Pharmaceutical Faculties.

★ 352 ★ American Association of Colleges of Podiatric Medicine (AACPM)

1350 Piccard Dr., Ste. 322
Rockville, MD 20850
Phone: (301)990-7400 **Free:** 800-922-9266
Fax: (301)990-2807
Email: aacpmas@aacpm.org
Website: http://www.aacpm.org
Moraith G. North, Interim

Fnded: 1932. **Mem:** 6. **Desc:** Professional organization of administrators, faculty, practitioners, students, and other individuals associated with podiatric medical education. Provides vocational guidance material for secondary schools and colleges. Conducts public affairs activities and legislative advocacy. Compiles statistics. **Frmly:** American Association of Colleges of

Chiropody; (1970) American Association of Colleges of Podiatry.

★ 353 ★ American Association for Community Dental Programs
3101 Burnet Ave.
Cincinnati, OH 45229-3014
Phone: (513)357-7380 **Fax:** (513)357-7385
Email: larry.hill@rcc.org
Lawrence F. Hill, DDS, MPH, Contact

Fnded: 1983. **Mem:** 200. **Desc:** Community dental programs. Provides or arranges for dental care for people with specific needs, eq. financial hardships, disabilities, and medical complications. **Pub:** *AACDP Newsletter.* Newsletter.

★ 354 ★ American Association of Community Psychiatrists (AACP)
c/o Frances M. Roton
PO Box 570218
Dallas, TX 75228-0218
Phone: (972)686-5227 **Fax:** (972)613-5532
Email: frda1@airmail.net
Website: http://www.communitypsychiatry.org/
Jacqueline M. Feldman, MD, Pres.

Fnded: 1984. **Mem:** 350. **Reg. Groups:** 7. **Desc:** Psychiatrists and psychiatry residents practicing in community mental health centers (CMHCs) or similar programs that provide care to populations of the mentally ill regardless of their ability to pay. Works to address issues faced by psychiatrists who practice within CMHCs, with the goal of ensuring quality patient care. Purposes are to: increase the number of psychiatrists who choose careers in community mental health; clarify and solve mutual problems regarding community mental health psychiatric practice; inform and educate the public about the community psychiatrist's role in treating the mentally ill; encourage research and training in psychiatry in the community mental health setting; establish liaison with similar professional associations and foster local and regional groups interested in public community psychiatry. Works to deal with issues such as professional burnout, the function of the psychiatrist within CMHCs, assuring relevant continuing medical education, and improving care in CMHCs. Proposes and promotes standards and guidelines of psychiatric practice and staffing in CMHCs; fosters a multidisciplinary approach to CMHC psychiatric care employing nurses, psychiatrists, psychologists, and social workers. Operates work groups in areas such as residency and fellowship training, standards of care, psychiatric leadership in community settings, and CMHCs and the homeless. Disseminates information on legislative activities, local and regional programs, treatment methods, and other matters relating to community psychiatry. **Pub:** *AACP Membership Directory*, annual. Membership Directory. • *Community Psychiatrist*, quarterly. Newsletter.

★ 355 ★ American Association for Continuity of Care (AACC)
PO Box 532
Dunedin, FL 34697-0532
Fax: (727)738-8099
Email: phudsonsommers@ij.net
Pat Hudson-Sommers, Pres.

Fnded: 1982. **Mem:** 500. **Reg. Groups:** 6. **Desc:** Health care professionals involved in discharge planning, social work, hospital administration, home care, long-term care, home health agencies, and continuity of care. Studies and researches issues; proposes and supports legislation concerning Medicare changes and home health care. Maintains speakers' bureau. **Pub:** *ACCESS*, bimonthly. Newsletter. Includes calendar of events, regional reports, member notes, and committee reports. *Price:* Included in membership dues. • *American Association for Continuity of Care–Membership Directory*, annual. Membership Directory. *Price:* Included in membership dues.

★ 356 ★ American Association of Critical-Care Nurses (AACN)
101 Columbia
Aliso Viejo, CA 92656-4109
Phone: (949)362-2000 **Free:** 800-899-AACN
Fax: (949)362-2020
Email: info@aacn.org
Website: http://www.aacn.org
Connie Barden, RN, Pres.

Fnded: 1969. **Mem:** 65,000. **Local Groups:** 275. **Desc:** Professional critical care nurses. Established to provide continuing education programs for nurses specializing in critical care and to develop standards of nursing care of critically ill patients. Conducts educational programs. Offers certification program for critical care nurses through AACN Certification Corporation. Seeks liaison with other professional nursing organizations and related health agencies. **Pub:** *AACN Clinical Issues*, quarterly. Journal. Contains peer-reviewed articles on clinically relevant topics. *Price:* $49.30/year for members; $58/year for nonmembers; $90/year for institutions. • *American Journal of Critical Care*, bimonthly. Journal. Covers original research in critical care. Contains directory of educational programs. *Price:* Included in membership dues; $45/year for nonmembers; $110 for institutions. • *Core Curriculum for Critical-Care Nursing.* • *Critical Care Nurse*, bimonthly. Clinical, peer-reviewed magazine focusing on critical care clinical practice. Contains listing of educational programs. *Price:* Included in membership dues; $27/year for nonmembers; $45/year for institutions. **Frmly:** (1970) American Association of Cardiovascular Nurses.

★ 357 ★ American Association of the Deaf-Blind (AADB)
814 Thayer Ave., Ste. 302
Silver Spring, MD 20910-4500
Fax: (301)495-4404
Email: info@aadb.org
Website: http://www.tr.wou.edu/dblink/aadb.htm
Jamie McNamara, Exec. Dir.

Fnded: 1937. **Mem:** 600. **Desc:** Deaf-blind persons and individuals directly concerned with their well-being, including spouses, children, friends, and health care professionals. Seeks to encourage independent living for deaf-blind individuals. Provides basic services to members, such as print-to-braille or braille-to-print transcription of personal papers, shopping services, loan of braille books and other necessitites. **Pub:** *Deaf-Blind American*, quarterly. Magazine. In large print and braille. *Price:* $15. **Frmly:** (1937) American League for Deaf-Blind.

★ 358 ★ American Association of Dental Examiners (AADE)
211 E Chicago Ave., Ste. 760
Chicago, IL 60611
Phone: (312)440-7464 **Fax:** (312)440-3525
Email: info@aadexam.org
Website: http://www.aadexam.org
Molly Nadler, Exec. Dir.

Fnded: 1883. **Mem:** 850. **Desc:** Present and past members of state dental examining boards and board administrators. To assist member agencies with problems related to state dental board examinations and licensure, and enforcement of the state dental practice act. Conducts research; compiles statistics. **Pub:** *American Association of Dental Examiners Bulletin*, quarterly, 3-4/year. Newsletter. *Price:* Available to members and related organizations. • Proceedings, annual. **Frmly:** National Association of Dental Examiners.

★ 359 ★ American Association for Dental Research (AADR)
1619 Duke St.
Alexandria, VA 22314-3406
Phone: (703)548-0066 **Fax:** (703)548-1883
Email: research@iadr.org
Website: http://www.iadr.com/IADR_AADR/About/AADR/default.htm
Robert Collins, DDS, Interim Exec. Dir.

Fnded: 1972. **Mem:** 4,500. **Reg. Groups:** 40. **Desc:** A division of the International Association for Dental Research. Dentists, researchers, dental schools, and dental products manufacturing companies. Seeks to promote better dental health and research activities. Presents current research information at annual meeting. Sponsors competitions; sponsors seminars. **Pub:** *Advances in Dental Research*, periodic. • *Journal of Dental Research*, monthly, 16/year. Journal. Provides information on all sciences relevant to dentistry and to the oral cavity and associated structures in health and disease. *Price:* $70/year for members; $25/year for student members; $390 institutions.

★ 360 ★ American Association of Diabetes Educators (AADE)
100 W Monroe, Ste. 400
Chicago, IL 60603-1901
Phone: (312)424-2426 **Free:** 800-338-3633
Fax: (312)424-2427
Email: aade@aadenet.org
Website: http://www.aadenet.org
Chris Laxton, Exec. Dir.

Fnded: 1973. **Mem:** 10,000. **Local Groups:** 105. **Desc:** Nurses, dietitians, social workers, physicians, pharmacists, podiatrists, and others involved in teaching diabetes self-management to diabetics. Purposes are: to provide educational opportunities for the professional growth and development of members; to promote the development of quality diabetes education for the diabetic consumer; to foster communication and cooperation among individuals and organizations involved in diabetes patient education. Offers continuing education programs for diabetes educators. **Pub:** *AADE FYI*, quarterly. Newsletter. Includes calendar of events, and articles on diabetes education and practice. *Price:* Included in membership dues. • *AADE Member Resource Guide*, annual. Membership Directory. • *Core Curriculum for Diabetes Education.* • *The Diabetes Educator*, bimonthly. Journal. Contains original articles from all disciplines regarding diabetes and diabetes patient education. Includes advertisers index and book reviews. *Price:* Included in membership dues; $45/year for nonmembers. • Also publishes position statements and various guidelines for diabetes education.

★ 361 ★ American Association of Directors of Psychiatric Residency Training (AADPRT)
Executive Office
University of Connecticut Health Center
Department of Psychiatry
263 Farmington Ave., LG066
Farmington, CT 06030-1935
Phone: (860)679-8112 **Fax:** (860)679-1246
Email: aadprt@psychiatry.uchc.edu
Website: http://www.aadprt.org
David Goldberg, MD, Exec. Dir.

Fnded: 1973. **Mem:** 428. **Desc:** Creates, Reviews and maintains standards for Psychiatric residency training programs **Pub:** *Academic Psychiatry*, quarterly. • Newsletter, quarterly.

★ 362 ★ American Association of Drugless Practitioners (AADP)
708 Madalaine Dr.
Gilmer, TX 75644
Phone: (903)843-6401 **Free:** 888-764-AADP
Email: join@aadp.net
Website: http://www.aadp.net
Donald A. Rosenthal, PhD, Dir.

Fnded: 1990. **Mem:** 1,000. **Desc:** Health care professionals including physicians, chiropractors, nurses, and herbalists. Promotes drugless health care and the professional advancement of members. Serves as a clearinghouse on drugless health care; sponsors educational and training programs for health care professionals interested in drugless practice. Conducts examinations and bestows certification upon qualified drugless practitioners.

★ 363 ★ American Association of Electrodiagnostic Medicine (AAEM)
421 1st Ave., SW, Ste. 300 East
Rochester, MN 55902
Phone: (507)288-0100 **Fax:** (507)288-1225
Email: aaem@aaem.net
Website: http://www.aaem.net
Shirlyn A. Adkins, J.D., Exec. Dir.

Fnded: 1953. **Mem:** 4,414. **Desc:** M.D.'s and D.O.'s or equivalent foreign degrees who practice or are interested in electrodiagnostic medicine. Objective is to increase and extend knowledge of electromyography and electrodiagnostic medicine, and to improve patient care. **Pub:** *AAEM Case Reports*, periodic. Monograph. *Price:* $8 for members; $10 for nonmembers. • *AAEM Minimonographs*, 2-3/year. Monograph. *Price:* $10 for members; $15 for nonmembers. • *American Association of Electrodiagnostic Medicine–Membership Directory*, annual. Membership Directory. *Price:* Included in membership dues; $50 for nonmembers. • *Guidelines*, periodic. *Price:* $75 for members; $150 for nonmembers; $10 each, for individual chapters to members; $20 each, for individual chapters to nonmembers. • *Muscle & Nerve*, monthly. *Price:* Included in fellow/associate membership. • Also publishes course syllabi. **Frmly:** (1990) American Association of Electromyography and Electrodiagnosis.

★ 364 ★ American Association of Endodontists (AAE)
211 E Chicago Ave., Ste. 1100
Chicago, IL 60611-2691
Phone: (312)266-7255 **Free:** 800-872-3636
Fax: (312)266-9867
Email: info@aae.org
Website: http://www.aae.org
James M. Drinan, Exec. Dir.

Fnded: 1943. **Mem:** 5,800. **Desc:** Endodontic specialists and other interested professionals. (Endodontics is a branch of dentistry that deals with the soft tissues inside the tooth.) Seeks to promote the exchange of ideas, to stimulate research, and to encourage the highest standard of quality care in the practice of endodontics. **Pub:** *Appropriateness of Care and Quality Assurance Guidelines.* • *Communique*, quarterly. Newsletter. • *Endodontics: Collegues for Excellence*, semiannual. Newsletter. • *Glossary: Contemporary Terminology for Endodontics.* • *Journal of Endodontics*, monthly. Journal. • *Membership Roster*, annual. • *Tooth Pain Guide.* Brochure. • *Your Guide to Cracked Teeth.* Brochure. • *Your Guide to Endodontic Retreatment.* Brochure. • *Your Guide to Endodontic Surgery.* Brochure. • *Your Guide to Endodontic Treatment.* Brochure. • *Your Guide to Traumatic Dental Injuries.* Brochure. • Brochure. • Brochure.

★ 365 ★ American Association of Equine Practitioners (AAEP)
4075 Iron Works Parkway
Lexington, KY 40511
Phone: (859)233-0147 **Free:** 800-443-0177
Fax: (859)233-1968
Email: aaepoffice@aaep.org
Website: http://www.aaep.org
David L. Foley, Exec. Dir.

Fnded: 1954. **Mem:** 6,500. **Desc:** Veterinarians who specialize in equine medicine and surgery. Disseminates the latest scientific information relative to the practice of equine medicine; promotes research on horses. Maintains 10 professional committees. **Pub:** *AAEP Report*, monthly. Newsletter. • *Annual Convention Proceedings*, annual. Proceedings. *Price:* $37 for members; $74 for nonmembers. • Directory, annual.

★ 366 ★ American Association of Eye and Ear Hospitals (AAEEH)
1100 Wilson Blvd. Ste. 1200
Arlington, VA 22209
Phone: (703)243-8848 **Fax:** (703)243-8664
Email: rbetz@aaeeh.org
Website: http://www.aaeeh.org
Robert Betz, PhD, Exec. Dir.

Fnded: 1983. **Mem:** 13. **Desc:** Chief executive officers and administrators of eye and ear specialty hospitals. Seeks to advance, at the federal level, fair economic treatment for eye and ear specialty hospitals; to share business functions such as purchasing, planning, and information and data collection. Compiles statistics. **Pub:** *Washington Eyeline*, monthly. Newsletter.

★ 367 ★ American Association of Feline Practitioners (AAFP)
200 4th Ave. N, No. 900
Nashville, TN 37219
Phone: (615)257-7788 **Free:** 800-204-3514
Fax: (615)254-7047
Email: aafp@walkermgmt.com
Website: http://www.aafponline.org
Dr. Joanna Guglielmino, Pres.

Fnded: 1970. **Mem:** 1,400. **Desc:** Doctors of veterinary medicine who specialize or have a general interest in the field of feline medicine and surgery. Works to promote the interests and improve the public stature of feline practice and to increase the knowledge of veterinarians in the field. Cooperates with other veterinary and cat fancier organizations. **Pub:** Newsletter, semiannual.

★ 368 ★ American Association for Functional Orthodontics (AAFO)
106 S Kent St.
Winchester, VA 22601
Phone: (540)662-2200 **Free:** 800-441-3850
Fax: (540)665-8910
Email: info@aafo.org
Website: http://www.aafo.org
Dr. Craig C. Stoner, Co-Founder

★ 369 ★ American Association for Geriatric Psychiatry (AAGP)
7910 Woodmont Ave., Ste. 1050
Bethesda, MD 20814-3004
Phone: (301)654-7850 **Fax:** (301)654-4137
Email: main@aagpgpa.org
Website: http://www.aagpgpa.org
David Greenspan, MD, Sec.

Fnded: 1978. **Mem:** 1,468. **Desc:** Psychiatrists interested in promoting better mental health care for the elderly. Maintains placement service and speakers' bureau. **Pub:** *AAGP Membership Directory*, annual. Membership Directory. • *American Journal of Geriatric Psychiatry*, quarterly. Journal. • *Geriatric Psychiatry News*, bimonthly. Newsletter. Provides brief articles on psychiatric topics and case reports pertaining to elderly patients; includes association news, and employment listings. • *Growing Older and Wiser.* Covers consumer and general public information. *Price:* 14.

★ 370 ★ American Association of Gynecological Laparoscopists (AAGL)
13021 E Florence Ave.
Santa Fe Springs, CA 90670-4505
Phone: (562)946-8774 **Free:** 800-554-2245
Fax: (562)946-0073
Email: generalmail@aagl.com
Website: http://www.aagl.com
Linda Michels, Exec. Dir.

Fnded: 1972. **Mem:** 7,200. **Desc:** Physicians who specialize in obstetrics and gynecology and who are interested in gynecological endoscopic procedures. Purposes are to: teach; demonstrate; exchange ideas; distribute literature; stimulate interest in gynecological laparoscopy; maintain and improve medical standards in medical schools and hospitals regarding gynecological laparoscopy; maintain and improve the ethics, practice, and efficiency of the medical practice pertaining to obstetrics and laparoscopy. Conducts seminars and workshops. **Pub:** *Endoscopic Female Sterilization.* Book. Covers methods, complications, legal implications, and comparisions of endoscopic female tubal stevailization. *Price:* $35. • *Endoscopy in Gynecology.* Book. *Price:* $45. • *Hysteroscopy: Principles and Practice.* Book. Covers many aspects of hysteroscopy. *Price:* $50. • *Manual of Endoscopy.* Book. *Price:* $90. • *Microsurgery in Gynecology.* Book. Contains proceedings from the AAGL First Seminar in Laparoscopy and Tubal Reconstsruction by Microsurgery. *Price:* $35. • *Microsurgery in Gynecology II.* Book. *Price:* $45.

★ 371 ★ American Association for Hand Surgery (AAHS)
20 N Michigan Ave., Ste. 700
Chicago, IL 60602
Phone: (312)236-3307 **Fax:** (312)782-0553
Email: contact@handsurgery.org
Website: http://www.handsurgery.org
Laura Downes Leeper, CAE, Asst. VP

Fnded: 1970. **Mem:** 1,081. **Desc:** Plastic, orthopedic, general surgeons, and physical and occupational therapists having a specific interest in hand surgery; individuals in the medical profession, basic sciences, or allied services interested in the improvement of hand surgery. Purpose is to advance hand surgery. Conducts symposia; offers specialized education. **Pub:** *Annual Program.* • *Hand Surgery Newsletter*, quarterly. Newsletter. *Price:* Included in membership dues.

★ 372 ★ American Association of Healthcare Consultants (AAHC)
5 Revere Dr., Ste. 200
Northbrook, IL 60062
Phone: (847)657-6964 **Free:** 888-350-2242
Fax: (847)350-2241
Email: info@aahc.net
Website: http://www.aahc.net
Jim Morell, FAAHC, Chm.

Fnded: 1949. **Mem:** 200. **Desc:** Professional association of individuals (185) and firms (50) exclusively devoted to health care consultation. Serves as a resource for health care providers; offers continuing education to members. Provides information concerning the role of health consulting. **Pub:** Membership Directory, annual. **Frmly:** (1984) American Association of Hospital Consultants.

★ 373 ★ American Association for Health Education (AAHE)
1900 Association Dr.
Reston, VA 20191
Phone: (703)476-3437 **Free:** 800-213-7193
Fax: (703)476-6638
Email: aahe@aahperd.org
Website: http://www.aahperd.org/aahe
Becky J. Smith, PhD, Exec. Dir.

Fnded: 1937. **Mem:** 7,500. **Desc:** Professionals who have responsibility for health education in schools, colleges, communities, hospitals and clinics, and industries. Purposes are advancement of health education through program activities and federal legislation; encouragement of close working relationships between all health education and health service organizations; achievement of good health and well-being for all Americans automatically, without conscious thought and endeavor. Member of the American Alliance for Health, Physical Education, Recreation and Dance. **Pub:** *Directory of Institutions Offering Undergraduate and Graduate Degree Programs in Health Education*, biennial. Directory. Features appearence in the Journal of Health Education. • *HE-XTRA*, 5/year. Reports on health education programs across the nation. Includes association news and research updates. *Price:* Included in membership dues. • *Journal of Health Education*, bimonthly. Journal. • Books. • Handbooks. • Reports. • Videos. • Also publishes guides and educational packets, and produces microcomputer software. **Frmly:** (1974) School Health Division of American Association for Health, Physical Education and Recreation; (1997) Association for the Advancement of Health Education.

★ 374 ★ American Association for Health Freedom

PO Box 458
Great Falls, VA 22066
Phone: (703)759-0662 **Free:** 800-230-2762
Fax: (703)759-6711
Email: aahf@healthfreedom.net
Website: http://www.healthfreedom.net
Candace Campbell, Exec. Dir.

Fnded: 1992. **Mem:** 500. **Desc:** Non-profit advocacy organization dedicated to promoting health care freedom and to protecting practitioners offering complementary and alternative therapies. **Pub:** *Directors Report*, monthly. Newsletter. *Price:* Free to members. **Frmly:** (2002) American Preventive Medical Association.

★ 375 ★ American Association of Health Plans (AAHP)

1129 20th St. NW, Ste. 600
Washington, DC 20036-3421
Phone: (202)778-3200 **Fax:** (202)331-7487
Email: aahp@aahp.org
Website: http://www.aahp.org
Karen Ignagni, Pres.

Fnded: 1959. **Mem:** 1,000. **Desc:** Supports the managed health care industry. Lobbies; conducts research programs and workshops; Maintains placement service. **Pub:** *healthplan*, bimonthly. Magazine. *Price:* $75/year.

★ 376 ★ American Association of Healthcare Administrative Management (AAHAM)

11240 Waples Mill Rd., Ste. 200
Fairfax, VA 22030
Phone: (703)281-4043 **Fax:** (703)359-7562
Email: debra@statmarketing.com
Website: http://www.aaham.org
Sharon Rosenblatt Galler, Exec. Dir.

Fnded: 1968. **Mem:** 2,600. **State Groups:** 39. **Desc:** Business offices, credit and collection managers, and admitting officers for hospitals, clinics, and other health care organizations. To educate members, exchange information and techniques, and keep members abreast of new regulations relating to their field. Seeks proper recognition for the financial aspect of hospital and clinic management. Offers certification program. Administers examinations in April and October for qualification as Certified Patient Account Manager (CPAM) and Certified Clinic Account Manager (CCAM). Maintains placement services; sponsors seminars and workshops on a local, regional, and national level. Operates speakers' bureau. **Pub:** *Journal of Healthcare Administrative Management*, quarterly. Journal. Lists employment opportunities; includes industry news. *Price:* Included in membership dues; $30/year for nonmembers. **Frmly:** (1981) American Guild of Patient Account Managers; (1999) American Guild of Patient Account Management.

★ 377 ★ American Association of Hip and Knee Surgeons (AAHKS)

704 Florence Dr.
Park Ridge, IL 60068-2104
Phone: (847)698-1200 **Fax:** (847)825-9294
Email: helpdesk@aahks.org
Website: http://www.aahks.org
Priscilla Majewski, Exec. Dir.

Fnded: 1991. **Mem:** 814. **Nat'l Groups:** 1. **Desc:** Provides current educational, research and communication opportunities to promote quality management of arthritic disorders of the hip and knee. **Pub:** Newsletter, quarterly. Contains association information for members. *Price:* included in membership dues.

★ 378 ★ American Association of Homes and Services for the Aging (AAHSA)

2519 Connecticut Ave. NW
Washington, DC 20008-1520
Phone: (202)783-2242 **Fax:** (202)783-2255
Email: info@aahsa.org
Website: http://www.aahsa.org
Bruce Rosenthal, Dir. Media Relations

Fnded: 1961. **Mem:** 5,600. **Reg. Groups:** 3. **State Groups:** 40. **Desc:** Committed to advancing the vision of healthy, affordable, ethical aging services for America. Represents 5,600 mission-driven, not-for-profit nursing homes, continuing care retirement communities, assisted living and senior housing facilities, and community service organizations. Serves its members through interaction with Congress and Federal agencies. Strives to enhance the professionalism of practitioners and facilities through the certification program for retirement housing professionals, the Continuing Care Accreditation Commission, conferences and programs, and publications representing current thinking in the long-term care and retirement housing fields. Seeks to enhance its members' financial strength through group purchasing and the AAHSA Development Council. **Pub:** *American Association of Homes and Services for the Aging Publications Catalog*, 2/year. Catalog. • *Best Practices*, bimonthly. Magazine. • *Directory of Members*, annual. Membership Directory. • *Washington Report*, biweekly. Report. Provides legislative and regulatory highlights. *Price:* Included in membership dues. **Frmly:** American Association of Homes for the Aging.

★ 379 ★ American Association of Hospital Podiatrists (AAHP)

8508 18th Ave.
Brooklyn, NY 11214
Phone: (718)259-1822 **Fax:** (718)259-4002
Frank Rinaldi, Exec. Dir.

Fnded: 1950. **Mem:** 800. **Desc:** A general specialty group of the American Podiatric Medical Association (see separate entry). Podiatrists (trained and certified persons dealing in the care and diseases of the foot) who are affiliated with hospitals. Seeks to: elevate the standards of podiatry practices in hospitals and health institutions; standardize hospital podiatry procedures, charting, recording forms, and methods; promote understanding among personnel in podiatry, medicine, and allied health professions; aid podiatrists in attaining institutional affiliations; assist in the educational and teaching programs of health institutions and hospitals; foster the development of podiatric internships and residencies in hospitals and institutions. Compiles statistics. **Pub:** *The Hospital Podiatrist*, annual. • Newsletter, annual.

★ 380 ★ American Association of Immunologists (AAI)

9650 Rockville Pike
Bethesda, MD 20814-3994
Phone: (301)530-7178 **Fax:** (301)571-1816
Email: infoaai@aai.faseb.org
Website: http://mercury.faseb.org/aai/default.asp
M. Michele Hogan, PhD, Contact

Fnded: 1913. **Mem:** 5,500. **Desc:** Scientists engaged in immunological research including aspects of virology, bacteriology, biochemistry, genetics, and related disciplines. Goals are to advance knowledge of immunology and related disciplines and to facilitate the interchange of information among investigators in various fields. Promotes interaction between laboratory investigators and clinicians. Conducts training courses, symposia, workshop, and lectures. Compiles statistics. **Pub:** *AAI Newsletter*, bimonthly. Newsletter. *Price:* included in membership dues. • *Journal of Immunology*, semimonthly. Journal. Reports on original research efforts on cellular immunology; clinical immunology and immunopathology; cytokines, mediators, and regulatory molecules. *Price:* Included in membership dues; $200 for nonmembers in USA.

★ 381 ★ American Association of Industrial Veterinarians (AAIV)

PO Box 488
Oskaloosa, KS 66066-0488
Phone: (785)863-2389 **Fax:** (785)863-3141
Email: aaiv@rualnet.com
Peggy Miller, Admin. Coord.

Fnded: 1954. **Mem:** 450. **Desc:** Veterinarians, many of whom are members of the American Veterinary Medical Association and are employed in a professional capacity in industrial activities, for example, with drug and chemical firms, in livestock and poultry enterprises, or in independent research. Holds workshops. **Pub:** *AAIV Highlights*, semiannual. Newsletter. Membership activities newsletter. Includes member biographical sketches. *Price:* Included in membership dues. • Directory, annual. **Frmly:** Industrial Veterinarians Association.

★ 382 ★ American Association of Integrated Healthcare Delivery Systems

4435 Waterfront Dr., Ste. 101
PO Box 4913
Glen Allen, VA 23058-4913
Phone: (804)747-5823 **Fax:** (804)747-5316
Email: sreed@aaihds.org
Website: http://www.aaihds.org
Sloane J. Reed, Chm.

Fnded: 1993. **Mem:** 1,000. **Desc:** Dedicated to the educational advancement of provider-based managed care professionals involved in integrated healthcare delivery. **Pub:** *Integrated Healthcare Delivery System*, quarterly. Newsletter. **Frmly:** (1998) American Association of Physician-Hospital Organizations.

★ 383 ★ American Association for International Aging (AAIA)

3800 N Fairfax Dr., Ste. 1001
Arlington, VA 22203
Phone: (703)525-9755
Ambassador John W. McDonald, Pres.

Fnded: 1983. **Desc:** Advocates for the aged; organizations, corporations, foundations, and individuals concerned about the interests and needs of the aged worldwide, particularly in the Third World. Seeks to improve the socioeconomic conditions of older, low-income persons in developing countries through self-help, mutual support, and economic development activities. Sponsors international developmental education programs for retired Americans. Provides small grants assistance to economic-development projects for Third World aging; sponsors an information exchange program. **Pub:** *Aging and the Global Agenda for Women: Conversations in Nairobi.* • *American Association for International Aging Reports*, quarterly. Newsletter. Highlights activities benefiting aging persons worldwide. • *International Directory of Organizations in Aging.* Directory. • *Retired Americans Look at International Development.*

★ 384 ★ American Association of Kidney Patients (AAKP)

3505 E Frontage Rd., Ste. 315
Tampa, FL 33607
Phone: (813)636-8100 **Free:** 800-749-2257
Fax: (813)636-8122
Email: info@aakp.org
Website: http://www.aakp.org
Kris Robinson, Exec. Dir.

Fnded: 1969. **Mem:** 10,000. **Nat'l Groups:** 16. **Reg. Groups:** 16. **State Groups:** 16. **Local Groups:** 16. **Desc:** Works to improve the lives of fellow kidney patients and their families by helping them deal with the physical, emotional and social impact of kidney disease; provides educational and supportive programs and reading materials. **Pub:** *AAKPRENALIFE*, bimonthly. Magazine. Provides articles, news and healthcare information of interest to kidney patients. *Price:* included in membership dues. • *Americans with Disabilities Act of 1990.* Brochure. Explains the Americans with Disabilities Act. • *Blood Chemistry Levels.* Brochure. • *Dietary Counters.* Brochure. • *Kidney Beginnings*, quarterly. Magazine. Features information on the kidneys and common questions about chronic kidney disease. *Price:* included in membership dues. • Also publishes other informational materials including care of the kidneys, treatment options and conditions that may affect the kidneys. **Frmly:** National Association of Patients on Hemodialysis; National Association of Patients on Hemodialysis and Transplantation.

★ 385 ★ American Association for Klinefelter Syndrome Information and Support (AAKSIS)

2945 W Farwell Ave.
Chicago, IL 60645-2925
Phone: (773)761-5298 **Free:** 888-466-5747
Fax: (773)761-5298
Email: aaksis@aol.com
Website: http://www.aaksis.org
Roberta Rappaport, Founding Pres.

Fnded: 1999. **Mem:** 750. **Reg. Groups:** 11. **Desc:** Volunteers, those affected by the genetic chromosomal condition and parents of those affected. Provides support, information and resources. Promotes public awareness. **Pub:** *KaleidoScope*, 3/year. Newsletter. Contains information, support, resources, and articles of interest on XXY/Klinefelter Syndrome. *Price:* included in membership dues. **AKA:** AAKSIS.

★ 386 ★ American Association for Laboratory Animal Science (AALAS)

9190 Crestwyn Hills Dr.
Memphis, TN 38125
Phone: (901)754-8620 **Fax:** (901)753-0046
Email: info@aalas.org
Website: http://www.aalas.org
Ann Tourigny Turner, PhD, Exec. Dir.

Fnded: 1950. **Mem:** 12,000. **Reg. Groups:** 8. **Local Groups:** 48. **Desc:** Persons and institutions professionally concerned with the production, use, care, and study of laboratory animals. Serves as clearinghouse for collection and exchange of information on all phases of laboratory animal care and management and on the care, use, and procurement of laboratory animals used in biomedical research. Conducts examinations and certification through its Animal Technician Certification Program. **Pub:** *American Association for Laboratory Animal Science–Reference Directory*, annual. Membership Directory. Arranged alphabetically by name and geographically. *Price:* Included in membership dues. • *Comparative Medicine*, bimonthly. Journal. Covers comparative and experimental medicine related to laboratory animal science. *Price:* $150 subscription rate. • *Contemporary Topics in Laboratory Animal Science*, bimonthly. Contains refereed papers covering topics in laboratory animal science; covers association activities. *Price:* Included in membership dues. • Also publishes educational materials. **Frmly:** (1967) Animal Care Panel.

★ 387 ★ American Association of Legal Nurse Consultants (AALNC)

4700 W Lake Ave.
Glenview, IL 60025-1485
Phone: (312)644-6610 **Free:** 877-402-2562
Fax: 877-734-8668
Email: aalnc@sba.com
Website: http://www.aalnc.org/
Pat Iyer, Pres.

Fnded: 1989. **Mem:** 3,600. **State Groups:** 48. **Desc:** Promotes the professional advancement of registered nurses consulting with the legal arena by providing a forum for education and exchange of information. Conducts annual educational program. **Pub:** *The Journal of Legal Nurse Consulting*, quarterly. Journal. Includes educational and legislative updates, and networking information. *Price:* Free to members. • *Legal Nurse Consulting: Principles and Practice*. *Price:* $95 for members; $100 non-members.

★ 388 ★ American Association of Managed Care Nurses (AAMCN)

4435 Waterfront Dr., Ste. 101
Glen Allen, VA 23060
Phone: (804)747-9698 **Fax:** (804)747-5316
Email: bwilliams@aamcn.org
Website: http://www.aamcn.org
W.C. (Bill) Williams, II, Sr. VP

Fnded: 1994. **Mem:** 2,500. **Desc:** Managed health care professionals, including registered nurses, licensed practical nurses, and nurse practitioners. Seeks to enhance the abilities of members to meet the future needs of the managed health care profession through education. Provides a home study program as a pre-requisite for the Certified Managed Care Nurse (CMCN) exam. **Pub:** *Nurses' Notes*, quarterly. Newsletter. *Price:* Included in membership dues.

★ 389 ★ American Association for Marriage and Family Therapy (AAMFT)

112 S Alfred St.
Alexandria, VA 22314
Phone: (703)838-9808 **Fax:** (703)838-9805
Email: exec@aamft.org
Website: http://www.aamft.org
Mary Hotvedt, PhD, Pres.

Fnded: 1942. **Mem:** 23,000. **Reg. Groups:** 53. **Desc:** Professional society of marriage and family therapists. Assumes a major role in developing & maintaining the highest standards of excellence in this field. Has 76 accredited training programs throughout the U.S. Sponsors educational and research programs. **Pub:** *Family Therapy Glossary*. Includes an overview of family therapy terms aimed at new MFTs. *Price:* $8.95. • *Family Therapy News*, bimonthly. Includes research news, interviews, reports on legislative and organization acivities, and activities calendar. *Price:* Included in membership dues; $25/year for nonmembers; $40/year for institutions. • *Journal of Marital and Family Therapy*, quarterly. Journal. Also includes articles on clinical practice, research, theory, and training. Includes book reviews. *Price:* Included in membership dues; $45/year for nonmembers; $75/year for institutions. • Also publishes other brochures and books; produces series of professional training videos. **Frmly:** (1970) American Association of Marriage Counselors; (1978) American Association of Marriage and Family Counselors.

★ 390 ★ American Association of Medical Assistants (AAMA)

20 N Wacker Dr., Ste. 1575
Chicago, IL 60606-2963
Phone: (312)899-1500 **Free:** 800-228-2262
Fax: (312)899-1259
Website: http://www.aama-ntl.org
Donald A. Balasa, Exec. Dir.

Fnded: 1956. **Mem:** 20,000. **State Groups:** 46. **Desc:** Medical assistants are allied health professionals who work primarily in anbilatory (out patient) settings and perform clinical and administrative procedures. Activities include a certification program consisting of study and an examination, passage of which entitles the individual to become credentialed as a Certified Medical Assistant. Conducts accreditation of one- and two-year programs in medical assisting in conjunction with the commission on Accreditation of Allied Health Education Programs. Provides assistance and information to institutions of higher learning desirous of initiating courses for medical assistants. Awards continuing education units for selected educational programs. **Pub:** *Accounts Receivable and Collection for the Medical Practice. Price:* $20 for members; $30 for nonmembers. • *AIDS Concepts for Medical Assistnts – Part I. Price:* $15 for member; $25 for nonmember. • *Human Relations for the Medical Office. Price:* $30 for member; $50 for nonmember. • *Law for the Medical Office. Price:* $30 for member; $50 for nonmember. • *Managing Managed Care. Price:* $15 for member; $25 for nonmember. • *Medical Office Management – Part I. Price:* $22 for member; $32 for nonmember. • *PMA*, bimonthly. Journal. Includes association news, index of advertisers, continuing education articles, and calendar of events. *Price:* Included in membership dues; $30/year for nonmembers and students. • *Urinalysis Today. Price:* $30 for member; $50 for nonmember. • Brochures. • Pamphlets.

★ 391 ★ American Association of Medical Milk Commissions (AAMMC)

c/o Paul Fleiss, M.D.
1824 N Hillhurst Ave.
Los Angeles, CA 90027
Phone: (323)664-1977 **Fax:** (323)664-0870
Email: fleiss@hsc.usc.edu
Paul Fleiss, MD, Pres.

Fnded: 1907. **Mem:** 35. **Desc:** Professional society of physician members of local Medical Milk Commissions, including veterinarians, sanitarians, and bacteriologists who supervise production of certified milk (milk from dairies conforming to official standards of sanitation). **Pub:** *Methods and Standards for the Production of Certified Milk*, annual.

★ 392 ★ American Association of Medical Society Executives (AAMSE)

611 East Wells St.
Milwaukee, WI 53202
Phone: (414)221-9275 **Fax:** (414)276-3349
Email: aamse@aamse.org
Website: http://www.aamse.org
Irene Sjostedt, Exec. Dir.

Fnded: 1947. **Mem:** 1,200. **Desc:** Professional society of executives of national, state, regional, or county medical and specialty societies. Conducts continuing education seminars. Makes available management resources and operational evaluations. **Pub:** *Hotline*, monthly. • *Who's Who in Medical Society Management*, annual. **Frmly:** Medical Society Executives Association.

★ 393 ★ American Association for Medical Transcription (AAMT)

100 Sycamore Ave.
Modesto, CA 95354-0550
Phone: (209)527-9620 **Free:** 800-982-2182
Fax: (209)527-9633
Email: aamt@aamt.org
Website: http://www.aamt.org
Kimberly Andosca, CEO

Fnded: 1978. **Mem:** 7,000. **State Groups:** 26. **Local Groups:** 86. **Desc:** Medical transcriptionists, their supervisors, teachers and students of medical transcription, owners and managers of medical transcription services, and other interested health personnel. Purpose is to provide information about the profession of medical transcription and to provide continuing education for medical transcriptionists. (Medical transcriptionists translate patients' records of medical care and treatment from oral dictation to printed form.) Advocates professional recognition of medical transcriptionists in county, state, and national medical societies and in health care facilities nationwide. Sponsors voluntary certification/credentialing program. Offers updates on developments in medicine and curricula, and on new transcription methods and equipment; sponsors and encourages research in the field. Establishes guidelines for education of medical transcriptionists. Fosters positive relations among medical transcriptionists, the public, members of allied health services, and the legislature. **Pub:** *The AAMT Book of Style for Medical Transcription, 2nd Ed.*. Book. *Price:* $79. • *AAMT Insights*, monthly. Newsletter. • *Journal of the American Association for Medical Transcription*, bimonthly. Journal. Offers guidance in quality assurance for medical transcription, medical and nonmedical educational articles, word lists, and technology updates. *Price:* Included in membership dues; $225/year for nonmembers; $40/issue. • *The Leading Edge*, monthly. Newsletter. • Also publishes medical transcription modules and medical transcription video programs.

★ 394 ★ American Association of Mental Health Professionals in Corrections (AAMHPC)

PO Box 160208
Sacramento, CA 95816-0208
Fax: (916)649-1080
Email: corrmentalhealth@aol.com
J.S. Zil, MD, JD, National Pres.

Fnded: 1940. **Mem:** 2,000. **Nat'l Groups:** 1. **Desc:** Psychiatrists, psychologists, social workers, nurses, and other mental health professionals; individuals working in correctional settings. Fosters the progress of behavioral sciences related to corrections. Goals are: to improve the treatment, rehabilitation, and care of the mentally ill, mentally retarded, and emotionally disturbed; to promote research and professional education in psychiatry and allied fields in corrections; to advance standards of correctional services and facilities; to foster cooperation between individuals concerned with the medical, psychological, social, and legal aspects of corrections; to share knowledge with other medical practitioners, scientists, and the public. Conducts scientific meetings to contribute to the advancement of the therapeutic community in all its institutional settings, including correctional institutions, hospitals, churches, schools, industry, and the family. **Pub:** *Corrective and Social Psychiatry*, quarterly. Journal. Includes book reviews, calendar of events, and research reports. *Price:* Included in membership dues; $35/year for nonmembers. • Papers. **Frmly:** (1978) Medical Correctional Society of the American Correctional Association.

★ 395 ★ American Association on Mental Retardation (AAMR)

444 N Capitol St. NW, Ste. 846
Washington, DC 20001-1512
Phone: (202)387-1968 **Free:** 800-424-3688
Fax: (202)387-2193
Email: dcroser@aamr.org
Website: http://www.aamr.org
Ms. M. Doreen Croser, Exec. Dir.

Fnded: 1876. **Mem:** 9,500. **Reg. Groups:** 9. **State Groups:** 40. **Desc:** Physicians, educators, administrators, social workers, psychologists, psychiatrists, students, and others interested in the general welfare of persons with mental retardation and the study of the cause, treatment, and prevention of mental retardation. Maintains 17 divisions and subdivisions. **Pub:** *American Journal of Mental Retardation*, bimonthly. Journal. Research in the Biological Sciences. *Price:* $175. • *Innovations: A Research to Practice Series*, 3/year. • *Mental Retardation*, bimonthly. Journal. Contains a journal of policy, practices, and perspectives. *Price:* 149. • *Mental Retardation: Definition, Classification, and Systems of Supports*. Manual. Contains terminology and classification in mental retardation. • *News and Notes*, bimonthly. • Monograph. • Also publishes testing materials. **Frmly:** (1906) Association of Medical Officers of American Institutions of Idiotic and Feebleminded Children; (1933) American Association for the Study of the Feebleminded; (1987) American Association on Mental Deficiency.

★ 396 ★ American Association of Naturopathic Physicians (AANP)

3201 New Mexico Ave., NW Ste. 350
Washington, DC 20016
Phone: (202)895-1392 **Free:** (866)538-2267
Fax: (202)274-1992
Email: member.services@naturopathic.org
Website: http://www.naturopathic.org
Michael Traub, Pres.

Fnded: 1986. **Mem:** 1,300. **State Groups:** 29. **Desc:** Naturopathic physicians. Unites naturopathic physicians and represents their legislative interests; promotes high educational standards and uniform criteria for licensing; increases public awareness of naturopathic medicine. **Pub:** *AANP Quarterly Newsletter*, quarterly. Newsletter. *Price:* Included in membership fee. • *Journal of Naturopathic Medicine*. Journal.

★ 397 ★ American Association of Neurological Surgeons (AANS)

5550 Meadowbrook Dr.
Rolling Meadows, IL 60008
Phone: (847)378-0500 **Free:** 888-566-2267
Fax: (847)378-0600
Email: info@aans.org
Website: http://www.aans.org
Julian T. Hoff, MD, Chmn.

Fnded: 1931. **Mem:** 6,000. **State Groups:** 50. **Desc:** Neurological surgeons united to promote excellence in neurological surgery and its related sciences. Provides funding to foster research in the neurosciences. Conducts specialized education. The largest publisher of neurosurgical books in the world. **Pub:** *AANS Membership Directory of Neurological Surgery*, annual. Membership Directory. Electronic directory on CD-ROM. *Price:* $50 for members. • *American Association of Neurological Surgeons Bulletin*, quarterly. Magazine. *Price:* Included in membership dues. • *Journal of Neurosurgery*, monthly. Journal. *Price:* $100/year for members; $110/year for nonmembers; $60/year for residents. • *Journal of Neurosurgery: Spine*, bimonthly. Journal. • *Neurosurgical Focus*, bimonthly. Journal. Electronic journal. • *Neurosurgical Operative Atlas*. Booklets. • *Neurosurgical Topics*, quarterly. Books. *Price:* $85 for members; $95 for nonmembers; $75 for residents. • *Neurosurgical Topics Series*. Books. **Frmly:** (1966) Harvey Cushing Society.

★ 398 ★ American Association of Neuropathologists (AANP)

c/o J.E. Parisi, MD
Department Lab Med & Pathology
Mayo Clinic
200 First St. SW
Rochester, MN 55905
Phone: (507)284-3394 **Fax:** (507)284-1599
Email: aanp@mayo.edu
Website: http://www.aanp-jnen.com
Dr. Joseph Parisi, Sec. -Treas.

Fnded: 1959. **Mem:** 800. **Desc:** Promotes neuropathology, especially the study of diverse aspects of diseases of the nervous system including changes at tissue, cellular, subcellular, and molecular levels with consideration of etiology and pathophysiology, genetics, epidemiology and clinical manifestations of such diseases. **Pub:** *Journal of Neuropathology and Experimental Neurology*, monthly. Journal. • Membership Directory, annual. **Frmly:** (1932) Club of Neuropathologists.

★ 399 ★ American Association of Neuroscience Nurses (AANN)

4700 W Lake Ave.
Glenview, IL 60025
Phone: (847)375-4733 **Free:** 888-557-2266
Fax: 877-734-8677
Email: info@aann.org
Website: http://www.aann.org
Diane Simmons, RN,CAE, Exec. Dir.

Fnded: 1968. **Mem:** 4,000. **State Groups:** 50. **Desc:** Registered nurses engaged in or primarily interested in neurosurgical or neurological nursing. Objectives are to: foster interest, education, and high standards of practice in the field of neuroscience nursing; encourage continuing growth in the field; provide a medium for communication among neuroscience nurses in the U.S. and Canada. Has developed core curriculum for neuroscience nursing practice. **Pub:** *American Association of Neuroscience Nurses Synapse*, bimonthly. Newsletter. Includes calendar of events, continuing education course listings, employment listings, and information on new members and publications. *Price:* Included in membership dues. • *Core Curriculum for Neuroscience Nursing*. • *Journal of Neuroscience Nursing*, bimonthly. Journal. Includes book reviews, pharmacology update, and research reports. *Price:* Included in membership dues; $110/year for nonmembers; $135/year for institutions.

★ 400 ★ American Association of Nurse Anesthetists (AANA)

222 S Prospect Ave.
Park Ridge, IL 60068
Phone: (847)692-7050 **Fax:** (847)692-6968
Email: info@aana.com
Website: http://www.aana.com
Jeffery M. Beutler, Exec. Dir.

Fnded: 1931. **Mem:** 27,222. **State Groups:** 52. **Desc:** Active registered professional nurses who have successfully completed an accredited program in nurse anesthesia and passed a national examination for certification. Advances the art and science of anesthesiology; promotes research in anesthesia; develops educational standards and techniques for the administration of anesthesia. Sponsors continuing education; promotes biennial recertification. **Pub:** *AANA Journal*, bimonthly. Journal. Contains clinical, practical, theoretical, and research articles. Includes advertisers' index, and alphabetical inex by organization. *Price:* Included in membership dues; $24/year for nonmembers. • *AANA News Bulletin*, monthly. Bulletin. Contains legislative news, president's message, calendar of events, and employment listings. *Price:* Included in membership dues. • *American Association of Nurse Anesthestists List of Recognized Educational Programs*, semiannual. Arranged by state.

★ 401 ★ American Association of Nurse Attorneys (TAANA)

7794 Grow Dr.
Pensacola, FL 32514
Phone: (850)474-3646 **Free:** 877-532-2262
Fax: (850)484-8762
Email: taana@puetzamc.com
Website: http://www.taana.org
Belinda E. Puetz, RN,PhD, Exec. Dir.

Fnded: 1982. **Mem:** 400. **Local Groups:** 24. **Desc:** Nurse attorneys, nurses in law school, and attorneys in nursing school. Aims to better nurse attorneys and inform the public on matters of nursing, health care, and law. Goals are to facilitate communication and information sharing between professional groups; to establish an employment network; to assist new and potential nurse attorneys; to develop the profession; to promote the image of nurse attorneys as experts and consultants in nursing and law. Maintains educational foundation. **Pub:** *Demonstrating Financial Responsibility in Nursing Practice*. Brochure. Contains information for nurses considering the purchase of professional liability insurance. *Price:* $2. • *Inside TAANA*, 3/year. Newsletter. Contains reports from committees and chapters, legislative information, and member notes. *Price:* Included in membership dues. • *Journal of Nursing Law*, quarterly. Journal. • *Making the Transition: From Nursing to the Law*. • *Model Curriculum for Legal Content in Nursing Education*. • *On Becoming A Nurse Attorney*.

★ 402 ★ American Association of Nutritional Consultants (AANC)

400 Oak Hill Dr.
Winona Lake, IN 46590
Free: 888-828-2262 **Fax:** (219)269-4060
Email: registrar@aanc.net
Website: http://www.aanc.net
Wilma Johnson, Asst. Admin.

Fnded: 1980. **Mem:** 5,000. **Desc:** Professional nutritional consultants. Seeks to create a forum for exchange of nutritional information. Offers benefits such as car rental and laboratory discounts. **Pub:** *HealthKeepers Journal*, quarterly. Journal. Focuses on innovation in the field of professional nutritional counseling, and vitamin, mineral, and food therapies. Includes nutrition digest. *Price:* Available to members only. • Membership Directory.

★ 403 ★ American Association of Occupational Health Nurses (AAOHN)

2920 Brandy Wine Rd., Ste. 100
Atlanta, GA 30341
Phone: (770)455-7757 **Fax:** (770)455-7271
Email: aaohn@aaohn.org
Website: http://www.aaohn.org
Susan A. Randolph, VP

Fnded: 1942. **Mem:** 12,500. **Reg. Groups:** 1. **State Groups:** 34. **Local Groups:** 138. **Desc:** Registered professional nurses employed by business and industrial firms; nurse educators, nurse editors, nurse writers, and others interested in occupational health nursing. Promotes and sets standards for the profession. Provides and approves continuing education; maintains governmental affairs program; offers placement service. **Pub:** *AAOHN Core Curriculum Study Guide*. Includes guidelines of Occupational Health & Safety Services. • *AAOHN Journal*, monthly. Journal. • *AAOHN News*, monthly. Newsletter. • *SuccessTools: Strategies for Thriving & Surviving in Business*. Includes guidelines for Occupational Health & Safety Services. **Frmly:** (1977) American Association of Industrial Nurses.

★ 404 ★ American Association of Office Nurses (AAON)
109 Kinderkamack Rd.
Montvale, NJ 07645
Phone: (201)391-2600 **Free:** 800-457-7504
Fax: (201)573-8543
Email: aaonmail@aaon.org
Website: http://www.aaon.org
Michelle Aronowitz, Dir.

Fnded: 1988. **Mem:** 2,000. **Reg. Groups:** 21. **Desc:** Nurses working primarily in physicians' offices. Promotes improvement of the image of the office nurse. Encourages professional growth and development; facilitates exchange of information among members. Provides continuing education opportunities. Issues publications. **Pub:** *NEON*, quarterly. Newsletter. *Price:* included in membership dues.

★ 405 ★ American Association of Oral and Maxillofacial Surgeons (AAOMS)
9700 W Bryn Mawr Ave.
Rosemont, IL 60018-5701
Phone: (847)678-6200 **Free:** 800-822-6637
Fax: (847)678-6286
Email: inquiries@aaoms.org
Website: http://www.aaoms.org
Dr. Robert Rinaldi, Asst. Exec. Dir.

Fnded: 1918. **Mem:** 6,100. **Reg. Groups:** 9. **State Groups:** 53. **Desc:** Dentists specializing in disease diagnosis and surgical, adjunctive, and esthetic treatment of diseases, injuries, and defects of the oral and maxillofacial region (jaw deformities, dental implants, infections, and oral cancer). **Pub:** *AAOMS Digest*, bimonthly. Newsletter. Contains association news and events. • *AAOMS Directory*, annual. Directory. • *AAOMS Forum*, quarterly. • *Journal of Oral Maxillofacial Surgery*, monthly. Journal. • *Office Anesthesia Evaluation Manual*. Manual. • *Report of Annual Meeting*. Report. • *Surgical Update*, 3/year. • Annual Report. **Frmly:** (1944) American Society of Exodontists; (1977) American Society of Oral Surgeons.

★ 406 ★ American Association of Oriental Medicine (AAOM)
5530 Wisconsin Ave., Ste. 1210
Chevy Chase, MD 20815
Phone: (301)941-1063 **Free:** 888-500-7999
Fax: (301)986-9313
Email: info@aaom.org
Website: http://www.aaom.org
Andrew Avery, Exec. Dir.

Fnded: 1981. **Mem:** 2,600. **Reg. Groups:** 32. **State Groups:** 32. **Desc:** Professional acupuncturists and Oriental Medicine Practitioners. Seeks to: elevate the standards of education and practice of acupuncture and oriental medicine; establish laws governing acupuncture; provide a forum to share information on acupuncture techniques; increase public awareness of acupuncture; support research in the field. Conducts educational programs; compiles statistics. Operates speakers' bureau. **Pub:** *AAOM Membership Directory*, annual. Membership Directory. Contains listing of U.S. acupuncture and oriental medicine practitioners. *Price:* $12/copy. • *American Acupuncturist Newsletter*, semiannual. Newsletter. Contains political and educational news and information. • *American Acupuncturist Update*, quarterly. Newsletter. Contains political & educational news and info. **Frmly:** (1996) American Association for Acupuncture and Oriental Medicine.

★ 407 ★ American Association of Orthodontists (AAO)
401 N Lindbergh Blvd.
Saint Louis, MO 63141-7816
Phone: (314)993-1700 **Free:** 800-424-2841
Fax: (314)997-1745
Email: info@aaortho.org
Website: http://www.aaortho.org
Thomas Watters, Exec. Dir.

Fnded: 1901. **Mem:** 14,300. **Nat'l Groups:** 1. **Reg. Groups:** 8. **State Groups:** 54. **Desc:** Professional society of orthodontists. To advance the art and science of orthodontics through continuing education, encouragement of research and cooperation with other health groups. Maintains museum. **Pub:** *AAO Bulletin*, bimonthly. Newsletter. Includes meetings schedules. *Price:* Included in membership dues. • *American Association of Orthodontists Membership Directory*, biennial. Membership Directory. *Price:* $55 for members; $110 for nonmembers. • *American Journal of Orthodontics and Dentofacial Orthopedics*, monthly. Journal. *Price:* Included in membership dues. • Pamphlets. • Also publishes administration guide kits. **Frmly:** American Society of Orthodontists.

★ 408 ★ American Association of Orthopedic Medicine (AAOM)
30897 CR 356-3
PO Box 4997
Buena Vista, CO 81211-4997
Phone: (719)475-0032 **Free:** 800-992-2063
Fax: (719)395-5615
Email: aaom@aaomed.org
Website: http://www.aaomed.org
Jeff Peterson, DO, Contact

Fnded: 1982. **Mem:** 450. **Desc:** Physicians and allied health professionals interested in the advancement of knowledge, diagnosis, and nonsurgical treatment of musculoskeletal and related disorders. Seeks to: advance the standards of practice and quality of service in the field of orthopedic medicine; unite the common interests and skills of medicine and osteopathy; serve as a forum of learning for all of the specialties that deal with pain and dysfunction in the neural, muscular, skeletal, and vascular systems. Encourages research and the dissemination of results. Provides training and continuing medical education in orthopedic medicine; conducts regional seminars every two to three months. **Pub:** *AAOM Membership Directory*, annual. Membership Directory. • *AAOM News*, quarterly. • *The Journal of Orthopaedic Medicine*, 3/year. Journal. Contains scientific papers and articles, editorials, and book reviews. *Price:* Included in membership dues.

★ 409 ★ American Association of Pathologists' Assistants (AAPA)
Rosewood Office Plaza
1711 W County Rd. B, Ste. 300 N
Roseville, MN 55113-4036
Phone: (651)697-9264 **Free:** 800-532-AAPA
Fax: (651)635-0307
Email: oei@assocmgmt.org
Website: http://www.pathologistsassistants.org
Jon Wagner, Pres.

Fnded: 1972. **Mem:** 750. **Desc:** Pathologists' assistants and individuals qualified by academic and practical training to provide service in anatomic pathology under the direction of a qualified pathologist who is responsible for the performance of the assistant. Promotes the mutual association of trained pathologists' assistants and informs the public and the medical profession concerning the goals of this profession. Compiles statistics on salaries, geographic distribution, and duties of pathologists' assistants. Sponsors a continuing medical education program; offers a job hotline for members only. **Pub:** *AAPA Newsletter*, quarterly. Newsletter. Includes employment and educational opportunity listings. *Price:* Included in membership dues. • Membership Directory, biennial.

★ 410 ★ American Association for Pediatric Ophthalmology and Strabismus
PO Box 193832
San Francisco, CA 94119
Phone: (415)561-8505 **Fax:** (415)561-8531
Email: aapos@aao.org
Website: http://med-aapos.bu.edu/
Sue A. Brown, Admin.

Fnded: 1974. **Mem:** 844. **Desc:** Ophthalmologists who limit their practice largely to children. Encourages quality eye care for children by establishing high ethical standards of practice, supporting educational training programs for pediatric ophthalmologists, and promoting basic research in children's eye diseases. Conducts research programs. **Pub:** Journal, bimonthly. • Membership Directory, annual. **Frmly:** (1978) American Association of Pediatric Ophthalmology.

★ 411 ★ American Association of People with Disabilities (AAPD)
1819 H St. NW, Ste. 330
Washington, DC 20006
Phone: (202)457-0046 **Free:** 800-840-8844
Fax: (202)457-0473
Email: aapd@aol.com
Website: http://www.aapd-dc.org
Helena Berger, COO

Fnded: 1995. **Mem:** 28,000. **Nat'l Groups:** 1. **Desc:** Promotes economic and political empowerment of persons with disabilities; educating businesses and general public about disability issues. **Pub:** *AAPD News*, quarterly. Newsletter. Also available in Braille. *Price:* included in membership dues.

★ 412 ★ American Association of Pharmacy Technicians (AAPT)
PO Box 1447
Greensboro, NC 27402
Phone: (336)333-9356 **Free:** 877-368-4771
Fax: (336)333-9068
Email: felt@pulse.net
Website: http://www.pharmacytechnician.com/
Bobbie Craddock, Pres.

Desc: Pharmacy technicians. Promotes professional advancement of members. Represents members before health care and public organizations; conducts continuing professional development courses; publicizes the role of the pharmacy technician as an "integral part of the patient care team."

★ 413 ★ American Association of Physician Specialists (AAPS)
2296 Henderson Mill Rd., Ste. 206
Atlanta, GA 30345
Phone: (770)939-8555 **Free:** 800-447-9397
Fax: (770)939-8559
Email: wcarbone@aapsga.org
Website: http://www.aapsga.org
William J. Carbone, Exec. Dir.

Fnded: 1952. **Mem:** 2,500. **Desc:** Represents twelve major specialties and twelve sub-specialties of medicine. Accepts qualified physicians into membership with either an allopathic (M.D.) or osteopathic (D.O.) degree. Official headquarters for 12 academies of medicine and boards of certification in the following specialties: anesthesiology, dermatology, emergency medicine, family practice, internal medicine, geriatric medicine, neurology/psychiatry, obstetrics/gynecology, orthopedic surgery, plastic/reconstructive surgery, radiology, surgery. **Pub:** *AAPS Directory*, annual. Directory. Provides alphabetical and geographical list of members. *Price:* Included in membership dues. • *The American Journal of Clinical Medicine (AJCM)*, quarterly. • *Member Notes*, quarterly. Newsletter. **Frmly:** American Association of Osteopathic Specialists; (1984) American Academy of Osteopathic Surgeons.

★ 414 ★ American Association of Physicians of Indian Origin (AAPI)
17W300 22nd St., Ste. 300A
Oakbrook Terrace, IL 60181-4490
Phone: (630)530-2277 **Fax:** (630)530-2475
Email: info@aapiusa.net
Website: http://www.aapiusa.org/aapi.nsf
S. Jay Jayasankar, MD, Pres.

Fnded: 1984. **Mem:** 100. **Desc:** Serves as a forum to facilitate and enable Indian American physicians to excel in patient care, teaching and research. **Pub:** *AAPI Journal*, quarterly. Journal. Contains articles on medical and social matters related to Indian physicians and public health.

★ 415 ★ American Association of Physicists in Medicine (AAPM)
One Physics Ellipse
College Park, MD 20740-3846
Phone: (301)209-3350 **Fax:** (301)209-0862
Email: aapm@aapm.org
Website: http://www.aapm.org
Sal Trofi, Jr., Exec. Dir.

Fnded: 1958. **Mem:** 4,500. **Reg. Groups:** 20. **Desc:** Persons professionally engaged in application of physics to medicine and biology in medical research and educational institutions; encourages interest and training in medical physics and related fields; promotes high professional standards; disseminates technical information. Maintains placement service. Conducts research programs. Member society of American Institute of Physics. **Pub:** *American Association of Physicists in Medicine–Membership Directory*, annual. Membership Directory. *Price:* Included in membership dues, Free. For members only. • *Medical Physics*, monthly. Journal. Contains articles broadly concerned with the relationship of human biology and medicine. *Price:* included in membership dues; $390 for nonmembers; $430 library.

★ 416 ★ American Association of Plastic Surgeons (AAPS)
c/o R. Barrett Noone, M.D.
444 E Algonquin Rd.
Arlington Heights, IL 60005
Phone: (847)228-9900 **Free:** 888-475-2784
Fax: (847)228-9131
Email: executivewsecretary@aaps1921.org
Website: http://www.aaps1921.org
R. Christie Wray, Jr.,MD, Pres.

Fnded: 1921. **Mem:** 425. **Desc:** Professional society of plastic surgeons. **Frmly:** (1942) American Association of Oral and Plastic Surgeons.

★ 417 ★ American Association of Podiatric Physicians and Surgeons (AAPPS)
1328 Southern Ave. SE, Ste. 200
Washington, DC 20032
Phone: (202)562-2777 **Fax:** (202)562-5351
Email: rsbenjamin@aol.com
Website: http://www.theaapps.com
Richard S. Benjamin, DPM, Exec. Sec.

Fnded: 1979. **Mem:** 1,500. **State Groups:** 14. **Desc:** Podiatrists. Seeks to represent members' interests and educate podiatrists and the public. Provides training and certification for podiatry and podiatric surgery. Offers accreditation to agencies providing podiatric services, education, or training; also provides podiatric peer review. Operates speakers' bureau and placement service; compiles statistics. **Pub:** *AAPPS Newsletter*, annual. Newsletter.

★ 418 ★ American Association of Poison Control Centers (AAPCC)
3201 New Mexico Ave. NW, Ste. 310
Washington, DC 20016
Phone: (202)362-7217
Email: aapcc@poison.org
Website: http://www.aapcc.org
R. A. Soloway, Pres.

Fnded: 1958. **Mem:** 1,400. **Reg. Groups:** 70. **Desc:** ""–4 Individuals and organizations engaged in operation of poison control centers and/or interested in poison prevention. Has established standards for poison information, control centers and specialists in poison information. Compiles statistics about poison exposures in the United States. Coordinates nationwide toll-free poison emergency hotline. **Pub:** *Annual Report of the American Association of Poison Control Centers Toxic Exposure Surveillance System*, annual. Article. Journal article in American Journal of Emergency Medicine. *Price:* $10 reprint.

★ 419 ★ American Association of Preferred Provider Organizations
PO Box 429
Jeffersonville, IN 47131-0429
Phone: (812)246-4376 **Free:** 800-642-2515
Fax: (812)246-4630
Email: kgreenrose@aappo.org
Website: http://www.aappo.org
Karen Greenrose, Pres.

Fnded: 1983. **Mem:** 1,100. **Reg. Groups:** 4. **State Groups:** 9. **Desc:** Seeks to advance the development, growth and success of network-based managed health care organizations(PPOs PSOs IPAs, etc.). Provides its members with a variety of educational and networking opportunities. Advocates the needs and interests of its members before local, state and federal legislators and regulators. Promotes network-based managed health care to payors, employers and the general public through a variety of media outlets. **Pub:** *AAPPO Legislative Bulletin*, periodic. Newsletter. Provides information on legislation and regulations affecting the PPO industry. *Price:* Free to members; $75/year for nonmembers. • *Directory of Operational PPOs*, annual. Directory. Contains information on approximately 1000 PPO organizations and products. *Price:* Free to organizational members; $225 for individual members; $425 for nonmembers. • *Health Care Innovations*, bimonthly. Magazine. Contains information on product innovations, systems, trends, and individuals in the managed care field. *Price:* Included in membership dues; $50/year for nonmembers. • *PPO Market Report*, annual. Provides summary data and charts on the PPO industry. *Price:* Free to organizational members; $62.50 for individual members; $125 for nonmembers. **Frmly:** (1999) Association of Managed Healthcare Organizations.

★ 420 ★ American Association of Professional Hypnotherapists (AAPH)
4149A El Camino Way
Palo Alto, CA 94306-4036
Phone: (650)323-3224
Email: josie@deepideas.com
Website: http://www.aaph.org
Josie Hadley, Exec. Dir.

Fnded: 1980. **Mem:** 1,525. **Desc:** Hypnotherapists, marriage and family therapists, psychologists, clinical social workers, physicians, pastoral counselors, and others trained and experienced in hypnosis therapy. Promotes public awareness of hypnosis as applied to personal motivation and improvement, habit control, and assisting the healing process. Acts as forum for the exchange of ideas and techniques; encourages a high level of professional ethics; promotes positive image of hypnotherapy. **Pub:** *Hypnotherapy Today*, quarterly. Newsletter. Covers techniques, new theories and innovations, case descriptions, and new uses of hypnotherapy. *Price:* Included in membership dues. • *National Register of Professional Hypnotherapists*, annual. Arranged by state and country. *Price:* Included in membership dues.

★ 421 ★ American Association of Professional Ringside Physicians (AAPRP)
40 Heights Rd.
Darien, CT 06820-4132
Phone: (914)699-2020 **Fax:** (914)699-2025
Email: mcs@clnn.com
Website: http://www.aaprp.org
Mana Camille Sclafani, Exec. Dir.

Fnded: 1997. **Desc:** Physicians who provide ringside services during boxing matches. Seeks to create and develop protocols and guidelines for ringside physicians; works to ensure the safety and protection of professional boxers. Facilitates communication and cooperation among members; develops standards of practice for ringside physicians; serves as a clearinghouse on the medical aspects of boxing.

★ 422 ★ American Association of Psychiatric Administrators (AAPA)
c/o Frances Roton, Exec. Dir.
PO Box 570218
Dallas, TX 75357-0218
Free: 800-650-5888 **Fax:** (972)613-5532
Email: frdal@airmail.net
Website: http://www.psychiatricadministrators.org/
Frances Roton, Exec. Dir.

Fnded: 1960. **Mem:** 300. **Reg. Groups:** 3. **State Groups:** 6. **Desc:** Psychiatrists who occupy the position of chief administrative or clinical officer of a public or private neuropsychiatric hospital or clinic. Provides for the efficient consolidation and dissemination of information concerning the treatment, care, and rehabilitation of the mentally ill or handicapped; the effective application of training and research; and the development of the highest standards and qualifications for administrators of public neuropsychiatric hospitals. Conducts educational programs. Acts as a forum through which the common voice of the membership may be expressed and publicized. **Pub:** *Journal of American Association of Psychiatric Administrators*, periodic. Journal. • *List of Members*, biennial. Membership Directory. • Newsletter, quarterly. **Frmly:** (1975) Association of Medical Superintendents of Mental Hospitals.

★ 423 ★ American Association of Psychiatric Technicians (AAPT)
2000 "O" St., Ste. 250
Sacramento, CA 95814-5286
Phone: (916)443-1701 **Free:** 800-391-7589
Fax: (916)329-9145
Email: appt@psych-health.com
Website: http://www.psychtechs.org
Keith Hearn, Exec. Dir.

Fnded: 1991. **Mem:** 2,500. **Desc:** Administers the Nationally Certified Psychiatric Technician examination to non-licensed direct-care workers in the fields of mental illness, developmental disabilities and substance abuse.

★ 424 ★ American Association of Public Health Dentistry (AAPHD)
1224 Centre W, Ste. 400B
Springfield, IL 62704
Phone: (217)391-0218 **Fax:** (217)793-0041
Email: natoff@aaphd.org
Website: http://www.aaphd.org
William R. Maas, DDS, Pres.

Fnded: 1937. **Mem:** 900. **Desc:** Professional society of dentists, dental hygienists, health educators, and others actively engaged in dental public health. Sponsors competitions. **Pub:** *American Association of Public Health Dentistry–Communique*, quarterly. Newsletter. *Price:* Included in membership dues; $20/year for nonmembers. • *Journal of Public Health Dentistry*, quarterly. Journal. Covers fluoridation, sealants, demographics, and utilization of dental services. Includes research reports and book reviews. *Price:* Included in membership dues; $100/year for nonmembers in U.S.; $100/year for nonmembers outside U.S.; $135/year airmail. **Frmly:** (1983) American Association of Public Health Dentists.

★ 425 ★ American Association of Public Health Physicians (AAPHP)
1300 W Belmont Ave.
Chicago, IL 60657
Phone: (630)604-3256 **Fax:** (630)604-3256
Email: aaphp@iname.com
Website: http://www.aaphp.org
Mary Ellen Bradshaw, MD, Pres.

Fnded: 1954. **Mem:** 200. **Desc:** Physicians actively engaged in public health. Promotes leadership in the field of public health; speaks for its membership on proposed health legislation at various levels; supports coordination of public health responsibilities in a variety of agencies. Conducts or cosponsors educational seminars. **Pub:** *American Association of Public Health Physicians–Bulletin*, quarterly. Newsletter. *Price:* Included in membership dues.

★ 426 ★ American Association of Public Health Veterinarians (AAPHV)
c/o Dr. Joe Horman
5649 Horman Ln.
Frederick, MD 21701
Fax: (410)333-6333
Email: jthdvmmph@aol.com
Website: http://www.avma.org/aaphv
Dr. Joe Horman, Treas.

Fnded: 1953. **Mem:** 100. **Desc:** Executive veterinary public health administrators in each state. Work to guide and develop veterinary public health programs in the states and on the national level. **Pub:** *Annual National Compendium of Animal Rabies Control*, annual. **Frmly:** (1968) Association of State Public Health Veterinarians; (1979) Association of State and Territorial Public Health Veterinarians; (1984) National Association of State and Territorial Public Health Veterinarians; (2002) National Association of State Public Health Veterinarians.

★ 427 ★ American Association for Respiratory Care (AARC)
11030 Ables Ln.
Dallas, TX 75229-4593
Phone: (972)243-2272 **Fax:** (972)484-2720
Email: info@aarc.org
Website: http://www.aarc.org
Michael T. Amato, Chair

Fnded: 1947. **Mem:** 35,000. **Nat'l Groups:** 4. **State Groups:** 50. **Desc:** Allied health society of respiratory therapists and other respiratory caregivers employed by hospitals, skilled nursing facilities, home care companies, group practices, educational institutions, and municipal organizations. Encourages, develops, and provides educational programs for persons interested in the profession of respiratory care; and advances the science of respiratory care. **Pub:** *AARC Times: The Magazine for the Respiratory Care Professional*, monthly. Magazine. Includes advertisers' index, calendar of events, employment opportunities, and legislative update. *Price:* Included in membership dues; $75/year for nonmembers in the U.S.; $90/year for nonmembes outside the U.S. • *Respiratory Care*, monthly. Provides original studies, case reports, and method/device evaluations in cardiopulmonary clinical medicine. *Price:* Included in membership dues; $75/year for nonmembers in the U.S.; $5/copy; $90/year for nonmembers outside the U.S. **Frmly:** (1954) Inhalation Therapy Association; (1967) American Association of Inhalation Therapists; (1973) American Association for Inhalation Therapy; (1986) American Association for Respiratory Therapy.

★ 428 ★ American Association of Retired Veterinarians
PO Box 4826
Ithaca, NY 14852
Phone: (607)533-4114
Dr. Walter J. Martin, Jr., Pres.

Fnded: 1986. **Mem:** 425. **Desc:** Individuals with a degree in veterinary medicine who are retired or considering retiring, and their spouses. Seeks to advance the science and art of veterinary medicine. Encourages friendship among those in the profession. Promotes social and professional lives of retired veterinarians. Attempts to assist future retirees in achievement of their goals in retirement life. Organizes group trips and cruises. **Pub:** *AARV Newsletter*. Newsletter. • Membership Directory, periodic.

★ 429 ★ American Association of Sex Educators, Counselors and Therapists (AASECT)
PO Box 5488
Richmond, VA 23220-0488
Phone: (804)644-3288 **Fax:** (804)644-3290
Email: aasect@aasect.org
Website: http://www.aasect.org
Stephen Conley, PhD, Exec. Dir.

Fnded: 1967. **Mem:** 1,700. **Reg. Groups:** 7. **Desc:** Professionals concerned with sex education, counseling, and therapy; students pursuing degrees in the field. Certifies sex educators, counselors, and therapists. Provides educational services. Acts as a referral service for the general public. **Pub:** *Contemporary Sexuality*, monthly. Newsletter. *Price:* $42. • *Journal of Sex Education and Therapy*, quarterly. Journal. *Price:* $40 U.S.; $50 outside U.S. **Frmly:** (1976) American Association of Sex Educators and Counselors.

★ 430 ★ American Association of Small Ruminant Practitioners (AASRP)
1910 Lyda Ave., No. 200
Bowling Green, KY 42104
Phone: (270)793-0781 **Fax:** (270)782-0188
Email: aasrp@assrp.org
Website: http://www.aasrp.org
Richard W. Stobaeus, Jr., Pres.

Fnded: 1968. **Mem:** 1,200. **Desc:** Practicing veterinarians and veterinary students; associate members are producers, feeders, hobbyists, and others interested in sheep, goats, llamas, deer, and exotic small ruminants. Aims are to: elevate standards of practice in the field; further research programs that will assist in solving small ruminant health problems; foster communication between veterinarians, owners, and researchers in order to improve small ruminant health management programs. Sponsors specialized education programs. Conducts educational programs. Maintains speakers' bureau. **Pub:** *AASRP Newsletter (Wool & Wattles)*, quarterly. Newsletter. *Price:* Included in membership dues. • *Proceedings of Symposium on Health and Disease of Small Ruminants*, annual. Proceedings. *Price:* Included in membership dues. • Also publishes fact sheets and abstracts. **Frmly:** (1988) American Association of Sheep and Goat Practitioners.

★ 431 ★ American Association of Spinal Cord Injury Nurses (AASCIN)
75-20 Astoria Blvd.
East Elmhurst, NY 11370-1177
Phone: (718)803-3782 **Fax:** (718)803-0414
Email: aascin@epva.org
Website: http://www.aascin.org
Sara Lerman, MPH, Prog. Mgr.

Fnded: 1983. **Mem:** 1,200. **Desc:** Nurses who care for patients with spinal cord impairment; nurses interested in the field of spinal cord impairment; persons who have provided extraordinary service to improve the quality of life for spinal cord impairment patients. Purposes are to: promote and improve nursing care of spinal cord impairment patients; develop and advance related education and research; recognize nurses whose careers are devoted to the problems of spinal cord impairment; keep medical personnel informed of state-of-the-art techniques. Focuses on topics such as sexuality and spinal cord impairment, care of respiratory dependent spinal cord impairment patients, alcohol and drug dependent spinal cord impairment patients, and planning for care in the community. Monitors and participates in legislative and regulatory activities affecting spinal cord impairment and professional nursing practice. Conducts research and educational programs. **Pub:** *Clinical Practice Guideline: Autonomic Dysreflexia*. Pamphlet. *Price:* $10. • *SCI Nursing*, quarterly. Journal. Contains articles on all facets on spinal cord injury patient care and association news. • *Standards of Spinal Cord Injury Nursing Practice*. Pamphlet. *Price:* $6.

★ 432 ★ American Association of Spinal Cord Injury Psychologists and Social Workers (AASCIPSW)
75-20 Astoria Blvd.
Jackson Heights, NY 11372
Phone: (718)803-3782 **Fax:** (718)803-0414
Email: aascipsw@epva.org
Website: http://www.aascipsw.org
Dr. Vivian Beyda, DrPH, Assoc. Exec. Dir.

Fnded: 1986. **Mem:** 430. **Desc:** Psychologists and social workers who treat patients with spinal cord impairment; others interested in the spinal injury field. Promotes improved psychsocial care of spinal cord injury patients; develops and enhances related education and research programs. Focuses on topics such as sexuality and spinal cord injury, alcohol and drug dependent spinal cord injury patients, adjusting to spinal cord injuries, and planning for care in the community. Sponsors research grant program. **Pub:** *SCI Psychosocial Process*, quarterly. Journal. *Price:* Included in membership dues. • Also publishes suggested reading list and practice guidelines.

★ 433 ★ American Association for the Study of Liver Diseases (AASLD)
1729 King St.
Alexandria, VA 22314
Phone: (703)299-9766 **Fax:** (703)299-9622
Email: aasld@aasld.org
Website: http://www.aasld.org
Sherrie H. Cathcart, Exec. Dir.

Fnded: 1950. **Mem:** 2,400. **Nat'l Groups:** 1. **Desc:** Medical society focused solely on the science and practice of hepatology, promoting liver wellness and high-quality, cost-effective, compassionate care of patients with hepatobiliary diseases. **Pub:** *Hepatology*, monthly. Journal. • *Liver Transplantation and Surgery*, monthly. Journal. • Newsletter, bimonthly.

★ 434 ★ American Association of Suicidology (AAS)
4201 Connecticut Ave. NW, Ste. 408
Washington, DC 20008
Phone: (202)237-2280 **Fax:** (202)237-2282
Email: info@suicidology.org
Website: http://www.suicidology.org
Dr. Alan Berman, Exec. Dir.

Fnded: 1968. **Mem:** 1,100. **Reg. Groups:** 5. **Desc:** Psychologists, psychiatrists, social workers, nurses, health educators, physicians, directors of suicide prevention centers, clergy, and others from various disciplines and fields of experience who share a common interest in the advancement of studies of suicide prevention and life-threatening behavior. Seeks to recognize and encourage suicidology (the study of suicide, suicide prevention, and related phenomena of self-destruction). Advances education, disseminates information through programs and publications, and cooperates with other organizations in suicidology. **Pub:** *AAS Membership Roster*, periodic. Arranged by state and region. *Price:* $10/copy. • *American Association of Suicidology–Newslink*, quarterly. Newsletter. Includes association news and calendar of events. *Price:* Included in membership dues. • *Crisis Center Directory*, periodic. Directory. Lists approximately 600 suicide prevention and crisis intervention agencies in the United States. *Price:* $20/copy. • *Directory of Survivors of Suicide Support Groups*, periodic. Directory. *Price:* $10. • *Proceedings of Annual Meeting*. *Price:* $30. • *Suicide and Life-Threatening Behavior*, quarterly. Journal. *Price:* available to members only. • *Surviving Suicide*, quarterly. Newsletter. *Price:* $20/year.

★ 435 ★ American Association for the Surgery of Trauma (AAST)
Department of Surgery
UCLA Medical Center
10833 LeConte Ave. CHS 72-178
Los Angeles, CA 90024
Phone: (310)825-5981 **Fax:** (310)206-2472
Email: hcryer@mednet.ucla.edu
Website: http://www.aast.org

Fnded: 1938. **Mem:** 844. **Desc:** Professional society of surgeons interested in the cultivation and improvement of the science and art of the surgery of trauma and allied sciences. **Pub:** *Journal of Trauma*, monthly. Journal.

★ 436 ★ American Association of Surgical Physician Assistants (AASPA)
PO Box 867
Bernardsville, NJ 07924
Free: 888-882-2772 **Fax:** (732)805-9582
Email: theaaspa@aol.com

Website: http://www.aaspa.com
Susan E. Lusty, Exec. Dir.

Fnded: 1973. **Mem:** 600. **Nat'l Groups:** 1. **Desc:** Surgical physician assistants, students in accredited physician assistant programs, and allied health professionals. Purposes are to promote academic and clinical excellence among members, to respond to the needs of surgical physician assistants, and to educate the medical community and the public about the role of surgical physician assistants in health care. **Pub:** *Surgical Physician Assistant*, monthly. Journal. • *The Sutureline*, quarterly. Newsletter. *Price:* Included in membership dues. **Frmly:** (1996) American Association of Surgeon Assistants.

★ 437 ★ American Association of Swine Veterinarians (AASV)

902 1st Ave.
Perry, IA 50220-1703
Phone: (515)465-5255 **Fax:** (515)465-3832
Email: aasv@netins.net
Website: http://www.aasv.org
Dr. Tom Burkgren, Exec. Dir.

Fnded: 1969. **Mem:** 1,550. **Desc:** Veterinarians concerned with swine health and nutrition. To improve public stature and increase the knowledge of veterinarians in the field of swine practice. **Pub:** *Proceedings*, annual. *Price:* $60 plus s/h. • *Swine Health and Production*, bimonthly. Journals. *Price:* $85/year.

★ 438 ★ American Association for Therapeutic Humor (AATH)

1951 W Camelback Rd., Ste. 445
Phoenix, AZ 85015-3498
Phone: (602)995-1454 **Fax:** (602)995-1449
Email: office@aath.org
Website: http://www.aath.org
April Becerra, Exec. Dir.

Fnded: 1987. **Mem:** 500. **Desc:** Health care providers, clergy, and educators; other interested individuals. Promotes the use of humor as a therapeutic technique; disseminates public information about laughter and humor; offers networking service to further understanding of therapeutic humor; conducts research programs that incorporate therapeutic uses of humor. Maintains speakers' bureau. **Pub:** *Laugh It Up*, quarterly. Newsletter. • *Laugh It Update*, bimonthly. Monograph. • Bibliographies. • Also makes available tapes.

★ 439 ★ American Association for Thoracic Surgery (AATS)

13 Elm St.
Manchester, MA 01944
Phone: (978)526-8330 **Fax:** (978)526-7521
Email: aats@prri.com
Website: http://www.aats.org
Fred A. Crawford, Chm.

Fnded: 1917. **Mem:** 1,200. **Desc:** Specialists in surgery of the chest region, including cardiovascular surgeons. Encourages investigation and study of intrathoracic physiology, pathology, and therapy. **Pub:** *Journal of Thoracic and Cardiovascular Surgery*, monthly. Journal. • Membership Directory, annual.

★ 440 ★ American Association of Tissue Banks (AATB)

1350 Beverly Rd., Ste. 220-A
Mc Lean, VA 22101
Phone: (703)827-9582 **Free:** 800-635-2282
Fax: (703)356-2198
Email: aatb@aatb.org
Website: http://www.aatb.org
Samuel H. Doppeit, MD, Pres.

Fnded: 1976. **Mem:** 1,200. **Desc:** Goals are to encourage the development of regional tissue banks and the establishment of guidelines and standards for the retrieval, preservation, storage, and distribution of tissues for transplantation. **Pub:** *AATB Membership Directory*, annual. Membership Directory. Lists individuals and institutions. *Price:* Included in membership dues. • *AATB Newsletter*, quarterly. Newsletter. *Price:* Available to members only. • *American Association of Tissue Banks–Technical Manual*, periodic. • *Standards for Tissue Banking*, periodic.

★ 441 ★ American Association of Veterinary Clinicians (AAVC)

37 W Broad St., Ste. 480
Columbus, OH 43215-4132
Phone: (614)228-6599 **Fax:** (614)241-2215
Website: http://www.craiggroup.com/Welcome.htm

Fnded: 1958. **Desc:** Veterinary clinicians engaged in teaching and/or research at the professional, graduate or postgraduate level. Strives to enhance the quality of teaching, service and research, provides a forum for exploration and creative resolution of clinical issues. Hosts annual meetings, educational programs and sponsors achievement awards.

★ 442 ★ American Association of Veterinary Immunologists (AAVI)

c/o Dr. Will Goff
USDA, ARS
3003 ADBF
Washington State University
Pullman, WA 99164-6630
Phone: (509)335-6029 **Fax:** (509)335-8328
Email: wgoff@vetmed.wsu.edu
Website: http://www.cvm.missouri.edu/aavi
Will Goff, Sec. -Treas.

Fnded: 1979. **Mem:** 260. **Desc:** Holders of BS or DVM degrees with an interest in veterinary immunology. Promotes development and dissemination of knowledge in the field of veterinary immunology. Conducts research and educational programs. **Pub:** *AAVI Newsletter*, periodic. Newsletter.

★ 443 ★ American Association of Veterinary Laboratory Diagnosticians (CAHFS:SVM)

c/o UC Davis
PO Box 1770
Davis, CA 95617
Phone: (530)754-9719 **Fax:** (530)752-5680
Email: aaardans@ucdavis.edu
Website: http://www.aavld.org
Dr. Alex Ardans, Sec. -Treas.

Fnded: 1957. **Mem:** 1,200. **Desc:** Each state has an official delegate and alternate to the association's executive board. Individual membership is open to persons active in veterinary laboratory diagnostic medicine. Disseminates information on diagnosis of animal disease; coordinates diagnostic activities of regulatory, research, and service laboratories; establishes uniform diagnostic techniques; seeks to improve existing diagnostic techniques and facilitate the development of new ones; establishes guides for personnel qualifications and facilities; acts as consultant to the U.S. Animal Health Association on uniform diagnostic criteria. **Pub:** *AAVLD Newsletter*, 3/year. Newsletter. Contains association news and information on employment opportunities. *Price:* Included in membership dues. • *Journal of Veterinary Diagnostic Investigation*, bimonthly. Journal. *Price:* Included in membership dues.

★ 444 ★ American Association of Veterinary State Boards (AAVSB)

3100 Main St., Ste. 208
Kansas City, MO 64111-1918
Phone: (816)931-1504 **Free:** 877-698-8482
Fax: (816)931-1604
Email: info@aavsb.org
Website: http://www.aavsb.org
Charlotte P. Ronan, Exec. Dir.

Fnded: 1957. **Mem:** 56. **Desc:** State boards of examiners in veterinary medicine. Aids state boards of veterinary medicine in the protection of the public health and welfare. Acts as a clearing house for research, collects and disseminates information about legal regulation of the veterinary profession. Works to simplify and standardize licensing and certification processes for veterinarians and veterinary technicians. Interacts with other veterinary organizations; legislative, judicial, regulatory, and executive governmental bodies; and other associations whose areas of interest may coincide. Assists member boards in fulfilling statutory, public, and ethical obligations in legal regulation and enforcement. Cooperates with the National Board Examination Committee in the design and use of entry level, relicensure and disciplinary examinations regarding the practice of veterinary medicine and regulation. Collects and disseminates information regarding disciplinary actions taken by member boards. Provides veterinary medical educational programs. **Frmly:** (1968) Association of American Board of Examiners in Veterinary Medicine; (1974) American Association State Boards, Veterinary.

★ 445 ★ American Association of Wildlife Veterinarians (AAWV)

c/o Dr. Kirsten Gilardi
Wildlife Health Center
University of California
1 Shields Ave.
Davis, CA 95616
Phone: (530)752-4896 **Fax:** (530)752-3318
Email: kvgilardi@ucdavis.edu
Website: http://www.aawv.net
Dr. Kirsten Gilardi, Sec.

Fnded: 1979. **Mem:** 350. **Desc:** Veterinarians in state and federal wildlife resource agencies, universities, private practice, public health service agencies, agricultural agencies, and diagnostic laboratories; veterinary students; and interested individuals. To deal with problems confronting veterinarians who work with free-ranging wildlife. Encourages colleges of veterinary medicine to increase emphasis on management of and preventive medicine for free-ranging species; educates governmental agencies and wildlife resource interest groups; promotes utilization of veterinarians in the field of wildlife resource management and research; encourages cooperation among resource management professionals and wildlife veterinarians; promotes continuing education programs for wildlife veterinarians; emphasizes interrelationships of man, domestic animals, and wildlife with disease; encourages recognition of disease syndromes as potentially influenced by habitat succession, alteration, and pollution. **Pub:** *AAWV Newsletter*, quarterly. Newsletter. • Membership Directory, periodic.

★ 446 ★ American Association of Women Dentists (AAWD)

330 S Wells St., Ste. 1110
Chicago, IL 60606
Phone: (312)280-9296 **Free:** 800-920-2293
Fax: (830)612-3067
Email: info@womendentists.org
Website: http://www.womendentists.org
Dr. Rise' Lyman, Pres.

Fnded: 1921. **Nat'l Groups:** 1. **Reg. Groups:** 17. **Desc:** Dental students or dentists who are interested in dentistry and advancing women in dentistry. AAWD dedicates itself to enhancing and promoting unique participation and leadership for women in organized dentistry. **Pub:** *AAWD Membership Directory*, annual. Directory. • *The Chronicle/Women's Dental Journal*, bimonthly. Journal. Includes member activities at the local and national level, scientific and technical news, upcoming events and a list of various jobs. *Price:* Included in membership dues; $30/year for nonmembers. **Frmly:** (1978) Association of American Women Dentists.

★ 447 ★ American Association of Women Emergency Physicians (AAWEP)

c/o American College of Emergency Physicians
1125 Executive Cir.
Irving, TX 75038-2522
Phone: (972)550-0911 **Free:** 800-798-1822
Fax: (972)580-2816
Email: info@aawep.org

Website: http://www.acep.org/1.3071.0.html
John Walker, Exec. Dir.

Fnded: 1983. **Mem:** 400. **Desc:** Women engaged in the practice of emergency medicine. Promotes professional advancement of members. Provides support and guidance to female emergency physicians; conducts leadership skills development programs for female emergency physicians, residents, and medical students. Maintains speakers' bureau. **Pub:** *Epic Quarterly Newsletter*, periodic. Directory. • Newsletter, periodic.

★ 448 ★ American Association for Women Podiatrists (AAWP)

c/o Dr. Marlene Reid, DPM, Pres.
6601 S Cass Ave.
Westmont, IL 60559
Phone: (630)852-8640 **Fax:** (630)852-8612
Email: rwoodfoot@aol.com
Website: http://www.aawpinc.com
Dr. Marlene Reid, DPM, Pres.

Fnded: 1965. **Mem:** 997. **Reg. Groups:** 14. **Desc:** Promotes the advancement of the educational, political, financial and social well-being of members. Provides networking opportunities, consulting and financial assistance to student members. Maintains speakers' bureau **Pub:** *AAWP Newsletter*, quarterly. Newsletter. *Price:* Included in membership dues; Free to students.

★ 449 ★ American Association for Women Radiologists (AAWR)

4550 Post Oak Pl., Ste. 342
Houston, TX 77027
Phone: (713)623-8335 **Fax:** (713)960-0488
Email: admin@aawr.org
Website: http://www.aawr.org
Darcee Brown, Acct. Exec.

Fnded: 1981. **Mem:** 1,400. **Local Groups:** 3. **Desc:** Physicians involved in diagnostic or therapeutic radiology, nuclear medicine, or radiologic physics. Facilitates exchange of knowledge and information as it relates to women in radiology; encourages publication of materials on radiology and medicine by members; supports women who are training in the field and encourages women at all levels to participate in radiological societies. Maintains ad hoc committees on affirmative action, radiation therapists, and policy on pregnancy. **Pub:** *AAWR Focus*, quarterly. Newsletter. *Price:* Free, to members only. • *AAWR Membership Directory*, annual. Membership Directory. *Price:* Free, to members only. • *Survival Guide for Women Radiologists: The AAWR Pocket Mentor. Price:* Free; available to members only. **Frmly:** (1991) American Association of Women Radiologists.

★ 450 ★ American Association for World Health (AAWH)

1825 K St., NW, Ste. 1208
Washington, DC 20006
Fax: (202)466-5896
Email: staff@aawnworldhealth.org
Richard L. Wittenberg, Pres. & CEO

Fnded: 1953. **Mem:** 1,200. **Desc:** Individuals and organizations interested in strengthening U.S. commitment to world health. To inform Americans about world health issues and to strengthen public support for activities and programs that improve health conditions worldwide. Supports programs of the World Health Organization, Pan American Health Organization, and other agencies. Sponsors: World Health Day in U.S.; World AIDS Day, and World No-Tobacco Day. **Pub:** *AAWH Quarterly*, quarterly. Newsletter. Covering international health policy issues; includes news of the AAWH and WHO. *Price:* Included in membership dues. • *Tobacco Alert*, annual. Newsletter. *Price:* Free. • *World AIDS Day Action Kit*, annual. Booklet. *Price:* First copy free. • *World Health Day Planning Kit*, annual. Booklet. *Price:* First copy free. **AKA:** U.S. Committee for the World Health Organization. **Frmly:** (1966) National Citizens Committee for the World Health Organization.

★ 451 ★ American Association of Zoo Veterinarians (AAZV)

c/o Dr. Wilbur Amand
6 N Pennell Rd.
Media, PA 19063
Phone: (610)892-4812 **Fax:** (610)892-4813
Email: aazv@aol.com
Website: http://www.aazv.org/aazv_001.htm
Dr. Wilbur Amand, Exec. Dir.

Fnded: 1947. **Mem:** 1,200. **Desc:** Veterinarians actively engaged in the practice of zoo and wildlife medicine for at least four years; veterinarians who do not qualify for active membership; persons interested in diseases of wildlife; students of veterinary medicine in any accredited veterinary school. Purposes are to: advance programs for preventive medicine, husbandry, and scientific research dealing with captive and free-ranging wild animals; provide a forum for the presentation and discussion of problems related to the field; enhance and uphold the professional ethics of veterinary medicine. **Pub:** *Conference Proceedings*, annual. Proceedings. Contains papers presented at the annual conference. *Price:* $45. • *Journal of Zoo and Wildlife Medicine*, quarterly. Journal. Contains original manuscripts, book and paper reviews and research notes/case reports. *Price:* Included in membership dues. • *Zoo Vet News*, quarterly. Newsletter. • Membership Directory, annual.

★ 452 ★ American Auditory Society (AAS)

352 Sundial Ridge Cir.
Dammeron Valley, UT 84783-5196
Phone: (435)574-0062 **Fax:** (435)574-0063
Email: amaudsoc@aol.com
Website: http://www.amauditorysoc.org
Wayne J. Staab, PhD, Sec. -Treas.

Fnded: 1973. **Mem:** 2,000. **Desc:** Audiologists, otolaryngologists, scientists, hearing aid industry professionals, and educators of hearing impaired people; individuals involved in industries serving hearing impaired people, including the amplification systems industry. Works to increase knowledge and understanding of: the ear, hearing, and balance; disorders of the ear, hearing, and balance; prevention of these disorders; habilitation and rehabilitation of individuals with hearing and balance dysfunction. **Pub:** *The Bulletin of the AAS*, 3/year. Newsletter. *Price:* included in membership dues. • *Ear and Hearing*, bimonthly. Journal. Includes periodic supplements. • *Peer Reviewed Clinical Research Publication. Price:* $77 in U.S. personal; $112 outside U.S. personal; $145 in U.S. institution; $180 outside U.S. institution. **Frmly:** (1982) American Audiology Society.

★ 453 ★ American Autoimmune Related Diseases Association (AARDA)

22100 Gratiot Ave.
East Detroit, MI 48021-2227
Phone: (586)776-3900 **Free:** 800-598-4668
Fax: (586)776-3903
Email: aarda@aarda.org
Website: http://www.aarda.org
Virginia Ladd, Exec. Dir.

Fnded: 1991. **Mem:** 4,000. **Desc:** Promotes national focus and collaborative efforts among state and national volunteer health groups on autoimmunity, the major cause of serious chronic diseases. Offers research and educational programs; maintains speakers' bureau. **Pub:** *InFocus*, quarterly. Newsletter. Includes research updates and national autoimmune activities designed primarily for lay membership. *Price:* $24/year.

★ 454 ★ American Back Society (ABS)

2647 International Blvd., Ste. 401
Oakland, CA 94601
Phone: (510)536-9929 **Fax:** (510)536-1812
Email: info@americanback.org
Website: http://www.americanbacksoc.org/contact.html

Desc: Orthopedic and neurological surgeons, physical therapists, chiropractors, and other health care professionals with an interest back and spinal health. Promotes continuing professional development of members; seeks to advance the prevention, diagnosis, and treatment of back and spinal disorders. Serves as a clearinghouse on spinal health; sponsors research and educational programs; facilitates exchange of information among members.

★ 455 ★ American Behcet's Disease Association (ABDA)

PO Box 19952
Amarillo, TX 79114-9952
Free: 800-723-4238
Email: bbailey@behcct.com
Website: http://www.behcets.com
Bettina Bailey, Pres.

Fnded: 1986. **Mem:** 1,000. **Local Groups:** 25. **Desc:** Gathers statistics on people with Behcet's syndrome; educates the public and medical community about the disease. (Behcet's syndrome is characterized by painful oral ulcers which often resolve spontaneously, but recur at unpredictable intervals. Other symptoms include recurring genital lesions, skin lesions, blurred vision, pain and redness of the eyes, and nervous system abnormalities. The disease is most common among young adults, and methods of treatment are varied and controversial.) Conducts educational programs; maintains speakers' bureau. **Pub:** *ABDA Flame*, biennial. Newsletter. Contains news on research projects, treatments, patients, and organizational activities. *Price:* $35. • *Behcet's Disease and Your Eyes*. Brochure. • *Behcet's Disease and Your Nervous System*. Brochure. • *Behcet's Disease: What You Should Know*. Brochure. • *Only Hope*. Brochure. **Frmly:** (1995) American Behcet's Association.

★ 456 ★ American Blind Bowling Association (ABBA)

6317 Phillips Ave.
Pittsburgh, PA 15217-1807
Phone: (412)421-1861
Judith A. Fitzpatrick, Sec. -Treas.

Fnded: 1951. **Mem:** 2,000. **Reg. Groups:** 4. **State Groups:** 125. **Local Groups:** 140. **Desc:** Legally blind men and women, 18 years of age and older, competing in organized tenpin bowling. Promotes bowling as a recreational activity for adult blind persons. Sanctions member leagues; sponsors annual mail-o-graphic. Presents awards. **Pub:** *The Blind Bowler*, 3/year.

★ 457 ★ American Blind Skiing Foundation (ABSF)

163 Walnut St.
Elmhurst, IL 60126
Phone: (847)255-1739
Email: absf@bigfoot.com
Website: http://www.absf.org/
Sam Skobel, Founder

Fnded: 1972. **Mem:** 175. **Desc:** Volunteers who teach downhill and cross-country recreational and competitive skiing to the blind and visually handicapped. Holds giant slalom, downhill, and cross-country races; awards trophies. Travels with blind skiers to skiing areas in Colorado, Wisconsin, and Michigan. Sponsors international races in Canada, World Cup for Disabled in Switzerland, and Olympics for Disabled in Austria.

★ 458 ★ American Board of Abdominal Surgery (ABAS)

675 Main St.
Melrose, MA 02176
Phone: (617)665-6102 **Fax:** (617)665-4127
Email: office@abdominalsurg.org
Website: http://www.abdominalsurg.org
Louis F. Alfano, MD, Exec. Sec.

Fnded: 1957. **Mem:** 2,402. **Desc:** Specialists in abdominal surgery. Improves the quality of graduate education for abdominal surgery. Establishes minimum educational and training standards for the specialty. Determines whether candidates have received adequate preparation as defined by the board. Provides comprehensive examinations to determine the ability and fitness of candidates. Certifies surgeons who have satisfied the requirements of the board as a protection to the public and the profession. Gives oral and written examinations in abdominal surgery. **Pub:** *ASAS Journal*, annual. Journal. *Price:* for members. • *Surgeon*, semiannual. *Price:* for members.

★ 459 ★ American Board of Allergy and Immunology (ABAI)

510 Walnut, Ste. 1701
Philadelphia, PA 19106-3699
Phone: (215)592-9466 **Fax:** (215)592-9411
Email: abai@abai.org
Website: http://www.abai.org
John W. Yunginger, Jr., Exec. Sec.

Fnded: 1971. **Mem:** 4,859. **Desc:** Examining and credentialing body whose primary function is to establish qualifications and examine physician candidates who meet the requirements for training and experience and grant certification to those who pass the examination. Does not recommend specialists and cannot offer advice on individual allergic or immunologic problems. Member board of the American Board of Medical Specialties and conjoint board of the American Board of Internal Medicine and the American Board of Pediatrics. **Pub:** *Policies and Procedures*, biennial.

★ 460 ★ American Board of Alternative Medicine (ABAM)

c/o Dr. B. Alli
16126 E Warren
PO Box 24224
Detroit, MI 48224-0224
Phone: (313)882-0641
Dr. B. Alli, Contact

Fnded: 1994. **Mem:** 800. **Desc:** Practitioners of alternative medicine. Promotes increased use of alternative treatments including mind-body intervention, bioelectromagnetic therapy, and herbal medicines. Conducts research and educational programs; maintains hall of fame. **Pub:** *Newsletter of the American Board of Alternative Medicine*, periodic. Newsletter. *Price:* $120 for members only.

★ 461 ★ American Board of Anesthesiology (ABA)

4101 Lake Boone Trail, Ste. 510
Raleigh, NC 27607-7506
Phone: (919)881-2570 **Fax:** (919)881-2575
Website: http://www.abanes.org
Francis P. Hughes, PhD, Exec. VP

Fnded: 1938. **Mem:** 15. **Desc:** Certification board which seeks to elevate and maintain the standards of the practice of anesthesiology and to establish criteria of fitness for the designation of a certified specialist in this field. Advises the Accreditation Council for Graduate Medical Education concerning training of individuals seeking certification. Arranges and conducts examinations to determine whether physicians who apply meet its standards; issues certificates to those who meet the required standards. **Pub:** *American Board of Anesthesiology–Booklet of Information*, annual. Booklet. Describes the examination system and the policies and regulations governing the board's examination and certification process. *Price:* Free.

★ 462 ★ American Board of Bariatric Medicine (ABBM)

5453 E Evans Pl.
Denver, CO 80222-5234
Phone: (303)779-0279 **Fax:** (303)779-0965
Email: abbm@qwest.net
Website: http://www.abbmcertification.org

Desc: Works to certify physicians in the field of bariatric medicine through comprehensive testing and review process.

★ 463 ★ American Board of Cardiovascular Perfusion (ABCP)

207 N 25th Ave.
Hattiesburg, MS 39401
Phone: (601)582-2227 **Fax:** (601)582-2271
Email: abcp@abcp.org
Website: http://www.abcp.org
Drs. Mark and Beth Richmond, Exec. Dirs.

Fnded: 1975. **Mem:** 3,400. **Desc:** Certified clinical perfusionists. Seeks to protect the public through the establishment and maintenance of standards in the field. Has established qualifications for examination and procedures for recertification. Administers annual board examinations.

★ 464 ★ American Board for Certification in Orthotics and Prosthetics (ABC)

330 John Carlyle St., Ste. 210
Alexandria, VA 22314
Phone: (703)836-7114 **Fax:** (703)836-0838
Email: lhoxie@abcop.org
Website: http://www.abcop.org
Lance O. Hoxie, Exec. Dir.

Fnded: 1948. **Mem:** 6,200. **Desc:** Certification board to establish qualifications, conduct examinations, and certify individuals (5000) and facilities (1200) whom board standards deem qualified to practice orthotics and prosthetics (the science of making and fitting artificial limbs and braces). **Pub:** *Mark of Merit*, bimonthly. Newsletter. • *O&P Almanac*, monthly. Magazine. • *Practice Analysis Report On the Scope of Practice in Prosthetics and Orthotics.*. Report. • *Registry of Board-Credentialed Orthotic and Prosthetic Professionals and Facilities*, annual. Directory. Contains lists all certified orthotists & prosthetists, registered technicians, and accredited facilities. *Price:* $20 for libraries; $75 for general public.

★ 465 ★ American Board of Chelation Therapy (ABCT)

1407-½ N Wells St.
Chicago, IL 60610-1305
Free: 800-356-2228 **Fax:** (312)266-3685
Email: jackhank@mindspring.com
Website: http://www.abct.info
Jack Hank, Exec. Dir.

Fnded: 1982. **Mem:** 220. **Desc:** Works to define and establish qualifications required of licensed physicians and surgeons for certification in the field of chelation therapy. (Chelation therapy is used in cases of blood poisoning and involves the use of metal binding and bio-inorganic agents intravenously infused into the bloodstream to "pick up" and remove calcium, lead, or other toxic heavy metals and restore cellular homeostasis. Because of lack of controlled studies for conditions other than calcinosis, digitalis toxicity, and excessive body storage of heavy metals, chelation therapy is not considered standard medical procedure.) Stresses that proper use of chelation therapy requires knowledge of nutrition and exercise and expertise in assisting patients in implementing lifestyle changes. Refers candidate physicians to sponsor inorganizations for teaching workshops, audio and video learning aids, and reading and study materials. Has created series of testing procedures designed to be comprehensive and unbiased. Administers oral and written examinations and conducts reviews of candidates' background experience and patient records. Maintains standards through process of recertification and reexamination. Sponsored by the American Holistic Medical Association, American College for Advancement in Medicine, Great Lakes Association of Clinical Medicine, and the International Oxidative Medical Association.

★ 466 ★ American Board of Colon and Rectal Surgery (ABCRS)

20600 Eureka Rd., Ste. 600
Taylor, MI 48180
Phone: (734)282-9400 **Fax:** (734)282-9402
Email: admin@abcrs.org
Website: http://www.abcrs.org
Irene Babcock, Exec. Asst.

Fnded: 1934. **Desc:** Certification board established to investigate qualifications, administer examinations, and provide certification as diplomates for medical doctors specializing in colon and rectal surgery. **Pub:** *American Board of Colon and Rectal Surgery–Newsletter to Diplomates*, annual. Newsletter. Includes research updates. *Price:* Included in membership dues. **Frmly:** American Board of Proctology.

★ 467 ★ American Board of Dental Public Health (ABDPH)

c/o Stanley Lotzkar, D.D.S.
1321 NW 47th Ter.
Gainesville, FL 32605
Phone: (352)378-6301 **Fax:** (352)367-8430
Email: slotzkar@yahoo.com
Website: http://www.pitt.edu/
Dr. Caswell Evans, Jr., Pres.

Fnded: 1950. **Mem:** 5. **Desc:** Board whose purpose is to investigate the qualifications of, administer examinations to, and certify as diplomates, dentists specializing in dental public health. Sponsored by American Association of Public Health Dentistry. **Pub:** *ABDPH Membership Directory*, triennial. Directory. • Newsletter, annual.

★ 468 ★ American Board of Dermatology (ABD)

Henry Ford Health System
1 Ford Pl.
Detroit, MI 48202-3450
Phone: (313)874-1088 **Fax:** (313)872-3221
Email: abderm@hfhs.org
Website: http://www.abderm.org
Antoinette F. Hood, MD, Exec. Dir.

Fnded: 1932. **Mem:** 16. **Desc:** Examining and certifying body. Seeks to assure provision of competent care for patients with cutaneous diseases, via capable board representation. Establishes requirements of postdoctoral training. Creates and conducts annual comprehensive examination to determine the competence of physicians who meet the requirements for examination by the board. Issues appropriate certificate to those who satisfactorily complete examination. Member of American Board of Medical Specialties . **Pub:** *Booklet of Information*, annual. Describes requirements for certification. *Price:* Free.

★ 469 ★ American Board of Disability Analysts (ABDA)

345 24th Ave. N, Ste. 200
Park Plaza Medical Bldg.
Nashville, TN 37203
Phone: (615)327-2984 **Fax:** (615)327-9235
Email: americanbd@aol.com
Alexander E. Horwitz, MD, Exec. Officer

Fnded: 1989. **Mem:** 7,600. **Desc:** Physicians, nurses, speech therapists, psychologists, physical therapists, osteopaths, occupational therapists, chiropractors, case managers, rehabilitation counselors, professional counselors, dentists, insurance claims adjusters, educators, economists, attorneys, engineers, and correctional specialists. Serves as a multidisciplinary credentialing association for all disciplines dealing with the physically and/or mentally disabled. Provides continuing education programs. **Pub:** *The Catastrophic Injury Handbook (2003). Price:* $95. • *Disability Analysis Handbook (1996).* Newsletter. *Price:* $65. • *Disability Analysis in Practice (1999). Price:* $70. • *The Disability Analyst*, 3/year. Journal. *Price:* $18. • *National Directory of Disability Analysts.* Directory.

★ 470 ★ American Board of Emergency Medicine (ABEM)

3000 Coolidge Rd.
East Lansing, MI 48823-6319
Phone: (517)332-4800 **Fax:** (517)332-2234
Email: abem@abem.org
Website: http://www.abem.org
Mary Ann Reinhart, PhD, Exec. Dir.

Fnded: 1976. **Desc:** Seeks to: improve the quality of emergency medical care; establish and maintain high standards of excellence in the specialty of emergency medicine and its approved subspecialties; improve medical education and facilities for training emergency physicians and subspecialist in approved ABEM subspecialties; evaluate specialists in emergency medicine and subspecialist in approved ABEM subspecialties applying for certification and recertification; serve the public, subcertification physicians, hospitals, and medical schools by furnishing lists of those diplomats certified by ABEM. **Pub:** *ABEM Annual Report*, annual. Annual Report. Includes summary of current year's events and activities, volunteers, and exam statistics. • *ABEM Policies and Procedures*, annual. Booklet. *Price:* Free. • *ABEMemo*, semiannual. Newsletter. For diplomates and organizations associated with ABEM.

★ 471 ★ American Board of Endodontics (ABE)

211 E Chicago Ave., Ste. 1100
Chicago, IL 60611-2691
Phone: (312)266-7255 **Free:** 800-872-3636
Fax: (312)266-9867
Email: info@aae.org
Website: http://www.aae.org/ABE1.html
Dr. Gerald N. Glickman, Pres.

Desc: Dentists who have successfully completed study and training in an advanced endodontics education program that is accredited by the Commission on Dental Accreditation of the American Dental Association . Primary objective is to protect the public by raising the standards of endodontic practice and requiring candidates for diplomate status to show strong evidence of specialized skills and knowledge in endodontics. Administers examinations and certifies dentists who successfully complete the examinations. **Pub:** *Membership Roster*, annual. Published in conjunction with American Association of Endodontists.

★ 472 ★ American Board of Examiners of Psychodrama, Sociometry, and Group Psychotherapy (ABEPSGP)

PO Box 15572
Washington, DC 20003
Phone: (202)483-0514
Dale Richard Buchanan, PhD, Exec. Dir.

Fnded: 1975. **Mem:** 389. **Desc:** Certifying body for professionals in the fields of group psychotherapy, psychodrama, and sociometry. (Psychodrama was developed by Dr. Jacob L. Moreno, 1889-1974, and is used to afford catharsis and social relearning. Sociometry studies interpersonal relationships in groups of people.) Works to establish and maintain national professional standards. Administers annual exam which includes on-site observation. Compiles statistics. **Pub:** *Board News*, semiannual. *Price:* available to members only. • Directory, annual. *Price:* Free. • Also publishes standards for psychodramatists.

★ 473 ★ American Board of Facial Plastic and Reconstructive Surgery (ABFPRS)

115C S Asaph St.
Alexandria, VA 22314
Phone: (703)549-3223 **Fax:** (703)549-3357
Email: tshill@abfprs.org
Website: http://www.abfprs.org/
Wayne F. Larrabee, Jr.,MD, Pres.

Fnded: 1986. **Desc:** Dedicated to improving the quality of facial plastic surgery available to the public.

★ 474 ★ American Board of Family Practice (ABFP)

2228 Young Dr.
Lexington, KY 40505-4294
Phone: (859)269-5626 **Free:** 888-995-5700
Fax: (859)335-7501
Email: general@abfp.org
Website: http://www.abfp.org
Robert F. Avant, MD, Exec. Dir.

Fnded: 1969. **Desc:** Certifying board for physicians specializing in family practice. Conducts certification/recertification examinations. **Pub:** *Journal of the American Board of Family Practice*, bimonthly. Journal. *Price:* $60 institution; $35 physician.

★ 475 ★ American Board of Forensic Anthropology (ABFA)

c/o Dr. Frank P. Saul
Lucas County Coroner's Office
2595 Arlington Ave.
Toledo, OH 43614-2674
Phone: (419)213-3908 **Fax:** (419)223-3941
Email: saul@dmort.org
Website: http://www.csuchico.edu/anth/ABFA
Dr. Frank P. Saul, PhD, Contact

Fnded: 1977. **Mem:** 50. **Desc:** Board for certification of physical anthropologists who wish to become forensic anthropologists. (Forensic anthropology refers to application of the science of physical anthropology in assistance of law enforcement agencies; forensic anthropologists identify and glean information from human remains.) Promotes improvement in the practice of forensic anthropology and encourages adherence to high standards in the field. Conducts written and practical examinations for prospective forensic anthropologists; awards certificates of qualification. Compiles statistics. **Pub:** *Diplomates, American Board of Forensic Anthropology Directory*, annual. Directory. Contains listings of current diplomates in forensic anthropology.

★ 476 ★ American Board of Forensic Odontology (ABFO)

c/o The Forensic Sciences Foundation
PO Box 669
Colorado Springs, CO 80901-0669
Phone: (719)636-1100
Website: http://www.abfo.org/

Fnded: 1976. **Desc:** Works to establish, enhance, and revise as necessary, standards of qualifications for those practicing forensic odontology and certify qualified specialists.

★ 477 ★ American Board of Genetic Counseling (ABGC)

9650 Rockville Pike
Bethesda, MD 20814-3998
Phone: (301)634-7300 **Fax:** (301)634-7320
Email: tvogel@genetics.faseb.org
Website: http://www.abgc.net
Sharon Robinson, Admin.

Fnded: 1993. **Mem:** 1,400. **Desc:** Individuals who have passed the Board examination. Certifies individuals for the delivery of genetic counseling services; accredits genetic counseling master's degree granting programs. **Pub:** *American Board of Genetic Counseling–Membership Directory*, free online. Membership Directory. Includes the ABGC, Genetics Society of America, American Society of Human Genetics, American College of Medical Genetics, and the American Board of Medical Genetics. *Price:* Included in membership dues.

★ 478 ★ American Board of Hair Restoration Surgery (ABHRS)

c/o The American Board of Cosmetic Surgery
18525 S Torrence Ave.
Lansing, IL 60438
Phone: (708)474-2600
Website: http://www.regrowth.com
Dr. Matt Leavitt, VP

Fnded: 1996. **Desc:** Promotes hair restoration surgery; grants certification.

★ 479 ★ American Board of Health Physics (ABHP)

1313 Dolley Madison Blvd., Ste. 402
Mc Lean, VA 22101-3926
Phone: (703)790-1745 **Fax:** (703)790-2672
Email: aahp@burkinc.com
Website: http://www.aahp-abhp.org
Nancy Johnson, Exec. Sec.

Fnded: 1960. **Mem:** 8. **Desc:** Certifying body. Promotes the health physics profession by establishing standards and procedures for certification and conducting certification examinations. Issues written proof of certification.

★ 480 ★ American Board of Industrial Hygiene (ABIH)

6015 W St. Joseph, Ste. 102
Lansing, MI 48917
Phone: (517)321-2638 **Fax:** (517)321-4624
Email: abih@abih.org
Website: http://www.abih.org/
Lynn C. O'Donnell, CIH, Exec. Dir.

Fnded: 1960. **Mem:** 19. **Desc:** Certifies industrial hygienists and promotes high standards within the profession. Maintains a record of holders of certificates. **Pub:** *ABIH Candidate Handbook*. • *ABIH News*, Biannual. Newsletter. • *Roster of the American Board of Industrial Hygiene*, annual.

★ 481 ★ American Board of Internal Medicine (ABIM)

501 Walnut St., Ste. 1700
Philadelphia, PA 19106-3699
Phone: (215)446-3500 **Free:** 800-441-2246
Fax: (215)446-3470
Email: request@abim.org
Website: http://www.abim.org
Harry R. Kimball, Pres.

Fnded: 1936. **Desc:** Certification board for doctors of internal medicine and the subspecialties of internal medicine. Assesses the qualifications of, and administers examinations to, general internists and sub-specialists. Certification is granted to those doctors meeting its standards of cognitive knowledge and clinical competence. Board members are elected from certified leaders in internal medicine. The board has certified approximately 150,000 internists and 65,000 sub-specialist diplomates and issued 15,000 recertification certificates. **Pub:** *ABIM Perspectives*, quarterly. Newsletter. • *Policies and Procedures*, annual.

★ 482 ★ American Board of Managed Care Nursing (ABMCN)

4435 Waterfront Dr., Ste. 101
Glen Allen, VA 23060-3393
Phone: (804)527-1905 **Fax:** (804)747-5316
Email: amason@aamcn.org
Website: http://www.abmcn.org
Andrea Mason, Contact

Fnded: 1998. **Desc:** Seeks to advance the study, teaching, and practice of managed care nursing. Conducts examinations and bestows certification upon qualified nurses.

★ 483 ★ American Board of Medical Genetics (ABMG)

9650 Rockville Pike
Bethesda, MD 20814-3998
Phone: (301)634-7300 **Fax:** (301)634-7320
Email: srobinson@genetics.faseb.org
Website: http://www.faseb.org/genetics/abmg/abmg-menu.htm
Roberta A. Pagon, MD, Pres.

Fnded: 1981. **Mem:** 2,000. **Desc:** Certifies individuals and accredits training programs in the field of human genetics.

★ 484 ★ American Board of Medical Psychotherapists and Psychodiagnosticians (ABMPP)

345 24th Ave. North, Ste. 200
Park Plaza Medical Bldg.
Nashville, TN 37203-1520
Phone: (615)327-2984 **Fax:** (615)327-9235
Email: americanbd@aol.com
Alex Horowitz, MD, Exec. Officer

Fnded: 1982. **Mem:** 2,900. **Desc:** Psychiatrists, psychologists, social workers, and psychiatric nurses working in public or private facilities. Promotes high standards of professional practice of medical psychotherapy. (Medical psychotherapy is the treatment of psychiatric and/or medical disorders from a mental health perspective.) Offers certification review and continuing education programs. Compiles statistics. **Pub:** *Advances in Medical Psychotherapy and Psychodiagnosis Volume 10*, annual. Journal. Scholarly articles of interest to mental health practitioners. *Price:* $48/volume. • *Medical Psychotherapist*, semiannual. Newsletter. Includes listing of board certification recipients; activities and announcements of general interest for members. *Price:* $20/year. • *National Directory of Medical Psychotherapists*, annual. Directory. Includes geographic index. *Price:* $32/copy.

★ 485 ★ American Board of Medical Specialties (ABMS)

1007 Church St., Ste. 404
Evanston, IL 60201-5913
Phone: (847)491-9091 **Fax:** (847)328-3596
Email: info@abms.org
Website: http://www.abms.org
Stephen H. Miller, MD, MPH, Exec. VP

Fnded: 1933. **Mem:** 32. **Desc:** Primary medical specialty boards and conjoint boards; organizations with related interests are associate members. Acts as spokesman for approved medical specialty boards as a group; is actively concerned with the establishment, maintenance, and elevation of standards for the education and qualification of physicians recognized as specialists through the certification procedures of its members; cooperates with other groups concerned in establishing standards, policies, and procedures for ensuring the maintenance of continued competence of such physicians. Compiles statistics. **Pub:** *ABMS Directory of Board Certified Medical Specialists*, annual. Directory. Four volumes listing over 500,000 specialists certified by 24 U.S. medical specialty boards. Arranged by specialty, name, and location. *Price:* $525/copy; $1200 CD-ROM. • *ABMS Record*, quarterly. Newsletter. Reports on events related to medical certification and education. Includes meeting reports. *Price:* Free. • *American Board of Medical Specialties–Annual Report and Reference Handbook*, annual. Guide to medical specialty boards and specialty certification. *Price:* $10. • Also publishes text publications on evaluating physicians.

★ 486 ★ American Board of Medical Specialties in Podiatry

1350 Broadway, Ste. 1705
New York, NY 10018
Phone: (212)356-0690 **Free:** 888-852-1442
Fax: (212)356-0678
Email: abmsp@ptcny.com
Website: http://www.abmsp.org
Leonard Feigenblatt, Admin.

Fnded: 1986. **Mem:** 600. **Desc:** Seeks to insure high standards of training, ethics, and practice in the field of podiatric medicine, podiatric surgery and the prevention and treatment of diabetic foot wounds. Facilitates professional advancement of members. **Pub:** Newsletter, periodic. • Directory, annual. • Brochure, periodic. **Frmly:** (2000) American Podiatric Medical Specialties Board.

★ 487 ★ American Board of Neurological Surgery (ABNS)

6550 Fannin St., No. 2139
Houston, TX 77030-2722
Phone: (713)790-6015 **Fax:** (713)794-0207
Email: abns@tmb.tmc.edu
Website: http://www.abns.org
Mary Louise Sanderson, Admin.

Fnded: 1940. **Desc:** Certification board to investigate qualifications of, administer examinations to, and certify as diplomates medical doctors specializing in neurological surgery. Works to stimulate development of adequate training facilities and aids in evaluating residencies under consideration by the Accreditation Council on Graduate Medical Education of the American Medical Association. **Pub:** *Newsletter to Diplomates*, annual. Newsletter. *Price:* Free.

★ 488 ★ American Board of Neuroscience Nursing (ABNN)

4700 W Lake Ave.
Glenview, IL 60025
Phone: (847)375-4733 **Free:** 888-557-2266
Fax: 877-734-8677
Email: info@aann.org
Website: http://www.AANN.org
Louise S. Miller, Dir. of Certification

Fnded: 1978. **Mem:** 1,500. **Desc:** Certifying body for registered nurses who have passed a written examination demonstrating achievement in neuroscience nursing. Objective is to promote excellence in the field by encouraging professional growth and individual study; granting neuroscience nursing certification; measuring knowledge and level of theory required for certification; establishing certification standards. Administers certifying examination. **Frmly:** (1984) Neurosurgical Nurses.

★ 489 ★ American Board of Nuclear Medicine (ABNM)

900 Veteran Ave., Rm. 13-152
Los Angeles, CA 90024-2703
Phone: (310)825-6787 **Fax:** (310)794-4821
Website: http://www.abnm.org
Lawrence E. Holder, MD, Ch.

Fnded: 1971. **Mem:** 12. **Desc:** A primary medical specialty board and member of the American Board of Medical Specialties. Provides educational standards and evaluates the competence of physicians in nuclear medicine; establishes requirements for certification. Conducts examinations and issues certification. Maintains registry of certificate holders. Aids in the assessment and accreditation of nuclear medicine programs in hospitals and institutions offering graduate training. **Pub:** *American Board of Nuclear Medicine Information, Policies and Procedures*, annual. Brochure. Provides information on the annual certifying examination. *Price:* Free.

★ 490 ★ American Board of Nursing Specialties (ABNS)

610 Thornhill Ln.
Aurora, OH 44202
Phone: (330)995-9172 **Fax:** (330)995-9743
Email: EDatABNS@aol.com
Website: http://www.nursingcertification.org
Sharon Kemerer, Pres.

Fnded: 1991. **Mem:** 25. **Desc:** National nursing certification boards and nursing organizations concerned with nursing credential issues. National peer review program for specialty nursing certification bodies.

★ 491 ★ American Board of Nutrition (ABN)

University of Alabama at Birmingham
1675 University Blvd./WEBB 232
Department of Nutrition Sciences
Birmingham, AL 35294-3360
Phone: (205)975-5564 **Fax:** (205)934-7049
Email: joness@shrp.uab.edu
Website: http://www.uab.edu/nusc/abn.htm
Donna Swaggerty, Contact

Fnded: 1948. **Mem:** 524. **Desc:** Physicians qualified to treat nutritional and metabolic disorders; doctoral recipients working on problems of human nutrition and nutrient requirements. Establishes standards for qualification of persons as specialists in the field of clinical human nutrition; holds examinations and certifies those who meet its qualifications. **Pub:** *Directory of Diplomates in Human Nutrition and Clinical Nutrition*, biennial. Directory. *Price:* Free.

★ 492 ★ American Board of Obstetrics and Gynecology (ABOG)

2915 Vine St.
Dallas, TX 75204
Phone: (214)871-1619 **Fax:** (214)871-1943
Email: info@abog.org
Website: http://www.abog.org
Norman F. Gant, MD, Exec. Dir.

Fnded: 1930. **Mem:** 35,277. **Desc:** Certification board to establish qualifications, conduct examinations, and certify as diplomates those doctors whom the board finds qualified to specialize in obstetrics and gynecology. **Pub:** Bulletin, annual.

★ 493 ★ American Board for Occupational Health Nurses (ABOHN)

201 E Ogden Ave., Ste. 114
Hinsdale, IL 60521-3652
Phone: (630)789-5799 **Free:** 888-842-2646
Fax: (630)789-8901
Email: info@abohn.org
Website: http://www.abohn.org
Mary Amann, RN,MSN, Exec. Dir.

Fnded: 1972. **Mem:** 6,600. **Desc:** Occupational health nurses. Establishes standards and confers initial and ongoing certification in occupational health nursing. Conducts semiannual certification examination. **Pub:** *The ABOHN Report*, semiannual. Newsletter. • *Directory of Certified Occupational Health Nurses*, annual. Directory. Contains contact information for certified occupational health nurses. • *Reference Guide for Examination Preparation*. • Also publishes position papers on occupational health nursing issues.

★ 494 ★ American Board of Ophthalmology (ABO)

111 Presidential Blvd., Ste. 241
Bala Cynwyd, PA 19004-1075
Phone: (610)664-1175 **Fax:** (610)664-6503
Email: info@abop.org
Website: http://www.abop.org
Denis O'Day, MD, Exec. Dir.

Fnded: 1916. **Mem:** 17. **Desc:** Medical specialty board to determine the adequacy of training, the professional preparation, and ophthalmic knowledge of ophthalmologists who wish to be certified. Works to improve the standards of graduate medical education and the facilities for special ophthalmic training. **Pub:** *Qualifications Brochure*, annual. Brochure. **Frmly:** (1933) American Board for Ophthalmic Examinations.

★ 495 ★ American Board of Opticianry (ABO)

6506 Loisdale Rd., Ste. 209
Springfield, VA 22150-1815
Phone: (703)719-5800 **Free:** 800-296-1379
Fax: (703)719-9144
Email: mail@abo-ncle.org
Website: http://www.abo.org
Michael H. Robey, Exec. Dir.

Fnded: 1979. **Mem:** 38,000. **Desc:** Provides uniform standards for dispensing opticians by administering the National Opticianry Competency Examination and by issuing the Certified Optician Certificate to those passing the exam. Also administers the Master in Ophthalmic Optics Examination and issues certificates to opticians at the advanced level passing the exam. Maintains records of persons certified for competency in eyeglass dispensing. Adopts and enforces continuing education requirements; assists and encourages state licensing boards in the use of the National Opticianry Competency Examination for licensure purposes.

★ 496 ★ American Board of Oral and Maxillofacial Pathology

625 N Michigan Ave., No. 1820
Chicago, IL 60611
Phone: (312)642-0070 **Fax:** (312)642-8584
Email: cefilas@aboms.org
Website: http://www.aboms.org/
Cheryl E. Mounts, Exec. Sec.

Fnded: 1948. **Mem:** 260. **Desc:** Works to encourage the study and promote and improve the practice of oral pathology; arrange, conduct, and control examinations to determine the competence of applicants; grant and issue certificates. **Frmly:** American Board of Oral Pathology.

★ 497 ★ American Board of Oral and Maxillofacial Surgery (ABOMS)
625 N Michigan Ave., Ste. 1820
Chicago, IL 60611
Phone: (312)642-0070 **Fax:** (312)642-8584
Email: CPena@aboms.org
Website: http://www.aboms.org
James R. Hupp, DDS, Pres.

Fnded: 1946. **Mem:** 3,580. **Desc:** Certification board to establish qualifications, conduct examinations, and certify surgeons whom the board finds qualified to practice oral and maxillofacial medicine, including diagnostic, surgical, and adjunctive treatment of the diseases, injuries, and defects of the oral and maxillofacial regions. **Frmly:** (1978) American Board of Oral Surgery.

★ 498 ★ American Board of Orthodontics (ABO)
401 N Lindbergh Blvd., Ste. 308
Saint Louis, MO 63141
Phone: (314)432-6130 **Fax:** (314)432-8170
Email: info@americanboardortho.com
Website: http://www.americanboardortho.com
Christine L. Eisenmayer, Exec. Sec.

Fnded: 1929. **Nat'l Groups:** 1. **Reg. Groups:** 8. **Desc:** Certification board to investigate the qualifications of, administer examinations to, and certify as diplomats dentists specializing in orthodontics (prevention and correction of irregularities and faulty positions of the teeth). Sponsored by the American Association of Orthodontists. **Frmly:** (1938) American Board of Orthodontia.

★ 499 ★ American Board of Orthopaedic Surgery (ABOS)
400 Silver Cedar Ct.
Chapel Hill, NC 27514
Phone: (919)929-7103 **Fax:** (919)942-8988
Website: http://www.abos.org
Dr. G. Paul DeRosa, Exec. Dir.

Fnded: 1934. **Mem:** 12. **Desc:** Certification board to establish qualifications, conduct annual examinations, and certify as diplomates those whom the board finds qualified to practice orthopaedic surgery. **Pub:** *Directory of Diplomates*, annual. Directory. *Price:* $25 plus shipping and handling.

★ 500 ★ American Board of Otolaryngology (ABO)
3050 Post Oak Blvd. Ste.1700
Houston, TX 77056
Phone: (713)850-0399 **Fax:** (713)850-1104
Email: czw@aboto.org
Website: http://www.aboto.org
Gerald B. Healy, MD, Exec. VP

Fnded: 1924. **Desc:** Purposes are to: elevate standards of practice in otolaryngology (the medical specialty dealing with ear, nose, throat, head, and neck surgery); hold examinations and certify qualified otolaryngologists; advance the cause of the field. Conducts annual in-training, written and oral examinations. **Pub:** Newsletter, semiannual.

★ 501 ★ American Board of Pain Medicine
4700 W Lake Ave.
Glenview, IL 60025-1485
Phone: (847)375-4726 **Fax:** (847)375-6326
Email: info@abpm.org
Website: http://www.abpm.org
Michael Decker, Pres.

Fnded: 1991. **Mem:** 1,335. **Desc:** Develops and administers practice-related examinations in the field of pain medicine. Awards certification to physicians successfully completing the examination and credentialing process. **Frmly:** American College of Pain Medicine.

★ 502 ★ American Board of Pathology (ABP)
PO Box 25915
Tampa, FL 33622-5915
Phone: (813)286-2444 **Fax:** (813)289-5279
Website: http://www.abpath.org/
William H. Hartmann, MD, Exec. VP

Fnded: 1936. **Mem:** 12. **Desc:** Seeks to: encourage study of pathology; maintain profesional standards and advance practice in the field; maintain registry of certified pathologists; participate in the evaluation and review of graduate medical education programs in pathology. Examines doctors of medicine or osteopathy who have had three to five years postgraduate training in laboratory medicine and pathology. Certifies qualified and successful applicants as specialists in pathology. **Pub:** *The American Board of Pathology*, 2-3/year. Newsletter. • *Information Booklet*, annual. Booklet.

★ 503 ★ American Board of Pediatric Dentistry (ABPD)
325 E Washington St., Ste. 101
Iowa City, IA 52240
Phone: (319)341-8488 **Free:** 800-410-1250
Fax: (319)341-9499
Email: info@abpd.org
Website: http://www.abpd.org
Arthur Nowak, DMD, Exec. Dir.

Fnded: 1940. **Mem:** 1,222. **Desc:** Certification board whose purpose is to investigate the qualifications of, administer examinations to, and certify as diplomates, dentists specializing in the care of children. Sponsored by American Academy of Pediatric Dentistry. **Pub:** *Directory of Diplomates*, biennial. Directory. Lists all board certified pediatric dentists. *Price:* $28. **Frmly:** (1986) American Board of Pedodontics.

★ 504 ★ American Board of Pediatrics (ABP)
111 Silver Cedar Ct.
Chapel Hill, NC 27514
Phone: (919)929-0461 **Fax:** (919)929-9255
Email: abpeds@abpeds.org
Website: http://www.abp.org
James A. Stockman, MD, Pres.

Fnded: 1933. **Mem:** 250. **Desc:** Certification board to establish qualifications, conduct examinations, and certify as diplomates those whom the board finds qualified as specialists in pediatrics. **Pub:** *American Board of Pediatrics–Booklet of Information*, annual. Booklet. Outlines requirements for admission to certifying examinations; includes details of examinations. *Price:* Free. • *American Board of Pediatrics–Informal Newsletter to Members*, periodic. Newsletter. • *American Board of Pediatrics–Newsletter for Diplomates*, annual. Newsletter. *Price:* Free. • *Newsletter to Pediatric Training Program Directors*. Newsletter. *Price:* Free.

★ 505 ★ American Board of Perianesthesia Nursing Certification (ABPANC)
475 Riverside Dr., 6th Fl.
New York, NY 10115-0089
Phone: (212)367-4253 **Free:** 800-622-7262
Fax: (212)367-4256
Email: abpanc@proexam.org
Website: http://www.cpancapa.org
Bonnie Niebuhr, MS, RN, CAE, Exec. Dir.

Fnded: 1985. **Desc:** Administers examination to individuals wishing to attain perianesthesia nursing certification. **Pub:** *Certification Newsletter*. Newsletter. *Price:* Free.

★ 506 ★ American Board of Periodontology (ABP)
4157 Mountain Rd.
PBN 249
Pasadena, MD 21122
Phone: (410)437-3749 **Fax:** (410)437-4021
Email: abperio@msn.com
Website: http://www.perio.org/amboard
Dr. Gerald Bowers, Contact

Fnded: 1939. **Mem:** 1,500. **Desc:** Conducts examinations to determine the qualifications and competence of periodontists who voluntarily apply for certification as diplomates in the field of periodontology. Maintains registry of holders of diplomate certificates.

★ 507 ★ American Board of Physical Medicine and Rehabilitation (ABPMR)
21 1st St. SW, Ste. 674
Rochester, MN 55902-3092
Phone: (507)282-1776 **Fax:** (507)282-9242
Email: info@abpmr.org
Website: http://www.abpmr.org/
Nicholas E. Walsh, MD, Chair

Fnded: 1947. **Mem:** 6,515. **Desc:** Certification board to establish qualifications, conduct examinations, and certify physicians who have completed the requirements in physical medicine and rehabilitation. **Pub:** Booklet, annual. *Price:* Free.

★ 508 ★ American Board of Plastic Surgery (ABPS)
7 Penn Center, Ste. 400
1635 Market St.
Philadelphia, PA 19103-2204
Phone: (215)587-9322 **Fax:** (215)587-9622
Email: info@abplsurg.org
Website: http://www.abplsurg.org
Dr. R. Barrett Noone, Exec. Dir.

Fnded: 1937. **Mem:** 20. **Desc:** Certification board established to investigate the qualifications of, administer examinations to, and certify as diplomates medical doctors specializing in the entire field of plastic and reconstructive surgery. **Pub:** *Booklet of Information*, annual.

★ 509 ★ American Board of Podiatric Orthopedics and Primary Podiatric Medicine (ABPOPPM)
22910 Crenshaw Blvd., Ste. B
Torrance, CA 90505
Phone: (310)891-0100 **Fax:** (310)891-0500
Email: admin@abpoppm.org
Website: http://www.abpoppm.org/
Gerald A. Weber, DPM, Pres.

Fnded: 1975. **Mem:** 3,000. **Desc:** Podiatrists who have taken a competency exam prepared by the board. Offers certifying examinations in podiatric orthopedics and primary podiatric medicine aims at improving public health by encouraging and elevating standards for practicing podiatrics. **Pub:** *ABPOPPM Newsletter*, semiannual. Newsletter. *Price:* Free w/ membership. • *Directory of Diplomates*, annual. Membership Directory. Includes alphabetical and geographical listing of members. *Price:* Free. **Frmly:** American Board of Podiatric Orthopedics; (2003) American Board of Podiatric Orthopedics and Primary Medicine.

★ 510 ★ American Board of Podiatric Surgery (ABPS)
445 Fillmore St.
San Francisco, CA 94117-3404
Phone: (415)553-7800 **Fax:** (415)553-7801
Email: info@abps.org
Website: http://www.abps.org
James A. Lamb, Exec. Dir.

Fnded: 1975. **Mem:** 5,800. **Desc:** Podiatrists certified as diplomates. Objectives are: to protect and improve public health by advancing the science of foot surgery and by encouraging the study and evaluation of standards of foot surgery; to act upon application for certification of legally licensed podiatrists to ascertain their competency in foot surgery; to grant certificates to candidates who have met all qualifications.

★ 511 ★ American Board of Preventive Medicine (ABPM)
330 S Wells St., Ste. 1018
Chicago, IL 60606
Phone: (312)939-2276 **Fax:** (312)939-2218
Email: abpm@abprevmed.org
Website: http://www.abprevmed.org
James M. Vanderploeg, MD,MPH, Exec. Dir.

Fnded: 1948. **Mem:** 11. **Desc:** Determines requirements, administers examinations, and certifies qualified physicians in the specialty areas of public health and general preventive medicine, aerospace medicine, and occupational medicine. **Pub:** *ABPM Booklet of Information*. Booklet. Covers board requirements. *Price:* Free. • *Study Guide*. Includes outlines of examinations. **Frmly:** (1952) American Board of Preventive Medicine and Public Health.

★ 512 ★ American Board of Professional Neuropsychology
John Heinz Institute of Rehabilitation Medicine
150 Mundy St.
Wilkes Barre Township, PA 18702
Phone: (570)826-3771 **Fax:** (570)826-3898
Website: http://abpn.net
Michael J. Raymond, PhD., Exec. Sec.

Desc: Professional neuropsychologists.

★ 513 ★ American Board of Professional Psychology (ABPP)
514 E Capitol Ave.
Jefferson City, MO 65101-3008
Phone: (573)634-5607 **Free:** 800-255-7792
Fax: (573)634-7157
Email: office@abpp.org
Website: http://www.abpp.org
Ted Packard, PhD, Pres.

Fnded: 1947. **Mem:** 3,950. **Nat'l Groups:** 11. **Desc:** Certification board which conducts oral examinations and awards diplomas to advanced specialists in 11 professional specialties: psychoamalysis, rehabilitation psycholgy, behavioral psychology, clinical psychology, industrial and organizational psychology, forensic psychology, counseling psychology, clinical neuropsychology, family psychology, health psychology, and school psychology. Candidates must have three years of qualifying experience in psychological practice. **Pub:** *American Board of Professional Psychology–Diplomat*, semiannual. Newsletter. *Price:* Included in membership dues. • *Directory of Diplomats*, biennial. Directory. • *Manual for Oral Examinations*, annual. • *Policies and Procedures*, annual. **Frmly:** (1968) American Board of Examiners in Professional Psychology.

★ 514 ★ American Board of Prosthodontics (ABP)
PO Box 271894
West Hartford, CT 06127
Phone: (860)679-2649 **Fax:** (860)679-1370
Email: ttaylor@nso.uchc.edu
Website: http://www.prosthodontics.org/abp
Dr. Thomas D. Taylor, Exec. Dir.

Desc: Seeks to advance the science and art of prosthodontics by encouraging its study and improving its practice. Certifies dentists who specialize in the field of fixed, removable, and maxillofacial prosthodontics. Approved by the American Dental Association and the Council on Dental Education.

★ 515 ★ American Board of Psychiatry and Neurology (ABPN)
500 Lake Cook Rd., Ste. 335
Deerfield, IL 60015-5249
Phone: (847)945-7900 **Fax:** (847)945-1146
Email: webmaster@abpn.com
Website: http://www.abpn.com
Edgar J. Kenton, III, Pres.

Fnded: 1934. **Desc:** Physicians with specialized training in psychiatry, neurology, child neurology, child adolescent psychiatry, clinical neurophysiology, and geriatric psychiatry. Determines eligibility requirements, administers examinations, and certifies physicians.

★ 516 ★ American Board of Psychological Hypnosis (ABPH)
c/o Samuel M. Migdole, Ed.D., ABPH
North Shore Counseling Center
23 Broadway
Beverly, MA 01915
Phone: (978)922-2280 **Fax:** (978)927-1758
Email: pres.abph@prodigy.net
Samuel M. Migdole, Ed.D., Pres.

Fnded: 1959. **Desc:** Awards specialty diplomas to qualified licensed doctoral level psychologists in experimental and clinical hypnosis. Purpose is to raise the standards of individuals conducting research in hypnosis and those using it in clinical practice by requiring specialized training and experience in the field as evidenced by advanced educational credentials in psychology, published research, written and oral examinations, and recommendations of colleagues. **Frmly:** American Board of Examiners in Psychological Hypnosis; American Board of Professional Psychology in Hypnosis.

★ 517 ★ American Board of Quality Assurance and Utilization Review Physicians (ABQAURP)
2120 Range Rd.
Clearwater, FL 33765-2125
Phone: (727)298-8777 **Free:** 800-998-6030
Fax: (727)449-0555
Email: abqaurp@abqaurp.org
Website: http://www.abqaurp.org
Arthur I. Border, MD, Chair

Fnded: 1977. **Mem:** 6,351. **Desc:** Seeks to maintain and improve the process of health care quality and management through development, administration, and supervision of a certification program in the field. Provides continuing education for physicians, RNs and other health care professionals and makes available study material. **Pub:** *Diplomat Focus*, quarterly. Newsletter. Contains information on ABQAURP and issues important to diplomats. *Price:* Free with diplomat status. • *Journal of Quality Health Care*, quarterly. Journal. Contains information on ABQAURP and issues important to diplomats. *Price:* included in membership dues; $49 subscription. • Books.

★ 518 ★ American Board of Radiology (ABR)
5441 E Williams Blvd., Ste. 200
Tucson, AZ 85711
Phone: (520)790-2900 **Fax:** (520)790-3200
Email: info@theabr.org
Website: http://www.theabr.org/
Dr. Robert R. Hattery, Exec. Dir.

Fnded: 1934. **Mem:** 23. **Desc:** Certification board to establish qualifications, conduct examinations, and certify physicians in the specialty of radiation oncology, diagnostic radiology and radiological physics (science dealing with X-rays or rays from radioactive substances for medical use). **Pub:** Booklets.On examinations in diagnostic radiology, radiological physics, radiation oncology, special competence in nuclear radiology, subspecialty radiology.

★ 519 ★ American Board of Registration of EEG and EP Technologists (ABRET)
1904 Croyden Dr.
Springfield, IL 62703
Phone: (217)553-3758 **Fax:** (217)585-6663
Email: abreteo@aol.com
Website: http://www.abret.org
Janice Walbert, Exec. Dir.

Fnded: 1964. **Desc:** Determines the competency of electroneurodiagnostic technologists through administration of written and oral examinations. **Frmly:** (1992) American Board of Registration of EEG Technologists.

★ 520 ★ American Board of Science in Nuclear Medicine (ABSNM)
c/o Sandra Fenton
1850 Samuel Morse Dr.
Reston, VA 20190
Phone: (703)708-9000 **Fax:** (703)708-9013
Email: vpappas@snm.org
Website: http://www.absnm.org
Virginia Pappas, Contact

Fnded: 1976. **Desc:** Certifies scientists in nuclear medicine; promotes nuclear medicine science, including nuclear medicine physics and instrumentation, nuclear pharmaceutical science, radiochemistry and radiation protection.

★ 521 ★ American Board of Sleep Medicine
One Westbrook Corporate Ctr., Ste. 920
Westchester, IL 60154
Phone: (708)492-1290 **Fax:** (708)492-0943
Website: http://www.absm.org/
Joshua N. Aaron, Contact

Fnded: 1991. **Desc:** Works to encourage the study and elevate the standards of sleep medicine. Offers certification in sleep medicine to licensed physicians and individuals with Ph.D.s in health related fields. **Pub:** Brochure.Contains information for applicants.

★ 522 ★ American Board of Surgery (ABS)
1617 John F. Kennedy Blvd., Ste. 860
Philadelphia, PA 19103
Phone: (215)568-4000 **Fax:** (215)563-5718
Website: http://www.absurgery.org
Dr. Wallace P. Ritchie, Jr., Exec. Dir.

Fnded: 1937. **Mem:** 29. **Desc:** Examining and certifying board in general surgery; also certifies in Pediatric Surgery, Vascular Surgery, Surgical Critical Care, and Hand Surgery. Membership is drawn from 23 national and regional surgical and specialty societies and organizations. Currently offers Recertification in General Surgery, Pediatric Surgery, Vascular Surgery, and Surgical Critical Care. **Pub:** *ABMS Directories of Certified Specialists*. Directory. • *Directory of Medical Specialists*. • *Service Booklets of Information*, annual.

★ 523 ★ American Board of Thoracic Surgery (ABTS)
1 Rotary Center, Ste. 803
Evanston, IL 60201
Phone: (847)475-1520 **Fax:** (847)475-6240
Email: abts_evanston@msn.com
Website: http://www.abts.org/
William A. Gay, Jr. MD, Sec. -Treas.

Fnded: 1948. **Desc:** Medical certification board that certifies surgeons specializing in thoracic surgery. **Frmly:** Board of Thoracic Surgery.

★ 524 ★ American Board of Tropical Medicine (ABTM)
PO Box 24224
Detroit, MI 48224
Phone: (313)882-0641 **Fax:** (313)882-5110
Dr. Ben Alli, Assoc. Dir.

Fnded: 1980. **Mem:** 2,100. **State Groups:** 2. **Desc:** Physicians including pediatricians, dermatologists, surgeons, professionals of public health and preventive medicine, and pathologists interested in tropical medicine. United to preserve the quality of care in tropical medicine. Investigates qualifications and determines the competency of candidates applying for membership and provides continuing medical education programs to specialists in tropical medicine. Issues certificate as evidence of meeting continuing medical education requirements. Compiles statistics. **Pub:** Newsletter, annual. *Price:* $100. • Publishes *Directory of Specialists in Tropical Medicine*. **AKA:** American College of Tropical Medicine.

★ 525 ★ American Board of Urology (ABU)
2216 Ivy Rd., Ste. 210
Charlottesville, VA 22903
Phone: (434)979-0059 **Fax:** (434)979-0266
Website: http://www.abu.org
Stuart S. Howards, MD, Exec. Sec.

Fnded: 1935. **Mem:** 12. **Desc:** Conducts examinations and certifies physicians in the specialty of urology (branch of medicine that is concerned with the genito-urinary tract). **Pub:** *Information for Applicants and Candidates*, annual. Handbook. Includes certification details and schedule of exams. *Price:* Free.

★ 526 ★ American Board of Veterinary Practitioners (ABVP)
200 4th Ave. N, Ste. 900
Nashville, TN 37219
Phone: (615)254-3687 **Fax:** (615)254-7047
Email: abvp@walkermgt.com
Website: http://www.abvp.com
Dee Ann Walker, CAE, Exec. Officer

Fnded: 1978. **Mem:** 750. **Desc:** Veterinarians. Seeks to recognize excellence in clinical, species-oriented specialty practice. Works to insure delivery of superior, comprehensive, multidisciplinary veterinary services. Confers certification; conducts educational programs. **Pub:** *ABVP News*, quarterly. Newsletter. Includes directory.

★ 527 ★ American Board of Veterinary Specialties (ABVS)
c/o American Veterinary Medical Association
1931 N Meacham Rd., Ste. 100
Schaumburg, IL 60173-4360
Phone: (847)925-8070 **Fax:** (847)925-1329
Email: avmainfo@avma.org
Website: http://www.avma.org
Beth A. Sabin, DVM, Asst. Dir.,Educ. &Res.

Fnded: 1959. **Mem:** 22. **Desc:** A board of the American Veterinary Medical Association. Organization of veterinarians with advanced training in one or more specialty areas of veterinary practice, research, or study whose purpose is to recognize and supervise organizations that provide certification to qualified specialists. **Pub:** *Policies and Procedures Manual*, periodic. Manual. *Price:* First copy free; $1/additional copy. **Frmly:** Advisory Board on Veterinary Specialties.

★ 528 ★ American Board of Veterinary Toxicology (ABVT)
School of Veterinary Medicine
382 W St. Rd.
Kennett Square, PA 19348
Phone: (610)444-5800 **Fax:** (610)925-8117
Email: roder@cox-internet.com
Website: http://www.abvt.org
Robert H. Poppenga, Pres.

Fnded: 1967. **Mem:** 100. **Desc:** Seeks to: further education and scientific progress in veterinary toxicology; encourage research and training; establish and maintain the highest possible standards of training and experience for qualification in toxicology; recognize qualified specialists through certification. Conducts annual examination. **Pub:** *American Board of Veterinary Toxicology–Directory of Diplomates*, annual. Directory. Lists diplomates certified as veterinary toxicologists by the board.

★ 529 ★ American Bone Marrow Donor Registry (ABMDR)
PO Box 8841
Mandeville, LA 70470-8841
Phone: (504)626-1749 **Free:** 800-745-2452
Fax: (504)626-7414
Email: jakardna@neosoft.com
Website: http://www.abmdr.org
Joan Keller, Dir.

Fnded: 1984. **Desc:** Committed to keeping donor files accessible to any medically viable candidate for a marrow transplant being treated at an accredited bone marrow transplant center.

★ 530 ★ American Brain Tumor Association (ABTA)
2720 River Rd., Ste. 146
Des Plaines, IL 60018
Phone: (847)827-9910 **Free:** 800-886-2282
Fax: (847)827-9918
Email: info@abta.org
Website: http://www.abta.org
Naomi Berkowitz, Exec. Dir.

Fnded: 1973. **Desc:** Seeks to eliminate brain tumors through research and meet the needs of brain tumor patients and their families. **Pub:** *Building Knowledge Series*. Pamphlets. A Brain Tumor-Sharing Hope (also in Spanish); Dictionary for Brain Tumor patients; Living with a Brain Tumor; A Primer of Brain Tumors. *Price:* Free. • *Connections - A Pen Pal Program*. Pamphlet. • *Focusing on Treatment Series*. Pamphlets. Pamphlet titles include: Gene Therapy; Radiation Therapy of Brain Tumors: A Basic Guide; Stereotactic Radiosurgery. • *Focusing on Tumors Series*. Pamphlets. Ependymoma; Glioblastoma Multiforme & Anaplastic Astrocytoma; Medullobblastoma; Meningioma; Metastatic Brain Tumors; Oligodendroglioma. • *For & About Children Series*. Pamphlets. Titles include: Alex's Journey: The Story of a Child with a Brain Tumor for ages 9-13, video and booklet format; When Your Child Returns to School. **Frmly:** (1992) Association for Brain Tumor Research.

★ 531 ★ American Broncho-Esophagological Association (ABEA)
c/o Kim Davis, MD, Sec.
Division of Otolaryngology
University of Utah
50 N Medical Cr., 3C120SOM
Salt Lake City, UT 84132-0002
Phone: (801)587-7678 **Fax:** (801)585-5744
Email: peak.woo@mountsinai.org
Website: http://www.abea.net/
Peak Woo, Pres.

Fnded: 1917. **Mem:** 386. **Desc:** Professional society of otolaryngologists, chest specialists, thoracic surgeons, and gastroenterologists engaged in the practice of broncho-esophagology (diseases and injuries of the respiratory system and upper digestive tract). Conducts program on study of foreign bodies. **Pub:** *Annals of Otology, Rhinology and Laryngology*. Proceedings. • *Transactions*, annual. **Frmly:** (1928) American Bronchoscopic Society.

★ 532 ★ American Bureau for Medical Advancement in China (ABMAC)
45 John St. No.1100
New York, NY 10038
Phone: (212)233-0608 **Fax:** (212)233-0614
Email: phyllis@abmac.org
Website: http://www.abmac.org
Phyllis Scarnozzino, Exec. Dir.

Fnded: 1937. **Mem:** 52. **Desc:** Cooperates with medical and health personnel to support a broad program of medical and health services for the Chinese people. Provides, upon request from Republic of China institutions, consultants for development projects and visiting specialists for longer term teaching and clinical assignments in Taiwan. Sponsors Republic of China postgraduate fellowships for study, research, and observation in the U.S. Organizes research projects for treatment of diseases prevalent in Southeast Asia. Offers placement services for Chinese doctors and nurses interested in postgraduate study in the U.S.

★ 533 ★ American Burn Association (ABA)
c/o National Headquarters Office
625 N Michigan Ave., Ste. 1530
Chicago, IL 60611
Phone: (312)642-9260 **Free:** 800-548-2876
Fax: (312)642-9130
Email: info@ameriburn.org
Website: http://www.ameriburn.org
Marion H. Jordan, MD, Pres.

Fnded: 1967. **Mem:** 3,500. **Desc:** Physicians, nurses, physical therapists, occupational therapists, dietitians, biomedical engineers, social service workers, and researchers interested in the care of burn injuries. Objective is the improvement of the care and treatment of burns, which includes a program of prevention of burn injuries. Sponsors visiting professorship, education, and awards. **Pub:** *American Burn Association–Book of Abstracts*, annual. Journal. *Price:* Included in membership dues; $15/copy for nonmembers. • *American Burn Association–Membership Directory*, annual. Directory. *Price:* Included in membership dues. • *Burn Care Services in North America*, annual. Directory. Lists specialized burn care facilities in the United States and Canada. *Price:* Included in membership dues; $50/copy for nonmembers. • *Journal of Burn Care and Rehabilitation*, bimonthly. Journal. Covers burn injuries and their treatment. Includes a list of employment opportunities, research reports, and statistics. *Price:* Included in membership dues; $35/year for nonmembers; $52/year for institutions.

★ 534 ★ American Cancer Society (ACS)
2200 Century Pky., Ste. 950
Atlanta, GA 30345
Phone: (404)816-4994 **Free:** 800-ACS-2345
Fax: (404)315-9348
Website: http://www.cancer.org
John R. Seffrin, PhD, CEO

Fnded: 1913. **Reg. Groups:** 17. **Local Groups:** 3400. **Desc:** The American Cancer Society is the nationwide, community-based, voluntary health organization dedicated to eliminating cancer as a major health problem by preventing cancer, saving lives and diminishing suffering from cancer, through research, education, advocacy, and service. **Pub:** *American Cancer Society*. Annual Report. *Price:* Free. • *CA-A Cancer Journal for Clinicians*, bimonthly. Covers cancer treatment, prevention, and diagnosis. *Price:* Free for health professionals. • *Cancer*, semimonthly. Medical journal covering cancer prevention, research, diagnosis, and treatment. Includes proceedings supplements covering ACS conferences. *Price:* $219/year for individuals; $437/year for institutions. • *Cancer Facts and Figures*, annual. Report providing statistical information on the major sites of cancer including incidence, mortality and survival rates, and risk factors. *Price:* Free. **Frmly:** (1944) American Society for the Control Cancer.

★ 535 ★ American Canine Sports Medicine Association (ACSMA)
PO Box 82433
Baton Rouge, LA 70884
Email: postmaster@acsma.org
Website: http://www.acsma.org
Robert L. Gillette, Contact

Fnded: 1991. **Mem:** 200. **Desc:** Promotes interests of members. Conducts research and educational programs. **Pub:** *Newsletter of the ACSMA*, quarterly. Newsletter. *Price:* Included in membership dues.

★ 536 ★ American Celiac Society/Dietary Support Coalition (ACS/DSC)
PO Box 23455
New Orleans, LA 70183
Phone: (973)325-8837 **Fax:** (973)669-8808
Email: amerceliacsoc@netscape.net
Annette Bentley, Exec. Off.

Fnded: 1970. **Mem:** 7,000. **Nat'l Groups:** 4. **Reg. Groups:** 76. **Local Groups:** 57. **Desc:** Individuals interested in a gluten-free diet; physicians who diagnose and care for individuals with gluten-sensitive intestinal disease, dietitians, nutritionists, and agencies that serve or have an interest in individuals with gluten-sensitive enteropathy, also known as celiac sprue. Provides information on how to follow a gluten-free diet; assists members in locating specialty foods that are gluten-free; encourages retailers to make gluten-free products available. Coordinates activities with other international celiac societies. Maintains speakers' bureau for patients and health care professionals. **Pub:** *Whoo's Report*, 3/year. Newsletter. **Frmly:** (1990) America Celiac Society.

★ 537 ★ American Center for the Alexander Technique (ACAT)

39 W 14th St. No. 507
New York, NY 10011
Phone: (212)633-2229
Email: acatusa@aol.com
Website: http://www.acatnyc.org
Jane Tomkiewicz, Exec. Dir.

Fnded: 1964. **Mem:** 100. **Desc:** Promotes the Alexander Technique, an educational technique that enables individuals to use their bodies with ease, grace, flexibility, and freedom from strain in any physical activity. Formed to assure further development of the technique in this country and to maintain its standards. Answers requests for information and refers interested people to certified teachers. Sponsors Teacher Certification Program consisting of 1600 hours over nine ten-week terms, the last a teaching apprenticeship, to certify students who have demonstrated, to the satisfaction of the faculty, a high standard both of teaching skills and of personal use. **Pub:** *ACAT News*, periodic. Newsletter. • *Annual Certified Member/Teacher List*.

★ 538 ★ American Central European Dental Institute (ACEDI)

60 Federal St.
Boston, MA 02110-2510
Phone: (617)423-6165 **Fax:** (617)426-0006
Email: info@watkinosorio.com
Dr. Arnold Watkin, Chm.

Fnded: 1991. **Mem:** 2. **Desc:** Dentists and others serving in capacities related to the dental profession. Seeks to advance standards in the profession of dentistry. Conducts educational programs; maintains speakers' bureau. **Pub:** *ACEDI*, annual. Newsletter.

★ 539 ★ American Chinese Pharmaceutical Association (ACPA)

PO Box 2623
Cherry Hill, NJ 08034
Phone: (609)394-6121
Email: clau@chsnj.org
Website: http://www.geocities.com/acpa_rx

Fnded: NNas. **Mem:** soci,ate. **Desc:** Pharmacists and pharmaceutical scientists. Seeks to advance the professional well being of pharmacists and pharmaceutical scientists of Chinese heritage; encourages exchange of ideas; provides educational opportunities; promotes health-related issues to the Chinese community. Encourages development of pharmacy practice in China, Taiwan, and Hong Kong. **Pub:** Newsletter, quarterly. Contains organization's events, activities and membership news. • Membership Directory.

★ 540 ★ American Chiropractic Association (ACA)

1701 Clarendon Blvd.
Arlington, VA 22209
Phone: (703)276-8800 **Free:** 800-986-4636
Fax: (703)243-2593
Email: memberinfo@amerchiro.org
Website: http://www.amerchiro.org
Garrett F. Cuneo, HCD, Exec. VP

Fnded: 1930. **Mem:** 18,000. **Desc:** Enhances the philosophy, science, and art of chiropractic, and the professional welfare of individuals in the field. Promotes legislation defining chiropractic health care and improves the public's awareness and utilization of chiropractic. Conducts chiropractic survey and statistical study; maintains library. Sponsors Correct Posture Week in May and Spinal Health Month in October. Chiropractic colleges have student ACA groups. **Pub:** *ACA/Today*, monthly. Newsletter. Covers the issues facing the profession and the association. *Price:* Included in membership dues. • *American Chiropractic Association Membership Directory*, annual. Directory. • *Journal of the American Chiropractic Association*, monthly. Journal. Provides information on the progress of chiropractic procedures and research, and developments in other fields of interest to chiropractors. *Price:* Included in membership dues; $3/year for student members; $80/year for nonmembers; $150/year for international members. **Frmly:** (1963) National Chiropractic Association.

★ 541 ★ American Chiropractic Association - Council on Sports Injuries and Physical Fitness (ACA)

303 Beach Dr.
Annapolis, MD 21403
Phone: (410)990-1112 **Free:** 800-593-3222
Fax: (410)990-1134
Website: http://www.acasc.org
Tim Ray, Pres.

Desc: Active chiropractors. Promotes the treatment of athletes; works closely with athletic organizations and health professionals to promote better understanding of chiropractic care as valuable in athletic training and treatment.

★ 542 ★ American Chiropractic College of Radiology (ACCR)

PO Box 1151
Lombard, IL 60148
Phone: (630)372-7260
Email: dacbr219@hotmail.com
Website: http://www.accr.org/
J. Todd Knudsen, Sec. /Treas.

Desc: Seeks to educate the chiropractic and health care communities.

★ 543 ★ American Chiropractic Registry of Radiologic Technologists (ACRRT)

2330 Gull Rd.
Kalamazoo, MI 49048
Phone: (616)343-6666 **Fax:** (616)343-7236
Website: http://www.acrrt.com
Dr. Edward Maurer, Exec. VP

Fnded: 1982. **Mem:** 2,000. **Desc:** Chiropractic assistants and radiologic technologists employed in chiropractic offices. Educates the general public concerning the importance of having highly skilled radiologic technologists (those who administer X-rays) in chiropractic offices. Serves as a national certifying agency for individuals in the field; maintains registry of certified chiropractic radiologic technologists. **Pub:** *Wavelengths*, bimonthly. Newsletter.

★ 544 ★ American Chronic Pain Association (ACPA)

PO Box 850
Rocklin, CA 95677
Phone: (916)632-0922 **Free:** 800-533-3231
Fax: (916)632-3208
Email: acpa@pacbell.net
Website: http://www.theacpa.org
Penney Cowan, Exec. Dir.

Fnded: 1980. **Nat'l Groups:** 450. **Desc:** Individuals suffering from chronic pain; health care professionals. Mutual support organization that works to help individuals suffering from chronic pain (pain lasting more than six months) learn positive ways to deal with pain and become involved in their own recovery. Fosters the managing of pain through methods such as exercise, assertiveness, self-awareness, and relaxation techniques. Consults with health care facilities in developing and upgrading pain management units; disseminates guidelines for selecting pain management facilities. (The organization stresses that it provides no medical advice or treatment.) Operates speakers' bureau; conducts charitable program. program. **Pub:** *ACPA Chronicle*, quarterly. Newsletter. • *ACPA Facilitation Guide*, periodic. Directory. Features how-tos for ACPA group development and ongoing resources. • *Family Manual*. A handbook for caregivers. • *From Patient to Person: First Steps*, periodic. • *Reflections of You*. A daily meditation and personal journal. • *Staying Well: Advanced Pain Management for Members Workbook*. Handbook.

★ 545 ★ American Cleft Palate-Craniofacial Association (ACPA)

104 S Estes Dr., Ste. 204
Chapel Hill, NC 27514-2866
Phone: (919)933-9044 **Fax:** (919)933-9604
Email: info@cleftpalate-craniofacial.org
Website: http://www.cleftpalate-craniofacial.org
Nancy Smythe, Exec. Dir.

Fnded: 1943. **Mem:** 2,700. **Desc:** Physicians, dentists, speech pathologists, audiologists, surgeons, psychologists, nurses and others surgeons actively engaged in the care of individuals with cleft lip and palate and associated craniofacial anomalies. Works to extend and improve the understanding of the scientific and clinical problems involved in the habilitation of patients with cleft lip and palate, and to stimulate professional and public interest in the field. Conducts educational programs. **Pub:** *American Cleft Palate-Craniofacial Association Membership and Team Directory*, annual. Membership Directory. *Price:* available to members only. • *American Cleft Palate-Craniofacial Association Newsletter*, quarterly. Newsletter. *Price:* Included in membership dues. • *Cleft Palate-Craniofacial Journal*, bimonthly. Journal. Includes research reports, book reviews, and commentaries. *Price:* Included in membership dues; $110 for nonmembers; $145 for institutions. **Frmly:** American Association for Cleft Palate Rehabilitation; (1949) American Academy of Cleft Palate Prosthesis; (1988) American Cleft Palate Association.

★ 546 ★ American Clinical and Climatological Association (ACCA)

Univ. of Cincinnati Medical Center
231 Albert Sabin Way
PO Box G70557
Cincinnati, OH 45267-0557
Phone: (513)558-4231 **Fax:** (513)558-0852
Dr. Robert Luke, Sec/Treas.

Fnded: 1884. **Mem:** 375. **Desc:** Internists interested in the clinical study of disease. **Pub:** *Transactions*, annual.

★ 547 ★ American Clinical Laboratory Association (ACLA)

1250 H St. NW, Ste. 880
Washington, DC 20005
Phone: (202)637-9466 **Fax:** (202)637-2050
Email: chawk@clinical-labs.org
Website: http://www.clinical-labs.org
David N. Sundwall, MD, Pres.

Fnded: 1971. **Desc:** Corporations, partnerships, or individuals owning or controlling one or more independent clinical laboratory facilities operating for a profit and licensed under the Clinical Laboratories Improvement Act of 1967 or the Clinical Laboratories Improvement Amendment of 1988, or accredited by the Medicare program. Promotes the development of uniformly high quality laboratory testing; eliminates the present inequalities in the standards applied to different segments of the clinical laboratory market; discourages the enactment of restrictive legislative or regulatory policies that may impede the free flow of commerce or operate to the detriment of the public. Examines federal and state health care and laboratory regulatory and legislative proposals and submi ts comments and opinions to the appropriate agencies or legislative bodies.

★ 548 ★ American Clinical Neurophysiology Society

PO Box 30
Bloomfield, CT 06002
Phone: (860)243-3977 **Fax:** (860)286-0787
Email: acns@ssmgt.com
Website: http://www.acns.org/
Jacquelyn T. Coleman, Exec. Dir.

Fnded: 1946. **Mem:** 1,450. **Desc:** Professional society of electroencephalographers and neurophysiologists. Offers clinical course annually. **Pub:** *Journal of Critical Neurophysiology*, bimonthly. Journal. **Frmly:** (1997) American Electroencephalographic Society.

★ 549 ★ American College of Addiction Treatment Administrators (ACATA)

c/o Ronald J. Hunsicker, D.Min.
313 W Liberty St., Ste. 129
Lancaster, PA 17603
Phone: (717)392-8480 **Fax:** (717)392-8481
Email: rhunsicker@naatp.org
Ronald Hunsicker, Pres. /CEO

Fnded: 1984. **Mem:** 250. **Desc:** Administrators of addiction treatment facilities. Promotes educational and professional standards in the field of addiction treatment administration. Encourages continuing education and training of members. Recognizes individuals who have provided outstanding service in the field. Seeks to educate members and the public on issues surrounding the administration of treatment programs. Sponsors workshops. **Pub:** *Visions*, monthly. Newsletter.

★ 550 ★ American College for Advancement in Medicine (ACAM)

23121 Verdugo Dr., Ste. 204
Laguna Hills, CA 92653
Phone: (949)583-7666 **Fax:** (949)455-9679
Email: acam@acam.org
Website: http://www.acam.org
Edward A. Shaw, PhD, Exec. Officer

Fnded: 1973. **Mem:** 535. **Desc:** Physicians organized for the promotion of preventive medicine throughout the world. Conducts research and educational programs in the fields of chelation therapy, nutritional medicine, and other preventive modalities. Maintains physician referrals. Offers specialized education program; compiles statistics. **Pub:** *ACAM Update*, monthly. Newsletter. Contains abstracts on issues and developments in preventive medicine. Includes book reviews and calendar of events. *Price:* Included in membership dues. • *Journal of Advancement in Medicine*, quarterly. Journal. Covers research and clinical applications pertaining to preventive and nutritional medicine. *Price:* Included in membership dues. • Membership Directory, annual. **Frmly:** (1987) American Academy of Medical Preventics.

★ 551 ★ American College of Allergy, Asthma and Immunology (ACAAI)

85 W Algonquin Rd., Ste. 550
Arlington Heights, IL 60005-4425
Phone: (847)427-1200 **Fax:** (847)427-1294
Email: mail@acaai.org
Website: http://www.allergy.mcg.edu
James R. Slawny, Exec. Dir.

Fnded: 1942. **Mem:** 4,300. **Desc:** Practicing allergists, educators, researchers, and clinical immunologists united to: encourage the study, improve the practice, and advance the cause of clinical immunology and allergy; promote association of and highest possible standards among medical scientists and physicians specializing in clinical immunology and in research, teaching, and treatment of allergy; promote dissemination of information regarding clinical immunology and allergy. Maintains a special program for allergy assistants such as nurses, technologists, and clinic aides of lectures, conferences, seminars, participatory workshops, peer-group discussions, poster programs, and technical and scientific exhibits. **Pub:** *ACAAI News*, bimonthly. Newsletter. • *Annals of Allergy, Asthma and Immunology*, 12/year. Journal. Includes original articles by experts in the field, abstracts, reviews, and editorials. *Price:* $50/year for individuals; $75/year for institutions; $78/year outside the U.S. • Membership Directory, biennial. **Frmly:** (1996) American College of Allergy and Immunology.

★ 552 ★ American College of Angiology (ACA)

295 Northern Blvd., Ste. 104
Great Neck, NY 11021-4701
Phone: (516)466-4055 **Fax:** (516)466-4099
Email: aca@collegeofangiology.org
Website: http://www.collegeofangiology.org
H. E. Shaftel, MD, Meeting Chm.

Fnded: 1959. **Mem:** 1,700. **Desc:** Scientists from 27 countries interested in the field of vascular medicine and surgery and dedicated to scientific advancement and continued education in angiology (the study of the circulatory, or vascular system). Seeks to: define, represent, and foster the growth and development of the specialty practice of angiology; improve patient care by advising physicians on recent developments in the field; provide a common forum for the exchange of ideas, technical research, and clinical experiences. Conducts continuing medical education programs. Disseminates original research findings related to cerebrovascular, cardiovascular, and peripheral vascular diseases, diagnostic methods, therapeutic procedures, clinical and laboratory research, and case reports. Holds clinical, diagnostic, and therapeutic symposia and seminars. **Pub:** *The Journal of the American College of Angiology*, bimonthly. Journal.

★ 553 ★ American College of Apothecaries (ACA)

2830 Summer Oaks Dr.
Bartlett, TN 38134-3811
Phone: (901)383-8119 **Fax:** (901)383-8882
Email: acainfo@acaresourcecenter.org
Dr. D. C. Huffman, Jr., Exec. VP

Fnded: 1940. **Mem:** 1,000. **Reg. Groups:** 13. **State Groups:** 24. **Desc:** Professional society of pharmacists owning and operating ethical prescription pharmacies, including hospital pharmacists, pharmacy students, and faculty of colleges of pharmacy. Primary objective is the translation, transformation, and dissemination of knowledge, research data, and recent developments in the pharmaceutical industry and public health. Offers continuing education courses and certificate program. Conducts research programs; sponsors charitable program; compiles statistics; operates speakers' bureau. **Pub:** *American College of Apothecaries–Directory*, annual. Membership Directory. *Price:* Included in membership dues. • *American College of Apothecaries Newsletter*, monthly. Newsletter. Covers membership activities and developments affecting the profession. *Price:* Included in membership dues. • *American College of Apothecaries–Patron's Newsletter*, monthly. Newsletter. Provides tips on health and medications for patrons of member pharmacists. *Price:* Included in membership dues. • *American College of Apothecaries–Physician's Newsletter*, monthly. Newsletter. Provides health tips on the use of drugs and medications. *Price:* Included in membership dues. • *Voice of the Pharmacist*, quarterly. Newsletter. Provides information on issues affecting pharmacy practice, including legislative developments. *Price:* Included in membership dues; $40/year for nonmembers. • Books. • Handbooks. • Also publishes bylaws.

★ 554 ★ American College of Cardiology (ACC)

9111 Old Georgetown Rd.
Bethesda, MD 20814-1699
Phone: (301)897-5400 **Free:** 800-253-4636
Fax: (301)897-9745
Email: exec@acc.org
Website: http://www.acc.org
Christine W. McEntee, CEO

Fnded: 1949. **Mem:** 26,000. **State Groups:** 37. **Desc:** Professional society of physicians, surgeons, and scientists specializing in cardiology (heart) and cardiovascular (circulatory) diseases. Operates Heart House Learning Center. Maintains numerous committees. **Pub:** *ACC Current Journal Review*, bimonthly. Journal. Provides abstracts and reviews of pertinent clinical articles. *Price:* Included in membership dues; $105 for individuals; $185 for institutions; $60 for interns. • *ACCEL*, monthly. Journal. On audiocassette. Contains 15 to 20 interviews with leaders in the field of cardiovascular medicine. *Price:* $165/year for members; $200/year for nonmembers. • *Affiliates in Training*, bimonthly. Newsletter. Provides information of the association pertinent to the Affiliate-In-Training category. Includes list of employment opportunities. *Price:* Included in membership dues; $20/year for nonmembers. • *Cardiology*, monthly. Newsletter. Contains information on clincal cardiology practice. Covers health care issues, legislative and socioeconomic activities, and education opportunities. *Price:* Included in membership dues; $59/year. • *Journal of the American College of Cardiology*, monthly. Journal. Covers original clinical and experimental papers on cardiovascular disease featuring reports on medical and surgical therapy, and other subjects. *Price:* Included in membership dues; $152/year for nonmember individuals; $236/year for institutions; $92/year for interns, residents, health professionals. • Also publishes self-study materials.

★ 555 ★ American College of Cardiovascular Administrators (ACCA)

701 Lee St., Ste. 600
Des Plaines, IL 60016
Phone: (847)759-8601 **Fax:** (847)759-8602
Email: info@aameda.org
Website: http://www.aameda.org
Renee S. Schleicher, Contact

Fnded: 1986. **Mem:** 900. **Reg. Groups:** 7. **State Groups:** 50. **Desc:** A specialty college of the American Academy of Medical Administrators. Upperand middle-level managers of health care professionals in the cardiovascular health care field; associate members are junior supervisors, salespersons, and individuals. Represents members within the medical industry; provides credentialing of cardiology administrators. Serves as a forum for the exchange of information. Conducts educational programs. **Pub:** *Journal of Cardiovacular Management*, bimonthly. Journal. *Price:* included in membership dues.

★ 556 ★ American College of Chest Physicians (ACCP)

3300 Dundee Rd.
Northbrook, IL 60062
Phone: (847)498-1400 **Free:** 800-343-ACCP
Fax: (847)498-5460
Email: accp@chestnet.org
Website: http://www.chestnet.org
Alvin Lever, Exec. VP/CEO

Fnded: 1935. **Mem:** 15,000. **Desc:** Professional society of physicians and surgeons specializing in diseases of the chest (heart and lungs). Promotes undergraduate and postgraduate medical education and research in the field. Sponsors forums. Maintains placement service; conducts educational programs. **Pub:** *American College of Chest Physicians Membership Directory*, annual. Membership Directory. Arranged geographically and by specialty. *Price:* Included in membership dues. • *Chest: The Pulmonary and Critical Care Journal*, monthly. Journal. Presents clinical investigations and case reports in cardiopulmonary medical and surgical specialties. Contains author and subject indexes. *Price:* Included in membership dues; $132/year for nonmembers; $162/year for institutions. • Books. • Brochures.On smoking and health, bronchitis, and asthma. • Also publishes self-teaching series on pulmonary and critical care medicine.

★ 557 ★ American College of Chiropractic Consultants (ACCC)

1720 Washington Rd., Ste. 201
Pittsburgh, PA 15241
Fax: (412)833-6320
Email: willtell@usaor.net
Website: http://www.accc-chiro.com/
William Tellin, DC, Pres.

Fnded: 1980. **Desc:** Independent contractors providing advisory consulting services to insurance carriers and health care organizations, and other entities sponsoring chiropractic benefits. Promotes adherence to high standards of ethics and practice among chiropractors. Establishes chiropractic standards and conducts certification examinations; sponsors continuing professional development courses for chiropractors.

★ 558 ★ American College of Chiropractic Orthopedists (ACCO)
c/o Dr. Jesse Rothenberger
1030 Broadway, Ste. 101
El Centro, CA 92243
Phone: (760)370-9106
Website: http://www.accoweb.org
Dr. Jesse Rothenberger, Pres.

Fnded: 1964. **Mem:** 730. **Desc:** Certified (426) and noncertified (304) chiropractic orthopedists; students enrolled in a postgraduate chiropractic orthopedic program (100). Seeks to establish and maintain optimal educational and clinical standards within the field of chiropractic orthopedics. Sponsors educational programs. **Pub:** *Journal of the American College of Chiropractic Orthopedists*, semiannual. Journal. *Price:* available to members only. • Membership Directory, annual. • Also publishes orthopedic and neurologic tests booklets. **AKA:** American College of Chiropractic Specialists.

★ 559 ★ American College of Clinical Pharmacology (ACCP)
3 Ellinwood Ct.
New Hartford, NY 13413-1105
Phone: (315)768-6117 **Fax:** (315)768-6119
Email: accp1ssu@aol.com
Website: http://www.accp1.org
Susan S. Ulrich, Exec. Dir.

Fnded: 1969. **Mem:** 1,000. **Local Groups:** 2. **Desc:** Strives to be the premier professional society with the size, influence, and diversity of membership consistent with the breadth of the discipline of clinical pharmacology. Provides educational programs and forum for membership, health professionals, students, and the public. Assists in the development and dissemination of basic and clinical knowledge to improve rational drug use and patient outcomes. Serves as a forum for active public debate to influence scientific, regulatory, and public health policy issues. Provides opportunities to influence future directions of the College. Supports and encourages the discovery and development efforts designed to provide improved therapeutic modalities. **Pub:** *ACCP Newsletter*, 3/year. Newsletter. *Price:* Free for members. • *American College of Clinical Pharmacology–Directory*, annual. Membership Directory. *Price:* Included in membership dues. • *Journal of Clinical Pharmacology*, monthly. Journal. *Price:* Included in membership dues; $295 for nonmembers in the U.S.; $365 for nonmembers outside the U.S.

★ 560 ★ American College of Clinical Pharmacy (ACCP)
3101 Broadway, Ste. 650
Kansas City, MO 64111
Phone: (816)531-2177 **Fax:** (816)531-4990
Email: accp@accp.com
Website: http://www.accp.com
Robert M. Elenbaas, Exec. Dir.

Fnded: 1979. **Mem:** 6,900. **Reg. Groups:** 16. **Desc:** Clinical pharmacists dedicated to: promoting rational use of drugs in society; advancing the practice of clinical pharmacy and interdisciplinary health care; assuring high quality clinical pharmacy by establishing and maintaining standards in education and training at advanced levels. Encourages research and recognizes excellence in clinical pharmacy. Offers educational programs, symposia, research forums, fellowship training, and college-funded grants through competitions. Maintains placement service. **Pub:** *ACCP Report*, monthly. Newsletter. *Price:* Free. • *Pharmacotherapy: The Journal of Human Pharmacology and Drug Therapy*, monthly. Journal. *Price:* Included in membership dues. • *Residency and Fellowship Programs Offered by ACCP Members*, annual. Directory of training programs in clinical pharmacy. *Price:* Free.

★ 561 ★ American College of Dentists (ACD)
839-J Quince Orchard Blvd.
Gaithersburg, MD 20878-1614
Phone: (301)977-3223 **Fax:** (301)977-3330
Email: info@facd.org
Website: http://www.facd.org
Dr. Stephen A. Ralls, Exec. Dir.

Fnded: 1920. **Mem:** 7,000. **Reg. Groups:** 8. **State Groups:** 48. **Desc:** Dentists and others serving in capacities related to the dental profession. Seeks to advance the standards of the profession of dentistry. Conducts educational and research programs. Maintains speakers' bureau and charitable programs. **Pub:** *American College of Dentists News and Views*, quarterly. Newsletter. *Price:* Included in membership dues. • *Journal of the American College of Dentists*, quarterly. Journal. Includes news and research reports. *Price:* Included in membership dues; $40/year for nonmembers.

★ 562 ★ American College of Domiciliary Midwives (ACDM)
3889 Middlefield Rd.
Palo Alto, CA 94303-4718
Phone: (650)328-8491
Email: info@collegeofmidwives.org
Website: http://www.collegeofmidwives.org
Faith Gibson, Exec. Dir.

Fnded: 1993. **Mem:** 75. **State Groups:** 2. **Desc:** Strives to preserve lawful access to home-based maternity care as provided by community midwives and family-practice physicians. **Pub:** *International Journal of Domiciliary Midwifery*, quarterly. Journal. Includes historical and contemporary articles on the history, politics, and practice of independent midwifery. *Price:* Free.

★ 563 ★ American College of Emergency Physicians (ACEP)
1125 Executive Cir.
Irving, TX 75038-2522
Phone: (972)550-0911 **Free:** 800-798-1822
Fax: (972)580-2816
Email: info@acep.org
Website: http://www.acep.org
Dr. Colin C. Rorrie, Jr., Exec. Dir.

Fnded: 1968. **Mem:** 21,971. **State Groups:** 53. **Desc:** Supports quality emergency medical care and promotes the interests of emergency physicians. Represents more than 22,000 members and is the emergency medicine specialty society recognized by organized medicine. **Pub:** *ACEP News*, monthly. Newsletter. Discusses socioeconomic issues affecting emergency medicine. *Price:* Included in membership dues; $20/year for nonmembers. • *Annals of Emergency Medicine*, monthly. Journal. Covers emergency medicine and emergency health services. Includes abstracts of emergency medical literature, book reviews, and calendar of events. *Price:* Included in membership dues. • *Foresight*, 3/year. Newsletter. Covers emergency medicine risk management. • *Physicians Evaluation and Education Review.* • Also publishes a homestudy series, and reference manuals on diagnosis and procedure coding, quality assurance, independent contractor status, EMS medical direction, working with managed care plans, patient transfer, risk management, developing and negotiating contracts, and advanced pediatric life support.

★ 564 ★ American College of Epidemiology (ACE)
1500 Sunday Dr., Ste. 102
Raleigh, NC 27607
Phone: (919)861-5573 **Fax:** (919)787-4916
Email: info@acepidemiology.org
Website: http://www.acepidemiology.org
Peter Kralka, Exec. Dir.

Fnded: 1979. **Mem:** 960. **Desc:** Medical professionals involved in the field of epidemiology. (Epidemiology is the study of the causes of human disease and the pattern of disease in human populations.) Promotes education in the practice of epidemiology and maintains professional standards in the field. Relates epidemiological issues to public policy. **Pub:** *Annals of Epidemiology*, monthly. • Newsletter, quarterly.

★ 565 ★ American College of Eye Surgeons (ACES)
2265 Oak Ridge Court, Ste. A
Fort Myers, FL 33901
Phone: (239)275-8881 **Free:** 888-335-0077
Fax: (239)275-9969
Email: quality@aces-abes.org
Website: http://www.aces-abes.org
Brenda S. Sheets, Exec. Dir.

Fnded: 1986. **Mem:** 700. **Desc:** Ophthalmic surgeons. Promotes and seeks to "sustain excellence in eye surgery while supporting self-direction and selfregulation" in the field of ophthalmic surgery. Works to ensure the quality and availability of ophthalmic health and surgical services. Conducts examinations and certifies qualified surgeons in ophthalmic surgical subspecialties; conducts continuing professional education courses for members; serves as a clearinghouse on emerging ophthalmic surgical techniques and technologies. **Pub:** *American Board of Eye Surgery Directory*, annual. Directory. *Price:* $2. • *Synergism*, periodic. Newsletter.

★ 566 ★ American College of Foot and Ankle Orthopedics and Medicine (ACFAOM)
3525 Ellicott Mills Dr., Ste. N
Ellicott City, MD 21043
Free: 800-265-8263 **Fax:** 888-336-6832
Email: info@acfaom.org
Website: http://www.acfaom.org/
Annemarie Edwards, DPM, Pres.

Fnded: 1949. **Mem:** 1,300. **Desc:** Professional society of podiatrists sanctioned as specialists to practice foot orthopedics (deformities and diseases of bones, joints, and muscles of the foot) and primary podiatric medicine. **Pub:** *ACFAOM News*, quarterly. Newsletter. *Price:* included in membership dues; $5 for nonmembers. **Frmly:** (1993) American CLG of Foot Orthopedists.

★ 567 ★ American College of Foot and Ankle Pediatrics (ACFAP)
6477 College Park Sq.
Virginia Beach, VA 23464
Phone: (757)523-0414 **Fax:** (757)523-2047
Patrick Agnew, DPM, Pres.

Fnded: 1977. **Mem:** 200. **Desc:** Podiatric physicians and surgeons, general physicians and surgeons, psychologists, and physical therapists. Seeks to bring together all professionals interested in children's foot health. Goals are to: disseminate information; consider all forms of therapy of value in foot and ankle pediatrics; bring to all those interested the most advanced and valuable forms of therapy through publications, seminars, and research sessions; establish teaching courses on foot and ankle pediatrics so that more podiatric students will consider specializing in the field. Encourages individual research projects; maintains speakers' bureau. **Pub:** *ACP Abstracts*, bimonthly. Newsletter. • Newsletter, annual. **Frmly:** (1993) American College of Podopediatrics.

★ 568 ★ American College of Foot and Ankle Surgeons (ACFAS)
515 Busse Hwy.
Park Ridge, IL 60068
Phone: (847)292-2237 **Free:** 800-421-2237
Fax: (847)292-2022
Email: mail@acfas.org
Website: http://www.acfas.org/
Thomas R. Schedler, CAE, Exec. Dir.

Fnded: 1942. **Mem:** 5,000. **Reg. Groups:** 14. **Desc:** Objectives are to: promote and disseminate information on podiatric surgery among the public, podiatric surgeons, and other health professionals; encourage and publish research findings and related literature; provide intensive programs for clinical and experimental research to improve podiatric surgery and to promote our members' professional and socioeconomic activities. **Pub:** *American College of Foot and Ankle Surgeons–Newsletter*, bimonthly. Bulletin. *Price:* Included in membership dues. • *Complications in Foot* and Ankle Surgery. • *Journal of Foot and Ankle Surgery*, bimonthly. Journal. Includes book reviews and journal abstracts. *Price:* Included in membership dues; $73/year for nonmember individuals; $97/year for nonmember institutions. • *Membership Roster*, annual. Membership Directory. **Frmly:** (1993) American College of Foot Surgeons.

★ 569 ★ American College of Gastroenterology (ACG)

4900B S 31st St.
Arlington, VA 22206-1656
Phone: (703)820-7400 **Fax:** (703)931-4520
Email: orders@acg.gi.org
Website: http://www.acg.gi.org
Frank L. Lanza, Pres.

Fnded: 1932. **Mem:** 7,000. **Desc:** Professional society of physicians and surgeons specializing in diseases and disorders of the gastrointestinal tract and accessory organs of digestion, including disorders due to nutrition. **Pub:** *American Journal of Gastroenterology*, monthly. Journal. **Frmly:** (1934) Society for the Advancement of Gastroenterology; (1954) National Gastroenterological Association.

★ 570 ★ American College Health Association (ACHA)

PO Box 28937
Baltimore, MD 21240-8937
Phone: (410)859-1500 **Fax:** (410)859-1510
Email: pcrone@sacha.org
Website: http://www.acha.org
Col. Doyle E. Randol, MS, Exec. Dir.

Fnded: 1920. **Mem:** 3,438. **Local Groups:** 11. **Desc:** Institutions (930) and individuals (2500). Provides an organization in which institutions of higher education and interested individuals may work together to promote health in its broadest aspects for students and all other members of the college community. Offers continuing education programs for health professionals. Maintains placement listings for physicians and other personnel seeking positions in college health. Compiles statistics. Conducts seminars and training programs. **Pub:** *ACHA Action*, quarterly. Newsletter. Includes calendar of events, college health resource listings, annual report, and leadership directory. *Price:* included in membership dues. • *Health Information Series*. Pamphlets. • *Journal of American College Health*, bimonthly. Journal. • *Membership Profile Directory*, periodic. Directory. • Catalog.Lists publications. • Monographs. • Reports. • Also publishes guidelines. **Frmly:** American Student Health Association.

★ 571 ★ American College of Health Care Administrators (ACHCA)

300 N Lee St., No. 301
Alexandria, VA 22314
Phone: (703)739-7900 **Free:** 888-88-ACHCA
Fax: (703)739-7901
Email: mtn@achca.org
Website: http://www.achca.org
Mary Tellis-Nayak, Pres. & CEO

Fnded: 1962. **Mem:** 6,360. **Reg. Groups:** 11. **State Groups:** 48. **Desc:** Persons actively engaged in the administration of long-term care facilities, such as nursing homes, retirement communities, assisted living facilities, and subacute care programs. ACHCA administers professional certification programs for assisted living, subacute and nursing home administrators. Works to elevate the standards in the field and to develop and promote a code of ethics and standards of education and training. Seeks to inform allied professions and the public that good administration of long-term care facilities calls for special formal academic training and experience. Encourages research in all aspects of geriatrics, the chronically ill, and administration. Maintains placement service. Holds special education programs; facilitates networking among administrators. **Pub:** *Balance*, bimonthly. Journal. Contains original research and practical applications, commentaries, and book reviews. *Price:* included in membership dues. • *E-Compass*, bimonthly. Newsletter. Contains information on initiatives and industry updates. *Price:* included in membership dues. • Also publishes educational materials. **Frmly:** American College of Nursing Home Administrators.

★ 572 ★ American College of Healthcare Executives (ACHE)

1 N Franklin, Ste. 1700
Chicago, IL 60606-3491
Phone: (312)424-2800 **Fax:** (312)424-0023
Email: ache@ache.org
Website: http://www.ache.org
Thomas C. Dolan, PhD,, FACHE, CAE, Pres. and CEO

Fnded: 1933. **Mem:** 30,000. **Local Groups:** 110. **Desc:** Healthcare executives. Conducts credentialing and educational programs and an annual Congress on Healthcare Management. Conducts ground-breaking research and career development and public policy programs. Publishing division, Health Administration Press, publishes books and journals on health services management and textbooks for use in college and university courses. Works toward goal of improving the health status of society by advancing healthcare leadership management excellence. Works toward goal of improving the health status of society by advancing healthcare management excellence. by advancing healthcare management excellence. **Pub:** *Frontiers of Health Services Management*, quarterly. Journal. Contains articles debating current healthcare topics and commentaries from outstanding scholars and practitioners in the field. *Price:* $75/year; in U.S. • *Healthcare Executive*, bimonthly. Magazine. Provides in-depth analysis of emerging trends in healthcare management and includes strategies for confronting healthcare management issues. *Price:* $118/year outside U.S. institution; $75/year outside U.S.; $65/year in U.S. • *Journal of Healthcare Management*, bimonthly. Journal. Provides healthcare management research and articles on topics such as leadership and managed care. *Price:* $85/year outside U.S.; $75/year (U.S.). • *Member Directory*. Directory. Available online, free of charge to members. • Also publishes case studies, books, journals, manuals, and newsletters; offers cassette tapes. **Frmly:** (1985) American College of Hospital Administrators.

★ 573 ★ American College of Home Obstetrics (ACHO)

2821 Rose St.
Franklin Park, IL 60131
Phone: (847)455-2030
Gregory White, MD, Pres.

Fnded: 1978. **Mem:** 30. **Desc:** Physicians interested in cooperating with families who wish to give birth in the home. Objective is to accumulate and exchange data on home birth. Maintains speakers' bureau; compiles statistics. Plans to conduct research. **Pub:** Newsletter, periodic. • Also publishes statement of purpose.

★ 574 ★ American College of International Physicians (ACIP)

c/o Sally Askew, Exec.Dir.
370 S Lowe Ave., Ste. A-309
Cookeville, TN 38501
Phone: (931)526-8675 **Fax:** (931)525-6769
Email: acip@citlink.net
Website: http://www.acip.org
Sally Askew, Exec. Dir.

Fnded: 1975. **Mem:** 1,200. **State Groups:** 8. **Desc:** Physicians and surgeons interested in initiatives to promote national efforts in international health, education, research, training, and welfare. Promotes the betterment of the health of all peoples and seeks to advance the art and science of medicine. Emphasizes the international character of medicine and the education of international physicians. Seeks parity for foreign medical graduates. Supports relief programs to areas struck by natural calamities or epidemic diseases. **Pub:** *International Medical Journal*, semiannual. Newsletter. • *The International Physician*, quarterly. Newsletter.

★ 575 ★ American College of Laboratory Animal Medicine (ACLAM)

c/o Dr. Melvin W. Balk
96 Chester St.
Chester, NH 03036
Phone: (603)887-2467 **Fax:** (603)887-0097
Email: mwbaclam@gsinet.net
Website: http://www.aclam.org
Dr. Melvin W. Balk, Exec. Dir.

Fnded: 1957. **Mem:** 360. **Desc** Veterinarians specializing in laboratory animal medicine. Establishes standards of training and experience for qualification of specialists in the field, administers examinations, and certifies eligible specialists. Encourages education, training, and research in laboratory animal medicine. Sponsors symposia on infectious and metabolic diseases of laboratory animals. Conducts continuing education forums for diplomates on topics including quality assurance, biohazards, and animal production. **Pub:** *The Biology of the Laboratory Rabbit*. • *Membership Directory*, annual. Directory. • Newsletter, 4/year. **Frmly:** American Board of Laboratory Animal Medicine.

★ 576 ★ American College of Legal Medicine (ACLM)

1111 N Plaza Dr., Ste. 550
Schaumburg, IL 60173
Phone: (847)969-0283 **Free:** 800-433-9137
Fax: (847)517-7229
Email: info@aclm.org
Website: http://www.aclm.org
Miles Zaremski, Pres.

Fnded: 1960. **Mem:** 1,450. **Desc:** Persons who hold degrees in medicine, dentistry, law and nursing. Promotes and advances the field of legal medicine or medical jurisprudence; arranges for meetings with medical, legal, and professional groups and legislative, judicial, and enforcement bodies interested in any province where law and medicine are contiguous; fosters and encourages centers for study and research in the field of legal medicine and publishes materials pertaining to legal medicine. **Pub:** *American College of Legal Medicine–Newsletter*, quarterly. Newsletter. Contains basic news and information of the College. *Price:* Included in membership dues. • *College of Legal Medicine Membership Directory*, annual. Membership Directory. *Price:* Included in membership dues; $50/copy for nonmembers. • *Journal of Legal Medicine*, periodic. Journal. Offers discussion of topics of interest in legal medicine, health law, food and drug law, and medicolegal research and education. *Price:* Included in membership dues; $134/year for nonmembers. • *Legal Medicine Perspectives*, bimonthly. • *Medical Legal Lessons*, bimonthly. Includes summaries of prominent cases and discussions of recent statutes.

★ 577 ★ American College of Managed Care Administrators (ACMCA)

701 Lee St., No. 600
Des Plaines, IL 60016-4516
Phone: (847)759-8601 **Fax:** (847)759-8602
Email: info@aamed.org
Website: http://www.aameda.org
Lt. Col. A. Adolphe Edward, Pres.

Fnded: 1994. **Mem:** 600. **Reg. Groups:** 7. **State Groups:** 50. **Desc:** Specialty college of the American Academy of Medical Administrators. Managers of professionals who are directly or indirectly providing managed healthcare. Works to promote the advancement of members' professional standing, education, and personal achievement and develop innovative concepts in managed care administration. Conducts an employment referral and educational programs. **Pub:** *Executive*, bimonthly. Journal.

★ 578 ★ American College of Managed Care Medicine (ACMCM)

4435 Waterfront Dr., Ste. 101
PO Box 4765
Glen Allen, VA 23060
Phone: (804)527-1906 **Fax:** (804)747-5316

Email: info@acmcm.org
Website: http://www.acmcm.org
Dr. W.C. Williams, III,MD, Contact

Fnded: 1995. **Mem:** 2,000. **Desc:** Physicians and other health care providers working for managed care organizations. Seeks to advance the effectiveness of managed care health services. Conducts continuing professional development courses for health care providers and prepares members for a managed care certificate examination; facilitates exchange of information among members; sponsors research; maintains speakers' bureau. **Pub:** *American Journal of Integrated Health Care*, quarterly. Journal.

★ 579 ★ American College of Medical Administrators (ACMA)

701 Lee St., Ste. 600
Des Plaines, IL 60016
Phone: (847)759-8601 **Fax:** (847)759-8602
Email: info@aameda.org
Website: http://www.aameda.org
Nancy Anderson, Contact

Fnded: 1991. **Mem:** 225. **Reg. Groups:** 7. **State Groups:** 50. **Desc:** Specialty College of the American Academy of Medical Administrators. Healthcare information leaders serving in management positions. Works to promote the advancement of members' knowledge, professional standing, credentialing, and personal achievements in information technology, management, and strategic planning. Conducts educational programs. **Pub:** *Executive*, bimonthly. Journal. *Price:* included in membership dues.

★ 580 ★ American College of Medical Genetics (ACMG)

9650 Rockville Pike
Bethesda, MD 20814
Phone: (301)634-7127 **Fax:** (301)571-0677
Email: acmg@faseb.org
Website: http://www.asmg.net
Charles J. Epstein, MD, Pres.

Fnded: 1991. **Mem:** 1,230. **Desc:** Physicians and others with an interest in genetics and the delivery of medical genetics services to the public. Works to insure the availability of genetic services without regard to considerations of race, gender, sexual orientation, disability, or ability to pay. Promotes and supports genetics research. Establishes and maintains scientific and professional standards for medical genetics education, research, and practice. Lobbies for effective and fair health policies and legislation; provides information and technical assistance to government agencies engaged in health care regulation or policy formation. Makes available continuing professional education programs; represents members' interests. Conducts advocacy campaigns for people with genetic problems; sponsors public education programs. **Pub:** *Genetics in Medicine; Standards and Guidelines*, bimonthly. Journal. *Price:* $215/yr. US individual; $435/yr. US in training; $85/yr. Outside US.

★ 581 ★ American College of Medical Physics (ACMP)

11250 Roger Bacon Dr., Ste. 8
Reston, VA 20190-5202
Phone: (703)481-5001 **Fax:** (703)435-4390
Email: lrowland@drohanmgmt.com
Website: http://www.acmp.org
Laureen Rowland, Exec. Dir.

Fnded: 1982. **Mem:** 450. **Reg. Groups:** 9. **Desc:** Covers socioeconomic aspects of practice, management issues, reimbursement, licensure, and practice standards. **Pub:** *Diagnostic Radiology*. Report. *Price:* $25 for nonmembers. • *Magnetic Resonance Imaging*. Report. *Price:* $25 for nonmembers. • *Mammography*. Report. *Price:* $25 for nonmembers. • *Medical Laser Systems*. Report. *Price:* $25 for nonmembers. • *Nuclear Medicine*. Report. *Price:* $25 for nonmembers. • *Radiation Oncology*. Report. *Price:* $25 for nonmembers. • Newsletter, 3-4/year.

★ 582 ★ American College of Medical Practice Executives (ACMPE)

104 Inverness Ter. E
Englewood, CO 80112-5306
Free: 877-275-6462 **Fax:** (303)643-4439
Email: acmpe@mgma.com
Website: http://www.mgma.com/acmpe
Andrea M. Rossiter, FACMPE, Sr. VP

Fnded: 1956. **Mem:** 5,000. **Desc:** Professional credentialing organization. Membership is drawn from Medical Group Management Association and beyond. Works to encourage medical group practice administrators to improve and maintain their proficiency and to provide appropriate recognition; to establish a program with uniform standards of admission, advancement, certification and fellowship in order to achieve the highest possible standards in the profession of medical group practice administration; to participate in the development of educational and research programs for the advancement of the profession; to inform the medical profession and the public of the value of trained and experienced men and women in the management of the administrative affairs of all forms of group practice; to instill in its membership a constant awareness of the high ideals and traditions of the medical profession and medical group administration so that its members will conduct themselves in such a manner as to augment those ideals and traditions. Conducts educational programs such as Management Education Programs and Group Practice Governance Leadership Institute. **Pub:** *College Review*, semiannual. Professional manuscripts submitted to the College for advancement to fellow status; arranged by subject and author. *Price:* $10/copy to members; $16/copy to affiliates; $22/copy to nonmembers. • *Your Pathway to Excellence*. Brochure. Provides general information regarding ACMPE membership application. **Frmly:** (1976) American College of Clinic Managers; (1993) American College of Medical Group Administrators.

★ 583 ★ American College of Medical Quality (ACMQ)

4334 Montgomery Ave.
Bethesda, MD 20814
Phone: (301)913-9149 **Free:** 800-924-2149
Fax: (301)913-9142
Email: ACMQ@acmq.org
Website: http://www.acmq.org
Bridget Brodie, Exec. VP

Fnded: 1973. **Mem:** 1,000. **Reg. Groups:** 4. **Desc:** Physicians, affiliates, and institutions. Seeks to educate and set standards of competence in the field of quality improvement and management. Offers a core curriculum in quality. Maintains speakers' bureau. **Pub:** *American College of Medical Quality Newsletter - Focus*, bimonthly. Newsletter. Includes topical articles and college and chapter news. *Price:* Included in membership dues. • *American Journal of Medical Quality*, bimonthly. Journal. Covers topics concerning evaluation of quality in health care, DRGs, Medicare and Medicaid, risk management, and other areas of interest. *Price:* Included in membership dues; $151/year for nonmembers. **Frmly:** (1988) ACURP.

★ 584 ★ American College of Medical Toxicology (ACMT)

PO Box 356
Hershey, PA 17033
Phone: (602)239-2353 **Free:** 888-633-5784
Fax: (425)645-6139
Email: hmiller@pamedsoc.org
Website: http://www.acmt.net
Michael J. Kosnett, Pres.

Fnded: 1993. **Mem:** 282. **Desc:** Seeks to advance the science, study and practice of medical toxicology by fostering the development of medical toxicology in its provision of emergency, consultation, forensic, legal, community and industrial services; and by otherwise striving to advance and elevate the science, study and practice of medical toxicology. **Pub:** *Internet Journal of Medical Toxicology*. Journal. • Newsletter, 3/year. *Price:* for members only. **Frmly:** American Board of Medical Toxicology.

★ 585 ★ American College of Mental Health Administration (ACMHA)

324 Freeport Rd.
Pittsburgh, PA 15238-3422
Phone: (412)820-0670 **Fax:** (412)820-0669
Email: lawhel@aol.com
Website: http://www.acmha.org
Dr. Lawrence A. Heller, PhD, Exec. Dir.

Fnded: 1980. **Mem:** 200. **Desc:** Mental health clinician administrators. **Pub:** *ACMHA Newsletter*, quarterly. Newsletter. Includes organization news and critical essays. *Price:* $12/year.

★ 586 ★ American College of MOHS Micrographic Surgery and Cutaneous Oncology (ACMMSCO)

611 E Wells St.
Milwaukee, WI 53202
Phone: (414)347-1103 **Free:** 800-500-7224
Fax: (414)272-6070
Email: bpaez@aad.org
Website: http://www.mohscollege.org
Janet Arnold-Grych, Exec. Dir.

Fnded: 1967. **Mem:** 600. **Desc:** Physicians, dermatologists, surgeons, plastic surgeons, and other specialists who have had a minimum of one year of training in Mohs surgery at an approved institution. (Mohs surgery is used for the microscopically controlled excision of skin cancer.) Provides a means for recognition of physicians who have become proficient in the method; to facilitate education and the exchange of ideas. **Frmly:** (1987) American College of Chemosurgery.

★ 587 ★ American College of Neuropsychiatrists (ACN)

28595 Orchard Lake Rd., Ste. 200
Farmington Hills, MI 48334
Phone: (248)553-0010 **Fax:** (248)553-0818
Email: acn-aconp@msn.com
Louis E. Rentz, Exec. Dir.

Fnded: 1937. **Mem:** 420. **Desc:** Psychiatrists, neurologists, physicians in training, and persons in interrelated professions. Promotes study and research in neurology and psychiatry in the osteopathic profession. Maintains specialized education programs. **Pub:** *Journal of the American College of Neuropsychiatrists*, semiannual. Journal. Reports information on medical developments, case studies, and analysis of political actions. Includes calendar of events and research updates. *Price:* Included in membership dues. • Directory, annual.

★ 588 ★ American College of Neuropsychopharmacology (ACNP)

2014 Broadway, Ste. 320
Nashville, TN 37203
Phone: (615)322-2075 **Fax:** (615)343-0662
Email: acnp@acnp.org
Website: http://www.acnp.org
Ronnie Wilkins, EdD, Exec. Dir.

Fnded: 1961. **Mem:** 735. **Desc:** Experienced investigators whose work is related to neuropsychopharmacology. Promotes and encourages the scientific study and application of neuropsychopharmacology. Conducts study groups and plenary sessions. **Pub:** *Mailings*, monthly. Journal. • *Neuropsychopharmacology*, monthly. Journal. Focuses on clinical and basic science contributions to neuropharmacology. *Price:* Included in membership dues. • *Roster*, annual.

★ 589 ★ American College of Nuclear Medicine (ACNM)

PO Box 175
Landisville, PA 17538
Phone: (717)898-5008 **Fax:** (717)898-2555
Email: rpowell2248@aol.com
Website: http://www.acnucmed.org/
Robert Powell, Contact

Fnded: 1972. **Mem:** 500. **Desc:** Physicians and medical scientists in nuclear medicine united to: advance the science of nuclear medicine; improve its benefits to patients; study the socioeconomic aspects of the practice of nuclear medicine; encourage improved and continuing education for practitioners in this and allied fields. **Pub:** *ACNM Directory*, biennial. Directory. • *ACNM Report*, bimonthly. Newsletter.

★ 590 ★ American College of Nuclear Physicians (ACNP)

1850 Samuel Morse Dr.
Reston, VA 20190-5316
Phone: (703)326-1190 **Fax:** (703)708-9015
Email: grobinson@snm.org
Website: http://www.acnponline.org/
Gregg Robinson, Assoc. Exec. Dir.

Fnded: 1974. **Mem:** 1,600. **Desc:** Nuclear medicine physicians, scientists, and corporations. Objectives are: to foster the highest standards of nuclear medicine service and consultation to the public, hospitals, and referring physicians; to advance the science of nuclear medicine and improve nuclear medicine consultation and service through study, education, and improvement of the socioeconomic aspects of the practice of nuclear medicine; to promote the continuing competence of practitioners of nuclear medicine. Problem-solving areas include: unnecessary and costly regulations and restrictions; public fear, lack of understanding, and misinformation; complex state and federal legislation; transportation difficulties involving nuclear medicine supplies; previous lack of cohesive effort in attacking such problems. Conducts educational seminars and continuing education program; maintains speakers' bureau. **Pub:** *Scanner*, 10/year. • Directory, annual.

★ 591 ★ American College of Nurse-Midwives (ACNM)

818 Connecticut Ave., Ste. 900
Washington, DC 20006
Phone: (202)728-9860 **Fax:** (202)289-9897
Email: info@acnm.org
Website: http://www.midwife.org
Deanne Williams, Exec. Dir.

Fnded: 1955. **Mem:** 6,200. **Reg. Groups:** 6. **Local Groups:** 53. **Desc:** Seeks to develop and support the profession of certified nurse-midwives in order to promote the health and well-being of women and infants within their families and communities. A CNM is a licensed health care practitioner educated in the two disciplines of nursing and midwifery. Provides gynecological services and care of mothers and babies throughout the maternity cycle; members have completed an ACNM accredited program of study and clinical experience in midwifery and passed a national certification exam. Cooperates with allied groups to enable nurse-midwives to concentrate their efforts in the improvement of services for mothers and newborn babies. Seeks to identify areas of nurse-midwifery practices as they relate to the total service and educational aspects of maternal and newborn care. Studies and evaluates activities of nurse-midwives in order to establish qualifications; cooperates in planning and developing educational programs. conducts research and continuing education workshops. sponsors research. Compiles statistics. Maintains speakers' bureau and archives; offers placement service. **Pub:** *American College of Nurse-Midwives Membership Directory Supplement*, annual. Directory. *Price:* Included in membership dues. • *Directory of Nurse-Midwifery Practices*, annual. Directory. Computer listing of certified nurse-midwives by state. *Price:* Included in membership dues; $10 for nonmembers. • *Journal of Nurse-Midwifery*, bimonthly. Journal. Covers topics relevant to maternal and newborn health, obstetrics, well-woman gynecology, family planning, and midwifery education. *Price:* Included in membership dues; $48/year for nonmembers; $69/year for institutions. • *Quickening*, bimonthly. Newsletter. Includes activities, calendar of events, employment listings, and legislative updates. *Price:* Included in membership dues. • Also publishes pamphlets and brochures. **Frmly:** (1969) American College of Nurse-Midwifery.

★ 592 ★ American College of Nurse Practitioners (ACNP)

1111 19th St. NW, Ste. 404
Washington, DC 20002
Phone: (202)659-2190 **Fax:** (202)659-2191
Email: acnp@nurse.org
Website: http://www.nurse.org/acnp
Eric G. Scharf, CAE, Exec. Dir.

Fnded: 1993. **Mem:** 2,800. **Desc:** Licensed and student nurse practitioners; state and national associations representing nurse practitioners. Seeks to strengthen the voice of nurse practitioners within the medical profession; promotes advancement in the study, teaching, and practice of nursing. ACNP's mission is to unite and represent nurse practitioners on policy and professional issues, in order to ensure an appropriate, prevention-based health care system that meets the needs of individuals, families and communities. ACNP provides advocacy on federal policy issues, publishes newsletters and continuing education materials, sponsors conferences and symposia and provides a range of professional networking opportunities. **Pub:** *Forum*, quarterly. Newsletter. • *Nurse Practitioner World News*, periodic. Newsletter. • *Washington Word*, monthly. Newsletter.

★ 593 ★ American College of Nutrition (ACN)

300 S Duncan Ave., Ste. 225
Clearwater, FL 33755
Phone: (727)446-6086 **Fax:** (727)446-6202
Email: office@am-coll-nutr.org
Website: http://www.am-coll-nutr.org
Stanley Wallach, MD, Exec. Dir.

Fnded: 1959. **Mem:** 1,170. **Nat'l Groups:** 1. **Reg. Groups:** 1. **Desc:** Physicians, research scientists, nutritionists, dietitians, allied health personnel, and postbaccalaureate students and trainees in these fields. Provides education on clinical, scientific, and experimental developments in the field of nutrition. Stimulates the exchange of information between nutrition scientists and physicians interested in applying research findings to the care of patients; encourages nutrition education in medical schools; provides for continuing education of physicians and other scientists on nutritional subjects. Sponsors a postgraduate course on nutritional problems. Advises physicians on nutrition developments of clinical importance. Certifies credentials of professional nutritionists, including by formal examination. **Pub:** *ACN Newsletter*, quarterly. Newsletter. Contains member news, calendar of events, and nutritional articles. *Price:* Free. • *Journal of the American College of Nutrition*, bimonthly. Journal. Contains peer-reviewed articles. *Price:* Included in membership dues; $70/year for U.S. nonmembers; $160/year for U.S. institutions; $100/year for nonmembers outside the U.S.

★ 594 ★ American College of Obstetricians and Gynecologists (ACOG)

409 12th St. SW
PO Box 96920
Washington, DC 20090-6920
Phone: (202)638-5577 **Fax:** (202)484-8107
Email: mgraves@acog.org
Website: http://www.acog.org
Ralph Hale, MD, Exec. VP

Fnded: 1951. **Mem:** 41,000. **Reg. Groups:** 10. **State Groups:** 50. **Desc:** Physicians specializing in childbirth and the diseases of women. Sponsors continuing professional development program. **Pub:** *ACOG Newsletter*, monthly. Newsletter. • *Committee Opinions, Educational Bulletins, Practice Bulletins, and Criteria sets* ., periodic. Bulletin. Includes technical information. • *Obstetrics and Gynecology*, monthly. Journal. *Price:* $70 med. students/residents; $160 personal; $255 libraries. • Manuals. **Frmly:** (1956) American Academy of Obstetrics and Gynecology.

★ 595 ★ American College of Occupational and Environmental Medicine (ACOEM)

1114 N Arlington Hts. Rd.
Arlington Heights, IL 60004-4770
Phone: (847)818-1800 **Fax:** (847)818-9266
Email: acoeminfo@acoem.org
Website: http://www.acoem.org
Barry S. Eisenberg, Exec. Dir.

Fnded: 1916. **Mem:** 7,000. **Reg. Groups:** 31. **Desc:** Physicians specializing in occupational and environmental medicine. Promotes maintenance and improvement of the health of workers; works to increase awareness of occupational medicine as a medical specialty. Sponsors educational programs; maintains placement service. **Pub:** *ACOEM Report*, monthly. Newsletter. Covers Occupational Safety and Health Administration rulings. *Price:* Included in membership dues. • *American College of Occupational and Environmental Medicine–Membership Directory*, annual. Membership Directory. Arranged alphabetically, geographically, and by affiliation. *Price:* Included in membership dues; $150/copy for nonmembers. • *Journal of Occupational and Environmental Medicine*, monthly. Journal. Contains book reviews, calendar of events, and employment listings. • *MRO Update*, 10/year. Newsletter. Designed for medical review officers and provides latest information on alcohol and drug testing. *Price:* $200 members; $225 nonmembers. **Frmly:** (1992) American College of Occupational Medicine.

★ 596 ★ American College of Oncology Administrators (ACOA)

701 Lee St., Ste. 600
Des Plaines, IL 60016-4516
Phone: (847)759-8601 **Fax:** (847)759-8602
Email: info@aameda.org
Website: http://www.aameda.org
Joseph M. Spallina, Pres.

Fnded: 1991. **Mem:** 500. **Reg. Groups:** 7. **State Groups:** 50. **Desc:** Specialty College of the American Academy of Medical Administrators. Oncology administrators, managers and consultants. Brings together all components of oncology management to develop creative strategies, quality programs, and sound evaluation mechanisms. Promotes advancement of members through continuing education and research in oncology management. Conducts educational programs. **Pub:** *Journal of Oncology Management*, bimonthly. Journal. Contains information and ideas for professionals involved in managing cancer programs. *Price:* included in membership dues.

★ 597 ★ American College of Oral and Maxillofacial Surgeons (ACOMS)

c/o Emelie C. Schnettler
1100 NW Loop 410, Ste. 420
San Antonio, TX 78213-2266
Phone: (210)344-5674 **Free:** 800-522-6676
Fax: (210)344-9754
Email: info@acoms.org
Website: http://www.acoms.org
Daniel Lanka, Exec. Dir.

Fnded: 1975. **Mem:** 2,500. **Desc:** Diplomates of the American Board of Oral and Maxillofacial Surgery who practice oral and maxillofacial surgery. To advance the integrity of the profession through continuing education, exchange of ideas, certification procedures, and cooperation with allied groups. **Pub:** *ACOMS Review*, quarterly. **Frmly:** (1975) Association of Diplomates of the American Board of Oral Surgery.

★ 598 ★ American College of Orgonomy (ACO)

PO Box 490
Princeton, NJ 08542
Phone: (732)821-1144 **Fax:** (732)821-0174
Email: aco@orgonomy.org
Website: http://www.orgonomy.org
Gary A. Karpf, MD, Pres.

Fnded: 1968. **Mem:** 12. **Desc:** Physicians and social scientists seeking to promote and advance the science of orgonomy. (Orgonomy is derived from the theory formulated by Wilhelm Reich, M.D. "that all space is filled with a specific form of energy called orgone energy which accounts for life and living functions.") Provides training in medical orgonomy and character analysis for physicians. Sponsors training and research for physicians and scientists in orgone physics, orgone biology, and weather control. Holds laboratory workshops for physicians and scientists. Offers referral service. Conducts specialized education. **Pub:** *Journal of Orgonomy*, semiannual. Journal. Contains articles on scientific topics related to Orgonomy, sociopolitical and case studies. *Price:* $40/year in the U.S. and Canada; $45/year outside the U.S. and Canada, surface rate; $55/year outside the U.S. and Canada, airmail. • *Man in the Trap.* • *Orgonomic Medicine.*

★ 599 ★ American College of Osteopathic Emergency Physicians (ACOEP)

142 E Ontario St., Ste. 1250
Chicago, IL 60611
Phone: (312)587-3709 **Free:** 800-521-3709
Fax: (312)587-9951
Email: jwachtler@acoep.org
Website: http://www.acoep.org
Janice Wachtler, Exec. Dir.

Fnded: 1975. **Mem:** 1,500. **Desc:** Provides and evaluates postdoctoral and continuing education for osteopathic emergency physicians; encourages and implements the training of emergency physicians; promotes the coordination of community emergency care facilities and personnel. Sponsors Emergency Medicine CME Program for Accreditation. Conducts research and educational programs. Maintains speakers' bureau. **Pub:** *ACOEP Newsletter*, quarterly. Newsletter. *Price:* included in membership dues; $25 / year for nonmembers. • *Member Directory.* • *Student's Guide to AOA Approved Emergency Medicine Residency Programs.*

★ 600 ★ American College of Osteopathic Family Physicians (ACOFP)

330 E Algonquin, Ste. 1
Arlington Heights, IL 60005
Free: 800-323-0794 **Fax:** (847)228-9755
Email: membership@acofp.org
Website: http://www.acofp.org
Peter L. Schmelzer, CAE, Exec. Dir.

Fnded: 1950. **Mem:** 20,000. **State Groups:** 35. **Desc:** Provides information, education and advocacy for osteopathic physicians practicing family medicine. **Pub:** *Osteopathic Family Physician News*, monthly. Journal. Includes calendar of events and member news. *Price:* Free. **Frmly:** (1993) American College of General Practitioners in Osteopathic Medicine and Surgery.

★ 601 ★ American College of Osteopathic Internists (ACOI)

3 Bethesda Metro Ctr., Ste.508
Bethesda, MD 20814
Phone: (301)656-8877 **Free:** 800-327-5183
Fax: (301)656-7133
Email: bjd@acoi.org
Website: http://www.acoi.org
Robert J. Stomel, DO, Pres.

Fnded: 1943. **Mem:** 1,300. **Desc:** Osteopathic doctors who limit their practice to internal medicine and various subspecialties and who intend, through postdoctoral education, to qualify as certified specialists in the field. Aims to provide educational programs and to improve educational standards in the field of osteopathic internal medicine. Sponsors competitions. Compiles statistics; offers placement service. **Pub:** Directory, annual. • Newsletter, monthly.

★ 602 ★ American College of Osteopathic Neurologists and Psychiatrists (ACONP)

28595 Orchard Lake Rd., Ste. 200
Farmington Hills, MI 48334
Phone: (248)553-0010 **Fax:** (248)553-0818
Email: acn-aconp@msn.com
Louis Rentz, DO, Exec. Dir.

Fnded: 1937. **Desc:** Osteopathic neurologists and psychiatrists. Promotes adherence to high standards of training, ethics, and practice within the fields of osteopathic neurology and psychiatry. Conducts examinations and confers certification upon qualified osteopathic neurologists and psychiatrists; sponsors continuing professional development courses.

★ 603 ★ American College of Osteopathic Obstetricians and Gynecologists (ACOOG)

900 Auburn Rd.
Pontiac, MI 48342-3365
Phone: (248)332-6360 **Free:** 800-875-6360
Fax: (248)332-4607
Email: acoog@acoog.com
Website: http://www.acoog.com
Jaki K. Holzer, Admin.

Fnded: 1934. **Mem:** 1,100. **Desc:** Osteopathic physicians and surgeons specializing in obstetrics and gynecology. Conducts educational programs, and reviews osteopathic obstetric and gynecologic residency training programs. Holds annual postgraduate course and annual convention. **Pub:** *ACOOG Newsletter*, quarterly. Newsletter. Includes legislative news, calendar of events, employment listings, and lists of residents completing training and newly certified physicians. *Price:* Free. • *American College of Osteopathic Obstetricians and Gynecologists Membership Directory*, annual. Membership Directory. *Price:* Included in membership dues. • Also publishes medical education brochures.

★ 604 ★ American College of Osteopathic Pain Management and Sclerotherapy (ACOPMS)

303 S Ingram Ct.
Middletown, DE 19709
Phone: (302)376-8080 **Free:** 800-471-6114
Fax: (302)376-8081
Email: admin@acopms.com
Website: http://acopms.com
Linda J. Pavina, Exec. Sec.

Fnded: 1938. **Desc:** Osteopathic medical therapists. Seeks to improve the practice of and disseminate knowledge about Sclerotherapy. Supports research and education.

★ 605 ★ American College of Osteopathic Pediatricians (ACOP)

142 E Ontario St.
Chicago, IL 60611
Free: 877-231-ACOP **Fax:** (312)202-8224
Website: http://www.acopeds.org
Stephen M. Syder, DO, Pres.

Fnded: 1940. **Mem:** 365. **Desc:** Osteopathic physicians who have received or are receiving advanced training in pediatrics and who are specializing in pediatric practice. **Pub:** *ACOP Pulse*, quarterly. Newsletter. Reports on new regulations and sources of information in the field of osteopathic pediatrics. *Price:* $10/year. • Membership Directory, annual.

★ 606 ★ American College of Osteopathic Surgeons (ACOS)

123 N Henry St.
Alexandria, VA 22314-2903
Phone: (703)684-0416 **Fax:** (703)684-3280
Email: info@theacos.org
Website: http://www.facos.org
Guy D. Beaumont, Jr., Exec. Dir.

Fnded: 1927. **Mem:** 1,700. **Desc:** Professional society of osteopathic physicians specializing in surgery and surgical specialties. Maintains placement service; conducts seminars in continuing surgical education. **Pub:** *ACOS News*, monthly. Newsletter. Covers association activities and legislative and regulatory issues affecting osteopathic surgeons. Includes calendar of events. *Price:* Included in membership dues.

★ 607 ★ American College of Phlebology (ACP)

100 Webster St., Ste. 101
Oakland, CA 94607-3724
Phone: (510)834-6500 **Fax:** (510)832-7300
Email: acp@amsinc.org
Website: http://www.phlebology.org
Bruce A. Sanders, Exec. Dir.

Fnded: 1985. **Mem:** 1,050. **Nat'l Groups:** 1. **Desc:** Physicians and medical students with an interest in the evaluation and management of patients with varicose veins, thrombophlebitis, thrombosis, and venous leg ulcers. Seeks to advance the study, teaching, and practice of phlebology; promotes continuing professional development of members. Serves as a network facilitating cooperation and exchange of information among medical professionals with an interest in phlebology; conducts educational programs; functions as a clearinghouse on medical techniques and technologies applicable to the practice of phelbology. **Pub:** *Journal of Dermatologic Surgery*, monthly. Journal. • *Vein Line*, quarterly. Newsletter. **Frmly:** (1997) North American Society of Phlebology.

★ 608 ★ American College of Physician Executives (ACPE)

4890 W Kennedy Blvd., Ste. 200
Tampa, FL 33609
Phone: (813)287-2000 **Free:** 800-562-8088
Fax: (813)287-8993
Email: acpe@acpe.org
Website: http://www.acpe.org
Roger S. Schenke, Exec. VP

Fnded: 1974. **Mem:** 10,000. **Desc:** Physicians whose primary professional responsibility is the management of health care organizations. Provides for continuing education and certification of the physician executive and the advancement and recognition of the physician executive and the profession. Offers specialized career planning, counseling, recruitment and placement services, and research and information data on physician managers. **Pub:** *American College of Physician Executives–Membership Registry*, annual. Membership Directory. *Price:* Included in membership dues. • *The Ethics of the Ordinary in Healthcare: Concepts & Cases.* Book. *Price:* $52 for members; $57 for nonmembers. • *Fundamentals of Medical Management: A Guide for the Physician Executive.* Book. Includes discussion of organizational theory, effective communication, negotiating skills, conflict management, and organizational politics. *Price:* $48 for members; $58 for nonmembers. • *Get the Job You Want and the Money You're Worth, 2nd Ed..* Book. Guide to successful opportunities. *Price:* $20 for members; $25 for nonmembers. • *The Higher Ground: Biomedical Ethics & the Physician Executive.* Book. *Price:* $10. • *Hope for the Future: A Career Development Guide for Physician Executives.* Book. Provides a list of techniques for prospering in the environment in which health care organizations operate, audiotapes included. *Price:* $40 for members; $48 for nonmembers. • *Managed Care Ethics: Essays on the Impact of Managed Care on Traditional Medical Ethics.* Book. *Price:* $30 for members; $35 for nonmembers. • *Managing in an Academic Health Care Environment.* Book. Provides an overview of managing in this unique environment. *Price:* $15 for members; $15 for nonmembers. • *Mastering the Negotiation Process: A Practical Guide for the Healthcare Executive.* Book. *Price:* $50 for members; $55 for nonmembers. • *MD/MBA: Physicians on the New Frontier of Medical Management.* Book. Guidance in assessing professional and personal strengths and more. *Price:* $35 for members; $45 for nonmembers. • *New Leadership in Health Care Management–The Physician Executive.* Book. Outlines the knowledge base physician executives must master in order to effectively compete and succeed. *Price:* $40 for members; $45 for nonmembers. • *Physician Executive: Journal of Management*, bimonthly. Journal. Includes recurring columns on health economics and health law. *Price:* Included in members.

★ 609 ★ American College of Physicians-American Society of Internal Medicine (ACP-ASIM)
190 N Independence Mall West
Philadelphia, PA 19106-1572
Phone: (215)351-2400 **Fax:** (215)351-2799
Email: interpub@mail.acponline.org
Website: http://www.acponline.org

Fnded: 1915. **Mem:** 85,000. **Desc:** Professional society of medical doctors specializing in internal medicine and closely related specialties such as dermatology, neurology, psychiatry, cardiology, gastroenterology, and public health. Sponsors annual postgraduate courses for practicing physicians. Sponsors teaching and research scholarship competition. **Pub:** *ACP Journal Club*, bimonthly. • *Annals of Internal Medicine*, biweekly. Journal. *Price:* $131/year. • *Medical Knowledge Self-Assessment*, triennial. • *Observer*, monthly. • Directory, periodic. **Frmly:** (2003) American College of Physicians.

★ 610 ★ American College of Podiatric Medical Review (ACPMR)
c/o Dr. Craig Gastwirth, Secretary
3800 Woodward Ave., Ste. 318
Detroit, MI 48201
Phone: (313)833-3090 **Fax:** (313)833-7843
Email: craiggastwrith@aol.com
Website: http://www.acpmr.org
Marc Borovoy, DPM, Pres.

Mem: 60. **Desc:** Licensed podiatric professionals. Works to elevate standards, improve education, standardize guidelines, develop universal methods for peer and claims review. Clearinghouse and liaison for the podiatric medical profession, the public and government agencies.

★ 611 ★ American College of Podiatric Radiologists (ACPR)
VA Medical Ctr.
Rte. 9
Martinsburg, WV 25401
Irving H. Block, D.P.M., Sec. -Treas.

Fnded: 1944. **Mem:** 80. **Desc:** Professional society of podiatrists interested in the use and interpretation of X-rays in treating ailments of the lower extremities. Sponsors postgraduate seminars on podiatric radiology; supports research. Makes available 1400 volume archives to members. Maintains speakers' bureau. **Pub:** *Post Convention Reports*, 1-2/year. • Newsletter, 2-4/year. **Frmly:** (1962) American College of Chiropodial Roentgenologists; (1974) American College of Foot Roentgenologists.

★ 612 ★ American College of Preventive Medicine (ACPM)
1307 New York Ave. NW, No. 200
Washington, DC 20005
Phone: (202)466-2044 **Fax:** (202)466-2662
Email: info@acpm.org
Website: http://www.acpm.org
Jordan Richard, Exec. Dir.

Fnded: 1954. **Mem:** 2,200. **Desc:** Professional society of medical doctors specializing in preventive medicine, public health, aerospace medicine, and occupational medicine. Sponsors educational programs. **Pub:** *ACPM News*, quarterly. Newsletter. Reports on continuing medical education, legislative activities, and programs of the college. Includes calendar of events and research updates. *Price:* Included in membership dues; $25/year for nonmembers. • *American Journal of Preventive Medicine*, bimonthly. Journal. • *Careers in Preventive Medicine*. • *Directory of Residency Programs*, periodic. Directory.

★ 613 ★ American College of Prosthodontists (ACP)
211 E Chicago Ave., Ste. 1000
Chicago, IL 60611-2616
Phone: (312)573-1260 **Free:** 800-378-1260
Fax: (312)573-1257
Email: acp@prosthodontics.org
Website: http://www.prosthodontics.org
Edward J. Cronin, Jr., Exec. Dir.

Fnded: 1970. **Mem:** 2,800. **Reg. Groups:** 40. **Desc:** Dentists specializing in prosthetics who are either board certified, board eligible, or under training in approved graduate or residency programs. Seeks to improve prosthodontic treatment for patients by encouraging educational activities designed to bring new ideas, techniques, and research into clinical practice. Sponsors annual prosthodontic research competition. **Pub:** *Journal of Prosthodontics*, quarterly. Journal. • *Journal of Prosthodontics–Clinical Journal*. Articles. • Newsletter, 4/year. ACP Messenger–Membership Newsletter. *Price:* Included in membership dues. • Also publishes study guide.

★ 614 ★ American College of Psychiatrists (ACP)
732 Addison St., Ste. C
Berkeley, CA 94710
Phone: (510)704-8020 **Fax:** (510)704-0113
Email: aliceacp@aol.com
Website: http://www.acpsych.org
Jack W. Bonner, III, Pres.

Fnded: 1963. **Mem:** 1,000. **Desc:** Established to honor men and women who have made a significant contribution to psychiatry. Members, in turn, invite into membership younger psychiatrists whose scholarly work and demonstrated clinical excellence indicate that they show promise of becoming leaders in the field. **Pub:** *ACP News*, quarterly. Newsletter. • Handbook. • Membership Directory, annual.

★ 615 ★ American College of Psychoanalysts (ACPA)
520 Breck Ct.
Benicia, CA 94510-1372
Phone: (707)745-2070 **Fax:** (707)746-7677
Email: amercolpsa@aol.com
Angela Clark, Exec. Sec.

Fnded: 1969. **Mem:** 240. **Desc:** Physician psychoanalysts. Honorary, scientific, and professional organization. Goal is to contribute to the development of psychoanalysis. Provides professional leadership and supports high standards in the practice of psychoanalysis. Offers a scientific forum for theoretical points of view and encourages the understanding, acceptance, and constructive utilization of sound analytic concepts by an informed public. Offers specialized education program. **Pub:** Bulletin, biennial.

★ 616 ★ American College of Radiation Oncology (ACRO)
4350 East West Hwy., No. 401
Bethesda, MD 20814
Phone: (301)718-6519 **Fax:** (301)656-0989
Email: information@acro.org
Website: http://www.acro.org
Norman Wallis, PhD, Sec.

Fnded: 1989. **Mem:** 1,500. **Desc:** Radiation oncologists, physicists, and administrators. Seeks to ensure that regulatory legislation is fair to radiation oncologists. Lobbies on behalf of radiation oncology physicians. Represents physicians in fee disputes with Medicare. **Pub:** *ACRO Bulletin*, quarterly. Newsletter. *Price:* Included in membership dues.

★ 617 ★ American College of Radiology (ACR)
1891 Preston White Dr.
Reston, VA 20191-4397
Phone: (703)648-8900 **Free:** 800-ACR-LINE
Fax: (703)295-6773
Email: info@acr.org
Website: http://www.acr.org
John J. Curry, Exec. Dir.

Fnded: 1923. **Mem:** 32,000. **State Groups:** 53. **Desc:** Principal organization serving radiologists with programs which focus on the practice of radiology and the delivery of comprehensive radiological health services. These programs in medical sciences, education, and in practice management, serve the public interest and the interests of the medical community in which radiologists serve in both diagnostic and therapeutic roles. Seeks to "advance the science of radiology, improve radiologic service to the patient, study the economic aspects of the practice of radiology, and encourage imrooved and continuing education for radiologists and allied professional fields". **Pub:** Booklets. • Books. • Bulletin, monthly. • Directory, annual. • Pamphlets. • Also publishes textbooks, reprints, kits, and slides.

★ 618 ★ American College of Rheumatology (ACR)
1800 Century Pl., Ste. 250
Atlanta, GA 30345
Phone: (404)633-3777 **Fax:** (404)633-1870
Email: acr@rheumatology.org
Website: http://www.rheumatology.org
Mark Andrejeski, Exec. VP

Fnded: 1934. **Mem:** 8,200. **Desc:** Rheumatologists and rheumatology health professionals. Provides unified leadership in research, education, and the care of people with rheumatic diseases. **Pub:** *ACR Membership Directory*, annual. Membership Directory. • *ACR Scientific Program*, annual. • *Arthritis and Rheumatism*, monthly. Journal. Covers research and trends in the treatment and investigation in the field. Includes book reviews, calendar of events, and employment opportunities. *Price:* $325/year for individuals; $699/year for institutions. • *Arthritis Care and Research*, quarterly. Journal. For health professionals interested in the rheumatic diseases. **Frmly:** (1989) American Rheumatism Association.

★ 619 ★ American College of Sports Medicine (ACSM)
401 W Michigan St.
Indianapolis, IN 46202-3233
Phone: (317)637-9200 **Fax:** (317)634-7817
Email: jgavm@acsm.org
Website: http://www.acsm.org
James R. Whitehead, Exec. VP

Fnded: 1954. **Mem:** 20,000. **Reg. Groups:** 12. **Desc:** Promotes and integrates scientific research, education, and practical applications of sports medicine and exercise science to maintain and enhance physical performance, fitness, health, and quality of life. Certifies fitness leaders, fitness instructors, exercise test technologists, exercise specialists, health/fitness program directors, and U.S. military fitness personnel. Grants continuing medical education (CME) and continuing education credits (CEC). Operates more than 50 committees. **Pub:** *ACSM Fitness Book*. Book. Gives Guidelines on Daily Fitness Programs and Training Regimens. *Price:* $15. • *ACSM's Guidelines for Exercise Testing and Prescription, 6th Ed.*. • *ACSM's Health/Fitness Facility Standards and Guidelines*. • *ACSM's Resource Manual for Guidelines for Exercise Testing and Prescription*. Manual. • *American College of Sports Medicine Directory of Graduate Programs in Sports Medicine and Exercise Science*, annual. Directory. Lists graduate programs in fields related to exercise science and sports medicine at North American institutions. *Price:* $20. • *American College of Sports Medicine Guidelines for the Team Physician*. • *Exercise and Sport Sciences Reviews*, annual. Monographs. *Price:* Included in membership dues; $88/year for nonmembers. • *Medicine and Science in Sports and Exercise*, monthly. Journal. *Price:* Included in membership dues; $303/year for nonmembers. • *Medicine and Science in Sports and Exercise Cumulative Index*. • *Sports Medicine Bulletin*, bimonthly. Magazine. Covers association activities and professional topics. Includes book reviews, calendar of events, and information on membership and fellowship. *Price:* Included in membership dues. • Also publishes position stands, current comments and health and fitness brochures.

★ 620 ★ American College of Surgeons (ACS)

633 N Saint Clair St.
Chicago, IL 60611-3211
Phone: (312)202-5000 **Fax:** (312)202-5001
Email: postmaster@facs.org
Website: http://www.facs.org
Thomas R. Russell, MD, Exec. Dir.

Fnded: 1913. **Mem:** 63,400. **Local Groups:** 67. **Desc:** Professional association of surgeons worldwide organized primarily to improve the quality of care for surgical patients by elevating the standards of surgical education and practice. Conducts nationwide programs to improve emergency medical services and hospital cancer programs. Sponsors continuing education and self-assessment courses for surgeons in practice. **Pub:** *ACS Publications and Services Catalog*, annual. Catalog. Lists ACS publications. *Price:* Free. • *American College of Surgeons Yearbook*, triennial. Yearbook. Lists ACS fellows. *Price:* Free. For members only. • *Bulletin of the American College of Surgeons*, monthly. Bulletin. Includes ACS and Washington news. *Price:* Included in membership dues. • *Journal of the American College of Surgeons*, monthly. Journal. Includes The Surgeon at Work Section, collective literature reviews, and book reviews. • *Resources for Optimal Care of the Injured Patient*. *Price:* $15. • *Surgical Forum*, annual. Abstracts of research papers presented during clinical congress. *Price:* $25/issue.

★ 621 ★ American College of Theriogenologists

PO Box 3065
Montgomery, AL 36109
Phone: (334)395-4666 **Fax:** (334)270-3399
Email: franzc@cs.com
Website: http://www.theriogenology.org
Dr. Dale Paccamonti, Pres.

Fnded: 1970. **Mem:** 350. **Desc:** Veterinarians specializing in animal reproduction. Advances knowledge, education, and services in theriogenology. Acts as certifying agency for theriogenologists. Sponsors scientific programs. Conducts educational programs. **Pub:** *Newsletter of ACT*, bimonthly. Newsletter. *Price:* Free. • Directory, annual.

★ 622 ★ American College of Veterinary Anesthesiologists (ACVA)

c/o Jana L. Jones, AVCA-Exec. Sec. & Dir.
3524 Circle Lake Ln.
Knoxville, TN 37920
Fax: (405)744-6265
Email: execdir@acva.org
Website: http://www.acva.org
Sheilah Robertson, Pres.

Fnded: 1975. **Desc:** Veterinary anesthesiologists and other individuals with an interest in the field. Promotes high standards of practice in veterinary anesthesiology; facilitates continuing professional development of members. Establishes practice guidelines and certification criteria; conducts examinations; bestows certification. Advises the American Veterinary Medical Association regarding accreditation of veterinary anesthesiology training programs.

★ 623 ★ American College of Veterinary Dermatology (ACVD)

c/o Alexis Borich, Exec. Sec.
5610 Kearny Mesa Rd., Ste. B
San Diego, CA 92111
Phone: (858)560-9393 **Fax:** (858)560-0206
Website: http://www.acvd.org
Dr. Donna W Angarano, Pres.

Fnded: 1982. **Mem:** 133. **Desc:** Specialists in veterinary dermatology who have satisfied examination requirements; individuals with national reputation and standing are charter diplomates. promotes veterinary dermatology enhances the competency of professionals in the field. Seeks to develop guidelines for postdoctoral education and to establish experience prerequisites for certification in veterinary dermatology. Administers examinations and certifies veterinarians as veterinary dermatology specialists. Encourages research and other contributions in areas of pathogenesis, diagnosis, therapy, prevention, and control of diseases affecting the skin of animals. Authorizes training programs in the field.

★ 624 ★ American College of Veterinary Internal Medicine (ACVIM)

1997 Wadsworth
Lakewood, CO 80214
Phone: (303)231-9933 **Free:** 800-245-9081
Fax: (303)231-0880
Email: acvim@acvim.org
Website: http://www.acvim.org
Dr. Guy Pidgeon, Pres.

Fnded: 1972. **Mem:** 1,277. **Desc:** Veterinarians certified in internal medicine and related specialties such as cardiology, neurology, and oncology. Works to advance the scope and ideals of veterinary internal medicine and to increase the competence of those practicing in the field. Issues certifying diplomas. **Pub:** *ACVIM Proceedings*, annual. Proceedings. Contains papers submitted by speakers at annual conference. *Price:* $49 in U.S.; $49 outside U.S. • *Journal of Veterinary Internal Medicine*, bimonthly. Journal.

★ 625 ★ American College of Veterinary Ophthalmologists (ACVO)

PO Box 1311
Meridian, ID 83680
Phone: (208)898-0275 **Fax:** (208)846-9826
Email: acvo@mtgs-etc.com
Website: http://www.acvo.com
Dr. Mary B. Glaze, Sec. -Treas.

Fnded: 1969. **Mem:** 166. **Desc:** Veterinarians certified by examination in veterinary ophthalmology. Purposes are: continuing education, research, and practice in veterinary ophthalmology; establishment of standards of training and experience; recognition of individuals who have fulfilled such standards; certification of qualified veterinarians. **Pub:** *Directory of Diplomates*, quinquennial. Directory. *Price:* $10.

★ 626 ★ American College of Veterinary Pathologists (ACVP)

7600 Terrace Ave., No. 203
Middleton, WI 53562-3174
Phone: (608)833-8725 **Fax:** (608)831-5122
Email: info@acvp.org
Website: http://www.acvp.org/
Mary Schumacher, Exec. Dir.

Fnded: 1948. **Mem:** 1,200. **Desc:** Professional society of specialists in veterinary pathology (origin, nature, and course of diseases in animals). Aims to further scientific progress in the specialty of veterinary pathology; to establish standards of training and experience for qualification of specialists in veterinary pathology; to further the recognition of such qualified specialists by suitable certification and other means. Recognized as the certifying agency for the specialty of veterinary pathology in the U.S. and Canada. Conducts specialized education programs and certifying exams. **Pub:** *American College of Veterinary Pathologists–Newsletter*, bimonthly. Newsletter. Covers developments in veterinary pathology; also includes association news, calendar of events, obituaries, and listing of employment opportunities. *Price:* Included in membership dues. • *Membership List*, annual. Directory. • *Veterinary Pathology: An International Journal of Natural and Experimental Disease in Animals*, bimonthly. Includes book reviews and periodic special supplements on a scientific topic. *Price:* $75/year. • Proceedings, annual.

★ 627 ★ American College of Veterinary Radiology (ACVR)

c/o Dr. M. Bernstein
PO Box 87
Glencoe, IL 60022
Phone: (847)251-5517 **Fax:** (847)446-8618
Email: tgnyland@usdavis.edu
Website: http://www.acvr.ucdavis.edu/
Dr. M. Bernstein, Exec. Dir.

Fnded: 1964. **Mem:** 215. **Desc:** Diplomate members (215) are veterinarians certified by the college in veterinary radiology; associate members (6) are individuals distinguished in radiological science but who are not certified veterinary radiologists. Educational association working to advance the art and science of radiology. Certifies candidates who have demonstrated proficiency in veterinary radiology. Encourages the development of teaching personnel and training facilities in veterinary radiology. Aids in the evaluation of residencies and fellowships in veterinary radiology under consideration by the Council on Education of the American Veterinary Medical Association. Advises veterinarians who desire certification in veterinary radiology. Conducts continuing education seminars in conjunction with other veterinary organizations. **Pub:** *Veterinary Radiology and Ultrasound*, bimonthly. Journal. Covers diagnostic and therapeutic radiology, ultrasound, MR, CT, and scintigraphy. *Price:* Included in membership dues; $78/year for institutions. • Brochure. **Frmly:** (1969) American Board of Veterinary Radiology.

★ 628 ★ American College of Veterinary Surgeons (ACVS)

4401 E W Hwy., No. 205
Bethesda, MD 20814-4523
Phone: (301)913-9550 **Fax:** (301)913-2034
Email: acvs@aol.com
Website: http://www.acvs.org
Ann Loew, Exec. Dir.

Fnded: 1965. **Mem:** 978. **Desc:** Acts as certification board for veterinary surgeons. **Pub:** *ACVS Newsletter*, 3/year. Newsletter. *Price:* included in membership dues. • *American College of Veterinary Surgeons–Directory of Diplomates*, biennial. Membership Directory. Includes photographic and biographical information on each member; includes alphabetical name and geographic region indexes. *Price:* Included in membership dues. • *Veterinary Surgery*, bimonthly. Journal. Presents clinical and research papers on veterinary surgery; topics include surgical techniques and management of the surgical patient. *Price:* $156/year for individuals; $256/year for institutions.

★ 629 ★ American Conference of Governmental Industrial Hygienists (ACGIH)

1330 Kemper Meadow Dr., Ste. 600
Cincinnati, OH 45240
Phone: (513)742-2020 **Fax:** (513)742-3355
Email: mail@acgih.org
Website: http://www.acgih.org
A. Anthony Rizzuto, Exec. Dir.

Fnded: 1938. **Mem:** 5,500. **Desc:** Professional society of occupational and environmental safety and health professionals. Devoted to the development of administrative and technical aspects of worker health protection. Functions mainly as a medium for the exchange of ideas and the promotion of standards and techniques in industrial health. Compiles statistics; conducts educational programs. **Pub:** *Air Sampling Instruments*. • *Applied Occupational and Environmental Hygiene*, monthly. Journal. Includes book reviews, peer-reviewed scientific/technical articles and columns, employment listings and information on new products and literature. *Price:* Included in membership dues; $118/year for nonmembers; $204 for institutions. • *Guidelines for the Assessment of Bioaerosols in the Indoor Environment*. • *Industrial Ventilation–A Manual of Recommended Practice*. • *Threshold Limit Values and Biological Exposure Indices*. • *Ventilation System Testing*. • Also publishes other manuals, guides, and studies. **Frmly:** (1945) National Conference of Governmental Industrial Hygienists.

★ 630 ★ American Congress of Rehabilitation Medicine (ACRM)

6801 Lake Plz. Dr., No. B-205
Indianapolis, IN 46220-4049
Phone: (317)915-2250 **Fax:** (317)915-2245

Email: acrm@acrm.org
Website: http://www.acrm.org
Ric Morgan, MBA, Exec. Dir.

Fnded: 1923. **Mem:** 1,100. **Desc:** Physicians, nurses, physical therapists, psychologists, occupational therapists, social workers, speech/language pathologists, and other allied health specialists active in and contributing to advancement in the field of medical rehabilitation. **Pub:** *ACRM Membership Directory*, annual. Membership Directory. • *Archives of Physical Medicine and Rehabilitation*, monthly. Journal. • *Rehabilitation Outlook*, quarterly. Newsletter. **Frmly:** American Congress of Physical Medicine; American Congress of Physical Medicine and Rehabilitation.

★ 631 ★ American Contact Dermatitis Society (ACDS)

233 E Erie, No. 700
Chicago, IL 60611
Phone: (312)988-7700 **Fax:** (312)988-7759
Email: info@contactderm.org
Website: http://www.contactderm.org/about.html

Mem: 500. **Desc:** Promotes information about contact dermatitis and occupational skin disease. **Pub:** *American Journal of Contact Dermatitis*. Journal. *Price:* included in membership dues.

★ 632 ★ American Correctional Health Services Association (BCHSA)

250 Gatsby Pl.
Alpharetta, GA 30022-6161
Free: 877-918-1842 **Fax:** (770)650-5789
Email: achsa@mindspring.com
Website: http://www.corrections.com/achsa
Willma Miles, Exec. Dir.

Fnded: 1975. **Mem:** 1,100. **State Groups:** 8. **Desc:** Health care providers, individuals, or organizations interested in improving the quality of correctional health services. Aims are: to promote the provision of health services to incarcerated persons consistent in quality and quantity with acceptable health care practices; to promote and encourage continuing education and provide technical and professional guidance for correctional health care personnel; to establish a forum for the sharing and discussion of correctional health care issues. Conducts conferences on correctional health care management, nursing, mental health, juvenile corrections, dentistry, and related subjects. Maintains placement service. **Pub:** *CORHEALTH*, bimonthly. Newsletter. Includes book reviews, conference calendar, list of new members, and chapter news. *Price:* Included in membership dues. • Brochures.Provides information on policy matters.

★ 633 ★ American Council on Alcohol Problems (ACAP)

2376 Lakeside Dr.
Birmingham, AL 35244
Phone: (205)989-8177 **Fax:** (205)985-9015
Email: dliacap@aol.com
Dr. D.L. Ireland, contact

Fnded: 1895. **Desc:** Federation of 36 state affiliates and 22 denominational judicatories; 1000 associate members. Seeks long-range solutions to the problems posed by alcohol. Employs educational, and legislative approaches for the prevention of alcoholism and other alcohol-related problems. Coordinates the work of state affiliates who carry on their programs under provisions of the 21st Amendment, putting alcohol control largely at state level. Denominations channel their cooperative social concerns through elected directors who guide the program and activities of ACAP. **Pub:** *The American Issue*, quarterly. • Directory, annual. **Frmly:** (1948) Anti-Saloon League of America; (1950) Temperance League of America; (1964) National Temperance League.

★ 634 ★ American Council on Alcoholism (ACA)

PO Box 25126
Arlington, VA 22202
Phone: (703)248-9005 **Free:** 800-527-5344
Fax: (703)248-9007
Email: aca2@earthlink.net
Website: http://www.aca-usa.org

Fnded: 1953. **Mem:** 400. **Desc:** Works to educate the public about the effects of alcohol, alcoholism, alcohol abuse, and the need for prompt, effective, affordable, and available treatment. Provides a toll-free Helpline for alcoholism treatment and recovery referral and assistance. **Pub:** *Frequently Asked Questions About Alcoholism*. • *Recovery*, quarterly. Newsletter. Publicizes issues concerning alcoholism; promotes the understanding that alcoholism is a treatable disease; contains research results. *Price:* Included in membership dues. • *Teenage Drinking*. **Frmly:** Maryland Society on Alcoholism; (1974) Baltimore Area Council on Alcoholism.

★ 635 ★ American Council of Applied Clinical Nutrition (ACACN)

PO Box 509
Florissant, MO 63032
Phone: (314)921-3997 **Free:** 800-826-5366
Fax: (314)921-8485
Clarence T. Smith, PhD, Pres.

Fnded: 1974. **Mem:** 500. **Desc:** Clinical nutrition specialists. Offers structured academic course and certification; conducts research.

★ 636 ★ American Council of the Blind (ACB)

1155 15th St. NW, Ste. 1004
Washington, DC 20005
Phone: (202)467-5081 **Free:** 800-424-8666
Fax: (202)467-5085
Email: info@acb.org
Website: http://www.acb.org
Charles Crawford, Exec. Dir.

Fnded: 1961. **Mem:** 20,000. **Nat'l Groups:** 19. **State Groups:** 51. **Desc:** Blind and visually impaired persons. Serves as a national information clear Security and supplemental security income programs, radio reading services, special library services, eye research, and low vision technology. Offers group insurance plans, professional assistance in public interest, class action litigation, and public education about blindness and the abilities of visually impaired people. **Pub:** *Braille Forum*, monthly. Newsletter. Concerned with legislative developments, new products and services, medical and technological advances, and human interest stories for the blind. *Price:* Free for individuals in U.S.; $25/yr. for organizations & international subscribers.

★ 637 ★ American Council of the Blind Enterprises and Services (ACBES)

120 S 6th St., Ste. 1005
Minneapolis, MN 55402-1839
Phone: (612)332-3242 **Free:** 800-866-3242
Fax: (612)332-7850
Email: acbesall@ix.netcom.com
Website: http://www.acb.org
James R. Olsen, CFO

Fnded: 1978. **Mem:** 16. **Desc:** Board of directors of the American Council of the Blind. Owns and operates 10 ACB thrift stores which help finance ACB and its programs and aid the blind and visually impaired in leading productive and independent lives.

★ 638 ★ American Council of Blind Lions (ACBL)

PO Box 2312
Fort Collins, CO 80522
Phone: (970)484-2598
Email: jabeatty1@yahoo.com
Website: http://www.acb.org/acbl
Alan Beatty, Pres.

Fnded: 1970. **Mem:** 141. **Desc:** Legally blind members of Lions Clubs International. Informs the public of the needs and capabilities of blind persons; exchanges information on club activities benefiting work for the blind; encourages blind people to join Lions Clubs and other civic organizations. Supports speakers' bureau. **Pub:** Newsletter, quarterly. **Frmly:** (1985) World Council of Blind Lions; (1986) Council of Blind Lions.

★ 639 ★ American Council of Certified Podiatric Physicians and Surgeons

6421 Inkster Rd., Ste. 102
Bloomfield Hills, MI 48301
Phone: (248)855-7740 **Fax:** (248)855-7743
Email: accpps1@juno.com
Website: http://www.accpps.com
Howard L. Lazar, DPM,JD, Exec. Dir.

Fnded: 1982. **Mem:** 650. **Desc:** Promotes the profession of podiatric medicine and surgery. Gains equal acceptance for all podiatrists by hospitals and managed care organizations.

★ 640 ★ American Council for Drug Education (ACDE)

164 W 74th St.
New York, NY 10023
Free: 800-488-DRUG **Fax:** (212)595-2553
Email: acde@phoenixhouse.org
Website: http://www.acde.org
Robert Balster, PhD, Advisor

Fnded: 1977. **Desc:** Doctors, mental health counselors, teachers, clergymen, policymakers, school librarians, parent groups, industry leaders, and concerned individuals. Disseminates information and research on all drugs of abuse. Makes available resource information kits that include both written and audiovisual materials. Provides prevention materials such as "How to Speak to Your Kids about Marijuana." **Pub:** *Free Catalog*. For parents, children, schools, and other professionals. • Brochures. • Handbooks. **Frmly:** (1983) American Council on Marijuana and Other Psychoactive Drugs.

★ 641 ★ American Council on Exercise (ACE)

4851 Paramount Dr.
San Diego, CA 92123
Phone: (858)279-8227 **Free:** 800-825-3636
Fax: (858)279-8064
Email: kristiep@acefitness.org
Website: http://www.acefitness.org
Kristie Paterson, PR Mgr.

Fnded: 1985. **Desc:** Certifies fitness professionals and non-profit organization. Keeps them aware of new information in the health and fitness industry. Offers continuing education programs. Sponsors children's services. Provides consumers with health and fitness research and information. **Pub:** *ACE Certified News*, bimonthly. Newsletter. For ACE-certified fitness professional. • *ACE Faculty Network*. • *Ace Fitness/Matters*, bimonthly. Magazine. *Price:* $25/year; $60/3 years; $33/year in North America; $49 outside North America.

★ 642 ★ American Council for Headache Education (ACHE)

19 Mantua Rd.
Mount Royal, NJ 08061
Phone: (856)423-0258 **Free:** 800-255-ACHE
Fax: (856)423-0082
Email: achehq@talley.com
Website: http://www.achenet.org
Linda McGillicuddy, Exec. Dir.

Fnded: 1990. **Mem:** 5,000. **Desc:** Headache sufferers and physicians dedicated to advancing treatment and management of headache; promotes public awareness. **Pub:** *Headache*, quarterly. Newsletter. Provides current information on new treatments and management strategies. *Price:* Included in membership dues.

★ 643 ★ American Council of Hypnotist Examiners (ACHE)

700 S Central Ave.
Glendale, CA 91204
Phone: (818)242-1159 **Fax:** (818)247-9379

Email: hypnotismla@earthlink.net
Gil Boyne, Exec. Dir.

Fnded: 1980. **Mem:** 8,200. **Nat'l Groups:** 4. **Reg. Groups:** 8. **State Groups:** 1. **Local Groups:** 1. **Desc:** Educates, examines, and awards certification in the field of hypnotherapy. Maintains speakers' bureau. Sponsors educational programs. **Pub:** *American Hypnotherapy Report*, annual. Report. Contains news and information on the hypnotherapy profession. *Price:* Included in membership dues. • *Directory of Certified Members*, periodic. Membership Directory. • *International Hypnotherapy Report*, quarterly. Magazine. *Price:* Free to members. • Newsletter, periodic. *Price:* Free to members. **AKA:** Hypnotists Examining Council.

★ 644 ★ American Council on Pharmaceutical Education (ACPE)

20 N Clark St., Ste. 2500
Chicago, IL 60602-5109
Phone: (312)664-3575 **Fax:** (312)664-4652
Email: pvlasses@acpe-accredit.org
Website: http://www.acpe-accredit.org
Peter H. Vlasses, PharmD, Exec. Dir.

Fnded: 1932. **Desc:** National agency for accreditation of professional degree programs in pharmacy and providers of continuing pharmaceutical education, including certificate programs in pharmacy. **Pub:** *Accredited Professional Programs of Colleges and Schools of Pharmacy*, annual. Directory. • *Accredited Providers of Continuing Pharmaceutical Education*, annual. Directory.

★ 645 ★ American Council on Science and Health (ACSH)

1995 Broadway, 2nd Fl.
New York, NY 10023-5860
Phone: (212)362-7044 **Fax:** (212)362-4919
Email: acsh@acsh.org
Website: http://www.acsh.org
Dr. Elizabeth M. Whelan, Pres.

Fnded: 1978. **Mem:** 2,000. **Desc:** Provides consumers with scientifically balanced evaluations of food, chemicals, the environment, and human health. Council personnel participate in government regulatory proceedings, congressional hearings, appear on radio and television programs, and public debates and forums. **Pub:** *Cigarettes: What the Warning Label Doesn't Tell You.* • *Directory of Scientific Advisors*, triennial. Directory. • *Media Update*, semiannual. • *News From ACSH*, semiannual. • *Priorities*, quarterly. Magazine. Health and environmental reports for consumers. *Price:* $6.25 single copy; $25 annual subscription. • Papers. • Reports.On health risks and benefits associated with public health and environmental issues.

★ 646 ★ American CranioSacral Therapy Association (ACSTA)

c/o Upledger Institute
11211 Prosperity Farms Rd., Ste. D-325
Palm Beach Gardens, FL 33410
Phone: (561)622-4334 **Fax:** (561)622-4771
Email: acsta@acsta.com
Website: http://www.acsta.com/
John Matthew, Dir.

Desc: CranioSacral Therapy practitioners and proponents of the modality. Represents the CranioSacral Therapy profession; creates understanding and acceptance of CST within legislative, insurance, public, media, and medical arenas; supports educational and competency standards; monitors insurance and public policy.

★ 647 ★ American Cryonics Society (ACS)

1901 Old Middlefield Way, Ste. 1
Mountain View, CA 94043
Phone: (650)254-2001 **Free:** 800-523-2001
Fax: (408)253-0444
Email: cryonics@americancryonics.org
Website: http://pweb.jps.net/~cryonics
Edgar Swank, Pres.

Fnded: 1969. **Mem:** 500. **Desc:** Individuals interested in life extension through cryonics (the practice of freezing a clinically dead human in hopes of bringing the person back to life when resuscitation or reconstruction is possible). Promotes education and provides information about cryonic suspension, suspended animation, and low-temperature medicine. Enables individuals to arrange for their own cryonic suspension. Sponsors research into suspended animation, life extension sciences, and low temperature medicine. Conducts programs to freeze tissue samples from endangered species for possible future cloning. Maintains library; operates speakers' bureau; conducts charitable programs. **Pub:** *American Cryonics*, semiannual. Journal. Synopsis of research, national news and editorials affecting cryonics field. • *American Cryonics News*, bimonthly. Newsletter. Covers cryonics and life extension. Includes calendar of events and research reports. *Price:* Included in membership dues; $35/year for nonmembers. • *The Immortalist*, monthly. Contains articles on cryonics, health, aging research, and science. **Frmly:** (1985) Bay Area Cryonics Society.

★ 648 ★ American Dance Therapy Association (ADTA)

2000 Century Plz., Ste. 108
Columbia, MD 21044
Phone: (410)997-4040 **Fax:** (410)997-4048
Email: info@adta.org
Website: http://www.adta.org
Elissa Q. White, Pres.

Fnded: 1966. **Mem:** 1,200. **Desc:** Individuals professionally practicing dance therapy, students interested in becoming dance therapists, university departments with dance therapy programs, and individuals in related therapeutic fields. Purpose is to establish and maintain high standards of professional education and competence in dance therapy. Acts as information center; develops guidelines for educational programs and for approval of programs; maintains registry of qualified dance therapists. Maintains Marian Chace Memorial Fund to be used for educational, literary, or scientific projects related to dance in the field of mental health. **Pub:** *American Journal of Dance Therapy*, semiannual. Journal. • *Conference Proceedings.* Proceedings. • *Dance Therapy Bibliography.* Bibliography. • Membership Directory, annual. • Monographs. • Newsletter, quarterly.

★ 649 ★ American Dental Assistants Association (ADAA)

35 E Wacker Dr., No. 1730
Chicago, IL 60601-2211
Phone: (312)541-1550 **Fax:** (312)541-1496
Email: adaa1@aol.com
Website: http://www.dentalassistant.org
Lawrence H. Sepin, Exec. Dir.

Fnded: 1923. **Mem:** 15,000. **State Groups:** 50. **Local Groups:** 125. **Desc:** Individuals employed as dental assistants in dental offices, clinics, hospitals, or institutions; instructors of dental assistants; dental students. Sponsors workshops and seminars; maintains governmental liaison. Offers group insurance; maintains scholarship trust fund. Dental Assisting National Board examines members who are candidates for title of Certified Dental Assistant. **Pub:** *The Dental Assistant*, bimonthly. Journal. Features articles pertaining to dental assisting. *Price:* included in membership dues; $20/yr. for nonmembers. • Also publishes educational materials.

★ 650 ★ American Dental Association (ADA)

211 E Chicago Ave.
Chicago, IL 60611
Phone: (312)440-2500 **Fax:** (312)440-2800
Email: publicinfo@ada.org
Website: http://www.ada.org
James Bramson, Exec. Dir.

Fnded: 1859. **Mem:** 144,510. **State Groups:** 54. **Local Groups:** 535. **Desc:** Professional society of dentists. Encourages the improvement of the health of the public and promotes the art and science of dentistry in matters of legislation and regulations. Inspects and accredits dental schools and schools for dental hygienists, assistants, and laboratory technicians. Conducts research programs at ADA Foundation Research Institute. Produces most of the dental health education material used in the U.S. Sponsors National Children's Dental Health Month. Compiles statistics on personnel, practice, and dental care needs and attitudes of patients with regard to dental health. Sponsors 13 councils. **Pub:** *ADA News*, biweekly. *Price:* $61 for nonmembers. • *Journal of the American Dental Association*, monthly. Journal. *Price:* $100 for nonmembers. **Frmly:** (1922) National Dental Association.

★ 651 ★ American Dental Education Association

1625 Massachusetts Ave. NW, Ste. 600
Washington, DC 20036-2212
Phone: (202)667-9433 **Fax:** (202)667-0642
Email: adea@adea.org
Website: http://www.adea.org/
Dr. Richard Valachovic, Exec. Dir.

Fnded: 1923. **Mem:** 3,600. **Desc:** Individuals interested in dental education; schools of dentistry, graduate dentistry, and allied dental education in the U.S., Canada, and Puerto Rico; affiliated institutions of the federal government. To promote better teaching and education in dentistry and dental research and to facilitate exchange of ideas among dental educators. Sponsors meetings, conferences, and workshops; conducts surveys, studies, and special projects and publishes their results. Maintains 39 sections representing teaching and administrative areas of dentistry. **Pub:** *Bulletin of Dental Education*, monthly. Newsletter. Provides information, grant and fellowship announcements, legislation updates, news, member activities. *Price:* included in membership dues. • *Directory of Institutional Members*, annual. Directory. • *Journal of Dental Education*, monthly. Journal. *Price:* included in membership dues. • *Official Guide to United States and Canadian Dental Schools*, annual. Catalog. Helps students decide on a career in dentistry, and explains how to go about it. *Price:* $35. • *Opportunities for Minority Students in U.S. Dental Schools*, semiannual. Catalog. *Price:* $10. • Proceedings, annual. *Price:* $10. **Frmly:** (2000) American Association Dental Schools.

★ 652 ★ American Dental Hygienists' Association (ADHA)

444 N Michigan Ave., Ste. 3400
Chicago, IL 60611
Phone: (312)440-8911 **Free:** 800-243-ADHA
Fax: (312)467-1806
Email: exec.office@adha.net
Website: http://www.adha.org
Stanley B. Peck, Exec. Dir.

Fnded: 1923. **Mem:** 35,000. **Nat'l Groups:** 1. **Reg. Groups:** 12. **State Groups:** 53. **Local Groups:** 360. **Desc:** Professional organization of licensed dental hygienists possessing a degree or certificate in dental hygiene granted by an accredited school of dental hygiene. Makes available scholarships, research grants, and continuing education programs. Maintains accrediting service through the American Dental Association's Commission on Dental Accreditation. Compiles statistics. **Pub:** *American Dental Hygienists' Association Access*, 10/year. Magazine. Covers current dental hygiene topics, regulatory and legislative developments, and association news. Includes membership profiles. *Price:* Included in membership dues; $30/year for nonmembers. • *Journal of Dental Hygiene*, quarterly. Journal. Includes association news, book reviews, abstracts, government news, and information on research and new products. *Price:* Included in membership dues; $40/year for nonmembers.

★ 653 ★ American Dental Society of Anesthesiology (ADSA)
211 E Chicago Ave., Ste. 780
Chicago, IL 60611
Phone: (312)664-8270 **Free:** 800-722-7788
Fax: (312)642-9713
Email: adsahome@cs.com
Website: http://www.adsahome.org
Jeffrey D. Bennett, DMD, Pres.

Fnded: 1953. **Mem:** 3,200. **State Groups:** 21. **Desc:** Dentists and physicians. Encourages study and progress in dental anesthesiology. **Pub:** *ADSA Directory*, annual. Directory. • *ADSA Pulse*, bimonthly. Newsletter. Includes society news, calendar of events, and research updates. *Price:* Included in membership dues; $5/year for nonmembers. • *Anesthesia Progress*, bimonthly. *Price:* $30/year for members; $35/year for nonmembers; $55/year for institutions.

★ 654 ★ American Dental Society of Europe (ADSE)
c/o Lloyd Searon
2 Harcourt House
19A Cavendish Sq.
London W1M 9AB, United Kingdom
Phone: 44 207 6374518 **Fax:** 44 207 6291869
Email: lloydsearson@compuserve.com

Fnded: 1873. **Mem:** 250. **Lang(s):** English. **Desc:** Graduates of North American schools of dentistry who practice in Europe. Seeks the interchange of dental information and the advancement of the profession. Offers scholarship for European dentists to study in the United States.

★ 655 ★ American Diabetes Association (ADA)
1701 N Beauregard St.
Alexandria, VA 22311
Phone: (703)549-1500 **Free:** 800-DIABETES
Fax: (703)549-6995
Email: askada@diabetes.org
Website: http://www.diabetes.org
John H. Graham, IV, CEO

Fnded: 1940. **Mem:** 280,000. **State Groups:** 53. **Local Groups:** 800. **Desc:** Physicians, laypersons, and health professionals interested in diabetes mellitus. Promotes research, information and advocacy to find a prevention and cure for diabetes and to improve the lives of all people with diabetes. Promotes public awareness of diabetes as a serious disease. Conducts educational programs and provides information to people with diabetes and the health professionals who care for them. Administers research grants. **Pub:** *Clinical Diabetes*, bimonthly. Newsletter. Provides current scientific information about diabetes and its treatment to the primary care provider. *Price:* $15/year member; $30/year nonmember; $40/year institution. • *Diabetes*, monthly. Contains original research papers on the physiology and pathophysiology of diabetes mellitus and related disorders. *Price:* $75/year members; $135/year nonmembers; $200/year institution. • *Diabetes Care*, monthly. Journal. Covers original clinical research and commentaries primarily directed toward improving the medical management of people with diabetes mellitus. *Price:* $75/year members; $100/year nonmembers; $150/year institution. • *Diabetes Forecast*, monthly. Magazine. Healthy life styles magazine for people with diabetes. Provides in fo. about diabetes, self-care exercise, diet, travel, and personal development. *Price:* Included in membership dues. • *Diabetes Reviews*, quarterly. Journal. Provides comprehensive reviews of basic science and clinical issues in diabetes. *Price:* $45/year for members; $85/year for nonmembers; $125/year for institutions. • *Diabetes Spectrum: From Research to Practice*, quarterly. Journal. *Price:* Included in membership dues; $30/uear member; $45/year nonmember. • Videos. • Publishes a catalog of publications available.

★ 656 ★ American Dietetic Association (ADA)
120 S Riverside Plz.
Chicago, IL 60606
Phone: (312)899-0040 **Free:** 800-877-1600
Fax: (312)899-1979
Email: membrshp@eatright.org
Website: http://www.eatright.org
Ronald Moen, CEO

Fnded: 1917. **Mem:** 67,000. **State Groups:** 52. **Desc:** Food and nutrition professionals. Promotes nutrition, health and well-being. **Pub:** *Journal of the American Dietetic Association*, monthly. Journal. Contains research and practice articles, association news, literature abstracts, and a list of new publications. *Price:* Included in membership dues; $98/year for nonmembers.

★ 657 ★ American Disability Association
2201 Sixth Ave. South
Birmingham, AL 35233
Phone: (205)328-9090 **Fax:** (205)251-7417
Email: adanet@adanet.org
Website: http://www.adanet.org
Bill Freeman, Pres.

Fnded: 1991. **Mem:** 60,000. **Reg. Groups:** 20. **State Groups:** 40. **Desc:** Serves as a support group for individuals with disabilities. Provides exchange of information on disability issues. Makes available children's services, educational and research programs, and charitable services. **Pub:** *Journal of the American Disability Association*, monthly. Journal. *Price:* Free.

★ 658 ★ American Disabled for Attendant Program Today (ADAPT)
201 S Cherokee St.
Denver, CO 80223-1836
Phone: (303)733-9324 **Fax:** (303)733-6211
Email: adapt@adapt.org
Website: http://www.adapt.org/
Babs Johnson, Dir.

Fnded: 1983. **Mem:** 5,000. **Nat'l Groups:** 1. **State Groups:** 34. **Local Groups:** 50. **Desc:** Promotes federal funding of in-home support services for the elderly and disabled in an effort to decrease the number of individuals being placed in nursing homes. **Pub:** *Incitement*, 6/year. Newsletter. **Frmly:** (1991) American Disabled for Accessible Public Transit.

★ 659 ★ American Electrology Association (AEA)
106 Oakridge Rd.
Trumbull, CT 06611
Phone: (203)374-6667 **Free:** 877-746-9723
Fax: (203)372-7134
Email: infoaea@electrology.com
Website: http://www.electrology.com
Teresa E. Petricca, Exec. Dir.

Fnded: 1958. **Mem:** 2,000. **Nat'l Groups:** 2. **State Groups:** 27. **Desc:** Electrologists united for education, professional advancement, protection of public welfare. Promotes uniform legislative standards throughout the states. Coordinates efforts of affiliated associations in dealing with problems of national scope. Sponsors the International Board of Electrologist Certification and Council on Accreditation of Electrology Schools/Programs. Maintains referral, reference, advisory, and consulting services. **Pub:** *American Electrology Association–Roster*, annual. Membership Directory. Arranged geographically. Includes modalities used. *Price:* Included in membership dues. • *Direct Line*, periodic. Bulletin. Provides communication between AEA executives and board members. Includes meeting minutes, committee reports, and program status reports. *Price:* Available to board members and committee chairs. • *Electrolysis World*, quarterly. Newsletter. Includes calendar of events. *Price:* available to members only. • *Infection Control Standards for the Practice of Electrology*. • *Journal of the American Electrology Association*, semiannual. Journal. Includes case studies. *Price:* $10/issue. • *Medical/Professional News*, semiannual. • Brochures. **Frmly:** (1986) American Electrolysis Association.

★ 660 ★ American Endodontic Society (AES)
1321 N Harbor Blvd., No. 201
Fullerton, CA 92835
Phone: (714)870-5590 **Fax:** (714)526-2818
Email: amendsoc@aol.com
Website: http://www.aesoc.com
Dr. Ramon Werts, Exec. Dir.

Fnded: 1969. **Mem:** 10,000. **Desc:** Dentists united to promote and provide educational and scientific information on simplified root canal therapy for the general practitioner. Conducts research programs. **Pub:** *American Endodontic Society Newsletter*, quarterly. Newsletter. Contains society news, member profiles, and instructional articles. • *Hotline*, periodic.

★ 661 ★ American Environmental Health Foundation (AEHF)
8345 Walnut Hill Ln., Ste. 225
Dallas, TX 75231
Phone: (214)361-9515 **Free:** 800-428-2343
Fax: (214)361-2534
Email: aehf@aehf.com
Website: http://www.aehf.com/aboutaehf.htm

Fnded: 1975. **Desc:** Provides research and education into chemical sensitivity.

★ 662 ★ American Epilepsy Society (AES)
342 N Main St.
West Hartford, CT 06117-2507
Phone: (860)586-7505 **Fax:** (860)586-7550
Email: info@aesnet.org
Website: http://www.aesnet.org
M. Suzanne C. Berry, CAE, Exec. Dir.

Fnded: 1946. **Mem:** 3,000. **Desc:** Clinicians, scientists investigating basic and clinical aspects of epilepsy, and related professional workers with an active interest in seizure disorders. Seeks to promote interdisciplinary communication, scientific investigation and exchange of clinical information about epilepsy. Works to prevent and treat epilepsy. **Pub:** *Epilepsia*, monthly. Journal. Published in conjunction with the International League Against Epilepsy. *Price:* Included in membership fee. • Also publishes Epilepsy Research incorporating the Journal of Epilepsy **Frmly:** (1959) American League Against Epilepsy.

★ 663 ★ American Equilibration Society (AES)
8726 N Ferris Ave.
Morton Grove, IL 60053
Phone: (847)965-2888 **Fax:** (847)965-4888
Email: aesdental@sprynet.com
Website: http://www.occlusion-tmj.org/
Shel Marcus, Exec. Dir.

Fnded: 1955. **Mem:** 1,100. **Desc:** Dentists, orthodontists, oral surgeons, and physicians interested in study and proficiency in the diagnosis and treatment of occlusal and temporomandibular joint disorders. Bestows Student Recognition Certificates annually to outstanding graduating students. **Pub:** *American Equilibration Society Newsletter*, 3/year. Newsletter. *Price:* Included in membership dues. • *Roster*, annual. • *TMJ Update*, bimonthly. *Price:* Included in membership dues.

★ 664 ★ American Federation for Aging Research (AFAR)
70 W 40th St.
New York, NY 10018
Phone: (212)703-9977 **Free:** 800-330-4660
Fax: (212)997-0330
Email: amfedaging@aol.com
Website: http://www.afar.org
Hadley C. Ford, Chair

Fnded: 1981. **Reg. Groups:** 1. **Desc:** Physicians, scientists, and other individuals involved or interested in research in aging and associated diseases. Purpose is to stimulate and fund research on aging. Facilitates communication among scientists in the field. Fosters public education regarding the need for support of related research. **Pub:** *AFAR Newsletter*, biennial. Newsletter. Includes profiles of members. *Price:* Free. • *The Paul Besson Physician Faculty Scholars in Aging Research Report*, annual. Reprint. Contains scientific research projects of physician scientists.

★ 665 ★ American Federation for Medical Research

13 Elm St.
Manchester, MA 01944
Phone: (978)526-8330 **Fax:** (978)526-1703
Email: afmr@prri.com
Website: http://www.afmr.org
Jane E.B. Reusch, Pres.

Fnded: 1940. **Mem:** 6,000. **Reg. Groups:** 4. **Local Groups:** 19. **Desc:** Provides a forum for young clinical scientists (under 43); promotes and encourages original research in clinical and laboratory medicine. Offers specialized education program; maintains information services on membership status, files, and National Abstracting Processing. Annual scientific program presents sections on: Cardiovascular; Dermatology; Endocrinology; Gastroenterology; Genetics; Hematology; Immunology and Connective Tissue; Infectious Disease; Metabolism; Neoplastic Disease; Patient Care; Pulmonary; Renal and Electrolytes. **Pub:** *Journal of Investigative Medicine*, bimonthly. Journal. **Frmly:** (1998) American Federation for Clinical Research.

★ 666 ★ American Fibromyalgia Syndrome Association (AFSA)

6380 E Tanque Verde, Ste. D
Tucson, AZ 85715
Phone: (520)733-1570
Website: http://www.afsafund.org/
Kristin Thorson, Pres.

Fnded: 1994. **Desc:** Dedicated to research, education and patient advocacy for fibromyalgia syndrome (FMS) and chronic fatigue syndrome (CFS). Provides phone service "warm line" for patients and physicians. Sponsors information booths at major medical conferences. **Pub:** *AFSA Update.*

★ 667 ★ American Foundation for Aging Research (AFAR)

North Carolina State University
Biochemistry Department
128 Polk Hall
Raleigh, NC 27695-7622
Phone: (919)515-5679 **Fax:** (919)515-2047
Email: afar_office@ncsu.edu
Website: http://www4.ncsu.edu/unity/users/a/agris/afar/afar.htm
Dr. Paul F. Agris, Pres.

Fnded: 1979. **Mem:** 375. **Desc:** Supports basic research and educational opportunities for the study of age-related diseases and the biology of aging. Supports projects emphasizing modern biological, genetic, biochemical, and biophysical techniques and approaches to the problems of age-associated diseases and the understanding of aging. **Pub:** *The Newsletter of the American Foundation for Aging Research*, quarterly. Newsletter. *Price:* Included in membership dues.

★ 668 ★ American Foundation for AIDS Research (amfAR)

120 Wall St., 13th floor
New York, NY 10005-3902
Phone: (212)806-1600 **Free:** 800-39-AMFAR
Fax: (212)806-1601
Email: teresa.coffey@amfar.org
Website: http://www.amfar.org
William F. Zabel, Secretary

Fnded: 1985. **Reg. Groups:** 2. **Desc:** Dedicated to the support of AIDS research and prevention, treatment education, and advocacy of AIDS-related public policy. **Pub:** *amfAR Treatment Insider*, bimonthly. Reprint. • *HIV/AIDS Treatment Directory*, semiannual. Directory. *Price:* Most distributed free. • Bulletin, periodic.

★ 669 ★ American Foundation for the Blind (AFB)

11 Penn Plz., Ste. 300
New York, NY 10001
Phone: (212)502-7600 **Free:** 800-232-5463
Fax: (212)502-7777
Email: afbinfo@afb.net
Website: http://www.afb.org
Carl R. Augusto, Pres.

Fnded: 1921. **Desc:** Mission is to eliminate the inequities faced by the ten million Americans who are blind or visually impaired; Helen Keller dedicated 40 years of her life to the organization. Develops, collects, and disseminates information that benefits people who are blind or visually impaired, their families and friends, professionals in the blindness field, and the general public. Takes a leadership role in identifying issues critical to people who are blind or visually impaired; conducts research, and acts as a catalyst for change. Educates the public and policymakers as to the needs and capabilities of people who are blind or visually impaired; records and duplicates Talking Books for the Library of Congress and other audio materials for various corporations and organizations; and develops public education programs. Maintains offices in Atlanta, Chicago, Dallas and San Francisco, and a governmental relations office in Washington, DC. **Pub:** *AFB Directory of Services for Blind and Visually Impaired Persons in the U.S. and Canada.* Directory. Lists over 3000 local, state, regional, and national services, including educational, informational, rehabilitative, low-vision, and aging services. *Price:* $100/copy. • *AFB News*, semiannual. Newsletter. Covers programs and activities of the AFB. *Price:* Free. • *Journal of Visual Impairment and Blindness*, monthly. Journal. Contains articles on research and practice in the areas of rehabilitation, psychology, education, legislation, medicine, and sensory devices. *Price:* $74/year for individuals in the U.S. and Canada; $99/year for individuals outside the U.S. and Canada; $104/year for institutions in the U.S. and Canada; $129/year for institutions outside the U.S. and Canada. • Also publishes textbooks, training manuals, and resource guides, videos, and educational materials for teachers.

★ 670 ★ American Foundation for Health (AFH)

2107 Dwight Way
Berkeley, CA 94704
Phone: (510)644-3366
Molleen Matsumura, Exec. Dir.

Fnded: 1979. **Mem:** 17,,000. **Desc:** Individuals interested in improving the delivery of health care services. Encourages recording of personal medical data. Conducts educational research projects and activities. **Pub:** *Health Features*, periodic. Newsletter.

★ 671 ★ American Foundation for Maternal and Child Health (AFMCH)

439 E 51st St., 8th Fl.
New York, NY 10022
Phone: (212)759-5510 **Fax:** (212)935-0191
Doris Haire, Pres.

Fnded: 1972. **Desc:** Serves as a clearinghouse for interdisciplinary research on maternal and child health; focuses on the perinatal or birth period and its effect on infant development. Sponsors medical research designed to improve application of technology in maternal and child health; conducts educational programs; compiles statistics. Operates extensive reference library.

★ 672 ★ American Foundation for Pharmaceutical Education (AFPE)

1 Church St., Ste. 202
Rockville, MD 20850-4158
Phone: (301)738-2160 **Fax:** (301)738-2161
Email: afpe@worldnet.att.net
Website: http://www.afpenet.org
Robert M. Bachman, Pres.

Fnded: 1942. **Mem:** 40. **Desc:** Established by pharmaceutical and drug trade associations to improve pharmaceutical education, colleges of pharmacy, and pharmacy student performance. Accepts and administers gifts, legacies, bequests, and funds and makes disbursements for fellowships and the promotion of pharmaceutical education. **Pub:** *Annual Progress Report*, annual. Report. Reports on contributions and programs. *Price:* Free.

★ 673 ★ American Foundation for Suicide Prevention (AFSP)

120 Wall St., Fl. 22
New York, NY 10005
Phone: (212)363-3500 **Free:** 888-333-AFSP
Fax: (212)363-6237
Email: inquiry@afsp.org
Website: http://www.afsp.org
Robert Gebbia, Exec. Dir.

Fnded: 1987. **Mem:** 1,500. **Reg. Groups:** 12. **Desc:** Medical professionals, community leaders, and suicide survivors. Provides funding for research on the causes and prevention of suicide. Trains professionals in the treatment of suicidal individuals; offers support programs for suicide survivors. **Pub:** *Lifesavers*, quarterly. Newsletter. *Price:* Included with membership dues. **Frmly:** (1998) Maryland Suicide Foundation.

★ 674 ★ American Foundation for Surgery of the Hand (AFSH)

6300 N River Rd., Ste. 600
Rosemont, IL 60018-4256
Phone: (847)384-8300 **Fax:** (847)384-1435
Email: info@hand-surg.org
Website: http://www.assh.org
Mark Anderson, Exec. Dir.

Fnded: 1986. **Desc:** Awards grants to medical, educational, research, and public education programs related to the field of hand and upper extremity surgery.

★ 675 ★ American Foundation for Urologic Disease (AFUD)

1128 N Charles St.
Baltimore, MD 21201
Phone: (410)468-1800 **Free:** 800-242-2383
Fax: (410)468-1808
Email: admin@afud.org
Website: http://www.afud.org
Thomas Bruckman, Exec. Dir.

Fnded: 1987. **Desc:** Medical research and education organization working to broaden the base of urological research and enhance public and health care providers awareness of urologic disease in the U.S. Conducts public educational programs on topics including childhood urological problems, prostate disease, and bladder disorders. Encourages advocacy among prostate cancer survivors. Makes available research fellowships and grants. **Pub:** *Family Urology*, quarterly. Magazine. Includes information about latest treatments. *Price:* included in membership dues. • *Foundation Focus.* Newsletter. *Price:* included in membership dues.

★ 676 ★ American Foundation for Vision Awareness (AFVA)

243 N Lindbergh Blvd.
Saint Louis, MO 63141
Free: 800-927-2382 **Fax:** (314)991-4101
Email: afva@aol.com

Fnded: 1927. **Mem:** 5,000. **Desc:** Seeks to educate people of all ages about their vision; to create awareness of quality eye and vision care; and to support vision-related scientific research. **Pub:** *In Focus*, quarterly. **Frmly:** (1970) Women's Auxiliary to the American Optometric Association; (1989) Auxiliary to the American Optometric Association.

★ 677 ★ American Fracture Association (AFA)
20 N Michigan Ave., Ste. 700
Chicago, IL 60602
Phone: (312)263-7150 **Fax:** (312)782-0553
Website: http://www.afa4docs.org
Raymond O. Pierce, MD, Pres.

Fnded: 1938. **Mem:** 500. **Desc:** Orthopedic, general, industrial, plastic, traumatic, and dental surgeons and physicians interested in the care and treatment of fractures. Seeks to further and create interest in the study of the various accepted types of bone fracture therapy. **Pub:** *Orthopedic Transactions*, annual. • Directory, periodic. **Frmly:** American Ambulatory Fracture Association.

★ 678 ★ American Gastroenterological Association (AGA)
7910 Woodmont Ave., 7th Fl.
Bethesda, MD 20814
Phone: (301)654-2055 **Fax:** (301)652-3890
Email: webinfo@gastro.org
Website: http://www.gastro.org
Robert Greenberg, Exec. VP

Fnded: 1897. **Mem:** 8,600. **Desc:** Physicians of internal medicine certified in gastroenterology; radiologists, pathologists, surgeons, and physiologists with special interest and competency in gastroenterology. Studies normal and abnormal conditions of the digestive organs and problems connected with their metabolism; conducts scientific research; offers placement services. **Pub:** *AGA News*, monthly. *Price:* Included in membership dues. • *Directory of Researchers in Gastroenterology*, annual. Directory. • *Gastroenterology*, monthly. *Price:* $135 for individuals; $212 for institutions.

★ 679 ★ American Geriatrics Society (AGS)
350 5th Ave., Ste. 801
New York, NY 10118
Phone: (212)308-1414 **Free:** 800-247-4779
Fax: (212)832-8646
Email: info.amger@americangeriatrics.org
Website: http://www.americangeriatrics.org
Linda Hiddemen Barondess, Exec. VP

Fnded: 1942. **Mem:** 6,022. **Reg. Groups:** 3. **State Groups:** 23. **Desc:** Professional society of physicians and other health care professionals interested in problems of the aged. Encourages and promotes the study of geriatrics; stresses the importance of medical research in the field of aging. Conducts seminars. **Pub:** *AGS Newsletter*, bimonthly. Newsletter. Includes information on public policy issues of concern to members, upcoming courses, events, publications, and annual meeting. *Price:* Free. • *Annals of Long-Term Care*, monthly. Journal. Contains articles, abstracts and meeting notices. *Price:* included in membership dues; $60 for medical students; $95 for nonmembers. • *Geriatrics Review Syllabus: A Core Curriculum in Geriatric Medicine. Price:* Call for information. • *Journal of the American Geriatrics Society*, monthly. Journal. Includes original articles, abstracts of geriatric literature, book reviews, employment listings, and notices of meetings, courses, and symposia. *Price:* Included in membership dues; $175/year for nonmembers in U.S.; $313/year for institutions in U.S.; $80/year for nonmember residents and interns in U.S.

★ 680 ★ American Group Psychotherapy Association (AGPA)
25 E 21st St., 6th Fl.
New York, NY 10010
Phone: (212)477-2677 **Free:** 877-668-2472
Fax: (212)979-6627
Email: info@agpa.org
Website: http://www.agpa.org
Marsha S. Block, CAE, CEO

Fnded: 1942. **Mem:** 4,500. **Reg. Groups:** 40. **Desc:** Psychiatrists, psychologists, social workers, psychiatric nurses, and other mental health professionals who meet specific educational and professional requirements. Sponsors educational and research programs. **Pub:** *The Group Circle*, bimonthly. Newsletter. • *Group Works!*, quarterly. Brochure. Information about group psychotherapy. *Price:* Included in membership dues. • *Guidelines for Training of Group Psychotherapists*, quarterly. Journal. Includes calendar of events and research updates. *Price:* Included in membership dues. • *International Journal of Group Psychotherapy*, quarterly. Journal. • Membership Directory, biennial.

★ 681 ★ American Guild of Hypnotherapists (AGH)
2200 Veterans Blvd., No. 108
Kenner, LA 70062-4005
Phone: (504)468-3223 **Fax:** (504)468-3213
Email: drreg@southwest.edu
Reg Sheldrick, PhD, Pres.

Fnded: 1975. **Mem:** 685. **Desc:** Hypnotherapists and professional hypnotists; mental health, medical, dental, and chiropractic professionals who use hypnosis in their practices. Offers home study course in hypnosis/hypnotherapy. Is approved by many state licensing boards as a provider of continuing education credit. **Pub:** *Journal of Hypnotherapy*, quarterly. Journal. • Newsletter, periodic.

★ 682 ★ American Guild for Infant Survival (AGIS)
301 Eastwood Cir., Ste. 200
Virginia Beach, VA 23454-4014
Phone: (757)463-3845
Email: afgisinc@ivilliage.com
Scott Hessek, Pres.

Fnded: 1972. **Mem:** 170. **Nat'l Groups:** 1. **Reg. Groups:** 1. **Local Groups:** 2. **Desc:** Works to reduce infant mortality, especially Sudden Infant Death Syndrome. Develops low-tech innovations to reduce infant mortality, such as the AFGIS test, which scores risk categories of infants and fetuses. Promotes the home monitoring program. Conducts educational and research programs. Compiles statistics. Maintains speakers' bureau. Offers children's services. **Pub:** *The Baby and Family Newspaper*, semiannual. Newspaper. • Brochures. • Directory. **AKA:** American Forces Guild for Infant Survival; Tidewater Guild for Infant Survival, Inc.

★ 683 ★ American Gynecological and Obstetrical Society (AGOS)
University of Utah
50 N Medical Dr.
Salt Lake City, UT 84132
Phone: (801)581-5501 **Fax:** (801)581-7199
Paul B. Underwood, Jr., Sec.

Fnded: 1981. **Mem:** 243. **Desc:** Works to cultivate and promote knowledge concerning obstetrics and gynecology. **Pub:** *Transactions*, annual.

★ 684 ★ American Hair Loss Council (AHLC)
125 17th St. Ste 625
Pittsburgh, PA 15222
Phone: (412)765-3666 **Fax:** (412)765-3669
Email: ahlc@ahlc.org
Website: http://www.ahlc.org
Penny Bell, Pres.

Fnded: 1985. **Mem:** 420. **Desc:** Dermatologists, plastic surgeons, cosmetologists, barbers, and interested others. Provides nonbiased information regarding treatments for hair loss in both men and women. Facilitates communication and information exchange between professionals in different areas of specialization. Conducts educational programs; compiles statistics. **Pub:** *AHLC News*, quarterly. Brochures. A newsletter for members only (association & industry news). *Price:* Free for members.

★ 685 ★ American Head and Neck Society (AHNS)
601 N Caroline, Rm. 6221
Baltimore, MD 21287
Phone: (412)647-2227 **Fax:** (412)647-8944
Email: rwagner@pitt.edu
Website: http://www.headandneckcancer.org
Paul A. Levine, MD, Pres.

Fnded: 1959. **Mem:** 1,635. **Desc:** Otolaryngologists and other physicians with board certification whose primary interest is head and neck oncology. Associate membership is for other other practioners who treat head and neck cancer. Seeks to advance knowledge relevant to treatment of diseases of the head and neck, including reconstruction and rehabilitation. Promotes development of programs of training in head and neck oncology. **Pub:** *Head and Neck Cancer Practice Guidelines.* Practice Guidelines for Head and Neck Oncology. *Price:* $5 members; $10 non-members. **Frmly:** (1998) Society of Head and Neck Surgeons; (1999) American Society for Head and Neck Surgery; (2000) American Society of Head and Neck Surgeons.

★ 686 ★ American Headache Society (AHS)
19 Mantua Rd.
Mount Royal, NJ 08061
Phone: (856)423-0043 **Fax:** (856)423-0082
Email: ahshq@talley.com
Website: http://www.ahsnet.org
Linda McGillicuddy, Exec. Dir.

Fnded: 1959. **Mem:** 2,000. **Desc:** Professional society of health care providers dedicated to the study and treatment of headache and face pain. Objectives are to promote the exchange of information and ideas concerning the causes and treatments of headache and related painful disorders, to educate physicians, health professionals and the public, and to encourage research. **Pub:** *Headache: The Journal of Head and Face Pain*, 10/year. Journal. Presents papers concerning basic research and clinical studies. Includes book reviews. *Price:* Included in membership dues; $40/year for medical students, interns, and residents; $95/year for U.S. nonmembers; $110/year for nonmembers outside U.S. **Frmly:** (2001) American Association for the Study of Headache.

★ 687 ★ American Health Assistance Foundation (AHAF)
22512 Gateway Center Dr.
Clarksburg, MD 20871-2005
Phone: (301)948-3244 **Free:** 800-437-2423
Fax: (301)258-9454
Email: aphillips@ahaf.org
Website: http://www.ahaf.org
Angelia Ragsdale, Head Receptionist

Fnded: 1973. **Desc:** Established to support medical research. Four programs within the foundation are Alzheimer's Family Relief Program, Coronary Heart Disease Research, National Glaucoma Research, and Alzheimer's Disease Research. **Pub:** *Alzheimer's Research Review*, quarterly. Newsletter. Updates the work of Alzheimer's disease researchers. Provides tips for families with members who have the disease.

★ 688 ★ American Health Care Association (AHCA)
1201 L St. NW
Washington, DC 20005
Phone: (202)842-4444 **Fax:** (202)842-3860
Website: http://www.ahca.org
Dr. Charles H. Roadman, II, CEO

Fnded: 1949. **Mem:** 12,000. **State Groups:** 50. **Desc:** Federation of state associations of long-term health care facilities. Promotes standards for professionals in long-term health care delivery and quality care for patients and residents in a safe environment. Focuses on issues of availability, quality, affordability, and fair payment. Operates as liaison with governmental agencies, Congress, and professional associations. Compiles statistics. **Pub:** *AHCA Notes*, monthly. Newsletter. Covers legislation and regulations. *Price:* Included in membership dues. • *Provider: For Long Term Care Professionals*, monthly. Magazine. Includes buyers' guide, news reports, advertisers' index, a listing of new products and services, and calendar of events. *Price:* Free to long-term health care professionals; $48/year for nonmembers and libraries. • Also produces audio-visual aids. **Frmly:** (1975) American Nursing Home Association.

★ 689 ★ American Healthcare Radiology Administrators (AHRA)

490-B Boston Post Rd., Ste. 101
Sudbury, MA 01776
Phone: (978)443-7591 **Free:** 800-334-2472
Fax: (978)443-8046
Email: info@ahraonline.org
Website: http://www.ahraonline.org
Mary S. Reitter, Exec. Dir.

Fnded: 1973. **Mem:** 4,000. **Desc:** Promotes leaders in radiology and imaging sciences, including administrators and managers of imaging services in hospitals, imaging centers, and physician practices. Publishes benchmarking research studies that include compensation and benefits, utilization of imaging staff, image management, and patient care quality. Awards Certified Radiology Administrator credential to individuals meeting eligibility and examination requirements. **Pub:** *Link*, monthly. Newsletter. *Price:* for members. • *Online Membership Directory*, annual, updated weekly. Membership Directory. • *Radiology Management*, bimonthly. **Frmly:** (1986) American Hospital Radiology Administrators.

★ 690 ★ American Health Decisions (AHD)

The Hastings Center
21 Malcolm Gordon Rd.
Garrison, NY 10524
Phone: (845)424-0005
Email: jennings@thehastingscenter.org
Website: http://www.ahd.org/
David Clarke, Chm.

Fnded: 1989. **Mem:** 13. **State Groups:** 13. **Desc:** Confederation of state health programs. Assists in establishing public education programs about health care and policy; works to increase availability of quality medical care. Promotes personal autonomy on ethical issues, such as patients making the decision to refuse or accept treatment. Addresses problems arising from ethical conflicts over new medical technologies and disease prevention. Maintains research and educational programs; disseminates information.

★ 691 ★ American Health Information Management Association (AMRA)

233 N Michigan Ave., Ste. 2150
Chicago, IL 60601-5800
Phone: (312)233-1100 **Fax:** (312)233-1500
Email: info@ahima.org
Website: http://www.ahima.org
Barbara A. Siegel, Pres.

Fnded: 1928. **Mem:** 40,000. **State Groups:** 52. **Desc:** Registered record administrators; accredited record technicians with expertise in health information management, biostatistics, classification systems, and systems analysis. Sponsors Independent Study Programs in Medical Record Technology and coding. Conducts annual qualification examinations to credential medical record personnel as Registered Record Administrators (RRA), Accredited Record Technicians (ART) and Certified Coding Specialists (CCS). Maintains Foundation of Research and Education Library, Scholarships and loans. **Pub:** *From the Couch: Official Newsletter of the Mental Health Record Section of the American Medical Record Association*, quarterly. Newsletter. *Price:* Included in membership dues. • *Journal of AHIMA*, 10/year. Journal. Contains articles on the theory, practice, and current issues in health information management. Includes book reviews and calendar of events. *Price:* $72. • *Leader: AHIMA Volunteer*, quarterly. Newsletter. *Price:* Included in membership dues. • *QA Section Connection*, bimonthly. Newsletter. Provides educational information on the management and methodology of health care quality assurance programs. Includes annual subject index. *Price:* Included in membership dues. • *Spectrum*, quarterly. Newsletter. *Price:* Included in membership dues. • Also publishes guides, workbooks, and other materials on medical record management and related subjects. **Frmly:** (1928) American Association of Medical Record Librarians; (1938) Association of Record Librarians of North America; (1991) American Medical Records Association.

★ 692 ★ American Health Planning Association (AHPA)

7245 Arlington Blvd., Ste. 300
Falls Church, VA 22042
Phone: (703)573-3103 **Fax:** (703)573-1276
Email: tpiper@mail.state.mo.us
Website: http://www.ahpanet.org/
Dean Montgomery, Contact

Fnded: 1970. **Desc:** State and local health planning agencies and affiliated organizations and individuals. Conducts research; disseminates information; serves as clearinghouse for health planning activities and concepts; sponsors programs of technical assistance; provides continuing education. **Pub:** *National Directory of Health Planning, Policy, and Regulatory Agencies*, annual. Directory. *Price:* $125. • *TODAY in Health Planning*, quarterly. **Frmly:** (1977) American Association for Comprehensive Health Planning.

★ 693 ★ American Health Quality Association (AHQA)

1140 Conneticut Ave. NW, Ste. 1050
Washington, DC 20036
Phone: (202)331-5790 **Fax:** (202)331-9334
Email: info@ahqa.org
Website: http://www.ahqa.org
Amanda D. Scott, Admin. Asst.

Fnded: 1973. **Mem:** 1,400. **State Groups:** 53. **Local Groups:** 11. **Desc:** Institutions and individuals. Purpose is to develop communications programs for physicians, institutions, and others interested in peer review organizations (PROs). Provides a national forum for the interchange of ideas, techniques, and information relating to medical quality assessment. Conducts courses and on-site educational programs to increase physicians' involvement and leadership in PROs, improve practice patterns through review, understand and use PRO data to improve service delivery, pre-admission review, profile analysis, retrospective review, and organizational development. Sponsors placement service; maintains a speakers' bureau and a library. **Pub:** *AHQA Bulletin*, periodic. Bulletin. Covers medical regulatory and legislative developments. *Price:* Included in membership dues. • *Legislative Monitor*, periodic. *Price:* Free, available to members only. • *Physician Advisor Manual.* • *Quality Advocate*, quarterly. Newsletter. Includes Policy Outlook, Innovation, Washington Update, Legislative Update, Calendar of Events columns and job announcements. *Price:* Included in membership dues; $75/year for nonmembers. • *Resource Document and Private Review Manual.* • *Tapes of Conference Programs.* • Membership Directory, annual. **Frmly:** (1982) American Association of Professional Standards Review Organizations; (1997) American Medical Peer Review Association.

★ 694 ★ American Hearing Impaired Hockey Association (AHIHA)

1143 W Lake St.
Chicago, IL 60607
Phone: (312)226-5880 **Fax:** (312)829-2250
Stan Mikita, Pres.

Fnded: 1973. **Mem:** 80. **Desc:** Hearing impaired boys and men, aged 5 to 26, who wish to play ice hockey. Seeks to develop members' skills and self-confidence, both as hockey players and as individuals, through participation in the annual Stan Mikita Hockey School for the Hearing Impaired. **Pub:** *Locker Room Briefs*. Newsletter.

★ 695 ★ American Hearing Research Foundation (AHRF)

8 S Michigan Ave., Ste. 814
Chicago, IL 60603-4539
Phone: (312)726-9670 **Fax:** (312)726-9695
Email: blederer@american-hearing.org
Website: http://www.american-hearing.org/
William L. Lederer, Exec. Dir.

Fnded: 1956. **Mem:** 1,585. **Desc:** Works to encourage and support medical research, education, and public information concerning deafness and other hearing disorders. Produces scientific exhibits and film exhibits for professional and public audiences. **Pub:** *American Hearing Research Foundation Newsletter*, 3/year. Newsletter. Reviews developments in hearing research and education. *Price:* Free. • *Hearing Health*. Brochure. • *Progress Report*, semiannual. Report. • Also publishes research papers.

★ 696 ★ American Heart Association (AHA)

7272 Greenville Ave.
Dallas, TX 75231-4596
Phone: (301)223-2307 **Free:** 800-242-8721
Website: http://www.americanheart.org
M. Cass Wheeler, CEO

Fnded: 1924. **Mem:** 26,000. **Reg. Groups:** 15. **State Groups:** 56. **Desc:** Physicians, scientists, and laypersons. Supports research, education, and community service programs with the objective of reducing premature death and disability from cardiovascular diseases and stroke; coordinates the efforts of physicians, nurses, health professionals, and others engaged in the fight against heart and circulatory disease. Financed entirely by voluntary contributions of the public, principally during the Heart Campaign held in February. **Pub:** *Arteriosclerosis, Thrombosis, and Vascular Biology*, monthly. Journal. Contains findings of basic and clinical research related to vascular biology and related topics. *Price:* $227/year for individuals; $363/year for institutions. • *Circulation*, weekly. Journal. Covers clinical research, including clinical studies and trials, and advances in cardiovascular medicine. *Price:* $223/year for individuals; $396/year for institutions. • *Circulation Research*, biweekly. Journal. Covers basic cardiovascular research in the areas of biology, biochemistry, biophysics, microbiology, cellular biology, genetics, molecular biology. *Price:* $267/year for individuals; $487/year for institutions. • *Currents in Emergency Cardiac Care*, quarterly. Newsletter. Offers scientific information about ideas, development, and trends in emergency cardiac care; published in conjunction with the Citizen CPR Foundation. *Price:* Free. • *Hypertension*, monthly. Journal. Reports clinical and laboratory investigations in blood pressure regulation and pathophysiological mechanisms underlying the hypertensive diseases. *Price:* $213/year for individuals; $302/year for institutions. • *Stroke–A Journal of Cerebral Circulation*, monthly. Journal. Provides information on the prevention, diagnosis, treatment, and rehabilitation of cerebrovascular disease. *Price:* $213/year for individuals; $299/year for institutions.

★ 697 ★ American Heartworm Society (AHS)

Executive Office
PO Box 667
Batavia, IL 60510-0667
Phone: (630)844-9676 **Fax:** (630)892-0818
Email: heartwormsociety@aol.com
Website: http://www.heartwormsociety.org
Eve C. Larocca, Admin.

Fnded: 1974. **Mem:** 1,200. **Desc:** Veterinarians, physicians, parasitologists, and other scientists. Promotes scientific programs for the study of heartworm disease, caused by the filarial parasite, dilofilaria immitis. Encourages standardization of procedures for diagnosis, treatment, and prevention of heartworm disease. Keeps members abreast of current research and recent developments concerning the disease. **Pub:** *AHS Bulletin*, quarterly. Bulletin. Contains topical commentary, synopsis of clinical and scientific literature and society news. *Price:* Included in membership dues; $38/year for nonmembers. • *Recent Advances in Heartworm Disease: Symposium '98*. Proceedings.

★ 698 ★ American Hepato-Pancreato-Biliary Association (AHPBA)
c/o Vanderbilt Transplant Center
Oxford House, Ste. 801
Nashville, TN 37232
Phone: (615)343-2735 **Fax:** (615)343-5365
Email: hannah.wilson@vanderbilt.edu
Website: http://www.ahpba.org
Steven Strasberg, Pres.

Fnded: 1978. **Mem:** 2,000. **Desc:** Endoscopists, hepatologists, radiologists, and surgeons in 25 countries. Provides a forum for the presentation of papers concerning diagnostic and treatment modalities of lymphatic, pancreatic, and biliary disorders. Promotes exchange of ideas, reviews current standards of practice, and seeks to establish prospective controlled protocols in the field. Initiates research regarding factors involved in biliary, pancreatic, and liver diseases. **Frmly:** International Hepato-Biliary Pancreatic Association; (1988) International Biliary Association; (2003) International Hepato-Pancreato-Biliary Association.

★ 699 ★ American Herbalists Guild (AHG)
1931 Gaddis Rd.
Canton, GA 30115
Phone: (770)751-6021 **Fax:** (770)751-7472
Email: ahgoffice@earthlink.net
Website: http://www.americanherbalistsguild.com
Aviva Romm, Pres.

Fnded: 1989. **Mem:** 750. **State Groups:** 3. **Desc:** Promotes research and education in the field of herbal medicine. Works to establish high standards for the professional practice of herbalism. Provides a forum for the exchange of information in the field. **Pub:** *Directory of Herbal Education Programs. Price:* $7.95. • *The Herbalist*, quarterly. Newsletter. • *Recommended Reading List. Price:* $2.

★ 700 ★ American Hernia Society (AHS)
PO Box 536544
Orlando, FL 32853-6544
Phone: (407)898-1695 **Fax:** (407)894-2312
Email: wilkesmgmt@aol.com
Website: http://www.americanherniasociety.org
Shelburn M. Wilkes, Exec. Dir.

Fnded: 1997. **Mem:** 400. **Desc:** Surgeons interested in the management of hernias. Seeks to advance the diagnosis and treatment of hernias; promotes continuing professional development of members. Serves as a forum for the exchange of information among members; gathers and disseminates information on emerging methods of hernia surgery and management. **Pub:** *Hernia*, quarterly. Journal. *Price:* $35.

★ 701 ★ American Holistic Health Association
PO Box 17400
Anaheim, CA 92817
Phone: (714)779-6152
Email: mail@ahha.org
Website: http://ahha.org
Ms. Suzan Walter, MBA, Pres.

Fnded: 1989. **Desc:** Seeks to further the understanding of holistic health care, a concept that stresses the integration of physical, mental, emotional, and spiritual concerns with environmental harmony.

★ 702 ★ American Holistic Medical Association (AHMA)
12101 Menaul Blvd. NE, Ste. C
Albuquerque, NM 87112
Phone: (505)292-7788 **Fax:** (505)293-7570
Email: info@holisticmedicine.org
Website: http://www.holisticmedicine.org
Amy Driggs, Assoc. Dir.

Fnded: 1978. **Mem:** 1,000. **Reg. Groups:** 11. **Desc:** Licensed medical doctors, doctors of osteopathy, and students enrolled in medical or osteopathic programs who are interested in furthering the practice of holistic health care, a concept that stresses the integration of physical, mental, emotional, and spiritual concerns with environmental harmony. Medical education is provided in these areas through the association's conference. **Pub:** *AHMA Member Directory*, annual. Membership Directory. *Price:* available to members only. • *Members Brochures*. Brochures. • *National Referral Directory of Holistic Practitioners*. Directory. *Price:* $15. • *Newsletter to Members*. Newsletter.

★ 703 ★ American Holistic Nurses Association (AHNA)
PO Box 2130
Flagstaff, AZ 86003-2130
Phone: (520)526-2196 **Free:** 800-278-2462
Fax: (520)526-2752
Email: communications@ahna.org
Website: http://www.ahna.org
Michael French, Communications Admin.

Fnded: 1981. **Mem:** 2,700. **State Groups:** 11. **Local Groups:** 63. **Desc:** The AHNA is a 501(c) (3) nonprofit educational organization whose membership is open to nurses and other individuals interested in holistically-oriented health care practices throughout the United States and the world. ASHNA supports the education of nurses, allied health practitioners, and the general public on health-related issues. The American Holistic Nurses' Association embraces nursing as a lifestyle and a profession and provides a means to create bonds within the nursing community. Because true healing comes from within, the AHNA recognizes that nurses must first heal themselves before they can facilitate the healing of others. **Pub:** *Beginnings*, bimonthly. Newsletter. Covers membership activities. Includes calendar of events, tape and book reviews, and regional reports. *Price:* Included in membership dues; $25/year for nonmembers. • *Come Home to the Heart of Nursing*. Brochure. • *Journal of Holistic Nursing*, quarterly. Journal. Presents academic and scholarly works from the field of holistic nursing practice; includes research news. *Price:* Included in membership dues; $28.80/year for nonmembers; $60/year for institutions. • Also publishes membership directory.

★ 704 ★ American Holistic Veterinary Medical Association (AHVMA)
2218 Old Emmorton Rd.
Bel Air, MD 21015
Phone: (410)569-0795 **Fax:** (410)569-2346
Email: ahvma82@cs.com
Website: http://www.ahvma.org
Dr. Carvel G. Tiekert, Exec. Dir.

Fnded: 1982. **Mem:** 1,000. **Desc:** Veterinarians and others interested in exploring alternative approaches in veterinary medicine, including clinical nutrition, homeopathy, and herbal medicine. **Pub:** *Journal of the AHVMA*, quarterly. Journal. Includes association news and book reviews. *Price:* Included in membership dues. **Frmly:** (1985) American Veterinary Holistic Medical Association.

★ 705 ★ American Horticultural Therapy Association (AHTA)
909 York St.
Denver, CO 80206
Phone: (303)370-8087 **Free:** 800-634-1603
Fax: (303)331-5776
Email: ahtaadmin@earthlink.net
Website: http://www.ahta.org
Stephanie Shulman, Admin. Dir.

Fnded: 1973. **Mem:** 800. **Reg. Groups:** 12. **Desc:** Professional horticultural therapists and rehabilitation specialists; horticultural therapy students; institutions and commercial organizations. Promotes and encourages the development of horticulture and related activities as a therapeutic and rehabilitative medium. Coordinates efforts of professional and educational organizations and conducts regional workshops and seminars. Provides resource information; offers papers at various conferences. Registers professional horticultural therapists. **Pub:** *AHTA Annual Membership Directory*, annual. Membership Directory. *Price:* Free for members; $35 for nonmembers. • *Journal of Therapeutic Horticulture*, annual. Journal. Contains research and programmatic articles. *Price:* $12 for members; $15 for nonmembers. • *Newsletter American Horticulture Therapy Association*, biennial. Newsletter. Includes association news, program features, horticultural therapy activities, and member profiles. *Price:* $35/year; $3/issue.

★ 706 ★ American Hospital Association (AHA)
1 N Franklin
Chicago, IL 60606-3421
Phone: (312)422-3000 **Fax:** (312)422-4796
Email: hromero@aha.org
Website: http://www.aha.org
Richard J. Davidson, PhD, Pres.

Fnded: 1898. **Mem:** 54,500. **Desc:** Health care provider organizations. Seeks to advance the health of individuals and communities. Leads, represents, and serves health care provider organizations that are accountable to the community and committed to health improvement. **Pub:** *AHANews*, weekly. • *Guide to the Health Care Field*, annual. • *Hospital Statistics*, annual. • *Hospitals and Health Networks*, biweekly. **Frmly:** (1906) Association of Hospital Superintendents of U.S. and Canada.

★ 707 ★ American Hypnosis Association (AHA)
18607 Ventura Blvd., Ste. 310
Tarzana, CA 91356
Fax: (818)344-2262
Email: info@hypnosismotivation.com
Website: http://www.hypnosismotivation.com
George Kappas, Pres.

Fnded: 1972. **Mem:** 1,000. **State Groups:** 2. **Desc:** Professionals and paraprofessionals in hypnotherapy. Acts as a resource center for members. **Pub:** *American Hypnotherapist*, quarterly. Newsletter.

★ 708 ★ American Independent Dentist's Association (AIDA)
c/o K. Randall Groh
336 Alhambra Cir.
Coral Gables, FL 33134
Email: feeforserv@aol.com
Website: http://www.dentalbeacon.org/
K. Randall Groh, DDS, Acting Chm.

Desc: Promotes traditional fee-for-service dentistry as an option that requires representation at all levels of organized dentistry and civil government.

★ 709 ★ American Industrial Hygiene Association (AIHA)
2700 Prosperity Ave., Ste. 250
Fairfax, VA 22031
Phone: (703)849-8888 **Fax:** (703)207-3561
Email: infonet@aiha.org
Website: http://www.aiha.org
Steven Davis, Atg. Exec. Dir.

Fnded: 1939. **Mem:** 12,000. **Reg. Groups:** 76. **Local Groups:** 70. **Desc:** Professional society of industrial hygienists. Promotes the study and control of environmental factors affecting the health and well-being of workers. Sponsors continuing education courses in industrial hygiene, government affairs program, and public relations. Accredits laboratories. Maintains 40 technical committees and a foundation. Operates placement service. Conducts educational and research programs. **Pub:** *The AIHA Journal*, bimonthly. Journal. Includes peer-reviewed technical and scientific articles. • *The Synergist*, monthly, update online. Includes news magazine covering occupational and environmental health and safety issues. *Price:* $65/year in U.S.; $90/year international. • *Who's Who in Industrial Hygiene*, annual. Directory. • Books. • Manuals. • Videos.

★ 710 ★ American Institute of Biomedical Climatology (AIBC)
1050 Eagle Rd.
Newtown, PA 18940-2818
Phone: (215)968-4483
Email: info@aibc.cc
Website: http://www.aibc.cc
George W.K. King, Sec. -Treas.

Fnded: 1958. **Mem:** 45. **Desc:** Meteorologists, biologists, epidemiologists, physicians, atmospheric physicists, engineers, architects, physiologists, climatologists, and other professionals interested in investigating the influence of the outdoor and indoor environment on the health and diseases of man. Areas of interest include: global warming, indoor and outdoor air pollution, biological effects of electromagnetic fields, power lines, cell phones and cell towers, and beneficial and detrimental effects of climate and weather on health. **Pub:** *AIBC News Med-Clime Currents*. Newsletter. Contains news concerning new publications and research studies. Available via member contributions. *Price:* Included in membership dues. • *Membership List*. Available to members only. • Also publishes scientific papers. **Frmly:** (1988) American Institute of Medical Climatology.

★ 711 ★ American Institute for Cancer Research (AICR)
1759 R St., NW
Washington, DC 20009
Phone: (202)328-7744 **Free:** 800-843-8114
Fax: (202)328-7226
Email: aicrweb@aicr.org
Website: http://www.aicr.org

Fnded: 1983. **Desc:** Fosters research on diet, nutrition and cancer prevention and educates the public about the results. **Pub:** Newsletter, quarterly. *Price:* Free.

★ 712 ★ American Institute of the History of Pharmacy (AIHP)
777 Highland Ave.
Madison, WI 53705
Phone: (608)262-5378
Email: aihp@aihp.org
Website: http://www.aihp.org
Gregory J. Higby, Dir.

Fnded: 1941. **Mem:** 1,000. **Desc:** Pharmacists, firms, and organizations interested in historical and social aspects of the pharmaceutical field. Maintains pharmaceutical Americana collection; conducts research programs. **Pub:** *AIHP Notes*, quarterly. Newsletter. *Price:* Included in membership dues. • *Pharmacy in History*, quarterly. Journal. Contains writings on the history of pharmaceutical practice, including drugs and therapeutics and related facets of the medical sciences. *Price:* Included in membership dues. • Booklets.

★ 713 ★ American Institute of Homeopathy (AIH)
801 N Fairfax St., Ste. 306
Alexandria, VA 22314
Phone: 888-445-9988
Email: aih@homeopathyusa.org
Website: http://www.homeopathyusa.org
Jennifer Jacobs, MPH, Pres.

Fnded: 1844. **Mem:** 160. **Desc:** Professional society of medical doctors, osteopaths, and dentists practicing homeotherapeutics according to the three natural laws of cure propounded by German physician Samuel C. F. Hahnemann (1755-1843). Promotes research and quality homeopathic health care. **Pub:** *Homeopathy Notes*, monthly. Newsletter. • *Journal of the American Institute of Homeopathy*, quarterly. Journal. *Price:* $12/each; $35/year (inside North America); $45/year (outside North America).

★ 714 ★ American Institute of Oral Biology (AIOB)
PO Box 7184
Loma Linda, CA 92354-7184
Phone: (909)558-4671 **Fax:** (909)558-0285
Email: jbarrientos@sd.llu.edu
Website: http://www.aiob.org
June J. Barrientos, Exec. Sec.

Fnded: 1943. **Mem:** 150. **Desc:** Dental and medical health professionals united for continuing education. Conducts lectures. **Pub:** *AIOB Proceedings Manual*, annual. *Price:* $75.

★ 715 ★ American Institute for Preventive Medicine
30445 Northwestern Hwy., Ste. 350
Farmington Hills, MI 48334
Phone: (248)539-1800 **Free:** 800-345-2476
Fax: (248)539-1808
Email: aipm@healthy.net
Website: http://www.healthylife.com
Dr. Don R. Powell, Pres.

Fnded: 1983. **Desc:** Not an association. Consulting firm. Conducts educational programs. Maintains speakers' bureau. **Pub:** *A Year of Health Hints - 365 Practical Ways to Feel Better and Live Longer*. *Price:* $23.95. • *Being a Wise Healthcare Consumer*. • *Guide to Mental Fitness*. • *Guide to Self Care*. • *Health at Home: Your Complete Guide to Symptoms, Solutions, and Self Love*. Book. *Price:* $17.95. • *Healthy Self: The Guide to Self Care and Wise Consumers*. Book. *Price:* $7.95. • *Hotlines to Health Directory*, annual. Directory. *Price:* $2.95. • *Self Care: Your Family Guide to Symptoms and How to Treat Them*. Book. *Price:* $14.95. • *Seniors Health at Home*. Book. *Price:* $19.95.

★ 716 ★ American Institute of Stress (AIS)
124 Park Ave.
Yonkers, NY 10703
Phone: (914)963-1200 **Fax:** (914)965-6267
Email: stress124@earthlink.net
Website: http://www.stress.org
Paul J. Rosch, MD, Pres. & Chm.

Fnded: 1979. **Mem:** 2,000. **Desc:** Physicians, health professionals, scholars, and others from varied disciplines constitute board of trustees. Explores the personal and social consequences of stress. Compiles research data on topics such as: relationships between emotional factors and cardiovascular disease; stress and the immune system with specific emphasis on cancer; stress reduction programs for industry; occupational stress (for example, that of law enforcement officers or air traffic controllers); executive stress ("burn out"); and pharmacological and holistic methods of stress reduction. Seeks a definition of health that recognizes the need for harmony between the individual and the physical and social environments as well as the effects of positive emotions such as creativity, faith, and humor on health. Evaluates ongoing research efforts and stress management programs in the U.S. and abroad. Disseminates information to individuals, institutions, and organizations. Serves as a network for rapid communication among individuals in different disciplines. Sponsors consulting services. **Pub:** *Health and Stress: The Newsletter of the American Institute of Stress*, monthly. Newsletter. *Price:* $35 in U.S.; $45 outside U.S. • *Readings in Oncology*. Book. • Also publishes papers and speeches and issues reprints on stress.

★ 717 ★ American Institute for Stuttering Treatment and Professional Training
c/o Catherine Montgomery
27 W 20th St., Ste. 1203
New York, NY 10011-3707
Phone: (212)633-6400 **Free:** 877-378-8883
Fax: (212)220-3922
Email: ais@stutteringtreatment.org
Website: http://www.stutteringtreatment.org
Catherine Montgomery, Exec. Dir.

Fnded: 1995. **Desc:** Facility offers both intensive and non-intensive treatment options for people of all ages who stutter, while also providing clinical training to both new and established speech-language pathologists. **Frmly:** (1998) Total Immersion Fluency Training.

★ 718 ★ American Institute for Teen AIDS Prevention
PO Box 395
Oberlin, OH 44074-0395
Phone: (440)774-5411 **Fax:** (440)233-6455
Email: TeenAIDS@msn.com
Duane Crumb, Exec. Dir.

Fnded: 1987. **Desc:** Provides HIV/STD education programs to schools and churches. Maintains speakers' bureau. Develops and distributes HIV/STD education materials. **Pub:** *Developing Your Church AIDS Policy*. Book. Leads church leaders through the process of researching, drafting, and implementing an AIDS policy. *Price:* $8. • *Don't Let AIDS Catch You!*. Brochure. HIV/AIDS education for teens. • *Guide to Positive HIV/AIDS Education*. Book. • *It's Your Choice*. Video. • *Making Love without Doing It*. Brochure. **Frmly:** American Institute for Teen Aids Prevention.

★ 719 ★ American Institute of Ultrasound in Medicine (AIUM)
14750 Sweitzer Ln., Ste. 100
Laurel, MD 20707-5906
Phone: (301)498-4100 **Free:** 800-638-5352
Fax: (301)498-4450
Email: admin@aium.org
Website: http://www.aium.org
Carmine M. Valente, PhDCAE, CEO

Fnded: 1952. **Mem:** 9,500. **Desc:** A multidisciplinary organization dedicated to advancing the art and science of ultrasound in medicine through its educational, scientific, literary and professional activities. Membership comprises professionals from many medical specialties, as well as basic scientists, engineers, manufacturers, nurses, physicists, radiologic technologists, sonographers and veterinarians involved with diagnostic medical ultrasound. **Pub:** *Acoustic Output Labeling Standard for Diagnostic Ultrasound Equipment*, monthly. Newsletter. Covers institute activities and developments in diagnostic ultrasound. Includes listing of continuing education courses and employment opportunities. *Price:* $15 for members; $30 for nonmembers. • *Acoustic Output Measurement Standard for Diagnostic Ultrasound Equipment*, monthly. Journal. Contains research papers and case reports covering all aspects of diagnostic ultrasound, advances in instrumentation, and biological effects. *Price:* $22 for members; $44 for nonmembers; $190/year for institutions. • *AIUM Sound Waves*, 10/year. Newsletter. Covers institute activities and developments in diagnostic ultrasound. *Price:* Included in membership dues. • *Bioeffects & Safety of Diagnostic Ultrasound*. Videos. *Price:* $17 for members; $34 for nonmembers. • *Evaluation of Research Reports: Bioeffects Literature Reviews 1985-1991*. *Price:* $16 for members; $30 for nonmembers. • *Evaluation of Research Reports: Bioeffects Literature Reviews 1962-1982*. *Price:* $9 for members; $16 for nonmembers. • *Journal of Ultrasound in Medicine*, monthly. Journal. Contains research papers and case reports covering all aspects of diagnostic ultrasound, advances in instrumentation, and biological effects. *Price:* Included in membership dues; $265/year for nonmembers; $295/year for institutions. • *Mechanical Bioeffects from Diagnostic Ultrasound: AIUM Consensus Statements*. *Price:* $25. • *Medical Ultrasound Safety*. *Price:* $10 for members; $19 for nonmembers. • *Obstetrical Measurements Used in A Routine Examination*. *Price:* $20 for members; $40 for nonmembers. • *Perf. Criteria & Measurements for Doppler U/S Devices: Tech. Discussions-2nd Ed.*. *Price:* $18 for members; $36 for nonmembers. • Videos. • *AIUM Annual Convention Proceedings*. *Price:* $12/copy for members; $22/copy for nonmembers. • *Is Sonography the Career for You?*. *Price:* $55 for members, bulk; $120 for nonmembers, bulk.

★ 720 ★ American International Health Alliance (AIHA)
1212 New York Ave. NW, Ste. 750
Washington, DC 20005
Phone: (202)789-1136 **Fax:** (202)789-1277
Email: aiha@aiha.com
Website: http://www.aiha.com
James Smith, Exec. Dir.

Fnded: 1992. **Desc:** Institutional health care providers. Promotes increased availability of health care services in previously underserved areas worldwide. Creates partnerships between hospitals in the United States and their counterparts abroad to facilitate sharing of technology and expertise; sponsors educational programs; serves as a clearinghouse on international health issues and emerging medical technologies and practices. **Pub:** *Commonhealth*, monthly. Newsletter. Focuses on topics of concern to healthcare providers/practitioners in the countries of the former Soviet Union and Central and Eastern Europe. *Price:* Free.

★ 721 ★ American In-Vitro Allergy/Immunology Society
PO Box 341461
Bethesda, MD 20827-1461
Phone: (301)263-0703 **Fax:** (301)263-0776
Email: aiais@erols.com
Website: http://www.invitroallergy.org
Barbara Buchman, Admin.

Fnded: 1988. **Mem:** 210. **Desc:** Physicians, scientists, and other health professionals who study or use in-vitro technology in the diagnosis and treatment of allergic and immunologic disorders; individuals engaged in activities related to the treatment of allergies or the advancement of immunological science. Promotes the appropriate use of in-vitro procedures in allergy and immunology; explores and refines allergy and immunology in-vitro techniques; fosters research in and development of in-vitro procedures that enhance the diagnosis and management of allergy or immune dysfunction. Acts as forum on information regarding new scientific information, research, and application of in-vitro techniques in allergy and immunology practice; represents members in professional and public relations; operates physician referral service. Offers services in third party payer negotiation and in-vitro testing standardization. Conducts continuing medical education. **Pub:** Brochure. • Newsletter, quarterly.

★ 722 ★ American Israeli Lighthouse (AIL)
276 5th Ave, Rm. 713
New York, NY 10001-4509
Phone: (212)838-5322
Mrs. Leonard F. Dank, Pres.

Fnded: 1927. **Mem:** 1,500. **State Groups:** 8. **Local Groups:** 7. **Desc:** Works to raise funds for the maintenance of a rehabilitation center in Kiriat Haim, Israel for adult blind and physically handicapped persons. Promotes research in the development of techniques in education, vocational training, and rehabilitation. **Pub:** *The Tower*, annual.

★ 723 ★ American-Israeli Ophthalmological Society
130 E 67th St., Ste. 1C
New York, NY 10021-6136
Fax: (212)734-2682
Dr. Albert Hombless, Contact

Fnded: 1974. **Mem:** 450. **Nat'l Groups:** 1. **Desc:** Ophthalmologists. Seeks to facilitate communication between American and Israeli ophthalmologists. Provides training for Israeli opthalmologists in the United States. Organizes conventions.

★ 724 ★ American Joint Committee on Cancer (AJCC)
633 North St. Clair St.
Chicago, IL 60611
Phone: (312)202-5313 **Fax:** (312)202-5009
Email: sburkhardt@facs.org
Website: http://www.cancerstaging.org
Susan Burkhardt, AJCC Admin.

Fnded: 1959. **Mem:** 40. **Desc:** Surgeons, physicians, radiologists, pathologists, American Cancer Society representatives, and National Cancer Institute representatives. Formulates and publishes systems of classification for cancer staging and end results reporting for the purpose of selecting the most effective treatment, determining prognosis, and continuing evaluation of cancer control measures. Promotes the use of developed systems of classification of cancer and evaluates systems of recording and reporting data. **Pub:** *AJCC Manual for Staging of Cancer, 6th ed.*, quadrennial. Manual. Includes classification for cancer staging & end results reporting for selecting treatment, determining prognosis and evaluating cancer. *Price:* $59.95. **Frmly:** (1981) American Joint Committee for Cancer Staging and End Results Reporting.

★ 725 ★ American Juvenile Arthritis Organization (AJAO)
1330 W Peachtree St.
Atlanta, GA 30309
Phone: (404)872-7100 **Free:** 800-283-7800
Fax: (404)872-9559
Website: http://www.arthritis.org/communities/about_ajao.asp
Dave Anderson, Sr. VP

Fnded: 1980. **Mem:** 3,000. **State Groups:** 58. **Desc:** Parents, health care professionals, and others interested in the problems of juvenile arthritis. Serves as advocate for the needs of those affected by juvenile arthritis. A council of the Arthritis Foundation. **Pub:** *Arthritis in Children.* Brochure. • *Decision Making for Teens.* Brochure. • *Educational Rights for Children with Arthritis: A Manual for Parents.* Manual. • *Kids Get Arthritis, Too,* bimonthly. Newsletter. Covers AJAO activities, current research, legislative topics, and medical and scientific updates. *Price:* $20 for nonmembers; Free, for members. • *When Your Student.* Brochure.

★ 726 ★ American Kidney Fund (AKF)
6110 Executive Blvd., Ste. 1010
Rockville, MD 20852
Phone: (301)881-3052 **Free:** 800-638-8299
Fax: (301)881-0898
Email: helpline@akfinc.org
Website: http://www.akfinc.org
Karen M. Sendelback, CFRE, Exec. Dir.

Fnded: 1971. **Reg. Groups:** 1. **Desc:** Works to alleviate the financial burdens caused by kidney disease; improve the quality of life for kidney patients; promote kidney health care nationwide. Provides direct financial assistance to needy kidney disease victims with costs specific to their treatment. Funds are raised through direct mail from the public. Supports dialysis center emergency funds. Programs include: American Kidney Fund Clinical Scientist in Nephrology program, which provides assistance to nephrology students pursuing scholarship in the provision of clinical care; patient and community services; public and professional education; kidney donor development; and clinical research. **Pub:** *American Kidney Fund–Annual Report*, annual. Annual Report. *Price:* Free. • *Clinical Strategies Newsletter for Health Professionals*, semiannual. Newsletter. *Price:* Free. • Brochures.

★ 727 ★ American Kinesiotherapy Association (AKTA)
PO Box 1390
Hines, IL 60141-1390
Free: 800-296-AKTA **Fax:** (312)202-7960
Email: ccbkt@aol.com
Website: http://www.akta.org
Michael Westmoreland, Pres.

Fnded: 1946. **Mem:** 450. **Reg. Groups:** 7. **State Groups:** 50. **Desc:** Professional society of kinesiotherapists, and associate and student members with interest in physical and mental rehabilitation and adapted physical education. (Kinesiology is the study of human movement; kinesiotherapists use kinesiology to design and implement therapeutic exercise to meet the rehabilitative needs of persons with disease, injury, and/or physical disorders.) Goal is to promote the profession of kinseotheraphy by working toward public recognition of kinesiotherapy and to pursue and support legislative concerns of the profession. Works to maintain and advance the standard of care through educational opportunities. **Pub:** *Career in Kinesiology.* Brochure. • *Cinical Kinesiology*, quarterly. Journal. Publishes manuscripts of professional and scientific nature in disciplines relates to kinesiotherapy. *Price:* $25 individuals; $45 library or institution. • *Mobility*, quarterly. Newsletter. • Also publishes rehabilitation brochures. **Frmly:** (1968) Association for Physical and Mental Rehabilitation; (1987) American Corrective Therapy Association.

★ 728 ★ American Laryngeal Papilloma Foundation (ALPF)
PO Box 6108
Spring Hill, FL 34611-6108
Phone: (352)686-8583 **Fax:** (352)684-7191
Email: alpf@atlantic.net
Website: http://www.alpf.org
William Lazar, Pres.

Fnded: 1991. **Mem:** 1,000. **Reg. Groups:** 6. **Desc:** Individuals and families affected by laryngeal papillomatosis (LP), a rare disease in which tumors grow inside the trachea or larynx preventing normal breathing. Also known as recurrent respiratory papillomatosis. Promotes the health and welfare of victims. Seeks to increase public awareness, solicit donations, and support research efforts. Conducts a vitamin program; maintains national register of those afflicted with the disease. Provides children's services and educational programs; compiles statistics. **Pub:** *ALPF*, annual. Brochure. *Price:* Free. • *ALPF National Newsletter*, semiannual. Newsletter. *Price:* Free. **Frmly:** (1992) Christina Lazar Foundation for Juvenile Papillomatosis; (1995) Christina Lazar Foundation for Laryngeal Papillomatosis.

★ 729 ★ American Laryngological Association (ALA)
c/o Robert H. Ossoff, D.M.D., M.D.
Vanderbilt University Medical Ctr.
Medical Center North
S-2100 MCN
Nashville, TN 37232-2559
Phone: (615)322-6326 **Fax:** (615)343-7604
Email: robert.ossoff@vanderbuilt.edu
Website: http://www.alahns.org
Stanley M. Shapshay, MD, Pres.

Fnded: 1879. **Mem:** 232. **Desc:** Professional medical society of otorhinolaryngologists (specialists in ear, nose, and throat diseases). Works to advance research in medicine and surgery, with emphasis on the upper aerodigestive tract. **Pub:** *Transactions*, annual.

★ 730 ★ American Laryngological, Rhinological and Otological Society (ALROS)
c/o Boy's Town National Research Hosp.
555 N 30th St.
Omaha, NE 68131
Phone: (402)346-5500 **Fax:** (402)346-5300
Email: info@triological.org
Website: http://www.triological.org/
Patrick E. Brookhouser, MD, Exec. Sec.

Fnded: 1896. **Mem:** 1,300. **Reg. Groups:** 4. **Desc:** Professional society of medical specialists dealing with the ear, nose, and throat. **Pub:** *Laryngoscope*, monthly. Journal. Covers annual meeting; includes membership list. *Price:* Included in membership dues. • *The Laryngoscope Journal*, monthly. **AKA:** Triological Society.

★ 731 ★ American Lebanese Medical Association (ALMA)
3654 E Imperial Hwy.
Lynwood, CA 90262

Phone: (617)937-3071 Fax: (617)937-3081
Email: eayoub@hotmail.com
Website: http://www.ALMAmater.org/ALMA/Default.html
Joe F. Jabre, MD, Contact

Fnded: 1994. **Desc:** Health care professionals with Lebanese heritage, or with and interest in providing assistance to the people of Lebanon. Promotes increased access to improved health care for all religious and cultural communities in Lebanon. Fosters development of medical education institutions and health care facilities in Lebanon. Gathers and distributes Lebanese medical and scientific publications; conducts continuing professional education programs for members. Plans to operate library in conjunction with the Lebanese Medical Association.

★ 732 ★ American Lebanese Syrian Associated Charities (ALSAC)

501 St. Jude Pl.
PO Box 3704
Memphis, TN 38103
Free: 800-877-5833
Website: http://comnet.org/MECS/directory/national/alsac.html

Desc: Dedicated to treatment, research of catastrophic childhood diseases, helping children with diseases like acute lymphocytic leukemia, acute myeloid leukemia, pediatric AIDS.

★ 733 ★ American Leprosy Missions (ALM)

1 ALM Way
Greenville, SC 29601
Phone: (864)271-7040 **Free:** 800-543-3135
Fax: (864)271-7062
Email: amlep@leprosy.org
Website: http://www.leprosy.org
David Galvin, Org. /Donor Svcs. Mgr.

Fnded: 1906. **Desc:** Provides medical, rehabilitative, and social care for people with leprosy, also known as Hansen's disease, in over 20 countries. Conducts specialized training for medical workers; supports medical and social rehabilitation; provides special literature on leprosy to medical personnel abroad. Sponsors research in the U.S., Brazil and India. Assists the national leprosy control programs of Brazil, Angola, Myanmar, Mexico and the Philippines. Provides management assistance for the International Journal of Leprosy. **Pub:** *Word and Deed*, quarterly. Newsletter. Includes ALM news. *Price:* Free.

★ 734 ★ American Licensed Practical Nurses Association (ALPNA)

1090 Vermont Ave. NW, Ste. 800
Washington, DC 20005
Phone: (202)682-9000 **Fax:** (202)682-0168
Email: ptendler@tendler.com
Paul M. Tendler, Exec. Dir.

Fnded: 1984. **Mem:** 6,200. **Desc:** Licensed practical nurses. Promotes the practical nursing profession; lobbies and maintains relations with the government on issues and legislation that may have an impact on LPNs. Conducts continuing education classes. Facilitates discussion of issues affecting the nursing and health professions. **Pub:** Pamphlets.Contain information on legislation and nursing standards. • Papers.

★ 735 ★ American Lithotripsy Society (ALS)

305 Second Ave., Ste. 200
Waltham, MA 02451
Phone: (781)895-9098 **Fax:** (781)895-9088
Email: als@lithotripsy.org
Website: http://www.lithotripsy.org
Kenneth G. Scholl, Jr., Pres.

Fnded: 1987. **Mem:** 1,207. **Desc:** Promotes trade and public awareness of Lithotripsy. (Lithotripsy is a noninvasive procedure to treat kidney stones and gall stones.) Disseminates information; conducts educational programs, quality improvement and certification programs. **Pub:** *ALS Quarterly*, quarterly. Newsletter.

★ 736 ★ American Liver Foundation (ALF)

75 Maiden Ln., Ste. 603
New York, NY 10038
Phone: (212)668-1000 **Free:** 800-223-0179
Fax: (212)483-8179
Email: info@liverfoundation.org
Website: http://www.liverfoundation.org
Alan P. Brownstein, Pres. /CEO

Fnded: 1976. **Mem:** 24,000. **Desc:** Health agency working to fund research, promote the understanding and prevention of hepatitis and other liver diseases, and find cures for hepatitis and other liver diseases. Disseminates public and patient information on liver diseases, liver functions, and preventive measures. Provides information about support groups for liver disease patients and their families. Offers physician referral service. Sponsors seminars on disease diagnosis and management for physicians and other health professionals. Sponsors programs, which enables liver disease patients and concerned individuals to meet specialists and learn of recently developed information on treatment and research. Operates continuing organ donor awareness campaign in order to increase the number of organs available for transplant; monitors legislation (nationally and regionally) in areas affecting liver patients. Serves as trustee of funds raised to cover costs related to liver transplant surgery. Sponsors Corporate Wellness Program to provide information on liver disease for use in employee publications. **Pub:** *American Liver Foundation–Annual Report. Price:* Free. • *American Liver Foundation–Progress*, 3/year. Newsletter. Covers foundation programs; reports on research, news of liver diseases. *Price:* Included in membership dues. • *Liver Update: Function and Disease*, semiannual. Newsletter. *Price:* Included in membership dues. • Also publishes brochures, leaflets, and information sheets.

★ 737 ★ American Lung Association (ALA)

61 Broadway, 6th Fl.
New York, NY 10006
Phone: (212)315-8700 **Free:** 800-LUN-GUSA
Fax: (212)315-8872
Email: info@lungusa.org
Website: http://www.lungusa.org
John L. Kirkwood, CEO

Fnded: 1904. **Local Groups:** 78. **Desc:** Committed to fighting Big Tobacco, Bad Air and the Asthma Epidemic through research, education and advocacy in an effort to prevent lung disease and promote lung health. **Frmly:** (1918) National Association for the Study and Prevention of Tuberculosis; (1968) National Tuberculosis Association; (1973) National Tuberculosis and Respiratory Disease Association.

★ 738 ★ American Lyme Disease Foundation (ALDF)

Mill Pond Offices
293 Rte. 100
Somers, NY 10589
Phone: (914)277-6970 **Free:** 800-876-LYME
Fax: (914)277-6974
Email: inquire@aldf.com
Website: http://www.aldf.com
David L. Weld, Contact

Fnded: 1990. **Nat'l Groups:** 1. **Desc:** Health care professionals and other individuals with an interest in Lyme Disease, a disorder transmitted to humans by the deer tick. Works to control the spread of Lyme Disease, and to improve treatments for the disorder. Maintains physician referral service; produces educational materials and conducts public and professional education programs; supports Lyme Disease research. **Pub:** Newsletter, periodic. *Price:* Included in membership dues. • Video.Educational videos for use in schools, libraries, and camps.

★ 739 ★ American Managed Behavioral Healthcare Association (AMBHA)

c/o Pamela Greenberg, Exec.Dir.
1101 Pennsylvania Ave., Ste. 600
Washington, DC 20004
Phone: (202)756-7726 **Fax:** (202)756-7308
Website: http://www.ambha.org
Pamela Greenberg, MPP, Exec. Dir.

Fnded: 1994. **Mem:** 10. **Desc:** Managed behavioral healthcare organizations. Works to advance the value of managed behavioral healthcare and promotes the inclusion of mental illnesses and addiction disorders in benefit coverage. **Pub:** *Catalog of Special Reports*. Catalog.

★ 740 ★ American Massage Therapy Association (AMTA)

820 Davis St., Ste. 100
Evanston, IL 60201-4444
Phone: (847)864-0123 **Free:** 888-843-2682
Fax: (847)864-1178
Email: info@amtamassage.org
Website: http://www.amtamassage.org
Ronald Precht, Communications Mgr.

Fnded: 1943. **Mem:** 46,000. **State Groups:** 52. **Desc:** Massage therapists and massage schools. Promotes standards for the profession, has a Code of Ethics, and supports chapter efforts for state regulation of massage. Sponsors National Massage Therapy Awareness Week to promote public education on the benefits of massage; offers educational literature. Supports research on the efficacy of massage. Offers free Find A Message Therapists National locater service to help consumers and healthcare professionals find qualified, professional massage therapists. **Pub:** *AMTA's Find a Massage Therapist/Experience the Benefits of Massage*. Brochure. • *Hands On*, bimonthly. Newsletter. Features association and member news. *Price:* Free for members. • *Massage Therapy*. Brochure. • *Massage Therapy Journal*, quarterly. Journal. Contains scholarly articles on massage therapy. *Price:* $25/year in U.S.; $70/year outside U.S. • *Sports Massage*. Brochure. • *Stress*. Brochure. • Product brochure of AMTA products and publications. **Frmly:** (1983) American Massage and Therapy Association.

★ 741 ★ American Medical Association (AMA)

515 N State St.
Chicago, IL 60610
Phone: (312)464-5000 **Free:** 800-AMA-3211
Fax: (312)464-4184
Website: http://www.ama-assn.org/
Dr. Yank D. Coble, Jr., Pres.

Fnded: 1847. **Mem:** 297,000. **State Groups:** 54. **Desc:** County medical societies and physicians. Disseminates scientific information to members and the public. Informs members on significant medical and health legislation on state and national levels and represents the profession before Congress and governmental agencies. Cooperates in setting standards for medical schools, hospitals, residency programs, and continuing medical education courses. Offers physician placement service and counseling on practice management problems. Operates library which lends material and provides specific medical information to physicians. Ad-hoc committees are formed for such topics as health care planning and principles of medical ethics. **Pub:** *American Medical News*, weekly. Newspaper. Covers news and opinions on key issues of political, social, and economic significance concerning the practice and delivery of medical care. *Price:* Included in membership dues; $99/year for nonmembers; $49.50/year for medical students, interns, and residents. • *Archives of Dermatology*, monthly. Journal. Oriented to the dermatologic clinician. Includes book reviews, employment opportunity listings, annual index, and index of advertisers. *Price:* $67.50/year for members; $135/year for nonmembers; $67.50/year for residents and medical students. • *Archives of Family Medicine*, monthly. Oriented to physicians in family and general practice. *Price:* $47.50 for members; $95 for nonmembers. • *Archives of General Psychiatry*, monthly. Journal. Oriented toward the psychiatric clinician. Includes employment opportunity listings, book reviews, annual index, and index of advertisers. *Price:* $47.50/year for members; $95/year for nonmembers; $47.50/year for residents and medical students. • *Archives of Internal Medicine*, semimonthly. Journal. Oriented toward physicians in internal medicine. Includes employment opportunity listings, annual index, and index of advertisers. *Price:* $57.50/year for members; $115/year for nonmembers; $57.50/year for residents and medical students. • *Archives of Neurology*, monthly. Journal. Oriented toward the neurologic clinician. Includes employment opportunity listings, annual index, and index of advertisers. *Price:* $72.50/year for members; $145/year for nonmembers; $72.50/year for residents and medical students. • *Archives of Ophthalmology*, monthly. Journal. Includes employment opportunity listings, case reports, book reviews, annual index, and index of advertisers. *Price:* $55/year for members; $110/year for nonmembers; $55/year for residents and medical students. • *Archives of Otolaryngology–Head and Neck Surgery*, monthly. Journal. Ori.

★ 742 ★ American Medical Association Alliance (AMAA)

515 N State St.
Chicago, IL 60610-0174
Phone: (312)464-4470 **Fax:** (312)464-5020
Email: amaa@ama-assn.org
Website: http://www.ama-assn.org/ama/pub/category/2109.html
Gay Bowman, Pres.

Fnded: 1922. **Mem:** 70,000. **Nat'l Groups:** 100. **State Groups:** 46. **Local Groups:** 815. **Desc:** Physicians' spouses. Serves as the volunteer arm of the American Medical Association. Promotes the goals of the medical profession and works to meet public health needs. Raises more than $2 million annually for the American Medical Association Education and Research Foundation (see separate entry), which provides assistance to medical schools and students. Sponsors the Shape Up for Life Campaign, a nationwide auxiliary program to promote good health. Maintains Project Bank, an information clearinghouse of community projects initiated by auxiliaries across the country. Implements community health projects on such concerns as child abuse prevention, adolescent health, family violence, AIDS education, seatbelt usage, pre- and postnatal care, drug abuse, suicide prevention, proper nutrition, drunk driving prevention, venereal disease awareness, and services to the aging. Works with the AMA to promote sound health legislation; conducts public education programs, letter-writing campaigns, and personal interviews with legislators involved in health matters. **Pub:** *Facets Magazine*, bimonthly. Magazine. Includes information on community health projects, public health issues, socioeconomic health care issues, and physician family concerns. *Price:* Included in membership dues; $7/year for nonmembers. • *Horizons Newsletter*, bimonthly. Newsletter. Covers topics of concern to the families of resident physicians and medical students. *Price:* Free to resident physicians and medical students. • *Newsline*, bimonthly. Includes information on health periodicals and health projects. *Price:* Included in membership dues. **Frmly:** (1975) Women's Auxilliary to the American Medical Association; (1993) American Medical Association Auxilliary.

★ 743 ★ American Medical Association Foundation

515 N State St.
Chicago, IL 60610
Phone: (312)464-4543 **Fax:** (312)464-5973
Website: http://www.amafoundation.org
Kathleen MacArthur, Exec. Dir.

Fnded: 1962. **Desc:** Foundation managed by Directors of the American Medical Association . Receives and distributes funds to benefit medical education in U.S. medical schools and to support education, research and service progams within the community of medicine. Foundation funds consist of contributions from physicians, medical societies and auxiliaries, of other foundations, private industry, and the public. Accepts bequests and other gifts for allocation to various projects in medicine. **Frmly:** (1999) American Medical Association Education and Research Foundation.

★ 744 ★ American Medical Directors Association (AMDA)

10480 Little Patuxent Pky., Ste. 760
Columbia, MD 21044
Phone: (410)740-9743 **Free:** 800-876-2632
Fax: (410)740-4572
Email: info@amda.com
Website: http://www.amda.com
Lorraine Tarnove, Exec. Dir.

Fnded: 1975. **Mem:** 8,000. **State Groups:** 35. **Desc:** Physicians providing care in long-term facilities including nursing homes. Sponsors continuing medical education in geriatrics and medical administration. Promotes improved long term care. **Pub:** *AMDA Reports*, bimonthly. Newsletter. Includes calendar of events, reviews of articles, publications, and other resources. *Price:* available to members only. • *Nursing Home Medicine: The Annals of Long Term Care*, 10/year. Journal. *Price:* Free for members; $2/single issue. • Audiotapes.Related to medical direction. • Videos.Related to long term care issues such as restraints, CPT coding, and advance directions.

★ 745 ★ American Medical Electroencephalographic Association (AMEEGA)

PO Box 757
Pewaukee, WI 53072-0757
Fax: (414)782-8788
Email: medassn@aol.com
Michael J. Herzog, Contact

Fnded: 1964. **Mem:** 700. **Desc:** Works to advance clinical electroencephalography and to promote the development of clinical and technical training programs. **Pub:** *Clinical EEG*, quarterly.

★ 746 ★ American Medical Equestrian Association (AMEA)

PO Box 130848
Birmingham, AL 35213-0848
Free: (866)441-2632 **Fax:** (866)441-2632
Email: amea@charter.net
Website: http://www.ameaonline.org
Rusty Lowe, Exec. Dir.

Fnded: 1990. **Mem:** 175. **Nat'l Groups:** 1. **Desc:** Physicians, health personnel, and individuals interested in equestrian safety. Seeks to decrease accidents related to horseback riding through education and awareness programs. Advocates use of headgear for riders. Offers recommendations, consultations, and leadership to equestrian organizations. Conducts studies and surveys. Compiles statistics. **Pub:** *AMEA News*, quarterly. Newsletter. Includes articles and statistics on horse-related human injuries. *Price:* Included in membership dues. • *Planning Event Coverage*. Booklet. • *When Can My Child Ride a Horse*. Brochure.

★ 747 ★ American Medical Group Association (AMGA)

1422 Duke St.
Alexandria, VA 22314-3430
Phone: (703)838-0033 **Fax:** (703)548-1890
Email: roconnor@amga.org
Website: http://www.amga.org
Dr. Donald W. Fisher, CAE, Pres. /CEO

Fnded: 1949. **Mem:** 300. **Desc:** Trade association for medical groups and integrated delivery systems and IPAS representing more than 65,000 physicians. Provides public policy advocacy, compiles statistics on group practice, sponsors research, patient education, insurance programs. **Pub:** *Group Practice Journal*, 10/year. Journal. Covers market trends, health care policy and legislation, and management topics affecting the medical profession. Includes advertiser index. *Price:* Included in membership dues; $87/year for nonmembers. **Frmly:** American Group Practice Association; (1974) American Association of Medical Clinics.

★ 748 ★ American Medical Informatics Association (AMIA)

4915 St. Elmo Ave., Ste. 401
Bethesda, MD 20814
Phone: (301)657-1291 **Fax:** (301)657-1296
Email: mail@mail.amia.org
Website: http://www.amia.org
Ina King, Mgr. Admin.

Fnded: 1990. **Mem:** 3,200. **Nat'l Groups:** 1. **Desc:** Medical personnel, physicians, physical scientists, engineers, data processors, researchers, educators, hospital administrators, nurses, medical record administrators, and computer professionals. Objectives are: to apply advanced systems and information technologies to scientific, literary, and educational activities; to promote excellence in health care; to promote patient care, teaching, research, and health administration. **Pub:** *Journal of the American Medical Informatics Association*, bimonthly. Journal. • *Proceedings of Annual Symposium*, annual. Book. Contains abstracts of sessions of the association's annual symposium. *Price:* $95 plus shipping and handling.

★ 749 ★ American Medical Network

15429 N Florida Ave.
Tampa, FL 33613
Free: (866)346-2354 **Fax:** (813)264-0647
Email: benefits@americanmednetwork.com
Website: http://www.americanmednetwork.com

Fnded: 1996. **Desc:** Practicing physicians. Represents doctors' concerns for their patients; establishes a national quality database for use in negotiating managed care contracts; educates laymen and policy makers on quality of care issues; and influences health care policy.

★ 750 ★ American Medical Rehabilitation Providers Association (AMRPA)

1710 N St. NW
Washington, DC 20036
Phone: (202)223-1920 **Free:** 888-346-4624
Fax: (202)223-1925
Email: czollar@amrpa.org
Website: http://www.amrpa.org
Kenneth W. Aitchison, Pres.

Fnded: 1997. **Mem:** 300. **State Groups:** 29. **Desc:** Rehabilitation facilities in the U.S. and Canada; agencies operating established medical, residential and vocational rehabilitation facilities. Promotes expansion and improvement of rehabilitation services to disabled persons as provided in rehabilitation facilities. Represents the concerns of rehabilitation providers before Congress and government agencies. Is concerned with quality operation of rehabilitation centers and facilities. Conducts research and development programs in national rehabilitation policy. Sponsors seminars and provides specialized education programs. **Pub:** *Rehabilitation Insurance Report*, monthly. Newsletter. Analyzes insurance issues relevant to rehabilitation services. *Price:* $50/year to members; $65/year to nonmembers. • *Rehabilitation Review*, weekly. Newsletter. Monitors developments in the rehabilitation industry. Includes research updates and a calendar of events. *Price:* Included in membership dues; $125/year for nonmembers. • Books. • Monographs. • Videos. **Frmly:** (1975) International Association of Rehabilitation Facilities; (1980) Association of Rehabilitation Facilities; (1994) National Association of Rehabilitation Facilities; (1998) American Rehabilitation Association.

★ 751 ★ American Medical Resources Foundation (AMRF)

PO Box 3609
Brockton, MA 02304-3609
Phone: (508)580-3301 **Fax:** (508)580-3306
Email: info@amrf.com
Website: http://www.amrf.com

Fnded: 1988. **Desc:** Donates used, but fully functional, medical equipment to hospitals and clinics serving the poor in Third World and developing nations. The equipment is donated to AMRF by over 300 hospitals and industries in the U.S. and by private physicians and dentists. Donated equipment includes beds and patient transports; through monitors; x-rays; infant warmers; infant transformers; patient handling equipment; pulmonary, cardiac or ultrasonic diagnostic equipment; and diverse equipment for general and specialized use in prenatal, natal, pediatric and adult departments. Coordinates volunteer procedures and assists in the setting up and calibration of all equipment at the recipient hospitals. Provides training for the hospital biomedical technicians. **Pub:** *AMRF News*, quarterly. Newsletter.

★ 752 ★ American Medical Society for Sports Medicine (AMSSM)

11639 Earnshaw
Overland Park, KS 66210
Phone: (913)327-1415 **Fax:** (913)327-1491
Email: office@amssm.org
Website: http://www.amssm.org

Fnded: 1991. **Desc:** Sports medicine specialists. Provides a forum specific for primary care non-surgical sports medicine physicians.

★ 753 ★ American Medical Student Association (AMSA)

1902 Association Dr.
Reston, VA 20191
Phone: (703)620-6600 **Free:** 800-767-2266
Fax: (703)620-5873
Email: amsa@www.amsa.org
Website: http://www.amsa.org
Eric Hodgson, Pres.

Fnded: 1950. **Mem:** 35,000. **Local Groups:** 140. **Desc:** Medical students; local, state, and national organizations; premedical students, interns, and residents. Seeks to improve medical education by making it relevant to today's needs and by making the process by which physicians are trained more humanistic. Contributes to the improvement of health care of all people; involves its members in the social, moral, and ethical obligations of the profession of medicine. Serves as a mechanism through which students may actively participate in the fields of community health through various student health programs. Addresses political issues relating to the nation's health care delivery system and other medical and health issues. Maintains action committees and interest groups which publish newsletters, organize educational workshops, and initiate special projects. **Pub:** *The New Physician*, 9/year. Magazine. *Price:* included in membership dues; $25/year. **Frmly:** (1975) Student American Medical Association.

★ 754 ★ American Medical Technologists (AMT)

710 Higgins Rd.
Park Ridge, IL 60068-5765
Phone: (847)823-5169 **Free:** 800-275-1268
Fax: (847)823-0458
Email: mail@amt1.com
Website: http://www.amt1.com
Christopher A. Damon, J.D., Exec. Dir.

Fnded: 1939. **Mem:** 25,000. **State Groups:** 38. **Desc:** National professional association and certifying body for medical laboratory technologists, technicians, medical assistants, dental assistants, and phlebotomists. Maintains job information service. Sponsors AMT Institute for Education, evaluates and recommends continuing education programs. **Pub:** *AMT Events and Continuing Education Supplement*, 6/yr. Journal. Includes book reviews and legislative updates. *Price:* Included in membership dues; $35/year for nonmembers in the U.S.; $45/year for foreign nonmembers.

★ 755 ★ American Medical Women's Association (AMWA)

801 N Fairfax St., Ste. 400
Alexandria, VA 22314
Phone: (703)838-0500 **Fax:** (703)549-3864
Email: info@amwa-doc.org
Website: http://www.amwa-doc.org
Elinor T. Christriansen, MD, Pres.

Fnded: 1915. **Mem:** 10,000. **Reg. Groups:** 10. **Local Groups:** 160. **Desc:** Women holding a M.D. or D.O. degree from approved medical colleges; women interns, residents, and medical students. Promotes women's health issues in medical education and public policy. Seeks to find solutions to problems common to women studying or practicing medicine, such as career advancement and the integration of professional and family responsibilities. Provides student members with educational loans and personal counseling. Sponsors continuing medical education programs. **Pub:** *What's Happening in AMWA*, semiannual. Newsletter. *Price:* Included in membership dues. • Journal, quarterly. • Newsletter, quarterly.

★ 756 ★ American Mental Health Counselors Association (AMHCA)

801 N Fairfax, Ste. 304
Alexandria, VA 22314
Phone: (703)548-6002 **Free:** 800-326-2642
Fax: (703)548-5233
Email: mhamilton@amhca.org
Website: http://www.amhca.org
W. Mark Hamilton, Phd.D., Exec. Dir.

Fnded: 1976. **Mem:** 7,000. **State Groups:** 50. **Desc:** Professional counselors employed in mental health services; students. Aims to: deliver quality mental health services to children, youth, adults, families, and organizations; improve the availability and quality of counseling services through licensure and certification, training standards, and consumer advocacy. Supports specialty and special interest networks. Fosters communication among members. A division of the American Counseling Association. **Pub:** *Advocate*, 6/year. Newsletter. Contains current information on the mental health profession. *Price:* Included in membership dues; $25 nonmembers. • *Journal of Mental Health Counseling*, quarterly. Journal. • *Mental Health Brights*. Brochures. Contains information on divorce, eating disorders, child abuse, parenting young children, handling conflict, caring for aging parents.

★ 757 ★ American Motility Society (AMS)

230 E Ohio St., Ste. 400
Chicago, IL 60611-3265
Phone: (312)644-0828 **Fax:** (312)644-8557
Email: ams@bostrom.com
James Ryan, PhD, Treas.

Fnded: 1980. **Mem:** 220. **Desc:** Professionals interested in the study of gastrointestinal (GI) motility. Promotes basic science and clinical research on the neural, humoral, and paracrine control of GI tract motility in health and disease.

★ 758 ★ American Music Therapy Association (AMTA)

8455 Colesville Rd., Ste. 1000
Silver Spring, MD 20910
Phone: (301)589-3300 **Fax:** (301)589-5175
Email: info@musictherapy.org
Website: http://www.musictherapy.org
Dr. Andrea Farbman, Exec. Dir.

Fnded: 1950. **Mem:** 4,000. **Reg. Groups:** 8. **Desc:** Supports the therapeutic use of music in hospital, rehabilitation, educational and community settings. Monitors the clinical practice of music therapy to insure the services provided to persons with disabilities are the highest quailty possible. Serves as the national voice advocating for the development and expansion of music therapy services and programs. **Pub:** *AMTA Membership Sourcebook*, annual. Membership Directory. Contains statistical information and association documents. *Price:* Included in membership dues; $50/year for nonmembers. • *Journal of Music Therapy*, quarterly. Journal. *Price:* Included in membership dues. • *Music Therapy Clinical Training Facilities Handbook*. Handbook. Lists approved facilities and programs offering music therapy internships, available on Website. • *Music Therapy Matters*, quarterly. Newsletter. *Price:* Included in membership dues. • *Music Therapy Perspectives*, semiannual. *Price:* Included in membership dues. **Frmly:** (1998) National Association for Music Therapy; (2001) American Association for Music Therapy.

★ 759 ★ American Naprapathic Association (ANA)

c/o Roy P. Krueger, D.N.
5913 W Montrose Ave.
Chicago, IL 60634
Phone: (773)685-6020
Roy P. Krueger, D.N., Corr. Sec.

Fnded: 1909. **Mem:** 300. **Desc:** Professional society of naprapathic physicians. (Naprapathy is the science and system of therapeutic manipulation of tissue structures that have become damaged due to stress and strain.) Promotes and publishes the principles of natural healing; seeks to further legislation and recognition of the system of treatment based on the belief that many functional disorders are caused by abnormal connective tissue and ligamentous changes and can be corrected by manipulation. Sponsors Naprapathic Education and Research Foundation. Conducts seminars and educational programs. Maintains speakers' bureau. **Pub:** *Back Pain*. • *Headache: A Warning*. • *Naprapathy: A Scientific Approach to Natural Healing*. • *The Three Facets of Naprapathy*. • *Voice of Naprapathy*. Booklet. Includes articles on nutrition and health topics. *Price:* Free. • *Why Manipulation?*. • Directory, periodic.

★ 760 ★ American Naturopathic Association

PO Box 78600
North Capitol Station
Washington, DC 20013-8600
Dr. George A. Freibott, Pres.

Fnded: 1896. **Mem:** 5,000. **Nat'l Groups:** 1. **Reg. Groups:** 7. **State Groups:** 32. **Local Groups:** 15. **Desc:** Students, laypeople, and naturopathic physicians. Promotes the practice and education of naturopathy. Operates a national training center and university; offers public awareness and wellness programs. Conducts research; provides statistics; maintains a museum, Hall of Fame, and speakers' bureau. **Pub:** *Naturopath and Herald of Health*, monthly. Journal. *Price:* $5/each.

★ 761 ★ American Naturopathic Medical Association (ANMA)

PO Box 96273
Las Vegas, NV 89193
Phone: (702)897-7053 **Fax:** (702)897-7140
Website: http://www.anma.com/frontpg.htm

Fnded: 1981. **Mem:** 3,000. **Desc:** Dedicated to exploring new frontiers of mind, body, medicine and health. **Pub:** *ANMA Monitor Online*.

★ 762 ★ American Nephrology Nurses' Association (ANNA)

Box 56, E Holly Ave.
Pitman, NJ 08071
Phone: (856)256-2320 **Free:** 888-600-2662
Fax: (856)589-7463
Email: anna@ajj.com
Website: http://www.annanurse.org
Mike Cunningham, Exec. Dir.

Fnded: 1969. **Mem:** 11,500. **Reg. Groups:** 4. **Local Groups:** 106. **Desc:** Registered nurses; physicians, dietitians, social workers, and technicians. Promotes continuing education of members at national, regional, and local levels. **Pub:** *Building Your Career in Dialysis*. Video. *Price:* $29. • *Contemporary Nephrology Nursing Textbook*. Book. *Price:* $88 members; $103 nonmembers. • *Core Curriculum for Nephrology Nursing*. *Price:* $70 member; $90 non-member. • *Nephrology Nursing: A Guide to Professional Development*. *Price:*

$35 member; $50 non-member. • *Nephrology Nursing Certification Review Guide. Price:* $20 members; $30 non-members. • *Nephrology Nursing Journal.* Journal. *Price:* $36 individual; $54 individual outside USA; $50 institution; $68 institution outside USA. • *RPA Shared Decision-Making in the Appropriate Initiation of and Withdrawal from Dialysis. Price:* $10 members. • *Standardized Training Program for the Patient Care Technician in Hemodialysis - Instructor's Guide. Price:* $18. • *Standardized Training Program for the Patient Care Technician in Hemodialysis - Learner's Guide. Price:* $28. • *Standards and Guidelines of Clinical Practice for Nephrology Nursing. Price:* $35 members; $50 non-members. • *Standards of Clinical Practice for Continuous Renal Replacement Therapy.* This publication is included in Standards of Clinical Practice for Nephrology Nursing. *Price:* $10 members; $15 non-members. **Frmly:** (1984) American Association of Nephrology Nurses and Technicians.

★ 763 ★ American Neurological Association (ANA)

5841 Cedar Lake Rd. S, Ste. 204
Minneapolis, MN 55416-1491
Phone: (952)545-6284 **Fax:** (952)545-6073
Email: lindawilkerson@llmsi.com
Website: http://www.aneuroa.org
Linda J. Wilkerson, Exec. Dir.

Fnded: 1875. **Mem:** 960. **Desc:** Physicians and scientists interested in the form, functioning, and disorders of the nervous system. Conducts research programs. **Pub:** *Annals of Neurology*, monthly. Journal. Includes book reviews. *Price:* Included in membership dues; $68/year for nonmembers; $84/year for institutions; $52.50/year for students.

★ 764 ★ American Neuropsychiatric Association (ANPA)

c/o Sandra Bornstein
700 Ackerman Rd., Ste. 550
Columbus, OH 43202
Phone: (614)447-2077 **Fax:** (614)263-4366
Email: anpa@osu.edu
Website: http://www.neuropsychiatry.com
Sandra Bornstein, Contact

Fnded: 1987. **Mem:** 425. **Desc:** Conducts educational and research programs. **Pub:** *Journal of Neuropsychiatry and Clinical Neurosciences.* Journal.

★ 765 ★ American Neurotology Society (ANS)

c/o Paul Lambert, MD, Chairman
Medical University of South Carolina
Box 250582
Charleston, SC 29425
Phone: (843)792-7161 **Fax:** (843)792-0546
Email: lambert@musc.edu
Website: http://itsa.ucsf.edu/~ajo/ANS/ANS.html
Newton J. Coker, MD, Pres.

Fnded: 1965. **Mem:** 500. **Desc:** Physicians and audiologists interested in the diagnosis and treatment of hearing and balance disorders. Promotes education and research in the field of neurotology. **Pub:** Directory, annual. Published in conjunction with American Academy of Otolaryngology - Head and Neck Surgery. **Frmly:** (1965) ENG Study Group.

★ 766 ★ American Nouthetic Psychology Association (ANPA)

PO Box 801
Hardwick, GA 31034
Email: biblespy@alltel.net
Website: http://www.alltel.net/~biblepsy
Dr. David M. Carnrike, Pres.

Fnded: 1986. **Mem:** 800. **Reg. Groups:** 7. **State Groups:** 50. **Desc:** Psychologists and other individuals with an interest in nouthetic psychology. Promotes high standards of training, ethics, and practice in the field. Conducts research and educational programs.

★ 767 ★ American Nurses Association (ANA)

600 Maryland Ave. SW, Ste. 100 W
Washington, DC 20024-2571
Phone: (202)651-7000 **Free:** 800-274-4262
Fax: (202)651-7001
Email: memberinfo@ana.org
Website: http://www.nursingworld.org
Barbara A. Blakeney, Pres.

Fnded: 1896. **Mem:** 210,000. **State Groups:** 53. **Local Groups:** 860. **Desc:** Membership association representing registered nurses. **Pub:** *The American Nurse*, monthly. Newspaper. Includes employment listings. *Price:* Included in membership dues; $20/year for nonmembers; $10/year for full-time nursing students. • *Proceedings of the House of Delegates*, periodic. Proceedings. • Catalog, annual. • Also publishes nursing standards and professional literature. **Frmly:** (1911) Nurses Associated Alumnae of United States and Canada.

★ 768 ★ American Nurses Foundation (ANF)

600 Maryland Ave. SW, Ste. 100W
Washington, DC 20024-2571
Phone: (202)651-7227 **Fax:** (202)651-7354
Email: anf@ana.org
Website: http://www.nursingworld.org/anf
Leo Schargorodski, Dir.

Fnded: 1955. **Desc:** Research, education, and charitable arm of the American Nurses' Association. Promotes nursing and consumers wherever nurses practice. Mission accomplished through four major functions: fundraising, Nursing Research Grants, grant development and management, and American Nurses Publishing. **Pub:** Books.

★ 769 ★ American Nursing Informatics Association (ANIA)

PMB 105
10808 Foothill Blvd., Ste. 160
Rancho Cucamonga, CA 91730
Email: mbrs@ania.org
Website: http://www.ania.org
Anna L. Easter, PhD, Pres.

Fnded: 1992. **Mem:** 350. **Desc:** Licensed nurses, nursing students, and individuals involved with clinical, administrative and educational aspects of healthcare information systems. Provides networking, education, and information resources to members; serves as a forum for the advancement of nursing and nursing professionals in informatics. Makes available discounts on professional program attendance and conference tuition to members. **Pub:** *Input-Output*, periodic. Newsletter. *Price:* Free to members.

★ 770 ★ American Obesity Association (AOA)

1250 24th St., NW
No. 300
Washington, DC 20037
Phone: (202)776-7711 **Free:** 800-986-2373
Fax: (202)776-7712
Email: executive@obesity.org
Website: http://www.obesity.org
Morgan Downey, Exec. Dir.

Fnded: 1995. **Mem:** 450. **Desc:** Health professionals. Supports research and education about obesity including the discrimination against the obese. Actively seeks government funding and is an advocate for insurance coverage for the obese. **Pub:** *AOA Report*, quarterly. Newsletter.

★ 771 ★ American Occupational Therapy Association (AOTA)

4720 Montgomery Ln.
PO Box 31220
Bethesda, MD 20824-1220
Phone: (301)652-2682 **Free:** 800-377-8555
Fax: (301)652-7711
Email: praota@aota.org
Website: http://www.aota.org
Joseph C. Isaacs, Exec. Dir.

Fnded: 1917. **Mem:** 41,000. **Desc:** Occupational therapists and occupational therapy assistants who provide services to people whose lives have been disrupted by physical injury or illness, developmental problems, the aging process, or social or psychological difficulties. Occupational therapy focuses on the active involvement of the patient in specially designed therapeutic tasks and activities to improve function, performance capacity, and the ability to cope with demands of daily living. **Pub:** *American Journal of Occupational Therapy*, bimonthly. Journal. • *OT Practice*, biweekly. • *Publications Catalog.* Catalog. • Also publishes more than 100 single titles. **Frmly:** National Society for the Promotion of Occupational Therapy.

★ 772 ★ American Occupational Therapy Foundation (AOTF)

4720 Montgomery Lane
PO Box 31220
Bethesda, MD 20824-1220
Phone: (301)652-6611 **Fax:** (301)656-3620
Email: aotf@aotf.org
Website: http://www.aotf.org
Martha Kirkland, Exec. Dir.

Fnded: 1965. **Desc:** Encourages practice, research and scholarship in occupation and occupational therapy. Educates the public and professionals about occupation and occupational therapy. **Pub:** *Occupation, Participation and Health.* Journal. • *The Occupational Therapy Journal of Research*, quarterly. Journal. Features a peer-reviewed journal.

★ 773 ★ American Ophthalmological Society (AOS)

PO Box 19340
San Francisco, CA 94119-3940
Phone: (415)561-8578 **Fax:** (415)561-8531
Email: admin@aosonline.org
Website: http://www.aosonline.org
Charles P. Wilkinson, MD, Sec. Treas.

Fnded: 1864. **Mem:** 325. **Desc:** Professional honorary society of physicians specializing in the functions and treatment of the eye. **Pub:** *Transactions of the American Ophthalmological Society*, annual. Journal. Contains papers presented at annual meeting and accepted theses. *Price:* $55.

★ 774 ★ American Optometric Association (AOA)

243 N Lindbergh Blvd.
Saint Louis, MO 63141
Phone: (314)991-4100 **Fax:** (314)991-4101
Website: http://www.aoanet.org/
Michael D. Jones, Exec. Dir.

Fnded: 1898. **Mem:** 32,000. **State Groups:** 53. **Local Groups:** 500. **Desc:** Professional association of optometrists, students of optometry, and paraoptometric assistants and technicians. Purposes are: to improve the quality, availability, and accessibility of eye and vision care; to represent the optometric profession; to help members conduct their practices; to promote the highest standards of patient care. Monitors and promotes legislation concerning the scope of optometric practice, alternate health care delivery systems, health care cost containment, Medicare, and other issues relevant to eye/vision care. Supports the International Library, Archives and Museum of Optometry which includes references on ophthalmic and related sciences with emphasis on the history and socieconomic aspects of optometry. Operates Vision U.S.A. program, which provides free eye care to the working poor. Conducts specialized education programs; operates placement service; compiles statistics. Maintains museum. Conducts Seal of Certification and Acceptance Program. **Pub:** *American Optometric Association–News*, semimonthly. Magazine. Includes employment listings, classified ads, promotional news, and obituaries. *Price:* $80/year for nonmembers; $95 in Canada; $103 outside U.S. and Canada. • *Optometry: Journal of the American Optometric Association*, monthly. Journal. Includes research articles, book reviews, calendar of events, legislative news, new products information, and advertisers' index. *Price:* $95/year for nonmembers; $130/year in Canada; $145/year outside U.S. and Canada. **Frmly:** (1903) American Optical Association.

★ 775 ★ American Optometric Foundation (AOF)
6110 Executive Blvd., Ste. 506
Rockville, MD 20852
Phone: (301)984-4734 **Free:** 800-368-6AOF
Fax: (301)984-4737
Email: christine@aapotom.org
Website: http://www.aaopt.org/aof/about/index.asp
Christine Armstrong, Dir.

Fnded: 1947. **Desc:** Optometrists, optometric organizations, corporations, and the public. Promotes research, education, literature, and professional advancement in the visual sciences. Supports fellowships in graduate research. **Pub:** *The Torch*, quarterly. Newsletter. Updates on foundation's activities. *Price:* Free.

★ 776 ★ American Optometric Student Association (AOSA)
243 N Lindbergh
Saint Louis, MO 63141
Phone: (314)991-4100 **Fax:** (314)991-4101
Website: http://www.theaosa.org/frameset2.htm
Ryan Parker, Pres.

Fnded: 1972. **Mem:** 5,600. **Nat'l Groups:** 1. **Local Groups:** 19. **Desc:** Optometric students, state optometric associations, and family members of optometric students. Collects updated information on progress in the optometry field. Provides members with opportunities to work in areas of health care need such as local community health projects, school curriculum changes, and health manpower legislation. Works to improve optometric education and health care for the general population. Maintains active liaison with other optometric associations. Conducts communications program. **Pub:** *AOSA Foresight: Optometry Looking Forward*, semiannual. Reports information concerning scholarships, grants, internships, and other educational issues related to the study of optometry. *Price:* Included in membership dues. • *Communicator*, 9/year. Newsletter.

★ 777 ★ American Organization for Bodywork Therapies of Asia (AOBTA)
1010 Haddonfield-Berlin Rd., STe 408
Voorhees, NJ 08043-3514
Phone: (856)782-1616 **Fax:** (856)782-1653
Email: aobta@prodigy.net
Website: http://www.aobta.org
Debra Howard, Pres.

Fnded: 1984. **Mem:** 1,500. **Reg. Groups:** 3. **Desc:** Professional oriental bodyworkers and teachers; interested individuals. (Oriental bodywork is a form of massage which includes soft tissue and myofascial manipulation and techniques used in acupuncture.) Identifies qualified practitioners; serves as a legal entity representing members when dealing with the government, especially in terms of establishing professional status. Sets teaching standards for all styles of oriental bodywork including acupressure, five element shiatsu, macrobiotic shiatsu, nippon, and zen. Sponsors speakers' bureau; conducts educational programs. **Pub:** *AOBTA Directory*, annual. Membership Directory. Lists members of the association. • *PULSE Newsletter*, quarterly. Newsletter. **Frmly:** (1990) American Shiatsu Association; (1991) American Association of Oriental Healing Arts; (2001) American Oriental Bodywork Therapy Association.

★ 778 ★ American Organization of Nurse Executives (AONE)
325 Seventh St. NW
Washington, DC 20004
Phone: (202)626-2240 **Fax:** (202)638-5499
Email: aone@aha.org
Website: http://www.aone.org
Pamela Thompson, RN, Exec. Dir.

Fnded: 1967. **Mem:** 4,000. **State Groups:** 69. **Desc:** Provides leadership, professional development, advocacy, and research to advance nursing practice and patient care, promote nursing leadership and excellence, and shape healthcare public policy. Supports and enhances the management, leadership, educational, and professional development of nursing leaders. Offers placement service through Career Development and Referral Center. **Pub:** *AONE Updates*, 3/weeks. Newsletter. Bulleted update of information related to nursing administration. • Books. • Membership Directory, annual. *Price:* Included in membership dues. • Monographs. • Videos. **Frmly:** (1977) American Society for Hospital Nursing Service Administrators; (1984) American Society for Nursing Service Administrators.

★ 779 ★ American Orthodontic Society (AOS)
11884 Greenville Ave., No. 112
Dallas, TX 75243-3537
Phone: (972)234-4000 **Free:** 800-448-1601
Fax: (972)234-4290
Email: tchapman@orthodontic.com
Tom Chapman, Exec. Dir.

Fnded: 1974. **Mem:** 1,900. **Desc:** General and pediatric dentists. Objectives are: to make orthodontic information readily available to any ethical dentist; to zealously protect the right of members to pursue orthodontic knowledge; to keep a watchful eye on third party services and government programs. Offers courses in orthodontic techniques. Conducts educational programs. **Pub:** *American Orthodontic Society Newsletter*, quarterly. Newsletter. Provides information on the society's seminars and conventions and news of interest to members. *Price:* Included in membership dues. • *American Orthodontic Society Technique Directory*, biennial. Membership Directory. Lists members by city and state; includes the type of orthodontic technique used by listee. *Price:* $150. • Brochures.

★ 780 ★ American Orthopaedic Association (AOA)
6300 N River Rd., Ste. 505
Rosemont, IL 60018-4263
Phone: (847)318-7330 **Fax:** (847)318-7339
Email: info@aoassn.org
Website: http://www.aoassn.org
Thomas E. Stautzenbach, Exec. Dir.

Fnded: 1887. **Mem:** 10,000. **Desc:** Professional society of bone and joint surgeons. Seeks to further knowledge in the diagnosis and treatment of crippling diseases. **Pub:** *American Orthopedic Association–Newsletter*, 3/year. Journal. • *Journal on Bone and Joint Surgery*, 8/year. Journal.

★ 781 ★ American Orthopaedic Foot and Ankle Society (AOFAS)
2517 Eastlake Ave. E, Ste. 200
Seattle, WA 98102
Phone: (206)223-1120 **Free:** 800-235-4855
Fax: (206)223-1178
Email: aofas@aofas.org
Website: http://www.aofas.org
Richard Cantrall, Exec. Dir.

Fnded: 1969. **Mem:** 1,800. **Desc:** Members of American Academy of Orthopaedic Surgeons interested in research on, education in, and care of the foot and ankle. Sponsors continuing medical education courses. **Pub:** *A Guide to Children's Shoes*. Pamphlet. • *The Adult Foot*. Pamphlet. • *The Child's Foot*. Pamphlet. • *The Diabetic Foot*. Pamphlet. • *Foot and Ankle International*, monthly. Journal. *Price:* Included in membership dues; $149/year for nonmembers; $180/year for institutions; $11/copy. **Frmly:** (1983) American Orthopaedic Foot Society.

★ 782 ★ American Orthopaedic Society for Sports Medicine (AOSSM)
6300 N River Rd., Ste. 200
Rosemont, IL 60018
Phone: (847)292-4900 **Free:** 877-321-3500
Fax: (847)292-4905
Email: irv@aossm.org
Website: http://www.sportsmed.org
Irvin E. Bomberger, Exec. Dir.

Fnded: 1972. **Mem:** 1,600. **Desc:** Promotes sports medicine education, research, communication and fellowship; disseminates information to orthopaedic surgeons working in sports medicine. **Pub:** *American Journal of Sports Medicine*, bimonthly. Journal. Reports on the diagnosis, treatment, prevention, and rehabilitation of sports-related injury and disease; also includes society news and book reviews. *Price:* $80/year for individuals; $100/year for institutions; $30/year students.

★ 783 ★ American Orthopsychiatric Association (ORTHO)
330 7th Ave., 18th Fl.
New York, NY 10001-3010
Phone: (212)564-5930 **Fax:** (212)564-6180
Email: amerortho@aol.com
Website: http://www.amerortho.org
Lisa Shuger Hublitz, Exec. Dir.

Fnded: 1924. **Mem:** 4,500. **Desc:** Psychiatrists, psychologists, social workers, and educators; psychiatric nurses and lawyers; others in related fields, including anthropology, sociology, and economics. Seeks to unite and provide a common meeting ground for those engaged in the study and treatment of problems of human behavior. Fosters research and disseminates information concerning scientific work in the field of mental health. **Pub:** *American Journal of Orthopsychiatry*, quarterly. Journal. Covers therapeutic work with children and adults, community mental health, studies in interpersonal relations, and other related topics. *Price:* Included in membership dues; $60/year for nonmember individuals; $85/year for institutions. • *Readings: A Journal of Reviews and Commentary in Mental Health*, quarterly. Journal. *Price:* Included in membership dues; $25/year for nonmember individuals; $35/year for institutions. • Books. • Catalog. • Monographs.

★ 784 ★ American Orthoptic Council (AOC)
c/o Leslie France
3914 Nakoma Rd.
Madison, WI 53711
Phone: (608)233-5383 **Fax:** (608)263-4247
Email: lwfranceco@att.net
Website: http://www.orthoptics.org
Dr. George S. Ellis, Jr.,MD, Pres.

Fnded: 1935. **Mem:** 20. **Desc:** Ophthalmologists and orthoptists. Directs practice of orthoptists; determines qualifications of candidates; regulates training and certification of orthoptists; supervises the practice of orthoptists after certification. **Pub:** *A Career in Orthoptics*, annual. Pamphlet. Contains list of current programs and general description of profession. *Price:* Free. • *American Orthoptic Journal*, annual. Journal. Covers ocular motility and visual physiology. Contains abstracts of ophthalmic literature. *Price:* Included in membership dues; $20/year for nonmembers; $35/year for institutions. • *Orthoptic Training Centers*, annual. Pamphlet.

★ 785 ★ American Osler Society (AOS)
c/o Charles S. Bryan
University of South Carolina School of Medicine
2 Medical Park, Ste. 502
Columbia, SC 29203
Phone: (803)540-1000 **Fax:** (803)540-1075
Email: trout@abanet.org
Website: http://www.americanosler.org/
Charles S. Bryan, Sec. -Treas.

Fnded: 1970. **Mem:** 135. **Desc:** Physicians, librarians, and scientists united to further a humanistic approach to the study and practice of medicine as exemplified in the life work of Sir William Osler (1849-1919). **Pub:** *Osler Biographical Directory*, annual. Directory. • *The Persisting Osler*. Book. • *The Persisting Osler II*. Book. • Also publishes books on Sir William Osler, medical humanism, and the history of medicine.

★ 786 ★ American Osteopathic Academy of Addiction Medicine

142 E Ontario St.
Chicago, IL 60611
Phone: (312)202-8163 **Free:** 800-621-1773
Fax: (312)202-8224
Email: nvidmer@aoa-net.org
Nina Vidmer, Asst. Dir.

Fnded: 1986. **Mem:** 100. **Desc:** Physicians. Conducts research into the diagnosis, intervention, and treatment of substance abuse problems. Seeks to educate society, and to influence the passage of legislation regarding drug abuse. Provides seminars and lectures to students, physicians, medical and dental societies, civic groups, religious organizations, bar associations, and law enforcement bodies. **Pub:** *AOAAM News and Advocate*, quarterly. Newsletter. **Frmly:** (1996) American Osteopathic Academy Addictionology.

★ 787 ★ American Osteopathic Academy of Orthopedics (AOAO)

PO Box 291690
Davie, FL 33329-1690
Phone: (954)262-1700 **Free:** 800-741-2626
Fax: (954)262-1748
Email: mmorris@noa.edu
Website: http://www.aoao.org
Morton Morris, DOJD, Exec. Dir.

Fnded: 1941. **Mem:** 851. **Desc:** Professional society of osteopathic orthopedic surgeons. **Pub:** *American Osteopathic Academy of Orthopedics–Membership Roster*, annual. Membership Directory. Arranged alphabetically and geographically; also lists resident candidates and AOAO-approved residency programs. *Price:* Free. • *AOAO Newsletter*, 3/year. Newsletter. *Price:* included in membership dues. • *Orthopod*, semiannual. *Price:* Included in membership dues.

★ 788 ★ American Osteopathic Academy of Sports Medicine (AOASM)

7600 Terrace Ave., Ste. 203
Middleton, WI 53562-3174
Phone: (608)831-4400 **Fax:** (608)831-5485
Email: info@aoasm.org
Website: http://www.aoasm.org/
Susan M. Reese, Exec. Dir.

Fnded: 1975. **Mem:** 500. **Desc:** Members of the American Osteopathic Association and students enrolled in approved colleges of osteopathic medicine. Objectives are to promote education, development of high ethical standards, communication, and research in the field of sports medicine. Conducts study programs, lectures, forums, and seminars. Encourages publication of articles and dissertations in scientific and professional journals. Sponsors student academy organizations at osteopathic education institutions. Maintains speakers' bureau. **Pub:** *Sport Medicine Today*, quarterly. Newsletter. Reviews research and educational programs in sports medicine. Contains calendar of events. *Price:* Included in membership dues. • Membership Directory, annual.

★ 789 ★ American Osteopathic Association (AOA)

142 E Ontario St.
Chicago, IL 60611
Phone: (312)202-8000 **Free:** 800-621-1773
Fax: (312)202-8200
Email: info@aoa-net.org
Website: http://www.aoa-net.org
John B. Crosby, JD, Exec. Dir.

Fnded: 1897. **Mem:** 23,000. **State Groups:** 50. **Desc:** Osteopathic physicians, surgeons, and graduates of approved colleges of osteopathic medicine. Associate members include teaching, research, administrative, and executive employees of approved colleges, hospitals, divisional societies, and affiliated organizations. Forms (with its affiliates) an officially recognized structure of the osteopathic profession. Promotes the public health, to encourage scientific research, and to maintain and improve high standards of medical education in osteopathic colleges. Inspects and accredits colleges and hospitals; conducts a specialty certification program; sponsors a national examining board satisfactory to state licensing agencies; maintains mandatory program of continuing medical education for members. Compiles statistics on location and type of practice of osteopathic physicians. Sponsors research activities through Bureau of Research in osteopathic colleges and hospitals. Maintains Physician Placement Service. Produces public service radio and television programs; maintains 2000 item library and biographical archives on osteopathic medicine and history. Offers speakers' bureau. **Pub:** *American Osteopathic Association Yearbook and Directory*. Directory. • *The D.O.*, monthly. • *Journal of AOA*, monthly. Journal. • Brochures.

★ 790 ★ American Osteopathic Board of Emergency Medicine (AOBEM)

c/o Josette Fleming
142 E Ontario St.
Chicago, IL 60611
Phone: (312)335-1065 **Fax:** (312)335-5489
Email: jfleming@aobem.org
Website: http://www.aobem.org
Josette M. Fleming, Admin.

Fnded: 1980. **Mem:** 9. **Desc:** Seeks to improve the quality of emergency medical care, to establish and maintain high standards of excellence in the specialty of emergency medicine, to improve medical education and facilities for training emergency physicians, to evaluate specialists in emergency medicine applying for certification and recertification, and to serve the public, physicians, hospitality, and medical schools by furnishing lists of medical schools by furnishing lists of those diplomates certified by the board. **Pub:** *American Osteopathic Association Yearbook and Directory of Osteopathic Physicians*. Directory.

★ 791 ★ American Osteopathic Board of Family Physicians (AOBFP)

330 E Algonquin Rd., Ste. 6
Arlington Heights, IL 60005
Phone: (847)640-8477 **Free:** 800-390-5801
Website: http://www.aobfp.org
Carol A. Thoma, Exec. Dir.

Fnded: 1972. **Desc:** Certifying board for osteopathic physicians. Prepares and administers semiannual certification examination and annual recertification exam. **Frmly:** (1993) American Osteopathic Board of General Practice.

★ 792 ★ American Osteopathic Board of Pediatrics (AOBP)

142 E Ontario St., 6th Fl.
Chicago, IL 60645
Phone: (312)202-8267
Email: rmcclary@aoa-net.org
Website: http://www.aobp.org
Robbin McClary, Coord.

Desc: Certification board for osteopathic pediatricians. Standards are formulated by the American Osteopathic Association. Certification is conducted by annual examination.

★ 793 ★ American Osteopathic College of Anesthesiologists (AOCA)

6500 NW Tower Dr., Ste. 103
Kansas City, MO 64151-4414
Phone: (816)373-4700 **Free:** 800-842-2622
Fax: (816)373-1529
David Bitonte, Pres.

Fnded: 1952. **Mem:** 500. **Desc:** Members of American Osteopathic Association who are engaged in the practice of anesthesiology. **Pub:** Membership Directory, annual. • Newsletter, 3/year. **Frmly:** (1952) American Osteopathic Society of Anesthesiologists.

★ 794 ★ American Osteopathic College of Dermatology (AOCD)

PO Box 7525
1501 E Illinois St.
Kirksville, MO 63501-7525
Phone: (660)665-2184 **Free:** 800-449-2623
Fax: (660)627-2623
Email: execdirector@aocd.org
Website: http://www.aocd.org
Rebecca A. Mansfield, Exec. Dir.

Fnded: 1958. **Mem:** 300. **Desc:** Members of the osteopathic profession certified or involved in dermatology. Conducts specialized education programs. **Pub:** *American Osteopathic College of Dermatology Annual Membership Directory*, annual. Directory. *Price:* Free. • Newsletter, quarterly.

★ 795 ★ American Osteopathic College of Occupational and Preventive Medicine (AOCOPM)

PO Box 2606
Leesburg, VA 20177
Free: 800-558-8686 **Fax:** (703)443-0567
Email: aocopm@starpower.net
Website: http://www.aocopm.org/homepage.htm

Fnded: 1995. **Desc:** Designed to promote the public health and practice of preventive medicine in order to create a better understanding of the relationship of health and prevention in regard to the wellness of the population. Provides a three-part basic course in occupational/environmental medicine.

★ 796 ★ American Osteopathic College of Ophthalmology and the American Osteopathic College of Otolaryngology-Head and Neck Surgery (AOCOO-HNS)

405 W Grand Ave.
Dayton, OH 45405
Phone: (937)222-8820 **Free:** 800-455-9404
Fax: (937)222-8840
Email: info@aocoohns.org
Website: http://www.aocoohns.org
Debra L. Bailey, Admin. Dir.

Fnded: 1918. **Mem:** 670. **Desc:** Osteopathic ophthalmologists and osteopathic otolaryngologists/facial plastic surgeons. Created to improve quality of training, education and practice of osteopathic ophthalmologists and facial plastic surgeons. Provides "members only" access for a wealth of information.

★ 797 ★ American Osteopathic College of Pathologists (AOCP)

142 E Ontario St.
Chicago, IL 60611
Phone: (312)202-8197 **Fax:** (312)202-8224
Website: http://www.aocp-net.org
Kristen Smith, Exec. Dir.

Fnded: 1954. **Mem:** 180. **Desc:** Osteopathic physicians who have completed residency training programs in pathology and clinical pathology; candidate members are in residency training in pathology. Establishes guidelines for training programs in pathology and clinical pathology for osteopathic physicians; maintains standards in residency training programs. Offers placement service and mid-year tutorial program. Maintains collection of slide study sets. **Pub:** *American Osteopathic College of Pathologists Directory*, annual. Directory. • *Nova*, monthly. Newsletter. Includes reports on employment opportunities and topics of interest. *Price:* Included in membership dues.

★ 798 ★ American Osteopathic College of Physical Medicine and Rehabilitation (AOCPMR)

PO Box 732
Dover, NH 03821-0732
Phone: (603)343-1937 **Fax:** (603)343-1938
Email: executive.director@aocpmr.org
Website: http://www.aocpmr.org/
Peter G. Markos, DO, Exec. Dir.

Fnded: 1954. **Mem:** 225. **Desc:** Osteopathic physicians with a strong interest in physical and rehabilitation medicine as a specialty. Active members are those certified in the specialty by the American Osteopathic Board of Rehabilitation Medicine of Physical Medicine & Rehabilitation, an affiliate of the American Osteopathic Association. To stimulate study, extend knowledge, and improve practice in rehabilitation medicine. Cosponsors training programs; sponsors competitive writing for predoctoral osteopathic medical students, interns, and residents. **Pub:** Directory, annual. • Newsletter, periodic. **Frmly:** (1955) American Osteopathic Academy of Physical Medicine and Rehabilitation; (1970) American Osteopathic College of Physical Medicine and Rehabilitation; (2001) American Osteopathic College of Rehabilitation Medicine.

★ 799 ★ American Osteopathic College of Preventive Medicine (AOCPM)

PO Box 2606
Leesburg, VA 20177
Free: 800-558-8686 **Fax:** (703)443-0576
Email: aocpm@starpower.net
Website: http://www.aocpm.org/
James T. Alexander, Sec.

Fnded: 1982. **Mem:** 160. **Desc:** Osteopathic doctors. Prepares and educates doctors of osteopathy who wish to specialize in aerospace medicine, occupational/environmental medicine, or public health preventive medicine. Seeks to foster an understanding of these fields of study among osteopathic doctors and the public. Provides consultant services to other physicians. Maintains speakers' bureau. Conducts studies. **Pub:** Directory, annual. • Newsletter, quarterly.

★ 800 ★ American Osteopathic College of Proctology (AOCPr)

9948 State Rte. 682
Athens, OH 45701-5090
Fax: (740)594-5090
Dr. Zolton Brody, Exec. Officer

Mem: 155. **Desc:** Osteopathic physicians and surgeons specializing in treatment of diseases of the anus, rectum, and colon.

★ 801 ★ American Osteopathic College of Radiology (AOCR)

119 E 2nd St.
Milan, MO 63556
Phone: (660)265-4011 **Fax:** (660)265-3494
Email: aocr@nemr.net
Website: http://www.aocr.org/
Pamela A. Smith, Exec. Dir.

Fnded: 1941. **Mem:** 730. **Desc:** Certified radiologists, residents-in-training, and others active in the field of radiology. **Pub:** *Viewbox*, quarterly. Newsletter. • Membership Directory, annual.

★ 802 ★ American Osteopathic Colleges of Ophthalmology and Otolaryngology-Head and Neck Surgery (AOCOO-HNS)

320 W Grand Ave.
Dayton, OH 45405
Phone: (937)222-8820 **Free:** 800-455-9404
Fax: (937)222-8840
Email: info@aocoohns.org
Website: http://www.aocoohns.org
Dr. Alvin Dubin, Exec. VP

Fnded: 1916. **Mem:** 670. **Desc:** Osteopathic physicians who have completed formal specialty training or are acquiring such training in ophthalmology, otorhinolaryngology, and facial plastic surgery, and those who are certified specialists in one or more of the above named areas. Develops application of osteopathic concepts in this specialty; determines minimum standards of education at undergraduate and postgraduate levels. Sponsors research programs. **Pub:** *American Osteopathic Colleges of Ophthalmology and Otolaryngology Head & Neck Surgery–News Letter*, quarterly. Newsletter. *Price:* Included in membership dues. • *AOCOO-HNS*, annual. Journal. • Directory, periodic. • Also publishes collected papers. **Frmly:** Osteopathic College of Ophthalmology and Otorhinolaryngology.

★ 803 ★ American Osteopathic Foundation (AOF)

c/o Leda Hanin
142 East Ontario
Chicago, IL 60611
Phone: (312)202-8230 **Free:** 800-621-1773
Fax: (312)202-8216
Email: Sdowney@aoa-net.org
Website: http://www.osteopathic.org
Steve Downey, Deputy Dir.

Fnded: 1949. **Mem:** 9,300. **Desc:** Osteopathic physicians and laypersons interested in raising and administering funds for osteopathic medical education, research, colleges, and hospitals. Functions as philanthropic affiliate of the American Osteopathic Association; seeks to foster understanding of osteopathic principles and practice. **Pub:** *AOF In Touch*, triennial. Newsletter. *Price:* Free. For members only. **Frmly:** (1960) Osteopathic Foundation; (1998) National Osteopathic Foundation.

★ 804 ★ American Osteopathic Healthcare Association (AOHA)

5550 Friendship Blvd., Ste., 300
Chevy Chase, MD 20815
Phone: (301)968-2642 **Fax:** (301)968-4195
Email: aoha@osteohdq.org
David Kushner, Pres. & CEO

Fnded: 1934. **Mem:** 160. **Reg. Groups:** 6. **Desc:** AOHA's mission is to serve its members by promoting the health and welfare of the American public through effective leadership; serving as the unified voice in areas of common interest for the advancement of osteopathic health care; and providing advocacy and eduation to ensure members' success. **Pub:** *Osteopathic Membership Directory*, annual. Membership Directory. Lists osteopathic hospitals; contains statistical data. *Price:* Included in membership dues; $125 for non-members. • *Osteopathic Progress*, monthly. Newsletter. *Price:* Included in membership dues. **Frmly:** (1993) American Osteopathic Hospital Association.

★ 805 ★ American Otological Society (AOS)

2720 Tartan Way
Springfield, IL 62707
Phone: (217)483-6966 **Fax:** (217)483-6966
Email: segossard@aol.com
Website: http://www.americanotologicalsociety.org
Dr. Clough Shelton, Sec. -Treas.

Fnded: 1868. **Mem:** 294. **Desc:** Otologists and contributors to the advancement of otology. Encourages study and research in otology (the science of the ear and its diseases). Objectives are to advance and promote medical and surgical otology, including the rehabilitation of the hearing impaired, and to encourage and promote research in otology and related disciplines. Maintains research fund for advanced studies of otosclerosis. **Pub:** *Otology & Neurotology*. Journal.

★ 806 ★ American Outreach Association (AOA)

PO Box 25042
Colorado Springs, CO 80936
Phone: (719)592-1134
Email: info@americanoutreach-org
Website: http://www.americanoutreach.org
Charles Prusch, Dir.

Fnded: 1989. **Reg. Groups:** 5. **Desc:** Collects and disseminates information on subjects such as alcoholism, drug abuse, inhalants, and smoking to the public. Organizes community awareness activities and presentations. Reviews drug policies, programs, and educational material. Assists business and industry in establishing drug-free work environments. Sponsors Project HOLD, a program that fosters a change of attitudes, values, and behaviors in the home away from drug abuse. Operates placement service; maintains speakers' bureau. **Pub:** *Health Watch*, quarterly. Newsletter. • *Mommy, What are Drugs?.* • *Mommy What are Inhalants?.* • *Mommy, What is Alcohol?.* • *Mommy, What is Smoking?.* • *Mother Earth, What is Cultural Diversity?.*

★ 807 ★ American Pain Society (APS)

4700 W Lake Ave.
Glenview, IL 60025
Phone: (847)375-4715 **Fax:** 877-734-8758
Email: info@ampainsoc.org
Website: http://www.ampainsoc.org
Richard Payne, MD, Pres.

Fnded: 1977. **Mem:** 3,500. **Reg. Groups:** 6. **Desc:** Physicians, dentists, psychologists, nurses, and other health professionals interested in the study and treatment of pain. Purposes are to: promote control, management, and understanding of pain through scientific meetings and research activities; develop standards for training and ethical management of pain patients. Conducts scientific conferences. **Pub:** *APS Bulletin*, bimonthly. Newsletter. • *Guideline for the Management of Acute & Chronic Pain in Sickle Cell Disease.* • *Guideline for the Management of Cancer Pain in Adults and Children (2003).* • *Guideline for the Management of Pain in Osteoarthritis, Rheumatoid Arthritis, and Juvenile Chronic Arthritis (2nd Ed.).* • *Pain Facilities Directory.* Directory. • *The Pain Journal*, quarterly. Journal. • *Principles of Analgesic Use in the Treatment of Acute Pain and Cancer Pain (4th edition)*, periodic.

★ 808 ★ American Paraplegia Society (APS)

75-20 Astoria Blvd.
Jackson Heights, NY 11372
Phone: (718)803-3782 **Fax:** (718)803-0414
Email: aps@epva.org
Website: http://www.apssci.org
DrPH Vivian Beyda, Assoc. Exec. Dir.

Fnded: 1954. **Mem:** 550. **Desc:** Physicians and researchers in the spinal cord injury field. Purpose is to advance and foster improved health care of spinal cord injury patients, and develop and promote education and research in the neuroscience fields. Sponsors seminars; maintains library. Conducts annual educational program. **Pub:** *Journal of Spinal Cord Medicine*, quarterly. Journal.

★ 809 ★ American Parkinson's Disease Association (APDA)

1250 Hylan Blvd., Ste. 4B
Staten Island, NY 10305-1946
Phone: (718)981-8001 **Free:** 800-223-2732
Fax: (718)981-4399
Email: apda@apdaparkinson.org
Website: http://www.apdaparkinson.com
Joel Gerstel, Exec. Dir.

Fnded: 1961. **Mem:** 2,000. **Reg. Groups:** 90. **Local Groups:** 400. **Desc:** Works to find the cure for Parkinson's disease and to alleviate the suffering of its victims by subsidizing information and referral centers and providing funds for research. Offers counseling services to patients and their families. Maintains 51 information and referral centers and more than 800 support groups. Conducts symposia. **Pub:** *American Parkinson Disease Association–Newsletter*, quarterly. Newsletter. Includes association and research news, and calendar of events. *Price:* Free. • *Be Active! A Suggested Exercise Program for People with Parkinson's Disease.* Booklet. • *Be Independent! To Help the Patient with Parkinson's Disease in the Activities of Daily Living.* Booklet. • *Coping With Parkinson's Disease.* Booklet. • *Let's Communicate: Speech Problems and Swallowing Problems in Parkinson's Disease.* Booklet. • *Parkinson's Disease Handbook.* Booklet. • Annual Report. • Also publishes educational supplements.

★ 810 ★ American Pathology Foundation (APF)

1202 Allanson Rd.
Mundelein, IL 60060
Phone: (847)949-6055 **Free:** 877-993-9935
Fax: (847)566-4580
Email: mbuckley2@covad.net
Website: http://americanpathologyfoundation.org
Edward J. Stygar, Jr., Exec. Dir.

Fnded: 1959. **Mem:** 750. **Desc:** Board-certified pathologists. Objectives are: to promote the practice of pathology in private laboratories; to provide for exchange of information that will improve anatomic and clinical pathology; to cooperate in the development of the art and sciences of medicine and pathology. Compiles statistics. **Pub:** Directory, annual. • Newsletter, quarterly. **Frmly:** Private Practitioners of Pathology Foundation.

★ 811 ★ American Pediatric Society (APS)

3400 Research Forest Dr., Ste. B7
The Woodlands, TX 77381-4259
Phone: (281)419-0052 **Fax:** (281)419-0082
Email: info@aps-spr.org
Website: http://www.aps-spr.org
Kathy A. Cannon, Assoc. Exec. Dir.

Fnded: 1888. **Mem:** 1,500. **Desc:** Professional academic society of M.D. educators and researchers interested in the study of children and their diseases, prevention of illness, and promotion of health in childhood. Maintains archives. **Pub:** *Pediatric Research*, monthly. Journal. • *Program and Abstracts of Annual Meeting.*

★ 812 ★ American Pediatric Surgical Association (APSA)

60 Revere Dr., Ste. 500
Northbrook, IL 60062
Phone: (847)480-9576 **Fax:** (847)480-9282
Email: eapsa@eapsa.org
Website: http://www.eapsa.org
Melanie Stanton, Exec. Dir.

Fnded: 1970. **Mem:** 488. **Desc:** Pediatric surgeons who are certified by the American Board of Surgery for competence in dealing with surgical problems of infancy and childhood. Seeks to provide competent medical care for children. Serves as a forum for discussion of ethics involving child care. Presents new concepts and advances in surgical care of infants and children. **Pub:** *Annual Program Booklet*, annual. Booklet. • *APSA Membership Directory*, annual. Membership Directory. • *Business Meeting Minutes*, annual. • *Cancer Newsletter*, annual. Newsletter. • *Journal of Pediatric Surgery*, monthly. Journal. • Newsletter, semiannual.

★ 813 ★ American Pediatric Surgical Nurses Association (APSNA)

PO Box 200585
Boston, MA 02120
Phone: (203)457-1275
Email: info@apsna.com
Website: http://www.apsna.com/
Laura Flanigan, RN, Pres.

Fnded: 1992. **Mem:** 200. **Desc:** Supports the practice of pediatric surgical nurses through continuing education, networking and mentoring.

★ 814 ★ American Pharmaceutical Association - Academy of Pharmacy Practice and Management (APHA-APPM)

c/o Anne Burns
2215 Constitution Ave. NW
Washington, DC 20037-2985
Phone: (202)628-4410 **Free:** 800-237-APHA
Fax: (202)783-2351
Email: apha-appm@aphanet.org
Website: http://www.aphanet.org
Anne Burns, Dir., Practice Development and Research

Fnded: 1965. **Mem:** 26,000. **Desc:** Pharmacists concerned with rendering professional services directly to the public, without regard for status of employment or environment of practice. Purposes are to provide a forum and mechanism whereby pharmacists may meet to discuss and implement programs and activities relevant and helpful to the practitioner of pharmacy; to recommend programs and courses of action which should be undertaken or implemented by the profession; to coordinate academy efforts so as to be an asset to the progress of the profession. Provides and cosponsors continuing education meetings, seminars, and workshops; produces audiovisual materials. **Frmly:** (1966) General Practice Section of APhA; (1975) Academy of General Practice of Pharmacy; (1987) Academy of Pharmacy Practice; (1995) Academy of Pharmacy Practice and Management.

★ 815 ★ American Pharmaceutical Association Academy of Students of Pharmacy (APhA-ASP)

2215 Constitution Ave., NW
Washington, DC 20037
Phone: (202)429-7559 **Free:** 800-237-APHA
Fax: (202)628-0443
Email: APhA-ASP@APhAnet.org
Website: http://www.aphanet.org/students/students-new.htm
Val Peteet, Contact

Fnded: 1954. **Mem:** 18,000. **Reg. Groups:** 8. **Local Groups:** 79. **Desc:** A division of the American Pharmaceutical Association, the national professional society of pharmacy students. Keeps members informed of the affairs of the APhA and the profession. Provides a forum for the expression of student opinion on activities and policies. Seeks to strengthen the program whereby student members, upon graduation, become active members of the APhA. Encourages participation by pharmacy students in interdisciplinary projects that attempt to find solutions to social problems; works in community-oriented drug education programs; supports interdisciplinary clinical training for pharmacists. **Pub:** *Academy of Students of Pharmacy–Chapter Management*, monthly. Newsletter. For chapter presidents only. • *The Pharmacy Student*, bimonthly. Magazine. *Price:* Included in membership dues; $25/year for nonmembers. **Frmly:** (1969) American Pharmaceutical Association Student Section; (1988) Student American Pharmaceutical Association; (2003) Academy of Students of Pharmacy.

★ 816 ★ American Physical Therapy Association (APTA)

1111 N Fairfax St.
Alexandria, VA 22314-1488
Phone: (703)684-2782 **Free:** 800-999-2782
Fax: (703)684-7343
Email: giniblodgett@apta.org
Website: http://www.apta.org
Ben F. Massey, Jr., Pres.

Fnded: 1921. **Mem:** 68,000. **Nat'l Groups:** 18. **Reg. Groups:** 52. **State Groups:** 52. **Desc:** Professional organization of physical therapists and physical therapist assistants and students. Fosters the development and improvement of physical therapy service, education, and research; evaluates the organization and administration of curricula; directs the maintenance of standards and promotes scientific research. Acts as an accrediting body for educational programs in physical therapy and is responsible for establishing standards. Offers advisory and consultation services to schools of physical therapy and facilities offering physical therapy services; provides placement services at conference. **Pub:** *Physical Therapy*, monthly. Journal. Features peer-reviewed scientific and professional articles, continuing education course listings, abstracts of current literature, and book reviews. *Price:* Included in membership dues; $80/year for nonmembers; $10/single issue. • *PT Bulletin Online*, weekly. Newsletter. Includes public affairs and member news, plus information on upcoming seminars. *Price:* Included in membership dues. • *PT Magazine*, monthly. Journal. Features columns on risk management and reimbursement strategies. Contains advertisers' index and information on new products and literature. *Price:* Included in membership dues; $70/year for nonmembers; $10/copy. • Brochures. • Monographs. • Also issues bulletins to chapters and publishes anthologies, handbooks, and educational resource guides. **Frmly:** (1921) American Women's Physical Therapeutic Association; (1947) American Physiotherapy Association.

★ 817 ★ American Physicians Association of Computer Medicine (APACM)

4579 Corrientes Cir. S
Jacksonville, FL 32217-4330
Phone: (904)730-7306
Lawrence B. Tilis, MD, Pres.

Fnded: 1984. **Mem:** 350. **Desc:** Physicians, interns, and medical students. Encourages the use of computers in medicine. Seeks to inform physicians about the computer and its applications in patient care, education, and research. Conducts lectures.

★ 818 ★ American Podiatric Circulatory Society (APCS)

c/o Dr. Stanley Goldstein
5704 18th Ave.
Brooklyn, NY 11204
Phone: (718)236-7952 **Fax:** (718)236-7953
Email: 72167.345@compuserve.com
Dr. Stanley Goldstein, Pres.

Fnded: 1979. **Mem:** 900. **Desc:** Podiatrists. Disseminates information on the Suffuse Osmotic Chemisorb Asphyxiation (SOCA) therapy, now known as the Tereno Method, devised by Dr. Isaac Tereno for treatment of geriatric patients suffering from arterial blockage in their limbs. (The Tereno Method uses vitamins to enrich the blood and enlarge subcutaneous capillaries and lymph vessels, thus creating an alternate circulatory network which bypasses blocked arteries. It is an alternative to major surgery and/or amputation in geriatric patients with poor circulation in their limbs.) Conducts research; maintains speakers' bureau. **Pub:** *American Podiatric Circulatory Society Bulletin*, quarterly. Bulletin. Contains case studies of patients treated using the Tereno Method.

★ 819 ★ American Podiatric Medical Association (APMA)

9312 Old Georgetown Rd.
Bethesda, MD 20814-1621
Phone: (301)581-9200 **Free:** 800-ASK-APMA
Fax: (301)530-2752
Email: askapma@apma.org
Website: http://www.apma.org
Glenn B. Gastwirth, DPM

Fnded: 1912. **Mem:** 10,500. **State Groups:** 53. **Desc:** Professional society of doctors of podiatric medicine. **Pub:** *APMA News*, monthly. Magazine. Includes calendar of events, research updates, and statistics. *Price:* Included in membership dues; $50/year for nonmembers. • *Desk Reference of the APMA*, annual. • *Journal of the American Podiatric Medical Association*, monthly. Journal. *Price:* Included in membership dues; $90 for non-members. • Also publishes foot health literature. **Frmly:** (1958) National Association of Chiropodists; (1984) American Podiatry Association.

★ 820 ★ American Podiatric Medical Students Association (APMSA)

9312 Old Georgetown Rd.
Bethesda, MD 20814
Phone: (301)493-9667
Website: http://www.apmsa.org/
Jennifer Wiggins, Exec. Dir.

Fnded: 1954. **Mem:** 2,000. **Desc:** Podiatric medical students enrolled at seven podiatric schools in the U.S. Purpose is to represent the interests of podiatric medical students in legislative, professional, and educational programs. Cosponsors seminars and writing contests. Compiles statistics. **Pub:** *First Step*, quarterly. Newsletter. • *Graduation Handbook*, annual. Reference guide. **Frmly:** American Podiatric Students Association.

★ 821 ★ American Podiatric Medical Writers Association (APMWA)

PO Box 750129
Forest Hills, NY 11375
Phone: (718)897-9700 **Fax:** (718)896-5747
Email: bblock@prodigy.net
Dr. Barry H. Block, Exec. Dir.

Fnded: 1985. **Mem:** 100. **Desc:** Podiatric medical writers. Promotes the improvement of writing on podiatric topics. **Pub:** *American Podiatric Medical Writers Association–Membership Directory*, annual. Membership Directory. *Price:* Free. • *American Podiatric Medical Writers Association–Newsletter*, quarterly. Newsletter. Lists new members. *Price:* Free with self-addressed stamped envelope.

★ 822 ★ American Polarity Therapy Association (APTA)

PO Box 19858
Boulder, CO 80308
Phone: (303)545-2080 **Fax:** (303)545-2161
Email: hq@polaritytherapy.org
Website: http://www.polaritytherapy.org
Ellie Simmons, RPP, Exec. Dir.

Fnded: 1984. **Mem:** 1,200. **State Groups:** 6. **Desc:** Dedicated to the advancement of polarity therapy. (Polarity therapy is a non-diagnostic holistic health system supplementing and supporting medical treatment. Polarity techniques include bodywork, diet, exercise and self awareness for health maintenance.) Develops and disseminates educational and support materials; registers practitioners; holds competitions. **Pub:** *Energy*, quarterly. Newsletter. *Price:* included in membership dues. • Books.

★ 823 ★ American Polocrosse Association (APA)

PO Box 915
New Hampton, NY 10958
Phone: (914)856-4265
Email: bhu@cbsnews.com
Website: http://www.americanpolocrosse.org/sport.php3

Fnded: 1984. **Desc:** Promotes the sport of polocrosse. Provides club insurance, umpire training and certification, instructional clinics, sanctions tournaments, selection of teams. **Pub:** Newsletter.

★ 824 ★ American Porphyria Foundation (APF)

PO Box 22712
Houston, TX 77227
Phone: (713)266-9617 **Fax:** (713)871-1788
Email: porphyrus@aol.com
Website: http://www.porphyriafoundation.com/
Yvette Strange, Office Admin.

Fnded: 1981. **Mem:** 1,900. **Desc:** Persons interested in advancing awareness and treatment of the porphyrias; affected patients. Porphyria is a class of seven rare (and usually inherited) metabolic disorders of varying severity affecting the nervous system or the skin. It is characterized by a deficiency of an enzyme used in making heme (a ring-shaped molecule called a porphyrin), which in turn is used in making hemoglobin. One of porphyria's recurrent though not requisite symptoms is purple-red urine. The foundation's purposes are to: provide financial support for researchers in porphyria; improve the diagnosis and treatment of porphyria through educational programs; locate porphyria patients. Maintains a lending library of videotapes, papers, and pamphlets. **Pub:** *American Porphyria Foundation–Newsletter*, quarterly. Newsletter. Contains educational information. *Price:* Included in membership dues. • Pamphlets. • Also compiles list of physicians with experience in treating porphyria.

★ 825 ★ American Printing House for the Blind (APH)

PO Box 6085
1839 Frankfort Ave.
Louisville, KY 40206-0085
Phone: (502)895-2405 **Free:** 800-223-1839
Fax: (502)899-2274
Email: info@aph.org
Website: http://www.aph.org
Dr. Tuck Tinsley, III, Pres.

Fnded: 1858. **Desc:** Produces literature in all media (braille, large type, recorded, computer disc) for the blind. Manufactures special products for use by visually impaired students and adults, such as preschool and vocational materials and talking software. Conducts ongoing educational research program. Conducts art contest, tours of the plant and of the APH Museum of artifacts from the education of the blind field. **Pub:** *APH Slate*, quarterly. Newsletter. Provides information on new products for the visually impaired; also includes organization news and activities. *Price:* Free. • *APH Technology Update: Technology for People Who Are Visually Impaired*, annual. Newsletter. Covers computer and other high-tech products designed for blind persons. *Price:* Free. • Makes available Newsweek, Readers Digest, and Weekly Reader in braille, tape, or large type.

★ 826 ★ American Professional Practice Association (APPA)

Hillsboro Executive Center N
350 Fairway Dr., Ste. 200
Deerfield Beach, FL 33441-1834
Phone: (954)571-1877 **Free:** 800-221-2168
Fax: (954)571-8582
Email: membership@assnservices.com
Website: http://www.appa-assn.com
Joseph P. Santol, Jr., Mgr., Membership Services

Fnded: 1963. **Mem:** 70,000. **Desc:** Provides physicians with economic benefits and financial services including the following: unsecured loan plans; group insurance discounts; accounts receivable collections; electronic credit services; continuing medical education. **Pub:** *Association's Digest*, semiannual. Newsletter. Provides business advice on private practice; also covers APPA activities. *Price:* Included in membership dues.

★ 827 ★ American Prostate Society

PO Box 870
Hanover, MD 21076
Phone: (410)859-3735 **Free:** 800-308-1106
Fax: (410)850-0818
Email: ameripros@mindspring.org
Website: http://www.ameripros.org
Claude Gerard, Chm.

Fnded: 1991. **Mem:** 51,000. **Nat'l Groups:** 1. **Local Groups:** 1. **Desc:** Works to increase the public's awareness of prostate disease. Encourages men to get annual exams. Aids hospitals and other health care facilities that are dedicated exclusively to detection and treatment of prostate disease. Sponsors Prostate Awareness Week. Conducts speakers' bureau. Sponsors educational programs. **Pub:** *Update*, quarterly. Newsletter. Review and special reports on developments in prostate disease. *Price:* Free. • Brochures, annual.

★ 828 ★ American Prosthodontic Society (APS)

426 Hudson St.
Hackensack, NJ 07601
Phone: (201)440-8144 **Free:** 877-499-3500
Fax: (201)440-7963
Email: aps@prostho.com
Website: http://www.prostho.com
Dr. Alan C. Keyes, DDS, Exec. Dir.

Fnded: 1928. **Mem:** 800. **Nat'l Groups:** 1. **Desc:** Dentists interested in the discipline of prosthodontics (the art and science of replacing missing teeth and supporting structures). **Pub:** *Journal of Prosthetic Dentistry*, monthly. Journal. Published in conjunction with 21 other prosthodonic organizations. *Price:* Included in membership dues.

★ 829 ★ American Psychiatric Association (APA)

1000 Wilson Blvd., Ste. 1825
Arlington, VA 22209-3901
Phone: (703)907-7300 **Free:** 888-357-7924
Fax: (703)907-7322
Email: apa@psych.org
Website: http://www.psych.org
Richard K. Harding, Pres.

Fnded: 1844. **Mem:** 40,000. **Reg. Groups:** 77. **Desc:** Psychiatrists. Seeks to further the study of the nature, treatment, and prevention of mental disorders. Assists in formulating programs to meet mental health needs; compiles and disseminates facts and figures about psychiatry; furthers psychiatric education and research. **Pub:** *American Journal of Psychiatry*, monthly. Journal. Includes book reviews. *Price:* Included in membership dues; $60/year for nonmembers; $30/year for students; $90/year for institutions. • *Psychiatric News*, semimonthly. • *Psychiatric Services*, monthly. Journal. Covers the delivery of mental health services in organized setings. Includes book reviews and research reports. *Price:* $40/year for members; $20/year for students; $60/year for institutions. • Books. • Membership Directory, biennial. • Pamphlets. **Frmly:** (1892) Association of Medical Superintendents of American Institutions for Insane; (1921) American Medico Psychological Association.

★ 830 ★ American Psychoanalytic Association (APsaA)

309 E 49th St.
New York, NY 10017
Phone: (212)752-0450 **Fax:** (212)593-0571
Email: central.office@apsa.org
Website: http://www.apsa.org/
Ellen B. Fertig, Admin. Dir.

Fnded: 1911. **Mem:** 3,500. **Local Groups:** 43. **Desc:** Psychoanalysts who have graduated from or are currently attending an accredited institute. Seeks to establish and maintain standards for the training of psychoanalysts and for the practice of psychoanalysis; fosters the integration of psychoanalysis with other branches of medicine; encourages research. Conducts educational programs. **Pub:** *The American Psychoanalyst*, quarterly. Newsletter. • *Journal of the American Psychoanalytic Association*, quarterly. Journal. • *Roster*, biennial. • *Title Key Word and Author Index to Psychoanalytic Journals.* • Also publishes material on psychoanalytic education and research.

★ 831 ★ American Psychoanalytic Foundation (APF)

1636 Connecticut Ave. NW, 2nd Fl.
Washington, DC 20009
Phone: (202)667-6363 **Fax:** (202)667-4477
Email: apf@cyberpsych.org
Website: http://www.cyberpsych.org/apf/contactus.htm

Desc: Dedicated to the advancement of psychoanalysis through community outreach, education, research, clinical programs.

★ 832 ★ American Psychological Association (APA)

750 First St. NE
Washington, DC 20002-4242
Phone: (202)336-5500 **Free:** 800-374-2721
Fax: (202)336-6069
Email: mhonaker@apa.org
Website: http://www.apa.org/
L. Michael Honaker, PhD, CEO

Fnded: 1892. **Mem:** 154,000. **Reg. Groups:** 7. **State Groups:** 58. **Desc:** Scientific and professional society of psychologists. Students participate as affiliates. Works to advance psychology as a science, a profession, and as a means of promoting human welfare. **Pub:** *American Psychologist*, monthly. Journal. Publishes articles on current issues in psychology as well as empirical, theoretical, and practical articles on broad aspects of psychology. *Price:* Included in membership dues; $180/year for nonmembers in the U.S.; $220/year for nonmembers outside the U.S.; $332/year for institutions in the U.S. • *APA Monitor*, monthly. Newspaper. Reports on the science, profession, and social responsibility of psychology, plus legislative developments affecting mental health and education. *Price:* Included in membership dues; $30/year for nonmembers in the U.S.; $48/year for institutions in the U.S.; $35/year for nonmembers outside the U.S. • *Behavioral Neuroscience*, bimonthly. Journal. Publishes original research papers in the broad field of the biological bases of behavior. Includes reviews and theoretical articles. *Price:* $83/year for members; $166/year for nonmembers in the U.S.; $186/year for nonmembers outside the U.S.; $332/year for institutions in the U.S. • *Clinician's Research Digest*, monthly. Newsletter. Contains selections and summaries of articles from clinical research journals. *Price:* $46/year for U.S. members; $83/year for U.S. nonmembers; $123/year for nonmembers outside of the U.S.; $110/year for U.S. institutions. • *Contemporary Psychology*, monthly. Journal. Contains critical reviews of books, films, tapes, and other media relevant to psychology. *Price:* $73/year for members; $145/year for nonmembers in the U.S.; $185/year for nonmembers outside the U.S.; $291/year for institutions in the U.S. • *Developmental Psychology*, bimonthly. Journal. Publishes articles that advance knowledge and theory about human development across the life span. *Price:* $72/year for members; $144/year for nonmembers in the U.S.; $164/year for nonmembers outside the U.S.; $284/year for institutions in the U.S. • *Directory of the American Psychological Association*, quinquennial. Me.

★ 833 ★ American Psychological Association Division of Independent Practice (APADIP)

750 First St., NE
Washington, DC 20002-4242
Phone: (202)336-5500 **Free:** 800-374-2721
Fax: (202)336-5997
Email: div42apa@mindspring.com
Website: http://www.apa.org/about/division/div42.html
Jean A. Carter, Pres.

Fnded: 1982. **Mem:** 8,600. **Desc:** Members of the American Psychological Association (APA) engaged in independent practice. Works to insure that the needs and concerns of independent psychology practitioners are considered by the APA. Gathers and disseminates information on legislation affecting the practice of psychology, managed care and other developments in the health care industries, office management, malpractice risk and insurance, hospital management. Offers continuing professional education programs. **Pub:** *Independent Practitioner*, quarterly. Bulletin.

★ 834 ★ American Psychological Association - Division of Psychotherapy

Division 29 Central Office
Tracey Martin
6557 E Riverdale St.
Mesa, AZ 85215
Phone: (602)363-9211 **Fax:** (480)854-8966
Email: assnmgmt@aol.com
Website: http://www.apa.org/about/division/div29.html
Patricia M. Bricklin, PhD, Pres.

Fnded: 1964. **Mem:** 6,500. **Desc:** A division of the American Psychological Association. Psychologists and psychotherapists interested in exchanging scientific and technical information about psychotherapy. Conducts continuing education workshops. **Pub:** *Psychotherapy Bulletin*, quarterly. Bulletin. • *Psychotherapy Journal*, quarterly. Journal.

★ 835 ★ American Psychological Society (APS)

1010 Vermont Ave. NW, Ste. 1100
Washington, DC 20005-4907
Phone: (202)783-2077 **Fax:** (202)783-2083
Email: akraut@aps.washington.dc.us
Website: http://www.psychologicalscience.org
Alan G. Kraut, Exec. Dir.

Fnded: 1988. **Mem:** 15,000. **Desc:** Scientists and academics. Works for the advancement of the discipline of psychology and the promotion of human welfare through research and application. Conducts research programs; educates policy makers on the role human behavior plays in societal problems; offers liability insurance plans. **Pub:** *APS Observer*, monthly. Newsletter. Features current society activities and world events affecting noteworthy research. • *Current Directions in Psychological Science*, bimonthly. Journal. Provides informative reviews on important trends and controversies in psychological research. • *Psychological Science*, bimonthly. Journal. • *Psychological Science in the Public Interest.* Monographs.

★ 836 ★ American Psychopathological Association (APPA)

Department of Psychiatry
Washington University School of Medicine
4940 Children's Pl.
Saint Louis, MO 63110
Email: zorumskc@psychiatry.wustl.edu
Website: http://www.appassn.org
Chuck Zorumski, MD, Pres.

Fnded: 1912. **Mem:** 500. **Desc:** Physicians and scientists interested in the field of psychopathology. To investigate scientific problems of abnormal psychology including: study of phenomena arising from abnormal mental processes; study of organic pathological conditions directly connected with abnormal mental processes; study of means which may remove or modify social or individual factors operating in the production of mental disease; study of relationship between psychopathological and social or cultural problems. **Pub:** *Comprehensive Psychiatry*, quarterly. Journal. General psychiatry journal. • *Proceedings of Annual Meeting.*

★ 837 ★ American Psychosomatic Society (APS)

6728 Old McLean Village Dr.
Mc Lean, VA 22101
Phone: (703)556-9222 **Fax:** (703)556-8729
Email: info@psychosomatic.org
Website: http://www.psychosomatic.org
Laura Degnon, Assoc. Exec. Dir.

Fnded: 1943. **Mem:** 900. **Desc:** Promotes scientific understanding of interrelationships among biological, psychological, social and behavioral factors in human health and disease, and the integration of the fields of science that separately examine them, fosters this understanding in education and improved health care. **Pub:** *APS Newsletter*, semiannual. Newsletter. • *Psychosomatic Medicine*, 6/year. Journal. **Frmly:** (1948) American Society for Research in Psychosomatic Problems.

★ 838 ★ American Psychotherapy Association (APA)

2750 E Sunshine
Springfield, MO 65804
Phone: (417)823-0173 **Free:** 800-205-9165
Fax: (417)823-9959
Email: member@americanpsychotherapy.com
Website: http://www.americanpsychotherapy.com
Brent McCoy, Ch. Assoc. Off.

Fnded: 1997. **Mem:** 5,000. **Desc:** Counselors, social workers, marriage and family therapists, psychologists, psychiatrists, psychoanalysts, pastoral counselors and nurse psychotherapists. Seeks to enhance public perception of psychotherapy. Serves as a forum for the discussion, development, and dissemination of ethical and professional standards for psychotherapists. Works to establish guidelines, promotes education and training confirm the professional identity of members, educate the public about benefits of psychotherapy; provides networking and resource development. Operates library and biographical archives. Compiles statistics; sponsors competitions. Maintains Board of Examiners in Psychotherapy to evaluate training, experience, and professional excellence of individuals. **Pub:** Journal.Peer-reviewed journal.

★ 839 ★ American Public Health Association (APHA)

800 I St., NW
Washington, DC 20001-3710
Phone: (202)777-2742 **Fax:** (202)777-2534
Email: comments@apha.org
Website: http://www.apha.org
Mohammad Akhter, MD, Exec. Dir.

Fnded: 1872. **Mem:** 32,000. **Desc:** Professional organization of physicians, nurses, educators, academicians, environmentalists, epidemiologists, new professionals, social workers, health administrators, optometrists, podiatrists, pharmacists, dentists, nutritionists, health planners, other community and mental health specialists, and interested consumers. Seeks to protect and promote personal, mental, and environmental health. Services include: promulgation of standards; establishment of uniform practices and procedures; development of the etiology of communicable diseases; research in public health; exploration of medical care programs and their relationships to public health. Sponsors job placement service. **Pub:** *American Journal of Public Health*, monthly. Journal. Includes news briefs and annual leadership directory. *Price:* Included in membership dues; $125/year for nonmembers. • *The Nation's Health*, 11/year. Reports on current and proposed legislation, regulations, and policy issues affecting public health; includes reports on current health issues. *Price:* Included in membership dues; $25/year for nonmembers. • Also publishes books, manuals, and pamphlets; maintains publications service.

★ 840 ★ American Radiological Nurses Association (ARNA)

7794 Grow Dr.
Pensacola, FL 32514
Phone: (850)474-7292 **Free:** (866)486-2762
Fax: (850)484-8762
Email: arna@puetzamc.com
Website: http://www.arna.net
Belinda Puetz, Exec. Dir.

Fnded: 1981. **Mem:** 1,426. **Nat'l Groups:** 24. **Desc:** Radiological nurses. Seeks to provide, promote, and maintain continuity of quality patient care through education, standards of care, professional growth, and collaboration with other health care providers. **Pub:** *Images*, quarterly. Journal. Conveys news related to developments in practice, technology, and research. Prints timely papers. *Price:* Free to members; $15/copy; $50/year. • *RN News*, quarterly. Newsletter. Conveys news of the association. *Price:* Free to members.

★ 841 ★ American Radium Society (ARS)

15048 S Cicero Ave.
Oak Forest, IL 60452
Phone: (708)687-1034 **Fax:** (708)687-1072
Email: info@americanradiumsociety.org
Website: http://www.americanradiumsociety.org
Catherine Carey, Exec. Dir.

Fnded: 1916. **Mem:** 800. **Desc:** Professional, multidisciplinary society promoting the study of cancer in all its aspects, including the scientific study of the treatment of cancer patients. Encourages liaison among medical specialists and allied scientists concerned with cancer treatment. **Pub:** *American Radium Society–Membership Directory*, annual. Directory. *Price:* Included in membership dues. • *The Cancer Journal.* Journal.

★ 842 ★ American Reflexology Certification Board (ARCB)
PO Box 740879
Arvada, CO 80006-0879
Phone: (303)933-6921 **Fax:** (303)904-0460
Email: arcbnet@aol.com
Website: http://www.arcb.net/
George S. Balut, Pres.

Fnded: 1992. **Desc:** Works to protect the public; promotes advancement of field through recognition of competent reflexologists meeting national standards; provides National Board Certified Reflexologist certification. **Pub:** Newsletter, semiannual.

★ 843 ★ American Registry of Diagnostic Medical Sonographers (ARDMS)
51 Monroe St., Plz. East One
Rockville, MD 20850-2400
Phone: (301)738-8401 **Free:** 800-541-9754
Fax: (301)738-0312
Email: administration@ardms.org
Website: http://www.ardms.org
Dale R. Cyr, MBA, Exec. Dir.

Fnded: 1975. **Mem:** 40,000. **Desc:** Administers examinations in the field of diagnostic medical sonography and vascular technology throughout the U.S. and Canada and registers candidates passing those exams in the specialties of their expertise. Maintains central office for administering examination plans and schedules and assisting registered candidates and those interested in becoming registered. **Pub:** *American Registry of Diagnostic Medical Sonographers Directory*, annual. Directory. *Price:* Free. • *Continuing Competency Requirements*. Brochure. • *Examination Information and Application Booklet*. Booklet. • *Informational Brochure*, annual. Brochure. • *Mailing List Brochure*. Brochure.

★ 844 ★ American Registry of Medical Assistants (ARMA)
69 Southwick Rd.
Westfield, MA 01085-4729
Phone: (413)562-7336 **Free:** 800-527-2762
Fax: (413)562-9021
Annette H. Heyman, Dir.

Fnded: 1950. **Mem:** 10,000. **Desc:** Medical assistants who have completed an accredited medical assistant training course or who have trained with a physician for a minimum of three years. Objectives are to: establish and maintain high training standards for medical assistants; promote greater efficiency within the profession; raise awareness of medical assistants within the medical community. **Pub:** *The Medical Assistant*, annual. Journal. Information of interest to the medical community. *Price:* included in membership dues. • *Registry Connection*, quarterly. • *200 Ways to Put Your Talent To Work in the Health Field*. Pamphlet. *Price:* Free. • Brochures.*Price:* Included in application fee and annual fee of; Members.

★ 845 ★ American Registry of Pathology (ARP)
c/o Armed Forces Institute of Pathology
14th St. & Alaska Ave. NW
Washington, DC 20306-6000
Phone: (202)782-2143 **Fax:** (202)782-4567
Website: http://www.afip.org/ARP/arp.html
Dr. William Gardner, Exec. Dir.

Fnded: 1976. **Desc:** Engages in cooperative enterprises in medical research and education with the Armed Forces Institute of Pathology. Functions as a fiscal agent in the management of research grants and monies derived from tuition fees, publications, and contributions. Serves as a link between, and encourages cooperation among, the military and civilian medical, dental, and veterinary communities for the mutual benefit of military and civilian medicine. Provides personnel and other services in support of research. Offers 38 continuing medical education courses annually. Bestows annual John Hill Brinton Award in recognition of outstanding young researcher, John Shaw Billings Lifetime Achievement Award to senior AFIP staff member, Callender-Binford fellowships.

★ 846 ★ American Registry of Radiologic Technologists (ARRT)
1255 Northland Dr.
Saint Paul, MN 55120-1155
Phone: (651)687-0048
Website: http://www.arrt.org
Darrell E. McKay, Pres.

Fnded: 1922. **Mem:** 223,000. **Desc:** Radiologic technologist certification board that administers examinations, issues certificates of registration to radiographers, nuclear medicine technologists, and radiation therapists, and investigates the qualifications of practicing radiologic technologists. Governed by trustees appointed from American College of Radiology and American Society of Radiologic Technologists. **Pub:** *ARRT Annual Report*. Annual Report. • *Educator Update*, 2/year. Newsletter. **Frmly:** American Registry of X-Ray Technicians; (1936) American Registry of Radiological Technicians.

★ 847 ★ American Rehabilitation Counseling Association (ARCA)
c/o American Counseling Association
5999 Stevenson Ave.
Alexandria, VA 22304-3300
Phone: (703)823-9800 **Free:** 800-545-2223
Fax: (703)823-0252
Website: http://www.nchrtm.okstate.edu/arca/
Ellen Fabian, Pres.

Fnded: 1958. **Mem:** 2,329. **Desc:** A division of the American Counseling Association. Rehabilitation counselors and interested professionals and students. Purpose is to improve the rehabilitation counseling profession and its services to individuals with disabilities. Promotes high standards in rehabilitation counseling, practice, research, and education. Encourages the exchange of information between rehabilitation professionals and consumer groups. Serves as liaison among members and public and private rehabilitation counselors across the country. Sponsors educational and training programs. **Pub:** *ARCA News*, quarterly. Newsletter. Provides information on the procedures and problems involved in rehabilitation counseling and special education for the disabled and the aged. *Price:* Included in membership dues. • *Rehabilitation Counseling Bulletin*, quarterly. Journal. *Price:* Included in membership dues; $18/year for nonmembers.

★ 848 ★ American Rehabilitation Economics Association (AREA)
127 N Westwind Dr.
El Cajon, CA 92020-2955
Free: 800-317-AREA **Fax:** (619)593-9989
Email: areaorg@cox.net
Website: http://www.a-r-e-a.org
Margy Ashby, Sec. -Treas.

Fnded: 1989. **Mem:** 105. **Nat'l Groups:** 1. **Desc:** Forensic specialists with expertise in evaluating the medical, vocational, and economic aspects of injury. Strives to bring recognition to the combined use of vocational rehabilitation and earnings loss assessment as a distinct discipline. Also provides a peer-exchange forum for vocational, economic, and legal experts who practice in this field. **Pub:** *The Earnings Analyst*, annual. Journal. *Price:* $25.

★ 849 ★ American Reiki Master Association (ARMA)
PO Box 130
Lake City, FL 32056-0130
Phone: (904)755-9638
Email: arma@atlantic.net
Website: http://www.atlantic.net/~arma/
Cheri L. Robertson, Pres.

Desc: Promotes the Reiki therapy technique as a method of natural healing; offers training and certification.

★ 850 ★ American Rhinologic Society (ARS)
c/o Marvin P. Fried, MD
Montefiore Medical Center Department of Otolaryngology
3400 Bainbridge Ave.
3rd Fl. MAP
Bronx, NY 10467
Phone: (718)675-6262 **Free:** 888-520-9585
Fax: (718)675-6260
Email: info@american-rhinologic.org
Website: http://www.american-rhinologic.org
Marvin P. Fried, MD, Sec.

Fnded: 1954. **Mem:** 1,087. **Desc:** Physicians who are diplomates of the American Board of Otolaryngology, the American Board of Plastic Surgery, and other boards and who have had additional training and interest in the study of medical and surgical rhinology. Works to advance knowledge of rhinology (branch of medicine that relates to the nose and its diseases) internationally through short, frequent teaching courses at universities in conjunction with their faculties. Conducts research in nasal physiology, rhinomanometry, and anatomy. **Pub:** *American Journal of Rhinology*, bimonthly. Journal. • Membership Directory, biennial. • Newsletter, 4-5/year.

★ 851 ★ American Roentgen Ray Society (ARRS)
44211 Slatestone Ct.
Leesburg, VA 20176-5109
Phone: (703)729-3353 **Free:** 800-438-2777
Fax: (703)729-4839
Email: rdunnick@umich.edu
Website: http://www.arrs.org
N. Reed Dunnick, Pres.

Fnded: 1900. **Mem:** 14,000. **Desc:** Trade association for radiologists worldwide. Offers many educational programs. **Pub:** *American Journal of Roentgenology*, monthly, Peer reviewed.Journal. *Price:* $210/year. • *ARRS Memo*, quarterly. Newsletter. • *Categorical Course Syllabi*. **Frmly:** (1906) Roentgen Society of the U.S.

★ 852 ★ American Samoa Planned Parenthood Association
PO Box 1043
Pago Pago, American Samoa

Lang(s): English. **Desc:** Promotes responsible parenthood and family planning as a means to improve the quality of life for people living in American Samoa. Advocates family planning as a basic human right. Sponsors programs in sex education, family planning, and health. Provides contraceptive and health care services.

★ 853 ★ American School Health Association (ASHA)
PO Box 708
7263 State Route 43
Kent, OH 44240
Phone: (330)678-1601 **Free:** 800-445-2742
Fax: (330)678-4526
Email: asha@ashaweb.org
Website: http://www.ashaweb.org
Susan Wooley, Exec. Dir.

Fnded: 1927. **Mem:** 2,500. **State Groups:** 16. **Desc:** School physicians, school nurses, dentist, nurses, nutritionists, health educators, dental hygienist, school-based professionals and public health workers. Promotes coordinated school health programs that include health education, health services, a healthful school environment, physical education, nutrition services, and psycho-social health services offered in schools collaboratively with families and other members of the community. Offers professional reference materials. Conducts pilot programs that inform materials development, provides technical assistance to school professionals, advocates for school health, and complies statistics. **Pub:** *A Comprehensive Approach to Reduce Pregnancy & the Spread of HIV*. Book. An advocacy kit with workbook. *Price:* $25. • *Building Effective Coalitions to Prevent the Spread of HIV.*

Book. *Price:* $18 for nonmembers; $16 for members. • *Guide to Developing and Evaluating Medicine Education Programs.* *Price:* $7 for members; $10 for nonmembers. • *Guidelines for Protecting Confidential Student Health Information.* Book. *Price:* $13 for members; $19 for nonmembers. • *Health Counseling.* Book. • *Health in Action*, quarterly. *Price:* $20/year for members; $10/year, student member; $40 for nonmembers; Included in Associate membership. • *Health is Academic: A Guide to Coordinated School Health Programs.* Book. *Price:* $25. • *How Physicians Work & How to Work with Physicians.* Booklet. *Price:* $11. • *Introductory Guide to Advocacy.* Booklet. *Price:* $15. • *Journal of School Health*, 10/year. Journal. Includes articles, research papers, reports, commentaries, teaching techniques, and health service application. *Price:* included in membership dues; $145/year for institutions; $165/year outside U.S.; $10/copy for members. • *National Health Education Standards: Achieving Health Literacy.* Booklet. *Price:* $8. • *The PULSE*, quarterly. *Price:* $12 for members; Included in membership. • *The Role of the Nurse in the School Setting: A Historical Perspective.* Book. • *Roll Up Both Sleeves: Vaccinating Students & Staff at School.* Book. Book & video. *Price:* $15. • *School Health: Findings form Evaluated Programs, 2nd Ed..* Book. *Price:* $18. • *School Health in America.* Survey. *Price:* $20. • *Scope & Standards of Professional School Nursing Practice.* Book. *Price:* $15. • *Sexuality Education Within Comprehensive School Health Education.* Book. *Price:* $15. • *Tell Me About AIDS.* Curricular materials for grades K-1, 2-3, 4-5, & 6. • *Topical Packages of Articles From the Journal*, annual. Book. *Price:* $22. **Frmly:** (1936) American Association of School Physicians.

★ 854 ★ American Senior Citizens Association (ASCA)

PO Box 41
Fayetteville, NC 28302
Phone: (910)323-3641 **Free:** 800-323-6525
Fax: (910)323-4343
Ben Sutton, Exec. VP

Fnded: 1982. **Mem:** 35,000. **Desc:** Currently Inactive. Senior citizens. Purpose is to promote the physical, mental, emotional, and economic well-being of senior citizens. Believes that senior citizens have a right to live with competence, security, and dignity. Promotes activities that help senior citizens to be active participants in their communities. Seeks affiliations with state senior citizens associations. **Pub:** *Senior Citizens Voice*, quarterly. Newspaper. *Price:* included in membership dues.

★ 855 ★ American Shoulder and Elbow Surgeons (ASES)

c/o American Academy of Orthopaedic Surgeons
6300 N River Rd., Ste. 727
Rosemont, IL 60018-4226
Phone: (847)698-1629 **Fax:** (847)823-0536
Email: leffevt@mqh.harvard.edu
Website: http://www.aaos.org/wordhtml/ases/homeases.htm
Karen Jared, Dir.

Fnded: 1982. **Mem:** 146. **Desc:** Orthopedic surgeons. Purpose is to promote the exchange and dissemination of information on shoulder and elbow surgery and treatment. Sponsors educational courses.

★ 856 ★ American Sickle Cell Anemia Association (ASCAA)

10300 Carnegie Ave.
Cleveland Clinic/East Office Bldg. (EEb18)
Cleveland, OH 44106
Phone: (216)229-8600 **Fax:** (216)229-4500
Email: irabragg@ascaa.org
Website: http://ascaa.org
Ira Bragg-Grant, Exec. Dir.

Fnded: 1971. **Desc:** Ensures the availability and accessibility of quality, comprehensive sickle cell services. Provides quality and quantity counseling, education, testing services, and promotes public professional awareness about sickle cell anemia and its hemoglobin diseases and trait variants. **Frmly:** (2001) American Sickle Cell Society; (2002) American Sickle Cell Anemia Society.

★ 857 ★ American Skin Association (ASA)

346 Park Ave. S
New York, NY 10010
Phone: (212)889-4858 **Free:** 800-499-SKIN
Email: info@skinassn.org
Website: http://www.americanskin.org

Fnded: 1987. **Mem:** 200. **Desc:** Supports research on all skin diseases. Promotes public education on prevention and treatment of skin disorders. Created School Skin Health Education Program, K-12, with the New York Academy of Medicine. **Pub:** *Childhood Skin Diseases.* Brochure. • *Healthy Skin and Gardening.* Brochure. • *Melanoma.* Brochure. • *Outdoor Sports and Your Skin.* Brochure. • *Skin Facts*, quarterly. Newsletter. • *The Sun, Your Skin, and Your Health.* Brochure. • *Your Newborn's Skin and the Sun.* Brochure.

★ 858 ★ American Sleep Apnea Association (ASAA)

1424 K St. NW, Ste. 302
Washington, DC 20005
Phone: (202)293-3650 **Fax:** (202)293-3656
Email: asaa@sleepapnea.org
Website: http://www.sleepapnea.org
Christin Engelhardt, Exec. Dir.

Fnded: 1990. **Mem:** 5,000. **Local Groups:** 225. **Desc:** Individuals affected by sleep apnea; health care professionals. Promotes public awareness of sleep apnea; encourages research on the causes and treatments of breathing abnormalities during sleep. Sponsors educational programs and support groups through the A.W.A.K.E. Network. Serves as an advocate for people with sleep apnea.. **Pub:** *Get the Facts about Sleep Apnea.* Brochure. • *Wake Up Call The Wellness Letter for Snoring and Apnea*, bimonthly. Newsletter. Articles of interest to people affected by sleep apnea. *Price:* With membership. • Choosing a CPAP, Choosing a Mask and Headgear, Sleep and the Internet, Sleep Apnea and Driving, Reprints of newsletter articles.

★ 859 ★ American Social Health Association (ASHA)

PO Box 13827
Research Triangle Park, NC 27709
Phone: (919)361-8400 **Fax:** (919)361-8425
Email: phidra@ashastd.org
Website: http://www.ashastd.org
William C. Parra, CEO

Fnded: 1914. **Desc:** A national voluntary health agency dedicated to stopping sexually transmitted diseases and their harmful consequences to individuals, families and communities. Works to expand biomedical research, provide information and education programs, upgrade clinical care, and improve public policy. Provides leadership in public policy issues. Supplies public health agencies with patient education materials. Engages directly in biomedical research through its ASHA Research Fund. Operates Herpes Resource Center, a national program for those infected with the genital herpes virus, and HPV Support Program, a national program for those infected with the human papilloma virus. **Pub:** *Helper*, quarterly. Newsletter. Reports on the latest research on the herpes simplex virus; includes information on strategies for coping with the virus and on treatments. *Price:* $25/yr. • *HPV News*, quarterly. Includes latest research on HPV/genital warts and information on coping strategies. *Price:* $25/yr. • *Managing Herpes.* *Price:* $19.75 includes shipping and handling. • Brochures. • Pamphlets. **Frmly:** (1959) American Social Hygiene Association.

★ 860 ★ American Society of Abdominal Surgeons (ASAS)

675 Main St.
Melrose, MA 02176
Phone: (781)665-6102 **Fax:** (781)665-4127
Email: office@abdominalsurg.org
Website: http://www.abdominalsurg.org
Louis F. Alfano, MD, Exec. Sec.

Fnded: 1959. **Mem:** 2,842. **Desc:** Medical doctors specializing in abdominal surgery. Sponsors extensive program of surgical education including study courses, postgraduate programs, lectures, and demonstrations. **Pub:** *American Society of Abdominal Surgeons*, annual. Journal. *Price:* available to members only. • *The Surgeon*, semiannual. Newsletter. Includes calendar of events. *Price:* available to members only. • Books.

★ 861 ★ American Society of Addiction Medicine (ASAM)

4601 N Park Ave., Arcade Ste. 101
Chevy Chase, MD 20815
Phone: (301)656-3920 **Fax:** (301)656-3815
Email: email@asam.org
Website: http://www.asam.org
Dr. James F. Callahan, Exec. VP/CEO

Fnded: 1954. **Mem:** 3,000. **State Groups:** 28. **Desc:** Physicians with special interest and experience in the field of alcoholism and other drug dependencies and who wish to share this experience with other professionals in order to extend their knowledge of addictive diseases; promote dissemination of that knowledge; enlighten the public regarding these problems; advance education and research in the field of addiction. Holds annual Ruth Fox Course for Physicians, annual Medical-Scientific Conference and five other conferences/courses. **Pub:** *ASAM News*, bimonthly. Newsletter. *Price:* $25. • *ASAM Patient Placement Criteria for the Treatment of Substance-Related Disorders.* • *Guidelines for Facilities Treating Chemically Dependent Patients at Risk for AIDS.* • *Journal of Addictive Diseases*, quarterly. Journal. • *Principles of Addiction Medicine.* *Price:* $155. **Frmly:** (1967) New York City Medical Society on Alcoholism; (1989) American Medical Society on Alcoholism and Other Drug Dependencies.

★ 862 ★ American Society for Adolescent Psychiatry (ASAP)

PO Box 570218
Dallas, TX 75357-0218
Phone: (972)686-6166 **Fax:** (972)613-5532
Email: info@adolpsych.org
Website: http://www.adolpsych.org
Frances M. Roton, Exec. Dir.

Fnded: 1967. **Mem:** 800. **Reg. Groups:** 20. **Desc:** Qualified psychiatrists concerned with the behavior of adolescents. Provides for the exchange of psychiatric knowledge; encourages the development of adequate standards and training facilities; stimulates research in the psychopathology and treatment of adolescents. Consults with national organizations interested in the welfare of youth and adolescence. **Pub:** *Adolescent Psychiatry*, annual. Journal. Contains articles and case studies on adolescent psychiatry. *Price:* included in membership dues. • *American Society for Adolescent Psychiatry–Newsletter*, quarterly. Newsletter. Includes society news, calendar of events, and research updates. *Price:* Included in membership dues; $10/year for nonmembers. • *ASAP Membership Directory*, biennial. Membership Directory. • *Journal of Youth and Adolescence*, bimonthly. Journal.

★ 863 ★ American Society for Advancement of Anesthesia and Sedation in Dentistry (ASAAD)

6 East Union Ave.
Bound Brook, NJ 08805
Phone: (732)469-9050 **Fax:** (732)271-1985
Email: info@sedation4dentists.com
Website: http://www.sedation4dentists.com
Dr. David Crystal, Contact

Fnded: 1925. **Mem:** 200. **Desc:** Dentists and physicians interested in dental anesthesia. Studies new anesthetics and chemicals; researches pain control methods. Organized and sponsored international congresses on modern pain control in dentistry in Latin America, Europe, and Japan. Advances education opportunities for dentists using sedation and anesthesia. Maintains speakers' bureau. **Pub:** *Modern Anesthesia in Dentistry*. Book. • *Modern Dental Anesthesia*. Book. • *Modern Pain Control*, biennial. • *Pain Control in Dentistry*, semiannual. Journal. Covers and promotes the use of dental anesthesia. *Price:* Included in membership dues. • *Transcripts*, semiannual. **Frmly:** (1975) American Society for Advancement of General Anesthesia in Dentistry; (2001) American Society for Advancement of Anesthesia in Dentistry.

★ 864 ★ American Society for Aesthetic Plastic Surgery (ASAPS)

11081 Winners Cir.
Los Alamitos, CA 90720-2813
Phone: (562)799-2356 **Fax:** (562)799-1098
Email: asaps@surgery.org
Website: http://www.surgery.org
Sue Dykema, Dep. Exec. Dir.

Fnded: 1964. **Mem:** 1,800. **Desc:** Board-certified plastic surgeons. Provides continuing education to members in the area of aesthetic plastic surgery, through presentation of papers, study sessions, and scientific sessions. Provides speakers; conducts research programs. **Pub:** *Aesthetic Society News*, quarterly. Newsletter. • *Aesthetic Surgery Journal*, bimonthly. Journal. Reviews developments in the field and research results; includes society news. *Price:* Included in membership dues.

★ 865 ★ American Society on Aging (ASA)

833 Market St., Ste. 511
San Francisco, CA 94103-1824
Phone: (415)974-9600 **Fax:** (415)974-0300
Email: info@asaging.org
Website: http://www.asaging.org
Gloria H. Cavanaugh, Exec. Dir.

Fnded: 1954. **Mem:** 10,000. **Desc:** Health care and social service professionals, educators, researchers, administrators, businesspersons, students, and senior citizens. Works to enhance the well-being of older individuals and to foster unity among those working with and for the elderly. Offers 25 continuing education programs for professionals in aging-related fields. **Pub:** *Aging Today*, bimonthly. Newspaper. Tabloid covering critical events and issues in the field of aging, including legislative news, new products and designs, and research. *Price:* Included in membership dues; $14.95/year for nonmembers. • *Generations*, quarterly. Journal. Provides practical, current information in the field of aging, with emphasis on medical and social practice, research, and policy. *Price:* Included in membership dues; $38/year for nonmember individuals; $50 for institutions. **Frmly:** (1985) Western Gerontological Society.

★ 866 ★ American Society for the Alexander Technique (AMSAT)

PO Box 60008
Florence, MA 01062-0008
Phone: (413)584-2359 **Free:** 800-473-0620
Fax: (413)584-3097
Email: alexandertech@earthlink.net
Website: http://www.amsat.ws
Indrani Kowlessar Gallagher, Exec. Admin.

Fnded: 1987. **Mem:** 600. **Desc:** Individuals who have completed a three-year training course and have been certified by AMSAT; students currently enrolled in an approved AMSAT teacher training course. Promotes and trains teachers of the Alexander Technique. (Created by Australian actor F. M. Alexander (1863-1955), the technique employs reeducation of habitual movement patterns so the body is used efficiently with the least amount of "wear and tear.") Seeks to: promote proficiency, knowledge, and skill in the field of psycho-physical reeducation; encourage education and study in the Alexander Technique; approve the establishment and continuation of teacher training courses. Promotes communication and the interchange of skills and information between the society and other organizations of teachers in the Alexander Technique; works to achieve reciprocal memberships between such organizations. Promotes and conducts research. Compiles information regarding teacher members and members of affiliated societies and disseminates this information to the public. Maintains speakers' bureau. **Pub:** *AMSAT News*, quarterly. Newsletter. *Price:* $30/year. • *List of Certified Training Courses*, semiannual. • *Teaching Members List*, semiannual.

★ 867 ★ American Society of Alternative Therapists (ASAT)

PO Box 703
Rockport, MA 01966
Phone: (978)281-4400 **Fax:** (978)546-2905
Email: asat@asat.org
Website: http://www.asat.org
Dr. Martin Hart, Pres.

Fnded: 1990. **Mem:** 1,700. **Desc:** CORE counselors. Seeks to advance CORE counseling training and services; promote continuing professional development of members. Conducts educational programs to raise public awareness and acceptance of CORE counseling methods; sponsors training programs for CORE counselors; holds examinations and bestows CORE counseling certification upon qualified individuals; establishes and monitors CORE counseling guidelines.

★ 868 ★ American Society of Andrology (ASA)

111 N Plaza Dr., Ste. 550
Schaumburg, IL 60173
Phone: (847)619-4909 **Fax:** (847)517-7229
Email: asa@wjweiser.com
Website: http://www.andrologysociety.com
Jon L. Pryor, MD, Pres.

Fnded: 1975. **Mem:** 800. **Desc:** Individuals interested in andrology, the science and medicine of the male reproductive system. Promotes advancement of knowledge of the male reproductive system and its diseases. Fosters interdisciplinary communication within the field of andrology; cooperates with other organizations holding similar interests. Conducts educational programs. **Pub:** *Handbook of Andrology*, periodic. Handbook. • *Journal of Andrology*, periodic. Journal.

★ 869 ★ American Society of Anesthesia Technologists and Technicians (ASATT)

PO Box 2588
Mission, KS 66201
Phone: (913)262-2249 **Fax:** (913)262-0174
Email: asil@dir.net
Frank Bistrom, Exec. Dir.

Fnded: 1989. **Mem:** 1,048. **Reg. Groups:** 7. **Desc:** Anesthesia technicians and technologists, medical technology students, and other individuals, organizations, and corporations with an interest in the field of anesthesiology. Promotes continuing professional development of members. Conducts continuing education programs for anesthesiology technicians and technologists; represents members' interests at the national level in the United States; maintains certification program and develops standards of ethics and practice. **Pub:** *Sensor*, quarterly. Newsletter.

★ 870 ★ American Society of Anesthesiologists (ASA)

520 N Northwest Hwy.
Park Ridge, IL 60068-2573
Phone: (847)825-5586 **Fax:** (847)825-1692
Email: mail@asahq.org
Website: http://www.asahq.org
Ronald A. Burns, Exec. Dir.

Fnded: 1905. **Mem:** 38,000. **State Groups:** 50. **Desc:** Professional society of physicians specializing or interested in anesthesiology. Seeks "to develop and further the specialty of anesthesiology for the general elevation of the standards of medical practice." Encourages education, research, and scientific progress in anesthesiology. Conducts refresher courses and other postgraduate educational activities. Maintains placement service. **Pub:** *Anesthesiology*, monthly. Journal. *Price:* $246/year for individuals; $445/year for institutions. • *ASA Newsletter*, monthly. Newsletter. Reports on the educational and scientific work of ASA. Contains calendar of events. *Price:* Included in membership dues; $36/year for nonmembers. **Frmly:** (1911) Long Island Society of Anesthetists; (1936) New York Society of Anesthetists; (1945) American Society of Anesthetists.

★ 871 ★ American Society for Apheresis (ASFA)

3900 E Timrod
Tucson, AZ 85711
Phone: (520)327-8584 **Fax:** (520)322-6778
Email: asfa@azstarnet.com
Website: http://www.apheresis.org
Phillip Gutt, Contact

Fnded: 1981. **Mem:** 800. **Desc:** Physicians, nurses, technologists, scientists, and other allied health professionals active in the field of apheresis, the separation and removal of components from blood. Aims to: promote training and research in apheresis therapy for patients; improve the care and management of apheresis donors; encourage the use of apheresis technology; assist in forming standards and regulations in the field of apheresis. Provides opportunity for the exchange of experiences and opinions through discussions, presentations, and publications; offers consulting on problems in the practice of apheresis. Conducts studies and courses. Plans to establish a central registry of apheresis information. **Pub:** *ASFA Newsletter*, periodic. Newsletter. • *Journal of Clinical Apheresis*, quarterly. Journal. *Price:* $124/year.

★ 872 ★ American Society of Bariatric Physicians (ASBP)

5453 E Evans Pl.
Denver, CO 80222-5234
Phone: (303)770-2526 **Fax:** (303)779-4834
Email: info@asbp.org
Website: http://www.asbp.org
Beth A. Little, CAE, Interim Exec. Dir.

Fnded: 1950. **Mem:** 1,000. **Nat'l Groups:** 1. **State Groups:** 2. **Desc:** Physicians with a special interest in the study and treatment of obesity and associated conditions. Encourages excellence in the practice of bariatric medicine through exchange of information, research, and continuing education. Sponsors regional courses and clinical research programs. Offers a physician referral service. **Pub:** *The Bariatrician*, quarterly. Journal. Includes articles on health, fitness, nutrition, and current treatments for obesity. *Price:* $48/year in U.S.; $72/year outside U.S. • *Membership Directory*, annual. Membership Directory. • *News from ASBP*, bimonthly. Newsletter. *Price:* available to members only. • Manuals. • Pamphlets. **Frmly:** (1972) The Obesity Foundation.

★ 873 ★ American Society for Bariatric Surgery (ASBS)

7328 W University Ave., Ste. F
Gainesville, FL 32607
Phone: (352)331-4900 **Fax:** (352)331-4975
Email: info@asbs.org
Website: http://www.asbs.org
Georgeann Mallory, Exec. Dir.

Fnded: 1983. **Mem:** 1,000. **Desc:** Works to advance the art and science of bariatric surgery. Supports clinical and laboratory investigations; promotes guidelines for ethical patient care; conducts educational programs for physicians, paramedicals and lay people; provides a forum for the exchange of ideas. **Pub:** *ASBS Newsletter*, periodic. Newsletter. • *Obesity Surgery*, bimonthly. Journal. International, interdisciplinary forum for communicating latest research and surgical techniques. *Price:* $350/institute; $180/personal.

★ 874 ★ American Society Bioethics and Humanities
4700 W Lake Ave.
Glenview, IL 60025-1485
Phone: (847)375-4745 **Free:** 877-734-9385
Fax: 877-734-9385
Email: info@asbh.org
Website: http://www.asbh.org
Richard G. Muir, Exec. Dir.

Fnded: 1998. **Mem:** 1,500. **Desc:** Promotes the exchange of ideas and fosters multidisciplinary, interdisciplinary, and interprofessional scholarship, research, teaching, policy development, professional development, and collegiality among people engaged in all of the endeaavors related to clinical and academic bioethics and the health-related humanities. **Pub:** *Core Competencies for Health Care Ethics Consultation*. Report. *Price:* $12.00. • Membership Directory, annual.

★ 875 ★ American Society for Blood and Marrow Transplantation (ASBMT)
85 W Algonquin Rd., Ste. 550
Arlington Heights, IL 60005
Phone: (847)427-0224 **Fax:** (847)427-9656
Email: mail@asbmt.org
Website: http://www.asbmt.org
Alan K. Leahigh, Exec. Dir.

Fnded: 1993. **Mem:** 1,000. **Desc:** Individuals, organizations, and corporations with an interest in blood and marrow transplantation. Seeks to advance blood and marrow transplantation techniques; promotes professional advancement of physicians and support personnel engaged in blood and marrow transplantations. Facilitates exchange of information among members; serves as a clearinghouse on blood and marrow transplantation; sponsors educational programs. **Pub:** *ASBMT News*, quarterly. Newsletter. • *Biology of Blood and Marrow Transplantation*, monthly. Journal. • *Blood and Marrow Transplantation Reviews*, quarterly. Bulletin.

★ 876 ★ American Society for Bone and Mineral Research (ASBMR)
2025 M St. NW, Ste. 800
Washington, DC 20036-3309
Phone: (202)367-1161 **Fax:** (202)367-2161
Email: asbmr@dc.sba.com
Website: http://www.asbmr.org
Joan R. Goldberg, Exec. Dir.

Fnded: 1977. **Mem:** 3,100. **Desc:** Physicians, dentists, veterinarians, clinical investigators, and researchers interested in bone and mineral metabolism. Provides placement service. Is a member of FASEB. **Pub:** *Journal of Bone and Mineral Research*, monthly. Journal. • *Primer on the Metabolic Bone Diseases and Disorders of Mineral Metabolism*. • Membership Directory, annual.

★ 877 ★ American Society of Breast Disease
PO Box 140186
Dallas, TX 75214
Phone: (214)368-6836 **Fax:** (214)368-5719
Email: asbd1@aol.com
Website: http://www.asbd.org
Debu Tripathy, MD, Contact

Fnded: 1976. **Mem:** 850. **Nat'l Groups:** 1. **Desc:** Physicians and nurses, primarily those engaged in the fields of obstetrics and gynecology, surgery, radiology, family practice, and medical and radiation oncology. Seeks to further the study of diseases of the breast and to inform physicians and other health care professionals of developments in the diagnosis and treatment of breast cancer and benign diseases of the breast. Serves as a forum for discussion among members. Encourages research pertaining to breast disease. **Pub:** *ASBD Advisor*, quarterly. Newsletter. • *The Breast Journal*, bimonthly. **Frmly:** (1994) Society for the Study of Breast Disease.

★ 878 ★ American Society of Cataract and Refractive Surgery (ASCRS)
4000 Legato Rd. No., 850
Fairfax, VA 22033
Phone: (703)591-2220 **Fax:** (703)591-0614
Email: ascrs@ascrs.org
Website: http://www.ascrs.org
Marguerite B. McDonald, MD, Pres.

Fnded: 1974. **Mem:** 8,000. **Desc:** Ophthalmologists interested in anterior segment surgery and refractive corneal surgery. Offers continuing medical education to ophthalmologists on cataract and refractive surgery techniques, intraocular lens designs, and related research areas; assists allied health care professionals in ophthalmology on medical and surgical care of pseudophakic (lens implant) patients. Works to improve public education in the field of eye care. Conducts research in ocular pathology in cataract and refractive surgery. Compiles statistics. **Pub:** *Administrative Eyecare*, quarterly. *Price:* Included in membership dues; $60/year for nonmembers. • *ASCRS Roster*, biennial. Membership Directory. *Price:* Free for members. • *Journal of Cataract and Refractive Surgery*, bimonthly. Journal. *Price:* Included in membership dues; $149/year for nonmembers. • Newsletter, monthly. **Frmly:** (1986) American Intra-Ocular Implant Society.

★ 879 ★ American Society of Childbirth Educators (ASCE)
PO Box 2282
Sedona, AZ 86339
Phone: (928)284-9897 **Fax:** (928)284-9897
Email: jsasmor@sedona.net
Dr. James C. Sasmor, Corporate Sec.

Fnded: 1972. **Desc:** Seeks to provide a medium for the exchange and dissemination of information relating to prepared childbirth as a shared family experience and disseminate information to qualified professionals regarding standards, techniques, and skills relevant to the concept of prepared birth. Presently inactive.

★ 880 ★ American Society for Clinical Evoked Potentials (ASCEP)
c/o Mrs. S. Moss
14 Soundview Ave., No. 51
White Plains, NY 10606
Phone: (914)761-4713
Mrs. S. Moss, Exec. Sec.

Fnded: 1981. **Mem:** 410. **Desc:** Physicians in physical medicine and rehabilitation, neurology, neurosurgery, ophthalmology, and anesthesiology. Purpose is to study the central nervous system's transmissions and to teach electrodiagnostic reading of evoked potentials. (Evoked potential is the sum of the stimulus-evoked bioelectrical potentials from the peripheral nerve, retina, or cochlear mechanism, from the spinal cord or central conduction pathways, and from cortical and subcortical structures.) Teaches and encourages the practice of and research in the clinical application of evoked potentials for the betterment of patient care. Conducts seminars and workshops; maintains speakers' bureau. **Pub:** Membership Directory, periodic. • Journal.

★ 881 ★ American Society of Clinical Hypnosis (ASCH)
140 N Bloomingdale Rd.
Bloomingdale, IL 60108-1017
Phone: (630)980-4740 **Fax:** (630)351-8490
Email: asch@asch.net
Website: http://www.asch.net
John E. Kasper, PhD, Exec. VP

Fnded: 1957. **Mem:** 3,000. **Reg. Groups:** 36. **State Groups:** 17. **Local Groups:** 19. **Desc:** Physicians, dentists, psychologists with doctoral or masters degrees, and clinical social workers and counselors, and nurses with master's degrees. Brings together professional people in medical, dental, and psychological fields using hypnosis; sets up standards of training; conducts teaching sessions and workshops at basic and advanced levels. Offers instruction on clinical hypnosis and various simple forms of psychotherapy and psychodynamics. Cooperates with all scientific disciplines with regard to use of hypnosis. Maintains speakers' bureau. **Pub:** *American Journal of Clinical Hypnosis*, quarterly. Journal. *Price:* $88. • *American Society of Clinical Hypnosis–Newsletter*, quarterly. Promotes the acceptance of hypnosis as a tool in clinical medicine and scientific research. Includes member news and calendar of events. *Price:* Included in membership dues. • Directory, annual.

★ 882 ★ American Society of Clinical Hypnosis - Education and Research Foundation (ASCH-ERF)
140 N Bloomingdale Rd.
Bloomingdale, IL 60108-1017
Phone: (630)980-4740 **Fax:** (630)351-8490
Email: info@asch.net
Website: http://www.asch.net
Philip R. Appell, PhD, Pres.

Fnded: 1957. **Mem:** 2,400. **Desc:** Teaching and research arm of the American Society of Clinical Hypnosis. Physicians, dentists, and psychologists. Underwrites workshops in the U.S. and Canada to train professionals in hypnosis and broaden their knowledge of psychotherapy. Basic section is designed to familiarize physicians, psychologists, and dentists with hypnosis and its applications to problems of the psychologically normal patient including preparation for childbirth, comfort in the dental chair, and other problems and complaints complicated by emotional conflicts, such as smoking and obesity. Advanced section deals with techniques that can be used in addition to hypnotherapy in treating patients. **Frmly:** (1962) Seminars on Hypnosis Foundation.

★ 883 ★ American Society for Clinical Investigation (ASCI)
35 Research Dr., Ste. 300
Ann Arbor, MI 48103
Phone: (734)222-6050 **Fax:** (734)222-6058
Email: asci@the-jci.org
Website: http://www.asci-jci.org
Dr. Chi Van Dang, Pres.

Fnded: 1909. **Mem:** 2,600. **Desc:** Physician scientists with meritorious original clinical investigations. Active members are doctors under age 50; senior members are those over age 50. Promotes cultivation of clinical research by methods of natural sciences, correlation of science with the art of medical practice, encouragement of scientific investigation by medical practitioners, and publication of papers on the methods and results of clinical research. **Pub:** *Journal of Clinical Investigation*, biweekly. Journal. • Newsletter, quarterly.

★ 884 ★ American Society for Clinical Laboratory Science (ASCLS)
6701 Democracy Blvd., Ste. 300
Bethesda, MD 20817
Phone: (301)657-2768 **Fax:** (301)657-2909
Email: ascls@ascls.org
Website: http://www.ascls.org
Elissa Passiment, EdM, Exec. VP

Fnded: 1932. **Mem:** 13,000. **Reg. Groups:** 10. **State Groups:** 50. **Desc:** Primarily clinical laboratory personnel who have an associate or baccalaureate degree and clinical training and specialists who hold at least a master's degree in one of the major fields of clinical laboratory science such as bacteriology, mycology, or biochemistry; also includes technicians, specialists, and educators with limited certificates and students enrolled in approved programs of clinical laboratory studies and military medical technology schools. Promotes and maintains high standards in clinical laboratory methods and research and advances standards of education and training of personnel. Conducts educational program of seminars and workshops. Sponsors award competition to encourage the writing of scientific papers. Approves programs of continuing education and maintains records on participation in continuing education programs for members. **Pub:** *ASCLS Today*, monthly. Newsletter. *Price:* Included in membership dues. • *Clinical Laboratory Science*, quarterly. Journal. *Price:* Included in membership dues; $40 for individuals; $60 for corporations. • Books. • Brochures. • Manuals. • Videos. **Frmly:** American Society of Medical Technologists; (1936) American Society of Clinical Laboratory Technicians; (1993) American Society for Medical Technology.

★ 885 ★ American Society for Clinical Nutrition (ASCN)

9650 Rockville Pike
Bethesda, MD 20814-3998
Phone: (301)530-7110 **Fax:** (301)571-1863
Email: secretar@ascn.faseb.org
Website: http://www.faseb.org/ascn
Sandra A. Schlicker, PhD, Exec. Dir.

Fnded: 1959. **Mem:** 1,565. **Desc:** Physicians and scientists actively engaged in clinical nutrition research. Promotes teaching, research, and reporting of progress in clinical nutrition. Offers annual postgraduate course. **Pub:** *The American Journal of Clinical Nutrition*, monthly. Journal. Contains original research findings. Includes book reviews, commentaries, letters to the editor, and editorials. *Price:* $60/year for members; $120/year for nonmembers in U.S.; $140/year for nonmembers outside U.S.; $50/year for students. • Publishes 6-8 supplements per year. **Frmly:** (1997) American Institute of Nutrition.

★ 886 ★ American Society of Clinical Oncology (ASCO)

1900 Duke St., Ste. 200
Alexandria, VA 22314
Phone: (703)299-0150 **Fax:** (703)299-1044
Email: asco@asco.org
Website: http://www.asco.org
Charles M. Balch, Exec. VP/CEO

Fnded: 1964. **Mem:** 15,400. **Desc:** Physicians who treat people with cancer. Sets the standard for patient care worldwide, and leads the fight for more effective cancer treatments, increased funding for clinical and translational research. **Pub:** *ASCO News*, quarterly. Newsletter. • *Journal of Clinical Oncology*, monthly. Journal. • Directory, annual. • Proceedings, annual.

★ 887 ★ American Society for Clinical Pathology (ASCP)

2100 W Harrison
Chicago, IL 60612
Phone: (312)738-1336 **Free:** 800-621-4142
Fax: (312)738-1619
Email: info@ascp.org
Website: http://www.ascp.org
Nadine M. Filipiak, Dir./Comm. & Membership

Fnded: 1922. **Mem:** 150,000. **Desc:** Works to promote public health and safety by the appropriate application of pathology and laboratory medicine. Provides educational programs for pathologists and laboratory professionals throughout the year, certification for laboratory professionals, and publishes scientific journals and reference textbooks. **Pub:** *American Journal of Clinical Pathology*, monthly. Journal. • *ASCP Member News*, monthly. Newsletter. • *Laboratory Medicine*, monthly. Journal. • *Pathology Patterns*, semiannual. • Membership Directory, triennial. **Frmly:** (2002) American Society of Clinical Pathologists.

★ 888 ★ American Society for Clinical Pharmacology and Therapeutics (ASCPT)

528 N Washington St.
Alexandria, VA 22314-2314
Phone: (703)836-6981 **Fax:** (703)836-5223
Email: info@ascpt.org
Website: http://www.ascpt.org
Donna Krupa, Pres. /CEO

Fnded: 1900. **Mem:** 2,150. **Desc:** Works to "promote and advance the science of human pharmacology and therapeutics and in so doing to maintain the highest standards of research, education, and exchange of scientific information." Provides a Medical Education Program of Continuing Education for practicing physicians. **Pub:** *Clinical Pharmacology and Therapeutics*, monthly. Journal. *Price:* Included in membership dues.

★ 889 ★ American Society of Clinical Psychopharmacology (ASCP)

PO Box 2257
New York, NY 10116
Phone: (212)696-1088 **Free:** 800-248-4344
Fax: (212)696-0563
Website: http://www.ascpp.org
J. Craig Nelson, MD, Pres.

Fnded: 1992. **Mem:** 1,200. **Nat'l Groups:** 1. **Desc:** Works to encourage clinical research in psychopharmacology and provide continuing education for members. Sponsors research; facilitates exchange of information; conducts professional educational programs and; provides educational programs on the treatment of psychiatric disorders for patients and families; develops relationships with mental health advocacy groups; advocates public policies which promote research and the delivery of high quality care. **Pub:** *ASCP Update*, quarterly. Newsletter. *Price:* Free for members. • *Progress Notes*, quarterly. Newsletter.

★ 890 ★ American Society of Colon and Rectal Surgeons (ASCRS)

85 W Algonquin Rd., Ste. 550
Arlington Heights, IL 60005
Phone: (847)290-9184 **Fax:** (847)290-9203
Email: ascrs@execadmin.com
Website: http://www.fascrs.org/
Richard Billingham, MD, Pres.

Fnded: 1899. **Mem:** 2,100. **Reg. Groups:** 20. **Desc:** Professional society of surgeons specializing in the diagnosis and treatment of diseases of the colon, rectum, and anus. Offers placement service; conducts research programs. **Pub:** *Diseases of the Colon and Rectum*, monthly. Journal.

★ 891 ★ American Society for Colposcopy and Cervical Pathology (ASCCP)

20 W Washington St., Ste. 1
Hagerstown, MD 21740
Phone: (301)733-3640 **Free:** 800-787-7227
Fax: (301)733-5775
Website: http://www.asccp.org
Kathleen G. Poole, Exec. Dir.

Fnded: 1964. **Mem:** 3,500. **Desc:** Gynecologists, family physicians, pathologists, nurses, and other individuals interested in promoting the accurate and ethical application of colposcopy (the examination of the lower genital tract by means of a colposcope). Organizes and approves training programs and audio visual materials in the diagnosis and management of lower genital tract disease. Conducts accredited postgraduate courses. **Pub:** *A Classical Approach to Vulvar Disease*. *Price:* $150 for members; $170 for nonmembers. • *Advanced Colposcopy CD-ROM 2002*. Video. 30-minute videotape on colposcopy, LGSIL, HGSIL, and cancer. *Price:* $175 for members; $195 for nonmembers. • *ASCCP Algorithms form the Consensus Guidelines for the Management of Women with Cervical Cytological Abnormalities*. Booklet. Algorithm booklet with Algorithm wall chart. *Price:* $4/booklet (non-government); $2/booklet (government); $8/wall chart (non-government); $4/wall chart (government). • *ASCCP Patient Education*, quarterly. Pamphlets. Topics include Cervical Cryotherapy, Genital Warts, HIV-AIDS, Human Papillomavirus (HPV), The Pap Smear, Sexuality and Pain: A Real Challenge, etc. *Price:* $25 50 pamphlets/pack. • *ASCCP Videoguide to Colposcopy*. Video. 30-minute videotape on colposcopy, LGSIL, HGSIL, and cancer. *Price:* $40 in U.S. • *Colposcopy Image Library CD-ROM 2003*. *Price:* $200 for members; $250 for nonmembers. • *Comprehensive Colposcopy Review*. *Price:* $150 for members; $180 for non-members. • *Home Study Program*, quarterly. *Price:* $165/year. • *Journal of Lower Genital Tract Disease*, quarterly. **Frmly:** American Society for Colposcopy and Colpomicroscopy.

★ 892 ★ American Society of Consultant Pharmacists (ASCP)

1321 Duke St.
Alexandria, VA 22314-3563
Phone: (703)739-1300 **Free:** 800-355-2727
Fax: (703)739-1321
Email: info@ascp.com
Website: http://www.ascp.com
R. Timothy Webster, Exec. Dir.

Fnded: 1969. **Mem:** 7,000. **State Groups:** 20. **Desc:** Provides leadership, education, advocacy, and resources to advance the practice of senior care pharmacy practice. welfare. Conducts surveys of long-term care pharmacy operations. Sponsors educational and research programs. Maintains information center, hall of fame, and speakers' bureau; operates placement service; compiles statistics. **Pub:** *UPDATE*, bimonthly. Newsletter. *Price:* Included in membership dues. • Also publishes books and manuals.

★ 893 ★ American Society of Contemporary Ophthalmology (ASCO)

820 N Orleans, Ste. 208
Chicago, IL 60610
Phone: (312)440-0699 **Free:** 800-621-4002
Fax: (312)440-0580
Email: iaos@aol.com
Website: http://www.ASCMSO.com
Randall T. Bellows, MD, Dir.

Fnded: 1966. **Mem:** 800. **Desc:** Ophthalmologists interested in promoting clinical investigative advances in ophthalmology. Offers continuing medical education courses approved by the American Council for Continuing Medical Education (ACCME) on new ophthalmic developments in medical, therapeutic, diagnostic, and surgical procedures. **Pub:** *Annals of Ophthalmology*, 3/year. Journal. Includes book reviews and information on educational activities and new products. A continuing medical education publication for ophthalmologist. *Price:* $160. **Frmly:** (1970) Society for Cryo-Opthamology.

★ 894 ★ American Society of Critical Care Anesthesiologists (ASCCA)

520 N Northwest Hwy.
Park Ridge, IL 60068-2573
Phone: (415)476-1977 **Fax:** (415)476-3683
Email: cohenn@medsch.ucsf.edu
Website: http://gasnet.med.yale.edu/societies/ascca/
Neal H. Cohen, MD, Pres.

Fnded: 1986. **Mem:** 900. **Desc:** Provides for the specialized needs of intensivists as well as the broader needs of practicing anesthesiologists. **Pub:** *The Interchange*, quarterly. Newsletter. Disseminates thought & information about various topics including historical aspects of anesthesiology, ethically controversial issues, surveys. • Membership Directory.

★ 895 ★ American Society of Cytopathology (ASC)

400 W 9th St., Ste. 201
Wilmington, DE 19801
Phone: (302)429-8802 **Fax:** (302)429-8807
Email: asc@cytopathology.org
Website: http://www.cytopathology.org
Elizabeth A. Jenkins, Exec. Admin.

Fnded: 1951. **Mem:** 3,500. **Desc:** Physicians, Cytotechnologists and scientists dedicated to the cytologic method of diagnostic pathology. **Pub:** *Acta Cytologica*, bimonthly. Journal. • *The ASC Bulletin*, 8/year. Bulletin. • *Consider a Career in Cytotechnology*. Brochure. • *Cytopathology Review Course Syllabus*. **Frmly:** Inter-Society Cytology Council; American Society of Cytology.

★ 896 ★ American Society for Cytotechnology (ASCT)

1500 Sunday Dr., Ste. 102
Raleigh, NC 27607
Phone: (919)787-5181 **Free:** 800-948-3947
Fax: (919)787-4916
Email: info@asct.com

Website: http://www.asct.com
Kathleen Norris, Exec. Dir.

Fnded: 1979. **Mem:** 1,500. **Reg. Groups:** 10. **Desc:** Cytotechnologists (technologists trained in the identification of cells and cellular abnormalities such as cancer), students of cytotechnology, and medical doctors in the field of cytopathology. Seeks to: enhance the role of the cytotechnologist in the health care system; stimulate communication and cooperation among cytotechnologists and other health professionals; inform members of current legislative and legal issues pertaining to the profession of cytotechnology and other related professions; support and promote educational opportunities. Urges participation in educational programs available through the American Society of Cytopathology. **Pub:** *ASCT News*, 8/year. Newsletter. Covers educational, legislative, and other developments affecting the profession. Includes book reviews, calendar of events and employment listings. *Price:* available to members only.

★ 897 ★ American Society for Deaf Children (ASDC)

PO Box 3355
Gettysburg, PA 17325
Phone: (717)334-7922 **Free:** 800-942-ASDC
Fax: (717)334-8808
Email: asoc1@aol.com
Website: http://www.deafchildren.org/
Natalie Long, Pres.

Fnded: 1965. **Mem:** 1,300. **Local Groups:** 93. **Desc:** Parents of deaf and hard of hearing children; researchers, professionals, and others interested in the welfare of deaf and hard of hearing children and their families. Seeks to provide parent-to-parent support to help improve the education, recreation, health, and employment opportunities of deaf and hard of hearing children and youth. Promotes "total communication" as a way of life for deaf and hard of hearing children and their families. Assists other organizations in locating parents for seminars, workshops, and learning sessions regarding parental needs and the education of deaf and hard of hearing children. Provides speakers for meetings, seminars, and conventions. **Pub:** *The Endeavor*, quarterly. Newsletter. *Price:* Included in membership dues. **Frmly:** (1984) International Association of Parents of the Deaf.

★ 898 ★ American Society for Dental Aesthetics (ASDA)

635 Madison Ave., 13th Fl.
New York, NY 10022
Phone: (212)751-3263 **Free:** 800-454-ASDA
Fax: (212)755-3263
Email: info@asdatoday.com
Website: http://www.asdatoday.com
Irwin Smigel, DDS, Pres.

Fnded: 1978. **Mem:** 175. **Desc:** Accredited dentists practicing aesthetic concepts in dentistry, including porcelain lamination (a technique where porcelain veneer is chemically fused to teeth to lengthen them, close spaces, or recontour the entire mouth). Dentists must have 5 years experience and submit 5 "before and after" photos of their work in aesthetic dentistry to qualify for membership. Promotes development, research, and teaching of aesthetic concepts in dentistry. Although centered in New York City, the group promotes expansion of aesthetic dentistry concepts in other states and abroad. Sponsors educational programs on tooth and crown repair, aesthetic fillings, orthodontics, periodontics, implantology, and other topics. **Pub:** *ASDA Today*, semiannual. Journal. Promotes development, teaching & research of aesthetic dentistry. *Price:* Free.

★ 899 ★ American Society of Dentist Anesthesiologists (ASDA)

c/o Dr. Lee Lichtenstein
723 N Beers St.
Holmdel, NJ 07733
Fax: (732)739-6288
Website: http://www.asdahq.org/about.html
Dr. Lee Lichtenstein, Contact

Desc: Strives to make the full spectrum of anesthesia care available to dental patients; train dentists in anesthesia care.

★ 900 ★ American Society of Dentistry for Children (ASDC)

211 E Chicago Ave., Ste. 700
Chicago, IL 60611-2663
Phone: (312)337-2169 **Fax:** (312)337-6329
Email: asdckids@aol.com
Website: http://asdckids.org
Carol Teuscher, Asst. Exec. Dir.

Fnded: 1927. **Mem:** 3,000. **State Groups:** 50. **Desc:** General practitioners and specialists interested in dentistry for children. Conducts specialized education and research programs. **Pub:** *ASDC News*, quarterly. Newsletter. Contains news about children's dental health concerns. Includes scientific references and governmental activities related to children's health. *Price:* Included in membership dues. • *Directory of the Membership of the American Society of Dentistry for Children.* Membership Directory. • *Journal of Dentistry for Children*, bimonthly. Journal.

★ 901 ★ American Society for Dermatologic Surgery (ASDS)

5550 Meadowbrook Dr., No. 102
Rolling Meadows, IL 60008
Phone: (847)956-0900 **Free:** 800-441-2737
Fax: (847)956-0999
Email: info@aboutskinsurgery.com
Website: http://www.asds-net.org
Roy G. Geronemus, MD, Pres.

Fnded: 1970. **Mem:** 2,500. **Desc:** Physicians specializing in dermatologic surgery. Purpose is to maintain the highest possible standards in medical education, clinical practice, and patient care. Seeks to promote high standards in allied health professions and services as they relate to dermatology. **Pub:** *Dermatologic Surgery Journal*, monthly. Journal. *Price:* included in membership dues. • *Roster*, annual.

★ 902 ★ American Society of Dermatology (ASD)

2721 Capital Ave.
Sacramento, CA 95816-6004
Phone: (916)446-5054 **Fax:** (916)446-0500
Website: http://www.asd.org
M. John Hanni, Jr., C, Exec. Dir.

Desc: Dermatologists. Committed to make dermatology care available to everyone in the U.S.

★ 903 ★ American Society of Dermatopathology (ASDP)

60 Revere Dr., Ste. 500
Northbrook, IL 60062
Phone: (847)400-5820 **Fax:** (847)480-9282
Email: info@asdp.org
Website: http://www.asdp.org
Leah McCrackin, Acct. Mgr.

Fnded: 1962. **Mem:** 1,024. **Desc:** Seeks to: improve the quality of dermatopathology (the study of abnormal skin conditions, especially the structural and functional changes produced by disease); aid in the dissemination of information; encourage continuing education and research. **Pub:** *Journal of Cutaneous Pathology*, 10/year. Journal. • Membership Directory, semiannual.

★ 904 ★ American Society of Echocardiography (ASE)

1500 Sunday Dr., Ste. 102
Raleigh, NC 27607
Phone: (919)861-5574 **Fax:** (919)787-4916
Email: rbarry@asecho.org
Website: http://www.asecho.org
Robin L. Barry, Exec. Dir.

Fnded: 1976. **Mem:** 7,000. **Desc:** Physicians and sonographers specializing in ultrasound heart imaging and diagnosis. Promotes excellence in the ultrasonic examination of the heart and assists in establishing standards for education of physicians and cardiac-sonographers in echocardiography. Sponsors educational activities including distribution of self-testing materials, continuing education calendar, and annual scientific sessions. Maintains liaison with governmental agencies and other professional groups. **Pub:** *American Society of Echocardiography Standards Documents*, periodic. • *ASE Membership Directory*, biennial. Membership Directory. • *Journal of the American Society of Echocardiography*, monthly. Journal. For physicians and sonographers covering echocardiography. Includes legislative and membership updates. • Also publishes standards documents and number news briefs.

★ 905 ★ American Society of Electroneurodiagnostic Technologists (ASET)

426 West 42nd St.
Kansas City, MO 64111
Phone: (816)931-1120 **Fax:** (816)931-1145
Email: sheila@aset.org
Website: http://www.aset.org
Sheila R. Navis, CAE, Exec. Dir.

Fnded: 1959. **Mem:** 2,750. **Desc:** Persons engaged in clinical electroencephalographic (EEG) technology, evoked potential responses, nerve conduction studies, and polysomnography (sleep studies). Objective is the advancement of electroneurodiagnostic technology education and practice standards. **Pub:** *American Journal of Electroneurodiagnostic Technology*, quarterly. Journal. Covers EEG, evoked potentials, polysomnography, nerve conduction, and related electroneurodiagnostics. *Price:* Included in membership dues; $40/year for nonmembers in U.S.; $55/year for nonmembers outside U.S.; $80/year for institutions in U.S. • *ASET Newsletter*, quarterly. Newsletter. Includes calendar of events, local, state, and regional society news and workshop and seminar news. *Price:* Included in membership dues. • *Who's Who in Electroneurodiagnostics–Membership Directory*, annual. Membership Directory. Provides product listings for suppliers. Member listings are arranged alphabetically and geographically. *Price:* Included in membership dues. • Monographs.Provides information on selected END technology and related management subjects. • Books. • Also publishes study materials and guides. **Frmly:** (1985) American Society of Electroencephalographic Technologists.

★ 906 ★ American Society of Emergency Radiology (ASER)

820 Jorie Blvd.
Oak Brook, IL 60523
Phone: (630)368-3765 **Fax:** (630)571-7837
Email: aser@comresource.net
Website: http://www.erad.org/

Fnded: 1988. **Desc:** Seeks to advance the quality of diagnosis and treatment of acutely ill or injured patients by means of medical imaging, enhance teaching and research. **Pub:** *ASER Newsletter.* Newsletter. • Membership Directory.

★ 907 ★ American Society for Experimental Neuro Therapeutics (ASENT)

611 E Wells St.
Milwaukee, WI 53202
Phone: (414)273-8290 **Fax:** (414)276-3349
Email: info@asent.org
Website: http://www.asent.org
Kay Whalen, Exec. Dir.

Fnded: 1997. **Mem:** 225. **Desc:** Neurologists and other medical professionals with an interest in experimental neuro therapeutics. Seeks to advance the development of improved therapies for diseases and disorders of the nervous system; promotes professional advancement of members. Serves as a forum for the exchange of information among those concerned with the development of neuro therapeutics; works to maintain friendly and cooperative relationships between members and government agencies and industries with an interest in neurology; assists in the formulation of public policies affecting experimental neuro therapeutics; provides support to health care professionals and research scientists pursuing careers in neuro therapeutics. **Pub:** *ASENT Membership Directory*, annual. Directory.

★ 908 ★ American Society of Extra-Corporeal Technology (AmSECT)

503 Carlisle Dr. No. 125
Herndon, VA 20170-4838
Phone: (703)435-8556 **Fax:** (703)435-0056
Email: gcate@amsect.org
Website: http://www.amsect.org
George M. Cate, Exec. Dir.

Fnded: 1964. **Mem:** 3,000. **Reg. Groups:** 11. **Desc:** Perfusionists, technologists, doctors, nurses, and others actively employed and using the applied skills relating to the practice of extracorporeal technology (involving heart-lung machines); student members. Disseminates information necessary to the proper practice of the technology. Conducts programs in continuing education and professional-public liaison and hands-on workshops. Maintains placement service. **Pub:** *AMSECT Today*, 11/year. Magazine. Includes calendar of events, reading and employment opportunities lists, and reports of regional events. *Price:* Included in membership dues; $55/year for nonmembers. • *Journal of Extra-Corporeal Technology*, quarterly. Journal. Covers dialysis, hemodynamics, organs and tissues , oxygenation, and research. Includes book reviews, case studies and membership directory. *Price:* Included in membership dues; $70/ year for nonmembers. • Also publishes self-study modules and monographs. **Frmly:** (1968) American Society of Extracorporeal Circulation Technicians.

★ 909 ★ American Society of Forensic Odontology (ASFO)

c/o Dr. Susan Rivera
11 Tiffany Pl.
Saratoga Springs, NY 12866-9050
Phone: (518)584-2342 **Fax:** (518)584-9706
Email: skrivera@global2000.net
Website: http://www.asfo.org
Dr. Susan Rivera, Sec. -Treas.

Fnded: 1970. **Mem:** 1,013. **Reg. Groups:** 1. **Desc:** Individuals interested in furthering the field of forensic dentistry. Conducts research and specialized education programs. Maintains library. **Pub:** *The Manual of Forensic Odontology, Third Edition.* Book. • Membership Directory, annual. • Newsletter, 3/year.

★ 910 ★ American Society for Gastrointestinal Endoscopy (ASGE)

1520 Kensington Rd., Ste. 202
Oak Brook, IL 60523
Phone: (630)573-0600 **Free:** (866)353-ASGE
Fax: (630)573-0691
Email: info@asge.org
Website: http://www.asge.org
Patricia V. Blake, Exec. Dir.

Fnded: 1941. **Mem:** 7,500. **Desc:** Gastroenterologists, internists, and surgeons who perform gastroscopic, esophagoscopic, coloscopic, and peritoneoscopic examinations. Works to further the knowledge of digestive disease by endoscopic methods (visual inspection of the intestinal tract). **Pub:** *ASGE News*, bimonthly. Newsletter. Includes member and specialty news. *Price:* included in membership dues. • *Gastrointestinal Endoscopy*, bimonthly. Journal. Includes index, book reviews, case reports, and new materials and methods. *Price:* Included in membership dues. **Frmly:** American Gastroscopic Club; American Gastroscopic Society.

★ 911 ★ American Society of Gene Therapy

611 E Wells St.
Milwaukee, WI 53202
Phone: (414)278-1341 **Fax:** (414)276-3349
Email: info@asgt.org
Website: http://www.asgt.org
Elizabeth Dooley, CAE, Exec. Dir.

Fnded: 1996. **Mem:** 3,000. **Desc:** Medical professional organization representing researchers and scientists dedicated to discovering new gene therapies. Committed to promoting and fostering exchange and dissemination of information and ideas related to gene therapy; encourages the general field of research involving gene therapy; promotes professional and public education in all areas of gene therapy. **Pub:** *The Journal of Molecular Therapy*, monthly. Journal. Contains scientifically meritorious papers on primary research and methodological advances in general areas of gene transfer, gene and cell therapy.

★ 912 ★ American Society of General Surgeons

4200 Commercial Way
Glenview, IL 60025
Phone: (847)391-9770 **Free:** 800-998-8322
Fax: (847)391-9711
Email: asgs-info@theasgs.org
Website: http://www.theasgs.org
L. Jack Carow, III, Exec. Dir.

Fnded: 1993. **Mem:** 3,600. **Desc:** Board certified general surgeons who perform procedures within the scope of general surgery. **Pub:** *Surgfax*, monthly. Features timely updates on current issues.

★ 913 ★ American Society of Group Psychotherapy and Psychodrama (ASGPP)

301 N Harrison St., Ste. 508
Princeton, NJ 08540
Phone: (609)452-1339 **Fax:** (609)936-1659
Email: asgpp@asgpp.org
Website: http://www.asgpp.org
Eduardo Garcia, Exec. Dir.

Fnded: 1942. **Mem:** 650. **Nat'l Groups:** 4. **State Groups:** 8. **Local Groups:** 6. **Desc:** Social workers, psychologists, psychiatrists, clergy members, nurses, and others interested in group psychotherapy, psychodrama, and sociometry. Conducts educational programs; compiles statistics. **Pub:** *The International Journal of Action Methods, Psychodrama Skill Training and Role Playing*, quarterly. Journal. Application of Action methods to the fields of psycotherapy, counseling, education & organizational development. • *Psychodrama Network News*, quarterly. Newsletter.

★ 914 ★ American Society of Hair Restoration Surgery (ASHRS)

c/o American Academy of Cosmetic Surgery
737 N Michigan Ave., Ste. 820
Chicago, IL 60611
Phone: (312)981-6760 **Fax:** (312)981-6787
Email: info@cosmeticsurgery.org
Website: http://www.cosmeticsurgery.org
Jeffrey P. Knezovich, Exec. VP

Fnded: 1985. **Mem:** 1,800. **Desc:** Dedicated to fostering the growth and quality of hair restoration surgery worldwide; promotes exchange of information among surgeons and allied professionals in the area of hair restoration surgery; advances the latest scientific data and techniques in clinical practice.

★ 915 ★ American Society of Hand Therapists (ASHT)

401 N Michigan Ave.
Chicago, IL 60611-4267
Phone: (312)321-6866 **Fax:** (312)673-6670
Email: asht@sba.com
Website: http://www.asht.org
Lisa Keckich, Exec. Dir.

Fnded: 1977. **Mem:** 2,700. **Desc:** Registered and licensed occupational and physical therapists specializing in hand therapy and committed to excellence and professionalism in hand rehabilitation. Purposes are to promote research, publish information, improve treatment techniques, and standardize hand evaluation and care. Fosters education and communication between therapists in the U.S. and abroad. Compiles statistics; conducts research and education programs and continuing education seminars. **Pub:** *ASHT Times*, quarterly. Newsletter. *Price:* Included in membership dues. • *Journal of Hand Therapy*, quarterly. Journal. *Price:* Included in membership dues.

★ 916 ★ American Society of Handicapped Physicians (ASHP)

3424 S Culpepper Ct.
Springfield, MO 65804
Phone: (417)881-1570 **Fax:** (417)887-9830
Jericho Peden, Contact

Fnded: 1981. **Mem:** 1,200. **Desc:** Handicapped physicians and others concerned with the problems faced by handicapped physicians. Acts as a forum to address the needs of physically disabled physicians. Works against discrimination of the handicapped and serves as a support group and legal and career counselor. Disseminates information about resources for handicapped physicians. Plans to offer rehabilitation services. Maintains speakers' bureau and placement service; compiles statistics; offers specialized education. Founded by the late Spencer B. Lewis, M.D. and Terry Winkler, M.D. **Pub:** *American Society of Handicapped Physicians–SYNAPSE*, quarterly. Includes book reviews and research updates. *Price:* Free. • Directory, annual.

★ 917 ★ American Society for Healthcare Central Service Professionals (ASHCSP)

c/o American Hospital Association
1 N Franklin, No. 2800
Chicago, IL 60606
Phone: (312)422-3750 **Fax:** (312)422-4572
Email: pcostello@aha.org
Website: http://www.ashcsp.org
Virginia Sylvestri, Exec. Dir.

Fnded: 1967. **Mem:** 1,000. **Reg. Groups:** 6. **State Groups:** 20. **Local Groups:** 48. **Desc:** Managers, directors, technicians and supervisors of central service-supply distribution and sterile processing of medical devices and instrumentation. Certification, education and training. **Pub:** *Healthcare Central Service*, bimonthly. Newsletter. *Price:* available to members only. • Also publishes technical materials and training manuals. **Frmly:** (1987) American Society for Hospital Central Service Personnel.

★ 918 ★ American Society for Healthcare Engineering of the American Hospital Association (ASHE)

c/o American Hospital Association
One N Franklin, 28th Fl.
Chicago, IL 60606
Phone: (312)422-3800 **Fax:** (312)422-4571
Email: ashe@aha.org
Website: http://www.ashe.org
Albert J. Sunseri, PhD, Exec. Dir.

Fnded: 1962. **Mem:** 5,500. **Local Groups:** 75. **Desc:** Hospital engineers, facilities managers, directors of buildings and grounds, assistant administrators, directors of maintenance, directors of clinical engineering, design and construction professionals, and safety officers. Works to: promote better patient care by encouraging and assisting members to develop their knowledge and increase their competence in the field of facilities management; cooperate with hospitals and allied associations in matters pertaining to facilities management; bring about closer cooperation among members; provide contractors a medium for interchange of material relative to facilities management. Maintains library; conducts educational programs. Offers Actions for Professional Excellence Recognition Program (APEx) and the Certified Healthcare Facility Manager (CHFM) Designation. **Pub:** *American Society for Healthcare Engineering–Management Monograph Series*, quarterly. Report. Covers a specific topic in clinical/biomedical engineering, facilities management engineering, or design and construction. • *ASHE Fire, Electrical & Life Safety Compendium.* Book. *Price:* $65 for members; $85 for nonmembers. • *Emergency Management Handbook.* Handbook.

Price: $85 for members; $125 for nonmembers. • *The Guidelines for Design & Construction of Hospital & Health Care Facilities 2001 Ed.*. *Price:* $65 for members; $75 for nonmembers. • *Health Facilities Management Magazine*, monthly. Journal. Lists books, films, tapes, documents, and publications available from the society. *Price:* Free. • *Inside ASHE Magazine*, monthly. Journal. • *Preparing for the Certified Healthcare Facility Manager Exam...A Compendium of Resources.* Book. *Price:* $75 for members, plus shipping and handling; $95 for nonmembers, plus shipping and handling. • *Publications Catalog*, semiannual. Lists books, films, tapes, documents, and publications available from the society. *Price:* Free. • *Space Planner Toolkit 2002 Ed.*. Book. Arranged alphabetically by name, hospital, and city and state; includes vendor directory. *Price:* $495. • *Waste Management Issues for Health Care Facilities.* Book. *Price:* $85 for members; $125 for nonmembers. • Also publishes books. **Frmly:** American Society for Hospital Engineering.

★ 919 ★ American Society for Healthcare Environmental Services of the American Hospital Association (ASHES)
1 N Franklin St.
Chicago, IL 60606
Phone: (312)422-3860 **Fax:** (312)422-4572
Email: ashes@aha.org
Website: http://www.hospitalconnect.com
Patti Costello, Exec. Dir.

Fnded: 1986. **Mem:** 1,600. **Nat'l Groups:** 1. **Reg. Groups:** 16. **Desc:** Managers and directors of hospital environmental services, laundry and linen services, as well as housekeeping departments and waste management (non-hazardous and hazardous), in government or university settings. Provides a forum for discussion among members of common challenges, Professional development, and career advancement. Maintains liaison between members and governmental and standards setting bodies. Bestows Accolades Awards, Phoenix Award, Years of Service Award. Certified Healthcare Environmental Services Professional (CHESP) available through education and Examination. **Pub:** *PhoenixNewsletter*, quarterly. Newsletter. • *Professional Development Series*, quarterly. • Multiple publications related to env. svc. and technical issues.

★ 920 ★ American Society for Healthcare Food Service Administrators (ASHFSA)
One N Franklin
Chicago, IL 60606
Phone: (312)422-3870 **Fax:** (312)422-4581
Email: ashfsa@aha.org
Website: http://www.ashfsa.org
Patricia Burton, Exec. Dir.

Fnded: 1967. **Mem:** 1,200. **Local Groups:** 50. **Desc:** Serves individuals with healthcare food service management responsibilities, educators, suppliers and consultants to the profession, is the driving force in the healthcare food service industry and provides healthcare professionals with the resources to compete and succeed. **Pub:** *Healthcare Food Service TRENDS*, quarterly. Magazine. • Video.Cassette recordings of ASHFSA Internet-based conferences. • Also publishes food service reference works on administration, budgeting, cafeteria and financial management, and hospital food service system planning. **Frmly:** American Society for Hospital Food Service Administrators.

★ 921 ★ American Society for Healthcare Human Resources Administration (ASHHRA)
c/o American Hospital Association
One N Franklin, 31st Fl.
Chicago, IL 60606
Phone: (312)422-3725 **Fax:** (312)422-4577
Email: ashhra@aha.org
Website: http://www.ashhra.org
Mary Anne Kelly, Exec. Dir.

Fnded: 1964. **Mem:** 2,400. **Desc:** Purposes are: to provide effective and continuous leadership in the field of health care human resources administration; to promote cooperation with hospitals and allied associations in matters pertaining to hospital human resources administration; to further the professional and educational development of members; to encourage and promote research; to encourage and assist local groups in chapter formation through regular programs and institutes on health care human resources issues. Offers placement service. **Pub:** *Directory of Health Care Human Resources Consultants*, annual. Directory. • *Hospitals*, bimonthly. • *The Pulse*, quarterly. Journal. Reports on professional ethics and legislative activity. Includes calendar of events and chapter and member news. *Price:* Included in membership dues. • *Roster of Membership*, annual. Membership Directory.

★ 922 ★ American Society for Healthcare Risk Management (ASHRM)
One N Franklin
Chicago, IL 60606
Phone: (312)422-3989 **Fax:** (312)422-4580
Email: esummy@aha.org
Website: http://www.ashrm.org
Elizabeth Summy, Exec. Dir.

Fnded: 1980. **Mem:** 4,300. **State Groups:** 47. **Desc:** Employees actively involved in the risk management functions of hospitals or other health care providers, and others involved in insurance, brokerage, and consulting. Purposes are to: promote professional development of hospital risk managers; provide educational resources and programs on healthcare risk management; address risk management issues affecting the health care industry, particularly patient safety and risk financing. **Pub:** *Journal of Healthcare Risk Management*, quarterly. Journal. Covers research, trends, and new developments in the field of healthcare risk management. Includes educational program calendar and legal update. *Price:* Included in membership dues; $80/year for nonmembers.

★ 923 ★ American Society of Health System Pharmacists (ASHP)
7272 Wisconsin Ave.
Bethesda, MD 20814
Phone: (301)657-3000 **Fax:** (301)664-8867
Email: ahfs@ashp.org
Website: http://www.ashp.org
Henri R. Manasse, Jr., Exec. VP

Fnded: 1942. **Mem:** 30,000. **State Groups:** 50. **Desc:** Professional society of pharmacists employed by hospitals, HMOs, clinics, and other health systems. Provides personnel placement service for members; sponsors professional and personal liability program. Conducts educational and exhibit programs. Has 30 practice interest areas, special sections for home care practitioners and clinical specialists, and research and education foundation. **Pub:** *AHFS Drug Information*, annual. *Price:* $163/year. • *American Journal of Health System Pharmacy*, semimonthly. Journal. *Price:* Included in membership dues; $137/year for nonmembers (U.S.). • *ASHP Newsletter*, monthly. Newsletter. Covers developments in pharmacy and health care. Includes information on legislation and regulations and association news. *Price:* Included in membership dues. • *Handbook on Injectable Drugs*, biennial. *Price:* $158. • *International Pharmaceutical Abstracts*, semimonthly. *Price:* $100/year for members; $425/year for nonmembers (U.S.); $450/year for nonmembers (outside U.S.); $20 for single copy. • Books. • Videos. • Also publishes user manuals and aids, and produces software, CD-ROMS, and training programs.

★ 924 ★ American Society of Hematology (ASH)
1900 M St., NW, Ste. 200
Washington, DC 20036
Phone: (202)776-0544 **Fax:** (202)776-0545
Email: ash@hematology.org
Website: http://www.hematology.org
Martha Liggett, Exec. Dir.

Fnded: 1958. **Mem:** 9,500. **Desc:** Hematologists (specialists in the study of blood) and other persons holding doctorate degrees with an interest in the field. Promotes exchange of information and ideas related to blood and blood-forming tissues and investigation of hematologic problems. Offers educational programs. **Pub:** *ASH News*, 3/year. Newsletter. • *Blood*, bimonthly. Journal. • *Meeting Program*, annual.

★ 925 ★ American Society for Histocompatibility and Immunogenetics (ASHI)
1700 Commerce Pky., Ste. C
Mount Laurel, NJ 08054
Phone: (856)638-0428 **Fax:** (856)439-0525
Email: info@ashi-hla.org
Website: http://www.ashi-hla.org
Steve Echard, Exec. Dir.

Fnded: 1968. **Mem:** 1,000. **Desc:** Scientists, physicians, and technologists involved in research and clinical activities related to histocompatibility testing (a state of mutual tolerance that allows some tissues to be grafted effectively to others). Conducts proficiency testing and educational programs. Maintains liaison with regulatory agencies; offers placement services and laboratory accreditation. Has co-sponsored development of histocompatability specialist and laboratory certification program. **Pub:** *ASHI Quarterly*, quarterly. Includes calendar of events, employment listings, certification data, and notices of awards. *Price:* Included in membership dues; $30/year for nonmembers. • *Human Immunology*, monthly. Journal. • *Laboratory Procedures Manual.* Manual. Covers laboratory procedures. • Membership Directory. • Papers. • Proceedings. **Frmly:** American Association for Clinical Histocompatibility Testing.

★ 926 ★ American Society of Hypertension (ASH)
148 Madison Ave., 5th Fl.
New York, NY 10016
Phone: (212)696-9099 **Fax:** (212)696-0711
Email: ash@ash-us.org
Website: http://www.ash-us.org
Torry Mark Sansone, Exec. Dir.

Fnded: 1985. **Mem:** 4,000. **Reg. Groups:** 6. **Desc:** To organize and conduct educational activities designed to promote and encourage the development, advancement and exchange of scientific information in all aspects of research, diagnosis and treatment of hypertension and related cardiovascular diseases. **Pub:** *American Journal of Hypertension*, monthly. Journal. A peer-review, available in print or online. *Price:* $120. • *ASH Membership Directory.* Membership Directory.

★ 927 ★ American Society for Investigative Pathology (ASIP)
9650 Rockville Pke.
Bethesda, MD 20814-3993
Phone: (301)634-7130 **Fax:** (301)634-7990
Email: asip@asip.org
Website: http://www.asip.org
Mark E. Sobel, MD,PhD, Exec. Off.

Fnded: 1976. **Mem:** 2,000. **Desc:** Experimental research pathologists who have made significant contributions to the knowledge of disease. **Pub:** *The American Journal of Pathology*, monthly. Journal. Research papers in experimental pathology. Covers cell injury and death, inflammatory reactions, disturbances in circulation, and neoplastic growth. *Price:* Included in membership dues; $195/year for nonmembers; $350/year for institutions. • *ASIP Bulletin*, quarterly. Newsletter. Contains articles on public policy issues and research opportunities. Includes new members and personnel promotions and appointments. *Price:* Included in membership dues. • *The Journal of Molecular Diagnostics*, quarterly. Journal. Research papers in experimental pathology. Covers cell injury and death, inflammatory reactions, disturbances in circulation, and neoplastic growth. *Price:* Included in membership dues; $195/year for nonmembers; $350/year for institutions. • Membership Directory, annual. **Frmly:** (1992) American Association of Pathologists.

★ 928 ★ American Society for Laser Medicine and Surgery (ASLMS)
2404 Stewart Ave.
Wausau, WI 54401
Phone: (715)845-9283 **Fax:** (715)848-2493
Email: information@aslms.org
Website: http://www.aslms.org
Richard O. Gregory, MD, Sec.

Fnded: 1980. **Mem:** 3,325. **Desc:** Physicians, physicists, and other scientists; nurses, dentists, podiatrists, veterinarians, and other paramedical personnel; technicians and commercial representatives concerned with the medical applications of lasers. Facilitates exchange of information concerning lasers. **Pub:** *Lasers in Surgery and Medicine*, bimonthly. Journal. *Price:* Included in membership dues. • *Official ASLMS Newsletter*, periodic. Newsletter.

★ 929 ★ American Society of Law, Medicine and Ethics (ASLME)
765 Commonwealth Ave., Ste. 1634
Boston, MA 02215
Phone: (617)262-4990 **Fax:** (617)437-7596
Email: info@aslme.org
Website: http://www.aslme.org
Benjamin W. Moulton, Exec. Dir.

Fnded: 1972. **Mem:** 4,500. **Desc:** Physicians, attorneys, health care management executives, nurses, insurance company personnel, members of the judiciary, and others interested in medicolegal relations, health law, and ethics. Purpose is to provide opportunities for continuing education through publications, conferences, and information clearinghouse. Maintains speakers' bureau. **Pub:** *American Journal of Law & Medicine*, quarterly. Journal. Health care law review containing annotations of recent court decisions, book releases, and student case and note section. *Price:* $115 /year for individuals; $215 /year for institutions. • *Journal of Law, Medicine & Ethics*, quarterly. Journal. Reports on medically related legal and social issues such as managed care, genetics, pain management, physician-assisted suicide. Peer reviewed. *Price:* $115 /year for individuals; $215 /year for institutions. **Frmly:** (1911) Massachusetts Society of Examing Physicians; (1973) Massachusetts Society of Law and Medicine; (1993) American Society of Law and Medicine.

★ 930 ★ American Society of Lipo-Suction Surgery (ASLSS)
737 N Michigan Ave., Ste. 820
Chicago, IL 60611-6659
Phone: (312)981-6760 **Fax:** (312)981-6787
Email: info@cosmeticsurgery.org
Website: http://www.cosmeticsurgery.org
Jeffery P. Knezozich, Exec. VP

Fnded: 1982. **Mem:** 400. **Desc:** Surgeons specializing in dermatology, general surgery, gynecology, otolaryngology, plastic and reconstructive surgery, and cosmetic surgery. Trains surgeons in the art and methods of lipo-suction surgery. (Lipo-suction surgery is a procedure wherein fatty tissue is removed from the body by suction. It is not meant to reduce weight but to adjust body contours. Lipo-suction surgery is not currently part of the ordinary medical school curriculum.) Conducts workshops and seminars. **Pub:** *American Journal of Cosmetic Surgery*, quarterly. Journal. *Price:* $128 U.S.; $154 Intl. • *Membership Roster*, annual. Membership Directory. • *Newsline*, bimonthly. Newsletter.

★ 931 ★ American Society of Master Dental Technologists (ASMDT)
PO Box 640248
Oakland Gardens, NY 11364
Phone: (718)347-1239 **Fax:** (718)347-3113
Email: info@asmdt.com
Website: http://www.asmdt.com
Sue Heppenheimer, Exec. Sec.

Fnded: 1976. **Mem:** 125. **Desc:** Dental lab technicians. Dedicated to the upgrading of dental technology. Seeks to provide educational resources such as texts, instructors, and guidance for technicians interested in becoming master dental technologists. Conducts associate and master level courses in conjunction with New York University School of Dentistry, Dept. of Continuing Education.

★ 932 ★ American Society of Maxillofacial Surgeons (ASMS)
4900B S 31st. St.
Arlington, VA 22206-1656
Phone: (703)820-7400 **Fax:** (703)931-4520
Email: admin@maxface.org
Website: http://www.maxface.org
Thomas F. Fise, Exec. Dir.

Fnded: 1947. **Mem:** 385. **Desc:** Professional society of doctors of medicine and doctors of dental surgery who have at least five years of recognized graduate training and experience in maxillofacial surgery. Seeks to stimulate and advance knowledge of the science and art of maxillofacial surgery and improve and elevate the standard of practice. **Pub:** *Maxillofacial News*, quarterly. Newsletter.

★ 933 ★ American Society for Medicine and Science (ASMS)
875 Providence Hwy.
Dedham, MA 02026-6868
Phone: (781)326-7800 **Free:** 800-972-7777
Fax: (781)326-2921
Email: medical@colpittswt.com
Alan M. Krensky, Contact

Desc: Not an association. Organizes medical and scientific conventions worldwide for nonprofit organizations. **Frmly:** (1998) American Academy of Medicine and Science.

★ 934 ★ American Society of Minority Health and Transplant Professionals (ASMHTP)
4208 22nd St. NE
Washington, DC 20018
Phone: (202)269-3853 **Free:** 800-633-6562
Email: webmaster@mail.lifegift.org

Desc: Promotes organ and tissue donation and transplantation among minorities.

★ 935 ★ American Society of Nephrology (ASN)
1725 I St. NW, Ste. 510
Washington, DC 20006
Phone: (202)659-0599 **Fax:** (202)659-0709
Email: email@asn-online.org
Website: http://www.asn-online.org/
Karen Campbell, PhD, Exec. Dir.

Fnded: 1966. **Mem:** 7,500. **Desc:** Nephrologists united for the exchange of scientific information. Seeks to contribute to the education of members and to improve the quality of patient care. Conducts educational courses. Maintains placement service. **Pub:** *Abstracts and Program*, annual. Journal. Program and abstracts for annual scientific meeting. *Price:* $35. • *ASN Highlights*, quarterly. Newsletter. • *Journal of the American Society of Nephrology*, monthly. Journal. • *Member Resource Directory*, periodic. Membership Directory.

★ 936 ★ American Society of Neuroimaging (ASN)
c/o B. Todd Troost, MD
Department of Neurology
Wake Forest University School of Medicine
Medical Center Blvd.
Winston Salem, NC 27157-1068
Phone: (336)716-3429 **Fax:** (336)716-9489
Email: reneemolstad@llmsi.com
Website: http://www.asnweb.org
Todd Troost, VP

Fnded: 1977. **Mem:** 800. **Desc:** Neurologists, neurosurgeons, neuroradiologists, and scientists. Promotes the development of computerized tomography (CT scanning), magnetic resonance imaging (MRI), neurosonology, and other neurodiagnostic techniques for clinical service, teaching, and research. Encourages the collaboration of members to improve techniques through educational programs and scientific research. Holds annual certification exam in MRI and neurosonology. **Pub:** *Journal of Neuroimaging*, quarterly. Journal. • Newsletter, semiannual. **Frmly:** (1980) Society for Computerized Tomography and Neuroimaging.

★ 937 ★ American Society of Neuroradiology (ASNR)
2210 Midwest Rd., Ste. 207
Oak Brook, IL 60523
Phone: (630)574-0220 **Fax:** (630)574-0661
Email: jgantenberg@asnr.org
Website: http://www.asnr.org
James B. Gantenberg, Exec. Dir. /CEO

Fnded: 1962. **Mem:** 2,905. **Desc:** Neuroradiologists who spend at least half of their time practicing neuroradiology. Fosters education, basic science research, and communication in neuroradiology. **Pub:** *American Journal of Neuroradiology*, 10/year. Journal. *Price:* Included in membership dues; $210/year for nonmembers; $270/year for nonmembers outside the U.S.; $90 in training. • *Membership Roll*, annual.

★ 938 ★ American Society of Neurorehabilitation
5841 Cedar Lk. Rd., Ste. 204
Minneapolis, MN 55416
Phone: (952)545-6324 **Fax:** (952)545-6073
Email: reneemolstad@llmsi.com
Website: http://www.asnr.com
Lori Anderson, Exec. Dir.

Fnded: 1990. **Mem:** 500. **Desc:** Neurologists, neurosurgeons, psychiatrists, pediatricians, and other medical professionals interested in disorders of the nervous system. Rehabilitates and monitors patients with neurological disabilities. Acts as an advocate for patients; liases with other neurological organizations. Promotes research. **Pub:** *Neurorehabilitation and Neural Repair*, quarterly. Journal. • Newsletter, semiannual.

★ 939 ★ American Society of Nuclear Cardiology (ASNC)
9111 Old Georgetown Rd.
Bethesda, MD 20814-1699
Phone: (301)493-2360 **Fax:** (301)493-2376
Email: admin@asnc.org
Website: http://www.asnc.org
Ernest V. Garcia, Pres.

Fnded: 1993. **Mem:** 4,100. **Reg. Groups:** 28. **Desc:** Physicians, scientists, technologist, biomedical engineers and health care workers. Seeks to foster optimal delivery of nuclear cardiology services and promote research. Provides continuing medical education opportunities; establishes guidelines and standards for training and practice; provides information on licensure requirements. **Pub:** *Journal of Nuclear Cardiology*, bimonthly. Journal. • Membership Directory, biennial.

★ 940 ★ American Society for Nutritional Sciences (ASNS)
9650 Rockville Pke.
Bethesda, MD 20814-3990
Phone: (301)634-7050 **Fax:** (301)571-1892
Email: sec@asns.org
Website: http://www.asns.org
Richard G. Allison, PhD, Exec. Off.

Fnded: 1928. **Mem:** 3,100. **Desc:** Professional society of nutrition research scientists from universities, government, and industry. **Pub:** *Journal of Nutrition*, monthly. Journal. Peer-reviewed research papers covering all aspects of experimental nutrition, critical reviews, biographies, and commentaries on controversial issues. *Price:* Included in membership dues; $125/year for non-members; $145/year outside the U.S.; $30/year for students. • *Nutrition Notes*, quarterly. Newsletter. Provides information about the Institute's activities as well as topical national and international issues in nutrition. *Price:* Included in membership dues; $30/year for nonmembers. **Frmly:** (1997) American Institute of Nutrition.

★ 941 ★ American Society of Ocularists (ASO)
PO Box 7342
Charlottesville, VA 22906-7342
Phone: (434)973-4066
Email: aso@ocularist.org
Website: http://www.ocularist.org

Fnded: 1957. **Desc:** Technicians specializing in artificial eyes. Promotes research in the field of ophthalmic prosthetics and provides education and support to their members. **Pub:** *Journal of Ophthalmic Prosthetics*, annual. Journal. Published in conjunction with the ABI Professional Publications. *Price:* $35 in North America; $45 outside North America.

★ 942 ★ American Society of Ophthalmic Administrators (ASOA)
4000 Legato Rd., No. 850
Fairfax, VA 22033
Phone: (703)591-2220 **Free:** 800-451-1339
Fax: (703)591-0614
Email: asoa@asoa.org
Website: http://www.asoa.org
Lucy Santiago, Exec. Dir.

Fnded: 1986. **Mem:** 2,000. **Desc:** A division of the American Society of Cataract and Refractive Surgery . Persons involved with the administration of an ophthalmic office or clinic. Facilitates the exchange of ideas and information in order to improve management practices and working conditions. Offers placement services. **Pub:** *A Manager's Survival Guide to Employee Rights.* • *Administrative Eyecare*, quarterly. Magazine. • *Effective Interviews for Every Situation.* • *Federal Employment Law. Price:* $95 for members; $125 for nonmembers. • *Guidebook to Medical Practice Finances Reporting.* • *Managed Care and Contracting.* Manual. *Price:* $150 for members; $225 for nonmembers. • *Marketing Ophthalmology.* • *Ophthalmic Practice Management I & II.* • *Ophthalmic Regulatory Manual.* Handbook. *Price:* $100 for members; $150 for nonmembers. • *Ophthalmic Reimbursement Manual.* Manual. *Price:* $90 for members; $145 for nonmembers. • *Performance Appraisals: The Latest Legal Nightmare.*

★ 943 ★ American Society of Ophthalmic Plastic and Reconstructive Surgery (ASOPRS)
1133 W Morse Blvd., Ste. 201
Winter Park, FL 32789
Phone: (407)647-8839
Website: http://www.asoprs.org
Barbara Beatty, Exec.

Fnded: 1969. **Mem:** 400. **Desc:** Physicians specializing in ophthalmic plastic and reconstructive surgery. Seeks to "advance education, research, and the quality of clinical practice in the fields of plastic and reconstructive surgery involving the eyelids, orbits, and lacrimal system." Facilitates exchange of information among members; conducts fellowship training programs.

★ 944 ★ American Society of Ophthalmic Registered Nurses (ASORN)
PO Box 193030
San Francisco, CA 94119
Phone: (415)561-8513 **Fax:** (415)561-8531
Email: asorn@aao.org
Website: http://www.asorn.org
Lisa Brown, Admin.

Fnded: 1976. **Mem:** 1,100. **Local Groups:** 27. **Desc:** Registered nurses and other ophthalmic medical personnel specializing in the field of ophthalmology. Promotes excellence in ophthalmic nursing for the best and safest care of patients with eye disorders or injuries. Facilitates continuing education through the study, discussion, and exchange of knowledge, experience, and ideas in the field. Represents members' interests before governmental agencies, hospitals, industries, research organizations, technical societies, universities, and other professional associations. Conducts educational programs. **Pub:** *Insight, The Journal of the American Society of Ophthalmic Registered Nurses*, quarterly. Journal. Covers trends in ophthalmology, standards of care, and legislative issues. Includes society news, calendar of events, and chapter news. *Price:* Included in membership dues; $48 nonmember; $64.20 Canada; $60 outside U.S. and Canada. • Ophthalmic Procedures, A Nursing Perspective - Office & Clinic; Ophthalmic Procedures, A Nursing Perspective - Operating Room. Core curriculum for Ophthalmic Nursing; Care & Handling of Ophthalmic Microsurgical Instruments; Standards of Ophthalmic Clinical Nursing Practice. Recommended Practices in Laser Refractive Surgery.

★ 945 ★ American Society of Orthopaedic Physician's Assistants (ASOPA)
6300 N River Rd., Ste. 727
Rosemont, IL 60018-4226
Free: 800-998-6022 **Fax:** (847)823-0536
Email: asopa@aaos.org
Website: http://www.asopa.org

Desc: Physician's assistants who specialize in orthopaedic board-certified surgery. Aims to enhance the quality of medical treatment of orthopaedic patients. Provides information on advances in the field through continuing education, certification, publications and meetings.

★ 946 ★ American Society of Orthopedic Professionals (ASOP)
PO Box 7440
Seminole, FL 33775
Website: http://www.asop.org/

Desc: Promotes continuing education for members and raises awareness of the orthopedic allied professional. **Pub:** Newsletter, bimonthly.

★ 947 ★ American Society of Pain Management Nurses
7794 Grow Dr.
Pensacola, FL 32514
Phone: (850)473-0233 **Free:** 888-342-7766
Fax: (850)484-8762
Email: aspmn@puetzamc.com
Website: http://www.aspmn.org

Fnded: 1990. **Mem:** 1,600. **Nat'l Groups:** 26. **Desc:** Professional nurses. Dedicated to promoting and providing optimal care of patients with pain. **Pub:** *Pain Management*, quarterly. Journal. • *Pathways*, bimonthly. Newsletter.

★ 948 ★ American Society for Parenteral and Enteral Nutrition (ASPEN)
8630 Fenton Ste., No. 412
Silver Spring, MD 20910-3805
Phone: (301)587-6315 **Fax:** (301)587-2365
Email: aspen@nutr.org
Website: http://www.nutritioncare.org
Robin Kriegel, Exec. Dir.

Fnded: 1975. **Mem:** 6,000. **State Groups:** 49. **Desc:** Physicians, dietitians, nurses, pharmacists, and members of the industry. Works to promote quality patient care, education, and research in the field of nutrition and metabolic support in all health care settings. Educates health care professionals. Conducts postgraduate courses and research programs; compiles statistics. **Pub:** *Journal of Parenteral and Enteral Nutrition*, bimonthly. Journal. Includes current research, book reviews, case reports, and citations from world literature. *Price:* Included in membership dues; $45/year for students; $151 for institutions; $90 for individuals. • *Nutrition in Clinical Practice*, bimonthly. Journal. Contains abstracts of literature in the field from other publications, ASPEN news, case reports, legislative news, and a list of new products. *Price:* Included in membership dues; $25/year for students; $88 for institutions; $42 for individuals. • *Nutrition Support Practice Manual.* Manual. Covers product resources. • Monographs. • Also publishes course syllabi on a variety of clinical nutrition topics, self-assessment programs, and reference anthologies.

★ 949 ★ American Society of Pediatric Hematology/Oncology (ASPHO)
4700 W Lake Ave.
Glenview, IL 60025-1485
Phone: (847)375-4716 **Fax:** 877-734-9557
Email: info@aspho.org
Website: http://www.aspho.org
Cynthia Porter, Exec. Dir.

Fnded: 1981. **Mem:** 1,020. **Desc:** Dedicated to promoting optimal care of children and adolescents with blood disorders and cancer by advancing research, education, treatment and professional practice. scientists, and others interested in comprehensive care or research in the field. Purpose is to promote the knowledge, understanding, and management of disorders of the blood and of cancer in children. Seeks improvements in the total care of children with these diseases through the fostering of education and all relevant clinical and basic research. Provides a forum for the exchange of ideas on issues in the field. Cooperates with other societies concerned with the field. scientists, and others interested in comprehensive care or research in the field. Purpose is to promote the knowledge, understanding, and management of disorders of the blood and of cancer in children. Seeks improvements in the total care of children with these diseases through the fostering of education and all relevant clinical and basic research. Provides a forum for the exchange of ideas on issues in the field. Cooperates with other societies concerned with the field. **Pub:** *Directory of Members*, annual. Membership Directory. • *Journal of Pediatric Hematology/Oncology*, 9/year. Journal. • *President's Letter*, bimonthly. Newsletter. News of the society, members, committees, etc, sent via email.

★ 950 ★ American Society of Pediatric Nephrology
c/o James Whitcomb Riley Hospital for Children
Wells Research Center, 2600A
702 Barnhill Dr.
Indianapolis, IN 46202
Phone: (317)278-0854 **Fax:** (317)278-3599
Email: kmatteso@lupul.edu
Website: http://www.aspneph.com
Kristie Matteson, Off. Coord.

Fnded: 1969. **Mem:** 500. **Desc:** Committed to optimal are for children with renal disease and to disseminate advances in the clinical practice and basic science of pediatric nephrology.

★ 951 ★ American Society of Pediatric Neuroradiology
2210 Midwest Rd., Ste. 207
Oak Brook, IL 60523-8205
Phone: (630)574-0220 **Fax:** (630)574-0661
Website: http://www.asnr.org/aspnr/
Ken Cammarata, Bus. Mgr.

Fnded: 1993. **Mem:** 346. **Desc:** Promotes the profession of pediatric neuroradiology.

★ 952 ★ American Society of PeriAnesthesia Nurses (ASPAN)
10 Melrose Ave., Ste. 110
Cherry Hill, NJ 08003-3696
Phone: (856)616-9600 **Free:** 877-737-9696
Fax: (856)616-9601
Email: aspan@aspan.org
Website: http://www.aspan.org
Kevin Dill, CEO

Fnded: 1980. **Mem:** 10,000. **Nat'l Groups:** 3. **Reg. Groups:** 40. **Local Groups:** 100. **Desc:** Nurses practicing in all phases of ambulatory surgery, preanesthesia and post anesthesia care. Promotes quality and cost effective care for patients, their families, and the community through public and professional education, research and standards of practice. Offers continuing education programs. **Pub:** *Breathline*, bimonthly.

Newsletter. • *The Journal of PeriAnesthesia Nursing*, bimonthly. Journal. • Also publishes a manual of forms and the Core Curriculum for Post Anesthesia Nursing Practice. **Frmly:** (2001) American Society of Post Anesthesia Nurses.

★ 953 ★ American Society of Pharmacognosy (ASP)

c/o David J. Slatkin, Treas.
Midwestern University
College of Pharmacy
19555 N 59th Ave.
Glendale, AZ 85308
Phone: (623)572-3500 **Fax:** (623)572-3510
Email: dslatk@arizona.midwestern.edu
Website: http://www.phcog.org
William Gerwick, PhD, Pres.

Fnded: 1959. **Mem:** 1,200. **Desc:** Professional society of pharmacognosists (persons engaged in the study of drugs from a natural origin) and others interested in the plant sciences and natural products. **Pub:** *ASP Newsletter*, quarterly. Newsletter. • *Journal of Natural Products*, monthly. Journal.

★ 954 ★ American Society for Pharmacology and Experimental Therapeutics (ASPET)

9650 Rockville Pike
Bethesda, MD 20814-3995
Phone: (301)634-7060 **Fax:** (301)634-7061
Email: info@aspet.org
Website: http://www.aspet.org
Christine K. Carrico, PhD, Exec. Officer

Fnded: 1908. **Mem:** 4,400. **Desc:** Scientific society of investigators in pharmacology and toxicology interested in research and promotion of pharmacological knowledge and its use among scientists and the public. **Pub:** *Clinical Pharmacology and Therapeutics*, monthly. • *Drug Metabolism and Disposition*, monthly. Journal. • *Journal of Pharmacology and Experimental Therapeutics*, monthly. Journal. • *Molecular Interventions*, monthly. Journal. • *Molecular Pharmacology*, monthly. • *Pharmacological Reviews*, quarterly. • *Pharmacologist*, quarterly. Brochures. • Brochures. • Also distributes listings of schools of medicine and pharmacy.

★ 955 ★ American Society for Pharmacy Law (ASPL)

1224 Centre W, Ste. 200B
Springfield, IL 62704
Phone: (217)391-0219 **Fax:** (217)793-0041
Email: bobplye@assn-srvs.com
Website: http://www.aspl.org
Pamela Tolson, CAE, Interim Exec. Dir.

Fnded: 1974. **Mem:** 1,000. **Desc:** Pharmacists, lawyers, and students. Purposes are to: further legal knowledge; communicate accurate legal information to pharmacists; foster knowledge and education pertaining to the rights and duties of pharmacists; distribute information of interest to members; provide a forum for exchange of information pertaining to pharmacy law. **Pub:** *Pharmacy Law Annual*, annual. Membership Directory. Contains legal pharmacy law articles. • *RX Ipsa Loquitur*, monthly.

★ 956 ★ American Society for Philosophy Counseling and Psychotherapy (ASPCP)

c/o Dr. Kenneth F.T. Cust
Central Missouri State University
Center for Applied & Professional Ethics
Warrensburg, MO 64093
Phone: (660)543-4268 **Fax:** (660)543-8544
Email: kencust@philosophical-services.com
Website: http://www.aspcp.org
Dr. Kenneth F.T. Cust, Interim Exec. Dir.

Desc: Promotes both the professional and academic sides of philosophical counseling and philosophy as a private practice profession. **Pub:** Newsletter.*Price:* included in membership dues.

★ 957 ★ American Society of Plastic Surgeons and Plastic Surgery Education Foundation (ASPRS)

444 E Algonquin Rd.
Arlington Heights, IL 60005
Phone: (847)228-9900 **Free:** 888-4-PLASTIC
Fax: (847)228-9131
Website: http://www.plasticsurgery.org
James Wells, MD, Pres.

Fnded: 1931. **Mem:** 5,000. **Reg. Groups:** 29. **State Groups:** 35. **Desc:** Professional society of plastic surgeons. Works in cooperation with the Plastic Surgery Educational Foundation to promote optimal care for plastic surgery patients through research, service, and education activities. Sponsors public/patient education program, clinical symposia, and professional development workshops. Acts as a liaison between members and government and medical organizations. Conducts charitable activities; maintains speakers' bureau; compiles statistics. **Pub:** *American Society of Plastic and Reconstructive Surgeons Combined Roster*, annual. Directory. Administrative, member alpha/geo, bylaws and related organization listing. *Price:* First copy free to members; $35 additional copies; $750 nonmembers. • *Journal of Plastic and Reconstructive Surgery*, monthly. Journal. Includes research reports and book reviews. *Price:* Free to members; $303 for nonmembers. • *Plastic Surgery News*, monthly. Tabloid including information on employment opportunities and current events. *Price:* Free to members; $75 for nonmembers. **Frmly:** (2000) American Society of Plastic and Reconstructive Surgeons.

★ 958 ★ American Society of Plastic Surgical Nurses (ASPSN)

E Holly Ave.
Box 56
Pitman, NJ 08071
Phone: (856)256-2340 **Fax:** (856)589-7463
Email: asprsn@ajj.com
Rick Grimes, Exec. Dir.

Fnded: 1975. **Mem:** 1,830. **Reg. Groups:** 4. **State Groups:** 30. **Desc:** Registered nurses, licensed practical nurses, and licensed vocational nurses working with plastic surgeons or interested in plastic and reconstructive nursing. Objectives are: to enhance leadership qualities of nurses in the field of plastic surgery; to increase the skills, knowledge, and understanding of personnel in plastic surgery nursing through continuing education; to study existing practices and new developments in the field; to encourage participation and interest in professional organizations; to cooperate with others in the profession. **Pub:** *ASPRS News*, bimonthly. Newsletter. *Price:* available to members only. • *ASPRSN Membership Directory*, annual. Membership Directory. • *Core Curriculum for Plastic and Reconstructive Surgical Nursing.* • *Plastic Surgical Nursing*, quarterly. Journal. **Frmly:** (2001) American Society of Plastic and Reconstructive Surgical Nurses.

★ 959 ★ American Society of Podiatric Dermatology (ASPD)

c/o Dr. Steven Berlin
1901 Sulfer Spring Rd.
Baltimore, MD 21227-0378
Fax: (410)247-7329
Dr. Richard Chase, Contact

Fnded: 1914. **Mem:** 260. **Desc:** Doctors of podiatric medicine with demonstrated expertise in foot dermatology (100); candidates for D.P.M. degrees in colleges of podiatric medicine (400). Fosters research in podiatric dermatology; supports college-affiliated study groups; conducts semiannual continuing education programs; sponsors student affiliates. Maintains speakers' bureau; conducts research programs; sponsors competitions. **Pub:** Monographs. • Newsletter, quarterly. Includes book reviews, information on new products, and obituaries. *Price:* Free. **Frmly:** (1973) American Board of Chiropodical Dermatology.

★ 960 ★ American Society of Podiatric Medical Assistants (ASPMA)

2124 S Austin Blvd.
Cicero, IL 60804
Phone: (708)863-6303 **Free:** 888-88ASPMA
Fax: (708)863-5375
Email: mmalone@aspma.org
Website: http://www.aspma.org
Sandra Lohrentz, PMAC, Exec. Dir.

Fnded: 1964. **Mem:** 1,350. **Nat'l Groups:** 1. **Reg. Groups:** 14. **Desc:** Podiatric assistants. Purposes are to hold educational seminars and to administer certification examinations. **Pub:** Journal, quarterly. *Price:* Free to members.

★ 961 ★ American Society of Podiatric Medicine (ASPM)

c/o Dr. Warren L. Simmonds
1111 Kane Concourse Ste. 111
Miami, FL 33154-2039
Dr. Warren L. Simmonds, Sec.

Fnded: 1944. **Mem:** 110. **Desc:** Promotes research in podiatry. Sponsors postgraduate courses and presents scientific programs at annual meeting. Focuses on aging and diabetes. Maintains collection of material presented by candidates for fellowship. Maintains speakers' bureau; conducts research programs. **Frmly:** American Academy of Chiropody.

★ 962 ★ American Society of Podiatrists and Chiropractors (ASPC)

PO Box 35215
Chicago, IL 60707-0215
Phone: (708)453-0080 **Fax:** (708)453-0083
Email: aspc@rentamark.com
Website: http://www.rentamark.com/aspc/
L. Stroller, Contact

Fnded: 1975. **Mem:** 58,989. **Nat'l Groups:** 1. **Desc:** Podiatrists and chiropractors. Seeks to increase members' public visibility and professional influence. Provides trademark licensing and product and service endorcement services to support members' activities. A platform to network Podiatrists and Chiropractors with patients on the net. **Pub:** *ASPC Journal*. Journal. Online journal. *Price:* included in membership dues.

★ 963 ★ American Society of Preventive Oncology (ASPO)

c/o Dr. Richard R. Love
256 WARF Bldg.
610 Walnut St.
Madison, WI 53705
Phone: (608)263-9515 **Fax:** (608)263-4497
Email: hasahel@facstaff.wisc.edu
Website: http://www.aspo.org
Heidi Sahel, Exec. Dir.

Fnded: 1976. **Mem:** 420. **Desc:** Professionals in clinical, educational, or research disciplines concerned with the field of cancer prevention. Promotes the exchange of information and ideas relating to cancer prevention and the causes of human cancer, including environmental exposures and lifestyles; encourages research. Works to implement programs for the prevention and early detection of cancer. Evaluates programs intended to reduce cancer incidence, mortality, and morbidity. Encourages professional and public education regarding cancer prevention. Maintains communication and liaison with other oncological societies. Provides expert advice to scientific, public health, and governmental organizations and agencies. **Pub:** *Cancer Epidemiology, Biomarkers, and Prevention*, monthly. Journal. *Price:* included in membership dues.

★ 964 ★ American Society of Psychoanalytic Physicians (ASPP)

4804 Jasmine Dr.
Rockville, MD 20853
Phone: (301)929-1470 **Fax:** (301)929-1491
Email: cheesick@casbah.acns.nwu.edu

Website: http://pubweb.northwestern.edu/~chessick/aspp.htm
Janice S. Wright, Exec. Dir.

Fnded: 1985. **Mem:** 275. **Desc:** Physicians, psychiatrists, and psychoanalysts united to: foster a wider understanding and utilization of psychoanalytic concepts; provide an opportunity to study psychoanalytic theory from all schools of thought; encourage clinical and didactic research; promote social and professional fraternalism among members in the field and maintain good relationships with other professional groups. Offers lectures on therapy that combines psychoanalytic orientation with other disciplines. **Pub:** *The Bulletin*, semiannual. Bulletin. *Price:* Included in membership dues.

★ 965 ★ American Society of Psychopathology of Expression (ASPE)

c/o Dr. Irene Jakab
74 Lawton St.
Brookline, MA 02446
Phone: (617)738-9821 **Fax:** (617)975-0411
Dr. Irene Jakab, Pres.

Fnded: 1964. **Mem:** 137. **Desc:** Psychiatrists, psychologists, art therapists, sociologists, art critics, artists, social workers, linguists, educators, criminologists, writers, and historians. At least two-thirds of the members must be physicians. Fosters collaboration among specialists in the United States who are interested in the problems of expression and in the artistic activities connected with psychiatric, sociological, and psychological research. Disseminates information about research and clinical applications in the field of psychopathology of expression. Sponsors consultations, seminars, and lectures on art therapy. **Pub:** *American Society of Psychopathology of Expression–Newsletter*, semiannual. Newsletter. Includes obituaries and book reviews. *Price:* Included in membership dues. • *Art Media as a Vehicle of Communication. Price:* $33. • *The Personality of the Therapist.* • *The Role of the Imagination in the Healing Process.* • *Stress Management Through Art. Price:* $18. • Proceedings, annual.

★ 966 ★ American Society of Radiologic Technologists (ASRT)

15000 Central Ave. SE
Albuquerque, NM 87123
Phone: (505)298-4500 **Free:** 800-444-2778
Fax: (505)298-5063
Email: customerservices@asrt.org
Website: http://www.asrt.org
Joan Parsons, Exec. VP, Operations

Fnded: 1920. **Mem:** 100,000. **Reg. Groups:** 10. **State Groups:** 50. **Desc:** Professional society of diagnostic radiography, radiation therapy, ultrasound, and nuclear medicine technologists. Advances the science of radiologic technology; establishes and maintains high standards of education; evaluates the quality of patient care; improves the welfare and socioeconomics of radiologic technologists. Operates ASRT Education and Research Foundation, which provides educational materials to radiologic technologists. **Pub:** *ASRT Scanner*, monthly. Magazine. Includes calendar of events, member profiles, state affiliate news, educational opportunities, and research updates. *Price:* Included in membership dues. • *Radiation Therapist*, semiannual. Journal. *Price:* Included in membership dues; $25/year for nonmembership in U.S.; $50/year for nonmembers outside U.S. • *Radiologic Technology*, bimonthly. Journal. Includes advertisers and cumulative annual author and title indexes, book reviews, literature abstracts, and calendar of events. *Price:* Included in membership dues; $49/year for nonmembers; $75/year for nonmembers outside the U.S.; $29.50/year for students. **Frmly:** (1934) American Society of Radiographers; (1964) American Society of X-Ray Technicians.

★ 967 ★ American Society for Reconstructive Surgery (ASRM)

20 N Michigan Ave., Ste. 700
Chicago, IL 60602
Phone: (312)456-9579 **Fax:** (312)782-0553
Email: contact@microsurg.org
Website: http://www.microsurg.org
Erika Monroe Kane, Exec. Dir.

Desc: Healthcare professionals. Strives to facilitate information flow for reconstructive microsurgery professionals. **Pub:** Newsletters. • Membership Directory.

★ 968 ★ American Society of Regional Anesthesia and Pain Medicine (ASRA)

2209 Dickens Rd.
PO Box 11086
Richmond, VA 23230-1086
Phone: (804)282-0010 **Fax:** (804)282-0090
Email: asra@societyhq.com
Website: http://www.asra.com
James C. Eisenach, MD, Pres.

Fnded: 1974. **Mem:** 8,000. **Desc:** Physicians and research Ph.D.s. Conducts educational workshops. Sponsors annual refresher course. **Pub:** *ASRA Newsletter*, quarterly. Newsletter. *Price:* Included in membership dues. • *Regional Anesthesia and Pain Medicine*, bimonthly. Journal. *Price:* Included in membership dues. **Frmly:** (2002) American Society of Regional Anesthesia and Pain Practice.

★ 969 ★ American Society for Reproductive Medicine (ASRM)

1209 Montgomery Hwy.
Birmingham, AL 35216-2809
Phone: (205)978-5000 **Fax:** (205)978-5005
Email: asrm@asrm.com
Website: http://www.asrm.com/
Dr. Robert W. Rebar, MD, Exec. Dir.

Fnded: 1944. **Mem:** 10,500. **Desc:** Gynecologists, obstetricians, urologists, reproductive endocrinologists, veterinarians, research workers, and others interested in reproductive health in humans and animals. Seeks to extend knowledge of all aspects of fertility and problems of infertility and mammalian reproduction; provides a rostrum for the presentation of scientific studies dealing with these subjects. Offers patient resource information and placement service. **Pub:** *American Fertility Society–Membership Directory*, biennial. Membership Directory. Arranged alphabetically and geographically. *Price:* Included in membership dues. • *Fertility and Sterility*, monthly. Journal. Includes book reviews and announcements of meetings, courses, services, and employment opportunities. *Price:* Included in membership dues; $135/year nonmembers; $220/year institutions. • *Fertility News*, quarterly. Newsletter. Includes new member and regional postgraduate course listings. *Price:* Included in membership dues. • Also publishes syllabi used for postgraduate courses. **Frmly:** American Fertility Society; (1966) American Society for the Study of Sterility.

★ 970 ★ American Society of Spine Radiology (ASSR)

2210 Midwest Rd., Ste. 207
Oak Brook, IL 60523-8205
Phone: (630)574-0220 **Fax:** (630)574-0661
Email: kcammarata@asnr.org
Website: http://www.asnr.org/assr
Ken Cammarata, Bus. Mgr.

Fnded: 1993. **Mem:** 500. **Desc:** Radiologists. Provide support and exchange ideas and information concerning spine radiology. Hold meetings, lectures and discussions. **Pub:** *The Myelon*, quarterly. Newsletter.

★ 971 ★ American Society for Stereotactic and Functional Neurosurgery (ASSFN)

c/o Andres Lozano MD, PhD
STE 2-433 McLaughlin Pav.
399 Bathurst St., Western Div.
Toronto, ON, Canada
Phone: (416)603-6200 **Fax:** (416)603-5298
Email: lozano@uhnres.utoronto.ca

Fnded: 1968. **Mem:** 300. **Lang(s):** English. **Desc:** Neurosurgeons practicing stereotactic surgery united to promote communication in the field. (Stereotactic surgery utilizes a technique for inserting delicate instruments in precise areas of the nervous system.) Compiles statistics. Plans to establish museum. **Pub:** *Stereotactic and Functional Neurosurgery*, bimonthly. Journal. **Frmly:** (1972) International Society for Research in Stereoencephalotomy, American Branch.

★ 972 ★ American Society for the Study of Orthodontics (ASSO)

70-15 164th St.
Flushing, NY 11365
Phone: (718)591-6411 **Fax:** (718)591-5424
Dr. Milton Bloch, Pres.

Fnded: 1945. **Mem:** 100. **Desc:** Members of the American Dental Association or other societies, with special interest in orthodontics but not limited to those who practice in the field. Purposes are to: preserve the highest ideals in orthodontics and in dentistry; encourage and assist the diffusion of orthodontic knowledge to all dentists who include orthodontics as an integral part of their health service or limit their practice to orthodontics; institute an intensive program of fundamental and advanced studies and guidance for its members in theoretical, didactic, and applied orthodontics; encourage the orthodontic departments of university dental schools to provide both short and extended courses in orthodontics; to establish discussion and clinical study groups throughout the U.S. Conducts lectures, panel discussions, postgraduate seminars, table clinics, and consultation service. **Pub:** *ASSO Newsletter*, quarterly. Newsletter. • *International Journal of Orthodontics*, 3/year. Journal. **Frmly:** (1962) New York Society for the Study of Orthodontics.

★ 973 ★ American Society for Surgery of the Hand (ASSH)

6300 N River Rd., Ste. 600
Rosemont, IL 60018-4256
Phone: (847)384-8300 **Fax:** (847)384-1435
Email: info@assh.org
Website: http://www.assh.org
Mark Anderson, Exec. Dir.

Fnded: 1946. **Mem:** 2,000. **Desc:** Surgeons specializing in surgery of the hand. Funds research in the field of hand surgery. Sponsors educational programs. Maintains a website that offers information on common hand problems **Pub:** *Essentials of Hand Surgery.* Book. • *Global Service Information for Hand Surgery.* Manual. • *Hand Surgery Guide to the ICD-9-CM-Second Edition.* Book. • *Hand Surgery Update.* Book. • *Hand Surgery Update 2.* Booklet. • *The Journal of Hand Surgery*, bimonthly. Journal. • *Patient Education Brochures.* Brochures. Series of 16 brochures with information for patients. • *Self-assessment Examination in Hand Surgery*, annual.

★ 974 ★ American Society for Therapeutic Radiology and Oncology (ASTRO)

12500 Fair Lakes Cir., Ste. 375
Fairfax, VA 22033-3882
Phone: (703)502-1550 **Free:** 800-962-7876
Fax: (703)502-7852
Email: webmaster@astro.org
Website: http://www.astro.org
Laura I. Thevenot, Exec. Dir.

Fnded: 1958. **Mem:** 7,200. **Desc:** Physicians who limit their practice to radiation therapy; associate members are scientists and health care personnel who have a major interest "in furthering the aims of the society"; junior members are residents who have completed one year of training in radiation therapy. Aim is "to extend the benefits of radiation therapy to patients with cancer or other disorders, to advance its scientific basis, and to provide for the education and professional fellowship of its members." **Pub:** *ASTRO News*, quarterly. Magazine. *Price:* Included in membership dues. • *The International Journal of Radiation Oncology, Biology, and Physics*, 15/year. Journal. **Frmly:** (1983) American Society of Therapeutic Radiologists.

★ 975 ★ American Society of Transplant Surgeons
1020 N Fairfax St., No. 200
Alexandria, VA 22314-1537
Phone: (703)684-5990 **Free:** 888-990-2787
Fax: (703)684-6303
Email: shaked@mail.med.upenn.edu
Arthur J. Matas, MD, Sec.

Fnded: 1975. **Mem:** 850. **Desc:** Surgeons specializing in transplantation. Promotes and encourages education and research, especially in transplantation surgery; collaborates with public and private organizations; participates and assists in developing programs and coordinates efforts on projects that will benefit organ recipients. **Pub:** *Chimera*, quarterly. • *Transplantation*, monthly.

★ 976 ★ American Society of Transplantation (ASTA)
17000 Commerce Pkwy., Ste. C
Mount Laurel, NJ 08054
Phone: (856)439-9986 **Fax:** (856)439-9982
Email: ast@ahint.com
Website: http://www.a-s-t.org/
Susan J. Nelson, MD, Exec. Dir.

Fnded: 1982. **Mem:** 1,300. **Desc:** Promotes and encourages education and research with respect to transplantation medicine and immunology; provides a forum for exchange of scientific information related to transplantation across solid organ specialties. **Pub:** *AST Newsletter*, quarterly. Newsletter. *Price:* Included in membership dues. • *AST Primer on Transplantation*. • *AST Washington Round-Up*, monthly.

★ 977 ★ American Society of Tropical Medicine and Hygiene (ASTMH)
60 Revere Dr., Ste. 500
Northbrook, IL 60062
Phone: (847)480-9592 **Fax:** (847)480-9282
Email: astmh@astmh.org
Website: http://www.astmh.org
Kevin Hacke, Exec. Dir.

Fnded: 1951. **Mem:** 3,000. **Desc:** Professional society of physicians and scientists interested in tropical medicine and hygiene, including the areas of arbovirology, entomology, medicine, nursing, parasitology, immunology, infectious disease, and travelers' health. **Pub:** *American Journal of Tropical Medicine and Hygiene*, monthly. Journal. *Price:* included in membership dues; $400/yr North America; $450/yr outside North America. • *Health Hints for the Tropics*. • *Tropical Medicine and Hygiene News*, bimonthly.

★ 978 ★ American Society of Veterinary Ophthalmology (ASVO)
1416 W Liberty Ave.
Stillwater, OK 74075
Phone: (405)377-4388
Email: membership@asvo.org
Website: http://www.asvo.org/
Dr, Virginia Schultz, D.V.M., Sec. -Treas.

Fnded: 1957. **Mem:** 250. **Desc:** Veterinarians with a special interest in ophthalmology (the science of the eye and its diseases). Sponsors research proposal competition. **Pub:** Directory, annual. • Newsletter, periodic. • Proceedings, annual.

★ 979 ★ American Speech Language Hearing Association
10801 Rockville Pike
Rockville, MD 20852
Free: 800-638-8255 **Fax:** (301)897-7355
Email: actioncenter@asha.org
Website: http://www.asha.org
Frederick Samphor, Exec. Dir.

Fnded: 1919. **Desc:** Consumers of speech, language, and hearing services and their families. Provides educational and referral information on speech, language, and hearing disabilities. **Pub:** Pamphlets.Covers a wide range of communication disorders and development of speech, language, and hearing in children. **Frmly:** (1922) American Association for the Hard of Hearing; (1935) American Federation of Organizations for the Hard of Hearing; (1946) American Society for the Hard of Hearing; (1966) American Hearing Society; (1974) National Association of Hearing and Speech Agencies; (1999) National Association for Hearing and Speech Action.

★ 980 ★ American Spinal Injury Association (ASIA)
345 E Superior, Rm. 1436
Chicago, IL 60611
Phone: (312)238-1242 **Fax:** (312)238-0869
Email: mars@northwestern.edu
Website: http://www.asia-spinalinjury.org
Marianne G. Kaplan, Exec. Sec.

Fnded: 1973. **Mem:** 500. **Desc:** Medical doctors and Allied Health Care professionals who have been trained in the care of spinal injury patients and who are either actively engaged in the field and acknowledged to be competent by their peers or who have made a significant contribution to the advancement of the basic sciences or one of the clinical fields of practice as they are applicable to the treatment of spinal cord injury. Purposes are to: develop knowledge and investigation of the causes, cure, and prevention of spinal injury and related trauma; pursue excellence in spinal injury patient care; promote and exchange ideas between professionals in the field; standardize medical terminology in spinal cord injury; foster and encourage basic research in the field; develop teaching and educational material; foster education of the medical profession and laity in the prevention and proper management of spinal injury, including the necessity for specialized regional spinal injury centers, provision for educational and vocational training, removal of architectural barriers, and promotion of a society more sensitive to the physically inconvenienced individual, including adequate housing and transportation; establish criteria for centers and/or systems of total spinal injury management so as to provide optimal care of the spinal injured person. Conducts annual scientific sessions. Sponsors G. Heiner Sell Distinguished Lectureship. **Pub:** *International Standards of Neurological Classification of Spinal Injuries*. A teaching package which includes videos and manuals.

★ 981 ★ American Sports Medicine Association Board of Certification (ASMA)
660 W Duarte Rd.
Arcadia, CA 91007
Phone: (626)445-1978 **Fax:** (625)574-1999
Email: americansportsmedicine@hotmail.com
Joe S. Borland, Bd. Chm.

Fnded: 1978. **Mem:** 1,400. **Desc:** Verifies and qualifies the educational competency of active athletic trainers and sports medicine trainers for certification. Establishes competency standards of education required for the prevention and care of athletic injuries and sports medicine. Maintains speakers' bureau. **Pub:** *ASMA News*, quarterly. Newsletter. *Price:* Included in membership dues. • *Special Bulletin*, periodic. Bulletin. • *Why be a Sport Medicine Trainer*. Brochure.

★ 982 ★ American Sports Medicine Institute (ASMI)
1313 13th St. S
Birmingham, AL 35205
Phone: (205)918-0000 **Fax:** (205)918-0800
Website: http://www.asmi.org/

Desc: Committed to improving understanding, prevention, and treatment of sports-related injuries through research and education. **Pub:** *American Journal of Sports Medicine*. Journal. • *Sports Engineering*.

★ 983 ★ American Stroke Association
National Center
7272 Greenville Ave.
Dallas, TX 75231
Free: 888-478-7653
Website: http://www.strokeassociation.org

Fnded: 1998. **Desc:** Committed to reducing disability and death from stroke through research, education, fundraising, and advocacy. **Pub:** *Stroke Connection*, bimonthly. Magazine. *Price:* included in membership dues. • *Stroke: Journal of the American Heart Association*. Journal.

★ 984 ★ American Student Dental Association (ASDA)
211 E Chicago Ave., Ste. 1160
Chicago, IL 60611
Phone: (312)440-2795 **Free:** 800-621-8099
Fax: (312)440-2820
Email: asda@asdanet.org
Website: http://www.asdanet.org/
Cynthia Airhart, Exec. Dir.

Fnded: 1971. **Mem:** 15,000. **Local Groups:** 54. **Desc:** Predoctoral and postdoctoral dental students organized to improve the quality of dental education and to promote the accessibility of oral health care. Additional membership categories include predental, postdoctoral, international and associate. Represents dental students before legislative bodies, organizations, and associations that affect dental students. Disseminates information to dental students. Sponsors advocacy program and "externships" inc luding Washington National Helath Policy, Chicago Administrative, State Governm ent Affairs, and Research. **Pub:** *ASDA Handbook*, annual. Handbook. Contains annual reference volumes, with information on applying to dental school, financial aid, membership benefits, post-doctoral opportunities. *Price:* $25 in U.S.; $40 outside U.S. • *ASDA News*, monthly. • *Dentistry*, quarterly. • Also publishes a series of guides to postgraduate programs in dentistry and reprints of National Board Examinations. **Frmly:** (1971) Student American Dental Association.

★ 985 ★ American Sudden Infant Death Syndrome Institute (ASIDSI)
2480 Windy Hill Rd., Ste. 380
Marietta, GA 30067
Phone: (770)612-1030 **Free:** 800-232-SIDS
Fax: (770)612-8277
Email: prevent@sids.org
Website: http://www.sids.org
Dr. Betty McEntire, Exec. Dir.

Fnded: 1983. **Reg. Groups:** 1. **Desc:** Participants include health care professionals, researchers, and laypeople concerned about sudden infant death syndrome (SIDS); families who have lost babies to SIDS. Works to identify the cause and cure of SIDS. Promotes infant health through research, clinical services, education, and support for SIDS families. Conducts research on siblings of SIDS babies; sponsors research programs seeking the cause and cure of SIDS. Conducts seminars for health care professionals and laypeople; maintains speakers' bureau. **Pub:** Brochures. • Also publishes research results. **AKA:** American SIDS Institute.

★ 986 ★ American Surgical Association (ASA)
c/o Robert P. Jones, Jr., Ed.D.
13 Elm St.
Manchester, MA 01944-1314
Phone: (978)526-8330 **Fax:** (978)526-7521
Email: asa@prri.com
Carlos A. Pellegrini, MD, Sec.

Fnded: 1880. **Mem:** 949. **Desc:** Surgeons organized to promote the science and art of surgery. Bestows medallion for scientific achievement. **Pub:** *Annals of Surgery*, monthly. • *Transactions*, annual.

★ 987 ★ American Syringomyelia Alliance Project (ASAP)
PO Box 1586
Longview, TX 75606-1586
Phone: (903)236-7079 **Free:** 800-ASAP-282
Email: info@asap.org

Website: http://www.syringo.org
Patricia Maxwell, Oper. Admin.

Fnded: 1988. **Mem:** 4,000. **Nat'l Groups:** 1. **Desc:** Seeks to increase awareness of and promote research on syringomyelia, a rare spinal disorder. Conducts fundraising activities and children's services. **Pub:** *Syringomyelia Connections*, bimonthly. Newsletter. • *What Is Syringomyelia.* Brochure.

★ 988 ★ American Therapeutic Recreation Association (ATRA)

1414 Prince St., Ste. 204
Alexandria, VA 22314
Phone: (703)683-9420 **Fax:** (703)683-9431
Email: membership@atra-tr.org
Website: http://www.atra-tr.org/atra.htm
Ann D. Huston, Exec. Dir.

Fnded: 1984. **Mem:** 3,750. **Reg. Groups:** 25. **Desc:** Therapeutic recreation professionals and students; interested others. (Therapeutic recreation is often referred to as recreational therapy and uses treatment modalities to improve the physical, mental, and emotional functions of persons with illnesses or disabling conditions.) Promotes the use of therapeutic recreation in hospitals, mental rehabilitation centers, physical rehabilitation centers, senior citizen treatment centers, and other public health facilities. Conducts discussions on certification and legislative and regulatory concerns that affect the industry. Sponsors seminars and workshops; conducts research. **Pub:** *Annual in Therapeutic Recreation*, annual. Journal. Published in conjunction with American Association for Leisure and Recreation. *Price:* Included in membership dues. • *ATRA Newsletter*, bimonthly. Newsletter. *Price:* Included in membership dues. • *Employment Update*, monthly. Features employment and internship opportunities for therapeutic recreation professionals. *Price:* Included in membership dues. • *Evaluation of Therapeutic Recreation through Quality Assurance.* • *Risk Management in Therapeutic Recreation.*

★ 989 ★ American Thoracic Society (ATS)

61 Broadway
New York, NY 10006
Phone: (212)315-8600 **Fax:** (212)315-8651
Email: nblack@thoracic.org
Website: http://www.thoracic.org
Carl Booberg, Exec. Dir.

Fnded: 1905. **Mem:** 13,300. **State Groups:** 43. **Desc:** International Educational and scientific Society for respiratory and critical care medicine. Seeks to prevent and fight respiratory diseases through research, education and patient advocacy. **Pub:** *American Journal of Respiratory and Critical Care Medicine*, semimonthly. Journal. Includes society news, book reviews, and case reports. *Price:* Included in membership dues. • *American Journal of Respiratory Cell and Molecular Biology*, monthly. Journal. *Price:* included in membership dues. • *ATS News*, monthly. Newsletter. Includes summary of health legislation and annual index. *Price:* Included in membership dues. • Membership Directory, biennial. **Frmly:** (1939) American Sanatorium Association; (1960) American Trudeau Society.

★ 990 ★ American Thyroid Association (ATA)

6066 Leesburg Pike, Ste. 650
Falls Church, VA 22041
Phone: (703)998-8890 **Free:** 800-THY-ROID
Fax: (703)998-8891
Email: admin@thyroid.org
Website: http://www.thyroid.org
Barbara Smith, Exec. Dir.

Fnded: 1923. **Mem:** 650. **Desc:** Endocrinologists, surgeons, pathologists, radiologists, and research scientists interested in the thyroid gland and its disorders. **Pub:** *Thyroid*, periodic. Journal. • Membership Directory, annual. **Frmly:** (1948) American Association for the Study of Goiter; (1961) American Goiter Association.

★ 991 ★ American Tinnitus Association (ATA)

PO Box 5
Portland, OR 97207-0005
Phone: (503)248-9985 **Free:** 800-634-8978
Fax: (503)248-0024
Email: Tinnitus@ata.org
Website: http://www.ata.org
Cheryl McGinnis, Exec. Dir.

Fnded: 1971. **Mem:** 18,000. **Nat'l Groups:** 1. **State Groups:** 42. **Desc:** Dedicated to tinnitus research and educating patients, and professionals through conferences, books, brochures, videos and the quarterly journal Tinnitus Today. ATA is the national champion of tinnitus awareness, prevention and treatment. Under its guiding principles - Education, Advocacy, Research and Support - the ATA offers prevention programs in schools, urges governmental and private organizations to support hearing conservation, funds the nation's brightest researchers and facilitates self-help groups around the country. **Pub:** *Coping With the Stress of Tinnitus.* Brochure. • *If You Have Tinnitus - The First Steps To Take.* Brochure. • *Information About Tinnitus.* Brochure. • *Noise - Its Effects on Hearing and Tinnitus.* Brochure. • *Tinnitus Bibliography.* Bibliography. • *Tinnitus Today*, quarterly, March, July, September, December. Journal. Includes book reviews, calendar of events, research updates, and statistics. *Price:* $35/year. • *Tinnitus Treatments - What's New, What Works.* Brochure. • *Understanding Tinnitus - Advice for Family & Friends.* Brochure.

★ 992 ★ American Transplant Association (ATA)

980 N Michigan Ave., Ste. 1400
Chicago, IL 60611
Free: 800-494-4527 **Fax:** 800-494-4527
Email: ata@americantransplant.org
Website: http://www.americantransplant.org/
John Butorac, Exec. Dir.

Fnded: 1995. **Mem:** 1,200. **Desc:** Provides patient-oriented education, services and support to transplant patients and their families and friends. **Pub:** *A Patient's Guide to Transplantation.* Book. *Price:* included in membership dues; $10 non-member. • *reOrganized!*, monthly. Newsletter. *Price:* included in membership dues. • *Transcend*, 3/year. Newsletter. For contributors and supporters.

★ 993 ★ American Trauma Society (ATS)

8903 Presidential Pky., Ste. 512
Upper Marlboro, MD 20772
Phone: (301)420-4189 **Free:** 800-556-7890
Fax: (301)420-0617
Email: atstrauma@aol.com
Website: http://www.amtrauma.org
John W. Ashworth, III, Exec. VP/COO

Fnded: 1968. **Mem:** 3,000. **State Groups:** 22. **Desc:** Physicians, nurses, EMT personnel, other healthcare professionals, institutions, corporations, and interested individuals. Seeks to: prevent trauma situations; improve trauma care through professional and paraprofessional education; educate the public through campaigns and dissemination of information. **Pub:** *Promotional Media Resource Catalog.* Catalog. • *Traumagram Newsletter*, 4/year. Newsletter. Includes prevention activities, news on the annual meeting, and legislative and research updates. *Price:* Included in membership dues for institutions. • *TraumaView Newsletter.* Newsletter. *Price:* Included in membership dues.

★ 994 ★ American Urogynecologic Society (AUGS)

2025 M St. NW, Ste. 800
Washington, DC 20036
Phone: (202)367-1167 **Fax:** (202)367-2167
Email: augs@dc.sba.com
Website: http://www.augs.org
Steven C. Kemp, Exec. Dir.

Fnded: 1979. **Mem:** 1,000. **Desc:** Physicians and health professionals actively engaged in providing quality urogynecologic care to women. Dedicated to research and education in urogynecology and to improved care for women with lower urinary tract disorders. **Pub:** *Quarterly Report*, quarterly. Newsletter. Describe Case Reports-Articles. *Price:* $30/subscription.

★ 995 ★ American Urological Association (AUA)

1120 N Charles St.
Baltimore, MD 21201
Phone: (410)727-1100 **Fax:** (410)223-4370
Email: aua@auanet.org
Website: http://www.auanet.org
G. James Gallagher, Exec. Dir.

Fnded: 1902. **Mem:** 13,000. **Reg. Groups:** 8. **Desc:** Professional society of physicians specializing in urology. Provides education and formulation of health casre policy for urologists. **Pub:** *AUA News*, monthly. Magazine. • *Health Policy Brief*, monthly. Newsletter. • *Journal of Urology*, monthly. Journal. • *Membership Roster*, biennial.

★ 996 ★ American Venous Forum (AVF)

c/o Robin Hoyle, J.D.
13 Elm St.
Manchester, MA 01944
Phone: (978)526-8330 **Fax:** (978)526-8330
Email: avf@prri.com
Website: http://www.venous-info.com
Robin Hoyle, Exec. Dir.

Fnded: 1988. **Mem:** 225. **Desc:** Board-certified vascular surgeons. Provides a forum intent on improving the quality care to patients suffering venous and lymphatic disorders. Assists in research and offers guidelines for clinical trials.

★ 997 ★ American Veterinary Chiropractic Association

442154 E 140 Rd.
Bluejacket, OK 74333
Phone: (918)784-2231 **Fax:** (918)784-2675
Email: amvetchiro@aol.com
Website: http://www.animalchiropractic.org/
Paul D. Rowan, DVM, Contact

Fnded: 1989. **Mem:** 350. **Desc:** Professional association, sets animal chiropractic education standards, board examinations, legislative issues.

★ 998 ★ American Veterinary Dental Society (AVDS)

200 4th Ave. North, Ste. 900
Nashville, TN 37219
Phone: (615)251-0082 **Free:** 800-332-2837
Fax: (615)254-7047
Email: avds@walkermgt.com
Dee Ann Walker, Exec. Sec.

Fnded: 1976. **Mem:** 1,000. **Reg. Groups:** 1. **Desc:** Dentists, veterinarians, and others dedicated to the scientific advancement of dentistry for animals. Conducts continuing education seminars on veterinary dentistry; serves as a forum for exchange of experience and ideas. **Pub:** *Journal of Veterinary Dentistry*, quarterly. Journal. Includes association news and clinical reports. *Price:* Included in membership dues. • *Membership List*, periodic.

★ 999 ★ American Veterinary Medical Association (AVMA)

1931 N Meacham Rd., Ste. 100
Schaumburg, IL 60173-4360
Phone: (847)925-8070 **Free:** 800-248-2862
Fax: (847)925-1329
Email: avmainfo@avma.org
Website: http://www.avma.org
Bruce Little, DVM, Contact

Fnded: 1863. **Mem:** 67,000. **State Groups:** 52. **Local Groups:** 433. **Desc:** Professional society of veterinarians. Conducts educational and research programs. Provides placement service. Sponsors American Veterinary Medical Association Foundation (also known as AVMF Foundation) and Educational Commission for Foreign Veterinary Graduates. Compiles statistics. Accredits veterinary medical education programs and veterinary technician education programs. **Pub:** *American Journal of Veterinary Research*, monthly. Journal. • *AVMA Animal Welfare Forum*, annual. Book. • *AVMA Convention Notes*, annual. • *AVMA Disaster Preparedness & Response Guide*. Handbook. • *Economic Report on Veterinarians and Veterinary Practices*, semiannual. Report. • *Journal of the AVMA*, semimonthly. Journal. • *US Pet Ownership and Demographic Sourcebook*, semiannual. Book. • Directory, annual. **Frmly:** (1988) United States Veterinary Medical Association.

★ 1000 ★ American Veterinary Society of Animal Behavior (AVSAB)

c/o Steven Feldman
1535 Rugby Cir.
Thousand Oaks, CA 91360
Email: avsabe@yahoo.com
Website: http://www.avma.org/avsab/
Steve Feldman, Sec. /Treas.

Fnded: 1975. **Mem:** 440. **Desc:** Veterinarians and veterinary students. Promotes inquiry and research into animal behavior. Seeks to advance ethological knowledge regarding the care and utilization of captive, domesticated, and free-living animals. Promotes and facilitates the exchange of information among those concerned with animal behavior and well-being; encourages discussion on veterinary aspects of animal behavior and the publication of materials in the field. **Pub:** *American Veterinary Society of Animal Behavior*, quarterly. Newsletter. *Price:* Included in membership dues; $30/year for nonmembers. **Frmly:** (1984) American Society of Veterinary Ethology.

★ 1001 ★ American Wheelchair Bowling Association (AWBA)

6264 North Andrews Ave.
Fort Lauderdale, FL 33309-2129
Phone: (727)734-0023
Email: bowlawba@juno.com
Website: http://www.awba.org/
George H. Snyder, Exec. Sec. -Treas.

Fnded: 1962. **Mem:** 600. **Reg. Groups:** 12. **Desc:** Male and female athletes with permanent disabilities who are confined to wheelchairs. To organize and promote wheelchair bowling and regulate rules. Provides information about wheelchair bowling. Conducts state and national wheelchair bowling tournaments. Maintains hall of fame and museum; compiles statistics. **Pub:** *The 11th Frame*, bimonthly. • *Wheelchair Bowling*. Book.

★ 1002 ★ American Women's Hospitals Service Committee of AMWA (AWHS/AMWA)

801 N Fairfax St., Ste. 400
Alexandria, VA 22314
Phone: (703)838-0500 **Fax:** (703)549-3864
Email: info@amwa-doc.org
Website: http://www.amwa-doc.org
Marie P. Glanz, Dir. Special Programs

Fnded: 1917. **Desc:** A project of the American Medical Women's Association Foundation. International philanthropic medical relief service that supports medical and hospital services conducted by women doctors and nurses for the care of the indigent sick and prevention of disease. Currently supports nine clinics in the U.S. and abroad, including Haiti and India. **Frmly:** (1959) American Women's Hospitals; (1982) American Women's Hospitals Service.

★ 1003 ★ Americans for Better Care of the Dying

4125 Albemarle St. NW, Ste. 210
Washington, DC 20016
Phone: (202)895-9485 **Fax:** (202)895-9484
Email: info@abcd-caring.org
Website: http://www.abcd-caring.org
Joanne Lynn, Pres.

Fnded: 1997. **Mem:** 500. **Desc:** Strives to improve the experience of the last phase of life for all Americans. Advocates the interests of patients and families. Works to improve communication between providers and patients.

★ 1004 ★ Americans for Free Choice in Medicine (AFCM)

1525 Superior Ave., Ste. 100
Newport Beach, CA 92663
Phone: (949)645-2622 **Fax:** (949)645-4624
Email: mail@afcm.org
Website: http://www.afcm.org

Fnded: 1993. **Desc:** Patients, Medicare recipients, physicians, nurses and health care professionals, insurance industry professionals, pharmacists and pharmaceutical industry professionals, financial services professionals, businessmen, employee benefits professionals, and hospital staff. Promote the philosophy of individual rights, personal responsibility and free market economics in the health care industry. Sponsors educational programs, lectures and town hall meetings, as well as "The Andrew Lewis Show", a weekly radio show.

★ 1005 ★ Americans for Medical Progress Educational Foundation (AMPEF)

908 King St., Ste. 301
Alexandria, VA 22314-3067
Phone: (703)836-9595 **Free:** 800-426-7872
Fax: (703)836-9594
Email: info@amprogress.org
Website: http://www.amprogress.org
Jacqueline Calnan, Pres.

Fnded: 1990. **Mem:** 3,000. **Desc:** Works to ensure the public supports the role of animals in medical research. Supports scientists' ability to search for cures and treatments for injury, illness, and disease. **Pub:** *News and Notes*, quarterly. Newsletter. *Price:* Included in membership dues. • Brochures. • Also, publishes bimedical research fact sheets and other educational materials.

★ 1006 ★ Americans for Nonsmokers' Rights American Nonsmokers' Rights Foundation (ANR)

2530 San Pablo Ave., Ste. J
Berkeley, CA 94702
Phone: (510)841-3032 **Fax:** (510)841-3060
Email: anr@no-smoke.org
Website: http://www.no-smoke.org
Cynthia Hallett, Exec. Dir.

Fnded: 1976. **Mem:** 15,000. **Desc:** Seeks to protect the rights of nonsmokers in the workplace and other public settings. Maintains American Nonsmokers' Rights Foundation, which promotes smoking prevention, educational programs, and public education about secondhand smoke issues. **Pub:** *ANR Materials*. • *ANR Update*, quarterly. Newsletter. Provides information on issues important to nonsmokers. *Price:* included in membership dues. • *Clearing the Air*. Book. • *Secondhand Smoke*. Manual. • *Teens Take Action Guidebook: How to Butt In*. Book. • *Tobacco Smoke and the Non-Smoker*. Brochure. **Frmly:** (1976) California Group Against Smoking Pollution; (1986) Californians for Nonsmokers' Rights; (2001) Americans for Nonsmokers' Rights.

★ 1007 ★ Americans With Disabilities Act (ADA)

10765 SW 104 St.
Miami, FL 33176
Phone: (305)271-0012 **Fax:** (305)273-1221
Email: ergobob@consultant.com
Website: http://www.rehabserv.com
Robert L. Lessne, PhD, Contact

Fnded: 1990. **Mem:** 100. **Desc:** Individuals and organizations united to ensure compliance with the Americans With Disabilities Act of 1992. Compiles statistics; sponsors competitions; maintains speakers' bureau; and operates a museum with cones for visually impaired individuals. **Pub:** *ADA Compliance Kit*. Booklet. • *ADA Compliance Sourcebook*.

★ 1008 ★ America's Athletes with Disabilities (AAD)

National Headquarters
8630 Fenton St., Ste. 920
Silver Spring, MD 20910
Phone: (301)589-9042 **Free:** 800-238-7632
Fax: (301)589-9052
Website: http://www.americasathletes.org/

Desc: Strives to promote and sponsor sports, recreation, fitness and leisure events for children and adults with physical disabilities. Maintains a National Athlete Registry. **Pub:** *Victory Voice*. Newsletter.

★ 1009 ★ America's Blood Centers

725 15th St. NW, Ste. 700
Washington, DC 20005
Phone: (202)393-5725 **Free:** 888-USB-LOOD
Fax: (202)393-1282
Email: bthaler@americasblood.org
Website: http://www.americasblood.org
Brooke Thaler, Contact

Fnded: 1962. **Mem:** 75. **Desc:** Independent, nonprofit, federally licensed blood centers serving defined geographic areas that collectively provide about half of the nation's volunteer donor blood supply. Purpose is to ensure an optimal supply of blood, blood components, and blood derivatives and the development of a comprehensive range of the highest quality blood services to meet the needs of the American people. Compiles data and statistics; conducts research concerning organizational, administrative, fiscal, and operational phases of blood banking; establishes liaison and conducts cooperative activities of all kinds with national, regional, and local associations, groups, and organizations having a relationship of any kind to the drawing, processing, storing, or distribution of blood. **Pub:** *ABC Membership Directory*, semiannual. Membership Directory. • *ABC Newsletter*, weekly. Newsletter. Includes calendar of events and list of employment opportunities. *Price:* Free to members; $480/year in North America; $576/year outside North America; $336/year email. **Frmly:** (1971) Community Blood Bank Council; (1998) Council of Community Blood Centers.

★ 1010 ★ Amputee Coalition of America (ACA)

900 E Hill Ave., Ste. 285
Knoxville, TN 37915-2568
Phone: (865)524-8772 **Free:** 888-AMP-KNOW
Fax: (865)525-7917
Email: acainfo@amputee-coalition.org
Website: http://www.amputee-coalition.org
Pat Isenberg, COO

Fnded: 1989. **Desc:** Information clearinghouse and cooperative program of the Centers for Disease Control & Prevention and the Amputee Coalition of America. Serves people who have limb differences, their families, and friends, healthcare providers, and the general public. Provides information on adapting to limb loss, directs referrals to groups/agencies and programs. Offers informative resources, technical assistance and education for consumer and professional groups. **Pub:** *First Step - A Guide For Adapting To Limb Loss*, biennial. Magazine. *Price:* Shipping & handling costs only. • *inMotion*, bimonthly. Magazine. • Books. • Videos.

★ 1011 ★ Amyotrophic Lateral Sclerosis Association (ALSA)

27001 Agoura Rd. Suite 150
Calabasas Hills, CA 91301-5104
Phone: (818)880-9007 **Free:** 800-782-4747
Fax: (818)880-9006
Email: alsinfo@alsa-national.org
Website: http://www.alsa.org
Michael W. Havlicek, Pres. /CEO

Fnded: 1985. **Mem:** 250,000. **Reg. Groups:** 135. **Desc:** Patients; relatives and friends of patients;

doctors, neurologists, physical therapists, nurses, and professional organizations dedicated to finding the cause, prevention, and cure for amyotrophic lateral sclerosis (ALS). Offers help and information to ALS patients and their families. Funds ALS-specific research at major medical institutions. Works with other agencies, including the government, to increase their involvement on a priority basis in ALS research. Conducts patient meetings. **Pub:** *Amyotrophic Lateral Sclerosis Association–Link*, quarterly. Newspaper. Includes book reviews and research and chapter news. *Price:* Free. • Also publishes fact sheets and pamphlets on ALS and patient care. **AKA:** ALS Association.

★ 1012 ★ Amyotrophic Lateral Sclerosis Society of Canada (Societe Canadienne de la Sclerose Laterale Amyotrophique)

265 Yorkland Blvd., Ste. 300
Toronto, ON, Canada M2J 1S5
Phone: (416)497-2267 **Free:** 800-267-4257
Fax: (416)497-1256
Email: alscanada@als.ca
Website: http://www.als.ca

Fnded: 1977. **Nat'l Groups:** 1. **Reg. Groups:** 11. **Lang(s):** English, French. **Desc:** Health care professionals; individuals with amyotrophic lateral sclerosis (ALS) and their families. Promotes advancement in the diagnosis of ALS and seeks to find a cure for the disease; works to improve the quality of life for people with ALS and their families. Provides support and services to people with ALS and their families: sponsors research and educational programs. **Pub:** *Coast to Coast*, bimonthly. Newsletter. Contains items of interest to the ALS Canada Network.

★ 1013 ★ Anaesthetic Research Society (ARS)

Univ. Department of Anaesthesia & Intensive Care
Queen's Medical Centre
Nottingham NG7 2UH, United Kingdom
Phone: 44 115 9709229 **Fax:** 44 115 9700739
Email: ravi.mahajan@nottingham.ac.uk
Website: http://www.ars.ac.uk/

Fnded: 1958. **Mem:** 660. **Lang(s):** English. **Desc:** Facilitates the presentation of members' research in anesthesiology (clinical or experimental, completed or in progress). **Pub:** *Proceedings*, 3/year. Journal. Included in the *British Journal of Anaesthesia*.

★ 1014 ★ Anatomical Society (AS) (Anatomische Gesellschaft — AG)

c/o Wolfgang Kuhnel, M.D.
Ratzeburger Allee 160
D-23538 Lubeck, Germany
Phone: 49 451 5004030 **Fax:** 49 451 5004034
Email: kuehnel@anat.mu-luebeck.de
Website: http://www.anat.mu-luebeck.de/anatges.html

Fnded: 1886. **Mem:** 1,056. **Lang(s):** English, French, German. **Desc:** Anatomists, histochemists, histologists, biologists. **Pub:** *Annals of Anatomy*. Journal. • *Verhandlungen der Anatomischen Gesellschaft*, annual. Proceedings.

★ 1015 ★ Anatomical Society of Great Britain and Ireland

c/o Prof. J.P. Fraher
Department of Anatomy
University College
Cork, Ireland
Phone: 353 21 4902115 **Fax:** 353 21 4902246
Email: j.fraher@ucc.ie
Website: http://www.anatsoc.org.uk

Fnded: 1887. **Mem:** 650. **Lang(s):** English. **Desc:** Individuals involved in anatomical science. Promotes development and advancement in anatomy and related science through research and education. Offers program for graduate students. **Pub:** *Journal of Anatomy*, 12/year. Journal. Contains research information in the anatomical sciences.

★ 1016 ★ Anatomical Society of Paris (Societe Anatomique de Paris)

45, rue des Saints-Peres
F-75270 Paris, France
Phone: 33 1 42862259 **Fax:** 33 1 42863366
Email: josiane.bargain@biomedicale.univ-paris5.fr
Website: http://www.biomedicale.univ-paris5.fr/anat/

Fnded: 1802. **Mem:** 120. **Lang(s):** French. **Desc:** Promotes exchange between members on all subjects concerning anatomy; fosters studies on anatomy.

★ 1017 ★ Anatomical Society of Southern Africa (ASSA) (Anatomiese Vereniging van Suider-Afrika)

c/o Prof. H. B. Groenewald
Faculty of Veterinary Science
Private Bag X04
Onderstepoort 0110, Republic of South Africa
Phone: 27 12 5298247 **Fax:** 27 12 5298320
Email: hgroenew@op.up.acza

Fnded: 1969. **Mem:** 200. **Lang(s):** Afrikaans, English. **Desc:** Individuals from 5 countries interested in the study of anatomy. Aims to: promote the study of anatomy; encourage anatomical research; represent anatomists of Southern Africa at the international level. Organizes seminars and workshops. Bestows awards. **Pub:** *Newsletter of the ASSA*, semiannual. Newsletter. • *Proceedings*, annual.

★ 1018 ★ Andean Rural Health Care (ARHC)

224 E Martin St.
Raleigh, NC 27601-1818
Phone: (828)452-3544 **Fax:** (828)452-7790
Email: sarale@haywood.main.nc.us
David Shanklin, Exec. Dir.

Desc: Volunteers united to improve the health care available to people living in rural areas of Bolivia. Collaborates with Bolivian health organizations and government agencies to develop and expand health care services. Trains indigenous people to operate and maintain public health services. Conducts research to determine health care needs in rural Bolivia. Maintains home visitation programs; sponsors volunteer work teams from the U.S. to support Bolivian health care services.

★ 1019 ★ Andorran College of Dentists

La Llacuna, 2, 2n
Andorra, Andorra
Phone: 376 824118 **Fax:** 376 824229
Email: coea@andorra.ad

Fnded: 1991. **Mem:** 45. **Desc:** Represents dentists and the field of dentistry in Andorra.

★ 1020 ★ Anesthesia Patient Safety Foundation (APSF)

4246 Colonial Park Dr.
Pittsburgh, PA 15227-2621
Phone: (412)882-8040
Email: info@apsf.org
Website: http://gasnet.med.yale.edu/apsf/

Fnded: 1984. **Desc:** Promotes safer anesthesia, fosters investigations to provide understanding of preventable anesthetic injuries. **Pub:** *Anesthesia Patient Safety, A Modern History*. Book. Contains substantive articles from the APSF Newsletter. *Price:* $25 includes postage. • Newsletter, quarterly. Contains information on issues pertaining to anesthesia safety.

★ 1021 ★ Aneurysm Outreach Inc. (AOI)

17222 Hwy. 929
Prairieville, LA 70769
Phone: (225)622-1577 **Fax:** (225)622-1577
Email: AOI@alink.org
Website: http://www.alink.org
Sheila G. Arrington, Pres.

Fnded: 1999. **Nat'l Groups:** 1. **Local Groups:** 1. **Desc:** Volunteers, family and friends affected or at risk. Provide a support network. Promote public awareness; funds research through advocacy and tax-deductible donations. Coordinates a free community abdominal aorta aneurysm screening program quarterly in the Baton Rogue area and participates in area health fairs.

★ 1022 ★ Anglo-European College of Chiropractic (AECC)

13-15 Parkwood Rd.
Bournemouth BH5 2DF, United Kingdom
Phone: 44 1202 436200 **Fax:** 44 1202 436312
Email: aecc@aecc.ac.uk
Website: http://www.aecc.ac.uk

Fnded: 1965. **Mem:** 25. **Lang(s):** English. **Desc:** Chiropractic practitioners, educators, and students. Seeks to advance the study, teaching, and practice of chiropractic. Facilitates communication among members; sponsors research and educational programs. **Pub:** Newsletter, semiannual.

★ 1023 ★ Animal Assisted Therapy Foundation (Therapet)

PO Box 1696
Whitehouse, TX 75791-1696
Email: therapet@juno.com
Website: http://www.therapet.com/

Desc: Facilitates the use of animals in healing and rehabilitation of acute and chronically ill individuals.

★ 1024 ★ Animal Care College

Ascot House
High St.
Ascot SL5 7JG, United Kingdom
Phone: 44 1344 628269 **Fax:** 44 1344 622771
Email: admin@rtc-associates.freeserve.co.uk
Website: http://www.corsini.co.uk/animalcare/

Fnded: 1980. **Desc:** Open to all those who have gained certification in course recognized by the Animal Care College. To improve the quality of training in and standards of animal care. **Pub:** *Dogs Monthly*, monthly. Magazine.

★ 1025 ★ Animal Health Distributors Association (AHDA)

Gable Court
8 Parsons Hill
Hollesley
Woodbridge IP12 3RB, United Kingdom
Phone: 44 1394 410444 **Fax:** 44 1394 410455
Email: info@ahda.org.uk
Website: http://www.ahda.org.uk

Fnded: 1985. **Mem:** 150. **Desc:** Agricultural Merchants who are registered and qualified to distribute animal medicines to farmers and horse owners together with several wholesalers of such products. Aims to prevent the EC legislating members out of business and to ensure an appropriate number of animal medicines are classified for distribution by registered distributors and that new products are so classified. **Pub:** Newsletter, monthly.

★ 1026 ★ Animal Health Foundation (AHF)

3615 Bassett Rd.
Pacific, MO 63069
Website: http://www.animalhealthfoundation.com

Fnded: 1984. **Mem:** 1,000. **Desc:** Individuals interested in finding the causes, treatments, and cure for the crippling equine disease laminitis/founder syndrome. (Laminitis is an inflammation of the laminae, the semi-rigid internal supporting structures of the horse's foot; founder is the crippling result of laminitis in which the coffin bone in the horse's foot puts pressure on the sole of the foot, and sometimes actually penetrates the sole.) These ailments affect horses of any age or breed, and are counted by the AHF as the second ranking disease leading to the need to euthanize horses. Supports extensive research and collects a range of related data. **Pub:** *AHF Newsletter*, periodic. Newsletter. • Brochure.

★ 1027 ★ Animal Health Information Specialists (AHIS)

c/o Tom Roper
RCVS Library and Information Service
Belgravia House
62-64 Horseferry Rd.
London SW1P 2AF, United Kingdom
Phone: 44 20 72222021 **Fax:** 44 20 72222004
Email: t.roper@rcvs.org.uk
Website: http://www.ahis.org

Desc: Fosters cooperation and exchange among individuals interested in animal health information.

★ 1028 ★ Animal Health Trust

Lanwades Park
Kentford
Newmarket CB8 7UU, United Kingdom
Phone: 44 8700 502424 **Fax:** 44 8700 502425
Email: info@aht.org.uk
Website: http://www.aht.org.uk

Fnded: 1942. **Reg. Groups:** 15. **Desc:** Aims to push back the frontiers of veterinary science. Develops new technology and knowledge for the better diagnosis, prevention and cure of disease. Provides a referral service for veterinary surgeons in practice. **Pub:** *AHT News*, quarterly. Newsletter. Update on the work of the Trust. • *Annual Review*, annual. Annual Report. • *Scientific Report*, triennial. Report.

★ 1029 ★ Animals First

153 E 18th St., Ste. 22
New York, NY 10003
Phone: (212)505-1073
John Zeigler, Exec. Dir.

Fnded: 1972. **Nat'l Groups:** 1. **Desc:** Seeks to demonstrate to nations that their interests are best served by putting the rights of animals first. Believes that if the needs of animals are addressed as the first priority, a saner and more humane civilization would then be closer to eradicating overpopulation and environmental destruction. **Frmly:** (2000) Speak Out!.

★ 1030 ★ Anne Sullivan Foundation for Deafblind

40 Lower Drumcondra Rd.
Dublin 9, Ireland
Phone: 353 1 8300562 **Fax:** 353 1 8603199
Email: info@annesullivan.ie
Website: http://www.annesullivan.ie

Fnded: 1989. **Desc:** Irish national agency formed to help people who are both deaf and blind, and particularly those who are also low-functioning. Operates a residential center, a home for life, for young congenital deaf and blind people. Provides outreach services to other agencies.

★ 1031 ★ Anorexia Bulimia Nervosa Association (ABNA)

Woodwards House, 1st Fl.
47-49 Waymouth St.
Adelaide, SA 5000, Australia
Phone: 61 8 82121644 **Fax:** 61 8 82127991
Email: mail@abnasa.asn.au

Fnded: 1983. **Desc:** Individuals with eating disorders, their families, and friends. Promotes prevention and effective treatment of eating disorders

★ 1032 ★ Anorexia Nervosa and Related Eating Disorders (ANRED)

PO Box 5102
Eugene, OR 97405
Phone: (541)344-1144 **Free:** 800-931-2237
Email: jarinor@rio.com
Website: http://www.anred.com
Dr. J. Bradley Rubel, Pres.

Fnded: 1979. **Mem:** 20,000. **Desc:** Provides comprehensive information about anorexia nervosa, bulimia, binge eating disorder, and other lesser known eating disorders. eating, and compulsive exercising. eating, and compulsive exercising. **Pub:** Pamphlets. • Also publishes resource material and fact sheets.

★ 1033 ★ Anthroposophical Medical Association

35 Park Rd.
London NW1 6XT, United Kingdom

Fnded: 1968. **Desc:** Acts as a professional association of registered doctors practicing in the field of anthroposophical medicine.

★ 1034 ★ Anthroposophical Nurses Association of America

1923 Geddes Ave.
Ann Arbor, MI 48104
Phone: (734)761-5172 **Fax:** (734)761-6617
Email: artemisia@anthroposophy.org
Website: http://www.artemisia.net/anaa/
Rise Smythe-Freed, Pres.

Fnded: 1985. **Mem:** 90. **Desc:** Seeks to further the practice of anthroposophical nursing in the U.S. (Anthroposophy is a 20th century body of knowledge centering on human development.) Encourages nurses to apply their knowledge of humankind to nursing practices. Promotes members' continued education. **Pub:** Newsletter, annual. *Price:* $12.

★ 1035 ★ Anti-Tuberculosis Association Afghanistan Programme (ATA)

35/E Canal Rd.
University Town
Peshawar, Afghanistan
Phone: 92 91 840126

Fnded: 1990. **Desc:** Works to control the spread of tuberculosis in Afghanistan. Operates tuberculosis clinics. Makes available medications.

★ 1036 ★ Antigua and Barbuda Association of Persons with Disabilities (ABAPD)

PO Box W123
Woods Centre
Saint Johns, Antigua-Barbuda
Phone: (268)461-7260 **Fax:** (268)461-7260
Email: info@abapd.org
Website: http://www.abapd.org/

Fnded: 1995. **Desc:** Promotes the rights and needs of persons with disabilities; provides support and services where possible. Sponsors Essay Competition to raise awareness.

★ 1037 ★ Antigua Planned Parenthood Association (APPA)

Bishopgate St.
PO Box 419
Saint Johns, Antigua-Barbuda
Phone: (268)462-1187 **Fax:** (268)560-2297
Email: appa@candw.ag

Fnded: 1970. **Mem:** 52. **Lang(s):** English. **Desc:** Promotes family planning and maternal and infant health care as a way to improve the quality of life for individuals living in Antigua Barbuda. Seeks to reduce the number of unwanted pregnancies and abortions. Provides contraceptive services for men and women. Sponsors programs on family plannng and sex education. Acts as an advocate for family planning on the national level. Conducts research. **Pub:** *Family Fare*. Newsletter. Covers reproductive health issues, family planning and family life education issues.

★ 1038 ★ Aplastic Anemia and MDS International Foundation (AAFA)

PO Box 613
Annapolis, MD 21404-0613
Free: 800-747-2820 **Fax:** (410)867-0240
Email: help@aamds.org
Website: http://www.aplastic.org
Marilyn Baker, Exec. Dir.

Fnded: 1983. **Mem:** 15,000. **Desc:** Serves as an information source for persons with aplastic anemia and myelodysplastic syndromes. (Aplastic anemia is an often fatal disease in which the bone marrow fails to produce new blood cells.) Provides free educational materials and medical information. Financially supports research. Hosts annual International Patient Conferences presenting the latest in medical research findings and networking opportunities for patients and their families. **Pub:** *Aplastic Anemia and MDS International Foundation*, quarterly. Newsletter. Provides information on aplastic and other bone marrow failure dise s. *Price:* Free. • *Aplastic Anemia: MDS Basic Explanations*, periodic. Describes the course of the disease and current treatment options. Includes glossary of medical terms. *Price:* Free. • *Communicating Patient and Family Needs to the Medical Care Team.* • *Families Coping with Hospital Life*, periodic. • Booklets. • Brochures. • Newsletter, quarterly. **Frmly:** (1999) Aplastic Anemia Foundation of America.

★ 1039 ★ Aplastic Anemia and Myelodysphasia Association of Canada (AAAC)

22 Aikenhead Rd.
Etobicoke, ON, Canada M9R 2Z3
Phone: (416)235-0468 **Free:** 888-840-0039
Email: aamac@canada.com
Website: http://www.aplastic.ualberta.ca

Fnded: 1987. **Mem:** 1,200. **Reg. Groups:** 3. **State Groups:** 3. **Lang(s):** English, French. **Desc:** Individuals with aplastic anemia or myelodysplasia; health care professionals, family members of people with aplastic anemia or myelodysplasia, and others with an interest in this condition. Promotes research into the cause, treatment, and cure of aplastic anemia and myelodysplasia. Conducts charitable and educational programs. **Pub:** *Aplastic Anemia & Myelodysplasia Association of Canada Newsletter*, quarterly. Newsletter. **Frmly:** (1999) Aplastic Anemia of Canada.

★ 1040 ★ Applied Research Ethics National Association (ARENA)

132 Boylston St., 4th Fl.
Boston, MA 02116
Phone: (617)423-4112 **Fax:** (617)423-1185
Email: info@arena.org
Website: http://www.arena.org
Joan Rachlin, Exec. Dir.

Fnded: 1986. **Mem:** 1,500. **Reg. Groups:** 6. **Desc:** Professionals concerned with ethical issues related to humans and animal subject research. Promotes the protection of humans and the humane care and treatment of animals. Sponsors national and regional meetings, disseminates research information and assists with the development of regional networks.

★ 1041 ★ Applied Vision Association

c/o The College of Optometrists
42 Craven St.
London WC2N 5NG, United Kingdom
Phone: 44 20 78396000 **Fax:** 44 20 78396800
Email: ndebrunner@college-optometists.org
Website: http://www.dmu.ac.uk/ava/

Fnded: 1975. **Mem:** 240. **Desc:** Works to advance, promote, develop and improve the study and knowledge of human vision including medical problems relating to vision. **Pub:** *Bulletin of the Applied Vision Association*, quarterly. Newsletter.

★ 1042 ★ Arab Thoracic Association

c/o Dr. Abdullah Al-Qudah
PO Box 13255
Amman, Jordan
Phone: 962 6 5512606 **Fax:** 962 6 5512616
Email: arab_thoracic_association@hotmail.com
Website: http://www.arabthoracic.org/

Fnded: 1997. **Nat'l Groups:** 14. **Desc:** Provides forum for information exchange for Arab thoracic physicians and surgeons; works to unify the teaching of thoracic medicine and surgery in the Arab world;

provides training. **Pub:** *Arab Thoracic Association Journal*. Journal.

★ 1043 ★ Archaeus Project (AP)
PO Box 7079
Kamuela, HI 96743
Phone: (808)887-1280 **Fax:** (808)885-9013
Email: dstillings@archaeusproject.com
Website: http://www.fivemtn.org
Dennis Stillings, Dir.

Fnded: 1981. **Desc:** Business, medical, academic, and engineering professionals, scientists, psychologists, psi researchers, and interested others. Investigates the effects of ordinary and altered states of consciousness on conditions of health and disease; studies the relationships between the mind, body, and matter, and the implications of these relationships for medicine. Sponsors lecture series, seminars, and workshops; conducts cyberphysiology (science of self-regulation in physiology) research. **Pub:** *Healing Island*, quarterly. Journal. Contains items on health care, health care costs, and the integration of alternative with mainstream medicine, Hawaii as a health/healing destination. *Price:* Free on request at present. • *Project 2010*. Monograph. • *Tape Catalog*. Catalog.

★ 1044 ★ L'Arche Australia (AA)
PO Box 312
Burwood, NSW 1805, Australia
Phone: 61 2 97475858 **Fax:** 61 2 97475858
Website: http://www.larche.net/

Fnded: 1989. **Mem:** 9. **Local Groups:** 3. **Lang(s):** English. **Desc:** Individuals and corporate members. Advocates a holistic approach to human development through the establishment of L'Arche communities for intellectually disabled individuals in neighborhood homes. Promotes a Christian perspective in L'Arche communities in Australia and abroad. **Pub:** *L'Arche Australia Newsletter*, quarterly. Provides news of Australian L'Arche communities. • *Letters of L'Arche*, quarterly. Journal. Includes articles about life in L'Arche communities and issues concerning persons with intellectual disabilities.

★ 1045 ★ Argentine Academy of Surgery (Academia Argentina de Cirugia)
Marcelo T. de Alvear 2415
1122 Buenos Aires, Argentina
Phone: 54 1 9253649
Fnded: 1911.

★ 1046 ★ Argentine Association of Biology and Nuclear Medicine (Asociacion Argentina de Biologia y Medicina Nuclear)
Bulnes 1878 6 to.23
1425 Buenos Aires, Argentina
Fax: 54 11 48272340
Email: correo@aabymn.org.ar
Website: http://www.aabymn.org.ar
Fnded: 1963.

★ 1047 ★ Argentine Association of Mycology (Asociacion Argentina de Micologia)
Paraguay 2155
1121 Buenos Aires, Argentina
Phone: 54 1 9627274 **Fax:** 54 1 9625404
Fnded: 1960.

★ 1048 ★ Argentine Orthopedic and Traumatology Association (A.A.O.T.) (Asociacion Argentina de Ortopedia y Traumatologia)
Vicente Lopez 1878
1128 Buenos Aires, Argentina
Phone: 54 1 48012320 **Fax:** 54 1 48017703
Fnded: 1936.

★ 1049 ★ Argentine Society of Endocrinology and Metabolism (Sociedad Argentina de Endocrinologia y Metabolismo)
Diaz Velez 3889
Buenos Aires, Argentina
Fnded: 1941.

★ 1050 ★ Argentine Society of Experimental Pharmacology (Asociacion Argentina de Farmacologia Experimental — SAFE)
c/o Dr. Luis Malgor
Catedra de Farmacologia
Facultad de Medicina
Universidad National de Nordeste
3400 Morenco, Argentina
Phone: 54 3783 432902 **Fax:** 54 3783 432902
Email: lmalgor@med.unne.edu.ar

Mem: 325. **Desc:** Promotes experimental pharmacology in Argentina.

★ 1051 ★ Argentine Society of Gastroenterology (Sociedad Argentina de Gastroenterologia)
Santa Fe 1171
1059 Buenos Aires, Argentina
Phone: 54 1 411633
Fnded: 1927.

★ 1052 ★ Argentine Society of Hematology (SAH) (Sociedad Argentina de Hematologia)
Av Angel Gallardo 899
1405 Buenos Aires, Argentina
Fnded: 1948.

★ 1053 ★ Argentine Society of Opthalmology (Sociedad Argentina de Oftalmologia)
Santa Fe 1171
1059 Buenos Aires, Argentina
Phone: 54 1 2410392
Fnded: 1920.

★ 1054 ★ Argentine Society of Pediatrics (Sociedad Argentina de Pediatria)
Coronel Diaz 1971
1425 Buenos Aires, Argentina
Phone: 54 1 8242063
Fnded: 1911.

★ 1055 ★ Argentine Society of Physiological Sciences (SACF) (Sociedad Argentina de Ciencias Fisiologicas)
Solis 453
1078 Buenos Aires, Argentina
Phone: 54 1 3831110 **Fax:** 54 1 3810323
Fnded: 1950.

★ 1056 ★ Argentine Society of Psychology (Sociedad Argentina de Psicologia)
Callao 435
1022 Buenos Aires, Argentina
Phone: 54 1 4323760
Fnded: 1930.

★ 1057 ★ Argentine Society of Psychosomatic Obstetrics and Gynaecology
c/o Lic. Silvina Ramos
Cedes
Sanchez de Bustamante 27
1173 Buenos Aires, Argentina
Fax: 54 11 8620805
Email: arcoiris@clacso.edu.ar
Website: http://www.ispog.org

Desc: Promotes the study of psychobiological and psychosocial, ethical and cross-cultural problems in the fields of obstetrics and gynaecology, women's health and reproductive health; facilitates the dissemination of new information in these fields. **Pub:** *Journal of Psychosomatic Obstetrics and Gynecology*. Journal.

★ 1058 ★ Argentinian Association of Dermatology (AAD) (Asociacion Argentina de Dermatologia — AAD)
Mexico 1720
1100 Buenos Aires, Argentina
Phone: 54 1 3812737 **Fax:** 54 1 3812737
Email: info@aad.org.ar
Website: http://www.aad.org.ar

Fnded: 1907. **Mem:** 950. **Reg. Groups:** 5. **State Groups:** 14. **Local Groups:** 6. **Lang(s):** English, Spanish. **Desc:** Dermatologists in Argentina. Bestows awards; provides educational programs. **Pub:** *Indice General*, periodic. Journal. Contains dermatological articles. • *Journal of Argentine Dermatology*. Journal. • *Revista Argentina de Dermatologia*, quarterly. Includes summary in English.

★ 1059 ★ Armed Forces Institute of Pathology (AFIP)
6825 16th St. NW
Washington, DC 20306-6000
Phone: (202)782-2111 **Fax:** (202)782-9376
Email: draleyd@afip.osd.mil
Website: http://www.afip.org/
Captain Glenn N. Wagner, Dir.

Fnded: 1862. **Mem:** 842. **Desc:** Chartered by the Department of Defense to: maintain a consultation service for the diagnosis of pathologic material; conduct experimental, statistical, and morphological research in pathology; provide instruction in advanced pathology and related subjects; prepare, procure, and duplicate teaching aids; operate the AFIP Repository and Research Services; maintain the National Museum of Health and Medicine of the AFIP and a Visual Information Service for the collection, preparation, duplication, reference, and filing of medical illustrative material. Sponsors a series of courses. **Pub:** *AFIP Letter*, bimonthly. Newsletter. Third series, containing 30 separate fascicles, with international distribution. • *Atlas of Tumor Pathology*. **Frmly:** (1949) Army Medical Museum.

★ 1060 ★ Armenian Pharmacological Society
c/o Prof. E. Gabrielian
Department of Pharmacology
Yerevan Medical University
Yerevan, Armenia

Mem: 85. **Desc:** Promotes pharmacology in Armenia.

★ 1061 ★ Armenian Society of Cardiology
Institute of Cardiology
5 P Sevak St.
375044 Yerevan, Armenia
Phone: 374 1 288942 **Fax:** 374 1 588751
Email: grigor@card.iiap.sci.am
Website: http://www.escardio.org/society/natsoc/armenia.htm

Fnded: 1996. **Mem:** 56. **Lang(s):** English, Russian. **Desc:** Promotes the study of cardiology in Armenia.

★ 1062 ★ Army Nurse Corps Association (ANCA)
PO Box 39235, Serna Sta.
San Antonio, TX 78218-1235

Phone: (210)650-3534 **Fax:** (210)650-3534
Email: anca@e-anco.org

Fnded: 1977. **Mem:** 2,100. **Desc:** Army Nurse Corps officers from active, or retiree status or those serving honorably for shorter periods, or reserve duty. Provides educational and social opportunities for members; disseminates information to the public. Seeks to preserve history of the U.S. Army Nurse Corps. **Pub:** *Connection*, quarterly. Newsletter. **Frmly:** (2001) Retired Army Nurse Corps Association.

★ 1063 ★ Aromatherapy Organisation Council
PO Box 19834
London SE25 6WF, United Kingdom
Phone: 44 208 2517912 **Fax:** 44 208 2517942
Email: secretary@aocuk.net
Website: http://www.aocuk.net

Fnded: 1991. **Desc:** Voluntary, regulatory body for the aromatherapy profession. Seeks to establish common standards of training. Offers mediation and arbitration services in disputes involving aromatherapy. Sponsors research.

★ 1064 ★ Arthritis Care (AC)
18 Stephenson Way
London NW1 2HD, United Kingdom
Phone: 44 207 3806500 **Fax:** 44 207 3806505
Email: lizziee@arthritiscare.org.uk
Website: http://www.arthritiscare.org.uk

Fnded: 1948. **Mem:** 66,000. **Nat'l Groups:** 3. **Reg. Groups:** 7. **Local Groups:** 520. **Lang(s):** English. **Desc:** Individuals with arthritis and concerned others. Seeks to: increase awareness of the problems associated with rheumatic diseases; disseminate information; establish a nationwide network of branches; improve welfare facilities; provide information, advice and practical aid. Maintains hotels. **Pub:** *Arthritis News*, bimonthly. Magazine. **Frmly:** British Rheumatism and Arthritis Association.

★ 1065 ★ Arthritis Foundation (AF)
PO Box 7669
Atlanta, GA 30357-0669
Phone: (404)872-7100 **Free:** 800-283-7800
Fax: (404)872-0457
Website: http://www.arthritis.org
Mr. Tino Mantello, CEO/Pres.

Fnded: 1948. **Mem:** 700,000. **Local Groups:** 71. **Desc:** Seeks to: discover the cause and improve the methods for the treatment and prevention of arthritis and other rheumatic diseases; increase the number of scientists investigating rheumatic diseases; provide training in rheumatic diseases for more doctors; extend knowledge of arthritis and other rheumatic diseases to the lay public, emphasizing the socioeconomic as well as medical aspects of these diseases. **Pub:** *Arthritis Today*, bimonthly. Magazine. Includes research reports and selfhelp tips from readers. *Price:* Included in membership dues. • *Bulletin on the Rheumatic Diseases*, bimonthly. Bulletin. Contains articles on developments in research and management of rheumatic diseases; geared for the nonrheumatologist. *Price:* Free. • *Index of Rheumatology*, annual. **Frmly:** Arthritis and Rheumatism Foundation.

★ 1066 ★ Arthritis and Muscoskeletal Alliance (ARMA)
41 Eagle St.
London WC1R 4AR, United Kingdom
Phone: 44 20 8415191 **Fax:** 44 20 72423277
Email: arma@rheumatology.org.uk

Fnded: 1972. **Mem:** 26. **Reg. Groups:** 15. **Desc:** Umbrella organization of national societies concerned with rheumatic and musculoskeletal diseases. Has developed patient-centered standards for the care of individuals with arthritis. Conducts audits of current levels of support and care. Aims to raise awareness of the need for high quality services for those with rheumatic and musculoskeletal diseases. Promotes the development of prevention, treatment, rehabilitation, and relief from the disease. Fosters cooperation, understanding, and mutual support between individuals and organizations concerned with rheumatic diseases. Provides a forum for the exchange of ideas and information. **Pub:** *BLAR Purchaser's Pack*. Contains guidelines for providing the best service for people with rheumatic diseases. • *Disability & Arthritis*. Report. Discusses the impact of osteoarthritis and rheumatoid arthritis on quality of life. **Frmly:** (2002) British League Against Rheumatism.

★ 1067 ★ Arthritis Research Campaign
Copeman House
St. Mary's Court
St. Mary's Gate
Chesterfield S41 7TD, United Kingdom
Phone: 44 1246 558033 **Fax:** 44 1246 558007
Email: info@arc.org.uk
Website: http://www.arc.org.uk

Fnded: 1936. **Mem:** 40,000. **Desc:** Voluntary helpers, donators and support staff. Conducts research and education to find the cause of rheumatic disease. In pursuit of these objectives mounts a wide ranging research program involving people, projects and centers - usually at university medical schools. Currently running at over 20 million pounds per year. The income raised to meet this commitment comes entirely from voluntary donations. **Pub:** *Arthritis Today*, quarterly. Booklets. • Booklets. **Frmly:** Arthritis and Rheumatism Council for Research.

★ 1068 ★ Arthritis and Rheumatism Natural Therapy Research Association
c/o Ken Wright, Sec.
12 Clive Rd.
West Duluich
London SE21 8BY, United Kingdom
Phone: 44 208 6703763 **Fax:** 44 208 6703763
Email: renewnham@aol.com

Fnded: 1994. **Mem:** 220. **Nat'l Groups:** 1. **Desc:** Seeks to educate people about arthritic diseases. Conducts research into the causes and cures of arthritis. **Pub:** *ARNTRA*, quarterly. Newsletter. • *Arthritis Without Drugs*. Book.

★ 1069 ★ Arthritis Society
393 University Ave., Ste. 1700
Toronto, ON, Canada M5G 1E6
Phone: (416)979-7228 **Free:** 800-321-1433
Fax: (416)979-8366
Email: info@arthritis.ca
Website: http://www.arthritis.ca/

Reg. Groups: 1000. **Desc:** Committed to funding and promoting arthritis research, programs, education, and patient care. Sponsors awareness and fundraising events. Celebrates Arthritis Month every September to increase awareness of the impact of arthritis. **Pub:** *Arthritis News*. Magazine.

★ 1070 ★ Arthritis Society of Ireland (ASI)
1 Clanwilliam Sq.
Grand Canal Quay
Dublin 2, Ireland
Phone: 353 1 6618188 **Fax:** 353 1 6618261

Lang(s): English, Irish. **Desc:** Individuals and organizations with an interest in arthritis. Seeks to improve the quality of life of people with arthritis; promotes advancement in the diagnosis and treatment of arthritis. Serves as a clearinghouse on arthritis, its treatment, and services available to people with arthritis; makes available aids and appliance to make life easier for people with arthritis; conducts educational programs; sponsors children's services; provides financial support to arthritis research programs. **Pub:** *Arthritis News*, quarterly. Newsletter.

★ 1071 ★ Arthroscopy Association of North America (AANA)
6300 N River Rd., Ste. 104
Rosemont, IL 60018
Phone: (847)292-2262 **Fax:** (847)292-2268
Email: moreinfo@aana.org
Website: http://www.aana.org
Edward A. Goss, Exec. Dir.

Fnded: 1982. **Mem:** 1,500. **Desc:** Orthopedic surgeons. To advance arthroscopy, a diagnostic or surgical procedure in which an arthroscope, is inserted into a joint. The surgeon can either look directly into the arthroscope or observe on a screen the view projected by the arthroscope. In this way the surgeon can diagnose a condition using only a small incision for insertion of the arthroscope. The arthroscope also allows certain surgical procedures to be performed within viewing range of the scope. Sponsors research and continuing education programs. **Pub:** *AANA Membership Directory*, annual. Membership Directory. *Price:* Included in membership dues. • *Arthroscopy: The Journal of Arthroscopic and Related Surgery*, quarterly. Journal. *Price:* $170/year for individuals; $220/year for institutions. • *Inside AANA*, quarterly. Newsletter.

★ 1072 ★ ASEAN Association of Radiology (AAR)
2 Soi Soonvijai, New Petchburi
Bangkok 10320, Thailand
Fax: 66 2 7165964
Email: sissh@mahidol.ac.th

Fnded: 1979. **Desc:** Fosters all aspects of medical radiological sciences and imaging technologies particularly in the region of ASEAN.

★ 1073 ★ ASEAN Federation of Endocrine Societies
Philippine Diabetes Association
Unit 25 Facilities Center
Shaw Blvd.
Mandaluyong City, Philippines
Phone: 63 5311278 **Fax:** 63 5311278
Email: phildiab@pworld.net.ph
Website: http://www.diabetesphil.org

Fnded: 1958. **Reg. Groups:** 31. **Lang(s):** English, Filipino. **Desc:** Works for excellent diabetes care and prevention in the Philippines. **Pub:** *Diabetes Watch*, semiannual. Contains educational material for lay and paramedic; provides updates on diabetes mellitus and its management.

★ 1074 ★ ASEAN Federation of Plastic Surgeons
Sirindhorn Bldg.
Bangkok 10500, Thailand

★ 1075 ★ ASEAN Institute for Health Development
25/5 Phutthamonthon 4 Rd.
Salaya
Mahidol University
Nakorn Pathom 73170, Thailand
Phone: 66 2 4419040 **Fax:** 66 2 4419044
Email: www@mahidol.ac.th
Website: http://www.aihd.mahidol.ac.th

Fnded: 1982. **Lang(s):** English, Thai. **Desc:** International health agencies. Seeks to improve the availability and quality of primary health care services in Southeast Asia. Facilitates establishment of local health services and facilities; serves as a clearinghouse on public health policies and programs. **Pub:** *Journal of Primary Health Care*, quarterly. Journal. Articles/research on primary health care.

★ 1076 ★ ASEAN Neurological Association
Clinical Neuroscience Society - Singapore
c/o Department of Neurology
Singapore General Hospital
Outram Rd.
Singapore 169606, Singapore
Phone: 65 2223322 **Fax:** 65 2203321
Website: http://www.asean-neurology.org

Lang(s): Chinese, English. **Desc:** Health care professionals with an interest in neurology. Seeks to advance neurological study, teaching, and practice. Facilitates exchange of information among members; sponsors research and continuing professional development programs. **Frmly:** (2001) ASEAN Neurological Society.

★ 1077 ★ ASHP Foundation
7272 Wisconsin Ave.
Bethesda, MD 20814
Phone: (301)657-3000 **Fax:** (301)657-8817
Email: foundation@ashp.org
Website: http://www.ashpfoundation.org
Stephen J. Allen, Sec.

Fnded: 1968. **Desc:** Established for pharmaceutical care and research purposes. Offers research grants, awards; and anticoagulation, asthma, stem cell transplantation, diabetes, pain management, oncology, and traineeships. **Pub:** *Resource Book on Progressive Pharmaceutical Services.* **AKA:** American Society of Hospital Pharmacists Research and Education Foundation; ASHP Research and Education Foundation.

★ 1078 ★ Asia-Oceania Association for the Study of Obesity (AOASO)
Fac. of Allied Health Sciences, University Kebangsaan Malays
Jln. Raja Muda Abdul Aziz
50300 Kuala Lumpur, Malaysia
Phone: 60 3 40405679 **Fax:** 60 3 26941296
Email: mismail@medic.ukm.my
Website: http://www.iotf.org/oonet/aoaso.htm

Fnded: 1998.

★ 1079 ★ Asia and Oceania Society for Comparative Endocrinology (AOSCE)
College of Natural Sciences, Hanyang University
Seoul 133-791, Republic of Korea
Fax: 82 2 2993495
Email: ydyoon@email.hanyang.ac.kr

Desc: Provides a platform for exchange of ideas; fosters collaboration among comparative endocrinologists in the region.

★ 1080 ★ Asia and Oceania Thyroid Association (AOTA)
Department of Internal Medicine
Asian Medical Center
University of Ulsan
Songpa PO Box 145
Seoul 138-600, Republic of Korea
Phone: 82 2 30103244 **Fax:** 82 2 30106962
Email: ykshong@amc.seoul.kr
Website: http://aota.or.kr

Lang(s): English, Japanese. **Desc:** Endocrinologists and other medical professionals and scientists with an interest in the thyroid gland. Seeks to advance the understanding of the thyroid gland and its functions; works to improve the diagnosis and treatment of thyroid diseases. Gathers and disseminates endocrinological information pertaining to the thyroid gland; sponsors researcha and continuing professional development programs.

★ 1081 ★ Asia Pacific Academy of Ophthalmology (APAO)
Gleneagles Hospital
Annexe Block 02-38
6A Napier Rd.
Singapore 258500, Singapore
Phone: 65 4666666 **Fax:** 65 7333360

Lang(s): Chinese, English. **Desc:** Ophthalmologists. Seeks to advance ophthalmological study, teaching, and practice. Facilitates exchange of information among members; conducts continuing professional development courses.

★ 1082 ★ Asia Pacific Association for the Control of Tobacco (APACT)
12/F-3 No. 57, Fu Hsin N Rd.
Taipei 10559, Taiwan
Phone: 886 2 27734308 **Fax:** 886 2 27522455
Email: dyenjtfh@ms35.hinet.net

Fnded: 1989. **Mem:** 19. **Lang(s):** English, Mandarin. **Desc:** Working to create a "smoke-free Taiwan." Monitors advertising and government policy on tobacco trade. Campaigns for prohibition of cigarette advertising in Taiwan. **Pub:** *Health for All*, monthly. Magazine.

★ 1083 ★ Asia-Pacific Association of Psychotherapists (APAP)
4/4 Charles St.
Petersham, NSW 2049, Australia
Phone: 61 2 85851085 **Fax:** 61 2 85851010

Lang(s): English. **Desc:** Psychotherapists. Seeks to advance the study and practice of psychotherapy; promotes adherence to high standards of ethics and practice by members. Serves as a forum for the exchange of information among members; sponsors research and educational programs.

★ 1084 ★ Asia Pacific Clinical Nutrition Society (APCNS)
c/o Asia Pacific Health and Nutrition Centre
PO Box 11A
Monash University
Clayton, VIC 3800, Australia
Phone: 61 3 99058145 **Fax:** 61 3 99058146
Email: mark.wahlqvist@med.monash.edu.au

Lang(s): English. **Desc:** Nutritionists and other health care professionals with an interest in nutrition. Seeks to advance the study, teaching, and practice of nutrition. Serves as a clearinghouse on nutrition; sponsors research and continuing professional development programs.

★ 1085 ★ Asia-Pacific Council of Optometry (APCO)
c/o Prof. Willard B. Bleything, Sec.Gen.
2043 College Way
Forest Grove, OR 97116
Phone: (503)352-2170 **Free:** 877-722-8648
Fax: (503)352-2929
Email: bleythiw@pacificu.edu
Prof. Willard B. Bleything, Sec. Gen.

Fnded: 1978. **Mem:** 26. **Desc:** National associations of optometrists in 20 countries. Purpose is to improve the delivery of eye care and standards of visual welfare to people in the the Asian-Pacific region. **Frmly:** International Federation of Asian and Pacific Associations of Optometrists.

★ 1086 ★ Asia Pacific Deaf Sports Confederation (APDSC)
7B Kompleks Perniagaan Seri Selangor
Jln. San Peng
55200 Kuala Lumpur, Malaysia
Fax: 63 3 92226536
Email: deafsportsap@yahoo.com
Website: http://www.geocities.com/deafsportsap

Lang(s): English. **Desc:** Sports programs for people with impaired hearing; hearing impaired athletes. Promotes increased participation in athletics by people with impaired hearing. Facilitates communication and cooperation among members; sponsors competitions.

★ 1087 ★ Asia-Pacific Dental Students Association (APDSA)
c/o Dr. Yeo Kian Boon
No. 6, Jalan Waras 2
56000 Kuala Lumpur, Malaysia
Phone: 60 3 4532768 **Fax:** 60 3 4528486
Email: thiru@tm.net.my
Website: http://apdsa.ch-dental.co.kr/

Desc: Promotes dental education; represents dental students.

★ 1088 ★ Asia Pacific Endodontic Confederation (APEC)
c/o Dr. Phillipe Zimet, Sec.
77 Stud Rd.
Dandenong, Metro Manila 3175, Australia
Fax: 61 3 97940558
Email: sjlee@yumc.yonsei.ac.kr
Website: http://www.hku.hk/consden/apec

Lang(s): Chinese, English. **Desc:** Endodontists. Seeks to advance the study, teaching, and practice of endodontia. Serves as a forum for the exchange of information among members; sponsors research and continuing professional development programs.

★ 1089 ★ Asia-Pacific Implant Centre
Rm. 704 Takshing House
20 Des Voeux Rd.
Hong Kong, People's Republic of China
Phone: 852 25243559 **Fax:** 852 25243557
Email: info@implantecentre.com
Website: http://www.implantcentre.com

Desc: Dental and medical practitioners. Dedicated to the advancement of oral implantology in the Asia-Pacific region. Provides practicing clinicians with opportunities for professional education and training, as well as clinical facilities services for oral implant treatment. Fully equipped with educational, teaching, and clinical facilities.

★ 1090 ★ Asia Pacific Intraocular Implant Association (APIIA)
Annexe Block 02-38
Gleneagles Hospital
6A Napier Rd.
Singapore 258500, Singapore
Phone: 65 4666666 **Fax:** 65 7333360

Lang(s): Chinese, English. **Desc:** Ophthalmologists and ocular surgeons with an interest in intraocular implants. Seeks to advance the study, teaching, and practice of intraocular implantology. Facilitates exchange of information among members; sponsors research and continuing professional development programs.

★ 1091 ★ Asia Pacific Menopause Federation (APMF)
c/o Prof. Christopher Haines
The Prince of Wales Hospital Shatin, NT
Hong Kong, People's Republic of China
Phone: 852 26322800 **Fax:** 852 26360008
Email: info@apmf.net
Website: http://www.apmf.net/

Desc: Promotes the study of all aspects of menopause and aging in the Asia Pacific region. **Pub:** Reports.

★ 1092 ★ Asia-Pacific Network of People Living with HIV/AIDS
c/o Paul Toh, Sec.
62B Race Course Rd.
Singapore 218568, Singapore
Phone: 65 2951153 **Fax:** 65 2955567
Email: paultoh@pacific.net.sg
Website: http://www.xs4all.nl/~gnp/asap.html

Fnded: 1994. **Lang(s):** Chinese, English. **Desc:** People with AIDS and HIV and their families; organizations providing services to people with AIDS and HIV. Seeks to improve the quality of life of people with AIDS and HIV; promotes increased availability of social and medical services for people with AIDS and HIV. Coordinates members' programs; sponsors research on AIDS services.

★ 1093 ★ Asia Pacific Orthopaedic Association (APOA)
c/o Prof. David S.K. Choon
Department of Orthopaedic Surgery
Faculty of Medicine
University of Malaysia
50603 Kuala Lumpur, Malaysia
Phone: 60 3 79535643 **Fax:** 60 3 79535642

Email: secretariat@apoa-home.com
Website: http://www.apoa-home.com

Fnded: 1962. **Mem:** 1,602. **Reg. Groups:** 19. **Lang(s):** English. **Desc:** Orthopedic surgeons in 16 Asia countries. Facilitates the exchange of ideas and discuss new developments and methods relating to orthopedic surgery. Sponsors the Zimmer-WPOA Travelling Fellowship which enables young orthopedic surgeons to travel to academic training centers in the Asia Pacific region. **Pub:** *Journal of Orthopaedic Surgery*, 3/year. Journal. • *Newsletter of the Western Pacific Orthopaedic Association*, quarterly.

★ 1094 ★ Asia Pacific Public Health Nutrition Association (APPHNA)

Public Health Nutrition Program
421 Warren Hall
University of California
Berkeley, CA 94720-7360
Phone: (510)642-3852 **Fax:** (510)643-6981
Email: zaksabry@socrates.berkeley.edu
Website: http://www.monash.edu.au/APPHNA/
Zak Sabry, Contact

Desc: Public health practitioners and nutritionists. Promotes nutrition as a vital component of good health. Develops and implements national and international public health nutrition strategies; sponsors research and educational programs.

★ 1095 ★ Asia Pacific Society of Cornea and Refractive Surgery (APSCRS)

5-11-13 Sugano Ichikawa
Chiba 272, Japan
Phone: 81 473 220151 **Fax:** 81 212863
Email: vyb04652@niftyserve.or.jp

Fnded: 1998.

★ 1096 ★ Asia-Pacific Society of Impotence Research (APSIR)

c/o Dr. Tan Huimeng
c/o Subang Jaya Medical Centre
1, JLN ss 12/1A
47500 Suban Jaya, Malaysia
Email: aspirmal@tm.net.my

Fnded: 1987. **Mem:** 500. **Nat'l Groups:** 730. **Reg. Groups:** 78. **Lang(s):** English. **Desc:** Health care professionals with an interest in impotence. Seeks to advance the diagnosis and treatment of impotence. Serves as a forum for the exchange of information among members; sponsors research and continuing professional development programs. **Pub:** *AMSIR Book on ED*. Book. • Newsletter, monthly.

★ 1097 ★ Asia-Pacific Society of Travel Medicine (ASTM)

No. 252, Wu-Hsing St.
Taipei 110, Taiwan
Phone: 886 2 27362729 **Fax:** 886 27375412
Email: tonyfm@atsmail.tmch.org.tw

Desc: Promotes research in travel and provides a scientific focus for those interested in travel medicine; stimulates the practice of travel medicine at a high professional level.

★ 1098 ★ Asian Academy of Aesthetic Dentistry (AAAD)

268 Orchard Rd. 05-02
Singapore 238856, Singapore
Phone: 65 7343162 **Fax:** 65 7321979
Email: singdent@singnet.com.sg

Fnded: 1990. **Lang(s):** Chinese, English. **Desc:** Dentists practicing aesthetic dentistry. Seeks to advance the study, teaching, and practice of aesthetic dentistry. Gathers and disseminates information on aesthetic dentistry; sponsors research and Continuing professional development programs. **Pub:** *Asian Journal of Aesthetic Dentistry*, annual. Journal.

★ 1099 ★ Asian Association for Dynamic Osteosynthesis (AADO)

c/o Orthopedic Learning Centre
1/F Li Ka Shing Specialist Clinics
Prince of Wales Hospital
Shatin
Hong Kong, People's Republic of China
Phone: 852 26323482 **Fax:** 852 26477432
Email: info@aado.org
Website: http://www.aado.org

Lang(s): Chinese, English. **Desc:** Health care professionals with an interest in osteosynthesis. Seeks to advance the study, teaching, and practice of dynamic osteosynthesis; promotes professional development of members. Serves as a clearinghouse on osteosynthesis; sponsors research and educational programs.

★ 1100 ★ Asian Association of Occupational Health (AAOH)

420/1 Rajvidhi Rd.
Bangkok 10400, Thailand
Phone: 66 2 2457793 **Fax:** 66 2 2467765

Fnded: 1964.

★ 1101 ★ Asian Association of Social Psychology (AASP)

c/o Dr. Emi Kashima
Mail H24
Swinburne University of Technology
Hawthorn, VIC 3122, Australia
Phone: 61 3 92148206 **Fax:** 61 3 98190574
Email: ekashima@swin.edu.au
Website: http://www.sites.psych.unimelb.edu.au/aasp

Fnded: 1995. **Mem:** 200. **Lang(s):** English. **Desc:** Psychologists and other individuals with an interest in social psychology. Seeks to advance the study, teaching, and practice of social psychology. Serves as a forum for the exchange of information among members; sponsors research and educational programs. **Pub:** *Asian Journal of Social Psychology*, QRT. Journal.

★ 1102 ★ Asian Australasian Society of Neurological Surgeons (AASNS)

23, Bharathidasan Rd.
Teynampet
Chennai
Madras 600 018, India
Phone: 91 44 24364150 **Fax:** 91 44 4335050
Email: kganap@hotmail.com
Website: http://aasns.com

Mem: 15,000. **Lang(s):** English. **Desc:** Neurological surgeons. Seeks to advance the practice of neurological surgery; promotes continuing professional development among members. Serves as a clearinghouse on neurological surgery; sponsors training courses. **Pub:** Newsletter, annual.

★ 1103 ★ Asian - Australasian Society of Neurological Surgeons (AASNS)

23 Bharath Dasan Rd.
Teynampet
Chennai 600018, India
Phone: 91 44 24364150 **Fax:** 91 44 24335050
Email: kganap@vsnl.com
Website: http://aasns.com

Fnded: 1964. **Mem:** 5,000. **Nat'l Groups:** 16. **Lang(s):** English. **Desc:** Neurosurgeons seeking to advance neurosurgical studies and promote understanding between members from different countries. Conducts educational programs. **Pub:** Newsletter, annual.

★ 1104 ★ Asian Dermatological Association

c/o The Federation of Medical Societies of Hong Kong
Duke of Windsor Social Service Bldg., 4th Fl., Hennessy Rd.
Hong Kong, People's Republic of China
Phone: 852 25278898 **Fax:** 852 28650345
Email: info@fmshk.com.hk
Website: http://www.medicine.org.hk

Lang(s): Chinese, English. **Desc:** Dermatologists and medical students with an interest in dermatology. Seeks to advance the study, teaching, and practice of dermatology. Facilitates exchange of information among members; sponsors research and educational programs.

★ 1105 ★ Asian Federation for Medical Chemistry (AFMC)

c/o Korean Chemical Society
Science and Technology Bldg., Rm. 703
635-4 Yoksam-dong
Kangnam-gu
Seoul 135 703, Republic of Korea
Phone: 82 2 34533781 **Fax:** 82 2 34533785
Email: kcschem@neon.kcsnet.or.kr

Fnded: 1946. **Mem:** 5,000. **Reg. Groups:** 13. **Lang(s):** English, Korean. **Desc:** Chemists, physicians, and other scientists and health care personnel with an interest in medical chemistry. Promotes medical chemistry research and scholarship. Serves as a clearinghouse on medical chemistry; conducts research and educational programs. **Pub:** *Bulletin of the Korean Chemical Society*, monthly. Journal. • *Chemical Education*, quarterly. Magazine. • *ChemWorld*, monthly. Magazine. • *Journal of the Korean Chemical Society*, bimonthly. Journal.

★ 1106 ★ Asian Federation of Societies for Ultrasound in Medicine and Biology (AFSUMB)

Hiyoshi-cho, Funai-gun
Kyoto 629-0392, Japan
Phone: 81 771 721181 **Fax:** 81 771 720326

Fnded: 1986. **Desc:** Exchanges scientific research and education.

★ 1107 ★ Asian Foundation for the Prevention of Blindness (AFPB)

248 Nam Cheong St.
Shamshuipo
Hong Kong, People's Republic of China
Phone: 852 7788332 **Fax:** 852 7880040
Email: genadmin@hksb.org.hk

Lang(s): Chinese, English. **Desc:** Medical professionals and eye care institutions. Seeks to prevent blindness and improve the quality of life of people with impaired vision. Makes available visual health screening and other eye care services to needy individuals.

★ 1108 ★ Asian Health Institute (AHI)

987-30 Minamiyama
Komenogi
Nisshin, Aichi 470-0111, Japan
Phone: 81 5617 31950 **Fax:** 81 5617 31990
Email: ahi@jca.apc.org
Website: http://www.jca.apc.org/ahi/

Fnded: 1980. **Mem:** 7,000. **Lang(s):** English, Japanese. **Desc:** Promotes improved public health, particularly in Asia. Conducts public educational campaigns to create indigenous leadership for public health initiatives in the region. **Pub:** *Ajia no Kenko*, bimonthly. Magazine. Member Newsletter. • *Ajia no Kodomo*, semiannual. Magazine. Children's magazine on the lives of children in Asian countries. • *Asian Health Institute*, quarterly. Newsletter. Forum for training course alumni, grassroots health workers. Occasional reports on study tours, special research projects, retrospectives, and so on.

★ 1109 ★ Asian Hospital Federation (AHF)

Hospital Authority Bldg.
147B Argyle St.
Kowloon
Hong Kong, People's Republic of China
Phone: 852 23006555 **Fax:** 852 28907726
Email: info@cornhillpublications.com

Website: http://www.asianhf.com

Fnded: 1971. **Mem:** 5. **Desc:** National hospital federations in Indonesia, Japan, People's Republic of China, Philippines, and Republic of Korea. Promotes improved patient care and strives to achieve high standards of hospital administration. Encourages mutual assistance among members.

★ 1110 ★ Asian Oceania Society of Regional Anesthesia (AOSRA)

Philippine Society of Anaesthesiologists
PMA Bldg.
Quezon City, Metro Manila, Philippines
Phone: 63 3 9295852 **Fax:** 63 3 9295852
Email: psa@i.manila.com.ph

Fnded: 1951. **Mem:** 2,606. **Reg. Groups:** 13. **Lang(s):** English, Filipino. **Desc:** Anesthesiologists. Promotes increased use of regional anesthetics; seeks to advance anesthesiological study and practice. Serves as a clearinghouse on regional anesthesia; sponsors research and continuing professional development programs. **Pub:** *Philippine Journal of Anesthiology*, semiannual. Journal. • *The Pulse Monitor*, quarterly.

★ 1111 ★ Asian and Oceanian Epilepsy Organization (AOEO)

All India Institute of Medical Sciences
New Delhi 110 029, India
Phone: 91 11 26594210 **Fax:** 91 6521086 6521086
Email: satjain55@atshotmail.com

Fnded: 1991.

★ 1112 ★ Asian and Oceanian Society of Radiology

5 Lower Kent Ridge Rd.
Singapore 119074, Singapore
Phone: 65 7795555 **Fax:** 65 7778427

★ 1113 ★ Asian and Oceanian Thyroid Association (AOTA)

Songpa PO Box 145
Seoul 138-600, Republic of Korea
Phone: 82 2 30103244 **Fax:** 82 2 30106962
Email: ykshong@amc.seoul.kr
Website: http://www.aota.or.kr

Fnded: 1975. **Mem:** 400. **Nat'l Groups:** 20.

★ 1114 ★ Asian-Oceanic Glaucoma Society (AOGS)

Singapore National Eye Centre
11 Third Hospital Ave.
Singapore 168751, Singapore
Phone: 65 2277255 **Fax:** 65 2277290

Lang(s): Chinese, English. **Desc:** Ophthalmologists specializing in the treatment of glaucoma. Promotes early diagnosis and effective treatment of glaucoma; seeks to advance the science and practice of glaucomatology. Serves as a clearinghouse on the diagnosis and treatment of glaucoma; sponsors research and continuing professional development programs.

★ 1115 ★ Asian Ostomy Association (AOA)

c/o Stoma Care Society of Malaysia
190 Jalan C3 Taman Melawati
53100 Kuala Lumpur, Malaysia
Phone: 60 3 4081653

Lang(s): English, Malay. **Desc:** Physicians and other health care personnel with an interest in ostomy and the care of ostomy patients. Seeks to improve the quality of life of ostomy patients; promotes advancement in the practice of ostomy medicine. Serves as a clearinghouse on ostomy; sponsors research and continuing professional development programs.

★ 1116 ★ Asian-Pacific Association for Laser Medicine and Surgery (APALMS)

06-03 Mount Elizabeth Medical Centre
Singapore 0922, Singapore

★ 1117 ★ Asian Pacific Association for Medical Informatics (APAMI)

National University Hospital
Department of Community, Occupational and Family Medicine
Lower Kent Ridge Rd.
Singapore 0511, Singapore
Phone: 65 7724296 **Fax:** 65 7791489
Email: lunkc@nusvm.bitnet

Lang(s): Chinese, English. **Desc:** Medical information and information management organizations. Seeks to advance the practice of medical information management; promotes development and implementation of new medical informatics technologies. Serves as a clearinghouse on medical information management; sponsors research and educational programs.

★ 1118 ★ Asian Pacific Association for the Study of the Liver

62 Youido-gu
Seoul 150-010, Republic of Korea

★ 1119 ★ Asian and Pacific Cerebral Palsy Association (APCPA)

APCPA Secretariat
DEB Services
PO Box 315
Manly, NSW 2095, Australia
Phone: 61 2 99763595 **Fax:** 61 2 99778238
Website: http://www.dinf.ne.jp/doc/japanese/twg/eng/contact/apcpa.html

Lang(s): English. **Desc:** Physicians and other health care personnel with an interest in cerebral palsy; people with cerebral palsy and their families. Seeks to prevent cerebral palsy and to improve the quality of life of people with the disease. Serves as a clearinghouse on cerebral palsy; provides support and services to people with cerebral palsy and their families; sponsors research and educational programs.

★ 1120 ★ Asian Pacific Dental Federation/Asian Pacific Regional Organisation (APDF/APRO)

242 Tanjong Katong Rd.
Singapore 437030, Singapore
Phone: 65 3453125 **Fax:** 65 3442116
Email: bibi@pacific.net.sg

Fnded: 1955. **Mem:** 23. **Lang(s):** English. **Desc:** National dental associations in Australia, Bangladesh, Guam, Hong Kong, India, Figi, Jordan, Macau, Papua New Guines, Saudi Arabia, Indonesia, Japan, Malaysia, Mongolia, Myanmar, Nepal, New Zealand, Pakistan, Philippines, Republic of Korea, Singapore, Sri Lanka, Taiwan, and Thailand. Works to improve dental and general health in the Asia Pacific region. Encourages education and research links between national dental associations. **Pub:** *APDF/APRO Technical Report*, periodic. • *Dentistry in the Asian Pacific Region*, periodic.

★ 1121 ★ Asian Pacific Federation of Societies for Surgery of the Hand (APFSSH)

c/o Kwan-Chul Tark, MD
Plastic & Reconstructive Surgery
Yonsei University Medical Center
CPO Box 8044
Seoul, Republic of Korea
Phone: 82 2 3615694 **Fax:** 82 2 3936947
Email: kctark@yumc.yonsei.ac.kr
Website: http://www.apfssh.org

Fnded: 1995. **Mem:** 4,000. **Nat'l Groups:** 14. **Lang(s):** English. **Desc:** Orthopedic and plastic surgeons specializing in surgery on the hands. Seeks to advance the practice of hand surgery; promotes continuing professional development of members. Facilitates exchange of information among members; sponsors research and training programs. **Pub:** *Hand Surgery*. Journal.

★ 1122 ★ Asian and Pacific Islander American Health Forum

c/o Marnelle Marasigan
942 Market St. Ste 200
San Francisco, CA 94102
Phone: (415)954-9988 **Fax:** (415)954-9999
Email: hforum@apiahf.org
Website: http://www.apiahf.org
Tessie Guillermo, CEO

Fnded: 1986. **Mem:** 350. **Desc:** Promotes policy, program, and research efforts for the improvement of health status of all Asian and Pacific Islander Americans. Examines and review the distribution of factors associated with health problems and issues facing Asian and Pacific Islander Americans, including infectious diseases, diabetes, hypertension, cancer, HIV/AIDS, substance abuse, and mental health disorders. Compiles statistics. Conducts research programs. **Pub:** *APIAHF Focus*, quarterly. Newsletter. • *APITEN Newsletter*. Newsletter. • *Confronting Critical Health Issues of Asian and Pacific Islander Americans*. Book.

★ 1123 ★ Asian Pacific Neural Network Assembly (APNNA)

c/o Fanji Gu, Sec.
Center for Brain Science Research
Fudan University
Shanghai, People's Republic of China
Phone: 86 21 65298260
Email: yxzhong@ieee.org
Website: http://www.cse.cuhk.edu.hk/~apnna

Fnded: 1993. **Lang(s):** Chinese, English, Japanese, Korean. **Desc:** Researchers, scientists, and industry professionals with an interest in neural networks. Promotes more active interaction among members. Serves as a clearinghouse on neural networks; facilitates communication and cooperation among members.

★ 1124 ★ Asian-Pacific Resource and Research Centre for Women (ARROW)

Ground Floor, Block G
Anjung Felda
Jalan Maktab
54000 Kuala Lumpur, Malaysia
Phone: 60 3 26929913 **Fax:** 60 3 26929958
Email: arrow@arrow.po.my
Website: http://www.arrow.org.my

Fnded: 1993. **Lang(s):** English, Malay. **Desc:** Advocate to reorient health, population and reproductive health policies with women's gender perspectives and to ensure that health services are comprehensice, accessible and affordable for women in Malaysia. **Pub:** *Arrows for Change*, 3/year. Bulletin. Focuses on the gender dimension of women and health. • *Gender and Women's Health: Information Package, No. 2, 1997.* • *Reappraising Population Policies and Family Planning Programmes: An Annotated Bibliography Series 1, 1994.* • *Towards Women-Centered Reproductive Health: Information Package No. 1, 1994.* • *Women-Centered and Gender-Sensitive Experiences: Changing Our Perspectives, Policies, and Programmes on Womens Health in Asia and the Pacific Ref. Kit.*

★ 1125 ★ Asian Pacific Society of Atherosclerosis and Vascular Disease

c/o Department of Endocrinology
Singapore General Hospital
Outram Rd.
Singapore 169608, Singapore
Phone: 65 3214654 **Fax:** 65 2273576
Email: ce_tan@sgh.gov.sg

Lang(s): Chinese, English. **Desc:** Physicians and other health care personnel with an interest in atherosclerosis. Seeks to advance the prevention, diagnosis, and treatment of atherosclerosis; promotes continuing professional development of members. Gathers and disseminates information on atherosclerosis and related diseases; sponsors research and educational programs. **Frmly:** (2000) Asian Pacific Athersclerosis Society.

★ 1126 ★ Asian-Pacific Society of Cardiovascular and Interventional Radiology (APSCIR)
c/o Royal Melbourne Hospital
Department of Radiology
Grattan St.
Parkville, VIC 34052, Australia
Lang(s): English. **Desc:** Cardiovascular and interventional radiologists. Seeks to advance the study, teaching, and practice of radiology. Serves as a forum for the exchange of information among members; sponsors research and continuing professional development programs.

★ 1127 ★ Asian-Pacific Society of Digestive Endoscopy (APSDE)
Taimei Bldg. 22, 3-chome, Kanda, Ogawa-machi, Chiyoda-ku
Tokyo 101, Japan
Phone: 81 3 32914111 **Fax:** 81 3 32915568
Fnded: 1992. **Desc:** Fosters the exchange and diffusion of ideas relating to digestive endoscopy; encourages research and study; standardizes endoscopy methods and nomenclature.

★ 1128 ★ Asian Pacific Society for Digestive Endoscopy (APSDE)
c/o William S.C. Chao, MD
Rm. 3702-B, 37th Fl., Tower 2
Lippo Centre 89, Queen's Way
Hong Kong, People's Republic of China
Phone: 852 28681919
Email: wscchao@netvigator.com
Website: http://www.omed.org/membsocieties.htm
Desc: Works to promote the study and advancement of gastrointestinal endoscopy.

★ 1129 ★ Asian-Pacific Society of Nephrology (APSN)
Monash Medical Centre
246 Clayton Rd.
Clayton, VIC 3168, Australia
Lang(s): English. **Desc:** Nephrologists. Seeks to advance the study, teaching, and practice of nephrology. Facilitates exchange of information among members; sponsors research programs and continuing professional development courses.

★ 1130 ★ Asian Pacific Society of Respirology (APSR)
Yoshikawa No. 2 Bldg., 2nd Fl.
2-9-8 Hongo
Bunkyo-ku
Tokyo 113, Japan
Phone: 81 3 56843370 **Fax:** 81 3 56843382
Email: kyu00671@nifty.ne.jp
Website: http://www.apsresp.org
Fnded: 1985. **Mem:** 921. **Lang(s):** English, Japanese. **Desc:** Physicians specializing in the treatment of respiratory ailments. Seeks to advance the study, teaching, and practice of respirology. Facilitates exchange of information among members; conducts research and educational programs. **Pub:** *Respirology*, quarterly. Journal.

★ 1131 ★ Asian Pan-Pacific Society for Paediatric Gastroenterology, Hepatology and Nutrition (APPSGHAN)
Lower Kent Ridge Rd.
Singapore 119074, Singapore
Fnded: 1976. **Desc:** Promotes the knowledge of paediatric gastroenterology, hepatology and nutrition and stimulates research in these fields.

★ 1132 ★ Asian Pan-Pacific Society for Paediatric Gastroenterology and Nutrition (APPSPGAN)
Department of Pediatrics
National Taiwan University Hospital
Taipei, Taiwan
Email: tspgn@ms31.url.com.tw
Lang(s): English, Japanese. **Desc:** Pediatric gastroenterologists and nutritionists. Seeks to advance the study, teaching, and practice of pediatric gastroenterology and nutrition. Functions as a clearinghouse on pediatric gastroenterology and nutrition; sponsors research and educational programs.

★ 1133 ★ Asian Pediatric Nephrology Association
81 Kim Keat Rd.
Singapore 328836, Singapore
Phone: 65 2990200 **Fax:** 65 2993164

★ 1134 ★ Asian Sleep Research Society (ASRS)
c/o Tatsuro Ohta, Pres.
Konodai 1-7-3, Ichikawa
Nagoya University, School of Medicine
65 Tsuruma-cho
Showa-ku
Chiba 272-0827, Japan
Email: macoto@ncnp-k.go.jp
Website: http://www.wfsrs.org/iasrs.html
Fnded: 1994. **Mem:** 1,980. **Nat'l Groups:** 14. **Reg. Groups:** 14. **State Groups:** 14. **Local Groups:** 14. **Lang(s):** English. **Desc:** Promotes all aspects of sleep research; fosters training, education, dissemination of information, and establishment of fellowships and awards.

★ 1135 ★ Asian Society of Cardiothoracic Anaesthesia (ASCA)
c/o World Express
Singapore Society of Anaesthesiologists
114 Middle Rd., Ste. 05-01
Singapore 0718, Singapore
Phone: 65 3363875 **Fax:** 65 3397843
Lang(s): Chinese, English. **Desc:** Anesthesiologists specializing in cardiothoracic anesthesia. Seeks to advance the profession of cardiothoracic anesthesia; promotes continuing professional development among members. Serves as a forum for the exchange of information among members; sponsors research and training programs.

★ 1136 ★ Asian Society for Cardiovascular Surgery (ASCS)
c/o Department of Cardiac Surgery
University of Tokyo
7-3-1 Hongo
Bunkyo-ku
Tokyo 113-8655, Japan
Phone: 81 3 58008855 **Fax:** 81 3 58008854
Website: http://www.ascvs.org
Lang(s): English, Korean. **Desc:** Cardiovascular surgeons. Seeks to advance the practice of cardiovascular surgery; promotes continuing professional development among members. Facilitates exchange of information among members; sponsors research and educational programs.

★ 1137 ★ Asian Society of Pediatric Infectious Diseases
Rama VI Rd.
Bangkok 10400, Thailand
Phone: 66 2 2011674 **Fax:** 66 2 2462123

★ 1138 ★ Asian Society for Stereotactic Functional and Computer Assisted Neurosurgery
Functional and Gamma Knife Surgery Center
Nakao-machi
Takasaki 886, Japan
Phone: 81 272 3626201 **Fax:** 81 272 3628901
Fnded: 1994. **Mem:** 300. **Nat'l Groups:** 7. **Lang(s):** English, Japanese. **Desc:** Neurosurgeons. Promotes increased use of stereotactic and computer assisted neurosurgical techniques; seeks to advance surgical assistive technologies. Facilitates exchange of information among members; provides support to surgical technology research programs; sponsors continuing professional development courses. **Pub:** *Stereotactic and Functional Neurosurgery*, bimonthly. Journal. Special issues; proceedings of society meeting.

★ 1139 ★ Asian-South Pacific Association for Sport Psychology (ASPASP)
Beijing University
Beijing, People's Republic of China
Lang(s): Chinese, English. **Desc:** Sports psychologists. Promotes sports psychology as a means to the enhancement of athletic performance. Serves as a clearinghouse on sports psychology; provides services to athletes and athletic clubs; sponsors research and educational programs.

★ 1140 ★ Asian Surgical Association (ASA)
Department of Surgery
University of Hong Kong
Queen Mary Hospital
Hong Kong, People's Republic of China
Phone: 852 28554235 **Fax:** 852 28181186
Email: info@asiansurgassoc.org
Website: http://www.AsianSurgAssoc.org
Fnded: 1976. **Mem:** 1,030. **Lang(s):** Chinese, English. **Desc:** Surgeons. Seeks to advance surgical practice. Facilitates exchange of information among members; sponsors continuing professional development courses. **Pub:** *Asian Journal of Surgery*, quarterly. Journal. Includes original scientific contributions in clinical and experimental surgery, features the latest surgical advances and developments in Asia.

★ 1141 ★ Asociacion Argentina de Proteccion Familiar (AAPF)
Aguero 1355/59
Capital Federal
1425 Buenos Aires, Argentina
Phone: 54 11 48261216 **Fax:** 54 11 48248416
Email: info@aapf.com.ar
Website: http://www.aapf.com.ar
Fnded: 1966. **Mem:** 160. **Nat'l Groups:** 1. **Reg. Groups:** 6. **State Groups:** 154. **Local Groups:** 1. **Lang(s):** Spanish. Does not correspond in English. **Desc:** Works to improve the quality of family life in Argentina. Supports and promotes reproductive rights and equal parenting duties. Operates family planning centers; conducts research and educational programs on subjects including the importance of the father figure; sexual health and the transmission of STDs, and birth control methods. Offers training for health and professionals and social workers. Maintains speakers bureau. **Pub:** *Comunicaciones*, annual. Magazine.

★ 1142 ★ Asociacion de Bibliotecarios Graduados de la Republica Argentina (ABGRA)
Tucuman 1424 - 8 piso, D
C1050 AAB Buenos Aires, Argentina
Phone: 54 11 43715269 **Fax:** 54 11 43715269
Email: abgra@ciudad.com.ar
Website: http://abgra.sisbi.uba.ar/

Fnded: 1953. Desc: Represents professional librarians graduated from schools of Library Science in Argentina.

★ 1143 ★ Asociacion Demografica Costarricense (ADC)
La Uruca 300 metros al Norte y 100 metros al Este de la Fabrica de Galletas Pozuelo
Apartado Postal 10203
San Jose, Costa Rica
Phone: 506 2314430 **Fax:** 506 2314430
Email: adc@adc.or.cr
Website: http://www.adc.or.cr
Lang(s): Spanish. **Desc:** Advocates responsible parenthood and family planning in Costa Rica. Seeks to reduce the number of unwanted pregnancies and abortions. Encourages public awareness of contraception and methods of family planning. Offers contraceptive services. Sponsors programs in family planning, sex education, and awareness of sexually transmitted diseases, especially AIDS. Conducts research.

★ 1144 ★ Asociacion Dental Mexicana
Ezequiel Montes No. 29
Col. Revolucion Delegacion Cuahtemoc
Mexico City, Mexico
Fnded: 1942. **Mem:** 500. **Desc:** Promotes the dental sciences in Mexico.

★ 1145 ★ Asociacion Distrofia Muscular
Cordoba 5824
1414 Buenos Aires, Argentina
Phone: 54 11 9817522 **Fax:** 54 11 9561471
Email: dubro@interactive.com.ar
Desc: Individuals in Argentina who work toward the dissemination of information and research concerning muscular dystrophy, a hereditary disease characterized by progressive deterioration of muscles.

★ 1146 ★ Asociacion Espanola de Esclerosis Lateral Amiotrofica (ADELA)
C/Hierbabuena No. 12 Bajo
E-28039 Madrid, Spain
Phone: 34 91 2142142 **Fax:** 34 91 4593906
Email: adele@adelaweb.com
Fnded: 1990. **Mem:** 800. **Nat'l Groups:** 1. **Reg. Groups:** 3. **Desc:** Individuals in Spain affected by Amyotrophic Lateral Sclerosis (ALS), a muscle wasting condition. Offers home care services. Provides a forum for support and exchange of information.

★ 1147 ★ Asociacion Espanola de Esclerosis Multiple (AEDEM)
c/o Francisco Delgado Valcarcel
Modesto Lafuente
8-1 Centro Derecha
E-28010 Madrid, Spain
Phone: 34 914 481 261 **Fax:** 34 914 481 305
Email: aedem26884@teleline.es
Website: http://www.aedem.org
Fnded: 1984. **Reg. Groups:** 30. **Desc:** MS patients, families and professionals. Seeks to improve the quality of life for persons with multiple sclerosis and their families.

★ 1148 ★ Asociacion Hondurena de Planificacion de Familia (ASHONPLAFA)
Calle Principal, entre: Colonias Alameda y Ruben Dario
Apartado Postal 625
Tegucigalpa, Honduras
Phone: 504 323235 **Fax:** 504 325140
Email: central@ashonplafa.com
Fnded: 1963. **Mem:** 40. **Lang(s):** Spanish. **Desc:** Works to enhance the quality of life of people living in Honduras through the promotion of responsible parenthood and family planning. Advocates family planning as a basic human right. Seeks to reduce the number of unwanted pregnancies and abortions. Provides programs in family planning, sex education, and health.

★ 1149 ★ Asociacion para la Luch contra la Paralisis Infantil (ALPI)
Salguero 1639
1425 Buenos Aires, Argentina
Phone: 54 1 841034
Fnded: 1943. **Desc:** Devoted to rehabilitating adults and children with motor disabilities resulting from accidents or illness, furthers research in this field, especially complex cases of disability such as brain or spinal injuries.

★ 1150 ★ Asociacion Medica Argentina
Santa Fe 1171
1059 Buenos Aires, Argentina
Phone: 54 1 411633
Fnded: 1891.

★ 1151 ★ Asociacion Mexicana Contra Esclerosis Multiple
c/o Ian Thomas
Calzada de Tlalpan 4515
14050 Toriello, DF, Mexico
Phone: 52 5 550 9987 **Fax:** 52 5616 4509
Email: thomasi@infosel.net.mx
Fnded: 1984. **Reg. Groups:** 3. **Desc:** MS patients, families and professionals. Seeks to improve the quality of life for persons with multiple sclerosis and their families.

★ 1152 ★ Asociacion Mexicana de Facultades y Escuelas de Medicina
Apdo 836
San Luis Potosi, Mexico
Fnded: 1957.

★ 1153 ★ Asociacion Nacional Contra el Cancer (ANCEC)
Apdo 7358, Zona 5
Panama City, Panama
Phone: 507 2252512 **Fax:** 507 2255366
Website: http://www.panamatravel.com/ancec.htm
Fnded: 1970. **Mem:** 150. **Nat'l Groups:** 1. **Reg. Groups:** 21. **State Groups:** 9. **Lang(s):** Spanish. **Desc:** Works to educate Panamanian people on prevention and detection of cancer. Informs women on prevention, self-testing, and importance of regular gynecological examinations. Maintains clinics offering mammograms, Pap smears, and prostate examinations. **Pub:** *Revista ANCEC*, biennial. Magazine. Contains articles on cancer, ongoing activities, and projects.

★ 1154 ★ Asociacion Pro-Bienestar de la Familia Colombiana (PROFAMILIA)
Calle 34, Numero 14-52
Bogota, Colombia
Phone: 57 1 3390900 **Fax:** 57 1 2875530
Email: info@profamilia.org.co
Website: http://www.profamilia.org.co/
Fnded: 1965. **Mem:** 917. **State Groups:** 40. **Lang(s):** English, Spanish. **Desc:** Promotes sexual health and reproductive rights in Colombia. Seeks to: improve maternal and child health by increasing the time between pregnancies; foster awareness of the possible effects of demographics on the socio-economic development of Colombia. Operates 35 family planning clinics in Colombia offering legal, medical, and educational services. Has established the Population Management Training Centre for staff employed at the clinics. Provides continuing education programs for gynecologists, obstetricians, and other doctors. Conducts studies and surveys; sponsors lectures, seminars, and workshops. **Pub:** *Annual Report*, annual. Pamphlet. Lists accomplishments of previous year. • *Disfunciones Sexuales*. Booklet.

★ 1155 ★ Asociacion Pro-Bienestar de la Familia Ecuatoriana (APROFE)
Letamendi No. 602 y Noguchi
Apartado Postal 5954
Guayaquil, Ecuador
Phone: 593 4 2402991 **Fax:** 593 4 419667
Email: aprofe@aprofe.org.ec
Website: http://www.aprofe.org.ec
Fnded: 1965. **Mem:** 20. **Lang(s):** Spanish. **Desc:** Works to enhance the quality of life for people living in Ecuador through the promotion of responsible parenthood and family planning. Encourages public knowledge of family planning, contraception, AIDS, and other sexually transmitted diseases. Provides contraceptive and health care services. Sponsors educational programs. Conducts research. **Pub:** *Family Planning in Ecuador.* Reports. Features the history of Aprofe and information on family planning in Ecuador.

★ 1156 ★ Asociacion Pro-Bienestar de la Familia de Guatemala (APROFAM)
9a Calle 0-57, Zona 1
Apartado Postal 1004
Guatemala City, Guatemala
Phone: 502 2 305488 **Fax:** 502 2 514017
Email: info@aprofam.org.gt
Website: http://www.aprofam.org.gt
Fnded: 1964. **Mem:** 90. **Nat'l Groups:** 34. **Reg. Groups:** 1. **Local Groups:** 11. **Lang(s):** Spanish. **Desc:** Educators, doctors, social workers, and others interested in improving the quality of life through the promotion of family planning. Advocates family planning as a basic human right. Conducts family development program that stresses self-sufficiency and offers help in how to improve family income and health. Works to educate the public on family planning, contraception, AIDS, and other sexually transmitted diseases. Operates a clinic for women from which it provides contraceptive and health care services such as instruction in pre- and post-natal care; tests and treatment for infertility; tests to detect cervical and uterine cancer; coloscopies; and ultrasound. Conducts research. **Pub:** *Calendario Demografico*, annual. Journal. Contains information on demographics and the environment. • *Calendario Demografico*, annual.

★ 1157 ★ Asociacion Psiquiatrica de la America Latina (APAL)
Apdo 3380
Caracas, Venezuela
Fnded: 1951.

★ 1158 ★ Asociacion Venezolana de Facultades de Medicina (AVEFAM)
La Trinidad, Caracas
Urbanizacion Sorocaima 1080, Venezuela
Phone: 58 212 9450875 **Fax:** 58 212 9432840
Email: fepafempafams@cantv.net

★ 1159 ★ Asperger Syndrome Association of Ireland (ASPIRE)
Carmichael House
North Brunswick St.
Dublin 7, Ireland
Phone: 353 1 8780027 **Fax:** 353 1 8735737
Email: asperger@email.com
Website: http://www.aspire-irl.com
Fnded: 1995. **Mem:** 200. **Reg. Groups:** 1. **Lang(s):** English, Irish. **Desc:** People with Asperger's syndrome and their families; health care providers and other individuals providing support and services to people with Asperger's syndrome. Seeks to improve the quality of life of people with Asperger's syndrome. Functions as a support network for people with Asperger's syndrome and their families; facilitates research projects.

★ 1160 ★ Asperger Syndrome Coalition of the United States (ASC-US)
154 Blanchard Ln.
Martinsburg, WV 25401-5843

Free: (866)4AS-PRGR
Email: info@asc-us.org
Website: http://www.asperger.org/

Desc: Individuals, families, professionals such as doctors, psychologists, educators, therapists. Promotes understanding of Asperger Syndrome and related conditions, including pervasive developmental disorder, not otherwise specified; high functioning autism; nonverbal learning disability; semantic-pragmatic disorder, hyperlexia. Seeks to develop a nationwide support group assistance program, provide leadership training, and produce products, services and educational materials.

★ 1161 ★ Assistance Dogs of America (ADAI)

8806 State Rte. 64
Swanton, OH 43558
Phone: (419)825-3622 **Fax:** (419)825-3710
Email: adaifacili@aol.com
Website: http://www.assistancedogsofamerica.org/
Chris Diefenthaler, Exec. Dir.

Fnded: 1984. **Mem:** 4,500. **Desc:** Promotes increased independence for people with disabilities. Locates, trains, and places highly skilled service and therapy dogs with disabled adults and children. **Pub:** *Hearts in Harness*, 3/year. Newsletter. **Frmly:** (1989) Guide Dogs for the Handicapped, Inc.

★ 1162 ★ Assistance Dogs International (ADI)

PO Box 5174
Santa Rosa, CA 95402
Phone: (707)571-0427
Email: info@adionline.org
Website: http://www.adionline.org
Suzi Hall, Coord.

Fnded: 1986. **Mem:** 50. **Desc:** ADI is a coalition of not-for-profit organizations that train and place Assistance Dogs. Purpose is to improve the areas of training, placement, and utilization of Assistance Dogs, as well as staff and volunteer education. Members of ADI meet annually to share ideas, attend seminars and conduct business regarding such things as educating the public about Assistance Dogs, and the legal rights of people with disabilities partnered with Assistance Dogs, setting standards and establishing guidelines and ethics for the training of these dogs, and improving the utilization and bonding of each team.

★ 1163 ★ Associacao Brasileira de Esclerose Multipla (ABEM)

c/o Collete Levy
Rua Demostenes, 283
04614-011 Sao Paulo, Brazil
Phone: 55 11 5533 0582 **Fax:** 55 11 5533 3542
Email: abem@abem.org.br
Website: http://www.abem.org.br/

Fnded: 1984. **Mem:** 4,000. **Nat'l Groups:** 4100. **Reg. Groups:** 5. **State Groups:** 1765. **Local Groups:** 1096. **Desc:** MS patients, families and professionals. Seeks to improve the quality of life for persons with multiple sclerosis and their families; provides social care. **Pub:** *Vivabem*, trimester. Magazine.

★ 1164 ★ Associacao Medica Homeopatica Brasileira

SEPS 714/914 Ed. Santa Maria, Sala 312
70390-145 Brasilia, DF, Brazil
Phone: 55 61 3456077
Website: http://www.amhb.org.br

Fnded: 1951.

★ 1165 ★ Associacao Mocambicana dos Diabeticos

av Ho Chi Min No 1142
CP 2167
Maputo, Mozambique
Phone: 258 1 310389 **Fax:** 258 1 422698
Email: dalila@zebra.uem.mz
Website: http://www.diabetesafrica.com/idfmembers.html

Desc: Represents people with diabetes. Promotes research and support of those with diabetes in Mozambique.

★ 1166 ★ Associacao Mozambicana para o Desenvolimento da Familia (AMODEFA)

Av. Da Tanzania no. 40
50-Amodefa
PO Box 1535
Maputo, Mozambique
Phone: 258 1 405107 **Fax:** 258 1 405149
Email: manjos@amodefa.org

Fnded: 1989. **Lang(s):** Portuguese. **Desc:** Works to improve the quality of life for individuals living in Mozambique by promoting responsible parenthood and family planning. Attempts to stop the spread of AIDS and other sexually transmitted diseases. Offers programs in family planning, sex education, and health. Provides contraceptive and health care services. Acts as an advocate for family planning on a national level. Conducts research. **Pub:** *Crescer*, monthly. Magazine.

★ 1167 ★ Associacao Portuguesa de Miastenia Gravis e Doencas Neuromusculares (APMG-DNM)

Hospital de Santa Maria
P-1649-035 Lisbon, Portugal
Phone: 351 21 7805320 **Fax:** 351 21 7805630
Email: info@apmg-dnm.rcts.pt
Website: http://www.miastenia.co.pt

Fnded: 1989. **Mem:** 800. **Lang(s):** English. **Desc:** Promotes interest in neuromuscular diseases research among medical and scientific communities and the public in Portugal. Disseminates information. Provides medical and social support to patients and their families. **Pub:** *Boletim Informative*, quarterly. Journal. Contains news about neuromuscular dystrophy and information for patients.

★ 1168 ★ Associated Blind

110 William St., 9th Fl.
New York, NY 10011
Phone: (212)766-6800 **Fax:** (212)766-6809
Email: memberservices@esightcareers.net
Website: http://www.tabinc.org
Ruth-Ellen Simmonds, Exec. Dir.

Fnded: 1938. **Reg. Groups:** 1. **Local Groups:** 1. **Desc:** Provides employment and career management services for blind or visually impaired individuals through direct service programs and online. Assists corporations and other organizations with all accessibility consulting services, including Web accessibility and disability awareness and sensitivity training, and emergency preparedness. Conducts internship programs that enable blind and visually impaired colleges students to participate in national internships along with sighted peers. **Pub:** *eSight Careers Network*. An online service, at www.esightcareers.net, that is ongoing. • *eSight Job Alert*, weekly. An e-bulletin. • *eSight Net Works*, weekly. An e-newsletter.

★ 1169 ★ Associated Bodywork and Massage Professionals (ABMP)

1271 Sugarbush Dr.
Evergreen, CO 80439-9766
Free: 800-458-2267 **Fax:** 800-667-8260
Email: expectmore@abmp.com
Website: http://www.abmp.com
Katie Armitage, Exec. Dir.

Fnded: 1986. **Mem:** 40,000. **Nat'l Groups:** 1. **Desc:** Professional massage therapists and bodyworkers, sports massage therapists, skin care professionals, reflexologists, energy practitioners, etc.; massage therapy schools; affiliated organizations. Promotes massage and bodywork. Seeks to improve the image of massage therapy and bodywork, and to educate the public about its benefits. Fosters greater credibility and cooperation with the medical profession. Encourages ethical practices, high standards of professional conduct, and continuing education. Provides members with low-cost liability insurance coverage and product discounts. **Pub:** *ABMP Massage Marketplace*, annual. Directory. • *ABMP Successful Business Handbook*, annual. Handbook. • *ABMP Touch Resource Guide*. Directory. • *Massage and Bodywork*, bimonthly. *Price:* $26 included in membership dues. **Frmly:** (1988) Associated Professional Massage Therapists and Allied Health Practitioners International; (1990) Associated Professional Massage Therapists and Bodyworkers.

★ 1170 ★ Associated Medical Services (AMS)

162 Cumberland St., Ste. 228
Toronto, ON, Canada M5R 3N5
Phone: (416)924-3368 **Fax:** (416)323-3338
Email: ams@ams-inc.on.ca
Website: http://www.ams-inc.on.ca

Fnded: 1937. **Lang(s):** English, French. **Desc:** Health services. Promotes increased availability of quality health care. Facilitates communication and cooperation among members; represents members' interests before government agencies, professional medical organizations, and the public. **Pub:** *Corporate Report*, biennial. Report. • Newsletter, 3/year.

★ 1171 ★ Associated Professional Sleep Societies (APSS)

1 West Brook Corp. Ctr., Ste. 920
Westchester, IL 60154
Phone: (708)492-0930 **Fax:** (708)492-0943
Email: info@aasmet.org
Website: http://www.apss.org
Jerry Barrett, Exec. Dir.

Fnded: 1985. **Desc:** Members are the Sleep Research Society and American Academy of Sleep Medicine . Works to facilitate sleep research and development of sleep disorder medicine by encouraging cooperation and exchange of information among members. **Pub:** *SLEEP*, 8/year. Journal. *Price:* $129/year for individuals; $185/year for institutions; $159/year for foreign individuals; $220/year for foreign institutions. **Frmly:** Association of Professional Sleep Societies.

★ 1172 ★ Associated Services for the Blind (ASB)

919 Walnut St.
Philadelphia, PA 19107
Phone: (215)627-0600 **Fax:** (215)922-0692
Email: asbinfo@libertynet.org
Website: http://www.asb.org/
Patricia C. Johnson, Chief Exec. Officer

Fnded: 1984. **Desc:** Multiservice agency that provides services to blind and visually impaired people. Objective is to help blind and visually impaired people live independently. Activities include: operating a braille printing house that transcribes print materials into braille; radio reading service that reads newspapers and magazines over closed-circuit radio. Offers rehabilitation program, social services, and recorded periodicals. **Pub:** *ASB Visions*, 3/year. Newsletter. • Annual Report, annual. Reports on services, board, financials. • Brochure.

★ 1173 ★ Association of Academic Chairmen of Plastic Surgery (AACPS)

4900 B South 31st St.
Arlington, VA 22206
Phone: (703)820-7400 **Fax:** (703)931-4520
Email: aacps@mindspring.com
Website: http://www.aacplasticsurgery.org

Fnded: 1985. **Mem:** 270. **Desc:** Chairmen of plastic and reconstructive surgery education and residency programs. Seeks to advance the study and teaching of plastic and reconstructive surgery. Facilitates establishment of graduate medical education and residency programs in plastic and reconstructive surgery. Conducts educational programs.

★ 1174 ★ Association of Academic Health Centers (AHC)
1400 16th St. NW, Ste. 720
Washington, DC 20036
Phone: (202)265-9600 **Fax:** (202)265-7514
Email: ahc@acadhlthctrs.org
Website: http://www.ahcnet.org
Roger J. Bulger, MD, Pres.

Fnded: 1969. **Mem:** 102. **Desc:** Chief executive officers of university-based academic health centers in the U.S. and Canada. Interdisciplinary in focus, with a primary interest in total health manpower education. Sponsors task forces and forums to advance public policy dialogue on health and science issues. Develops research and education programs. Publishes, reports, books, and issues papers. **Pub:** *General Meetings*, periodic. • Directory, periodic. • Reports.Provides information on special projects. **Frmly:** Organization of University Health Center Administrators.

★ 1175 ★ Association of Academic Physiatrists (AAP)
1106 N Charles St., Ste. 201
Baltimore, MD 21201
Phone: (410)637-8300 **Fax:** (410)637-8399
Email: aap@physiatry.org
Website: http://www.physiatry.org
Carolyn L. Braddom, EdD, Exec. Dir.

Fnded: 1967. **Mem:** 1,400. **Desc:** Academic physicians practicing physical medicine and rehabilitation and certified by the American Board of Physical Medicine and Rehabilitation. Objectives are: to advance teaching and research in physical medicine and rehabilitation within the area of academic medicine; to promote the dissemination of information to future physicians planning to work in this field; to become involved in the exchange of information from other areas of medicine both in basic sciences and in the clinical areas of teaching and research. **Pub:** *AAP Newsletter*, quarterly. Newsletter. • *American Journal of Physical Medicine and Rehabilitation*, monthly. Journal. • *Residency Program Directory*, annual. Directory. • Membership Directory, annual.

★ 1176 ★ Association for Academic Surgery (AAS)
60 Revere Dr., Ste. 500
Northbrook, IL 60062
Phone: (847)509-1945 **Fax:** (847)480-9282
Email: aas@aasurg.org
Website: http://www.aasurg.org
Melanie Stanton, Exec. Dir.

Fnded: 1966. **Mem:** 2,736. **Desc:** Active (700) and senior (1250) surgeons with backgrounds in all surgical specialties in academic surgical centers at chief resident level or above. Encourages young surgeons to pursue careers in academic surgery; supports them in establishing themselves as investigators and educators by providing a forum in which senior surgical residents and junior faculty members may present papers on subjects of clinical or laboratory investigations; promotes interchange of ideas between senior surgical residents, junior faculty, and established academic surgeons; facilitates communication among academic surgeons in all surgical fields. Maintains placement service. service. service. **Pub:** *Journal of Surgical Research*, monthly. Journal. *Price:* Included in membership dues; $65 for candidate and senior.

★ 1177 ★ Association for Addiction Professionals (NAADAC)
901 N Washington St., Ste. 600
Alexandria, VA 22314
Phone: (703)741-7686 **Free:** 800-548-0497
Fax: (703)741-7698
Website: http://naadac.org/documents/index.php?CategorID=1
Pat Ford-Roegner, Exec. Dir.

Fnded: 1972. **Mem:** 14,000. **State Groups:** 47. **Desc:** Serves counselors specializing in addiction treatment, focusing on alcohol and drug addiction. **Pub:** *Counselor*, monthly. Magazine. • Newsletter, monthly.

★ 1178 ★ Association of Adult Day Support Programs (AADSP)
9735 80th Ave.
Edmonton, AB, Canada T6E 1S8
Phone: (780)434-4747 **Fax:** (780)433-3758
Email: iheemeryck@worldgate.com
Website: http://www.greynuns.ab.ca/adult-day.htm

Fnded: 1979. **Mem:** 160. **Desc:** Educational and recreational programs for adults with disabilities living in non-institutional settings. Promotes an improved quality of life for adults with disabilities that prevent them from participating in mainstream recreational activities. Facilitates communication and cooperation among members; provides educational and recreational programs to adults with disabilities.

★ 1179 ★ Association for Advanced Training in the Behavioral Sciences (AATBS)
5126 Ralston St.
Ventura, CA 93003
Free: 800-472-1931 **Fax:** (805)676-3033
Website: http://www.aatbs.com/

Desc: Aims to produce study materials in order to provide education and training for psychologists, marriage and family therapists, social workers, mental health counselors and alcohol/drug counselors to pass professional exams.

★ 1180 ★ Association for the Advancement of Applied Sport Psychology
801 Main St., Ste. 010
Louisville, CO 80027
Phone: (303)494-5931
Website: http://www.aaasponline.org
Linda Petlichkoff, Pres.

Fnded: 1986. **Mem:** 1,300. **Desc:** Promotes the development of research, theory, and intervention strategies in sport psychology. Concerned with ethical and professional issues related to the development of sport psychology and to the provision of psychological services in sport and exercise settings. Sponsors research and educational programs. **Pub:** *AAASP Newsletter*, 3/year. Newsletter. Contains professional articles, organization information, and book reviews. • *Journal of Applied Sport Psychology*, quarterly. Journal.

★ 1181 ★ Association for Advancement of Behavior Therapy (AABT)
305 7th Ave., Ste. 16A
New York, NY 10001-6008
Phone: (212)647-1890 **Free:** 800-685-AABT
Fax: (212)647-1865
Email: mjeimer@aabt.org
Website: http://www.aabt.org/
Mary Jane Eimer, CAE, Exec. Dir.

Fnded: 1966. **Mem:** 4,500. **Desc:** Psychologists primarily, but also psychiatrists, social workers, counselors, physicians, dentists, nurses, students, and other professionals interested in the issues, problems, and development of the field of behavior therapy and cognitive behavior therapy, with specific emphasis on research and clinical applications. Sponsors training programs and lectures for professionals; maintains speakers' bureau; handles referrals for the public to locate behavior therapists in their area; facilitates communication between behavior therapists interested in specific problems or information. AABT local affiliates hold training meetings, workshops, seminars, case demonstrations, and discussion groups. discussion groups. **Pub:** *The Behavior Therapist*, 10/year. Newsletter. Reports the latest research and includes book reviews, association news, professionals and legislative issues reports, training updates, job listings. *Price:* Included in membership dues; $60/year for nonmembers. • *Behavior Therapy*, quarterly. Journal. An international journal devoted to the application of behavioral and cognitive sciences to clinical problems. *Price:* $75/year for nonmembers; $145/year for institutions. • *Cognitive and Behavioral Practice*, quarterly. Journal. Integrates behavior therapy principles and research with clinical practice techniques. *Price:* $75/ for nonmembers; $145/for institutions. • *Directory of Graduate Training in Behavior Therapy and Experimental-Clinical Psychology*, biennial. Lists over 300 psychology, special education, and counseling programs that offer training in behavior therapy. *Price:* $20 for members; $25 for non-members. • *Directory of Psychology Internships: Programs Offering Behavioral Training*, periodic. Contains information on admission requirements, application deadlines, and program structure; statistics. *Price:* $20 for members; $25 for nonmembers. • Videos.For training purposes. *Price:* Included in membership dues; $50 for nonmembers. • Also publishes a series of Fact Sheets to educate lay audiences about a variety of psychological disorders, including panic attacks, obsessive-compulsive disorder, post-traumatic stress syndrome, depression, eating disorders, and more. Call for a complete list of available titles. **Frmly:** (1968) Association for Advancement of the Behavioral Therapies.

★ 1182 ★ Association for the Advancement of Blacks in Health Sciences (AABHS)
42 Charles St. E
Toronto, ON, Canada M4Y 1T4
Phone: (416)928-9201 **Fax:** (416)928-3325

Fnded: 1993. **Desc:** Health care professionals, researchers, graduate, undergraduate students, non-health professionals. Promotes the pursuit of higher education in health science fields to black youth; strives to optimize health care services and information to black community. Supports the following initiatives: Health Sciences Summer Mentorship Program, Visions of Science Forums, Camp Jumoke, Black Medical Student Association (BMSA), and community outreach programs.

★ 1183 ★ Association for the Advancement of Blind and Retarded (AABR)
PO Box 560247
College Point, NY 11356
Phone: (718)321-3800 **Fax:** (718)321-8688
Email: aabr1@aol.com
Website: http://aabr.org
Christopher Weldon, Jr., Exec. Dir.

Fnded: 1955. **Desc:** Community groups and individuals interested in multi-handicapped blind and severely retarded adults. Operates 19 group residences providing intermediate care and individual residential alternative facilities for blind and retarded adults; two treatment centers for blind, multi-handicapped, and severely retarded adults; NYS approved special education program for autistic children from pre-school to school age. Provides information and referral services. **Pub:** *AABR Newsletter*, 3/year. Newsletter. Contains donor update letter. *Price:* Free. **Frmly:** (1974) Association for Advancement of Blind Children.

★ 1184 ★ Association for the Advancement of Gestalt Therapy (AAGT)
c/o Carol Brockmon
7861 Spring Ave.
Elkins Park, PA 19027
Phone: (215)782-1484 **Fax:** (215)635-2391
Email: info@aagt.org
Website: http://www.aagt.org
Carol Brockmon, VP

Desc: Psychiatrists, psychologists, social workers, teachers, academics, writers, artists, performers, organizational consultants and political and social analysts, activists, and students. Seeks to advance theory, philosophy, practice and research in Gestalt Therapy and its various applications, including but not limited to, personal growth, mental health, education, organization and systems development, political and social development and change, and the fine and performing arts.

★ 1185 ★ Association for Advancement of Psychoanalysis (of the Karen Horney Psychoanalytic Institute and Center) (AAP)
329 E 62nd St.
New York, NY 10021
Phone: (212)838-8044 **Fax:** (212)888-1610
Email: karenhorneyctr@aol.com
Website: http://www.karenhorneycenter.org
Judith Fox-Fliesser, MD, Pres.

Fnded: 1941. **Mem:** 80. **Desc:** Certified psychoanalysts interested in encouraging training in psychoanalysis and disseminating psychoanalytic principles to the medical-psychiatric profession and the general community. Conducts scientific meetings. Maintains a consultation and referral service, placement service, and speakers' bureau. Supports research programs; sponsors public educational lectures; maintains library of 4000 volumes. **Pub:** *The American Journal of Psychoanalysis*, quarterly. Journal. Includes book reviews. *Price:* $24 for individuals; $50 for libraries and institutions. • Newsletter, semiannual.

★ 1186 ★ Association for the Advancement of Psychological Understanding of Human Nature (VPM)
Postfach 2161
CH-8033 Zurich, Switzerland
Phone: 41 1 2610031 **Fax:** 41 1 2610561
Email: vpm@compuserve.com

Fnded: 1986. **Mem:** 700. **Lang(s):** English, French, German, Italian. **Desc:** Psychologists and other scientists with an interest in human behavior. Seeks to advance scholarship on the psychological components of human behavior. Facilitates exchange of information among members; sponsors research and educational programs.

★ 1187 ★ Association for Advancement of Psychology (AAP)
PO Box 38129
Colorado Springs, CO 80937
Phone: (719)520-0688 **Free:** 800-869-6595
Fax: (719)520-0375
Email: smpfeiffer@aapnet.org
Website: http://www.aapnet.org/
Stephen M. Pfeiffer, PhD, Exec. Dir.

Fnded: 1974. **Mem:** 6,000. **Desc:** Members of the American Psychological Association or other national psychological associations, students of psychology, and organizations with a primarily psychological focus. Purposes are to advance psychology and represent the interests of all psychologists (professional, social, and scientific) in the public policy arena. Maintains Psychologists For Legislative Action Now, a political action and education committee. **Pub:** *Association for Advancement of Psychology–Advance*, quarterly. Newsletter. Includes calendar of events and research updates. *Price:* Included in membership dues.

★ 1188 ★ Association for the Advancement of Psychotherapy (AAP)
c/o T. Byram Karasu, M.D.
Albert Einstein College of Medicine
Belfer Education Center, Rm. 405
1300 Morris Park Ave.
Bronx, NY 10461-1602
Phone: (718)430-3503 **Fax:** (718)430-8907
Email: info@ajp.org
Website: http://www.ajp.org
T. Byram Karasu, MD, Editor-in-Chief

Fnded: 1939. **Desc:** Works to create a forum where all concepts of psychotherapeutic thought can be aired for the advancement of psychotherapy in practice, research, and training. **Pub:** *American Journal of Psychotherapy*, quarterly. Journal. Includes book reviews and software reviews. *Price:* $70 for individuals; $100 for institutions; $78 for individuals in Canada; $108 for institutions in Canada.

★ 1189 ★ Association for the Advancement of Wound Care (AAWC)
83 General Warren Blvd., Ste. 100
Malvern, PA 19355
Phone: (610)560-0484 **Free:** (866)AAWC-999
Fax: (610)560-0502
Email: aawchelp@voicenet.com
Website: http://www.aawcone.com
Tina Thomas, Assoc. Liaison

Fnded: 1996. **Mem:** 900. **Desc:** Works to advance the cause of wound care through education, research, clinical practice and public policy. Provides a forum for communication and partnership among all people involved in wound care. **Pub:** *AAWC Newsletter*, quarterly. Newsletter. Contains updates on wound care. *Price:* Free for members. • *Ostomy/Wound Management*, monthly. Journal. *Price:* Free for members. • *Wound Care Clinic Directory*, annual. Directory. *Price:* $10 for members; $20 for nonmembers. • *Wounds*, bimonthly. Journal. *Price:* Free for members.

★ 1190 ★ Association of African Optometric Educators (AAOE)
Morny Optical Centre
PO Box 1814
Kumasi, Ghana
Phone: 233 51 22511 **Fax:** 233 51 25306
Email: mornyko@africaonline.com.gh

Fnded: 1992. **Mem:** 179. **Nat'l Groups:** 10. **Reg. Groups:** 4. **State Groups:** 4. **Local Groups:** 10. **Lang(s):** English. **Desc:** Optometry educators. Seeks to advance optometric scholarship and practice. Sponsors training programs for optometric personnel; makes available continuing professional development courses for members. **Pub:** *Nuclus*, semiannual. Journal. Contains research findings.

★ 1191 ★ Association of Air Medical Services (AAMS)
526 King St., Ste. 415
Alexandria, VA 22314-3143
Phone: (703)836-8732 **Fax:** (703)836-8920
Email: information@aams.org
Website: http://www.aams.org
Dawn Mancuso, CAE, Exec. Dir. /CEO

Fnded: 1980. **Mem:** 400. **Reg. Groups:** 10. **Desc:** Air medical transport providers; manufacturers and distributors of air medical transport equipment and supplies. Objective is to provide quality medical care during rapid air transport. Seeks to develop standards for aircraft configuration, minimum professional and educational requirements for personnel on board, medical and communications equipment, and operations. **Pub:** *AAMS News & Views*, monthly. Newsletter. For members only. • *AAMS Resource Guide*, annual. Membership Directory. • *Air Medical Journal*, bimonthly. Magazine. Published in conjunction with several other Associations. *Price:* Included in membership dues. **Frmly:** (1988) American Society of Hospital-Based Emergency Air Medical Services.

★ 1192 ★ Association Alzheimer Suisse (ALZ)
Rue des Pecheurs 8
CH-1400 Yverdon-les-Bains, Switzerland
Phone: 41 24 4262000 **Fax:** 41 24 4262167
Email: alz@bluewin.ch
Website: http://www.alz.ch

Fnded: 1988. **Mem:** 5,500. **Nat'l Groups:** 1. **State Groups:** 18. **Local Groups:** 82. **Lang(s):** English, French, German, Italian. **Desc:** Individuals and organizations. Seeks to improve the quality of life of people with Alzheimer's disease and their families. Makes available support and services; facilitates research on Alzheimer's disease and related disorders; conducts educational programs. **Pub:** *Alzheimer Info*, 3/year. Magazine.

★ 1193 ★ Association for Ambulatory Behavioral Healthcare
11240 Waples Mill Rd., Ste. 200
Fairfax, VA 22032
Phone: (703)934-0160 **Fax:** (703)359-7562
Email: info@aabh.org
Website: http://www.aabh.org
Jerry Galler, Exec. Dir.

Fnded: 1965. **Mem:** 250. **Reg. Groups:** 20. **Desc:** Individuals interested in the development and improvement of the continuum of psychiatric treatment. To support, encourage, and stimulate the expansion of ambulatory behavioral health services. Sponsors educational discussions on partial hospitalization, intensive outpatient and rehabilitative services including clinical research and administrative issues. Provides consultation services to stimulate and support the study, evaluation, and implementation of ambulatory behavioral health services. Collaborates with other groups in establishing standards of operation and performance in the field. Monitors local and national legislative activity directly related to behavioral healthcare. **Pub:** *Insurance and Partial Hospitalization*. • *Milieu*, bimonthly. Newsletter. • *Standards and Guidelines for Child and Adolescent Partial Hospitalization*. • *Standards and Guidelines for Partial Hospitalization*. **Frmly:** (1975) Partial Hospitalization Study Group; (1979) Federation of Partial Hospitalization Study Groups; (1996) American Association for Partial Hospitalization.

★ 1194 ★ Association of Ambulatory Vaginal and Incontinence Surgeons (AAVIS)
c/o Dr. Bruce Farnsworth, Sec.
PO Box 438
Edgecliff 2027, Australia
Phone: 61 4 27424195 **Fax:** 61 2 94494274
Email: brucef@midcoast.com.au
Website: http://www.aavis.org/

Desc: Pelvic surgeons interested in conservative treatment methods and day-stay surgery for vaginal prolapse and incontinence, particularly new keyhole surgical techniques.

★ 1195 ★ Association of American Cancer Institutes (AACI)
c/o Dr. Edwin A. Mirand
200 Lathrop St.
Iroquois Bldg., No. 305
Pittsburgh, PA 15213
Phone: (412)647-2076 **Fax:** (412)647-3659
Website: http://www.roswellpark.org
Barbara Duffy Stewart, Exec. Dir.

Fnded: 1959. **Mem:** 85. **Desc:** Directors of cancer centers. Informs members of important legislative and program developments in the field. Promotes discussion among cancer center leadership throughout the world; fosters collaboration between members on research, education, and service programs; works to further educational and training opportunities in related biomedical sciences; advises federal, state, and local governments, and private and civic organizations concerning cancer research and related health topics. **Pub:** *AACI Newsletter*, periodic. Newsletter. *Price:* Free. **Frmly:** (1968) Association of Cancer Institute Directors.

★ 1196 ★ Association of American Indian Physicians (AAIP)
1225 Sovereign Row, Ste. 103
Oklahoma City, OK 73108-1854
Phone: (405)946-7072 **Fax:** (405)946-7651
Email: aaip@aaip.com
Website: http://www.aaip.com
Ben Muneta, MD, Pres.

Fnded: 1971. **Mem:** 270. **Desc:** Physicians (M.D. or D.O.) of American Indian descent. Encourages American Indians to enter the health professions. Provides a forum for the interchange of ideas and information of mutual interest to physicians of Indian descent. Establishes contracts with government agencies to provide consultation and other expert opinion regarding health care of American Indians and Alaskan Natives; receives contracts and grant monies and other forms of assistance from these sources. Supports and encourages all other agencies and organizations, Indian and non-Indian, working to improve health conditions of American Indians and Alaskan Natives. Locates scholarship funds for Indian professional students; provides counseling assistance; preserves American Indian culture. Conducts seminars for students interested in health careers and for counselors in government and other schools where American Indian children are taught. **Pub:** Newsletter, quarterly.

★ 1197 ★ Association of American Medical Colleges (AAMC)

2450 N St. NW
Washington, DC 20037-1136
Phone: (202)828-0400 **Fax:** (202)828-1125
Email: amcas@aamc.org
Website: http://www.aamc.org
Jordan J. Cohen, MD, Pres.

Fnded: 1876. **Mem:** 2,200. **Desc:** Medical schools, graduate affiliate medical colleges, academic societies, teaching hospitals, and individuals interested in the advancement of medical education, biomedical research, and healthcare. Provides centralized application service. Offers management education program for medical school deans, teaching hospital directors, department chairmen, and service chiefs of affiliated hospitals. Develops and administers the Medical College Admissions Test (MCAT). Operates student loan program. Maintains information management system and institutional profile system. Compiles statistics. **Pub:** *Academic Medicine*, monthly. Journal. Provides scholarly articles on physician education and workforce issues. *Price:* $120/year in U.S.; $180 Canada and foreign. • *Directory of American Medical Education*, annual. Directory. • *Medical School Admission Requirements*, annual. • Reports, annual. • Reports, semiannual.

★ 1198 ★ Association of American Medical Colleges-Women in Medicine Program (AAMC-WIM)

c/o Janet Bickel
2450 N St. NW
Washington, DC 20037-1126
Phone: (202)828-0521 **Fax:** (202)828-1125
Email: jbickel@aamc.org
Website: http://www.aamc.org/members/wim/start.htm
Janet Bickel, MA, Assoc. VP & Dir.

Desc: Dedicated to increasing women's leadership in academic medicine. **Pub:** *Membership Directory*. • *Women in Medicine Update*, quarterly.

★ 1199 ★ Association of American Physicians and Surgeons (AAPS)

1601 N Tucson Blvd., Ste. 9
Tucson, AZ 85716
Phone: (520)327-4885 **Free:** 800-635-1196
Fax: (520)326-3529
Email: jorient@mindspring.com
Website: http://www.aapsonline.org/
Jane M. Orient, MD, Exec. Dir.

Fnded: 1943. **Mem:** 4,500. **Desc:** Physicians dedicated to preserving and promoting quality medical care. Represents physicians in the socioeconomic and legal aspects of medical practice such as medical economics, public relations, and legislation. Makes available legal consultation services. **Pub:** *AAPS News*, monthly. Newsletter. Covers developments affecting health care and the profession. Includes legislative news, calendar of events, and health law commentary. *Price:* Included in membership dues; $35/year for nonmembers. • *The Medical Sentinel*, quarterly. Journal. Peer-reviewed journal. • Audiotapes.

★ 1200 ★ Association of Anaesthetists of Great Britain and Ireland

21 Portland Pl.
London W1B 1PY, United Kingdom
Phone: 44 207 6318801 **Fax:** 44 207 6314352
Email: members@aagbi.org
Website: http://www.aagbi.org

Fnded: 1932. **Mem:** 7,000. **Lang(s):** English. **Desc:** Ordinary Members, Trainee Members and Associate Members. Aims to promote education and research in anaesthesia and to bring together as many members as is possible at the three annual meetings to disseminate relevant information both at home and abroad. Fosters research in anaesthesia and allied subjects; encourages collaborative ventures involving members; represents members' interests. **Pub:** *Anaesthesia*, monthly. Journal.

★ 1201 ★ Association for Applied Hypnosis (AAH)

21B High Holme Rd.
Louth LN11 0EX, United Kingdom
Phone: 44 1507 607336

Fnded: 1980.

★ 1202 ★ Association for Applied Poetry (AAP)

60 N Main St.
Johnstown, OH 43031-1015
Phone: (740)967-6060
Email: pudding@johnstown.net
Website: http://www.puddinghouse.com
Jennifer Bosveld, pres.

Fnded: 1984. **Desc:** Poets, teachers, therapists, social workers, creative artists, librarians, and interested individuals. Promotes the application of poetry and creative writing to human services, healing, and self-awareness and self-actualization. Conducts support groups and tutorials. Operates Pudding House Bed and Breakfast retreat at Puddings House Wrtiters Resource Center. Maintains speakers'bureau. Conducts educational programs. **Pub:** *Pudding Magazine: The International Journal of Applied Poetry*, periodic. Journal. Contains poetry essays and reviews applicable to education and human services and art. *Price:* Included with membership. • *Topics for Getting in Touch: A Poetry Therapy Sourcebook*. • Also publishes articles, chapbooks, and educational materials.

★ 1203 ★ Association for Applied Psychophysiology and Biofeedback (AAPB)

10200 W 44th Ave., Ste. 304
Wheat Ridge, CO 80033
Phone: (303)422-8436 **Free:** 800-477-8892
Fax: (303)422-8894
Email: fbutler@resourcecenter.com
Website: http://www.aapb.org
Francine Butler, PhD, Pres.

Fnded: 1969. **Mem:** 2,000. **State Groups:** 35. **Desc:** Persons interested in the "interrelationship of external feedback systems, states of consciousness, and the physiological mechanisms involved." Promotes rapid interchange of ideas and information among members. Offers Continuing Education Training Programs. Maintains numerous committees. **Pub:** *Applied Psychophysiology and Biofeedback*, quarterly. Journal. Study of physiological systems and social environmental health. *Price:* included in membership dues. • *Biofeedback News magazine*, quarterly. Newsletter. • *Proceedings of Annual Meeting*. Proceedings. **Frmly:** (1976) Biofeedback Research Society; (1988) Biofeedback Society of America.

★ 1204 ★ Association of Aromatherapists Southern Africa (AOASA)

PO Box 23924
Claremont 7735, Republic of South Africa
Phone: 27 21 5317314

Desc: Represents the professional interests of all its members nationally and internationally, as well as educational government level.

★ 1205 ★ Association of Asian/Pacific Community Health Organizations (AAPCHO)

429 23rd St.
Oakland, CA 94612-2025
Phone: (510)272-9536 **Fax:** (510)272-0817
Email: jeffc@aapcho.org
Website: http://www.aapcho.org
Jeffrey B. Caballero, Exec. Dir.

Fnded: 1987. **Mem:** 14. **Desc:** Works to improve access to culturally and linguistically appropriate health care in order to improve the health status of Asians and Pacific Islanders with a special focus on the medically underserved. **Pub:** *Hepatitis B*. Brochure. • *Parent's Guide to Common Childhood Illnesses*. Brochure. • *Thalassemia Among Asians*. Brochure.

★ 1206 ★ Association for Assessment and Accreditation of Laboratory Animal Care International (AAALAC)

11300 Rockville Pike, Ste. 1211
Rockville, MD 20852-3035
Phone: (301)231-5353 **Free:** 800-926-0066
Fax: (301)231-8282
Email: accredit@aaalac.org
Website: http://www.aaalac.org
Dr. John G. Miller, DVM, Exec. Dir.

Fnded: 1965. **Mem:** 50. **Desc:** Promotes the humane treatment of animals in science thourgh a voluntary accrediation program. More than 600 institutions around the world have earned AAALAC International accreditation, demonstrating their commitment to responsible animal care and use. **Pub:** *AAALAC Connection*, 4/year. Newsletter. **Frmly:** American Association for Accreditation of Laboratory Animal Care.

★ 1207 ★ Association of Behavioral Healthcare Management (ABHM)

12300 Twinbrook Pkwy, Ste. 320
Rockville, MD 20852
Phone: (301)984-6200 **Fax:** (301)881-7159
Email: davids@nccbh.org
Website: http://www.nccbh.org/abhm/index.htm
Ann L. Brand, PhD, Ch.

Fnded: 1959. **Mem:** 600. **Desc:** Administrators of services for the emotionally disturbed, mentally ill, mentally retarded, developmentally disabled, and those with problems of alcohol and substance abuse. Objectives are to: further the education of administrators; develop criteria for and certify the competence of administrators; promote adherence to a code of ethics. Aids in developing professional administrative skills and administration of services. Sponsors educational workshops. **Pub:** *ABHM Leader*, quarterly. Newsletter. Current news and information on mental health administration issues. *Price:* $90/year. • *Journal of Behavioral Health Services & Research*, quarterly. Journal. Covers management practice, research, and policy issues in the mental health field. **Frmly:** (1969) American Society of Mental Health Business Administrators; (1997) Association of Mental Heath Administrators.

★ 1208 ★ Association of Biomedical Communication Directors (ABCD)

c/o Beverly E. Hill Ed. D
Medical Educational Resources Program
Indiana University School of Medicine
1226 W Michigan St., BR 156
Indianapolis, IN 46202-5178
Fax: (317)274-4638
Beverly E. Hill, Ed.D., Sec.

Fnded: 1972. **Mem:** 87. **Desc:** Individuals with common managerial concerns in health science communications, such as persons with direct administrative responsibility for operations of a biomedical communications facility in a school or academic health science center. Provides a forum for the sharing and dissemination of information, materials, and ideas. Promotes research and education in administrative practices with regard to health sciences communications. Works to develop information materials such as surveys and profiles helpful in the management of biomedical communications. **Pub:** *Exchange*, quarterly. • *Journal of Biocommunication*, quarterly. Journal. • *Membership Roster*, annual. • *Report of Annual Survey of The Directors of Biomedical Communications*.

★ 1209 ★ Association for Birth Psychology (ABP)
444 E 82nd St.
New York, NY 10028
Phone: (212)988-6617
Website: http://birthpsychology.org
Leslie Feher, PhD, Exec. Dir.

Fnded: 1978. **Mem:** 352. **Desc:** Obstetricians, pediatricians, midwives, nurses, psychotherapists, psychologists, counselors, social workers, sociologists, and others interested in birth psychology, a developing discipline concerned with the experience of birth and the correlation between the birth process and personality development. Seeks to promote communication among professionals in the field; encourage commentary, research, and theory from different points of view; establish birth psychology as an autonomous science of human behavior; develop guidelines and give direction to the field. **Pub:** *Birth Psychology Bulletin*, semiannual. Journal. Covers conception to the first year of life. Includes book reviews, research reports, calendar of events, and case reports. *Price:* Included in membership dues; $20/year for nonmembers. • Books.

★ 1210 ★ Association of Black Cardiologists (ABC)
6849-B2 Peachtree Dunwoody Rd. NE
Atlanta, GA 30328
Phone: (678)302-4222 **Free:** 888-874-6559
Fax: (678)302-4223
Email: jbutts@abcardio.org
Website: http://www.abcardio.org
B. Waine Kong, PhD, CEO

Fnded: 1974. **Mem:** 800. **Desc:** Physicians and other health professionals interested in lowering mortality and morbidity resulting from cardiovascular diseases. Seeks to improve prevention and treatment of cardiovascular diseases. Conducts educational and research programs; maintains speakers' bureau. **Pub:** *ABC*, quarterly. Newsletter. *Price:* Free. • *The Digest of Urban Cardiology*, periodic. Journal. *Price:* included in membership dues.

★ 1211 ★ Association of Black Nursing Faculty (ABNF)
5823 Queens Cove
Lisle, IL 60532
Phone: (630)969-3809 **Fax:** (630)969-3895
Email: stewarth@wt.net
Website: http://abnfinc.org
Barbara Broome, Pres.

Fnded: 1987. **Mem:** 127. **State Groups:** 25. **Desc:** Black nursing faculty teaching in nursing programs accredited by the National League for Nursing. Works to promote health-related issues and educational concerns of interest to the black community and ABNF. Serves as a forum for communication and the exchange of information among members; develops strategies for expressing concerns to other individuals, institutions, and communities. Assists members in professional development; develops and sponsors continuing education activities; fosters networking and guidance in employment and recruitment activities. Promotes health-related issues of legislation, government programs, and community activities. Supports black consumer advocacy issues. Encourages research. Maintains speakers' bureau and hall of fame. Offers charitable program and placement services. Compiles statistics. Is establishing a computer-assisted job bank; plans to develop bibliographies related to research groups. **Pub:** *ABNF Journal*, bimonthly. Journal. Includes research reports and scholarly papers. *Price:* $300/year. • *ABNF Newsletter*, quarterly. Newsletter. Includes member profiles and activities, research abstracts, conference information, job opportunities, and fellowship information. *Price:* Included in membership dues; $25/year. • *Membership Directory of the ABNF*, annual. Membership Directory.

★ 1212 ★ Association of Black Psychologists (ABPsi)
PO Box 55999
Washington, DC 20040-5999
Phone: (202)722-0808 **Fax:** (202)722-5941
Email: info@abpsi.org
Website: http://www.abpsi.org
Harvette Grey, PhD, Exec. Dir.

Fnded: 1968. **Mem:** 1,400. **Reg. Groups:** 4. **State Groups:** 29. **Local Groups:** 35. **Desc:** Professional psychologists and others in associated disciplines. Aims to: enhance the psychological well-being of black people in America; define mental health in consonance with newly established psychological concepts and standards; develop policies for local, state, and national decision-making that have impact on the mental health of the black community; support established black sister organizations and aid in the development of new, independent black institutions to enhance the psychological, educational, cultural, and economic situation. Offers training and information on AIDS. Conducts seminars, workshops, and research. **Pub:** *Association of Black Psychologists Publications Manual*. Manual. • *Journal of Black Psychology*, quarterly. Journal. Provides research results. Includes book reviews. *Price:* $30/year for individuals; $50/year for institutions. • *Monographs From the Journal of Black Psychology*, biennial. Monographs. • *Proceedings of Annual Convention*. Proceedings. • *Psych Discourse*, monthly. Journal. Includes calendar of events and research updates. *Price:* Included in membership dues; $95/year for nonmembers. • *Resource Manual for Black Psychology Students*. Manual. • *Sourcebook on the Teaching of Black Psychology*. • Also publishes brochures, bulletins, and research projects; distributes videotapes on issues in black psychology.

★ 1213 ★ Association of Blind and Partially Sighted Teachers and Students
BM Box 6727
London WC1N 3XX, United Kingdom

Fnded: 1970. **Mem:** 350. **Nat'l Groups:** 1. **Desc:** Visually impaired teachers, trainers, students, people looking for work or who have an interest in education. Provides mutual support through the exchange of ideas and experience of education and employment, promotes the needs and strengths of visually impaired teachers and students, and campaigns on relevant issues. **Pub:** *ABAPSTS Bulletin*, monthly. Bulletin. Features education employment issues.

★ 1214 ★ Association of Blind Piano Tuners (ABPT)
31 Wyre Cres.
Lynwood
Darwen BB3 0JG, United Kingdom
Phone: 44 1254 776148 **Fax:** 44 1254 773158
Email: info@uk-piano.org
Website: http://www.uk-piano.org

Fnded: 1954. **Mem:** 110. **Desc:** Serves the professional and particular needs of blind and partially sighted piano tuners. **Pub:** Newsletter, quarterly.

★ 1215 ★ Association of Bone and Joint Surgeons (ABJS)
6300 N River Rd., Ste. 727
Rosemont, IL 60018-4226
Phone: (847)698-1636 **Fax:** (847)823-4921
Email: abjs@aaos.org
Website: http://www.abjs.org
Colette I. Hohimer, Exec. Dir.

Fnded: 1947. **Mem:** 265. **Desc:** Orthopedic surgeons interested in clinical aspects of orthopedics and in training of leaders in the specialty. **Pub:** *Clinical Orthopaedics and Related Research*, monthly. Journal. **Frmly:** ABJS.

★ 1216 ★ Association of Brethren Caregivers (ABC)
1451 Dundee Ave.
Elgin, IL 60120
Phone: (847)742-5100 **Free:** 800-323-8039
Fax: (847)742-5160
Email: abc@brethren.org
Website: http://www.brethren.org/abc/
Steve Mason, Exec. Dir.

Fnded: 1968. **Mem:** 24. **Desc:** Develops resources, leadership, and programs within the caring ministries of the Church of the Brethren and the wider community. **Pub:** *Caregiving*, quarterly. Newsletter. Contains information for the Church of the Brethren on caregiving issues. *Price:* $10/year. **Frmly:** (1989) Church of the Brethren Homes and Hospitals Association; (1990) Board of Brethren Homes and Older Adult Ministries; (1993) Brethren Homes and Older Adult Ministries.

★ 1217 ★ Association of British Neurologists
Ormond House, 4th Fl.
27 Boswell St.
London WC1N 3JZ, United Kingdom
Phone: 44 207 4054060 **Fax:** 44 207 4054070
Email: abn@abnoffice.demon.co.uk
Website: http://www.theabn.org

Fnded: 1933. **Mem:** 1,000. **Desc:** Trainee and consultant in the neurological sciences. To promote the advancement of the neurological sciences, including the practice of neurology in the British Isles. **Pub:** Newsletter, quarterly.

★ 1218 ★ Association of British Veterinary Acupuncture
c/o Bishopton Veterinary Group
Moor Farm
Morchard Bishop
Crediton EX17 6RX, United Kingdom
Phone: 44 1363 877636 **Fax:** 44 1363 877471
Email: robert.vere@farmline.com

Fnded: 1987. **Mem:** 70. **Desc:** Ordinary members are veterinary surgeons. To further advancement of veterinary acupuncture in the UK. **Pub:** *Newsletter*, semiannual. Newsletter.

★ 1219 ★ Association of Camp Nurses (ACN)
8630 Thorsonveien NE
Bemidji, MN 56601
Phone: (218)586-2633 **Fax:** (218)586-8771
Email: acn@campnurse.org
Website: http://www.campnurse.org
Linda Ebner Erceg, RN, Exec. Dir.

Fnded: 1990. **Mem:** 500. **Nat'l Groups:** 2. **Reg. Groups:** 9. **Desc:** Works to promote and develop the nursing practice in the camp community. Maintains resource center; provides consulting services; supports camp nursing research; conducts educational programs. **Pub:** *Compass Point*, quarterly. Newsletter.

★ 1220 ★ Association of Canadian Academic Healthcare Organizations (Association Canadienne des Institutions de Sante Universtaires)
4500 Oak St., Rm. E405
Vancouver, BC, Canada V6H 3N1
Phone: (604)875-3468 **Fax:** (604)872-3290
Email: secretariat@acaho.org
Website: http://www.acaho.org

Fnded: 1973. **Mem:** 16. **Lang(s):** English, French. **Desc:** Teaching hospitals. Promotes advancement of medical education and residency. Represents the interests of medical residents and teaching hospitals; sponsors research and conducts educational programs. **Frmly:** (2000) Association of Canadian Teaching Hospitals.

★ 1221 ★ Association of Canadian Ergonomists (ACE)
(l'Association canadienne d'ergonomie)
c/o Andrew Parr
1304 - 2 Carlton St.
Toronto, ON, Canada M5B 1J3
Phone: (416)979-3946 **Free:** 888-432-2223
Fax: (416)979-1144
Email: info@ace.ergonomist.ca
Website: http://www.ace-ergocanada.ca/
Fnded: 1968. **Mem:** 650. **Nat'l Groups:** 1. **Reg. Groups:** 6. **Lang(s):** French. **Desc:** Promotes interest in ergonomics.

★ 1222 ★ Association of Canadian Faculties of Dentistry (ACFD)
(Association des Facultes Dentaires du Canada — AFDC)
100 Bronson St.
Ottawa, ON, Canada K1R 6G8
Phone: (613)237-6505 **Fax:** (613)236-8386
Email: director@acfd.ca
Website: http://www.acfd.ca
Lang(s): English, French. **Desc:** Dental school faculties. Promotes improvement of dental education; seeks to advance the teaching, study, and practice of dentistry. Conducts research and educational programs; facilitates exchange of information among members.

★ 1223 ★ Association of Canadian Medical Colleges (ACMC)
(Association des Facultes de Medecine du Canada — AFMC)
774 Echo Dr.
Ottawa, ON, Canada K1S 5P2
Phone: (613)730-0687 **Fax:** (613)730-1196
Email: cjuneau@acmc.ca
Website: http://www.acmc.ca
Lang(s): English, French. **Desc:** Colleges of medicine. Promotes excellence in the study and teaching of medicine; seeks to advance the profession of medicine through improved medical education. Conducts research and educational programs; facilitates exchange of information among members.

★ 1224 ★ Association of Cancer Executives (ACE)
475 S Frontage Rd., Ste. 101
Burr Ridge, IL 60527
Phone: (630)323-1170 **Fax:** (630)323-6989
Email: info@cancerexecutives.org
Website: http://www.cancerexecutives.org/
Shirley A. Johnson, RN,MBA, Pres.
Desc: Promotes the advancement of professional standing and personal achievement in oncology management, research, strategic planning, program development. **Pub:** *ACE Newsletters*, bimonthly. Newsletter. *Price:* included in membership dues.

★ 1225 ★ Association of Cancer Online Resources (ACOR)
173 Duane St., Ste. 3A
New York, NY 10013-3334
Phone: (212)226-5525
Website: http://www.acor.org/about/about.html
Fnded: mail. **Mem:** ing li,sts. **Reg. Groups:** rces. **Desc:** Provides information and support cancer patients and those who care for them through creation and maintenance of cancer-related Internet mailing lists and Web-based resources. **Pub:** *Abstracts*. Contains abstracts of new knowledge about cancer, treatment, side effects and more.

★ 1226 ★ Association of Cardiologists of Bosnia and Herzegovina
Josipa Stadlera 6
Sarajevo, Bosnia-Hercegovina
Phone: 387 33 251253 **Fax:** 387 33 251257
Email: rik@bih.net.ba
Website: http://www.escardio.org/society/natsoc/bosnia.htm
Mem: 107. **Desc:** Promotes the study of cardiology in Bosnia & Herzegovina. **Pub:** Book. Contains abstracts of papers. • Papers.

★ 1227 ★ Association of Cardiothoracic Anaesthetists
21 Portland Pl.
London W1B 1PY, United Kingdom
Phone: 44 20 76311650 **Fax:** 44 20 7614352
Email: info@aagbi.org
Website: http://www.acta.org.uk
Fnded: 1984. **Mem:** 326. **Desc:** Consultants who are currently engaged in the practice of cardiothoracic anaesthesia. To further the development of the art and science of caring for patients undergoing heart and chest surgery. **Pub:** Articles. Produced in association with the British Journal of Intensive Care.

★ 1228 ★ Association of Caribbean Occupational Therapists (ACOT)
PO Box 8677
CSO
Kingston, Jamaica
Phone: (876)928-1380 **Fax:** (876)928-1236
Email: leanycam@hotmail.com
Fnded: 1991. **Mem:** 25. **Lang(s):** English. **Desc:** Occupational therapists. Seeks to advance the practice of occupational therapy; promotes adherence to high standards of professional conduct and ethics by members. Facilitates exchange of information among members; sponsors continuing professional development courses. **Pub:** *Association of Caribbean Occupational Therapists' Scientific Conferen ce*, biannual. Newsletter.

★ 1229 ★ Association Centrafricaine pour le Bien-Etre Familial (ACABEF)
BP 1366
Bangui, Central African Rèpublic
Phone: 236 615435 **Fax:** 236 616700
Fnded: 1987. **Mem:** 537. **Lang(s):** English, French. **Desc:** Promotes and supports the use of family planning techniques for citizens of the Central African Republic. Fosters family welfare through educational programs and counseling.

★ 1230 ★ Association for Chemoreception Sciences (AChemS)
744 Duparc Cir.
Tallahassee, FL 32312-1409
Phone: (850)531-0854
Email: achems@achems.org
Website: http://achems.org
Dr. Stuart J. Firestein, Past Pres.
Fnded: 1979. **Mem:** 700. **Desc:** Research scientists, experimental psychologists, and industrial researchers. Purpose is to study chemoreception (the physiological reception of chemical stimuli) by the senses of taste and smell. Conducts research on the differences in human and animal perception of chemical stimuli in taste and smell. Offers seminars, fellowships, and workshops. Maintains placement service. Bestows annual Best Student Presentation at conference. **Pub:** Newsletter, biennial.

★ 1231 ★ Association for Child Psychoanalysis (ACP)
PO Box 253
Ramsey, NJ 07446
Phone: (201)825-3138 **Fax:** (201)825-3138
Email: childanalysis@compuserve.com
Nancy Hall, Admin.
Fnded: 1965. **Mem:** 650. **Desc:** Child psychoanalysts united to provide a forum for discussion and dissemination of information in their field. Conducts national and international scientific meetings. **Pub:** *Abstracts*, triennial. • *Association for Child Psychoanalysis–Newsletter*, semiannual. Newsletter. Covers child analysis methods, child psychoanalysis training, and the treatment and education of children throughout the world. *Price:* Included in membership dues. • *Membership Roster*, biennial. **Frmly:** (1971) American Association for Child Psychoanalysis.

★ 1232 ★ Association for Child Psychology and Psychiatry (ACPP)
Child Clinical Psychology Service, Mary Sheridan Centre for
St. Savlors House
39/41 Union St.
London SE1 1SD, United Kingdom
Phone: 44 207 4037458 **Fax:** 44 207 4037081
Email: acpp@acpp.org.uk
Website: http://www.acpp.org.uk/
Fnded: 1956. **Mem:** 2,750. **Nat'l Groups:** 15. **Lang(s):** English. **Desc:** Professionals working in the field of child mental health. Encourages dissemination of scientific research and information. **Pub:** *Child Psychology and Psychiatry Review*, quarterly. • *Journal of Child Psychology and Psychiatry*, 8/year. Journal.

★ 1233 ★ Association of Child Psychotherapists (ACP)
120 West Heath Rd.
London NW3 7TU, United Kingdom
Phone: 44 208 4581609
Email: acp@dial.pipex.com
Fnded: 1949. **Mem:** 597. **Desc:** Safeguards the interests of psychotherapists and fosters the exchange of information on the treatments of psychological disturbances of behavior, thinking, and feeling. Provides a forum for discussion. **Pub:** *Journal of Child Psychotherapy*, 3/year. Journal. • Bulletin, monthly.

★ 1234 ★ Association for Childbirth at Home, International (ACHI)
14140 Magnolia Blvd.
Sherman Oaks, CA 91423
Phone: (818)386-1082 **Fax:** (818)386-9374
Email: nbwc@ix.netcom.com
Tonya Brooks, Founder & Pres.
Fnded: 1972. **Mem:** 30,000. **Reg. Groups:** 9. **State Groups:** 40. **Local Groups:** 120. **Desc:** Parents, midwives, doctors, childbirth educators, other professionals, and interested individuals, all of whom support childbirth at home. Purposes are to bring accurate information and competent support to parents seeking home birth and safe hospital birth; to identify and implement correct obstetrical and pediatric practice. Offers parent education classes, leader training programs, international resource and referral service, and professional education seminars and programs; instructs parents, childbirth educators, midwives, and physicians in safe home birth and noninterventive alternative techniques. Conducts research; compiles statistics. Maintains speakers' bureau. **Pub:** *Birth Notes*, quarterly. Newsletter. *Price:* $25/year. • *Founders Letter*, 6/year. • *Giving Birth at Home*. Handbook. • Brochures. **Frmly:** Association for Childbirth at Home.

★ 1235 ★ Association for Childbirth and Parenthood
c/o Dr. James McIntyre
Department of Obstetrics and Gynaecology
Baragwanath Hospital
Bertsham 2013, Republic of South Africa
Fax: 27 11 9381534
Email: mcintyre@pixie.co.za
Website: http://www.ispog.org
Desc: Promotes the study of psychobiological and psychosocial, ethical and cross-cultural problems in the fields of obstetrics and gynaecology, women's health and reproductive health; facilitates the dissemination of new information in these fields. **Pub:** *Journal of Psychosomatic Obstetrics and Gynecology*. Journal.

★ 1236 ★ Association for Children with a Disability (ACD)
590 Orrong Rd.
Armidale, VIC 3143, Australia
Phone: 61 3 95001232 **Fax:** 61 3 95001240
Email: mail@acd.org.au
Website: http://www.acd.org.au

Fnded: 1980. **Mem:** 3,500. **Lang(s):** English. **Desc:** Provides information, support, and advocacy for families of children with a disability in Victoria, Australia. Engages in a range of community education and systemic advocacy work.

★ 1237 ★ Association of Children's Prosthetic-Orthotic Clinics (ACPOC)
6300 N River Rd., No. 727
Rosemont, IL 60018-4226
Phone: (847)698-1637 **Fax:** (847)823-0536
Email: king@aaos.org
Website: http://www.acpoc.org
Sheril B. King, Soc. Dir.

Fnded: 1980. **Mem:** 450. **Desc:** Prosthetic-orthotic clinics for children. Promotes the exchange of information concerning children's prosthetic-orthotic devices. Fosters cooperative research development and evaluative efforts among member clinics. Seeks to improve care in member clinics. **Pub:** Newsletter, quarterly.

★ 1238 ★ Association of Chiropractic Colleges (ACC)
c/o David S. O'Bryon
4424 Montgomery Ave., Ste. 102
Bethesda, MD 20814
Phone: (301)652-5066 **Fax:** (301)913-9146
Email: Info@ChiroColleges.org
Website: http://www.chirocolleges.org
David S. O'Bryon, CAE, Exec. Dir.

Fnded: 1977. **Mem:** 18. **Desc:** Presidents of chiropractic colleges that are members of the Council on Chiropractic Education. Objective is to provide a cooperative base that assists members in the search for and promotion of the practices and concepts most effective in the academic and continuing education of doctors of chiropractic. Serves as a clearinghouse for information related to opportunities and advancement in research as they affect chiropractic education and health care. Seeks to enhance services to the consumer of chiropractic education and to the public. **Pub:** *Journal of Chiropractic Education*, quarterly. Journal. **Frmly:** (1985) Association of Chiropractic College Presidents.

★ 1239 ★ Association des Chirurgiens Dentistes du Benin (ACDB)
BP 04
Cadjehoun
Cotonou, Benin
Phone: 229 332105 **Fax:** 229 332105
Email: e.china@intnet.bj

Fnded: 1987. **Mem:** 55. **Desc:** Promotes dentistry in Benin.

★ 1240 ★ Association of Clinical Pathologists (ACP)
189 Dyke Rd.
Hove BN3 1TL, United Kingdom
Phone: 44 1273 775700 **Fax:** 44 1273 773303
Website: http://www.pathologists.org.uk

Fnded: 1927. **Mem:** 2,000. **Reg. Groups:** 12. **Lang(s):** English. **Desc:** Promotes the study and practice of clinical pathology. Offers courses. **Pub:** *ACP News*, quarterly. Newsletter. • *ACP Yearbook*. Directory. Includes transcripts of speeches delivered at the annual meeting. • *Journal of Clinical Pathology*, monthly. Journal.

★ 1241 ★ Association of Clinical Research Professionals (ACRP)
500 Montgomery St., Ste. 800
Alexandria, VA 22314
Phone: (730)254-8100 **Fax:** (202)737-8101
Email: office@acrpnet.org
Website: http://www.acrpnet.org
Tom Adams, CEO

Fnded: 1976. **Mem:** 18,000. **Desc:** Individuals engaged in clinical pharmacology and other related research professions, including clinical monitors and research associates, nurses, pharmacists, pharmacologists, physicians, and regulatory professionals. Promotes professional growth in the field through the dissemination of information, the exchange of ideas, and the development of educational programs. Provides continuing education credits to pharmacy and nursing professionals through the American Council on Pharmaceutical Education and the American Nurses Association. **Pub:** *ACRP Membership Directory*, annual. Membership Directory. *Price:* Free. For members only. • *Monitor*, quarterly. Magazine. Includes activities information and committee reports, industry news, calendar of events, clinical research articles. *Price:* Free. For members only. **Frmly:** (1999) Associates of Clinical Pharmacology.

★ 1242 ★ Association of Clinical Scientists
PO Box 1287
Middlebury, VT 05753
Phone: (802)462-2507 **Fax:** (802)462-2673
Email: clinsci@sover.net
Website: http://www.clinicalscience.org
Robert E. Brown, MD, Pres.

Fnded: 1949. **Mem:** 500. **Desc:** Professional society of physicians and scientists working in various fields of laboratory medicine. Seeks to promote education and research in clinical science by practical methods; maintain and improve the accuracy of measurements in clinical laboratories and promote uniformity in clinical laboratory procedures; encourage cooperation between physicians and nonphysicians concerned with the application of scientific methods to medical practice. **Pub:** *Annals of Clinical and Laboratory Science*, quarterly. Journal. Scientific peer-reviewed journal. *Price:* Included in membership dues; $130 / year for nonmembers. • *Clinical Science Trumpet*, bimonthly. Newsletter. • Membership Directory, annual. **Frmly:** (1956) Clinical Science Club.

★ 1243 ★ Association of Coloprociology of Great Britain and Ireland
c/o The Royal College of Surgeons of England
35-43 Lincoln's Inn Fields
London WC2A 3PE, United Kingdom
Phone: 44 20 79730307 **Fax:** 44 20 74309235
Email: acpgbi@asgbi.org.uk
Website: http://www.acpgbi.org.uk

Fnded: 1990. **Mem:** 1,300. **Reg. Groups:** 20. **Lang(s):** English. **Desc:** A multidisciplinary association to promote standards and training in coloproctology. **Pub:** *Colorectal Disease*, bimonthly. Journal. • *Guidelines for the Management of Colorectal Cancer*. Handbook. • *Resources for Coloproctology*. Handbook.

★ 1244 ★ Association for Common European Nursing Diagnoses, Interventions and Outcomes (ACENDIO)
Royal College of Nursing
20 Cavendish Sq.
London W1M 0AB, United Kingdom
Email: alex.westbrook@chelwest.nhs.uk

Fnded: 1995. **Lang(s):** English. **Desc:** Nurses and nursing organizations. Network and development of resources towards standards supporting sharing and comparison of data about nursing.

★ 1245 ★ Association of Community Cancer Centers (ACCC)
11600 Nebel St., Ste. 201
Rockville, MD 20852
Phone: (301)984-9496 **Fax:** (301)770-1949
Website: http://www.accc-cancer.org
Edward L. Braud, MD, Pres.

Fnded: 1974. **Mem:** 6,000. **State Groups:** 23. **Desc:** Institutions (680) and 23 state oncology societies involved in the provision of community cancer care. Fosters communication among providers of community cancer care; seeks to improve the quality of care available to cancer patients in community settings; encourages clinical research utilizing the community as a setting. **Pub:** *Community Cancer Programs in the U.S.*, annual. Reference guide to freestanding and hospital-based cancer programs. *Price:* $50 non-profit organizations; $150 others. • *Compendia-Based Drug Bulletin*, quarterly. Bulletin. • *Critical Pathways*, periodic. • *Oncology Issues*, bimonthly. Journal. Provides information on community cancer programs for association members, who are physicians, nurses, social workers, and other health professionals. *Price:* $60/ year. • *Standards for Cancer Programs*, periodic.

★ 1246 ★ Association of Community Health Councils for England and Wales (ACHCEW)
Earlsmead House
30 Drayton Park
London N5 1PB, United Kingdom
Phone: 44 20 76098405 **Fax:** 44 207 7001152
Email: mailbox@achcew.org.uk
Website: http://www.achcew.org.uk

Fnded: 1977. **Mem:** 204. **Desc:** Community Health Councils set up to monitor the National Health Service. Provides forum for member CHCs, provides information and advisory services to CHCs and represents the user of health services at a national level. **Pub:** *CHC News*, 10/year. • *Factsheets for the Public*, periodic. • *Health News Briefings*, 10/year. • *Perspectives - Brief Topic Papers*, 10/year. Papers.

★ 1247 ★ Association of Community Health Nursing Educators
7794 Grow Dr.
Pensacola, FL 32514
Phone: (850)474-8821 **Fax:** (850)484-8762
Email: achne@nysna.org
Belinda E. Puetz, Exec. Dir.

Mem: 350. **Reg. Groups:** 5. **Desc:** Nurses and graduate students. Committed to "excellence in community and public health nursing education, research, and practice." **Pub:** Newsletter, quarterly. *Price:* included in membership dues.

★ 1248 ★ Association for Comprehensive Energy Psychology (ACEP)
c/o Dr. Dorothea Hover-Kramer
12307 Oak Knoll Rd.
Poway, CA 92064
Phone: (858)748-5963 **Fax:** (858)673-9825
Email: acep@energypsych.org
Website: http://www.energypsych.org/
Dr. Dorothea Hover-Kramer, Contact

Fnded: 1999. **Mem:** 600. **Reg. Groups:** 11. **Desc:** Professionals in psychotherapeutic practice, allied health professionals, researchers, organizations, students, and interested laypersons. Promotes understanding of energy psychology in order to establish the field's credibility among health professionals, particularly psychotherapists; creates collegial atmosphere for collaboration in order to produce treatments for the public. **Pub:** *The Energy Field*, quarterly. Newsletter. *Price:* included in membership dues.

★ 1249 ★ Association for Comprehensive NeuroTherapy (ACN)
c/o Latitudes
PO Box 210848
Royal Palm Beach, FL 33421-0848
Phone: (561)798-0472 **Fax:** (561)798-9820
Email: acn@latitudes.org
Website: http://www.latitudes.org
Sheila Rogers, Dir.

Desc: Practitioners and lay persons. Dedicated to exploring advanced and complementary treatments for neurological conditions, focusing on autism, Tourette syndrome, attention deficit disorder/hyperactivity, obsessive compulsive disorder, and learning disabilities. Articles, editorials, and letters, as well as a survey on Tourette Syndrome, are available through their website. **Pub:** *ACN Today*. Newsletter. *Price:* Free. • *Latitudes*, quarterly. Magazine. Contains articles, research updates, and clinical findings about autism, Tourette syndrome, attention disorders and learning problems. *Price:* $45.

★ 1250 ★ Association for Continence Advice (ACA)
102a Astra House
Arklow Rd.
New Cross
London SE14 6EB, United Kingdom
Phone: 44 20 86924680 **Fax:** 44 20 86926217
Email: info@aca.uk.com
Website: http://www.aca.uk.com/mainindex.html

Fnded: 1981. **Mem:** 755. **Reg. Groups:** 14. **Desc:** Professionals with an interest in the health and social care of people with continence problems. Aims to provide a means of communication and support between members and other interested groups; to promote educational activities; to produce and distribute a newsletter; to promote research activities and disseminate research findings; to liaise and maintain dialogue with relevant manufacturers; to promote public awareness and positive attitudes within society. **Pub:** *Continence*, quarterly. Journal. • Pamphlets.

★ 1251 ★ Association for Dance Movement Therapy - United Kingdom (ADMTUK)
c/o Quaker Meeting House
Wedmore Vale
Bristol BS3 5HX, United Kingdom
Email: query@admt.org.uk
Website: http://www.admt.org.uk

Fnded: 1982. **Mem:** 200. **Lang(s):** English. **Desc:** Individuals united to promote dance movement therapy. Monitors and promotes training. Offers professional services. Organizes summer schools, workshops and seminars. **Pub:** *ADMTUK Quartly - "E-Motion"*, quarterly. Newsletter. • Articles, periodic. • Pamphlets, periodic.

★ 1252 ★ Association of Danish Pharmacists
Rygards Alle 1
DK-2900 Hellerup, Denmark
Phone: 45 39463600 **Fax:** 45 39463639
Email: df@pharmaceut.dk
Website: http://www.pharmaceut.dk

Fnded: 1873. **Mem:** 3,500. **Reg. Groups:** 10. **State Groups:** 5. **Lang(s):** English. **Desc:** Pharmaceutical executives and editors of pharmaceutical journals of Denmark, Finland, Iceland, Norway, and Sweden. Promotes members' interests. Encourages cooperation among members. **Pub:** *Farmaceuten*, every second week. Journal. **Frmly:** Union of Nordic Pharmacists.

★ 1253 ★ Association of the Deaf in Israel (ADI) (Agudat Hachershim Beisrael)
Helen Keller Center
13 Yad Lebanim Blvd.
PO Box 9001
IL-61090 Tel Aviv, Israel
Phone: 972 3 7303355 **Fax:** 972 3 7396419
Email: deaf-isr@zahav.net.il
Website: http://www.deaf.org.il

Fnded: 1944. **Mem:** 2,200. **Reg. Groups:** 19. **Lang(s):** English, Hebrew. **Desc:** Works toward the cultural, social, and professional rehabilitation of the deaf in Israel.

★ 1254 ★ Association of Deans of Pharmacy of Canada (ADPC) (Association des Doyens de Pharmacie du Canada — ADPC)
College of Pharmacy and Nutrition
University of Saskatchewan
110 Science Pl.
Saskatoon, SK, Canada S7N 5C9
Phone: (306)966-6327 **Fax:** (514)343-2102
Email: cwloomis@morgan.ucs.mun.ca

Lang(s): English, French. **Desc:** Deans of pharmacy. Promotes excellence in pharmacy education. Facilitates communication among schools of pharmacy and among members; conducts research and educational programs.

★ 1255 ★ Association of Democratic Pharmacists (Verein Demokratischer Pharmazeutinnen und Pharmazeuten)
Fleming-Apotheke
Grindelallee 182
D-20144 Hamburg, Germany
Phone: 49 40 458768 **Fax:** 49 40 458768
Email: geschaeftsstelle@vdpp.de
Website: http://www.vdpp.de

Fnded: 1989. **Mem:** 160. **Desc:** Promotes the interests of registered pharmacists in Germany. Concerned with issues focusing on environmental and public health policies. **Pub:** *VDPP-Rundbrief*, bimonthly. Journal.

★ 1256 ★ Association Dentaire Francaise (ADF)
c/o Michel Chabre
7, rue Mariotte
F-75017 Paris, France
Phone: 33 1 58221710 **Fax:** 33 1 58221740
Email: adf@adf.asso.fr
Website: http://www.adf.asso.fr

Fnded: 1970. **Mem:** 33,000. **Lang(s):** French. **Desc:** Federation of dental associations in France. Promotes and defends the dental profession; works for the evaluation and standardization of dental products. Organizes an annual conference for continuing education. **Pub:** *Les Cahiers de F A.D.F*, quarterly. Journal.

★ 1257 ★ Association of Dental Dealers in Europe (ADDE)
Moosstrasse 2
PO Box 29
CH-3073 Bern, Switzerland
Phone: 41 31 9527892 **Fax:** 41 31 9527683
Email: uwanner@swissonline.ch

Mem: 16. **Lang(s):** English, French, German, Italian. **Desc:** Manufacturers of dental equipment and supplies. Promotes growth and development of members' businesses; seeks to advance dental technologies. Represents members' interests before labor, industrial, and professional organizations, government agencies, and the public; sponsors research and development programs. **Pub:** *Economic Survey 2000 on the European Dental Trade*, annual. Survey.

★ 1258 ★ Association for Dental Education in Europe (ADEE)
Malmo University
Carl Gustafs vag 34
S-21421 Malmo, Sweden
Phone: 46 40 6658410 **Fax:** 46 40 6658549
Email: Madeleine.rohlin@od.mah.se
Website: http://tmk.odont.ku.dk/adee

Fnded: 1975. **Mem:** 85. **Lang(s):** English. **Desc:** Teachers of dentistry. Objectives are: to further dental education in Europe; to evaluate the goals and methods of dental education; to assess training programs for teachers; to promote ties among dentistry teachers. Holds lectures, seminars, and working discussion groups in conjunction with annual meeting. **Pub:** *European Journal of Dental Education*, quarterly. Journal.

★ 1259 ★ Association for Dental Education in Europe (ADEE)
Faculdad de Odontologia, Universidad
Madrid, Spain
Phone: 34 913941906 **Fax:** 34 913941910
Email: marsan@atseucmax.sim.ucm.es

Fnded: 1975.

★ 1260 ★ Association of Dental Hospitals of the UK
Birmingham Dental Hospital
St. Chad's Queensway
Birmingham B4 6NN, United Kingdom
Phone: 44 121 2368611 **Fax:** 44 121 2372750

Fnded: 1952. **Mem:** 32. **Desc:** Open only to representatives of Dental Hospitals and Schools.

★ 1261 ★ Association des Diabete du Gabon
c/o Dr. Epigat-Apinda
BP 7369
Libreville, Gabon
Phone: 241 737345
Website: http://www.diabetesafrica.com/idfmembers.html

Desc: Represents people with diabetes. Promotes research and support of those with diabetes in Gabon.

★ 1262 ★ Association des Diabetiques de Cote D'Ivoire (ADIACI)
c/o Prof. Adrien Lokrou
01 BP 4241
Abidjan 01, Cote d'Ivoire
Phone: 225 471072
Email: mseabe@abidjan.bceao.int
Website: http://www.diabetesafrica.com/idfmembers.html

Desc: Represents people with diabetes. Promotes research and support of those with diabetes in Cote d'Ivoire.

★ 1263 ★ Association of Disabled Professionals (ADP)
BCM ADP
London WC1N 3XX, United Kingdom
Phone: 44 208 7785008 **Fax:** 44 208 92241420
Email: assdisprof@aol.com
Website: http://www.adp.org.uk

Fnded: 1971. **Mem:** 230. **Lang(s):** English. **Desc:** Professionals and students with disabilities. Offers advice and information especially on employment issues. Provides means to disabled professionals and those in managerial positions to network and offer advice and support. Maintains liaisons with government authorities. **Pub:** *ADP Quarterly*, quarterly.

★ 1264 ★ Association of Doctors for the Environment - ISDE Italy
Via della Fioraia, 17/19
I-52100 Arezzo, Italy
Phone: 39 0575 22256 **Fax:** 39 0575 28676
Email: isde@ats.it

Fnded: 1989. **Mem:** 4,200. **Desc:** Promotes environmentally focused research related to illness and disease. **Pub:** *Inquinamento Atmosferico e Salute (Atmospheric Pollution & Health)*. • *ISDE Italia News*, semiannual.

★ 1265 ★ Association for Education in Healthcare Information Technology
4500 Hugh Howell Rd., Ste. 340
Tucker, GA 30084
Phone: (770)270-9611 **Fax:** (770)270-0632
Email: insight@pami.org
Website: http://www.insight-net.org
J.W. Holderfield, Exec. Dir.

Desc: Employees, consultants in healthcare industry. Works to provide its members with information on the healthcare industry and related information technology issues.

★ 1266 ★ Association for Education and Rehabilitation of the Blind and Visually Impaired (AERBVI)
4600 Duke St., Ste. 430
Alexandria, VA 22304-9239
Phone: (703)823-9690 **Fax:** (703)823-9695
Email: aer@aerbvi.org
Website: http://www.aerbvi.org
Mark Richert, Exec. Dir.

Fnded: 1984. **Mem:** 5,000. **State Groups:** 44. **Desc:** Provides support and assistance to professionals "who work in all phases of education and rehabilitation of blind and visually impaired persons of all ages." **Pub:** *AER Report*, quarterly, plus annual year end edition. Newsletter. For professionals in the field of service to blind and visually impaired persons; includes legislative and membership news. *Price:* Included in membership dues. • *Association for Education and Rehabilitation of the Blind and Visually Impaired–Job Exchange*, monthly. Bulletin. Lists job openings in the field of services to blind and visually impaired children and adults. *Price:* Free to members online. • *Re:View*, quarterly. Journal.

★ 1267 ★ Association of Emergency Physicians (AEP)
127 Branchaw Blvd.
New Lenox, IL 60451
Free: 800-449-4237 **Fax:** (815)463-9230
Email: aep@interaccess.com
Website: http://www.aep.org/
Atwood L. Rice, MD, Pres.

Fnded: 1991. **Desc:** Represents emergency physicians who practice clinical emergency medicine.

★ 1268 ★ Association for Equine Sports Medicine (AESM)
3579 E Foothill Blvd., No. 288
Pasadena, CA 91107
Phone: (909)869-4849 **Fax:** (909)869-6788
Email: aesm@relaypoint.net
Holly M. Greene, M.S., Exec. Dir.

Fnded: 1982. **Mem:** 400. **Desc:** Members are veterinarians, sports physiology researchers, other health professionals, or anyone who has special interest in understanding and/or application of scientific knowledge in the area of equine sports medicine and who will promote the well being of the athletic horse. **Pub:** *Equine Review*, quarterly. Newsletter. • *Proceedings of Annual Conference.*

★ 1269 ★ Association of European Cancer Leagues (ECL)
c/o Swiss Cancer League
Effingerstrasse 40
CH-3008 Bern, Switzerland
Phone: 41 31 3899121 **Fax:** 41 31 3899160
Email: lenz@swisscancer.ch
Website: http://www.swisscancer.ch

Fnded: 1980. **Mem:** 39. **Lang(s):** English. **Desc:** Promotes information exchange to carry out joint campaigns; advocates for common aims in various fields of cancer control. Main areas of activity include cancer prevention, tobacco control, public education, professional education, service and rehabilitation, fundraising and advocacy. Coordinates annual health promotion campaign European Week Against Cancer.

★ 1270 ★ Association of European Coeliac Societies (AOECS)
Ave. Louis Bertrand 100, Boite A20
B-1030 Brussels, Belgium
Phone: 32 2 2168347 **Fax:** 32 2 2168347

Fnded: 1987. **Mem:** 120. **Lang(s):** English. **Desc:** Health care professionals with an interest in coeliac disease and related disorders; individuals with coeliac disease and their families. Promotes improved diagnosis and treatment of coeliac disease; seeks to improve the quality of life of people with coeliac disease. Facilitates exchange of information among health researchers and practitioners working with coeliac disease; provides support and services to people with coeliac disease.

★ 1271 ★ Association for European Paediatric Cardiology (AEPC)
c/o Dr. Ingrid Oberhaensli-Weiss
Hopital Cantonal Universitaire de Geneve
Paediatric Cardiology Unit
6, rue Willy Donze
CH-1211 Geneva 14, Switzerland
Phone: 41 22 3824583 **Fax:** 41 22 3824546
Email: secr@aepc.org
Website: http://www.aepc.org

Fnded: 1963. **Mem:** 620. **Reg. Groups:** 30. **Lang(s):** English, French. **Desc:** Physicians specializing in pediatric cardiology. Seeks to advance pediatric cardiological study, teaching, and practice. Serves as a clearinghouse on pediatric cardiology; conducts research and continuing professional development programs, and courses in pediatric cardiology. **Pub:** *Cardiology in the Young*, biweekly. Newsletter.

★ 1272 ★ Association of European Psychiatrists (AEP)
Clinique Psychiatrique
CHU
1, Place de l'Hopital
F-67091 Strasbourg Cedex, France
Phone: 33 3 88115406 **Fax:** 33 3 88116189
Email: aep.strasbourg@wanadoo.fr
Website: http://www.aep.lu

Fnded: 1983. **Mem:** 1,200. **Lang(s):** English, French. **Desc:** Psychiatrists. Seeks to advance psychiatric scholarship and practice. Facilitates communication and cooperation among members; sponsors research and continuing professional development programs. **Pub:** *European Psychiatry*, 8/year, plus supplements. Journal.

★ 1273 ★ Association of the European Self-Medication Industry (AESGP) (Europaischer Fachverband der Arzneimittel-Hersteller)
7, ave. de Tervuren
B-1040 Brussels, Belgium
Phone: 32 2 7355130 **Fax:** 32 2 7355222
Email: info@aesgp.be
Website: http://www.aesgp.be

Fnded: 1964. **Mem:** 25. **Lang(s):** English. **Desc:** National European proprietary medicines associations. (Proprietary medicines are packaged, over-the-counter drugs.) Advocates self-medication, defined as the therapeutic use of drugs that are safe, effective, and available without prescription. Objectives are to: encourage the involvement of the pharmaceutical industry in European national health care systems; promote and maintain high standards of production, distribution, and advertising of proprietary drugs; ensure that the interests of the proprietary drug industry are recognized by institutions responsible for health legislation; enhance cooperation and the exchange of information among members, and with international professional, industrial, and governmental organizations; represent member associations in World Self-Medication Industry (WSMI). Compiles statistics. **Pub:** *Annual Meeting Proceedings.* • *Developing Self-Medication in Central and Eastern Europe.* • *Self-Medication and the Pharmacist*, periodic. • *Summary of Product Characteristics for Non-Prescription Medicines in the EC.*

★ 1274 ★ Association of European Toxicologists and European Societies of Technology (EUROTOX)
c/o Christian Hodel
Hovat Pharma Consulting
Neubadstrasse 83
CH-4054 Basel, Switzerland
Phone: 41 61 4821455 **Fax:** 41 61 4821440
Email: eurotox@hodel.net
Website: http://www.eurotox.com

Fnded: 1962. **Mem:** 6,500. **Nat'l Groups:** 30. **Lang(s):** English. **Desc:** Industrial, university, and government toxicology researchers in 50 countries. Purpose is to encourage and advance research in the field of drug toxicity and in other areas of toxicology. Fosters exchange of information concerning problems in toxicology. Topics of interest have included the effects of drugs on the human fetus, toxicological methods and their reliability, toxicity problems of organs such as the liver and the nervous system, carcinogenesis, and sensitization. Sponsors working groups and training courses in toxicology. **Pub:** *EUROTOX*, 3/year. Newsletter. Contains news and views on a variety of toxicological issues. • *EUROTOX Membership Directory*, periodic. Directory. Contains names and addresses of members. • *Proceedings of the Annual Meeting.*

★ 1275 ★ Association of Faculties of Pharmacy of Canada (AFPC)
2609 Eastview
Saskatoon, SK, Canada S7J 3G7
Phone: (306)374-6327 **Fax:** (306)374-0555
Email: jblackburn@sasktel.net
Website: http://www.afpc.info

Fnded: 1944. **Mem:** 250. **Lang(s):** English, French. **Desc:** Educators engaged in postsecondary pharmacy programs. Promotes excellence in pharmacy education; encourages continuing professional development among members. Facilitates exchange of information among members; conducts research and educational programs. **Pub:** *AFPC Communications*, quarterly. Newsletter.

★ 1276 ★ Association of Family Practice Administrators (AFPA)
11400 Tomahawk Creek Parkway
Leawood, KS 66211
Phone: (913)906-6000 **Free:** 800-274-2237
Fax: (913)906-6092
Email: dsexton@aafp.org
Website: http://www.afpa.net
Dawn Sexton, Exec. Sec.

Fnded: 1984. **Mem:** 375. **Nat'l Groups:** 1. **Desc:** Administrators and coordinators of family practice residency training programs. Promotes professionalism in family practice administration. Serves as a network for sharing of information and fellowship among members. Provides technical assistance to members; functions as a liaison to related professional organizations. **Pub:** *Connections*, quarterly. Newsletter.

★ 1277 ★ Association of Family Practice Residency Directors (AFPRD)
11400 Tomahawk Creek Pkwy.
Leawood, KS 66211
Phone: (913)906-6000 **Free:** 800-274-2237
Fax: (913)906-6105
Email: afprd@aafp.org
Website: http://www.afprd.org
Stacy Singleton, Mgr.

Fnded: 1990. **Mem:** 406. **Desc:** Promotes excellence in family practice graduate education. Provides representation for residency directors at a national level and provides a political voice for them in appropriate arenas. Promotes cooperation and communication between residency programs and different branches of the family practice specialty. Dedicated to improving of education of family physicians. Provides a network for mutual assistance among FP. residency directors. **Pub:** *Highlights*, quarterly. Newsletter. *Price:* Free for members.

★ 1278 ★ Association France Alzheimer (AFA)
21, boulevard Montmartre
F-75002 Paris, France
Phone: 33 1 803802806 **Fax:** 33 1 42960470
Email: cd.fralzheimer@wanadoo.fr

Website: http://www.maladie-alzheimer.com

Lang(s): English, French. **Desc:** Individuals and organizations. Seeks to improve the quality of life of people with Alzheimer's disease and their families. Makes available support and services; facilitates research on Alzheimer's disease and related disorders; conducts educational programs.

★ 1279 ★ Association of Freestanding Radiation Oncology Centers (AFROC)

1875 Eye St. NW, 12th Fl.
Washington, DC 20006
Free: 888-334-4542 **Fax:** (202)466-5938
Email: info@afroc.org
Website: http://www.afroc.org
Sheila Gell, Exec. Dir.

Fnded: 1986. **Mem:** 200. **Desc:** Freestanding radiation oncology center employees; radiologists; oncologists; physicists; radiation therapists; laboratory clinicians. Promotes the interests of freestanding radiation oncology centers to insure high quality care for patients. Upgrades management services offered. Represents members in legal matters and to other associations. **Pub:** Directory, annual.

★ 1280 ★ Association of French Language Epidemiologists (AFLE) (Association des Epidemiologistes de Langue Francaise — ADELF)

INSERM U 88
Hopital Nationale de Saint Maurice
14, rue du Val d'Osne
F-94410 Saint Maurice, France
Phone: 33 1 45183850 **Fax:** 33 1 45183889
Email: adelf@st_maurice.inserm.fr

Fnded: 1976. **Mem:** 510. **Lang(s):** French. **Desc:** Epidemiologists, doctors, surgeons, veterinarians, biologists, medical and social science educators, and public health planners. Facilitates communication among epidemiologists. Develops and provides information on epidemiological methods. Promotes epidemiological research. **Pub:** *ADELF-Info*, bimonthly. Newsletter.

★ 1281 ★ Association of French-Language Leprologists (AFLL) (Association des Leprologues de Lange Francaise — ALLF)

4 rue Jean Jacques Bel
F-33000 Bordeaux, France
Phone: 33 5 56523214 **Fax:** 33 5 56523214
Email: pibobin@fr.packardbell.org

Fnded: 1984. **Mem:** 500. **Lang(s):** English, French. **Desc:** Health care professionals with an interest in leprosy and Buruli Ulcer. Promotes advancement in the prevention, diagnosis, and treatment of leprosy; seeks to improve the quality of life of people with leprosy. Facilitates communication and cooperation among members; serves as a clearinghouse on leprosy and its treatment; sponsors research; makes available services to people with leprosy. **Pub:** *Bulletin de l'ALLF*, semiannual. Journal. Information and continuous training about Leprosy and Buruli Ulcer.

★ 1282 ★ Association of French-Speaking Dermatologists (AFSD) (Association des Dermatologistes Francophone — ADF)

Dermotologie Hospital Michallon, BP 217X
F-38013 Grenoble Cedex, France
Phone: 33 4 76765508 **Fax:** 33 4 76765558
Email: pierre.amblard@ujf-grenoble.fr

Lang(s): English, French. **Desc:** Dermatologists and dermatology students and educators. Seeks to advance the study, teaching, and practice of dermatology. Establishes standards for dermatological certification and practice; sponsors continuing professional development courses.

★ 1283 ★ Association of French-Speaking Physicians of Canada (AFSPC) (Association des Medicins de Langue Francaise du Canada — AMLFC)

8355 Boulevard Saint-Laurent
Montreal, QC, Canada H2P 2Z6
Phone: (514)388-2228 **Free:** 800-387-2228
Fax: (514)388-5335
Email: info@amlfc.org
Website: http://www.amlfc.org

Fnded: 1902. **Mem:** 5,000. **Lang(s):** English, French. **Desc:** French-speaking physicians practicing in Canada. Seeks to increase availability and quality of health care in French-speaking areas of Canada; promotes professional advancement of members. Makes available health services in underserved areas; facilitates communication and cooperation among members.

★ 1284 ★ Association of Gastrointestinal Motility Disorders (AGMD)

11 North St.
Lexington, MA 02420
Phone: (781)861-3874 **Fax:** (781)861-7834
Email: AGMDInc@aol.com
Website: http://www.agmd-gimotility.org
Mary-Angela DeGrazia-DiTucci, Pres. -CEO

Fnded: 1991. **Mem:** 550. **Desc:** Non-profit international organization which serves as an integral educational resource concerning digestive motility disorders. Also functions as an important information base for members of the medical community. **Pub:** *AGMD Beacon*, quarterly. Newsletter. Updates members about organization and medical alerts. *Price:* included in membership dues. • *AGMD GI Compass*, quarterly. Forum of articles by physicians, scientists and general members. *Price:* included in membership dues. • *AGMD Search and Research*, quarterly. Newsletter. Poses questions from members and provides responses. • Also publishes educational materials concerning digestive motility disorders and diseases. **Frmly:** (2000) American Society of Adults with Pseudo-Obstruction.

★ 1285 ★ Association for Genito Urinary Medicine (AGUM)

c/o Dr. I.H. Ahmed-Jusuf, Hon.Sec.
Department of Genito-Urinary Medicine
Nottingham City Hospital NHS Trust
Hucknall Rd.
Nottingham NG5 1PD, United Kingdom
Phone: 44 115 9627746 **Fax:** 44 115 9627684
Email: imtyazahmed@hotmail.com
Website: http://www.agum.org.uk/

Fnded: 1992. **Desc:** Represents and promotes the medical specialty for genitourinary medicine; developed a set of guidelines for commissioners on genitourinary medicine service specifications and the management of sexually transmitted infections.

★ 1286 ★ Association for Genito-Urinary Medicine

Department of Genito-Urinary Medicine
Nottingham City Hospital
Hucknall Rd.
Nottingham CH2 1UL, United Kingdom
Phone: 44 1244 363091 **Fax:** 44 1244 636095
Website: http://www.agum.org.uk

Fnded: 1992.

★ 1287 ★ Association of German Dental Manufacturers (Verband der Deutschen Dental-Industrie — VDDI)

Postfach 40 06 63
D-50836 Cologne, Germany
Phone: 49 221 9486280 **Fax:** 49 221 2824942
Email: info@vddi.de
Website: http://www.vddi.de

Fnded: 1917. **Mem:** 200. **Lang(s):** German. **Desc:** Companies manufacturing dental equipment and supplies. Establishes international standards and technical harmonization for dental equipment. Represents members' interests before government bodies, international agencies, and the public. Maintains liaison with organizations representing dentists, dental technicians, and dental supply dealers and distributors. Compiles statistics. **Pub:** *The German Dental Industry*, biennial. Brochure.

★ 1288 ★ Association of German Urologists (Berufsverband der Deutschen Urologen)

Erdinger Str. 19
D-84405 Dorfen, Germany
Phone: 49 8081 41313 **Fax:** 49 8081 4468
Email: bdu@bdurol.de

Fnded: 1956. **Mem:** 2,980. **State Groups:** 19. **Desc:** Urologists practicing in Germany. Promotes the advancement of the field of urology. **Pub:** *Urologeb*, bimonthly. Journal. • *Urotelegramm*, bimonthly. Newsletter.

★ 1289 ★ Association of Gerontology (India) (AGI)

Biochemistry & Molecular Biology Laboratory
Department of Zoology
Banaras Hindu University
Varanasi 221 005, Uttar Pradesh, India
Phone: 91 542 2317649 **Fax:** 91 542 368174
Email: agi@banaras.ernet.in

Fnded: 1982. **Mem:** 205. **Reg. Groups:** 6. **Lang(s):** English. **Desc:** Health care professionals treating the elderly; scientists and clinicians with an interest in the aging process and diseases of the aged. Works to insure high standards of research and practice in gerontology, and to maximize availability of gerontological services. Conducts research in biological, clinical and psycho-social aspects of gerontology. **Pub:** Newsletter, semiannual.

★ 1290 ★ Association for Glycogen Storage Disease

1 Cridlands
Lydiard St. Lawrence
Taunton TA4 3RZ, United Kingdom
Phone: 44 161 9807303 **Fax:** 44 161 2263813
Email: info@agsd.org.uk
Website: http://www.agsd.org.uk

Mem: 150. **Desc:** Provides contacts and support for all persons with Glycogen Storage Disease. Encourages the provision of Specialist Centres for the diagnosis, monitoring and treatment of GSD affected persons, both children and adults. Provides a focus for scientific, educational and charitable activities concerning GSD. Encourages the formation and interaction of GSD families and professionals around the world.

★ 1291 ★ Association for Glycogen Storage Disease (AGSD)

PO Box 896
Durant, IA 52747
Phone: (563)785-6038 **Fax:** (563)785-6038
Email: maryc@agsdus.org
Website: http://www.agsdus.org
Hollie Swain, Pres.

Fnded: 1979. **Mem:** 400. **Desc:** Individuals afflicted with glycogen storage disease; families of GSD sufferers; health care professionals. (GSD is a hereditary condition characterized by a lack of or deficiency in any of the enzymes used by the body to break down glycogen, resulting in hypoglycemia and related disorders, and requiring diet modifications and frequent or continual feeding, and in extreme cases resulting in death.) Acts as a forum for the discussion of GSD, its treatment, and the problems faced by parents raising children with GSD. Disseminates medical information; fosters communication between the families of GSD patients and health care professionals. Conducts fundraising drive. Aids members in obtaining equipment necessary for home care of GSD patients; provides referral services for individuals seeking GSD treatment facilities. **Pub:** *Could Someone You Know* *be Affected?*. Brochures. *Price:* Free. • *Parent Handbook*. Book. *Price:* $10. • *The Ray*, quarterly. Newsletter. *Price:* Free.

★ 1292 ★ Association for Group and Individual Psychotherapy

1 Fairbridge Rd.
London N19 3EW, United Kingdom
Phone: 44 207 2727013

★ 1293 ★ Association of Halfway House Alcoholism Programs of North America (AHHAP)

860 N Center St.
Mesa, AZ 85201
Phone: (480)610-8300 **Free:** 800-861-0599
Fax: (480)964-2004
Email: ahhap@aol.com
Website: http://www.ahhap.org
John Curtiss, Pres.

Fnded: 1965. **Mem:** 450. **Reg. Groups:** 13. **State Groups:** 50. **Desc:** Halfway house corporations, staff, board members, and individuals closely related to the halfway house movement. Charitable organization dedicated to educating and serving halfway house programs through technical assistance, consultant services, workshops, conferences, and related services. Operates placement service. Disseminates information and materials. **Pub:** *AHHAP Membership Directory*, annual. Membership Directory. • *Communications and Services Newsletter*, quarterly. Newsletter. • *Conference Proceedings*, annual. Proceedings.

★ 1294 ★ Association of the Handicapped Children of Romania

Str. Gral Haralambie 36, Sector 4
Bucharest, Romania
Phone: 40 1 3371875 **Fax:** 40 1 3371875
Email: aschfr@ant.ro

Fnded: 1990. **Mem:** 2,500. **Reg. Groups:** 7. **Lang(s):** English, Romanian. **Desc:** Promotes improved quality of life for children with physical disabilities in Romania. Conducts educational and instructional programs for children with physical handicaps and their teachers and family members; makes available physical therapy and other treatment programs. **Pub:** *Informative Bulletin*, semiannual. Newsletter. Information bulletin.

★ 1295 ★ Association of Healthcare Internal Auditors (AHIA)

PO Box 449
Onsted, MI 49265-0449
Phone: (517)467-7729 **Fax:** (517)467-6104
Email: ahia@ahia.org
Website: http://www.ahia.org
Pat Bogusz, Exec. Dir.

Fnded: 1981. **Mem:** 1,000. **Desc:** Health care internal auditors and other interested individuals. Promotes cost containment and increased productivity in health care institutions through internal auditing. Serves as a forum for the exchange of experience, ideas, and information among members; provides continuing professional education courses and informs members of developments in health care internal auditing. Offers employment clearinghouse services. **Pub:** *New Perspectives on Healthcare Auditing*, quarterly. Journal. Contains book reviews, audit findings, and local and regional group news. **Frmly:** (1989) Healthcare Internal Audit Group.

★ 1296 ★ Association for Healthcare Philanthropy (AHP)

313 Park Ave., Ste. 400
Falls Church, VA 22046
Phone: (703)532-6243 **Fax:** (703)532-7170
Email: bill@go-ahp.org
Website: http://www.go-ahp.org
Dr. William C. McGinly, Pres.,CEO

Fnded: 1967. **Mem:** 2,800. **Reg. Groups:** 7. **Desc:** Persons employed by healthcare organizations in the field of healthcare resource development and fundraising; hospital administrators and trustees; hospitals; interested individuals. Purposes are to create a cohesive body of healthcare development executives to advance the interests and knowledge of healthcare fund development; to encourage and stimulate better understanding of healthcare needs; to accomplish common goals through an exchange of ideas and information. Conducts educational programs. Holds regional seminars. Compiles statistics; conducts research; sponsors competitions. Maintains library. **Pub:** *AHP Connect*, 8/year. Newsletter. • *Association for Healthcare Philanthropy–Directory*, annual. Directory. Lists members and allied firms. Includes calendar of events. *Price:* Included in membership dues. • *Association for Healthcare Philanthropy–Journal*, semiannual. Journal. *Price:* Included in membership dues; $38/year for nonmembers. • *Report on Giving*. • *Salary and Benefits*. **Frmly:** (1967) Developartners; (1991) National Association for Hospital Development.

★ 1297 ★ Association for Healthcare Resource and Materials Management (AHRMM)

c/o American Hospital Association
1 N Franklin
Chicago, IL 60606
Phone: (312)422-3840 **Fax:** (312)422-4573
Email: ahrmm@aha.org
Website: http://www.ahrmm.org
Deborah Sprindzunas, Exec. Dir.

Fnded: 1962. **Mem:** 2,950. **Local Groups:** 45. **Desc:** Individuals active in the field of purchasing, inventory and distribution, and materials management as performed in hospitals, related patient care institutions, or government and voluntary health organizations, and who are employed by an organization eligible for institutional membership in the American Hospital Association; associate members are individuals active in the areas of health care supply manufacturing, distributing, and consulting. Purposes are to: assist members with their responsibilities; provide access to the latest ideas, methods, developments, information, and techniques in the field of hospital purchasing and materials management; establish associations with others in the profession; provide recognition in the profession through participation in policy-making; provide a link with the AHA. Conducts certification program in health care management. **Pub:** *Association for Healthcare Resource & Materials Management–Conference Proceedings*, annual. Proceedings. Presents case studies. *Price:* $45/year for members; $65/year for nonmembers. • *Association for Healthcare Resource & Materials Management–Membership Roster*, annual. Membership Directory. *Price:* Included in membership dues. • *Healthcare Resource & Materials Management News*, bimonthly. Newsletter. Contains reviews of educational programs, current legal and legislative problems, new resources and materials management techniques, and assoc. news. *Price:* Included in membership dues. • *Resource Catalog*, annual. **Frmly:** (1976) American Society for Hospital Purchasing Agents; (1983) American Society for Hospital Purchasing and Materials Management; (1994) American Society for Hospital Materials Management; (1998) American Society for Healthcare Materials Management.

★ 1298 ★ Association of Health Facility Survey Agencies (AHFSA)

Missouri Department of Health
Bureau of Health Facility Regulation
912 Wildwood Dr.
PO Box 570
Jefferson City, MO 65102
Phone: (573)751-6302 **Fax:** (573)526-3621
Shanna E. Schopp, Interim Admin.

Fnded: 1968. **Mem:** 51. **Desc:** Directors of state or territorial health facility licensure and certification programs; staff members of a state or territorial health facility licensure and certification agency; employees of the federal Health Care Financing Administration; interested individuals. (The term health facilities refers to health/medical institutions including hospitals, nursing homes, rehabilitation centers, reproductive health centers, independent clinical laboratories, hospices, and ambulatory surgical centers.) Purposes are to exchange information among members and between members and the Association of State and Territorial Health Officials; constitute a "reservoir of expertise" to aid in the guidance of ASTHO; improve the quality of health facility licensure and certification programs; provide a forum for state and territorial issues at the national level. Has a representative on an ASTHO standing committee and liaises with the federal Department of Health and Human Services and the HCFA. Has developed new training programs with the HHS and testified before the U.S. Senate Special Committee on Aging on survey and certification procedures. Bestows annual Surveyor of the Year Award. **Pub:** *AHFSA Directory*, annual. Directory. • *Association of Health Facility Survey Agencies Newsletter*, semiannual. Newsletter. Reports on the quality of health facility licensure and certification programs and related issues. Includes calendar of events. *Price:* Included in membership dues. • Papers. **Frmly:** (1991) Association of Health Facility Licensure and Certification Directors.

★ 1299 ★ Association of Health Insurance Advisors

2901 Telestar Ct.
Falls Church, VA 22042
Phone: (703)770-8200 **Fax:** (703)770-8201
Email: ahia@naifa.org
Website: http://www.ahia.net
Michael L. Kerley, Exec. VP

Fnded: 1990. **Mem:** 5,000. **Desc:** Insurance agents and advisors specializing in health, disability, long term care insurance and/or employee benefits. **Pub:** *Health Insurance Matters*, biweekly. *Price:* included in membership dues.

★ 1300 ★ Association of Healthcare Philanthropy (AHP)

c/o St. Joseph's Health Centre Foundation
30 The Queen's Way
Toronto, ON, Canada M6R 1B5
Phone: (416)530-6392 **Fax:** (416)530-6836
Email: gamacl@stjoe.on.ca
Website: http://www.ahpcanada.com/

Mem: 3,100. **Desc:** Promotes healthcare fundraising professionals; dedicated to supporting members ability to perform philanthropic work for healthcare organizations; develops career opportunities.

★ 1301 ★ Association for the Help of Retarded Children

200 Park Ave. S
New York, NY 10003
Phone: (212)780-2500
Email: sbstein@ahrcnyc.org
Website: http://www.ahrcnyc.org

Fnded: 1949. **Mem:** 12,000. **Desc:** Developmentally disabled children and adults; their families; interested individuals. Provides support services, training programs, clinics, schools, and residential facilities to the developmentally disabled. **Pub:** *The Chronicle*, monthly. Newsletter.

★ 1302 ★ Association for Higher Education Access and Disability (AHEAD)

Newman House
86 St., Stephen's Green
Dublin 2, Dublin, Ireland
Phone: 353 1 4752386 **Fax:** 353 1 4752387
Email: ahead@iol.ie
Website: http://www.ahead.ie

Fnded: 1989. **Mem:** 70. **Lang(s):** English, Irish. **Desc:** Individuals and organizations. Promotes increased access to higher education for people with disabilities. Lobbies for more stringent statutes mandating accessibility of educational institutions; represents the interests of people with disabilities before institutions of higher education.

★ 1303 ★ Association on Higher Education and Disability (AHEAD)
University of Massachusetts Boston
100 Morrissey Blvd.
Boston, MA 02125-3393
Phone: (617)287-3880 **Fax:** (617)287-3881
Email: stephan.smith@umb.edu
Website: http://www.ahead.org
Stephan J. Smith, Exec. Dir.

Fnded: 1977. **Mem:** 2,000. **Desc:** Individuals interested in promoting the equal rights and opportunities of disabled postsecondary students, staff, faculty, and graduates. Provides an exchange of communication for those professionally involved with disabled students; collects, evaluates, and disseminates information; encourages and supports legislation for the benefit of disabled students. Conducts surveys on issues pertinent to college students with disabilities; offers resource referral system and employment exchange for positions in disability student services. Conducts research programs; compiles statistics. **Pub:** *ALERT*, quarterly. Newsletter. • *Journal of Postsecondary Education & Disability*. Journal. • Membership Directory, ongoing. **AKA:** AHEAD.

★ 1304 ★ Association of Hispanic Healthcare Executives (AHHE)
PO Box 230832
Ansonia Station
New York, NY 10023
Phone: (212)877-1615 **Fax:** (212)877-2406
Email: ahheinnyc@aol.com
Website: http://www.ahhe.org/
George A. Zeppenfeldt-Cestero, Pres.

Fnded: 1988. **Mem:** 215. **Nat'l Groups:** 1. **Reg. Groups:** 2. **State Groups:** 13. **Desc:** Seeks to foster programs and policies to increase presence of Hispanics in health administration professions. **Pub:** Reports.

★ 1305 ★ Association for the History of Chiropractic (AHC)
c/o Alana Callender
1000 Brady St.
Davenport, IA 52803
Phone: (563)884-5245 **Fax:** (563)884-5616
Email: callender_a@palmer.edu
Website: http://chirohistory.com
Alana Callender, Exec. Dir.

Fnded: 1980. **Mem:** 340. **Nat'l Groups:** 2. **Desc:** Chiropractors, students, educators, and writers; chiropractic colleges; organizations. Researches and records the history of the chiropractic profession and disseminates information on the subject. Maintains speakers' bureau. **Pub:** *AHC Bulletin*, 3/year. Newsletter. *Price:* Included in membership dues. • *Association for the History of Chiropractic Membership Directory*, periodic. Membership Directory. Includes association bylaws. *Price:* available to members only. • *Chiropractic History: The Archives and Journal of the Association of the History of Chiropractic*, semiannual. Magazine. Includes association news. Index available. *Price:* Included in membership dues; $35 for nonmembers. • *Style Manual for Authors*. Manual.

★ 1306 ★ Association for Holotropic Breathwork International (AHBI)
PO Box 7169
Santa Cruz, CA 95061-7169
Phone: (650)325-4254 **Fax:** (650)325-4254
Email: office@breathwork.com
Website: http://www.breathwork.com/
Sarah Brudge, Coord.

Desc: Works to preserve and enhance the principles of holotropic breathwork. **Pub:** *The Inner Door*, quarterly. *Price:* included in membership dues.

★ 1307 ★ Association of Hong Kong Nursing Staff (AHKNS)
Hing Wan Commercial Bldg., 3/F
25-27 Parkes St.
Jordan
Kowloon
Hong Kong, People's Republic of China
Phone: 852 23146900 **Fax:** 852 27366020
Email: info@nurse.org.hk
Website: http://www.nurse.org.hk

Fnded: 1977. **Mem:** 18,500. **Lang(s):** Chinese, English. **Desc:** Registered, enrolled, and student nurses. Seeks to advance the nursing profession; promotes professional development of members. Represents members' legal and professional interests. Conducts continuing professional education and training courses; makes available to members services including legal advice and travel and merchandise discounts. **Pub:** *AHKNS Newsletter*, quarterly. Newsletter. **Frmly:** (1990) Association of Government Nursing Staff.

★ 1308 ★ Association for Hospital Medical Education (AHME)
419 Beulah Rd.
Pittsburgh, PA 15235
Phone: (412)244-9302 **Free:** (866)617-4780
Fax: (412)243-4693
Email: info@ahme.org
Website: http://ahme.org
Margie Kleppick, Exec. Dir.

Fnded: 1956. **Mem:** 683. **Desc:** Dedicated to the comprehensive support of medical education professionals; supports continuum if medical education. **Pub:** *AHME Membership Directory*, annual. Membership Directory. Online version, updated continuously. • *AHME News*, semiannual. Newsletter. • *Guide to Graduate Medical Education (Guide I and II)*. Guide III will be posted online as articles become available. *Price:* $35 Guide II. • *The Purple Book Online*, annual. • *Resource and Reference Center*. **Frmly:** (1968) Association of Hospital Directors of Medical Education.

★ 1309 ★ Association for Humanistic Psychology (AHP)
1516 Oak St., No. 320A
Alameda, CA 94501-2947
Phone: (510)769-6495 **Fax:** (510)769-6433
Email: ahpoffice@aol.com
Website: http://www.ahpweb.org
Leland Baggett, Pres.

Fnded: 1962. **Mem:** 2,000. **Nat'l Groups:** 2. **State Groups:** 1. **Local Groups:** 2. **Desc:** Psychologists, social workers, clergy, educators, psychiatrists, and others engaged in humanistic practice. Functions as an international community of people who are dedicated to the exploration, healing, and expansion of the human mind, body and soul, and to building a society that advances our ability to choose, to grow, and to create. Aims to realize a vision of the possible for humanity. **Pub:** *AHP Perspective*, bimonthly. Newsletter. Covers growth therapies, holistic education, interdisciplinary humanistic practices, and social concerns. Includes calendar of events. *Price:* Included in membership dues. • *Journal of Humanistic Psychology*, quarterly. Journal. **Frmly:** American Association for Humanistic Psychology.

★ 1310 ★ Association of Humanistic Psychology Practitioners (AHPP)
BCM AHPP
London WC1N 3XX, United Kingdom
Phone: 44 8457 660326
Email: admin.ahpp@btinternet.com
Website: http://www.ahpp.org/

Fnded: 1980. **Mem:** 250. **Lang(s):** English, French, German, Italian, Swedish. **Desc:** Provides accreditation of humanistic psychotherapists as member organization of the U.K. Council for Psychotherapy and for other therapists and counsellors; makes available referral services; conducts training and professional development programs. Disseminates information to members.

★ 1311 ★ Association of Independent Care Advisors
6 West Mount Close
Southwick
Brighton BN42 4SR, United Kingdom
Phone: 44 1483 203066 **Fax:** 44 1483 202535
Website: http://www.aica.org.uk

Fnded: 1994. **Mem:** 8. **Nat'l Groups:** 1. **Desc:** Members provide advice to individuals about their care options, either in their own homes or in residential homes.

★ 1312 ★ Association of Independent Physical Therapists (Bundesverband Selbstaendiger PhysiotherapeutInnen)
Konigsallee 178A
D-44799 Bochum, Germany
Phone: 49 234 977450 **Fax:** 49 234 9774545
Email: ifk@ifk.de
Website: http://www.IFK.de

Fnded: 1981. **Mem:** 3,500. **Lang(s):** English. **Desc:** Physical therapists in Germany. Promotes the physical therapy industry. Represents the interests of freelance physical therapists. **Pub:** *KG-Intern*, bimonthly. Magazine.

★ 1313 ★ Association of Industrial Laser Users (AILU)
100 Ock St.
Abingdon OX14 5DH, United Kingdom
Phone: 44 1235 539595 **Fax:** 44 1235 550499
Email: admin@ailu.org.uk
Website: http://www.ailu.org.uk

Fnded: 1995. **Mem:** 270. **Desc:** Aims to foster cooperation and collaboration on non-competitive technical matters and provide a forum and mechanisms for sharing experience and expertise. Represents and promotes the interests of industrial laser users. Disseminates professional and other information to members. Promotes the best practice in the industrial applications of lasers in materials processing and allied technologies. Supports the maintenance and improvement of standards of safety and performance in the industrial user of lasers.

★ 1314 ★ Association of Institutions Teaching Veterinary Medicine Totally or Partially in the French Language (Association des Etablissements d'Enseignement Veterinaire Totalement ou Partiellement de Langue Francaise)
Faculte de Medicine Veterinaire
Universite de Montreal
Campus St.-Hyacinthe
CP 5000
St.-Hyacinthe, QC, Canada J2S 7C6
Phone: (514)343-6111 **Fax:** (514)778-8101
Email: raymond.s.roy@umontreal.ca

Lang(s): English, French. **Desc:** Institutions offering veterinary medical education programs in French. Promotes excellence in French-language veterinary medical education. Facilitates communication and exchange among members; conducts training programs for veterinary medical educators.

★ 1315 ★ Association of Institutions for Tropical Veterinary Medicine (AITVM)
c/o Secretariat
Faculty of Veterinary Medicine
Office for International Co-operation
PO Box 80.163
NL-3508 TD Utrecht, Netherlands
Phone: 31 30 2532116 **Fax:** 31 30 2531815
Email: aitvm@vet.uu.nl
Website: http://aitvm.vet.uu.nl/

Desc: Works to improve human health and quality of life through safe food production in tropical regions by enhancing research, training and education in veterinary medicine and livestock production within the framework of sustainable development.

★ 1316 ★ Association for International Cancer Research (AICR)
Madras House
South St.
North Haugh
Saint Andrews KY16 9EH, United Kingdom
Phone: 44 1334 477910 **Fax:** 44 1334 478667
Email: jane.wilson@aicr.org.uk
Website: http://www.aicr.org.uk/

Fnded: 1979. **Mem:** 14. **Desc:** Funds cancer research. Disseminates research results. **Pub:** *Progress*, 3/year.

★ 1317 ★ Association of International Health Researchers (AIHR)
2665 Pleasant Valley Rd.
Mobile, AL 36606
Phone: (251)473-3946
Dr. Roy E. Kadel, Pres.

Fnded: 1982. **Mem:** 123. **Reg. Groups:** 5. **Desc:** Individuals interested in quality health research. Works to: promote a better understanding of scientifically effective research techniques and methodologies; encourage interaction among individuals in international health research. Compiles statistics.

★ 1318 ★ Association Internationale Francophone des Aines (AIFA)
39 rue Dalhousie
Quebec, QC, Canada G1K 8R8
Phone: (418)646-9117 **Fax:** (418)644-7670
Email: cvfa@cvfa.ca
Website: http://www.cvfa.ca

Fnded: 1981. **Mem:** 125. **Lang(s):** French. **Desc:** Individuals in 9 countries belonging to associations or organizations that provide services to senior citizens. Aims to: unite associations of senior citizens in French-speaking areas; encourage participation by senior citizens in social life; foster independent living; promote the use of French and an understanding of francophone culture; encourage information exchange and visits to French-speaking areas. **Pub:** *Maturite*, quarterly.

★ 1319 ★ Association Internationale de Psychologie du Travail de Langue Francaise (AIPTLF)
Universite Lille 3
Pr Claude Lemoine, AIPTLF
UFR Psychologie
BP 149
F-59653 Villeneuve d'Ascq Cedex, France
Phone: 33 3 20416315 **Fax:** 33 3 20416324
Email: lemoine@univ-lille3.fr
Website: http://www.psp.ucl.ac.be/aiptlf2002

Fnded: 1980. **Mem:** 1,000. **Nat'l Groups:** 1. **Reg. Groups:** 3. **Lang(s):** French. Does not correspond in English. **Desc:** Doctors, personnel directors, industrial psychologists, and sociologists in 30 countries. Promotes the French language within the field of industrial psychology. Seeks to keep members informed and to aid in the perfection of their work. Facilitates the exchange of current research and information among members. **Pub:** *Actes de Congres*, biennial. Journal. • *Psychologie du Travail et des Organisations*, quarterly. Journal. **Frmly:** French-Language Association of Work Psychology.

★ 1320 ★ Association Ivoirienne de Bien-Etre Familial (AIBEF)
Adjame vers l'Institut National de la Sante Publique
Bd. Giscard d'Estaing
01 BP 5315
Abidjan 01, Cote d'Ivoire
Phone: 225 251811 **Fax:** 225 251868
Email: aibef@africaonline.co.ci

Fnded: 1979. **Mem:** 650. **Lang(s):** French. **Desc:** Promotes advances in women's health care and family planning programs. X

★ 1321 ★ Association of Jewish Aging Services (AJAS)
316 Pennsylvania Ave. SE, Ste. 402
Washington, DC 20003
Phone: (202)543-7500 **Fax:** (202)543-4090
Email: ajas@ajas.org
Website: http://ajas.org
Harvey Tillipman, Exec. Dir.

Fnded: 1960. **Mem:** 200. **Desc:** Nonprofit charitable Jewish homes and nursing homes; retirement and housing units; independent and assisted living, geriatric hospitals, and special facilities for Jewish aged and chronically ill. Conducts institutes and conferences; undertakes legislative activities; compiles statistics. **Pub:** *Escribe Newsletter*, quarterly. Newsletter. • Membership Directory, annual. **Frmly:** (1982) National Association of Jewish Homes for the Aged; (1998) North American Association of Jewish Homes and Housing for the Aging.

★ 1322 ★ Association of Labor Assistants and Childbirth Educators (ALACE)
PO Box 390436
Cambridge, MA 02139
Phone: (617)441-2500
Website: http://www.alace.org/

Desc: Provides pregnant women with information and alternatives for childbirth. **Pub:** *Special Delivery*, quarterly. Journal. Provides information on pregnancy and birth, midwifery, women's health issues, breastfeeding, parenting, childbirth education, labor assisting. *Price:* included in membership dues; $4 non-member, sample issue.

★ 1323 ★ Association of Late-Deafened Adults (ALDA)
1131 Lake St., No. 204
Oak Park, IL 60301
Free: 877-907-1738 **Fax:** 877-907-1738
Email: board@alda.org
Website: http://www.alda.org
Mary Clark, Pres.

Fnded: 1987. **Mem:** 1,500. **Reg. Groups:** 25. **Desc:** People who have become deaf adventitiously and rely on visual systems to communicate effectively. Provides information, support, and social opportunities through selfhelp groups, general membership meetings, and social events. Advocates for the needs of late-deafened people. Conducts and participates in surveys, workshops, and seminars on late-deafness. Maintains speakers' bureau and biographical archives. **Pub:** *ALDA News*, quarterly. Newsletter. Includes pen pal section. *Price:* Included in membership dues. • *Proceedings of ALDAcon*. Monograph.

★ 1324 ★ Association of Lesbian, Gay, and Bisexual Psychologists - Europe (ALGPE)
c/o Dr. Melanie Steffens
F BI-Psychologie
Universitaet Trier
D-54286 Trier, Germany
Phone: 49 651 2012017 **Fax:** 49 651 2012955
Email: steffens@cogpsy.uni-trier.de
Website: http://www.psychologie.uni-trier.de/projects/ALGP/algphome.html

Lang(s): English, German. **Desc:** Gay and lesbian psychologists. Promotes adherence to high standards of ethics and practice among members. Facilitates communication and cooperation among members; sponsors continuing professional development courses.

★ 1325 ★ Association of Life Insurance Medicine of Japan (Nihon Hoken Igakkai)
3-4-1 Marunouchi, Chiyoda-ku
Tokyo, Japan
Phone: 81 3 2862735
Fnded: 1901.

★ 1326 ★ Association of Local Public Health Agencies (ALPHA)
425 University Ave., Ste. 502
Toronto, ON, Canada M5G 1T6
Phone: (416)595-0006 **Fax:** (416)595-0030
Email: mail@alphaweb.org
Website: http://www.alphaweb.org

Lang(s): English, French. **Desc:** Local public health agencies. Promotes increased availability and effectiveness of public health programs. Lobbies for improved legislation governing public health; facilitates communication and cooperation among members; publicizes public health programs. **Pub:** *Canadian Directory of Public Health Agencies*, annual. Directory. Directory listing of all public health units in Canada, cross-referencing by provinces. **Frmly:** (1997) Association of Local Official Health Agencies.

★ 1327 ★ Association for Low Flow Anaesthesia
c/o Dr. Mike Logan
Department of Anaesthesia
Royal Infirmary of Edinburgh
Edinburgh EH3 9YW, United Kingdom
Phone: 44 131 5363652 **Fax:** 44 131 5363672
Email: mikel@srv1.med.ed.ac.uk
Website: http://www.alfanaes.freeserve.co.uk/alfa-1.htm

Fnded: 1995. **Desc:** Promotes the use and understanding of methods of inhalational anesthesia involving recirculation of exhaled gases and reduced fresh gas input. Fosters continuing education for anesthesiologists. Conducts research.

★ 1328 ★ Association malienne de Lutte contre le Diabete (AMLD)
c/o Centre Hospitalo-Universitaire Gabriel Toure
Bamako, Mali
Phone: 223 230780 **Fax:** 223 226090
Email: dr.a.nientao@ifrance.com
Website: http://www.diabetesafrica.com/idfmembers.html

Desc: Represents people with diabetes. Promotes research and support of those with diabetes in Mali.

★ 1329 ★ Association Luxembourg Alzheimer (ALA)
Boite Postale 5021
L-1050 Luxembourg, Luxembourg
Phone: 352 4216761 **Fax:** 352 42167630
Email: ala@sl.lu

Lang(s): English, French, German. **Desc:** Individuals and organizations. Seeks to improve the quality of life of people with Alzheimer's disease and their families. Makes available support and services; facilitates research on Alzheimer's disease and related disorders; conducts educational programs.

★ 1330 ★ Association Luxembourgeoise de Gerontologie/Geriatrie
c/o Jean Hamen, Sec.
20, rue de Contern
Itzig, Luxembourg
Phone: 352 26821 **Fax:** 352 26822240
Email: jean-claude.leners@chnp.lu

Fnded: 1985. **Mem:** 120. **Desc:** Represents all professionals working in the field of gerontology/geriatrics, including senior citizen associations.

★ 1331 ★ Association for Macular Diseases (AMD)
210 E 64th St., 8th Fl.
New York, NY 10021
Phone: (212)605-3719 **Fax:** (212)605-3795
Email: association@retinalresearch.org
Website: http://www.macula.org/
Nikolai Stevenson, Pres.

Fnded: 1977. **Mem:** 8,000. **Desc:** Individuals afflicted with macular diseases, and their families. (The macula of the eye is the posterior middle portion of the retina responsible for central vision. Disorders involving the macula include inflammations, tumors, retinal growths, and degenerative problems.) Purposes are to: disseminate information on available resources such as recorded material and low vision aids; promote public awareness of macular diseases; encourage growth of research into the causes, treatment, and possible prevention of macular diseases; inform the public of the need for postmortem donation of eyes having a history of macular disease and advise on procedures for making such a donation. Provides counseling programs and group sharing for afflicted persons and their families. **Pub:** *Eyes Only*, quarterly. Newsletter. *Price:* $20 included in membership dues. **Frmly:** Association for Mascular Degeneration.

★ 1332 ★ Association of Managed Care Dentists (AMCD)

1223 Wilshire Blvd., Ste. 483
Santa Monica, CA 90403
Phone: (310)453-3439 **Free:** 800-864-6848
Fax: (310)453-7895
Email: jmaguire@dentalgroup.com
Website: http://www.amcd.org
Bonnie Ross, Contact

Desc: Dentists participating in managed dental care programs. Seeks to advance the provision of managed dental care. Serves as liaison linking members with government agencies and dental plan administrators; sponsors educational programs. **Pub:** *News Flash*, periodic. Newsletter. **Frmly:** (2000) Association of Managed Care Providers.

★ 1333 ★ Association of Massage Therapists Australia (AMTA)

PO Box 358
Prahran, VIC 3181, Australia
Phone: 61 3 95103930 **Fax:** 61 3 95213209
Email: amta@amta.asn.au
Website: http://www.amta.asn.au

Fnded: 1989. **Mem:** 1,750. **Reg. Groups:** 9. **State Groups:** 7. **Lang(s):** English. **Desc:** Professional massage therapists and those studying professional massage. Promotes the professional interests of massage therapists in Australia. **Pub:** *AMTA Journal*, quarterly. Journal. Features issues affecting the industry and members.

★ 1334 ★ Association of Maternal and Child Health Programs (AMCHP)

1220 19th St. NW, Ste. 801
Washington, DC 20036
Phone: (202)775-0436 **Fax:** (202)775-0061
Email: info@amchp.org
Website: http://www.amchp.org
Christopher Kus, MD, Pres.

Fnded: 1944. **Mem:** 450. **Desc:** Individuals responsible for or involved in the Administration of state and territorial maternal and child health programs and programs for children with special health care needs. Seeks to: inform public and private sector decision makers of the health care needs of mothers and children; develop and recommend maternal and child health policies and programs; develop coalitions with other interested organizations. Promotes exchange of ideas and experiences among members; studies and reports on the health of and services for mothers and children; develops models and standards for and provides technical assistance to maternal and child health programs. **Pub:** *Abstinence Education in the States: Implementation of the 1996 Abstinence Education Law.* • *AMCHP Updates*, bimonthly. Newsletter. *Price:* Included in membership dues. • *Caring for Mothers and Children: A Report of a Survey of 1987 State MCH Program Activities.* • *Dedicated to Care for Children: A Report on States Use of OBRA 1986 Earmarked Title V Funds.* • *Home Visiting: An Effective Strategy for Improving the Health of Mothers and Children.* • *The Impact of the State Child Health Insurance Program (CHIP) on Title V Children with Special Health Care Needs Programs.* • *Smoking Cessation Makes Cents: The Cost-Effectiveness of Tobacco Interventions.* • Magazines. • Proceedings. • Reports. • Also publishes cost-based reimbursement studies and health care reform studies. **Frmly:** Association of State and Territorial Maternal and Child Health and Crippled Children's Directors.

★ 1335 ★ Association for Medical Deans in Europe (AMDE)

Grosvenor Rd.
Belfast BT12 6HJ, United Kingdom
Phone: 44 28 90240503 **Fax:** 44 28 90240899

Fnded: 1979.

★ 1336 ★ Association of Medical Doctors of Asia (AMDA)

310-1 Narazu
Okayama 701-1202, Japan
Phone: 81 86 2847730 **Fax:** 81 86 2848959
Email: member@amda.or.jp
Website: http://www.amda.or.jp

Fnded: 1984. **Mem:** 665. **Reg. Groups:** 30. **Lang(s):** English, French, Japanese, Spanish. **Desc:** Physicians, medical students, and organizations are members; nurses and other health care personnel and organizations are associate members. Promotes and works to strengthen partnership among Asian doctors. Seeks to insure adequate medical care for people in underserved areas. Conducts emergency relief and rehabilitation operations in areas affected by natural disasters or human conflicts; implements community health development programs in rural areas; facilitates continuing professional education and training of members. **Pub:** *AMDA International*, quarterly. Newsletter. • *Harukanaru Yume.* Book. • *International Collaboration of Medical Care*, monthly. Journal. • *International Medical Cooperation - Proceedings of the Hayabashibara Forum 1993.* Proceedings. • *Proceedings of the 1994 Okayama NGO Summit.* Proceedings. • *Ruwandakarano Shogen.* Book. • *Tobidase! AMDA.* Report.

★ 1337 ★ Association for Medical Education in the Eastern Mediterranean Region (AMEEMR)

Jordan University of Science and Technology
PO Box 3030
Irbid, Jordan
Phone: 962 2 7095111 **Fax:** 962 2 7095123
Email: hijazi@just.edu.jo

Lang(s): English. **Desc:** Medical schools, educators, and students. Seeks to advance medical scholarship and practice. Serves as a clearinghouse on medical education; encourages communication and cooperation among members; sponsors research programs and continuing professional development courses.

★ 1338 ★ Association for Medical Education in Europe (AMEE)

Centre for Medical Education
University of Dundee
Tay Park House
484 Perth Rd.
Dundee DD2 1LR, United Kingdom
Phone: 44 1382 631953 **Fax:** 44 1382 645748
Email: amee@dundee.ac.uk
Website: http://www.amee.org

Lang(s): English. **Desc:** Medical schools, educators, and students. Seeks to advance medical scholarship and practice. Serves as a clearinghouse on medical education; encourages communication and cooperation among members; sponsors research programs and continuing professional development courses. **Pub:** *Medical Teacher*, bimonthly. Journal.

★ 1339 ★ Association of Medical Education and Research in Substance Abuse (AMERSA)

125 Whipple, 3rd Fl., Ste. 300
Providence, RI 02908
Phone: (401)349-0000 **Fax:** 877-418-8769
Email: isabel@amersa.org
Website: http://www.amersa.org
Isabel Vieira, Co-Dir.

Fnded: 1976. **Mem:** 300. **Desc:** Multidisciplinary organization of health care professionals dedicated to improving education in the care of individuals with substance abuse problems. **Pub:** *Substance Abuse*, quarterly. Journal. *Price:* Included in membership dues; $40/year for nonmembers. • Membership Directory, biennial.

★ 1340 ★ Association for Medical Education in the Western Pacific Region (AMEWPR)

Seoul National University
College of Medicine
28 Yong-Dong, Chongno-Gu
Seoul 110-799, Republic of Korea
Phone: 82 2 7602552 **Fax:** 82 2 7476779
Email: kimyi@plaza.snu.ac.kr

Lang(s): English, Japanese. **Desc:** Medical schools, educators, and students. Seeks to advance medical scholarship and practice. Serves as a clearinghouse on medical education; encourages communication and cooperation among members; sponsors research programs and continuing professional development courses.

★ 1341 ★ Association for Medical Education in the Western Pacific Region - Malaysia (AMEWPR)

Jalan Raja Muda Abdul Aziz
50300 Kuala Lumpur, Malaysia
Phone: 60 3 2923066 **Fax:** 60 3 2912659

Fnded: 1988.

★ 1342 ★ Association of Medical Illustrators (AMI)

5475 Mark Dabling Rd., Ste. 108
Colorado Springs, CO 80918-3847
Phone: (719)598-8622 **Fax:** (719)599-3075
Email: ami@capsys.com
Website: http://www.ami.org
Janet McAndless, Exec. Dir.

Fnded: 1945. **Mem:** 1,000. **Desc:** Medical illustrators and individuals engaged in related pursuits. Promotes the study and encourages the advancement of medical illustration and allied fields of visual education. Works to advance medical education and to promote understanding and cooperation with medical and related professions; accredits six postgraduate medical illustration programs. Offers continuing education program; provides professional certification; compiles statistics. **Pub:** *Journal of Biocommunication*, quarterly. Journal. • *Medical Illustration Sourcebook*, annual. • Directory, annual. • Newsletter, bimonthly.

★ 1343 ★ Association of Medical Instrumentation

2 Prannok Rd.
Bangkok 10700, Thailand

★ 1344 ★ Association of Medical Microbiologists

c/o Dr. Beryl Oppenheim
Public Health Laboratory
Birmingham Heartlands Hospital
Bordesley Green East
Birmingham B9 5SS, United Kingdom
Phone: 44 121 4243240 **Fax:** 44 121 7726229
Website: http://www.amm.co.uk

Fnded: 1983. **Mem:** 500. **Desc:** Scientists, academics, consultants, and others interested in medical microbiology. Professional body concerned with all aspects of medical microbiology. Promotes high quality training in medical microbiology.

★ **1345** ★ **Association of Medical Physicists of India**
Bhabba Atomic Research Centre
Bombay 400 085, India
Phone: 91 22 2556060 **Fax:** 91 5560750 5560750
Fnded: 1976.

★ **1346** ★ **Association for Medical Physics Technology (AMPT)**
30 Burnham Ave.
Ickenham, United Kingdom
Fnded: 1952.

★ **1347** ★ **Association of Medical Professionals with Hearing Losses**
c/o Danielle N. Rastetter
3709 Waterbridge Ln.
Miamisburg, OH 45342-6728
Email: drastet@attglobal.net
Website: http://www.amphl.org
Danielle N. Rastetter, Pres.
Fnded: 1999. **Desc:** Provides information, promotes advocacy and mentorship. Creates a network for individuals with hearing losses interested in or working in health care fields.

★ **1348** ★ **Association of Medical Research Charities (AMRC)**
61 Gray's Inn Rd.
London WC1X 8TL, United Kingdom
Phone: 44 20 72698820 **Fax:** 44 20 72698821
Email: info@amrc.org.uk
Website: http://www.amrc.org.uk
Fnded: 1987. **Mem:** 111. **Lang(s):** English. **Desc:** Represents medical research charities. Furthers the advancement of medical research in the United Kingdom. Focuses attention on the collective effectiveness of members. Provides information, advice and guidance to members and others. **Pub:** *Handbook*, annual. Booklet. Lists member charities that award funding for medical research. • Newsletter. Features member information.

★ **1349** ★ **Association of Medical School Pediatric Department Chairs (AMSPDC)**
c/o Jean Bartholomew
111 Silver Cedar Ct.
Chapel Hill, NC 27514-1651
Phone: (919)942-1993 **Fax:** (919)929-9255
Email: jbartholomew@abpeds.org
M. Douglas Jones, MD, Sec. -Treas.
Fnded: 1961. **Mem:** 147. **Desc:** Chairmen of the department of pediatrics of each accredited medical school in the United States and Canada. Fosters education and research in the field of child health and human development. Is cooperating with other national pediatric groups to consider problems of pediatric education, research, and care. **Pub:** *AMSPDC Membership List*, annual.

★ **1350** ★ **Association of Medical Schools in Europe (AMSE)**
University of Vienna
Wahringerstrabe 13
A-1090 Vienna, Austria
Phone: 43 1 4088366 **Fax:** 43 1 40480224
Fnded: 1979. **Lang(s):** English. **Desc:** Deans of medical schools; representatives of medical deans in 25 countries. Provides a forum for the exchange of ideas and information. Objectives are: to address important questions concerning medical education, with special emphasis on policies affecting the future of medical education in Europe; to discuss practical issues such as admission criteria and organizational problems; to analyze the relationship between medical schools and health service organizations; to assess the impact of medical science on medical education. **Pub:** *AMSE Newsletter*, quarterly. Newsletter. **Frmly:** (1992) Association of Medical Deans in Europe.

★ **1351** ★ **Association of Military Surgeons of the U.S. (AMSUS)**
9320 Old Georgetown Rd.
Bethesda, MD 20814
Phone: (301)897-8800 **Free:** 800-761-9320
Fax: (301)530-5446
Email: amsus@amsus.org
Website: http://www.amsus.org
RADM Frederic G. Sanford, MC USN, Ret. Contact
Fnded: 1891. **Mem:** 11,000. **Nat'l Groups:** 1. **Local Groups:** 10. **Desc:** Physicians, dentists, veterinarians, nurses, pharmacists, dietitians, therapists, and others of commissioned rank (or grades E5 through E9) or equivalent in the Army, Navy, Air Force, Public Health Service, and Veterans Administration; Reserve and National Guard officers are also eligible for membership. Advances all phases of federal medicine and allied sciences related to federal health services. Provides group insurance. **Pub:** *AMSUS Newsletter*, quarterly. Newsletter. • *Military Medicine*, monthly.

★ **1352** ★ **Association of Minority Health Professions Schools (AMHPS)**
507 Capitol Court, Ste. 200
Washington, DC 20002
Phone: (202)544-7499 **Fax:** (202)546-7105
Dale P. Dirks, Wash. Rep.
Fnded: 1978. **Mem:** 11. **Desc:** Predominantly black health professions schools. Seeks to: increase the number of minorities in health professions; improve the health of blacks in the U.S.; increase the federal resources available to minority schools and students. Provides information to the U.S. Congress; conducts educational programs. **Pub:** *Study of the Health Status of Minorities in the U.S.*, periodic.

★ **1353** ★ **Association for Molecular Pathology (AMP)**
9650 Rockville Pike
Bethesda, MD 20814-3993
Phone: (301)634-7939 **Fax:** (301)634-7990
Email: amp@asip.org
Website: http://www.ampweb.org/
Mark E. Sobel, MD,PhD, Exec. Off.
Fnded: 1995. **Mem:** 870. **Desc:** Individuals interested in, or engaged in the practice of, molecular pathology. Promotes clinical practice, basic research, and education in the field. Represents members' interests within the health care industry. Develops and maintains liaison with other organizations and agencies concerned with molecular pathology; serves as a forum for the exchange of ideas and information among members. Participates in the development of regulatory and credentialing policies applied to molecular pathology; promulgates guidlines for molecular pathology training programs. Conducts educational programs to increase public awareness of molecular pathology. **Pub:** *AMP Membership Directory*, annual. Directory. • Newsletter, periodic.

★ **1354** ★ **Association of Morphologists**
c/o Prof. J.P. Barbet
Laboratorie d'Histologie-Embryologie
Faculte de medicine
24, rue de Faubaurg St. Jacques
Cochin Port Royal
F-75014 Paris, France
Phone: 33 1 40488233
Email: jp.barbet@pop3.teso.net
Fnded: 1899. **Lang(s):** English, French. **Desc:** Encourages discussion and publication of papers on anatomy, histology, embryology, and odontology.

★ **1355** ★ **Association of Multiple Sclerosis Therapy Centres - Scotland (AMSTCS)**
MS Therapy Centre
1 Burnett Rd.
Inverness IV1 1FT, United Kingdom
Phone: 44 1463 240365
Fnded: 1992. **Mem:** 12. **Lang(s):** English. **Desc:** Multiple sclerosis therapy centers. Seeks to advance the treatment of multiple sclerosis; promotes an improved quality of life for people with multiple sclerosis and their families. Facilitates communication and cooperation among members; conducts research and educational programs; participates in charitable activities; compiles statistics.

★ **1356** ★ **Association of National, European and Mediterranean Societies of Gastroenterology (Association des Societes Nationales, Europeennes et Mediterraneennes de Gastroenterologie — ASNEMGE)**
c/o Andrea Bauer, Sec.
Vereinsmanagement
Lassingleithnerplatz 2/3
A-1020 Vienna, Austria
Phone: 43 1 5333542 **Fax:** 43 1 5351045
Email: info@asnemge.org
Website: http://www.asnemge.org
Fnded: 1947. **Mem:** 37. **Reg. Groups:** 1. **Lang(s):** English, French, German. **Desc:** A branch of the World Organization of Gastroenterology. National societies for gastroenterology in 37 European and Mediterranean countries. Promotes the exchange of scientific information in the field of gastroenterology and co-organizer of yearly United European Gastroenterology week. **Pub:** Proceedings, quadrennial.

★ **1357** ★ **Association Nationale du Diabete de la Republique Democratique du Congo**
16 Ave. Miabi
Quartier Righini - Zone de Lemba
BP 123
Kinshasa XI, Republic of the Congo
Email: cerdadkandjingu@yahoo.fr
Website: http://www.diabetesafrica.com/idfmembers.html
Desc: Represents people with diabetes. Promotes research and support of those with diabetes in Democratic Republic of Congo.

★ **1358** ★ **Association of Native American Medical Students (ANAMS)**
1225 Sovereign Row, Ste. 103
Oklahoma City, OK 73108
Phone: (405)946-7072 **Fax:** (405)946-7651
Email: aaip@aaip.com
Website: http://www.aaip.com/anams
Margaret Knight, Exec. Dir.
Nat'l Groups: 1. **Desc:** Committed to Native American medical students.

★ **1359** ★ **Association for the Neurologically Disabled of Canada (AND) (Association Canadienne pour les Handicapes Neurologiques — ACHN)**
59 Clement Rd.
Etobicoke, ON, Canada M9R 1Y5
Phone: (416)244-1992 **Free:** 800-561-1497
Fax: (416)244-4099
Email: info@and.ca
Website: http://www.and.ca
Fnded: 1983. **Mem:** 150. **Desc:** Individuals with neurological disabilities and their families; health care professionals working with people with neurological disabilities. Seeks to improve the quality of life of people with neurological disabilities and their families; promotes advancement in the treatment of neurological disabilities. Provides support and services to people with neurological disabilities and their families. **Pub:** *AND...Now*, quarterly. Newsletter.

★ 1360 ★ Association des Neurologues Liberaux de Langue Francaise (ANLLF)
39, blvd. du Roi
F-78000 Versailles, France
Phone: 33 1 39532064 **Fax:** 33 1 39519244
Website: http://www.anllf.asso.fr/

Fnded: 1987. **Mem:** 560. **Reg. Groups:** 8. **Local Groups:** 3. **Lang(s):** English, French. **Desc:** French-speaking clinical neurologists working in the private sector. Provides for information exchange and organizes post-university teaching adapted to meet the needs of members. Makes arrangements for follow-up treatment of patients who have relocated. **Pub:** *Journal Faxe de Neurologie*, weekly. Journal. • *Neurologie Liberale*, quarterly. Journal.

★ 1361 ★ Association of Neuromuscular Disorders
Hatboyu cad. No. 12
Yesilkoy
34800 Istanbul, Turkey
Phone: 90 212 5730975 **Fax:** 90 212 6630168
Email: kashasder@turk.net

Fnded: 1978. **Mem:** 1,000. **Reg. Groups:** 5. **Lang(s):** English. **Desc:** Promotes study and research of neurological muscle diseases. Works as a support group for individuals suffering with muscle disorders. Conducts educational programs. **Pub:** *Hope and Life*, quarterly. Journal. Provides information about neuromuscular disorders and activities. • Pamphlets.

★ 1362 ★ Association of Neuroscience Departments and Programs (ANDP)
41218 Roundup Rd.
Magnolia, TX 77354
Phone: (281)259-6737 **Fax:** (281)356-2837
Email: andp@andp.org
Website: http://www.andp.org

Desc: Association of neuroscience departments and programs; works to advance education and research in neuroscience. **Pub:** *Survey Report*. Report.

★ 1363 ★ Association of Neurosurgical Physician Assistants (ANSPA)
PO Box 559
Bernardsville, NJ 07924
Free: 888-94A-NSPA **Fax:** (732)805-9582
Email: TheANSPA@aol.com
Website: http://www.anspa.org
Susan Lusty, Exec. Dir.

Fnded: 1990. **Mem:** 250. **Desc:** Physicians assistants active in the field of neurosurgery; students enrolled in accredited physicians assistant education programs. Promotes professional advancement of members. Represents members before medical organizations; conducts continuing professional development and educational and training programs. **Pub:** *Surgical Physician Assistant*, periodic. Journal. *Price:* $110/year.

★ 1364 ★ Association of Nigerian Physicians in the Americas (ANPA)
6876 Indiana Ave., Ste. F
Riverside, CA 92501-4010
Phone: (909)778-0716 **Fax:** (909)778-0717
Email: dokita@anpa.org
Website: http://www.anpa.org
Alphonsus Obayuwana, Pres.

Fnded: 1995. **Desc:** Physicians and surgeons of Nigerian descent practicing in the United States and Canada. Promotes professional advancement of members; seeks to stimulate interest in matters affecting the health of people of Nigerian descent; encourages adherence to high standards of professional ethics and practice by members. Serves as a clearinghouse on professional opportunities available to physicians of Nigerian descent in North America; conducts charitable, social, educational, and scientific activities. **Pub:** *Directory of Nigerian Physicians in the United States and Canada*, annual. Directory. • *Quarterly News Bulletin*, quarterly. Newsletter.

★ 1365 ★ Association of Nursery Training Colleges
Montessori Centre International
18 Balderton St.
London W1K 6TJ, United Kingdom
Phone: 44 118 9471847 **Fax:** 44 118 9463218
Email: info@chilterncollege.com

Fnded: 1931. **Mem:** 5. **Desc:** Private colleges providing nursery nurse training. Aims to foster co-operation between like minded organizations, to exchange information and promote interest in the training of a nursery nurse.

★ 1366 ★ Association of Nurses in AIDS Care (ANAC)
80 S Summit St.
500 Courtyard Sq.
Akron, OH 44308
Phone: (330)762-5739 **Free:** 800-260-6780
Fax: (330)762-5813
Email: anac@anacnet.org
Website: http://www.anacnet.org/
Adele Webb, Exec. Dir.

Fnded: 1987. **Mem:** 2,800. **Nat'l Groups:** 1. **State Groups:** 52. **Desc:** Nurses and other health care professionals involved in caring for people who are HIV-infected or have AIDS. Functions as a network and provides leadership and educational services for members. Promotes public awareness of AIDS issues; advocates for HIV-infected individuals. Plans to develop a national standard for care of people with AIDS. **Pub:** *ANACdotes*, quarterly. Newsletter. • *Journal of the Association of Nurses in AIDS Care*, bimonthly. Journal. • Also publishes position papers.

★ 1367 ★ Association of Nurses Endorsing Transplantation (ANET)
PO Box 320669
Cocoa Beach, FL 32932-0669
Phone: (321)458-3777 **Fax:** (321)868-2703
Email: stwbear@cfl.rr.com
Website: http://www.anetonline.org
Judi Cavazos, RN, Exec. Dir.

Fnded: 1983. **Mem:** 75. **Desc:** Registered nurses, LVNs, LPNs, student nurses, chaplains, social workers, hospitals, health care facilities and individuals interested in the promotion of organ and tissue donation for transplantation and research. **Pub:** *ANET Newsletter*, quarterly. Newsletter. • *Handbook*, annual. **Frmly:** (1983) Consortium of Registered Nurses for Eye Acquisition.

★ 1368 ★ Association of Obstetrics and Gynecology of the Republic of China
201 Shihpai Rd., Section 2
Taipei, Taiwan
Fax: 886 2 8739512
Fnded: 1961.

★ 1369 ★ Association of Occupational and Environmental Clinics (AOEC)
1010 Vermont Ave. NW, Ste. 513
Washington, DC 20005
Phone: (202)347-4976 **Fax:** (202)347-4950
Email: aoec@aoec.org
Website: http://www.aoec.org
Katherine H. Kirkland, Exec. Dir.

Fnded: 1987. **Mem:** 324. **Desc:** Seeks to enhance the practice of occupational and environmental medicine. Shares information. Provides educational and research programs. **Pub:** *AOEC News*, quarterly. Newsletter.

★ 1370 ★ Association of Occupational Health Professionals in Healthcare (AOHP)
500 Commonwealth Dr.
Warrendale, PA 15086
Free: 800-362-4347 **Fax:** (724)772-8349
Email: info@aohp.org
Website: http://www.aohp.org
MaryAnne Gruden, Exec. Pres.

Mem: 1,000. **Reg. Groups:** 5. **Desc:** Occupational health professionals. **Pub:** *The Journal*, quarterly.

★ 1371 ★ Association of Operating Department Practitioners (AODP)
Lewes Enterprise Centre
112 Malling St.
Lewes BN7 2RJ, United Kingdom
Phone: 44 870 7460984 **Fax:** 44 870 7460985
Email: office@aodp.org
Website: http://www.aodp.org

Fnded: 1945. **Mem:** 7,500. **Desc:** Seeks to maintain quality standards among operating department practitioners. **Pub:** *Technic*, monthly. Journal.

★ 1372 ★ Association of Optometric Educators (AOE)
NSU College of Optometry
1001 N Grand Ave.
Tahlequah, OK 74464-7017
Phone: (918)456-5511 **Fax:** (918)458-2104
Website: http://www.nsuok.edu
Dr. George Foster, Dean

Fnded: 1972. **Mem:** 100. **Desc:** Teachers in schools and colleges of optometry. Works to enhance the professional and academic status and conditions of service of optometric educators and to promote communication among members. Concerned with faculty welfare, faculty-administration relations, faculty-student relations, and faculty-professional relations.

★ 1373 ★ Association of Optometrists
61 Southwark St.
London SE1 0HL, United Kingdom
Phone: 44 20 72619661 **Fax:** 44 20 72610228
Email: postbox@assoc-optometrists.org
Website: http://www.assoc-optometrists.org

Fnded: 1946. **Mem:** 7,000. **Desc:** Optometrists and dispensing opticians and students. Aims to support, promote and protect interests of members individually and corporately; to encourage high standards of practice; to make suitable arrangements for the defence of members in disciplinary and professional matters. Advises on commercial, legal and administrative aspects of practice. **Pub:** *Optometry Today*. Journal.

★ 1374 ★ Association of Organ Procurement Organizations (AOPO)
1364 Beverly Rd., Ste. 100
Mc Lean, VA 22101
Phone: (703)556-4242 **Fax:** (703)556-4852
Email: organdonation@aopo.org
Website: http://www.aopo.org
Paul M. Schwab, Exec. Dir.

Fnded: 1984. **Mem:** 59. **Desc:** Works to represent and serve organ procurement organizations to maximize the availability of organs and tissues and enhance the quality and effectiveness of the donation process. Establishes organizational and ethical standards for OPOs; offers accreditation; provides status reports of federal legislative activities; disseminates information on federal policies and technical advancements; conducts educational programs. **Pub:** *AOPO Update*, monthly. Newsletter. • Membership Directory.

★ 1375 ★ Association of Orthopaedic Foot and Ankle Surgeons (AOFAS)
c/o J. Adam Speer, Exec.Dir.
2517 Eastlake Ave. E, Ste. 200
Seattle, WA 98102
Phone: (206)223-1582
Website: http://www.footdocs.org/factsheet.html
J. Adam Speer, Exec. Dir.

Desc: Promotes the orthopaedic surgeon as premier provider of foot and ankle care. **Pub:** *Foot & Ankle International*. *Price:* included in membership dues.

★ 1376 ★ Association of Osteopathic Directors and Medical Educators (AODME)
142 E Ontario
Chicago, IL 60611
Phone: (312)202-8170 **Fax:** (312)202-8224
David Kushner, CMP, Exec. Dir.

Mem: 250. **Reg. Groups:** 8. **Desc:** Provides leadership for the development, improvement, and evaluation of education and training of osteopathic physicians at all levels in order to further the quality of the osteopathic profession. Offers educational programs. **Pub:** *Osteopathic Progress.* Newsletter.

★ 1377 ★ Association of Osteopathic State Executive Directors (AOSED)
c/o American Osteopathic Association
142 East Ontario St.
Chicago, IL 60611
Phone: (312)202-8000 **Free:** 800-621-1773
Fax: (312)202-8200
Email: info@aaoa-net.org
Website: http://www.aoa-net.org/AffiliatedOrgs/AOSED/aosed.htm
Lynette McClain, Exec. Dir.

Fnded: 1919. **Mem:** 75. **Desc:** Divisional and affiliated societies of the American Osteopathic Association. Objectives are: to promote and improve associations and procedures among members; to examine and develop procedures and policies that will bring about an efficient unit of operation within the divisional societies; to disseminate information on the activities of members and foster and participate in the objects of the AOA. **Pub:** *Association of Osteopathic State Executive Directors.* Newsletter. • *Directory of Osteopathic Publications*, biennial. Directory.

★ 1378 ★ Association of Otolaryngology Administrators (AOA)
c/o Concepts in Meetings and Events
1805 Ardmore Blvd.
Pittsburgh, PA 15221
Phone: (412)243-5156 **Fax:** (412)243-5160
Email: conceptsmtg@ol.com
Website: http://www.oto-online.org
Robert Glazer, Pres.

Fnded: 1983. **Mem:** 730. **Reg. Groups:** 8. **Desc:** Persons employed in a managerial capacity for private or academic group medical practices specializing in otolaryngology (the study of the ear, nose, and throat). Seeks to: promote the concept of professional management in otolaryngology; provide a forum for interaction and exchange of information between otolaryngological managers; present educational programs. Maintains data exchange service for members researching specific topics. **Pub:** *Oto's Scope*, 3/year.

★ 1379 ★ Association of Paediatric Anaesthetists of Great Britain and Ireland (APA)
c/o Dr. G. H. Meakin
University Department of Anaesthesia
Royal Manchester Childrens Hospital
Manchester M30 9HF, United Kingdom
Phone: 44 161 7272291 **Fax:** 44 161 7272291
Email: george.meakin@man.ac.uk
Website: http://www.apagbi.org.uk

Fnded: 1973. **Mem:** 550. **Lang(s):** English. **Desc:** Pediatric anesthetists practicing in Great Britain and Ireland and outside the British Isles. Promotes the study of pediatric anesthesiology. Collects and disseminates information; conducts research; advises other professional bodies on matters pertaining to pediatric anesthesiology. **Pub:** *Paediatric Anaesthesia*, bimonthly. • *Yearbook.*

★ 1380 ★ Association of Pakistani Physicians of North America (APPNA)
6414 S Cass Ave.
Westmont, IL 60559
Phone: (630)968-8585 **Fax:** (630)968-8677
Email: appna@appna.org
Website: http://www.appna.org
Dr. Raana Akbar, MD, Pres.

Fnded: 1976. **Mem:** 1,200. **Desc:** Physicians and dentists who are native to Pakistan but now live and practice in North America. Purposes are: to support medical education and research and advance the interests of medicine and medical organizations; to foster scientific development and education in order to improve the quality of medicine and health care; to facilitate better relations among Pakistani physicians and between them and the people of North America. Assists Pakistani physicians newly arrived in North America in orientation and adjustment. Arranges for donation of medical literature and medical supplies to Pakistan, and for lecture tours, medical conferences, and seminars to be held there. Participates in medical relief and charitable activities in Pakistan and North America; cooperates with other medical organizations in North America. Offers scientific programs for which continuing medical education credits are awarded. **Pub:** Bulletin, monthly. • Newsletter, quarterly. **Frmly:** (2003) Association of Pakistani Physicians.

★ 1381 ★ Association for Palliative Medicine of Great Britain and Ireland
11 Westwood Rd.
Southampton SO17 1DL, United Kingdom
Phone: 44 23 80672888 **Fax:** 44 23 80672888
Email: apmsecretariat@claranet.co.uk
Website: http://www.palliative-medicine.org

Fnded: 1985. **Mem:** 760. **Desc:** Aims to promote the advancement and development of palliative medicine and is recognized as representing physicians at all grades who work in palliative medicine and those with an interest in the specialty.

★ 1382 ★ Association of Pathology Chairs (APC)
c/o Gretchen Bretsch, Admin.
9650 Rockville Pike
Bethesda, MD 20814-3993
Phone: (301)634-7880 **Fax:** (301)634-7990
Email: apc@asip.org
Website: http://www.apcprods.org/
Mary F. Lipscomb, MD, Pres.

Fnded: 1967. **Mem:** 148. **Reg. Groups:** 4. **Desc:** Chairs of medical school departments of pathology. Acts as a communications center for exchange of information and for workshops on innovations for teaching and resident training, department administration, and relationships with governmental and other non-university agencies. Compiles statistics. **Pub:** Newsletter, semiannual. *Price:* available to members only. **Frmly:** (1970) American Association of Chairmen of Medical School Departments of Pathology; (1993) Association of Pathology Chairmen.

★ 1383 ★ Association for Pediatric Education in Europe (APEE)
Pl Amelie-Raba-Leon
F-33076 Bordeaux, France
Phone: 33 5 56795539 **Fax:** 33 5 57820007
Email: Claude.Billeaud@atsneonata.u-bordeaux2.Fr
Website: http://www.atinternet.com/apee/

Fnded: 1970. **Lang(s):** English, French. **Desc:** Fosters research and advances in pediatric education.

★ 1384 ★ Association of Pediatric Oncology Nurses (APON)
4700 W Lake Ave.
Glenview, IL 60025-1485
Phone: (847)375-4724 **Fax:** 877-734-8755
Email: info@apon.org
Website: http://www.apon.org/
CJ Hutto, RNCPON, Pres.

Fnded: 1973. **Mem:** 2,000. **Reg. Groups:** 37. **Desc:** Scientific and educational association seeking to establish lines of communication among nurses caring for children and adolescents with cancer. Encourages updating of literature and development of standards of care for children with cancer. Plans annual conference. **Pub:** *APON Counts*, quarterly. Newsletter. • *Essentials of Pediatric Oncology Nursing: A Core Curriculum*, quarterly. Newsletter. *Price:* $70 for members; $84 for nonmembers. • *Journal of Pediatric Oncology Nursing*, bimonthly. • *Pain Management in Children with Cancer. Price:* $5 for members; $9 for nonmembers. • *Pediatric Tumor Series: Handbooks for Families. Price:* $5 for members; $10 for nonmembers. • *Scope of Practice and Outcome Standard of Practice for Pediatric Oncology Nurses. Price:* $12 for members; $15 for nonmembers. • *When Your Child Has Cancer*, bimonthly. *Price:* $165 for members; $250 for nonmembers. • *Cancer Treatment Fact Sheets. Price:* $20 members; $35 nonmembers.

★ 1385 ★ Association of Pediatric Oncology Social Workers (APOSW)
c/o Nancy Barbach
Schneider Children's Hospital
Pediatric Hemotology Oncology
300 Community Dr.
Manhasset, NY 11030
Phone: (516)562-4634 **Fax:** (516)562-4747
Email: nanbarcsw@aol.com
Website: http://www.aposw.org
Nancy Barbach, Pres.

Fnded: 1977. **Mem:** 200. **Desc:** Social workers involved with pediatric cancer patients in medical settings nationwide. Purposes are to: advance the practice, enhance knowledge, and develop policy and programs of pediatric oncology social work; foster quality and effectiveness of the social work practice of pediatric oncology; promote solidarity among social workers; provide community and professional education; formulate and record local and federal legislation related to pediatric oncology. **Pub:** Brochure. • Newsletter, quarterly.

★ 1386 ★ Association of Pediatric Program Directors (APPD)
6728 McLean Village Dr.
Mc Lean, VA 22101
Phone: (703)556-9222 **Fax:** (703)556-8729
Email: info@appd.org
Website: http://www.appd.org
Laura E. Degnon, Exec. Dir.

Fnded: 1984. **Mem:** 1,024. **Desc:** Directors of accredited pediatric residency programs. Seeks to advance the study, teaching, and practice of pediatrics. Facilitates communication and cooperation among members; supports research in clinical medicine as it relates to resident education.

★ 1387 ★ Association of Pediatric Societies of the Southeast Asian Region (APSSEAR)
c/o Prof. Perla D. Santos Ocampo
Ste. 326, Medical Center of Manila
1122 General Luna St.
PO Box EA 100
Manila, Philippines
Phone: 63 2 5247874 **Fax:** 63 2 7216569
Email: hclue@ha.mc.ntu.edu.tw

Fnded: 1974. **Mem:** 20. **Lang(s):** English. **Desc:** Pediatrics societies in Asian countries and the Pacific region. Works to disseminate information for the benefit of children and child health in the Southeast Asian region and surrounding countries. Encourages research. **Pub:** *Association of Pediatric Societies of the Southeast Asian Region*, quarterly. Bulletin. • *State of Asian Children.* Report.

★ 1388 ★ Association for Pediatric Therapists (APT)
c/o Natalie Ward
2784 Lantz Ave.
San Jose, CA 95124
Phone: (408)377-3345
Email: otdave@ix.netcom.com
Natalie Ward, Contact

Desc: Occupational, physical, and speech therapists, certified assistants, and students. Promotes continuing professional development of members. Functions as a communication network linking members. Cooperates with other organizations representing professionals in related fields. Conducts continuing professional education programs. **Pub:** *Resource Directory*, annual. Directory. • Newsletter, monthly.

★ 1389 ★ Association of PeriOperative Registered Nurses (AORN)

2170 S Parker Rd., Ste. 300
Denver, CO 80231-5711
Phone: (303)755-6300 **Free:** 800-755-2676
Fax: (303)755-4511
Email: clindmar@aorn.org
Website: http://www.aorn.org/
Tom Cooper, Exec. Dir.

Fnded: 1949. **Mem:** 41,000. **Local Groups:** 350. **Desc:** Professional perioperative (operating room) nurses. Provides education, representation, and standards for quality patient care. **Pub:** *AORN Journal*, monthly. Journal. Includes film and book reviews, educational opportunities, employment listings, and legislation. *Price:* Included in membership dues; $80/year for domestic nonmembers; $90/year for foreign nonmembers. • *SSM*, bimonthly. Contains information about trends in management and the surgical environment, changing policies & regulations, clinical practice, and other issues. **Frmly:** (1999) Association of Opertating Room Nurses.

★ 1390 ★ Association of Philippine Physicians in America (APPA)

PO Box 452164
Los Angeles, CA 90045
Fax: (310)889-7131
Email: masmd@aboutappa.org
Website: http://www.aboutappa.org/
Alfonso Nillas, MD, Pres.

Fnded: 1972. **Mem:** 3,000. **Nat'l Groups:** 27. **State Groups:** 27. **Desc:** Individuals from the Philippines who are licensed to practice medicine in the U.S. Seeks to: render free medical care to indigent persons; establish a continuing medical education program for physicians; provide aid for education of physicians; support medical research. Sends medical missions to the Philippines. Provides medical residency program placement service. Maintains speakers' bureau; compiles statistics. **Pub:** *Directory of Physicians*, biennial. Directory. • *Leadership Roster of Officers*, annual. • *Philippine Physician*, periodic. Association and professional newsletter. *Price:* Free. • Also publishes CME abstracts; plans to publish journal of medicine. **Frmly:** (1986) Association of Philippine Practicing Physicians in America.

★ 1391 ★ Association of Physician Assistant Programs (APAP)

950 N Washington St.
Alexandria, VA 22314-1552
Phone: (703)548-5538 **Fax:** (703)684-1924
Website: http://www.apap.org
David P. Asprey, Pres.

Fnded: 1972. **Mem:** 123. **Reg. Groups:** 6. **Desc:** Represents physician assistant (PA) educational programs in the United States. Assists PA educational programs-institutions with training programs for physician assistants to primary care and surgical physicians. Assists in the development and organization of educational curricula for PA programs to assure the public of competent PAs. Contributes to defining the roles of PAs in the field of medicine to maximize their benefit to the public; serves as a public information center on the profession; coordinates program logistics such as admissions and career placements; and is currently initiating a centralized application service for PA applicants. Sponsors the Annual Survey of Physician Assistant Educational Programs in the United States. Conducts and sponsors research projects; compiles statistics; offers ongoing training for PA leadership and faculty. **Pub:** *Annual Report on Physician Assistant Education in the U.S.*, annual. Report. Provides data on physician assistant education, employment, and trends affecting the profession. Includes statistics. *Price:* $50/copy. • *APAP Update*, monthly. Newsletter. For physician assistant program faculty and others concerned with curricula and government/legislative developments affecting the profession. *Price:* Included in membership dues. • *Physician Assistant Programs Directory*, annual. Directory. Describes curriculum, university and institutional affiliations, entrance requirement's, selection factors, credentials awarded, and financial aid. *Price:* $35/copy.

★ 1392 ★ Association of Physician Assistants in Cardiovascular Surgery (APACVS)

PO Box 4834
Englewood, CO 80155
Phone: (303)221-5651 **Free:** 877-221-5651
Fax: (303)771-2550
Email: carol@goddardassociates.com
Website: http://www.apacvs.org
Joseph H. Cooper, Pres.

Fnded: 1981. **Mem:** 600. **Desc:** Physician assistants who work with cardiovascular surgeons. Objective is to assist in defining the role of physician assistants in the field of cardiovascular surgery through educational forums. **Pub:** *CardioVision*, quarterly. Newsletter. • *Salary and Benefits Survey*, annual. Survey. • Membership Directory, annual.

★ 1393 ★ Association for Play Therapy

2050 N Winery Ave., Ste. 101
Fresno, CA 93703
Phone: (559)252-2278 **Fax:** (559)252-2297
Email: info@a4pt.org
Website: http://www.a4pt.org
William M. Burns, Exec. Dir.

Fnded: 1982. **Mem:** 4,400. **Desc:** Promotes play therapy; addresses the professional needs of members. **Pub:** *Association for Play Therapy Newsletter*, quarterly. Newsletter. *Price:* Included in membership dues. • *International Journal of Play Therapy*, semiannual. Journal. *Price:* Included in membership dues.

★ 1394 ★ Association of Police Surgeons

1 Tennant Ave.
College Milton South
East Kilbride
Glasgow G74 5NA, United Kingdom
Phone: 44 1355 244101
Email: aps@glasconf.demon.co.uk
Website: http://www.apsweb.org.uk

Fnded: 1951. **Mem:** 1,050. **Desc:** Members are medical practitioners who regularly assist or advise the police in medical or forensic cases. To promote the best interests of police surgeons; advancement of medico legal knowledge in all its aspects; liaison between appointed police surgeons and other medical practitioners; practical and theoretical study of the subject by lectures, discussions, correspondence and any other means.

★ 1395 ★ Association of Polysomnographic Technologists (APT)

PO Box 14861
Lenexa, KS 66285-1991
Phone: (913)541-1991 **Fax:** (913)599-5340
Email: soneal@goamp.com
Website: http://www.aptweb.org
Sheila O'Neal, Exec. Dir.

Fnded: 1978. **Mem:** 2,600. **Desc:** Individuals who practice polysomnography in research or clinical settings. (Polysomnographic technology deals with the measurement and recording of multiple physiological activity, such as eye movement and heart rate, during sleep.) Seeks to establish standards for polysomnographic technology and provide education and training for people entering in the field. Acts as a forum for communication among members. **Pub:** *A2ZZZ Newsletter*, quarterly. Newsletter.

★ 1396 ★ Association of Port Health Authorities

Dutton House
46 Church St.
Runcorn WA7 1LL, United Kingdom
Phone: 44 8707 444505 **Fax:** 44 1928 581596
Email: apha@cieh.org.uk
Website: http://www.apha.org.uk

Fnded: 1899. **Mem:** 65. **Lang(s):** English. **Desc:** Local authorities, port health authorities in the United Kingdom, Ireland and the Channel Islands. Promoting the health and safety of seafarers, discussing issues on imported food, environmental health, etc. with central government, EU organisations, etc. **Pub:** *Lookout Newsletter*, monthly. Newsletter. • *Port Health Handbook*. Handbook.

★ 1397 ★ Association for Post Natal Illness (APNI)

145 Dawes Rd.
Fulham
London SW6 7EB, United Kingdom
Phone: 44 20 73860868
Email: info@apni.org
Website: http://www.apni.org/

Fnded: 1979. **Desc:** Provides support to mothers suffering from post-natal illness; strives to promote public awareness of post-natal illness; encourages research into post-natal illness. **Pub:** Brochures. Contain information about post-natal illness. • Newsletter.

★ 1398 ★ Association Pour La Lutte Contre Le Psoriasis (APLCP)

Contre Le Psoriasis
1 allee du stade
95610 Eragny, France
Phone: 33 1 34641768 **Fax:** 33 1 30374581
Email: michele.corvest@wanadoo.fr
Website: http://www.aplcp.org

Fnded: 1983. **Mem:** 1,400. **Nat'l Groups:** 1. **Reg. Groups:** 12. **Lang(s):** English. **Desc:** National psoriasis organizations. Acts as advisory, consulting, and coordinating body for member groups implementing medical, social, and psychological research into psoriasis. Seeks to influence related social legislation and to collect all available information on psoriasis. Promotes public awareness of psoriasis and works to remove the social stigma associated with skin conditions. **Pub:** *PSO Magazine*, quarterly. Magazine.

★ 1399 ★ Association of Professional Music Therapists

26 Hamlyn Rd.
Glastonbury BA6 8HT, United Kingdom
Phone: 44 1458 834919 **Fax:** 44 1458 834919
Email: apmtoffice@aol.com
Website: http://www.apmt.org.uk

Fnded: 1976. **Mem:** 500. **Reg. Groups:** 12. **Lang(s):** French. **Desc:** Professional music therapists and music therapy students. To fulfill the needs of qualified music therapists in Great Britain. Focuses on employment and sharing of information. Works to protect music therapists already in work and to assist in the creation of new posts. Sets standards of practice and training. **Pub:** *APMT Newsletter*, quarterly. Newsletter. • *British Journal of Music Therapy*, semiannual. Journal. • *Job List*, monthly.

★ 1400 ★ Association for Professionals in Infection Control and Epidemiology (APIC)

1275 K St. NW, Ste. 1000
Washington, DC 20005
Phone: (202)789-1890 **Fax:** (202)789-1899
Email: apicinfo@apic.org
Website: http://www.apic.org
James Masland, Exec. Dir.

Fnded: 1972. **Mem:** 11,800. **Nat'l Groups:** 1. **State Groups:** 50. **Local Groups:** 112. **Desc:** Physicians, microbiologists, nurses, epidemiologists, medical technicians, sanitarians, and pharmacists. Purpose is to improve patient care by improving the profession of infection control through the development of educational programs and standards. Promotes quality research and standardization of practices and procedures. Develops communications among members, and assesses and influences legislation related to the field. Conducts seminars at local level. **Pub:** *American Journal of Infection Control*, 8/year. Journal. Academic Peer Reviewed Journal. *Price:* $99/year. • *APIC News*, bimonthly. Newsletter. **Frmly:** (1997) Association for Practitioners in Infection Control.

★ 1401 ★ Association Professionelle des Opticiens et Optometristes de Belgique

rue Capitaine Crespel 26
B-1050 Brussels, Belgium
Phone: 32 2 5125526 **Fax:** 32 2 5023402
Email: apob@apob.be
Website: http://www.apoob.be

Fnded: 1923. **Desc:** Promotes the profession of optometry. Provides educational opportunities for optometrists. **Pub:** *Optonagazine*, bimonthly. Magazine.

★ 1402 ★ Association of Professors of Cardiology (APC)

9111 Old Georgetown Rd.
Bethesda, MD 20814-1699
Phone: (301)493-2330 **Fax:** (301)897-9745
Email: sthayer@cardiologyprofessors.org
Website: http://www.cardiologyprofessors.org
Susan C. Thayer, Contact

Fnded: 1990. **Mem:** 115. **Desc:** Directors or acting directors of divisions of cardiology in accredited medical schools in the U.S. and Puerto Rico. Conducts educational and scientific programs with respect to cardiology.

★ 1403 ★ Association of Professors of Gynecology and Obstetrics (APGO)

2130 Priest Bridge Dr., Ste. 7
Crofton, MD 21114
Phone: (410)451-9560 **Fax:** (410)451-9568
Email: djohnson@apgo.org
Website: http://www.apgo.org
Donna Wachter, Exec. Dir.

Fnded: 1962. **Mem:** 1,500. **Desc:** Departments of obstetrics and gynecology in approved medical schools in the U.S. and Canada, and in non-university teaching hospitals with active educational program for undergraduate medical students in OB/GYN. Works to consider problems relating to the departments of obstetrics and gynecology; to advance and improve the study of gynecology and obstetrics; to provide a means of exchanging information relating to the programs of study, teaching methods, and research activities of such departments. Compiles statistics. **Pub:** *Academic Position Report*, 3/year. Report. Job openings in the academic OB/GYN community. *Price:* $5. • *APGO Membership Directory*, annual. Membership Directory. *Price:* $20. • *The APGO Reporter.* Newsletter. • *Medical Student Educational Objectives and Basic Science Prerequisites. Price:* $20 per copy; $17.50 2-49 copies. • *Women's Health Issues. Price:* $30.

★ 1404 ★ Association of Professors of Medicine (APM)

2501 M St. NW, Ste. 550
Washington, DC 20037-1308
Phone: (202)861-7700 **Fax:** (202)861-9731
Email: apm@im.org
Website: http://www.im.org/apm
Tod Ibrahim, Exec. VP

Fnded: 1954. **Mem:** 152. **Desc:** Heads of departments of internal medicine in medical schools. Conducts educational programs; compiles statistics. **Pub:** *APM Update*, quarterly. Newsletter. • *Federal Health Policy Update*, quarterly. • Directory, annual. **Frmly:** Academic Medicine Club.

★ 1405 ★ Association of Program Directors in Endocrinology, Diabetes and Metabolism

8401 Connecticut Ave., Ste. 900
Chevy Chase, MD 20815
Phone: (301)941-0243 **Fax:** (301)941-0259
Email: staff@apdem.org
Website: http://www.apdem.org
Nancy Chill, Association Mgr.

Fnded: 1996. **Mem:** 160. **Desc:** Founded to benefit and aid the education, research and patient care missions of subspecialty training programs in endocrinology, diabetes and metabolism. Supports new initiative in educational and public research and patient care. **Frmly:** (2002) Association of Program Directors in Endocrinology and Metabolism.

★ 1406 ★ Association of Program Directors in Internal Medicine (APDIM)

2501 M St. NW Ste. 550
Washington, DC 20037
Phone: (202)887-9450 **Free:** 800-622-4558
Fax: (202)887-9447
Email: jpearson@im.org
Website: http://apdim.med.edu
Julia Pearson, Membership

Fnded: 1977. **Mem:** 1,400. **Desc:** Physicians in internal medicine including departmental chairmen and directors of internal medicine, directors of residency training programs, associate program directors, medical education directors, and chiefs of medical service. Advances medical education through assisting accredited hospital internal medicine residency training programs in the United States and Puerto Rico. Conducts annual course for chief residents and program directors. Offers consulting services. **Pub:** *APDIM Directory*, annual. Membership Directory. • *Careers in Internal Medicine*, quarterly. • Membership Directory, annual. • Newsletter, quarterly. Profiles successful residency programs and summarizes developments in the field of internal medicine. *Price:* Included in membership dues.

★ 1407 ★ Association of Program Directors in Radiology (APDR)

820 Jorie Blvd.
Oak Brook, IL 60523
Phone: (630)368-3737 **Fax:** (630)571-7837
Email: apdr@rsna.org
Website: http://www.apdr.org
Josette Szalko, Acct. Exec.

Fnded: 1993. **Mem:** 402. **Desc:** Directors, associate directors, assistant directors, and coordinators of medical residency and fellowship programs in radiology. Promotes the "advancement of the art and science of radiology." Facilitates communication and cooperation among members; sponsors research and educational programs.

★ 1408 ★ Association of Program Directors in Surgery

4900B 31st St.
Arlington, VA 22206
Phone: (703)820-7400 **Fax:** (703)931-4520
Email: veldenz@jax.ufl.edu
Website: http://www.apds.org
Thomas F. Fise, Contact

Fnded: 1978. **Mem:** 507. **Desc:** Program directors in surgery. Conducts educational programs and scientific meetings. **Pub:** *Current Surgery*, 9/year. *Price:* $40 for members.

★ 1409 ★ Association for Psychoanalytic Medicine (APM)

4560 Delafield Ave.
Bronx, NY 10471-3905
Phone: (718)548-6088 **Fax:** (718)548-8302
Email: gsagi@aol.com
Website: http://theapm.org
Dr. George Sagi, Treas.

Fnded: 1945. **Mem:** 241. **Desc:** Organization of physicians who are psychoanalysts. Provides forum on psychoanalytic developments for membership and community. Conducts postgraduate seminars. Sponsors speakers for community or medical groups. Is conducting research on psychoanalytic involvement in social issues. **Pub:** *Between Analyst and Patient.* Book. • *The Psychology of Men.* Book. • *Roster*, biennial. • Bulletin, every 9 months. **Frmly:** (1946) Association for Psychoanalytic and Psychosomatic Medicine.

★ 1410 ★ Association for Psychological Type (APT)

4700 W Lake Ave.
Glenview, IL 60025
Phone: (847)375-4717 **Fax:** (847)375-4777
Email: info@aptcentral.org
Website: http://www.aptcentral.org
Daniel Robinson, Pres.

Fnded: 1979. **Mem:** 5,000. **Reg. Groups:** 7. **Local Groups:** 60. **Desc:** Individuals involved in organizational development, religion, management, education, and counseling, and who are interested in psychological type, the Myers-Briggs Type Indicator, and the works of Carl G. Jung (1875-1961). Purpose is to bring together and share ideas related to the uses of MBTI and the application of psychological type theory in any area; promotes research, development, and education in the field. Sponsors seminars conferences and training sessions on the use of psychological type. **Pub:** *Bulletin of Psychological Type*, quarterly. Bulletin. Covers interest area issues, upcoming events, and book reviews. *Price:* Included in membership dues. • *Journal of Psychological Type*, semiannual. Journal. Discusses type theory and research. *Price:* Included in membership dues.

★ 1411 ★ Association of Psychology Postdoctoral and Internship Centers (APPIC)

10 G St., NW Ste. 750
Washington, DC 20002
Phone: (202)589-0600 **Fax:** (202)589-0603
Email: appic@aol.com
Website: http://www.appic.org
Emil Rodolfa, Chm.

Fnded: 1968. **Mem:** 550. **Desc:** Veterans Administration hospitals, medical centers, state hospitals, university counseling centers, and other facilities that provide internship and postdoctoral programs in professional psychology. Promotes activities that assist in the development of professional psychology training programs. Serves as a clearinghouse to provide Ph.D. candidates with internship placement assistance at member facilities. Conducts workshops and seminars on training procedures in clinical psychology at the Ph.D. level. **Pub:** *APPIC Newsletter*, semiannual. Newsletter. *Price:* $10 free for members. • *Internship and Postdoctoral Programs in Professional Psychology*, annual. Directory. **Frmly:** (1991) Association of Psychology Internship Centers.

★ 1412 ★ Association of Public Health Laboratories (APHL)

2025 M St. NW, Ste. 550
Washington, DC 20036-3320
Phone: (202)822-5227 **Fax:** (202)887-5098
Email: info@aphl.org
Website: http://www.aphl.org
Scott J. Becker, Exec. Dir.

Fnded: 1989. **Mem:** 386. **Desc:** Represents national, state and local public health laboratories. Collaborates with partners in private and public sectors, advocating and formulating sound public health and partners in private and public sectors advocating and formulating sound public health and environmental health policies, and providing technical assistance and training. **Pub:** *APHL Washington Bulletin*, monthly. Report. Features legislation update.

★ 1413 ★ Association for Public Health Statistics and Information Systems
801 Roeder Rd., No. 650
Silver Spring, MD 20910
Phone: (301)563-6001 **Fax:** (301)563-6012
Email: hq@napshis.org
Website: http://www.naphsis.org
Alvin Onaka, Pres.

Fnded: 1933. **Mem:** 300. **Desc:** Officials of state and local health agencies responsible for registration, tabulation, and analysis of births, deaths, fetal deaths, marriages, divorces, and other health statistics. **Pub:** Journal, bimonthly. **Frmly:** (1958) American Association of Registration Executives; (1980) American Association for Vital Records and Public Health Statistics; (1997) Association for Vital Records and Health Statistics.

★ 1414 ★ Association of Qualified Curative Hypnotherapists (AQCH)
PO Box 9989
Birmingham B14 4WA, United Kingdom
Phone: 44 121 6931223
Email: info@aqch.org
Website: http://www.aqch.org

Fnded: 1985. **Mem:** 60. **Nat'l Groups:** 1. **Local Groups:** 5. **Desc:** Curative hypnotherapists. Maintains and advances the standards of hypnotherapy. Promotes professional development and training programs. Registered charity. **Pub:** *Hypnotherapy Journal*, semiannual. Journal. Continuing professional development.

★ 1415 ★ Association of Radical Midwives (ARM)
62 Greetby Hill
Ormskirk L39 2DT, United Kingdom
Phone: 44 1695 572776 **Fax:** 44 1695 572776
Email: arm@radmid.demon.co.uk
Website: http://www.radmid.demon.co.uk

Fnded: 1976. **Mem:** 1,700. **Local Groups:** 50. **Lang(s):** English. **Desc:** Midwives, mothers, health professionals, and interested individuals. Supports the interests of midwives. Provides supportive services and information to women experiencing difficulty in securing adequate and sympathetic maternity care. **Pub:** *Choices in Childbirth*. Booklet. • *Midwifery Matters*, quarterly. Magazine. "What is a Midwife?" Leaflet in English, sponsored. No further advertising. Free single distribution, bulk orders for postage costs only.

★ 1416 ★ Association pour la Recherche sur la Sclerose Laterale Amyotrophique (ARS)
75 avenue de la republique
F-75011 Paris, France
Phone: 33 1 43389989 **Fax:** 33 1 43383159
Email: contact@greenwich.fr
Website: http://www.ars.asso.fr

Fnded: 1985. **Mem:** 4,000. **Nat'l Groups:** 1. **Reg. Groups:** 19. **State Groups:** 1. **Local Groups:** 43. **Desc:** Promotes interest in amyotropic lateral sclerosis or ALS (a rare progressive degenerative disease of the motor neurons, characterized by atrophy of the muscles of the hands, forearms, and legs spreading to involve most of the body; also called Lou Gehrig's Disease) research among medical and scientific communities and the public. Faciliates exchange of information with ALS patients, researchers, clinics, and discussion/support groups. **Pub:** Booklets. • Magazine, annual. • Newsletter, quarterly. • Reports.

★ 1417 ★ Association of Recovering Motorcyclists (ARM)
1503 Market St.
La Crosse, WI 54601
Phone: (608)784-8462 **Fax:** (608)784-9085
Email: armintl86@aol.com
Website: http://arm-intl.com
Jerry Scudder, Pres.

Fnded: 1985. **Mem:** 500. **State Groups:** 44. **Desc:** Support group for motorcyclists who are recovering from alcohol or drug addiction. Helps members enjoy the hobby of motorcycling; tries to eliminate the notion of motorcycling as a negative lifestyle. Sponsors motorcycle runs, picnics, and dances. Operates speakers' bureau. **Pub:** *ARM Newsletter*, quarterly. Newsletter. *Price:* Free to inmates; Included in membership dues. • Directory, periodic.

★ 1418 ★ Association of Reflexologists
27 Old Gloucester St.
London WC1N 3XX, United Kingdom
Phone: 44 870 5673320 **Fax:** 44 1989 567676
Email: aor@assocmanagement.co.uk
Website: http://www.aor.org.uk

Fnded: 1984. **Mem:** 6,700. **Reg. Groups:** 43. **Desc:** Promotes reflexology to the public. **Pub:** *Reflexions*, quarterly. Journal.

★ 1419 ★ Association of Regulatory Boards of Optometry (ARBO)
1750 S Brentwood Blvd., Ste. 503
Saint Louis, MO 63144
Phone: (314)785-6000 **Fax:** (314)785-6002
Email: arbo@arbo.org
Website: http://www.arbo.org
Thomas Eichhorst, Exec. Dir.

Fnded: 1919. **Mem:** 56. **Nat'l Groups:** 4. **State Groups:** 50. **Desc:** ARBO's members are North American regulatory boards of optometry; our mission is to represent and assist member licensing agencies in regulating the practice of optometry for the public welfare. **Pub:** *ARBO Greensheet*, 3/year. Newsletter. • *Directory of Boards of Optometry*, annual. Directory. Lists members of state boards with addresses and phone/fax. *Price:* $50/copy. **Frmly:** (1999) International Association of Boards of Examiners in Optometry.

★ 1420 ★ Association for the Rehabilitation of the Brain Injured (ARBI)
3412 Spruce Dr. SW
Calgary, AB, Canada T3C 3A4
Phone: (403)242-7116 **Fax:** (403)242-7478
Email: arbi@cadvision.com
Website: http://www.arbi.ca

Lang(s): English, French. **Desc:** Individuals with brain injuries and their families; health care professionals working with people with brain injuries. Seeks to improve the quality of life of people with brain injuries and their families; promotes advancement in the treatment of brain injuries. Makes available support and services to people with brain injuries and their families.

★ 1421 ★ Association of Rehabilitation Nurses (ARN)
4700 W Lake Ave.
Glenview, IL 60025-1485
Phone: (847)375-4710 **Free:** 800-229-7530
Fax: 877-734-9384
Email: info@rehabnurse.org
Website: http://www.rehabnurse.org
Paul Nathenson, Pres.

Fnded: 1974. **Mem:** 6,000. **Local Groups:** 80. **Desc:** Registered nurses concerned with or actively engaged in the practice of rehabilitation nursing; others interested in rehabilitation. Works to advance the quality of rehabilitation nursing practice through educational opportunities and to facilitate the exchange of ideas. Committees involve members in issues of organizational, local, and national importance and provide an avenue to effect change. Has formed the Rehabilitation Nursing Foundation to promote, develop, and engage in scientific research in the rehabilitation field. **Pub:** *ARN Network*, 6/year. Newsletter. • *Rehabilitation Nursing*, bimonthly. Journal. • Membership Directory, annual.

★ 1422 ★ Association of Rehabilitation Programs in Computer Technology (ARPCT)
503 S York St.
Denver, CO 80209-4640
Phone: (303)733-2111 **Fax:** (303)733-2225
Email: info@arpct.org
Website: http://www.arpct.org
Steven C. Lawrence, Pres.

Fnded: 1978. **Mem:** 70. **Desc:** Rehabilitation training programs; business and community leaders and rehabilitation trainers are associate members. Dedicated to providing data processing as a career path for handicapped persons. Purposes are to: promote communications among the programs designed to train and place handicapped persons in the data processing field; foster and provide assistance for new projects and programs; establish standards and procedures for programs to ensure the maximum benefit for the disabled persons served. Promotes the involvement of the education and research communities. Offers professional training; compiles statistics; sponsors competitions. **Pub:** *Handbook for Implementing New Projects*. • *Viewpoint*, quarterly. Newsletter. • Membership Directory, annual. **Frmly:** (1996) Association of Rehabiliation Programs in Data Processing.

★ 1423 ★ Association for Repetitive Motion Syndromes (ARMS)
PO Box 471973
Aurora, CO 80047-1973
Phone: (303)369-0803
Email: arms@lightspeed.net
Website: http://www.certifiedpst.com/arms
Stephanie S. Barnes, Exec. Dir.

Fnded: 1990. **Nat'l Groups:** 1. **Reg. Groups:** 1. **State Groups:** 1. **Desc:** Individuals suffering from repetitive motion injuries; other interested individuals and organizations. Promotes the welfare of persons at risk of developing repetitive motion injuries. Works to increase public awareness of repetitive motion injuries and prevention and treatment. Develops and implements occupational safety standards and educational programs. Compiles, analyzes, and disseminates data; conducts research programs; and clearinghouse. **Pub:** *ARMS News*, quarterly. Newsletter. *Price:* $20 individual; $75 professional; $150 organization membership.

★ 1424 ★ Association of Reproductive Health Professionals (ARHP)
2401 Pennsylvania Ave. NW, Ste. 350
Washington, DC 20037-1718
Phone: (202)466-3825 **Fax:** (202)466-3826
Email: arhp@arhp.org
Website: http://www.arhp.org
Wayne C. Shields, Pres. /CEO

Fnded: 1963. **Mem:** 2,000. **Desc:** Professionals in reproductive health, including obstetricians, gynecologists, family practitioners, pediatricians, nurse clinicians, researchers, educators, counselors, and administrators. Interested in contraception, sexually transmitted diseases, HIV/AIDS, menopause, urogenital disorders, sexuality, cancer prevention/detection, abortion and infertility. Maintains speakers' bureau; sponsors clinical and public educational programs. **Pub:** *Clinical Proceedings*. Proceedings. • *Health and Sexuality*, quarterly. Newsletter. • Journal, bimonthly. • Journals. • Videos. **Frmly:** (1973) American Association of Parenthood Physicians; (1982) Association of Planned Parenthood Physicians; (1987) Association of Planned Parenthood Professionals.

★ 1425 ★ Association of Reptilian and Amphibian Veterinarians (ARAV)
c/o Wilbur B. Amand
Box 605
Chester Heights, PA 19017
Phone: (610)892-4812 **Fax:** (610)892-4813
Email: aravets@aol.com
Website: http://www.arav.org
Wilbur B. Amand, VMD, Exec. Dir.

Fnded: 1991. **Mem:** 1,250. **Desc:** Veterinarians specializing in the treatment of reptiles and amphibians. Seeks to advance the study and practice of reptilian and amphibian veterinary medicine; promotes ongoing professional development of members. Serves as a clearinghouse on reptilian and amphibian veterinary medicine; sponsors educational programs; facilitates communication and cooperation among members. **Pub:** *Journal of Herpetological Medicine and Surgery*, quarterly. Journal. *Price:* included in membership dues. • *Membership Directory*. Directory. *Price:* included in membership dues.

★ 1426 ★ Association for Research of Childhood Cancer (AROCC)

PO Box 251
Buffalo, NY 14225-0251
Phone: (716)681-4433
Email: odonnell@msn.com
Website: http://www.arocc.org
Ann O'Donnell, Pres.

Fnded: 1971. **Mem:** 1,000. **Reg. Groups:** 2. **Desc:** Parents who have lost children to various pediatric cancers; persons supporting cancer research. Seeks to fund the expansion and continuation of research in pediatric cancer centers and to provide seed money for pilot projects in cancer research. Offers support to parents of children with cancer. Bestows research and clinical investigation grants; offers research and medical student fellowships. **Pub:** *AROCC–Newsletter*, quarterly. Newsletter. Contains book reviews; donations list; memorial list. *Price:* included in membership dues. • *Parent/Child Handbook*.

★ 1427 ★ Association for Research in Nervous and Mental Disease (ARNMD)

c/o Weill Medical College of Cornell University
1300 York Ave., Box 171, Rm. F-1231
New York, NY 10021
Phone: (570)839-0296 **Fax:** (570)839-0297
Email: amgoder@med.cornell.org
Website: http://www.arnmd.org/arnmd/
Annlouise R. Goodermuth, Exec. Dir.

Fnded: 1920. **Mem:** 950. **Desc:** Individuals engaged in the practice or research of neurology, neurosurgery, or psychiatry who are members of neurologic or psychiatric societies. **Pub:** *Proceedings*, annual. **Frmly:** (1922) Neuropsychiatric Research Society.

★ 1428 ★ Association for Research in Otolaryngology (ARO)

c/o Susan Whitehouse
19 Mantua Rd.
Mount Royal, NJ 08061
Phone: (856)423-0041 **Fax:** (856)423-3420
Email: headquarters@aro.org
Website: http://www.aro.org
Darla Dobson, Headquarter Admin. Mgr.

Fnded: 1973. **Mem:** 2,300. **Desc:** Medical professionals, scientists, and researchers with an interest in otolaryngology. Promotes increased understanding of basic science and clinical practice associated with hearing, speech, balance, the senses of taste and smell, and diseases of the head and neck. Conducts educational programs; facilitates exchange of information among members. **Pub:** *Journal of the Association for Research in Otolaryngology (JARO)*, quarterly. Journal. • *Membership Directory*, annual. Directory. Contains membership information.

★ 1429 ★ Association for Research into Restricted Growth (ARRG)

5 Teak Walk
Witham CM8 2SX, United Kingdom
Fnded: 1970.

★ 1430 ★ Association for Research and Training on Integration in Europe (ARTI) (Association de Recherche et Formation pour l'Insertion — ARFI)

38, rue de Fontenay
F-94130 Nogent-sur-Marne, France
Phone: 33 1 48862365 **Fax:** 33 1 48862365
Email: jsarfaty@free.fr
Website: http://www.arfie.org

Fnded: 1987. **Mem:** 15. **Lang(s):** English, French. **Desc:** Promotes and conducts multidisciplinary research on the incorporation of disabled persons into mainstream society and other issues impacting the disabled. Organizes reflection groups. Interacts with related associations elsewhere in Europe. Conducts research and educational programs.

★ 1431 ★ Association for Research in Vascular Surgery (ARVS) (Association de Recherche en Chirurgie Vasculaire — ARCV)

Clinique de Franciscaines
9, impasse Jean-Bouin
F-30000 Nimes, France
Phone: 33 66 766048 **Fax:** 33 66 269812
Email: jeanmariecardon@hotmail.com

Fnded: 1986. **Mem:** 30. **Lang(s):** French. **Desc:** Vascular and cardiac surgeons, vascular radiologists, and anesthesiologists. Conducts research in the field, particularly on the uses of endovascular devices. Members exchange information on technological advancement in the field.

★ 1432 ★ Association for Research in Vision and Ophthalmology (ARVO)

12300 Twinbrook Pkwy., Ste. 250
Rockville, MD 20852-1606
Phone: (240)221-2900 **Fax:** (240)221-0370
Email: arvo@arvo.org
Website: http://www.arvo.org
Joanne G. Angle, Exec. Dir.

Fnded: 1928. **Mem:** 10,500. **Desc:** Professional society of researchers in vision and ophthalmology. To encourage ophthalmic research in the field of blinding eye disease. Operates placement service. Maintains 13 scientific sections. **Pub:** *Investigative Ophthalmology and Visual Science*, monthly. Includes announcements and information for authors. *Price:* Included in membership dues for qualified members. • Also publishes membership brochure; makes available posters. **Frmly:** (1970) Association for Research in Ophthalmology.

★ 1433 ★ Association of Residents in Radiation Oncology (ARRO)

12500 Fair Lakes Circle, Ste. 375
Fairfax, VA 22033
Phone: (703)502-1550 **Free:** 800-962-7876
Fax: (703)502-7852
Email: arro@astro.org
Website: http://www.arro.org/
Nancy Crum, Mgr.

Fnded: 1983. **Mem:** 550. **Desc:** Medical residents in the field of radiation oncology. Seeks to "formalize resident input into professional organizations affecting radiation oncology residents." Serves as a clearinghouse on radiation oncology; fosters communication and cooperation among members.

★ 1434 ★ Association of Rheumatology Health Professionals (ARHP)

1800 Century Pl. Ste. 250
Atlanta, GA 30345
Phone: (404)633-3777 **Fax:** (404)633-1870
Email: acr@rheumtalogy.org
Website: http://www.rheumatology.org/arhp/
Mark Andrejeski, Exec. VP

Fnded: 1965. **Mem:** 1,000. **Nat'l Groups:** 1. **Desc:** Advanced practice nurses, physician assistants, nurses, occupational and physical therapists, social workers, psychologists, vocational counselors, pharmacists, and other health professionals concerned with the practice, education, and research of rheumatic diseases. Seeks to establish a scientific base of knowledge to improve the quality and provision of health services to individuals with rheumatic diseases. Disseminates information regarding the study and treatment of rheumatic diseases. Develops and implements medical and scientific programs in the field of rheumatology. A division of the American College of Rheumatology. **Pub:** *ARHP News*, 4/year. Newsletter. *Price:* Included in membership dues. • *Arthritis Care and Research*, bimonthly. Journal. • *Book for Clinicians*, periodic. Book. Includes research updates. *Price:* Included in membership dues. • *Clinical Care in the Rheumatic Diseases*, periodic. Book. **Frmly:** (1993) Arthritis Health Professions Association.

★ 1435 ★ Association of Schools of Allied Health Professions (ASAHP)

1730 M St. NW, Ste. 500
Washington, DC 20036
Phone: (202)293-4848 **Fax:** (202)293-4852
Email: asahp3@asahp.org
Website: http://www.asahp.org
Thomas W. Elwood, PhD, Exec. Dir.

Fnded: 1967. **Mem:** 750. **Desc:** National allied health professional membership organizations, clinical service programs, academic institutions, and other institutions and organizations whose interests include the advancement of allied health education, research, and service delivery. Aims include: to provide communication among schools and colleges of allied health professions; to promote development of new programs; to encourage research and to provide liaison with other health organizations, professional groups, and educational and governmental institutions. Sponsors short-term institutes for allied health education, administration, and practice. Conducts research programs. programs. **Pub:** *Allied Health Trends*, monthly. Newsletter. *Price:* $55. • *Journal of Allied Health*, quarterly. Journal. *Price:* $75. • Directory, annual. **Frmly:** (1974) Association of Schools of Allied Health Professions; (1992) American Society of Allied Health Professions.

★ 1436 ★ Association of Schools and Colleges of Optometry (ASCO)

6110 Executive Blvd., Ste. 510
Rockville, MD 20852
Phone: (301)231-5944 **Fax:** (301)770-1828
Email: mwall@opted.org
Website: http://www.opted.org
Martin A. Wall, CAE, Exec. Dir.

Fnded: 1941. **Mem:** 23. **Desc:** Committed to achieving excellence in optometric education and to helping its member schools/colleges prepare well-qualified graduates for entrance into the profession of optometry. Mission is to serve the American public through the continued advancement and promotion of all aspects of academic optometry. **Pub:** *Faculty Directory*. Directory. Online directory. • *Faculty Survey Report*, annual. Report. A survey report. • *Optometric Education*, quarterly. Journal. • *Residency Online Directory*. Directory. • *Student Survey Report*, annual. Report.

★ 1437 ★ Association of Schools of Public Health (ASPH)

1101 15th St. NW, Ste. 910
Washington, DC 20005
Phone: (202)296-1099 **Fax:** (202)296-1252
Email: info@asph.org
Website: http://www.asph.org
R. Palmer Beasley, MD, Chair

Fnded: 1941. **Mem:** 28. **Desc:** Accredited graduate schools of public health. Provides focus for the enhancement of academic public health programs. Serves as an information center for governmental and private groups, and individuals whose concerns overlap those of higher education for public health. **Pub:** *Gerontology Programs and Curricula in U.S. Schools of Public Health*. • *Public Health Career Information*. • *Reach*.

★ 1438 ★ Association of Schools of Public Health in the European Region (ASPHER)
(Association des Ecoles de Sante Publique de la Regional Europeenne)
c/o Hospital National de Saint Maurice
14, rue du val d'Onse
F-94415 Saint Maurice Cedex, France
Phone: 33 1 43966459 **Fax:** 33 1 43966463
Email: aspher@aspher.ensp.fr
Website: http://www.ensp.fr/aspher

Fnded: 1966. **Mem:** 57. **Lang(s):** English, French, German, Spanish. **Desc:** Schools of public health and other institutions offering graduate instruction in public health. Promotes the study and development of education in public health and health services. Conducts workshops and seminars. Organizes exchange of students and staff between member schools. **Pub:** Newsletter, monthly. Contains information about the association's activities.

★ 1439 ★ Association of the Scientific Medical Societies of Germany
(Arbeitsgemeinschaft der Wissenschaftlichen Medizinischen Fachgesellschaften — AWMF)
Moorenstr 5
D-40225 Dusseldorf, Germany
Phone: 49 211 312828 **Fax:** 49 211 316819
Email: awmf@awmf.org
Website: http://www.awmf.org

Fnded: 1962. **Mem:** 141. **Desc** Advises on matters and tasks of fundamental and interdisciplinary interest in medicine.

★ 1440 ★ Association Senegalaise de Soutien aux Diabetiques
Immeuble Pasteur-3 eme etage
BP 6151
Dakar-Etoile, Senegal
Phone: 221 8234427 **Fax:** 221 8228187
Email: sndiop@ucad.sn
Website: http://www.diabetesafrica.com/idfmembers.html

Desc: Represents people with diabetes. Promotes research and support of those with diabetes in Senegal.

★ 1441 ★ Association of SIDS and Infant Mortality Programs
c/o MNSID Center, Children's Hospitals and Clinics
2525 Chicago Ave. So.
Minneapolis, MN 55404
Phone: (612)813-6285 **Fax:** (612)813-7344
Email: kathyfountain@adph.state.al.us
Kathleen L. Fernbach, Pres.

Fnded: 1987. **Mem:** 110. **Desc:** Health and human services professionals who provide support services to those affected by Sudden Infant Death Syndrome (SIDS). Represents SIDS information and counseling services at the national, state, and international levels. Acts as an advocate for continued developmental and expansion of SIDS and bereavement services. Organizes activities which promote professional growth, develops practice standards and links together practitioners working with SIDS families. Supports research. **Pub:** *SIDs and Sleeping Position: Counseling Implications*, annual. Newsletter. • *Standards of Service.* **Frmly:** (1998) Association for SIDS Program Professionals.

★ 1442 ★ Association for Spina Bifida and Hydrocephalus (ASBAH)
ASBAH House
42 Park Rd.
Peterborough PE1 2UQ, United Kingdom
Phone: 44 1733 555988 **Fax:** 44 1733 555985
Email: postmaster@asbah.org
Website: http://www.asbah.org

Fnded: 1966. **Nat'l Groups:** 1. **Reg. Groups:** 4. **Desc:** Provides help and information to individuals/families with spina bifida and/or hydrocephalus in England, Wales and Northern Ireland; trained advisers visit families; team of specialist advisers in continence, education, mobility etc. Organises study days for professionals and families. Produces factsheets and magazines. **Pub:** *LINK*, bimonthly.

★ 1443 ★ Association of State Drinking Water Administrators (ASDWA)
1025 Connecticut Ave. NW, Ste. 903
Washington, DC 20036-3902
Phone: (202)293-7655 **Fax:** (202)293-7656
Email: asdwa@erols.com
Website: http://www.asdwa.org
Jay Rutherford, Pres.

Fnded: 1984. **Mem:** 56. **Desc:** Managers of state and territorial drinking water programs; state regulatory personnel. Works to meet communication and coordination needs of state drinking water program managers; facilitates the exchange of information and experience among state drinking water agents. Acts as a collective voice for the protection of public health through assurance of high quality drinking water; oversees the implementation of the Safe Drinking Water Act. Liaises with Congress and the Environmental Protection Agency. Holds training sessions. **Pub:** *ASDWA Update*, bimonthly. Newsletter. For state drinking water administrators, water industry personnel, and all others interested in the latest issues related to drinking water. *Price:* Included in membership dues; $40/year for nonmembers.

★ 1444 ★ Association of State and Provincial Psychology Boards
c/o Randolph P. Reaves
PO Box 241245
7177 Halcyon Summit Dr.
Montgomery, AL 36124
Phone: (334)832-4580 **Free:** 800-448-4069
Fax: (334)269-6379
Email: asappb@asppb.org
Website: http://www.asppb.org
Randolph P. Reaves, J.D., Exec. Off.

Fnded: 1961. **Mem:** 62. **Desc:** State boards of psychology from across the U.S. and Canada. Promotes the development and administration of the national EPPP examination for certification for the practice of psychology. Provides legal counsel to the member boards as well as keeping them abreast of changes in the field of psychology. Provides Certificate of Professional Qualification in Psychology (CPQ) to qualified psychologists for licensure in multiple jurisdictions. **Pub:** *ASPPB*, quarterly. Newsletter. *Price:* $8/year. **Frmly:** American Association of State Psychology Boards.

★ 1445 ★ Association of State and Territorial Dental Directors (ASTDD)
322 Cannondale Rd.
Jefferson City, MO 65109
Phone: (573)636-0453
Email: astdd@socket.net
Website: http://www.astdd.org
M. Dean Perkins, DDS, Exec. Dir.

Mem: 53. **Desc:** Directors of state and territorial dental programs. Provides a forum for consideration of dental health administrative problems and policies on the state and territorial level; promotes constructive plans for better administrative procedures.

★ 1446 ★ Association of State and Territorial Directors of Public Health Education (ASTDHPPHE)
1101 5th St., NW, Ste. 601
Washington, DC 20005
Phone: (202)659-2230 **Fax:** (202)659-2339
Email: director@astdhpphe.org
Website: http://www.astdhpphe.org
Rose Marie Matulionis, Exec. Dir.

Fnded: 1946. **Mem:** 175. **Desc:** Directors of public health education in state and territorial departments of health and Indian health service areas. Seeks to improve the quality of public health education practice; promote information exchange and advocacy. Develops practice guidelines and supports collection and dissemination of data and information relevant to public health education. **Pub:** *Conference Call*, quarterly. Newsletter. • *Roster of Members*, quarterly. • Proceedings, annual. **Frmly:** (1989) Conference of State and Territorial Directors of Public Health Education.

★ 1447 ★ Association of State and Territorial Health Officials (ASTHO)
1275 K St., NW, Ste. 800
Washington, DC 20005-4006
Phone: (202)371-9090 **Fax:** (202)371-9797
Email: ghardy@astho.org
Website: http://www.astho.org
George E. Hardy, Jr., Exec. Dir.

Fnded: 1942. **Mem:** 57. **Desc:** Represents the executive officer of the department of public health of each of the U.S. states, territories and possessions and is engaged in a wide range of legislative, educational, scientific and programmatic issues and activities on behalf of public health. Seeks to"formulate and influence sound national public health policy and to assist state health officials in the development and implementation of programs and policies to promote health and prevent disease, injury and disability." Serves as a primary information resource to state health agencies on a wide range of issues, including HIV/AIDS, immunizations, tobacco-use control, primary care, maternal and child health, school health and the environment. Its sixteen affiliate organizations represent state public health specialty associations for chronic disease programs, dental health, emergency medical services, epidemiology, health facility survey agencies, HIV/AIDS, local health liaisons, maternal and child health programs, nursing services, nutrition services, public health laboratories, public health promotion and education, public health statistics and information systems, social work and vector control services. **Pub:** *ASTHO Annual Report*, annual. Annual Report. *Price:* Free. • *Conference Proceedings*, annual. Proceedings. • *State Public Health Agencies*, biennial. Directory. Lists state health departments. *Price:* $150. • Membership Directory, biennial. • Newsletter, periodic. **Frmly:** (1975) Association of State and Territorial Health Officers.

★ 1448 ★ Association of Stress Consultants
BSY Group
Stanhope Sq.
Holsworthy EX22 6DF, United Kingdom
Phone: 44 1409 259214 **Free:** 800-731-9271
Fax: 44 1409 259215
Email: info@bsygroup.co.uk
Website: http://www.bsygroup.co.uk

Fnded: 1946. **Desc:** Stress consultants.

★ 1449 ★ Association of Stress Therapists
8 Greenriggs
Wigmore
Luton LU29TQ, United Kingdom
Phone: 44 1582 452964
Email: associationofstresstherapists@groups.msn.com
Website: http://uk.msnusers.com/AssociationofStressTherapists

Fnded: 1991. **Mem:** 30. **Local Groups:** 1. **Desc:** Promotes stress therapy as a complementary therapy used to alleviate the physical and mental symptoms caused by stress.

★ 1450 ★ Association for the Study of Dreams (ASD)
PO Box 1592
Merced, CA 95341-1592

Phone: (209)724-0889 **Fax:** (209)724-9319
Email: asdcentraloffice@aol.com
Website: http://www.asdreams.org
Sue Moreno, Contact

Fnded: 1984. **Mem:** 900. **Desc:** Medical professionals, sociologists, counselors, educators, researchers, students, and others whose disciplines are involved in the study of dreams and dreaming. Provides an international interdisciplinary forum for the promotion and public dissemination of information regarding research into the physiological and therapeutic aspects of dreams and their interpretation. **Pub:** *Dream Time*, quarterly. Magazine. Contains research reports, clinical reports, interviews, case studies, and book reviews. *Price:* Included in membership dues. • *Dreaming*, quarterly. Journal. Contains scholarly articles on every aspect of dreams and dreaming. Includes book reviews. • Audiotapes.Contains conference lectures.

★ 1451 ★ Association for the Study of Medical Education (ASME)

12 Queen St.
Edinburgh EH2 1JE, United Kingdom
Phone: 44 131 2259111 **Fax:** 44 131 2259444
Email: info@asme.org.uk

Fnded: 1957. **Mem:** 970. **Lang(s):** English. **Desc:** Individuals engaged in medical education at the undergraduate, postgraduate, and continuing professional development levels. Promotes "knowledge and expertise in medical education." Facilitates information exchange and the establishment of formal networks linking members; serves as a forum for the debate of issues impacting the field of medical education. **Pub:** *ASME Bulletin*, bimonthly. Newsletter. • *Journal of Medical Education*, monthly. Journal.

★ 1452 ★ Association for the Study of Obesity (ASO)

20 Brook Meadow Close
Woodford Green IG8 9NR, United Kingdom
Phone: 44 20 85032042 **Fax:** 44 20 85032042
Email: chris@aso.ndo.co.uk
Website: http://www.aso.org.uk

Fnded: 1967. **Mem:** 420. **Nat'l Groups:** 1. **Lang(s):** English. **Desc:** Scientists, researchers, dieticians, health education workers, and students in England. Promotes information exchange between members; promotes research into the causes, prevention and treatment of obesity; seeks to encourage action to reduce the prevalence of obesity and to enhance treatment.

★ 1453 ★ Association de la Suisse Romande et Italienne Contre les Myopathies (ASRIM)

Chemin de la Traverse 12
PO Box 179
Aubonne, Switzerland
Phone: 41 21 8087411 **Fax:** 41 21 8088111
Email: asrim@planet.ch
Website: http://www.asrim.ch

Fnded: 1977. **Mem:** 850. **Lang(s):** English, German. **Desc:** Individuals in Switzerland affected by neuromuscular disorders. Provides a forum for support and exchange of information. Makes available research funding and other financial support. **Pub:** *Revue Medicale*, quarterly. Newsletter.

★ 1454 ★ Association of Supervisors of Midwives

c/o James Paget Hospital
Corporate Services
Lowestoft Rd.
Gorleston
Great Yarmouth NR31 6LA, United Kingdom
Phone: 44 1493 452269 **Fax:** 44 1493 452078
Email: elayne.guest@jpaget.nhs.uk

Fnded: 1910. **Mem:** 350. **Desc:** Qualified midwives nominated as Supervisors of Midwives. Promotes a high standard of Supervision of Midwives in the practice and teaching of midwifery. Offers support to members and represents the interests of Supervisors of Midwives at national and international levels. **Pub:** *Risk Management in Midwifery Practice.* • Annual Report, annual.

★ 1455 ★ Association for Support of Social and Community Integration (ASSCI)

(Espaco t)
Centro Comercial Capitolio-lojs 5, 22e23
Av. Franca n0 256
P-4050 Porto, Portugal
Phone: 351 22 8302432 **Fax:** 351 22 8305593
Email: espacot@espacot.pt
Website: http://www.espacot.pt

Fnded: 1994. **Mem:** 396. **Lang(s):** English, Portuguese. **Desc:** Individuals and organizations working with people with disabilities. Promotes integration of people with disabilities into mainstream society. Conducts programs in the arts, martial arts, theater, and language to better equip people with disabilities for integration into society. Makes available counseling, support, and services to people with disabilities and to people suffering from addictions, psychological disorders, and health problems. **Pub:** *Contacto*, semiannual. Magazine.

★ 1456 ★ Association of Surgeons of Great Britain and Ireland

c/o The Royal College of Surgeons of England
35-43 Lincoln's Inn Fields
London WC2A 3PN, United Kingdom
Phone: 44 20 79730303 **Fax:** 44 20 74309235
Email: admin@asgbi.org.uk
Website: http://www.asgbi.org.uk

Fnded: 1920. **Mem:** 2,000. **Lang(s):** English. **Desc:** General surgeons. Concerned with the advancement of the science and art of surgery and the promoting of friendship amongst surgeons. The Association is the specialty association for general surgery and is recognized as such by Government as well as by the profession. **Pub:** *British Journal of Surgery*, monthly. Journal.

★ 1457 ★ Association of Surgeons of India

Adams Rd., Chepauk
Madras 600 005, India
Phone: 91 44 2567095

Fnded: 1938.

★ 1458 ★ Association of Surgeons of South Africa

PO Box 52027, Saxonwold
Johannesburg 2132, Republic of South Africa
Phone: 27 11 8371011

Fnded: 1945.

★ 1459 ★ Association for Surgical Education (ASE)

SIU School of Medicine
Department of Surgery
PO Box 19655
Springfield, IL 62794-9655
Phone: (217)545-3835 **Fax:** (217)545-2431
Email: membershipo@surgicaleducation.com
Website: http://www.surgicaleducation.com
Susan Kepner, Exec. Dir.

Fnded: 1980. **Mem:** 850. **Desc:** Surgeons and individuals involved or interested in undergraduate surgical education. Purpose is to develop and disseminate information on motivation, techniques, research, and applications for presenting curricula in undergraduate surgical education. Acts as forum for research in surgical education; serves as information clearinghouse. Compiles statistics; maintains speakers' bureau. Conducts educational programs. **Pub:** *Focus on Surgical Education*, quarterly. Journal. *Price:* Included in membership dues.

★ 1460 ★ Association of Surgical Technologists (AST)

7108-C S Alton Way
Englewood, CO 80112-2106
Phone: (303)694-9130 **Fax:** (303)694-9169
Email: bteutsch@ast.org
Website: http://www.ast.org
William J. Teutsch, Exec. Dir.

Fnded: 1969. **Mem:** 17,700. **Desc:** Individuals who have received specific education and training to deliver surgical patient care in the operating room. Membership categories are available for both certified and student surgical technologists. Emphasis is placed on encouraging members to participate actively in a continuing education program. Aims are: to study, discuss, and exchange knowledge, experience, and ideas in the field of surgical technology; to promote a high standard of surgical technology performance in the community for quality patient care; to stimulate interest in continuing education. Local groups sponsor workshops and institutes. Conducts research. **Pub:** *AST Core Curriculum for Surgical First Assisting.* Book. • *AST Core Curriculum for Surgical Technology.* Book. • *The Surgical Technologist*, monthly. Journal. Covers surgical procedures and equipment, aseptic techniques, medical law, and legislation. Also includes association news, and annual subject index. *Price:* Included in membership dues; $36/year for nonmembers. • *Surgical Technologist Certifying Exam Study Guide.* Book. **Frmly:** (1978) Association of Operating Room Technicians.

★ 1461 ★ Association of Systematic Kinesiology (ASK)

19 Westfield Ln.
Saint Leonards-on-Sea TN37 7NE, United Kingdom
Phone: 44 1424 753375
Email: marie.cheshire@hotmail.com
Website: http://www.kinesiology-uk.com

Fnded: 1988. **Mem:** 250. **Pub:** Newsletter, quarterly.

★ 1462 ★ Association of Teachers of Lipreading to Adults

PO Box 506
Hanley
Stoke-On-Trent ST2 9RE, United Kingdom
Fax: 44 870 7062916
Email: atla@lipreading.org.uk
Website: http://www.lipreading.org.uk

Fnded: 1975. **Mem:** 340. **Desc:** To promote understanding of the needs of people with an acquired hearing loss. To advance the awareness of the benefits of lipreading and other communication skills in the rehabilitation of people with an acquired hearing loss. **Pub:** *Catchword*, semiannual. Magazine.

★ 1463 ★ Association of Teachers of Preventive Medicine (ATPM)

1660 L St. NW, Ste. 208
Washington, DC 20036
Phone: (202)463-0550 **Free:** (866)474-ATPM
Fax: (202)463-0555
Email: info@atpm.org
Website: http://www.atpm.org
Barbara J. Calkins, MA, Exec. Dir.

Fnded: 1942. **Mem:** 900. **Desc:** Dedicated to advancing individual and community health promotion and disease prevention in the education of physicians and other health professionals. Individual members are teachers, researchers, practitioners, administrators, residents and students. Institutional members include preventive medicine and related departments in medical schools, schools and graduate programs in public health and preventive medicine, other health professions schools and various health agencies. **Pub:** *American Journal of Preventive Medicine*, bimonthly. Journal. • *ATPM News Now!*, weekly. Newsletter. An electronic newsletter. • *ATPM Quarterly*, quarterly. Newsletter. • *Directory and Profile of Academic Units in Preventive Medicine*, periodic. Directory. **Frmly:** (1955) Conference of Professors of Preventive Medicine.

★ 1464 ★ Association for Teaching Psychology
c/o British Psychological Society
48 Princess Rd., E
Leicester LE1 7DR, United Kingdom
Phone: 44 116 2549568
Website: http://www.theatp.org

Mem: 1,000. **Desc:** Teachers of psychology in Secondary Schools, Further Education Colleges and Colleges of Higher Education. Supports teachers of psychology at pre-degree level. Provides help and advice. Organizes an annual updating conference for members and distributes resources produced by teachers for teachers. **Pub:** *Psychology Teaching Journal*, annual. Journal.

★ 1465 ★ Association of Technical Personnel in Ophthalmology (ATPO)
2025 Woodlane Dr.
Saint Paul, MN 55125
Phone: (651)731-7239 **Fax:** (651)731-0410
Email: atpomembership@jcahpo.org
Website: http://www.atpo.org
Jennifer Anderson Warwick, Mgr.

Fnded: 1969. **Mem:** 1,200. **Nat'l Groups:** 1. **State Groups:** 4. **Desc:** Ophthalmic assistants, technicians, technologists, surgical and keratorefractive techs, photographers, nurses, and orthoptists. Promotes high standards and professional ethics dedicated to quality ophthalmic medical care under the direction of an ophthalmologist. Recognizes the utilization of ophthalmalic medical personnel to perform certain non-medical procedures or tests as a means of enhancing the productivity of ophthalmologists and thereby increasing the availability of ophthalmologists to provide the highest level of medical service and comprehensive vision care to their patients. **Pub:** *Viewpoints*, quarterly. Newsletter. *Price:* Free for members. **Frmly:** (1989) American Association of Certified Allied Health Personnel in Ophthalmology.

★ 1466 ★ Association of Telemedicine Service Providers (ATSP)
4702 SW Scholls Ferry Rd., No. 400
Portland, OR 97225-2008
Phone: (503)222-2406 **Fax:** (503)223-7581
Email: info@atsp.org
Website: http://www.atsp.org

Desc: Companies providing telemedical services. Seeks to advance the practice of telemedicine and to stimulate the development of more effective telemedical technologies. Provides educational, business leadership, and marketing services to members; facilitates networking among members; makes available discounts on products and services to members; represents members before government agencies, industry organizations, and the public. **Pub:** *ATSP Annual Survey*, annual. Report.

★ 1467 ★ Association of Therapeutic Communities (ATC)
Bams Centre
Church Ln.
Toddington
Glos
Cheltenham GL54 5DQ, United Kingdom
Phone: 44 1242 620077 **Fax:** 44 1242 620077
Email: post@therapeuticcommunities.org
Website: http://www.therapeuticcommunities.org

Fnded: 1972. **Mem:** 200. **Desc:** Nurses, social workers, researchers, psychologists, creative therapists, managers, residential care staff, teachers, psychotherapists, psychiatrists, and academics. Conducts training and education programs. **Pub:** *Therapeutic Communities Journal*, quarterly. Journal.

★ 1468 ★ Association for Therapeutic Philosophy (ATP)
33 Marlborough Rd.
Swindon SN3 1PH, United Kingdom
Phone: 44 1793 538586 **Fax:** 44 1793 538586
Email: psycountrg@aol.com
Website: http://members.aol.com/psycountrg

Fnded: 1983. **Mem:** 450. **Desc:** Seeks to develop therapeutic philosophy concepts and treatment type. **Frmly:** (2001) Association of Psychological Counselling and Training.

★ 1469 ★ Association Togolaise du Diabete
PO Box 3278
Lome, Togo
Phone: 228 274304 **Fax:** 228 213675
Email: atdiabete@yahoo.fr
Website: http://www.diabetesafrica.com/idfmembers.html

Desc: Represents people with diabetes. Promotes research and support of those with diabetes in Togo.

★ 1470 ★ Association Tunisienne du Planning Familial (ATPF)
9, rue Essoyouti
El Menzah
TN-1004 Tunis, Tunisia
Phone: 216 1 232419 **Fax:** 216 1 767263
Email: atpf@planet.tn

Fnded: 1968. **Mem:** 1,200. **Nat'l Groups:** 23. **Reg. Groups:** 450. **State Groups:** 104. **Local Groups:** 1500. **Lang(s):** Arabic, French. **Desc:** Advocates family planning as a basic human right. Works to reduce the number of unwanted pregnancies and abortions. Attempts to stop the spread of AIDS and other sexually transmitted diseases. Offers programs in sex education, family planning, and health. Provides contraceptive and health care services. Acts as an advocate for family planning on the national level. **Pub:** *Bulletin de l'Association*, quarterly. Newsletter.

★ 1471 ★ Association of University Anesthesiologists (AUA)
520 N Northwest Hwy.
Park Ridge, IL 60068-2573
Phone: (847)825-5586 **Fax:** (847)825-5658
Email: aua@asahq.org
Website: http://www.auahq.org
Steven J. Baker, PhD, Sec.

Fnded: 1953. **Mem:** 700. **Desc:** Academic anesthesiologists from medical school faculties. Encourages members to pursue original investigations in the clinic and the laboratory; develops methods of teaching anesthesiology. **Pub:** Directory, annual. **Frmly:** (1990) Association of University Anesthetists.

★ 1472 ★ Association of University Professors of Ophthalmology (AUPO)
PO Box 420369
San Francisco, CA 94142-0369
Phone: (415)561-8548 **Fax:** (415)561-8531
Email: aupo@aao.org
Steve M. Podos, MD, Exec. VP

Fnded: 1966. **Mem:** 246. **Desc:** Heads of departments or divisions of ophthalmology in accredited medical schools throughout the U.S. and Canada; directors of ophthalmology residency programs in institutions not connected to medical schools. Promotes medical education, research, and patient care relating to ophthalmology. Operates Ophthalmology Matching Program and faculty placement service, which aids ophthalmologists interested in being associated with university ophthalmology programs to locate such programs. **Pub:** *News & Views*, quarterly. • Membership Directory, annual.

★ 1473 ★ Association of University Programs in Health Administration (AUPHA)
730 11th St. NW, Fl. 4
Washington, DC 20001-4510
Phone: (202)638-1448 **Fax:** (202)638-3429
Email: aupha@aupha.org
Website: http://www.aupha.org
Jeptha W. Dalston, Ph.D., FACHE, Pres. /CEO

Fnded: 1948. **Mem:** 1,200. **Desc:** Universities offering graduate and undergraduate study in health services and hospital administration. To improve the quality of education in health services administration. Undertakes research and educational programs, such as studies of the criteria used for selection of students and curriculum patterns adopted by various universities. Conducts faculty institutes on topics relating to health administration. Compiles statistics. **Pub:** *AUPHA Exchange*, bimonthly. Newsletter. • *Health Services Administration Education*, biennial. Directory. • *Journal of Health Administration Education*, quarterly. Journal. **Frmly:** (1973) Association of University Programs in Hospital Administration.

★ 1474 ★ Association of University Radiologists (AUR)
820 Jorie Blvd.
Oak Brook, IL 60523
Phone: (630)368-3730 **Fax:** (630)571-7837
Email: aur@rsna.org
Website: http://www.aur.org/
Josette Szalko, Exec.

Fnded: 1953. **Mem:** 4,000. **Desc:** Physician and non-physician scientists who have been appointed to a university faculty. Seeks to: encourage excellence in laboratory and clinical investigation, teaching, and clinical practice; stimulate interest in academic radiology as a medical career; advance radiology as a medical science; provide a forum for university based radiologists to present and discuss results of research, teaching, and administrative issues. **Pub:** *Academic Radiology*, monthly. Journal. • Also publishes award and scientific papers.

★ 1475 ★ Association of Vascular and Interventional Radiographers
820 Jorie Blvd.
Oak Brook, IL 60523
Phone: (630)571-2266 **Fax:** (630)571-7837
Email: avir@rsna.org
Website: http://www.avir.org
Betty Rohr, Exec. Sec.

Fnded: 1988. **Mem:** 1,100. **Desc:** Cardiovascular and interventional radiographers and allied health care professionals. **Pub:** *AVIR Interventional Informer*, quarterly. Newsletter. *Price:* included in membership dues; $35 for nonmembers.

★ 1476 ★ Association of Veterinary Anaesthetists
Animal Health Trust
Landvades Park
Kentford
Newmarket CB8 7UU, United Kingdom
Phone: 44 1638 555651
Email: dave.brodbelt@aht.org.uk
Website: http://www.ava.eu.com/

Fnded: 1964. **Mem:** 400. **Desc:** Veterinary surgeons; medics, anaesthetists, those with medical university qualifications and scientists, Animal technicians and veterinary nurses. Furthers teaching and research in veterinary anaesthetics. **Pub:** *Journal of Veterinary Anaesthesia and Analgesia*, quarterly. Journal. **Frmly:** Association of Veterinary Anaesthetists of Great Britian and Ireland.

★ 1477 ★ Association for Veterinary Clinical Pharmacology and Therapeutics
Pfizer Central Research
Sandwich CT13 9NJ, United Kingdom
Phone: 44 1304 646160 **Fax:** 44 1304 651251
Email: avcpt@avcpt.org
Website: http://www.avcpt.org

★ 1478 ★ Association of Veterinary Teachers and Research Workers
Department of Veterinary Pathology
Glasgow University Veterinary School

Bearsden Rd.
Glasgow G61 1QH, United Kingdom
Phone: 44 141 3305783 **Fax:** 44 141 3305602
Email: a.williams@vet.gla.ac.uk
Website: http://www.avtrw.org

Fnded: 1946. **Mem:** 800. **Reg. Groups:** 4. **Lang(s):** English. **Desc:** Individuals engaged primarily in veterinary teaching and research in UK and Eire. To further contact between research workers and teachers in animal research; promote and influence veterinary education; provide for and maintain the technical excellence of veterinary teaching and research. **Pub:** *AVT and RW Annual Conference*, annual. Proceedings. • Proceedings.

★ 1479 ★ Association of Visually Impaired Chartered Physiotherapists
c/o Guildford Physiotherapy and Sports Clinic
Matthews House
85 Epsom Rd.
Guildford GU1 3PA, United Kingdom
Phone: 44 1483 575876 **Fax:** 44 1483 302691

Fnded: 1919. **Mem:** 125. **Desc:** Visually impaired chartered physiotherapists. To supply support and encouragement and benefits to its members. **Pub:** *Physiotherapist*, monthly. Audiotapes.

★ 1480 ★ Association for Women in Psychology (AWP)
c/o Cassandra Nichols, AWP Treas.
PO Box 641065
Pullman, WA 99164-1065
Email: support@awpsych.org
Website: http://www.awpsych.org
Dr. Susan Rose, Contact

Fnded: 1969. **Mem:** 2,400. **Desc:** Seeks to: end the role that the association feels psychology has had in perpetuating unscientific and unquestioned assumptions about the "natures" of women and men; encourage unbiased psychological research on sex and gender in order to establish facts and expose myths; encourage research and theory directed toward alternative sex-role socialization, child rearing practices, life-styles, and language use; educate and sensitize the science and psychology professions as well as the public to the psychological, social, political, and economic rights of women; combat the oppression of women of color; encourage research on issues of concern to women of color; achieve equality of opportunity for women and men within the profession and science of psychology. Conducts business and professional sessions at meetings of regional psychology associations. Maintains Hall of Fame and speakers' bureau. Monitors sexism in the American Psychological Association. **Pub:** *AWP Membership Directory*, annual. Membership Directory. *Price:* Free with membership. • *AWP Newsletter*, quarterly. Newsletter. **Frmly:** (1970) Association for Women Psychologists.

★ 1481 ★ Association of Women Surgeons (AWS)
414 Plaza Dr., Ste. 209
Westmont, IL 60559
Phone: (630)655-0392 **Fax:** (630)655-0391
Email: info@womensurgeons.org
Website: http://www.womensurgeons.org
Judith Keel, Exec. VP

Fnded: 1981. **Mem:** 1,600. **Desc:** Women surgeons, interns, and residents; retired women surgeons; women in medical school interested in a career in surgery; interested individuals. Promotes the professional and personal goals of women surgeons and women involved and interested in the medical profession. Encourages interaction between women surgeons internationally. Serves as a network for the exchange of ideas and information. **Pub:** *AWS Connections*, quarterly. Newsletter. Includes notice of meetings, lists employment opportunities, profiles of outstanding women surgeons. • *Pocket Mentor*. Handbook. Features information for residents and interns. • *Resource Manual*, biennial. Membership Directory. Serves as a networking device among members.

★ 1482 ★ Association for Women Veterinarians (AWV)
c/o Magnolia Association Management Affiliates
310 North Indian Hill Blvd., Box 337
Claremont, CA 91711-4611
Email: lapancho@ra.msstate.edu
Website: http://www.awv-women-veterinarians.org
Dr. Marilyn Waldhalm, Exec. Sec.

Fnded: 1947. **Mem:** 400. **Desc:** Works to support veterinary medicine by providing leadership in women's issues. **Pub:** *AWV Bulletin*, quarterly. Bulletin. *Price:* Included in membership dues; $10/year for nonmembers. • *Roster of Women Veterinarians*, periodic. **Frmly:** (1981) Women's Veterinary Medical Association.

★ 1483 ★ Association of Women's Health, Obstetric and Neonatal Nurses (AWHONN)
2000 L St. Nw, Ste. 740
Washington, DC 20036
Phone: (202)261-2400 **Free:** 800-673-8499
Fax: (202)728-0575
Email: gailk@awhonn.org
Website: http://www.awhonn.org
Gail Kincaide, Exec. Dir.

Fnded: 1969. **Mem:** 22,000. **Reg. Groups:** 10. **State Groups:** 62. **Desc:** Members are registered nurses; associate members are allied health workers with an interest in obstetric, women's health, and neonatal (OGN) nursing. Promotes and establishes the highest standards of OGN nursing practice, education, and research; cooperates with all members of the health team; stimulates interest in OGN nursing. Sponsors educational meetings, audiovisual programs, and continuing education courses. **Pub:** *AWHONN Lifelines*, bimonthly. Magazine. Includes annual index, calendar of events, employment opportunity listings, and legislative news. *Price:* $26/yr. for individuals. • *Journal of Obstetric, Gynecologic, and Neonatal Nursing*, bimonthly. Journal. Includes advertisers' index and annual subject and author index. Contains book reviews, case studies, and employment opportunity listings. *Price:* $50/year for individuals; $170/year for institutions. • Also publishes manual of standards and OGN nursing practice resources. **Frmly:** Nurses Association of the American College of Obstetricians and Gynecologists; (1993) NAACOG: The Organization of Obstetric, Gynecologic, and Neonatal Nurses.

★ 1484 ★ Association of Workers for Children with Emotional and Behavioural Difficulties
Charlton Ct.
East Sutton
Maidstone ME17 3DQ, United Kingdom
Phone: 44 1622 843104 **Fax:** 44 1622 844220
Email: awcebd@mistral.co.uk
Website: http://www.awcebd.co.uk

Fnded: 1953. **Mem:** 1,000. **Reg. Groups:** 6. **Desc:** All professions involved in work with children and young people with emotional and behavioural difficulties and those who are involved in training. Promotes meeting the needs of children and young people with emotional and/or behavioural difficulties, in a variety of settings including education. **Pub:** *Emotional and Behavioral Difficulties*, 3/year. Journal. Multidisciplinary practitioners journal. • Newsletter, semiannual.

★ 1485 ★ Association of Zoo Veterinary Technicians
White Oak Conservation Center
3823 Owens Rd.
Yulee, FL 32097
Phone: (336)879-7636 **Fax:** (336)879-7637
Email: cheryl_purnell@ncmail.net
Website: http://www.AZVT.org
Cheryl Purnell, Exec. Dir.

Fnded: 1981. **Mem:** 350. **Nat'l Groups:** 1. **Desc:** Zoo veterinary technicians. **Pub:** *AZVT News*, quarterly. Newsletter. *Price:* included in membership dues.

★ 1486 ★ Associazione Italian Sclerosi Laterale Amiotrofica (AISLA)
Via Roma 32
I-28100 Novara, NO, Italy
Phone: 39 0321 499727 **Fax:** 39 0321 499719
Email: segreteria@aisla.it
Website: http://www.aisla.it

Fnded: 1983. **Reg. Groups:** 11. **Desc:** Individuals in Italy affected by Amyotrophic Lateral Sclerosis (ALS), a muscle wasting condition. Provides a forum for support and exchange of information. Funds research. **Pub:** *Notiziario AILSA*, quarterly. Bulletin.

★ 1487 ★ Associazione Italiana di Anestesia Odonto-Stomatologica (AINOS)
Colonia Servizi Italia
Via Altinate, 125
I-35121 Padua, Italy
Phone: 39 049 3766097 **Fax:** 39 049 8776917
Email: colonna.servizi@tim.it

Fnded: 1972. **Mem:** 60. **State Groups:** 1. **Lang(s):** Italian. **Desc:** Physicians concerned with dental anesthesiology. Sponsors educational and research programs. **Pub:** *Giornale di Anestesia Stomatologica*, semiannual. Magazine.

★ 1488 ★ Associazione Italiana Biblioteche (AIB)
c/o Biblioteca nazionale centrale
viale Castro Pretorio 105
I-00185 Rome, Italy
Phone: 39 06 4463532 **Fax:** 39 06 4441139
Email: aib@aib.it
Website: http://www.aib.it

Desc: Represents and supports librarians in Italy.

★ 1489 ★ Associazione Italiana Sclerosi Multipla (AISM)
c/o Dr. Mario Alberto Battaglia
Vico Chiuso Paggi 3
I-16128 Genoa, Italy
Phone: 39 010 27131 **Fax:** 39 010 2470226
Email: aism@aism.it
Website: http://www.aism.it

Fnded: 1968. **Reg. Groups:** 86. **Desc:** MS patients, families and professionals. Seeks to improve the quality of life for persons with multiple sclerosis and their families.

★ 1490 ★ Associazione la Nostra Famiglia (LNF)
Via don Luigi Monza 1
I-22037 Ponte Lambro, Italy
Phone: 39 031 625111 **Fax:** 39 031 625243
Email: info@pl.lnf.it
Website: http://www.lanostrafamiglia.it/

Fnded: 1947. **Mem:** 150. **Lang(s):** English, Italian. **Desc:** Association, based on evangelical principles, devoted to the social and physical rehabilitation of disabled children and young adults. Particular emphasis is placed on individuals with physical neuromotor and sensorial dysfunctions. Maintains more than 30 rehabilitation centers throughout Italy; also operates work centers and family homes providing social and educational training. Manages developing cooperation projects in Sudan, Brazil, and Ecuador and collaborates with projects in China and Palestina. Offers training and continuing education courses to specialists in the field. Sponsors seminars; maintains the Eugenio Medea Scientific Institute for hospitalization and treatment. Conducts research; compiles statistics. Maintains a clinic. **Pub:** *Notiziario d'Informazione*, quarterly. Newsletter. • *SAGGI-Child Development and Disabilities*, bimonthly. Journal. Scientific magazine.

★ 1491 ★ Asthma and Allergy Foundation of America (AAFA)
1233 Twentieth St. NW, Ste. 402
Washington, DC 20036
Phone: (202)466-7643 **Free:** 800-7-ASTHMA
Fax: (202)466-8940
Email: info@aafa.org
Website: http://www.aafa.org
William McLin, Exec. Dir.

Fnded: 1953. **Reg. Groups:** 12. **Desc:** Dedicated to finding a cure for and controlling asthma and allergic diseases. AAFA serves the estimated 50 million Americans with asthma and allergic diseases through the support of research, patient and public education programs, public and governmental advocacy, and a nationwide network of chapters and education/support groups. **Pub:** *ADVANCE*, bimonthly. Newsletter. • Also publishes educational pamphlets. **Frmly:** (1957) American Foundation for Allergic Diseases; (1978) Allergy Foundation of America.

★ 1492 ★ Asthma Society of Canada
130 Bridgeland Ave., Ste. 425
Toronto, ON, Canada M6A 1Z4
Phone: (416)787-4050 **Free:** 800-787-3880
Fax: (416)787-5807
Email: info@asthma.ca
Website: http://www.asthmasociety.com

Fnded: 1974. **Desc:** Dedicated to the treatment and prevention of asthma. Conducts educational and research programs; provides counseling. **Pub:** *Helping People Breathe Easier*, quarterly. Newsletter. • *Living Well with Asthma.*

★ 1493 ★ Asthma Society of Ireland (ASI)
Eden House
15-17 Eden Quay
Dublin 1, Ireland
Phone: 353 1 8788511 **Fax:** 353 1 8788128
Email: asthma@indigo.ie
Website: http://www.asthmasociety.ie

Fnded: 1973. **Mem:** 5,000. **Nat'l Groups:** 1. **Reg. Groups:** 5. **State Groups:** 1. **Local Groups:** 5. **Lang(s):** English, Irish. **Desc:** Individuals with asthma; health care personnel and other individuals providing support and services to people with asthma. Seeks to improve the quality of life of people with asthma. Serves as a clearinghouse on asthma and its treatment; supports health professionals treating people with asthma. **Pub:** *Asthma Society News*, 3/year. Magazine. Contains 64 full colour pages highlighting asthma issues.

★ 1494 ★ Ataxia Telangiectasia Children's Project
668 S Military Tr.
Deerfield Beach, FL 33442
Email: info@atcp.org
Website: http://www.atcp.org/mission_of_the_a.htm

Fnded: 1993. **Desc:** Supports laboratory research to accelerate the discovery of a cure or possible therapies for Ataxia Telangiectasia; develops and maintains international registry of A-T patients; supports and oversees clinical center and information clearinghouse; maintains a tissue/cell bank; develops quantitative endpoints for measuring the rate and severity of the symptoms of A-T.

★ 1495 ★ Ataxia-Telangiectasia Society
IACR - Rothamsted
Harpenden AL5 2JQ, United Kingdom
Phone: 44 582 760733 **Fax:** 44 582 760162
Email: atcharity@aol.com
Website: http://www.atsociety.org.uk

Fnded: 1989. **Mem:** 110. **Desc:** Seeks to alleviate the suffering caused by Ataxia-Telangiectasia by supporting families, raising awareness of the disease and funding research. Conducts fund-raising activities. **Pub:** *A-T Society News*, semiannual. Newsletter.

★ 1496 ★ Ataxia - UK
10 Winchester House
Kennington Park
Cranmer Rd.
London SW9 6EJ, United Kingdom
Phone: 44 207 5821444 **Fax:** 44 207 5829444
Email: office@ataxia.org.uk
Website: http://www.ataxia.org.uk

Fnded: 1965. **Mem:** 2,700. **Reg. Groups:** 8. **Lang(s):** English. **Desc:** Fundraising organization supporting research into Friedreich's, Cerebellar, and other ataxias (hereditary spinal diseases which cause the loss of muscular coordination). Offers support services for ataxia sufferers and their families. **Pub:** *Ataxian*, quarterly. Magazine. • Brochures, periodic. • Newsletter, quarterly.

★ 1497 ★ Athletics and Entertainers for Kids
3337 Colorado St.
Long Beach, CA 90814
Phone: (562)438-5905 **Free:** 800-933-KIDS
Fax: (562)438-9175
Elise Kim, Exec. Dir.

Fnded: 1986. **State Groups:** 5. **Desc:** Participants include individuals and corporations concerned about children with catastrophic illnesses, particularly AIDS. Seeks to bring hope to seriously ill children. Provides services to children and their families including: counseling and referral services; community outings; educational rallies. Provides AIDS education and awareness programs and presentations. Conducts hospital and charitable programs; provides placement and children's services. Sponsored by Athletes and Entertainers for Kids. **Pub:** *Financial Report*, annual. Report. • *Heros*, quarterly. Newsletter. **Frmly:** (1998) Ryan White National Teen Education Program.

★ 1498 ★ Attention Deficit Information Network (AD-IN)
58 Prince St.
Needham, MA 02492
Phone: (781)455-9895
Email: adin@gis.net
Website: http://www.addinfonetwork.com
Libby Ostrofsky, Contact

Fnded: 1988. **Reg. Groups:** 41. **State Groups:** 20. **Desc:** People with Attention Deficit Disorders (ADD), their families, and other individuals with an interest in ADD. Promotes improved quality of life for people with ADD. Works to expand home, school, and work-based strategies for aiding people with ADD; advocates for improved responsiveness to the needs of people with ADD by schools, businesses, and organizations. Provides support and information to families of people with ADD; conducts educational programs; maintains speakers' bureau. **Pub:** *AD-IN*. Brochure.

★ 1499 ★ Australasian College of Dermatologists
PO Box B65
Boronia Park, NSW 2111, Australia
Phone: 61 2 98796177 **Fax:** 61 2 98161174
Email: admin@dermcoll.asn.au
Website: http://www.dermcoll.asn.au/

Fnded: 1966. **Desc:** Aims to train dermatologists and to promote dermatology.

★ 1500 ★ Australasian College for Emergency Medicine (ACEM)
17 Grattan St.
Carlton, VIC 3053, Australia
Phone: 61 3 96633800 **Fax:** 61 3 96638013
Email: admin@acem.org.au
Website: http://www.acem.org.au

Fnded: 1984. **Mem:** 510. **Reg. Groups:** 6. **Lang(s):** English. **Desc:** Provides the training and examination of specialist emergency physicians. **Pub:** *Emergency Medicine*, quarterly. Journal. Peer-reviewed scientific journal.

★ 1501 ★ Australasian College of Sexual Health Physicians
GPO Box 1614
Sydney, NSW 2001, Australia
Phone: 61 2 93827457 **Fax:** 61 2 93827475
Email: secretariat@acshp.org.au
Website: http://www.acshp.org.au

Fnded: 1988. **Mem:** 207. **Reg. Groups:** 6. **Lang(s):** English. **Desc:** Physicians engaged in the practice of reproductive medicine and other specialties related to sexual health. Seeks to advance the study, teaching, and practice of sexual health medicine; promotes the prevention and control of sexually transmitted diseases. Establishes standards for sexual health medicine training and practice; holds examinations and accredits qualifying sexual health physicians; conducts continuing professional development courses for members. Makes available consulting services.

★ 1502 ★ Australasian College of Tropical Medicine (ACTM)
POB 123
Red Hill, QLD 4059, Australia
Phone: 61 7 38722246 **Fax:** 61 7 38564727
Email: actm@tropmed.org
Website: http://www.tropmed.org

Fnded: 1991. **Mem:** 400. **Desc:** Encourages education and exchange of knowledge in tropical medicine; promotes research. **Pub:** *Annals of the ACTM*, semiannual. Journal. • *Briefcase*, quarterly. Newsletter. • *Bulletin*, quarterly. Newsletter.

★ 1503 ★ Australasian Lymphology Association
Reul-Hirche
Physiotherapist Department
Royal Brisbane Hospital
Herston, QLD 4029, Australia
Email: lymphology@sapro.com.au

★ 1504 ★ Australasian Menopause Society (AMS)
PO Box 1228
Buderim, QLD 4556, Australia
Phone: 61 7 54562660 **Fax:** 61 7 54562661
Email: ams@netlink.com.au
Website: http://www.menopause.org.au

Mem: 700. **Lang(s):** English. **Desc:** Doctors, nurses, paramedical and community workers, and those with an interest in menopause. Seeks to improve the quality of life of women during and after menopause.

★ 1505 ★ Australasian Pharmaceutical Science Association (APSA)
Department of Pharmacy
University of Sydney
Sydney, NSW 2007, Australia
Phone: 61 2 93512320 **Fax:** 61 2 93512320

Fnded: 1960.

★ 1506 ★ Australasian Society of Clinical and Experimental Pharmacologists and Toxicologists (ASCEPT)
c/o Catherine Kennedy, Sec.
145 Macquarie St.
Sydney, NSW 2000, Australia
Phone: 61 2 92565406 **Fax:** 61 2 92520294
Email: ascept@hcn.net.au
Website: http://www.ascept.org

Mem: 881. **Desc:** Promotes experimental pharmacology and toxicology in the Australasian region.

★ 1507 ★ Australasian Society of Clinical and Experimental Pharmacologists and Toxicologists New Zealand Section (ASCEPT/NZ)
c/o Dr. Evan Begg
Department of Clinical Pharmacology
Christchurch School of Medicine

PO Box 4345
Christchurch, New Zealand
Phone: 64 3 3641055 **Fax:** 64 3 3641055
Email: evan.begg@chmeds.ac.nz

Mem: 85. **Desc:** Promotes clinical and experimental pharmacology and toxicology in New Zealand.

★ 1508 ★ Australasian Society for HIV Medicine (ASHM)

Locked Mail Bag 5057
Darlinghurst, NSW 1300, Australia
Phone: 61 2 93682700 **Fax:** 61 2 93809528
Email: ashm@ashm.org.au
Website: http://www.ashm.org.au

Fnded: 1989. **Mem:** 750. **Lang(s):** English. **Desc:** Physicians, medical scientists, health care professionals, and other individuals involved in the field of HIV/AIDS medicine. Seeks to advance the study, teaching, and practice of HIV/AIDS medicine; works to stop the spread of AIDS. Serves as a clearinghouse on HIV/AIDS medicine; maintains journal club; conducts lobbying campaigns; sponsors national HIV Education Program for Australasian Doctors; develops and distributes educational materials. Facilitates establishment of international HIV/AIDS medical networks. Advises government agencies responsible for public health and other policies relating to HIV/AIDS. **Pub:** *ASHM Journal Club*, bimonthly. Newsletter. • *ASHM News*, bimonthly. Newsletter. • *Directory of Australasian HIV, Hepatitis and Related Services*, annual. Directory.

★ 1509 ★ Australasian Society for Human Biology (ASHB)

School of Anatomy & Human Biology
University of Western Australia
35 Stirling Hwy.
Crawley, WA 6009, Australia
Phone: 61 8 93802671 **Fax:** 61 8 93801051
Email: maciej.henneberg@adelaide.edu.au
Website: http://www.anhb.uwa.edu.au/ASHB

Fnded: 1987. **Mem:** 250. **Nat'l Groups:** 3. **Reg. Groups:** 3. **State Groups:** 4.

★ 1510 ★ Australasian Society of Oral Medicine and Toxicology (ASOMAT)

PO Box A860
Sydney, NSW 2000, Australia
Phone: 61 2 98671111 **Fax:** 61 2 92832230
Email: asomat@asomat.com

Lang(s): English. **Desc:** Medical professionals working in the fields of oral medicine and toxicology. Promotes "concepts of "Bio-Compatible Dentistry which are supported by scientific, peer reviewed research. Serves as a clearinghouse on research in oral medicine, toxicology, and natural therapies.

★ 1511 ★ Australasian Society for the Study of Obesity (ASSO)

c/o Dr. Tim Gill
Human Nutrition Unit
University of Sydney
Sydney, NSW 2006, Australia
Phone: 61 2 93513758 **Fax:** 61 2 93516022
Email: office@asso.org.au
Website: http://www.asso.org.au/

Fnded: 1991. **Mem:** 550. **Desc:** Works to improve the management and prevention of obesity in Australasia; promotes public awareness and understanding and improved research on obesity.

★ 1512 ★ Australasian Society for Traumatic Stress Studies (ASTSS)

PO Box 5
Kettering, TAS 7155, Australia
Phone: 61 3 62674877
Email: i.p.b.watson@utas.edu.au
Website: http://www.astss.org.au

Fnded: 1990. **Lang(s):** English. **Desc:** Scientists and health care professionals with an interest in traumatic stress. Promotes "advancement of knowledge about the nature, consequences, treatment and prevention of highly stressful experiences." Gathers and disseminates information on traumatic stress and its diagnosis and treatment; sponsors research and educational programs.

★ 1513 ★ Australasian Society for Ultrasound in Medicine

2/181 High St.
Willoughby
Sydney, NSW 2068, Australia
Phone: 61 2 99587655 **Fax:** 61 2 99588002
Email: asum@asum.com.au
Website: http://www.asum.com.au

Fnded: 1975. **Mem:** 2,500. **Desc:** Doctors, scientists, medical specialists, sonographers, trainee sonographers/radiographers and corporations in ultrasound field. **Pub:** *Australasian Society for Ultrasound in Medicine*, quarterly. Bulletin.

★ 1514 ★ Australian Association of the Deaf (AAD)

149 Castlereagh St., Ste. 513
Sydney, NSW 2000, Australia
Phone: 61 2 92863944 **Fax:** 61 2 92863955
Email: aad@aad.org.au
Website: http://www.aad.org.au

Fnded: 1986. **State Groups:** 6. **Lang(s):** English. **Desc:** Deaf people who use Australian Sign Language (Auslan). Educates the Deaf community about their basic rights and obligations under the law and promotes public awareness about issues relating to deafness. **Pub:** *AAD Outlook*, quarterly. Magazine. • *Lookout*. Bulletin.

★ 1515 ★ Australian Association of Gerontology (AAG-IAG)

Centre for Ageing Studies
Mark Oliphant Bldg.
Laffer Dr.
Bedford Park, SA 5042, Australia
Phone: 61 8 82017552 **Fax:** 61 8 82017551
Email: aag.secre@flinders.edu.au
Website: http://www.aag.asn.au

Fnded: 1961. **Mem:** 950. **Desc:** Focuses on issues related to aging and the aging process. **Pub:** Newsletter, quarterly.

★ 1516 ★ Australian Association of Neurologists

AAN Secretariat
145 Macquarie St.
Sydney, NSW 2000, Australia
Phone: 61 2 92565443 **Fax:** 61 2 92414083
Email: aansyd@hotkey.net.au
Website: http://www.medeserv.com.au/aan

Fnded: 1950. **Mem:** 450. **Lang(s):** English. **Desc:** Neurologists and researchers and scientists with an interest in neurology. Seeks to "ensure that high standards of clinical neurology are practised in Australia." Develops standards of neurological training and practice; conducts research and continuing professional development programs; functions as a clearinghouse on neurology. **Pub:** Newsletter, 3/year.

★ 1517 ★ Australian Association of Occupational Therapists (AAOT)

97 Grange Rd.
Alphington, VIC 3078, Australia
Fnded: 1945.

★ 1518 ★ Australian Association of Practice Managers (AAPM)

PO Box 2477
Fortitude Valley, QLD 4006, Australia
Email: national@aapm.org.au
Website: http://www.aapm.org.au

Fnded: 1979. **Mem:** 1,500. **Lang(s):** English. **Desc:** Practice managers in the healthcare industry. Promotes professional excellence in healthcare practice management. **Pub:** *The Practice Manager*, quarterly. Journal.

★ 1519 ★ Australian College of Health Service Executives (ACHSE)

PO Box 341
North Ryde, NSW 1670, Australia
Phone: 61 2 98785088 **Fax:** 61 2 98782272
Email: achse@achse.org.au
Website: http://www.achse.org.au

Fnded: 1945. **Mem:** 3,000. **Lang(s):** English. **Desc:** Aims to develop and foster excellence in Health Service Management through education and ongoing professional development of existing and potential health service managers.

★ 1520 ★ Australian College of Obstetricians and Gynaecologists (ACOG)

8 La Trobe St.
Melbourne, VIC 3000, Australia
Fnded: 1978.

★ 1521 ★ Australian College of Occupational Health Nurses (ACOHN)

PO Box 1205
Tullamarine, VIC 3043, Australia
Phone: 61 3 93352577 **Fax:** 61 3 93353454
Email: admin@acohn.com.au
Website: http://www.acohn.com.au

Fnded: 1976. **Mem:** 400. **Lang(s):** English. **Desc:** Registered nurses and nurses in training working in occupational health and safety or in a relevant discipline. Promotes occupational health; promotes high standards and encourage excellence in the practice of occupational health; supports education for nurses who practice in occupational health; encourages research by nurses in the field.

★ 1522 ★ Australian College of Pharmacy Practice (ACPP)

PO Box 7007
Canberra Mail Centre
Canberra, ACT 2610, Australia
Phone: 61 2 62738989 **Fax:** 61 2 62738988
Email: info@acpp.edu.au
Website: http://www.acpp.edu.au

Fnded: 1983. **Mem:** 1,124. **Lang(s):** English. **Desc:** Provides postgraduate pharmacy educational opportunities for pharmacists throughout the world via distance learning. **Pub:** *Pharmacy Risins*, quarterly. Newsletter.

★ 1523 ★ Australian Council for Health, Physical Education and Recreation (ACHPER)

214 Port Rd.
PO Box 304
Hindmarsh, SA 5007, Australia
Phone: 61 8 83403388 **Fax:** 61 8 83403399
Email: achper@achper.org.au
Website: http://www.achper.org.au

Mem: 3,300. **State Groups:** 8. **Desc:** Professionals dedicated to healthy lifestyles. Promotes healthy lifestyles in schools and the community; develops public awareness through political process and media; supports research and projects aimed at creating healthy lifestyle awareness. **Pub:** *Active & Healthy*. Magazine. • *Australian Journal of Science and Medicine in Sport*. Journal.

★ 1524 ★ Australian Deaf Sports Federation (ADSF)

101-117 Wellington Parade South
East Melbourne, VIC 3002, Australia
Phone: 61 3 96502524 **Fax:** 61 3 96542868

Email: dsa@deafsports.org.au
Website: http://www.deafsports.org.au

Fnded: 1954. **Lang(s):** English. **Desc:** Encourages an increased level and standard of sports participation and performance for all Deaf Australians.

★ 1525 ★ Australian Dental Association (ADA)
75 Lithgow St.
Saint Leonards, NSW 2065, Australia
Phone: 61 2 99064412 **Fax:** 61 2 99064917
Email: adainc@ada.org.au
Website: http://www.ada.org.au

Fnded: 1928. **Mem:** 7,500. **State Groups:** 7. **Lang(s):** English. **Desc:** Dentists, specialists, and dental students. Represents dentists' interests nationally and internationally. Seeks to improve the dental health of the community. Sponsors educational and research programs; cosponsors the Australian Dental Research Fund. **Pub:** *ADA Dental Directory*, biennial. Directory. • *ADA News Bulletin*, 11/year. • *Australian Dental Journal*, quarterly. • *Facts and Figures - Australian Dentistry*, annual.

★ 1526 ★ Australian Drug Foundation (ADF)
409 King St.
PO Box 818
North Melbourne, VIC 3051, Australia
Phone: 61 3 92788100 **Fax:** 61 3 93283008
Email: adf@adf.org.au
Website: http://www.adf.org.au

Fnded: 1959. **Lang(s):** English. **Desc:** Educators, journalists, librarians, health workers, and researchers. Seeks to prevent and reduce alcohol and other drug problems in the Australian community through the provision of quality information and practical assistance in a professional manner. Assists in the development of school and community programs; conducts research and training; and sponsors art and sporting events as part of outreach efforts.

★ 1527 ★ Australian Federation for Medical and Biological Engineering
Biomedical Engineering Services
Queen Elizabeth Hospital
Woodville Rd.
Woodville, SA 5011, Australia
Phone: 61 8 82226533 **Fax:** 61 8 82226031

Fnded: 1959.

★ 1528 ★ Australian Hypnotherapists' Association
19 Macleay St.
Wahroongah, NSW 2076, Australia
Phone: 61 2 94186730 **Fax:** 61 2 94890158

Fnded: 1949. **Mem:** 65. **State Groups:** 2. **Local Groups:** 1. **Lang(s):** English. **Desc:** Seeks to further the art of hypnotherapy and maintains a high level of standards and education for members. Lobbies health funds and the government for recognition; works to increase public awareness of hypnotherapy and its practitioners.

★ 1529 ★ Australian Infection Control Association (AICA)
PO Box 322
Wilston Brisbane, QLD 4051, Australia
Phone: 61 4 14422307
Email: aica@ozemail.com.au
Website: http://www.aica.org.au/

Desc: Represents specialist practitioners in infection control; works to develop best practice in infection management and prevention.

★ 1530 ★ Australian Institute of Radiography (AIR)
PO Box 1169
Collingwood, VIC 3066, Australia
Phone: 61 3 94193336 **Fax:** 61 3 94160783
Email: info@a-i-r.com.au
Website: http://www.a-i-r.com.au

Fnded: 1950. **Mem:** 3,800. **Nat'l Groups:** 1. **Reg. Groups:** 13. **State Groups:** 6. **Local Groups:** 1. **Lang(s):** English. **Desc:** Diagnostic radiographers, radiation therapists, and sonographers in Australia. Fosters cooperation and exchange of information between members. Conducts educational and research projects; prepares guidelines and policies for the practice of radiography in Australia. Encourages high professional standards. Disseminates information; offers educational programs and seminars. **Pub:** *Radiographer*, 3/year, April, August, December. Journal. • *Spectrum*, 10/yr. **Frmly:** Australasian Institute of Radiography.

★ 1531 ★ Australian Medical Association (AMA)
42 Macquarie St.
PO Box E115
Kingston, ACT 2604, Australia
Phone: 61 2 62705400 **Fax:** 61 2 62705499
Email: ama@ama.com.au
Website: http://www.ama.com.au/

Fnded: 1962.

★ 1532 ★ Australian Medical Council (AMC)
PO Box 4810
Kingston, ACT 2604, Australia
Phone: 61 2 62709777 **Fax:** 61 2 62709799
Email: amc@amc.org.au
Website: http://www.amc.org.au

Fnded: 1984. **Lang(s):** English. **Desc:** Academic and governmental groups associated with Australian medical standards. Functions as a national standards body for primary medical training. Advises and makes recommendations to State and Territory Medical Boards; maintains a national network of medical registers; provides advice to the Australian Health Ministry Advisory Council.

★ 1533 ★ Australian Medical Students' Association (AMSA)
Level 1, Hunstanton
88 L'Estrange Tee
Herston, QLD 4006, Australia
Phone: 61 7 38722275 **Fax:** 61 7 38722282
Email: mail@amsa.org.au
Website: http://www.amsa.org.au

Fnded: 1960. **Mem:** 8,500. **State Groups:** 11. **Lang(s):** English. **Desc:** Medical students in Australia. Provides social activities, supplements members' intellectual development, and offers support for discovering life in the workforce; provides political representation. **Pub:** *Antics*, 3/year. Magazine.

★ 1534 ★ Australian Music Therapy Association (AMTA)
PO Box 79
Turramurra, NSW 2074, Australia
Phone: 61 2 94495279 **Fax:** 61 2 99883856
Email: info@austmta.org
Website: http://www.austmta.org.au

Fnded: 1975. **Mem:** 450. **State Groups:** 3. **Lang(s):** English. **Desc:** Registered music therapists, students, and interested others. Promotes the theory and practice of music therapy. Offers registration accreditation of training program and in-service education for other professional groups; provides printed resources; conducts research. **Pub:** *Australian Journal of Music Therapy*, annual. Journal. Contains clinical documentation and research information. • *Bulletin*, 3/year. Newsletter. • *Network*, 3/year. Newsletter. For RMTs only.

★ 1535 ★ Australian National Council on AIDS, Hepatitis C and Related Diseases (ANCAHRD)
GPO Box 9848
Mail Drop 13
Department of Health and Family Services
Canberra, ACT 2601, Australia
Phone: 61 2 62897029 **Fax:** 61 2 62898098
Website: http://www.ancahrd.org

Fnded: 1988. **Mem:** 27. **Lang(s):** English. **Desc:** Provides independent and expert advice to the Minister of Health on the implementation of the National HIV/AIDS Strategy. Identifies national objectives and priorities. Disseminates information to increase community understanding. **Pub:** Bulletin, periodic. **Frmly:** (1998) Australian National Council on AIDS.

★ 1536 ★ Australian and New Zealand Forensic Medicine Society (ANZFMS)
57 Kavanagh St.
Southbank 3006, Australia
Email: morriso@vifp.monash.edu.au
Website: http://www.nifs.com.au/ANZFMS/ANZFMS.html

Mem: 100.

★ 1537 ★ Australian and New Zealand Society of Nuclear Medicine (ANZSNM)
PO Box 7108
Upper Fern Tree Gulley, VIC 3156, Australia
Phone: 61 3 97560128 **Fax:** 61 3 97536372
Email: anzsnm@21century.com.au
Website: http://www.anzsnm.org.au

Fnded: 1969.

★ 1538 ★ Australian Nursing Federation (ANF)
Unit 3
28 Eyre St.
Kingston, ACT 2604, Australia
Phone: 61 2 62326533 **Fax:** 61 2 62326610
Email: cathy@anf.org.au
Website: http://www.anf.org.au

Fnded: 1924. **Mem:** 115,000. **Reg. Groups:** 8. **Lang(s):** English. **Desc:** Nurses in both the public and private sectors in Australia. Provides industrial and professional representation of nurses and pursues improved public policy on health and related issues. Participates in the development of policy in nursing, nursing regulation, community services, veterans' affairs, education, training, occupational health and safety, industrial matters, immigration and law reform. **Pub:** *Australian Journal of Advanced Nursing (AJAN)*, quarterly. Journal. Includes peer reviewed research. • *Australian Nursing Journal (ANJ)*, monthly. Journal. Includes clinical articles and latest nursing news.

★ 1539 ★ Australian Orthopaedic Association
Level 12, Culwulla Chambers
67 Castlereagh St.
Sydney, NSW 2000, Australia
Phone: 61 2 92333018 **Fax:** 61 2 92218301
Email: admin@aoa.org.au
Website: http://www.aoa.org.au/

Fnded: 1936.

★ 1540 ★ Australian Physiotherapy Association
Level 3, 201 Fitzroy St.
St. Kilda
Melbourne, VIC 3182, Australia
Phone: 61 3 95349400 **Fax:** 61 3 95349199
Email: national.office@physiotherapy.asn.au
Website: http://www.physiotherapy.asn.au

Mem: 10,200. **Nat'l Groups:** 11. **Lang(s):** English. **Desc:** Physiotherapists. Seeks to improve public health through advancing the science and practice of physiotherapy. Establishes standards of ethics, training, and practice for physiotherapists. Represents members' interests within the national health care system; supports research; conducts continuing professional development courses.

★ 1541 ★ Australian Private Hospitals Association (APHA)
Level 1
25 Napier Close
Deakin, ACT 2600, Australia
Phone: 61 2 62852716 **Fax:** 61 2 62852243
Email: info@apha.org.au
Website: http://www.apha.org.au

Lang(s): English. **Desc:** Represents private hospitals in Australia.

★ 1542 ★ Australian Psychological Society
PO Box 38
Flinders Ln. PO
Melbourne, VIC 8009, Australia
Phone: 61 3 86623300 **Fax:** 61 3 96636177
Email: contactus@psychsociety.com.au
Website: http://www.psychsociety.com.au/

Fnded: 1966. **Mem:** 13,000. **Lang(s):** English. **Desc:** Psychologists. Seeks to "represent, promote and advance psychology and psychologists within the context of improving community well-being and scientific knowledge." Develops and maintains standards of training and practice; lobbies government agencies on matters of social_welfare, justice, education, and health; conducts educational programs for members and the public. **Pub:** *In Psych*, bimonthly. Magazine.

★ 1543 ★ Australian Quadriplegic Association (AQA)
1 Jennifer St.
Little Bay, NSW 2036, Australia
Phone: 61 2 96618855 **Fax:** 61 2 96619598
Email: aqa@aqa.org.au
Website: http://www.aqa.com.au

Fnded: 1967. **Lang(s):** English. **Desc:** People with severe physical disabilities and their families. Seeks to enable people with severe physical disabilities to achieve maximum independence through a rehabilitation perspective in all its services. Provides community support and counseling, peer support, advocacy, and disability awareness training. **Pub:** *QUAD WRANGLE*, quarterly. Journal.

★ 1544 ★ Australian Reproductive Health Alliance (ARHA)
PO Box 3937
Weston, ACT 2611, Australia
Phone: 61 2 62874422 **Fax:** 61 2 62873532
Email: arha@arha.org.au
Website: http://www.arha.org.au/committee.htm

Desc: Works for the improvement in the well being and status of women and development of reproductive health in families and individuals, particularly the development of family planning and other reproductive health services with focus on needs of indigenous people within Australia and internationally.

★ 1545 ★ Australian Rheumatology Association (ARA)
145 Macquarie St.
Sydney, NSW 2000, Australia
Phone: 61 2 9256 5458 **Fax:** 61 2 9252 3310
Email: robynm@racp.edu.au
Website: http://www.medeserv.com.au/ara/

Lang(s): English. **Desc:** Physicians who specialize in the assessment and management of musculoskeletal and inflammatory diseases. Promotes rheumatology as a state-of-the-art, evidenced-based discipline and advances research in the field. Supports grant allocating bodies.

★ 1546 ★ Australian Self-Medication Industry
140 Arthur St., Level 4
North Sydney, NSW 2060, Australia
Phone: 61 2 99225111 **Fax:** 61 2 99593693
Email: juliet@asmi.com.au
Website: http://www.asmi.com.au

Fnded: 1974. **Mem:** 56. **Desc:** Manufacturers nonprescription medicines, also know as over the counter medicines. Seeks to ensure the safe and effective over the counter medications are readily available at a reasonable to cost. Serves as a source of information on responsible and cost-effective self medication. Represents members before parliament and government and industry organizations. Commissions research. **Pub:** *One Voice, STAR, Re: Claim*. Contains industry, scientific and regulatory news and information. **Frmly:** (2000) Proprietary Medicine Association of Australia.

★ 1547 ★ Australian Sleep Association
GPO Box 295
Sydney, NSW 1043, Australia
Phone: 61 500 500701 **Fax:** 61 500 500702
Email: sleepaus@ozemail.com.au
Website: http://www.sleepaus.on.net

Desc: Represents clinicians, scientists, and researchers. Oversees training in the area of clinical sleep medicine. Provides quality assurance through credentialing of sleep laboratories. **Pub:** Newsletter, periodic.

★ 1548 ★ Australian Small Animal Veterinary Association (ASAVA)
PO Box 674
Surry Hills, NSW 2010, Australia
Phone: 61 2 92118899 **Fax:** 61 2 92118851
Email: asava@ava.com.au
Website: http://www.ava.com.au/

Fnded: 1968. **Mem:** 950. **Desc:** Represents small animal practitioners; works to advance veterinary science; promotes high quality companion animal practice. **Pub:** *Australian Veterinary Practitioner*, quarterly. Journal. Presents papers, case reports and other material of interest. • Pamphlets.

★ 1549 ★ Australian Society of Anaesthetists (ASA)
Ste. 603 Eastpoint Tower
180 Ocean St.
Edgecliff, NSW 2027, Australia
Phone: 61 2 93274022 **Fax:** 61 2 93277666
Email: asa@fed.asa.org.au
Website: http://www.asa.org.au

Fnded: 1934. **Lang(s):** English. **Desc:** Anaesthetists and medical practitioners with an interest in anaesthesia. Represents members' interests and promotes public awareness of anaesthesia.

★ 1550 ★ Australian Society for Biomaterials
PO Box 743
Brunswick Lower, VIC 3056, Australia
Phone: 61 3 96627239 **Fax:** 61 3 96627218
Website: http://www.biomaterials.org.au/Information.html

Fnded: 1989. **Desc:** Promotes research, education, development and regulation of biomaterials and medical devices.

★ 1551 ★ Australian Society of Clinical Hypnotherapists
PO Box 471
Eastwood, NSW 2122, Australia
Phone: 61 2 98742776 **Fax:** 61 2 98742776
Email: referrals@asch.com.au
Website: http://www.asch.com.au/

Fnded: 1974. **Mem:** 390. **Nat'l Groups:** 1. **State Groups:** 3. **Lang(s):** English. **Desc:** Clinical hypnotherapists. Seeks to maintain high ethical and professional standards in the practice of clinical hypnotherapy. Promotes advancement of hypnotherapeutic techniques. Informs members about developments in clinical hypnotherapy; conducts continuing professional education programs; operates referral service. **Pub:** *The Australian Journal of Clinical Hypnotherapy and Hypnosis*, biennial. Journal.

★ 1552 ★ Australian Society of Hypnosis
PO Box 5114
Alphington, VIC 3078, Australia
Phone: 61 3 94585133 **Fax:** 61 3 94585399
Email: hypnosis@alphalink.com.au

Fnded: 1971. **Mem:** 1,000. **State Groups:** 6. **Lang(s):** English. **Desc:** Promotes training and research in hypnosis for health professionals in Australia.

★ 1553 ★ Australian Society for Medical Research (ASMR)
145 Macquarie St.
Sydney, NSW 2000, Australia
Phone: 61 2 92565450 **Fax:** 61 2 92520294
Email: asmr@world.net
Website: http://www.asmr.org.au

Fnded: 1961. **Mem:** 1,200. **Lang(s):** English. **Desc:** Persons who are or have been engaged in the practice of medical research, including postgraduate students. Fosters excellence in Australian health and medical research and promotes community understanding and support. **Pub:** Newsletter, 3/year.

★ 1554 ★ Australian Society of Orthodontists
Private Bag No. 1
Darlinghurst, NSW 2010, Australia
Phone: 61 2 93316920 **Fax:** 61 2 93317296
Email: aso@apcasyd.com
Website: http://www.aso.org.au/

Fnded: 1927. **Mem:** 500.

★ 1555 ★ Australian Society of Otolaryngology Head and Neck Surgery (ASOHNS)
level 4, 68 Alfred St., Ste. 403
Missions Pointe, NSW 2061, Australia
Phone: 61 2 99545856 **Fax:** 61 2 99576863
Email: enquiries@asohns.org.au
Website: http://www.asohns.org.au

Fnded: 1950. **Mem:** 427. **Nat'l Groups:** 1. **State Groups:** 6. **Lang(s):** English. **Desc:** Ear, nose, and throat surgeons. Represents member interests. Provides registrar training. **Pub:** *Australian Journal of Oto-Laryngology*, semiannual. Journal. • *Australian Otolaryngology*, quarterly. Newsletter.

★ 1556 ★ Australian Society of Plant Scientists
c/o Prof. Hans Lambers
School of Plant Biology
Faculty of Natural & Agricultural Sciences
University of Western Australia
Crawley, WA 6009, Australia
Phone: 61 8 93807381 **Fax:** 61 8 93801108
Email: hlambers@cyllene.uwa.edu.au
Website: http://www.plantsci.org.au/

Fnded: 1958.

★ 1557 ★ Australian Society for Reproductive Biology
c/o Dr. Michael Sinosich, Communication Officer
Royal North Shore Hospital
Saint Leonards, NSW 2065, Australia
Phone: 61 2 99267408 **Fax:** 61 2 99061872
Email: msino@med.usyd.edu.au

Fnded: 1969.

★ 1558 ★ Australian Sonographers Association (ASA)
PO Box 709
Cheltenham, VIC 3192, Australia
Phone: 61 3 95852996 **Fax:** 61 3 95852331
Website: http://www.a-s-a.com.au/

Fnded: 1992. **Mem:** 920. **Desc:** Works to advance the practice of sonography; promotes education and research in diagnostic medical sonography; disseminates information; assists in guidelines for the competent practice of diagnostic medical sonography. **Pub:** *Sound Effects*, quarterly. Encourages sonographers to express views, provides forum for education and discussion.

★ 1559 ★ Australian Teratology Society (ATS)
c/o Dr. Tricia Woodman
Department of Biomedical Sciences
University of Sydney
Lidcombe, NSW 2141, Australia
Phone: 61 2 93519256 **Fax:** 61 2 93519520
Email: p.woodman@cchs.usyd.edu.au

Fnded: 1983. **Desc:** Professionals interested in the causes and prevention of birth defects. **Pub:** Newsletter. Incorporates a teratogen update, reviews and opinions.

★ 1560 ★ Australian-Traditional Medicine Society (ATMS)
PO Box 1027
Meadowbank, NSW 2114, Australia
Phone: 61 2 98096800 **Fax:** 61 2 98097570
Website: http://www.atms.com.au/body.htm

Fnded: 1984. **Mem:** 8,963. **Desc:** Represents complementary medicine practitioners in Australia.

★ 1561 ★ Australian Vascular Biology Society
c/o Dr. Levon Khachigian
Center for Thrombosis & Vascular Research
School of Pathology
University of New South Wales
Kensington, NSW 2052, Australia
Email: robert.andrews@baker.edu.au
Website: http://www.baker.edu.au/avbs

Fnded: 1993. **Desc:** Works to advanced concepts in vascular biology.

★ 1562 ★ Australian Vascular Ultrasound Accreditation Board
PO Box 709
Cheltenham, VIC 3192, Australia
Phone: 61 3 95852996
Email: trevaskis@hotkey.net.au

Desc: Works towards a standard of quality for the utilization of vascular ultrasound by implementing a professional accreditation structure.

★ 1563 ★ Australian Veterinary Association (AVA)
PO Box 371
Artarmon, NSW 1570, Australia
Phone: 61 2 94112733 **Fax:** 61 2 94115089
Email: avahq@ava.com.au
Website: http://www.ava.com.au

Fnded: 1921. **Mem:** 4,500. **State Groups:** 8. **Local Groups:** 52. **Lang(s):** English. **Desc:** Graduates of Australian veterinary schools; graduates of overseas veterinary schools qualified for registration in Australia; veterinary students; associate members are non-veterinarians with close ties to the veterinary profession. Promotes the professional practice of veterinary medicine; seeks improvements in the areas of animal health, productivity, and welfare. Represents members' interests; lobbies governmental bodies on matters related to animal welfare, quarantine, and agricultural problems. Maintains 23 special interest groups offering continuing education programs. Maintains museum. **Pub:** *Australian Veterinary Journal*, monthly. Journal. • *Members Directory and Policy Compendium*, triennial. Directory. • Report, annual.

★ 1564 ★ Australian Women's Health Network (AWHN)
c/o Dr. Helen Keleher
29/219 Auburn Rd.
Hawthorn, VIC 3122, Australia
Phone: 61 3 92446688 **Fax:** 61 3 92446017
Website: http://www.awhn.org.au/

Fnded: 1986. **Desc:** Aims to maintain and increase a national focus on women's health issues. Aims to be a national advocacy and information sharing organization.

★ 1565 ★ Austrian Neuroscience Association (ANA) (Osterreichische Gesellschaft fuer Neurowissenschaften)
Department of Experimental and Clinical Pharmacology
University of Graz
Universitaetplatz 4
A-8010 Graz, Austria
Phone: 43 316 3804314 **Fax:** 43 316 3809645
Email: peter.holzer@kfunigraz.ac.at
Website: http://www.univie.ac.at/ANA/anahome.htm

Fnded: 1993. **Desc:** Promotes neuroscience in Austria. **Pub:** *OGN-Newsletter*. Newsletter.

★ 1566 ★ Austrian Pharmacological Society (APHAR)
c/o Prof. Gunther Sperk
Institut fur Pharmakologie
Universitat Innsbruck
Peter-Mayer-Strasse 1a
A-6020 Innsbruck, Austria
Phone: 43 512 5073710 **Fax:** 43 512 5072868
Email: guenther.sperk@uibk.ac.at
Website: http://www.uibk.ac.at/aphar

Mem: 94. **Desc:** Promotes pharmacology in Austria.

★ 1567 ★ Austrian Society of Acupuncture (ASA) (Osterreichische Gesellschaft fur Akupunktur — OGA)
Kaiserin-Elisabeth Hospital
Huglgasse 1-3
A-1150 Vienna, Austria
Phone: 43 1 981045758 **Fax:** 43 1 981045759
Email: aku@kes.magwien.gv.at
Website: http://www.akupunktur.at

Fnded: 1954. **Mem:** 2,147. **Lang(s):** Chinese, English, French, Italian. **Desc:** Promotes the acceptance of acupuncture as a recognized healing method in the western medical world. Works in conjunction with the World Health Organization to disseminate and standardize nomenclature. Offers training course.

★ 1568 ★ Austrian Society of Cardiology
Klinik fur Innere Medizin II
Abteilung fur Kardiologie
Wahringer Gurtel 18-20
A-1090 Vienna, Austria
Phone: 43 1 404004616 **Fax:** 43 1 4081148
Email: edith.tanzl@akh-wein.ac.at
Website: http://www.atcardio.at

Fnded: 1971. **Mem:** 1,008. **Nat'l Groups:** 17. **Lang(s):** German. **Desc:** Promotes the study of cardiology in Austria. **Pub:** *Mitteilungen*. Newsletter.

★ 1569 ★ Austrian Society for Geriatrics and Gerontology
Sophienspital
Apollogasse 19
A-1070 Vienna, Austria
Phone: 43 1 52103 **Fax:** 43 1 52103
Email: franz.boehmer@sop.magwien.gv.at

Fnded: 1995. **Mem:** 400. **Lang(s):** German. **Desc:** Promotes gerontological research, training in the field of aging, and interests of gerontological organizations in international affairs. **Pub:** *Geriatric Praxis*, bimonthly. Journal.

★ 1570 ★ Austrian Society of Psychosomatics in Gynaecology and Obstetrics
c/o Dr. Peter Kemeter
Hadikgasse 82
A-1140 Vienna, Austria
Fax: 43 1 894636018
Email: p-kem@asog.co.at

Desc: Promotes the study of psychobiological and psychosocial, ethical and cross-cultural problems in the fields of obstetrics and gynaecology, women's health and reproductive health; faciliates the dissemination of new information in these fields. **Pub:** *Journal of Psychosomatic Obstetrics and Gynecology*. Journal. **Frmly:** Austrian Society of Psychomatic Obstetrics and Gynaecology.

★ 1571 ★ Autism-Europe
Ave. E Van Becelaere 26b, Bte 21
B-1170 Brussels, Belgium
Phone: 32 2 6757505 **Fax:** 32 2 6757270
Email: president@autismeurope.org
Website: http://www.autismeurope.org

Fnded: 1982. **Mem:** 40. **Lang(s):** English, French. **Desc:** National and regional associations of parents of children with autism in 21 European countries. Seeks to improve the lives of those whose existence is affected by autism. Works to advance research on the causes of autism and its prevention and treatment; ensures effective liaison between various associations, governments, European and international exchange programs involved with autism; works to provide a charter of rights for people with autism. **Pub:** *LINK*. Journal.

★ 1572 ★ Autism Independent UK
199-205 Blandford Ave.
Kettering NN16 9AT, United Kingdom
Phone: 44 1536 523274 **Fax:** 44 1536 523274
Email: autism@rmplc.co.uk
Website: http://www.autismuk.com/

Fnded: 1987. **Mem:** 4,000. **Lang(s):** English. **Desc:** Individuals with autism and their families. Seeks to increase awareness of autism; promotes development of improved diagnosis and treatment of people with autism. Works to improve the quality of life of people with autism. Serves as a nonmedical information center on autism and its treatment; sponsors research and educational programs; provides support and services to people with autism and their families. Maintains Diagnosis and Assessment Resource Centre, where interested individuals can access information on autism and its treatment. Collaborates with county agencies in the development of public health policies impacting people with autism. **Frmly:** (2000) Society of the Austically Handicapped.

★ 1573 ★ Autism Initiatives
7 Chesterfield Rd.
Crosby
Liverpool L23 9XL, United Kingdom
Website: http://www.autisminitiatives.org/

Desc: Provides information on autism from behavior management to diagnosis.

★ 1574 ★ Autism Network International (ANI)
PO Box 35448
Syracuse, NY 13235-5448
Phone: (315)476-2462 **Fax:** (315)425-1978
Email: jisincla@mailbox.syr.edu
Website: http://www.ani.ac
Jim Sinclair, Coord.

Fnded: 1992. **Mem:** 400. **Desc:** Autistic-run self-help and advocacy organization for autistic individuals.

Seeks to provide a forum for autistic people to share information and tips for coping and problem-solving; advocates for appropriate services and civil rights for all autistic people at all levels of functioning. Provides information and referrals for parents and teachers of autistic people; sponsors group lobbying and educational campaigns. Serves as a support group.

★ 1575 ★ Autism Research Institute (ARI)

4182 Adams Ave.
San Diego, CA 92116
Phone: (619)281-7165 **Fax:** (619)563-6840
Website: http://www.autismresearchinstitute.com

Fnded: 1967. **Desc:** Committed to conducting and disseminating research on the causes of autism and methods of preventing, diagnosing and treating autism and other severe behavioral disorders of childhood. **Pub:** *The Autism Research Review International*, quarterly. Newsletter.

★ 1576 ★ Autism Services Center (NAH)

605 9th St.
PO Box 507
Huntington, WV 25710-0507
Phone: (304)525-8014 **Fax:** (304)525-8026
Website: http://www.autismservices.com
Dr. Ruth C. Sullivan, PhD, Exec. Dir.

Fnded: 1979. **Desc:** Service agency for individuals with autism and other developmental disabilities, and their families. (Autism is a disorder of communication and behavior which often manifests itself in social isolation, severe language deficiency, and compulsive insistence on routine and ritual in daily activities.) Assists families and agencies attempting to meet the unique needs of individuals with autism and other developmental disabilities; makes available technical assistance in designing programs. Provides supervised apartments, group homes, respite services, independent living services, and job-coached employment. Conducts workshops and consulting in autismD-isseminates information regarding autism and its treatment. **Frmly:** (1993) National Autism Hotline.

★ 1577 ★ Autism Society of America (ASA)

7910 Woodmont Ave., Ste. 300
Bethesda, MD 20814-3067
Phone: (301)657-0881 **Free:** 800-3AU-TISM
Fax: (301)657-0869
Email: info@autism-society.org
Website: http://www.autism-society.org/
Robert L. Beck, Pres.

Fnded: 1965. **Mem:** 23,000. **Local Groups:** 230. **Desc:** Parents, teachers, psychologists, speech therapists, pediatricians, neurologists, and others interested in the welfare of children with severe disorders of communication and behavior. Informs the public of the symptoms and problems of children and adults with autism; promotes better understanding of the condition in general; aids physicians in making earlier and more accurate diagnoses. Committed to the alleviation of this disorder through support of research, public and professional education, and development of habilitative services. Sponsors two mail-order book stores with over 100 titles on autism. **Pub:** *Advocate*, quarterly. Magazine. Promotes better understanding of autism by informing the public of the symptoms and problems of children and adults with autism. *Price:* Included in membership dues. • Proceedings, annual. • Reprints. **Frmly:** (1981) National Society for Autistic Children; (1987) NSAC, The National Society for Children and Adults with Autism.

★ 1578 ★ Autism Society of Canada (ASC) (Societe Canadienne de l'Autisme — SCA)

PO Box 65
Orangeville, ON, Canada L9W 2Z5
Phone: (519)942-8720 **Free:** (866)874-3334
Fax: (519)942-8720
Email: info@autismsocietycanada.ca
Website: http://autismsocietycanada.ca

Lang(s): English, French. **Desc:** People with autism and their families; health care professionals, educators, therapists, and others working with people with autism. Promotes advancement in the diagnosis and treatment of autism; seeks to improve the quality of life of people with autism and their families. Provides support and services to people with autism and their families; serves as a clearinghouse on autism and its diagnosis and treatment; conducts educational programs.

★ 1579 ★ Autism Treatment Services of Canada (ATSC)

404 94th Ave. SE
Calgary, AB, Canada T2J 0E8
Phone: (403)253-6961 **Fax:** (403)253-6974
Email: atsc@autism.ca
Website: http://www.autism.ca

Lang(s): English, French. **Desc:** Organizations providing treatment services to people with autism and their families. Seeks to advance the treatment of autism. Serves as a clearinghouse on the treatment of autism; provides support and services to people with autism and their families; conducts research and educational programs.

★ 1580 ★ Autistic Association - Singapore

Blk 381, Clementi Ave. 5, No. 01-398
Singapore 120381, Singapore
Phone: 65 7746649 **Fax:** 65 7746957
Email: autism@singnet.com.sg

Lang(s): English. **Desc:** Parents, caregivers, and professionals who are concerned with autism in Singapore. Works to assist people with autism, their parents and caregivers, and professionals involved in the field of autism. Provides resources, training, and information about autism.

★ 1581 ★ Autonomous Group of Analytical Psychology (Gruppo Autonomo di Psicologia Analitica — GAPA)

Via della Consulta, 50
I-00184 Rome, Italy
Phone: 39 06 4885304

Fnded: 1971. **Desc:** organizes teaching and training courses in analytical psychology (C.G. Jung); promotes research in the Jungian textual field; publishes texts by Jungian authors.

★ 1582 ★ Auxiliary to the American Osteopathic Association (AAOA)

142 E Ontario St.
Chicago, IL 60611
Phone: (312)202-8192 **Free:** 800-621-1773
Fax: (312)202-8218
Email: bprice@aoa-net.org
Website: http://www.aux-aoa.org
Bridget L. Price, Exec. Dir.

Fnded: 1940. **Mem:** 5,000. **Desc:** Immediate family members of osteopathic physicians; spouses of students of osteopathic medicine. Promotes public health education; provides funds for scholarships for the training of osteopathic physicians and surgeons, and for research and other activities at osteopathic colleges; encourages establishment and continuation of volunteer service organizations in nonprofit osteopathic hospitals; participates in national and community health programs. Sponsors summer seminars. **Pub:** *AAOA Accent*, quarterly. Newsletter. Covers osteopathic medicine and related subjects such as safety projects, public health information, and osteopathic college scholarship awards. *Price:* Included in membership dues. • *Newsbriefs*, bimonthly. • *Roster of Affiliates*, annual. • Annual Report. • Also publishes handbooks.

★ 1583 ★ Auxiliary to the National Medical Association (ANMA)

1012 10th St. NW
Washington, DC 20001
Phone: (202)371-9008 **Fax:** (202)289-2662
Email: info@anma-online.org
Website: http://www.anma-online.org
Mrs. Maurce W. Ayton, Pres.

Fnded: 1935. **Mem:** 1,000. **Reg. Groups:** 6. **State Groups:** 14. **Local Groups:** 40. **Desc:** Spouses of active members of the National Medical Association; widows and widowers of former members. Purposes are to: create a greater interest in the NMA; assist and encourage the medical profession in its efforts to educate and serve the public in matters of sanitation and health; develop and promote a national program on health and education with subcategories in community needs, legislation, and human relations. Conducts workshops on teenage pregnancy, breast self-examinations, high blood pressure screening, and sickle cell anemia screening. Plans and implements an annual youth forum under the auspices of the March of Dimes Birth Defects Foundation . Provides youth with professional guidance and the opportunity for peer exchange in the areas of mental and physical health; deals with the health of newborns, health services, nutrition, and teenage pregnancy. Also conducts programs for youth on parenting, socially transmitted diseases, nutrition, birth defects, and continued education after pregnancy. **Pub:** Book.Covers standard procedures. • Membership Directory, periodic. *Price:* available to members only. • Newsletter, quarterly. **Frmly:** (1975) Women's Auxiliary to the National Medical Association.

★ 1584 ★ Avenues, National Support Group for Arthrogryposis Multiplex Congenita

c/o Mary Anne Schmidt
PO Box 5093
Sonora, CA 95370
Phone: (209)928-3688 **Free:** 888-SONNET-1
Fax: (209)533-9778
Email: avenues@sonnet.com
Website: http://www.sonnet.com/avenues/
Mary Anne Schmidt, Dir.

Fnded: 1980. **Mem:** 1,200. **Desc:** Individuals with arthrogryposis multiplex congentia (AMC), their families and friends, and interested professionals. (AMC, a birth defect, is a muscle and/or nerve syndrome affecting some or all of the body's limbs.) Purpose is to share positive attitudes and selfhelp ideas for the handicapped and for all who deal with them. **Pub:** *Avenues*, semiannual. Newsletter. Lists doctors and families interested in corresponding with others about arthrogryposis. *Price:* Included in membership dues; $10 annual donation requested for members in U.S.; $15 annual donation requested for members outside U.S. • Audiotapes. • Bibliography. • Pamphlet.*Price:* $1. • Also a $3.00 Resource Packet for Doctors, Therapists, Pen Pals Families, Clinics, Support Groups.

★ 1585 ★ AVERT

4 Brighton Rd.
Horsham RH13 5BA, United Kingdom
Phone: 44 1403 210202 **Fax:** 44 1403 211001
Email: info@avert.org
Website: http://www.avert.org

Fnded: 1986. **Lang(s):** English. **Desc:** Seeks to improve the quality of life for persons with AIDS. Conducts research and educational programs. Provides free information on AIDS, both within the U.K. and overseas. **Pub:** Booklets. Various booklets on HIV/AIDS and sex education. **Frmly:** (2002) AIDS Education and Research Trust.

★ 1586 ★ Azerbaijan Stomatological Association

Tabriz St. 102
370033 Baku, Azerbaijan
Phone: 994 12 412081 **Fax:** 994 12 412081
Email: asa@aznetmail.com

Fnded: 1997. Mem: 500. Desc: Medical professionals performing stomatological procedures.

★ 1587 ★ BACCHUS and Gamma Peer Education Network
National Headquarters
PO Box 100430
Denver, CO 80250
Phone: (303)871-0901 **Fax:** (303)871-0907
Email: admin@bacchusgamma.org
Website: http://www.bacchusgamma.org
Drew Hunter, Exec. Dir.

Fnded: 1975. **Mem:** 24,500. **Nat'l Groups:** 3. **Reg. Groups:** 13. **State Groups:** 49. **Local Groups:** 750. **Desc:** Students, advisors, faculty, and staff of colleges and universities in the U.S., Canada, and Mexico. Primary mission is to deliver alcohol abuse prevention and health education to college students and their communities. Promotes responsible decisions and healthy lifestyles and discourages irresponsible or illegal use of alcohol. Encourages year-round prevention and education programs and activities. Operates: Project GAMMA (Greeks Advocating Mature Management of Alcohol), a cooperative effort between BACCHUS and national greek-letter organizations to increase undergraduate participation in alsohol education programs; National Collegiate Alcohol Awareness Week; and Safe Spring Break. Offers the Certified Peer Educator Training Progam, a skill-based training curriculum for students. (Bacchus is the acronym for Boost Alcohol Consciousness Concerning the Health of University Students and the name of the Roman god of wine.) **Pub:** *The Bacchus Beat*, monthly. Newsletter. *Price:* Free for members. • *CPE Training Series*. • Catalog.Lists educational materials. • Newsletter, 10/year. • Pamphlets. • Videos. **Frmly:** (1993) BACCHUS of the U.S.

★ 1588 ★ BackCare, The Charity for Healthy Backs
16 Elmtree Rd.
Teddington TW11 8ST, United Kingdom
Phone: 44 208 9775474 **Fax:** 44 208 9435318
Email: website@backcare.org.uk
Website: http://www.backcare.org.uk

Fnded: 1968. **Mem:** 6,000. **Local Groups:** 50. **Lang(s):** English. **Desc:** Back pain sufferers, osteopaths, chiropractors, medical doctors, and safety and training officers in 12 countries. Sponsors research on the causes and treatment of back pain. Teaches individuals to use their bodies sensibly in order to prevent spinal damage. Promotes the formation of local branches. Keeps back pain sufferers informed on current developments in research, education, treatment and equipment. **Pub:** *A Carer's Guide to Moving and Handling Patients*. Manual. • *Guide to the Handling of Patients*. Fourth edition. • *Safer Handling of People in the Community*. Manual. • *TalkBack*, quarterly. Magazine. **Frmly:** (2000) National Back Pain Association.

★ 1589 ★ Bahrain Diabetic Association
PO Box 29080
Bahrain, Bahrain
Phone: 973 252822 **Fax:** 973 400488
Email: fzurba@batelco.com.bh

Desc: Individuals in Bahrain with diabetes. Seeks to assist and inform diabetic individuals. Furthers public understanding of diabetes by disseminating information.

★ 1590 ★ Balearic Association of Stutterers Association
c/o Marina Llobera-Martorell
Rector Vives 133
E-07015 Palma de Mallorca, Spain
Phone: 34 971 402237 **Fax:** 34 971 718730
Email: marina@arrakis.es

Desc: Works to find a cure for stuttering in Spain.

★ 1591 ★ Balkan Academy of Cosmetic Surgery
c/o Dr. Nikolay P. Serdev, Chm.
Medical Centre - Aesthetic Surgery
Aesthetic Medicine
11 20th April St.
BG-1606 Sofia, Bulgaria
Phone: 359 2 9524652 **Fax:** 359 2 9515668
Email: nserdev@infocom.bg
Website: http://www.ijacbs.com/index.htm

Desc: Represents physicians and dentists residing in the Balkan region countries performing cosmetic surgery procedures.

★ 1592 ★ Bangladesh Dental Society
PO Box 4168
Dhaka 1000, Bangladesh
Phone: 880 2 418469 **Fax:** 880 2 2837718

Fnded: 1977. **Mem:** 800. **Lang(s):** Bangla, English. **Desc:** Dental surgeons. Promotes prevention, treatment, and reduction of oral and dental disease. Works to improve the standard of dental practice and to enhance the professional standing of members. Conducts charitable, educational, and children's programs. **Pub:** *Bangladesh Dental Journal*, quarterly. Journal.

★ 1593 ★ Bangladesh Medical Association of North America (BMA)
c/o S. Hasan
43700 Woodward, Ste. 210
Bloomfield Hills, MI 48302
Fax: (248)338-9520
Website: http://www.heartburnnet.com
F. Hasan, MD, Sec.

Fnded: 1982. **Mem:** 200. **Desc:** Physicians who are from Bangladesh or have graduated from a medical college in Bangladesh. Seeks to bring together and improve communication between physicians who are of Bangladeshi origin or have trained in Bangladesh, and are currently residents of the United States or Canada, and other physicians. Assists medical students and physicians in obtaining specialized medical training and in post-training job placement in North America.

★ 1594 ★ Bangladesh Medical Studies and Research Institute (BMSRI)
35 H Rd., No. 14 A
Dhanmondi Residential Area
Dhaka, Bangladesh
Phone: 880 2 9120792 **Fax:** 880 2 9125655
Email: bmch@bangla.net

Fnded: 1984. **Mem:** 15. **Lang(s):** English. **Desc:** Promotes medical studies and research with the object of raising the standard of medical education in Bangladesh. Encourages growth in Bangladesh's pharmaceutical, medical, and surgical instrument industries. Conducts research in disease prevention and treatment and on medical applications of indigenous plants and herbs. Offers refresher courses and monthly academic seminar; organizes conferences, lectures, seminars, and study groups. Operates speakers' bureau. Maintains the Bangladesh Medical College which grants degrees in medicine and surgery and the Dental College which grants degrees in dentistry. **Pub:** *Annual Report and Prospectus*, annual. Directory. • *Bangladesh Medical College*, quarterly. Journal.

★ 1595 ★ Barbados Association of Medical Practitioners (BAMP)
c/o Dr. Ermine Belle, Pres.
BAMP Complex
Spring Garden
Saint Michael, Barbados
Phone: (246)429-7569 **Fax:** (246)435-2328
Email: bamp@sunbeach.net
Website: http://www.bamp.org.bb

Mem: 375. **Desc:** Promotes the medical and allied sciences and better health education of the community. Aims to maintain the honor and interests of the medical profession.

★ 1596 ★ Barbados Cancer Society (BCS)
Henry's Ln.
Collymore Rock
Saint Michael, Barbados
Phone: (246)436-8888 **Fax:** (246)429-3227
Email: info@barbacan.com
Website: http://www.barbadoscancersociety.com

Fnded: 1980. **Mem:** 2,500. **Local Groups:** 1. **Lang(s):** English. **Desc:** Doctors, nurses, social workers, and other concerned individuals. Researches cancer prevention methods and treatment strategies for cancer patients. Assists in coordinating efforts to reduce Barbadian mortality from cancer. Provides occupational therapy, transportation, and early detection services. Encourages efforts to educate the public in the problems, symptoms, and treatment of cancer; disseminates information. Aids in establishing and furthering cancer research activities. Sponsors researchers to attend international conferences and training sessions. Visits schools and distributes literature; offers financial assistance to children who have lost a parent to cancer. Maintains speakers' bureau. Works in cooperation with the American Cancer Society. Maintains facilities for mammography, ultrasound, biopsies, and tobacco control program. **Pub:** *Newsletter*, 3/year. Newsletter.

★ 1597 ★ Barbados Dental Association (BDA)
17 Pine Rd., Belleville
Saint Michael, Barbados
Phone: (246)228-6488 **Fax:** (246)429-8483

Fnded: 1965. **Mem:** 34. **Local Groups:** 1. **Lang(s):** English. **Desc:** Promotes dentistry and the interests of dental professionals in Barbados; works to improve the dental and general health of the public. Conducts educational programs at schools. Offers competitions for school children to foster dental health awareness.

★ 1598 ★ Barbados Family Planning Association (BFPA)
Bay St.
Saint Michael, Barbados
Phone: (246)426-2027 **Fax:** (246)427-6611
Email: bfpa@mail.sunbeach.net

Fnded: 1954. **Lang(s):** English. **Desc:** Promotes family planning as a basic human right. Encourages family planning activities in Barbados. Offers educational programs in family planning, sexually transmitted diseases, and health care. Provides contraceptive services. Acts as an advocate for family planning on a national level. **Pub:** *Annual Report*, annual, always May. • *Family*, semiannual. Newsletter.

★ 1599 ★ Baromedical Nurses Association (BNA)
PO Box 18994
Denver, CO 80218-0994
Phone: (303)918-9686 **Fax:** (303)282-7031
Website: http://www.hyperbaricnurses.org
Harry Vincent, Pres.

Fnded: 1985. **Mem:** 160. **Reg. Groups:** 6. **Desc:** Registered nurses practicing baromedicine (hyperbaric medicine), involved in research related to baromedical nursing, completing basic orientation in baromedicine, or contributing to literature on baromedicine or baromedical nursing. Defines, develops, and promotes the status and standards of baromedical nursing. Facilitates professional activities and continuing education programs. Provides a forum for the exchange of ideas, information, and support; maintains speakers' bureau. **Pub:** *BNA Update*, quarterly. Newsletter. Includes research findings, safety and educational information, and upcoming events. *Price:* Free. For members only. • Membership Directory, periodic.

★ 1600 ★ Bates Association for Vision Education
Savoy Court Hotel
11-15 Cavendish Pl.
Eastbourne BN1 3EJ, United Kingdom

Fax: 44 870 2417458
Email: info@seeing.org
Website: http://www.seeing.org

Fnded: 1954. **Mem:** 28. **Lang(s):** English. **Desc:** Teachers of Bates Method vision education. To advance the knowledge and practice of vision education. **Pub:** *Vision Education News*, quarterly. Newsletter. **Frmly:** (1989) London Association of Eyesight Training; (1999) Bates Association of Great Britain.

★ 1601 ★ Bath Institute for Rheumatic Diseases

Trim Bridge
Bath BA1 1HD, United Kingdom
Phone: 44 1225 448444 **Fax:** 44 1225 336809

Desc: Promotes the study of rheumatic diseases.

★ 1602 ★ Batten Disease Support and Research Association (BDSRA)

120 Humphries Dr., Ste. 2
Reynoldsburg, OH 43068
Phone: (740)927-4298 **Free:** 800-448-4570
Email: bdsra1@bdsra.org
Website: http://www.bdsra.org
Lance W. Johnson, Exec. Dir.

Fnded: 1987. **Mem:** 900. **State Groups:** 18. **Desc:** Families of children afflicted with Batten Disease; health care professionals; interested others. (Batten Disease, is a degenerative neurological disease affecting children, causing seizures, dementia, loss of motor skills, and blindness.) Represents the interest of individuals with Batten; seeks to educate the public and professional community concerning the needs of Battens Disease patients. Provides information and referral services. Conducts support group activities. Maintains registry. **Pub:** *Family Directory*, annual. Directory. *Price:* Free; available to member families only. • *Illuminator*, quarterly. Newsletter. Provides information on research, education, meetings, and other topics of interest. *Price:* Free.

★ 1603 ★ BC Wheelchair Sports Association

1367 W Broadway, Ste. 224
Vancouver, BC, Canada V6H 4A9
Phone: (604)737-3090 **Free:** 877-737-3090
Fax: (604)737-6043
Email: info@bcwheelchairsports.com
Website: http://www.bcwheelchairsports.com

Fnded: 1967. **Mem:** 800. **Reg. Groups:** 5. **Local Groups:** 5. **Lang(s):** English, French. **Desc:** Assists wheelchair sport development through advocacy, marketing, and providing information and resources. Works in close partnership with community groups and agencies to ensure that there are opportunities for participation. Supports participation froma recreational to elite level in a wide variety of sports. **Pub:** *The Newswheel*, 3/year. Newsletter. **Frmly:** (1996) Canadian Wheelchair Sports Association.

★ 1604 ★ Beckwith-Wiedemann Support Network (BWSN)

2711 Colony Rd.
Ann Arbor, MI 48104
Phone: (734)973-0263 **Free:** 800-837-2976
Fax: (734)973-9721
Email: a800bwsn@aol.com
Website: http://www.beckwith-wiedemann.org
Susan Fettes, Pres.

Fnded: 1989. **Mem:** 500. **Desc:** Patients with Beckwith-Wiedemann Syndrome and their families; health care professionals; interested others. Works to provide information and peer support to individuals and families affected by Beckwith-Wiedemann Syndrome (BWS). (BWS is a congenital growth-related disorder. Patients are at risk for developing hypoglycemia and various tumors.) Seeks to increase public and professional awareness of BWS. Encourages research on the cause, early detection, and treatment of BWS as well as Simpson Golabi-Belomel Syndrome. **Pub:** *Beckwith Wiedeman Support Network Newsletter*, 3/year. Newsletter. *Price:* included in membership dues. • *Family Directory for Parent Members*. Directory. • *What Is Beckwith-Wiedemann Syndrome*. Brochure.

★ 1605 ★ Befrienders International (BI)

c/o The Samaratans
Upper Mill
Kingston Rd.
Ewell KT1 1JH, United Kingdom
Phone: 44 208 5414949 **Fax:** 44 208 5411544
Email: jo@samaritans.org
Website: http://www.befrienders.org

Fnded: 1974. **Mem:** 30,000. **Nat'l Groups:** 34. **Reg. Groups:** 7. **Local Groups:** 318. **Lang(s):** English. **Desc:** Mission is to build effective suicide prevention services resourced by volunteers throughout the world. **Pub:** *Befriending Worldwide*, quarterly. Newsletter. **Frmly:** (1991) Befrienders International Samaritans Worldwide.

★ 1606 ★ Behavior Genetics Association (BGA)

c/o Deborah Finkel
Indiana University SE
Department of Psychology
New Albany, IN 47150
Phone: (812)941-2668 **Fax:** (812)941-2591
Email: nancy.pedersen@mep.ki.se
Website: http://www.bga.org
Nancy Pedersen, Pres.

Fnded: 1971. **Mem:** 400. **Desc:** Individuals engaged in teaching or research in some area of behavior genetics. Purposes are: to promote the scientific study of the interrelationship of genetic mechanisms and human and animal behavior through sponsorship of scientific meetings, publications, and communications among and by members; to encourage and aid the education and training of research workers in the field of behavior genetics; to aid in public dissemination and interpretation of information concerning the interrelationship of genetics and behavior and its implications for health, human development, and education. **Pub:** *Behavior Genetics*, bimonthly. Journal. Includes research reports. *Price:* Included in membership dues; $240/year for nonmembers in the U.S.; $267/year for nonmembers outside the U.S.

★ 1607 ★ Belgian Federation of Psychologists

Galerie Agora, Office 421
rue du Marche aux Herbes 105/18
B-1000 Brussels, Belgium
Phone: 32 2 5147509 **Fax:** 32 2 5147510
Email: bfp@skynet.be
Website: http://www.bfp-fbp.be

Desc: Umbrella organization for psychological societies in Belgium.

★ 1608 ★ Belgian Royal Society of Dermatology and Venerology (BSD) (Societe Royale Belge de Dermatologie et Venerologie)

Av. E Demot 14 69
B-1000 Brussels, Belgium
Phone: 32 2 6475399 **Fax:** 32 2 6466227

Fnded: 1901. **Mem:** 600. **Lang(s):** Dutch, English, French. **Desc:** Dermatologists and other scientists interested in dermatology. Conducts biennial postgraduate course. **Pub:** *Dermatology*, 10/year.

★ 1609 ★ Belgian Society of Cardiology

Elyzeese-Veldenstraat
43 rue des Champs Elysees
B-1050 Brussels, Belgium
Phone: 32 2 6446232 **Fax:** 32 2 6444830
Email: lisa.hobbs@bvc-sbc.be
Website: http://www.bscardio.be

Fnded: 1936. **Mem:** 400. **Desc:** Promotes the study of cardiology in Belgium. **Pub:** *ActaCardiologica*. Journal.

★ 1610 ★ Belgian Society of Fundamental and Clinical Physiology and Pharmacology (Societe Belge de Physiologie et de Pharmacologie Fondamentales et Cliniques)

c/o Philippe Lebrun
Universite Libre de Bruxelles
Lab. Pharmacodynamie et Therapeutique
Faculte de Medecine
route de Lennik 808, bat G
B-1070 Brussels, Belgium
Phone: 32 2 5556221 **Fax:** 32 2 5556356
Email: plebrun@ulb.ac.be

Mem: 305. **Desc:** Promotes fundamental and clinical physiology and pharmacology in Belgium.

★ 1611 ★ Belgian Society of Gerontology and Geriatrics

Nieuwpoort Steenweg 57
B-8400 Oostende, Belgium
Phone: 32 59553404 **Fax:** 32 59519943
Email: jpbaeyens@skynet.be
Website: http://www.geriatrie.be

Desc: Promotes gerontological research, training in the field of aging, and interests of gerontological organizations in international affairs.

★ 1612 ★ Belgian Veterinary Association (Union Syndicat Veterinaire Belge — USVB)

c/o Prof. P.L. Leroy
Department of Genetics
Faculty of Veterinary Medicine
University of Liege
B-1060 Liege, Belgium
Phone: 32 4 3664120 **Fax:** 32 4 3664122
Email: leroy@stat.fmv.ulg.ac.be
Website: http://www.ulg.ac.be/fmv/bvca/

Lang(s): Dutch, English, French. **Desc:** Representatives from all branches of veterinary science. Represents and protects the interests of veterinarians. **Pub:** *Veterinaria*, monthly.

★ 1613 ★ Belize Family Life Association (BFLA)

Old Hospital Bldg.
Eve St., PO Box 529
Belize City, Belize
Phone: 501 2 31018 **Fax:** 501 2 32667
Email: bfla@btl.net

Fnded: 1985. **Mem:** 5,000. **Lang(s):** English. **Desc:** Works to enhance the quality of life in Belize through promotion of family planning and maternal and infant health care. Encourages public awareness of methods of contraception. Offers educational programs in family planning, sex education, and health care. Conducts AIDS education and counselling. Provides contraceptive services. Also provides diagnosis and treatment of STDs, testing for cervical cancer, and counselling and support (including pre-natal education and post-natal services) for young parents. **Pub:** *Annual Report*, annual. Report. • *Information Sheets*. • *Journey*, quarterly. Newsletter. • Brochures.

★ 1614 ★ Bellwoods Centres for Community Living (BCCL)

789 Don Mill Rd., Ste. 701
Toronto, ON, Canada M3C 1T5
Phone: (416)696-9663 **Fax:** (416)696-9481
Email: hapurre@bellwoodscentres.org

Lang(s): English, French. **Desc:** Community living centers serving adults with physical disabilities. Seeks to improve the quality of life of individuals with physical disabilities residing in community living facilities. Provides support and services to increase the self-reliance of people with physical disabilities; facilitates communication and cooperation among members.

★ 1615 ★ Belorussian Scientific Society of Cardiologists
Belorussian Research Institute of Cardiology
110 Luxembourg St.
220036 Minsk, Belarus
Phone: 375 172 567634 **Fax:** 375 172 567634
Email: pharm@bcsmi.minsk.by
Website: http://www.escardio.org/society/natsoc/Belorussia.htm

Fnded: 1964. **Mem:** 50. **Reg. Groups:** 6. **Desc:** Promotes the study of cardiology in Belarus, including instrumental investigation methods on cardiology, cardiosurgery, coronary heart disease, and drug therapy and nonmedicamentous treatment of arterial hypertension. **Pub:** Reports.

★ 1616 ★ BeNeLux Association of Bariatric Surgeons (BABS)
Vromenhove 13
B-2070 Zwijdrecht, Belgium
Phone: 32 3 2528103 **Fax:** 32 3 2528103
Email: luc.lemmens@pandora.be
Website: http://www.babsweb.org/

Fnded: 1996. **Mem:** 100. **Desc:** Promotes discussion on surgical treatment; brings together health care specialists of all disciplines to improve treatment; provides standards and guidelines of treatment.

★ 1617 ★ Benign Essential Blepharospasm Research Foundation (BEBRF)
PO Box 12468
Beaumont, TX 77726-2468
Phone: (409)832-0788 **Fax:** (409)832-0890
Email: bebrf@ih2000.net
Website: http://www.blepharospasm.org/
Bob Campbell, Contact

Fnded: 1981. **Mem:** 8,900. **Reg. Groups:** 4. **State Groups:** 50. **Local Groups:** 170. **Desc:** Victims of benign essential blepharospasm (BEB), a rare disorder of unknown cause characterized by an involuntary forcible closure of the eyelids. Purpose is to undertake, promote, and develop research into the cause and cure of BEB and related disorders and infirmities of the facial musculature, such as Meige's Syndrome (involving muscle spasms of the eyes, lower face, mouth, tongue, throat, and respiratory system). Seeks to foster public awareness of the disorder in order to guarantee detection at the onset of symptoms. Encourages continuity and cooperation among neurologists, neuro-ophthalmologists, ophthalmologists, plastic surgeons, psychologists, psychiatrists, and other medical professionals in rendering correct diagnoses, implementing effective treatment, improving surgical procedure, and discovering a cure. Organizes seminars, clinical studies, and other programs in continuing education; sponsors fundraising activities. Endeavors to locate sufferers of the disorder and to compile data in order to determine the incidence of BEB and to advise on available treatment. Carries out research activities in areas such as brain tissue collection and experimental treatments. **Pub:** *BEBRF Newsletter*, bimonthly. Newsletter. Includes research reports and statistics, medical articles, patient stories. *Price:* $15/year. • *Blepharospasm and Related Disorders. Price:* $16. • *Physician Reprint Articles.* Articles. • Pamphlets.

★ 1618 ★ Benjamin Franklin Literary and Medical Society (BFLMS)
1100 Waterway Blvd.
Indianapolis, IN 46202
Phone: (317)636-8881 **Fax:** (317)639-0126
Email: satevepst@aol.com
Website: http://www.satevepost.org
Dr. Cory SerVaas, Pres. /CEO

Fnded: 1976. **Mem:** 2300,000. **Desc:** Individuals, industries, and businesses united to support research and promote sciences, literature, and the arts in order to achieve greater public understanding of science and the humanities. Major emphasis is on the dissemination of health, preventive medicine, and nutrition information to the health community and the public. Advocates a preventive approach to health care including proper nutrition, daily exercise, and good health habits. Offers training in cardiopulmonary resuscitation and other life-saving skills; conducts health education programs. Sponsors the Children's Better Health Institute, which publishes material designed to educate children of preschool through elementary school levels on health, nutrition, safety, and exercise, and provides parents with medical information concerning infants and children. Operates Medical Education and Research Foundation, which disseminates medical information in lay terms, covering concepts and developments in preventive medicine, safety procedures and techniques, health dangers, proper dietary habits, and reports on new and developing treatments and medications for cancer patients and techniques used for early detection of cancer. Sponsors the Saturday Evening Post Society which conducts national health surveys; publicizes advances in science, medicine, nutrition, and preventive medicine; funds research projects; and encourages commercial manufacturers to produce innovative health equipment. Is named for Benjamin Franklin (1706-90), who founded the Pennsylvania Gazette in 1728, which eventually became the Saturday Evening Post. (The society purchased this magazine from the Curtis Publishing Company in 1982.) Franklin was also a strong supporter of the arts and sciences. **Pub:** *Child Life*, 8/year. Magazine. Promotes reading and good health habits in children between the ages of seven and nine. Includes "Ask the Doctor" column, poems, and short stories. *Price:* $14.95/year. • *Children's Digest*, 8/year. Magazine. Promotes reading and good health habits in children between the ages of eight and ten. Includes book reviews. *Price:* $14.95/year. • *Children's Playmate Magazine*, 8/year. Magazine. Promotes reading and good health habits for children between the ages of five and seven. Includes book reviews. *Price:* $14.95/year. • *Humpty Dumpty*, 8/year. Magazine. Promotes reading and good health habits for children between the ages of four and six. *Price:* $14.95/year. • *Jack and Jill*, 8/year. Magazine. Promotes reading and good health habits for children between the ages of six and eight. *Price:* $14.95/year. • *Mecidal Update Newsletter*, monthly. Newsletter. Includes foundation news and research updates. *Price:* $12/year. • *Saturday Evening Post*, bimonthly. • *Turtle Magazine for Preschool Kids*, 8/year. Magazine. Promotes reading and good health, safety, and nutrition habits for children between the ages of two and five. Includes book reviews. *Price:* $14.95/year.

★ 1619 ★ Bermuda Dental Association (BDA)
c/o Dr. Laidlaw Fraser-Smith
PO Box HM 3059
Hamilton HM NX, Bermuda
Phone: (441)295-2452 **Fax:** (441)292-7678
Email: bdadental@ibl.bm
Website: http://www.bermudadental.bm/

Mem: 25. **Lang(s):** English. **Desc:** Dentists in Bermuda. Promotes dentistry; represents members' interests. Sponsors study club.

★ 1620 ★ Berufsverband der Pharmaberater (BP)
Europahaus
Postfach 18 30
D-67547 Worms, Germany
Phone: 49 6241 24239 **Fax:** 49 6241 24239
Email: bdp-wo@t-online.de
Website: http://www.pharmaberater-bdp.de

Fnded: 1973. **Mem:** 1,500. **Lang(s):** German. **Desc:** Medical advisers. Promotes professional advancement of members. Represents members' interests before industrial organizations, government agencies, and the public.

★ 1621 ★ Better Hearing Australia (BHA)
5 High St.
Prahran, VIC 3181, Australia
Phone: 61 3 95101577 **Fax:** 61 3 95106076
Email: bhavic@betterhearing.org.au
Website: http://www.betterhearing.org.au

Fnded: 1940. **Mem:** 3,000. **Local Groups:** 18. **Desc:** Adults with acquired deafness. Works toward the rehabilitation of the deaf; represents the hearing impaired before government. Provides hearing education and rehabilitation activities. **Pub:** *Better Hearing*, quarterly.

★ 1622 ★ Better Hearing Institute (BHI)
515 King St., Ste. 420
Alexandria, VA 22314
Phone: (703)684-3391 **Free:** 800-EAR-WELL
Fax: (703)684-6048
Email: mail@betterhearing.org
Website: http://www.betterhearing.org
John T. Olive, Jr., Exec. Dir.

Fnded: 1973. **Desc:** Professionals and others dedicated to helping persons with impaired hearing. Purpose is to inform the public about the nature of hearing loss and the available medical, surgical, rehabilitative, and amplification help. Methods of communication used include television and radio public service announcements, films, speakers' bureaus, booklets, editorial publicity, and exhibits. Produces general information and education kits of communication tools. Maintains telephone service that provides information on hearing loss and help to callers from anywhere in the United States and Canada. **Pub:** Pamphlets.

★ 1623 ★ Better Sleep Council (BSC)
501 Wythe St.
Alexandria, VA 22314
Phone: (703)683-8371 **Fax:** (703)683-4503
Email: bsc@sleepproducts.org
Website: http://www.bettersleep.org
Nancy Blatt, Exec. Dir.

Fnded: 1978. **Desc:** Bedding manufacturers and suppliers organized to increase public awareness of the importance of sleep to good health, quality of life, and the role of the sleep system in pursuit of a good night's sleep. **Pub:** *Better Sleep Guide.* Brochure. A consumer guide to sleep and mattresses. • Also publishes press kits. **Frmly:** (1987) Better Sleep Council (of the National Association of Bedding Manufacturers); (1993) Better Sleep Council (of the International Sleep Products Association).

★ 1624 ★ Better Vision Institute (BVI)
1700 Diagonal Rd., Ste. 500
Alexandria, VA 22314
Phone: (703)548-4560 **Free:** 877-642-3253
Fax: (703)548-4580
Email: vca@visionsite.org
Website: http://www.visionsite.org
Joe LaMountain, VP of Strategic Commun.

Fnded: 1929. **Mem:** 500. **Desc:** Advisory council of the Vision Council of America. Carried out in consultation with a board of eye care professionals who inform the public of the need for more adequate vision care. **Pub:** *BVI News Bureau*, periodic. Contains press releases of various eyecare and eyewear information. *Price:* Free. • *Perspective.* Article. • Pamphlets. • Also publishes charts, posters, and press releases; produces school kits and counter displays for vision care practitioners, schools, and the public.

★ 1625 ★ Beverly Foundation (BF)
566 El Dorado St., No. 100
Pasadena, CA 91101-2560
Phone: (626)792-2292 **Fax:** (626)792-6117
Email: bf3@ix.netcom.com
Website: http://www.beverlyfoundation.org/
Helen Kerschner, Pres.

Fnded: 1978. **Desc:** Develops education and research programs and policy studies to facilitate long-term health care and supportive services and life quality of people with chronic-care needs, particularly older adults, their families, and caregivers. The focus is on optimal functional independence and an informed public. Unrestricted income is derived from product sales, interest, dividends, donations, and grants. Restricted funds are sought to support new program developments which focus on improving service systems and methods of long-term care. Sells educational materials to health care industry. Maintains library. **Pub:** *Pioneering Times*, biennial. Newsletter. *Price:* Free.

★ 1626 ★ Big Picture Alliance
1315 Walnut St., Ste. 1616
Philadelphia, PA 19107-4716
Phone: (215)735-5750 **Fax:** (215)735-9291
Email: BPAinfo@aol.com
Website: http://www.bigpicturealliance.com/newsite/frame/index_2.html
Jeffrey A. Seder, Exec. Dir.

Fnded: 1976. **Mem:** 50. **Desc:** Supports projects on anti-violence. Conducts research; compiles statistics. Supports vocational education in media field in inner-city minority communities via a project called "The Childrens Film Festival". **AKA:** (1995) Association for The Advancement of Social Potential. **Frmly:** (1997) Association for the Advancement of Sports Potential.

★ 1627 ★ Bill and Melinda Gates Foundation
PO Box 23350
Seattle, WA 98102
Phone: (206)709-3140
Email: libraryinfo@gatesfoundation.org
Website: http://www.gatesfoundation.org
Richard Akeroyd, Exec. Dir.

Desc: Strives to help improve people's lives through health and learning and looks for strategic opportunities to extend the benefits of modern science and technology to people around the world.

★ 1628 ★ BioCommunications Association (BCA)
220 Southwind Ln.
Hillsborough, NC 27278
Phone: (919)245-0906 **Fax:** (919)245-0906
Email: bcaoffice@aol.com
Website: http://bca.org
Nancy Hurtgen, Central Office Admin.

Fnded: 1931. **Mem:** 350. **Local Groups:** 29. **Desc:** Photographers, technicians, doctors, scientists, educators, and others concerned with photography in the health sciences and related fields. Seeks to advance the techniques of biophotography and biomedical communications through meetings, seminars, and workshops. Has established Board of Registry to offer qualifying examinations for Registered Biological Photographer. **Pub:** *Journal of Biocommunication.* Journal. Published jointly with two other associations. **Frmly:** (2001) Biological Photographic Association.

★ 1629 ★ Biofeedback Certification Institute of America (BCIA)
10200 W 44th Ave., Ste. 310
Wheat Ridge, CO 80033-2840
Phone: (303)420-2902 **Fax:** (303)422-8894
Email: bcia@resourcenter.com
Website: http://www.bica.org/

Fnded: 1981. **Desc:** Committed to establish and maintain professional standards for the provision of biofeedback services and to certify those who meet the standards.

★ 1630 ★ Biofeedback Foundation of Europe (BFE)
PO Box 75416
NL-1070 AK Amsterdam, Netherlands
Phone: 31 20 4422631 **Fax:** 31 20 4422632
Email: mail@bfe.org
Website: http://www.bfe.org

Fnded: 1996. **Lang(s):** Dutch, English. **Desc:** Health professionals and clinicians with an interest in biofeedback. Seeks to advance the study, teaching, and practice of biofeedback techniques. Conducts training and continuing professional development courses; serves as a clearinghouse on biofeedback. **Pub:** *Psychophysiology and Biofeedback Journal*, periodic. Journal.

★ 1631 ★ Biomagnetic Therapy Association (BTA)
PO Box 394
Lyons, CO 80540
Phone: (303)823-0307
Email: info@biomagnetic.org
Website: http://www.biomagnetic.org
Suzy Balliett, Contact

Fnded: 1995. **Mem:** 150. **Desc:** Health care professionals and other individuals with an interest in biomagnetic therapy. Biomagnetic therapy is the art and science of applying and removing magnetic fields for health benefits. Seeks to advance the study and practice of biomagnetic therapy; promotes increased use of biomagnetic therapy in the treatment of a wide variety of disorders. Serves as a clearinghouse on biomagnetic and related therapies; conducts continuing professional education programs; sponsors research. **Pub:** *Biomagnetic Therapy Association Newsletter*, quarterly. *Price:* $45/year.

★ 1632 ★ Biomedical Engineering Association of Ireland (BEAI)
c/o Patrick Pentony
St. Vincents University Hospital
Department of Clinical Engineering
Elm Park 2, Dublin, Ireland
Phone: 353 1 2094073
Email: p.pentony@st-vincents.ie
Website: http://www.beai.org/

Fnded: 1990. **Nat'l Groups:** 1. **Reg. Groups:** 4. **Local Groups:** 6. **Lang(s):** English. **Desc:** Promotes biomedical and clinical engineering in Ireland. **Pub:** *Spectrum*, quarterly.

★ 1633 ★ Biomedical Engineering Society of South Africa
Medical School, Department of Biomedical Engineering
Observatory 7925, Republic of South Africa
Phone: 27 21 4066235 **Fax:** 27 21 4483291
Email: dbee@cormack.uct.ac.za

★ 1634 ★ Biomedical Research and Union University Experimental Therapeutics Society of Singapore (BRETSS)
c/o Prof. Vernon Oh Min Sen
Department of Medicine
National University Hospital
5 Lower Kent Ridge Rd.
Singapore 119074, Singapore
Phone: 65 7724355 **Fax:** 65 7794112
Email: mdcohms@nus.edu.sg
Website: http://www.bretss.org

Mem: 180. **Desc:** Promotes biomedical research and experimental therapeutics in Singapore.

★ 1635 ★ Biotech Medical Management Association (BMMA)
10592 Perry Hwy., No. 300
Wexford, PA 15090
Free: 888-990-2662 **Fax:** (724)934-8449
Email: contactus@bioastec.com
Website: http://www.bmma.org
Mark G. Fuller, MD, Contact

Fnded: 1993. **Desc:** Physicians and pharmacists involved in managed care insurance programs; insurance companies, pharmaceutical manufacturers, and other firms with an interest in managed care medicine; academic institutions, medical and insurance consultants, and health care representatives. Promotes establishment of national standards regulating medical and drug policies and the administration of medical and pharmacy benefits. Represents members before government agencies, industrial organizations, and the public; facilitates communication between biotechnology manufacturers and health care payers and providers; supports pharmaceutical research; conducts educational programs. **Pub:** *Journal of the Biotech Medical Management Association*, quarterly. Journal. Dedicated to new developments in biotechnology. *Price:* $120/yr.

★ 1636 ★ Birth Defect Research for Children (BDRC)
930 Woodcock Rd., Ste. 225
Orlando, FL 32803
Phone: (407)895-0802 **Fax:** (407)895-0824
Email: staff@birthdefects.org
Website: http://www.birthdefects.org
Betty Mekdeci, Exec. Dir.

Fnded: 1982. **Desc:** A national clearinghouse to provide services to parents and professionals caring for children with disabilities. Services include the collection of data on over 300 categories of birth defects and developmental disabilities, search for links between birth defects and the mother's/father's exposure to drugs or environmental agents, matching families of children with similar birth defects for mutual sharing and support, support group information, newsletters, a medical/scientific database, literature and research findings. **Pub:** *Birth Defect Fact Sheets.* Offers diagnosis, treatment, and support group information. • *Birth Defects News*, monthly. Newsletter. Electronic. Includes parent-to-parent column and a birth defects registry. *Price:* Free. • *Special Reports.* Reports. Comprehensive reports on important environmental birth defect issues. • *Why My Child?.* Videos. **Frmly:** (1982) Association of Benedictin Children; (2000) Association of Birth Defect Children.

★ 1637 ★ Black Coalition for AIDS Prevention (BCAP)
110 Spadina Ave., Ste. 207
Toronto, ON, Canada M5V 2K4
Phone: (416)977-9955 **Fax:** (416)977-7664
Email: blackcap@black-cap.com

Lang(s): English, French. **Desc:** Individuals concerned about the spread of HIV and AIDS in African Canadian communities. Promotes increased awareness of AIDS prevention techniques. Conducts educational programs; serves as a clearinghouse on AIDS prevention.

★ 1638 ★ Black Mental Health Alliance (BMHA)
733 W 40th St., Ste. 10
Baltimore, MD 21211
Phone: (410)338-2642 **Fax:** (410)338-1771
Email: bhealthall@aol.com
Website: http://bmhaec.org
Tracee E. Bryant, Exec. Dir.

Fnded: 1984. **Mem:** 250. **Reg. Groups:** 1. **State Groups:** 1. **Local Groups:** 1. **Desc:** Seeks to increase clinicians, clergy, educators, and social service professionals awareness of African-Americans mental health needs and concerns on issues including stress, violence, racism, substance abuse, and parenting. Provides consultation, public information, and resource referrals. Conducts a public awareness campaign; educates the community about available resources; develops programs that benefit African-American children and families. Offers training to human service workers, teachers, police officers, and other service providers who work with culturally diverse populations. Maintains speakers' bureau. The support group provides emotional support, education and interaction for family members experiencing the stresses of caring for and/or living with a mentally ill relative. Provides a resource referral service; maintains an extensive list of African American mental health professionals who are sensitive to and appreciate cultural differences. Offers programs that invest in the needs of African American adult and adolescent females who are at risk of, or have, HIV or AIDS. Offers the "Free Yourself Stop Smoking and Prevention" program. **Pub:** *Visions*, quarterly. Newsletter. Contains updates, information, employment opportunities, community service information, and calendar. *Price:* Included in membership dues.

★ 1639 ★ Blair Chiropractic Society
c/o Todd A. Hubbard, D.C.
610 Plaza Dr., Ste. 2
Sycamore, IL 60178
Free: 877-732-6300
Email: hubchiro@tbcnet.com
Website: http://www.blairchiropracticsoc.org
Todd A. Hubbard, D.C., Contact

Desc: For practitioners using the Blair method of upper cervical chiropractic.

★ 1640 ★ Blind Children's Fund (BCF)
311 W Broadway St., Ste. 1
Mount Pleasant, MI 48858
Phone: (517)347-1357 **Fax:** (517)347-1459
Email: blindchildren@aol.com
Website: http://www.blindchildrensfund.org
Karla B. Storrer, Exec. Dir.

Fnded: 1978. **Mem:** 1,300. **Reg. Groups:** 1. **Desc:** Parents and teachers of visually handicapped children from birth to seven years old. Provides parents and professionals information, materials, and resources that help them successfully teach and nurture blind, visually impaired and multi-impaired children. **Pub:** *Get A Wiggle On*. Booklet. For parents of blind or visually impaired infants with suggestions for assisting development form birth to the walking stage. *Price:* $5. • *Get Ready. . .Get Set. . .Go!*. Teaches techniques for the parent or educator of the blind child, focusing on self-help skills. *Price:* $7. • *Learning to Look*. Book. For parents of severely visually impaired children. Contains specific suggestions on how to help your child use what vision she/he has or may have. *Price:* $9. • *Move It*. Booklet. Contains suggestions for the development of a preschool blind or visually impaired child from walking to school entrance age. *Price:* $5. • *Movement Education*. A movement curriculum for preschoolers. *Price:* $13. • *Parent Packet #1*. Booklet. Includes activities to teach skills at home, toys to make, how to stimulate language, and readings on blindness for parents and children. *Price:* $7. • *Our Kids Are Great!*. Parents of visually impaired children share short stories about what their children can do because of their help, love, and attention. *Price:* $3. • *VIP Newsletter*, quarterly. Newsletter. Contains information and articles for parents of blind or visually impaired children. *Price:* $10/year; $15/year outside of US. • *Watch Me Grow*. Book. Contains month by month suggestions for assisting the development of a blind or visually impaired infant from birth to age three. *Price:* $12. **Frmly:** (1987) International Institute for Visually Impaired.

★ 1641 ★ Blind Citizens Australia (BCA)
87 High St.
Prahran, VIC 3181, Australia
Phone: 61 3 95213433 **Fax:** 61 3 95213732
Email: bca@bca.org.au
Website: http://www.bca.org.au

Fnded: 1975. **Mem:** 3,000. **Reg. Groups:** 5. **State Groups:** 7. **Lang(s):** English. **Desc:** Blind and vision impaired people in Australia. Seeks to achieve equity and equality by empowering members, by promoting positive community attitudes, and by striving for high quality and accessible services. Provides advocacy, information dissemination, peer support, and consultancy and advice to governments, corporations and the community. **Pub:** *Blind Citizens News*, quarterly. Newsletter. Also available in Braille.

★ 1642 ★ Blind Service Association (BSA)
22 W Monroe, 11th Fl.
Chicago, IL 60603
Phone: (312)236-0808 **Fax:** (312)236-8679
Email: blindsrvc@aol.com
Debbie Grossman, Exec. Dir.

Fnded: 1924. **Mem:** 550. **Desc:** Organization that has supported the independence of blind and partially blind Chicago residents since 1924. The association maintains reading rooms for daily oral readings of textbooks and work-related material primarily to blind students, senior citizens, and business and professional people; records textbooks on cassette tapes for blind people's home, study, work and leisure needs; supplies visual aids, field trips, and other assistance to blind and visually handicapped children in Chicago, IL schools; operates senior program and a consortium of blind computer users.

★ 1643 ★ Blinded Veterans Association (BVA)
477 H St. NW
Washington, DC 20001
Phone: (202)371-8880 **Free:** 800-669-7079
Fax: (202)371-8258
Email: bva@bva.org
Website: http://www.bva.org
Thomas H. Miller, Exec. Dir.

Fnded: 1945. **Mem:** 10,000. **Reg. Groups:** 51. **Desc:** Veterans who lost their sight as a result of military service in the armed forces of the U.S.; associate members are veterans whose loss of sight was not connected with military service. Assists blinded veterans in attaining benefits and employment and with reestablishing themselves as adjusted, active, and productive citizens in their communities. Offers placement service; supports research programs; compiles statistics. Constructs initiatives designed to improve blind rehabilitation programs for veterans. **Pub:** *BVA Bulletin*, bimonthly. Newsletter. Reports on legislation, benefits, and Department of Veterans Affairs programs affecting blind veterans; also includes association news. *Price:* Free to blind veterans.

★ 1644 ★ Blue Cross and Blue Shield Association (BCBSA)
225 N Michigan Ave.
Chicago, IL 60611
Phone: (312)297-6000 **Fax:** (312)297-6609
Website: http://www.bluecares.com
Patrick G. Hays, Pres. and CEO

Fnded: 1982. **Desc:** Local Blue Cross and Blue Shield Plans in the U.S., and other licensees in Europe, Japan, and Jamaica. To promote the betterment of public health and security; to secure the widest public acceptance of voluntary nonprofit, prepayment of health services; to provide services to Blue Cross and Blue Shield Plans and licensees. Contracts with federal government as administrative agency for federal health progams; sponsors and conducts programs on health care and prepayment issues. Also publishes reports and pamphlets.

★ 1645 ★ Blue Heron Support Services Association (BHSSA)
PO Box 4238
Barrhead, AB, Canada T7N 1A2
Phone: (780)674-4944 **Fax:** (780)674-6294
Email: admin@bhssa.com
Website: http://www.bhssa.com

Lang(s): English, French. **Desc:** Rehabilitation centers. Seeks to advance rehabilitative therapies; promotes increased availability of rehabilitation services. Represents members' interests; conducts research and educational programs.

★ 1646 ★ Board for Certification in Pedorthics (BCP)
2517 Eastlake Ave. E, Ste. 200
Seattle, WA 98102
Phone: (206)329-0309 **Free:** 888-530-2733
Fax: (206)223-1178
Email: info@cpeds.org
Website: http://www.cpeds.org
David L. Stumph, CAE, Exec. Dir.

Fnded: 1958. **Mem:** 1,400. **Desc:** Certified Pedorthists. (Pedorthists fit and provide prescription footwear, footwear modifications and foot orthoses to clients referred by physicians.) Sponsors certification program; sets standards of practice in pedorthics and requires continuing education of certificants to maintain certification. **Pub:** *Pedorthic Candidate's Handbook*, annual. • *Study Guide for Pedorthic Skills Examination.*

★ 1647 ★ Board of Nephrology Examiners Nursing and Technology (BONENT)
PO Box 15945-282
Lenexa, KS 66285
Phone: (913)541-9077 **Fax:** (913)541-0156
Email: rjpcht@aol.com
Website: http://www.goamp.com/bonent/
RJ Picciano, Pres.

Fnded: 1974. **Mem:** 1,900. **Desc:** Registered nurses, licensed practical nurses, licensed vocational nurses, and dialysis technicians. Provides nephrology nursing and technology certification examinations. Through certification, seeks to ensure: safe, competent practitioners in nephrology nursing and technology; excellence in the quality of care of the nephrology patient; the continued study and advance of the science of nursing and technological fields in nephrology. Compiles statistics. **Pub:** *Bonent Update*, quarterly. Newsletter. *Price:* Included in membership dues. **Frmly:** (2002) Board of Nephrology Examiners - Nursing and Technology.

★ 1648 ★ Board for Orthotist/Prosthetist Certification
c/o Dr. D.O. Fedder, CEO
515 W Lombard St., 1st Fl.
Baltimore, MD 21201-1715
Phone: (410)539-3910 **Free:** 877-776-2200
Fax: (410)706-0869
Email: info@bocusa.org
Website: http://www.bocusa.org
Dr. D.O. Fedder, CEO

Fnded: 1984. **Desc:** Certifies orthotists and prosthetists based on comprehensive performance and examinations. Also accredits orthotic and prosthetic facilities and maintains a registry of Orthotic Fitters and Mastectomy Fitters. **Pub:** *BOC Report*, quarterly. Newsletter. • *Candidate Handbook*, annual. Handbook.

★ 1649 ★ Bockus International Society of Gastroenterology (BISG)
300 Community Dr.
Manhasset, NY 11030
Phone: (516)562-4281 **Fax:** (516)562-1688
Email: dbernste@nshs.edu
Dr. David Bernstein, Sec. Gen.

Fnded: 1958. **Mem:** 440. **Nat'l Groups:** 1. **Desc:** Physicians in 22 countries specializing in gastroenterology (the study of the anatomy, physiology, and pathology of the stomach and intestines). Furthers scientific advances in gastroenterology worldwide. (The society is named for noted gastroenterologist H.L. Bockus of Philadelphia, PA.) **Pub:** Proceedings, biennial.

★ 1650 ★ Body Positive
19 Fulton St., Ste. 308B
New York, NY 10038
Phone: (212)566-7333 **Free:** 800-566-6599
Fax: (212)566-4539
Email: bodypositive@bodypos.org
Website: http://www.thebody.com/bp/bp.html
Michael Dentato, Exec. Dir.

Fnded: 1987. **Mem:** 15,000. **Desc:** Provides support services for people who are HIV-infected or have AIDS, and their families and friends. Organizes seminars on treatment issues and socials. Provides outreach programs and recreational services. **Pub:** *Body Positive*, monthly. Newsletter. *Price:* $35 invidual. • *Positive Options*. Book. Book for people living with HIV/AIDS. • *Resource Directory*, 2/year. • *SIDA*, 6/year.

★ 1651 ★ BODYWHYS: Help, Support, Understanding for Anorexia and Bulimia Nervousa
PO Box 105
Blackrock, Dublin, Ireland
Phone: 353 1 2834963 **Fax:** 353 1 2834963
Email: info@bodywhys.ie
Website: http://www.bodywhys.ie

Fnded: 1995. **Local Groups:** 5. **Desc:** Offers support to people with/affected by eating disorders. Disseminates information to promote a better understanding of eating disorders. Runs self-help and support groups. Operates telephone helpline.

★ 1652 ★ Bone Marrow Donors Worldwide
Plesmanlaan 1B
NL-2333 BZ Leiden, Netherlands
Phone: 31 71 5685300 **Fax:** 31 71 5210457
Email: bmdw@europdonor.nl
Website: http://www.bmdw.org

Fnded: 1989. **Mem:** 80. **Desc:** Umbrella organization for bone marrow and cord blood registries. Promotes unrelated bone marrow and cord blood donation worldwide.

★ 1653 ★ Bone Marrow Foundation
337 E 88th St., Ste. 1B
New York, NY 10128
Phone: (212)838-3029 **Free:** 800-365-1336
Email: thebmf@bonemarrow.org
Website: http://www.bonemarrow.org/index.cfm?action=test&area=1
Christina Merrill, Exec. Dir.

Fnded: 1992. **Nat'l Groups:** 1. **Desc:** Works to improve quality of life for bone marrow and stem cell transplant patients and their families through financial aid, education, emotional support.

★ 1654 ★ Bones Society
6300 N River Rd., Ste. 727
Rosemont, IL 60018-4226
Free: 800-247-9699 **Fax:** (847)823-4921
Email: bones@aaos.org
Website: http://www.bonessociety.org

Fnded: 1969. **Mem:** 1,400. **Desc:** Solo practitioners, private group practices and university-affiliated groups of all sizes. Dedicated to the professional development of the orthopaedic practice administrator through educational and research programs and peer interaction.

★ 1655 ★ Boston International Foundation for Medical Exchange
c/o Joseph J. Vitale, MD
784 Massachusetts Ave.
Boston, MA 02118-2317
Phone: (617)414-4829
Email: jjvitale@bu.edu
Website: http://www.bifme.org
Joseph J. Vitale, Chm.

Fnded: 1996. **Mem:** 6. **Desc:** Supports senior medical students, medical and surgical residents and junior faculty from Harvard, Tufts and Boston University, who successfully complete a minimum two to six month elective at a foreign medical center acceptable to the respective medical school administration and the foundation. Support is intended to defray travel and living expenses. Believes this experience provides useful and practical insight into cultural, moral and ethnic perceptions of health care in our multi-ethnic and multi-cultural society.

★ 1656 ★ Boston Women's Health Book Collective/Our Bodies, Ourselves (OBOS)
34 Plympton St.
Boston, MA 02118
Phone: (617)451-3666 **Fax:** (617)451-3664
Email: office@bwhbc.org
Website: http://www.ourbodiesourselves.org
Judy Norsigian, Exec. Dir.

Fnded: 1969. **Desc:** Promotes increased awareness of women's health issues among health care professional and the public. Gathers and disseminates information on health topics of concern to women. Maintains speakers' bureau. **Pub:** *Nuestros Cuevpos, Nuestras Videas.* Book. Our Bodies Ourselves adapted for Latinas. *Price:* $24. • *Our Bodies, Ourselves for the New Century.* Book. Contains comprehensive information regarding women's health. *Price:* $24. **Frmly:** BWHBC; (2003) Boston Women's Health Book Collective.

★ 1657 ★ Braille Authority of North America (BANA)
919 Walnut St.
Philadelphia, PA 19107
Phone: (215)627-0600 **Free:** 800-223-1839
Fax: (215)922-0692
Email: dfgodz@asb.org
Website: http://www.brailleauthority.org/
Eileen Curran, Chairperson

Fnded: 1976. **Mem:** 12. **Desc:** Braille publishers, producers, and transcribers; representatives of consumer groups; educators of the visually handicapped; professional organizations. To promote and facilitate the use, teaching, and production of braille texts and other braille items. Promulgates rules, makes interpretations, and renders opinions concerning literary and technical braille codes and related forms and formats of embossed materials for the blind. **Pub:** *Braille Textbook Code Formats and Techniques.* Book. • *English Braille, American Edition.* • *Learning the Nemeth Code.* • *Nemeth Code of Braille Mathematics and Scientific Notation.* • Directory, annual.

★ 1658 ★ Braille Foundation of Uruguay (Fundacion Braille del Uruguay — FBU)
Durazno 1772
Blanes 1132
11200 Montevideo, Uruguay
Phone: 598 2 4095943 **Fax:** 598 2 4000789
Email: fbu@fbraille.com.uy
Website: http://www.fbraille.com.uy

Fnded: 1978. **Lang(s):** English, Spanish. **Desc:** Braille publishers, producers, transcribers, and others with an interest in the production of reading materials for the blind. Promotes the use, teaching, and production of braille texts and other braille items. Works to insure availability of braille materials nationwide.

★ 1659 ★ Braille Revival League (BRL)
57 Grandview Ave.
Watertown, MA 02472
Phone: (617)926-9198 **Free:** 800-424-8666
Fax: (617)923-0004
Email: kimcharlson@earthlink.net
Kim Charlson, Contact

Fnded: 1981. **Mem:** 1,000. **State Groups:** 6. **Desc:** Blind and visually impaired persons; professionals interested in promoting the use, production, and teaching of Braille. Encourages blind people to read and write in Braille; advocates the mandatory use of Braille instruction in educational facilities for the blind; promotes use of Braille material available through libraries and printing houses. Lends support to the Braille Authority of North America. Conducts research into Braille efficiency. **Pub:** *BRL Memorandum*, quarterly. Newsletter. Volumes are in Braille, large print, and computer diskette.

★ 1660 ★ Brain Injury Association of America
105 N Alfred St.
Alexandria, VA 22314
Phone: (703)236-6000 **Free:** 800-444-6443
Fax: (703)236-6001
Email: publicrelations@biausa.org
Website: http://www.biausa.org/Pages/splash.html
Allan I. Bergman, Pres. & CEO

Fnded: 1980. **Mem:** 43. **State Groups:** 43. **Local Groups:** 575. **Desc:** National organization working for and with people with brain injury and their families. Seeks to create a better future through brain injury prevention, research, education and advocacy. **Pub:** *Brain Injury Association CER Catalogue of Educational Resources*, annual. Catalog. Includes listings of books, articles, videotapes, audiocassette tapes, booklets, and other materials on head injury available through BIA. *Price:* Free. • *Brain Injury Awareness Presentation Kit.* Handbook. *Price:* $175. • *The Brain Injury Source*, quarterly. Magazine. *Price:* $32 annually. • *National Directory of Rehabilitation Services*, annual. Directory. *Price:* $16. • *TBI Challenge!*, bimonthly. Newsletter. *Price:* $25/year. **Frmly:** National Head Injury Foundation; (2002) Brain Injury Association.

★ 1661 ★ Brain Research Society of Finland (BRSF)
c/o Prof. Esa R. Korpi
University of Turku
Department of Pharmacology & Clinical Pharmacology
Itainen Pitkakatu 4
FIN-20520 Turku, Finland
Email: esa.korpi@utu.fi
Website: http://brain.utu.fi/

Mem: 200. **Desc:** Basic and clinical neuroscientists. Promotes basic and clinical research into the neurosciences.

★ 1662 ★ Brain Tumor Foundation of Canada (BTFC) (La Fondation Canadienne des tumeurs cerebrales)
650 Waterloo St., Ste. 100
London, ON, Canada N6B 2R4
Phone: (519)642-7755 **Free:** 800-265-5106
Fax: (519)642-7192
Email: btfc@btfc.org
Website: http://www.braintumour.ca

Fnded: 1982. **Desc:** Provides support services to those affected by brain tumors; promotes public awareness, education and funding. **Pub:** Handbooks.

★ 1663 ★ The Brain Tumor Society (TBTS)
124 Watertown St., Ste. 3-H
Watertown, MA 02472
Phone: (617)924-9997 **Free:** 800-770-8287
Fax: (617)924-9998
Email: info@tbts.org
Website: http://www.tbts.org
Neal P. Levitan, Exec. Dir.

Fnded: 1989. **Desc:** Strives to improve the quality of life of brain tumor patients by providing support for them and their families. Raises funds for research in order to find a cure for brain tumors. **Pub:** *Color Me Hope.* A Resource Guide for patients and families. *Price:* Free.

★ 1664 ★ Brainwave The Irish Epilepsy Association (BIEA)
249 Crumlin Rd.
Dublin 12, Ireland
Phone: 353 1 4557500
Email: info@epilepsy.ie
Website: http://www.epilepsy.ie

Fnded: 1967. **Mem:** 1,500. **Reg. Groups:** 9. **Lang(s):** English, Irish. **Desc:** Individuals and organizations. Seeks to improve the quality of life of people with epilepsy; promotes advancement in the diagnosis and treatment of epilepsy. Serves as a clearinghouse on epilepsy; provides support and assistance to people with epilepsy and their families and caregivers working with people with epilepsy. **Pub:** *Epilepsy News*, bimonthly. Magazine.

★ 1665 ★ Brazilian Association of Amyotrophic Lateral Sclerosis (Associacao Brasileira de Esclerose Lateral Amiotrofica)
Rua Pedro de Toledo 377
Villa Clementino
04039-000 Sao Paulo, SP, Brazil
Phone: 55 11 55792668 **Fax:** 55 11 55792668
Email: capovilla@usp.br
Website: http://www.alsmndalliance.org/directory/brazil.html

Fnded: 1998. **Reg. Groups:** 2. **State Groups:** 2. **Lang(s):** Portuguese. **Desc:** Individuals in Brazil affected by Amyotrophic Lateral Sclerosis (ALS), a muscle wasting condition. Provides a forum for support and exchange of information. Conducts research into development of multimedia communication systems for patients with severe motor and speech impairments.

★ 1666 ★ Brazilian Association of the Medical and Dental Equipment Industry (Associacao Brasileira da Industria de Artigos Equipamentos Medicos, Odontologicos Hospitalares e de Laboratorios — ABIMO)
Sala 806, Av. Paulista 1313
01311-923 Sao Paulo, Brazil
Phone: 55 11 2850155 **Fax:** 55 11 2850018

Nat'l Groups: s Medi. **State Groups:** iacao. **Local Groups:** ria de. **Lang(s):** , , , , , , , , ,.

★ 1667 ★ Brazilian Association for the Promotion of Appropriate Technology in Health Care (Associacao Brasileira de Tecnologia Alternativa na Promocao da Saude — TAPS)
Caixa Postal 11363
05422-970 Sao Paulo, SP, Brazil
Phone: 55 19 38263860 **Fax:** 55 19 38263860
Email: info@taps.org.br
Website: http://www.taps.org.br

Fnded: 1981. **Mem:** 40. **Lang(s):** Portuguese. **Desc:** Promotes primary health care in Brazil with emphasis on improving health through lifestyle and nutrition. Functional in the following areas: health and nutrition; publications, Website and counseling.

★ 1668 ★ Brazilian Genetics Society (Sociedade Brasileira de Genetica)
Departamento de Genetica
Faculdade de Medicina, USP
14049 Ribeirao Preto, Brazil
Phone: 55 16 6331610

Fnded: 1955.

★ 1669 ★ Brazilian Interdisciplinary AIDS Association (ABIA) (Associacao Brasileiar Interdisciplinar de AIDS)
Rua da Candelaria 79, Andar 10
20050-000 Rio de Janeiro, RJ, Brazil
Phone: 55 21 2231040 **Fax:** 55 21 22538495
Email: abia@abiaids.org.br
Website: http://www.alternex.com.br/~abia/

Fnded: 1986. **Mem:** 17. **Lang(s):** English, Portuguese, Spanish. **Desc:** Advocates a multidisciplinary approach to issues raised by AIDS. Assesses AIDS-related government initiatives and works to develop adequate prevention, education, and information policies. Studies the social impact of AIDS in Brazil; compiles and disseminates updated information on HIV-infection prevention and control; critiques available information and works to lessen the spread of misinformation; provides consultancy and advisory services. Serves as a clearing house and resource center; maintains database in cooperation with the Brazilian Institute of Social and Economic Analyses. Conducts seminars on ethical, moral, and social aspects of the disease and educational and research programs. **Pub:** *ABIA Bulletin*, quarterly. Newsletter. • *Acao Anti AIDS*, bimonthly. Magazine. • *AIDS in Brazil*. Book. • Books.

★ 1670 ★ Brazilian Muscular Dystrophy Association (Associacao Brasileira de Distrofia Muscular)
rua Eng. Teixeira Soares, 715
05505-030 Butanta, SP, Brazil
Phone: 55 11 38148562 **Fax:** 55 11 38148562
Email: abdim@sili.com.br
Website: http://www.abdim.org.br

Fnded: 1981. **Desc:** Promotes interest in muscular dystrophy research among medical and scientific communities and the public in Brazil. Disseminates information. **Pub:** *Revista da ABDIM*, every 3 months. Magazine. Contains Muscular Dystrophy interests like researches, treatments, and work with children and adolescents from Brazil.

★ 1671 ★ Brazilian Society of Aesthetic Medicine (Sociedade Brasileira de Medicina Estetica)
Av Rio Branco, 257 Suite 906
20040-009 Rio de Janeiro, Brazil
Phone: 51 21 25244401 **Fax:** 51 21 22202555
Email: sbme@congregare.com.br
Website: http://www.sbme.org.br

Fnded: 1987. **Desc:** Organizes post-graduate courses of aesthetic medicine in association with the School of Medicine "Souza Marques" in Rio de Janeiro and Sao Paulo.

★ 1672 ★ Brazilian Society of Dermatology (SBD)
CP 389
20001-970 Rio de Janeiro, Brazil
Phone: 55 21 2536747

Fnded: 1912.

★ 1673 ★ Brazilian Society of Pharmacology and Experimental Therapeutics (Sociedade Brasileira de Farmacologia e Terapeutica Experimental — SBFTE)
c/o Dr. Antonio Jose Lapa
Department of Pharmacology
Escola Paulista de Medicina
Universidade Federal de Sao Paulo
Rua Tres de Maio 100
04044-020 Sao Paulo, SP, Brazil
Phone: 55 11 55764447 **Fax:** 55 11 55764499
Email: ajlapa.farm@infar.epm.br
Website: http://www.sbfte.org.br

Mem: 750. **Desc:** Promotes pharmacology and experimental therapeutics in Brazil.

★ 1674 ★ Breast Cancer Action (BCA)
55 New Montgomery St., Ste. 323
San Francisco, CA 94105
Phone: (415)243-9301 **Free:** 877-278-6722
Fax: (415)243-3996
Email: info@bcaction.org
Website: http://www.bcaction.org/
Barbara Brenner, Exec. Dir.

Fnded: 1990. **Mem:** 8,500. **Nat'l Groups:** 1. **Reg. Groups:** 1. **Desc:** Women living with breast cancer. Seeks to carry "the voices of people affected by breast cancer to inspire and compel the changes necessary to end the breast cancer epidemic." Monitors and publicizes developments in breast cancer detection and treatment; sponsors lobbying programs; advocates for increased access to breast cancer screening and treatment services; facilitates environmental protection initiatives; works to ensure accurate reporting of breast cancer issues in public media. **Pub:** *Breast Cancer Action Newsletter*, bimonthly. Newsletter. Information on developments in treatment, research, detection and politics of breast-cancer. *Price:* $35 per year.

★ 1675 ★ Breast Cancer Care
Kiln House
210 New Kings Rd.
London SW6 4NZ, United Kingdom
Phone: 44 207 3842984 **Fax:** 44 207 3843387
Email: info@breastcancercare.org.uk
Website: http://www.breastcancercare.org.uk

Fnded: 1973. **Reg. Groups:** 3. **Lang(s):** English. **Desc:** Provides information and support to those affected by breast cancer. Operates advice line, one-to-one volunteer support, and aftercare services, including prosthesis fitting. **Pub:** Books. • Newsletter, quarterly. • Pamphlets. Contains information on breast cancer awareness and breast cancer treatments. **Frmly:** (1993) Breast Care and Masectomy Association.

★ 1676 ★ Breast Cancer Society
401 St. Clair St.
Point Edward, ON, Canada N7V 1P2
Phone: (519)336-0746 **Free:** 800-567-8767
Fax: (519)336-5725
Email: bcsc@bcsc.ca
Website: http://www.bcsc.ca/

Fnded: 1991. **Desc:** Private charity dedicated to funding breast cancer research to improve the detection, prevention, and treatment, and ultimately a cure for the disease. Sponsors golf tournaments, fashions shows, and other fundraising events, as well as the sale of pins to show support.

★ 1677 ★ Breast Cancer Support Service - Northern Ireland
c/o Ulster Cancer Foundation
40-42 Eglantine Ave.
Belfast BT9 6DX, United Kingdom
Phone: 44 2890 663281 **Fax:** 44 2890 660081
Email: info@ulstercancer.org
Website: http://www.ulstercancer.co.uk

Fnded: 1974. **Reg. Groups:** 13. **Local Groups:** 18. **Desc:** Promotes awareness of breast care and early detection of breast cancer. Supports the rehabilitation of women who have breast cancer and breast surgery. **Pub:** *Coping with Breast Cancer*. Booklet. **Frmly:** Breast Care and Mastectomy Support Service.

★ 1678 ★ Britain - Nepal Medical Trust (BNMT)
c/o Export House
130 Yale Rd.
Tonbridge TN9 1SP, United Kingdom
Phone: 44 1732 360284 **Fax:** 44 1732 363876

Fnded: 1968. **Lang(s):** English. **Desc:** Health care professionals and health organizations. Seeks to improve the health of the people of Nepal. Works with Nepalese government agencies to increase delivery of health services in underserved areas. Evaluates health programs and makes recommendations for their improvement; distributes medical equipment, medications, and other supplies.

★ 1679 ★ British Acupuncture Association and Register (BAAR)
34 Alderney St.
London SW1V 4EU, United Kingdom
Phone: 44 171 8346229

Fnded: 1962. **Mem:** 320. **Lang(s):** English. **Desc:** British acupuncturists. **Pub:** *BAAR Journal*, semiannual. Journal. • *Directory*, periodic. Directory. • Books, periodic. • Papers, periodic.

★ 1680 ★ British Acupuncture Council
63 Jeddo Rd.
London W12 9HQ, United Kingdom
Phone: 44 208 7350400 **Fax:** 44 208 7350404
Email: info@acupuncture.org.uk
Website: http://www.acupuncture.org.uk

Fnded: 1995. **Mem:** 2,000. **Lang(s):** English. **Desc:** Practitioners of acupuncture who have completed at least three year's training in traditional acupuncture and western medical sciences appropriate to the practice of acupuncture. Promotes the use of traditional Chinese acupuncture. Maintains standards of education, ethics, discipline, and practice to ensure the health and safety of the public. Encourages exchange of ideas among members. Disseminates information local practitioner members and accredited training courses. **Pub:** *BAcC News*, bimonthly. Newsletter. • *Register of Members*, semiannual. Membership Directory. **Frmly:** Traditional Acupuncture Society.

★ 1681 ★ British Andrology Society
Reproductive & Dev. Med.
Sheffield University
Level 4, Jessop Wing, Tree Root Walk
Sheffield S10 2SF, United Kingdom
Phone: 44 114 2268195 **Fax:** 44 114 2268538
Email: a.fazeli@sheffield.ac.uk
Website: http://www.britishandrology.org.uk

Fnded: 1977. **Desc:** Scientists and clinicians working in the fields of human and mammalian reproduction with an interest in the male. Promotes the interests of members. Research is an important activity in the organization.

★ 1682 ★ British Association for Accident and Emergency Medicine
c/o Royal College of Surgeons of England
35-43 Lincoln's Inn Fields
London WC2A 3PE, United Kingdom
Phone: 44 207 8319405 **Fax:** 44 207 4050318
Email: baem@emergencymedicine.uk.net
Website: http://www.baem.org.uk

Fnded: 1967. **Mem:** 1,500. **Desc:** Membership of the British Association for Accident and Emergency Medicine is available to any registered medical practitioner who has an interest in Accident and Emergency Medicine. Concerned with the development of the specialty of Accident and Emergency Medicine and, in particular, to achieve a minimum of one Accident and Emergency Consultant in every major Accident and Emergency Department. It has a network of Regional Representatives who are available to advise Districts on the establishment of Accident and Emergency Consultant posts, staffing issues, design of Accident and Emergency Departments, etc. **Pub:** *Emergency Medicine*, bimonthly. Journal.

★ 1683 ★ British Association of Aesthetic Plastic Surgeons (BAAPS)
Royal College of Surgeons of England
35-43 Lincoln's Inn Fields
London WC2A 3PE, United Kingdom
Phone: 44 207 4052234 **Fax:** 44 207 4301840
Email: info@baaps.org.uk
Website: http://www.baaps.org.uk

Fnded: 1980. **Mem:** 140. **Lang(s):** English. **Desc:** Fosters exchange of information among surgeons for the advancement of aesthetic plastic surgery. Encourages specialized training among plastic surgeons. Develops and advocates high standards of professional conduct; advises, promotes, and disseminates information on aesthetic plastic surgery. Provides educational programs for general practitioners and the press; conducts semiannual educational program for trainees and consultants.

★ 1684 ★ British Association of Art Therapists
c/o Mary Ward House
5 Tavistock Pl.
London WC1H 9SN, United Kingdom
Phone: 44 207 3833774 **Fax:** 44 207 3875513
Email: baat@ukgateway.net
Website: http://www.baat.org

Fnded: 1964. **Desc:** Art therapists. **Pub:** *Art Therapy in Education*. Brochure. • *Code of Ethics*. • *Inscape*, semiannual. Journal. • *Register of Therapists*. • Brochure. Discusses art therapy as a profession in Great Britain.

★ 1685 ★ British Association of Audiological Physicians
c/o Dr. Ewa Raglan
St. George's Hospital
Blackshaw Rd.
London SW17 0QT, United Kingdom
Phone: 44 208 7251988 **Fax:** 44 208 7251874
Email: info@baap.org.uk
Website: http://www.baap.org.uk/

Fnded: 1977. **Mem:** 100. **Desc:** Consultant physicians practising in audiology. Concerned with the diagnosis and care/management of adults and children suffering from disorders of balance and hearing; the promotion of education (postgraduate) and standards of medical practice; also concerned with training and educational issues of junior doctors. **Pub:** *Policy Document 2002: Audiological Medicine in a Modern NHS*.

★ 1686 ★ British Association of Behavioral Optometrists
Greygarth
Littleworth
Winchcombe
Cheltenham GL54 5BT, United Kingdom
Phone: 44 1242 602689 **Fax:** 44 1242 602689
Email: greygarth@compuserve.com
Website: http://www.babo.co.uk

Fnded: 1990. **Mem:** 93. **Reg. Groups:** 6. **Desc:** Seeks to improve understanding of Behavioral Optometry, through continuing education and training and by providing an accredited list of trained optometrists.

★ 1687 ★ British Association for Behavioural and Cognitive Psychotherapies
Globe Centre
PO Box 9
Accrington BB5 2GD, United Kingdom
Phone: 44 1254 875277 **Fax:** 44 1254 239114
Email: babcp@babcp.com
Website: http://www.babcp.org.uk

Fnded: 1972. **Mem:** 2,000. **Lang(s):** English. **Desc:** Health, Social Service, education staff and therapists in private practice; individuals interested in psychotherapies and accredited/registered psychotherapists. Promotion of behavioural and cognitive therapy approaches in health, educational and social problem areas. **Pub:** *BABCP Newsletter*, 3/year. Newsletter. • *Behavioural & Cognitive Psychotherapy Journal*, quarterly. Journal.

★ 1688 ★ British Association for Cancer Research (BACR)
Institute of Cancer Research
15 Cotswold Rd.
Sutton SM2 5NG, United Kingdom
Phone: 44 208 7224208 **Fax:** 44 208 7701395
Email: bacr@icr.ac.uk
Website: http://www.icr.ac.uk/bacr

Fnded: 1960. **Mem:** 1,300. **Lang(s):** English. **Desc:** Laboratory and clinical cancer research workers. Conducts and promotes research into the prevention, causes, treatment, and cure of cancer. **Pub:** *British Journal of Cancer*, monthly. Journal.

★ 1689 ★ British Association of Clinical Anatomists (BACA)
School of Biomedical Sciences
University of Leeds
Leeds LS2 9JT, United Kingdom
Phone: 44 113 2334296

Fnded: 1977.

★ 1690 ★ British Association and College of Occupational Therapists
106-114 Borough High St.
London SE1 1HL, United Kingdom
Phone: 44 207 3576480 **Fax:** 44 207 4502299
Email: beryl.steeden@cot.co.uk
Website: http://www.cot.org.uk

Fnded: 1932. **Mem:** 23,000. **Reg. Groups:** 20. **Desc:** State registered Occupational Therapists, Occupational Therapy Helpers and Technical Instructors. Acts as a professional association in the field of rehabilitative medicine; promotion of occupational therapy education; honourable practice, repression of malpractice and to provide the facilities for the advancement of the science of occupational therapy. BAOT is also the Trade Union for the members. **Pub:** *British Journal of Occupational Therapy*, monthly. Journal. Contains articles on clinical, educational, research, and management aspects of occupational therapy. • *Occupational Therapy News*, monthly. Magazine.

★ 1691 ★ British Association of Cosmetic Surgeons
17 Harley St.
London W1N 1DA, United Kingdom
Phone: 44 207 3235728

Fnded: 1980. **Mem:** 20. **Desc:** All members are cosmetic surgeons, carrying out cosmetic surgery in private practice. Maintains and improves the standards of cosmetic surgery in Britain and interchanges information between members. Informs the public. **Pub:** *Basic Account of Cosmetic Surgery*. Booklet.

★ 1692 ★ British Association for Counselling and Psychotherapy (BACP)
1 Regent Pl.
Rugby CV21 2PJ, United Kingdom
Phone: 44 870 4 435252 **Fax:** 44 870 4 435160
Email: bacp@bacp.co.uk
Website: http://www.counselling.co.uk

Fnded: 1977. **Mem:** 17,000. **Desc:** Individual or organisational membership for those working as counsellors or those using counselling skills as part of their role. Aims to promote awareness of counselling internationally and raise standards of training and practice through its Ethical Framework for Good Practice in Counselling and Psychotherapy. It provides support for members including an information service for members and the public, divisions for special interest groups and local affiliated groups. **Frmly:** (2001) British Association for Counselling.

★ 1693 ★ British Association of Day Surgery
35-43 Lincoln's Inn Fields
London WC2A 3PN, United Kingdom
Phone: 44 207 9730308 **Fax:** 44 207 9730314
Email: bads@bads.co.uk
Website: http://www.bads.co.uk

Fnded: 1990. **Mem:** 720. **Lang(s):** English. **Desc:** Nurses, managers, surgeons and anaesthetists. To encourage the expansion of day surgery and to promote education, research and high-quality treatment in this field. Organizes seminars, meetings and holds an annual conference. Advice is provided to Royal Colleges, NHS Executive, regional commissions and trusts including private health organizations. **Pub:** *Journal of One Day Surgery*, quarterly. Journal.

★ 1694 ★ British Association of Dental Nurses
11 Pharos St.
Fleetwood FY7 6BG, United Kingdom
Phone: 44 1253 778631 **Fax:** 44 1253 773266
Email: admin@badn.org.uk

Fnded: 1940. **Lang(s):** English. **Desc:** Professional association representing dental nurses in the UK and overseas as well as other members of the dental industry. Represents members working in specialist areas such as training, orthodontics, special care, and the armed forces. Aims to support, encourage, and provide advice to dental nurses; to develop and maintain nationally recognised standards; to protect the professional status of the dental nurse; and to maintain contact with the necessary bodies to achieve the above. **Pub:** *The British Dental Nurses Journal*, quarterly, always March, June, September, and December. Journal. **Frmly:** (1994) ABDSA.

★ 1695 ★ British Association of Dermatologists (BAD)
19 Fitzroy Sq.
London W1T 6EH, United Kingdom
Phone: 44 207 3830266 **Fax:** 44 207 3885263
Email: admin@bad.org.uk
Website: http://www.bad.org.uk

Fnded: 1921. **Mem:** 946. **Nat'l Groups:** 6. **Lang(s):** English. **Desc:** Medical professionals united to further the knowledge and teaching of dermatology. Promotes the interests of members and their patients. Conducts medical and scientific research; disseminates information. **Pub:** *British Journal of Dermatology*, monthly. Journal. Also publishes results of research projects.

★ 1696 ★ British Association for Dramatherapists
41 Broomhouse Ln.
London SW6 3DP, United Kingdom
Phone: 44 207 7310160
Email: gllian@demon.co.uk

Fnded: 1976. **Mem:** 630. **Desc:** Aims to: educate the public about dramatherapy, support dramatherapists wherever they work and increase the availability of properly-trained and supervised dramatherapists. Also aims to ensure that high standards are maintained and to implement Equal Opportunities policies. It responds to increasing demands for information and represents dramatherapy at a national and international level. **Pub:** *Dramatherapy*, quarterly. Newsletter. • *The Journal of Dramatherapy*, 3/year. Journal. Also publishes an information pack.

★ 1697 ★ British Association in Forensic Medicine
Department of Forensic Pathology
University of Sheffield
Sheffield S3 7ES, United Kingdom
Phone: 44 141 3304574 **Fax:** 44 141 3304602
Email: p.d.lumb@sheffield.ac.uk
Website: http://www.shef.ac.uk/~bafm

Fnded: 1950. **Mem:** 200. **Desc:** Promotes the specialty of forensic pathology. Represents members' interests.

★ 1698 ★ British Association of Head and Neck Oncologists (BAHNO)
Queen Victoria Hospital
Maxillofacial Head & Neck Unit
East Grinstead RH19 3DZ, United Kingdom
Phone: 44 1342 410210 **Fax:** 44 1342 328339
Email: andrew.brown@qvh-tr.sthames.nhs.uk

Fnded: 1968.

★ 1699 ★ British Association of Homoeopathic Pharmacists (BAHP)
c/o Ainsworth Homeopathic Pharmacy
36 New Cavendish St.
London W1G 8UF, United Kingdom
Phone: 44 20 79355330 **Fax:** 44 20 74864313

Fnded: 1980.

★ 1700 ★ British Association of Homoeopathic Veterinary Surgeons (BAHVS)
Chinham House
Stanford-in-the-Vale SN7 8NQ, United Kingdom
Phone: 44 1367 718115 **Fax:** 44 1367 718243
Email: enquiries@bahvs.com
Website: http://www.bahvs.com

Fnded: 1981.

★ 1701 ★ British Association for Immediate Care (BASICS)
Turret House, Turret Ln.
Ipswich IP4 1DL, United Kingdom
Phone: 44 870 1654999 **Fax:** 44 870 1654949
Email: admin@basics.org.uk
Website: http://www.basics.org.uk

Fnded: 1977. **Mem:** 2,500. **Local Groups:** 87. **Desc:** Medical practitioners and non-medical practitioners (e.g., ambulance, nurse, emergency planning personnel) involved in pre-hospital immediate medical care. Aims to foster co-operation between existing Immediate Care Schemes and to encourage and aid the formation and extension of schemes in the UK; to develop and strengthen co-operation between all services in dealing with emergencies and to encourage and assist research into all aspects of pre-hospital immediate medical care and accident prevention. **Pub:** Newsletter, 3/year.

★ 1702 ★ British Association for Lung Research (BALR)
St. Thomas' Hospital
London SE1 7EH, United Kingdom
Phone: 44 20 79228155 **Fax:** 44 20 79280658

Fnded: 1982.

★ 1703 ★ British Association of Medical Managers
Petersgate House, 3rd Fl.
St. Petersgate
Stockport SK1 1HE, United Kingdom
Phone: 44 161 4741141 **Fax:** 44 161 4747167
Email: bamm@bamm.co.uk
Website: http://www.bamm.co.uk

Fnded: 1991. **Mem:** 1,800. **Desc:** Doctors from all specialties and at all levels of interest in management are invited to apply for membership. Junior doctors are warmly welcomed and non medical managers are welcome to apply for associate membership. Concerned with the promotion of quality healthcare by improving and supporting the contribution of doctors in management. Unites doctors with an interest in healthcare management. Members are keen to learn from, and work with each other to ensure a meaningful and effective contribution to the management of organisations. **Pub:** *Clinician in Management*, bimonthly. • Newsletter.

★ 1704 ★ British Association of Neuroscience Nurses
c/o Neuro ICU
Radcliff Infirmary
Woodstock Rd.
Oxford OX2 6HE, United Kingdom
Phone: 44 28 94461203
Email: admin@bann.org.uk
Website: http://www.bann.org.uk

Fnded: 1971. **Mem:** 310. **Desc:** Promotes the highest standards of patient care in the Neurosciences field. Provides opportunities for knowledge transfer between neuroscience nurses. Encourages clinical research and promotes interest in the neuroscience area.

★ 1705 ★ British Association of Occupational Therapists
106-114 Borough High St.
Southwark
London SE1 1LB, United Kingdom
Phone: 44 207 3576480 **Fax:** 44 207 4502299
Email: cot@cot.co.uk
Website: http://www.cot.co.uk

Fnded: 1974. **Mem:** 25,000. **Reg. Groups:** 8. **Desc:** Promotes high standards among occupational therapists. Supports the provision of efficient, reliable, and effective services that benefit all users of occupational therapy. Encourages personal and intellectual development of occupational therapists and support staff. **Pub:** *British Journal of Occupation Therapy*, monthly. Journal. • *OT News*, monthly. Magazine.

★ 1706 ★ British Association of Oral and Maxillofacial Surgeons
c/o Royal College of Surgeons of England
35-43 Lincoln's Inn Fields
London WC2A 3PN, United Kingdom
Phone: 44 20 74058074 **Fax:** 44 20 74309997
Email: office@baoms.org.uk
Website: http://www.baoms.org.uk

Fnded: 1962. **Mem:** 1,200. **Desc:** Aims to promote the advancement of education and research into the development of oral and maxillofacial surgery in the British Isles; to encourage, and assist postgraduate education, study and research in oral and maxillofacial surgery. Arranges regular meetings at which lectures and demonstrations will be given. **Pub:** *British Journal of Oral & Maxillofacial Surgery*, bimonthly. Journal.

★ 1707 ★ British Association of Orthodontists (BAO)
16 Castle Hill
Maidenhead SL6 4JJ, United Kingdom
Phone: 44 1628 23279

Fnded: 1965.

★ 1708 ★ British Association of Otorhinolaryngologists - Head and Neck Surgeons
c/o Royal College of Surgeons
35-43 Lincoln's Inn Fields
London WC2A 3PE, United Kingdom
Phone: 44 20 74048373 **Fax:** 44 20 74044200
Email: orl@bao-hns.demon.co.uk
Website: http://www.orl-baohns.org

Fnded: 1943. **Mem:** 1,111. **Lang(s):** English. **Desc:** Consultant ENT and head and neck surgeons, consultant audiological physicians as well as medical practitioners engaged in the practice of otorhinolaryngology and head and neck surgery in grades other than that of consultant. Aims to support and encourage education, research, development, and audit in otorhinolaryngology, head and neck surgery. Promotes the highest standards or medical and surgical practice within otorhinolarynglogy, head and neck surgery, for the benefit of patients. **Pub:** *Clinical Otolaryngology*, bimonthly. • Newsletter, bimonthly.

★ 1709 ★ British Association for Paediatric Nephrology
c/o Dr. Lesley Rees
Renal Office
St. Ormond St. Hospital fo Children
London WC1N 3JH, United Kingdom
Phone: 44 207 8138346 **Fax:** 44 207 8298841
Email: reesl@gosh.nhs.uk
Website: http://www.uwcm.ac.uk/uwcm/ch/bapn

Fnded: 1973. **Mem:** 60. **Desc:** Paediatricians participating in the care of children with kidney diseases. Aims to promote policies concerning the care of children with renal disease, to conduct scientific meetings, to consider manpower and training issues and to conduct multicentre trials and other collaborative research.

★ 1710 ★ British Association of Paediatric Surgeons (BAPS)
c/o Royal College of Surgeons of England
35-43 Lincoln's Inn Fields
London WC2A 3PH, United Kingdom
Phone: 44 20 78696915 **Fax:** 44 20 78696919
Email: adminsec@baps.org.uk
Website: http://www.baps.org.uk

Fnded: 1953. **Mem:** 700. **Lang(s):** English. **Desc:** Pedriatric surgeons, consultants, and trainees. Works to improve the techniques of study, practice, and research in pediatric surgery; fosters professional relations among pediatric surgeons. Sponsors training program. **Pub:** *Journal of Pediatric Surgery*, periodic.

★ 1711 ★ British Association of Perinatal Medicine (BAPM)
c/o Prof. David Field, Hon.Sec.
Leicester Royal Infirmary
Leicester LE1 5WW, United Kingdom
Phone: 44 1162 587707 **Fax:** 44 1162 585502
Website: http://www.bapm-london.org/

Desc: Works to improve the standard of perinatal care in the British Isles.

★ 1712 ★ British Association of Plastic Surgeons
The Royal College of Surgeons
35-43 Lincoln's Inn Fields
London WC2A 3PE, United Kingdom
Phone: 44 20 78315161 **Fax:** 44 20 78314041
Email: secretariat@baps.co.uk
Website: http://www.baps.co.uk

Fnded: 1946. **Mem:** 650. **Desc:** Plastic Surgeons. Promotes and directs the development of plastic surgery and aims to foster and co-ordinate education, study and research in plastic surgery. **Pub:** *British Journal of Plastic Surgery*, 8/year. Journal.

★ 1713 ★ British Association of Prosthetists and Orthotists (BAPO)
Sir James Clark Bldg.
Abbey Mills Business Centre
Paisley PA1 1TJ, United Kingdom
Phone: 44 141 5617217 **Fax:** 44 141 5617218
Email: admin@bapo.com
Website: http://www.bapo.com

Lang(s): English. **Desc:** Orthotists and prosthetists. Seeks to "protect the prosthetic and orthotic profession with regard to its status and interests." Encourages high standards of ethics and practice among members; conducts continuing professional education and training programs; serves as a clearinghouse on orthotics and prosthetics; provides advice and assistance to members. **Pub:** *BAPOMAG*, periodic. Magazine.

★ 1714 ★ British Association for Psychopharmacology (BAP)
c/o Susan Chandler
36 Cambridge Pl.
Hills Rd.
Cambridge CB2 1NS, United Kingdom
Phone: 44 1223 358395 **Fax:** 44 1223 321268
Email: susan@bap.org.uk

Fnded: 1974. **Mem:** 1,200. **Lang(s):** English. **Desc:** Psychopharmacologists, psychiatrists, neuropharmacologists, psychologists, and neurochemists. Brings together scientists working in academic, clinical, and industrial applications of psychopharmacology. Arranges scientific meetings, study groups, and seminars; encourages basic research and pharmaceutical development. Offers professional guidance to the public on matters related to psychopharmacology. **Pub:** *Journal of Psychopharmacology*, bimonthly. Journal. • Monographs, periodic.

★ 1715 ★ British Association of Psychotherapists (BAP)
37 Mapesbury Rd.
London NW2 4HJ, United Kingdom
Phone: 44 20 84529823 **Fax:** 44 20 84525182
Email: mail@bap-psychotherapy.org
Website: http://www.bap-psychotherapy.org

Fnded: 1951. **Mem:** 500. **Desc:** Full, Associate and Student Members, trained and qualified by BAP in either adult or child psychotherapy. Aims to promote the knowledge and application of psychotherapy and the training of both Adult and Child Psychotherapists. External courses were begun in 1989 for the benefit of interested members of the helping professions. A clinical service is also operated to help people find a qualified psychotherapist. An Msc. Training is also available. **Pub:** Journal, semiannual.

★ 1716 ★ British Association for Sexual and Relationship Therapy
PO Box 13686
London SW20 9ZH, United Kingdom
Email: info@basrt.org.uk
Website: http://www.basrt.org.uk

Fnded: 1975. **Mem:** 700. **Desc:** Professional psychosexual therapists/clinicians/medics working in the field of sexual and marital therapy. Aims to advance the education and training of persons engaged in sexual, marital and relationship therapy; to promote research in this field; to advance public education about sexual, marital and relationship therapy. **Pub:** *Sexual and Marital Therapy*, quarterly. Journal. **Frmly:** (2000) British Association for Sexual and Marital Therapy.

★ 1717 ★ British Association of Skin Camouflage
c/o Resources for Business
South Park Rd.
Macclesfield SK11 6SH, United Kingdom
Phone: 44 1625 267880 **Fax:** 44 1625 267879
Email: thorpm@resources.demon.co.uk
Website: http://www.skin-camouflage.net

Fnded: 1986. **Mem:** 100. **Desc:** Trains professionals. Encourages and supports members. Informs and provides remedial camouflage service for patients. **Pub:** Newsletter, 3/year.

★ 1718 ★ British Association of Sport and Medicine (BASM)
67 Springfield Lane
Eccleston WA10 5HB, United Kingdom
Phone: 44 1744 28198 **Fax:** 44 1744 28198

Fnded: 1952.

★ 1719 ★ British Association of Surgical Oncology (BASO)
c/o Royal College of Surgeons
35-43 Lincoln's Inn Fields
London WC2A 3PE, United Kingdom
Phone: 44 20 74055612 **Fax:** 44 20 74046574

Fnded: 1973.

★ 1720 ★ British Association of Teachers of the Deaf
21 The Haystacks
High Wycombe
Buckinghamshire HP13 6PY, United Kingdom
Phone: 44 1494 464190 **Fax:** 44 1494 464190
Email: secretary@batod.org.uk
Website: http://www.batod.org.uk

Fnded: 1976. **Mem:** 1,750. **Reg. Groups:** 7. **Local Groups:** 7. **Desc:** Qualified teachers of the deaf; Associate membership available to persons not qualified as teachers of the deaf. Represents the interests of all teachers of the hearing-impaired in Britain. It exists to promote the education of all hearing impaired persons and to promote and safeguard the interests and status of all teachers of the hearing-impaired **Pub:** *Association Magazine*, 5/year. Magazine. Contains articles related to teaching deaf children. • *The Journal of the British Association of Teachers of the Deaf-Deafness and Education International*, 3/year. Journal. Also publishes booklets and leaflets relating to the education of deaf people.

★ 1721 ★ British Association of Urological Surgeons
c/o Royal College of Surgeons of England
35-43 Lincoln's Inn Fields
London WC2A 3PE, United Kingdom
Phone: 44 20 78696950 **Fax:** 44 20 74045048
Email: pneville@baus.org.uk
Website: http://www.baus.org.uk

Fnded: 1945. **Mem:** 1,400. **Desc:** Urological surgeons from the UK and overseas. Medical practitioners in other specialties with an interest in urology. Aims to promote a high standard in the practice of urology. **Pub:** *Members Handbook*. Handbook.

★ 1722 ★ British Biophysical Society
Gunnels Wood Rd.
Stevenage SG1 2NY, United Kingdom
Phone: 44 1438 763367 **Fax:** 44 1438 764865
Email: rc8817@glaxowellcome.co.uk
Website: http://www.cryst.bbk.ac.uk/BBS/bbs.html

Fnded: 1960.

★ 1723 ★ British Blind Sport
4-6 Victoria Terr.
Leamington Spa CV31 3AB, United Kingdom
Phone: 44 8700 789000 **Fax:** 44 8700 789001
Email: info@britishblindsport.org.uk
Website: http://www.britishblindsport.org.uk/

Fnded: 1975. **Desc:** Committed to encouraging blind and partially sighted children and adults to participate in sports at all levels, from grassroots to Paralympic representation. Sports include archery, cricket, football, goalball, judo, martial arts, swimming, and ten-pin bowling, with an interest in chess, golf, riding, sailing and skiing. Organizes rifle shooting fundraising events and National Championships. **Pub:** *Target*, bimonthly. Newsletter.

★ 1724 ★ British Blood Transfusion Society (BBTS)
Plymouth Grove
Manchester M13 9LL, United Kingdom
Phone: 44 161 2514300 **Fax:** 44 161 2514331
Email: bbts@bbts.org.uk
Website: http://www.bbts.org.uk

Fnded: 1983. **Mem:** 1,520. **Pub:** *Transfusion Medicine*, bimonthly. Journal.

★ 1725 ★ British Burn Association
BBA Secretariat
Burn Centre, Acute Block
Wythenshawe Hospital
Southmoor Rd.
Manchester M23 9LT, United Kingdom
Phone: 44 161 2916323 **Fax:** 44 161 2916823
Email: bba@smuth.nwest.nhs.uk

★ 1726 ★ British Cardiac Society
Unit D1
2 Station Rd.
Swave Sey CB4 5QJ, United Kingdom
Email: admin@bcpa.co.uk

Fnded: 1937.

★ 1727 ★ British Cattle Veterinary Association
c/o BCVA Office
The Green
Frampton-on-Severn
Gloucester GL2 7EP, United Kingdom
Phone: 44 1452 740816 **Fax:** 44 1452 741117
Email: office@cattlevet.co.uk
Website: http://www.bcva.org.uk

Fnded: 1967. **Mem:** 1,500. **Desc:** Veterinary surgeons, research workers; mostly professional veterinary surgeons in practice. Concerned with education; promotion; research into cattle topics; promotion of cattle veterinarian; political opinion on cattle matters; source of information and reference on cattle topics. **Pub:** *Cattle Practice*, quarterly. Journal. • Newsletters, quarterly.

★ 1728 ★ British Chiropractic Association
Blagrave House
17 Blagrave St.
Reading RG1 1QB, United Kingdom
Phone: 44 118 9505950 **Fax:** 44 118 9588946
Email: enquiries@chiropractic-uk.co.uk
Website: http://www.chiropractic-uk.co.uk

Fnded: 1925. **Mem:** 860. **Desc:** Complementary medicine practitioners/chiropractors. Concerned with treatment of spinal disorders by specialised manipulative techniques. **Pub:** *Contact*, quarterly. • *In Touch*, monthly. Newsletter.

★ 1729 ★ British Colostomy Association
15 Station Rd.
Reading RG1 1LG, United Kingdom
Phone: 44 118 9391537 **Fax:** 44 118 9569095
Email: sue@bcass.org.uk
Website: http://www.bcass.org.uk

Fnded: 1967. Mem: 16,000. Reg. Groups: 26. Lang(s): English. Desc: Anyone who has a colostomy and/or their carer. Exists to offer help and encouragement to anyone who has had or is about to have a colostomy. Home and hospital visits by arrangement. Pub: *Living With a Colostomy*. Booklet. • *Tidings*, semiannual. Newsletter.

★ 1730 ★ British Computer Association of the Blind (BDS)
c/o RNIB
58-72 John Bright St.
Birmingham B1 1BN, United Kingdom
Phone: 44 121 6654256
Email: info@bcab.org.uk
Website: http://www.bcab.org.uk

Fnded: 1969. **Mem:** 230. **Desc:** Provides general assistance and advice on information technology issues for blind and visually impaired persons. Organizes training courses. Engages in lobbying. **Pub:** Newsletter, quarterly.

★ 1731 ★ British Council of Disabled People (BCODP)
Litchurch Plaza
Litchurch Ln.
Derby DE24 8AA, United Kingdom
Phone: 44 1332 295551 **Fax:** 44 1332 295580
Email: info@bcodp.org.uk
Website: http://www.bcodp.org.uk

Fnded: 1981. **Mem:** 140. **Reg. Groups:** 123. **Desc:** Organizations controlled by disabled people and individual membership is now available to all disabled people and their supporters. The national umbrella organisation representing groups controlled by disabled people. Current concern is to secure anti-discrimination legislation. Has begun a 3-year group development programme to actively support the growth of regional organisations controlled by disabled people. **Pub:** *Activate*. Newsletter. • *Personal Assistance Users Newsletter*. Newsletter. • *Update*, monthly. Newsletter. **Frmly:** (1999) British Council of Organisations of Disabled People.

★ 1732 ★ British Deaf Association
1-3 Worship St.
London EC2A 2AB, United Kingdom
Phone: 44 207 5883520 **Fax:** 44 207 5883527
Email: helpline@bda.org.uk
Website: http://www.bda.org.uk

Fnded: 1890. **Mem:** 6,500. **Desc:** Mainly profoundly deaf people who use sign language as their means of communication. Aims to serve and protect the deaf community. **Pub:** *British Deaf News*, monthly.

★ 1733 ★ British Deaf Sports Council
PO Box 2232
Leagrave LU3 2YU, United Kingdom
Phone: 44 1943 850214 **Fax:** 44 1582 613938
Email: enquiries@britishdeafsportscouncil.org.uk
Website: http://www.britishdeafsportscouncil.org.uk

Fnded: 1930. **Mem:** 4,500. **Reg. Groups:** 8. **Desc:** Deaf people interested in sport. **Pub:** Yearbook.

★ 1734 ★ British Dental Association (BDA)
64 Wimpole St.
London W1G 8YS, United Kingdom
Phone: 44 207 9350875 **Fax:** 44 207 4875232
Email: enquiries@bda-dentistry.org.uk
Website: http://www.bda-dentistry.org.uk

Fnded: 1880. **Mem:** 20,000. **Reg. Groups:** 21. **Local Groups:** 130. **Lang(s):** English. **Desc:** Professional association and trade union for dental surgeons in the United Kingdom. Promotes dentistry and the provision of dental services to the public. Represents members' interests individually and collectively before the government. **Pub:** *BDA News*, monthly. Newsletter. • *British Dental Journal*, bimonthly. Journal.

★ 1735 ★ British Dental Hygienists Association (BDHA)
13 Yatton Ridge
Yatton
Bristol BS49 4DG, United Kingdom
Phone: 44 1934 876389 **Fax:** 44 1934 876389

Fnded: 1949.

★ 1736 ★ British Dental Practice Managers Association
Osprey House
Primett Rd.
Stevenage SGI 3EE, United Kingdom
Phone: 44 870 8400341 **Fax:** 44 870 8400342
Email: info@bdpma.org.uk
Website: http://www.bdpma.org.uk

Fnded: 1992. **Mem:** 400. **Reg. Groups:** 10. **Desc:** Promote co-operation and provide a way to communicate and support those actively involved in Dental Practice Management. **Pub:** *Networking*, quarterly. Newsletter.

★ 1737 ★ British Dental Trade Association (BDTA)
Mineral Ln.
Chesham HP5 1NL, United Kingdom
Phone: 44 1494 782873 **Fax:** 44 1494 786659
Email: admin@bdta.org.uk
Website: http://www.bdta.org.uk

Fnded: 1923. **Mem:** 116. **Lang(s):** English. **Desc:** Companies manufacturing dental equipment and supplies. Establishes international standards and technical harmonization for dental equipment. Represents members' interests before government bodies, international agencies, and the public. Maintains liaison with organizations representing dentists, dental technicians, and dental supply dealers and distributors. Compiles statistics. **Pub:** *Dental Trader*, quarterly. Journal.

★ 1738 ★ British Dietetic Association (BDA)
Charles House, 5th Fl.
148/9 Great Charles St. Queensway
Birmingham B3 3HT, United Kingdom
Phone: 44 121 2008080 **Fax:** 44 121 2008081
Email: info@bda.uk.com
Website: http://www.bda.uk.com

Fnded: 1936. **Mem:** 4,000. **Local Groups:** 11. **Lang(s):** English. **Desc:** Professional registered dietitians. Promotes advancement of the science and practice of dietetics and related subjects. Sponsors training and educational programs. Arranges meetings, refresher courses, and study conferences. Provides liaison between dietitians in the United Kingdom and other countries. **Pub:** *Adviser Magazine*, quarterly. • *Journal of Human Nutrition and Dietetics*, bimonthly. • *Members' Newsletter*, monthly. Newsletter.

★ 1739 ★ British Disabled Water Ski Association
Tony Edge National Centre
Heron Lake
Hythe TW19 6HW, United Kingdom
Phone: 44 1784 483664 **Fax:** 44 1784 482747
Email: southern@bdwsa.org.uk
Website: http://www.bdwsa.org.uk

Fnded: 1979. **Reg. Groups:** 4. **Desc:** Disabled full members and able-bodied helpers associate members. Teaches people with a disability to water ski and trains drivers, observers and instructors.

★ 1740 ★ British Dyslexia Association
98 London Rd.
Reading RG1 5AU, United Kingdom
Phone: 44 118 9668271 **Fax:** 44 118 9351927
Email: admin@bda-dyslexia.demon.co.uk
Website: http://www.bda-dyslexia.org.uk/

Fnded: 1972. **Mem:** 10,000. **Local Groups:** 96. **Desc:** Acts as an umbrella organization for dyslexia in the UK. **Pub:** *Contact*. Magazine. • *Dyslexia*. Journal.

★ 1741 ★ British Endodontic Society (BES)
PO Box 707
Gerrards Cross SL9 0DR, United Kingdom
Phone: 44 1494 581542 **Fax:** 44 1494 581542

Fnded: 1963.

★ 1742 ★ British Epilepsy Association
New Anstey House
Gate Way Dr.
Yeadon
Leeds LS19 7XY, United Kingdom
Phone: 44 113 2108800 **Fax:** 44 113 3910300
Email: epilepsy@epilepsy.org.uk
Website: http://www.epilepsy.org.uk

Fnded: 1950. **Mem:** 20,000. **Reg. Groups:** 140. **Desc:** Association is owned by its members. Provides care in the community for the country's estimated 420,000 people with epilepsy. Publications on all aspects of epilepsy counselling, advice, information and support and the National Epilepsy Helpline. Around 140 regional groups and branch - regional office in Belfast. National information centre provides extensive service to public and professionals. **Pub:** *Epilepsy Today*, quarterly. Magazine. • *Seizure*, quarterly. Journal.

★ 1743 ★ British Equine Veterinary Association
Wakefield House
46 High St.
Sawston CB2 4BG, United Kingdom
Phone: 44 1223 836970 **Fax:** 44 1223 835287
Email: info@beva.org.uk
Website: http://www.beva.org.uk

Fnded: 1961. **Mem:** 1,400. **Desc:** Practising equine vets, members of academia, Veterinary universities and members of pharmaceutical companies, home and overseas. Promotes the cultural, scientific and professional activities of veterinary surgeons and others interested in equine practice, welfare, teaching and research. **Pub:** *Equine Veterinary Education*, bimonthly. Journal. • *Equine Veterinary Journal*, bimonthly. Journal. • *Supplement*, periodic.

★ 1744 ★ British False Memory Society
Bradford-on-Avon BA15 1NF, United Kingdom
Phone: 44 1225 868682 **Fax:** 44 1225 862251
Email: bfms@bfms.org.uk
Website: http://www.bfms.org.uk

Fnded: 1993. **Mem:** 1,200. **Desc:** Seeks to raise awareness of the dangers of recovered memory therapy. Collaborates with associated organizations. Offers telephone support to family members falsely accused of childhood sexual abuse. Fosters research. **Pub:** *BFMS Newsletter*, 2-3/year. Newsletter.

★ 1745 ★ British Fertility Society
c/o Helen Gregson
16 The Courtyard
Woodlands
Bradley Stoke BS32 4NQ, United Kingdom
Phone: 45 1454 642217 **Fax:** 45 1454 642222
Email: bfs@bioscientifica.com
Website: http://www.britishfertilitysociety.org.uk

Fnded: 1973. **Mem:** 800. **Desc:** Promotes the practice, training, education and research in the field of infertility and reproductive medicine.

★ 1746 ★ British Fluoridation Society
5th Fl., Dental School
University of Liverpool
PO Box 147, Pembroke Pl.
Liverpool L69 3GN, United Kingdom
Phone: 44 151 7065216 **Fax:** 44 151 7065845
Email: bfs@liv.ac.uk

Website: http://www.liv.ac.uk/bfs

Fnded: 1969. **Desc:** Promotes fluoridation of the water supplies to improve dental health and reduce health inequalities.

★ 1747 ★ British Geriatrics Society
Marjory Warren House
31 St. John's Sq.
London EC1M 4DN, United Kingdom
Phone: 44 20 76081369 **Fax:** 44 20 76081041
Email: info@bgs.org.uk
Website: http://www.bgs.org.uk

Fnded: 1947. **Mem:** 2,500. **Reg. Groups:** 17. **Lang(s):** English. **Desc:** Consultant geriatricians and other doctors, scientists, and professionals with an interest in geriatric medicine and care of older individuals. To promote scientific developments of geriatric medicine, improve medical and social services for older individuals and promote measures which will improve health throughout adult life to ensure better fitness on achieving old age. **Pub:** *Age and Ageing*, bimonthly. Journal. Medical journal.

★ 1748 ★ British Healthcare Business Intelligence Association (BHBIA)
c/o Steven Gibson
Merck Sharp & Dohme Pharmaceuticals
Hertford Rd.
Hoddesdon EN11 9BU, United Kingdom
Phone: 44 1992 467272 **Fax:** 44 1992 470191
Email: admin@bhbia.org.uk
Website: http://www.bhbia.org.uk/

Pub: Journal. • Handbook, semiannual. Contains membership details.

★ 1749 ★ British Heart Foundation (BHF)
14 Fitzhardinge St.
London W1H 6DH, United Kingdom
Phone: 44 207 9350185 **Fax:** 44 207 4865820
Email: internet@bhf.org.uk
Website: http://www.bhf.org.uk

Fnded: 1961. **Reg. Groups:** 9. **Local Groups:** 430. **Lang(s):** English. **Desc:** Funds research into the causes and prevention diagnosis and treatment of cardiovascular disease. Sponsors postgraduate medical education; distributes fellowships and research funds. Organizes symposia, and workshops for health care and research professionals. Provides cardiac equipment for hospitals and ambulance services. Supports heart patients through rehabilitation programmes, heart support groups and BHF nurses. Conducts fundraising events. Compiles statistics. **Pub:** *BHF Heart News*, bimonthly. Newsletter. Magazine for heart patients.

★ 1750 ★ British Holistic Medical Association
59 Landsdowne Place
East Sussex
Hove BN3 1FL, United Kingdom
Phone: 44 1273 725951 **Fax:** 44 1273 725951
Email: admin@bhma.org
Website: http://www.bhma.org

Fnded: 1983. **Mem:** 900. **Desc:** Professional corporate/associate membership (for the lay public) nurse/student membership and overseas membership. To educate doctors and other healthcare professionals in the principles and practice of holistic medicine, to encourage research studies and publication of work carried out in the field of holistic medicine and to bring together holistic healthcare practitioners for mutual support and further personal and professional development. **Pub:** Newsletter, quarterly.

★ 1751 ★ British Homeopathic Association
15 Clerkenwell Close
London EC1R 0AA, United Kingdom
Phone: 44 207 5667800 **Fax:** 44 207 5667815
Email: info@trusthomeopathy.org
Website: http://www.homeopathy.org

Fnded: 1902. **Mem:** 3,000. **Desc:** The Association is a registered charity supported by a membership of people who, being convinced of the efficacy of the homoeopathic system of medicine, give regular subscriptions or donations for its maintenance. Aims to support, extend and develop homoeopathy. Puts the general public in touch with homoeopathic doctors, veterinary surgeons and pharmacies. Also book publishers, maintaining in print a number of books on various aspects of homoeopathy as well as the magazine. **Pub:** *Health & Homoeopathy*, quarterly. Journal. • Books.

★ 1752 ★ British Hypertension Society (BHS)
127 High St
Teddington TW11 8HH, United Kingdom
Phone: 44 20 89770011 **Fax:** 44 20 89770055
Email: hmc@hamptonmedical.com
Website: http://www.bhsoc.org

Fnded: 1981. **Mem:** 250. **Desc:** Investigates all aspects of research in hypertension and related vascular disease.

★ 1753 ★ British In-Vitro Diagnostics Association (BIVDA)
1 Queen Anne's Gate
London SW1H 9BT, United Kingdom
Phone: 44 207 9574633 **Fax:** 44 207 9574644
Email: enquiries@bivda.co.uk
Website: http://www.bivda.co.uk

Fnded: 1992. **Mem:** 107. **Desc:** National trade association for companies with major involvement and interest in the In-Vitro Diagnostics industry.

★ 1754 ★ British Infection Society
Infectious Disease Unit, Ward 38
Leicester Royal Infirmary
Infirmary Sq.
Leicester LE1 5WW, United Kingdom
Phone: 44 116 2586952 **Fax:** 44 116 2585067
Email: martin.wiselka@uhl-tr.nhs.uk
Website: http://www.britishinfectionsociety.org

Fnded: 1997. **Mem:** 900. **Desc:** Members of the medical profession and others working in related spheres which are relevant to the society's objectives. Established to relieve sickness by the study of all aspects of infection and to promote the wide dissemination of relevant knowledge. **Pub:** *The Journal of Infection*, bimonthly. Journal. **Frmly:** (1997) British Society for the Study of Infection.

★ 1755 ★ British Institute of Dental and Surgical Technologists
c/o Prof. A.C. Roberts, Pres.
4 Thompson Green
Shipley BD17 7PR, United Kingdom
Phone: 44 1274 532303
Website: http://www.bidst.mmu.ac.uk

Fnded: 1935. **Mem:** 300. **Desc:** Maintains standards as a professional institute for dental and surgical technicians. **Pub:** *Journal of the British Institute of Surgical Technologists*, annual. Journal. **Frmly:** (1998) British Institute of Surgical Technologists.

★ 1756 ★ British Institute of Industrial Therapy
243 Shelley Rd.
Wellingborough NN8 3EN, United Kingdom
Phone: 44 1933 675327 **Fax:** 44 1933 675327

Fnded: 1970. **Mem:** 59. **Desc:** Directors and managers of services and units providing industrial therapy for those working in the mental health field. Provides information regarding developments in industrial therapy and work schemes as appropriate to those working in the field of training people who are suffering or recovering from mental illness so that they may remain in sheltered or open employment. **Pub:** *Focus*, monthly.

★ 1757 ★ British Institute of Learning Disabilities (BILD)
Campion House
Green St.
Kidderminster DY10 1JL, United Kingdom
Phone: 44 1562 723010 **Fax:** 44 1562 723029
Email: enquiries@bild.org.uk
Website: http://www.bild.org.uk

Fnded: 1972. **Mem:** 2,000. **Desc:** Works towards improving the quality of life of people with learning disabilities, by the promotion and provision of education and training; information; research; books and journals. Provides consultancy. **Pub:** *British Journal of Learning Disabilities*, quarterly. Journal. • *Current Awareness Service*, monthly. • *Good Autism Practice*, semiannual. Journal. • *Journal of Applied Research in Intellectual Disability*, quarterly. Journal. • *Learning Disability Bulletin*, quarterly. Bulletin. • *SLD Experience*, quarterly. Journal.

★ 1758 ★ British Institute of Musculoskeletal Medicine
34 The Ave.
Watford WD17 4AH, United Kingdom
Phone: 44 1923 220999 **Fax:** 44 1923 249037
Email: info@bimm.org.uk
Website: http://www.bimm.org.uk

Fnded: 1992. **Mem:** 360. **Desc:** Doctors involved in musculoskeletal medicine. Concerned with the furtherance of knowledge and expertise in musculoskeletal medicine which includes treatment of sports injuries, backpain and other conditions of the locomotor system. By osteopathy, injections and other physical modalities. **Pub:** *Journal of Orthopaedic Medicine*, quarterly. Journal.

★ 1759 ★ British Institute of Radiology (BIR)
c/o Mary-Anne Piggott
36 Portland Pl.
London W1B 1AT, United Kingdom
Phone: 44 207 3071400 **Fax:** 44 207 3071414
Email: admin@bir.org.uk
Website: http://www.bir.org.uk

Fnded: 1897. **Mem:** 2,000. **Reg. Groups:** 1. **Local Groups:** 4. **Lang(s):** English. **Desc:** Medical radiologists, scientists, and allied professionals in 55 countries. Conducts seminars; bestows awards. **Pub:** *British Journal of Radiology*, monthly. Journal. Multidisciplinary research. • Membership Directory, periodic.

★ 1760 ★ British Leprosy Relief Association (LEPRA)
Fairfax House, 3rd Fl.
Causton Rd.
Essex
Colchester CO1 1PU, United Kingdom
Phone: 44 1206 562286 **Fax:** 44 1206 762151
Email: lepra@lepra.org.uk
Website: http://www.lepra.org.uk

Desc: Seeks to restore health, hope and dignity to people affected by leprosy. Offers social and economic rehabilitation programs. Sponsors research into the causes, prevention, and treatment of leprosy and allied diseases.

★ 1761 ★ British Lung Foundation (BLF)
78 Hatton Garden
London EC1n 8LD, United Kingdom
Phone: 44 20 78315831
Email: general@britishlungfoundation.com
Website: http://www.lunguk.org/

Fnded: 1984. **Mem:** 75,000. **Lang(s):** English. **Desc:** Individuals and organizations. Seeks to advance the prevention, diagnosis, and treatment of lung diseases. Maintains support groups for people with lung disease; provides financial and other assistance to lung disease research; conducts educational programs; participates in charitable activities; compiles statistics. **Pub:** *Breathe Easy*, quarterly. Newsletter.

★ 1762 ★ British Medical Acupuncture Society
12 Marbury House
Higher Whitley
Warrington WA4 4QW, United Kingdom
Phone: 44 1925 730727 **Fax:** 44 1925 730492
Email: admin@medical-acupuncture.org.uk
Website: http://www.medical-acupuncture.co.uk
Fnded: 1980. **Mem:** 2,000. **Reg. Groups:** 11. **Desc:** Medically qualified practitioners. Concerned with the training of medical practitioners in acupuncture. Geographic listings of medically qualified practitioners of acupuncture. **Pub:** *Acupuncture in Medicine*, quarterly. Journal.

★ 1763 ★ British Medical Association (BMA)
Tavistock Sq.
London WC1H 9JP, United Kingdom
Phone: 44 20 73874499 **Fax:** 44 20 73836400
Email: info.web@bma.org.uk
Website: http://www.bma.org.uk
Fnded: 1832. **Mem:** 124,000. **Local Groups:** 202. **Lang(s):** English. **Desc:** Doctors' trade union. A scientific and educational body and a publishing house. **Pub:** *BMA News Review*, monthly. Magazine. • *BMJ Specialist Journals*. Journal. • *British Medical Journal*, weekly. Journal. • *Student BMJ*. Journal. Reports and recommendations.

★ 1764 ★ British Medical Laser Association (BMLA)
Ninewells Hospital and Medical School
Dundee DD1 9SY, United Kingdom
Phone: 44 1382 632240 **Fax:** 44 1382 646047
Email: h.moseley@dundee.ac.uk
Website: http://www.bmla.co.uk/
Fnded: 1983.

★ 1765 ★ British Medical Ultrasound Society (BMUS)
36 Portland Pl.
London W1N 3DG, United Kingdom
Phone: 44 207 6363714 **Fax:** 44 207 3232175
Email: secretariat@bmus.org
Website: http://www.bmus.org
Fnded: 1969. **Mem:** 2,230. **Lang(s):** English. **Desc:** Medical practitioners, physicists/scientists, sonographers radiographers, veterinarians, and manufacturers of sonographic equipment. Seeks to advance the science and technology of ultrasound and to improve education in the field. **Pub:** *BMUS Bulletin*, quarterly. Newsletter. • *BMUS Membership Register*, triennial. • *Proceedings of Annual Meeting*, annual. Published in the British Journal of Radiology. **Frmly:** (1984) British Medical Ultrasound Group.

★ 1766 ★ British Menopause Society (BMS)
36 West St.
Marlow SL7 2NB, United Kingdom
Phone: 44 1628 890199 **Fax:** 44 1628 474042
Fnded: 1989.

★ 1767 ★ British Microcirculation Society (BMS)
c/o Dr. David Bates
Microvascular Research Laboratories
Department of Physiology
Preclinical Veternary School
University of Bristol
Bristol BS2 8EJ, United Kingdom
Phone: 44 171 9289818 **Fax:** 44 171 9288151
Email: dave.bates@bris.ac.uk
Website: http://www.microcirculation.org.uk
Fnded: 1963. **Mem:** 220. **Lang(s):** English. **Desc:** Individuals interested in the study of microcirculation and endothelium. Conducts clinical and scientific research.

★ 1768 ★ British Natural Hygiene Society (BNHS)
Shalimar, 3 Harold Grove
Frinton-on-Sea CO13 9BD, United Kingdom
Phone: 44 1255 672823
Website: http://members.rotfl.com/bnhs
Fnded: 1959. **Desc:** Promotes holistic and complementary health care as an alternative to conventional medical approaches to health disease.

★ 1769 ★ British Neuropathological Society (BNS)
Beach Hill Rd.
Sheffield S10 2RX, United Kingdom
Phone: 44 114 2712949
Email: secretary@bns.org.uk
Website: http://www.bns.org.uk
Fnded: 1950. **Mem:** 250. **Nat'l Groups:** 1. **Desc:** Promotes science and clinical practice related to neuropathology and diseases of the nervous system and skeletal muscle.

★ 1770 ★ British Neuroscience Association (BNA)
The Sherrington Bldg.s
Ashton St.
Liverpool L69 3GE, United Kingdom
Phone: 44 151 7945449 **Fax:** 44 151 7945516
Email: bna@liv.ac.uk
Website: http://www.bna.org.uk/
Desc: Promotes study of the structure and functions of the nervous system.

★ 1771 ★ British Nuclear Medicine Society (BNMS)
291 Kirkdale
London SE26 4QD, United Kingdom
Phone: 44 20 86767864 **Fax:** 44 20 86768417
Email: office@bnms.org.uk
Website: http://www.bnms.org.uk
Fnded: 1969.

★ 1772 ★ British Nutrition Foundation
High Holborn House
52-54 High Holborn
London WC1V 6RQ, United Kingdom
Phone: 44 207 4046504 **Fax:** 44 207 4046747
Email: postbox@nutrition.org.uk
Website: http://www.nutrition.org.uk
Fnded: 1967. **Mem:** 41. **Desc:** No individual members. Corporate membership open to any organisation, company or corporation (except trade associations) interested or concerned in achieving the objectives of the Foundation (which are listed in the Annual Report). Provides reliable information and scientifically based advice on nutrition and related health matters. Aims to help individuals understand how they may best match their diet with their lifestyle. Produces a wide range of publications on many aspects of diet and health. **Pub:** *BNF Bulletin*, 3/year. Bulletin. • *Food: A Fact of Life*. Nutrition program for schools. • *Proceedings of Annual Conference*, annual. • Papers. Briefing papers.

★ 1773 ★ British Occupational Hygiene Society (BOHS)
Georgian House, Ste. 2
Great Northern Rd.
Derby DE1 1LT, United Kingdom
Phone: 44 1332 298101 **Fax:** 44 1332 298099
Email: admin@bohs.org
Website: http://www.bohs.org/
Fnded: 1953. **Mem:** 1,000. **Local Groups:** 7. **Lang(s):** English. **Desc:** Individuals and companies. Promotes public and professional awareness of occupational and environmental hygiene practices and standards. **Pub:** *Annals of Occupational Hygiene*, 8/year. Journal. • *Directory*, annual. Directory. • *Occupational Hygiene Newsletter*, quarterly. Newsletter.

★ 1774 ★ British Oncological Association (BOA)
c/o Institute of Cancer Research
15 Cotswold Rd.
Sutton
Belmont SM2 5NG, United Kingdom
Phone: 44 20 86438901 **Fax:** 44 20 86436940
Email: pamela@lcr.ac.uk
Fnded: 1985.

★ 1775 ★ British Orthodontic Society
291 Gray's Inn Rd.
London WC1X 8QJ, United Kingdom
Phone: 44 207 8372193 **Fax:** 44 207 8372193
Website: http://www.bos.org.uk
Fnded: 1994. **Mem:** 1,600. **Desc:** Persons interested in orthodontics eligible for membership. Members (normally resident in the UK), honorary members, life members, international members, associate members, retired members, laboratory and trades members. Concerned with the promotion of the study and practice of orthodontics. Orthodontics is a speciality of dentistry and involves the treatment of abnormalities of jaw size and dental arch relationship and irregularities of tooth position. **Pub:** *BOS Newsletter*, 3/year. Newsletter. • *British Journal of Orthodontics*, quarterly. Journal.

★ 1776 ★ British Orthopaedic Association
c/o Royal College of Surgeons
35-43 Lincoln's Inn Fields
London WC2A 3PN, United Kingdom
Phone: 44 207 4056507 **Fax:** 44 207 8312676
Email: secretary@boa.ac.uk
Website: http://www.boa.ac.uk
Fnded: 1918. **Mem:** 2,700. **Desc:** Practising orthopaedic surgeons, orthopaedic surgeons in training, retired orthopaedic surgeons, orthopaedic surgeons resident abroad who have done all or part training in the United Kingdom. Concerned with the advancement of the science, art and practice of orthopaedic surgery with the aim of bringing relief to patients of all ages suffering from the effects of injury or disease to the musculo-skeletal system. **Pub:** *British Orthopaedic News*, semiannual.

★ 1777 ★ British Orthopaedic Foot Surgery Society (BOFSS)
c/o British Orthopaedic Association
35-43 Lincoln's Inn Fields
London WC2A 3PN, United Kingdom
Phone: 44 20 74056507
Fnded: 1978.

★ 1778 ★ British Orthoptic Society
Tavistock House North
Tavistock Sq.
London WC1H 9HX, United Kingdom
Phone: 44 207 3877992 **Fax:** 44 207 3872584
Email: bos@orthoptics.org.uk
Website: http://www.orthoptics.org.uk
Fnded: 1937. **Mem:** 1,200. **Desc:** Orthoptists, including students and retired orthoptists. Members work in both NHS and private practice. **Pub:** *British Orthoptic Journal*, annual. Journal.

★ 1779 ★ British Osteopathic Association
Langham House West
Luton LU1 2NA, United Kingdom
Phone: 44 158 2488455 **Fax:** 44 158 2481533
Email: enquiries@osteopathy.org
Website: http://www.osteopathy.org
Fnded: 1911. **Mem:** 1,600. **Desc:** Provides independent representation, care and support. **Pub:** Directory, annual. Membership information.

★ 1780 ★ British Paralympic Association (BPA)
Norwich Union Bldg., 9th Fl.
69 Park Ln.
Croydon CR9 1BG, United Kingdom
Phone: 44 20 76628882 **Fax:** 44 20 76628310
Website: http://www.paralympics.org.uk

Desc: Selects, prepares, enters, funds, and manages British teams at the Paralympic Games and Paralympic Winter Games. The Paralympic games take place once every four years, with the Winter Games two years after each summer event of the games.

★ 1781 ★ British Performing Arts Medicine Trust
196 Shaftesbury Ave.
London WC2H 8JL, United Kingdom
Phone: 44 20 72403331 **Fax:** 44 20 72403335
Email: bpamt@dial.pipex.com
Website: http://www.bpamt.co.uk

Fnded: 1987. **Mem:** 700. **Reg. Groups:** 2. **Desc:** Provides helpline and free assessment and diagnosis for performers with performance-related injuries and illnesses. **Frmly:** (2001) British Association for Performing Arts Medicine.

★ 1782 ★ British Pharmacological Society
16, Angel Gate
City Rd.
London EC1V 2SG, United Kingdom
Phone: 44 20 74170113 **Fax:** 44 20 74170114
Email: admin@bps.ac.uk
Website: http://www.bps.ac.uk/BPS.html

Fnded: 1931. **Mem:** 2,500. **Lang(s):** English. **Desc:** Pharmacologists and clinical pharmacologists in academia and industry in 20 countries. Conducts educational symposia and lectures; makes available travel bursaries. **Pub:** *British Journal of Clinical Pharmacology*, monthly. Journal. • *British Journal of Pharmacology*, 2x/mo. Journal.

★ 1783 ★ British Photodermatology Group (BPG)
St. Thomas Hospital
London SE1 7EH, United Kingdom
Phone: 44 20 79289292

★ 1784 ★ British Psychoanalytical Society (BP-AS)
Byron House
112A Shirland Rd.
London W9 2EQ, United Kingdom
Phone: 44 20 7563 5000 **Fax:** 44 20 7563 5001
Email: editors@psychoanalysis.org.uk
Website: http://www.ijpa.org

Fnded: 1919. **Mem:** 500. **Lang(s):** English. **Desc:** Psychoanalysts in the United Kingdom. Offers instructional programs. Promotes members' interests. **Pub:** *International Journal of Psychoanalysis*, 6/year. Journal. Peer-reviewed journal covering research and applied psychoanalysis, its history and film and book reviews. • Newsletter. Also publishes calendar of events.

★ 1785 ★ British Psychodrama Association
Flat 1/1
105 Hyndland Rd.
Glasgow G12 9JD, United Kingdom
Phone: 44 141 3390141
Website: http://www.psychodrama.org.uk

Fnded: 1984. **Mem:** 250. **Desc:** Promotes the use of psychodrama and sociodrama as a creative and effective approach to working with a wide range of people in a variety of different settings. Psychodrama, sociometry, and group psychotherapy developed from the work of Jacob Levy Moreno (1889-1974). **Pub:** Journal, semiannual. • Bulletin, quarterly.

★ 1786 ★ British Psychological Society (BPS)
St. Andrews House
48 Princess Rd. E
Leicester LE1 7DR, United Kingdom
Phone: 44 116 2549568 **Fax:** 44 116 2470787
Email: enquiry@bps.org.uk
Website: http://www.bps.org.uk

Fnded: 1901. **Mem:** 34,600. **Nat'l Groups:** 24. **Local Groups:** 7. **Lang(s):** English. **Desc:** Academic, research, and all branches of applied psychology. Promotes the advancement of psychological study and works to ensure high standards of professional education and conduct. Offers courses. **Pub:** *British Journal of Clinical Psychology*, quarterly, in February, May, September, and November. Journal. • *British Journal of Developmental Psychology*, quarterly, in March, June, September, and November. Journal. • *British Journal of Health Psychology*, quarterly, in February, May, September, and November. Journal. • *British Journal of Mathematical and Statistical Psychology*, semiannual, in May and November. Journal. • *British Journal of Psychology*, quarterly, in February, May, August, and November. Journal. • *British Journal of Social Psychology*, quarterly, in March, June, September, and December. Journal. • *Journal of Occupational and Organizational Psychology*, quarterly, in March, June, September, and December. Journal. • *Psychology and Psychotherapy: Theory, Research and Practice*, quarterly, in March, June, September, and December. Journal.

★ 1787 ★ British Reflexology Association
Monks Orchard
Whitbourne
Worcester WR6 5RB, United Kingdom
Phone: 44 1886 821207 **Fax:** 44 1886 822017
Email: bra@britreflex.co.uk
Website: http://www.britreflex.co.uk

Fnded: 1985. **Mem:** 750. **Lang(s):** English. **Desc:** Reflexology practitioners and students training to become reflexology practitioners. Representative body for persons practising the method of reflexology as a profession and for students training in the method. The official teaching body of the BRA is the Bayly School of Reflexology. **Pub:** *Footprints*, quarterly. Newsletter. • *Register of Members*, annual.

★ 1788 ★ British Retinitis Pigmentosa Society
PO Box 350
Buckingham MK18 1GZ, United Kingdom
Phone: 44 1280 860363 **Fax:** 44 1280 815900
Email: info@brps.org.uk
Website: http://www.brps.org.uk

Fnded: 1976. **Mem:** 3,000. **Desc:** RP sufferers and their families and interested multidisciplinary members. Aims to help RP sufferers and their families cope with living with RP and to raise money for medical research. **Pub:** Handbook, annual. • Newsletter, quarterly.

★ 1789 ★ British Ski Club for the Disabled (BSCD)
Randlehayes Farm
Aylesbeare Exeter
Devon UB8 1NR, United Kingdom
Phone: 44 1395 239088

Desc: Promotes skiing for the disabled in Great Britain.

★ 1790 ★ British Small Animal Veterinary Association (BSAVA)
Woodrow House
1 Telford Way
Waterwells Business Pk.
Quedgeley
Gloucester GL2 4AB, United Kingdom
Phone: 44 1452 726700 **Fax:** 44 1452 726701
Email: adminoff@bsava.com
Website: http://www.bsava.com

Fnded: 1957. **Mem:** 5,500. **Reg. Groups:** 13. **Local Groups:** 13. **Lang(s):** English. **Desc:** Veterinarians in 20 countries. Operates speakers' bureau; sponsors educational programs. Compiles statistics. Sponsors competitions; conducts charitable activities. **Pub:** *BSAVA Handbook*, annual. Handbook. • *BSAVA News*, monthly. Newsletter. • *Journal of Small Animal Practice*, monthly. Journal.

★ 1791 ★ British Society for Allergy and Clinical Immunology (BSACI)
66 Weston Park
Thames Ditton K17 0HL, United Kingdom
Phone: 44 20 83989240 **Fax:** 44 20 83982766
Email: sduff@compuserve.com

Fnded: 1948.

★ 1792 ★ British Society for Allergy, Environmental and Nutritional Medicine (BSAENM)
PO Box 7
Knighton LD7 1WT, United Kingdom
Phone: 44 1547 550378 **Fax:** 44 1547 550339

Fnded: 1981.

★ 1793 ★ British Society for Antimicrobial Chemotherapy (BSAC)
11 The Wharf
16 Bridge St.
Birmingham B1 2JS, United Kingdom
Phone: 44 121 6330410 **Fax:** 44 121 6439497
Email: enquiries@bsac.org.uk
Website: http://www.bsac.org.uk

Fnded: 1971. **Mem:** 770. **Lang(s):** English. **Desc:** Individuals in 33 countries working in the field of antimicrobial chemotherapy. Furthers research and understanding of chemotherapy. **Pub:** *Journal of Antimicrobial Chemotherapy*, monthly. Journal.

★ 1794 ★ British Society of Audiology
80 Brighton Rd.
Reading RG6 1PS, United Kingdom
Phone: 44 118 9660622 **Fax:** 44 118 9351915
Email: ann@b-s-a.demon.co.uk
Website: http://www.b-s-a.demon.co.uk

Fnded: 1968. **Mem:** 1,400. **Reg. Groups:** 4. **Desc:** Anyone with an interest in audiology. To promote the science of audiology (i.e. the study of hearing and balance) and the diagnosis, alleviation and prevention of hearing and balance impairment. The advancement of education in audiology and the furtherance of research in audiology and the publication of the results of such research. **Pub:** *BSA News*, 3/year. Magazine. • *International Journal of Audiology*, bimonthly. Journal.

★ 1795 ★ British Society for Clinical Cytology (BSCC)
PO Box 352
Oxbridge OB10 9TX, United Kingdom
Phone: 44 1895 274080

Fnded: 1962.

★ 1796 ★ British Society for Clinical Neurophysiology
Department of Clinical Neurophysiology
Middlesex Hospital
Mortimer St.
London W1N 8AA, United Kingdom
Email: secretariat@bscn.org.uk
Website: http://www.bscn.org.uk

Fnded: 1942. **Mem:** 350. **Desc:** Medical practitioners, scientists and technologists. Medical and scientific study of electrical activity which can be recorded from the nervous system. **Pub:** Papers. Presents abstracts of scientific papers. **Frmly:** (1992) EEG Society.

★ 1797 ★ British Society for Dental and Maxillofacial Radiology
Department of Dental Radiology
University of British Dental School & Hospital
Lower Mardlen St.
Bristol BS1 2LY, United Kingdom
Phone: 44 113 2336209 **Fax:** 44 113 2336165
Email: jane.luker@nbht.swcst.nhi.uk
Website: http://www.bsdmfr.org.uk

Mem: 150. **Desc:** Dental radiologists. Offers educational and public service programs. Conducts research. **Pub:** Newsletter, semiannual.

★ 1798 ★ British Society for Dental Research (BSDR)
c/o Prof. Angus Walls, Sec.
The Dental School
Framington Pl.
Newcastle upon Tyne NE2 4BW, United Kingdom
Phone: 44 191 2227823 **Fax:** 44 191 2228191
Email: a.w.g.walls@newcastle.ac.uk
Website: http://www.bsdr.org.uk

Lang(s): English. **Desc:** Individuals engaged in all aspects of dental research. Seeks to "advance research and increase knowledge for the improvement of oral health worldwide." Provides support and assistance to the oral health research community; facilitates dissemination of new research findings. Conducts continuing professional development programs for members. Works closely with international public health and dental organizations.

★ 1799 ★ British Society of Experimental and Clinical Hypnosis
c/o Phyllis A. Alden, Hon.Sec.
Psychology Consultancy
District General Hospital
Scartho Rd.
Grimsby DN33 2BA, United Kingdom
Phone: 44 1472 873423 **Fax:** 44 1472 879238
Email: honsec@bsech.demon.co.uk
Website: http://www.alden-residence.demon.co.uk

Fnded: 1977. **Mem:** 300. **Lang(s):** English. **Desc:** Medical doctors, dentists, psychologists, other health service personnel. A learned society for doctors, dentists, psychologists and other health care professionals interested in theory, research and therapeutic applications of hypnosis. It organizes meetings, training events and an annual conference. **Pub:** *Contemporary Hypnosis*, quarterly. Journal.

★ 1800 ★ British Society of Gastroenterology
3 St Andrews Pl.
London NW1 4LB, United Kingdom
Phone: 44 20 73873534 **Fax:** 44 20 74873734
Email: bsg@mailbox.ulcc.ac.uk
Website: http://www.bsg.org.uk

Fnded: 1937. **Mem:** 2,500. **Reg. Groups:** 16. **Desc:** Physicians and surgeons with a special interest in gastroenterology. Associate nurse/clinical members. Concerned with the advancement of gastroenterology and the promotion of friendship amongst those who have a special interest in the subject. **Pub:** *Gut*, monthly.

★ 1801 ★ British Society of Gerontology (BSG)
c/o Prof. Mary Gilhooly
Centre of Gerontology & Health Studies
University of Paisley
Paisley PA1 2BE, United Kingdom
Phone: 44 141 8483771
Email: m.gilhooly@paisley.ac.uk
Website: http://www.britishgerontology.org

Desc: Promotes understanding of human aging and later life through research and communication in order to improve quality of life in old age. **Pub:** *Ageing and Society.*

★ 1802 ★ British Society of Gynaecological Endoscopy (BSGE)
Duckworth Lane
Bradford BD9 6RJ, United Kingdom
Phone: 44 1274 364618 **Fax:** 44 1274 366690

Fnded: 1989.

★ 1803 ★ British Society for Haematology
2 Carlton House Terr.
London SW1Y 5AF, United Kingdom
Phone: 44 208 6437305 **Fax:** 44 208 7700933
Email: janice@bshhya.demon.co.uk
Website: http://www.blackwell-science.com/uk/society/bsh/

Fnded: 1960. **Mem:** 1,251. **Lang(s):** English. **Desc:** Committed to advancing the practice and study of haematology; promotes good haematological practice and communication. **Pub:** *British Journal of Haematology*, 25/year. Journal. • *BSH Bulletins*, quarterly. Bulletins.

★ 1804 ★ British Society of Hearing Aid Audiologists
9 Lukins Dr.
Great Dunmow
Essex CM6 1XQ, United Kingdom
Phone: 44 1371 876623 **Fax:** 44 1371 876623
Email: secretary@bshaa.com
Website: http://www.bshaa.com

Fnded: 1957. **Mem:** 700. **Desc:** Educational and trade association for private hearing aid dispensers. Promotion of ethical standards through training, examination and codes of practice. **Pub:** *BSHAA News*, quarterly. Newsletter. **Frmly:** BSHAA.

★ 1805 ★ British Society for Human Genetics (BSHG)
Edgbaston
Birmingham B15 2TG, United Kingdom
Phone: 44 121 6272634 **Fax:** 44 121 6272634
Email: bshg@bshg.org.uk
Website: http://www.bshg.org.uk

Fnded: 1996. **Desc:** Aims to advance the science of human genetics, to promote research and public awareness of human genetics related to health and disease, to guide professionals contributing to genetics in healthcare and to offer informed opinion on issues of public interest.

★ 1806 ★ British Society of Hypnotherapists
37 Orbain Rd.
London SW6 7JZ, United Kingdom
Phone: 44 207 73851166 **Fax:** 44 207 73851166
Email: sy@bsh1950.fsnet.co.uk
Website: http://www.bsh1950.fsnet.co.uk

Fnded: 1950. **Mem:** 20. **Desc:** Specialising in the treatment of nervous disorders and addictions. Provides information service for public; conducts research on behalf of members and distributes information to them.

★ 1807 ★ British Society for Immunology
Triangle House
Broomhill Rd.
London SW18 4HX, United Kingdom
Phone: 44 208 8752400 **Fax:** 44 181 8752424
Email: bsi@immunology.org
Website: http://immunology.org

Fnded: 1956. **Mem:** 4,000. **Reg. Groups:** 18. **Lang(s):** English. **Desc:** Immunologists. To advance the science of immunology for the benefit of the public. **Pub:** *Clinical & Experimental Immunology*, monthly. Journal. • *Immunology*, monthly. Journal. • *Immunology News*, bimonthly. Newsletter.

★ 1808 ★ British Society of Medical and Dental Hypnosis
The National Secretary
28 Dale Park Gardens
Leeds LS16 7PT, United Kingdom
Phone: 44 7000 560309 **Fax:** 44 7000 560309
Email: secretary@bsmdh.org
Website: http://www.bsmdh.com

Fnded: 1952. **Mem:** 369. **Reg. Groups:** 7. **Desc:** Qualified doctors, dentists and other registered health professionals Promotes the study and training in the principles and practice of hypnosis. It encourages research and publication of work relating to hypnosis. **Pub:** Journal, annual. • Newsletter, 3/year. **Frmly:** British Society of Dental Hypnosis; The Dental and Medical Society for the Study of Hypnosis.

★ 1809 ★ British Society for Medical Mycology (BSMM)
Mycology Reference Centre
Department of Microbiology
Leeds General Infirmary
Leeds LS1 3EX, United Kingdom
Phone: 44 113 3923390 **Fax:** 44 113 3435640
Email: h.r.ashbee@leeds.ac.uk
Website: http://www.bsmm.org

Fnded: 1965. **Mem:** 250. **Pub:** Newsletter, 3/year.

★ 1810 ★ British Society for Music Therapy
25 Rosslyn Ave.
East Barnet
Barnet EN4 8DH, United Kingdom
Phone: 44 208 3688879 **Fax:** 44 208 3688879
Email: denize@bsmt.demon.co.uk
Website: http://www.bsmt.org

Fnded: 1958. **Mem:** 800. **Lang(s):** English. **Desc:** Open to all interested in music therapy. Promotes the use and development of music therapy in treatment, and rehabilitation of children and adults suffering from emotional, physical or mental handicap. Holds meetings and conferences. **Pub:** *British Journal of Music Therapy*, semiannual. Journal. • *BSMT Bulletin*, 3/year. • Papers. Related to conference proceedings. • Newsletter, periodic.

★ 1811 ★ British Society for Oral Medicine
c/o Dr. David Felix
Glasgow Dental Hospital and School
Glasgow G2 3JE, United Kingdom
Phone: 44 114 2717956 **Fax:** 44 114 2717894
Website: http://www.bsom.org.uk/

Fnded: 1967.

★ 1812 ★ British Society of Periodontology
44 Pool Rd.
Hartley Wintney
Hook RG27 8RD, United Kingdom
Phone: 44 1252 843598 **Fax:** 44 1252 844018
Email: bspadmin@btinternet.com
Website: http://www.bsperio.org

Fnded: 1949. **Mem:** 800. **Desc:** Members are dental surgeons. To promote for the benefit of the public the art and science of dentistry and in particular the art and science of periodontology. **Pub:** *Journal of Clinical Periodontology*, monthly. Journal.

★ 1813 ★ British Society of Psychosomatic Obstetrics, Gynaecology and Andrology
c/o Dr. Ian Allen
Wishaw General Hospital
50 Netherton St.
Wishaw ML2 0DP, United Kingdom
Email: kenbidgood@bspoga.org
Website: http://www.bspoga.ukgateway.net/

Fnded: 1988. **Desc:** Promotes the study of psychobiological and psychosocial, ethical and cross-cultural problems in the fields of obstetrics and gynaecology, women's health and reproductive health; facilitates the dissemination of new information in these fields. **Pub:** *Journal of Psychosomatic Obstetrics and Gynecology*. Journal.

★ 1814 ★ British Society of Rehabilitation Medicine (BSRM)
11 St. Andrews Place
London NW1 4LE, United Kingdom
Phone: 44 1992 638865 **Fax:** 44 1992 638905
Email: admin@bsrm.co.uk
Website: http://www.bsrm.co.uk

Fnded: 1984.

★ 1815 ★ British Society for Research on Ageing (BSRA)
PO Box 2316
Cardiff CF23 5YY, United Kingdom
Phone: 44 29 20744847 **Fax:** 44 29 20744276
Email: info@bsra.org.uk
Website: http://www.bsra.org.uk

Fnded: 1945. **Mem:** 150. **Lang(s):** English. **Desc:** Biological scientists and clinicians involved in the study of aging. Promotes knowledge of the biology of aging and effective treatment of age-related diseases. Works to increase public awareness of the aging process. Sponsors annual postgraduate award competition. **Pub:** *Lifespan*, semiannual. Newsletter. • *Newsletter*, periodic. Newsletter.

★ 1816 ★ British Society for Restorative Dentistry (BSRD)
Turner Dental School
University Dental Hospital Manchester
Manchester M15 6FH, United Kingdom
Phone: 44 161 2756797 **Fax:** 44 161 2756797
Email: ann.shearer@man.ac.uk

Fnded: 1968.

★ 1817 ★ British Society for Rheumatology
41 Eagle St.
London WC1R 4TL, United Kingdom
Phone: 44 207 2423313 **Fax:** 44 207 2423277
Email: bsr@rheumatology.org.uk
Website: http://www.rheumatology.org.uk

Fnded: 1984. **Mem:** 1,500. **Lang(s):** English. **Desc:** Hospital doctors, non-clinical scientists, general practitioners, other professions allied to medicine. Promotes the treatment and prevention of rheumatic diseases, education and research. **Pub:** *Rheumatology*, monthly. Journal.

★ 1818 ★ British Society for the Study of Prosthetic Dentistry
University Dental School and Hospital
Wilton, Cork, Ireland
Phone: 353 21 4901141 **Fax:** 353 21 4345737
Email: finbarrallen@hotmail.com
Website: http://www.bsspd.org

Fnded: 1953. **Mem:** 490. **Desc:** Ordinary and Honorary Members. Ordinary membership shall be available to those dentists, doctors or scientists who profess an interest in prosthetic dentistry and shall be by election. Established to advance education in prosthetic dentistry for the benefit of the public. **Pub:** *BSSPD Proceedings*, annual. Proceedings.

★ 1819 ★ British Society for Surgery of the Hand
The Royal College of Surgeons of England
35-43 Lincoln's Inn Fields
London WC2A 3PE, United Kingdom
Phone: 44 20 78315162 **Fax:** 44 20 78314041
Email: secretariat@bssh.ac.uk
Website: http://www.bssh.ac.uk

Fnded: 1970. **Mem:** 653. **Desc:** The membership is drawn from the two major parent specialties of orthopedic and plastic surgery; all members share an interest in the hand. To promote and direct the development of hand surgery and to foster and coordinate education, study and research in hand surgery including the dissemination and diffusion of knowledge of hand surgery among members of the Society and the medical profession. **Pub:** *Journal of Hand Surgery*, bimonthly. Journal.

★ 1820 ★ British Society of Toxicological Pathologists (BSTP)
PO Box 222
Horrogate HG2 9XL, United Kingdom
Phone: 44 1423 870045 **Fax:** 44 1423 870045
Email: bstp@msn.com
Website: http://www.bstp.org.uk

Fnded: 1985.

★ 1821 ★ British Stammering Association
15 Old Ford Rd.
Bethnal Green
London E2 9PJ, United Kingdom
Phone: 44 181 9831003 **Fax:** 44 181 9833591
Email: mail@stammering.org
Website: http://www.stammering.org

Fnded: 1978. **Mem:** 1,600. **Lang(s):** English. **Desc:** Self-help organization aimed at assisting individuals with stammering speech patterns. Conducts free information and advice service for all stammerers and parents/teachers with stammering children. Operates facilities and activities for members. Projects on early referral to speech therapy for dysfunctional children, and stammering pupils project. **Pub:** *Annual Report*. • *Speaking Out*, quarterly. • Pamphlets, periodic. Offers guidance to stutterers.

★ 1822 ★ British Support Group - Inter-African Committee Against Harmful Traditional Practices
Russell Lodge
Parkend
Lydney GL15 4HS, United Kingdom
Phone: 44 1594 562617
Email: johnholman@namloh.fsnet.co.uk

Fnded: 1990. **Lang(s):** English. **Desc:** Expresses solidarity with African women who struggle against traditional health practices which are harmful to their lives, health, and personal dignity. Raises funds and conducts research. Arouses public awareness through the media. Offers educational programs related to the population in Africa and African immigrants in Britain. **Pub:** Newsletter, bimonthly.

★ 1823 ★ British Tinnitus Association
Acorn Business Pk.
Ground Fl., Unit 5
Woodseats Close
Sheffield S8 0%B, United Kingdom
Phone: 44 114 2509922 **Fax:** 44 114 2557059
Email: info@tinnitus.org.uk
Website: http://www.tinnitus.org.uk

Fnded: 1979. **Mem:** 9,000. **Reg. Groups:** 80. **Desc:** Individual Members or via a network of 80 local self-help groups and contacts. Offers information about tinnitus and helps to found and implement self-help groups to provide mutual support and varying degrees of counselling. BTA campaigns for better services for people with tinnitus and for more tinnitus clinics. A national conference is held annually. **Pub:** *BTA Information Pack*. Journal. • *QUIET*, quarterly.

★ 1824 ★ British Toxicology Society (BTS)
PO Box 249
Macclesfield SK11 6FT, United Kingdom
Phone: 44 1625 267881 **Fax:** 44 1625 267879
Email: secretariat@thebts.org
Website: http://www.thebts.org

Fnded: 1979. **Desc:** Promotes the science of toxicology through epidemiological evaluation of the prevalence of the chemical toxicity, bioanalysis of exposure to potentially harmful chemicals, and prediction of the toxicity of chemicals.

★ 1825 ★ British Transplantation Society (BTS)
Broomhill Rd.
Triangle House
London SW18 4HX, United Kingdom
Phone: 44 20 88752430 **Fax:** 44 20 88742421
Email: secretariat@bts.org.uk

Fnded: 1971.

★ 1826 ★ British Veterinary Association (BVA)
7 Mansfield St.
London W1G 9NQ, United Kingdom
Phone: 44 207 6366541 **Fax:** 44 207 4362970
Email: bvahq@bva.co.uk
Website: http://www.bva.co.uk

Fnded: 1882. **Mem:** 10,000. **Nat'l Groups:** 20. **Local Groups:** 31. **Desc:** Veterinarians and veterinary students. Promotes interests of members and the animals in their care. Monitors activities of, provides advice to, and develops and maintains contact with organizations interested in animal health including government agencies, local authorities, professional societies, animal rights groups, and universities. Disseminates information to the public and the media. Conducts charitable programs. Sponsors seminars and symposia. Maintains 20 specialist divisions. **Pub:** *Annual Report*, annual. • *In Practice*, monthly. • *Journal of Small Animal Practice*. Journal. • *Veterinary Nursing*. • *Veterinary Record*, weekly. • *You and Your Vet*, quarterly. **Frmly:** (1952) National Veterinary Medical Association.

★ 1827 ★ British Veterinary Nursing Association
Terminus House, Level 15
Terminus St.
Harlow CM20 1XA, United Kingdom
Phone: 44 1279 450567 **Fax:** 44 1279 420886
Email: bvna@bvna.co.uk
Website: http://www.bvna.org.uk

Fnded: 1965. **Mem:** 4,500. **Reg. Groups:** 34. **State Groups:** 1. **Desc:** Full membership qualified veterinary nurses; students; associate; supporter. To foster and promote the status of the veterinary nurse; representation on associated professional committees, and government committees. Gives advice on a career as a veterinary nurse. Membership benefits include an employment register, annual congress, reduced entry into BVNA regional and national meetings and BVNA Educational Courses. **Pub:** *Veterinary Nurse Journal, bimonthly, through membership or subscription*, bimonthly. Journal.

★ 1828 ★ British Wheelchair Sports Foundation
Guttmann Rd.
Stoke Mandeville HP21 9PP, United Kingdom
Phone: 44 1296 395995 **Fax:** 44 1296 424171
Email: enquiries@britishwheelchairsports.org
Website: http://www.britishwheelchairsports.org

Fnded: 1952. **Mem:** 2,500. **Desc:** Promotes wheelchair sports. **Pub:** *Annuae Handbook*, quarterly. Newsletter.

★ 1829 ★ Brittle Bone Society
30 Guthrie St.
Dundee DD1 5BS, United Kingdom
Phone: 44 1382 204446 **Fax:** 44 1382 206771
Email: bbs@brittlebone.org
Website: http://www.brittlebone.org

Fnded: 1972. **Mem:** 2,000. **Nat'l Groups:** 1. **Desc:** Supports research into osteogenesis imperfecta and related conditions. Supplies or identifies alternative sources of accurate information on genetics and other medical issues associated with OI. **Pub:** Newsletter, quarterly.

★ 1830 ★ Bulgarian Anatomical Society
c/o Dr. A. Bojilova-Pastitrova
Department of Anatomy
Medical University
BG-6003 Sofia, Bulgaria
Phone: 359 2 514274
Email: botzilovns@medfac.acad.bg

Fnded: 1962. **Mem:** 52. **Desc:** Fosters research in histochemistry and elctronic microscopy.

★ 1831 ★ Bulgarian Association on Aging
Blvd. Vitosha 36
BG-1000 Sofia, Bulgaria
Phone: 359 2 9876877 **Fax:** 359 2 874145
Email: medlib@sun.medun.acad.bg

Desc: Promotes gerontological research, training in the field of aging, and interests of gerontological organizations in international affairs.

★ 1832 ★ Bulgarian Dermatological Society (BDS)
(Balgarsko Dermatologichno Drujestvo — BDD)
c/o Dr. Nikolai Tsankov, Pres.
Georgi Sofiisky St. 1
University of Medicine
BG-1431 Sofia, Bulgaria
Phone: 359 2 9522774 **Fax:** 359 2 9522774
Email: tsankn@medfac.acad.bg

Fnded: 1923. **Mem:** 400. **Reg. Groups:** 1. **Local Groups:** 7. **Lang(s):** Bulgarian, English, French. **Desc:** Dermatologists and individuals interested in furthering the development of dermatology in Bulgaria. Coordinates efforts in combatting the spread of skin and venereal diseases. Furthers post-graduate education. Conducts educational and research programs. **Pub:** *Dermatologia i Venerologia Bulgaran*, quarterly. Journal. • Books. • Monographs.

★ 1833 ★ Bulgarian Family Planning and Sexual Health Association (BFPA)
67 Knyaz Dondukov
BG-1504 Sofia, Bulgaria
Phone: 359 2 9433052 **Fax:** 359 2 9433710
Email: bfpa@online.bg
Website: http://www.bfpa-bg.org

Fnded: 1986. **Mem:** 450. **Desc:** Sponsors reproductive health projects and health and sexuality education for various groups including young people, health and helping professions professionals, minority groups, special needs groups, and young offenders. Promotes training for all aspect of NGO and other management and training programs for trainers. Fosters research in parenting and family development.

★ 1834 ★ Bulgarian Neuromuscular Disease Association
90 Pilska St., Entr. 2, App. 4
7004 Rousse, Bulgaria
Phone: 359 82 237045 **Fax:** 359 82 452055

Desc: Individuals in Bulgaria affected by Amyotrophic Lateral Sclerosis (ALS), a muscle wasting condition. Provides a forum for support and exchange of information.

★ 1835 ★ Bulgarian Pediatric Association
I. Geshiv 11
BG-1606 Sofia, Bulgaria
Phone: 359 2 594128 **Fax:** 359 2 9521650
Email: pediatr@internet-bg.net

Fnded: 1961. **Mem:** 960. **Reg. Groups:** 20. **Lang(s):** English. **Desc:** Fosters research in pediatrics, including Immunological, diabetological, neonatological, oncochematology, cardiological and neurological. **Pub:** *Pediatria*, quarterly. Journal. Discusses scientific and practical problems in pediatrics. **Frmly:** Scientific Society of Pediatrics.

★ 1836 ★ Bulgarian Pharmacological Society
(Societe Bulgare de Pharmacologie)
c/o Ivan M. Krushkov, Pres.
Medical University Sofia
Medical Faculty
Department of Pharmacology and Toxicology
2 Zdrave St.
BG-1431 Sofia, Bulgaria
Phone: 359 2 518782 **Fax:** 359 2 544643
Email: krushkov@medfac.acad.bg

Mem: 146. **Desc:** Promotes pharmacology in Bulgaria.

★ 1837 ★ Bulgarian Scientific Dental Association
1 G. Sofilski St.
BG-1431 Sofia, Bulgaria
Phone: 359 2 542669 **Fax:** 359 2 9520559
Email: dental@sum.medum.acad.bg

Fnded: 1905. **Mem:** 112. **Desc:** Promotes the dental sciences in Bulgaria.

★ 1838 ★ Bulgarian Society of Aesthetic Surgery and Aesthetic Medicine
c/o Dr. Nikolay P. Serdev
11, 20th April Str.
Medical Centre - Aesthetic Surgery
BG-1606 Sofia, Bulgaria
Phone: 359 2 9524652 **Fax:** 359 2 9515668
Email: nservdev@infocom.bg

Fnded: 1993. **Mem:** 47. **Lang(s):** Bulgarian, English. **Desc:** Fosters research in aesthetic, comestic surgery and medicine.

★ 1839 ★ Bulgarian Society of Cardiology
National Heart Hospital
65 Koniovitsa Str.
BG-1309 Sofia, Bulgaria
Phone: 359 2 229388 **Fax:** 359 2 229388
Email: nhh@tea.bg
Website: http://www.escardio.org/society/natsoc/bulgaria.htm

Mem: 116. **Desc:** Promotes the study of cardiology in Bulgaria. **Pub:** *Bulgarian Cardiology*. Journal. Contains abstracts in Bulgarian and English.

★ 1840 ★ Bulgarian Society of Endocrinology
Bolnitsa po Endokrinologia
Dame Gruev 6
BG-1303 Sofia, Bulgaria
Phone: 359 2 9871497 **Fax:** 359 2 9874145
Email: dimitar@medicalnet-bg.org

Fnded: 1973. **Mem:** 170. **Nat'l Groups:** 1. **Reg. Groups:** 3. **State Groups:** 1. **Local Groups:** 3. **Lang(s):** English. **Desc:** Fosters research in endocrinology. **Pub:** *Journal of Endocrinology: Endocrinologia*, quarterly. Journal. **Frmly:** (1997) Scientific Society of Endocrinology.

★ 1841 ★ Bulgarian Society for Immunology of Reproduction (IBIR-BAN)
c/o Bulgarian Academy of Sciences
73, Tzangradsko Chaussee Blvd.
BG-1113 Sofia, Bulgaria
Phone: 359 2 720925 **Fax:** 359 2 720925

Fnded: 1989. **Mem:** 32. **Desc:** Conducts research in reproduction immunology.

★ 1842 ★ Bulgarian Society of Opthalmology
c/o Eye Clinic, Fifth City Clinical Hospital
Stolebov 67 - A
1233 Sofia, Bulgaria
Phone: 359 2 9268195 **Fax:** 359 2 9808546
Email: oftalmo@cbo.com.br

Fnded: 1927. **Mem:** 300. **Local Groups:** 5. **Lang(s):** English, French, Russian. **Desc:** Ophthalmologists. Fosters research in fundamental ophtalmic studies. **Pub:** *Bulgarian Review of Opthalmology*, 3/year. Journal.

★ 1843 ★ Bulgarian Society of Sport Medicine and Kinestherapy
k. Lulin, Bl. 333-b, ap. 17
BG-1336 Sofia, Bulgaria
Phone: 359 2 279282 **Fax:** 359 2 894145
Email: ivan_topouzov@yahoo.com

Fnded: 1953. **Mem:** 140. **State Groups:** 1. **Lang(s):** English. **Desc:** Fosters research in sport medicine and kinestherapy. **Pub:** *Sport i Nauka*. • *Vaprosi na Fizicheskata Kultura*, quarterly. Journal. Features information on sports and nauka.

★ 1844 ★ Bulimia Anorexia Nervosa Association (BANA)
300 Cabana Rd. E
Windsor, ON, Canada N9G 1A3
Phone: (519)969-2112 **Fax:** (519)969-0227
Email: info@bana.ca
Website: http://www.bana.ca

Fnded: 1982. **Mem:** 200. **Lang(s):** English, French. **Desc:** Individuals with eating disorders; health care professionals and others with an interest in the treatment of people with eating disorders; interested others. Promotes prevention and effective treatment of eating disorders. Conducts therapy groups for people with eating disorders; sponsors research and educational programs; makes available children's services; maintains speakers' bureau. **Pub:** *Apple Bytes*, quarterly. Directory.

★ 1845 ★ Bureau of Professional Education of the American Osteopathic Association (BPEAOA)
American Osteopathic Association
142 E Ontario St.
Chicago, IL 60611
Phone: (312)202-8048 **Free:** 800-621-1773
Fax: (312)202-8202
Email: kretz@aoa-net.org
Website: http://www.aoa-net.org
Konrad C. Miskowicz-Retz, PhD, Sec.

Mem: 13. **Desc:** Membership comprises American Osteopathic Associations representatives from other AOA affiliates, and public representatives. Approves policy regarding new and/or different intern and residency training programs in approved osteopathic hospitals. Serves as accrediting agency for colleges of osteopathic medicine. Oversees osteopathic continuing medical education activities. **Pub:** *Accreditation of Colleges of Osteopathic Medicine*. Handbook. Contains accreditation standards, policies and procedures, and administrative handbook.

★ 1846 ★ Burns United Support Groups (BUSG)
PO Box 36416
Detroit, MI 48236
Phone: (313)881-5577 **Fax:** (313)417-8702
Email: burnsunited@hotmail.com
Donna Schneck, Exec. Off.

Fnded: 1986. **Mem:** 150. **Nat'l Groups:** 2. **Reg. Groups:** 4. **State Groups:** 4. **Local Groups:** 3. **Desc:** Burn survivors and their families. Provides support services and information on burn care and prevention. Conducts educational programs and childrens' services. Operates speakers' bureau. **Pub:** Newsletter.

★ 1847 ★ Byelorussian Anatomical Society
c/o Prof. Dr. P.I. Lobko
Department of Anatomy
Byelorussian State Medical University
Dzerzinskogo 83
Minsk, Belarus
Phone: 375 17 2726597 **Fax:** 375 17 2726197

Email: lobkopeter@tut.by

Fnded: 1947. **Mem:** 136. **Desc:** Disseminates information on anatomical and morphological research in Belarus.

★ 1848 ★ C. G. Jung Foundation for Analytical Psychology
28 E 39th St.
New York, NY 10016
Phone: (212)697-6430 **Fax:** (212)953-3989
Email: cgjungny@aol.com
Website: http://www.cgjungny.org
Janet M. Careswell, Exec. Dir.

Fnded: 1963. **Mem:** 1,000. **Desc:** Analysts who follow the precepts of Carl G. Jung (1875-1961), Swiss psychologist; persons interested in analytical psychology. Provides information on analytical psychology. Sponsors public lectures, films, continuing education courses and professional seminars. Operates book service which provides publications on analytical psychology and related topics, and lectures on audiocassettes. **Pub:** *Quadrant*, semiannual. Journal. • Annual Report.

★ 1849 ★ C/SEC
22 Forest Rd.
Framingham, MA 01701
Phone: (508)877-8266
Norma Shulman, Dir.

Fnded: 1972. **Mem:** 2,000. **Desc:** Childbirth groups, doctors, laypersons, and nurses. Established out of concern for the lack of resources available to couples who anticipate or have had a cesarean delivery. Goals are to: improve the cesarean childbirth experience and make the cesarean delivery a good and meaningful childbirth experience for each couple; provide information and promote education on cesarean prevention and vaginal birth after cesarean; change attitudes and policies that affect the cesarean childbirth experience. Offers support for cesarean couples through informal discussion meetings, telephone contact, and personal reply to letters. Provides information on many aspects of cesarean childbirth in order to make couples aware of exactly what the procedure entails and what o ptions are available. Works with doctors, hospitals, childbirth educators, and others in the medical community to effect policy changes and to promote family-centered maternity care for cesarean couples. Conducts in-service programs for hospital staffs and has spoken at conventions and workshops on childbirth. Acronym C/SEC stands for Cesareans/Support, Education and Concern. **Pub:** *Frankly Speaking*. Book. Discussion of cesarean birth. *Price:* $4. • *Preventing Unnecessary Cesareans: A Guide to Labor Management and Detailed Bibliography*. Pamphlet. Outlines avoidable factors which may lead to preventable cesareans. *Price:* $2. **Frmly:** (1976) C/SEC (Cesarean Sections: Education and Concern).

★ 1850 ★ Caesarean Support Network
55 Cooil Dr.
Douglas
Isle of Man IM2 2HF, United Kingdom
Phone: 44 1624 661269

Desc: Provides support and information on caesarean birth. Promotes improved maternal and child health-care services.

★ 1851 ★ Caitlin Raymond International Registry
University of Massachusetts Medical Center
55 Lake Ave. N
Worcester, MA 01655
Phone: (508)334-8969 **Free:** 800-726-2824
Fax: (508)334-8972
Email: info@crir.org
Website: http://www.crir.org/

Fnded: 1986. **Desc:** Works as a comprehensive resource for patients and physicians conducting a search for unrelated bone marrow or cord blood donor.

★ 1852 ★ Cajal Club (CC)
c/o Henry J. Ralston, MD
Department of Anatomy
University of California
San Francisco, CA 94143-0452
Phone: (415)476-1861
Email: hjr@phy.ucsf.edu
Website: http://www.anatomy.org/anatomy/cajal-club.htm
Dr. Henry J. Ralston, MD, Contact

Fnded: 1947. **Mem:** 450. **Desc:** Neuroanatomists who meet for discussion and the presentation of papers on prospective research, technique, and history of neurology. (Club is named after Sr. Don Santiago Ramon y Cajal, a founder of and Nobel laureate for the science of neuroanatomy.) **Pub:** *History of Cajal Club*, quinquennial. • Proceedings, periodic.

★ 1853 ★ Calix Society (CS)
2555 Hazelwood Ave.
Saint Paul, MN 55109-2030
Phone: (651)773-3117 **Free:** 800-398-0524
Website: http://www.calixsociety.org
Jim Billigmeier, Pres.

Fnded: 1947. **Mem:** 3,000. **State Groups:** 14. **Local Groups:** 22. **Desc:** Catholic alcoholics who are maintaining sobriety through their own participation in Alcoholics Anonymous. Non-Catholic alcoholics and interested individuals are welcome. Promotes total abstinence for Catholic alcoholics and encourages their spiritual development. ("Calix" means "chalice" in Latin and refers to the society's belief in "substituting the cup that sanctifies for the cup that stupefies.") **Pub:** *Calix and the Twelve Steps*. Book. *Price:* $7. • *The Chalice*, bimonthly. Newsletter. Contains contributed stories regarding spiritual and physical recovery. Includes book reviews, obituaries, research reports, and statistics. *Price:* $15/year. • *Directory of Calix Units in the U.S. and Canada*, periodic. Directory. • *The Light of Faith*. Book. *Price:* $7. • *What and Why*. Brochure.

★ 1854 ★ Cameroon National Association for Family Welfare (CAMNAFAW)
BP 11994
Yaounde, Cameroon
Phone: 237 2236230 **Fax:** 237 2236230
Email: camnafaw@iccnet.cm

Fnded: 1987. **Mem:** 2,000. **Reg. Groups:** 7. **Lang(s):** English, French. **Desc:** Those involved in the domain of reproductive health. Encourages public awareness of family planning and responsible parenthood through youth programs in Cameroon. Works to reduce the number of unwanted pregnancies and abortions and STI/HIV/AIDS. Advocates family planning as a basic human right. Sponsors programs in sex education, family planning, and health. Provides contraceptive services. **Pub:** *CAMNAFAW - The Road so Far*, periodic. Brochure. Containing information on youth and planning issues. • *Youth and Sexuality*. Booklet. • *Youth Prepare for Responsible Parenthood*. Booklet.

★ 1855 ★ Canada Academy and Association of Chinese Acupuncture
c/o Dr. Peter Yea, Ch. Off.
3852 Finch Ave. E, No. 407
Toronto, ON, Canada M1T 3T6
Phone: (416)298-3070

Fnded: 1994. **Mem:** 150. **Desc:** Promotes Chinese acupuncture.

★ 1856 ★ Canada's Association for the Fifty-Plus (CARP)
27 Queen St. E, Ste. 1304
Toronto, ON, Canada M5C 2M6
Phone: (416)363-8748 **Free:** 800-363-9736
Fax: (416)363-8747
Email: carp@50plus.com
Website: http://www.fifty-plus.net

Fnded: 1976. **Mem:** 380,000. **Reg. Groups:** 8. **Lang(s):** English. **Desc:** Canadians who are at least 50 years old. Promotes the rights and seeks to improve the quality of life of older people. Provides products and services to members; represents members in public forums. **Pub:** *CARPNEWS*, bimonthly. Magazine. **Frmly:** (1999) Canadian Association of Retired Persons.

★ 1857 ★ Canada's Health Informatics Association (COACH)
2 Carlton St., Ste. 1304
Toronto, ON, Canada M5B 1J3
Phone: (416)979-5551 **Free:** 888-253-8554
Fax: (416)979-1144
Email: info@coachorg.com

Fnded: 1975. **Mem:** 850. **Lang(s):** English. **Desc:** Health care and information systems professionals. Promotes education and the exchange of ideas in the field of medical information systems. **Pub:** *Guidelines for the Protection of Health Information*. Book. Contains a framework for developing and implementing security and privacy programs. **Frmly:** (1999) Canadian Organization for Advancement of Computers in Health.

★ 1858 ★ Canadian Academy of Denturism (CAD)
2 Athabascan Ave., Ste. 200
Sherwood Park, AB, Canada T8A 4E3
Phone: (780)467-5541 **Fax:** (780)467-9263

Mem: 90. **Lang(s):** English, French. **Desc:** Dentists and related health professionals. Promotes advancement in the study and practice of denturism. Conducts continuing professional education programs. Sponsors research. **Pub:** *Academy Report*, annual. Journal.

★ 1859 ★ Canadian Academy of Endodontics (CAE) (Academie Canadienne d'Endodontie — ACE)
Dental Clinic Bldg.
Univ. of Saskatchewan
105 Wiggins Rd.
Saskatoon, SK, Canada S7N 5E4
Phone: (306)966-5089 **Fax:** (306)966-5018
Email: teplitsky@skyfox.usask.la
Website: http://www.caendo.ca

Fnded: 1965. **Mem:** 200. **Lang(s):** English, French. **Desc:** Member dentists of the Canadian Dental Association or other Canadian national dental associations who have been graduated for at least 3 years or have earned recognition by graduate or postgraduate training, teaching, or research. Works to maintain and improve public health through the advancement of endodontics. Sponsors competitions and bestows awards; maintains speakers' bureau; compiles statistics. **Pub:** *Roster*, annual. • Newsletter, 2-3/year.

★ 1860 ★ Canadian Academy of Facial, Plastic and Reconstructive Surgery (Academie Canadienne de Chirurgie Plastique et Reconstructive Faciale)
2150 Burnhamthorpe Rd. W
PO Box 98013
Mississauga, ON, Canada L5L 5V4
Phone: (905)569-6965 **Fax:** (905)569-6965
Email: info@facialcosmeticsurgery.org
Website: http://www.facialcosmeticsurgery.org

Fnded: 1981. **Mem:** 50. **Lang(s):** English, French. **Desc:** Plastic and reconstructive surgeons specializing in facial procedures. Seeks to advance the practice of facial cosmetic surgery. Facilitates exchange of information among members; conducts continuing professional education courses. **Frmly:** CAFPRS.

★ 1861 ★ Canadian Academy of the History of Pharmacy (CAHP) (Academie Canadienne d'Histoire de la Pharmacie — ACHP)
Faculty of Pharmacy
University of Toronto

19 Russell St.
Toronto, ON, Canada M5S 2S2
Phone: (416)978-2889 **Fax:** (416)978-8511
Email: wayne.hindmarsh@utoronto.ca
Website: http://www.utoronto.ca

Lang(s): English, French. **Desc:** Pharmacists, historians, and other individuals with an interest in the history of pharmacy. Promotes historical research. Provides support and assistance to pharmaceutical historians; conducts educational programs; serves as a clearinghouse on pharmacy history.

★ 1862 ★ Canadian Academy of Oral and Maxillofacial Radiology (Academie Canadienne de Radiologie Buccale et Maxillofaciale)

c/o Richard Bohay
School of Dentistry
University of Western Ontario
London, ON, Canada N6A 5C1
Phone: (519)661-3327 **Fax:** (519)850-2316
Email: rbohay@uwo.ca

Lang(s): English, French. **Desc:** Oral radiologists. Seeks to advance the study, teaching, and practice of oral radiology. Conducts research; makes available continuing professional education courses. **Frmly:** (2000) Canadian Academy of Oral Radiology.

★ 1863 ★ Canadian Academy of Periodontology (CAP) (Academie Canadienne de Parodotologie)

1815 Alta Vista Dr., Unit 105
Ottawa, ON, Canada K1G 3Y6
Phone: (613)523-9800 **Fax:** (613)523-1968
Email: central-office@cap-acp.ca
Website: http://www.cap-acp.ca

Mem: 300. **Lang(s):** English, French. **Desc:** Periodontologists, educators, and students. Promotes advancement in the practice and teaching of periodontology. Conducts continuing professional education courses for members. Maintains speakers' bureau. **Pub:** *CAPsule*, 3/year. Newsletter. • Directory, annual.

★ 1864 ★ Canadian Academy of Sport Medicine (CASM)

1010 Poytek St., Unit 14
Gloucester, ON, Canada K1J 9H9
Phone: (613)748-5851 **Free:** 877-585-2394
Fax: (613)748-5792
Email: jburke@casm-acms.org
Website: http://www.casm-acms.org

Fnded: 1970. **Mem:** 500. **Lang(s):** English, French. **Desc:** Physicians committed to excellence in the practice of medicine as it applies to all aspects of physical activity. Seeks to be a leader in advancing the art and science of sport medicine, including health promotion and disease prevention, for the benefit of all Canadians through programs of education, research, and service. **Pub:** *Clinical Journal of Sport Medicine*, quarterly. Journal.

★ 1865 ★ Canadian Adult Congenital Heart Network

c/o BB&C Association Management Services
2121 Argentia Rd., Ste. 404
Mississauga, ON, Canada L5N 2X4
Phone: (416)417-6523 **Fax:** (416)340-5014
Email: gwebb77452@aol.com
Website: http://www.cachnet.org/cachn.html

Fnded: 1992. **Mem:** 86. **Reg. Groups:** 15. **Lang(s):** English, French. **Desc:** Represents the interests of Canadian adults who were born with heart defects. Encourages efforts to educate the public on the problems and treatment of heart disease. Works as a support network for congenital heart patients. **Pub:** *CACH News*, quarterly. Newsletter.

★ 1866 ★ Canadian AIDS Society (CAS)

309 Cooper St., 4th Fl.
Ottawa, ON, Canada K2P 0G5
Phone: (613)230-3580 **Fax:** (613)563-4998
Email: casinfo@cdnaids.ca
Website: http://www.cdnaids.ca

Fnded: 1986. **Mem:** 103. **Nat'l Groups:** 62. **Reg. Groups:** 98. **Local Groups:** 36. **Lang(s):** English, French. **Desc:** National coalition of over one hundred community-based AIDS organizations across Canada. **Pub:** *Quarterly Update*, quarterly. Newsletter.

★ 1867 ★ Canadian AIDS Treatment Information Exchange (CATIE)

555 Richmond St. W, Ste. 505
Box 1104
Toronto, ON, Canada M5V 3B1
Phone: (416)203-7122 **Free:** 800-263-1638
Fax: (416)203-8284
Email: info@catie.ca
Website: http://www.catie.ca

Fnded: 1991. **Mem:** 700. **Lang(s):** English, French. **Desc:** Seeks to assist people with AIDS and health care providers in making informed treatment decisions. Gathers and disseminates information on AIDS treatments. Facilitates access by health care professionals to the latest information on advances in AIDS care. Conducts educational programs. **Pub:** *Factsheet*, periodic. Pamphlet. • *HIV+ Peers as Treatment Information Counselors*. Handbook. • *HIV-Related Clinical Trials in Ontario*, periodic. Directory. • *Hooking Up to Social Services*. Report. • *InfoCATIE*, quarterly. Newsletter. • *Managing Your Health*. Book. • *TreatmentUpdate*, 8/year. Journal.

★ 1868 ★ Canadian Alliance of British Pensioners (CABP)

605 Royal York Rd., Ste. 202
Toronto, ON, Canada M8Y 4G5
Phone: (416)253-6402 **Fax:** (416)253-6402
Email: info@britishpensions.com
Website: http://www.britishpensions.com

Fnded: 1991. **Lang(s):** English. **Desc:** Senior citizens and British expatriates in Canada. Works to safeguard the interests of senior citizens. Campaigns to end pension discrimination such as freezing of British pension for those residents in Canada. **Pub:** *Quarterly View*, quarterly. Newsletter. **Frmly:** British Pensioners Association.

★ 1869 ★ Canadian Alliance of Physiotherapy Regulators

1243 Islington Ave., Ste. 501
Etobicoke, ON, Canada M8X 1Y9
Phone: (416)234-8800 **Fax:** (416)234-8820
Website: http://www.alliancept.org/

Desc: Advocates on national regulatory issues for physiotherapy regulators; seeks to develop a national consistency of registration requirements, national consistency of standards, and to have the Physiotherapy National Exam used throughout Canada. **Pub:** Annual Report. • Bulletin.

★ 1870 ★ Canadian Amputee Sports Association (Association Canadienne des Sports pour Amputes)

1185 Eglinton Ave. E, Ste. 102
Toronto, ON, Canada M3C 3C6
Phone: (416)426-7187 **Fax:** (416)426-7361
Email: ampsport@interlog.com
Website: http://www.interlog.com/~ampsport/can_amputee.html

Fnded: 1977. **Mem:** 160. **State Groups:** 5. **Lang(s):** English, French. **Desc:** Amputees and other individuals with an interest in sports for people with disabilities. Seeks to increase the availability of sports programs for amputees. Conducts athletic and other recreational programs.

★ 1871 ★ Canadian Anesthesiologists' Society (CAS) (Societe Canadienne des Anesthesiologistes — SCA)

1 Eglinton Ave. E, Ste. 208
Toronto, ON, Canada M4P 3A1
Phone: (416)480-0602 **Fax:** (416)480-0320
Email: anesthesia@cas.ca
Website: http://www.cas.ca

Fnded: 1920. **Mem:** 2,500. **Nat'l Groups:** 10. **Local Groups:** 10. **Lang(s):** English, French. **Desc:** Professional anesthesiologists and students. Promotes the art and science of anesthesia in Canada. Advocates measures designed to improve health care in Canada and hospital standards regarding anesthesia. Works in conjunction with the Canadian Medical Association. Conducts discussion sessions, panels, refresher courses, and workshops. Maintains C.A.S. International Education Fund for aid to developing countries and the Canadian Anesthesia Research Foundation for the promotion of anesthesia research in Canada. **Pub:** *Canadian Journal of Anesthesia*, 10/year. Journal. • *CAS Guidelines to the Practice of Anesthesia*, annual. Directory. • *CAS-SCA Newsletter*, quarterly. Newsletter. • *CJA Annual Meeting Supplement*, annual. Refresher courses and abstracts. **Frmly:** (1924) Canadian Society of Anaesthetists; (1943) Anaesthesia Section of the Canadian Medical Association; (1998) Canadian Anaesthetists' Society.

★ 1872 ★ Canadian Animal Health Institute (CAHI)

160 Research Lane, Ste. 102
Guelph, ON, Canada N1G 5B2
Phone: (519)763-7777 **Fax:** (519)763-7407
Email: cahi@cahi-icsa.ca
Website: http://www.cahi-icsa.ca

Fnded: 1968. **Mem:** 60. **Lang(s):** English, French. **Desc** Trade association representing companies that develop and manufacture pharmaceuticals, biologicals, feed additives, and animal pesticides used in veterinary medicine and livestock production. Member firms collectively manufacture approximately 90 percent of all animal health products manufactured in Canada. **Pub:** *Inforum*, bimonthly. Bulletin. Deals with current issues in the animal health industry.

★ 1873 ★ Canadian Apheresis Group (CAG) (Groupe Canadien d' Apherese — GCA)

435 St. Laurent Blvd., Ste. 199
Ottawa, ON, Canada K1K 2Z8
Phone: (613)748-9613 **Fax:** (613)748-6392
Email: cag@magi.com
Website: http://www.pheresis.org/orgs.html

Fnded: 1980. **Lang(s):** English, French. **Desc:** Apheresis practitioners. Seeks to advance the study and practice of apheresis. Conducts research and educational programs.

★ 1874 ★ Canadian Association for Adolescent Health (CAAH) (Association canadienne pour la sante des adolescents — ACSA)

Sainte-Justine Hospital
3175 Cote Ste-Catherine, 7th Fl., 2nd Block
Montreal, QC, Canada H3T 1C5
Phone: (514)345-9959 **Fax:** (514)345-4778
Email: acsacaah@microtec.ca
Website: http://www.acsa-caah.ca/

Fnded: 1993. **Mem:** 900. **Desc:** Professionals, students, community workers and organizations. Promotes health, education and well-being of adolescents in Canada at the regional and national level; provides self-advocacy among adolescents or serves as an advocate for adolescent health issues. **Pub:** *Pro-Ado*, 3/year. Journal. • *Pro-Teen*, 3/year. Journal. Contains articles of scientific events, description of programs, news, research summaries, clinical facts, original articles, section on ethics.

★ 1875 ★ Canadian Association of Advanced Practice Nurses
c/o Rosemary Kohr
London Health Sciences Centre
E-510-375 South St.
London, ON, Canada N6A 4G5
Phone: (519)685-8500
Email: rkohr@lhsc.on.ca
Website: http://www.caapn.com

Lang(s): English, French. **Desc:** Nurses engaged in clinical practice. Promotes professional development of members; seeks to advance the practice of clinical nursing. Facilitates communication and cooperation among members; sponsors continuing professional education courses. **Frmly:** (1999) Canadian Clinical Nurse Specialist Group.

★ 1876 ★ Canadian Association for Anatomy, Neurobiology and Cell Biology (CAANCB)
Department of Anatomy and Cell Biology
Faculty of Medicine and Dentistry
University of Western Ontario
London, ON, Canada N6A 5C1
Phone: (519)661-2111 **Fax:** (519)661-3936
Email: ahrycysh@uwo.ca

Fnded: 1957. **Mem:** 125. **Desc:** Represents members' interests. **Pub:** *Bulletin of the CAANCB/ACANBC*, annual. Bulletin.

★ 1877 ★ Canadian Association of Blue Cross Plans (CABCP) (Association Canadienne des Croix Bleue)
185 The West Mall, Ste. 600
Etobicoke, ON, Canada M9C 5P1
Phone: (416)626-1688 **Fax:** (416)626-6445
Email: gerry.devlin@ont.bluecross.ca
Website: http://www.bluecross.ca

Fnded: 1955. **Mem:** 6. **Lang(s):** English, French. **Desc:** Independent Blue Cross health plans. Seeks to promote, enhance and protect association trademarks and trade names across Canada; facilitates communication and cooperation among members in support of regional and national growth and development.

★ 1878 ★ Canadian Association of Burn Nurses (CABN)
48 Strath Ln.
Dartmouth, NS, Canada B2X 1Z3
Phone: (902)474-0300

Lang(s): English, French. **Desc:** Nurses specializing in the treatment of burns. Promotes professional advancement of members. Facilitates exchange of information among members; conducts continuing professional education programs.

★ 1879 ★ Canadian Association of Cardiac Rehabilitation (CACR)
1390 Taylor Ave.
Winnipeg, MB, Canada R3M 3V8
Phone: (204)488-5854 **Fax:** (204)488-4819
Email: info@cacr.ca
Website: http://www.cacr.ca/

Fnded: 1991. **Mem:** 450. **Nat'l Groups:** 1. **Desc:** Promotes leadership in clinical practice, research and advocacy in cardiac disease prevention and rehabilitation in order to improve and maintain the cardiovascular health of Canadians. **Pub:** *CACR Newsbeat*, quarterly. Newsletter. Contains information about cardiac rehabilitation and related topics. • *Canadian Guidelines for Cardiac Rehabilitation & Secondary Prevention*, annual. Book. Resource for professionals within the field of cardiovascular health and rehabilitation.

★ 1880 ★ Canadian Association of Cardio-Pulmonary Technologists (CACPT)
PO Box 848, Sta. A
Toronto, ON, Canada M5W 1G3
Phone: (403)670-1190
Email: contactus@cacpt.ca
Website: http://cacpt.ca

Fnded: 1970. **Mem:** 240. **Lang(s):** English, French. **Desc:** Medical technologists specializing in cardiopulmonary practice. Promotes professional advancement of members. Supports cardio-pulmonary research; conducts continuing professional education programs. **Pub:** *CP-Update*, quarterly. Newsletter.

★ 1881 ★ Canadian Association of Centers for the Management of Hereditary Metabolic Diseases (Association Canadienne des Centres de Traitement pour les Malades Metaboliques Hereditaires)
c/o Health Sciences Ctr., Section of Genetics Metabolism
FE229-820 Sherbrook St.
Winnipeg, MB, Canada R3A 1R9
Phone: (204)787-2711 **Fax:** (204)787-1419
Email: cgroenberg@hsc.mb.ca
Website: http://www.garrod.ca/

Lang(s): English, French. **Desc:** Medical centers specializing in the treatment of people with hereditary metabolic disorders. Seeks to advance the diagnosis and treatment of hereditary metabolic disorders. Facilitates exchange of information among members; serves as a clearinghouse on hereditary metabolic disorders.

★ 1882 ★ Canadian Association for Child Neurology (CACN) (Association Canadienne de Neurologie Pediatrique — ACNP)
c/o Canadian Congress of Neurological Sciences
PO Box 5456, Station A.
Calgary, AB, Canada T2H 1X8
Phone: (403)229-9544 **Fax:** (403)229-1661
Email: brains@ccns.org
Website: http://www.ccns.org/

Fnded: 1991. **Mem:** 110. **Lang(s):** English, French. **Desc:** Neurologists with an interest in neurological disorders in children. Seeks to advance the practice of child neurology; promotes professional development of members. Serves as a clearinghouse on child neurology; conducts continuing professional education courses; provides support and assistance to research projects. **Pub:** *Canadian Journal of Neurological Sciences*, quarterly. Journal. Contains papers from all branches of neuroscience.

★ 1883 ★ Canadian Association for Children of Alcoholics (CACA) (Association Canadienne pour Enfants d'Alcoholiques — ACEA)
Hospital for Sick Children
555 University Ave.
Toronto, ON, Canada M5G 1X8
Phone: (416)813-1500

Lang(s): English, French. **Desc:** Individuals providing services to alcoholics and their families; children of alcoholics. Promotes increased awareness of issues faced by children of alcoholics and other substance abusers. Encourages research; advocates for expansion of services available to children of substance abusers.

★ 1884 ★ Canadian Association for Clinical Microbiology and Infectious Diseases (CACMID) (Association Canadienne de Microbiologie Clinique et des Maladies — ACMCM)
c/o Astrid Petrich
L424, Microbiology
St. Joseph's Healthcare
50 Charlton Ave. E
Hamilton, ON, Canada L8N 4A6
Phone: (905)522-1155 **Fax:** (905)521-6083
Email: petricha@mcmaster.ca
Website: http://www.cacmid.ca

Fnded: 1980. **Mem:** 250. **Lang(s):** English, French. **Desc:** Microbiologists and other scientists and medical professionals engaged in the clinical study of infectious diseases. Seeks to advance the biological and medical sciences; promotes professional development of members. Serves as a clearinghouse on the clinical study of infectious diseases; facilitates exchange of information among members; conducts research and educational programs. **Pub:** *CACMID Contact*, quarterly. Newsletter.

★ 1885 ★ Canadian Association for Community Care (CACC) (Association Canadienne de Soins et Services Communautaires — ACSSC)
1 Nicholas St., Ste. 712
Ottawa, ON, Canada K1N 7B7
Phone: (613)241-7510 **Fax:** (613)241-5923
Email: info@cacc-acssc.com
Website: http://www.cacc-acssc.com

Fnded: 1980. **Mem:** 300. **Lang(s):** English, French. **Desc:** Home health care services and long-term care facilities. Promotes development of a "range of high-quality, flexible, responsive and accessible community care services" in Canada. Serves as a clearinghouse on community care services; conducts public advocacy on behalf of members, consumers, and researchers; develops standards of practice and facilities in community care; serves as liaison between members and government, consumers, and related organizations. **Frmly:** HomeSupport Canada; Canadian Long Term Care Association.

★ 1886 ★ Canadian Association of Critical Care Nurses (CACCN)
PO Box 25322
London, ON, Canada N6C 6B1
Phone: (519)649-5284 **Fax:** (519)649-1458
Email: caccn@caccn.ca
Website: http://www.caccn.ca/

Fnded: 1985. **Mem:** 1,050. **Reg. Groups:** 10. **Lang(s):** English, French. **Desc:** Critical care nurses. Promotes professional advancement of members and improvement in the practice of critical care nursing. Conducts continuing professional education programs for members. **Pub:** *Dynamics Official Journal of the CACCN*, quarterly. Journal. • *Standards for Critical Care Nursing Practice (2nd Edition)*. • *Study Guide for Critical Care Nursing Certification Examination (2nd Edition)*.

★ 1887 ★ Canadian Association of the Deaf (CAD)
203-251 Bank St.
Ottawa, ON, Canada K2P 1X3
Phone: (613)565-2882 **Fax:** (613)565-1207
Email: cad@cad.ca
Website: http://www.cad.ca

Fnded: 1940. **Mem:** 44. **Lang(s):** English, French. **Desc:** Regional and local organizations for the deaf. Promotes interests of the deaf through advocacy; provides educational and support facilities. Maintains speakers' bureau; conducts research; compiles statistics. **Pub:** *CAD Chat*, quarterly. Newsletter.

★ 1888 ★ Canadian Association for Dental Research (CADR) (Association Canadienne de Recherches Dentaires — ACRD)
c/o Dr. Charles Smith
IADR Canadian Division
McGill University, Faculty of Dentistry
3640 University St.
Montreal, QC, Canada H3A 2B2
Phone: (403)491-1624

Email: cesmith@med.mcgill.ca
Website: http://www.iadr.com

Lang(s): English, French. **Desc:** Dentists, dental schools, and dental research facilities. Seeks to advance the practice of dentistry. Sponsors dental research projects; conducts continuing professional education courses.

★ 1889 ★ Canadian Association for Disabled Skiing (CADS) (Association Canadienne des Sports pour Skieurs Handicapes — ACSSH)
PO Box 307
Kimberly, BC, Canada V1A 2Y9
Phone: (250)427-7712 **Fax:** (250)427-7715
Email: cads@rockies.net
Website: http://www.disabledskiing.ca

Fnded: 1976. **Mem:** 3,000. **Nat'l Groups:** 10. **Lang(s):** English, French. **Desc:** People with disabilities. Promotes participation in skiing by members. Provides skiing opportunities for people with disabilities. **Pub:** Newsletter, semiannual.

★ 1890 ★ Canadian Association of Electroneurophysiology Technologists (Association Canadienne des Technologues en Electroneurophysiologie)
c/o Tajsha Neuls, Sec.
6110 Kitchener St.
Burnaby, BC, Canada V5B 2J4
Phone: (604)298-1311 **Fax:** (604)291-5877
Email: caet@canada.com
Website: http://www.caet.org

Lang(s): English, French. **Desc:** Medical technologists specializing in electroneurophysiology. Promotes professional advancement of members; works to advance the practice of electroneurophysiology. Represents members' interests; conducts continuing professional development courses.

★ 1891 ★ Canadian Association of Emergency Physicians (Association Canadienne des Medecins d'Urgence)
1785 Alta Vista Dr., Ste. 104
Ottawa, ON, Canada K1G 3Y6
Phone: (613)523-3343 **Free:** 800-643-1158
Fax: (613)523-0190
Email: admin@caep.ca
Website: http://www.caep.ca

Fnded: 1978. **Mem:** 1,650. **Lang(s):** English, French. **Desc:** National, voluntary, charitable organization dedicated to excellence in providing emergency health care. Promotes education for health professionals involved in emergency health care as well as providing leadership in the advancement of knowledge through research in emergency medicine. **Pub:** *Canadian Journal of Emergency Medicine*, quarterly. Journal.

★ 1892 ★ Canadian Association for Entrostomal Therapy (CAET)
PO Box 48069
60 Dundas St., E
Mississauga, ON, Canada L5A 1W4
Phone: (905)270-8433 **Fax:** (905)270-8963
Email: caet@on.aibn.com
Website: http://www.caet.ca

Fnded: 1979. **Mem:** 309. **Reg. Groups:** 5. **Lang(s):** English, French. **Desc:** Health care professionals and medical facilities providing enterostomal therapy. Seeks to advance the practice of enterostomal therapy. Serves as a clearinghouse on enterostomal therapy; conducts continuing professional education courses. **Pub:** *Link*. Newsletter. Includes updates of focus groups and regional or membership news.

★ 1893 ★ Canadian Association of Familial Ataxia (Association Canadienne des Ataxies Familiales)
5620, rue C.A. Jobin
Montreal, QC, Canada H1P 1H8
Phone: (514)321-8684 **Free:** 800-222-3968
Fax: (514)321-2957
Email: acaf@cam.org
Website: http://www.cam.org/~acaf

Fnded: 1972. **Mem:** 1,500. **Local Groups:** 2. **Lang(s):** English, French. **Desc:** Individuals with Friedreich's Ataxia (a muscular disorder which results in an inability to coordinate voluntary muscular movements). Encourages exchange between families of ataxic persons. Raises funds for medical research; offers social services to victims; recruits volunteer support. Facilitates contact with medical specialists and disseminates information about the disease. **Pub:** *Eldorado*, quarterly. Newsletter. **Frmly:** Canadian Association of Friedreich's Ataxia.

★ 1894 ★ Canadian Association of Gastroenterology (CAG) (Association Canadienne de Gastroenterologie — ACG)
2902 S Sheridan Way
Oakville, ON, Canada L6J 7L6
Phone: (905)829-2504 **Free:** 888-780-0007
Fax: (905)829-0242
Email: cagoffice@cag-acg.org
Website: http://www.cag-acg.org

Lang(s): English, French. **Desc:** Gastroenterologists and other health care professionals with an interest in gastroenterology. Seeks to advance gastroenterological practice. Conducts continuing professional education programs.

★ 1895 ★ Canadian Association of General Surgeons (CAGS)
774 Promenade Echo Dr.
Ottawa, ON, Canada K1S 5N8
Phone: (613)730-6280 **Fax:** (613)730-1116
Email: cags@rcpsc.edu
Website: http://cags.medical.org

Lang(s): English, French. **Desc:** General surgeons. Promotes professional development of members; seeks to advance the practice of general surgery. Represents members' collective interests; conducts continuing professional education courses.

★ 1896 ★ Canadian Association of Gerontology (CAG)
824 Meath St., Ste. 100
Ottawa, ON, Canada K1Z 6E8
Phone: (613)728-9347 **Fax:** (613)728-8913
Email: info@cagacg.ca
Website: http://www.cagacg.ca

Fnded: 1973. **Mem:** 1,000. **Desc:** Focuses on the problems and process of aging. **Pub:** *CAG Newsletter*, quarterly. Newsletter. • *Canadian Journal on Aging*, quarterly. Journal.

★ 1897 ★ Canadian Association of Independent Living Centers (CAILC)
1104-170 Laurier Ave. W
Ottawa, ON, Canada K1P 5V5
Phone: (613)563-2581 **Fax:** (613)563-3861
Email: cailc@magma.ca
Website: http://www.cailc.ca

Fnded: 1986. **Mem:** 24. **Nat'l Groups:** 1. **Lang(s):** English, French. **Desc:** Promotes and fosters the development of Independent Living Resource Centres in Canada. Fosters full integration of people with disabilities into society.

★ 1898 ★ Canadian Association of Internes and Residents (CAIR)
151 Slater St., Ste. 412
Ottawa, ON, Canada K1P 5H3
Phone: (613)234-6448 **Fax:** (613)234-5292
Email: cair@magma.ca
Website: http://www.cair.ca

Fnded: 1973. **Mem:** 6,000. **Lang(s):** English, French. **Desc:** Medical residents, interns, and other physicians-intraining. Promotes professional advancement of members. Represents members' interests before medical organizations, government agencies, and the public in matters including medical education, licensure, certification, and entry into practice.

★ 1899 ★ Canadian Association of Medical Microbiologists (CAMM) (Association Canadienne des Medecins Microbiologistes — ACMM)
London, ON, Canada N6A 5A5
Email: gdelage@hema-quebec.qc.ca

Lang(s): English, French. **Desc:** Medical microbiologists. Seeks to advance the science of medical microbiology; promotes professional advancement of members. Facilitates communication and cooperation among members; conducts research and educational programs.

★ 1900 ★ Canadian Association of Medical Radiation Technologists (CAMRT) (Association Canadienne des Technologues en Radiation Medicale — ACTRM)
130 Albert St., Ste. 1510
Ottawa, ON, Canada K1P 5G4
Phone: (613)234-0012 **Fax:** (613)234-1097
Email: skamble@camrt.ca
Website: http://www.camrt.ca

Fnded: 1942. **Mem:** 10,100. **Lang(s):** English, French. **Desc:** Certifies medical radiation technologists in the fields of radiography, radiation therapy, nuclear medicine, and magnetic resonance imaging. Provides standards in the training and certification of members; promotes and maintains code of ethics. Participates in the accreditation of medical radiation technologist training programs; organizes continuing education programs. Advises private and governmental organizations involved in the fields of health and education. Provides placement assistance, professional liability insurance and numerous other member benefits. **Pub:** *CAMRT News*, quarterly. Newsletter. Contains activity information and education programmes. • *Canadian Journal of Medical Radiation Technology*, quarterly. Journal.

★ 1901 ★ Canadian Association for Music Therapy (CAMT) (Association de Musicotherapie du Canada — AMC)
Wilfrid Laurier University
Waterloo, ON, Canada N2L 3C5
Phone: (519)884-1970 **Free:** 800-996-CAMT
Fax: (519)886-9351
Email: camt@musictherapy.ca
Website: http://www.musictherapy.ca

Fnded: 1974. **Mem:** 400. **Reg. Groups:** 6. **Local Groups:** 1. **Lang(s):** English, French. **Desc:** Promotes the use and development of music for health and well-being in prevention and treatment with all age groups. Establishes, maintains, and improves standards of treatment and service in music therapy; encourages and develops research. Acts as a forum for the exchange of ideas, advice, guidance, and professional experience. Represents the interests of music therapists in matters relating to governmental legislation, jobs, and salary scales. Offers professional accreditation to music therapists. **Pub:** *CAMT Newsletter*, 3/year. Newsletter. News on professional issues concerning music therapists. • *Canadian Journal of Music Therapy*, annual. Journal. • *Conference Proceedings*, published from 1979-1992. • *Membership Directory*, annual.

★ 1902 ★ Canadian Association of Nephrology Nurses and Technologists
336 Yonge St., Ste. 322
Barrie, ON, Canada L4N 4C8
Phone: (705)720-2819 **Fax:** (705)720-1451
Email: cannt@cannt.ca
Website: http://www.cannt.ca

Lang(s): English, French. **Desc:** Nephrology nurses and technicians. Promotes professional development of members; seeks to advance the treatment of individuals with nephrological conditions. Serves as a clearinghouse on nephrology treatment centers; conducts continuing professional education courses.

★ 1903 ★ Canadian Association of Neuropathologists (CAND) (Association Canadienne de Neuropathologistes — ACN)
c/o Department of Pathology & Lab Medicine
University of Alberta Hospital
5B4.16 Mackenzie Health Sciences Centre
Edmonton, AB, Canada T6G 2B7
Phone: (780)407-8952 **Fax:** (780)407-3009
Email: edwardj@ualberta.ca
Website: http://canp.medical.org

Fnded: 1960. **Mem:** 100. **Lang(s):** English, French. **Desc:** Neuropathologists and other health care professionals with an interest in the field. Promotes professional development of members; seeks to advance the practice of neuropathology. Facilitates exchange of information among members; conducts continuing professional education programs.

★ 1904 ★ Canadian Association of Neuroscience Nurses (CANN) (Association Canadienne des Infirmieres en Sciences Neurologiques — ACISN)
1818 W 6th Ave., Ste. 205
Vancouver, BC, Canada V6J 1R6
Email: birwin@cw.bc.ca
Website: http://www.cann.ca

Lang(s): English, French. **Desc:** Neuroscience nurses. Seeks to advance the practice of neuroscience nursing; promotes professional development of members. Facilitates exchange of information among members; conducts continuing professional development courses.

★ 1905 ★ Canadian Association of Nurses in AIDS Care (Association Canadienne des Infirmieres et Infirmiers en Sidologie)
250 Frechett St., Ste. 2
Ottawa, ON, Canada K1L 7T4
Fax: (613)746-5420
Email: info@canac.org
Website: http://www.canac.org

Lang(s): English, French. **Desc:** Nurses engaged in the care of people with AIDS and HIV. Seeks to improve the quality of life of people with AIDS and HIV, and to advance the prevention and treatment of autoimmune diseases. Provides support and services to people with AIDS and HIV; makes available continuing professional development programs.

★ 1906 ★ Canadian Association of Nurses in Oncology (CANO) (Association canadienne des infirmieres en oncologie)
329 March Rd., No. 232
PO Box 11
Kanata, ON, Canada K2K 2E7
Phone: (613)270-0711
Email: canacio@igs.net

Fnded: 1985. **Mem:** 850. **Lang(s):** English, French. **Desc:** Registered nurses in independent practice. Promotes improved public access to health care; seeks to increase the role of nurses in the delivery of health care services. Develops business and practice guidelines for members. Provides support and assistance to members; conducts educational programs to raise public awareness of nursing and other health care services; sponsors business and continuing professional development courses for members. Conducts lobbying activities; undertakes research projects; compiles statistics. **Pub:** *Visions*, quarterly. Newsletter. • Brochure. • Directory, periodic.

★ 1907 ★ Canadian Association of Occupational Therapists (CAOT) (Association Canadienne des Ergotherapeutes — ACE)
CTTC Bldg., Ste. 3400
1125 Colonel By Dr.
Ottawa, ON, Canada K1S 5R1
Phone: (613)523-2268 **Fax:** (613)523-2552
Email: sdokuchie@caot.ca
Website: http://www.caot.ca

Fnded: 1926. **Mem:** 6,400. **Lang(s):** English, French. **Desc:** Occupational therapists. Promotes professional development of members; seeks to advance the practice of occupational therapy. Facilitates communication among members; makes available continuing professional development programs.

★ 1908 ★ Canadian Association of Optometrists (CAO)
234 Argyle Ave.
Ottawa, ON, Canada K2P 1B9
Phone: (613)235-7924 **Fax:** (613)235-2025
Email: reception@opto.ca
Website: http://www.opto.ca

Fnded: 1948. **Mem:** 3,100. **Reg. Groups:** 10. **Lang(s):** English, French. **Desc:** Optometrists, educators, and students. Promotes professional advancement of members and improvement in the teaching and practice of optometry. Conducts research and educational programs; compiles statistics. **Pub:** *CJO*, quarterly. Journal. • *FYI*, quarterly. Newsletter. • Directory, annual.

★ 1909 ★ Canadian Association of Oral and Maxillofacial Surgeons (CAOMS) (Association canadienne des specialistes en chirurgie buccale et maxillo-faciale — ACSCBMF)
174 Colonnade Rd., Unit 26
Ottawa, ON, Canada K2E 7J5
Phone: (613)721-1816 **Free:** 888-369-5641
Fax: (613)721-3581
Email: info@caoms.com
Website: http://www.caoms.com

Lang(s): English, French. **Desc:** Promotes and represents oral and maxillofacial surgeons in Canada.

★ 1910 ★ Canadian Association of Orthodontists (CAO) (Association Canadienne des Orthodontistes — ACO)
2175 Sheppard Ave. E, Ste. 310
North York, ON, Canada M2J 1W8
Phone: (416)491-3186 **Free:** 877-CAO-8800
Fax: (416)491-1670
Email: cao@taylorenterprises.com
Website: http://www.cao-aco.org

Lang(s): English, French. **Desc:** Orthodontists. Promotes excellence in the practice of orthodonture. Conducts continuing professional development courses for members.

★ 1911 ★ Canadian Association of Paediatric Surgeons (CAPS) (Association Canadienne de la Chirurgie Pediatrique — ACCP)
c/o Dr. Peter Fitzgerald
Division of Pediatric Surgery, Rm. 4E2
McMaster Children's Hospital
1200 Main St. W
Hamilton, ON, Canada L8N 3Z5
Phone: (905)521-2100 **Fax:** (905)521-9992
Email: fitzger@mcmaster.ca
Website: http://www.caps.ca

Lang(s): English, French. **Desc:** Pediatric surgeons and other health care professionals with an interest in the field. Seeks to advance the practice of pediatric surgery; promotes professional development of members. Facilitates communication and cooperation among members; makes available continuing professional education courses.

★ 1912 ★ Canadian Association of Pathologists (CAP) (Association Canadienne des Pathologistes — ACP)
774 Echo Dr.
Ottawa, ON, Canada K1S 5N8
Phone: (613)730-6230 **Free:** 800-668-3740
Fax: (613)730-1116
Email: cap@rcpsc.edu
Website: http://cap.medical.org

Lang(s): English, French. **Desc:** Pathologists and other health care professionals with an interest in pathology. Promotes professional development of members; seeks to advance the study and practice of pathology. Facilitates communication and cooperation among members; conducts continuing professional education programs.

★ 1913 ★ Canadian Association of Pediatric Nurses (CAPN) (Association canadienne des infirmieres et infirmiers en pediatrie)
10413 Town line, RR1
Acton, ON, Canada L7J 2L7
Phone: (905)878-1732

Lang(s): English, French. **Desc:** Nurses specializing in pediatrics. Promotes professional development of members; seeks to advance the practice of pediatric nursing. Encourages exchange of information among members; makes available continuing professional education courses.

★ 1914 ★ Canadian Association for People Who Stutter (CAPS)
PO Box 444
Branch NDG
Montreal, QC, Canada H9B 3P8
Free: 888-788-8837
Email: caps@stutter.ca
Website: http://www.stutter.ca

Fnded: 1991. **Mem:** 7. **Lang(s):** English. **Desc:** Individuals who stutter and self-help groups for people who stutter. Provides coordination for a national network of autonomous Canadian self-help groups that serve people who stutter and their families. Works closely with speech professionals and treatment centers; seeks to increase public awareness and acceptance of people who stutter. **Pub:** Newsletter, quarterly. Contains stuttering information, personal stories about stuttering.

★ 1915 ★ Canadian Association of Pharmacy in Oncology (CAPhO)
10660 11th Ave.
Edmonton, AB, Canada T6J 6H4
Website: http://capho.ca

Lang(s): English. **Desc:** Pharmacists and other health care professionals interested in the practice of oncology pharmacy in Canada. Represents the professional interests and issues of oncology pharmacy at a national level.

★ 1916 ★ Canadian Association of Pharmacy Technicians (CAPT)
PO Box 1271 Station F,
Toronto, ON, Canada M4Y 2V8
Phone: (416)410-1142
Email: contact@capt.ca
Website: http://www.capt.ca

Fnded: 1983. **Mem:** 600. **Lang(s):** English. **Desc:** Pharmacy technicians in Canada. Seeks to improve the communication, education, and recognition of pharmacy technicians. **Pub:** Newsletter, bimonthly.

★ 1917 ★ Canadian Association of Physical Medicine and Rehabilitation (CAPM&R)

774 Echo Dr.
Ottawa, ON, Canada K1S 5N8
Phone: (613)730-6245 **Fax:** (613)730-1116
Email: capmr@rcpsc.edu
Website: http://capmr.medical.org

Fnded: 1952. **Mem:** 300. **Lang(s):** English, French. **Desc:** Organizes scientific retreats. **Pub:** *CAPM&R Newsletter*, 3/year. Newsletter.

★ 1918 ★ Canadian Association of Physicians of Indian Origin

1920 Ellesmere Rd., No. 204
Toronto, ON, Canada
Phone: (416)289-1999

Fnded: 1993. **Mem:** 600. **Desc:** Strives to gather and discuss issues related to people of Indian origin in Canada regarding health matters.

★ 1919 ★ Canadian Association of Poison Control Centres

Children's Hospital
840 Sherbrook St.
Winnipeg, MB, Canada R3A 1S1
Phone: (204)787-2444

Fnded: 1981. **Lang(s):** English, French. **Desc:** Poison control centers. Promotes increased public awareness of poisoning prevention and the steps to take in case of poisoning. Facilitates communication and cooperation among members; conducts educational and promotional programs.

★ 1920 ★ Canadian Association of Pre-Retirement Planners (CAPP)

289 Greenwood Dr.
Stratford, ON, Canada N5A 7K6
Phone: (519)273-5616 **Fax:** (519)273-6097
Email: cappnational@cyg.net
Website: http://www.retirementplanners.ca

Fnded: 1981. **Mem:** 200. **Nat'l Groups:** 1. **Reg. Groups:** 6. **Lang(s):** English. **Desc:** Organizations that provides pre- or post-retirement services, seminars or workshops, and individuals who are lifestyle planners, human resource personnel, financial planners, counselors, adult educators, health professionals, leisure and fitness personnel, program planners, gerontologists, and others. Promotes the retirement planning industry. Provides information and networking opportunities; encourages high standards of performance and ethical behavior; seeks to improve public awareness; encourages members to become registered with the Professional Retirement Planners Registry.

★ 1921 ★ Canadian Association of Prosthetists and Orthotists (Association Canadienne des Prothesistes et Orthesistes)

303-267 Edmonton St.
Winnipeg, MB, Canada R3C 1S2
Phone: (204)949-4972 **Fax:** (204)947-3627
Email: capo@mb.sympatico.ca
Website: http://www.pando.ca

Lang(s): English, French. **Desc:** Organizations and individuals engaged in the production and fitting of orthotic and prosthetic devices. Seeks to advance the science and practice of orthotics and prosthetics; facilitates professional development of members. Sponsors research and educational programs; serves as a clearinghouse on orthotics and prosthetics. **Pub:** *Alignment*, annual. Magazine.

★ 1922 ★ Canadian Association of Psychoanalytic Child Therapists

42 Brookmount Rd.
Toronto, ON, Canada M4L 3N2
Phone: (416)690-5464 **Fax:** (416)690-2746
Email: capct@interlog.com
Website: http://www.interlog.com/~capct/

Mem: 65. **Lang(s):** English, French. **Desc:** Child therapists specializing in psychoanalysis. Promotes use of psychoanalysis in child therapy; encourages professional advancement of members. Serves as a forum for the exchange of information among members; conducts continuing professional development courses.

★ 1923 ★ Canadian Association of Psychological Oncology (Association Canadienne d'Oncologie Psychosociale)

c/o Tom Baker Cancer Centre
Department of Psychosocial Resources
29 St. NW
Calgary, AB, Canada R2N 4N2
Phone: (403)944-1768 **Fax:** (403)283-6032
Website: http://www.capo.ca

Lang(s): English, French. **Desc:** Oncologists and psychologists with an interest in oncology. Promotes improved care of oncology patients through interdisciplinary use of oncological and psychological treatment strategies. Sponsors research and educational programs.

★ 1924 ★ Canadian Association of Public Health Dentistry (L'Association Canadienne des Dentistes en Sante Communautaire)

c/o Dr. Dan Otchere, Sec.
44 Peel Centre Dr., Ste. 102
Brampton, ON, Canada L6T 4B5
Phone: (905)791-7800 **Fax:** (905)791-2697
Email: info@caphd-acsdp.org
Website: http://www.caphd-acsdp.org

Lang(s): English, French. **Desc:** Public health dentists. Seeks to advance the practice of public health dentistry; encourages continuing professional development of members. Sponsors research and educational programs.

★ 1925 ★ Canadian Association of Radiation Oncologists (CARO) (Association Canadienne des Radio-Oncologues)

600 W 10th Ave.
Vancouver, BC, Canada V5Z 4E6
Phone: (604)877-6193 **Fax:** (604)877-0505
Email: sbroadbe@caro-acro.ca
Website: http://www.caro-acro.ca

Fnded: 1986. **Mem:** 300. **Lang(s):** English, French. **Desc:** Radiation oncologists and oncology residents and fellows. Promotes advancement of the science and practice of radiation oncology. Seeks to facilitate professional advancement of members. Conducts continuing professional education programs. **Pub:** Newsletter, quarterly.

★ 1926 ★ Canadian Association of Radiologists (CAR) (Association canadienne des radiologistes)

1740 Cote Vertu Blvd.
St.-Laurent, QC, Canada H4L 2A4
Phone: (514)738-3111 **Fax:** (514)738-5199
Email: info@car.ca
Website: http://www.car.ca

Fnded: 1937. **Mem:** 1,300. **Reg. Groups:** 10. **Lang(s):** English, French. **Desc:** Physicians specializing in radiology and medical imaging. Seeks to advance the practice of radiology; promotes continuing professional development of members. Represents the medical, scientific, and economic interests of radiologists; sponsors research and educational programs. **Pub:** *CAR Journal*, 3/year. Journal.

★ 1927 ★ Canadian Association of Rehabilitation Professionals (CARP)

201 Consumers Rd., Ste. 302
Toronto, ON, Canada M2J 4G8
Phone: (416)494-4700 **Free:** 888-876-9992
Fax: (416)494-9139
Email: info@carpnational.org

Fnded: 1970. **Mem:** 2,600. **Reg. Groups:** 7. **Lang(s):** English, French. **Desc:** Professional association for people working in the field of rehabilitation. Promotes excellence in rehabilitation education, training, and practice. Formulates and enforces Code of Ethics. Facilitates communication to its members and stakeholders. Responsible for professional development, promotion of the Canadian Certified Rehabilitation Counselling (CCRC), Certified Vocational Evaluator (CVE), and the granting of the Registered Rehabilitation Professional (RRP) designation to qualified members. **Pub:** *Rehab Review*, quarterly. Newsletter. • *Rehabilitation Journal*, quarterly. Journal. Two international and two Canadian publication per year. **Frmly:** (1995) Canadian Association of Rehabilitation Personnel.

★ 1928 ★ Canadian Association for School Health (CASH)

2835 Country Woods Dr.
Surrey, BC, Canada V4P 9P9
Phone: (604)535-7664 **Fax:** (604)531-6454
Email: dmccall@netcom.ca
Website: http://www.schoolfile.com/CASH.htm

Lang(s): English, French. **Desc:** School health services. Promotes increased availability and quality of school health programs. Serves as a clearinghouse on school health services; facilitates communication and cooperation among members.

★ 1929 ★ Canadian Association of Schools of Nursing (CASN) (Association Canadienne des Ecoles de sciences infirmieres — ACESI)

15-15A Fifth Ave. Crt.
99 Fifth Ave.
Ottawa, ON, Canada K1S 5K4
Phone: (613)235-3150 **Fax:** (613)235-4476
Email: inquire@casn.ca
Website: http://www.casn.ca

Fnded: 1942. **Mem:** 87. **Reg. Groups:** 4. **State Groups:** 10. **Lang(s):** English, French. **Desc:** University schools of nursing. Promotes excellence in the study, teaching, and practice of nursing. Facilitates communication and cooperation among members; sponsors research and educational programs.

★ 1930 ★ Canadian Association of Speech-Language Pathologists and Audiologists (Association Canadienne des Orthophonistes et Audiologistes)

200 Elgin, Ste. 401
Ottawa, ON, Canada K2P 1L5
Phone: (613)567-9968 **Free:** 800-259-8519
Fax: (613)567-2859
Email: caslpa@caslpa.ca
Website: http://www.caslpa.ca

Fnded: 1964. **Mem:** 4,300. **Lang(s):** English, French. **Desc:** Audiologists, speech and language pathologists, and other individuals with an interest in speech and hearing. Seeks to increase availability and effectiveness of treatment programs for people with communication disabilities. Makes available programs and services for people with speech and language disorders; conducts continuing professional development courses for members. **Pub:** *Journal of Speech-Language Pathology and Audiology*. Journal.

★ 1931 ★ Canadian Association for Suicide Prevention (CASP)
(Association Canadienne pour la Prevention du Suicide — ACPS)
11456 Jasper Ave, Ste. 301
Edmonton, AB, Canada T5K 0M1
Phone: (780)482-0198 **Fax:** (780)488-1495
Email: casp@suicideprevention.ca
Website: http://www.suicideprevention.ca

Fnded: 1985. **Mem:** 300. **Lang(s):** English, French. **Desc:** Individuals and organizations. Seeks to reduce the incidence of suicide through advocacy, support, and advising. **Pub:** *CASP News*, 3/year. Newsletter.

★ 1932 ★ Canadian Athletic Therapists Association (CATA)
(Association Canadienne des Therapeutes du Sport — ACTS)
902 11th Ave. SW, Ste. 312
Calgary, AB, Canada T2R 0E7
Phone: (403)509-2282 **Fax:** (403)509-2280
Email: cata12@telusplanet.net
Website: http://www.athletictherapy.org

Fnded: 1965. **Mem:** 1,200. **Reg. Groups:** 7. **Lang(s):** English, French. **Desc:** Athletic therapists and other individuals engaged in the practice of sports medicine. Promotes advancement of the study and practice of sports medicine and athletic therapy; seeks to enhance the professional status of members. Encourages adoption of healthy and active lifestyles. Facilitates communication among members. Develops standards of conduct and practice and bestows certification in athletic therapy. Delivers sports medical services to grass roots sports organizations throughout Canada. Conducts educational programs; maintains hall of fame. **Pub:** *Canadian Athletic Therapists Association*, quarterly. Newsletter. • Directory, periodic.

★ 1933 ★ Canadian Bacterial Diseases Network (CBDN)
Heritage Medical Research Bldg., Rm. 282
3330 Hospital Dr. NW
Calgary, AB, Canada T2N 4N1
Phone: (403)220-2562 **Fax:** (403)283-5241
Email: info@cbdn.ca
Website: http://www.cbdn.ca

Fnded: 1989. **Mem:** 50. **Lang(s):** English. **Desc:** Canadian researchers from 15 universities whose focus is on bacterial diseases that affect humans, animals, fish, plants and the environment. Seeks to advance scientific knowledge and enhance Canada's economic competitiveness through networking, excellence in fundamental research on bacterial diseases and collaboration with industry through a virtual research network.

★ 1934 ★ Canadian Brain Tissue Bank (CBTB)
(Banque Canadienne de Tissue du Cerveau — BCTC)
University of Toronto
UHN-Toronto Western Hospital
399 Bathurst St., Fell Wing 5-222 A&B
Toronto, ON, Canada M5T 2S8
Phone: (416)978-5490 **Fax:** (416)978-7935
Email: cbtb@uhn.on.ca

Lang(s): English, French. **Desc:** Neurologists, psychiatrists, and other individuals with an interest in the structure and function of the brain. Seeks to advance understanding of the brain and its function; promotes professional development of members. Maintains brain tissue bank for research and study; provides support and assistance to brain research programs; conducts educational programs.

★ 1935 ★ Canadian Breast Cancer Foundation
790 Bay St., Ste. 1000
Toronto, ON, Canada M5G 1N8
Phone: (416)596-6773 **Free:** 800-387-9816
Fax: (416)596-7857
Email: emills@cbcf.org
Website: http://www.cbcf.org

Fnded: 1986. **Reg. Groups:** 4. **Lang(s):** English. **Desc:** Health care professionals, women with breast cancer, their families, and others interested in breast cancer issues. Promotes the advancement of breast cancer research, education, diagnosis and treatment through various programs and fundraising events.

★ 1936 ★ Canadian Burn Survivors Association (BSA)
c/o Ross Tilley Burn Centre
Sunnybrook & Women's College Health Centre
247 Willow St.
Truro, NS, Canada B2N 5A3
Phone: (902)895-4895
Email: burnsurvivors@hotmail.com

Fnded: 1999. **Mem:** 642. **Nat'l Groups:** 118. **Reg. Groups:** 13. **Local Groups:** 2. **Lang(s):** English, French. **Desc:** People who have suffered burns. Seeks to improve the quality of life of burn survivors. Facilitates communication among members; makes available support and services to burn survivors. **Pub:** *Abilities Magazine*. Magazine. • *IBSS News*.

★ 1937 ★ Canadian Cancer Society (CCS)
10 Alcorn Ave., Ste. 200
Toronto, ON, Canada M4V 3B1
Phone: (416)961-7223 **Fax:** (416)961-4189
Email: ccs@cancer.ca
Website: http://www.cancer.ca

Fnded: 1938. **Lang(s):** English, French. **Desc:** Community-based volunteers. Promotes research into the causes, detection, and cure of cancer; seeks to improve the quality of life of people with cancer. Conducts fundraising activities benefitting cancer research; sponsors volunteer training programs; makes available educational courses. **Pub:** *Progress Against Cancer*, 3/year. Magazine.

★ 1938 ★ Canadian Cardiovascular Society (CCS)
(Societe Canadienne de Cardiologie — SCC)
222 Queen St., Ste. 1403
Ottawa, ON, Canada K1P 5V9
Phone: (613)569-3407 **Fax:** (613)569-6574
Email: ccsinfo@ccs.ca
Website: http://www.ccs.ca

Fnded: 1946. **Mem:** 1,200. **Lang(s):** English, French. **Desc:** Physicians, surgeons, and scientists practicing or conducting research in cardiology and related fields. Works to advance the cardiovascular health and care of Canadians through leadership on professional development, advocacy, and the promotion, dissemination of research.

★ 1939 ★ Canadian Celiac Association (CCA)
(L'Association Canadienne de la Maladie Coeliaque — ACMC)
5170 Dixie Rd., Ste. 204
Mississauga, ON, Canada L4W 1E3
Phone: (905)507-6208 **Free:** 800-363-7296
Fax: (905)507-4673
Email: celiac@look.ca
Website: http://www.celiac.ca

Fnded: 1926. **Mem:** 6,000. **Nat'l Groups:** 1. **Reg. Groups:** 25. **Lang(s):** English, French. **Desc:** Individuals with celiac sprue; health care professionals with an interest in gastrointestinal diseases. Seeks to improve the quality of life of people with celiac sprue and related disorders; promotes advancement in the diagnosis and treatment of gastrointestinal maladies. Provides support and assistance to people with celiac sprue and related disorders; conducts research and educational programs. **Pub:** *Celiac News*, 3/year. Newsletter.

★ 1940 ★ Canadian Centre for Stress and Well-Being/Stress Management Center
1 Yonge St., Ste. 1801
Toronto, ON, Canada M5E 1W7
Phone: (416)363-6204 **Fax:** (416)369-0515
Email: smeen@yahoo.com

Lang(s): English, French. **Desc:** Individuals suffering from stress; health care professionals and organizations with an interest in stress. Seeks to advance the diagnosis and treatment of stress and related disorders; works to improve the quality of life of people suffering from stress. Provides support and assistance to victims of stress and their families; sponsors research and educational programs.

★ 1941 ★ Canadian Centre on Substance Abuse (CCSA)
(Centre Canadien de lutte contre l'alcoolisme et les toxicomanies — CCLCAT)
75 Albert St., Ste. 300
Ottawa, ON, Canada K1P 5E7
Phone: (613)235-4048 **Fax:** (613)235-8101
Email: info@ccsa.ca
Website: http://www.ccsa.ca

Fnded: 1988. **Lang(s):** English, French. **Desc:** Individuals and organizations. Seeks to prevent substance abuse; promotes recovery among substance abusers. Seeks to raise awareness of substance abuse issues among policy makers and the public; makes available support and services to substance abusers and their families. **Pub:** *Action News*, quarterly. Newsletter.

★ 1942 ★ Canadian Cerebral Palsy Sports Association (CCPSA)
(L'Association canadienne des sports pout paralytiques cerebraux)
1010 Polytek St., Unit 2, 2nd Fl.
Gloucester, ON, Canada K1G 9H9
Phone: (613)748-1430 **Fax:** (613)748-1335
Email: ccpsa@cyberus.ca
Website: http://www.ccpsa.ca

Fnded: 1985. **Mem:** 2,000. **Reg. Groups:** 7. **Lang(s):** English, French. **Desc:** Individuals with cerebral palsy and their families; volunteer officials and organizers. Promotes participation in competitive sports, such as boccia, cycling, athletics, and powerlifting by people with cerebral palsy. Conducts training programs; sponsors competitions. **Pub:** *Canadian Cerebral Palsy Sports Association*. Brochure.

★ 1943 ★ Canadian Child Care Federation (CCCF)
(Federation Canadienne des Services de Garde a l'Enfance — FCSGE)
201-383 Parkdale Ave.
Ottawa, ON, Canada K1Y 4R4
Phone: (613)729-5289 **Free:** 800-858-1412
Fax: (613)729-3159
Email: info@cccf-fcsge.ca
Website: http://www.cfc-efc.ca

Fnded: 1986. **Mem:** 8,000. **Lang(s):** English, French. **Desc:** Child care services and their employees. Promotes increased availability and improved quality of child care services. Provides support and services to members.

★ 1944 ★ Canadian Chiropractic Association (CCPA)
(L'Association de Protection Chiropratique Canadienne)
1396 Eglinton Ave. W
Toronto, ON, Canada M6C 2E4
Phone: (416)781-5656 **Free:** 800-668-2076
Fax: (416)781-7344
Email: ccachiro@ccachiro.org
Website: http://www.ccachiro.org

Lang(s): English, French. **Desc:** Chiropractors. Promotes professional advancement of members; seeks to increase public awareness of chiropractic. Conducts promotional and educational programs.

★ 1945 ★ Canadian Chiropractic Examining Board (CCE B)
1144 29th Ave. NE, Ste. 103
Calgary, AB, Canada T2E 7P1
Phone: (403)230-5997 **Fax:** (403)230-3221
Email: drlawson@cceb.ca
Website: http://www.cceb.ca

Fnded: 1962. **Lang(s):** English, French. **Desc:** Chiropractic practitioners and educators. Promotes excellence in the practice of chiropractic. Conducts examinations and bestows certification upon chiropractic practitioners; develops standards of practice for chiropractors.

★ 1946 ★ Canadian Coalition for High Blood Pressure Prevention and Control (Coalition Canadienne pour la Prevention et le Controle de l'Hypertension Arterielle)
c/o Dr. Robert Petrella
Centre for Activity and Ageing, Rm. 208A
1490 Richmond St. N
London, ON, Canada N6G 2M3
Phone: (519)661-1610 **Fax:** (519)661-1635
Email: petrella@julian.uwo.ca
Website: http://www.canadianbpcoalition.org

Lang(s): English, French. **Desc:** Individuals with high blood pressure; health care professionals with an interest in hypertension. Seeks to advance the diagnosis and treatment of high blood pressure. Sponsors research; conducts educational programs; serves as a clearinghouse on hypertension and its treatment.

★ 1947 ★ Canadian Coalition for the Prevention of Developmental Disabilities (CCPDD)
384 Banks St. Ste. 300
Ottawa, ON, Canada K2P 1Y4
Phone: (613)230-8838 **Fax:** (613)230-6654
Email: cich@cich.ca

Lang(s): English, French. **Desc:** Health care professionals and other individuals with an interest in developmental disabilities. Seeks to advance understanding of the causes and prevention of developmental disabilities. Facilitates interdisciplinary exchange of information among scientists and medical professionals studying developmental disabilities; sponsors research and educational programs.

★ 1948 ★ Canadian College of Health Service Executives
350 Sparks St., Ste. 402
Ottawa, ON, Canada K1R 7S8
Phone: (613)235-7218 **Fax:** (613)235-5451
Email: cchse@cchse.org
Website: http://www.cchse.org

Fnded: 1970. **Mem:** 3,000. **Reg. Groups:** 20. **Desc:** Health service executives in Canada. **Pub:** *Healthcare Management Forum*, quarterly, always March, June, September, and December. Journal. Contains articles on innovations in health services.

★ 1949 ★ Canadian College of Medical Geneticists (CCMG) (College Canadien de Geneticiens Medicaux — CCGM)
c/o Royal College of Physicians and Surgeons of Canada
774 Echo Dr.
Ottawa, ON, Canada K1S 5N8
Phone: (613)730-6250 **Fax:** (613)730-1116
Email: ccmg@rcpsc.edu
Website: http://ccmg.medical.org

Fnded: 1975. **Mem:** 180. **Lang(s):** English, French. **Desc:** Physicians and other health care professionals with an interest in genetics. Promotes professional development of members; seeks to advance medical genetic research and practice. Facilitates exchange of information among members; conducts research and educational programs.

★ 1950 ★ Canadian College of Naturopathic Medicine (CCNM)
1255 Sheppard Ave. E
Toronto, ON, Canada M2K 1E2
Phone: (416)498-1255 **Free:** (866)241-2266
Fax: (416)498-1576
Email: info@ccnm.edu
Website: http://www.ccnm.edu

Fnded: 1978. **Lang(s):** English. **Desc:** Promotes naturopathic medical education, clinical practice, and research. Operates an accredited four-year, fulltime professional program in naturopathic medicine.

★ 1951 ★ Canadian Confederation of Ambulance Service Associations (CCASA)
PO Box 129
Rodney, ON, Canada N0L 2C0
Phone: (519)785-0318 **Fax:** (519)785-2002
Email: oaoa@mco.net

Lang(s): English. **Desc:** Ambulance operators in Canada. Works to improve the standard of emergency prehospital care for Canadians.

★ 1952 ★ Canadian Congress of Neurological Sciences (CCNS)
PO Box 5456, Sta. A
Calgary, AB, Canada T2H 2X8
Phone: (403)229-9544 **Fax:** (403)229-1661
Email: brains@ccns.org
Website: http://www.ccns.org

Fnded: 1989. **Mem:** 1,100. **Lang(s):** English, French. **Desc:** Represents and promotes adult and child neurologists, neurosurgeons and clinical neurophysiologists in Canada. **Pub:** *Canadian Journal of Neurological Sciences*, quarterly. Journal.

★ 1953 ★ Canadian Continence Foundation
PO Box 30
Victoria Branch
Westmount, QC, Canada H3Z 2V4
Phone: (514)488-8379 **Fax:** (514)488-1379
Email: help@continence-fdn.ca
Website: http://www.continence-fdn.ca

Fnded: 1986. **Mem:** 14,000. **Lang(s):** English, French. **Desc:** People suffering from incontinence, health care professionals, and other individuals with an interest in incontinence and related health problems. Seeks to improve the quality of life of people with incontinence. Facilitates formation of support groups; conducts research and educational programs; participates in charitable activities. **Pub:** *Informer*, 3/year. Newsletter. **Frmly:** Simon Foundation - Canada.

★ 1954 ★ Canadian Council for Accreditation of Pharmacy Programs (CCAPP) (Le Conseil canadien de l'agrement des programmes de pharmacie — CCAPP)
Thorvaldson Bldg., Rm. 123
110 Science Pl.
Saskatoon, SK, Canada S7N 5C9
Phone: (306)966-6388 **Fax:** (306)966-6377
Email: schnell@sask.usask.ca

Lang(s): English, French. **Desc:** Promotes excellence in the study and teaching of pharmacy. Formulates and enforces standards for pharmacy training programs; examines pharmacy programs and bestows accreditation.

★ 1955 ★ Canadian Council of the Blind (CCB) (Conseil Canadien des Aveugles — CCA)
396 Cooper St., Ste. 401
Ottawa, ON, Canada K2P 2H7
Phone: (613)567-0311 **Free:** 877-304-0968
Fax: (613)567-2728
Email: ccb@ccbnational.net

Fnded: 1944. **Mem:** 4,000. **Local Groups:** 95. **Lang(s):** English, French. **Desc:** National consumer organization representing legally blind and vision impaired individuals in Canada. Offers support through social and recreational activities. Represents members' interests in relation to government, business and industry. **Pub:** *CCB Newsletter*, monthly. Newsletter.

★ 1956 ★ Canadian Council of Cardiovascular Nurses (CCCN) (Conseil Canadien des Infirmieres en Nursing Cardiovasculaire — CCINC)
222 Queen St., Ste. 1402
Ottawa, ON, Canada K1P 5V9
Phone: (613)569-4361 **Fax:** (613)569-3278
Email: cccnmail@hsf.ca
Website: http://www.cardiovascularnurse.com

Fnded: 1973. **Mem:** 650. **Lang(s):** English, French. **Desc:** Nurses specializing in cardiovascular practice. Promotes advancement of cardiovascular nursing; facilitates continuing professional development of members. Serves as a forum for the exchange of information among members; conducts educational and training programs. **Pub:** *Canadian Journal of Cardiovascular Nursing*, quarterly. Journal. Science-based peer reviewed journal.

★ 1957 ★ Canadian Council on Continuing Education in Pharmacy (CCCEP)
3861 Athol St.
Regina, SK, Canada S4S 3J2
Phone: (306)584-5703 **Fax:** (306)584-5703
Email: nmcbean@accesscomm.ca
Website: http://www.cccep.org

Lang(s): English. **Desc:** Pharmacists, educators, and educational institutions. Promotes professional development of pharmacists; seeks to advance the accreditation standards and criteria and accredit continuing professional education courses for pharmacists.

★ 1958 ★ Canadian Council on Health Services Accreditation (CCHSA)
1730 St. Laurent Blvd., Ste. 100
Ottawa, ON, Canada K1G 5L1
Phone: (613)738-3800 **Fax:** (613)738-1244
Email: nowl@cchsa.ca
Website: http://www.cchsa.ca

Fnded: 1958. **Mem:** 1,541. **Lang(s):** English, French. **Desc:** Agencies and organizations accrediting health care services including mental health care, cancer treatment centers, home health care, and community health. Seeks to ensure high standards of ethics, practice, and equipment and facilities among Canadian health services. Formulates and enforces standards; conducts research and educational programs. **Pub:** *The Accreditation Standard*, quarterly. Newsletter. • *Standards*. Manual. • Annual Report. • Reports. **Frmly:** (1995) Canadian Council on Health Facilities Accreditation.

★ 1959 ★ Canadian Council on Multicultural Health (CCMH) (Conseil Canadien de la Sante Multiculturelle — CCSM)
1450 St. George St.
University of Toronto
Toronto, ON, Canada M5S 3G6
Phone: (416)978-3234

Lang(s): English, French. **Desc:** Health care professionals and other individuals with an interest in public health. Promotes increased availability of health care services among previously underserved populations.

Serves as a clearinghouse on multicultural health and related issues; makes available support and assistance to health care services.

★ 1960 ★ Canadian Council on Rehabilitation and Work (CCRW)
(Conseil Canadien de la Readaptation et du Travail — CCRT)
500 University Ave., Ste. 302
Toronto, ON, Canada M5G 1V7
Phone: (416)260-3060 **Free:** 800-664-0925
Fax: (416)260-3093
Email: info@ccrw.org
Website: http://www.ccrw.org
Fnded: 1976. **Lang(s):** English, French. **Desc:** Promotes and supports the meaningful employment of persons with disabilities. **Pub:** *Ability & Enterprise*, every 6-8 weeks. Newsletter.

★ 1961 ★ Canadian Council for Tobacco Control (CCTC)
75 Albert St., Ste. 508
Ottawa, ON, Canada K1P 5E7
Phone: (613)567-3050 **Fax:** (613)567-2730
Email: info-services@cctc.ca
Website: http://www.cctc.ca
Fnded: 1974. **Lang(s):** English, French. **Desc:** Seeks to raise public awareness regarding the dangers of smoking. Lobbies for reduced tobacco use in Canada; assists those wishing to quit smoking. Disseminates information. **Frmly:** Canadian Council on Smoking and Health.

★ 1962 ★ Canadian Counselling Association (CCA)
116 Albert St., Ste. 702
Ottawa, ON, Canada K1P 5G3
Phone: (613)237-1099 **Free:** 877-765-5565
Fax: (613)237-9786
Email: info@ccacc.ca
Website: http://www.ccacc.ca
Fnded: 1965. **Mem:** 1,900. **Nat'l Groups:** 5. **Reg. Groups:** 3. **Lang(s):** English, French. **Desc:** Professionally trained counselors in the fields of education, employment and career development, social work, business, industry, mental health, public service agencies, government, and private practice. Promotes the counseling profession in Canada.

★ 1963 ★ Canadian Critical Care Society (CCCS)
(La Societe Canadienne de Soins Intensifs — SCSI)
9 Eaton North, Rm. 242
Toronto General Hospital
Toronto, ON, Canada M5G 2C4
Phone: (416)340-3573 **Fax:** (416)595-9486
Email: deborah.wilson@uhn.on.ca
Website: http://www.canadiancriticalcare.org
Lang(s): English, French. **Desc:** Health care professionals specializing in the provision of critical care. Seeks to advance the practice of critical and intensive care; promotes ongoing professional development of members. Serves as a forum for the exchange of information among members; conducts continuing professional education courses.

★ 1964 ★ Canadian Cultural Society of The Deaf (CCSD)
House 144, 11337 - 61 Ave.
Edmonton, AB, Canada T6H 1M3
Phone: (780)436-2599 **Fax:** (780)430-9489
Email: ccsd@connect.ab.ca
Website: http://www.ccsdeaf.com
Fnded: 1970. **Desc:** Deaf and hard of hearing people. Promotes the use of American Sign Language (ASL) and Langue des Signes Quebecois (LSQ). Promotes fellowship in the deaf community and deaf culture. Encourages new and developing forms of creativity, research, participation, and interests in the arts, humanities, and social sciences. Promotes improved understanding between deaf and hearing populations. Advocates for progress in literacy at all levels and promotes bilingual bicultural education of deaf children. **Pub:** *Canadian Dictionary of ASL*. Book. • *Deaf People Are Like You But....* Manual.

★ 1965 ★ Canadian Cystic Fibrosis Foundation (CCFF)
(Fondation canadienne de la fibrose kystique — FCFK)
2221 Yonge St., Ste. 601
Toronto, ON, Canada M4S 2B4
Phone: (416)485-9149 **Free:** 800-378-2233
Fax: (416)485-0960
Email: info@cysticfibrosis.ca
Website: http://www.cysticfibrosis.ca
Fnded: 1960. **Lang(s):** English, French. **Desc:** Individuals with cystic fibrosis and their families, health care and other professionals working with people with cystic fibrosis. Promotes CF research in Canadian universities and hospitals by funding research grants and major research development programs and gives special grants for training and research to students, fellows, scholars and visiting scientists skilled in such areas as respiratory, pediatrics and gastroenterology. Promotes the regular exchange of information among researchers, scholars and clinical personnel and offers incentive grants to Canadian cystic fibrosis clinics. Provides support and services to people with cystic fibrosis and their families; sponsors research and educational programs. **Pub:** *Candid Facts*, quarterly. Newsletter.

★ 1966 ★ Canadian Deaf Curling Association (CDCA)
c/o Bradford Bentley
Vancouver, BC, Canada
Email: president-cdca@home.com
Website: http://www.canadiandeafcurlingassociation.com
Desc: Promotes participation among deaf and hard of hearing adults in the sport of curling across Canada.

★ 1967 ★ Canadian Deaf Sports Association (CDSA)
(Association des Sports des Sourds du Canada — ASSC)
4545 ave. Pierre du coubertin
CP 1000, succ. M
Montreal, QC, Canada H1V 3R2
Phone: (514)252-3069 **Free:** 800-855-0511
Fax: (514)252-3213
Email: office@assc-cdsa.com
Website: http://www.assc-cdsa.com
Lang(s): English, French. **Desc:** Individuals with impaired hearing who participate in athletics; sports organizations. Promotes increased participation in athletics by people with impaired hearing. Organizes athletic leagues and competitions for people with impaired hearing.

★ 1968 ★ Canadian Deafblind and Rubella Association (CDBRA)
350 Brant Ave.
Brantford, ON, Canada N3T 3J9
Phone: (519)754-0729 **Fax:** (519)754-5400
Email: cdbra.nat@sympatico.ca
Website: http://www.cdbra.ca
Fnded: 1975. **Mem:** 485. **Nat'l Groups:** 1. **State Groups:** 6. **Lang(s):** English, French. **Desc:** Professional intervenors, deafblind individuals and their families, volunteer service providers. Seeks to ensure availability of services to enable deafblind individuals to participate in society to the fullest of their capabilities. Provides lifelong intervention and educational services; conducts training programs for individuals wishing to work with the deafblind. Sponsors advocacy campaigns on behalf of deafblind individuals; facilitates cooperation between government agencies and programs assisting the deafblind. **Pub:** *Intervention*, semiannual. Magazine. • Brochure.

★ 1969 ★ Canadian Dental Assistants Association (CDAA)
1750 Courtwood Cres.
Ste. 208
Ottawa, ON, Canada K2C 2B5
Phone: (613)521-5495 **Fax:** (613)521-5572
Email: info@cdaa.ca
Website: http://www.cdaa.ca
Reg. Groups: 10. **Lang(s):** English. **Desc:** Dental assistants in Canada. Fosters opportunities for growth in the field in of dental assisting and represents members' interests.

★ 1970 ★ Canadian Dental Association (CDA)
(Association Dentair Canadienne — ADC)
1815 Alta Vista Dr.
Ottawa, ON, Canada K1G 3Y6
Phone: (613)523-1770 **Free:** 800-267-6354
Fax: (613)523-7736
Email: reception@cda-adc.ca
Website: http://www.cda-adc.ca
Lang(s): English, French. **Desc:** Dentists. Seeks to advance the profession of dentistry. Facilitates exchange of information among members; sponsors continuing professional education courses.

★ 1971 ★ Canadian Dental Hygienists' Association (CDHA)
96 Centerpointe Dr.
Ottawa, ON, Canada K2G 6B1
Phone: (613)224-5515 **Free:** 800-267-5235
Fax: (613)224-7283
Email: info@cdha.ca
Lang(s): English, French. **Desc:** Dental hygienists. Promotes development of standards of ethics and practice in the field of dental hygiene; facilitates professional advancement of members. Provides dental hygiene services to previously underserved populations; conducts educational programs.

★ 1972 ★ Canadian Dental Protective Association (CDPA)
2175 Sheppard Ave. E
Ste. 310
Toronto, ON, Canada M2J 1W8
Phone: (416)491-5932 **Free:** 800-876-2372
Fax: (416)491-1670
Email: cdpa@taylorenterprises.com
Website: http://www.cdpa.com
Lang(s): English. **Desc:** Dentists in Canada. Cares for the risk management needs of its members. Sponsors legal benefits insurance plan for members and their families.

★ 1973 ★ Canadian Dermatology Association (CDA)
774 Echo Dr., Ste. 521
Ottawa, ON, Canada K1S 5N8
Phone: (613)730-6262 **Fax:** (613)730-8262
Email: contact.cda@dermatology.ca
Website: http://www.dermatology.ca
Fnded: 1925. **Mem:** 600. **Lang(s):** English, French. **Desc:** Certified dermatologists and related professionals interested in the professional advancement of dermatology. Promotes continuing education programs in dermatology. Provides public education program on skin cancer prevention. Holds an annual National Sun Awareness Week. Recognizes sun protection products. **Pub:** *Canadian Dermatology Association Bulletin*, 3/year. Bulletin. Contains Association news for members. • *Journal of Cutaneous Medicine and Surgery*, quarterly. Journal. • Directory, annual.

★ 1974 ★ Canadian Diabetes Association (CDA)
(Association Canadienne du Diabete — ACD)
15 Toronto St., Ste. 800
Toronto, ON, Canada M5C 2E3
Phone: (416)363-3373 **Free:** 800-BAN-TING
Fax: (416)363-3393
Email: info@diabetes.ca
Website: http://www.diabetes.ca
Lang(s): English, French. **Desc:** People with diabetes and their families; health care professionals with an interest in diabetes. Seeks to advance the prevention, diagnosis, and treatment of diabetes. Provides support and services to people with diabetes and their families; sponsors research and educational programs.

★ 1975 ★ Canadian Diabetes Association - Diabetes Educator Section
15 Toronto St., Ste. 800
Toronto, ON, Canada M5C 2E3
Phone: (416)363-0177 **Free:** 800-226-8464
Fax: (416)363-7465
Email: info@diabetes.ca
Website: http://www.diabetes.ca
Fnded: 1973. **Mem:** 2,200. **Local Groups:** 43. **Lang(s):** English, French. **Desc:** Health professionals with an interest in diabetes. Seeks to advance the prevention and management of diabetes. Conducts research and educational programs. **Pub:** *Canadian Journal of Diabetes*, quarterly. Journal. • *Diabetes Quarterly*, quarterly. Newsletter.

★ 1976 ★ Canadian Down Syndrome Society (CDSS)
14th St. NW, Ste. 811
Calgary, AB, Canada T2N 2A4
Phone: (403)270-8500 **Free:** 800-883-5608
Fax: (403)270-8291
Email: dsinfo@cdss.ca
Website: http://www.cdss.ca
Fnded: 1987. **Mem:** 2,000. **Local Groups:** 50. **Lang(s):** English, French. **Pub:** *Babies with Down syndrome*. • *CDSS Quarterly*, quarterly. Newsletter.

★ 1977 ★ Canadian Dyslexia Association (CDA)
(Association Canadienne de la Dyslexie)
290 Picton Ave.
Ottawa, ON, Canada K1Z 8P8
Phone: (613)722-2699 **Fax:** (613)722-7881
Email: info@dyslexiaassociation.ca
Website: http://www.dyslexiaassociation.ca
Lang(s): English, French. **Desc:** Promotes awareness of dyslexia and seeks to develop and implement specialized methods to improve the quality of life for Canadian s who have dyslexia.

★ 1978 ★ Canadian Ehlers Danlos Association (CEDA)
88 De Rose Ave.
Bolton, ON, Canada L7E 1A8
Phone: (905)857-0172 **Free:** (866)999-2332
Email: office@ceda.ca
Website: http://www.ceda.ca
Fnded: 1996. **Reg. Groups:** 6. **Lang(s):** English. **Desc:** People who suffer from Ehlers-Danlos Syndrome (EDS), their families, and other interested individuals. Works to enhance the lives of all persons affected by EDS. Increases public awareness, provides information resources, works to establish EDS self-help groups. **Pub:** Newsletter, quarterly.

★ 1979 ★ Canadian Epilepsy Consortium (CEC)
55 Queen St. E
9th Fl., Ste. 921
Toronto, ON, Canada M5C 1R6
Phone: (416)864-5506 **Fax:** (416)864-5636
Email: cec-hq@egroups.com
Website: http://www.epilepsyconsortium.ca
Fnded: 1996. **Mem:** 40. **Lang(s):** English. **Desc:** Licensed neurologists residing in Canada who specialize in treating and/or researching pediatric and/or adult patients with epilepsy. Works to develop and promote multi-centre epilepsy research projects in Canada. Partners with industry to evaluate and execute clinical trials of new agents.

★ 1980 ★ Canadian Federation of Aromatherapists (CFA)
Administrative Office
843479 Oxford R. 84, RR No. 3
Lakeside, ON, Canada N0M 2G0
Phone: (519)537-2099 **Free:** 888-340-4445
Fax: (519)537-2887
Email: officemanager@cfacanada.com
Website: http://www.cfacanada.com/
Fnded: 1993. **Desc:** Fosters growth and high standards of education within the profession of aromatherapy, aromatherapy products and services.

★ 1981 ★ Canadian Federation of Mental Health Nurses (CFMHN)
1185 Eglington Ave. E, Ste. 104
Toronto, ON, Canada M3C 3C6
Phone: (416)426-7029
Email: info.mental.health@firststageinc.com
Website: http://www.cfmhn.org
Fnded: 1988. **Mem:** 1,000. **Nat'l Groups:** 1. **Lang(s):** English, French. **Desc:** Nurses engaged in mental health practice. Promotes professional development of members; seeks to advance the practice of mental health nursing. Facilitates communication and cooperation among members; sponsors continuing professional education activities.

★ 1982 ★ Canadian Federation of Nurses Unions (CFNU)
(Federation Canadienne des Syndicats d'Infirmieres et Infirmiers — FCSII)
2841 Riverside Dr.
Ottawa, ON, Canada K1V 8X7
Phone: (613)526-4661 **Free:** 800-321-9821
Fax: (613)526-1023
Email: cfnu@nursesunions.ca
Website: http://www.nursesunions.ca
Fnded: 1981. **Mem:** 123,000. **Reg. Groups:** 10. **Lang(s):** English, French. **Desc:** Canadian nurses. Promotes nurses and the nursing profession. Lobbies the federal government; represents the profession in dealings with the media; provides information resources. **Pub:** *Nurses' Voice*, biweekly. Newsletter.

★ 1983 ★ Canadian Fertility and Andrology Society
2065 Alexandre-de-Seve. Ste. 409
Montreal, QC, Canada H2L 2W5
Phone: (514)524-9009 **Fax:** (514)524-2163
Email: christine.lajeunesse@cfas.ca
Website: http://www.cfas.ca
Fnded: 1954. **Mem:** 530. **Desc:** Medical professionals, scientists, and others with an interest in human fertility and andrology. Serves as a forum for exchange of information.

★ 1984 ★ Canadian Fitness and Lifestyle Research Institute (CFLRI)
(Institut Canadien de la Recherche sur la Condition Physique et le Mod e de Vie — ICRCP)
185 Somerset St. W, Ste. 201
Ottawa, ON, Canada K2P 0J2
Phone: (613)233-5528 **Fax:** (613)233-5536
Email: info@cflri.ca
Website: http://www.cflri.ca
Fnded: 1980. **Mem:** 5. **Lang(s):** English, French. **Desc:** Conducts research on physical activities in Canada and distributes information about physical activity. **Pub:** *Physical Activity Monitor*, annual. Report. • *The Research File*, 4/year. Contains summaries of research on physical activity.

★ 1985 ★ Canadian Foundation for AIDS Research (CANFAR)
(Fondation canadienne de recherche sur le SIDA — FCRS)
165 University Ave., Ste. 901
Toronto, ON, Canada M5H 3B8
Phone: (416)361-6281 **Free:** 800-563-2873
Fax: (416)361-5736
Email: cure@canfar.com
Website: http://www.canfar.com
Fnded: 1988. **Mem:** 75. **Lang(s):** English, French. **Desc:** Seeks to advance AIDS and HIV research and services. Provides support and assistance to Canadian AIDS and HIV research projects; conducts educational programs to raise public awareness of AIDS and HIV. **Pub:** *Catalyst*, semiannual. Newsletter.

★ 1986 ★ Canadian Foundation for Dietetic Research (CFDR)
(La Fondation Canadienne de la Recherche en Dietetique — FCRD)
480 University, Ste. 604
Toronto, ON, Canada M5G 1V2
Phone: (416)596-0857 **Fax:** (416)596-0603
Email: cfdr@dietitians.ca
Website: http://www.dietitians.ca/cfdr
Fnded: 1991. **Lang(s):** English, French. **Desc:** Dietitians and other individuals with an interest in nutrition. Seeks to advance dietetic research. Provides support and assistance to nutrition research projects; conducts educational programs. **Pub:** Report, annual.

★ 1987 ★ Canadian Foundation for Pharmacy (CFP)
(Fondation Canadienne pour la Pharmacie — FCP)
15 Sawyer Crescent
Markham, ON, Canada L3P 5V2
Phone: (905)201-9559 **Fax:** (905)201-0717
Email: da-browns@home.com
Fnded: 1947. **Lang(s):** English, French. **Desc:** Pharmacists and other health care personnel. Seeks to advance pharmaceutical practice and research. Provides support and assistance to pharmacy research projects; conducts continuing professional education courses.

★ 1988 ★ Canadian Foundation for Physically Disabled Persons (CFPDP)
731 Runnymede Rd.
Toronto, ON, Canada M6N 3V7
Phone: (416)760-7351 **Fax:** (416)760-9405
Email: whynot@sympatico.ca
Website: http://www3.sympatico.ca/whynot/
Fnded: 1987. **Lang(s):** English. **Desc:** Works to bring public attention to the needs and accomplishments of people with physical disabilities. Creates public awareness in public, business, and government on issues of housing, employment, education, accessibility, sports and recreation, and research. Provides financial assistance to organizations that share concerns for adults with physical disabilities.

★ 1989 ★ Canadian Foundation for the Study of Infant Deaths (CFSID)
586 Eglinton Ave. E, Ste. 308
Toronto, ON, Canada M4P 1P2
Phone: (416)488-3860 **Free:** 800-END-SIDS
Fax: (416)488-3864
Email: sidsinfo@sidscanada.org
Fnded: 1973. **Mem:** 125. **Local Groups:** 10. **Lang(s):** English, French. **Desc:** Health care providers, families who have lost a child to sudden infant death syndrome, and other individuals with an interest in SIDS. Provides emotional support to families that have experienced the loss of a child to SIDS. Operates network of support groups; serves as a clearinghouse

on SIDS and grief; provides educational programs for general public; conducts fundraising activities benefitting SIDS research projects. **Pub:** *Baby's Breath*, quarterly. Newsletter.

★ 1990 ★ Canadian Friends of the American-Israel Medical Foundation (CFAIMF)
600 University Ave., Ste. 474
Toronto, ON, Canada M5G 1X5
Phone: (416)586-4473 **Fax:** (416)586-4507

Lang(s): English, French, Hebrew. **Desc:** Supporters of the American-Israel Medical Foundation and its programs. Seeks to advance the practice of medicine. Provides support and assistance to the programs of the American-Israel Medical Foundation.

★ 1991 ★ Canadian Friends of the Bene Berak Hospital (CRBBH)
579 Old Orchard Grove
Toronto, ON, Canada M5M 2H2
Phone: (416)783-5773 **Fax:** (416)537-0437

Fnded: 1979. **Lang(s):** English, French. **Desc:** Individuals and organizations. Promotes continuation and expansion of the activities of the Bene Berak Hospital. Conducts fundraising activities; sponsors charitable programs. **Pub:** Brochure, periodic.

★ 1992 ★ Canadian Friends of Bikur Cholim Hospital of Jerusalem
579 Old Orchard Grove
Toronto, ON, Canada M5M 2H2
Phone: (416)783-5773 **Fax:** (416)537-0487

Fnded: 1976. **Lang(s):** French. **Desc:** Solicits and collects donations to help support the Bikur Cholim Hospital. **Pub:** Newsletter.

★ 1993 ★ Canadian Genetic Diseases Network
2150 Western Pkwy., Ste. 201
Vancouver, BC, Canada V6T 1V6
Phone: (604)221-7300 **Fax:** (604)221-0778
Email: info@cgdn.generes.ca
Website: http://www.cgdn.generes.ca/

Fnded: 1990. **Mem:** 112. **Reg. Groups:** 13. **Lang(s):** English, French. **Desc:** Canadian scientists and health care professionals engaged in medical genetic research. Works to develop and commercialize basic research in genetically related diseases including cancer, cystic fibrosis, myotonic dystrophy, and huntington's disease. Forms partnerships with industry to develop basic research technologies; trains students in genetic research, with particular focus on the graduate and post-doctoral levels. **Pub:** *The Scanner*, semiannual. Newsletter. Relates advances in genetically related disease research for members, related industries and government agencies.

★ 1994 ★ Canadian Geriatrics Society (Societe Canadienne de Geriatrie — SCG)
Health Sciences Centre
Calgary, AB, Canada T2N 4N1
Phone: (403)220-4578

Fnded: 1980. **Mem:** 200. **Lang(s):** English, French. **Desc:** Health care professionals with an interest in geriatric medicine. Seeks to advance the practice of gerontology; promotes ongoing professional development of members. Facilitates exchange of information among members; conducts continuing professional education courses. **Frmly:** (2001) Canadian Society of Geriatric Medicine.

★ 1995 ★ Canadian Gerontological Nursing Association (CGNA) (Association Canadienne des Infirmiers et Infirmieres en Gerontologie — ACIG)
c/o South Granville Business Services
101-1001 W Broadway Department 370
Vancouver, BC, Canada V6H 4E4
Phone: (250)769-0664 **Fax:** (604)734-0778
Email: cgna@home.com
Website: http://www.cgna.net

Lang(s): English, French. **Desc:** Nurses specializing in gerontological practice. Promotes professional development of members; seeks to advance the practice of gerontological nursing. Serves as a forum for the exchange of information among members; conducts continuing professional education programs.

★ 1996 ★ Canadian Guide Dogs for the Blind (Chiens Guides Canadiens pour Aveugles)
PO Box 280
4120 Rideau Valley Dr. N
Manotick, ON, Canada K4M 1A3
Phone: (613)692-7777 **Fax:** (613)692-0650
Email: cgdb@sympatico.ca
Website: http://www.guidedogs.ca

Fnded: 1984. **Lang(s):** English, French. **Desc:** Works to assist visually impaired Canadians with their mobility by providing and training them in the use of professionally trained guide dogs.

★ 1997 ★ Canadian Hard of Hearing Association (CHHA)
2435 Holly Ln., Ste. 205
Ottawa, ON, Canada K1V 7P2
Phone: (613)526-1584 **Free:** 800-263-8068
Fax: (613)526-4718
Email: chhanational@chha.ca
Website: http://www.chha.ca

Fnded: 1982. **Mem:** 2,100. **Lang(s):** English, French. **Desc:** Individuals with or without hearing impairments. Seeks to raise public awareness of issues of concern to members; promotes full integration into society of people with hearing loss. Identifies and works to remove barriers to full social and economic participation by people with hearing impairments; conducts educational programs. **Pub:** *Listen*, quarterly. Magazine.

★ 1998 ★ Canadian Health Coalition (CHC) (Coalition Canadienne de la Sante — CCS)
2841 Riverside Dr.
Ottawa, ON, Canada K1V 8X7
Phone: (613)521-3400 **Fax:** (613)521-9638
Email: info@healthcoalition.ca
Website: http://www.healthcoalition.ca

Lang(s): English, French. **Desc:** Individuals and organizations with an interest in health care. Promotes increased availability and quality of health services. Monitors the performance of health care facilities and services and makes recommendations for their improvement.

★ 1999 ★ Canadian Health Economics Research Association (CHERA) (Association Canadienne pour la Recerche en Economie de la Sante — ACRES)
Abramsky Hall, 3rd Fl.
Queen's University
Kingston, ON, Canada K7L 3N6
Phone: (613)533-6675 **Fax:** (613)533-6353
Email: swanb@post.queensu.ca
Website: http://www.chera.ca

Fnded: 1983. **Mem:** 330. **Desc:** Economists, administrators, political scientists, sociologists, social workers, policymakers, and other individuals with an interest in the economics of health care. Facilitates communication and exchange of information among members. Gathers and disseminates health economics information. Promotes quality research in health economics and related fields. Maintains registry of health economics researchers and research projects in Canada. Maintains Internet server. **Pub:** *CHERAction*, quarterly. Newsletter. • *Membership Registry*, annual. Directory.

★ 2000 ★ Canadian Health Record Association (CHRA) (College des Archivists Medicale du Canada — CAMC)
1090 Don Mills Rd., Ste. 501
Don Mills, ON, Canada M3C 3R6
Phone: (416)447-4900 **Fax:** (416)447-4598
Email: info@chra.ca
Website: http://www.chra.ca

Fnded: 1942. **Mem:** 3,000. **Lang(s):** English, French. **Desc:** Librarians, archivists, and other individuals engaged in the maintenance of medical records. Promotes excellence in the practice of medical records management. Facilitates communication and cooperation among members; sponsors continuing professional development courses for medical records managers. **Pub:** *CHRA Source*, quarterly. Newsletter.

★ 2001 ★ Canadian Healthcare Association
17 York St.
Ottawa, ON, Canada K1N 9J6
Phone: (613)241-8005 **Fax:** (613)241-5055
Email: info@cha.ca
Website: http://www.cha.ca/

Fnded: 1931. **Mem:** 13. **State Groups:** 13. **Lang(s):** French. **Desc:** Promotes a humane, effective, efficient health system of the highest quality. **Pub:** *Guide to Canadian Healthcare Facilities*, annual. Directory. Lists health care facilities in Canada.

★ 2002 ★ Canadian Healthcare Engineering Society (CHES) (Societe Canadienne d'Ingenierie des Services de Sante — SCIH)
The Woolen Mill
4 Cataraqui St., Ste. 310
Kingston, ON, Canada K7K 1Z7
Phone: (613)531-2661 **Fax:** (613)531-0626
Email: info@ches.org
Website: http://www.ches.org

Lang(s): English, French. **Desc:** Hospital maintenance engineers and other individuals responsible for the physical plant of health care facilities. Promotes excellence in hospital engineering. Serves as a forum for the exchange of information among members; sponsors educational and training programs. **Frmly:** (2000) Canadian Hospital Engineering Society.

★ 2003 ★ Canadian Hearing Society (CHS) (La Societe Canadienne de l'Ouie)
271 Spadina Rd.
Toronto, ON, Canada M5R 2V3
Phone: (416)928-2500 **Fax:** (416)928-2525
Email: info@chs.ca
Website: http://www.chs.ca

Fnded: 1940. **Lang(s):** English, French. **Desc:** Those who are deaf or experience hearing loss, and their families; health care and other professionals; and educators. Provides services that enhance the independence of deaf, deafened, and hard of hearing people and encourages the prevention of hearing loss. **Pub:** *Vibes*, quarterly. Magazine.

★ 2004 ★ Canadian Hematology Society (CHS) (Societe Canadienne d'Hematologie — SCH)
206-435 St. Laurent Blvd.
Ottawa, ON, Canada K1K 2Z8
Phone: (613)748-9613 **Fax:** (613)748-6392
Email: armand.keating@uhn.on.ca
Website: http://www.CanadianHematologySociety.com

Lang(s): English, French. **Desc:** Hematologists and other scientists and health care professionals with an interest in hematology. Seeks to advance the study, teaching, and practice of hematology. Serves as a forum for the exchange of information among members; conducts continuing professional education courses. **Pub:** *Canadian Hematology Society*, 3/year. Newsletter.

★ 2005 ★ Canadian Hemochromatosis Society (CHS)

272-7000 Minoru Blvd.
Richmond, BC, Canada V6Y 3Z5
Phone: (604)279-7135 **Free:** 877-223-4766
Fax: (604)279-7138
Email: office@cdnhemochromatosis.ca
Website: http://www.cdnhemochromatosis.ca

Fnded: 1982. **Mem:** 900. **Lang(s):** English, French. **Desc:** People with hemochromatosis and their families; health care providers with an interest in metabolic and genetic disorders. Promotes early diagnosis, and treatment of hemochromatosis. Operates national support group network. Conducts educational programs to raise awareness of hemochromatosis. **Pub:** *Among Ourselves*, biennial. Newsletter. Provides information about hemochromatosis and the activities of the society. Information packages; "The Bronze Killer" (book).

★ 2006 ★ Canadian Hemophilia Society (CHS)
(Societe Canadienne de l'Hemophilie — SCH)

625 President Kennedy Ave., Ste. 1210
Montreal, QC, Canada H3A 1K2
Phone: (514)848-0503 **Free:** 800-668-2686
Fax: (514)848-9661
Email: chs@hemophilia.ca
Website: http://www.hemophilia.ca

Fnded: 1953. **Mem:** 2,500. **Nat'l Groups:** 1. **Reg. Groups:** 5. **State Groups:** 10. **Lang(s):** English, French. **Desc:** People with hemophilia and their families; health care professionals with an interest in hematological disorders. Seeks to advance the diagnosis and treatment of hemophilia; promotes improvement in the quality of life of people with hemophilia. Provides support and services to people with hemophilia and their families; conducts educational programs. **Pub:** *Hemophilia Today*, quarterly. Newsletter.

★ 2007 ★ Canadian Hispanic Senior Services (CHSS)

1829 54th St. SE, Ste. 200
Calgary, AB, Canada T2B 1N5
Phone: (403)569-0133 **Fax:** (403)569-0133

Lang(s): English, French. **Desc:** Individuals and organizations providing services to senior citizens. Promotes increased availability of senior services among Canadians of Hispanic descent. Provides support and services to Hispanic Canadians.

★ 2008 ★ Canadian HIV/AIDS Legal Network
(Reseau juridique canadien VIH/sida)

417 Saint-Pierre St., Ste. 408
Montreal, QC, Canada H2Y 2M4
Phone: (514)397-6828 **Fax:** (514)397-8570
Email: info@aidslaw.ca
Website: http://www.aidslaw.ca

Fnded: 1992. **Mem:** 300. **Lang(s):** English, French. **Desc:** Legal professionals and other individuals with an interest in the legal rights and status of people with HIV and AIDS. Promotes increased respect for the civil and human rights of people with HIV and AIDS. Conducts research and educational programs. **Pub:** *Canadian HIV/AIDS Policy and Law Review*, 3/year. Journal. Summarizes developments in HIV/AIDS policy and law in Canada and internationally.

★ 2009 ★ Canadian Holistic Nurses Association (CHNA)
(Association Canadienne des Informieres en Approches Holistiques de Soins)

50 Driveway
Ottawa, ON, Canada K2P 1E2
Phone: (613)237-2133 **Free:** 888-910-9998
Fax: (613)237-3520
Email: pdownton@nfld.com
Website: http://mypage.direct.ca/h/hutchings/chna.html

Fnded: 1988. **Mem:** 140. **Lang(s):** English, French. **Desc:** Registered nurses are members; health care providers including registered psychiatric nurses, massage therapists, physiotherapists, nursing students, and chiropractors are associate members. Seeks to further the development of the field of holistic nursing. Promotes use of a conceptual framework based on nursing principles and human environmental field theory in the treatment of patients; encourages employment of noninvasive strategies for promoting health and wellness. Promulgates and enforces standards of practice in holistic nursing; provides consulting services and other support to members; interacts with health care consumer and provider organizations to influence health policy formation. **Pub:** Newsletter, semiannual.

★ 2010 ★ Canadian Home Care Association (CHCA)
(Association Canadienne de Soins et Services a Domicile — ACSSD)

17 York St., Ste. 401
Ottawa, ON, Canada K1N 9J6
Phone: (613)569-1585 **Fax:** (613)569-1604
Email: chca@cdnhomecare.on.ca
Website: http://www.cdnhomecare.on.ca

Lang(s): English, French. **Desc:** Providers of home health care services. Promotes excellence in the practice of home care. Represents members' interests before medical organizations, government agencies, and the public. Conducts continuing professional development courses for home care personnel. Sponsors promotional programs. **Pub:** *Cnez Nous, At Home*, quarterly. Newsletter.

★ 2011 ★ Canadian Hyperlexia Association (CHA)

300 John St.
PO Box 87673
Thornhill, ON, Canada L3T 7R3
Phone: (905)886-9163 **Fax:** (905)886-4624
Email: cha@ican.net
Website: http://home.ican.net/~cha

Desc: Parents and professionals promoting awareness of the hyperlexia syndrome; provides information regarding the syndrome.

★ 2012 ★ Canadian Hypertension Society (CHS)
(Societe Canadienne d'Hypertension Arterielle — SCHA)

c/o Dr. Venkat Gopal, Sec.
Department of Pharmacology
College of Medicine
University of Saskatchewan
Saskatoon, SK, Canada S7N 5E5
Phone: (306)966-6294 **Fax:** (306)966-6220
Email: gopal@sask.usask.ca
Website: http://www.chs.md

Lang(s): English, French. **Desc:** Health care professionals and other individuals with an interest in hypertension. Seeks to advance the prevention, diagnosis, and treatment of high blood pressure. Conducts educational programs to raise public awareness of hypertension prevention; sponsors research and continuing professional development programs.

★ 2013 ★ Canadian Infectious Disease Society (CIDS)
(Societe Canadienne de Maladies Infectieuses — SCMI)

2197 promenade Riverside Dr.
Ste./piece 504
Ottawa, ON, Canada K1H 7X3
Phone: (613)260-3233 **Fax:** (613)260-3235
Email: cids@magma.ca

Lang(s): English, French. **Desc:** Promotes excellence in the prevention, diagnosis, and management of human infectious diseases. **Pub:** *The Canadian Journal of Infectious Diseases*, bimonthly. Journal.

★ 2014 ★ Canadian Institute of Child Health (CICH)
(Institut Canadien de la Sante Infantile — ICSI)

384 Bank St., Ste. 300
Ottawa, ON, Canada K2P 1Y4
Phone: (613)230-8838 **Fax:** (613)230-6654
Email: cich@cich.ca
Website: http://www.cich.ca

Fnded: 1977. **Mem:** 600. **Lang(s):** English, French. **Desc:** Health care providers and other individuals and organizations with an interest in child health. Promotes increased access to quality health services for all children. Serves as a clearinghouse on child health, health services, and related topics; sponsors educational and advocacy activities in areas including children's health, pregnancy, and childbirth.

★ 2015 ★ Canadian Institute of Health Care and Business (CIHCB)

No. 7 Hayden St., Ste. 303
Toronto, ON, Canada M4Y 2P2
Phone: (416)925-4417 **Fax:** (905)731-2771
Email: can_inst@istar.ca
Website: http://www.nacc.ca/2355.htm

Lang(s): English, French. **Desc:** Business professionals working in the field of health care. Promotes effective application of business principles within the health care industries. Sponsors continuing professional education courses for members.

★ 2016 ★ Canadian Institute for Health Information (CIHI)

377 Dalhousie St., Ste. 200
Ottawa, ON, Canada K1N 9N8
Phone: (613)241-7860 **Fax:** (613)241-8120
Email: communications@cihi.ca

Fnded: 1994. **Lang(s):** English, French. **Desc:** Working to improve the health of Canadians and the health care system, provides quality health information, committed to safeguarding the privacy and confidentiality of personal health information. Seeks to coordinate the development and maintenance of a common approach to health information for Canada, provides accurate and timely information that needed to establish sound health policies, manages the Canadian health system effectively and creates public awareness of factors affecting good health.

★ 2017 ★ Canadian Institute of Hypnotism (CIH)

110 rue Greystone
Pointe Claire, QC, Canada H9R 5T6
Phone: (514)426-1010 **Fax:** (514)426-4680
Email: mmker@qc.aibn.com

Fnded: 1953. **Mem:** 486. **Nat'l Groups:** 1. **Reg. Groups:** 2. **Lang(s):** English, French. **Desc:** Health care professionals making use of hypnosis in their practices. Promotes improved training in and application of hypnosis as a medical care technique. Conducts research and educational programs; makes available children's services; maintains speakers' bureau. **Pub:** *Newsletter of CIH*, quarterly. Newsletter. Classical Format. • Bulletin, periodic. • Brochure.

★ 2018 ★ Canadian Institute of Public Health Inspectors (CIPHI)
(Institut Canadien des Inspecteurs en Hygiene Publique — ICIHP)
15180 N Bluff Rd.
PO Box 75264
White Rock, BC, Canada V4B 5L4
Phone: (604)543-0935 **Free:** 888-245-8180
Fax: (604)543-0936
Email: president@ciphi.ca
Website: http://www.ciphi.ca

Fnded: 1934. **Mem:** 1,000. **Lang(s):** English. **Desc:** Public health inspectors. Seeks to advance the profession of public health inspection; promotes adherence to high standards of ethics and practice among members. Conducts advocacy campaigns to increase public appreciation of the role of public health inspectors; sponsors educational and training programs. **Pub:** *Environmental Health Review*, quarterly. Journal.

★ 2019 ★ Canadian Institute of Stress (CIS)
Medcan Clinic Office
Ste. 1500, 150 York St.
Toronto, ON, Canada M5H 3S5
Phone: (416)236-4218
Email: earle@stresscanada.org
Website: http://www.stresscanada.org

Fnded: 1979. **Lang(s):** English. **Desc:** Works to educate workplaces, communities, and individuals in change-abilities and risk management strategies for successful, not stressful transitions. Provides clinical assessment, counseling, and coaching; develops specialized change and risk management services; conducts research; and sponsors professional certification programs.

★ 2020 ★ Canadian Intramural Recreation Association (CIRA)
2197 Riverside Dr., No. 403
Ottawa, ON, Canada K1H 7X3
Phone: (613)523-1348 **Fax:** (613)523-1206
Email: cira@intramurals.ca
Website: http://www.intramurals.ca

Fnded: 1977. **Mem:** 800. **Lang(s):** English, French. **Desc:** Seeks to encourage, promote and develop active living, healthy lifestyle and personal growth through intramural and recreational programs within the educational community. **Pub:** Catalog, periodic. Contains more than 160 resources. • Bulletin, 8/year.

★ 2021 ★ Canadian Intravenous Nurses Association (CINA)
PO Box 66572
685 McCowan Rd.
Toronto, ON, Canada M1J 3N8
Phone: (416)696-7761 **Fax:** (416)696-8437
Email: cina@cina.ca
Website: http://www.cina.ca

Fnded: 1975. **Mem:** 774. **Local Groups:** 6. **Lang(s):** English. **Desc:** Registered nurses specializing in intravenous therapy or employed in supervisory, educational, or administrative positions related to intravenous therapy. Works to establish and promote standards of intravenous therapy. Offers educational programs designed to enhance patient care and safety. Facilitates discussion of intravenous therapy issues. **Pub:** *CINA Journal*, annual. Journal. • *CINA Mainliner*, quarterly. Newsletter. • *I.V. Therapy Guidelines*.

★ 2022 ★ Canadian Liver Foundation (CLF)
2235 Sheppard Ave. E, Ste. 1500
Toronto, ON, Canada M2J 5B5
Phone: (416)491-3353 **Free:** 800-563-5483
Fax: (416)491-4952
Email: clf@liver.ca
Website: http://www.liver.ca

Fnded: 1969. **Lang(s):** English, French. **Desc:** Health care professionals and researchers with an interest in hepatic diseases. Promotes increased understanding of the causes, prevention, and treatment of diseases of the liver; facilitates professional advancement of members. Works to lessen the incidence of hepatic disease through public education; provides support and services to people with hepatic diseases and their families; funds medical research. Conducts charitable programs; maintains speakers' bureau. **Pub:** Pamphlets.

★ 2023 ★ Canadian Lung Association (CLA)
(Association Pulmonaire du Canada — APC)
National Office
3 Raymond st., Ste. 300
Ottawa, ON, Canada K1R 1A3
Phone: (613)569-6411 **Fax:** (613)569-8860
Email: info@lung.ca
Website: http://www.lung.ca

Fnded: 1900. **Mem:** 10. **State Groups:** 10. **Lang(s):** English, French. **Desc:** Individuals and organizations with an interest in lung disease. Seeks to raise public awareness of lung disease and its causes; promotes advancement in the diagnosis, prevention, and treatment of lung disease. Sponsors educational programs; conducts fundraising activities; provides support to research and treatment projects. **Pub:** *Cybersn zz*, bimonthly. Newsletter.

★ 2024 ★ Canadian Marfan Association (CMA)
Central Plaza Postal Outlet
128 Queen St. S
PO Box 42257
Mississauga, ON, Canada L5M 4Z0
Phone: (905)826-3223 **Fax:** (905)826-2125
Email: info@marfan.ca
Website: http://www.marfan.ca

Fnded: 1986. **Mem:** 600. **Reg. Groups:** 4. **Lang(s):** English, French. **Desc:** People with Marfan Syndrome (a genetic disorder of the connective tissue), their families, and health care providers and other individuals with an interest in the disorder. Promotes an improved quality of life for people with Marfan Syndrome; seeks to prove diagnostic techniques and treatments of Marfan. Serves as a clearinghouse on Marfan Syndrome; provides support and services to people with Marfan and their families; conducts educational campaigns to raise public awareness of the disorder. Maintains network of local Marfan support groups. **Pub:** *Newslinks*, 3/year. Newsletter.

★ 2025 ★ Canadian Massage Therapist Alliance (CMTA)
344 Lakeshore Rd. E, Ste. B
Oakville, ON, Canada L6J 1J6
Phone: (905)849-7606 **Fax:** (905)849-8606
Email: info@cmta.ca
Website: http://www.cmta.ca

Fnded: 1991. **Mem:** 4,000. **Lang(s):** English. **Desc:** Alliance of provincial associations for massage therapists. Seeks to advance the practice of therapeutic massage; promotes professional development of members. **Pub:** *Hand in Hand*, semiannual. Newsletter.

★ 2026 ★ Canadian Medical Association
1867 Alta Vista Dr.
Ottawa, ON, Canada K1G 3Y6
Free: 800-457-4205 **Fax:** (613)236-8864
Email: cmamsc@cma.ca
Website: http://www.cma.ca

Desc: Seeks to improve medical care for persons living in Canada. Works to maintain high standards of hospital care and health related services. Encourages constant improvement in the medical profession.

★ 2027 ★ Canadian Medical Malpractice Prevention Association (CMMPA)
2900 Warden Ave. No. 92093
Toronto, ON, Canada M1W 3Y8
Phone: (416)969-1587

Fnded: 1987. **Lang(s):** English, French. **Desc:** Individuals with an interest in medical malpractice and related issues. Promotes effective medical treatment and reform of legal medical malpractice procedures. Maintains speakers' bureau.

★ 2028 ★ Canadian Medical Protective Association (CMPA)
(Association Canadienne de Protection Medicale — ACPM)
PO Box 8225, Sta. T
Ottawa, ON, Canada K1G 3H7
Phone: (613)725-2000 **Free:** 800-267-6522
Fax: (613)725-1300
Website: http://www.cmpa.org

Fnded: 1901. **Mem:** 61,000. **Lang(s):** English, French. **Desc:** Defense organization for physicians practicing in Canada.

★ 2029 ★ Canadian MedicAlert Foundation (CMAF)
(La Fondation Canadienne MedicAlert — FCMA)
2005 Sheppard Ave. E, Ste. 800
Toronto, ON, Canada M2J 5B4
Phone: (416)696-0267 **Free:** 800-668-1507
Fax: 800-392-8422
Email: medinfo@medicalert.ca
Website: http://www.medicalert.ca

Fnded: 1961. **Mem:** 1000,000. **Lang(s):** English, French. **Desc:** Provides life-long access to personal and medical information in order to protect and save member's lives; offers immediate access to medical information in emergencies, unlimited record updates, a MedicAlert bracelet or necklet (engraved with ID number, 24-hour emergency hotline number and specific medical conditions) and a wallet card with additional medical data. A complete record is available to emergency responders and medical professionals worldwide in 140 languages on the 24-hour hotline, in order to assist in making accurate diagnosis and to administer proper treatment. **Pub:** *MedicAlert Connects*, semiannual. Newsletter. Provides information to members and donors regarding CMAF activities, accomplishments, etc.

★ 2030 ★ Canadian Mental Health Association
(Association Canadienne pour la Sante Mentale)
8 King St. E, Ste. 810.
Toronto, ON, Canada M5C 1B5
Phone: (416)484-7750 **Fax:** (416)484-4617
Email: national@cmha.ca
Website: http://www.cmha.ca

Fnded: 1918. **Local Groups:** 135. **Lang(s):** English, French. **Desc:** Mental health professionals and other individuals with an interest in community mental health. Works to enable individuals, groups, and communities to increase control over and enhance their mental health. Serves as a social advocate to encourage public action to strengthen community mental health services; conducts lobbying activities. Promotes mental health research; organizes and operates grass roots programs to help people whose mental health is at risk make use of the services available to them. Sponsors educational programs. **Pub:** Newsletter, quarterly. • Pamphlets.

★ 2031 ★ Canadian National Institute for the Blind (CNIB)
(L'Institut National Canadien pour les Aveugles — INCA)
1929 Bayview Ave.
Toronto, ON, Canada M4G 3E8
Phone: (416)480-2500 **Free:** 800-513-7813
Fax: (416)480-7677
Website: http://www.cnib.ca

Fnded: 1918. **Mem:** 100,000. **Nat'l Groups:** 2. **Reg. Groups:** 9. **Local Groups:** 57. **Lang(s):** English,

French. **Desc:** Rehabilitation organization serving people with visual impairment. Seeks to improve the quality of life of people with visual impairment and their families. Promotes full integration of people with visual impairment into Canadian society. Makes available support and assistance to people with visual impairment; conducts educational programs. **Pub:** *CNIB Vision Magazine*, semiannual. Magazine. Provides publications in Braille, on tape, and in large print.

★ 2032 ★ Canadian Natural Health Association (CNHA)
2219 Queen St. E Rear
Toronto, ON, Canada M4E 1E8
Phone: (416)686-7056

Fnded: 1960. **Mem:** 900. **Lang(s):** English. **Desc:** Holistic health care educators. Seeks to raise public awareness of holistic health care and the importance of a healthy lifestyle. Conducts educational programs; provides referral services; disseminates information on holistic health. **Pub:** *Natural Living Directory*, annual. Directory. • *Vegetarian Persuasion*. Book. textbooks and placemats. **Frmly:** (1995) Canadian Natural Hygiene Society.

★ 2033 ★ Canadian Naturopathic Association (CNA)
(Association Canadienne de Naturopathie — ACN)
1255 Sheppard Ave. E
North York, ON, Canada M2K 1E2
Phone: (416)496-8633 **Free:** 800-551-4381
Fax: (416)496-8634
Email: info@naturopathicassoc.ca
Website: http://www.naturopathicassoc.ca

Fnded: 1953. **Mem:** 600. **Reg. Groups:** 6. **Lang(s):** English, French. **Desc:** Naturopathic medical practitioners. Promotes excellence in the practice of naturopathic medicine; encourages professional development of members. Gathers and disseminates information on naturopathic medicine; sponsors research and educational programs. **Pub:** *Vital Link*, quarterly. Newsletter.

★ 2034 ★ Canadian Network for Asthma Care (CNAC)
6 Forest Laneway, Ste. 1607
North York, ON, Canada M2N 5X9
Phone: (416)224-9221 **Fax:** (416)224-9220
Email: ased@cnac.net
Website: http://www.cnac.net/

Desc: Dedicated to the promotion of asthma care and education in Canada; strives to reduce illness and death caused by this disease. Provides Asthma Educators Certification program.

★ 2035 ★ Canadian Neurosurgical Society (CNSS)
(Societe Canadienne de Neurochirurgie — SCN)
c/o Canadian Congress of Neurological Sciences
PO Box 5456, Sta. A
Calgary, AB, Canada T2H 1X8
Phone: (403)229-9544 **Fax:** (403)229-1661
Email: brains@ccns.org
Website: http://www.ccns.org

Fnded: 1948. **Mem:** 300. **Lang(s):** English, French. **Desc:** Neurosurgeons, neurologists, and other individuals with an interest in neurosurgery. Seeks to improve neurosurgical techniques; promotes professional development of members. Sponsors research and educational programs; facilitates communication and cooperation among members. **Pub:** *Canadian Journal of Neurosurgical Sciences*, quarterly. Journal. Peer-reviewed international journal specializing in neurology, neurosurgery, and related neuroscience.

★ 2036 ★ Canadian Nurses Association (CNA)
(Association des Infirmieres et Infirmiers du Canada — AIIC)
50 Driveway
Ottawa, ON, Canada K2P 1E2
Phone: (613)237-2133 **Free:** 800-361-8404
Fax: (613)237-3520
Email: dross@cna-aiic.ca
Website: http://www.cna-nurses.ca

Fnded: 1908. **Mem:** 111,708. **Local Groups:** 11. **Lang(s):** English, French. **Desc:** Works to advance the quality of nursing in the interests of the public. Promotes high standards of nursing practice, education, research, and administration in order to achieve quality nursing care in the public interest. Also promotes uniform and high quality regulatory practices in the public interest and in collaboration with nursing regulatory bodies. Acts in the public interest for Canadian nursing and nurses, providing national and international leadership in nursing and health issues. **Pub:** *Canadian Nurse/Infirmiere Canadienne*, 10/year. Journal. • Monograph, periodic.

★ 2037 ★ Canadian Nurses Foundation (CNF)
(Fondation des Infirmieres et Infirmiers du Canada — FIIC)
50 Driveway
Ottawa, ON, Canada K2P 1E2
Phone: (613)237-2133 **Fax:** (613)237-3520
Email: info@cnursesfdn.ca
Website: http://www.canadiannursesfoundation.com

Fnded: 1961. **Mem:** 678. **Lang(s):** English, French. **Desc:** Promotes health and patient care in Canada; fosters excellence in nursing through nursing research grants, scholarships, specialty certification, and financial support for other educational purposes. **Pub:** *Foundation Focus*, 3-4/year. Newsletter.

★ 2038 ★ Canadian Nurses Protective Society (CNPS)
50 Driveway
Ottawa, ON, Canada K2P 1E2
Phone: (613)237-2092 **Free:** 800-267-3390
Fax: (613)237-6300
Email: info@cnps.ca
Website: http://www.cnps.ca

Fnded: 1988. **Lang(s):** English. **Desc:** Provides legal liability protection related to nursing practice to eligible registered nurses in Canada by providing information, education, and financial and legal assistance. Also offers a group insurance plan.

★ 2039 ★ Canadian Nurses Respiratory Society (CNRS)
(Societe Canadienne des Infirmieres en Sante Respiratoire — SCISR)
300-3 Raymond St.
Ottawa, ON, Canada K1R 1A3
Phone: (613)569-6411 **Fax:** (613)569-8860
Email: info@lung.ca
Website: http://www.lung.ca/resp

Fnded: 1977. **Mem:** 125. **Lang(s):** English, French. **Desc:** Nurses specializing in the treatment of respiratory diseases. Promotes excellence in the practice of nursing; encourages professional development of members. Serves as a forum for the exchange of information among members; sponsors research and educational programs. **Pub:** *Bulletin*, 3/year. Newsletter.

★ 2040 ★ Canadian Occupational Health Nurses Association (COHNA)
(Association Canadienne des Infirmieres et Infirmiers en Sante du Travail — ACIST)
PO Box 383
CBS
Mauels, NL, Canada A1W 1M9
Phone: (709)778-1561
Email: president@cohna-aciist.ca
Website: http://www.cohna-aciist.ca

Fnded: 1992. **Mem:** 2,000. **Reg. Groups:** 9. **Lang(s):** English, French. **Desc:** Nurses specializing in occupational health. Seeks to advance the study and practice of occupational health nursing. Facilitates communication among members; sponsors research and educational programs on a national basis.

★ 2041 ★ Canadian Occupational Therapy Foundation (COTF)
(Fondation Canadienne d'Ergotherapie — FCE)
150 Eglinton Av, Ste. 207
Toronto, ON, Canada M4P 1E8
Phone: (416)487-5438 **Fax:** (416)487-5407
Email: pat@cotfcanada.org
Website: http://www.cotfcanada.org

Fnded: 1983. **Lang(s):** English, French. **Desc:** Occupational therapists and other health care professionals. Seeks to advance the study and practice of occupational therapy. Conducts fundraising activities; provides support and assistance to occupational therapy research programs; sponsors educational courses.

★ 2042 ★ Canadian Oncology Society (COS)
(Societe d'Oncologie du Canada — SOC)
82-84 Barrie St.
Kingston, ON, Canada K7L 3N6
Phone: (613)533-6430 **Fax:** (613)533-2941
Email: bvandersluis@ctg.queensu.ca
Website: http://www.cos.ca

Lang(s): English, French. **Desc:** Oncologists and other health care professionals with an interest in oncology. Seeks to advance the study and practice of oncology. Serves as a clearinghouse on oncology; sponsors research and educational programs.

★ 2043 ★ Canadian Ophthalmological Society (COS)
(Societe Canadienne d'Ophthalmologie — SCO)
1525 Carling Ave., Ste. 610
Ottawa, ON, Canada K1Z 8R9
Phone: (613)729-6779 **Free:** 800-267-5763
Fax: (613)729-7209
Email: cos@eyesite.ca
Website: http://www.eyesite.ca

Fnded: 1937. **Mem:** 950. **Nat'l Groups:** 1. **Lang(s):** English, French. **Desc:** Ophthalmologists and ophthalmology students. Seeks to advance the study and practice of ophthalmology. Facilitates exchange of information among members; sponsors research and educational programs. **Pub:** *Canadian Journal of Ophthalmology*, 7/year. Journal.

★ 2044 ★ Canadian Organization for Rare Disorders (CORD)
PO Box 814
Coaldale, AB, Canada T1M 1M7
Phone: (403)345-4544 **Free:** 877-302-7273
Fax: (403)345-3948
Email: office@cord.ca
Website: http://www.cord.ca

Fnded: 1987. **Mem:** 35. **Lang(s):** English. **Desc:** People suffering from rare disorders and their families. Works to enhance the lives of all persons affected by rare disorders through an educational and informational support network. Provides information on more than 6,000 rare disorders. **Pub:** *The Link*, semiannual. Newsletter. Contains updates on organization and progress among other rare disorder groups in Canada.

★ 2045 ★ Canadian Orthopaedic Association (COA)
(Association Canadienne d'Orthopedie — ACO)
1440 St. Catherine St. W, Ste. 718
Montreal, QC, Canada H3G 1R8
Phone: (514)874-9003 **Fax:** (514)874-0464
Email: info@coa-aco.org
Website: http://www.coa-aco.org
Fnded: 1945. **Mem:** 1,200. **Lang(s):** English, French. **Desc:** Orthopedic surgeons. Seeks to advance the study and practice of orthopedics. Facilitates exchange of information among members; sponsors research and educational programs. **Pub:** *COA Bulletin*, quarterly. Magazine.

★ 2046 ★ Canadian Orthopaedic Foundation (COF)
1 First Canadian Pl., Ste. 5100
Toronto, ON, Canada M5X 1K2
Free: 800-461-3639 **Fax:** 800-244-8825
Email: mailbox@canorth.org
Website: http://www.canorth.org
Lang(s): English, French. **Desc:** Health care professionals specializing in orthopedics. Seeks to advance orthopedic research, study, and practice. Serves as a clearinghouse on orthopedices; provides support and assistance to medical students; sponsors educational programs.

★ 2047 ★ Canadian Orthopaedic Nurses Association (CONA)
(Association Canadienne des Infirmieres et Infirmiers en Orthopedie — ACIO)
258 Vancouver St.
London, ON, Canada N5W 4R8
Phone: (519)685-8500
Email: terrylyne@sympatico.ca
Website: http://www.cona-nurse.org
Lang(s): English, French. **Desc:** Nurses specializing in orthopedic practice. Promotes advancement of the profession of orthopedic nursing. Sponsors continuing professional development courses for members. **Pub:** *Orthoscope*, quarterly. Newsletter.

★ 2048 ★ Canadian Orthopractic Manual Therapy Association (COMTA)
No. 207, 11520-100 Ave.
Edmonton, AB, Canada T5K 0J7
Phone: (780)482-7428 **Fax:** (780)488-2463
Email: info@orthopractic.org
Website: http://orthopractic.org
Lang(s): English. **Desc:** Professional groups that support orthopractic philosophy, including clinical specialists, basic scientists, and educators. Works to provide the public, healthcare professionals, government and funding agencies with guidelines on the provision of safe and effective manual therapy, including mobilization and manipulation.

★ 2049 ★ Canadian Orthoptic Council (COC)
(Conseil Canadien d'Orthoptique — CCO)
506 71st Ave. SW, Ste. 5
Calgary, AB, Canada T2V 4V4
Fax: (403)259-6784
Website: http://www.chebucto.ns.ca/Health/TCOS/COC-e.html
Lang(s): English, French. **Desc:** Health care professionals specializing in orthoptics and occular surgery. Seeks to advance the study and practice of orthoptics. Serves as a forum for the exchange of information among members; sponsors research and educational programs.

★ 2050 ★ Canadian Osteopathic Aid Society (COAS)
(Societe Canadienne d'Assistance Osteopathique — SCAO)
PO Box 24081
London, ON, Canada N6H 5C4
Phone: (519)681-1500 **Fax:** (519)681-1500
Email: coas@rogers.com
Website: http://coas.ca
Lang(s): English, French. **Desc:** Osteopathic physicians. Seeks to advance the study and practice of osteopathic medicine. Facilitates communication and cooperation among members; provides support and assistance to osteopathic medical students.

★ 2051 ★ Canadian Osteopathic Association (COA)
PO Box 24081
London, ON, Canada N6H 5C4
Phone: (519)681-1500 **Fax:** (519)681-1500
Email: coas@rogers.com
Website: http://coas.ca
Lang(s): English, French. **Desc:** Osteopathic physicians and students of osteopathy. Seeks to advance the study and practice of osteopathic medicine. Serves as a clearinghouse on osteopathy; sponsors research and educational programs.

★ 2052 ★ Canadian Paediatric Society (CPS)
(Societe Canadienne de Pediatrie — SCP)
100-2204 Walkley Rd.
Ottawa, ON, Canada K1G 4G8
Phone: (613)526-9397 **Fax:** (613)526-3332
Email: info@csp.ca
Website: http://www.cps.ca
Fnded: 1922. **Mem:** 1,954. **Lang(s):** English, French. **Desc:** Professional organization of pediatricians serving on committees and sections focusing on adolescent medicine, bioethics, drug therapy, hazardous substances, fetus and newborns, Indian and Inuit health, infectious disease and immunization, injury prevention, paediatric practice, nutrition, and psychological paediatrics. Provides services to Canadian children and to its membership. Serves as an advocate on issues relating to child health and welfare. Provides continuing education for the maintenance of competence of its members. Establishes Canadian standards/guidelines for paediatric care and practice, and promotes the interest of pediatricians. **Pub:** *Clinical Practice Guidelines*, periodic. Paper. • *CPS News*, bimonthly. Newsletter. • *Paediatrics & Child Health*, bimonthly. Journal. • *Well Beings*. Book. • *Your Child's Best Shot: A Parent's Guide to Vaccination*. Book. • Reports. **Frmly:** (1951) Canadian Society for the Study of Diseases of Children.

★ 2053 ★ Canadian Pain Society (CPS)
268 Grosvenor St.
London, ON, Canada N6A 4L6
Phone: (519)646-6388 **Fax:** (519)646-6376
Email: jenn.ronald@sjhc.london.on.ca
Website: http://www.medicine.dal.ca/cps
Fnded: 1982. **Lang(s):** English, French. **Desc:** Health care professionals and medical and pharamceutical researchers with an interest in pain and its alleviation. Fosters research on the causes of pain; seeks improved methods of pain management. Facilitates communication and cooperation among pain researchers and clinicians; sponsors educational and research programs. **Pub:** *Pain Research and Management*, quarterly. Journal.

★ 2054 ★ Canadian Paralympic Committee (CPC)
(Comite Paralympique du Canada — CPC)
1400-85 Albert St.
Ottawa, ON, Canada K1P 6A4
Phone: (613)569-4333 **Fax:** (613)569-2777
Email: reachus@paralympic.ca
Website: http://www.paralympic.ca
Fnded: 1993. **Nat'l Groups:** 28. **Lang(s):** English, French. **Desc:** Works to develop and promote the paralympic movement in Canada. Dedicated to supporting the achievement of excellence in paralympic sport; ; empowers persons with disabilities through sport. Sends Canadian Teams to the Paralympic Games.

★ 2055 ★ Canadian Paraplegic Association (CPA)
230-1101 Prince of Wales Dr.
Ottawa, ON, Canada K2C 3W7
Phone: (613)723-1033 **Free:** 800-720-4933
Fax: (613)723-1060
Email: info@canparaplegic.org
Website: http://www.canparaplegic.org
Fnded: 1945. **Lang(s):** English, French. **Desc:** To assist persons with spinal cord injuries and other physical disabilities to achieve independence, self-reliance and full community participation. **Pub:** *Total Access*, quarterly. Journal.

★ 2056 ★ Canadian Pharmacists Association (CPhA)
(Association des Pharmaciens du Canada — APhC)
1785 Alta Vista Dr.
Ottawa, ON, Canada K1G 3Y6
Phone: (613)523-7877 **Fax:** (613)523-0445
Email: info@pharmacists.ca
Website: http://www.pharmacists.ca
Fnded: 1907. **Mem:** 9,000. **Lang(s):** English, French. **Desc:** Pharmacists in Canada. Works to provide leadership for the pharmacy profession. Monitors government health care policies and legislation; lobbies for the interests of pharmacists. Maintains liaison with government departments, pharmaceutical manufacturers, and health care organizations. Conducts education and research programs. Bestows awards. **Pub:** *Annual Report*, annual. • *Canadian Pharmaceutical Journal*, 10/year. • *Compendium of Pharmaceuticals and Specialties*, annual. **Frmly:** Canadian Pharmaceutical Association.

★ 2057 ★ Canadian Physiotherapy Association (CPA)
(Association Canadienne de Physiotherapie — ACP)
2345 Younge St., Ste. 410
Toronto, ON, Canada M4P 2E5
Phone: (416)932-1888 **Free:** 800-387-8679
Fax: (416)932-9708
Email: information@physiotherapy.ca
Website: http://www.physiotherapy.ca
Lang(s): English, French. **Desc:** Physiotherapists and educational institutions. Seeks to advance the study, teaching, and practice of physiotherapy. Facilitates communication and cooperation among members; sponsors research and educational programs.

★ 2058 ★ Canadian Physiotherapy Cardio-respiratory Society (CPCRS)
(Societe Canadienne de physiotherapie cardio-respiatoire)
300-3 Raymond St.
Ottawa, ON, Canada K1R 1A3
Phone: (613)569-6411 **Fax:** (613)569-8860
Email: info@lung.ca
Website: http://www.lung.ca/physio
Mem: 300. **Lang(s):** English. **Desc:** Promotes cardio-pulmonary research. Administers Canadian Lung Association research funds. Promotes cardio-pulmonary physiotherapy care and education. **Pub:** *Bulletin*, 3/year. Newsletter.

★ 2059 ★ Canadian Play Therapy Institute (CPTI)
PO Box 2153
Kingston, ON, Canada K7L 5J9

Phone: (613)634-3125
Website: http://www.playtherapy.org

Fnded: 1990. **Mem:** 700. **Lang(s):** English. **Desc:** Play therapists, psychologists, and others with an interest in play therapy. Promotes excellence in the practice of play therapy; seeks to advance the profession of child psychology. Facilitates exchange of information among members; sponsors research and continuing professional development programs.

★ 2060 ★ Canadian Podiatric Medical Association (CPMA) (Association Medicale Podiatrique Canadienne — AMPC)

900 - 45 Sheppard Ave. E
Toronto, ON, Canada M2N 5W9
Phone: (416)927-9111 **Free:** 888-220-3338
Fax: (416)733-2491
Email: info@podiatrycanada.org
Website: http://www.podiatrycanada.org

Fnded: 1924. **Mem:** 220. **Nat'l Groups:** 1. **State Groups:** 6. **Lang(s):** English, French. **Desc:** Aims to serve and provide guidance to the podiatry profession in Canada. **Pub:** *Podiatry*, semiannual. Newsletter. Features president's message, provincial reports, educational activities.

★ 2061 ★ Canadian Porphyria Foundation

PO Box 1206
Neepawa, MB, Canada R0J 1H0
Phone: (204)476-2800 **Fax:** (204)476-2800
Email: porphyria@cpf-inc.ca
Website: http://www.cpf-inc.ca

Fnded: 1988. **Mem:** 2,000. **Nat'l Groups:** 1. **Lang(s):** English. **Desc:** Porphyria patients and their families. Works to improve the quality of life for people affected by prophyria. **Pub:** *A Guide to Diet In Porphyria*, biennial. Newsletter. • Newsletter, semiannual.

★ 2062 ★ Canadian Post-MD Education Registry (CAPER)

774 Echo Dr.
Ottawa, ON, Canada K1S 5P2
Phone: (613)730-1204 **Fax:** (613)730-1196
Email: caper@acmc.ca
Website: http://www.caper.ca

Fnded: 1986. **Lang(s):** English, French. **Desc:** National data source concerning post-MD (residency) training. Provides information concerning the number and type of residents in Canadian training programs. **Pub:** *CAPER Annual Census of Post-M.D. Trainees*, annual. Directory. Contains data pertaining to residency training in Canada.

★ 2063 ★ Canadian Psoriasis Foundation (CPF)

100A-824 Meath St.
Ottawa, ON, Canada K1Z 6E8
Phone: (613)728-4000 **Fax:** (613)728-8913
Email: cpf-fcp@psoriasis.ca

Fnded: 1983. **Mem:** 1,200. **Lang(s):** English, French. **Desc:** People with psoriasis and their families; health care providers with an interest in dermatology. Promotes an improved quality of life for people with psoriasis; seeks advancement in the prevention and treatment of psoriasis and related disorders. Maintains support groups; conducts research and educational programs. **Pub:** *CPF Newsletter*, 3/year. Newsletter. • Brochure.

★ 2064 ★ Canadian Psychiatric Association (CPA) (Association des Psychiatres du Canada — APC)

260-441 MacLaren St.
Ottawa, ON, Canada K2P 2H3
Phone: (613)234-2815 **Fax:** (613)234-9857
Email: cpa@cpa-apc.org
Website: http://www.cpa-apc.org

Fnded: 1951. **Mem:** 2,800. **State Groups:** 10. **Lang(s):** English, French. **Desc:** Works to improve mental health and psychiatric care delivery systems in Canada. Fosters high standards among Canadian psychiatrists; promotes continuing education of members; encourages and participates in educational programs for patient care providers; promotes research into psychiatric disorders; advocates for mental health system reforms and on related issues affecting the practice of psychiatry. **Pub:** *Canadian Journal of Psychiatry*, 11/year. Journal. • *CPA Bulletin*, bimonthly.

★ 2065 ★ Canadian Psychoanalytic Society (CPS) (Societe et Institut Canadiens de Psychanalyse — SICP)

7000 Cote Des Neiges
Montreal, QC, Canada H3S 2C1
Phone: (514)738-6105 **Fax:** (514)738-6393
Email: psyanal@qc.aira.com
Website: http://www.psychoanalyst.ca

Fnded: 1967. **Mem:** 405. **Reg. Groups:** 7. **Lang(s):** English, French. **Desc:** Psychoanalysts and other mental health professionals with an interest in psychoanalysis. Seeks to advance the study, teaching, and practice of psychoanalysis. Serves as a forum for the exchange of information among members; conducts educational and continuing professional development courses; sponsors research. **Pub:** *Canadian Journal of Psychoanalysis/Revue Canadienne de Psychanalyse*, semiannual. Journal. Contains manuscripts and book reviews.

★ 2066 ★ Canadian Psychological Association (CPA) (Societe Canadienne de Psychologie — SCP)

151 Slater St., Ste. 205
Ottawa, ON, Canada K1P 5H3
Phone: (613)237-2144 **Fax:** (613)237-1674
Email: cpa@cpa.ca
Website: http://www.cpa.ca

Fnded: 1939. **Mem:** 5,000. **Lang(s):** English, French. **Desc:** Psychologists and other individuals with an interest in psychology. Seeks to advance the study, teaching, and practice of psychology; promotes ongoing professional development of members. Facilitates exchange of information among members. **Pub:** *Canadian Journal of Behavioral Science*, quarterly. Journal. • *Canadian Journal of Experimental Psychology*, quarterly. Journal. • *Canadian Psychology*, quarterly. Journal. • *Psynopsis*, quarterly. Newsletter.

★ 2067 ★ Canadian Public Health Association

Ste. 400
1565 Carling Ave.
Ottawa, ON, Canada K1Z 8R1
Phone: (613)725-3769 **Fax:** (613)725-9826
Email: info@cpha.ca
Website: http://www.cpha.ca

Fnded: 1912. **Mem:** 1,600. **Lang(s):** English, French. **Desc:** Works to mobilize national charitable and volunteer resources to address public health concerns worldwide. Conducts immunization, maternal and child health, and HIV/AIDS programs in at-risk areas.

★ 2068 ★ Canadian Register of Health Service Providers in Psychology (CRHSPP) (Repertoire Canadien des Psychologues Offrant des Services de Sante — RCPOSS)

368 Dalhousie St., Ste. 300
Ottawa, ON, Canada K1N 5P4
Phone: (613)562-0900 **Fax:** (613)562-0902
Email: info@crhspp.ca
Website: http://www.crhspp.ca

Fnded: 1985. **Mem:** 3,000. **Lang(s):** English, French. **Desc:** Provides psychologists' credentials. Promotes increased availability of psychological services. Serves as a clearinghouse on psychological and related services; sponsors research and educational programs.

★ 2069 ★ Canadian Reiki Association (CRA)

PO Box 74072, Hillcrest RPO
Vancouver, BC, Canada V5V 5C8
Phone: (604)669-9049 **Free:** 800-835-7525
Fax: (604)521-9557
Email: reiki@reiki.ca
Website: http://www.reiki.ca/

Desc: Promotes Reiki practitioners and teachers. Provides the public with referrals to registered practitioners and registered teachers, promotes ethical practice and teaching, encourages educational standards, informs and protects the public, provides national voice for members.

★ 2070 ★ Canadian Rheumatology Association (CRA) (La Societe Canadienne de Rhumatologie — SCR)

43 Lundys Lane
Newmarket, ON, Canada L3Y 3R7
Phone: (905)952-0698 **Fax:** (905)952-0708
Website: http://www.cra.ucalgary.ca

Lang(s): English, French. **Desc:** Rheumatologists, people with rheumatic diseases, and other individuals with an interest in rheumatology. Seeks to advance rheumatological study and practice. Serves as a clearinghouse on rheumatology; sponsors research and educational programs.

★ 2071 ★ Canadian Schizophrenia Foundation (CSF)

16 Florence Ave.
Toronto, ON, Canada M2N 1E9
Phone: (416)733-2117 **Fax:** (416)733-2352
Email: centre@orthomed.org
Website: http://www.orthomed.org/csf/csf.htm

Fnded: 1969. **Lang(s):** English. **Desc:** People with schizophrenia and their families, mental health professionals, and others with an interest in schizophrenia and related conditions. Promotes an improved quality of life for people with schizophrenia; seeks to identify more effective treatments for the disorder. Facilitates communication among mental health professionals studying schizophrenia; sponsors research. **Pub:** *Nutrition and Mental Health*, quarterly. Newsletter.

★ 2072 ★ Canadian Sickle Cell Society (CSCS) (La Societe de l'Anemie Falciforme du Canada — SAFC)

6999 Cote-Des-Neiges Rd., Ste. 33
Montreal, QC, Canada H3S 2B8
Phone: (514)735-5109 **Fax:** (514)735-5100
Email: cslaf@total.net

Lang(s): English, French. **Desc:** People with sickle cell anemia and their families; health care professionals with an interest in sickle cell anemia. Seeks to improve the quality of life of people with sickle cell anemia; promotes advancement in the prevention and treatment of the disease. Provides support and assistance to people with sickle cell anemia and their families; sponsors research and educational programs.

★ 2073 ★ Canadian Sleep Society (CSS)

School of Psychology
Laval University
Laval, QC, Canada G1K 7P4
Phone: (418)656-2131 **Fax:** (418)656-5152
Email: celyne.bastien@css.to
Website: http://www.css.to

Fnded: 1986. **Mem:** 226. **Lang(s):** English, French. **Desc:** Scientists, health care professionals, students, and other individuals with an interest in sleep; corporations manufacturing sleep-related products. Promotes increased understanding of sleep and sleep disorders and their treatment. Sponsors research and educational programs. **Pub:** *Vigilance*, 3/year. Newsletter. • Brochure.

★ 2074 ★ Canadian Society for Aesthetic (Cosmetic) Plastic Surgery (CSACPS)
2334 Heska Rd.
Pickering, ON, Canada L1V 2P9
Phone: (905)831-7750 **Fax:** (905)831-7248
Email: information@csaps.ca
Website: http://www.csaps.ca

Fnded: 1972. **Mem:** 136. **Lang(s):** English, French. **Desc:** Educates plastic surgeons and residents, in the United States and Canada, on cosmetic surgery techniques. Conducts educational programs.

★ 2075 ★ Canadian Society of Allergy and Clinical Immunology (CSACI)
774 Echo Dr.
Ottawa, ON, Canada K1S 5N8
Phone: (613)730-6272 **Fax:** (613)730-1116
Email: csaci@rcpsc.edu
Website: http://csaci.medical.org

Fnded: 1945. **Mem:** 342. **Lang(s):** English, French. **Desc:** Allergists, immunologists, and others with an interest in the diagnosis and treatment of allergic and immunological disorders. Seeks to advance the understanding and treatment of allergic and immunological diseases. Conducts continuing professional education courses; sponsors research. **Pub:** *Canadian Journal Allergy and Clinical Immunology*, periodic. Journal. • Newsletter, periodic.

★ 2076 ★ Canadian Society of Atherosclerosis, Thrombosis and Vascular Biology (CSATVB)
Centre des Maladies Lipidiques, Bureau TR-93
CHUQ pavillon CHUL
2705 Blvd. Laurier
Ste.-Foy, QC, Canada G1V 4G2
Phone: (418)525-4444 **Fax:** (418)654-2145
Email: jshill@interchange.ubc.ca
Website: http://www.csatvb.ca

Fnded: 1983. **Mem:** 275. **Lang(s):** English, French. **Desc:** Canadian scientists and physicians specializing in atherosclerosis, thrombosis and vascular biology. Promotes in Canada the advancement of science, research, and teaching related to the fields of atherosclerosis, thrombosis and vascular biology.

★ 2077 ★ Canadian Society for Biomechanics (CSB)
c/o Dr. Darren J. Stefanyshyn, Sec.
Faculty of Kinesiology
University of Calgary
2500 University Dr. NW
Calgary, AB, Canada T2N 1N4
Phone: (403)220-8637 **Fax:** (403)284-3553
Email: darren@kin.ucalgary.ca
Website: http://www.health.uottawa.ca/biomech/csb/

Fnded: 1973. **Desc:** Fosters research and the interchange of information on the biomechanics of human physical activity. **Pub:** Newsletter. • Proceedings.

★ 2078 ★ Canadian Society for Brain, Behaviour and Cognitive Science (CSBBCS) (Societe Canadienne des Sciences du Cerveau, du Comportement et de la Cognition — SCSCCC)
Department of Psychology
McMaster University
1280 Main St. W
Hamilton, ON, Canada L8S 4K1
Email: bbcs@mcmaster.ca
Website: http://psych.mcmaster.ca/bbcs/index.html

Lang(s): English, French. **Desc:** Canadian scientists actively engaged in brain, behaviour, and cognitive science research. Promotes Canadian research in experimental psychology and behavioral neuroscience. Works with federal and provincial funding agencies and science ministries with a view to influencing science policy and funding.

★ 2079 ★ Canadian Society of Cardiology Technologists (CSCT) (Societe Canadienne des Technologistes en Cardiologie — SCTC)
PO Box 3121
Winnipeg, MB, Canada R3C 4E6
Email: info@csct.ca
Website: http://www.csct.ca

Lang(s): English, French. **Desc:** Cardiology technologists. Seeks to advance the practice of cardiology; promotes professional development of members. Facilitates exchange of information among members; sponsors research and educational programs.

★ 2080 ★ Canadian Society of Clinical Neurophysiologists (CSCN) (Societe Canadienne de Neurophysiologistes Cliniques — SCNC)
c/o Canadian Congress of Neurological Sciences
709 7015 Macleod Tr. SW
Calgary, AB, Canada T2H 2K6
Phone: (403)229-9544 **Fax:** (403)229-1661
Email: brains@ccns.org

Fnded: 1990. **Mem:** 200. **Lang(s):** English, French. **Desc:** Neurophysiologists and other individuals with an interest in the field. Seeks to advance the study and practice of neurophysiology. Facilitates exchange of information among members. **Pub:** *Canadian Journal of Neurological Sciences*, quarterly. Journal.

★ 2081 ★ Canadian Society for Clinical Pharmacology (CSCP)
105 Main St. E, Level P1
Hamilton, ON, Canada L8N 1G6
Phone: (905)522-1155 **Fax:** (905)528-7386
Email: gaebk@mcmaster.ca
Website: http://www.cscp.net

Fnded: 1978. **Lang(s):** English, French. **Desc:** Clinical pharmacologists and other health care professionals and scientists with an interest in therapeutics. Seeks to advance the study, teaching, and practice of clinical pharmacology. Serves as a network linking members; sponsors research and educational programs.

★ 2082 ★ Canadian Society of Diagnostic Medical Sonographers (CSDMS)
PO Box 1220
Kemptville, ON, Canada K0G 1J0
Phone: (613)258-0855 **Free:** 888-273-6746
Fax: (613)258-0899
Email: info@csdms.com
Website: http://www.csdms.com

Fnded: 1981. **Mem:** 1,700. **Lang(s):** English. **Desc:** Ultrasound professionals from all specialty areas of Diagnostic Medical Ultrasound, as well as technical representatives, physicians, educators, and students. Fosters excellence in patient care and professional interaction and promotes the highest level of professional standards of practice for sonographers in Canada.

★ 2083 ★ Canadian Society of Endocrinology and Metabolism (CSEM) (Societe canadienne d'endocrinologie et metabolisme — SCEM)
c/o Dr. Lenore Beitel
Lady Davis Institute
3755 Cote St. Catherine Rd.
Montreal, QC, Canada H3T 1E2
Phone: (514)340-8222 **Fax:** (514)340-7502
Email: lenore.beitel@mcgill.ca
Website: http://www.csem.mcgill.ca

Fnded: 1973. **Mem:** 280. **Lang(s):** English, French. **Desc:** Endocrinologists and other health care professionals with an interest in metabolism. Seeks to advance the study of metabolism and the practice of endocrinology; promotes ongoing professional development of members. Serves as a forum for the exchange of information among members; sponsors research and educational programs.

★ 2084 ★ Canadian Society of Gastroenterology Nurses and Associates (CSGNA)
27 Nicholson Dr.
Lakeside, NS, Canada B3T 1B3
Phone: (902)473-4006 **Fax:** (902)473-4406
Email: ednalang@hotmail.com
Website: http://www.csgna.com

Fnded: 1985. **Mem:** 510. **Reg. Groups:** 14. **Lang(s):** English, French. **Desc:** Gastroenterology nurses, medical technicians, and sales representatives of medical equipment and pharmaceutical manufacturers. Promotes excellence in the teaching and practice of gastroenterological nursing. Facilitates communication among members; produces patient education materials. Conducts continuing professional education programs; maintains speakers' bureau. **Pub:** *Guiding Light*, 3/year. Newsletter.

★ 2085 ★ Canadian Society of Hospital Pharmacists (CSHP) (Societe Canadienne des pharmaciens d'Hopitaux — SCPH)
1145 Hunt Club Rd., Ste. 350
Ottawa, ON, Canada K1V 0Y3
Phone: (613)736-9733 **Fax:** (613)736-5660
Email: lcarquez@cshp.ca
Website: http://www.cshp.ca

Fnded: 1947. **Mem:** 2,400. **State Groups:** 8. **Lang(s):** English, French. **Desc:** Hospital pharmacists, graduate pharmacists, and students. Promotes safe and effective drug therapy in organized health care settings. Provides leadership to members in institutional pharmacy practice. Evaluates and accredits postgraduate training programs in hospital pharmacy through the Canadian Hospital Pharmacy Residency Board. Enhances the visibility of hospital pharmacy in the health care field through public relations activities and meetings with government and health care associations. Promotes programs of continuing education; operates the CSHP Research and Educational Foundation. Maintains committees and task forces to recommend development of areas of interest and need to members; promotes funding and research programs. **Pub:** *Canadian Journal of Hospital Pharmacy*, bimonthly. Journal. • *Employment Opportunities Bulletin*, biweekly. Bulletin. • *Pharmascope*, bimonthly. Newsletter.

★ 2086 ★ Canadian Society for Immunology (CSI) (Societe Canadienne d'Immunologie — SCI)
795 McDermot Ave.
Winnipeg, MB, Canada R3E 0W3
Phone: (204)789-3316 **Fax:** (204)789-3921
Email: michael.ratcliffe@utoronto.ca
Website: http://www.csi.ucalgary.ca

Fnded: 1980. **Mem:** 300. **Lang(s):** English, French. **Desc:** Immunologists and other health care professionals and scientists with an interest in immunology. Seeks to advance immunological study, research, and practice. Promotes ongoing professional development of members. Serves as a network linking members; sponsors research and educational programs.

★ 2087 ★ Canadian Society of Internal Medicine (CSIM) (Societe canadienne de medecine interne — SCMI)
774 Echo Dr.
Ottawa, ON, Canada K1S 5N8

Phone: (613)730-6244 **Fax:** (613)730-1116
Email: csim@rcpsc.edu
Website: http://www.csim.medical.org

Fnded: 1984. **Mem:** 700. **Lang(s):** English, French. **Desc:** Represents the interests of general internists; promotes and provides leadership in the areas of clinical practice, education and research. **Pub:** *The General Internist*, 3/year. Newsletters.

★ 2088 ★ Canadian Society for International Health (SCIH) (Societe Canadienne de Sante Internationale — SCSI)

1 Nicholas St., Ste. 1105
Ottawa, ON, Canada K1N 7B7
Phone: (613)241-5785 **Fax:** (613)241-3845
Email: csih@csih.org
Website: http://www.csih.org

Fnded: 1977. **Mem:** 600. **Lang(s):** English, French. **Desc:** Health care services and individuals and organizations with an interest in global public health. Promotes increased availability and quality of health services in previously underserved areas worldwide. Advocates for health policy and programming that contributes to global objectives of health for all; equity, and social justice through partnership building with Canadian and other institutions and organizations. **Pub:** *Online Synergy*, weekly. Newsletter. • *PAHO News*, weekly.

★ 2089 ★ Canadian Society for Medical Laboratory Science

PO Box 2830 LCD 1
Hamilton, ON, Canada L8N 3N8
Phone: (905)528-8642 **Fax:** (905)528-4968
Email: toupitch@csmls.org
Website: http://www.csmls.org

Fnded: 1937. **Mem:** 14,000. **Lang(s):** English, French. **Desc:** Laboratory technologists in 20 countries. Seeks to maintain high standards of medical laboratory technology to insure effective and economical laboratory services. Promotes the interests of medical laboratory technologists. Emphasizes the importance of continuing education; sponsors courses. Communicates with government authorities concerning issues affecting members. Offers insurance program to members. Organizes national medical laboratory week annually. Bestows awards. **Pub:** *Annual Roster*. • *Canadian Journal of Medical Laboratory Science*, bimonthly. Journal. • *Catalogs of Continuing Education*. • *Guidelines for Laboratory Safety*. Manual.

★ 2090 ★ Canadian Society for Mucopolysaccharide and Related Diseases

PO Box 64714
Unionville, ON, Canada L3R 0M9
Phone: (905)479-8701 **Free:** 800-667-1846
Fax: (905)479-8701
Email: lori@mpssociety.ca
Website: http://www.mpssociety.ca

Fnded: 1984. **Lang(s):** English. **Desc:** Families whose children are affected with lysosomal storage diseases, and other interested individuals. Works to increase public awareness of lysosomal storage diseases. Raises funds for research; provides support for affected families. **Pub:** *The Connection*, quarterly. Newsletter.

★ 2091 ★ Canadian Society of Nuclear Medicine (CANM)

c/o Dr. Michael Chamberlain
Division of Nuclear Med.
Ottawa Hospital - Civic Site
1053 Carling Ave.
Ottawa, ON, Canada K1Y 4E9
Phone: (613)761-5265 **Fax:** (613)761-4041
Email: mchamberlain@civich.ottawa.on.ca
Website: http://www.csnm.medical.org/foundation_e.html

Lang(s): English, French. **Desc:** Physicians and other health care professionals with an interest in nuclear medicine. Seeks to advance the practice of nuclear medicine; promotes professional development of members. Sponsors research; conducts continuing professional education programs.

★ 2092 ★ Canadian Society for Nutritional Sciences (CSNS) (Societe Canadienne des Sciences de la Nutrition — SCSN)

c/o School of Dieticians and Human Nutrition
MacDonald Campus
McGill University
21111 Lakeshore
Ste.-Anne-de-Bellevue, QC, Canada H9X 3V9
Phone: (514)398-7547 **Fax:** (514)398-7739
Email: jonesp@macdonald.mcgill.ca

Lang(s): English, French. **Desc:** Dieticians and other scientists and health care professionals with an interest in nutrition. Seeks to advance the study and practice of the nutritional sciences. Serves as a forum for the exchange of information among members; sponsors research and educational programs.

★ 2093 ★ Canadian Society of Orthopaedic Technologists (CSOT) (Societe Canadienne des Technologistes en Orthopedie — SCTO)

18 Wynford Dr., No. 715A
North York, ON, Canada M3C 3S2
Phone: (416)445-4516
Email: csot@look.ca
Website: http://www.pappin.com/csot

Fnded: 1972. **Mem:** 325. **Reg. Groups:** 7. **Lang(s):** English. **Desc:** Individuals employed in the application of plaster casts and traction assemblies; associate members are persons working in related fields; industrial members are those engaged in the manufacture or sale of orthopedic equipment or supplies. Promotes and develops uniform training programs and examinations that contribute to the science of medicine. Facilitates cooperation between orthopedic technologists and the medical profession. **Pub:** *Body Cast*, quarterly. Journal. • *News Cast*, quarterly.

★ 2094 ★ Canadian Society of Otolaryngology - Head and Neck Surgery

221 Millford Cres.
Elora, ON, Canada N0B 1S0
Phone: (519)846-0630 **Free:** 800-655-9533
Fax: (519)846-9529
Email: cso.hns@sympatico.ca
Website: http://www.csohns.com

Fnded: 1947. **Mem:** 650. **Nat'l Groups:** 1. **Lang(s):** English, French. **Desc:** Professional society of practicing and retired otolaryngologists; otolaryngology residents join as associates. Provides for the discussion of professional issues. Arranges educational programs and competitions. **Pub:** *Canadian Journal of Otolaryngology*, bimonthly. • Brochure, annual. • Membership Directory, periodic. • Newsletter, semiannual.

★ 2095 ★ Canadian Society of Plastic Surgeons (CSPS)

30 St. Joseph Blvd. E, No. 917
Montreal, QC, Canada H2T 1G9
Phone: (514)843-5415 **Fax:** (514)843-7005
Email: csps_sccp@sympatico.ca
Website: http://www.plasticsurgery.ca

Fnded: 1947. **Mem:** 503. **Lang(s):** English, French. **Desc:** Plastic surgeons, medical educators, and students. Seeks to advance the study and practice of cosmetic surgery. Serves as a clearinghouse on plastic surgery. **Pub:** *CSPS News*, 3/year. Newsletter.

★ 2096 ★ Canadian Society for Psychomotor Learning and Sport Psychology (Societe Canadienne d'Apprentissage Psychomoteur et de Psychologie du Sport)

School of Human Kinetics
University of British Columbia
6081 University Blvd., Ste. 210
Vancouver, BC, Canada V6T 1Z1
Phone: (403)492-2187 **Fax:** (403)492-2364
Email: webmaster@scapps.org
Website: http://www.scapps.org

Lang(s): English, French. **Desc:** Health care professionals and other individuals with an interest in psychomotor learning and sports psychology. Seeks to advance the study and practice of sports psychology. Gathers and disseminates information; sponsors research and educational programs.

★ 2097 ★ Canadian Society of Respiratory Therapists (CSRT) (Societe Canadienne des Therapeutes Respiratoires — SCTR)

1785 Alta Vista Dr., Ste. 102
Ottawa, ON, Canada K1G 3Y6
Phone: (613)731-3164 **Free:** 800-267-3422
Fax: (613)521-4314
Email: info@csrt.com
Website: http://www.csrt.com

Fnded: 1964. **Mem:** 2,700. **Reg. Groups:** 8. **Lang(s):** English, French. **Desc:** Respiratory therapists. Seeks to advance the study and practice of respiratory therapy; promotes ongoing professional development of members. Facilitates exchange of information among members; sponsors training programs. **Pub:** *Canadian Journal of Respiratory Therapy*, 5/year. Journal. Contains research, clinical information, and association news.

★ 2098 ★ Canadian Sport Massage Therapists Association

1849 Yonge St., Ste. 814
Toronto, ON, Canada M4S 1Y2
Phone: (416)488-4414 **Fax:** (416)488-3079
Email: natoffice@csmta.ca
Website: http://www.csmta.ca

Fnded: 1987. **Mem:** 80. **Nat'l Groups:** 1. **Reg. Groups:** 4. **Desc:** Works to enhance the health care of Canadian athletes through the affective application of sport massage during all phases of athletic training, performance and competition. Promotes a professional climate for the growth of sport massage therapy in Canada. **Pub:** *CSMTA*, semiannual, spring and fall. Newsletter. Contains news, education and advertising.

★ 2099 ★ Canadian Thoracic Society (CTS) (Societe Canadienne de Thoracologie — SCT)

3 Raymond St., Ste. 300
Ottawa, ON, Canada K1R 1A3
Phone: (613)569-6411 **Fax:** (613)569-8860
Email: info@lung.ca
Website: http://www.lung.ca/cts

Fnded: 1958. **Mem:** 400. **Lang(s):** English, French. **Desc:** Physicians, PhD trained other health care professionals, and PhD trained scientists with an interest in respiratory health care and research. **Pub:** *Canadian Respiratory Journal*, 8/year. Journal. Peer-reviewed journal in respiratory medicine. • *Canadian Tuberculosis Standards, Cybersnewzzz Apnea Handbook*. Handbook.

★ 2100 ★ Canadian Urologic Oncology Group (CUOG)

c/o Dr. Fred Saad, Sec.-Treas.
1560, rue Sherbrooke E
Montreal, QC, Canada H2L 4M1
Phone: (514)890-8000 **Fax:** (514)412-7620
Email: fred.saad@ssss.gouv.qc.ca

Website: http://www.cuog.org/

Desc: Devoted to the medical specialty of urologic oncology; promotes clinical trials in uro-oncology.

★ 2101 ★ Canadian Urological Association (CUA) (Association Canadienne d'Urologie — ACU)

c/o Dr. Michael Leonard, Sec.
CHEO
401 Smyth
Ottawa, ON, Canada K1H 8L1
Phone: (613)738-3600 **Fax:** (613)738-4840
Email: cua@cua.org
Website: http://www.cua.org

Lang(s): English, French. **Desc:** Urologists, scientists, and other health care professionals with an interest in urology. Seeks to advance the study and practice of urology. Facilitates exchange of information among members; sponsors research and educational programs.

★ 2102 ★ Canadian Veterinary Medical Association (CVMA) (Association Canadienne des Medecins Veterinaires — ACMV)

339 Booth St.
Ottawa, ON, Canada K1R 7K1
Phone: (613)236-1162 **Fax:** (613)236-9681
Email: info@canadianveterinarians.net
Website: http://www.cvma-acmv.org

Fnded: 1948. **Mem:** 4,300. **Lang(s):** English, French. **Desc:** Veterinarians in Canada. Encourages excellence in the field of veterinary medicine; seeks to increase awareness of the importance of animals; represents the interests of members. **Pub:** *Canadian Journal of Veterinary Research*, quarterly. • *Canadian Veterinary Journal*, monthly. • *CVMA Directory*, annual.

★ 2103 ★ Canadian Women's Health Network (CWHN)

419 Graham Ave., Ste. 203
Winnipeg, MB, Canada R3C 0M3
Phone: (204)942-5500 **Free:** 888-818-9172
Fax: (204)989-2355
Email: cwhn@cwhn.ca
Website: http://www.cwhn.ca

Fnded: 1993. **Mem:** 70. **Desc:** Committed to sharing information, resources and strategies to better women's health; promotes women's involvement in health research. **Pub:** *Network*, quarterly. Magazine.

★ 2104 ★ Canadians for Health Research (CHR) (Canadiens pour la Recherche Medicale — CRM)

PO Box 126
Westmount, QC, Canada H3Z 2T1
Phone: (514)398-7478 **Fax:** (514)398-8361
Email: info@chrcrm.org
Website: http://www.chrcrm.org

Fnded: 1976. **Mem:** 400. **Lang(s):** English, French. **Desc:** Health care professionals and scientists with an interest in health research. Seeks to advance medical research; promotes continuing professional development of members. Serves as a forum for the exchange of information among members; sponsors research and educational programs. **Pub:** *Future Health/Perspectives Sante*, quarterly. Magazine. Contains Canadian health research news.

★ 2105 ★ Canadians for Safe and Sober Driving

PO Box 397
Post Sta. "A"
Brampton, ON, Canada L6V 2L3
Phone: (905)793-4233 **Fax:** (905)793-7035
Email: cssd@safeandsober.ca
Website: http://www.add.ca

Fnded: 1983. **Lang(s):** English, French. **Desc:** Seeks to promote public safety and eliminate deaths and injuries caused by impaired or drunk driving. Conducts educational programs to raise public awareness of the dangers of driving while intoxicated. **Frmly:** (2000) Against Drunk Driving.

★ 2106 ★ Cancer Association of South Africa

PO Box 2121
Bedfordview 2008, Republic of South Africa
Phone: 27 11 6167662 **Fax:** 27 11 6223424
Website: http://www.cansa.org.za

Fnded: 1931. **Desc:** Seeks to prevent and fight cancer and its consequences in partnership with all South African communities by providing direction for, and by supporting health promotion, patient service and research.

★ 2107 ★ Cancer Care (CC)

275 7th Ave.
New York, NY 10001-6708
Phone: (212)712-8400 **Free:** 800-813-4673
Fax: (212)712-8495
Email: info@cancercare.org
Website: http://www.cancercare.org/
Diane Blum, Exec. Dir.

Fnded: 1944. **Mem:** 80,000. **Local Groups:** 38. **Desc:** The oldest and largest national non-profit agency dedicated to providing emotional support, information and practical help to people with cancer, and their loved ones. Has assisted over two million people nationwide through telephone counseling, referral services, teleconference programs, office-based services, and via the internet. All services are provided free of charge and are available to people of all ages, with all types of cancer, at any stage of the disease. All services, including cancer awareness initiatives, extend also to family members, caregivers and professionals. **Pub:** *Cancer Care*. Annual Report. *Price:* Free. • *Currents*, quarterly. Newsletter. • Also publishes symposia proceedings, social research studies, professional papers, and brochures; distributes films and videotapes. **Frmly:** (1986) National Cancer Foundation; (1991) National Cancer Care Foundation.

★ 2108 ★ Cancer Control Society (CCS)

2043 N Berendo St.
Los Angeles, CA 90027
Phone: (323)663-7801
Email: cancercontrol@cox.net
Website: http://www.cancercontrolsociety.com
Norman Fritz, Pres.

Fnded: 1973. **Mem:** 5,500. **Desc:** Cancer patients, doctors, and interested individuals. Educates the public on the prevention and control of cancer and other diseases through nutrition, tests, and nontoxic alternative therapies, such as Laetrile, Gerson, Hoxsey, Koch, Enzymes, Wheat Grass, Immunology, Mega-Vitamins and Minerals, Detoxification and Nutrition, and DMSO and Chelation Therapy. Provides information through a 12-hour telephone hot line, direct mail, doctor and patient lists, speakers, films, cancer clinic tours, and Cancer Book House. **Pub:** *Cancer Book House List*, biennial. • *Cancer Control Journal*, periodic. Journal. Reports on one specific cancer-related topic in each issue. *Price:* Included in membership dues. • *Doctor and Clinic Directory*, 6/year. Directory. • *Patient Directory*, 6/year. Directory.

★ 2109 ★ Cancer Council Australia

GPO Box 4708
Sydney, NSW 2001, Australia
Phone: 61 2 90363100 **Fax:** 61 2 90363101
Email: info@cancer.org.au
Website: http://www.cancer.org.au

Fnded: 1999. **Frmly:** (2003) Australian Cancer Society.

★ 2110 ★ Cancer Federation (CFI)

PO Box 1298
Banning, CA 92220-0009
Phone: (909)849-4325 **Free:** 800-207-2873
Fax: (909)849-0156
Email: cancerfederation@yahoo.com
Website: http://www.cancerfed.com
Karen Alene, Admin.

Fnded: 1977. **Mem:** 1,500. **Desc:** Physicians, scientists, nurses, and laymen (both cancer patients and nonpatients). Promotes research and education in the field of cancer immunology. Seeks to discover appropriate cancer therapies using natural biological modifiers. Funds research at major centers throughout the U.S., including the University of California (Riverside and Santa Barbara), University of Hawaii, and University of Pittsburgh, on biological modifiers, such as lymphokines; killer cells; Interleukin I and II; diet; and psychological aspects of cancer. Compiles statistics; conducts research and education in cancer therapy, including vaccines, and in psychological programming for patients. Offers counseling program for cancer patients and their families. Sponsors public medical conferences and in-service courses for nurses on the psychology of cancer, and research projects at many universities and hospitals in the field of immunology. Sponsors charitable program. **Pub:** *Challenge of the Cancer Federation*, quarterly. Newsletter. Provides general information on cancer research and treatments. Contains information on federation activities and book reviews. *Price:* Included in membership dues. • Audiotapes. • Booklets. • Books. • Monographs. • Videos.

★ 2111 ★ Cancer Information Service (CIS)

c/o National Cancer Institute
STe. 3036 A, 6116 Exec. Blvd. MSC 8322
Bethesda, MD 20892-8322
Free: 800-4-CANCER
Website: http://cis.nci.nih.gov/
Mary Bright, Program Dir.

Fnded: 1975. **Reg. Groups:** 19. **Desc:** Funded by the National Cancer Institute. Trained counselors provide information about cancer causes, prevention, detection, diagnosis, rehabilitation, and research. Provides technical assistance to state and regional organizations conducting cancer education activities. Serves the entire United States, Puerto Rico, the U.S. Virgin Islands and the Pacific territories through a network of regional offices.

★ 2112 ★ Cancer Registry of Norway

Montebello
N-0310 Oslo, Norway
Phone: 47 22451300 **Fax:** 47 22451370
Email: kreftregisteret@kreftregisteret.no
Website: http://www.kreftregisteret.no

Lang(s): English, Norwegian. **Desc:** National cancer registries. Promotes availability of data on cancer patients; seeks to advance the prevention, diagnosis, and treatment of cancer. Serves as a clearinghouse on cancer and its treatment; sponsors health screenings and other services; conducts research. **Frmly:** (1999) Norweigan Cancer Registry.

★ 2113 ★ Cancer Research Foundation of America

1600 Duke St., Ste. 110
Alexandria, VA 22314
Phone: (703)836-4412 **Free:** 800-227-2732
Fax: (703)836-4413
Website: http://www.preventcancer.org

Fnded: 1985. **Desc:** Foundations, individuals and companies. Aims to prevent cancer through research and education. Sponsors grants and fellowships, publishes educational materials.

★ 2114 ★ Cancer Research Society (CRS)
(Societe de Recherche sur le Cancer — SRC)
402 - 625 Ave Du President-Kennedy
Montreal, QC, Canada H3A 3S5
Phone: (514)861-9227 **Free:** 888-766-2262
Fax: (514)861-9220
Email: info@cancerresearchsociety.ca
Website: http://www.cancer-research-society.ca

Fnded: 1946. **Lang(s):** English, French. **Desc:** Health care professionals and research scientists with an interest in cancer. Seeks to advance cancer research. Serves as a forum for the exchange of information among members; sponsors research and educational programs; provides financial support to cancer research and treatment institutions.

★ 2115 ★ Candlelighters Childhood Cancer Foundation (CCCF)
3910 Warner St.
Kensington, MD 20895
Phone: (301)962-3520 **Free:** 800-366-2223
Fax: (301)962-3521
Email: info@candlelighters.org
Website: http://www.candlelighters.org
Ruth Hoffman, Exec. Dir.

Fnded: 1970. **Mem:** 50,000. **Nat'l Groups:** 1. **Local Groups:** 400. **Desc:** Educates, supports, serves and advocates for children and adolescents with cancer, their family members, survivors of childhood cancer, and professionals who work with them. Coordinates a network of more than 400 peer support groups and contacts for parents of children/adolescents with cancer. Offers newsletters, other publications, literature and searches. Makes referrals to volunteers who can assist with health insurance problems, second opinions, and employment issues. Local groups offer meetings at which parents share information and emotional support and hear speakers. Referrals for parent-to-parent visitation, transportation, blood or wig banks, speakers' bureaus, meetings for young people, and bereavement groups. Named for the Chinese proverb, "It is better to light one candle than to curse the darkness." **Pub:** *Bone Marrow Transplant Guide.* Handbook. *Price:* $7.50; Free to families with children with cancer. • *CCCF Bibliography and Resource Guide*, annual. Bibliography. Annotated reviews of books, articles, pamphlets, and videos. *Price:* $5 in U.S.; $8 in Canada and Mexico; $12 all other countries; Free to families with children with cancer. • *CCCF Quarterly Newsletter*, quarterly. Newsletter. Articles, poetry, and reviews pertaining to living with and treating childhood cancer. *Price:* Free-families and health/education professionals. • *Educating the Child with Cancer.* Handbook. *Price:* $7.50; Free to families with children with cancer. • *Know before You Go, The Childhood Cancer Journey.* Handbook. • *The Phoenix*, periodic. Newsletter. For adult survivors of childhood cancer. • *You are not Alone, A Sourcebook for Support Groups for Families of Children with Cancer.* Handbook. • Also publishes basic family library, publications list, guide to the Americans with Disabilities Act, camp list, and wish fulfillment organizations list. **Frmly:** (1984) Candlelighters Foundation.

★ 2116 ★ Canine Companions for Independence (CCI)
PO Box 446
Santa Rosa, CA 95402-0446
Phone: (707)577-1700 **Free:** 800-572-2275
Fax: (707)577-1712
Email: info@caninecompanions.org
Website: http://www.caninecompanions.org/
Mr. Corey Hudson, Exec. Dir.

Fnded: 1975. **Nat'l Groups:** 1. **Reg. Groups:** 5. **State Groups:** 3. **Desc:** Provides to people with disabilities, specially-bred and trained dogs enabling them to lead more personally fulfilling and socially productive lives. Believes that human attendant care is reduced with the aid these dogs provide. Provides four types of Canine Companions: Hearing Dogs trained to alert the hearing-impaired to sounds such as the doorbell, smoke alarm, or a baby's cry; skilled companion dogs used for children and adults with disabilities, people with developmental disabilities, or anywhere the supervision of a third party is required; Service Dogs trained to provide physical assistance, such as retrieving dropped objects, operating elevator buttons and light switches, and pulling wheelchairs and Facility dogs placed with professionals in facilities where interaction with a dog will be beneficial to the mental or physical health of those in their care. Works to expand services to aid more persons with disabilities. Sponsors puppy raising programs where puppies are placed and raised in volumteer homes for 13 months; advanced training takes about 6-8 months to master over 60 required working commands. Conducts ongoing research in canine breeding, training, and nutrition. **Pub:** *Canine Companion Courier*, quarterly. Newsletter. *Price:* Free. • Annual Report. • Brochures. • Manuals.

★ 2117 ★ CAPCOM
PO Box 149
Mc Lean, VA 22101-0149
Phone: (703)749-1876 **Fax:** (703)544-8911
Email: signlanguagelesa@worldnet.att.net
Richard F. Rosen, PhD, Exec. Dir.

Fnded: 1982. **Desc:** Board of directors (3) comprising hearing impaired or physically handicapped individuals and senior citizens. Conducts research on the special needs of the hearing impaired, including senior citizens. Presents workshops on law and the deaf and on promoting productive working relationships for the hearing impaired employees of agencies and corporations. Maintains speakers' bureau and file of publications from organizations serving the deaf. Serves as a center for interpreter referrals. **Pub:** *CAPCOM Reports*, semiannual. **AKA:** Capital Communications Service for the Hearing-Impaired.

★ 2118 ★ Carcinoid Cancer Foundation
333 Mamaroneck Ave., No. 492
White Plains, NY 10605
Phone: (212)722-3132 **Free:** 888-722-3132
Fax: (914)683-5919
Email: mewarner@carcinoid.org
Website: http://www.carcinoid.org/
Monica Warner, Res. Coord.

Fnded: 1968. **Desc:** Promotes research and education on carcinoid tumors and related neuro-endocrine neoplasms. Provides general information for general public and health care professionals regarding special carcinoid-related events.

★ 2119 ★ Cardiac Arrhythmias Research and Education Foundation (CARE)
2082 Michelson Dr., No. 301
Irvine, CA 92612
Phone: (949)752-2273 **Free:** 800-404-9500
Fax: (949)752-9119
Email: care@longqt.org
Website: http://www.longqt.org/
Doris Goldman, National Dir.

Fnded: 1995. **Desc:** Dedicated to research and education about cardiac arrhythmias that cause sudden death. **AKA:** Care Foundation.

★ 2120 ★ Cardiac Society of Australia and New Zealand
145 Macquarie St
Sydney, NSW 2000, Australia
Phone: 61 2 92565452 **Fax:** 61 2 92477916
Email: csanz@racp.edu.au
Website: http://www.csanz.edu.au

Fnded: 1951. **Desc:** Promotes advancement of knowledge of the cardiovascular system, maintenance of professional and ethical standards; promotion of good fellowship among those in the practice of cardiovascular medicine or surgery, or in research in these or allied subjects. **Pub:** *On the Pulse.* Newsletter.

★ 2121 ★ Cardiovascular Credentialing International (CCI)
Thalia Landing Offices, Bldg. 2
4356 Bonney Rd., Ste. 103
Virginia Beach, VA 23452
Phone: (757)497-3380 **Free:** 800-326-0268
Fax: (757)497-3491
Email: ccij@widowmaker.com
Website: http://www.cci-online.org/
Randy Christian, Exec. Dir.

Fnded: 1988. **Mem:** 26,000. **Desc:** Cardiovascular technologists involved in the allied health professions. Conducts testing of allied health professionals throughout the U.S. and Canada. Provides study guides and reliability and validity testing. Compiles statistics. **Pub:** *Pulse*, quarterly. Newsletter. For Level II registered cardiovascular technologists. *Price:* Included in membership dues; $25/year for nonmembers. • Directory, biennial. **Frmly:** (1984) National Board for Cardiopulmonary Credentialing; (1986) National Board for Cardiovascular and Pulmonary Credentialing; (1991) Cardiovascular Credentialing International/Board of Cardiovascular Technology.

★ 2122 ★ Cardiovascular and Interventional Radiological Society of Europe (CIRSE)
Bellerivestr. 42
CH-8008 Zurich, Switzerland
Phone: 41 1 3849330 **Fax:** 41 1 3849339
Email: office@cirse.org
Website: http://www.cirse.org

Fnded: 1985. **Mem:** 1,350. **Lang(s):** English, French, German, Italian, Portuguese. **Desc:** Cardiologists, radiologists, and other health care personnel with an interest in cardiology and interventional radiology. Seeks to advance cardiological and radiological study, teaching, and practice. Sponsors continuing professional development courses for members; serves as a clearinghouse on cardiology and interventional radiology. **Pub:** *Cardio Vacular and Interventional Radiology.* Newsletter.

★ 2123 ★ Care Ministries
PO Box 1830
Starkville, MS 39760-1830
Phone: (662)323-4999 **Free:** 800-336-2232
Email: care@careministries.org
Website: http://www.careministries.org/
B.J. LeJeune, Dir.

Fnded: 1989. **Desc:** Provides information, spiritual support, community resources to blind and visually impaired. **Pub:** *Our Daily Bread*, monthly. Devotional and the Evangelical Sunday School Teachers Edition of lessons on cassette tape. • Catalog.Cassette catalog containing a variety of Christian materials, Bible studies and publications on cassette tape.

★ 2124 ★ Carers Association
Metropole Centre
James St.
Kilkenny, Kilkenny, Ireland
Website: http://www.carersireland.com

Fnded: 1987. **Mem:** 8,000. **Reg. Groups:** 42. **Desc:** Care-givers who provide high levels of care in their own homes for family members and neighbors. Provides home-based respite services. Disseminates information; conducts educational programs. **Pub:** Journal, quarterly.

★ 2125 ★ Carers Northern Ireland
11 Lower Crescent
Belfast BT7 1NR, United Kingdom
Phone: 44 28 90439843 **Fax:** 44 28 90329299
Email: info@carersni.org

Lang(s): English. **Desc:** Individuals and organizations involved in caring. Seeks to raise the awareness of the needs of carers. Works with all levels of government and society to inform, support and advise.

★ 2126 ★ Carers UK
Ruth Pitter House
20-25 Glass House Yard
London EC1A 4JS, United Kingdom
Phone: 44 207 4908818 **Fax:** 44 207 4908824
Email: info@ukcarers.org
Website: http://www.carersonline.org.uk

Fnded: 1988. **Mem:** 12,000. **Reg. Groups:** 120. **Desc:** Provides information and support to carers, persons who provide assistance and support to ill, disabled, or elderly individuals. Encourages carers to recognize and work towards meeting their own needs as caregivers through actively participating in social issues and legislative development that affects care givers and recipients. Offers training programs for professionals. **Pub:** *The Carer*, quarterly. Newsletter. • Brochures, bimonthly. **Frmly:** (2001) Carers National Association.

★ 2127 ★ CARF, The Rehabilitation Accreditation Commission (CARF)
4891 E Grant Rd.
Tucson, AZ 85712
Phone: (520)325-1044 **Fax:** (520)318-1129
Email: info@carf.org
Website: http://www.carf.org
Brian J. Boon, Pres.

Fnded: 1966. **Desc:** Sponsored by rehabilitation organizations. The commission is the standard setting and accrediting authority for organizations providing rehabilitation services. Encourages development and improvement of uniformly high standards of performance for all organizations serving individuals with developmental, physical, or emotional disabilities. Surveys and accredits rehabilitation organizations; conducts research and educational activities related to standards for organizations offering programs in comprehensive inpatient rehabilitation, spinal cord injury, chronic pain management, brain injury, outpatient medical rehabilitation, work hardening, infant and early childhood development, vocational evaluation, work adjustment, occupational skill training, job placement, work services, supported employment, industry-based programs, community living, psychosocial programs, respite programs, alcoholism and other drug abuse rehabilitation programs, and community mental health programs. Accreditation Program is administered by a 53-member appointed board of trustees. **Pub:** *CARF Connection*, semiannual. Covers commission activities. *Price:* Free. • *Standards Manual for Employment Community Services*, annual. Describes accreditation standards for programs providing services to the disabled; includes glossary. *Price:* $90/year. **Frmly:** (1998) Commission on Accreditation of Rehabilitation.

★ 2128 ★ Caribbean Family Planning Affiliation (CFPA)
PO Box 3386
Saint Johns, Antigua-Barbuda
Phone: (268)462-4170 **Fax:** (268)462-4171
Email: kadax@candw.ag

Fnded: 1971. **Mem:** 18. **Lang(s):** English. **Desc:** Family planning associations in Caribbean countries. Works to increase awareness and acceptance of family planning in the region. Advocates family planning as a basic human right and assists member governments in incorporating family planning into maternal and child health care services. Develops training programs for adolescents and young mothers. Studies demographic, sociological, and health issues. Offers training to teachers, family planning workers, and clinicians. Produces and distributes audiovisual educational materials. Compiles statistics. Offers research programs; sponsors competitive. Operates Documentation Centre for students, teachers, and researchers. Offers educational programs.

★ 2129 ★ Carroll Center for the Blind (CCB)
770 Centre St.
Newton, MA 02458
Phone: (617)969-6200 **Free:** 800-852-3131
Fax: (617)969-6204
Email: intake@carroll.org
Website: http://www.carroll.org
Rachel Ethier Rosenbaum, Pres.

Fnded: 1936. **Desc:** Rehabilitation center that specializes in services for adults ages 16 and up who have become blind. Provides programs for resident and commuter clients. Offers diagnostic evaluation, personal adjustment training, low vision, and children's services. Trains professionals in work with the blind through supervision of student internships and seminars for workers in the field. Maintains information and referral service. Offers computer training in specialized access devices for blind and job training. Operates charitable program. Manages statewide materials center of books in braille and large print, books for ages Kindergarten through 12th grade. **Pub:** *Blindness: What It Is, What It Does, and How to Live With It. Price:* $15. • *Carroll Center for the Blind–Focus*, semiannual. Newsletter. Covers membership activities. Includes information for donors and new program information. *Price:* Free. • *Computer Access, Resource Manual. Price:* $20. • *Educational Software, Compiled Listing. Price:* $5. • *Facing the Wind. Price:* $25. • *Mapping. Price:* $15. • *Medical Transcription Training Manual. Price:* 125. • *Resource Manual for Teaching Blind Persons to Use Computers*, annual. *Price:* $20/year; $10 for tape. • *Selected Exercises in Sensory Training. Price:* $15. • *Sensory Training, Principles of. Price:* $15. • *Videation and Spatial Orientation, Vols. I & II. Price:* $50. **Frmly:** (1972) Catholic Guild for All the Blind; (1974) Carroll Rehabilitation Center for the Visually Impaired.

★ 2130 ★ Case Management Society of America (CMSA)
8201 Cantrell Rd., Ste. 230
Little Rock, AR 72227
Phone: (501)225-2229 **Fax:** (501)221-9068
Email: cmsa@cmsa.org
Website: http://www.cmsa.org
Anne Llewellyn, Pres.

Fnded: 1990. **Mem:** 7,500. **State Groups:** 1. **Local Groups:** 72. **Desc:** Case management and allied healthcare professionals. Offers members a voice in the future through opportunities for professional leadership and networking opportunities, case management legislative impact and visibility, publications, educational workshops, seminars, conferences, recognition and fellowship opportunities. **Pub:** *The Case Manager*, bimonthly. Journal. • *Case Report*, bimonthly. Newsletter. Published in The Case Manager, CMSA's official journal. • *Standards of Practice.* • Brochure, annual. • Membership Directory, annual.

★ 2131 ★ Catholic Association of Persons With Visual Impairment (CAPVI)
c/o Msgr. Paul M. Lackner
111 Perrymont Ave.
Pittsburgh, PA 15237
Phone: (412)687-1409 **Fax:** (412)826-8377
Msgr. Paul Lackner, Pres.

Fnded: 1984. **Mem:** 150. **Desc:** To assist, support, and further the vocational, spiritual, and social integration of blind and visually impaired persons in local parishes and in the community. CAPVI focuses on: raising awareness of the ability and spiritual needs, promotes active participation in the spiritual and social life of the church and within the community; exchanges ideas, resources and other pertinent information, assists in obtaining religious material in accessible format; and works toward establishing programs within dioceses to serve this group. activities; instructs volunteers to act as guides. Assists in obtaining audiotapes and religious materials printed in Braille and large type. large type. A national CAPVI office is open in New York City. **Pub:** *CAPVI Newsletter*, quarterly. Newsletter. Contains information regarding visually impaired persons active in the life of the church. Printed in large type, cassettes and Braille upon request. *Price:* Free.

★ 2132 ★ Catholic Health Association of Canada
1247 Kilborn Pl.
Ottawa, ON, Canada K1H 6K9
Phone: (613)731-7148 **Fax:** (613)731-7797
Email: chac@web.ca
Website: http://www.chac.ca

Fnded: 1939. **Lang(s):** English, French. **Desc:** Works to administer Christian principles within the Canadian healthcare system. Fosters competent and efficient health care services. Disseminates health information. **Pub:** *CHAC Review*, 3/year. Journal. Contains in-depth articles.

★ 2133 ★ Catholic Health Association of the United States (CHA)
4455 Woodson Rd.
Saint Louis, MO 63134-3797
Phone: (314)427-2500 **Fax:** (314)427-0029
Email: webmaster@chausa.org
Website: http://www.chausa.org
Rev. Michael D. Place, Pres. & CEO

Fnded: 1915. **Mem:** 2,000. **Desc:** Supports and strengthens the Catholic health ministry in the U.S. by uniting members to advance selected strategic ministry issues addressed, rather than as individual organizations. **Pub:** *Catholic Health World*, biweekly, except Jan. and Aug.Newspaper. Reports on the health care ministry. Includes *Catholic Health Association Assembly. Price:* Included in membership dues; $35/year for nonmembers. • *Catholic Long-Term Care Facilities and Services Online Directory*, periodic. Directory. Online directory that details current list of facilities and services for long term care needs. • *Health Progress*, bimonthly. Journal. Addresses the administrative, ethical, financial, legal, and political problems faced by Catholic health care administrators. *Price:* Included in membership dues; $50/year for nonmembers. **Frmly:** Catholic Hospital Association of U.S. and Canada; (1979) Catholic Hospital Association.

★ 2134 ★ Catholic Medical Association (CMA)
2020 Pennsylvania Ave. NW, Ste. 864
Washington, DC 20006
Free: 877-228-4362 **Fax:** (703)830-1308
Email: adelong02@aol.com
Website: http://www.cathmed.org
Michael J. Herzog, Exec. Dir.

Fnded: 1932. **Mem:** 3,500. **Local Groups:** 90. **Desc:** Catholic physicians and dentists dedicated to upholding the principles of the Catholic faith in the practice of medicine. **Pub:** *The Linacre Quarterly*, quarterly. Journal. Bioethics journal. **Frmly:** (1998) National Federation of Catholic Physicians Guilds.

★ 2135 ★ CAVDA-Citizens AIDS Project (CAP)
Ste. 128
800 W Central Rd.
Mount Prospect, IL 60056
Phone: (847)398-3378 **Fax:** (847)398-7309
Email: cavdarx@earthlink.net
Howard A. Mirsky, Dir.

Fnded: 1986. **Mem:** 125. **Desc:** A project of the Citizens Alliance for VD Awareness. Physicians, pharmacists, nurses, health professionals, and interested others. Seeks to provide information and educational programs to professionals and the public in order to dispel myths associated with sexually transmitted diseases and Acquired Immune Deficiency Syndrome. Conducts research programs and disseminates information and surveys through media and group presentations. Compiles statistics; maintains speakers' bureau. **Pub:** *STD Spotlight*, quarterly. Newsletter. *Price:* $30/year. • Pamphlets.

★ 2136 ★ CCHS Family Network
71 Maple St.
Oneonta, NY 13820
Phone: (607)432-8872 **Fax:** (607)431-4351
Email: vanderlaanm@hartwick.edu

Website: http://www.cchsnetwork.org
Mary Vanderlaan, Founder/Dir.

Fnded: 1990. **Mem:** 300. **Desc:** Seeks to provide support to families with a CCHS child. Supports CCHS research; shares information on ventilation methods and technologies and home care issues; collects data on CCHS. **Pub:** *CCHS Family Newsletter*, 3/year. Newsletter. Shares news on research/technology development and family stories. **Frmly:** (1998) CCHS Family Network.

★ 2137 ★ CDC National Prevention Information Network (NPIN)

PO Box 6003
Rockville, MD 20849-6003
Phone: 800-458-5231 **Free:** 800-243-7012
Fax: (301)562-1050
Email: info@cdcnpin.org
Website: http://www.cdcnpin.org
Jesse Milan, Jr., Project Dir.

Fnded: 1987. **Desc:** A service of the Centers for Disease Control and Prevention. Collects, analyzes, and disseminates information on HIV/AIDS, STDs, and TB primarily for healthcare professionals, educators, social service workers, attorneys, employers and human resource professionals, state HIV/AIDS programs, community organizations, and service associations. Responds to the information needs of health professionals. Offers referral service, and Business and Labor Resource Service (BLRS). **Pub:** *List of Materials*, quarterly. Booklet. • Brochures. **Frmly:** (1991) National AIDS Information Clearinghouse; (1992) National AIDS Clearinghouse.

★ 2138 ★ Celiac Disease Foundation (CDF)

13251 Ventura Blvd., Ste. 1
Studio City, CA 91604-1838
Phone: (818)990-2354 **Fax:** (818)990-2379
Email: cdf@celiac.org
Website: http://www.celiac.org
Elaine Monarch, Exec. Dir.

Fnded: 1990. **Desc:** Provides services and support for persons with Celiac Disease/Dermatitis Herpetiformis (CD/DH) through programs of education advocacy, and research; telephone information and referral services; medical advisory board; and special educational seminars and general meetings. (CD is a digestive disorder found in genetically susceptible individuals, in which the surface of the small intestine is damaged by the ingestion of food products containing proteins commonly known as gluten. Toxic glutens are found in all forms of wheat, rye, barley, and possibly oats.) **Pub:** *Celiac Disease Foundation Newsletter*, quarterly. Newsletter. Includes information about the disease, treatment, nutrition, food and drug updates, support articles, and recipes. *Price:* Included in membership dues.

★ 2139 ★ Celiac Sprue Association/ United States of America (CSA/USA)

PO Box 31700
Omaha, NE 68131-0700
Phone: (402)558-0600 **Fax:** (402)558-1347
Email: celiacs@csaceliacs.org
Website: http://www.csaceliacs.org
Mary Schluckebier, Exec. Dir.

Fnded: 1986. **Mem:** 9,143. **Nat'l Groups:** 1. **Reg. Groups:** 6. **State Groups:** 6. **Local Groups:** 93. **Desc:** Individuals with the conditions of celiac sprue and dermatitis herpetiformis; parents of celiac children. (Celiac sprue is a genetic disorder resulting in digestive malabsorption of the protein portion of wheat, rye, and other cereal grains, causing symptoms such as intestinal lesions, diarrhea, vomiting, weight loss, and abdominal discomfort; dermatitis herpetiformis is a gluten-related skin disorder. Successful treatment usually calls for removing all gluten-containing cereal grains and their derivatives from the diet.) Serves as a vehicle for the provision of mutual support groups and facilitates interaction with other organizations involved in digestive disorders. Encourages and supports research on celiac disease. Disseminates educational materials on gluten-free foods and research on results; exchanges information on maintaining a gluten-free diet. **Pub:** *Cookbooks for Diets Free of Cereal Grains*. Books. • *Lifeline*, quarterly. Newsletter. • *On the Celiac Condition: A Handbook for Celiacs and Their Families, 2nd Ed.*. Handbook. • Brochures. • Pamphlets. **Frmly:** (1979) Midwestern Celiac Sprue Association.

★ 2140 ★ Center for Advocacy for the Rights and Interests of the Elderly (CARIE)

100 N 17th St., Ste. 600
Philadelphia, PA 19103
Phone: (215)545-5728 **Free:** 800-356-3606
Fax: (215)545-5372
Email: duncan@carie.org
Website: http://www.carie.org/
Jill Duncan, Dir. of Fin. & Admin.

Fnded: 1977. **Desc:** Dedicated to improving the quality of life for vulnerable older people. Maintains speaker's bureau. **Pub:** Brochures. • Newsletter, periodic.

★ 2141 ★ Center for Applications of Psychological Type (CAPT)

2815 NW 13th St., Ste. 401
Gainesville, FL 32609
Phone: (352)375-0160 **Free:** 800-777-2278
Fax: (352)378-0503
Email: info@capt.org
Website: http://www.capt.org
Elizabeth Styron, Pres.

Fnded: 1975. **Desc:** Works to disseminate information on Isabel Briggs Myers' works and encourage practical applications of Carl G. Jung's (1875-1961) theory of psychological types; seeks to foster understanding and constructive use of personality differences. Primary focus is on the theory of psychological types utilizing the Myers-Briggs Type Indicator (for young people and adults, created by Myers and her mother, Katharine Briggs) and the Murphy-Meisgeier Type Indicator For Children to identify Jungian types. (Jung's theory states that seemingly random variations in behavior are actually consistent and orderly if one understands differences in the ways people process information and make decisions.) Conducts introductory and advanced training through workshops, consultation, and other training sessions for psychologists in the areas of counseling, education, religion, organizations, and research; offers continuing education courses. Sponsors research and offers research consultation; provides computer scoring of MBTI forms to professionally qualified users. Provides consultation on the applications of the MBTI and on-site development of MBTI skills of qualified personnel. Operates the Isabel Briggs Myers Memorial Library containing MBTI- and Jungian-related material. Distributes teaching aids, question booklets, answer sheets, scoring keys, and computer software for MBTI analyses. Sponsors exhibits on professional conferences. Works closely with Association for Psychological Type. **Pub:** *Atlas of Type Tables*. • *Bibliography of the MBTI*, semiannual. Bibliography. • Books. • Reports. • Also publishes papers, training exercises, and other materials.

★ 2142 ★ Center for Attitudinal Healing (CAH)

33 Buchanan Dr.
Sausalito, CA 94965
Phone: (415)331-6161 **Fax:** (415)331-4545
Email: home123@aol.com
Website: http://www.healingcenter.org
Don Goewey, Exec. Dir.

Fnded: 1975. **Mem:** 12,000. **Desc:** Nonsectarian organization established to supplement traditional health care by offering free services in attitudinal healing for both children and adults with life-threatening illnesses, loss, or other crises. (The concept of attitudinal healing is based on the belief that it is possible to choose peace rather than conflict, and love rather than fear; the center defines health as inner peace and healing as the process of letting go of fear.) Offers support groups and arranges home and hospital visits for children, youth, and adults. Offers volunteer training program. Maintains speakers' bureau; conducts educational programs and charitable activities. **Pub:** *Advice to Doctors and Other Big People*. Book. • *Another Look at the Rainbow*. Book. • *Rainbow Connection*, 3/year. Newsletter. • *There is a Rainbow Behind Every Dark Cloud*. Book.

★ 2143 ★ Center for Biologics Evaluation and Research (CBER)

Food & Drug Administration
1401 Rockville Pike
Rockville, MD 20852-1448
Phone: (301)827-1800 **Free:** 800-835-4709
Fax: (301)827-0440
Email: octma@cber.fda.gov
Website: http://www.fda.gov/cber/about.htm
Kathryn C. Zoon, PhD, Dir.

Desc: Advances public health through innovated regulations that ensure safety, effectiveness, timely delivery to patients of biological products including blood, vaccines, tissue, allergenics, biological therapeutics.

★ 2144 ★ Center for Craniofacial Development and Disorders (CCDD)

Childrens Medical & Surgical Center, Rm. 1004
The Johns Hopkins Hospital
600 N Wolfe St.
Baltimore, MD 21287-3914
Phone: (410)614-9245 **Fax:** (410)955-0484
Email: ccdd@lists.jhmi.edu
Website: http://www.hopkinsmedicine.org/craniofacial/
Ethylin Wang, MD, Dir.

Desc: Seeks to increase understanding of normal and abnormal craniofacial development, including cleft lip and palate, craniosynostosis, Apert and Crouzon syndromes. **Pub:** Brochure.

★ 2145 ★ Center for Health Design

3478 Buskirk Ave., Ste. 1000
Pleasant Hill, CA 94523
Phone: (925)746-7188 **Fax:** (925)746-7101
Email: admin@healthdesign.org
Website: http://www.healthdesign.org/
Debra J. Levin, Exec. VP

Fnded: 1988. **Desc:** Works to create a future where healthcare environments enhance healing and promote well-being for patients, staff, and visitors through research, design, architecture. Conducts fundraisers. **Pub:** Reports.

★ 2146 ★ Center for Health and the Global Environment

Harvard Medical School
333 Longwood Ave., Ste. 640
Boston, MA 02115
Phone: (617)432-0493 **Fax:** (617)432-2595
Email: chge@hms.harvard.edu
Website: http://www.med.harvard.edu/chge/the-center.html

Fnded: 1996. **Desc:** Promotes human health consequences of global environmental change. **Pub:** *Biodiversity: Its Importance to Human Health*. Report. • *Biological & Physical Signs of Climate Change: Focus on Mosquito-Borne Diseases*. Report. • *Climate Change & U.S. Agriculture: The Impacts of Warming & Extreme Weather Events on Productivity, Plant Diseases, & Pests*. Report. • *Environment & Health: Species Loss & Ecosystem Disruption - the Implications for Human Health*. Report. • *Is Global Warming Harmful to Health?*. Report. • *Marine Ecosystems: Emerging Diseases as Indicators of Change*. Report. • *Oil: A Life Cycle Analysis of its Health & Environmental Impacts*. Report. • *The Quarterly Review*. Contains the latest findings in the field of human health and global environment.

★ 2147 ★ Center on Human Policy (CHP)
Syracuse University
School of Education
805 S Crouse Ave.
Syracuse, NY 13244-2280
Phone: (315)443-3851 **Free:** 800-894-0826
Fax: (315)443-4338
Email: thechp@sued.syr.edu
Website: http://soeweb.syr.edu/thechp
Steven Taylor, PhD, Dir.

Fnded: 1971. **Desc:** Consumers and students; parents of persons with disabilities; human services administrators and staff members; professionals in psychology, special education, rehabilitation, sociology, law, social work, and planning. Goal is to promote the inclusion of persons with severe disabilities into the mainstream of society. Disseminates information to families, human services professionals, and others on laws, regulations, and programs affecting children and adults with disabilities, focusing on those with developmental disabilities. Provides speakers to professional gatherings and parents' groups. Documents outstanding community living and educational programs and assists in creating exemplary services. Evaluates public policies to determine their impact on people with disabilities. Participates in public forums, legislative hearings, national conventions, and other community events involving issues relating to people with disabilities. Operates National Resource Center on Supported Living and Choice for people with developmental disabilities. Offers technical assistance, consultation, and training on service system issues to local, regional, state, and national organizations and agencies. Conducts research related to community inclusion.

★ 2148 ★ Center for Humane Options in Childbirth Experiences (CHOICE)
3474 N High St.
Columbus, OH 43214
Phone: (614)263-2229 **Fax:** (614)449-0140
Email: shortstork@aol.com
Website: http://choicemidwives.org
Abby Kinne, Dir.

Fnded: 1977. **Mem:** 1,200. **Local Groups:** 1. **Desc:** Medical professionals, paraprofessionals, and interested individuals. Purpose is to teach and encourage parents, parents-to-be, groups, and interested individuals working in family-oriented childbirth in hospital birth centers and out-of-hospital situations. Trains and certifies attendants to attend or coach births. Acts as consumer advocate for hospital births. Services include medical referrals, childbirth education classes, and supplementary prenatal care. Sponsors community educational programs; operates speakers' bureau; compiles statistics.

★ 2149 ★ Center for Medical Consumers (CMC)
130 MacDougal St.
New York, NY 10012-5030
Phone: (212)674-7105 **Fax:** (212)674-7100
Email: medconsumers@earthlink.net
Website: http://www.medicalconsumers.org
Arthur Aaron Levin, Dir.

Fnded: 1976. **Desc:** Advocacy group on health and medical information at the state and local legislative level. **Pub:** *HealthFacts*, monthly. Newsletter. Helps consumers determine the risks and effectiveness of common medical procedures. Presents all treatment options, including nonmedical. *Price:* $25/year. • Reports. **Frmly:** (1998) Center for Medical Consumers and Health Care Information.

★ 2150 ★ Center for Medicare Advocacy
PO Box 350
Willimantic, CT 06226
Phone: (860)456-7790 **Free:** 800-262-4414
Website: http://www.medicareadvocacy.org/
Judith Stein, Exec. Dir.

Fnded: 1986. **Desc:** Provides education, advocacy, legal assistance to help elders and people with disabilities obtain necessary healthcare.

★ 2151 ★ Center for Organ Recovery and Education (CORE)
204 Sigma Dr.
Ridc Park
Pittsburgh, PA 15238
Free: 800-366-6777 **Fax:** (412)963-3563
Email: pkornick@core.org
Website: http://www.core.org
Pat Kornick, VP, Corporate Development

Fnded: 1977. **Desc:** Manages organ, tissue and eye donation activities. Offers families the opportunity to donate; coordinates the surgical recovery of the organs, tissue and eyes, and facilitates the computerized matching of donating organs and placement of corneas. Maintains permanent tribute to donors. Sponsors continuing education programs for health professionals in regional hospitals and associations. Also provides speakers for presentation to civic organizations and schools or corporations. **Pub:** *The CORE-nection*, quarterly. Newsletter. • Pamphlets. • Also publishes protocols. **Frmly:** (1984) Transplant Organ Procurement Organization; (1992) Pittsburgh Transplant Foundation.

★ 2152 ★ Center Perzent
PO Box 27
Karakalpakstan
12 Nukus 742012, Uzbekistan
Phone: 998 61 2223417 **Fax:** 998 61 2222794
Email: perzent@online.ru

Fnded: 1992. **Mem:** 1,000. **Lang(s):** English, Uzbekistani. **Desc:** Environment and health professionals. Seeks to research the impact of environmental degradation on reproductive health; encourages improvement of the status of women and children in the Aral Sea region of the former Soviet Union. Conducts environmental mitigation programs around the Aral Sea, which has suffered a collapse due to overuse as a source of water for agricultural irrigation; seeks to raise public awareness of public health issues arising from the demise of the Aral Sea. **Pub:** *Perzent*, monthly. Bulletin.

★ 2153 ★ Center for Professional Well-Being (CWBHP)
21 W Colony Pl., Ste. 150
Durham, NC 27705
Phone: (919)489-9167 **Fax:** (919)419-0011
Email: cpwb@mindspring.com
Website: http://www.cpwb.org
Margaret Seeman, Program Dir. /Office Mgr.

Fnded: 1979. **Mem:** 800. **Nat'l Groups:** 1. **Reg. Groups:** 1. **Desc:** Society serving health and other professional associations. Promotes the well-being of health professionals and their families through: preventive education on manifestations of disabilities; increased awareness about the stresses inherent in the system of providing health services; efforts to improve and maintain effectiveness. Conducts research and supports efforts to study the incidence and causes of professional impairment, with prevention as a goal. Maintains speakers' bureau; provides individual consulting and counseling. Offers workshops on The Joy of Medicine, Physician Burnout, and Preventive Malpractice Strategies; sponsors retreats, seminars, and lectures. **Pub:** *Being Well: Bulletin of the Society for Professional Well-Being*, quarterly. Bulletin. *Price:* Included in membership dues; $55. • Booklets. • Monographs. • Videos. **Frmly:** (1993) Center for the Well-Being of Health Professionals.

★ 2154 ★ Center for Psychological and Spiritual Health (CPSH)
1782 Church St.
San Francisco, CA 94103
Phone: (415)575-6299
Email: cpsh@ciis.org
Website: http://www.senatciis.org/
Christina Grot, Founder

Fnded: 1980. **Mem:** 10,000. **Desc:** Seeks to develop an expanded model of mental health care to help people in crisis by using scientific and spiritual assistance. Operates an information and referral service. Offers educational programs. Maintains speakers' bureau. **Pub:** *Spiritual Emergence Network Newsletter*, 2-3/year. Newsletter. • *Spiritual Emergency*. Book. • Brochure. **Frmly:** (2003) Spiritual Emergence Network.

★ 2155 ★ Center for Reproductive and Family Health
63, Ln. 35, Cat Linh St.
Dong Da
Hanoi, Vietnam
Phone: 84 4 8234288 **Fax:** 84 4 8234288
Email: rafh@hn.vnn.vn
Website: http://www.rafh-vie.org

Fnded: 1993. **Mem:** 12. **Nat'l Groups:** 1. **Reg. Groups:** 2. **Local Groups:** 1. **Lang(s):** English, French, Vietnamese. **Desc:** Promotes availability of family planning and reproductive health services throughout Vietnam, and particularly in rural areas. Does both research and intervention on reproductive health, disadvantaged women, and children. Increases awareness and knowledge of community people on gender equality, sexuality, and reproductive rights. Provides assistance to rural development programs operating in Vietnam; works to integrate population control and family planning activities into development programs. **Pub:** *Midwife*. Booklet. • *Reproductive Health*, quarterly. Magazine. • *Women's health Rain Drops - STDs Prevention What's cannot poured out*, annual. Video. Also publishes leaflets and posters. **Frmly:** (2001) Center for Reproductive Health and Family Health.

★ 2156 ★ Center for Research in Ambulatory Health Care Administration (CRAHCA)
104 Inverness Ter. E
Englewood, CO 80112-5306
Phone: (303)397-7897 **Fax:** (303)397-1827
Email: gtn@mgma.com
Website: http://www.mgma.com
Glenn T. Hammons, MD, VP

Fnded: 1973. **Desc:** Seeks to advance the art and science of medical group practice management to improve the health of our communtities. Vision is to be the source of excellence and innovation as the leading association in providing quality and timely services and resources for medical practice management and leadership. Develops and advances research-based knowledge in the field of ambulatory health care by improving education, management technology, publications, and database services. Research is directed toward health care economics, policy development and analysis, alternative organizational models for health care delivery, evaluation methodologies, models of provider team leadership, and the social aspects of health services organizations and the communities in which they serve. Research interests include provider reimbursement and the analysis of ambulatory health care and medical practice costs. The evolution and impact of integrated and managed care systems and the role of access and quality in the production and management of ambulatory care services will be examined. The impact of these areas on health system reform will be studied. **Pub:** *Actuarial Issues in the Fee-for-Service/Prepaid Medical Group*. Book. *Price:* $32/copy. • *Case Management in Primary Care*. Manual. *Price:* $24/copy. • *Geriatric Collaborative Care Model*. Book. *Price:* $17/copy. • *Getting Started in Geriatrics*. Handbook. *Price:* $29/copy. • *Health Information Management Medical Record Processes in Group Practice*. Book. *Price:* $39/copy. • *Integrated Health Care*. Book. *Price:* $44/copy. • *Making Integrated Care Work*. Book. *Price:* $49/copy. • *Medical Group Practice Chart of Accounts*. Book. *Price:* $49/copy. • *Performance Efficiency Evaluation*, annual. Report. *Price:* $695/year. • *Prepare for Eldercare*. Handbook. *Price:* $14/copy. • *Quality Improvement*. Book. *Price:* $39/copy. **AKA:** CRAHCA.

★ 2157 ★ The Center for Social Gerontology (TCSG)
2307 Shelby Ave.
Ann Arbor, MI 48103
Phone: (734)665-1126 **Fax:** (734)665-2071
Email: tcsg@tcsg.org
Website: http://www.tcsg.org
Clifford Douglas, Pres.

Fnded: 1971. **Desc:** Purpose is to advance the well-being of older people in the U.S. through research, education, technical assistance, and training. Focuses primarily on legal rights, guardianship and alternative protective services, delivery of legal services, and issues of tobacco and older persons. Provides consulting services. Develops and researches standards for the provision of guardianship services for older people; works to improve the court processes for determining the need for guardianship through development and evaluation of a new model. Conducts periodic training on Legal rights and Legal resources, for legal advocates, nonlawyers who work with the elderly, and older consumers. **Pub:** *Adult Guardianship Mediation.* Manuals. • *Adult Guardianship Mediation: An Introduction.* Videos. • *Best-Practice Notes on Delivery of Legal Services to Older Persons*, quarterly. Bulletin. • *Comprehensive Guide to Delivery of Legal Assistance to Older Persons.* • *Guidelines for Planning and Evaluating Legal Assistance Programs Funded Under the Older Americans Act.* • Audiotapes. • Reports. • Adult Guardianship Mediation Manual, Guardianship & Alternatives: A Guide to Personal, Health Care & Financial Management Options, and National Study of Guardianship Systems: Findings & recommendations. **Frmly:** (1985) International Center for Social Gerontology.

★ 2158 ★ Center for Sports and Osteopathic Medicine (CDM)
c/o Dr. Richard Bachrach
317 Madison Ave.
New York, NY 10017
Phone: (212)685-8113 **Fax:** (212)697-4541
Email: richardbachrach@bonesdoctor.com
Website: http://www.bonesdoctor.com/
Richard M. Bachrach, Pres.

Fnded: 1978. **Desc:** Educates dancers about their bodies and preventive medicine in order to help them avoid injuries. Activities are currently concentrated in New York City area. **Frmly:** (1997) CTR for Dance Medicine.

★ 2159 ★ Center for the Study of Aging of Albany (CSA)
706 Madison Ave.
Albany, NY 12208
Phone: (518)465-6927 **Fax:** (518)462-1339
Email: apaas@aol.com
Website: http://www.rit.edu/~pjr0120/csa/iapaas/main.html
Norm Thompson, Dir. Office of Mgmt.

Fnded: 1957. **Desc:** Participants include behavioral scientists, educators, gerontologists, physicians, and other health professionals. Promotes education, research, and training; provides leadership in the field of health and fitness for older people. Includes: programs for volunteers and professionals in aging, gerontology, geriatrics, wellness, physical fitness, and mental health; consultant services include adult day care, nutrition, physical and mental fitness, nursing home, housing, and retirement; speakers' bureau. Develops national and international conferences on health, fitness, and prevention. Provides expert assistance in research, institutional and community program development, planning, and organization; offers consultation addressing the development of library resource centers and collections of books on aging. Conducts seminars and offers information and referral services. **Pub:** *Classics in Aging.* Book. • *Environment and Aging.* Book. • *Physical Activity, Aging and Sports - Volume I: Scientific and Medical Research.* • *Physical Activity, Aging and Sports - Volume II: Practice, Program, and Policy.* • *Physical Activity Aging and Sports - Volume III: International Perspectives Toward Healthy Aging, Part I Physiological and Biomedical Aspects.* • *Physical Activity, Aging and Sports - Volume IV: Toward Healthy Aging, Part 2 Psychology, Motivation and Programs.* • *Safe Therapeutic Exercise for the Frail Elderly: An Introduction.* Manual. • *Senior Citizen School Volunteer Program: A Manual for Program Implementation.* • *Series: Life Long Health and Fitness-Volume I-Prevention and Human Aguiy*, annual. Bibliographies. Covers health and fitness. • *Who? Me!? Exercise: Safe Exercise for Over Fifty.* 48 pp. exercises illustrations. • Books. **AKA:** International Association of Physical Activity.

★ 2160 ★ Center for Study of Multiple Birth (CSMB)
333 E Superior St., Ste. 464
Chicago, IL 60611
Phone: (312)908-7532 **Fax:** (312)908-8500
Email: lgk395@nwu.edu
Website: http://www.multiplebirth.com
Louis Keith, MD, Pres.

Fnded: 1977. **Desc:** Medical research foundation concerned with the study of multiple birth and the care of multiple birth children. Disseminates information on the medical risks of multiple birth. Encourages funding for the support of medical and social research. Serves as resource center for the media and the public through informative website. **Frmly:** (1981) Center for Study of Multiple Gestation.

★ 2161 ★ Center for Studying Health System Change (HSC)
600 Maryland Ave. SW, No. 550
Washington, DC 20024
Phone: (202)484-5261 **Fax:** (202)484-9258
Email: hscinfo@hschange.org
Website: http://www.hschange.com/
Paul B. Ginsburg, Pres.

Desc: Works to inform health care decision makers about changes in health care system at local and national levels, and effects of such changes on people. **Pub:** *Issue briefs.* • Reports.Community and tracking reports.

★ 2162 ★ Center for Substance Abuse Prevention (CSAP)
c/o Training System Technical Assistance to Communities Project
1010 Wayne Ave., Ste. 850
Silver Spring, MD 20910
Phone: (301)459-1591 **Fax:** (301)495-2919
Email: dbanks@prevline.health.org
Website: http://www.covesoft.com/csap.html

Desc: Works to disseminate information, increase dialog, and promote community empowerment to combat alcohol and other drug problems. Maintains speakers bureau.

★ 2163 ★ Center for Veterinary Medicine (CVM)
c/o Food & Drug Administration
Communications Staff
7519 Standish Pl., HFV-12
Rockville, MD 20855
Phone: (301)827-3800
Email: cvmhomep@cvm.fda.gov
Website: http://www.fda.gov/cvm/aboutcvm/aboutcvm.html

Desc: Regulates manufacture and distribution of food additives and drugs given to animals, including animals used for human foods, food additives, drugs for pets. **Pub:** *The Green Book*, annual. Book. *Price:* $85 first copy; $60 additional copies to same name and address; $105 first copy outside U.S.; $60 additional copies to same name and address outside U.S.

★ 2164 ★ Center for the Well Being of Health Professionals
21 W Colony Pl., Ste. 150
Durham, NC 27705-5589
Phone: (919)489-9167 **Fax:** (919)419-0011
Email: cpwb@mindspring.com
Website: http://www.cpwb.org
John-Henry Pfifferling, PhD, Founder & Dir.

Desc: Offers presentations on all areas relevant to professional well-being. Works to find a balance between personal and professional lives.

★ 2165 ★ Center for Workers with Disabilities
c/o APHSA
810 1st St., Ste. 500
Washington, DC 20002
Phone: (202)682-0100 **Fax:** (202)682-3706
Email: mcheek@aphsa.org
Website: http://www.nasmd.org/disabilities/

Fnded: 2001. **Desc:** Aids participating states to implement provisions of "Ticket to Work and Work Incentives Improvement Act of 1999".

★ 2166 ★ Centra-Cam Vocational Training Association (CCVTA)
PO Box 1443
Camrose, AB, Canada T4V 1X4
Phone: (780)672-9995 **Fax:** (780)672-0534
Email: cctva@centracam.ca

Fnded: 1979. **Mem:** 25. **Lang(s):** English, French. **Desc:** Individuals with an interest in the vocational training of adults with disabilities. Seeks to improve the quality of life of people with disabilities; encourages employers to hire qualified people with disabilities. Assists in the integration of adults with disabilities into society; sponsors training programs for people providing vocational education to individuals with disabilities.

★ 2167 ★ Central Africa Diabetes Association (Association des Diabetiques en Centrafrique)
BP 2726
Bangui, Central African Republic
Phone: 236 618626 **Fax:** 236 610137
Website: http://www.diabetesafrica.com/idfmembers.html

State Groups: des Di. **Local Groups:** rique. **Desc:** Represents people with diabetes. Promotes research and support of those with diabetes in Central African Republic.

★ 2168 ★ Central American Health Institute (ICAS)
PO Box 6-2010
Zapote
San Jose, Costa Rica
Phone: 506 221 5278 **Fax:** 506 258 3943
Email: costarica@icas.net
Website: http://www.icas.net

Fnded: 1993. **Mem:** 25. **Reg. Groups:** 3. **Lang(s):** English, Spanish. **Desc:** Promotes improvement to the health of the population of Central America.

★ 2169 ★ Central Institute of Medical Medicinal and Aromatic Plants (CIMAP)
c/o Dr. Ashok Sharma, Coord.
Kukrail Picnic Spot Rd.
PO Box CIMAP
Lucknow 226 015, Uttar Pradesh, India
Phone: 91 522 2357133 **Fax:** 91 522 344159
Email: ashoksharma@cimap.org

Desc: Promotes research and development in the field of medicinal and aromatic plants, especially the biopreservation of medicinal and aromatic plants; conservation and molecular documentation of genetic diversity in medicinal and aromatic plants; screening of phytochemicals for biological activity; conservation, genetics, breeding and genetic engineering, characterization and employment of genetic resources of medicinal and aromatic plants of economic value. **Pub:** *Bioprospection of Medicinal Plants - Vol. I.* Book. Contains information covering 54 medicinal plants.

★ 2170 ★ Centre for African Family Studies (CAFS) (Centre d'Etudes de la Famille Africaine — CEFA)

Pamstech House
Woodvale Grove
Westlands
PO Box 60054
Nairobi, Kenya
Phone: 254 20 4448618 **Fax:** 254 20 4448621
Email: info@cafs.org
Website: http://www.cafs.org

Fnded: 1975. **Lang(s):** English, French. **Desc:** Dedicated to strengthening the capacities of organizations and individuals working in the field of reproductive health and population and development in order to contribute to improving the quality of life of families in sub-Saharan Africa. Provides training, technical assistance and research in reproductive health and population and development. **Pub:** *CAFS Information Brochure*, annual. Brochure. • *CAFS News*, semiannual. Newsletter. Includes family planning issues. • *Programme of Activities*, annual. • *Research Reports*, periodic. Reports. • Annual Report.

★ 2171 ★ Centre for Arctic Medicine

c/o University of Oulu/Thule Institute
PO Box 5000
90014 University of Oulu
FIN-90220 Oulu 22, Finland
Phone: 358 8 5376200 **Fax:** 358 8 5376203
Email: juhani.hassi@oulu.fi
Website: http://arctichealth.oulu.fi

Fnded: 1969. **Lang(s):** English, Finnish, Swedish. **Desc:** Promotes research into arctic medicine; encourages cooperation among researchers. Disseminates reports and other information to persons engaged in arctic medicine. **Pub:** *International Journal of Circumpolar Health*, quarterly. Journal. • Monographs. • Proceedings. **Frmly:** Nordic Council for Artic Medical Research; Institute of Arctic Medicine.

★ 2172 ★ Centre for Deaf Studies

8 Woodland Rd.
Bristol BS8 1TN, United Kingdom
Phone: 44 117 9546900 **Fax:** 44 117 9546921
Email: coursesecretary-cds@bris.ac.uk
Website: http://www.bris.ac.uk/deaf/

Fnded: 1978.

★ 2173 ★ Centre for Development and Population Activities - Egypt (CEDPA)

53 Manial St., Ste. 500
Manial El Rodah
Cairo 11451, Egypt
Phone: 20 2 3654565 **Fax:** 20 2 3654568
Email: cedpaegypt@cedpa.org.eg
Website: http://www.cedpa.org

Fnded: 1975. **Lang(s):** Arabic, English. **Desc:** Seeks to enhance the managerial and technical capabilities of family planning, health, and development professionals. Conducts reproductive health programs focusing on the need of women and youth. Facilitates creation of primary health care services in rural and developing areas; makes available financial assistance to local health and development initiatives. Sponsors training programs for health and development personnel.

★ 2174 ★ Centre for Development and Population Activities - Nigeria (CEDPAN)

18 A&B Temple Rd.
Off Kingsway Rd.
Ikoyi, Lagos, Nigeria
Phone: 234 1 2600020 **Fax:** 234 1 2600022
Email: cedpa_nigeria@usips.org
Website: http://www.cedpa.org/aboutus/field_offices.html

Fnded: 1996. **Local Groups:** 34. **Lang(s):** English. **Desc:** National branch of the international organization. Seeks to improve the technical and managerial capacities of indigenous planning, health, and development professionals. Promotes empowerment of women. Provides training and technical assistance to development, reproductive health, family planning, and environmental protection programs. Conducts educational programs to raise public awareness of population, reproductive health, and development issues. **Pub:** *CEDPA News*, quarterly. Contains articles of interest on activities and events. • *Small Doctors.* Booklet. • *Women on the Move*, periodic. Journal. • *Women Politicians on the Move.* Produces videotapes.

★ 2175 ★ Centre for Health Education, Training and Nutrition Awareness (CHETNA)

Lilavatiben Laibhai's Bungalow
Civil Camp Rd.
Shahibaug
Ahmedabad 380 004, Gujarat, India
Phone: 91 79 2866695 **Fax:** 91 79 2866513
Email: chetna@iccnet.net.in
Website: http://indianngos.com/chetna/

Fnded: 1980. **Lang(s):** English, Gujarati, Hindi. **Desc:** Promotes development of regional health programs with a feminist perspective. Works to expand understanding of women's health beyond matters of maternal and child health; examines gender relations as they impact on women's health; develops local health care capabilities through encouragement of appropriate traditional treatments; trains women to manage local and regional health care programs. Main program areas include: early childhood care and development; school health; adolescent health; women's health and development; promotion of traditional health practices; and gender and development. Activities include: training; documentation of innovative efforts; creating educational material, and networking and advocacy. **Pub:** *CHETNA News*, quarterly. Newsletter. Contain current activity profiles. • *List of Material.* Directory. • Manual. Also publishes manuals, posters, and charts.

★ 2176 ★ Centre for Indian Medical Heritage (CIMH)

Ayurbedic Trust Campus
Trichy Rd.
PO Box 7102
Ramanathapuram
Coimbatore 641 045, Tamil Nadu, India
Phone: 91 422 2311095 **Fax:** 91 422 314953
Email: cimh@sify.com

Fnded: 1985. **Mem:** 1,214. **Lang(s):** English, Hindi. **Desc:** Village healers, midwives, folk practitioners, and other individuals interested in traditional healing methods. Seeks to revitalize folk traditions in areas including: childcare, nutrition, and home remedies for common ailments. Encourages the integration of folk medicine and organized health care systems in India. Cultivates medicinal gardens, forests, and nurseries. Fosters communication among members; gathers and disseminates information. **Pub:** *CIMH Newsletter*, quarterly. Newsletter.

★ 2177 ★ Centre Muraz

01 Boite Postale 153
Bobo-Dioulasso 01, Burkina Faso
Phone: 226 970102 **Fax:** 226 970457
Email: direction.muraz@fasonet.bf
Website: http://www.multimania.com/centremuraz

Lang(s): English, French. **Desc:** Medical researchers and health care professionals. Promotes improved diagnostic techniques and treatments of common diseases. Conducts research and educational programs; makes available health services.

★ 2178 ★ Centre for Policy on Ageing (CPA)

19-23 Ironmonger Row
London EC1V 3QP, United Kingdom
Phone: 44 207 5536500 **Fax:** 44 207 5536501
Email: cpa@cpa.org.uk
Website: http://www.cpa.org.uk

Fnded: 1947. **Mem:** 90. **Lang(s):** English. **Desc:** Health care professionals; social workers; academics. Promotes policies in England which will result in higher standards of care and a better lifestyle for the elderly. Encourages informed debate about issues affecting older people and stimulates public awarenesss of their needs. Conducts studies and makes recommendations to policy makers. Maintains CPA Information Service which keeps readers abreast of trends in policy, practice, and research development. Areas of interest include residential care policy, educational and recreational activities for the elderly, and elderly people in ethnic minorities. Strives to address the needs of housebound and vulnerable elderly people and integrate all older people into the community. Currently investigating possible methods of providing for homeless elderly people. **Pub:** *Age Info CD-ROM.* CD-Rom which provides information from 3 different databases, covering all aspects of aging. • *Aging and Society*, quarterly. • *CPA Papers*, periodic. • *CPA Report*, periodic. • *New Literature on Old Age*, bimonthly. • *Old Age: A Register of Social Research*, periodic. • *Policy Studies in Ageing*, periodic.

★ 2179 ★ Centre for Women's Health

6 Sandyford Pl.
Sauchiehall St.
Glasgow G3 7NB, United Kingdom
Phone: 44 141 2116700 **Fax:** 44 141 2116702
Email: cwh@glacomen.scot.nhs.uk
Website: http://www.sandyford.org

Fnded: 1994. **Desc:** Seeks to promote women's health. Offers counseling services and groups for women. Provides a training center and meeting place. Conducts studies on the quality of existing women's health services. Disseminates information and provides an extensive information an library service and links to health service and local authority prevision.

★ 2180 ★ Cerebral Palsy International Sports and Recreation Association (CP-ISRA)

Postbus 16
NL-6666 ZG Heteren, Netherlands
Phone: 31 26 4722593 **Fax:** 31 26 4723914
Email: cpisra_nl@hotmail.com
Website: http://www.cpisra.org

Fnded: 1978. **Mem:** 60. **Lang(s):** English. **Desc:** Organizations in 60 countries interested in sports and recreation for the cerebral palsied. Provides greater opportunities for the cerebral palsied to participate in a wide variety of sports and recreational activities. Assists members in developing sports and recreation programs through demonstrations, courses, films, and seminars; provides means for communication and dissemination of information among members. **Pub:** *Classification and Sport Rules Manual.* Manual. • *Classification Video.* Video. • *News*, semiannual. Newsletter.

★ 2181 ★ Certification Board for Music Therapists (CBMT)

506 E Lancaster Ave., Ste. 102
Downingtown, PA 19335
Phone: (610)269-8900 **Free:** 800-765-CBMT
Email: info@cbmt.com
Website: http://www.cbmt.com
Joy S. Schneck, Exec. Dir.

Fnded: 1982. **Mem:** 3,330. **Desc:** Board-certified professional music therapists. Certifies and recertifies (every 5 years) professional music therapists through examination and continuing professional education. Monitors competence and professional growth of certificants. **Pub:** *BC-Status*, semiannual. Newsletter. Includes list of new members and updates on recertification process. *Price:* Free for members. • *Candidate Handbook.* Handbook. • *Recertification Manual.* Manual. • *Recertification, Self-Growth, and You.*

★ 2182 ★ Certification Board Perioperative Nursing (CBPN)
c/o Shannon Carter
2170 S Parker Rd., Ste. 295
Denver, CO 80231
Phone: (303)369-9566 **Free:** 888-257-2667
Fax: (303)695-8464
Email: webmaster@certboard.org
Website: http://www.certboard.org
Shannon S. Carter, Exec. Dir.

Fnded: 1979. **Mem:** 30,000. **Desc:** Works to promote surgical services registered nurses. Offers certification programs for nurses practicing in the operating room and assist in surgeries. **Frmly:** (2001) National Certification Board Perioperative Nursing.

★ 2183 ★ Certification Board for Urologic Nurses and Associates
East Holly Ave., Box 56
Pitman, NJ 08071-0056
Phone: (856)256-2351 **Fax:** (856)589-7463
Email: cbuna@ajj.com
Website: http://www.suna.org
Karen Graf, Pres.

Fnded: 1972. **Mem:** 500. **Desc:** Conducts certification exam for urological professionals. **Frmly:** American Board of Urologic Allied Health Professionals.

★ 2184 ★ Certifying Board of Gastroenterology Nurses and Associates (CBGNA)
3525 Ellicott Mills Dr., Ste. N
Ellicott City, MD 21043-4547
Phone: (410)418-4808 **Free:** 800-245-SGNA
Fax: (410)418-4805
Email: info@cbgna.org
Website: http://www.cbgna.org
Nancy Bellas, RN, Pres.

Desc: Maintains and improves the knowledge, understanding and skill of nurses in the fields of gastroenterology and gastroenterology endoscopy; administers certification program.

★ 2185 ★ Cervical Spine Research Society (CSRS)
c/o Peggy Wlezien
6300 N River Rd., Ste. 727
Rosemont, IL 60018-4226
Phone: (847)698-1628 **Fax:** (847)823-0536
Email: wlezien@aaos.org
Website: http://www.csrs.org/
Peggy Wlezien, Mgr.

Fnded: 1973. **Desc:** Promotes the exchange and development of ideas and philosophy regarding the diagnosis and treatment of cervical spine injury and disease.

★ 2186 ★ CFIDS Association of America
PO Box 220398
Charlotte, NC 28222-0398
Free: 800-442-3437 **Fax:** (704)365-9755
Email: cfids@cfids.org
Website: http://www.cfids.org
Jon Sterling, Chm.

Fnded: 1986. **Mem:** 23,000. **Desc:** Individuals with chronic fatigue and immune dysfunction syndrome (chronic viral illness associated with dysfunction of the immune system; formerly called chronic Epstein-Barr virus); doctors, nurses, and government officials. Advocates continued research into the cause and cure of the syndrome. Funds pilot medical research projects. **Pub:** *The CFIDS Chronicle*, quarterly. Journal. Contains research and medical articles, advocacy efforts reports, practical tips on living with CFIDS and book and media reviews. *Price:* Included in membership dues. • *Research Review*, semiannual. • Also publishes patient guide and other educational materials. **Frmly:** (1994) CFIDS Association.

★ 2187 ★ Chad Association for the Fight against Diabetes (Association Tchadienne de lutte contre le Diabete)
BP 703
N'Djamena, Chad
Phone: 235 534008
Email: cssiitsn@intnet.td
Website: http://www.diabetesafrica.com/idfmembers.html

State Groups: Tchadi. **Local Groups:** le Di. **Desc:** Represents people with diabetes. Promotes research and support of those with diabetes in Chad.

★ 2188 ★ Challenge Aspen at Snowmass
PO Box M
Aspen, CO 81612-9119
Phone: (970)923-0578 **Fax:** (970)923-7338
Email: possibilities@challengeaspen.com
Website: http://www.challengeaspen.com
Sarah Williams, Prog. Dir.

Fnded: 1995. **Desc:** Persons with a physical or mental disability. Assists in appreciating outdoor recreation. Operates on the "can-do" theory for people. Provides volunteer guides to help enjoy the outdoors by skiing, skating, hiking, fishing, horseback riding, swimming, and biking. Designs and conducts training courses for activity leaders in downhill skiing. **Frmly:** (2000) Blind Outdoor Leisure Development; (2000) BOLD/Challenge Aspen.

★ 2189 ★ Challenge International
1204 Ina Ln.
Mc Lean, VA 22102-1704
Phone: (703)821-3385 **Fax:** (703)790-1791
Email: mndoremus@msn.com
Mary Nemec Doremus, Pres. & Exec. Dir.

Fnded: 1983. **Desc:** A media awareness campaign designed to make disability a familiar and comfortable issue by closing the communication gap between the public and the disabled community. Purposes are to: serve the disabled community by changing the way in which Americans perceive disability and disabled individuals; promote positive images of disabled persons in the media through newspaper articles, radio and television news reports, television shows, motion pictures, and advertisements; educate the public about disability issues; serve as clearinghouse on the needs of the disabled and the organizations that represent them; assist the media so that they report realistically and positively on disability and disabled persons; encourage the acceptance of people with disabilities, thus enabling them to become more productive, contributing members of society. Other activities include: providing internships for qualified disabled persons to pursue careers in media-related fields; establishing a speakers' bureau; designing school programs and educational materials. **Frmly:** (1985) National Challenge Committee of the Disabled; (1988) National Challenge Committee on Disability.

★ 2190 ★ Challenged Conquistadors
c/o Shaun Best
Rt2 Box 32
Hampton, AR 71744
Phone: (870)798-4558
Email: shaun_best_2000@yahoo.com
Website: http://www.SpeakersQuest.com/speakers/Best.htm
Shaun Best, Pres. & Founder

Fnded: 1993. **Mem:** 10,000. **Local Groups:** 1. **Desc:** Works to increase self preservation, reduce dependency, and eradicate negative stereotypes, myths, and stigmas. Targets active, positive, challenged role models to show others that success is obtainable. Reinforces individual empowerment and capabilities to reveal the talents inherent in all challenged individuals and reap rewards as opposed to the "stagnation and destruction that many social programs have achieved." Offers educational and research programs.

★ 2191 ★ Charcot-Marie-Tooth Association (CMTA)
2700 Chestnut St.
Chester, PA 19013-4867
Phone: (610)499-9264 **Free:** 800-606-CMTA
Fax: (610)499-9267
Email: cmtassoc@aol.com
Website: http://www.charcot-marie-tooth.org/site/content
Ann L. Beyer, Chair

Fnded: 1983. **Mem:** 14,000. **Nat'l Groups:** 1. **Reg. Groups:** 25. **Desc:** Charcot-Marie-Tooth patients and their families, medical professionals treating the disorder, and interested individuals. (Charcot-Marie-Tooth Disease, also known as peroneal muscular atrophy or hereditary motor sensory neuropathy, is a progressive neurological disorder beginning in childhood or adult life with weakness and muscle wasting in feet, legs, hands, and arms.) Works to inform and educate patients and their families, the medical community, and the public about medical treatment for CMT. Offers support groups for patients and their families; disseminates educational materials; encourages and funds research; sponsors lay and professional symposia. Makes available videotapes; maintains speakers' bureau. **Pub:** *A Physician's Guide to CMT Disorder*. Handbook. *Price:* $20. • *Charcot-Marie-Tooth Disorders*. Pamphlets. • *CMT Facts I*, periodic. Booklets. *Price:* $3. • *CMT-Facts II*, periodic. Booklets. *Price:* $5. • *CMT Facts III*, periodic. Booklets. Containing articles on CMT topics, research news, patient profiles, and meeting and program announcements. *Price:* $5 with membership. • *CMT-Facts IV*, periodic. Booklets. *Price:* $8. • *CMTA Report*, bimonthly. Newsletter. Containing articles on CMT topics, research news, patient profiles, and meeting and program announcements. *Price:* With membership. **Frmly:** (1990) National Foundation for Peroneal Muscular Atrophy.

★ 2192 ★ Chartered Institute of Environmental Health
Chadwick Court
15 Hatfields
London SE1 8DJ, United Kingdom
Phone: 44 207 9286006 **Fax:** 44 207 8275866
Email: information@cieh.org
Website: http://www.cieh.org

Fnded: 1883. **Mem:** 9,800. **Nat'l Groups:** 1. **Reg. Groups:** 15. **State Groups:** 2. **Local Groups:** 54. **Lang(s):** English, French, German. **Desc:** The majority of its members are employed by local government to enforce a wide range of legislation on issues such as food safety, pollution, housing standards, safety at work and to educate the public on matters of hygiene and safety. An increasing number of its members are working in the commercial sector either for individual companies or as private environmental health consultants. Responsible for the training and professional development of over 8000 environmental health officers. Its primary objective is the promotion of environmental health and the dissemination of knowledge about environmental health issues. The CIEH represents the views of its members on environmental and public health issues and is independent of central and local government. **Pub:** *Environmental Health*, monthly. Journal. • *Environmental Health News*, weekly. • *Food Forum*, quarterly. • *Health and Housing Insight*, quarterly. • *Pollution Control Bulletin*, quarterly. Bulletin. **Frmly:** Institution of Environmental Health Offices.

★ 2193 ★ Chartered Society of Physiotherapy (CSP)
14 Bedford Row
London WC1R 4ED, United Kingdom
Phone: 44 207 3066666 **Fax:** 44 207 3066611
Email: csp@csp.org.uk
Website: http://www.csp.org.uk

Fnded: 1894. **Mem:** 40,000. **Desc:** The professional association, educational body and trade union of the United Kingdom's 39,000 chartered psychotherapists, physical students and assistants. Aims to protect member's interests and help them to achieve the best possible patient care. **Pub:** *Frontline*, bimonthly. • *Physiotherapy Journal*, monthly. Journal.

★ 2194 ★ Chemotherapy Foundation (CF)
183 Madison Ave., Rm. 403
New York, NY 10016
Phone: (212)213-9292 **Fax:** (212)213-3831
Email: scox@chemotherapyfoundation.org
Shirley Cox, Exec. Dir.

Fnded: 1968. **Mem:** 3,500. **Desc:** Supports laboratory and clinical research for the control, cure, and prevention of cancer through innovative medical therapies; conducts professional symposia to enable oncologists to incorporate advances in cancer treatment into the care of their patients; distributes free educational literature. Grant allocations currently include five major metropolitan medical centers. **Pub:** *The Breast Cancer Epidemic in the United States - How 15,000 More Lives Can Be Saved Each Year.* Booklet. Provides educational information for patients and the public; updated as necessary. *Price:* Free. • *Chemotherapy - Your Weapon Against Cancer.* Booklet. Contains educational material for patients and the public. *Price:* Free. • *Major Research Achievements of the Chemotherapy Foundation Grant Programs 1968-2002.* Booklet. *Price:* Free. • *Souvenir Journal*, annual. Book. Updates status of chemotherapy, foundation activities, and studies being conducted by its research recipients. • *Symposium Abstracts*, annual, For medical oncologists.Booklet. *Price:* $15 per copy. • *What Every Man Should Know About Prostate Cancer.* Booklet. Contains educational material for patients and the public. *Price:* Free. • *What Every Woman and Her Doctor Should Discuss About Ovarian Cancer.* Booklet. Contains educational material for patients and the public. *Price:* Free. • Newsletter, semiannual. Includes research reports and membership activities.

★ 2195 ★ CHERUBS - Association of Congenital Diaphragmatic Hernia Research (CDH)
c/o Dawn M. Torrence
1109 Williamsboro St.
Oxford, NC 27565
Phone: (919)693-8158 **Free:** (866)603-1944
Fax: (707)924-1114
Email: info@cherubs-cdh.org
Website: http://www.cherubs-cdh.org/
Dawn M. Torrence, Pres.

Mem: 650. **Nat'l Groups:** 27. **State Groups:** 50. **Desc:** Parents, grandparents, foster parents, pediatric surgeons, genetic counselors, pediatricians, nurses, ECMO directors, respiratory therapists, and epidemiologists. Dedicated to helping families of children born with Congenital Diaphragmatic Hernia (CDH); promotes research into possible causes and better treatments.

★ 2196 ★ Cheshire Foundation in Ireland (CFI)
1-4 Adelaide Rd.
Glasthule, Dublin, Ireland
Phone: 353 1 2804879 **Fax:** 353 1 2804954
Email: info@cheshire-foundation.ie
Website: http://www.cheshire-foundation.ie

Lang(s): English, Irish. **Desc:** Individuals and organizations. Seeks to improve the quality of life of people with disabilities. Provides housing and support and services to people with disabilities and their families.

★ 2197 ★ Chi Delta Mu
PO Box 1
River Edge, NJ 07661-0001
Phone: (202)842-1111 **Free:** 800-484-7593
Fax: (202)842-0222
Email: mollynj@hotmail.com
Website: http://www.geocities.com/westhollywood/heights/7396/
Tracy M. Walton, Jr., Sec.

Fnded: 1913. **Mem:** 650. **State Groups:** 7. **Desc:** To improve relationships among physicians, dentists, and pharmacists so that they may better serve their respective communities. Maintains revolving loan funds. **Pub:** *Chi Delta Mu News*, quarterly. Newsletter. • *Dragon*, annual. Magazine. • Proceedings, annual.

★ 2198 ★ Chi Eta Phi Sorority
3029 13th St. NW
Washington, DC 20009
Phone: (202)232-3858 **Fax:** (202)232-3460
Email: chietaphi@erols.com
Website: http://www.chietaphi.com
Carolyn Mosley, Pres.

Fnded: 1932. **Mem:** 8,000. **Desc:** Professional sorority - registered and student nurses. Objectives are to: encourage continuing education; stimulate friendship among members; develop working relationships with other professional groups for the improvement and delivery of health care services. Sponsors leadership training seminars every two years and holds additional seminars at the local, regional, and national levels. Offers educational programs for entrance into nursing and allied health fields. Maintains health screening and consumer health education programs; volunteers assistance to senior citizens; sponsors recruitment and retention programs for minority students in nursing. Operates speakers' bureau on health education. **Pub:** *Chi Line*, semiannual. Newsletter. Includes membership activities. *Price:* available to members only. • *The Directory*, biennial. Directory. • *Glowing Lamp - Journal of Chi Eta Phi Sorority*, annual. Journal. *Price:* $15. • *History of Chi Eta Phi Sorority, Inc.* • *Mary Eliza Mahoney, America's First Black Professional Nurse.*

★ 2199 ★ Child Aid
2902 SW Fairmount Blvd.
Portland, OR 97201
Phone: (503)223-3008 **Free:** 888-881-8241
Fax: (503)223-3008
Email: childaid@attbi.com
Website: http://www.child-aid.org
Richard Carroll, Exec. Dir.

Fnded: 1988. **Desc:** Individuals who volunteer to aid hearing impaired children in Mexico and Guatemala. Promotes increased access to audiological aids and services among Mexican, Guatemalan, and Turkish children. Provides audiological and educational services to indigent children with impaired hearing; provides funds and assistance to organizations pursuing similar goals; conducts fundraising programs; recruits and trains volunteers. Supports literacy, education and health programs in Latin America. **Frmly:** (2001) SoundAid.

★ 2200 ★ Child Care Action Campaign (CCAC)
330 7th Ave., 17th Fl.
New York, NY 10001
Phone: (212)239-0138 **Fax:** (212)268-6515
Email: info@childcareaction.org
Website: http://www.childcareaction.org
Elinor Guggenheimer, Founder

Fnded: 1983. **Mem:** 3,500. **Desc:** Individuals and organizations interested and active in child care; corporations and financial institutions; labor organizations; editors of leading magazines; leaders in government and representatives of civic organizations. Purposes are to alert the country to the problems of and need for child care services; prepare and disseminate information responsive to inquiries resulting from publicity; analyze existing services and identify gaps; work directly with communities to stimulate the development of local task forces and long-range plans for improved and coordinated services. Promotes development of language skills in child care settings. Has worked to help make liability insurance available for child care providers. **Pub:** *An Employer's Guide to Child Care Consultants.* Focuses on the reasons for using a child care consultant, services that consultants can offer, and how to choose the child care consultant for you. *Price:* $10 for members; $15 for nonmembers. • *Building Links: Developer Initiatives for Financing Child Care.* Covers financing alternatives for child care and examines the ways in which communities have begun to involve real estate developers in child care. *Price:* $15 for members; $25 for nonmembers. • *Child Care ActioNews*, bimonthly. Newsletter. Covers innovations in the field of child care for working parents. Includes calendar of events, legislative update, and resource information. *Price:* Included in membership dues. • *Investing in the Future: Child Care Financing Options for the Public and Private Sectors.* Highlights successful financing models, including grants and loans, bank reinvestment strategies, community initiatives, bonds and pension funds. *Price:* $15 for members; $25 for nonmembers. • *Not Too Small to Care: Small Businesses and Child Care.* Profiles 29 small businesses that have implemented child care benefits: on-or-near-site child care centers, employee subsidies, and parental leave. *Price:* $15 for members; $25 for nonmembers. • *Where They Stand: A Digest of Organizational Policies on Child Care and Education.* Provides a guide to 45 national organizations' policy positions on quality child care, early childhood education, and education reform. *Price:* $15 for members; $25 for nonmembers. • Also publishes resource guides for parents who need help finding appropriate child care services.

★ 2201 ★ Child Care Law Center (CCLC)
221 Pine St., 3rd Fl.
San Francisco, CA 94104
Phone: (415)394-7144 **Fax:** (415)394-7140
Email: info@childcarelaw.org
Website: http://www.childcarelaw.org
Nancy Strohl, Exec. Dir.

Fnded: 1978. **Desc:** Provides legal services, technical assistance, and training programs to attorneys and others working to improve child care for low-income families. Develops legislative and regulatory policies; monitors legislative issues. **Pub:** *The ADA and Child Care: Information for Parents of Children with Disablilities.* • *Caring for Children with HIV or AIDS in Child Care.* • *Caring for Children with Special Needs: The ADA and Child Care.* • *Child Care Contracts: Information for Parents.* • *Child Care Contracts: Information for Providers.* • *The Child Care Tax Credit: A Booklet for Parents.* Booklet. • *Employing People with Disabilities: The ADA and Child Care.* • *Family Day Care Zoning Advocacy Guide.* • *Legal Update*, quarterly. Newsletter. • *Liability Insurance: Insuring Your Program.* • *Working For Change*, quarterly. • Offers various additional publications.

★ 2202 ★ Child Health Association (CHA)
PO Box 366
Rosny Park, TAS 7018, Australia
Phone: 61 3 62314765 **Fax:** 61 3 62314749

Fnded: 1917. **Mem:** 450. **State Groups:** 34. **Lang(s):** English. **Desc:** Network of parent groups who work with and for the family, child, and youth health service in Tasmania, Australia. Aims to support parents and enhance the health and wellbeing of children and families. Offers friendship and support; provides information and resources; actively participates and advocates within health services organizations; sponsors pram walking groups, nutrition programs, and playgroups; conducts fundraising for children's items. **Pub:** *Child Health*, bimonthly. Newsletter.

★ 2203 ★ Child Health Foundation (ICHF)
10630 Little Patuxat Pkwy., Ste. 126
Columbia, MD 21044
Phone: (301)596-4514 **Fax:** (410)992-5641
Email: chf@erols.com
Website: http://www.childhealthfoundation.org
Eric Marler, MD Chm.

Fnded: 1985. **Desc:** Addresses significant health issues of children and families, primarily in developing countries and medically underserved populations in the U.S. Focuses on diarrheal diseases, related social and medical problems of malnutrition, and poverty. Develops and encourages use of simple, low-cost technologies. Conducts health programs in research training in oral rehydration therapies, nutrition, breastfeeding and other lowcost approaches to better health. Operates programs to strengthen research capabilities of institutions in developing countries to enable them to develop and perform research on diseases most prevalent in their own countries. Conducts educational training programs and workshops for: volunteers in disease prevention and simple treatments effective in rural and urban areas. Conducts charitable activities;

maintains speakers' bureau. **Pub:** *Cereal-Based Oral Rehydration Therapy Symposium Proceedings.* Journal. • *Child Health Foundation Newsletter*, quarterly. Newsletter. Includes research summaries and foundation information. • *Food-based Oral Rehydration Therapy Report.* • *Proper Nutrition and Hygiene.* • *Training Manual for Treatment and Prevention of Childhood Diarrhea with Oral Rehydration Therapy.* • Annual Report. **Frmly:** International Child Health Foundation; (1994) International Child Health Foundation.

★ 2204 ★ Child Life Council (CLC)

11820 Parklawn Dr., Ste. 202
Rockville, MD 20852-2529
Phone: (301)881-7090 **Free:** 800-CLC-4515
Fax: (301)881-7092
Email: clcstaff@childlife.org
Website: http://www.childlife.org
Deborah E. Brouse, Exec. Dir.

Fnded: 1982. **Mem:** 2,200. **Desc:** Professional organization representing child life personnel, patient activities specialists, and students in the field. Promotes psychological well-being and optimum development of children, adolescents, and their families in health care settings. Works to minimize the stress and anxiety of illness and hospitalization. Addresses professional issues such as program standards, competencies, and core curriculum. Provides resources and conducts research and educational programs. Offers a Job Bank Service listing employment openings. **Pub:** *Child Life Council Bulletin*, quarterly. Bulletin. • *Child Life Programs*, biennial. Directory. • *Making Ethical Decisions in Child Life Practice.* • *Official Documents of the Child Life Council.* • *Program Review Guidelines.* • *Psychosocial Care of Children in Hospitals: A Clinical Practice Manual.* **Frmly:** (1975) Child Life Specialist Committee; (1979) Child Life Activity Study Section; (1982) Child Life Task Force.

★ 2205 ★ Childbirth Without Pain Education Association (CWPEA)

20134 Snowden
Detroit, MI 48235
Phone: (313)341-3816
Email: cat-flora@juno.com
Flora Hommel, Exec. Dir. /Founder

Fnded: 1958. **Mem:** 2,000. **Nat'l Groups:** 8. **Reg. Groups:** 3. **State Groups:** 3. **Local Groups:** 1. **Desc:** Former and current students of the Lamaze-Pavlov (psychoprophylactic) method of painless childbirth; physicians, nurses, midwifes, students, former students and interested individuals. Sponsors classes and films for women with or without partners, nurses, midwifes and medical and lay groups about the method, which is based on conditioned reflexes to help prevent pain, thus allowing for normal, usually drug- and intervention free childbirth. Works to provide a method-trained person (monitrice) in attendance at the birth where possible. Collects data for further development of the method; surveys maternity services. Sponsors childbirth teacher and monitrice training and certification nationally with workshops. Provides teen pregnancy programs. Offers some referral service. **Pub:** *Childbirth Without Pain Education Association Memo*, bimonthly. Newsletter. Includes association news and book reviews, and current practices and research. *Price:* Included in membership dues; $50/year for physicians; $35/year for nurses and nonmembers; $16/year for alumni. **AKA:** Lamaze Birth Without Pain Education Association.

★ 2206 ★ Childhood Brain Tumor Foundation

20312 Watkins Meadow Dr.
Germantown, MD 20876
Phone: (301)515-2900 **Free:** 877-217-4166
Email: cbtf@childhoodbraintumor.org
Website: http://www.childhoodbraintumor.org/
Jeanne Young, Pres.

Fnded: 1994. **Desc:** Committed to raising funds for scientific research and public awareness of brain tumors in children; works to improve prognosis and quality of life. **Pub:** *The Neurotransmitter*, triennial. Newsletter. Contains educational articles, personal stories and updates.

★ 2207 ★ Childhood Cancer Foundation - Candelighters Canada

55 Eglinton Ave. E, Ste. 401
Toronto, ON, Canada M4P 1G8
Phone: (416)489-6440 **Free:** 800-363-1062
Fax: (416)489-9812
Email: staff@candlelighters.ca
Website: http://www.candlelighters.ca

Fnded: 1987. **Local Groups:** 50. **Lang(s):** English, French. **Desc:** Volunteers. Seeks to improve the quality of life of children with cancer and their families. Provides assistance to children with cancer and their families; maintains support groups; sponsors educational and recreational programs. **Pub:** *Contact*, every 6 months. Newsletter.

★ 2208 ★ Children and Adults With Attention Deficit/Hyperactivity Disorder (CHADD)

8181 Professional Pl., Ste.201
Landover, MD 20785
Phone: (301)306-7070 **Free:** 800-233-4050
Fax: (301)306-7090
Email: national@chadd.org
Website: http://www.chadd.org
E. Clarke Ross, DPA, CEO

Fnded: 1987. **Mem:** 20,000. **Local Groups:** 250. **Desc:** Works to improve the lives of people affected by AD/HD through collaborative leadership, advocacy, research, education and support. Provides support network for parents and caregivers, a forum for continuing education; works to be a community resource, disseminates accurate evidence-based information about AD/HD to parents, educators, adults, professionals and the media; promotes ongoing research; advocated on behalf of AD/HD community. **Pub:** *ATTENTION*, bimonthly. Magazine. • Booklets. • Brochures. • Also publishes fact sheets. **Frmly:** (1993) Children with Attention-Deficit Disorders; (2001) Children and Adults With Attention Deficit Disorder.

★ 2209 ★ Children of Aging Parents (CAPS)

Woodbourne Office Campus, Ste. 302A
1609 Woodbourne Rd.
Levittown, PA 19057-1511
Phone: (215)945-6900 **Free:** 800-227-7294
Fax: (215)945-8720
Email: caps4caregivers@aol.com
Website: http://www.caps4caregivers.org/
Lorraine Sailor, Contact

Fnded: 1977. **Mem:** 1,300. **Desc:** National information and referral service for caregivers of the elderly. Provides a speakers bureau as part of its educational outreach mission to churches, service clubs, schools, hospitals, TV/radio and colleges. Conducts workshops, seminars, and conferences for lay individuals and professionals in the field of aging. Publishes a bimonthly newsletter and numerous fact sheets on various topics of interest to caregivers. Organizes and promotes caregivers' support groups, and responds to requests for assistance nationally. **Pub:** *The Capsule*, bimonthly. Newsletter. Reports on concerns of elderly persons and their families. Includes publications listing, book reviews, and research news. *Price:* Included in membership dues. • *Guide to Selecting a Nursing Home.* • *How to Start A Self Group for Caregivers.* • *Instant Aging–Sensory Deprivation Manual.* Manual. • Bibliographies. • Publishes fact sheets on caregiving issues.

★ 2210 ★ Children of Alcoholics Foundation (COAF)

164 W 74th St.
New York, NY 10023-2301
Phone: (212)595-5810 **Free:** 800-488-3784
Fax: (212)595-2553
Email: coaf@phoenixhouse.org
Website: http://www.coaf.org

Fnded: 1982. **Desc:** Seeks to educate the public and professionals about children of substance abusers and the effects of parental substance abuse, and stimulate interest in seeking solutions to their problems. Promotes research, educational and informational programs, and public discussion on alcoholism, substance abuse, and its effects on children; disseminates reports and research results; investigates the effectiveness of public policies, programs, and laws; encourages participation and assists government and community agencies in providing assistance to children of substance abusers and seeking solutions to the problems of these children. Facilitates research and educational and informational programs on other aspects of childhood, the parent-child relationship, physiological and psychological aspects of human development, child abuse and neglect, and substance abuse of other psychoactive substances. **Pub:** *Free Catalog.* Catalog.

★ 2211 ★ Children of Deaf Adults (CODA)

Box 30715
Santa Barbara, CA 93130
Phone: (805)682-0997
Email: coda@coda-international.org
Website: http://www.coda-international.org
Millie Brother, Founder

Fnded: 1983. **Mem:** 500. **Desc:** Hearing children of deaf parents who are interested in sharing experiences with others of similar backgrounds. Provides information to professional organizations, libraries, community agencies, researchers, and other interested persons. Acts upon issues regarding deafness; provides support to deaf parent/hearing child families. Serves as clearinghouse for deaf parent/hearing children families. **Pub:** *CODA Connection*, quarterly. Newsletter. For the adult hearing children of deaf parents. Reports on national and international meetings and resources. Includes association news. *Price:* Included in membership dues. • *Hearing Children/Deaf Parents.* Bibliography. • *Proceedings from Annual Conferences.* Proceedings.

★ 2212 ★ Children of the Night (CN)

14530 Sylvan St.
Van Nuys, CA 91411
Phone: (818)908-4474 **Free:** 800-551-1300
Fax: (818)908-1468
Email: cotnll@aol.com
Website: http://www.childrenofthenight.org
Dr. Lois Lee, Pres. /Founder

Fnded: 1979. **Desc:** Provides assistance to children between the ages of 11-17 who are sexually abused and are forced to prostitute on the streets. Children of the night's goal is to mainstream street children into the larger society. Operates a 24-hour toll-free hotline and a 24-bed home that also features a private school approved by the California Department of Education. **Pub:** Brochures.

★ 2213 ★ Children's AIDS Fund

PO Box 16433
Washington, DC 20041
Phone: (703)433-1560 **Free:** (866)829-1560
Fax: 800-577-8529
Email: info@childrensaidsfund.org
Website: http://www.childrensaidsfund.org
Anita M. Smith, Pres.

Fnded: 1987. **Desc:** Serves children and families who are HIV impacted through direct assistance referrals, counseling, and resource materials. Advisory board of doctors, public health professionals, legislators, educators, and clergy assisting in the formulation of a sound public policy on HIV/AIDS that will be understood and promoted by the public. Encourages the public to react compassionately toward persons affected, infected, or ill with HIV or AIDS. Advocates early diagnosis; promotes reducing transmission of the epidemic through public health intervention strategies such as confidential and voluntary partner notification. Supports development of treatments, diagnostics, vaccines, and an eventual cure for the disease.

Promotes health care access for individuals infected with HIV and AIDS. Testifies before national, state, and local government agencies. Operates speakers' bureau. **Pub:** *AIDS/HIV News*, bimonthly. *Price:* $25/year. • *The Church's Response to the Challenge of AIDS/HIV.* Compiled in conjunction with MAP International. • *Guide to Federal Funding of HIV Disease*, periodic. • Audiotapes. • Brochures. • Videos. • Also issues literature, conference transcripts, and testimonies. **Frmly:** (1993) Americans for a Sound AIDS Policy; (1998) Americans for a Sound AIDS/HIV Policy.

★ 2214 ★ Children's Blood Foundation (CBF)
333 E 38th, Room 830
New York, NY 10016
Phone: (212)297-4336 **Fax:** (212)297-4340
Email: info@childrensbloodfoundation.org
Website: http://www.childrensbloodfoundation.org
Theodora Ziongas, Exec. Dir.

Fnded: 1952. **Reg. Groups:** 1. **Desc:** Seeks to raise funds to combat diseases of the blood in children, such as leukemia, hemophilia, thalassemia (Cooley's anemia), childhood cancers, sickle cell, and other anemias and diseases of the immune system, and AIDS. Supports a total patient care center in the New York Hospital-Cornell Medical Center, which includes diagnostic and treatment clinics, progressive research laboratories, and intensive training of physicians in the specialty of pediatric hematology/oncology. Also sponsors specialized social events.

★ 2215 ★ Children's Brain Tumor Foundation (CBTF)
274 Madison Ave., No. 1301
New York, NY 10016
Phone: (212)448-9494 **Free:** (866)228-HOPE
Fax: (212)448-1022
Email: info@cbtf.org
Website: http://www.cbtf.org
Judy Hurley, Exec. Dir.

Fnded: 1988. **Desc:** Works to improve the outlook for children with brain and spinal cord tumors. Raises funds for research; provides counseling, education and support services for families and survivors. **Pub:** *A Resource Guide for Parents of Children with Brain and Spinal Cord Tumors.* Booklet. Contains technical and practical information for parents. *Price:* Free. • *The Challenge.* Newsletter.

★ 2216 ★ Children's Craniofacial Association (CCA)
13140 Coit Rd., Ste. 307
Dallas, TX 75240
Phone: (214)570-9099 **Free:** 800-535-3643
Fax: (972)566-8489
Email: contactCCA@ccakids.com
Website: http://www.ccakids.com
Charlene Smith, Exec. Dir.

Fnded: 1989. **Desc:** Participants include craniofacial surgeons and others wishing to aid individuals with craniofacial deformities. Promotes increased awareness of craniofacial deformities and their treatment among health care professionals and the public. Provides financial assistance to craniofacially deformed patients for costs related to treatment such as food, travel and lodging. Functions as a networking and referral service for patients. Makes referrals to qualified centers. Conducts craniofacial family workshops. **Pub:** Booklets.Provides information on craniofacial conditions and their treatment. • Films. • Videos. • Also publishes materials for health care professionals, government officials, and parents of craniofacially deformed children. **Frmly:** (1992) International Craniofacial Foundations.

★ 2217 ★ Children's Environmental Health Network (CEHN)
110 Maryland Ave. NE, Ste. 511
Washington, DC 20002
Phone: (202)543-4033 **Fax:** (202)543-8797
Email: cehn@cehn.org
Website: http://www.cehn.org/
Daniel J. Swartz, Exec. Dir.

Desc: Promotes the development of sound public health and child-focused national policy for children affected by exposures to environmental hazards.

★ 2218 ★ Children's Healthcare Is a Legal Duty (CHILD)
PO Box 2604
Sioux City, IA 51106
Phone: (712)948-3500 **Fax:** (712)948-3704
Email: childinc@netins.net
Website: http://www.childrenshealthcare.org
Dr. Rita Swan, Pres.

Fnded: 1983. **Mem:** 450. **Desc:** Advocate for the provision of healthcare for all children; opposes child abuse and neglect related to religion or cultural tradition. **Pub:** *CHILD, Inc. Newsletter*, quarterly. Newsletter. *Price:* Included in membership dues; $25/year for nonmembers. • *Children, Medicine, Religion and the Law.* Reprint. *Price:* $5. • *Cry, the Beloved Children.* Booklet. *Price:* $2. **AKA:** CHILD, Inc.

★ 2219 ★ Children's Health Fund
317 E 64th St.
New York, NY 10021
Phone: (212)452-3340 **Free:** 800-535-7448
Fax: (212)861-0235
Email: development@chfund.org
Website: http://www.childrenshealthfund.org
Irwin Redlener, MD, Pres.

Fnded: 1987. **Desc:** Supports pediatric programs for children who are homeless, poor, or have no other access to medical care. Maintains Children's Health Projects in urban and rural areas throughout the United States. Provides mobile medical units in order to bring health care to underserved children.

★ 2220 ★ Children's Heart Association for Support and Education (CHASE)
Hospital for Sick Children
Cardiac Clinic
Division of Cardiology
Toronto, ON, Canada M5G 1X8
Phone: (416)410-2427
Email: kidheart@angelfire.com
Website: http://www.angelfire.com/on/chase

Fnded: 1983. **Mem:** 550. **Lang(s):** English, French. **Desc:** Parents of children with congenital heart defects. Works to improve the quality of life of children with cardiological problems and their families. Maintains network of support groups for members; encourages exchange of information among members and between members and cardiologists; conducts social and educational activities; works to increase public awareness of pediatric cardiology. Provides support and assistance to the Hospital for Sick Children's Division of Pediatric Cardiology. **Pub:** *Straight from the Heart*, monthly. Newsletter.

★ 2221 ★ Children's HeartLink (CHL)
5075 Arcadia Ave.
Minneapolis, MN 55436
Phone: (952)928-4860 **Fax:** (952)928-4859
Email: info@childrensheartlink.org
Website: http://www.childrensheartlink.org
Elizabeth Bickel, Pres.

Fnded: 1969. **Reg. Groups:** 1. **Desc:** Medical charity and service agency. Advocates the prevention and treatment of heart disease in needy children throughout the world; helps selected developing countries expand and improve their cardiac services for children. Provides: treatment for needy children with heart disease; support for rheumatic fever prevention programs; education and training opportunities for foreign physicians, nurses, and other medical professionals; technical advice and problem-solving assistance; medical equipment and supplies. Organizes fund-raising events. **Pub:** *Heartbeat*, 3/year. Newsletter. *Price:* Free. **Frmly:** (1994) Children's Heart Fund.

★ 2222 ★ Children's Hospice International (CHI)
901 N Pitt St., No. 230
Alexandria, VA 22314
Phone: (703)684-0330 **Free:** 800-24-CHILD
Fax: (703)684-0226
Email: chiorg@aol.com
Website: http://www.chionline.org
Ann Armstrong Dailey, Founding Dir.

Fnded: 1983. **Mem:** 700. **Desc:** Physicians, nurses, teachers, social workers, clergy, psychologists, art and music occupational therapists, volunteers, and students who work or are interested in hospice programs. Objectives are to: promote hospice support through pediatric care facilities; encourage the inclusion of children in existing and developing hospices and home care programs; include hospice perspectives in all areas of pediatric care and education. Supports health care agencies that engage in the treatment of terminally ill children and their families. Disseminates information concerning support groups and research, education, and training programs. Children's hospice care involves an interdisciplinary team of physicians, social workers, nurses, clergy, therapists, teachers and trained volunteers; parents act as primary caregivers. **Pub:** *Approaching Grief.* Pamphlet. • *Children's Hospice/Home Care.* Manual. • *Children's Hospice International–Newsletter*, quarterly. Newsletter. Contains calendar of events and list of resources. *Price:* Included in membership dues; $20/year for nonmembers. • *Home Care for Seriously Ill Children: A Manual for Parents.* Manual. • *Palliative Pain and Symptom Management for Children and Adolescents.* • *The Psychological Aspects of Pain and Symptom Management.* • Audiotapes. • Videos.

★ 2223 ★ Children's Leukemia Research Association (NLA)
585 Stewart Ave., Ste. LL18
Garden City, NY 11530
Phone: (516)222-1944 **Fax:** (516)222-0457
Email: clra@erols.com
Website: http://www.childrensleukemia.org/
Allan D. Weinberg, Exec. Dir.

Fnded: 1965. **Desc:** Promotes leukemia research and public awareness of the disease. Provides financial aid to leukemia patients and their families, based on need. **Frmly:** (1994) National Leukemia Association.

★ 2224 ★ Children's Medical Ministries (CMM)
PO Box 3382
Crofton, MD 21114
Phone: (301)261-3211 **Fax:** (301)721-4647
Email: childmed@olg.com
Website: http://www.childmed.org/

Fnded: 1988. **Mem:** 700. **Desc:** Committed to serving the poor and needy children by offering health care, nutritional support, and dental care.

★ 2225 ★ Children's Organ Transplant Association (COTA)
2501 COTA Dr.
Bloomington, IN 47403
Phone: (812)336-8872 **Free:** 800-366-2682
Fax: (812)336-8885
Email: jennifer@cota.org
Website: http://www.cota.org/
Richard E. Lofgren, Pres.

Fnded: 1986. **Mem:** 700. **Desc:** Dedicated to ensuring that no U.S. child is ever denied a life-saving transplant, or access to a transplant waiting list, due solely to lack of funds; promotes organ donations and provides public education on all aspects of the organ donation process. **Pub:** *Life-Giving Report*, quarterly. Newsletter.

★ 2226 ★ Children's PKU Network (CPN)
3790 Via De La Valle, Ste. 120
Del Mar, CA 92014
Phone: (858)509-0767 **Free:** 800-377-6677
Fax: (858)509-0768

Email: pkunetwork@aol.com
Website: http://www.pkunetwork.org

Fnded: 1991. **Mem:** 8. **Nat'l Groups:** 1. **Desc:** Works to address the special needs of all people involved in the treatment of Phenylketonuria (PKU), a genetic metabolic disease whereby the body is unable to process the amino acid phenylalanine. Networks families and individuals with each other; provides discount dietary aids; offers financial assistance and support groups; provides crisis intervention; advocates mandatory guidelines for insurance carriers to cover expenses of medical food treatment of PKU individuals; conducts fundraisers; endows research benefiting PKU and other metabolic disorders. **Pub:** *UPDATE*, semiannual. Newsletter.

★ 2227 ★ Chilean Gerontological Study Group (CGSG)

Avenida Presidente Riesco 6007
Classifiacdor 1
Correo 27
Santiago, Chile

Lang(s): English, Spanish. **Desc:** Health care professionals treating the elderly; scientists and clinicians with an interest in the aging process and diseases of the aged. Promotes gerontological research and increased availability of gerontological care; facilitates training of gerontology specialists. Represents the interests of gerontologists and gerontological organizations.

★ 2228 ★ Chilean Society of Cardiology and Cardiovascular Surgery (Sociedad Chilena de Cardiologia y Cirugia Cardiovascular)

Esmeralda 678
Santiago, Chile

Fnded: 1949.

★ 2229 ★ Chilean Society of Obstetrics and Gynecology (Sociedad Chilena de Obstetricia y Ginecologia)

Roman Diaz 205, Of 205, Providencia
Santiago, Chile
Phone: 56 2 2350133 **Fax:** 56 2 2351294
Email: sochog@entelchile.net
Website: http://www.sochog.cl

Fnded: 1935.

★ 2230 ★ Chilean Society of Pharmacology

c/o Dr. Gonzalo Bustos
Laboratory of Biochemical Pharmacology
Department of Cell & Molecular Biology
Catholic University of Chile
PO Box 114D
Santiago, Chile
Phone: 56 2 6862654 **Fax:** 56 2 6862660
Email: gbustos@genes.bio.puc.cl
Website: http://sbch.conicyt.cl:9090/sociedad/farmac01.htm

Mem: 100. **Desc:** Promotes pharmacology in Chile.

★ 2231 ★ China Academy of Traditional Chinese Medicine

18 Beixincang, Dongzhimennai
Beijing 100900, People's Republic of China
Phone: 86 10 446661

★ 2232 ★ China AIDS Network (CAN)

5 Dong Dan San Tiao
Peking Union Medical College
Beijing 100005, People's Republic of China
Phone: 86 10 65288167 **Fax:** 86 10 65288170
Email: klzhang@bj.col.com.cn

Desc: Works to minimize the incidence of AIDS through education. Develops and distributes materials on AIDS and its transmission.

★ 2233 ★ China Anticancer Association (CACA)

52 Fucheng Rd.
Beijing 100036, People's Republic of China
Phone: 86 22 3359958 **Fax:** 86 22 23526512
Email: xuzhigang@caca.or.cn
Website: http://www.caca.org.cn

Fnded: 1985. **Mem:** 20,000. **Nat'l Groups:** 1. **Reg. Groups:** 3. **State Groups:** 26. **Local Groups:** 33. **Lang(s):** Chinese, English. **Desc:** Physicians, researchers, and interested individuals in the People's Republic of China. Conducts research programs concentrating on the prevention of cancer. Sponsors research exchange with cancer experts in other countries. Maintains 23 academic commissions. Offers educational programs; disseminates information to the public about cancer prevention. Organizes academic conferences and symposia. **Pub:** *Cancer Research on Prevention and Treatment*, quarterly. Journal. • *Chinese Journal for Cancer Research*, quarterly. Journal. • *Chinese Journal of Clinical Oncology*, monthly. Journal. Includes English abstracts.

★ 2234 ★ China Family Planning Association (CFPA)

35 Shaoyaoju Chaoyang District
Beijing 100029, People's Republic of China
Phone: 86 10 84657811 **Fax:** 86 10 84657975
Email: cfpa@public.fhnet.cn.net

Fnded: 1980. **Reg. Groups:** 29. **Lang(s):** Chinese, English. **Desc:** Works to enhance the quality of life for individuals living in China by promoting family planning. Works to reduce the number of unwanted pregnancies and abortions. Provides contraceptive and health care services. Sponsors programs in family planning, sex education, and health. **Pub:** *Life*, monthly. Magazine.

★ 2235 ★ China Leprosy Association

126 Gulou Xidajie
Xicheng District
Beijing 100009, People's Republic of China
Phone: 86 10 64033787 **Fax:** 86 10 64033787
Email: cla2000@163.com
Website: http://skinstd.com.cn

Fnded: 1985. **Mem:** 9,192. **State Groups:** 23. **Lang(s):** English. **Desc:** Individuals (9192) and organizations (23) in the People's Republic of China. Seeks to prevent leprosy; works to develop advanced treatment methods. Fosters exchange and cooperation with leprosy organizations in other countries. Conducts research and educational programs. **Pub:** *China Leprosy and Skin Diseases Journal*, quarterly. Journal. Contains scientific reports and papers on operational activities related to leprosy skin diseases and STD control in China. • *Selected Papers of Foreign Leprosy Journals*. Translated in Chinese. • Films.

★ 2236 ★ China Medical Board of New York (CMBNY)

750 3rd Ave., 23rd Fl.
New York, NY 10017-2703
Phone: (212)682-8000 **Fax:** (212)949-8726
Email: administrator@chinamedicalboard.org
Website: http://www.chinamedicalboard.org/
M. Roy Schwarz, MD, Pres.

Fnded: 1928. **Desc:** Purpose is to support programs of medical, nursing, and public health education and research. Assists institutions in East and Southeast Asia in improving the health levels and services in Asian societies. Seeks to improve the quality and increase the numbers of appropriate health practitioners in these societies. Has programs in Korea, Taiwan, Hong Kong, the Philippines, Thailand, Malaysia, Myanmar, Singapore, Indonesia, Mongolia, Vietnam, Laos, and China. Endowed by the Rockefeller Foundation and controlled by an independent board of trustees who serve without compensation. Formerly devoted entire income to support of Peking Union Medical College, nationalized in 1949 by People's Republic of China. **Pub:** *China Medical Board of New York–Annual Report*. Includes list of grants and endowments made during year of report. *Price:* Free.

★ 2237 ★ China Optometric and Optical Association (COOA)

No. 6, East Changan St.
Beijing 100740, People's Republic of China
Phone: 86 10 63022411 **Fax:** 86 10 63185325
Email: optics@public.bta.net.cn
Website: http://www.chinaoptics.com

Fnded: 1985. **Lang(s):** English. **Desc:** Manufacturers, optometrists, research institutes, and other companies and organizations within the optical industry. Represents and promotes the optical industry in China. **Pub:** *China Glasses Science and Technology*. Magazine.

★ 2238 ★ China Spiritual Therapy Study Association

5 Alley 11, Lane 131, Olung St.
Taipei, Taiwan

Fnded: 1926.

★ 2239 ★ Chinese American Medical Society (CAMS)

c/o Dr. H.H. Wang
281 Edgewood Ave.
Teaneck, NJ 07666
Phone: (201)833-1506 **Fax:** (201)833-8252
Email: hw5@columbia.edu
Website: http://www.camsociety.org
Dr. Daisy Saw, MD, Pres.

Fnded: 1963. **Mem:** 850. **Reg. Groups:** 4. **Desc:** Physicians of Chinese origin residing in the U.S. and Canada. Seeks to advance medical knowledge, scientific research, and interchange of information among members and to promote the health status of Chinese Americans. Conducts educational meetings; supports research. Maintains placement service. Sponsors limited charitable program. **Pub:** *Chinese American Medical Society–Newsletter*, 3-4/year. Newsletter. Includes membership news, announcements, and calendar of events. *Price:* Included in membership dues. • Membership Directory, annual. **Frmly:** (1985) American Chinese Medical Society.

★ 2240 ★ Chinese Anti-Tuberculosis Society

42 Dung-si-xi-da St.
Beijing, People's Republic of China
Phone: 86 10 553685

★ 2241 ★ Chinese Association of Animal Science and Veterinary Medicine

33 Dongdaqiao Nongfengli, Chao Yang District
Beijing 10020, People's Republic of China
Phone: 86 10 65066533 **Fax:** 86 10 65005670

★ 2242 ★ Chinese Association of Integrated Traditional and Western Medicine

18 Beixincang, Dongzhimennei
Beijing, People's Republic of China
Phone: 86 10 64010688 **Fax:** 86 10 64010688
Email: caim@medboo.com

★ 2243 ★ Chinese Association for Mental Health

5 An Kang Hutong
Desheng Men Wai
Beijing 100088, People's Republic of China
Phone: 86 10 62359838 **Fax:** 86 10 62359838

Fnded: 1985. **Mem:** 20,000. **Local Groups:** 26. **Lang(s):** Chinese. **Desc:** Physicians, psychologists, sociologists. Seeks to increase people's psychological health, to elevate their social adaptation ability, and to prevent psychological disorders.

★ 2244 ★ Chinese Association for Physiological Sciences
42 Dongsixidajie
Beijing 100710, People's Republic of China
Email: lingxiao12341@sina.com
Website: http://www.caps-china.org

★ 2245 ★ Chinese Association of Psychological Testing (CAPT)
162 Sec. 1 Hoping E Rd.
Taipei 10610, Taiwan

Fnded: 1951. **Desc:** Assists members in conducting educational research; designs and develops assessments for educational planning; encourages members in data collection related to testing; supplies schools and organizations with testing materials; provides consultation services on testing questions.

★ 2246 ★ Chinese Association on Smoking and Health
907, Bldg. 16
Anhuidongli
Chaoyang District
Beijing 100101, People's Republic of China
Phone: 86 10 64892695 **Fax:** 86 10 64983805
Email: cash@mx.cei.gov.cn
Website: http://www.cash-prc.com

Fnded: 1990. **Mem:** 50,000. **Nat'l Groups:** 1. **State Groups:** 28. **Local Groups:** 300. **Lang(s):** English. **Desc:** National academic and non-governmental organization in China promoting smoking cessation and tobacco control. Conducts research and educational programs; compiles statistics. Offers consulting services. **Pub:** *Smoking and Health in China*, quarterly. Newsletter.

★ 2247 ★ Chinese Association of Sports Medicine
11 Tiyuguan Rd.
Beijing 100061, People's Republic of China
Phone: 86 10 7120239 **Fax:** 86 10 4912129

★ 2248 ★ Chinese Association of Urine Therapy
72 Wu Kon Lio Rd.
Wuki Industrial Park
Taipei, Taiwan
Phone: 886 2 22988446 **Fax:** 886 2 22996990
Email: webmaster@autourine.com

Desc: Promotes urine therapy and medical research on urine therapy. **Pub:** *Urine Therapy Association Magazine*, quarterly. Magazine.

★ 2249 ★ Chinese Medical Association
42 Dongsi Xidajie
Beijing 100710, People's Republic of China
Phone: 86 10 65250394 **Fax:** 86 10 65123754
Email: infor@chinamed.com.cn
Website: http://www.chinamed.com.cn

Fnded: 1915. **Mem:** 250,000. **Desc:** Physicians in the People's Republic of China. Promotes the advancement of medical science and technology. Conducts information exchanges among physicians in China and in other countries. Conducts and analyzes medical research programs. Gathers and disseminates medical data. Develops and approves medical terminology. Offers training programs to members.

★ 2250 ★ Chinese Medical Association
201 Shih-Pai Rd., Section 2
Taipei, Taiwan
Phone: 886 10 551943

Fnded: 1915.

★ 2251 ★ Chinese National Association for Mental Hygiene
National Taiwan University Hospital, 1 Changteh St.
Taipei, Taiwan

Fnded: 1936.

★ 2252 ★ Chinese Nursing Association
42 Dongsi Xi Da Jie
Beijing 100710, People's Republic of China
Phone: 86 10 65265331 **Fax:** 86 10 65123754

Fnded: 1909. **Mem:** 240,000. **Lang(s):** English, Japanese. **Desc:** Nurses and nursing attendants in the People's Republic of China. Promotes research and advanced technological developments in the nursing profession; represents members' interests. Conducts educational programs. **Pub:** *Chinese Journal of Nursing*, monthly. Journal.

★ 2253 ★ Chinese Nutrition Society
29 Nanwei Rd.
Beijing 100050, People's Republic of China
Phone: 86 10 63043472 **Fax:** 86 10 63011875

★ 2254 ★ Chinese Pharmaceutical Association
A38 Lishi Rd. N
Beijing 100810, People's Republic of China
Phone: 86 10 88385405 **Fax:** 86 10 88385405
Email: sinopharmacy@163.net

Fnded: 1907. **Mem:** 10,000. **Pub:** *Chinese Pharmaceutical Journal*, monthly. Journal.

★ 2255 ★ Chinese Pharmacological Society
c/o Prof. J-T Zhang
1 Xian Nong Tan St.
Institute of Materia Medica, CAMS
Beijing 100050, People's Republic of China
Phone: 86 10 3013366 **Fax:** 86 10 3017757
Email: zhxd@imm.ac.cn
Website: http://www.cnphars.org/

Fnded: 1985. **Mem:** 3,303. **Lang(s):** English, Japanese. **Desc:** Pharmacologists and interested individuals in the People's Republic of China. Promotes the study of pharmacology. Conducts research programs. Fosters exchange among members and pharmacologists in other countries. Provides consulting services. **Pub:** *China Journal of Pharmacology and Toxicology*, periodic. Journal. • *Chinese Pharmacological Bulletin*. Newsletter. • *Chinese Pharmacology and Clinical Application*, periodic. Journal. • *Pharmacologica Sinica*, periodic. Journal. • *Pharmacology and Clinics of Chinese Materia Medica*. Directory.

★ 2256 ★ Chinese Psychological Association (CPA)
National Taiwan University
Taipei 106, Taiwan
Phone: 886 2 3630231 **Fax:** 886 2 3629909

Fnded: 1962.

★ 2257 ★ Chinese Psychological Society
Institute of Psychology
Chinese Academy of Sciences
10A Datun Rd.
Beijing 100101, People's Republic of China
Phone: 86 10 64888946 **Fax:** 86 10 64855830
Email: xuehui@psych.ac.cn
Website: http://www.cpsbeijing.org

Fnded: 1921. **Mem:** 4,000. **Desc:** Promotes academic communication through congresses, conferences, meetings, organizing research projects, publishing books, providing counseling services and suggestions to related institutions and departments. **Pub:** *Progresses of Psychology in China*. Book.

★ 2258 ★ Chinese Society for Anatomical Sciences
c/o Xu Qunyuan, Pres.
42 Dongsi Xidajie
Beijing 100710, People's Republic of China
Phone: 86 10 65133311 **Fax:** 86 10 65123754
Email: csas@public.bta.net.cn

Mem: 7,000. **Desc:** Seeks to enhance the friendship and cooperation between anatomists not only domestic but also international members and groups, to promote the development of the Anatomical Sciences.

★ 2259 ★ Chinese Society of Veterinary Science
PO Box 23, Chunan
Miaoli 350, Taiwan
Phone: 886 37 672352 **Fax:** 886 37 692806

★ 2260 ★ ChiroFeed International
300 Vine St., Ste. 18
Seattle, WA 98121
Phone: (206)448-2004
Email: julianemes@reachone.com

Fnded: 1998. **Desc:** Chiropractors. Provide chiropractic exams and care to underprivileged people.

★ 2261 ★ Chiropractic Association of South Africa (CASA) (Chiropraktiese Vereniging van Suid-Afrika)
PO Box 706
Bethlehem 9700, Republic of South Africa
Phone: 27 58 3034571 **Fax:** 27 58 3091480
Email: drreg@mweb.co.za
Website: http://www.chiropractic.co.za

Fnded: 1970. **Mem:** 195. **Nat'l Groups:** 1. **Reg. Groups:** 4. **State Groups:** 1. **Local Groups:** 4. **Lang(s):** Afrikaans, English. **Desc:** Seeks to: heighten public awareness of the chiropractic system of therapy and educational standards; improve medical insurance coverage of such treatment. Offers training curricula; conducts periodic seminars. **Pub:** *Inter-Association Newsletter*, periodic. Newsletter. Membership. • *Newswire*, periodic. Newsletter.

★ 2262 ★ Chiropractic Doctors' Association of Hong Kong (CDAHK)
Hong Kong, People's Republic of China
Phone: 852 81085688
Email: chairman@cda.org.hk
Website: http://www.cda.org.hk

Fnded: 2000. **Desc:** Promotes Chiropractic in Hong Kong; aims to educate the general public on spinal health care.

★ 2263 ★ Chiropractors' Association of Australia (CAA)
148 Station St., Ste. 4
PO Box 6246
South Penrith, NSW 2750, Australia
Phone: 61 2 47318011 **Fax:** 61 2 47318088
Email: nhq@caa.asn.au
Website: http://www.chiropractors.asn.au

Desc: Works to achieve a fundamental paradigm shift in healthcare direction where Chiropractic is recognized as the most cost efficient and effective and accessible health regime to all people.

★ 2264 ★ CHOICE
1233 Locust St., Ste. 301
Philadelphia, PA 19107
Phone: (215)985-3355 **Fax:** (215)985-2838
Email: info@choice-phila.org
Website: http://www.choice-phila.org
Trina Johnston, Exec. Dir.

Fnded: 1971. **Desc:** Dedicated to increasing awareness of and access to sexual and reproductive health services, especially among underserved minority populations who experience barriers to care. **Pub:** *Changes: You and Your Body*, periodic. Directory. Directory of sexual and reproductive health services for teens. • *Where to Find*, periodic. Directory. Lists family planning services. *Price:* Free. **AKA:** Concern for Health Options - Information, Care and Education.

★ 2265 ★ Christian Addiction Rehabilitation Association (CARA)
c/o Dr. Robert A. Emberger
Whosoever Gospel Mission and Rescue Home
101 E Chelten Ave
Philadelphia, PA 19144
Website: http://www.iugm.org/cara.html
Dr. Bob Emberger, Contact
Fnded: 1967. **Mem:** 48. **Desc:** Provides support and serves as a clearinghouse of information for individuals involved in ministry to addicts. Conducts two conferences per year. **Pub:** Newsletter, monthly. *Price:* Free w/membership. **Frmly:** Christian Alcoholic Rehabilitation Association.

★ 2266 ★ Christian Association of Primetimers
PO Box 777
Saint Charles, IL 60174
Phone: (630)443-0050 **Free:** 800-443-0227
Fax: (630)444-0087
Email: email@christianprimetimers.org
Website: http://christianprimetimers.org
Roland Johnson, Pres.
Fnded: 1993. **Mem:** 40,000. **Desc:** Seeks to improve, encourage and provide a better quality of life to those ages 50 and older; offers discount travel and volunteer opportunities. **Pub:** *PrimeTimer Newsletter*, bimonthly. Newsletter. Provides updates on new benefits, travel opportunities, and CAP activities.

★ 2267 ★ Christian Association for Psychological Studies (CAPS)
c/o Dr. Randolph K. Sanders
PO Box 310400
New Braunfels, TX 78131-0400
Phone: (830)629-2277 **Fax:** (830)629-2342
Email: capsintl@compuvision.net
Website: http://www.caps.net
Dr. Randolph K. Sanders, PhD, Exec. Dir.
Fnded: 1956. **Mem:** 2,100. **Reg. Groups:** 7. **Local Groups:** 65. **Desc:** Psychologists, marriage and family therapists, social workers, educators, physicians, nurses, ministers, researchers, pastoral counselors, and rehabilitation workers and others professionally engaged in the fields of psychology, counseling, psychiatry, pastoring, and related areas. Association is based upon a genuine commitment to superior clinical, pastoral, and scientific enterprise in the theoretical and applied social sciences and theology, assuming persons in helping professions will be guided to professional and personal growth and a greater contribution to others in this way. Aims to help members cooperatively as Christians to explore the fields of psychology, pastoring, and psychotherapy for a better insight into personality and interpersonal relations and to articulate and promote the lordship of Christ in these scientific disciplines. **Pub:** *CAPS Report*, quarterly. Newsletter. Includes information on membership activities and schedule of events. *Price:* Free. • *Christian Monograph Series*, periodic. Monograph. • *International Directory of the Christian Association for Psychological Studies*, annual. Membership Directory. Arranged geographically, with separate listings for libraries. *Price:* $10. • *Journal of Psychology and Christianity*, quarterly. Journal. Contains articles on clinical and theoretical topics. Includes book reviews and professional employment opportunities. *Price:* Included in membership dues; $40/year for nonmembers; $50/year for libraries.

★ 2268 ★ Christian Blind Mission International (CBMI)
450 E Park Ave.
PO Box 19000
Greenville, SC 29601
Phone: (864)239-0065 **Free:** 800-YES-CBMI
Fax: (864)239-0069
Email: info@cbmi-usa.org
Website: http://www.cbmi-usa.org/
Alan Harkey, Dir.
Fnded: 1908. **Mem:** 7. **Nat'l Groups:** 12. **Desc:** Interdenominational Christian organization dedicated to service of the blind, visually impaired, and physically handicapped in more than 100 countries. Supports national activities of missions, churches, and voluntary organizations in developing countries with financial aid to cover operational expenses and the provision of equipment, drugs, medicines, and instruments. Fosters prevention of visually disabling ailments such as glaucoma, trachoma, and blinding cataracts. Assists in education and rehabilitation of all disabled indiviudals through establishment of vocational training centers and a corps of community volunteers to coordinate and stimulate project participation. Contributes to international efforts in the battle against blindness; conducts research on onchocerciasis, xerophthalmia, and glaucoma. Sponsors rural education programs on personal and environmental hygiene and nutrition. **Pub:** *CBMI Report*, annual. Report. • *Human Interest Stories*, monthly. • *Light*, quarterly. Newsletter.

★ 2269 ★ Christian Council on Persons with Disabilities (CCPD)
1100 W 42nd St., Ste. 223
Indianapolis, IN 46208
Phone: (317)923-2273 **Fax:** (317)923-2273
Email: info@ccpd.org
Website: http://www.ccpd.org/
LisaRose Hall, Exec. Dir.
Fnded: 1988. **Desc:** Christian disability advocacy organization promoting the spiritual well-being of people with physical, mental or emotional disabilities. **Pub:** *CCPD News*, quarterly. Newsletter. Contains information in the field of Christian disability ministry and developments in the U.S. and worldwide. Available in Braille and large print.

★ 2270 ★ Christian Dental Society (CDS)
PO Box 296
Sumner, IA 50674
Phone: (563)578-8887 **Fax:** (563)578-8887
Email: cdssent@iowatelecom.net
Website: http://www.christiandental.org
Jim Jespersen, DDS, contact
Fnded: 1962. **Mem:** 900. **Desc:** Encourages dentists to donate their professional services to Christian schools, clinics, and hospitals. Members also supply materials and equipment to missions. Maintains speakers' bureau. **Pub:** *CDS News Update*, monthly. Newsletter. • *CDS Newsletter*, quarterly. Newsletter. • *Portable Mission Dentistry*. **Frmly:** (1962) Presbyterian Missionary Committee.

★ 2271 ★ Christian Health Association of Kenya (CHAK)
PO Box 30690
Nairobi, Kenya
Phone: 254 20 441920 **Fax:** 254 20 440306
Email: chak@insightkenya.com
Fnded: 1930. **Mem:** 230. **Reg. Groups:** 4. **Lang(s):** English. **Desc:** Fosters improved health in Kenya through programs in health education. Compiles statistics on youth and population. Disseminates information. Organizes training courses in health, AIDS/HIV prevention, essential drugs program and family planning. Provides forum for members to network. Acts as advocate with the government Ministry of Health and donors on behalf of members. **Pub:** *AIDS for Health Workers*. Manuals. • *CHAK Quarterly News*, quarterly. Newsletter.

★ 2272 ★ Christian Medical Commission (Commission Medicale Chretienne — CMC)
CP 2100
CH-1211 Geneva, Switzerland
Phone: 41 22 916111 **Fax:** 41 22 7910361
Fnded: 1967.

★ 2273 ★ Christian Medical and Dental Associations (CMDA)
PO Box 7500
Bristol, TN 37621
Phone: (423)844-1000
Email: main@cmdahome.org
Website: http://www.cmdahome.org
David Stevens, MD, Exec. Dir.
Fnded: 1931. **Mem:** 15,000. **Reg. Groups:** 6. **Desc:** Serves as a voice and ministry for Christian doctors. Its mission is to "change the heart of healthcare." Promotes positions and addresses policies on health care issues; conducts overseas and domestic medical mission projects; coordinates a network of Christian doctors for fellowship and professional growth; sponsors student ministries in medical and dental schools; distributes educational and inspirational resources; holds marriage and family conferences; provides Third World missionary doctors with continuing education resources; and conducts academic exchange programs overseas. **Pub:** *Christian Doctor's Digest*, 8/year. Magazine. *Price:* included in membership dues. • *Today's Christian Doctor*, quarterly. Journal. Contains articles on medical and ethical issues. *Price:* Included in membership dues. • Brochure. • SCAN is distributed free to doctors serving in foreign countries; public service announcements - CMDS Healthwise (quarterly, CD format). **Frmly:** (1988) Christian Medical Society; (1998) Medical Group Missions of the Christian Medical and Dental Society; (2000) Christian Medical and Dental Society; (2000) Global Health Outreach of the Christian Medical and Dental Society.

★ 2274 ★ Christian Medical and Dental Society of Canada (CMDS)
30 5155 Spectrum Way
Mississauga, ON, Canada L4W 5A1
Phone: (905)625-4457 **Free:** 888-256-8653
Fax: (905)625-1812
Email: main@cmds-emas.ca
Website: http://www.cmds-emas.ca
Fnded: 1970. **Mem:** 1,450. **Reg. Groups:** 14. **Lang(s):** English, French. **Desc:** Christian physicians, dentists, and medical and dental students. Seeks to present "a positive witness of God our Father and our Saviour, Jesus Christ, to the medical and dental professions and to the recipients of health care." Serves as a Christian voice within the medical community and before government agencies, medical and dental associations, policy makers, and patients. Facilitates communication among members; makes available to members opportunities for overseas voluntary service; sponsors social and fellowship activities. **Pub:** *Focus*, 3/year. Magazine. • *NUCLEUS*, quarterly. Journal. • *Spotlight*, periodic. Newsletter.

★ 2275 ★ Christian Medical Foundation International (CMF)
730 Emma St.
PO Box 152136
Tampa, FL 33684-2136
Phone: (813)932-3688 **Fax:** (813)232-4745
Email: cmfintl@aol.com
Website: http://www.wwmedical.com/cmf/
William S. Reed, MD, MS, Pres.
Fnded: 1962. **Mem:** 4,854. **State Groups:** 4. **Desc:** Physicians, nurses, clergy, and laity. Seeks to: investigate and promote the Christian spiritual care of those who are ill; educate doctors, nurses, and medical students regarding Christian medical and ethical principles. Maintains speakers' bureau, placement service, biographical archives, and 2500 volume library; sponsors charitable programs. **Pub:** *Progress Notes*, bimonthly. • Also publishes books and monographs.

★ 2276 ★ Christian Overcomers (CO)
c/o Debbie Neillyh
PO Box 2007
Garfield, NJ 07026
Phone: (973)253-2343 **Fax:** (973)253-2351
Website: http://www.gracechurchweb.org/missions/missionaries/overcomers.htm
Debbie Neilley, Exec. Dir.
Fnded: 1977. **Desc:** Individuals with physical disabilities and volunteers. Provides holistic physical and spiritual guidance to help members live with their disabilities. Sponsors camp program that provides

Bible study, worship, recreational and social activities, and encourages "commitment to Jesus Christ and each other." Functions as a resource for local groups that wish to conduct activities including athletic events, outings, dinners, and other socially oriented educational programs for physically disabled individuals. Maintains speakers' bureau. Provides volunteer training. **Pub:** *Library Catalog*, annual. Catalog. • *The Overcomer*, quarterly. Newsletter. • Brochure.

★ 2277 ★ Christian Pharmacists Fellowship International (CPFI)
PO Box 1717
501 5th St.
Bristol, TN 37621-1717
Phone: (423)764-6000 **Free:** 888-253-6885
Fax: (423)764-4490
Email: info@cpfi.org
Website: http://www.cpfi.org
Allan Sharp, P.D., Admin. Dir.

Fnded: 1984. **Mem:** 1,200. **Reg. Groups:** 3. **State Groups:** 3. **Local Groups:** 7. **Desc:** To promote and maintain fellowship among Christian pharmacists. Establishes clubs and chapters at universities, colleges, schools, hospitals, and in communities; sponsors activities and retreats for Christian pharmacists and their families. Encourages active Christian witness and evangelism; teaches pharmacists how to share and present the Gospel of Jesus Christ in their practice; disseminates information among Christian pharmacists; identifies areas of service for pharmacists in missions worldwide and sponsors missionaries in the field. Provides and promotes Christian pharmacist-speakers. speakers at state and national pharmacy meetings. **Pub:** *Christian Pharmacists Fellowship International–Newsletter*, bimonthly. Newsletter. Reports on the activities of members and the fellowship, as well as Christian events in pharmacy. Includes book reviews and directory. *Price:* Free. • *Christianity and Pharmacy*. Journal. Official journal of chrisitian Pharmacists Fellowship International. • Membership Directory, biennial.

★ 2278 ★ Christian Record Services (CRS)
4444 S 52nd St.
Lincoln, NE 68516-1302
Phone: (402)488-0981 **Fax:** (402)488-7582
Email: info@christianrecord.org
Website: http://www.christianrecord.org
Ron Bowes, Contact

Fnded: 1899. **Desc:** Assists blind, visually impaired individuals. Sponsors Bible correspondence courses. Representatives visit about 40,000 blind people annually. Conducts glaucoma screening clinics in cooperation with local physicians and organizations; provides home visitation program. Sponsors National Camps for Blind Children; maintains speakers' bureau. **Pub:** *Christian Record*, quarterly. In braille; for adults. • *Christian Record Talking Magazine*, quarterly. Magazine. On cassette; for adults. • *Encounter*, bimonthly. On cassette; for late teens and adults. • *Lifeglow*, quarterly. In large print; for adults. • *The Student*, monthly. In braille and on cassette. • *Young and Alive*, quarterly. In braille and large print; for teenagers/young adults. • Also publishes braille cards. **Frmly:** Christian Record Benevolent Association; (1989) Christian Record Braille Foundation.

★ 2279 ★ Christian Record Services (CRS)
1300 King St. E, Ste. 119
Oshawa, ON, Canada L1H 8N9
Phone: (905)436-6938 **Fax:** (905)436-7102
Email: crs-ncb@oix.com
Website: http://www.crsblindservices.ca

Fnded: 1899. **Lang(s):** English, French. **Desc:** Volunteers. Seeks to "enrich the lives of blind, deaf, and physically handicapped individuals." Provides services including reading, braille materials and personal visitations to people with physical disabilities. Maintains National Camps for the Blind; conducts educational programs to raise public awareness on meeting the needs of blind people. **Pub:** *NCB News*, annual. Newsletter. • Brochure.

★ 2280 ★ Christian Services for the Blind
1124 Fair Oaks Ave.
PO Box 26
South Pasadena, CA 91031-0026
Phone: (626)799-3935 **Free:** 888-511-3935
Fax: (626)403-9460
Email: frank@csbonline.org
Website: http://www.csbonline.org
Dr. Franklin D. Tucker, Exec. Dir.

Fnded: 1949. **Nat'l Groups:** 1. **Local Groups:** 1. **Desc:** Makes available books on cassette for blind and braille books for deaf-blind individuals. **Pub:** *Bartimaeus Review*, 3/year. Newsletter. *Price:* Free. **Frmly:** Christian Fellowship for the Blind.

★ 2281 ★ Christian Veterinary Missions of Canada (CVM Canada)
PO Box 31059
Guelph, ON, Canada N1H 8K1
Phone: (905)304-6146
Email: cvandij@attglobal.net
Website: http://www.cvmcanada.org/

Desc: Committed to the empowerment of veterinarians, technicians and veterinary students to Christian ministry through veterinary profession.

★ 2282 ★ Christina Noble Children's Foundation - Vietnam (CNF)
PO Box 386
Saigon Post Office Centre
Ho Chi Minh City, Vietnam
Phone: 84 8 9326484 **Fax:** 84 8 9327276
Email: vietnan@cncf.org
Website: http://www.cncf.org

Fnded: 1991. **Desc:** Individuals interested in child health. Seeks to improve the quality of life of children in Vietnam. Makes available primary health care services; conducts nutrition programs; sponsors educational and vocational training programs. Maintains center for abandoned children.

★ 2283 ★ Christoffel Blindenmission (CBM)
Nibelungenstr. 124
D-64625 Bensheim, Germany
Phone: 49 6251 131131 **Fax:** 49 6251 131122
Email: overseas@cbm-i.org
Website: http://www.christoffel-blindenmission.de

Fnded: 1908. **Mem:** 60. **Lang(s):** English, French, German, Spanish. **Desc:** Seeks to prevent and cure blindness and improve the quality of life for blind and partially sighted people. Represents the interests of visually impaired people; works to combat discrimination. Seeks to educate and rehabilitate blind and other handicapped persons. **Pub:** *Blickkontakt*, bimonthly. Magazine. • *Freundesbrief*, quarterly. Newsletter. **Frmly:** Christian Blind Mission International.

★ 2284 ★ Christopher Reeve Paralysis Foundation
500 Morris Ave.
Springfield, NJ 07081
Phone: (973)379-2690 **Free:** 800-225-0292
Fax: (973)912-9433
Website: http://www.christopherreeve.org
David R. Landrey, Chair/Exec. Committee

Fnded: 1982. **Nat'l Groups:** 1. **Reg. Groups:** 1. **Desc:** Seeks to encourage and support research to find a cure for paralysis caused by spinal cord injury and other central nervous system disorders. **Pub:** *American Paralysis Association Progress in Research*, semiannual. Newsletter. • *Annual Review*. • *Progress in Research*, 2-3/year. • *Walking Tomorrow*, semiannual. Newsletter. **Frmly:** (1981) Kent Waldrep International Spinal Cord Research Foundation; (2002) American Paralysis Association.

★ 2285 ★ Chromosome Deletion Outreach (CDO)
c/o Linda Sorg
PO Box 724
Boca Raton, FL 33429-0724
Phone: (561)395-4252 **Fax:** (561)395-4252
Email: lindasorg@hotmail.com
Website: http://www.chromodisorder.org
Linda Sorg, Contact

Fnded: 1992. **Mem:** 1,800. **Desc:** Promotes research and understanding of chromosome disorders, including partial duplications (trisomies), inversions, translocations, rings and sex chromosome disorders; provides support to families of children born with these rare disorders; gathers and disseminates information; promotes research and a positive community understanding of these disorders. **Pub:** *Chromosome Deletion Outreach*, quarterly. Newsletter. Contains articles submitted by members and a column offering advice from doctors. *Price:* included in membership dues.

★ 2286 ★ Chromosome 18 Registry and Research Society
c/o Jannine D. Cody
6302 Fox Head
San Antonio, TX 78247
Phone: (210)657-4968 **Fax:** (210)657-4968
Email: office@chromosome18.org
Website: http://www.chromosome18.org
Jannine Cody, PhD, Pres.

Fnded: 1990. **Mem:** 500. **Reg. Groups:** 12. **Desc:** Individuals with the chromosome 18 disorder, their families, and physicians. (Chromosome 18 anomalies cover a wide range of disorders, including: Trisomy 18, 18q-, 18p-, and Ring 18.) Purposes are: to locate persons with chromosome 18 anomalies; to educate the families, as well as the public about the prognoses and treatments of these disorders; to encourage, conduct, and publish research into areas that impact these families; and to link affected families and their physicians to the research community. Offers educational programs. **Pub:** *Chromosome 18 Communique*, quarterly. Newsletter. • Brochure.

★ 2287 ★ Chromosome 9P Network (9P)
393 N Grass Valley Rd.
Pine Valley, UT 84781
Phone: (435)574-1121 **Fax:** (435)574-2000
Email: beverly.udell@9pminus.org
Website: http://www.9pminus.org
Beverly Udell, Pres.

Fnded: 1984. **Mem:** 210. **Desc:** Parents and caregivers of children that have Monosomy 9P (also known as 9P-; Alfi's Syndrome; Ring 9; 9PDeletion; Trisomy 9P). Offers support to families. (Monosomy 9P is a rare chromosome disorder in which a piece of the 9th chromosome pair is broken off. It results in mental retardation, physical deformity, and triganocephaly of the forehead.) Acts as a clearinghouse for information on the disorder. Maintains a roster of families having a child with Monosomy 9P. Partakes in research, and holds an annual conference. **Pub:** Newsletter, quarterly. • Brochures. **Frmly:** (1999) Support Groups for Monosomy 9P.

★ 2288 ★ Chronic Fatigue Syndrome Association (Associazione Italiana Sindrome da Fatica Cronica)
Via Pedemontana Occidentale, 12
I-33081 Aviano, Italy
Phone: 39 0434660277 **Fax:** 39 0434659531
Email: cfs@cro.it

Fnded: 1991. **Desc:** Major tasks are: to create awareness and understanding that CFS is a very real, and for many, a very debilitating illness; to publicise and create awareness of the consequences of living with CFS for the sufferer and relatives and to highlight their needs.

★ 2289 ★ Chronic Granulomatous Disease Association
c/o Mary Hurley
2616 Monterey Rd.
San Marino, CA 91108-1646
Phone: (626)441-4118
Email: cgda@socal.rr.com
Website: http://www.cgdassociation.org
Mary Hurley, Pres.

Fnded: 1982. **Desc:** Seeks to improve the quality of life of people with chronic granulomatous disease (CGD) and their families (CGD is characterized by the presence of multiple granulomas, or nodular inflammatory lesions). Provides support and services to people with CGD; assists in the formation of support networks for people with CGD; maintains international registry of CGD patients; compiles statistics. **Pub:** Newsletter, semiannual. • Brochures.

★ 2290 ★ Chronic Pain Support Group (CPSG)
PO Box 148
Peninsula, OH 44264
Email: cps.group@cpsg.22n.com
Website: http://www.chronicpainsupport.org/
Raggedy Anne, Contact

Fnded: 1985. **Desc:** Individuals suffering from chronic pain and their families and friends. Provides a forum for pain sufferers to help themselves through communication with other members. Promotes public awareness of chronic pain and its victims; encourages medical research on causes and treatments. Operates speakers' bureau; conducts educational programs. **Pub:** *Stop Pain*, monthly. Newsletter. Covers coping skills. *Price:* $25/year.

★ 2291 ★ Churches Medical Council (CMC)
PO Box 3269
Boroko, Papua New Guinea
Phone: 675 3252362 **Fax:** 675 3013898
Email: cmcpng@datron.com.pg

Fnded: 1960. **Mem:** 24. **Nat'l Groups:** 1. **Reg. Groups:** 4. **State Groups:** 18. **Lang(s):** English. **Desc:** Health care programs and services operated by religious organizations. Promotes effective delivery of health care to previously underserved populations. Facilitates communication and cooperation among members. Sponsors public health and educational programs; makes available health services.

★ 2292 ★ Citizen Advocacy Center (CAC)
1400 16th St. NW, Ste. 330
Washington, DC 20036
Phone: (202)462-1174 **Fax:** (202)265-6564
Website: http://www.cacenter.org/
David A. Swankin, Pres.

Desc: Provides training and support for public members serving on health care regulatory agencies, governing boards, advisory bodies representing consumer interests. **Pub:** *Citizen Advocacy News & Views*. • Reports.

★ 2293 ★ Citizens Alliance for VD Awareness (CAVDA)
Ste. 128
800 W Central Rd.
Mount Prospect, IL 60056
Phone: (847)398-3378 **Fax:** (847)398-7309
Email: cavdarx@earthlink.net
Howard A. Mirsky, Pres.

Fnded: 1972. **Mem:** 125. **Desc:** Businessmen, corporations, social service agencies, public health agencies, physicians, nurses, and pharmacists. Provides information to the public, especially to high incidence groups, about symptoms, treatment, and prevention of sexually transmitted diseases, including AIDS (acquired immune deficiency syndrome). Seeks to increase commitment of health professionals and the public to venereal disease and AIDS control. Conducts demonstrations, public service messages, and surveys. **Pub:** *STD Spotlight: Dedicated to Thought and Activity in STD Information-Education Programs*, quarterly. Newsletter. *Price:* $30/year. • Pamphlets. • Also publishes fact sheets.

★ 2294 ★ Citizens for Health
5 Thomas Cir., NW, Ste. 500
Washington, DC 20005
Free: 800-357-2211
Email: info@citizens.org
Website: http://www.citizens.org
Jim Turner, Chm.

Fnded: 1992. **Local Groups:** 150. **Desc:** Committed to protecting and expanding consumers natural health choices. Initiates and monitors legislation with the goal of ensuring access to health information and the freedom to choose from a broad range of health options. **Pub:** *Action Alert*, periodic. Bulletin. • *FAX Hotline*. • *The Natural Activist*, bimonthly. Newsletter. *Price:* Included in full member dues.

★ 2295 ★ Citizens for Midwifery
PO Box 82227
Athens, GA 30608
Free: 888-CFM-4880
Email: info@cfmidwifery.org
Website: http://www.cfmidwifery.org

Fnded: 1996. **Desc:** Works to ensure that the Midwives Model of Care is available to all childbearing women and recognized as best care for pregnancy and birth; endorses Mother-Friendly Childbirth Initiative. **Pub:** Newsletter.*Price:* included in membership dues; $15 for nonmembers.

★ 2296 ★ City of Hope National Medical Center (COH)
1500 E Duarte Rd.
Duarte, CA 91010
Phone: (626)359-8111 **Free:** 800-826-HOPE
Fax: (626)301-8115
Email: egoehner@coh.org
Website: http://www.cityofhope.org
Elaine Goehner, Contact

Fnded: 1913. **Desc:** This center and Beckman Research Institute is an innovative biomedical research, treatment, and educationl institution, dedicated to the prevention and cure of cancer, diabetes, HIV/AIDS and other life-threatening diseases. Guided by a "compassionate patient-centered philosophy". Has 244 chartered auxiliaries in 163 cities, donations from top corporations, national foundations, philanthropic agencies, industries, celebrities and individuals in every state of the nation. **Pub:** *Chapters*, biennial. Magazine. • *City News*, quarterly. Magazine. • *eHope*, monthly. Newsletter. Delivered through email. **Frmly:** (2003) City of Hope.

★ 2297 ★ CityMatch
c/o Magda G. Peck
University of Nebraska Medical Center
Department of Pediatrics
982170 Nebraska Medical Center
Omaha, NE 68198-2170
Phone: (402)561-7500 **Fax:** (402)561-7525
Email: citymch@unmc.edu
Website: http://www.citymatch.org/
Magda G. Peck, SC.D., Exec. Dir. /CEO

Fnded: 1989. **Mem:** 142. **Nat'l Groups:** 11. **Reg. Groups:** 10. **Local Groups:** 11. **Desc:** City and county health departments, leaders representing urban communities in the United States, and interested others. Seeks to provide optimal health care for children and families in urban areas. Gives particular attention to increasing racial disparities in infant mortality, inadequate access to prenatal care, substance abuse in pregnancy, and interpersonal violence. Provides children's services; compiles statistics. **Pub:** *CityLights*, quarterly. Newsletter. • *Technical Reports.* • *What Works: 1990 Urban MCH Programs.* Directory. Maternal and Child health programs in major urban health departments.

★ 2298 ★ Civil Aviation Medical Association (CAMA)
PO Box 23864
Oklahoma City, OK 73123-3864
Phone: (405)840-0199 **Fax:** (405)848-1053
Email: jmlharris@aol.com
Website: http://www.civilavmed.com
Robin Dodge, MD, Pres.

Fnded: 1948. **Mem:** 800. **Desc:** Aviation medical examiners, physicians who are pilots, aviation medical educators, flight instructors, fixed base operators, NASA physicians, and airline medical department physicians. Purposes are to: ascertain the basic mental and physical requirements of civil airmen and the proper methods for the physical assessment of airmen engaged in civil aviation; review continuously the scientific status of civil aviation medicine and advance and disseminate the information by which civil aviation medicine safeguards public safety; sponsor basic and advanced training in civil aviation medicine; foster international fellowship among members, allied medical and technical groups, and students of aviation medicine; unite the designated civil aviation medical examiners of the world into an effective medical body dedicated to the promotion and practice of aviation safety for the public benefit. Maintains speakers' bureau; compiles statistics. **Pub:** *FlightPhysician*, every other month. Newsletter. Covers membership activities. Contains meetings calendar and promotion of members and medical information on all topics relative to aviation medicine. *Price:* $5/issue. **Frmly:** (1955) Airline Medical Examiners Association.

★ 2299 ★ Clearinghouse on Disability Information (CDI)
Office of Special Educ. and Rehabilitative Services
Switzer Bldg., Rm. 3132
Washington, DC 20202-2524
Phone: (202)205-8241 **Fax:** (202)401-2608
Website: http://www.health.gov/nhic/NHICScripts/Entry.cfm?RCode=hR0035
Carolyn Corlett, Tech. Asst.

Fnded: 1973. **Desc:** Responds to inquiries on topics concerning federally-funded programs serving disabled persons and federal legislation affecting the disabled community. Researches and documents information providers serving the handicapped. Makes resource referrals. **Pub:** *Pocket Guide to Federal Help for Individuals With Disabilities*. **Frmly:** (1989) Clearinghouse on the Handicapped.

★ 2300 ★ Cleft Lip and Palate Association (CLPA)
235-237 Finchley Rd.
London NW3 6LS, United Kingdom
Phone: 44 20 74310033 **Fax:** 44 20 74318881
Email: info@clapa.fsnet.co.uk
Website: http://www.clapa.com/

Fnded: 1979. **Reg. Groups:** 60. **Lang(s):** English. **Desc:** Local groups comprising parents of children with cleft lips or palates and health care professionals. Seeks to improve treatment of cleft lips and palates; promotes an improved quality of life for children with cleft lips and palates. Provides support to children with cleft lips and palates and their parents; supports research into the causes and treatment of cleft lips and palates; conducts educational programs; undertakes fundraising campaigns. Maintains specialist service for parents having difficulty feeding children with cleft lips or palates. **Pub:** Pamphlets.

★ 2301 ★ Cleft Lip and Palate Association of Ireland (CLAPAI)
c/o Ms. Libby O'Brien, Hon.Sec.
Station Rd.
Ballyshannon, Donegal, Ireland
Phone: 353 72 58026
Email: dulaing@cleft.ie
Website: http://www.cleft.ie/

Desc: Provides support and information for parents and children affected by cleft lip and palate; provides support to new parents and advice on feeding and ongoing medical care throughout treatment.

★ 2302 ★ Cleft Palate Foundation
104 S Estes Dr., Ste. 204
Chapel Hill, NC 27514-2866
Phone: (919)933-9044 **Free:** 800-242-5338
Fax: (919)933-9604
Email: info@cleftline.org
Website: http://www.cleftline.org
Nancy C. Smythe, Exec. Dir.

Fnded: 1973. **Desc:** Enhances the quality of life for individuals with facial birth defects through education, research support, and facilitation of family-centered care. Provides research programs and information services. **Pub:** *As You Get Older: Information for the Teenager Born with a Cleft Lip and/or Palate*. Booklet. *Price:* 2.00. • *Audiovisual & Supplemental Resource Catalog*. Catalog. • *Cleft Lip and Cleft Palate: The First Four Years*. Booklet. *Price:* $2.00. • *Cleft Lip and Cleft Palate - The School-Aged Child*. Booklet. *Price:* $2.00. • *Cleft Lip & Palate: The Adult Patient*. Booklet. • *Cleft Palate-Craniofacial Journal*, bimonthly. Journal. • *Cleft Palate & Hearing Loss*. Booklet. • *Cleft Surgery*. Booklet. • *Feeding an Infant with a Cleft*. Booklet. • *For Parents of Newborn Babies with Cleft Lip/Palate*. Brochure. *Price:* $.25. • *The Genetics of Cleft Lip and Palate: Information for Families*. Booklet. *Price:* $2.00. • *Hemangiomas & Vascular Malformations*. Booklet. • *Information About Choosing a Cleft Palate or Craniofacial Team*. *Price:* Free. • *Information About Choosing a Cleft Palate or Craniofacial Team*. • *Information About Crouzon's Disease*. *Price:* Free. • *Information About Dental Care*. *Price:* Free. • *Information about Dental Care*. • *Information About Financial Assistance*. *Price:* Free. • *Information About Pierre Robin Malformation Sequence*. *Price:* Free. • *Information About Submucous Cleft Palate*. *Price:* Free. • *Information About Teacher Collins Syndrome*. *Price:* Free. • *Information About Treatment for Adults with Cleft Lip and Palate*. *Price:* Free. • *Parameters for Evaluation and Treatment of Patients with Cleft Lip/Palate or other Craniofacial Conditions*. **Frmly:** (2000) American Cleft Palate Educational Foundation.

★ 2303 ★ Clerkship Directors of Internal Medicine (CDIM)
2501 M St. NW, Ste. 550
Washington, DC 20037-1308
Phone: (202)861-8600 **Fax:** (202)861-9731
Email: cdim@im.org
Website: http://www.im.org/cdim/
Julia Pearson, Membership Asst.

Desc: Promotes education in the core clerkship in internal medicine at accredited medical schools in the U.S., Puerto Rico, and Canada. **Pub:** *CDIM News*. • Membership Directory.

★ 2304 ★ Clinical Cytometry Society (CCS)
PO Box 25456
Colorado Springs, CO 80936
Phone: (719)590-1620 **Fax:** (719)590-1619
Email: admin@cytometry.org
Website: http://www.cytometry.org/

Desc: Fosters the development and implementation of cytometry in relation to human pathology. **Pub:** *Clinical Cytometry*, bimonthly. Journal. • Newsletter.

★ 2305 ★ Clinical Dental Technicians Association
7 The Studios
The Row
New Ash Green
Longfield DA3 8JL, United Kingdom
Phone: 44 1474 879430 **Fax:** 44 1474 872086
Email: cdta@btinternet.com
Website: http://www.cdta.org.uk

Fnded: 1950. **Mem:** 115. **Desc:** Dental technicians seeking legal status in the United Kingdom to train and qualify to make and fit dentures directly with the public under Act of Parliament. **Pub:** *The Denturist*, monthly. Newsletter. **Frmly:** Association for Denture Prosthesis.

★ 2306 ★ Clinical Directors Network (CDN)
54 W 39TH St Fl 11
New York, NY 10018-3808
Phone: (212)382-0699 **Fax:** (212)382-0669
Email: info@cdnetwork.org
Website: http://www.cdnetwork.org
Jonathan N. Tobin, Exec. Dir.

Fnded: 1985. **Mem:** 15. **Desc:** Provides clinical leaders and staff at community, migrant, HIV and homeless health centers with educational meetings and peer support activities. Also, improves access of minority communities to clinical research. **Pub:** Annual Report, annual. • Brochure, annual.

★ 2307 ★ Clinical Genetics Society (CGS)
c/o British Society for Human Genetics
Birmingham Women's Hospital
Edgabston
Birmingham B15 2TF, United Kingdom
Email: bshg@bshg.org.uk
Website: http://www.bshg.org.uk

Fnded: 1970.

★ 2308 ★ Clinical Immunology Society (CIS)
611 E Wells St.
Milwaukee, WI 53202
Phone: (414)224-8095 **Fax:** (414)272-6070
Email: cis@execinc.com
Website: http://www.clinimmsoc.org
Lynda J. Patterson, CAE, Exec. Dir.

Fnded: 1986. **Mem:** 840. **Desc:** Investigators and clinicians concerned with immunologic diseases. Promotes research on: the causes and mechanisms of immunologic diseases; improved treatment, evaluation, and prevention of diseases related to immunity. Facilitates exchange of ideas and findings; fosters excellence in research and medical practice. Works to increase public awareness and knowledge of immunologically-mediated diseases. Conducts scientific, educational programs. **Pub:** *Clinical Immunology*, monthly. Journal. *Price:* Included with membership.

★ 2309 ★ Clinical Laboratory Management Association (CLMA)
989 Old Eagle School Rd., Ste. 815
Wayne, PA 19087
Phone: (610)995-9580 **Fax:** (610)995-9568
Email: rneri@lcma.org
Website: http://www.clma.org
Robert A. Neri, Exec. VP

Fnded: 1976. **Mem:** 6,500. **Nat'l Groups:** 90. **Local Groups:** 103. **Desc:** Individuals holding managerial or supervisory positions with clinical laboratories; persons engaged in education of such individuals; manufacturers or distributors of equipment or services to clinical laboratories. Objectives are: to enhance management skills and promote more efficient and productive department operations; to further exchange of professional knowledge, new technology, and colleague experience; to encourage cooperation among those engaged in management or supervisory functions. Activities include: workshops, seminars, and expositions; dissemination of information about legislation and other topics. **Pub:** *Clinical Laboratory Management Association–Membership Directory*, annual. Directory. Arranged alphabetically and geographically. *Price:* Included in membership dues, online for members. • *Clinical Laboratory Management Review*, bimonthly. Journal. Covers concepts and techniques of management and issues and trends in health care that affect the clinical laboratory. *Price:* Included in membership dues; $130/year for nonmembers; $176/year for U.S. institutions. • *CLMA Vantage Point*, monthly. Newsletter. Contains articles on time management, employee performance appraisals, selecting a laboratory, information system and communication skills. *Price:* Included in membership dues. **Frmly:** (1976) American Association of Clinical Laboratory Supervisors and Administrators.

★ 2310 ★ Clinical Ligand Assay Society (CLAS)
3139 S Wayne Rd.
Wayne, MI 48184
Phone: (734)722-6290 **Fax:** (734)722-7006
Email: clas@clas.org
Website: http://www.clas.org
Daisy S. McCann, PhD, Exec. Dir.

Fnded: 1976. **Mem:** 400. **Nat'l Groups:** 1. **Reg. Groups:** 12. **State Groups:** 8. **Desc:** Seeks to establish and promote high standards in the science and application of ligand assay technology by encouraging research, education practitioners, and fostering communication and cooperation among individuals in laboratories in medicine, academia, and industry. Sponsors job placement service. **Pub:** *Journal of Clinical Ligand Assay*, quarterly. Journal. Contains reviews and articles on clinical ligand assay techniques. Includes bibliography of recent articles and manufacturers' directory. *Price:* Included in membership dues. • Directory, biennial. • Also publishes syllabi for annual meeting, and a newsletter. **Frmly:** (1981) Clincial Radioassay Society.

★ 2311 ★ Clinical Magnetic Resonance Society (CMRS)
4550 Post Oak Pl., Ste. 342
Houston, TX 77027
Phone: (713)623-8336 **Free:** 877-841-2522
Fax: (713)960-0488
Email: cmrs@one.net
Website: http://www.cmrs.com
Darcee Brown, Acct. Exec.

Fnded: 1995. **Mem:** 1,000. **Desc:** Offers experience-based credentialing for physicians who practice MRI. Provides a forum for networking among members. Defines procedure protocols and safety information. **Pub:** *CMRS Vision*, quarterly. Newsletter. Contains information on new developments in magnetic resonance imaging. *Price:* included in membership dues.

★ 2312 ★ Clinical Orthopaedic Society (COS)
PO Box 531823
Indianapolis, IN 46253-1823
Phone: (317)388-0329 **Free:** 800-843-9735
Fax: (317)388-8984
Email: clinicalorthosoc@aol.com
Website: http://www.cosociety.org
J. Donald Opgrande, MD, Pres.

Fnded: 1912. **Mem:** 700. **Desc:** Orthopedic surgeons practicing in cities of the Midwest. **Pub:** Directory, annual.

★ 2313 ★ Clinical Pathology Accreditation
45 Rutland Park
Botanical Gardens
Sheffield S10 2PB, United Kingdom
Phone: 44 114 2515800 **Fax:** 44 114 2515801
Email: office@cpa-uk.co.uk
Website: http://www.cpa-uk.co.uk/

Fnded: 1992. **Desc:** Provides a means to accredit clinical pathology services, including external audits and peer review.

★ 2314 ★ Clowns Without Borders
Payasos Sin Fronteras
c/Roser, 74
08004 Barcelona, Spain
Phone: 34 93 3248420 **Fax:** 34 93 4412099
Email: coordinacion@clowns.org
Website: http://www.clowns.org

Fnded: 1993. **Mem:** 700. **Desc:** Seeks to improve the psychological condition of populations living in refugee camps and areas of conflict, by organising volunteer artist preformances and sociocultural workshops; and to raise our society's awareness of the situation of affected populations and to promote a spirit of solidarity.

★ 2315 ★ Co-Anon Family Groups
PO Box 12722
Tucson, AZ 85732
Free: 800-898-9985
Email: info@co-anon.org
Website: http://www.co-anon.org/

Fnded: 1985. **Nat'l Groups:** 28. **Desc:** Spouses, relatives, and friends of people who are chemically dependent. Seeks to help individuals affected by another's cocaine addiction by applying the Twelve Steps and Twelve Traditions of Alcoholics Anonymous. Assists in the formation of Co-Anon groups. **Pub:** Brochure.

★ 2316 ★ Coalition for Education and Self-help Training Advocates (C'esta)
c/o John-Paul LeBlanc
52 Faith Ln.
PO Box 6368
Manchester, NH 03108-6368
Phone: (603)627-5656 **Fax:** (603)679-4693
John-Paul LeBlanc, Pres. -Dir.

Fnded: 1993. **Desc:** Disabled individuals, their families, and advocates. Provides public, educational, and information services. Strives to help increase independent skills regardless of disability. **Pub:** Newsletter, monthly. *Price:* Free. • Journal, annual. *Price:* Free.

★ 2317 ★ Coalition For Heritable Disorders Of Connective Tissue
23 Mountain Rd.
Sharon, MA 02067
Phone: (781)784-6672
Email: info@chdct.org
Website: http://www.chdct.org
Sharon Terry, Pres.

Fnded: 1989. **Desc:** Strives to bring about greater awareness of heritable disorders of connective tissue in the medical professions and in the public; encourages teaching about these conditions in medical schools; encourages the training of health practitioners to identify, diagnose and treat various heritable connective tissue disorders; fosters research.

★ 2318 ★ Coalition for Healthy Korean Americans (COHKA)
196 Harvard Ave., Ste. 4
Allston, MA 02134
Email: sonnykim@cohka.org

Desc: Promotes better health through education. Health care services include cancer screening and dental care. Also offers health insurance, HIV prevention, immunization, and smoking cessation programs.

★ 2319 ★ Coalition of National Health Education Organizations (CNHEO)
c/o Ellen M. Capwell, PhD, CHES
Otterbein College
Department of Health & Physical Education
Rike Center
Westerville, OH 43081
Phone: (614)823-3535 **Fax:** (614)823-1965
Email: ecapwell@otterbein.edu
Website: http://hsc.usf.edu/CFH/cnheo/
Ellen M. Capwell, PhD, Coordinator

Fnded: 1972. **Mem:** 9. **Desc:** Nine national health education organizations, each represented by a delegate and an alternate. Facilitates coordination, collaboration and communication among the member organizations, to identify and discuss profession wide issues. Formulates recommendations, takes appropriate action, communicates information to the health education field, and serves as a focus for collaborative initiatives.

★ 2320 ★ Coalition for Nonprofit Health Care Research and Development (CNHCRD)
c/o T.J. Sullivan
1301 K St. NW, Ste. 900E
Washington, DC 20005-3317
Phone: (202)230-5070 **Fax:** (202)230-5570
Email: info@cnhc.org
Website: http://www.cnhc.org
James W. Varnum, Ch.

Fnded: 1997. **Mem:** 27. **Desc:** Nonprofit health care institutions and systems. Seeks to "ensure the continued survival of a primarily nonprofit, tax exempt health care delivery system." Works to improve communication between health care providers, plans, community organizations, and government agencies. Conducts grass roots public education programs; sponsors advocacy campaigns; undertakes research projects. **Pub:** *Coalition for Nonprofit Health Care.* Brochure.

★ 2321 ★ Cocaine Anonymous World Services (CAWS)
3740 Overland Ave., Ste. C
Los Angeles, CA 90034
Phone: (310)559-5833 **Free:** 800-347-8998
Fax: (310)559-2554
Email: cawso@ca.org
Website: http://www.ca.org
Mary Hukill, Dir. of Operations

Fnded: 1982. **Mem:** 15,000. **Reg. Groups:** 2000. **Desc:** Fellowship of men and women who share their experience, strength, and hope with each other that they may solve their common problem and help others to recover from addiction, remaining free from cocaine and all other mind-altering drugs. Applies the Alcoholics Anonymous World Services' 12-step approach to persons addicted to cocaine. **Pub:** *A Guide to the Twelve Steps.* Pamphlet. *Price:* $.15. • *A Higher Power.* Pamphlet. *Price:* $.15. • *And All Other Mind Altering Substances.* Pamphlet. *Price:* $.15. • *Choosing Your Sponsor.* Pamphlet. *Price:* $.15. • *Crack.* Pamphlet. *Price:* $.15. • *The First 30 Days.* Pamphlet. *Price:* $.15. • *Hope, Faith, and Courage.* Book. *Price:* $12.95 hard cover; $9.95 soft cover. • *The Newsgram,* quarterly. Newsletter. *Price:* Free. • *Self Test for Cocaine Addiction.* Pamphlet. *Price:* $.15. • *Suggestions for Relapse Prevention and Recovery.* Pamphlet. *Price:* $.15. • *Tips on Staying Clean and Sober.* Pamphlet. *Price:* $.15. • *To the Newcomer.* Pamphlet. *Price:* $.15. • *Tools of Recovery.* Pamphlet. *Price:* $.15. • *What Is C.A.?.* Pamphlet. *Price:* $.15.

★ 2322 ★ Cochlear Implant Association
5335 Wisconsin Ave. NW, Ste. 440
Washington, DC 20015-2052
Phone: (202)895-2781 **Fax:** (202)895-2782
Email: info@cici.org
Website: http://www.cici.org
John McCelland, Pres.

Fnded: 1981. **Mem:** 1,500. **Local Groups:** 38. **Desc:** Cochlear implant users, candidates for cochlear implant, and their families and friends; and health care professionals. Provides support services including advocacy for the hearing impaired. Promotes improved cochlear implant technology and research on hearing impairment. Serves as an information clearinghouse. Conducts educational programs and childrens' services; operates speakers' bureau. **Pub:** *Contact,* quarterly. Magazine. Covers current research, legislation, insurance issues, association activities, and coping advice. *Price:* Included in membership dues.

★ 2323 ★ Coeliac Society of Ireland
4 N Brunswick
Carmichael House
Dublin 7, Ireland
Phone: 353 1 8721471
Email: coeliac@iol.ie
Website: http://www.coeliac.ie

Fnded: 1970. **Mem:** 2,500. **Reg. Groups:** 8. **State Groups:** 1. **Desc:** Promotes, safeguards, and protects the interests of our members in relation to coeliac disease. Produces a list of gluten free foods, information leaflets, and cook books. **Pub:** Newsletter, semiannual.

★ 2324 ★ Coeliac Society of the United Kingdom (CSUK)
Box 220
High Wycombe HP11 2HY, United Kingdom
Phone: 44 1494 437278 **Fax:** 44 1494 474349
Email: admin@coeliac.co.uk
Website: http://www.coeliac.co.uk

Fnded: 1968. **Mem:** 55,000. **Local Groups:** 55. **Desc:** National support organisation for people with intolerance to Gluten. **Pub:** *Gluten Free Food & Drink Directory,* annual. Directory.

★ 2325 ★ Coffin-Lowry Syndrome Foundation
3045 255th Ave. SE
Sammamish, WA 98075
Phone: (425)427-0939
Email: clsfoundation@yahoo.com
Website: http://clsfoundation.tripod.com
Mary Hoffman, Chair

Fnded: 1991. **Desc:** Serves as a clearinghouse for information on Coffin-Lowry Syndrome. (CLS is an inherited syndrome causing retardation, developmental delay, dysmorphic features, and skeletal anomolies.) Offers support services for families dealing with CLS. **Pub:** *CLSF News,* monthly. Newsletter. *Price:* Free.

★ 2326 ★ College of American Pathologists (CAP)
325 Waukegan Rd.
Northfield, IL 60093-2750
Phone: (847)832-7000 **Free:** 800-323-4040
Fax: (847)832-8000
Website: http://www.cap.org
Nick Norris, Exec. VP

Fnded: 1947. **Mem:** 15,467. **Desc:** Physicians practicing the specialty of pathology (diagnosis, treatment, observation, and understanding of the progress of disease or medical condition) obtained by morphologic, microscopic, chemical, microbiologic, serologic, or any other type of laboratory examination made on the patient. Fosters improvement of education, research, and medical laboratory service to physicians, hospitals, and the public. Provides job placement information for members. Conducts laboratory accreditation program and laboratory proficiency testing surveys. Maintains spokespersons network; provides free health information to the public; compiles statistics; sponsors educational programs. **Pub:** *Archives of Pathology and Laboratory Medicine,* monthly. Journal. *Price:* Free to members; $185 US and Canada; $270 other countries. • *CAP TODAY,* monthly. Magazine. Includes scientific abstracts. *Price:* included in membership dues; $60 US; $75 US possessions and the rest of North America; $130 other Countries. • *College of American Pathologists–Directory,* annual. Directory. *Price:* Included in membership dues. • *College of American Pathologists-Positions Listing Service.* Provides job listings. *Price:* included in membership dues, for members only. • Also publishes other materials of interest to pathologists and the public.

★ 2327 ★ College of Diplomates of the American Board of Orthodontics (CDABO)
6 Woods Trail Ct.
Saint Charles, MO 63303
Phone: (636)928-3700 **Fax:** (636)688-1650
Email: cdabo@charter.net
Website: http://www.cdabo.org/
Karen Seiler, Exec. Dir.

Mem: 1,726. **Desc:** Members are diplomates of the American Board of Orthodontics who pass qualifying examinations. Promotes self-evaluation and ongoing professional improvement among orthodontists. Conducts seminars. **Pub:** *The Diplomate,* semiannual. Newsletter. *Price:* For members only.

★ 2328 ★ College of Family Physicians of Canada (CFPC)
(College des Medecins de Famille du Canada — CMFC)
2630 Skymark Ave.
Mississauga, ON, Canada L4W 5A4
Phone: (905)629-0900 **Free:** 800-387-6197
Fax: (905)629-0893
Email: ocfp@cfpc.ca
Website: http://www.cfpc.ca

Fnded: 1954. **Mem:** 15,000. **State Groups:** 10. **Lang(s):** English, French. **Desc:** National medical association of family physicians and general practitioners. Members must maintain a minimum of 50 hours of continuing medical education credits annually. Works to maintain standards of family medicine training in the 16 Canadian medical schools through support of the Departments of Family Medicine and the accreditation of family practice residency programs. Administers certification examinations in emergency medicine and family medicine. Runs practice assessment program. Offers public education programs on family medicine topics. **Pub:** *Canadian Family Physician*, monthly. Journal. • *CFPC-Liaison Newsletter*, quarterly. Newsletter. • *Self-Evaluation*, bimonthly. Home study program.

★ 2329 ★ College of Optometrists
42 Craven St.
London WC2N 5NG, United Kingdom
Phone: 44 207 8396000 **Fax:** 44 207 8396800
Email: optometry@college-optometrists.org
Website: http://www.college-optometrists.org

Fnded: 1980. **Mem:** 10,560. **Desc:** Consists of Fellows and Members, both home and overseas, Associate Members who do not hold full qualifications, non-practising Fellows, Honorary and Life Fellows. Concerned with the improvement and conservation of human vision, advancement for the public benefit of the study of and research into optometry and publication of the results, promotion of the science and practice of optometry and encouragement of the highest possible standards of professional competence and conduct for the public benefit. **Pub:** *Ophthalmic and Physiological Optics*, bimonthly. **Frmly:** British College of Optometrists.

★ 2330 ★ College of Optometrists in Vision Development (COVD)
243 N Lindbergh Blvd., Ste. 310
Saint Louis, MO 63141
Phone: (314)991-4007 **Free:** 888-COVD-770
Fax: (314)991-1167
Email: info@covd.org
Website: http://www.covd.org
Stephen C. Miller, O.D., Exec. Dir.

Fnded: 1970. **Mem:** 1,600. **Reg. Groups:** 3. **State Groups:** 50. **Desc:** Optometrists involved in orthoptics and optometric vision therapy with emphasis on visual information processing in visually related learning problems. Seeks to establish a body of practitioners who are knowledgeable in functional and developmental concepts of vision, to insure that the public will receive continually improving vision care; to promote, foster, and engage in interdisciplinary cooperation; to enable members to maintain the highest standards of professional knowledge and competency; to educate and encourage optometrists to qualify for membership and fellowship in the college; to certify optometrists skilled in this specialty. Conducts national educational programs and public information programs. **Pub:** *College of Optometrists in Vision Development–Membership Directory*, annual. Directory. Listings of associate and fellow members. *Price:* Included in membership dues; $3.50/copy for nonmembers. • *Journal of Optometric Vision Development*, quarterly. *Price:* $65/year. • *Visions Newsletter*, bimonthly. Newsletter. *Price:* Included in membership dues. • Brochures. • Monographs. • Also publishes research reviews.

★ 2331 ★ College of Osteopathic Healthcare Executives (COHE)
5550 Friendship Blvd., Ste. 300
Chevy Chase, MD 20815-7201
Fax: (301)968-4195
David L. Kushner, Pres.

Fnded: 1954. **Mem:** 124. **Desc:** Executives and other employees of osteopathic hospitals. To encourage development of hospital administration; to set criteria of competency; to assist in educational programs; to contribute to advancement of efficient hospital administration. **Pub:** *Osteopathic Membership Directory*, annual. Directory. • *Osteopathic Progress*, bimonthly. Newsletter. *Price:* Included in membership dues. **Frmly:** (1986) American College of Osteopathic Hospital Administrators.

★ 2332 ★ College of Phytotherapy
Bucksteep Manor
Bodle St. Green
Hailsham BN27 4RJ, United Kingdom
Phone: 44 1323 834800 **Fax:** 44 1323 834801
Email: medherb@pavilion.co.uk.school

Fnded: 1982. **Mem:** 500. **Desc:** Runs a training school for practitioners of phytotherapy (herbal medicine) incorporating a 4 year Bachelor of Science degree course, a 5-year BSC Degree Distance Learning Course, specially structured course for practising general practitioners, plus a one-year basic home study course. **Pub:** *British Journal of Phytotherapy*, semiannual. Journal. • *Training for a Career in Herbal Medicine*, annual.

★ 2333 ★ Colleges of Medicine of South Africa (CMSA)
17 Milner Rd
Rondebosch 7700, Republic of South Africa
Phone: 27 21 6899533 **Fax:** 27 21 6853766
Email: cmsa-adm@iafrica.com
Website: http://www.collegemedsa.ac.za

Fnded: 1955. **Mem:** 7,800. **Desc:** Provides postgraduate examinations in all branches of medicine for all doctors and dentists in South Africa. **Pub:** *TRANSACTIONS: Journal of the College of Medicine of South Africa*, semiannual. Journal.

★ 2334 ★ Collegium Internationale Neuro-Psychopharmacologicum (CINP)
c/o Oakley Ray, PhD
2014 Broadway, Ste. 372
Nashville, TN 37203
Phone: (615)343-2068 **Fax:** (615)343-2069
Email: cinp@cinp.org
Website: http://www.cinp.org
Oakley Ray, PhD, Exec. Sec.

Fnded: 1957. **Mem:** 1,000. **Desc:** Individuals engaged in experimental and clinical neuropsychopharmacological research and teachers in this field. Purposes are to advance the experimental and clinical aspects of the neuropsychopharmacological sciences; facilitate international relations between branches of the neuropsychopharmacological disciplines; further the international exchange of information and promote personal relations; consider the medico-social problems of psychopharmacology. **Pub:** *Mailings*, periodic. Journal. • Proceedings.Covers symposia and congresses. • Reports. • Also publishes abstracts.

★ 2335 ★ Colombian Association of Bioengineering and Medical Electronics
Technological Specialization on electromedical Instruments
Technologies Units of Santander
Apartado Aereo 40253
Bucaramanga, Colombia
Phone: 57 7 6342225 **Fax:** 57 7 6437752
Email: ingelmed@bioingenieros.com
Website: http://www.ifmbe.org/members_directory/Affiliated%20organisations.htm

★ 2336 ★ Colombian Association of Psychiatry
(Asociacion Colombiana de Psiquiatria)
Carrera 18 No. 84-87, Of. 403
Bogota, Colombia
Phone: 57 1 2561148 **Fax:** 57 1 6162706
Email: asocopsi@col1.telecom.com.co

Fnded: 1961.

★ 2337 ★ Colombian Institute of Pediatric Oncology
(Instituto Colombiano de Oncologia Pediatrica)
Calle 120, No 8-23
Bogota, Colombia
Phone: 57 1 2133067

Fnded: 1982.

★ 2338 ★ Colombian Pharmacological Association
(Asociacion Colombiana de Farmacologia — ACF)
c/o Dr. Jorge E. Olarte Caro, Pres.
AA 94733
Bogota, Colombia
Phone: 57 1 2719811 **Fax:** 57 1 5302961
Email: jolartec@hotmail.com

Mem: 110. **Desc:** Promotes pharmacology in Colombia.

★ 2339 ★ Colombian Society of Cardiology
(Sociedad Colombiana de Cardiologia)
Apdo Aereo 1875
Bogota, Colombia
Phone: 57 1 2191388 **Fax:** 57 1 2191399

Fnded: 1950.

★ 2340 ★ Colombian Society of Obstetrics and Gynecology (SCOG)
Apdo Aereo 34188
Bogota, Colombia
Phone: 57 1 2681485

Fnded: 1943.

★ 2341 ★ Coma Recovery Association (CRA)
807 Carman Ave.
Westbury, NY 11590-6429
Phone: (516)997-1826 **Fax:** (516)997-1613
Email: office@comarecovery.org
Website: http://www.comarecovery.org
Florence Manginaro, Pres.

Fnded: 1980. **Mem:** 1,056. **Reg. Groups:** 1. **State Groups:** 2. **Local Groups:** 1. **Desc:** Coma and head injury survivors and their families; medical professionals; interested persons. Goal is to provide support to and assist families of coma and head injury survivors. Provides information and referrals regarding treatment, rehabilitation, and socialization options. Represents the common needs of families and patients before legislative bodies. Offers Medicaid case management services. **Pub:** *Coma Recovery Association Newsletter*, quarterly. Newsletter. *Price:* Included in membership dues.

★ 2342 ★ ComCARE Alliance
888 17th St., NW, 12th Fl.
Washington, DC 20006
Phone: (202)429-0574 **Fax:** (202)296-2962
Email: info@comcare.org
Website: http://www.comcare.org
Alan Kitey, Exec. Dir.

Fnded: 1998. **Mem:** 90. **Desc:** Emergency doctors and nurses, state and local public safety officials, departments of transportation, citizen organizations, wireless transportation and technology companies committed to improving emergency communications and response. **Pub:** *ComCARE Insider*, monthly. Newsletter.

★ 2343 ★ Comissao Nacional de Luta Contra a SIDA (CNLCS)
Palacio Bensaude
Estrada da Luz 153
P-1600-153 Lisbon, Portugal
Phone: 351 21 7220820 **Fax:** 351 21 7220822
Email: cnlcs@cnlcs.min-saude.pt

Fnded: 1985. **Reg. Groups:** 20. **Lang(s):** English, French, Portuguese, Spanish. **Desc:** Works to prevent the spread of HIV and AIDS. Advises governmental and nongovernmental agencies. Conducts educational programs, compiles and disseminates information. Coordinates health care and social support activities, screening, and viral load testing. Offers financial support to NGO's. **Pub:** *Contra Sida*, quarterly. Bulletin. Contains epidemiological data on AIDS in Portugal and Europe. • Pamphlets.

★ 2344 ★ Commission for Certification in Geriatric Pharmacy (CCGP)
1321 Duke St.
Alexandria, VA 22314
Phone: (703)535-3038 **Fax:** (703)739-1500
Email: info@ccgp.org
Website: http://www.ccgp.org

Fnded: 1997. **Desc:** Working to promote excellence in Geriatric Health Care through education and certification.

★ 2345 ★ Commission on Graduates of Foreign Nursing Schools (CGFNS)
3600 Market St., Ste. 400
Philadelphia, PA 19104
Phone: (215)222-8454 **Fax:** (215)662-0425
Email: info@cgfns.org
Website: http://www.cgfns.org
Barbara Nichols, RN,MSN, CEO

Fnded: 1977. **Desc:** Established to help ensure safe nursing and other health care for the American public while assisting health care professionals educated outside the United States in assessing their ability to become licensed, as well as to practice, in the U.S. Offers a certification program with credentials review and exam of nursing knowledge and English-language proficiency for foreign-educated registered nurses. Administers the Visascreen: Visa credentials assessment through its division, the International Commission on Healthcare Professions, which meets federal requirements for a screening and assessment service for foreign-born healthcare professionals seeking certain occupational visas in the U.S. Provides the CGFNS Credentials Evaluation Service which can evaluate any health care professional's academic records and registration/licensure in terms of U.S. comparability. Conducts studies and surveys; participates in policy discussions concerning international nursing education, licensure, and practice. **Pub:** *An Assessment of North American Nursing*. Book. • *Characteristics of Foreign Nurse Graduates in the U.S Workforce 2000-2001*. • *How to Study: Preparing for the CGFNS Qualifying Exam & the NCLEX-RN Examination*. Book. • *How To Take Tests: Strategies for the CGFNS Qualifying Exam & The NCLEX-RN Examination*. Book. • *Official Study Guide for the CGFNS Qualifying Exam, 4th Ed.*. Book. • *Practice English Audio Tape & Booklet - Series I*. Booklet. Includes audiotape. • *Practice English Audio Tape & Booklet - Series 2*. Booklet. Includes audio tape. • *Western Regional Directory of U.S. Hospitals, Nursing Licensure Agencies & INS Offices*. Book.

★ 2346 ★ Commission on Opticianry Accreditation (COA)
PO Box 3073
Merrifield, VA 22116-3073
Email: coa@erols.com
Website: http://www.coaccreditation.com
Amy J. Hammer, Dir. of Accreditation

Fnded: 1979. **Mem:** 26. **Desc:** Accrediting agency for ophthalmic dispensing and ophthalmic laboratory technology programs in postsecondary institutions. Conducts an evaluator's workshop to train on-site evaluators. **Pub:** *Accreditation Guide for Laboratory Technician Programs*. Manual. *Price:* $10. • *Accreditation Guide for Ophthalmic Dispensing Programs*. Manual. *Price:* $10. • *Essentials of an Accredited Educational Program for Ophthalmic Laboratory Technician Programs*. Handbook. • *Essentials of an Accredited Educational Program for Opticianry Programs*. Handbook. • *Evaluator's Checklist for Ophthalmic Dispensing Programs*. Manual. • *Evaluator's Checklist for Ophthalmic Laboratory Technology Programs*. Manual. • *Evaluator's Handbook for Ophthalmic Dispensing Programs*. Handbook. • *Evaluator's Handbook for Ophthalmic Laboratory Technology Programs*. Handbook. • *Self-Study Report Format for Ophthalmic Dispensing Programs*. Manual. • *Self-Study Report Format for Ophthalmic Laboratory Technology Program*. Manual.

★ 2347 ★ Commissioned Officers Association of the United States Public Health Service (COA)
8201 Corporate Dr., Ste. 560
Landover, MD 20785
Phone: (301)731-9080 **Fax:** (301)731-9084
Email: gfarrell@coausphs.org
Website: http://www.coausphs.org
Jerry Farrell, Exec. Dir.

Fnded: 1910. **Mem:** 6,700. **Local Groups:** 52. **Desc:** Commissioned officers of the U.S. Public Health Service; includes career active duty, retired, and inactive reserve officers who are physicians, dentists, scientists, engineers, pharmacists, nurses, and other types of professional personnel. Acts as an official spokesperson for the Commissioned Corps, as an information center for its members, and "as a sounding board where views and concerns of the Corps may be brought to the proper authorities for official action." **Pub:** *Frontline*, 10/year. Bulletin. *Price:* included in membership dues. • *Proceedings of Annual Meeting*. Proceedings.

★ 2348 ★ Committee on Accreditation of Medical Transport Systems (CAMTS)
PO Box 1305
Anderson, SC 29622
Phone: (864)287-4177 **Fax:** (864)287-4251
Email: efrazer@camts.org
Website: http://www.camts.org/

Desc: Works to advance professionals involved with air medical services and ground interfacility transport services.

★ 2349 ★ Committee on Accreditation for Respiratory Care (COARC)
1248 Harwood Rd.
Bedford, TX 76021-4244
Phone: (817)283-2835 **Free:** 800-874-5615
Fax: (817)354-8519
Email: info@coarc.com
Website: http://www.coarc.com
Richard T. Walker, Exec. Dir.

Fnded: 1963. **Mem:** 13. **Desc:** Physicians (6); respiratory therapists (6); public representative (1). Purposes are to develop standards and requirements for accredited educational programs of respiratory therapy for recommendation to the American Medical Association; to conduct evaluations of educational programs that have applied for accreditation of the AMA and to make recommendations to the AMA's Committee on Allied Health Education and Accreditation; to maintain a working liaison with other organizations interested in respiratory therapy education and evaluation. Publishes lists of programs. **Frmly:** (1970) Board of Schools of Inhalation Therapy; (1998) Joint Review Committee for Respiratory Therapy Education.

★ 2350 ★ Committee for Freedom of Choice in Medicine (CFCM)
1180 Walnut Ave.
Chula Vista, CA 91911
Phone: (619)429-8200 **Free:** 800-227-4473
Fax: (619)429-8004
Email: cfcm@americanbiologics.com
Website: http://www.americanbiologies.com
Robert W. Bradford, DSC, Founder/Pres.

Fnded: 1972. **Mem:** 30,000. **Local Groups:** 30. **Desc:** Purpose is to support freedom of choice for any therapy which shows clear evidence of efficacy and to prohibit the interference of government or any third party in the relationship between an informed patient and his or her physician. Activities include publishing information to keep members apprised of the latest developments in research and treatment, directing people with questions concerning alternative therapy to physicians in their areas, maintaining an information service for physicians interested in expanding their knowledge of metabolic/nutritional treatment, and providing educational exhibits for programs and seminars being conducted by various medical groups. Conducts research; compiles statistics on people with degenerative diseases who have been treated with metabolic therapy. Operates speakers' bureau. **Pub:** *Choice Magazine*, quarterly. Magazine. Includes science corner and heart, cancer, drug, and court watch sections. *Price:* Included in membership dues. • Audiotapes. • Books. • Brochures. • Pamphlets. • Reprints. • Videos. **Frmly:** (1985) Committee for Freedom of Choice in Cancer Therapy.

★ 2351 ★ Committee of Interns and Residents (CIR)
520 8th Ave., Rm. 1200
New York, NY 10018-4181
Phone: (212)725-5500 **Free:** 800-247-8877
Fax: (212)779-2413
Email: info@cirseiu.org
Website: http://www.cirseiu.org
Mark Levy, Exec. Dir.

Fnded: 1957. **Mem:** 11,000. **Desc:** Medical and dental interns, residents, chief residents, and fellows (collectively referred to as house staff officers) at 60 member hospitals located in California, Florida, New York, New Jersey, and Washington, DC. Purposes include representing house staff in matters pertaining to compensation, benefits, hours, working conditions, and other issues affecting their employment, education, training, and the quality of health services and patient care. **Pub:** *CIR News*, quarterly. Newsletter. **Frmly:** (1974) Committee of Interns and Residents in New York City.

★ 2352 ★ Committee of Ministers
c/o Council of European
Palais de l'Europe
Ave. de l'Europe
F-67075 Strasbourg, France
Phone: 33 3 88412000 **Fax:** 33 3 88412781
Website: http://www.coe.int

Desc: Makes recommendations to member states of the Council of Europe. Supervises judgments of the European Court of Human Rights.

★ 2353 ★ Committee for the Promotion of Medical Research
191 Hayward St.
Yonkers, NY 10704
Ellen M. Cosgrove, Exec. Sec.

Fnded: 1944. **Desc:** Is concerned with the administration of medical research grants.

★ 2354 ★ Committee on the Rehabilitation and Integration of People with Disabilities
Council of Europe
F-67075 Strasbourg Cedex, France
Phone: 33 3 88412600 **Fax:** 33 3 88412732
Email: thorsten.afflerbach@coe.int

Website: http://www.coe.int/T/E/Social_Cohesion/soc-sp/

Fnded: 1959. **Mem:** 50. **Nat'l Groups:** 25. **Lang(s):** English, French. **Desc:** Promotes rehabilitation for persons with disabilities and their integration into society. **Pub:** *Legislation to Counter Discrimination Against Persons with Disabilities.* Book. • *Recommendation, No. R(92) on a Coherent Policy for People with Disabilities.* Book.

★ 2355 ★ Committee for Truth in Psychiatry (CTIP)

PO Box 1214
New York, NY 10003
Phone: (212)665-6587
Email: ctip@erols.com
Website: http://dspace.dial.pipex.com/comcare/cftip.html
Linda Andre, Dir.

Fnded: 1984. **Mem:** 500. **Desc:** Former psychiatric patients who have had electroconvulsive therapy (ECT), working to bring about truthfully informed consent to shock treatment. Works to retain ECT's current FDA classification as a high-risk procedure. Has submitted a proposal to the Food and Drug Administration regarding a statement of information about ECT that would be given to patients before they give consent for treatment. Seeks endorsements for the CTIP statement. Also has petitioned the FDA for an animal and human CAT scan study of ECT. Provides counseling for individuals/families facing a decision about ECT, or recovering from ECT. **Pub:** *A Synopsis of the Conflict Over ECT at the FDA.* Pamphlet. *Price:* Free. • *FDA's Regulatory Proceedings Concerning ECT.* Pamphlet. *Price:* Free. • *Shockwaves,* quarterly. Newsletter. *Price:* $10/year for survivors and supporters; $5/year for low-income subscribers; $25/year for professionals, agencies, institutions. • *What You Need to Know about ECT. Price:* Free.

★ 2356 ★ Commonwealth Association for Mental Handicap and Developmental Disabilities (CAMHDD)

36A Osberton Pl.
Sheffield S11 8XL, United Kingdom
Phone: 44 114 2682695 **Fax:** 44 114 2678883

Fnded: 1980. **Mem:** 200. **Nat'l Groups:** 1. **Lang(s):** English. **Desc:** Interested individuals and professionals in 30 countries employed in fields dealing with mental handicaps and developmental disability working to prevent mental retardation, especially in the developing countries. Promotes better health for the handicapped. Works to prevent mental handicaps through early detection of disabilities and to establish intervention programs in developing countries. Holds workshops and symposia; plans to organize a training course in developmental pediatrics. Sponsors children's services and charitable program; maintains speakers' bureau; compiles statistics. **Pub:** *CAMHDD Directory,* semiannual. Directory. • *Manual on Prevention of Handicap.* Book.

★ 2357 ★ Commonwealth Dental Association (CDA)

13 Rodney House
12/13 Pembridge Cres.
London W11 3DY, United Kingdom
Phone: 44 20 72293931 **Fax:** 44 20 76812758
Email: juliacampion@cdauk.com
Website: http://www.cdauk.com

Fnded: 1991. **Mem:** 44. **Lang(s):** English. **Desc:** Local dental associations. Serves as a forum for discussion of matters of interest to members; works to coordinate members' activities. Promotes dental hygiene and oral health. Develops primary preventive dental strategies; conducts training programs for dental health workers; provides technical support to members in implementing programs. Holds educational courses. **Pub:** *CDA Bulletin,* semiannual. Newsletter.

★ 2358 ★ The Commonwealth Fund

1 E 75th St.
New York, NY 10021
Phone: (212)606-3800 **Fax:** (212)606-3500
Email: cmwf@cmwf.com
Website: http://www.cmwf.org/
Karen Davis, Pres.

Desc: Social scientists, health care professionals, and other individuals and organizations with an interest in health and social issues. Seeks to improve the quality and availability of health care services in the United States, particularly among elderly, minority, and economically disadvantaged communities. Conducts research on health and social issues; assists government agencies and health care organizations seeking to reform public health policies and delivery systems in the United States.

★ 2359 ★ Commonwealth Medical Association (CMA)

BMA House
Tavistock Sq.
London WC1H 9JP, United Kingdom
Email: office@commat.org
Website: http://www.commedas.org

Fnded: 1962. **Mem:** 37. **Nat'l Groups:** 37. **Reg. Groups:** 6. **Lang(s):** English. **Desc:** National medical associations in Commonwealth countries. Provides technical assistance and cooperation to the national medical associations of Commonwealth developing countries. Conducts projects in areas such as reproductive health, women's health, youth health, medical ethics and human rights. Acts as a clearinghouse for news and information. **Pub:** *Manual on Ethics and Human Rights Standards for Health Professionals.*

★ 2360 ★ Commonwealth Nurses Federation (CNF)

c/o International Office
Royal College of Nursing
20 Cavendish Sq.
London W1G 0RN, United Kingdom
Phone: 44 20 76473593 **Fax:** 44 20 76473413
Email: cnf@rcn.org.uk
Website: http://www.commonwealthnurses.org

Fnded: 1973. **Mem:** 54. **Nat'l Groups:** 54. **Reg. Groups:** 6. **Lang(s):** English. **Desc:** Organization of national nurses associations in Commonwealth countries. Strives to further the development of nursing and midwifery for the benefit of the community in Commonwealth nations. Promotes cooperation and coordinated activities among member associations. Liaises with governmental and health agencies to facilitate the delivery of appropriate health services. Disseminates professional information, advice, and assistance. Supports regional and pan-Commonwealth educational nursing projects. **Pub:** *CNF Newsletter,* semiannual. Newsletter. • *Directory of Nursing Associations and Chief Nursing Officers in Countries of the Commonwealth,* periodic. Directory. • *Reports of Workshops,* periodic. Reports.

★ 2361 ★ Commonwealth Pharmaceutical Association (CPA)

1 Lambeth High St.
London SE1 7JN, United Kingdom
Phone: 44 207 7522364 **Fax:** 44 207 7522508
Email: bfalconbridge@rpsgb.org.uk

Fnded: 1970. **Mem:** 550. **Nat'l Groups:** 39. **Reg. Groups:** 6. **Lang(s):** English. **Desc:** Pharmaceutical organizations in 39 Commonwealth countries; pharmacists. Objectives are to: maintain the honor and traditions of the profession and promote high standards of conduct, practice, and education at all levels; encourage close links among members in the profession and facilitate personal contacts between pharmacists and students; disseminate information about the professional practice of pharmacy and the pharmaceutical sciences. **Pub:** *Newsletter,* quarterly. Newsletter.

★ 2362 ★ Commonwealth Society for Deaf Charity (CSD)

Sound Seekers
34 Buckingham Palace Rd.
London SW1W 0RE, United Kingdom
Phone: 44 20 72335700 **Fax:** 44 20 72335800
Email: sound.seekers@btinternet.com
Website: http://www.sound-seekers.org.uk

Fnded: 1959. **Mem:** 102. **Lang(s):** English. **Desc:** Works for the deaf, especially children, in developing Commonwealth countries. In conjunction with governmental and voluntary organizations, deploys working parties of ENT Surgeons/Audiologists who are volunteers; trains technicians to support audiologists, and to maintain and repair electronic equipment; provides equipment for use by schools for the deaf. Conducts research into the prevention of deafness and compiles statistics on such research; has studied the incidence and causes of deafness in Gambia, Nigeria, and Botswana. Maintains contact with and disseminates information about schools, societies, and government councils for the deaf throughout the Commonwealth. **Pub:** *Newsletter,* annual. Newsletter. Provides information documents to supporters. • *Sound Seekers Zutomation Leaflet,* periodic. Brochure. • Annual Report, annual.

★ 2363 ★ Commonwealth Veterinary Association (CVA)

c/o Centre for Animal and Plant Health
93 Mount Edward Rd.
Charlottetown, PE, Canada C1A 5T1
Phone: (902)368-0950 **Fax:** (902)368-0960
Email: stevensonr@inspection.gc.ca
Website: http://www.commonwealthvetassoc.org

Fnded: 1967. **Mem:** 50. **Reg. Groups:** 6. **Lang(s):** English. **Desc:** National veterinary medical associations of Commonwealth countries. Promotes the veterinary profession through "encouraging the highest professional standards of education, ethics, and service." Seeks to advance animal health. Facilitates communication and cooperation among members; sponsors continuing professional education courses for veterinarians; serves as a clearinghouse on veterinary medicine. **Pub:** *CVA News,* semiannual. Journal.

★ 2364 ★ Communication Independence for the Neurologically Impaired (CINI)

116 John St., Ste. 1304
New York, NY 10038
Phone: (212)385-8045 **Fax:** (212)385-9724
Email: cini@cini.org
Website: http://www.cini.org/

Desc: Works to improve quality of life for those with ALS/MND (Lou Gehrig's Disease).

★ 2365 ★ Community Anti-Drug Coalitions of America (CADCA)

901 N Pitt St., Ste. 300
Alexandria, VA 22314
Free: 800-54-CADCA **Fax:** (703)706-0565
Email: info@cadca.org
Website: http://www.cadca.org

Fnded: 1992. **Mem:** 5,000. **Desc:** Working to create and strengthen the capacity of new and existing coalitions to build safe, healthy and drug-free communities.

★ 2366 ★ Community and District Nursing Association

Westel House
32-38 Uxbridge Rd.
Ealing
London W5 2BS, United Kingdom
Phone: 44 20 82805342

★ 2367 ★ Community Dreamsharing Network (CDN)

PO Box 8032
Hicksville, NY 11802-8032
Phone: (516)735-1969

Website: http://yalenewhavenhealth.org/Library/HealthGuide/SelfHelp/Topic.asp?hwid=shc63dre

Fnded: 1982. **Mem:** 600. **Nat'l Groups:** 150. **Reg. Groups:** 7. **State Groups:** 5. **Local Groups:** 10. **Desc:** Social groups of individuals interested in discussing and understanding their dreams. Works to organize local dreamsharing groups which meet weekly and encourages networking between these groups. Refers qualified dreamsharing activity helpers to schools and groups. Trains elementary and high school teachers in using the dreams of students. Sponsors training sessions in dream understanding methods; conducts research. Maintains speakers' bureau and placement service. Maintains a database of dreamsharing groups. **Pub:** *Dream Switchboard*, quarterly. Newsletter. Includes networking notices. *Price:* $15 /year for individuals. **Frmly:** (1970) Center for Dream Drama; (1982) New York/New Jersey DreamSharing Network; (1988) Dreamsharing Grassroots Network.

★ 2368 ★ Community Guidance Service (CGS)

133 E 73rd St.
New York, NY 10021
Phone: (212)724-1091 **Fax:** (212)724-1091
Alphrodite Clamar, PhD, Dir.

Fnded: 1953. **Desc:** Service agency providing low-cost psychotherapy services at private offices throughout the New York City area. Staff includes psychiatrists, psychologists, and social workers. **Frmly:** Group for Community Guidance Centers.

★ 2369 ★ Community Health Nurses Association of Canada (CHNAC)

19 Melrose Ave., S
Hamilton, ON, Canada L8M 2Y4
Phone: (905)543-9474 **Fax:** (905)545-1568

Fnded: 1989. **Mem:** 2,500. **Lang(s):** English, French. **Desc:** Community health nurses and provincial organizations. Seeks to advance the practice of community health nursing and enhance members' professional status. Represents members' interests before government agencies and medical associations; provides support, services, and assistance to members. **Pub:** *CHNAC*, quarterly. Newsletter.

★ 2370 ★ Community and Hospital Infection Control Association - Canada (CHICA)

PO Box 46125
RPO Westdale
Winnipeg, MB, Canada R3R 3S3
Phone: (204)897-5990 **Fax:** (204)895-9595
Email: chicacanada@mts.net
Website: http://www.chica.org

Fnded: 1971. **Mem:** 800. **Lang(s):** English, French. **Desc:** Health care professionals engaged in the prevention and control of infections. Seeks to improve the health of Canadians by promoting excellence in the practice of infection prevention and control. Serves as a clearinghouse on infection control standards and practices; facilitates communication and exchange of information among members; conducts continuing professional education programs for members. Collaborates with government agencies responsible for public health in the formulation and enforcement of certification standards and in the development of public policies. Provides advice and assistance to organizations and agencies concerned with specific diseases, including AIDS. Maintains speakers' bureau. **Pub:** *Canadian Journal of Infection Control*, quarterly. Journal.

★ 2371 ★ Community Hospitals Association

Meadow Brow
Broadway Rd.
Ilminster TA19 9RG, United Kingdom
Phone: 44 1460 55951 **Fax:** 44 1460 3207
Email: irh@rural-health.ac.uk
Website: http://www.rural-health.ac.uk/ruralhealthworld/cha.php

Fnded: 1969. **Mem:** 409. **Desc:** Community hospitals within and outside the NHS. Works towards developing the range and continuing improvement of services provided by community hospitals. Gathers and disseminates information on all aspects of work carried out in community hospitals; gives help and advice to members in furthering the interests of community hospitals. **Pub:** *Community Hospital Association Newletter*, quarterly.

★ 2372 ★ Community Systems Foundation (CSF)

1310 Hill St.
Ann Arbor, MI 48104
Phone: (734)761-1357 **Fax:** (734)761-1356
Email: williamddrake@cs.com
Website: http://www-personal.umich.edu/~wddrake/csf/
William D. Drake, Pres.

Fnded: 1963. **Mem:** 10. **Desc:** Organization committed to improving the quality of life through applied research and direct assistance to communities, governmental agencies, and service-oriented entities in the private sector. Focuses on community learning and encourages citizen involvement. Is working to develop systems for evaluating, monitoring, and implementing programs of nutrition and family planning such as UNICEF's ChildInfo System. **Pub:** *Research Reports*. Reports.

★ 2373 ★ Complementary Medicine Association (CMA)

c/o Mary Wolken
4649 E Malvern
Tucson, AZ 85711-4249
Fax: (520)323-0264
Email: compmeded@aol.com
Website: http://www.compmed.com
Mary Wolken, Exec. Dir.

Fnded: 1990. **Mem:** 80. **Desc:** Provides education and supports cooperation between all medical disciplines. Fosters and teaches cost effective and more natural systems of medicine to professionals and the public. Focuses on homeopathic, acupuncture, herbal medicines, kinesiology and learning/memory improvement research and education. **Pub:** *Complementary Health*, annual. Journal. Holistic scientific publication.

★ 2374 ★ Comprehensive Health Education Foundation (CHEF)

22419 Pacific Hwy. S
Seattle, WA 98198
Phone: (206)824-2907 **Free:** 800-323-2433
Fax: (206)824-3072
Email: chefstaff@chef.org
Website: http://www.chef.org
Larry Clark, Pres. & CEO

Fnded: 1974. **Desc:** Encourages and supports improvement of health through education. Seeks to improve health education in the schools and community, enhance the public image of health educators, and stimulate community support of health education. Produces and disseminates health education information and materials. Initiates and supports innovations in health education. Supports the Health Education Fund, which sponsors pilot programs, offers scholarships for health education studies, and bestows leadership/recognition and professional enrichment awards.

★ 2375 ★ Computerized Medical Imaging Society (CMIS)

c/o Natl. Biomedical Research Foundation
Georgetown Univ. Med. Center
3900 Reservoir Rd. NW
Washington, DC 20007
Phone: (202)687-2121 **Fax:** (202)687-1662
Email: ledlex@nbrf.georgetown.edu
Robert S. Ledley, Editor-in-Chief

Fnded: 1976. **Mem:** 350. **Desc:** Physicians and other medical personnel concerned with computerized tomography (a diagnostic technique using X-ray photographs in which the shadows of structures before and behind the section under scrutiny do not show), and other radiological diagnostic procedures. Provides a forum for the exchange of information concerning the medical use of computerized tomography in radiological diagnosis. **Pub:** *Computerized Medical Imaging and Graphics*, bimonthly. **Frmly:** (1983) Computerized Tomography Society; (1988) Computerized Radiology Society.

★ 2376 ★ Concern Foundation

8383 Wilshire Blvd., Ste. 337
Beverly Hills, CA 90211
Phone: (310)724-5333 **Fax:** (310)858-1474
Email: info@concernfoundation.org
Website: http://www.concernfoundation.org/

Fnded: 1968. **Desc:** Dedicated to funding basic cancer research. **Pub:** Journal.

★ 2377 ★ Confederation of Dental Employers (CODE)

c/o CODE Office
5a Stanhope Sq.
Holsworthy EX22 6AP, United Kingdom
Phone: 44 1409 254354 **Fax:** 44 1409 254364
Email: info@codeuk.com
Website: http://www.codeuk.com

Fnded: 1978. **Mem:** 450. **Lang(s):** English. **Desc:** Owners of dental practices. Promotes success of dental businesses; seeks to advance the profession of dentistry. Develops codes of business ethics and standards of professional practice for members; conducts research and advises members on business issues including taxation, business management, and the law. Implements discount care schemes for promotional use by members. **Pub:** *Dentistry Opportunities*, quarterly. Magazine.

★ 2378 ★ Confederation of European National Societies of Anaesthesiology (CENSA)

9 Bedford Sq.
London WC1B 3RA, United Kingdom
Phone: 44 20 76311650
Email: davidwilkinson1@compuserve.com

★ 2379 ★ Confederation of European Specialists in Pediatrics (CESP)

Av. Couronne, 20
B-1050 Brussels, Belgium
Phone: 32 2 4775172 **Fax:** 32 2 4775179
Email: pedrtj@az.vub.ac.be
Website: http://www.uems.be

Fnded: 1959. **Mem:** 90. **Nat'l Groups:** 15. **Lang(s):** English, French. **Desc:** Representatives of professional associations of member nations of the European Union and EFTA countries. Purpose is to coordinate the practice of and training in pediatric medicine within the EEC; promotes development of the European Academy of Pediatrics. **Pub:** *Report of Annual Meeting*. • Newsletter, 3/year.

★ 2380 ★ Confederation of Latin American Societies of Anesthesiology (CLASA) (Confederacion Latinoamericana de Sociedades de Anestesiologia)

c/o CLASA Admin. Office
Aranguren 1323 piso 3
1405 Buenos Aires, Argentina
Phone: 54 11 44312547 **Fax:** 54 11 44312463
Email: clasa@satlink.com
Website: http://www.clasa-anestesia.org

Fnded: 1962.

★ 2381 ★ Confederation of Medical Associations in Asia and Oceania (CMAAO)
173 Dinsor Rd., Phranakom District
Bangkok 10200, Thailand
Phone: 66 2 2264871 **Fax:** 66 2 2214866
Email: wonchats@health.moph.go.th
Fnded: 1956.

★ 2382 ★ Conference of Educational Administrators of Schools and Programs for the Deaf (CEASD)
c/o Joseph P. Finnegan, Jr.
PO Box 1778
Saint Augustine, FL 32085-1778
Phone: (904)810-5200 **Fax:** (904)810-5525
Email: email@ceasd.org
Website: http://www.ceasd.org
Joseph P. Finnegan, Jr., Exec. Dir.
Fnded: 1868. **Mem:** 355. **Desc:** Executive heads of public, private, and denominational schools for the deaf in the U.S. and Canada. Coordinates research on the problems of deafness. Compiles statistics on pupils, teachers, and programs from schools for the deaf. **Pub:** *American Annals of the Deaf*, 5/year. • Newsletter, bimonthly. **Frmly:** Association of Superintendents and Principals of American Schools for the Deaf; (1980) Conference of Executives of American Schools for the Deaf; (2000) Conference of Eduaction-al Administrators Serving the Deaf.

★ 2383 ★ Conference of Research Workers in Animal Diseases (CRWAD)
c/o Dr. Robert Ellis
Colorado State University
Department of Microbiology, Immilology & Pathology
Microbiology Bldg., Rm. A 102
Fort Collins, CO 80523-1677
Phone: (970)491-5740 **Fax:** (970)491-1815
Email: robert.ellis@colostate.edu
Website: http://www.cvmbs.colostate.edu/microbiology/crwad/crwad.htm
Dr. Robert P. Ellis, Exec. Dir.
Fnded: 1920. **Mem:** 550. **Desc:** Research workers in animal diseases. **Pub:** *Proceedings of the Annual Meeting–CRWAD*, annual. Journal. Contains abstracts presented at annual meeting. *Price:* $15/year.

★ 2384 ★ Congres Des Psychoanalyses De Langue Francaise (CPLF)
187, rue St.-Jacques
F-75005 Paris, France
Phone: 33 1 43296670 **Fax:** 33 1 44070744
Mem: 500. **Lang(s):** French. **Desc:** Psychoanalysts and students of the International Psycho-Analytical Association. Sponsors research work groups, plenary sessions, and meetings. **Frmly:** Congress of Romance Language Psychoanalysts.

★ 2385 ★ Congress of Chiropractic State Associations (COCSA)
PO Box 2054
Lexington, SC 29071
Phone: (803)356-6809 **Fax:** (803)356-6826
Email: cocsa@sc.rr.com
Website: http://www.cocsa.org
Janet Jordan, Exec. Dir.
Fnded: 1968. **Mem:** 69. **Nat'l Groups:** 8. **Reg. Groups:** 5. **State Groups:** 54. **Desc:** State chiropractic associations. Seeks to "provide an apolitical forum for the promotion and advancement of the chiropractic profession." Works to advance the study, teaching, and practice of chiropractic and natural health; serves as a clearinghouse on problems facing the chiropractic profession; provides support and services to members.

★ 2386 ★ Congress of Lung Association Staff (CLAS)
1726 M St. NW, Ste. 902
Washington, DC 20036-4502
Phone: (202)785-3355 **Fax:** (202)452-1805
Website: http://www.lungusa.org
Janet Widmer, Exec. Dir.
Fnded: 1912. **Mem:** 800. **Desc:** Professional society of executives and staff members of the American Lung Association. Sponsors network opportunities and staff development and training programs. **Pub:** *CLAS Action Report*, quarterly. • Booklets. • Membership Directory, annual. **Frmly:** National Conference of Tuberculosis Secretaries; (1968) National Conference of Tuberculosis Workers; (1973) National Respiratory Disease Conference.

★ 2387 ★ Congress of Neurological Surgeons (CNS)
10 N Martingale Rd., Ste. 190
Schaumburg, IL 60173
Phone: (847)240-2500 **Free:** 877-517-1267
Fax: (847)240-0804
Email: info@1cns.org
Website: http://www.neurosurgery.org
Gerald E. Rodts, Jr., Sec.
Fnded: 1951. **Mem:** 3,500. **Desc:** Professional society of neurological surgeons in the United States and 55 other countries who meet annually to express their views on various aspects of the principles and practice of neurological surgery; to exchange technical information and experience; to join study of the developments in scientific fields allied to neurological surgery. Promotes interest of neurological surgeons in their practice; provides placement service; honors a living leader in the field of neurological surgery annually. **Pub:** *Clinical Neurosurgery*, annual. • *Neurosurgery*, monthly. • *U.S. and Canada Directory*, annual. Directory. • *World Directory*, biennial. Directory. • Newsletter, quarterly.

★ 2388 ★ Consejo General de Colegios Oficiales de Odontologos y Estomatologos de Espana
c/Alcala 79, 2 planta
E-28009 Madrid, Spain
Phone: 34 914264410 **Fax:** 34 915770639
Email: consejo@infomed.es
Website: http://www.consejodentistas.org
Desc: Represents the dental profession in Spain.

★ 2389 ★ Conservative Orthopedics International Association (COIA)
2547 Monroe St.
Dearborn, MI 48124
Phone: (313)563-0360 **Fax:** (248)669-0636
Dr. Stephen R. Castor, Pres.
Fnded: 1982. **Mem:** 4,222. **Desc:** Medical doctors, osteopaths, chiropractors, orthopedists, psychiatrists, and physical therapists. Promotes continuing education, research, and practice of conservative orthopedics. (Conservative orthopedics concentrates on non-operative, nonradical, preventive and rehabilitive treatment of musculoskeletal disorders.) Seeks to advance the science and art of conservative orthopedics as they relate to the whole person. Operates charitable program; compiles statistics. Maintains speakers' bureau; offers educational and research programs. Sponsors hall of fame. **Pub:** *Conservative Orthopedics International Bulletin*, annual. Bulletin. • *Updates*, periodic. • Membership Directory, periodic. • Newsletter, quarterly.

★ 2390 ★ Consortium of Behavioral Health Nurses and Associates
PMB 1214
1733 H St., Ste. 330
Blaine, WA 98230
Phone: (360)332-9105 **Free:** 800-87-NCCDN
Fax: (360)332-2280
Randy Bryson, Exec. Dir.
Fnded: 1987. **Mem:** 1,000. **Reg. Groups:** 21. **State Groups:** 21. **Desc:** Professional nurses specializing in behavioral health with focus on chemical dependency. Goals are: to increase the effectiveness of nursing services for behavioral health; to establish a professional standard in chemical dependency nursing through a system of competency-based testing and programs of professional development and certification. Aims to increase public awareness of the need for chemical dependency treatment and nurses specializing in this field. Encourages the growth of knowledge, skills, and competency in chemical dependency nursing. Offers certification exam for nurses with 4000 hours experience in the previous 5 years and 30 hours of chemical dependency coursework; conducts educational programs. Maintains speakers' bureau. **Pub:** *CD Nurse Briefing*, quarterly. Newsletter. Covers issues of interest of NCCDN membership. *Price:* available to members only. • Pamphlets. **Frmly:** (2003) National Consortium of Chemical Dependency Nurses.

★ 2391 ★ Consortium of Institutes of Higher Education in Health and Rehabilitation in Europe (COHEHRE)
Elfde Liniestraat 24
B-3500 Hasselt, Belgium
Phone: 32 11 238615
Email: cohehre@phlimburg.be
Website: http://www.cohehre.org
Fnded: 1990. **Mem:** 39. **Nat'l Groups:** 15. **Desc:** Promotes the development and quality of higher education for health care professions. **Pub:** Reports. • Manual.

★ 2392 ★ Consultant Dietitians in Health Care Facilities (CDHCF)
2219 Cardinal Dr.
Waterloo, IA 50701
Phone: (319)235-0991 **Fax:** (319)235-7224
Email: cdhcf@cdhcf.org
Website: http://www.cdhcf.org
Marolyn Steffani, RD, LD, Chm.
Fnded: 1975. **Mem:** 6,100. **Reg. Groups:** 7. **State Groups:** 50. **Desc:** A special interest group of the American Dietetic Association. Dietitians employed in extended care facilities, nursing homes, homecare, and a variety of food service operations. Disseminates information; assists in solving their problems in the field. Conducts workshops; offers networking opportunities for professionals. **Pub:** *The Consultant Dietitian*, quarterly. Newsletter. *Price:* $25/year. • *Dining Skills*. • *Inservice Manual*. • *Pocket Resource for Nutrition Assessment*. • *Tool Box (Adults with Developmental Disabilities)*. • *Video Tapes on Dining Skills*. **Frmly:** Consultant Dieticians Special Interest Group.

★ 2393 ★ Consumer Coalition for Quality Health Care
1275 K St. NW, Ste. 602
Washington, DC 20005
Phone: (202)789-3606 **Fax:** (202)898-2389
Email: bwlind@erols.com
Website: http://www.consumers.org/
Brian W. Lindberg, Exec. Dir.
Fnded: 1993. **Desc:** Consumer groups dedicated to protecting and improving quality of health care for all Americans. **Pub:** *The Quality Connection*. Newsletter. Alerts activists to campaigns in other states and lists resources. • *White Papers*. Papers.

★ 2394 ★ Consumers' Health Forum of Australia (CHF)
PO Box 170
Curtin, ACT 2605, Australia
Phone: 61 2 6281 0811 **Fax:** 61 2 6281 0959
Email: info@chf.org.au
Website: http://www.chf.org.au
Fnded: 1987. **Mem:** 250. **Desc:** Health organizations. Promotes public and preventative health perspective; encourages development of health services; promotes consumer rights in the area of health care. **Pub:** *The*

Australian Health Consumer, 3/year. Promotes debate on health care issues.

★ 2395 ★ Contact Lens Association of Ophthalmologists (CLAO)

c/o John S. Massare, PhD
721 Papworth Ave., Ste. 206
Metairie, LA 70005
Phone: (504)835-3937 **Fax:** (504)833-5884
Email: eyes@clao.org
Website: http://www.clao.org
John S. Massare, PhD, Exec. Dir.

Fnded: 1963. **Mem:** 1,500. **Desc:** To advance quality medical eyecare for the public by providing comprehensive ophthalmologists and other eye care professionals with education and training in contact lenses, refractive surgery, and related eyecare science. **Pub:** *CLAO Journal*, quarterly. Journal. • *CLAOgram Online*, bimonthly. Bulletin. • *Who's Who in CLAO*, biennial. Membership Directory. *Price:* included in membership dues; $24.95 for nonmembers. • Report. • Also publishes Contact Lenses: The CLAO Guide to Basic Science and Clinical practice Third Edition, and The CLAO Pocket Guide to Contact Lens Fitting and patient information pamphlets.

★ 2396 ★ Contact Lens Council (CLC)

8201 Corporate Dr., Ste. 850
Landover, MD 20785
Phone: (301)459-2618 **Fax:** (301)459-1802
Email: clc@us.net
Website: http://www.contactlenscouncil.org

Desc: Working to promote the safe use of contact lenses and provide opportunities for both current and prospective contact lens consumers to learn about the variety of lens options available to meet their vision and lifestyle needs.

★ 2397 ★ Continence Restored, Inc. (CRI)

407 Strawberry Hill Ave.
Stamford, CT 06902
Phone: (203)348-0601
Email: smith_younganne@hotmail.com
Anne Smith-Young, Pres.

Fnded: 1985. **State Groups:** 2. **Desc:** Participants are people with bladder control problems and interested individuals. Organizes support groups. Provides information on incontinence devices and treatment; offers referrals. Compiles statistics.

★ 2398 ★ Continuing Care at Home Association

Churchview
Sunningwell Willage
Abingdon OX13 6RD, United Kingdom
Phone: 44 1865 326595 **Fax:** 44 1865 326595
Email: avis@concah.demon.co.uk
Website: http://www.concah.demon.co.uk/

Fnded: 1992. **Desc:** Health and social service professionals. To improve the relief at home of those people suffering from chronic illness and disability, and to advance the learning and understanding of those caring for such persons

★ 2399 ★ Convention of American Instructors of the Deaf (CAID)

PO Box 377
Bedford, TX 76095-0377
Phone: (817)354-8414
Email: caid@swbell.net
Website: http://www.caid.org/
Dr. Liz O'Brien, Pres.

Fnded: 1850. **Mem:** 1,200. **Desc:** Professional organization of teachers, administrators, and professionals in allied fields related to education of the deaf and hard-of-hearing. Objectives are: to provide opportunities for a free interchange of views concerning methods and means of educating the deaf and hard-of-hearing; to promote such education by the publication of reports, essays, and other information; to develop more effective methods of teaching deaf and hard-of-hearing children. **Pub:** *American Annals of the Deaf*, quarterly. Journal. Includes scholarly articles on deafness. *Price:* Included in membership dues; $50/year for nonmembers. • *News 'N' Notes*, quarterly. Newsletter. Includes articles on education of the deaf and organization activities. *Price:* Free. For members only. • *Reference Issue of the American Annals of the Deaf*. Directory. • Proceedings. **AKA:** American Instructors of the Deaf.

★ 2400 ★ Cook Islands Family Welfare Association (CIFWA)

PO Box 109
Rarotonga, Cook Islands
Phone: 682 23420 **Fax:** 682 23421
Email: cifwa@oyster.net.ck

Lang(s): English. **Desc:** Works to enhance the quality of life for individuals living in the Cook Islands by promoting responsible parenthood and family planning. Advocates family planning as a basic human right. Sponsors programs in sex education, family planning, and health. Provides contraceptive and health care services.

★ 2401 ★ Cooleycare

Centro Trasfusionale e di Immunologia dei Trapianti
Ospedale Policlinico
Via Francesco Sforza 35
I-20122 Milan, Italy
Phone: 39 02 55034012 **Fax:** 39 02 5458129
Email: info@ctit.org

Fnded: 1984. **Mem:** 36. **Lang(s):** English. **Desc:** Hematologists and specialists dealing with thalassemia-related problems. (Thalassemia, also known as Cooley's Anemia, is a dysfunction of the red blood cells that occurs in individuals of Mediterranean descent.) Promotes regular studies on thalassemia; provides children's services. Offers professional training. **Pub:** *Meeting Proceedings*, biennial. Proceedings. • *Thalassemia Today*, periodic. Journal.

★ 2402 ★ Cooley's Anemia Foundation (CAF)

129-09 26th Ave., No. 203
Flushing, NY 11354
Phone: (718)321-2873 **Free:** 800-522-7222
Fax: (718)321-3340
Email: info@cooleysanemia.org
Website: http://www.cooleysanemia.org
Jayne Restivo, National Exec. Dir.

Fnded: 1954. **Mem:** 8,000. **Nat'l Groups:** 16. **State Groups:** 4. **Local Groups:** 6. **Desc:** Dedicated to advancing the treatment and cure of Coley's Anemia (also known as Thalassemia). Conducts national programs that provide medical research patient services, awareness and education. Sponsors the Thalassemia Action Group, a support group for patients and families. Provides information about the condition referrals to local medical sources, brochures, newsletters and other information. Provides medical supplies to patients in need. anemia or other thalassemias. Sponsors Thalassemia Action Group, a networking task force of young adult victims of thalassemia. Operates speakers' bureau. Conducts blood drives. **Pub:** *CAF Medical Update*, semiannual. Newsletter. • *Lifeline*, semiannual. Newsletter. • Also publishes 'What is Thalassemia Trait?', 'Desferal Q&A' and 'What Is Cooley's Anemia. **Frmly:** (1977) Cooley's Anemia Blood and Research Foundation for Children.

★ 2403 ★ Cooper Institute for Aerobics Research

12330 Preston Rd.
Dallas, TX 75230
Phone: (972)341-3200 **Free:** 800-635-7050
Fax: (972)341-3227
Email: courses@cooperinst.org
Website: http://www.cooperinst.org
Kenneth H. Cooper, MD, Pres.

Fnded: 1970. **Desc:** Goals are to promote understanding of the relationship between living habits and health, to provide leadership in enhancing the physical and emotional well-being of individuals, and to promote participation in aerobics. Seeks to increase the quality and quantity of fitness programs within major institutions. Conducts innovative studies on health and living habits and methods of facilitating changes in living habits; promotes the awareness and skills needed to develop a positive life-style. Sponsors workshops and seminars; conducts weekly training course and certification testing of fitness leaders in education, government, human services, and corporate sectors. **Frmly:** (2000) Institute for Aerobics Research.

★ 2404 ★ Cord Blood Donor Foundation (CBDF)

1200 Bayhill Dr., Ste. 301
San Bruno, CA 94066
Phone: (650)635-1452 **Fax:** (650)635-1428
Email: information@cordblooddonor.org
Website: http://www.cordblooddonor.org

Desc: Promotes education awareness and further research in the use of cord blood stem cells. Cord blood is blood that remains in the umbilical cord and placenta following birth. Cord blood stem cells are used to treat life-threatening diseases including leukemia, other cancers and blood and immune disorders.

★ 2405 ★ Cornea Research Foundation of America

c/o Susan P. Simon, Devel.Dir.
9002 N Meridian St., Ste. 212
Indianapolis, IN 46260
Phone: (317)844-5610 **Free:** 800-255-6520
Fax: (317)814-2806
Website: http://www.cornea.org
Susan P. Simon, Devel. Dir.

Fnded: 1988. **Desc:** Works to restore and preserve vision through clinical research and educational programs that relate to eye disorders and diseases. **Pub:** *Visionary*, semiannual. Newsletter. Provides news and information to donors, patients, friends. • Papers.

★ 2406 ★ Cornelia de Lange Syndrome Foundation (CdLSF)

302 W Main St., No. 100
Avon, CT 06001
Phone: (860)676-8166 **Free:** 800-223-8355
Fax: (860)676-8337
Email: info@cdlsusa.org
Website: http://www.cdlsusa.org
Julie Mairano, Exec. Dir.

Fnded: 1977. **Mem:** 5,000. **Desc:** Cornelia de Lange Syndrome is a rare birth defect thought to be genetic in origin. A child with this syndrome develops mentally and physically, at a slower rate. The CDLS foundation seeks to ensure early and accurate diagnosis of the syndrome and to enable families, friends, and professionals to make informed decisions and plans for the affected person. Provides updates on the medical aspects of CdLS and responds to correspondences and members' inquiries on an individual basis. Support research programs. **Pub:** *CdLS Foundation - Album*, periodic. Yearbook. Lists families and professionals interested in providing mutual support. *Price:* $25. • *Facing the Challenges: A Parent's Guide to CdLS*. Book. • *Facts about Cornelia de Lange Syndrome*. Pamphlet. • *Reaching Out*, bimonthly. Newsletter. Provides articles of general interest dealing with the complexities of raising a handicapped child. Includes medical column. • Videos. **Frmly:** (1981) Cornelia de Lange Parents Group.

★ 2407 ★ Cornell Feline Health Center

c/o Dr. James R. Richards Dir.
New York State College of Veterinary Medicine
Cornell University
Ithaca, NY 14853
Phone: (607)253-3414 **Fax:** (607)253-3419

Website: http://web.vet.cornell.edu/Public/FHC/FelineHealth.html
Dr. James R. Richards, Dir.

Fnded: 1975. **Mem:** 6,000. **Desc:** Professionals devoted to cats. Seeks to unravel the mysteries of feline health, nutrition, and behavior. Works to educate veterinarians and cat owners, and to aid veterinarians when new or unknown diseases occur. Provides educational programs. **Pub:** *CatWatch*, monthly. Newsletter. Informs cat fanciers of news on cat diseases and activities at the center. • *The Cornell Book of Cats, Second Edition.* • *Feline Health Topics.*

★ 2408 ★ Coronary Artery Disease Research Association (CORDA)
121 Sydney St.
London SW3 6NR, United Kingdom
Phone: 44 20 73498686 **Fax:** 44 20 73499414
Email: corda@rbh.nthames.nhs.uk
Website: http://www.corda.org.uk

Fnded: 1975.

★ 2409 ★ Coronary Club (CC)
9500 Euclid Ave.
Mailcode EE-37
Cleveland, OH 44195
Fax: (216)444-9385
Kathryn E. Ryan-Muldoon, Adm. Asst.

Fnded: 1969. **Mem:** 9,000. **Desc:** Heart patients, doctors, nurses, therapists, educators, and other health professionals involved in cardiac care. **Pub:** *Heartline*, monthly. Newsletter. Covers heart care and rehabilitation. Includes surgery, medication, diet, exercise, depression, stress management, and new research developments. *Price:* $29/year.

★ 2410 ★ Corporacion Chilena de Prevencion del SIDA (CChPS)
Casilla 49, Correo 22
General Jofre 179
Santiago, Chile
Phone: 56 2 2225255 **Fax:** 56 2 2228356
Email: chilaids@cchps.mic.cl

Fnded: 1987. **Mem:** 125. **Lang(s):** English, Spanish. **Desc:** Promotes AIDS awareness, operating safe-sex educational programs and distributing information on the facts of AIDS. Conducts HIV testing and research programs. Offers counseling and referral to medical and social services. Maintains speakers' bureau. Organizes HIV-positive persons to advocate for improved services. **Pub:** *Rapport Annuel*, annual. Report. De Amores y Sombras: Poblaciones y Culturas Homo y Bisexuales de Hombres en Santiago **Frmly:** Corporacion Chilena contra el SIDA; Comite Nationale de Lutte contre le SIDA.

★ 2411 ★ Corporate Angel Network (CAN)
Westchester County Airport
One Loop Rd.
White Plains, NY 10604
Phone: (914)328-1313 **Free:** (866)328-1313
Fax: (914)328-3938
Email: info@corpangelnetwork.org
Website: http://www.CorpAngelNetwork.org
Bonnie LeVar, Exec. Dir.

Fnded: 1981. **Mem:** 500. **Desc:** Arranges free air transportation for cancer patients traveling to and from recognized cancer treatment centers, using empty seats on corporate aircraft. All ambulatory cancer patients and bone marrow donors not needing onboard care are eligible. **Pub:** *FlightLines*, quarterly. Newsletter.

★ 2412 ★ Corp. for Menke's Disease (CMD)
5720 Buckfield Ct.
Fort Wayne, IN 46804
Phone: (219)436-0137 **Fax:** (219)436-0137
Email: bjswiss@aol.com
Jane Swiss, Pres.

Mem: 86. **Desc:** Families with children born with Menke's disease; medical professionals. (Menke's disease is a terminal genetic disorder, primarily found in males, in which the body is unable to process copper.) Supports research; promotes experimental treatments. **Pub:** Newsletter, annual.

★ 2413 ★ Costa Rican Gerontology Association (CRGA) (Asociacion Gerontological Costarricense — AGECO)
Apartado Postal 5956-100
San Jose 1000, Costa Rica
Phone: 506 2210310 **Fax:** 506 2220348
Email: agecocr@racsa.co.cr
Website: http://www.agecocr.com

Fnded: 1980. **Mem:** 54. **Nat'l Groups:** 120. **Reg. Groups:** 40. **Local Groups:** 80. **Lang(s):** Spanish. **Desc:** Health care professionals treating the elderly; scientists and clinicians with an interest in the aging process and diseases of the aged. Promotes gerontological research and increased availability of gerentological care; facilitates training of gerontology specialists. Represents the interests of gerontologists and gerontological organizations. **Pub:** *Ejercicios en la Tercera Edad*, biennial. Manual. • *Envejecer Sano Con Una Buena Allimentacion*, biennial. Bulletin. • *La Voz de Ageco*, biennial. Bulletin. • *Manual de Consejos Practicos en la III Edad Y Otros*, biennial. Bulletin.

★ 2414 ★ Council for Accreditation in Occupational Hearing Conservation (CAOHC)
611 E Wells St.
Milwaukee, WI 53202-3816
Phone: (414)276-5338 **Fax:** (414)276-2146
Email: info@caohc.org
Website: http://www.caohc.org
Larri Bass, Contact

Fnded: 1973. **Mem:** 22,000. **Desc:** To establish and maintain standards for the training of audiometric technicians (persons certified to conduct pure tone air conduction hearing tests and related duties as part of an occupational hearing conservation program). Approves courses in occupational hearing conservation and certifies those who pass these courses. Council members represent professional associations in the hearing conservation field. **Pub:** *CABLE*, semiannual. Newsletter. Newsletter to course directors. • *Occupational Hearing Conservation Manual, 4th Ed.*. Manual. Contains information on the hearing conservationist's mission, training, and role; and federal and state regulations. *Price:* $55/each. • *The Update*, 3/year. Newsletter.

★ 2415 ★ Council for the Advancement of Communication with Deaf People
Durham University Science Park
Block 4
Stockton Rd.
Durham DH1 3UZ, United Kingdom
Phone: 44 191 3831155 **Fax:** 44 191 3837914
Email: durham@cacdp.org.uk
Website: http://www.cacdp.org.uk

Fnded: 1982. **Mem:** 1,000. **Desc:** Aims to improve communication between deaf and hearing people by the development of curricula and examinations in communication skills. Offers certification in British Sign Language, Lipspeaking. Communicating with Deafblind people and Deaf Awareness, and carries out the selection, training, monitering and registration of examiners. **Pub:** *CACDP Directory*, annual. Book. • *CACDP Standard Newsletter*, quarterly. Newsletter.

★ 2416 ★ Council for Affordable Health Insurance (CAHI)
112 S West St., Ste. 400
Alexandria, VA 22314
Phone: (703)836-6200 **Fax:** (703)836-6550
Email: mail@cahi.org
Website: http://www.cahi.org

Fnded: 1992. **Mem:** 200. **Desc:** Companies and individuals with an interest in the health care financing system in the United States. Promotes health care reform that "enact positive, market-based reforms that preserve freedom of choice for individuals and encourage a competitive health care market." Devises model health care reform plans; conducts lobbying and advocacy campaigns; sponsors educational programs.

★ 2417 ★ Council on Arteriosclerosis, Thrombosis and Vascular Biology of the American Heart Association
c/o American Heart Association National Center
7272 Greenville Ave.
Dallas, TX 75231
Free: 800-242-8721
Email: karen.modesitt@heart.org
Website: http://www.americanheart.org/presenter.jhtml?identifier=1201
Elizabeth G. Nabel, MD, Chairperson

Fnded: 1946. **Mem:** 1,014. **Desc:** Professional society of physicians and others interested in cardiovascular diseases, especially arteriosclerosis (hardening of the arteries). **Pub:** *Arteriosclerosis and Thrombosis - A Journal of Vascular Biology*, bimonthly. Journal. • Newsletter, semiannual. **Frmly:** (1959) American Society for the Study of Arteriosclerosis; (1997) Council on Arteriosclerosis of the American Heart Association.

★ 2418 ★ Council on Certification of Nurse Anesthetists (CCNA)
222 S Prospect Ave.
Park Ridge, IL 60068
Phone: (847)692-7050 **Fax:** (847)692-7082
Email: chodson@aana.com
Website: http://www.catinc.com/clients/ccna.htm
Susan S. Caulk, Dir., Certification

Fnded: 1975. **Mem:** 11. **Desc:** Sets certification standards and policies; confers certification upon entry-level nurse anesthetists. Conducts research. Works within the framework of the American Association of Nurse Anesthetists.

★ 2419 ★ Council on Chiropractic Education (CCE)
8049 N 85th Way
Scottsdale, AZ 85258-4321
Phone: (480)443-8877 **Fax:** (480)483-7333
Email: cce@cce-usa.org
Website: http://www.cce-usa.org
Paul D. Walker, PhD, Exec. VP

Fnded: 1971. **Mem:** 13. **Desc:** Advocates high standards in chiropractic education; establishes criteria of institutional excellence for educating chiropractic physicians; acts as national accrediting agency for chiropractic colleges. Conducts workshops for college teams, consultants, and chiropractic college staffs. **Pub:** *CCE Board of Directors*, annual. • *Educational Standards for Chiropractic Colleges*, semiannual. • Newsletter, periodic. • Also publishes pamphlets, news releases, and lists of institutions conforming to its standards and policies.

★ 2420 ★ Council on Chiropractic Orthopedics (CCO)
4409 Sterling Ave.
Kansas City, MO 64133
Phone: (816)358-5100 **Fax:** (816)358-6565
Email: gcdc7@earthlink.net
Website: http://www.ccodc.org/
Gary L. Carver, Pres.

Fnded: 1967. **Mem:** 750. **Desc:** Licensed doctors of chiropractic who have completed 360 hours of postgraduate courses in orthopedics (690); chiropractic physicians with an interest in orthopedics (60). Objectives are: to assist in the advancement of chiropractic as a science and healing art; to protect the welfare and interests of members; to encourage and maintain the highest standards of moral and ethical conduct; to romote research; to encourage the standardization of terminology; to disseminate information; to encourage the teaching of chiropractic orthopedics at all levels.

Reviews and revises postgraduate courses in chiropractic. Fosters seminars and courses in personal, athletic, and industrial injuries; provides consulting. Maintains American Board Board of Chiropractic Orthopedists which serves as an examining body for certification. Certified orthopedists comprise the Academy of Chiropractic Orthopedists. A division of the American Chiropractic Association. **Pub:** *Orthopedic Briefs*, bimonthly. • Brochure. • Directory, annual.

★ 2421 ★ Council on Chiropractic Physiological Therapeutics and Rehabilitation (CCPT)
c/o Donald Fedoryk
7 Mystic Ln.
Malvern, PA 19355
Phone: (908)722-9075 **Fax:** (908)722-1144
Email: jsharpdc@aol.com
Website: http://www.ccptr.org/
Jan Sharp, VP

Fnded: 1920. **Mem:** 200. **Desc:** Chiropractors who use physiotherapy in their practice and are dedicated to furthering the extended use of physiotherapy in the chiropractic field. Plans to provide a diplomate or certification program. **Pub:** *Physiotherapy Briefs*, periodic. **Frmly:** (1985) American Council on Chiropractic Physiotherapy.

★ 2422 ★ Council of Citizens With Low Vision (CCLV)
c/o American Council of the Blind
1155 15th St. NW, Ste. 1004
Washington, DC 20005
Phone: (202)467-5081 **Free:** 800-733-2258
Email: badkron@aol.com
Website: http://www.cclvi.org
Ken Stewart, Pres.

Fnded: 1978. **Mem:** 2,000. **State Groups:** 11. **Desc:** Partially sighted and low-vision individuals, their families, and professional workers. Provides a vehicle through which partially sighted people may voice their needs, preferences, and interests. Promotes the concept that partially sighted and low-vision individuals are not blind and that they have the right to maximize the use of residual vision through the use of any visual aid, service, or technology. Keeps abreast of all developments benefiting partially sighted persons. Promotes educational, engineering, medical, rehabilitative, scientific, and social research that facilitates the lives of individuals with residual vision. Supports the development of pre-service professional training programs for the establishment and expansion of multidisciplinary low-vision services. Strives to educate the public about the existence, capabilities, and needs of such individuals. Establishes outreach programs to insure access to available services for partially sighted persons. Maintains speakers' bureau. **Pub:** *Vision Access*, quarterly. Newsletter. Reports on research and resources. Available on audiocassete and in large print. *Price:* Included in membership dues.

★ 2423 ★ Council of Colleges of Acupuncture and Oriental Medicine (CCAOM)
7501 Greenway Center Dr., Ste. 820
Greenbelt, MD 20770
Phone: (301)313-0870 **Fax:** (301)313-0869
Email: ccaom@compuserve.com
Website: http://www.ccaom.org
David Sale, Exec. Dir.

Fnded: 1982. **Mem:** 45. **Desc:** Acupuncture and oriental medicine colleges. Purposes are: to advance the status of acupuncture and oriental medicine through educational programs; to provide high-quality classroom and clinical instruction; to promote the improvement of research and teaching methods. **Pub:** Newsletter, annual. **Frmly:** (1992) National Council of Acupuncture Schools and Colleges.

★ 2424 ★ Council on Diagnostic Imaging
PO Box 567
Wake Forest, NC 27588
Phone: (919)562-6570
Email: dacbrnc@aol.com
Dr. Kathy Thorn, Sec. -Treas.

Fnded: 1936. **Mem:** 2,000. **Desc:** Professional society of chiropractic roentgenologists, educators, students, and chiropractors interested in roentgenology. **Pub:** *Topics in Diagnostic Radiology and Advanced Imaging*, quarterly. Journal. Covers diagnostic radiology, advanced imaging, thermology, and case studies. *Price:* $50; $75 only in U.S.A.; $100 outside of U.S.A. **Frmly:** (1963) National Council of Chiropractic Roentgenologists; (1968) American Council on Chiropractic Roentgenology; (1970) American Chiropractic Council on Roentgenology; (1983) Council on Roentgeneology to the American Chiropractic Association.

★ 2425 ★ Council on Education of the Deaf (CED)
c/o Department of Administration; Gallaudet University
800 Florida Ave. NE, FH 209
Washington, DC 20002-3695
Phone: (202)651-5525 **Fax:** (202)651-5749
Email: roz.rosen@gallaudet.edu
Website: http://www.deafed.net
Roz Rosen, EdD, Exec. Dir.

Fnded: 1930. **Nat'l Groups:** 6. **Desc:** Representatives from the Alexander Graham Bell Association for the Deaf, the Conference of Educational Administrators Serving the Deaf, the Convention of American Instructors of the Deaf. Association of College Educators; Deaf and Hard of Hearing, National Association of the Deaf and The American Society for Deaf Children. Certifies teachers and accredits university teacher training programs specializing in deaf education and the related. Seeks to improve educational opportunities for deaf and hard of hearing children through cooperation in publication practices, liaison with lay and peripheral groups, teacher certification, public information, and research. Provides certification programs for educators and professionals. Establishes, evaluates, accredits, and maintains certification standards for teacher education programs. **Pub:** *Certification Standards Document.* • *Standards for Evaluation of Programs.*

★ 2426 ★ Council on Education for Public Health (CEPH)
800 Eye St., NW Ste. 202
Washington, DC 20001-3710
Phone: (202)789-1050 **Fax:** (202)789-1895
Email: patevans@ceph.org
Website: http://www.ceph.org
Patricia P. Evans, Exec. Dir.

Fnded: 1974. **Mem:** 2. **Desc:** Participants are professional associations representing public health practice (American Public Health Association) and public health education (Association of Schools of Public Health). Seeks to strengthen educational programs in schools of public health and graduate public health programs through accreditation, consultation, research, and other appropriate services; and to encourage the development of experimental and innovative programs which will ensure educational quality. **Pub:** *Manuals for Accreditation of Graduate Schools of Public Health and Graduate Public Health Programs.* Manuals.

★ 2427 ★ Council of Families with Visual Impairment (CFVI)
c/o American Council of the Blind
6212 W Franklin St.
Richmond, VA 23226
Phone: (202)467-5081 **Free:** 800-424-8666
Fax: (202)467-5085
Email: info@acb.org
Website: http://www.acb.org/affiliates/
Roy Ward, Contact

Fnded: 1979. **Mem:** 400. **Desc:** Sighted parents of blind and visually impaired children; blind and visually impaired parents, professionals, and interested individuals. Offers forum for support and outreach, sharing of experiences in parent-child relationships, and educational and cultural information about child development. Monitors developments in technical and legislative arenas. **Pub:** *Reflections*, 3/year. Newsletter. Published in large print. *Price:* $6; $8 for tape. **Frmly:** (1990) American Council of the Blind Parents.

★ 2428 ★ Council on Health Information and Education (CHIE)
2272 Colorado Blvd., No. 1228
Los Angeles, CA 90041
Fax: (323)344-8594
D. Andre, Dir.

Fnded: 1978. **Desc:** Promotes health and fitness of Americans through the dissemination of information on health care, nutrition, and exercise. Warns against fads in health and nutrition; conducts research on health and exercise products; reviews books on health, fitness, nutrition, sexuality, and sports. **Pub:** Pamphlets.

★ 2429 ★ Council on Health Research for Development (Conseil de la recherch en sante pur le development)
c/o Dr. Yvo Nuyens, UNDP
Ch des anemones 11
CH-1219 Chatelaine, Switzerland
Phone: 41 22 5918900 **Fax:** 41 22 5918910
Email: cohred@cohred.ch
Website: http://www.cohred.ch/

Fnded: 1993. **Desc:** Works with countries that wish to implement Essential National Health Research; provides national strategy for health research management in order to achieve better health.

★ 2430 ★ Council for International Organizations of Medical Sciences (CIOMS) (Conseil des Organisations Internationales des Sciences Medicales)
World Health Org.
Ave. Appia
CH-1211 Geneva 27, Switzerland
Phone: 41 22 7913406 **Fax:** 41 22 7913111
Email: cioms@who.ch
Website: http://www.cioms.ch

Fnded: 1949. **Mem:** 90. **Lang(s):** English, French. **Desc:** International organizations of medical sciences. Promotes and coordinates medical and scientific activities of member associations and national institutions affiliated with the council. Maintains collaborative relations with the World Health Organization and United Nations Educational, Scientific and Cultural Organization. Serves the scientific interests of the international biomedical community.

★ 2431 ★ Council of Medical Specialty Societies (CMSS)
51 Sherwood Ter., Ste. M
Lake Bluff, IL 60044-2232
Phone: (847)295-3456 **Fax:** (847)295-3759
Email: mailbox@cmss.org
Website: http://www.cmss.org
Walter J. McDonald, MD, Exec. VP

Fnded: 1965. **Mem:** 17. **Desc:** National medical specialty societies representing 325,000 physicians. Purpose is to improve the quality of medical care in the United States and to foster excellence in the education of physicians. Provides a forum for discussion by specialty societies of national issues affecting the practice and teaching of medicine. Promotes communication among specialty organizations involved in the principal disciplines of medicine. **Frmly:** Tri-College Council.

★ 2432 ★ Council of Musculoskeletal Special Societies (COMSS)
c/o Richard B. Welch, MD
6300 N River Rd., Ste. 727
Rosemont, IL 60018-4226

Phone: (847)698-1629 **Fax:** (847)823-8125
Email: jones@aaos.org
Website: http://www.aaos.org/
Richard B. Welch, MD, Ch.

Desc: Advocates the interests of its orthopedic specialty societies while promoting and encouraging orthopedic unity among the specialty societies and the American Academy of Orthopedic Surgeons and the American Association of Orthopedic Surgeons.

★ 2433 ★ Council for the National Register of Health Service Providers in Psychology (CNRHSPP)

1120 G St. NW, Ste. 330
Washington, DC 20005
Phone: (202)783-7663 **Fax:** (202)347-0550
Email: judy@nationalregister.org
Website: http://www.nationalregister.org
Judy E. Hall, PhD, Contact

Fnded: 1974. **Mem:** 14,000. **Desc:** Psychologists who are licensed or certified by a state/provincial/territorial board of examiners of psychology and who have met council criteria as health service providers in psychology. **Pub:** *Designated Doctoral Programs in Psychology.* • *National Register of Health Service Providers in Psychology*, annual. • *The Register Report*, semiannual. Magazine. Includes current issues in practice.

★ 2434 ★ Council of Occupational Therapists for the European Countries (COTEC)

106-114 Borough High St.
London SE1 1LB, United Kingdom
Phone: 44 171 3576480 **Fax:** 44 171 4502349
Email: beryl.steeden@cot.co.uk
Website: http://www.cotec-europe.org

Fnded: 1986. **Mem:** 20. **Lang(s):** English. **Desc:** Works to enable national associations in European countries to develop, harmonize, and improve standards of professional practice and education, as well as to advance the theory of occupational therapy throughout Europe.

★ 2435 ★ Council on Podiatric Medical Education (CPME)

9312 Old Georgetown Rd.
Bethesda, MD 20814-1621
Phone: (301)571-9200 **Free:** 800-275-2762
Fax: (301)530-2752
Email: sbsaylor@apma.org
Website: http://www.apma.org/CPME
Richard B. Viehe, Pres.

Fnded: 1918. **Mem:** 11. **Desc:** Accrediting agency for colleges of podiatric medicine, podiatric residency programs and continuing education programs in podiatry. Conducts in-service training programs for members engaged in accrediting activities. **Pub:** *Council on Podiatric Medical Education–Annual Report.* Annual Report. • *Standards and Requirements for Accreditation.* • Also publishes lists of accredited institutions and approved programs. **Frmly:** (1984) Council on Podiatry Education.

★ 2436 ★ Council for Professional Recognition

2460 16th St. NW
Washington, DC 20009-3575
Phone: (202)265-9090 **Free:** 800-424-4310
Fax: (202)265-9161
Email: webmaster@cdacouncil.org
Website: http://www.cdacouncil.org
Dr. Carol Brunson Day, Pres. and CEO

Fnded: 1985. **Desc:** Promotes availability of quality child care through the Child Development Associate National Credentialing Program. Credentials are awarded to family child care, center-based infant/toddler and preschool caregivers, and home visitors. Offers annual training program, the CDA Professional Preparation Program. **Pub:** *Council News and Views*, 3/year. Newsletter. • *Essentials.* • *Improving Child Care Through the Child Development Associate Program.* Book. **AKA:** CDA National Credentialing Program. **Frmly:** (1987) Child Development Associate National Credentialing Program; (1999) Council for Early Childhood Professional Recognition.

★ 2437 ★ Council for the Registration of Schools Teaching Dyslexic Pupils (CRESTED)

Greygarth
Littleworth
Winchcombe
Cheltenham GL54 5BT, United Kingdom
Phone: 44 1242 604852 **Fax:** 44 1242 604852
Email: crested@crested.org.uk
Website: http://www.crested.org.uk

Fnded: 1989. **Desc:** Offers guidance to parents seeking a school for their dyslexic child, providing a list of schools approved for their dyslexia provision. **Pub:** Directory, semiannual.

★ 2438 ★ Council on Rehabilitation Education (CORE)

1835 Rohlwing Rd., Ste. E
Rolling Meadows, IL 60008
Phone: (847)394-1785 **Fax:** (847)394-2108
Email: nchrtm@okstate.edu
Website: http://www.core-rehab.org
Donald C. Linkowski, Exec. Dir.

Fnded: 1972. **Mem:** 90. **Desc:** Sponsored by the American Rehabilitation Counseling Association, Council of State Administrators of Vocational Rehabilitation, American Rehabilitation Counseling Association, National Council on Rehabilitation Education, and the National Rehabilitation Counseling Association. Promotes effective delivery of rehabilitation services to people with disabilities. Surveys, critiques, and works to improve rehabilitation educational programs at the postgraduate level; bestows recognition on programs judged effective. **Pub:** *CORE News*, annual. Lists recognized rehabilitation counselor education programs.

★ 2439 ★ Council on Resident Education in Obstetrics and Gynecology (CREOG)

PO Box 96920
Washington, DC 20090-6920
Phone: (202)863-2554 **Fax:** (202)863-4994
Email: creog@acog.org
DeAnne Nehra, Assoc. Dir.

Fnded: 1967. **Mem:** 450. **Desc:** A semiautonomous nonregulatory organization founded by the American College of Obstetricians and Gynecologists and comprised of national specialty organizations. Works to promote and maintain high standards of resident training in obstetrics and gynecology. Services include: consultative site visits to residency programs; clearinghouse for residency positions; conferences; a resident data bank; national in-training examination. **Pub:** *A Design for Resident Education in Obstetrics and Gynecology.* • *Basic Science Monographs in Obstetrics and Gynecology*, periodic. Monograph. Covers metabolism, genetics, maternal physiology, pharmacology, microbiology, and other aspects of reproductive health. *Price:* $10 for members; $15 for nonmembers. • *Council on Resident Education in Obstetrics and Gynecology–Council News*, 3/year. Newsletter. Contains membership activities and *CREOG Directory of Obstetric and Gynecologic Residency Programs* update. • *CREOG Directory of Obstetric and Gynecologic Residency Programs and Directors*, annual. Directory. Lists accredited residency programs in the U.S. and Canada. *Price:* $10. • *Educational Objectives for Residents in Obstetrics and Gynecology.*

★ 2440 ★ Council for Responsible Nutrition (CRN)

1828 L St. NW, Ste. 900
Washington, DC 20036-5114
Phone: (202)776-7929 **Fax:** (202)204-4980
Email: webmaster@crnusa.org
Website: http://www.crnusa.org
John Cordaro, Pres. /CEO

Fnded: 1973. **Mem:** 100. **Desc:** Manufacturers, distributors, and other companies involved in the production and sale of nutritional supplements, including vitamins, minerals and herbal products. Seeks an improvement in the general health of the U.S. population through responsible nutrition, including the appropriate use of nutritional supplements. Acts as a liaison between vitamin and mineral products manufacturers and government regulatory agencies, such as the Food and Drug Administration, the Federal Trade Commission, and the U.S. Congress. Keeps members informed of relevant legislative developments. Provides a forum to review governmental actions and evaluate current nutrition information. Acts as a clearinghouse to keep members informed of new scientific developments in nutrient safety, health, and nutrition. **Pub:** *CRN News*, monthly. Newsletter. *Price:* For members only.

★ 2441 ★ Council for Sex Information and Education (CSIE)

2272 Colorado Blvd., No. 1228
Los Angeles, CA 90041
Joel Adams, Dir.

Fnded: 1977. **Desc:** A national clearinghouse for information on sexuality and related topics. Premise is that adequate knowledge and understanding of sexuality contributes not only to sexual well-being but to physical and emotional well-being and that helpful information should be readily available. **Frmly:** Sex Information Council of America.

★ 2442 ★ Council of State Administrators of Vocational Rehabilitation (CSAVR)

4733 Bethesda Ave., Ste. 330
Bethesda, MD 20814
Phone: (301)654-8414 **Fax:** (301)654-5542
Carl Suter, Exec. Dir.

Fnded: 1940. **Mem:** 81. **Reg. Groups:** 10. **State Groups:** 81. **Desc:** Administrators of state vocational rehabilitation agencies. Serves as an advisory body to federal agencies and the public in the development of policies affecting rehabilitation of handicapped persons; acts as a forum for discussion on the provision of quality rehabilitation services. Compiles statistics. **Pub:** *CSAVR Memorandum*, semimonthly. • *Proceedings of Conferences*, semiannual. • *State Rehabilitation Directors*, periodic. Directory. • Manuals. • Reports.

★ 2443 ★ Council of State and Territorial Epidemiologists (CSTE)

2872 Woodcock Blvd., No. 303
Atlanta, GA 30341-4015
Phone: (770)458-3811 **Fax:** (770)458-8516
Email: pmcconnon@cste.org
Website: http://www.cste.org
Pat McConnon, Exec. Dir.

Fnded: 1951. **Mem:** 435. **Reg. Groups:** 4. **Desc:** State epidemiologists. Works to establish closer working relationships among members; consults with and advises appropriate disciplines in other health agencies; provides technical advice and assistance to the Association of State and Territorial Health Officials; works closely with Centers for Disease Control on epidemiology, surveillance, and prevention activities. **Pub:** *CSTE Update*, quarterly. Newsletter. • *Minutes to State and Territorial Epidemiologists.* **Frmly:** (1986) Conference of State and Territorial Epidemiologists.

★ 2444 ★ Council of Teaching Hospitals (COTH)

c/o Association of American Medical Colleges
2450 N St. NW
Washington, DC 20037-1127
Phone: (202)828-0541 **Fax:** (202)828-1125
Email: kgserrin@aamc.org
Kevin Serrin, Contact

Fnded: 1965. **Mem:** 400. **Desc:** Teaching hospitals. Provides activities and programs relating to specific problems and opportunities in medical school-affiliated or university-owned teaching hospitals. Distributes communications analyzing congressional activities, Executive Branch actions, court decisions affecting teaching hospitals, and teaching hospital reimbursement regulations; disseminates special interest bibliographies, surveys of housestaff policies, comparative hospital financial data, and other materials. Appoints study groups and ad hoc advisory task forces. **Pub:** *COTH Report*, 8-10/year. Newsletter. Reviews current federal and state legislation and general activities of the association and its affiliates. *Price:* $30/year. • *Survey of House Staff Stipends, Benefits, and Funding*, annual.

★ 2445 ★ CPRI-HOST
4915 St. Elmo Ave., Ste. 401
Bethesda, MD 20814-6052
Phone: (301)657-5918 **Fax:** (301)657-1296
Email: administration@cpri-host.org
Website: http://www.cpri-host.org/
Patricia Wise, MA,MSN, Exec. Dir.

Fnded: 1992. **Desc:** Working to provide vision and leadership to promote the universal and effective use of electronic health care information systems to improve health and the delivery of health care. **Frmly:** (2002) Computer-based Patient Record Institute and Healthcare Open Systems and Trials.

★ 2446 ★ Cranial Academy (CA)
8202 Clearvista Parkway, No. 9-D
Indianapolis, IN 46256
Phone: (317)594-0411 **Fax:** (317)594-9299
Email: cranacad@aol.com
Website: http://www.cranialacademy.com
Patricia S. Crampton, Exec. Dir.

Fnded: 1947. **Mem:** 1,200. **Desc:** A component society of the American Academy of Osteopathy. Osteopathic physicians interested in study and development of osteopathic cranial concepts and techniques of diagnosis and treatment in structural manipulation of the body; members have taken a Cranial Academy approved basic course in Osteopathy in the cranial field. Promotes research programs. **Pub:** *Clinical Cranial Osteopathy*. Book. *Price:* $45 for members; $50 for nonmembers. • *The Cranial Bowl*. Book. *Price:* $15; $17 for nonmembers. • *The Cranial Bowl*. Brochure. *Price:* $.90 for members; $1 for nonmembers. • *The Cranial Concept*. Brochure. *Price:* $27/100 for members; $30/100 for nonmembers. • *The Cranial Letter*, quarterly. Newsletter. Contains articles related to new developments in cranial osteopathy. *Price:* $60/year. • *Journal of OCA 1948, 49, 54, 57, & 58*. *Price:* $18 for members; $20 for nonmembers. • *Manual of Cranial Technique*. Book. *Price:* $22.50 for members; $25 for nonmembers. • *Member Information Directory*, annual. Directory. *Price:* Included in membership dues. **Frmly:** (1960) Osteopathic Cranial Association.

★ 2447 ★ Craniofacial Foundation of America (CFA)
975 E 3rd St., Box 269
Chattanooga, TN 37403
Phone: (423)778-9192 **Free:** 800-418-3223
Fax: (423)778-8172
Email: farmertm@erlanger.org
Website: http://www.erlanger.org/craniofacial/found1.html
Dr. Larry A. Sargent, Med. Dir.

Desc: Dedicated to improving the lives of patients suffering from birth defects, tumors and trauma-related injuries affecting the shape and appearance of the face and skull.

★ 2448 ★ Craniosacral Therapy Association of North America (CSTNA)
12 Sato St.
Whitby, ON, Canada L1R 2E6
Email: info@craniosacraltherapy.org
Website: http://www.craniosacraltherapy.org

Fnded: 1998. **Mem:** 195. **Desc:** Craniosacral therapists and students. Maintains high professional standards for practitioners, teachers, and students of biodynamic craniosacral therapy. Offers referral service. **Pub:** Membership Directory. • Newsletter, periodic.

★ 2449 ★ Craniosacral Therapy Association of the UK
Monomark House
27 Old Gloucester St.
London WC1N 3XX, United Kingdom
Email: info@craniosacral.co.uk
Website: http://www.craniosacral.co.uk

Desc: Craniosacral therapy practitioners in the United Kingdom. **Pub:** *The Fulcrum*, periodic. Journal.

★ 2450 ★ Craniosynostosis and Positional Plagiocephaly Support (CAPPS)
c/o Jennifer Pitchke
6905 Xandu Ct.
Fredericksburg, VA 22407-2580
Free: 877-686-2277
Email: cappsorg@aol.com
Website: http://caps2000.org.cnchost.com/
Jennifer Pitchke, Pres. /Dir.

Fnded: 1999. **Desc:** Provides support and information to families with children suffering from craniosynostosis and positional plagiocephaly. Committed to increasing awareness through education, and to ensure proper diagnosis and appropriate treatment for children afflicted with these conditions.

★ 2451 ★ Cri du Chat Syndrome Mutual Help Group
c/o R. Clarke, Ph.D.
10640 SW 129th Ct.
Miami, FL 33186
R. Clarke, PhD, Contact

Fnded: 1997. **Nat'l Groups:** 1. **State Groups:** 1. **Local Groups:** 1. **Desc:** Family members of people with Cri du Chat Syndrome, a genetic disorder usually resulting in profound mental retardation. Promotes understanding of the syndrome and its manifestations. Facilitates communication and mutual support among members; conducts educational programs; makes available children's services. **Pub:** *Cri du Chat Newsletter*, periodic. Newsletter. *Price:* With membership.

★ 2452 ★ Croatian Cardiac Society
c/o University Hospital for Cardiovascular Diseases
Medical School
University of Zagreb-Rebro
Kispaticeva 12
HR-10000 Zagreb, Croatia
Phone: 385 1 2388483 **Fax:** 385 1 2312247
Email: d.milicic@mail.inet.hr
Website: http://www.escardio.org/society/natsoc/croatia.htm

Mem: 203. **Desc:** Promotes the study of cardiology in Croatia, including congestive heart failure and secondary prevention of coronary heart disease.

★ 2453 ★ Croatian Dental Society
Avenija Gojka Suska 6
CT-10040 Zagreb, Croatia
Phone: 385 1 2903565 **Fax:** 385 1 264250
Email: hsd@kbd.hr
Website: http://www.kbd.hr/hsd

Mem: 2,800. **Desc:** Dentists and others with an interest in providing dental care in Croatia. Represents members' interests.

★ 2454 ★ Croatian Pharmacological Society (Hrvatsko Drustvo Farmakologa)
c/o Prof. Z. Lackovic
Department of Pharmacology
Medical School
University of Zagreb
Salata 11
CT-10000 Zagreb, Croatia
Phone: 385 1 466843 **Fax:** 385 1 466843
Email: lac@mamef.mef.hr

Mem: 192. **Desc:** Promotes pharmacology in Croatia.

★ 2455 ★ Crohn's and Colitis Foundation of America (CCFA)
386 Park Ave. S, 17th Fl.
New York, NY 10016-8804
Phone: (212)685-3440 **Free:** 800-932-2423
Fax: (212)779-4098
Email: info@ccfa.org
Website: http://www.ccfa.org
Rodger L. DeRose, CEO

Fnded: 1967. **Mem:** 60,000. **State Groups:** 55. **Local Groups:** 300. **Desc:** Supports research to find the cause and cure of Crohn's Disease (ileitis) and ulcerative colitis. Provides educational programs for patients, physicians, and the public, support groups, chapter newsletters, a national magazine, informational brochures and books, professional medical forums, and research publications, and a website. **Pub:** *Foundation Focus*, 3/year. Magazine. Contains personal accounts of persons living with colitis and ileitis. *Price:* Included in membership dues. • *Inflammatory Bowel Disease: A Guide for Patients and Their Families*. Book. • *Inflammatory Bowel Diseases*, quarterly. Journal. • *Managing Your Child's Crohn's Disease or Ulcerative Colitis*. Book. • *The New People Not Patients: A Source Book for Living with IBD*. Book. **Frmly:** (1969) Foundation for Ileitis and Colitis; (1992) National Foundation for Ileitis and Colitis.

★ 2456 ★ Cushing's Support and Research Foundation (CSRF)
c/o Louise Pace
65 E India Row, Ste. 22-B
Boston, MA 02110
Phone: (617)723-3674
Email: cushinfo@csrf.net
Website: http://www.csrf.net
Louise Pace, Pres.

Fnded: 1995. **Mem:** 500. **Desc:** Provides information and support for Cushing's Disease and Cushing's Syndrome patients and their families; increases awareness, educates the public about Cushing's Disease and Cushing's Syndrome; provides information and support to health care professionals; raises and distribute funds for Cushing's Disease and Cushing's Syndrome research. **Pub:** Newsletter, quarterly.

★ 2457 ★ CVSA USA/Canada
3585 Cedar Hill Rd. NW
Canal Winchester, OH 43110
Phone: (614)837-2586 **Fax:** (614)837-2586
Email: waitesd@cvsaonline.org
Website: http://www.cvsaonline.org
Debra Waites, Exec. Dir.

Fnded: 1993. **Mem:** 1,000. **Reg. Groups:** 11. **Desc:** Individuals suffering from Cyclic Vomiting Syndrome (CVS), their families, and interested medical professionals. CVS is a rare disorder that usually affects children ages 3-7, and is characterized by recurrent, prolonged attacks of unexplained nausea and vomiting. Promotes medical research on CVS, and seeks to raise public awareness about CVS. Encourages support and information exchange among members. Acts as an information clearinghouse. **Pub:** Newsletter, semiannual. *Price:* Available to members only. **Frmly:** (1999) Cyclic Vomiting Syndrome Association.

★ 2458 ★ Cyclic Vomiting Syndrome Association USA/Canada (CVS)
3585 Cedar Hill Rd. NW
Canal Winchester, OH 43110
Phone: (614)837-2586 **Fax:** (614)837-2586
Email: waitesd@cvsaonline.org
Website: http://www.cvsaonline.org/
Debra Waites, Exec. Dir.
Fnded: 1993. **Mem:** 1,000. **Desc:** Provides patients, families and professionals opportunities to offer and receive support and share knowledge about CVS; promotes research.

★ 2459 ★ Cyprus Association of Medical Physics and Bio-Medical Engineering (CAMPBE)
c/o Dr. Stellos Christofides
Medical Physics Department
Nicosia General Hospital
Lefkosia
Nicosia 1450, Cyprus
Phone: 357 22 801771 **Fax:** 357 22 801773
Email: info@campbe.org
Website: http://www.campbe.org
Desc: Works to promote, develop and disseminate technology and science related to biomedical engineering and medical physics; enhance radiation protection; and encourage research in these fields. **Pub:** Newsletter. • Articles.

★ 2460 ★ Cyprus Medical Representatives Association (CMRA)
PO Box 2134
Nicosia, Cyprus
Phone: 357 2 377166
Lang(s): English, Greek, Turkish. **Desc:** Medical advisers. Promotes professional advancement of members. Represents members' interests before industrial organizations, government agencies, and the public.

★ 2461 ★ Cyprus Multiple Sclerosis Association
PO Box 26749
Nicosia 1647, Cyprus
Phone: 357 22 423644 **Fax:** 357 22 426697
Email: multips@logos.cy.net
Website: http://www.msif.org
Fnded: 1986. **Mem:** 200. **Reg. Groups:** 1. **Desc:** MS patients, families and professionals. Seeks to improve the quality of life for persons with multiple sclerosis and their families. Provides financial assistance, employment assistance, and organizes support groups. **Pub:** *Is Multiple Sclerosis your Problem?*.

★ 2462 ★ Cyprus Society of Cardiology
4 Stratigou Makrigianni Strasse
PO Box 57468
Lemesos CY-3022, Cyprus
Phone: 357 25 720554 **Fax:** 357 25 721644
Email: congress@congresswise.com
Website: http://www.escardio.org/society/natsoc/cyprus.htm
Desc: Promotes the study of cardiology in Cyprus, including coronary risk factors, desirable cholesterol levels in adults, and guidelines on hypertension. **Pub:** *Prevention of Coronary Heart Disease in Clinical Cardiology Practice*. Journal.

★ 2463 ★ Cystic Fibrosis Association of Ireland (CFAI)
CF House
24 Lower Rathmines Rd.
Dublin 6, Ireland
Phone: 353 1 4962433 **Fax:** 353 1 4962201
Email: info@cfireland.ie
Website: http://www.cfireland.ie
Fnded: 1963. **Mem:** 900. **Reg. Groups:** 8. **Lang(s):** English, Irish. **Desc:** People with cystic fibrosis and their families; individuals and organizations providing support and services to people with cystic fibrosis. Seeks to improve the quality of life of people with cystic fibrosis. Provides backup services for young people with cystic fibrosis. **Pub:** Magazine, annual.

★ 2464 ★ Cystic Fibrosis Foundation (CFF)
6931 Arlington Rd.
Bethesda, MD 20814
Phone: (301)951-4422 **Free:** 800-344-4823
Fax: (301)951-6378
Email: info@cff.org
Website: http://www.cff.org
Robert J. Beall, PhD, Pres. & CEO
Fnded: 1955. **Local Groups:** 85. **Desc:** Supports medical research, professional education, and care centers to benefit patients with cystic fibrosis (CF), an inherited fatal disease among children and adults. With this disease a thick mucus clogs the lungs, creating breathing difficulties and high susceptibility to infection; the digestive system and other organs are also affected. More than 113 care centers affiliated with the foundation provide patient services. Medical programs provide support for a national network of multidisciplinary basic and clinical research grants. **Pub:** *Commitment*, quarterly. Newsletter. Features updates on research news and fund-raising news. *Price:* Free. • Annual Report, annual. • Also publishes consumer fact sheets.

★ 2465 ★ Cystic Fibrosis Trust
11 London Rd.
Bromley BR1 1BY, United Kingdom
Phone: 44 208 4647211 **Fax:** 44 208 3130472
Email: enquires@cftrust.org.uk
Website: http://www.cftrust.org.uk
Fnded: 1964. **Mem:** 62,500. **Desc:** Individuals affected by Cystic Fibrosis. **Pub:** *CF News*, quarterly. Newsletter. Contains medical and clinical articles, experiences of people involved with cystic fibrosis, welfare issues. Publishes booklets, leaflets, and fact sheets.

★ 2466 ★ Cystinosis Foundation (CF)
604 Vernon St.
Oakland, CA 94610
Free: 800-392-8458 **Fax:** (209)222-7997
Email: jd2hotz@qnis.net
Website: http://www.cystinosisfoundation.org
Jean Hotz, Pres.
Fnded: 1983. **Mem:** 150. **Reg. Groups:** 20. **Desc:** Parents, relatives, and friends of cystinotic children; interested members of the medical community and the public. (Cystinosis is a genetic metabolic disease in which abnormal amounts of the amino acid cystine collect in the cells, leading to kidney failure.) Purposes are to increase public awareness about cystinosis; to act as a support group to parents of children with the disease; to raise funds for research. Maintains speakers' bureau. **Pub:** *Cystinosis Foundation Newsletter*, quarterly. Newsletter. • *Facts About Cystinosis*. Brochure. • *National Directory of Information*, periodic. Directory. For physicians engaged in cystinosis research. • Directory, periodic. For parents of children with cysinosis. **Frmly:** Alliance of Genetic Support Groups; (1986) Cystinosia Foundation of California.

★ 2467 ★ Czech Association for Family Planning and Sex Education (CAFPSE)
PO Box 399
Senovazna 2
111 21 Prague, Czech Republic
Phone: 42 2 24231524 **Fax:** 42 2 24224378
Email: planrod@centrobox.cz
Website: http://www.sexualnizdravi.info
Fnded: 1990. **Mem:** 180. **Reg. Groups:** 4. **Lang(s):** Czech, English. **Desc:** Health care professionals and other individuals and organizations with an interest in reproductive health, family planning, and population control. Promotes increased availability and improved access to sex education. Conducts educational programs to raise public awareness of population issues; lobbies for improved public policies governing reproductive health, sex education, and family planning services.

★ 2468 ★ Czech Dental Chamber (Ceska Stomatologicka Komora)
Jecna 3
CZ-120 00 Prague 2, Czech Republic
Phone: 42 2 24918611 **Fax:** 42 2 24917372
Email: csk@dent.cz
Desc: Represents dentists' interests.

★ 2469 ★ Czech Gynecological and Obstetrical Society (CGOS)
c/o Prof. Pavel Calda, MD
Department of Obstetrics & Gynaecology
Apolinarska 18
CS-128 51 Prague, Czech Republic
Phone: 42 296152 **Fax:** 42 291845
Email: calda@obgyn.anet.cz
Website: http://www.cgps.cz/english/history.htm
Desc: Promotes development of obstetrics and gynaecology in the prevention, diagnosis, treatment, and research of diseases in this field of medicine.

★ 2470 ★ Czech Medical Association (CzMA)
(Ceska Lekarska Spolecnost)
Sokolskoi 31
PO Box 88, Sokolska 31
CZ-120 26 Prague, Czech Republic
Phone: 42 2 24266223 **Fax:** 42 2 24266212
Email: crma@ds.cz
Website: http://www.cls.cz
Fnded: 1868. **Mem:** 32,000. **Reg. Groups:** 107. **Local Groups:** 40. **Lang(s):** English, French, German, Spanish. **Desc:** Physicians, pharmacists, and other medical personnel. **Pub:** *Medical Congresses and Symposia*, annual. • Journals, monthly. Twenty-nine various medical journals.

★ 2471 ★ Czech-Moravian Psychological Society
(Ceskomoravska psychologicka spolecnost)
Kladenska 48
CZ-160 00 Prague 6, Czech Republic
Phone: 42 2 35360477
Email: cmps@ecn.cz
Website: http://cmps.ecn.cz
Fnded: 1927. **Mem:** 1,050. **Nat'l Groups:** 1. **Reg. Groups:** 1. **Lang(s):** Czech, English. **Desc:** Psychologists in the Czech Republic. Promotes psychology as a field of knowledge and as a profession. Comments on psychological publications; promotes ethical practices and principles; provides information and counseling service. **Pub:** Bulletin, quarterly.

★ 2472 ★ Czech Multiple Sclerosis Society
c/o Jaroslav Zika
PO Box 38
CS-120 00 Prague 2, Czech Republic
Phone: 42 2 41728619 **Fax:** 42 2 66712511
Email: roska@roska-czmss.cz
Website: http://www.roska-czmss.cz
Fnded: 1992. **Mem:** 2,500. **Reg. Groups:** 33. **State Groups:** 1. **Desc:** MS patients, families and professionals. Seeks to improve the quality of life for persons with multiple sclerosis and their families. **Pub:** *Roska*, quarterly. Magazine. Contains specialized information on all fields of Multiple Sclerosis.

★ 2473 ★ Czech Radiological Society (CRS)
(Ceska Radiologicka Spolecnost — CRS)
c/o Dept. of Radiology
University
FNB Hospital

Jihlavska
CZ-63900 Brno 100, Czech Republic
Phone: 42 5 47193007 **Fax:** 42 5 47192383
Email: vlvalek@med.muni.cz
Website: http://www.crs.cz

Fnded: 1929. **Mem:** 340. **Nat'l Groups:** 1. **State Groups:** 1. **Local Groups:** 1. **Lang(s):** Czech. **Desc:** Diagnostic and interventional radiologists in the Czech Republic. Disseminates information on developments in diagnostic and interventional radiology. Acts as a forum for discussion among professionals. **Pub:** *Ceska Radiologie*, bimonthly. Journal. Covers all fields of interest in diagnostic radiology, radio-therapy and nuclear medicine.

★ 2474 ★ Czech Society of Cardiology
Faculty Hospital
FN U. Sv. Anny
Pekarska 53
CZ-656 91 Brno, Czech Republic
Phone: 42 5 43184230 **Fax:** 42 5 43184231
Email: cks@kardio-cz.cz
Website: http://www.kardio-cz.cz

Fnded: 1993. **Mem:** 364. **Desc:** Promotes the study of cardiology in the Czech Republic, including diagnosis and treatment of heart valve diseases, heart failure, hypertension, acute myocardial infarction and angina pectoris, chronic forms of ischemic heart disease, cerebral vascular accidents, arrhythmias, coronary heart disease and complications, pulmonary embolism, and infective endocarditis, as well as pacemaker and antiarrhythmic device implantation, coronarography, and stress tests. **Pub:** *Cor et Vasa*, 10/year. Journal. • *Kardio.* Newsletter. Copies are included in the Journal Cor et Vasa.

★ 2475 ★ Czech Society for Experimental and Clinical Pharmacology and Toxicology
(Ceska Spolecnost pro Experimentalni a Klinickou Farmakologii a Toxicologii)
Department of Pharmacology and Toxicology
Faculty of Medicine in Pilsen
Charles University in Prague
Karlovarska 48
CS-301 66 Pilsen, Czech Republic
Phone: 42 19 7597224 **Fax:** 42 19 7597217
Email: eybl@lfp.cuni.cz
Website: http://mednet.medicina.cz/farmspol/default.html

Mem: 276. **Desc:** Promotes experimental and clinical pharmacology and toxicology in the Czech Republic.

★ 2476 ★ Czech Society of Geronology and Geriatrics
Simunkova 1600
182 00 Prague 8, Czech Republic
Phone: 42 2 883676 **Fax:** 42 2 882788
Email: gerontocentrum@telecom.cz

Desc: Promotes gerontological research, training in the field of aging, and interests of gerontological organizations in international affairs.

★ 2477 ★ D.A.R.E. America
PO Box 512090
Los Angeles, CA 90051-0090
Website: http://www.dare.com/

Desc: Seeks to provide students with a knowledge base on the effects of drug abuse that go beyond the physical ramifications and extend to emotional, social, and economic aspects of life. Aims to build decision-making and problem solving skills and strategies to help students make informed decisions and resist drug use, peer pressure, and violence. Provides students with alternatives to drug use. Sponsors National D.A.R.E. Day. **Pub:** *Keeping Kids Drug Free: The Official Parents Guide.* Book.

★ 2478 ★ Damien Dutton Society for Leprosy Aid (DDSLA)
616 Bedford Ave.
Bellmore, NY 11710
Phone: (516)221-5829 **Fax:** (516)221-5909
Email: info@damienleprosysociety.org
Website: http://www.damienleprosysociety.org
Howard E. Crouch, Pres.

Fnded: 1944. **Mem:** 8,000. **Nat'l Groups:** 1. **Desc:** Religious leaders and laypeople interested in aiding victims of Hansen's disease (leprosy). Provides relief, research, and recreation to victims of leprosy all over the world regardless of race, color, or creed. **Pub:** *After Damien: Dutton.* Book. • *Brother Dutton of Molokai.* Book. • *Damien-Dutton Call*, quarterly. Newsletter. *Price:* available to members only. • *Once Over and Lightly.* Book. • *This One Is For Gussie.* Book. • *Two Hearts - One Fire.* Book. • *Two Josephs on Molokai.* Book. **Frmly:** (1972) Damien-Dutton Society.

★ 2479 ★ Damien Foundation - Belgium (DFB)
(Fondation Damien)
blvd. Leopold II 263
B-1081 Brussels, Belgium
Phone: 32 2 4225911 **Fax:** 32 2 4225900
Email: secret@damien-foundation.be
Website: http://www.fondationdamien.be

Fnded: 1964. **Mem:** 3,000. **Lang(s):** Dutch, English, French. **Desc:** Volunteers working to eradicate leprosy and tuberculosis. Promotes control of the disease through detection, treatment, training, and research. Supports field training as well as formal training in specialized institutions; maintains charitable programs. **Pub:** *Perspectives*, quarterly.

★ 2480 ★ Damon Runyon Cancer Research Foundation
675 3rd Ave., 25 Fl.
New York, NY 10017
Phone: (212)455-0500 **Free:** 800-445-2494
Fax: (212)455-0509
Email: info@drcrf.org
Website: http://www.drcrf.org
Lorraine W. Egan, Exec. Dir.

Fnded: 1946. **Desc:** Nonprofit organization dedicated to advancing cancer research through the funding of initial postdoctoral fellowships and junior faculty awards nationwide. Monies are raised through the Fund's Broadway Tickets theater service and the solicitation of individuals, foundations and corporations. **Pub:** Annual Report, annual. • Brochures. • Newsletter, 3/year. **Frmly:** Damon Runyon Foundation for Cancer Research; (1973) Damon Runyon Memorial Fund for Cancer Research; (1988) Damon Runyon - Walter Winchell Cancer Fund; (1993) Damon Runyon - Walter Winchell Cancer Research Fund.

★ 2481 ★ Dana-Farber Cancer Institute
44 Binney St.
Boston, MA 02115
Phone: (617)632-3000
Email: dana-farbercontact-us@dfci.harvard.edu
Website: http://www.dfci.harvard.edu

Fnded: 1947. **Desc:** Physicians and scientists. Disseminates innovative patient therapies and scientific discoveries worldwide to aid the fight against cancer and AIDS. Committed to providing compassionate care and support to both children and adults with cancer, AIDS, and related diseases.

★ 2482 ★ Danish Association of Medical Imaging
(Danske Radiologers Organisation — DRO)
Rontgenafdelingen
Centralsygehuset Noestved
DK-4700 Noestred, Denmark
Phone: 45 53721401 **Fax:** 45 53729859
Fnded: 1921.

★ 2483 ★ Danish Association of Sports Medicine
(Dansk Idraetsmedicinsk Selskab)
Ortopaedkirurgisk ambulatorium
Amager Hospital
Italiensvej 1
DK-2300 Copenhagen S, Denmark
Phone: 45 32343292 **Fax:** 45 32343964
Email: louice@ah.hosp.dk
Website: http://www.sportsmedicin.dk

★ 2484 ★ Danish Cancer Society
Strandboulevarden 49
DK-2100 Copenhagen O, Denmark
Phone: 45 35257500 **Fax:** 45 35257701
Email: info@cancer.dk
Website: http://www.cancer.dk

Fnded: 1928. **Mem:** 250,000. **Local Groups:** 260. **Lang(s):** Danish, English. **Desc:** Health care professionals and medical researchers and organizations with an interest in cancer; people with cancer and their families. Seeks to: prevent the development of cancer; improve the recovery rate of people with cancer; and limit the "physical, psychological, and social side-effects of cancer." Establishes "new, vital initiatives in the areas of prevention, research and patient support;" works to persuade public sector agencies to take over operation of these initiatives. Monitors existing treatment systems and makes recommendations for their improvement; provides support and services to people with cancer and their families. Maintains cancer registry.

★ 2485 ★ Danish Deaf Association
Postboks 704
Rantzausgade 60, 1
DK-2200 Copenhagen N, Denmark
Phone: 45 35240910 **Fax:** 45 35240920
Email: lf@deaf.dk
Website: http://www.deaf.dk

Fnded: 1935. **Mem:** 2,000. **Local Groups:** 17. **Lang(s):** Danish, English. **Desc:** Deaf people, their families, and health care and speech and hearing professionals. Works to improve the quality of life of deaf people. Works to insure that the legal and economic rights of deaf people are respected. Conducts research and educational programs on sign language and other means of nonverbal communication. Serves as a liaison with other national and international associations with similar aims. Assists members in obtaining assistive technologies including text telephones, alarm services, and TTD messages. **Pub:** *Dovebladet*, monthly. Magazine. **Frmly:** (2000) National Association for the Deaf in Denmark.

★ 2486 ★ Danish Dental Association (DDA)
(Dansk Tandlaegeforening — DTF)
Amaliegade 17
Postboks 143
DK-1004 Copenhagen K, Denmark
Phone: 45 70257711 **Fax:** 45 70251637
Email: dtf@dtf-dk.dk
Website: http://www.dtf-dk.dk

Fnded: 1873. **Mem:** 6,000. **Reg. Groups:** 11. **Lang(s):** Danish, English. **Desc:** Danish dentists. Represents members' interests; promotes dental health care in Denmark. Offers postgraduate training. Maintains placement services; compiles statistics. **Pub:** *Tandlaegebladet*, 18/year. Journal. Provides scientific information.

★ 2487 ★ Danish Dental Manufacturers
Borsen
DK-1217 Copenhagen K, Denmark
Phone: 45 70131200 **Fax:** 45 72255578
Email: dbf@hts.dk
Website: http://www.dentalbranchen.dk

Lang(s): Danish, English. **Desc:** Companies manufacturing dental equipment and supplies. Establishes international standards and technical harmonization for dental equipment. Represents members' interests before government bodies, international agencies, and the public. Maintains liaison with organizations representing dentists, dental technicians, and dental supply dealers and distributors. Compiles statistics.

★ 2488 ★ Danish Dermatological Society (DDS)
(Dansk Dermatologisk Selskab — DDS)
c/o Prof. G.L. Skovgaard
Bispebjerg Hospital
Department of Dermatology
Bispebjerg Bakke 23
DK-2400 Copenhagen NV, Denmark
Phone: 45 35313140 **Fax:** 45 35313113
Email: gls01@bbh.hosp.dk
Fnded: 1899. **Mem:** 295. **Lang(s):** English, German. **Desc:** Dermatologists in Denmark, Norway, and Sweden. Promotes advances in dermatology and venereology. Offers courses for members.

★ 2489 ★ Danish Epilepsy Society
(Dansk Epilepsiforening)
Dianalund Epilepsy Hospital
DK-4293 Dianalund, Denmark
Phone: 45 58264200 **Fax:** 45 58264461
Email: kfjral@vestamt.dk
Website: http://www.ilae-epilepsy.org/chapter/denmark.cfm
Fnded: 1970.

★ 2490 ★ Danish Gerontological Association (DGA)
Aurehojvej 24
DK-2900 Hellerup, Denmark
Phone: 45 39627627 **Fax:** 45 39626627
Email: dgs@geroinst.dk
Website: http://www.gerodan.dk
Lang(s): Danish, English. **Desc:** Health care professionals treating the elderly; scientists and clinicians with an interest in the aging process and diseases of the aged. Promotes gerontological research and increased availability of gerontological care; facilitates training of gerontology specialists. Represents the interests of gerontologists and gerontological organizations.

★ 2491 ★ Danish Medical Society
(Dansk Medicinsk Selskab — DMS)
Kristianiagade 14, 4 tv.
DK-2100 Copenhagen O, Denmark
Phone: 45 35448407 **Fax:** 45 35448408
Email: cs@dadl.dk
Website: http://www.dms.dk
Fnded: 1919. **Desc:** Promotes Danish medical research and represents 92 Danish scientific societies in the field of biomedicine.

★ 2492 ★ Danish Multiple Sclerosis Society
Mosedalvej 15
DK-2500 Valby, Denmark
Phone: 45 364 63646 **Fax:** 45 364 63677
Email: info@scleroseforeningen.dk
Website: http://www.scleroseforeningen.dk/
Fnded: 1957. **Reg. Groups:** 15. **Local Groups:** 33. **Desc:** MS patients, families and professionals. Seeks to improve the quality of life for persons with multiple sclerosis and their families.

★ 2493 ★ Danish Nurses' Organization
(Dansk Sygeplejeraad — DSR)
Vimmelskaftet 38
DK-1161 Copenhagen K, Denmark
Phone: 45 33151555 **Fax:** 45 33152455
Fnded: 1899. **Mem:** 65,985.

★ 2494 ★ Danish Occupational Therapy Association
c/o Scandinavian Journal of Occupational Therapy
Department of Social Medicine and Rehabilitation
Umea University
S-901 87 Umea, Sweden
Phone: 46 90 7869272 **Fax:** 46 90 7869267
Lang(s): Danish. **Desc:** Occupational therapists and other health care professionals engaged in occupational medicine in Denmark. Promotes scientific inquiry in the field of occupational therapy and serves as a forum for the dissemination of research results. Areas of inquiry include: physical disability; mental health and disabilities; therapeutic equipment, environments, and techniques; assessment and evaluation of disabilities; vocational and educational training.

★ 2495 ★ Danish Ophthalmological Society
(Dansk Oftalmologisk Selskab)
Frederiksberg Hospital
Ndr. Fasanvej 59
DK-2000 Frederiksberg, Denmark
Phone: 45 38163625 **Fax:** 45 38163639
Email: jens.c.norregaard@fh.hosp.dk
Website: http://www.dos.suite.dk
Fnded: 1901. **Mem:** 476. **Lang(s):** Danish. **Desc:** Supports developments in ophthalmology in Denmark.

★ 2496 ★ Danish Orthopedic Society
(Dansk Ortopaedisk Selskab — DOS)
Blegdamsvej
DK-2100 Copenhagen, Denmark
Email: dok@dadlnet.dk
Website: http://www.ortopaedi.dk
Fnded: 1946.

★ 2497 ★ Danish Psychologists' Association
(Dansk Psykolog Forening — DP)
Stockholmsgade 27
DK-2100 Copenhagen, Denmark
Phone: 45 35269955 **Fax:** 45 35259737
Email: dp@dp.dk
Website: http://www.dp.dk
Fnded: 1947. **Mem:** 6,898. **Pub:** *Psykolog Nyt.*

★ 2498 ★ Danish Society of Cardiology
Hauser Plads 10, 2nd Fl.
DK-1127 Copenhagen K, Denmark
Fax: 45 33917964
Email: dcs@dadlnet.dk
Website: http://www.cardio.dk
Fnded: 1960. **Mem:** 921. **Desc:** Promotes the study of cardiology in Denmark, including acute coronary syndrome, antithrombotic treatment in cardiovascular diseases, cardiac rehabilitation, cardiac risk in non-cardiac surgery, heart failure, driving and heart disease, dyslipidaemia and heart disease, ischaemic heart disease and stress tests, pulmonary embolism, stable angina pectoris, valvular heart disease, heart catheterization, coronary angiography and angioplasty, and pacemakers and implantable defibrillators. **Pub:** *Cardiologisk Forum*, quarterly. Journal. • Newsletter, quarterly.

★ 2499 ★ Danish Society of Gastroenterology
(Dansk Gastroenterologisk Selskab — DGS)
Kohenhavns Amts Sygehus Herlev
DK-2730 Herlev, Denmark
Fnded: 1970.

★ 2500 ★ Danish Society for Medical Physics
(Dansk Selskab for Medicinsk Fysik — DSMF)
c/o Dr. Jesper Carl, Radiofysisk Laboratorium
Hobrovej 18-22
DK-9100 Alborg, Denmark
Phone: 45 99322891 **Fax:** 45 99322904
Email: jcarl@aas.nja.dk
Website: http://www.efomp.org/members/denmark/denmark.html

★ 2501 ★ Danish Society for Neuroscience (DSfN)
(Dansk Selskab for Neurovidenskab — DSfN)
c/o Dr. Aase Frandsen
Institut for Farmakologi
Danmarks Farmaceutiske Universitet
Universitetsparken 2
DK-2100 Copenhagen O, Denmark
Phone: 45 35306307 **Fax:** 45 35306020
Email: dsfn@dsfn.dk
Website: http://www.dsfn.dk/
State Groups: Selsk. **Local Groups:** b. **Desc:** Promotes basic research in the field of neuroscience; provides educational activities.

★ 2502 ★ Danish Society of Obstetrics and Gynaecology (DSOG)
Clinic of Obstetrics & Gynaecology
University Hospital of Copenhagen
Frederiksberg Hospital
Nordre Fasanvej 57-59
DK-2000 Frederiksberg, Denmark
Phone: 45 38163427 **Fax:** 45 38163409
Email: cwj@dadlnet.dk
Website: http://www.dsog.dk/english/
Fnded: 1898. **Desc:** Promotes the professional and scientific fields of obstetrics and gynaecology in Denmark. **Pub:** Bulletin, bimonthly.

★ 2503 ★ Danish Society of Periodontology
Royal Dental College
Vennelyst Boulevard 9
DK-8000 Arhus, Denmark
Website: http://www.periodont.subnet.dk/pages/information.htm
Fnded: 1964. **Mem:** 409. **Lang(s):** Danish, English. **Desc:** Promotes and facilitates the development of periodontology in research and practice to the benefit of Danish people. **Pub:** *DPS-INFO*, 2-4/year. Newsletter. • *Journal of Clinical Periodontology.* Journal.

★ 2504 ★ Danish Society of Pharmacology and Toxicology
c/o Prof. Michael J. Mulvany
Department of Pharmacology
University of Aarhus
Universitetsparken 240
DK-8000 Arhus, Denmark
Phone: 45 89 421711 **Fax:** 45 89 128804
Email: mm@farm.au.dk
Website: http://www.dsft.dk
Mem: 277. **Desc:** Promotes pharmacology and toxicology in Denmark.

★ 2505 ★ Danish Veterinary History Society
(Dansk Veterinaerhistorisk Samfund)
Svalgaardsvej 20, Sjorring
DK-7700 Thisted, Denmark
Phone: 45 97971001 **Fax:** 45 97971701
Email: anton-rosenbom@post.tele.dk
Fnded: 1934. **Mem:** 300. **Nat'l Groups:** 1. **Lang(s):** English, German. **Desc:** Supports meetings, seminars, congresses, excursions relating to the history of veterinary medicine. **Pub:** *Dansk Veterinarhistorisk*

Arbog, biennial. Book. Contains veterinarian history, articles, obituaries on Danish vets.

★ 2506 ★ Dannemiller Memorial Educational Foundation (DMEF)

12500 Network Blvd., Ste. 101
San Antonio, TX 78249
Phone: (210)641-8311 **Free:** 800-328-2308
Fax: (210)641-8329
Email: editor@pain.com
Website: http://www.dannemiller.com
Alon P. Winnie, MD, Pres.

Fnded: 1971. **Mem:** 30. **Desc:** Conducts annual Anesthesia Review Course in June for M.D. anesthesiologists and in the fall for nurse anesthesiologists, and review course of current concepts in anesthesiology. Sponsors weekend anesthesia and pain management meetings. **Pub:** *AnalgesiaFile*, monthly. Journal. Contains abstracted articles monthly from leading journals on pain and pain management. *Price:* $225/year. • *Anesthesia File*, monthly. Journal. Contains abstracted articles on anesthesia. *Price:* $225/year. • *Progress In Anesthesiology*, monthly. Articles. *Price:* $295/year. **Frmly:** (1984) Society of Air Force Anesthesiologists.

★ 2507 ★ Danubian Psychiatric Association

c/o pro mente Oberosterreich
Figulystrasse 32
A-4020 Linz, Austria
Phone: 43 732 656103 **Fax:** 43 732 651321
Email: donausymposion@promenteooe.at

Fnded: 1964. **Mem:** 61. **State Groups:** 16. **Lang(s):** English. **Desc:** Provides international scientific contracts with psychiatrists. Organizes a biannual symposium of psychiatry in different countries.

★ 2508 ★ Dateable International

7830 Wisconsin Ave.
Bethesda, MD 20814
Phone: (301)656-8723 **Fax:** (301)657-4327
Email: robert@dateable.org
Website: http://www.dateable.org
Robert S. Watson, MSW, Exec. Dir.

Fnded: 1982. **Mem:** 600. **Local Groups:** 1. **Desc:** Purpose is to bring together persons with disabilities for love and friendship. Provides individual counseling and support network. **Pub:** *DateLine*, annual, 3-4/year. Newsletter. *Price:* Free. **Frmly:** (1994) Handicap Introductions; (1997) Date-Able/HI.

★ 2509 ★ Daughters of the Elderly Bridging the Unknown Together (DEBUT)

c/o Pat Meier
3616 E Homestead Dr.
Bloomington, IN 47401
Phone: (812)339-2092
Pat Meier, Facilitator

Fnded: 1981. **Mem:** 10. **Local Groups:** 1. **Desc:** Women involved in caring for elderly parents; individuals preparing for future roles as caregivers. Provides: nonjudgmental support; education in all areas of caring, coping, and in the complex process of aging. Stresses the importance of nursing center advocacy, community outreach, and intergenerational dialogue between adult children and their parents. Delivers presentations at local gerontological functions. **Pub:** *Daughters of the Elderly: Building Partnerships in Caregiving*. Book. *Price:* $9.95.

★ 2510 ★ Day-Break Geriatric Massage Institute

7434 King George Dr., Apt. A
Indianapolis, IN 46260-3447
Phone: (317)722-9896 **Fax:** (317)722-0511
Email: spuszko@juno.com
Website: http://www.daybreak-massage.com
Sharon Puszko, PhD, Contact

Fnded: 1981. **Desc:** Promotes geriatric massage to maintain health and regain physical capabilities that were thought permanently lost. **Pub:** Books. • Videos.

★ 2511 ★ Daycare Trust (NCCCDCT)

21 St. George's Rd.
London SE1 6ES, United Kingdom
Phone: 44 207 84033500 **Fax:** 44 207 8403355
Email: info@daycaretrust.org.uk
Website: http://www.daycaretrust.org.uk

Fnded: 1986. **Lang(s):** English. **Desc:** Promotes the development of quality, affordable, accessible, and equitable child care. Works to improve child care nationwide through: dissemination of information; negotiations with politicians, administrators, and trade unions; and cooperation with other voluntary organizations having similar goals. Provides free childcare information to parents. **Pub:** *Childcare Now*, quarterly. Magazine. • *Childwise*, periodic. Pamphlet. • Videos. **Frmly:** (2000) National Childcare Campaign/Daycare Trust.

★ 2512 ★ DB-Link

345 N Monmouth Ave.
Monmouth, OR 97361
Free: 800-854-7013
Email: dblink@tr.wou.edu
Website: http://www.tr.wou.edu/dblink/
Dr. John Reiman, Dir.

Fnded: 1992. **Desc:** Parents, service providers, administrators, and others interested in services. Identifies, coordinated, and disseminates information related to children and youth who are deaf-blind. Collaborative effort of the Helen Keller National Center, Perkins School for the Blind, and Teaching Research of Western Oregon University. **Pub:** *Deaf-Blind Perspectives*, 3/year. Newsletter. Available in standard print, Braille, large print and ASCII. *Price:* Free to subscribers. • Also publishes 10 fact sheets related to deaf-blindness. (7 of which are also in Spanish) Available full text also on web site.

★ 2513 ★ Deaf Education Through Listening and Talking (DELTA)

PO Box 20
Haverhill CB9 7BD, United Kingdom
Phone: 44 1440 783689 **Fax:** 44 1440 783689
Email: enquiries@deafeducation.org.uk
Website: http://www.deafeducation.org.uk

Fnded: 1980. **Mem:** 800. **Reg. Groups:** 6. **Lang(s):** English. **Desc:** Parents and teachers of children with hearing impairment; adults with hearing impairment. Promotes development of natural and effective spoken language among children with profound hearing impairment. Advocates use of the natural aural approach in teaching children with profound hearing impairment to use spoken language. Conducts workshops for teachers and families of children with profound hearing impairment; makes available teaching resources; sponsors research; provides children's services. **Pub:** *Chat*, semiannual. Newsletter. • *Chatting*, quarterly. Newsletter. • *Deaf Children*. Handbook. • *Deaf Children Talking*. Book. A guide for parents. • *Guide to the Natural Aural Approach*. Handbook. **Frmly:** (1995) National Aural Group.

★ 2514 ★ Deaf-REACH

3521 12th St. NE
Washington, DC 20017
Phone: (202)832-6681 **Fax:** (202)832-8454
Email: info@deafreach.org
Website: http://www.deaf-reach.org/otis.html
Sarah Brown, Exec. Dir.

Fnded: 1972. **Desc:** Committed to maximizing the self-sufficiency of deaf people needing special services by providing referral, education, advocacy, counseling, and housing. Seeks to establish residential homes and provide psychological, physical, spiritual, and social aid to deaf persons with mental and emotional problems. Operates Otis House and Kearny House, group homes for mentally ill deaf persons, designed to help meet the residents' emotional and social needs and teach them independent living skills. Administers the Community Housing for the Hearing Impaired Program which also provides a group home. Offers in-take, referral, housing placement assistance, and personal counseling; provides day-programs for learning disabled, deaf adults. Works in community advocacy for the mentally ill hearing impaired. **Pub:** Annual Report. *Price:* Free. • Brochure. • Newsletter, quarterly. **Frmly:** (1990) National Health Care Foundation for the Deaf.

★ 2515 ★ Deafblind Association

616 Riversdale Rd.
PO Box 1213
Camberwell, VIC 3124, Australia
Phone: 61 3 98827055 **Fax:** 61 3 98829210
Email: dba@internex.net.au
Website: http://www.dba.asn.au

Fnded: 1967. **Lang(s):** English. **Desc:** Deafblind people and their families. Represent the interests of people with a multi-sensory impairment; provides community support for them and their families; provides short term care and long term accommodation and respite care; educates the public about multi-sensory impairment; supports the rubella immunization campaign; offers an information resource about deafblindness; acts as a catalyst for the provision of services to the group of people it represents. Operates group homes for children and adults; provides respite care and counseling; provides community education and awareness.

★ 2516 ★ Deafblind International (Dbl)

c/o SENSE International
11-13 Clifton Terr.
London N4 3SR, United Kingdom
Phone: 44 20 72727774 **Fax:** 44 20 72726012
Email: dbi@sense.org.uk
Website: http://www.deafblindinternational.org

Fnded: 1976. **Mem:** 1,000. **Lang(s):** English. **Desc:** Serves as a network for deaf-blind people, their families, and professionals with an interest in their well-being. Seeks to develop public awareness of the needs and potential of deaf-blind people. Conducts charitable and educational programs. **Pub:** *DBI Review*, semiannual. Journal. **Frmly:** International Association for the Education of Deafblind People.

★ 2517 ★ Deafblind UK

100 Bridge St.
Peterborough PE1 1DY, United Kingdom
Phone: 44 1733 358100 **Fax:** 44 1733 358356
Email: info@deafblinduk.org.uk
Website: http://www.deafblinduk.org.uk

Fnded: 1928. **Mem:** 2,030. **Local Groups:** 24. **Lang(s):** English. **Desc:** Deafblind persons. Helps alleviate the isolation felt by those with dual sensory loss. Negotiates with government to secure better services and facilities for individuals with visual and hearing impairments. Conducts public service programs. Offers advice and financial consultation and some housing assistance. Organizes conferences, seminars, and communication courses. **Pub:** *The Rainbow*, quarterly. Available in large print, Braille, Moon, and cassette versions. • *Snippets*, weekly. Newspaper. Available in Braille, Moon, large print, and disk.

★ 2518 ★ Deafness Research Foundation (DRF)

1050 17th St. NW, Ste701
Washington, DC 20036
Phone: (202)289-5850 **Free:** 800-829-5934
Fax: (202)293-1805
Email: drf@drf.org
Website: http://www.drf.org
Kromeklia Bryant, Off. Mgr.

Fnded: 1958. **Mem:** 2,000. **Desc:** Participates in the National Temporal Bone and Balance Pathology Resource Registry Program of the National Institute on Deafness and Other Communication Disorders. Approximately 1000 physicians and other professionals in ear medicine and research and 52 medical societies underwrite the foundation's fundraising costs through membership in the Centurions of the Deafness Research Foundation; approximately 300 other interested individuals raise funds through membership in the Deafness Research Foundation Alliance. **Pub:** *Cochlear Implant: A Primer for Parents.* Booklet. • *Deafness Research Foundation Annual Report.* Annual Report. *Price:* Free. • Brochures.

★ 2519 ★ DEBRA European

c/o Debra House
13 Wellington Business Park
Duke's Ride
Crowthorne RG45 6LS, United Kingdom
Phone: 44 1344 771961 **Fax:** 44 1344 762661
Email: john.dart@btinternet.com
Website: http://www.debra-international.org

Fnded: 1992. **Mem:** 20. **Desc:** Umbrella organization of patient support groups for people whose lives have been affected by Epidemidysis Bullosa (EB). Activities include peer support, workshops, and dissemination of research findings. **Frmly:** (2001) EUR Network of EB Support Groups.

★ 2520 ★ DEBRA International

13 Wellington Business Pk.
Duke's Ride
Crowthorne RG45 6LS, United Kingdom
Phone: 44 1344 771961 **Fax:** 44 1344 762661
Email: john.dart@btinternet.com
Website: http://www.debra-international.org

Fnded: 1997. **Mem:** 29. **Desc:** Seeks to promote the well being of people with EB and to promote research in the area.

★ 2521 ★ DEBRA Ireland

10 Burgh Quay
Dublin 2, Ireland
Phone: 353 1 6776855 **Fax:** 353 1 6776875
Email: info@debraireland.org
Website: http://www.debraireland.org

Fnded: 1988. **Lang(s):** English, Irish. **Desc:** Individuals and organizations. Seeks to improve the quality of life of people with EB and their families. Makes available specialist care; conducts educational programs for health care personnel and the public.

★ 2522 ★ Delta Dental Plans Association (DDPA)

1515 W 22nd St., No. 1200
Oak Brook, IL 60523
Phone: (630)574-6001 **Fax:** (630)574-6999
Email: cs@ddpa.org
Website: http://www.deltadental.com
Kim Volk, Pres. /CEO

Fnded: 1965. **Mem:** 30. **Desc:** Active state dental service corporations; state dental societies; foreign dental service plans. Seeks to increase the availability of dental service to the public by assisting and coordinating the activities of dental service corporations and helping them in the development of dental care programs for application to multistate and national accounts. A dental service corporation (or dental service plan) refers to a nonprofit corporation organized by the dental profession to provide prepaid dental care coverage to the public on a group basis. Maintains speakers' bureau; conducts specialized education programs; compiles statistics. Holds marketing, management, financial, and educational workshops, seminars, and conferences. **Pub:** *The Communicator*, quarterly. Newsletter. Covers members news. • *Legal Briefs*, quarterly. Newsletter. Covers legislative issues. • Also publishes educational and promotional literature. **Frmly:** National Association of Dental Service Plans.

★ 2523 ★ Delta Omega

c/o Judy Peterson/Marsha Reinking
1101 15th St. NW, Ste. 910
Washington, DC 20005
Phone: (612)624-6669 **Free:** 800-774-8636
Fax: (612)626-3500
Email: ajf@asph.org
Website: http://www.deltaomega.org
Leonard Schuman, MD, Contact

Fnded: 1924. **Mem:** 4,000. **Reg. Groups:** 18. **Local Groups:** 18. **Desc:** Honorary society - men and women, public health. Promotes research and scholarly attainment; sponsors lectures.

★ 2524 ★ Delta Sigma Delta

296 15th Ave.
Nekoosa, WI 54457
Phone: (715)325-6320 **Free:** 800-335-8744
Fax: (715)325-3057
Email: supremescribe@deltsig.com
Website: http://www.deltsig.com
Dr. John H. Prey, Supreme Scribe

Fnded: 1882. **Mem:** 29,000. **Nat'l Groups:** 11. **State Groups:** 35. **Local Groups:** 34. **Desc:** Professional fraternity - dentistry. Maintains museum; offers educational programs. **Pub:** *Alumni Directory*, quadrennial. Directory. • *Desmos*, quarterly. Magazine. Includes chapter news, scientific articles, and announcements. *Price:* Free to members.

★ 2525 ★ Delta Society (DS)

580 Naches Ave. SW, No. 101
Renton, WA 98055
Phone: (425)226-7357 **Fax:** (425)235-1076
Email: info@deltasociety.org
Website: http://www.deltasociety.org
Michelle Cobey, Contact

Fnded: 1977. **Mem:** 6,000. **Desc:** Doctors, nurses, veterinarians, therapists, nursing home personnel, animal trainers and breeders, pet owners, academicians, and students of gerontology, psychology, therapeutic recreation, and other health fields. Assesses the role of animal companions in society and the effect of human-animal interaction on the mental and physical well-being of people. Seeks to establish an interdisciplinary approach to studying human-animal interactions, and to increase awareness of these interactions among health and social care professionals. Provides training to for persons seeking to establish and maintain programs that involve animals in animal-assisted activities/therapy. Operates National Service Dog Center serving people with disabilities in conjunction with the American Humane Association; and Pet Partners, a national registration for volunteers and animals involved in programs. Creating Service Dog Education System to train trainers of service dogs. Distributes information on research, programs, and legislation concerning human-animal relationships. Maintains collection of article reprints. **Pub:** *Alert*, bimonthly. Newsletter. • *InterActions*, quarterly. Magazine. • *Pet Partners Newsletter*, bimonthly. Newsletter. Includes practical information for volunteers in animal-assisted activities and therapy programs. • Journal.

★ 2526 ★ Democratic Nursing Organisation of South Africa (DENOSA)

PO Box 1280
Pretoria 0001, Republic of South Africa
Phone: 27 12 3432315 **Fax:** 27 12 3440750
Email: info@denosa.org.za
Website: http://www.denosa.org.za

Fnded: 1996. **Mem:** 75,000. **Frmly:** South African Nursing Association.

★ 2527 ★ Dental Assisting National Board (DANB)

676 N St. Clair, Ste. 1880
Chicago, IL 60611
Phone: (312)642-3368 **Free:** 800-FOR-DANB
Fax: (312)642-1475
Email: danbmail@danb.org
Website: http://www.danb.org
Cynthia C. Durley, Exec. Dir.

Fnded: 1948. **Desc:** Certifying agency that administers examinations to dental assistants. **Frmly:** Certifying Board of the American Dental Assistants Association.

★ 2528 ★ Dental Association of Malta

c/o Malta Federation of Professional Associations
The Professional Centre
Sliema Rd.
Gzira, Malta
Phone: 356 312888 **Fax:** 356 343002
Email: mfpb@maltanet.net

Fnded: 1945. **Mem:** 80. **Desc:** Represents dental surgeons in Malta. Conducts professional dental education programs.

★ 2529 ★ Dental Association of Russia

34 New Arbat St., Of. 201
121099 Moscow, Russia
Phone: 7 95 2053918 **Fax:** 7 95 2053918
Email: sadovski@dentist.ru

Desc: Represents the dental profession in Russia.

★ 2530 ★ Dental Association of Thailand (DAT)

71 Ladprao 95
Wangtonglhang
Bangkok 10310, Thailand
Phone: 66 2 5394748 **Fax:** 66 2 5141100
Website: http://www.welcome.to/thaidental

Fnded: 1947. **Mem:** 6,000. **Lang(s):** English, Thai. **Desc:** Licensed dentists. Promotes dental health and the advancement of the profession. **Pub:** *Journal of the Dental Association of Thailand*, bimonthly. Journal. With English abstracts. • *News Letter of the Dental Association of Thailand*, periodic.

★ 2531 ★ Dental Group Management Association (DGMA)

PO Box 42036
Phoenix, AZ 85080
Phone: (623)465-5691
Email: dreid@dentfirst.com
Website: http://www.dgma.org
Vince Cedola, Exec. Dir.

Fnded: 1951. **Mem:** 150. **Desc:** Dental group business managers and others interested in group practice management. **Pub:** *DGMA Communicator*, quarterly. Newsletter. Includes membership profiles. *Price:* Free.

★ 2532 ★ Dental Health Foundation

26 Harcourt St.
Dublin 2, Ireland
Phone: 353 1 4780466 **Fax:** 353 1 4780475
Email: info@dentalhealth.ie

Desc: Promotes oral health in Ireland.

★ 2533 ★ Dental Health International (DHI)

847 S Milledge Ave.
Athens, GA 30605
Phone: (706)546-1716 **Fax:** (706)546-1715
Email: bsdds@earthlink.com
Barry Simmons, D.D.S., Pres.

Fnded: 1973. **Desc:** Dentists, dental hygienists, dental technicians, and the International Association of Dental Students. Purposes are to promote dental health programs in developing countries; to provide general dental care using portable modular dental units in areas without electricity or water. Utilizes minimal fee structure to support projects; professionals in the field of dentistry donate their services for a period of 3 months. Volunteer dentists and dental technicians collect permanent non-obsolete dental equipment in their local areas and rendevous with the equipment in the host country and assist with the installation of it. Serves "pro-United States" countries.

★ 2534 ★ Dental Laboratories Association (DLA)
44-46 Wollaton Rd.
Nottingham NG9 2NR, United Kingdom
Phone: 44 115 9254888 **Fax:** 44 115 9254800
Email: info@dla.org.uk
Website: http://www.dla.org.uk

Fnded: 1961. **Mem:** 1,000. **Lang(s):** English. **Desc:** Seeks to advance the study, teaching, and practice of dental technology and the dental sciences. Represents members' commercial and professional interests; facilitates communication and cooperation among members; sponsors research and educational programs. **Pub:** *Dental Laboratory*, monthly. Magazine.

★ 2535 ★ Denturist Association of Canada
PO Box 46114, RPO Westdale
Winnipeg, MB, Canada R3R 3S3
Phone: (204)897-9092 **Fax:** (204)895-9595
Email: dentcda@mb.sympatico.ca
Website: http://www.denturist.org

Fnded: 1971. **Mem:** 1,800. **Lang(s):** English, French. **Desc:** Professional denturists, denturist students, and educators. Seeks to advance the profession of denturism and to establish educational standards in the field. Formulates standards of ethics and practice; represents members' interests before legislative bodies and the public; facilitates exchange of information among members; monitors advancements in the field of denturism. **Pub:** *Journal of Canadian Denturism*, quarterly. Journal.

★ 2536 ★ Depression Alliance
35 Westminster Bridge Rd.
London SE1 7JB, United Kingdom
Phone: 44 20 76330557 **Fax:** 44 20 76330559
Email: information@depressionalliance.org
Website: http://www.depressionalliance.org

Fnded: 1979. **Mem:** 3,000. **Reg. Groups:** 140. **Lang(s):** Welsh. **Desc:** Provides information and support to anyone affected by depression. Services include self-help groups, correspondence schemes and a unique range of literature. **Pub:** *A Single Step*, quarterly. Newsletter.

★ 2537 ★ Depression and Bipolar Support Alliance (DBSA)
730 N Franklin, Ste. 501
Chicago, IL 60610-7204
Phone: (312)642-0049 **Free:** 800-826-3632
Fax: (312)642-7243
Email: gpope@dbsalliance.org
Website: http://www.dbsalliance.org
Lydia Lewis, Pres.

Fnded: 1986. **Mem:** 65,000. **Reg. Groups:** 6. **Local Groups:** 1003. **Desc:** Seeks to educate patients, families, professionals, and the public concerning the nature of depressive and bipolar disorder as treatable medical diseases; to foster self-help for patients and families; to eliminate discrimination and stigma; to improve access to care; and to advocate for research toward the elimination of these illnesses. **Pub:** *A Guide to Depressive and Manic Depressive Illness: Diagnosis, Treatment and Support.* Pamphlet. Contains patient information on depression and bipolar illnesses. • *Dark Glasses and Kaleidoscopes: Living with Manic Depression.* Video. • *Outreach*, quarterly. Newsletter. Includes book reviews, calendar of events, articles on research and treatment, consumer awareness, and advocacy. **Frmly:** (1978) Manic Depressive and Depressive Association; (2003) National Depressive and Manic Depressive Association.

★ 2538 ★ Depression and Related Affective Disorders Association (DRADA)
Johns Hopkins Hospital Meyer 3-181
600 N Wolfe St.
Baltimore, MD 21287-7381
Phone: (410)955-4647 **Fax:** (410)614-3241
Email: drada@jhmi.edu
Website: http://www.drada.org
Cathy Pollock, Dir.

Fnded: 1986. **Mem:** 1,300. **Desc:** Individuals with affective disorders, their families and friends, and mental health professionals. (Affective disorders include depressive illnesses and manic-depression.) Provides support services including referrals, educational programs, networking, and consultation. Encourages and facilitates the formation of local support groups for those with affective disorders; provides training for support group leaders. Cosponsors with Johns Hopkins annual mood disorders symposium. Maintains speakers' bureau. **Pub:** *A Patients Perspective: Dick Cavett.* Video. • *A Patients Perspective: Mike Wallace.* Video. • *Day for Night: Recognizing Teenage Depression.* Video. • *Depressive Illness: What You Need to Know.* Video. • *Downtime: A Workplace Guide to Understanding Clinical Depression.* Video. • *DRADA Update*, bimonthly. Brochure. • *Manual for Affective Disorder Support Groups.* Manual. • *Smooth Sailing*, quarterly. Newsletter. *Price:* Included in membership dues.

★ 2539 ★ Depressives Anonymous: Recovery From Depression (DARFD)
4625 Douglas Ave.
Bronx, NY 10471
Phone: (718)796-0308
Dr. Helen DeRosis, Founder

Fnded: 1977. **Mem:** 3,000. **Desc:** Individuals suffering from depression or anxiety. A selfhelp organization which helps people deal with their anxiety or depression through weekly meeting and sharing of experiences. Conducts research; offers classes. Disseminates information. Interested people may send a SASE or ask for a collect call at the above number. **Pub:** Newsletter, 3-4/year. • Also publishes brochures and pamphlets.

★ 2540 ★ Dermatological Society of Malaysia (DSM)
(Persatuan Dermatologi Malaysia — PDM)
c/o Department of Dermatology
Hospital Kuala Lumpur
Jalan Pahang
50586 Kuala Lumpur, Malaysia
Phone: 60 3 26155251 **Fax:** 60 3 26985927
Email: dermal@tm.net.my
Website: http://www.dermatology.org.my

Fnded: 1976. **Mem:** 110. **Lang(s):** English. **Desc:** Dermatologists and other practitioners interested in dermatology. Promotes the research and development of dermatological medicine in Malaysia. Organizes scientific seminars and congresses. **Pub:** *Malaysian Journal of Dermatology*, annual. Journal.

★ 2541 ★ Dermatological Society of Singapore (DSS)
c/o National Skin Centre
1 Mandalay Rd.
Singapore 308205, Singapore
Phone: 65 2534455 **Fax:** 65 2533255

Fnded: 1972. **Mem:** 96. **Lang(s):** English. **Desc:** Dermatologists in Singapore. Holds clinico-pathological sessions and other academic meetings for dermatologists. Maintains research fund. **Pub:** *Proceedings of Dermatological Society of Singapore*, annual. Journal.

★ 2542 ★ Dermatology Foundation (DF)
1560 Sherman Ave., Ste. 870
Evanston, IL 60201-4808
Phone: (847)728-2256 **Fax:** (847)328-0509
Email: dfgen@dermatologyfoundation.org
Website: http://www.dermfnd.org/
Sandra Rahn Benz, Exec. Dir.

Fnded: 1964. **Mem:** 3,300. **Desc:** Members of national and regional dermatological societies; board-certified dermatologists. Raises funds for the control of skin diseases through research, improved education, and better patient care. Stimulates interest of graduate physicians in academic dermatology. Supports basic and clinical investigations. **Pub:** *Dermatology Focus*, quarterly. Newsletter. Covers membership activities. Includes research articles and lists recipients of foundation awards, fellowships, and grants. • *Progress in Dermatology*, quarterly. Bulletin. Bulletin containing research reports. *Price:* Included in membership dues. • *Stewardship Report.* Annual Report. *Price:* Free.

★ 2543 ★ Dermatology Nurses' Association (DNA)
E Holly Ave.
PO Box 56
Pitman, NJ 08071
Phone: (856)256-2330 **Free:** 800-454-4362
Fax: (856)589-7463
Email: dna@mail.ajj.com
Website: http://dna.inurse.com/
Cynthia Nowicki, Exec. Dir.

Fnded: 1982. **Mem:** 1,600. **Desc:** Addresses professional issues involving dermatology nurses; develops high standards of dermatologic nursing care; facilitates communication and interdisciplinary cooperation among members. Conducts educational meetings. **Pub:** *DNA Membership Directory*, annual. Directory. • *Product Guide*, annual. • Newsletter, bimonthly.

★ 2544 ★ DES Action Canada
5890 Monkland Ave., Ste. 203
Montreal, QC, Canada H4A 1G2
Phone: (514)482-3204 **Free:** 800-4821-DES
Fax: (514)482-1445
Email: desact@web.net
Website: http://www.web.net/~desact

Fnded: 1982. **Mem:** 1,000. **Reg. Groups:** 10. **Lang(s):** English, French. **Desc:** Persons who have been exposed to the drug DES (diethylstilbestrol) and/or concerned individuals. Seeks to detect, instruct, support, and defend the rights of people endangered by DES. Seeks to prevent health problems caused by DES and similar health concerns, especially in the field of reproductive health care. Provides informative written material as well as audio-visual aids for the general public and for health professionals. Offers physician referrals and peer counseling. **Pub:** *A New Look at Breast Cancer.* Booklet. A guide for women in need of Information about breast cancer and treatments related to it. • *Bulletin DES*, quarterly. Bulletin. • *DES Action Canada Newsletter*, quarterly. Newsletter. • *DES-General Info.* Pamphlet. • *DES-The Wonder Drug You Should Wonder About A Pamphlet for Sons.* Pamphlet. • *Direct-to-Consumer Prescription Drug Advertising.* Pamphlet. • *Fertility Issues Associates With DES-Exposure.* Booklet. • *How Safe Are Our Medicines?.* Pamphlet. • *Nursing Curriculum Unit.* Pamphlet.

★ 2545 ★ DES Action, U.S.A.
610 16th St., Ste. 301
Oakland, CA 94612
Phone: (510)465-4011 **Free:** 800-DES-9288
Fax: (510)465-4815
Email: desaction@earthlink.net
Website: http://www.desaction.org
Nora Cody, Exec. Dir.

Fnded: 1977. **Mem:** 3,000. **Reg. Groups:** 20. **Desc:** DES-exposed persons and others "working to try to ameliorate the problems caused by DES." DES (diethylstilbestrol) is a synthetic estrogen in use since 1938 and often prescribed for prevention of miscarriage, diabetes during pregnancy, difficulty in conceiving, staining during pregnancy, and cessation of premature labor. It has since been found that, in some cases, daughters born to women taking DES in the first five months of pregnancy have developed cervical and vaginal abnormalities, a very small percentage of which have resulted in cancer, and a greater number of DES daughters experience problems with pregnancies, including seven times the rate of tubal pregnancy and twice the rate of miscarriage. DES mothers have a higher risk of breast cancer. Goal is to reach DES-exposed persons and to stress to them the need for medical attention and monitoring; to educate professionals and the public. **Pub:** *DES Action Voice: A Focus on Diethylstilbestrol Exposure*, quarterly. Newsletter. Includes medical question and answer column; book reviews; legislation and litigation news; conference reports. *Price:* $35/year. • *Fertility and Pregnancy Guide for DES Daughters and Sons. Price:* $6. • Also publishes fact sheets, booklets and doctor referral sheet. **Frmly:** (1986) DES Action, National.

★ 2546 ★ Design Industries Foundation Fighting AIDS (DIFFA)
147 W 24th St., 7th Fl.
New York, NY 10011
Phone: (212)727-3100 **Fax:** (212)727-2574
Email: info@diffa.org
Website: http://www.diffa.org
David Sheppard, Exec. Dir.

Fnded: 1984. **Local Groups:** 15. **Desc:** Serves as a foundation bestowing grants to AIDS organizations and programs providing direct patient care and services; preventive, post-diagnostic, and community education; housing, meals, emergency assistance, and legal advocacy; treatment and community-based research. **Pub:** *Good Magazine*, quarterly. Magazine. Contains information on managing care and commerce. *Price:* $35. **Frmly:** Design Industries Foundation for AIDS.

★ 2547 ★ Deutsche Alzheimer Gesellschaft (DALEG)
Friedrichstrasse 236
D-10969 Berlin, Germany
Fax: 49 30 259379529
Email: info@deutsche-alzheimer.de
Website: http://www.deutsche-alzheimer.de

Lang(s): English, German. **Desc:** Individuals and organizations. Seeks to improve the quality of life of people with Alzheimer's disease and their families. Makes available support and services; facilitates research on Alzheimer's disease and related disorders; conducts educational programs.

★ 2548 ★ Deutsche Gesellschaft fur Muskelkranke
Im Moos 4
D-79112 Freiburg, Germany
Phone: 49 7665 94470 **Fax:** 49 7665 944720
Email: info@dgm.org
Website: http://www.dgm.org

Fnded: 1865. **Reg. Groups:** 15. **Desc:** Individuals in Germany affected by Amyotrophic Lateral Sclerosis (ALS), a muscle wasting condition. Provides a forum for support and exchange of information. **Pub:** *Muskelreport*.

★ 2549 ★ Deutsche Multiple Sklerose Gesellschaft (DMSG)
c/o Gottfried Milde Staatsminister
Kusterstr. 8
D-30519 Hannover, Germany
Phone: 49 511 96 83 40 **Fax:** 49 511 96 83 450
Email: dmsg@dmsg.de
Website: http://www.dmsg.de

Fnded: 1952. **Mem:** 43,957. **Reg. Groups:** 855. **State Groups:** 16. **Desc:** MS patients, families and professionals. Seeks to improve the quality of life for persons with multiple sclerosis and their families. **Pub:** *AKTIV*, quarterly. Magazine.

★ 2550 ★ Developmental Disabilities Nurses Association
PMB 1214
1733 H St., Ste. 330
Blaine, WA 98230-5107
Free: 800-888-6733 **Fax:** (360)332-2280
Email: ddnahq@aol.com
Website: http://www.ddna.org
Randy Bryson, RN, Exec. Dir.

Fnded: 1992. **Mem:** 1,100. **Reg. Groups:** 35. **State Groups:** 35. **Desc:** Dedicated to serving individuals with developmental disabilities, as well as having a certification program for RN's, and a developing program for LPN/LVN's.

★ 2551 ★ Diabetes Action Research and Education Foundation
426 C St. NE
Washington, DC 20002
Website: http://www.daref.org/
Pat DeVoe, Pres.

Desc: Works to improve quality of life for those affected by diabetes and its complications. **Pub:** *Managing Your Diabetes: Basics and Beyond*. Booklet. *Price:* Free.

★ 2552 ★ Diabetes Association of Nigeria
c/o Mr. Aminu Inuwa Muhammad
Department of Medicine
Aminu Kano Teaching Hospital
PMB 3452
Kano, Nigeria
Phone: 234 64 663383 **Fax:** 234 64 663354
Email: cmd@akth.org
Website: http://www.diabetesafrica.com/idfmembers.html

Desc: Represents people with diabetes. Promotes research and support of those with diabetes in Nigeria.

★ 2553 ★ Diabetes Association of Sri Lanka (DASL)
50 Sarana Mawatha
Kotte Rd.
Rajagiriya, Sri Lanka
Phone: 94 1 872951 **Fax:** 94 1 872951
Email: info@diabeteslanka.org

Fnded: 1984. **Desc:** Aims to prevent diabetes and its complications through ecuation, early detection, monitoring, control, and screening.

★ 2554 ★ Diabetes Association of Zambia
c/o Dr. Robert E. Mtonga
PO Box 109X Ridgeway
Lusaka, Zambia
Email: kkaonga@hotmail.com
Website: http://www.diabetesafrica.com/idfmembers.html

Desc: Represents people with diabetes. Promotes research and support of those with diabetes in Zambia.

★ 2555 ★ Diabetes Association of Zanzibar (DAZ)
PO Box 1902
Zanzibar, United Republic of Tanzania
Email: alisalum@hotmail.com
Website: http://www.diabetesafrica.com/idfmembers.html

Desc: Represents people with diabetes. Promotes research and support of those with diabetes in Tanzania.

★ 2556 ★ Diabetes Australia
Churchill House, 1st Fl.
218 Northbourne Ave.
Braddon, ACT 2612, Australia
Email: admin@diabetesaustralia.com.au
Website: http://www.diabetesaustralia.com.au/

Fnded: 1937. **Mem:** 12. **Desc:** Committed to minimizing the impact of diabetes in Australia.

★ 2557 ★ Diabetes Exercise and Sports Association (DESA)
PO Box 1935
Litchfield Park, AZ 85340
Phone: (623)535-4593 **Free:** 800-898-4322
Fax: (623)535-4741
Email: desa@diabetes-exercise.org
Website: http://www.diabetes-exercise.org
Paula Harper, RN, CDE, Pres.

Fnded: 1985. **Mem:** 3,500. **Reg. Groups:** 12. **Desc:** Individuals with diabetes and healthcare professionals. Promotes the participation of individuals with diabetes in sports activities. Provides a network and support group for athletes with diabetes. Conducts educational programs to increase self care skills for individuals with diabetes and counseling skills for healthcare professionals. Offers blood sugar screenings; sponsors volunteer services and speakers' bureau. Conducts children's services. **Pub:** *Challenge*, quarterly. Newsletter. Educational with inspiring stories of success with diabetes and exercise. *Price:* Free for members. • *Get Ready-Get Set-Go*. Pamphlet. **Frmly:** International Diabetic Athletes Association.

★ 2558 ★ Diabetes Federation of Ireland
76 Lower Gardiner St.
Dublin 1, Ireland
Phone: 353 1 8363022 **Fax:** 353 1 8365182
Email: info@diabetes.ie
Website: http://www.diabetesireland.ie

Fnded: 1967. **Mem:** 5,000. **Local Groups:** 21. **Desc:** Represents people with diabetes. Provides information, creates awareness encourages research and ongoing support of people with diabetes. **Pub:** *Identity*, quarterly. Magazine. Contains diabetes information.

★ 2559 ★ Diabetes New Zealand (DNZ)
Freepost 36
PO Box 54
Oamaru, New Zealand
Website: http://www.diabetes.org.nz

Fnded: 1962. **Mem:** 12,500. **Desc:** Provides support for members and health professionals involved with diabetes. Works to increase the general public's awareness of diabetes in order to reduce undiagnosed diabetes. Offers assistance to people with diabetes in their day to day management and control. Fosters research in the treatment, prevention and cure of diabetes. Liaises with other diabetes societies. Develops and distributes educational resources, including booklets, pamphlets, and videos.

★ 2560 ★ Diabetes Research Institute Foundation (DRIF)
3440 Hollywood Blvd., Ste. 100
Hollywood, FL 33021
Phone: (954)964-4040 **Free:** 800-321-3437
Fax: (954)964-7036
Website: http://www.drinet.org
Robert A. Pearlman, Pres.

Fnded: 1971. **Mem:** 10,000. **Reg. Groups:** 2. **Desc:** Works to improve the quality of life for individuals with diabetes and to find a cure for diabetes. Acts as an information clearinghouse. Offers referral services. Fosters research on diabetes. Conducts educational programs; maintains speakers' bureau. Compiles statistics. **Pub:** *Focus*, 3/year. Newsletter. Covers foundation events, research news, and donor profiles. *Price:* included in membership dues.

★ 2561 ★ Dietary Managers Association (DMA)
406 Surrey Woods Drive
Saint Charles, IL 60174
Phone: (630)587-6336 **Free:** 800-323-1908
Fax: (630)587-6308
Email: info@dmaonline.com
Website: http://www.dmaonline.org
Colleen A. Zenk, CFPP, Chair

Fnded: 1960. **Mem:** 14,000. **State Groups:** 50. **Desc:** Dietary managers united to maintain a high level of competency and quality in dietary departments through continuing education. Provides educational programs and placement service. **Pub:** *Diet Therapy for the Dietary Manager*. Book. *Price:* $47.50 for nonmembers. • *Dietary Manager*, bimonthly. Magazine. *Price:* $24/year. • *Managing Foodservice Operations*. Book. • *Professional Procurement Practices*.

Book. **Frmly:** Hospital, Institution and Educational Food Service Society.

★ 2562 ★ Dietitians Association of Australia (DAA)
1/8 Phipps Close
Deakin, ACT 2600, Australia
Phone: 61 2 62829555 **Fax:** 61 2 62829888
Email: nationaloffice@daa.asn.au
Website: http://www.daa.asn.au

Fnded: 1976. **Mem:** 2,200. **Nat'l Groups:** 1. **State Groups:** 8. **Lang(s):** English. **Desc:** Accredited dietitians, students, and other individuals with an interest in nutrition. Works to improve public health through establishment of healthier eating habits. Seeks to enhance the professional standing of members. Serves as a liaison linking members to related professional, governmental, industrial, and educational organizations. Provides technical and professional support to members; lobbies government agencies responsible for food and nutrition. **Pub:** *Nutrition & Dietetics*, quarterly. Journal. • *Vision and Strategic Direction Statement*. Brochure. • Annual Report. • Handbooks. • Newsletter, monthly. • Pamphlets. • Papers. • Proceedings.

★ 2563 ★ Dietitians of Canada (DC)
480 University Ave., Ste. 604
Toronto, ON, Canada M5G 1V2
Phone: (416)596-0857 **Fax:** (416)596-0603
Email: centralinfo@dietitians.ca
Website: http://www.dietitians.ca

Fnded: 1935. **Mem:** 5,000. **Lang(s):** English, French. **Desc:** Leads and supports members to promote health and well being through expertise in food and nutrition. **Pub:** *Canadian Journal of Dietetic Research and Practice*, quarterly. Journal.

★ 2564 ★ Digestive Disease National Coalition (DDNC)
507 Capital Court NE, Ste. 200
Washington, DC 20002
Phone: (202)544-7497 **Fax:** (202)546-7105
Website: http://www.ddnc.org
Dale P. Dirks, Washington Rep.

Fnded: 1979. **Mem:** 30. **Desc:** Lay and professional medical organizations concerned with digestive diseases. Objectives are to: inform the public and the health care community about digestive diseases and related nutrition; seek federal funding for research, education, and training. Represents members' interests regarding federal and state legislation that affects digestive diseases research, health care, and education. **Frmly:** (1986) Coalition of Digestive Disease Organizations.

★ 2565 ★ Digestive Disorders Foundation
3 St. Andrews' Place
London NW1 4LB, United Kingdom
Phone: 44 207 4860341 **Fax:** 44 20 72242012
Email: ddf@digestivedisorders.org.uk
Website: http://www.digestivedisorders.org.uk

Fnded: 1971. **Desc:** Aims to raise money for research into digestive disorders and diseases. Patient information leaflets are available on receipt of a stamped self-addressed envelope. These cover the most common digestive disorders. **Pub:** *Annual Review*, annual.

★ 2566 ★ Dinshah Health Society (DHS)
PO Box 707
Malaga, NJ 08328-0707
Phone: (856)692-4686 **Fax:** (856)696-7890
Email: dinshahhealth@aol.com
Website: http://www.dinshahhealth.org/
Darius Dinshah, Pres.

Fnded: 1975. **Mem:** 3,149. **Desc:** Health professionals and other interested individuals who use and promote chromopathy as a therapy. Chromopathy, or color therapy, involves the use of projected colors of light to treat specific health problems. Seeks to stimulate interest in and knowledge of chromopathy and other lesser-known therapies. **Pub:** *Let There Be Light*. Book. *Price:* $15. • Newsletter, 3-5/year.

★ 2567 ★ Disability Alliance
Universal House
89-94 Wentworth St.
London E1 7SA, United Kingdom
Phone: 44 20 72478776 **Fax:** 44 20 72478765
Email: office.da@dial.pipex.com
Website: http://www.disabilityalliance.org

Fnded: 1974. **Mem:** 380. **Desc:** Committed to breaking the link between poverty and disability by providing information to disabled people about entitlements; campaigns for improvements to social security system and for increases in disability benefits so persons can better reflect the real costs of disability. **Pub:** *AA Guide and Checklist*. Handbook. • *Disability Rights Handbook*, annual. Handbook. • *OLA Guide and Checklist*. Handbook. • Bulletin, 3/year. **Frmly:** (1999) Disability Alliance Education and Research Association.

★ 2568 ★ Disability Central
PO Box 8612
Long Beach, CA 90808-0612
Website: http://www.disabilitycentral.com

Desc: People with disabilities. Promote disability awareness. Provide information and resources.

★ 2569 ★ Disability Federation of Ireland (DFI)
2 Sandyford Office Park
Dublin 18, Ireland
Phone: 353 1 2959344 **Fax:** 353 1 2959346
Email: info@disability-federation.ie
Website: http://ireland.iol.ie/~dfi/

Fnded: 1960. **Mem:** 73. **Lang(s):** English, Irish. **Desc:** Voluntary and nonstatutory agencies providing support services to people with disabilities. Seeks to increase the availability and quality of services for people with disabilities; promotes development of the full potential of all people. Provides support and assistance to members; facilitates communication and networking among members; develops training programs for people providing services to people with disabilities; serves as a liaison linking members with public agencies responsible for statutes affecting people with disabilities. Makes available resource services; sponsors research and educational programs; conducts lobbying activities. **Pub:** *DFI Newsletter*, monthly. Newsletter. • *Disability Federation of Ireland Directory*, annual. Directory.

★ 2570 ★ Disability Resources
4 Glatter Ln.
Centereach, NY 11720-1032
Phone: (631)585-0290 **Fax:** (631)585-0290
Email: pubs@disabilityresources.org
Website: http://www.disabilityresources.org
Avery Klauber, Exec. Dir.

Fnded: 1993. **Desc:** Works to promote and improve awareness, availability and accessibility of information to help people with disabilities to live independently. Advises libraries, independent living centers, rehabilitation professionals, hospitals, health and social service organizations, and consumers of resources and publications concerning independent living. **Pub:** *Disability Information at Your Fingertips, 3rd Ed.*. Book. *Price:* $10. • *Disability Resources Monthly (DRM)*, monthly. Newsletter. Reports on and reviews resources for independent living. *Price:* $33/year.

★ 2571 ★ Disability Rights Center (DRC)
PO Box 2007
Augusta, ME 04338-2007
Phone: (207)626-2774 **Free:** 800-452-1948
Fax: (207)621-1419
Email: advocate@drcme.org
Website: http://www.drcme.org
Kim Moody, Exec. Dir.

Fnded: 1976. **Desc:** Public interest research group committed to educating society about the disability rights movement. Objectives are to inform the public, political activists, consumer activists, advocates, and students on the disability movement. Major current projects are disability photo project, capital ADAPT and using media effectively. Through its activities, the center seeks to involve as many disabled citizens as possible in processes that directly affect their lives, to work closely with other disability-related, consumer-based advocacy groups, and to educate the public in the legitimate demands and needs of the disabled. Through its activites, the center seeks to involve as many disabled citizens as possible in processes that directly affect their lives, to work closely wiht other disability-related, consumer-based advocacy groups, and to educate the public in the legitimate demands and needs of the disabled. Compiles statistics.

★ 2572 ★ Disability Rights Education and Defense Fund (DREDF)
2212 6th St.
Berkeley, CA 94710
Phone: (510)644-2555 **Fax:** (510)841-8645
Email: dredf@dredf.org
Website: http://www.dredf.org/
Beverly Bertaina, Pres.

Fnded: 1979. **Desc:** Dedicated to the principle that people with disabilities have the right to lead full and integrated lives, with the freedom of choice and dignity. Seeks to educate the public and policymakers in order to further the civil rights and liberties of people with disabilities. Educational activities include: training state and local government officials, attorneys, and judges on disability rights compliance requirements such as the Americans with Disabilities Act; preparing materials pertaining to the right of children with disabilities to a free and appropriate public education. Houses the Disability Rights Clinical Legal Education Program which educates law students about disability rights laws and represents people with disabilites who have experienced unlawful discrimination. Provides technical assistance. **Pub:** *Disability Rights News*, quarterly. • *Explanation of the Contents of the ADA*. Book. *Price:* $118. • Manuals.

★ 2573 ★ Disability Sport - England (DSE)
Unit 4G
784-788 High Rd.
Tottenham
London N17 0DA, United Kingdom
Phone: 44 208 8014466 **Fax:** 44 208 8016644
Email: info@dse.org.uk
Website: http://www.disabilitysport.org.uk

Fnded: 1961. **Mem:** 50,000. **Reg. Groups:** 10. **Desc:** Provides opportunities for persons with any kind of disability to enjoy and compete in physical recreation and sport. Promotes the benefits of physical fitness and encourages people with disabilities to participate in the organization and development of sports at all levels. Supports local clubs and groups in their provision of recreational and sporting opportunities. Educates the public, the sporting world, and the media of the sporting abilities and achievements of people with disabilities. Organizes 12 national championships and more than 200 regional events for persons with disabilities. **Pub:** *Disability View*, periodic. Brochures. • *Info Pack*, annual. Newsletter. • *Newsletter*, periodic. Newsletter. **Frmly:** British Sports Association for the Disabled.

★ 2574 ★ Disabled and Alone/Life Services for the Handicapped
c/o Roslyn Brilliant
352 Park Ave. S, 11th Fl.
New York, NY 10010
Phone: (212)532-6740 **Free:** 800-995-0066
Fax: (212)532-3588
Email: disabledandalone@aol.com
Roslyn Brilliant, Exec. Dir.

Fnded: 1988. **Mem:** 30. **Desc:** Helps families plan for the time when they will not be able to care for their disabled children. Functions as quasi/surrogate parents for disabled people whose families have left assets for their care. Conducts educational programs on lifetime planning for families with a disabled member. Maintains speakers' bureau. **Pub:** *How to be a Friend to the Handicapped.* Book. *Price:* $50 for a prepaid shipment of 10 books; $6.95 for 1 book including postage. • *Lifelines*, 3/year. Newsletter. Provides information about "lifetime care" (future care) planning for a person with a disability. *Price:* Free. • Also publishes brochures, prospectus, articles about "lifetime care" (future care) planning for a person with a disability. **Frmly:** (2000) Life Services for the Handicapped.

★ 2575 ★ Disabled Drivers' Association - England (DDA)

Ashwellthorpe
Norwich NR16 1EX, United Kingdom
Phone: 44 870 7703333 **Fax:** 44 1508 488173
Email: ddahq@aol.com
Website: http://www.dda.org.uk

Fnded: 1948. **Mem:** 26,500. **Local Groups:** 34. **Desc:** Available to all disabilities and also able bodied members. Offers advice and information, benefits and concessions with most ferry companies. Local and national campaigns.

★ 2576 ★ Disabled Drivers' Association of Ireland (DDA)

Ballindine, Mayo, Ireland
Phone: 353 9464054 **Fax:** 353 9464336
Email: ability@iol.ie
Website: http://www.iol.ie/~ability

Fnded: 1970. **Mem:** 4,500. **Reg. Groups:** 1. **Lang(s):** English, Irish, Russian. **Desc:** Individuals and organizations. Promotes improve mobility for people with disabilities. Lobbies to safeguard the right of people with disabilities to obtain drivers' licenses; conducts educational and training programs. **Pub:** *Steering Wheel*, annual. Magazine. Contains general interest information.

★ 2577 ★ Disabled Living Foundation

380-384 Harrow Rd.
London W9 2HU, United Kingdom
Phone: 44 207 2896111 **Fax:** 44 207 2662922
Email: advice@dlf.org.uk
Website: http://www.dlf.org.uk

Fnded: 1970. **Desc:** Provides impartial information on disability equipment for daily living.

★ 2578 ★ Disabled People's Association of Singapore (DPA)

150 A Pandan Gardens
No. 02-00 Day Care Center
Singapore 609342, Singapore
Phone: 65 68991220 **Fax:** 65 68991232
Email: dpa@dpa.org.sg
Website: http://www.dpa.org.sg

Fnded: 1986. **Mem:** 200. **Nat'l Groups:** 4. **Lang(s):** French, Malagasy. **Desc:** Physically, mentally, and sensorially disabled persons, their families, and other supporters. To empower disabled people to promote the changing of negative attitudes towards disability, advocacy and struggle for the equalization of opportunities in education, access to buildinga, information and documentation and income generation. All projects come under RRICCH - Resource and Research, Information Communications Centre of the Handicapped. Public education and awareness, disability groups, development and running of disability database - Enablenet - globally accessible through Internet. **Pub:** *Integrator*, quarterly. Newspaper. Contains news regarding disability issues locally, regionally and internationally.

★ 2579 ★ Disabled Peoples' International - Canada (DPI)

101-7 Evergreen
Winnipeg, MB, Canada R3L 2T3
Phone: (204)287-8010 **Fax:** (204)783-6270
Email: dpi@dpi.org
Website: http://www.dpi.org

Fnded: 1981. **Reg. Groups:** 5. **Lang(s):** English, French, Spanish. **Desc:** National organizations of physically or mentally disabled persons, their parents, and other advocates. Promotes equal opportunity and full participation of disabled people in all aspects of society as a matter of justice rather than charity and based on the principle of integration. Encourages unity among members and mutual cooperation, assistance, and understanding among all people. Is particularly concerned with developing organizations of disabled persons in the Third World and in developing selfhelp efforts in these countries. **Pub:** *Disability International*, quarterly. Magazine.

★ 2580 ★ Disabled Peoples' International - Jamaica (Organizacion Mundial de Peronas Impedidas)

PO Box 220
Liguarea
Kingston 6, Jamaica
Phone: (876)927-2537 **Fax:** (876)920-8989
Email: mmitchell@anngel.com.jm
Website: http://www.dpi.org

Desc: Promotes the interests of disabled individuals in Jamaica. **Pub:** *Statement on Equalization of Opportunities.* • *Vox Nostra.*

★ 2581 ★ Disabled Persons Assembly New Zealand (DPA)

PO Box 27524
Wellington 6035, New Zealand
Phone: 64 4 8019100 **Fax:** 64 4 8019565
Email: gen@dpa.org.nz
Website: http://www.dpa.org.nz

Fnded: 1983. **Mem:** 1,700. **Reg. Groups:** 20. **Lang(s):** English. **Desc:** People with disabilities, their families, and others with an interest in the rights of people with disabilities. Works to ensure that people with disabilities are considered in the formation of public policy; advocates to expand the rights of people with disabilities. **Pub:** *Able Update*, quarterly. Magazine. • *Blueprint for Change.* • *Guide to Access Legislation.* • Annual Report, annual. • Manual. Covers DPA policies. DPA Bites (all available on our website)

★ 2582 ★ Disabled Sports USA

451 Hungerford Dr., Ste. 100
Rockville, MD 20850
Phone: (301)217-0960 **Fax:** (301)217-0968
Email: kbauer@dsusa.org
Website: http://www.dsusa.org
Kirk M. Bauer, Exec. Dir.

Fnded: 1967. **Mem:** 20,000. **Reg. Groups:** 7. **Local Groups:** 86. **Desc:** Promotes sports and recreation opportunities for individuals with physical disabilities. Provides direct services to people with mobility impairments, including amputations, paraplegia, quadriplegia, spinal cord injuries, stroke, head injuries, cerebral palsy, polio, muscular dystrophy, multiple sclerosis, arthrogryposis, birth defects, neuromuscular disabilities, and visual impairments. Offers and sanctions recreational winter and summer programs, including learn-to-ski, learn-to-sail, and learn-to-race clinics, competitive alpine and nordic skiing, archery, basketball, cycling, lawnbowling, shooting, swimming, table tennis, track and field, volleyball, sailing, and weighlifting. Conducts special programs for children, women, and veterans with disabilities. Offers training and certification of adaptive fitness and adaptive ski instructors. Sponsors U.S. Disabled Ski Team, U.S. Amputee Summer Sports Team, and U.S. Disabled Sports Team. Maintains hall of fame. **Pub:** *Adaptive Ski Teaching Methods*, every 3/months. Newsletter. In two volumes. • *Aerobics for Amputees.* Video. • *Aerobics for Cerebral Palsy.* Video. • *Aerobics for Paraplegia.* Video. • *Aerobics for Quadriplegia.* Video. • *Disabled Children in Physical Education: Learning Through Movement.* Handbook. Overview of proper adapted physical education programs for disabled children. *Price:* $14.95. • *Fitness Programming and Physical Disabilities.* Manual. • *Manual for Adaptive Fitness Instructors.* Manual. • *Manual for Adaptive Ski Instructors.* Manual. • *Strengthen Flexibility Exercises for All Types of Disabilities.* Video. **Frmly:** (1972) National Amputee Skiers Association; (1977) National Inconvenienced Sportsmen's Association; (1989) National Handicapped Sports and Recreation Association; (1998) National Handicapped Sports.

★ 2583 ★ Disabled Women Union

Dachniy Ave. 7-5-23
Saint Petersburg, Russia
Phone: 7 812 1572937 **Fax:** 7 812 1572937

Fnded: 1990. **Mem:** 130. **Desc:** Disabled women. Promotes the interests of disabled women in Russia. Conducts charitable programs. **Frmly:** Disabled Women Foundation.

★ 2584 ★ Disabled Women's Network Canada

200 Bay St., Ste. 301
Ottawa, ON, Canada K1R 7W8
Phone: (613)235-4242 **Fax:** (613)235-3881
Email: kathy@dawncanada.net
Website: http://www.dawncanada.net

Fnded: 1985. **Mem:** 300. **Lang(s):** English, French. **Desc:** Women with disabilities, organizations concerned with disability issues, and non-disabled supporters. A feminist organization that recognizes and addresses issues of concern to women with disabilities such as: poverty; employment equity; violence against women; parenting; health; access to services; and education. Provides information regarding issues of concern to disabled women, women's organizations, and the government. Allows women with disabilities the opportunity to participate in the women's movement. Cooperates with other groups involved in the quest for social justice nationally and internationally. Offers role models to girls with disabilites. Participates in research. **Pub:** *Beating the Odds: Violence and Women with Disabilities.* Book. • *Different Therefore Unequal: Employment and Women with Disabilities.* Book. • *Meeting Our Needs: An Access Manual for Transition Houses.* Book. • *New Reproductive Technologies.* Book. • *The Only Parent in the Neighbourhood: Mothering and Women with Disabilities.* Book. • *Thriving*, quarterly. Newsletter. • *Who Do We Think We Are?: Self-Image and Women with Disabilities.* Book.

★ 2585 ★ Disabled Womyn's Educational Project

PO Box 8773
Madison, WI 53708-8773
Phone: (608)256-8883 **Fax:** (608)256-8883
Email: catherine-odette@juno.com
Catherine Odette, Exec. Officer

Fnded: 1988. **Desc:** Lesbians with disabilities. Promotes members' interests. Supports legislation sensitive to members' needs. Maintains speakers' bureau. **Pub:** *Building Community Through Access.* • *Dykes, Disability, and Stuff*, quarterly. Newsletter. Available in the format of audiocassette, braille, DOS diskette, large print, modem transfer, audio tape. • *Dykes, Disability & Stuff*, quarterly. Newsletter. *Price:* $25/year. • *The Time for Access is Now.*

★ 2586 ★ Disaster Psychiatry Outreach (DPO)

141 5th Ave., 3rd Fl.
New York, NY 10010
Phone: (212)598-9995 **Fax:** (212)598-5957
Email: info@disasterpsych.org
Website: http://www.disasterpsych.org
Anastasia Holmes, Exec. Dir.

Fnded: 1998. **Mem:** 1,100. **Desc:** Dedicated to providing high quality disaster mental health services.

★ 2587 ★ Disease Management Association of America (DMAA)
1129 20th St. NW, Ste. 850
Washington, DC 20036
Phone: (202)861-1490 **Fax:** (202)861-1477
Website: http://www.dmaa.org/
Warren E. Todd, Exec. Dir.

Fnded: 1999. **Desc:** Disease management through standardization of definitions, program components, outcome measures; promotes public awareness of importance of disease management to enhance health. **Pub:** *Disease Management*, quarterly. Journal. *Price:* included in membership dues.

★ 2588 ★ Disinfected Mail Study Circle (DMSC)
25 Sinclair Grove
London NW11 9JH, United Kingdom
Phone: 44 208 4559190
Email: vdvpratique@aol.com

Fnded: 1974. **Mem:** 140. **Lang(s):** English. **Desc:** Postal historians, doctors, researchers, libraries, and research foundations in 25 countries. Studies the historic treatment of mail so as to prevent the spread of contagious diseases. The study circle is continuing the research work of the late Dr. K. F. Meyer and his associates, many of whom are members. The study has been extended to include health certificates and passports, quarantine ephemera, anti-vaccination postal propaganda, and related subjects. Maintains speakers' bureau; conducts research programs. **Pub:** *Cumulative Indexes*, 3/year. Journal. • *Pratique*, 3/year. Magazine. Contains research articles and notices of meetings.

★ 2589 ★ Disorders of Chromosome 16 Foundation (DOC16)
c/o Karen Lange
331 Haddon Cir.
Vernon Hills, IL 60061
Phone: (847)816-0627 **Fax:** (847)367-4031
Email: kblange1@aol.com
Website: http://www.trisomy16.org
Karen Lange, Pres.

Desc: Promotes research into Disorders of Chromosome 16 and provides information on abnormalities; offers information, education and support to families of children living with the disorder and to expectant parents confronting a similar diagnosis; serves as a resource aiding families, friends, caregivers, and medical professionals in their supportive roles. Provides referrals and a database of registered families. **Pub:** Newsletter, quarterly.

★ 2590 ★ Division of Family Psychology
c/o American Psychological Association
750 First St. NE
Washington, DC 20002-4242
Phone: (202)336-6013 **Fax:** (202)218-3599
Email: brhamp@aol.com
Website: http://www.apa.org/divisions/div43
Nadine Kaslow, PhD, ABPP, Pres.

Fnded: 1984. **Mem:** 2,000. **Desc:** A division of the American Psychological Association. Psychologists interested in research, teaching, prevention, treatment, evaluation, and public interest initiatives in family psychology. seeks to promote human welfare through the development, dissemination, and application of knowledge about the dynamics, structure, and functioning of the family. Conducts research and specialized education programs. Maintains speakers' bureau. **Pub:** *The Family Psychologist*, quarterly. Bulletin.

★ 2591 ★ DKT International - Vietnam (DKTIVN)
8 Trang Thi St., Glass House No. 13-15
Hanoi, Vietnam
Phone: 84 4 8260043 **Fax:** 84 4 8260262
Email: larry@dktinternational.org
Website: http://www.dktinternational.org

Fnded: 1993. **Lang(s):** English, French, Vietnamese. **Desc:** Population and public health programs operating in Vietnam. Seeks to increase availability of primary health care and family planning services. Makes available health services; conducts educational programs to raise public awareness of population issues.

★ 2592 ★ Do It Now Foundation (DINF)
PO Box 27568
Tempe, AZ 85285
Phone: (480)736-0599 **Free:** 877-515-9411
Fax: (480)736-0771
Email: info@doitnow.org
Website: http://www.doitnow.org
James D. Parker, Exec. Dir.

Fnded: 1968. **Mem:** 40. **Nat'l Groups:** 1. **Desc:** Works to provide factual information to students and adults about prescription drugs, over-the-counter drugs, street drugs, alcohol, eating disorders, AIDS, and related health issues. Assists organizations engaged in alcohol and drug abuse education. Publishes educational materials; offers pamphlets, posters, books, and radio public service tapes in Spanish and English.

★ 2593 ★ Doctors for Disaster Preparedness (DDP)
1601 N Tucson Blvd Ste. 9
Tucson, AZ 85716
Phone: (520)325-2680 **Fax:** (520)326-3529
Website: http://www.oism.org/ddp
Jane Orient, MD, Pres.

Fnded: 1982. **Mem:** 200. **Desc:** Doctors, health professionals, medical students and interested individuals. Prepares physicians, health professionals, personnel, and the public for medical response in the case of natural or human-caused disaster. Seeks to prevent human suffering and death resulting from any catastrophe. Believes that "there is no disaster so great - including nuclear war - that the medical profession is not obliged to care for the survivors." Promotes accurate risk assessment. Supports civil defense measures; maintains no position on specific military or foreign policy measures, weapons systems, or arms control. Sponsors lectures for health professionals, government leaders, and the public concerning disaster preparedness. Compiles statistics; maintains speakers' bureau. **Pub:** *Civil Defense Perspectives*, bimonthly. Newsletter. *Price:* Included in membership dues. • *Doctors for Disaster Preparedness Newsletter*, bimonthly. Newsletter. *Price:* Included in membership fees. • Reprints.Consists of literature related to disaster preparedness.

★ 2594 ★ Doctors for the Environment - South Africa
c/o Heinz Niebuhr
PO Box 1616
Vryheid 3100, Republic of South Africa
Phone: 27 381 809151
Email: hfn@dorea.co.za
Website: http://www.isde.org/southafrica.html

Fnded: 1994. **Mem:** 30. **Desc:** Promotes the profession of environmental physician in South Africa.

★ 2595 ★ Doctors Ought to Care (DOC)
5615 Kirby Dr., Ste. 440
Houston, TX 77005
Phone: (713)528-1487 **Free:** 800-362-9340
Fax: (713)528-2146
Email: d-o-c@texas.net
Website: http://www.bcm.tmc.edu/doc
Eric Solberg, M.A., Pres.

Fnded: 1977. **Mem:** 1,374. **Local Groups:** 76. **Desc:** A physician-led organization of medical students, teachers, parents, and other concerned individuals working to counteract the promotion of unhealthy products, primarily tobacco and alcohol. Works through school programs, health professionals' offices, hospitals, media, and Super Health 2000, a health promotion effort which attempts to counter the effects of advertising unhealthy products. Seeks to launch a broad health promotion effort aimed at educating the public, particularly teenagers and children, on the "lethal" lifestyles of tobacco and alcohol use. Campaigns through television commercials, radio, sports events, posters and t-shirts, and its speakers' bureau to promote the image of good health through community-wide reinforcement of the positive role model of the health professional. Serves as a resource center on tobacco and alcohol issues. **Pub:** *The Journal of Medical Activism*, quarterly. Newsletter. Fights advertising and promotion of unhealthy products by the tobacco and alcohol industry. Includes information on the pro-health community. *Price:* included in membership dues.

★ 2596 ★ Dog Guides Canada
PO Box 907
Oakville, ON, Canada L6J 5E8
Phone: (905)842-2891 **Fax:** (905)842-3373
Email: info@dogguides.com
Website: http://www.dogguides.com

Lang(s): English, French. **Desc:** Breeders and trainers of hearing dogs. Promotes the use of special assistance dogs by people with disabilities. Breeds, raises, and trains hearing ear and seeing eye dogs; maintains registry of special assistance dogs for people with hearing and visual impairment.

★ 2597 ★ Dogs for the Deaf (DFD)
10175 Wheeler Rd.
Central Point, OR 97502
Phone: (541)826-9220 **Free:** 800-990-DOGS
Fax: (541)826-6696
Email: info@dogsforthedeaf.org
Website: http://www.dogsforthedeaf.org
Robin Dickson, CEO/Pres.

Fnded: 1977. **Mem:** 30,000. **Desc:** Trains hearing dogs to alert deaf persons to certain sounds. Dogs are chosen from pet adoption shelters and assigned on the basis of a prioritized waiting list. They undergo four to five months of training during which they are taught to alert their masters to the sounds of alarm clocks, smoke alarms, doorbells, oven timers, crying babies, and telephones. Deaf or severely hearing impaired persons are eligible to be recipients if they are old enough to assume responsibility for the care of the dog. When assigned, a trainer and the dog travel to the recipient's home for a week to teach the dog and recipient to work together. Costs of dog selection, veterinary care, housing, training, and placement are covered; recipients make a donation only if able. Trains individuals to be certified audio canine trainers. Has appeared on local and national television programs to present the hearing ear dog training process and the results of dog placement. **Pub:** *Canine Listener*, quarterly. Provides information on the Hearing Ear Dog Program for the deaf; includes profiles of dogs and owners. *Price:* Free.

★ 2598 ★ Donald W. Reynolds Foundation
1701 Village Center Cir.
Las Vegas, NV 89134
Phone: (702)804-6000 **Fax:** (702)804-6099
Email: generalquestions@dwrf.org
Website: http://www.dwreynolds.org

Desc: Works to provide support for cardiovascular clinical research and aging and quality of life programs.

★ 2599 ★ Doulas of North America (DONA)
PO Box 626
Jasper, IN 47547-0626
Free: 888-788-DONA
Email: doula@dona.org
Website: http://www.DONA.org
Kelly Livesay, Admin. Mgr.

Fnded: 1992. **Mem:** 3,500. **Reg. Groups:** 9. **State Groups:** 50. **Desc:** Seeks to help doulas provide quality labor support to birthing women. Offers certification program for doulas; provides continuing education opportnities; establishes standards of practice and code of ethics; compiles statistics. **Pub:** *DONA Referral Directory*. Directory. • *The International Doula*, quarterly. Newsletter. • *The International Doula Trainer*, quarterly. Newsletter. • *Introducing the Doula*. Video. *Price:* $15 for members; $25 for non-members.

★ 2600 ★ Down Syndrome Ireland (DSI)

30 Mary St.
Dublin 1, Ireland
Phone: 353 1 8730999 **Fax:** 353 1 8731064
Email: dsi@eircom.net
Website: http://www.downsyndrome.ie

Fnded: 1972. **Mem:** 2,650. **Reg. Groups:** 23. **Lang(s):** English, Irish. **Desc:** People with Down syndrome and their families; health care and service providers working with people with Down syndrome. Seeks to improve the quality of life of people with Down syndrome. Provides support and services to people with Down syndrome and their families; conducts educational programs. **Pub:** Magazine, quarterly. • Newsletter, 5/year.

★ 2601 ★ Down's Syndrome Association (DSA)

155 Mitcham Rd.
London SW17 9PG, United Kingdom
Phone: 44 208 6824001 **Fax:** 44 208 6824012
Email: info@downs-syndrome.org.uk
Website: http://www.dsa-uk.com

Fnded: 1970. **Mem:** 12,000. **Lang(s):** English. **Desc:** Provides information, advice, and support in England, Wales, and Northern Ireland on Down's Syndrome. Does this through its information service and helpline, regional offices, and parent-led local branches. Works toward creating the conditions whereby individuals with Down's Syndrome can receive necessary medical, educational, social, and financial support to develop to their full potential. **Pub:** Newsletter, quarterly. Contains information contributed by members and research updates.

★ 2602 ★ Drug and Alcohol Testing Industry Association (DATIA)

1600 Duke St., Ste. 220
Alexandria, VA 22314
Free: 800-355-1257 **Fax:** (703)519-1716
Email: datia@wpa.org
Website: http://www.datia.org
Dean Klassy, Chm.

Fnded: 1995. **Mem:** 1,000. **Desc:** Drug and alcohol service providers including collection sites, laboratories, consortiums/TPA's, MRO's and testing equipment manufacturers.

★ 2603 ★ Drug Free Kids: America's Challenge

PO Box 60865
Washington, DC 20039
Phone: (301)681-7861
Email: info@drugfreekids.org
Website: http://www.ourdrugfreekids.org
Joyce Nalepka, Pres.

Desc: Promote protection of children against drugs. Hold vigils and rallies.

★ 2604 ★ Drug Information Association (DIA)

800 Enterprise Rd., Ste. 200
Horsham, PA 19044
Phone: (215)442-6100 **Fax:** (215)442-6199
Email: dia@diahome.org
Website: http://www.diahome.org
Joseph R. Assenzo, PhD, Exec. Dir.

Fnded: 1965. **Mem:** 27,000. **Desc:** Provides neutral, global forum promoting exchange of information critical to professional performance and achievement in the discovery, development, regulation, surveillance, or marketing of pharmaceuticals or related products. **Pub:** *DIA Forum*, 3/year. Magazine. *Price:* included in membership dues. • *DIA Today*, quarterly. Newsletter. • *Drug Information Association–Membership Directory*, annual. Directory. *Price:* Included in membership dues; $100/copy for nonmembers. • *Drug Information Journal*, quarterly. Journal. *Price:* Included in membership dues.

★ 2605 ★ DrugScope

32-36 Loman St.
London SE1 0EE, United Kingdom
Phone: 44 20 79281211 **Fax:** 44 20 79281771
Email: info@drugscope.org.uk
Website: http://www.drugscope.org.uk

Fnded: 2000. **Mem:** 1,100. **Desc:** One of UK's leading centres of expertise on the misuse of drugs. Aims to inform policy development and reduce drug-related risk. Offers self-help information through website. **Pub:** Directories.

★ 2606 ★ Dual Disorders Anonymous

PO Box 681264
Schaumburg, IL 60168-1264
Phone: (847)490-9379
Email: pat63659@cs.com
Website: http://ourworld.cs.com/pat63659/myhomepage/business.html
Pat Kent, Pres.

Fnded: 1982. **Mem:** 500. **Nat'l Groups:** 20. **Reg. Groups:** 3. **State Groups:** 1. **Local Groups:** 21. **Desc:** Individuals with alcohol or drug addictions as well as mental or emotional disorders. Provides support group opportunities to emotionally or mentally disordered alcoholics and addicts; conducts volunteer programs for dually diagnosed patients. Utilizes the 12-step method of self-help. **Pub:** Booklet. • Brochures.

★ 2607 ★ Dutch Association of Abortion Doctors (Nederlands Genootschap van Abortusartsen — NGvA)

Postbox 113
NL-5660 AC Geldrop, Netherlands
Fax: 31 40 2851966
Email: mediscon@iae.nl
Website: http://www.ngva.net

Fnded: 1991. **Mem:** 60. **Lang(s):** Dutch, English, French, German. **Desc:** Physicians united to ensure the reproductive rights and health of women in the Netherlands. Conducts research and educational programs on the health, social, and psychological impact of abortion. **Pub:** *Practical Guide for Abortion Doctors*, annual. Handbook.

★ 2608 ★ Dutch Association of Environmental Medicine

c/o Peter Van den Hazel
PO Box 389
NL-6800 Arnhem, Netherlands
Phone: 31 26 3773915 **Fax:** 31 26 3773847
Email: p.j.van.den.hazel@inter.nl.net
Website: http://www.inter.nl.net/users/nvmm

Fnded: 1988. **Mem:** 150. **Desc:** Promotes the profession of environmental physician in the Netherlands. **Pub:** *Mededelingenblad*, bimonthly. • Brochures. Various brochures covering environmental topics, such as lead, indoor air pollution, etc.

★ 2609 ★ Dutch Council of the Chronically Ill and Disabled (DCD) (Federatie Nederlandse Gehandicaptenraad)

Postbus 169
NL-3500 AD Utrecht, Netherlands
Phone: 31 30 2916600 **Fax:** 31 30 2970111
Email: bureau@cg-raad.nl
Website: http://www.cg-raad.nl

Fnded: 1977. **Mem:** 75. **Lang(s):** Dutch, English. **Desc:** Physically handicapped individuals, their families, and affiliated organizations. Works for equality and full participation and opportunity for the disabled. Seeks to influence public policy toward the disabled in areas of: financial, social, technical, and infrastructural provisions; employment and volunteer work; education and educational services. Conducts educational programs. **Pub:** *Aan Zet*, monthly. • *Gehandicaptenraad Nieuws*, bimonthly. Newsletter. • *Norms and Values as a Handicap*. • Books, periodic.

★ 2610 ★ Dutch Deafship (Dovenschap)

PO Box 323
NL-3500 AH Utrecht, Netherlands
Fax: 31 30 2970030
Email: info@dovenschap.nl
Website: http://www.dovenschap.nl

Fnded: 1995. **Lang(s):** Dutch. **Desc:** Umbrella organization of associations for the hearing impaired. Encourages the emancipation and participation of the hearing impaired in society; disseminates information. Represents member organizations before government agencies and institutions; coordinates contact between members; works with other organizations concerned with the welfare of the deaf. **Frmly:** (1997) Dutch DeafAssociation.

★ 2611 ★ Dutch Dental Association (Nederlandsche Maatschappij tot Bevordering des Tandheelkunde — NMT)

PO Box 2000
NL-3430 CA Nieuwegein, Netherlands
Phone: 31 30 6076380 **Fax:** 31 30 6048994
Website: http://www.nmt.nl

Nat'l Groups: nde. **State Groups:** landsc. **Local Groups:** Bevord. **Desc:** Represents dentists and dental specialties, including dental surgeons and orthodontists, in the Netherlands.

★ 2612 ★ Dutch Pharmacological Society (Nederlandse Vereniging Voor Farmacologie)

c/o Prof. P.R. Saxena
Erasmus University
Institute of Pharmacology
PO Box 1738
NL-3000 Rotterdam, Netherlands
Phone: 31 10 4087537 **Fax:** 31 10 4089458
Email: saxena@farma.fgg.eur.nl

Mem: 320. **Desc:** Promotes pharmacology in the Netherlands.

★ 2613 ★ Dutch Society of Psychosomatic Obstetrics and Gynaecology

c/o Dr. E. Blokzijl
Department of Obstetrics & Gynaecology
Rijnstate Hospital
PO Box 9555
NL-6800 TA Arnhem, Netherlands
Fax: 31 26 3786892
Email: eblokzyl@knmg.nl
Website: http://www.ispog.org

Desc: Promotes the study of psychobiological and psychosocial, ethical and cross-cultural problems in the fields of obstetrics and gynaecology, women's health and reproductive health; facilitates the dissemination of new information in these fields. **Pub:** *Journal of Psychosomatic Obstetrics and Gynecology*. Journal.

★ 2614 ★ Dysautonomia Foundation

633 3rd Ave., 12th Fl.
New York, NY 10017
Phone: (212)949-6644 **Fax:** (212)682-7625
Email: dys212@aol.com
Website: http://www.familialdysautonomia.org/
Lenore F. Roseman, Exec. Dir.

Fnded: 1954. **Mem:** 14,000. **Desc:** Parents, relatives, friends, and benefactors of children afflicted with

Familial dysautonomia, a Jewish genetic disease of the autonomic nervous system. Now that the FD Gene has been located and there is a carrier available, we must now fund research into discovering the function the gene plays within the body. **Pub:** *DYS/COURSE*, semiannual. Newsletter. Includes research updates. *Price:* Free. • *Dysautonomia Foundation–Journal*, annual. Journal. *Price:* Free upon ad of $300 or more.

★ 2615 ★ Dyslexia Institute
Park House
Wick Rd.
Egham TW20 0HH, United Kingdom
Phone: 44 1784 222300 **Fax:** 44 1784 222333
Email: info@dyslexia-inst.org.uk
Website: http://www.dyslexia-inst.org.uk

Fnded: 1972. **Reg. Groups:** 25. **Desc:** Specializes in the development of individuals involved in the field of dyslexia; increases networking opportunities; broadens the sphere of influence, develops and maintains links with other bodies at all levels. **Pub:** *As We See It*, 3/year. Newsletter. • *Dyslexia Review*, 3/year. Journal. • *National DI Fee Guidelines.* • *Understanding Dyslexia*. Video. Contains practical advice and information including a guide for teachers and a guide for parents. Also publishes leaflets.

★ 2616 ★ Dyslexia Research Institute
5746 Centerville Rd.
Tallahassee, FL 32308
Phone: (850)893-2216 **Fax:** (850)893-2440
Email: dri@dyslexia-add.org
Website: http://www.dyslexia-add.org/
Patricia K. Hardman, PhD, Dir.

Fnded: 1975. **Desc:** Works to change the perception of learning differences, specifically in the area of dyslexia and attention deficit disorders (ADD).

★ 2617 ★ Dyspraxia Association of Ireland
c/o Communications House
Spruce Ave., Unit 58
Stillorgan Industrial Estate
Dublin, Ireland
Email: dyspraxiaireland@eircom.net
Website: http://indigo.ie/~dyspraxi/

Fnded: 1995. **Lang(s):** English. **Desc:** Parents of children with dyspraxia. Seeks to raise awareness of dyspraxia in Ireland and to create a better understanding of the difficulties children and parents face. Ensures adequate professional and medical resources are available to parents; provides information and a support network; works to improve diagnostic services.

★ 2618 ★ Dystonia Medical Research Foundation
1 E Wacker Dr., Ste. 2430
Chicago, IL 60601-1905
Phone: (312)755-0198 **Free:** 800-377-DYST
Fax: (312)803-0138
Email: dystonia@dystonia-foundation.org
Website: http://www.dystonia-foundation.org
Robert McAlister, PhD., Exec. Dir.

Fnded: 1977. **Mem:** 25,000. **Nat'l Groups:** 5. **Reg. Groups:** 8. **State Groups:** 100. **Local Groups:** 2. **Desc:** Dystonia patients and their families; medical personnel; health agencies; interested individuals. Promotes and funds research and encourages increased public awareness of dystonia, a neurologic muscular disorder causing muscles to jerk and contract into abnormal positions. Disseminates information concerning dystonia. Sponsors patient and family support groups. **Pub:** *Dystonia Dialogue*, 3/year. Newsletter. Includes foundation and chapter news and research updates. *Price:* Free. • Brochures.

★ 2619 ★ Dystrophic Epidermolysis Bullosa Research Association of America (DEBRA)
5 W 36th St., No. 404
New York, NY 10018
Phone: (212)868-1573 **Free:** (866)332-7276
Fax: (212)868-9296
Email: debra.nurse@mindspring.com
Website: http://www.debra.org
Martin Hassner, Exec. Dir.

Fnded: 1979. **Mem:** 5,000. **Desc:** People with Epidermolysis Bullosa and their families; other interested individuals. (Epidermolysis Bullosa represents a group of inherited disorders of the skin characterized by formation of blisters resulting from the most minimal trauma.) To raise funds to promote and support research into the cause, nature, and treatment of EB in all its forms; to relieve the physical and mental distress of victims by providing practical advice, guidance, support, and other assistance. Distributes educational material to the public and medical professionals. Works for federal funding for biomedical research of EB and related disorders. Offers children's services; conducts educational programs. conducts educational programs. **Pub:** *EB Currents*, semiannual. **AKA:** DEBRA of America.

★ 2620 ★ Dystrophic Epidermolysis Bullosa Research Association-Europe (DEBRA-Euro)
Duke's Ride
13 Wellington Business Park
Crowthorne RG11 6LS, United Kingdom
Website: http://www.debra.org.uk

★ 2621 ★ Ear Foundation (EF)
1817 Patterson St.
Nashville, TN 37203
Phone: (615)627-2724 **Fax:** (615)627-2728
Email: earfound@earfoundation.org
Website: http://www.theearfound.com
Suzane Wyatt, Exec. Dir.

Fnded: 1971. **Desc:** Benefactors dedicated to advance medical knowledge concerning ear diseases and to encourage public understanding of such disorders. Offers professional and public education programs; research directed towards Eustachian tube disorders, ear diseases, and related disorders such as hearing loss, tinnitus, and vertigo. **Pub:** Brochures. • Monographs. • Newsletter, periodic.

★ 2622 ★ East West Academy of Healing Arts (EWAHA)
117 Topaz Way
San Francisco, CA 94131
Phone: (415)288-9400 **Fax:** (415)647-5745
Email: eastwestqi@aol.com
Website: http://www.eastwestqi.com
Dr. Effie Chow, Founder

Fnded: 1973. **Desc:** Promotes holistic health, Qigong, and Oriental medicine. Sponsors educational and research programs; provides clinical services.

★ 2623 ★ Easter Seals
230 W Monroe St., Ste. 1800
Chicago, IL 60606
Phone: (312)726-6200 **Free:** 800-221-6827
Fax: (312)726-1494
Email: info@easter-seals.org
Website: http://www.easter-seals.org/

Desc: Provides children's services to help children with disabilities succeed in school, provides employment programs, physical medicine and rehabilitation services.

★ 2624 ★ Easter Seals National Headquarters
230 W Monroe, Ste. 1800
Chicago, IL 60606
Phone: (312)726-6200 **Free:** 800-221-6827
Fax: (312)726-1494
Email: info@easter-seals.org
Website: http://www.easter-seals.org
James E. Williams, Jr., Pres. /CEO

Fnded: 1919. **Mem:** 420. **Nat'l Groups:** 2. **State Groups:** 52. **Desc:** Provides services for children and adults with disabilities or special needs, and supports their families. Primary services include: medical rehabilitation, early intervention, physical therapy, occupational therapy, speech and hearing therapy, job training and employment, inclusive childcare, adult day services, camping and recreation. **Pub:** *Publications*. Catalog. **Frmly:** (1998) National Easter Seal Society.

★ 2625 ★ Eastern Branch of the Japan Endocrinological Society (Nippon Naibumpigaku-Kai Tobu-bukai)
School of Medicine, Gumma University
Maebashi, Japan
Fnded: 1954.

★ 2626 ★ Eating Disorders Association (EDA)
Wensum House, 1st Fl.
103 Prince of Wales Rd.
Norwich NR1 1DW, United Kingdom
Phone: 44 870 7703221 **Fax:** 44 1603 664915
Email: media@edauk.com
Website: http://www.edauk.com

Fnded: 1989. **Mem:** 3,500. **Local Groups:** 54. **Lang(s):** English. **Desc:** Individuals affected by anorexia, bulimia nervosa, and related eating disorders, their families, and friends. Offers information, help, and support. Seeks to enhance awareness and understanding of these illnesses. Communicates with related organizations and individuals in the medical and counseling professions. Disseminates information. Organizes regional support days. Offers training for professionals. **Pub:** *European Eating Disorders Review*, 5/year. Journal. • *Signpost*, quarterly. Magazine.

★ 2627 ★ Eating Disorders Northern Ireland
78 Glengoland Pk.
Belfast BT17 0JB, United Kingdom
Phone: 44 2890 621627

Fnded: 1992. **Mem:** 20. **Reg. Groups:** 2. **Local Groups:** 3. **Desc:** Support group for carers and sufferers of anorexia and other eating disorders. Disseminates information.

★ 2628 ★ Ebenezer Society (ES)
2722 Park Ave.
Minneapolis, MN 55407-1043
Mark Thomas, Pres.

Fnded: 1917. **Mem:** 45. **Desc:** Lutheran congregations and their delegates. Works to provide quality services and facilities for older people with varying needs; to make their lives more healthful, meaningful, and secure. Services are not limited to Lutheran clients. Offers nursing home care for low-income elderly; provides home services, including medical treatment, to help persons remain in their own homes as long as possible. Sponsors Ebenezer Center for Aging and Human Development which provides consultative services, conducts educational events and applied research, and issues publications. Maintains Ebenezer Foundation as the support arm of the society. Compiles research statistics; offers placement service. Ebenezer means "stone of help."

★ 2629 ★ Ecological Physicians Association (Okologischer Arztebund eV Ecological Physicians Association)
Bundesgeschaftsstelle
Fedelhoren 88
D-28203 Bremen, Germany
Phone: 49 421 4984251 **Fax:** 49 421 4984252
Email: oekologischer.aerztebund@t-online.de
Website: http://www.oekologischer-aerztebund.de

Fnded: 1987. **Mem:** 500. **Desc:** Promotes the return to a natural life existence as well as the preservation of human health. Provides information and treatment. Seeks to contribute to building ecological awareness. German section of the International Doctors for the Environment (ISDE). **Pub:** *Umwelt Medizin-Gesellschaft*, quarterly. Journal. Environment medicine society.

★ 2630 ★ ECRI

c/o Laurie D. Menyo, Communications Dept.
5200 Butler Pke.
Plymouth Meeting, PA 19462
Phone: (610)825-6000 **Fax:** (610)834-1275
Email: info@ecri.org
Website: http://www.ecri.org
Jeffrey C. Lerner, PhD, Pres. /CEO

Fnded: 1955. **Mem:** 5,000. **Desc:** Improves the safety, performance, reliability, and cost effectiveness of health care technology through research testing, and publication of results. Provides technical consulting and accident investigation and educational programs. Functions as a worldwide information clearinghouse for health care technology assessment and hazards and deficiencies in medical devices; sponsors seminars. Provides information and technical assistance for planning, procurement and management of medical equipment. Conducts research; compiles statistics and operates speakers' bureau. **Pub:** *Health Devices*, monthly. • *Health Devices Alerts*, weekly. • *Health Devices Sourcebook*, annual. Directory. • *Health Technology Trends*, monthly. Newsletter. • *Healthcare Environmental Management*, monthly. • *Healthcare Hazard Management Monitor*, monthly. Newsletter. • *Healthcare Product Comparison System*, monthly. • *Healthcare Risk Control*, monthly. • *Operating Room Risk Management*, bimonthly. • *Technology for Anesthesia*, periodic. Includes information on medical equipment and research updates. *Price:* $210/year. • *Technology for Cardiology*, monthly. Newsletter. Reports on ECRI comparative product evaluations; offers hazard reports on medical devices and device operation data. Includes research updates. *Price:* $210/year. • *Technology for Respiratory Therapy*, monthly. Newsletter. Evaluates medical devices and summarizes reported problems, hazards, and recalls. Includes research updates and health care technology abstracts. *Price:* $210/year. **Frmly:** (1955) Graduate Pain Research Foundation; (1968) Emergency Care Research Institute.

★ 2631 ★ Educational Audiology Association (EAA)

13153 N Dale Mabry Hwy., Ste. 105
Tampa, FL 33618-2410
Free: 800-460-7322 **Fax:** (813)968-3597
Email: eaa@l-tgraye.com
Website: http://www.edaud.org
Lois Kostroski, Exec. Dir.

Mem: 1,020. **Desc:** Audiologists and others with an interest in the field. Promotes advancement in the field of audiology and its educational applications. Conducts educational programs. **Pub:** *EAA Newsletter*, quarterly. Newsletter. • Journal, annual. Includes membership directory. **Frmly:** (1998) Educational Audiology Society.

★ 2632 ★ Educational Commission for Foreign Medical Graduates (ECFMG)

3624 Market St., 4th Fl.
Philadelphia, PA 19104-2685
Phone: (215)386-5900 **Fax:** (215)386-9196
Email: info@ecfmg.org
Website: http://www.ecfmg.org
Nancy E. Gary, MD, Pres. & CEO

Fnded: 1956. **Mem:** 20. **Desc:** Sponsoring organizations are American Board of Medical Specialties; American Medical Association; Association of American Medical Colleges; Association for Hospital Medical Education; the Federation of State Medical Boards of the U.S.; National Medical Association. Aims to provide information to graduates of foreign medical schools regarding entry into graduate medical education and the U.S. health care system; evaluate the qualifications of graduates of foreign medical schools; identify the cultural and professional needs of graduates of foreign medical schools and assist in the establishment of educational policies and programs; provides international access to testing and evaluation programs to meet theses needs. Sponsors exchange visitor program to enable physicians from other countries to participate in graduate medical education or training. Gathers and disseminates data about graduates of foreign medical schools. **Pub:** *Educational Commission for Foreign Medical Graduates–Annual Report*, annual. Annual Report. Details organizations history and programs. *Price:* Free. • *Educational Commission for Foreign Medical Graduates–Information Booklet*, annual. Booklet. Provides procedures for fulfilling ECFMG examination and certification requirements. *Price:* Free. **Frmly:** (1974) Educational Council for Foreign Medical Graduates.

★ 2633 ★ EFA

c/o Susana Palkonen
Allergia-ja Astnaliito
Pacuiksenkatu 19
FIN-00270 Helsinki, Finland
Phone: 358 9 47335303 **Fax:** 358 9 47335390
Email: susanna.palkonen@allergia.com

Fnded: 1991. **Desc:** Represents the interests of allergy patients in Europe.

★ 2634 ★ Egg Nutrition Center (ENC)

1050 17th St., NW, Ste. 560
Washington, DC 20036
Phone: (202)833-8850 **Fax:** (202)463-0102
Website: http://www.enc-online.org
Donald J. McNamara, PhD, Exec. Dir.

Fnded: 1984. **Desc:** Commercial egg producers and processors, health promotion agencies, and consumers. Provide scientifically accurate information on egg nutrition and the role of eggs in health and nutrition. Monitor nutrition research reports and nutrition policy development. **Pub:** *Nutrition Close-Up*, quarterly. Newsletter. Reviews and summarizes recent research reports.

★ 2635 ★ Egyptian Association for Psychological Studies (EAPS)

c/o Prof.Dr. Amal A.M. Sadek
Ain Shams University
Heliopolis
Cairo 11757, Egypt
Phone: 20 2 4515484 **Fax:** 20 2 6221642
Email: eapsegypt@hotmail.com
Website: http://eapsegypt.hypermart.net

Fnded: 1948. **Mem:** 750. **Desc:** Seeks to advance scholarship and research in psychology. **Pub:** *Arab Psychologist.* • *Egyptian Journal of Psychological Studies*, annual. Journal.

★ 2636 ★ Egyptian Autistic Society

9, Rd. 215
Degla
Maadi
Cairo, Egypt
Phone: 20 2 5199033 **Fax:** 20 2 5197055

Lang(s): English. **Desc:** Families with autistic children in Egypt. Works to increase awareness and understanding of autism. Provides a social club, workshops, summer camp, various forms of therapy; support groups, and training.

★ 2637 ★ Egyptian Orthopaedic Association (EOA)

c/o Hasan Elzaher Hassan, Pres.
16 Houda Shaarawi
Cairo 11111, Egypt
Phone: 20 2 3930013 **Fax:** 20 2 3930054
Email: eoa@starnet.com
Website: http://www.eoa.org.eg

Fnded: 1948. **Mem:** 2,000. **Lang(s):** English. **Desc:** Seeks to improve the knowledge of its members. Offers courses in orthopedics. **Pub:** *Egyptian Orthopaedic Journal*, semiannual. Journal.

★ 2638 ★ Egyptian Population Services Society (EPSS)

12 Sayem El Dahr St.
Rod El Faraq
Shoubra
Cairo, Egypt
Phone: 20 2 4573703

Fnded: 1989. **Mem:** 15. **Lang(s):** Arabic, English. **Desc:** Health care professionals and other individuals with an interest in family planning and related health services. Promotes increased availability primary health care in previously underserved areas. Makes available family planning, reproductive health, and pediatric health care services. Conducts surveys to determine medical needs of underserved communities.

★ 2639 ★ Egyptian Society of Cardiology

Egyptian Heart House
9 El-Saraya St.
Dokki
Giza EG-12311, Egypt
Phone: 20 2 3381308 **Fax:** 20 2 3381309
Email: seniors_ic@hotmail.com
Website: http://www.escardio.org/society/natsoc/egypt.htm

Fnded: 1951. **Mem:** 739. **Desc:** Promotes the study of cardiology in Egypt, including diagnosis and management of hypertension, and management of coronary heart disease. **Pub:** *Egyptian Heart*, 3/year. Journal. • *Pediatric Cardiology*, semiannual. Newsletter.

★ 2640 ★ Egyptian Society of Pharmacology and Experimental Therapeutics

c/o Prof. Essem E. Galal
20 El-Tayef St.
Mohandesseen
Cairo, Egypt
Phone: 20 2 3387739 **Fax:** 20 2 3387739

Mem: 240. **Desc:** Promotes pharmacology and experimental therapeutics in Egypt.

★ 2641 ★ Ehlers Danlos National Foundation (EDNF)

6399 Wilshire Blvd., Ste. 200
Los Angeles, CA 90048
Phone: (323)651-3038 **Free:** 800-956-2902
Fax: (323)651-1366
Email: staff@ednf.org
Website: http://www.ednf.org
Linda Neumann-Potash, Exec. Dir.

Fnded: 1985. **Mem:** 1,750. **Local Groups:** 25. **Desc:** Individuals who are affected with Ehlers Danlos Syndrome (EDS); medical professionals involved in the treatment of EDS. (Ehlers Danlos Syndrome, which is named after dermatologists Edward L. Ehlers (1863-1937) and Henri A. Danlos (1844-1912), is an inheritable connective tissue disorder characterized by fragile skin, hypermobile joints, and poor wound healing.) Provides networking among members for communication and support. Local branches and support groups throughout the U.S. provide support, educational material and public awareness to people affected by EDS, their families and health care professionals. **Pub:** *Emergency Room Physician's Guide to EDS Vascular Type*. Newsletter. • *The Facts about Ehlers Danlos Syndrome.* Brochures. Includes the types of Ehlers Danlos Syndrome and Genetic Inheritance Pattern to Ehlers Danlos Syndrome. • *Loose Connections*, quarterly. Newsletter. Includes medical updates on EDS, personal interest stories, local branch information. *Price:* Included in membership dues. • *The Types of Ehlers Danlos Syndrome.* Pamphlets.

★ 2642 ★ 800-COCAINE

c/o Jack Routleoge
Phoenix House

164 W 74th St.
New York, NY 10023
Phone: (212)595-5810 **Free:** 800-262-2463
Jack Routleoge, Contact

Desc: Provides general information about substance abuse, treatment referrals, and in emergency situations, crisis intervention. **Pub:** Pamphlets.

★ 2643 ★ Elder Craftsmen (EC)
610 Lexington Ave.
New York, NY 10022
Phone: (212)319-8128 **Fax:** (212)319-8141
Email: eldercraftsmen@mindspring.com
Website: http://www.eldercraftsmen.org/
Janet Langlois, Exec. Dir.

Fnded: 1955. **Desc:** Helps men and women 55 and older be creative, productive, and independent. Seeks broader recognition by the general public of the skills and capabilities of older people. Sponsors craft training workshops for representatives of Senior Centers. Sponsors community service projects with older adults making items for people in need. **Pub:** *Elder Craftnotes*, semiannual. Newsletter. • *What's This Got to do With Quilting: Nine Stories of Southern Women Quilters.* Booklet.

★ 2644 ★ Electrophysiological Technologists' Association (EPTA)
c/o Atkinson Morley's Hospital
31 Loppe Hill
Wimbledon
London SW20 0N6, United Kingdom
Fax: 44 20 87254637
Email: patricia.moore@lineone.net

Fnded: 1950. **Mem:** 600. **Lang(s):** English. **Desc:** Neurophysiology technicians; medical staff working in neurophysiology; individuals from commercial firms dealing with neurophysiology equipment. Promotes understanding of neurophysiology through preparation and presentation of scientific papers; oversees training of electrophysiology technology students. **Pub:** *Journal of Electrophysiological Technology*, 3/year. Journal. • *Newsletter*, periodic. Newsletter.

★ 2645 ★ Elizabeth Glaser Pediatric AIDS Foundation
2950 31st St., No. 125
Santa Monica, CA 90405
Phone: (310)314-1459 **Free:** 888-499-HOPE
Fax: (310)314-1469
Email: info@pedaids.org
Website: http://www.pedaids.org

Fnded: 1988. **Desc:** Devoted to pediatric AIDS research leading to new/better treatments and prevention of HIV infection in infants and children, to reduce and prevent HIV transmission from mother to child.

★ 2646 ★ Elliot Institute
PO Box 7348
Springfield, IL 62791-7348
Phone: (217)525-8202 **Fax:** (217)525-8212
Email: elliotinst@afterabortion.org
David C. Reardon, PhD, Dir.

Fnded: 1988. **Desc:** Seeks to promote post abortion healing and reconciliation through research and education on the after affects of abortion on women, men, children and society. Conducts educational and research programs; compiles statistics; maintains speakers' bureau. **Pub:** *The Post-Abortion Review*, quarterly. Newsletter. Original articles reporting on post-abortion research of trends in post-abortion healing & advocacy. *Price:* $20/yr. **AKA:** (1999) Elliot Institute for Social Sciences Research.

★ 2647 ★ Elton John AIDS Foundation (EJAIDSF)
PO Box 17139
Beverly Hills, CA 90209-3139
Phone: (310)535-1775
Email: AmgejAIDSF@ejaf.org
Website: http://ejaf.org
Alexandra Crane, Contact

Fnded: 1992. **Nat'l Groups:** 1. **Desc:** Individuals and organizations. Promotes increased access to, and improved quality of, patient care services for people with AIDS. Provides financial assistance to AIDS care programs and prevention projects; conducts fundraising activities.

★ 2648 ★ Emergency Medicine Foundation (EMF)
PO Box 619911
Dallas, TX 75261-9911
Phone: (972)550-0911 **Fax:** (972)580-2816
Email: emf@acep.org
Website: http://www.acep.org
Colin C. Rorrie, Jr., CAE Exec. Dir.

Fnded: 1972. **Desc:** Board of trustees is composed of representatives of American College of Emergency Physicians, Emergency Medicine Residents' Association, Emergency Nurses Association, Society for Academic Emergency Medicine . To promote and provide improved education and research in the field of emergency medicine in order to improve the availability and quality of emergency medical treatment. Conducts research programs. Funds hypothesis-based emergency medical research. **Pub:** *Scope*, semiannual. Newsletter. Donor newsletter that includes research funding information.

★ 2649 ★ Emergency Medicine Residents' Association (EMRA)
1125 Executive Cir.
Irving, TX 75038-2522
Phone: (972)550-0920 **Free:** 800-798-1822
Fax: (972)580-2829
Email: emra@emra.org
Website: http://www.emra.org
Liz McDonald, Exec. Dir.

Fnded: 1974. **Mem:** 4,500. **Desc:** Physicians enrolled in emergency medicine residency training programs; medical students. Purposes are to provide a unified voice for emergency medicine residents and encourage high standards in training and education for emergency physicians. Encourages research to improve emergency medicine education; promotes community, state, and national representation for emergency medicine in organized and academic medicine. **Pub:** *Career Development Guide.* • *EM Resident*, bimonthly. Newsletter. Focuses on issues such as residency issues, utilization of emergency department services, and educational opportunities. *Price:* Included in membership dues. • *Emergency Medicine in Focus: A Handbook for Medical Students and Prospective Residents.* Handbook. • *EMRA Job Catalog*, annual. Catalog. • *Outpatient Guide to Antibiotics.*

★ 2650 ★ Emergency Nurses Association (ENA)
915 Lee St.
Des Plaines, IL 60016
Phone: 800-900-9659 **Free:** 800-243-8362
Fax: (847)460-4001
Email: enainfo@ena.org
Website: http://www.ena.org
Donna Nowakowski, Exec. Dir.

Fnded: 1970. **Mem:** 23,000. **State Groups:** 50. **Local Groups:** 150. **Desc:** Registered nurses, licensed practical nurses, and licensed vocational nurses; emergency medical technicians or nurses and members of allied health fields engaged or interested in emergency patient care. Objectives are: to promote emergency nursing and to establish standards in the field; to work with other health-related organizations toward the improvement of emergency care; to serve as a resource for emergency nursing education and research. Seeks to identify and address emergency nursing issues. Disseminates educational and research information in the field. Sponsors: Emergency Nursing Core Curriculum; Standards of Emergency Nursing Practice; Emergency Nursing Pediatric Course; Trauma Nursing Core Course; Concepts in Advanced Trauma Nursing Course. **Pub:** *CEN Review Manual.* • *Connection*, 9/year. Newsletter. • *Emergency Nursing Core Curriculum.* • *Emergency Nursing Scope of Practice.* • *International Journal of Trauma Nursing*, quarterly. Journal. • *Journal of Emergency Nursing*, bimonthly. Journal. • *Leadership and Clinical Monograph Series.* • *Standards of Emergency Nursing Practice.* • *Triage: Meeting the Challenge.* **Frmly:** (1974) National Emergency Department Nurses Association; (1984) Emergency Department Nurses Association.

★ 2651 ★ Emotions Anonymous International Service Center (EA)
PO Box 4245
2233 University Ave. W, Ste. 402
Saint Paul, MN 55104-0245
Phone: (651)647-9712 **Fax:** (651)647-1593
Email: info@emotionsanonymous.org
Website: http://www.emotionsanonymous.org
Karen Mead, Exec. Dir.

Fnded: 1971. **Mem:** 5,000. **Nat'l Groups:** 1175. **State Groups:** 35. **Local Groups:** 20. **Desc:** "Fellowship of men and women who share their experience, strength, and hope with each other, that they may solve their common problem and help others recover from emotional illness." Uses the Twelve Steps of Alcoholics Anonymous World Services, adapted to emotional problems. Disseminates literature and information; provides telephone referrals to worldwide chapters. **Pub:** *Emotions Anonymous.* Book. Available in both soft and hard cover editions. *Price:* $15. • *The New Message*, quarterly. Magazine. Provides stories from EA members and their recovery through EA. • *Today.* Book.

★ 2652 ★ Employers' Managed Health Care Association (MHCA)
1129 20th St. NW, Ste. 850
Washington, DC 20036
Phone: (202)955-4380 **Fax:** (202)778-8506
Email: info@emhca.org

Fnded: 1989. **Desc:** Provides leadership role in driving high-quality, cost-effective, consumer-focused health care delivery systems. **Pub:** *The Employers' Guide to Medicare Managed Care in 1998 and Beyond.* Report.

★ 2653 ★ Endocrine Fellows Foundation
5959 W Century Blvd., Ste. 578
Los Angeles, CA 90045
Free: 877-877-6515
Email: endofellowsfnd@cs.com
Website: http://www.endocrinefellows.org
Marilyn Fishman, Exec. Dir.

Fnded: 1990. **Desc:** Endocrine fellows. Providing support to endocrine fellows in education, research grant funding and career guidance. Also, works to provide both fellows and endocrinology professionals with cutting-edge research results on developments in the fields of endocrinology, metabolism and diabetology.

★ 2654 ★ Endocrine Society (ES)
4350 East West Hwy., Ste. 500
Bethesda, MD 20814-4426
Phone: (301)941-0200 **Fax:** (301)941-0259
Email: endostaff@endo-society.org
Website: http://www.endo-society.org
Scott Hunt, Exec. Dir.

Fnded: 1915. **Mem:** 8,000. **Desc:** Promotes excellence in research, education, and clinical practice in endocrinology and related disciplines. Maintains placement service. **Pub:** *Endocrine News*, bimonthly. Newsletter. Includes calendar of events and listing of honors and awards recipients; legislative issues and clinical practice column. *Price:* Included in membership dues. • *Endocrine Reviews*, bimonthly. Journal. Covers clinical and experimental endocrinology; readers are encouraged to suggest prospective authors and to submit their own manuscripts. *Price:* $50 /year for members in U.S.; $115 /year for nonmembers in U.S.; $195 /year for institutions in U.S.; $85 for those in training in U.S. • *Endocrinology*, monthly. Journal. Covers current biomedical research for basic scientists. *Price:* $95/year for members in U.S.; $195 /year for nonmembers in U.S.; $410/year for institutions in U.S.; $125/year for those in training in U.S. • *Journal of Clinical Endocrinology and Metabolism*, monthly. Journal. Provides current information on the clinical applications of endocrine research for internists, pediatricians, and practicing obstetricians. *Price:* S85/year for members in U.S.; $180 /year for nonmembers in U.S.; $310/year for institutions in U.S.; $110/year for those in training in U.S. • *Molecular Endocrinology*, monthly. Journal. Covers the molecular mechanisms of cellular regulation and hormone action. *Price:* $80/ year for members in U.S.; $175 /year for nonmembers in U.S.; $295/year for institutions in U.S.; $110/year for those in training in U.S. **Frmly:** Association for Study of Internal Secretions.

★ 2655 ★ Endocrine Society of Australia (ESA)
145 Macquarie St.
Sydney, NSW 2000, Australia
Phone: 61 2 92565405 **Fax:** 61 2 92518174
Email: esa@racp.edu.au
Website: http://www.racp.edu.au/esa/

Fnded: 1958.

★ 2656 ★ Endometriosis Association (EA)
International Headquarters
8585 N 76th Pl.
Milwaukee, WI 53223
Phone: (414)355-2200 **Free:** 800-992-3636
Fax: (414)355-6065
Email: endo@endometriosisassn.org
Website: http://www.endometriosisassn.org
Mary Lou Ballweg, Exec. Dir.

Fnded: 1980. **Mem:** 1200,000. **Reg. Groups:** 200. **Desc:** Provides help and support to those affected by endometriosis; educates public and medical community about the disease. Promotes and funds research. **Pub:** *Are You a Teenager?*, bimonthly. Brochure. Available in 2 languages. *Price:* Included in membership dues. • *Endometriosis Association Newsletter*, 4-6/year. Newsletter. Includes news, tips, reviews, and research reports; also covers association and chapter news and activities. *Price:* Included in membership dues. • *The Endometriosis Sourcebook*. Book. • *Overcoming Endometriosis*. Book. • *Teens Speak Out on Endometriosis*. Video. • *Teensource*, quarterly. Newsletter. Includes information for teen/family members. • *What is Endometriosis?*. Brochure. Available in 28 languages. *Price:* Free.

★ 2657 ★ Endometriosis Association (Singapore) (EASe)
c/o Mt. Alvernia Hospital
820 Thomson Rd.
Singapore 574623, Singapore
Phone: 65 63476640 **Fax:** 65 62505138
Email: easespore@yahoo.co.uk
Website: http://sg.geocities.com/easespore/endoweek.html

Fnded: 1997. **Desc:** Support group for women suffering from endometriosis and pelvic pain. Sponsors Endometriosis Awareness Week. **Pub:** *EndoSource*, quarterly. Magazine. • *Pelvic Pain and Endometriosis Survey for Singapore*. Survey.

★ 2658 ★ Endometriosis Association of Victoria (Australia) (EAV)
28 Warrandyte Rd.
Ringwood, VIC 3134, Australia
Phone: 61 3 98792199 **Fax:** 61 3 98796519
Email: info@endometriosis.org.au
Website: http://www.endometriosis.org.au/

Desc: Provides support and information for women with endometriosis including counseling, public awareness, and research. Provides specialist clinic **Pub:** *Explaining Endometriosis*. Book. • Newsletter, quarterly.

★ 2659 ★ Energy Action (EA)
IDA Unit 14
Newmarket
Dublin 8, Ireland
Phone: 353 1 4545464 **Fax:** 353 1 4549797
Email: info@energyaction.ie
Website: http://www.energyaction.ie

Fnded: 1988. **Mem:** 14. **Reg. Groups:** 8. **Lang(s):** English, Irish. **Desc:** Individuals interested in meeting the energy needs of the elderly. Seeks to improve energy efficiency in the homes of elderly people. Provides home insulation services at no cost to elderly individuals. Trains unemployed people to install insulation in accordance with building codes and safety standards.

★ 2660 ★ EngenderHealth
440 9th Ave.
New York, NY 10001
Phone: (212)561-8000 **Fax:** (212)561-8067
Email: info@engenderhealth.org
Website: http://www.engenderhealth.org
Dr. Amy E. Pollack, Pres.

Fnded: 1943. **Mem:** 8,000. **Desc:** Seeks to provide women and men with access to voluntary and safe contraception. Helps countries and institutions develop, improve, and expand systems for the provision of clinic-based contraception services. Special expertise in female sterilization and vasectomy. **Pub:** *AVSC News*, quarterly. Newsletter. *Price:* Free. For members only and family planning community. • Brochures. • Also publishes clinical guides and resources for family planning professionals. **Frmly:** (1985) Association for Voluntary Sterilization; (1994) Association for Voluntary Surgical Contraception; (2001) AVSC International.

★ 2661 ★ English National Association of Visually Handicapped Bowlers
18 Hervey St.
Lowestoft NR32 2JG, United Kingdom
Phone: 44 1502 514700
Email: gailh@fish.co.uk

Fnded: 1974. **Mem:** 600. **Desc:** Males and females who are visually impaired, and sighted helpers. Promotes bowls throughout the UK and the international arena. **Pub:** Newsletter, quarterly.

★ 2662 ★ Entertainment Industries Council (EIC)
c/o Government Liaison and Administrative Office
1760 Reston Pky., Ste. 415
Reston, VA 20190-3303
Phone: (703)481-1414 **Fax:** (703)481-1418
Email: eic@eiconline.org
Website: http://eiconline.org
Brian Dyak, Pres.

Fnded: 1983. **Mem:** 130. **Desc:** Corporations and representatives of the entertainment industry including actors, agents, publicists, producers, directors, and writers. Goal is to utilize the power and influence of the entertainment industry in a national campaign to combat and deglamorize substance abuse, especially among young people. Seeks to identify and provide celebrity role models for young people. Hopes to increase youth awareness of drug abuse through television, radio, music, and motion pictures. Develops projects to aid in eliminating substance abuse problems within the entertainment industry. Conducts seminars and training sessions on drug abuse prevention; also conducts radio interview series, television specials, outreach programs, and employee assistance and fundraising programs. Collects and disseminates information on progress made by the entertainment industry in drug abuse prevention. In conjunction with IMMEDIA Foundation, coordinates network of 400 radio stations involved in public affairs projects designed to discourage substance abuse. Provides celebrity speakers' bureau on drug prevention, seat belt awareness, and intravenous drug use/AIDS. Bestows EIC Drug Prevention Award annually to a leader from entertainment industry contributing to drug awareness. **Pub:** *Profile*, monthly. • *Spotlight on Depiction*, annual. • Annual Report, quarterly.

★ 2663 ★ Environmental Health Accreditation Council (EHAC)
c/o National Environmental Health Association
720 S Colorado Blvd., Ste. 970
S Tower
Denver, CO 80246
Phone: (303)756-9090 **Fax:** (303)691-9490
Email: becky.roland@juno.com
Website: http://www.nea.org
Gary Smith, PhD, Contact

Fnded: 1969. **Mem:** 28. **Desc:** Purposes are: to establish a system for accreditation of environmental health curricula and related procedures; to accredit and carry out other responsibilities as may be essential to the accreditation of academic programs leading to baccalaureate and graduate degrees in environmental health. Assumes responsibility for all functions, related records, and correspondence pertaining to accreditation of environmental health curricula. Renders advice and counsel to institutions in the development of curricula and the conduct of educational programs in the environmental health sciences. Acts as clearinghouse for reports and information pertaining to the environmental health accreditation process and activities. **Frmly:** National Accreditation Council for Environmental Health Curricula; (1993) National Accreditation Council for Environmental Health Science and Protection; (1998) National Environmental Health Science and Protection Accreditation Council.

★ 2664 ★ Epilepsy Action Scotland (EAS)
48 Govan Rd.
Glasgow G51 1JL, United Kingdom
Phone: 44 141 4274911 **Fax:** 44 141 4191709
Email: enquiries@epilepsyscotland.org.uk
Website: http://www.epilepsyscotland.org.uk

Fnded: 1954. **Mem:** 600. **Reg. Groups:** 12. **Local Groups:** 1. **Lang(s):** English. **Desc:** Works to enable people with epilepsy to maximize their choices in life; lobbies for better services to meet local needs and campaigns against the stigma of epilepsy by raising public awareness. to members. **Pub:** *Epilepsy News*, semiannual. Newsletter. • Booklets. **Frmly:** Epilepsy Association of Scotland.

★ 2665 ★ Epilepsy Canada (EC)
1470 Peel St., Ste. 745
Montreal, QC, Canada H3A 1T1
Phone: (514)845-7855 **Free:** 877-734-0873
Fax: (514)845-7866
Email: epilepsy@epilepsy.ca
Website: http://www.epilepsy.ca

Fnded: 1966. **Lang(s):** English, French. **Desc:** People with epilepsy and their families; health care professionals with an interest in epilepsy and related disorders. Seeks to improve the quality of life of people affected by epilepsy through promotion and support of research. Offers education and awareness initiatives that build understanding and acceptance of epilepsy. **Pub:** *Lumina*, semiannual. Newsletter. • Brochure.

★ 2666 ★ Epilepsy Foundation (EFA)
4351 Garden City Dr.
Landover, MD 20785
Phone: (301)459-3700 **Free:** 800-332-1000
Fax: (301)577-4941
Email: postmaster@efa.org
Website: http://www.epilepsyfoundation.org/
Eric R. Hargis, Pres. /CEO

Fnded: 1967. **Mem:** 16,000. **Desc:** National voluntary health agency which serves as the "focal point for the fight against epilepsy in the United States." Augmented by 64 affiliates in the U.S. committed to preventing and controlling epilepsy and improving the lives of those who have it. Provides federal government liaison. The foundation supports medical, social, rehabilitational, legal, employment, and information, education, and advocacy programs. Sponsors research in causes of epilepsy, prevention, psychosocial needs, and improved methods of treatment. Provides research and training grants and fellowships to students and professionals. Assistance and counseling for epilepsy patients and their families is provided through local organizations and the National Information Center on Epilepsy. Annual projects include National Epilepsy Month (November), School Alert (a national educational program for schools), selection of the Epilepsy Poster Child, and a continuing professional and public education and information program. Maintains a resource center. Provides members with access to mail order pharmacy program. Compiles statistics; maintains placement program. **Pub:** *Between Us*, bimonthly. Magazine. Magazine for women. • *EpilepsyUSA*, bimonthly. Magazine. News magazine. • *In Touch*, quarterly. Newsletter. For adults with epilepsy. *Price:* Free. • *Kids News*, quarterly. Magazine. Magazine for children. • Also publishes pamphlets and makes available audiovisual material and informational/educational pieces for diversified audiences. **Frmly:** Epilepsy Foundation of America.

★ 2667 ★ Epilepsy Support Foundation

No. 3 Crocket Rd.
PO Box A104
Avondale
Harare, Zimbabwe
Phone: 263 4 571225 **Fax:** 263 4 571225

Fnded: 1990. **Mem:** 1,205. **Reg. Groups:** 3. **Lang(s):** English, Shona. **Desc:** Seeks to improve the quality of life for persons with epilepsy. Raises public awareness about epilepsy and its effects. Disseminates information. Makes available counseling services; maintains support groups; conducts rural outreach programs. **Pub:** *Epilepsy Back Up*, monthly. Newsletter. • Pamphlets, periodic. Contains information on epilepsy for patients, service providers, medical personnel, and various professionals.

★ 2668 ★ Episcopal Society for Ministry on Aging (ESMA)

PO Box 3065
Meridian, MS 39303
Phone: (601)485-0311
Email: info@esmanet.com
Website: http://www.episcopalchurch.org/episcopal-life/RetClose.html

Fnded: 1964. **Desc:** Develops and supports Episcopal Church by strengthening God's people for ministry throughout the entire life span. Publishes resources and provides education and training for clergy and lay leaders; offers consultations to seminaries on development of curricula in gerontology; develops Age in Action educational materials for parishes. Operates a national network of clergy and lay volunteers for the dissemination of information and for program development at grass-roots level. **Pub:** *Affirmative Aging*. Book. Includes study guide. • *Directory of Episcopal Related Housing for the Aging*. Directory. • *ESMA's Network News*, 3/year. Newsletter. • *Large Print Book of Common Prayer*. • *Older Adult Ministry: A Resource for Program Development*. • Distributes *(In)Diginity of Aging* (videotape).

★ 2669 ★ Erb's Palsy Association of Ireland

Canrawer
Oughterard, Galway, Ireland
Phone: 353 91 552623
Email: info@erbspalsy.ie
Website: http://www.erbspalsy.ie

Mem: 186. **Lang(s):** English. **Desc:** Parents of children born with Erb's Palsy. Seeks to raise awareness of and provide information on Erb's Palsy, a childbirth injury causing temporary and sometimes permanent paralysis in the arm. **Pub:** Newsletter, semiannual.

★ 2670 ★ Esclerosis Multiple Argentina

c/o Vernon R. Dougall
Uriarte 1465/69
1414 Buenos Aires, Argentina
Phone: 54 11 48316617 **Fax:** 54 11 48316786
Email: info@ema.org.ar

Fnded: 1968. **Mem:** 950. **Reg. Groups:** 2. **Desc:** MS patients, families and professionals. Seeks to improve the quality of life for persons with multiple sclerosis and their families. Provides self-help groups, physiotherapy, occupational therapy, and home visits.

★ 2671 ★ ESHEL - The Association for the Planning and Development of Services for the Aged in Israel (ESHEL)
(Haagudah Letichnun Vepituach Sherutim Lemaan Hazaken Beyisrael)

JDC Hill
PO Box 3489
IL-91034 Jerusalem, Israel
Phone: 972 2 6557128 **Fax:** 972 2 5662716
Email: eshelnet@jointnet.org.il
Website: http://www.jointnet.org.il/eshelnet/

Fnded: 1969. **Local Groups:** 115. **Lang(s):** Hebrew. **Desc:** Develops and plans services for the aged in Israel, including daycare centers, homes for the aged, sheltered housing projects, supportive neighborhoods, respite care centers, health promotion programs, volunteer-based services, and others. Conducts training programs for managers, professionals, paraprofessionals, and others who work with the aged in Israel and abroad. Develops computer based information services to improve access to information, products and services. Conducts research and develops products to improve the quality of life of the elderly in Israel. Publishes books and pamphlets and produces videos on aging. Provides consultation services to organizations around the world on the planning and development of services for the aged. **Pub:** *Aging as an Academic Field: Aging and SocioAnthropological Studies*. Book. • *The Association for the Elderly: A Guide for Establishing a Public Organization*. Book. • *Between Ourselves and Our Parents: A Reader on the Relationship betwe en Children and their Elderly Parents*. Book. • *Day Center for the Elderly*. Book. • *Guidelines for the Planning of Homes for the Aged in Israel*. Book. • *Suggested Activities for the Teaching of Aging as a High School Subject*. Book. • Audiotapes. • Pamphlets. • Videos.

★ 2672 ★ Esther A. and Joseph Klingenstein Fund

787 7th Ave., 6th Fl.
New York, NY 10019-6016
Phone: (212)492-6181 **Fax:** (212)492-7007
John Klingenstein, Pres.

Fnded: 1945. **Desc:** Works to support neuroscience research, especially in the area of epilepsy, independent school education, separation of Church and State, and animal-based research.

★ 2673 ★ Estonian Centre for Health Education and Promotion
(Eesti Tervisekasvatuse Keskus)

Ruutli St. 24
EE-0001 Tallinn, Estonia
Phone: 372 6 279280 **Fax:** 372 6 440800
Email: kadi@tervis.ee

Fnded: 1993. **State Groups:** 15. **Lang(s):** English, Finnish, Russian. **Desc:** Conducts health promotion and evaluation activities in Estonia to prevent disease. **Pub:** *Tervist*, monthly. Newsletter.

★ 2674 ★ Estonian Medical Association
(Eesti Arstide Liit)

Pepleri 32
EE-51010 Tartu, Estonia
Phone: 372 7 420029 **Fax:** 372 7 420029
Email: eal@arstideliit.ee
Website: http://www.arstideliit.ee

Fnded: 1921. **Mem:** 2,550. **Reg. Groups:** 20. **Desc:** Promotes the educational and professional interests of physicians. **Pub:** *Esti Arstide Liidu Teataja*, monthly. Journal. **Frmly:** Estonian Doctor's Association.

★ 2675 ★ Estonian Society of Cardiology
(Eesti Kardioloogide Selts)

North-Estonian Regional Hospital
Mustamae Hospital
19 Sutiste St.
EE-13419 Tallinn, Estonia
Phone: 372 6 971265 **Fax:** 372 6 971264
Email: margus.viigimaa@kliinikum.ee
Website: http://www.escardio.org/society/natsoc/estonia.htm

Fnded: 1963. **Mem:** 203. **Lang(s):** English. **Desc:** Physicians and scientists interested in the field of cardiology.

★ 2676 ★ Estonian Society of Pharmacology

c/o Prof. L. Rago
Department of Pharmacology
Faculty of Medicine
University of Tartu
Ulikooli 18
EE-2400 Tartu, Estonia
Phone: 372 7 441219 **Fax:** 372 7 441549
Email: lembit@sam.ee

Mem: 28. **Desc:** Promotes pharmacology in Estonia.

★ 2677 ★ Ethiopian Diabetes Association

c/o Dr. Ahmed Reja
PO Box 31840
Addis Ababa, Ethiopia
Phone: 251 1 625808
Email: areja@lycos.com
Website: http://www.diabetesafrica.com/idfmembers.html

Desc: Represents people with diabetes. Promotes research and support of those with diabetes in Ethiopia.

★ 2678 ★ Eurocare: Advocacy for the Prevention of Alcohol Related Harm in Europe

Rue des Confederes 96-98
B-1000 Brussels, Belgium
Phone: 32 2 7367351 **Fax:** 32 2 7360572
Email: eurocare@village.uunet.be
Website: http://www.eurocare.org/

Fnded: 1990. **Desc:** An alliance of agencies set up to tackle problems associated with alcohol use at European level, presenting its views to the European Commission and Parliament as well as decision making bodies of national member states.

★ 2679 ★ Eurolink Age - England

1268 London Rd.
London SW16 4ER, United Kingdom
Phone: 44 208 7657717 **Fax:** 44 208 6796727
Email: eurolink@ace.org.uk

Fnded: 1981. **Mem:** 100. **Lang(s):** English, French, German, Italian, Spanish. **Desc:** Works to improve the quality of life of the elderly. Gathers and disseminates information on issues including social benefits, pensions, and employment. **Frmly:** Eurolink Age - England.

★ 2680 ★ European Academy of Aesthetic Dentistry

47a Wimpole St.
London W1M 7DF, United Kingdom
Phone: 44 20 72241488 **Fax:** 44 20 71712241299

★ 2681 ★ European Academy of Allergology and Clinical Immunology (EAACI)
(Academie Europeenne d'Allergologie et d'Immunologie Clinique)

EAACI Executive Office
PO Box 24140
S-10451 Stockholm, Sweden

Phone: 46 8 4596623 **Fax:** 46 8 6633815
Email: executive.office@eaaci.org
Website: http://www.eaaci.org

Fnded: 1950. **Mem:** 3,500. **Nat'l Groups:** 38. **Lang(s):** English, French, German. **Desc:** Medical doctors in 38 countries. Facilitates the exchange of ideas and information in the field of allergy and clinical immunology; assists and promotes international initiatives among European workers in related fields. Conducts training courses. **Pub:** *Allergy - The European Journal of Allergy and Clinical Immunology*, monthly. Journal.

★ 2682 ★ European Academy of Andrology
c/o Prof. Rob F.A. Weber, Sec.
Erasmus MC
Department of Andrology
Dr Molewaterplein 40
NL-3015 Rotterdam, Netherlands
Phone: 31 10 4635767 **Fax:** 31 10 4635763
Email: weber@inw3.azr.nl

Desc: Promotes the study of male reproduction.

★ 2683 ★ European Academy of Childhood Disability (EACD)
Rte de Lennik 808
B-1070 Brussels, Belgium
Phone: 32 2 5553942 **Fax:** 32 2 5553429
Email: henri.szliwowski@ulb.ac.be

Fnded: 1989.

★ 2684 ★ European Academy of Craniomandibular Disorders (EACD)
Corso Buenos Aires, 18
I-20124 Milan, Italy
Fax: 39 022043465

Fnded: 1984. **Desc:** Promotes knowledge of etiology, diagnosis and treatment of orofacial and tempoRomendibular disorders.

★ 2685 ★ European Academy of Facial Plastic Surgery (EAFPS)
c/o British Association of Otothinolaryngologists - Head and Neck Surgeons
35-43 Lincoln's Inn Fields
London WC2A 3PN, United Kingdom
Phone: 44 20 74048373 **Fax:** 44 20 74044200
Email: eafps@bao-hns.demon.co.uk
Website: http://www.eafps.com

Fnded: 1977. **Mem:** 500. **Lang(s):** English. **Desc:** Practicing and student facial and neck surgeons. Aims to further plastic and reconstructive surgery by stimulating research in neurosurgery, ophthalmology, otorhinolaryngology, and maxillofacial surgery; encourages cooperation among members, particularly between surgeons working in different specialties. Offers program on techniques in reconstructive surgery. **Pub:** *Facial Plastic Surgery*, quarterly. Monograph. • *Membership List*, periodic. **Frmly:** Joseph Society.

★ 2686 ★ European Academy for Medicine of Ageing (EAMA)
CP 4176
CH-1950 Sion, Switzerland
Phone: 41 27 2037383 **Fax:** 41 27 2037384

Fnded: 1992. **Desc:** Performs EAMA study courses that aim to increase scientific, clinical, Educational and managerial competence in medical gerontology.

★ 2687 ★ European Academy of Nutritional Sciences (EANS)
c/o Secretariat
PO Box 114
NL-3130 AC Vlaardingen, Netherlands
Email: info@eans.net

Desc: Promotes the field of nutritional sciences.

★ 2688 ★ European Academy of Paediatric Dentistry
c/o Dr. Nick Lygidakis
2 Papadiamantopoulou St.
GR-115 28 Athens, Greece
Phone: 30 1 7211869 **Fax:** 30 1 7215384
Email: lygidakis@internet.gr
Website: http://www.eapd.gr

Fnded: 1990. **Desc:** Individuals whose primary concern is in the areas of practice, education, and research related to pediatric dentistry. Works to improve the oral health of children.

★ 2689 ★ European Addiction Training Institute
c/o Dr. Wim R. Buisman
Keizersgracht 582
NL-1017 Amsterdam, Netherlands
Phone: 31 20 6752041 **Fax:** 31 20 6764591
Email: info@eati.org
Website: http://www.eati.org

Desc: Works as an addiction training institute in Europe.

★ 2690 ★ European Aero-Medical Institute (EURAMI)
Raiffeisenstr. 32
D-70794 Filderstadt, Germany
Phone: 49 711 70073001 **Fax:** 49 711 70073009
Email: info@eurami.org
Website: http://www.eurami.net

Desc: Promotes the use of air rescue in Europe. Works to ensure a high level of medical care in all countries of the European Union.

★ 2691 ★ European Alliance Genetic Support Groups
31 Vredehofstraat
NL-3761 HA Soestdijk, Netherlands
Phone: 31 356034040 **Fax:** 31 356027440
Email: vsop@vsop.nl
Website: http://www.vsop.nl

Fnded: 1992. **Mem:** 30. **State Groups:** 15. **Desc:** Individuals with genetic disorders and their families. Promote services which meet the needs of those with genetic disorders and their families. Hold conferences, participate in patient organizations.

★ 2692 ★ European Alliance of Neuromuscular Disorders Associations (EANDA)
7-11 Prescott Pl.
London SW4 6BS, United Kingdom
Phone: 44 207 7208055 **Fax:** 44 207 7498963
Email: mail@eamda.sonnet.co.uk

Fnded: 1971. **Mem:** 33. **Lang(s):** English. **Desc:** Organizations representing people with neurmuscular disorders and health care professionals with an interest in neurological maladies. Seeks to improve the quality of life of people with neuromuscular disorders; promotes advances in the prevention, diagnosis, and treatment of neurological diseases. Facilitates exchange of information among members; serves as a clearinghouse on neuromuscular disorders; sponsors research and educational programs.

★ 2693 ★ European Association for Aviation Psychology (EAAP)
Sportallee 54a
D-22523 Hamburg, Germany
Fax: 49 40 51309660
Email: eaap@dlr.de
Website: http://www.eaap.net

Fnded: 1956.

★ 2694 ★ European Association for Body Psychotherapy (EABP)
Leidsestraat 106-108/2
NL-1017-PG Amsterdam, Netherlands
Phone: 31 20 3302703 **Fax:** 31 20 6257312
Email: eabpsecretariat@planet.nl
Website: http://www.eabp.org/

Fnded: 1988. **Desc:** Fosters dialogue and exchange of experience among members.

★ 2695 ★ European Association for Cancer Research (EACR)
c/o Paul Saunders
University of Nottingham
The Pharmacy School
Nottingham NG7 2RD, United Kingdom
Phone: 44 115 9515114 **Fax:** 44 115 9515115
Email: paul.saunders@nottingham.ac.uk
Website: http://www.eacr.org/

Fnded: 1968. **Mem:** 5,000. **Lang(s):** English. **Desc:** Persons who have worked actively in cancer research for at least 2 years and who have an academic degree or the equivalent; membership in 40 countries. Seeks to advance cancer research by facilitating communication among research workers, particularly by organizing meetings. Sponsors: EACR Travel Fellowship Program, awarding travel expenses for member researchers to and from host institutions. **Pub:** *Directory of the EACR*, biennial. Directory. • *EACR Newsletter*, semiannual. Newsletter. • *European Journal of Cancer and Clinical Oncology*, monthly. Journal.

★ 2696 ★ European Association for Cardio-Thoracic Surgery (EACTS)
The Cottage, 16 High St.
Windsor SL4 1LD, United Kingdom
Phone: 44 1753 832166 **Fax:** 44 1753 620407
Email: info@eacts.co.uk
Website: http://www.eacts.org

Fnded: 1986. **Desc:** Aims to advance education in the field of cardio-thoracic surgery. Promotes research into thoracic physiology, pathology and therapy.

★ 2697 ★ European Association of Centers of Medical Ethics (EACME)
Passeggiata di Ripetta, 11
I-00186 Rome, Italy
Phone: 39 06 32652401 **Fax:** 39 06 32652433
Email: iprs@mclink.it

Fnded: 1985.

★ 2698 ★ European Association of Centres of Medical Ethics (EACME)
c/o A. Heynen
PO Box 616
NL-6200 MD Maastricht, Netherlands
Phone: 31 43 3882145 **Fax:** 31 43 3884171
Email: secretariaat-ige@ige.unimaas.nl
Website: http://www.eacmeweb.com

Fnded: 1985. **Mem:** 59. **Lang(s):** English, French. **Desc:** Medical ethics centers. Promotes critical public and professional concern regarding ethical issues encountered in the practice of medicine. Gathers and disseminates information; conducts research and makes research tools available to members; coordinates collaborative research efforts among members. Encourages continuing ethical education for health care professionals. **Pub:** *EACME Newsletter*, 3/year. Bulletin.

★ 2699 ★ European Association of Clinical Anatomy
Institut fur Anatomie
Karl-Franzens-Universitat Graz
Harrarchgasse 21/1
A-8010 Graz, Austria
Phone: 43 316 3804210 **Fax:** 43 316 3809620
Email: friedrich.anderhuber@kfunigraz.ac.at
Website: http://www.eaca-aeac.org

Fnded: 1988. **Mem:** 200. **Desc:** Promotes anatomic research applied to everyday medical practice, surgery and medical imaging; facilitates the development of scientific relations. **Pub:** *Surgical & Radiological Anatomy*, bimonthly. Journal.

★ 2700 ★ European Association for Cranio-Maxillo-Facial Surgery (EACMFS)
Thomond House
North St.
Midhurst GU29 9DJ, United Kingdom
Phone: 44 1730 810951 **Fax:** 44 1730 812042
Email: ea.cms@virgin.net
Website: http://www.eacmfs.org
Fnded: 1970. **Mem:** 800. **Nat'l Groups:** 2. **Reg. Groups:** 5. **Lang(s):** English, French, German. **Desc:** Surgeons involved in oral and cranio-maxillofacial surgery. Encourages discussion and conducts medical courses on subjects such as orthognathic and temporomandibular joint surgery and plastic and aesthetic surgery. Maintains speakers' bureau. **Pub:** *Journal of Cranio-maxillo-facial Surgery*, bimonthly. Journal.

★ 2701 ★ European Association of Dental Graphology (Association Dentologique Europeene de Graphologues)
Cabinet d'etudes graphologique
rue de la Valle 67
B-1100 Brussels, Belgium
Phone: 32 2 7713645
Lang(s): English, French. **Desc:** Dental graphologists. Promotes adherence to high standards of ethics and practice by members. Establishes standards for dental graphology certification; sponsors continuing professional development courses.

★ 2702 ★ European Association for Dental Public Health
c/o Prof. Klaus Pieper
University of Marburg Dental School
George Voigt Str. 3
D-35033 Marburg, Germany
Fax: 49 6421 2866691
Website: http://www.dundee.ac.uk/eadph/
Desc: Promotes effective oral health care in Europe. Fosters research.

★ 2703 ★ European Association for Endoscopic Surgery and Other Interventional Techniques (EAES)
c/o Ria Palmen, Off.Mgr.
PO Box 335
NL-5500 Veldhoven, Netherlands
Phone: 31 40 2525288 **Fax:** 31 40 2523102
Email: info@eaes-eur.org
Website: http://www.eaes-eur.org
Desc: Promotes endoscopic surgery and other interventional medical techniques in Europe.

★ 2704 ★ European Association of Establishments for Veterinary Education (EAEVE) (Association Europeenne des Etablissements d'Enseignment Veterinaire)
c/o Prof. T.H. Fernandes
Universidade Tecnica de Lisboa
Polo da Ajuda
Rua Prof Cid dos Santos
P-1300-477 Lisbon, Portugal
Phone: 351 21 3652820 **Fax:** 351 21 3652889
Email: eaeve@ed.ac.uk
Fnded: 1987. **Mem:** 94. **Reg. Groups:** 9. **Desc:** Promotes veterinary education in Europe.

★ 2705 ★ European Association of Experimental Social Psychology (EAESP)
c/o Sibylle Classen
PO Box 420 143
D-48068 Muenster, Germany
Fax: 49 2533 281144
Email: sibylle@eaesp.org
Website: http://www.eaesp.org/
Fnded: 1964. **Mem:** 800. **Lang(s):** English. **Desc:** Individuals in 28 countries working in the field of experimental and theoretical social psychology. Promotes theoretical and experimental social psychology and arranges for the exchange of information among members and related associations worldwide. Conducts summer schools for young researchers. **Pub:** *European Bulletin of Social Psychology*, 3/year. Newsletter. • *European Journal of Social Psychology*, bimonthly. Journal. • *European Monographs*, periodic.

★ 2706 ★ European Association for Gastroenterology and Endoscopy (EAGE)
Leipziger Str 44
D-39120 Magdeburg, Germany
Phone: 49 3916 713100 **Fax:** 49 3916 713105
Fnded: 1970.

★ 2707 ★ European Association of Geriatric Psychiatry (Association europeenne de psychiatrie geriatrique)
c/o Prof. Lars Gustafson, Chm.
Department of Psychogeriatrics
University Hospital
SE-221 85 Lund, Sweden
Fax: 46 46 177457
Email: lars.gustafson@psykiatr.lu.se
Website: http://www.uni-duesseldorf.de/psychklinik-en/eag/index.htm
State Groups: europe. **Local Groups:** geriat. **Desc:** Promotes the field of geriatric psychiatry in Europe.

★ 2708 ★ European Association of Gynaecologists and Obstetricians (EAGO)
Klinikstr 28
D-38385 Gieben, Germany
Phone: 49 641 9945100 **Fax:** 49 641 9945109
Email: sybill.lenz@gyn.med.uni-giessen.de
Website: http://www.med.uni-giessen.de/eago/
Fnded: 1985.

★ 2709 ★ European Association of Hearing Aid Audiologists
16 Av General Jourdan
B-6220 Fleurus, Belgium
Fnded: 1968.

★ 2710 ★ European Association of Hearing Aid Dispensers (AEA) (Association Europeenne des Audioprothesistes — AEA)
Lepanto 190
1a la Planta
E-08013 Barcelona, Spain
Phone: 34 93 2318212 **Fax:** 34 93 2542422
Fnded: 1968. **Mem:** 14. **Lang(s):** Danish, English, French, German, Portuguese, Spanish. **Desc:** National associations representing hearing aid dispensers. Promotes the study and development of scientific knowledge in areas involving hearing aids. Defends the professional interests of members.

★ 2711 ★ European Association for the History of Medicine and Health (EAHMH)
4, rue Kirschleger
F-67085 Strasbourg, France
Fnded: 1991. **Desc:** Fosters research and education in the history of medicine and health; encourages scientific cooperation.

★ 2712 ★ European Association for the History of Psychiatry (EAHP)
Carmen Valiente, buzon 83
Facultad de Psicologia
Universidad de Complutense de Madrid
Campus de Somosaguas
E-28223 Madrid, Spain
Phone: 34 913942832 **Fax:** 34 913943189
Email: eahp_secretary@hotmail.com
Website: http://www.eahp.org/

★ 2713 ★ European Association of Hospital Pharmacists (EAHP) (Association Europeene des Pharmaciens des Hopitaux)
c/o Jacqueline Surugue, Pres.
Rte. de Spay, BP 4
F-72700 Allonnes, France
Phone: 33 2 43435116 **Fax:** 33 2 43435164
Email: info@eahponline.org
Website: http://www.eahponline.org
Fnded: 1972. **Mem:** 16,000. **Nat'l Groups:** 22. **Lang(s):** English, French, German. **Desc:** Individuals from 22 countries. Promotes and protects the interests of hospital pharmacists; disseminates information. **Pub:** *European Journal of Hospital Pharmacy*, periodic. Journal.

★ 2714 ★ European Association for Integrative Psychotherapy (EAIP)
Ealing
London W5 2QB, United Kingdom
Phone: 44 20 85792505
Fnded: 1993. **Desc:** Promotes and extends the practice of integrative psychotherapy in Europe.

★ 2715 ★ European Association for NeuroOncology (EANO)
c/o B. Mueller
Klinik Bavaria
An der Wodlfsschlucht 1-2
D-01731 Kreischa, Germany
Fax: 49 35 20662954
Email: mueller@eano.de
Website: http://www.eano.de
Fnded: 1990. **Mem:** 463. **Nat'l Groups:** 36. **Desc:** Physicians, epidemiologists, biostatisticians, scientists and health professionals worldwide with an interest in any field of neurooncology. Fosters international cooperation in neurooncologic research and clinical training. **Pub:** *Journal of Neuro-Oncology*. Journal. • Newsletter, periodic.

★ 2716 ★ European Association of Neurosurgical Societies (EANS) (Association europeene de societies de neurochirugie)
60 Cobden Ave.
Southampton SO18 1FT, United Kingdom
Phone: 44 23 80585115 **Fax:** 44 23 80585115
Email: stephanie.garfield@virgin.net
Website: http://www.eans.org/
Fnded: 1971. **Nat'l Groups:** 32. **Lang(s):** English. **Desc:** National European neurosurgical societies in 32 countries. Sponsors two training courses per year and various other activities and research projects. **Pub:** *Acta Neurochirurgica*, 3-4/year. Journal. • *EANS Newsletter*, semiannual. Bulletin. • Directory, annual. • Directory, annual.

★ 2717 ★ European Association of New Medical Techniques (EANMT) (Association Europeenne de Methodes Medicales Nouvelles — AEMMN)
Route d'Esch 7
L-1470 Luxembourg, Luxembourg
Phone: 352 250226
Email: grinberg@pt.lu
Fnded: 1987. **Mem:** 300. **Lang(s):** English, French, German. **Desc:** Physicians and other health care professionals. Promotes advancement of medical practice through the introduction of new techniques and technologies. Identifies and evaluates new medi-

cal methods and equipment; sponsors research; conducts training programs for health care personnel.

★ 2718 ★ European Association of Nuclear Medicine (EPRO)

c/o Sabine Zwetler
Altmannsdorfer Str. 91
A-1120 Vienna, Austria
Email: zwetler@okk.co.at
Website: http://www.epro-recycling.org/

Desc: Works to optimize recycling/recovery of plastics packaging to lowest possible costs using new technologies and increasing quality management to meet the EU directive's regulations.

★ 2719 ★ European Association for Nutrition and Child Development Studies (Association Europeene pour l'Etude de l'Alimentation et du Developpement de l'Enfant)

Hopital Trousseau
26 avenue Dr. Arnold Netter
F-75012 Paris, France
Phone: 33 1 43461390 **Fax:** 33 1 43467800

Lang(s): English, French, German, Polish. **Desc:** Physicians, nutritionists, and other individuals with an interest in nutrition and child development. Promotes increased understanding of the role played by nutrition in child development. Serves as a forum for the exchange of information among members; conducts public education courses to raise awareness of the importance of nutrition to health child development; sponsors research programs.

★ 2720 ★ European Association for Osseointegration (EAO)

c/o Annie Nagem
1 Wimpoe St.
London W1M 8AE, United Kingdom
Phone: 44 207 2903948 **Fax:** 44 207 2902989
Email: eao-office@roysocmed.ac.uk
Website: http://www.eao.org

Desc: Promotes the advancement of methods of treatment in reconstructive surgery and prosthetic rehabilitation based on the principles of osseointegration and related disciplines. Fosters research; disseminates information.

★ 2721 ★ European Association for Osseointegration (EAO)

Rosenkavallerplatz 18-IV
D-81925 Munich, Germany
Phone: 49 89 92878450 **Fax:** 49 89 92878411

★ 2722 ★ European Association for Palliative Care (EAPC)

Instituto Nazionale dei Tumori
Via Venezian 1
I-20133 Milan, Italy
Phone: 39 02 23903390 **Fax:** 39 02 23903393
Email: eapc@istitutotumori.mi.it
Website: http://www.eapcnet.org

Fnded: 1990. **Desc:** Specialists in palliative care and hospice services. Promotes palliative care to health authorities and other agencies. **Pub:** *European Journal of Palliative Care*, periodic. Journal.

★ 2723 ★ European Association of Perinatal Medicine (EAPM)

c/o Ricardo N. Laurini
Department of Obstetrics and Gynecology
University Hospital San Joao
Alameda Prof. H. Montiero
P-4200 Porto, Portugal
Phone: 351 22 5094958 **Fax:** 351 22 5505870
Email: rlaurini@hotmail.com
Website: http://www.krenet.it/A/EAPM/welcome.htm

Fnded: 1968. **Mem:** 900. **Lang(s):** English. **Desc:** Pediatricians, obstetricians, anesthesiologists, medical doctors, students, and nurses interested in perinatal medicine. Works to advance information and interest in perinatal medicine. **Pub:** *Perinatal Medicine*, biennial.

★ 2724 ★ European Association of Personality Psychology (EAPP)

University of Ghent
Henri Dunantlaan 2
B-9000 Gent, Belgium
Phone: 32 9 2646499 **Fax:** 32 9 2646499
Email: filip.defruyt@rug.ac.be
Website: http://allserv.rug.ac.be/~fdefruyt/eapp.html

Fnded: 1984. **Desc:** Develops empirical and theoretical personality psychology by exchange of information.

★ 2725 ★ European Association of Plastic Surgeons (EURAPS)

De Pintelaan 185
B-9000 Gent, Belgium
Fax: 32 9 2406356
Email: euraps@rug.ac.be
Website: http://www.euraps.org

Desc: Fosters communication and exchange among plastic surgeons in Europe.

★ 2726 ★ European Association of Poisons Centres and Clinical Toxicologists (EAPCCT) (Association Europeenne des Centres Anti-Poisons et de Toxicologie Clinique)

National Poisons Information Service, London
Guy's and St. Thomas' Hospital Trust
Medical Toxicology Unit
Avonley Rd.
London SE14 5ER, United Kingdom
Phone: 44 207 7715310 **Fax:** 44 207 7715309
Website: http://www.eapcct.org/

Fnded: 1964. **Mem:** 300. **Lang(s):** English. **Desc:** Physicians and scientists working in clinical toxicology and related fields. Association works to improve contacts between clinical toxicologists and poisons information specialists. Regularly organizes joint meetings with the World Health Organization and the European Commission. Is a member of the International Union on Toxicology (IUTOX). **Pub:** *Journal of Toxicology: Clinical Toxicology*, bimonthly. Journal. • *Newsletter*, quarterly. Newsletter. **Frmly:** (1990) European Association Poison COntrol Centres.

★ 2727 ★ European Association for Professions in Biomedical Science (EPBS)

c/o Gabriele Sander
Clinical Genetics
Mullerhauptotrasse 48
A-5020 Salzburg, Austria
Phone: 43 662 3804819 **Fax:** 43 662 44822621
Email: gabriele.sander@aon.at
Website: http://www.european-epbs.org

Fnded: 1998. **Mem:** 15. **Lang(s):** English. **Desc:** Professional organizations representing medical laboratory technologists in the European Community. Offers advice to the European Commission in matters concerning the medical laboratory technological profession. For those who work in the frontline of biomedical science in healthcare. EPBS is the organization to develop and promote cooperation in key areas such as education, continuing professional education, competencies and accreditation.

★ 2728 ★ European Association for the Promotion of the Hand Hygiene

46 Rue Lieutenant Liedel
B-1070 Brussels, Belgium
Fax: 32 2 5212099

Fnded: 1983.

★ 2729 ★ European Association of Psychological Assessment (EAPA)

c/o Dr. Maria Forns
Universidad de Barcelona
Dep. Personalidad, Evaluacion y Tratamiento Psicologico
Paseo Vall d'Hebron 171
E-08035 Barcelona, Spain
Phone: 34 92 3125115 **Fax:** 34 92 40211362
Email: mforns@psi.ub.es
Website: http://www.eapa.rwth-aachen.de

Fnded: 1990. **Desc:** Works to increase scientific interest in psychological assessment in Europe. Fosters communication and scientific exchange. **Pub:** *European Journal of Psychological Assessment*. Journal. • Newsletter, annual.

★ 2730 ★ European Association for Psychotherapy

c/o Dr. Alfred Pritz, Sec.
Krieglergasse 11/5
A-1030 Vienna, Austria
Phone: 43 1 7144243 **Fax:** 43 1 7159963
Email: eap.headoffice@magnet.at
Website: http://www.psychother.com/eap

Fnded: 1991. **Mem:** 650. **Desc:** Psychotherapists from 28 European countries. Fosters the free and independent practice of psychotherapy. Develops ethical guidelines for the protection of patients Promotes high training standards. **Pub:** *International Journal of Psychotherapy*. Journal.

★ 2731 ★ European Association of Radiology

c/o Prof.Dr. Peter Vock
Department of Diagnostic Radiology
Inselspital
Freiburger Str. 32
CH-3010 Bern, Switzerland
Phone: 41 31 6322435 **Fax:** 41 31 6324874
Email: peter.vock@insel.ch
Website: http://www.ear-online.org

Fnded: 1962. **Mem:** 40. **Nat'l Groups:** 40. **Lang(s):** English, French, German. **Desc:** National European societies of radiology representing 20,000 radiologists. Objectives are to: promote radiology as a unified scientific and clinical discipline; further and monitor the application of radiology in biology and medicine; investigate the theoretical and technical problems connected with different applications of radiation; coordinate study and examination programs in the field of radiology in member countries; standardize training for radiologists and nonmedical assistants; encourage a constructive rapport with scientific, professional, and industrial organizations; promote international exchange of medical and paramedical personnel. **Pub:** *European Radiology*, bimonthly. Newsletter. **Frmly:** (2001) Institute for Diagnostic Radiology.

★ 2732 ★ European Association of Schools of Occupational Medicine (EASOM)

c/o P.J. Kroon
Amsterdam School of Occupational Medicine Corvu
Meibergdreef 15
NL-1105 AZ Amsterdam, Netherlands
Phone: 31 20 5664949 **Fax:** 31 20 6975359
Email: p.j.kroon@amc.uva.nl
Website: http://www.medlav.unimo.it/easom/EASOM.htm

Desc: Promotes improvement in the training of doctors working in the field of occupational medicine in the European community.

★ 2733 ★ European Association of Senior Hospital Physicians
c/o Brigitte Jencik
Ave. de Cortenbergh 66
B-1000 Brussels, Belgium
Phone: 32 2 7366066 **Fax:** 32 2 7329972
Email: secretariat@aemh.org
Website: http://www.aemh.org

Desc: Hospital physicians in Europe. Fosters exchange of information on hospital-related topics. Works to improve the quality of hospital care. Maintains high ethical standards.

★ 2734 ★ European Association for Service Providers for Persons with Disability
(Asociacion Europea de Suministradores de Servicios para Personas con Minusvalias Disabilities)
c/o Katrijn Dekoninck
Oudergemlaan 63
B-1040 Brussels, Belgium
Phone: 32 2 2824610 **Fax:** 32 2 2307233
Email: easpd@skynet.be
Website: http://www.easpd.org

Mem: 5,500. **Nat'l Groups:** 19. **Desc:** Promotes the affairs of social firms and their umbrella associations who provide care services to persons with disabling conditions in Europe. Works to enhance the dignity, equality and citizenship of people with disabilities.

★ 2735 ★ European Association for Studies on Nutrition and Child Development (ADE)
(Association Europeenne pour l'Etude de l'Alimentation et du Developpement de l'Enfant — ADE)
4, Place du Breteuil
F-75015 Paris, France
Phone: 33 1 44736739 **Fax:** 33 1 44736739
Email: ade.paris@wanadoo.fr

Fnded: 1976. **Mem:** 120. **Nat'l Groups:** 4. **Lang(s):** English, French, German. **Desc:** Medical doctors, nutritionists, biologists, statisticians, and others working in related fields. Conducts surveys and research in nutrition and early childhood development; holds training sessions. Provides children's services. Humanitarian actions for children in distress, (orphans of war, street children). Ergotherapy by arts. Works in Sudan, Uganda, Poland, Russia, Georgia, China, and Albania. **Pub:** *Civil War: Children in International Conflict*, periodic. Book.

★ 2736 ★ European Association for the Study of Diabetes (EASD)
Rheindorfer Weg 3
D-40591 Dusseldorf, Germany
Phone: 49 221 7584690 **Fax:** 49 221 75846929
Email: secretariat@easd.org
Website: http://www.easd.org

Fnded: 1964. **Mem:** 5,500. **Lang(s):** English. **Desc:** Individuals and firms in over 100 countries. Promotes research into the disease of diabetes. Sponsors postgraduate education courses. **Pub:** *Diabetologia*, periodic. Journal. Scientific medical journal, containing diabetic research. • *Membership List*, triennial.

★ 2737 ★ European Association for the Study of Diabetic Eye Complications (EASDec)
Department of Ophthalmology
University of Udine
V.le Venezia, 410
I-33100 Udine, Italy
Phone: 39 432 239227 **Fax:** 39 432 239313
Email: francesco.bandello@dsc.uniud.it
Website: http://medweb.bham.ac.uk/easdec/index.html

Fnded: 1990. **Desc:** Organizes scientific meetings with ophthalmologists and diabetologists on issues of diabetic eye complications.

★ 2738 ★ European Association for the Study of Obesity
c/o Dr. Xavier Formiguera Sala
Obesity Unit
University Hospital Germans Trias I Pujol
Carretera de Canyet s/n
Catalonia
E-08916 Badalona, Spain
Phone: 34 93 4978912 **Fax:** 34 93 4978843
Email: xformig@ns.hugtip.scs.es
Website: http://www.iotf.org/oonet/easo/

Fnded: 1988. **Mem:** 2,500. **Nat'l Groups:** 27. **Desc:** Promotes study into the causes of obesity. **Pub:** *International Journal of Obesity*. Journal. • *Obesity Matters*.

★ 2739 ★ European Association of Surgical Sciences (EASS)
CP 2170
I-80100 Naples, Italy
Phone: 39 0815864320 **Fax:** 39 0815863606
Website: http://www.eass.it/

Desc: Supports the exchange of ideas and experience among surgeons.

★ 2740 ★ European Association of Transactional Analysis (EATO)
c/o Martine Huon
Les Toits de l'Aune Bat. E
3, rue Hugo Ely
F-13090 Aix-en-Provence, France
Email: info@eatanews.org

Desc: Promotes knowledge and research of transactional analysis. Seeks to develop standards of practice and certification. Conducts research; disseminates information. **Pub:** Newsletter, periodic.

★ 2741 ★ European Association of Trauma Emergency Surgery (EATES)
Chirrugia d'Urgenza
Universita Santa Chiara Hospital
I-56125 Pisa, Italy
Phone: 39 050 592423 **Fax:** 39 050 550593
Email: ecavina@dc.med.unipi.it

Fnded: 1973. **Lang(s):** English, French, Italian. **Desc:** Presidents and secretaries general of congresses of urgent surgery in 9 countries. Purpose is to organize and promote international congresses on urgent surgery. **Pub:** *Congress Abstracts*, biennial. • *Congress Proceedings*, biennial.

★ 2742 ★ European Association for the Treatment of Addiction - U.K. (EATA)
Waterbridge House
32-36 Loman St.
London SE1 0EE, United Kingdom
Phone: 44 20 79228753 **Fax:** 44 20 79284644
Email: secretariat@eata.org.uk
Website: http://www.box-1.freeserve.co.uk

Fnded: 1992. **Mem:** 80. **Lang(s):** English. **Desc:** Substance abuse treatment centers; health care and other professionals with an interest in the treatment of people who abuse substances. Seeks to advance the treatment of people with substance abuse problems; promotes increased understanding of the scientific, psychological, and medical aspects of substance abuse. Facilitates communication and cooperation among members; facilitates research and educational programs.

★ 2743 ★ European Association of Universities, Schools and Colleges of Optometry (AEUSCO)
(Association Europeene des Universites Ecoles et Colleges d'Optometrie — AEUSCO)
134, rte. de Chartres
F-91440 Bures-sur-Yvette, France
Phone: 33 1 64861213 **Fax:** 33 1 69284999
Email: ico.direction@wanadoo.fr
Website: http://www.ubi.pt/~aeusco

Fnded: 1979. **Mem:** 38. **Lang(s):** English, French. **Desc:** Schools in 16 countries providing education for optometrists and opticians. Promotes the development of optometry in Europe; seeks the standardization of optometric instruction and qualifications on a European level. Encourages cooperation and information exchange among teaching institutions. Compiles scientific and pedagogic documentation concerning optometric education in Europe. **Pub:** Newsletter, annual. **Frmly:** (1999) European Association of Schools and Colleges of Optometry.

★ 2744 ★ European Association of Urology (EAU)
PO Box 30016
NL-6803 AA Arnhem, Netherlands
Phone: 31 26 3890680 **Fax:** 31 26 3890674
Email: eau@uroweb.nl
Website: http://www.uroweb.org/

Desc: Promotes urology in Europe and worldwide; facilitates continued development of urology and all its sub-specialties. **Pub:** *European Urology*. Journal. • *European Urology Today*. Newsletter. Provides information about European urology in the broadest sense.

★ 2745 ★ European Association of Veterinary Anatomists (EAVA)
c/o Dr. Ignacio Salazar
Departmento de Anatomia y Embriologia
Facultad de Veterinaria
Universidad de Santiago de Compostela
E-27002 Lugo, Spain
Phone: 34 982 252239 **Fax:** 34 982 285939
Email: anigsabe@lugo.usc.es
Website: http://www.vetmed.uni-muenchen.de/anat1/eava/eava.html

Fnded: 1963. **Mem:** 270. **Lang(s):** English, French, German, Spanish. **Desc:** European and international veterinarians from 44 countries interested in morphologic research on domestic animals. **Pub:** *Vademecum of the European Association of Veterinary Anatomists*. Monographs.

★ 2746 ★ European Association of Veterinary Diagnostic Imaging (EAVDI)
c/o Kathrina Hittmair
Veterinarmedizinishe Universitat
Universitatsklinik fur Rontgenologiet
Veterinarplatz 1
A-1210 Vienna, Austria
Fax: 43 1250 775790
Email: katharina.hittmair@vu-wein.ac.at
Website: http://www.vet.gla.ac.uk/EVDI/eavdi.htm

Desc: Promotes the use of diagnostic imaging technology in veterinary medicine.

★ 2747 ★ European Association for Veterinary Pharmacology and Toxicology (EAVPT)
North Mymms
Hatfield AL9 7TA, United Kingdom
Phone: 44 1707 666294 **Fax:** 44 1707 666371
Email: plees@rvc.ac.uk

Fnded: 1978. **Desc:** Stimulates research and education in veterinary pharmacology and toxicology.

★ 2748 ★ European Association for Vision and Eye Research (EVER)
Postbus 74
B-3000 Leuven, Belgium
Phone: 32 1 6336785
Email: secretariat@ever.be
Website: http://www.ever.be/

Fnded: 1997. **Desc:** Encourages research and disseminates knowledge concerning eye and vision.

★ 2749 ★ European Atherosclerosis Society (EAS)
Institute of Medical Biochemistry & Molecular Biology
University Hospital Hamburg
Martinistrasse 52
D-20246 Hamburg, Germany
Phone: 49 40 428033017 **Fax:** 49 40 428034592
Email: beisiegel@uke.uni-hamburg.de
Website: http://www.elsevier.com/inca/homepage/sab/eas/menu.htm

Fnded: 1964. **Mem:** 127. **Lang(s):** English. **Desc:** Researchers in 24 countries of atherosclerosis (a disease characterized by the accumulation of fatty substances that have hardened inside the arteries). Purposes are to: exchange information concerning atherosclerosis and its causes and history; advance understanding of the treatment and prevention of atherosclerosis in humans and animals.

★ 2750 ★ European Bank of Frozen Blood of Rare Groups (EBFBRG) (Banque Europeenne de Sange Congele de Groupes Rares)
Sanquin Blood Supply Foundation
Plesmanlaan 125
NL-1066 CX Amsterdam, Netherlands
Phone: 31 20 5123373 **Fax:** 31 20 5123685
Email: m_overbeeke@clb.nl
Website: http://www.clb.nl

Fnded: 1969. **Mem:** 54. **Lang(s):** English, French, German. **Desc:** Individuals representing national blood banks and research centers.

★ 2751 ★ European Behavioral Pharmacology Society (EBPS)
Laboratory Neuro Cell et Function CNRS
31 Chemin Joseph-Arguier
F-12402 Marseille Cedex, France
Phone: 33 4 91164266 **Fax:** 33 4 91775083
Email: president@ebps.org
Website: http://www.ebps.org

Fnded: 1986. **Mem:** 250. **Desc:** Seeks to advance the development of behavioral pharmacology; disseminates research to members and non-members; assists practitioners of behavioral pharmacology to obtain knowledge extending into related disciplines.

★ 2752 ★ European Biomedical Research Association (EBRA)
58 Great Marlborough St.
London W1V 1DD, United Kingdom
Phone: 44 20 72872818 **Fax:** 44 20 72872627
Email: secretariat@ebra.org
Website: http://www.ebra.org/

Fnded: 1994. **Desc:** Promotes the best practice in animal research and high standards of laboratory animal welfare.

★ 2753 ★ European Blind Union (EBU) (Union Europeenne des Aveugles — UEA)
c/o Mokrane Boussaid
58 avenue Bosquet
F-75007 Paris, France
Phone: 33 1 47053820 **Fax:** 33 1 47053821
Email: ebu_uea@compuserve.com
Website: http://www.euroblind.org

Fnded: 1984. **Mem:** 44. **Lang(s):** English, Russian. **Desc:** European regional branch of the World Blind Union. Represents blind individuals in Europe, including those with additional handicaps. Promotes the prevention and cure of blindness. **Pub:** *EBU Newsletter*, quarterly. Newsletter.

★ 2754 ★ European Blue Cross Youth Association (EBY)
Lindenrain 5 a
CH-3001 Bern, Switzerland
Phone: 41 31 3005860 **Fax:** 41 31 3005869
Email: ifbc.bern@bluewin.ch

Fnded: 1979. **Mem:** 5. **Nat'l Groups:** 5. **Lang(s):** English. **Desc:** National societies in Germany, Great Britain, Norway, Sweden, and Switzerland representing 12,000 individuals. Purpose is to enhance cooperation among groups working with young people with substance abuse problems. Sponsors seminars, educational programs, camp sessions, student trips, and youth exchange programs.

★ 2755 ★ European Board of Cardiovascular Perfusion (EBCP)
c/o Kirk Graves
Department of Cardiovascular Surgery
Justus-Liebig-University
Rudolf-Buchheim-Strasse 7
D-35385 Giessen, Germany
Phone: 49 641 9944300 **Fax:** 49 641 9944329
Email: gravesebcp@gmx.net
Website: http://www.ebcp.org/

Desc: Works to develop, monitor and maintain standards in education and training of cardiovascular perfusion practice.

★ 2756 ★ European Board and College of Obstetrics and Gynecology (EBCOG)
Herestr 49
B-3000 Leuven, Belgium
Phone: 32 1 6344205 **Fax:** 32 1 6344208
Email: angele.lurquin@uz.kuleuven.ac.be
Website: http://www.ebcog.org

Fnded: 1996. **Mem:** 60. **Nat'l Groups:** 28. **Lang(s):** English, French. **Desc:** Enhances the health of women and their babies by promoting the highest possible standards of care in all European countries. **Pub:** *EBCOG Volumes.*

★ 2757 ★ European Board of Ophthalmology (EBO)
40a, av de Verdun
F-94010 Creteil, France
Phone: 33 1 45175222 **Fax:** 33 1 45175227
Email: 1063752207@compuserve.com

Fnded: 1992. **Mem:** 30. **Desc:** Works to Improve the training of ophthalmologists in Europe.

★ 2758 ★ European Board of Plastic, Reconstructive and Aesthetic Surgery (EBOPRAS)
3, rue du Languedoc
F-31100 Toulouse, France
Phone: 33 561 366988 **Fax:** 33 561 366969
Email: costagliola.m@wanadoo.fr
Website: http://www.uems.be/ebopras2.htm

Fnded: 1991. **Nat'l Groups:** 22. **Desc:** Guarantees highest standards of care in the field of plastic surgery.

★ 2759 ★ European Board for the Specialty of Cardiology (EBSC)
Papworth Everard
Cambridge CB3 8RE, United Kingdom
Phone: 44 1480 830541 **Fax:** 44 1480 831315

Fnded: 1992. **Desc:** Enhances the education and training of cardiologists in Europe.

★ 2760 ★ European Board of Urology (EBU)
PO Box 25285
NL-3001 HG Rotterdam, Netherlands
Phone: 31 10 4366665 **Fax:** 31 10 4366669
Email: ebu@ebu.com
Website: http://www.ebu.com/

Desc: Promotes optimal urological care to patients.

★ 2761 ★ European Board of Veterinary Specialization (EBVX)
c/o Federation of Veterinarians in Europe
Rue Defacqz 1
B-1000 Brussels, Belgium
Phone: 32 2 5337020 **Fax:** 32 2 5372828
Website: http://216.198.230.121/ebvs/about/

Desc: Promotes utilization and availability of veterinary specialty services. Maintains registry of veterinary specialists in Europe.

★ 2762 ★ European Brain and Behaviour Society (EBBS)
c/o Dr. Susan J. Sara
Institut des Neurosciences
9 quai St. Bernard
F-75005 Paris, France
Phone: 33 1 44273460 **Fax:** 33 1 44273251
Email: ebbs@hsantalucia.it
Website: http://www.ebbs-science.org/

Fnded: 1966. **Mem:** 550. **Lang(s):** Dutch, English, French. **Desc:** Scientists with an interest in the study of the brain and behavior. Promotes and facilitates exchange of information among members and between members and others working in related fields. Conducts research and and educational programs. **Pub:** Books, biennial. • Newsletter, periodic.

★ 2763 ★ European Brain Injury Consortium (EBIC)
c/o University Department of Neurosurgery
Institute of Neurological Science
Southern General Hospital
Glasgow G51 4TF, United Kingdom
Phone: 44 141 2012031
Website: http://homepages.ed.ac.uk/gdm/EBIC/

Desc: Promotes research aimed at improving the outcome of patients with acute brain injury. Fosters research.

★ 2764 ★ European Brain Injury Society (EBIS)
17, rue de Londres
B-1050 Brussels, Belgium
Phone: 32 2 5023488 **Fax:** 32 2 5022046
Email: ebis@euronet.be
Website: http://www.ebissociety.org/

Fnded: 1989.

★ 2765 ★ European Burns Association (EBA)
PO Box 1015
NL-1940 EA Beverwijk, Netherlands
Email: info@ebasecretariat.nl
Website: http://www.euroburn.nl/

★ 2766 ★ European Cancer Prevention Organization (ECP)
c/o M.C. Gueur
rue Martin V 40, Bte. 5
B-1200 Brussels, Belgium
Phone: 32 2 7790668 **Fax:** 32 2 7790668
Website: http://www.uicc.org/others/ecp/ecp.html

Fnded: 1983. **Mem:** 120. **Lang(s):** English. **Desc:** Scientists interested in cancer prevention research. Seeks to coordinate studies in cancer prevention and to inform the scientific community as well as the public. Conducts workshops. **Pub:** *ECP News*, quarterly. • *ECP Symposium Proceedings*, annual. • *European Journal of Cancer Prevention*, bimonthly. Journal.

★ 2767 ★ European Centre for Occupational Health, Safety and the Environment
c/o Dr. Charles Woolfson, Dir.
Faculty of Social Sciences
Lilybank House
University of Glasgow
Glasgow G1N 8RT, United Kingdom
Phone: 44 141 3304665 **Fax:** 44 141 3304665
Email: ecohse@socsci.gla.ac.uk
Website: http://www.gla.ac.uk/ecohse/
Desc: Promotes the exchange of academic, policy and practitioner experience in the fields of industrial relations and workplace health, safety and the environment.

★ 2768 ★ European Centre of Ophthalmology
99932 Rue du Meridien
B-1030 Brussels, Belgium
Fnded: 1990.

★ 2769 ★ European Charcot Foundation (Fondation Europeene Charcot)
c/o Mieke Friedrichs Bosmans
Heiweg 97
NL-6533 PA Nijmegen, Netherlands
Phone: 31 24 3561954 **Fax:** 31 24 3540920
Email: info@charcot-ms.org
Fnded: 1990. **Desc:** Fosters Multiple Sclerosis (MS) research in Europe. Recruits researchers. Coordinates funding of European MS research projects. Organizes treatment trials. **Pub:** Newsletter, periodic.

★ 2770 ★ European Chinese Society for Clinical Magnetic Resonance (ECSCMR)
c/o Prof. Dr. Juergen Hennig
Rontgendiagnostik Hugstetterstr. 55
D-79106 Freiburg, Germany
Phone: 49 761 2703836 **Fax:** 49 761 2703831
Email: hennig@nz11.ukl.uni-freiburg.de
Fnded: 1991. **Desc:** Fosters exchange of information between Europe and China on the application of magnetic resonance tomography.

★ 2771 ★ European College of Hypnotherapy
5 Schroder Ct.
Egham TW20 0EH, United Kingdom
Phone: 44 1784 479930
Email: principal@european-college.co.uk
Website: http://www.european-college.co.uk/
Desc: Promotes the development of new techniques in hypnotherapy, including the conversion of nightmares into pleasant dreams, externalizing hypnotic imagery, new pain-control procedures, and the concept of the virtual self. **Pub:** Articles.

★ 2772 ★ European College of Laboratory Animal Medicine (ECLAM)
c/o Vera Baumans, DVM
Department of Laboratory Animal Science
Universiteit Utrecht
PO Box 80.166
NL-3508 TD Utrecht, Netherlands
Fax: 31 30 2537997
Email: eclam.secretary@e-vet.com
Website: http://www.eclam.org/
Desc: Works to advance scientific progress in laboratory animal medicine.

★ 2773 ★ European College of Neuropsychopharmacology
PO Box 85410
NL-3508 AK Utrecht, Netherlands
Phone: 31 30 2538567 **Fax:** 31 30 2538568
Email: secretariat@ecnp.nl
Website: http://www.ecnp.nl/
Fnded: 1985.

★ 2774 ★ European College for the Study of Consciousness (ECSC)
c/o Dr. Michael Schlichting
Judenstr. 33
D-37073 Gottingen, Germany
Phone: 49 551 484463 **Fax:** 49 551 487487
Email: ecbsmschl@aol.com
Website: http://www.magnet.ch/ecbs/
Desc: Conducts research into the nature and qualities of consciousness. Disseminates information. Makes available advanced training for scientists and therapists.

★ 2775 ★ European College of Veterinary Diagnostic Imaging
c/o Martin Sullivan, Sec.
Division of Small Animal Studies
University of Glasgow
Bearsden Rd.
Bearsden
Glasgow G61 1QH, United Kingdom
Phone: 44 141 3305700 **Fax:** 44 141 9427215
Email: m.sullivan@vet.gla.ac.uk
Website: http://www.vet.gla.ac.uk/EVDI/ecvdi.htm
Fnded: 1993. **Mem:** 78. **Reg. Groups:** 3. **Desc:** Improves the quality of animal health care through specialized knowledge and skills in veterinary diagnostic imaging. **Pub:** *Veterinary Radiology & Ultrasound*, bimonthly. Journal.

★ 2776 ★ European College of Veterinary Internal Medicine - Companion Animals (ECVIN-CA)
c/o Dr. Cecile Clercx
Clin. Medicale des Petits Animaux
Faculty de Medecine Veterinaire
Sart Tilman Bat 44
B-4000 Liege, Belgium
Phone: 32 43 664200 **Fax:** 32 43 664240
Email: cclercx@ulg.ac.be
Website: http://www.ecvim-ca.org/
Fnded: 1994. **Desc:** Works to advance companion animal internal medicine in Europe.

★ 2777 ★ European College of Veterinary Ophthalmologists (ECVO)
Boxtelsebaan 6
NL-5061 VD Oisterwijk, Netherlands
Phone: 31 13 5285900 **Fax:** 31 13 5286667
Desc: Works to advance veterinary ophthalmology in Europe.

★ 2778 ★ European College of Veterinary Pathologists
c/o Dr. Ted van den Ingh, Sec.
Vakgroep Pathologie
Fakulteit Diergeneeskunde
Postbus 80 158
NL-3508 Utrecht, Netherlands
Phone: 31 30 2533195 **Fax:** 31 30 2534774
Email: thi@vet.uu.nl
Website: http://www.bris.ac.uk/Depts/PathAndMicro/eurovet/ecvpmain.html
Desc: Represents veterinary pathologists in Europe.

★ 2779 ★ European College of Veterinary Surgeons (ECVS)
Winterthurerstr 260
CH-8057 Zurich, Switzerland
Phone: 41 1 6358408 **Fax:** 41 1 3130384
Fnded: 1991. **Desc:** Promotes education in small and large animal surgery.

★ 2780 ★ European Committee of Private Hospitalization (ECPH) (Comite Europeen de l'Hospitalisation Privee — CEHP)
CEHP Registered Office
Ave. Alfred Solvay 5
B-1170 Brussels, Belgium
Phone: 32 2 6721350 **Fax:** 32 2 6729062
Fnded: 1977. **Mem:** 7. **Desc:** Promotes the private hospital industry in the European Community. Represents members' interests.

★ 2781 ★ European Committee on Radiopharmaceuticals
City Hospital NHS Trust
Birmingham B18 7QH, United Kingdom
Fax: 44 121 5075223

★ 2782 ★ European Committee for Treatment and Research in Multiple Sclerosis
Vanheylenstr 16
B-1910 Melsbroek, Belgium
Fax: 32 2 7518030

★ 2783 ★ European Communities Clinical Chemistry Committee
Piccadilly
London W1 0BN, United Kingdom
Phone: 44 20 74378656 **Fax:** 44 20 74378883
Fnded: 1973.

★ 2784 ★ European Confederation of Laboratory Medicine (ECLM)
Milngavie
Glasgow G62 8AW, United Kingdom
Phone: 44 141 9564573 **Fax:** 44 141 5639421
Email: robert.rowan@virgin.net
Website: http://www.inserm.fr
Fnded: 1993. **Desc:** Promotes the application of laboratory medicine to the provision of health services; supports European congresses of laboratory medicine and regional congresses and meetings of European scope and interest.

★ 2785 ★ European Confederation of Medical Devices Associations (EUCOMED)
Place St. Lambert 14
Woluwe
B-1200 Saint Lambert, Belgium
Phone: 32 2 7722212 **Fax:** 32 2 7713909
Email: eucomed@eucomed.be
Website: http://www.eucomed.be/
Fnded: 1999. **Desc:** Represents the interests of non-pharmaceutical European medical technology industries; works towards enhancing global market access.

★ 2786 ★ European Contact Dermatitis Society (ECDS)
Grosvenor Rd.
Belfast BT12 6BA, United Kingdom
Phone: 44 28 90240503

★ 2787 ★ European Contact Lens Society of Ophthalmologists (ECLSO)
2 Pl. Victor Hugo
F-38000 Grenoble, France
Phone: 33 4 76120211 **Fax:** 33 4 76120218
Email: eclso@tiscali.fr
Website: http://www.ophtalmo.net
Fnded: 1970. **Mem:** 3,000. **State Groups:** 20. **Desc:** Ophthalmologists in Europe. Provides information on contact lenses.

★ 2788 ★ European Council for Blood Pressure and Cardiovascular Research (ECCR)
127 High St.
Teddington TW11 8HH, United Kingdom
Phone: 44 20 89770011 **Fax:** 44 20 89770055
Email: eccr@hamptonmedical.com
Website: http://www.eccr.org
Fnded: 1997. **Mem:** 160. **Desc:** Promotes clinical and experimental research in hypertension and cardiovascular disease in Europe.

★ 2789 ★ European Council on Chiropractic Education
8, chemin de Tison
F-86000 Poitiers, France
Phone: 33 5 49415825

★ 2790 ★ European Council for Classical Homeopathy (ECCH)
Market Place
Kenninghall NR16 2AH, United Kingdom
Phone: 44 1953 888163 **Fax:** 44 888163
Email: ecch@homeopathy-ecch.org
Website: http://www.homeopathy-ecch.org/
Fnded: 1990. **Mem:** 8,000. **Nat'l Groups:** 17. **Desc:** Promotes and develops highest standards of homeopathic practice among the homeopathic profession.

★ 2791 ★ European Council of Coloproctology
24 Rue Micheli-du-Crest
CH-1211 Geneva, Switzerland
Phone: 41 22 3727901

★ 2792 ★ European Council on Eating Disorders (ECED)
Department of Psychiatry
St. George's Hospital Medical School
London SW17 0RE, United Kingdom
Phone: 44 208 7253489 **Fax:** 44 208 7253350
Email: eced@sghms.ac.uk
Fnded: 1989. **Mem:** 500. **Lang(s):** English. **Desc:** European medical clinicians and researchers with an interest in eating disorders. Seeks to advance the diagnosis and medical treatment of eating disorders. Facilitates exchange of information and clinical skills among members. **Pub:** Newsletter, periodic.

★ 2793 ★ European Council of Integrated Medicine (ECIM)
71 Rue des Echevins
1050 Brussels, Belgium
Fax: 32 2 6483480

★ 2794 ★ European Council of Legal Medicine
Institute of Legal Medicine
190 Winterthurstrasse
Bau 52
CH-8057 Zurich, Switzerland
Phone: 41 1 6355611 **Fax:** 41 1 6356815
Email: baer@irm.unizh.ch
Website: http://www.irm.unizh.ch/eclm
Fnded: 1992. **Mem:** 51. **Nat'l Groups:** 20. **Lang(s):** English, French, German, Italian. **Desc:** Representatives of member states of the European Free Trade Agreement in which legal medicine is recognized as a professional discipline. (Legal medicine refers to the medical examination of unexpected or unnatural deaths within the framework of the legal system.) Seeks to advance the study and practice of legal medicine. Represents the profession at the European level; serves as a clearinghouse on scientific, educational, and professional matters pertaining to legal medicine.

★ 2795 ★ European Council of Optics and Optometry (ECOO)
61 Southwark St.
London SE1 6LN, United Kingdom
Phone: 44 207 9289269 **Fax:** 44 207 6201140
Website: http://www.europtom.com
Fnded: 1960.

★ 2796 ★ European Cystic Fibrosis Society (ECSF)
Hyrdebakken 246
DK-8800 Viborg, Denmark
Phone: 45 8667 6260 **Fax:** 45 8667 6666
Email: info@ecfsoc.org
Website: http://www.ecfsoc.org
Fnded: 1969.

★ 2797 ★ European Cytoskeletal Club
1 Rue Michel Servet
CH-1211 Geneva, Switzerland
Fnded: 1980.

★ 2798 ★ European Dialysis and Transplant Nurses Association/ European Renal Care Association (EDTNA/ERCA)
Pilatusstrasse 35
Postfach 3052
CH-6002 Lucerne, Switzerland
Phone: 41 4407555 **Fax:** 41 4403962
Email: edtna_erca@compuserve.com
Website: http://www.edtna-erca.org
Fnded: 1972. **Mem:** 5,000. **Nat'l Groups:** 2. **Lang(s):** Dutch, English, French, German, Greek, Italian, Spanish. **Desc:** Promote renal care in Europe for patients and their families; updates standards for renal care; promotes renal care education and awareness of the social, cultural and ethical implications involved in the provision of care; promotes and conducts research in renal care. **Pub:** *Journal of the European Dialysis and Transplant Nurses Association/European Renal Care Association*, quarterly. Journal. Contains selected presentations made at the annual conference. • *Newsletter*, 3/yr. Newsletter.

★ 2799 ★ European Down's Syndrome Association (EDSA)
c/o Richard Bonjean
rue V. Close, 41
B-4800 Polleur-Verviers, Belgium
Phone: 32 87 223355 **Fax:** 32 87 220716
Desc: Professionals and family members of those with Down's syndrome. Promotes the right's and welfare of persons with Down's syndrome to receive health care and educational services; implements a network of local groups of parents and professionals; dedicated to the principles of normalization for those with Down's syndrome; strives to advance health programs for persons with Down's syndrome.

★ 2800 ★ European Dyslexia Association - International Organization for Specific Learning Disabilities (EDA)
46, av. de Port Royal des Champs
F-78320 Le Mesnil-Saint-Denis, France
Phone: 33 5 34619252
Fnded: 1987.

★ 2801 ★ European Dystonia Federation
69 East King St.
Helensburgh G84 7RE, United Kingdom
Phone: 44 143 6678799 **Fax:** 44 143 6678799
Email: sec@dystonia-europe.org
Website: http://www.dystonia-europe.org
Fnded: 1993. **Mem:** 19. **Nat'l Groups:** 19. **Desc:** National dystonia patient support groups of individual countries in Europe. **Pub:** Newsletter, semiannual.

★ 2802 ★ European Embryo Transfer Association (AETE) (Association europeene de transfert embryonnaire)
INRA-PRMD
F-37380 Nouzilly, France
Phone: 33 2 47427918 **Fax:** 33 2 47427743
Email: maugie@tours.inra.fr
Website: http://www.tours.inra.fr/aete/aeteeng.htm
Desc: Facilitates the diffusion and application of knowledge of embryo transfer in mammals.

★ 2803 ★ European Epilepsy Academy (EUREPA)
c/o Verena Hezser-v. Wehrs
Maraweg 21
D-33617 Bielefeld, Germany
Phone: 49 521 1444310 **Fax:** 49 521 1444311
Email: eurepa@owl-online.de
Website: http://www.epilepsy-academy.org
Fnded: 1996. **Desc:** Promotes advancements in the diagnosis and treatment of epilepsy. Conducts training programs.

★ 2804 ★ European Federation of the Associations of Dietitians (EFAD) (Federation Europeenne des Associations de Dieteticiens — FEAD)
Ziegeleiweg 4
D-46446 Emerich, Germany
Phone: 49 2822 63867 **Fax:** 49 2822 68358
Email: secretariat@efad.org
Website: http://www.efad.org/
Fnded: 1978. **Mem:** 22. **Lang(s):** English, French. **Desc:** National association of dietitians. Furthers dietetics as a scientific discipline and a profession. Objectives are: to improve the nutritional practices of European populations; to advance education in dietetics; to harmonize professional qualification criteria. Evaluates opportunities in the field.

★ 2805 ★ European Federation of Child Neurology Societies (EFCNS)
10 Av Hippocrate
1200 Brussels, Belgium
Phone: 32 2 7645231 **Fax:** 32 2 7641303
Fnded: 1970.

★ 2806 ★ European Federation of the Elderly (Federation Europeenne des Personnes Agees)
Secretariat General
Wielandgasse 9
A-8010 Graz, Austria
Phone: 43 316 814608 **Fax:** 43 316 814767
Email: eurag.europe@aon.at
Fnded: 1962. **Mem:** 350. **Lang(s):** English, French, German, Italian. **Desc:** Self-help groups working with older people; volunteers, physicians, psychologists, sociologists, social workers, researchers, and paramedical personnel helping the elderly in 33 countries. Promotes the well-being of the aged by working to improve their socioeconomic status; encourages the elderly to attain independence and become self-reliant by developing practical skills. Works to heighten public awareness of older people's needs. Cooperates with European organizations on questions regarding aging and the aged. Stimulates contacts and information exchange among members; compiles bibliographic information on aging. Sponsors colloquia. **Pub:** *EURAG Information*, monthly. • *EURAG Newsletter*, quarterly. **Frmly:** (1996) European Federation for the Welfare of the Elderly.

★ 2807 ★ European Federation of Endocrine Societies
c/o Prof. JMC Connell
British Endocrine Societies
17/18 The Courtyard

Woodlands
Bradley Stoke
Bristol BS32 4NQ, United Kingdom
Phone: 44 1454 642200 **Fax:** 44 1454 642222
Email: julie.cragg@endocrinology.org
Website: http://www.euro-endo.org

Fnded: 1984. **Desc:** Promotes endocrinology in Europe. Seeks to advance research and education in endocrinology. Organizes postgraduate courses.

★ 2808 ★ European Federation for Experimental Morphology (EFEM)

c/o Prof. Pierre Sprumont
Departement de medecine
Universite
Route Albert-Gockel 1
CH-1700 Fribourg, Switzerland
Phone: 41 26 3008450 **Fax:** 41 26 30009791
Email: pierre.sprumont@unifr.ch
Website: http://www.unifr.ch/efem

Fnded: 1989. **Mem:** 23. **Desc:** European scientific societies and groups concerned with morphology, anatomy, and related fields. Promotes exchange and dissemination of information.

★ 2809 ★ European Federation of Family Associations of People with Mental Illness (EUFAMI)

151 Groeneweg
B-3001 Heverlee, Belgium
Email: eufami@village.wwnet.org
Website: http://www.eufami.org

Fnded: 1992. **Mem:** 35. **Nat'l Groups:** 19. **Reg. Groups:** 16. **Lang(s):** English, French, German. **Desc:** Promotes the interests of people with mental illness and their careers. Works to remove the stigma surrounding mental illness by promoting a positive image to counteract misinformation. Lobbies for improved equality of legislation throughout Europe which benefits both the health and social care of people with mental illness and those who care for them. Sponsors research into the causes and treatments of mental illness. **Pub:** *Silent Partners*. Research document into careers' needs. • *Working Together*, 3/year. Newsletter. **Frmly:** (2001) European Federation of Associations of Families of Mentally Ill People.

★ 2810 ★ European Federation of Hereditary Ataxias (Euro-ATAXI)

Haagwindelaan 19
B-3090 Overijse, Belgium
Phone: 32 2 6571510 **Fax:** 32 2 6576176
Email: info@euro-ataxia.org
Website: http://www.euro-ataxia.org

Fnded: 1989.

★ 2811 ★ European Federation for Immunogenetics (EFI)

c/o Department of Immunohematology and Blood Transfusion
Leiden University Medical Centre
Bldg. 1 E3-Q
PO Box 9600
NL-2300 RC Leiden, Netherlands
Email: ihbsecr@euronet.nl

Fnded: 1985. **Mem:** 630. **Desc:** Individuals working in the field of immunogentics, histocompatibility testing, and transplantation. Seeks to advance the development of immunogenetics in Europe. Fosters the organization and and use of immunogenitic and histocompability databases. Provides a forum for the exchange of scientific information. **Pub:** Newsletter, quarterly.

★ 2812 ★ European Federation of Immunological Societies (EFIS)

c/o Anna Erdei, Sec.Gen.
Department of Immunology
Eotvos Lorand University
1/C Pazmany S
H-1117 Budapest, Hungary
Phone: 36 1 3812175 **Fax:** 36 1 3812176
Email: anna.erdei@freemail.hu
Website: http://www.efis.org

Fnded: 1975. **Mem:** 16,000. **Nat'l Groups:** 25. **Desc:** Immunological societies from around the world focusing on Europe. Promotes the advancement of research and education in immunology. **Pub:** *Immunology Letters*, monthly. Journal.

★ 2813 ★ European Federation of Internal Medicine (EFIM)

Eastern Rd.
Brighton BN2 5BE, United Kingdom
Phone: 44 1273 696955 **Fax:** 44 1273 684554
Email: info@efim.org
Website: http://www.efim.org/

Fnded: 1969. **Desc:** Promotes internal medicine at the scientific and professional level in the European Union.

★ 2814 ★ European Federation for Medicinal Chemistry (EFMC)

c/o Dr. Gerhard Ecker, Sec.
Institute of Pharmacological Chemistry
University of Vienna
Althanstr. 14
A-1090 Vienna, Austria
Phone: 43 1 313368571 **Fax:** 43 1 31336771
Email: gerhard.f.ecker@univie.ac.at
Website: http://www.efmc.ch/

Fnded: 1972.

★ 2815 ★ European Federation of National Associations of Orthopaedics and Traumatology (EFORT)

c/o Prof. George Bentley
Royal National Orthopedic Hospital
Stanmore HA7 4LP, United Kingdom
Phone: 44 208 9095532 **Fax:** 44 208 9543036
Email: office@efort.org
Website: http://www.efort.org/

Fnded: 1992. **Desc:** Promotes the exchange of knowledge and ideas in the field of prevention, the conservative and surgical treatment of diseases and injuries to the musculoskeletal symptom.

★ 2816 ★ European Federation of Neurological Societies (EFNS)

University Campus
Alser Strasse 4
A-1090 Vienna, Austria
Phone: 43 1 8890503 **Fax:** 43 1 889050313
Email: headoffice@efns.org
Website: http://www.efns.org

Fnded: 1991. **Mem:** 38. **Desc:** Promotes the advancement of neurological sciences, including the practice of neurology, in Europe. **Pub:** Newsletter, quarterly.

★ 2817 ★ European Federation of Nurse Educators

c/o Arne Kolsum
Eggervej 30
DK-2900 Hellerup, Denmark
Phone: 45 38 384422 **Fax:** 45 38 384400
Email: mjacquart@ulg.ac.be

Fnded: 1992. **Desc:** Promotes the continuing development of excellence of nurse education in Europe. Fosters quality assurance and professionalism in nurse education. Works to influence policy on the national and international levels in the European Union.

★ 2818 ★ European Federation of Organisations for Medical Physics (EFOMP)

BP 77980
F-21034 Dijon Cedex, France
Phone: 33 3 80737500 **Fax:** 33 3 80671915
Email: snaudy@dijon.fnclcc.fr
Website: http://www.efomp.org/

Fnded: 1980. **Desc:** Disseminates professional and scientific information through publications and meetings.

★ 2819 ★ European Federation of Orthodontic Specialist Associations (EFOSA)

c/o Dr. Wolfgang Schmiedel
Tempelhofer Damm 145
D-12099 Berlin, Germany
Phone: 49 30 7527015 **Fax:** 49 30 7529891
Email: dr.schmiedel@t-online.de
Website: http://www.efosa.org

Fnded: 1976. **Mem:** 8,000. **Nat'l Groups:** 20. **State Groups:** 20. **Lang(s):** English, French. **Desc:** Provides and promotes orthodontic treatment by orthodontic specialists of the highest quality; defends professional, political and economic interests of orthodontic specialists. **Pub:** *European Journal of Orthodontics*, bimonthly. Journal.

★ 2820 ★ European Federation of Periodontology (EFP)

Plaza Ramon y Cajal s/n
E-28040 Madrid, Spain
Phone: 34 913941905 **Fax:** 34 913941910
Email: marsan@eucmax.sim.ucm.es
Website: http://www.efp.net/

Fnded: 1987. **Desc:** Promotes and coordinates research on health and treatment needs in different countries and the impact on them of dental care systems.

★ 2821 ★ European Federation for Psychoanalytic Psychotherapy

5 Windsor Rd.
Finchley
London, United Kingdom
Phone: 44 20 84399873 **Fax:** 44 20 83433197
Email: joycepiper@compuserve.com

Desc: Umbrella organization that links together national networks of adult, child, and adolescent and group psychoanalytic psychotherapists, and psychoanalysts involved in public sector services.

★ 2822 ★ European Federation of Psychoanalytic Self-Psychology (EFPS)

Woerthstr 47
D-81667 Munich, Germany
Phone: 49 89 4482903 **Fax:** 49 89 2609740
Email: rbodansky@aol.com
Website: http://www.selfpsychology.org/europe/

★ 2823 ★ European Federation of Psychology Students' Associations (EFPSA)

Gallery Agora, B421
Grasmarkt 105/18
B-1000 Brussels, Belgium
Email: info@efpsa.intranets.com
Website: http://www.efpsa.org

Fnded: 1987. **Desc:** Promotes the exchange of social and ethical ideas among psychology students in Europe. Promotes scientific cooperation among psychology students.

★ 2824 ★ European Federation of Sexology (EFS)

Hannoversche Str 27
D-10115 Berlin, Germany
Phone: 49 30 45473665 **Fax:** 49 30 45473667
Email: HaeberleE@web.de
Website: http://www.geocities.com/HotSprings/Oasis/9249/

Fnded: 1988. **Desc:** Coordinates associations working in the field of sexology by encouraging research projects at a European level.

★ 2825 ★ European Federation of Sexology (EFS)
48 Boulevard Rodocanache
F-13008 Marseille, France
Phone: 33 4 91764489 **Fax:** 33 4 91770139
Fnded: 1988. **Reg. Groups:** 58. **Lang(s):** English, French, German. **Desc:** Scientific societies. Promotes study, research, and teaching in the field of sexology. Serves as a clearinghouse on sexology; sponsors research and educational programs.

★ 2826 ★ European Federation of Societies for Ultrasound in Medicine and Biology (EFSUMB)
Carpenters Court
4a Lewes Rd.
Bromley BR1 2RN, United Kingdom
Phone: 44 20 84028973 **Fax:** 44 20 84029344
Email: efsumb@efsumb.org
Website: http://www.efsumb.org/
Fnded: 1972. **Mem:** 13,500. **Nat'l Groups:** 26. **Lang(s):** English. **Desc:** Interdisciplinary national organizations and subgroups of bodies representing 26 countries. Members promote the application of ultrasound in biology and medicine or engage in research and development in the field. Proposes standards for ultrasound use and interpretation; arranges congresses and study and development meetings; promotes the exchange of information on ultrasound as applied to biology and medicine. Represents the European national societies in the World Federation of Societies for Ultrasound in Medicine and Biology. **Pub:** *European Journal of Ultrasound*, quarterly. Journal.

★ 2827 ★ European Federation of Sport Psychology (Federation europeenne de psychologie des sports et des activites corporelles — FEPSAC)
Box 213
S-221 00 Lund, Sweden
Phone: 46 46 2229115 **Fax:** 46 46 2224209
Email: Erwin.Apitzsch@psychology.lu.se
Website: http://www.psychology.lu.se/Fepsac/
Fnded: 1969. **Desc:** Organizes and coordinates scientific studies; establishes mutual scientific relations.

★ 2828 ★ European Federation of Sports Medicine (EFSM)
Via Saluzzo, 79
I-00182 Rome, Italy
Fnded: 1995.

★ 2829 ★ European Forum for Good Clincal Practice
Schoolberenstraat 47
B-3010 Kessel-Lo, Belgium
Phone: 32 16 350369 **Fax:** 32 16 350369
Email: info@efgcp.org
Website: http://www.efgcp.org
Fnded: 1995. **Mem:** 145. **Desc:** Individuals with a professional interest or involvement in clinical or biomedical research. Promotion of "good clinical practice" through education and to develop high quality standards in clinical research.

★ 2830 ★ European Generic Medicines Association (EGA)
PO Box 193
B-1040 Brussels, Belgium
Phone: 32 2 7368411 **Fax:** 32 2 7367438
Email: info@egagenerics.com
Website: http://www.egagenerics.com
Fnded: 1991. **Desc:** Maintains and develops the common scientific and technical interests of the generics branch of the pharmaceutical industry and manufactures of bulk chemicals destined for medicines.

★ 2831 ★ European Genetics Foundation (EGF)
c/o Lab. de Genetica Medica
Policlinico S Orsola-Malpighi pad. 11
Via Massarenti 9
I-40138 Bologna, Italy
Email: egf@eurogene.org
Website: http://www.eurogene.org
Lang(s): English, Italian. **Desc:** Professors, researchers, students, journalists, civil servants, and others interested in genetics. Promotes the training of young geneticists, continuing education in genetics, and the public understanding of genetics. Organizes and runs the European School of Genetic Medicine (ESGM) for postgraduate students.

★ 2832 ★ European Glaucoma Society
City Rd.
London EC1V 2PD, United Kingdom
Email: secretary@eugs.org
Website: http://www.eugs.org/
Fnded: 1979.

★ 2833 ★ European Health Management Association (EHMA)
Vergemount Hall
Clonskeagh
Dublin 6, Ireland
Phone: 353 1 2839299 **Fax:** 353 1 2838653
Email: marie@ehma.org
Website: http://www.ehma.org
Fnded: 1966. **Mem:** 200. **Lang(s):** English, French. **Desc:** Policy makers, senior managers, personnel directors, academic institutions, and research organizations in the healthcare sector. Seeks to improve healthcare in Europe by raising standards of managerial performance in the health sector. Fosters cooperation between health service organizations and institutions in the field of healthcare management education and training. Promotes the continuing education and development of healthcare managers. Offers advice and support to national governments in Europe; evaluates members' management development programs. **Pub:** *Conference Proceedings*, annual. Journal. • *Health Services Administration Education and Research*, annual. Directory. • *Management Development for Health Care: An International Perspective.* • *Management Education and Training in the Health Sector: A Perspective for Italy.* • Newsletter, bimonthly. **Frmly:** (1987) European Association of Programmes in Health Services Studies.

★ 2834 ★ European Health Psychology Society (EHPS)
Institute of Psychology
University of Greifswald
F.-Mehring-Str. 47
D-17487 Greifswald, Germany
Phone: 49 3834 863755 **Fax:** 49 3834 863755
Email: renner@uni-greifswald.de
Website: http://www.ehps.net/
Fnded: 1986. **Desc:** Promotes empirical and theoretical research in health psychology in Europe, in particular the study of behavior, health, illness and health care.

★ 2835 ★ European Heart Transplant Federation (EHTF)
BP 7 Anderlect ERASME
B-1070 Brussels, Belgium
Phone: 32 8 1460150 **Fax:** 32 8 1460157
Email: decannart@bigweb.be
Fnded: 1994. **Desc:** Encourages education and research relevant to organ transplantation.

★ 2836 ★ European Herbal Practitioners Association (EHPA)
45A Corsica St.
London N5 1JT, United Kingdom
Phone: 44 20 73455067 **Fax:** 44 20 73543605
Email: info@euroherb.com
Website: http://www.users.globalnet.co.uk/~ehpa/
Fnded: 1993. **Desc:** Herbal practitioners in Europe. Works to raise the standards of training and practice within the profession. Seeks to establish minimum standards of training and competence for herbal practitioners of all herbal traditions.

★ 2837 ★ European Hernia Society (Groupe de recherche europeen sur la paroi abdominale — GREPA)
74, rue Marcel Cachin
F-93017 Bobigny, France
Phone: 33 1 48369722 **Fax:** 33 1 48369731
Email: chevrel@compuserve.com
Fnded: 1978. **Desc:** Promotes research on all anatomic, physiologic and pathologic problems relating to the abdominal wall.

★ 2838 ★ European Histamine Research Society
Viale G B Morgagni, 65
I-50134 Florence, Italy
Phone: 39 0554237411 **Fax:** 39 0554361613
Fnded: 1972. **Desc:** Promotes experimental work in the area of histamine research.

★ 2839 ★ European Institute of Medicine
Karntner Ring 14/4
A-1010 Vienna, Austria
Phone: 43 1 5125760
Email: office@european-academy.at
Website: http://www.european-academy.at/en/index.html
Fnded: 1985. **Desc:** European scientists and artists concerned with problems and questions regarding medicine in Europe.

★ 2840 ★ European Kidney Research Association (EKRA)
Rue du Bugnon 27
CH-1005 Lausanne, Switzerland
Phone: 41 21 6925350 **Fax:** 41 21 6925355
Fnded: 2000. **Desc:** Promotes experimental nephrology in basic and clinical research.

★ 2841 ★ European Laryngological Society (ELS)
c/o Birgit Menzemer, Sec.
Hainbuchenstrasse 65
D-82024 Taufkirchen, Germany
Phone: 49 89 6126163 **Fax:** 49 89 6128176
Email: birgit.menzemer@escmid.org
Website: http://www.md.ucl.ac.be/els
Fnded: 1995. **Mem:** 200. **Lang(s):** Dutch, English, French, German. **Desc:** Physicians and researchers working in the field of laryngology. Promotes increased understanding of diseases of the neck and their treatments. Conducts research and continuing professional education programs. **Pub:** *European Archives of Otorhinolaryngology*, monthly. Journal.

★ 2842 ★ European Laser Association (ELA) (Association Europeenne du Laser — AEL)
Lund University Hospital
Department of Oncology
S-221 85 Lund, Sweden
Phone: 46 46 177520 **Fax:** 46 46 2223177
Email: info@ela-site.com
Fnded: 1981. **Mem:** 680. **Nat'l Groups:** 8. **Lang(s):** English, French. **Desc:** Physicians and surgeons in 15 countries concerned with laser medical instruments. Purpose is to advance the use of lasers in medicine. Conducts symposia and workshops. **Pub:** *Lasers in Medical Science*, periodic. Journal. • Newsletter, periodic.

★ 2843 ★ European League Against Rheumatism (EULAR)
(Ligue Europeenne Contre le Rhumatisme)
Witikonerstrasse 15
CH-8032 Zurich, Switzerland
Phone: 41 1 3839690 **Fax:** 41 1 3839810
Email: secretariat@eular.org
Website: http://www.eular.org

Fnded: 1947. **Mem:** 12,000. **Reg. Groups:** 4. **State Groups:** 3. **Lang(s):** English, French, German. **Desc:** Members of social and scientific organizations and pharmaceutical firms in 40 countries. Maintains small collection of rheumatology journals. **Pub:** *Annals of the Rheumatic Diseases*, monthly. Journal.

★ 2844 ★ European League of Stuttering Associations (ELSA)
Gereonswall 112
D-50670 Cologne, Germany
Phone: 49 221 1391106 **Fax:** 49 221 1391370
Email: elsa.europe@toalise.co.uk

Desc: Umbrella organization for stuttering associations throughout Europe. **Pub:** *Voice of ELSA*, semiannual. Newsletter.

★ 2845 ★ European Liaison Committee for Osteopaths (ELCO)
(Comite de Liaison Europeen des Osteopathes — CLEO)
116 Av. des Champs Elysee's
F-75008 Paris, France
Phone: 33 1 44218075

Fnded: 1978. **Mem:** 4. **Lang(s):** French. **Desc:** National associations in Belgium, England, France, and Greece. Seeks to protect the rights of osteopaths in the European Economic Community.

★ 2846 ★ European Lupus Erythematosus Federation (ELEF)
27-43 Eastern Rd.
St. James House
Romford RM1 3NH, United Kingdom
Phone: 44 1708 731251 **Fax:** 44 1708 731252
Website: http://www.elef.rheumanet.org/

Fnded: 1989. **Desc:** promotes research and improves the knowledge of Systematic Lupus Erythematosus.

★ 2847 ★ European Medical Association (EMA)
Place de Jamblinne de Meux 12
B-1030 Brussels, Belgium
Phone: 32 2 7342980 **Fax:** 32 2 7342135
Email: contact@emanet.org
Website: http://www.emanet.org

Fnded: 1991. **Desc:** Improves information and transparency; encourages collaboration and mobility for doctors; aims to influence actively the development of European health care.

★ 2848 ★ European Medical Laser Association (EMLA)
Lenzhalde 91
D-70192 Stuttgart, Germany
Email: laser@ticino.com
Website: http://www.emla-laser.com

Fnded: 1983. **Desc:** Promotes health care by high quality research and effective application of laser technologies in all fields of medicine.

★ 2849 ★ European Menopause and Andropause Society (EMAS)
Effingerstrasse 102
CH-3010 Bern, Switzerland
Phone: 41 31 6321010 **Fax:** 41 31 6321305

★ 2850 ★ European Midwives Liaison Committee (EMLC)
7 Dalestones
West Hunsbury NN4 9UU, United Kingdom
Phone: 44 1604 702121 **Fax:** 44 1604 285299
Email: mariannemead@compuserve.com

Fnded: 1968. **Mem:** 16.

★ 2851 ★ European Neural Network Society (ENNS)
p/a SNN, 231
University of Nijmegen
PO Box 9101
NL-6500 HB Nijmegen, Netherlands
Fax: 31 24 3541435
Email: enns@snn.kun.nl
Website: http://www.snn.kun.nl/enns

Fnded: 1991. **Desc:** Provides an interdisciplinary forum for researchers from different disciplinary backgrounds.

★ 2852 ★ European Neuroendocrine Association (ENEA)
Servicio de Endocrinologa
Hospital Sant Pau
Pare Claret 167
E-08025 Barcelona, Spain
Email: swebb@santpau.es
Website: http://www.eneassoc.org/

Fnded: 1984. **Desc:** Furthers development of research and clinical investigation in neuroendocrinology.

★ 2853 ★ European Neurological Society (ENS)
Hopital de Bicetre
F-94275 le Kremlin-Bicetre, France
Phone: 33 1 45212628 **Fax:** 33 1 46700931
Email: ensinfo@wanadoo.fr
Website: http://www.ensinfo.com

★ 2854 ★ European Oncology Nursing Society (EONS)
83 Ave. E Mounier
B-1200 Brussels, Belgium
Phone: 32 2 7799923 **Fax:** 32 2 7799937
Email: eons@village.uunet.be
Website: http://www.cancerworld.org

Fnded: 1987. **Mem:** 175. **Lang(s):** Dutch, English, French. **Desc:** Organizations, institutions, and individuals involved in cancer nursing. Seeks to promote and develop the practice of cancer nursing in Europe. Facilitates exchange of oncology nursing information; participates in European educational and research activities; makes available discounts on professional conference attendance fees to members. **Pub:** *Oncology Nurses Today*, periodic. Newsletter.

★ 2855 ★ European Ophthalmic Pathology Society (EOPS)
Ophthalmic Pathology Laboratory
Helsinki University, Central Hospital
Helsinki, Finland
Website: http://www.helsinki.fi/laak/silk/perus/eopshome.html

Fnded: 1962. **Desc:** Promotes knowledge in clinical and experimental ophthalmic pathology.

★ 2856 ★ European Opthalmological Society (EOS)
Moorfields Eye Hospital
City Rd.
London EC1V 2PD, United Kingdom
Phone: 44 171 2533411 **Fax:** 44 171 5662048

Fnded: 1956. **Nat'l Groups:** 45. **Lang(s):** English. **Desc:** National associations of ophthalmologists. Seeks to advance ophthalmological research, study, teaching, and practice. Promotes continuing professional development among ophthalmologists. Facilitates exchange of information among members; conducts research and educational programs.

★ 2857 ★ European Optical Society
Garbsener Landstrasse 10
D-30419 Hannover Cedex, Germany
Phone: 49 511 2771295 **Fax:** 49 511 277 1299
Email: eos@optecnet.de
Website: http://www.europeanopticalsociety.org

Fnded: 1991. **Mem:** 600. **Desc:** Contributes to programs in optics and related sciences, and to promote their applications at the European and international levels, by bringing together individuals and legal activities involved in these disciplines and their applications.

★ 2858 ★ European Organization for Caries Research (ORCA)
(Organisme Europeen de Recherche sur la Carie — ORCA)
c/o Prof. Lutz Stoesser
University of Jena
Preventive Dentistry
Nordhauser Str. 78
D-99089 Erfurt, Germany
Phone: 49 361 7411205 **Fax:** 49 361 7411105
Email: stoesser@zmkh.ef.uni-jena.de
Website: http://www.orca-caries-research.org

Fnded: 1953. **Mem:** 341. **Lang(s):** English. **Desc:** Scientists and organizations in 24 countries engaged in research on dental caries. Promotes research on dental caries and evaluates research findings. Establishes contact among organizations and individuals involved in similar research. **Pub:** *Caries Research*, bimonthly.

★ 2859 ★ European Organization for Research and Treatment of Cancer (EORTC)
(Organisation Europeenne pour la Recherche et le Traitement du Cancer)
83, ave. Mounier, bte. 11
B-1200 Brussels, Belgium
Phone: 32 2 7741611 **Fax:** 32 2 7723545
Email: eortc@eortc.be
Website: http://www.eortc.be

Fnded: 1962. **Mem:** 2,500. **Reg. Groups:** 36. **Lang(s):** English. **Desc:** Doctors, pharmacologists, clinicians, statisticians, computer analysts, and others in 25 countries involved in the development of anticancer therapies. Aims to develop cancer research in Europe through the coordination of joint research projects by hospitals and laboratories. Maintains screening program of potential anticancer agents and clinical research groups formed to carry out trials with new therapeutic agents. Maintains EORTC New Drug Development Program to coordinate the development of new anticancer medications; operates EORTC Central Office and Data Center to coordinate and conduct cancer clinical trials performed by a network of 2000 doctors in over 300 hospitals in Europe; conducts educational and research programs as well as health, economics, and quality of life studies. Compiles statistics. **Pub:** *EORTC Organisation, Activities and Current Research*, annual. Directory. • *European Journal of Cancer*, monthly.

★ 2860 ★ European Orthodontic Society (EOS)
49 Hallam St., Flat 20
London W1W 6JN, United Kingdom
Phone: 44 20 79352795 **Fax:** 44 20 73230410
Email: eoslondon@compuserve.com
Website: http://www.eoseurope.org

Fnded: 1907. **Mem:** 2,700. **Lang(s):** English. **Desc:** Orthodontists in 78 countries promoting the science of orthodontics. **Pub:** *European Journal of Orthodontics*, bimonthly. Journal. **Frmly:** (1935) European Orthodontia Society.

★ 2861 ★ European Ostomy Association
c/o Deutsche ILCO
PO Box 1265
D-85312 Freising, Germany
Phone: 49 8161 934301 **Fax:** 49 8161 934304
Email: info@ilco.de
Website: http://www.ilco.de

Fnded: 1990. **Mem:** 37. **Desc:** Umbrella ostomy Association that provides "member Associations information and management guidelines, helps to inform new ostomy Associations, and advocates on all related matters and policies."

★ 2862 ★ European Pediatric Neurology Society
48, bd Serrurier
F-75019 Paris, France
Phone: 33 1 40034773 **Fax:** 33 1 40034774

Fnded: 1970. **Desc:** Promotes development of knowledge in child neurology.

★ 2863 ★ European Pediatric Orthopedic Society (EPOS)
Weligerveld 1
3212 Pellenberg, Belgium
Phone: 32 1 6338803 **Fax:** 32 1 6338800
Email: michael.benson@doctors.org.uk
Website: http://ospiti.cilea.it/ortopedia/

Fnded: 1982. **Desc:** Promotes the advancement of pediatric orthopedics, particularly in the practice, scientific research and teaching of effects on the locomotor system during growth and of understanding of the bone pathology of the child.

★ 2864 ★ European Pineal and Biological Rhythm Society (EPBRS)
Bunteweg 17
D-30559 Hannover, Germany

Fnded: 1978. **Desc:** Promotes research on the pineal organ in its broadest

★ 2865 ★ European Prosthodontic Association (EPA)
Eastman Dental Hospital
256 Grays Inn Rd.
London WC1X 8LD, United Kingdom
Phone: 44 20 79151073 **Fax:** 44 20 79151246
Email: r.welfare@eastman.ucl.ac.uk
Website: http://www.eastman.ucl.ac.uk/~epa

Fnded: 1978. **Mem:** 528. **Lang(s):** English. **Desc:** Prosthodontists. Seeks to advance the profession of dentistry; promotes continuing professional development of members. Serves as a forum for the exchange of information among European prosthodontists; sponsors research and educational programs.

★ 2866 ★ European Psycho-Analytical Federation (EPF) (Federation Europeenne de Psychanalyse — FEP)
37 Wooddsome Rd.
London NW5 1SA, United Kingdom
Phone: 44 207 4857269 **Fax:** 44 207 2099963
Email: d.tuckett@ucl.ac.uk
Website: http://www.epf-eu.org

Fnded: 1969. **Reg. Groups:** 26. **Lang(s):** English, French, German. **Desc:** Psychoanalysts from 19 countries belonging to European psychoanalytical societies. Seeks to further psychoanalysis as a comprehensive theory of personality and therapeutic method based on the teachings of Sigmund Freud (1856-1939), Austrian neurologist and founder of psychoanalysis. Works to maintain and improve standards of education and scientific inquiry and to foster theoretical research. Disseminates information on theoretical and practical aspects of psychoanalysis. Stimulates communication among psychoanalysts; provides a forum for discussion of psychoanalytic and related topics. Encourages the integration of psychoanalysis and other disciplines. Organizes seminars and symposia. **Pub:** *Bulletin*, semiannual. • *Psychoanalytic Training in Europe: 10 Years of Discussion.* • *Pulsion de Mort.*

★ 2867 ★ European Public Health Alliance
33, rue de Pascale
B-1040 Brussels, Belgium
Phone: 32 2 2333880 **Fax:** 32 2 2333880
Email: epha@epha.org
Website: http://www.epha.org

Fnded: 1993. **Mem:** 82. **Lang(s):** Dutch, English, French, German, Italian, Spanish. **Desc:** Strives to improve public health in Europe through policy monitoring and development. Works to heighten public awareness on current public health reforms. Communicates with other organizations with similar interests. **Pub:** *Commercial Sponsorship and NGOs*. Booklet. Discusses the potential advantages and disadvantages of commercial sponsorship and NGOs. • *Creating a Citizen-centered EU Health Policy*. Paper. Position paper on the health strategy for the European union. • *European Health Directory*. Directory. Contains contact details of major European health stakeholders (NGOs and other not-for-profit associations). • *European Public Health Update*. Newsletter. • *Public Health and the EU - an Overview*. Book. Thirteen chapters introducing a range of health related EU policies. • *Research Priorities for Public Health in Europe*. The final report of a major EPHA conference held in Brussels, Belgium in July 1993.

★ 2868 ★ European Regional Organization of the World Dental Federation
c/o Marian Bader
Generalsekretariat ERO-FDI Koln
Ottostr 28
D-51427 Gladbach, Germany
Phone: 49 2204 427698 **Fax:** 49 2204 205316
Email: m.bader@bzaek.de
Website: http://www.fdiworldental.org/members/ero/

Fnded: 1955. **Mem:** 37. **Lang(s):** English, French, German. **Desc:** National dental associations in Europe belonging to the International Dental Federation. Works to establish common professional and health policies in European nations. Provides for the exchange of information; fosters cooperation among members. **Pub:** *ERO Circular Letter*, quarterly. Newsletter.

★ 2869 ★ European Research Group on Experimental Contact Dermatitis (ERGECD)
Alderley Park
Macclesfield SK10 4TJ, United Kingdom
Phone: 44 1625 590249

★ 2870 ★ European Research Organization of Genital Infection and Neoplasia (EUROGIN)
174, rue de Courcelles
F-75017 Paris, France
Phone: 33 1 47660529 **Fax:** 33 1 47667470

Desc: Stimulates research in the field of genital infections, pre-cancers and cancers.

★ 2871 ★ European Respiratory Society (ERS)
4, ave. Sainte-Luce
CH-1003 Lausanne, Switzerland
Phone: 41 21 2130101 **Fax:** 41 21 2130100
Email: info@ersnet.org
Website: http://www.ersnet.org

Mem: 5,000. **Nat'l Groups:** 81. **Lang(s):** English, Norwegian. **Desc:** Health care professionals and medical researchers with an interest in respiratory medicine. Seeks to advance the prevention, diagnosis, and treatment of respiratory disorders; promotes continuing professional development of members. Coordinates respiratory medical research efforts and facilitates exchange of information among members; conducts educational and training programs. Conducts promotional activities encouraging improved lung health in Europe; lobbies on public health issues including tobacco advertising. Operates European School of Respiratory Medicine. **Pub:** *European Respiratory Journal*, monthly. • Newsletter, periodic.

★ 2872 ★ European Rheumatoid Arthritis Surgical Society (ERASS)
Lengghalde 2
CH-8008 Zurich, Switzerland
Phone: 41 1 3857429 **Fax:** 41 1 3857599

Fnded: 1979. **Desc:** Promotes scientific and clinical work in rheumatoid arthritis surgery.

★ 2873 ★ European Rhinologic Society (ERS)
c/o Dr. K. Ingels
Dept of Otorhinolaryngology
Ph. Van Leydenlan 15
NL-6525 EX Nijmegen, Netherlands
Phone: 31 24 3614450 **Fax:** 31 24 3540251
Email: k.ingels@kno.azn.nl

Fnded: 1963. **Mem:** 700. **Lang(s):** English. **Desc:** Rhinosurgeons and otolaryngologists in 42 countries. Offers education and research in clinical, allergological, and immunological rhinology; provides training in functional and aesthetic rhinosurgery. Holds courses. **Pub:** *Rhinology*, quarterly. Journal.

★ 2874 ★ European Science Foundation (ESF)
1, quai Lezay Marnesia
F-67080 Strasbourg Cedex, France
Phone: 33 3 88767100 **Fax:** 33 3 88370532
Email: esf@esf.org
Website: http://www.esf.org

Fnded: 1974. **Mem:** 70. **Lang(s):** English. **Desc:** Association of 70 member organisations devoted to scientific research in 27 European countries. Core purpose is to promote high quality science at a European level. Committed to facilitating cooperation and collaboration in European science on behalf of its principal stakeholders. Combines both 'top-down' and 'bottom-up' approaches in the long-term development of science. Provides scientific leadership through its networking expertise and by ensuring that there is a European added value to all of its initiatives and projects. pertaining to research grants in those areas. pertaining to research grants in those areas. *Human Genome Research: A Review of European and International Contributions*, *Report on Genome Research*, and *Clinical Research Training in Europe*. **Frmly:** (2001) European Medical Research Councils.

★ 2875 ★ European Sleep Research Society (ESRS)
c/o Dr. Porkka-Heiskanen
Institute of Biomedicine
University of Helsinki, Biomedicum
PO Box 63
FIN-00014 Helsinki, Finland
Phone: 358 9 191 25317 **Fax:** 358 9 191 25302
Email: porkka@cc.helsinki.fi
Website: http://www.esrs.org

Fnded: 1972. **Mem:** 700. **Desc:** Those interested in sleep research. Promotes research on sleeping and other related disorders and to assist in the care of patients with sleeping disorders. Provides continuing education of all professional groups involved with this research and disseminates information regarding the disorder.

★ 2876 ★ European Society for Analytical Cellular Pathology (ESACP)
c/o H.E. Danielson
The Norwegian Radmium Hospital
Department of Pathology
Montebello
N-0310 Oslo, Norway

Phone: 47 22935617 Fax: 47 22935627
Email: hdaniels@labmed.uio.no

Lang(s): English, French. **Desc:** Scientists actively engaged in the field of analytical cellular pathology; health care professionals and scientists working in related fields; pharmaceutical manufacturers and biotechnology firms. Seeks to advance the study, teaching, and practice of analytical cellular pathology; promotes development of new technologies relevant to the field. Facilitates exchange of information among members; sponsors research and educational programs; serves as a clearinghouse on analytical cellular pathology. **Pub:** *Journal of Analytical Cellular Pathology*, bimonthly.

★ 2877 ★ European Society of Anesthesiologists (ESA)
Av de Tervuren 32, bte 30
B-1040 Brussels, Belgium
Phone: 32 2 7433290 **Fax:** 32 2 7433298
Email: secretariat.esa@euronet.be
Website: http://www.euroanesthesia.org/

Fnded: 1993. **Desc:** Provides continuous education and promotes organization, formation and improvement of qualifications of anesthetists in Europe.

★ 2878 ★ European Society for Artificial Organs - East European Office (ESAO)
c/o Prof. Jean Maria Wojcicki
Institute of Biocybernetics and Biomedical Engineering P.A.S
Trojedena 4
P-02-109 Warsaw, Poland
Phone: 48 22 6582875 **Fax:** 48 22 6597030
Email: jan.wojcicki@ibib.waw.pl
Website: http://www.esao.org/

Fnded: 1974. **Mem:** 450. **Lang(s):** English. **Desc:** Associations and individuals concerned with advancement in the creation of artificial organs. Promotes research. **Pub:** *International Journal of Artificial Organs*, monthly. Journal. Includes congress proceedings. • *Life Systems*, quarterly. Also publishes modifications.

★ 2879 ★ European Society of Biochemical Pharmacology (ESBP)
c/o Dr. Brian Burchell
University of Dundee
Department of Biochem. Med.
Ninewells Medical School
Dundee DD1 9SY, United Kingdom
Phone: 44 1382 632164 **Fax:** 44 1382 633952
Email: b.burchell@dundee.ac.uk
Website: http://www.geocities.com/ResearchTriangle/4787/welcome.htm

Desc: Researchers at academic institutions and in the pharmaceutical industry. Promotes advancements in the field of pharmacology.

★ 2880 ★ European Society for Biomedical Research on Alcoholism (ESBRA)
c/o Anita Riegler, c/o Prof. O.M. Lesch
Universite Klinik fuer Psychiatrie
Waehringerguertel 18-20
A-1090 Vienna, Austria
Phone: 43 676 6430320 **Fax:** 43 1 404003560
Email: office@esbra.com
Website: http://www.esbra.com

Fnded: 1987. **Desc:** Fosters biomedical research on alcoholism in Europe; assists in prevention and education in matters related to alcoholism.

★ 2881 ★ European Society of Breast Imaging (EUSOBI)
Neutorgasse 9/2a
A-1010 Vienna, Austria
Phone: 43 1 5358925 **Fax:** 43 1 5357037
Website: http://www.eusobi.org/

Desc: Promotes radiology training in the field of breast imaging and breast cancer screening with mammography, including interventional methods as well as new imaging breast cancer screening procedures.

★ 2882 ★ European Society of Cardiology
c/o The European Heart House
2035 Route des Colles
Les Templiers
Boite Postale 179
F-06903 Sophia Antipolis cedex, France
Phone: 33 4 92947600 **Fax:** 33 4 92947601
Email: webmaster@escardio.org
Website: http://www.escardio.org/

Fnded: 1950. **Mem:** 40,000. **Nat'l Groups:** 47. **Lang(s):** English, French. **Desc:** Cardiologists. Seeks to "improve the quality of life of the European population by reducing the impact of cardiovascular disease." Fosters interdisciplinary research and cooperation to advance the practice of cardiology; facilitates exchange of information among members and between members and individuals working in related fields; conducts public education programs. Serves as a clearinghouse on cardiovascular diseases and their prevention and treatment. **Pub:** *Cardiovascular Research*, monthly. Journal. • *European Heart Journal*, biweekly. Journal.

★ 2883 ★ European Society for Cardiovascular Surgery (ESCVS) (Societe Europeenne de Chirurgie Cardiovasculaire)
c/o Prof. C. Muneretto
Spedali Civili, U.D.A. Cardiochirurgia
P.le Spedali Civili 1
I-25123 Brescia, Italy
Phone: 39 030 3996400 **Fax:** 39 030 3996096
Email: webmaster@escvs.org
Website: http://www.escvs.org/

Fnded: 1952. **Mem:** 1,230. **Nat'l Groups:** 40. **Lang(s):** English. **Desc:** European Chapter of the International Society of Cardiovascular Surgery. Members are cardiac and vascular surgeons. Promotes the study of cardiovascular diseases; facilitates exchange of information and ideas concerning cardiovascular diseases. **Pub:** *Cardiovascular Surgery*, bimonthly. Journal.

★ 2884 ★ European Society for Cataract and Refractive Surgeons (ESCRS)
Temple House
Temple Rd.
Blackrock 2, Dublin, Ireland
Phone: 353 1 2091100 **Fax:** 353 1 2091112
Email: escrs@agenda-comm.ie
Website: http://www.escrs.com

Fnded: 1958. **Mem:** 3,000. **Lang(s):** English. **Desc:** Strives to advance scientific knowledge in the field of intraocular lens implantation and in the art and practice of such surgery.

★ 2885 ★ European Society of Child and Adolescent Psychiatry (ESCAP) (Societe Europeene de Psychiatrie de l'Enfant et de l'Adolescent — SEPEA)
Department Of Child and Adolescent Psychiatry
University Hospital Utrecht
Postbus 85500
NL-3508 GA Utrecht, Netherlands
Phone: 31 30 2506362 **Fax:** 31 30 2505444
Email: h.vanengeland@psych.azu.nl

Fnded: 1954. **Mem:** 28. **Lang(s):** English, French, German. **Desc:** National societies. **Pub:** *European Child and Adolescent Psychiatry*, quarterly. Journal.

★ 2886 ★ European Society for Classical Natural Medicine
Klinik Buchinger am Bodensee
D-101165 Eberlingen, Germany
Phone: 49 7551 8070 **Fax:** 49 7551 807889

Fnded: 1996. **Desc:** Fosters science, research and training in the field of classical natural medicine, including physiotherapy, nutrition, dietetics, fasting, phytotherapy, ordotherapy, psychotherapy.

★ 2887 ★ European Society of Clinical Microbiology and Infectious Diseases (ESCMID)
Postfach 6
CH-4005 Basel, Switzerland
Phone: 41 61 6867799 **Fax:** 41 61 6867798
Email: info@escmid.org
Website: http://www.escmid.org

Fnded: 1983. **Desc:** Promotes scientific and clinical excellence in microbiology and infectious diseases through postgraduate training, research and improvement of professional conditions across Europe. **Pub:** *Clinical Microbiology & Infection*, monthly. Journal.

★ 2888 ★ European Society of Clinical Microbiology and Infectious Diseases (ESCMID)
PO Box 11 31
D-82018 Taufkirchen, Germany
Phone: 41 61 6867799 **Fax:** 41 61 6867798
Email: info@escmid.org
Website: http://www.escmid.org

Fnded: 1983. **Mem:** 2,700. **Desc:** Professionals working in the fields of clinical microbiology and/or infectious diseases. **Pub:** *Clinical Microbiology and Infection.* Journal.

★ 2889 ★ European Society for Clinical Neuropharmacology (ESCNP)
Via Giustiniani, 5
I-35128 Padua, Italy
Phone: 39 0498213600 **Fax:** 39 0498751770
Email: segr.neurologia@unipd.it

Fnded: 1992. **Desc:** Maintains efficient collaboration with national and international societies, governmental organizations, professional Associations and individuals contributing to the progress in the field of clinical neuropharmacology.

★ 2890 ★ European Society of Clinical Pharmacy (ESCP)
Ave. des Gaulois, 7
B-1040 Brussels, Belgium
Phone: 32 2 7431542 **Fax:** 32 2 7431550
Email: escp@associationhq.com
Website: http://www.escp.nl

Fnded: 1979. **Mem:** 1,000. **Desc:** Seeks to develop and promote the rational and appropriate use of medicines. Provides a forum for the communication of new knowledge and new developments in clinical pharmacy. Plans, accredits, and develops educational and research programs in clinical pharmacy. Liaises with health care organizations worldwide. **Pub:** *Progress in Clinical Pharmacy*, annual. Proceedings. • Newsletter, bimonthly.

★ 2891 ★ European Society for Clinical Virology (ESCV)
Regional Public Health Laboratory
Department of Virology
van Ketwich Verschuurlaan 92
NL-9721 SW Groningen, Netherlands
Phone: 31 50 5215160 **Fax:** 31 50 5271488
Email: schirmjslg@compuserve.com
Website: http://www.escv.org

Fnded: 1997. **Mem:** 600. **Lang(s):** English, French. **Desc:** Virologists and other health care professionals; researchers and scientists with an interest in viruses. Seeks to advance the practice of virology and rapid viral diagnosis. Sponsors continuing professional education programs for virologists; conducts research. **Frmly:** (2000) European Group for Rapid Viral Diagnosis.

★ 2892 ★ European Society for Cognitive Psychology (ESCP)
c/o John Towse
Department of Psychology
Lancaster University
Bailrigg
Lancaster LA1 4YF, United Kingdom
Email: andre.vandierendonck@rug.ac.be
Website: http://www.escop.org

Fnded: 1985. **Mem:** 512. **Desc:** Stimulates research within the field of Cognitive Psychology and related subjects, particularly with respect to collaboration and exchange of information between researchers in different European countries. **Pub:** *European Journal of Cognitive Psychology*, quarterly. Journal.

★ 2893 ★ European Society for Communicative Psychotherapy
c/o The School of Psychotherapy and Counselling
Regent's College
Inner Cir.
Regent's Park
London NW1 4NS, United Kingdom
Phone: 44 20 78477584 **Fax:** 44 20 78477446
Email: info@escp.org
Website: http://www.escp.org

Desc: Psychiatrists and psychotherapists in Europe.

★ 2894 ★ European Society of Comparative Gastroenterology (ESCG)
50, rue Jeanne d'Arc
F-69003 Lyon, France

★ 2895 ★ European Society for Computing and Technology in Anaesthesia and Intensive Care (ESCTAIC)
c/o Lutz Krummereich
Draeger Medical
Moislinger Allee 53-55
D-23542 Lubeck, Germany
Phone: 49 451 8824316 **Fax:** 49 451 88274316
Email: treasurer@esctaic.org
Website: http://www.ESCTAIC.org

Fnded: 1989. **Mem:** 200. **Desc:** Fosters interchange of ideas among individuals as well as manufacturers in the field of computing and technology in anesthesia and intensive care medicine. Promotes exploration and innovation in medical technology.

★ 2896 ★ European Society of Contact Dermatitis (ESCD)
Occupational and Environmental Dermatology Unit
University Hospital
PO Box 30001
NL-9700 RB Groningen, Netherlands
Email: p.j.coenraads@med.rug.nl
Website: http://www.dermis.net/org/escd/index.htm

Lang(s): English, German. **Desc:** Dermatologists and other health care professionals and medical researchers with an interest in contact dermatitis and other environmental and occupational skin diseases. Seeks to advance the prevention, diagnosis, and treatment of environmental and occupational dermatological disorders. Facilitates exchanger of information among members; stimulates dermatological research; serves as a clearinghouse on contact dermatitis and related disorders; sponsors educational programs. **Pub:** *Contact Dermatitis*, periodic. Journal. • Newsletter, periodic.

★ 2897 ★ European Society for Dental Ergonomics (ESDE)
Kliniekstraat 9
B-3500 Hasselt, Belgium
Phone: 32 89412010 **Fax:** 32 11274490
Email: micholt-merchiers@pandora.be
Website: http://www.esde.org

Fnded: 1987. **Mem:** 80. **Desc:** Promotes the collection, analysis, following up, publication and archiving of scientific knowledge concerning dental ergonomics and dental practice.

★ 2898 ★ European Society for Dermatological Research (ESDR)
Department of Dermatology, Rm. 4-794
Geneva University Hospital
Rue Micheli du Crest 24
CH-1211 Geneva 14, Switzerland
Phone: 41 22 3729476 **Fax:** 41 22 37279475
Email: office@esdr.ch
Website: http://www.esdr.org/

Fnded: 1974. **Mem:** 800. **Reg. Groups:** 33. **Desc:** Promotes dermatological research in Europe.

★ 2899 ★ European Society for Developmental Pharmacology (ESDP)
82, av Denfert-Rochereau
F-75674 Paris, France
Fax: 33 1 40488328

Fnded: 1988. **Desc:** Promotes foetal, perinatal or pediatric pharmacology.

★ 2900 ★ European Society for Developmental Psychology (ESDP)
Loughborough University
Brighton LE11 3TU, United Kingdom
Phone: 44 1509 223037 **Fax:** 44 1509 223940
Email: m.c.hewitt1@iboro.ac.uk
Website: http://devpsy.lboro.ac.uk/eurodev/

Fnded: 1994. **Desc:** Advances education in developmental psychology for the public benefit; supports or conducts relevant research in the European context.

★ 2901 ★ European Society for Emergency Medicine (EuSEM)
c/o Francesco Della Corte, Sec.
Department of Emergency Medicine
University of Eastern Piedmont
Maggiore Hospital
Viale Mazzini 18
I-28100 Novara, Italy
Fax: 39 06 30113450
Email: fdcorte@tin.it
Website: http://www.diesis.com/eusem/

Fnded: 1994. **Desc:** Develops an integrated system of pre-hospital, in-hospital and inter-hospital emergency care.

★ 2902 ★ European Society for Emerging Infections (ESEI)
Rue Bruyns 2
B-1120 Brussels, Belgium
Phone: 32 2 2644048 **Fax:** 32 2 2644044
Email: jan.clement@msw.smd.be

Fnded: 1997. **Desc:** Determines infections affecting animals or humans which have emerged or are appearing with new, altered properties.

★ 2903 ★ European Society of Feline Medicine (ESFM)
Taeselbury High St.
Tisbury
Salisbury SP3 6LD, United Kingdom
Phone: 44 870 7422278
Email: esfm@fabcats.org
Website: http://www.fabcats.org/esfm.html

Lang(s): English. **Desc:** Veterinarians with an interest in feline medicine. Seeks to advance the medical treatment of cats; promotes continuing professional development of members. Facilitates exchange of information among veterinarians and researchers working in the field of feline medicine; sponsors educational courses. **Pub:** *Journal of Feline Medicine and Surgery*, quarterly.

★ 2904 ★ European Society of Gastrointestinal and Abdominal Radiology (ESGAR)
Neutorgasse 9/2A
A-1010 Vienna, Austria
Phone: 43 1 5358927 **Fax:** 43 1 5357037
Email: office@esgar.org
Website: http://www.esgar.org/

Desc: Radiologists interested in the imaging and treatment of patients with diseases of the gastrointestinal tract and associated abdominal organs.

★ 2905 ★ European Society for Gastrointestinal Endoscopy (ESGE)
c/o Prof. Guido Costamagna, Sec.
Policlinico A. Gemelli
Unita Operativa di Endoscopia Digestiva
L. go A. Gemelli 8
I-00168 Rome, Italy
Phone: 39 06 35511515 **Fax:** 39 06 35511515
Email: gcostamagna@rm.unicatt.it
Website: http://www.esge.com/

★ 2906 ★ European Society for Gender Specific Medicine (ESGSM)
c/o Prof. Weissenbaches
PF 702027
D-81320 Munich, Germany
Phone: 49 89 70954730 **Fax:** 49 89 70958884
Email: rainer.weissenbacher@helios.med.uni-muenchen.de
Website: http://www.esgsm.com

Lang(s): English, French, German, Italian. **Desc:** Promotes the study of gender-specific diseases and conditions such as sexually transmitted diseases, hormones, specific neoplasias, and pregnancy, among others.

★ 2907 ★ European Society of Gene Therapy (ESGT)
c/o Bernd Gansbacher
Experim. Onkologie & Therapieforschung
Klinikum r.d. Isar
Ismaninger Str. 22
D-81675 Munich, Germany
Phone: 49 89 41404451 **Fax:** 49 89 41404476
Email: b.gansbacher@lrz.tu-muenchen.de

Desc: Promotes clinical research in gene therapy. Fosters communication among members related to gene transfer and therapy. Liaises with regulatory bodies in Europe.

★ 2908 ★ European Society of Gene Therapy (ESGT)
School of Biological Sciences
Royal Holloway College
Egham Hill TW20 0EX, United Kingdom
Phone: 44 1784 443545 **Fax:** 46 1784 434326
Email: g.dickson@rhul.ac.uk

Fnded: 1992. **Desc:** Coordinates clinical and scientific on research gene therapy; acts as a scientific advisory board for the review of guidelines and clinical protocols.

★ 2909 ★ European Society of Gynaecological Oncology (ESGO)
Kenes International
17 rue du Cendrier
PO Box 1726
CH-1211 Geneva 1, Switzerland
Phone: 41 22 9080488 **Fax:** 41 22 7322850
Email: info@esgo.org

Fnded: 1983. **Mem:** 600. **Desc:** Promotes international communication in order to promote the improvement the standard of care in Gynecologic Oncology. Promotes clinical and basic research in Gynecologic Oncology. **Pub:** *International Journal of Gynaecological Cancer*, quarterly. Journal.

★ 2910 ★ European Society for Gynecological Endoscopy (ESGE)
Essenestraat 77
B-1740 Ternat, Belgium
Phone: 32 2 5820852 **Fax:** 32 2 5825515
Email: orgamed@pandora.be
Website: http://www.esge.org
Fnded: 1991. **Mem:** 600. **Desc:** Promotes study of gynecological surgical techniques using endoscopy; recommends standards of training in gynecological endoscopy.

★ 2911 ★ European Society of Gynecology (ESG)
c/o Dr. C. Pelissier
72, rue d'Auteuil
F-75016 Paris, France
Phone: 33 1 46511619 **Fax:** 33 1 47273261
Email: president@seg-weg.org
Website: http://www.seg-web.org
Desc: Fosters communication and exchange among gynecologists throughout Europe. Studies ethical and social issues in the field of gynecology.

★ 2912 ★ European Society for Haemapheresis and Haemotherapy (ESFH)
Abteilung fur Transfusionsmedizin der Universitat Marburg
D-35041 Marburg, Germany
Phone: 49 6421 2866283 **Fax:** 49 6421 2865655
Email: kretschv@post.med.uni-marburg.de
Website: http://www.esfh.de
Fnded: 1992. **Desc:** Promotes the field of medicine that uses extracorporeal blood circuitry for separation of blood components.

★ 2913 ★ European Society of Handwriting Psychology (ESHP) (Europaische Gesellschaft fur Schriftpsychologie und Schriftexpertise — EGS)
Klebestrasse 6
Postfach 2077
CH-8041 Zurich, Switzerland
Phone: 41 1 4816218 **Fax:** 41 1 4816288
Email: egs_sekretariat@web.de
Fnded: 1972. **Mem:** 468. **Nat'l Groups:** 10. **Lang(s):** English, French, German. **Desc:** Psychologists, psychiatrists, physicians, personnel consultants, criminal investigators, and university professors. **Pub:** *EGS-ESHP Bulletin*, annual. Newsletter.

★ 2914 ★ European Society of Head and Neck Radiology (ESHNR)
Hopital de Hautepierre
F-67098 Strasbourg, France
Fnded: 1987. **Desc:** Promotes knowledge in the field of head and neck diagnostic radiology, interventional radiology and diagnostic imaging; fosters research in head and neck radiology; improves methods of teaching radiologic diagnosis of diseases of the head and neck area.

★ 2915 ★ European Society of Human Reproduction and Embryology (ESHRE)
ESHRE Central Office
Van Akenstraat 41
B-1850 Grimbergen, Belgium
Phone: 32 2 2690969 **Fax:** 32 2 2695600
Email: herman.merckx@eshre.com
Website: http://www.eshre.com
Fnded: 1985. **Mem:** 3,839. **Desc:** Facilitates the study and discussion of all aspects of reproduction and embryology from before conception until the birth.

★ 2916 ★ European Society for Hyperthermic Oncology (ESHO)
Erasmus MC - Daniel den Hold Cancer Center
Groene Hilledijk 301
NL-3075 EA Rotterdam, Netherlands
Phone: 31 10 4391806 **Fax:** 31 10 4391022
Email: rhoon@hyph.azr.nl
Website: http://www.esho.info/
Fnded: 1987. **Mem:** 150. **Lang(s):** English. **Desc:** Oncologists and medical researchers with an interest in hyperthermic oncology. Promotes advancement in the techniques and technology of hyperthermic oncology. Facilitates "integration and exchange of information between different disciplines in the study of the biological effects of heat in the treatment of cancer." **Pub:** Newsletter, periodic.

★ 2917 ★ European Society for Immune Deficiencies (ESID)
Huddinge Hospital
S-14186 Huddinge, Sweden
Fax: 46 8 7745538
Email: edvard.smith@cbt.ki.se
Fnded: 1994. **Desc:** Facilitates exchange of ideas and information among physicians and other investigators concerned with immunodeficiency diseases.

★ 2918 ★ European Society for Immunodeficiencies (ESID)
c/o Dr. Bert Gerritsen
Medical Center Rynmond-S
Olympiaweg 350
NL-3078 HT Rotterdam, Netherlands
Phone: 31 10 2911911 **Fax:** 31 10 2911026
Email: gerritsene@mcrz.nl
Fnded: 1983. **Mem:** 200. **Desc:** Facilitates the exchange of immunological information among doctors, nurses, biomedical investigators, patients, and other individuals interested in immunodeficiency diseases. Fosters excellence in research and medical practice.

★ 2919 ★ European Society of Intensive Care Medicine (ESICM)
40 Ave. Joseph Wybran
B-1070 Brussels, Belgium
Phone: 32 2 5590350 **Fax:** 32 2 5270062
Email: public@esicm.org
Website: http://www.esicm.org
Fnded: 1982. **Mem:** 2,753. **Lang(s):** English, French. **Desc:** Physicians, nurses, physiotherapists, and students with an interest in intensive care medicine. Seeks to advance study, teaching, research, and practice in the field. Facilitates exchange of information among members; serves as a clearinghouse on intensive care medicine; conducts continuing professional development and other educational programs for members. Sponsors intensive care medical research; conducts examinations. **Pub:** *Intensive Care Medicine*, monthly. Journal. Includes original articles, pediatrics, experimental reports, and current topics.

★ 2920 ★ European Society of Intravenous Anaesthesia (EuroSIVA)
Forschstr 340
CH-8008 Zurich, Switzerland
Phone: 41 1 3863070 **Fax:** 41 1 3861609
Website: http://www.eurosiva.org

★ 2921 ★ European Society of Knee Surgery Sports Traumatology and Arthroscopy
7 Av. Krieg
case postale 139
CH-1211 Geneva 17, Switzerland
Phone: 41 22 7034808 **Fax:** 41 22 3474769
Email: esska200@gve.ch
Desc: Surgeons involved in sports traumatology, knee surgery, and arthroscopy. Fosters communication and exchange among members.

★ 2922 ★ European Society for Laboratory Animal Veterinarians (ESLAV)
BP 159
F-37401 Amboise, France
Email: pnowlan@tcd.ie
Fnded: 1996. **Desc:** Disseminates expert veterinary knowledge in the field of laboratory animal science.

★ 2923 ★ European Society for Laser Aesthetic Surgery (ESLAS)
23 Banbury Rd.
Oxford OX2 6NX, United Kingdom
Phone: 44 1865 244421 **Fax:** 44 1865 244421
Email: secretary@eslas.com
Website: http://www.eslas.com/
Desc: Promotes instruction, research and exchange of information related to the use of light and lasers for application in plastic and aesthetic surgery.

★ 2924 ★ European Society for Magnetic Resonance in Medicine and Biology (ESMRMB)
Neutorgasse 9/2A
A-1010 Vienna, Austria
Phone: 43 1 5351306 **Fax:** 43 1 5357041
Email: office@esmrmb.org
Website: http://www.esmrmb.org
Fnded: 1985. **Mem:** 500. **Lang(s):** English, German. **Desc:** Physicians, engineers, and scientists with an interest in the medical applications of magnetic resonance (MR) technologies. Promotes advancement of MR technologies and seeks to increase and improve their use by the medical profession. Conducts educational and training programs for physicians wishing to make use of MR; sponsors MR research and development programs; serves as a clearinghouse on MR technologies and their medical applications. **Pub:** *MAGMA*, bimonthly. Journal.

★ 2925 ★ European Society for Male Genital Surgery (ESMGS)
Via S Vittore, 12
I-20123 Milan, Italy
Phone: 39 0285994896 **Fax:** 39 0285994551
Email: ceresoli.md@homegate.it

★ 2926 ★ European Society of Mastology (EUSOMA)
Corso Italia, 16
I-20122 Milan, Italy
Phone: 39 02 89096008 **Fax:** 39 02 8909804
Email: secretariat@cusoma.org
Website: http://www.eusoma.org
Fnded: 1986. **Mem:** 450. **Lang(s):** English, Italian. **Desc:** Devoted to unifying and publicizing the results of scientific research in cancer and other diseases of the breast. **Pub:** *Journal of Cancer*, 18/year. Journal.

★ 2927 ★ European Society of Medical Hypnosis (ESMH)
D-200730 Munich, Germany
Phone: 49 89 555984 **Fax:** 49 89 555984

★ 2928 ★ European Society for Medical Oncology (ESMO)
Via la Santa 7
CH-6962 Viganello-Lugano Cedex, Switzerland
Phone: 41 91 9731900 **Fax:** 41 91 9731902
Email: andrea@esmo.org
Website: http://www.esmo.org/
Fnded: 1975. **Mem:** 520. **Lang(s):** English. **Desc:** Medical oncologists; associate members are biologists, surgeons, radiotherapists, and other specialists. Sponsors and contributes to education in oncology. **Pub:** *Proceedings of Meeting*, annual. Journal.

★ 2929 ★ European Society for Microcirculation (ESM)
Department of Physiology
Freie Universitat Berlin
Arnimallee 22
D-14195 Berlin, Germany
Phone: 49 30 84 451632 **Fax:** 49 30 84451634
Email: esmmail@zedat.fu-berlin.de
Website: http://www.medizin.fu-berlin.de/esm

Fnded: 1960. **Mem:** 386. **Lang(s):** English. **Desc:** Individuals from 27 countries involved in education, clinical medicine, and the pharmaceutical industry interested in the study of microcirculation. (Microcirculation is the flow of blood and other tissue fluids into small vessels.) Coordinates research among participating laboratories in areas directly affecting the development, application, and promotion of microcirculation methods that will benefit health care. **Pub:** *European Society for Microcirculation*, periodic. Directory. • *Journal of Vascular Research*, bimonthly. Journal. • *Newsletter*, periodic. Newsletter.

★ 2930 ★ European Society for Movement Analysis in Adults and Children (ESMAC)
Nuffield Orthopaedic Centre
Windmill Rd.
Headington OX3 7LD, United Kingdom
Phone: 44 1865 227609 **Fax:** 44 1865 227943
Email: tim.theologis@noc.anglox.nhs.uk
Website: http://www.esmac.org

Fnded: 1992. **Mem:** 97. **Lang(s):** English. **Desc:** Orthopedists and other health care professionals, researchers, and scientists with an interest in human gait and posture and their impact on overall health. Works to advance scientific knowledge in the field of movement analysis; promotes continuing professional development of members. Facilitates communication and cooperation among members; conducts educational programs and courses.

★ 2931 ★ European Society of Musculoskeletal Radiology (ESSR)
Department of Radiology, University Hospital
S-221 85 Lund, Sweden
Phone: 46 46 173000 **Fax:** 46 46 2116956

Fnded: 1993. **Desc:** Promotes musculoskeletal radiology in Europe with emphasis on education and research.

★ 2932 ★ European Society for Neurochemistry (ESN)
c/o Prof. Vera Adam-Vizi, Sec.
Department of Medical Biochemistry
Semmelweis University
Puskin St. 9
PO Box 262
H-1444 Budapest, Hungary
Phone: 36 1 2662773 **Fax:** 36 1 2670031
Email: av@puskin.sote.hu
Website: http://www.biokemia.sote.hu/ESN/esn.html

Fnded: 1976. **Mem:** 685. **Lang(s):** English. **Desc:** Researchers in 33 countries working in neurochemistry, neurology, molecular neurobiology, molecular neuropharmacology, and psychiatry. Works toward a greater understanding of the biochemical foundations of nervous activity and insight into neural and mental diseases. Conducts seminars and workshops. **Pub:** *ESN Directory*, periodic. Directory. • *Newsletter*, periodic. Newsletter. • *Proceedings of Biennial General Meetings*.

★ 2933 ★ European Society of Neurogastroenterology and Gastrointestinal Motility
Herestr 49
3000 Leuven, Belgium
Fax: 32 1 6345757
Email: theo.peeters@med.kuleuven.ac.be
Website: http://www.neurogastro.org/

Fnded: 1981. **Mem:** 250. **Nat'l Groups:** 10. **Desc:** Promotes research in the field of gastrointestinal motility; forum for presentation or discussion. **Pub:** *Neurogastroenterology & Motility*. Journal.

★ 2934 ★ European Society of Neuroradiology (ESNR)
c/o Prof. M. Leonardi
Servizio di Neuroradiologia
Ospedale Bellaria
Via Altura 3
I-40139 Bologna, Italy
Phone: 39 02 6225520 **Fax:** 39 02 6225785
Email: marco.leonardi@centauro.it
Website: http://www.esnr.org

Fnded: 1969. **Mem:** 650. **Lang(s):** English. **Desc:** Mission is accomplish the following: to promote neuroradiology in all its fields; to coordinate work and documents in neuroradiology and to ensure the circulation throughout Europe; to coordinate relations with general radiology and the clinical specialties concerning the nervous system; to contribute to the development of unified methods of teaching neuroradiology and unified standards for training and certification in neuroradiology; to promote and coordinate relations among the existing European national neuroradiological societies or national sections of the ESNR in countries where there are no existing societies; to form European research teams to deal with specific neuroradiological issues. **Pub:** *Neuroradiology*, monthly. Journal. • Directory, periodic.

★ 2935 ★ European Society of Neurosonology and Cerebral Hemodynamics
Mohlstr 28
D-81675 Munich, Germany
Phone: 49 89 41404668 **Fax:** 49 89 41404666

Desc: Promotes research and serves an advisory body for health policy and teaching standards.

★ 2936 ★ European Society for Noninvasive Cardiology
c/o Cardiology Department
UZ Gasthuisberg O/N
Herestraat 49
B-3000 Leuven, Belgium
Phone: 32 16 345840 **Fax:** 32 16 345846
Email: andre.aubert@med.kuleuven.ac.be

Fnded: 1979. **Mem:** 250. **Reg. Groups:** 3. **Desc:** Promotes noninvasive cardiology.

★ 2937 ★ European Society for Noninvasive Cardiovascular Dynamics (ESNICVD)
Institute of Physiology
Faculty of Medicine
Zaloska 4
SLO-1100 Ljubljana, Slovenia
Phone: 386 1 5437500 **Fax:** 386 1 5437501
Email: esnicvd@mf.uni-lj.si
Website: http://www2.mf.uni-lj.si/~esnicvd

Fnded: 1960. **Mem:** 86. **Lang(s):** English. **Desc:** Scientists and professionals in 17 countries active in fields such as biology, cardiology, physiology, sports science, hydraulics, and physics who seek better knowledge of the cardiovascular system. Promotes the exchange of ideas in noninvasive cardiovascular research. Fosters the study of cardiovascular function from a mechanical point of reference to gain knowledge applicable to medical practice and technical disciplines. Works to standardize methods used to study the mechanical activity of the cardiovascular system. **Pub:** *Bibliotheca Cardiologica*, periodic. • *Cardiovascular*, annual. Newsletter. Includes information on conferences, working groups, and ESNICVD. • *Proceedings of Congress*, biennial. **Frmly:** (1970) European Society for Ballistocardiographic Research; (1978) European Society for Ballistocardiography and Cardiovascular Dynamics.

★ 2938 ★ European Society of Ophthalmic Plastic and Reconstructive Surgery (ESOPRS)
c/o Prof. Rolph Guthoff
Univ. Rostock
Augenklinik
Postfach 10088
D-18055 Rostock, Germany
Phone: 49 381 4948501 **Fax:** 49 381 4948502
Email: rudolf.guthoff@med.uni-rostock.de

Fnded: 1981. **Mem:** 225. **Nat'l Groups:** 15. **Lang(s):** English. **Desc:** Coordinates activities in the field of plastic and reconstructive surgery of the eye. Disseminates information on the latest scientific advancements. **Pub:** *Orbit*, monthly. Journal.

★ 2939 ★ European Society of Paediatric Allergy and Clinical Immunology
University Children's Hospital
Augustenburger Platz 1
D-13353 Berlin, Germany
Phone: 49 30 45066643 **Fax:** 49 30 45066931
Email: brigitte.michel@charite.de

Fnded: 1988. **Desc:** Aims to promote the development of pediatric allergy and immunology by several means.

★ 2940 ★ European Society for Paediatric Endocrinology (ESPE)
St. Bartholomew's Hospital
London EC1A 7BE, United Kingdom
Phone: 44 20 76018468 **Fax:** 44 20 77262743
Email: research@eurospe.org
Website: http://www.eurospe.org

Fnded: 1962. **Desc:** Promotes research on paediatric endocrinology including metabolism, haematology, immunology, molecular biology, growth and development, nephrology, electrolytes and water metabolism.

★ 2941 ★ European Society of Paediatric Gastroenterology, Hepatology and Nutrition (ESPGHAN)
c/o Prof. Dr. M.J. Lentze
Children's Hospital Medical Center of the University of Bonn
Bonn, Germany
Phone: 49 228 2873213 **Fax:** 49 228 2873314
Email: lentze@mailer.meb.uni-bonn.de

Fnded: 1968. **Mem:** 300. **Desc:** Works to establish uniform nutrition standards for children in Europe. Fosters the improved treatment of gastrointestinal diseases of children. Promotes scientific exchange among research groups in Europe. Offers training programs and workshops for physicians.

★ 2942 ★ European Society for Paediatric Infectious Diseases (ESPID)
c/o Caroline Solway
Institute of Child Health
Education Centre
Royal Hospital for Children
Upper Maudlin St.
Bristol BS2 8BJ, United Kingdom
Email: espid-email@bristol.ac.uk
Website: http://www.e-luminaries.co.uk/espid/

Desc: Promotes the exchange of information among individuals with special experience in the field of paediatric infectious diseases, as well as research and training in PID. **Pub:** Proceedings.

★ 2943 ★ European Society for Paediatric Neurosurgery (ESPN)
Largo Gemelli, 8
I-00168 Rome, Italy

Fnded: 1967. **Desc:** Promotes pediatric neurosurgery and carries out research in the field.

★ 2944 ★ European Society of Paediatric Otorhinolaryngology
2 Via Belpoggio
I-34123 Trieste, Italy
Phone: 39 040 304798
Email: fiorfior@tin.it

Fnded: 1997. **Mem:** 250. **Lang(s):** English, French, German, Italian. **Desc:** Pediatric otorhinolaryngologists. Promotes the advancement of pediatric otorhinolaryngology (ORL), the prevention and control of disorders of the ear, nose, and throat. Conducts research and disseminates information. **Pub:** Newsletter, semiannual.

★ 2945 ★ European Society of Paediatric Radiology (ESPR)
c/o Freddy Avni, Gen.Sec.
Radiologie Pediatrique
Hospital Universitaire des Enfants Reine Fabiola
Ave. JJ Crocq, 15
B-1020 Brussels, Belgium
Phone: 32 2 5554273 **Fax:** 32 2 5554545
Email: favni@ulb.ac.be
Website: http://www.espr.org

Fnded: 1963. **Mem:** 471. **Lang(s):** English. **Desc:** Radiologists involved or interested in pediatric radiology. Seeks to contribute to the advancement of the clinical and scientific aspects of pediatric radiology in European countries through educational activities. Conducts Annual postgraduate courses; sponsors research programs. **Pub:** *Paediatric Radiology*, annual. • *Pediakic Radiology*, annual. Includes proceedings. • Bulletin, semiannual.

★ 2946 ★ European Society for Paediatric Research (ESPR)
Department of Pediatrics, Div. of Neonatology
Ulleval University Hospital
N-0514 Oslo, Norway
Phone: 47 23015537 **Fax:** 47 23015720
Email: t.a.stiris@ioks.ui.no
Website: http://www.espr.dk/

Fnded: 1968. **Desc:** Promotes pediatric research in Europe; fosters interchange of ideas among investigators in relevant subjects.

★ 2947 ★ European Society for Paediatric Urology (ESPU)
V Le Borri, 57
I-21100 Varese, Italy
Phone: 39 0332278207 **Fax:** 39 0332260520
Email: secretary@espu.org
Website: http://www.espu.org/

Fnded: 1989. **Desc:** Promotes paediatric urology in Europe as an independent and autonomous specialty.

★ 2948 ★ European Society of Parenteral and Enteral Nutrition (ESPEN)
Ospedale di Cattinara
I-34149 Trieste, Italy
Phone: 39 040910985 **Fax:** 39 0403994593
Email: gianfrang@clmed.univ.trieste.it

Fnded: 1980. **Desc:** Advances knowledge and its application in the field of parenteral and enteral nutrition, and related such as clinical nutrition and metabolism; fosters experimental and clinical research.

★ 2949 ★ European Society of Pathology (ESP)
c/o Prof. John M. Nesland
The Norwegian Radium Hospital-University Clinic
Department of Pathology
Montebello
N-0310 Oslo, Norway
Phone: 47 22 935620 **Fax:** 47 22 730164
Email: j.m.nesland@labmed.uio.no
Website: http://129.240.38.9/esp/

Fnded: 1964. **Mem:** 1,352. **Lang(s):** English, French, German, Italian, Russian, Spanish. **Desc:** Pathologists and other medical doctors in 49 countries with an interest in pathology. Fosters communication among pathologists; promotes publication of works on pathology and the development of a European school of pathology. **Pub:** *European Pathology Newsletter*, periodic. • *Virchows Archiv.*

★ 2950 ★ European Society of Pediatric and Neonatal Intensive Care (ESPNIC)
78, rue de General Leclerc
F-94275 Bicetre, France
Phone: 33 1 45213205 **Fax:** 33 1 45212255
Email: d.devictor@bct.ap-hop-paris.fr

Fnded: 1986. **Desc:** Stimulates pediatric and neonatal intensive care through promotion of activities, fostering research and education.

★ 2951 ★ European Society for Pediatric Nephrology (ESPN)
c/o Prof. Jochen Ehrich
Children's Hospital
Hanover Medical School
Carl Neuberg Str. 1
D-30625 Hannover, Germany
Phone: 49 5115323212 **Fax:** 49 5115323911
Email: ehrich.jochen@mh-hannover.de
Website: http://espn.uwcm.ac.uk

Fnded: 1967. **Mem:** 320. **Lang(s):** English. **Desc:** Pediatricians and medical scientists in 26 countries involved in pediatric nephrology. Promotes knowledge of and research on childhood renal disease. Coordinates international studies and disseminates information on pediatric nephrology. **Pub:** *Abstract of Communications*, annual. • *News Letter*, semiannual. • *Pediatric Nephrology.* Journal.

★ 2952 ★ European Society for Phenylketonuria and Allied Disorders (ESPKU)
Woestijne 16
9880 Aalter, Belgium
Phone: 32 5 3630657 **Fax:** 32 5 3622708

Desc: Promotes medical and scientific research in phenylketonuria; obliges the postnatal screening to detect the illness.

★ 2953 ★ European Society for Philosophy and Psychology (ESPP)
c/o Heather Jones
Department of Philosophy
Coventry CV4 7AL, United Kingdom
Email: h.a.jones@warwick.ac.uk
Website: http://www.eurospp.org/

Fnded: 1992.

★ 2954 ★ European Society for Pigment Cell Research (ESPCR)
St. George's Hospital Medical School
Cranmer Terrace SW17 OR5, United Kingdom
Phone: 44 20 87255202 **Fax:** 44 20 87253326
Email: dbennett@sghms.ac.uk
Website: http://www.ulb.ac.be/medecine/loce/espcr.htm

Fnded: 1985. **Desc:** Promotes interdisciplinary research on the pigmentary system, including normal and pathological conditions.

★ 2955 ★ European Society for Primary Care Gastroenterology
c/o Diana Balk
Department of General Practice
PO Box 85060
NL-3508 AB Utrecht, Netherlands
Phone: 31 30 2538188 **Fax:** 31 30 2539028
Email: secretariat@espcg.org
Website: http://www.espcg.org

Desc: Promotes high standards in the management of gastrointestinal problems in primary care throughout Europe.

★ 2956 ★ European Society for Psychosocial Oncology (ESPO)
Stanley House, Wilmslow Rd.
Withington M20 4BX, United Kingdom
Phone: 44 161 4463679 **Fax:** 44 161 4481655

★ 2957 ★ European Society of Public Health Ophthalmology (ESPHO)
Ecole de sante publique
United des deficiencies sensorielles
ULB, route de Lennik 808
B-1070 Brussels, Belgium
Phone: 32 2 5554070 **Fax:** 32 2 5554049

Fnded: 1996. **Mem:** 49. **Desc:** Aims to promote, in cooperation with affiliated members or institutions, studies on eye and vision related topics.

★ 2958 ★ European Society for Quality in Health Care
c/o Mary Halpin
Mid-Western Health Board
31-33 Catherine St.
Limerick, Ireland
Phone: 353 61 483389 **Fax:** 353 61 483211

Desc: Support quality improvement in European healthcare by creating a formal European Network of National Societies. Provides a forum for addressing issues of importance to quality health care.

★ 2959 ★ European Society of Regional Anaesthesia (ESRA) (Societe Europeenne d'Anesthesie Loco-Regionale)
Kempenlaan 12
B-2300 Turnhout, Belgium
Phone: 32 14 422773 **Fax:** 32 14 439284
Email: dionne@esraeurope.org
Website: http://www.esraeurope.org

Fnded: 1980. **Mem:** 2,200. **Reg. Groups:** 7. **Lang(s):** English, French. **Desc:** Doctors of medicine specializing in anesthesiology in 30 countries. Seeks to reduce the risks and heighten the effectiveness of anesthesia by improving techniques of anesthesiology. Provides professional training; conducts workshops and seminars. **Pub:** *International Monitor on Regional Anesthesia*, quarterly. • *Newsletter*, annual. Newsletter. • *Yearbook.*

★ 2960 ★ European Society of Reproductive and Development Immunology (ESRADI)
c/o Dr. M. Kurpisz
General Institute of Human Genetics
Polish Academy of Sciences
Strzeszynska 32
PL-60-479 Poznan, Poland
Fax: 48 61 8233235

Desc: Promotes fundamental and applied research concerning immunological processes in reproductive and developmental physiology and morphology, pathology and therapeutics. Fosters cooperation between laboratories involved in experimental and clinical research. Facilitates the exchange of research workers and training of students.

★ 2961 ★ European Society of Rheology (ESR)
c/o Prof. M.H. Wagner
Fasanenstr 90
D-10623 Berlin, Germany
Phone: 49 30 31424125 **Fax:** 49 30 31421108
Email: manfred.wagner@tu-berlin.de
Website: http://www.rheology-esr.com

Fnded: 1996. **Nat'l Groups:** 18. **Desc:** Encourages cooperation in all aspects of rheology.

★ 2962 ★ European Society for Sexual and Impotence Research (ESIR)
Reichskanzler Str. 8
D-22609 Hamburg, Germany
Phone: 49 40 35015916 **Fax:** 49 40 35015917
Email: essir@wtnet.de
Website: http://www.essir.org

★ 2963 ★ European Society for Stereotactic and Functional Neurosurgery (ESSFN)
Department of Neurosurgery
CHU Ranfueil
F-31054 Toulouse Cedex, France
Phone: 33 56 1322941 **Fax:** 33 56 1528350
Website: http://www.essfn.org
Fnded: 1970. **Desc:** Supports research and regulation of practice of stereotactic and functional neurosurgery.

★ 2964 ★ European Society for the Study and Prevention of Infant Death (ESPID)
Martinistr 52
D-20251 Hamburg, Germany
Phone: 49 40 47172900 **Fax:** 49 40 47175435
Fnded: 1991. **Desc:** Promotes research on all aspects of the prevention of infant death; provides a platform for exchange of information relating to research on infant deaths.

★ 2965 ★ European Society of Surgery
Nordre Ringgade 1
DK-8000 Arhus, Denmark

★ 2966 ★ European Society for Surgery of Shoulder and Elbow (ESSE)
50-52, av Chanoine Cartellier
F-69230 Saint-Genis-Laval, France
Fnded: 1987.

★ 2967 ★ European Society of Surgical Geriatrics
25, av Charles de Gaulle
F-91150 Etampes, France

★ 2968 ★ European Society of Surgical Oncology (ESSO)
Ave. E Mounier, 83
B-1200 Brussels, Belgium
Phone: 32 2 5373106 **Fax:** 32 2 5390374
Email: esso@esso-surgeonline.be
Website: http://www.esso-surgeonline.be
Fnded: 1981. **Mem:** 1,020. **Desc:** Surgical oncologists. Sponsors educational programs. Fosters multidisclipinary collaboration in the clinical management of cancer patients. **Pub:** *European Journal of Surgical Oncology*, monthly. Journal.

★ 2969 ★ European Society for Surgical Research (ESSR)
c/o Dr. Michael Menger, Pres.
Institute for Clinical and Experimental Surgery
University of Saarland
D-66421 Hamburg, Germany
Phone: 49 6841 1626550 **Fax:** 49 6841 1626553
Email: exmdme@med-rz.uni-saarland.de
Website: http://www.essr.info/
Fnded: 1966. **Desc:** Encourages scientific meetings and contacts between scientists on experimental surgery in Europe.

★ 2970 ★ European Society for Therapeutic Radiology and Oncology (ESTRO)
Av. E Mounier 83
B-1200 Brussels, Belgium
Phone: 32 2 7759340 **Fax:** 32 2 7795494
Email: info@estro.be
Website: http://www.estro.be
Fnded: 1980. **Mem:** 5,000. **Lang(s):** English. **Desc:** Individuals from 84 countries involved in the fields of radiotherapy and oncology. Works to improve standards of cancer treatment by fostering the exchange with other specialties involved in the treatment of cancer. Develops educational and training guidelines; makes available basic and continuing medical education courses. **Pub:** *ESTRO Newsletter*, periodic. Newsletter. Society's life. • *Journal of Radiotherapy and Oncology*, monthly. Journal.

★ 2971 ★ European Society of Thoracic Imaging (ESTI)
Herestr 49
3000 Leuven, Belgium
Phone: 32 1 6343782 **Fax:** 32 1 6343769
Email: johny.verschakelen@uz.kuleuven.ac.be
Website: http://www.esti-Society.org/
Fnded: 1993. **Desc:** Stimulates training and research in this radiology sub-specialty.

★ 2972 ★ European Society of Thoracic Surgeons (ESTS)
c/o ESTS Secretariat
PO Box 159
Stuttgart
Exeter EX2 5SH, United Kingdom
Phone: 44 1392 662727 **Fax:** 44 1392 662900
Email: sue@ests.org.uk
Desc: Thoracic surgeons in Europe. Seeks to improve the study and practice of thoracic surgery.

★ 2973 ★ European Society for Toxicology In Vitro (ESTIV)
Univ. of Surrey
Guildford GU2 5XH, United Kingdom
Phone: 44 1483 259204 **Fax:** 44 1483 300374
Email: d.benford@surrey.ac.uk
Desc: Promotes in vitro toxicology, scientifically and educationally.

★ 2974 ★ European Society of Urogenital Radiology (ESUR)
c/o Sameh K. Morcos, MD, Sec.-Treas.
Department of Diagnostic Radiology
Northern General Hospital
Herries Rd.
Sheffield S5 7AU, United Kingdom
Phone: 44 114 2434343 **Fax:** 44 114 2560472
Email: sameh.morcos@northngh-tr.trent.nhs.uk
Website: http://www.esur.org/
Desc: Promotes advancement of uro-genital imaging and intervention; stimulates the study of normal and abnormal kidney, urinary tract and genital organs with emphasis on integration of roentgenology, ultrasonography, computed tomography, magnetic resonance, nuclear medicine, and new imaging techniques as well as research on contrast media.

★ 2975 ★ European Society of Urological Oncology (ESUOE)
Hufelandstr 55
D-45122 Essen, Germany

★ 2976 ★ European Society for Vascular Surgery (ESVS)
University of Bath, Rm. L2.27
Clavertown Down
Bath BA2 7AY, United Kingdom
Phone: 44 1225 323770 **Fax:** 44 1225 323669
Email: s.needham@bath.ac.uk
Website: http://www.esvs.org
Fnded: 1987. **Lang(s):** English. **Desc:** Vascular surgeons and national vascular societies. Seeks to advance vascular surgical techniques; promotes continuing professional development among vascular surgeons. Serves as a clearinghouse on vascular surgery; facilitates exchange of information among members; sponsors research and educational programs. **Pub:** *European Journal of Vascular and Endovascular Surgery*, monthly.

★ 2977 ★ European Society of Veterinary Cardiology (ESVC)
Via Conte Rosso, 3
I-10121 Turin, Italy
Phone: 39 011 6709082 **Fax:** 39 011 6709083
Email: mboresvc@tin.it
Fnded: 1981. **Mem:** 120. **Desc:** Promotes the knowledge of veterinary cardiology. **Pub:** *Journal of Veterinary Cardiology*, semiannual. Journal.

★ 2978 ★ European Society of Veterinary Clinical Ethology (ESVCE)
11 Cotebrook Dr.
Upton CH2 1RA, United Kingdom
Phone: 44 1244 377365 **Fax:** 44 1244 399228
Email: heath@vetethol.demon.co.uk
Website: http://www.esvce.org/
Fnded: 1994. **Desc:** Promotes scientific progress in veterinary and comparative clinical ethology; furthers education in veterinary clinical ethology and behavior medicine, facilitates exchange of information.

★ 2979 ★ European Society of Veterinary and Comparative Nutrition (ESVCN)
Veterinarstr 13
D-80539 Munich, Germany
Phone: 49 89 21803549 **Fax:** 49 89 21803208
Fnded: 1991. **Desc:** Supports interaction of European veterinary nutritionists; advances applied and scientific veterinary nutrition.

★ 2980 ★ European Society of Veterinary Dermatology (ESVD)
43, av Aristide-Briand
F-94110 Arcueil, France
Fax: 33 1 49858301
Email: secretary@www.esvd.org
Website: http://www.esvd.org
Fnded: 1984. **Mem:** 550. **Desc:** Fosters exchange of information with veterinary dermatologists; promotes veterinary dermatology in Europe. **Pub:** Journal, bimonthly.

★ 2981 ★ European Society of Veterinary Nephrology and Urology (ESVNU)
Postboks 8146 DEP
N-0033 Oslo, Norway
Phone: 47 22964500 **Fax:** 47 22964962
Email: Lars.Moe@atsveths.no

★ 2982 ★ European Society of Veterinary Orthopaedics and Traumatology (ESVOT)
c/o Aldo Vezzoni, Sec.
Via Massarotti 24
I-26100 Cremona, Italy
Fax: 39 037220074
Email: avezzoni@scivac.it
Website: http://www.digicolor.net/esvot/

★ 2983 ★ European Society of Veterinary Orthopaedics and Traumatology (ESVOT)
c/o Dr. Herman A.W. Hazewinkel
Faculty of Veterinary Medicine
University of Utrecht
NL-3508 TD Utrecht, Netherlands
Desc: Disseminates basic principles of veterinary orthopedics and traumatology through continuing education programs.

★ 2984 ★ European Society of Veterinary Pathology (ESVP)
c/o Dr. Manfred Reinacher, Sec.
Institute for Veterinary Pathology
Der Justus-Liebeg University
Frankfurter Str. 96
D-35302 Giessen, Germany
Email: manfred.reinacher@vetmed.uni-giessen.de
Website: http://bris.ac.uk/pathandmicro/eurovet/eurovet.htm

Fnded: 1952. **Mem:** 500. **Lang(s):** English, French, German. **Desc:** Veterinary pathologists in 33 countries. Promotes the exchange of information and research findings. **Pub:** *European Journal of Veterinary Pathology*, 3/year. Journal.

★ 2985 ★ European Society of Veterinary Virology
c/o Moredun Research Institute
Pentlands Science Park, Bush Loan.
Edinburgh EH2 6OPZ, United Kingdom
Phone: 44 131 4455111 **Fax:** 44 131 4456111
Email: nettp@mri.sari.ac.uk
Website: http://www.ploufragan.afssa.fr/esvv/fee_member.html

Fnded: 1985. **Mem:** 250. **Desc:** Researchers and teachers in veterinary virology. Seeks to further progress in veterinary virology. Fosters communication and exchange between members. **Pub:** Newsletter, annual.

★ 2986 ★ European Strabismological Association (ESA) (Association strabismologique europeene)
c/o University Eye Clinic
Schleichstrasse 12
D-72078 Tubingen, Germany
Phone: 49 7071 2983738 **Fax:** 49 7071 293749

Fnded: 1960. **Mem:** 250. **Lang(s):** English, French, German. **Desc:** Physicians in 21 countries interested in strabismology and neuro-ophthalmology. (Strabismology is the study of the condition known as strabismus, in which an individual is unable to fix both eyes on a single point due to muscular imbalance. Neuro-ophthalmology refers to visual representation in the central nervous system.) **Pub:** *Proceedings*, annual.

★ 2987 ★ European Study Group on Lysosomal Diseases (ESGLD)
c/o Professor B. Winchester
Institute of Child Health, University of London
Biochemistry, Endocrinology and Metabolism Unit
30 Guilford St.
London WC1N 1EH, United Kingdom
Phone: 44 20 79052114 **Fax:** 44 20 74046191
Email: b.winchester@ich.ucl.ac.uk
Website: http://www.technothesp.co.uk/esgld

Fnded: 1978. **Mem:** 90. **Lang(s):** English. **Desc:** Laboratories in 22 countries conducting research on lysosomal storage diseases. (Lysosomal storage diseases are hereditary disorders, resulting from defects in lysosomal enzymes or membrane components, characterized by accumulation of partially digested metabolites in tissues and excretion in urine.) Promotes research; encourages exchange of ideas and personnel among member laboratories. **Pub:** *Register of Laboratories*, biennial.

★ 2988 ★ European Thrombosis Research Organization (ETRO)
Consorzio 'Mario Negri Sud'
I-66030 Santa Maria Imbaro, Italy
Phone: 39 08725701 **Fax:** 39 087257112
Email: degaetano@cmns.mnegri.it

Fnded: 1972. **Desc:** Promotes fundamental research in thrombosis and haemostasis; facilitates scientific exchange.

★ 2989 ★ European Thyroid Association (ETA) (Association Europeenne Thyroide — AET)
c/o Prof. J.J. Orgiazzi
Service de Endocrinologie Centre
Hospitalier Lyon Sud
Pierre Benite
F-69495 Lyon, France
Phone: 33 4 78509515 **Fax:** 33 4 78778612
Email: jacques.orgiazzi@chu-lyon.fr

Fnded: 1967. **Mem:** 365. **Lang(s):** English, French. **Desc:** Physicians and research scientists in 37 countries with an interest in the thyroid gland. Promotes research; works to improve knowledge of the thyroid gland and its diseases. **Pub:** *Abstracts From Annual Meeting.*

★ 2990 ★ European Transplant Coordinators Organization (ETCO)
Steenveldstraat 18
B-3210 Linden, Belgium
Phone: 32 16 622110 **Fax:** 32 16 622981
Email: etco.trekels@unicall.be
Website: http://www.etco.org

Fnded: 1983. **Mem:** 450. **Lang(s):** English. **Desc:** Professionals working in the field of tissue procurement and transplantation; other interested individuals. Seeks to increase the availability of human tissues and organs for transplantation; promotes professional advancement of members. Serves as a clearinghouse on tissue procurement and transplantation; facilitates communication and cooperation among members; sponsors educational programs; compiles statistics. **Pub:** Journal, periodic.

★ 2991 ★ European Underwater and BaroMedical Society (EUBS)
Benview
Prospect Terrace
Port Elphinstone
Inverurie AB51 3UN, United Kingdom
Phone: 44 1467 620408 **Fax:** 44 1467 620408
Email: secretary@eubs.org
Website: http://www.eubs.org

Mem: 390. **Lang(s):** English. **Desc:** Professionals and students interested in undersea medicine and related fields. Provides a forum for scientific communication among those interested in undersea medicine; encourages cooperation with related scientific disciplines. Strives to improve the safety of underwater activities by providing expert advice and educational programs; promotes undersea medicine. Holds workshops on topics concerning medical aspects of diving. **Pub:** *Long Term Neurological Consequences of Deep Diving.* • *Newsletter*, quarterly. Newsletter.

★ 2992 ★ European Union of Clinicians in Implant Dentistry (EUCID)
Rue Leon Mignon 21
4000 Liege, Belgium
Phone: 32 4 2210654 **Fax:** 32 4 2237556

Fnded: 1989. **Desc:** supports clinical and statistical studies and their application in the odonto-stomatological practice; provides information of patients and of the concerned bodies

★ 2993 ★ European Union of the Deaf (EUD)
Coupure Rechts 314
B-9000 Gent, Belgium
Phone: 32 9 2240817 **Fax:** 32 9 2240831
Email: info@eudnet.org
Website: http://www.eudnet.org

Fnded: 1985. **Desc:** Coordination of activities on a pan-European level, which includes dissemination of information, policy development, advice, lobbying and promoting use of the indigenous sign languages of Europe and recognition of the deaf culture.

★ 2994 ★ European Union of Dentists (Europaische Union der Zahnarzte)
62B Northgate
Regent's Park
London NW8 7EH, United Kingdom
Phone: 44 207 5864056 **Fax:** 44 207 5864096

Fnded: 1973. **Mem:** 1,000. **Desc:** Works to provide dental services to the socially and economically disadvantaged. Promotes solidarity and friendship among dentists of the EC.

★ 2995 ★ European Union of General Practitioners (Europaische Vereinigung der Allgemeinartze)
FNOMCEO
Piazza Cola di Rienzo 80/A
I-00192 Rome, Italy
Phone: 39 05 5284011 **Fax:** 39 05 5284038
Email: cricelli@dada.it
Website: http://www.uemo.org

Fnded: 1967. **Lang(s):** English, French, German, Italian, Spanish. **Desc:** National European medical organizations. Promotes the educational and professional interests of general practitioners and defends their professional independence. Fosters unity among general practitioners. Advocates high standards in medical training and patient care.

★ 2996 ★ European Union of Independent Hospitals (Union Europeenne de l'Hopitalisation Privee — UEHP)
5 Av. Alfred Solvay
B-1170 Watermael-Boitsfort, Belgium
Phone: 32 2 6603550 **Fax:** 32 2 6729062

Fnded: 1991. **Mem:** 12.

★ 2997 ★ European Union of Medical Specialists (UEMS)
20, ave. de la Couronne
B-1050 Brussels, Belgium
Phone: 32 2 6495164 **Fax:** 32 2 6403730
Email: uems@skynet.be
Website: http://www.uems.be

Fnded: 1958. **Nat'l Groups:** 25. **Lang(s):** English, French. **Desc:** Representative national associations of medical specialists in all European countries. Works to ensure high quality care for patients. Fosters communication among members; promotes members' interests.

★ 2998 ★ European Union of Medical Specialties
c/o Dr. C.C. Leibrandt
Ave. de la Couronne, 20
B-1050 Brussels, Belgium
Phone: 32 2 6495164 **Fax:** 32 2 6403730
Email: uems@skynet.be
Website: http://www.uems.be/eaccme.htm

Desc: Works to improve the quality of specialist medical care in Europe. Fosters continuing medical education.

★ 2999 ★ European Union of Paediatric Surgical Associations (EUPSA)
Division of Pediatric Surgery
Academic Hospital Free University de Brussels
B-1090 Brussels, Belgium
Phone: 32 2 4776061 **Fax:** 32 2 4776074
Email: hlkdbra@az.vub.ac.be

Fnded: 1972. **Mem:** 24. **Lang(s):** English. **Desc:** National associations of pediatric surgeons. Promotes high standards of practice. Works to: standardize educational requirements in pediatric surgery; define the scope of pediatric surgery. Participates in the exchange of trainees among member associations.

★ 3000 ★ European Union of Veterinary Practitioners
(Union europeenne des veterinaires praticiens — UEVP)
Dorpstraat 15
NL-3223 GZ Hellevoestsluis, Netherlands
Fnded: 1970. **Desc:** Coordinates the work of European veterinary practitioners, relations with farmers, consumers and the European courts.

★ 3001 ★ European Venous Forum (EVF)
c/o Beaumont Associates
PO Box 172
Greenford UB6 92D, United Kingdom
Phone: 44 20 85757044 **Fax:** 44 20 85757044
Email: evenousforum@aol.com
Website: http://www.europeanvenousforum.org
Fnded: 2000. **Mem:** 150. **Lang(s):** English. **Desc:** Developes scientific knowledge, research, clinical expertise, training and education and aims to establish standards in the fields of venous disease; promotes collaboration between phlebological and vascular societies, health agencies and authorities at national and European levels.

★ 3002 ★ European Veterinary Dental College
Fraz ternavasso
I-10046 Poirino, Italy
Phone: 39 0119453232 **Fax:** 39 0119453436
Email: deavet@tin.it

★ 3003 ★ European Veterinary Dental Society (EVDS)
309 The Ridge
Hastings TN34 2RA, United Kingdom
Phone: 44 1424 751595 **Fax:** 44 1424 756378
Email: pcooper@vetdent.softnet.co.uk
Website: http://www.vetdent.org
Fnded: 1985. **Desc:** Supports education in and promotion of clinical excellence in veterinary dentistry.

★ 3004 ★ European Veterinary Libraries Group (EVLG)
c/o Karen Beijer
ICP-NTI
PO Box 2313
NL-1100 DS Amsterdam, Netherlands
Phone: 31 20 5662095 **Fax:** 31 20 6963228
Email: eahil@amc.uva.nl
Fnded: 1994. **Desc:** Represents and promotes professionals in the field of animal health information. **Pub:** Newsletter.

★ 3005 ★ European Veterinary Society for Small Animal Reproduction (EVSSAR)
c/o Prof. John Verstegen
Bd Colonster 20, B44
University of Liege
B-4000 Liege, Belgium
Phone: 32 4 3664231 **Fax:** 32 4 3664236
Email: j.verstegen@ulg.ac.be
Website: http://www.ulg.ac.be/fmv/EVSSAR/
Desc: Promotes research of small animal reproduction.

★ 3006 ★ European Wound Management Association (EWMA)
PO Box 864
London SE1 8TT, United Kingdom
Phone: 44 207 8483496
Email: ewma@kcl.ac.uk
Website: http://www.ewma.org
Fnded: 1991. **Lang(s):** English. **Desc:** Health care professionals, scientists, and pharmaceutical manufacturers with an interest in wound healing. Seeks to "address clinical and scientific issues associated with wound healing," in areas including the native epidemiology, pathology, diagnosis, prevention, and management of wounds. Serves as a clearinghouse on wound healing; facilitates exchange of information among members; sponsors research and educational programs. **Pub:** *EWMA Journal*, quarterly. Journal.

★ 3007 ★ Eurotransplant International Foundation (EIF)
c/o Mrs. V. Diepeveen, Sec.
PO Box 2304
NL-2301 CH Leiden, Netherlands
Phone: 31 71 5795795 **Fax:** 31 71 5790057
Email: verena@eurotransplant.nl
Website: http://www.eurotransplant.nl
Fnded: 1967. **Lang(s):** English. **Desc:** International non-profit organ exchange organization. **Pub:** *Eurotransplant Newsletter*, monthly.

★ 3008 ★ Evans Syndrome Research and Support Group
c/o Lou Addington
PO Box 290203
Port Orange, FL 32119
Phone: (386)322-2656 **Fax:** (386)760-5583
Email: info@legalnurseassociates.com
Website: http://www.legalnurseassociates.com
Lou Addington, Pres.
Fnded: 1992. **Desc:** Provides mutual support and ongoing research for parents and concerned friends and caregivers of children with Evans Syndrome. (Evans Syndrome is a rare autoimmune disease.) Facilitates networking and exchange of information. Distributes literature. Developing a group of interested physicians in immunology, genetics, and hematology/oncology. Works to formulate questions for caregivers/patients to ask their doctors.

★ 3009 ★ Every Child By Two (ECBT)
c/o Amy Pisani
666 11th St., NW, Ste. 202
Washington, DC 20001-4542
Phone: (202)783-7034 **Fax:** (202)783-7042
Email: info@ecbt.org
Website: http://www.ecbt.org
Amy Pisani, Exec. Dir.
Fnded: 1981. **Desc:** Campaigns for early immunization. Visit health departments, hospitals, and schools nationwide to promote timely immunizations. Works to raise awareness and foster a systematic way to ensure the health of all America's children. Targets community leaders of service organizations for assistance. Compiles statistics. Sponsors educational programs and children's services. **Pub:** *Every Child By Two*, bimonthly. Newsletter.

★ 3010 ★ Exercise Safety Association (ESA)
PO Box 547916
Orlando, FL 32854-9716
Phone: (352)683-5246 **Fax:** (407)246-5090
Email: askesa@aol.com
Website: http://www.exercisesafety.com
Sharon Foy, Dir.
Fnded: 1978. **Mem:** 20,000. **Local Groups:** 150. **Desc:** Fitness instructors, personal trainers, health spas, YMCAs, community recreation departments, and hospital wellness programs. Purposes are: to improve the qualifications of exercise instructors; to train instructors to develop safe exercise programs that will help people avoid injury while exercising; to prepare instructors for national certification. Offers training in aerobics and exercise and on the physiological aspects of exercise. Conducts exercise safety and research programs. Sponsors charitable program; maintains speakers' bureau. Offers instructor placement services. **Pub:** *ESA Member Directory*, annual. Membership Directory. • *Exercise Safety Association Newsletter*, bimonthly. Newsletter. Provides exercise information based on current scientific research. Includes schedule of upcoming programs. *Price:* Included in membership dues. **Frmly:** Exer-Safety Association; (1985) International Exer-Safety Association.

★ 3011 ★ EXIT
17 Hart St.
Edinburgh EH1 3RN, United Kingdom
Phone: 44 131 5564404
Email: exit@euthanasia.org
Website: http://www.euthanasia.org
Fnded: 1980. **Desc:** Aims to make dying with dignity an option available to anyone, to protect patients and doctors alike in upholding the humanity of dying well, to seek legal reform, where necessary, and to introduce safeguards regarding voluntary euthanasia. **Frmly:** (2002) Voluntary Euthanasia Society of Scotland.

★ 3012 ★ Exodus Trust (ET)
1523 Franklin St.
San Francisco, CA 94109
Phone: (415)928-1133 **Fax:** (415)928-8061
Ted McIlvenna, Pres.
Fnded: 1968. **Desc:** Established to: educate and train professionals interested in sex counseling, therapy, education, or research; provide sex education, counseling, and therapy for adults; research human sexuality; produce films, slides, and literature for use in sex counseling, therapy, and education. Conducts continuing education programs for physicians and nurses, and workshops and counseling programs for professional and laypeople in San Francisco, CA and other cities. **Frmly:** (1989) National Sex Forum.

★ 3013 ★ Exotic Pathology Society (EPS)
(Societe de Pathologie Exotique)
Institut Pasteur
25, rue du Docteur-Roux
F-75724 Paris Cedex 15, France
Phone: 33 1 45668869 **Fax:** 33 1 45664485
Email: socpatex@pasteur.fr
Website: http://www.pasteur.fr/sante/socpatex/pages
Fnded: 1908. **Mem:** 550. **Lang(s):** French. **Desc:** Doctors, bacteriologists, biologists, entomologists, epidemiologists, parapsychologists, pharmacists, veterinarians, and virologists. Promotes the study of tropical diseases. Provides a forum for the presentation and discussion of research findings in the field. **Pub:** *Annuaire*, quadrennial. Yearbook. • *Bulletin de la Societe de Pathologie Exotique*, quarterly. Newsletter.

★ 3014 ★ Experimental Psychology Society (EPS)
Earley Gate, Whiteknights
Reading RG6 6AL, United Kingdom
Phone: 44 118 9875123 **Fax:** 44 118 9314404
Email: e.a.gaffan@reading.ac.uk
Website: http://www.eps.ac.uk
Fnded: 1946. **Desc:** Furthers scientific enquiry within the field of psychology and cognate subjects; disseminates information and educational material made available as a consequence of psychological research.

★ 3015 ★ Extensions for Independence (EI)
c/o The Mouthstick Connection
555 Saturn Blvd., No. B-368
San Diego, CA 92154
Phone: (619)423-7709 **Free:** (866)632-7149
Fax: (619)423-7709
Email: info@mouthstick.net
Website: http://www.mouthstick.net
Arthur Heyer, Contact
Fnded: 1976. **Desc:** Develops, manufactures, and markets vocational equipment for the physically handicapped. Promotes improvements in design, materials, production, and quality of products while maintaining affordable prices. Products include the Multi-Tip Telescoping H-A Modular Mouthstick which enables individuals to talk and swallow while drawing, turning pages, loading and unloading computer software, and performing other tasks.

★ 3016 ★ Eye Bank Association of America (EBAA)
1015 18th St., NW, Ste. 1010
Washington, DC 20036
Phone: (202)775-4999 **Fax:** (202)429-6036
Email: patricia@restoresight.org
Website: http://www.restoresight.org
Patricia Aiken-O'Neill, Pres.

Fnded: 1961. **Mem:** 109. **Desc:** Eye banks working to restore sight through the promotion and advancement of eye banking. Makes possible over 46,000 corneal transplants annually. Establishes standards for the procurement and distribution of eyes and corneal tissue. Offers training and certification programs for eye banking personnel. Compiles statistics; maintains speakers' bureau. Conducts research and educational programs. **Pub:** *Eye Bank Association of America–Eye Bank Statistics Report*, annual. Annual Report. Includes statistics on eye donations and corneal transplants. • *Eye Bank Association of America–Insight*, periodic. Newsletter. Contains association and industry news. • *Eye Bank Association of America–Membership Directory*, annual. Membership Directory. Lists member eye banks; listed geographically by state. • *Guidelines and Resources for Successful Public and Professional Relations and Development.*

★ 3017 ★ Eye-Bank for Sight Restoration (EBSR)
120 Wall St., 3rd Fl.
New York, NY 10005-3902
Phone: (212)742-9000 **Fax:** (212)269-3139
Email: info@ebsr.org
Website: http://www.eyedonation.org
Patricia Dahl, Exec. Dir. /CEO

Fnded: 1944. **Desc:** Collects and distributes healthy corneal tissue obtained from individuals who have arranged to donate their eyes, or whose relatives have authorized such donation, at the time of death. Provides speakers to explain the eye-bank program to hospital, professional, and civic groups. **Pub:** *Eye-Bank for Sight Restoration–Eye to Eye*, 3/year. Newsletter. Includes annual report. *Price:* Free.

★ 3018 ★ The Eyecare Trust
PO Box 131
Lincolnshire
Market Rasen LN8 5TS, United Kingdom
Phone: 44 1673 857847 **Fax:** 44 1673 857696
Email: eis@btinternet.com

Fnded: 1993. **Desc:** Individual optometrists and dispensing opticians, multiples, manufacturing and importing companies, who subscribe voluntarily to fund the EIS's public relations work. Concerned with the generic promotion of eyecare services and products available from professionally qualified, registered UK optical practitioners. **Frmly:** (2002) Eyecare Information Service.

★ 3019 ★ FACES: The National Craniofacial Association
PO Box 11082
Chattanooga, TN 37401
Phone: (423)266-1632 **Free:** 800-332-2373
Fax: (423)267-3124
Email: faces@faces-cranio.org
Website: http://www.faces-cranio.org
Lynne G. Mayfield, Pres.

Fnded: 1969. **Desc:** Provides financial assistance for travel expenses to individuals with severe facial deformities resulting from congenital defects or accidents. Provides a resource file of available treatment centers, support groups, and general information concerning severe facial deformities. Is currently involved in an extensive fundraising campaign in order to increase awareness of the organization and to broaden its base of support. **Pub:** *FACES*, quarterly. Newsletter. Provides information and support for craniofacially handicapped persons. Includes updates on clients and medical updates. *Price:* Free. • *FACES Brochure*. Brochure. Provides information on the organization. • *So Brightly Within*. Video. *Price:* $20 donation. **Frmly:** (1977) Debbie Fox Foundation for Treatment of Cranio-Facial Deformities; (1985) Debbie Fox Foundation; (1998) National Association for the Craniofacially Handicapped.

★ 3020 ★ Facioscapulohumeral (FSH) Society
3 Westwood Rd.
Lexington, MA 02420
Phone: (781)860-0501 **Fax:** (781)860-0599
Email: info@fshsociety.org
Website: http://www.fshsociety.org
Daniel Paul Perez, Pres.

Fnded: 1992. **Mem:** 1,000. **Reg. Groups:** 6. **Desc:** Individuals, families, and medical and business professionals interested in Facioscapulohumeral Muscular Dystrophy. (FSHD is an inheritable disease that causes a progressive loss of skeletal muscle with weakness of facial, scapular, and upper arm muscles.) Promotes research, solicits contributions and grants, and disperses information on FSHD. Offers support groups, acts as clearinghouse for researchers, clinicians and patients to facilitate participation in FSHD studies. Funds Research on FSHD. **Pub:** *FSH WATCH*, quarterly. Newsletter. Contains updates on FSHD Internationally and cites current research articles. • Also publishes a patient brochure in English and Spanish.

★ 3021 ★ Faculty of Dental Surgery (FDS)
c/o The Royal College of Surgeons of England
35-43 Lincoln's Inn Fields
London WC2A 3PE, United Kingdom
Phone: 44 20 78696810 **Fax:** 44 20 78696816
Email: fds@rcseng.ac.uk
Website: http://www.rcseng.ac.uk/dental/fds

Fnded: 1947. **Mem:** 2,500.

★ 3022 ★ Faculty of Homeopathy
c/o British Homeopathic Association
15 Clerkenwell Close
London EC1R 0AA, United Kingdom
Phone: 44 20 75667800 **Fax:** 44 20 75667815
Email: info@trusthomeopathy.org
Website: http://www.trusthomeopathy.org

Fnded: 1950. **Mem:** 1,200. **Desc:** Professional body responsible for regulating the education, training and practice of homeopathy by medically qualified doctors, veterinary surgeons, dentists, pharmacists and other statutorily registered health care professionals. Accredited post-graduate training courses lead to the LFHom qualification and, for doctors and vets, medical/veterinary membership of the faculty. **Pub:** *Homeopathy*, quarterly. Journal.

★ 3023 ★ Faculty of Occupational Medicine
c/o Royal College of Physicians
6 St. Andrews Pl.
Regent's Park
London NW1 4LB, United Kingdom
Phone: 44 207 3175890 **Fax:** 44 207 3175899
Website: http://www.facoccmed.ac.uk/

★ 3024 ★ Faculty of Public Health Medicine
4 St Andrew's Pl.
London NW1 4LB, United Kingdom
Phone: 44 20 79350243 **Fax:** 44 20 72246973
Email: enquiries@fphm.org.uk
Website: http://www.fphm.org.uk

Fnded: 1972. **Mem:** 3,000. **Desc:** Principally trainees and consultants in public health medicine. To promote, for the public benefit, the advancement of education in the field of public health medicine; and to develop public health medicine with a view to maintaining the highest possible standards of professional competence and practice, and act as an authoritative body for the purpose of consultation in matters of education or public interest concerning public health medicine. **Pub:** *Journal of Public Health Medicine*, quarterly. Journal. • *ph.com*, quarterly. • Reports.

★ 3025 ★ Familiares y Amigos de Enfermos de la Neurona Motora (FYADENMAC)
Enrique Farman 169-B
Col. Ampliacion Civil
15740 Mexico City, DF, Mexico
Phone: 52 5 1151285 **Fax:** 52 5 1151286
Email: fyadermac@yahoo.com

Fnded: 1982. **Mem:** 96. **Lang(s):** English, German. **Desc:** Promotes interest in motor neurone disease (MND) research among medical and scientific communities and the public in Mexico. Offers support services to MND sufferers and their families. Disseminates information about the disease.

★ 3026 ★ Families of Adults Afflicted with Asperger's Syndrome (FAAAS)
PO Box 514
Centerville, MA 02632-0514
Phone: (508)790-1930 **Fax:** (508)790-1930
Email: faaas@faaas.org
Website: http://www.faaas.org/
Karen E. Rodman, Pres. /Founder

Fnded: 1997. **Desc:** Provides support to family members of adult individuals afflicted with the neurological disorder, Asperger's Syndrome. Promotes public awareness to families and medical communities.

★ 3027 ★ Families Anonymous (FA)
PO Box 3475
Culver City, CA 90231-3475
Phone: (310)815-8010 **Free:** 800-736-9805
Fax: (310)815-9682
Email: famanon@familiesanonymous.org
Website: http://www.familiesanonymous.org

Fnded: 1971. **Nat'l Groups:** 300. **Desc:** Twelve-step groups of parents, relatives, and friends concerned about drug abuse, alcoholism, or related behavioral problems. Self-supported, self-help modeled after Al-Anon Family Groups and Alcoholics Anonymous programs. Assists families in overcoming over-protectiveness of substance abusers and developing a better understanding of their problems, thereby improving interfamily relationships. Aids in establishing community meetings; makes referrals to other agencies. Can provide speakers on request. **Pub:** *Today A Better Way*. Book. FA's daily thought book, written entirely by the fellowship. *Price:* $9/copy. • *The Twelve Step Rag: For Relatives and Friends Concerned about the Use of Drugs or Related Behavioral Problems*, bimonthly. Newsletter. Contains articles, poetry and organizational information. *Price:* Free to FA groups; $4.50/year for individuals; $8.50/2 yrs.; $12/3 yrs. • Catalog. • Directory, periodic. • Pamphlets. • Publishes over 80 items of literature for member inspiration and recovery. Prices vary by size and pages.

★ 3028 ★ Families of S.M.A. (FSMA)
PO Box 196
Libertyville, IL 60048-0196
Phone: (847)367-7620 **Free:** 800-886-1762
Fax: (847)367-7623
Email: sma@fsma.org
Website: http://www.fsma.org
Audrey Lewis, Exec. Dir.

Fnded: 1985. **Mem:** 3,500. **Reg. Groups:** 1. **State Groups:** 21. **Local Groups:** 22. **Desc:** Individuals with Spinal Muscular Atrophy; their families; medical professionals; and interested others. Major funder of SMA research. Promotes public awareness. SMA diseases include: Infantile Progressive SMA (Werdnig-Hoffman Disease), Juvenile Progressive SMA (Kugelberg-Welander Disease) and Adult Progressive SMA (Aran-Duchenne Type). Offers support to families. **Pub:** *Direction*, quarterly. Newsletter. Includes research updates and information network. *Price:* $25/year for families in U.S.; $35/year for professionals in U.S.; $40/year outside U.S. • *Living with SMA*. Video. • *Understanding Muscular Atrophy.*

★ 3029 ★ Families U.S.A. Foundation
1334 G St. NW
Washington, DC 20005
Phone: (202)628-3030 **Fax:** (202)347-2417
Email: info@familiesusa.org
Website: http://www.familiesusa.org
Ron Pollack, Exec. Dir.

Fnded: 1981. **Desc:** Issues reports and other materials on health care and long term care for use by consumer organizations, policymakers, the media, and state-based coalitions working on health care and long term care reform. **Pub:** *Crossing to Mexico: Priced Out of American Health Care.* Survey. Surveys Mexican doctors and American consumers about the reasons Americans go to Mexico for routine medical care. *Price:* $5. • *The Crunch: The Health Insurance Crisis Comes to America's Charities.* Covers the problems of the small business market for health insurance by examining the experiences of 500 nonprofit groups surveyed. *Price:* $5. • *Half of Us: Families Priced Out of Health Protection.* Provides an analysis of government survey data. *Price:* $10. • *The Health Cost Squeeze on Older Americans.* Provides an analysis of elderly out-of-pocket health care costs; compares current costs to those prior to the enactment of Medicare. *Price:* $5. • *The Heavy Burden of Home Care.* Provides an analysis of home care expenditures and the high out-of-pocket costs consumers pay to provide home care. *Price:* $5. • *Making Them Wait For Social Security Disability Benefits.* Provides an analysis of the waiting times and backlogs for people applying for Social Security and SSI Disability benefits. *Price:* $5. • *The Medicare Buy-in: A Promise Unfulfilled.* Describes the Medicare buy-in benefits, the Qualified Medicare Beneficiary and Specified Low-income Medicare Beneficiary. *Price:* $5. • *No Sale: The Failure of Barebones Insurance.* Examines state barebones policies and their ability to provide affordable coverage and to expand insurance to the uninsured population. *Price:* $15. • *Nursing Home Insurance: Who Can Afford It?.* Provides an analysis of the affordability of providing nursing home insurance policies for today's elderly population. *Price:* $5. • *Prescription Costs: America's Other Drug Crisis.* Provides an analysis (for years 1985-1991) of the prices of America's 20 top selling drugs and the pharmaceutical companies' profits. *Price:* $5. • *They Make That Much.* Survey. Contains salaries of medical specialists, CEOs of dru. **Frmly:** (1989) Villers Foundation.

★ 3030 ★ Family Care International (FCI)
588 Broadway Ste. 503
New York, NY 10012
Phone: (212)941-5300 **Fax:** (212)941-5563
Email: info@familycareintl.org
Website: http://familycareintl.org/

Fnded: 1986. **Nat'l Groups:** 170. **Desc:** Works to improve women's sexual and reproductive health and rights in developing countries, especially safer pregnancy and childbirth.

★ 3031 ★ Family Council on Drug Awareness (FCDA)
PO Box 1716
El Cerrito, CA 94530
Phone: (510)215-8326 **Fax:** (510)215-8326
Email: director@fcda.org
Website: http://www.fcda.org
Chris Conrad, Dir.

Fnded: 1989. **Desc:** Promotes "legal reforms that recognize human rights, encourage responsible behavior, separate cannabis from hard drugs, and protect children from the unregulated and indiscriminate market of illegal drugs." Serves as an information clearinghouse on medical marijuana, illegal substances and drug law reform; distributes educational materials and supports 18 years, age of consent, for cannabis use. **Pub:** Brochures.

★ 3032 ★ Family of the Future Health Care (Banja la Mtsogolo)
PO Box 3008
Blantyre, Malawi
Phone: 265 677671 **Fax:** 265 677859
Email: banja@malawi.net

Fnded: 1987. **Lang(s):** English. **Desc:** Promotes population control, family planning, and reproductive health. Makes available reproductive health care services in urban and rural areas; conducts campaigns encouraging male factory workers to participate in family planning and population control programs. Emphasizes dual protection and gives out information on HIV/AIDS prevention.

★ 3033 ★ Family Health Care Association of America
c/o James Mark Reynolds
PO Box 222
Jamestown, NC 27282
Phone: (336)987-0108
Email: jmreynolds@justice.com
James Mark Reynolds, Sr., Pres.

Fnded: 1996. **Mem:** 4,401. **Reg. Groups:** 1. **State Groups:** 1. **Desc:** Provides educational, charitable, and research programs. Also offers a speakers bureau.

★ 3034 ★ Family Health International (FHI)
PO Box 13950
Research Triangle Park, NC 27709
Phone: (919)544-7040 **Fax:** (919)544-7261
Email: services@fhi.org
Website: http://www.fhi.org
Albert J. Siemens, CEO

Fnded: 1971. **Mem:** 300. **Desc:** Biomedical researchers and technical assistants. Promotes increased availability, safety, effectiveness, acceptability, and ease of using family planning methods. Works to improve the delivery of voluntary fertility planning and primary health care services, and reduce the spread of sexually transmitted diseases, especially HIV infection. Conducts, analyzes, and disseminates research on contraception and distribution of family planning services. Supports a program of contraceptive safety and health records. Maintains library of 8000 monographs, journals, and reports. Operates computerized services. **Pub:** *Family Health International–Network,* quarterly. Bulletin. Covers reproductive health and family planning for health care personnel and policymakers in developing countries. *Price:* Free. **Frmly:** (1982) International Fertility Research Program.

★ 3035 ★ Family and Health Section of the National Council on Family Relations (FHS)
3989 Central Ave. NE, Ste. 550
Minneapolis, MN 55421
Phone: (763)781-9331 **Free:** 888-781-9331
Fax: (763)781-9348
Email: tjulian@otterbein.edu
Website: http://www.ncfr.org
Theresa Julian, Ch.

Fnded: 1984. **Mem:** 345. **Desc:** A section of the National Council on Family Relations. Health and education professionals. Serves as a forum for all professionals involved in interdisciplinary work in the family and health fields. Presents clinical research and educational programs at NCFR conferences. **Pub:** *Family Health News,* periodic. Newsletter. **Frmly:** (1991) Family and Health Section.

★ 3036 ★ Family Life Association of Swaziland (FLAS)
PO Box 1051
Manzini, Swaziland
Phone: 268 53586 **Fax:** 268 53191
Email: khetsiwe@org.sz
Website: http://www.flas.org.sz

Fnded: 1979. **Mem:** 200. **Lang(s):** English, SiSwati. **Desc:** Promotes family planning programs in Swaziland. Works for the improvement of maternal, child, and family health. **Pub:** Newsletter, bimonthly.

★ 3037 ★ Family Planning Association (FPA)
2-12 Pentonville Rd.
London N1 9FP, United Kingdom
Phone: 44 20 78375432 **Fax:** 44 20 78373042
Email: melissad@fpa.org.uk
Website: http://www.fpa.org.uk

Fnded: 1930. **Desc:** Improves the sexual health and reproductive rights of all people throughout the UK.

★ 3038 ★ Family Planning Association of Albania
c/o Valentina Leskaj
Rr. Marsel Kashen pallatet e Lanes
Pall. 1
Shk1 Ap. 1
Tirana, Albania
Phone: 355 42 26256 **Fax:** 355 42 24269
Email: postmaster@fpa.tirana.al
Website: http://www.popin.org/~unpopdir/files/data/d0001880.htm

Fnded: 1992. **Mem:** 254. **Local Groups:** 15. **Lang(s):** English. **Desc:** Works on issues of reproductive health and rights. **Pub:** *Reproductive Health,* quarterly. Newsletter.

★ 3039 ★ Family Planning Association of Cyprus (CFPA)
25 Bouboulina St.
Nicosia 1061, Cyprus
Phone: 357 22 751093 **Fax:** 357 22 757495
Email: famplan@spidernet.com.cy

Fnded: 1971. **Mem:** 300. **Lang(s):** English, Greek. **Desc:** Promotes the sexual and reproductive rights of women, men, and young people, including the right to family planning, sex education and access to affordable and high quality services. Provides medical and counseling services to the public. Runs information and awareness campaigns on sexual and reproductive health issues. **Pub:** *Family Law in Cyprus.* Booklet. A series of sex education leaflets in Greek; booklets on contraception and reproductive rights, some information material is also in English

★ 3040 ★ Family Planning Association - England
2-12 Pentonville Rd.
London N1 9FP, United Kingdom
Phone: 44 20 78375432 **Fax:** 44 171 8373042
Website: http://www.fpa.org.uk

Fnded: 1936. **Mem:** 2,000. **Lang(s):** English. **Desc:** Promotes family planning and sexual health in England. Conducts public education programs; conducts research. Provides helpline and reference library. **Pub:** *Contraceptive Education Bulletin,* quarterly. Newsletter. **Frmly:** (2001) Family Planning Association.

★ 3041 ★ Family Planning Association of Estonia (FPA)
Kotka 2
EE-11315 Tallinn, Estonia
Phone: 372 6 552755 **Fax:** 372 6 552755
Email: eppl@amor.ee
Website: http://www.amor.ee

Fnded: 1994. **Mem:** 117. **Lang(s):** English, Estonian, Finnish, Russian. **Desc:** Works to improve reproductive health and family planning services and to increase the availability of such services. Conducts research and educational programs; organizes youth services. **Pub:** *Bulletin of FPA of Estonia,* biennial. Bulletin. Covers important areas of sexuality, health and education. Educational materials for youth on sexual and reproductive health.

★ 3042 ★ Family Planning Association of Hong Kong

Southorn Centre, 10/F
130 Hennessy Rd.
Hong Kong, People's Republic of China
Phone: 852 25754477 **Fax:** 852 28346767
Email: fpahk@famplan.org.hk
Website: http://www.famplan.org.hk

Fnded: 1950. **Mem:** 1,000. **Lang(s):** Chinese, English. **Desc:** To advocate, promote and provide information, education and services in sexual and reproductive health and responsible parenthood for the community. **Pub:** *Contraceptive Methods.* Video. • *Family Life Education Handbook for Teachers.* Book. • *Marriage: Crisis and Future in the Modern World.* Book. • *Puberty News.* Video. Appendix

★ 3043 ★ Family Planning Association of India (FPAI)

Bajaj Bhavan
Nariman Point
Bombay 400 021, Maharashtra, India
Phone: 91 22 2029080 **Fax:** 91 22 2029038
Email: fpai@giasbm01.vsnl.net.in
Website: http://www.fpaindia.com

Fnded: 1949. **Mem:** 2,979. **Lang(s):** English, Hindi Suriname Hindustanti. **Desc:** Works to improve the quality of life for people living in India by promoting family planning and responsible parenthood. Advocates family planning as a basic human right. Works to reduce the number of unwanted pregnancies and abortions. Provides contraceptive and health care services including maternal and child health services. Offers programmes in family life and sexuality education and counselling. Conducts research and training of health professionals, NGOs and other categories of personnel.

★ 3044 ★ Family Planning Association of Kenya (FPAK)

PO Box 30581
Nairobi, Kenya
Phone: 254 20 603923 **Fax:** 254 20 603928
Email: info@fpak.org
Website: http://www.fpak.org

Fnded: 1961. **Mem:** 6,000. **Local Groups:** 50. **Lang(s):** English. **Desc:** Seeks to help all Kenyans, especially young people, live quality healthy lives. Provides leadership and plays a pioneering role in offering sustainable, innovative and holistic services in response to health and socio-economic needs of all Kenyans. Aims at being a regional centre of excellence that assists in capacity building for other organizations serving young people. Particularly committed to championing sexual and reproductive health and other rights and the empowerment of Kenya's young people. Believes in upholding human rights to good health and social development through providing high quality gender sensitive services and information, advocating for freedom of choice, access to quality, appropriate and acceptable services, and promoting dialogue with key stake holders and beneficiaries.

★ 3045 ★ Family Planning Association New Zealand (FPA)

PO Box 11515
Wellington, New Zealand
Phone: 64 4 3844349 **Fax:** 64 4 3828356
Email: national@fpanz.org.nz
Website: http://www.fpanz.org.nz

Fnded: 1936. **Mem:** 300. **Nat'l Groups:** 1. **Reg. Groups:** 3. **State Groups:** 33. **Local Groups:** 12. **Lang(s):** English. **Desc:** Promotes a positive view of sexuality to enable people to make informed choices about their sexual health. Works to reduce the number of unintended pregnancies and abortions. Attempts to stop the spread of AIDS and other sexually transmitted diseases through education and contraceptive services. **Pub:** *Forum*, quarterly. Newsletter.

★ 3046 ★ Family Planning Association of Sri Lanka (FPASL)

37/27, Bullers Ln.
Colombo 7, Sri Lanka
Phone: 94 1 584157 **Fax:** 94 1 580915
Email: dayaabey@fpasl.org

Fnded: 1953. **Mem:** 350. **Local Groups:** 17. **Lang(s):** Sinhalese, Tamil. **Desc:** Advocates family planning as a basic human right and as a means to enhance the quality of life for individuals living in Sri Lanka. Works to reduce the number of unwanted pregnancies and abortions. Offers programs in sex education, family planning, and health. Provides contraceptive and health care services. Conducts research. Promotes the empowerment of women and gender equality and reproductive and sexual health for youth. **Pub:** *Annual Report*, annual. Magazine. Contains reports of the year's activities.

★ 3047 ★ Family Planning Association of Trinidad and Tobago (FPATT)

79 Oxford St.
Port of Spain, Trinidad and Tobago
Phone: (868)623-4764 **Fax:** (868)625-2256
Email: fpattrep@wow.net

Fnded: 1956. **Mem:** 15. **Reg. Groups:** 2. **Lang(s):** English. **Desc:** Works toward the following goals: to respond to the need for improved sexual and reproductive health among the underserved population with particular emphasis on young people; to further develop the financial and human resources of the association to boost its efforts; to advocate responsible sexual and reproductive health practices as a catalyst for the improvement of living standards. **Pub:** *Myths, Perceptions, Mistakes. A Study of Trinidadian Adolsecents.* Survey. Identifies the problems of pregnancy, child caring, and attitudes among teenagers in Trinidad. • *The Sexual Health Needs of Youth in Tobago.* Surveys. Assesses the social, economic and political factors that impact the lives and sexual health of youth in Tobago. • *Teenage Sexuality, Perceptions, and Attitudes of the Youth of Tobago.* Survey. Identifies the problems of pregnancy and child bearing among teenagers in Tobago. • *Trinidad and Tobago Demographic and Health Survey.* Survey. Provides detailed information about fertility, family planning, and child health for use in program planning and evaluaton.

★ 3048 ★ Family Planning Association of Turkey (Turkiye Aile Planlamasi Dernegi)

Atac Sokak 73/3
TR-06420 Ankara, Turkey
Phone: 90 312 4318355 **Fax:** 90 312 4342946
Email: tapd@adanet.tr

Fnded: 1963. **Mem:** 1,500. **Lang(s):** English. **Desc:** Promotes enhanced awareness of family planning rights and services throughout Turkey. Advocates reproductive health including family planning as a basic human right. Disseminates information. Works for the advancement of women's studies, health, and rights. **Pub:** *Islam and Family Planning.* Booklet. • Books. • Newsletters. • Brochures. Additional publications available on request.

★ 3049 ★ Family Planning Australia (FPA)

Ste. 4, Level 1
Construction House
217 Northbourne Ave.
Turner, ACT 2612, Australia
Phone: 61 2 62305255 **Fax:** 61 2 62305344
Email: fpa@fpa.net.au
Website: http://www.fpa.net.au

Mem: 7. **State Groups:** 7. **Lang(s):** English. **Desc:** Seeks to heighten governmental and public awareness of the population problems of local communities and the world. Believes that the availability and use of contraceptives is a basic human right. Makes available sexual and reproductive health services; conducts educational programs for the public and for health care providers. **Frmly:** (1992) Family Planning Federation of Australia.

★ 3050 ★ Family Planning International Assistance - Kenya (FPIA)

Box 53538
Nairobi, Kenya
Phone: 254 20 2727049 **Fax:** 254 20 2717013
Email: fpia@nbi.ispkenya.com

Fnded: 1971. **Lang(s):** English, French, Kiswahili. **Desc:** Family planning organization that works to improve reproductive health in developing countries.

★ 3051 ★ Family Planning International Assistance - USA (FPIA)

c/o Planned Parenthood Federation of America
810 7th Ave.
New York, NY 10019
Phone: (212)541-7800 **Free:** 800-230-PLAN
Fax: (212)247-6274
Email: fpia@ppfa.org
Website: http://www.plannedparenthood.org/fpia
Allie Stickney, Contact

Fnded: 1971. **Desc:** Provides financial, technical, and commodity assistance to organizations in developing countries interested in reproductive health programs.

★ 3052 ★ Family Planning Organization of the Philippines (FPOP)

50 Dona M. Hemady St.
New Manilla
Quezon City, Metro Manila 1112, Philippines
Phone: 63 2 7217302 **Fax:** 63 2 7214067
Email: fpop@fastmail.i-next.net

Lang(s): English, Filipino. **Desc:** Advocates family planning and responsible parenthood as a basic human right and a means to enhance the quality of life for individuals living in the Philippines. Attempts to stop the spread of AIDS and other sexually transmitted diseases through education and contraceptive services. Provides programs in family planning and health care. Conducts research.

★ 3053 ★ Family Planning and Sexual Health Association (FPSHA)

58 Saltoniskiu
2600 Vilnius, Lithuania
Phone: 370 52 790319 **Fax:** 370 52 790319
Email: lithfpa@delfi.lt
Website: http://www.spa.lt

Fnded: 1995. **Mem:** 250. **Local Groups:** 5. **Lang(s):** English, Lithuanian, Russian. **Desc:** Health care professionals with an interest in reproductive medicine; individuals interested in family planning and sexual health. Seeks to avoid unwanted pregnancies and to eliminate the spread of sexually transmitted diseases. Promotes increased availability of reproductive health services; facilitates advancement of reproductive medicine. Serves as a clearinghouse on family planning and sexual health; conducts public education programs; sponsors continuing professional development courses; lobbies for improved public policies dealing with reproductive health issues. **Pub:** Brochure. • Bulletin.

★ 3054 ★ Family Research Institute (FRI)

PO Box 62640
Colorado Springs, CO 80962-2640
Phone: (303)681-3113 **Fax:** (303)681-3427
Website: http://familyresearchinst.org
Dr. Paul Cameron, Exec. Officer

Fnded: 1982. **Mem:** 1,900. **Desc:** Promotes information about sexual, family, and substance abuse issues. Conducts research and educational programs. Maintains speakers' bureau; compiles statistics. **Pub:** *Family Research Report*, 8/year. Newsletter. *Price:* $25/year.

★ 3055 ★ Family Resource Center on Disabilities (FRCD)

c/o Charlotte Des Jardins
20 E Jackson Blvd., Rm. 300
Chicago, IL 60604

Phone: (312)939-3513 **Free:** 800-952-4199
Fax: (312)939-7297
Email: frcdptiil@ameritech.net
Website: http://www.frcd.org
Charlotte Des Jardins, Exec. Dr

Fnded: 1969. **Desc:** Parents, professionals, and volunteers seeking to improve services for all children with disabilities. Originally organized as a result of the 1969 Illinois law mandating the education of all children with disabilities, FRCD operates as a coalition to inform and activate parents. Provides information and referral services, individualized support services for low-income Chicago families, transition services, and special education rights training. **Pub:** *How to Get Services by Being Assertive*. Manual. *Price:* $10 plus shipping and handling. • *How to Organize an Effective Parent/Advocacy Group and Move Bureaucracies*. Manual. *Price:* $10 plus shipping and handling. • *Rehabilitation Act Manual*. Manual. *Price:* $25 plus shipping and handling. • Also publishes pamphlets. **Frmly:** Coordinating Council for Handicapped Children.

★ 3056 ★ Family Therapy Section of the National Council on Family Relations (FTSNCFR)

3989 Central Ave. NE, No. 550
Minneapolis, MN 55421
Phone: (763)781-9331 **Free:** 888-781-9331
Fax: (763)781-9348
Email: kbriggs@okstate.edu
Website: http://www.oakland.edu/~blume/ncfr/
Kathleen Briggs, Ch.

Fnded: 1955. **Mem:** 400. **Desc:** A section of the National Council on Family Relations. Practicing family therapists and family therapy supervisors, educators, and researchers. Seeks to improve the practice of family therapy through the development of theory, research, and training. Promotes communication between family therapy researchers and clinicians; functions as a network for family therapy research projects; conducts educational programs. **Frmly:** (1991) National Council on Family Relations Family Therapy Section.

★ 3057 ★ Famplan Jamaica

PO Box 92
St. Ann's Bay
Saint Ann, Jamaica
Phone: (876)972-2515 **Fax:** (876)972-2224
Email: famplan@cwjamaica.com

Fnded: 1957. **Mem:** 110. **Lang(s):** English. **Desc:** National affiliate of the International Family Planning Federation. Promotes availability of family planning services; advocates on behalf of family planning. Maintains clinics; conducts educational programs. **Pub:** Newsletter, quarterly. **Frmly:** (1990) Jamaica Family Planning Association.

★ 3058 ★ Fanconi Anemia Research Fund (FARF)

1801 Willamette St., Ste. 200
Eugene, OR 97401
Phone: (541)687-4658 **Free:** 800-828-4891
Fax: (541)687-0548
Email: info@fanconi.org
Website: http://www.fanconi.org
Mary Ellen Eiler, Exec. Dir.

Fnded: 1989. **Mem:** 2,000. **Nat'l Groups:** 13. **Desc:** Families with children afflicted with Fanconi anemia, a genetic disorder. Seeks to offer support to families, help them network, and keep them apprised of research relating to Fanconi anemia; assists research on this disorder. Operates support group. Conducts fundraising for research through public awareness programs and special projects. Funds research projects. **Pub:** *FA Family Directory*, annual. Directory. *Price:* $5 in US; $7 all other countries. • *FA Family Newsletter*, semiannual. Newsletter. • *Fanconi Anemia: A Handbook for Families and Their Physicians*. Handbook. **Frmly:** (1989) Fanconi's Anemia Support Group.

★ 3059 ★ FDI World Dental Federation

13 chemin du levant
l'Avant Centre
F-01210 Ferney-Voltaire, France
Phone: 33 4 50405050 **Fax:** 33 4 50405555
Email: info@fdiworldental.org
Website: http://www.fdiworldental.org

Fnded: 1900. **Mem:** 700,000. **Nat'l Groups:** 129. **Reg. Groups:** 5. **Lang(s):** French, German, Japanese, Spanish. **Desc:** National Dental Associates and individual dentists worldwide. A federation of National Dental Association and individual member dentists with the aim of helping to promote oral health worldwide. **Pub:** *Community Dental Health*, quarterly. Magazine. • *The European Journal of Prosthodontics and Restorative Dentistry*, quarterly. Journal. • *International Dental Journal*, bimonthly. Magazine.

★ 3060 ★ Federal Physicians Association (FPA)

9001 Braddock Rd., No. 380
Springfield, VA 22151
Phone: (703)323-9888 **Free:** 800-403-3374
Fax: 800-528-3492
Email: info@fedphy.org
Website: http://www.fedphy.org
Dennis W. Boyd, Exec. Dir.

Fnded: 1978. **Mem:** 500. **Nat'l Groups:** 1. **Reg. Groups:** 1. **State Groups:** 1. **Desc:** Physicians employed by or retired from the federal government. Objectives are: to improve the health care of patients served by federal physicians; to advance the practice of medicine within the federal government; to better the working conditions and benefits of federal physicians. Conducts specialized education programs. **Pub:** *The Federal Physician*, bimonthly. Newsletter. *Price:* $37.50/year. **Frmly:** (1982) American Academy of Federal Civil Service Physicians.

★ 3061 ★ Federated Ambulatory Surgery Association (FASA)

700 N Fairfax St., No. 306
Alexandria, VA 22314
Phone: (703)836-8808 **Fax:** (703)549-0976
Email: fasa@fasa.org
Website: http://www.fasa.org
Kathy Bryant, Exec. Dir.

Fnded: 1974. **Mem:** 1,220. **Desc:** Physicians, nurses, health administrators, and other individuals representing more than 1,100 outpatient surgery centers. Promotes the concept of ambulatory (outpatient) surgical care. Facilitates exchange of knowledge and ideas regarding the care of ambulatory surgical patients. Represents members' interests at national level. Provides information to members, other organizations, and the public regarding government activities, legislation, statistical studies, group purchase programs, and the availability of malpractice insurance. Sponsors seminars, educational programs, and panel discussions; conducts studies and surveys in the field. **Pub:** *FASA Update*, bimonthly. Newsletter. • Membership Directory, annual. **Frmly:** Society for the Advancement of Freestanding Ambulatory Surgical Care; (1986) Freestanding Ambulatory Surgery Association.

★ 3062 ★ Federation for Accessible Nursing Education and Licensure (FANEL)

PO Box 1418
Lewisburg, WV 24901
Phone: (304)645-4357 **Fax:** (304)645-4357
Email: fedaccnsgedlic@hotmail.com
Twyla Wallace, Pres.

Fnded: 1983. **Desc:** Registered nurses, licensed practical nurses, educators, health organizations, schools, and hospital administrators seeking to maintain licensure through current educational programs for RNs and LPNs. **Pub:** Brochures. • Newsletter, biennial.

★ 3063 ★ Federation of Active Retirement Association (FARA)

Shamrock Chambers
59-61 Dame St.
Dublin 2, Ireland
Phone: 353 1 6792142 **Fax:** 353 1 6792142

Fnded: 1995. **Mem:** 110,000. **Reg. Groups:** 65. **Local Groups:** 69. **Desc:** Retired individuals over 55 years of age. Encourages member to "lead a full, happy and healthy retirement." Organizes outings, social activities, sports activities, educational programs, and community service activities. **Pub:** Bulletin, monthly.

★ 3064 ★ Federation of American Hospitals (FAH)

801 Pennsylvania Ave. NW, Ste. 245
Washington, DC 20004-2604
Phone: (202)624-1500 **Fax:** (202)737-6462
Email: info@americashospitals.com
Website: http://www.americashospitals.com
Charles N. Kahn, III, Pres.

Fnded: 1966. **Mem:** 1,000. **Desc:** Privately- or investor-owned (for-profit) hospitals. **Pub:** *Hospital Outlook*, bimonthly. Newsletter. Monitors health legislation, regulatory and reimbursement matters and developments in the health care industry. *Price:* Included in membership dues; $150/year for nonmembers. **Frmly:** (2001) Federation of American Health Systems.

★ 3065 ★ Federation of Asia-Oceania Perinatal Societies

246 Clayton Rd.
Clayton, VIC 3168, Australia
Phone: 61 3 95945191 **Fax:** 61 3 95946115

Fnded: 1980. **Desc:** Promotes the science and art of perinatology, maternal, fetal, and neonatal welfare; encourages cooperation with international bodies; provides expert advice to governmental and other bodies.

★ 3066 ★ Federation of Asian Nutrition Societies (FANS)

134 Shinchon-don, Sudaemun-ku
Seoul 120-749, Republic of Korea
Phone: 82 2 3613090 **Fax:** 82 2 3125229
Email: ycleekim@atsbubble.yonsie.ac.kr

Desc: Promotes international fellowship and cooperation among nutrition scientists in Asia.

★ 3067 ★ Federation of Asian and Oceanian Physiological Societies

GPOB 2609
Sydney, NSW 2001, Australia
Phone: 61 2 92411478 **Fax:** 61 2 92513552
Email: physiol98@icmsaust.com.au

★ 3068 ★ Federation of Asian Veterinary Associations (FAVA)

c/o AusVet Animal Health Services
PO Box 3180
South Brisbane, QLD 4101, Australia
Phone: 61 7 32551712 **Fax:** 61 7 32781953
Email: ausvet@eis.net.au

Mem: 75,000. **Desc:** Works to enhance the quality of life for those living in the Asia-Pacific region through responsible animal care and welfare.

★ 3069 ★ Federation of Associations of Regulatory Boards (FARB)

1603 Orrington Ave., Ste. 2080F
Evanston, IL 60201
Phone: (847)328-7909 **Fax:** (847)864-0588
Email: farb@farb.org
Website: http://www.farb.org
Dale Atkinson, Contact

Fnded: 1973. **Mem:** 13. **Desc:** National associations of regulatory boards united to exchange information and engage in programs and joint activities relating to the education and licensing of professionals and to cooperate in solving the mutual problems of members. Conducts attorney certification course. **Pub:** *FARB Facts*, periodic. **Frmly:** (1985) Federation of Associations of Health Regulatory Boards.

★ 3070 ★ Federation of Chiropractic Licensing Boards (FCLB)
901 54th Ave., Ste. 101
Greeley, CO 80634-4400
Phone: (970)356-3500 **Fax:** (970)356-3599
Email: fclb@fclb.org
Website: http://www.fclb.org
Donna M. Liever, Exec. Dir.

Fnded: 1926. **Desc:** Dedicated to protecting the public promoting excellence in chiropractic regulation. **Pub:** *Chiropractic Licensure and Practice Statistics*, annual. Directory.

★ 3071 ★ Federation of European Cancer Societies (FECS)
Ave. E Mounier 83
B-1200 Brussels, Belgium
Phone: 32 2 7750201 **Fax:** 32 2 7750200
Email: info@fecs.be
Website: http://www.fecs.be

Fnded: 1981. **Lang(s):** Dutch, English, French, Italian, Spanish. **Desc:** European societies active in the fields of clinical and experimental oncology and oncology nursing. Promotes collaboration among members; seeks to advance the prevention, diagnosis, and treatment of cancer. Encourages international cooperation in oncology research; represents members' interests at the European level. **Pub:** *European Journal of Cancer*, periodic.

★ 3072 ★ Federation of the European Dental Industry (Federation de l'Industrie Dentaire en Europe — FIDE)
Kirchweg 2
D-50858 Cologne, Germany
Phone: 49 221 9486280 **Fax:** 49 221 483428

Fnded: 1957. **Mem:** 10. **Lang(s):** English. **Desc:** National associations of companies engaged in the manufacture of dental instruments and supplies. Functions as a platform for coordination of development and works to harmonize international standards within the industry; represents members' interests before government and European Community agencies. Promotes environmental protection, bar coding (HIBC), market statistics (project). **Pub:** *FIDE - European Dental Industry*, biennial. Brochure. Membership brochure. • *FIDE News*, 1-2/year. Newsletter.

★ 3073 ★ Federation European Menopause Societies (FEMS)
15, rue Daru
F-75008 Paris, France
Phone: 33 1 42677747 **Fax:** 33 1 46222072
Email: henri.rozenbaum@wanadoo.fr

Fnded: 1999. **Mem:** 400. **Lang(s):** French, Italian, Spanish. **Pub:** *Menopause Review*, bimonthly.

★ 3074 ★ Federation of European Neuroscience Societies - Milan (FENS)
c/o Prof./Dr. Monica Di Luca
University Milan
Department of Pharmacological Sciences
via Balzaretti 9
I-20133 Milan, Italy
Phone: 39 02 50318374 **Fax:** 39 02 50318284
Email: diluca@mailserver.unimi.it
Website: http://www.fens.org/

Desc: Neuroscience societies and those in the field of neurosciences. Promotes the neurosciences in Europe. Organizes Winter and Summer Schools.

★ 3075 ★ Federation of European Pharmacological Societies (EPHAR)
9 Via Balzaretti
I-20133 Milan, Italy
Phone: 39 0229488314 **Fax:** 39 0229404961
Email: flaminio.cattabeni@unimi.it

Fnded: 1989. **Desc:** Promotes research and education in pharmacology; stimulates cooperation between national/regional pharmacological societies in Europe.

★ 3076 ★ Federation of European Societies for Surgery of the Hand (FESSH)
Via Candiani 8
I-20025 Legnano, Italy
Phone: 39 0331454094
Email: fessh@thehand.com

★ 3077 ★ Federation of European Societies for Tropical Medicine and International Health (FESTMIH)
25, rue du Docteur Roux
F-75724 Paris, France
Phone: 33 1 45668869 **Fax:** 33 1 45664485
Email: socpatex@club-internet.fr

Fnded: 1995. **Desc:** Fosters cooperation between societies dedicated to tropical medicine and international health.

★ 3078 ★ Federation of European Veterinarians in Industry and Research (FEVIR)
Pfizer Animal Health SA.
Mercuriusstraat 20
B-1930 Zaventem, Belgium

Fnded: 1975. **Nat'l Groups:** 7. **Lang(s):** English, French. **Desc:** Organizations representing 4000 veterinarians working in industry and research. Represents members before the Federation of Veterinarians in Europe and provides expert opinions to European Economic Community groups. Works to improve the status of salaried veterinarians. Maintains a file on positions available for veterinarians in Europe. Conducts seminars and symposia.

★ 3079 ★ Federation of Families for Children's Mental Health (FFCMH)
1101 King St., Ste. 420
Alexandria, VA 22314
Phone: (703)684-7710 **Fax:** (703)836-1040
Email: ffcmh@ffcmh.org
Website: http://www.ffcmh.org
Barbara Huff, Exec. Dir.

Fnded: 1987. **Mem:** 6,300. **Nat'l Groups:** 125. **Reg. Groups:** 125. **State Groups:** 27. **Desc:** Parents, children, and mental health and related professionals. Seeks to ensure the rights to full citizenship, support, and access to services for children and youth with mental disorders and their families. Provides leadership in the field of children's mental health care and services; works to address the needs of children and youth with emotional, behavioral, and mental disorders. Gathers and disseminates information on mental illness and mental health care and services; conducts educational and training programs; makes available support, referral, and transition services to children and youth with mental disorders and their families. Maintains speakers' bureau. **Pub:** *Claiming Children*, quarterly. Newsletter.

★ 3080 ★ Federation of Family Planning Associations of Malaysia (FFPAM)
81-B Jalan SS 15/5A
Subang Jaya
47500 Petaling Jaya, Malaysia
Phone: 60 3 7337514 **Fax:** 60 3 7346638
Email: ffeam@po.jaring.mg

Lang(s): Malay. **Desc:** Promotes and advocates family health including family planning, women's development, family life education, youth sexuality, AIDS and sexually transmitted disease prevention, through service, research training and activities. Thus, improving the quality of life of individuals living in Malaysia.

★ 3081 ★ Federation of French-Language Gynecologists and Obstetricians (Federation des Gynecologues et Obstetriciens de Langue Francaise — FGOLF)
c/o Prof. Jean Rene Zorn
Clinique Universitaire Baudelocque
123, blvd. de Port-Royal
F-75674 Paris Cedex 14, France
Phone: 33 1 42341143 **Fax:** 33 1 42341231

Fnded: 1950. **Mem:** 700. **Lang(s):** French. **Desc:** French-speaking gynecologists and obstetricians. Purpose is to promote scientific study in the French language of all aspects of the biology of human reproduction. Conducts training sessions and travel and exchange programs. Maintains permanent committees to deal with special topics. **Pub:** *Journal de Gynecologie Obstetrique et Biologie de la Reproduction*, bimonthly. Journal.

★ 3082 ★ Federation of German Psychological Associations
Heilsbachstr 22-24
D-53123 Bonn, Germany
Phone: 49 228 987310 **Fax:** 49 228 9873170
Email: info@bpd-verband.org

★ 3083 ★ Federation of Hungarian Medical Societies (Magyar Orvostudomanyi Tarsasagok es Egyesuletek Szovetsege — MOTESZ)
Nador v. 36
H-1051 Budapest, Hungary
Phone: 36 1 3123807 **Fax:** 36 1 3837918
Email: motesz@doki.net
Website: http://www.motesz.hu

Fnded: 1966. **Mem:** 93. **Lang(s):** English, German, Hungarian. **Desc:** Medical and Dental professionals. Works to enhance the medical sciences in Hungary. Encourages the development of Hungarian health care, medical, dental and closely related social sciences. Promotes the development of international relations in the field of health. Conducts educational programs. **Pub:** *MOTESZ Calendar*, annual. Brochure. Information on Medical Congresses. • *MOTESZ Magazine*, monthly. Journal of Medical Scientific and Medical Policy issues.

★ 3084 ★ Federation of Immunological Societies of Asia-Oceania (FIMSA)
Ansari Nagar
New Delhi 110 029, India
Phone: 91 11 26967588 **Fax:** 91 11 6862663
Email: nkmehra@medinst.ernet.in

Fnded: 1992. **Desc:** Facilitates exchange of scientific information and personnel, organizes workshops and conferences.

★ 3085 ★ Federation Laique de Centres de Planning Familial
34, rue de la Tulipe
B-1050 Brussels, Belgium
Phone: 32 2 5028203 **Fax:** 32 2 5025613
Email: pascale@planningfamilial.net
Website: http://www.planningfamilial.net

Fnded: 1963. **Mem:** 37. **Lang(s):** French. **Desc:** Advocates family planning as a basic human right. Works to reduce the number of unwanted pregnancies and abortions. Attempts to stop the spread of AIDS and other sexually transmitted diseases through education and contraceptive services. Sponsors programs in family planning and health. Acts as an advocate for family planning on a national and international level. **Pub:** *En Question*, semiannual. Newsletter. **Frmly:** (2000) Federation Francophone Belge pour le Planning Familial et l'Education Sexuelle.

★ 3086 ★ Federation of Latin American Cancer Societies (Federacion Latinoamericana de Sociedades de Cancerologia — FLASCA)
Rebsamen 1142, Col Del Valle
03100 Mexico City, Mexico
Fnded: 1965. **Desc:** Coordinates the scientific aspects of the fight against cancer in Latin America, academic interchange, and permanent relations with medical groups, hospitals and research centers.

★ 3087 ★ Federation of Medical Societies of Hong Kong
Duke of Windsor Social Service Bldg., 4/F
15 Hennessy Rd.
Hong Kong, People's Republic of China
Phone: 852 25278898 **Fax:** 852 28650345
Email: info@fmshk.com.hk
Website: http://www.fmshk.com.hk
Fnded: 1965. **Mem:** 115. **Lang(s):** Chinese, English. **Desc:** Medical and dental associations and related professional organizations. Promotes advancement of the medical, dental, and related sciences. Represents the interests of the medical community. Coordinates activities of members; conducts educational programs. **Pub:** *Hong Kong Medical Diary*, monthly. Bulletin. • *Medical and Dental Directory of Hong Kong*, quadrennial. Directory.

★ 3088 ★ Federation of Medicinal Chemistry (EFMC)
c/o Dr. Gerhard Ecker
Austrian Chemical Society
Medicinal Chemistrt Institute of Pharm. Chemistry
University of Vienna
A-1090 Vienna, Austria
Phone: 43 1 313368571 **Fax:** 43 1 31336771
Email: gerhard.f.ecker@univie.ac.at
Website: http://www.efmc.ch
Fnded: 1962. **Mem:** 19. **Lang(s):** English. **Desc:** National medicinal chemistry societies. Works to advance the science of medicinal chemistry by promoting cooperation among member societies.

★ 3089 ★ Federation of Natural Medicine Users in North America
c/o Christine Murphy
PO Box 140
Monsey, NY 10952-0140
Phone: (845)268-2627 **Fax:** (845)268-2764
Website: http://fonmuna.org
Christine Murphy, Contact
Fnded: 1995. **Desc:** Supports and expands education and research into health care practices using an anthroposophical, or holistic approach. Liaison among health professionals. Studies groups in various geographical areas. Provides self-help instruction for lay people.

★ 3090 ★ Federation of Nurses and Health Professionals (FNHP)
555 New Jersey Ave. NW
Washington, DC 20001
Phone: (202)879-4491 **Free:** 800-238-1133
Fax: (202)879-4597
Email: healthcare@aft.org
Website: http://www.aft.org/newmembers/fnhp/about.html
Gary Stevenson, Dir.
Fnded: 1978. **Mem:** 54,000. **Nat'l Groups:** 1. **Local Groups:** 95. **Desc:** AFL-CIO. A division of the American Federation of Teachers. Collective bargaining organization of registered nurses, licensed practical nurses, and other professional and technical employees in the health field. Works to improve members' professional standards through promoting continuing education, advancing their economic status, and securing working conditions conducive to optimum performance and the most effective delivery of health care. Seeks to have an impact on legislation affecting national health insurance, cost containment, utilization of manpower resources, consumer health education, health personnel training funds, allocation of health research grants, and other national health issues. Maintains legal defense fund to provide assistance to members whose legal or contractual rights have been violated. **Pub:** *Healthwire*, bimonthly. Newsletter. Includes book reviews. *Price:* Included in membership dues.

★ 3091 ★ Federation of Obstetric and Gynecological Societies of India
6th F, Cama and Albless Hospital
Mahapalika Marg.
Bombay 400 001, India
Phone: 91 22 2672033 **Fax:** 91 22 2676405
Email: fogsi@bom7.vsnl.net.in
Website: http://www.fogsi.org/
Fnded: 1950.

★ 3092 ★ Federation of Podiatric Medical Boards (FPMB)
c/o Larry Shane, Exec.Dir.
PO Box 880187
Boca Raton, FL 33488-0187
Phone: (561)477-3060
Website: http://www.fpmb.org/
Larry I. Shane, Exec. Dir.
Fnded: 1936. **Mem:** 45. **State Groups:** 52. **Desc:** State boards of podiatry examiners. Goals are to: serve as a repository for information relating to common problems among boards of podiatry examiners; promote competency examinations with national standards to be utilized by examining boards; monitor and catalog legislation pertaining to podiatry. Conducts business sessions and educational programs on topics concerning the licensure and regulation of health professions. Compiles statistics. **Pub:** *Disciplinary Data Reports*, semiannual. **Frmly:** (1985) Federation of Podiatry Boards; (1986) Federation of Podiatry Medical Boards.

★ 3093 ★ Federation of State Medical Boards of the United States (FSMB)
PO Box 619850
Dallas, TX 75261-9850
Phone: (817)868-4000 **Fax:** (817)868-4099
Email: fsmb@fsmb.org
Website: http://www.fsmb.org
Dale L. Austin, MA, Dep. Exec. Pres. /COO
Fnded: 1912. **Mem:** 70. **State Groups:** 69. **Desc:** State medical examining and licensing boards (including fourteen osteopathic boards). **Pub:** *Exchange*, triennial. Journal. Listing of MD and DO licensing requirements in each state of US. *Price:* $25 each volume; $60 for set of three volumes. • *Federation Journal*, quarterly. Journal. • *FSMB NewsLine*, monthly. • *Handbook*, annual. Directory.

★ 3094 ★ Federation of Straight Chiropractors and Organizations (FSCO)
2276 Wassergass Rd.
Hellertown, PA 18055
Phone: (610)838-3030 **Free:** 800-521-9856
Fax: (610)838-3031
Email: fsco@straightchiropractic.com
Website: http://www.straightchiropractic.com
Dr. Richard Plummer, Chm.
Fnded: 1978. **Mem:** 600. **State Groups:** 5. **Desc:** Individuals and organizations in the chiropractic field. Promotes the practice of straight (traditional) chiropractic. Conducts lobbying and educational programs. **Pub:** *FSCO Insider*, bimonthly. Reports on current organization news and professional information. • *President's Update*, bimonthly. **Frmly:** Federation of Straight Chiropractic Organizations.

★ 3095 ★ Federation of the Trade Unions in Health Care
Maria Luiza 45
BG-1202 Sofia, Bulgaria
Phone: 359 2 9882097 **Fax:** 359 2 9831814
Email: fsz_citub@mail.orbitel
Fnded: 1990. **Mem:** 18,000. **Nat'l Groups:** 326. **Reg. Groups:** 28. **State Groups:** 34. **Local Groups:** 448. **Lang(s):** English, French, Russian. **Desc:** Defends and represents members' interests.

★ 3096 ★ Federation of Trade Unions of Health Services
Blvd. Maria Louisa 45
BG-1202 Sofia, Bulgaria
Phone: 359 2 882097 **Fax:** 359 2 831814
Fnded: 1990. **Mem:** 70,000.

★ 3097 ★ Federation of Veterinarians of Europe (FVE)
1 rue Defacqz
B-1000 Brussels, Belgium
Phone: 32 2 5337020 **Fax:** 32 2 5372828
Email: info@fve.org
Website: http://www.fve.org
Fnded: 1961. **Mem:** 42. **Lang(s):** Dutch, English, French, German. **Desc:** Professional organizations of veterinarians and interested individuals in more than 30 countries. Serves as a liaison to the European Economic Community. Works toward the unification of veterinary programmes in member countries of the EU and its observers. **Pub:** *FVE Newsletter*, quarterly. Newsletter. • *Good Veterinary Practice*. Manual. • *Prudent Use of Antibiotics*. • *Stable to Table; Food Safety*.

★ 3098 ★ Federation of Women's Health Councils - New Zealand
103 Old Porirua Rd.
Ngaio
Wellington, New Zealand
Phone: 64 4 4795852 **Fax:** 64 4 4795752
Email: teenah@handiside.wn.planet.gen.nz
Fnded: 1990. **Reg. Groups:** 15. **Lang(s):** English. **Desc:** Women's health councils united to develop a national health policy for women. Coordinates information sharing and networking among member organizations. Monitors the provision of women's health care services to ensure that doctors and health professionals are accountable to consumers. Defends women's rights to control their bodies; supports access to free abortions. Fosters research activities. **Pub:** *Accident Compensation: A Women's Issue*. Monograph. • *Consumer Consultation, Representation and Participation*. Monograph. • *Ensuring the Cervical Screening Programme Survives the Health Changes*. Monograph. • Newsletter, bimonthly.

★ 3099 ★ Federazione Alzheimer Italia (FAI)
Via T. Marino 7
I-20121 Milan, Italy
Phone: 39 2 809767 **Fax:** 39 2 875781
Email: alzit@tin.it
Website: http://www.alzheimer.it
Fnded: 1993. **Local Groups:** 47. **Lang(s):** English, Italian. **Desc:** Individuals and organizations. Seeks to improve the quality of life of people with Alzheimer's disease and their families. Makes available support and services; facilitates research on Alzheimer's disease and related disorders; conducts educational programs.

★ 3100 ★ Feingold Association of the United States (FAUS)
127 E Main St., Ste. 106
Riverhead, NY 11901
Phone: (631)369-9340 **Free:** 800-321-3287
Fax: (631)369-2988
Email: info@feingold.org

Website: http://www.feingold.org
Jane Hersey, Dir.

Fnded: 1976. **Mem:** 30,000. **Reg. Groups:** 7. **Local Groups:** 30. **Desc:** Committed to helping people determine if certain foods or synthetic food additives are triggering various learning, health, or behavior problems. Program eliminates synthetic dye, artificial flavor, and three preservatives. Provides comprehensive materials to assist people in finding suitable brand-name products. Disseminates information, including medical studies that link diet to behavior and health problems. **Pub:** *Healthier Food for Busy People: 20 little rules to help you navigate the supermarket.* Book. • *Pure Facts*, 10/year. Newsletter. *Price:* Included in membership dues; $38/year for nonmembers. • *School Year Calendar*, annual. • *What are all those funny things in food?...and should I eat them?*. Audiotape. • *Why Can't My Child Behave?*. Book. Provides guidance to parents through process of using diet to help children. *Price:* $38.

★ 3101 ★ Feline Advisory Bureau (FABCFFS)

Taeselbury,
High St.
Tisbury
Tisbury SP3 6LD, United Kingdom
Phone: 44 870 7422278 **Fax:** 44 1747 871873
Email: information@fabcats.org
Website: http://www.fabcats.org

Fnded: 1958. **Mem:** 3,000. **Lang(s):** English. **Desc:** Veterinary surgeons, cat breeders, and pet owners. Promotes humane behavior toward cats and provides information on feline health and care. Raises funds for feline clinical research. Provides cat boarding information service. **Pub:** *Fab Journal*, quarterly. Journal. Information, news articles, scientific articles, letters. • *Journal of Feline Medicine and Surgery*, quarterly. Journal.

★ 3102 ★ Fellowship of Associates of Medical Evangelism (FAME)

PO Box 34800
Indianapolis, IN 46234
Phone: (317)272-5937 **Free:** 800-379-4351
Fax: (317)272-5940
Email: medicalmissions@fameworld.org
Website: http://www.fameworld.org
Rick Wolford, Exec. Dir.

Fnded: 1970. **Desc:** Builds hospitals and clinics and provides mobile medical units for Christian missionaries outside the U.S.; secures and ships medicine and medical supplies. Conducts charitable programs; maintains speakers' bureau. **Pub:** *Spreading the Fame of Christ*, quarterly. Newsletter.

★ 3103 ★ Fellowship of Sports Masseurs and Therapists

BM Soigneur
London WC1N 3XX, United Kingdom
Phone: 44 1992 537778
Email: admin@fsmt-uk.org

Fnded: 1975. **Mem:** 500. **Desc:** Sports masseurs and therapists having produced evidence of skills and knowledge in dealing with sports persons in competition, industry, rehabilitation. Sets and maintains standards in sports massage and therapy; advises on courses, helps to set up specific courses for national sports governing bodies, educational establishments sports centres and local authorities. **Pub:** Newsletter, quarterly.

★ 3104 ★ Fenway Community Health Center

Lesbian/Gay Family & Parenting Services
7 Haviland St.
Boston, MA 02115-2608
Phone: (617)267-0900 **Free:** 888-242-0900
Email: drockwell@fenwayhealth.org
Website: http://www.fenwayhealth.org

Desc: Strives to treat every client as a whole and unique person to receive the best health care available, including HIV prevention, treatment, and research; women's health, particularly understanding the needs of lesbians; and the health care needs of gays and lesbians.

★ 3105 ★ Fertility Research Foundation (FRF)

877 Park Ave.
New York, NY 10021
Phone: (212)744-5500 **Free:** 888-439-2999
Fax: (212)744-6536
Email: info@frfbaby.com
Website: http://www.frfbaby.com
Masood A. Khatamee, MD, Exec. Dir.

Fnded: 1962. **Mem:** 500. **Nat'l Groups:** 1. **Desc:** Specializes in human reproduction. Provides therapeutic, diagnostic, and consultation service for childless couples. Conducts comprehensive infertility surveys which include: endoscopy, sperm antibodies determination, bacteriological assessment, endocrine studies, laboratory facilities for complete hormone assays, surgical correction of genital diseases, artificial donor insemination, and ovulation induction. Maintains research projects in human reproduction pertaining to: the study of influence of mycoplasma on infertility; the relationship of prostaglandins and infertility; the study of genetic defects and dermatoglyphics; immunology research; sperm physiology and migration; ovum transplantation. Conducts educational programs for practicing physicians, residents, and medical students in infertility and education of the public about the human reproductive processes. **Pub:** *Fertility Sourcebook.* Book. **Frmly:** (1967) New York Fertility Institute; (1981) New York Fertility Research Foundation.

★ 3106 ★ Fidelco Guide Dog Foundation (FGDF)

PO Box 142
Bloomfield, CT 06002
Phone: (860)243-5200 **Fax:** (860)243-7215
Email: training@fidelco.org
Website: http://www.fidelco.org
George Salpietro, Exec. Dir.

Fnded: 1960. **Mem:** 25,000. **Desc:** Purpose is to breed, train, and place Fidelco German shepherd guide dogs with blind persons (the Fidelco shepherd is a special breed ideally suited for guide work because of its intelligence, strength, health, and stability). Provides "In-Community" training services to blind persons; reviews performance of the guide dog teams (dog and blind individual) to see that satisfactory level of achievement is maintained; utilizes genetic processes and clinical methods to improve and refine the breed; maintains an ongoing program for development and improvement of training methods. Fidelco puppies are raised in a volunteer family for the first 12-14 months, then trained by FGDF staff for six months before final introduction to and training in the workplace and home environment of the blind recipient with a trainer's help. Maintains speakers' bureau. **Pub:** *Fidelco Audio News*, 3/year. Newsletter. • *Fidelco News*, 4/year. Newsletter. • Annual Report, annual. **Frmly:** Fidelco Foundation; (1981) Fidelco Breeder's Foundation.

★ 3107 ★ Fiji Optometric Association (FOA)

GPO Box 1217
Suva, Fiji
Phone: 679 3311955 **Fax:** 679 3305408
Email: razak@is.com.fij

Fnded: 1982. **Mem:** 6. **Lang(s):** English. **Desc:** Optometrists. Promotes continuing professional development of members; seeks to advance the study and practice of optometry. Sponsors eye care programs; conducts educational courses for optometrists.

★ 3108 ★ Finnish Association for Mental Health (FAMH) (Suomen Mielenterveysseura)

Maistraatinportti 4 A
FIN-00240 Helsinki, Finland
Phone: 358 9 615516 **Fax:** 358 9 61551770
Website: http://www.mielenterveysseura.fi

Fnded: 1897. **Mem:** 3,000. **Local Groups:** 50. **Lang(s):** English, Finnish, German, Swedish. **Desc:** Voluntary organization for professional and lay people. Promotes mental health through programs of prevention. Introduces new procedures in voluntary and statutory mental health work. Provides support and crisis services; offers vocational training programs. Maintains 15 crisis centers. **Pub:** *Mielenterveys*, bimonthly. Magazine. • *Perheterapia*, quarterly. Provides family therapy information. • Books. • Journals. • Newsletter, annual.

★ 3109 ★ Finnish Cardiac Society (FCS) (Suomen Kardiologinen Seura — SKS)

PO Box 50
FIN-00621 Helsinki, Finland
Phone: 358 9 75275238 **Fax:** 358 9 75275233
Email: fcs@fimnet.fi

Fnded: 1967. **Mem:** 685. **Lang(s):** English, Finnish, Swedish. **Desc:** Physicians practicing in Finland. Encourages contact between cardiology specialists and doctors interested in the field. Organizes educational courses. **Pub:** *Sydanaani (Cardiac Sound)*, periodic. Newsletter.

★ 3110 ★ Finnish Dermatological Society (FDS) (Suomen Ihotautilaakariyhdistys Ry)

Department of Dermatology
PO Box 160
FIN-00029 Hyks, Finland
Phone: 358 9 471961639 **Fax:** 358 9 94716561

Fnded: 1916. **Mem:** 278. **Lang(s):** English, Finnish. **Desc:** Professional organization for dermatologists in Finland. Conducts educational programs. **Pub:** *Skinfo*, 4-6/year. Newsletter.

★ 3111 ★ Finnish Diabetes Association

Diabetes Center
Kirjoniementie 15
FIN-33680 Tampere, Finland
Phone: 358 3 2860111 **Fax:** 358 3 3600462
Email: diabetesliitto@diabetes.fi
Website: http://www.diabetes.fi/english/

Mem: 52,000. **Local Groups:** 109. **Desc:** Works to ensure quality care and quality of life for persons with diabetes. **Pub:** *Diabetes.* Magazine. Contains a medical supplement, "Diabetes & Physician".

★ 3112 ★ Finnish Federation of the Visually Impaired (Nakovammaisten Keskusliitto)

Makelankatu 50
FIN-00510 Helsinki, Finland
Phone: 358 9 396041 **Fax:** 358 9 39604200
Email: nkl@nkl.fi
Website: http://www.nkl.fi

Fnded: 1928. **Mem:** 25. **Local Groups:** 100. **Lang(s):** English, Finnish, German, Russian, Spanish, Swedish. **Desc:** Works to improve the quality of life of the blind and people with visual impairment. Promotes increased availability of services for people with visual impairment in Namibia, Zambia, Ecuador, Palestine, Estonia, and Russia. Conducts educational programs for personnel working with the blind; develops, produces, and distributes Braille and talking books. **Pub:** *AIRUT*, 33/year. Magazine. **Frmly:** Fissish Central Federation of the Visually Handicapped.

★ 3113 ★ Finnish Medical Association (Suomen Laakariliitto)
Makelankatu 2
PO Box 49
SF-00501 Helsinki, Finland
Phone: 358 9 393091 **Fax:** 358 9 3930794
Email: fma@fimnet.fi
Website: http://www.laakariliitto.fi

Fnded: 1910. **Mem:** 18,000. **Nat'l Groups:** 26. **State Groups:** 5. **Local Groups:** 60. **Lang(s):** English, Finnish, Swedish. **Desc:** Physicians' organizations to safeguard physicians' economic interests and working conditions. Promotes formation and implementation of effective national health policies. Develops and administers national training programs for physicians and confers professional certification. Conducts research on health systems and services. Facilitates international cooperation in the provision of health care in underserved areas. Aims at maintaining a high standard of professional ethics. **Pub:** *Finnish Medical Journal*, 36/year. Journal. • *Information Newsletter*, 15/year. Newsletter. • *Newsletter for the General Press*, 15/year. Newsletter. • Books. • Manuals. **Frmly:** (2000) Finnish Medical Association.

★ 3114 ★ Finnish MS Society
PO Box 15
SF-21251 Masku, Finland
Phone: 358 2 439 2111 **Fax:** 358 2 439 2133
Email: tiedotus@ms-liitto.fi
Website: http://www.ms-liitto.fi

Fnded: 1971. **Mem:** 10,000. **Local Groups:** 70. **Desc:** MS patients, families and professionals. Seeks to improve the quality of life for persons with multiple sclerosis and their families; promotes social justice and equality for members; strives to assist patients to maintain functional capacity in order to live independently. Established the MS Foundation to encourage research in medial and nursing sciences of MS and rare neurological diseases in Finland. **Pub:** *Avain - The Key*, 7/year. Newsletter. • Brochures. Contain information on disease and advice to overcome a handicap.

★ 3115 ★ Finnish Neuro-Muscular Disorders Association (FMD)
Lantinen Pitkakatu 35
SF-20100 Turku, Finland
Phone: 358 2 2739700 **Fax:** 358 2 2739701
Email: lihastautiliito@lihastautiliito.fi
Website: http://www.lihastautiliitto.fi

Fnded: 1972. **Reg. Groups:** 12. **Desc:** Individuals in Finland affected by Amyotrophic Lateral Sclerosis (ALS), a muscle wasting condition. Provides a forum for support and exchange of information. Offers educational programs.

★ 3116 ★ Finnish Occupational Therapy Association
c/o Scandinavian Journal of Occupational Therapy
Department of Social Medicine and yRehabilitation
Umea University
S-901 87 Umea, Sweden
Phone: 46 90 7869272 **Fax:** 46 90 7869267

Lang(s): Finnish. **Desc:** Occupational therapists and other health care professionals engaged in occupational medicine in Finland. Promotes scientific inquiry in the field of occupational therapy and serves as a forum for the dissemination of research results. Areas of inquiry include: physical disability; mental health and disabilities; therapeutic equipment, environments, and techniques; assessment and evaluation of disabilities; vocational and educational training.

★ 3117 ★ Finnish Pharmacological Society
c/o Dr. Raimo Tuominen
Division of Pharmacology & Toxicology
Department of Pharmacy
University of Helsinki
PO Box 56
FIN-00014 Helsinki, Finland
Phone: 358 9 19159469 **Fax:** 358 9 19159471
Email: rtuominen@sarka.helsinki.fi

Mem: 388. **Desc:** Promotes pharmacology in Finland.

★ 3118 ★ Finnish Society for Dermatopathology (FSD) (Suomen Dermatopatologiyhdistys)
c/o University Central Hospital
Department of Dermatology
Meilahdentie 2
FIN-00250 Helsinki, Finland
Phone: 358 9 47186263 **Fax:** 358 9 47186474

Fnded: 1984. **Mem:** 168. **Lang(s):** English, Finnish. **Desc:** Medical doctors. Promotes the study of dermatopathology.

★ 3119 ★ Finnish Veterinary Association (Finlands Veterinarforbund)
Makelank 2C
FIN-00520 Helsinki, Finland
Phone: 358 9 7011388 **Fax:** 358 9 7018397

Fnded: 1892. **Mem:** 1,350. **Lang(s):** English, Finnish, Swedish. **Desc:** Practitioners of veterinary medicine in Finland. Seeks to develop veterinary medicine in Finland. Encourages exchange and cooperation among members; promotes and represents the professional, social, and economic welfare of members. Makes recommendations to authorities on policy matters affecting veterinary medicine; fosters international contacts. Holds Annual veterinary seminar and talks and lectures. Conducts research. Operates charitable program. **Pub:** *Suomen Elainlaakarilehti*, monthly. Journal. Also publishes report of about 400 pages from lectures of the Finnish Veterinary Congress.

★ 3120 ★ First Steps to Freedom
7 Avon Ct.
School Lane
Kenilworth CV8 2GX, United Kingdom
Phone: 44 1926 864473 **Fax:** 44 1926 864473
Email: fstf1234@aol.com
Website: http://www.first-steps.org

Fnded: 1991. **Mem:** 1,500. **Desc:** People who suffer from phobias, panic attacks, general anxiety, obsessive compulsive disorders, and tranquilizer withdrawal. Makes available telephone help line, support groups, relaxation audio tapes. Conducts educational programs. **Pub:** *NWL*, quarterly.

★ 3121 ★ Fitness Industry Association
115 Eastbourne Mews
London W2 6LQ, United Kingdom
Phone: 44 207 2986730 **Fax:** 44 207 2986731
Email: info@fia.org.uk
Website: http://www.fia.org.uk

Fnded: 1989. **Mem:** 1,400. **Desc:** Operators, suppliers, educational establishments, and professionals in the fitness industry. Aims to raise standards across the industry via the publicising of the Code of Practice. **Pub:** *Club Business International*, monthly. Magazine. Provides health club industry news. • *Health Club Management*, monthly. • *Leisure Management Magazine*, monthly. Magazine. • *Leisure Opportunities*, bimonthly. Magazine.

★ 3122 ★ Fitness for Life (FFL)
5060 Cascade Rd. SE, Ste. A
Grand Rapids, MI 49546
Fax: (616)954-1728
Dan Distin, Contact

Fnded: 1984. **Desc:** Personal Fitness Training Massages. **Pub:** *On Purpose*, quarterly. Newsletter. • *On Purpose Manual*. Manual.

★ 3123 ★ Floating Hospital (FH)
Pier 11 Wall at South St.
New York, NY 10005
Phone: (212)514-7440 **Fax:** (212)785-0290
Ken Berger, Exec. VP & COO

Fnded: 1866. **Desc:** Provides medical, dental and health education services. Programs occur within a 4-deck ship, docked in the East River at Wall Street. Provides health services to homeless children and their families, children in kinship foster care and their kinship families, and adolescents who engage in high risk behaviors. Programs take place dockside and while sailing around New York harbor. The ship is open during day and evening hours, six days each week. All programs integrate health education and nutrition, the keys of disease prevention, with comprehensive and continuous primary care. **Frmly:** (1980) St. John's Guild - The Floating Hospital.

★ 3124 ★ Flower Essence Society (FES)
PO Box 459
Nevada City, CA 95959
Phone: (530)265-9163 **Free:** 800-736-9222
Fax: (530)265-0584
Email: mail@flowersociety.org
Website: http://www.flowersociety.org
Patricia A. Kaminski, Pres.

Fnded: 1979. **Mem:** 5,000. **Desc:** Project of Earth-Spirit Inc. Health centers, holistic health practitioners, and interested individuals. Seeks to increase public awareness of Nature and the evolving spiritual relationship between human beings and the earth. Promotes the use of flower essences as catalysts to health and important tools "for personal and planetary evolution." Seeks to establish a worldwide network among health practitioners and others using flower essences. Encourages intuitive and scientific investigation of the essences and the creation of a center for educational and research programs. Organizes introductory weekends and annual week-long intensives for professional and lay health practitioners. Sponsors lectures and research, educational, and experimental activities on topics concerning scientific and spiritual approaches to nature, preparation and use of flower essences, practical skills for flower essence practitioners, and recent developments in the field. Maintains library and referral service. Conducts seven-day professional training seminar and wildflower preservation and naturalist program. **Pub:** *Flower Essence Repertory*. Books. *Price:* $19.95. • *Flower Essence Society–Members' Newsletter*, 1-2/year. Newsletter. Includes book reviews, calendar of events, and research updates. *Price:* Included in membership dues. • *Member E-Bulletin*, quarterly. Bulletin. • Also publishes informational flyer series. **AKA:** Earth-Spirit, Inc.

★ 3125 ★ Flying Chiropractors Association (FCA)
2001 Bridgeway St.
Sausalito, CA 94965
Phone: (415)332-4304
Dr. Dwight A. Shaneyfelt, Contact

Fnded: 1968. **Mem:** 300. **Reg. Groups:** 9. **Desc:** Flying chiropractic physicians. Objectives are to: promote fellowship; seek designation as aviation medical examiners (doctors who examine pilots for their licensure); promote aviation safety. Conducts seminars. **Pub:** *D.C. Flyer*, quarterly.

★ 3126 ★ Flying Dentists Association (FDA)
10032 Wind Hill Dr.
Greenville, IN 47124-9673
Phone: (812)923-2100
Email: jsalis913@aol.com
Website: http://www.flyingdentists.org/
Bill Hohlt, Pres.

Fnded: 1960. **Mem:** 500. **Reg. Groups:** 4. **Desc:** Members of the American Dental Association who have an active aircraft pilot's license. Many members make use of private air travel in conducting their dental practice. **Pub:** *Flight Watch*, monthly.

★ 3127 ★ Flying Physicians Association (FPA)
PO Box 677427
Orlando, FL 32867

Phone: (407)359-1423 Fax: (407)359-1167
Email: fpahq@aol.com
Website: http://www.fpadrs.org
Lawrence O. Grahagan, MD, Pres.

Fnded: 1954. **Mem:** 1,200. **Reg. Groups:** 5. **Desc:** Doctors of medicine who have a current pilot certificate and are members of an ethical medical organization. Promotes the interests of medicine in aviation, safety, and education. **Pub:** *The Flying Physician*, quarterly. Magazine. For physicians with pilot's certificates covering medical and aviation topics; also includes association activities, book reviews, and calendar. *Price:* Included in membership dues; $50/year for nonmembers. • *Flying Physicians Association–Bulletin*, monthly. Newsletter. Membership activities newsletter. *Price:* Included in membership dues. • *Flying Physicians Association–Directory*, annual. Directory. *Price:* Included in membership dues.

★ 3128 ★ Flying Veterinarians Association (FVA)

101 Bingham Rd.
Columbia, MO 65203-3577
Phone: (573)449-4497 **Fax:** (573)449-4497
Email: mcclurer@missouri.edu
Robert C. McClure, D.V.M., Sec. -Treas.

Fnded: 1966. **Mem:** 328. **Desc:** Veterinarians holding valid private pilot certificates; individuals in the field who have an interest in flying; nonveterinarians who either teach in veterinary schools or who represent companies serving the veterinary industry. Promotes aviation safety through example and education; seeks to increase knowledge and proficiency in the operation of aircraft. Seeks to heighten awareness of and interest in aviation among young people. Emphasizes utilization of aircraft in veterinary practice. Sponsors two to four educational programs per year in conjunction with other professional veterinary medical meetings; organizes fly-ins. fly-ins. **Pub:** Directory, periodic. • Newsletter, periodic.

★ 3129 ★ Focus

c/o Marilyn T. Miller
1855 W Taylor St.
Chicago, IL 60612
Phone: (312)996-7445 **Fax:** (312)413-7895
Email: marimill@uic.edu
Marilyn T. Miller, MD, Contact

Fnded: 1961. **Mem:** 400. **Desc:** Volunteer eye surgeons. Allows American ophthalmologists the opportunity to represent their profession and country by working overseas in an area of desperate need. Doctors pay their own transportation and expenses, and contribute two working weeks of their vacation time to treating patients in Nigeria, where eye care would otherwise not be available. Medical equipment and drugs have been donated by U.S. drug and medical supply firms to the clinics operated by Focus in these countries. Group is unrelated to association of same name. **Pub:** Newsletter, 4-6/month.

★ 3130 ★ FOD Family Support Group

c/o Deb Lee Gould
805 Montrose Dr.
Greensboro, NC 27410
Phone: (336)547-8682
Email: deb@fodsupport.org
Website: http://www.fodsupport.org
Deb Lee Gould, Dir.

Fnded: 1991. **Mem:** 1,100. **Desc:** Seeks to provide emotional and practical support and medical information for families confronting fatty oxidation disorders (FOD), as well as interested professionals. **Pub:** *FOD Communication Network*, semiannual. Newsletter. Contains medical and pharmaceutical updates, family stories, questions and answers. Also available in hardcopy. *Price:* Free. **Frmly:** MCAD Family Support Group.

★ 3131 ★ Food Allergy and Anaphylaxis Network

10400 Eaton Pl., Ste. 107
Fairfax, VA 22030-2208
Phone: (703)691-3179 **Free:** 800-929-4040
Fax: (703)691-2713
Email: faan@foodallergy.org
Website: http://www.foodallergy.org

Fnded: 1991. **Mem:** 25,000. **Desc:** Individuals with food allergies; health care professionals with an interest in allergology. Seeks to increase public awareness of food allergies and their treatment. "Works with government agencies, health professionals, food manufacturers, restaurant associations, and schools to educate them about the needs of food allergic individuals." **Pub:** *Food Allergy News*, bimonthly. Newsletter. • *Food Allergy News for Kids*, bimonthly. Newsletter. **Frmly:** (2001) Food Allergy Network.

★ 3132 ★ Food and Nutrition Board (FNB)

2101 Constitution Ave. NW
Washington, DC 20418
Fax: (202)334-2316
Email: fnb@nas.edu
Allison Yates, Dir

Fnded: 1940. **Mem:** 13. **Desc:** Division of National Academy of Sciences - Institute of Medicine. Evaluates and offers advice to the federal government concerning the relationship between food consumption, nutritional status, and public health. **Pub:** Booklets. • Monographs.Covers nutrition, public health and food safety. • Report.

★ 3133 ★ Forbes Norris MDA-ALS Research Center (ALSNRF)

c/o California Pacific Medical Center
2324 Sacramento St., Ste. 150
San Francisco, CA 94115
Phone: (415)923-3604 **Fax:** (415)673-5184
Giovanna Kushner, Contact

Fnded: 1981. **Local Groups:** 3. **Desc:** Serves as clearinghouse for laboratory and clinical research into neuromuscular diseases, primarily Amyotrophic Lateral Sclerosis (Lou Gehrig's Disease). ALS is a paralytic and usually fatal disease of the motor neurons, nerves which innervate the muscles to allow movement. Although patients maintain their full intellectual capacities, they gradually lose their ability to move, talk, and breathe. Sponsors the ALS Research Center at the California Pacific Medical Center in San Francisco, CA and maintains an extensive bank of ALS patient information. Offers educational programs and a speakers' bureau. speakers' bureau. **Pub:** *Forbes Norris Research Center–Support Group Newsletter*, monthly. Newsletter. *Price:* Free. • Newsletter, semiannual. **Frmly:** (1994) ALS and Neuromuscular Research Foundation; (1999) ALS Forbes Norris Research Center.

★ 3134 ★ Foreign Pharmacy Graduate Examination Committee (FPGEC)

c/o Carmen A. Catizone
National Association of Boards of Pharmacy
700 Busse Hwy.
Park Ridge, IL 60068
Phone: (847)698-6227 **Fax:** (847)698-0124
Website: http://www.nabp.net
Carmen A. Catizone, Exec. Dir.

Fnded: 1982. **Desc:** A committee of the National Association of Boards of Pharmacy. Provides information to foreign pharmacy graduates regarding entry into the U.S. pharmacy profession and health care systems. Evaluates qualifications of foreign pharmacy graduates. Gathers and disseminates data on foreign graduates; maintains information on foreign pharmacy schools in order to produce an examination that measures academic competence with regard to U.S. pharmacy school standards. **Frmly:** (1988) Foreign Pharmacy Graduate Examination Commission.

★ 3135 ★ Forum for Medical Affairs (FORUM)

760 Riverside Ave.
Jacksonville, FL 32204-3335
Fax: (904)353-1247
Donald F. Foy, Sr., Exec. VP

Fnded: 1944. **Mem:** 800. **Desc:** Presidents, presidents-elect, and past presidents of state medical associations, members of the American Medical Association and the House of Delegates, editors of state medical association journals, executive directors of state medical associations, and representatives of AMA-recognized medical specialty societies. **Frmly:** (1972) Conference of Presidents and Officers of State Medical Associations.

★ 3136 ★ Forward Face

317 E 34th St., Ste. 901A
New York, NY 10016
Phone: (212)684-5860 **Fax:** (212)684-5864
Email: linda@forwardface.org
Website: http://www.forwardface.org/
Barbara Robertson, Pres.

Fnded: 1978. **Mem:** 900. **State Groups:** 1. **Desc:** Individuals with craniofacial disorders, their families and friends, and health care professionals. Provides medical, psychological, and financial support services. Facilitates communication and cooperation between patients and health care professionals; operates referral service. Offers workshops; conducts networking activities and children's services; Also includes a support group, Inner Faces, specifically for teenagers and young adults; activities include communications workshops theatre productions and social functions. Operates family assistance fund to assist families with expenses not covered by insurance, such as lodging and transportation. **Pub:** *Face Facts*. Videos. • *Forward Face Newsletter*, quarterly. Brochures. *Price:* Included in membership. • *Forward Face Newsletter*, quarterly. Newsletter. *Price:* $20/year. • My Face, book about a child with Mobius Syndrome.

★ 3137 ★ Foundation for Advancement in Cancer Therapy (FACT)

Box 1242, Old Chelsea Sta.
New York, NY 10113
Phone: (212)741-2790 **Fax:** (212)924-3634
Website: http://www.fact-ltd.org
Ruth Sackman, Pres.

Fnded: 1971. **Mem:** 2,500. **Reg. Groups:** 1. **Desc:** Believes that cancer is a symptom of imbalance in body chemistry; thus, to control the disease, not only must any tumors be destroyed, but the body must also be regenerated through the "total person approach" which emphasizes nutrition, detoxification, and mind-body cohesion. Asserts the right of the public to be informed of the "nontoxic biological" adjuncts and alternatives to surgery, chemotherapy, and radiotherapy, but cautions that patients be discriminating; disseminates information concerning only those preventive schemes and nontoxic therapies that have been verified as "safe" by long-term clinical tests. Does not intend to discredit traditional therapies, but to complement them; works cooperatively with established practitioners and instit utions. Seeks the elimination of carcinogens from the environment; supports cancer and nutrition research and compiles statistics; maintains speakers' bureau. **Pub:** *Cancer Forum*, bimonthly. Magazine. *Price:* included in membership dues. **Frmly:** (1988) Foundation for Alternative Cancer Therapies.

★ 3138 ★ Foundation for the Advancement of Chiropractic Tenets and Science (FACTS)

c/o International Chiropractors Association
1110 N Glebe Rd., Ste. 1000
Arlington, VA 22201
Phone: (703)528-5000 **Free:** 800-423-4690
Fax: (703)528-5023
Email: chiro@chiropractic.org
Website: http://www.chiropractic.org
Ronald Hendrickson, Exec. Dir.

Fnded: 1972. **Desc:** Dedicated to the improvement of human health through understanding and development of new chiropractic information. Offers financial aid for education and research programs in colleges and independent institutions; supports chiropractic research program at University of Colorado in Boulder. Has conducted extensive survey of the chiropractic profession for the federal government. Is approved by the National Institutes of Health of the U.S. Public Health Service. **Pub:** *Chiropractic Health Care.* **Frmly:** International Chiropractors Research Foundation.

★ 3139 ★ Foundation for the Advancement of Psychology
PO Box 92621
Bogota, Colombia
Phone: 57 1 2567527 **Fax:** 57 1 2567527
Email: psycholo@latino.net.co

Fnded: 1977. **Lang(s):** Spanish. **Desc:** Fosters research in basic and applied psychology. **Pub:** *Avances en Psicologia Clinica Latinoamericana*, periodic. Journal. • *Revista Latinoamericana de Psicologia*, periodic. Journal.

★ 3140 ★ Foundation for Advances in Medicine and Science (FAMS)
PO Box 832
Mahwah, NJ 07430-0832
Phone: (201)818-1010 **Free:** 800-443-0263
Fax: (201)818-0086
Email: scanning@fams.org
Website: http://www.scanning-fams.org/profile.html
Tony Bourgholtzer, Bd. Chm.

Fnded: 1983. **Mem:** 400. **Desc:** Clinical cardiologists, scientists, and scanning electron microscopists. Disseminates resource information in clinical medicine and science. Funds research projects. **Pub:** *Clinical Cardiology*, monthly. Journal. Contains peer-reviewed articles for practicing cardiologists. *Price:* $80/year in U.S.; $126.50/year outside U.S.; $15.50/single copy. • *Scanning*, 6/year. *Price:* $175/year in U.S.; $185/year outside U.S.; $325/year, institutional in the U.S.; $40/single copy. **Frmly:** (1990) Foundation for Advances in Clincal Medicine and Science.

★ 3141 ★ Foundation of American College of Health Care Administrators (FACHCA)
300 N Lee St., No. 301
Alexandria, VA 22314-2807
Phone: (703)739-7900 **Free:** 888-88A-CHCA
Fax: (703)739-7901
Email: mtn@achca.org
Website: http://www.achca.org
Mary Tellis-Nayak, Pres. /CEO

Fnded: 1962. **Mem:** 4,500. **Desc:** Individuals dedicated to the improvement of the administration of long-term care facilities. Conducts professional training programs and research in administration. **Pub:** *ACHCA Update*, bimonthly. Newsletter. **Frmly:** (1983) Foundation of American College of Nursing Home Administrators.

★ 3142 ★ Foundation for Biomedical Research (FBR)
818 Connecticut Ave. NW, Ste. 200
Washington, DC 20006
Phone: (202)457-0654 **Fax:** (202)457-0659
Email: info@fbresearch.org
Website: http://www.fbresearch.org
Ms. Frankie L. Trull, Pres.

Fnded: 1981. **Desc:** Individuals and organizations supporting humane animal research. Serves as public information and education program on what the foundation sees as the necessary and important role of laboratory animals in biomedical research and testing. Maintains speakers' bureau and public relations program. **Pub:** *Fact vs. Myth.* Brochure. • *FBRoadcast*, bimonthly. Newsletter. Includes foundation news and calendar of events. *Price:* Free. • *Hope!.* Film. • *Why I Should Stay Awake in Science Class.* Video.

★ 3143 ★ Foundation for the Children's Oncology Group (NCCF)
440 E Huntington Dr., Ste. 402
PO Box 60012
Arcadia, CA 91066-6012
Phone: (626)447-1674 **Free:** 800-458-6223
Fax: (626)447-6359
Email: info@conquerkidscancer.org
Website: http://www.conquerkidscancer.org

Desc: Physician-scientists. Supports a network of childhood cancer treatment and research institutions caring for infants, children, teens and young adults. **Frmly:** (2002) National Childhood Cancer Foundation.

★ 3144 ★ Foundation for Chiropractic Education and Research (FCER)
380 Wright Rd.
Norwalk, IA 50211
Phone: (515)981-9888 **Free:** 800-622-6309
Fax: (515)981-9427
Email: fcer@fcer.org
Website: http://www.fcer.org
DeAnna L. Beck, Dir.

Fnded: 1944. **Mem:** 3,000. **Desc:** Chiropractors and laymen. Provides funding for scientific research and research training that will "enhance the knowledge and practice of chiropractic as a conservative approach to health care restoration, maintenance, and disease prevention." **Pub:** *Chiropractic Healthways Newsletter*, bimonthly. Newsletter. Promotes health and fitness. Includes research updates. • *Foundation for Chiropractic Education and Research–Advance*, quarterly. Magazine. Foundation activities newsletter. *Price:* Free. • Also publishes pamphlets. **Frmly:** (1958) Chiropractic Research Foundation; (1967) Foundation for Accredited Chiropractic Education.

★ 3145 ★ Foundation for Digestive Health and Nutrition (FDHN)
7910 Woodmont Ave., Ste. 610
Bethesda, MD 20814-3015
Phone: (301)222-4002 **Fax:** (301)222-4010
Email: info@fdhn.org
Website: http://www.fdhn.org
David Lee, Dir. Operations

Fnded: 2001. **Desc:** FDHN is the foundation of the American Gastroenterological Association. The goal of the FDHN is to be the largest source of funds for research and public education in digestive diseases. **Frmly:** (2001) American Digestive Health Foundation.

★ 3146 ★ Foundation Fighting Blindness (FFB)
11435 Cronhill Dr.
Owings Mills, MD 21117-2220
Phone: (410)568-0150 **Free:** 800-683-5555
Fax: (410)363-2393
Email: info@blindness.org
Website: http://www.blindness.org
Mitsy Palmer, Constituent Serv. Coord.

Fnded: 1971. **Mem:** 65,000. **Local Groups:** 35. **Desc:** Works to fund research on causes, treatments, preventive methods and cures for Retinitis Pigmentosa, macular degeneration, Usher Syndrome, Stargardt disease, and the entire spectrum of retinal degenerative diseases. Provides information and referral services; promotes public awareness; sponsors research programs; conducts fundraisers. **Pub:** *Fighting Blindness News*, semiannual. Newsletter. Includes articles on coping, Foundation activites and research updates. *Price:* Free. • *Macular Update*, 3/year. Newsletter. Includes informational articles and research updates on macular degeneration. *Price:* Free. • Also disseminates comprehensive information kits or retinitis pigmentosa (RP), macular degeneration and Usher Syndrome. **Frmly:** RP Foundation Fighting Blindness.

★ 3147 ★ Foundation for Hand Research and Education
8501 Harcourt Rd.
PO Box 80434
Indianapolis, IN 46280-0434
Phone: (317)471-4340 **Free:** 800-888-HAND
Fax: (317)876-0462
Email: information@indianahandcenter.com
Website: http://www.indianahandcenter.com
Tony O'Connell, MALS, Fnd. Mgr.

Fnded: 1988. **Desc:** Promotes the advancement of hand surgery and research. Aims to improve the quality of life of persons with injuries or disorders of the hands and upper extremities. Conducts educational programs. **Pub:** *Indiana Hand Center Newsletter*, 3/year. Newsletter. Full color descriptions of hand surgery and rehabilitation. *Price:* $75/year. **Frmly:** Indiana Foundation for Hand Surgical Research.

★ 3148 ★ Foundation for Health (FFH)
337 East Ave.
Watertown, NY 13601-3829
Phone: (315)782-6664 **Free:** 800-724-7460
Fax: (315)782-6664
Email: gbonadio@imcnet.net
George Bonadio, Exec. Dir.

Fnded: 1972. **Desc:** Gathers and disseminates information regarding health; seeks to publicize "natural" laws of health in an effort to make excellent health and long, useful lives common throughout the world. Proclaims the simplicity and inexpensiveness of maintaining one's health in contrast to the complexity and expense of disease. Researches and develops nutrition and health related projects and programs. **Pub:** *Ask the Nutritionist*, weekly. Newspaper. • *Seven Disciplines of Health.* • Also contributes weekly health column to newspapers; plans to publish book.

★ 3149 ★ Foundation for Hospital Art
120 Stonemist Ct.
Roswell, GA 30076
Phone: (770)645-1717 **Fax:** (770)645-1720
Email: johnfeight@hospitalart.org
Website: http://www.hospitalart.org/about.html
John Feight, Founder

Fnded: 1984. **Desc:** Dedicated to involving patients and volunteers to create colorful, soothing artwork donated to hospitals to help soften the stressful hospital experience.

★ 3150 ★ Foundation for Ichthyosis and Related Skin Types (FIRST)
650 N Cannon Ave., Ste. 17
Lansdale, PA 19446
Phone: (215)631-1411 **Free:** 800-545-3286
Fax: (215)631-1413
Email: info@scalyskin.org
Website: http://www.scalyskin.org
Jean R. Pickford, Exec. Dir.

Fnded: 1981. **Mem:** 3,300. **Reg. Groups:** 10. **Desc:** Dedicated to helping persons affected with ichthyosis, a rare genetic skin disease characterized by dry, cracked, scaling and thickened skin, and related diseases. **Pub:** *A Handbook for Teachers of Children with Ichthyosis.* Handbook. Tool for parents to help make the transition to the school environment for children with ichthyosis. *Price:* $5. • *Butterflies: The Children of Ichthyosis.* Video. • *Ichthyosis: An Overview. Price:* Free. For members only; $1 for nonmembers; Free for members. • *Ichthyosis Focus*, quarterly. Newsletter. Features medical news, tips for day-to-day coping, and correspondence column for members who would like to exchange letters. *Price:* Free. For members only. • *Ichthyosis: The Genetics of Its Inheritance.* Booklet. Description of the genetic inheritance patterns for the different forms of ichthyosis. *Price:* Free. For members only; $1 for nonmembers; Free, available to members only. • *Release The Butterfly: A Handbook for Parents and Caregivers of Children with Ichthyosis.* Handbook. Covers care, medication, therapy, and nutrition for child with ichthyosis. *Price:* $5. **Frmly:** (1986) National Ichthyosis Foundation.

★ 3151 ★ Foundation for Informed Medical Decision Making (FIMDM)
40 Court St., 2nd Fl.
Boston, MA 02108
Phone: (617)367-2000
Email: smbagley@fimdm.org
Shannon Bagley, Off. Mgr.

Fnded: 1989. **Desc:** Gathers and contributes scientific research information for use in videotape programs on shared decision making topics. **Pub:** Video.

★ 3152 ★ Foundation for Innovation in Medicine (FIM)
411 North Ave. E
Cranford, NJ 07016
Phone: (908)272-2967 **Fax:** (908)272-4583
Email: fimdefelice@aol.com
Website: http://www.fimdefelice.org/
Stephen L. DeFelice, MD, Chair

Fnded: 1976. **Desc:** Seeks to regenerate interest in medical discovery and innovation, which the foundation believes flourished in the U.S. in the 1940s and 1950s, but has since declined despite "vastly increased public and private expenditures in research and development." Intends to monitor the state of innovation by conducting seminars and conferences. Encourages clinical research on natural substances and substances with little commercial value. **Pub:** *From Oysters to Insulin: Nature and Medicine at Odds.* Book. *Price:* $15.95. • *Nutraceutical White Paper. Price:* $10.

★ 3153 ★ Foundation for International Self Help Development (FISH)
19 Gordon Town Rd.
Kingston, Jamaica
Phone: (809)927-6715 **Fax:** (809)927-2757
Email: fish.jam@yahoo.com

Fnded: 1985. **Lang(s):** English. **Desc:** Seeks to improve the health and nutrition of the needy in Jamaica. Maintains medical, dental, and eye care clinic. Plans to operate programs in areas including community development, reforestation, and energy conservation and alternative fuels.

★ 3154 ★ Foundation for Pet Provided Therapy
PO Box 6308
Oceanside, CA 92058
Phone: (760)630-4824
Email: info@fppt.org
Website: http://fppt.org
Liz Palika, Founder

Desc: Promotes positive interaction between pets and people.

★ 3155 ★ Foundation for Physical Therapy (FPT)
c/o American Physical Therapy Association
1111 Fairfax St.
Alexandria, VA 22314-1488
Phone: (703)683-6743 **Free:** 800-875-1378
Fax: (703)684-7343
Email: foundation@apta.org
Website: http://www.apta.org/Foundation
Christine A. Williams, COO

Fnded: 1979. **Nat'l Groups:** 1. **Desc:** Supports the physical therapy profession's research needs by funding scientific and clinically-relevant physical therapy research.

★ 3156 ★ Foundation for the Promotion of Responsible Parenthood - Aruba (FPRP)
PO Box 2256
San Nicolas, Aruba
Phone: 297 8 48833 **Fax:** 297 8 41107
Email: arfamplan@setarnet.aw

Fnded: 1970. **Lang(s):** Dutch. **Desc:** Works to improve the quality of life of people living in Aruba through promotion of family planning and maternal and infant health care. Sponsors programs in family planning, sex education, and basic health care. Offers contraceptive services. Conducts research.

★ 3157 ★ Foundation for the Promotion of Responsible Parenthood Netherlands Antilles (FPRP) (Fundashon Famia Plania)
PO Box 308
Curacao, Netherlands Antilles
Phone: 599 9 4611323 **Fax:** 599 9 4611024

Mem: 11. **Lang(s):** Dutch. **Desc:** Advocates sexual and reproductive health, responsible parenthood and family planning. Seeks to reduce the number of unwanted pregnancies and abortions. Encourages public knowledge of AIDS and other sexually transmitted diseases. Offers educational programs on sexual and reproductive health, family planning and maternal and infant health care.

★ 3158 ★ Foundation for Revitalization of Local Health (FRLHT)
50 MSH Layout, 2nd Stage, 3rd Main
Anandnagar
Bangalore 560 024, Karnataka, India
Phone: 91 80 23336909 **Fax:** 91 80 3334167
Email: root@frlht.ernet.in

Fnded: 1991. **Lang(s):** English, Hindi. **Desc:** Promotes traditional medicine as an integral part of public health programs in developing areas. Facilitates international cooperation in understanding the theoretical foundation and epistemology of traditional medical practices; works to preserve the biodiversity upon which traditional medicine depends. Gathers and disseminates information on medicinal plants. Promotes development of traditional medical centers. **Pub:** *Amruth*, bimonthly. Magazine.

★ 3159 ★ Foundation for Science and Disability (FSD)
236 Grand St.
Morgantown, WV 26501-7509
Phone: (304)293-5201 **Fax:** (304)293-6363
Email: ekeller@wvu.edu
Website: http://www.as.wvu.edu/~scidis/organize/fsd.html
E. C. Keller, Jr., Treas.

Fnded: 1978. **Mem:** 206. **Nat'l Groups:** 1. **Desc:** Disabled scientists and interested individuals. Offers consultation and advice concerning problems faced by persons with disabilities in scientific fields. **Pub:** *The Abled Disabled in Science*, periodic. Book. • *Newsletter of FSD*, semiannual. Newsletter. *Price:* available to members only. **Frmly:** (1993) Foundation for Science and the Handicapped.

★ 3160 ★ Foundation for the Support of International Medical Training (FSIMT)
417 Center St.
Lewiston, NY 14092
Phone: (716)754-4883
Email: iamat@sentex.net
Mrs. M. A. Uffer, Pres.

Fnded: 1960. **Mem:** 6000,000. **Desc:** Individuals and corporations organized to provide information regarding the availability of competent medical care overseas and information concerning sanitary conditions, health hazards, and climatic conditions in various parts of the world. Offers detailed guidance on vaccination and immunization requirements and tropical diseases. **Pub:** *Be Aware of Schistosomiasis.* • *How to Protect Yourself Against Malaria*, annual. • *Immunization Chart*, annual. • *Set of 24 World Climate Charts*, annual. • *Traveller Clinical Chart*, annual. • *When Hiking Through Latin America, Be Alert to Chagas' Disease*, annual. • *World Malaria Risk Chart*, annual. • *World Schistosomiasis Risk Chart*, annual. • Brochure, annual. • Directory, annual.

★ 3161 ★ Foundation for Women's Health Research and Development (FORWARD)
40 Eastbourne Terrace
London W2 3QR, United Kingdom
Phone: 44 171 7252606 **Fax:** 44 171 7252796
Email: forward@forwarduk.org.uk
Website: http://www.forwarduk.org.uk

Fnded: 1983. **Mem:** 951. **Nat'l Groups:** 10. **Reg. Groups:** 10. **Lang(s):** English. **Desc:** Promotes the studies of women's health research and development throughout Europe and other western countries and Africa. Supports the rights of women and children. Promotes the prevention of early childhood marriage that contributes to VVF and RVF. Protects women and children from becoming victims of abuse. Opposes and fights for the elimination of the practice of genital mutilation of young girls. Disseminates information. Conducts training programs. **Pub:** *Another Form of Physical Abuse: Prevention of Female Genital Mutilation in the United Kingdom.* Video. • *Child Protection and Female Genital Mutilation: Advice for Health, Education, and Social Work Professionals.* Book. • *Cutting the Rose: Female Genital Mutilation - The Practice and its Prevention.* • *Female Genital Mutilation Proposals for Change.* • *Holistic Care for Women: A Practical Guide for Midwives.* Offers detailed advice for midwives caring for women affected by FGM. • *Out of Sight, Out of Mind?.* Report of a survey into interagency policies and procedures relating to female genital mutilation in England and Wales. • *Report on the First Study Conference on Genital Mutilation of Girls in Europe July 1992 in London.* Position papers and reports.

★ 3162 ★ Fragile X Society
c/o Mrs. Lesley Walker
53 Winchelsea Lane
Hastings TN35 4LG, United Kingdom
Phone: 44 142 4813147
Email: lesley@fragilex.force9.co.uk
Website: http://www.fragilex.org.uk

Fnded: 1990. **Mem:** 1,400. **Desc:** Aims to provide support and comprehensive information to families whose children and adult relatives have fragile X syndrome, to raise awareness of fragile X and to encourage research. **Pub:** Newsletter, 3/year.

★ 3163 ★ Freedom From Fear (FFF)
308 Seaview Ave.
Staten Island, NY 10305
Phone: (718)351-1717 **Fax:** (718)667-8893
Website: http://www.freedomfromfear.org/
Mary Guardino, Founder/Exec. Dir.

Fnded: 1984. **Desc:** Seeks to provide better understanding of the causes and treatments of mental illnesses.

★ 3164 ★ Freeman-Sheldon Parent Support Group (FSPSG)
509 E Northmont Way
Salt Lake City, UT 84103-3324
Phone: (801)364-7060
Email: fspsg@aol.com
Website: http://www.fspsg.org
Joyce Dolcourt, Exec. Dir.

Fnded: 1982. **Mem:** 150. **Nat'l Groups:** 1. **Desc:** Families affected by Freeman-Sheldon Syndrome; interested health professionals. (Freeman-Sheldon Syndrome, also known as Whistling Face Syndrome and Cranio-Carpo-Tarsal Dysplasia, is a disorder characterized by a flat, stiff, immobile face with excessively bulging cheeks, resembling that seen when whistling; retarded growth, flexion contraction of the fingers and thumbs, walking difficulties, and speech impairment may also be experienced. The syndrome is believed to be transmitted genetically.) Compiles information on the growth and development of individuals with Freeman-Sheldon Syndrome; disseminates information for parents of afflicted children. Operates referral services; promotes medical research. **Pub:** *FSPSG Newsletter*, annual. Newsletter. Updates members on research and news. • Also publishes brochures. Bibliography of Medical Literature on Freeman-Sheldon syndrome.

★ 3165 ★ French Committee of the World Veterinary Association (FCWVA) (Comite Francais de l'Association Mondiale Veterinaire — CFAMV)
Ecole Natl. Veterinaire d'Alfort
F-94704 Maisons-Alfort Cedex, France
Phone: 33 1 43967021 **Fax:** 33 1 43967022
Email: cfamv@vet-alfort.fr
Fnded: 1964. **Desc:** No further information was available for this edition.

★ 3166 ★ French Diabetes Association (FDA) (Association Francaise des Diabetiques — AFD)
58, rue Alexandre Dumas
F-75544 Paris Cedex 11, France
Phone: 33 1 40092425 **Fax:** 33 1 40092030
Email: afdsiege@noos.fr
Website: http://www.afd.asso.fr
Fnded: 1938. **Mem:** 30,000. **Reg. Groups:** 130. **Local Groups:** 130. **Lang(s):** English, French. **Desc:** Individuals with diabetes in France. Works to inform, assist, and defend diabetics. Furthers public understanding of diabetes by disseminating information to the public and medical specialists. **Pub:** *Equilibre*, quarterly. Magazine. • *Medical and Informations sur le Diabete*, periodic.

★ 3167 ★ French-Language Association of Scientific Psychology (Association de Psychologie Scuentifique de Langue Francaise — APSLF)
29, av R Schumann
F-13621 Aix-en-Provence, France
Fax: 33 4 542590312
Fnded: 1950. **Desc:** Stimulates contacts between psychologists using the French language.

★ 3168 ★ French-Language Association for the Study of Diabetes and Metabolic Disorders (Association de Langue Francaise pour l'Etude du Diabete et des Maladies Metaboliques — ALFEDIAM)
58, rue Alexandre Dumas
F-75011 Paris, France
Phone: 33 1 40098907 **Fax:** 33 1 40092914
Email: alfediam@magic.fr
Website: http://www.alfediam.org
Fnded: 1954. **Mem:** 1,150. **Lang(s):** English, French. **Desc:** Health care professionals and researchers with an interest in diabetes and other metabolic disorders. Seeks to advance the prevention, diagnosis, and treatment of metabolic disorders. Provides support and services to people with diabetes and their families; serves as a clearinghouse on research on metabolic disorders; sponsors research and continuing professional development programs. **Pub:** *Diabetes and Metabolism*, bimonthly. Magazine.

★ 3169 ★ French-Language Society of Medical Psychology
95, bd Pinel
F-69677 Bron, France
Phone: 33 4 72358694 **Fax:** 33 4 72358593
Fnded: 1960.

★ 3170 ★ French-Language Society of Nutrition and Dietetics (Societe de Nutrition et de Dietetique de Langue Francaise — SNDLF)
Hopital Bichat
F-75877 Paris, France
Phone: 33 1 40257200 **Fax:** 33 1 40258783
Fnded: 1963.

★ 3171 ★ French Pharmacology Society (Societe Francaise de Pharmacologistes)
c/o Philippe Lechat
Department of Pharmacology
Hopital Pitie Salpetriere
47 Boulevard de l'Hopital
F-75013 Paris, France
Phone: 33 1 42161682 **Fax:** 33 1 42161688
Email: philippe.lechat@psl.ap-hop-paris.fr
Website: http://www.pharmacol-fr.org
Mem: 1,017. **Desc:** Promotes pharmacology in France.

★ 3172 ★ French Society of Cardiology
15 rue Cels
F-75014 Paris, France
Phone: 33 1 43223333 **Fax:** 33 1 43226361
Email: contact@cardio-sfc.org
Website: http://www.sfcardio.net
Mem: 1,873. **Desc:** Promotes the study of cardiology in France.

★ 3173 ★ French Society of Genetics (SFG)
3b, rue de la Ferollerie
F-45071 Orleans, France
Phone: 33 2 38515438
Fnded: 1987.

★ 3174 ★ French Society of Gerontology (FSG) (Societe Francaise de Gerontologie — SFG)
Faculte de Medecine Pite-Salpetriere - 91
Boulevard de l'Hopital
F-75013 Paris, France
Phone: 33 1 40779645 **Fax:** 33 1 40779644
Email: michel-frossard@umpf.grenoble.fr
Fnded: 1961. **Lang(s):** French. **Desc:** Health care professionals treating the elderly; scientists and clinicians with an interest in the aging process and diseases of the aged. Works to insure high standards of research and practice in gerontology, and to maximize availability of gerontological services. Conducts research and educational activities.

★ 3175 ★ French Society of History of Ophthalmology (Societe francophone d'histoire de l'ophtalmologie — SFHO)
4, rue Ferroussat
F-69630 Chaponost, France
Email: heitz@sdv.fr
Website: http://www.histoph.org
Fnded: 1980. **Mem:** 150.

★ 3176 ★ French Society of Manual Medicine, Orthopedic and Osteopathics (Societe Francaise de Medecine Manuelle Orthopedique et Osteopathique — SOFMMOO)
56, av Joseph Giordan
F-06200 Nice, France
Phone: 33 4 93211043 **Fax:** 33 4 93216547
Fnded: 1968. **Desc:** Promotes and teaches orthopedic medicine and manual medicine.

★ 3177 ★ French Society of Psychosomatic Obstetrics and Gynaecology
c/o Dr. Sylvain Mimoun
45 rue de Maubeuge
F-75009 Paris, France
Fax: 33 1 42802512
Email: sylvain.mimoun@free.fr
Website: http://sfgop.free.fr
Desc: Promotes the study of psychobiological and psychosocial, ethical and cross-cultural problems in the fields of obstetrics and gynaecology, women's health and reproductive health; faciliates the dissemination of new information in these fields. **Pub:** *Journal of Psychosomatic Obstetrics and Gynecology*. Journal.

★ 3178 ★ French-Speaking Association of Surgical Endocrinology (FSASE) (Association Francophone de Chirurgie Enocrinienne — AFCE)
Hopital de la Timone
Service de Chirurgie Generale et Endocrinienne
Centre Hospitalier Reg Universite de Lyon
1, rue de l'Antiquaille
F-69321 Lyon Cedex 5, France
Phone: 33 4 72385036 **Fax:** 33 4 72386540
Fnded: 1988. **Mem:** 125. **Lang(s):** English, French. **Desc:** Surgical endocrinologists. Seeks to advance the study, teaching, and practice of surgical endocrinology. Sponsors research programs and continuing professional development courses. **Pub:** *Anales de chisurgie*, 10/year. Journal.

★ 3179 ★ French-Speaking Neuropsychological Society (Societe de Neuropsychologie de Langue Francaise)
Hopital Purpan
place de Dr. Baylac
F- 31059 Toulouse Cedex, France
Phone: 33 5 61779505 **Fax:** 33 5 61499524
Email: agniel@purpan.inserm.fr
Website: http://www.ulg.ac.be/neuropsy/snlf/
Fnded: 1977. **Mem:** 450. **Lang(s):** French. **Pub:** *Revue de Neuropsychologie*, quarterly.

★ 3180 ★ Friedreichs Ataxia Society of Ireland (FASI)
San Martino
Mart Ln.
Foxrock
Dublin 18, Ireland
Phone: 353 1 2894788 **Fax:** 353 1 2898845
Email: fasi@eircom.net
Website: http://www.fasi.ie
Fnded: 1980. **Mem:** 250. **Nat'l Groups:** 1. **Lang(s):** English. **Desc:** Individuals and organizations. Seeks to improve the quality of life of people with Friedreich's ataxia and their families. Makes available support and services; conducts educational and advocacy campaigns. **Pub:** *FASI Newsletter*, annual. Newsletter.

★ 3181 ★ Friendly Hand Foundation (FHF)
347 S Normandie
Los Angeles, CA 90020
Phone: (213)389-9964 **Fax:** (213)389-9747
Email: friendlyhous@aol.com
Peggy Albrecht, Exec. Dir.
Fnded: 1951. **Desc:** Operates Friendly House, a home to aid in the recovery of alcoholic women. Provides a home-like setting, love and understanding, and the companionship of individuals in similar situations to women recovering from alcohol dependence. Not officially affiliated with Alcoholics Anonymous World Services, but women in the home learn the principles of AA as part of group and individual therapy; the average stay at Friendly House is four weeks. Supported by contributions and through projects undertaken by affiliated groups of alcoholic and nonalcoholic women in California (known as Sweet Hearts and Grateful Hearts).

★ 3182 ★ Friends of Celiac Disease Research
8832 N Port Washington Rd., No. 204
Milwaukee, WI 53217
Phone: (414)540-6679 **Fax:** (414)540-0587

Email: friends@aero.net
Website: http://www.friendsofceliac.com
Dana Tehako-Esser, Exec. Dir.
Fnded: 1999. **Desc:** Devoted to assisting people with celiac disease and dermatitis herpetiformis; supports research and education.

★ 3183 ★ Friends of the Jose Carreras International Leukemia Foundation
1100 Fairview Ave. N, D5-100
PO Box 19024
Seattle, WA 98109-1024
Phone: (206)667-7108 **Fax:** (206)667-6498
Email: friendsjc@carrerasfoundation.org
Website: http://www.carrerasfoundation.org
Jose Carreras, Pres.
Fnded: 1990. **Desc:** Raises funds for fellowship awards focused on research into the treatment and cure of leukemia and related blood disorders. **Pub:** *Friends to Friends*, 3/year. Newsletter. Current news about the Foundation.

★ 3184 ★ Friends of the National Institute of Dental and Craniofacial Research
1555 Connecticut Ave. NW, Ste. 200
Washington, DC 20036
Phone: (202)483-1057 **Fax:** (202)462-9043
Email: alec@fnider.org
Website: http://www.fnidcr.org
Alec Stone, Exec. Dir.
Fnded: 1998. **Mem:** 250. **Desc:** Individuals, institutions, and corporations with an interest in dental research. Believes dental, oral and craniofacial health are of critical importance to the well-being of society. **Pub:** *Online Update!*, monthly. Newsletter. • *Update!*, semiannual. Newsletter.

★ 3185 ★ Friends of the National Library of Medicine
1555 Connecticut Ave., NW, Ste. 200
Washington, DC 20036
Phone: (202)462-0992 **Fax:** (202)462-9043
Email: info@fnlm.org
Website: http://www.fnlm.org
Alec Stone, Exec. Dir.
Fnded: 1986. **Mem:** 500. **Desc:** Seeks to improve health by increasing the use of the latest, most effective medical and scientific information by health care professionals, scientists, and the general public. Strives to educate the health, corporate, and public communities about the National Library of Medicine by building a coalition of financial and others supporters.

★ 3186 ★ Friends of St. Luke's Hospital
c/o St. Luke's Hospital
Highfield Rd.
Rathgar
Dublin 6, Ireland
Phone: 353 1 4065102 **Fax:** 353 1 4065237
Email: info@friendsofstlukes.ie
Website: http://www.friendsofstlukes.ie
Fnded: 1981. **Mem:** 15. **Desc:** Seeks to enhance the care, comfort and management of cancer patients at Dublin's St. Luke's Hospital. Works to ensure that patients benefit to the fullest extent from the advances in techniques and equipment.

★ 3187 ★ Friends of Temperance (FT) (Raittiuden Ystavat — RY)
Annankatu 29 A 9
FIN-00100 Helsinki, Finland
Phone: 358 9 54209522 **Fax:** 358 9 54209555
Email: ry@raitis.fi
Website: http://www.raitis.fi
Fnded: 1853. **Mem:** 10,000. **Local Groups:** 100. **Lang(s):** English, Finnish, Swedish. **Desc:** Temperance and substance abuse prevention and treatment organizations. Promotes increased involvement in temperance issues by the public and by development organizations worldwide. Conducts temperance education courses; facilitates cooperation among temperance organizations. **Pub:** *Ystavien Kesken*, QRT. Newsletter.

★ 3188 ★ Friends: The Association of Young People Who Stutter
1220 Rosita Rd.
Pacifica, CA 94044-4223
Free: (866)866-8335
Email: jtahlbach@aol.com
Website: http://www.friendswhostutter.org
John Ahlbach, Contact
Fnded: 1998. **Desc:** Children and teenagers who stutter; family members of young people who stutter; professionals working with people who stutter. Seeks to create a network of love and support for members; promotes increased self-esteem among young people who stutter. Facilitates communication among members. **Pub:** *Reaching Out*, 9/year. Journal.

★ 3189 ★ Frontier Nursing Service (FNS)
132 FNS Dr.
Wendover, KY 41775
Phone: (606)672-2317 **Fax:** (606)672-3022
Website: http://www.frontiernursing.org
Barb Gibson, Exec. Asst.
Fnded: 1925. **Mem:** 15. **Desc:** Provides health care to persons in approximately 1000 square miles of eastern Kentucky using a 40-bed hospital, two primary care centers, three rural health clinics, and a home health agency. Operates Frontier School of Midwifery and Family Nursing. Provides social and ancillary services; conducts research on health services; compiles statistics; offers educational programs. Maintains a hall of fame and museum. **Pub:** *Quarterly Bulletin*. Bulletin. *Price:* $5 for individuals; $10 for institutions. • Brochure, annual. For Christmas appeal.

★ 3190 ★ Fund for Podiatric Medical Education (FPME)
9312 Old Georgetown Rd.
Bethesda, MD 20814
Phone: (301)581-9200 **Fax:** (301)530-2752
Email: mpgaujean@apma.org
Website: http://www.apma.org/fpme/fundmain.htm
Steven J. Berlin, Pres.
Fnded: 1959. **Desc:** Open to all People who wish to join. Offers financial support to third and fourth year podiatric medical students. Awards scholarships.

★ 3191 ★ Fundacion ALFA-1 de Puerto Rico
PO Box 6729
Bayamon, PR 00960-9007
Phone: (787)743-0268 **Fax:** (787)743-0268
Email: fundacion.alfa1@alfa1.org
Website: http://www.alfa1.org
Elaine Alfonzo, Coord.
Fnded: 1996. **Desc:** Offers support and education for the Spanish speaking Alpha 1-Antitrypsin Deficiency patients and their families. Distributes Spanish educational materials. Works to increase awareness about Alpha 1-Antitrypsin Deficiency and the importance of early detection and treatment. **Frmly:** (1999) Puerto Rico Alpha 1 Support Group.

★ 3192 ★ Fundacion Alzheimer Espana (FAE)
c/Pedro Muguruza, 1 6o C
E-28036 Madrid, Spain
Phone: 34 91 3431165 **Fax:** 34 91 3595450
Email: alzheuro@yahoo.es
Fnded: 1991. **Lang(s):** English, Spanish. **Desc:** Individuals and organizations. Seeks to improve the quality of life of people with Alzheimer's disease and their families. Makes available support and services; facilitates research on Alzheimer's disease and related disorders; conducts educational programs.

★ 3193 ★ Fundacion Antidrogas de El Salvador
71 S Ave. and Olympic Ave. No. 3718
Colonia Step.
San Salvador, El Salvador
Phone: 503 982233 **Fax:** 503 234873
Email: fundasalva@ejje.com
Fnded: 1989. **Mem:** 50. **Lang(s):** Spanish. **Desc:** Works to prevent substance abuse among at-risk children and youths. Conducts activities for at-risk youths in urban areas; makes available services for young people attempting to quit abusing substances.

★ 3194 ★ G-Jo Institute
PO Box 1460
Columbus, NC 28722-1460
Phone: (828)863-4660
Email: office@g-jo.com
Website: http://www.g-jo.com
Michael Blate, Exec. Dir.
Fnded: 1977. **Mem:** 3,000. **Desc:** People interested in "self-health" techniques that are natural, require no drugs or medications, and are based on traditional Oriental healing philosophies, especially acupuncture and acupressure. Objective is to promote the use of self-health techniques. Makes available charts and teaching guides. Provides classes in self-health methods and natural (vegetarian) cooking. Conducts radio program and research on natural health and healing. Sponsors Vegetarian Gourmet Society. Institute derives name from G-Jo, the easiest form of acupressure. Publishes self-health reports.

★ 3195 ★ Gambia Diabetes Association
c/o Mr. Momodou Lamin Jaiteh
PO Box 1853
Banjul, Gambia
Phone: 220 228223 **Fax:** 220 225909
Email: balamere@qanet.gm
Website: http://www.diabetesafrica.com/idfmembers.html
Desc: Represents people with diabetes. Promotes research and support of those with diabetes in Gambia.

★ 3196 ★ Gastro-Intestinal Research Foundation (GIRF)
c/o Joseph B. Kirsner, M.D.
70 E Lake St., Ste. 1015
Chicago, IL 60601-5907
Phone: (312)332-1350
Email: girf@girf.org
Website: http://www.girf.org
Joseph B. Kirsner, MD, Contact
Fnded: 1967. **Desc:** Physician-clinicians and physician-scientists. Committed to the goal of solving the problems of digestive diseases.

★ 3197 ★ Gauchers Association (GA)
25 W Cottages
London NW6 1RJ, United Kingdom
Phone: 44 207 4331121
Email: office@gauchersassociation.org.uk
Website: http://www.gaucher.org.uk
Fnded: 1991. **Lang(s):** English. **Desc:** Individuals with Gaucher's disease. (Gaucher's disease is a genetic disorder resulting in enzyme deficiency, producing symptoms including anemia, fatigue, bone pain and degeneration, easy bruising, and a tendency to bleed. The rare Type 2 and Type 3 forms of Gaucher's disease can also cause various neurological problems.) Seeks to improve the quality of life of people with Gaucher's disease; encourages medical research on the diagnosis, prevention, and treatment of the disease. Serves as a support group for people with Gaucher's disease; works to increase the availability of enzyme treatments; facilitates contact among the families of people with Gaucher's disease in the UK.

★ 3198 ★ Gay and Lesbian Medical Association (GLMA)
459 Fulton St., Ste. 107
San Francisco, CA 94102
Phone: (415)255-4547 **Fax:** (415)255-4784
Email: info@glma.org
Website: http://www.glma.org
Maureen S. O'Leary, Exec. Dir.

Fnded: 1981. **Mem:** 2,000. **Desc:** Physicians and allied health professionals. Seeks elimination of discrimination on the basis of gender identity and sexual orientation in the health professions; promotes unprejudiced medical care for gay and lesbian patients through advocacy and education. Maintains a referral and support program for HIV infected health care workers. Sponsors annual continuing medical education (CME, CEU) symposium on lesbian and gay health issues. Offers support to lesbian, gay, bisexual, and transgendered health care workers; encourages research into the health needs of gays and lesbians. Maintains liaison with medical schools and other organizations concerning needs of gay patients and professionals; fosters communication and cooperation among members and other groups and individuals supportive of gay and lesbian physicians. Sponsors Lesbian Health Fund for researching lesbian health needs. **Pub:** *GLMA Report*, quarterly. Newsletter. Covers the activities of the association, the medical community, and the public regarding lesbian and gay health issues. *Price:* Included in membership dues. • *Journal of the Gay and Lesbian Medical Association*, quarterly. Journal. **Frmly:** American Association of Physicians for Human Rights.

★ 3199 ★ Gay Men's Health Crisis (GMHC)
119 W 24th St.
The Tisch Bldg.
New York, NY 10011-1913
Phone: (212)367-1000 **Free:** 800-243-7692
Fax: (212)367-1236
Email: hotline@gmhc.org
Website: http://www.gmhc.org
Ana Oliveira, Exec. Dir.

Fnded: 1982. **Mem:** 14,000. **Desc:** GMHC is "the world's most experienced and comprehensive not-for-profit AIDS service organization." Provides direct social services to people coping with HIV/AIDS, educates the public about HIV, and advocates at all levels of government for sound AIDS policies. **Pub:** *Program Service News*, monthly. Newsletter. • *Treatment Issues*, monthly. Newsletter. *Price:* $55 individuals; $95 physicians/institutions/international; Sliding scale for HIV-positive and/or low-income. • *The Volunteer*, bimonthly. Newsletter. Updates medical, clinical, political, and referral information on AIDS. Includes calendar of events. *Price:* Free. • Catalog.Contains marketed education materials. • Pamphlets.Prevention of AIDS materials.

★ 3200 ★ Gazette International Networking Institute (GINI)
4207 Lindell Blvd., No. 110
Saint Louis, MO 63108-2915
Phone: (314)534-0475 **Fax:** (314)534-5070
Email: gini_intl@msn.com
Website: http://www.post-polio.org
Joan L. Headley, Dir.

Fnded: 1958. **Mem:** 6,500. **Desc:** Polio survivors, ventilator users, other individuals with neuromuscular diseases, health care personnel, insurance agencies, government agencies, independent living centers, and interested others. Works to inform, encourage, dignify, and sustain people with disabilities. Seeks to create a communications network to provide information on issues related to disabilities. Serves as clearinghouse for information on polio, ventilators, neuromuscular diseases, and independent living. Sponsors seminars. Coordinates International Polio Network and International Ventilator Users Network. **Pub:** *Handbook on the Late Effects of Poliomyelitis for Physicians and Survivors.* Handbook. *Price:* $18.50/copy. • *IUUN Resource Directory*, annual. Directory. *Price:* $5/copy. • *IVUN News*, semiannual. Newsletter. Includes information for those interested in home mechanical ventilation. *Price:* $17/year. • *Polio Network News*, quarterly. Contains information about the late effects of polio and topics related to disability. *Price:* $20/year for institutions/individuals. • *Post Polio Directory*, annual. Directory. Lists self-identified clinics, health professionals, and support groups knowledgeable about the late effects of polio. *Price:* $5/copy for individuals. • *Rehabilitation Gazette*, semiannual. Journal. Written by persons with disabilities. *Price:* $12. • *Rehabilitation into Independent Living.* **Frmly:** (1983) Rehabilitation Gazette.

★ 3201 ★ General Association of Municipal Health and Technical Experts (GAMHTE)
(Association Generale des Hygienistes et Techniciens Municipaux — AGHTM)
83 Av. Foch
BP 3916
F-75761 Paris cedex 16, France
Phone: 33 1 53701353 **Fax:** 33 1 53701340
Email: aghtm@aghtm.org
Website: http://www.aghtm.org

Fnded: 1905. **Mem:** 3,500. **Local Groups:** 5. **Lang(s):** French. **Desc:** Engineers, engineering consultants, technicians, architects, scientists, administrators, and municipal and private services in 32 countries. Objectives are to: stimulate fundamental and applied research on urban and rural public hygiene; disseminate findings of such research; encourage the exchange of information and ideas among members. Areas of interest include city planning, energy management, traffic problems, and pollution prevention. Operates information service; organizes field tours.

★ 3202 ★ General Chiropractic Council (GCC)
344-354 Gray's Inn Rd.
London WC1X 8BP, United Kingdom
Phone: 44 20 77135155 **Fax:** 44 20 77135844
Email: enquiries@gcc-uk.org
Website: http://www.gcc-uk.org/

Fnded: 1999. **Desc:** Aims to protect the public by regulating Chiropractors; set standards of chiropractic education, practice and conduct.

★ 3203 ★ General Council and Register of Naturopaths
Goswell House
2 Goswel Rd.
Somerset BA16 0JG, United Kingdom
Phone: 44 870 7456984 **Fax:** 44 870 7456985
Email: admin@naturopathy.org.uk
Website: http://www.naturopathy.org.uk

Fnded: 1964. **Mem:** 325. **Desc:** Fully qualified naturopathic practitioners. Maintains educational, professional and ethical standards and the safe practice of naturopathy for the benefit and protection of the public. **Pub:** Membership Directory, annual.

★ 3204 ★ General Dental Council (GDC)
c/o Antony Townsend, Chief Exec./Registrar
37 Wimpole St.
London W1G 8DQ, United Kingdom
Phone: 44 207 8873800 **Fax:** 44 207 2243294
Email: information@gdc-uk.org
Website: http://www.gdc-uk.org

Fnded: 1956. **Mem:** 29. **Desc:** Regulatory body of the dental profession; registers all qualified dentists, dental hygienists and dental therapists. **Pub:** *Dentists Register*, annual. • *Maintaining Standards.* • *Minutes of Meeting of the Council and Professional Conduct Committee*, annual. Proceedings. • *Rolls of Dental Auxiliaries*, annual. • *Specialist Lists*, annual.

★ 3205 ★ General Dental Practitioners Association
Victoria House
Victoria Rd.
Barnsley S70 2BB, United Kingdom
Phone: 44 1226 299020 **Fax:** 44 1226 299629

★ 3206 ★ General Hypnotherapy Register (GHR)
PO Box 204
Lymington S041 6WP, United Kingdom
Phone: 44 1590 683770 **Fax:** 44 1590 683770
Email: admin@general-hypnotherapy-register.com
Website: http://www.general-hypnotherapy-register.com

Fnded: 2000. **Mem:** 1,000. **Desc:** Counselors and therapists, mainly offering short-term treatment in private practice. Most members offer hypnotherapy as their main method of treatment. To represent and protect the interests of independent therapists and hypnotherapists. To provide referrals lists of practitioners in which the public may have full confidence by maintaining high standards of practice and conduct among members. Provides register of practitioners. **Pub:** Bulletin, bimonthly. **Frmly:** (1997) National Council of Psychotherapists and Hypnotherapy Register; (2000) National Council of Psychotherapists.

★ 3207 ★ General Medical Council
178 Great Portland St.
London W1N 5JE, United Kingdom
Phone: 44 207 5807642 **Fax:** 44 207 9153641
Email: gmc@gmc.uk.org

Fnded: 1858. **Mem:** 102. **Desc:** Doctors elected by UK doctors or appointed by UK universities with medical schools and by Royal Colleges. Lay members nominated by Privy Council. Protects the public by overseeing medical education, keeping a register of qualified doctors and taking action where a doctor's fitness to pratise is in doubt. **Pub:** *Duties of a Doctor - Guidance on Professional Ethics.* • *GMC News Review*, semiannual. Newsletter. • *Medical Register*, annual. • Annual Report, annual.

★ 3208 ★ General Osteopathic Council (GOsC)
Osteopathy House
176 Tower Bridge Rd.
London SE1 3LU, United Kingdom
Phone: 44 171 3576655
Email: concerns@osteopathy.org.uk
Website: http://www.osteopathy.org.uk/index.htm

Desc: Promotes the profession of Osteopathy in the United Kingdom; provides a Code of Practice which sets out standards of conduct and practice for all osteopaths. **Pub:** *The Osteopath*, monthly. Journal. Includes registrar's report, book reviews, letters, media reviews.

★ 3209 ★ General Trade Union of Health Services
22 El-Sheikh Kamar St.
El-Sakakiny
Cairo, Egypt
Mem: 56,000.

★ 3210 ★ Genetic Alliance (GA)
4301 Connecticut Ave. NW, Ste. 404
Washington, DC 20008
Phone: (202)966-5557 **Free:** 800-336-4363
Fax: (202)966-8553
Email: info@geneticalliance.org
Website: http://www.geneticalliance.org
Mary E. Davidson, MSW, Exec. Dir.

Fnded: 1986. **Mem:** 884. **Desc:** Voluntary genetic organizations; professionals and other interested individuals. Promotes the health and well-being of individuals and families affected by genetic disorders. Provides a forum for the discussion of cross-disability similarities and the identification of available resources. Fosters a partnership among consumers and professionals to enhance education and service for and represent the needs of individuals affected by genetic disorders. Supports networking efforts of members with government agencies, professional groups, service providers, and organizations. Provides technical assistance to genetic support groups. Disseminates information to the public on available resources and referrals. Makes available traveling educational exhibit for member organizations. **Pub:** *Alliance Alert*, monthly. Newsletter. Includes announcements, calendar of events, and membership information. *Price:* For members only. • *Alliance Health Insurance Resource Guide.* • *Informed Consent: Participation in Genetic Research Studies.* • *International Directory of Genetic Advocacy Organizations and Related Resources.* Directory. • *Media Reporting in the Genetic Age.* • Brochures. **Frmly:** (2001) Alliance of Genetic Support Groups.

★ 3211 ★ Genetic and Inherited Disorders Organization (GIDO)

Carmichael House
N Brunswick St.
Dublin 7, Ireland
Phone: 353 1 8721501
Email: inherited.disorders@ireland.com

Fnded: 1989. **Lang(s):** English, Irish. **Desc:** An umbrella organization for voluntary organizations in Ireland involved with genetic disorders.

★ 3212 ★ Genetics Society of Australia (GSA)

Department of Genetics
University of Melbourne
Parkville, VIC 3052, Australia
Phone: 61 3 83445137 **Fax:** 61 3 83445139
Email: p.batterham@genetics.unimelb.edu.au
Website: http://gsa.angis.org.au

Fnded: 1954. **Desc:** Fosters genetic research in Australia.

★ 3213 ★ Genetics Society of China

917 Datun Rd., Andingmenwai
Beijing 100101, People's Republic of China
Phone: 86 10 64919944 **Fax:** 86 10 64914896

★ 3214 ★ Georgian Association of Cardiology

National Center of Therapy
4 Ljubljana St.
380059 Tbilisi, Georgia
Phone: 995 32 942544 **Fax:** 995 32 955114
Email: cardiosociety@myoffice.net
Website: http://www.escardio.org/society/natsoc/georgia.htm

Mem: 96. **Desc:** Promotes the study of cardiology in Georgia.

★ 3215 ★ Georgian Gerontology and Geriatrics Society

4, Chachava St.
380059 Tbilisi, Georgia
Phone: 995 32 227630 **Fax:** 995 32 230147
Email: nodarkip@hotmail.com

Fnded: 1965. **Mem:** 50. **Lang(s):** English. **Desc:** Promotes gerontological research, training in the field of aging, and interests of gerontological organizations in international affairs.

★ 3216 ★ German Academy for Psychoanalysis (GAP) (Deutsche Akademie fur Psychoanalyse — DAP)

c/o Dr. Maria Ammon
Kantstr. 120/121
D-10625 Berlin, Germany
Phone: 49 30 3132893 **Fax:** 49 30 3132698
Email: dapberlin@aol.com
Website: http://www.dapberlin.de

Fnded: 1969. **Mem:** 100. **Lang(s):** English, German. **Desc:** Psychoanalysts, psychiatrists, and psychotherapists in Germany. Promotes training and research in psychoanalysis and psychotherapy within the framework of "dynamic psychiatry" as developed by the group's former president, Gunter Ammon. **Pub:** *Dynamic Psychiatry*, bimonthly. Journal. • *Handbook of Dynamic Psychiatry.* Handbook.

★ 3217 ★ German Association of Biologists (Verband Deutscher Biologen e.V. — VDBiol)

Von-Melle-Park 8
D-20146 Hamburg, Germany

★ 3218 ★ German Association of Dietitians (AGD) (Verband der Diatassistenten - Deutscher Bundesverband — VDDe.v.)

Postfach 10 51 12
D-40042 Dusseldorf, Germany
Phone: 49 211 162175 **Fax:** 49 211 357389
Email: vdd-duesseldorf@t-online.de
Website: http://www.vdd.de

Fnded: 1957. **Mem:** 3,800. **Lang(s):** English, German. **Desc:** Dietitians in Germany working to improve nutritional practices. Represents interests of members. Provides a forum for information exchange among dieticians, doctors, and other medical workers. Supports training of dietitians. Affiliated with the European Federation of the Associations of Dietitians (EFAD) and with the International Confederation of Dietetic Associations (ICDA). **Pub:** *Diet & Information*, bimonthly. Journal. • *Ernahrungs Umschau*, annual. Journal.

★ 3219 ★ German Association for Music Therapy (Deutsche Gesellschaft fur Musiktherapie e.V. — DGMT)

Libauer Str 17
D-10245 Berlin, Germany
Phone: 49 30 29492493 **Fax:** 49 30 29492494
Email: info@musiktherapie.de
Website: http://www.musiktherapie.de

★ 3220 ★ German Association for Physiotherapy (Deutscher Verband fur Physiotherapie)

Deutzer Freiheit 72-74
D-50679 Cologne, Germany
Phone: 49 221 9810270 **Fax:** 49 221 98102725
Email: info@zvk.org

Fnded: 1949. **Mem:** 32,000. **Nat'l Groups:** 16. **Reg. Groups:** 15. **Lang(s):** English, French. **Desc:** Promotes physical therapy education. Maintains contacts with medical and scientific associations. Represents the interests of physical therapists. Contracts with national health organizations (HMO's). **Pub:** *Curriculum, 4 vols.*. Journal. • *Krankengymnastik*, monthly. Brochure. Includes news from the Association. Provides summaries in English and French. • *Physiotherapy Profession.* Brochure. Special information brochures and sheets.

★ 3221 ★ German Association of Sport Psychology

c/o Prof. Dr. Henning Allmer
Deutsche Sprothochschule
Psychologisches Institut
Carl-Diem-Weg 6
D-50933 Cologne, Germany
Phone: 49 221 4982571 **Fax:** 49 221 4982817
Email: info@asp-sportpsychologie.de
Website: http://www.asp-sportpsychologie.org

Fnded: 1969. **Mem:** 250. **Desc:** Promotes and furthers development of sport psychology through research, teaching, and application. Fosters communication and exchange among members. **Pub:** *Psychologie & Sport*, quarterly. Journal.

★ 3222 ★ German Cardiac Society

Goethestrasse 38A
DE-40237 Dusseldorf, Germany
Phone: 49 211 6006920 **Fax:** 49 211 60069210
Email: info@dgkardio.de
Website: http://www.dgkardio.de

Fnded: 1927. **Mem:** 4,025. **Desc:** Promotes the study of cardiology in Germany. **Pub:** *Basic Research in Cardiology*, bimonthly. Journal. • *Cardio News*, monthly. Journal. • *Zeitschrift fur Kardiologie*, monthly. Journal.

★ 3223 ★ German Centre of Gerontology (Deutsches Zentrum fur Altersfragen e.V.)

Manfred-von-Richthofen-Str 2
D-12101 Berlin, Germany
Phone: 49 30 78604260 **Fax:** 49 30 7854350
Email: dza@dza.de
Website: http://www.dza.de

Fnded: 1973. **Desc:** Examines and evaluates continuous and new social policy issues of old age and aging and social policy measures of national importance; promotes research in the fields of employment and social security, life situations and life styles, social relationships and social participation, structures of health care and care delivery for the aged.

★ 3224 ★ German Dental Association (BundeszahnArztekammer-BZAK)

Kassenzahnarztliche
Bundesrereinigung
Universitatsstr. 73
D-50931 Cologne, Germany
Phone: 49 221 40010 **Fax:** 49 221 404035
Email: post@kzbv.de
Website: http://www.kzbv.de

Fnded: 1953. **State Groups:** 17. **Desc:** Promotes the dental sciences in Germany and represents German dentistry internationally. Promotes dental education and continuing education. Represents the interests of members to authorities, associations, and the public. Promotes quality assurance, is ethical body. **Pub:** *Zahnarztlidie Mi*, bimonthly. Journal. Contains professional and scientific papers and political statements on dentistry. **Frmly:** National Association of German Dentists; Bundesverband der Deutschen Zahnarzte.

★ 3225 ★ German Dermatological Society (GRS) (Deutsche Dermatologische Gesellschaft — DDG)

c/o Prof. Dr. Gernot Rassner
Department of Dermatology
Univ. of Tuebingen
Liebermeisterstr. 25
D-72076 Tubingen, Germany
Phone: 49 2151 523850 **Fax:** 49 7071 295113
Website: http://www.derma.de

Fnded: 1888. **Mem:** 1,800. **Lang(s):** English, German. **Desc:** Individuals united to promote dermatology. Conducts educational and research programs. **Pub:** *Der Hautarzt*, periodic.

★ 3226 ★ German Group Psychotherapeutic Society (GGPS) (Deutsche Gruppenpsychotherapeutische Gesellschaft — DGG)

c/o Dr. Dorothy Doldinger
Kantstrabe 120-121
D-10625 Berlin, Germany
Phone: 49 30 3132698 **Fax:** 49 30 3136959
Email: dgg@dynpsych.de

Fnded: 1968. **Mem:** 150. **Lang(s):** German. **Desc:** Group psychotherapists and experts in group dynamics. Practices in the field of prevention based on the concept of psychoanalytical group dynamics of the Berlin School founded by Dr. G. Ammon. Conducts research and therapy sessions; provides training to individuals interested in group dynamics. Holds group dynamic weekends. **Pub:** *Dynamic Psychiatry*, bimonthly.

★ 3227 ★ German Hospital Federation (GHF)
(Deutsche Krankenhausgesellschaft — DKG)
Strasse des 17. Juni 114
D-10623 Berlin, Germany
Phone: 49 30 39801 502 **Fax:** 49 30 39801 502
Email: berlinmail@dkgev.de
Website: http://www.dkgev.de

Fnded: 1949. **Mem:** 28. **Nat'l Groups:** 12. **Reg. Groups:** 16. **State Groups:** 12. **Lang(s):** English, French. **Desc:** Federal state hospital associations and welfare federations in Germany. Publicizes members' accomplishments in public health. Works to maintain and improve the performance of hospitals; fosters exchange of information among members. Serves as liaison between members and government and other organizations; makes recommendations to legislative bodies. **Pub:** *das Krankenhaus*, monthly. Magazine. **Frmly:** (1998) German Hospital Association.

★ 3228 ★ German Interdisciplinary Association of Critical Care Medicine
(Deutsche Interdisziplinare Vereinigung fur Intensiv- und Notfallmedizin — DIVI)
Koppensteinstr. 1
D-50935 Cologne, Germany
Phone: 49 221 436326 **Fax:** 49 221 436328
Email: a.karimi@uni-koeln.de
Website: http://www.divi-org.de

Fnded: 1989. **Desc:** Promotes the science of intensive and emergency medicine and their application.

★ 3229 ★ German Neuroscience Society
(Neurowissenschaftliche Gesellschaft e.V.)
c/o Meino Alexandra Gibson, Sec.
Max Delbruck Center for Moleculare Medizin
Robert Rossle Str. 10
D-13092 Berlin, Germany
Phone: 49 30 94063133 **Fax:** 49 30 94063819
Email: gibson@mdc-berlin.de
Website: http://nwg.glia.mdc-berlin.de

Fnded: 1993. **Mem:** 1,600. **Desc:** Supports research and education in the field of neuroscience; establishes political concepts; partners with industry; offers methodological courses and educational programs for teachers. **Pub:** *Neuroforum*, quarterly. Journal. Contains review articles, book reviews, historical and methodological articles, information on grants programs, prizes and more.

★ 3230 ★ German Nutrition Society
(Deutsche Gesellschaft fur Ernahrung e.V. — DGE)
Godesberger Allee 18
D-53175 Bonn, Germany
Phone: 49 228 3776600
Website: http://www.dge.de

Fnded: 1953. **Desc:** Supports nutritional scientific research; collects and evaluates results of related disciplines, and publishes them in a documentation.

★ 3231 ★ German Ophthalmological Society
(Deutsche Ophthalmologische Gesellschaft Heidelberg e.V. — DOG)
Berliner Str. 14
D-69120 Heidelberg, Germany
Phone: 49 6221411787 **Fax:** 49 6221484616
Email: dog-hd@t-online.de
Website: http://www.dog.org
Fnded: 1857.

★ 3232 ★ German Sleep Society
(Deutsche Gesellschaft fur Schlafforschung und Schlafmedizin e.V. — DGSM)
Schimmelpfengstr 2
D-34613 Schwalmstadt, Germany
Phone: 49 66912733 **Fax:** 49 66912823
Email: dgsm.mayer@t-online.de
Website: http://www.dgsm.de

Fnded: 1982. **Desc:** Fosters research on sleep and sleep disorders as well as development of clinical diagnosis and therapy of sleep-wake disorders.

★ 3233 ★ German Society of Anaesthesiology and Intensive Care Medicine (GSAIM)
(Deutsche Gesellschaft fur Anaesthesiologie und Intensivmedizin — DGAI)
Roritzerstrasse 27
D-90419 Nuremberg, Germany
Phone: 49 911 933780 **Fax:** 49 911 3938195
Email: dgai@dgai-ev.de
Website: http://www.dgai.de

Fnded: 1953. **Mem:** 9,600. **Desc:** Promotes scientific advancement and high standards of practice in anesthesiology and intensive care medicine. **Pub:** *Anaesthesie, Intensivmedizin, Notfallmedizin, Schmerztherapie*, periodic. Journal. • *Anaesthesiologie und Intensivmedizin*, periodic. • *Der Anaesthesist*, periodic.

★ 3234 ★ German Society for Aviation and Space Medicine (DGLRM)
(Deutsche Gesellschaft fur Luft- und Raumfahrtmedizin)
Konigswinter Strasse 522-524
D-53227 Bonn, Germany
Phone: 49 228 447528 **Fax:** 49 228 447707
Email: michael.reichert@dlr.de
Website: http://www.kp.dlr.de/DGLR

Fnded: 1963. **Mem:** 700. **Lang(s):** English, German. **Desc:** Scientists and physicians. Supports scientific work in the fields of aviation and space medicine. Conducts work group studies on ergonomics, the history of aviation medicine, and related subjects. Participates in the presentation of educational courses in aviation medicine for physicians. **Pub:** *Mitteilungen*, bimonthly.

★ 3235 ★ German Society for Disaster Medicine
(Deutsche Gesellschaft fur Katastrophenmedizin e.V. — DGKM)
Kafkastr 62
D-81737 Munich, Germany
Phone: 49 89 4147209 **Fax:** 49 89 67974368
Email: dgkm@dgkmev.de
Website: http://www.dgkmev.de

Desc: Promotes and supports the advancement of scientific and applied disaster medicine, including emergency medicine.

★ 3236 ★ German Society for Experimental and Clinical Pharmacology and Toxicology
(Deutsche Gesellschaft fur Experimentelle und Klinische Pharmakologie und Toxikologie e.v.)
c/o Prof. Kay Brune
Institut fur Exp. Und Klinische Pharmakologie und Toxikologi
Universitat Erlangen Nurnberg
Fahrstrasse 17
D-91054 Erlangen, Germany
Phone: 49 91 318522292 **Fax:** 49 91 318522774
Email: brune@pharmakologie.uni-erlangen.de
Website: http://www.dgpt-online.de

Mem: 2,600. **Desc:** Promotes experimental and clinical pharmacology and toxicology in Germany.

★ 3237 ★ German Society for Fat Science
(Deutsche Gesellschaft fur Fettwissenschaft e.V. — DGF)
Varrentrappstr 40-42
D-60486 Frankfurt am Main, Germany
Phone: 49 69 7917529 **Fax:** 49 69 7917564
Email: info@dgfett.de
Website: http://www.dgfett.de

Fnded: 1936. **Mem:** 350. **Desc:** Promotes scientific and applications-oriented research; supports the creation of a stimulating community where experts from research, technology and business have the opportunity to communicate their ideas and to learn from each other.

★ 3238 ★ German Society of Gerontology and Geriatrics
Schiffgraben 43
D-30175 Hannover, Germany
Phone: 49 40 65761660 **Fax:** 49 40 65761666
Email: info@dggg-online.de

Fnded: 1990. **Mem:** 1,250. **Desc:** Geriatricians, scientists, and other professionals with an interest in geriatric medicine. Works to improve health and welfare of elderly people.

★ 3239 ★ German Society for Hematology and Oncology
(Deutsche Gesellschaft fur Hamatologie und Onkologie e.V.)
Ernst-Heydemann-Str 6
Universitat zu Rostock
D-18057 Rostock, Germany
Phone: 49 381 4947420 **Fax:** 49 381 4947422
Email: sekretaer@dgho.de
Website: http://www.dgho.de

Desc: Promotes research, diagnostics and treatment of hematologic diseases and solid tumors.

★ 3240 ★ German Society of Neurogenetics
(Deutsche Gesellschaft fur Neurogenetik)
c/o Dr. Ulrich Mueller
Institut fur Humangenetik der Universitat
Shlangenzahl 14
D-35392 Giessen, Germany
Phone: 49 641 9041600 **Fax:** 49 641 9941609
Email: ulrich.mueller@humangenetik.med.uni-giessen.de

Fnded: 1994. **Desc:** Works to enhance scientific exchange between those disciplines involved in genetics of normal and abnormal function of the nervous system, including biophysics, human genetics, cell biology, neuroanatomy, neurosurgery, neurology, neuropathology, and psychiatry. **Pub:** Newsletter, semiannual.

★ 3241 ★ German Society for Physical Medicine and Rehabilitation
(Deutsche Gesellschaft fur Physikalische Medizin und Rehabilitation — DGPMR)
Carl-Neuberg-Str 1
D-30625 Hannover, Germany
Phone: 49 511 5324124 **Fax:** 49 511 5328124
Email: gutenbrunner.christoph@mh-hannover.de
Website: http://www.dgpmr.de

Desc: Aims to maintain and to promote the development of physical medicine, including balneology and medical climatology in research and practice under consideration of preventive, curative and rehabilitative demands.

★ 3242 ★ German Society of Plastic and Reconstructive Surgery (Deutsche Gesellschaft fur Plastische und Wiederherstellungschirurgie e.V. — DGPW)
Elise-Averdieck-Str 17
D-27342 Rotenburg, Germany
Phone: 49 4261 772127 **Fax:** 49 4261 772128
Email: info@dgpw.de
Website: http://www.dgpw.de
Fnded: 1961. **Desc:** Promotes interdisciplinary exchange of clinical and scientific knowledge and application in plastic and reconstructive surgery.

★ 3243 ★ German Society of Psychosomatic Obstetrics and Gynaecology
c/o Prof.Dr. Heribert Kentenich
DRK Kliniken Westend
Frauenklinik
Spandauer Damm 130
D-14050 Berlin, Germany
Phone: 49 30 30354405 **Fax:** 49 30 30354409
Email: frauenklinik@drk-kliniken-westend.de
Desc: Promotes the study of psychobiological and psychosocial, ethical and cross-cultural problems in the fields of obstetrics and gynaecology, women's health and reproductive health; faciliates the dissemination of new information in these fields. **Pub:** *Journal of Psychosomatic Obstetrics and Gynecology*. Journal.

★ 3244 ★ German Society for Sex Research (GSSR) (Deutsche Gesellschaft fuer Sexualforschung — DGSF)
c/o Universitaets-Klinikum Hamburg-Eppendorf
Klinik fur Psychiatrie und Psychotherapie
Abteilung fur Sexualforschung und Forensik
Martinistr 52
D-20246 Hamburg, Germany
Phone: 49 40 428032225 **Fax:** 49 40 428036406
Email: hrichter@uke.uni-hamburg.de
Website: http://www.klinik.uni-frankfurt.de/zpg/sexualwissenschaft/dgfsa.htm
Fnded: 1952. **Mem:** 225. **Reg. Groups:** 4. **Desc:** Conducts research in sexology. **Pub:** *Beitrage zur Sexualforschung*, periodic. Journal. • *Zeitschrift fur Sexualforschung*, quarterly. Journal. Also publishes research findings.

★ 3245 ★ German Society for Social Scientific Sexuality Research (Deutsche Gesellschaft fur Sozialwissenschaftliche Sexualforschung e.V. — DGSS)
Gerresheimer Str 20
D-40211 Dusseldorf, Germany
Phone: 49 211 354591 **Fax:** 49 211 360777
Email: sexualforschung@sexologie.org
Website: http://www.sexologie.org
Fnded: 1971. **Desc:** Organizes and promotes sexuality research through social sciences.

★ 3246 ★ German Society of Speech, Language, and Voice-Pathology (Deutsche Gesellschaft fur Sprach- und Stimmheilkunde e.V.)
c/o Dr. Rainer Schonweiler
University of Lubeck
Lubeck, Germany
Phone: 49 451 5003485 **Fax:** 49 451 5006792
Email: webmaster@dgss-ev.org
Website: http://www.dgss-ev.org
Fnded: 1925. **Mem:** 200. **Desc:** Concentrates on interdisciplinary cooperation in speech-language-voice research.

★ 3247 ★ German Society of Visceral Surgery (Deutsche Gesellschaft fur Viszeralchirurgie e.V. — DGVC)
Luisenstr 58/59
D-10117 Berlin, Germany
Fnded: 1998.

★ 3248 ★ German Women Physicians Association (Deutscher Arztinnenbund)
Herbert-Lewin-Str. 1
D-50931 Cologne, Germany
Phone: 49 221 4004540 **Fax:** 49 221 4004541
Email: gsdaeb@aol.com
Fnded: 1924. **Mem:** 2,200. **Reg. Groups:** 33. **Lang(s):** Dutch, English, Portuguese. **Desc:** Promotes solidarity among women doctors. Represents members' interests in the medical sphere. Cultivates international contacts. **Pub:** *Aerztin*, bimonthly. Magazine.

★ 3249 ★ Gerontological Association of Malaysia (GeM) (Persatuan Gerontologi Malaysia)
Jabatan Pengajian Pembangunan Keluarga
Fakulti Ekologi Manusia
Serdang
Selangor D
43400 Ehsan, Malaysia
Phone: 60 3 78750076 **Fax:** 60 3 78749208
Email: philip@ummc.edu.my
Fnded: 1989. **Mem:** 110. **Desc:** Works to promote awareness on various aspects of aging and the elderly in Malaysia.

★ 3250 ★ Gerontological Association of Slovenia
Teslova, 17
61000 Ljubljana, Slovenia
Phone: 386 61 322536 **Fax:** 386 61 1741511
Desc: Promotes gerontological research, training in the field of aging, and interests of gerontological organizations in international affairs.

★ 3251 ★ Gerontological Society of America (GSA)
1030 15th St. NW, Ste. 250
Washington, DC 20005-1503
Phone: (202)842-1275 **Fax:** (202)842-1150
Email: cschutz@geron.org
Website: http://www.geron.org
Carol A. Schutz, Exec. Dir.
Fnded: 1945. **Mem:** 5,000. **Desc:** Physicians, physiologists, psychologists, anatomists, biochemists, sociologists, social workers, psychiatrists, pharmacologists, nurses, geneticists, zoologists, endocrinologists, economists, administrators, and other professionals interested in improving the well-being of older people by promoting scientific study of the aging process, publishing information for professionals about aging, and bringing together groups interested in aging research. Encourages research and education on the aging process. **Pub:** *Aging and Sensory Change: An Annotated Bibliography*. Bibliography. • *CommonStake*. • *The Gerontologist*, bimonthly. Journal. Includes book and media reviews and abstracts of papers to be presented at the annual meeting. *Price:* included in membership dues; $77/year for nonmembers in U.S.; $145/year for institutions in U.S. • *Gerontology News*, monthly. Newsletter. Includes employment listings, information on fellowship opportunities and new books, and conference calendar. *Price:* Included in membership dues; $50/year for nonmembers. • *Journal of Gerontology - Series B*, bimonthly. Journal. *Price:* $73 included in membership dues; $85/year for domestic nonmembers; $175/year for domestic institutions. • *Journals of Gerontology - Series A*, monthly. Journal. Contains two individual journals entitled *Biological Sciences, Medical Sciences*. *Price:* Included in membership dues; $161/year for domestic nonmembers; $350/year for domestic institutions. • Membership Directory, periodic. **Frmly:** (1980) Gerontological Society.

★ 3252 ★ Gerontological Society of the Russian Academy of Sciences
NN Petrov Research Institute of Oncology, 68 Leningradskaya St., Pesochny-2
197758 Saint Petersburg, Russia
Phone: 7 812 5968607 **Fax:** 7 812 5968947
Email: aging@mail.ru
Website: http://www.gerontology.spb.ru
Fnded: 1994. **Mem:** 1,500. **Reg. Groups:** 40. **Desc:** Facilitates research in Russian gerontological science and related fields of physiology and biology. Liaises with other scientific gerontological organizations. **Pub:** *Advances in Gerontology*, 1-3/year. Journal. Contains peer-reviewed articles about gerontology. • *Herald of Gerontological Society*, monthly. Newsletter.

★ 3253 ★ Gerson Institute (GI)
1572 Second Ave.
San Diego, CA 92101
Phone: (619)685-5353 **Free:** 888-4-GERSON
Fax: (619)685-5359
Email: mail@gerson.org
Website: http://www.gerson.org
Charlotte Gerson, Pres.
Fnded: 1977. **Mem:** 3,000. **Desc:** Individuals interested in health information. Purpose is to educate the public on nutritional health and to disseminate information about the Gerson therapy for healing. (The Gerson therapy was developed by Max Gerson, M.D., and seeks to prevent disease as well as to restore the natural healing mechanism in patients suffering from cancer and other degenerative diseases without the use of standard toxic therapies. Therapy includes a detoxification program to help the body eliminate toxins and waste materials that interfere with metabolism and healing and an intensive nutrition program.) Acts as consultant to operating physicians at hospital near Tijuana, Mexico; assists and trains physicians who want to learn the Gerson therapy. Presents lectures on health; conducts medical and nutritional research. **Pub:** *A Cancer Therapy - Results of 50 Cases*. Includes historical reviews and therapy details. *Price:* $25/year inside U.S.; $30/year outside U.S. • *Censored for Curing Cancer*. • *Healing Newsletter*, bimonthly. Newsletter. • Videos.

★ 3254 ★ Ghana Diabetes Association
c/o Charles L. Mingle
PO Box KB 68
Korle-Bu
Accra, Ghana
Phone: 233 21 668219 **Fax:** 233 21 668219
Email: fofei@africaonline.com.gh
Website: http://www.diabetesafrica.com/idfmembers.html
Desc: Represents people with diabetes. Promotes research and support of those with diabetes in Ghana.

★ 3255 ★ Gift from the Heart Foundation
2653 N Narragansett
Chicago, IL 60639
Phone: (773)237-4800 **Fax:** (773)237-1221
Email: giftheart@att.net
Website: http://www.giftfromtheheart.org
Krystyna B. Pasek, Pres.
Fnded: 1988. **Nat'l Groups:** 1. **Local Groups:** 1. **Desc:** Works to assist seriously ill children around the world by obtaining information regarding medical care. Provides food, lodging, transportation, and interpreters for children and their accompanying parents. Purchases rehabilitation equipment. Provides charitable programs and various social activities. **Pub:** *Gift From the Heart Foundation*, triennial. Brochure. Regular charitable organization's pamphlet. *Price:* Free. • *Gift from the Heart Foundation's Newletter*, semiannual. Newsletter. **Frmly:** (1992) Dar Serca.

★ 3256 ★ Gilda Radner Familial Ovarian Cancer Registry
c/o Cathy Fahey
Roswell Park Cancer Institute
Elm & Carlton Sts.
Buffalo, NY 14263-0001
Phone: (716)845-4503 **Free:** 800-682-7426
Fax: (716)845-8266
Email: gradner@roswellpark.org
Website: http://www.ovariancancer.com/grwp.html
Cathy Fahey, Mgr.

Fnded: 1990. **Desc:** Committed to the identification of new genes associated with familial ovarian cancer, thereby improving genetic and psychosocial counseling for individuals and families. Characterizes lifestyle choices (i.e., oral contraceptive use, hormone replacement therapy, number of pregnancies) that reduce ovarian cancer risk in women who may be susceptible to the disease. Strives for better methods for detecting ovarian cancer, for reliable predictive testing for cancer predisposition and prevention.

★ 3257 ★ Gilda's Club
322 8th Ave., Ste. 1402
New York, NY 10001
Phone: (917)305-1200 **Free:** 888-GILDA-4-U
Fax: (917)305-0549
Email: info@gildasclub.org
Website: http://www.gildasclub.org
Joyce Bichler, Contact

Fnded: 1995. **Mem:** 20,000. **Reg. Groups:** 16. **Desc:** Provides places where people with cancer and their families and friends join with others to build social and emotional support as a supplement to medical care. The free program consists of The Basic III: I. Support and Networking groups; II. Lectures and Workshops; and III. Social Activities.

★ 3258 ★ Girls and Boys Town
c/o Father Val. J. Peter
Boys Town Center
Boys Town, NE 68010
Free: 800-448-3000
Website: http://www.girlsandboystown.org/hotline/index.htm
Father Val J. Peter, Contact

Desc: Provides a 24-hour hotline available to children and parents.

★ 3259 ★ Glasgow Obstetrical and Gynaecological Society
Royal Maternity Hospital
Glasgow G4 0NA, United Kingdom
Phone: 44 141 5522435

Fnded: 1886.

★ 3260 ★ Glaucoma Foundation
116 John St., Ste. 1605
New York, NY 10038
Phone: (212)285-0080 **Fax:** (212)651-1888
Email: info@glaucomafoundation.org
Website: http://www.glaucomafoundation.org/
Scott R. Christensen, Pres. /CEO

Fnded: 1984. **Desc:** Individuals who have been affected by glaucoma and interested others. Works to increase public awareness and to provide research funding. Provides information about glaucoma to the medical and lay communities. Targets and funds the following areas for research: optic nerve regeneration; molecular genetics. Sponsors scientific research. **Pub:** *Doctor, I Have a Question....* Booklet. Answers the basic questions about glaucoma and treatments. • *Eye to Eye*, quarterly. Newsletter. Provides up to date information on advances in research and development. • *Glaucoma: What You Need To Know.* Brochure. • *You and Your Medication.* Brochure.

★ 3261 ★ Glaucoma Research Foundation
490 Post St., Ste. 1427
San Francisco, CA 94102
Phone: (415)986-3162 **Free:** 800-826-6693
Fax: (415)986-3763
Email: info@glaucoma.org
Website: http://www.glaucoma.org
Rita Loskill, Dir. of Education

Fnded: 1978. **Desc:** Dedicated to protecting the sight and independence of individuals with glaucoma through research and education, with the ultimate goal of finding a cure. Funds pilot project grants. **Pub:** *Childhood Glaucoma.* Provides information for people with glaucoma and their families. *Price:* Free. • *Gleams*, quarterly. Newsletter. Includes research updates, foundation news, and medical column. *Price:* Free. • *Living With Glaucoma.* Reference guides for people with glaucoma. • *Understanding and Living with Glaucoma. Price:* Free. **Frmly:** (1993) Foundation for Glaucoma Research.

★ 3262 ★ Glaucoma Society of the International Congress of Ophthalmology
Tsukasa-machi 40
Gifu 500, Japan
Phone: 81 582 659012 **Fax:** 81 582 659012
Email: yoshikit-gif@umin.u-tokyo.ac.jp

Fnded: 1980. **Desc:** Promotes the study of glaucoma.

★ 3263 ★ Glenkirk
3504 Commercial Ave.
Northbrook, IL 60062
Phone: (847)272-5111 **Fax:** (847)272-7350
Email: info@glenkirk.org
Website: http://www.glenkirk.org
John Manchester, Chief Info. Officer

Desc: Advocacy for, and support and service to empower individuals with developmental disabilities in order for them to participate fully in all areas of life, including day and residential services.

★ 3264 ★ Global Alliance for Women's Health
823 UN Plaza, Ste. 712
New York, NY 10017
Phone: (212)286-0424 **Fax:** (212)286-9561
Email: webmaster@gawh.org
Website: http://www.gawh.org
Elaine M. Wolfson, PhD, Pres.

Desc: Individuals and organizations working to improve the quality of women's health worldwide. Gathers and disseminates information on topics including primary health care, education of health care providers, cultural practices affecting the health of women and girls, occupational health and safety, sexually transmitted diseases, domestic violence, and mental health. Develops model health programs addressing women's needs. Conducts research; compiles statistics. **Pub:** *Women's Health Compendium.* Book.

★ 3265 ★ Global Health Action (GHA)
2250 N Druid Hills Rd., Ste. 130
Atlanta, GA 30329-3118
Phone: (404)634-5748 **Fax:** (404)634-9685
Email: gha@globalhealthaction.org
Website: http://www.globalhealthaction.org
Robin C. Davis, Exec. Dir.

Fnded: 1972. **Desc:** Provides health education and leadership and management training for participants from more than 88 countries worldwide. Programs include: health management and leadership courses; community health worker, goat farmer, and maternal health training programs in Haiti; HIV/AIDS programs in Africa, China and India; U.S.-based community empowerment programs; organizational capacity building in Haiti and India; and custom-designed training courses and workshops held throughout the world. Participants include health and development professionals, community health workers and community health leaders from the U.S. and abroad. **Pub:** *A Great and Mighty Tree.* Video. • *Global Health Action Annual Report*, annual. Annual Report. Provides donor education and publicity. • *Global Health Action General Brochure*, annual. Brochure. Provides donor education and publicity. • *Global Health Action Newsletter*, semiannual. Newsletter. Primarily for donor education and publicity. **Frmly:** (1985) International Nursing Services Association; (1993) INSA, The International Service Association for Health.

★ 3266 ★ Global Health Council
1701 K St. NW, Ste. 600
Washington, DC 20006-1503
Phone: (202)833-5900 **Fax:** (202)833-0075
Email: ghc@globalhealth.org
Website: http://www.globalhealth.org/

Fnded: 1971. **Mem:** 1,600. **Desc:** Membership organization made up of private voluntary organizations, health and medical associations, universities, government agencies, foundations, corporations, consulting firms, and individuals interested in promoting greater and more effective U.S. participation in practical international health and development programs. Seeks to strengthen U.S. public and private sector participation in international health activities. Areas of concern include: HIV/AIDS; women's health; improving primary health care worldwide; environmental health; population and family planning; tropical and preventive medicine; appropriate health technology. Supports improved health and development legislation. Conducts career service in conjunction with annual conference. **Pub:** *AIDS Link*, bimonthly. Newsletter. Contains the latest global information on HIV/AIDS issues. • *Career Network*, monthly. Bulletin. Contains listings of employment opportunities in International Health. • *Directory of U.S.-Based Agencies Involved in International Health Assistance*, periodic. Directory. Lists geographical areas served and types of workers sought by U.S. health agencies. *Price:* $60 non-members; $30 members. • *Global Learning for Health.* Paper. *Price:* $16.95 for members; $26.95 for non-members. • *Healthlink*, 10/year. Contains information on international health policy issues and calendar of events. *Price:* available to members only. • *NCIH Membership Directory*, periodic. Membership Directory. Contains individual and organizational members with phone numbers and key contacts. **Frmly:** (1999) National Council for International Health.

★ 3267 ★ Global Health Ministries (GHM)
7831 Hickory St. NE
Minneapolis, MN 55432-2500
Phone: (763)586-9590 **Fax:** (763)586-9591
Email: ghm@cs.com
Website: http://www.ghm.org/
Rev. Timon C. Iverson, Exec. Dir.

Fnded: 1987. **Desc:** Provides Lutheran health care work overseas; gathers and sends medical supplies around the world, recruits health related personnel; funds training of national health care givers. **Pub:** *Global Health*, bimonthly. Newsletter. • Annual Report.

★ 3268 ★ Global Human Research Foundation (GHR)
14-4-14 Satyakrishna Nivas
Kolagatlavari St.
Vizianagaram 535 002, Andhra Pradesh, India
Phone: 91 2892227283 **Fax:** 91 892227283

Fnded: 1991. **Mem:** 6. **Lang(s):** English, Hindi. **Desc:** Seeks to curtail the spread of infectious diseases, with particular emphasis on slowing the AIDS epidemic. Conducts preventive health education programs; serves as a clearinghouse for development organizations interested in public health issues. Makes available health care services.

★ 3269 ★ Global Vaccine Awareness League (GVAL)
25422 Trabuco Rd., Ste. 105-230
Lake Forest, CA 92630-2797
Email: michelle@gval.com
Website: http://www.gval.com/
Michelle Helms, Founder

Fnded: 1995. **Mem:** 160. **Desc:** Dedicated to disseminating information on the serious side effects of government sponsored vaccinations. Conducts educational programs; promotes parents right to choose whether or not to vaccinate their children; supports research; conducts fundraising events. **Pub:** Newsletter.

★ 3270 ★ Gluten Intolerance Group of North America (GIGNA)
15110 10th Ave., SW
Ste. A
Seattle, WA 98116-1820
Phone: (206)246-6652 **Fax:** (206)246-6531
Email: info@gluten.net
Website: http://www.gluten.net
Cynthia Kupper, CRD, CDE, Exec. Dir.

Fnded: 1974. **Mem:** 2,000. **Local Groups:** 2. **Desc:** Persons with gluten-sensitive enteropathy (celiac sprue) or dermatitis herpetiformis, family members, physicians, dietitians, and celiac sprue societies. (Gluten is a protein found in wheat, rye, oats, and barley. Gluten-sensitive enteropathy is an inherited disorder characterized by gluten-related destruction of the small intestine. Symptoms include diarrhea, weight loss, fatigue, and anemia.) Works to educate patients, health care personnel, and the public; to offer psychological support to celiac sprue patients and their families in dealing with the adjustment and nutritional limitations of the disease; to conduct research into the causes. Promotes practical application in specific food research, such as recipe development and information on gluten content of products. Offers children's services and group and individual counseling. **Pub:** *GIG Cookbook*. Book. Contains instructions for a gluten-free diet. *Price:* $22.50. • *GIG Newsletter*, quarterly. Newsletter. Provides book reviews, product information, recipes, and research reports to help in monitoring diets for persons with celiac sprue and dermatitis. *Price:* $30/year in U.S. • Videos. • Also publishes cookbook and fact sheets. **Frmly:** (1985) Gluten Intolerance Group.

★ 3271 ★ Goat Veterinary Society
c/o John Matthews
The Limes
Chalk St.
Rettendon Common
Chelmsford CM3 5DA, United Kingdom
Phone: 44 1245 353741 **Fax:** 44 1245 348564
Email: goatvetsoc@vetweb.co.uk
Website: http://www.vetweb.co.uk/sites/goatsoc1.htm

Fnded: 1979. **Desc:** Works to improve knowledge about goats in the veterinary profession. **Pub:** *The Goat Veterinary Society Journal*, periodic. Journal.

★ 3272 ★ Gonstead Clinical Studies Society
2778 Cumberland Blvd., No. 230
Smyrna, GA 30080
Free: 888-556-4277 **Fax:** 888-556-4277
Email: gcsschiro@aol.com
Website: http://www.gonstead.com

Desc: Promotes awareness of the Gonstead System of chiropractic and its record of safety and effectiveness in correcting vertebral subluxation.

★ 3273 ★ Goodwill Industries International (GII)
9200 Rockville Pike
Bethesda, MD 20814
Phone: (240)333-5200
Email: contactus@goodwill.org
Website: http://www.goodwill.org
George W. Kessinger, Pres. & CEO

Fnded: 1902. **Mem:** 226. **Reg. Groups:** 7. **State Groups:** 12. **Desc:** Federation of Goodwill Industries organizations across North America and the world are concerned primarily with providing employment, training, evaluation, counseling, placement, job training, and other vocational rehabilitation services and opportunities for individual growth for people with disabilities and other special needs. Member Goodwill Industries organizations collect donated goods and sell them in Goodwill retail stores as a means of providing employment and generating income. Conducts seminars and training programs; compiles statistics. **Pub:** *Corporate Brochure*, annual. Brochure. • *Internal Membership Directory*, annual. Membership Directory. • *Working!*, quarterly. Magazine. • Annual Report. • Also publishes promotional materials. **Frmly:** (1910) Morgan Memorial and Cooperative Industries and Stores; (1946) National Association of Goodwill Industries; (1994) Goodwill Industries of America.

★ 3274 ★ Goodwill Industries of Venezuela (Industrias Venezolanas de Buena Voluntad)
Sabana Grande
Apartado 50074
Caracas 1050-A, Venezuela
Phone: 58 12 9444555 **Fax:** 58 12 9444815
Email: buenavoluntad@cantv.net
Website: http://www.goodwill.org

Fnded: 1964. **Mem:** 14. **Lang(s):** English, Spanish. **Desc:** Provides vocational training, employment, and rehabilitation services to people with disabilities. Promotes economic and social self-sufficiency for people with disabilities; maintains social worker visitation program.

★ 3275 ★ Goodwill Industries Volunteer Services (GIVS)
c/o Goodwill Industries International Inc.
9200 Rockville Pike
Bethesda, MD 20814
Phone: (301)530-6500 **Fax:** (301)530-1516
Email: contactus@goodwill.org
Website: http://www.goodwill.org

Fnded: 1933. **Mem:** 3,000. **Nat'l Groups:** 1. **Local Groups:** 71. **Desc:** Persons interested in volunteer work in programs serving people with disabilities or other barriers to employment. Supports the efforts of national and local Goodwill Industries International, Inc., programs through volunteer services. Programs vary according to local needs and include such activities as direct program services, fundraising, and public relations. **Pub:** *Giving*, quarterly. Directory. • *Goodwill Volunteer Services Directory*, annual. Manual. • *Goodwill Volunteer Services Handbook*, annual. • Annual Report, annual. **Frmly:** National Auxiliary of Goodwill Industries; National Women's Auxiliary to the Goodwill Industries.

★ 3276 ★ Goodwill - The Amity Group
34 Ottawa St. N
Hamilton, ON, Canada L8H 3Y7
Phone: (905)526-8481 **Fax:** (905)526-9342
Email: amity@amity.on.ca
Website: http://www.amity.on.ca

Fnded: 1935. **Lang(s):** English, French. **Desc:** Individuals with disabilities. Promotes employment and full participation in society by members. Operates businesses providing employment to people with disabilities; provides support and services to industries employing people with disabilities.

★ 3277 ★ Gospel Association for the Blind (GAB)
PO Box 1162
Bunnell, FL 32110
Phone: (386)586-5885
George Montanus, Pres.

Fnded: 1947. **Desc:** Religious corporation supported by contributions "to evangelize the physically blind by presenting the Gospel of the Lord Jesus Christ." Provides counseling; summer camp. **Pub:** *Jottings*, monthly. Newsletter. Christian-oriented; includes profiles of blind people. *Price:* Free. • *"The Gospel Messenger"*, monthly. Newsletter. Carries the message of the Gospel to the blind. Contains religious stories, poems, and articles. Available on cassette. *Price:* Free to the blind.

★ 3278 ★ Grace and Compassion Benedictines
St. Benedict's Generalate
1 Manor Rd.
Kemp Town
Brighton BN2 5EA, United Kingdom
Phone: 44 1273 680720 **Fax:** 44 1273 680527
Email: generalate@graceandcompassion.co.uk
Website: http://www.dabnet.org/gcb.htm

Fnded: 1954. **Mem:** 201. **Reg. Groups:** 14. **Lang(s):** English. **Desc:** Individuals, Benedictine congregations, and long-term care facilities for the elderly. Seeks to improve the quality of life of elderly people requiring residential care and other living assistance. Maintains network of nursing homes, group residences, and shelters for the elderly. Provides charitable assistance to the elderly, frail and sick. **Pub:** *Our Lady's Newsletter*, quarterly. Newsletter.

★ 3279 ★ Graves' Disease Foundation (NGDF)
PO Box 1969
Brevard, NC 28712-1969
Phone: (828)877-5251 **Fax:** (828)885-7122
Email: ngdf@citcom.net
Website: http://www.ngdf.org
Nancy H. Patterson, PhD, Exec. Dir.

Fnded: 1990. **Mem:** 1,400. **State Groups:** 19. **Local Groups:** 25. **Desc:** People with Graves' disease; families of those affected; physicians and other professionals. Facilitates establishments of support groups for members in all states. Fosters public awareness and education on the causes, effects, and treatment of Grave's disease, a result of hyperthyroidism (the excess production by the body of thyroxine and triiodothyronine) in which the thyroid gland may be slightly enlarged, and symptoms such as a rapid heartbeat, eye problems, weight loss, or fatigue may occur. Participates in research on Graves' disease. **Pub:** Bulletin, periodic. • Newsletter, quarterly. **AKA:** National Graves' Disease Foundation.

★ 3280 ★ Gray Panthers (GP)
733 15th St. NW, Ste. 437
Washington, DC 20005
Phone: (202)737-6637 **Free:** 800-280-5362
Fax: (202)737-1160
Email: info@graypanthers.org
Website: http://www.graypanthers.org
Tim Fuller, Exec. Dir.

Fnded: 1970. **Mem:** 40,000. **Local Groups:** 60. **Desc:** Consciousness-raising activist group of older adults and young people. Aims to combat ageism - the discrimination against persons on the basis of chronological age. Believes that both the old and the young have much to contribute to make our society more just and humane. Advises, acts as acatalyst for, and organizes local groups of young, middle-aged, and older persons to work on issues of their choosing. Conducts work on eight national interests: national health care, affordable housing, environmental preservtion, peace, ending discrimination, education, economic and tax justice, and social justice. **Pub:** *Gray Panther Network*, bimonthly. Newsletter. Contains articles on ageism, health care, housing, disarmament, and other intergenerational issues. *Price:* Included in membership dues; $20/year for nonmembers; $35/year for organizations. • *Network Newsletter*, bimonthly. Covers national Gray Panther issues like housing, health care, and environmental protection. **AKA:** Gray Panthers Project Fund.

★ 3281 ★ Great Britain Wheelchair Basketball Association
Hemel Hempstead Sports Centre
Park Rd.
Hemel Hempstead HP1 1JS, United Kingdom
Phone: 44 1442 228793
Email: c.bethel@gbwba.org.uk
Website: http://www.gbwba.org.uk

Fnded: 1981. **Mem:** 800. **Reg. Groups:** 10. **Desc:** Persons with a physical (lower limb) disability. Develops and promotes wheelchair basketball in the UK.

Administers the national leagues and non-league clubs to enhance, through sport, the lives and lifestyles of physically disabled people. Administers and runs national teams, senior men's, juniors and women. **Pub:** *GBWBA Handbook*, annual. Handbook. • *GBWBA Newsletter*, quarterly. Newsletter.

★ 3282 ★ Greek Alzheimer's Association (GAA)

Charisio Old People's Home
Terma Dimitriou Charisi
A. Toumba
Thessaloniki
GR-54352 Hellas, Greece
Phone: 30 2310 925802 **Fax:** 30 2310 283973
Email: alzhass@med.auth.gr
Website: http://www.alzheimer-hellas.gr

Fnded: 1995. **Mem:** 1,000. **Reg. Groups:** 20. **Lang(s):** English, Greek. **Desc:** Individuals and organizations. Seeks to improve the quality of life of people with Alzheimer's disease and their families. Makes available support and services; facilitates research on Alzheimer's disease and related disorders; conducts educational programs. **Pub:** *Living With Alzheimer Disease.*

★ 3283 ★ Greek Dietetic Association

Erythrou Stavrou 8-10 St.
GR-115 26 Athens, Greece
Phone: 30 2 106984400 **Fax:** 30 2 106984400
Email: nutritio@otenet.gr
Website: http://www.hda.gr

Fnded: 1969. **Mem:** 330. **Lang(s):** Greek. **Desc:** Professional dietitians. Promotes advancement in the study and application of dietetics; advises government agencies and the public regarding a healthy diet. Conducts research and educational programs. **Pub:** *Journal of Nutrition and Dietetics*, quarterly. Journal.

★ 3284 ★ Greek Multiple Sclerosis Society

c/o Yiannis Kotsirilos
2-4 Faethonos Str.
GR-543 51 Thessaloniki, Greece
Phone: 30 23109 49909 **Fax:** 30 23109 49909
Email: mssoc@hol.gr
Website: http://www.msif.org

Fnded: 1993. **Mem:** 1,700. **Reg. Groups:** 3. **Desc:** MS patients, families and professionals. Seeks to improve the quality of life for persons with multiple sclerosis and their families. Provides telephone consultations, social advice, psychological treatment, home visits, and physiotherapy.

★ 3285 ★ Greek Society of Pharmacology (Ellhnikh Etaireia Farmakologias)

c/o Prof. Kyriaki Thermos
University of Crete
Faculty of Medicine
Department of Basic Sciences, Laboratory of Pharmacology
Heraklion
GR-71 110 Crete, Greece
Phone: 30 81 394533 **Fax:** 30 81 394530
Email: thermos@med.uoc.gr

Mem: 163. **Desc:** Promotes pharmacology in Greece.

★ 3286 ★ Greek Society of Psychosomatic Obstetrics and Gynaecology

c/o Prof. Papadakis
Ravine 24
GR-115 21 Athens, Greece
Fax: 30 12 6830559
Email: mitera@otenet.gr
Website: http://www.ispog.org

Desc: Promotes the study of psychobiological and psychosocial, ethical and cross-cultural problems in the fields of obstetrics and gynaecology, women's health and reproductive health; facilitates the dissemination of new information in these fields. **Pub:** *Journal of Psychosomatic Obstetrics and Gynecology*. Journal.

★ 3287 ★ Greek Stammering Association

c/o Jorge Perdikis V
Eptalofu 3
Nea Smirni
GR-171-22 Athens, Greece
Website: http://www.europe.is/elsa/members/m_greece.html

Desc: Works to find a cure for stuttering in Greece.

★ 3288 ★ Grenada Planned Parenthood Association (GPPA)

Deponthieu St.
PO Box 127
Saint George's, Grenada
Phone: (473)440-3341 **Fax:** (473)440-8071
Email: gppa@caribsurf.com

Fnded: 1964. **Mem:** 26. **Lang(s):** English. **Desc:** Advocates responsible parenthood and family planning. Promotes family planning as a basic human right. Encourages public awareness of contraception, family planning, and sexually transmitted diseases. Provides contraceptive health care services. Sponsors educational programs. Conducts research. **Pub:** Annual Report.

★ 3289 ★ Group for the Advancement of Psychiatry (GAP)

PO Box 570218
Dallas, TX 75357-0218
Phone: (972)613-3044 **Fax:** (972)613-5532
Website: http://www.groupadpsych.org/
Frances Roton, Contact

Fnded: 1946. **Mem:** 300. **Desc:** Independent group of psychiatrists organized in working committees interested in applying the principles of psychiatry toward the study of human relations. Works closely with specialists in many other disciplines. Investigates such subjects as school desegregation, use of nuclear energy, religion, psychiatry in the armed forces, mental retardation, cross-cultural communication, medical uses of hypnosis, and the college experience. Maintains 25 committees. **Pub:** Reports.

★ 3290 ★ Group Against Smokers' Pollution (GASP)

PO Box 632
College Park, MD 20741-0632
Email: gaspamerica@aol.com
Willard K. Morris, Sec.

Fnded: 1971. **Mem:** 10,000. **Nat'l Groups:** 1. **State Groups:** 10. **Local Groups:** 100. **Desc:** Nonsmokers who are adversely affected by tobacco smoke united to promote the rights of nonsmokers, educate the public about the problems of second-hand smoke, and regulate smoking in places where nonsmokers are exposed. Supports the establishment and enforcement of laws and other public policy measures which reduce environmental tobacco smoke. Provides information and referral services; distributes educational literature, buttons, posters, and bumper stickers. Helps members find local GASP chapters or establish a chapter. **Pub:** *Nonsmokers' Bill of Rights.* • *The Nonsmokers' Liberation Guide*. Handbook. • Booklets. • Pamphlets. **AKA:** GASP of America.

★ 3291 ★ Group-Analytic Society

258 Belize Rd.
London NW6 4BT, United Kingdom
Phone: 44 207 3161824 **Fax:** 44 207 3161880
Email: groupanalytic.society@virgin.net
Website: http://www.groupanalyticsociety.org/

Fnded: 1952. **Mem:** 600. **Desc:** Group-analysts, doctors, psychiatrists, professors, educationalists, caring professions. Receives and administers funds to be used for the promotion and development of group analysis as a treatment, prophylaxis and science; its advancement through study, research and teaching, and the provision of advisory services, lectures and publications. **Pub:** *Journal - Group Analysis*, quarterly. Journal.

★ 3292 ★ Group B Strep Association

PO Box 16515
Chapel Hill, NC 27516
Website: http://www.groupbstrep.org
Gina Burns, Pres.

Fnded: 1990. **Mem:** 3,000. **Nat'l Groups:** 1. **Desc:** Seeks to educate the public about Group B Strep (GBS) infections during pregnancy. Promotes screening of mothers and the development of a vaccine. Seeks to control the disease which is a leading cause of life-threatening infections in newborns. Acts as a support group; provides educational programs. **Pub:** *GBSA Public Education Packet.* • Also provides GBSA Public Education Packet, medical contacts and legislation information.

★ 3293 ★ Guam Lytico and Bodig Association

PO Box 1458
Hagatna, GU 96932
Phone: (671)477-2293 **Fax:** (671)477-2294
Email: lyticobodig@hotmail.com
Website: http://lytico.tripod.com/
Madeleine Z. Bordallo, Pres.

Fnded: 1983. **Mem:** 18. **Desc:** Provides supportive services and information to individuals stricken with disease.

★ 3294 ★ Guardians of Hydrocephalus Research Foundation (GHRF)

2618 Ave. Z
Brooklyn, NY 11235-2023
Phone: (718)743-4473 **Fax:** (718)743-1171
Email: ghrf2618@aol.com
Katherine Soriano, VP

Fnded: 1977. **Mem:** 5,000. **State Groups:** 11. **Local Groups:** 2. **Desc:** Hydrocephalics and their families, health care professionals, and other concerned individuals. Seeks to find the cause and cure of hydrocephalus. (Hydrocephalus is the buildup of cerebrospinal fluid in the brain cavity, which can cause brain damage or death if untreated.) Disseminates information on hydrocephalus; conducts public awareness and fundraising projects. Plans to conduct research and educational programs, and to operate computerized services. **Pub:** *An Introduction to Hydrocephalus.* • *Journal Ad Book*, annual. Journal. • Newsletter, quarterly. Includes news briefs and fundraising and project information. *Price:* Included in membership dues. • Makes available documentary film.

★ 3295 ★ Guide Dog Foundation for the Blind (GDFB)

371 E Jericho Tpke.
Smithtown, NY 11787
Phone: (631)265-2121 **Free:** 800-548-4337
Fax: (631)361-5192
Email: info@guidedog.org
Website: http://www.guidedog.org
Wells B. Jones, CAE, CEO

Fnded: 1946. **Mem:** 160,000. **Desc:** Works to provide independence and mobility for qualified blind applicants free of charge. Dogs are raised in volunteer homes for the first year, then trained for an additional four to six months with qualified instructor. Conducts 25-day residential training program for blind persons and guide dogs at Smithtown, NY. **Pub:** *Guideways*, 3-5/year. Newsletter. Updates the foundation's activities. *Price:* Free. • Annual Report, annual. **AKA:** Second Sight; Guiding Eyes; Guide Dog Foundation.

★ 3296 ★ Guide Dog Users, Inc. (GDUI)

14311 Astrodome Dr.
Silver Spring, MD 20906
Phone: (301)598-5771 **Free:** 888-858-1008
Fax: (301)871-7591
Email: info@gdui.org

Website: http://www.gdui.org
Jane Sheehan, Off. Mgr.

Fnded: 1969. **Mem:** 1,000. **State Groups:** 15. **Desc:** Persons who are visually handicapped or blind and who use guide dogs; other interested individuals. Conducts seminars, workshops, and public relations programs. Encourages promotion of aids for mobility skills and employment of the blind; promotes self-help concept for blind persons. Operates speakers' bureau. **Pub:** *Pawtracks*, quarterly. Newsletter. Provides medical, legal, financial information on canine maintenance, on audiocassette and compact disk; specific emphasis on needs of guide dogs. *Price:* Included in membership dues; $25/year for nonmembers. • Brochures.

★ 3297 ★ Guide Dogs of America (GDA)

13445 Glenoaks Blvd.
Sylmar, CA 91342
Phone: (818)362-5834 **Free:** 800-459-4843
Fax: (818)362-6870
Email: mail@guidedogsofamerica.org
Website: http://www.guidedogsofamerica.org
Jay A. Bormann, Pres. /Dir.

Fnded: 1948. **Desc:** GDA breeds, raises and trains guide dogs for legally blind men and women throughout the U.S. and Canada and provides instruction in the use of these "special" dogs for safe mobility. All GDA services which include guide dog, specially designed harness, individualized 28 day in-residence training, and life-time follow up is free of charge. GDA is supported by donations from individuals, companies, foundations, organizations, and service clubs. Maintains speakers' bureau. Tours available by appointment. **Pub:** *Partners*, quarterly. Newsletter. **AKA:** (2001) International Guiding Eyes. **Frmly:** (1993) International Guiding Eyes.

★ 3298 ★ Guide Dogs for the Blind (GDB)

PO Box 151200
San Rafael, CA 94915-1200
Phone: (415)499-4000 **Free:** 800-295-4050
Fax: (415)499-4035
Email: information@guidedogs.com
Website: http://www.guidedogs.com
Bob Phillips, Pres. /CEO

Fnded: 1942. **Desc:** Provides guide dogs and training on their use to visually impaired people throughout the U.S. and Canada; services are free to those served through the generosity of donors and support volunteers. **Pub:** *Guide Dog News*, quarterly. Newsletter. Available in Braille, and available on tape. *Price:* $12/year.

★ 3299 ★ Guide Dogs for the Blind Association

Hillfields
Burghfield Common
Reading RG7 3YG, United Kingdom
Phone: 44 118 9835555 **Fax:** 44 118 9835433
Email: guidedogs@gdba.org.uk
Website: http://www.guidedogs.org.uk

Fnded: 1934. **Mem:** 5,000. **Local Groups:** 450. **Lang(s):** English. **Desc:** Provides guide dogs, mobility and other rehabilitation services that meet the needs of blind and partially sighted people. **Pub:** *FORWARD*, quarterly. Magazine. Also available in Braille and on audiotape.

★ 3300 ★ Guiding Eyes for the Blind (GEB)

611 Granite Springs Rd.
Yorktown Heights, NY 10598
Phone: (914)245-4024 **Free:** 800-942-0149
Fax: (914)245-1609
Email: webmaster@guidingeyes.org
Website: http://guidingeyes.org
William D. Badger, Pres. /CEO

Fnded: 1954. **Desc:** Breeds and provides fully trained guide dogs and instruction in their use to visually impaired and blind individuals including special needs students with additional challenges. Conducts 3-year course for instructors and 4-week training programs for blind persons in proper use and care of guide dogs at Yorktown Heights, NY. Provides in-service education for staff and seminars for orientation and mobility instructors and other rehabilitation professionals. Maintains speakers' bureau of program graduates; provides home training. **Pub:** *Guide Lines*, quarterly. Newsletter. • *Insight*, biennial. Magazine. • *Lions Connection*, quarterly.

★ 3301 ★ Guild of Psychotherapists

47 Nelson Sq.
London SE1 02A, United Kingdom
Phone: 44 20 74013260
Email: guild@psycho.org.uk
Website: http://www.psycho.org.uk

Fnded: 1974. **Mem:** 190. **Lang(s):** French, German, Greek, Hebrew, Spanish. **Desc:** Qualified and registered psychoanalytic psychotherapists practising in London and all parts of the country. Aims to train psychoanalytic psychotherapists and to offer a clinical referral service with qualified psychotherapists in all areas of the country. Reduced fees available.

★ 3302 ★ Guild for Structural Integration (GSI)

PO Box 1559
Boulder, CO 80306
Phone: (303)447-0122 **Free:** 800-447-0150
Fax: (303)447-0180
Email: gsi@rolfguild.org
Website: http://www.rolfguild.org/
Richard Stenstavold, Pres.

Fnded: 1989. **Desc:** Dedicated to the teaching of Dr. Ida P. Rolf, a ten-session sequence of structural, fascial and educational goals establishing order in human structures. **Pub:** *Guild Online*. Newsletter. Provides exchange of information. • Catalog.

★ 3303 ★ Guillain-Barre Syndrome Foundation International (GBSFI)

PO Box 262
Wynnewood, PA 19096
Phone: (610)667-0131 **Fax:** (610)667-7036
Email: info@gbfi.com
Website: http://www.webmast.com/gbs/
Estelle L. Benson, Exec. Dir.

Fnded: 1980. **Mem:** 15,000. **Reg. Groups:** 148. **Desc:** Individuals concerned with Guillain-Barre syndrome (Acute Idiopathic Polyneuritis), a rare, paralyzing, potentially catastrophic disorder of the peripheral nerves. Objectives are to: educate the public and medical community about the availability of support groups and maintain their awareness of the disorder; foster research on cause, prevention, and treatment; encourage financial support for research; develop nationwide support groups. Arranges for recovered or recovering patients to visit patients in acute care and rehabilitation hospitals; assists patients in dealing with disabilities should complete recovery not occur. Maintains steering committee of physicians, some of who have had the disorder. **Pub:** *Communicator*, quarterly. Newsletter. • *Guide for Caregivers*. Handbook. • *Guillain-Barre Syndrome, an Overview for the Layperson*. Booklet. **Frmly:** (1988) Guillian-Barre Syndrome Support Group; (1990) Guillian-Barre Syndrome Support Group International.

★ 3304 ★ Guinean Association for the Education and Help to Diabetic (Association Guineenne d'Education et d'aide Diabetiques)

BP 1206
Conakry, Guinea
Phone: 224 414336 **Fax:** 224 414336
Email: naby@mirinet.net.gn
Website: http://www.diabetesafrica.com/idfmembers.html

State Groups: Guinee. **Local Groups:** Diabe. **Desc:** Represents people with diabetes. Promotes research and support of those with diabetes in Guinea.

★ 3305 ★ Guyana Responsible Parenthood Association (GRPA)

70 Quamina St.
South Cummingsburg
Georgetown, Guyana
Phone: 592 2253286 **Fax:** 592 2252144
Email: grpafpa@sdnp.org.gy
Website: http://www.sdnp.org.gy/grpafpa/

Fnded: 1973. **Desc:** Promotes family life education and family planning issues focusing on its importance to an improved quality of life and national development. Provides clinical services for family planning.

★ 3306 ★ Gynaecological Cancer Society

c/o John Gower, Ch. Exec.
100 Kilkivan Ave.
Kenmore, QLD 4069, Australia
Phone: 61 7 38784790 **Fax:** 61 7 38788451
Email: j.gower@gcs.org.au
Website: http://www.gcsq.org.au/

Desc: Provides information on a wide range of gynecological cancer specialty areas.

★ 3307 ★ Gynecologic Oncology Group (GOG)

PO Box 60167
Philadelphia, PA 19103
Phone: (215)854-0770 **Free:** 800-225-3053
Email: cgaloppo@agog.org
Website: http://www.gog.org
Philip J. Disaia, Chm.

Fnded: 1970. **Mem:** 65. **Desc:** Institutions and teaching hospitals conducting research in gynecological oncology. Sponsored by the American College of Obstetricians and Gynecologists.

★ 3308 ★ Gynecologic Surgery Society (GSS)

2440 M St., NW Ste. 801
Washington, DC 20037
Phone: (202)293-2046 **Fax:** (202)778-6195
Email: information@gynecologicsurgerysociety.org
Website: http://www.gynecologicsurgerysociety.org
John Marlow, MD, Chm.

Fnded: 1979. **Mem:** 700. **Desc:** Individuals interested in gynecologic surgery. Facilitates communication among members. Conducts educational programs and demonstrations of new surgical techniques. **Pub:** *Journal of Gynecologic Surgery*, periodic. Journal. • Newsletter, periodic.

★ 3309 ★ Haitian Coalition on AIDS (HCA)

50 Court St., Ste. 1010
Brooklyn, NY 11201
Phone: (718)855-7275 **Fax:** (718)852-5377
Email: info@haitiancenterscouncil.org
Website: http://www.haitiancenterscouncil.org/programs.htm
Henry Frank, Exec. Dir.

Fnded: 1983. **Mem:** 70. **Reg. Groups:** 8. **State Groups:** 7. **Local Groups:** 6. **Desc:** Community centers; professional groups of doctors, journalists, lawyers, nurses, social workers, and civil rights and media representatives. Purpose is to educate the public concerning what the coalition feels is the discriminatory classification of Haitians as an ethnonational group that runs a high risk of contracting AIDS. Seeks to heighten AIDS awareness within the Haitian community. Offers social services and placement for persons with AIDS; provides counseling to their families. Sponsors conferences and seminars at churches and universities. Compiles statistics; maintains speakers' bureau.

★ 3310 ★ Handicap International (HI)

14, ave. Berthelot
F-69361 Lyon Cedex 07, France
Phone: 33 4 78697979 **Fax:** 33 4 78697994
Email: contact@handicap-international.org
Website: http://www.handicap-international.org

Fnded: 1982. **Mem:** 56,000. **Lang(s):** English, French, Portuguese, Spanish. **Desc:** Works for the rehabilitation of physically disabled persons in Third World countries. Trains local technicians in appropriate technologies to create small prosthetics and physical rehabilitation units. Offers charitable programs. **Pub:** *L'Enfant Handicape et Village*. Book. • *Operations Handicap International*, quarterly. • Books. Contains translations of text from other languages.

★ 3311 ★ Handicapped Scuba Association (HSA)
1104 El. Prado
San Clemente, CA 92672-4637
Phone: (949)498-4540 **Fax:** (949)498-6128
Email: hsa@hsascuba.com
Website: http://www.hsascuba.com
Jim Gatacre, Pres.

Fnded: 1975. **Mem:** 2,000. **Nat'l Groups:** 34. **Reg. Groups:** 30. **State Groups:** 50. **Desc:** Individuals with handicaps and interested others. Purpose is to advance and promote scuba diving among the handicapped. Seeks to enhance the self-image of handicapped divers by emphasizing their abilities rather than their disabilities. Stresses the importance of education and safety procedures in diving; maintains training agency for handicapped divers. Offers training and certification worldwide for scuba diving instructors in teaching the handicapped. Holds monthly diving excursion and lectures, and conducts four diving vacations per year. Offers instructor referrals worldwide. **Pub:** *Freedom in Depth*. Film. • *Getting Down Scuba News*, annual. *Price:* $20. • *Instructor Training Manual*. Manual. • *To Fly in Freedom*. Film. • Also is producing a film about the association with the Cousteau Society. To fly in freedom IS with Cousteau.

★ 3312 ★ Handidactis
146 Haslam St.
Toronto, ON, Canada M1N 3N7
Phone: (416)267-5939 **Fax:** (416)267-8183
Email: handidac@idirect.com
Website: http://www.handidactis.com/ontario/index.html

Fnded: 1986. **Reg. Groups:** 2. **Lang(s):** English, French. **Desc:** Promotes awareness of the needs of people with disabilities among employers and service providers. Seeks to ensure full integration of workplaces with employees with disabilities while maintaining excellence in customer service. Conducts customized cross-disability awareness training programs; sponsors educational courses. Develops and delivers site audits to remove barriers at work, home, recreational sites.

★ 3313 ★ Harvard Injury Control Research Center (HICRC)
Harvard School of Public Health
677 Huntington Ave., 3rd Fl.
Boston, MA 02115
Phone: (617)432-3420 **Fax:** (617)432-3699
Email: hicrc@hsph.harvard.edu
Website: http://www.hsph.harvard.edu/hicrc
David Hemenway, PhD, Dir.

Fnded: 1998. **Desc:** A comprehensive CDC-funded Center. Primary activity is the interdisciplinary study of the causes and etiology of injury among vulnerable populations and applications for primary prevention and intervention strategies and policy. Areas of focus are violence - primarily youth and family violence - and cross-cutting issues - including alcohol and drug use, firearm use and treatment setting. Also offers graduate courses, internships, conferences, trainings, grand rounds, and a Seminar Series, and provides technical assistance to State Health Departments and Regional Networks. **Frmly:** (1998) Injury Control Center; (2001) Injury Control Research Center.

★ 3314 ★ Harveian Society of London
c/o Neil Douglas
Department of Medicine
Royal Infirmary
Edinburgh EH3 9YW, United Kingdom

Fnded: 1831. **Mem:** 350. **Lang(s):** English. **Desc:** Promotes discussion of the medical, surgical, and philosophical subjects connected with medical subjects.

★ 3315 ★ Harvey Society (HS)
c/o Dr. Savio L.C. Woo
Mt. Sinai School of Medicine
Institute of Gene Therapy
1425 Madison Ave., PO Box 1496
New York, NY 10029
Phone: (212)659-8260 **Fax:** (212)849-2572
Email: Savio.Woo@mssm.edu
Dr. Savio Woo, Prof. /Dir.

Fnded: 1905. **Mem:** 1,600. **Desc:** Persons with a Ph.D. or M.D. degree active or interested in making contributions to the literature of medical and biological science. Seeks to disseminate knowledge and promote the development of the biomedical sciences. Sponsors a series of public lectures delivered by leaders in the field. Society is named after William Harvey (1578-1657), who identified the circulation of blood. **Pub:** *Harvey Lectures*, annual. Book. Contains lectures given during the year.

★ 3316 ★ Hazelden Foundation (HF)
15245 Pleasant Valley Rd.
PO Box 11
Center City, MN 55012-0011
Phone: (651)213-4000 **Free:** 800-257-7800
Fax: (651)213-4544
Email: info@hazelden.org
Website: http://www.hazelden.org
Nick Hilger, Pres. /CEO

Fnded: 1949. **Desc:** Provides treatment, recovery, education, and professional services for chemical dependency and other addictive behaviors. Operates: Hazelden Foundation Center, a treatment center; Fellowship Club in New York, St. Paul and West Palm Beach, Florida, an intermediate care facility; Hazelden Center for Youth and Families for adolescents and young adults; Hazelden Renewal Center for individuals recovering from addictive behaviors and their families; Hanley-Hazelden Center in West Palm Beach, Florida, for inpatient and outpatient treatment; Also provides: aftercare therapy; counselor training; 5-7 day, live-in family program that acquaints relatives and other associates of chemically-dependent individuals with problems of chemical dependency; continuing education programs for professionals; and communities. **Pub:** *Hazelden Voice*, semiannual. Newsletter. Provides information on health and recovery from addictive behavior. • *Publishing Catalog*, monthly. Catalog. • Books. • Pamphlets. • Makes available educational and audiovisual materials.

★ 3317 ★ Head Injury Hotline (PP)
c/o Constance Miller
212 Pioneer Bldg.
Seattle, WA 98104-2221
Phone: (206)621-8558 **Fax:** (206)624-4961
Email: brain@headinjury.com
Website: http://www.headinjury.com
Constance Miller, Contact

Fnded: 1985. **Desc:** A non profit clearinghouse founded and operated by head injury activists since 1985. It is a place where visitors can get information, join a discussion group, build advocacy skills, and self-care skills. The site integrates resources from diverse organizations including support groups, rehabilitation, and research sites, as well as lay and professional journals and more. Maintains speakers' bureau. **Pub:** *From the Ashes: A Head Injury Self-Advocacy Guide*, periodic. Contains worksheets to assist in locating and assessing doctors and therapists; self-assessment inventories; glossary of commonly-used phrases. *Price:* $20/copy; $5 shipping and handling. **Frmly:** (1993) Phoenix Project.

★ 3318 ★ Headway Ireland - National Association for Acquired Brain Injury (HINHIA)
101 Parnell St.
Dublin 1, Ireland
Phone: 353 1 8729222 **Fax:** 353 1 8729590
Email: services@headwayireland.ie
Website: http://www.headwayireland.ie

Fnded: 1993. **Mem:** 800. **Reg. Groups:** 8. **Lang(s):** English, Irish. **Desc:** Individuals and organizations. Seeks to improve the quality of life of people with head injuries and their families. Makes available support and services; conducts educational and advocacy campaigns; sponsors training programs for providers of care and services to people with head injuries.

★ 3319 ★ Healing Touch International
12477 W Cedar Dr., Ste. 202
Lakewood, CO 80228
Phone: (303)989-7982 **Fax:** (303)980-8683
Email: htiheal@aol.com
Website: http://www.healingtouch.net/
Lisa Anselme, Exec. Dir.

Fnded: 1996. **Mem:** 3,000. **Desc:** Promotes the practice and teaching of Healing Touch. **Pub:** *Healing Touch*, bimonthly. Newsletter. *Price:* included in membership dues.

★ 3320 ★ Health Academy (HA)
c/o Public Relations Society of America
33 Irving Pl.
New York, NY 10003-2376
Phone: (212)995-2230 **Fax:** (212)995-0757
Email: hq@prsa.org
Website: http://www.healthacademy.prsa.org/
David Henry, Chair

Fnded: 1989. **Mem:** 600. **Nat'l Groups:** 1. **Desc:** A professional section of the Public Relations Society of America. Senior public relations professionals working in hospitals, multi-hospital systems, medical and dental organizations, insurance companies and Health Maintenance Organizations, foundations, rehabilitation facilities, pharmaceutical firms, government health care units, or health education and research organizations; public relations consultants working in the health care industry. Seeks to enhance the quality and stature of health care public relations. Conducts professional development seminars. **Pub:** *By-laws and Membership Directory*, annual. Directory. *Price:* included in membership dues. • *Health Academy News*, bimonthly. • Monographs.

★ 3321 ★ Health and Allied Workers' Union
PO Box 47011
Greyville 4023, Republic of South Africa
Phone: 27 11 3063993

★ 3322 ★ Health Benefits Coalition for Affordable Choice and Quality
1201 F St. NW, Ste. 200
Washington, DC 20004
Website: http://www.hbcweb.com/

Mem: 3000,000. **Desc:** Employers providing health care coverage. Promotes affordable, quality health care, through broader coverage, choice and competition in the marketplace, rather than government mandates.

★ 3323 ★ Health Care Compliance Association (HCCA)
1211 Locust St.
Philadelphia, PA 19107
Phone: (215)545-3334 **Free:** 888-580-8373
Fax: (215)545-8107
Email: info@hcca-info.org
Website: http://www.hcca-info.org
Bill Ward, Contact

Fnded: 1997. **Mem:** 3,200. **Nat'l Groups:** 1. **Reg. Groups:** 10. **Desc:** Healthcare professionals involved in compliance in the health care industry. Promotes quality compliance programs in health care. Offers educational programs, professional network and discussion groups. **Pub:** *Compliance Today*, monthly. Magazine.

★ 3324 ★ Healthcare Financial Management Association (HFMA)
2 Westbrook Corporate Financial Center, Ste. 700
Westchester, IL 60154-5700
Phone: (708)531-9600 **Free:** 800-252-HFMA
Fax: (708)531-0032
Email: tarya@hfma.org
Website: http://www.hfma.org
Richard L. Clarke, Pres. & CEO

Fnded: 1946. **Mem:** 34,000. **State Groups:** 70. **Desc:** Financial management professionals employed by hospitals and long-term care facilities, public accounting and consulting firms, insurance companies, medical groups, managed care organizations, government agencies, and other organizations. Conducts conferences, including annual conference in late June, audio teleconferences. Publishes books on healthcare financial issues. A Fellowship in Healthcare Financial Management (FHFMA) as well as the Certified Healthcare Professional (CHFP) in Fianace and Accounting, Financial Management of Physician Practices, Managed Care, and Patient Financial Services are offered. **Pub:** *Healthcare Financial Management*, monthly. Magazine. Includes industry news, articles on financial management in all types of facilities across the healthcare continuum. *Price:* $82 /year for nonmembers. • *Notes from National*, monthly. Newsletter. *Price:* Included in membership dues. • *Patient Accounts*, monthly. Newsletter. Covers the financial operations of business office and patient accounting functions, including preadmission information gathering. *Price:* $60/year for members; $108/year for nonmembers. • Books. • Videos. **Frmly:** (1968) American Association of Hospital Accountants; (1982) Hospital Financial Management Association.

★ 3325 ★ Healthcare Financing Study Group (HFSG)
1666 K St. NW, Ste. 500
Washington, DC 20006
Fax: (202)466-3215

Fnded: 1973. **Mem:** 40. **Desc:** Investment banking, law, consulting, and accounting firms involved in providing capital financing for health care institutions. Analyzes legislative and regulatory proposals from the standpoint of the health care financial community. Provides forum for exchange of information concerning health care financing. **Pub:** Bulletin, periodic. • Newsletter, monthly. **Frmly:** (1981) Hospital Financing Study Group.

★ 3326 ★ Healthcare Information and Management Systems Society (HIMSS)
230 E Ohio St., Ste. 500
Chicago, IL 60611-3269
Phone: (312)664-4467 **Fax:** (312)664-6143
Email: himss@himss.org
Website: http://www.himss.org/
H. Stephen Lieber, CAE, Pres.

Fnded: 1961. **Mem:** 13,500. **Reg. Groups:** 40. **Desc:** Persons who, by education and/or appropriate experience, are professionally qualified to engage in the analysis, design, and operation of health care information systems, management engineering, telecommunications, and clinical systems professions. Also, corporate members include companies with information technology solutions for health care organizations. Provides leadership in health care for the management of systems, information, and change, while striving for high quality, efficient and effective patient care through analysis and technology implementation. Maintains speakers' bureau. Offers placement service. **Pub:** *Annual Conference*, annual. Proceedings. • *HIMSS News*, monthly. Newsletter. *Price:* Included in membership dues. • *Journal of Healthcare Information Management*, quarterly. Journal. Technical peer reviewed journal. *Price:* Included in membership dues. • Monographs, periodic. • Books, periodic. • Handbooks, periodic. **Frmly:** (1987) Hospital Management Systems Society.

★ 3327 ★ Health Care Liability Alliance (HCLA)
PO Box 19008
Washington, DC 20036-9008
Phone: (202)293-4255 **Fax:** (202)296-7689
Website: http://www.hcla.org/

Desc: Medical organizations. Dedicated to improving America's health care system through reform.

★ 3328 ★ Health Care Supplies Association
32 Eton Close
Chester House
Datchet
Slough SL3 9BE, United Kingdom
Phone: 44 1753 580176 **Fax:** 44 1753 580176

Fnded: 1960. **Mem:** 490. **Desc:** To promote maintain and seek continuously to improve professional standards and training relating to supplies and associated services within the healthcare sector. To establish and maintain a professional link with appropriate statutory bodies. To liaise with professional and other organizations. Activities include two annual training schools for junior grades in the supplies discipline and an annual conference. **Pub:** *Official Procurement Guide*, annual. Book.

★ 3329 ★ Health Connection
55 W Oak Ridge Dr.
Hagerstown, MD 21740
Phone: (301)393-3267 **Free:** 800-548-8700
Fax: 888-294-8405
Email: sales@healthconnection.org
Website: http://www.healthconnection.org
Larry Macomber, Supvr.

Fnded: 1954. **Desc:** Promotes nationwide education for the prevention of drug addiction and alcoholism through direct mailings of materials to schools, churches, and civic organizations. Participates, through exhibits, in conferences and conventions of teachers and school personnel. **Pub:** *Catalogue*, annual. • *Listen*, monthly. Magazine. • *Teaching Guide to Winner Magazine*, 9/year. Magazine. • *Winner*, 9/year. • Books. • Films. • Pamphlets. • Reprints. • Videos. • Also publishes teaching aids, posters, and filmstrips. Distributes puppets/puppet programs. **Frmly:** (1993) Narcotics Education.

★ 3330 ★ Health and Development International (HDI)
PO Box 382077
Cambridge, MA 02238-2077
Phone: (617)864-2042 **Fax:** (617)864-7757
Email: anders@hdi.no
Website: http://www.hdi.no/
Dr. Anders R. Seim, Founder

Desc: Works to free the world of guinea worm and lymphatic filariasis (elephantiasis).

★ 3331 ★ Health Education Foundation (HEF)
2600 Virginia Ave. NW, Ste. 502
Washington, DC 20037
Phone: (202)338-3501 **Fax:** (202)965-6520
Email: hefmona@erols.com
Morris E. Chafetz, MD, Pres.

Fnded: 1975. **Desc:** Seeks to develop cost-effective health promotion programs for government, industry, and the business community; helps people make informed decisions about their physical and mental health; participates in research for analysis and development of standards and programs to meet public health needs. **Pub:** *Conference Proceedings*, periodic. Proceedings. • *Health Fact Tips*, semiannual. • *HEF News: Perspectives on Health, Behavior, and Lifestyle*, quarterly. Newsletter. *Price:* $15/year. • Monograph. • Pamphlets.

★ 3332 ★ Health Industry Business Communications Council (HIBCC)
2525 E Arizona Biltmore Clr., Ste. 127
Phoenix, AZ 85016-2129
Phone: (602)381-1091 **Fax:** (602)381-1093
Email: info@hibcc.org
Website: http://www.hibcc.org/
Robert A. Hankin, PhD, Pres.

Fnded: 1984. **Mem:** 1,000. **Desc:** Individuals and companies in the health care industry. To improve the quality and economic efficiency of health care by instituting and overseeing a uniform system of computer bar coding (for identification of health care equipment) and by promoting the use of this and other automated technologies in the health care industry. **Pub:** *Health Industry Lines*, quarterly. Newsletter. *Price:* Included in membership dues. • *Standards*, periodic. **Frmly:** (1987) Health Industry Bar Code Council.

★ 3333 ★ Health Industry Group Purchasing Association (HIGPA)
1100 Wilson Blvd., Ste. 1200
Arlington, VA 22209
Phone: (703)243-9262 **Fax:** (703)243-8664
Email: info@higpa.org
Website: http://www.higpa.org

Fnded: 1990. **Desc:** For-profit and not-for-profit corporations, purchasing groups, associations, multi hospital systems and health care provider alliances. **Pub:** *CapitoLine*. Newsletter. *Price:* included in membership dues.

★ 3334 ★ Health Information Resource Center (HIRC)
c/o Carole Klein-Alexander
1850 W Winchester Rd., Ste. 213
Libertyville, IL 60048
Phone: (847)816-8660 **Free:** 800-828-8225
Fax: (847)816-8662
Email: info@healthawards.com
Website: http://www.healthawards.com
Patricia Henze, Exec. Dir.

Fnded: 1993. **Desc:** Clearinghouse for consumer health information. Provides information and referral services to many organizations that use or produce consumer health information materials. Conducts market research. **Pub:** *Consumer Health Information Online*, annual. *Price:* $29.95. • *Consumer Health Information: The Professional Guide to the Nations Best Consumer Health Information Programs and Materials*, annual. • *Health and Medical Media '99*, annual. Sourcebook of health and medical media contacts. *Price:* $149. • *The Health Events Calendar*, annual. Planning guide to national health events. *Price:* $19.95.

★ 3335 ★ Health Ministries (HM)
Board for Human Care Ministries
1333 S Kirkwood Rd.
Saint Louis, MO 63122-7295
Free: 888-843-5267 **Fax:** (314)965-0277
Email: healthministries@lcms.org
Website: http://humancare.lcms.org/hm/hm.htm
Bruce M. Hartung, PhD, Dir.

Desc: Consultants to all boards and commissions of the Lutheran Church-Missouri Synod having a relationship to the "healing mission" of the church and health issues of professional church workers. **Pub:** *AIDS Alert*. Newsletter. • *Cross and Caduceus*, 3/year. Newsletter. Focuses on health and wellness issues. *Price:* Free. • *Gesundheit*. Newsletter. • *Parish Nurse*, quarterly. Newsletter. **Frmly:** (1969) Council for Christian Medical Work; (1981) Commission on Health and Healing; (1986) Health and Healing Ministries.

★ 3336 ★ Health Occupations Students of America (HOSA)
6021 Morris Rd., No. 111
Flower Mound, TX 75028
Free: 800-321-HOSA **Fax:** (972)874-0063
Email: info@hosa.org

Website: http://www.hosa.org
Dr. Jim Koeninger, Exec. Dir.

Fnded: 1975. **Mem:** 52,000. **State Groups:** 36. **Local Groups:** 2100. **Desc:** Secondary and postsecondary students enrolled in health occupations education programs; health professionals and others interested in assisting and supporting the activities of HOSA; alumni of health occupations education programs and individuals who have made significant contributions to the field. Primary aim is to improve the quality of healthcare for all Americans by urging members to develop self-improvement skills. Operates within health occupation education programs in public high schools and postsecondary institutions. Encourages members to develop an understanding of current healthcare issues, environmental concerns, and survival needs worldwide. Conducts programs to help individuals improve their occupational skills and develop leadership qualities. Conducts exhibits, management workshops, and medical facility tours; provides social and recreational activities. Maintains speakers' bureau; compiles statistics. **Pub:** *HOSA Leaders Directory*, annual. Directory. • *HOSA Leaders' Update*, quarterly. • *HOSA News Magazine*, quarterly. Magazine. • *Story of HOSA*. Video. • Brochure. • Handbook. • Also publishes recruitment package. **AKA:** National HOSA.

★ 3337 ★ Health Optimizing Institute (HOI)

PO Box 1233
Del Mar, CA 92014
Phone: (858)481-7751 **Fax:** (858)481-7751
Email: year2020vision@earthlink.net
Dr. Howard Hunt, Exec. Officer

Fnded: 1978. **Desc:** Disseminates information on holistic and alternative health therapies aimed at building the human immune system and reversing the aging process. Conducts research and training programs in energy medicine. **Pub:** *Chronicle of Holistic Health*. Journal. **Frmly:** National Center for the Exploration of Human Potential.

★ 3338 ★ Health Physics Society (HPS)

1313 Dolley Madison Blvd., Ste. 402
Mc Lean, VA 22101-3926
Phone: (703)790-1745 **Fax:** (703)790-2672
Email: hps@burkinc.com
Website: http://www.hps.org/
Richard J. Burk, Jr., Exec. Sec.

Fnded: 1956. **Mem:** 6,890. **Local Groups:** 41. **Desc:** Persons engaged in some form of activity in the field of health physics (the profession devoted to radiation protection). To improve public understanding of the problems and needs in radiation protection; to promote health physics as a profession. Maintains Elda E. Anderson Memorial Fund to be used for teachers, researchers, and others. Provides placement service at annual meeting. Cosponsors American Board of Health Physics for certification of health physicists. **Pub:** *Health Physics Journal*, monthly. Journal. • *Health Physics Society–Membership Handbook*, annual. • *Health Physics Society–Newsletter*, monthly. Newsletter.

★ 3339 ★ Health in Prisons Project (ICPMS) (Conseil International des Services Medicaux Penitentiaires)

Wicken House, Weston Rd.
Aston Clinton
Buckinghamshire HP22 5EP, United Kingdom
Phone: 44 1296 630448 **Fax:** 44 1296 632448
Email: england&wales@hipp-europe.org

Fnded: 1976. **Mem:** 200. **Nat'l Groups:** 1. **Lang(s):** English, French, Spanish. **Desc:** Medical and health care professionals; associate members are administrators of prison health care agencies. Promotes discussion among prison health professionals. Strives to improve health care worldwide; encourages postgraduate training for doctors working in prison settings. **Pub:** Proceedings.

★ 3340 ★ Health Professions Authority Zimbabwe

PO Box A410 Avondale
Harare, Zimbabwe
Phone: 263 754930 **Fax:** 263 756731

Lang(s): English. **Desc:** Statutory body registering health practitioners. Promotes and coordinates members' activities; facilitates communication among members. Issues certification; formulates and enforces standards of conduct and practice among members.

★ 3341 ★ Health Promotion Institute (HPI)

c/o National Council on the Aging
300 D St. SW, Ste. 801
Washington, DC 20024
Phone: (202)479-1200 **Fax:** (202)479-0735
Email: info@ncoa.org
Website: http://www.ncoa.org
Glendale Johnson, Contact

Fnded: 1986. **Mem:** 700. **Desc:** A program of the National Council on the Aging. Seeks to aid professionals who are interested in developing and implementing health promotion programs for senior citizens and serving older consumers. Promotes optimal quality of life for older adults, including physical, emotional, and mental health as well as social and spiritual well-being. Advocates for and empowers older adults to achieve health and well-being through a multidisciplinary approach. Provides information and materials on health promotion programs. **Frmly:** (1991) National Center for Health Promotion and Aging.

★ 3342 ★ Health Research Board

73 Lower Baggot St.
Dublin 2, Ireland
Phone: 353 1 6761176 **Fax:** 353 1 6612335
Email: hrb@hrb.ie
Website: http://hrb2002.healthnet.ie/

Fnded: 1987. **Desc:** Promotes, assists, commissions or conducts medical, epidemiological, health and health services research.

★ 3343 ★ Health Research Council of New Zealand (HRC)

PO Box 5541
Wellesley St.
Auckland, New Zealand
Phone: 64 9 3798227 **Fax:** 64 9 3779988
Email: bcrocker@hrc.govt.nz
Website: http://www.hrc.govt.nz

Fnded: 1990. **Mem:** 12. **Desc:** Initiates and supports general health-related research, including the biomedical, public health, Maori, and clinical fields in New Zealand. Coordinates health research on a national basis and administers and disburses government research funding. Bestows awards. **Pub:** *HRC Annual Report*. Annual Report. • *HRC Newsletter*, quarterly. Newsletter. Contains information on health research in New Zealand. • *Maori Health Research Newsletter*, semiannual. Newsletter. **Frmly:** (1937) Medical Research Council of New Zealand.

★ 3344 ★ Health Research and Educational Trust (HRET)

c/o American Hospital Association
1 N Franklin
Chicago, IL 60606
Phone: (312)422-3000 **Fax:** (312)422-4568
Email: mpittman@aha.org
Website: http://www.hospitalconnect.com/aha/hret/
Mary A. Pittman, Dr.PH, Pres.

Fnded: 1944. **Desc:** Encourages and engages in educational, research, and demonstration activities to improve the management of hospital and health services. **Pub:** *Health Services Research*, bimonthly. • Books. • Manuals. • Monographs. **Frmly:** (1959) Educational Trust of the American Hospital Association; (2002) Hospital Research and Educational Trust.

★ 3345 ★ Health Sciences Communications Association (HESCA)

39 Wedgewood Dr., Ste. A
Jewett City, CT 06351
Phone: (860)376-5915 **Fax:** (860)376-6621
Email: hesca@hesca.org
Website: http://www.hesca.org/
Ronald Sokolowski, Exec. Dir.

Fnded: 1959. **Mem:** 400. **Reg. Groups:** 9. **Desc:** Media managers, graphic artists, biomedical librarians, producers, faculty members of health science and veterinary medicine schools, health professional organizations, and industry representatives. Acts as a clearinghouse for information used by professionals engaged in health science communications. Coordinates Media Festivals Program which recognizes outstanding media productions in the health sciences. Offers placement service. **Pub:** *Feedback*, 5/year. Provides members with information on the field of biocommunications and on work of colleagues. Includes employment listings and regional news. *Price:* Included in membership dues; $30/year for nonmembers. • *Health Sciences Communications Association–Who's Who*, annual. Membership Directory. *Price:* Included in membership dues. • *HESCA Learning Resources Center Catalog*, annual. Catalog. • *Journal of Biocommunication*, quarterly. Journal. Includes abstracts of biocommunication literature, gallery of medical art, and video and other media reviews. *Price:* Included in membership dues; $25 for nonmembers; $28 for institutions; $20 for students. • *Patient Education Sourcebook*. • Brochures. • Monographs. • Also publishes indexes; distributes audiovisual materials. **Frmly:** (1972) Council on Medical Television.

★ 3346 ★ Health Services Union of Australia (HSUA)

171 Drummond St.
Carlton, VIC 3053, Australia
Phone: 61 3 93413328 **Fax:** 61 3 96542386
Email: hsua@hsua.asn.au
Website: http://www.hsua.asn.au

Mem: 90,000. **Lang(s):** English. **Desc:** Workers in the health care industries. Seeks to advance the economic well-being and improve the conditions of employment of members. Represents members in negotiations with employers.

★ 3347 ★ Health and Social Policy Corp. (Corporacion de Salud y Politicas Sociale — CORSAPS)

Roman Diez 228 Of. 401
Providencia
Santiago, Chile
Phone: 56 2 2641261 **Fax:** 56 2 2352312
Email: corsaps@reuna.cl

Fnded: 1990. **Lang(s):** English, Spanish. **Desc:** Promotes health reform and the development of related social policy for the citizens of Chile. Focuses primarily on the health concerns of young people and women. Supports applied research.

★ 3348 ★ Health Systems Trust - South Africa (HNSA)

PO Box 808
Durban 4000, Republic of South Africa
Phone: 27 31 3072954 **Fax:** 27 31 3040775
Email: hst@healthlink.org.za
Website: http://www.hst.org.za

Lang(s): Afrikaans, English. **Desc:** Hospitals, clinics, and other health care facilities; telecommunications and satellite communications networks. Promotes improved communication and cooperation among health care facilities. Serves as a clearinghouse on medicine and telecommunications; maintains electronic network linking members; conducts educational and training programs for health care and telecommunications professionals.

★ 3349 ★ Health Workers Union of the Russian Federation
Lenin Ave. 42
117119 Moscow, Russia
Phone: 7 95 9388443 **Fax:** 7 95 9388134
Email: ckprz@online.ru

Fnded: 1990. **Mem:** 3100,022. **Reg. Groups:** 78. **Local Groups:** 23094. **Lang(s):** English, Russian. **Desc:** Physicians, nurses, pharmacists, paramedical personnel, and medical students and trainees. Promotes professional advancement of members; works to maintain high standards of practice and ethics in the field of medicine. Represents members' interests before government agencies; promulgates and enforces standards of practice and conduct. **Pub:** *Profsoiuznaya Tema*, quarterly. Information on protection of health workers' rights and interests.

★ 3350 ★ Healthcare Billing and Management Association
1540 S Coast Hwy., No. 203
Laguna Beach, CA 92651
Free: 877-640-4262 **Fax:** (949)376-3456
Email: info@hbma.com
Website: http://www.hbma.com
Sanford J. Hill, Pres.

Desc: Companies who provide third paty medical billing services.

★ 3351 ★ HealthCare Compliance Packaging Council (HCPC)
252 N Washington St., Ste. A
Falls Church, VA 22046
Phone: (703)538-4030 **Fax:** (703)538-6305
Email: pgmayberry@aol.com
Website: http://www.unitdose.org
Peter G. Mayberry, Exec. Dir.

Fnded: 1990. **Mem:** 80. **Desc:** Promotes the use of "unit-dose blister packaging" for pharmaceutical as a means of insuring better patient compliance with drug regimens. Sponsors research and provides educational programs. **Pub:** *Compliance News and Views*, quarterly. Newsletter. • *Unit Dose Alert*, bimonthly. Newsletter.

★ 3352 ★ Healthcare Financial Management Association (HFMA)
1301 Connecticut Ave., NW, Ste. 300
Washington, DC 20036-3417
Phone: (202)296-2920 **Free:** 800-252-HFMA
Fax: (202)223-9771
Email: webmaster@hfma.org
Website: http://www.hfma.org
Terry Arya, Contact

Mem: 33,000. **Desc:** Healthcare management associates. Strives to help its members excel in their jobs and careers. Hosts seminars and conferences. **Pub:** *Healthcare Financial Management*, monthly. Magazine. Contains information related to the healthcare industry. • *HFMA Express News*, weekly. Newsletter. E-mailed to members. *Price:* included in membership dues. • *HFMA Wants You to Know*, biweekly. Newsletter. Available via e-mail to members and public. *Price:* Free. • *Patient Accounts*, monthly. Newsletter. Contains information related to patient financial services.

★ 3353 ★ Healthcare Forum
180 Montgomery St., Ste. 1520
San Francisco, CA 94104-4230
Kathryn E. Johnson, CEO & Pres.

Fnded: 1927. **Mem:** 1,100. **Desc:** Healthcare leaders and executives. Promotes visionary leadership and motivation in healthcare. Conducts leadership development education programs; produces computer based educational materials. Sponsors research activities. **Pub:** *Healthcare Forum Journal*, bimonthly. Journal. *Price:* $55.

★ 3354 ★ Healthcare Leadership Council (HLC)
900 17th St. NW, Ste. 600
Washington, DC 20006
Phone: (202)452-8700 **Fax:** (202)296-9561
Email: dwiermanski@hlc.org
Website: http://hlc.org
Mary Grealey, Pres.

Fnded: 1988. **Desc:** Health care industry executives. Promotes the advancement of a market-based health care system that values innovation and provides affordable, high-quality health care; presents its system idea to Congress, administration, media, the research community and the public.

★ 3355 ★ HealthCare Ministries (HCM)
521 W Lynn St.
Springfield, MO 65802
Phone: (417)866-6311 **Fax:** (417)866-4711
Email: ivainio@hcmdfm.org
Website: http://www.healthcareministries.org

Desc: Medical missions arm of the Assemblies of God Foreign Missions. Strives to demonstrate and teach love and compassion in all aspects of the ministry. Conducts seminars, short-term medical evangelism teams and teaches health education.

★ 3356 ★ Healthlink Worldwide
Cityside
40 Adler St.
London E1 1EE, United Kingdom
Phone: 44 20 75391570 **Fax:** 44 20 75391580
Email: info@healthlink.org.uk
Website: http://www.healthlink.org.uk

Fnded: 1977. **Mem:** 70. **Lang(s):** English. **Desc:** Works in partnership with organisations in developing countries seeking to improve the health and well-being of poor and vulnerable communities by strengthening the provision, use, and impact of information. Offers expertise in various aspects of health and disability-related communications, including development of print and electronic materials, resource centre, and database development. **Pub:** *AIDS Action*, quarterly. Newsletter. • *Annual Report.* • *Child Health Dialogue*, quarterly. Newsletter. • *Disability Dialogue*, quarterly. Newsletter. **Frmly:** Appropriate Health Resources and Technologies Action Group.

★ 3357 ★ HealthNet Zimbabwe (HZ)
Computer Science Department
University of Zimbabwe
Harare, Zimbabwe
Phone: 263 4 303211 **Fax:** 263 4 333407
Email: borland@healthnet.zw

Lang(s): English. **Desc:** Health care professionals. Promotes increased use of electronic communications to advance the practice of health care. Serves as a clearinghouse on medicine.

★ 3358 ★ HEAR Center (HEAR)
301 E Del Mar Blvd.
Pasadena, CA 91101
Phone: (626)796-2016 **Fax:** (626)796-2320
Email: auditory@mindspring.com
Website: http://www.hearcenter.org
Josephine F. Wilson, MA, Exec. Dir.

Fnded: 1954. **Desc:** Auditory and verbal program designed to help hearing impaired children, infants, and adults lead normal and productive lives. Seeks to develop auditory techniques to aid people who have communication problems due to deafness. Primary objectives include early identification of hearing loss in infants and children and early amplification. Operates a program involving: binaural hearing aids where appropriate; continuous exposure to sound; development of auditory perception; wide-range amplification; environmental stimulation. Provides services in: diagnosis and audiological evaluation; hearing aid evaluation and trial use; development of listening skills and articulation; speech therapy; hearing aid dispensing; parent counseling. **Pub:** *Conquering Childhood Deafness*. Book. • *Effectiveness of Early Detection and Auditory Stimulation on the Speech and Language of Hearing Impaired Children.* • *Hear: A Four Letter Word*. Book. • *HEAR Center Proceedings*, periodic. Proceedings. • *The Listener*, quarterly. Newsletter. Covers topics of interest to the hearing and speech impaired community, as well as services and activities of the center. *Price:* Free. **Frmly:** (1975) Hearing Education Through Auditory Research Foundation.

★ 3359 ★ Hear Now (HN)
6700 Washington Ave. S
Eden Prairie, MN 55344-3405
Phone: 800-648-4327 **Free:** 800-648-HEAR
Fax: (952)828-6946
Email: joanita@sotheworldmayhear.org
Website: http://www.sotheworldmayhear.org
Joanita Stelter, Prog. Dir.

Fnded: 1988. **Desc:** Provides hearing aids for very low income hard of hearing individuals of all ages. Offers financial and fund raising assistance for hard of hearing and deaf individuals who need cochlear implants. Collects broken and used hearing aids through its HEAR-O Recycling Program to support assistance programs. Also publishes information packet.

★ 3360 ★ Hearing Concern
7/11 Armstrong Rd.
London W3 7JL, United Kingdom
Phone: 44 181 7429151 **Fax:** 44 181 7429043
Email: info@hearingconcern.org.uk
Website: http://www.hearingconcern.org.uk

Fnded: 1947. **Mem:** 3,000. **Nat'l Groups:** 1. **Reg. Groups:** 180. **Lang(s):** English, Welsh. **Desc:** Dedicated to improving the quality of life for those who are hard of hearing. Provides advice, information and support, as well as communication access and raises public and professional awareness of the issues associated with hearing loss. **Pub:** *Hearing Concern*, quarterly. Magazine. **Frmly:** Hearing Concern, British Association of the Hard of Hearing; (1993) British Association of the Hard of Hearing.

★ 3361 ★ Hearing Education and Awareness for Rockers (HEAR)
PO Box 460847
San Francisco, CA 94146-0847
Fax: (415)409-5683
Email: orders@hearnet.com
Website: http://www.hearnet.com
Kathy Peck, Exec. Dir.

Fnded: 1988. **Desc:** Musicians, music industry professionals, and music lovers. Seeks to prevent hearing loss and Tinnitus by promoting public awareness regarding the dangers of over amplified music and noise. Promotes the use of hearing protection and enhancement devices, especially among young people. Produces public service announcements recording artists, school programs, distributes ear protection and information at music events, conducts free hearing screening programs and provides hearing information and resources and H.E.A.R. Affiliate referrals via HEARNET.COM. **Pub:** *Can't Hear You Knocking*. Video. *Price:* $39.95. • *HEAR Information Packet*. *Price:* $10.

★ 3362 ★ Hearing Instrument Manufacturer's Software Association
c/o Scott Peterson
2550 University Ave. W, Ste. 241N
Saint Paul, MN 55114
Phone: (651)644-2921 **Free:** 800-435-9246
Fax: (651)644-3046
Email: himsa@himsa.com
Website: http://www.himsa.com/
Scott Peterson, Contact

Fnded: 1993. **Desc:** Works to develop, market and support NOAH, one standard for integrated hearing care software. **Pub:** *HIMSA News*, quarterly. Newsletter. Contains recent information on the organization and products.

★ 3363 ★ Heart Disease Research Foundation (HDRF)
50 Court St.
Brooklyn, NY 11201
Phone: (718)649-6210
Dr. Yoshiaki Omura, MD, Dir., Med. Research

Fnded: 1962. **Desc:** Promotes research aimed at the prevention, early diagnosis, and treatment of cardiovascular disease and related medico-social problems. Supports and conducts research, both basic and clinical, in the early diagnosis, prevention, and treatment of cardiovascular diseases using a multidisciplinary approach. Studies include the effects of acupuncture and electrotherapeutics on blood chemistry and the cardiovascular system, the clinical applications of these methods, and the noninvasive early diagnostic methods of cardiovascular diseases. Sponsors postgraduate continuing medical educational courses for physicians, dentists, and medical researchers. Conducts public education programs on the heart and heart disease. Answers questions from the public and professionals; supplies available educational information on cardiovascular diseases and research.

★ 3364 ★ Heart Foundation of Australia
Corner of Denison St. and Gelis Ct.
Deakin, ACT 2600, Australia
Email: heartlinesa@heartfoundation.com.au

Fnded: 1961. **Desc:** Works to improve the heath of Australians and to reduce disability and death from heart and blood vessel disease. Fosters research into heart health and blood vessel diseases. Promotes behaviors which improve heart health through educational programs for health professionals, people with heart disease, and others.

★ 3365 ★ Heart and Stroke Foundation of Canada (HSFC)
222 Queen St., Ste. 1402
Ottawa, ON, Canada K1P 5V9
Phone: (613)569-4361 **Fax:** (613)569-3278
Website: http://ww1.heartandstroke.ca

Desc: Seeks to improve the health of Canadians by preventing and reducing disability and death from heart disease and stroke through research, health promotion, and advocacy. Fosters pioneering diagnostic techniques. Advocates for healthy public policies, including review of Canadian food labeling legislation and smoking cessation legislation.

★ 3366 ★ Heartbeat
2015 Devon St.
Colorado Springs, CO 80909
Phone: (719)596-2575
Email: archlj@msn.com
LaRita Archibald, Founder

Fnded: 1980. **Desc:** Persons who have lost a loved one due to suicide. Provides an atmosphere whereby grieving participants receive support, understanding, direction, and encouragement from those who have successfully resolved their grief. Offers "postvention" education program aimed at preventing the suicide of survivors. Maintains speakers' bureau. **Pub:** *Forming Heartbeat Chapters.* Manual. **Frmly:** Heartbeat/Survivors After Suicide.

★ 3367 ★ HEATH Resource Center (GWHRC)
George Washington University
2121 K St. NW, Ste. 220
Washington, DC 20037
Phone: (202)973-0904 **Free:** 800-544-3284
Fax: (202)973-0908
Email: askheath@heath.gwu.edu
Website: http://www.heath.gwu.edu
Pamela Ekpone, Dir.

Fnded: 1977. **Desc:** National information Clearinghouse. Works to aid in the postsecondary education of people who are disabled. Provides information on educational support services, procedures, policies, adaptations, campus opportunities, vocational technical schools, adult education programs, and independent living centers. **Pub:** *Fact Sheet*, quarterly. Newsletter. • *Information*, 3/year. Directory. • *Resource Directory*, semiannual. Directory. • Also publishes topical informational materials.

★ 3368 ★ Helen Keller International - Asia-Pacific Regional Office (HKII)
Jl. Bungur Dalam 23A-B
Kemang
12730 Jakarta, Indonesia
Phone: 62 21 7198147 **Fax:** 62 21 7198148
Email: info@hkiasiapacific.org
Website: http://www.hkiasiapacific.org

Desc: National branch of the international organization. Fosters community-based blindness prevention and rehabilitation programs and services. Provides technical assistance and materials for the design and implementation of eye care within the existing primary health care system. Conducts projects and disseminates information on: preventing nutritional blindness; reducing cataract blindness; combatting onchocerciasis ("river blindness"); and improving the quality of life of the blind. Distributes medicine for eye disease treatment. Offers educational services.

★ 3369 ★ Helen Keller International - Morocco (HKI)
3, rue Sekkoura
Rabat, Morocco
Phone: 212 7 756636
Email: info@hkworld.org
Website: http://www.hki.org

Fnded: 1915. **Lang(s):** Arabic, French. **Desc:** Fosters community-based blindness prevention and rehabilitation programs and services. Provides technical assistance and materials for the design and implementation of eye care within the existing primary health care system. Conducts projects and disseminates information on: preventing nutritional blindness; reducing cataract blindness; combatting onchocerciasis ("river blindness"); and improving the quality of life of the blind. Distributes medicine for eye disease treatment. Offers educational services.

★ 3370 ★ Helen Keller International - Nepal (HKIN)
Jl Bungur Dalam 23A-B
Jakarta 12730, India
Phone: 62 21 27198147 **Fax:** 62 21 7198148
Email: info@hkiasiapacific.org
Website: http://www.hkiasiapacific.org

Fnded: 1988. **Desc:** Works to prevent blindness; provides rehabilitative services to the blind. Cooperates with nongovernment agencies to devise and implement vision care initiatives. Programs focus on preventing nutritional and other preventable forms of blindness. Makes available routine eye care services; collaborates with government and nongovernment agencies to reduce micronutrient deficiencies which lead to an increase in morbidity and mortality in women and children.

★ 3371 ★ Helen Keller National Center for Deaf-Blind Youths and Adults (HKNC)
111 Middle Neck Rd.
Sands Point, NY 11050
Phone: (516)944-8900 **Fax:** (516)944-7302
Email: hkncdir@aol.com
Website: http://helenkeller.org/national/
Joseph J. McNulty, Exec. Dir.

Fnded: 1969. **Reg. Groups:** 10. **Desc:** Provides diagnostic evaluations, comprehensive vocational and personal adjustment training, job preparation and placement for people who are deaf-blind from every state and territory. Field services include information and referral and advocacy and technical assistance to professionals, consumers, and families. Sponsors annual National Helen Keller Deaf-Blind Awareness Week. **Pub:** *Giving.* Newsletter. • *Guidelines for Helping Deaf-Blind Persons.* Brochure. • *HKNC Description of Services.* Booklet. • *Nat-Cent News*, periodic. Magazine. • *National Family Association for the Deaf-Blind Newsletter*, periodic. Newsletter. • *Older Adult Program.* Brochure. • Also publishes many other free materials about the annual Deaf-Blind Awareness week. **Frmly:** National Rehabilitation of Deaf-Blind Adults.

★ 3372 ★ Helen Keller Worldwide (HKW)
352 Park Ave. S, Ste. 1200
New York, NY 10010
Phone: (212)532-0544 **Free:** 877-535-5374
Fax: (212)532-6014
Email: info@hkworld.org
Website: http://www.hkworld.org
John M. Palmer, Pres.

Fnded: 1915. **Desc:** Assists governments and voluntary agencies throughout Asia, Africa, and the Americas (including the United States) to establish and integrate, into their national health and welfare systems, services to prevent or cure eye diseases and blindness and to rehabilitate and educate visually disabled persons. Focuses on programs in the prevention and treatment of blindness caused by malnutrition, trachoma, onchocerciasis and cataracts. Trains health workers at all levels in the use of specially developed materials to diagnose and treat eye problems and to refer patients to hospitals. Conducts courses for teachers of blind children and for vocational and mobility instructors of blind adults; offers training for indigenous field workers who instruct the rural blind in daily living skills and provide vocational education. Provides information on programs and services on the problem of blindness throughout the world. Compiles statistics. Provides free prescription eyeglasses to junior high school students through the Childsight Program. **Pub:** *Helen Keller Annual Report*, annual. Annual Report. *Price:* Free. • *Insight*, 4/year. Newsletter. *Price:* Free. • Also publishes fact sheets, technical reports, training materials on nutritional blindness detection and treatment, and educational materials. **Frmly:** (1925) Permanent Blind Relief War Fund; (1946) American Braille Press for War and Civilian Blind; (1977) American Foundation for Overseas Blind; (1999) Helen Keller International; (2000) Helen Keller Worldwide; (2002) Helen Keller International.

★ 3373 ★ Helene Fuld Health Trust
452 Fifth Ave., 17th Fl.
New York, NY 10018
Phone: (212)525-2418 **Fax:** (212)681-1335
Email: www.mail@fuldtrust.org
Website: http://www.fuldtrust.org
Jina Piak, Grants Mgr.

Desc: Strives to support the improvement of the health, welfare, and education of student nurses.

★ 3374 ★ Hellenic American Dental Society (HADS)
PO Box 4803
Oak Brook, IL 60523-4803
Phone: (773)763-3600
Email: info@hads.com
Website: http://www.hads.com/
Dr. Athina Danigeles, Pres.

Desc: Dentists, dental hygienists and dental technicians of Greek descent, promoting Hellenic heritage. **Pub:** Newsletter, periodic. *Price:* included in membership dues.

★ 3375 ★ Hellenic Association of Dermatology and Venereology
5 I. Dragoumi St.
GR-161 21 Athens, Greece
Phone: 30 1 7239611 **Fax:** 30 1 7211122
Email: info@edae.gr
Website: http://www.edae.gr

Mem: 600. **Lang(s):** English, Greek. **Desc:** Offers awards; Conducts educational programs; compiles statistics. Maintains museum. **Pub:** *Hellenic Dermato-Venereological Review*, quarterly. **Frmly:** (2000) Hellenic Society of Dermatology and Venereology.

★ 3376 ★ Hellenic Association of Gerontology and Geriatrics (HAGG)
Kaningos 23
GR-10677 Athens, Greece
Phone: 30 21 3811612 **Fax:** 30 21 3840317
Email: hagg@compulink.gr
Website: http://www.gerontology.gr

Fnded: 1977. **Mem:** 168. **Nat'l Groups:** 1. **Lang(s):** English, French, Greek. **Desc:** Focuses on the problems and the process of aging. **Pub:** *Alzheimer's Disease*. Booklet. • *Depression for the Elderly*. Booklet. Guides to geriatric health and nutrition. **Frmly:** (1994) Hellenic Association for Geronontoolgy and Geriatrics.

★ 3377 ★ Hellenic Cardiological Society
6 Potamianou St.
GR-115 28 Athens, Greece
Phone: 30 1 7221633 **Fax:** 30 1 7226139
Email: hcs@eexi.gr
Website: http://www.hcs.gr

Fnded: 1927. **Mem:** 1,633. **Desc:** Promotes the study of cardiology in Greece, including electrophysiologic studies and ablation techniques, pacemakers and defibrillators, echocardiography, cardiac MRI, nuclear cardiology procedures and applications, exercise stress tests, and cardiac rehabilitation. **Pub:** *Hellenic Journal of Cardiology*. Journal. Contains articles on aspects of cardiovascular disease.

★ 3378 ★ Hellenic Psychological Society (HPS)
Psychological Laboratory
Aristotle University of Thessaloniki
GR-540 06 Thessaloniki, Greece
Phone: 30 31 997374 **Fax:** 30 31 997384
Email: efklides@psy.auth.gr

Fnded: 1990. **Mem:** 300. **Desc:** Psychologists in Greece. Promotes the advancement of psychological science. **Pub:** *Psychology: The Journal of the Hellenic Psychological Society*, quarterly. Journal.

★ 3379 ★ Hellenic Radiological Society
P. Kyriakou 21
GR-115 21 Athens, Greece
Phone: 30 1 6451489
Email: info@helrad.org
Website: http://www.helrad.org/whoweare/whoweare.htm

Fnded: 1933. **Desc:** Works to promote and develop standards of radiology, scientific information exchange in all fields of radiology and related sciences through education and research. **Pub:** *Hellenic Radiology Journal*, quarterly. Journal. Covers all technical and clinical aspects of diagnostic imaging and intervention.

★ 3380 ★ Help the Aged
1300 Carling Ave., Ste. 205
Ottawa, ON, Canada K1Z 7L2
Phone: (613)232-0727 **Free:** 800-648-1111
Fax: (613)232-7625
Email: info@helptheaged.ca
Website: http://www.helptheaged.ca

Fnded: 1975. **Mem:** 10,000. **Lang(s):** English, French. **Desc:** Individuals and organizations united to provide assistance to the destitute elderly. Works to increase public awareness of issues facing older people in Canada and in the developing world. **Pub:** *Agecare*, annual. Newspaper.

★ 3381 ★ HELP - Institute for Body Chemistry (HELP)
PO Box 1338
Bryn Mawr, PA 19010
Phone: (610)525-1225
Email: ekrimmel2@earthlink.net
Edward & Patricia Krimmel, Dirs.

Fnded: 1979. **Mem:** 2,500. **Desc:** Health professionals and interested individuals. Promotes public awareness of body chemistry problems within the context of general health. Seeks to collect, verify, and distribute information related to body chemistry especially hypoglycemia (low blood sugar), Celiac Disease, and cholesterol management. Conducts seminars regarding nutrition, exercise, life style, and emotional stability. Develops support groups and encourages communication among members. **Pub:** *Advocate*. Newsletter. Includes information on body chemistry, nutrition, and related medical research. • *Cholesterol Control Handbook and Cookbook*. • *Low Blood Sugar Cookbook*. • *Low Blood Sugar Handbook*. • *Vital Health Facts and Composition of Foods*.

★ 3382 ★ Helpage International
PO Box 32832
London N1 9UZ, United Kingdom
Phone: 44 207 2787778 **Fax:** 44 207 7137993
Email: hai@helpage.org

Fnded: 1983. **Mem:** 65. **Reg. Groups:** 5. **Lang(s):** English, French, Russian, Spanish. **Desc:** Works with and for disadvantaged older people worldwide, to achieve lasting improvement in the quality of their lives. Supports the development of "grass roots" activity and the growth of local organisations working with older people. Projects focus on health, social services, residential, community and home care, income generation, advocacy, training and organisational development. **Pub:** *Adding Health to Years*. Handbook. • *Helpage International News*, 3/year. Newsletter. • *Opening a Residential Home for Elderly People*. Handbook.

★ 3383 ★ Helpage International - Thailand
c/o Asia/Pacific Regional Development Centre
Faculty of Nursing
Chiang Mai University
Chiang Mai 50200, Thailand
Phone: 66 53 894895 **Fax:** 66 53 358142
Email: helpage@helpageasia.com

Fnded: 1988. **Mem:** 16. **Lang(s):** English. **Desc:** Works to improve quality of life of older persons. Initiates and supports programs worldwide designed to help older persons meet their financial, material, medical, and social needs. **Pub:** *New Age Asia*, semiannual. Newsletter. A contact point for the network of members and non-member organisations of HelpAge International in order to promote age care in Asia region. • *Withichiwit (Thai Ageways)*, quarterly. Magazine. Magazine with pratical information on ageing issues for those working with older people.

★ 3384 ★ Helpage Latin America
c/o Valerie Mealla
Regional Centre for Latin America
Casilla 2217
La Paz, Bolivia
Phone: 591 2 2410583 **Fax:** 591 2 2410957
Email: helpage.bolivia@unete.com

Fnded: 1991. **Desc:** Works with groups and associations of older people worldwide to defend their rights and achieve lasting changes in their quality of life, promoting older people as development agents and achieving inclusion of aging as a development issue. **Pub:** *Latin America Quarterly Magazine*, quarterly. Magazine. Features information about the exchange of experiences at the regional level.

★ 3385 ★ Hemochromatosis Foundation (HF)
c/o Margit A. Krikker, MD
PO Box 8569
Albany, NY 12208-0569
Phone: (518)489-0972 **Fax:** (518)489-0227
Website: http://www.hemochromatosis.org
Margit A. Krikker, MD, Med. Dir. /Founder

Fnded: 1982. **Mem:** 4,000. **Reg. Groups:** 8. **State Groups:** 6. **Local Groups:** 4. **Desc:** Physicians and other individuals concerned with hereditary hemochromatosis. (Hereditary hemochromatosis is a disorder of iron metabolism in which dietary iron absorption exceeds body needs. If not diagnosed and treated, the accumulating iron may result in one or more complications: liver enlargement, heart irregularities and failure, diabetes and other hormonal deficiencies, arthritis, and early death.) Seeks to increase public and professional awareness of hereditary hemochromatosis and of the hazards of supplemental iron. Encourages routine use of screening tests by physicians, conducts screening studies of apparently healthy blood donors. Assists public, patients, families, and physicians with HH diagnosis, treatment, and genetic counseling and in forming regional support networks. Sponsors periodic teaching day for physicians and patients and their families. Conducts research programs. Plans to establish a central registry of persons with the disorder. **Pub:** *Family Teaching Conference 1992 at Cleveland Clinic*. Video. • *Hemochromatosis Awareness: A Quarterly Update on Hereditary and Acquired Iron-Overload*. Newsletter. Includes calendar of events and information on available services. *Price:* Free. • Booklets. **Frmly:** (1992) Hemochromatosis Research Foundation.

★ 3386 ★ Hepatitis Foundation International
c/o Martha Young
504 Blick Dr.
Silver Spring, MD 20904
Phone: (301)622-4200 **Free:** 800-891-0707
Fax: (301)622-4702
Email: hfi@comcast.net
Website: http://www.hepfi.org
Thelma King Thiel, Chm. and C. E. O.

Fnded: 1994. **Mem:** 50,000. **Local Groups:** 425. **Desc:** Individuals concerned about those with hepatitis. Provides education and information for distribution to the general public, patients, educators, and medical professionals about the diagnosis, treatment, and prevention of viral hepatitis. Maintains database of hepatitis support groups and website information. Conducts train-the-trainer programs for those interested in the topic. **Pub:** *Hepatitis Alers*, quarterly. Newsletter. Contains current articles about the latest research and developments in combating viral hepatitis.

★ 3387 ★ Herbal Association of South Africa (HAOSA)
PO Box 1831, Escourt
Kwazulu 3310, Republic of South Africa
Phone: 27 33 2631227 **Fax:** 27 33 2631227
Email: jinxsnuf@futurest.co.za

Fnded: 1991. **Desc:** Aims to provide an umbrella body. Provides an educational forum by teaching about herbs. Reduces the high cost of healthcare. Unites those interested in herbs.

★ 3388 ★ Hereditary Disease Foundation (HDF)
1303 Pico Blvd.
Santa Monica, CA 90405-1553
Phone: (310)450-9913 **Fax:** (310)450-9532
Email: cures@hdfoundation.org
Website: http://www.hdfoundation.org
Leslie P. Weiner, Chair

Fnded: 1968. **Desc:** To fund basic biomedical research on the causes, prevention, diagnosis, treatment, and cure of genetic disorders and in particular Huntington's Disease, an inherited neurological disorder. Maintains grant programs to support scientific projects in major medical and basic science laboratories throughout the U.S. Offers grants and postdoctoral fellowships. Sponsors a series of interdisciplinary workshops to stimulate new ideas and approaches to understanding hereditary problems. Helps maintain two tissue banks for research purposes. Disseminates information to organizations and individuals. **Pub:** *Hereditary Disease Foundation*, 4/yr.Newsletter. *Price:* Free.

★ 3389 ★ Herpes Resource Center - American Social Health Association (HRC)
PO Box 13827
Research Triangle Park, NC 27709

Phone: (919)361-8488 **Fax:** (919)361-8425
Email: phidra@ashastd.org
Website: http://www.ashastd.org/hrc

Fnded: 1979. **Local Groups:** 98. **Desc:** Individuals with recurrent genital herpes infections; individuals interested in the dissemination of information about genital herpes. (Herpes is a sexually transmitted disease which is as yet incurable.) Works to give emotional support to individuals, and to provide current information about herpes. Maintains the National HPV Hotline. Offers referrals to local support groups (HELP) throughout the U.S. and Canada for people living with herpes; HELP groups provide a safe, confidential environment in which to obtain accurate information about HPV and share experiences with other people concerned about herpes. Compiles statistics. **Pub:** *The Helper*, quarterly. Journal. *Price:* $25/yr. • *Herpes: Questions & Answers*. Pamphlet. *Price:* Free. • *Managing Herpes: How to Live and Love with a Chronic STD*. Book. *Price:* $27. • *Understanding Herpes*. Booklet. *Price:* $6.

★ 3390 ★ Herpes Viruses Association
41 North Rd.
London N7 9DP, United Kingdom
Phone: 44 207 6099061
Email: info@herpes.org.uk
Website: http://www.herpes.org.uk

Fnded: 1985. **Mem:** 1,300. **Local Groups:** 7. **Lang(s):** English, French, Spanish. **Desc:** Provides accurate information on herpes simplex virus (to counteract the "herpes hype"), to the media, health professionals and the public. **Pub:** *Sphere*, quarterly. Journal.

★ 3391 ★ Herpetological Association of Africa (HAA)
PO Box 13147
Port Elizabeth 6013, Republic of South Africa
Phone: 27 41 561051 **Fax:** 27 41 562175

★ 3392 ★ Hesperian Foundation (HF)
1919 Addison St., Ste. 304
Berkeley, CA 94704
Phone: (510)845-1447 **Fax:** (510)845-9141
Email: hesperian@hesperian.org
Website: http://www.hesperian.org
Sarah Shannon, Exec. Dir.

Fnded: 1973. **Desc:** Promotes good health in the developing world and in poor communities in the U.S. through community-based, informed self-care. Fosters constructive dialogue on health care and social change. Originally established to help launch Project Piaxtla, a health care network, and Project Projimo, a community-based rehabilitation center for spinal cord injuries, in western Mexico. The foundation now focuses on publishing community self-help health care books that are used throughout the world. Analyzes and criticizes existing social, political, and economic systems that prevent the poor from obtaining adequate standards of life and health. Operates gratis book fund, in which third world health care workers in the developing world receive Hesperian publications at no charge. **Pub:** *A Book for Midwives*. Book. *Price:* $22. • *Disabled Village Children*. Book. *Price:* $22. • *Helping Children Who Are Blind*. Book. *Price:* $12. • *Helping Health Workers Learn*. Book. *Price:* $20. • *Where There Is No Dentist*. Book. *Price:* $12. • *Where There Is No Doctor*. Book. *Price:* $17. • *Where Women Have No Doctor*. Book. *Price:* $20. • *The Women's Health Exchange*, quarterly. Newsletter. *Price:* Free.

★ 3393 ★ HHT Foundation International
PO Box 8087
New Haven, CT 06530
Phone: (410)357-9932 **Free:** 800-448-6389
Fax: (410)357-9931
Email: hhtinfor@hht.com
Website: http://www.hht.org

Fnded: 1991. **Mem:** 300. **Reg. Groups:** 3. **State Groups:** 3. **Desc:** Patients and their families; physicians, counselors, and health administrators; interested others. Promotes research into the treatment, causes, and cure of hereditary hemmorrhagic telangiectasia (HHT), also known as Osler-Weber-Rendu Syndrome. A rare genetic blood vessel disorder, HHT causes malformations of arteries and veins; hemorrhaging from the nose and intestine is also common. Malformations in the lungs cause shortness of breath, stroke, and brain abscess. Provides information exchange. Raises funds for research and patient service programs. Sponsors support groups. **Pub:** *HHT Newsletter*, quarterly. Newsletter. • *Our Blood Vessels*. Pamphlet. • Brochures. • Newsletter, semiannual.

★ 3394 ★ HIKE Fund
c/o Shirley R. Terrill
10115 Cherry Hill Pl.
Spring Hill, FL 34608-7116
Phone: (352)688-2579 **Fax:** (352)688-2579
Email: ceterrilli@aol.com
Website: http://www.missouriiojd.org/MO-HIKE/HIKE.htm
Carol Mentges, Pres.

Fnded: 1985. **Mem:** 15. **Desc:** Supported by the International Order of Job's Daughters. Works for complete equality and integration of the hearing impaired in society. Provides support and information services. Provides hearing devices for children (up to the age of 20) with financial need. **AKA:** Hearing Impaired Kids Endowment Fund.

★ 3395 ★ The Hip Society
c/o Karen V. Andersen
951 Old County Rd., No. 182
Belmont, CA 94002
Phone: (650)596-6190 **Fax:** (650)508-2039
Website: http://www.hipsoc.org/
Karen V. Andersen, Exec. Dir.

Fnded: 1968. **Desc:** Dedicated to the advancement of knowledge relating to the hip joint.

★ 3396 ★ Hispanic Dental Association
188 W Randolph St., Ste. 415
Chicago, IL 60601
Phone: (312)577-4013 **Free:** 800-852-7921
Fax: (312)577-4013
Email: hdassoc@aol.com
Website: http://www.hdassoc.org
Sandy Reed, Exec. Dir.

Fnded: 1990. **Mem:** 2,500. **Reg. Groups:** 31. **Desc:** Provides leadership and represents professionals who share a common commitment to improve the oral health of the Hispanic community. **Pub:** *HDA News & Reports*, quarterly. Newsletter.

★ 3397 ★ Hispanic-Serving Health Professions Schools
c/o Elena Rios, MD
1411 K St., NW, Ste. 200
Washington, DC 20005
Phone: (202)783-5262 **Fax:** (202)628-5898
Email: hishps@aol.com
Website: http://www.hshps.com
Elena Rios, MD, Dir.

Fnded: 1996. **Mem:** 22. **Desc:** Represents 16 medical schools. Seeks to strengthen the nation's capacity to educate and increase then numbers of high-quality Hispanic health care providers to serve and improve the health status of Hispanics and other populations. Develops educational opportunities in health professions schools in curriculum, research, and clinical experiences that will enable Hispanic and non-Hispanic health professions students to provide excellent health care to Hispanic populations. Promotes collaboration at the regional and national levels between educational institutions, communities, and other partners. **Frmly:** (2003) National Association of Hispanic-Serving Health Professions Schools.

★ 3398 ★ Histiocytosis Association of America
72 E Holly Ave., Ste. 101
Pitman, NJ 08071
Phone: (856)589-6606 **Fax:** (856)589-6614
Email: histiocyte@aol.com
Website: http://www.histio.org/association/index.shtml
Jeffrey M. Toughill, Pres.

Fnded: 1985. **Mem:** 5,200. **Desc:** Patients, families, and friends of those suffering from histiocytic disorders; physicians, oncologists, and hematologists working in the field of histiocytosis research. (Histiocytosis is a rare disease that causes histiocytes, a type of white blood cell, to multiply and attack organs, body systems, or bones.) Works to provide support for patients and their families and friends. Funds research on the cause and treatment of histiocytosis. Acts as a referral service. Maintains speakers' bureau. **Pub:** *The Facts About HLH/FHL*. Brochure. *Price:* Free. • *The Facts about Langerhans Cell Histiocytosis*. Brochure. *Price:* Free. • *The Facts about Langerhans Cell Histiocytosis and Diabetes Insipidus*. Brochure. • *Patient Directory*, periodic. Directory. • Newsletter, quarterly. Reports on histiocytosis patients, their families, physicians, researchers, and other interested parties. *Price:* Free. **Frmly:** (1987) Histiocytosis-X Association of America.

★ 3399 ★ Histochemical Society (HCS)
University Station
PO Box 85630
Seattle, WA 98145-1630
Phone: (206)616-5895 **Fax:** (206)616-5842
Email: mail@histochemicalsociety.org
Website: http://www.histochemicalsociety.org
Elizabeth Unger, Pres.

Fnded: 1950. **Mem:** 450. **Desc:** Physicians and scientists who employ hisotchemical and cytochemical techniques in their research. **Pub:** *The Journal of Histochemistry and Cytochemistry*, monthly. Journal. • Newsletter, semiannual.

★ 3400 ★ HIV/AIDS Prevention Grants Program
c/o United States Conference of Mayors
1620 Eye St. NW
Washington, DC 20006
Phone: (202)293-7330 **Fax:** (202)293-2352
Email: jobrien@usamayors.org
Website: http://www.usmayors.org
Thomas M. Menino, Pres.

Fnded: 1983. **Desc:** AIDS prevention program of the United States Conference of Mayors. Acts as a forum for information exchange among members; provides policy information to the media. Operates speakers' bureau and conducts educational programs. **Pub:** *AIDS Information Exchange*, bimonthly. Newsletter. • *Local AIDS Policy*. • *Local AIDS Services: A National Directory*, periodic. Directory. **Frmly:** (2003) HIV/AIDS Program.

★ 3401 ★ HIV/AIDS Treatment Information Service (ATIS)
PO Box 6303
Rockville, MD 20849-6303
Phone: (301)519-0459 **Free:** 800-448-0440
Fax: (301)519-6616
Email: atis@hivatis.org
Website: http://hivatis.org/

Desc: Provides bilingual health information regarding HIV/AIDS treatment options.

★ 3402 ★ Holistic Dental Association (HDA)
c/o Dr. Paul Plowman
PO Box 5007
Durango, CO 81301
Phone: (970)259-1091 **Fax:** (970)259-1091
Email: hda@frontier.net
Website: http://www.holisticdental.org
Dr. Dick Shepard, Exec. Dir.

Fnded: 1980. Mem: 200. Desc: Dentists, chiropractors, dental hygienists, physical therapists, and medical doctors. Goals are: to provide a holistic approach to better dental care for patients; to expand techniques, medications, and philosophies that pertain to extractions, anesthetics, fillings, crowns, and orthodontics. Encourages use of homeopathic medications, acupuncture, cranial osteopathy, nutritional techniques, and physical therapy in treating patients in addition to conventional treatments. Sponsors training and educational seminars. **Pub:** *Communicator*, quarterly. Newsletter. Includes calendar of events and research updates. *Price:* Included in membership dues. **Frmly:** Holistic Dental Association International.

★ 3403 ★ Home Birth Association of Ireland
36 Springlawn Ct.
Blachardstown
Dublin 15, Ireland
Phone: 353 1 8206940
Email: homebirth@eircom.net
Website: http://www.homebirth.ie

Fnded: 1982. **Mem:** 210. **Reg. Groups:** 22. **Lang(s):** English, Galician, Irish. **Desc:** Those interested in homebirthing. Seeks to increase the awareness of birth as a normal physiological process, while incorporating homebirthing into mainstream maternity services. Produces information booklets, midwives' directory, and holds conferences and support group meetings. **Pub:** Newsletter, quarterly.

★ 3404 ★ Home Healthcare Nurses Association (HHNA)
228 Seventh St. SE
Washington, DC 20003
Phone: (202)546-4754 **Free:** 800-558-4462
Fax: (202)547-3540
Email: hhna-info@nahc.org
Website: http://www.hhna.org
Margaret J. Cushan, Exec. Dir.

Fnded: 1999. **Mem:** 800. **Local Groups:** 10. **Desc:** Works to develop and promote the specialty of home healthcare nursing. Provides a forum for members to exchange information; influences public policy affecting the practice; fosters excellence in practice. **Pub:** *Home Healthcare Nurse*, 10/year. Journal. Published by Lippincott.

★ 3405 ★ Homeopathic Pharmacopoeia of the U.S.
PO Box 2221
Southeastern, PA 19399-2221
Phone: (610)783-5124 **Fax:** (610)783-5180
Website: http://www.hpus.com
John A. Borneman, III, Pres.

Fnded: 1980. **Mem:** 75. **Desc:** Prepares, publishes and distributes the Homeopathic Pharmacopoeia of the US. **Pub:** *Homeopathic Pharmacopoeia of the U.S.*.

★ 3406 ★ Homoeopathic Medical Association (HMA)
6 Livingstone Rd.
Gravesend DA12 5DZ, United Kingdom
Phone: 44 1474 560336 **Fax:** 44 1474 327431
Email: info@the-hma.org
Website: http://www.the-hma.org

Fnded: 1985. **Mem:** 300. **Desc:** Develops, supports and encourages the practice of homeopathic medicine in the UK and in other countries; increase public awareness and acceptance of homeopathy. **Pub:** *Homeopathy International*, quarterly. Journal. • *Register of Qualified Homeopathic Practitioners.*

★ 3407 ★ Hong Kong Alzheimer's Disease and Brain Failure Association
c/o GF Wang Lai House
Wang Tau Hom Estate
Kowloon
Hong Kong, People's Republic of China
Phone: 852 27943010 **Fax:** 852 23384820

Fnded: 1995. **Lang(s):** English. **Desc:** Advocates improvement in services and resources for patients affected by dementia and their families. Works to increase public awareness; assists and provides sponsorship for local research.

★ 3408 ★ Hong Kong Anti-Cancer Society (HKACS)
8/F, Comprehensive Services Block
Nam Long Hospital
30 Nam Long Shan Rd.
Hong Kong, People's Republic of China
Phone: 852 28140950 **Fax:** 852 28731405
Email: admin@hkacs.org.hk
Website: http://www.hkacs.org.hk

Fnded: 1963. **Mem:** 140. **Lang(s):** Chinese, English. **Desc:** Coordinates and promotes activities against cancer. Seeks to identify the causes of cancer and educate the public regarding cancer prevention. Sponsors cancer research and organizes educational programs.

★ 3409 ★ Hong Kong Association of Blood Transfusion and Haematology
15 King's Park Rise
Kowloon
Hong Kong, People's Republic of China
Phone: 852 27101271 **Fax:** 852 27804151
Email: ckleea@ha.org.hk
Website: http://www.fmshk.com.hk/hkabth

Fnded: 1992. **Mem:** 140. **Lang(s):** Chinese, English. **Desc:** Health care professionals operating in the fields of hematology and blood transfusion; corporations and organizations with an interest in hematology. Seeks to advance the practice of hematology and transfusion. Establishes and enforces standards of practice and professional conduct for members; serves as a forum for discussion of developments in hematology and transfusion; facilitates formation of contacts between members and their counterparts worldwide. **Pub:** Newsletter, 3/year.

★ 3410 ★ Hong Kong Association of Dental Surgery Assistants (HKADSA)
6/F Prince Philip Dental Hospital
34 Hospital Rd., Sai Ying Pun
Hong Kong, People's Republic of China
Phone: 852 28590325 **Fax:** 852 25470164
Email: lkleung@hkucc.hku.hk
Website: http://www.fmshk.com.hk/hkadsa/

Fnded: 1987. **Mem:** 120. **Lang(s):** Putonghua. **Desc:** Dental surgery assistants and trainees. Promotes the study and practice of dental surgery assistance; seeks to further the professional development of members. Serves as a clearinghouse on dental surgery assistance. Facilitates exchange of information among members; conducts educational and continuing professional development courses; sponsors social activities; maintains speakers' bureau. **Pub:** Newsletter, monthly.

★ 3411 ★ Hong Kong Association of Gerontology
GPO Box 10020
Hong Kong, People's Republic of China
Phone: 852 25581181 **Fax:** 852 27755586
Email: hkag@netvigator.com
Website: http://www.hkag.org

Fnded: 1987. **Mem:** 850. **Lang(s):** Chinese, English. **Desc:** Health care professionals treating the elderly; scientists and clinicians with an interest in the aging process and diseases of the aged. Works to insure high standards of research and practice in gerontology, and to maximize availability of gerontological services. Conducts research and educational activities. **Pub:** *Hong Kong Journal of Gerontology*, biennial. Journal.

★ 3412 ★ Hong Kong Association of Sports Medicine and Sports Science
Department of Physical Education
Hong Kong Baptist University
224 Waterloo Rd.
Kowloon Tong
Hong Kong, People's Republic of China
Phone: 852 26816368 **Fax:** 852 34115757
Email: raymonds@hksi.org.hk
Website: http://www.fmshk.com.hk/hkasmss/

Fnded: 1988. **Desc:** Promotes and advances the practice, education and research of medicine and science in relation to sports and exercise.

★ 3413 ★ Hong Kong Cancer Chemotherapy Society
810 Melbourne Plz.
33 Queens Rd.
Central
Hong Kong, People's Republic of China
Phone: 852 25861726 **Fax:** 852 25960802
Email: shiucho@hkstar.com
Website: http://www.fmshk.com.hk/hkccs

Fnded: 1990. **Mem:** 81. **Lang(s):** Chinese, English. **Desc:** Physicians practicing cancer chemotherapy. Seeks to advance the study and practice of chemotherapy; promotes continuing professional development of members. Facilitates exchange of knowledge, skill, and experience among members.

★ 3414 ★ Hong Kong College of Obstetricians and Gynaecologists
c/o Ms. Winnie Choi
Hong Kong Academy of Medicine Jockey Club, 8th Fl.
Bldg. 99
Wong Chuk Hang Rd.
Hong Kong, People's Republic of China
Phone: 852 28718700 **Fax:** 852 28964902
Email: admin@hkcog.org.hk
Website: http://www.hkcog.org.hk

Desc: Works to encourage the study and advancement of obstetrics and gynecology in Hong Kong; promotes highest professional standards.

★ 3415 ★ Hong Kong College of Radiologists
Rm. 909, 9/F Hong Kong Academy of Medicine Jockey Club Bldg.
99 Wong Chuk Hang Rd.
Aberdeen
Hong Kong, People's Republic of China
Phone: 852 28718788 **Fax:** 852 25540739
Email: enquiries@hkcr.org
Website: http://www.hkcr.org

Fnded: 1991. **Mem:** 362. **Desc:** Encourages the study and advancement of the science and practice of diagnostic and therapeutic radiology in Hong Kong. Seeks to develop and maintain high professional standards of competence and ethical integrity. **Pub:** *Journal of the Honk Kong College of Radiologists*, quarterly. Journal. • Newsletter, quarterly.

★ 3416 ★ Hong Kong Dental Association
8/F Duke of Windsor Social Service Bldg.
15 Hennesey Rd.
Hong Kong, People's Republic of China
Phone: 852 25285327 **Fax:** 852 25290755
Email: hkda@hkda.org
Website: http://www.hkda.org

Fnded: 1950. **Mem:** 1,339. **Lang(s):** Chinese, English. **Desc:** Dentists, orthodontists, and others with an interest in the provision of dental care in Hong Kong. Promotes the welfare of the dental profession; encourages continuing professional education of members. Represents members' interests before government agencies and the public. Conducts research to advance dental practice; disseminates information to encourage public dental health maintenance. Maintains liaison with other dental organizations worldwide. Operates speakers' bureau; sponsors competitions; compiles statistics. **Pub:** *Hong Kong Dental Associa-*

tion Newsletter, bimonthly. Newsletter. • *Hong Kong Dental Association Yearbook*, annual. Yearbook.

★ 3417 ★ Hong Kong Dental Hygienists' Association (HKDHA)
GPO Box 706
Centralital Rd.
Hong Kong, People's Republic of China
Phone: 852 28590299 **Fax:** 852 28587874

Fnded: 1981. **Mem:** 60. **Lang(s):** Chinese, English. **Desc:** Dental hygienists and students of dental hygiene. Promotes the study and practice of dental hygiene. Represents the dental hygiene profession; serves as a clearinghouse for government agencies and public and private organizations with an interest in dental hygiene. Conducts educational programs. **Pub:** *HKDHA Newsletter*, quarterly. Newsletter.

★ 3418 ★ Hong Kong Gynaecological Endoscopy Society (HKGES)
Department of Obstetrics and Gynaecology
Prince of Wales Hospital
30-32 Ngan Shing St.
Hong Kong, People's Republic of China
Phone: 852 26322810 **Fax:** 852 26360008
Email: pmyuen@cuhk.edu.hk
Website: http://www.fmshk.com.hk/hkges

Fnded: 1994. **Mem:** 60. **Lang(s):** Chinese, English. **Desc:** Gynecological endoscopists and other health care professionals. Promotes advancement of the practice of gynecological endoscopy. Conducts continuing professional education programs. **Pub:** *Endovision*, quarterly. Newsletter.

★ 3419 ★ Hong Kong Institute of Family Medicine
18 Fu Kin St.
Tai Wai
Shatin
Hong Kong, People's Republic of China
Phone: 852 26083311 **Fax:** 852 26053334
Email: chm@union.org

Fnded: 1994. **Lang(s):** Chinese, English. **Desc:** Seeks to advance the study, theory, and practice of family medicine; encourages professional advancement of individuals engaged in the provision of family medical services. Conducts research and continuing professional development programs.

★ 3420 ★ Hong Kong Medical Association
Duke of Windsor Social Service Bldg., 5/F
15 Hennessy Rd.
Hong Kong, People's Republic of China
Phone: 852 25278285 **Fax:** 852 28650943
Email: hkma@hkma.org
Website: http://www.hkma.org

Fnded: 1920. **Mem:** 5,800. **Lang(s):** Chinese, English. **Desc:** Physicians and other health care professionals. Seeks to advance the profession and practice of medicine. Promotes professional advancement of members. Represents members' interests before government agencies and the public. Conducts continuing professional development courses; sponsors research projects; holds social and charitable activities. **Pub:** *HK Medical Journal*, quarterly. Journal. Features official journal of Hong Kong Medical Association and Hong Kong Academy of Medicine. • *HKMA News*, monthly. Newsletter. **Frmly:** (1970) Hong Kong Chinese Medical Association.

★ 3421 ★ Hong Kong Occupational Therapy Association (HKOTA)
Haven of Hope Nursing Home Rehabilitation Department
23 Haven of Hope Rd.
Tseung Kwan 0
Kowloon, People's Republic of China
Fax: 852 29840581
Email: samuelycchan@ctimail3.com
Website: http://www.fmshk.com.hk/hkota/home.htm

Fnded: 1981. **Mem:** 500. **Lang(s):** Chinese, English. **Desc:** Occupational therapists and students. Seeks to insure high standards of practice in the field of occupational therapy. Serves as a forum for exchange of information among members; represents members' interests; conducts continuing professional development programs. **Pub:** *Hong Kong Journal of Occupational Therapy*, annual. Journal. • *Hong Kong Occupational Therapy Newsletter*, 3/year.

★ 3422 ★ Hong Kong Paediatric Haematology and Oncology Study Group (HKPHOSG)
c/o Dr. Chi Wai Anselm Lee
Department of Pediatrics
Tuen Mun Hospital
Tuen Mun, NT.
Hong Kong, People's Republic of China
Phone: 852 24685111 **Fax:** 852 24569111
Email: aclee@netvigator.com
Website: http://www.fmshk.com.hk/hkphosg

Fnded: 1993. **Mem:** 43. **Lang(s):** Chinese, English. **Desc:** Physicians with an interest in pediatric hematology and oncology. Seeks to advance methods of diagnosis and treatment of pediatric hematological and oncological problems. Conducts educational and continuing professional development courses for members. Compiles statistics. **Pub:** Newsletter, monthly.

★ 3423 ★ Hong Kong PHAB Association
75 Pokfulam Reservoir Rd.
Hong Kong, People's Republic of China
Phone: 852 25514161 **Fax:** 852 28751401
Email: hq@hkphab.org.hk
Website: http://www.hkphab.org.hk

Fnded: 1972. **Mem:** 6,000. **Lang(s):** Chinese, English. **Desc:** Works to integrate people with and without disabilities of all ages in the community through social, recreational, educational and developmental programs. **Pub:** *PHAB News*, 3/year. Newsletter.

★ 3424 ★ Hong Kong Pharmacology Society (HKPS)
c/o Prof. Robert Jones
Department of Pharmacology
Faculty of Medicine
The Chinese University of Hong Kong
Shatin
Hong Kong, NT, People's Republic of China
Phone: 852 26096820 **Fax:** 852 26035139
Email: rljones@cuhk.edu.hk

Mem: 90. **Desc:** Promotes pharmacology in Hong Kong.

★ 3425 ★ Hong Kong Psychologcial Society
Pokfulam Rd.
Department of Psychology
University of Hong Kong
Hong Kong, People's Republic of China
Phone: 852 25490364 **Fax:** 852 28583518
Email: general_secretary@hkps.org.hk
Website: http://www.hkps.org.hk/

Fnded: 1994.

★ 3426 ★ Hong Kong Sex Education Association (HKSEA)
PO Box 50419
Sai Ying Pun
Hong Kong, People's Republic of China
Phone: 852 28554166 **Fax:** 852 28551345
Email: hksea@hksea.org
Website: http://www.hksea.org

Fnded: 1985. **Mem:** 100. **Lang(s):** Chinese, English. **Desc:** Individuals working in the fields of sex education, family planning, social work, psychology, and medicine; students. Promotes availability of quality educational programs dealing with sexuality, which the group defines as "those aspects of the human body that relate specifically to being male or female." Conducts research and educational programs; gathers and disseminates information. **Pub:** *Sex Forum*, semiannual. Newsletter. • Bulletin.

★ 3427 ★ Hong Kong Society of Certified Prosthetist-Orthotists
Hong Kong Polytechnic University
Hung Hom, Kowloon
Hong Kong, People's Republic of China
Phone: 852 27667676 **Fax:** 852 23624365
Email: rcaaron@polyu.edu.hk
Website: http://www.polyu.edu.hk/~hkscpo

Fnded: 1995. **Mem:** 90. **Lang(s):** Chinese, English. **Desc:** Individuals who have successfully completed an accredited program in prosthetics and orthotics and have passed the organization's examination. Promotes high standards of ethics and professional practice in the field of orthotics and prosthetics. Conducts continuing professional development and scientific education programs; makes available certification examinations.

★ 3428 ★ Hong Kong Society for the Deaf (HkS.D)
Duke of Windsor Social Service Bldg., Rm. 903
15 Hennessy Rd.
Hong Kong, People's Republic of China
Phone: 852 25278969 **Fax:** 852 25293316
Email: headoffice@deaf.org.hk
Website: http://www.deaf.org.hk

Fnded: 1968. **Mem:** 4,656. **Lang(s):** Chinese, English. **Desc:** Seeks to undertake projects of publicity, education, recreation, counseling, clinical, audio logical and medical services for the hearing impaired: and to assist or cooperate with any institutions, organizations or individuals to improve the services for the hearing impaired to work towards improving the educational standards for the hearing impaired, to provide scholarship and special equipment for the hearing impaired as well as to provide guidance for the parents of hearing-impaired children to inform the public about the problems and needs of hearing impaired, to give necessary information to hearing-impaired persons and their families about institutions and services available to them, and to exchange information among institutions serving the hearing impaired. **Pub:** Newsletter, monthly.

★ 3429 ★ Hong Kong Society of Dermatology and Venereology (HKSD)
c/o Social Hygiene Service
Sai Ying Pun Jockey Club Clinic, 3rd Fl.
Queen's Rd. W
Hong Kong, People's Republic of China
Phone: 852 25409804 **Fax:** 852 25409804
Email: lychong@cuhk.edu.hk
Website: http://www.medicine.org.hk/hksdv/

Fnded: 1983. **Mem:** 150. **Lang(s):** English. **Desc:** Dermatologists and physicians in Hong Kong. Stimulates interest in dermatology; promotes exchange and cooperation among members; encourages discussions to address problems in the field. Inspires high standards of dermatological care. Fosters international contacts; disseminates information.

★ 3430 ★ Hong Kong Society of Gastroenterology (HKSG)
Room 1203, Bank of America Tower
12 Harcourt Rd. Central
Hong Kong, People's Republic of China
Phone: 852 28695933 **Fax:** 852 28699533
Email: gastro@netvigator.com
Website: http://www.fmshk.com.hk/hksg

Fnded: 1981. **Mem:** 155. **Lang(s):** Chinese, English. **Desc:** Gastroenterologists and other individuals with an interest in gastroenterology. Seeks to advance gastroenterological research, teaching, and practice; promotes continuing professional development among members. Serves as a clearinghouse on gastroenterology; sponsors research and educational programs.

★ 3431 ★ Hong Kong Society of Health Services Executives
PO Box 70875
Kowloon Central Post Office
Hong Kong, People's Republic of China
Email: chengmy@ha.org.hk
Website: http://www.fmshk.com.hk/hkshse

Mem: 200. **Desc:** Promotes the professional advancement of health service management. Seeks to achieve excellence in health care service in Hong Kong through the advancement of professional and ethical standards in service management. Organizes educational activities.

★ 3432 ★ Hong Kong Society for Infectious Diseases
c/o Dept. of Pediatrics
Princess Margaret Hospital
Lai Chi Kok
Hong Kong, People's Republic of China
Phone: 852 29903771 **Fax:** 852 29903333
Email: somkt@ha.org.hk
Website: http://www.fmshk.com.hk/hksid/home.htm

Fnded: 1995. **Mem:** 100. **Lang(s):** Chinese, English. **Desc:** Health care professionals, researchers, scientists, medical practitioners and other persons who are interested in infectious diseases. The objectives are to promote the study of infectious diseases. Conducts public education programs and continuing professional development courses; sponsors research projects. **Pub:** *Bulletin of the Hong Kong Society for Infectious Diseases*, quarterly. Bulletin. Includes Scientific articles and calendar of local and international meetings on infectious diseases. • *Bulletin of the Hong Kong Society for Infectious Diseases*, quarterly. Newsletter.

★ 3433 ★ Hong Kong Society of Medical Genetics (HKSMG)
c/o Clinical Genetic Service
2 Kwong Lee Rd., 3/F
Sham Shui Po Kowloon
Hong Kong, People's Republic of China
Phone: 852 23605479 **Fax:** 852 27291440
Email: wkchan@vol.net
Website: http://www.fmshk.com.hk/hksmg

Fnded: 1986. **Lang(s):** Chinese, English. **Desc:** Geneticists and health care personnel working in the field of genetics. Seeks to advance the study and practice of medical genetics. Facilitates exchange of information among members; conducts research and educational programs; maintains speakers' bureau.

★ 3434 ★ Hong Kong Society of Medical Informatics (HKSMI)
c/o Dr. C.P. Wong
Ruttonjee Hospital
266 Queen's Rd. E
Hong Kong, People's Republic of China
Phone: 852 22911345 **Fax:** 852 22911335
Email: cpwong@ha.org.hk
Website: http://www.hksmi.org

Fnded: 1986. **Mem:** 250. **Lang(s):** Chinese, English. **Desc:** Medical practitioners. Promotes the use of medical informatics in health care. Sponsors research and educational programs.

★ 3435 ★ Hong Kong Society of Minimal Access Surgery
c/o Dr. Siu Wing Tai
Department of Surgery
Pamela Youde Nethersole Eastern Hospital
3 Lok Man Rd.
Chai Wan
Hong Kong, People's Republic of China
Email: info@hksmas.org

Fnded: 1992. **Mem:** 369. **Lang(s):** Chinese, English. **Desc:** Medical practitioners, scientists and researchers, and other individuals with an interest in laparoscopy and other minimal access surgical techniques. Seeks to advance the practice of minimal access surgery. Promotes continuing professional advancement of members. Conducts public education programs and continuing professional development courses; facilitates international exchange among minimal access surgeons; sponsors research projects; makes available scholarships and other assistance to minimal access surgery students. Provides charitable medical care; assists in the development of hospitals and other health care facilities. **Pub:** *Elsa Journal*, quarterly. Journal.

★ 3436 ★ Hong Kong Society of Nephrology
Department of Medicine
Prince of Wales Hospital
Hong Kong, People's Republic of China
Fax: 852 26 375396
Email: philipli@cuhk.edu.hk
Website: http://www.fmshk.com.hk/hksnephrol

Fnded: 1979. **Mem:** 606. **Lang(s):** Chinese, English. **Desc:** Doctors of medicine specializing in nephrology (157) are full members; nurses, other health care professionals, and students with an interest in nephrology (583) are associate members. Seeks to advance the study and practice of nephrology; encourages professional development of members. Promotes organ donation. Serves as a forum for discussion of nephrology and related medical and scientific topics; functions as liaison linking members with related scientific and professional bodies; holds interhospital renal meetings. Conducts research and educational programs. Sponsors competitions and charitable, recreational, and social activities. **Pub:** *Hong Kong Journal of Nephrology*, semiannual. Journal. • Newsletter, quarterly.

★ 3437 ★ Hong Kong Society for Nursing Education
PO Box 98898
Tsimshatsui Post Office
Hong Kong, People's Republic of China
Phone: 852 26096222 **Fax:** 852 23148550
Email: sallychan@uhk.edu.hk
Website: http://www.medicine.org.hk/hksne/home.htm

Fnded: 1985. **Mem:** 200. **Lang(s):** Chinese, English. **Desc:** Nurses and nursing educators. Promotes excellence in nursing education; seeks to advance the practice of nursing. Represents the interests of the nursing profession; facilitates communication among nurses and nursing educators; conducts continuing professional development courses; sponsors research; maintains liaison with nursing education organizations worldwide. **Pub:** *Newsletter of the Hong Kong Society for Nursing Education*, 3/year. Newsletter.

★ 3438 ★ Hong Kong Society of Oral Implantology
Takshing House, Rm. 704
20 Des Voeux Rd.
Central
Hong Kong, People's Republic of China
Phone: 852 25225571 **Fax:** 852 25243557
Email: info@oralimplant.org.hk
Website: http://www.oralimplant.org.hk

Fnded: 1995. **Mem:** 100. **Lang(s):** Chinese, English. **Desc:** Registered dental and medical practitioners; dental and medical students. Seeks to advance the practice of oral implantology; promotes professional development of members. Establishes standards of professional conduct and practice; conducts research, educational, and continuing professional development courses; makes available to members technical and other assistance. **Pub:** *Newsletter of the Hong Kong Society of Oral Implantology*, quarterly. Newsletter.

★ 3439 ★ Hong Kong Society of Professional Optometrists
PO Box 98603
Tsimshatsui Post Office
Hong Kong, People's Republic of China
Fax: 852 27826755
Email: query@hkspo.org.hk
Website: http://www.hkspo.org.hk

Fnded: 1982. **Mem:** 250. **Lang(s):** Chinese, English. **Desc:** Optometrists. Seeks to insure high standards of ethics and practice in optometry; facilitates professional advancement of members. Conducts continuing professional education courses; sponsors research; makes available optometric services. Participates in charitable activities; maintains speakers' bureau; compiles statistics. **Pub:** Newsletter, quarterly.

★ 3440 ★ The Hong Kong Society for Rehabilitation (HKSR)
7 Sha Wan Dr.
Hong Kong, People's Republic of China
Phone: 852 28176277 **Fax:** 852 28551947
Email: hksr@rehabsociety.org.hk

Fnded: 1959. **Mem:** 120. **Lang(s):** Chinese, English. **Desc:** Works to restore victims of physical or visceral disability brought on by disease or injury to economic self-sufficiency. Promotes continued professional advancement by members. Conducts research, educational, and charitable programs. **Pub:** Pamphlet, periodic. • Report, periodic.

★ 3441 ★ Hong Kong Society of Rheumatology
c/o Dr. T.H. Chan
1501 Prince's Bldg.
Central
Hong Kong, People's Republic of China
Phone: 852 25212567 **Fax:** 852 28681238
Email: jhksr@fmshk.com.hk
Website: http://www.fmshk.com.hk/hksr

Fnded: 1987. **Mem:** 150. **Desc:** Promotes interest in and understanding of rheumatology in Hong Kong. Conduct research in prevention, treatment, and patient care.

★ 3442 ★ Hong Kong Stoma Association
14-15 Lung Fook House, Ground Fl.
Lower Wong Tai Sin Estate
Kowloon
Hong Kong, People's Republic of China
Phone: 852 28346096 **Fax:** 852 28383873
Email: hksa@stoma.org.hk
Website: http://www.ostomyinternational.org/regionasia.htm

Fnded: 1979. **Mem:** 1,500. **Lang(s):** Cantonese, English. **Desc:** Individuals with stoma (small surgical openings in their gastrointestinal systems allowing for the elimination of urine and feces when the body's normal excretory functions are impaired) are members. Seeks to improve the quality of life of people with stoma. Provides support, information, and counseling for people planning on undergoing stoma surgery; conducts educational and support group meetings for members. **Pub:** Newsletter, bimonthly.

★ 3443 ★ Hong Kong Thoracic Society
Department of Medicine
Prince of Wales Hospital
Shatin
New Territories
Hong Kong, People's Republic of China
Phone: 852 26322195 **Fax:** 852 26489957
Website: http://www.fmshk.com.hk/hkts

Fnded: 1987. **Mem:** 800. **Lang(s):** Chinese, English. **Desc:** Thoracic physicians, surgeons, and other medical personnel. Seeks to improve the study and practice of thoracic surgery and related disciplines. Conducts research and educational programs. **Pub:** *HKTS/ACCP Joint Newsletter*, periodic. Newsletter.

★ 3444 ★ Hong Kong Tuberculosis, Chest and Heart Diseases Association
266 Queen's Rd. E
Wanchai
Hong Kong, People's Republic of China
Phone: 852 25723466 **Fax:** 852 28340711
Email: antitb@ha.org.hk

Website: http://www.ha.org.hk/org/antitb/default.htm

Fnded: 1948. **Mem:** 50. **Lang(s):** Chinese, English. **Desc:** Health care professionals and other individuals with an interest in respiratory diseases and cardiology. Seeks to advance the study and treatment of respiratory and cardiac diseases. Encourages professional development of members. Conducts research and educational programs. Maintains sanitarium, clinics, and home for the elderly. **Pub:** *Health Information*, periodic. Brochure.

★ 3445 ★ Hong Kong Urological Association

c/o Dr. Bth Wong
Department of Surgery
Queen Elizabeth Hospital
Kowloon
Hong Kong, People's Republic of China
Phone: 852 29586006 **Fax:** 852 29586076
Website: http://www.fmshk.com.hk/hkua/home.htm

Fnded: 1987. **Desc:** Promotes the medical specialty of urology in Hong Kong; works to improve and set the standard of urological care in Hong Kong.

★ 3446 ★ Hong Kong Veterinary Association (HKVA)

c/o Secretary
Laboratory Animal Services Centre
Chinese University
Hong Kong, People's Republic of China
Phone: 852 26096036 **Fax:** 852 26035723
Email: tonyjames@cuhk.edu.hk
Website: http://www.hkva.org

Fnded: 1982. **Mem:** 100. **Lang(s):** Cantonese, Chinese, English. **Desc:** Veterinary surgeons. Fosters advancement in the field of veterinary science. Sponsors clinical lectures. Seeks to liaise with veterinary surgeons registration board on matters affecting veterinary science in Hong Kong. **Pub:** *HKVA Newsletter*, quarterly. Contains news, reports, and abstract reprints.

★ 3447 ★ Hospice Association of America (HAA)

228 Seventh St., SE
Washington, DC 20003
Phone: (202)547-7424 **Fax:** (202)547-3540
Email: exec@nahc.org
Website: http://www.nahc.org

Desc: Home care, hospice and home care aide services. Working to heighten the public visibility of hospice services, to affect legislative and regulatory processes impinging on hospice services. To promote hospice care as a viable component of the health care delivery system. To provide an organized and unified voice for hospice providers, to disseminate information and provide for the exchange of information, to collaborate with state organizations representing hospice interests and initiate, sponsor and promote research related to hospice services.

★ 3448 ★ Hospice Education Institute (HEI)

3 Unity Sq.
PO Box 98
Machiasport, ME 04655-0098
Phone: (207)255-8800 **Free:** 800-331-1620
Fax: (207)255-8008
Email: hospiceall@aol.com
Website: http://www.hospiceworld.org
Michal Galazka, Exec. Dir.

Fnded: 1985. **Desc:** Provides educational and informational services to health professionals and the public on subjects such as hospice and palliative care, death and dying, and bereavement counseling. Encourages educational exchange among hospice and palliative care professionals and volunteers. Offers advice and support to persons working to open local hospice programs. Organizes continuing education seminars on hospice care throughout the U.S. and abroad. **Pub:** *Notes on Symptom Control in Hospice and Palliative Care*. Book. *Price:* $30. • Booklets.

★ 3449 ★ Hospice Foundation of America (HFA)

2001 S St. NW, Ste. 300
Washington, DC 20009
Free: 800-854-3402 **Fax:** (202)638-5312
Email: david@hospicefoundation.org
Website: http://www.hospicefoundation.org
David Abrams, Pres.

Fnded: 1982. **Desc:** Works to promote the philosophy and application of hospice care for terminally ill people and improve the American health system. Advocates the hospice concept of care; offers professional development and educational programs; sponsors research on ethical issues; participates in public policy initiatives; provides technical assistance to hospices **Pub:** *Choosing Hospice*. Booklet. Provides consumer information on Hospices. *Price:* Free. • *Hospice Care and the Military Family*. Brochure. • *Hospice Forum*, bimonthly. Newsletter. Provides information on research, regulatory issues, public policy, legislation, and state hospice programs. *Price:* $105/year for nonmembers; included in membership dues. • *Volunteering in Hospice*. Booklet. *Price:* Free.

★ 3450 ★ Hospice and Palliative Nurses Association (HPNA)

Penn Center W One, Ste. 229
Pittsburgh, PA 15276
Phone: (412)787-9301 **Fax:** (412)787-9305
Email: hpna@hpna.org
Website: http://www.hpna.org
Judy Lentz, Exec. Dir.

Fnded: 1985. **Mem:** 5,000. **Reg. Groups:** 10. **Desc:** Registered nurses engaged in end of life care in all settings. Promotes excellence in the specialties of hospice and palliative nursing. Conducts education and research programs. Has the only certification boards in hospice and palliative nursing. **Pub:** *Core Curriculum for the Generalist Hospice and Palliative Nurse*. • *Core Curriculum for the Hospice and Palliative Nursing Assistant*. • *Journal of Hospice and Palliative Nursing*, quarterly. Journal. *Price:* $50. • *Study Guide for the Generalist Hospice and Palliative Nurse*. • *Study Guide for the Generalist Hospice & Palliative Nurse*. **Frmly:** (1998) Hospice Nurses Association.

★ 3451 ★ Hospital-Based Massage Network (HBMN)

PO Box 1038
Olympia, WA 98507-1038
Phone: (360)754-9799 **Free:** 800-754-9790
Fax: (360)705-3864
Email: info@info4people.com
Website: http://www.HBMN.com
Laura Koch, Founder/Dir.

Fnded: 1995. **Desc:** Promotes integration of complementary health care into mainstream medicine supporting massage and touch therapists working with ill, recovering, elderly, hospitals, medical centers, nursing homes. **Pub:** Books.*Price:* $80 for one book; $140 for 2 books; $200 for all 3 books.

★ 3452 ★ Hospital Consultants and Specialists Association (HCSA)

1 Kingsclere Rd.
Overton
Basingstoke RG25 3JA, United Kingdom
Phone: 44 1256 771777 **Fax:** 44 1256 770999
Email: enquiries@hcsa.com

Fnded: 1948. **Desc:** Membership is open to hospital consultants, associate specialists, senior registrars, and staff grade doctors working in the National Health Service. Concerned with the interests of senior hospital doctors and their patients. Aims to improve the conditions of service of members, informing them on matters affecting their practice and endeavouring to ensure that key health decisions are taken with due regard to their views. **Pub:** *The Consultant*, annual. • *Consultant Newsletter*, 10/year. Newsletter. • Yearbook.

★ 3453 ★ Hospital Infection Society (HIS)

University of Leeds
Leeds LS2 9JT, United Kingdom
Email: markwi@pathology.leeds.ac.uk
Website: http://www.his.org.uk/

Desc: Furthers medical knowledge and disseminates information on the subject of Hospital associated infection.

★ 3454 ★ Hospital Organisation of Pedagogues in Europe (HOPE)

c/o Christian Lieutenant, Pres.
Av. Hippocrate 10, bte. 8510
B-1200 Brussels, Belgium
Phone: 32 2 7644799 **Fax:** 32 2 7648915
Email: cogels@pedi.ucl.ac.be
Website: http://www.connect-to-hope.org

Fnded: 1994. **Mem:** 9. **Nat'l Groups:** 30. **Lang(s):** English, French, German, Italian. **Desc:** Aims to establish the rights of children in hospitals to receive an appropriate education to their individual needs, in a suitable adapted environment. Ensures the continuity of this education during convalescent. **Pub:** Newsletter, quarterly.

★ 3455 ★ Hospitalized Veterans Writing Project (HVWP)

5920 Nall, Rm. 105
Mission, KS 66202
Phone: (913)432-1214
Barbara Sauvan, Pres.

Fnded: 1946. **Desc:** Individuals and organizations united to encourage hospitalized U.S. veterans to write for pleasure and rehabilitation during their hospital stay. Maintains speakers' bureau and slide program with commentary. Conducts writing sessions in hospitals. **Pub:** *Veterans' Voices*, 3/year. Magazine. Contains prose, poetry, artwork, and cartoons submitted by hospitalized veterans. *Price:* $8/year for hospitalized veterans and outpatients; $15/year for others.

★ 3456 ★ House Ear Institute (HEI)

2100 W 3rd St.
Los Angeles, CA 90057
Phone: (213)483-4431 **Fax:** (213)483-8789
Email: webmaster@hei.org
Website: http://www.hei.org
James Boswell, CEO

Fnded: 1946. **Desc:** Develops conceptual and technically feasible approaches to resolving hearing and balance disorders through applied research. Conducts research on subjects including hearing aids, auditory implants, aging ear, brain mapping, neuroanatomy, infant hearing diagnosis, and acoustic tumor. Offers seminars and classes for senior residents and practicing physicians. Operates children's center to serve profoundly deaf children and their families. Maintains library of 2700 volumes and 180 journal titles on otology. Sponsors videotape seminars and conducts courses on the use of hearing devices and how to evaluate hearing disorders. Provides support for parents raising a deaf or hard of hearing child. Compiles statistics; offers children's services; maintains speakers' bureau and library. **Pub:** *House Calls*, semiannual. Magazine. News magazine. • Annual Report. • Manuals. • Monographs. • Papers. • Brochures. **Frmly:** (1972) Los Angeles Foundation of Otology; (1981) Ear Research Institute.

★ 3457 ★ Howard Hughes Medical Institute (HHMI)

4000 Jones Bridge Rd.
Chevy Chase, MD 20815-6789
Phone: (301)215-8500
Email: webmaster@hhmi.org
Website: http://www.hhmi.org

Desc: Works to help enhance biomedical science education at all levels. Conducts research.

★ 3458 ★ HPV Support Program - American Social Health Association
PO Box 13827
Research Triangle Park, NC 27709
Phone: (919)361-8400 **Fax:** (919)361-8425
Email: bonrei@ashastd.org
Website: http://www.ashastd.org

Fnded: 1991. **Local Groups:** 15. **Desc:** Disseminates information and educational materials about human papillomavirus (HPV). Offers assistance to local support groups and/or people living with HPV. **Pub:** *HPV News*, quarterly. Journal. Covers medical and psychosocial information about HPV and genital warts. *Price:* $25/yr. • *HPV Questions and Answers*. Pamphlet.

★ 3459 ★ Human Ecology Action League (HEAL)
PO Box 29629
Atlanta, GA 30359
Phone: (404)248-1898 **Fax:** (404)248-0162
Email: healnatnl@aol.com
Website: http://members.aol.com/HEALNatnl
Muriel A. Dando, Pres.

Fnded: 1977. **Mem:** 10,000. **Nat'l Groups:** 1. **Local Groups:** 50. **Desc:** Individuals and organizations interested in the study of human ecology and multiple chemical sensitivities, specifically how human health may be affected by synthetic and natural substances in the environment. Objectives are: to collect and disseminate information on human ecology and ecological illness to persons suffering from such illness, and to government agencies, scientists, and health care professionals; to raise public awareness about potential dangers from substances in the environment. **Pub:** *Chemicals and Health*. Brochure. • *Electromagnetic Fields: Investigations into the Biological Activity of Low Frequency Electromagnetic Fields*. • *Fragrance and Health*. Book. *Price:* $12 members in the U.S.; $15 members in Canada; $20 members in other countries. • *Hospitality Directory*, periodic. Directory. Lists environmentally safe lodgings in the United States for allergic and chemical-sensitive travelers; arranged by state. • *How Chemicals In Your Environment Can Effect Your Health*. Brochure. • *Human Ecologist*, quarterly. Journal. Includes association news, book and video reviews, environmental health tips for children, and pesticide update. *Price:* $24/copy; $26/year for low-income Individuals; $20 in Canada; $38 included in membership dues. • *Multiple Chemical Sensitivities and the Americans with Disabilities Act: A Guide to Accommodation*. *Price:* $26; $20/year for low-income individuals; $38 international. • *Perspectives on Pesticides*. • *Selected Bibliography: Chemicals and Health*. Bibliography. • *Selected Bibliography: Perspectives on Pesticides and Human Health 1983-1993*. Bibliography. • *Service List/Back Issue Guide*, periodic.

★ 3460 ★ Human Genome Organization (HUGO)
144 Harley St.
London W1G 7LD, United Kingdom
Phone: 44 20 79358085 **Fax:** 44 20 79358341
Email: hugo@hugo-International.org
Website: http://www.gene.ucl.ac.uk/hugo

★ 3461 ★ Human Growth Foundation (HGF)
997 Glen Cove Ave.
Glen Head, NY 11545-1584
Free: 800-451-6434 **Fax:** (516)671-0455
Email: hgf1@hgfound.org
Website: http://www.hgfound.org/
Patricia D. Costa, Exec. Dir.

Fnded: 1965. **Mem:** 1,000. **Nat'l Groups:** 30. **Desc:** Families of children with physical growth problems and interested persons united to help medical science better understand the process of growth. Distributes money for basic and clinical growth research. Disseminates informative literature and presents educational programs to families and physicians. **Pub:** *Fourth Friday*, quarterly. Newsletter. • *Growth Series*. Brochure. **Frmly:** (1971) Human Growth.

★ 3462 ★ Hungarian Anatomical Society
c/o Prof. Dr. Guyla Lazar
Department of Anatomy
University pf Pecs Medical
Szigeti ut 12
Pecs, Hungary
Phone: 36 72 536392 **Fax:** 36 72 536393
Email: gyula.lazar@aok.pte.hu

Fnded: 1966. **Mem:** 103. **Desc:** Seeks to broaden members' knowledge of anatomical, histological, embyrological, and histochemical sciences. Disseminates information on Hungarian Morphological research. Works to improve teaching methods.

★ 3463 ★ Hungarian Association of Gerontology
Semmelweis University
Fac. Health Sciences 1st
Department Medicine & Geriatrics
Szabolcs utca 35
H-1135 Budapest, Hungary
Phone: 36 1 3294630 **Fax:** 36 1 3291206
Email: csaszalb@hiete.hu

Desc: Promotes gerontological research, training in the field of aging, and interests of gerontological organizations in international affairs.

★ 3464 ★ Hungarian Dermatological Society (HDS)
(Magyar Dermatologiai Tarsulat — MDT)
c/o Prof. Attila Horvath
Department of Dermatology
Semmelweis University Budapest
Faculty of Medicine
Maria str. 41
H-1085 Budapest, Hungary
Phone: 36 1 2660471 **Fax:** 36 1 2676974
Email: aurelius@bor.sote.hu
Website: http://www.derma.hu

Fnded: 1928. **Mem:** 550. **Local Groups:** 3. **Lang(s):** English, Hungarian. **Desc:** Promotes dermatological practice and research. Monitors progress in the field of dermatology. Participates in international forums. **Pub:** *Borgyogyaszati es Venerologiai Szemle*, bimonthly. Journal. Accepts English and German papers. Contains English abstracts. • *Progress of Dermatology and Venereology*. Yearbook.

★ 3465 ★ Hungarian Gerontological Association (HGA)
PO Box 45
H-1428 Budapest, Hungary
Phone: 36 1 3294630 **Fax:** 36 1 3291206
Email: csaszalb@hiete.hu

Fnded: 1966. **Mem:** 215. **Local Groups:** 5. **Lang(s):** English, German, Hungarian. **Desc:** Health care professionals treating the elderly; scientists and clinicians with an interest in the aging process and diseases of the aged. Promotes gerontological research and increased availability of gerontological care; facilitates training of gerontology specialists. Represents the interest of gerontologists and gerontological organizations, and civil organizations of the Pensioners and Elderly.

★ 3466 ★ Hungarian Multiple Sclerosis Society
c/o Central Hospital of County
Fejer Department of Neurology
Seregelyesi ut. 3
H-8001 Szekesfehervar, Hungary
Phone: 36 22 316001 **Fax:** 36 22 314198

Fnded: 1984. **Mem:** 2,400. **Reg. Groups:** 22. **Desc:** MS patients, families and professionals. Seeks to improve the quality of life for persons with multiple sclerosis and their families. Provides home services.

★ 3467 ★ Hungarian Psychological Association
Victor Hugo u. 18-22 I/122
H-1132 Budapest, Hungary
Phone: 36 1 2796090 **Fax:** 36 1 2796090
Email: mpt@mtapi.hu
Website: http://www.mpt.hu

Desc: Fosters increased knowledge regarding psychology through educational programs and conferences.

★ 3468 ★ Hungarian Society of Allergology and Clinical Immunology
c/o National Institute Rheumatology
PO Box 54
H-1525 Budapest, Hungary
Phone: 36 1 3350915 **Fax:** 36 1 3350915
Email: nekamkr.allergy@mail.datanet.hu

Fnded: 1989. **Mem:** 400. **Lang(s):** English, German. **Desc:** Incorporates all health providers interested and active in diagnosis, therapy, prevention, epidemiology, rehabilitation, under- and post-graduate education, national and international basic and clinical research in the field of allergology and clinical immunology. **Pub:** *Nutrition - Allergy - Diet*, bimonthly. Journal.

★ 3469 ★ Hungarian Society of Cardiology (HSC)
(Magyar Kardiologusok Tarsasaga — MKT)
Chazar A. u. 19 1/3
PO Box 24
HU-1406 Budapest, Hungary
Phone: 36 1 3429746 **Fax:** 36 1 3429746
Email: mkt@mail.matav.hu
Website: http://www.mkardio.hu

Fnded: 1955. **Mem:** 1,200. **Local Groups:** 17. **Lang(s):** English, Hungarian. **Desc:** Cardiologists and other medical specialists. Promotes development of cardiology; facilitates scientific exchanges of information among members. Monitors standards in cardiology training programs; provides cardiologists with ethical advice. Conducts educational, research, and public service programs. **Pub:** *Cardiologia Hungarica*, quarterly. Journal.

★ 3470 ★ Hungarian Society for Experimental and Clinical Pharmacology (MFT)
(Magyar Kiserletes es Klinikai Farmakologiai Tarsasag)
c/o Prof. E. Sylvester Vizi
Institute of Experimental Medicine
Hungarian Academy of Sciences
Szigony u.43
H-1450 Budapest, Hungary
Phone: 36 1 2109421 **Fax:** 36 1 2109423
Email: esvizi@koki.hu

Mem: 500. **Desc:** Promotes experimental and clinical pharmacology in Hungary.

★ 3471 ★ Hungarian Society of Human Genetics
c/o Dr. Peter Maroy
Department of Genetics
Jozsef Attila University
Kozepfasor 52
H-6726 Szeged, Hungary
Phone: 36 62 454268 **Fax:** 36 62 432485
Email: maroy@sol.cc.u-szeged.hu

Mem: 260. **Desc:** Researchers, teachers, and students interested in the study of genetics.

★ 3472 ★ Hungarian Society of Nutrition (HSN)
(Magyar Taplalkozastudomanyi Tarsasag — MTT)
c/o Prof. Dr. Barna Maria
Gyali ut. 3/a
H-1085 Horanszky, Hungary

Phone: 36 1 4864820 **Fax:** 36 1 4862761
Email: drbarnam@hotmail.com

Fnded: 1966. **Mem:** 270. **Lang(s):** Hungarian. **Desc:** Promotes the study of general and clinical nutrition. Researches medical aspects of food production and consumption. Conducts periodic discussion groups on nutrition related issues and problems; offers postgraduate training courses. **Pub:** *Tapallkozas, Allergia, Dieta*, bimonthly. Journal. Contains reviews, experimental studies, and information on scientific meetings. Comes with English summary. **Frmly:** Hungarian Society of Nutritional Sciences.

★ 3473 ★ Hungarian Society of Psychosomatic Obstetrics and Gynaecology

c/o Dr. Peter Szeverinyi
Department of Obstetrics & Gynaecology
University of Debrecen
PO Box 37
H-4012 Debrecen, Hungary
Fax: 36 52 414577
Email: szepi@jaguar.dote.hu
Website: http://www.hspog.dote.hu/

Desc: Promotes the study of psychobiological and psychosocial, ethical and cross-cultural problems in the fields of obstetrics and gynaecology, women's health and reproductive health; facilitates the dissemination of new information in these fields. **Pub:** *Journal of Psychosomatic Obstetrics and Gynecology*. Journal.

★ 3474 ★ Huntington Society of Canada (HSC)

151 Frederick St., Ste 400
Kitchener, ON, Canada N2H 2M2
Phone: (519)749-7063 **Free:** 800-998-7398
Fax: (519)749-8965
Email: info@hsc-ca.org
Website: http://www.hsc-ca.org

Fnded: 1973. **Mem:** 8,000. **Nat'l Groups:** 1. **Reg. Groups:** 60. **Lang(s):** English, French. **Desc:** Individuals with Huntington disease (a hereditary neurological disorder) and their families; health care professionals and others with an interest in Huntington disease and related disorders. Seeks to identify the cause and find a cure for Huntington disease; promotes an improved quality of life for people with Huntington disease. Serves as a clearinghouse on Huntington disease; conducts educational programs; funds research; maintains speakers' bureau. **Pub:** *Horizon*, quarterly. Newsletter.

★ 3475 ★ Huntington's Disease Association (HDA)

108 Battersea High St.
London SW11 3HP, United Kingdom
Phone: 44 207 2237000 **Fax:** 44 207 2239489
Email: info@hda.org.uk
Website: http://www.hda.org.uk

★ 3476 ★ Huntington's Disease Association of Ireland (HDAI)

Carmichael House
N Brunswick St.
Dublin 7, Ireland
Phone: 353 1 8721303 **Fax:** 353 1 8729931
Email: hdai@indigo.ie
Website: http://indigo.ie/~hdai

Lang(s): English, Irish. **Desc:** Individuals and organizations. Seeks to improve the quality of life of people with Huntington's disease and their families. Makes available support and services; conducts educational and advocacy campaigns; serves as a clearinghouse on Huntington's disease.

★ 3477 ★ Huntington's Disease Society of America (HDSA)

158 W 29th St., 7th Fl.
New York, NY 10001-5300
Phone: (212)242-1968 **Free:** 800-345-4372
Fax: (212)239-3430
Email: hdsainfo@hdsa.org
Website: http://www.hdsa.org
Barbara T. Boyle, Exec. Dir., CEO

Fnded: 1986. **Mem:** 50,000. **Reg. Groups:** 34. **Local Groups:** 3331. **Desc:** Individuals and groups of volunteers concerned with Huntington's disease, an inherited and terminal neurological condition causing progressive brain and nerve deterioration. Goals are to: identify HD families; educate the public and professionals, with emphasis on increasing consumer awareness of HD; promote and support basic and clinical research into the causes and cure of HD; maintain patient services program, coordinated with various community services, to assist families in meeting the social, economic, and emotional problems resulting from HD. Is working to change the attitude of the working community toward the HD patient, enhance the HD patient's lifestyle, and promote better health care and treatment, both in the community and in facilities. Has launched nationwide campaign in support of federal and state legislation establishing clinics, genetic counseling and screening centers, and diagnostic and treatment centers for HD patients and those suffering from other chronic, debilitating diseases. Actively cooperates with researchers in ongoing studies; cosponsors and supports workshops and symposia; provides grants to individual researchers; sponsors brain donor program. Crisis intervention and other support services are available. **Pub:** *Huntington's Disease Society of America-The Marker*, semiannual. Magazine. *Price:* Free. • *Toward A Cure*, semiannual. Newsletter. • Booklets. • Pamphlets. • Videos.

★ 3478 ★ Hydrocephalus Association (HA)

870 Market St., Ste. 705
San Francisco, CA 94102
Phone: (415)732-7040 **Free:** 888-598-3789
Fax: (415)732-7044
Email: info@hydroassoc.org
Website: http://www.hydroassoc.org
Emily Fudge, Exec. Dir.

Fnded: 1983. **Mem:** 2,000. **Desc:** People with hydrocephalus and their families, health care professionals with an interest in hydrocephalus, and interested businesses and foundations. Works to improve the quality of life of people with hydrocephalus through education. Conducts training for families of people with hydrocephalus; sponsors social gatherings; facilitates networking among families of people with hydrocephalus and between organizations representing people with hydrocephalus. **Pub:** *About Hydrocephalus - A Book for Parents*. Booklet. • *About Normal Pressure Hydrocephalus-A book for Adults and their families*. Booklet. • *Directory of Hydrocephalus Support Groups*, periodic. Directory. • *Directory of Neurosurgeons for Adult Hydrocephalus*. Directory. • *Directory of Pediatric Neurosurgeons*. Directory. Lists 130 neurosurgeons geographically and alphabetically. • *Fact Sheet 12 Different Topics*. Pamphlet. • *Hydrocephalus Diagnosed in Young & Middle-Aged Adults*. Booklet. • *Prenatal Hydrocephalus A Book for Parents*. Booklet. • *Quarterly Newsletter*, quarterly. Newsletter. • *Resource Guide*. Bibliography. Includes over 600 published articles regarding hydrocephalus. • *Teachers Guide to Hydrocephalus*. Book.

★ 3479 ★ Hypnotherapy Association

14 Crown St.
Chorley
Lancashire PR7 1DX, United Kingdom
Phone: 44 1257 262124 **Fax:** 44 1257 262124
Email: bha@lineone.net
Website: http://www.zednet.co.uk/bhahypnotherapy/

Fnded: 1958. **Mem:** 483. **Lang(s):** Spanish. **Desc:** Practitioners with at least 4 years post graduate of training in psychotherapy and hypnotherapy who comply with the Association's code of competence and ethics. Concerned with professional standards in the treatment of nervous disorders by trained psychotherapists who use hypnosis when appropriate to facilitate recall by the patient, as well as using other methods proven by research into long-term results. Referrals, research, lectures, broadcasts, talks, papers, articles, books and seminars arranged.

★ 3480 ★ Hysterectomy Educational Resources and Services Foundation (HERS)

422 Bryn Mawr Ave.
Bala Cynwyd, PA 19004
Phone: (610)667-7757 **Free:** 888-750-HERS
Fax: (610)667-8096
Email: hersfdn@earthlink.net
Website: http://www.uterinearteryembolization.com
Nora W. Coffey, Pres.

Fnded: 1982. **Desc:** Helps women make informed decisions regarding hysterectomy and alternatives to surgery. Provides medical journal articles and other educational materials concerning hysterectomy and alternative procedures, networking with other women on a one to one basis, referral to physicians and telephone counseling by appointment. **Pub:** *HERS Annual Hysterectomy Conference Proceedings*. Proceedings. • *HERS Newsletter*, quarterly. Newsletter. Contains book reviews, medical and scientific literature reviews, writer's chronicle of journal, and letters from readers. *Price:* $20/year. • *Hysterectomy Pamphlet*. Pamphlet. • Reprints. • Also makes available reading list and copies of medical journal articles; distributes audio cassettes and other related materials. **AKA:** HERS Foundation.

★ 3481 ★ I CAN

4 Dyer's Bldg.s
Holborn
London EC1N 2QP, United Kingdom
Phone: 44 870 104066 **Fax:** 44 870 104067
Email: info@ican.org.uk
Website: http://www.ican.org.uk

Fnded: 1888. **Lang(s):** English. **Desc:** Works as charity helping children with speech and language difficulties. Services include three residential schools, an early years program, mainstream support language resources in secondary schools, and a national training program for professionals. **Pub:** *Annual Report*, annual.

★ 3482 ★ I-ANON

119 S Ruth St.
Maryville, TN 37803
Free: 800-669-1603
Email: info@impotenceworld.org
Eileen V. MacKenzie, Founder and Conslt.

Fnded: 1982. **State Groups:** 100. **Local Groups:** 3. **Desc:** Concerned partners of impotent males. Seeks to provide information and group support to members. Refers members to doctors who treat impotence. Supplies patients with information on prosthetic implants, and other forms of treatment. **Pub:** *Answers to the Most Often Asked Questions About Impotence*. • *Impotence Worldwide*, quarterly. • *Its Not All in Your Head: A Couple's Guide to Overcoming Impotance*.

★ 3483 ★ Ibero-American Equine Veterinary Association (Asociacion Ibero-Americana Veterinaria Equina)

R Nicolau Maeder 330/62
Curitiba, Brazil
Phone: 55 41 3664492
Email: arsvet@bsi.com.br

State Groups: acion. **Local Groups:** rinari.

★ 3484 ★ Ibero-Latin American College of Dermatology (ILACD) (Colegio Ibero-Latino-Americano de Dermatologia — CILAD)

Av. Callao 852, Piso 2
1023 Buenos Aires, Argentina
Phone: 54 11 49590392 **Fax:** 54 11 48117581
Email: cilad@cilad.org.ar

Fnded: 1948. **Mem:** 2,210. **Lang(s):** Portuguese, Spanish. **Desc:** Iberian or Latin American doctors in 29 countries working in various fields related to dermatology including mycology (the study of fungi), venereology (the study of sexually transmitted diseases), the treatment of leprosy, dermatologic surgery, and criosurgery. Seeks to foster a working relationship between Ibero-Latin American specialists and those in other countries. **Pub:** *Boletin del CILAD*, quarterly. Bulletin. Contains information about the activities of the college. • *Ciladerma*, bimonthly. Magazine. • *Medicina Cutanea Ibero-Latino-Americana*, bimonthly. • Directory, periodic. • Monographs, periodic.

★ 3485 ★ Ibero-Latin American Federation of Plastic Surgery (Federacion Iber-Latinoamericana de Cirugia Plastica — FILACP)

P Viviana 32, Parques Herradura, Huixquilucan
Mexico City, Mexico
Phone: 52 56521543 **Fax:** 52 52910064
Email: mgavel@dfl.telmex.net.mx
Website: http://filacp.org/

Fnded: 1974.

★ 3486 ★ Icelandic Cardiac Society (ICS) (Hjartasjukdomafelag Islenskra Laekna — HIL)

Department of Medicine
Division of Cardiology
Landspitalinn 101
PO Box 10
IS-121 Reykjavik, Iceland
Phone: 354 5601000 **Fax:** 354 5601287
Email: ragnarda@rsp.is
Website: http://www.escardio.org/society/natsoc/iceland.htm

Fnded: 1968. **Mem:** 33. **Nat'l Groups:** 1. **Lang(s):** Danish, English, Finnish, Icelandic, Norwegian, Swedish. **Desc:** Physicians and scientists interested in the field of cardiology.

★ 3487 ★ Icelandic Nurses' Association (Felag Islenskra Hjukrunarfraedinga)

Sudurlandsbraut 22
IS-108 Reykjavik, Iceland

Fnded: 1994. **Mem:** 2,700.

★ 3488 ★ Icelandic Occupational Therapy Association

c/o Scandinavian Journal of Occupational Therapy
Department of Social Medicine and Rehabilitation
Umea University
S-901 87 Umea, Sweden
Phone: 46 90 7869272 **Fax:** 46 90 7869267

Lang(s): Icelandic. **Desc:** Occupational therapists and other health care professionals engaged in occupational medicine in Iceland. Promotes scientific inquiry in the field of occupational therapy and serves as a forum for the dissemination of research results. Areas of inquiry include: physical disability; mental health and disabilities; therapeutic equipment, environments, and techniques; assessment and evaluation of disabilities; vocational and educational training.

★ 3489 ★ IDEA, The Health and Fitness Source

6190 Cornerstone Ct. E, Ste. 204
San Diego, CA 92121-3773
Phone: (619)535-8979 **Free:** 800-999-IDEA
Fax: (858)535-8234
Email: member@ideafit.com
Website: http://www.ideafit.com
Kathie Davis, Exec. Dir.

Fnded: 1982. **Mem:** 23,000. **Desc:** Provides continuing education for fitness professionals including; fitness instructors, personal trainers, program directors, and club/studio owners. Offers workshops for continuing education credits. **Pub:** *Gearing Up: How to Evaluate and puchase Quality Home Exercise Equipment*. Brochure. • *Get Active: How to Make Activity A Habit and Change Your Life*. Brochure. • *Get Real: A Personal Guide to Real-Life Weight Management*. Book. Contains information on weight management. • *Get Real: 8 Keys to Healthy Sensible Weight Management*. Brochure. • *IDEA Fitness Manager*, 5/yr.Newsletter. • *IDEA Health & Fitness Source*, 10/year. Magazine. Includes articles on exercise science, teaching techniques, and business management. Also includes annual index to articles and calendar of events.. *Price:* Included in membership dues. • *IDEA Personal Trainer*, 10/year. Magazine. Includes marketing client relationship and business information. • *Personal Best: How to Choose the Personal Trainer Who's Right For You*. Brochure. • *Young At Heart: How to Preserve Your Health with Active Living at any Age!*. Brochure. • Brochures. • Pamphlets. • Videos. **Frmly:** (1982) IDEA: International Dance Exercise Association; (1989) IDEA: The Association for Fitness Professionals; (1997) Idea, The Health & Fitness Source.

★ 3490 ★ Ileostomy and Internal Pouch Support Group

Peverill House
1-5 Mill Rd.
County Antrim
Ballyclare BT39 9DR, United Kingdom
Phone: 44 28 93344043 **Fax:** 44 289 3324606
Email: info@the-ia.org.uk
Website: http://www.ileostomypouch.demon.co.uk

Fnded: 1956. **Mem:** 9,636. **Desc:** To help people who have had or are about to have their colon removed, to return to a fully active and normal life as soon as possible. The activities of IA include hospital and home visiting, members' meetings, equipment exhibitions, medical research, stoma-care clinics, advisory services, lectures and demonstrations. **Pub:** *IA Journal*, quarterly. Journal.

★ 3491 ★ Imagine World Health (IWH)

105 E Dolphin Blvd.
Ponte Vedra Beach, FL 32082-1714
Phone: (904)285-0240
Email: imagineuldhealth@aol.com
Website: http://www.imagineworldhealth.org
David Stearns, Contact

Fnded: 1998. **Desc:** Strives to educate and promote good health and fitness in mind, body and spirit.

★ 3492 ★ Immune Deficiency Foundation (IDF)

40 W Chesapeake Ave., Ste. 308
Towson, MD 21204
Phone: (410)321-6647 **Free:** 800-296-4433
Fax: (410)321-9165
Email: idf@primaryimmune.org
Website: http://www.primaryimmune.org
Thomas L. Moran, Pres.

Fnded: 1980. **Mem:** 11,500. **State Groups:** 19. **Local Groups:** 14. **Desc:** Immune deficiency patients, their families, and medical professionals. Promotes education and research in primary immune deficiency diseases. Holds medical symposia; bestows patient scholarship and research awards. **Pub:** *Guide for Nurses*. • *IDF Newsletter*, quarterly. Newsletter. Contains announcements of patient scholarship and research awards. Includes health insurance information and calendar of events. *Price:* Free. • *Our Immune System*. • *Patient and Family Handbook*. • *Primer for Physicians*.

★ 3493 ★ Immunization Action Coalition (IAC)

1573 Selby Ave., Ste. 234
Saint Paul, MN 55104
Phone: (651)647-9009 **Fax:** (651)647-9131
Email: admin@immunize.org
Website: http://www.immunize.org
Deborah L. Wexler, MD, Exec. Dir.

Fnded: 1990. **Desc:** Works to boost immunization rates. Promotes awareness of and responsibility for immunization of all people against all vaccine-preventable diseases. Conducts educational and outreach programs; develops print and audiovisual educational materials. Facilitates communication concerning issues of safety efficacy and the use of vaccines. **Pub:** *IAC Express*, weekly. Newsletter. Provides timely immunization news to health professionals and others interested in immunization issues. • *Needle Tips and the Hepatitis B Coalition News*, semiannual. Newsletter. Discuss all vaccine-preventable diseases and hepatitis B. *Price:* Free. • *Vaccinate Adults!*, semiannual. Newsletter. *Price:* Free. • *Vaccinate Women*, semiannual. Newsletter. *Price:* Free.

★ 3494 ★ Impaired Physician Program (IPP)

c/o Georgia Impaired Health Professionals Program
5448 Yorketown Dr.
Atlanta, GA 30349
Phone: (770)994-0185 **Free:** 800-445-4232
Fax: (770)994-2024
Website: http://www.talbottcampus.com
G. Douglas Talbott, MD, Founder & Dir.

Fnded: 1975. **Desc:** Purpose is to provide assistance to physicians, other health professionals, and their spouses with problems such as alcoholism, substance abuse, or codependence; seeks to locate and identify persons in need of help and to provide assistance. Conducts in- and outpatient treatment programs. Offers counseling; maintains advocacy program to assist physicians and other health professionals in reentering their profession. Maintains speakers' bureau.

★ 3495 ★ Implanted Defibrillator Association of Scotland (IDAS)

10 Selkirk Ave.
Paisley PA2 8JF, United Kingdom
Phone: 44 1505 813995
Email: hanheart@aol.com
Website: http://www.hermit1960.pwp.blueyonder.co.uk

Fnded: 1994. **Mem:** 104. **Reg. Groups:** 4. **Lang(s):** English. **Desc:** Individuals with implanted defibrillating devices and their families. Promotes and improved quality of life for people with implanted defibrillators. Sponsors support groups for members; advocates on behalf of members before medical organizations and the public; conducts educational programs; participates in charitable activities. **Pub:** *Vital Spark*, quarterly. Newsletter.

★ 3496 ★ Impotence Association

c/o Ann Tailor
PO Box 10296
London SW17 9WH, United Kingdom
Phone: 44 20 87677791 **Fax:** 44 20 85167725
Email: info@impotence.org.uk
Website: http://www.impotence.org.uk

Fnded: 1995. **Mem:** 1,300. **Desc:** Raises awareness among the public and health professionals on impotence. Offers free advice and information via a telephone hotline. Maintains up to date information on the causes and treatments available for impotence.

★ 3497 ★ Impotence Institute of America (IIA)

119 S Ruth St.
Maryville, TN 37803
Free: 800-669-1603
Email: info@impotenceworld.org
Eileen MacKenzie, Founder & Chm.

Fnded: 1983. **Desc:** Urologists, psychiatrists, psychologists, sex therapists and counselors, and plastic surgeons; manufacturers of penile implant devices and other productsused in the treatment of impotence; impotent men and their partners; hospitals and other institutions that offer assistance and meeting facilities for Impotents Anonymous (IA) and I-ANON. Informs and educates the public on the subject of impotence and its causes and treatments. Provides information on various programs and organizations that can assist individuals concerned about impotence. Aids other charitable, educational, and social welfare organizations. Compiles statistics. **Pub:** *Answers to the Most Often Asked Questions about Impotence.* • *It's Not all in Your Head - A Couple's Guide to Overcoming Impotence.*

★ 3498 ★ In Touch Networks (ITN)
15 W 65th St.
New York, NY 10023
Phone: (212)769-6270 **Fax:** (212)769-4148
Website: http://www.intouchnetworks.net
Pete Williamson, Gen. Mgr.
Fnded: 1974. **Mem:** 1000,000. **Desc:** Volunteer service that allows blind or physically impaired people to listen to readings of articles from more than 100 newspapers and magazines via closed-circuit radio. Broadcasts nationally accessible on Galaxy 4 satellite. **Pub:** *Program Guide*, annual.

★ 3499 ★ Incontinentia Pigmenti International Foundation (IPIF)
c/o Susanne Bross Emmerich
30 E 72nd St.
New York, NY 10021
Phone: (212)452-1231 **Fax:** (212)452-1406
Email: ipif@ipif.org
Website: http://imgen.bcm.tmc.edu/IPIF/
Susanne Bross Emmerich, Exec. Dir.
Fnded: 1995. **Desc:** Patients, physicians, educators, parents, relatives, volunteers. Strives to support research, education and funding for Incontinentia Pigmenti; provides family support and education; seeks to develop accurate and safe prenatal diagnostic testing; and develop database to assess clinical variation, natural history, and prognostic indicators. **Pub:** Newsletter, annual. • Reports. **Frmly:** (2003) National Incontinentia Pigmenti Foundation.

★ 3500 ★ Incurably Ill for Animal Research (IIFAR)
PO Box 27454
Lansing, MI 48909
Phone: (517)887-1141 **Fax:** (517)887-1550
Email: info@iifar.org
Website: http://www.iifar.org/
Gregory A. Maas, CEO
Fnded: 1985. **Mem:** 2,500. **Local Groups:** 18. **Desc:** Persons who have health problems and interested individuals who are concerned that animal research for medical purposes will be stopped or severely limited due to the efforts of animal rights activists. Supports the use of animals for the purpose of medical research, teaching, and testing. Seeks to educate the public regarding the role animals serve in biomedical research and improving human and animal health. Maintains speakers' bureau. **Pub:** *Have You Benefited?*. Brochure. • *How Can You Show Your Support?*. Brochure. • *iiFAR Update*, monthly. Includes local chapter news and information on legislation and the activities of animal rights activists. • *iiFARsighted Report*, quarterly. Report. • *Why Should You Care?*. Brochure. • Also distributes educational literature and student information packets.

★ 3501 ★ INDENT, Dutch Dental Association
Postbus 190
NL-2700 AD Zoetermeer, Netherlands
Phone: 31 79 3531269 **Fax:** 31 79 3531365
Email: indent@fme.nl
Fnded: 1978. **Mem:** 24. **Lang(s):** Dutch. **Desc:** Companies manufacturing dental equipment and supplies. Establishes international standards and technical harmonization for dental equipment. Represents members' interests before government bodies, international agencies, and the public. Maintains liaison with organizations representing dentists, dental technicians, and dental supply dealers and distributors. Compiles statistics. **Pub:** *INDENT Export Group, the Netherlands*. Brochure. Contains information regarding products and activities of members of the INDENT export group. **Frmly:** (1993) VNFTP.

★ 3502 ★ Independent Association of German Dentists (Freier Verband Deutscher Zahnarzte)
Mallwitzstr. 16
D-53177 Bonn, Germany
Phone: 49 228 85570 **Fax:** 49 228 347967
Email: ms@fvdz.de
Website: http://www.fvdz.de
Fnded: 1955. **Mem:** 24,000. **Nat'l Groups:** 1. **Reg. Groups:** 60. **State Groups:** 17. **Lang(s):** English. **Desc:** Represents and promotes the professional interests of German dentists. **Pub:** *Der Freie Zahnarzt*, monthly. Magazine. Informs members of relevant politics, science, technologies, and service supplies of the association.

★ 3503 ★ Independent Citizens Research Foundation for the Study of Degenerative Diseases (ICRFSDD)
PO Box 97
Ardsley, NY 10502
Phone: (914)591-4374 **Fax:** (914)591-7090
Mark Bereday, Exec. Dir.
Fnded: 1957. **Desc:** Individuals united to seek and publish information of aid to those affected by degenerative diseases. Makes available in bulletin form documented information on the multiple and contributing causes of degenerative diseases, testing procedures for their early detection, and possible approaches to therapy and prevention. Seeks out factors in the environment that are detrimental to health. Supports research on calibrated transcutaneous electric nerve stimulation and preventive medicine techniques. Maintains 400 volume library on maintenance of health and prevention of disease. Seeks out factors in the environment that are detrimental to health. **Pub:** Newsletter, bimonthly. • Also publishes authorized transcripts of radio lectures on nutrition.

★ 3504 ★ Independent Healthcare Association
Westminster Tower
3 Albert Embankment
London SE1 7SP, United Kingdom
Phone: 44 20 77934620 **Fax:** 44 20 78203738
Email: info@iha.org.uk
Website: http://www.iha.org.uk
Fnded: 1987. **Mem:** 1,000. **Desc:** Independent hospitals and homes registered under the 1984 Registered Homes Act. The representative body for independently-owned healthcare providers, whether voluntary or private, funded largely by member subscriptions based on a fee per bed. Its charitable status derives from its objectives to promote high standards of care in the independent sector. **Pub:** *Focus*, quarterly. • Bulletin, monthly.

★ 3505 ★ Independent Hospitals' Association of Ireland
41 Fitzwilliam Pl
Dublin 2, Ireland
Phone: 353 1 6768550 **Fax:** 353 1 6768554

★ 3506 ★ Independent Living Centre
St. Loyes Foundation
Topsham Rd.
Exeter EX2 6EP, United Kingdom
Phone: 44 1392 286239 **Fax:** 44 1392 286239
Fnded: 1986. **Lang(s):** English. **Desc:** Provides a permanent exhibition and demonstration centre of equipment for people of all ages with a variety of needs and disabilities providing information to their families, carers, health professionals, students and the general public. **Pub:** Brochure.

★ 3507 ★ Independent Midwives Association
1 The Great Quarry
Guildford
Surrey GU1 3XN, United Kingdom
Phone: 44 1483 821104
Email: info@independentmidwives.org.uk
Website: http://www.independentmidwives.org.uk
Fnded: 1982. **Mem:** 60. **Lang(s):** English. **Desc:** Midwives practicing in England. Promotes the involvement of midwives in childbirth, doing mainly home births. Promotes education in midwifery. Represents members' interests.

★ 3508 ★ Indian Association of General Practitioners (IAGP)
c/o Mohan's Clinic
No. 613, 2nd Main
1 Stage, Indirangar
Bangalore 560 038, Karnataka, India
Email: docmohan@vsnl.com
Fnded: 1979. **Mem:** 500. **Desc:** Represents the interests of family physicians in India. Works to strengthen partnership between Indian doctors. **Pub:** Journal, bimonthly.

★ 3509 ★ Indian Association of Paediatric Surgeons (IAPS)
Department of Paediatric Surgery
B.J. Wadia Hospital for Children
Parel
Bombay 400 012, Maharashtra, India
Phone: 91 22 24172543 **Fax:** 91 22 4143435
Email: santoshjk@yahoo.com
Website: http://www.iapsindia.com
Fnded: 1965. **Mem:** 600. **Desc:** Pediatric surgeons in India. Promotes continuing professional advancement of members. **Pub:** Journal, periodic.

★ 3510 ★ Indian Association of Parasitologists
110 Chittaranjan Av
Calcutta 700 012, India

★ 3511 ★ Indian Association of Surgical Oncology (IASO)
c/o Dr. Ravi Kent
Department of Surgery
Maulana Azad Medical College
New Delhi 110 002, Delhi, India
Phone: 91 11 24353320 **Fax:** 91 11 3230316
Email: ravibina@hotmail.com
Website: http://www.indiandoctors.com/iaso
Fnded: 1977. **Mem:** 500. **Nat'l Groups:** 1. **Desc:** Cancer surgeons, radiologists, pathologists, and biochemists. Promotes advancement and practice of surgical oncology. **Pub:** Annual Report. • Journal, periodic. • Newsletter, semiannual. Contains academic and association news.

★ 3512 ★ Indian Brain Research Association
35 Ballygunge Circular Rd.
Calcutta 700 019, India
Fnded: 1964.

★ 3513 ★ Indian Cancer Society
c/o Lady Ratan Tata Medical and Research Centre
74 Jerbai Wadia Rd.
Parel, Bhoiwada
Bombay 400 021, Maharashtra, India
Phone: 91 22 2029941 **Fax:** 91 22 2048742
Fnded: 1951. **Local Groups:** 30. **Desc:** Provides educational, diagnostic, therapeutic, and related services relating to cancer. Promotes cancer detection, treatment, and prevention through mobile cancer detection service. Offers rehabilitation services. Sponsors public and professional educational programs.

★ 3514 ★ Indian Council of Medical Research (ICMR)
V. Ramalingaswami Bhawan
Ansari Nagar
New Delhi 110 029, India
Phone: 91 11 26588895 **Fax:** 91 11 26588662
Email: icmrhqds@sansad.nic.in
Website: http://icmr.nic.in
Fnded: 1911.

★ 3515 ★ Indian Dental Association (IDA)
c/o Dr. V.M. Veerabahu
83 Dewan Bahadur Rd.
R S Puram
Coimbatore 641 002, Tamil Nadu, India
Phone: 91 422 2453684 **Fax:** 91 442 449555
Website: http://www.dentalhealthindia.com
Fnded: 1945. **Mem:** 14,000. **State Groups:** 22. **Local Groups:** 176. **Lang(s):** English. **Desc:** Dental surgeons; dental students. Promotes the dental profession and educates the public concerning the contributions of dental professionals. Offers educational and public service programs; conducts research programs. **Pub:** *Journal of IDA*, monthly. Journal. • Directory, annual.

★ 3516 ★ Indian Dental Association U.S.A.
3540 82nd St.
Jackson Heights, NY 11372
Phone: (718)639-0192 **Fax:** (718)639-8122
Dr. Parikh Amrish, Pres.
Fnded: 1983. **Mem:** 345. **State Groups:** 5. **Desc:** Dentists in the U.S. who are of Asian-Indian descent. Seeks to further the professional education of members. Conducts social events. **Pub:** *IDA Newsletter*, monthly. Newsletter.

★ 3517 ★ Indian Muscular Dystrophy Association (IMDA)
MIG 72
APHB Colony
Machilipatnam 521 001, India
Phone: 91 8 26722817
Fnded: 1982. **Mem:** 850. **Nat'l Groups:** 3. **State Groups:** 7. **Lang(s):** English. **Desc:** Individuals in India who work toward the dissemination of information and research concerning muscular dystrophy, a hereditary disease characterized by progressive deterioration of muscles. **Pub:** *Bridge*, quarterly. Newsletter. • *Varadhi.*

★ 3518 ★ Indian Optometric Association
Laxmi Rd.
Pune 411 030, India
Fnded: 1961.

★ 3519 ★ Indian Pharmacological Society
c/o Department of Pharmacology and Therapeutics
Patna Medical College
Patna 800 014, Bihar, India
Desc: Fosters the science of pharmacology. Promotes research in pharmacology and allied disciplines with reference to current health needs in India and national health policy. Collects, evaluates, and disseminates scientific knowledge about drugs. **Pub:** *IPS Newsletter*, periodic. Newsletter. • Journal, periodic.

★ 3520 ★ Indian Psychological Association
J.L. Nehru Marg
New Delhi 110 002, India
Phone: 91 11 26447189
Email: satsang@mailcity.com

★ 3521 ★ Indian Public Health Association
110 Chittaranjan Av
Calcutta 700 073, India

★ 3522 ★ Indian Society of Anesthetists
Parel
Bombay 400 012, India
Fnded: 1947.

★ 3523 ★ Indian Society of Critical Care Medicine (ISCCM)
c/o Dr. Sandhya Talekar
Prayag Hospital
1247 Deccan Gymkhana
Pune 411 004, Maharashtra, India
Phone: 91 20 25532812 **Fax:** 91 20 5534448
Email: drsandhya@hotmail.com
Website: http://www.isccm.org
Fnded: 1993. **Desc:** Physicians, anesthetists, and surgeons interested in intensive care medicine. Promotes high quality critical care in India. **Pub:** *Indian Journal of Critical Care Medicine*, quarterly. Journal.

★ 3524 ★ Indian Society of Human Genetics (ISHG)
c/o Dr. V.R. Rao
Scientist E11,
Centre for Cellular and Molecular Biology
Rm. E406, 3rd Fl.
Uppal Rd.
Hyderabad 500 007, Andhra Pradesh, India
Phone: 91 40 27192655 **Fax:** 91 40 7171195
Email: raovr@ccmb.res.in
Website: http://www.ishg.org
Desc: Fosters growth and dissemination of knowledge of human genetics and related fields. Promotes awareness of current developments in the field. **Pub:** *Indian Journal of Human Genetics*. Journal.

★ 3525 ★ Indian Society for Medical Statistics (ISMS)
c/o Indian Council of Medical Research
Ansari Nagar
New Delhi 110 029, India
Phone: 91 11 26516003 **Fax:** 91 11 6856713
Email: padamsingh@icmr.dehli.nic.in
Fnded: 1983. **Desc:** Facilitates communication among those engaged in medical research and teaching of medical statistics; enhances the development and use of statistics in medicine and public health.

★ 3526 ★ Indian Society of Nephrology (ISN)
c/o Department of Nephrology
Sir Ganga Ram Hospital
Rajinder Nagar
New Delhi 110 060, Delhi, India
Phone: 91 11 25758660 **Fax:** 91 11 5812727
Email: dsrana@bol.net.in
Website: http://www.isn-india.com
Fnded: 1970. **Mem:** 732. **Desc:** Physicians specializing in nephrology. Fosters professional development of members. **Pub:** *Indian Journal of Nephrology*, quarterly. Journal.

★ 3527 ★ Indian Society for Parenteral and Enteral Nutrition (ISPEN)
C-13 Qutab Institutional Area
New Delhi 110 016, Delhi, India
Email: crnss@hotmail.com
Fnded: 1994. **Desc:** Promotes advancement in the study and application of parenteral and enteral nutrition.

★ 3528 ★ Indian Society of Psychosomatic Obstetrics and Gynaecology
c/o Dr. P.K. Khan
6c Middleton Rd.
Calcutta 700 071, India
Fax: 91 33 2493578
Email: khanpk@rediffmail.com
Website: http://www.ispog.org
Desc: Promotes the study of psychobiological and psychosocial, ethical and cross-cultural problems in the fields of obstetrics and gynaecology, women's health and reproductive health; faciliates the dissemination of new information in these fields. **Pub:** *Journal of Psychosomatic Obstetrics and Gynecology*. Journal.

★ 3529 ★ Indian Society of Vascular and Interventional Radiology (ISVIR)
c/o Dr. Sanjiv Sharma
Department of Cardiac Radiology
Cardiothoracic Centre
All India Institute of Medical Science
New Delhi 110 029, India
Email: meetisv@nda.vsnl.net.in
Website: http://www.isvir.org/
Fnded: 1997. **Desc:** Promotes the practice of cardiovascular and interventional radiology in India, including streamlining availability of devices in different regions. **Pub:** Newsletter, quarterly.

★ 3530 ★ Indians Into Medicine (INMED)
University of North Dakota
School of Medicine and Health Services
PO Box 9037
Grand Forks, ND 58202-9037
Phone: (701)777-3037 **Fax:** (701)777-3277
Email: inmed@medicine.nodak.edu
Website: http://www.med.und.edu/depts/inmed/home.htm
Eugene DeLorme, JD, Dir.
Fnded: 1973. **Desc:** Support program for American Indian students. Seeks to: increase the awareness of and interest in healthcare professions among young American Indians; recruit and enroll American Indians in healthcare education programs; place American health professionals in service to Indian communities. Coordinates financial and personal support for students in healthcare curricula. Provides referral and counseling services. Maintains 2000 volume library. Provides summer enrichment sessions at the junior high, high school and pre-medical levels as well as academic year support for college and professional level students. **Pub:** *Serpent, Staff and Drum*, quarterly. Newsletter. *Price:* Free. • Also publishes program information and motivational materials.

★ 3531 ★ Indonesian Planned Parenthood Association (IPPA)
Jalan Hang Jebat III/F3
PO Box 6017
Kebayoran Baru
12120 Jakarta, Indonesia
Phone: 62 21 7394123 **Fax:** 62 21 7253172
Email: pkbinet@link.net.id
Fnded: 1957. **Mem:** 1,500. **Nat'l Groups:** 1. **Reg. Groups:** 24. **Local Groups:** 150. **Lang(s):** English, Indonesian. **Desc:** Works to improve the quality of life for individuals living in Indonesia through responsible parenthood and family planning. Advocates family planning as a basic human right. Offers programs in family planning, sex education, and reproductive and family health care. Provides contraceptive and reproductive and general care services. Conducts research. **Pub:** *IPPA's News Letter*, semiannual. Newsletter. • *Kabar*, quarterly. Magazine. • Brochures.

★ 3532 ★ Indonesian Psychologist Association (Himpsi)
Kebayoran Centre A16
12240 Jakarta, Indonesia
Phone: 62 21 7254040 **Fax:** 62 21 7254040
Email: pusat@himpsi.org
Fnded: 1959. **Mem:** 6,500. **Reg. Groups:** 10. **Lang(s):** English, Indonesian. **Desc:** Professors, researchers, and graduate students in psychology as well as psychologists in the Republic of Indonesia. Promotes the development of psychological sciences and professions in Indonesia.

★ 3533 ★ Indonesian Society of Gerontology
Jalan Iskandarsyah Raya 7
12160 Jakarta, Indonesia
Lang(s): English, Indonesian. **Desc:** Health care professionals treating the elderly; scientists and clinicians with an interest in the aging process and diseases of the aged. Works to insure high standards of research and practice in gerontology, and to maximize availability of gerontological services. Conducts research and educational activities.

★ 3534 ★ Indonesian Society for Perinatology (PERINASIA) (Perkumpulan Perinatologi Indonesia — PERINASIA)
Jalan Tebet Utara IA/22
12820 Jakarta, Indonesia
Phone: 62 21 8281243 **Fax:** 62 21 8281243
Email: perinasi@centrin.net.id
Fnded: 1981. **Mem:** 1,104. **Local Groups:** 19. **Lang(s):** English, Indonesian. **Desc:** Obstetricians, gynecologists, pediatricians, midwives, and interested others. Strives to reduce the perinatal mortality rate; works to improve prenatal, natal, and postnatal health care; seeks improved medical facilities. Holds workshops, congresses, seminars, and symposia on perinatal health care and related subjects. Advocates research in safe birth practices; promotes the use of preventive medicine in prenatal care. Encourages community participation in health care improvement programs. Offers technical assistance to government authorities. Cooperates with similar international organizations. Conducts surveys. Disseminates information. **Pub:** *Perinasia Bulletin*, quarterly. Bulletin. • Proceedings, periodic.

★ 3535 ★ Indoor Sports Club (ISC)
16 Liberty St.
Larkspur, CA 94939
Phone: (415)924-3549 **Fax:** (415)927-9556
Email: russab@earthlink.net
Russ Bohlke, Exec. Sec.
Fnded: 1930. **Mem:** 500. **Reg. Groups:** 6. **Local Groups:** 17. **Desc:** Social, benevolent, educational, and rehabilitative organization for persons with physical disabilities. Provides entertainment and amusement for disabled persons and shut-ins; seeks aid for needy disabled persons; provides opportunities for active participation in civic affairs; and promotes a better understanding and acceptance of the seriously disabled by the able-bodied. **Pub:** *National Hookup*, bimonthly. Newsletter. *Price:* $6.50/year.

★ 3536 ★ Infection Control Association of Southern Africa (ICASA)
24 Finsbury Rd.
Auckland Park 2096, Republic of South Africa
Phone: 27 11 4890341 **Fax:** 27 11 4890883
Email: infect@mweb.co.za
Website: http://www.wits.ac.za/ic/icasa/
Fnded: 8621. **Mem:** 200. **Desc:** Nurses, microbiologists, physicians, pharmacists, and other individuals interested in infection control. Supports the education and training of infection control practitioners. Provides consulting services. **Pub:** *Infection Control Journal of South Africa*, quarterly. Journal.

★ 3537 ★ Infection Control Nurses' Association
Freepost
Drumcross Hall
Bathgate EH48 4BR, United Kingdom
Phone: 44 1506 811077 **Fax:** 44 1506 811477
Email: info@fitwise.co.uk
Website: http://www.icna.co.uk
Fnded: 1969. **Mem:** 1,079. **Nat'l Groups:** 8. **Reg. Groups:** 11. **Desc:** Infection control nurses and allied professionals. Concerned with the education of public and health care staff in infection. **Pub:** *British Journal of Infection Control*, quarterly. Journal.

★ 3538 ★ Infectious Diseases Society of Southern Africa (IDSSA) (Aansteeklike Siektesvereniging van Suider Afrika — ASVSA)
Department of Medical Microbiology
Observatory
Cape Town 7925, Republic of South Africa
Phone: 27 21 4045137 **Fax:** 27 21 4045190
Email: steve@medmicro.uct.ac.za
Website: http://www.idlinks.com/international_id/idafrica.html
Fnded: 1983. **Mem:** 150. **Lang(s):** English. **Desc:** Health care professionals including doctors, medical researchers and technologists, and trade representatives in 4 countries. Stimulates interest among doctors in infectious disease; seeks to alleviate the current shortage of infectious disease specialists in southern Africa. Compiles statistics. **Pub:** *Infectious Diseases Update*, 3/month. • *Southern African Journal of Epidemiology and Infection*, quarterly.

★ 3539 ★ Infertility Awareness Association of Canada (IAAC) (Association Canadienne de Sensibilisation a l'Infertilite)
PO Box 23025
Ottawa, ON, Canada K2A 4E2
Phone: (613)244-7222 **Free:** 800-263-2929
Fax: (613)244-8908
Email: info@iaac.ca
Website: http://www.iaac.ca
Fnded: 1990. **Mem:** 600. **Reg. Groups:** 5. **Lang(s):** English, French. **Desc:** Individuals and organizations working to increase the awareness and understanding of the causes, treatments, and the emotional impact of infertility. Represents the interests of those with infertility concerns. Collaborates with infertility support groups to advance the organization's agenda. Disseminates information through media interviews, seminars, and educational materials. Maintains resource center and speakers' bureau. **Pub:** *Infertility Awareness*, bimonthly. Newsletter.

★ 3540 ★ Inflammation Research Association (IRA)
c/o Richard J. Griffiths, Secretary
Pfizer Global R&D
Eastein Point Rd.
Groton, CT 06340
Phone: (860)441-6124 **Fax:** (860)441-0510
Email: richard_J_Griffiths@groton.pfizer.com
Website: http://www.inflammationresearch.org
Richard D. Dyer, PhD, Pres.
Fnded: 1970. **Desc:** Brings together scientists with an interest in inflammation research. Encourages the communication and discussion of science. **Pub:** *IRA Newsletter*, quarterly. Newsletter. Exchanges information between the Association and its members. • *Official Journal: Inflammation Research*. Journal.

★ 3541 ★ Informed Homebirth/Informed Birth and Parenting (IH/IBP)
PO Box 1733
Fair Oaks, CA 95628
Phone: (916)961-6923 **Fax:** (916)961-6923
Email: ihibp@aol.com
Rahima Baldwin Dancy, Pres.
Fnded: 1977. **Desc:** Expectant and new parents, childbirth educators, midwives, nurses, preschool and elementary school teachers, and others interested in safe childbirth alternatives. Seeks to provide information on alternatives in childbirth methods, parenting, and developmental education. Childbirth Educator Training Program leading to certification as Childbirth Educator; Childbirth Assistant Training emphasizing practical skills to help the birthing woman and the primary caregiver. **Frmly:** (1981) Informed Homebirth.

★ 3542 ★ Infoshare International (II)
584 Castro St., Ste. 671
San Francisco, CA 94114
Fax: (415)843-4066
Email: infoshare1@aol.com
Website: http://www.spiral.com/infoshare/welcome.html
Julie Stachowiak, Exec. Dir.
Fnded: 1993. **Desc:** AIDS organizations in Russia and the United States. Promotes increased public awareness of AIDS and HIV and their prevention and treatment. Serves as a clearinghouse on AIDS and HIV; provides clothing, food, and support services to people with HIV and their families; makes available technical and administrative assistance to grass roots AIDS organizations; conducts educational programs.

★ 3543 ★ Infusion Nurses Society (INS)
220 Norwood Park S
Norwood, MA 02062
Phone: (781)440-9408 **Fax:** (781)440-9409
Email: chris.hunt@ins1.org
Website: http://www.ins1.org
Mary Alexander, CEO
Fnded: 1973. **Mem:** 5,300. **Reg. Groups:** 62. **Local Groups:** 62. **Desc:** Registered nurses involved in infusion therapy; licensed practical nurses and pharmacists. Works to promote the education of individuals practicing infusion therapy. Conducts certification program for nurses and advanced studies program in infusion nursing. Maintains speakers' bureau; compiles statistics. **Pub:** *Infusion Nursing Standards of Practice*, periodic. Journal supplement. *Price:* $15 for members; $45 for nonmembers. • *Journal of Infusion Nursing*, bimonthly. Journal. Includes information on meetings, clinical manuscripts, products, and certification and recertification exams. *Price:* Included in membership dues; $102 year for nonmembers; $256 year for institutions; $42 year for students. • *Newsline*, bimonthly. Newsletter. Includes convention news, legislative network information, chapter agendas, and calendar of events. • *Policies and Procedures for Infusion Nursing*, periodic. • Also publishes news releases and nursing standards. **Frmly:** (2002) Intravenous Nurses Society.

★ 3544 ★ Inspiration Ministries (CLH)
PO Box 948
Corner State Rd. 67 and County F
Walworth, WI 53184-0948
Phone: (262)275-6131 **Fax:** (262)275-3355
Email: tschnake@inspirationministries.org
Website: http://www.inspirationministries.org
Tim Schnake, VP Resident Services
Fnded: 1948. **Mem:** 90. **Desc:** Seeks to provide fully accessible, permanent residence with attendant care in room and board facility for physically disabled adults. Conducts summer camping program for disabled persons and retreat opportunities for groups. **Pub:** *Seasons*, quarterly. Newsletter. *Price:* Free. **Frmly:** (2001) Christian League for the Handicapped.

★ 3545 ★ Institut Pierre Richet
Boite Postale 1500
Bouake, Cote d'Ivoire
Phone: 225 31633746 **Fax:** 225 632738
Email: ipr@ird.ci
Website: http://www.ird.ci/ird/richet.html
Lang(s): English, French. **Desc:** Medical researchers and health care professionals. Promotes improved diagnostic techniques and treatments of common diseases. Conducts research and educational programs; makes available health services.

★ 3546 ★ Institute for Advanced Research in Asian Science and Medicine (IARASM)
PO Box 555
Garden City, NY 11530
Email: admin@AJCM.org
Dr. John J. Kao, MD, Contact
Fnded: 1972. **Desc:** Purpose is to advance international understanding between Asia and the West in the areas of science, medical systems, and health care delivery. Serves as a clearinghouse for international

scholarly efforts in the comparative study of science and medicine. Provides consulting services and mediation of scientific and biomedical exchange with Asian countries. Assists in generating innovative curricula in medical education; translates contemporary and classical Asian scientific and medical literature; provides training for medical professionals in acupuncture therapeutics. **Pub:** *American Journal of Chinese Medicine*, bimonthly. Journal. Publishes original articles and essays related to traditional or ethnomedicine of all cultures. *Price:* $240 subscription price for 2003 vol. 31.

★ 3547 ★ Institute for the Advancement of Human Behavior (IAHB)
4370 Alpine Rd., Ste. 209
Portola Valley, CA 94028
Phone: (650)851-8411 **Free:** 800-258-8411
Fax: (650)851-0406
Website: http://www.iahb.org
G. W. Piaget, Pres.

Fnded: 1977. **Desc:** Continuing educational organization for health care professionals. Provides training opportunities in behavioral topics such as: the psychology of health care; human sexuality; brief therapy, PTSD, couples therapy, maintaining long-term health behaviors, and the role of imagery in health care. **Pub:** Audiotapes, periodic. **AKA:** Institute for Behavioral Healthcare.

★ 3548 ★ Institute for Applied Psychology (IAP)
Av de Stalingrad 23
1000 Brussels, Belgium
Phone: 32 2 5112411 **Fax:** 32 2 5117181
Email: kvonvietinghoff@skynet.be

Fnded: 1993.

★ 3549 ★ Institute of Athletic Motivation (IAM)
2308 Crystal Ct.
Antioch, CA 94509
Phone: (925)754-2828 **Free:** 800-288-2992
Fax: (925)978-1503
Email: winslowwri@aol.com
Website: http://www.winslowresearch.com
William J. Winslow, Pres.

Fnded: 1962. **Desc:** Originated by sports psychologists to: enhance the performance of athletes in competitive and recreational sports; enable coaches to better understand and coach athletes; provide athletes with self-knowledge for self-improvement and development. Prepares reports on athletic attitudes of athletes based on results of Athletic Motivation Inventory and Athletic Success Profile, written questionnaires prepared specifically for sports to measure 11 traits related to success: agressiveness, drive, determination, responsibility, leadership, self-confidence, emotional control, mental toughness, coachability, conscientiousness, and trust. Markets programs to high schools, colleges, amateur athletes, professional teams, and recreational athletes. Maintains software licensing program for sports organizations and consultants. Operates speakers' bureau. **AKA:** (2001) Athletic Success Institute. **Frmly:** (1971) Institute for the Study of Athletic Motivation; (1998) Institute for the Study of Athletic Motivation and Institute of Athletic Motivation.

★ 3550 ★ Institute for Cancer Prevention
390 5th Ave.
New York, NY 10018
Phone: (212)953-1900 **Fax:** (212)687-2339
Email: Vbaker60@yahoo.com
Jeffrey Rosoff, Admin.

Fnded: 1969. **Desc:** Devoted to promoting preventive medicine, emphasizing four major fields: research (nutrition, environmental carcinogenesis, molecular biology, experimental pathology, and epidemiology); clinical research and service for children (through screening and intervention); public health action (educating laymen and medical and government personnel in the principles of preventive medicine); health economics research (investigating direct and indirect costs of major diseases and comparing them with preventive approaches). in New York City. in New York City. **Pub:** *Preventive Medicine*, monthly. Journal. Contains scientific, preventive medicine and public health information. *Price:* $264 institutional subscription; $132 personal subscription. **Frmly:** (1968) Environmental Health Foundation; (2003) American Health Foundation.

★ 3551 ★ Institute of Certified Healthcare Business Consultants (ICHBC)
307 N Michigan Ave., Ste. 800
Chicago, IL 60601-5309
Phone: (312)360-0384 **Free:** 800-447-1684
Fax: (312)360-0388
Email: info@ichbc.org
Website: http://www.ichbc.org
Barbara Boden, Exec. Dir.

Fnded: 1975. **Mem:** 295. **Desc:** Individuals providing business advisory services to physicians, dentists, and other healthcare professionals. Maintains code of ethics, rules of professional conduct, and certification program; administers examination and conducts review course. Membership by successful completion of certification examination only. **Pub:** *Institute of Certified Healthcare Business Consultants–Certified News*, quarterly. Newsletter. *Price:* available to members only. **Frmly:** (1999) Institute of Certified Professional Business Consultants.

★ 3552 ★ Institute of Chiropodists and Podiatrists
27 Wright St.
Southport PR9 0TL, United Kingdom
Phone: 44 1704 546141 **Fax:** 44 1704 500477
Email: editor@inst-chiropodist.org.uk
Website: http://www.inst-chiropodist.org.uk

Fnded: 1938. **Mem:** 2,500. **Local Groups:** 31. **Desc:** State registered and non-state registered chiropodists. Members governed by strict code of ethics. Third party surgery risks insurance provided for members. **Pub:** *Chiropody Review*, bimonthly. Journal. Journal for chiropodists and podiatrists. **Frmly:** (1997) Institute of Chiropodists.

★ 3553 ★ Institute for Complementary Medicine (ICM)
PO Box 194
London SE16 7QZ, United Kingdom
Phone: 44 207 2375165 **Fax:** 44 207 2375175
Email: info@icmedicine.co.uk
Website: http://www.icmedicine.co.uk

Fnded: 1982. **Mem:** 6,000. **Lang(s):** English. **Desc:** Registered charity of individuals united to promote the practice of alternative medicine. Seeks to establish educational standards for practitioners and to establish ties between therapy groups, organizations, teachers, and practitioners. Cooperates with the British government to develop natural therapy curricula. Maintains British Register of Complementary Practitions. Conducts research; disseminates information. Advises groups establishing healing practices on legal, organizational, and practical matters. **Pub:** *Journal for Complementary Medicine*, semiannual. Journal. • *Newsletter*, quarterly. Newsletter. Supplement to journal.

★ 3554 ★ Institute for the Development of Emotional and Life Skills/National Institute of Relationship Enahancement (IDEALS)
4400 East- West Hwy., Ste. 28
Bethesda, MD 20814
Phone: (301)986-1479 **Free:** 800-THE-NIRE
Fax: (301)680-3756
Email: niremd@nire.org
Website: http://www.nire.org
Dr. William Nordling, Exec. Dir.

Fnded: 1972. **Mem:** 12. **Desc:** Strives to develop and research effective programs for improving emotional and interpersonal skills and providing high-quality training and supervision for mental health professionals, managers, workers, and the public. Conducts training programs for professionals in the areas of mental health, health care, human services, education, and business; sponsors training programs for laypeople in the areas of improving interpersonal relations, problem solving, and effective functioning in family and in business settings. Offers programs for workers and managers in communication, goal planning, motivation, negotiation, stress and time management, personnel management, and supervision. **Pub:** *A Scriptural Guide to a Fulfilling Marriage.* • *Parenting: A Skills Training Manual.* • *Relationship Skills Manual.* • Bibliography.Contains training programs, research articles, books and films. **Frmly:** (2000) Institute for the Development of Emotional and Life Skills.

★ 3555 ★ Institute for a Drug-Free Workplace
1225 I St. NW, Ste. 1000
Washington, DC 20005-3914
Phone: (202)842-7400 **Fax:** (202)842-0022
Email: pizanias@drugfreeworkplace.org
Website: http://www.drugfreeworkplace.org/
Mark A. de Bernardo, Exec. Dir.

Fnded: 1989. **Mem:** 90. **Desc:** Businesses, organizations, and individuals united to preserve the rights of employers and employees involved in corporate drug abuse prevention programs. Seeks to influence public policy pertaining to drug-abuse prevention in the workplace. Conducts surveys. **Pub:** *Avoiding Legal Liability: The 25 Most Common Employer Mistakes in Addressing Drug Abuse.* Book. *Price:* $40. • *Does Drug Testing Work?*. Book. *Price:* $36. • *Drug and Alcohol Abuse Prevention and the ADA: An Employer's Guide.* Book. *Price:* $32. • *Drug Testing in the Workplace: Basic Issues, Answers, and Options for Employees.* Booklet. *Price:* $4.50. • *Employee Assistance Programs: An Employer's Development and Implementation Guide.* Booklet. *Price:* $4.50. • *Employee Drug Education and Awareness and Supervisor Training: An Employer's Development and Implementation Guide.* Booklet. *Price:* $4.50. • *Guide to Dangerous Drugs.* Booklet. *Price:* $2.40. • *Guide to State and Federal Drug Testing Laws*, annual. Book. *Price:* $345. • *International Guide to Workplace Substance Abuse Prevention.* Book. *Price:* $80. • *Policy on Drug and Alcohol Abuse Prevention: An Employer's Development and Implementation Guide.* Booklet. *Price:* $4.50. • *What Every Employee Should Know About Alcohol Abuse: Answer to 25 Good Questions.* Booklet. *Price:* $2.30.

★ 3556 ★ Institute for Expressive Analysis (IEA)
205 W 89th
New York, NY 10024
Phone: (212)362-2167
Joel Gavriele Gold, Exec. Dir.

Fnded: 1976. **Mem:** 64. **Local Groups:** 1. **Desc:** Practicing art, dance, and music therapists, social workers, art teachers, and psychotherapists trained in expressive analysis (a psychotherapy that strives to develop the left and right brain activities to achieve body-mind integration and the mobilization of creative energies). Sponsors lectures and workshops for the public and professionals. Provides advanced courses leading to certification as associate, fellow, or full member of the institute. Maintains educational and counseling center. **Pub:** Journal, annual. **Frmly:** Center for Expressive Analysis; Center for Expressive Psychotherapy.

★ 3557 ★ Institute for Female Alternative Medicine
1500 S Central Ave., Ste. 214
Glendale, CA 91204
Phone: (818)956-3391 **Free:** 800-505-IFAM
Fax: (818)956-0545
Email: doctor@drdeljuncojr.com
Website: http://www.drdeljuncojr.com
Dr. Tirso del Junco, Jr., Founder

Desc: Focusing on alternative surgical procedures for the treatment of benign female pathologies, ie: fibroids, ovarian cystic disease, endometriosis. Philosophy is "reconstructive" with extensive use of lasers, not removal of pelvic organs. **Pub:** *Women's Health quarterly*, quarterly. **Frmly:** (1998) Institute for Reproductive Health.

★ 3558 ★ Institute of Group Analysis

1 Daleham Gardens
London NW3 5BY, United Kingdom
Phone: 44 20 74312693 **Fax:** 44 20 74317246
Email: iga@igalondon.org.uk
Website: http://www.igalondon.org.uk

Fnded: 1971. **Mem:** 300. **Desc:** Counsellors, social workers, psychologists, psychiatrists, caring professionals, probation officers. Responsible for the establishment of a widely recognised professional qualification in group-analytic psychotherapy. The principal aim is to promote and forward the selection, education and training of persons in order to qualify them for the conduct and study of group analysis and related forms of psychotherapy. **Pub:** *Dialogue*, quarterly. Newsletter.

★ 3559 ★ Institute for Health Care Management

Postbus 9697
NL-3506 GR Utrecht, Netherlands
Phone: 31 30 2739700 **Fax:** 31 30 2739560
Email: nzi@nzi.nl

Fnded: 1968. **Local Groups:** 7. **Lang(s):** Dutch, English, French, German. **Desc:** Seeks to develop a "sound, humane, and financially feasible health service" in the Netherlands. Conducts scientific research; offers advisory services; maintains educational programs. Disseminates information to health institutions and health care services. **Pub:** *NZI Notities*, bimonthly. Magazine. **Frmly:** (1999) Institute for Health Management.

★ 3560 ★ Institute of Health Promotion and Education

University Dental Hospital
Department of Oral Health and Development
Higher Cambridge St.
Manchester M15 6FH, United Kingdom
Phone: 44 161 2756610 **Fax:** 44 161 2756299
Email: anthony.blinkhorn@man.ac.uk
Website: http://www.ihpe.org.uk

Fnded: 1962. **Mem:** 1,000. **Desc:** Members are individuals concerned with the promotion of health and the prevention of illness in all sections of the community at home, school, work and leisure. **Pub:** *International Journal of Health Promotion and Education*, quarterly. Journal.

★ 3561 ★ Institute of Healthcare Management - United Kingdom

46 Grosvenor Gardens
London SW1, United Kingdom
Phone: 44 207 8819235 **Fax:** 44 207 8819236
Email: enquiries@ihm.org.uk
Website: http://www.ihm.org.uk

Fnded: 1902. **Mem:** 8,000. **Reg. Groups:** 8. **State Groups:** 3. **Desc:** Those involved in the management and administration of health care. To promote excellence in health services management and the development of good managers, to affect health services policy and its implementation and to create and sustain a professional community of health services managers. It is a forum, network and management development association for individuals both inside and outside the NHS. **Pub:** *Health Management*, monthly. Magazine. Contains in-house journal for IHM members. • *The IHSM Health and Social Services Yearbook*, annual. Book. **Frmly:** (2000) Institute of Health Services Management.

★ 3562 ★ Institute of Holistic Therapies

PO Box 37
Scarborough YO11 1AR, United Kingdom
Phone: 44 1723 378573 **Fax:** 44 1723 378573
Email: lnroche@talk21.com

Fnded: 1989. **Mem:** 1,200. **Nat'l Groups:** 1. **Desc:** Qualified holistic practitioners only. Provides indemnity and malpractice insurance cover and a register of all qualified professional holistic therapists who have satisfactorily completed a recognised study course worldwide.

★ 3563 ★ Institute for Integral Development (IID)

PO Box 2172
Colorado Springs, CO 80901
Phone: (719)634-7943 **Free:** 800-544-9562
Fax: (719)630-7025
Email: iidevo@aol.com
Website: http://www.institutefortraining.com
Dan Barmettler, MA, Dir.

Fnded: 1977. **Desc:** Provides a forum for discussion of issues pertaining to alcoholism and other addictions; seeks to train educators, medical professionals, and mental health practitioners in understanding and assisting addicted individuals. Sponsors seminars and workshops; provides educational audiotapes; offers consulting services. Maintains speakers' bureau; operates small library.

★ 3564 ★ Institute for Labor and Mental Health (ILMH)

3137 Telegraph Ave.
Oakland, CA 94609
Phone: (510)653-6166
Dr. Richard Epstein, Dir.

Fnded: 1977. **Mem:** 50. **Desc:** Purpose is to help working people with problems related to the workplace. Seeks to identify conditions at work that cause stress; believes that education and communication about common work problems are the first steps in dealing with job stress. Assists unions in handling grievances and stress-related disabilities; provides counseling to union members and their families; offers legal and worker compensation assistance to working people. Provides consultation to government and businesses on ways to reduce stress. Develops ongoing stress programs; operates summer institute on occupational stress. **Pub:** *Occupational Stress*, bimonthly. Newsletter. • *Occupational Stress: A Union Based Approach.* • *Occupational Stress: The Inside Story.* • *Surplus Powerlessness.* Book. • Directory, periodic.

★ 3565 ★ Institute for Laboratory Animal Research (ILAR)

National Research Council
2101 Constitution Ave. NW
Washington, DC 20418
Phone: (202)334-2590 **Fax:** (202)334-1687
Email: ilar@nas.edu
Website: http://www.national-academies.org/ilar
Joanne Zurlo, PhD, Dir.

Fnded: 1952. **Desc:** Organized under the auspices of the National Academy of Sciences. Acts in an advisory capacity to the federal government, upon request, and to other public and private agencies. Maintains information center and answers inquiries concerning animal models for biomedical research, location of unique animal colonies, availability of genetically defined animals from those colonies and from animal breeders, and nonanimal alternatives. Committees develop guidelines on breeding, conservation, and humane care and use of animals, including species-specific documents on cats, nonhuman primates, and rodents. Also prepares documents on guidelines and policy issues of biotechnology and use of animals in precollege education, facilities, disease prevention, and other topics in laboratory animal science. Sources of financial support include government agencies and private organizations. Maintains advisory council and several committees comprising scientists from universities, research organizations, and medical schools. **Pub:** *Guide for the Care and Use of Laboratory Animals.* Book. • *ILAR Journal*, quarterly. • Proceedings. • Reports.Laboratory animal management documents. **Frmly:** (1997) Institute of Laboratory Animal Resources.

★ 3566 ★ Institute for Medical Quality (IMQ)

PO Box 7690
San Francisco, CA 94120-7690
Phone: (415)882-5151 **Fax:** (415)882-5149
Email: jsilverman@imq.org
Website: http://www.imq.org
Jill K. Silverman, MSPH, Pres. /CEO

Desc: Devoted to improving quality of care to patients across the continuum of health care.

★ 3567 ★ Institute for Mental Health Initiatives (IMHI)

2175 K St., NW, Ste. 700
Washington, DC 20037
Phone: (202)467-2285 **Fax:** (202)467-2289
Email: imhi-info@gwumc.edu
Website: http://www.gwumc.edu/sphhs/imhi/
Suzanne Stutman, Dir.

Fnded: 1982. **Desc:** Uses a public health approach to promote mental health and prevent emotional disorders. Seeks to transform complex mental health concepts into positive models of human interaction. Gathers knowledge derived from clinical and research findings on good mental health, which it then adapts for use by the media, educators, health and mental health professionals, community leaders, and parents. Conducts meetings and workshops; consults with media professionals; creates training videos, discussion guides, and public service announcements. Works to influence perceptions and attitudes through the power of commercial mass media. **Pub:** *Dialogue*, quarterly. Newsletter. Provides information on human emotions for media professionals. *Price:* $30. • *Exploring First Feelings.* Video. • *Intiatives*, quarterly. Newsletter. Reports on current issues and new developments in mental health. • *The Rethink Workout for Teens: Learning to Manage Anger.* Video. • *Take Another Look: Learning to Rethink Anger.* Video. • *The Violence Framework: Guidelines for Understanding, Reporting, and Portraying Violence.* Handbook. • *What Do You Tell the Children? How to Help Children Deal with Disasters.* Handbook.

★ 3568 ★ Institute of Mental Health Research and Postgraduate Training

35 Poplar Rd.
Parkville, VIC 3052, Australia
Phone: 61 3 83468215 **Fax:** 61 3 93479099
Email: hkrstev@unimelb.edu.au
Website: http://www.eppic.org.au/graddip.html

Fnded: 1955.

★ 3569 ★ Institute of Nutrition of Central America and Panama (INCAP) (Instituto de Nutricion de Centro America y Panama — INCAP)

Calzada Roosevelt, Zona 11
Apartado Postal 1188
01901 Guatemala City, Guatemala
Phone: 502 2 4715655 **Fax:** 502 2 4756529
Email: hdelgado@incap.org.gt
Website: http://www.incap.org.gt

Fnded: 1949. **Nat'l Groups:** 7. **Lang(s):** English, Spanish. **Desc:** Representatives of Belize, Costa Rica, El Salvador, Guatemala, Honduras, Nicaragua, and Panama. Advises members on policies concerning nutrition in their countries. Encourages technical cooperation by coordinating available resources and promoting exchange of information and personnel in areas such as food and nutrition surveillance, maternal-infant nutrition, food aid programs, food and nutrition in school programs, improvement of basic grains, development of food resources, and nutritional fortification of foods. Conducts research in the areas of food sciences, food technology, and agro-industrial activities. Provides specialized training courses for professional, technical, and auxiliary personnel. Sponsors tutorial training programs for all levels in related fields; offers postgraduate courses in food and nutrition, health, and food sciences and technology. Conducts periodic conferences, seminars, and workshops. Compiles statistics. Administered by the Pan American Health Organization.

★ 3570 ★ Institute of Occupational Medicine (IOM)

8 Roxburgh Pl.
Edinburgh EH8 9SU, United Kingdom
Phone: 44 131 6675131 **Fax:** 44 131 6670136
Email: info@iomhq.org.uk
Website: http://www.iom-world.org

Fnded: 1969. **Desc:** Major independent centre of scientific excellence in the fields of occupational and environmental health, hygiene and safety. We aim to provide quality research, consultancy and training to help ensure that peoples health is not damaged by conditions at work or in the environment. **Pub:** *COSHH - A Helpful Guide.* • *COSHH - Making an Assessment.* • *NORSE - A Helpful Guide.* • *Technical Memoranda*, 10/year. Reports. • *Thermal Environment.*

★ 3571 ★ Institute of Ophthalmology

Bath St.
London EC1V 9EL, United Kingdom
Phone: 44 207 6086800 **Fax:** 44 207 6086852
Email: k.bonstein@ucl.ac.uk
Website: http://www.ucl.ac.uk/ioo

Fnded: 1948. **Desc:** Promotes research into eye diseases and other causes of blindness.

★ 3572 ★ Institute on Psychiatric Services/American Psychiatric Association

1400 K St. NW
Washington, DC 20005
Phone: (202)682-6314 **Free:** 888-357-7924
Fax: (202)682-6850
Email: apa@psych.org
Website: http://www.psych.org
Jill L. Gruber, Coord.

Fnded: 1949. **Desc:** Annual meeting sponsored by the American Psychiatric Association. Open to employees of all psychiatric and related health and educational facilities. Includes lectures by experts in the field and workshops and accredited courses on problems, programs, and trends. Offers on-site Job Bank, which lists opportunities for mental health professionals. Organized scientific exhibits. **Pub:** *Psychiatric Services*, monthly. Journal. *Price:* $45/individuals; $75/institutions; $22.50/students. **Frmly:** (1995) Institute on Hospital and Community Psychiatry.

★ 3573 ★ Institute of Psychiatry

c/o Kings College London
De Crespigny Park
Denmark Hill
London SE5 8AF, United Kingdom
Phone: 44 20 78365454
Email: enquiries@iop.kcl.ac.uk
Website: http://www.iop.kcl.ac.uk/iop/home.shtml

Fnded: 1948. **Desc:** To promote excellence in the research, development and teaching of psychiatry and its allied subjects and to apply and disseminate this knowledge through the development of treatment for the relief of suffering. **Pub:** Annual Report, annual. • Papers, periodic.

★ 3574 ★ Institute of Psychosexual Medicine

12 Chandos St.
Cavendish Sq.
London W1G 9DR, United Kingdom
Phone: 44 207 5800631 **Fax:** 44 207 5800631
Email: ipm@ipm.org.uk
Website: http://www.ipm.org.uk

Fnded: 1974. **Mem:** 450. **Desc:** Medical practitioners only. Seeks to promote the study and practice of psychosexual medicine through seminar training and research. **Pub:** *Journal of the Institute of Psychosocial Medicine*, 3/year. Journal.

★ 3575 ★ Institute for Research in Hypnosis and Psychotherapy (IRHP)

1991 Broadway, Apt. 18B
New York, NY 10023
Phone: (212)874-5290 **Fax:** (212)874-5290
Website: http://www.hypnosis-institute.org
Dr. Milton V. Kline, Dir.

Fnded: 1954. **Desc:** Psychologists, psychiatrists, physicians, and social workers trained in clinical hypnosis, hypnotherapy, and hypnoanalysis. Sponsors research in clinical and experimental hypnosis; offers postgraduate training in hypnosis and its applications; develops standards and procedures for advanced education in clinical and experimental hypnosis. Operates Morton Prince Centers, low-cost treatment centers for outpatients who cannot afford hypnotherapy or hypnoanalysis in private practice. Conducts consulting and educational training services. Compiles statistics; maintains databases and speakers' bureau. **Frmly:** (1982) Institute for Research in Hypnosis.

★ 3576 ★ Institute for Research on Women's Health

c/o Deborah Brower
PMB 4013
1825 I St., Ste. 400
Washington, DC 20006
Phone: (202)429-2025 **Fax:** (301)564-0184
Email: djbrower2@earthlink.net
Website: http://www.geocities.com/IRWH/IRWH1.htm
Deborah J. Brower, Exec. Dir.

Fnded: 1984. **Desc:** Scholarly research, education, and policy work related to the health of women. Promotes work related to the physical and mental health of women.

★ 3577 ★ Institute of Sterile Services Management

c/o Frank Waller
2 Grange Close
Winchester SO23 9RS, United Kingdom
Phone: 44 1962 843988
Email: frank_waller@yahoo.co.uk
Website: http://www.issm.org.uk

Desc: Different grades of membership - Fellow, Member, Student member, Associate, Corporate, Honorary, Associate Technician. Aims to organise and initiate training programmes for members/students, with the object of achieving high professional standards; provides a forum for members through regional branches to consider and discuss matters relating to sterilization and disinfection and promotes and encourages research and development in the world of sterile service. **Pub:** *The ISSM Journal*, quarterly. Journal. • *Official Reference Book*, annual. • *Training Handbook for Steril Service Personnel.*

★ 3578 ★ Institute of Transactional Analysis

3 Kents Ln.
Soham
Ely CB7 5DX, United Kingdom
Phone: 44 1353 724982 **Fax:** 44 1353 724982
Email: admin@ita.org.uk
Website: http://www.ita.org.uk

Fnded: 1973. **Mem:** 1,100. **Reg. Groups:** 75. **Desc:** Professional members, qualified to teach and supervise the practice of TA. Certified TA analysts and trainee TA analysts. Also those interested in TA. Promotes and maintains the practice of TA, sets and maintains standards of professional practice and training. **Pub:** *ITA News*, bimonthly. Newsletter. • *Transactions*, semiannual. Journal.

★ 3579 ★ Institute of Trichologists (IT)

20/22 Queensberry Place
London SW7 2D2, United Kingdom
Phone: 44 870 6070602 **Fax:** 44 115 9384303
Email: trichologists@ambernet.co.uk
Website: http://www.trichologists.org.uk/

Fnded: 1902. **Mem:** 240. **Lang(s):** English. **Desc:** Promotes study, research, and application in the treatment and care of human scalp and hair. Provides scientific training of individuals qualified to advise and offer treatment of hair and scalp disorders and serves as an examining body for students of trichology. Provides centers for clinical study. Maintains Scalp and Hair Hospital where students conduct clinical observations and gain practical experience. Bestows awards; sponsors charitable program; maintains speakers' bureau. **Pub:** *Membership Directory*, annual. Membership Directory. • *Monograph*, periodic. • *Update*, 3/year. Journal. • Newsletter, 3/year.

★ 3580 ★ Instituto Nacional de Higiene

Calzada, Mariano Escobedo 20
Mexico City, Mexico
Fax: 52 5276693

Fnded: 1904.

★ 3581 ★ Instituto Peruano de Paternidad Responsable (INPPARES)

Gregorio Escobedo 115
Jesus Maria, Peru
Phone: 51 1 2615522 **Fax:** 51 1 2617885
Email: postmast@inppares.org.pe
Website: http://www.inppares.org.pe

Fnded: 1976. **Mem:** 140. **State Groups:** 14. **Local Groups:** 5. **Lang(s):** Spanish. **Desc:** Works to improve the quality of life for people living in Peru through the promotion of information and services related to sexual and reproductive health. Maintains programs in 14 cities. Works with local governments and community leaders to promote gender equality, the empowerment of women, prevention of unsafe abortions, and the prevention and control of sexually transmitted diseases, especially HIV and AIDS. **Pub:** *Information Bulletin*, periodic. Newsletter.

★ 3582 ★ Insulin-Free World Foundation

677 Craig Rd., Ste. 105
Saint Louis, MO 63141-7115
Phone: (314)468-2439 **Free:** 888-746-4439
Fax: (314)468-2444
Email: action@fasttrackcure.org
Website: http://www.insulin-free.org/
Deb Butterfield, Founder/Exec. Dir.

Fnded: 1996. **Desc:** Facilitates the exchange of information in the diabetes community. Corresponds with diabetes researchers and clinicians at 200 prominenet academic institutions. Gathers research articles, facts and statistics, scientific abstracts, human-interest stories, insurance advice, pharmaceutical counsel, and as much information as possible about advances in insulin-free treatments and cures for diabetes. This information is redistributed through InsulinFree.org, Insulin-Free Times, on-line interviews through its sister-site, Diabetes Station, and other publications. Has created the "definitive on-line directory of pancreas and islet transplant specialists". **Pub:** *Insulin-Free Times*, quarterly. Magazine. Integrates information about advances toward curing diabetes. • *Showdown with Diabetes.* Book.

★ 3583 ★ Integral Health for Women (Salud Integral para la Mujer — SIPAM)

Vista Hermosa 89
Col. Portales
C.P. 03300
Mexico City, DF, Mexico
Phone: 52 55 55398703 **Fax:** 52 55 55398703
Email: sipam@laneta.apc.org

Fnded: 1987. **Lang(s):** English, Spanish. **Desc:** Feminist and citizens' organization that contributes to the full and pleasant exercise of women's sexuality and the enjoyment of their sexual and reproductive health as axles for the personal, cultural, and political transformation of Mexican society. Made up of women from various backgrounds and professional fields. Promotes the knowledge and exercise of women's sexual and reproductive rights. Makes conceptual and methodological proposals and influences public policies to create favorable conditions for the exercise of these rights. Contributes to strengthen organized civil society and the public projection of its proposals and promotes the citizens' participation of women and contributes to the construction of a democratic civil society with equality and respect for plurality and diversity from a gender perspective. Aims to achieve its objectives through communicative efforts and actions to influence the public opinion, research and systemization, education and training, and the design and development of proposals for public policies.

★ 3584 ★ Intensive Care Society (ICS)
29 B Montague St., 3rd Fl.
London WC1B 5BH, United Kingdom
Phone: 44 20 72910690 **Fax:** 44 20 75800689
Email: marie@ics.ac.uk
Website: http://www.ics.ac.uk

Fnded: 1970. **Mem:** 2,000. **Lang(s):** English. **Desc:** Medical and scientific specialists in the field of intensive care. Seeks to provide the scientific and professional basis necessary for the research activities related to intensive care issues, and to make advice and information available to interested parties. Promotes communication among related organizations. **Pub:** *Fire Safety in the Intensive Care Unit.* Book. • *ICS Newsletter*, quarterly. Newsletter. • *Recommendations for Training in Intensive Care.* Book. • *Transport of the Critically Ill.* Book.

★ 3585 ★ Inter-African Bureau for Animal Resources (IBAR)
PO Box 30786
Nairobi, Kenya
Phone: 254 20 338544 **Fax:** 254 20 332046

Fnded: 1951. **Mem:** 53. **Reg. Groups:** 5. **Lang(s):** Arabic, English, French, Portuguese. **Desc:** Countries belonging to the Organization of African Unity. Aims to control widespread animal diseases; seeks improvements in animal health and production in Africa. **Pub:** *Bulletin of Animal Health and Production in Africa*, quarterly. Bulletin. • *Information Leaflet*, weekly. • *Proceedings of ISCTRC Meeting*, biennial. **Frmly:** (1960) Inter-American Bureau for Epizootic Diseases.

★ 3586 ★ Inter-American Society of Cardiology (ISC) (Sociedad Interamericana de Cardiologia)
Instituto Nacional de Cardiologia
Calle Jaun Bardiano 1
14080 Mexico City, DF, Mexico
Phone: 52 5 5732911 **Fax:** 52 5 55135177
Email: soimca@mail.cpesa.com.mx
Website: http://www.soinca.org

Fnded: 1944. **Mem:** 23. **Lang(s):** English, French, Portuguese, Spanish. **Desc:** National societies of cardiology from the Americas; medical doctors; individuals who have made outstanding contributions in the cardiovascular and allied fields. Purpose is to unite members for the development and advancement of cardiology and related fields, particularly by promoting the association of physicians, surgeons, and scientists with cardiovascular specialties. Fosters cooperation and exchange of information, medical specialists, and scientists at national, regional, and world levels; provides advice to governments seeking counsel. Sponsors exchange programs. **Pub:** *News Bulletin*, periodic. Bulletin.

★ 3587 ★ Inter-American Society for Chemotherapy (IASC)
Azcuenaga 769, Piso 2, Apt 7
1029 Buenos Aires, Argentina
Phone: 54 11 49542365 **Fax:** 54 1 49528255

Fnded: 1983. **Desc:** Promotes acquisition and dissemination of knowledge in chemotherapy and related areas.

★ 3588 ★ Inter American Society of Digestive Endoscopy (Sociedad Interamericana de Endoscopia Digestiva — SIED)
Calle 11, no 1129 1e A
1900 La Plata, Argentina
Phone: 54 21 241991 **Fax:** 54 1 225111
State Groups: dad In. **Local Groups:** scopia.

★ 3589 ★ Inter-Association Task Force on Alcohol and Other Substance Abuse Issues (IATF)
c/o Bacchus and Gamma Peer Education Network
PO Box 100430
Denver, CO 80250
Phone: (303)871-0901 **Fax:** (303)871-0907
Email: dhunter@du.edu
Website: http://www.iatf.org
Drew Hunter, Convener

Fnded: 1983. **Mem:** 20. **Desc:** Associations of college professionals and student leaders. Purposes are to enhance the development and implementation of alcohol and other substance abuse education activities in institutions of higher education throughout the U.S. and to encourage collaboration among professionals and student associations. Sponsors National Collegiate Alcohol Awareness Week and National Collegiate Health and Wellness Week. **Pub:** *First National Conference on Alcohol Policy Initiatives.* • *Guidelines for Marketing of Alcohol Beverage on Campus.* Pamphlet. • *National Collegiate Alcohol Awareness Week Mailing Handbook.* Handbook. **Frmly:** Inter-Association Task Force on Alcohol Issues; (2002) Inter-Association Task Force on Campus Alcohol and Other Substance Abuse Issues.

★ 3590 ★ Interagency Coalition on AIDS and Development
1 Nicholas St., Ste. 726
Ottawa, ON, Canada K1N 7B7
Phone: (613)233-7440 **Fax:** (613)233-8361
Email: info@icad-cisd.com
Website: http://www.icad-cisd.com

Fnded: 1990. **Mem:** 117. **Lang(s):** French. **Desc:** Seeks to lessen the impact of HIV/AIDS in resource-poor communities and countries. We are a coalition of Canadian international development organizations, AIDS service organizations and other interested organizations and individuals. **Pub:** *ICAD Member News*, quarterly. Newsletter. Contains articles, Internet sites, and upcoming events.

★ 3591 ★ Interamerican Association of Pediatric Otolaryngology (IAPO)
c/o Dr. Eavey
243 Charles St.
Boston, MA 02114-3002
Dr. Eavey, Contact

Fnded: 1996. **Mem:** 2,000. **Desc:** Pediatric Otolaryngologists.

★ 3592 ★ Interamerican College of Physicians and Surgeons (ICPS)
233 Broawway, Rm. 771
New York, NY 10279-0711
Phone: (212)777-3642 **Fax:** (212)777-5000
Email: icps@icps.org
Website: http://www.icps.org
Dr. Rene F. Rodriguez, MD, Pres.

Fnded: 1979. **Mem:** 4,000. **Desc:** Physicians in countries of the Americas. Encourages understanding and communication among members concerning all aspects of medical practice. Promotes health education in Hispanic communities in the Western Hemisphere. Maintains library of Spanish language medical books. **Pub:** *Interamerican Medical Directory*, biennial. Directory. • *Medico Interamericano*, monthly. Journal.

★ 3593 ★ InterAmerican Heart Foundation (IAHF)
7272 Greenville Ave.
Dallas, TX 75231-4596
Phone: (214)706-1218 **Fax:** (214)373-0268
Email: beatrizc@ix.netcom.com
Javier Valenzuela, PhD, Office Coordinator

Fnded: 1992. **Mem:** 31. **Desc:** The InterAmerican Heart Program was created in September, 1992 under the auspices of the International Society and Federation of Cardiology with the support of the American Heart Association, the InterAmerican Society of Cardiology and heart foundations and societies throughout the American continent. **Pub:** *Heart of the Americas*, quarterly. Newsletter. *Price:* Free. **Frmly:** International Cardiology Foundation; (1998) Interamerican Heart Cardiology Foundation.

★ 3594 ★ Interamerican Medical and Health Association (IMHA)
7900 Los Pinos Cir.
Coral Gables, FL 33143-6472
Phone: (305)666-9222 **Fax:** (561)483-3239
Dr. Maurizio Luca-Moretti, Pres.

Fnded: 1989. **Mem:** 4,000. **Desc:** Academicians of national academies of medicine, deans of medical facilities, and professors of medical science. Promotes the work of biomedical and health scientists and the effectiveness of science in the promotion of human welfare. Facilitates networking among members and their institutions. Conducts research programs on medical and public health issues; current research focuses on nutrition and AIDS. **Pub:** *Journal of the Interamerican Medical and Health Association*, 3/year. Journal. *Price:* $60/year for institutions in North America; $60/year for institutions in Europe and Japan; $30/year for individuals in North America; $30/year for individuals in Europe and Japan.

★ 3595 ★ Intercare
900 Wilshire Blve., Ste. 500
Los Angeles, CA 90017
Phone: (213)627-8878 **Fax:** (213)627-9183
Email: info@intercare.com
Website: http://www.intercare.com/
Theodore Carcich, Jr., Pres.

Fnded: 1976. **Mem:** 600. **Desc:** Individuals involved or interested in the long-term health care of the chronically ill. Works to improve long-term health care; to encourage high standards of professional care and administration; to interact with professional groups, academic institutions, and governmental agencies; to provide opportunities for individual research; to discover solutions to the problems of the aged, chronically ill, and disabled; to establish a clearinghouse of research findings and resources. Maintains speakers' bureau. Provides semi-quarterly educational program in various countries. **Pub:** *Intercare, International Directory*, annual. Directory. • Journal, quarterly.

★ 3596 ★ Interchurch Medical Assistance (IMA)
College Ave. at Blue Ridge
Box 429
New Windsor, MD 21776
Phone: (410)635-8720 **Fax:** (410)635-8726
Email: imainfo@interchurch.org
Website: http://www.interchurch.org
Paul Derstine, Pres.

Fnded: 1961. **Mem:** 12. **Desc:** Denominational-founded autonomous organization for the solicitation, collection, and distribution of pharmaceutical, medical, dental, and hospital supplies for use in the overseas charity medical programs of American Protestant churches, relief agencies, and other American charitable organizations. **Pub:** *Interchurch Medical Newsletter*, monthly. Newsletter. Electronic newsletter. • Annual Report, annual.

★ 3597 ★ Intergovernmental Health Policy Project (IHPP)
444 N Capital St. Ste 515
Washington, DC 20001
Phone: (202)624-8698 **Fax:** (202)737-1069
Email: dick.merritt@ncsl.org
Richard E. Merritt, Dir.

Fnded: 1979. **Desc:** Health policy researchers. Provides information on state health legislation and programs to state executive officials, legislators, legislative staff, and others. Serves as information clearinghouse; responds to specific information requests on state programs. Compiles statistics. Offers a customized legislative tracking service to customers. **Pub:** *State Health Notes*, semimonthly. Newsletter. *Price:* $297. • Newsletter, bimonthly. • Newsletter, 10/year. • Monograph, annual. Summarizes state legislation relating to health care.

★ 3598 ★ Intermed International
420 Lexington Ave., Ste. 2331
New York, NY 10170
Phone: (212)687-3620 **Fax:** (212)599-6137
Email: dooleyfdn@aol.com
Verne Chaney, MD, Founder & Pres.

Fnded: 1961. **Desc:** Assists Third World countries in the development of medical care systems through self-help projects in disease prevention, health education, personnel development, and research and medical aid to refugees. Presently operates programs in Laos, Honduras, Nepal, and Nicaragua. **Pub:** *Intermed Journal*, semiannual. Brochure. • *INTERMED Journal*, semiannual. Journal. **Frmly:** Dooley Foundation/INTERMED; (1962) Dr. Thomas A. Dooley Foundation; (1978) Thomas A. Dooley Foundation; (1980) Thomas A. Dooley Foundation/INTERMED U.S.A.

★ 3599 ★ International Academy of Aviation and Space Medicine (IAASM) (Academie Internationale de Medecine Aeronautique et Spatiale — AIMAS)
c/o Dr. George Takahashi
21 Antares Dr., Ste. 112
Nepean, ON, Canada K2E 7T8
Phone: (613)228-9345 **Fax:** (613)228-0242
Email: g.takahashi@sympatico.ca
Website: http://www.iaasm.org

Fnded: 1955. **Mem:** 225. **Lang(s):** English, French. **Desc:** Doctors over 40 years of age who have specialized in aerospace medicine for at least 10 years; associate members may have another qualification or equivalent scientific title in a related field and must be at least 30 years of age and have sufficient qualifications in aviation medicine. Promotes development of science and fosters research in biology, aviation, and space medicine; seeks to improve the teaching of these sciences and their corollaries and to foster the training of experts in aviation and space medicine. Offers scholarships through the Aerospace Medicine Trust.

★ 3600 ★ International Academy of Chest Physicians and Surgeons of the American College of Chest Physicians, Republic of China Chapter
1 Changteh St
Taipei, Taiwan
Phone: 886 2 3123456

Fnded: 1969.

★ 3601 ★ International Academy for Child Brain Development (IACBD)
8801 Stenton Ave.
Glenside, PA 19038
Phone: (215)233-2050 **Fax:** (215)233-1530
Email: institutes@iahp.org
Website: http://www.iahp.org
Neil Harvey, PhD, Sec.

Fnded: 1985. **Desc:** Professionals from a variety of disciplines including physicians, psychologists, and anthropologists, who are interested in the physical and psychological processes involved in child brain development. Seeks to gain recognition for the study of child brain development as a discipline in itself and establish criteria for the certification of child brain developmentalists. Provides a forum for presentation of scholarly works in the field; offers courses in child-brain development; conducts field research and prepares reports of results. **Pub:** *The In-Report*, quarterly. Journal.

★ 3602 ★ International Academy of Compounding Pharmacists (IACP)
PO Box 1365
Sugar Land, TX 77487
Free: 800-927-4227 **Fax:** (281)495-0602
Email: iacpinfo@iacprx.org
Website: http://www.iacprx.org
L.D. King, Exec. Dir.

Fnded: 1991. **Mem:** 1,600. **Desc:** Pharmacists who compound custom medications to meet unique patient needs. Seeks to "enhance credibility and respect of the compounding pharmacy practice to the health care community and its patients"; promotes empowerment of compounding pharmacists. Develops and enforces codes of ethics and practice for members; facilitates cooperation and exchange of information among members; sponsors research and educational programs. **Pub:** *The Pharmacists Link*, quarterly.

★ 3603 ★ International Academy of Cosmetic Dermatology
c/o Timothy C. Flynn, Md
1430 Tulane Ave., Ste. Sl73
New Orleans, LA 70112-2699
Phone: (504)588-5114 **Fax:** (504)587-7382
Website: http://www.dermato.med.br/iacd/
Larry Millikan, MD, Sec. Treas.

Desc: Cosmetic dermatologists.

★ 3604 ★ International Academy of Cosmetic Surgery (IACS)
Via della Camilluccia 643
I-00135 Rome, Italy
Phone: 39 06 36303204 **Fax:** 39 06 36304165

Fnded: 1970. **Mem:** 410. **Desc:** Cosmetic and reconstructive surgeons. Conducts training programs for doctors from underdeveloped countries. **Pub:** *Bulletin*, quarterly. Bulletin.

★ 3605 ★ International Academy of Cytology (IAC)
Department of Obstetrics and Gynecology
University of Freiburg
Burgunderstr. 1
D-79104 Freiburg, Germany
Phone: 49 761 2923802 **Fax:** 49 761 2923802
Email: centraloffice@cytology-iac.org
Website: http://www.cytology-iac.org

Fnded: 1957. **Mem:** 1,900. **Lang(s):** English, French, German, Japanese, Spanish. **Desc:** Doctors of medicine concerned with research in clinical cytology (the scientific study of the structure, organization, and function of cells, particularly for cancer diagnosis); cytotechnologists actively engaged in the practice of cytodiagnosis and research. Encourages cooperation among persons engaged in the practice of clinical cytology; facilitates international exchange of information on specialized problems in this field; standardizes terminology; stimulates development of all phases of clinical cytology and encourages research. **Pub:** *Acta Cytologica*, bimonthly. • *Analytic and Quantitative Cytology and Histology*, bimonthly. • Newsletter, periodic.

★ 3606 ★ International Academy of Gnathology-American Section (IAG)
3868 Riviera Dr.
San Diego, CA 92109-6351
Dr. James M. Benson, Sec. -Treas.

Fnded: 1964. **Mem:** 200. **Desc:** Dentists and educators interested in the science of gnathology. (Gnathology is the science that treats the biology of chewing and the jaws and cheeks as related to the rest of the body.) Areas of concern include morphology, anatomy, psychology, physiology, pathology, and therapy of the mouth. **Pub:** *Journal of Gnathology*, annual. Journal.

★ 3607 ★ International Academy of Health Care Professionals (IAHCP)
333 Glen Cove Rd., Ste. 180
Old Brookville, NY 11545
Phone: (516)759-4630 **Fax:** (516)931-3163
Dr. Henry H. Reiter, Pres.

Fnded: 1984. **Mem:** 38. **Desc:** Nurses, psychologists, social workers, and medical and health care professionals. Provides for educational exchange among members. Offers research and educational materials to Third World health care institutions. **Pub:** *Membership Brochure*. Brochure. • Newsletter, periodic.

★ 3608 ★ International Academy of Myodontics (IAM)
c/o Dr. Harry Cooperman D.D.S.
777 Ferry Rd. P-6
Doylestown, PA 18901
Phone: (215)345-1149 **Fax:** (215)609-2588
Email: myodont@comcat.com
Website: http://www.comcat.com/~myodont/
Harry N. Cooperman, D.D.S., Pres.

Fnded: 1970. **Mem:** 1,100. **Reg. Groups:** 2. **Desc:** Dentists who specialize in the treatment of head and neck syndromes that cause dental or oral malfunction. Works with physicians and dentists in the field of myodontics, especially those working on the treatment of Cooperman-Muira Syndrome, also known as uvulatongue malposture syndrome.

★ 3609 ★ International Academy of Olympic Chiropractic Officers (IAOCO)
c/o Dr. Stephen J. Press
546 Broad Ave.
Englewood, NJ 07631
Phone: (201)569-1444
Website: http://www.iaoco.org/
Dr. Stephen J. Press, Chm.

Desc: Honorary society for Doctors of Chiropractic who have been officially credited as team doctors in the Olympic games.

★ 3610 ★ International Academy of Oral Medicine and Toxicology (IAOMT)
PO Box 608531
Orlando, FL 32860-8531
Phone: (407)298-2450 **Fax:** (407)298-3075
Email: mziff@iaomt.org
Website: http://www.iaomt.org
Michael F. Ziff, D.D.S., Exec. Dir.

Fnded: 1984. **Mem:** 1,000. **Nat'l Groups:** 11. **Desc:** Dentists, physicians, and medical scientists. Encourages, sponsors, and disseminates scientific research on the biocompatibility of materials used in dentistry. Offers educational programs; maintains speakers' bureau. **Pub:** *Bio-Probe Newsletter*, bimonthly. Newsletter. Review of scientific literature and legislative activities. *Price:* Included in membership dues. • *IN VIVO*, quarterly. Newsletter. Available to members only. *Price:* Included in membership dues. • Membership Directory.Indexed alphabetically and geographically.

★ 3611 ★ International Academy of Osteopathy
Schipholpoort 100
NL-2034 MC Haarlem, Netherlands
Phone: 31 23 5300485 **Fax:** 31 23 5300437
Website: http://www.iao.be

★ 3612 ★ International Academy of Pathology (IAP)
c/o Florabel G. Mullick
Armed Forces Institute of Pathology
Center for Advanced Pathology
14th St. & Alaska Ave. NW
Washington, DC 20306-6000
Phone: (202)782-2550 **Fax:** (202)782-7166
Email: mullick@email.afp.osd.mil
Website: http://www.afip.org/iap/
Florabel G. Mullick, Sec.

Fnded: 1906. **Mem:** 8,300. **Reg. Groups:** 32. **Desc:** Professional society of pathologists and medical scientists. Aim is to improve methods of teaching pathology. Coordinates anatomical pathology, pathologic physiology, and comparative pathology; promotes research in pathology in medical schools, laboratories, hospitals, and medical museums. **Pub:** *International Pathology*, quarterly. Newsletter. *Price:* Included in membership dues. **Frmly:** (1954) International Association of Medical Museums.

★ 3613 ★ International Academy of Periodontology
5 Battery Green Rd.
Lowestoft NR32 1DE, United Kingdom
Phone: 44 1502 511522 **Fax:** 44 1502 583152
Email: perioiap@btclick.com
Website: http://www.perioiap.org

★ 3614 ★ International Academy for Sports Dentistry (IASD)
118 Faye St.
Farmersville, IL 62533
Phone: (217)227-3431 **Free:** 800-273-1788
Fax: (217)227-3438
Email: iasdsportsdentistry@cillnet.com
Website: http://www.acadsportsdent.org/
Shelly Lott, Exec. Sec.

Fnded: 1983. **Mem:** 750. **Nat'l Groups:** 1. **Desc:** Dentists, dental students, physicians, athletic trainers, and others interested in the study and prevention of dental injuries incurred during sports participation. Purpose is to foster research, development, and education in all sciences related to sports dentistry and its relationship to the body as a whole. Encourages utilization of this knowledge in promoting better approaches to the prevention and treatment of athletic injuries and oral disease. Facilitates the exchange of ideas and experience among members. **Pub:** *ASD Newsletter*, 2-3/year. Newsletter. Provides information on the use of craniofacial protection such as helmets, mouthguards, and faceguards. *Price:* Included in membership dues. **Frmly:** (2002) Academy for Sports Dentistry.

★ 3615 ★ International Academy of Sports Vision (NASV)
3721 Redmont Rd.
Birmingham, AL 35213
Email: nasv@mindspring.com
Dr. A. I. Garner, Exec. Dir.

Fnded: 1984. **Mem:** 1,000. **Desc:** Optometrists and opthalmologists; athletic trainers, team physicians, coaches, and students; educational institutions and eyewear manufacturers. Purpose is to: provide comprehensive vision care for individuals active in sports and fitness programs; foster the promotion and advancement of research, development, and education in the field; facilitate the design, development, and fitting of both protective and corrective contact lenses and eyewear for athletes; advance and enhance the role of the sports specialist to the public through a public relations program. Acts as a forum for the discussion and exchange of information in the areas of developmental vision, vision training, and therapy. Offers referral services. **Pub:** *Journal of the International Academy of Sports Vision*. Journal. • *SportsVision*, quarterly. Magazine. • *Update*, quarterly. • Audiotapes. • Membership Directory, annual. • Videos. **Frmly:** (1991) National Academy of Sports Vision.

★ 3616 ★ International Acupuncture Institute
301 Nathan Rd., Rm. 1304
Hong Kong, People's Republic of China
Phone: 852 27711066 **Fax:** 852 23888836

Fnded: 1978. **Mem:** 700. **Nat'l Groups:** 2. **Lang(s):** Chinese, English. **Desc:** Acupuncturists and other health care professionals; individuals with an interest in acupuncture. Promotes effective practice of acupuncture; devises and maintains standards of practice. Conducts research and educational programs. **Pub:** *Clinical Acupuncture*. Book.

★ 3617 ★ International Adhesions Society (IAS)
c/o David Wiseman
Synechion, Inc.
6757 Arapaho Rd., Ste. 711 No. 238
Dallas, TX 75248
Phone: (972)931-5596 **Fax:** (972)931-5476
Email: david.wiseman@adhesions.org
Website: http://www.adhesions.org
Dr. David Wiseman, Contact

Fnded: 1996. **Desc:** Promotes treatment for adhesions and chronic pelvic pain. Adhesions are scars that form an abnormal connection between two parts of the body, including non-surgical insults such as endometriosis, infection, chemotherapy, radiation and cancer, or from surgical procedures. Assists formation of support groups. **Pub:** Audiotapes.Set of lecture tapes from the March 12, 2001 IAS conference held in Detroit, Michigan. *Price:* Included with $50 member donation.

★ 3618 ★ International Agency for the Prevention of Blindness (IAPB)
c/o Dr. Gullapalli N. Rao, Sec.Gen.
LV Prasad Eye Institute
LV Prasad Marg
Banjara Hills
Hyderabad 500034, India
Phone: 91 40 23545389 **Fax:** 91 40 3548271
Email: iapb@lvpeye.stph.net

Fnded: 1975. **Lang(s):** English. **Desc:** Ophthalmic societies and societies for the prevention of blindness whose members include ophthalmologists, public health officers, nutritionists, geneticists, and other health workers. Coordinates international research into the causes of impaired vision or blindness; promotes measures calculated to eliminate such causes; disseminates knowledge worldwide on preventing blindness and on matters pertaining to care of the eyes. Cooperates with the World Health Organization, United Nations Children's Fund, and other international agencies. **Pub:** *IAPB Fifth General Assembly*. Proceedings document. • *IAPB News*. Newsletter. • *World Blindness and Its Prevention Vols. 1-4*. Proceedings. Based on proceedings of respective General Assemblies.

★ 3619 ★ International Agency for Research on Cancer (IARC) (Centre International de Recherche sur le Cancer — CIRC)
150, cours Albert Thomas
F-69372 Lyon, France
Phone: 33 4 72738485 **Fax:** 33 4 72738575
Email: lastname@iarc.fr
Website: http://www.iarc.fr

Fnded: 1965. **Mem:** 16. **Lang(s):** English, French. **Desc:** Cancer research arm of the World Health Organization. Representatives of nations involved in international collaboration in cancer research. Generates and disseminates information on the causes and prevention of cancer; conducts research in the field of cancer epidemiology, biostatistics, and environmental carcinogenesis. Evaluates and examines populations with unusually high or low frequencies of cancer and identifies the role of environmental factors including cultural and dietary habits and chemicals. Assists governments in cancer control programs. Maintains laboratories and collaborates with scientists working in national laboratories. Organizes training courses; compiles statistics. **Pub:** *Directory of On-Going Research in Cancer Epidemiology*, biennial. • *Technical Report Series*, periodic.

★ 3620 ★ International AIDS Society (IAS)
Karolinska Institute
Berzeliusvag 8
S-171 77 Stockholm, Sweden
Phone: 46 8 50884640 **Fax:** 46 8 50884664
Email: secretariat@ias.se
Website: http://www.ias.se/

Fnded: 1988. **Mem:** 5,700. **Desc:** Promotes the study of AIDS internationally. **Pub:** *IAS Membership Directory*. Newsletter. • *IAS Newsletter*, 3/year.

★ 3621 ★ International AIDS Vaccine Initiative (IAVI)
110 William St.
New York, NY 10038-3901
Phone: (212)847-1111 **Fax:** (212)847-1112
Email: info@iavi.org
Website: http://www.iavi.org

Fnded: 1996. **Desc:** Works to speed the development and distribution of preventative AIDS vaccines.

★ 3622 ★ International Alliance of Healthcare Educators (IAHE)
11211 Prosperity Farms Rd., Ste. D-325
Palm Beach Gardens, FL 33410
Phone: (561)622-4334 **Fax:** (561)622-4771
Email: iahe@iahe.com
Website: http://www.iahe.com
Kathy Wall, Dir.

Fnded: 1996. **Desc:** Health care instructors and curriculum developers; seeks to advance innovative therapies through continuing education.

★ 3623 ★ International and American Association of Clinical Nutritionists (IAACN)
16775 Addison Rd., Ste. 102
Addison, TX 75001
Phone: (972)407-9089 **Fax:** (972)250-0233
Email: ccnl990ccn@msn.com
Website: http://www.iaacn.org
Winna C. Henry, Exec. Dir.

Fnded: 1971. **Mem:** 400. **State Groups:** 7. **Desc:** Physicians (medical, osteopathic, chiropractic), dentists, veterinarians, clinical nutritionists, pharmacists, nurses and scientists. Practitioners hold accredited undergraduatiate, graduate or professional degrees in science and/or nutrition, or in fields related to nutrition with the addition of required core courses. IAACN sponsors the Certified Clinical Nutritionist (CCN) credential under the responsibility of the Clinical Nutrition Certicication Board (CNCB). Members work in the U.S. and other countries to stimulate and encourage research in the nutritional aspects of disease, promote the science and study of nutrition and complementary therapies in medical and dental schools, hospitals, colleges and research institutions. Provides a referral service for people seeking nutrition/preventive health care providers. Holds an annual scientific symposium with world-class faculty. **Pub:** *Journal of Applied Nutrition*, quarterly. Journal. *Price:* $67/year for members; $90/year for nonmembers and institutions; $40/year for students; $110/year outside U.S. • *Your Health*, bimonthly. Newsletter. Includes information on nutrition and preventative medicine applied to a variety of health issues. *Price:* Included in membership dues. **Frmly:** (1998) International Academy of Nutrition and Preventitive Medicine.

★ 3624 ★ International Anesthesia Research Society (IARS)
2 Summit Park Dr., Ste. 140
Cleveland, OH 44131-2571
Phone: (216)642-1124 **Fax:** (216)642-1127
Email: iarshq@iars.org

Website: http://www.iars.org

Fnded: 1922. **Mem:** 15,000. **Desc:** Anesthesiologists and other doctors of medicine and dentistry interested in the specialty of anesthesiology; associate members are registered nurses, physician assistants, and respiratory therapists. Fosters progress and research in all phases of anesthesiology. **Pub:** *Anesthesia & Analgesia*, monthly. Journal. Contains research articles and clinical reports on anesthesia and anesthesia-related subjects. Includes book reviews and employment listings. *Price:* $120/year for members; $440/year for nonmember institutions.

★ 3625 ★ International Aromatherapy and Herb Association

c/o Jeffrey Schiller
3541 W Acapulco Ln.
Phoenix, AZ 85053-4625
Phone: (602)938-4439
Email: jeffreys@aztec.asu.edu
Website: http://aztec.asu.edu/makingscents/
Jeffrey Schiller, Pres.

Fnded: 1996. **Mem:** 300. **Desc:** People interested in aromatherapy, herbs and natural health. **Pub:** *Making Scents*, semiannual. Magazine. Includes article of interest, resource lists, and book and product reviews. *Price:* included in membership dues.

★ 3626 ★ International Association for Adolescent Health (IAAH)

c/o Section Medecine de l'Adoescence
Hopital Sainte-Justine
3175 Cote Ste.-Catherine
Montreal, QC, Canada H3T 1C5
Fax: (514)345-4778
Email: president@iaah.org
Website: http://www.iaah.org/

Fnded: 1987. **Mem:** 330. **Desc:** Aims to foster wider understanding of the importance of youth health in each region of the world; to encourage interaction and co-operation between youth and non-youth and between organizations and individuals on youth health issues. **Pub:** Newsletter, 3/year.

★ 3627 ★ International Association of Agricultural Medicine and Rural Health (IAAMRH) (Association Internationale de Medecine Agricole et de Sante Rurale)

ul. Marszalkowska 82
PL-00-517 Warsaw, Poland
Phone 48 22 6236551 **Fax:** 48 22 6236568
Email: pmt@pravara.ren.nic.in
Website: http://www.iaamrh.org

Fnded: 1961. **Mem:** 450. **Nat'l Groups:** 4. **Reg. Groups:** 3. **Lang(s):** English, French, German, Polish, Russian. **Desc:** Independent association for agricultural and rural professionals in over 40 countries. Studies agricultural medicine and rural health around the world. Strives to improve the health of rural communities and to protect the health of agricultural workers. Studies agricultural and rural health in association with other sciences and provides scientific information and advice. Cooperates with other branches of medicine, health, agricultural, environmental and other related sciences. Studies the effects of social, physical and environmental conditions on human health. **Pub:** *Agricultural Medicine and Rural Health*, semiannual. Journal.

★ 3628 ★ International Association of ALS/MND Associations

PO Box 246
Northampton NN1 2PR, United Kingdom
Phone: 44 1604 611821 **Fax:** 44 1604 611852
Email: alliance@alsmndalliance.org

Fnded: 1992. **Desc:** Umbrella organization for Amyotrophic Lateral Sclerosis (ALS) and Motor Neruone Disease (MND) associations. ALS and MND are muscle-wasting conditions. Provides a forum for support and exchange of information for ALS and MND associations worldwide. **Pub:** Directory.

★ 3629 ★ International Association for Ambulatory Surgery

Ave du Duc Jean 71-73
1083 Brussels, Belgium
Phone: 32 2 4257076 **Fax:** 32 2 4224271
Email: c.delathouwer@baas.be
Website: http://www.iaas-med.org/

Fnded: 1995. **Desc:** Promotes exchange of information on and advancement of ambulatory surgery; encourages its high quality development and expansion; fosters education and research in the field and disseminates research results; establishes close relations with relevant organizations and stimulates development of national societies in the field.

★ 3630 ★ International Association of Applied Psychology (IAAP) (Association Internationale de Psychologie Appliquee — AIPA)

Compultense University
Faculty of Psychology
Department of Individual Differences and Work Psychology
Somosaguas
E-28223 Madrid, Spain
Phone: 34 91 3510091 **Fax:** 34 91 3510091
Email: iaap@psi.ucm.es
Website: http://www.iaapsy.org

Fnded: 1920. **Mem:** 3,000. **Lang(s):** English, French. **Desc:** Specialists in applied psychology from 90 countries. Seeks to establish contact between persons who engage in scientific work in various fields of applied psychology; studies ways to contribute to scientific and social development in these fields. Organizes parallel research and experiments in different countries. **Pub:** *Applied Psychology: An International Review*, quarterly. • *Newsletter*, semiannual. Newsletter.

★ 3631 ★ International Association for Aquatic Animal Medicine (IAAAM)

c/o Donald W. Stremme, VMD
1129 Pine St.
Philadelphia, PA 19107-6035
Phone: (215)928-9289 **Fax:** (215)925-1510
Email: donstremme@aol.com
Website: http://iaaam.org
Donald W. Stremme, VMD, Sec. -Treas.

Fnded: 1969. **Mem:** 450. **Desc:** Veterinarians, PhDs, and marine biologists involved in aquatic animal medicine and husbandry. Objectives are: to advance the art of aquatic animal medicine; to promote the free exchange of knowledge in the interest of improving the health care and husbandry of domestic aquatic animals and the proper management of aquatic animal resources in the wild; to provide an organization in which interested and professionally qualified individuals can work together to achieve these objectives; to provide a setting in which the development of the practice of aquatic animal medicine may be facilitated and enhanced; to promote the application of veterinary medical principles to aquatic animal disease problems. **Pub:** *IAAAM Conference Proceedings*, annual. Contains Annual Conference abstracts. *Price:* included in membership dues; $40 for nonmembers. • *IAAAM Directory*, annual. Directory. Included in proceedings book. *Price:* for members only. • *IAAAM News*, 3/year. Newsletter. Includes association news, book reviews, calendar of events, and research updates. *Price:* Included in membership dues.

★ 3632 ★ International Association of Asthmology (INTERASMA) (Asociacion Internacional de Asmologia — INTERASMA)

c/o Gianni Ralzano, Enrico Melillo Foundation
Via Bagni Vecchi
I-82037 Telese Terme, BN, Italy
Phone: 39 082 4909111 **Fax:** 39 082 4909614
Email: emelillo@fsm.it
Website: http://www.asmanet.com/interasma.html

Fnded: 1954. **Mem:** 1,200. **Reg. Groups:** 12. **Lang(s):** English, French, German, Russian, Spanish. **Desc:** Doctors and other individuals interested in asthmology. Promotes a broadening of knowledge of bronchial asthma and related diseases, especially with regard to their etiology, pathological mechanisms, patho-physiology, therapy, epidemiology, rehabilitation, and prevention. Sponsors specialized training in allergology. **Pub:** *INTERASMA Membership Directory*, triennial. Directory. • *Journal of Investigational Allergology and Clinical Immunology*, bimonthly. Journal. • *Newsletter of Interasma*, quarterly. Newsletter.

★ 3633 ★ International Association of Audio Information Services (IAAIS)

c/o WVTF Radio Reading Service
4235 Electric Rd. NW, Ste. 105
Roanoke, VA 24014
Phone: (540)989-8900 **Free:** 800-280-5325
Fax: (540)776-2727
Email: aiblink@ak.net
Website: http://www.iaais.org
Ben Martin, Pres.

Fnded: 1977. **Mem:** 140. **Desc:** Helps members provide access to current printed information not available to print disabled people. Volunteers broadcast daily newspapers, community news updates, grocery ads, and death notices. Advocates access to printed material as a key issue under the Americans with Disabilities Act and that the Internet needs to be accessible to people with disabilities. Compiles statistics; holds competitions; maintains speakers' bureau. **Pub:** *Directory of Radio Reading Services*, annual. Directory. *Price:* $150. • *HEARSSAY*, quarterly. Newsletter. • *IAAIS Newsletter*, quarterly. Newsletter. Audio information industry news. *Price:* Free. • *Members*, annual. Directory. **Frmly:** National Association of Radio Reading Services.

★ 3634 ★ International Association of Biomedical Gerontology (IABG)

c/o Denham Harman, MD
Department of Medicine
84635 Nebraska Medical Center
Omaha, NE 68198-4635
Phone: (402)559-4416 **Fax:** (402)559-7330

Fnded: 1985. **Mem:** 200. **Desc:** Promtoes the study of biomedical gerontology.

★ 3635 ★ International Association of Biomedical Laboratory Science (Association Internationale des Technologistes de Laboratoire Medical)

PO Box 2830, LCD 1
Hamilton, ON, Canada L8N 3N8
Phone: (905)528-8642 **Fax:** (905)528-4968
Email: office@ifbls.org

Fnded: 1954. **Mem:** 39. **Reg. Groups:** 1. **State Groups:** 39. **Lang(s):** English, French, German. **Desc:** Member of the World Health Organization. National societies united to provide a means of communication among medical laboratory technologists in 39 countries. Promotes the continued education of health laboratory workers; plans curriculum for courses in health laboratory technology and management. Advises governments and governmental agencies on these matters and on validation of examinations leading to qualifications in medical laboratory. Maintains science development fund. **Pub:** *Curriculum for a Course in Health Safety*. Journal. • *International Directory of Medical Laboratory Science Education*, periodic. Directory. Details medical lab education worldwide. • *MedTec International*, semiannual. Journal. Covers information for medical laboratory technologists. **Frmly:** (2002) International Association of Medical Laboratory Technologists.

★ 3636 ★ International Association of Cancer Registries (IACR) (Association Internationale des Registres du Cancer)
c/o International Agency for Research on Cancer
150, cours Albert Thomas
F-69372 Lyon Cedex 08, France
Phone: 33 4 72738485 **Fax:** 33 4 72738575
Email: whelan@iarc.fr
Website: http://www.iacr.com.fr

Fnded: 1966. **Mem:** 410. **Lang(s):** English. **Desc:** Population-based cancer registries in 100 countries. Encourages the development and application of cancer registration and morbidity techniques to studies of defined populations. Endeavors to increase global awareness of the importance of producing accurate and comparable morbidity and mortality data which can be used to generate etiological hypotheses for cancer and as a basis for epidemiological studies, health planning, and other aspects of cancer control. **Pub:** *Cancer Incidence in Five Continents*, 5/year. Book. • *International Association of Cancer Registries' Newsletter*, biennial. Newsletter.

★ 3637 ★ International Association of Cancer Victors and Friends (IACVF)
5336 Harwood Rd.
San Jose, CA 95124-5711
Phone: (408)448-4094 **Free:** 888-613-6733
Fax: (408)264-9659
Email: cmckenna@best.com
Website: http://www.cancervictors.org
C. McKenna, Coord.

Fnded: 1963. **Mem:** 4,000. **Nat'l Groups:** 10. **Reg. Groups:** 13. **State Groups:** 2. **Desc:** Encourages independent research on cancer therapies and disseminates information on "nontoxic" chemotherapies. Works directly with cancer patients providing one-on-one services. Offers educational programs on topics including carcinogens in air, food, and water and nutrition in relation to cancer. **Pub:** *Cancer Victors Journal*, quarterly. Journal. Provides news on nontoxic cancer treatments and breakthroughs in cancer research; includes studies on carcinogenic conditions. *Price:* Included in membership dues. • Audiotapes. • Books. • Pamphlets. • Reprints. **Frmly:** (1985) International Association of Cancer Victims and Friends.

★ 3638 ★ International Association for Child and Adolescent Psychiatry and Allied Professions (IACAPAP)
PO Box 207900
New Haven, CT 06520-7900
Phone: (203)785-5759 **Fax:** (203)785-7402
Email: donald.cohen@yale.edu
Website: http://www.iacapap.org
Donald J. Cohen, MD, Pres.

Fnded: 1948. **Mem:** 50. **Nat'l Groups:** 50. **Desc:** National societies; others in the field of child and adolescent psychiatry and allied professions. Promotes collaboration among related professions including pediatrics, psychology, public health, social work, education, nursing, and others involved in research and practice in the field of child and adolescent psychiatry. **Pub:** *IACAPAP Newsletter*, quarterly. Newsletter. • Monograph, semiannual. **AKA:** Association Internationale de Psychiatrie de l'Enfant et de l'Adolescent et des Professions Associees. **Frmly:** (1978) International Association for Child Psychiatry and Allied Professions.

★ 3639 ★ International Association for Child and Adolescent Psychiatry and Allied Professions - Germany (IACAPAP)
c/o Ian Goodyer. Sec.
Hans-Sachs-Str. 6
Douglas House
186 Trumpington Rd.
D-35039 Marburg, Germany
Phone: 49 6421 2866260 **Fax:** 49 6421 2868975
Email: remschm@post.med.uni-marburg.de
Website: http://www.iacapap.org

★ 3640 ★ International Association of Colon Therapy (I-ACT)
c/o A.R. Hoenninger III, N.D.
PO Box 461285
San Antonio, TX 78246-1285
Phone: (210)366-2888 **Fax:** (210)366-2999
Email: iact@healthy.net
Website: http://www.iact.org
A.R. Hoenninger, PhD, Exec. Dir.

Fnded: 1988. **Mem:** 2,500. **Reg. Groups:** 15. **Desc:** Professional colon hydrotherapists and other health care practitioners. Works to unite the community of colon hydrotherapy professionals and increase visibility and recognition in the health care industry. Promotes the establishment of uniform guidelines and standards of practice and the establishment of accredited colon hydrotherapy schools. Conducts research and educational programs; plans to operate referral service. Maintains library. **Pub:** *I-ACT Newsletter*, quarterly. Newsletter. Provides organization updates, convention schedule, and continuing education course schedule. *Price:* Included in membership dues. **Frmly:** (1993) American Colon Therapy Association.

★ 3641 ★ International Association for Comparative Research on Leukemia and Related Diseases (IACRLRD)
c/o The de Burlo Group
50 Federal St.
Boston, MA 02110
Phone: (617)483-0275 **Fax:** (617)338-6077
Email: deBurlo@erols.com
C. Russell de Burlo, PhD, Treas.

Fnded: 1963. **Mem:** 500. **Desc:** Promotes cooperation and coordination of basic and clinical research on leukemia and related diseases. Emphasizes comparative aspects of different disciplines in order to develop new hypotheses and introduce comparable working methods. Sponsors educational programs. **Pub:** *Symposium Proceedings*, biennial. Proceedings. *Price:* Free for members only; $35/issue for nonmembers.

★ 3642 ★ International Association of Contact Lens Educators (IACLE)
PO Box 6328
Randwick
Sydney, NSW 1466, Australia
Phone: 61 2 93857466 **Fax:** 61 2 93857467
Email: iacle@iacle.org
Website: http://www.iacle.org

Fnded: 1979. **Mem:** 534. **Nat'l Groups:** 8. **Reg. Groups:** 5. **Lang(s):** Bahasa Indonesia, Chinese, English, Spanish. **Desc:** Optometrists, Ophthalmologists, Opticians and Contactologists from 60 countries who are involved either full-time or part-time in contact lens education. Also includes staff members of recognized teaching institutions. Works to raise the standard of contact lens education worldwide and promotes the widespread, safe use of contact lenses. Provides educational infrastructure; cooperates with any organization that advances ophthalmic education.

★ 3643 ★ International Association of Coroners and Medical Examiners (IACME)
PO Box 899
Mansfield, LA 71052
Fax: (318)872-4495
Jack Grindle, MD, Contact

Fnded: 1938. **Mem:** 335. **Desc:** Educational seminar involving all aspects of death investigation such as pathology, autopsy, crime scene investigation, mass disasters and anthropology. Offers continuing medical education credit. **Pub:** *RECAP*, quarterly. Newsletter. *Price:* Included in membership dues.

★ 3644 ★ International Association of Counselors and Therapists (IACT)
10915 Bonita Beach Rd., Ste. 1101
Bonita Springs, FL 34135-9049
Phone: (941)498-9710 **Fax:** (941)498-1215
Email: iactnow@aol.com
Website: http://www.iact.org
Jillian R. LaVelle, Pres/CEO

Fnded: 1990. **Mem:** 7,000. **Desc:** Mental health professionals, medical professionals, social workers, clergy, educators, hypnotherapists, counselors, and individuals interested in the helping professions. Promotes enhanced professional image and prestige for complementary therapy. Provides a forum for exchange of information and ideas among practitioners of traditional and nontraditional therapies and methodologies; fosters unity among "grassroots" practitioners and those with advanced academic credentials. Facilitates the development of new therapy programs. Conducts educational, research, and charitable programs. Awards credits for continuing education. Maintains speakers' bureau and library; operates referral and placement services; compiles statistics. Assists in the development of local chapters. **Pub:** *Unlimited Human!*, quarterly. Magazine. Includes health and wellness articles. *Price:* Included in membership dues.

★ 3645 ★ International Association of Craniofacial Identification
Oxford Rd.
Manchester M13 9PT, United Kingdom
Email: rneave@fs2.scg.man.ac.uk

★ 3646 ★ International Association for Cross-Cultural Psychology (IACCP)
c/o Klaus Boehnke, Sec.Gen.
International University Bremen
Campus Ring 1
D-28759 Bremen, Germany
Phone: 49 421 2003401 **Fax:** 49 421 200493401
Email: k.boehnke@iu-bremen.de
Website: http://www.iaccp.org

Fnded: 1972. **Mem:** 700. **Lang(s):** English. **Desc:** Serves as a forum for exchanges among psychologists and other researchers who are interested in comparative research into human behavior and experience. Pursues the universal validity of psychological theories in all branches of psychology and related disciplines. **Pub:** *Cross-Cultural Psychology Bulletin*, quarterly. Bulletin. Contains news of IACCP, brief reports, and other items of interest. • *Journal of Cross-Cultural Psychology*, bimonthly. Journal. • Proceedings, biennial.

★ 3647 ★ International Association for Dance Medicine and Science (IADMS)
1214 University of Oregon
Department of Dance
Eugene, OR 97403-1214
Phone: (541)465-1763 **Fax:** (541)465-1763
Email: executivedirector@iadms.org
Website: http://www.iadms.org
Steven J. Chatfield, PhD, Exec. Dir.

Fnded: 1990. **Mem:** 600. **Desc:** Serves as a forum for reeducation, promotion of research and public services in the field of dance medicine and science. Committed to providing continuing education for the dance and medical communities as well as the public regarding appropriate training for dance. Offers educational programs. **Pub:** *The Dance Medicine/Science Bibliography*. Bibliography. Listing of all English language dance medicine articles (from 1975 to the present). *Price:* $45. • *IADMS Newsletter*, quarterly. Newsletter. Offers information of recent activities both within the organization and the dance medicine field in general. • *Journal of Dance Medicine/Science*, quarterly. Journal. Peer-reviewed medical journal.

★ 3648 ★ International Association for Dental Research (IADR)
1619 Duke St.
Alexandria, VA 22314

Phone: (703)548-0066 Fax: (703)548-1883
Email: research@iadr.org
Website: http://www.iadr.com
Robert Collins, DDS, Interim Exec. Dir.

Fnded: 1920. **Mem:** 10,000. **Reg. Groups:** 20. **Desc:** Individuals engaged or interested in advancing research in the various aspects of dental and related sciences. **Pub:** *Abstracts, A Special Issue of Journal of Dental Research*, quarterly. Journal. • *Advances in Dental Research*, periodic. Journal. Covers developments in dental research and the chemistry, biology, and function of the oral cavity. Also includes conference proceedings. • *Critical Reviews in Oral Biology and Medicine*, bimonthly. • *Journal of Dental Research*, monthly. Journal. Disseminates new information and knowledge on all sciences relevant to dentistry, the oral cavity, and associated structures in health and disease.

★ 3649 ★ International Association of Dental Students (IADS)

c/o FDI World Dental Federation
13 Chemin du Levant l'Avant Centre
F-01210 Ferney-Voltaire, France
Phone: 33 4 50405050 **Fax:** 33 4 50405555
Email: gsecretary@iads-web.org
Website: http://www.iads-web.org

Fnded: 1951. **Mem:** 52. **Nat'l Groups:** 47. **Local Groups:** 5. **Lang(s):** English. **Desc:** Coordinating body between National Association of Dental students. Association members in 52 countries. Promotes international contact among dental students; facilitates exchange of students between member countries; develops international programs. Organises annual concerts. Conducts competitions. **Pub:** *ADS Newsletter*, semiannual. Newsletter. • *IADS Exchange Guide*. Manual.

★ 3650 ★ International Association of Dental Traumatology

517 St. Kilda Rd.
Melbourne 3004, Australia
Website: http://www.iadt-dentaltrauma.org/

Fnded: 1989. **Desc:** Furthers clinical, experimental research in dental traumatology; promotes integrated education and treatment in dental trauma; fosters public awareness for the purpose of prevention of dental trauma.

★ 3651 ★ International Association for Disability and Oral Health (IADH)

c/o Dr. Jan Andersson-Norinder
Mun-H-Center
Odontologen
Medicinaregatan 12 A
413 90 Goteborg, Sweden
Phone: 46 31 7952952 **Fax:** 46 31 7951800
Email: jan.andersson-norinder@vgregion.se
Website: http://www.iadh.org

Lang(s): English. **Desc:** Promotes oral health care for people with disabilities.

★ 3652 ★ International Association of Eating Disorders Professionals (IAEDP)

PO Box 1295
Pekin, IL 61555-1295
Phone: (309)346-3341 **Free:** 800-800-8126
Email: info@iaedp.com
Website: http://www.iaedp.com

Fnded: 1985. **Mem:** 800. **Desc:** Eating disorders counselors, specialists, and associates. Establishes and develops curricula; operates and implements a system for certifying eating disorders specialists and associates; provides public education and information on eating disorders. Offers professional consulting and assistance to the medical community, hospitals, courts, law enforcement agencies, schools, churches, and social welfare agencies. Facilitates networking among members; makes available employment opportunity information. Sponsors workshops; maintains speakers' bureau and annual symposia. **Pub:** *Clinical Quorum*. *Price:* Included in membership dues. • Bulletin, monthly. Contains association news and activities and certification update. *Price:* included in membership dues. • Also publishes certification manual and curriculum for higher education.

★ 3653 ★ International Association for Education to a Life Without Drugs - Norway

Odinsvei 13
N-4846 Arendal, Norway
Email: dag-magne.johannessen@tyholmen.vgs.no

Lang(s): Norwegian. **Desc:** National branch of the international organization. Individuals and organizations interested in preventing substance abuse among youth. Promotes international cooperation among alcohol and drug abuse education programs. Gathers and disseminates information on drug abuse and youth; facilitates contact among members and between members and organizations with similar goals worldwide. Conducts educational programs.

★ 3654 ★ International Association of Endocrine Surgeons (IAES)

Department of Surgery, University Hospital
S-75185 Uppsala, Sweden

★ 3655 ★ International Association of Equine Dental Technicians (IAEDT)

c/o Richard Miller, DVM
23411 Via Alondra
Coto de Caza, CA 92679
Phone: (828)883-2230 **Fax:** (828)883-4610
Email: rqhydedvm@anent.com
Website: http://www.iaeqd.org/
Doug Smith, Pres.

Fnded: 1987. **Mem:** 60. **Desc:** Equine dental technicians, veterinarians, and others interested in equine dental maintenance. Promotes the health and welfares of horses, and high standards and recognition in the field of equine dentistry. Acts as a forum for the exchange of information and experiences in the field. Sponsors educational programs. Offers certification program and testing. Maintains hall of fame. **Pub:** *IAEDT Newsletter*, quarterly. Newsletter. *Price:* Included in membership dues.

★ 3656 ★ International Association of Forensic Nurses (IAFN)

PO Box 56, East Holly Ave.
Pitman, NJ 08071-0056
Phone: (856)256-2425 **Fax:** (856)589-7463
Email: iafn@ajj.com
Website: http://www.forensicnurse.org
Kim Marrero, Exec. Sec.

Fnded: 1992. **Mem:** 2,050. **State Groups:** 15. **Desc:** The IAFN is a professional association of registered nurses working in the medico-legal arena whose purpose is to develop, promote, and disseminate information about the science of forensic nursing internationally. IAFN works with other nursing organizations to set standards of practice and strives to foster growth and development of forensic nursing as an emerging area of nursing expertise. IAFN also promotes the exchange of ideas and the transmission of developing knowledge among its members and with other interested professionals. **Pub:** *On the Edge*, quarterly. Newsletter. *Price:* included in membership dues. • Membership Directory, annual. *Price:* included in membership dues.

★ 3657 ★ International Association for Forensic Psychotherapy (IAFP)

Cranmer Terrace
London SW17 0RE, United Kingdom
Phone: 44 20 87255568 **Fax:** 44 20 87252475
Email: gmcgaule@sghms.ac.uk

Fnded: 1991. **Desc:** Promotes scientific research into causes and prevention of crime; establishes observation centres and clinics for diagnosis and treatment of delinquency and crime; secures cooperation between all bodies engaged in similar work.

★ 3658 ★ International Association of French-Language Labor Psychology (Association Internationale de Psychologie du Travail de Langue Francais — AIPTLF)

Pr. Claude Lemoine-Aiptlf
Universite Lille 3, UFR Psychologie
BP 149
F-76821 Villeneuve d'Ascq Cedex, France
Phone: 33 3 20416315 **Fax:** 33 3 20416324
Email: lemoine@univ-lille3.fr
Website: http://www.psp.ucl.ac.be/aiptlf2002

Fnded: 1980. **Lang(s):** English, French. **Desc:** French-speaking psychologists specializing in labor psychology. Seeks to advance scholarship and practice in the field of labor psychology. Facilitates exchange of information among members; sponsors research and training programs. **Pub:** *Psychologie du Travail et des Organisations*, quarterly. Journal. • *Top-Actualite*. Newsletter.

★ 3659 ★ International Association for Gastrointestinal Motility in Children (GIMIC)

Av de la Cote de Nacre
F-14033 Caen, France

Fnded: 1989. **Desc:** Promotes Research on gastrointestinal motility in children and its disturbances.

★ 3660 ★ International Association of Gerontology (IAG)

Secretariat: Gerontology Research Centre
Simon Fraser University
2800 - 515 W Hastings St.
Vancouver, BC, Canada V6B 5K3
Phone: (604)268-7972 **Fax:** (604)291-5066
Email: iag@sfu.ca
Website: http://www.sfu.ca/iag

Fnded: 1950. **Mem:** 46,000. **Nat'l Groups:** 65. **Lang(s):** English. **Desc:** National gerontological societies. Promotes basic and applied research on aging and the aged and members interests on international issues. Fosters training of highly qualified personnel. Organizes a World Congress every four years and auspices other events. Has a consultative status with the UN and collaborates regularly with the UN's Programme on Aging, the WHO's Ageing and Life Course Programme and with other international agencies concerned with the well being of aging persons. **Pub:** *IAG Newsletter*, semiannual. Newsletter.

★ 3661 ★ International Association of Gerontology European Region (IAG)

c/o Dr. Francisco G. Llera, Sec.
Hospital Universitario de Getafe Servicio de Geriatria
Ctra. Toledo, Km. 12, 5 Getafe
E-28905 Madrid, Spain
Phone: 34 91 6833241 **Fax:** 34 91 6839748
Email: fguillenl@segg.org
Website: http://www.sfu.ca/iag

Desc: Gerontology research, including biological, medical, behavioral, and social. Provides training in fields of aging.

★ 3662 ★ International Association of Group Psychotherapy (IAGP)

c/o D. Mattke
Auf Der Steige 5
D-53129 Bonn, Germany
Phone: 49 228 232897 **Fax:** 49 228 232897
Email: djmattke@aol.com
Website: http://www.iagpweb.org

Fnded: 1954. **Mem:** 800. **Desc:** Physicians, psychologists, social workers, nurses, and mental health workers in 32 countries interested in group psychotherapy. Seeks to further communication and education between professionals in the practice and study of group psychotherapy. **Pub:** *Forum*, quarterly. Articles and member information. • Directory, triennial.

★ 3663 ★ International Association for Handicapped Divers Foundation
Hazelaarlaan 47
1775 EE Middenmeer, Netherlands
Phone: 31 227 503631 **Fax:** 31 227 503729
Email: klaas@iahd.org
Website: http://www.iahdeurope.org

Fnded: 1993. **Mem:** 500. **Nat'l Groups:** 35. **Reg. Groups:** 3. **Lang(s):** Dutch, English, German. **Desc:** Scuba diving instructors, divemasters, and underwater assistants trained to meet the specific needs of divers with physical handicaps. Encourages divers with disabilities to assume a role of leadership in diving. Promotes participation in diving by people with disabilities as a means to better physical fitness and increased self-esteem. Conducts training programs for divemasters, instructors, and assistants wishing to work with people with disabilities. **Pub:** Newsletter, quarterly. Contains member information.

★ 3664 ★ International Association of Healthcare Central Service Materiel Management (IAHCSMM)
213 W Institute Pl., Ste. 307
Chicago, IL 60610
Phone: (312)440-0078 **Free:** 800-962-8274
Fax: (312)440-9474
Email: mailbox@iahcsmm.com
Website: http://www.iahcsmm.com
Betty Hanna, Exec. Dir.

Fnded: 1958. **Mem:** 9,000. **State Groups:** 35. **Desc:** Professional personnel responsible for management and distribution of supplies from central service materiel management departments of a hospital. Works to improve the quality of central service materiel management departments in hospitals; share information and ideas; research hospital central service materiel management methods and practices; conduct and promote continuing education programs. Sponsors management correspondence courses, technician training and materials management courses through Purdue University in Indiana. Has established a certification program to recognize exceptional achievement. Maintains technician registry and placement service. Surveys salaries. Conducts research programs; compiles statistics. Maintains 23 committees. **Pub:** *Communique*, bimonthly. • Also publishes technical management and training manuals. **Frmly:** (1969) National Association of Hospital Central Service Personnel; (1989) International Association of Hospital Central Service Management.

★ 3665 ★ International Association for Healthcare Security and Safety (IAHSS)
PO Box 637
Lombard, IL 60148
Phone: (630)871-9936 **Free:** 888-353-0990
Fax: (630)871-9938
Email: nancy@iahss.org
Website: http://www.iahss.org
Carl Mogavero, Pres.

Fnded: 1968. **Mem:** 1,700. **Reg. Groups:** 17. **Local Groups:** 53. **Desc:** Administrative and supervisory personnel in the field of hospital security and safety. To develop, promote, and coordinate better security/safety programs in medical care facilities. Offers placement services; conducts specialized education programs. **Pub:** *Healthcare Protection Management*, semiannual. Journal. • Membership Directory, annual. • Newsletter, quarterly. **Frmly:** (1990) International Association for Hospital Security.

★ 3666 ★ International Association of Healthcare Practitioners (IAHP)
11211 Prosperity Farms Rd., Ste. D-325
Palm Beach Gardens, FL 33410
Phone: (561)622-4334 **Free:** 800-233-5880
Fax: (561)622-4771
Email: iahp@iahp.com
Website: http://www.iahp.com
Kathy Woll, Dir.

Fnded: 1996. **Mem:** 50,000. **Desc:** Osteopathic physicians, medical doctors, doctors of Chiropractic, doctors of Oriental medicine, naturopathic physicians, nurses, psychiatric specialists, psychologists, dentists, speech pathologists, physical acupuncturists, massage therapists and other professional bodyworkers. Dedicated to offering innovative therapies and solutions in healthcare; provides a united voice to legislative bodies, insurance regulators, patients, clients and other healthcare providers. **Pub:** *IAHP Connections*, annual. Newsletter. • Directories, annual. Contains member listing. *Price:* $7. **AKA:** Upledger's International Association of Healthcare Practitioners.

★ 3667 ★ International Association for the History of Psychoanalysis (IAHP) (Association internationale d'histoire de l Psychanalys)
8, rue du Commandant Mouchotte
F-75014 Paris, France
Phone: 33 1 40478933 **Fax:** 33 1 40470449
Email: aihpsy@wanadoo.fr
Website: http://www.aihp-iahp.com/

Fnded: 1985. **Mem:** 250. **Lang(s):** English, French. **Desc:** Promotes a thorough knowledge of the history of psychoanalysis and of its founder; bridges differences among national approaches to psychoanalysis and overcomes them through exposure. **Pub:** *Journal of the IAHP*, semiannual. Newsletter.

★ 3668 ★ International Association of Holistic Medicine
BernaDean University
4842 Whitsett Ave.
Valley Village, CA 91607-3544
Adele Kadans, Pres.

Fnded: 1954. **Desc:** Works to: establish standards for public retreats for the study of health practices; operate health havens as pilot studies; approve and supervise retreats operated by others. **Pub:** *Holistic Health Quarterly*, quarterly. Journal. **Frmly:** (1998) Holistic Health Havens.

★ 3669 ★ International Association for Hospice and Palliative Care (IAHPC)
c/o Josefina B. Magno
5535 Memorial Dr., Ste. F-PMB 509
Houston, TX 77007
Phone: (713)880-2940 **Fax:** (713)880-2948
Email: info@iahpc.com
Website: http://www.hospicecare.com/
Liliana DeLima, MHA, Exec. Dir.

Fnded: 2000. **Mem:** 400. **Desc:** Promotes availability and access to high quality hospice and palliative care for patients and families in order to alleviate physical and psychosocial suffering associated with progressive, incurable illness throughout the world. Provides communication and education for patients, professionals, health care providers and policy makers. **Pub:** Reports.

★ 3670 ★ International Association of Human-Animal Interaction Organizations (IAHAIO)
c/o Linda Hines
580 Naches Ave. SW, No. 101
Renton, WA 98055
Phone: (425)226-7357 **Fax:** (425)235-1076
Email: info@deltasociety.org
Website: http://www.iahaio.org
Linda M. Hines, Sec. -Treas.

Fnded: 1990. **Mem:** 22. **Nat'l Groups:** 22. **Desc:** Provides a forum for exchange of ideas and information among organizations concerned with the study of the mutual welfare of people and animals. Encourages research and promotes educational and practical developments in the field of human-animal interactions. Hosts and international conference every three years. **Pub:** *Proceedings of International Conference*, triennial. Proceedings. Includes papers presented at international conference. • Also contributes to and distributes *Anthrozoos: Journal of the Delta Society*. **Frmly:** (1990) International Society for the Study of the Human-Companion Animal Bond.

★ 3671 ★ International Association of Hydatidology (Asociacion Internacional de Hidatologie)
Florida 460, 3o piso
1005 Buenos Aires, Argentina
Phone: 54 11 43244700 **Fax:** 54 11 43258231

Lang(s): English, Spanish. **Desc:** Physicians and other health care professionals. Seeks to increase understanding of the hydatid and its diseases. (The hydatid is a vestigal organ present in both the male and female reproductive systems.) Promotes exchange of information on the hydatid; sponsors research and educational programs.

★ 3672 ★ International Association of Hygienic Physicians (IAHP)
4620 Euclid Blvd.
Youngstown, OH 44512
Phone: (330)788-0526 **Fax:** (330)788-0093
Email: boar_mah@access-k12.org
Website: http://free.freespeech.org/nhn/iahp/
Mark A. Huberman, Sec. -Treas.

Fnded: 1978. **Mem:** 45. **Desc:** Doctors of medicine, osteopathy, chiropractic, and naturopathy who specialize in the supervision of therapeutic fasting as part of a natural hygiene regimen. Promotes clinical advancement and ethical responsibility. Works for the health freedom of members. Provides certification for professionals and accreditation for schools and training programs; offers internship programs. Funds research. **Pub:** *IAHP Newsletter*, quarterly. Newsletter. Includes association news, bibliography, book reviews, case studies, Medical journal reviews, and reports from foreign countries. *Price:* Included in membership dues. **Frmly:** (1995) International Association of Professional Natural Hygienists.

★ 3673 ★ International Association of Individual Psychology (IAIP)
Via Assalini 35
I-42100 Reggio Emilia, Italy
Phone: 39 0522 285882 **Fax:** 39 0522 285882
Email: gsmazzoli@libero.it
Website: http://www.iaiponline.org

Fnded: 1954. **Mem:** 26. **Lang(s):** English, French, German, Italian. **Desc:** Societies, associations, and institutes of Adlerian or Individual Psychology. Seeks to expand and deepen the scientific and practical aspects of Alfred Adler's (1870-1937) theory of Individual Psychology. Fosters cooperation and information exchange among members. **Pub:** *Directory and Constitution*, triennial. Directory.

★ 3674 ★ International Association of Infant Massage (IAIM)
1891 Goodyear Ave., Ste. 622
Ventura, CA 93003
Phone: (805)644-8524 **Free:** 800-248-5432
Fax: (805)644-7699
Email: iaim4us@aol.com
Website: http://www.iaim-us.com
Susan Campbell, Business Admin.

Fnded: 1986. **Mem:** 3,000. **Nat'l Groups:** 1. **Reg. Groups:** 4. **Desc:** Parents, caregivers. Works to promote nurturing touch, positive interactive contact, and communication through massage. Trains and certifies individuals to teach parents and caregivers to massage their babies. **Pub:** *Tender Loving Care*, semiannual. Newsletter. Features articles on infant massage. *Price:* included in membership dues. **Frmly:** (1989) International Association of Infant Massage Instructors.

★ 3675 ★ International Association of Laryngectomees (IAL)
8900 Thornton Rd.
Box 99311
Stockton, CA 95209
Free: (866)425-3678 **Fax:** (209)472-0516
Email: ial@larynxlink.com
Website: http://www.larynxlink.com
Jack Henslee, Exec. Dir.

Fnded: 1952. **Nat'l Groups:** 275. **Desc:** Persons who have had their larynx removed; physicians, surgeons, speech therapists, rehabilitation experts, nurses, and others interested in the rehabilitation of laryngectomees. Encourages exchange of ideas and methods for training and teaching of alaryngeal methods of communication. Fosters recognized standards for the rehabilitation of laryngectomees. Maintains the Voice Rehabilitation Institute for training teachers of alaryngeal voice and the Lost Chord Clubs. Organizes support groups for laryngectomes and their families. **Pub:** *IAL News*, 3/year. Newsletter. *Price:* Free. • Directory, annual. • Films.Provides information on first aid and post-laryngectomy speech. • Pamphlets.Provides information on laryngectomees, esophageal voice, and rehabilitation.

★ 3676 ★ International Association of Logopedics and Phoniatrics (IALP)

c/o Prof. Dolores Battle
141 South Ln.
Orchard Park, NY 14127
Phone: (716)878-6210 **Fax:** (716)878-6234
Email: battlede@buffalostate.edu
Website: http://www.ialp.info
Prof. Harm Schutte, Pres.

Fnded: 1924. **Mem:** 450. **Nat'l Groups:** 59. **Reg. Groups:** 55. **Desc:** Phoniatricians (voice disorder specialists), logopedists (speech-language defect therapists), and audiologists (hearing specialists) from 55 affiliated societies in 38 countries. Fosters and conducts scientific study of disorders in human communication. **Pub:** *Folia Phoniatrica et Logopaedica*, bimonthly. Journal. • *Folia Phoniatrica et Logopedica*, bimonthly. Journal. Professional scientific journal. • *IALP Directory*, triennial. Directory.

★ 3677 ★ International Association for Malacology

Crowell Rd.
London SW7 5BD, United Kingdom
Phone: 44 20 79425210 **Fax:** 44 20 79425054
Email: pbm@nhm.ac.uk
Website: http://www.ucmp.berkeley.edu/mologis/mollia.html

★ 3678 ★ International Association for Maternal and Neonatal Health (IAMENEH)

Aeschengraben 16
CH-4051 Basel, Switzerland
Phone: 41 61 2056080 **Fax:** 41 61 2717900
Email: info@iamaneh.ch
Website: http://www.iamaneh.ch

Fnded: 1977. **Mem:** 4,500. **Nat'l Groups:** 39. **Lang(s):** English, French. **Desc:** Medical professionals and individuals interested in improving maternal and neonatal care throughout the world, especially at the primary health care level. Objectives are to: promote basic and applied research in the field of human reproduction and publish and distribute the findings; improve the standards of medical and paramedical care in the field of obstetrics and gynecology; foster research programs on social problems related to maternal and perinatal health; purpose curriculum on improving maternal and perinatal health to higher education institutions; disseminate scientific information concerning women, mothers, fetuses, newborns, and children. **Pub:** *High Risk Mothers and Newborns - Detection, Management and Prevention.* Book. • *Maternal and Child Care in Developing Countries - Assessment, Promotion and Implementation.* Book. • *Maternal and Infant Mortality.* Book. • *Primary Maternal and Neonatal Health - A Global Concern.* Book. **Frmly:** (1994) Mother and Child International.

★ 3679 ★ International Association of Medical Equipment Remarketers (IAMER)

183 Lucy Ln.
Wylie, TX 75098-7244
Phone: 877-304-2637 **Fax:** (480)575-0891
Email: radlady@att.net
Website: http://www.iamers.org/
Tom Norman, Pres.

Fnded: 1994. **Mem:** 150. **Desc:** Dealers, lessors, refurbishers, and services of medical equipment. Promotes ethical business practices and delivers high quality previously owned medical equipment. Offers educational and research programs and maintains a speakers bureau. **Pub:** Newsletter. • Directory. • Brochure.

★ 3680 ★ International Association for Medical Research and Cultural Exchange (AIRMEC) (Association Internationale pour la Recherche Medicale et les Echanges Culturels — AIRMEC)

2, blvd. Pershing
F-75017 Paris, France
Phone: 33 1 55379015 **Fax:** 33 1 55379040

Fnded: 1956. **Mem:** 2,000. **Lang(s):** French. **Desc:** Medical and pharmaceutical professionals. Fosters and participates in the development of medical research. Initiates scientific exchange among members throughout the world. Organizes activities such as conferences, conventions, and workshops to facilitate medico-pharmaceutical comparison. Promotes and contributes to postgraduate medical and pharmaceutical study. **Pub:** *Medecine d'Afrique Noire*, monthly.

★ 3681 ★ International Association of Medical Science Educators (IAMSE)

One Crested Butte Dr., Ste. 100
Huntington, WV 25705
Phone: (304)733-1270 **Fax:** (304)733-6203
Email: julie@iamse.org
Website: http://www.iamse.org
Julie Hewett, Bus. Mgr.

Fnded: 1997. **Mem:** 390. **Desc:** Dedicated to sharing experiences and strategies for teaching the fundamental sciences of medicine. **Pub:** *Basic Science Educator*, semiannual. Journal. Written specifically for medical science educators. *Price:* included in membership dues.

★ 3682 ★ International Association of Medicine and Biology of Environment (IAMBE) (Association Internationale de Medecine et de Biologie de l'Environnement — AIMBE)

115, rue de la Pompe
F-75116 Paris, France
Phone: 33 1 45534504 **Fax:** 33 1 45534175
Email: aimbe.world@free.fr

Fnded: 1971. **Lang(s):** English, French, Spanish. **Desc:** Individuals, associations, and firms in 79 countries concerned with ecological medicine and biology. Purpose is to study the adaptation of mankind to the environment and to study and treat sicknesses resulting from this adaptation. Examines natural cycles and balances; promotes research in ecological medicine and biology and corollary sciences; collects and disseminates information concerning the protection of mankind and the environment. Facilitates contacts with persons who deal professionally with problems related to the protection of humans and their surroundings. Organizes symposia and congresses; conducts courses and seminars.

★ 3683 ★ International Association of Neuromuscular Neurologists

Queen's University
Belfast BT7 1NN, United Kingdom

★ 3684 ★ International Association of Ocular Surgeons (IAOS)

820 N Orleans St., Ste. 208
Chicago, IL 60610
Phone: (312)440-0699 **Free:** 800-621-4002
Fax: (312)440-0580
Email: iaos@aol.com
Website: http://www.ascmso.com
Randall T. Bellows, MD, Dir.

Fnded: 1981. **Mem:** 900. **Desc:** A division of the American Society of Contemporary Ophthalmology. Seeks to develop a global community of ophthalmic surgeons who examine and deliberate on all aspects of ocular surgery; encourage information exchange among members; and disseminate information about contemporary diagnostic and surgical procedures. **Pub:** *Annals of Ophthalmology*, 3/year. Journal. Continuing medical education for ophthalmologists. *Price:* $160.

★ 3685 ★ International Association of Optometric Executives (IAOE)

1505 Price, Ste. 3
Alexandria, VA 22314
Phone: (703)739-9200 **Free:** 800-678-9262
Fax: (703)739-9497
Email: khipp@theaoa.org
Website: http://www.aoanet.org
Kelly Hipp, Contact

Mem: 75. **Desc:** Executives of optometric associations in 10 countries. Promotes continuing education in optometric association management. **Frmly:** Society of Association Optometric Executives.

★ 3686 ★ International Association of Oral and Maxillofacial Surgeons (IAOMS)

9700 W Bryn Mawr, Ste. 210
Rosemont, IL 60018-5701
Phone: (847)678-9370 **Fax:** (847)878-9380
Email: lsayler@iaoms.org
Website: http://www.iaoms.org/
Victor Moncarz, Exec. Dir.

Fnded: 1965. **Mem:** 4,000. **Nat'l Groups:** 63. **Desc:** Seeks to improve the quality of healthcare worldwide through the advancement of patient care, education, and research in oral and maxillofacial surgery. **Pub:** *I.A.O.M.S.*, semiannual. Newsletter. • *International Journal of Oral and Maxillofacial Surgery*, bimonthly. Journal. • *Registry of Fellows.* • *Rules and Regulations of the IAOMS.*

★ 3687 ★ International Association of Oral Pathologists (IAOP)

Eastman Dental Institute for Oral Health Care Sciences
University College London
256 Gray's Inn Rd.
London WC1X 8LD, United Kingdom
Phone: 44 20 79151000 **Fax:** 44 20 79151039
Email: academic@eastman.ucl.ac.uk
Website: http://www.eastman.ucl.ac.uk

Fnded: 1976. **Mem:** 380. **Lang(s):** English. **Desc:** Dentists who have had postgraduate instruction in pathology. Seeks to advance the science of oral pathology; works to foster international cooperation in the field. **Pub:** *Journal of Oral Pathology and Medicine*, 10/year. Journal. • *Membership List*, periodic.

★ 3688 ★ International Association on Oro-Facial Pain and Temporomandibular Disorder

Yongon-dong, Chongno-gu
Seoul 110-744, Republic of Korea
Phone: 82 2 7602610 **Fax:** 82 2 7449135

★ 3689 ★ International Association of Orthodontics (IAO)

c/o Detlef B. Moore
735 N Water St., Ste. 617
Milwaukee, WI 53202
Phone: (414)272-2757 **Free:** 800-447-8770
Fax: (414)272-2754
Email: worldheadquarters@iaortho.org

Website: http://www.iaortho.org
Detlef B. Moore, Exec. Dir.

Fnded: 1961. **Mem:** 3,600. **Reg. Groups:** 15. **Local Groups:** 80. **Desc:** Dentists. Promotes the study and dissemination of information on the cause, control, treatment, and prevention of malocclusion of the teeth; facilitates exchange of ideas and experiences, based on a biomechanical approach, between the various fields of dentistry related to orthodontics. **Pub:** *IAO Straight Talk*, quarterly. Newsletter. Provides information on membership activities. *Price:* Included in membership dues; $15/year for nonmembers. • *International Association of Orthodontics–Directory of Members*, annual. Directory. *Price:* Included in membership dues; $150 for nonmembers. • *International Journal of Orthodontics*, quarterly. Journal. Contains clinical articles on orthodontics, self-assessment, troubleshooting, and new products. *Price:* $40/year. **Frmly:** International Academy of Orthodontics.

★ 3690 ★ International Association for Oxygen Therapy (IAOT)

PO Box 1360
Priest River, ID 83856
Phone: (208)443-4319 **Fax:** (208)443-4319
Email: info@oxytherapies.com
Website: http://www.oxytherapies.com
Nicole S. Sacks, Contact

Fnded: 1898. **Mem:** 3,500. **Nat'l Groups:** 1. **Reg. Groups:** 12. **State Groups:** 24. **Local Groups:** 150. **Desc:** Oxidation therapists. Promotes the use of oxidation enhancing therapies to physicians and the general public. Compiles statistics. Conducts research, educational, and charitable programs. Maintains museum and speakers' bureau. **Pub:** *IAOT Newsletter (Oxidation News)*, quarterly. Newsletter. Features international journal of WNHO. *Price:* Free sample; included in membership dues.

★ 3691 ★ International Association of Paediatric Dentistry (IAPD)

123 Gray's Inn Rd.
London WC1X 8WD, United Kingdom
Phone: 44 20 79051251 **Fax:** 44 20 79051285
Email: iapd@eastman.ucl.ac.uk
Website: http://www.iapd.org.uk

Fnded: 1969. **Mem:** 700. **Lang(s):** English, French. **Desc:** Dentists, dental and medical libraries, bookshops, and research institutions in 36 countries. Encourages research and foster progress in the field of children's dental health. Provides a forum for the exchange of information concerning children's dentistry worldwide. **Pub:** *International Journal of Paediatric Dentistry.*, quarterly. Journal. • *Newsletter*, semiannual. Newsletter.

★ 3692 ★ International Association of Parents and Professionals for Safe Alternatives in Childbirth (NAPSAC)

Rte. 4, Box 646
Marble Hill, MO 63764-9418
Phone: (573)238-2010 **Fax:** (573)238-2010
Email: napsac@clas.net
Website: http://www.napsac.org
Lee Stewart, Pres.

Fnded: 1975. **Mem:** 1,000. **Nat'l Groups:** 20. **Local Groups:** 20. **Desc:** Parents, midwives, physicians, nurses, health officials, social workers, and childbirth educators in 10 countries who are "dedicated to exploring, examining, implementing, and establishing family-centered childbirth programs which meet the needs of families as well as provide the safe aspects of medical science." Promotes education concerning the principles of natural childbirth; facilitates communication and cooperation among parents, medical professionals, and childbirth educators; assists in the establishment of maternity and childbearing centers. Provides educational opportunities to parents and parents-to-be, enabling them to assume more personal responsibility for pregnancy, childbirth, infant care, and child rearing. **Pub:** *Childbirth Activists Handbook*. Book. *Price:* $15.95. • *Emergency Childbirth. Price:* $18.95. • *Five Standards for Safe Childbearing. Price:* $19.95. • *NAPSAC News*, quarterly. Newsletter. Includes association news, book reviews, and calendar of events. *Price:* Included in membership dues. • *Safe Alternatives in Childbirth. Price:* $12.95. • *Transitions. Price:* $10.95. • *21st Century Obstetrics Now. Price:* $14.95/2 vol. **Frmly:** (1979) National Association of Parents and Professionals for Safe Alternatives in Childbirth.

★ 3693 ★ International Association of Physicians in AidS Care (IAPAC)

33 N LA Salle St. Ste. 1700
Chicago, IL 60602-2601
Phone: (312)795-4930 **Fax:** (312)795-4938
Email: iapac@iapac.org
Website: http://www.iapac.org
Jose M. Zuniga, Pres. /CEO

Fnded: 1995. **Mem:** 12,000. **Reg. Groups:** 2. **Desc:** Provides educational programs to caregivers, physicians and patients. Promotes public policy reform and research. **Pub:** *JIAPAC*, quarterly. Journal. Clinical and Social Articles-peer reviewed. *Price:* $60/year. • Also publishes IAPAC monthly AIDS public policy and medical conference coverage.

★ 3694 ★ International Association of Physicians in Audiology (IAPA)

c/o Prof. Dr. K. Schorn
ENT - University Hospital
Kinikum Grosshadern
Marchioninistrasse15
D-81377 Munich, Germany
Website: http://www.iapa-online.org/

Fnded: 1980. **Mem:** 200. **Lang(s):** English. **Desc:** Practitioners of medical audiology in 35 countries. Promotes the field of medical audiology and practitioners' interests worldwide. **Pub:** *Journal of Audiological Medicine*, 3/year. Journal.

★ 3695 ★ International Association of Physicians in Audiology (IAPA)

c/o Konrad Konradsson, Sec.
Department of Audiology
University Hospital
S-22185 Lund, Sweden
Fax: 34 946172912
Email: secretary@iapa-online.org
Website: http://www.iapa-online.org

Fnded: 1980. **Desc:** Promotes world wide discussion of problems of mutual interest to audiological physicians.

★ 3696 ★ International Association of Physicians and Health Care Professionals

PO Box 13089
Tallahassee, FL 32317
R.S. Rhinehart, Pres. /CEO

Fnded: 1996. **Mem:** 85. **Desc:** Organization for physicians and allied health care workers.

★ 3697 ★ International Association for the Psychology of Food and Nutrition (IAPFoN)

Edgbaston
Birmingham B15 2TT, United Kingdom
Phone: 44 121 4144932 **Fax:** 44 121 4144897
Email: d.a.booth@bham.ac.uk
Website: http://www.westenhoefer.de/iapfon/Welcome.html

Fnded: 1992. **Desc:** Brings together basic and applied psychologists in research and practice on food and nutrition.

★ 3698 ★ International Association of Psychosocial Rehabilitation Services (IAPSRS)

601 N Hammonds Ferry Rd., Ste. A
Linthicum, MD 21090
Phone: (410)789-7054 **Fax:** (410)789-7675
Email: general@iapsrs.org
Website: http://www.iapsrs.org
Ruth A. Hughes, PhD, CEO

Fnded: 1976. **Mem:** 1,900. **Nat'l Groups:** 2. **Reg. Groups:** 2. **State Groups:** 32. **Local Groups:** 32. **Desc:** Individuals (1200) and organizations (700) serving adults with a psychiatric disability. Promotes the advancement of the role, scope, and quality of service designed to facilitate the readjustment into the community of the adults with psychiatric disabilities. Provides a forum for the exchange of ideas, experiences, and contributions to the field. Offers technical assistance to organizational members; sponsors regional training conferences. **Pub:** *PSR Connection*, quarterly. Newsletter. *Price:* Included in membership dues. • *Psychosocial Rehabilitation Journal*, quarterly. Journal. Includes calendar of events and research reports. *Price:* Included in membership dues. • *Weekly Email Report: What's New in Psyciatric Rehabilitation*. Newsletter. • Also publishes legislative bulletins, documents, and professional information.

★ 3699 ★ International Association of Radiopharmacology (IAR)

c/o Dr. Steve McQuarrie
Faculty of Pharmacy and Pharmaceutical Sciences
University of Alberta
Edmonton, AB, Canada T6G 2N8
Phone: (403)492-2905 **Fax:** (403)492-1217
Email: smcquarrie@pharmacy.ualberta.ca
Website: http://www.pharmacy.ualberta.ca/iar

Fnded: 1980. **Desc:** Represents members' interest. **Pub:** *Symposium Proceedings*, biennial.

★ 3700 ★ International Association for Regression Research and Therapies (IARRT)

PO Box 20151
Riverside, CA 92516
Phone: (909)784-1570 **Fax:** (909)784-8440
Email: info@iarrt.org
Website: http://www.iarrt.org
Connie Brooks, Exec. Dir.

Fnded: 1980. **Mem:** 800. **State Groups:** 20. **Desc:** Psychiatrists, psychologists, counselors, and students; organizations and individuals interested in past-life regression therapy. Promotes past-life therapy as a means of helping individuals realize their capacity to change and improve their lives. Works for progressive application of the therapy and the establishment of clinical standards for training therapists. Acts as a communications network for the exchange of information and experiences. Disseminates information to the public about benefits of the therapy. Registers therapists. Promotes research in the field. **Pub:** *Journal of Regression Therapy*, annual. Journal. *Price:* $26/volume. • *Past Life Research and Therapies*, quarterly. Newsletter. Contains editorials, Open Forum, reviews, and calender of events. *Price:* $10/year. • Audiotapes. • Directory, periodic. • Videos. **Frmly:** Association for Past Life Research and Therapies; (1991) Association for Past-Life Research and Therapy; (2002) Association for Past-Life Research and Therapies.

★ 3701 ★ International Association of Rehabilitation Professionals (IARP)

3540 Soqel Ave., Ste. A
Santa Cruz, CA 95062-1769
Free: 800-240-9059
Email: gzimmermann@rehabpro.org
Website: http://www.rehabpro.org
Glenn Zimmermann, Exec. Dir.

Mem: 2,800. **Desc:** Members of the rehabilitation industry. Promotes effective interdisciplinary rehabilitation, disability management and return-to-work services for the disabled and disadvantaged. Provides continuing education and career enhancement programs for members. Works to influence government and industry policy.

★ 3702 ★ International Association for Research on Epstein Barr Virus
080
F-94800 Villejuif, France

★ 3703 ★ International Association for Research in Favour of Persons with Mental Handicaps (AIRHM)
(Association Internationale de recherche scientifique en faveur des personnes handicapees mentales)
CP 70
CH-1000 Lausanne, Switzerland
Phone: 41 21 6516200 **Fax:** 41 21 6516288
Fnded: 1988. **Desc:** Furthers francophone study and research on mental deficiency; encourages cooperation between researchers; exchanges information with organizations in similar fields.

★ 3704 ★ International Association for the Scientific Study of Intellectual Disabilities (IASSID)
Moore Abbey
Monasterevan, Ireland
Phone: 353 45 525327 **Fax:** 353 45 525251
Email: 101720.3537@compuserve.com
Website: http://www.iassid.org/
Fnded: 1964. **Mem:** 430. **Reg. Groups:** 2. **Local Groups:** 10. **Desc:** Scientific study of mental deficiency by means of a multidisciplinary approach. **Pub:** *Journal of Intellectual Disability Research*, biennial. Journal. • Newsletter, quarterly.

★ 3705 ★ International Association for the Scientific Study of Intellectual Disabilities (IASSID)
c/o Association De Villepinte
28 rue de L'eglise
F-93420 Villepinte, France
Phone: 33 1 43851206 **Fax:** 33 1 49361154
Email: njross@compuserve.com
Website: http://www.iassid.org
Fnded: 1964. **Nat'l Groups:** 50. **Reg. Groups:** 1. **Lang(s):** English, French, Spanish. **Desc:** National associations representing 15,000 scientists and clinicians in 40 countries working in the field of intellectual disabilities. Encourages research in the field of intellectual disabilities, including its causes, prevention, diagnosis, evaluation, therapy, and rehabilitation, management, education, and social inclusion. **Pub:** *IASSID*, biennial. Newsletter. • *JIDR - Journal of Intellectual Disability Research*. Journal. • Proceedings, quadrennial. Printed in specialized journals. **Frmly:** (1995) International Association for the Scientific Study of Mental Deficiency.

★ 3706 ★ International Association of Specialised Kinesiologists (IASK)
Hauptstr 35
CH-4102 Binningen, Switzerland
Website: http://www.iask.ch/ziele.html

★ 3707 ★ International Association of Spiritual Psychiatry (IASP)
c/o Association Essence
Villa Alcedonia, 486, Chemin des Combattants AFN
F-06140 Vence, France
Phone: 33 4 93581654 **Fax:** 33 1 93581654
Email: info@essence-euro.org
Website: http://essence-euro.org
Fnded: 1994. **Mem:** 200. **Lang(s):** English, French. **Desc:** Integrates the spiritual dimension in medicine, psychology and psychiatry. **Pub:** *Internet Journal*, daily. Journal.

★ 3708 ★ International Association for the Study of the Liver (IASL)
(Association Internationale pour l'Etude du Foie)
c/o Jenny Heathcote
Toronto Western Hospital
399 Bathhurst St., 6BF, Rm. 170
Toronto, ON, Canada M5T 2S8
Phone: (416)603-5914 **Fax:** (416)603-7175
Email: elise_iasl@hotmail.com
Fnded: 1958. **Mem:** 879. **Lang(s):** English. **Desc:** Members of regional societies for the study of the liver representing 67 countries. Supports the training of experts in hepatology; encourages basic and clinical research on the liver and its diseases; acts to facilitate prevention, recognition, and treatment of diseases of the liver. **Pub:** Newsletter, biennial.

★ 3709 ★ International Association for the Study of Lung Cancer
National University Hospital
Finsen Center 5072
9 Blegdamsvej
DK-2100 Copenhagen, Denmark
Phone: 45 35454090 **Fax:** 45 35356906
Email: lungcancer@iaslc.org
Website: http://www.iaslc.org/
Fnded: 1974. **Mem:** 1,500. **Desc:** Promotes the study of prevention, diagnosis, treatment, and all aspects of lung cancer. **Pub:** *Lung Cancer*, monthly. Journal.

★ 3710 ★ International Association for the Study of Obesity (IASO)
231 North Gower St.
London NW1 2NS, United Kingdom
Phone: 44 207 3876033 **Fax:** 44 207 6911914
Email: kate.baillie@iaso.org
Website: http://www.iaso.org
Fnded: 1986. **Desc:** Improves prevention, management and treatment of obesity worldwide by promoting medical research, extending and disseminating knowledge, facilitating contact between investigators and promoting public education.

★ 3711 ★ International Association for the Study of Pain (IASP)
909 NE 43rd St., Ste. 306
Seattle, WA 98105-6020
Phone: (206)547-6409 **Fax:** (206)547-1703
Email: iaspdesk@juno.com
Website: http://www.iasp-pain.org
Louisa E. Jones, Exec. Off.
Fnded: 1973. **Mem:** 7,000. **Nat'l Groups:** 61. **Reg. Groups:** 61. **Desc:** Scientists, physicians, and other health professionals interested in pain research and therapy. Encourages research on pain mechanisms and syndromes; seeks to improve management of patients with acute and chronic pain. Promotes education and training in the field of pain; informs the public of results of current research. Fosters development of an international data bank, adoption of a uniform classification and definition regarding pain and pain syndromes, and creation of a uniform records system on information relating to pain mechanisms, syndromes, and management. Promotes the formation of national associations for the study and treatment of pain. **Pub:** *A Virtual Pocket Dictionary of Pain Terms*. Online only. • *Abstracts - 9th World Congress on Pain*. Book. • *Acute and Procedure Pain in Infants and Children*. Book. • *Assessment and Treatment of Cancer Pain - 1998*. Book. • *The Child With Headache: Diagnosis and Treatment*. Book. • *Chronic and Recurrent Pain in Children and Adolescents*. Book. • *Classification of Chronic Pain, 2nd ed. 1994*. Book. • *Complex Regional Pain Syndrome*. Book. • *Curriculum on Pain for Students in Psychology*. • *Desirable Characteristics for Pain Treatment Facilities*. • *Epidemiology of Pain*. Book. • *Ethical Guidelines for Investigations of Experimental Pain in Conscious Animals*. • *Ethical Guidelines for Pain Research in Humans*. • *IASP Pain Terminology*. • *Manual de Farmacoes Utilizados en el Tratamiento del Dolor Cronico*. Book. • *Measurement of Pain in Infants and Children*. Book. • *Molecular Neurobiology of Pain*. Book. • *Neuropathic Pain: Pathophysiology and Treatment*. Book. • *Opiod Sensitivity of Chronic Noncancer Pain*. Book. • *Outline Curriculum on Pain for Medical Schools*. • *Outline Curriculum on Pain for Schools of Nursing*. • *Outline Curriculum on Pain for Schools of Occupational Therapy and Physical Therapy*. • *Outline Curriculum on Pain for Schools of Pharmacy*. • *Pain*, 15/year. Journal. • *Pain and Suffering*. Book. • *Pain: Clinical Updates*, quarterly. Newsletter. • *Pain Imaging*. Book. • *Pain in the Elderly*. Book. • *Pain 1999 - An Updated Review (Refresher Course Syllabus) 1999*. Book. • *Pain Treatment Centers at a Crossroads: A Practical and Conceptual Reappraisal*. Book. • *Pharmacological Approaches to the Treatment of Chronic Pain*. Book. • *Proceedings*.

★ 3712 ★ International Association for Surgical Metabolism and Nutrition (IASMEN)
Postfach 1527
CH-4133 Pratteln, Switzerland
Phone: 41 61 8159666 **Fax:** 41 61 8114775
Email: surgery@iss-sic.ch
Fnded: 1993. **Mem:** 112. **Desc:** Promotes research on all aspects of surgical nutrition as a field of primary importance in surgical care. **Pub:** *World Journal of Surgery*. Journal.

★ 3713 ★ International Association of Therapeutic Drug Monitoring and Clinical Toxicology (IATDMCT)
PO Box 1570
4 Cataraqui St., Ste. 310
Kingston, ON, Canada K7L 5C8
Phone: (613)531-8166 **Fax:** (613)531-0626
Email: office@iatdmet.org
Website: http://www.iatdmct.org
Desc: Professionals with an interest in either therapeutic drug monitoring and clinical toxicology, physicians, clinical chemists, pharmacologists, medical technologists, toxicologists and environmental analysts. Aims are to promote the knowledge and understanding of clinical drug analysis and interpretation of results. Enhances communication between scientists and physicians of all disciplines involved in therapeutic drug monitoring and clinical toxicology. Encourages the effective application of therapeutic drug monitoring and clinical toxicology.

★ 3714 ★ International Association of Trichologists (IAT)
185 Elizabeth St., Ste. 919
Sydney, NSW 2000, Australia
Phone: 61 2 92671384 **Fax:** 61 8 82968450
Email: dsalinger@ozemail.com.au
Website: http://www.trichology.edu.au
Fnded: 1973. **Mem:** 125. **Nat'l Groups:** 3. **Lang(s):** English. **Desc:** Individuals licensed to practice or perform manipulative, electrical, light, or cosmetic therapy upon the scalp. Promotes the study, research, and legitimate practice of the treatment and care of the human hair and scalp. Prescribes and administers course of study of trichology. Conducts testing; grants certification; offers placement service. Has established code of ethics. **Pub:** *Guide to Hair Loss*. Book. • *Picture Guide to Scalp & Hair Problems*. Book. • Newsletter, bimonthly.

★ 3715 ★ International Atherosclerosis Society (IAS)
6550 Fannin, Ste. 1211
Houston, TX 77030-2704
Phone: (713)797-9620 **Fax:** (713)797-9507
Email: ias@bcm.tmc.edu
Website: http://www.athero.org
Ann S. Jackson, MBA, Exec. Dir.
Fnded: 1979. **Mem:** 9,500. **Nat'l Groups:** 36. **Desc:** Scientists and other professionals involved in research in the field of atherosclerosis; corporations and firms supporting aims of the IAS. Promotes the advance-

ment of science, research, and teaching in the field of atherosclerosis throughout the world. (Atherosclerosis is a form of arteriosclerosis characterized by the deposition of fatty substances in and fibrosis of the inner layer of the arteries.) Advocates an interdisciplinary approach to the study of atherosclerosis and related diseases. Facilitates international communication and exchange of knowledge among scientists in the field. Assists in the organization of exchange visits among scientists at various research centers. Fosters and encourages young researchers by arranging contacts, and offering travel support to world gatherings in the field. Coordinates activities in atherosclerosis research. **Pub:** *Proceedings of Symposia*, triennial. Proceedings. • *Roster of Member Societies.* • Newsletter, semiannual.

★ 3716 ★ International Autistic Research Organization (IARO)
49 Orchard Ave.
Croydon CR0 7NE, United Kingdom
Phone: 44 20 87770095 **Fax:** 44 20 87762362
Email: iaro@autismresearchww.freeservice.co.uk
Website: http://www.charitynet.org/~iaro

Fnded: 1981. **Mem:** 300. **Lang(s):** Czech, English, French, German. **Desc:** Provides information about scientific research into autism. **Pub:** Magazine, quarterly.

★ 3717 ★ International Balint Federation (IBF)
(Federation Internationale Balint)
c/o Dr. David Watt
Tollgate Health Ctr., 220
Tollgate Rd.
London E64 JS, United Kingdom
Phone: 44 20 89042844
Email: jvsalinsky@aol.com
Website: http://www.balint.co.uk/international.html

Fnded: 1975. **Lang(s):** English, French. **Desc:** Groups and corresponding members in 34 countries. Promotes group training and practice according to the principles of Michael Balint (1896-1970), psychiatrist and author. Studies the patient-physician relationship on a psychosocial level and encourages improved psychological training and research in practice. **Pub:** *Balint*, quarterly. Journal.

★ 3718 ★ International Behavioural and Neural Genetics Society (IBANGS)
c/o Mara Dierssen, Pres.
Center for Genomic Regulation Research
Paseig Maritim, 37-49
E-08003 Barcelona, Spain
Email: mdierssen@iro.es
Website: http://www.ibngs.org/

Fnded: 1996. **Mem:** 500. **Desc:** Scientists and students in the field of behavioural neurogenetics. Promotes excellence in the field of neurobehavioural genetics. **Pub:** *Genes, Brain and Behavior.*

★ 3719 ★ International Behavioural and Neural Genetics Society (IBANGS)
Viale Regina Elena, 299
I-00161 Rome, Italy
Phone: 39 06 49902352
Email: alleva@iss.it
Website: http://www.ibngs.org/

Desc: Advances neuro-behavioral genetic studies both in animal and in humans.

★ 3720 ★ International Blind Sports Federation (IBSA)
(Association Internationale pour le Sport des Aveugles)
c/Jose Ortega y Gasset, 18
E-28006 Madrid, Spain
Phone: 34 91 4365335 **Fax:** 34 91 4365354
Email: ibsa@ibsa.es
Website: http://www.ibsa.es

Fnded: 1981. **Mem:** 100. **Reg. Groups:** 5. **Lang(s):** English, French, Spanish. **Desc:** National organizations, institutions, and committees involved in sports for the blind. Objectives are to: involve and inspire blind persons in regular sports activities; encourage friendship among blind athletes; promote and disseminate the ideas of competitive sport and recreational sport for the blind; uphold the Olympic ideal and act in accordance with its principles. Plans, promotes and coordinates international sports events for the blind; registers records and best performances. Sponsors competitions. **Frmly:** International Blind Sports Association.

★ 3721 ★ International Board of Environmental Medicine (IBEM)
65 Wehrle Dr.
Buffalo, NY 14225
Phone: (716)837-1320 **Fax:** (716)833-2244
Website: http://www.medical-library.net
Dr. Kalpana Patel, Pres.

Fnded: 1988. **Mem:** 110. **Desc:** An accrediting agency for physicians and osteopaths working in related environmental professions. Examines licensed practitioners, facilities, and relevant training programs. Offers programs to evaluate qualifications of healthcare professionals, their training programs, and those facilities offering special types of treatment. Plans and supervises accrediting examinations. **Pub:** *Register of the International Board of Environmental Medicine*, annual. Directory. Contains names of diplomates. *Price:* $25.

★ 3722 ★ International Board for Regression Therapy (IBRT)
9091 Beach Rd.
Canastota, NY 13032
Email: freedman@dreamscape.com
Website: http://www.ibrt.org
Russell Davis, PhD, Contact

Desc: Therapists, researchers, training programs. Provide documentation, training and certificates. Promote public awareness of regression therapy.

★ 3723 ★ International Bone Marrow Transplant Registry (IBMTR)
8701 Watertown Plank Rd.
PO Box 26509
Milwaukee, WI 53226
Phone: (414)456-8325 **Fax:** (414)456-6530
Email: ibmtr@mcw.edu
Website: http://www.ibmtr.org
Mary M. Horowitz, MD, MS, Scientific Dir.

Fnded: 1972. **Mem:** 450. **Desc:** Voluntary organizations of basic and clinical scientists. Working to address important issues in blood and marrow transplantation. Gathers information on results of blood and marrow transplants; Information is used to guide clinical decisions and identify the most effective treatment strategies for individual patients based on a number of variables including age, disease type and stage, prior treatment, etc. **Pub:** *IBMTR/ABMTR Newsletter*, semiannual. Newsletter.

★ 3724 ★ International Brain Injury Association
c/o Stig Tomasen
Hjerneskadeforeningen
Brondby Mollevej 8
DK-2605 Brondby, Denmark
Phone: 45 43 432433 **Fax:** 45 43 422430
Email: info@hjerneskadeforeningen.dk
Website: http://www.hjerneskadeforeningen.dk

Fnded: 1985. **Mem:** 1,500. **Reg. Groups:** 10. **State Groups:** 1. **Lang(s):** English. **Desc:** Supports those with brain injuries and their families in the rehabilitation process of resuming normal activities.

★ 3725 ★ International Brain Research Organization (IBRO)
(Organisation Internationale de Recherche sur le Cerveau)
51, Blvd. de Montmorency
F-75016 Paris, France
Phone: 33 1 46479292 **Fax:** 33 1 45206006
Email: admin@ibro.org
Website: http://www.ibro.org

Fnded: 1960. **Mem:** 50,000. **Nat'l Groups:** 33. **Lang(s):** English, French. **Desc:** Scientists working in neuroanatomy, neuroendocrinology, the behavioral sciences, neurocommunications and biophysics, brain pathology, and clinical and health-related sciences. Works to promote international cooperation in research on the nervous system. Sponsors fellowships, exchange of scientific workers, and traveling teams of instructors to supplement local teachings. Organizes international neuroscience symposia and workshops. **Pub:** *Directory of Members.* Directory. • *Neuroscience*, bimonthly. • *News*, annual.

★ 3726 ★ International Bronchoesophagological Society (IBES)
Mayo Clinic Scottsdale
13400 E Shea Blvd.
Scottsdale, AZ 85259
Phone: (480)301-7149 **Fax:** (480)301-4869
Email: dsanderson@mayo.edu
Richard A. Helmers, MD, Exec. Sec. -Treas.

Fnded: 1951. **Mem:** 400. **Desc:** Endoscopists from varying disciplines. Fosters advances in laryngology, bronchoscopy, upper gastrointestinal endoscopy, diagnostic techniques, and endoscopic therapy. Encourages exchange of ideas; conducts original investigations and research.

★ 3727 ★ International Bundle Branch Block Association (IBBBA)
6631 W 83rd St.
Los Angeles, CA 90045-2899
Phone: (310)670-9132
Rita Kurtz Lewis, Exec. Dir.

Fnded: 1979. **Desc:** Individuals with bundle branch block (BBB), concerned professionals, and laypersons. (BBB is a rare heart condition caused by an "electrical malfunction".) Objectives are: to increase public awareness of BBB; to disseminate information on the disease; to answer inquiries of members; to serve as a forum for sharing information and experiences; to maintain a bank of information to aid professional research on BBB. Compiles statistics. Plans to conduct specialized education and research programs. **Pub:** *Heartbeat*, quarterly. Provides professional replies to readers' medical questions, reprints from other publications, and names and addresses of members. *Price:* Included in membership dues.

★ 3728 ★ International Bureau for Epilepsy (IBE)
(Bureau International pour l'Epilepsie)
PO Box 21
NL-2100 AA Heemstede, Netherlands
Phone: 31 23 5291019 **Fax:** 31 23 5470119
Email: ibe@sein.nl

Fnded: 1961. **Mem:** 96. **Nat'l Groups:** 62. **Lang(s):** English. **Desc:** National organizations and individuals interested in the medical, social, and scientific aspects of epilepsy. Focuses on aspects of daily life with epilepsy. Facilitates exchange of information and experience regarding the care of persons with epilepsy. Provides material on how to organize and finance non-medical societies. Organizes training sessions. Works to build an international film library on epilepsy. **Pub:** *Employing People with Epilepsy: Principles for Good Practice.* Handbook. • *International Epilepsy News*, quarterly. Magazine. Contains information on epilepsy.

★ 3729 ★ International Cardiac Doppler Society (ICDS)
Viamonte 1336, Piso 9, Of 52/53
1053 Buenos Aires, Argentina
Phone: 54 11 43749911 **Fax:** 54 11 43749911
Email: sppi@movi.com.ar

★ 3730 ★ International Center for the Health Sciences (ICHS)
Barracks Hill
PO Box 4744
Charlottesville, VA 22904-4744
Phone: (804)971-7605 **Fax:** (804)971-7605
Email: info@ichsciences.org
Website: http://www.ichsciences.org
Warren E. Grupe, Medical Dir.
Fnded: 1991. **Desc:** Works to improve the health of all people through creative health education programs designed to meet the unique needs and capabilities of communities around the world. Sponsors collaborative research; develops and strengthens current preventative and curative care; manages and implements health science education programs in cooperation with US institutions in Central America, Africa and the former Soviet Union; advocates for the health care needs of all people.

★ 3731 ★ International Center of Medical and Psychological Hypnosis (ICMPH) (Centro Internazionale di Ipnosi Medica e Psicologica)
Istituto di Indagini Psicologiche
Corso XXII Marzo 57
I-20129 Milan, Italy
Phone: 39 02 7388427 **Fax:** 39 02 7491051
Email: uim.psico@tin.it
Website: http://www.uim-psico.org
Fnded: 1969. **Mem:** 340. **Reg. Groups:** 15. **Desc:** Physicians, psychologists, and teachers of psychology and psychiatry at universities. Seeks to advance the knowledge of hypnosis and its applications. Organizes courses in psychosomatic medicine and medical and psychological hypnosis for physicians and psychologists. Conducts research on hypnosis, hypnoanesthesia, hypnotherapy, hypnotic eugenics, childbirth, and hypnotic contraception. Holds seminars and workshops. Also handles courses in psychology of handwriting, expert analysis for handwriting or forensic issues, autogenous training, and naturopathy. **Pub:** *Literature*, semiannual. Also publishes *Dictionary of Hypnopsychology and Handwriting Psychology*.

★ 3732 ★ International Center for the Study of Psychiatry and Psychology (ICSPP)
1036 Park Ave., Ste. 1B
New York, NY 10028
Phone: (212)585-3758
Email: email@icspp.org
Website: http://www.icspp.org
David Cohen, PhD, Pres.
Fnded: 1971. **Desc:** A nonprofit research and educational network whose focus is the critical study of the mental health movement. Founded by Dr. Peter Breggin, ICSSP is concerned with the impact of mental health theories on public policy and the effects of therapeutic practices upon individual well-being, personal freedom, and community and family values. Members include psychiatrists, psychologists, social workers, philosophers, counselors, therapists and psychiatric victims and survivors worldwide, and includes journalists, editors, academics, practitioners and interested lay people. **Pub:** *Ethical Human Sciences and Services (EHSS)*, quarterly. Journal. **Frmly:** (1995) Center for the Study of Psychiatry; (2003) Center for the Study of Psychiatry and Psychology.

★ 3733 ★ International Cerebral Palsy Society (ICPS)
19 St. Mary's Grove
London W4 3LL, United Kingdom
Phone: 44 208 9946386 **Fax:** 44 208 7478528
Email: a.loring@easynet.co.uk
Website: http://www.icps.org.uk
Fnded: 1969. **Mem:** 317. **Lang(s):** English. **Desc:** Professionals, parents, handicapped persons, and organizations in 60 countries. Seeks to stimulate research in cerebral palsy and promote related improvements and developments in early diagnosis, methods of treatment, and appropriate teaching and rehabilitation programs. Acts as the international coordinating organization for collection, distribution, and exchange of specialized information on cerebral palsy. Disseminates information about: architectural design for the handicapped; operation and equipment of a mobile visiting aid unit; aids and appliances; how to obtain entry visas for handicapped children emigrating with their families; medical matters; sex education; research on integration; publications for parents; alternative forms of physiotherapy; employment opportunities. Offers consulting services and referrals. **Pub:** *Bulletin*, 3/year. Bulletin.

★ 3734 ★ International Cesarean Awareness Network (ICAN)
1304 Kingsdale
Redondo Beach, CA 90278
Phone: (310)542-6400 **Fax:** (310)542-5368
Email: info@ican-online.org
Website: http://www.ican-online.org
Anita Woods, Pres.
Fnded: 1982. **Mem:** 600. **Reg. Groups:** 15. **Desc:** Men and women and birth professionals concerned with the increasing rate of cesarean births. Objectives are: to oppose and lower through education the high cesarean rate currently prevalent and to offer encouragement, information and support to those women who wish to have a vaginal birth after previous cesarean(s) or VBAC. ICAN shall endeavor to share information about the prevention of unnecessary cesareans and to encourage vaginal birth; to encourage positive birthing assistance that is non-interventive in nature; to refer mothers desiring a VBAC to birth attendants who will assist them; to inform the public as to VBAC option; and to offer direct encouragement, counseling and support to women pursuing a VBAC. ICAN shall assist and encourage the establishment of local associations, committees, and support groups to further the purposes outlined above. Promote the safety of vaginal birth vs. cesarean section through printed and other media nationwide. Provide information on cesarean and VBAC issues via our website and through printed media. Active ICAN chapters throughout the US sand Internationally. **Pub:** *The Clarion*, quarterly. Newsletter. Includes research and informational articles, book reviews and chapter news. *Price:* Included in membership dues; One free copy for nonmembers. **Frmly:** (1992) Cesarean Prevention Movement.

★ 3735 ★ International Child Care - Canada (ICC)
2476 Argentia Rd., Ste. 113
Mississauga, ON, Canada L5N 6M1
Phone: (905)821-6318 **Free:** 888-72-CHILD
Fax: (905)821-6319
Email: canada@intlchildcare.org
Website: http://www.gospelcom.net/icc/
Fnded: 1966. **Mem:** 200. **Lang(s):** English, French. **Desc:** Health care personnel. Promotes global availability of community-based health care, with emphasis on the prevention of tuberculosis, maternal and child health, and provision of primary health care services. Cooperates with local administrative bodies to strengthen public health programs in the Dominican Republic and Haiti. Conducts primary health care and immunization services. Sponsors health care training courses for people living in underserved areas.

★ 3736 ★ International Child Neurology Association (ICNA)
Via di Torvergata, 135
I-00133 Rome, Italy
Phone: 39 03358348921 **Fax:** 39 065917415
Email: icna@atsmf.uni-lj.si
Website: http://www.child-neuro.net
Fnded: 1973. **Desc:** Promotes child neurology.

★ 3737 ★ International Childbirth Education Association (ICEA)
PO Box 20048
Minneapolis, MN 55420-0048
Phone: (952)854-8660 **Fax:** (952)854-8772
Email: info@icea.org
Website: http://www.icea.org/
Cheryl Coleman, Pres.
Fnded: 1960. **Mem:** 12,000. **Local Groups:** 275. **Desc:** Purposes are: to further the educational, physical, and emotional preparation of expectant parents for childbearing and breastfeeding; to increase public awareness on current issues related to childbearing; to cooperate with physicians, nurses, physical therapists, hospitals, health, education, and welfare agencies, and other individuals and groups interested in furthering parental participation and minimal obstetric intervention in uncomplicated labors; to promote development of safe, low-cost alternatives in childbirth that recognize the rights and responsibilities of those involved. Develops, publishes, and distributes literature pertaining to family-centered maternity care. Offers a teacher certifi cation program for childbirth educat ors. Conducts workshops. Operates mail order book store in Minneapolis, MN which makes available literature on all aspects of childbirth education and family-centered maternity care. **Pub:** *ICEA Bookmarks*, 4/year. • *International Journal of Childbirth Education*, 4/year. Journal. • Membership Directory, annual. • Also publishes pamphlets.

★ 3738 ★ International Chiropractic Pediatric Association (ICPA)
5295 Hwy. 78, Ste. D362
Stone Mountain, GA 30087-3414
Phone: (610)565-2360 **Free:** 800-670-KIDS
Fax: (770)736-1651
Email: info@icpa4kids.com
Fnded: 1996. **Mem:** 1,200. **Desc:** Chirpractors and chiropractic students with an interest in the treatment of pediatric patients. Seeks to advance the study, teaching, and practice of pediatric chiropractic; promotes continuing professional development of members. Serves as a clearinghouse on pediatric health; sponsors research and educational programs; formulates standards of practice for pediatric chiropractic and conducts certification examinations. **Pub:** Newsletter, bimonthly.

★ 3739 ★ International Chiropractors Association (ICA)
1110 N Glebe Rd., Ste. 1000
Arlington, VA 22201
Phone: (703)528-5000 **Free:** 800-423-4690
Fax: (703)528-5023
Email: chiro@chiropractic.org
Website: http://www.chiropractic.org/
Ronald Hendrickson, Exec. Dir.
Fnded: 1926. **Mem:** 6,000. **Desc:** Professional society of chiropractors, chiropractic educators, students, and laypersons. Sponsors professional development programs and practice management seminars. **Pub:** *Congressional Directory*, annual. Directory. • *ICA Today*, bimonthly. Newsletter. Covers membership and association activities; includes legislative information and research updates. *Price:* Included in membership dues. • *International Chiropractors Association Membership Directory*, annual. Directory. • *International Review of Chiropractic*, bimonthly. • Also publishes materials on patient education. **Frmly:** (1941) Chiropractic Health Bureau.

★ 3740 ★ International Christian Leprosy Mission (ICLM)
PO Box 596
Forest Grove, OR 97116
Phone: (503)285-9098 **Fax:** (503)285-6535
Email: HealingHands8414@aol.com

Website: http://www.christian-relief.org
Dr. Daniel Pulliam, Pres.

Fnded: 1943. **Mem:** 12. **Reg. Groups:** 3. **Desc:** Carries on evangelical missionary work and assists in physical treatment of people with leprosy and their children. **Pub:** *Global Missions*, quarterly. Newsletter. *Price:* Free. • *KLM Healing Hands*, monthly. Newsletter. *Price:* Free.

★ 3741 ★ International Clinical Epidemiology Network (INCLEN)

1420 Market St., No. 411
Philadelphia, PA 19102-4003
Phone: (215)222-7700 **Fax:** (215)222-7741
Email: inclen@inclen.org
Website: http://www.inclen.org/

Desc: Physicians, statisticians, social scientists. Seeks to improve the health of individuals; promotes clinical practice, research and medical education. **Pub:** Brochure.

★ 3742 ★ International College of Angiology

5 Daremy Ct.
Nesconset, NY 11767-1547
Phone: (631)366-1429 **Fax:** (631)366-3609
Email: denisemrossignol@cs.com

Fnded: 1958. **Desc:** Dedicated to advancement and education in angiology, the study of the circulatory and vascular system. **Pub:** *International Journal of Angiology*, quarterly. Journal. Promotes multi-disciplinary approaches to all aspects of vascular disease.

★ 3743 ★ International College of Applied Kinesiology - U.S.A. (ICAK-U.S.A.)

6405 Metcalf Ave., Ste. 503
Shawnee Mission, KS 66202-3929
Phone: (913)384-5336 **Fax:** (913)384-5112
Email: icak@dci-kansascity.com
Website: http://www.icakusa.com
Andria Dibbern, Membership Services

Fnded: 1975. **Mem:** 700. **Desc:** Promotes the science of applied kinesiology. Applied Kinesiology is the system of evaluating the structural, chemical, and mental aspect of human heath, involving muscle health, nutrition, manipulation, diet, acupressure, and exercise. Conducts educational programs, research programs, and training seminars. **Pub:** *International Journal*, semiannual. Journal. • *International Journal*, semiannual. Directory. • *Membership Directory*, annual. *Price:* $16/issue.

★ 3744 ★ International College of Cranio-Mandibular Orthopedics

c/o Hallie Truswell
619 N 35th St., Ste. 307
Seattle, WA 98103
Phone: (206)633-4355 **Free:** 800-446-1763
Fax: (206)633-4352
Email: hallie@tmj-iccmo.org
Website: http://tmj-iccmo.org
Hallie Truswell, Exec. Dir.

Fnded: 1979. **Mem:** 550. **Desc:** Cranio-mandibular orthopedists. Seeks to advance the study and practice of cranio-mandibular orthopedics. Conducts continuing professional development courses for members. **Pub:** *ICCMO Newsletter*, 3/year. Newsletter. • *Journal of Craniomandibular Orthopedics*, 3/year. Journal.

★ 3745 ★ International College of Dentists (ICD)

51 Monroe St., Ste. 1400
Rockville, MD 20850-2408
Phone: (301)251-8861 **Fax:** (301)738-9143
Email: reg-sg@icd.org
Website: http://www.icd.org
Minoru Horiuchi, Pres.

Fnded: 1928. **Mem:** 9,200. **Desc:** Dentists who have made outstanding contributions to the profession. Acclaims meritorious service to dentistry; fosters growth and diffusion of dental information; upholds high standards in dental education. Supports the Dental Career Option Seminar for Students. Promotes continuing education through the International Clinicians Program. Operates charitable programs. **Pub:** *Globe*, annual. Journal. • *Key*, annual. Magazine. • *Keynotes*, semiannual. Newsletter. • *Roster*, periodic.

★ 3746 ★ International College for Health Cooperation in Developing Countries - Italy (CUAMM - Medici con l'Africa)

Via San Francesco 126
I-35121 Padua, Italy
Phone: 39 049 8751649 **Fax:** 39 049 8574738
Email: cuamm@cuamm.org
Website: http://www.cuamm.org

Fnded: 1950. **Mem:** 378. **Local Groups:** 15. **Lang(s):** English, Italian. **Desc:** Works to improve public health and increase the availability of health care services and preventive medical programs in developing countries. Facilitates cooperation among international development agencies with health-related programs. Conducts educational and training programs in health related areas including community development and water supply and sanitation. Makes available emergency medical relief services. **Pub:** *Salute E Sviluppo*, quarterly. Journal.

★ 3747 ★ International College of Nuclear Medicine Physicians

c/o Carlos M. Duncker, MD, PhD
Zacatecas 230-502
Colonia Roma
06700 Mexico City DF, DF, Mexico
Fax: 52 55 744885
Email: medicina_molecular@hotmail.com
Website: http://www.icnmp.edu.mx

Desc: Nuclear medicine physicians, general physicians and other medical specialists and health care professionals. Promotes current knowledge in nuclear medicine.

★ 3748 ★ International College of Prosthodontists

PO Box 99119
San Diego, CA 92169-1119
Phone: (858)270-1814
Email: res-inc@msn.com
Website: http://www.icp-org.com
Eben Yancy, Exec. Dir.

Mem: 750. **Desc:** Prosthodontists.

★ 3749 ★ International College of Psychosomatic Medicine (ICPM)

Roehampton
London SW15 5JJ, United Kingdom
Phone: 44 20 83924227 **Fax:** 44 20 83922632

Fnded: 1970. **Desc:** Advances principles of psychosomatic medicine worldwide, achieves highest standards of research.

★ 3750 ★ International College of Surgeons (ICS)

1516 N Lake Shore Dr.
Chicago, IL 60610
Phone: (312)642-3555 **Fax:** (312)787-1624
Email: max@icsglobal.org
Website: http://www.icsglobal.org
Max C. Downham, Exec. Dir.

Fnded: 1935. **Mem:** 10,000. **Nat'l Groups:** 70. **Reg. Groups:** 6. **Desc:** General surgeons and surgical specialists in 110 countries maintaining official relations with the World Health Organization. Promotes the universal teaching and advancement of surgery and its allied sciences. Maintains International Museum of Surgical Sciences containing specialty rooms showing the growth and perfection of many surgical specialties. Maintains library open to researchers, individuals working in the profession, and the public. Organizes postgraduate clinics around the world; conducts lecture series and periodic congresses; offers grants, scholarships, and loans for residencies, research, and advanced study in surgery. Sends surgical teaching teams to developing countries. Bestows honorary fellowship. **Pub:** *International College of Surgeons Newsletter*, quarterly. Newsletter. Covers college news and business. • *International Surgery*, quarterly. Journal. Presents papers on clinical, experimental, cultural, and historical topics pertinent to surgery and related fields. Contains book reviews. *Price:* $25/year for members; $50/year for nonmembers.

★ 3751 ★ International Color Vision Society

c/o Prof. J.D. Mollon
Department of Experimental Psychology
University of Cambridge
Downing St.
Stafford CB2 3EB, United Kingdom
Phone: 44 1782 583060 **Fax:** 44 7071 295038
Email: anne.kurtenbach@uni-tuebingen.de
Website: http://orlab.optom.unsw.edu.au/icvs

Fnded: 1971. **Mem:** 200. **Lang(s):** English. **Desc:** Ophthalmologists, optometrists, physicists, physiologists, psychologists, and zoologists. Seeks to collaborate on the study of congenital and acquired color vision deficiencies. **Pub:** *Daltoniana*, quarterly. Newsletter. • *Proceedings of the IRGCVD Symposia*, biennial. **Frmly:** (2000) International Research Group on Coloru Vision Deficiencies.

★ 3752 ★ International Commission on Biological Effects of Noise (ICBEN)

c/o Prof. Soames Job
School of Psychology
University of Sydney
Sydney, NSW 2006, Australia
Phone: 61 2 93512859 **Fax:** 61 2 93512603
Email: soamesj@psych.usyd.edu.au

Fnded: 1973. **Mem:** 500. **Nat'l Groups:** 10. **Desc:** Encourages international cooperation in the study of the biological effects of noise; promotes communication among research scientists, governmental agencies, industrial workers and managers, and other parties and entities concerned with noise effects.

★ 3753 ★ International Commission on Occupational Health (Commission Internationale de la Sante au Travail)

c/o Prof. Chia Kee Seng
Department of Community, Occupational, and Family Medicine
National University of Singapore
16 Medical Dr.
Singapore 117597, Singapore
Phone: 65 68744971 **Fax:** 65 67791489
Email: icohsg@singnet.com.sg
Website: http://www.icoh.org.sg/

Fnded: 1906. **Mem:** 2,000. **Lang(s):** English, French. **Desc:** Physicians specializing in occupational medicine and other individuals with an interest in occupation safety and health. Seeks to advance the study, teaching, and practice of occupational medicine. Serves as a forum for the exchange of information among members; sponsors research and educational programs.

★ 3754 ★ International Commission for the Prevention of Alcoholism and Drug Dependency (ICPA)

12501 Old Columbia Pike
Silver Spring, MD 20904
Phone: (301)680-6719 **Fax:** (301)680-6707
Email: 74617.1663@compuserve.com
Dr. Peter N. Landless, Exec. Dir.

Fnded: 1952. **Desc:** Representatives of national public health committees and other individuals interested in the physical and social effects of alcoholism and drug dependency. Fosters the scientific study of alcohol and drugs, their effects on the physical, mental, and moral powers of the individual, and their effects on social, economic, political, and religious life. Encourages preventive education; disseminates information on drug and alcohol abuse. Serves as a liaison with similar groups around the world. Sponsors exchange and research programs. Conducts film shows, forums, and radio and television events. **Pub:** *ICPA Dispatch*, periodic. • *ICPA Reporter*, periodic. Newsletter. Describes worldwide activities of ICPA and local communities. **Frmly:** (1982) International Commission for the Prevention of Alcoholism.

★ 3755 ★ International Commission on Protozoology (ICOP)

Institute of Tropical Medicine
First Miliatary Medical University
Tonghe
Guangzhou 510515, People's Republic of China
Phone: 86 20 61648305 **Fax:** 86 20 61648324
Email: tropmed@fimmu.edu.cn

Desc: Promotes the exchange of ideas among protozoologists throughout the world, and helps to arrange periodic International Congresses of Protozoology.

★ 3756 ★ International Committee Against Mental Illness (ICAMI)

PO Box 1921, Grand Central Sta.
New York, NY 10163-1921
Phone: (212)263-6214 **Fax:** (212)263-8135
Email: rc31@nyu.edu
Dr. Robert Cancro, Pres.

Fnded: 1958. **Desc:** Fosters psychosocial rehabilitation and mental health research, services, and information systems. Provides technical assistance to professional rehabilitation organizations in expanding or installing computer information systems in psychiatry and in planning workshops, symposia, and conferences. Organizes international consortium of voluntary agencies and rehabilitation groups. Conducts research; operates speakers' bureau. Has worked on projects in Colombia, Indonesia, Iran, Israel, Kuwait, Liberia, Nepal, Pakistan, and Yugoslavia. The committee is a direct outgrowth of a pioneering psychiatric treatment project in Haiti that is now operated by the Haitian government.

★ 3757 ★ International Committee on Food Microbiology and Hygiene

13-17 Setembro
NL-1999 Veldhoven, Netherlands
Email: leon.gorris@unilever.com

Fnded: 1953. **Desc:** Aims at improving the control of diseases of microbial etiology transmitted by foods and of food spoilage.

★ 3758 ★ International Committee of Homeopathic Pharmacists (Comite International des Pharmaciens Homeopathiques — CIPH)

c/o Emile Devey
Laboratories Boiron
Avenida Valdelaparra 27
Alcobendas
E-28108 Madrid, Spain
Phone: 34 91 4840438

Fnded: 1955. **Mem:** 121. **Lang(s):** English, French, German. **Desc:** Homeopathic pharmacists in 21 countries. **Pub:** *Annual Report*. • *Circular Letter*, semiannual. • *Draft of an International Homeopathic Pharmacopeia*.

★ 3759 ★ International Committee for Life Disability and Health Assurance Medicine

c/o Hannover RE
7, rue montauvet
F-75008 Paris, France
Phone: 33 1 42668778 **Fax:** 33 1 42668798
Email: christianearry@hanover.re.com
Website: http://www.iclam2004.com

Fnded: 1899. **Mem:** 77. **Lang(s):** English. **Desc:** Medical doctors working in life insurance and reinsurance companies in 41 countries. Promotes fraternal benefit life insurance; facilitates contact and cooperation among members. Establishes societies of life assurance medicine in countries where they do not exist. **Pub:** *Annals of Life Assurance Medicine*, triennial. Newsletter.

★ 3760 ★ International Committee of Military Medicine (ICMM) (Comite International de Medecine Militaire — CIMM)

Queen Astrid Military Hospital
B-1120 Brussels, Belgium
Phone: 32 2 2644348 **Fax:** 32 2 2644367
Email: cimm.icmm@smd.be
Website: http://www.cimm-icmm.org

Fnded: 1921. **Mem:** 96. **Lang(s):** English, French. **Desc:** Medical representatives of the military forces of nations worldwide. Works to encourage and maintain professional cooperation among those in various countries whose mission is to care for the sick and wounded of the armed forces. Aims to improve such care by standardization of related disciplines and techniques, complete documentation and dissemination of military-medical information, and development of an international medical law. Conducts courses. **Pub:** *International Review of the Armed Forces Medical Services*, quarterly. Journal. **Frmly:** (1990) International Committee of Military Medicine and Pharmacy.

★ 3761 ★ International Committee of Sports for the Deaf (CISS)

7310 Grove Rd., Ste. 106
Frederick, MD 21704
Fax: (301)620-2990
Email: info@ciss.org
Website: http://www.ciss.org
Dr. Donalda K. Ammons, Sec. Gen.

Fnded: 1924. **Mem:** 77. **Reg. Groups:** 4. **Desc:** National athletic organizations for the deaf. Provides an international sports competition for the deaf patterned after the International Olympic Games. Promotes and develops physical education and the practice of sports among the deaf. Encourages friendly relations between countries with programs in silent sports and countries without programs for deaf athletes. Holds Summer World Games and Winter Games alternately at 2-year intervals for competitors with hearing loss of 55 decibels or more. The committee is recognized by the International Olympic Committee. **Pub:** *Bulletin*, quarterly. Magazine. *Price:* $20/year. • *Handbook*, periodic. **AKA:** (2000) Deaf Olympics.

★ 3762 ★ International Committee on Veterinary Gross Anatomical Nomenclature (Committee Internationale de la Nomeclature Macroanatomique Veterinaire)

Department of Veterinary Anatomy
Anatomisches Institut
Tierarfliche Hochschule
Binchofsholer Damm 15
D-30173 Hannover, Germany

Lang(s): English, French, German, Italian. **Desc:** Veterinarians. Promotes international standardization of veterinary anatomical nomenclature. Develops standard nomenclature; sponsors research; facilitates cooperation among veterinary anatomists worldwide.

★ 3763 ★ International Confederation of Midwives (ICM) (Confederation Internationale des Sages-Femmes — CISF)

Eisenhowerlaan 138
NL-2517 KN The Hague, Netherlands
Phone: 31 70 3060520 **Fax:** 31 70 3555651
Email: info@internationalmidwives.org
Website: http://www.internationalmidwives.org

Fnded: 1919. **Mem:** 82. **Reg. Groups:** 4. **Lang(s):** English, French, Spanish. **Desc:** National midwives' associations in 75 countries. Seeks to improve the standard of care provided to mothers, babies, and the family by promoting midwifery education and disseminating information about the art and science of midwifery. **Pub:** *A Birthday for Midwives - Seventy Five Years of International Collaboration*. Book. • *International Code of Ethics for Midwives, 1993*. Book. • *International Midwifery Matters*, semiannual. Newsletter. • *Planning for Action for Midwives*.

★ 3764 ★ International Confederation for Plastic, Reconstructive and Aesthetic Surgery (IPRAS)

4 Exec. Pk. Dr.
Albany, NY 12203
Phone: (518)438-1434 **Fax:** (518)489-1205
Email: ipras@ipras.org
Website: http://www.ipras.org
Dr. James G. Hoehn, MD, Gen. Sec.

Fnded: 1955. **Mem:** 91. **Nat'l Groups:** 91. **Reg. Groups:** 3. **Desc:** National associations representing 13000 plastic surgeons. Promotes plastic surgery both clinically and scientifically. Encourages closer relationships between international members and direct contact between national societies. Disseminates information on developments in other countries. Seeks to widen the scope of understanding and knowledge in the field and reinforce the worldwide fraternity of plastic surgeons. **Pub:** *Globe Plast*, 3/year. Newsletter. *Price:* Free to members.

★ 3765 ★ International Confederation for Plastic Reconstructive and Aesthetic Surgery Asian-Pacific Section

22/23, Bhaktawar Annexe 22
Narayan Dabholkar Rd.
Bombay 400006, India
Phone: 91 22 23675431 **Fax:** 91 22 3686368
Website: http://worldplasticsurgery.org

Fnded: 1970. **Mem:** 2,282. **Nat'l Groups:** 18. **Lang(s):** English. **Desc:** Plastic and reconstructive surgeons who are members of national societies of the International Confederation for Plastic, Reconstructive and Aesthetic Surgery. Promotes high standards of practice and continuing education for members. **Pub:** *Newsletter of the Asian Pacific Section*, annual. Newsletter.

★ 3766 ★ International Congress of Oral Implantologists (ICOI)

248 Lorraine Ave., Ste. 3
Upper Montclair, NJ 07043
Phone: (973)783-6300 **Free:** 800-442-0525
Fax: (973)783-1175
Email: icoi@dentalimplants.com
Website: http://www.dentalimplants.com
R. Craig Johnson, Exec. Dir.

Fnded: 1975. **Mem:** 6,000. **Desc:** Dentists and oral surgeons dedicated to the teaching of and research in oral implantology (branch of dentistry dealing with dental implants placed into or on top of the jaw bone). Offers fellowship and course certification programs. Compiles statistics and maintains registry of current research in the field. Sponsors classes, seminars, and workshops at universities, hospitals, and societies worldwide. Provides consultation and patient information/referral services. **Pub:** *ICOI News*, quarterly. Newsletter. *Price:* Included in membership dues. • *Implant Dentistry*, quarterly. Journal. Includes scientific manuscripts, new product reports, membership updates, and calendar of seminars. *Price:* Included in membership dues; $76 for nonmembers; $95 for nonmembers outside U.S. • Membership Directory, annual. **Frmly:** (1976) International College of Oral Implantologists.

★ 3767 ★ International Contact Dermatitis Research Group (ICDRG)
c/o Prof. Jean-Marie Lachapelle
Clos Chapelle aux Champs 30
Louvain University, UCL 3033
B-1200 Brussels, Belgium
Phone: 32 2 7643324 **Fax:** 32 2 7643334
Email: jean-marie.lachapelle@derm.ucl.ac.be
Website: http://www.med.nagoya-u.ac.jp/Environderm/icdrg.htm
Fnded: 1967. **Desc:** Encourages research into skin problems related to the environment.

★ 3768 ★ International Continence Society (ICS)
c/o Victoria Rees, Admin.
Southmead Hospital
Bristol BS10 5NB, United Kingdom
Phone: 44 117 9503510 **Fax:** 44 117 9503469
Email: vicky@icsoffice.org
Website: http://www.icsoffice.org
Fnded: 1971. **Mem:** 1,500. **Lang(s):** English. **Desc:** Physicians, surgeons, nurses, physicists, physiotherapists, bio-engineers, and scientists. Promotes the study of the storage and voiding function of the lower urinary tract, its diagnosis, and the management of lower urinary tract dysfunction. Encourages research into pathophysiology, diagnostic techniques, and treatment. **Pub:** *Neurourology and Urodynamics*, bimonthly. Journal.

★ 3769 ★ International Correspondence Society of Allergists and Clinical Immunologists (ICSA)
4601 W 109 St.
Shawnee Mission, KS 66211
Phone: (913)469-4043 **Fax:** (913)469-6580
Email: jebaptist@worldnet.att.net
Dr. Jeremy E. Baptist, PhD, Exec. Dir.
Fnded: 1936. **Mem:** 204. **Desc:** Physicians who specialize in research and treatment of allergies. Exchanges of technical information and experiences are conducted via letters. **Pub:** *Allergy Letters*, monthly. Newsletter. Includes case reports, comments, questions and answers, and related material. *Price:* Included in membership dues. **Frmly:** (1995) International Correspondence Society of Allergists.

★ 3770 ★ International Correspondence Society of Obstetricians and Gynecologists (ICSOG)
12693 Tamiami Tr. E, No. 213
Naples, FL 34113
Fax: (941)417-2780
Email: dmlassoc@mediaone.net
Dean M. Laux, Exec. Sec.
Fnded: 1960. **Mem:** 2,600. **Desc:** Physicians concerned with obstetrics and gynecology and related surgery; medical schools and libraries; civilian and military hospitals; others with research or clinical interests. **Pub:** *The Collected Letters*, monthly. Newsletter. *Price:* $119.

★ 3771 ★ International Council on Alcohol and Addictions (ICAA) (Conseil International sur les Problemes de l'Alcoolisme et des Toxicomanies — CIPAT)
Case Postale 189
CH-1001 Lausanne, Switzerland
Phone: 41 21 3209865 **Fax:** 41 21 3209817
Email: secretariat@icaa.ch
Website: http://www.icaa.de/
Fnded: 1907. **Mem:** 450. **Lang(s):** English, French, German, Spanish. **Desc:** Persons and organizations interested in or working with problems of alcoholism or drug addiction in 80 countries. Encourages interdisciplinary exchange of information and experience in research, prevention, treatment, and rehabilitation for alcoholism and drug addiction. Organizes international conferences on the prevention and treatment of alcohol and drug dependence. Also focusses on issues related to tobacco dependence and gambling. **Pub:** *Alcoholism*, semiannual. Journal. • *ICAA News*, quarterly. **Frmly:** (1935) International Bureau Against Alcoholism; (1968) International Union Against Alcoholism.

★ 3772 ★ International Council on Alcohol, Drugs and Traffic Safety (ICADTS)
Mississippi State, MS 39762
Phone: (601)325-7959 **Fax:** (601)325-7966
Email: bwparker@ssrc.msstate.edu
Barry M. Sweedler, Pres.
Fnded: 1950. **Mem:** 150. **Desc:** Working to reduce mortality and morbidity brought about by misuse of alcohol and drugs by operators of vehicles in all modes of transportation. Sponsors international and regional conferences to collect, disseminate and share essential information among professionals in the fields of law, medicine, public health, economics, law enforcement, public information and education, human factors and public policy. **Pub:** *ICADTS Reporter*, quarterly. Newsletter. • *Journal of Traffic Medicine*, quarterly. Journal. *Price:* included in membership dues.

★ 3773 ★ International Council for the Control of Iodine Deficiency Disorders - Australia (ICCIDD)
c/o Dr. Basil Hetzel
8th Fl., Samuel Way Bldg.
Women's and Children's Hospital
North Adelaide, SA 5006, Australia
Phone: 61 8 81617021 **Fax:** 61 8 816170221
Email: iccidd@a011.aone.net.au
Website: http://www.people.virginia.edu/~jtd/iccidd
Fnded: 1986. **Desc:** Promotes development of national iodine deficiency disorders, assists and promotes adaptive research, practical validation and transfer of technology.

★ 3774 ★ International Council for Education of People with Visual Impairment (ICEVI)
c/o M. Mani, Sec. Gen.
IHRDC Campus
Ramakrishna Mission Vidyalaya
Penang 641 020, Tamil Nadu, India
Phone: 91 422 2697530 **Fax:** 91 422 2692353
Email: sgicevi@vsnl.net
Website: http://www.icevi.org
Fnded: 1952. **Reg. Groups:** 8. **Lang(s):** English, Spanish. **Desc:** Teachers and educators of the visually handicapped and other interested persons. Advocates education of the visually handicapped worldwide; works to improve existing facilities through training programs for teachers, refresher courses, and provision of teaching materials. Offers assistance for professional training. Conducts teacher training courses in developing countries. **Pub:** *The Educator*, semiannual. Journal. • *International Resource Directory*. Book. **Frmly:** International Council for Education of the Visually Handicapped; (1972) International Conference of Educators of Blind Youth.

★ 3775 ★ International Council of Nurses (ICN) (Conseil International des Infirmieres — CII)
3, place Jean-Marteau
CH-1201 Geneva, Switzerland
Phone: 41 22 9080100 **Fax:** 41 22 9080101
Email: icn@icn.ch
Website: http://www.icn.ch
Fnded: 1899. **Mem:** 124. **Nat'l Groups:** 112. **Lang(s):** English, French, Spanish. **Desc:** Federation of national nurses' associations, representing nurses in more than 120 countries. World's first and widest reaching international organisation for health professionals. Operated by nurses for nurses working to ensure quality nursing care for all, sound health policies globally, the advancement of nursing knowledge, and the presence worldwide of a respected nursing profession and a competent and satisfied nursing workforce. **Pub:** *International Nursing Review*, bimonthly. Journal. Contains information on nursing and health issues. • Brochures, periodic.

★ 3776 ★ International Council for Physical Activity and Fitness Research (ICPAFR)
Faculty of Physical Education & Physiotherapy
Katholieke Universitet Leuven
Tervuursevest 101
B-3001 Leuven, Belgium
Phone: 32 16 329083 **Fax:** 32 16 329197
Email: albrecht.claessens@flok.kuleuven.ac.be
Website: http://www.unipd.it/esterni/wwwmedic/Servizi.htm
Fnded: 1964. **Mem:** 140. **Nat'l Groups:** 36. **Lang(s):** English. **Desc:** Medical doctors, physiologists, anthropologists, biochemists, physical educators, and psychologists in 30 countries who have done substantial research on physical fitness. Promotes international comparative studies on the effect of physical fitness upon the welfare of children, adults, and the aged. Works toward establishing standardized physical fitness assessment and measurement procedures. Operates speakers' bureau. Maintains advisory committees for the establishment of a sports research center and for the facilitation of scientific cooperation in the preparation, execution, and publication of comparative studies. **Pub:** *Nutrition and Physical Activity*. • *Physical Fitness and the Ages of Man*. • *Physical Fitness Assessment: Principles, Practices and Application*. **Frmly:** (1978) International Committee on Physical Fitness Research; (1992) International Council for Physical Fitness Research.

★ 3777 ★ International Council of Reflexologists (ICR)
PO Box 78060
Hamilton, ON, Canada L9C 7N5
Fax: (905)387-6199
Email: icr@mountaincable.net
Website: http://www.icr-reflexology.org/
Fnded: 1990. **Nat'l Groups:** 22. **Desc:** Works to establish reflexology as a self-regulating profession, ensure public safety and promote study and exchange of knowledge and art of reflexology within the profession. **Pub:** Newsletter, quarterly.

★ 3778 ★ International Council for the Study of Virus and Virus-like Diseases of the Grapevine
Chemin de Trembley 27
CH-1197 Prangins, Switzerland
Fnded: 1964.

★ 3779 ★ International Cranial Association
478 Baker St.
Middlesex
Enfield EN1 3QS, United Kingdom
Phone: 44 20 83675561 **Fax:** 44 20 82026686
Fnded: 1965. **Mem:** 84. **Desc:** Osteopaths, chiropractors, manipulative therapists. Holds a register of members for enquiries from the public; provides a training course each year; holds an annual conference for members and the public; provides a code of ethics. **Pub:** Newsletter, quarterly. **Frmly:** (1999) Cranial Osteopathic Association.

★ 3780 ★ International Cystic Fibrosis-Mucoviscidosis Association (ICFMA)
Avda Campanar 106, 3, 6
E- 46015 Valencia, Spain
Phone: 34 963461414 **Fax:** 34 963494047
Email: fq@vic.servicom.es

Fnded: 1964. Desc: Promotes research on cystic fibrosis among medical professionals, governments and the general public.

★ 3781 ★ International Cytokine Society (ICS)

Biotech Park, Ste. 9
1021 15th St.
Augusta, GA 30901
Phone: (706)722-7511 **Fax:** (706)722-7515
Email: menachem.rubenstein@weizmann.ac.il
Website: http://bioinformatics.weizmann.ac.il/cyto-kine/
Dr. Menachem Rubenstein, Contact

Fnded: 1978. **Mem:** 700. **Desc:** Physicians and scientists associated with universities; private, industrial, and government institutes; hospital clinics; and the pharmaceutical industry. Promotes research into and awareness of the health importance of shock and trauma; fosters the dissemination and application of information in these fields; provides a forum for the multidisciplinary integration of current and basic clinical knowledge and concepts in the study of shock and trauma. **Pub:** *Advances in Shock Research*. Book. • *American Society for Photobiology–Directory and Constitution*, biennial. Directory. • *Cytokine*, monthly. Journal. • *Directory and Constitution*, biennial. Directory. • Newsletter, quarterly. **Frmly:** (2001) Shock Society.

★ 3782 ★ International Dalkon Shield Victims Education Association (IDEA)

212 Pioneer Bldg.
Seattle, WA 98104
Phone: (206)329-1371 **Fax:** (206)624-4961
Constance Miller, Treas.

Fnded: 1986. **Mem:** 2,000. **State Groups:** 2. **Desc:** Women who have contracted illnesses and/or been disabled through use of the Dalkon Shield intrauterine contraceptive device; their supporters. Promotes public education about the dangers of using the Dalkon Shield. Disseminates information regarding Dalkon Shield injuries, claim resolution, and related topics. Offers seminars. Maintains speakers' bureau.

★ 3783 ★ International Dental Federation (IDF)

7 Carlisle St.
London W1V 5RG, United Kingdom
Fnded: 1900.

★ 3784 ★ International Dental Health Foundation (IDHF)

2414 Black Cap Ln., Ste. L-1
Reston, VA 20191
Phone: (703)860-9244 **Free:** 800-368-3396
Fax: (703)860-9245
Email: idhf@aol.com
Website: http://members.aol.com/idhf/
Patricia L. Cartwright, Exec. Dir.

Fnded: 1981. **Mem:** 450. **Desc:** Dentists, dental hygienists, and other dental professionals. Advocates a method of treating periodontal disease that deemphasizes cleaning and surgery and instead concentrates on eliminating the disease-causing bacteria. **Pub:** *Annotations*, bimonthly. Newsletter. *Price:* Included in membership dues. • *Seminar Brochures*. • Brochures.

★ 3785 ★ International Diabetes Federation (IDF)
(Federation Internationale du Diabete — FID)

1, rue Defacqz
B-1000 Brussels, Belgium
Phone: 32 2 5385511 **Fax:** 32 2 5385114
Email: idf@idf.org

Fnded: 1949. **Mem:** 1,100. **Nat'l Groups:** 156. **Reg. Groups:** 7. **Lang(s):** English, French, Spanish. **Desc:** National diabetes associations; diabetes sections of national academies; endocrinology, metabolic, and diabetes societies; diabetes supplies companies are supporting members; association represents over one million individuals through its national associations. Objectives are: to improve the quality of life in the global diabetic community; to promote the exchange of information; to improve standards of treatment; to develop educational methods designed to patients a better understanding of there disease; to educate the public in the early recognition of the disease and the importance of its medically supervised treatment; to encourage medical, scientific, and socioeconomic research. Maintains liaison with the World Health Organization. Compiles statistics. **Pub:** *Diabetes Voice*, quarterly. Journal. • *The Economics of Diabetes & Diabetes Care: Costing Diabetes, the cause for Prevention*. • *IDF Bulletin*, quarterly. Journal. • *IDF Diabetes Voice*, 3/year. • *Triennial Report*.

★ 3786 ★ International Doctors in Alcoholics Anonymous (IDAA)

3311 Brookhill Cir.
Lexington, KY 40503
Phone: (859)277-9379 **Fax:** (859)278-6128
Email: idaaghyde@aol.com
Website: http://www.idaa.org
Gordon L. Hyde, MD, Exec. Dir.

Fnded: 1949. **Mem:** 4,200. **Nat'l Groups:** 1. **Desc:** Doctorate level health care professionals interested in Alcoholics Anonymous. Seeks to exchange knowledge and experience in the recovery from and management of alcoholism for members and persons who fall within their sphere of influence. Supports AA-type group activities. **Pub:** *International Doctors in Alcoholics Anonymous–Newsletter*, semiannual. Newsletter. *Price:* Included in membership dues. • *Letter*, semiannual.

★ 3787 ★ International Drug Strategy Institute

901 Garfield
Topeka, KS 66606
Email: cvoth@stormontvail.org
Website: http://www.estreet.com/orgs/dsi/
Eric A. Voth, Chm.

Mem: 40. **Desc:** Works to develop effective international policies and strategies to discourage drug use and legalization of illicit drugs. Disseminates accurate scientific information on drugs.

★ 3788 ★ International Dyslexia Association (IDA)

8600 LaSalle Rd.
Chester Bldg., Ste. 382
Baltimore, MD 21286-2044
Phone: (410)296-0232 **Free:** 800-ABCD-123
Fax: (410)321-5069
Email: info@interdys.org
Website: http://www.interdys.org
J. Thomas Viall, Exec. Dir.

Fnded: 1949. **Mem:** 13,000. **Reg. Groups:** 44. **Desc:** Offers free information to the public and referrals for diagnosis and treatment. Membership includes professionals in the fields of neurology, pediatrics, psychiatry, education, social work, and psychology; parents; other persons interested in the study, treatment, and prevention of the problems of specific language disability, often called developmental dyslexia or simply dyslexia. Provides a focal point for activities and ideas generated in various fields as they relate to problems of language development and learning. IDA is founded in memory of Dr. Samuel T. Orton, a pioneer in the field of dyslexia. Disseminates materials. Offers support groups. Presents seminars and conferences around the U.S. Advocates for appropriate educational policies. **Pub:** *Annals of Dyslexia*, annual. Journal. Peer-reviewed journal with current research on dyslexia. *Price:* Free with membership; $35. • *Orton Emeritus Series*. Monographs. Series 12 of 26 published. • *Perspectives*, quarterly. Magazine. • Also issues reprints of papers. **Frmly:** (1981) Orton Society; (1998) Orton Dyslexia Society.

★ 3789 ★ International Electrology Educators (IEE)

c/o SCME
132 Great Rd., No. 200
Stow, MA 01775
Fax: (617)237-9039
Email: mmeyer@tconl.com
Website: http://www.scmhr.org/ieeabou.htmiee
Marilyn Meyer, Contact

Fnded: 1979. **Mem:** 55. **Desc:** Electrology schools and teachers. Purposes are to instruct teachers and standardize the curriculum and teaching of electrology. Conducts educational programs and regional educational conferences for electrology educators. **Pub:** *IEE Directory of Schools*, periodic. Directory. • *Perspectives*, quarterly. **Frmly:** (1982) National Electrology Educators; (1985) International Electrology Educators; (1993) Institute of Electrology Educators.

★ 3790 ★ International Embryo Transfer Society (IETS)

1111 N Dunlap Ave.
Savoy, IL 61874
Phone: (217)356-3182 **Fax:** (217)398-4119
Email: iets@assochq.org
Website: http://www.iets.org
Carol L. Keefer, Pres.

Fnded: 1974. **Mem:** 1,100. **Desc:** Veterinarians; researchers in reproductive physiology, animal science, genetics, endocrinology, and immunology; representatives of regulatory agencies such as government agencies and breed associations; sales representatives of drugs or equipment; students. Works to disseminate scientific and educational information; to promote more effective research; to foster and maintain high standards of education and ethics. Conducts Code Numbers to Identify Units Freezing Embryos Program, through which containers of frozen embryos are labeled with a permanent, recognized identification number. Sponsors exhibits of drugs and equipment used in embryo transfer. Conducts student competition to promote excellence in research. Maintains speakers' bureau. **Pub:** *IETS Manual*. Manuals. Covers information on minimum sanitary standards for embryo transfer procedures. *Price:* $35. • *IETS Newsletter*, quarterly. Newsletter. • *Proceedings of Annual Symposium and Conference*.

★ 3791 ★ International Enneagram Association (IEA)

PO Box 78008
San Francisco, CA 94107-8008
Phone: (408)971-5905 **Fax:** (408)999-0344
Email: ieastaff@intl-enneagram-assn.org
Website: http://www.internationalenneagram.org/
Debi Goddard, Adm.

Desc: Working to promote the highest human values through the insights of the Enneagram. Sponsors open and constructive interactions among various schools of Enneagram thought; encourages innovative application of the Enneagram and builds community through grass roots regional participation.

★ 3792 ★ International Epidemiological Association (IEA)

c/o Prof. Ahmed Mandil
38, Ismailiah St., Apt. 201
Mostafa Kamel
Alexandria, Egypt
Email: ieasecretariat@link.net
Website: http://www.dundee.ac.uk/iea/

Fnded: 1950. **Mem:** 2,250. **Lang(s):** English. **Desc:** Individuals interested in epidemiology (science dealing with incidence, distribution, and control of disease in populations). Studies methods and applications of disease control, clinical medicine, and health services. Conducts seminars and workshops. Encourages epidemiologic research. **Pub:** *Dictionary of Epidemiology*. • *International Journal of Epidemiology*, bimonthly. Journal. • Manuals. • Membership Directory, triennial. • Monographs.

★ 3793 ★ International Essential Tremor Foundation (IETF)
PO Box 14005
Lenexa, KS 66285-4005
Phone: (913)341-3880 **Free:** 888-387-3667
Fax: (913)341-1296
Email: staff@essentialtremor.org
Website: http://www.essentialtremor.org
Catherine S. Rice, Exec. Dir.

Fnded: 1988. **Mem:** 25,000. **State Groups:** 54. **Desc:** Provides services, support, research, funds, and education to families, friends, and individuals suffering from Benign Essential Tremor. Current treatment includes drug therapy and surgical intervention. Provides patient information and referrals to physicians who specialize in Essential Tremor. **Pub:** Newsletter, quarterly. Includes research reports and networking information. *Price:* Included in membership dues. **Frmly:** (2003) International Tremor Foundation.

★ 3794 ★ International Eye Foundation (IEF)
10801 Connecticut Ave.
Kensington, MD 20895-2134
Phone: (301)290-0264 **Fax:** (301)290-0269
Email: ief@iefusa.org
Website: http://www.iefusa.org
Victoria M. Sheffield, Exec. Dir.

Fnded: 1961. **Desc:** Works to restore sight and prevent blindness in poor countries around the world. Focuses on making eye clinics financially self-sufficient. Developed eye health services. Trains ophthalmologists and para-medicals, and fights vitamin A deficiency, trachoma and river blindness. Strives to help clinics become less dependent on outside donors and government funds. **Pub:** *International Eye Foundation–Eye to Eye*, semiannual. Newsletter. Concerned with the prevention of blindness in the developing countries; includes information on foundation programs. *Price:* Free. • Annual Report, annual. • Also publishes fact sheets. Primary Eye Care Manual Eye Care in Developing Nations

★ 3795 ★ International Federation on Ageing (IFA)
c/o Mr. Ivan Hale
425 Viger Ave. W, Ste. 520
Montreal, QC, Canada H2Z 1X2
Phone: (514)396-3358 **Fax:** (514)396-3378
Email: ifa@citenet.net
Website: http://www.ifa-fiv.org

Fnded: 1973. **Mem:** 215. **Nat'l Groups:** 1. **Reg. Groups:** 1. **Lang(s):** English, French, Spanish. **Desc:** Federation of voluntary organizations from close to 50 countries that represents the elderly as their advocate and/or provide services to them. Purposes are: to serve as an international advocate for the aging; to exchange information on a cross-national level of developments in aging of primary interest to the practitioner. **Pub:** *An Older World: Reflections on the Second World Assembly on Ageing and NGO Forum.* Book. • *EAGLE*, 3/year. Bulletin. Covers legal issues and related policy questions affecting older people around the world. • *Empowering Older People.* Book. • *IFA Journal on Ageing*, quarterly. Journal. Contains news about older persons around the world. Provides coverage of trends; contains international conference calendar. • *Network News*, semiannual. Newsletter. Contains information about midlife and older women. Includes reviews of publications and calendar.

★ 3796 ★ International Federation on Aging - European Office (IFA)
1268 London Rd.
London SW16 4EJ, United Kingdom
Phone: 44 20 86798000 **Fax:** 44 20 86796069
Fnded: 1973.

★ 3797 ★ International Federation of Anti-Leprosy Associations (ILEP) (Federation Internationale des Associations Contre la Lepre — ILEP)
234 Blythe Rd.
London W14 0HJ, United Kingdom
Phone: 44 20 76026925 **Fax:** 44 20 73711621
Email: ilep@ilep.org.uk
Website: http://www.ilep.org.uk

Fnded: 1966. **Mem:** 16. **Lang(s):** English, French, German. **Desc:** International federation of autonomous non-governmental anti-leprosy organizations, most of which generate their income by raising funds from private donors to support more than a thousand projects in more than 90 countries. Members support medical, scientific, social, and humanitarian activities throughout the world to cure and rehabilitate people affected by leprosy and to prevent and eventually eradicate the disease. **Pub:** *ILEP Connect*, quarterly. Newsletter.

★ 3798 ★ International Federation of Aromatherapists (Australian Branch)
PO Box 786
Templestowe, VIC 3106, Australia
Phone: 61 3 98509254 **Fax:** 61 3 98505730
Email: ifa-aus@bigpond.com
Website: http://www.ifa.org.au/

Fnded: 1989. **Mem:** 400. **Desc:** Dedicated to the preservation of health through aromatherapy. Aromatherapy is the therapeutic treatment using essential oils with specialized message. Provides courses and study programs. **Pub:** Journal. • Articles.

★ 3799 ★ International Federation of Associations of Pharmaceutical Physicians (IFAPP)
Rendementsweg 24 E-I
NL-3641 SL Mijdrecht, Netherlands
Phone: 31 297 285144 **Fax:** 31 297 256046
Email: ifapp@planet.nl
Website: http://www.ifapp.org

Fnded: 1975. **Mem:** 25. **Nat'l Groups:** 25. **Lang(s):** English. **Desc:** National organizations representing 6000 physicians in 25 countries specializing in pharmaceutical medicine. Encourages contact among members. **Pub:** *International Journal of Pharmaceutical Medicine: IFAPP Section*, bimonthly. Newsletter.

★ 3800 ★ International Federation of Blood Donor Organizations (IFBDO) (Federazione Internazionale delle Organizzazioni dei Donatori di Sangue)
c/o Ms. Nicole Patterson
34 place Raoul-Dautry
F-75748 Paris Cedex 15, France
Phone: 33 1 45387193

Fnded: 1955. **Mem:** 43. **Lang(s):** English, French, Spanish. **Desc:** National voluntary blood donor associations united to promote voluntary blood giving. Considers problems of common interest such as voluntary donations from which all political and religious considerations are excluded, and medical progress of blood transfusions. Seeks laws related to voluntary blood giving and governmental action prohibiting blood commerce. Exchanges information; acts as liaison with the European Council, League of Red Cross and Red Crescent Societies, United Nations Educational, Scientific and Cultural Organization, and World Health Organization. Provides specialized education. **Pub:** *FIODS Revue*, quarterly.

★ 3801 ★ International Federation of the Blue Cross (IFBC) (Federation Internationale de la Croix-Bleue — FICB)
Lindenrain 5A
PO Box 6813
CH-3001 Bern, Switzerland
Phone: 41 31 3005860 **Fax:** 41 31 3005869
Email: ifbc.bern@bluewin.ch
Website: http://www.eurocare.org/bluecross/

Fnded: 1877. **Mem:** 72,946. **Nat'l Groups:** 33. **Reg. Groups:** 2170. **Lang(s):** English, French, German, Portuguese. **Desc:** National societies and local groups representing individuals in 50 countries. Works to help alcoholics and drug addicts. Disseminates information concerning alcoholism. Operates cure homes and clinics. **Pub:** *Editorial*, bimonthly. Newsletter. • *INFO*, semiannual. **Frmly:** (1983) International Federation of the Temperance Blue Cross Societies.

★ 3802 ★ International Federation for Cervical Pathology and Colposcopy (IFCPC) (Federacion Internacional de Patologia Cervical y Colposcopia)
c/o Giuseppe De Palo, M.D.
Instituto Nazionale Tumori
Via Venezian, 1
I-20133 Milan, Italy
Phone: 39 02 2390324 **Fax:** 39 02 23903345
Email: depalo@istitutotumori.mi.it
Website: http://www.ifcpc.org

Fnded: 1972. **Mem:** 34. **Nat'l Groups:** 34. **Lang(s):** English, French, German, Spanish. **Desc:** Federation of national societies encouraging basic and applied research and the dissemination of information concerning uterine cervical pathology and colposcopy.

★ 3803 ★ International Federation of Clinical Neurophysiology (Federation Internationale de Neurophysiologie Clinique)
c/o IFCN Secretariat
42 Canham Rd.
London W3 7SR, United Kingdom
Phone: 44 208 7433106 **Fax:** 44 208 7431010
Email: ifcn@ifcn.info
Website: http://www.ifcn.info

Fnded: 1951. **Mem:** 55. **Lang(s):** English, Japanese. **Desc:** Neurologists, physiologists, and other medical professionals; scientists and researchers. Seeks to advance knowledge in clinical neurophysiology and related fields; promotes development of more effective neurological diagnostic and surgical procedures. Serves as a clearinghouse on neurophysiology; conducts educational, training, and continuing professional development courses.

★ 3804 ★ International Federation of Comparative Endocrinological Society (IFCES)
c/o Dr. Hubert Vaudry
European Institute for Peptide Research
Department of Cellular and Molecular Neuroendocrinology
University of Rouen
Mont-Saint-Aignan, France
Phone: 33 235 146624 **Fax:** 33 235 146946
Email: hubert.vaudry@univ-rouen.fr

Mem: 1,500. **Nat'l Groups:** 6. **Lang(s):** English. **Desc:** Constituent societies include the Asia and Oceania Society for Comparative Endocrinology, European Society for Comparative Endocrinology, Division of Comparative Endocrinology of the American Society of Zoologists, Japan Society for Comparative Endocrinology, the Indian Society of General and Comparative Endocrinology, and the Endocrine and Osmoregulation Groups of the Society for Experimental Biology. Promotes and advances research in comparative endocrinology and facilitates the interchange of ideas among scientists worldwide.

★ 3805 ★ International Federation of Dental Anesthesiology Societies (IFDAS)
13 Corinna Chambers
Corinna St.
Woden, ACT 2606, Australia
Phone: 61 2 62822605 **Fax:** 61 2 62815321
Email: jameskg@ozenail.com.au

Fnded: 1982. **Nat'l Groups:** 16. **Lang(s):** English. **Desc:** Societies of dental and medical practitioners in 14 countries. Promotes and encourages the study and practice of improved methods for administering anesthesia, analgesia, and sedation in dentistry and its related branches. Works to bring the benefits of these methods to people throughout the world. Facilitates the international exchange of information, research, and technology in the field. **Pub:** *IFDAS Newsletter*, semiannual. Newsletter.

★ 3806 ★ International Federation of Denturists
RPO Westdale
Winnipeg, MB, Canada R3R 3S3
Phone: (204)897-9092 **Free:** 800-773-0099
Fax: (204)895-9595
Email: ifdenturist@mts.net
Website: http://www.international-denturist.org

Fnded: 1985. **Mem:** 8,000. **Nat'l Groups:** 8. **Desc:** International voice of denturism; facilitates communication among member nations; promotes denturism and legislation for denturism throughout the world.

★ 3807 ★ International Federation of Fertility Societies (IFFS)
c/o Bernard Hedon, Pres. Elect
CSI
337 rue de la Combe Caude
F-34090 Montpellier, France
Phone: 33 4 67585903 **Fax:** 33 4 67583160
Email: algcsi@mnet.fr

Fnded: 1953. **Lang(s):** English. **Desc:** National fertility and sterility societies. Conducts congresses to study human reproduction and problems relating to fertility and sterility in humans and animals. **Pub:** *International Journal of Fertility*, quarterly. Journal.

★ 3808 ★ International Federation of Gynecology and Obstetrics (FIGO) (Federation Internationale de Gynecologie et d'Obstetrique — FIGO)
70 Wimpole St.
London W1G 8AX, United Kingdom
Phone: 44 207 2243270 **Fax:** 44 207 9350736
Email: figo@figo.org
Website: http://www.figo.org

Fnded: 1954. **Mem:** 102. **Lang(s):** English, French, Spanish. **Desc:** Objectives are to: promote and assist in the development of scientific and research work relating to all facets of gynecology and obstetrics; improve the physical and mental health of women, mothers, and their children; provide an exchange of information and ideas; improve teaching standards; promote international cooperation among medical bodies. Acts as liaison with World Health Organization and other international organizations. **Pub:** *Figo Annual Report on the Results of Treatment of Gynecologic Cancer*, annual. Annual Report. Provides results of treatment in gynecological cancer. • *Figo Newsletter*, 3/year. Newsletter. • *International Journal of Gynecology and Obstetrics*, monthly. Journal.

★ 3809 ★ International Federation of Hard of Hearing People (IFHOH)
c/o Darja Holec, Sec.
Head Office
Drenikova 24
Ljubljana, Slovenia
Phone: 386 31316921
Email: maghani@unive.at
Website: http://www.ifhoh.org

Fnded: 1977. **Mem:** 40. **Lang(s):** English. **Desc:** National organizations for individuals with acquired deafness representing 24 countries. Objectives are to: improve the standards of technical and social provisions for the hearing impaired; increase the understanding of the problems and needs of the hard of hearing; stimulate research into hearing impairment and the development of facilities for the hearing impaired; improve communication between the hard of hearing and among organizations for the hearing impaired. Coordinates the work of member organizations. Cooperates with governments and organizations for the prevention and cure of hearing impairments. Collects research data, public relations materials, and technical aids. **Pub:** *Congress and Symposia Proceedings*, quadrennial. Proceedings. • *Congress Report*. Report. • *IFHOH Journal*, 3/year. Journal. • *Working for the Hard of Hearing Within the IFHOH*. Brochure. **Frmly:** International Federation of the Hard of Hearing.

★ 3810 ★ International Federation of Hard of Hearing Young People (IFHOHYP)
c/o Vanessa Migliosi
Via Oriola 12
I-38100 Trento, Italy
Phone: 39 0461 236966 **Fax:** 39 0461 236966
Email: vanessamigliosi@tin.it
Website: http://www.ifhohyp.dk

Fnded: 1968. **Mem:** 15. **Lang(s):** English, German. **Desc:** National organizations; hearing impaired individuals under the age of 30 living in countries where no organizations for the hearing impaired exist. Encourages friendship between individuals of different nationalities. Objectives are to: increase understanding of the problems and needs of the hard of hearing; improve self-confidence of young hearing impaired people. Supervises annual summer camps. **Pub:** *The Ear Talking*, quarterly. Magazine. • *IFHOHYP Annual Report*, annual. Annual Report. • *IFHOHYP Newsletter*, quarterly. Newsletter. **Frmly:** (1994) International Committee of Hard of Hearing Young People.

★ 3811 ★ International Federation of Health Plans (IFHP)
46 Grosvenor Gardens
London SW1W 0EB, United Kingdom
Phone: 44 20 78819281 **Fax:** 44 20 77309234
Email: maria@ifhp.com
Website: http://www.ifhp.com

Fnded: 1968. **Mem:** 100. **Lang(s):** English. **Desc:** Nongovermental organizations involved in the execution of independent health care finance (100); associations of health funds (11) and individuals (26) in 20 countries. Promotes the study and development of independent health care services. Encourages research and the exchange of information. Operates conferences and meetings; information and research; sharing of information in cohesive network of member health funds. Offers study tours and educational programmes. **Pub:** *Conference Proceedings*, biennial. • *Membership Directory*, annual. Directory. • *Newsletter*, quarterly. Newsletter. • Booklets, periodic. **Frmly:** (1989) International Federation of Voluntary Health Service Funds; (1999) International Federation of Health Funds.

★ 3812 ★ International Federation of Health Records Organizations (IFHRO)
c/o Philip Roxborough
2/365 Richardson Rd.
Mount Roskill
Auckland, New Zealand
Phone: 64 9 6267975 **Fax:** 64 9 6267975
Email: philipr@ahsl.co.az

Fnded: 1968. **Mem:** 200. **Nat'l Groups:** 2. **Lang(s):** English. **Desc:** Organizations in 21 countries working in the health records field; persons involved in the field of health records in countries where no national organizations exist are associate members; individuals who have made significant contributions to the federation are honorary members. Objectives are to: improve health records standards in hospitals, dispensaries, and various health and medical institutions; promote efficient methods of health records in patient care, statistics, research, and teaching; provide a worldwide forum for individuals working in the health records field; encourage the international exchange of education requirements and training programs in the field of health records. Works closely with the World Health Organization and jointly sponsors workshops and research and educational projects in the health records field. **Pub:** *International Health Records*, quarterly. Newsletter.

★ 3813 ★ International Federation for Hydrocephalus and Spina Bifida (IFHSB)
Cellebroerstr 16
B-1000 Brussels, Belgium
Phone: 32 2 5020413 **Fax:** 32 2 5021129
Email: if@wanadoo.be
Website: http://www.ifglobal.org

Fnded: 1981. **Desc:** Disseminates information and expertise throughout the world to families, individuals, professionals and volunteers involved in the Hydrocephalus and Spina Bifida field, stimulates research; encourages cooperation between organizations; stimulates international discussion on ethics.

★ 3814 ★ International Federation of Infantile and Juvenile Gynecology (IFIJG) (Federation Internationale de Gynecologie Infantile et Juvenile — FIGIJ)
c/o George Creatsas
9 Kanari St.
GR-106 71 Athens, Greece
Phone: 30 1 7286353 **Fax:** 30 1 7233330
Email: geocze@azetaieio.uooc.gz

Fnded: 1972. **Mem:** 3,850. **Nat'l Groups:** 40. **Lang(s):** English, French, German. **Desc:** Gynecologists and pediatricians in 43 countries. Promotes the diagnosis and treatment of gynecological problems during childhood and adolescence. Maintains the FIGO Joint Committee for the Study of Gynecological Problems in Childhood and Adolescence. **Pub:** *Gynecologie*, periodic. Magazine. • *Pediatric and Adolescent Gynecology*, periodic. Newsletter.

★ 3815 ★ International Federation of Infection Control (IFIC)
c/o Moira Walker, Sec.
Division of Microbiology and Infection Control
Vancouver General Hospital
899 W 12th Ave.
Vancouver, BC, Canada V5Z 1M9
Phone: (604)875-4002 **Fax:** (604)875-4359
Email: mwalker@vanhosp.bc.ca
Website: http://www.ific.narod.ru/

Fnded: 1987. **Desc:** Umbrella organization for societies and organizations; seeks to reduce or minimize nosocomial infections worldwide; aims to develop network of infection control organizations; promotes education and training programs; serves as liaison with the World Health Organization and other organizations. **Pub:** *Educational Programme for Infection Control Basic Concepts and Training*. Booklet. • *IFIC Newsletter*, semiannual. Newsletter. Provides members and individuals in countries without infection control societies with articles on infection control.

★ 3816 ★ International Federation of the Little Brothers of the Poor (IFLBP) (Federation Internationale des Petits Freres des Pauvres — FIPFP)
c/o Dr. R. Scott Walker
33, ave. Parmentier
F-75011 Paris, France
Phone: 33 1 49231300 **Fax:** 33 1 47009466
Email: federation@petits-freres.org

Fnded: 1979. **Mem:** 8. **Nat'l Groups:** 8. **Lang(s):** English, French, Spanish. **Desc:** National Little Brothers organizations from Canada, France, Germany, Mexico, Morocco, Spain, Republic of Ireland, and the United States. Provides material and emotional support to older people who are handicapped, isolated, or destitute. Believes that old age should not prevent people from leading satisfying and fulfilling lives. Coordinates the efforts of volunteers and professionals to assist the elderly in areas such as housing, travel, and social and cultural activities.

★ 3817 ★ International Federation of Manual/Musculoskeletal Medicine
c/o Dr. Michel Dedee
Their Saive 49
B-4608 Warsage, Belgium
Phone: 32 4 3766438 **Fax:** 32 4 3766528
Email: michel.dedee@skynet.be
Website: http://www.fimm-online.org

Fnded: 1965. **Mem:** 26. **Nat'l Groups:** 26. **Lang(s):** English, French, German. **Desc:** National organizations of musculoskeletal medicine from countries throughout the world. Promotes scientific research in the field of musculoskeletal medicine. Provides including quality management, education, legal representation in dealing with official authorities.

★ 3818 ★ International Federation for Medical and Biological Engineering (IFMBE) (Federation Internationale de Genie Medical et Biologique)
c/o Dr. Heikki Terio, Dir.
Department of Biomedical Engineering
Huddinge University Hospital
S-141 86 Huddinge, Sweden
Phone: 46 8 58580852 **Fax:** 46 8 58586290
Email: heikki.terio@mta.hs.sll.se
Website: http://www.ifmbe.org/

Fnded: 1959. **Lang(s):** English. **Desc:** Medical and biological engineers and others involved in the field. Encourages and fosters research in the field of medical and biological engineering. Promotes international cooperation; disseminates scientific information; cooperates with developing countries to encourage training of health personnel in maintenance and repair of laboratory and other equipment. **Pub:** *Medical and Biological Engineering and Computing*. Journal.

★ 3819 ★ International Federation of Ophthalmological Societies (IFOS)
c/o Bruce E. Spivey. MD, Sec.-General
945 Green St.
San Francisco, CA 94133
Phone: (415)409-8410 **Fax:** (415)409-8400
Email: bruce@spivey.org
Website: http://www.icoph.org
Bruce E. Spivey, MD, Sec. -Gen.

Fnded: 1857. **Mem:** 120. **Nat'l Groups:** 125. **Reg. Groups:** 5. **Desc:** ICO (the executive body of IFOS) represents opthalmologic organizations throughout the world. Dedicated to international exchange in ophthalmology. Encourages the study and improvement of ophthalmologic education; formulates international standards. Advocates the prevention and treatment of preventable blindness in developing nations, particularly Africa. Supports the International Agency for the Prevention of Blindness.

★ 3820 ★ International Federation of Oto-Rhino-Laryngological Societies (IFOS) (Federation Internationale des Societes Oto-Rhino-Laryngologiques)
PO Box 124
ZK 1135 Edam, Netherlands
Phone: 31 299 373733 **Fax:** 31 299 373723
Email: ifos@cest-bien.com
Website: http://www.ifosworld.org

Fnded: 1965. **Mem:** 105. **Reg. Groups:** 6. **Lang(s):** English, French, German, Japanese, Spanish. **Desc:** National (105) and international otorhinolaryngological societies (12) in 140 countries. Works to identify critical global ORL care needs and communication disorders, to propose ways to prevent and treat them and to set priorities among these needs according to their impact on society. Promotes the advancement of otorhinolaryngology (ORL), the prevention and control of diseases and disorders of the ear, nose, and throat, and the training of otorhinolaryngologists. Participates, as an affiliate to the World Health Organization, in the Worldwide Prevention Action on Hearing Impairment. Encourages international cooperation between otorhinolaryngologists and members. **Pub:** *IFOS Newsletter*, quarterly. Newsletter. • Films, periodic. • Reports, periodic. • Videos, periodic.

★ 3821 ★ International Federation of Persons with Physical Disabilities (Federation Internationale des Personnes Handicapees Physiques)
Plittersdorfer Strasse 103
D-53173 Bonn, Germany
Phone: 49 228 9359191 **Fax:** 49 228 9359192
Email: fimitic@t-online.de
Website: http://www.fimitic.org

Fnded: 1953. **Mem:** 5000,000. **Lang(s):** English, French, German. **Desc:** National organizations in 28 countries united to promote physical and vocational rehabilitation and full employment for the disabled. Seeks to foster international cooperation in the development of rehabilitation services; sponsors the International Day of the Disabled. Holds seminars. Acts as clearinghouse. **Pub:** *Congress Reports*. • *Nouvelles*, quarterly. Bulletin. **Frmly:** (2000) International Federation of Disabled Workers and Civilan Handicapped.

★ 3822 ★ International Federation of Placenta Associations (IFPA)
c/o Prof. Greg Rice, Sec.
Mercy Perinatal Research Centre
Mercy Hospital for Women
126 Clarendon St.
East Melbourne, VIC 3002, Australia
Phone: 61 3 92702553
Email: ger@placenta.cc
Website: http://www.placenta.cc

Fnded: 1994. **Desc:** Promotes research and development in the area of placentology and trophoblast science.

★ 3823 ★ International Federation of Practitioners of Natural Therapeutics (IFPNT)
21 Bingham Pl.
London W1M 3FH, United Kingdom
Phone: 44 20 79356933

Fnded: 1963.

★ 3824 ★ International Federation of Professional Aromatherapists
82 Ashby Rd.
Leicestershire
Hinckley LE10 1SN, United Kingdom
Phone: 44 1455 637987 **Fax:** 44 1455 890956
Email: admin@ifparoma.org
Website: http://www.ifparoma.org

Fnded: 1990. **Mem:** 2,300. **Nat'l Groups:** 1. **Desc:** Various categories of membership, the main group of which has trained with or meet the high standards required by ISPA accredited schools. Only full membership, members are entitled to use the letter MISPA. To develop and stimulate high professional standards, through qualification and practice. Accredited schools across the country. Local practitioner lists and public hot-line service. **Pub:** *Aromatherapy World*, quarterly. Journal. Also publishes conference transcripts.

★ 3825 ★ International Federation of Psoriasis Associations (IFPA)
6600 SW 92nd, Ste. 300
Portland, OR 97223-7195
Phone: (503)244-7404 **Free:** 800-723-9166
Fax: (503)245-0626
Email: info@ifpa-pso.org
Website: http://www.ifpa-pso.org
Lars Ettarp, Chair

Fnded: 1968. **Mem:** 37,000. **Desc:** Individuals suffering from psoriasis, or psoriatic arthritis, their families and friends. Supports research at various university research centers. Facilitates communication through pen pal programs, group sessions, and other activities. Testifies annually to Congress for psoriasis research. Provides literature to schools and libraries; works with the media to disseminate information on psoriasis. Compiles physician directory. Sponsors regional educational symposia. Established and maintains a public tissue bank for gene research in psoriasis and psoriatic arthritis. **Pub:** *National Psoriasis Foundation–Annual Report*. Annual Report. *Price:* Included in membership dues. • *National Psoriasis Foundation–Bulletin*, bimonthly. Newsletter. Covers psoriasis treatment and research. Includes doctor's question and answer column. *Price:* Included in membership dues. • *National Psoriasis Foundation–Psoriasis Rsource*, 3/year. *Price:* Included in membership dues. • *Psoriasis Forum*, quarterly. Newsletter. Published for medical professionals. *Price:* Included in dues. • Brochures. • Pamphlets. **Frmly:** (2000) National Psoriasis Foundation.

★ 3826 ★ International Federation of Psychoanalytic Societies (IFPS)
c/o Dr. Sonia Gojman
Callejon del Horno No. 6
04000 Villa Coyoacan, Mexico
Phone: 52 55 55546383 **Fax:** 52 55 55540925
Email: sgojman@yahoo.com
Website: http://www.ifp-s.org

Fnded: 1962. **Mem:** 23. **Lang(s):** English, German, Spanish. **Desc:** Psychoanalytic societies in 14 countries. Promotes interest in psychoanalytic theory; encourages information exchange and discussion; fosters practice of psychoanalytic theory. **Pub:** *International Federation of Psychoanalytic Societies–Membership Directory*, periodic. Directory. • *International Forum of Psychoanalysis*, quarterly. Journal. • *Papers*, periodic.

★ 3827 ★ International Federation of Reflexologists
Croydon CRO 1EF, United Kingdom
Phone: 44 181 6679458 **Fax:** 44 181 6499291
Email: ifr44@aol.com
Website: http://www.reflexology-ifr.com

Desc: Promotes reflexology therapist profession enforcing a code of ethics and practice.

★ 3828 ★ International Federation of Societies for Hand Therapy
c/o Corrianne van Velze
PO Box 846
Groenkloof
Pretoria 0027, Republic of South Africa
Phone: 27 12 3462700 **Fax:** 27 12 3462700
Email: vanvelze@afnca.com
Website: http://www.ifsht.org

Fnded: 1985. **Mem:** 26. **Desc:** Works to develop the field of hand therapy. Promotes continuing education, training and networking among members.

★ 3829 ★ International Federation of Societies for Histochemistry and Cytochemistry (IFSHC)
c/o Dr. Denis G. Baskin
Department of Biological Structure
Univ. of Washington
PO Box 357420
Seattle, WA 98195-9420
Phone: (206)616-5894 **Fax:** (206)616-5842
Email: baskindg@u.washington.edu
Website: http://www.ifshc.org
Prof.Dr. Denis G. Baskin, Sec. Gen.

Fnded: 1960. **Mem:** 22. **Nat'l Groups:** 22. **Desc:** National societies for histochemistry and cytochemistry. Seeks to promote communication and cooperation among scientists throughout the world and establish histochemistry and cytochemistry institutes. Promotes histochemistry and cytochemistry as basic, independent sciences and advocates their teaching in universities. Appoints committees for the study of scientific matters requiring international collaboration. **Pub:** *Proceedings*, quadrennial. • Also publishes scientific journals.

★ 3830 ★ International Federation of Societies for Surgery of the Hand (IFSSH)
c/o Dr. James R. Urbaniak
PO Box 2912
Duke University Medical Center
Durham, NC 27710
Phone: (919)684-5388 **Fax:** (919)681-7378
Email: urban006@mc.duke.edu
Website: http://www.handlibrary.org/handsocieties/ifssh/ifsshmain.html
James R. Urbaniak, MD, Sec. Gen.

Fnded: 1966. **Mem:** 5,000. **Reg. Groups:** 43. **Desc:** Individuals involved in hand surgery. Coordinates activities by maintaining liaison among member societies; promotes the exchange of information; attempts to improve opportunities for study and observation on an international level. Establishes and recommends standards of nomenclature, classification of malformations, and disability evaluation; promotes a bibliography of world literature on surgery of the hand. Conducts scientific sessions; maintains committees to develop standards and agreements on special areas of hand surgery. **Pub:** Newsletter, annual.

★ 3831 ★ International Federation of Societies for Surgery of the Hand (IFSSH)
4, bd du President Edwards
F-67000 Strasbourg, France
Phone: 33 3 88354500 **Fax:** 33 3 88240707
Email: ifssh@handlibrary.org

Fnded: 1966. **Desc:** Exchanges knowledge, improving education and research, furthering availability of hand surgery and cooperation among hand surgeons.

★ 3832 ★ International Federation of Sports Chiropractic (FICS)
Chemin de la Joliette 5
CH-1006 Lausanne, Switzerland
Phone: 41 21 6172933 **Fax:** 41 21 6173016
Email: admin@fics-ch.org
Website: http://www.fics-ch.org/

Desc: Works for the promotion of sports chiropractic; promotes chiropractic as an independent health profession.

★ 3833 ★ International Federation for the Surgery of Obesity (IFSO)
c/o Mervyn Deitel, MD, Exec.Dir.
3100 Bayview Ave., Unit 4
Toronto, ON, Canada M2N 5L3
Phone: (416)750-9608 **Fax:** (416)750-9051
Email: journal@obesitysurgery.com
Website: http://www.obesity-online.com/ifso/

Fnded: 1996. **Mem:** 640. **Nat'l Groups:** 31. **Desc:** Promotes the practice of surgery for obesity. **Pub:** *Obesity Surgery Journal*. Journal.

★ 3834 ★ International Federation of Surgical Colleges (IFSC)
c/o SWA Gunn, MD, MS, FRCSC, Hon. Sec.-Gen.
CH-1279 Bogis-Bossey, Switzerland
Phone: 41 22 7762161 **Fax:** 41 22 7766417
Email: donna.muldoon@uphs.upenn.edu

Fnded: 1958. **Mem:** 795. **Nat'l Groups:** 77. **Lang(s):** English. **Desc:** National colleges, academies, and associations of surgery in 77 countries. Works to improve standards of surgery throughout the world. Promotes cooperation and exchange of medical and surgical information among surgical institutions. Encourages high standards of education, training, and research in surgery and its allied sciences. Supports clinical and scientific congresses in the surgical community. Fosters cooperation in developing the best possible standards of surgical facilities and treatment, and in providing appropriate scholarships and surgical training in countries requesting aid. Collaborates with the World Health Organization to strengthen rural surgical health services in developing countries; maintains distribution facility for journals to Third World nations. **Pub:** *IFSC News*, biennial. Newsletter. • *World Journal of Surgery*, monthly. Journal. Additional publications include collected papers.

★ 3835 ★ International Federation of Teratology Societies (IFTS)
Department of Anatomy & Developmental Biology
St. George's Hospital Medical School
University of London
Cramner Terrace
London SW17 0RE, United Kingdom
Phone: 44 208 7252830 **Fax:** 44 208 6727098
Email: ifts@sghms.ac.uk

Fnded: 1983. **Mem:** 2,600. **Reg. Groups:** 4. **Lang(s):** English. **Desc:** Individuals from the European Teratology Society, Teratology Society, Japanese Teratology Society, and Australian Teratology Society. Fosters international cooperation, increased understanding, and a greater interest in the global aspects of teratology. (Teratology is the study of congenital malformations and serious deviations from normal characteristics.) Encourages information exchange and collaboration with health and charitable agencies. Provides education to organizations and individuals interested in prevention and treatment of birth defects. Supports research in the area of teratology.

★ 3836 ★ International Federation for Tropical Medicine
Keppel St.
London WC1E 7HT, United Kingdom
Phone: 44 20 76368739
Email: g.targett@lshtm.ac.uk
Website: http://www.iftm.org

★ 3837 ★ International Fibrodysplasia Ossificans Progressiva Association (IFOPA)
PO Box 196217
Winter Springs, FL 32719-6217
Phone: (407)365-4194 **Fax:** (407)365-3213
Email: together@ifopa.org
Website: http://www.ifopa.org
Jeannie L. Peeper, Pres.

Fnded: 1988. **Mem:** 300. **Desc:** Individuals affected by FOP, their families and friends, and health care professionals. (FOP, also known as fibrodysplasia ossificans progressiva, is a rare genetic disorder in which normal bone is produced in abnormal locations, causing joints to become rigid and immobile. Onset usually occurs during childhood and may eventuate in the complete immobilization of nearly every joint in the body. The cause is currently unknown.) Provides support services to those affected by FOP, including medical resources. Encourages and funds medical research into causes of FOP and other bone-related disorders; promotes public education regarding the disorder and its effects. Facilitates communication among those affected by FOP. **Pub:** *FOP Connection*, quarterly. Newsletter. Including articles on daily coping skills new members, research updates. *Price:* Included in membership dues. **AKA:** International FOP Association.

★ 3838 ★ International Foundation for Functional Gastrointestinal Disorders (IFFGD)
PO Box 170864
Milwaukee, WI 53217
Phone: (414)964-1799 **Free:** 888-964-2001
Fax: (414)964-7176
Email: iffgd@iffgd.org
Website: http://www.iffgd.org

Desc: Promotes gastrointestinal disorders research and provides a voice for patients. **Pub:** *Participate*, quarterly. Offers state-of-the-art information about functional GI disorders.

★ 3839 ★ International Foundation for Stutterers (IFS)
PO Box 462
Belle Mead, NJ 08502
Phone: (609)275-3806
Website: http://www.medhelp.org/amshc/amshc701.htm
Elliot Dennis, Contact

Fnded: 1980. **Mem:** 1,100. **Desc:** Individuals who stutter, their families, speech therapists, and other interested persons. Goal is to provide for the treatment and cure of stuttering through speech therapy in conjunction with selfhelp groups. Believes it is imperative for stutterers to reinforce techniques learned through speech therapy in an atmosphere outside of clinics and with the support of other stutterers. Establishes, maintains, and encourages formation of regional selfhelp groups for individuals undergoing therapy. Aims to make the public aware of the availability of professional treatment for stutterers. Conducts research to examine the causes and treatments of stuttering and to provide findings to the public. Sponsors seminars for speech therapists. Maintains speakers' bureau. **Pub:** *Look Who's Talking*, quarterly. Newsletter. *Price:* $18/year.

★ 3840 ★ International French-Speaking Association of Paraplegic Therapy Groups (Association Francophone Internationale des Groupes d'Animation de la Paraplegie — AFIGAP)
Service de Reeducation Foutionelle
C.H.U. de Nantes
F-44093 Saint Jacques, France
Phone: 33 1 64422081 **Fax:** 33 1 64422082

Fnded: 1976. **Mem:** 180. **Reg. Groups:** 6. **Lang(s):** French. **Desc:** Doctors, nurses, physical therapists, occupational therapists, social workers, and others who have an interest in the treatment and rehabilitation of paraplegics. Purpose is to study and develop all means of advancing the knowledge and treatment of paraplegia. Provides for the exchange of information, publications, and research. Organizes professional training for nurses, physiotherapists, and occupational therapists. **Pub:** *Annuales de Medecine de Reeducation, Readaptation, et Medecin Physique*, periodic. • *Congress Proceedings*, annual. • *Early Treatment of Paraplegia*. Book. • Brochures, periodic.

★ 3841 ★ International Gastric Cancer Association (IGCA)
1-37-1 Kami-ikebukuro, Toshima-ku
Tokyo 170, Japan
Phone: 81 3 39180111 **Fax:** 81 3 39180167

Fnded: 1995.

★ 3842 ★ International Glaucoma Association (IGA)
108C Warner Rd.
Camberwell Hill
London SE5 9HQ, United Kingdom
Phone: 44 20 77373265 **Fax:** 44 20 73465929
Email: info@iga.org.uk
Website: http://www.iga.org.uk

Fnded: 1974. **Mem:** 14,500. **Lang(s):** English. **Desc:** Glaucoma patients. Seeks to educate the public about glaucoma, its causes, detection, and treatment. Provides patients, doctors, opticians, optometrists, and others a forum for the exchange of ideas on glaucoma. Supports research; bestows grants. Conducts surveys; disseminates information. **Pub:** *Glaucoma 98 - A Guide for Patients*, annual. Booklet. • Newsletter, semiannual. • Pamphlets. Leaflets. **Frmly:** (1974) Glaucoma Association.

★ 3843 ★ International Group for Research on Drug Abuse (GRITO)
21, rue d'Assas
F-75270 Paris, France
Phone: 33 1 44395227 **Fax:** 33 1 44395228

Email: fiuc@club-internet.fr

★ 3844 ★ International Guild of Professional Electrologists (IGPE)

803 N Main St., Ste. A
High Point, NC 27262
Phone: (336)841-6631 **Free:** 800-830-3247
Fax: (336)841-5187
Email: igpc@northstate.net
Website: http://www.igpe.org
Trudy Brown, Pres.

Fnded: 1978. **Mem:** 2,200. **Reg. Groups:** 5. **Desc:** Electrologists; electrology schools; manufacturers and suppliers of electrolysis equipment. Works to improve the image of electrolysis and promote it as an acceptable allied health profession. Promotes licensing of electrologists. Provides referral service. Conducts seminars. **Pub:** *A Complete Guide to Hair Removal.* Brochure. • *A Doctor Answers Questions About Hair Removal.* Brochure. • *Consumer Health Guidelines.* Brochure. • *Everything You Ever Wanted to Know About Hair Removal But Were Afraid to Ask.* Brochure. • *International Directory*, annual. Directory. • *International Guild of Professional Electrologists*, quarterly. Newsletter. Includes biennial conference reports. *Price:* Free to members. • *Physical Methods for the Management of Hirsutism.* Brochure. • *Selecting an Electrologist: Thermolysis for Permanent Hair Removal.* Brochure.

★ 3845 ★ International Headache Society (IHS)

Oakwood
9 Willowmead Dr.
Prestbury SKIO 4BU, United Kingdom
Phone: 44 1625 828663 **Fax:** 44 1625 828494
Email: rosemary@ihs.u-net.com
Website: http://www.i-h-s.org

Fnded: 1982. **Desc:** Conducts research into the causes, mechanisms, treatment and other aspects of headache.

★ 3846 ★ International Healthcare Safety Professional Certification Board (IHSPCB)

8009 Carita Ct.
Bethesda, MD 20817
Phone: (301)469-0648
Email: info@chcm-chsp.org
Website: http://www.chcm-chsp.org
Harold M. Gordon, Exec. Dir.

Fnded: 1978. **Desc:** Individuals working or consulting in hospitals or healthcare facilities who are responsible for the handling and control of hazardous materials. Areas of concern include: emergency and disaster planning; biological, chemical, and physical hazards; ventilation; fire prevention and protection; maintenance and engineering; personal protective equipment; sanitation; life safety code. Grants affiliate, associate, and executive level distinctions for the title of Certified Healthcare Safety Professional. Encourages exchange of ideas and technology to improve performance. Sponsors HSP Academy, which conducts professional development activities. **Pub:** *Directory of Certified Healthcare Safety Professionals*, annual. Directory. • Brochure.

★ 3847 ★ International Health Evaluation Association (IHEA)

846 S Hotel St., Ste. 303
Honolulu, HI 96813-2583
Phone: (808)524-4411 **Fax:** (808)524-5559
Website: http://www.ihea.net
Vicki Shambaugh, Exec. VP

Fnded: 1971. **Mem:** 300. **Reg. Groups:** 3. **Desc:** Users, suppliers, and manufacturers of computer-based health evaluation systems including clinics, hospitals, physicians, medical students, and research institutions. Is dedicated to the improvement of health care through: the advancement of computer-based health testing and evaluation techniques; the refinement of associated data-processing systems and biomedical devices; the development of a low-cost, high-quality health programs. Believes the technique of computer-based health evaluation can be used in the areas of testing industrial workers and others exposed to environmental hazards, mandatory tests conducted by governmental agencies, and pre-admission hospital testing. Sponsors seminars on clinical preventive medicine for the discussion of medical results, operational techniques, new applications, and cost-effectiveness data. Conducts research; compiles statistics; maintains library; operates speakers' bureau. **Pub:** *Proceedings of Annual Symposia*, quarterly. Proceedings. *Price:* Free. • *Regional Newsletter*, periodic. Newsletter. • Newsletter, quarterly.

★ 3848 ★ International Health and Safety Association for Radio and Television (IHSART)

c/o Andre Vincke
VRT-2N20
52, Auguste Reyers
B-1043 Brussels, Belgium
Phone: 32 2 7413681 **Fax:** 32 2 7349351
Email: aslak.savolainen@yle.fi

Fnded: 1980. **Mem:** 14. **Lang(s):** English, French. **Desc:** Broadcasting corporations; organizations and individuals interested in the radio and television fields. Seeks to: improve the physical and mental health of radio and television employees; promote safety, hygiene, and preventive medicine as well as better working facilities for radio and television personnel; advance ergonomics, rehabilitation for the handicapped, and the disciplines of industrial medicine. Encourages the collection of statistical and nosological information on the health of television and radio personnel. Conducts research on ergonomics and occupational therapy and medicine. **Pub:** *Newsletter*, annual. Newsletter. • Papers, periodic. Containing information on science and applied medical and paramedical technology. **Frmly:** International Medical Association for Radio and Television.

★ 3849 ★ International Hearing Dog (IHDI)

5901 E 89th Ave.
Henderson, CO 80640
Phone: (303)287-3277 **Fax:** (303)287-3425
Email: ihdi@aol.com
Website: http://www.ihdi.org/
Valerie Foss-Brugger, Pres.

Fnded: 1979. **Desc:** An independent organization formed to train and place dogs, free of cost, with the deaf. Hearing dogs are trained to alert the hearing impaired to important sounds that occur in the owners' environment, such as a door knock or bell, a baby crying, a smoke alarm, an alarm clock, a telephone, a security buzzer, and other sounds which might indicate danger. Presents public awareness demonstrations. **Pub:** *Paws for Silence*, 3/year. Newsletter. Reports on the group's current activities and includes stories about hearing dog recipients. *Price:* Free. **Frmly:** (1981) Hearing Dogs.

★ 3850 ★ International Hearing Society (IHS)

16880 Middlebelt Rd.
Livonia, MI 48154-3367
Phone: (734)522-7200 **Free:** 800-521-5247
Fax: (734)522-0200
Email: rclowers@ihsinfo.org
Website: http://www.ihsinfo.org/
Robin Clowers, BC-HIS, Exec. Dir.

Fnded: 1951. **Mem:** 3,000. **State Groups:** 54. **Desc:** Hearing aid specialists who test hearing for the selection, adaptation, fitting, adjusting, servicing, and sale of hearing aids. Members counsel the hearing impaired and instruct them in care and use of hearing aids. Activities include: administration of a qualification program for screening persons designated as Hearing Instrument Specialists; administration of a consumer information program; publication of information and research concerning hearing health care; establishment of standards of education, equipment, and techniques in the fitting of hearing aids; cooperation with other professional organizations engaged in hearing health care; cooperation and consultation with government officials and agencies in the development of policies and legislation. Accredits seminars and workshops for the education of hearing aid specialists. Maintains the National Institute for Hearing Instruments Studies as the educational arm of the society. **Pub:** *The Hearing Professional*, bimonthly. Journal. Contains technical articles, business information, and news for hearing health professionals. Includes annual index, chapter news, and book reviews. *Price:* Free to members; $45/year for others; $35 foreign. • *International Hearing Society–Directory of Members*, annual. Membership Directory. Arranged geographically and alphabetically. Includes supplemental directory of manufacturers, suppliers, hearing aid designers, and others. • *International Hearing Society-Professional Association of Hearing Instrument Specialists.* Brochures. • *World of Sound.* Pamphlets. • Books. • Brochures. • Also publishes bylaws and code of ethics. **Frmly:** (1966) Society of Hearing Aid Audiologists; (1990) National Hearing Aid Society.

★ 3851 ★ International Homeopathic Medical League

c/o Ulrich Fischer, Sec.
Grunwalderstrasse 10-14
D-79098 Freiburg, Germany
Email: generalsecretary@lmhi.net
Website: http://www.lmhi.org.mx

Fnded: 1925. **Desc:** Creates links between homeopathic trained doctors, surgeons and pharmacists. Promotes scientific research.

★ 3852 ★ International Hospital Federation (IHF) (Federacion Internacional de Hospitales)

Immeuble JB SAY
13 Chemin de Levant
F-01210 Ferney-Voltaire, France
Phone: 33 450426000 **Fax:** 33 450426001
Email: info@ihf-fih.org
Website: http://www.hospitalmanagement.net

Fnded: 1929. **Mem:** 1,694. **Reg. Groups:** 1. **Lang(s):** English, French, Spanish. **Desc:** Individuals (1117); organizations (388); professional firms (114); government representatives (75). Promotes improvement in the planning and management of hospitals and health services through study tours, publications, and research and development projects. Serves as an advocate for hospitals and related health service organizations in world health affairs. Sponsors regional conferences and courses for senior hospital and health services managers from developing countries. Compiles statistics. **Pub:** *Health Service International*, quarterly. Newsletter. • *Hospitals International*, quarterly. Newsletter. • *World Hospitals*, 3/year. Journal. Includes summaries in French and Spanish.

★ 3853 ★ International Huntington Association (IHA)

Callunahof 8
NL-7217 ST Harfsen, Netherlands
Phone: 31 573 431595 **Fax:** 31 573 431719
Email: iha@huntington-assoc.com
Website: http://www.huntington-assoc.com

Fnded: 1974. **Mem:** 52. **Nat'l Groups:** 41. **Lang(s):** Dutch, English, German. **Desc:** National health agencies concerned about Huntington's disease. (Huntington's disease is an inherited neurological disorder causing physical, emotional, and cognitive deterioration.) Promotes international cooperation in efforts to find a cure for Huntington's disease. Serves as a clearinghouse on Huntington's disease and related research. Maintains liaison with scientists and scientific organizations engaged in work pertaining to Huntington's disease worldwide. Assists in the establishment of new Huntington's disease associations and in the establishment of international collaborative research efforts to find a cure for the disease. Provides support and services to people with Huntington's disease and their families; conducts educational programs for health care professionals treating people with Huntington's disease and the public. **Pub:** *Living With HD Your Guide to Effective Eating and Diet.* Brochures. • *Nutrition and Huntington's Disease.* Books.

★ 3854 ★ International Institute on Ageing
c/o United Nations - Malta
117 St. Paul's St.
Valletta VLT 07, Malta
Phone: 356 21 243044 **Fax:** 356 21 230248
Email: info@inia.org.mt
Website: http://www.inia.org.mt

Fnded: 1988. **Lang(s):** English. **Desc:** Gerontologists and other individuals with an interest in the aging process. Seeks to advance medical understanding of aging; promotes development of new gerontological practices to improve the quality of life of the elderly. Serves as a forum for the exchange of information among members; sponsors research and educational programs. **Pub:** *BOLD*, quarterly. Journal. Contains scientific articles by international scholars/experts in the field of aging.

★ 3855 ★ International Institute for Bioenergetic Analysis (IIBA)
Steinackerstrasse 10
Udorf
CH-8902 Zurich, Switzerland
Phone: 41 43 4559152 **Fax:** 41 43 4559154
Email: iiba.schweiz@bluewin.ch
Website: http://www.bioenergetic-therapy.com

Fnded: 1956. **Mem:** 1,700. **Reg. Groups:** 50. **Lang(s):** English, French, Italian, Portuguese, Spanish. **Desc:** Works to promote research and education in the fields of mental and physical health as they relate to biological energy processes. Areas of interest include: the role of muscle tension in emotional and physical illness, relationship of body structure and body movement, energy dynamics, disturbances in motility as a factor in illness, genetic factors, principles and methods of therapy, and growth and development of the child in response to patterns of child rearing. Conducts lectures, 1-day patient workshops, professional weekend workshops, seminars, and exercise classes. **Pub:** *Bioenergetic Analysis*, periodic. Journal. • Books. • Brochures. • Membership Directory, periodic. • Papers. **Frmly:** (1979) Institute for Bioenergetic Analysis.

★ 3856 ★ International Institute of Concern for Public Health (IICPH)
2300 Lawrence Ave. E
Toronto, ON, Canada M1P 4Z5
Phone: (416)755-3685
Email: info@iicph.org
Website: http://www.iicph.org

Fnded: 1984. **Mem:** 80. **Lang(s):** English, French, Spanish. **Desc:** Promotes dissemination of information on public health and related topics including environmental and occupational health and human rights. Serves as a clearinghouse on international public health and related issues; assists in the development of model health-related human rights legislation. Conducts research and educational programs; compiles statistics; maintains speakers' bureau. Provides support and assistance to communities wishing to maintain their own public health databases. **Pub:** *International Perspectives in Public Health*, annual. Journal. • Newsletter, bimonthly. Contains articles relating to the environment, work and health.

★ 3857 ★ International Institute of Reflexology
5650 1st Ave. N
PO Box 12642
Saint Petersburg, FL 33733-2642
Phone: (727)343-4811 **Fax:** (727)381-2807
Email: iir@tampabay.rr.com
Website: http://www.reflexology-usa.net/

Fnded: whic. **Mem:** h corre,spo. **Reg. Groups:** rgans,. **State Groups:** f the. **Desc:** Promotes the ancient art of reflexology, scientifically based on the premise that there are zones and reflex areas in the feet and hands which correspond to all glands, organs, parts and systems of the body.

★ 3858 ★ International Institute of Reflexology (IIR)
255 Turleigh
Bradford-on-Avon BA15 2HG, United Kingdom
Phone: 44 1225 865899 **Fax:** 44 1225 865899
Email: reflexology_uk@hotmail.com
Website: http://www.reflexology-uk.co.uk

Desc: Dedicated to professional standards in reflexology based on the Ingham Method of Foot Reflexology.

★ 3859 ★ International Iridology Practitioner's Association (IIPA)
c/o Central Office
PO Box 3334
Escondido, CA 92033
Free: 888-682-2208 **Fax:** 888-682-2208
Email: iridology@ssn.org
Website: http://www.iridologyassn.org
Dr. Ellen Tart-Jensen, Pres.

Fnded: 1982. **Mem:** 300. **Desc:** Organization for professional Iridologists who study the eye for indications of body stresses that may influence health. Offers members educational classes and information, conventions, research and certification. **Pub:** *IIPA Insights*, quarterly. Newsletter. Contains news in the field of iridology. *Price:* included in membership dues. • *The Iridology Review*, quarterly. Article. Presents research in Iridology. **Frmly:** (1999) National Iridology Reserach Association; (2002) International Iridology Research Association.

★ 3860 ★ International Lawyers in Alcoholics Anonymous (ILAA)
c/o Ben Graham
PO Box 552212
Las Vegas, NV 89155-2212
Phone: (702)870-5466 **Fax:** (702)455-9597
Email: grahamr@co.clark.nv.us
Website: http://www.ilaa.org
Ben Graham, Sec.

Fnded: 1975. **Mem:** 1,300. **Desc:** Alcoholic lawyers who are seeking sobriety through their affiliation with Alcoholics Anonymous World Services. Seeks to: spread the message of AA to alcoholic attorneys; work to educate the judiciary and lawyers on the problem of alcoholism; support attorneys in their recovery. **Pub:** *ILAA*, 3-4/year. Newsletter.

★ 3861 ★ International League Against Epilepsy (ILAE)
Ave. Marcel Thiry 204
B-1200 Brussels, Belgium
Phone: 32 2 7749547 **Fax:** 32 2 7749690
Email: dsartiaux@ilae-epilepsy.org
Website: http://www.ilae-epilepsy.org

Fnded: 1909. **Mem:** 84. **Lang(s):** Dutch, English, French, German. **Desc:** National organizations united to encourage scientific research on epilepsy, and to promote optimal treatment and rehabilitation of epileptic patients. Fosters development of and cooperation among associations with common interests. **Pub:** *Epigraph*, 2/year. Newsletter. • *Epilepsia*, monthly. Journal. Contains scientific papers and meeting abstracts for professional researchers in the field of epilepsy. Includes book reviews and research reports.

★ 3862 ★ International League of Associations for Rheumatology (ILAR)
c/o Prof. Tahsin El-Hadidi
38, Kambiz St.
Dokki
Cairo 12311, Egypt
Phone: 20 2 760 9344
Email: thadidi@ilarportal.org
Website: http://www.ilar.org

Fnded: 1927. **Mem:** 12,000. **Nat'l Groups:** 63. **Reg. Groups:** 3. **Lang(s):** English. **Desc:** Physicians interested in rheumatism. Promotes research and education in rheumatic disease. Facilitates communication among members and with United Nations Educational, Scientific and Cultural Organization and World Health Organization. **Pub:** *Handbook*, quadrennial. Also publishes proceedings. **Frmly:** (2002) International League Against Rheumatism.

★ 3863 ★ International League of Dermatological Societies (ILDS)
PO Box 35069
Sarasota, FL 34242
Phone: (941)346-1226 **Fax:** (941)927-1936
Email: mtgmgr@gte.net
Website: http://www.ilds.org/
Barbara Nichols, Admin. Officer

Fnded: 1957. **Mem:** 102. **Nat'l Groups:** 102. **Desc:** Works to stimulate cooperation between dermatology societies and encourage worldwide advancement of the profession. Promotes personal and professional relations among the dermatologists of the world. Provides educational programs; represents dermatology in commissions and health organizations. **Pub:** Directory, annual. • Newsletter, quarterly.

★ 3864 ★ International Leprosy Association (Societe Internationale Contre la Lepre)
Royal Tropical Institute
135 Wibautstraat
NL-1097 DN Amsterdam, Netherlands
Phone: 31 20 6939297 **Fax:** 31 20 6680823

Lang(s): Dutch, English. **Desc:** Health care professionals and medical researchers. Seeks to lessen the incidence of leprosy worldwide; promotes development of more effective leprosy treatments. Serves as a clearinghouse on leprosy and its prevention, diagnosis, and treatment. Sponsors research; conducts educational programs.

★ 3865 ★ International Life Sciences Institute - North America (ILSINA)
One Thomas Cir. NW, 9th Fl.
Washington, DC 20005
Phone: (202)659-0074 **Fax:** (202)659-3859
Email: ilsi@ilsi.org
Website: http://www.ilsi.org
PhD Richard Black, PhD, Exec. Dir.

Fnded: 1985. **Mem:** 44. **Desc:** Advances the understanding of scientific issues related to the nutritional quality and safety of the food supply, as well as health issues related to consumer self-care products. Sponsors relevant research programs, professional education programs and workshops, seminars, and publications, as well as providing a neutral forum for government, academic, and industry scientists to discuss and resolve scientific issues of common concern for the well-being of the general public. Fosters career development of outstanding new scientists. Programs are supported primarily by its industry membership. Also publishes monographs, reprints, scientific reports, and educational materials. **Frmly:** (1991) International Life Sciences Institute - Nutrition Foundation.

★ 3866 ★ International Liver Transplantation Society (ILTS)
17000 Commerce Pkwy, Ste. C
Mount Laurel, NJ 08054
Phone: (856)439-0500 **Fax:** (856)439-0525
Email: ilts@ahint.com
Website: http://www.ilts.org
Michael F. Sorrell, MD, Pres.

Fnded: 1992. **Mem:** 700. **Desc:** Individuals interested in liver transplantation. Seeks to educate members on liver transplantation. Offers post graduate courses and mini-symposia. **Pub:** *Liver Transplantation and Surgery*, bimonthly. Journal.

★ 3867 ★ International Maritime Health Association (IMHA)
Italielei 51
B-2000 Antwerp, Belgium
Phone: 32 3 2250015 **Fax:** 32 3 2252038
Email: imha@online.be
Website: http://www.imha.net/

Fnded: 1997. **Desc:** Fosters scientific research and the quality of maritime medicine worldwide; creates a forum for people, ideas, efforts, research and questions regarding maritime health.

★ 3868 ★ International Massage Association (IMA)
PO Drawer 421
Warrenton, VA 20188
Phone: (540)351-0800 **Free:** 800-933-7113
Fax: (540)351-0816
Email: info@imagroup.com
Website: http://www.imagroup.com
Will Green, Pres.

Fnded: 1994. **Mem:** 48,000. **Desc:** Professional massage practitioners and massage schools. Promotes unification of massage practitioners, regardless of technique or training. Provides services to members including credit card merchant accounts, industry discounts, personal business assistance and free internet advertising. Makes available professional insurance policies and health care plan to members. **Pub:** *IMA Success*. Newsletter.

★ 3869 ★ International Medical and Dental Hypnotherapy Association (IMDHA)
4110 Edgeland, Ste. 800
Royal Oak, MI 48073-2285
Phone: (248)549-5594 **Fax:** (248)549-5421
Email: aspencer@infinityinst.com
Website: http://www.infinityinst.com
Anne H. Spencer, PhD, Exec. Dir.

Fnded: 1987. **Mem:** 1,500. **State Groups:** 18. **Local Groups:** 2. **Desc:** Certified hypnotherapists; associate members are non-certified hypnotherapists and individuals interested in hypnosis. Hypnotherapists help to mentally prepare patients to deal with the stress and pain involved with medical and dental procedures. Offers certification courses. Maintains an International Referral Directory which lists certified members. Maintains speakers' bureau and library on hypnosis and mind development. Offers educational programs. Has affiliate Hypnosis training schools. Has free Email Hypnosis and Holistic Living Journal written monthly. Offers Specialty Certifications to certified members at annual Educational Conference. **Pub:** *Hypnosis and Holistic Health*. Journal. • *Subconsciously Speaking: You Can Change Your Life Through the Powers of Your Mind*, bimonthly. Newsletter. Contains articles of interest including hypnosis, imagery, holistic health, and consciousness. *Price:* Included in membership dues; $14/year to nonmembers in U.S. • Articles.

★ 3870 ★ International Medical Informatics Association (IMIA)
5782 172th St.
Edmonton, AB, Canada T6M 1B4
Phone: (780)489-4531 **Fax:** (780)489-3290
Email: info@imia.org
Website: http://www.imia.org

Fnded: 1978. **Mem:** 78. **Nat'l Groups:** 45. **Reg. Groups:** 4. **Lang(s):** English. **Desc:** National organizations in the field of medical and health informatics. Objective is the international exchange of knowledge concerning health care and biomedical research through medical informatics. Sponsors conferences. **Pub:** *IMIA Yearbook*, annual. Yearbook.

★ 3871 ★ International Medical Informatics Association for Latin America and the Caribbean (IMIA-LAC)
PO Box 6005
13081-970 Campinas, Brazil
Phone: 55 19 2899800 **Fax:** 55 19 2894959
Email: sabbatin@nib.unicamp.br

Fnded: 1983.

★ 3872 ★ International Medical Services for Health (INMED)
45449 Severn Way, Ste. 161
Sterling, VA 20166
Phone: (703)444-4477 **Free:** 800-521-1175
Fax: (703)444-4471
Email: contact@inmed.org
Website: http://www.inmed.org
Linda Pfeiffer, PhD, Pres.

Fnded: 1986. **Desc:** Works to help disadvantaged people worldwide to improve the health of their families and communities. Assists community based programs in 98 countries to achieve lasting changes for better health. Operates MotherNet America, a lay home visiting program to reduce infant mortality, low birthweight, child abuse and neglect and other risks facing disadvantaged families; conducts the Children as Agents of Change treatment and education program; links businesses and non-profit organizations in strategic alliances; provides access to medicine for non-profit organizations; offers technical assistance and training. **Pub:** *InScope*, quarterly. Newsletter.

★ 3873 ★ International Medical Society for Bio-Physical Information-Therapy Association (Internationale Arzte-Gesellschaft fur Biophysikalische Informations-Therapie e.V.)
Sandstr 19
D-72104 Freiburg, Germany
Phone: 49 761 53380 **Fax:** 49 761 57522
Email: info@bit-org.de
Website: http://www.bit-org.de

Desc: Promotes research and practice of magnetic field therapy.

★ 3874 ★ International Menopause Society
c/o Monique Boulet chez Maitre M. Steyaert
3/1 Av. des Cattleyas
B-1150 Brussels, Belgium
Phone: 32 2 7722183 **Fax:** 32 2 7624295
Email: imsociety@filink.net
Website: http://www.imsociety.org

Fnded: 1978. **Mem:** 800. **Nat'l Groups:** 30. **Lang(s):** English. **Desc:** Medical doctors, sociologists, psychologists, anthropologists, and others in 42 countries interested in basic research and clinical work in the field of menopause and climacteric. Objectives are to promote study of medical, sociological, and psychological aspects of the climacteric, or menopausal stage in men and women and to advance international exchange of information and research plans. Studies subjects such as anatomy, gynecology, biochemistry, cardiology, etc...and psychology as they relate to the aging process; examines methods of management, preventive measures, and therapeutic problems related to aging. **Pub:** *Climacteric*, quarterly. Journal. • *Newsletter*, 4/year. Newsletter. • *Proceedings of World Congress*, triennial.

★ 3875 ★ International Microsurgical Society
Via Sabbioni, 10
I-25050 Rome, Italy
Fax: 39 06 6852516

★ 3876 ★ International MS Support Foundation (IMSSF)
9420 E Golf Links Rd., No. 291
Tucson, AZ 85720-1340
Website: http://www.msnews.org/

Desc: Dedicated to providing support, education and resources to individuals, families and friends of those suffering from Multiple Sclerosis.

★ 3877 ★ International Musculoskeletal Laser Society (IMLAS)
The Arbury Centre
Manchester Rd.
Rochdale OL11 4LZ, United Kingdom
Phone: 44 1706 358229 **Fax:** 44 1706 353166
Email: imlas@imlas.org
Website: http://www.imlas.org/

Fnded: 1993. **Mem:** 350. **Nat'l Groups:** 27. **Desc:** Advances the development of medical laser techniques, mainly in the muscoloskeletal system.

★ 3878 ★ International Myeloma Foundation (IMF)
12650 Riverside Dr., Ste. 206
North Hollywood, CA 91607
Phone: (818)487-7455 **Free:** 800-452-CURE
Fax: (818)487-7454
Email: theimf@myeloma.org
Website: http://www.myeloma.org
Susie Novis, Pres.

Fnded: 1990. **Mem:** 95,000. **Local Groups:** 57. **Desc:** The International Myeloma Foundation is a non-profit organization dedicated to the education, treatment and research of multiple myeloma, a little-known cancer of the bone marrow. We provide a variety of patient and physician education and support programs and services. **Pub:** *A Concise Review of the Disease and Treatment Options*. Book. • *Myeloma Today*, bimonthly. Newsletter. *Price:* Free for U.S. subscribers; $15 international subscribers. • *Patient Handbook*. Book. • *"So You're Considering..."*. Brochure.

★ 3879 ★ International Myopain Society (IMS)
c/o Barbara Runnels
PO Box 690402
San Antonio, TX 78269
Phone: (210)567-4661 **Fax:** (210)567-6669
Email: russell@uthscsa.edu
Website: http://www.myopain.org/
Robert M. Bennett, MD, Pres.

Desc: Research scientists, physicians, other health care professionals, individuals in training toward a health-related career, institutions, foundations, and commercial companies. Promotes information exchange, research, and education about soft tissue pain syndrome such as myofascial pain syndrome and fibromyalgia syndrome. **Pub:** *Journal of Musculoskeletal Pain*, quarterly. Journal. Devoted to the topic of soft tissue pain.

★ 3880 ★ International Nanny Association (INA)
191 Clarksville Rd.
Princeton Junction, NJ 08550
Fax: (856)858-2519
Email: ina@nanny.org
Website: http://www.nanny.org
Pat Cascio, Pres.

Fnded: 1985. **Mem:** 700. **Nat'l Groups:** 1. **Desc:** An educational association for nannies and those who educate, place, employ, and support professional in-home child care. Membership is open to those who are directly involved with the in-home child care profession, including nannies, nanny employers, nanny placement agency owners (and staff), nanny educators, and providers of special services related to the nanny profession. **Pub:** *A Nanny for Your Family*. Brochure. *Price:* $0.30/each for members; $0.40/each for nonmembers. • *Beyond Peanut Butter and Jelly*. *Price:* $19.95 + 4.95 shipping. • *Directory of Nanny Placement Agencies, Training Programs and Special Services*, annual. Directory. *Price:* $19.95/year. • *Family and Nanny Agreement*. *Price:* $50. • *INA Vision*. Newsletter. *Price:* Included in membership dues. • *Recommended Competencies for the Education of Nurses*. • *Recommended Practices for Nannies*. • *Recommended Practices for Nanny Placement Agencies*. • *So You Want to Be a Nanny*. Brochure. *Price:* $0.30/each for members; $0.40/each for nonmembers.

★ 3881 ★ International Network for Cancer Treatment and Research (INCTR)
Institut Pasteur
Rue England 642
B-1180 Brussels, Belgium
Phone: 32 2 3739323 **Fax:** 32 2 3739313
Email: edupont@inctr.de
Website: http://www.inctr.org/

Fnded: 1998. **Desc:** Seeks to build capacities for cancer treatment and research in countries where such capacities are currently limited. **Pub:** Newsletter, quarterly.

★ 3882 ★ International Network for the History of Public Health (INHPH)
c/o Marie C. Nelson
The Tema Institute
Linkoping University
S-58183 Linkoping, Sweden
Phone: 46 13 282808 **Fax:** 46 13 281843
Email: marne@tema.liu.se
Website: http://www.liu.se/tema/inhph

Fnded: 1992. **Mem:** 332. **Lang(s):** English. **Desc:** Scholars throughout the world who are interested in history of public health. Promotes the study of the history of the collective efforts for the improvement of the health of populations from antiquity to modern times. Seeks to improve communication among scholars in the field and promotes comparative research efforts. **Pub:** *Hygiea Internationalis: An Interdisciplinary Journal for the History of Public Health.* Journal. Refereed electronic journal with limited paper copies.

★ 3883 ★ International Network Towards Smoke-free Hospitals
c/o John Bickerstaff, Gen.Sec.
45 Brookscroft
Linton Glade
Croydon CR0 9NA, United Kingdom
Phone: 44 20 86515436 **Fax:** 44 20 86513428
Email: jbickerstaff@cix.co.uk

Fnded: 1991. **Lang(s):** English. **Desc:** Physicians, nurses, hospital administrators, healthcare workers, and other interested parties. Seeks to protect, preserve, and improve the health of patients, visitors, and person working in hospitals or in connection with health services, in the U.K. and overseas, by promoting smoke-free environments in hospitals and other healthcare facilities. Provides advice and briefings to hospitals wishing to become smoke-free. **Pub:** *Making Hospitals Smoke Free.* • *Smoke-Free Hospitals International.*

★ 3884 ★ International Neural Network Society (INNS)
19 Mantua Rd.
Mount Royal, NJ 08061
Phone: (856)423-0162 **Fax:** (856)423-3420
Email: innshq@talley.com
Website: http://www.inns.org
Lee Feldkamp, Pres.

Fnded: 1987. **Mem:** 1,000. **Desc:** Individuals interested in theoretical and computational understanding of the brain. Provides a forum for neurocomputing and theoretical approaches to neuroscience. Promotes research into behavioral processes and models of the brain. Encourages development of computing applications which use neural modeling concepts. **Pub:** *INNS Newsletter*, 9/year. Newsletter. Includes calendar of events and special interest group information. • *Neural Networks*, bimonthly. Journal.

★ 3885 ★ International Neuro-Linguistic Programming Association (INLPA)
42 Spruce Ridge
Route 9P
Saratoga Springs, NY 12866
Phone: (518)587-3478
Email: info@inlpa.org
Website: http://www.inlpa.org
Laura Shaw, Mgr.

Fnded: 1983. **Mem:** 1,300. **Reg. Groups:** 9. **Desc:** Certified neuro-linguistic programming practitioners and programmers (355); certified master programmers (393); certified NLP trainers (152); individuals with some training in NLP (400). (NLP is a discipline that examines the structure of human thought and response and is used in counseling, psychotherapy, and business applications.) Provides an international network for the exchange of ideas, materials, and services. Sets standards for the ethical use of NLP and for NLP training and certification. Encourages and supports research and development; fosters utilization of new technologies in NLP; seeks to integrate the skills and ideas of other disciplines with those of NLP. Promotes greater public understanding of NLP and its objectives. Sponsors NLP workshops. Cooperates with other professional organizations. **Pub:** *IANLP*, annual. Membership Directory. • Newsletter, bimonthly. **Frmly:** (1991) International Association for Neuro-Linguistic Programming; (1993) International Association of Neuro-Linguistic Programming; (1995) North American Association of Neuro-Linguistic Programming; (2003) International Association of Neuro-Linguistic Programming.

★ 3886 ★ International Neuromodulation Society
c/o Tia Sofatzis
2000 Van Ness Ave., Ste. 402
San Francisco, CA 94109
Phone: (415)567-1219 **Fax:** (415)567-2534
Email: tiasofatzis@aol.com
Website: http://www.neuromodulation.com
Tia Sofatzis, Contact

Fnded: 1994. **Mem:** 400. **Nat'l Groups:** 1. **Reg. Groups:** 5. **Desc:** Individuals with an interest in implantable technologies that impact on the nervous system. Promotes advancement of neuromodulation technologies and techniques; encourages continuing professional development of members. Serves as a forum for the exchange of scientific information on neuromodulation; conducts research and educational programs. **Pub:** *Neuromodulation*, quarterly. Journal. *Price:* included in membership dues.

★ 3887 ★ International Neuromodulation Society (INS)
Swiss Paraplegic Centre
CH-6207 Nottwil, Switzerland
Phone: 41 41 4603010 **Fax:** 41 41 4603033

★ 3888 ★ International Nurses Anonymous (INA)
c/o Kathy Kavanaugh R.N.
68 Farrington Rd.
Croton on Hudson, NY 10520
Phone: (914)271-3517
Email: wkavanaugh@aol.com
Website: http://members.aol.com/IntNursesAnon
Kathy Kavanaugh, Sec. -Treas.

Fnded: 1988. **Mem:** 500. **Desc:** Nurses, nursing students, and former nurses who are involved in a 12-step recovery program. Provides mutual support and networking; serves as a resource for newly recovering nurses. **Pub:** *INA Newsletter*, semiannual. Newsletter. *Price:* Free to members.

★ 3889 ★ International Nurses Society on Addictions (NNSA)
PO Box 10752
Raleigh, NC 27605
Phone: (919)821-1292 **Fax:** (919)833-5743
Email: snow@uta.edu
Website: http://www.intnsa.org
Diane Snow, Pres.

Fnded: 1975. **Mem:** 800. **Reg. Groups:** 10. **Desc:** Promotes quality nursing care for persons addicted to alcohol and other drugs, and their families. Fosters continuing education and development of skills among nurses involved in the field; works to enhance the professional image of addictions nurses. Participates in public policy and social issues related to alcohol or chemical abuse. Serves as liaison between members and professional groups with common goals. Represents members' interests before national organizations. Regional groups sponsor workshops. Provides certification program. **Pub:** *The Care of Clients with Addictions: Dimensions of Nursing Practice and Standards of Addictions.* Book. • *The Core Curriculum of Addictions Nursing.* Book. • *NNSA Today*, quarterly. Newsletter. Includes articles on clinical and research areas of addictions field. *Price:* Available to members only. • *Nursing Care Planning with the Addicted Client.* Book. • *Nursing Practice with Selected Diagnoses and Criteria.* Book. • Booklets. • Monographs. • Papers. **Frmly:** (1983) National Nurses Society on Alcoholism; (2001) National Nurses Society on Addictions.

★ 3890 ★ International Ocular Inflammation Society (IOIS)
Avda de Denia, III
E-03015 Alicante, Spain
Phone: 34 96 5150025 **Fax:** 34 96 5151501
Email: secretariat@iois.org
Website: http://www.iois.org

★ 3891 ★ International Organization Against Trachoma (IOAT) (Organisation Internationale pour la Lutte Contre le Trachome)
Hospital de Creteil
Universite de Paris-Val de Marne
40, ave. de Verdun
F-94010 Creteil, France
Phone: 33 1 45175225 **Fax:** 33 1 45175227
Email: gabriel.coscas@libertysurf.fr

Fnded: 1923. **Mem:** 1,200. **Lang(s):** English, French. **Desc:** Circulates information in 20 countries on current trachoma research (trachoma is a chronic, contagious eye disease) and supplies the latest information on etiology, diagnosis, epidemiology, prevention, and treatment, thus providing a scientific basis for the fight against the disease. Promotes research on trachoma; facilitates the adoption of sanitary and other regulations aimed at implementing the fight against trachoma. Maintains close contact with the World Health Organization and other institutions engaged in the fight against trachoma. **Pub:** *Revue Internationale du Trachome*, semiannual. Journal.

★ 3892 ★ International Organization for Cooperation in Health Care (IOCHC) (Medicus Mundi International — MMI)
64, rue des Deux Eglises
B-1210 Brussels, Belgium
Phone: 32 2 2310605 **Fax:** 32 2 2311852
Email: info@medicusmundi.be
Website: http://www.medicusmundi.org

Fnded: 1963. **Mem:** 11. **Nat'l Groups:** 8. **Lang(s):** English, French. **Desc:** National branches and organizations of physicians and paramedical personnel. Promotes the fields of health care and disease prevention as a necessary part of development of all nations. Encourages primary health care through comprehensive, integrated, long-term health programs. Documents socio-medical information on developing countries to assess the medical needs and demands of those countries. Other aims include: encouraging dialogue with the Third World; strengthening relations between national branches and European governments; profiling experts serving IOHC; providing field workers with practical conclusions, recommendations, and moral support regarding new strategies, methods, or operations. Offers training programs. **Pub:** Newsletter, quarterly. • Proceedings, periodic. Contains meeting reports.

★ 3893 ★ International Organization for Forensic Odonto-Stomatology (IOFOS)
c/o Tore Solheim
Department of Pathology
Boks 1109
Blindern
N-0317 Oslo, Norway

Phone: 47 22852359 **Fax:** 47 22852351
Email: solheim@odont.uio.no

Fnded: 1973. **Mem:** 1,500. **Nat'l Groups:** 30. **Lang(s):** English. **Desc:** National professional societies active in the field of forensic odonto-stomatology. Promotes forensic dentistry worldwide. Fosters cooperation among members; collects and disseminates information and ideas on forensic dentistry. Compiles statistics. Supports educational and research programs. **Pub:** *Forensic Odontology, Its Scope and History*. Book. Out of Print, but obtainable through co. Pres. • *International Journal of Forensic Odonto-Homatology*. Journal. • *IOFOS Newsletter*, 3/year. Newsletter. • *The Journal of Forensic Odonto-Stomatology*, semiannual. **Frmly:** (1981) International Society of Forensic Odonto-Stomatology.

★ 3894 ★ International Organization for Medical Physics (IOMP)
c/o Gary D. Fullerton, PhD
Department of Radiology
MSC 7800
7703 Floyd Curl Dr.
San Antonio, TX 78229-3900
Phone: (210)567-5551 **Fax:** (210)567-5549
Email: fullertson@uthscsa.edu
Website: http://www.iomp.org/
Gary D. Fullerton, PhD, Sec. Gen.

Fnded: 1963. **Mem:** 56. **Desc:** A member of the International Union of Physical and Engineering Sciences in Medicine. National organizations of medical physics representing 10,000 individuals. Fosters international cooperation in medical physics; promotes communication between various branches of medical physics and allied subjects. Conducts training programs. Has established 43 libraries in developing countries. **Pub:** *Clinical Physics and Physiological Measurement*, bimonthly. • *Medical Physics World*, semiannual. • *Physics in Medicine and Biology*, monthly.

★ 3895 ★ International Organization of Psychophysiology (IOP) (Organisation Internationale de Psychophysiologie — IOP)
Douglas Hospital, McGill University
6875 LaSalle Blvd.
Montreal, QC, Canada H4H 1R3
Phone: (514)761-6131 **Fax:** (514)762-3031
Email: iop@iop-world.org
Website: http://www.iop-world.org

Fnded: 1982. **Nat'l Groups:** 45. **Lang(s):** English, French. **Desc:** Scientists who hold a Ph.D., M.D., or equivalent degree and who specialize in psychophysiology or one of the neurosciences. (Psychophysiology is the study of the physiology of the psychic functions through the brain-body-behavior interrelationships of the living organism in conjunction with the environment.) Undertakes and promote psychophysiological research, teaching, and applications worldwide. Seeks to develop guidelines for the improvement of the human psychophysiological condition throughout the world. Disseminates information on subjects including aggression and defense, evolution and development of behavior, information processing, interhemispneric relations, learning and memory, motivation and emotion, and psychophysiological disorders. Collaborates with the United Nations and its specialized agencies with the aim of reinforcing international scientific cooperation in psychophysiology and related fields for the good of the human race. Maintains International Centre of Psychophysiology, providing research, practice, and training opportunities for qualified graduates. **Pub:** *International Journal of Psychophysiology*, monthly. Journal. • *IOP Newsletter*, quarterly. Newsletter.

★ 3896 ★ International Orthoptic Association (IOA)
c/o Mrs. Bronia Unwin
Moorfields Eye Hospital
Orthoptic Department
City Rd.
London EC1B 2PD, United Kingdom
Phone: 44 171 5662163 **Fax:** 44 171 3885066
Website: http://home.vicnet.net.au/~ioaorth/

Fnded: 1967. **Mem:** 4,000. **Lang(s):** English. **Desc:** Orthoptists in 22 countries certified to treat defects in binocular vision, faulty visual habits, and low visual acuity. Organizes and conducts an international congress of orthoptists; shares information through newsletters. **Pub:** *Abstracts of Congress*, quadrennial. Journal. • *Newsletter*, annual. Newsletter.

★ 3897 ★ International Osteoporosis Foundation - France (IOF)
71, cours Albert-Thomas
F-69447 Lyon Cedex 03; France
Phone: 33 4 72914177 **Fax:** 33 4 72369052
Email: info@osteofound.org
Website: http://www.osteofound.org/iof

Fnded: 1987. **Mem:** 240. **Desc:** Works to advance the understanding of osteoporosis; promotes prevention, diagnosis and treatment of the disease worldwide. Lobbies for policy changes.

★ 3898 ★ International Ostomy Association (IOA)
c/o British Colostomy Association
15 Station Rd.
Reading RG1 1LG, United Kingdom
Phone: 44 1189 391537 **Fax:** 44 1189 569095
Email: sue@bcass.org.uk
Website: http://www.ostomyinternational.org

Fnded: 1975. **Desc:** Aims to provide information and management guides lines to its Member Associations. Helps to form new Ostomy Associations. Represents worldwide the interests of all ostomoates and those with related surgeries by advocating on all Ostomy-related matters and policies. **Pub:** *Ostomy International*, semiannual. Magazine.

★ 3899 ★ International Paediatric Pathology Association
c/o Dr. A.J. Bourne
Women's and Children's Hospital
North Adelaide, SA 5006, Australia
Phone: 61 8 81617318 **Fax:** 61 8 81617022
Email: bournet@wch.sa.gov.au

Fnded: 1976. **Mem:** 700. **Reg. Groups:** 5. **Desc:** Works throughout the world to facilitate increased knowledge of diseases of the embryo, fetus, infant, and child.

★ 3900 ★ International Palmtherapy Association
PO Box 7453
Van Nuys, CA 91409-7453
Phone: (661)944-4909
Email: info@palmtherapy.com
Website: http://www.palmtherapy.com

Fnded: 1995. **Desc:** Dedicated to the research of the "hand/mind connection". Palm therapy is the art and practice of "enhancing optimum potential, self-growth, fulfillment and success in all aspects of life through the massage stimulation of specific lines and areas of the hand". Offers seminars.

★ 3901 ★ International Pancreas and Islet Transplant Association (IPITA)
John Radcliffe Hosp Headington
Oxford 0X3 9DU, United Kingdom
Phone: 44 1865 225092 **Fax:** 44 1865 225616
Email: derek.gray@nds.ox.ac.uk
Website: http://www.ipita.org/

Fnded: 1993. **Desc:** Encourages research and training relevant to transplantation of insulin producing tissue in the treatment of diabetes mellitus; promotes and encourages contacts between clinical and experimental researchers from different institutions.

★ 3902 ★ International Pediatric Endosurgery Group (IPEG)
2716 Ocean Park Blvd., Ste. 3000
Santa Monica, CA 90405
Phone: (310)314-2536 **Fax:** (310)314-2589
Email: admin@ipeg.org
Website: http://www.ipeg.org
Erin Simmons, Contact

Desc: Doctors, surgeons, pediatricians, and those in the medical field. Present materials and articles keeping up to date on pediatric endosurgery and endoscopy, offer open forum for discussions and ideas, and extend support.

★ 3903 ★ International Pediatric Nephrology (IPNA)
c/o F. Bruder Stapleton, MD
Children's Hospital and Regional Medical Center
CH-65
4800 Sand Point Way, NU
Seattle, WA 98105
Phone: (206)526-2150 **Fax:** (206)527-3836
Email: bstaplet@u.washington.edu
F. Bruner Stapleton, MD, Treas.

Fnded: 1973. **Mem:** 1,752. **Reg. Groups:** 7. **Desc:** Specialists in children's kidney disease. Purpose is to promote communication and disseminate information among pediatric nephrologists. Maintains training facilities. **Pub:** *Pediatric Nephrology*, monthly. Journal. Peer review journal, peer reviewed original research, clinical data. *Price:* Included with membership dues. • *Proceedings*, triennial. Book.

★ 3904 ★ International Pemphigus Foundation
Atrium Plz., Ste. 203
828 San Pablo Ave.
Albany, CA 94706
Phone: (510)527-4970 **Fax:** (510)527-8497
Email: pvnews@aol.com
Website: http://www.pemphigus.org
Janet Segall, Exec. Dir.

Fnded: 1994. **Desc:** Provides information and support for people living with pemphigus and their families, friends and the general public. Information forum for medical community and general public, provides general support and counseling for those in need, raises funds for research. **Pub:** Newsletter, quarterly. **Frmly:** (2003) National Pemphigus Foundation.

★ 3905 ★ International Perimetric Society (IPS)
c/o Dr. Richard P. Mills
Department of Ophthalmology, Kentucy Clinic
801 Rose St.
Lexington, KY 40536-0284
Email: vpm@pop.uky.edu
Website: http://www.perimetry.org
Michael Wall, MD, Pres.

Fnded: 1974. **Mem:** 200. **Desc:** Ophthalmologists, scientists, and technicians in 20 countries working in the field of perimetry (visual field testing) and related areas. Promotes the study of normal and abnormal visual function and encourages worldwide cooperation and friendship among those working in the field. **Pub:** *Perimetry Update*, biennial. Proceedings.

★ 3906 ★ International Pharmaceutical Federation (IPF) (Federation Internationale Pharmaceutique — FIP)
PO Box 84200
NL-2508 AE The Hague, Netherlands
Phone: 31 70 3021970 **Fax:** 31 70 3021999
Email: fip@fip.org
Website: http://www.fip.org

Fnded: 1912. **Mem:** 4,700. **Lang(s):** English, French, German, Spanish. **Desc:** Worldwide organization of pharmacists and pharmaceutical scientists. Objectives are to: develop pharmacy at the international level in professional and scientific fields; development and standardization of professional standards; extend the role of the pharmacist in the health care field; foster communication among members; act as a clearinghouse; collaborate with efforts to improve pharmaceutical structures in various countries; advocate and support measures to ensure distribution, dispensation, and proper use of medicines. Exchanges opinions on professional and ethical issues; develops research and study programs; fosters cooperation among pharmacists, teachers, research workers, and the practitioners in the field of drug information; improves methods for assembling, selecting, summarizing, indexing, storing, classifying, and analyzing clinical and social surveys. Subjects studied include biopharmaceutics, pharmacokinetics and drug metabolism, administrative and social pharmacy, pharmacognosy, and the history of pharmacy. Collaborates with World Health Organization. **Pub:** *International Pharmacy Journal*, semiannual. • *Scientific Congress Proceedings*, biennial. Also publishes abstracts.

★ 3907 ★ International Photodynamic Association (IPA)

c/o Prof. Harubumi Kato, MD
Tokyo Medical University
Department of Surgery
6-7-1 Nishishinjuku
Shinjuku-ku
Tokyo 160-0023, Japan
Fax: 81 3 32637537
Email: imcc@tokyo-med.ac.jp
Website: http://www.tokyo-med.ac.jp/surg1/ipa/index.htm

Fnded: 1986. **Mem:** 300. **Lang(s):** English. **Desc:** Clinicians and scientists worldwide involved in photodynamic therapy and photodiagnosis. Promotes the study of diagnosis and treatment using light and sensitizers and disseminates information to the medical community and the general public. Provides training.

★ 3908 ★ International Phototherapy Association (IPA)

c/o Judy Weiser
PhotoTherapy Centre
1300 Richards St., Ste. 205
Vancouver, BC, Canada V6B 3G6
Phone: (604)689-9709 **Fax:** (604)633-1505
Email: jweiser@phototherapy-centre.com
Website: http://www.phototherapy-centre.com

Fnded: 1981. **Mem:** 225. **Lang(s):** English. **Desc:** Art therapists, psychologists, social workers, psychiatric nurses, other human service professionals (150), and students (75) in 9 countries. Fosters the development and use of still photographs, films, videotapes, discs, and holography in human service interventions including mental health and social welfare services. Seeks to: increase the effectiveness of phototherapy through research and practice; train and supervise students and professionals in behavioral and psychological phototherapy. Conducts training workshops. **Pub:** Booklets, annual.

★ 3909 ★ International Planned Parenthood Federation - Africa Regional Office

Madison Insurance House
Upper Hill Rd./Ngong Rd.
Nairobi, Kenya
Phone: 254 20 720280 **Fax:** 254 20 726596
Email: info@ippfaro.org
Website: http://www.ippf.org

Fnded: 1971. **Lang(s):** English, French. **Desc:** Coordinates activities of Planned Parenthood member associations operating in sub-Saharan Africa. Advocates family planning as a basic human right. Works to heighten governmental and public awareness of the population problems of local communities in Africa. Seeks to extend and improve family and sexual and reproductive health planning services. Conducts research on human fertility and contraception. **Pub:** *Adam & Eve and the Serpent*. Book. • *Africa Link*, semiannual. Magazine. Reports on sexual and reproductive health programmes of family planning associations in the region and provides related information on global events. • *Contraceptive Update: A Handbook for Health Workers*. Handbook. • *Legal and Policy Barriers Affecting Sexual and Reproductive Health Service in: Burkina Faso, Senegal, Swaziland, Zambia*. • *Regional Conference of Women, Islam and Family Planning, Niamey, Niger*. Report.

★ 3910 ★ International Planned Parenthood Federation - East and Southeast Asia and Oceania Regional Office

246 Jalan Ampang
50450 Kuala Lumpur, Malaysia
Phone: 60 3 42566122 **Fax:** 60 3 42566386
Email: rkarim@ippfeseaor.org
Website: http://www.ippf.org/regions/

Fnded: 1952. **Mem:** 19. **Lang(s):** Malay. **Desc:** Works to co-ordinate activities for Planned Parenthood offices operating in the Asia and Oceania region. Advocates family planning as a basic human right. Works to increase governmental and public awareness of population problems in local regions. Promotes effective family planning programs. Conducts research on human fertility and contraception. **Pub:** *People and Development Challenges*, semiannual. Magazine.

★ 3911 ★ International Planned Parenthood Federation - Tunis

Arab World Regional Office
2, Place Virgile
Notre Dame
TN-1082 Tunis, Tunisia
Phone: 216 1 847344 **Fax:** 216 1 788661
Email: awro@ippf.intl.tn

Lang(s): Arabic, French. **Desc:** Advocates family planning as a basic human right. Works to increase governmental and public awareness of population problems. Promotes effective family planning services. Conducts research on human fertility and contraception.

★ 3912 ★ International Planned Parenthood Federation - United Kingdom (IPPF) (Federation Internationale pour la Planification Familiale)

Regent's College
Inner Circle
Regent's Park
London NW1 4NS, United Kingdom
Phone: 44 20 74877900 **Fax:** 44 20 74877950
Email: info@ippf.org
Website: http://www.ippf.org

Fnded: 1952. **Mem:** 147. **Nat'l Groups:** 180. **Reg. Groups:** 6. **Lang(s):** Arabic, English, French, Spanish. **Desc:** Initiates and supports worldwide sexual and reproductive health searvices, including family planning, HIV prevention and care and support programs. **Pub:** *Family Planning Handbook for Health Professionals*, periodic. Handbook. • *IPPF Annual Report*. Annual Report. • *IPPF Directory of Hormonal Contraceptives*, periodic. • *IPPF Medical Bulletin*, bimonthly. Bulletin.

★ 3913 ★ International Planned Parenthood Federation, Western Hemisphere Region (IPPF/WHR)

120 Wall St., 9th Fl.
New York, NY 10005
Phone: (212)248-6400 **Fax:** (212)248-4221
Email: info@ippfwhr.org
Website: http://www.ippfwhr.org
Zhenja La Rosa, Communications Mgr.

Fnded: 1952. **Mem:** 44. **Desc:** A division of the International Planned Parenthood Federation. Provides more than 9 million sexual and reproductive health services and information each year to men, women and youth throughout North and Latin America, and the Caribbean. **Pub:** *Forum*, quarterly. Magazine. Includes calendar of events. Distributed primarily to affiliated family planning programs. • Annual Report. • Also publishes occasional monographs, studies, and position papers.

★ 3914 ★ International Polio Network (IPN)

4207 Lindell Blvd., No. 110
Saint Louis, MO 63108
Phone: (314)534-0475 **Fax:** (314)534-5070
Email: gini_intl@msn.com
Website: http://www.post-polio.org
Joan L. Headley, Dir.

Fnded: 1985. **Mem:** 6,500. **Desc:** Individuals who have had polio; rehabilitation health professionals. Promotes networking and the exchange of information among the post-polio community; encourages research into the long-term effects of polio. **Pub:** *Handbook on the Late Effects of Poliomyelitis for Physicians and Survivors (Revised Edition)*. Handbook. *Price:* $12. • *Polio Network News*, quarterly. Newsletter. *Price:* $22. • *Post-Polio Directory*, annual. Directory. Contains directory of clinics, health professionals, and support groups. *Price:* $8. • *Rehabilitation Gazette, Int'l Ventilator Users Network (IVUN) News*.

★ 3915 ★ International Prader-Willi Syndrome Organization (IPWSO)

Via Bartolomeo Bizio, 1
I-36023 Costozza, Italy
Phone: 39 0444555557 **Fax:** 39 0444555557
Email: president@ipwso.org
Website: http://www.ipwso.org

Fnded: 1991. **Mem:** 56. **Nat'l Groups:** 56. **Desc:** Stimulates International co-operation on PWS research projects on the origins, management and prevents of the Prader-Willi syndrome; encourages national Associations to exchange and share their PWS projects and experiences; fosters the foundation and development of new national PWS associations. **Pub:** *Wavelength*, 3/year. Newsletter.

★ 3916 ★ International Professional Surrogates Association (IPSA)

3428 Motor Ave.
Los Angeles, CA 90034
Phone: (323)469-4720
Email: ipsa1@aol.com
Website: http://www.ipsa.us
Vena Blanchard, Pres.

Fnded: 1973. **Mem:** 50. **Nat'l Groups:** 1. **Local Groups:** 1. **Desc:** IPSA is non-profit professional organization of Surrogate Partners and Therapists. IPSA provides referrals to therapists seeking trained, ethical professional surrogate partners and referrals to clients seeking therapists with expertise in surrogate partner therapy. IPSA sponsors training for surrogate partners, and provides continuing education to sex therapists, psychotherapists, and surrogate partners, and recently began offering personal enrichment courses for individuals and couples. IPSA's Code of Ethics helped to establish and maintain the highest professional standards within the field of surrogate partner therapy. **Pub:** *Code of Ethics*. Brochure. • *IPSA Training*. Brochure. • *Surrogate Partner Therapy*. • Brochures, semiannual. Informational brochures. *Price:* Available to members only. • Newsletter, semiannual. *Price:* Available to members only.

★ 3917 ★ International Programme on Chemical Safety (IPCS) (Programme International sur la Securite des Substances Chimiques — PISSC)

c/o World Health Organization
Ave. Appia 20
CH-1211 Geneva 27, Switzerland
Phone: 41 22 7913592 **Fax:** 41 22 7914848
Email: ipcsmail@who.int
Website: http://www.who.int/pcs/

Fnded: 1980. **Mem:** 33. **Lang(s):** English, French. **Desc:** States belonging to the World Health Organization, the International Labour Organization, and the United Nations Environment Programme. Evaluates the health risks posed to humans and the environment by exposure to chemicals. Proposes methods and guidelines for measuring chemical exposure and for assessing health risks. Encourages the use and improvement of methods for laboratory testing and epidemiological studies. Provides guidelines on safe levels of chemical exposure through daily intake of food additives and pesticide and veterinary drug residues. Disseminates information regarding diagnosis and treatment of chemical poisoning; promotes international cooperation in dealing with chemical emergencies. Seeks to enhance the sci entific basis for health risk assessment for determination of chemical hazards controls. Conducts training courses on subjects such as ecotoxicology, clinical toxicology, the detection of mutagenesis, and occupational hazards and human reproduction; coordinates international research programs; maintains expert advisory groups and offers advisory services for technical cooperation in regulation and control of chemicals. Organizes symposia and workshops on chemical safety. **Pub:** *Environmental Health Criteria Document*, 15/year. • *Health and Safety Guides*, 20/year. • *IPCS Newsletter*, 2-3/year. Newsletter. • *Poison Information Monographs*, periodic. • *Technical Document on Food Additives and on Pesticide Residues*, periodic.

★ 3918 ★ International Psycho-Oncology Society (IPOS)
1242 Second Ave.
New York, NY 10021
Phone: (212)673-8768 **Fax:** (212)717-3763
Email: info@ipos-aspboa.org
Website: http://www.ipos-aspboa.org
Uwe Koch, MD,PhD, Contact

Desc: Addresses the two major psychological dimensions of cancer: the psychological response of patients to cancer and the behavioral and social factors that influence risk, detection and survival.

★ 3919 ★ International Psychoanalytical Association (IPA)
(Association Psychanalytique Internationale)
Broomhills
Woodside Ln.
London N12 8UD, United Kingdom
Phone: 44 208 4468324 **Fax:** 44 208 4454729
Email: ipa@ipa.org.uk
Website: http://www.ipa.org.uk

Fnded: 1910. **Mem:** 10,700. **Nat'l Groups:** 62. **Reg. Groups:** 1. **Lang(s):** English, French, German, Spanish. **Desc:** Organizations in 30 countries involved in psychoanalysis. Encourages communication among members and promotes high educational standards. Organizes training programs, conferences, and gives research grants. **Pub:** *Bulletin*, annual. Bulletin. • *Information Booklet*, periodic. Booklet. • *Newsletter*, semiannual. Newsletter. • *Roster*, annual. • Monographs, annual.

★ 3920 ★ International Psychoanalytical Association Trust
Broomhills, Woodside Ln.
London N12 8UD, United Kingdom
Phone: 44 20 84468324 **Fax:** 44 20 84454724
Email: ipa@ipa.org.uk
Website: http://www.ipa.org.uk/

Fnded: 1910. **Mem:** 10,800. **Lang(s):** English, French, German, Spanish. **Desc:** Promotes communication among psychoanalysts and psychoanalytic component organizations; supports development of psychoanalytical organizations.

★ 3921 ★ International Psychogeriatric Association (IPA)
Ste. 340 5215 Old Orchard Rd.
Skokie, IL 60077
Phone: (847)663-0574 **Fax:** (847)663-0591
Email: ipa@ipa-online.org
Website: http://www.ipa-online.org
Alistar Burns, Pres.

Fnded: 1981. **Mem:** 1,500. **Reg. Groups:** 2. **Desc:** To improve the mental health of the aging world population through information dissemination, research, professional development, advocacy and service development. Multidisciplinary health care professionals and scientists from 70 countries with an interest in the behavioral and biological aspects of mental in the elderly. Works to keep members abreast of developments in research and clinical practice in the field of geriatric mental health. **Pub:** *International Psychogeriatrics*, quarterly. Journal. *Price:* available to members only. • *IPA Bulletin*, quarterly. Newsletter. • Books. • Pamphlets.

★ 3922 ★ International Regional Organization of Plant Protection and Animal Health
(Organismo Internacional Regional de Sanidad Agropecuaria — OIRSA)
No 14 Colonia San Francisco
San Salvador, El Salvador
Phone: 503 2631123 **Fax:** 503 2631128
Website: http://www.oirsa.org.sv

Fnded: 1953. **Mem:** 9. **Lang(s):** Spanish. **Desc:** Ministries of agriculture and livestock from the countries of Costa Rica, Dominican Republic, El Salvador, Guatemala, Honduras, Mexico, Belize, Nicaragua, and Panama. Objective is to prevent epidemics and exotic diseases among crops and farm animals in Central America. Informs and advises members and coordinates their activities. Special programs include: plant and animal quarantine; a regional effort to prevent Foot and Mouth Disease and a joint effort with Honduras and Guatemala to control Coffee Berry Borer; and a cooperative. Cooperative projects with the United States Department of Agriculture include identification and classification of fruit flies and the eradication of the Africanized bee. Presents national and international courses on the quarantining of cattle. **Pub:** *Animal Health*. Bulletin. • *NOTI-OIRSA*, bimonthly. Bulletin. Contains technical information.

★ 3923 ★ International Rehabilitation Council for Toture Victims (IRCT)
(Det Internationale Rehabiliteringsrad for Torturofre)
Borgergade 13
PO Box 9049
DK-1022 Copenhagen K, Denmark
Phone: 45 33 760600 **Fax:** 45 33 760500
Email: irct@irct.org
Website: http://www.irct.org

Fnded: 1982. **Desc:** Medical doctors, nurses, psychologists, social workers, physiotherapists, interpreters and administrative staff. Studies and develops optimal treatment and rehabilitation programs for victims of torture. Provides, on outpatient basis, traditional medical treatment and personal and social counseling. Participates in information campaigns against torture. Sponsors seminars and symposia. Maintains documentation center. **Pub:** *Annual Report*, annual. • *Torture*, quarterly. Journal. Includes information on rehabilitation of torture victims and prevention of torture. **Frmly:** (2002) Rehabilitation and Resource Centre for Torture Victims.

★ 3924 ★ International Rescue and Emergency Care Association (IRECA)
PO Box 13527
Charleston, SC 29422-3527
Free: 800-221-3435
Email: tannerc@cpchem.com
Website: http://www.ireca.org
Randy Tanner, Pres.

Fnded: 1948. **Mem:** 3,000. **Local Groups:** 500. **Desc:** Organized volunteers and paid industrial rescue and emergency squads, ambulance and first aid crews, fire departments, military personnel, and other units equipped with rescue equipment and emergency care supplies which can be carried in mobile units; county, state, and other associations and individuals interested in rescue and emergency patient care. To cooperate in, foster, and conduct research designed to advance the science and art of rescue and emergency care and to encourage standardization of practice and equipment. Sponsors seminars. **Pub:** *International Rescuer*, quarterly. • Also publishes and endorses the publication of emergency care and rescue training information. **Frmly:** (1978) International Rescue and First Aid Association.

★ 3925 ★ International Research Council of Neuromuscular Disorders (IRCND)
1434 Pleasantville Rd.
Lancaster, OH 43130
Phone: (740)653-1098 **Fax:** (740)653-3121
James R. Grilliot, D.C., Exec. Dir.

Fnded: 1982. **Mem:** 82. **Desc:** Health professionals interested in neuromuscular diseases of the human body. Purpose is to advance and disseminate information on the causes, effects, occurrence, cure, and prevention of neuromuscular disorders and associated topics related to the human spine. Coordinates and encourages basic research and the exchange of ideas and related materials between professionals in the field. Prepares teaching and educational materials. Compiles statistics for distribution; sponsors seminars and speakers' bureau. Is currently developing a library. **Pub:** *Information/Newsletter*, annual. Newsletter.

★ 3926 ★ International Research Group on Biochemistry of Exercise
Av Paul Heger 28
1000 Brussels, Belgium
Phone: 32 2 6504209 **Fax:** 32 2 6502195
Email: jrpoortma@ulb.ac.be

★ 3927 ★ International REST Investigators Society (IRIS)
c/o Thomas H. Fine
Medical College of Ohio
Department of Psychiatry
Toledo, OH 43614
Phone: (419)383-5695 **Fax:** (419)383-3031
Email: tfine@mco.edu
Thomas H. Fine, Pres.

Fnded: 1983. **Desc:** Scientists and individuals interested in exploring the psychophysiological effects of floating. Serves as an information exchange for researchers, therapists, and individuals interested in restricted environmental stimulation techniques (REST). (Restricted environmental stimulation techniques include methods of producing a relaxed environment to create changes in consciousness and behavior such as floatation or isolation tanks.) Clinically, REST is being used in conjunction with relaxation training, biofeedback, psychotherapy, and a variety of stress-related disorders. Organizes meetings where members and other interested individuals can communicate current interests, exchange ideas and suggestions, and form collaborative research groups. **Pub:** *REST and Self-Regulation Conference Proceedings*, periodic. • Bulletin, 3/year. • Also publishes bibliography.

★ 3928 ★ International Rett Syndrome Association (IRSA)
9121 Piscataway Rd.
Clinton, MD 20735
Phone: (301)856-3334 **Free:** 800-818-RETT
Fax: (301)856-3336
Email: irsa@rettsyndrome.org
Website: http://www.rettsyndrome.org
Kathy Hunter, Pres.

Fnded: 1985. **Mem:** 3,500. **State Groups:** 20. **Desc:** Parents of children with Rett Syndrome; interested professionals and supporters. (A child afflicted with Rett Syndrome, which strikes predominately in females, seems normal until 7 to 18 months of age, when a regression leads to loss of psychomotor and communication skills. Autistic-like withdrawal often sets in; though this symptom eases in time, higher brain functions are compromised. The child also loses purposeful use of her hands, wringing them in a constant "hand-washing" movement in front of the face or chest. The syndrome is named for Dr. Andreas Rett, of Vienna, Austria, who described it in 1966. The cause of Rett Syndrome has been traced to a defective gene, called the MeCP2 on the X chromosome.) Provides support to parents; encourages research; collects and disseminates information. Assists in identifying patients; conducts activities aimed at the prevention, treatment, and eventual eradication of Rett Syndrome. **Pub:** *A Closer Look at Rett Syndrome.* Video. • *International Rett Syndrome Association–Newsletter Rett Gazette*, quarterly. Newsletter. *Price:* Included in membership dues. • *Rett Sydrome: A Physician's Approach.* Video. • *Rett Syndrome: A Conversation with Families.* Video. • *Rett Syndrome: A Therapeutic Approach.* Video. • *Rett Syndrome Handbook.* Handbook. *Price:* $15 members; $29.95 nonmembers. • *Silent Angels: The Rett Syndrome Story.* Video. **Frmly:** (1985) International Rett's Syndrome Association.

★ 3929 ★ International Rorschach Society (IRS)
(Societe Rorschach Internationale)

c/o Anne Andronikof - Sanglade, Sec.
Laboratoire IPSe
Universite Paris X
200, Ave. de la Republique
F-92001 Nanterre, France
Phone: 33 3 44497881 **Fax:** 33 3 44491831
Email: andronik@u-paris10.fr
Website: http://www.rorschach.com

Fnded: 1948. **Mem:** 1,700. **Lang(s):** English, French, Italian, Spanish. **Desc:** Societies (12) and individuals (76). Develops international contacts between Rorschach specialists and other interested individuals; promotes theoretical and practical knowledge of Rorschach and other projective techniques. (Rorschach test, named after Hermann Rorschach, a Swiss psychiatrist, is a test in which personality characteristics are made accessible to analysis by the subject's interpretation of the nature and meaning of a series of standard inkblot patterns.) Organizes regional and international meetings. Conducts research. **Pub:** *Bulletin of the International Rorschach Society*, annual. Bulletin. • *Rorschachiana*, triennial. Yearbook. Includes congress proceedings.

★ 3930 ★ International School Psychology Association

Hans Knudsens Plads 1A
DK-2100 Copenhagen, Denmark
Phone: 45 44982106 **Fax:** 45 39293700
Email: info@ispaweb.org
Website: http://www.ispaweb.org/

Fnded: 1974. **Desc:** Promotes communication between professionals committed to improvement of mental health of children.

★ 3931 ★ International Skeletal Society (ISS)

c/o Harry K. Genant, M.D.
University of California San Francisco
San Francisco, CA 94143-0628
Phone: (415)476-4864 **Fax:** (415)476-8550
Email: harry.genant@oarg.ucsf.edu
Website: http://www.intskelsoc.com
Michael J. Pitt, MD, Pres.

Fnded: 1973. **Mem:** 500. **Desc:** Physicians and scientists interested in skeletal muscle disease. Seeks to advance the science of skeletal radiology; brings together radiologists and individuals in related disciplines; provides continuing education courses. **Pub:** *Skeletal Radiology*, 8/year. Journal. Contains scientific articles and case reports. *Price:* Included in membership dues. • Membership Directory, annual. • Newsletter, semiannual.

★ 3932 ★ International Society for Adult Congenital Cardiac Disease

c/o Pamela D. Sproul
9111 Old Georgetown Rd.
Bethesda, MD 20814-1616
Phone: (919)787-5181 **Fax:** (919)787-4916
Email: isaccd@olsonmgmt.com

Fnded: 1992. **Mem:** 200. **Desc:** Seeks to achieve and promote execellence in the care of adolescents and adults with contgenital cardiac disease. **Pub:** *ISACCD Update*, quarterly. Newsletter.

★ 3933 ★ International Society of Andrology (ISA)

c/o Hector E. Chemes, Pres.
Department of Endocrinology
Buenos Aires Children's Hospital
Gallo 1330
1425 Buenos Aires, Argentina
Phone: 54 11 49635931 **Fax:** 54 11 49635930
Email: president@andrology.org
Website: http://andrology.org

Fnded: 1981. **Mem:** 8,000. **Desc:** Aims to serve Andrology and andrologists world-wide through its Newsletter.

★ 3934 ★ International Society for Applied Ethology (ISAE)
(Societe International d'Ethologie Applie)

c/o Dr. Ute Knierim
International Animal Hygiene Welfare & Farm Animal Behavior
Buenteweg 17p
D-30559 Hannover, Germany
Phone: 49 511 9538449 **Fax:** 49 511 9538588
Email: ute.knierim@tiho-hannover.de
Website: http://www.applied-ethology.org

Fnded: 1966. **Mem:** 655. **Lang(s):** English. **Desc:** Veterinarians; scientists and individuals with special knowledge of ethology, the study of animal behavior. Purpose is to advance the study of ethology as it affects animal health and welfare. Seeks to: stimulate ethological teaching and research in the veterinary and related professions; encourage discussion among members and publication of original works; further ethological knowledge on domesticated, captive, and wild animals; acts as clearinghouse for veterinarians and other interested individuals. **Pub:** *ISAE Newsletter*, semiannual. Newsletter. • *Proceedings.* **Frmly:** (1991) Society for Veterinary Ethology; (1993) Societe d'Ethologie Veterinaire.

★ 3935 ★ International Society of Art and Psychopathology
(Societe Internationale de Psychopathologie de l'Expression — SIPE)

27, rue du Marechal Joffre
F-64000 Pau, France
Phone: 33 5 9276974 **Fax:** 33 5 9276974

Fnded: 1959.

★ 3936 ★ International Society of Arthroscopy, Knee Surgery and Orthopaedic Sports Medicine (ISAKOS)

145 Town and Country Dr., Ste. 106
Danville, CA 94526-3963
Phone: (925)314-7920 **Fax:** (925)314-7922
Email: isakos@isakos.com
Website: http://www.isakos.com
Barry R. Tietjens, Pres.

Fnded: 1978. **Mem:** 1,100. **Desc:** Orthopaedic surgeons specializing in problems of the knee, arthoscopy, orthopaedic sports medicine. **Pub:** *The Journal of Athroscopic and Related Surgery.* Journal. • Newsletter, semiannual. **Frmly:** International Arthroscopy Association; (1995) International Society of the Knee.

★ 3937 ★ International Society of Behavioral Medicine

Department of Medical Sociology
University of ULM
Am Hochstrass 8
D-89077 Ulm, Germany
Phone: 49 731 5025626 **Fax:** 49 731 5025632
Email: richard.peter@medizin.uni-ulm.de
Website: http://www.isbm.miami.edu/

★ 3938 ★ International Society for Bioengineering and the Skin

c/o Peter Elsner, Sec.
Department of Dermatology
University of Jena
Erfurter Str. 35
D-07743 Jena, Germany
Fax: 49 3641 937343
Email: randy.wickett@uc.edu
Website: http://pharmacy.uc.edu/isbs/default.html

Fnded: 1993. **Mem:** 120. **Lang(s):** English. **Desc:** Promotes development of instrumentation and standardized methods for measuring the properties of skin. Develops techniques and instruments for diagnosis and treatment of skin diseases; promotes the study and development of synthetic materials for skin grafting and as dressings for wounds. **Pub:** *Skin Research and Technology*, quarterly. Journal.

★ 3939 ★ International Society of Biomechanics (ISB)

c/o Julie Steele, Sec.Gen.
Biomechanics Research Laboratory
Department of Biomedical Science
University of Wollongong
Northfields Ave.
Wollongong, NSW 2522, Australia
Phone: 61 2 42231881 **Fax:** 61 2 42214096
Email: julie_steele@uow.edu.au
Website: http://www.isbweb.org

Fnded: 1973. **Mem:** 1,000. **Desc:** Scientists from a variety of disciplines which include anatomy, physiology, engineering (mechanical, industrial aerospace, etc.), orthopedics, rehabilitation medicine, sport science and medicine, ergonomics, electro-physiological kinesiology and others. Promotes the study of biomechanics, especially the biomechanics of human movement. **Pub:** *Conference proceedings.* Proceedings. • Newsletter, quarterly. Contains Calendar of Scientific Events, thesis abstracts, and special feature articles.

★ 3940 ★ International Society for Biomedical Research on Alcoholism (ISBRA)

PO Box 202332
Denver, CO 80220-8332
Phone: (303)355-6420 **Fax:** (303)355-1207
Email: isbra@usa.net
Website: http://www.isbra.com
Phillipe De Witte, Pres.

Fnded: 1980. **Mem:** 730. **Reg. Groups:** 3. **Desc:** Physicians, psychologists, biologists, and other scientists in over 20 countries who conduct research on biological factors in the etiology and treatment of alocholism and its medical complications. Official collaborating agency of the World Health Organization. Conducts international collaborative research projects and training courses. **Pub:** *Advances in Biomedical Alcohol Research*, biennial. Book. Contains proceedings of the biennial congresses. • *Alcoholism: Clinical and Experimental Research*, bimonthly. Journal. *Price:* $55 members; $110 nonmembers.

★ 3941 ★ International Society of Blood Purification

c/o Prof. Thomas A. Golper
S-3301 MCN
Vanderbilt University Medical Center
Nashville, TN 37232
Phone: (615)343-2220 **Fax:** (615)343-7156
Dr. Michael J. Lysaght, Contact

Fnded: 1982. **Mem:** 140. **Desc:** Blood purification professionals.

★ 3942 ★ International Society of Blood Transfusion (ISBT) (Societe Internationale de Transfusion Sanguine — SITS)

Jan van Goyenkade 11
NL 1075 HP Amsterdam, Netherlands
Phone: 31 20 6793411 **Fax:** 31 20 6737306
Email: isbt@eurocongress.com
Website: http://www.isbt-web.org

Fnded: 1937. **Mem:** 1,300. **Nat'l Groups:** 105. **Lang(s):** English, French. **Desc:** Members of national blood bank societies in 105 countries. Works toward solving the scientific, technical, social, and ethical problems related to the transfusion of blood. Encourages closer relations among individuals dealing with such problems; standardizes methods and equipment. Facilitates the exchange of information among members. **Pub:** *Transfusion Today*, quarterly. • *Vox Sanguinis*, quarterly. Also publishes congress proceedings and technical guides.

★ 3943 ★ International Society for Brain Electromagnetic Topography (ISBET)

Lenggstr 31
CH-8029 Zurich, Switzerland
Fax: 41 1 3843396

Fnded: 1989. **Desc:** Stimulates research on electric and magnetic fields of the brain.

★ 3944 ★ International Society for Burn Injuries (ISBI)

c/o Dr. Ronald Tompkins
Massachusetts General Hospital
55 Fruit St.
Boston, MA 02114-2696
Phone: (617)726-3442 **Fax:** (617)367-8936
Email: rtompkins@partners.org
Website: http://www.worldburn.org
Dr. Ronald Tompkins, MD, Sec. -Treas.

Fnded: 1965. **Mem:** 1,740. **Desc:** Physicians, surgeons, nurses, scientists, and other interested medical and non-medical personnel who are engaged in the care and research of burns. Seeks to disseminate knowledge and stimulate prevention in the field of burns. Promotes and coordinates scientific, clinical, and social research in burns; promotes first aid, nursing, and other types of education in all phases of burn care. **Pub:** *BURNS*, 8/year. Journal. *Price:* Free to members. • Membership Directory, annual.

★ 3945 ★ International Society of Cardiovascular Pharmacotherapy (ISCP)

Austin Hospital
University of Melbourne
Melbourne, VIC 3084, Australia

★ 3946 ★ International Society for Cardiovascular Surgery (ISCVS)

13 Elm St.
Manchester, MA 01944-1314
Phone: (978)526-8330 **Fax:** (978)526-7521
Email: iscvs@prri.com
David Cloud, Exec. Dir.

Fnded: 1951. **Mem:** 2,500. **Desc:** Encourages exchange and cooperation between cardiovascular specialists. Promotes discussion of ideas pertinent to the cardiovascular disease field and stimulates investigation and study of cardiovascular diseases. **Pub:** *Cardiovascular Surgery*, bimonthly. Journal. **Frmly:** (1983) International Cardiovascular Society.

★ 3947 ★ International Society of Chemotherapy (ISC) (Societe Internationale de Chimiotherapie)

c/o Dr. Faridah Moosdeen
31 St. Olav's Ct.
City Business Centre
25 Lower Rd.
London SE16 2XB, United Kingdom
Phone: 44 20 72312944 **Fax:** 44 20 72312124
Email: moosdeen@ischemo.demon.co.uk
Website: http://www.ischemo.org

Fnded: 1961. **Mem:** 16,000. **Nat'l Groups:** 64. **Reg. Groups:** 5. **Lang(s):** English. **Desc:** Societies or specialized groups within societies that are concerned with chemotherapy; scientists and clinicians working in chemotherapy. (Chemotherapy is the use of chemical agents in the treatment or control of infectious and neoplastic diseases and immunological disorder.) Promotes the development of chemotherapy through scientific and educational means. Encourages cooperation between members and scientists in related fields. Urges formation of new societies in countries where such groups do not exist. Promotes and/or sponsors formation of international working groups and training projects in the field of antimicrobial, antiparasitic, and antineoplastic chemotherapy; coordinates their activities. Appoints commissions for special activities. **Pub:** *Antibiotics Chemotherapy*, quarterly. Newsletter. • *Congress Proceedings*, biennial. • *International Journal of Antimicrobial Agents*, monthly. Journal.

★ 3948 ★ International Society for Child and Adolescent Injury Prevention (ISCAIP)

c/o Child Accident Prevention Trust
18-20 Farringdon Ln.
London EC1R 3AU, United Kingdom
Email: iscaip@capt.demon.co.uk
Website: http://www.iscaip.org/

Fnded: 1993. **Desc:** Persons with interest or involvement in prevention of childhood and adolescent injuries. Promotes reduction and severity of injury to children and adolescents; provides multi-disciplinary forum; provides advocacy at national and international levels; fosters national injury prevention initiatives; disseminates research findings and funding opportunities; proposes policy on international basis. **Pub:** *Injury Prevention*. Journal. • Newsletter. Contains information about professional meetings, specialists, and research.

★ 3949 ★ International Society for Clinical Electrophysiology of Vision

c/o Prof. Colin Barber
Medical Physics Department
Queens Medical Ctr.
Nottingham NG7 2UH, United Kingdom
Phone: 44 115 9709131 **Fax:** 44 115 9422745
Email: colin.barber@nottingham.ac.uk
Website: http://www.iscev.org

Fnded: 1962. **Mem:** 700. **Nat'l Groups:** 34. **Reg. Groups:** 5. **State Groups:** 34. **Local Groups:** 34. **Lang(s):** English, Japanese. **Desc:** Ophthalmologists and other individuals with an interest in the electrophysiology of vision. Seeks to advance understanding of the mechanics of vision; promotes development of new ophthalmologic techniques and technologies. Functions as a clearinghouse on the electrophysiology of vision; facilitates cooperation and communication among workers in the field of the clinical and basic electrophysiology of vision; formulates standards of terminology, research, and practice in the field. **Pub:** *Documents of Ophthalmology*, annual. Newsletter.

★ 3950 ★ International Society for Clinical Haemorheology (ISCH)

Bldg. South Kensington
London SW7 2AZ, United Kingdom
Phone: 44 20 75943187 **Fax:** 44 20 75943100
Email: m.rampling@ic.ac.uk

Fnded: 1993. **Desc:** Advances study of clinical haemorheology.

★ 3951 ★ International Society for Comparative Psychology (ISCP)

c/o Dr. Ty Partridge
Department of Psychology
71 W Warren
Detroit, MI 48202
Phone: (313)577-2813 **Fax:** (313)577-7636
Email: tpartridge@sun.science.wayne.edu
Website: http://www.comparativepsychology.org/
Robert M. Murphey, Sec.

Fnded: 1983. **Mem:** 80. **Desc:** Psychologists, biologists, anthropologists, and neuroscientists who work in or are interested in comparative psychology. Aims: to promote the international development of comparative psychology; establish worldwide communication among comparative psychologists; encourage the study of the development and evolution of behavior. **Pub:** *Advances in Comparative Psychology*, semiannual. *Price:* $35. • *International Journal of Comparative Psychology*, quarterly. Journal. *Price:* Free to members; $95. • *ISCP Newsletter*, bimonthly. Newsletter.

★ 3952 ★ International Society for Computerized Electrocardiology (ISCE)

11495 Emmanuel Way, No. 518
Solomons, MD 20688-3031
Phone: (301)855-1004 **Fax:** (410)394-3219
Email: mrh@chesapeake.net
Website: http://www.isce.org/

Fnded: NNal. **Mem:** l other, co. **Reg. Groups:** al. **Desc:** Promotes advancement of the science of electrocardiology. **Pub:** *Journal of Electrocardiology*. Journal.

★ 3953 ★ International Society of Contact Lens Specialists

c/o Dr. Theo F. Gumpelmayer
Landstr. 49
A-4020 Linz, Austria
Phone: 43 70 773660 **Fax:** 43 70 7736703

Fnded: 1952. **Mem:** 74. **Lang(s):** German. **Desc:** Contact lens specialists.

★ 3954 ★ International Society of Craniofacial Surgery (ISCFS)

Tung Hwa N Rd.
Taipei, Taiwan
Phone: 886 3 3281200 **Fax:** 886 3285507
Email: uraychen@adm.cgmh.com.tw
Website: http://www.craniofaciaal.com/isoc.html

Fnded: 1983. **Desc:** Fosters advances in craniofacial surgery; stimulates research, investigation and teaching in methods of preventing and correcting congenital and acquired craniofacial deformities.

★ 3955 ★ International Society of Cryosurgery (ISC)

Via Ospedali, 14
I-12038 Savigliano, Italy
Phone: 39 0172719418 **Fax:** 39 0172711701

Fnded: 1975. **Desc:** Promotes exchange of scientific knowledge and application of cryosurgery.

★ 3956 ★ International Society for Cutaneous Lymphomas (ISCL)

c/o Dr. Nicola Pimpinelli
Department Dermatological Sciences
University of Florence Medical School
Via degli Alfani 37
I-50121 Florence, Italy
Phone: 39 055 2344422 **Fax:** 39 055 2758757
Email: pimpi@unifi.it
Website: http://www-usz.unizh.ch/iscl/isclhome.htm

Fnded: 1992. **Mem:** 225. **Nat'l Groups:** 32. **Lang(s):** English. **Desc:** Fosters communication and cooperation among individuals and groups interested in the diagnosis, treatment, and investigation of primary cutaneous lymphomas.

★ 3957 ★ International Society of Dacryology
Fleminggatan 22
S-11282 Stockholm, Sweden
Fax: 46 8 6723070

Fnded: 1982. **Desc:** Understanding the health and fighting the disease of the lachrymal system.

★ 3958 ★ International Society for Dermatologic Surgery (ISDS)
930 E Woodfield Rd.
Schaumburg, IL 60173-4729
Phone: (847)330-9830 **Fax:** (847)330-1135
Email: info@isdsworld.org
Website: http://www.isdsworld.org
Perry Robins, Founder-Pres.

Fnded: 1976. **Mem:** 1,200. **Desc:** Dermatologists, otolaryngologists, plastic surgeons, and skin surgery specialists. Goals are to: promote high standards of patient care; provide for continuing education and research in dermatologic surgery; encourage public interest in the field. Provides a forum for the exchange of ideas and methodology in dermatologic surgery and related basic sciences. **Pub:** Directory, annual.

★ 3959 ★ International Society of Dermatology (ISD)
930 E Woodfield Rd.
Schaumburg, IL 60173
Phone: (847)330-9830 **Fax:** (847)330-1135
Email: info@intsocdermatol.org
Website: http://www.intsocdermatol.org
Coleman Jacobson, MD, Pres.

Fnded: 1957. **Mem:** 2,000. **Desc:** Dermatologists and general physicians. Promotes interest, education, and research in dermatology with international meetings, publications, and scholarships. **Pub:** *International Journal of Dermatology*, monthly. Journal. **Frmly:** (1984) International Society of Tropical Dermatology; (1997) International Society of Dermatology: Tropical, Geographic, and Ecologic.

★ 3960 ★ International Society for Developmental Psychobiology (ISDP)
c/o Dr. Robert Lickliter
Virginia Tech
Blacksburg, VA 24061-0436
Phone: (540)231-5346 **Fax:** (540)231-3652
Email: rsullivan@ou.edu
Website: http://www.isdp.org
Regina Sullivan, Sec.

Fnded: 1967. **Mem:** 335. **Desc:** Research scientists in the field of developmental psychobiology; biology and psychology students. Promotes research in the field of developmental psychobiology, the study of the brain and behavior throughout the life span and in relation to other biological processes. Stimulates communication and interaction among scientists in the field. Provides the editorship for the journal, *Development Psychobiology*. Compiles statistics. **Pub:** *Developmental Psychobiology*, bimonthly. Journal. Addresses the anatomical, physiological, biochemical, hormonal, pharmacological, genetic, and evolutionary aspects of behavioral development. *Price:* Included in membership dues. • Membership Directory, every 1-2 years. • Newsletter, 2-3/year.

★ 3961 ★ International Society for Diagnostic Quantitative Pathology (ISDQP)
Grosvenor Rd.
Belfast BT12 6BL, United Kingdom
Phone: 44 1232 263115 **Fax:** 44 1232 233643
Email: p.hamilton@qub.ac.uk

Fnded: 1994. **Desc:** Furthers the development and application of quantitative methodology in pathological research, practice and education.

★ 3962 ★ International Society for Digestive Surgery
900 Cummings Center, Ste. 221-U
Beverly, MA 01915
Phone: (978)927-8330 **Fax:** (978)524-8890
Email: isds@prri.com
Website: http://www.isds-cicd.org
Carlos A. Pellegrini, Pres.

Fnded: 1969. **Mem:** 1,205. **Desc:** Dedicated to presenting current information to the medical world concerning advances in gastrointestinal surgery, to permit the free exchange of new knowledge, to allow comparison of experiences, to stimulate clinical studies, and to seek improved diagnostic and therapeutic measures. **Pub:** *Digestive Surgery*, bimonthly. Journal. Contains information concerned with diseases of the alimentary tract.

★ 3963 ★ International Society for Diseases of the Esophagus (ISDE) (Kokusai Shokudo Shikkan Kaigi)
Institute of Gastroentrology
Tokyo Women's Medical College
8-1, Kawada-cho
Shinjuku-ku
Tokyo 162-8666, Japan
Phone: 81 3 33581435 **Fax:** 81 3 33581424
Email: isde@home.email.ne.jp
Website: http://www.isde.net/

Fnded: 1979. **Mem:** 800. **Lang(s):** English. **Desc:** Physicians, researchers, and academicians devoted to esophageal diseases throughout the world. Purpose is to: promote the exchange of scientific and medical knowledge of the esophagus among specialists in the field including physicians, surgeons, basic scientists, and other professionals; maintain interchange with organizations interested in esophageal and related diseases; encourage basic and clinical research in fields related to the esophagus; promote the professional and educational development of individuals interested in the esophagus and related diseases and to encourage, represent, and sponsor individuals who have entered this field. Conducts scholastic meetings and symposia. **Pub:** *Disease of the Esophagus*, quarterly. Journal. • *ISDE News*, semiannual. Newsletter.

★ 3964 ★ International Society for Ecological Psychology (ISEP)
c/o William M. Mace
Department of Psychology
300 Summit St.
Hartford, CT 06106-3100
Phone: (860)297-2343 **Fax:** (860)297-2538
Email: william.mace@mail.trincoll.edu
William M. Mace, Contact

Fnded: 1981. **Mem:** 330. **Nat'l Groups:** 7. **Desc:** Promotes ecological psychology. **Pub:** *Ecological Psychology: The Journal*, quarterly. Journal. • *Resources for Ecological Psychology*.

★ 3965 ★ International Society of Electrocardiology (ISE)
c/o Prof. Peter W. Macfarlane
University Department of Medical Cardiology
Royal Infirmary
10 Alexandra Parade
Glasgow G31 2ER, United Kingdom
Phone: 44 141 2114724 **Fax:** 44 141 5526114
Email: peter.w.macfarlane@clinmed.gla.ac.uk
Website: http://www.electrocardiology.net

Fnded: 1994. **Mem:** 300. **Lang(s):** English. **Desc:** Researchers and physicians in 25 countries in cardiovascular physiology and pathology, cardiology, biomathematics, biophysics, and computer science who are interested in electrocardiology. Sponsors International Congress on Electrocardiology to develop professional programs. **Pub:** *Proceedings*, annual. Journal.

★ 3966 ★ International Society of Endocrinology (ISE)
c/o Prof. Lesley H. Rees
51-53 St. Bartholomew's Hospital
Bartholomew Close
London EC1A 7BE, United Kingdom
Phone: 44 207 6064012 **Fax:** 44 207 7964676
Email: l.h.rees@mds.gmw.ac.uk
Website: http://www.jingo.com/ise/

Fnded: 1966. **Mem:** 53. **Desc:** Federation of national endocrinology societies with 15,000 individual members. Disseminates information on endocrinology and facilitates collaboration between national endocrinological societies and persons interested in the field. **Pub:** *Abstracts of Congresses*, annual. Newsletter. • *Symposia Abstracts*, periodic.

★ 3967 ★ International Society of Endovascular Specialists (ISES)
1928 E Highland Ave., No. F104-605
Phoenix, AZ 85016
Phone: (602)240-5833 **Fax:** (602)266-6018
Email: admin@isesonline.org
Website: http://www.isesonline.org

Fnded: 1992. **Mem:** 2,300. **Desc:** Endovascular surgeons promoting the development of endovascular technologies and therapies. **Pub:** *Journal of Endovascular Therapy*. Journal.

★ 3968 ★ International Society of Exercise and Immunology (ISEI)
Warburger Str. 100
Institute of Sportsmedicine
University of Paderborn
D-33098 Paderborn, Germany
Phone: 49 5251 603200 **Fax:** 49 5251 603500
Email: berger@sportmed.upb.de
Website: http://www.isei.de/

Fnded: 1993. **Desc:** Promotes scientific research and education; disseminates scientific information.

★ 3969 ★ International Society for Experimental Hematology (ISEH)
2025 M St. NW, Ste. 800
Washington, DC 20036
Phone: (202)367-1183 **Fax:** (202)367-2183
Email: iseh@dc.sba.com
Website: http://www.iseh.org
Thomas Reiser, Exec. Dir.

Fnded: 1972. **Mem:** 1,400. **Desc:** Scientists and health care professionals in the field of experimental hematology. Seeks to advance the science and practice of hematology; promotes professional development of members. Serves as a forum for the exchange of information on experimental hematology and related topics; sponsors research and educational programs. **Pub:** *Experimental Hematology*, monthly. Journal. *Price:* included in membership dues. • *Membership Directory*, periodic. Directory.

★ 3970 ★ International Society of Gastroenterological Carcinogenesis (ISGC)
1-2-3 Kasumi, Minami-ku
Hiroshima 734, Japan
Phone: 81 82 2575146 **Fax:** 81 82 2575149
Email: wyasui@mcai.med.hiroshima-u.ac.jp

Fnded: 1996. **Desc:** Encourages research and communication in the areas of gastroenterological biology and oncology.

★ 3971 ★ International Society of Geographical and Epidemiological Ophthalmology (ISGEO)
c/o Kilimanjaro Centre for Community Ophthalmology
Tumaini University
PO Box 2254
Moshi, United Republic of Tanzania
Phone: 255 27 2753547 **Fax:** 255 27 2754890

Email: kcco@kcmc.ac.tz
Website: http://www.interchange.ubc.ca/bceio/isgeo/

Fnded: 1964. **Mem:** 150. **Desc:** Open to all professionals who have an interest in the scientific aspects of international ophthalmology in particular and epidemiology and geographical medicine in general. Aims to promote the science of geographic and epidemiological ophthalmology among all people and nations. **Pub:** *Ophthalmic Epidemiology*, quarterly. Journal. Scientific journal.

★ 3972 ★ International Society for Gerontology
Hermann Lingg Str 10
D-80336 Munich, Germany
Phone: 49 89 5441260 **Fax:** 49 89 54412611
Email: imu-nuernberg@imu-institut.de

Fnded: 1999.

★ 3973 ★ International Society for Gynaecologic Endoscopy (ISGE)
c/o Simone Wamsteker, Sec.
Department of OB/GYN
Spaarne Hospital
PO Box 1644
NL-2003 BR Haarlem, Netherlands
Phone: 31 23 5282686 **Fax:** 31 23 5470881
Email: isgeoff@euronet.nl
Website: http://www.isge.org/

Fnded: 1989. **Desc:** Provides an international forum to exchange information and new ideas between gynaecologic endoscopists of all nations; promotes development of new instrumentation, techniques and therapy.

★ 3974 ★ International Society for Gynecologic Endoscopy
c/o Simone Wamsteker, Sec.
Spaarne Hospital, Department Ob/Gyn
PO Box 1644
NL-2003 BR Haarlem, Netherlands
Phone: 31 23 5282686 **Fax:** 31 23 5470881
Email: isgeoff@euronet.nl
Website: http://isge.org

Desc: Aims to establish an international forum for the timely exchange of information and new ideas between gynecologic endoscopists of all nations.

★ 3975 ★ International Society of Gynecological Endocrinology (ISGE)
Lungarno Pacinotti, 43/44
I-56100 Pisa, Italy

Fnded: 1986.

★ 3976 ★ International Society of Hair Restoration Surgery (ISHRS)
930 E Woodfield Rd.
Schaumburg, IL 60173-4729
Free: 800-444-2737 **Fax:** (847)330-1135
Email: info@ishrs.org
Website: http://www.ishrs.org
Kim Hoarley, Dir.

Fnded: 1992. **Mem:** 700. **Desc:** Hair restoration specialists. Endeavors to advance the art and science of hair restoration. **Pub:** *Dermatologic Surgery*, monthly. Journal. *Price:* included in membership dues. • *Hair Transplant Forum International*, bimonthly. Newsletter. *Price:* included in membership dues.

★ 3977 ★ International Society for Heart and Lung Transplantation (ISHLT)
14673 Midway Rd., Ste. 200
Addison, TX 75001
Phone: (972)490-9495 **Fax:** (972)490-9499
Email: ishlt@ishlt.org
Website: http://www.ishlt.org
Amanda W. Rowe, Exec. Dir.

Fnded: 1981. **Mem:** 2,250. **Desc:** Medical doctors, Ph.D.s, nurses, researchers, and others interested in artificial hearts and in heart and heart-lung failure and transplantation. Provides a center for discussion, exchange of information, and activities that promote the interests of heart and lung transplantation. Seeks to heighten awareness of public and governmental agencies regarding developments in the field. Maintains the International Heart and Lung Transplantation Registry. **Pub:** *The Journal of Heart and Lung Transplantation*, monthly. Journal. **Frmly:** (1991) International Society for Heart Transplantation.

★ 3978 ★ International Society for Heart Research
c/o Division of Cardiology, ACB 3rd Fl.
Department of Medicine
University of Louisville Health Science Center
550 S Jackson
Louisville, KY 40292
Phone: (502)852-1837 **Fax:** (502)852-6474
Email: rbolli@louisville.edu
Website: http://www.ishrworld.org
Dr. Roberto Bolli, MD, Sec. Gen.

Fnded: 1967. **Mem:** 2,000. **Desc:** Professionals and investigators in the field of experimental cardiology united to foster multidisciplinary approaches for finding solutions to the problems of heart disease. Conducts research in cardiac metabolism. **Pub:** *Advances in Myocardiology*. Journal. • *Journal of Molecular and Cellular Cardiology*, monthly. Journal. **Frmly:** International Society for Cardiovascular Research.

★ 3979 ★ International Society of Hematology (ISH) (Societe Internationale d'Hematologie)
Diaz Ordaz 808, Anzures
72530 Puebla, Puebla, Mexico
Phone: 52 222 2438100 **Fax:** 52 222 2438428
Email: gruiz1@climicaruiz.com

Fnded: 1946. **Mem:** 3,000. **Reg. Groups:** 3. **Lang(s):** English. **Desc:** Doctors of medicine and persons holding Ph.D. degrees who have completed at least 5 years in the practice or research of hematology (branch of medical science dealing with the blood, its formation, functions, and diseases). Works to promote hematology research and the advancement and recognition of hematology as a biological science. **Pub:** *Membership List*, biennial. • Newsletter, semiannual.

★ 3980 ★ International Society of Hematology - European African Division
Hematology Laboratory Department
Hospital Clinic I Provincial
Calle Villarroel, 170
E-08036 Barcelona, Spain
Phone: 34 93 4548229 **Fax:** 34 93 4548229

Fnded: 1946. **Mem:** 1,300. **Nat'l Groups:** 45. **Reg. Groups:** 3. **State Groups:** 30. **Local Groups:** 140. **Lang(s):** English. **Desc:** Scientists and physicians in 85 countries with at least 5 years experience in the field of hematology. Promotes the exchange of ideas and information relating to blood and blood forming tissues; provides an international forum for the dissemination of new information concerning hematological problems. Aims to standardize hematological methods and nomenclature on an international scale and to heighten awareness of clinical hematological problems among scientific investigators while recognizing hematology as a legitimate branch of the biological sciences. Sponsors educational programs. **Pub:** *ISH*, biennial. Newsletter. • *ISH Newsletter*, semiannual. Newsletter.

★ 3981 ★ International Society for the History of Medicine (ISHM)
20, rue Armagis
F-78105 Saint Germain-en-Laye, France
Email: alain.lellouch@wanadoo.fr

★ 3982 ★ International Society for the History of Pharmacy (Internationale Gesellschaft fur die Geschichte der Pharmazie)
c/o Govi-Verlag
Carl-Mannich-Str 26
D-65760 Eschborn, Germany
Phone: 49 696 928262 **Fax:** 49 696 928203
Email: helmstaedter@em.uni-frankfurt.de
Website: http://www.govi.de/iggp.htm

Fnded: 1926. **Desc:** Forms an international centre for handling all matters of a pharmaceutical historical nature without commercial interests; endeavours to reach its goals by promoting research in writing and teaching history of pharmacy as well as disseminating knowledge and obtaining recognition for the discipline.

★ 3983 ★ International Society of Hypnosis
c/o Behavioural Medicine Unit
Austin and Repatriation Medical Centre
Repat Campus
Locked Bag 1
Heidelberg West, VIC 3081, Australia
Phone: 61 3 94964105 **Fax:** 61 3 94964107
Email: ish-central.office@medicine.unimelb.edu.au

Lang(s): English. **Desc:** Hypnotists and medical professionals. Promotes increased use of hypnosis in the treatment of diseases and as an adjunct to traditional medical therapies. Fosters interdisciplinary research into the medical benefits of hypnosis; facilitates exchange of information among members; sponsors training and continuing professional development programs.

★ 3984 ★ International Society for Immunology of Reproduction (ISIR)
c/o JNU Campus
Shahid Jeet Sing Marg
International Centre for Genetics, Engineering and Biotechno
New Delhi 110067, India
Phone: 91 11 26184446 **Fax:** 91 11 6184447
Email: talwar@icgebnd.erner.in

Fnded: 1976. **Mem:** 250. **Reg. Groups:** 12. **Lang(s):** English. **Desc:** Scientists and physicians interested in the immunological processes involved in all aspects of reproduction. Seeks to encourage and develop research on immunological processes through scientific publications, workshops, and colloquia. **Pub:** *American Journal of Reproductive Immunology*. Journal. • *ISIR Newsletter*, semiannual. Newsletter. Provides minutes of meetings, notices of upcoming meetings, and general news updates. • *Journal of Reproductive Immunology*. Journal.

★ 3985 ★ International Society of Integral Psychoanalysis (ISAT) (Sociedade Internacional de Trilogia Analitica)
Avenida Reboucas 3819
05401-450 Sao Paulo, SP, Brazil
Phone: 55 11 30323616
Email: sitaenk@trilogiaanalitica.com.br
Website: http://www.trilogiaanalitica.com.br

Fnded: 1970. **Mem:** 762. **Nat'l Groups:** 9. **Reg. Groups:** 6. **Lang(s):** English, French, German, Portuguese, Spanish. **Desc:** Accredited psychoanalysts having scientific training in Brazil, England, Finland, Portugal, and Sweden; individuals with a medical, human, or social science degree who are currently studying analytical trilogy; students working with accredited analysts. Promotes analytical trilogy, a form of psychoanalysis that uses dialogue to cure mental as well as physical illness through a technique called interiorization. (Also known as integral psychoanalysis, analytical trilogy was founded by Prof. Norberto R. Keppe as a continuation of the psychoanalytical discoveries of Sigmund Freud and his colleagues.) Conducts research and therapy for treatment of emotional and psychosomatic problems and encourages study of humanistic culture in all its forms including social, philosophical, religious, educational, and artistic. Promotes scientific investigation of psychoanalysis, philosophy, and theology. Fosters training in the integral psychoanalytical and trilogical fields. Activities include: group and individual analysis for treating neurosis, psychosis, and organic illness without drugs; children's services; radio and television programs; introductory courses for the public. Operates publishing company, bookshop, and cultural center. Is currently organizing a collection of case studies including written declarations, X-rays, medical examination data, and documented results obtained through the use of analytical trilogy. **Pub:** *Integral Psychoanalysis Magazine*, semiannual. Magazine. • *Trilogy*, quarterly. • Bulletin, monthly. Also publishes booklets and books. **Frmly:** (1982) Society of Integral Psychoanalysis.

★ 3986 ★ International Society of Internal Medicine (ISIM)
(Societe Internationale de Medecine Interne)
c/o Dr. Rolf A. Streuli
Regional Hospital
CH-4900 Langenthal, Switzerland
Phone: 41 62 9163102 **Fax:** 41 62 9164155
Email: r.streuli@sro.ch
Website: http://www.acponline.org/isim/

Fnded: 1948. **Mem:** 3,000. **Nat'l Groups:** 58. **Lang(s):** English. **Desc:** Internal medicine specialists. Promotes scientific knowledge in internal medicine; furthers the education of young internists; encourages friendship among physicians in all countries. Federation of Societies of Internal Medicine from 58 countries.

★ 3987 ★ International Society for the Investigation of Stress (ISIS)
Level 1
South Wing
A and RMC, Repat Campus
Heidelberg West, VIC 3081, Australia
Phone: 61 3 94964105 **Fax:** 61 3 94964107

★ 3988 ★ International Society of Lipo-Suction Surgery
Via della Camilluccia, 643
I-00135 Rome, Italy
Phone: 39 06 36304792
Email: giorgiofischer@atsflashnet.it

★ 3989 ★ International Society of Lymphology (ISL)
c/o M.H. Witte
University of Arizona
College of Medicine, Department. of Surgery
1501 N Campbell Ave.
PO Box 245063
Tucson, AZ 85724-5063
Phone: (520)626-6118 **Fax:** (520)626-0822
Email: lymph@u.arizona.edu
Website: http://www.u.arizona.edu/~witte/ISL.htm
M. H. Witte, MD, Sec. Gen.

Fnded: 1966. **Mem:** 385. **Nat'l Groups:** 9. **Desc:** Professionals active in the medical, biological, and technical sciences. Promotes the study of lymphology and seeks to advance and disseminate knowledge in the field. Activities include: stimulating and strengthening experimentation and clinical investigation in lymphology; establishing relations between researchers and clinicians in the different fields of lymphology; encouraging contact and exchange of ideas among members and national and international organizations. Organizes postgraduate courses. **Pub:** *Lymphology*, quarterly. Journal. *Price:* $75 with 10% discount for vendors. • *Progress in Lymphology*, biennial. Proceedings.

★ 3990 ★ International Society for Magnetic Resonance in Medicine
2118 Milvia St., Ste. 201
Berkeley, CA 94704
Phone: (510)841-1899 **Fax:** (510)841-2340
Email: info@ismrm.org
Website: http://www.ismrm.org
Jane Tiemann, Exec. Dir.

Fnded: 1994. **Mem:** 5,000. **Reg. Groups:** 2. **Desc:** Devoted to furthering the development and application of MRI and its techniques in medicine and biology. Sponsors educational and research programs. **Pub:** *Journal of Magnetic Resonance Imaging*, monthly. Journal. • *Magnetic Resonance in Medicine*, monthly. Journal. • Brochure. • Directory. **Frmly:** (1995) Society for Magnetic Resonance.

★ 3991 ★ International Society of Magnetic Resonance in Medicine - British Chapter (ISMRM)
c/o Prof. Peter Morris, Treas.
Magnetic Resonance Centre
University of Nottingham
University Park
Nottingham NG7 2RD, United Kingdom
Email: martin@icr.ac.uk
Website: http://www-ipg.umds.ac.uk/ismrm-bc/bylaws.html

Desc: Promotes communication, research, development, applications and availability of information on magnetic resonance in medicine and biology and other related topics.

★ 3992 ★ International Society for Magnetic Resonance in Medicine - German Chapter (ISMRM)
c/o Dr. Joachim Rother
Neurologische Universitatsklinik Eppendorf
Martinistrasse 52
D-20246 Hamburg, Germany
Phone: 49 40 428038164 **Fax:** 49 40 428035086
Email: roether@uke.uni-hamburg.de
Website: http://www.ismrm.de/

Fnded: 1997. **Mem:** 208. **Desc:** Promotes communication, research, development, applications and availability of information on magnetic resonance in medicine and biology and other related topics; provides support and encouragement to young scientists.

★ 3993 ★ International Society for Medical and Psychological Hypnosis (ISMPH)
(Centro Internazionale di Ipnosi Medica e Psicologica — CIIMP)
c/o Dr. Aurora Zavertanik, Sec.
Corso XXII Marzo 57
I-20129 Milan, Italy
Phone: 39 02 70126489 **Fax:** 39 02 7491051
Email: uimpsico@tin.it

Fnded: 1985. **Mem:** 172. **Reg. Groups:** 18. **Local Groups:** 15. **Lang(s):** English, Italian. **Desc:** Professional medical doctors and psychologists. Promotes the study and use of hypnotherapeutic treatments. Conducts annual courses for members.

★ 3994 ★ International Society for Medical and Psychological Hypnosis, U.S.A. Office (ISMPH)
1991 Broadway, Apt. 18B
New York, NY 10023
Phone: (212)874-5290 **Fax:** (914)764-1445
Website: http://www.hypnosis-institute.org
Dr. Milton V. Kline, Dir.

Fnded: 1982. **Mem:** 4,000. **Desc:** Health care professionals involved with medical and psychological hypnosis. Supports clinical research in hypnosis and research in psychotherapy strategies and tactics; offers advanced training and certification for hypnotherapists. Maintains speakers' bureau; compiles statistics. **Pub:** *Conference Proceedings*, annual. Proceedings. • *Morton Price Mental Health Center*, quarterly. Newsletter. Contains original research, membership news, book reviews, and conference reports.

★ 3995 ★ International Society of Mental Health Online (ISMHO)
6853 Tussic St.
Westerville, OH 43082
Email: ismho@ismho.org
Website: http://www.ismho.org
Martha Ainsworth, Pres.

Fnded: 1997. **Desc:** Mental health professionals. Works to promote the understanding, use, and development of online communication, information, and technology for the international mental health community. Hosts online discussion forums, annual dinners.

★ 3996 ★ International Society for Mental Training and Excellence (ISMTE)
CP 1807
Chelsea, QC, Canada J9B 1A1
Fax: (819)827-2652
Email: ismte@rems.net
Website: http://www.coach.ca/ismte/

Fnded: 1989. **Desc:** Promotes excellence in sport, performance, education, work, health and life in general; provides materials, educational opportunities, and consulting services. **Pub:** *Journal of Excellence*, semiannual. Journal. Devoted to nurturing excellence in human endeavors.

★ 3997 ★ International Society on Metabolic Eye Disease (ISMED)
1125 Park Ave.
New York, NY 10128
Phone: (212)427-1246 **Fax:** (212)360-7009
Heskel M. Haddad, MD, Sec. -Treas.

Fnded: 1971. **Mem:** 600. **Desc:** Ophthalmologists, pediatricians, endocrinologists, internists, and paramedical personnel in 20 countries. Promotes the study of metabolic eye problems and biochemical and genetic aspects of such problems. **Pub:** *Metabolic, Pediatric, and Systemic Ophthalmology*, quarterly. Journal. *Price:* $160/year. • Book.

★ 3998 ★ International Society for Minimal Intervention in Spinal Surgery
c/o Prof. Hansjoerg F. Leu, Sec.
Spital Neumunster
Prsima Spine Unit
Trichtenhauserstrasse 12
CH-8125 Zollikerberg, Switzerland
Fax: 41 1 3912646

Fnded: 1989. **Mem:** 361. **Reg. Groups:** 9. **State Groups:** 8. **Lang(s):** English. **Desc:** Promotes the development of minimally invasive spinal surgery.

★ 3999 ★ International Society for Minimally Invasive Cardiac Surgery (ISMICS)
13 Elm St.
Manchester, MA 01944
Phone: (978)526-0330 **Fax:** (978)526-4018
Email: ismics@prri.com
Website: http://www.ismics.org
Aurelie M. Alger, JD, Asst. Dir.

Fnded: 1997. **Mem:** 550. **Desc:** Concerned with patient outcomes, techniques, and progressive development of less invasive forms of heart surgery. **Pub:** *The Heart Surgery Forum*. Journal.

★ 4000 ★ International Society for Mountain Medicine (ISMM)
c/o Peter Hackett, MD
610 Sabeta Dr.
Ridgway, CO 81432-9335
Phone: (970)626-2477 **Fax:** (970)626-2467
Email: hackett@ismmed.org
Website: http://www.ismmed.org
Peter Hackett, MD, Contact

Fnded: 1985. **Mem:** 450. **Desc:** Brings together scientists and physicians, and allied trade professionals interested in mountain medicine. Encourages research on all aspects of mountains, mountain peoples and mountaineers. **Pub:** *High Altitude Medicine and Biology*, quarterly. Journal. Provides information about high altitude/mountain physiology and clinical medicine. *Price:* included in membership dues.

★ 4001 ★ International Society for Music in Medicine (ISMM) (Internationale Gesellschaft fur Musik in der Medizin)
Paulmannshoher Str. 17
D-58515 Ludenscheid, Germany
Phone: 49 2351 9452260 **Fax:** 49 2351 363035

Fnded: 1982. **Mem:** 80. **Reg. Groups:** 1. **Lang(s):** English. **Desc:** Medical doctors, scientists, and music therapists. Initiates and coordinates interdisciplinary research into the psychological and physiological basis for and applications of music in medicine. **Pub:** *International Journal of Arts Medicine*, quarterly. Journal. • *Music Medicine, Vol. I, 1993.* Book. • *Music Medicine, Vol. 2, 1996.* Book. • *Music Medicine Vol 3, 1998.* Book.

★ 4002 ★ International Society of Nephrology (ISN)
c/o Ms. Soha Fahmy, Office Mgr.
Cairo Kidney Center
3 Hussein El-Memar St., Antikhana
PO Box 91 El-Louk
Cairo 11513, Egypt
Phone: 20 2 5790267 **Fax:** 31 2 5790267
Email: isn@rusys.eg.net
Website: http://www.isn-online.org

Fnded: 1960. **Mem:** 8,715. **Desc:** Promotes the education, science and patient care in the field of nephrology. **Pub:** *Kidney International.* Journal.

★ 4003 ★ International Society for Neuroimmunomodulation
c/o Craig C. Smith
National Institute of Health
36 Convent Dr., Rm. 1A23/MSC 4020
Bethesda, MD 20892-4020
Phone: (301)496-4561 **Fax:** (301)496-6095
Email: ccs@codon.nih.gov
Website: http://www.isnim.org
Craig C. Smith, Exec. Dir.

Fnded: 1986. **Mem:** 150. **Desc:** Professional society for scientists involved in interdisciplinary research in the molecular and cellular aspects of neurobiology, neuroendocrinology, immunology, and the behavioral sciences. Interests focus on discerning the integrative elements underlying communication and modulation between the central nervous, endocrine, and immune systems, and upon related disease states. **Pub:** *NeuroImmunoModulation.* Journal.

★ 4004 ★ International Society for Neuronal Regulation (ISNR)
394 Rd. 34
Merino, CO 80741
Free: 800-488-3867 **Fax:** (775)305-9379
Email: office@snr-jnt.org
Website: http://www.snr-jnt.org/
Darlene Nelson, Exec. Dir.

Fnded: 1995. **Mem:** 500. **Nat'l Groups:** 1. **Desc:** Promotes professionals in the fields of neurotherapy, neurofeedback, training and research. **Pub:** *Journal of Neurotherapy*, quarterly. Journal. *Price:* included in membership dues. **Frmly:** (1999) Society for the Study of Neuronal Regulation; (2003) Society for Neuronal Regulation.

★ 4005 ★ International Society of Neuropathology (Societe Internationale de Neuropathologie)
c/o Hannu Kalimo, Sec.Gen.
Department of Pathology
Turku University Hospital
FIN-20520 Turku, Finland
Phone: 358 2 2611685 **Fax:** 358 2 3337459
Email: hkalim@mailhost.utu.fi
Website: http://brainpath.medsch.ucla.edu/isn/isnhome.htm

Fnded: 1972. **Mem:** 2,500. **Lang(s):** English. **Desc:** Members of national societies of neuropathology in 30 countries. Works to foster the formation of national and regional societies of neuropathology and to promote cooperation among these societies. Maintains liaison with international organizations in various fields of neurological sciences. Encourages the exchange of information and persons engaged in neuropathology. Initiates research projects. **Pub:** *Brain Pathology*, quarterly. Journal. • *Membership Directory*, periodic. Directory.

★ 4006 ★ International Society of Neurovirology
c/o Brian Wigdahl, Dept. of Microbiology and Immunology Penn State College of Medicine
500 University Dr.
PO Box 850
Hershey, PA 17033
Phone: (717)531-8258 **Fax:** (717)531-5580
Email: bwigdahl@psu.edu
Website: http://www.isnv.org
Brian Wigdahl, PhD, Pres.

Fnded: 1998. **Mem:** 245. **Nat'l Groups:** 1. **Desc:** Neurovirologists. **Pub:** *Journal of NeuroVirology*, bimonthly. Journal. Scholarly journal, basic and clinical research in neurovirology. *Price:* $240 for nonmembers; included in membership dues.

★ 4007 ★ International Society of Noninvasive Cardiology (ISCN)
Herestr 49
3000 Leuven, Belgium
Phone: 32 1 6345844 **Fax:** 32 1 6345840
Email: andre.aubert@med.kuleuven.ac.be

Fnded: 1980. **Mem:** 250. **Nat'l Groups:** 27. **Desc:** Promotes research on the heart and the circulation by non-invasive means.

★ 4008 ★ International Society of Nurses in Cancer Care (ISNCC)
PO Box 297
Macclesfield SK11 7FZ, United Kingdom
Phone: 44 1625 669588 **Fax:** 44 1625 428128
Email: secretariat@isncc.org
Website: http://www.isncc.org

Fnded: 1984. **Mem:** 90. **Nat'l Groups:** 35. **Desc:** Provides communication network for cancer nursing societies and professionals; works as resource for nurses working in clinical practice, education, research and management for cancer nursing and the nurse's role in cancer care. **Pub:** *Directory of Oncology Nurse Researchers.* Directory. • *International Cancer Nursing News*, quarterly. Directory. Contains a listing of nurses worldwide who are engaged in oncology nursing research. • *Palliative Care Curriculum.*

★ 4009 ★ International Society of Nurses in Genetics (ISONG)
c/o Jean Anderson, RN, MA, CPNP
2593 W 15th St. S
Newton, IA 50208
Phone: (641)831-9230
Email: janderson@isong.us
Website: http://www.isong.org
Jean Anderson, RN,MA, Exec. Dir.

Fnded: 1988. **Mem:** 300. **Desc:** Case managers, administrators, coordinators of public and private programs, educators in the field of nursing and/or genetics, genetic counselors, researchers. Committed to incorporating the knowledge of human genetics into nursing practice, education and research activities. **Pub:** Newsletter, 3/year. • Membership Directory.

★ 4010 ★ International Society for Oncodevelopmental Biology and Medicine (ISOBM)
Department of Immunology
Umea University
S-901 85 Umea, Sweden
Phone: 46 90 7852345 **Fax:** 46 90 7852250
Email: sten.hammarstrom@climi.umu.se
Website: http://www.med.uio.no/dnr/ISOBM/ISOBMhome.htm

Fnded: 1972.

★ 4011 ★ International Society for Oneiric Mental Imagery Techniques (ISMIT) (Societa Internazionale per le Techniche d'Imagerie Mentale Onirique)
c/o Chez Mme. Odile Dorkel, Pres.
56 rue Sedaine
F-52110 Daillancourt, France
Phone: 33 1 0147001663
Email: odile.dorkel@wanadoo.fr
Website: http://www.arbrevert.org

Fnded: 1966. **Mem:** 80. **Desc:** Fosters inquiry and interaction among researchers and practitioners of mental imagery techniques in psychotherapy. Conducts research on mental imagery psychotherapy; disseminates research results. Organizes seminars on psychotherapeutic practice. **Pub:** *Decentration*, periodic. • *Mental Imagery.* • *Vocabulary of Psychotherapies.* Additional publications available on request.

★ 4012 ★ International Society of Oriental Medicine (ISOM)
965-1 Chegi 2-dong, Dongdaemun-ku
Seoul 130-060, Republic of Korea
Phone: 82 2 9597344 **Fax:** 82 2 9597347
Email: isom@chollian.net

Desc: Promotes research exchange and cooperation required for the development of oriental medicine.

★ 4013 ★ International Society for Orthomolecular Medicine
16 Florence Ave.
Toronto, ON, Canada M2N 1E9
Phone: (416)733-2117 **Fax:** (416)733-2352
Email: centre@orthomed.org
Website: http://www.orthomed.org/isom/isom.htm

Fnded: 1994. **Desc:** Aims to further the advancement of Orthomolecular medicine throughout the world, to raise awareness of this rapidly growing and cost effective practice of health care, and to unite the many and various groups already operating in this field.

★ 4014 ★ International Society of Orthopaedic Surgery and Traumatology (Societe Internationale de Chirurgie Orthopedique et de Traumatologie — SICOT)
40, rue Washington, bte. 9
B-1050 Brussels, Belgium
Phone: 32 2 6486823 **Fax:** 32 2 6498601
Email: hq@sicot.org
Website: http://www.sicot.org

Fnded: 1929. **Mem:** 3,000. **Nat'l Groups:** 108. **Lang(s):** English, French. **Desc:** Orthopaedic surgeons in 108 countries united to contribute to the progress of science by conducting studies related to orthopedic surgery and traumatology. **Pub:** *International Orthopedics*, bimonthly. Journal. Includes Newsletter.

★ 4015 ★ International Society for Pediatric and Adolescent Diabetes (ISPAD)
c/o Dr. Peter G.F. Swift
Children's Hospital
Leicester Royal Infirmary
LE1 5WW Leicester, Norway
Phone: 44 116 2541414 **Fax:** 44 116 2587637
Email: peter.swift3@networld.com
Website: http://www.ispad.org
Fnded: 1974. **Mem:** 700. **Lang(s):** Dutch, English, Finnish, Japanese, Norwegian. **Desc:** Health professionals worldwide who study and treat juvenile diabetes. Promotes improvements in research and clinical care of children and adolescents with diabetes.

★ 4016 ★ International Society for Pediatric Neurosurgery (ISPN)
Universitatsklinik fur Neurchirurgie
Landeskrankenhaus
A-8036 Graz, Austria
Fnded: 1972. **Mem:** 160. **Desc:** Physicians specializing in pediatric neurosurgery. Objective is to contribute to the advancement of the specialty. Activities include the study of the most recent advancements in the field. **Pub:** *Child's Nervous System*, bimonthly. Journal.

★ 4017 ★ International Society of Pediatric Oncology (SIOP) (Societe Internationale d'Oncologie Pediatrique — SIOP)
c/o IMEDEX
Bruistensingel 360
PO Box 3283
NL-5203 DG Hertogenbosch, Netherlands
Phone: 31 73 6462929
Email: administrator@siopbrain.org
Fnded: 1969. **Mem:** 955. **Lang(s):** English. **Desc:** Pediatric oncologists, pediatric surgeons involved in oncology, pathologists, radiotherapists, researchers, and others interested in malignant tumors in children. Purpose is to promote research, treatment, and clinical review of cancerous growths in children. Facilitates collaboration and exchange of information among members and others in the field. Organizes and participates in controlled therapeutic trials. **Pub:** *Medical and Pediatric Oncology*, monthly. Journal. • *SIOP Newsletter*, semiannual. Newsletter. • Brochure, periodic.

★ 4018 ★ International Society for Peritoneal Dialysis (ISPD)
c/o Dr. Sarah Prichard, Pres.
Royal Victoria Hospital
687 Pine Ave. W
Montreal, QC, Canada H3A 1A1
Email: jwinch@ix.netcom.com
Website: http://www.ispd.org
Fnded: 1984. **Mem:** 1,500. **Lang(s):** English. **Desc:** Physicians, nurses, and biomedical engineers involved in peritoneal dialysis, a procedure similar to artificial kidney machine dialysis but involving insertion of a tube into the abdomen to cleanse blood within the body. Seeks to advance knowledge of peritoneal dialysis through exchange and research. **Pub:** *Peritoneal Dialysis International*, bimonthly. Journal.

★ 4019 ★ International Society for Pharmacoeconomics and Outcomes Research (ISPOR)
3100 Princeton Pke., Bldg 3, Ste. E
Lawrenceville, NJ 08648
Phone: (609)219-0773 **Fax:** (609)219-0774
Email: info@ispor.org
Website: http://www.ispor.org
Marilyn Dix Smith, Exec. Dir.
Fnded: 1995. **Mem:** 2,000. **Nat'l Groups:** 13. **Reg. Groups:** 3. **Desc:** Researchers who study the cost effectiveness of treatments. Researchers and users of cost-effectiveness information, health care decision makers. **Pub:** *ISPOR News*, bimonthly. Newsletter. Pharmacoeconomic news articles. • *Value in Health*, bimonthly. Journal. Provides information on pharmacoeconomic and outcomes research; health policy development. Now indexed in "Index Medicus/Medline". *Price:* $165 per year.

★ 4020 ★ International Society for Phosphoinositide Metabolism and Signaling
2-1 Seiryo-cho, Aoba-ku
Sendai 980 0872, Japan
Phone: 81 22 7178031 **Fax:** 81 22 7178035
Email: hkondo@mail.cc.tohoku.ac.jp

★ 4021 ★ International Society of Physical Medicine and Rehabilitation
c/o Werner Van Cleemputte
Medicongress
28-34 Waalpoel
B-9960 Assenede, Belgium
Phone: 32 9 3443959 **Fax:** 32 9 3444010
Email: isprm@medicongress.com
Website: http://www.isprm.org
Fnded: 1950. **Mem:** 40. **Lang(s):** English. **Desc:** National societies of physical medicine and rehabilitation composed of qualified physicians and surgeons, and approved by the Federation's Board of Governors. Promotes high standards in education and training and the importance of physical medicine and rehabilitation; encourages the exchange of information between medical and nonmedical workers in the field of rehabilitation. Collects and distributes data on rehabilitation; encourages contact between members. **Pub:** *Regulations and List of Members*, quadrennial. Directory. • *White Book on Education and Training*, periodic. Book.

★ 4022 ★ International Society for Plastination (ISP)
c/o R.W. Henry
University of Tennessee
College of Veterinary Medicine
2407 River Dr.
Knoxville, TN 37996
Fax: (865)974-5640
Email: rhenry@utk.edu
Website: http://www.kfunigraz.ac.at/anawww/plast/index.htm
Robert W. Henry, DVMPhD, Treas.
Fnded: 1984. **Mem:** 200. **Desc:** Anatomists, pathologists, and technologists. Seeks to share information about plastination, a means of infiltrating biological specimens with curable polymers. **Pub:** *Journal of the International Society for Plastination*, semiannual. Journal. *Price:* $40/year.

★ 4023 ★ International Society of Political Psychology (ISPP)
c/o Dana Ward, Exec. Dir.
ISPP Central Office
Pitzer College
1050 N Mills Ave.
Claremont, CA 91711
Phone: (909)621-8442 **Fax:** (928)395-2224
Email: ispp@pitzer.edu
Website: http://ispp.org/ispp/centraloffice.html
Dana Ward, Exec. Dir.
Fnded: 1978. **Mem:** 1,400. **Nat'l Groups:** 3. **Reg. Groups:** 8. **Desc:** Psychologists, psychiatrists, psychoanalysts, political scientists, historians, sociologists, economists, anthropologists, media representatives, and government officials. Promotes understanding and scientific interest in the relationship between psychological, political, social, and economic processes. Seeks to facilitate communication among members and to increase the quality and application of work in political psychology. Examines relationships between psychological and political events. Areas of interest include: political violence and terrorism; socialization and the media; human rights conflict resolution; bureaucracy negotiation and mediation; totalitarianism. Sponsors the Summer Institute in Political Psychology in conjunction with Ohio State University. Conducts panel discussions. **Pub:** *ISPPNews*, semiannual. Newsletter. Contains information on activities and news of the organization; includes availability of fellowships, grants, and visiting scholar programs. *Price:* Free for members. • *Political Psychology*, quarterly. Journal. Covers classics in political psychology, interdisciplinary foundations of political psychology, and issues in professional development.

★ 4024 ★ International Society of Prenatal and Perinatal Psychology and Medicine (ISPPM)
c/o A. & J. Bischoff
Friedhofweg 8
D-69118 Heidelberg, Germany
Phone: 49 6221 892729 **Fax:** 49 6221 892730
Email: secretary@isppm.de
Website: http://www.isppm.de/
Fnded: 1971. **Desc:** Devoted to the initial phase of human development, prenatal and perinatal life. Works to improve the quality of life of the human being through research and practice. **Pub:** *International Journal of Prenatal and Perinatal Psychology and Medicine*, quarterly, March, June, September, December. Journal.

★ 4025 ★ International Society for Preventive Oncology (ISPO)
c/o Bloodline
55 Lake Ave. North, Box 20
Worcester, MA 01655
Phone: (508)856-1822 **Fax:** (508)856-1824
Email: editor@cancerprev.org
Website: http://www.bloodline.net/stories/storyreader$2126
J. Kirby Robinson, Ed.
Fnded: 1980. **Mem:** 400. **Desc:** Physicians and other professionals at the doctoral level; individuals with professional equivalence who are actively engaged in preventive oncology. Promotes the prevention of cancer through the identification and control of cancer causing factors; fosters secondary prevention through detection and treatment of cancer in its earliest, most curable stages. Sponsors basic research on cancer prevention and early detection and provides a forum for information exchange between scientists engaged in research and those working on preventive and clinical oncology. Conducts workshops. **Pub:** *Cancer Detection and Prevention*, 6/year. • *Proceedings of International Symposium on Immunobiology of Cancer and Allied Immune Dysfunctions*, biennial. • *Proceedings of the International Conference on Human Tumor Markers*, biennial. • *Proceedings of the International Symposium on Prevention and Detection of Cancer*, biennial.

★ 4026 ★ International Society for Prosthetics and Orthotics (ISPO) (Societe Internationale de Prothese et Orthese)
Borgervaenget 5
DK-2100 Copenhagen, Denmark
Phone: 45 39207260 **Fax:** 45 39207501
Email: ispo@ispo.ws
Website: http://www.ispo.ws
Fnded: 1970. **Mem:** 2,900. **Nat'l Groups:** 35. **Lang(s):** English. **Desc:** Medical and paramedical professionals in 83 countries interested in prosthetics, orthotics, and other fields of rehabilitation engineering. Promotes improvements in the care of people with neuromuscular and skeletal impairments. Serves as nonpolitical coordinating and advisory organization on prosthetics, orthotics, rehabilitation engineering, and other matters related to the neuromuscular and skeletal system. Promotes and guides programs in research, development, and evaluation regarding prosthetics and orthotics. Fosters quality practice and develops standards for nomenclature, device design, techniques, processes, and patient care. Sponsors exhibits, conferences, regional and international courses, seminars, and symposia; supports education and training in the field. **Pub:** *CAD CAM in Prosthetics*

& Orthotics. Report. • *The Deformed Foot & Orthopaedic Footwear.* Report. • *Prosthetics & Orthotics in the Developing World with Respect to Training Education & Clinical Services.* Report. • *Training & Education in Prosthetics & Orthotics for Developing Countries.* Report.

★ 4027 ★ International Society for Prosthetics and Orthotics - United Kingdom (ISPO)

131 St. James Rd.
Glasgow G4 OLS, United Kingdom
Phone: 44 141 5524049 **Fax:** 44 141 5521283
Email: l.mclachlan@strath.ac.uk

Fnded: 1970.

★ 4028 ★ International Society of Psychiatric Mental Health Nurses (ISPN)

1211 Locust St.
Philadelphia, PA 19107
Phone: (215)545-2843 **Free:** 800-826-2950
Fax: (215)545-8107
Email: ispn@nursecominc.com
Website: http://www.ispn-psych.org
Joseph Broden, Exec. Dir.

Fnded: 1999. **Mem:** 900. **Local Groups:** 25. **Desc:** Psychiatric and mental health nurses. Seeks to advance the study, teaching, and practice of psychiatric and mental health nursing. Represents members' professional and economic interests. **Pub:** *Archives of Psychiatric Nursing*, quarterly. Journal. *Price:* $43/year for nonmembers; included in membership dues. • *ISPN Connections*, 3/year. Newsletter. *Price:* Included in membership dues; $20 for nonmembers. • *Journal of Child and Adolescent Psychiatric Nursing*, quarterly. Journal. *Price:* Included in membership dues; $43 for nonmembers. **Frmly:** (1992) Advocates for Child Psychiatric Nursing; (1999) Association of Child and Adolescent Psychiatric Nurses.

★ 4029 ★ International Society of Psychology of Handwriting (ISPH) (Societa Internazionale di Psicologia della Scrittura — SIPS)

Istituto di Indagini Psicologiche
Corso XXII Marzo 57
I-20129 Milan, Italy
Phone: 39 02 70126489 **Fax:** 39 02 7491051
Email: uimpsico@tin.it
Website: http://www.psicoprofili.it

Fnded: 1961. **Mem:** 192. **Reg. Groups:** 12. **Lang(s):** English, German, Spanish. **Desc:** Physicians, psychologists, psychiatrists, teachers, and others. Promotes study and research in the psychology of handwriting. Has prepared documentaries on the subject for classroom and public instruction. Offers children's services. **Pub:** *Albo dei Docenti e Specialisti dell'UIM*, semiannual. Newsletter. Contains information on activities, research, schedule of courses, and professional updates. • *Catalog of Publications.* Catalog. • Directory.

★ 4030 ★ International Society for Psychophysics (ISP)

c/o Prof. Ana Garriga-Trillo
Psychology Faculty
UNED
Ciudad Universitaria
E-28040 Madrid, Spain
Phone: 34 91 3730997 **Fax:** 34 91 3864461
Email: agarriga@psi.uned.es
Website: http://www.psychology.adelaide.edu.au/psychophysics/

Fnded: 1985. **Mem:** 114. **Lang(s):** English. **Desc:** Promotes research in psychophysics. **Pub:** *Fechner Day*, annual, same year as meeting. Book. Contains all contributions to the yearly meetings.

★ 4031 ★ International Society of Psychosomatic Obstetrics and Gynaecology (ISPOG)

c/o Berit Sjogren, MD, Sec.Gen.
Department of Obstetrics & Gynaecology
Karolinska Hospital
S-171 76 Stockholm, Sweden
Email: berit.sjogren@ks.se
Website: http://www.ispog.org/

Desc: Promotes the study of psychobiological and psychosocial, ethical and cross-cultural problems in the fields of obstetrics and gynecology, women's health and reproductive health; promotes education, research, and training. **Pub:** *Journal of Psychosomatic Obstetrics and Gynecology.* Journal.

★ 4032 ★ International Society for Radiation Oncology (ISRO)

Av E Mounier 83-4
1200 Brussels, Belgium
Phone: 32 2 7759342 **Fax:** 32 2 7795494
Email: info@isro.be
Website: http://www.isro.be

Fnded: 1981. **Mem:** 86. **Nat'l Groups:** 81. **Reg. Groups:** 5. **Desc:** Fosters the fields of radiotherapy and oncology, by promoting studies and research.

★ 4033 ★ International Society of Radiographers and Radiological Technologists (ISRRT) (Societe Internationale des Radiographes et Techniciens de Radiologie)

143 Bryn Pinwydden
Pentwyn
Cardiff CF23 7DG, United Kingdom
Phone: 44 2920 745075 **Fax:** 44 2920 540551
Email: isrrt.yule@btopenworld.com
Website: http://www.isrrt.org

Fnded: 1959. **Mem:** 78. **Nat'l Groups:** 72. **Reg. Groups:** 3. **Lang(s):** English. **Desc:** National radiographic societies and other organizations having radiographers as members. Objectives are to: advance the science and practice of radiography, radiotherapy, and allied subjects by promoting improved standards of training and research in technical aspects of radiation medicine and protection; make results of research and experience available to practitioners; raise funds to further these objectives. Compiles statistics and maintains museum. Has established educational trust fund. Conducts teachers' seminars. **Pub:** *Health and Safety Manual*, periodic. Proceedings. • *Quality Control Handbook.* **Frmly:** International Society of Radiographers and Radiological Technicians.

★ 4034 ★ International Society of Radiolabeled Blood Elements (ISORBE)

c/o Dr. Margarida Rodrigues
Department of Nuclear Medicine
University of Vienna
Waehringer Guertel 18-20
A-1090 Vienna, Austria
Phone: 43 1 4020902 **Fax:** 43 1 4029292
Email: rodriguesradischat@hotmail.com
Website: http://www.isorbe.org

Fnded: 1990. **Mem:** 201. **State Groups:** 28. **Lang(s):** English. **Desc:** Scientists working in the field of labeled blood cells. Seeks to promote the study of radiolabeled blood elements. Protects archives and promotes standardization.

★ 4035 ★ International Society of Radiology (ISR)

7910 Woodmont Ave., Ste. 400
Bethesda, MD 20814
Phone: (301)657-2652 **Fax:** (301)907-8768
Email: isr@isradiology.org
Website: http://www.his.com/~isr/
O.W. Linton, MSJ, Exec. Dir.

Fnded: 1953. **Mem:** 69. **Nat'l Groups:** 69. **Reg. Groups:** 4. **Desc:** National radiological associations. Seeks to promote medical radiology worldwide through the work of its sections and international commissions. Undertakes business referred to it by member societies. Provides financial support for the work of its commissions. **Pub:** *Congress Programs*, biennial. • *Reports of Commissions of ISR*, periodic. • Newsletter, semiannual.

★ 4036 ★ International Society of Refractive Surgery (ISRS)

1180 Springs Centre South Blvd., No. 116
Altamonte Springs, FL 32714-1954
Phone: (407)786-7446 **Fax:** (407)786-7447
Email: isrshq@isrs.org
Website: http://www.isrs.org
Julia Lewis, Exec. Dir.

Fnded: 1979. **Mem:** 4,000. **Desc:** Eye care professionals. Provides scientific research, knowledge, and information to all individuals who are interested in refractive surgery. The association is committed to supporting and advancing the ethical practice of refractive surgery by providing quality education, stimulating information exchange, and promoting scientific research worldwide. **Pub:** *Journal of Refractive Surgery*, 6/yr.Journal. Features original research and a review of refractive and corneal surgical procedures. *Price:* $125 per year. **Frmly:** (1996) International Society Refractive Keratplasty.

★ 4037 ★ International Society of Reproductive Medicine (ISRM)

c/o Donald C. McEwen, M.D.
336 W Main St.
Bound Brook, NJ 08805-1840
Donald C. McEwen, MD, Sec.

Fnded: 1968. **Mem:** 300. **Desc:** Research specialists in reproductive medicine, obstetrics/gynecology, and endocrinology; associate members are laypersons interested in world population problems. Encourages basic and clinical research on the physiology of reproduction with special emphasis on the normal reproductive process, methods for enhancement of fertility, conception control, the pharmacology of steroids and polypeptides, and the immunology of reproduction. Fosters discussion and evaluation of new concepts, controversies in management of patients with reproductive disorders, and clinical relevance of advances in reproductive biology. Disseminates information and promotes continuing education for physicians and scientists. **Pub:** *Annual Proceedings.* **Frmly:** (1970) Family Planning Association of the Americas; (1980) International Family Planning Research Association.

★ 4038 ★ International Society for Research in Human Milk and Lactation

c/o Frank R. Greer
Meriter Hospital
Perinatal Center
202 S Park St.
Madison, WI 53715
Phone: (608)262-6561 **Fax:** (608)267-6377
Email: frgreer@facstaff.wisc.edu
Website: http://www.isrhml.org/
Dr. Frank R. Greer, Sec. Treas.

Fnded: 1984. **Mem:** 200. **Desc:** Promotes research and dissemination of findings in the field of human milk and lactation. Establishes liaisons with government agencies, public health authorities, industry, and other organizations; provides listserver for communication of information among members.

★ 4039 ★ International Society for Respiratory Protection (ISRP)

8598 Kingcome Cr.
Sidney, BC, Canada V8L 5C7
Email: rwono@cdc.gov

Fnded: 1982. **Mem:** 400. **Lang(s):** English. **Desc:** Technical and professional people involved with all aspects of nonmedical occupational respiratory protection. Seeks to advance knowledge of respiratory protection for firefighters, commercial divers, persons working in and around foundries, coke ovens, and mines, and other individuals exposed to airborne particles and other unsuitable breathing conditions. **Pub:** *ISRP Journal*, quarterly. Journal. Includes scientific articles. • *Special Conference Proceedings*, biennial. Proceedings. • Membership Directory, annual.

★ 4040 ★ International Society for Sexual and Impotence Research

c/o Jo-Els van de Woude
Postbus 97
NL-3950 AB Maarn, Netherlands
Phone: 31 343 443888 **Fax:** 31 343 442043
Email: secretariat@issir.org
Website: http://www.issir.org

Fnded: 1982. **Mem:** 600. **Reg. Groups:** 4. **Lang(s):** English. **Desc:** Seeks to establish a scientific society to benefit the public y encouraging the highest standards of practice, education, and research in the field of human sexuality. Develops scientific methods for the diagnosis, prevention, and treatment of conditions affecting human sexual function.

★ 4041 ★ International Society for Ski Traumatology and Medicine of Winter Sports (Societe Internationale de Traumatologie du Ski et de Medecine des Sports d'Hiver)

c/o Dr. M.H. Binet
Centre Medical
F-74110 Avoriaz, France
Phone: 33 4 50740542 **Fax:** 33 4 50740758
Email: binet@mdem.org

Fnded: 1956. **Lang(s):** English, French, German, Italian, Spanish. **Desc:** Encourages an international exchange of medical experiences and ideas on the treatment of injuries resulting from mountaineering and other winter sports. **Pub:** *Congress Reports*, biennial.

★ 4042 ★ International Society for Skin Imaging (ISSI)

Gudrunstr 56
Dermatological Clinic
Ruhr-University Bochum
D-44791 Bochum, Germany
Fax: 49 234 5093409
Email: office@issi.de
Website: http://www.issi.de/

Fnded: 1990.

★ 4043 ★ International Society of Sports Psychology (ISSP)

c/o Gershon Tenenbaum
Department of Educational Psychology & Learning Systems
Florida State University
307 Stone Bldg.
Tallahassee, FL 32306
Phone: (850)644-8780 **Fax:** (850)644-8776
Email: tenenbaum@mail.coe.fsu.edu
Website: http://www.issponline.org
Gershon Tenenbaum, Past Pres.

Fnded: 1965. **Mem:** 1,000. **Nat'l Groups:** 10. **State Groups:** 5. **Desc:** Professionally qualified individuals in 47 countries interested in sports psychology. Supports and promotes scientific research and professional relations between scholars in the field; participates in information and documentation services in sports psychology; advises and facilitates the establishment of other continental, regional, and national societies of sport psychology. Provides the International Olympic Committee and United States Olympic Committee with information on sport psychology services. Maintains speakers' bureau. **Pub:** *International Journal of Sport & Exercise Psychology*, quarterly. Journal. Reports scientific and applied issues in sport and exercise psychology. *Price:* $80/year. • *ISSP Newsletter*, semiannual. Newsletter. Covers professional issues in sports psychology; includes conference reports, employment opportunities, and membership list. *Price:* Included in membership dues. • Also publishes proceedings.

★ 4044 ★ International Society for the Study of Dissociation (ISSD)

60 Revere Dr., Ste. 500
Northbrook, IL 60062
Phone: (847)480-0899 **Fax:** (847)480-9282
Email: issd@issd.org
Website: http://www.issd.org
Richard Chefetz, MD, Pres.

Fnded: 1982. **Mem:** 1,200. **Desc:** Promotes research and training in the identification and treatment of dissociative disorders. Supports international communications and cooperation among professional clinicians and investigators working in the field of dissociation. **Pub:** *ISSD Membership Directory*, periodic. Membership Directory. Ongoing electronic directory. • *ISSD News*, bimonthly. Newsletter. • *The Journal of Trauma and Dissociation*, quarterly. Journal. • *Standards of Practice Guidelines for treating Dissociative Identity Disorder in Adults. Price:* Included in membership dues; $5/additional copy for members; $10 for nonmembers. **Frmly:** International Society for the Study of Multiple Personalities and Dissociation.

★ 4045 ★ International Society for the Study of Hypertension in Pregnancy

Royal Victoria Infirmary
Newcastle upon Tyne NE1 4LP, United Kingdom

Fnded: 1978. **Desc:** Conducts research in the field of hypertension in pregnancy; advances education in the field.

★ 4046 ★ International Society for the Study of the Lumbar Spine

2075 Bayview Ave., Room MG323
Toronto, ON, Canada M4N 3M5
Phone: (416)480-4833 **Fax:** (416)480-6055
Email: shirley.fitzgerald@swchsc.on.ca
Website: http://www.issls.org

Fnded: 1974. **Mem:** 346. **Desc:** Aims to bring together those individuals throughout the world, who, by their contributions and activities both in the area of research and clinical study, have, or are indicating interest in the lumbar spine in health and in disease.

★ 4047 ★ International Society for the Study of Subtle Energies and Energy Medicine (ISSSEEM)

c/o C. Penny Hiernu
11005 Ralston Rd., Ste. 100D
Arvada, CO 80004
Phone: (303)425-4625 **Fax:** (303)425-4685
Email: issseem@cs.com
Website: http://www.issseem.org
C. Penny Hiernu, CEO

Fnded: 1989. **Mem:** 1,400. **Desc:** Individuals interested in the study of human capacities and the role of consciousness in Nature. Offers educational programs. **Pub:** *Bridges*, quarterly. Magazine. Written for clinicians. *Price:* $50. • *Subtle Energies and Energy Medicine*, 3/year. Journal.

★ 4048 ★ International Society for the Study of Tension in Performance

c/o 28 Emperor's Gate
Kingston University
School of Music
London SW7 4HS, United Kingdom
Phone: 44 207 3737307 **Fax:** 44 207 3735440
Email: carogrindea@yahoo.com

Fnded: 1981. **Mem:** 360. **Nat'l Groups:** 3. **Lang(s):** English, Russian, Spanish. **Desc:** Musicians, actors, dancers, medical practitioners, consultants, psychologists, physiotherapists, Alexander Technique, yoga, Feldenkrais disciplines teachers and practitioners and others interested in the subject and in the problems created by muscular and nervous tensions, physical injuries, among instrumentalists. Aims to collect and disseminate information regarding the debilitating effects of excess anxiety and tensions experienced by musicians, actors, dancers, public speakers, sportsmen, etc; to foster research and related activities; to provide advisory service for members and to assist performers with their physical or psychological problems offering free consultations. **Pub:** Journal, annual.

★ 4049 ★ International Society of Surgery (ISS) (Societe Internationale de Chirurgie — SIC)

Netzibodenstr. 34
PO Box 1527
CH-4133 Pratteln, Switzerland
Phone: 41 61 8159666 **Fax:** 41 61 8114775
Email: surgery@iss-sic.ch
Website: http://www.iss-sic.ch

Fnded: 1902. **Mem:** 3,700. **Nat'l Groups:** 105. **Lang(s):** English. **Desc:** Surgeons from 105 countries wishing to contribute to the progress of science by researching and discussing surgical problems at congresses and general assemblies. **Pub:** *ISS/SIC*, 2-3/year. Newsletter. Contains membership information. • *Membership Booklet*, biennial. Booklet. • *World Journal of Surgery*, monthly. Scientific publication on general surgery.

★ 4050 ★ International Society of Technology Assessment in Health Care (ISTAHC)

PO Box 1390
Montreal, QC, Canada H3B 3L2
Phone: (514)844-3033 **Fax:** (514)844-3823
Email: gtombs@istahc.org

Fnded: 1985. **Desc:** Aims to lead the world in partnering for research and education on the clinical, economic and social implications of health technologies.

★ 4051 ★ International Society for Telemedicine (IST)

c/o Arvid Overgard
PO Box 1233
N-9262 Oslo, Norway
Phone: 47 77 638460 **Fax:** 47 77 610866
Email: isft.coordinator@trollnet.no
Website: http://www.isft.org

Desc: Aims to promote the development of telemedicine, telecare and telehealth around the world. Seeks to work with existing national telemedicine societies, and encourage the formation of new national societies where they do not currently exist. **Frmly:** (2000) International Conference on the Medical Aspects of Telemedicine.

★ 4052 ★ International Society of Theoretical and Experimental Hypnosis (ISTEH)

Corso XXII Marzo, 57
I- 20129 Milan, Italy
Phone: 39 0270126489 **Fax:** 39 027491051

Fnded: 1988.

★ 4053 ★ International Society on Thrombosis and Haemostasis (ISTH)

CB 7035
UNC Medical School
Chapel Hill, NC 27599-7035
Phone: (919)929-3807 **Fax:** (919)929-3935
Email: headquarters@isth.org
Website: http://www.isth.org
Cathy Cole, Exec. Sec.

Fnded: 1969. **Mem:** 2,600. **Desc:** Biomedical scientists in over 50 countries interested in thrombosis (the presence of a clot in a blood vessel) and hemostasis (the arrest of bleeding). Engages in research and education concerning thrombosis, hemostasis, blood clotting, and vascular biology. **Pub:** *Thrombosis and Haemostasis*, monthly. Journal. • Abstracts of congressional proceedings and lectures published as special issues of journal, and annual reports of SSC Scientific subcommittees. **Frmly:** (2002) International Society on Thrombosis and Hemostasis.

★ 4054 ★ International Society for Traumatic Stress Studies (ISTSS)

60 Revere Dr., Ste. 500
Northbrook, IL 60062
Phone: (847)480-9028 **Fax:** (847)480-9282
Email: istss@istss.org
Website: http://www.istss.org
Rick Koepke, Exec. Dir.

Fnded: 1985. **Mem:** 2,500. **Desc:** Professionals who treat individuals suffering from traumatic stress. (Traumatic stress is a medical term applied to persons who experience severe mental or emotional reactions to extraordinary stressful situations such as war, crime, natural disasters, and high-stress occupations.) Conducts research in the treatment of these cases; disseminates information. Holds seminars. Bestows awards. **Pub:** *Journal of Traumatic Stress*, bimonthly. Journal. Reports on the latest findings and innovations in the study and treatment of those affected by traumatic stress. • *Membership List*, periodic. *Price:* $500 flat fee. • *Traumatic Stress Points*, quarterly. Newsletter. Contains book reviews, topical articles, and association news. *Price:* Included in membership dues; Included in membership dues. **Frmly:** Society for Traumatic Stress Studies.

★ 4055 ★ International Society for Twin Studies (ISTS) (Societe Internationale d'Etudes Gemellaires)

c/o Jennifer Harris, Sec.
The Norwegian Institute of Public Health
PO Box 404
N-0403 Nydalen, Norway
Phone: 47 23 408214 **Fax:** 47 23 408252
Email: jennifer.harris@fhi.no
Website: http://www.ists.qimr.edu.au

Fnded: 1974. **Mem:** 272. **Desc:** Professionals and lay persons interested in twin research; national or large local organizations of twins or mothers of twins. Purposes are to advance twin research as applied to a variety of biomedical and psychological disciplines and to promote high standards of medical and psychosocial management of twin pregnancy and development. Assists researchers in contacting twins through twin clubs and mothers of twins clubs; advises and assists lay organizations conducting surveys or research about twins. Holds workshops. **Pub:** *Acta Geneticae Medicae et Gemellologiae/Twin Research*, quarterly. • *Twins*, 1-2/year. Newsletter.

★ 4056 ★ International Society on Ultrasonic Diagnostics in Ophthalmology (Societas Internationalis pro Diagnostica Ultrasonica in Ophthalmologia — SIDUO)

Landshuterstr 9
D-93047 Regensburg, Germany
Phone: 49 941 50430 **Fax:** 49 941 5043180
Website: http://www.echography.com/siduo.html

Fnded: 1964. **Desc:** Stimulates scientific work in the physical principles, technical developments, modes of examination and measurement, and diagnostic and therapeutic capabilities of ultrasound in ophthalmology.

★ 4057 ★ International Society of Ultrasound in Obstetrics and Gynecology

Unit 4
Blythe Mews
Blythe Rd.
London W14 OHW, United Kingdom
Phone: 44 20 74719955 **Fax:** 44 20 74719959
Email: info@isuog.org
Website: http://obg.med.wayne.edu/ISUOG/home.htm

Fnded: 1991. **Mem:** 2,000. **Desc:** Healthcare practitioners in the field of ultrasound in obstetrics and gynecology. Fosters scientific and educational advancements in ultrasound technology in obstetrics and gynecology. Conducts training programs. **Pub:** *Ultrasound in Obstetrics and Gynecology*, monthly. Journal. • Newsletter, semiannual.

★ 4058 ★ International Society for the Understanding, Prevention and Treatment of Mental Illness Relating to Child Bearing

Goldhawk Rd.
London W6 0XG, United Kingdom
Phone: 44 20 87417407 **Fax:** 44 20 87411948
Email: marcesoc@rpms.ac.uk

Desc: Organizes research conferences.

★ 4059 ★ International Society of Veterinary Ophthalmology (ISVO)

Via Nizza, 52
I-10126 Turin, Italy
Phone: 39 0116698828 **Fax:** 39 0116502687

★ 4060 ★ International Spa Association

2365 Harrodsburg Rd., Ste. A325
Lexington, KY 40504
Phone: (859)226-4326 **Free:** 888-651-4772
Fax: (859)226-4445
Email: ispa@hostcommunications.com
Website: http://www.experienceispa.com
Lynne Walker, Exec. Dir.

Fnded: 1991. **Mem:** 1,450. **Reg. Groups:** 2. **Desc:** Professional association and voice of the spa industry. Forms and maintains alliances that educate, set standards, provide resources, influence policy and build coalitions for the industry. Raises awareness of the spa industry and educates the public and industry professionals about the benefits of the spa experience.

★ 4061 ★ International Spinal Cord Society

c/o National Spinal Injuries Centre
Stoke Mandeville Hospital
Aylesbury HP21 8AL, United Kingdom
Phone: 44 1296 315866 **Fax:** 44 1296 315870
Email: admin@iscos.org.uk
Website: http://www.iscos.org.uk

Fnded: 1961. **Mem:** 1,200. **Desc:** Qualified medical practitioners with an interest and activity in research or treatment and rehabilitation of spinal cord afflictions. To study all problems concerning traumatic and non-traumatic problems of the spinal cord. To advance research, treatment and prevention; social integration of paraplegics - encourage medical services throughout the world especially in developing countries. To sponsor young specialists to attend annual scientific meetings and undertake research work. **Pub:** *Spinal Cord*, monthly. Journal. **Frmly:** (2002) International Medical Society of Paraplegia.

★ 4062 ★ International Spinal Injection Society (ISIS)

10 Edgehill Way
San Francisco, CA 94127
Phone: (415)661-6177 **Free:** 888-255-0005
Fax: (415)661-6179
Website: http://www.spinalinjection.com/ISIS/

Desc: Physicians interested in development, implementation, standardization of percutaneous techniques for the precision diagnosis of spinal pain.

★ 4063 ★ International Spinal Research Trust (ISRT)

River Front
Enfield EN1 3TR, United Kingdom
Phone: 44 20 83673555 **Fax:** 44 20 83667999
Email: isrt@isrthq.demon.co.uk

Fnded: 1980.

★ 4064 ★ International Sports Massage Federation (ISMF)

2156 Newport Blvd.
Costa Mesa, CA 92627
Phone: (949)642-0735 **Fax:** (949)642-1729
Email: doctorh@aimt-inc-smti.com
Website: http://www.aimt-inc-smti.com
M. K. Hungerford, PhD, Dir.

Fnded: 1989. **Mem:** 43. **Desc:** National sports massage federations. Facilitates exchange of techniques and ideas among members; emphasizes improving relations between Socialist and non-Socialist countries. Conducts international exchange programs. Plans to publish newsletter and hold annual meeting. **Pub:** *Sports Massage Journal*, quarterly. Journal. *Price:* $35/year.

★ 4065 ★ International Sports Organisation for the Disabled (ISOD) (Federation Internationale de Sport pour Handicapes)

c/o Alan Dean
353 Ontario St.
Newmarket, ON, Canada L3Y 2K2
Phone: (905)898-3661 **Fax:** (905)895-5527

Fnded: 1963. **Mem:** 52. **Lang(s):** English, French, German, Spanish. **Desc:** National federations in countries concerned with development of sports for the disabled. Encourages international cooperation among national organizations in the field of sports for the disabled; coordinates international activities of members. Sponsors training and education seminars and world championship Olympic games for the physically handicapped. **Pub:** *Circular*, semiannual. Newsletter. • *ISOD Handbook*, periodic.

★ 4066 ★ International Standing Committee of the International Congress on Animal Reproduction (ICAR)

c/o Prof. Gareth Evans
Faculty of Veterinary Science
University of Sydney
Sydney, NSW 2006, Australia
Phone: 61 2 93513363 **Fax:** 61 2 93513957
Email: garethe@vetsci.usyd.edu.au
Website: http://www.vetsci.usyd.edu.au/icar/

Fnded: 1948. **Lang(s):** English. **Desc:** Scientists from 50 countries. Primary activity is to conduct an international congress dealing with agricultural problems such as the fundamental study and practical application of reproduction in farm animals. Congresses concentrate on physiology, pathology, and biotechnology. Other discussion topics include: techniques of artificial insemination and embryo transfer; intensification of animal reproduction; and the control and prevention of animal diseases. Fosters information exchange among scientists on an international level. **Pub:** *Congress Proceedings*, quadrennial. • *Report Booklet*, periodic. Booklet. **Frmly:** International Standing Committee of the International Congress of Physiology and Pathology of Animal Reproduction; International Standing Committee of International Congress on Animal Reproduction and Artificial Insemination.

★ 4067 ★ International Stoke Mandeville Wheelchair Sports Federation (ISMWSF)

Olympic Village
Guttmann Rd.
Aylesbury HP21 9PP, United Kingdom
Phone: 44 1296 436179 **Fax:** 44 1296 436484
Email: info@wsw.org.uk

Fnded: 1952. **Mem:** 80. **Desc:** National organizations concerned with development of sport for paralyzed and other disabled individuals. Promotes sports activities and competitions to foster self-confidence in disabled individuals. **Pub:** Newsletter, 3/year. **Frmly:** (1991) International Stoke Mandeville Games Federation.

★ 4068 ★ International Stroke Society
5-7-1 Fujishirodai Suita
Osaka 565-8565, Japan
Phone: 81 6 8335012 **Fax:** 81 6 8727483
Email: iss@skyblue.ocn.ne.jp

Fnded: 1989. **Desc:** Encourages dissemination of scientific information; promotes professional and cultural exchange of scientists

★ 4069 ★ International Study Group for Steroid Hormones (ISGSH) (Gruppo di Studio Internazionale degli Ormoni Steroidei)
Dip di Fisipatologia medica
Universita degli Studi
Viale Policlinico
I-00161 Rome, Italy
Phone: 39 06 490465 **Fax:** 39 06 49970560

Fnded: 1961. **Mem:** 350. **Lang(s):** English. **Desc:** Researchers, physicians, and professors in medical specialties such as endocrinology, urology, oncology, and gynecology, whose main scientific activity concerns steroid hormones; pharmaceutical firms. Strives to encourage and advance steroid hormone studies and research. Promotes education and training in steroid assays. **Pub:** *Abstracts of the Meeting*, biennial. • *Research on Steroids*, biennial. Contains proceeding. • *Steroids*. Journal.

★ 4070 ★ International Thai Therapists Association (ITTA)
3600 S 60th Ave.
Shelby, MI 49455
Email: itta@megsinet.net
Website: http://www.spiritcafe.com/itta/ittaindex.html
Anthony B. James, Pres.

Desc: Promotes the needs and concerns of students, practitioners, teachers and schools of Nuat Thai and Thai Style therapeutic massage and body work. **Pub:** *ThaiMassage.com*. Contains articles on techniques, business practices, upcoming events and training.

★ 4071 ★ International Traffic Medicine Association (ITMA)
973 Saterlee Rd.
Bloomfield Hills, MI 48304-3153
Phone: (248)203-6417 **Fax:** (248)203-6417
Email: le@scienceservingsociety.com
Website: http://www.TrafficMedicine.org
Dr. Leonard Evans, Pres.

Fnded: 1960. **Mem:** 120. **Reg. Groups:** 7. **Desc:** Devoted to the reduction of harm caused by traffic crashes. **Pub:** *Congress Proceedings*. Proceedings. • *Traffic Injury Prevention*, quarterly. Journal. *Price:* $85; Free to members.

★ 4072 ★ International Transactional Analysis Association (ITAA)
436 14th St. Ste. 1301
Oakland, CA 94612-2710
Phone: (510)625-7720 **Fax:** (510)625-7725
Email: itaa@itaa-net.org
Website: http://www.itaa-net.org
Gordon B. Hewitt, PhD, Pres.

Fnded: 1958. **Mem:** 2,500. **Desc:** Educational corporation of persons in medical and behavioral sciences, including psychiatrists, psychologists, social workers, nurses, educators, marriage and family counselors, clergy, and organizational consultants. Maintains standards of practice and teaching of transactional analysis, which involves group therapy, social dynamics, and personality theory based on analysis of the "transactions" or interactions between persons. (The book, *Games People Play*, covers basic transactional analysis theory; its author, Dr. Eric Berne, was ITAA founder.) **Pub:** *International Transactional Analysis Association Membership Directory*, annual. Contains alphabetical and geographical listing of members. *Price:* $10. • *ITAA Membership Directory*, annual. Membership Directory. • *Script*, 9/year. Newsletter. • *Transactional Analysis Journal*, quarterly. Journal. **Frmly:** (1961) San Francisco Social Psychiatry Seminar.

★ 4073 ★ International Transplant Coordinators Society (ITCS)
Steenveldstraat 18
B-3210 Linden, Belgium
Phone: 32 16 622110 **Fax:** 32 16 622981
Email: itcs@online.be
Website: http://www.kuleuven.ac.be/facdep/medicine/itcs/Home.html

Desc: Creates a structure that could respond to transplant coordination issues at international meetings.

★ 4074 ★ International Transplant Nurses Society (ITNS)
1739 E Carson St., No. 351
PO Box 351
Pittsburgh, PA 15203-1700
Free: (412)343-ITNS **Fax:** (412)343-3959
Email: itns@msn.com
Website: http://www.itns.org
Beth Kassalen, MBA, Exec. Dir.

Fnded: 1992. **Mem:** 850. **Reg. Groups:** 16. **Local Groups:** 17. **Desc:** Nurses, LVNs, LPNs, and others involved in patient care for organ transplantation. Works to encourage cooperation among all medical disciplines involved in transplantation, disseminate information, and establish certification for this nursing specialty. **Pub:** *ITNS Newsletter*, quarterly. Newsletter. Contains clinical transplant articles, society updates. *Price:* Included in membership dues. • *Progress in Transplantation*, quarterly. Journal. *Price:* $55 annually.

★ 4075 ★ International Trauma Anesthesia and Critical Care Society (ITACCS)
PO Box 4826
Baltimore, MD 21211
Fax: (410)235-8084
Email: info@nwas.com
Website: http://www.trauma.itaccs.com
Christopher M. Grande, MD,MPH, Exec. Dir.

Fnded: 1988. **Mem:** 2,000. **Desc:** Healthcare professionals involved in trauma and critical care anesthesiology. Works to gain recognition for trauma anesthesiology as a discipline within anesthesiology and critical care medicine. Promotes cooperation and information sharing among healthcare professionals. Sponsors seminars and workshops; conducts research and educational programs; provides children's services; holds competitions; maintains speakers' bureau and placement service. **Pub:** *Textbook of Trauma Anesthesia and Critical Care*. Book. • *Trauma Care*, biennial. Magazine. *Price:* Free.

★ 4076 ★ International Union Against Cancer (UICC) (Union Internationale Contre le Cancer)
3, rue du Conseil General
CH-1205 Geneva, Switzerland
Phone: 41 22 8091811 **Fax:** 41 22 8091810
Email: info@uicc.org
Website: http://www.uicc.ch/

Fnded: 1933. **Mem:** 286. **Lang(s):** English. **Desc:** Voluntary cancer leagues and societies, national organizations, private or public cancer research institutions, and ministries of health in 86 countries. Promotes a comprehensive international campaign against cancer. Directs activities in fields of prevention, research, and treatment; sponsors special projects in fields including cervical cancer, head and neck cancer, and exchange of information on unproven methods in cancer treatment. Facilitates training courses for researchers and health professionals; makes available advisory visits by cancer experts. **Pub:** *International Calendar of Meetings on Cancer*, semiannual. • *International Journal of Cancer and Predictive Oncology*, 30/year. Journal. • *UICC International Directory of Cancer Institutes and Organizations*, quadrennial. Directory. • *UICC News*, quarterly. Also publishes monographs, reports, publication lists, and new book announcements; produces cancer education packs and workshop guidelines.

★ 4077 ★ International Union Against Sexually Transmitted Infections - Australia
135 Hutt St.
Adelaide, SA 5000, Australia
Phone: 61 8 82324511 **Fax:** 61 8 823796145

Lang(s): English. **Desc:** Medical and public health professionals and other individuals with an interest in sexually transmitted diseases. Seeks to minimize the incidence of sexually transmitted disease and improve their diagnosis and treatment. Conducts educational programs to raise public awareness of sexually transmitted diseases and their prevention; sponsors training courses for health care workers serving people with sexually transmitted diseases; serves as a clearinghouse on sexually transmitted diseases and their prevention.

★ 4078 ★ International Union Against Sexually Transmitted Infections, Regional Office for North America
c/o Jonathon Zenilman
Johns Hopkins Hospital - Division of ID
1159 Ross Research Bldg.
720 Rutland Ave.
Baltimore, MD 21205
Phone: (410)955-7636 **Fax:** (410)614-9775
Email: jzenilma@jhmi.edu
Website: http://www.iusti.org
Jonathan Zenilman, Pres.

Fnded: 1923. **Desc:** U.S. office of the International Union Against Sexually Transmitted Diseases. Governmental and nongovernmental agencies and individuals working in the field of venereal disease control. Encourages campaigns, both medical and social, against venereal diseases and treponematoses. **Pub:** Proceedings, biennial. **Frmly:** (1998) International Union Against the Veneral Diseases and the Treponematoses, Regional Office for North America.

★ 4079 ★ International Union Against Sexually Transmitted Infections - United Kingdom (IUSTI)
c/o Dr. Raj Patel
Royal South Hants Hospital
Brintons Terrace
South Hampton SE1 7EH, United Kingdom
Phone: 44 207 9289292 **Fax:** 44 207 4036459
Email: raj.patel@iusti.org
Website: http://www.iusti.org

Fnded: 1923. **Lang(s):** English, French, Spanish. **Desc:** Promotes international cooperation in the control of sexually transmitted diseases, including HIV infection, with an emphasis on the medical, social, and epidemiological aspects.

★ 4080 ★ International Union Against The Venereal Diseases and The Treponematoses (IUVDT)
Saint Mary's Hospital
London W2 1NY, United Kingdom
Phone: 44 20 72621123

Fnded: 1923.

★ 4081 ★ International Union Against Tuberculosis and Lung Disease (IUATLD) (Union Internationale Contre la Tuberculose et les Maladies Respiratoires — UICTMR)
68, blvd. St. Michel
F-75006 Paris, France
Phone: 33 1 44320360 **Fax:** 33 1 43299087
Email: union@iuatld.org
Website: http://www.iuatld.org

Fnded: 1920. **Mem:** 4,000. **Reg. Groups:** 6. **Lang(s):** English, French, Spanish. **Desc:** National associations, physicians, and other individuals worldwide dedicated to the fight against tuberculosis and other respiratory diseases. Promotes community health and, within its framework, the delivery of preventive, diagnostic, and therapeutic measures against tuberculosis. Aids governmental efforts to improve health services; helps countries formulate, prepare, and execute national tuberculosis control programs. Provides training, advice, antituberculosis drugs and vaccines, medical equipment, and transportation. Encourages community participation. Activities include: dissemination of scientific knowledge; exchange of experience and conferences; operational and applied research; field projects under the Mutual Assistance Programme. Acts as liaison with the World Health Organization and other organizations. **Pub:** *The International Journal of Tuberculosis and Lung Disease*, monthly. Journal. With summaries in French and Spanish. • *IUATLD Newsletter*, 3/year. Newsletter. Contains news and reports on the activities of the IUATLD and information on conferences and courses. • *Management of the Child with Cough or Difficult Breathing.* • *Tuberculosis Guide for Low Income Countries.* **Frmly:** (1986) International Union Against Tuberculosis.

★ 4082 ★ International Union of Angiology (IUA)

1, av J Poulhes
F-31403 Toulouse Cedex 04, France
Phone: 33 5 61552637 **Fax:** 33 5 61322634
Email: angio@wanadoo.fr
Website: http://www.i.u.angiology.org/

Fnded: 1958. **Desc:** Stimulates scientific knowledge in the whole field of angiology and diseases of blood vessels.

★ 4083 ★ International Union for Health Promotion and Education (IUHPE) (Union Internationale de Promotion de la Sante et d'Education pour la Sante — UIPES)

2, rue Auguste Comte
F-92170 Vanves, France
Phone: 33 1 46450059 **Fax:** 33 1 46450045
Email: mclamarre@iuhpe.org
Website: http://www.iuhpe.org

Fnded: 1951. **Mem:** 2,000. **Reg. Groups:** 6. **Lang(s):** English, French, Spanish. **Desc:** Promotes global health and contributes to the achievement of equity in health among all countries of the world. Builds and operates an independent, global professional network of individuals and institutions to encourage free exchange of ideas, knowledge, and development of relevant collaboration at the global and regional levels. **Pub:** *Conference Proceedings*, triennial. • *The Evidence of Health Promotion Effectiveness*, periodic. Report. Report for the European Commission on the health, social, economic, and political impacts of health promotion. • *Promotion & Education*, quarterly. Journal. Contains articles on the theory and practice of health promotion and health education as well as international news about major events. • Brochure, periodic. • Newsletters, periodic.

★ 4084 ★ International Union of Immunological Societies (IUIS)

c/o Dr. Fritz Melchers
Basel Institute for Immunology
Postfach
Grenzacherstrasse 487
CH-4005 Basel, Switzerland
Phone: 41 61 6051237 **Fax:** 41 61 6051300
Email: iuispres@bii.ch
Website: http://www.qimr.edu.au/iuis/

Fnded: 1969. **Mem:** 53. **Reg. Groups:** 4. **Lang(s):** English. **Desc:** National professional societies of basic and applied immunologists. Encourages the orderly development and utilization of the science of immunology. Promotes the application of new developments to clinical and veterinary problems and standardizes reagents and nomenclature. Conducts educational symposia and scientific meetings. **Pub:** *The Immunologist*, bimonthly. Journal.

★ 4085 ★ International Union of Medical Advisers Associations (IUMAA) (Union Internationale des Associations de Delegues Medicaux — UIADM)

c/o Angelo De Rita
Via F. Turati, 19
I-50136 Florence, Italy
Phone: 39 055 691166 **Fax:** 39 055 650736

Fnded: 1974. **Lang(s):** French. **Desc:** Medical advisers and related scientific and medical personnel. Promotes professional advancement of members; seeks to facilitate medical and scientific research. Represents the interests of medical advisers before industrial organizations, government agencies, scientific and medical bodies, and the public. Formulates codes of ethics and practice for members.

★ 4086 ★ International Union of Nutritional Sciences (IUNS)

c/o Prof. Osman M. Galal
UCLA School of Public Health
International Health Program
PO Box 951772
Los Angeles, CA 90095-1772
Phone: (310)206-9639 **Fax:** (310)794-1805
Email: ogalal@ucla.edu
Website: http://www.iuns.org
Prof. O.M. Galal, Sec. Gen.

Fnded: 1946. **Mem:** 70. **Desc:** National nutritional societies. Promotes international cooperation in the scientific study of nutrition and its applications. Encourages research and the exchange of scientific information. Cooperates with the Food and Agriculture Organization of the United Nations, the United Nations Educational, Scientific and Cultural Organization, and the World Health Organization. Maintains 9 task forces. **Pub:** *Annual Report.* • *Directory*, quadrennial. Directory. • *Newsletter*, 1-2/year. Newsletter.

★ 4087 ★ International Union of Pharmacology (IUPHAR)

c/o Prof. P.M. Vanhoutte
University of Strathclyde
204 George St.
Glasgow G1 1XW, United Kingdom
Email: vanhoutt@servier.fr

Fnded: 1966. **Mem:** 52. **Nat'l Groups:** 52. **Lang(s):** English. **Desc:** National and international societies in pharmacology and related disciplines representing approximately 30,000 individuals. Purpose is to promote cooperation between pharmacological societies and encourage free international exchange of ideas and research. Acts as a forum for participation between related scientific bodies. Works to standardize the use of drugs worldwide and rationally define the receptors and ion channels on which they act. **Pub:** *Congress Proceedings*, quadrennial. • *Directory of IUPHAR*, annual. • *Pharmacology International*, semiannual. Newsletter.

★ 4088 ★ International Union of Physiological Sciences (IUPS)

c/o Ole Peterson, Sec.
Physiological Laboratory
University of Liverpool
Crown St.
Liverpool L69 3BX, United Kingdom
Phone: 44 151 7945342 **Fax:** 44 151 7945323
Email: o.h.peterson@liverpool.ac.uk
Website: http://www.iups.org

Fnded: 1929. **Mem:** 71. **Nat'l Groups:** 53. **Reg. Groups:** 5.

★ 4089 ★ International Union of Psychological Science (IUPsyS)

School of Psychology
University of Ottawa
145 Jean-Jacques Lussier
C.P. 450, Sta. A
Ottawa, ON, Canada K1N 6N5
Phone: (613)562-5800 **Fax:** (613)562-5169
Email: pritchie@uottawa.ca
Website: http://www.iupsys.org

Fnded: 1951. **Mem:** 66. **Lang(s):** English, French. **Desc:** National psychological societies and committees united for: the development of psychological science through exchange of ideas and scientific information; the exchange of scholars and students; the organization of international congresses of psychology; publication and documentation; cooperation with related scientific groups interested in the development of psychology as a discipline and a profession. Conducts educational programs and international research network project. **Pub:** *International Directory of Psychologists*, quinquennial. Directory. • *International Journal of Psychology*, bimonthly. Journal. Peer reviewed scholarly journal including International Platform.

★ 4090 ★ International Union of Therapeutics (Union Therapeutique Internationale)

c/o Prof. A. Pradalier
Hopital Universitaire Louis Mourier
178, rue des Renouillers
F-92701 Colombes Cedex, France
Phone: 33 47 606705 **Fax:** 33 47 606072
Email: secretariat.medecine4@lmr.ap-hop-paris.fr

Fnded: 1934. **Mem:** 350. **Lang(s):** English, French. **Desc:** International organizations in 22 countries interested in the development of therapeutics. Conducts training, research, and exchange programs. **Pub:** *Abstracts or Communications' Book of the Congress*, biennial.

★ 4091 ★ International Veterinary Acupuncture Society (IVAS)

PO Box 271395
Fort Collins, CO 80527-1395
Phone: (970)266-0660 **Fax:** (970)266-0777
Email: office@ivas.org
Website: http://www.ivas.org/
Edward C. Boldt, Jr., Exec. Dir.

Fnded: 1974. **Nat'l Groups:** 6. **Desc:** Veterinarians and veterinary students. Encourages knowledge and research of the philosophy, technique, and practice of veterinary acupuncture. Fosters high standards in the field; promotes scientific investigation. Accumulates resources for scientific research and education; collects data concerning clinical and research cases where animals have been treated with acupuncture; disseminates information to veterinary students, practitioners, other scientific groups, and the public. Offers 100 contact hour basic veterinary acupuncture course; administers certification examination. **AKA:** IVAS.

★ 4092 ★ International Vitamin A Consultative Group (IVACG)

c/o ILSI Human Nutrition Institute
One Thomas Cir. NW, 9th Fl.
Washington, DC 20005
Phone: (202)659-9024 **Fax:** (202)659-3617
Email: hni@ilsi.org
Website: http://www.ilsi.org
Veronica Triana, MPH, Project Mgr.

Fnded: 1974. **Desc:** Offers consultation and guidance to operating and donor agencies that are seeking to reduce vitamin A deficiencies. Prepares guidelines and recommendations for assessing the regional distribution and magnitude of vitamin A deficiency, developing intervention methods and strategies against the deficiency, evaluating the effectiveness of implemented programs, and conducting research needed to support the assessment of intervention. Holds international meeting every 18 months. Publishes and distributes technical references which are used globally; conducts task forces. globally; conducts task forces. **Pub:** *A Brief Guide to Current Methods of Assessing Vitamin A Status. Price:* $4. • *The Bioavailability of Dietary Carotenoids: Current Concepts. Price:* $4. • *Biochemical Methodology for the Assess-*

ment of Vitamin A Status, and Reprints of Selected Methods for the Analysis of Vitamin A and Carotenoids. Book. • Combining Vitamin A Distribution with EPI Contacts. Price: $4. • Delivery of Vitamin A Supplements with DPT/Polio and Measles Immunization. Price: $4. • IVACG Meeting Reports. Report. Price: Free. • IVACG Policy Statement on Vitamin A, Diarrhea and Measles. Price: $4. • IVACG Policy Statement on Vitamin A Status and Childhood Mortality. Price: $4. • IVACG Statement on Clustering of Xerophthalmia and Vitamin A Deficiency Within Communities and Families. Price: $4. • IVACG Statement on Maternal Night Blindness: Extent and Associated Risk Factors. Price: $4. • IVACG Statement on Safe Doses of Vitamin A During Pregnancy and Lactation. Price: $4. • IVACG Statement on Vitamin A and Iron Interactions. Price: $4. • Nutrition Communications in Vitamin A Programs: A Resource Book. Price: $4. • The Safe Use of Vitamin A. Price: $4. • The Safe Uses of Vitamin A by Women During the Reproductive Years. Price: $4. • Status of the Studies on Vitamin A and Human Immunodeficiency Virus Infection. Price: $4. • Strategic Placement of IVACG in the Evolving Micronutrient Field. Price: Free. • Vitamin A Conversions to SI. Price: Free. • Vitamin A Supplements: A Guide to their Use in the Treatment and Prevention of Vitamin A Deficiency and Xerophthalmia. Price: $4. • Also publishes monographs, guidelines, and books.

★ 4093 ★ International Wheelchair Road Racers Club (IWRRC)

c/o Joseph M. Dowling
30 Myano Ln., Box 3
Stamford, CT 06902
Phone: (203)967-2231 **Fax:** (203)327-7999
Email: dowling007@aol.com
Joseph M. Dowling, Pres.

Fnded: 1981. **Mem:** 200. **Desc:** Disabled persons, able-bodied persons, rehabilitation institutes, and major road race organizations interested in health and physical fitness for the disabled. Promotes wheelchair road racing in the U.S.; assists road race organizations in incorporating wheelchair divisions. Provides educational and technical assistance to race directors and road racers; maintains communications network concerning multi-sports for the disabled. Governs the sport of wheelchair road racing. **Pub:** Newsletter, semimonthly.

★ 4094 ★ International Women's Health Coalition (IWHC)

24 E 21st St.
New York, NY 10010
Phone: (212)979-8500 **Fax:** (212)979-9009
Email: info@iwhc.org
Website: http://www.iwhc.org
Ellen Sweet, VP Public Affairs

Fnded: 1980. **Desc:** Guided by the principle that global well-being and social and economic justice can only be achieved by ensuring women's rights. Committed to three main goals: comprehensive sexuality education and services for adolescents, worldwide access to safe abortion, and expansion of sexual rights for women and girls. Provides technical and financial support to local organizations and networks in Africa, Asia and Latin America working to promote these rights. Advocates directly for women's health and rights on an international level: informs public debate at home and abroad through its multilingual publications, media involvement, web site, and videos; collaborates with UN agencies, donor governments, and private foundations on health sector reform and global health initiatives; participates in major UN conferences on health, population, women and children. **Pub:** *The Sexuality Connection in Reproductive Health*. Report. Explores the importance of the study of sexuality and gender-based power relations to reproductive health policies and programs. • *Special Challenges in Third World Women's Health: Reproductive Tract Infections, Cervical Cancer, and Contraceptive Safety*. Report. • *Women's Political Action and Population Policy in Three Developing Countries*. Report. • Reports. **Frmly:** (1980) National Women's Health Coalition.

★ 4095 ★ Interplast

300-B Pioneer Way
Mountain View, CA 94041-1506
Phone: (650)962-0123 **Free:** 888-467-5278
Fax: (650)962-1619
Email: ipnews@interplast.org
Website: http://www.interplast.org
Susan W. Hayes, Pres. /CEO

Fnded: 1969. **Desc:** Provides free reconstructive plastic surgery for needy children around the world, with more than 47,000 free surgeries performed since 1969. Seeks to ensure access to reconstructive plastic surgery in developing countries worldwide by sending teams of medical volunteers overseas and providing advanced medical training and support to host-country medical partners. **Pub:** *Healing Hands*, semiannual. Newsletter. Highlights photos and stories of programs. *Price:* Free.

★ 4096 ★ Interprofessional Fostering of Ophthalmic Care for Underserved Sectors (InFOCUS)

327 Tealwood Dr.
Houston, TX 77024
Phone: (713)468-3040 **Fax:** (713)468-7704
Email: infocus@houston.rr.com
Website: http://www.infocusonline.org
Barbara Kazdan, Dir.

Fnded: 1988. **Desc:** Works in cooperation with eye care specialists, public health care professionals, health care providers and humanitarian organizations to develop sustainable eye care practices in areas with underserved populations; encourages community self-reliance. Conducts educational and charitable programs; sponsors research on appropriate technology for primary eye care.

★ 4097 ★ Intersocietal Commission for the Accreditation of Vascular Laboratories (ICAVL)

8840 Stanfod Blvd., Ste. 4900
Columbia, MD 21045-5852
Phone: (410)872-0100 **Fax:** (410)872-0030
Email: morales@intersocietal.org
Website: http://www.icavl.org
Sandra Katanick, Exec. Dir.

Fnded: 1994. **Desc:** Establishes industry standards. **Frmly:** (2000) Intersocietal Commission for the Accreditation of Vascular Laboratories.

★ 4098 ★ Intersociety Committee on Pathology Information (ICPI)

9650 Rockville Pike
Bethesda, MD 20814-3993
Phone: (301)634-7200 **Fax:** (301)634-7990
Email: icpi@asip.org
Website: http://www.pathologytraining.org
Gretchen Bretsch, Admin.

Fnded: 1957. **Mem:** 5. **Desc:** One representative from each sponsoring society: American Society for Investigative Pathology; American Society for Clinical Pathology; Association of Pathology Chairs; College of American Pathologists; U.S. & Canadian Academy of Pathology. Disseminates information about the medical practice and research achievements of pathology. Produces career information, especially training of residents and postdoctoral fellows in pathology. **Pub:** *Directory of Pathology Training Programs: Residencies and Fellowships in US and Canada*, annual. Directory. *Price:* $25; $5 for medical students/residents; Free to medical schools/medical libraries/teaching; Hospital. • *Pathology as a Career in Medicine*. Brochure.

★ 4099 ★ Interstate Postgraduate Medical Association of North America (IPMANA)

PO Box 5474
Madison, WI 53705
Phone: (608)231-9045 **Fax:** (608)231-9045
Email: ipma@chorus.net
Mary W. Ales, Exec. Dir.

Fnded: 1916. **Desc:** Presents annual four-day teaching program in various branches of medicine and medical research, aimed at the family practitioner who must keep up with new developments in a short time away from his practice.

★ 4100 ★ Interstitial Cystitis Association (ICA)

110 N Washington St., No. 340
Rockville, MD 20850-2239
Phone: (301)610-5300 **Free:** 800-HEL-PICA
Fax: (301)610-5308
Email: icamail@ichelp.org
Website: http://www.ichelp.org
Nicole Mehall, Admin. Mgr.

Fnded: 1984. **Desc:** Support network for patients suffering or suspected of suffering from interstitial cystitis, an inflammation of the bladder wall that primarily affects women; its cause and cure are unknown. Works to inform the public and especially the medical profession about the seriousness of IC. Raises funds for research into treatments and cures; maintains a medical advisory board. Is establishing a national registry to record facts about IC. **Pub:** *ICA Update*, quarterly. Newsletter. Covers IC research and political and educational activities of the ICA. *Price:* $45/year.

★ 4101 ★ Intestinal Disease Foundation

Landmarks Bldg., Ste. 525
100 W Station Sq. Dr.
Pittsburgh, PA 15219-1122
Phone: (412)261-5888 **Free:** 877-587-9606
Fax: (412)471-2722
Email: intdis@stargate.net
Website: http://www.intestinalfoundation.org
Linda E. Schorr, MSEd, Exec. Dir.

Fnded: 1986. **Mem:** 1,200. **Local Groups:** 1. **Desc:** Works to improve the quality of life of adults and children affected by chronic digestive illness through information, guidance and support. These illnesses include inflammatory bowel disease (Crohn's disease and ulcerative colitis), diverticular disease, short-bowel syndrome, irritable bowel syndrome (IBS) and other functional gastrointestinal disorders. **Pub:** *Intestinal Fortitude*, quarterly. Newsletter. Provides most current information on medical and surgical treatments, coping techniques, and inspiration for living better with chronic illness. *Price:* Free. For members only.

★ 4102 ★ Iranian Society of Physiology and Pharmacology

c/o Dr. Fereshteh Motamedi
Department of Physiology
Shaheed Beheshti University of Medical Sciences
PO Box 19835-181
Tehran, Iran
Phone: 98 21 2414131 **Fax:** 98 21 2400681
Email: afshar@khayam.ut.ac.ir

Mem: 200. **Desc:** Promotes physiology and pharmacology in Iran.

★ 4103 ★ Irish Association for Nurses in Oncology (IANO)

PO Box 1499
Dublin 4, Ireland
Phone: 353 1 2310529
Email: mkennedy@irishcancer.ie
Website: http://www.iano.ie/

Desc: Provides education and information exchange for members of the nursing profession, particularly those caring for people with cancer.

★ 4104 ★ Irish Association of the Sovereign Military Order of Malta (IASMOM)

St. John's House
32 Clyde Rd.
Ballsbridge
Dublin 4, Ireland
Phone: 353 1 6684891 **Fax:** 353 1 6685288

Email: smom@orderofmalta.ie
Website: http://www.orderofmalta.ie

Fnded: 1934. **Mem:** 4,000. **Nat'l Groups:** 1. **Reg. Groups:** 6. **Local Groups:** 80. **Lang(s):** English, Irish. **Desc:** Volunteers committed to serving those in need. Seeks to increase the availability of emergency services. Operates ambulance corps.

★ 4105 ★ Irish Association for Spina Bifida and Hydrocephalus (IASBH)
Old Nangor Rd.
Clandalkin
Dublin 22, Ireland
Phone: 353 1 4572329 **Fax:** 353 1 4572328

Lang(s): English, Irish. **Desc:** Individuals and organizations. Seeks to improve the quality of life of people with spina bifida or hydrocephalus and their families. Makes available support and services; conducts educational and advocacy campaigns.

★ 4106 ★ Irish Association of Suicidology (IAS)
St. Mary's Hospital
Castlebar, Mayo, Ireland
Phone: 353 94 21333 **Fax:** 353 94 27904
Email: info@ias.ie
Website: http://www.ias.ie/

Fnded: 1996. **Desc:** Works to facilitate communication between clinicians, volunteers, survivors, and researchers in all matters relating to suicide and suicide behavior; promotes public awareness of problems of suicide and suicidal behavior.

★ 4107 ★ Irish Cancer Society (ICS)
5 Northumberland Rd.
Dublin 4, Ireland
Phone: 353 1 2310500 **Fax:** 353 1 2310555
Email: reception@irishcancer.ie
Website: http://www.irishcancer.ie

Lang(s): English, Irish Gaelic. **Desc:** National cancer societies. Promotes advancement in the prevention, diagnosis, and treatment of cancer; seeks to improve the quality of life of people with cancer and their families. Facilitates communication and cooperation among members; sponsors research and educational programs; provides support and services to people with cancer.

★ 4108 ★ Irish Cardiac Society
4 Clyde Rd.
Ballsbridge
Dublin 4, Ireland
Phone: 353 1 6685001 **Fax:** 353 1 6685896
Email: irishcardiac@eircom.net
Website: http://www.irishcardiacsociety.org

Mem: 135. **Desc:** Promotes the study of cardiology in Ireland.

★ 4109 ★ Irish Deaf Society (IDS)
c/o National Association of the Deaf
30 Blessington St.
Dublin 7, Ireland
Phone: 353 1 8601878 **Fax:** 353 1 8601960
Email: ids@indigo.ie

Fnded: 1981. **Mem:** 300. **Reg. Groups:** 20. **Lang(s):** English, Irish. **Desc:** A representative organization of Deaf people, seeks recognition of Irish sign language and conducts various educational and advocacy campaigns. **Pub:** *Irish Deaf Journal*, quarterly. Magazine. Covers deaf news in Ireland and abroad.

★ 4110 ★ Irish Dental Association (IDA)
Clonskeagh Rd.
Dublin 14, Ireland
Phone: 353 1 2830499
Email: info@irishdentalassoc.ie
Website: http://www.dentist.ie

Fnded: 1922.

★ 4111 ★ Irish Diabetes Association
76 Lower Gardiner St.
Dublin, Ireland
Phone: 353 1 8363022
Website: http://www.iol.ie/diabetes/

Desc: Supports individuals with diabetes and diabetes research.

★ 4112 ★ Irish Ergonomics Society
c/o Manufacturing & Operations Engineering
University of Limerick
Limerick, Ireland
Phone: 353 61 202900 **Fax:** 353 61 202913
Website: http://www.ul.ie/~ies/

Desc: Professionals involved in the ergonomics field promoting the discovery and exchange of knowledge concerning the characteristics of human beings that are applicable to the design of systems and devices of all kinds.

★ 4113 ★ Irish Family Planning Association (IFPA)
Solomons House
42A Pearse St.
Dublin 2, Ireland
Phone: 353 1 4740944 **Fax:** 353 1 4740945
Email: post@ifpa.ie
Website: http://www.ifpa.ie

Fnded: 1969. **Nat'l Groups:** 1. **Lang(s):** English. **Desc:** Works to improve the quality of life for individuals living in Ireland by promoting family planning and responsible parenthood. Advocates family planning as a basic human right. Offers programs in sex education, family planning, and health. Provides contraceptive and health care services. Conducts research.

★ 4114 ★ Irish Fragile X Society
5 Fitzwilliam Pl.
Dublin 2, Ireland
Email: info@fragilex-ireland.org
Website: http://www.fragilex-ireland.org/pages/app.htm

Desc: Works to improve the quality of life of all people affected by Fragile X syndrome; provides mutual support and information to families, promotes public awareness of Fragile X syndrome.

★ 4115 ★ Irish Gerontological Society (IGS)
Department Age-Related Healthcare
Adelaide & Health Hospital
Tallaght
Tallaght 24, Dublin, Ireland
Phone: 353 1 4143215
Email: des.oneill@amnch.ie

Fnded: 1952. **Mem:** 300. **Nat'l Groups:** 1. **State Groups:** 1. **Desc:** Health care professionals treating the elderly; scientists and clinicians with an interest in the aging process and diseases of the aged. Promotes gerontological research and increased availability of gerontological care; facilitates training of gerontology specialists. Represents the interests of gerontologists and gerontological organizations.

★ 4116 ★ Irish Guide Dogs for the Blind (IGDB)
Model Farm Rd.
Cork, Cork, Ireland
Phone: 353 21 4878200 **Fax:** 353 21 4874152
Email: info@guidedogs.ie
Website: http://www.guidedogs.ie

Lang(s): English, Irish. **Desc:** Dog trainers and individuals providing support and services to people with impaired vision. Seeks to improve the quality of life of people with impaired vision. Makes available trained guide dogs to people with impaired vision; conducts training programs for people wishing to use guide dogs.

★ 4117 ★ Irish Haemophilia Society (IHS)
Iceland House
Arran Ct.
Arran Quay
Dublin 7, Ireland
Phone: 353 1 8724466 **Fax:** 353 1 8724494
Email: info@haemophilia-society.ie
Website: http://www.haemophilia-society.ie

Fnded: 1968. **Mem:** 300. **Nat'l Groups:** 1. **Lang(s):** English, Irish. **Desc:** Individuals and organizations. Seeks to improve the quality of life of people with hemophilia and their families. Makes available support and services; conducts educational and advocacy campaigns; supports hematological research. **Pub:** Newsletter, annual, 3 monthly.

★ 4118 ★ Irish Hard of Hearing Association
c/o Emma McAuley
35 N Frederick St.
Dublin 1, Ireland
Phone: 353 1 8723800 **Fax:** 353 1 8723816
Email: info@ihha.ie
Website: http://www.ihha.ie/homepage.html

Fnded: 1986. **Desc:** Hearing impaired persons holding social evenings to share problems and fears and offer support. Offers lip reading courses, family information nights, one-to-one counseling, coping strategies, technical aids, and more. **Pub:** *Hearsay*, 3/year. Magazine.

★ 4119 ★ Irish Hospital Consultants' Association
Lowell House
Herbert Ave.
Dublin 4, Ireland
Phone: 353 1 2838461
Email: ihca@indigo.ie

★ 4120 ★ Irish Kidney Association (IKA)
Donor House
43A Park W
Dublin 12, Ireland
Phone: 353 1 6689788 **Fax:** 353 1 6683820
Email: info@ika.ie
Website: http://www.ika.ie

Fnded: 1978. **Mem:** 2,200. **Reg. Groups:** 23. **Lang(s):** English, Irish. **Desc:** Provides support for those with end-stage renal disease and kidney transplants. Prints and distributes Organ Donor Cards. Irish representative of the World Transplant Games; maintains five-apartment Holiday Centre in Tramore for all kidney patients; offers counseling and financial assistance. The Renal Support Centre on the grounds of Beaumont Hospital, the only transplant center in Ireland, provides accommodation and support to family members of inpatients while in hospital. **Pub:** *Support*, quarterly. Magazine.

★ 4121 ★ Irish Medical Association (IMA)
10 Fitzwilliam Pl.
Dublin 2, Ireland
Phone: 353 1 6767273 **Fax:** 353 1 6612758
Email: im@101.ie

Fnded: 1936.

★ 4122 ★ Irish Medical Organisation (IMO)
10 Fitzwilliam Pl.
Dublin 2, Ireland
Phone: 353 1 6767273 **Fax:** 353 1 6612758
Email: imo@imo.ie
Website: http://www.imo.ie

Mem: 5,000. **Lang(s):** English, Irish. **Desc:** Physicians and medical students and their families. Seeks to develop a "caring, efficient and effective health service." Serves as a professional body representing physicians in Ireland; facilitates exchange of information among members; encourages medical research. **Pub:** *Irish Medical Journal*. Journal.

★ 4123 ★ Irish Motor Neurone Disease Association
Coleraine House
Coleraine St.
Dublin 7, Ireland
Phone: 353 1 8730422 **Fax:** 353 1 8731409
Email: info@imnda.ie

Fnded: 1985. **Desc:** Promotes interest in motor neurone disease (MND) research among medical and scientific communities and the public in Ireland. Offers support services to MND sufferers and their families. Disseminates information about the disease. **Pub:** *IMNDA Newsletter*, quarterly. Newsletter.

★ 4124 ★ Irish Nutrition and Dietetic Institute (INDI)
Ashgrove House
Kill Ave.
Dun Laoghaire, Dublin, Ireland
Phone: 353 1 2804839 **Fax:** 353 1 2804299
Email: info@indi.ie
Website: http://www.indi.ie

Fnded: 1968. **Mem:** 350. **Lang(s):** English. **Desc:** Professional dietitians. Promotes growth in the number of dietary and nutrition-related positions in the Republic of Ireland. Represents the interests of members. **Pub:** Papers. Contain information on diet, health, and food for sport.

★ 4125 ★ Irish Pharmaceutical Healthcare Association (IPHA)
Franklin House
140 Pembroke Rd.
Dublin, Ireland
Phone: 353 1 6603350 **Fax:** 353 1 6686672
Email: info@ipha.ie
Website: http://www.ipha.ie/

Desc: Promotes the economic and political environment of the pharmaceutical industry in Ireland in order to provide quality medicines and healthcare to patients.

★ 4126 ★ Irish Psycho-Analytical Association
89 Grosvenor Sq.
Rathmines
Dublin 6, Ireland
Phone: 353 1 4967288 **Fax:** 353 1 4978766

Fnded: 1942. **Mem:** 21. **Lang(s):** English. **Desc:** Practicing psychoanalysts and psychoanalytic psychotherapists. Represents members in dealings with government agencies, both Irish and within the European Union, and maintains standards of psychoanalytic practice in Ireland in conjunction with sister organizations.

★ 4127 ★ Irish Raynaud's and Scleroderma Society (IRSS)
PO Box 2958
Foxrock
Dublin 18, Ireland
Phone: 353 1 2350900 **Fax:** 353 1 2350900
Email: irss@indigo.ie

Fnded: 1988. **Mem:** 400. **Nat'l Groups:** 1. **State Groups:** 1. **Lang(s):** English, Irish. **Desc:** Individuals and organizations. Seeks to improve the quality of life of people with Raynaud's disease or scleroderma and their families. Promotes better physician-patient communication. Makes available support and services; conducts educational and advocacy campaigns. **Pub:** Newsletter, semiannual.

★ 4128 ★ Irish Society for Autism (ISA)
Unity Bldg.
16 Lower O'Connell St.
Dublin 1, Ireland
Phone: 353 1 8744684 **Fax:** 353 1 8744224
Email: autism@isa.iol.ie
Website: http://www.iol.ie/~isa1

Fnded: 1963. **Lang(s):** English, Irish. **Desc:** Individuals and organizations. Seeks to improve the quality of life of people with autism and their families. Makes available support and services; conducts educational and advocacy campaigns. **Pub:** Newsletter, bimonthly.

★ 4129 ★ Irish Society of Chartered Physiotherapists
Royal College of Surgeons
St. Stephen's Green
Dublin 2, Ireland
Phone: 353 1 4022148 **Fax:** 353 1 4022160
Email: info@iscp.ie
Website: http://www.iscp.ie

Fnded: 1983. **Mem:** 1,600. **Reg. Groups:** 8. **Desc:** Physiotherapists.

★ 4130 ★ Irish Society of Homeopaths (ISHom)
Ruxton Ct.
35-37 Dominick St.
Galway, Ireland
Phone: 353 91 565040 **Fax:** 353 91 565040
Email: ishom@eircom.net
Website: http://www.irishsocietyofhomeopaths.com/

Fnded: 1990. **Mem:** 297. **Desc:** Represents lay homeopaths in Ireland. Works to make homeopathy accessible to all, increase awareness and understanding about Homeopathy, regulate standards and ethics of professional practice, provide continuing professional development, and work towards integration of Homeopathy within the Irish health care system.

★ 4131 ★ Irish Society of Human Genetics (ISHG)
c/o Dr. David Croke
Department of Biochemistry
Royal College of Surgeons in Ireland
Dublin 2, Ireland
Email: dtcroke@rcsi.ie
Website: http://www.iol.ie/~ishg/

Desc: Geneticists, molecular biologists, medical doctors, laboratory scientists, epidemiologists, ethicists, and lawyers. Promotes study and research in human genetics as it relates to health and disease. Conducts research; disseminates information.

★ 4132 ★ Irish Society of Occupational Medicine (ISOM)
c/o Dr. Dominick Natin, Hon.Sec.
PO Box 7453
Malahide
Dublin, Ireland
Email: isom@eircom.net
Website: http://www.iol.ie/~isom/

Mem: 270. **Desc:** Occupational physicians and doctors promoting occupational medicine in Ireland.

★ 4133 ★ Irish Society of Periodontology
c/o Dr. Anne O'Donoghue
108 Merrion Rd.
Ballsbridge 4, Dublin, Ireland
Phone: 353 1 2692985 **Fax:** 353 1 2837818
Website: http://www.iol.ie/~perio/

Desc: Works as professional organization that brings together Irish dentists to promote excellence in dentistry and the importance of periodontology in dental health.

★ 4134 ★ Irish Society for Quality in Healthcare (ISQH)
PO Box 6448
Dublin 9, Ireland
Phone: 353 1 8092585 **Fax:** 353 1 8093318
Email: secretary@isqh.net
Website: http://www.isqh.net/

Fnded: 1995. **Desc:** Promotes quality healthcare in Ireland.

★ 4135 ★ Irish Society for Rheumatology
c/o Dr. Paul O'Connell
Beaumont Hospital
Dublin, Ireland
Website: http://www.isr.ie/about_isr.htm

Mem: 60. **Desc:** Promotes the specialty medical field of rheumatology in Ireland.

★ 4136 ★ Irish Sports Medicine Association
Trinity College
Dublin 2, Ireland
Phone: 353 1 6081182 **Fax:** 353 1 6790119

★ 4137 ★ Irish Stammering Association (ISA)
Carmichael House
North Brunswick St.
Dublin 7, Ireland
Phone: 353 1 8735702 **Fax:** 353 1 5735737
Website: http://www.europe.is/elsa/members/m_ireland.html

Desc: Works to find a cure for stuttering in Ireland.

★ 4138 ★ Irish Sudden Infant Death Association (ISIDA)
Carmichael House
4 N Brunswick St.
Dublin 7, Ireland
Phone: 353 1 8732711 **Fax:** 353 1 8726056
Email: kibnsidr@iol.ie
Website: http://www.iol.ie/~isidansr/main.htm

Desc: Provides information and support to families bereaved by sudden infant death and others affected by it; supports research into the causes and prevention of sudden infant death syndrome. Offers bereavement group therapy, befriending service, annual memorial service, SIDS Model of Care, speakers' bureau. **Pub:** *A Book of Remembrance*. Book. Commemorates babies and young children who have died suddenly and unexpectedly. • *A Precious Past, A Hopeful Future*. Handbook.

★ 4139 ★ Irish Veterinary Association
53 Lansdowne Rd.
Ballsbridge 4, Dublin, Ireland

Fnded: 1888. **Desc:** Promotes the veterinary profession.

★ 4140 ★ Irish Wheelchair Association (IWA)
Aras Chuchulainn
Blackheath Dr.
Clontarf
Dublin 3, Ireland
Phone: 353 1 8186400 **Fax:** 353 1 8333873
Email: info@iwa.ie
Website: http://www.iwa.ie

Fnded: 1960. **Mem:** 20,000. **Reg. Groups:** 8. **Local Groups:** 50. **Lang(s):** English, Irish. **Desc:** Individuals and organizations. Seeks to improve the social, economic, and legal status of people with disabilities. Makes available support and services; conducts educational and advocacy campaigns. **Pub:** *Spokeout*, quarterly. Magazine. Lifestyle magazine.

★ 4141 ★ Iron Overload Diseases Association (IOD)
433 Westwind Dr.
North Palm Beach, FL 33408-5123
Phone: (561)840-8512 **Fax:** (561)842-9881
Email: iod@ironoverload.org
Website: http://www.ironoverload.org
Roberta Crawford, Pres.

Fnded: 1981. **Mem:** 8,000. **Desc:** Physicians and patients. Purposes are to: serve hemochromatosis patients and families; encourage research and public information; press for earlier diagnosis and more effective treatment. (Hemochromatosis is a genetic condition of iron overload in which excess iron damages organs and tissues, producing varying late-stage symptoms including liver cirrhosis, diabetes, heart failure, arthritis, and skin pigmentation, leading to death unless diagnosed early and treated adequately.) Specific plans are: to develop a public relations plan, television interviews, and press releases; to sponsor screening programs and patient referral service; prepare diagnosis sheets for doctors and medical schools. Current emphasis is on alerting the public to the dangers of excess iron, since the disease is more prevalent than previously believed, and most susceptible individuals are unaware of the hazard. Authorities believe that five in 1000 carry both genes and that one in eight carries a single gene. Acts as a clearinghouse for doctors to call on for research materials. Sponsors fundraising program. Is also in the process of setting up an index of laboratory research in progress. Conducts programs; compiles statistics; maintains speakers' bureau; conducts research programs. **Pub:** *Ironic Blood*, bimonthly. Newsletter. Information on iron overload. *Price:* Free. • *Overload: An Ironic Disease.* Booklet.

★ 4142 ★ Islamic Medical Association of North America (IMANA)

950 75th St.
Downers Grove, IL 60516
Phone: (630)852-2122 **Fax:** (630)435-1429
Email: imana@aol.com
Website: http://www.imana.org
Abdul Rauf Mir, MD, Pres.

Fnded: 1967. **Mem:** 6,000. **Desc:** Muslim physicians and allied health professionals. Unites Muslim physicians and allied health professionals in the U.S. and Canada for the improvement of professional and social contact; provides assistance to Muslim communities worldwide. Charitable programs include: donation of books, journals, and educational and research materials to medical institutions; donation of medical supplies and equipment to charity medical institutions in Muslim countries. Maintains speakers' bureau to present Islamic viewpoints on medical topics; sponsors placement service; offers assistance in orientation. **Pub:** *Al-Itiknga*, quarterly. Newsletter. • *The Journal of IMA*, quarterly. Journal. *Price:* $50/year. • *The Mediview*, quarterly. Newsletter. **Frmly:** (2001) Islamic Medical Association.

★ 4143 ★ Islamic Organization for Medical Sciences (IOMS)

PO Box 31280
Sulaibekhat 90803, Kuwait
Phone: 965 4834984 **Fax:** 965 4837854
Email: info@islamset.com
Website: http://www.islamset.com

Fnded: 1984. **Mem:** 432. **Reg. Groups:** 6. **Lang(s):** English. **Desc:** Promotes human health standards through collaborative activities in Islamic countries and Muslim communities throughout the world, focusing on medical ethics, healthy lifestyles, and herbal medicine, as well as the fight against endemic and emerging diseases.

★ 4144 ★ Israel Cancer Association (ICA) (Haagudah Lemilchama Besartan Beyisrael)

7 Revivim St.
PO Box 437
IL-53104 Givatayim, Israel
Phone: 972 3 5721616 **Fax:** 972 3 5719578
Email: info@cancer.org.il
Website: http://www.cancer.org.il

Fnded: 1952. **Local Groups:** 52. **Lang(s):** Arabic, English, Hebrew, Russian. **Desc:** Encourages and facilitates research on cancer prevention and early diagnosis. Supports cancer medical treatment services, and finances rehabilitation and social welfare programs for cancer patients. Provides educational programs. **Pub:** *Adcan*, semiannual. • *Bama*, periodic. Journal. Includes information on medical, psychosocial, and welfare aspects of cancer.

★ 4145 ★ Israel Family Planning Association

9 Rambam St.
65601 Tel Aviv, Israel
Phone: 972 3 5101511 **Fax:** 972 3 5102589
Email: ippf@post.com
Website: http://www.opendoor.org.il

Fnded: 1966. **Mem:** 250. **Lang(s):** Arabic, Hebrew. **Desc:** Promotes healthy and responsible sexual behavior as a means to enhance the quality of life for individuals living in Israel. Works to stop the spread of AIDS and other sexually transmitted diseases through education and contraceptive services. Advocates women's empowerment through programs enhancing their self image. Operates 14 "Open-Door" sexual counseling clinics. Offers programs in sex education, family planning, and health. Acts as an advocate for family planning on the national level.

★ 4146 ★ Israel Gerontological Society (IGS)

PO Box 2371
IL-55000 Kiryat Ono, Israel
Phone: 972 3 5357161 **Fax:** 972 3 6359399
Email: igs@netvision.net.il

Fnded: 1956. **Mem:** 520. **Lang(s):** English, Hebrew. **Desc:** Health care professionals treating the elderly; scientists and clinicians with an interest in the aging process and diseases of the aged. Works to insure high standards of research and practice in gerontology, and to maximize availability of gerontological services. Conducts research and educational activities.

★ 4147 ★ Israel Heart Society

2 Twin Towers
35 Jabotinsky Str.
IL-52511 Ramat Gan, Israel
Phone: 972 3 6122577 **Fax:** 972 3 6122588
Email: ihs@israel-heart.org.il
Website: http://www.israel-heart.org.il

Mem: 497. **Desc:** Promotes the study of cardiology in Israel. **Pub:** *Journal of the Israel Heart Society*. Includes review articles and abstracts.

★ 4148 ★ Israel Multiple Sclerosis Society

c/o Michael Sela
75 Yehuda Halevi St.
65796 Tel Aviv, Israel
Phone: 972 3 560 9222 **Fax:** 972 3 560 9224

Fnded: 1976. **Nat'l Groups:** 1. **Desc:** MS patients, families and professionals. Seeks to improve the quality of life for persons with multiple sclerosis and their families.

★ 4149 ★ Israel Physiological and Pharmacological Society

c/o Prof. Arie Moran
Department of Physiology
Faculty of Health Sciences
Ben-Gurion University of the Negev
IL-84105 Beer-Sheva, Israel
Phone: 972 7 6477331 **Fax:** 972 7 6477628
Email: arie@bgumail.bgu.ac.il

Mem: 250. **Desc:** Promotes physiology and pharmacology in Israel.

★ 4150 ★ Israel Psychological Association (IPA)

PO Box 11497
IL-61114 Tel Aviv, Israel
Phone: 972 3 5239393 **Fax:** 972 3 5230763
Email: psycho@zahav.net.il
Website: http://psychology.org.il

Fnded: 1958. **Mem:** 2,900. **Lang(s):** Hebrew. **Desc:** Psychologists in Israel. Promotes high ethical standards in patient treatment. Represents members' interests; disseminates information. **Pub:** *Psychologia*, semiannual. Journal. Contains local articles and publications.

★ 4151 ★ Israel Society of Anesthesiologists (ISA)

c/o Dr. Leonid Eidelman, Pres.
Department of Anesthesiology
Rabin Hospital
Campus Beilinson
Petach-Tiqva, Israel
Email: leidelman@clalit.org.il
Website: http://www.isranest.org.il

Fnded: 1952. **Mem:** 600. **Lang(s):** English. **Desc:** Specialists and residents in training in the field of anesthesiology. Promotes the profession of anesthesiology in Israel and works to enhance the status of its members. Develops professional guidelines and standards.

★ 4152 ★ Israel Society on Calcified Tissues Research

c/o Metabolic Diseases
Beilison Medical Center
49100 Petah Tikva, Israel
Phone: 972 3 376124 **Fax:** 972 3 376143

Fnded: 1971. **Mem:** 120. **Lang(s):** English. **Desc:** Physicians and graduate students in Israel engaged in the clinical research on calcified tissues. Seeks to advance knowledge in the field of bone and mineral metabolism.

★ 4153 ★ Israel Society for Microbiology (ISM)

c/o Unitours Israel
PO Box 3190
IL-61031 Tel Aviv, Israel
Phone: 972 3 5209975 **Fax:** 972 3 5239099
Email: ism@unitours.co.il
Website: http://ism.md.huji.ac.il

Lang(s): English, Hebrew. **Desc:** Microbiologists in Israel. Seeks to unite its members to ensure the scientific and professional standards are upheld; advances the science of microbiology and its research. Strengthens ties with similar societies.

★ 4154 ★ Israel Society for Neuroscience

PO Box 666
IL-75106 Rishon Le Zion, Israel
Phone: 972 2 6758731 **Fax:** 972 2 6758741
Email: martar@cc.huji.ac.il
Website: http://isfn.org.il

Lang(s): English. **Desc:** Promotes neuroscience in Israel.

★ 4155 ★ Israel Society for the Prevention of Alcoholism (ISPA)

c/o Israeli Residential Treatment Center for Alcoholics
13 Nordau St.
IL-52464 Ramat Gan, Israel
Phone: 972 3 6724128 **Fax:** 972 3 6724120
Email: marketch@netvision.net.il
Website: http://www.ias.org.uk/ispa/

Fnded: 1976. **Lang(s):** English, Hebrew. **Desc:** Psychiatrists, physicians, nurses, social workers, recovering alcoholics. Works to develop and advance research, prevention and treatment of alcoholism in Israel. Participates in the "Drugs and Alcohol" committee in the Israeli parliament; offers advice to police on the enforcement of alcohol regulations. **Pub:** *Alcohol in Israel*, semiannual. Journal. Contains summaries in English. • *ISPA Bulletin*, quarterly. Bulletin.

★ 4156 ★ Israeli Association of Creative and Expressive Therapies (ICET)

c/o Hava Kamerinsky
PO Box 49002
IL-91491 Jerusalem, Israel
Phone: 972 2 5817232 **Fax:** 972 2 5817232
Email: micnelso@isdn.net.il

Website: http://www.yahat.org

Fnded: 1971. **Mem:** 1,700. **Local Groups:** 4. **Lang(s):** Hebrew. **Desc:** Music, dance movement, and art therapists. Fosters public awareness of the use of art therapies in the treatment and prevention of various dysfunctions. Provides educational and growth opportunities for therapy professionals. Establishes training standards; conducts workshops and lectures; maintains placement service; offers childrens' services. **Pub:** *ICET Information Bulletin*, periodic. Bulletin. Includes yearly directory. • *Therapy Through Arts*, 2-3/year. • Brochure. Yearly calendar and diary including phone directory. **Frmly:** (1997) Israeli Association of Creative-Extensive Therapy.

★ 4157 ★ Israeli Foundation for Osteoporosis and Bone Diseases

PO Box 1513
IL-37000 Pazdes Hanna, Israel
Phone: 972 4 6274549 **Fax:** 972 4 6274549
Email: lfob@internet-zahav.net.il

Fnded: 1998. **Mem:** 4,000. **Nat'l Groups:** 1. **State Groups:** 1. **Local Groups:** 5. **Lang(s):** English. **Desc:** Promotes the education of the medical profession, patients, and the general public on osteoporosis and bone disease. Conducts political lobbying. **Pub:** *Bone-Tone*, quarterly. Newsletter.

★ 4158 ★ Israeli Society of Psychosomatic Obstetrics and Gynaecology

c/o Dr. Dalia Merari
Sackler Faculty of Medicine
Department of Occupational Therapy
Tel Aviv University
PO Box 39040
IL-69978 Ramat Aviv, Israel
Fax: 972 3 6409933
Email: zdvir@post.tau.ac.il
Website: http://www.ispog.org

Desc: Promotes the study of psychobiological and psychosocial, ethical and cross-cultural problems in the fields of obstetrics and gynaecology, women's health and reproductive health; facilitates the dissemination of new information in these fields. **Pub:** *Journal of Psychosomatic Obstetrics and Gynecology*. Journal.

★ 4159 ★ ISSUE, the National Fertility Association

114 Lichfield St.
West Midlands
Walsall WS1 1SZ, United Kingdom
Phone: 44 1922 722888 **Fax:** 44 1922 640070
Email: info@issue.co.uk
Website: http://www.issue.co.uk

Fnded: 1976. **Mem:** 6,000. **Lang(s):** English. **Desc:** Infertile women and men. Disseminates information and provides support and offers telephone counseling to infertile individuals on all aspects of infertility. **Pub:** *ISSUE*, quarterly. Magazine.

★ 4160 ★ Italian Association for the Fight against Parkinson's Disease, Extrapyramidal Disorders and Dementia (Lega Italiana per la Lotta contro la Malattia di Parkinson, le Sindromi Extrapiramidali e le Demenze — LIMPE)

Viale dell' Universita 30
I-00185 Rome, Italy
Phone: 39 06 4455618 **Fax:** 39 06 4455618
Email: limpe@interfree.it
Website: http://www.parkinson-limpe.it

Fnded: 1983. **Desc:** Promotes the exchange of scientific knowledge; encourages continuing medical education for neurologists in the field of neurodegenerative diseases.

★ 4161 ★ Italian Association of Friends of Raoul Follereau (IAFRF) (Associazione Italiana Amici di Raoul Follereau — AIFO)

Via Borselli 4-6
I-40135 Bologna, Italy
Phone: 39 051 433402 **Fax:** 39 051 434046
Email: info@aifo.it
Website: http://www.aifo.it

Fnded: 1961. **Lang(s):** English, French, Portuguese. **Desc:** Promotes increased availability of medical services and assistance for people with disabilities in developing areas worldwide. Provides medical supplies and equipment to development projects; makes available technical assistance to health and rehabilitation services. Conducts educational and training programs to enhance local administrative capabilities and ensure sustainability and autonomy of health services. Sponsors educational campaigns to raise public awareness in Italy of global health and development issues. **Pub:** *Amici dei Lebbrosi*, monthly. Magazine. • *Quaderni di Cooperazione Sanitaria (Health Cooperation papers)*, periodic. Report. • Books.

★ 4162 ★ Italian Association of Gestalt Psychotherapy (Societa Italiana Psicoterapia Gestalt)

Via Alaimo da Lentini, 2
I-96100 Siracusa, Italy
Phone: 39 093135207 **Fax:** 39 0931442734
Email: training@gestalt.it
Website: http://www.gestalt.it

Fnded: 1987. **Desc:** Promotes Gesalt psychotherapy in the fields of psychotherapies, culture and politics; advances research and training in Gesalt psychotherapy.

★ 4163 ★ Italian Association for Inflammatory Bowel Diseases (Associazione per le Malattie Infiammatorie Croniche dell'Intestino — AMICI)

Via Adolfo Wildt, 19/4
I-20131 Milan, Italy
Phone: 39 022893673 **Fax:** 39 0226822670
Email: amicilombardia@iol.it
Website: http://www.amicilom.org

Fnded: 1989.

★ 4164 ★ Italian Association of Pediatric Hematology and Oncology (Associazione Italiana di Ematologia ed Oncologia Pediatrica — AIEOP)

Via Giustiniani, 3
I-35128 Padua, Italy
Phone: 39 0498211111 **Fax:** 39 0498213510
Website: http://www.sameint.it/AIEOP

Fnded: 1981. **Desc:** Promotes exchange of scientific knowledge in the pediatric hematology-oncology field.

★ 4165 ★ Italian Association of Physics in Medicine (Associazione Italiana di Fisica in Medicina — AIFM)

Viale Borri, 57
I- 21100 Varese, Italy
Phone: 39 0332278459 **Fax:** 39 0332278279
Email: leopcon@tin.it

★ 4166 ★ Italian Federation of Cardiology

c/o Cardio Thoracic Department
Universita degliStudi di Pisa
Via Paradisa 2
IT-56124 Pisa, Italy
Phone: 39 050 542929 **Fax:** 39 050 542947
Email: fedcard@docline.it

Mem: 5,506. **Desc:** Promotes the study of cardiology in Italy. **Pub:** *The Italian Heart Journal*.

★ 4167 ★ Italian Neuroscience Society (Societa Italiana di Neuroscienze)

Ospedale S Eugenio, Piazzale dell'Umanesimo, 10
I-00144 Rome, Italy
Phone: 39 06 59044402

★ 4168 ★ Italian Pharmacological Society (Societa Italiana di Farmacologia)

c/o Prof. Vincenzo Cuomo
Department of Pharmacology and Human Physiology
Section of Pharmacology
University of Bari
Piazza Giulio Cesare
I-70124 Bari, Italy
Phone: 39 080 5478439 **Fax:** 39 080 5478444
Email: cuomo@cimedoc.uniba.it
Website: http://farmacologiasif.unito.it/

Mem: 1,058. **Desc:** Promotes pharmacology in Italy.

★ 4169 ★ Italian Society of Anatomy (ISA) (Societa Italiana di Anatomia — SIA)

Dipartimento di Anatomia, Istologia e Medicina Legale
Sezione "E Allara" Viale Pieraccini 6
I-50139 Florence, Italy
Phone: 39 055 4271389 **Fax:** 39 055 4271385
Email: paolo.romagnoli@unifi.it

Fnded: 1929. **Mem:** 400. **Lang(s):** English, Italian. **Desc:** Fosters the study of anatomy, histology, and embryology in Italy. **Pub:** *Italian Journal of Anatomy and Embriology*, quarterly. Journal. • Papers, periodic.

★ 4170 ★ Italian Society of Artificial Organs (Societa Italiana Organi Artificiali)

Piazzale dell'Umanesimo, 10
I-00144 Rome, Italy
Phone: 39 06 51001 **Fax:** 39 06 5922681

★ 4171 ★ Italian Society for Endoscopic Surgery and New Technologies (Societa Italiana di Chirgugia Endoscopica e Nuove Tecnologie — SICE)

Viale del Policlinico, 155
I-00161 Rome, Italy
Phone: 39 06 49970204 **Fax:** 39 06 4465513
Email: segreteria@siceitalia.com
Website: http://www.siceitalia.com

Fnded: 1993. **Desc:** Promotes research, training and new technologies in the field of minimally-invasive surgery.

★ 4172 ★ Italian Society of Gerontology and Geriatrics (Societa Italiana di Gerontologia e Geriatria — SIGG)

Via G.C. Vanini, 5
I-50129 Florence, Italy
Phone: 39 055474330 **Fax:** 39 055461217
Email: sigg@sigg.it
Website: http://www.sigg.it

Fnded: 1950. **Desc:** Promotes scientific research into the fields of gerontology and geriatrics.

★ 4173 ★ Italian Society for Hospital Pharmacy (SIFO) (Societa Italiana di Farmacia Ospedaliera)

Viale Piceno, 18
I-20129 Milan, Italy
Fax: 39 0276110653
Email: dirfarmac@ospedaliriuniti.bergamo.it
Website: http://www.sifo.it

Fnded: 1952. **Desc:** Membership enables to participate in the updating courses, masters, workshops.

★ 4174 ★ Italian Society of Internal Medicine
(Societa Italiana di Medicina Interna — SIMI)
Viale dell University, 25
I-00183 Rome, Italy
Phone: 39 06 44340373 **Fax:** 39 06 44340474
Email: simimail@tin.it
Fnded: 1888.

★ 4175 ★ Italian Society of Neurosonology and Cerebral Hemodynamics
(Societa Italiana di Neurosonologia ed Emodinamica Cerebrale)
Via Altura, 3
I-40068 San Lazzaro di Savena, Italy
Phone: 39 0516225500 **Fax:** 39 0516564350
Fnded: 1970. **Desc:** Also acts as co-sponsor of neurosonological meetings in Italy.

★ 4176 ★ Italian Society of Psychosomatic Obstetrics and Gynaecology
c/o Dr. F. Facchinetti
Department of Obstetrics & Gynecology
University of Modena
Via del Pozzo 71
I-41110 Modena, Italy
Fax: 39 059 424394
Email: facchi@unimo.it
Website: http://www.ispog.org
Desc: Promotes the study of psychobiological and psychosocial, ethical and cross-cultural problems in the fields of obstetrics and gynaecology, women's health and reproductive health; facilitates the dissemination of new information in these fields. **Pub:** *Journal of Psychosomatic Obstetrics and Gynecology*. Journal.

★ 4177 ★ Italian Society for Research in Child Neurology
(Associazione Italiana per la Ricerca in Neurologia Infantile — AIRNI)
Via di Torvergata, 135
I-00133 Rome, Italy
Fnded: 1983. **Desc:** Promotes research in child neurology.

★ 4178 ★ Italian Society of Social Medicine
(Societa Italiana di Medicina Sociale — SIMS)
Corso Bramante, 83
I-10126 Turin, Italy
Phone: 39 011678282
Fnded: 1947.

★ 4179 ★ Italian Society of Social Psychiatry
(Societa Italiana di Psichiatria Sociale)
Via Adelaide Ristori, 36/A
I- 00197 Rome, Italy
Phone: 39 6 8083784

★ 4180 ★ Italian Society of Therapeutic Psychosynthesis
(Societa Italiana Psicosintesi Terapeutica — SIPT)
Via S Domenico, 16
I-50133 Florence, Italy
Phone: 39 055570140 **Fax:** 39 055570140
Email: istituto@psicosintesi.it
Website: http://www.psicosintesi.it/sipt/sipte.htm
Fnded: 1973. **Desc:** Diffuses therapeutical psychosynthesis, promotes psychotherapeutical training in psychosynthesis, fosters research and clinical practice, favours the cooperation between members and psychological organisations.

★ 4181 ★ Italian Union of the Blind
(Unione Italiana Ciechi — UIC)
via Borgognona 38
I-00187 Rome, Italy
Phone: 39 06 699881 **Fax:** 39 06 6786815
Website: http://www.uiciechi.it
Lang(s): English, Italian. **Desc:** Seeks to improve the quality of life of people with visual impairment in Italy. Represents the interests of people with visual impairment before government agencies and the public. Conducts health education programs. Sponsors projects in the Czech Republic.

★ 4182 ★ Italian Urological Association
(Societa Italiana di Urologia — SIU)
Largo Rodolfo Lanciani, 1
I-00162 Rome, Italy
Phone: 39 06 86202637 **Fax:** 39 06 86325073
Fnded: 1922.

★ 4183 ★ IUD Claims Information Source (ICIS)
PO Box 84151
Seattle, WA 98124
Phone: (206)329-1371 **Fax:** (206)624-4961
Constance Miller, Mng. Dir.
Fnded: 1989. **Desc:** Provides information and referrals to women filing lawsuits because of injuries sustained through use of an intrauterine contraceptive device (IUD). Offers professional seminars in claims filing and resolution. Maintains speakers' bureau. **Pub:** *Dalkon Shield Claims Guidebook*. • *Dalkon Shield Legal Guide*.

★ 4184 ★ Jacobs Institute of Women's Health
409 12th St. SW
Washington, DC 20024-2188
Phone: (202)863-4990 **Fax:** (202)488-4229
Website: http://www.jiwh.org/
Mem: 2,000. **Desc:** Works to improve health care for women through research, dialogue and education. **Pub:** *In Touch*, quarterly. Newsletter. *Price:* included in membership dues. • *Women's Health Data Book*. Book. Third edition.

★ 4185 ★ Jamaica Cancer Society (JCS)
16 Lady Musgrave Rd.
Kingston 5, Jamaica
Phone: (876)927-4265 **Fax:** (876)978-1918
Email: info@jamaicacancersociety.org
Website: http://www.jamaicacancersociety.org
Fnded: 1955. **Mem:** 1,200. **Nat'l Groups:** 1. **Reg. Groups:** 1. **Local Groups:** 1. **Desc:** Health care professionals, people with cancer and their families, and other interested individuals. Promotes and encourages research into the causes and cure of cancer, and improved treatments for people with cancer. Conducts public education programs on cancer detection and treatment; offers specialized training for cancer nurses. Operates cancer screening clinics for cervical, breast and prostate cancer. **Pub:** *Can Survive*, semiannual. Newsletter. • Brochure.

★ 4186 ★ Japan Amyotrophic Lateral Sclerosis Association
7-103 Nando-cho
Shinjuku
Tokyo 162-0837, Japan
Phone: 81 3 32676942 **Fax:** 81 3 32674123
Email: jalsa@jade.dti.ne.jp
Website: http://www.jade.dti.ne.jp/~jalsa
Desc: Individuals interested in amyotropic lateral sclerosis or ALS (also known as Lou Gehrig's Disease). Works to: heighten public awareness and understanding of the disease; encourage research among medical and scientific communities.

★ 4187 ★ Japan Association of Applied Psychology
(Nihon Oyo Shinri-gakkai)
3-25-40 Sakurajosui, Setagaya-ku
Tokyo, Japan
Phone: 81 3 3291151
Fnded: 1931.

★ 4188 ★ Japan Diabetes Society
(Nippon Tonyo-byo Gakkai)
3-38-11 Hongo, Bunkyo-ku
Tokyo, Japan
Fnded: 1958.

★ 4189 ★ Japan Gastroenterological Endoscopy Society
(Nihon Shokaki Naishikyo Gakkai)
Chiyoda-ku
Tokyo, Japan
Phone: 81 3 32914111 **Fax:** 81 3 32915568
Fnded: 1961.

★ 4190 ★ Japan Geriatrics Society
(Nihon Ronen Igakukai)
4-2-1 Yushima, Bunkyo-ku
Tokyo, Japan
Fnded: 1959.

★ 4191 ★ Japan Gerontological Society (JGS)
Kyorin Bldg., 702
4-2-1 Yushima
Bunkyo-ku
Tokyo 113, Japan
Lang(s): English, Japanese. **Desc:** Health care professionals treating the elderly; scientists and clinicians with an interest in the aging process and diseases of the aged. Promotes gerontological research and increased availability of gerontological care; facilitates training of gerontology specialists. Represents the interests of gerontologists and gerontological organizations.

★ 4192 ★ Japan Medical Association
(Nihon Ishi-Kai)
Honkomagome, Bunkyo-ku
Tokyo, Japan
Fnded: 1916.

★ 4193 ★ Japan Medical Women's Association
(Nihon Joi Kai)
3rd Floor, Aoyama-Shrinefield Bldg.
Shibuya 2-8-7
Shibuya-ku
Tokyo 150-0002, Japan
Phone: 81 3 34980571 **Fax:** 81 3 34988769
Email: jmwa@jade.dti.we.jp
Desc: Women working in the medical profession. Works to maintain high standards.

★ 4194 ★ Japan Multiple Sclerosis Society
c/o Kiyoaki Kikuchi
4-1-2 Kotobuki
Taito-Ku
Tokyo, Japan
Phone: 81 3 3847 3504 **Fax:** 81 3 3842 0289
Fnded: 1977. **Mem:** 31. **Reg. Groups:** 1. **Desc:** MS patients, families and professionals. Seeks to improve the quality of life for persons with multiple sclerosis and their families. **Pub:** *Seeking your Understanding of and Co-operation with the Japan MS Society (2000)*. • Newsletter.

★ 4195 ★ Japan Neuroscience Society (Nippon Shinkeikagaku Gakkai)
5-16-9 Honkomagome, Bunkyo-ku
Tokyo, Japan
Fnded: 1974. **Mem:** 4,000.

★ 4196 ★ Japan Neurosurgical Society (Nippon No-Shinkei Gek Gakkai)
5-27-8 Hongo, Bunkyo-ku
Tokyo, Japan
Phone: 81 3 38126226 **Fax:** 81 3 38122090
Email: jns@ssiij4u.ot.jp
Fnded: 1948. **Mem:** 7,733. **Pub:** *Neurologia medics - chirurgica*, monthly. Journal.

★ 4197 ★ Japan Optometric Association (JOA)
2-5-5 Izumi Higashiku
Nagoya 461-0001, Japan
Phone: 81 52 9320610 **Fax:** 81 52 9320629
Email: joa@pop01.odn.ne.jp
Fnded: 1979. **Mem:** 1,140. **Lang(s):** English, Japanese. **Desc:** Optometrists. Seeks to advance the study, teaching, and practice of optometry; promotes continuing professional development of members. Serves as a clearinghouse on optometry; sponsors research and educational programs. **Pub:** *Journal of the Japan Optometric Association*, semiannual. Journal.

★ 4198 ★ Japan Orthodontic Society (Nihon Kyosei Shikagakkai)
Toshima-ku
Tokyo, Japan
Phone: 81 3 39478891 **Fax:** 81 39478341
Fnded: 1932.

★ 4199 ★ Japan Overseas Christian Medical Cooperative Service (JOCS)
2-3-18-23 Nishiwaseda
Shinjuku-ku
Tokyo 169-0051, Japan
Phone: 81 3 32082416 **Fax:** 81 3 32326922
Email: info@www.jocs.or.jp
Website: http://www.jocs.or.jp/
Fnded: 1960. **Lang(s):** English, Japanese. **Desc:** Works to coordinate the efforts of Christian sects providing medical services in Bangladesh, Cambodia, India, Indonesia, Nigeria, Pakistan, and Taiwan. Organization believes that Japan is indebted to the rest of Asia due to atrocities committed during World War II. Does not conduct evangelical programs, providing medical services without reference to a patients race, religion, color, or creed.

★ 4200 ★ Japan Pediatric Society (Nihon Shonika Gakkai)
1-1-5, Koraku, Bunkyo-ku
Tokyo, Japan
Phone: 81 3 38180091
Fnded: 1896.

★ 4201 ★ Japan Prosthodontic Society (Nippon Hotetsu Shika Gakkai)
Toshima-ku
Tokyo, Japan
Fnded: 1931.

★ 4202 ★ Japan Public Health Association (Nippon Koshu-Eisei Kyokai)
Shinjuku 1-chome, Shinjuku-ku
Tokyo, Japan
Fnded: 1883.

★ 4203 ★ Japan Society of Blood Transfusion (JSBT)
The Japanese Red Cross, 4-1-31, Shibuya-ku
Tokyo, Japan
Phone: 81 3 54856020 **Fax:** 81 3 4067892
Email: shotyan@transf.med.kyushu-u.ac.jp
Website: http://www.yuketsu.gr.jp
Fnded: 1954. **Desc:** Promotes scientific activities on transfusion medicine through sharing and exchanging members' research outcomes; publishes journals and holds annual congresses and symposia; distributes guidelines and recommendations; educates individuals and medical institutions.

★ 4204 ★ Japan Society of Clinical Pathology (Nihon Rinsho Byori Gakkai)
2-11-10, Hongo, Bunkyo-ku
Tokyo, Japan
Fax: 81 3 8139998150
Fnded: 1951.

★ 4205 ★ Japan Society of Obstetrics and Gynecology
Hokenkaikan Bldg. Annex
Ichigaya-Sadoharacho 1-1
Shinjuku-ku
Tokyo 162-0842, Japan
Fax: 81 3 32692834
Fnded: 1957. **Pub:** *Journal of Obstetrics and Gynaecology Research*. Journal.

★ 4206 ★ Japan Surgical Society (Nippon Geka Gakkai)
2-3-10, Koraku, Bunkyo-ku
Tokyo, Japan
Fnded: 1899.

★ 4207 ★ Japanese Association for Acute Medicine (JAAM)
Department of Emergency Medicine
Osaka University School of Medicine
2-2 Yamadaoka
Suita City
Osaka 565, Japan
Phone: 81 6 8793331 **Fax:** 81 6 8783540
Desc: Medical practitioners involved in acute medicine. Represents members' interests. **Pub:** *Journal of he Japanese Association for Acute Medicine*. Journal.

★ 4208 ★ Japanese Association of Anatomists (Nippon Kaibo Gakkai)
5-16-9 Honkomagome, Bunkyo-ku
Tokyo, Japan
Fnded: 1893.

★ 4209 ★ Japanese Association for Dental Science (Nippon Shika Igakkai)
4-1-20 Kudan-kita, Chiyoda-ku
Tokyo, Japan
Phone: 81 3 32629214 **Fax:** 81 3 32629885
Fnded: 1949.

★ 4210 ★ Japanese Association on Disability and Handicap
Nishiwaseda Sekiguchi Bldg. 4F
2-15-10 Nishiwaseda
Shinjuku-ku
Tokyo 169-0051, Japan
Phone: 81 3 52852601 **Fax:** 81 3 52852603
Email: webmaster@nginet.or.jp
Desc: Seeks to protect the human rights of individuals with disabilities in Japan.

★ 4211 ★ Japanese Association of Educational Psychology (Nihon Kyoiku-shinri Gakkai)
Bunkyo-ku
Tokyo, Japan
Fnded: 1955.

★ 4212 ★ Japanese Association of Healthcare Information Systems Industry (JAHIS)
c/o Tranomon TBL Building
1-19-9, Toranomon
Minato-ku
Tokyo 105-0001, Japan
Phone: 81 3 35068010 **Fax:** 81 3 35068070
Website: http://www.jahis.gr.jp
Lang(s): English, Japanese. **Desc:** Corporations and organizations involved in the healthcare information system industry. Promotes the sound development of the healthcare information system industry and contributes to people's health, medical care, and welfare by improving technology and promoting the standardization of healthcare information systems. **Pub:** *JAHIS News*. Annual Report.

★ 4213 ★ Japanese Association for Infectious Diseases
Sankei 8 Bldg., 6F
1-8-7 Ebisu
Shibuya-ku
Tokyo 150-0013, Japan
Email: info@kansensho.or.jp
Desc: Healthcare professionals, researchers, and scientists working to advance the study and treatment of infectious diseases. **Pub:** Journal, periodic.

★ 4214 ★ Japanese Association of School Health (Nihon Gakko-hoken Gakkai)
7-3-1 Hongo, Bunkyo-ku
Tokyo 113, Japan
Phone: 81 3 38122111
Fnded: 1954.

★ 4215 ★ Japanese Cancer Association (Nippon Gan Gakkai)
Kami-Ikebukuro 1-37-1, Toshima-ku
Tokyo, Japan
Phone: 81 3 39180111 **Fax:** 81 3 39185776
Fnded: 1907.

★ 4216 ★ Japanese Chiropractic Association (JCA)
IK Bldg.
6-20-11 Shinbashi
Minato-ku
Tokyo 105-0004, Japan
Phone: 81 3 54010961 **Fax:** 81 3 54010956
Fnded: 1961. **Mem:** 170. **Desc:** Promotes the use of chiropractic therapy in Japan. Maintains and upholds standards of conduct of members. Conducts educational programs.

★ 4217 ★ Japanese College of Angiology
5-16-9, Honkomagome, Bunkyo-ku
Tokyo, Japan
Phone: 81 3 58145801 **Fax:** 81 3 58145820
Fnded: 1960.

★ 4218 ★ Japanese Dermatological Association (Nippon Hifuka Gakkai)
3-14-10 Hongo, Bunkyo-ku
Tokyo, Japan
Phone: 81 3 38115099 **Fax:** 81 3 38126790
Email: gakkai@dermatol.or.jp
Website: http://www.dermatol.or.jp

Fnded: 1901. **Mem:** 10,125. **Nat'l Groups:** 1. **Reg. Groups:** 4. **Local Groups:** 36. **Lang(s):** Japanese.

★ 4219 ★ Japanese Federation of Physical Fitness and Sports Medicine
Hon-Komagome, Bunkyo-ku
Tokyo 113-8622, Japan
Phone: 81 3 58145801 **Fax:** 81 3 58145820
Desc: Promotes the progress and development of research in physical fitness and sports medicine.

★ 4220 ★ Japanese Leprosy Association
(Nippon Hansen-byo Gakkai)
Higashimurayama-shi
Tokyo, Japan
Phone: 81 42 3918211 **Fax:** 81 42 3949092
Fnded: 1927. **Desc:** Promotes mutual exchange of research results on leprosy; cooperates with national and international associations.

★ 4221 ★ Japanese Nursing Association
Koubun-Kousan Bldg.
2-4-3 Hitotsubashi
Chiyoda-ku
Tokyo 101-0003, Japan
Phone: 81 3 52755896 **Fax:** 81 3 52755906
Email: intl@nurse.or.jp
Website: http://www.nurse.or.jp
Fnded: 1946. **Mem:** 420,000. **State Groups:** 47. **Desc:** Promotes the status of nurses in Japan. **Pub:** *Kyokai (Association) News*, monthly. Newsletter. Promotes and strengthens public relations.

★ 4222 ★ Japanese Ophthalmological Society
(Nippon Ganka Gakkai)
Chiyoda-ku
Tokyo, Japan
Fnded: 1897.

★ 4223 ★ Japanese Organization for International Cooperation in Family Planning (JOICFP)
Hoken Kaikan Shinkan Bldg.
1-10 Ichigaya Tamachi
Shinjuku-ku
Tokyo 162-0843, Japan
Phone: 81 3 32685875 **Fax:** 81 3 32357090
Email: info@joicfp.or.jp
Website: http://www.joicfp.or.jp
Fnded: 1968. **Mem:** 150. **Lang(s):** English, Japanese. **Desc:** Provides assistance to reproductive health and family planning programs in 12 countries worldwide. Works closely with Japanese government agencies and international development organizations including UNFPA and IPPF to devise projects and train staff. Promotes BCC using videotapes and films in reproductive health/family planning education programs. **Pub:** *Adolescent Women - Voices Unheard, Marian's Monolog*. Film. • *JOICFP News*, monthly. Newsletter. • *Sekaito Jinko*, monthly. Magazine. • Monographs.

★ 4224 ★ Japanese Orthopaedic Association
(Nippon Seikei Geka Gakkai)
40-17, Hongo 2-chome, Bunkyo-ku
Tokyo, Japan
Fax: 81 3 38182337
Fnded: 1926.

★ 4225 ★ Japanese Pharmacological Society
(Shadanhojin Nipon Yakurigakkai)
Office of the Japanese Pharmacological Society
2-4-16 Yayoi
Bunkyo-ku
Tokyo 113-0032, Japan
Phone: 81 3 38144818 **Fax:** 81 3 38144809
Email: pharmacology@hi-ho.ne.jp
Website: http://wwwsoc.nii.ac.jp/tjps
Mem: 6,500. **Desc:** Promotes pharmacology in Japan.

★ 4226 ★ Japanese Psychological Association
(Nihon Shinri Gakkai)
5-23-13-7F Hongo, Bungyo-ku
Tokyo 113-0033, Japan
Phone: 81 3 38143953 **Fax:** 81 3 38143954
Email: nisshin@mint.ocn.ne.jp

★ 4227 ★ Japanese Society of Adlerian Psychology (JSAP)
c/o Adler Guild
Futaba Bldg. 3F
5-12-15 Nishi-Nakajima, Yodogawa
Osaka 532-0011, Japan
Phone: 81 6 63064699 **Fax:** 81 6 63060160
Fnded: 1984. **Mem:** 1,200. **Desc:** Individuals interesting in studying and developing the psychology of Alfred Adler.

★ 4228 ★ Japanese Society of Allergology
(Nihon Arerugi Gakkai)
33-19-802, Hakusan-1, Bunkyo-ku
Tokyo, Japan
Phone: 81 3 8160280
Fnded: 1952.

★ 4229 ★ Japanese Society of Anesthesiologists
(Nihon Masuka Gakkai)
3-18-11 Hongo, Bunkyo-ku
Tokyo, Japan
Phone: 81 3 38150590 **Fax:** 81 3 38130464
Email: anesth@gamma.ocu.ne.jp
Website: http://www.anesth.or.jp
Fnded: 1954. **Mem:** 8,901. **Reg. Groups:** 8. **Lang(s):** English, Japanese. **Pub:** *Journal of Anesthesia*, quarterly. Magazine.

★ 4230 ★ Japanese Society for Artificial Organs
Society Center C21
5-16-9 honkomagome
Bunkyo-ku
Tokyo 113, Japan
Phone: 81 3 58145801 **Fax:** 81 3 58145820
Fnded: 1962. **Mem:** 4,000. **Desc:** Promotes the use of artificial organs in transplantation. **Pub:** *Journal of Artificial Organs*, semiannual. Journal.

★ 4231 ★ Japanese Society of Conservative Dentistry
c/o Kouku Hoken Kyoukai
Domagome TS Bldg.
1-43-9 Komagome
Toshimaku
Tokyo 170-0003, Japan
Phone: 81 3 39478891 **Fax:** 81 3 39478341
Email: gakkai8@kokuhoken.or.jp
Mem: 4,553. **Desc:** Specialists from all dental schools in Japan, individual dentists in private practice or hospitals. Areas of research interests include application of laser endodontics and immunological studies of periodontal diseases. **Pub:** *Japanese Journal of Conservative Dentistry*, bimonthly. Journal. Includes articles concerning operative dentistry, endodontics, and periodontics.

★ 4232 ★ Japanese Society for Dental Health
(Nihon Koku Eisei Gakkai)
1-chome, Toshima-ku
Tokyo, Japan
Fnded: 1952.

★ 4233 ★ Japanese Society of Dental Radiology
(Nippon Shika Hoshasen Gakkai)
Chiyoda-ku
Tokyo, Japan
Fnded: 1951.

★ 4234 ★ Japanese Society of Developmental Biologists
(Hassei Seibutsu Gakkai)
3-8-1 Komaba, Meguro-ku
Tokyo, Japan
Phone: 81 3 54542904
Fnded: 1968.

★ 4235 ★ Japanese Society of Environment Control in Biology
(Nihon Seibutsu Kankyo Chosetsu Kenkyukai)
University of Tokyo
Tokyo, Japan
Phone: 81 3 8122111
Fnded: 1969.

★ 4236 ★ Japanese Society of Hematology
(Nippon Ketsueki Gakkai)
14 Kawaramachi, Yoshida, Sakyo-ku
Kyoto 606-8305, Japan
Phone: 81 75 7518982 **Fax:** 81 75 7520761
Email: ijh-ind@umin.u-tokyo.ac.jp
Website: http://jshem.or.jp
Fnded: 1937. **Mem:** 6,000. **Local Groups:** 5. **Pub:** *International Journal of Hematology*, 10/year. Journal. Hematology-related articles.

★ 4237 ★ Japanese Society for Hygiene
(Nihon Eisei Gakkai)
Kita 15-jo, Kita-ku
Sapporo, Japan
Phone: 81 11 7065553 **Fax:** 81 11 7171140
Fnded: 1902.

★ 4238 ★ Japanese Society of Hypertension (JSH)
c/o Business Center for Academic Societies Japan
5-16-9 Honkomagome
Bunkyo-ku
Tokyo 113-8622, Japan
Phone: 81 3 58145810 **Fax:** 81 3 58145825
Email: jsh-qa@bcasj.or.jp
Website: http://www.bcasj.or.jp/hr
Fnded: 1978. **Mem:** 2,450. **Desc:** Studies the causes and prevention of hypertension. **Pub:** *Hypertension Research - Clinical and Experimental*, periodic. Journal. • Newsletter, semiannual.

★ 4239 ★ Japanese Society of Internal Medicine
(Nihon Naika Gakkai)
3-34-3 Hongo, Bunkyo-ku
Tokyo, Japan
Phone: 81 3 38135991
Fnded: 1903.

★ 4240 ★ Japanese Society of Legal Medicine (JSLM)
c/o Department of Forensic Medicine
Graduate School of Medicine
University of Tokyo
7-3-1 Hongo, Bunkyo-ku
Tokyo 113-0033, Japan
Phone: 81 3 58005416
Desc: Pathologists, toxicologists, lawyers, police criminalists, and professors of legal medicine in Japan. Conducts educational programs. **Pub:** Journal, periodic.

★ 4241 ★ Japanese Society of Medical Entomology and Zoology
(Nippon Eisei-Dobutsu Gakkai)
Bunkyo-ku
Tokyo, Japan
Phone: 81 3 58145801 **Fax:** 81 3 58145820
Fnded: 1943.

★ 4242 ★ Japanese Society of Medical Imaging Technology
c/o Quantum
YU Bldg., 3F
3-19-6 Hongou
Bunkyou-ku
Tokyo 113-0033, Japan
Phone: 81 3 56841636 **Fax:** 81 3 56841650
Email: office@jamit.jp
Website: http://www.jamit.jp
Desc: Fosters the advancement of medical imaging technology. **Pub:** *Medical Imaging Technology*, bimonthly. Journal.

★ 4243 ★ Japanese Society of Neurology
(Nippon Shinkei Gakkai)
Bunkyo-ku
Tokyo, Japan
Phone: 81 3 8151080 **Fax:** 81 3 8151931
Fnded: 1960.

★ 4244 ★ Japanese Society of Nuclear Medicine (JSNM)
2-28-45 Hon-Komagome, Bunkyo-ku
Tokyo 113-0021, Japan
Fax: 81 3 39472535
Fnded: 1964. **Desc:** Promotes the appropriate development of the application of radioactive substances and stable nuclides in medicine; furthers the exchange of ideas and information; researches nuclear medicine.

★ 4245 ★ Japanese Society for Oral and Maxillofacial Radiology
(Nihon Shika Hoshasen Gakkai)
1-8 Yamadaoka, Suita
Osaka, Japan
Phone: 81 6 8792967 **Fax:** 81 6 8755834
Fnded: 1951.

★ 4246 ★ Japanese Society of Oral Surgeons
(Nihon Koko Geka Gakkai)
10 Kawada-cho, Shinjuku-ku
Tokyo, Japan
Fnded: 1952.

★ 4247 ★ Japanese Society of Pathology
(Nippon Byori Gakkai)
2-40-9 Hongo Bunkyo-ku
Tokyo, Japan
Phone: 81 3 56846886 **Fax:** 81 3 56846936
Email: jsp@ma.kcom.ne.jp
Website: http://jsp.umin.ac.jp/
Fnded: 1911. **Mem:** 4,000. **Reg. Groups:** 7. **Pub:** *Pathology International*, monthly. Journal.

★ 4248 ★ Japanese Society of Pediatric Surgeons
(Nihon Shoni Geka Gakkai)
2-4-16 Yayoi, Bunkyo-ku
Tokyo, Japan
Fnded: 1964.

★ 4249 ★ Japanese Society of Psychiatry and Neurology
(Nihon Seishin Shinkei Gakkai)
3-chome, Hongo, Bunkyo-ku
Tokyo, Japan
Fnded: 1902.

★ 4250 ★ Japanese Society of Psychosomatic Obstetrics and Gynaecology
c/o Congress Corporation
Kosaikaikan Bldg.
5-1 Kojimachi
Chiyoda-ku
Tokyo 102-8481, Japan
Phone: 81 3 32631369 **Fax:** 81 3 32634033
Email: jimukyoku@jspog.com
Fnded: 1997. **Mem:** 500. **Nat'l Groups:** 1. **Lang(s):** Japanese. **Desc:** Promotes the study of psychobiological and psychosocial, ethical and cross-cultural problems in the fields of obstetrics and gynaecology, women's health and reproductive health; facilitates the dissemination of new information in these fields. **Pub:** *Journal of Japanese Society of Psychosomatic Obstetrics & Gynecology*, 3/year. Journal.

★ 4251 ★ Japanese Society of Social Psychology
(Nihon Shakai Shinri Gakkai)
Suginami-ku
Tokyo, Japan
Fnded: 1960.

★ 4252 ★ Japanese Society for Stereotactic and Functional Neurosurgery
30-1 Ohyaguchi Kamimachi, Itabashi-ku
Tokyo, Japan
Phone: 81 3 39728111 **Fax:** 81 3 35540425
Email: Youichik@bekkoame.or.jp
Fnded: 1963.

★ 4253 ★ Japanese Society for the Study of Pain
54 Kawahara-cho Syogoin, Sakyo-ku
Kyoto, Japan
Phone: 81 75 7513433 **Fax:** 81 75 7523259
Fnded: 1973.

★ 4254 ★ Japanese Society of Tropical Medicine
(Nihon Nettai Igakkai)
1-12-4 Sakamoto
Nagasaki, Japan
Phone: 81 95 8497804 **Fax:** 81 95 8497805
Website: http://www.tm.nagasaki-u.ac.jp/society/jstm/gkmain.html
Fnded: 1959. **Mem:** 579. **Nat'l Groups:** 1. **Reg. Groups:** 1. **Pub:** *Japanese Journal of Tropical Medicine & Hygiene*, quarterly. Journal.

★ 4255 ★ Japanese Society for Tuberculosis
(Nippon Kekkaku-byo Gakkai)
3-1-24 Matsuyama, Kiyose-shi
Tokyo 204, Japan
Phone: 81 424922091 **Fax:** 81 424918315
Fnded: 1925.

★ 4256 ★ Japanese Society of Veterinary Science
(Nihon Jui Gakkai)
1-37-20 Yoyogi, Shibuya-ku
Tokyo, Japan
Phone: 81 3 33790636 **Fax:** 81 3 3790636
Fnded: 1885.

★ 4257 ★ Japanese Urological Association
(Nihon Hinyokika Gakkai)
3-14-10 Hongo, Bunkyo-ku
Tokyo, Japan
Fnded: 1912.

★ 4258 ★ Jaw Joints and Allied Musculo-Skeletal Disorders Foundation (JJAMD)
c/o The Forsyth Institute
140 Fenway
Boston, MA 02115-3799
Phone: (617)266-2550 **Fax:** (617)267-9020
Email: tmjoints@aol.com
Website: http://www.tmjoints.org
Renee Glass, Co-Founder/Pres.
Fnded: 1982. **Desc:** Promotes public awareness of temporomandibular joint disorder (TMJ) and related musculoskeletal disorders. Provides information on prevention, treatment, and responsible diagnosis. Conducts research and educational programs; monitors legislative activities. Provides advocacy, networking, patients, professionals, governmental agencies, healthcare, academic, research communities, insurance providers, and support group activities. **Pub:** *Plain Talk Guide to TMJ; with Self-Help Tips to Keep Your Jaw Joints Healthy*. Pamphlet.

★ 4259 ★ JBI International - Jewish Braille Institute of America (JBI)
110 E 30th St.
New York, NY 10016
Phone: (212)889-2525 **Free:** 800-433-1531
Fax: (212)689-3692
Email: admin@jbilibrary.org
Website: http://www.jbilibrary.org
Dr. Ellen Isler, Exec. VP
Fnded: 1931. **Desc:** Jewish Braille Institute is the only library of Jewish interest in the world serving the cultural, religious, educational and communal needs of the visually impaired and blind in over 50 countries, including the U.S., Israel and the former Soviet Union, and in six languages (English, Russian, Hebrew, Hungarian, Yiddish, Polish). JBI materials are distributed free on audio cassette, in large print and in braille. Collection includes 10,000 titles covering fiction and non-fiction, liturgical materials, and 7 monthly magazines. JBI is an affiliated library of the United States Library of Congress and is accredited as a non-governmental organization of the United Nations. **Pub:** *Hebrew Braille Bible*. • *Hebrew Self-Taught*. Braille primer. • *JBI Voice*, 10/year. Magazine. Cassette format for non-braille reading blind and visually impaired. Includes articles on Jewish-related topics, politics, stories, and poetry. *Price:* Free to blind and visually impaired persons. • *Jewish Reference Calendar*, annual. Large print, 18-month with secular holidays and candle lighting times. • *Passover Haggadah*. Large print edition. • Also publishes prayer books and religious texts in Hebrew. **Frmly:** (2003) Jewish Braille Institute of America.

★ 4260 ★ Jean Piaget Society: Society for the Study of Knowledge and Development (JPSSSKD)
Human Development
Larsen Hall 702
Harvard GS Education
Cambridge, MA 02138
Phone: (617)495-3614 **Fax:** (617)495-3626
Email: kurt_fischer@harvard.edu
Website: http://www.piaget.org
Kurt Fischer, Contact
Fnded: 1970. **Mem:** 500. **Desc:** Scholars, teachers, and researchers interested in exploring the nature of the developmental construction of human knowledge. Purpose is to further research on knowledge and development, especially in relation to the work of Jean Piaget (1896-1980), a Swiss developmentalist noted for his work in child psychology, the study of human development, and the origin and growth of human

knowledge. Conducts small meetings and programs. **Pub:** *Genetic Epistemologist*, quarterly. Newsletter. Covers the nature of human knowledge. *Price:* Included in membership dues. • *Jean Piaget Symposium Series*, annual. *Price:* Included in membership dues; $80 for nonmembers. **Frmly:** (1989) Jean Piaget Society.

★ 4261 ★ Jeffrey Modell Foundation (JMF)

c/o Vicki Modell
747 3rd Ave.
New York, NY 10036
Phone: (212)819-0200 **Fax:** (212)764-4180
Email: info@jmfworld.org
Website: http://www.jmfworld.com/
Vicki Modell, Co-Founder

Desc: Devoted to primary immune deficiency, including research, physician and patient education, patient support, and public awareness.

★ 4262 ★ Jennifer Trust for Spinal Muscular Atrophy (JTSMA)

Elta House
Birmingham Rd.
Stratford-Upon-Avon CV37 0AQ, United Kingdom
Phone: 44 1789 267520 **Fax:** 44 1789 268371
Email: jennifer@jtsma.org.uk
Website: http://www.jtsma.org.uk

Fnded: 1985. **Mem:** 1,500. **Lang(s):** English. **Desc:** Offers support information and advice to all those whose lives have been affected by spinal muscular atrophy (SMA). **Pub:** *Holding Hands*, quarterly. Newsletter.

★ 4263 ★ Jewish Alcoholics, Chemically Dependent Persons and Significant Others (JACS)

850 Seventh Ave.
New York, NY 10019
Phone: (212)397-4197 **Fax:** (212)399-3525
Email: jacs@jacsweb.org
Website: http://www.jacsweb.org
Arnie Goldfein, Pres.

Fnded: 1980. **Mem:** 1,000. **State Groups:** 28. **Desc:** Jewish alcoholics and addicts, family members, and concerned friends. Acts as an additional resource to promote and enhance recovery from chemical dependency. Provides research and information on chemical addiction in the Jewish community. Maintains speakers' bureau. **Pub:** *JACS Journal*, annual. Journal. • *JACS Newsletter*, monthly. Newsletter. *Price:* Free.

★ 4264 ★ Jewish Association for Services for the Aged (JASA)

132 W 31st St., 15th Fl.
New York, NY 10001
Phone: (212)273-5272 **Fax:** (212)695-4206
David J. Stern, Exec. VP

Fnded: 1968. **Local Groups:** 61. **Desc:** Social welfare organization whose objective is to provide the services necessary to enable the older adult to remain in the community. Maintains 18 community service offices and 24 local senior citizens centers in New York City and Nassau and Suffolk Counties, NY. Services include: case management; information and referral to appropriate health, welfare, educational, social, recreational, and vacation services, and on government benefits and entitlements; personal counseling; financial assistance; health and medical service counsel; counsel on housing and long-term care; homemaker service; group educational and recreational activities through senior citizens centers; information and guidance for social action on legislative issues affecting the elderly; hot lunch programs; referral to summer camps; legal services; protective services; reaching out to the isolated; programs for independent senior clubs; volunteer service opportunities. Conducts programs for elderly Soviet Jewish immigrants. Operates home attendant agencies in Brooklyn and Queens, NY. Trains students from the New York University School of Social Work, Hunter College School of Social Work, Yeshiva University School of Social Work, and Adelphi University School of Social Work. **Pub:** *JPAC Action Memo/Senior Citizens Advocate*, 10/year. Addresses the issues of interest to senior citizens, especially those with low income. *Price:* Free.

★ 4265 ★ Jewish Guild for the Blind (JGB)

15 W 65th St.
New York, NY 10023
Phone: (212)769-6200 **Free:** 800-284-4422
Fax: (212)769-6266
Email: info@jgb.org
Website: http://www.jgb.org
Alan R. Morse, Pres. & CEO

Fnded: 1914. **Desc:** Medical and vision services for blind, visually handicapped, and multihandicapped people of all ages, races, and creeds. Provides social work, counseling, and AIDS case management; job development, placement, and training; support group services; rehabilitation, including vocational, high school equivalency training, orientation and mobility, activities of daily living, and computer training; adapted physical education; communication skills; adult day healthcare program, GuildCare, in New York City, Yonkers, Bronx, Buffalo, Niagara Falls, and Albany, New York. Operates Early Intervention Program for infants and preschoolers (up to age 5); school for multihandicapped children; state licensed psychiatric clinic for emotionally disturbed blind persons and their families; day treatment programs for multihandicapped blind adults; Low Vision Services; Comprehensive Outpatient Rehabilitation Facility (C.O.R.F.). J.G.B. Facilities Corporation, the residential health care affiliate, operates the Home for Aged Blind (a nursing home), the Newman Center for Alzheimer's Care, and Center for AIDS Care, a specialized facility for visually impaired persons with AIDS, in Yonkers, NY. Cosponsors health fairs/vision screenings for the community; operates GuildNet, a longterm managed healthcare program; a designated project library site, and SightCare, an education program for caregivers, and a center for diabetes care. **Pub:** *The Guild*, quarterly. Newsletter. Contains guild programs and events involving professional and volunteer supporters of Guild services. *Price:* Free. **Frmly:** (1960) New York Guild for the Jewish Blind.

★ 4266 ★ Jin Shin Do Foundation for Bodymind Acupressure (JSDF)

PO Box 416
Idyllwild, CA 92549
Phone: (909)659-5707 **Fax:** (909)659-5707
Email: teegers@earthlink.net
Website: http://www.jinshindo.org
Iona M. Teeguarden, Exec. Dir.

Fnded: 1982. **Mem:** 2,000. **Desc:** A referral and educational organization of teachers and practitioners of the Jin Shin Do acupressure method. (Jin Shin Do acupressure integrates a traditional Japanese acupressure technique with classical Chinese acutheory, Taoist philosophy and Qigong breathing exercises, and Western psychology.) Outlines tension points associated with common physical problems and distressing feelings, and teaches points and exercises that help release physical and emotional tensions. Conducts continuing education classes, practicums, and workshops for students. **Pub:** *A Complete Guide to Acupressure*. Book. • *Acupressure News*, annual. Newsletter. General association information; claps catalog; product catalog. *Price:* $2.50. • *The Acupressure Way of Health: Jin Shin Do*. Book. • *Directory of Registered Practitioners and Authorized Teachers*, annual. Directory. Includes listing of authorized basic, intermediate, and advanced teachers. *Price:* $1. • *Fundamentals of Self-Acupressure*. Booklet. • *Joy of Feeling: Bodymind Acupressure*. Book. • *JSD Strange Flows Wall Chart*.

★ 4267 ★ Job Accommodation Network (JAN)

WVU PO Box 6080
Morgantown, WV 26506-6080
Phone: (304)293-7186 **Free:** 800-526-7234
Fax: (304)293-5407
Email: jan@jan.icdi.wvu.edu
Website: http://www.jan.wvu.edu
D.J. Hendricks, Proj. Mgr.

Fnded: 1984. **Desc:** A service of U.S. Department of Labor's Office of Disability Employment Policy. An international toll-free consulting service that provides information about job accommodation and the employability of people with disabilities. Calls are answered by consultants who understand the limitations associated with disabilities and who have instant access to the most comprehensive and up-to-date information about accommodation methods, devices, and strategies.

★ 4268 ★ John A. Hartford Foundation

55 E 59th St., 16th Fl.
New York, NY 10022-1178
Phone: (212)832-7788 **Fax:** (212)593-4913
Email: mail@jhartford.org
Website: http://www.jhartfound.org
Corinne H. Rieder, Exec. Dir.

Fnded: 1929. **Desc:** Works to promote health care, training, research, and service related to older adults.

★ 4269 ★ John Milton Society for the Blind in Canada

40 St. Clair Ave. E, Ste. 202
Toronto, ON, Canada M4T 1M9
Phone: (416)960-3953 **Fax:** (416)960-3570
Email: admin@jmsblind.ca
Website: http://www.jmsblind.ca

Fnded: 1970. **Lang(s):** English. **Desc:** National ecumenical Organization. Provides Christian materials to blind, deafblind, and visually impaired Canadians. **Pub:** *In Touch*, quarterly. Newsletter. Braille newspaper. • *Insight*, bimonthly. Newsletter. • *Insound*, bimonthly. Audiotape.

★ 4270 ★ John Tracy Clinic (JTC)

806 W Adams Blvd.
Los Angeles, CA 90007
Phone: (213)748-5481 **Free:** 800-522-4582
Email: ewilson@johntracyclinic.org
Website: http://www.johntracyclinic.org
Eska Wilson, VP Finance & Admin.

Fnded: 1942. **Desc:** Offers parent-centered services to pre-school children with hearing loss, as well as advanced courses and an accredited Master's Degree (with USC) in Early Childhood Deaf Education. **Pub:** *The John Tracy Clinic Bulletin*, semiannual. Newsletter. Contains news of services, campaigns, and events. *Price:* Free.

★ 4271 ★ Join Together (JTO)

1 Appleton St.
Boston, MA 02116
Phone: (617)437-1500 **Fax:** (617)437-9394
Email: info@jointogether.org
Website: http://www.jointogether.org/about/

Fnded: 1991. **Desc:** Committed to reduce, prevent, and treat substance abuse. Offers reports, newsletters, and community action toolkits. Sponsors the National Leadership Fellows program.

★ 4272 ★ Joint Commission on Accreditation of Healthcare Organizations (JCAHO)

1 Renaissance Blvd.
Oakbrook Terrace, IL 60181
Phone: (630)792-5000 **Fax:** (630)792-5005
Email: doleary@jcaho.org
Website: http://www.jcaho.org
Dennis S. O'Leary, MD, Pres.

Fnded: 1951. **Desc:** Strives to improve the safety and quality of care provided to the public through the provision of health care accreditation and related services that support performance improvement in health care organizations. Evaluates and accredits nearly 20,000 health care organizations and programs in the United States, including hospitals, networks, home care, long term care, assisted living, behavioral health care, laboratory and ambulatory care services. **Pub:** *Accreditation Manuals for all Programs.* Manuals. • *Ambulatory Care Advisor.* Newsletter. Covers ambulatory care accreditation program, survey processes, standards and programs for ambulatory care. *Price:* Free. • *BHC Accreditation News,* 3/year. Newsletter. Covers the behavioral health care accreditation program. Includes information about survey processes for behavioral health care and substance abuse. *Price:* Free. • *Long Term Care Update,* 3/year. Newsletter. • *Sentinel Event Alert,* bimonthly. Newsletter. • *This Month,* monthly. Newsletter. • Also publishes educational materials, software, and videos. **Frmly:** (1987) Joint Commission on Accreditation of Hospitals.

★ 4273 ★ Joint Commission on Allied Health Personnel in Ophthalmology (JCAHPO)

2025 Woodlane Dr.
Saint Paul, MN 55125-2995
Phone: (651)731-2944 **Free:** 800-284-3937
Fax: (651)731-0410
Email: jcahpo@jcahpo.org
Website: http://www.jcahpo.org
Lynn D. Anderson, Exec. Dir.

Fnded: 1969. **Desc:** A certifying agency for allied health personnel. Objectives are: to encourage the establishment of medically oriented programs for training allied health personnel in ophthalmology; to develop standards of education and training in the field; to examine, certify, and recertify ophthalmic medical personnel, and encourage their continued occupational development. Conducts national certifying examinations. **Pub:** *Career of Ophthalmic Medical Assisting.* • *Certification - Why & How.* • *Criteria for Certification & Recertification - Ophthalmic Assistant, Ophthalmic Technician, Ophthalmic Medical Technologist.* • *Educational Programs for Ophthalmic Medical Personnel.* • *The President's Report,* annual. Annual Report. *Price:* Free. • *Viewpoints,* quarterly. Newspaper. *Price:* Free to certified ophthalmic medical personnel; $20/year.

★ 4274 ★ Joint Commission on Sports Medicine and Science (JCSMS)

401 W Michigan St.
Indianapolis, IN 46202-3233
Phone: (317)637-9200 **Fax:** (317)634-7817
Email: jwhitehead@acsm.org
James R. Whitehead, MD, Exec. Advisor

Fnded: 1966. **Desc:** Provides a forum and acts as a catalyst for the promotion of increased communication among the various organizations interested in the health and safety of sports participants and to help them convey to the public necessary information on that subject. Seeks to stimulate various organizations for continuous research on pertinent questions and problems in the field of sports injury prevention and care and for the acquisition of valid statistics on the incidence and epidemiology of injuries in sports activities. Also plays a role in helping corporations contact those sports organizations so that they can be of mutual benefit to each other. **Frmly:** (1988) Joint Commission on Competitive Safeguards and the Medical Aspects of Sports.

★ 4275 ★ Joint Council of Allergy, Asthma and Immunology (JCAAI)

50 N Brockway, Ste. 3-3
Palatine, IL 60067
Phone: (847)934-1918 **Fax:** (847)934-1820
Email: info@jcaai.org
Website: http://www.jcaai.org
J. Spencer Atwater, MD, Pres.

Fnded: 1975. **Mem:** 2,350. **Desc:** Physicians specializing in allergy or clinical immunology. Members must belong to the American Academy of Allergy and Immunology or the American College of Allergy and Immunology. Serves as political and socioeconomic arm for these sponsoring organizations. **Pub:** *JCAAI Reports,* periodic. Newsletter. **Frmly:** (1977) Joint Council of Socio Economics of Allergy.

★ 4276 ★ Joint Council for the Physically and Mentally Disabled - Hong Kong

Duke of Windsor Social Service Bldg., 12/F
15 Hennessy Rd.
Hong Kong, People's Republic of China
Phone: 852 28642931 **Fax:** 852 28642962
Email: rh@hkcss.org.hk
Website: http://www.hkcss.org.hk

Fnded: 1964. **Mem:** 130. **Lang(s):** Chinese, English. **Desc:** Organizations representing people with disabilities; interested individuals. Seeks to improve the quality of life of people with disabilities. Provides consulting to government agencies formulating legislation affecting people with disabilities; coordinates activities of members organizations and agencies. Conducts research and educational programs; participates in charitable activities; sponsors competitions. **Pub:** *Hong Kong Access Guide for Disabled Visitors,* periodic. Directory. • Brochure. • Reports.

★ 4277 ★ Jordanian Association for Family Planning and Protection (JAFPP)

Al Madina Area-Zomokhshary Str.
PO Box 8066
Amman, Jordan
Phone: 962 6 5160999 **Fax:** 962 6 5161020
Email: jafpp@nol.com.jo

Fnded: 1964. **Mem:** 200. **Local Groups:** 3. **Lang(s):** Arabic, English. **Desc:** Social workers and health care professionals in Jordan. Advocates responsible parenthood and family planning in Jordan. Operates family planning clinics and mobile units for rural areas. Offers advice to paretns on issues such as child spacing, marital problems, and child rearing; encourages couples to plan children according to financial means. Provides medical assistance to couples with infertility problems and helps them to overcome the social stigma attached to infertility through counseling services. Conducts annual family planning week. Organizes family planning courses for social workers and volunteers, lectures, workshops, siminar for targeting youth and women on the fields of reproductive health, commmunication skills, sexual health, population issues. Advocacy targeting decision makers. **Pub:** *Selected Lectures in Family Planning.* • Brochures, periodic.

★ 4278 ★ Josiah Macy, Jr. Foundation

44 E 64th St.
New York, NY 10021
Free: 800-521-0600
Website: http://www.josiahmacyfoundation.org
June E. Osborn, MD, Pres.

Desc: Strives to promote public health awareness. **Pub:** *Chairman's Summary of the Conference, Education for More Synergistic Practice of Medicine and Public Health.* Proceedings. Contains information on conference.

★ 4279 ★ Joslin Diabetes Center (JDC)

One Joslin Pl.
Boston, MA 02215
Phone: (617)732-2400 **Free:** 800-JOSLIN-1
Fax: (617)732-2562
Email: stephen.mally@joslin.harvard.edu
Website: http://www.joslin.org
Stephen M. Mally, Pres.

Fnded: 1898. **Desc:** An internationally recognized diabetes treatment, research and education institution affiliated with Harvard Medical School. Clinical programs include the Diabetes Outpatient Intensive Treatment (DO IT) Program, a three and a half day program designed to instruct and empower people with diabetes to better manage the disease. Other clinical services include internal medicine/endocrinology, ophthalmology, nephrology, pediatric endocrinology, pregnancy, mental health, nutrition and exercise physiology. The center also has affiliated treatment facilities in the Boston area and at prestigious hospitals from Florida to Washington state. Offers a disease management program as well as educational programs for health professionals, patients and corporations. **Pub:** *Joslin Magazine,* quarterly. Magazine. Provides information on diet, education, and research; also covers the activities of the center. *Price:* Included in membership dues. • Report, annual. • Newsletter. • Books. • Videos. **Frmly:** (1981) Joslin Diabetes Foundation.

★ 4280 ★ Joubert Syndrome Foundation

6931 S Carlinda Ave.
Columbia, MD 21046
Phone: (410)997-8084 **Fax:** (410)992-9184
Email: joubert@joubertsyndrome.org
Website: http://www.joubertsyndrome.org
Cheryl Duquette, Co-Founder & Family Resource Coordinator

Fnded: 1992. **Mem:** 375. **Nat'l Groups:** 1. **Reg. Groups:** 7. **Desc:** Support and information exchange group for families of people afflicted with Joubert's Syndrome, a genetically transmitted syndrome in which the cerebellar vermis, a section of the brain controlling balance and coordination, is partially or completely missing. Brain stem abnormality causes problems with breathing and eye movements. Physical manifestations of JS include disturbances in breathing patterns, ataxia (unsteadiness), abnormal eye movements, hypotonia, and possible mental retardation. Promotes continuing education for medical professionals. **Pub:** *Rainbow,* quarterly. Newsletter. • *Registry of Families.* **Frmly:** (1999) Joubert Syndrome Parents in Touch Network.

★ 4281 ★ Judaica Captioned Film Center (JCFC)

PO Box 21439
Baltimore, MD 21208-0439
Phone: (410)655-6767
Lois Lilienfeld-Weiner, Pres.

Fnded: 1983. **Desc:** Deaf, hearing impaired individuals, students of English as a second language and other users of captioned films. Locates, produces, and distributes captioned versions of films on Jewish subjects such as the Bible, archaeology, the Holocaust, and Israel. **Pub:** Newsletter, 1-4/year. *Price:* Free.

★ 4282 ★ Just One Break (JOB)

120 Wall St.
New York, NY 10005
Phone: (212)785-7300 **Fax:** (212)785-4513
Email: justonebreak@interactive.net
Website: http://www.justonebreak.com/
Kathryn Croft, Exec. Dir.

Fnded: 1947. **Desc:** Employment service for people with disabilities. Works to place job-ready people with disabilities into competitive employment. Concentrates efforts in New York, New Jersey, and Connecticut, but advises companies nationwide. Offers placement services, employment counseling, skills evaluation, college recruitment, a summer intern program, and an annual jobs fair. Conducts on-site Americans with Disabilities Act accessibility studies and advisory assistance for human resources managers to help them ease the transition of people with disabilities into their workforce. **Pub:** *Informational Brochure.* Brochure. • Annual Report, annual.

★ 4283 ★ Juvenile Diabetes Foundation in Israel (JDFI)

(Haagudah LeSukereth Neurim Beyisrael)
10 Blvd. Rothschild
IL-66881 Tel Aviv, Israel

Phone: 972 3 5160171 **Fax:** 972 3 5100724
Email: jdf_il@netvision.net.il

Fnded: 1981. **Mem:** 2,000. **Lang(s):** English, Hebrew. **Desc:** Strives to improve the situation of children and young adults with Juvenile diabetes in Israel. Conducts fundraising activities and research programs. **Pub:** *Ad-Kan*, semiannual. • *Update*, semiannual. • Newsletter, quarterly.

★ 4284 ★ Juvenile Diabetes Research Foundation

80-84 Chandos St., Level 4
Saint Leonards, NSW 2065, Australia
Phone: 61 2 996600400 **Fax:** 61 2 996600172
Email: info@jdrf.org.au
Website: http://www.jdrf.org.au

Fnded: 1982. **Mem:** 2,000. **Desc:** Committed to finding a cure for Type I diabetes and its complications, raise funds for research and educational programs. **Pub:** *Update*, quarterly. Magazine. **Frmly:** (2002) Juvenile Diabetes Foundation of Australia.

★ 4285 ★ Juvenile Diabetes Research Foundation - Hellas

PO Box 17177
GR-10024 Athens, Greece
Phone: 30 1 7796660 **Fax:** 30 1 3627777

Fnded: 1983. **Mem:** 1,300. **Desc:** Offers financial support (grants) to diabetes research scholarships to young investigators.

★ 4286 ★ Juvenile Diabetes Research Foundation International (JDFI)

120 Wall St.
New York, NY 10005-4001
Phone: (212)785-9500 **Free:** 800-533-CURE
Fax: (212)785-9595
Email: info@jdf.org
Website: http://www.jdrf.org
Peter Van Etten, Pres. /CEO

Fnded: 1970. **Mem:** 40,000. **Reg. Groups:** 114. **Desc:** World's leading nonprofit, nongovernmental funder of diabetes research. Mission is to find a cure for diabetes and its complications through the support of research. Sponsors international workshops and conferences for biomedical researchers. Individual chapters offer support groups and other activities for families affected by diabetes. **Pub:** *Countdown*, quarterly. Magazine. Covers diabetes treatment and research. *Price:* $25/year. • Also publishes pamphlets and brochures for diabetics, families, medical personnel, and teachers; produces videotapes. **Frmly:** (1983) Juvenile Diabetes Foundation.

★ 4287 ★ Juvenile Scleroderma Network (JSDN)

1204 W 13th St.
San Pedro, CA 90731
Phone: (310)519-9511 **Free:** 800-369-8309
Fax: (310)519-9511
Email: outreachjsdn@aol.com
Website: http://www.jsdn.org
Kathy Gaither, Contact

Desc: Children afflicted with scleroderma, parents and families, doctors. Provide online support, pen-pal programs, information, facts and literature.

★ 4288 ★ Kaiser Family Foundation

2400 Sand Hill Rd.
Menlo Park, CA 94025
Phone: (650)854-9400 **Fax:** (650)854-4800
Website: http://www.kff.org
Drew Altman, Pres.

Desc: Works to research and promote health care issues. Focuses on health policy, media and public education, and health and development in South Africa.

★ 4289 ★ Karen Horney Clinic (KHC)

329 E 62nd St.
New York, NY 10021
Phone: (212)838-4333 **Fax:** (212)838-7158
Email: karenhorneyclnic@aol.com
Website: http://www.karenhorneycenter.org
Dr. Giselle Galdi, Dir.

Fnded: 1955. **Desc:** Promotes psychoanalytic and psychotherapeutic treatment of individuals and groups focusing on the special problems of children, adolescents, victims of violent crimes, adult survivors of childhood sexual abuse, and persons with psychoneurotic and emotional problems. Named for Karen Horney (1885-1952), German/American psychoanalyst and author of several books on neurosis, psychoanalysis, and related topics. Conducts children's services. **Pub:** *American Journal of Psychoanalysis*, quarterly. Journal. • *Association for the Advancement of Psychoanalysis*, periodic. **Frmly:** (1979) Karen Horney Psychoanalytic Clinic.

★ 4290 ★ KDWB Variety Family Center

University of Minnesota Gateway
200 Oak St. SE, Ste. 160
Minneapolis, MN 55455-2002
Phone: (612)626-3087 **Free:** 800-276-8642
Fax: (612)624-0997
Email: kdwb-var@unm.edu
Website: http://www.allaboutkids.umn.edu/kdwbvfc/index.htm
Elizabeth Latts, Resource Coordinator

Desc: Provides family-centered services that promote physical, emotional, psychological and social health and well-being for children and youth at risk, including children and youth with disabilities. **Pub:** *Health Issues*, periodic. Newsletter. • Report, periodic. • Monograph, periodic.

★ 4291 ★ Kenya Dental Association (KDA)

00200 City Sq.
PO Box 20059
Nairobi, Kenya
Email: kda_nairobi@hotmail.com

Mem: 180. **Nat'l Groups:** 1. **Lang(s):** English. **Desc:** Dental surgeons in Kenya. Represents members' interests. Conducts educational programs in conjunction with the University of Kenya, works closely with International Association of Dental research; conducts charity work in Kenya. **Pub:** *Newsletter*, quarterly. Newsletter.

★ 4292 ★ Kenya Diabetes Association

PO Box 55098
Nairobi, Kenya
Phone: 254 20 336725 **Fax:** 254 20 340740
Website: http://www.diabetesafrica.com/idfmembers.html

Desc: Represents people with diabetes. Promotes research and support of those with diabetes in Kenya.

★ 4293 ★ Kenya Medical Association

PO Box 48502
Nairobi, Kenya
Phone: 254 20 714991 **Fax:** 254 20 717170
Email: kmanec@wananchi.com

Fnded: 1923. **Mem:** 1,200. **Desc:** Promotes health and well-being in Kenya.

★ 4294 ★ Kerato-Refractive Society (KRS)

PO Box 601149
Dallas, TX 75360-1149
Phone: (972)601-5750 **Fax:** (972)713-9722
Ronald A. Schachar, MD, Exec. Sec.

Fnded: 1979. **Mem:** 2,000. **Desc:** Ophthalmologists and scientists interested in the latest advances in keratorefractive and laser techniques. (Keratorefraction is a surgical procedure in which the shape of the cornea and iris is changed in order to correct nearsightedness and astigmatism. The procedure is now performed with a diamond knife; use of lasers is still in the investigational stage.) Purpose is to keep professionals and others informed of the most recent advances and developments in ophthalmologic care. Conducts research and raises funds. Sponsors training programs. **Pub:** *Keratorefraction*. Book. • *Radical Keratotomy*. Book. • *Refractive Keratoplasty*. Book. • *Refractive Modulation of the Cornea*. Book. • Newsletter, biennial.

★ 4295 ★ Keren-Or, Inc. (K-OI)

350 7th Ave., Rm. 200
New York, NY 10001
Phone: (212)279-4070 **Fax:** (212)279-4043
Email: kerenorinc@aol.com
Website: http://www.keren-or.org/
Albert Hornblass, MD, Pres.

Fnded: 1956. **Desc:** Maintains the Keren-Or Center for Multi-Handicapped Blind Children in Jerusalem which houses, rehabilitates, and trains over 70 severely disabled blind children and young adults. Funds acquired through public contributions and Israeli government funding. **Pub:** *InSights*, semiannual. Newsletter. **Frmly:** (1987) Jerusalem Institutions for the Blind.

★ 4296 ★ Kidney Cancer Association (KCA)

1234 Sherman Ave., Ste. 203
Evanston, IL 60202-1375
Phone: (847)332-1051 **Free:** 800-850-9132
Fax: (847)332-2978
Email: office@kidneycancerassociation.org
Website: http://www.kidneycancerassociation.org
Carl F. Dixon, Pres. /Exec. Dir.

Fnded: 1990. **Desc:** Provides a broad range of services related to kidney cancer, including patient meetings, annual convention for patients and doctors, sponsors research and advocates for changes.

★ 4297 ★ Kiribati Family Health Association

c/o Mrs. Katikova Amon
PO Box 345
Bikenibeh
Tarawa, Kiribati
Phone: 686 28749 **Fax:** 686 28728
Email: kfha@tski.net.ki

Fnded: 1992. **Mem:** 56. **Desc:** Promotes family planning and general health care. Offers health education programs for new mothers; provides PAP smears, breast exam, pregnancy testing, emergency contraception, STI/AIDS prevention, STI treatment.

★ 4298 ★ Klinefelter Syndrome and Associates (KSA)

PO Box 119
Roseville, CA 95678-0119
Phone: (916)773-2999 **Free:** 888-999-9428
Email: ksinfo@genetic.org
Website: http://genetic.org/ks/
Melissa Aylstock, Exec. Off.

Fnded: 1989. **Mem:** 2,000. **Reg. Groups:** 3. **Desc:** Individuals affected by Klinefelter Syndrome and their families. (Klinefelter syndrome is a genetic alteration, occurring only in males, identified by the presence of an extra "X" chromosome on the chromosome chain that determines gender.) Provides support services; facilitates networking and exchange of information. Conducts educational programs. **Pub:** *The Even Exchange*, periodic. Newsletter. • Brochure.Contains information Klinefelter Syndrome. **AKA:** KS and Associates.

★ 4299 ★ Klingenstein Third Generation Foundation

787 Seventh Ave., 6th Fl.
New York, NY 10019-6016
Phone: (212)492-6179 **Fax:** (212)492-7007
Email: sally@ktgf.org
Website: http://www.ktgf.org/
Sally Klingenstein, Exec. Dir.

Fnded: 1983. **Mem:** 7. **Desc:** Strives to improve the lives of families afflicted by clinical depressions; addresses childhood and adolescent depression as well as Attention Deficit/Hyperactivity Disorder.

★ 4300 ★ Klippel-Trenaunay Support Group (KTSG)
5404 Dundee Rd.
Edina, MN 55436
Phone: (952)925-2596 **Fax:** (612)925-4708
Email: contactkt@hotmail.com
Website: http://www.k-t.org/
Judy Vessey, Dir.

Fnded: 1986. **Mem:** 600. **Desc:** Support group for individuals affected by Klippel-Trenaunay Syndrome and their families. (Klippel-Trenaunay Syndrome is a congenital malformation of the extremities and is characterized by birth marks the color of port wine, excessive growth of the soft tissue and bone, and varicose veins. The cause is presently unknown but believed to be either genetic or the result of an intrauterine insult occuring between the third and sixth week of gestation.) Acts as a clearinghouse of information and correspondence between members. **Pub:** *K-T Newsletter*, quarterly. **AKA:** K-T Support Group.

★ 4301 ★ Korea Polio Foundation (KPF) (Chung Nip Hwe Gwan — CNHG)
c/o ChungNip Center
16-3 Gueui-Dong
KwangJin-Ku
Seoul 143-200, Republic of Korea
Phone: 82 2 4661237 **Fax:** 82 2 4542144

Fnded: 1965. **Mem:** 13,000. **Lang(s):** English, Japanese, Korean. **Desc:** Handicapped individuals and others in the Republic of Korea. Fosters the physical and mental development of the disabled. Strives to: increase awareness of the needs of the handicapped; promote and protect the rights of the disabled. Offers educational, vocational, and medical counseling and assistance. Cooperates with firms in sponsoring employment programs for the handicapped. Organizes collective living for the disabled; maintains specialized developmental camps. Operates the Institute of Sports Science for the Disabled. Sponsors athletic competitions; participates in the Paralympics (an athletic competition modeled after the Olympic Games and adapted to the handicapped). **Pub:** *Chung Nip Hwe Gwan Bulletin*, periodic. Bulletin. • *Chung Nip Newsletter*, periodic. Also publishes research reports, dissertations, and surveys.

★ 4302 ★ Korean Academy of Psychotherapists (KAP)
c/o Dr. Rhee Dongshick
178-23 Song-buk dong
Song-buk-ku
Seoul 136-020, Republic of Korea
Fax: 82 2 7659776
Email: kap8432@chollian.net
Website: http://www.daopsychotherapy.org

Fnded: 1974. **Mem:** 150. **Local Groups:** 1. **Lang(s):** English, Korean. **Desc:** Psychiatrists and psychologists united to study and integrate the principles of psychoanalysis and psychotherapy with those of Eastern Tao. (Eastern Tao is based on Taoist, Confucian, and Buddhist philosophies.) Operates training program. Conducts research; maintains speakers' bureau; compiles statistics. **Pub:** *Eastern Tao and Western Psychotherapy*. • *KAP Membership Directory*, annual. Directory. • *KAP Newsletter*, bimonthly. Newsletter. • *The Korean Journal of Psychotherapy*, semiannual. Journal. Korean, includes abstract in English. • *Psychotherapy Protocol*, monthly. Plans to publish case books.

★ 4303 ★ Korean Medical Association (KMA)
CPOB 2062
Seoul, Republic of Korea
Phone: 82 2 7942414 **Fax:** 82 2 7921296

★ 4304 ★ Korean Psychological Association
702-13 Yeoksam-Dong Kangnam-Ku
Seoul 135-080, Republic of Korea
Phone: 82 2 5670102 **Fax:** 82 2 5670103
Email: tyyoo@daisy.kwangwoon.ac.kr

★ 4305 ★ Korean Society of Anesthesiologists (KSA)
302-75, Korean Medical Association Bldg., Rm. 702
Ichon-Dong
Yoongsan-ku
Seoul 140-031, Republic of Korea
Phone: 82 2 7595129 **Fax:** 82 2 7924089
Email: anesthesia@kams.or.kr
Website: http://www.anesthesia.or.kr/english/eindex.htm

Fnded: 1956. **Mem:** 2,000. **Desc:** Represents and supports anesthesiologists in Korea.

★ 4306 ★ Korean Society for the Cerebral Palsied (KSCP)
771 Sanggye, 6-dong
Nowon-ku
Seoul 139-831, Republic of Korea
Phone: 82 2 9324292 **Fax:** 82 2 9324413
Email: webmaster@kscp.net
Website: http://www.kscp.net

Fnded: 1978. **Mem:** 23,000. **Local Groups:** 2. **Lang(s):** English, Korean. **Desc:** People who have a professional interest in rehabilitation for the people with cerebral palsy and their families. Promotes high quality care for people with cerebral palsy. Acts as a national coordinating body, provides guidance and seeking to achieve the optimal use of resources, acts as a vehicle for the exchange of information. Aims to provide rehabilitation services for people with cerebral palsy. **Pub:** *Newsletter of KSCP*, monthly. Newsletter.

★ 4307 ★ Korean Society for Clinical Neurophysiology
c/o Kwang-Woo Lee
Department of Neurology
College of Medicine
Seoul National University
28 Yongon-Dong, Chongno-Gu
Seoul 110-744, Republic of Korea
Phone: 82 2 7603215 **Fax:** 82 2 7441785

Fnded: 1996. **Reg. Groups:** 14. **Desc:** Fosters research and conducts patho-physiological experiments.

★ 4308 ★ Korean Society for Laboratory Medicine (SKLM)
KMA Bldg., Rm. 601
Ichon-ildong
Yongsan-Ku
Seoul, Republic of Korea
Phone: 82 2 7959914 **Fax:** 82 2 7904760

Fnded: 1946. **Mem:** 676. **Desc:** Promotes the field of Laboratory Medicine in Korea. **Pub:** Journal.

★ 4309 ★ Korean Society of Obstetricians and Gynecologists
14th Fl. Yuwon Bldg.
75-95 Seosomun-dong
Jung-gu
Seoul 100-814, Republic of Korea
Phone: 82 2 7793834 **Fax:** 82 2 7793837
Email: kaog@unitel.co.kr

Fnded: 1947. **Desc:** Represents all physicians of Korean in the field of obstetrics and gynecology.

★ 4310 ★ Korean Society of Pharmacology (KSP)
1st Fl., Eui-Hak Bldg.
448-13 Seokyo-dong, Mapo-gu
Seoul 121-841, Republic of Korea
Phone: 82 2 3260370 **Fax:** 82 2 3260371
Email: head@kosphar.org
Website: http://www.kosphar.or.kr

Fnded: 1947. **Mem:** 465. **Lang(s):** Korean. Does not correspond in English. **Desc:** Pharmacologists; interested others. Encourages growth in the industry through information exchange. Promotes advancement in the field through research and educational programs. Represents members' interests. **Pub:** *Korean Journal of Pharmacology*, 3/year. Journal. • *Pharmacology Experiments for Students*, periodic.

★ 4311 ★ Korean Society of Plastic and Reconstructive Surgery (KSPRS) (Dae Han Sung Hyung Owe Gua)
c/o Korean Medical Association Bldg. 601
302-75 Ichon-Dong Yongsan-ku
Seoul 140-30, Republic of Korea
Phone: 82 2 7901443 **Fax:** 82 2 7901442
Email: kprs@chollan.net
Website: http://www.plasticsurgery.or.kr

Fnded: 1966. **Mem:** 600. **Local Groups:** 5. **Lang(s):** Korean. **Desc:** Aims to: increase scientific knowledge in the field of plastic and reconstructive surgery; promote friendship and communication between surgeons. Conducts continuing medical education, resident teaching program, courses, and symposia. Sponsors research. **Pub:** *Journal of the Korean Society of Plastic and Reconstructive Surgery*, periodic. Journal. • *List of Members KSPRS*, periodic. • *Newsletter KSPRS*, quarterly.

★ 4312 ★ Korean Society of Sports Medicine
50 Ilwon Dong, Kangnam Ku
Seoul 135-230, Republic of Korea
Phone: 82 2 34103840 **Fax:** 82 2 34100054
Email: w.h.park@smc.sam.sung

★ 4313 ★ Korean Veterinary Medical Association
PO Box 463-050
Seongnam, Republic of Korea
Phone: 82 342 7028686 **Fax:** 82 342 7021020

★ 4314 ★ Kuwait Dental Association
PO Box 44563
Hawalli 32060, Kuwait
Phone: 965 5325094 **Fax:** 965 5316837
Email: asnandenta@yahoo.com

Fnded: 1974. **Mem:** 915. **Desc:** Represents the dental industry in Kuwait, including the specialties of endodontics, pedodontics, orthodontics, and oral and maxillofacial surgery. **Pub:** Articles. • Brochures.

★ 4315 ★ Kuwait Society for the Handicapped (KSH)
PO Box 6832
Hawalli 32043, Kuwait
Phone: 965 2631277 **Fax:** 965 2642630
Email: feedback@kshkw.com
Website: http://www.safat.com/modhi.html

Fnded: 1971. **Mem:** 250. **Local Groups:** 2. **Lang(s):** Arabic, English. **Desc:** Individuals dedicated to the care of the handicapped in Kuwait. Provides physical and psychological care for children who have not been accepted by other institutions; offers financial and moral support to the families of handicapped individuals; works to inform the public on the causes of handicaps. Conducts research. **Pub:** Magazine, quarterly. • Booklet, quinquennial. Also publishes pamphlets and offers posters and greeting cards.

★ 4316 ★ L. E. Support Club (LESC)
8039 Nova Ct.
North Charleston, SC 29420
Phone: (843)764-1769
Email: hbmesic@knology.net
Website: http://www.galaxymall.com/commerce/lupus/
Harriet B. Mesic, Dir. & Editor

Fnded: 1984. **Desc:** Individuals suffering from lupus erythematosus and other autoimmune diseases; friends and families of patients. Offers emotional support and selfhelp education to lupus patients through newsletters and personal correspondence; provides information on nutrition and medication. **Pub:** *Lupus Beacon*, 5/year. Newsletter. *Price:* Included in membership dues.

★ 4317 ★ La Leche League (LLL) (Ligue La Leche — LLL)

12 rue Quintal
Charlemagne, QC, Canada J5Z 1V9
Phone: (514)990-8917 **Fax:** (450)582-3536
Email: information@allaitement.ca
Website: http://www.allaitement.ca

Fnded: 1960. **Mem:** 802. **Lang(s):** French. **Desc:** French-speaking Canadians with an interest in breastfeeding. Promotes breastfeeding as the most healthy method of nourishing infants. Provides support and services to women wishing to breastfeed. Conducts charitable programs. **Pub:** *La Voie Lactee*, quarterly. Newsletter.

★ 4318 ★ Laboratory Animal Management Association (LAMA)

7300 Metro Blvd., Ste. 585
Edina, MN 55439
Phone: (952)250-6201 **Fax:** (952)835-4774
Email: imartinez@rcm.upr.edu
Website: http://www.lama-online.org
Ivette Martinez-Palma, Pres.

Fnded: 1984. **Mem:** 435. **Reg. Groups:** 3. **Desc:** Laboratory animal facility managers. Seeks to evaluate and update basic and advanced management techniques and to educate laboratory animal facility managers. Makes available resource material; coordinates exchange programs for management personnel. Offers consulting on management techniques. **Pub:** *LAMA Lines*, bimonthly. Includes branch news and a listing for employment opportunities. *Price:* Included in membership dues. • *Lama Review*, quarterly. Journal. • Membership Directory, annual. **Frmly:** Laboratory Animal Managers Association.

★ 4319 ★ LAM Foundation

10105 Beacon Hills Dr.
Cincinnati, OH 45241
Phone: (513)777-6899 **Fax:** (513)777-4109
Email: lamfoundtn@Juno.com
Website: http://lam.uc.edu/
Sue Byrnes, Exec. Dir.

Fnded: 1995. **Desc:** Works to find a cure for LAM (lymphangioleimyomatosis), a progressive, fatal lung disease that affects women. Provides information and support; conducts education programs; promotes and funds clinical research; sponsors a tissue bank; supports a national registry of LAM patients.

★ 4320 ★ Lamaze International

2025 M St., NW, Ste. 800
Washington, DC 20036
Phone: (202)367-1128 **Free:** 800-368-4404
Fax: (202)367-2128
Email: lamaze@dc.sba.com
Website: http://www.lamaze-childbirth.com
Linda L. Harmon, Exec. Dir.

Fnded: 1960. **Mem:** 5,000. **Local Groups:** 25. **Desc:** Physicians, nurses, nurse-midwives, certified teachers of psychoprophylatic (Lamaze) method of childbirth, other professionals, parents, and others interested in Lamaze childbirth preparation and family-centered maternity care. Disseminates information about the theory and practical application of psychoprophylaxis in obstetrics; administers teacher training courses and certifies qualified Lamaze teachers; provides educational lectures, public forums, films, and written materials; maintains national and local teacher and physician referral service. Also presents materials to prospective parents concerning the demands of childrearing. National office serves as information clearinghouse. **Pub:** *Genesis*, quarterly. Newsletter. Contains book and film reviews and calendar of events. *Price:* Included in membership dues. • *Journal of Perinatal Education*, quarterly. Journal. *Price:* Free for members; $55 for individual; $155 for institution. **Frmly:** (1998) American Society for Psychoprophylaxis in Obstetrics.

★ 4321 ★ Landmine Survivors Network (LSN)

1420 K St. NW, Ste. 650
Washington, DC 20005-3960
Phone: (202)464-0007 **Fax:** (202)464-0011
Email: lsn@landminesurvivors.org
Website: http://www.landminesurvivors.org

Fnded: 1997. **Desc:** Survivors of landmines.

★ 4322 ★ Late-Onset Tay-Sachs Foundation (LOTSF)

1303 Paper Mill Rd.
Erdenheim, PA 19038
Phone: (215)836-9426 **Free:** 800-672-2022
Website: http://www.lotsf.org/

Desc: Devoted to research and treatment of Late-onset Tay-Sachs disease, including clinical symptoms, molecular basis of the disease, and pattern of inheritance. **Pub:** *Horizon*. Newsletter.

★ 4323 ★ Latin American Association of Environmental Mutagens, Carcinogens and Teratogens (ALAMCTA) (Asociacion Latinoamericana de Mutagenesis, Carcinogenesis y Teratogenesis Ambiental)

Depto de Patologia, Faculdade de Medicina, UNESP, 18
618-000 Botucatu, Brazil
Phone: 55 14 8212116
Email: lribeiro@fmb.unesp.br

Fnded: 1980. **Desc:** Fosters scientific cooperation among Latin American researchers; supports research projects.

★ 4324 ★ Latin American Association for Genetics (Asociacion Latinoamericana de Genetica — ALAG)

University de Chile
Facultad de Medicine
Santiago, Chile

★ 4325 ★ Latin American Association of Medical Physics (Asociacion Latinoamericana de Fisica Medica — ALFIM)

Av San Fernando 22, Tlalpan
14000 Mexico City, Mexico
Fax: 52 55733627
Email: gaen1310@hp9000x0.uam.mx
Fnded: 1984.

★ 4326 ★ Latin American Association for Mycology (Asociacion Latinoamericana de Micologia — ALM)

Apdo 21827
Caracas 1020A, Venezuela
Phone: 58 212 5041040 **Fax:** 58 212 5041382
Email: gsanblas@pasteur.ivic.ve
Fnded: 1990.

★ 4327 ★ Latin American Association of Pharmacology (Asociacion Latinoamericana de Farmacologia — ALF)

c/o Dr. Jesualdo Fuentes Gonzalez
Jefe Departamento de Farmacologia y Toxicologia
Facultad de Medicina
Universidad de Antioquia
Medellin 1150, AA, Colombia
Phone: 57 4 5106020 **Fax:** 57 4 5106021
Email: farmacologia@medicina.udea.edu.co

Mem: 1,070. **Desc:** Promotes pharmacology in Latin American countries.

★ 4328 ★ Latin American Blind Union - Uruguay (LABU) (Union Latinoamericana de Ciegos — ULAC)

c/o Fundacion Braille del Uruguay
Duranzo 1772
Blanes 1132
11200 Montevideo, Uruguay
Phone: 598 2 4095943 **Fax:** 598 2 4000789
Email: fbu@fbraille.co.uy
Website: http://www.fbraille.com.uy

Fnded: 1985. **Mem:** 155. **Lang(s):** Spanish. **Desc:** Organizations of and for the blind in Latin American countries. Works for the prevention of blindness. Promotes the welfare of the blind and seeks to put them in control of their lives through the abolition of laws that discriminate against the visually handicapped. Sponsors educational programs in coordination with the International Agency for the Prevention of Blindness and the International Council for the Education of the Visually Handicapped. **Pub:** *America Latina*, quarterly. Newsletter.

★ 4329 ★ Latin American and Caribbean Women's Health Network

Casilla Postal 50610
Santiago 1, Chile
Phone: 56 2 2237077 **Fax:** 56 2 2231066
Email: redsalud@ctcreuna.cl
Website: http://www.reddesalud.web.cl

Fnded: 1984. **Mem:** 2,000. **Lang(s):** English, Spanish. **Desc:** Members include groups and organizations working directly or indirectly in fields related to women's health. Seeks to establish contacts among women and organizations active in women's health issues at the local, regional, and national levels. Promotes the sharing of information, experiences, and ideas through the development of communication networks. Coordinates common activities. Encourages informational campaigns on such subjects as reproductive rights, medicine, the environment, and other health topics of interest to women. Participates in conferences, seminars, and meetings. **Pub:** *Cuadernos Mujer Salud*, annual. Magazine. • *Revista Mujer Salud*, quarterly. Magazine. • *Women's Health Collection*, annual. Magazine.

★ 4330 ★ Latin American Club of Neuro Ophthalmology (Club Latinoamericano de Neuroftalmologia — CLAN)

Las Hualtatas 5951
Santiago, Chile
Phone: 56 2 3704600 **Fax:** 56 2 3718934
Email: apochile@entelchile.net

Fnded: 1989. **Mem:** 25. **Reg. Groups:** 4. **Desc:** Fosters communication among scientists concerned with neuroophthalmology.

★ 4331 ★ Latin American Confederation of Clinical Biochemistry (Confederacion Latinoamericana de Bioquimica Clinica — COLABIOCLI)

Paseo de la Reforma 2503, Dleg Miguel Hidalgo
11000 Mexico City, Mexico

Fnded: 1968. **Desc:** Promotes research and development in clinical laboratory sciences.

★ 4332 ★ Latin American Council of Ocular Ultra Sound
(Consejo Latinoamericano de Ecografia Ocular — CLEO)
Av PanteonSan Bernardino
Caracas, Venezuela
Phone: 58 212 5764228 **Fax:** 58 212 9798280

★ 4333 ★ Latin American Diabetes Association
(Asociacion Latinoamericana de Diabetes — ALAD)
Av potosi 425
San Luis Potosi, Mexico
Phone: 52 481 330050 **Fax:** 52 481 385260
Website: http://www.pitt.edu/~iml1/diabetes/ALAD.html
Desc: Promotes the study of diabetes. Works for the cure and prevention of diabetes.

★ 4334 ★ Latin American Federation of Sexology and Sexual Education Societies
(Federacion Latinoamericana de Sociedades de Sexologia y Educacion Sexual)
Sala 605-716 Sul
CEP 70 390 Brasilia, Brazil
Phone: 55 61 2452143
Email: secretariageneral@flasses.org
Website: http://www.flasses.org/english/apresentacao.htm

★ 4335 ★ Latin American Federation of Societies of Obesity (FLASO)
(Federacion Latinoamericana de Sociedades de Obesidad)
c/o Dr. Julio Montero, Pres.
JE Uriburu, 1312 Pta Baja A
1114 Buenos Aires, Argentina
Phone: 54 11 4904903 **Fax:** 54 11 49013272
Email: jcmontero@ciudad.com.ar
Website: http://www.iotf.org/oonet/flaso.htm
Fnded: 1990.

★ 4336 ★ Latin American Group of Angiography and Phacoemulsification (GLADAOF)
(Grupo Latino Americano de Angeografia Ocular y Facoemulsificacion)
Ayacucho 307, 1B
1025 Buenos Aires, Argentina
Phone: 54 11 48011486 **Fax:** 54 11 49536801

★ 4337 ★ Latin American Odontological Federation (FOLA)
(Federacion Odontologica Latinoamericana)
Riobamba 373 - 2D
1025 Buenos Aires, Argentina
Phone: 54 11 43722135
Email: fola@infovia.com.ar
Website: http://www.folaoral.org
Fnded: 1917.

★ 4338 ★ Latin American Society for Interventional Cardiology (SOLACI)
(Sociedad Latinoamericana de Cardiologia Intervencionista)
A Alsina 2653, Piso 2H
1090 Buenos Aires, Argentina
Phone: 54 11 49547173 **Fax:** 54 1 49547173
Email: solaci@satlink.com
Fnded: 1995. **Desc:** Seeks to improve and develop the practice of cardiovascular interventions in Latin America.

★ 4339 ★ Latin American Society of Nephrology and Hypertension
(Sociedad Latinoamericana de Nefrologia e Hipertension — SLANH)
Apdo Postal 67252
Caracas 1061-A, Venezuela
Phone: 58 212 6621845 **Fax:** 58 212 6614031
Email: ebellori@telcel.net.ve
Desc: 019030

★ 4340 ★ Latin American Society of Nutrition (SLAN)
(Sociedad Latinoamericana de Nutricion)
B De Irigoyen 240
1071 Buenos Aires, Argentina
Phone: 54 1 43341545 **Fax:** 54 1 43456011
Email: cesni@datamarkets.com.ar
Fnded: 1964.

★ 4341 ★ Latin American Society of Paraplegia (SLAP)
Triunvirato 5237, Dto G
Buenos Aires, Argentina
Fax: 54 1 45429338
Email: monisanchez@connmed.com.ar

★ 4342 ★ Latin American Society for Pediatric Gastroenterology and Nutrition
(Sociedad Latinoamericana de Gastroenterologia Pediatrica y Nutricion — SLAGPN)
Rua Pedro de Toledo 441
04039-031 Sao Paulo, Brazil
Phone: 55 11 5705834 **Fax:** 55 11 5705834
Email: slagpn@mandic.com.br
Fnded: 1974. **Desc:** Supports research of the functions of gastrointestinal tract, liver and nutrition in normal and abnormal conditions in children.

★ 4343 ★ Latin American Society for Pediatric Oncology
Avda Vollmer, San Bernardino
Caracas 1010, Venezuela
Phone: 58 212 5748278 **Fax:** 58 212 5781056
Email: oncoped@cantv.net

★ 4344 ★ Latin American Society for Stereotactic and Functional Neurosurgery (LSSFN)
(Sociedad Latinoamericana de Neurocirugia Funcional y Esterotaxia)
Puente de Piedra no 150-620
14050 Mexico City, Mexico
Phone: 52 57611079 **Fax:** 52 56060393

★ 4345 ★ Latin American Thoracic Association (ALAT)
(Asociacion Latinoamericana del Torax)
Rua Botucatu 740, 3o andar
04023-062 Sao Paulo, Brazil
Phone: 55 11 5756847
Email: josejardim@pneumo.epm.br
Website: http://www.alatorax.com
Fnded: 1996. **Desc:** Supports the development of thoracic medicine in Latin America.

★ 4346 ★ Latin American Thyroid Society (LATS)
Departamento de Fisiologia e Biofisica
ICB-USP
05508-900 Sao Paulo, Brazil
Phone: 55 11 36098845 **Fax:** 55 11 8187285
Email: hansgraf@bsi.com.br
Website: http://www.lats.org
Fnded: 1974. **Mem:** 488. **Lang(s):** English, Portuguese, Spanish.

★ 4347 ★ Latin American Union Against Sexually Transmitted Diseases
(Union Latinoamericana contra las Enfermedades de Transmision Sexual — ULACETS)
Rua Joao Obino 111
90470-150 Porto Alegre, Brazil
Phone: 55 51 3341126 **Fax:** 55 51 3341126
Email: pnaud@netmarket.com.br

★ 4348 ★ Latin American Vocational Rehabilitation Group
(Grupo Latinoamericano de Rehabilitacion Profesional — GLARP)
Carerra 21 No. 84-48
Apartado Aereo 56208
Bogota, Colombia
Phone: 57 1 6082255 **Fax:** 57 1 4811391
Email: glarp@cable.net.co
Fnded: 1977. **Mem:** 110. **Nat'l Groups:** 78. **Lang(s):** English, French, Portuguese, Spanish. **Desc:** Private institutions in 18 countries offering professional rehabilitation services. Promotes vocational rehabilitation and adjunctive professions throughout Latin America; encourages the growth of member groups. Coordinates projects in the interest of members, including courses, seminars, and consulting sessions; offers scholarships. Sponsors research and educational programs.

★ 4349 ★ Latin and Mediterranean Group for Sport Medicine (LMGSM)
(Groupement Latin et Mediterraneen de Medecine du Sport — GLMMS)
137 Chemin de St Etienne
F-06570 Saint Paul, France
Phone: 33 6 80305401 **Fax:** 33 4 93321494
Email: glmms@libertysurf.fr
Website: http://site.ifrance.com/glmms
Fnded: 1956. **Mem:** 2,000. **State Groups:** 27. **Lang(s):** English, French. **Desc:** Physicians in 27 Mediterranean countries interested in the medical study of sports and exercise. Objectives are to further sports medicine and to conduct studies on medical problems related to amateur and professional sports and physical activity in general. Offers continuing education classes to members. Operates speakers' bureau. **Pub:** *Apunto*, periodic. • *Archivos de Medicina del Deporte*, quarterly. • *Cinesiologie*, bimonthly. • *SMM Medecine du Sport*, bimonthly.

★ 4350 ★ Latino Gerontological Center
120 Wall St., 23rd Fl.
New York, NY 10005
Phone: (212)344-9636 **Fax:** (212)480-9734
Email: info@gerolatino.org
Website: http://www.gerolatino.org
Mario E. Tapia, Pres. & CEO
Fnded: 1991. **Mem:** 300. **Desc:** Works to improve the quality of life of Hispanic seniors. Provides Thanksgiving meals to needy families; operates cable television show in Manhattan, NY. Writes question and answer column in New York paper "El Diario" to provide information to hispanic seniors.

★ 4351 ★ Latvian Contraceptology Association (LCA)
c/o Mrs. Aija Tula
Health Rehabilitation Centre "Valeo"
8 Stirnu str., Rm. 447
LV-1080 Riga, Latvia
Phone: 371 7 210154 **Fax:** 371 2 593490
Fnded: 1995. **Reg. Groups:** 3. **Desc:** Devoted to the reduction in the number of abortions and to fight against legal abortion in Latvia. Works to ensure the protection of health for families, children and women; to promote and improve contraception methods to reduce unwanted pregnancies. **Pub:** Brochures. Six brochures on contraception.

★ 4352 ★ Latvian Society of Cardiology
P. Stradins Clinical University Hospital
Latvia Center of Cardiology
13 Pilsonu iela
LV-1002 Riga, Latvia
Phone: 371 7 613915 **Fax:** 371 7 613915
Email: cardio@mailbox.riga.lv
Website: http://www.escardio.org/society/natsoc/latvia.htm

Mem: 280.

★ 4353 ★ Latvian Society of Pharmacology (Latvijas Farmakologijas Biedriba)
Latvian Society of Pharmacology
Sarlotes St. 1A
LV-1001 Riga, Latvia
Phone: 371 9276263 **Fax:** 371 7366306
Email: vijaklus@acad.latnet.lv

Mem: 75. **Desc:** Promotes pharmacology in Latvia.

★ 4354 ★ Latvia's Association for Family Planning and Sexual Health Association
Caka Str. 83/83-22
LV-1011 Riga, Latvia
Phone: 371 7 242700 **Fax:** 371 7 293342
Email: lfpa@mailbox.riga.lv
Website: http://www.papardeszieds.lv

Fnded: 1994. **Mem:** 380. **Lang(s):** English, Latvian. **Desc:** Promotes family planning. Gathers and disseminates family planning information; conducts family planning education courses for health care professionals, educators, and social workers. **Pub:** *Abortion*. Brochure. • *Contraception*. Brochure. • *Happy Relations*. Brochure. • *Papardes Lapa*, semiannual. Newsletter. • *STD*. Brochure.

★ 4355 ★ Latvijas Multiplas Sklerozes Asociacijas
c/o Valerijs Ulmanis
Melidas Str 10
LV-1015 Riga, Latvia
Phone: 371 7351792 **Fax:** 371 7351792
Email: lmsa@lmsa.lv
Website: http://www.lmsa.lv

Fnded: 1995. **Mem:** 1,147. **Nat'l Groups:** 1. **Reg. Groups:** 31. **Lang(s):** English, German, Latvian, Russian. **Desc:** MS patients, families and professionals. Seeks to improve the quality of life for persons with multiple sclerosis and their families. **Pub:** *CERIBA (HOPE)*, quarterly. Newsletter.

★ 4356 ★ Laurence-Moon-Bardet-Biedl Syndrome Network (LMBBSN)
c/o Mary Morris
15205 W Port Royale Ln. Ave.
Surprise, AZ 85379
Phone: (301)863-5658
Email: josiahsmom@hotmail.com
Website: http://www.geocities.com/hotsprings/spa/1761/
Barbara Mielcarek, Contact

Fnded: 1984. **Desc:** Provides a network for individuals with Laurence-Moon-Bardet-Biedl syndrome, a genetic disorder. (Persons with LMBBS suffer from general developmental delay and exhibit symptoms of retinitis pigmentosa, a degenerative eye disease; hypogenitalism; polydactyly; obesity.) **Pub:** *LMBBS Network News*, periodic. Newsletter. Includes list of member families. **AKA:** Laurence-Moon-Biedl Syndrome Network; LMBS Network.

★ 4357 ★ Leader Dogs for the Blind (LDB)
PO Box 5000
Rochester, MI 48308
Phone: (248)651-9011 **Free:** 888-777-5332
Fax: (248)651-5812
Email: leaderdog@leaderdog.org
Website: http://www.leaderdog.org
William C. Hansen, Pres.

Fnded: 1939. **Desc:** Trains dogs to serve as guides for blind persons and conducts a supervised course of training to coordinate blind persons and their Leader Dogs as operating units; there is no charge for the service. Conducts research to determine the most satisfactory breed of dog for Leader Dog purposes. Places puppies into volunteer homes in preparation for formal adult dog training. Facilities include a dormitory, kennel, veterinary hospital, and training center. **Pub:** *Leader Dog Overview and Tour*. Videos. *Price:* Free. • *Leader Dog Update*, quarterly. Newsletter. Available in large print, braille, and tape. *Price:* Free. • *Orientation of Dog Guide Users to New Environments*. • Also produces taped cassettes of all written materials available to the visually impared. **Frmly:** Path-Finder Guide Dogs; (1952) Leader Dog League for the Blind.

★ 4358 ★ Leadership Council of Aging Organizations (LCAO)
c/o National Council of Senior Citizens
8403 Colesville Rd., Ste. 1200
Silver Spring, MD 20910-3314
Phone: (202)479-1200 **Fax:** (301)578-8999
Email: howard.bedlin@ncoa.org
Website: http://www.lcao.org
Howard Bedlin, Contact

Fnded: 1978. **Mem:** 37. **Desc:** Professional groups serving older persons. Objective is to further the public's understanding of the potential and needs of older persons. Responds to public or private initiatives concerning the aging. Acts as coordinating body in reviewing and acting on public policy issues. Compiles statistics on aging. **Pub:** Monographs. • Papers.

★ 4359 ★ Leadership Council for Mental Health, Justice and the Media
191 Presidential Blvd., Ste. C-132
Bala Cynwyd, PA 19004
Phone: (610)664-5007 **Fax:** (610)664-5279
Website: http://www.leadershipcouncil.org

Desc: Scientists, clinicians, educators, legal scholars, journalists and public policy analysts. Promote psychological science and provide current materials and information for mental health issues.

★ 4360 ★ League for the Hard of Hearing
71 W 23rd St.
New York, NY 10010-4162
Phone: (917)305-7700 **Fax:** (917)305-7888
Email: postmaster@lhh.org
Website: http://www.lhh.org/

Fnded: 1910. **Desc:** Dedicated to improve the life for infants, children and adults with all degrees of hearing loss.

★ 4361 ★ Learning Disabilities Association of Canada (LDAC) (Troubles d'Apprentissage - Association Canadienne)
323 Chapel St., Ste. 200
Ottawa, ON, Canada K1N 7Z2
Phone: (613)238-5721 **Fax:** (613)235-5391
Email: information@ldac-taac.ca
Website: http://www.ldac-taac.ca

Fnded: 1963. **Mem:** 10,000. **State Groups:** 12. **Local Groups:** 150. **Lang(s):** English, French. **Desc:** Parents of children with learning disabilities and individuals with learning disabilities; educators and administrators, psychologists, language experts, lawyers, and health care professionals. Works to advance the education, social development, legal rights, and general well-being of individuals with learning disabilities. Encourages early recognition, diagnosis, and treatment of individuals with learning disabilities. Develops educational, social, recreational, and career-oriented programs and promotes legislation, research, and training of personnel in the field. Initiates programs to increase public awareness and understanding of learning disabilities. Acts as an advocate for individuals before government and other agencies; develops parent support services to maximize parental involvement. **Pub:** *National*, quarterly. • Handbooks, periodic. • Papers, periodic. **Frmly:** (1986) Canadian Association for Children and Adults with Learning Disabilities.

★ 4362 ★ Lebanese Ostomy Association (LOA)
c/o Dr. Michel Daher, MD, FACS
PO Box 166378
St. George's Hospital
Beirut, Lebanon
Phone: 961 1 581714 **Fax:** 961 1 582560
Email: mndaher@inco.com.lb

Fnded: 1993. **Mem:** 43. **Lang(s):** Arabic, French. **Desc:** Medical professionals representing the interests of ostomy patients. Makes available training to nurses for ostomy care. Fosters communication and exchange.

★ 4363 ★ Lebanese Society of Cardiology
PO Box 6301
Beirut, Lebanon
Phone: 961 1 653414 **Fax:** 961 1 653411
Email: orca@cyberia.net.lb

Mem: 207. **Desc:** Promotes the study of cardiology in Lebanon. **Pub:** *The Lebanese Medical Journal*. • Newsletter, monthly.

★ 4364 ★ Lebanon Family Planning Association (LFPA)
Corniche Mazraa, Al Maskan Bldg.
PO Box 118240
Beirut, Lebanon
Phone: 961 1 311978
Email: fpaleb@inco.com.lb
Website: http://ippfnet.ippf.org

Lang(s): Arabic. **Desc:** Works to improve the quality of life for individuals living in Lebanon by promoting responsible parenthood and family planning. Advocates family planning as a basic human right. Offers programs in sex education, family planning, and health. Provides contraceptive and health care services. Conducts research.

★ 4365 ★ Legal Action for Women (LAW)
PO Box 11061
Pensacola, FL 32524
Phone: (334)962-3554 **Free:** 800-822-6783
Email: law@gulftel.com
Website: http://www.legalactionforwomen.org
Vicky Conroy, Contact

Fnded: 1985. **Desc:** Provides legal referral for women injured by abortions. Conducts research on medical malpractice; promotes action on abortion safety.

★ 4366 ★ Lemko Housing Organization (LHO)
603 S Ann St.
Baltimore, MD 21231
Phone: (410)342-7200 **Fax:** (410)276-1233
Dr. Ivan Dornic, Pres.

Desc: Individuals and organizations. Promotes availability of housing and living assistance for elderly people or people with disabilities of Slavic descent. Purchases property and constructs housing and assisted care facilities; provides programs and services to people with disabilities and the elderly.

★ 4367 ★ Leonard Cheshire International
30 Millbank
London SW1P 4QD, United Kingdom
Phone: 44 171 8028200 **Fax:** 44 171 8028275
Email: international@london.leonard-chesire.org.uk
Website: http://www.lcint.org.uk

Fnded: 1948. **Nat'l Groups:** 50. **Reg. Groups:** 9. **Local Groups:** 290. **Lang(s):** English, French, Spanish. **Desc:** Locally operated programs for people with disabilities and their families in 54 countries. Seeks to improve the quality of life of people with disabilities. Maintains rehabilitation centers, skills training centers, support for employment and education programs, independent living programs, community-based support and residential services. **Pub:** *COMPASS*, quarterly. Magazine. Contains news, featurs, and letters about Cheshire services. • *The Leonard Cheshire International*, periodic. Directory. • Handbooks. • Videos.

★ 4368 ★ Leonard Wood Memorial (American Leprosy Foundation) (LWM)
11600 Nebel St., Ste. 210
Rockville, MD 20852
Phone: (301)984-1336 **Fax:** (301)770-0580
Email: lwm-alf@erols.com
Website: http://www.ilep.org.uk/ilep_member_lwm.htm
Priscilla Reed, Administrative Dir.

Fnded: 1928. **Desc:** Health and research foundation concerned with microbiological research of Hansen's Disease (leprosy), and other related diseases. Conducts research programs in the U.S. and the Philippines. Supports clinical and basic laboratory research and epidemiological surveys. Sponsors exchange programs. Conducts collaborative studies with the Philippine Leprosy Mission, Culion Foundation, Colorado State University, Rockefeller University, the Delta Primate Center, American Leprosy Missions, International Sasakawa Memorial Health Foundation, Damien-Dutton Society, World Health Organization, UCLA School of Medicine, Ethiopia, India, Korea. **Pub:** Annual Report, annual. *Price:* Free. **AKA:** American Leprosy Foundation. **Frmly:** (1978) Leonard Wood Memorial for the Eradication of Leprosy.

★ 4369 ★ LEPRA - England
Fairfax House
Causton Rd.
Colchester CO1 1PU, United Kingdom
Phone: 44 1206 562286 **Fax:** 44 1206 762151
Email: lepra@lepra.org.uk
Website: http://www.lepra.org.uk

Fnded: 1924. **Mem:** 50. **Local Groups:** 2. **Lang(s):** English, French, Portuguese, Spanish. **Desc:** Objective is to eradicate leprosy throughout the world. Operates training programs for medical personnel. Supports research for the development of leprosy drugs and vaccines, and research projects of the World Health Organization. Concentrates efforts in Africa, Asia, and Brazil. Maintains special children's, eye, and hand remobilization funds. Investigates potential for treatment of leprosy in conjunction with that of other diseases. Sponsors competitions; bestows awards. **Pub:** *Leprosy Review*, quarterly. Journal.

★ 4370 ★ Leprosy Relief Association (LEPRA)
c/o Terry Vasey, Esq.
Fairfax House
Causton Rd.
Colchester CO1 1PU, United Kingdom
Phone: 44 1206 562286 **Fax:** 44 1206 762151
Email: terry_vasey@lepra.org.uk
Website: http://www.leprosy.org.uk

Desc: Works as medical development charity restoring health, hope and dignity to people affected by leprosy and other diseases of poverty.

★ 4371 ★ Lesbian Health Fund (LHF)
459 Fulton St., Ste. 107
San Francisco, CA 94102
Phone: (415)255-4547 **Fax:** (415)255-4784
Email: info@glma.org
Website: http://www.glma.org/

Fnded: 1992. **Desc:** Works to recognize the unique healthcare needs of lesbians; seeks to strengthen the health of lesbians and their families through health and medical research grants and education.

★ 4372 ★ Let's Face it USA (LFASU)
c/o Betsy Wilson
PO Box 29972
Bellingham, WA 98228-1972
Phone: (360)676-7325
Email: letsfaceit@faceit.org
Website: http://www.faceit.org
Betsy Wilson, Dir.

Fnded: 1987. **Desc:** A nonprofit information and support network for people who have or who care for those with facial disfigurement. Web site and annual publication with over 150 resources for professionals and families. Links to all related networks for specific conditions ie. Genetic Disorders, Burns, Cancer, etc. Resource can be downloaded in Adobe format from web site or send a self addressed 9" by 12" envelop stamped with a $2.00 stamp with a note telling of information need. **Pub:** *Resources for People with Facial Difference*, semiannual. Booklet.

★ 4373 ★ Leukemia and Lymphoma Society
1311 Mamaroneck Ave.
White Plains, NY 10605
Phone: (914)949-5213 **Free:** 800-955-4572
Fax: (914)949-6691
Email: infocenter@leukemia-lymphoma.org
Website: http://www.leukemia-lymphoma.org
Dwayne Howell, PhD, Pres. /CEO

Fnded: 1949. **Local Groups:** 59. **Desc:** Dedication to curing leukemia, lymphoma, Hodgkinson's disease and myeloma; seeks to improve the quality of life of patients and their families. Sponsors medical symposia and research; provides financial aid for patients; provides free information, support groups, teleconferences, and Web conferences for patients and families. **Pub:** *Educational Literature.* Brochures. Provides information about leukemia, lymphoma, myeloma, etc. *Price:* Free. • *The Leukemia & Lymphoma Society–Newsline*, quarterly. Newsletter. Provides information on advances in the research into leukemia, lymphoma, Hodgkin Disease and Myeloma. Includes research updates. *Price:* Free. **Frmly:** (1955) Robert Roesler de Villiers Foundation; (2000) Leukemia Society of America.

★ 4374 ★ Life and Liberty for Women
PMB 213
1015-M S Taft Hill Rd.
Fort Collins, CO 80521
Phone: (970)416-6872
Website: http://www.lifeandlibertyforwomen.org

Desc: Women. Advocates for safe abortion. Provides newsletters, research and information covering abortion issues.

★ 4375 ★ Life Works Institute (LWI)
14622 Ventura Blvd., No. 800
Sherman Oaks, CA 91403-3600
Phone: (818)386-9100 **Fax:** (818)386-9102
Email: lifeworks@lifeonnet.org
Website: http://lifeonnet.org/lifeworks.htm
Sanford Holst, Exec. Dir.

Fnded: 1996. **Desc:** Works to raise public awareness of life improvement and develop the belief that something can be done to make lives better. Develops and provides educational material and charitable services through others, and directly to the public, to begin improving people's lives. **Pub:** Newsletter. • Brochure.

★ 4376 ★ LifeBanc
20600 Chagrin Blvd., Ste. 350
Cleveland, OH 44122-5343
Phone: (216)752-5433 **Free:** 888-558-5433
Fax: (216)751-4204
Email: info@lifebanc.org
Website: http://www.lifebanc.org
Debbie May-Johnson, Exec. Dir.

Fnded: 1986. **Desc:** Responsible for all aspects of the organ and tissue donation process, as well as public and professional education programs, and bereavement services for donor families. Mission is to increase organ and tissue donation for those awaiting transplant, to provide community and professional education to people of all ages about the need for, and the benefits of, organ and tissue donation, and to respect and support those individuals and families whose generosity and compassion make it possible to improve and save the lives of others. **Pub:** Pamphlets.

★ 4377 ★ Lifegain Institute (LI)
115 Dunder Rd.
Burlington, VT 05401
Phone: (802)862-8855 **Fax:** (802)862-6389
Email: info@healthyculture.com
Website: http://www.healthyculture.com
Judd Allen, PhD, Pres.

Fnded: 1977. **Mem:** 600. **Desc:** People who work with health promotion programs in hospitals, corporations, colleges, and communities. Promotes healthy practices such as exercise, nutrition, safety, and the reduction or curtailment of smoking and alcohol consumption through health promotion programs that provide a supportive environment. Maintains speakers' bureau. Compiles data on improvements cultural support nationwide. **Pub:** *American Journal of Health Promotion*, quarterly. Journal. • *Lifegain: A Culture-Based Approach to Positive Health.* Book. • *Lifegain Healthy Communities System.* • Articles. • Also publishes support materials. **AKA:** Human Resources Institute.

★ 4378 ★ Lifespan Resources (LR)
1212 Roosevelt
Ann Arbor, MI 48104
Phone: (734)663-9891 **Fax:** (313)973-7645
Carol Tice, Pres.

Fnded: 1979. **Desc:** Designs, implements, and develops innovations for programs involving interaction between youth and senior citizens, emphasizing mentoring. Develops policy initiatives to assist states in determining their intergenerational program needs. Is concerned with multicultural issues and economic development for youth and senior citizens. Conducts surveys; operates speakers' bureau. **Pub:** *Guide for Mentoring At-risk Youths*, daily. Manuals. • *Guide to Intergenerational Programs.* Booklets. • *What We Have.* Film. • Reports. **Frmly:** (1990) New Age.

★ 4379 ★ Lighthouse International
111 E 59th St.
New York, NY 10022-1202
Phone: (212)821-9200 **Free:** 800-829-0500
Fax: (212)821-9707
Email: info@lighthouse.org
Website: http://www.lighthouse.org
Barbara M. Silverstone, Pres. /CEO

Fnded: 1906. **Desc:** Works to build confidence, independence, opportunity, quality of life and hope for people with impared vision. Provides information and resources to individuals and professionals. Operates the Lighthouse National Center for Vision and Aging and the Lighthouse National Center for Vision and Child Development; conducts continuing education programs for eye care providers; provides educational and advocacy services; offers training and employment to individuals with impaired vision; conducts laboratory research and studies on the consequences of vision impairment in everyday life. **Pub:** *Lighthouse News*, 3/year. Newsletter. *Price:* Free. • Annual Report; "Aging & Vision News"; literature on eye conditions and other aspects of vision loss.

★ 4380 ★ Ligue Francaise Contre la Sclerose en Plaques
40 rue Duranton
F-75015 Paris, France
Phone: 33 1 53989880 **Fax:** 33 1 53989888
Email: info@lfsep.asso.fr
Website: http://www.lfsep.com

Fnded: 1986. **Mem:** 4,500. **Reg. Groups:** 102. **Desc:** MS patients, families and professionals. Seeks to improve the quality of life for persons with multiple sclerosis and their families. **Pub:** *Courrier de la sclerose en plaques*, quarterly. Journal.

★ 4381 ★ Ligue Luxembourgeoise de la Sclerose en Plaques
c/o Pierre Wagner
Boite Postale 1444
L-1014 Luxembourg, Luxembourg
Phone: 352 40 08 44 **Fax:** 352 40 08 04

Fnded: 1980. **Mem:** 1,500. **Desc:** MS patients, families and professionals. Seeks to improve the quality of life for persons with multiple sclerosis and their families; offers occupational therapy and gymnastics.

★ 4382 ★ Ligue Nationale Belge de la Sclerose en Plaques
av. Eugene Plaskylaan, 173/11
B-1030 Brussels, Belgium
Phone: 32 2 7361638 **Fax:** 32 2 7323959
Email: ms.sep@ms-sep.be
Website: http://www.ms-sep.be

Desc: MS patients, families and professionals. Seeks to improve the quality of life for persons with multiple sclerosis and their families.

★ 4383 ★ Limbless Association
Rehabilitation Centre
Roehampton Ln.
London SW15 5PR, United Kingdom
Phone: 44 20 87881777 **Fax:** 44 20 87883444
Email: membership@limbless.association.org
Website: http://www.limbless-association.org

Fnded: 1983. **Mem:** 5,000. **Reg. Groups:** 2. **Lang(s):** English. **Desc:** Provides information and advice to people who have had amputations or who have been born without upper or lower limbs. Through a nationwide network of volunteer representatives who are all amputees themselves, offers support and encouragement to prospective amputees, careers, and those already trying to come to terms with limb loss or deficiency. **Pub:** *Step Forward*, quarterly. Magazine.

★ 4384 ★ Lithuanian Psychological Association
Didlaukio Str. 47
2057 Vilnius, Lithuania
Phone: 370 2 761581 **Fax:** 370 2 761890
Email: birute.pociute@fsf.vu.lt
Website: http://www.psd.fsf.vu.lt/lps

Fnded: 1958. **Mem:** 238. **Lang(s):** English, Russian. **Desc:** Psychologists promoting the development of professional activities in Lithuania for the good of all society.

★ 4385 ★ Lithuanian Society of Cardiology
Department of Cardiology
Vilnius University Hospital
Santariskiu Klinikos
Santariskiu 2
LT-2021 Vilnius, Lithuania
Phone: 370 2 365200 **Fax:** 370 2 365211
Email: cardio@cardio.lt
Website: http://www.escardio.org/society/natsoc/lithuania.htm

Mem: 401. **Desc:** Promotes the study of cardiology in Lithuania. **Pub:** *Lithuanian Journal of Cardiology*, 2-4/yr. Published jointly with the Institut of Cardiology. • *Seminars in Cardiology*, quarterly. Journal. Published jointly with the Lithuanian Heart Association.

★ 4386 ★ Lithuanian Stuttering Problem Club
Rasu 20
LT-2014 Vilnius, Lithuania
Phone: 370 2 614715 **Fax:** 370 2 614739
Email: dude@pub.osf.lt

Desc: Works to find a cure for stuttering in Lithuania.

★ 4387 ★ Little Brothers - Friends of the Elderly
954 W Washington Blvd., 5th Fl.
Chicago, IL 60607
Phone: (312)829-3055 **Fax:** (312)829-3077
Email: national@littlebrothers.org
Website: http://www.littlebrothers.org/
Roger Nash, Exec. Dir.

Fnded: 1959. **Mem:** 1,000. **Reg. Groups:** 7. **Desc:** Participants are individuals over 70 years old who live alone, have limited incomes, and do not receive emotional and physical support from relatives. Seeks to combat the isolation and loneliness often experienced by elderly people by providing friendship and special assistance. Sponsors visitation programs, holiday and birthday parties, and summer vacations. Provides transportation for shopping and doctor's visits, food packages, and other "special touches." Also offers information, referrals, and contacts with other public or private agencies. Maintains vacation homes. **Pub:** *Reaching Out*, 3/year. Newsletter. For donors and volunteers. • *Volunteer Newsletter*. Newsletter. • Annual Report. • Brochure. **AKA:** Little Brothers of the Poor.

★ 4388 ★ The Living Bank International (TLB)
PO Box 6725
Houston, TX 77265-6725
Phone: (713)961-9431 **Free:** 800-528-2971
Fax: (713)961-0979
Email: info@livingbank.org
Website: http://www.livingbank.org
Jon Eiche, Pres. /CEO

Fnded: 1968. **Mem:** 1850,000. **Desc:** Open to anyone who wishes to donate organs and/or tissues at time of death. Provides a centralized registry for people who want to donate organs/tissues at the time of death. Those interested in becoming donors can request donor registration forms on which they specify which organs and/or tissues they will donate and any limitations or special wishes. Document must be signed by two witnesses. Donors receive an organ donor card which is carried by the individual at all times and which indicates that the person is registered with The Living Bank. If death is imminent or has occurred, The Living Bank is notified and one of their staff members refers the situation to the closest organ procurement organization or other appropriate agency. The organ procurement organization makes the decision regarding what can and cannot be used for transplant. The major types of transplants that are currently being performed include cornea, skin, heart, liver, kidney, intestine, pancreas, and lung transplants. For individuals wishing to donate their whole bodies for anatomical research and study, they should contact The Living Bank for information on how to register with the nearest medical school. Due to many of the body donor programs being full, many medical schools now require that you be pre-registered. Operates speakers bureau in communities throughout the country. **Pub:** *Bank Account*, semiannual. Newsletter. Includes news updates on advances in the fields of organ donation and transplantation. *Price:* Free. • Brochures. • Also publishes educational and informational materials. **Frmly:** (2001) The Living Bank.

★ 4389 ★ LMBS Network
c/o Sonya Coster
124 Lincoln Ave.
Purchase, NY 10577
Phone: (914)251-1163
Email: josiahsmum@hotmail.com
Website: http://www.blindness.org
Sonya Coster, Contact

Fnded: 1980. **Mem:** 50. **Nat'l Groups:** 1. **Desc:** Individuals with LMBS and family members. Offers support to individuals and family members. **Pub:** *Network*, semiannual. Newsletter. Profiles and information. *Price:* Free. • Brochure, annual. Contains general information on disease, profile of cases, addresses of contacts.

★ 4390 ★ Logan Community Resources
PO Box 1049
1235 N Eddy St.
South Bend, IN 46624
Website: http://logancenter.org

Desc: Individuals, families, volunteers, neighbors, employers, donors. Strives to create opportunities for persons with developmental disabilities. Offers person directed planning.

★ 4391 ★ London Association of Primal Psychotherapists
West Hill House
6 Swains Ln.
London N6 6QS, United Kingdom
Phone: 44 207 2679616 **Fax:** 44 207 4820858
Email: info@lapp.org
Website: http://www.lapp.org

Fnded: 1986. **Mem:** 55. **Lang(s):** Croatian, French, German, Spanish. **Desc:** Student membership open to trainees; associate membership open to people with an interest in the field of psychotherapy; full membership open to those qualified to work as primal psychotherapists. Aims to refine and develop primal psychotherapy. To this end a four year training programme is run that is recognized by the United Kingdom Council for Psychotherapy. Also has a trust fund devoted to working with people facing life threatening illness.

★ 4392 ★ Long Term Care Campaign (LTCC)
PO Box 27394
Washington, DC 20038
Phone: (202)434-3744 **Fax:** (202)434-6403
Email: info@ltccampaign.org
Kevin Donnellan, Chair

Fnded: 1987. **Mem:** 143. **Nat'l Groups:** 143. **Desc:** Consumer, provider, business, labor, ciuk, older adult, and disability groups. Works to make long term health care accessible and affordable for all families. **Pub:** *The Campaigner*, quarterly. Newsletter. Long Term Care issues and legislative updates. • *The Time Is Now*. Videos.

★ 4393 ★ Long-term Medical Conditions Alliance (LMCA)
Unit 212
16 Baldwins Gardens
London EC1N 7RJ, United Kingdom
Phone: 44 2078133637 **Fax:** 44 2078133640
Email: info@lmca.org.uk
Website: http://www.lmca.demon.co.uk

Fnded: 1989. **Mem:** 115. **Desc:** Umbrella body working with member organisations towards better lives for people with long-term health conditions. Aims to gain recognition of people's needs and ensure resources are available to meet them, to campaign to achieve change in areas of common concern, to develop effective partnerships between service providers and service users, and to promote participation by individuals in their own care and treatment.

★ 4394 ★ Loops for Lupus
390 Hawk Ln.
Basalt, CO 81621-9788
Phone: (970)927-3983 **Fax:** (970)963-0590
Email: tommy@loopsforlupus.org
Website: http://www.loopsforlupus.org/

Desc: Committed to raising funds and heighten awareness about the disease Lupus.

★ 4395 ★ Lowe Syndrome Association (LSA)
222 Lincoln St.
West Lafayette, IN 47906
Phone: (765)743-3634
Email: info@lowesyndrome.org
Website: http://www.lowesyndrome.org
Kaye McSpadden, Dir. of Public & Scientific Affairs

Fnded: 1983. Mem: 400. Desc: Parents, friends, and relatives of individuals with Lowe syndrome; medical, educational, and social service professionals and agencies. Fosters communication among families; provides medical and educational information; promotes a better understanding of Lowe syndrome; supports and encourages medical research. **Pub:** *Living with Lowe Syndrome.* • *On the Beam*, 3/year. Membership newsletter for families affected by Lowe syndrome. *Price:* Included in membership dues.

★ 4396 ★ Lupus Foundation of America
1300 Piccard Dr., Ste. 200
Rockville, MD 20850-4303
Phone: (301)670-9292 **Free:** 800-558-0121
Fax: (301)670-9486
Email: lupusinfo@aol.com
Website: http://www.lupus.org
Sandra Reymond, Pres. /CEO

Fnded: 1977. **Local Groups:** 94. **Desc:** Works to increase knowledge and public awareness of lupus erythematosus, a noncontagious disease that may affect the skin alone or may manifest itself as a chronic, systemic, and inflammatory disease of the connective tissues. Assists lupus patients and their families, through chapters and patient support groups, to cope with the daily problems associated with lupus. Collects and distributes funds for research. Works to bring lupus to the attention of the public by encouraging the publication of articles on the disease by syndicated medical writers, national magazines, and newspapers, and by obtaining radio and television coverage. Has successfully worked for the establishment of an annual Lupus Awareness Month. Chapters hold patient meetings and occasional medical seminars. **Pub:** *Lupus Erythematosus.* Pamphlet. • *Lupus News*, quarterly. Newsletter. Reports current research both directly and indirectly related to lupus. *Price:* Free. For members only. • Also publishes other informational materials in Braille and Spanish.

★ 4397 ★ Lupus Information Network (LIN)
230 Ranch Dr.
Bridgeport, CT 06606-1747
Phone: (203)372-5795
Email: feedback@lupusinformationnetwork.org
Website: http://www.lupusinformationnetwork.org

Fnded: 1985. **Desc:** Educators, medical professionals, and individuals suffering from systemic lupus erythematosus. (Systemic lupus erythematosus is a chronic inflammatory disease of the connective tissue that affects the skin, joints, kidneys, nervous system, and mucous membranes.) Seeks to foster better understanding of the disease among patients, educators, and professionals through the distribution of information, both orthodox and alternative. **Pub:** *Introduction to Lupus.* Brochure. • Pamphlets. • Reprints. **Frmly:** (2001) Lupus Network.

★ 4398 ★ Lutheran Braille Evangelism Association (LBEA)
1740 Eugene St.
White Bear Lake, MN 55110
Phone: (651)426-0469
Email: lbea@qwest.net
Website: http://www.careministries.org/lbea.html
Rev. Dennis Hawkinson, Exec. Dir.

Fnded: 1952. **Mem:** 2,000. **Desc:** Fosters provision of religious material to the visually impaired in Braille, audio cassette, extra large print and digital formats. Supported by contributions of members. **Pub:** *Braille Evangelism Bulletin*, quarterly. Newsletter. Contains membership activities, and services and materials available. *Price:* Free. • *Christian Magnifier: A Christian Magazine in Magnified Print & Cassette*, monthly. Magazine. Contains large-print Christian inspirational readings. *Price:* $7/year. • *Tract Messenger*, monthly. Braille publication of Christian devotional readings and LBEA news. *Price:* Free to the blind. • Also provides religious material in braille, large print and audio cassette, such as the Holy Bible.

★ 4399 ★ Lutheran Braille Workers (LBW)
13471 California St.
PO Box 5000
Yucaipa, CA 92399
Phone: (909)795-8977 **Fax:** (909)795-8970
Email: lbw@lbwinc.org
Website: http://www.lbwinc.org
Loyd Coppenger, Exec. Dir.

Fnded: 1943. **Mem:** 7,000. **Nat'l Groups:** 206. **Desc:** Volunteers staffing 206 work centers worldwide, through which they seek to bring the Bible to the blind and visually impaired. Teaches sighted volunteers to transcribe printed material into Braille and large print. Produces and distributes free biblical and devotional material in Braille and large print in over 40 languages. Works to constantly upgrade the systems necessary for the production of Braille materials. **Pub:** *Lutheran Braille Workers–Newsletter*, quarterly. Newsletter. Covers association activities. *Price:* Free. • *Work Center Directory*, annual. Directory. • *Work Center Memo*, monthly. Newsletter. Provides information to LBW work centers.

★ 4400 ★ Luxembourg Dietetic Association (Association Nationale des Dieteticiens du Luxembourg)
Boite Postale 62
L-7201 Walferdange, Luxembourg
Phone: 352 26552728 **Fax:** 352 367684

Mem: 50. **Lang(s):** English, French, German. **Desc:** Professional dietitians. Promotes advancement in the study and application of dietetics; advises government agencies and the public regarding a healthy diet.

★ 4401 ★ Luxembourg Federation of Hospitals (Entente des Hopitaux Luxembourgeois — EHL)
13-15 rue Jean-Pierre Sauvage
L-2514 Luxembourg, Luxembourg
Phone: 352 424142 **Fax:** 352 425550
Email: marc.hastert@ehl.healthnet.lu
Website: http://www.ehl.org

Fnded: 1965. **Mem:** 26.

★ 4402 ★ Luz Social Services
2797 N Introspect Dr.
Tucson, AZ 85745
Phone: (520)882-6216 **Fax:** (520)623-9291
Email: pbarron@luzsocialservices.org
Website: http://www.luzsocialservices.org
Dr. Pepe Barron, PhD, CEO

Fnded: 1989. **Mem:** 18. **Desc:** Assists with family issues, specifically substance abuse. Maintains a speakers' bureau. Conducts research and educational programs. **Pub:** *Adelante Juntous*, monthly. Newsletter.

★ 4403 ★ Lyme Disease Foundation (LDF)
1 Financial Plz.
Hartford, CT 06103-2601
Phone: (860)525-2000 **Free:** 800-886-LYME
Fax: (860)525-8425
Email: lymefnd@aol.com
Website: http://www.lyme.org
John F. Anderson, Dir.

Fnded: 1988. **Local Groups:** 200. **Desc:** Seeks to educate medical professionals and the public about Lyme Borreliosis (Lyme disease), which is spread to humans by ticks with symptoms including rashes, joint swelling and pain, fever, severe headaches, and heart arrhythmia. Provides treatment protocols, diagnostic guidelines, and photographic case histories. Assists in the formation of support groups; offers referral service; maintains speakers' bureau. Sponsors medical seminars; provides videotape and slide programs; conducts research. Maintains registry of infected pregnant women and congenital cases. Works in cooperation with Congress, Centers for Disease Control, and National Institutes of Health. **Pub:** *Journal of Spirochetal and Tick Bourne Disease*, quarterly. Journal. *Price:* $75/year. • *Lymelight*, quarterly. Newsletter. *Price:* $30/year. • *Monthly Update. Price:* $50/year. • Pamphlets. **Frmly:** (1992) Lyme Borreliosis Foundation.

★ 4404 ★ Lymphatic Research Foundation (LRF)
39 Pool Dr.
Roslyn, NY 11576-2038
Phone: (516)625-9675 **Fax:** (516)625-9410
Email: lrf@lymphaticresearch.org
Website: http://www.lymphaticresearch.org
Wendy Chaite, Esq., Pres.

Fnded: 1998. **Desc:** Health care professionals, scientists, and researchers with an interest in lymphatic diseases and related disorders. Seeks to advance the prevention, diagnosis, and treatment of lymphatic diseases. Serves as a clearinghouse on lymphatic research; facilitates exchange of information among members; advocates the creation of a nationally supported lymphatic research program; functions as a liaison linking public and private-sector lymphatic research institutions and programs. **Pub:** *Lymphatic Research & Biology*, quarterly. Journal. *Price:* $163.

★ 4405 ★ Lymphoma Association
PO Box 386
Aylesbury HP20 2GA, United Kingdom
Phone: 44 1296 619400 **Fax:** 44 1296 619414
Email: support@lymphoma.org.uk
Website: http://www.lymphoma.org.uk

Fnded: 1986. **Mem:** 2,000. **Desc:** Provides information and emotional support for anyone affected by lymphoma. Provides a Help line; telephone links to helpers with similar experience of lymphoma; a network of regional support groups and a quarterly newsletter for members. **Pub:** *Fundraising News*, quarterly. • *Lymphoma News*, quarterly. Newsletter.

★ 4406 ★ Lymphoma Research Foundation (LRF)
8800 Venice Blvd., Ste. 207
Los Angeles, CA 90034
Phone: (310)204-7040 **Free:** 800-500-9976
Fax: (310)204-7043
Email: lrf@lymphoma.org
Website: http://www.lymphoma.org
Suzanne Buss, Exec. Dir.

Fnded: 2001. **State Groups:** 20. **Desc:** Provides support and information for lymphoma patients and their families regarding diagnosis, treatments, clinical trials, support services, literature, and physician referrals. Serves patients with a buddy support program. Supports lymphoma specific education for both patients and healthcare professionals. Promotes advocacy; funds research. **Pub:** *Lymphoma Update*, quarterly. Newsletter. Provides information about lymphoma and the Foundation, as well as current events.

★ 4407 ★ Macular Disease Society
Darwin House
13a Bridge St.
Andover SP10 1BE, United Kingdom
Phone: 44 1264 350836
Email: info@maculardisease.org
Website: http://www.maculardisease.org

Fnded: 1986. **Mem:** 12,000. **Local Groups:** 120. **Desc:** Aims to provide information, fellowship and support to those with macular disease.

★ 4408 ★ MAGIC Foundation (MAGIC)
c/o Mary Andrews
6645 W N Ave.
Oak Park, IL 60302
Phone: (708)383-0808 **Free:** 800-3MA-GIC3
Fax: (708)383-0899
Email: mary@magicfoundation.org
Website: http://www.magicfoundation.org
Mary Andrews, Exec. Dir.

Fnded: 1989. **Mem:** 10,000. **Local Groups:** 16. **Desc:** Provides support and assistance to families of children with physical growth related disorders. Sponsors educational programs, family networking, and Pen Pal for the Kids service. Maintains speakers' bureau **Pub:** *MAGIC Touch*, quarterly. Newsletter. *Price:* Free with membership. • Brochures. **Frmly:** Major Aspects of Growth in Children Foundation; (2003) MAGIC Foundation for Children's Growth.

★ 4409 ★ Make Early Diagnosis to Prevent Early Death (MEDPED)

University of Utah
410 Chipeta Way, Rm. 161
Salt Lake City, UT 84108
Free: 888-244-2465 **Fax:** (801)581-5402
Email: larrinaga-shum@hsc.utah.edu
Website: http://www.medped.org
Stacey Larrinaga-Shum, Prog. Mgr.

Fnded: 1989. **Desc:** Promotes early diagnosis, proper treatment, and prevention of premature deaths for people with inherited cholesterol disorders, specifically Familial Hypercholesterolemia (FH). **Frmly:** (2003) MedPed.

★ 4410 ★ Make Today Count (MTC)

1235 E Cherokee St.
Springfield, MO 65804-2203
Phone: (417)885-2588 **Fax:** (417)888-8761
Connie Zimmerman, Exec. Dir.

Fnded: 1974. **Mem:** 5,000. **Local Groups:** 200. **Desc:** Cancer patients and others with life-threatening illnesses, and their immediate families. Works to bring members and their neighbors together to discuss openly the false implications and the realities of life-threatening diseases. Takes a positive approach to the problems of serious illness in order to lessen the emotional trauma for all concerned. Assists professionals in communicating with and meeting the needs of seriously ill patients. Maintains speakers' bureau and referral service; plans educational programs, films, and tapes. **Pub:** *Chapter Directory*, annual. Directory. • *Make Today Count Newsletter*, bimonthly. Newsletter. Offers emotional support to people with cancer or other life-threatening illnesses, and to their family members, friends, and professionals. *Price:* $10/year. • *Make Today Count - Until Tomorrow Comes.*

★ 4411 ★ Malacological Society of China

2 Siangyang Rd.
Taipei, Taiwan

Fnded: 1970.

★ 4412 ★ Malawi Against Physical Disabilities (MAP)

PO Box 256
Blantyre, Malawi
Phone: 265 677951 **Fax:** 265 674604
Email: map@malawi.net

Fnded: 1980. **Mem:** 130. **Local Groups:** 300. **Lang(s):** English. **Desc:** Rehabilitation of people with physical disabilities caused by polio, burns, tuberculosis of the spine, amputations, congenital deformities, cerebral palsy, strokes etc. **Pub:** *Annual Report*, annual. • *Financial Report.* • *MAP Feedback.* • *MAP Newsletter.* Newsletter. • Journal, semiannual.

★ 4413 ★ Malaysian Association of Sports Medicine

Mezzanine Floor, Wisma OCM, Hang Jebat Rd.
50150 Kuala Lumpur, Malaysia
Phone: 60 3 7761469 **Fax:** 60 3 7750687
Email: ramlan@nsc.gov.my

★ 4414 ★ Malaysian Medical Association (MMA)

MMA House, 4th Fl.
124 Jalan Pahang
53000 Kuala Lumpur, Malaysia
Phone: 60 3 40411375 **Fax:** 60 3 40418187
Email: info@mma.org.my
Website: http://www.mma.org.my

Fnded: 1952. **Mem:** 8,000. **Lang(s):** English, Indonesian. **Desc:** Conducts educational programs for medical professionals; sponsors research and charitable activities. **Pub:** *Berita MMA*. Newsletter. • *Medical Journal of Malaysia*, quarterly. Journal.

★ 4415 ★ Malaysian Society of Anaesthesiologists

19 Jalan Folly Barat
50480 Kuala Lumpur, Malaysia
Phone: 60 3 2530100 **Fax:** 60 3 2530900
Email: acadmed@po.jaring.my

★ 4416 ★ Malaysian Society of Pharmacology and Physiology (Persatuan Farmakologi dan Fisiologi Malaysia)

c/o Dr. Harbindar Jeet Singh
Physiology Department
School of Medical Sciences
Universiti Sains Malaysia
Kubang Kerian
16150 Kelantan, Malaysia
Phone: 60 9 7651700 **Fax:** 60 9 7653370
Email: hjsingh@kb.usm.my
Website: http://www.members.tripod.com/~tekam/mspp/

Mem: 85. **Desc:** Promotes pharmacology and physiology in Malaysia.

★ 4417 ★ Malaysian Society of Radiographers (MSR) (Persatuan Juru X-Ray Malaysia — PJXM)

General Hospital
Department of Radiology
Jalan Pahang
50586 Kuala Lumpur, Malaysia
Phone: 60 3 2981044 **Fax:** 60 3 2984035
Email: krr@po.jaring.my
Website: http://www.angelfire.com/ms2/msr/

Fnded: 1968. **Mem:** 400. **Lang(s):** English, Malay. **Desc:** Radiographers working in diagnostic and radiotherapeutic specialties. Represents the interests of radiographers and allied practitioners through professional and social activities. Works to foster interest in radiography and radiotherapeutic technique and to improve the standards of practice. Operates a research program in radiation protection. Sponsors weekend lectures, technical sessions, seminars, symposia, workshops, and conferences. **Pub:** *Journal Majuray*, annual. Journal. Features writing pertaining to radiology. • *Newsletter*, quarterly. Newsletter.

★ 4418 ★ Malignant Hyperthermia Association (MHA)

Toronto General Hospital
200 Elizabeth St., EC-11-307
Toronto, ON, Canada M5G 2C4
Phone: (416)340-3238 **Fax:** (416)340-4960
Email: info@mhacanada.com
Website: http://www.mhacanada.org

Fnded: 1979. **Lang(s):** English, French. **Desc:** Individuals with malignant hyperthermia (high fever and muscle rigidity, usually brought on by a reaction to certain anesthetics, to which some individuals are genetically predisposed), their families, and interested health care professionals. Seeks to advance the prevention and treatment of malignant hyperthermia. Conducts research; operates charitable programs.

★ 4419 ★ Malignant Hyperthermia Association of the United States (MHAUS)

11 E State St.
PO Box 1069
Sherburne, NY 13460-1069
Phone: (607)674-7901 **Fax:** (607)674-7910
Email: info@mhaus.org
Website: http://www.mhaus.org
Dianne M. Daugherty, Exec. Dir.

Fnded: 1981. **Mem:** 2,500. **Desc:** Malignant Hyperthermia (MH) susceptible patients and health care providers. MH is a genetically transmitted, often fatal, muscular disorder triggered in susceptible individuals by certain general anesthetic agents. Objectives are to: save lives by making information about MH available; discuss problems that confront families affected by MH; fund research on the causes, detection, and management of MH; disseminate research information. **Pub:** *The Communicator*, quarterly. Newsletter. Contains MH updates for MHS patients and medical professionals. *Price:* $35 per year. • *Emergency Treatment for MH.* • *Malignant Hyperthermia, Four Cases (for medical professionals).* Video. • *Malignant Hyperthermia, Knowing Your Role (for medical professionals).* Video. • *Managing MH - Clinical Updates.* Pamphlet. • *MH Procedural Manuals w/video.* Hospital and Ambulatory versions. • *Preventing MH - An Anesthesia Protocol.* Pamphlet. • *Testing for Susceptibility to MH.* Pamphlet. • *Understanding MH.* Booklet.

★ 4420 ★ Malta Union of Professional Psychologists

PO Box 341
Valletta, Malta
Email: vcasl@educ.um.edu.mt

Desc: Psychologists in Malta. Promotes the advancement of psychological study.

★ 4421 ★ Malta Veterinary Association

PO Box 66
B'Kara, Malta

Fnded: 1990. **Mem:** 28. **Desc:** Veterinarians working to improve animal health and welfare in Malta.

★ 4422 ★ Maltese Association of Gerontology and Geriatrics

c/o Institute of Gerontology
University of Malta
Msida, Malta

Desc: Promotes professional and educational advancement of gerontologists and geriatricians, with emphasis on research based mutual education of members. The importance of all aspects of the elderly is stressed, including physical, spiritual, social and psychological.

★ 4423 ★ Management Society for Healthcare Professionals

88 Lockhart Rd., 8/F, Wanchai
Hong Kong, People's Republic of China
Phone: 852 28612668 **Fax:** 852 28610189
Email: enquiry@mshp.org.hk
Website: http://www.mshp.org.hk/english/f02.htm

Fnded: 1984. **Lang(s):** Chinese, English. **Desc:** Managerial and administrative staff of health care services; medical, paramedical, and nursing professionals. Promotes effective delivery of health care and patient care and management services. Seeks to facilitate the professional development of members. Represents members' interests; collaborates with government agencies in establishment of public health policies and programs; facilitates exchange of information among members. Conducts educational programs; sponsors social activities.

★ 4424 ★ MAP International (MAP)

2200 Glynco Pky.
PO Box 215000
Brunswick, GA 31521-6800
Phone: (912)265-6010 **Free:** 800-225-8550
Fax: (912)265-6170
Email: map@map.org
Website: http://www.map.org
Michael J. Nyenhuis, Pres. /CEO

Fnded: 1954. **Reg. Groups:** 5. **Desc:** Non-profit Christian relief and development organization that promotes the health of people living in the world's poorest communities. Works with partners in the areas of community health development, disease prevention and eradication, relief and rehabilitation and global health advocacy. Promotes access to health services and essential medicines in more than 100 countries each year. **Pub:** *MAP International Report*, bimonthly. Newsletter. • *Our Health*, semiannual. Magazine. • Annual Report. **Frmly:** (1976) Medical Assistance Programs.

★ 4425 ★ MAP International - Eastern Africa Office

3rd Fl. Studio House
Intersection of Argwings Kohdek and Chaka Rds.
PO Box 21663
Nairobi, Kenya
Phone: 254 20 727586 **Fax:** 254 20 714422
Email: mapesa@map.org
Website: http://www.map.org

Mem: 10. **Desc:** Provides training, consultancy, and health education services. Disseminates information about AIDS and other health issues. Provides a forum for the exchange of information. **Pub:** *A Pastoral Counselling Manual for AIDS*. Booklet. • *AIDS in Africa, the Churches Opportunity*. Booklet. • *AIDS in Your Community*. Booklet. • *Community Balanced Development*. Booklet. • *Facts and Feelings About AIDS*. Booklet. • *Giving and Getting AIDS*. Booklet. • *Growing Together*. Booklet. • *Helpers for a Healing Community*. Booklet. • *Patterns for Life*. Booklet. • *Springs of Life*. Video. Educational AIDS video for church leaders.

★ 4426 ★ Maple Syrup Urine Family Support Group

82 Ravine Rd.
Powell, OH 43065
Phone: (740)548-4475
Email: msud-support@characterlink.net
Website: http://www.msud-support.org
Sandra Bulcher, Contact

Fnded: 1982. **Desc:** Those affected by Maple Syrup Urine Disease (MSUD) and their families; health care professionals. (Maple Syrup Urine Disease usually occurs in infancy and is characterized by a strong odor of the urine, loss of sucking reflex, general listlessness, episodes of rigidity, and high-pitched crying. If undiagnosed, the condition can progress to seizures, coma and death. Symptoms sometimes do not occur for several months.) Gathers and distributes information on MSUD. Seeks to strengthen the liaison between families and health care professionals. Encourages increased research and newborn screening for MSUD. Sponsors education programs. **Pub:** Brochure. • Newsletter, semiannual. *Price:* $10. • Also publishes information packet. **Frmly:** Families with Maple Syrup Urine Disease; (2003) MSUD Family Support Group.

★ 4427 ★ March of Dimes Birth Defects Foundation (MDBDF)

1275 Mamaroneck Ave.
White Plains, NY 10605
Phone: (914)428-7100 **Free:** 888-663-4637
Fax: (914)428-8203
Website: http://www.marchofdimes.com
Dr. Jennifer L. Howse, Pres.

Fnded: 1938. **Reg. Groups:** 3. **State Groups:** 54. **Desc:** Founded by President Franklin D. Roosevelt as the National Foundation for Infantile Paralysis. Promotes prevention of birth defects by focusing on maternal and child health issues including low birthweight, infant mortality, prenatal care, and maternal substance abuse. Offers public and professional health education and community service programs to improve maternal and newborn health. Works with other national and local organizations to initiate and implement community programs of prenatal care education and service. Operates the Pregnancy and Newborn Health Education Center which provides information on pregnancy, birth defects, genetic disorders and related topics. Develops and distributes educational materials for health professionals and the public. **Frmly:** (1958) National Foundation for Infantile Paralysis; (1979) National Foundation - March of Dimes.

★ 4428 ★ Marie Curie Cancer Care (MCCC)

89 Albert Embankment
London SE1 7TP, United Kingdom
Phone: 44 207 5997777 **Fax:** 44 207 5997708
Email: info@mariecurie.org.uk
Website: http://www.mariecurie.org.uk

Fnded: 1948. **Lang(s):** English. **Desc:** Health care professionals working with people who have cancer. Seeks to improve the quality of life of people with cancer; promotes increased availability and effectiveness of cancer care. Operates nationwide network of Marie Curie Nurses in the community and operates ten hospices across England, Scotland, Wales, and Northern Ireland; provides specialist care for people with cancer; conducts cancer research. Conducts educational programs. **Pub:** *Marie Curie News*, quarterly. Newsletter. • Pamphlets.

★ 4429 ★ Marie Stopes International - United Kingdom (MSI)

153-157 Cleveland St.
London W1T 6QW, United Kingdom
Phone: 44 207 5747400 **Fax:** 44 207 5747417
Email: msi@stopes.org.uk
Website: http://www.mariestopes.org.uk

Fnded: 1975. **Desc:** Provides a wide range of maternal health and family planning services. Programs conducted include: contraceptive social marketing; male oriented services. Specializes in working with indigenous personnel to develop clinical family planning services and social marketing programs.

★ 4430 ★ Marie Stopes International - Vietnam (MSIVN)

Solday F2 No 1
Phuong, Bach Khoa
Hanoi, Vietnam
Phone: 84 4 8694356
Email: msihanoi@netnam.org.vn

Lang(s): English, French, Vietnamese. **Desc:** Maternal and child health organizations, health care providers, and other interested individuals. Seeks to increase access to health and family planning services among previously underserved populations. Conducts social marketing of contraceptives; sponsors male-oriented family planning campaigns. Develops locally administered family planning services and social marketing programs.

★ 4431 ★ Massage Therapy Association

c/o Sandra Williams
PO Box 53320
Kenilworth 7745, Republic of South Africa
Phone: 27 21 6715313
Email: aoasa@global.co.za

Fnded: 1989. **Desc:** Aims to ensure professional educational and training standards. Regulates the registration of certified therapists. Provides continued educational programs for certified therapists. Creates better public awareness and understanding of the benefits of massage.

★ 4432 ★ Maternity Alliance (MA)

2-6 Northburgh St., 3rd Fl. W
London EC1V 0AY, United Kingdom
Phone: 44 20 74907639 **Fax:** 44 20 70141350
Email: info@maternityalliance.org.uk
Website: http://www.maternityalliance.org.uk

Fnded: 1980. **Mem:** 70. **Lang(s):** English. **Desc:** Individuals and organizations concerned with rights and services for parents and babies. Campaigns for improvements in rights and services for mothers, fathers, and babies. Concerns include: improvement in health care before conception and the first year of life; financial support for low income families; protection of working mothers' rights; and availability of transportation and housing. Conducts research programs. **Pub:** *Maternity Action*, periodic. Bulletin. • *Money for Mothers and Babies*, periodic. • *Pregnant at Work 2003*, annual.

★ 4433 ★ Maternity Center Association (MCA)

281 Park Ave. S, 5th Fl.
New York, NY 10010
Phone: (212)777-5000 **Fax:** (212)777-9320
Email: info@maternitywise.org
Website: http://www.maternitywise.org
Maureen Corry, Exec. Dir.

Fnded: 1918. **Desc:** Laypersons, physicians, nurses, nurse-midwives, childbirth educators, and public health workers interested in improvement of maternity care, maternal and infant health, and family life. A national nonprofit health organization for over 800 years, MCA's goals are to expand access to family-centered maternity care through collaborative practice, education, publications, consultation services, public policy initiatives and demonstration programs. Sponsors research; administers nurse-midwifery student assistance fund. Co-sponsors community-based Nurse-Midwifery Education Program. Sponsors research; administers nurse-midwifery student assistance fund. Co-sponsors community-based Nurse-Midwifery Education Program. **Pub:** *Birth Atlas*. Book. Instructional Aide. • *Growing Uterus Chart Series*. • *Journey to Parenthood*. Booklets. • *Publications Catalog*, annual. Catalog. *Price:* Free. • Books. • Pamphlets. • Videos. • Also publishes teaching aids for health professionals, charts, and slides.

★ 4434 ★ Maternity Coalition

PO Box 1190
Blackburn, VIC 3130, Australia
Phone: 61 3 93802863 **Fax:** 61 3 93811362
Email: inquiries@maternitycoalition.org.au
Website: http://www.maternitycoalition.org.au

Fnded: 1989. **Mem:** 250. **State Groups:** 3. **Lang(s):** English. **Desc:** Midwives, educators and researchers in the area of childbirth and women's health, mothers and other interested individuals. Acts as an umbrella organization to bring together support groups and individuals for effective lobbying, information sharing, networking and support in maternity services. Works for the rights of mothers and seeks to improve maternity care for women during pregnancy, birth and beyond. Provides consumer information on choices for childbirth. **Pub:** *Birth Matters*, quarterly. Journal.

★ 4435 ★ Mature Market Resource Center (MMRC)

c/o Janet Jesse
1850 W Winchester Rd., Ste. 213
Libertyville, IL 60048
Phone: (847)816-8660 **Free:** 800-828-8225
Fax: (847)816-8662
Email: info@healthawards.com
Website: http://www.seniorprograms.com
Pat Ford, Assoc. Dir.

Fnded: 1992. **Desc:** Acts as a clearinghouse of resources for the mature market. Provides research and information on new trends and discoveries in senior health and fitness. Produces resource books. National Senior Health and Fitness Day and various Mature Fitness Awards USA. **Pub:** *Mature Market Calendar of Events*, annual. Directory. • *Mature Markets*, annual. Directory. • *Mature Markets Online*, annual. Directory. • *Resources for Senior Programs Catalog*, annual. • *What's New in senior Health and Fitness Action Cards*, annual.

★ 4436 ★ Mautner Project for Lesbians with Cancer

1707 L St. NW, Ste. 500
Washington, DC 20036
Phone: (202)332-5536 **Fax:** (202)332-0662
Email: mautner@mautnerproject.org
Website: http://www.mautnerproject.org/

Fnded: 1990. **Desc:** Dedicated to lesbians with cancer, their partners and caregivers; provides education and information to the lesbian community regarding cancer; promotes understanding to the health care community about special concerns of lesbians with cancer and their families; advocates for lesbian health issues in national arenas.

★ 4437 ★ Media Access Group at WGBH (NCAM)
PO Box 200
Boston, MA 02134
Phone: (617)300-5400 **Fax:** (617)300-1035
Email: access@wgbh.org
Website: http://www.wgbh.org/access

Desc: Dedicated to information equity to make media accessible to underserved populations such as disabled persons, minority-language users, and people with low literacy skills. **Pub:** *Media Access*, annual. Newsletter. **Frmly:** (2001) CPB/WGBH National CTR for Accessible Media.

★ 4438 ★ Medical Association of Jamaica (MAJ)
Paisley Ave.
Kingston 5, Jamaica
Phone: (876)927-2471
Email: medassnjam@kasnet.com

Fnded: 1967. **Mem:** 660. **Reg. Groups:** 5. **Lang(s):** English. **Desc:** Health care professionals. Works to ensure availability of medical care and to maintain high standards of practice in all medical specialties. Makes available professional and advisory services to members. Gathers and disseminates information.

★ 4439 ★ Medical Association of Malta
Federation of Professional Bodies
Alamein Rd.
Pembroke GZR 06, Malta
Phone: 356 312888 **Fax:** 356 331713
Email: mam@synapse.net.mt

Fnded: 1954. **Mem:** 700. **Lang(s):** English. **Desc:** Represents the interests of doctors and their patients in the differing spheres of professional activity at a national and international level.

★ 4440 ★ Medical Association of Thailand
3 Silom St.
Bangkok, Thailand

Fnded: 1921.

★ 4441 ★ Medical Benevolence Foundation (MBF)
PO Box 671226
Houston, TX 77267-1226
Free: 800-547-7627
Website: http://www.mbfoundation.org/
Jane L. Grant, Pres.

Desc: Medical mission providing support for medical personnel, as well as equipment and financial aid to hospitals, medical outposts and clinics outside the U.S. **Pub:** *Mission Connection*. Newsletter.

★ 4442 ★ Medical Council of India
Aiwan-e-Galib Marg
Kotla Rd.
New Delhi 110 002, India
Phone: 91 11 23232618 **Fax:** 91 11 23236604
Email: mci@del3.vsnl.net.in
Website: http://www.mciindia.org/

Fnded: 1933.

★ 4443 ★ Medical Defence Union (MDU)
230 Blackfriars Rd.
London SE1 8PJ, United Kingdom
Phone: 44 20 72021500 **Fax:** 44 20 72021667
Email: mdu@the-mdu.com
Website: http://www.the-mdu.com

Fnded: 1885.

★ 4444 ★ Medical Education for South African Blacks (MESAB)
120 Albany St., Ste. 810
New Brunswick, NJ 08901-2163
Phone: (732)745-1292 **Fax:** (732)745-9794
Email: mesab@mesab.org
Website: http://www.mesab.org/
James W. Scott, Pres.

Fnded: 1985. **Desc:** Supports the training of South African black health professionals to bring better health care to all South Africans. Provides scholarships for black students in the health professions at South African universities. Develops health-related training programs, rural outreach programs, and offers scholarship support for nurses enrolled in university-level nursing programs. **Pub:** *Annual Report*. • *MESAB News*, 1-2/year. Newsletter. Includes information about the organization and its programs. *Price:* Free.

★ 4445 ★ Medical Fitness Association
PO Box 73103
Richmond, VA 23235-8026
Phone: (804)327-0330 **Fax:** (804)327-1630
Email: mfacomm@aol.com
Website: http://medicalfitness.org
Cary Wing, EdD, Exec. Dir.

Fnded: 1991. **Mem:** 450. **Desc:** Hospitals, organizations, and medically based fitness and wellness center professionals. Seeks to reduce community health care costs through preventive care. Promotes strengthened operations and standards in fitness centers maintained by hospitals and organizations; works to improve the financial viability of fitness facilities. Serves as a network linking fitness professionals and facilities. Conducts research and educational programs; compiles statistics. **Pub:** *Medical Fitness Centers, 4th Edition*, biennial. Directory. Comprehensive Listing/Profile of Medical Fitness Centers In North America. *Price:* $295. • *Re:Source, Journal of the Medical Fitness Association*, quarterly. Journal. Contains industry news, center profiles, and programming ideas. **Frmly:** (1998) Association of Hospital Health and Fitness.

★ 4446 ★ Medical Foundation
Edward Ford Bldg., A27
University of Sydney
Sydney, NSW 2006, Australia
Phone: 61 2 93517315 **Fax:** 61 2 93513299
Email: medfdn@med.usud.edu.au
Website: http://www.medicalfoundation.usyd.edu.au

Fnded: 1958. **Desc:** Aims to improve the health of Australians of all ages. **Pub:** Annual Report.

★ 4447 ★ Medical Foundation for AIDS and Sexual Health
BMA House
Tavistock Sq.
London WC1H 9JP, United Kingdom
Phone: 44 20 73836345 **Fax:** 44 20 73882544
Email: enquiries.medfash@medfash.bma.org.uk
Website: http://www.medfash.org.uk

Desc: Works with policy-makers and health professional to promote excellence in the prevention and management of HIV and other sexually transmitted infections. Develops materials to support health professionals. **Pub:** *Standards for NHS Hospital HIV services*. Report. • *Take the HIV Test*. Pamphlet.

★ 4448 ★ Medical Group Management Association (MGMA)
104 Inverness Terr. E
Englewood, CO 80112-5306
Phone: (303)799-1111 **Free:** 877-275-6462
Fax: (303)643-4439
Email: infocenter@mgma.com
Website: http://www.mgma.com
William F. Jessee, MD, CEO

Fnded: 1926. **Mem:** 18,000. **Nat'l Groups:** 1. **Reg. Groups:** 4. **Desc:** For professionals involved in the business management of groups in medical practice. Products and services include education, benchmarking, surveys, national advocacy and networking opportunities for members. **Pub:** *Academic Practice Faculty Compensation and Production Survey Report*, annual. Report. A census of academic clinical science Departments designed to assist Department admins. in evaluating the scope of compensation and production of med. school fac. *Price:* $225/copy for members; $275/copy for affiliates; $375/copy for nonmembers. • *Academic Practice Management Compensation Survey Report*, annual. Report. A census of academic clinical science Departments and practice plans designed to provide comparative Information to academic medical practices and others. *Price:* $90/copy for members; $120/copy for affiliates; $150/copy for nonmembers. • *Ambulatory Surgery Center Performance Survey Report*, annual. Report. Provides comparative measures to assess annual ambulatory surgery center (ASC) financial and operational results. *Price:* $90/copy for members; $120/copy for affiliates; $150/copy for nonmembers. • *Cost Survey Report*, annual. Report. Covers every facet of medical group operating costs, bring over- and under-spending into sharp relief, enabling readers to right-size their practice. *Price:* $240/copy for members; $290/copy for affiliates; $450/copy for nonmembers. • *Management Services Organization Performance Survey Report*, annual. Report. Provides comparative measures useful in benchmarking annual MSO corporate financial and operational results. *Price:* $240/copy for members; $290/copy for affiliates; $450/copy for nonmembers. • *Physician Compensation and Production Survey*, annual. Report. **Frmly:** (1946) Association of Clinic Managers; (1963) National Association of Clinical Managers.

★ 4449 ★ Medical and Health Workers Union of Nigeria
PO Box 563
Lagos, Nigeria
Phone: 234 1 832274

★ 4450 ★ Medical Information Bureau (MIB)
PO Box 105, Essex Sta.
Boston, MA 02112
Phone: (781)329-4500
Email: infoline@mib.com
Website: http://www.mib.com
James F. Cook, Pres.

Fnded: 1902. **Mem:** 750. **Desc:** Life, health, and disability insurance companies. Seeks to reduce insurance fraud by providing member companies with information previous claims.

★ 4451 ★ Medical Letter (ML)
1000 Main St.
New Rochelle, NY 10801
Phone: (914)235-0500 **Free:** 800-211-2769
Fax: (914)632-1733
Email: custserv@themedicalletter.org
Website: http://www.medletter.com
Mark Abramowicz, MD, Ed.

Fnded: 1959. **Desc:** Gathers and publishes information on the therapeutic and side effects of drugs for the benefit of physicians and other members of the health professions. Emphasis is on new drugs. **Pub:** *Advice for Travelers*, semiannual. Provides quick access to information about specific countries, diseases and travel-related risks. *Price:* $139 20% discount for renewals. • *Handbook of Antimicrobial Therapy*. Handbook. • *Medical Letter: A Searchable Collection on CD-ROM*, annual. Permits users to quickly access, search and print articles. *Price:* $65. • *Medical Letter Handbook of Adverse Drug Interactions*. Handbook. *Price:* $22; $12 for members. • *Medical Letter on Drugs and Therapeutics*, biweekly. Newsletter. Evaluates drugs for physicians. *Price:* $49/year. **Frmly:** Drug and Therapeutic Information.

★ 4452 ★ Medical Mycological Society of the Americas (MMSA)
c/o Dr. James Harris
2501 Timberline Dr.
Austin, TX 78746
Phone: (512)458-7566 **Fax:** (512)458-7697
Email: jim.harris@tdh.state.tx.us
Dr. James L. Harris, Sec. Treas.

Fnded: 1966. **Mem:** 300. **Desc:** Medical professionals interested in fungi and fungal diseases. Seeks to exchange professional information; promotes continuing education in medical mycology in association with American Society for Microbiology. **Pub:** Bulletin, quarterly. • Directory, periodic.

★ 4453 ★ Medical Officers of Schools Association
21 St. Botorpa's Rd.
Sevenoaks TN13 3AQ, United Kingdom
Phone: 44 1732 459255 **Fax:** 44 1732 750586
Website: http://www.mosa.org.uk

Fnded: 1884. **Mem:** 440. **Desc:** School doctors and doctors with an interest in the health of the school child. To represent school doctors and those doctors with an interest in the health of the school child; to provide an advisory service for members, and nonmembers, on any aspect of school medicine. **Pub:** *Handbook of School Health*, quarterly. Handbook. • Newsletter, quarterly. • Report, annual.

★ 4454 ★ Medical Outcomes Trust
198 Tremont St., No. 503
Boston, MA 02116
Phone: (617)426-4046 **Fax:** (617)523-7322
Email: info@outcomes-trust.org
Website: http://www.outcomes-trust.org/

Fnded: 1992. **Desc:** Works to advance universal adoption of health outcomes assessment in health care to improve value of health care services.

★ 4455 ★ Medical Protection Society (MPS)
33 Cavendish Sq.
London W1G 0PS, United Kingdom
Phone: 44 207 3991300 **Fax:** 44 207 3991301
Email: info@mps.org.uk
Website: http://www.mps.org.uk/

Lang(s): English. **Desc:** Physicians, dentists, and other health care professionals. Seeks to assist members in protecting themselves from patient complaints and litigation. Provides technical and customer service assistance to members in matters involving disputes and litigation arising from patient care. Represents members before health boards, hospital inquiries, and other professional conduct or competence proceedings. Makes available legal and ethical advice to members.

★ 4456 ★ Medical Records Institute (MRI)
255 Washington St., Ste. 180
PO Box 600770
Newton, MA 02458
Phone: (617)964-3923 **Fax:** (617)964-3926
Email: cust_service@medrecinst.com
Website: http://www.medrecinst.com
C. Peter Waegemann, Exec. Dir.

Fnded: 1979. **Desc:** Conducts research and education in the fields of medical documentation and computerization of patient information. Maintains committees and network groups. Compiles statistics. **Pub:** *Handbook of Optical Memory Systems*. Handbook. Monthly updates available. *Price:* $100.50. • *Toward An Electronic Patient Record*, 10/year. *Price:* $145. • Proceedings. **Frmly:** (1988) Institute for Medical Record Economics.

★ 4457 ★ Medical Research Modernization Committee (MRMC)
PO Box 201791
Cleveland, OH 44120
Phone: (216)283-6702 **Fax:** (216)283-6702
Email: stkaufman@mindspring.com
Website: http://www.mrmcmed.org
Stephen R. Kaufman, MD, Co-Chair

Fnded: 1987. **Mem:** 1,000. **Desc:** Individuals, primarily scientists and clinicians, who evaluate the medical and/or scientific merit of research modalities in an effort to identify outdated research methods and to promote sensible, reliable, and efficient methods. Represents positions to the public, health care professionals, and government officials. Maintains speakers' bureau; distributes literature to the public. **Pub:** *A Critical Look at Animal Experimentation*, annual. Booklet. *Price:* Free to members; $1/copy for nonmembers. • *MRMC Report*, quarterly. Newsletter. *Price:* Free to members; $2/copy for nonmembers. • *Perspectives on Medical Research*, annual. Monograph. Includes essays and commentary. *Price:* $10/paperback; $16/hardback.

★ 4458 ★ Medical Research Society (MRS)
c/o Dr. A. Chaudhry, Sec.
Renal Unit, L Block
Hammersmith Hospital
DuCane Rd.
London W12 0NN, United Kingdom
Phone: 44 1438 314333 **Fax:** 44 7092 388555
Email: mrs@dial.pipex.com
Website: http://www.medres.org

Mem: 1,300. **Lang(s):** English. **Desc:** Individuals engaged in basic and clinical medical research. Facilitates interdisciplinary exchange of information and provides a forum for data presentations by biomedical researchers. **Pub:** *Clinical Science*, monthly. • *Clinical Science Abstracts*, semiannual.

★ 4459 ★ Medical Sciences Historical Society
117 Woodland Dr.
Cassiobury
Watford WD17 3DA, United Kingdom

Fnded: 1981. **Mem:** 60. **Desc:** Holds four annual meetings. Publishes two newsletters and a journal. **Pub:** Newsletter, semiannual. • Journal, periodic.

★ 4460 ★ Medical Society of Copenhagen (Det Medicinske Selskab i Copenhagen)
Trondhjemsgade 9
DK-2100 Copenhagen, Denmark
Phone: 45 31380984 **Fax:** 45 35448503

Fnded: 1772.

★ 4461 ★ Medical Society of London
11 Chandos St.
London W1M 0EB, United Kingdom
Phone: 44 20 75801043 **Fax:** 44 20 75805793
Email: mcisoc@telinco.co.uk

Fnded: 1773. **Mem:** 550. **Desc:** Promotes advancement of sciences of medicine. **Pub:** *Transactions of the Medical Society of London*, annual. Journal.

★ 4462 ★ Medical Society for the Study of Venereal Diseases
1 Wimpole St.
London W1M 8AE, United Kingdom
Phone: 44 20 72902968 **Fax:** 44 20 72902989
Email: mssvd@rsm.ac.uk
Website: http://www.mssvd.org.uk

Fnded: 1955.

★ 4463 ★ Medical Women's Federation
Tavistock House N
Tavistock Sq.
London WC1H 9HX, United Kingdom
Phone: 44 20 73877765 **Fax:** 44 20 73889216
Email: admin@mwfonline.org.uk
Website: http://www.mwfonline.org.uk

Fnded: 1917. **Mem:** 1,500. **Local Groups:** 20. **Desc:** Women doctors and medical students. The professional association of women doctors in the UK. **Pub:** *Medical Woman*, 3/year. Newsletter.

★ 4464 ★ Medical Women's International Association (MWIA)
Wilhelm-Brand-Str. 3
D-44141 Dortmund, Germany
Phone: 49 231 9432771 **Fax:** 49 231 9432773
Email: mwia@aol.com
Website: http://www.mwia.net

Fnded: 1919. **Mem:** 14,000. **Nat'l Groups:** 44. **Reg. Groups:** 8. **Lang(s):** English. **Desc:** Women involved in or interested in medicine in 70 countries. Provides women with an opportunity to exchange information about medical problems with worldwide implications; promotes friendship and understanding between women; secures members' cooperation in matters relating to international health. Seeks to encourage women to enter the field of medicine and allied sciences and to overcome discrimination against female physicians. Aids women in developing countries in obtaining fellowships and grants for research and travel; offers information and advice to members visiting other countries. **Pub:** *Congress Report*, triennial. Report. • *MWIA Update*, quarterly. Newsletter. • *Women Physicians of the World*. Book.

★ 4465 ★ MedicAlert Foundation (MAFI)
2323 Colorado Ave.
Turlock, CA 95382
Phone: (209)668-3333 **Free:** 888-633-4298
Fax: (209)669-2495
Email: customer_service@medicalert.org
Website: http://www.medicalert.org
Tanya J. Glazebrook, Pres. /CEO

Fnded: 1956. **Mem:** 4700,000. **Desc:** Medical information service open to all. Computerized, confidential medical file, MedicAlert emblem on pendant or bracelet engraved with primary medical condition and can call collect number to access 24-hour Emergency Response Center. Information is uses to speed diagnosis, accurate treatment and save lives. Conducts continuous public and professional education program. **Pub:** *MedicAlert Foundation*, semiannual. Newsletter.

★ 4466 ★ Medicare Rights Center
1460 Broadway, 17th Fl.
New York, NY 10036-7393
Phone: (212)869-3850 **Fax:** (212)869-3532
Email: info@medicarerights.org
Website: http://www.medicarerights.org
Robert Hayes, Pres.

Fnded: 1989. **Mem:** 29. **Desc:** Seeks to ensure the rights of senior citizens and people with disabilities to quality, affordable health care. Provides counseling services to people with Medicare with health insurance problems and questions; compiles information on inquiries to detect issues and systemic problems in Medicare claims administration. Educates consumers, advocates, providers, and social workers about developments in Medicare law and how to handle problems. Monitors trends and changes in Medicare laws, regulations, and guidelines. **Pub:** *"Lets Learn Medicare!" Training and Reference Manual.* A sense of Medicare educational materials for consumers and professionals. *Price:* $150 plus shipping and handling $15.00. • *The Medicare Survival Kit: Medicare Answers.* A sense of Medicare educational materials for consumers and professionals. *Price:* $25 plus shipping and handling $6.00. **Frmly:** (1997) Medicare Beneficiaries Defense Fund.

★ 4467 ★ Melpomene Institute
1010 University Ave.
Saint Paul, MN 55104
Phone: (651)642-1951 **Fax:** (651)642-1871
Email: health@melpomene.org
Website: http://www.melpomene.org
Anne Dimock, Pres. & CEO

Fnded: 1982. **Mem:** 1,350. **Desc:** Individuals professionally trained in healthcare, physical activity, and sports for girls and women. Conducts research and disseminates information on issues such as body image, osteoporosis, athletic amenorrhea, exercise and pregnancy, and aging. Offers undergraduate and graduate internships, and volunteer programs. Provides consulting services for program evaluations. Operates speakers' bureau. **Pub:** *The Bodywise Woman.* Book. Provides information for women on physical activity and health. *Price:* $16.95. • *Breast Cancer: A Handbook.* Book. • *Heroes: Growing Up Female and Strong.* Video. Concerns self-esteem in adolescent girls. *Price:* $19.95; $29.95 curriculum. • *HRT: Is It For Me?.* Booklet. Helps individuals make a more informed decision about Hormone Replacement Therapy. *Price:* $2.50. • *Let's Get Moving.* Booklet. Contains information about physical activity for women over 50. *Price:* $4.50. • *Melpomene Journal,* 3/year. Journal. Examines the relationship between physical activity and lifestyles. Features research reports, scientific bibliographies, and personal profiles. *Price:* Included in membership dues; $5/issue for nonmembers. • *Of Heroes, Hopes and Level Playing Fields.* Book. *Price:* $10. **Frmly:** (2002) Melpomene Institute for Women's Health Research.

★ 4468 ★ Men Against Breast Cancer (MABC)

2379 Lewis Ave.
Rockville, MD 20851-2335
Free: (866)547-6222 **Fax:** (301)770-5697
Email: info@menagainstbreastcancer.org
Website: http://www.menagainstbreastcancer.org/
Marc Heyison, Pres. /Co-Founder

Desc: Strives to eradicate breast cancer as a life-threatening disease by mobilizing and supporting men as active participants in the fight against the disease.

★ 4469 ★ Mended Hearts (MH)

7272 Greenville Ave.
Dallas, TX 75231-4596
Phone: (214)706-1442 **Free:** 888-HEART-99
Fax: (214)706-5231
Email: info@mendedhearts.org
Website: http://www.mendedhearts.org
Cathy Clapp, Exec. Asst.

Fnded: 1951. **Mem:** 25,000. **Local Groups:** 200. **Desc:** Persons who have heart disease; their families and friends. Works to: provide advice, encouragement, and services to heart disease patients and to their families; establish programs of assistance to surgeons, physicians, and hospitals. Conducts and assists in research programs designed to benefit heart patients. **Pub:** *Heartbeat,* quarterly. Magazine. **Frmly:** (1955) Mended Hearts Club.

★ 4470 ★ Meniere's Network (MN)

1817 Patterson St.
Nashville, TN 37203
Phone: (615)627-2724 **Free:** 800-545-HEAR
Fax: (615)627-2728
Email: ear@earfoundation.org
Bridget Lippard, Exec. Dir.

Fnded: 1987. **Mem:** 1,500. **Desc:** Persons suffering from Meniere's disease, an inner ear disorder of unknown cause that results in vertigo, tinnitus, and hearing fluctuation or loss. Seeks to develop a network of peer support groups to help integrate hearing- and balance-impaired people into mainstream society. Operates pen pals and "phone buddies" services; offers educational programs and materials. **Pub:** *A Dietary Guidebook for Meniere's Disease; An Introduction to Meniere's Disease; Meniere's Disease-Coping Skills.* Booklets. *Price:* $6.50 pack of 3. • *Steady,* quarterly. Newsletter. Provides medical information and lists selfhelp support groups, pen pals, "phone buddies" and "email buddies". *Price:* $25.

★ 4471 ★ Mental After Care Association (MACA)

Lincoln House, 1st Fl.
296-302 High Holborn
London WC1V 7JH, United Kingdom
Phone: 44 20 70613400 **Fax:** 44 20 70613401
Email: maca@maca.org.uk
Website: http://www.maca.org.uk

Fnded: 1879. **Mem:** 100. **Reg. Groups:** 3. **Lang(s):** English. **Desc:** MACA is a leading mental health charity providing high quality services in the community, hospitals and prisons. With more than 90 services throughout the country, we support more than 1,500 people with severe and enduring mental health needs and their carers. We work in partnership with health authorities, local authorities, housing associations and other voluntary agencies. **Pub:** *Annual Report.* • Pamphlets, periodic.

★ 4472 ★ Mental Health Corp.s of America (MHCA)

1876-A Elder Ct.
Tallahassee, FL 32308
Phone: (850)942-4900
Email: twilliams@mhca.com
Website: http://www.mhca.com/2WhatIsMHCA.htm

Desc: Behavioral healthcare organizations. Strives to enhance the business performance of members, while preserving its social mission.

★ 4473 ★ Mental Health Foundation

83 Victoria St., 7th Fl.
London SW1H 0HW, United Kingdom
Phone: 44 207 8020300 **Fax:** 44 207 8020301
Email: mhf@mhf.org.uk
Website: http://www.mentalhealth.org.uk

Fnded: 1949. **Desc:** Plays a vital role in pioneering new approaches to prevention, treatment and care. Allocates grants for research and community projects, contributes to public debate and strives to reduce the stigma attached to mental illness and learning disabilities.

★ 4474 ★ Mental Health Ireland

Mensana House
6 Adelaide St.
Dun Laoghaire, Dublin, Ireland
Phone: 353 1 2841166 **Fax:** 353 1 2841736
Email: mhai@iol.ie
Website: http://www.mentalhealthireland.ie

Local Groups: 90. **Lang(s):** English. **Desc:** Seeks to help those who are mentally ill and to promote positive mental health in Ireland. Works to provide various types of accommodation outside the hospital, to set-up workshops, to visit and befriend those affected, and to arrange social events.

★ 4475 ★ Mental Health Media

356 Holloway Rd.
London N7 6PA, United Kingdom
Phone: 44 20 77008171 **Fax:** 44 20 76860959
Email: info@mhmedia.com
Website: http://www.mhmedia.com

Fnded: 1965. **Lang(s):** German. **Desc:** Specializes in the use of the full range of communications media to promote understanding of mental health or learning difficulties issues from a user perspective in order to reduce discrimination and prejudice. Operates a media bureau, which supports mental health service users in working with journalists, writers, and broadcasters to improve their coverage of mental health issues. Also acts as a production house for a full range of information publications, including videos and CDs, about mental health and learning difficulties issues from the user perspective. **Frmly:** Mental Health Film Council; (1996) Mental Health Media Council.

★ 4476 ★ Mental Research Institute (MRI)

555 Middlefield Rd.
Palo Alto, CA 94301
Phone: (650)321-3055 **Fax:** (650)321-3785
Email: mri@mri.org
Website: http://www.mri.org
Wendel Ray, Dir.

Fnded: 1959. **Desc:** Psychiatrists, psychologists, and licensed therapists skilled in the disciplines related to the behavioral sciences. Conducts research, training, and service programs in the field of human behavior, with special emphasis on the family as a social unit. Research programs are primarily funded by foundation grants and private donations. Offers short-term residency programs, and short- and long-term workshops on family therapy, brief therapy, communication, and related subjects. Operates family-oriented and brief therapy-oriented sliding scale fee clinic, which also serves as a training and research base. Maintains speakers' bureau. Current research programs focus on longitudinal study of families of alcoholics, youth, violence, bullying, and pain management.

★ 4477 ★ Mercy Ships International Operations Center

PO Box 2020
Garden Valley, TX 75771-2020
Phone: (903)939-7000 **Free:** 800-MERCYSHIPS
Fax: (903)882-0336
Email: info@mercyships.org
Website: http://www.mercyships.org

Desc: Working to bring physical and spiritual healing to the poor and needy in port cities around the world.

★ 4478 ★ Metamorphic Association

PO Box 32368
London SW17 8YB, United Kingdom
Phone: 44 870 7707984
Website: http://www.metamorphicassociation.org.uk

Fnded: 1979. **Mem:** 200. **Lang(s):** French, German, Italian, Spanish. **Desc:** Promotion of good health and well-being through awareness, understanding and use of Metamorphic Technique in the UK and internationally, and to uphold standards and procedures and teaching the technique. **Pub:** *The Programme,* semiannual. Newsletter. Listing of practioners and teachers: details of courses and events, publication list.

★ 4479 ★ Mexican Academy of Dermatology (MAD) (Academia Mexicana de Dermatologia — AMD)

c/o Dr. Javier Ruiz-Avila
Georgia 114-503
Colonia Napoles
03810 Mexico City, DF, Mexico
Phone: 52 56 822545 **Fax:** 52 56 828963
Email: jraderma@yahoo.com
Website: http://www.amd.org.mx

Fnded: 1952. **Mem:** 300. **Nat'l Groups:** 1. **Reg. Groups:** 3. **Lang(s):** English, Spanish. **Desc:** Provides continuing medical education programs to members. Offers support to dermatology residents. **Pub:** *Dermatologia-Revista Mexicana,* monthly. Journal.

★ 4480 ★ Mexican Association for Promoting Kidney Transplant (Asociacio Mexicana Protransplante Renal — AMPRAC)

Yacatas 387
Col. Navarte
03020 Mexico City, Mexico
Phone: 52 55 435946 **Fax:** 52 55 432818

Fnded: 1997. **Desc:** Offers support to kidney patients and their families. Promotes organ donation. Disseminates information.

★ 4481 ★ Mexican Family Planning Association (MEXFAM) (Fundacion Mexicaca para la Planeacion Familiar)

Juarez 208
Tlalpan
14000 Mexico City, DF, Mexico

Phone: 52 55 54870030 **Fax:** 52 55 54870042
Email: mexinfo@mexfam.org.mx
Website: http://www.mexfam.org.mx

Lang(s): Spanish. **Desc:** Promotes responsible parenthood and family planning. Advocates family planning as a basic human right. Works to reduce the number of unwanted pregnancies and abortions. Encourages public awareness of family planning, contraception, and sexually transmitted diseases. Offers educational programs for teens and adults. Acts as an advocate for family planning on a national level. Conducts research.

★ 4482 ★ Mexican Society of Psychology (Sociedad Mexicana de Psicologia)

Indiana No 260-608, Col Napoles, Del Benito Juarez
03710 Mexico City, DF, Mexico
Phone: 52 55989566 **Fax:** 52 55636162
Email: sociedad@psicologia.org.mx
Website: http://www.psicologia.org.mx

Fnded: 1950.

★ 4483 ★ MHE Coalition

8838 Holly Lane
Olmsted Falls, OH 44138
Phone: (440)235-6325 **Fax:** (440)427-9032
Email: CheleZ1@aol.com
Website: http://www.geocities.com/mhecoalition
Chele Zelina, Pres.

Mem: 275. **Desc:** Support group for individuals and families affected by Multiple Hereditary Exostoses, encouraging research and services. **Pub:** *MHE Coalition Newsletter*, quarterly. Newsletter.

★ 4484 ★ Michael E. DeBakey International Surgical Society (MEDISS)

c/o Kenneth L. Mattox
1 Baylor Plz.
Department of Surgery
Houston, TX 77030
Phone: (713)798-4557 **Fax:** (713)796-9605
Email: mediss@aol.com
Website: http://www.debakeysoc.org/home.html
Kenneth L. Mattox, Sec. -Treas.

Fnded: 1976. **Mem:** 640. **Desc:** Physicians organized to encourage, advance, and promote scientific research relating to the treatment of general vascular, cardiac and cardiovascular defects and diseases through general vascular and cardiovascular surgery. **Frmly:** (1983) Michael E. DeBakey International Cardiovascular Society.

★ 4485 ★ Michael Fund (International Foundation for Genetic Research) (MF-IFGR)

4371 Northern Pike
Monroeville, PA 15146-2837
Phone: (412)374-0111
Email: randy@michaelfund.org
Website: http://www.michaelfund.org
Randy Engel, Exec. Dir.

Fnded: 1978. **Desc:** Intertwines the funding of scientific research on Down's Syndrome and related genetic disorders with a pro-life philosophy. Supports research on prevention, cure, or reduction of the effects of Down's Syndrome; enlists support from professionals; and advocates working in this field. Opposes intrauterine detection and abortion of the affected unborn as well as deliberate euthanasia of children and adults with birth defects. Aims to make research findings available to others conducting similar research and to advocate and encourage efforts to improve the care, treatment, education, evaluation and habilitation of children and adults with mental and physical handicaps, to the benefit of their families and communities. **Pub:** *Friends of the Michael Fund Newsletter*, semiannual. Newsletter. Contains topics on eugenics, genetics, prenatal diagnosis. *Price:* Donation.

★ 4486 ★ Microcirculatory Society (MCS)

Department of Veterinary and Biomedical Sciences
University of Missouri
Columbia, MO 65211
Phone: (573)882-7012
Email: gore@u.arizona.edu
Website: http://microcirc.org/
Dr. Robert W. Gore, Contact

Fnded: 1955. **Mem:** 450. **Desc:** Encourages the exchange and dissemination of information on microcirculation. **Pub:** *Microcirculatory Society Directory*, annual. Membership Directory. • *Microcirculatory Society Newsletter*, 3/year. Newsletter.

★ 4487 ★ Microsoft Healthcare Users Group (MS-HUG)

3300 Washtenaw Ave.
Ann Arbor, MI 48104
Phone: (734)973-1995 **Fax:** (734)973-1996
Email: kmalecki@ic.net
Website: http://www.mshug.org
Sue Dressel, Exec. Dir.

Desc: Forum for the exchange of ideas. Promotes learning, and sharing solutions for information systems using Microsoft technologies. "Works to provide industry leadership, drive appropriate standards and develop associated requirements in support of healthcare solutions."

★ 4488 ★ Mid-Atlantic States Association of Avian Veterinarians (MASAAV)

Memorial Bldg., Ste. 291
610 N Main St.
Blacksburg, VA 24060-3311
Phone: (540)951-2559 **Fax:** (540)953-0230
Email: office@masaav.org
Website: http://www.masaav.org
Keath L. Marx, DVM, Exec. Dir.

Fnded: 1979. **Mem:** 200. **Reg. Groups:** 1. **State Groups:** 9. **Desc:** Works to address the needs of the avian veterinarian and technicians. innovative veterinary medicine and surgery to improve the health of avian patients. Conducts educational programs; makes donations for avian research; keeps members informed regarding legislation of interest to the profession. **Pub:** *Conference Proceedings Book*, annual. Book. Annual conference, avian medicine and surgery. *Price:* $40; $56 overseas air. • *MASAAV Veterinary Directory for Pet Stores*, annual. Directory. • *MASAAView*, 3/year. Newsletter.

★ 4489 ★ Midwest Parentcraft Center (MPC)

5525 W Henderson
Chicago, IL 60641
Phone: (773)725-7767
Margaret Gamper, R.N., Exec. Dir.

Fnded: 1950. **Desc:** Prenatal instructors, parents, and professionals involved in parenting and pregnancy. To instruct and educate expectant mothers and others in the Gamper Method of childbirth. (The Gamper Method, based on the teachings of several 19th century physicians and developed by Margaret Gamper in 1946, is designed to prepare the prospective mother for childbirth by instilling self-determination and confidence in her ability to work with the physiological changes of her body during pregnancy, labor, and delivery.) Conducts prenatal and grandparenting classes and workshops; operates in-service programs for hospitals and clinics; sponsors programs on topics such as grieving and history of birth procedures. Disseminates teaching aids including slides, films, records, and tapes. Grants childbirth educator certificates to qualified applicants who have taught Gamper Method classes under the supervision of an instructor. Operates charitable program and speakers' bureau; maintains library of 6000 volumes on childbirth, midwifery, marriage, sex, and childcare. The center's activities are currently concentrated in Ohio, Illinois, Indiana, Wisconsin, and Michigan. **Pub:** *Heir Raising News*, quarterly. • *Preparation for the Heir Minded.*

★ 4490 ★ Midwestern Psychological Association (MPA)

c/o Ralph Erber
DePaul University
Department of Psychology
2219 N Kenmore
Chicago, IL 60614
Website: http://www.ssc.msu.edu/~mpa/

Mem: 3,000. **Desc:** Psychological association, with interests in the physiology of vision to social stereotyping, from political psychology to medical psychology, from organizational behavior to children's language development, from memory to depression, from sex roles to drug addiction.

★ 4491 ★ Midwives Alliance of North America (MANA)

4805 Lawrenceville Hwy., No. 116-279
Lilburn, GA 30047
Free: 888-923-6262 **Fax:** (801)720-3026
Email: info@mana.org
Website: http://www.mana.org
Diane Holzer, Pres.

Fnded: 1982. **Mem:** 1,000. **Reg. Groups:** 10. **Desc:** Midwives, student/apprentice midwives, and persons supportive of midwifery. Seeks to expand communication and support among midwives. Works to promote basic competency in midwives; develops and encourages guidelines for their education. Offers legal, legislative, and political information and resource referrals; conducts networking on local, state, and regional bases; compiles statistics. **Pub:** *MANA News*, bimonthly. • Brochures. • Also publishes information packets.

★ 4492 ★ Midwives Information and Resource Service (MIDIRS)

9 Elmdale Rd.
Clifton
Bristol BS8 1SL, United Kingdom
Phone: 44 117 9251791 **Fax:** 44 117 9251792
Email: sales@midirs.org
Website: http://www.midirs.org

Fnded: 1983. **Mem:** 14,000. **Lang(s):** English. **Desc:** Provides information for midwives and nurses who want to keep up-to-date with contemporary knowledge and thinking in the world of midwifery care, women's health, and care of new borns. Offers articles, books, and other information concerning midwifery. Conducts educational programs. **Pub:** *Directory of Maternity Organisations*, periodic. Directory. • *MIDIRS Midwifery Digest*, quarterly.

★ 4493 ★ Migraine Action Association

Oakley Hay Lodge Business Park, Unit 6
Great Folds Rd.
Great Oakley NN18 9AS, United Kingdom
Phone: 44 1536 461333 **Fax:** 44 1536 461444
Email: info@migraine.org.uk
Website: http://www.migraine.org.uk

Fnded: 1958. **Mem:** 17,000. **Desc:** Migraine sufferers, their families and friends, or anyone else who is interested, including medical professionals. Support for research into aspects of migraine, grants, information, understanding and encouragement to migraine sufferers. **Pub:** *Migraine Action News*, quarterly. Newsletter. • *The Migraine Handbook*. Handbook. **Frmly:** (1997) British Migraine Association.

★ 4494 ★ Migraine Association of Ireland

Senior House
All Hallows College
Gracepark Rd.
Drumcondra
Dublin 9, Ireland
Phone: 353 1 8064121 **Fax:** 353 1 8064122
Email: info@migraine.ie
Website: http://www.migraine.ie

Fnded: 1994. **Mem:** 1,700. **Nat'l Groups:** 1. **Reg. Groups:** 1. **State Groups:** 1. **Lang(s):** English. **Desc:** Seeks to share information and provide support for those affected by chronic migraine headaches in

Ireland. Encourages medical research; lobbies for a national headache/migraine specialist clinic in Ireland; maintains relationships with other related societies and associations. **Pub:** *Migraine Association of Ireland*, 3/year. Newsletter. Features information on migraine.

★ 4495 ★ Migraine Awareness Group: A National Understanding for "Migraineurs" (MAGNUM)

113 S Saint Asaph, Ste. 300
Alexandria, VA 22314
Phone: (703)739-9384 **Fax:** (703)739-2432
Email: magnumnonprofit@hotmail.com
Website: http://www.migraines.org
Michael John Coleman, Exec. V. P.

Fnded: 1994. **Desc:** Works to bring public and governmental awareness to the medical seriousness of the migraine disease. Provides information and support to migraine sufferers and their families.

★ 4496 ★ Milton H. Erickson Foundation (MHEF)

3606 N 24th St.
Phoenix, AZ 85016
Phone: (602)956-6196 **Fax:** (602)956-0519
Email: office@erickson-foundation.org
Website: http://www.erickson-foundation.org
Jeffrey K. Zeig, Dir.

Fnded: 1979. **Desc:** Seeks to promote and advance the contributions made to health sciences by Milton H. Erickson, M.D. (1901-1980), regarded as an authority on hypnotherapy and brief strategic therapy. Dedicated to the training of health and restricted to mental health professionals. **Pub:** *A Teaching Seminar with Milton H. Erickson, M.D.*. Book. Transcript with commentary of a one-week teaching seminar. • *Ericksonian Methods: The Essence of the Story.* Book. • *Ericksonian Monographs*, up to 3/year. Monographs. Contains selected articles on Ericksonian hypnosis and psychotherapy, including technique, theory, and research topics. • *M.H. Erickson Foundation Newsletter*, 3/year. Newsletter. Contains articles and notices relating to Ericksonian approaches to psychotherapy and hypnosis. *Price:* Optional donation, available to professionals. • *The Process of Hypnotic Induction: A Training Videotape Featuring Inductions Conducted by Milton H. Erickson in 1964.* Video. Discusses the process and describes the microdynamics of Erickson's techniques. • *Symbolic Hypnotherapy.* Video. Presents information regarding the use of symbols in psychotherapy and hypnosis. • *What Is Psychotherapy?: Contemporary Perspectives.* Book. Contains edited commentaries of eminent clinicians.

★ 4497 ★ Milton Helpern Institute of Forensic Medicine (MHIFM)

520 1st Ave.
New York, NY 10016
Phone: (212)447-2030 **Fax:** (212)447-2716
Dr. Charles S. Hirsch, Chief Med. Exam.

Fnded: 1968. **Mem:** 405. **Desc:** Operated by New York University and the city of New York to strengthen teaching and research in forensic medicine and forensic pathology. Trains postgraduate students; sponsors symposia, seminars, lectures, and courses; conducts research projects and undertakes investigations and related studies of sudden, suspicious, and violent deaths. Maintains Milton Helpern Library of Legal Medicine. **Frmly:** (1978) Institute of Forensic Medicine.

★ 4498 ★ MIND - Mental Health Charity

Granta House
15-19 Broadway
London E15 4BQ, United Kingdom
Phone: 44 20 85192122 **Fax:** 44 20 85221725
Email: contact@mind.org.uk

Fnded: 1948. **Mem:** 1,700. **Local Groups:** 208. **Lang(s):** English. **Desc:** Promotes mental health and encourages a better understanding of mental health problems. Seeks to eliminate the stigma associated with mental illness. Conducts research; disseminates information. Offers legal referral services. Sponsors charitable program. Maintains information service. Conducts training and educational courses and seminars. **Pub:** *Annual Report.* • *OpenMIND*, bimonthly. Magazine. • *Publications from MIND*, periodic. Catalog.

★ 4499 ★ Miracle Flights for Kids

2756 N Green Valley Pkwy., No. 115
Green Valley, NV 89014-2120
Phone: (702)261-0494 **Free:** 800-FLY-1711
Fax: (702)261-0497
Email: info@miracleflights.org
Website: http://www.miracleflights.org
Ann McGee, Pres.

Fnded: 1985. **Mem:** 500. **Desc:** Provides free air transportation to families who are unable to get to medical treatment centers far from home. **Pub:** Newsletter, quarterly. Includes safety and pilot news, flight updates, fundraising news, news about flights. *Price:* Free. **Frmly:** (1998) The Angel Planes.

★ 4500 ★ Miscarriage Association

c/o Clayton Hospital
Northgate
Wakefield WF1 3JS, United Kingdom
Phone: 44 1924 200799 **Fax:** 44 1924 298834
Email: info@miscarriageassociation.org.uk
Website: http://www.miscarriageassociation.org.uk

Fnded: 1982. **Mem:** 1,400. **Reg. Groups:** 50. **Lang(s):** English. **Desc:** Provides support and information for all on the subject of pregnancy loss. Gathers information about causes and treatments and promote good practice in the way pregnancy loss is managed in hospitals and in the community. **Pub:** Newsletter, quarterly.

★ 4501 ★ Miscarriage Association of Ireland

Carmichael Centre
N Brunswick St.
Dublin, Ireland
Phone: 353 1 8735702 **Fax:** 353 1 8735737
Website: http://www.coombe.ie/mai

Lang(s): English. **Desc:** Seeks to provide support to women (and men) who are dealing with miscarriage. **Pub:** Newsletter, semiannual.

★ 4502 ★ Miscarriage Infant Death Stillbirth Support Group (MIDS)

c/o Janet Tischler
180 Jillian Blvd.
Parsippany, NJ 07054-3444
Phone: (973)884-0061 **Fax:** (973)884-0062
Email: mids1982@yahoo.com
Website: http://www.kumc.edu/gec/support/miscarri.html
Janet Tischler, Founder/Pres.

Fnded: 1982. **Mem:** 700. **State Groups:** 2. **Local Groups:** 4. **Desc:** Offers friendship and support to parents who have experienced miscarriage, infant death, or stillbirth. Provides monthly meetings, friendships, in-hospital visits, workshops, and speakers. **Pub:** *MIDS Newsletter*, 4/year. Newsletter. *Price:* $18/year. • Brochure.

★ 4503 ★ Mitochondria Research Society (MRS)

c/o Keshav K. Singh
Johns Hopkins Oncology Center
School of Medicine
Bunting-Blaustein Cancer Research Bldg.
1650 Orleans St., Rm. 1-143
Baltimore, MD 21231-1000
Phone: (410)614-5128 **Fax:** (410)502-7234
Email: singhke@jhmi.edu
Website: http://www.mitoresearch.org
Keshav K. Singh, PhD, Contact

Desc: Scientists and physicians. Committed to finding a cure for mitochondrial diseases; promotes research on basic science of mitochondria, mitorchonrial pathogenesis, prevention, diagnosis and treatment throughout the world; fosters public education, training and provides a platform for communication and dissemination of knowledge among scientists, physicians and others interested in mitochondria. **Pub:** *Mitochondria Matters*, semiannual. Newsletter. Includes highlights of research, products, new developments in prevention, diagnosis and treatment of diseases associated with mitochondria. *Price:* included in membership dues. • *Mitochondrion.* Journal. *Price:* included in membership dues.

★ 4504 ★ Mobility International USA (MIUSA)

PO Box 10767
Eugene, OR 97440
Phone: (541)343-1284 **Fax:** (541)343-6812
Email: info@miusa.org
Website: http://www.miusa.org
Susan Sygall, Exec. Dir.

Fnded: 1981. **Mem:** 300. **Desc:** Strives to empower people with disabilities through international exchange opportunities. Organizes international exchange programs annually. Provides information on the range of international exchange opportunities available including work, study, research, and volunteering. Also provides information to international exchange organizations on accessibility, homestays, recruiting and inclusion in international development programs. **Pub:** *A World Awaits You: A Journal of Success of People with Disabilities in International Exchange.* Journal. *Price:* Free. • *A World of Options: A Guide to International Educational Exchange, Community Service, and Travel for Persons with Disabilities.* Book. *Price:* $35/individuals; $45/organizations. • *All Abroad!.* Video. Available with or without audio description and with captions. For People with Disabilities Interested in International Exchange. *Price:* $40 for members; $49 for nonmembers. • *Building Bridges: A Manual on Including People w/Disabilities in International Exchange Programs.* Manual. *Price:* $20. • *Building Bridges: A Training Video on Including People w/Disabilities in International Exchange Programs.* Video. Available with captions and with or without audio description. *Price:* $40 for members; $49 for nonmembers. • *Emerging Leaders.* Video. Available with or without captions. *Price:* $40 for members; $49 for nonmembers. • *Home Is in the Heart: Recruiting and Accommodating Persons with Disabilities into the Homestay Experience.* Video. Available with captions. *Price:* $40 for members; $49 for nonmembers. • *Loud, Proud and Passionate.* Video. Available with captions. *Price:* $40 for members; $49 for nonmembers. • *Loud, Proud and Passionate Including Women with Disabilities in International Development Programs*, quarterly. Book. Available with captions. *Price:* $18 for members; $25 for nonmembers. • *MIUSA's Global Impact*, semiannual. Newsletter. Also available on audio cassette. *Price:* Included in membership dues; $35/year for individual. • *Sustainable Transport*, semiannual. Available upon request. **Frmly:** (1989) Haitian Development Fund.

★ 4505 ★ Mobilization Against AIDS (MAA)

584 Castro St., No. 416
San Francisco, CA 94114-1465
Phone: (415)863-4676 **Fax:** (415)863-4740
Phillip Machingura, Prog. Asst.

Fnded: 1984. **Mem:** 1,000. **Local Groups:** 1. **Desc:** Individuals supporting increased government expenditure on AIDS research, treatment, and social services. Purposes are to: lobby Congress, the Food and Drug Administration, and the National Institutes of Health to provide support and funding to AIDS organizations; mobilize people into public expressions of support for persons with AIDS; oppose civil rights attacks on persons with AIDS. Organizes annual International AIDS candlelight vigil, marches, and the Just Sign IT postcard campaign. Provides speakers on the civil rights ramifications of the AIDS crisis. **Pub:** *Action Alert*, quarterly. Newsletter. *Price:* Included in membership. • *International AIDS Candlelight Memorial* and Mobilization. Booklet. **Frmly:** (1987) Mobilization Against AIDS; (1992) National Mobilization Against AIDS.

★ 4506 ★ Model Secondary School for the Deaf (MSSD)
Gallaudet University
800 Florida Ave. NE
Washington, DC 20002
Phone: (202)651-5031 **Fax:** (202)651-5109
Email: michael.peterson@gallaudet.edu
Website: http://clerccenter.gallaudet.edu/mssd/
Michael Peterson, Prog. Mgr.

Fnded: 1969. **Desc:** Authorized under Model Secondary School for the Deaf Act of 1966. An agreement between the Secretary of Health, Education, and Welfare and Gallaudet College provided for the establishment of the school. Operation was initiated in September 1969, with the intent to provide an exemplary program of instruction and construction of a facility which would exhibit excellence in both architecture and design and would include all innovative auditory and visual devices necessary for education of the deaf. The school's primary service area includes deaf residents of the District of Columbia, Maryland, Virginia, West Virginia, Delaware, and Pennsylvania. Students from all other states may also be accepted as space is available. Additional criteria for admission, such as age level, degree of hearing loss, and previous educational attainment are included in the agreement. U **Pub:** *Family Newsletter.* Newsletter. • *LRC Update*, monthly. Newsletter. Library newsletter. *Price:* Free. • *Perspectives.* Magazine. • *Preview.* Magazine. • *SAERIE.* Magazine. Features literary works by students. • Brochures.

★ 4507 ★ Moderation Management (MM)
c/o HRC
22 W 27th St.
New York, NY 10001
Phone: (212)871-0974 **Fax:** (212)213-6582
Email: mm@moderation.org
Website: http://www.moderation.org/

Fnded: NNsi. **Mem:** I,ver. **Desc:** People concerned about their drinking. Behavioral change program and national support group to aid people to reduce drinking and make positive lifestyle changes; empowers individuals to accept responsibility for their actions, whether its moderation or abstinence; promotes early self-recognition of risky drinking behavior.

★ 4508 ★ Moldavian Myopathy Association
Str. Bulgar 24
MD-2001 Kishinev, Moldova
Phone: 373 2 272687
Email: vtonu@mednet.md

Fnded: 1996. **Reg. Groups:** 4. **Desc:** Individuals in Moldova affected by neuromuscular disorders. Provides a forum for support and exchange of information.

★ 4509 ★ Moldavian Society of Cardiology
Moldavian Research Institute of Preventive & Clinical Medici
Cardiology Clinic
N Testemitsanu str. 20
MD-2025 Chisinau, Moldova
Phone: 373 2 727511 **Fax:** 373 2 739586
Email: mpopovici@madnet.md
Website: http://www.escardio.org/society/natsoc/moldavia.htm

Mem: 78. **Desc:** Promotes the study of cardiology in Moldavia.

★ 4510 ★ Moldova Family Planning Association (MFPA)
Armeneasca str. 47, office 68
MD-2005 Chisinau, Moldova
Phone: 373 2 541207 **Fax:** 373 2 541208
Email: fpam@cni.md

Fnded: 1992. **Lang(s):** English, Russian. **Desc:** Promotes population control through family planning. Gathers and disseminates information on family planning and reproductive health.

★ 4511 ★ Moroccan Society of Cardiology
BP 1326
Rabat, Morocco
Phone: 212 767 1549 **Fax:** 212 767 3232
Email: bcardio@arcnet.com.net.ma

Mem: 218. **Desc:** Promotes the study of cardiology in Morroco. **Pub:** *Bulletin de la societe marocaine de cardiology.* Journal.

★ 4512 ★ Moroccan Society for Rheumatology
Service de Rhumatologie B
Hopital el Ayachi CHU Rabat-Sali
Sali, Morocco
Phone: 212 37 781714 **Fax:** 212 37 883327
Email: nhh5@hotmail.com

Fnded: 1980. **Mem:** 150. **Desc:** Promotes interest and understanding of rheumatology in Morocco.

★ 4513 ★ Mothers Supporting Daughters with Breast Cancer (MSDBC)
c/o Charmayne Dierker
21710 Bayshore Rd.
Chestertown, MD 21620
Phone: (410)778-1982 **Fax:** (410)778-1411
Email: msdbc@dmv.com
Website: http://www.mothersdaughters.org
Charmayne Dierker, Pres.

Fnded: 1995. **Desc:** Assists mothers of daughters with breast cancer. Provides basic medical information about breast cancer as a disease and the various treatments that patients may receive. Also offers a local, regional, and national communication network for mothers and daughters. Our main goal is to offer emotional support to mothers of daughters newly-diagnosed with breast cancer. **Pub:** *Daughter's Brochure.* Brochure. Provides information about the difficulties a mother may be experiencing and how to help. *Price:* Free. • *Mother's Handbook.* Handbook. Prepared for mothers who have had a daughter diagnosed with breast cancer. Provides a list of free resources.

★ 4514 ★ Mothers' Voices
165 W 46th St., Ste. 701
New York, NY 10036
Phone: (212)730-2777 **Free:** 888-MVOICES
Fax: (212)730-4378
Email: ch@mvoices.org
Carol Henry, Exec. Dir.

Fnded: 1992. **Reg. Groups:** 5. **Desc:** Only national, grassroots, non-profit organizations mobilizing mothers as AIDS and sexual health educators and advocates. Provides resources for mothers to educate their children regarding sexuality and drug use, and how better understanding can help prevent HIV infection. **Pub:** *Speaking from the Heart*, quarterly. Newsletter.

★ 4515 ★ Motor Neurone Disease Association
PO Box 246
Northampton NN1 2PR, United Kingdom
Phone: 44 1604 250505 **Fax:** 44 1604 638289
Email: enquiries@mndassociation.org
Website: http://www.mndassociation.org

Fnded: 1979. **Mem:** 7,000. **Reg. Groups:** 85. **Local Groups:** 95. **Desc:** Aims to ensure that people affected by MND can secure the care and support needed; funds research into the disease. Services included a national telephone helpline, literature on all aspects of living with MND, free loan of specialist equipment, network of Regional Care Advisors, support groups and limited financial support to those with the disease. **Pub:** *Annual Review*, annual. Booklets. Information leaflets. • *Thumb Print*, quarterly. Magazine.

★ 4516 ★ Motor Neurone Disease Association of Australia
PO Box 359
Unley, SA 5061, Australia
Phone: 61 8 83570245 **Fax:** 61 8 83570265
Email: mndaa@mnd.asn.au
Website: http://home.vicnet.net.au/~mndaust/

Fnded: 1991. **Mem:** 7. **Nat'l Groups:** 7. **Desc:** Promotes interests in motor neurone disease (MND) research among medical and scientific communities and the public in Australia. Offers support services to MND sufferers and their families. Disseminates information about the disease.

★ 4517 ★ Motor Neurone Disease Association of India
40 Kologarh Rd.
St. No. 5
Rajendra Nagar 248 001, Delhi, India
Phone: 91 135 2754487
Email: nickleodeon@sancharnet.in

Fnded: 1993. **Mem:** 180. **Nat'l Groups:** 1. **Reg. Groups:** 1. **Local Groups:** 1. **Lang(s):** English, Hindi. **Desc:** Promotes interest in Motor Neurone Disease (MND) among medical and scientific communities and the public in India. Works as a support group to stimulate improvement in quality of life for people living with MND/ALS throughout the country. Promotes information exchange about the disease; provides counseling and loan of equipment. **Pub:** *MND Newsletter*, biennial. Newsletter. Provides news updates, research and management. Fundraising brochure containing comprehensive and general information on MND/ALS. **Frmly:** (1994) The MND Support Group of India.

★ 4518 ★ Motor Neurone Disease Association of New Zealand
PO Box 2129
Wellington, New Zealand
Phone: 64 4 4735555 **Fax:** 64 4 4735626
Email: mndanz@xtra.co.nz
Website: http://www.mndanz.org.nz

Fnded: 1985. **Local Groups:** 5. **Desc:** Supports people living with Motor Neurone Disease by providing emotional, social and practical support, advocacy, information, and by raising awareness. **Pub:** *MND Newsletter*, quarterly. Newsletter.

★ 4519 ★ Motor Neurone Disease Association of South Africa
PO Box 191
Milnerton 7435, Republic of South Africa
Phone: 27 21 5319744 **Fax:** 27 21 5316222
Email: mndaofsa@global.co.za

Fnded: 1991. **Nat'l Groups:** 2. **Reg. Groups:** 3. **Desc:** Promotes interests in motor neurone disease (MND) research among medical and scientific communities and the public in South Africa. Offers support services to MND sufferers and their families. Disseminates information about the disease. **Pub:** *Thumbs Up*, semiannual. Newsletter.

★ 4520 ★ Motor Neurone Disease Research Institute of Australia
PO Box 23
Canterbury, VIC 3126, Australia
Phone: 61 3 98302122 **Fax:** 61 3 98302228
Email: info@mndresearch.asn.au
Website: http://home.vicnet.net.au/~mndri/

Desc: Promotes interest in motor neurone disease (MND) and amyotrophic lateral sclerosis (ALS) research among medical and scientific communities and the public in Australia. Offers support services to MND sufferers and their families. Disseminates information about the disease.

★ 4521 ★ Mouvement Francais pour le Planning Familial (MFPF)
4, sq. St. Irenee
F-75011 Paris, France
Phone: 33 1 48072910 **Fax:** 33 1 47007977
Email: planfami@club-internet.fr

Fnded: 1956. **Mem:** 8,000. **Reg. Groups:** 20. **Local Groups:** 70. **Lang(s):** French. **Desc:** Works to enhance the quality of life for individuals living in France by promoting responsible parenthood and family planning. Advocates family planning as a basic human right and defends women's rights to contraception and abortion. Attempts to stop the spread of AIDS and other sexually transmitted diseases. Sponsors programs in sex education, family planning, and health. Provides contraceptive and health care services. Acts as an advocate for family planning on a national level. Conducts research.

★ 4522 ★ Movement Disorder Society (MDS)
611 E Wells St.
Milwaukee, WI 53202
Phone: (414)276-2145 **Fax:** (414)276-3349
Email: info@movementdisorders.org
Website: http://www.movementdisorders.org
Gail Bast, Exec. Dir.

Fnded: 1988. **Mem:** 1,746. **Desc:** Provides international forums and research to disseminate information on recent advances in clinical and basic science pertinent to movement disorders, enhance education of physicians and public, and enrich the quality of care to patients. **Pub:** *Movement Disorders*, monthly. Journal.

★ 4523 ★ Mozambique Association for Family Development (MAFD) (Asociacao Mocambicana para o Desenvolvimento da Familia — AMODEFA)
Av. da Tanzania No. 376
CP 1535
Maputo, Mozambique
Phone: 258 1 405107 **Fax:** 258 1 405149
Email: informe@amodefa.org.mz
Website: http://www.amodefa.org.mz

Fnded: 1989. **Mem:** 300. **Nat'l Groups:** 25. **Reg. Groups:** 4. **State Groups:** 19. **Local Groups:** 25. **Lang(s):** English, Portuguese. **Desc:** Promotes an improved quality of life for families. Sponsors reproductive health and family planning programs and services. Conducts public education campaigns; advocates on behalf of more effective public health policies. **Pub:** Newsletter, monthly. For youth.

★ 4524 ★ MS Felag Islands
c/o Gyda Olafsdottir
Slettluvegur 5
IS-103 Reykjavik, Iceland
Phone: 354 568 8620 **Fax:** 354 568 8688
Email: msfelag@mmedia.is

Fnded: 1968. **Mem:** 600. **Reg. Groups:** 2. **Desc:** MS patients, families and professionals. Seeks to improve the quality of life for persons with multiple sclerosis and their families.

★ 4525 ★ Multidisciplinary Association for Psychedelic Studies (MAPS)
2105 Robinson Ave.
Sarasota, FL 34232
Phone: (941)924-6277 **Free:** 888-868-6277
Fax: (941)924-6265
Email: info@maps.org
Website: http://www.maps.org
Dr. Rick Doblin, Pres.

Fnded: 1986. **Mem:** 1,800. **Desc:** Promotes the development of beneficial, socially sanctioned uses of psychedelic drugs and marijuana. Helps researchers design, obtain government approval for, fund, conduct and report on psychedelic research in human volunteers; funds MDMA psychotherapy studies; facilitates research and FDA approval for marijuana to be prescribed for medical uses. **Pub:** *Maps Bulletin*, quarterly. Magazine. Contains reports on MAPS activities, current research and feature articles. *Price:* $10/sample issue. • The Secret Chief: Conversations with a Pioneer of the Underground Psychedelic Therapy Movement.

★ 4526 ★ Multipel Sklerose Forbundet I Norge
c/o Gerd Hagen
Sorkedalsveien 3
N-0369 Oslo, Norway
Phone: 47 22 604960 **Fax:** 47 22 567695
Email: msfnorge@c2i.net

Fnded: 1966. **Mem:** 4,500. **Reg. Groups:** 45. **Desc:** MS patients, families and professionals. Seeks to improve the quality of life for persons with multiple sclerosis and their families; provides education to persons with MS. Sponsors MS Day. **Pub:** *MS Bladet 2001.* • *MS-En Veiledning For Helsepersonell.*

★ 4527 ★ Multiple Sclerose Vereniging Nederland (MSVN)
c/o Nina van 't Hof-Mennink
Laan van Meerdervoort 51
Postbus 30470
NL-2500 GL The Hague, Netherlands
Phone: 31 70 374 7777 **Fax:** 31 70 374 7770
Email: info@msvn.nl
Website: http://www.msweb.nl

Fnded: 1963. **Mem:** 12,000. **Reg. Groups:** 23. **Desc:** MS patients, families and professionals. Seeks to improve the quality of life for persons with multiple sclerosis and their families.

★ 4528 ★ Multiple Sclerosis Association of America (MSAA)
706 Haddonfield Rd.
Cherry Hill, NJ 08002-2652
Phone: (609)488-4500 **Free:** 800-532-7667
Fax: (856)661-9797
Email: msaa@msaa.com
Website: http://www.msaa.com
Douglas G. Franklin, Pres.

Fnded: 1970. **Mem:** 31,000. **Reg. Groups:** 5. **Desc:** Works to fulfill the daily needs of multiple sclerosis patients. Provides patient support, counseling, local transportation, therapeutic equipment, MRI scans for initial diagnosis and barrier-free housing. Conducts public education programs and symptom relief therapy research. **Pub:** *The Motivator*, bimonthly. Newsletter. *Price:* Free.

★ 4529 ★ Multiple Sclerosis Australia
Ste. 503, Level 5
157 Walker St.
North Sydney, NSW 2060, Australia
Phone: 61 2 99550700 **Fax:** 61 2 99550900
Email: infoline@mssociety.com.au
Website: http://www.mssociety.com.au

Desc: MS patients, families and professionals. Seeks to improve the quality of life for persons with multiple sclerosis and their families. **Frmly:** National Multiple Sclerosis Society Australia.

★ 4530 ★ Multiple Sclerosis Care Centre
Bushy Park House
65 Bushy Park Rd.
Rathgar
Dublin 6, Ireland
Phone: 353 1 1906234 **Fax:** 353 1 4906724
Email: msc@iol.ie

Fnded: 1989. **Desc:** Provides short-term respite care to people with Multiple Sclerosis and other neurological conditions. Assists people in dealing with disability and maintaining independence.

★ 4531 ★ Multiple Sclerosis Foundation (MSF)
6350 N Andrews Ave.
Fort Lauderdale, FL 33309-2130
Phone: (954)776-6805 **Free:** 800-225-6495
Fax: (954)938-8708
Email: admin@msfocus.org
Website: http://www.msfocus.org
Jules Kuperberg, National Dir.

Fnded: 1986. **Desc:** Dedicated to helping create "A Brighter Tomorrow" for those with MS, the foundation offers a wide array of free services, including: information and referral, subsidized home care and outreach, educational programs, free publications, a quarterly news magazine, and more to improve the quality of life for those affected by MS. **Pub:** *MS Fact Sheets.* Booklets. *Price:* Free. • *MSFocus Magazine*, quarterly. Magazine. • *MSFYi*, monthly. Newsletter. Internet newsletter. • *Multiple Sclerosis: Helpful Information for Patients and Families.* Booklet.

★ 4532 ★ Multiple Sclerosis International Federation
3rd. Fl., Skyline House
200 Union St.
London SE1 0LY, United Kingdom
Phone: 44 207 6201911 **Fax:** 44 207 6201922
Email: info@msif.org
Website: http://www.msif.org

Fnded: 1967. **Mem:** 36. **Lang(s):** English, French. **Desc:** Key aims are to stimulate scientific research at a global scale, disseminate information internationally, assist the development of national MS societies, and encourage full integration and participation of all people affected by MS. **Pub:** *Annual Report*, annual. Magazine. • *Federation Updates*, biennial. • *MS in Focus.* • *MS, The Guide to Treatment and Management.* **Frmly:** (2001) International Federation of Multiple Sclerosis Societies.

★ 4533 ★ Multiple Sclerosis Society of Canada
250 Bloor St. E, Ste. 1000
Toronto, Canada M4W 3P9
Phone: (416)922-6065 **Free:** 800-268-7582
Fax: (416)922-7538
Email: info@mssociety.ca
Website: http://www.mssociety.ca

Fnded: 1948. **Mem:** 28,000. **Lang(s):** English, French. **Desc:** Seeks to improve the quality of life for persons with multiple sclerosis and their families. **Pub:** *MS Canada*, quarterly.

★ 4534 ★ Multiple Sclerosis Society of Great Britain and Northern Ireland
MS National Centre
372 Edgware Rd.
Staples Corner
London NW2 6ND, United Kingdom
Phone: 44 208 4380700 **Fax:** 44 208 4380701
Email: info@mssociety.org.uk

Fnded: 1953. **Mem:** 60,000. **Reg. Groups:** 400. **Desc:** Persons with an interest in multiple sclerosis. Promoting and funding research to find the cause and cure of multiple sclerosis and the provision of a welfare and support service for anyone affected by MS. **Pub:** *MS Matters*, bimonthly. Magazine. Additional information on MS and living with Ms available upon request.

★ 4535 ★ Multiple Sclerosis Society of India
c/o N.S. Rao
Samata Sadan, 2nd Fl.
SH Paralkar Rd.
Shivaji Park
Dadar
Bombay 400 028, India
Phone: 91 22 24442067 **Fax:** 91 22 4442067
Email: mssindia@bom8.vsnl.net.in

Fnded: 1985. **Mem:** 1,005. **Reg. Groups:** 7. **Desc:** MS patients, families and professionals. Seeks to improve the quality of life for persons with multiple sclerosis and their families. Provides counseling services and home visits.

★ 4536 ★ Multiple Sclerosis Society of Ireland (MSSI)

Darmouth House
Grand Parade
Dublin 6, Ireland
Phone: 353 1 2694599 **Fax:** 353 1 2693746
Email: mscontact@ms-society.ie
Website: http://www.ms-society.ie

Fnded: 1961. **Mem:** 5,000. **Nat'l Groups:** 1. **Reg. Groups:** 8. **Local Groups:** 40. **Lang(s):** English, Irish. **Desc:** Individuals and organizations. Seeks to improve the quality of life of people with multiple sclerosis and their families. Makes available support and services; conducts educational and advocacy campaigns. **Pub:** *MS News*, quarterly. Magazine.

★ 4537 ★ Multiple Sclerosis Society of Malta

c/o Leslie N. Agius
PO Box 209
Valletta, Malta
Phone: 356 21 418066 **Fax:** 356 21 230538
Email: lagus@onvol.net

Fnded: 1997. **Mem:** 110. **Lang(s):** English, Maltese. **Desc:** MS patients, families and professionals. Seeks to improve the quality of life for persons with multiple sclerosis and their families. Provides physiotherapy and psychotherapy sessions for members. Conducts fund raisers and public awareness campaigns. **Pub:** Bulletin, quarterly.

★ 4538 ★ Multiple Sclerosis Society of New Zealand (MSSNZ)

PO Box 2627
Wellington, New Zealand
Phone: 64 4 499 4677 **Fax:** 64 4 499 4675
Email: info@mssocietynz.co.nz
Website: http://www.mssocietynz.co.nz

Fnded: 1968. **Reg. Groups:** 18. **Desc:** MS patients, families and professionals. Seeks to improve the quality of life for persons with multiple sclerosis and their families. Offers national support services program, national carers support network, MS support network, training video, and an education fund for children with MS. Hosts fundraisers, including Four Leaf Clover Raffle, Readathon, and the Great NZ Horse Trek. **Pub:** *MS Voice*, quarterly. Magazine. Updates management and research issues on MS.

★ 4539 ★ Multiple Sclerosis Society of Zimbabwe

PO Box BE1234
Belvedere
Harare, Zimbabwe
Phone: 263 4 740472 **Fax:** 264 4 740472
Email: pwmsic@ifmss.org.uk

Fnded: 1972. **Mem:** 50. **Nat'l Groups:** 1. **State Groups:** 9. **Desc:** Works to alleviate the suffering of persons with multiple sclerosis. Supports research to discover the cause of and cure for the disease. Offers financial assistance and counseling to individuals suffering from the disease. The society has just completed the constuction of a daycare/rehabilitation which will be geared to rehabilitate pwms, offer sympton management, carer & family training as well as support. **Pub:** *Missive*, monthly. Newsletter.

★ 4540 ★ Multiple Sclerosis South Africa

c/o Ellinor Galoway Greef
National Office
Auckland Park
PO Box 90177
Johannesburg 2006, Republic of South Africa
Phone: 27 11 6739643 **Fax:** 27 11 6739643
Email: ellinor@mssa.org.za
Website: http://www.kznms.org.za

Fnded: 1962. **Mem:** 1,900. **Reg. Groups:** 33. **Desc:** MS patients, families and professionals. Seeks to improve the quality of life for persons with multiple sclerosis and their families.

★ 4541 ★ MUMS National Parent-to-Parent Network (MUMS)

c/o Julie Gordon
150 Custer Ct.
Green Bay, WI 54301-1243
Phone: (920)336-5333 **Free:** 877-336-5333
Fax: (920)339-0995
Email: mums@netnet.net
Website: http://www.netnet.net/mums/
Julie Gordon, Pres.

Fnded: 1979. **Mem:** 18,000. **Nat'l Groups:** 1. **Reg. Groups:** 61. **State Groups:** 32. **Local Groups:** 28. **Desc:** Parents or care providers of a child with any disability, rare disorder, chromosomal abnormality or health condition. Seeks to provide support to parents in the form of a networking system that matches parents with other parents whose children have the same or similar condition, including rare disorders. Informs and updates families and professionals about services available. Refers parents to support groups & assists in forming new groups. **Pub:** *MUMS National Parent to Parent Network Matchmaker*, quarterly. Newsletter. **Frmly:** Mothrs United for Moral Support.

★ 4542 ★ Muscular Dystrophy Association (MDA)

3300 E Sunrise Dr.
Tucson, AZ 85718
Phone: (520)529-2000 **Free:** 800-572-1717
Fax: (520)529-5300
Email: mda@mdausa.org
Website: http://www.mdausa.org
Bob Mackle, Dir. Public Information

Fnded: 1950. **Local Groups:** 157. **Desc:** National voluntary health agency fostering research into the cause and cure of neuromuscular diseases in the following 8 categories. Muscular dystrophies: Becker; congenital; distal; Duchenne (pseudohypertrophic); Emery-Dreifuss; facioscapulohumeral (Landouzy-Dejerine); limb-girdle; myotonic (Steinert's disease); oculopharyngeal. Motor Neuron Diseases: adult spinal muscular atrophy (Aran-Duchenne type); amyotrophic lateral sclerosis (ALS); infantile progressive spinal muscular atrophy (type 1, Werdnig-Hoffmann disease); intermediate spinal muscular atrophy (type 2); juvenile spinal muscular atrophy (type 3, Kugelberg-Welander disease), Spinal Bulbar Muscular Atrophy (SBMA). Inflammatory Myopathies: dermatomyositis; polymyositis; inclusion body myositis. Diseases of Neuromuscular Junction: Eaton-Lambert (myasthenic) syndrome;congenital myasthenic syndrome; myasthenia gravis. Diseases of the Peripheral Nerve: Dejerine-Sottas disease; Friedreich's ataxia; Charcot-Marie-Tooth disease (peroneal muscular atrophy). Metabolic Diseases of Muscle: acid maltase deficiency (Pompe's disease); carnitine deficiency; carnitine palmityl transferase deficiency; Debrancher enzyme deficiency (Cori'sor Forbes' disease); lactate dehydrogenase deficiency; mitochondrial myopathy; myoadenylate deaminase deficiency; phosphofructokinase deficiency (Tarui's disease); phosphoglycerate kinase deficiency; phosphoglycerate mutase deficiency; phosphorylase deficiency (McArdle's disease). Myopathies due to Endocrine Abnormalities: hyperthyroid myopathy; hypothyroid myopathy. Other myopathies: central core disease; myotonia congenita; myotubular myopathy; nemaline myopathy; paramyotonia congenita; periodic paralysis. Supports international programs of some 350 research awards, major university-based neuromuscular disease research/clinical centers, and 230 outpatient clinics in hospitals in the U.S. and Puerto Rico. Awards grants for neuromuscular disease research to individual scientific investigators. Renders services to patients locally through its chapters, including: diagnostic examinations; follow-up medical evaluations; wheelchairs; leg braces; physical therapy; flu shots; summer camps. Maintains 28 centers across the nation offering research and care for persons affected by Lou Gehrig's disease. **Pub:** *Annual Report*, annual. Annual Report. • *The MDA/ALS Newsletter*, bimonthly. Newsletters. • *Quest*, bimonthly. Magazine. Contains stories, research updates, etc. of concern to those w/neuromuscular diseases. *Price:* Free to individuals served by MDA. • Booklets.Series of booklets, covering each disease in MDA's program. • Also publishes general and technical literature on muscular dystrophy and other neuromuscular diseases.

★ 4543 ★ Muscular Dystrophy Ireland (MDI)

c/o Coleraine House
Coleraine St.
Dublin 7, Ireland
Phone: 353 1 8721501 **Fax:** 353 1 8724482
Email: info@mdi.ie
Website: http://www.mdi.ie

Fnded: 1972. **Mem:** 500. **Reg. Groups:** 6. **Lang(s):** English. **Desc:** Provides support and information to individuals with muscular dystrophy and their families. Support services include family support, information, respite, youth activities and transportation. Funds research into the condition. **Pub:** *MDI News Update*, bimonthly. Newsletter.

★ 4544 ★ Musculoskeletal Tumor Society (MSTS)

PO Box 2217
Northbrook, IL 60065
Phone: (847)412-1780 **Fax:** (847)412-1781
Website: http://msts.org/
Frank J. Frassica, MD, Pres. -Elect

Desc: Seeks to advance the science of orthopaedic oncology and promote high standards of patient care.

★ 4545 ★ Museum of Menstruation (MUM)

Landover Hills Branch
Hyattsville, MD 20784-2398
Phone: (301)459-4450
Email: hfinley@mum.org
Website: http://www.mum.org
Barbara Czerwinski, Dir.

Fnded: 1994. **Mem:** 310. **Desc:** Seeks to educate the public on the cultural history of menstruation. Conducts research and statistical studies. Offers assistance to individuals conducting patent and advertising research, and scholarly work, musuem displays of advertising history and menstrual devices.

★ 4546 ★ Muskelsvindfonden

Kongsvang Alle 23
DK-8000 Arhus C, Denmark
Phone: 45 89482222 **Fax:** 45 89482212
Email: msfoplys@post1.tele.dk
Website: http://www.muskelsvindfonden.dk

Fnded: 1971. **Mem:** 1,800. **Desc:** Promotes the research of muscular diseases affecting individuals in Denmark. Fosters communication among members. Offers supportive services to patients and their families. **Pub:** *Muskelkraft*, 8/year. Magazine.

★ 4547 ★ Mutual Help Home Association (MHHA) (Association d'Entraide vive Chez Nous — AECN)

84 rue Principale
Saint Fidele, QC, Canada G0T 1T0
Phone: (418)434-2561

Lang(s): English, French. **Desc:** Individuals and organizations. Seeks to improve the quality of lives of elderly people living in nursing homes. Monitors conditions in nursing homes; provides support and services to the elderly.

★ 4548 ★ Myasthenia Gravis Association

Keynes House
Chester Pk.

Alfreton Rd.
Derby DE21 4AS, United Kingdom
Phone: 44 1332 290219 **Fax:** 44 1332 293641
Email: mg@mgauk.org.uk
Website: http://www.mgauk.org

Fnded: 1976. **Mem:** 1,125. **Reg. Groups:** 60. **Desc:** Supports research into the management and cure of Myasthenia. **Pub:** *MGA News*, quarterly. Newsletter.

★ 4549 ★ Myasthenia Gravis Foundation of America

5841 Cedar Lake Rd., Ste. 204
Minneapolis, MN 55416
Phone: (952)545-9438 **Free:** 800-541-5454
Fax: (952)545-6073
Email: myastheniagravis@msn.com
Website: http://www.myasthenia.org
Debora K. Boelz, CEO

Fnded: 1952. **Mem:** 30,000. **State Groups:** 36. **Desc:** Persons suffering from myasthenia gravis; their families, doctors, and nurses; others dedicated to the detection, treatment, and cure of MG. Raises funds for research and for professional and public education programs. Provides literature. Lay and professional materials available upon request. **Pub:** Brochures, annual. • Handbooks.For patients. • Manuals.For physicians and nurses. • Pamphlets. **Frmly:** (1998) Myasthenia Gracis Foundation.

★ 4550 ★ The Myositis Association (TMA)

755 Cantrell Ave., Ste. C
Harrisonburg, VA 22801
Phone: (540)433-7686 **Free:** 800-821-7356
Fax: (540)432-0206
Email: tma@myositis.org
Website: http://www.myositis.org
Bob Goldberg, Exec. Dir.

Fnded: 1993. **Mem:** 2,000. **Reg. Groups:** 65. **Desc:** Seeks to educate members in ways to avoid future degeneration process of myositis, give emotional support, investigate the different causes of the disease, act as a clearinghouse to physicians and scientists, and disseminate information to patients to inform on some of the known causes, pursue additional funding for research, investigate the most effective medical treatments available that have the least side effects and, most important, research a cure into these debilitating diseases. **Pub:** *Newsletter for Myositis*, quarterly. Newsletter. **Frmly:** (2002) Myositis Association of America.

★ 4551 ★ NAADAC The Association for Addiction Professionals (NAADAC)

901 N Washington St., Ste. 600
Alexandria, VA 22314
Phone: (703)741-7686 **Free:** 800-548-0497
Fax: (703)741-7698
Email: naadac@naadac.org
Website: http://www.naadac.org
Pat Ford Roegner, Exec. Dir.

Fnded: 1972. **Mem:** 14,000. **Reg. Groups:** 8. **State Groups:** 47. **Desc:** Counselors providing addiction treatment. Objective is to provide national representation for counselors as well as for their training and education. Works to gain public recognition of alcoholism as a disease. Seeks legislation establishing accreditation standards for counselors. Informs the public about chemical dependency and the availability of assistance. **Pub:** *Counseling Lesbian, Gay and Bisexual Persons with Alcohol and Drug Problems*. Papers. • *The Counselor*, bimonthly. Magazine. For counselors on alcohol and drug abuse. Includes book, pamphlet, and film list. Also contains notices of employment and educational opportunities. *Price:* Included in membership dues. • *NAADAC Ethical Standards*. • *NAADAC Newsletter*, bimonthly. Newsletter. *Price:* Included in membership. • *NAADAC Study Guide on Additional Counseling*. • Also publishes annual conference papers. **Frmly:** (2001) National Association of Alcoholism and Drug Abuse Counselors.

★ 4552 ★ NADD - An Association for Persons with Developmental Disabilities and Mental Health Needs

c/o Robert Fletcher
132 Fair St.
Kingston, NY 12401-4802
Phone: (845)331-4336 **Free:** 800-331-5362
Fax: (845)331-4569
Email: thenadd@aol.com
Website: http://www.thenadd.org
Dr. Robert Fletcher, Dir.

Fnded: 1983. **Mem:** 1,300. **State Groups:** 6. **Desc:** People with developmental disabilities and mental health care needs; mental health professionals; other interested individuals. Promotes public and professional interest in developmental disability; seeks to improve access to mental health care. Supports research programs; facilitates exchange of information among mental health professionals and consumers; conducts advocacy to insure implementation of effective public mental health policies and legislation. Holds educational programs; maintains speakers' bureau. **Pub:** *NADD Bulletin*, bimonthly. Journal. *Price:* included in membership dues. • Also publishes books, audio tapes, video tapes, and training materials. **Frmly:** (1997) National Association for the Dually Diagnosed.

★ 4553 ★ NAMDRC: Physician Advocacy for Excellence in the Delivery of Pulmonary and Critical Care

5454 Wisconsin Ave., Ste. 1270
Chevy Chase, MD 20815
Phone: (301)718-2975 **Fax:** (301)718-2976
Email: namdrc@erols.com
Website: http://www.namdrc.org
Phillip Porte, Exec. Dir.

Fnded: 1977. **Mem:** 650. **Desc:** Works to provide educational opportunities for pulmonologists and others involved in respiratory care. Interprets and advises on the changing healthcare delivery system and is a successfull advocate on regulatory and legislative issues affecting pulmonary and critical care medicine. Offers educational programs, publications and assistance regarding coding issues and federal reimbursement policies. **Pub:** *Clinical and Management Quarterly*, quarterly. Newsletter. • *Presidential Update*, biennial. • *Washington Watchline*, monthly. **Frmly:** (2003) National Association for Medical Direction of Respiratory Care.

★ 4554 ★ Names Project Foundation - AIDS Memorial Quilt (NPF)

PO Box 5552
Atlanta, GA 31107
Phone: (404)688-5500 **Fax:** (404)688-5552
Email: info@aidsquilt.org
Website: http://www.aidsquilt.org
Edward Gatta, Pres.

Fnded: 1987. **Nat'l Groups:** 38. **Local Groups:** 53. **Desc:** Promotes creation of AIDS Memorial Quilt as an "appropriate, compassionate response" to the AIDS epidemic. Goals of the project are to provide a creative means of remembrance and healing; to illustrate the enormity of the AIDS epidemic; to increase public awareness of AIDS; to assist with HIV prevention education; and to raise funds for community-based AIDS service organizations. The 25 acre quilt currently contains 43,000 panels from each of the 50 states and 39 foreign countries bearing the names of persons who have died as a result of AIDS. Among materials sewn into the panels are stuffed animals, merit badges, records, feather boas, and a baseball jersey. jersey. jersey. **Pub:** *A Promise To Remember*. Book. • *Always Remember*. Book. • *"On Display"*, quarterly. Newsletter. *Price:* Donation. • *The Quilt: Stories From the NAMES Project*. Book. • Also publishes fact sheets, flyers, and press releases. **Frmly:** Names Project.

★ 4555 ★ NANDA International

1211 Locust St.
Philadelphia, PA 19107
Phone: (215)545-8105 **Free:** 800-647-9002
Fax: (215)545-8107
Email: nanda@rmpinc.com
Website: http://www.nanda.org
Mary Ann Lavin, Pres.

Fnded: 1972. **Mem:** 400. **Desc:** Registered nurses; individuals interested in nursing language and informatics. Purpose is to develop, refine, and promote a taxonomy of nursing terminology for use by professional nurses. **Pub:** *NANDA Nursing Diagnoses: Definitions and Classification 2001-2002*, biennial. Book. *Price:* $19.95. • *Nursing Diagnoses and Critical Thinking*. Book. *Price:* $24.95. • *Nursing Diagnosis Journal*, quarterly. Journal. *Price:* $42/year; $54/year for members outside the U.S.; Included in membership. **AKA:** North American Nursing Diagnosis Association.

★ 4556 ★ Narcolepsy Association United Kingdom (UKAN)

Craven House, 1st Floor
121 Kingsway
London WC2B 6PA, United Kingdom
Phone: 44 20 77218904 **Fax:** 44 1322 863056
Email: info@narcolepsy.org.uk

Fnded: 1981. **Mem:** 700. **Reg. Groups:** 12. **Lang(s):** English. **Desc:** Narcoleptics, their relatives, and others interested in improving the lives of those afflicted with narcolepsy. Promotes awareness of narcolepsy and provides authoritative information about it to narcoleptics, the medical profession, and to the public. Supports the establishment of local self-help groups; encourages research; co-operates with narcolepsy associations overseas. **Pub:** *Catnap*, quarterly. Newsletter. Reports national and international developments in cause and treatment of narcolepsy.

★ 4557 ★ Narcolepsy Network

10921 Reed Hartman Hwy.
Cincinnati, OH 45242
Phone: (513)891-3522 **Fax:** (513)891-3836
Email: narnet@aol.com
Website: http://www.websciences.org/narnet
Robert L. Cloud, Exec. Dir.

Fnded: 1986. **Local Groups:** 60. **Desc:** Individuals with narcolepsy, their friends and families, sleep professionals, and interested others. Seeks to improve the quality of life of individuals who have narcolepsy. Works to educate members and the general public about narcolepsy. Fosters communication among members. Offers referral service. Supports research; disseminates information. **Pub:** *Narcolepsy: A Guide to Understanding*. • *The Network*, quarterly. Newsletter.

★ 4558 ★ Narcotic Educational Foundation of America (NEFA)

28245 Ave. Crocker, Ste. 230
Santa Clarita, CA 91355-1201
Phone: (661)775-6968 **Free:** 877-775-6272
Fax: (661)775-1648
Email: lwhite@cnoa.org
Website: http://www.cnoa.org/nefa.htm
Lorraine White, Exec. Sec.

Fnded: 1924. **Desc:** Conducts an education program revealing the dangers that result from the illicit and abusive use of narcotics and dangerous drugs, so that youth and adults will be protected from both mental and physical drug dependency and harm. **Pub:** *Alcohol-A Potent Drug*. Brochure. • *Am I Addicted or Dependent?*. • *Designer Drugs: The Analog Game*. • *The Heroin Story*. • *Huffing: Inhalants*. • *Lysergic Acid Diethylamide: Is it a Dream or Nightmare?*. • *The PCP Story*. • *Rohypnol: The Date Rape Drug*. • *Speed: Amphetamines*. • *The Story of Cocaine*. • *Tobacco: Smoke or Chew*. • *Understanding Anabolic Steroids*. • *Use of Marijuana as a 'Medicine'*. • *Valium & Other Depressants*. • *What About Marijuana?*.

★ 4559 ★ Narcotics Anonymous (NA)

PO Box 9999
Van Nuys, CA 91409
Phone: (818)773-9999 **Fax:** (818)700-0700

Email: fsmail@na.org
Website: http://www.na.org
Jeff Gershoff, Coordinator Svcs.

Fnded: 1953. **Mem:** 500,000. **Reg. Groups:** 105. **State Groups:** 50. **Local Groups:** 27400. **Desc:** Recovering addicts throughout the world meet to offer help to fellow addicts seeking recovery. Members meet regularly to facilitate and stabilize their recovery. Uses 12-step program adapted from Alcoholics Anonymous to aid in the recovery process. **Pub:** *It Works: How and Why*. Book. Guide to NA primary principles. • *Just For Today: Daily Meditations for Recovering Addicts*. Book. • *NA Way Magazine: The International Journal of the Fellowship of Narcotics Anonymous*, quarterly. Magazine. Recounts experiences of members during their recoveries. Includes calendar of events and annual index. *Price:* Free. • *Narcotics Anonymous*. Book. Basic textbook of NA. • *Narcotics Anonymous: It Works How and Why*. Books.

★ 4560 ★ National Ability Center (NAC)

PO Box 682799
Park City, UT 84068
Phone: (435)649-3991 **Fax:** (435)658-3992
Email: info@nac1985.org
Website: http://www.nationalabilitycenter.org/
Meeche White, Exec. Dir.

Fnded: 1985. **Mem:** 5,000. **Nat'l Groups:** 2. **State Groups:** 4. **Desc:** People with disabilities and their families. Promotes the development of lifetime skills for persons with disabilities and their families; works to increase the self-esteem of people with disabilities. Sponsors affordable sports and recreational activities, including cycling, skiing, challenge course, horseback riding, and river rafting, for members. **Pub:** *Ability Bulletin*, quarterly. Newsletter.

★ 4561 ★ National Abortion Federation (NAF)

1755 Massachusetts Ave. NW Ste 600
Washington, DC 20036
Phone: (202)667-5881 **Free:** 800-772-9100
Fax: (202)667-5890
Email: naf@prochoice.org
Website: http://www.prochoice.org
Vicki Saporta, Pres. /CEO

Fnded: 1977. **Mem:** 400. **Desc:** Abortion service providers (physician offices, clinics, feminist health centers, Planned Parenthood affiliates) and others committed to making safe, legal abortions accessible to all women. Unites abortion service providers into a professional community dedicated to health care; upgrades abortion services by providing continuing medical education, standards, and guidelines; serves as clearinghouse of information on variety and quality of services offered; keeps abreast of educational, legislative, and public policy developments in reproductive health care. Provides referrals. **Pub:** *A Clinician's Guide to Medical and Surgical Abortion*. Book. • *Clinical Training Curriculum in Abortion Practice*. Curriculum for residency training, medical reference. *Price:* $130. • *Unsure About Your Pregnancy? A Guide to Making the Right Decision for You*. • Bulletins. • Also publishes fact sheets, bulletins, and position papers on abortion, and resource materials for abortion praviders.

★ 4562 ★ National Abortion Rights Action League (NARAL)

1156 15th St. NW, Ste. 700
Washington, DC 20005
Phone: (202)973-3000 **Fax:** (202)973-3096
Email: comments@naral.org
Website: http://www.naral.org
Kate Michelman, Pres.

Desc: Politically involved in the pro-choice movement. Outspoken advocate of reproductive freedom and choice. Protects and preserves the right to choose. Promotes policies and programs to improve women's health. Seeks to make abortion less necessary.

★ 4563 ★ National Academies of Practice (NAP)

PO Box 1037
Edgewood, MD 21040
Phone: (410)676-3390
Website: http://www.nap.vcu.edu/memberinfo.htm
Hurdis Griffith, PhD,RN, Pres.

Fnded: 1981. **Mem:** 1,000. **Desc:** Devoted to promoting quality health care for all through interdisciplinary practice, education, research. **Pub:** *National Academies of Practice Forum*. Journal. Devoted to interdisciplinary issues in health care. • Papers.

★ 4564 ★ National Academy of Clinical Biochemistry (NACB)

c/o Charles D. Hawker
Laboratories
500 Chipeta Way
Salt Lake City, UT 84108
Phone: (801)584-5261 **Fax:** (801)584-5207
Email: hawkercd@aruplab.com
Website: http://www.nacb.org/

Desc: Dedicated to advancing the science and practice of clinical laboratory medicine through research, education, professional development. **Pub:** *Laboratory Medicine Practice Guidelines*. • *News & Views*. Newsletter.

★ 4565 ★ National Academy of Emergency Medical Dispatch (NAEMD)

139 E S Temple, N 530
Salt Lake City, UT 84111
Phone: (801)359-6916 **Free:** 800-960-6236
Fax: (801)359-0996
Website: http://www.naemd.org/
Robert L. Martin, Exec. Dir.

Fnded: 1988. **Mem:** 30,000. **Desc:** Works to advance public-safety emergency telecommunications professionals to ensure quality emergency, health and social services.

★ 4566 ★ National Academy of Medicine (Academia Nacional de Medicina)

Apdo Aereo 23224
Bogota, Colombia
Phone: 57 1 2493122
Fnded: 1890.

★ 4567 ★ National Academy of Neuropsychology (NAN)

2121 S Oneida St., Ste. 550
Denver, CO 80224-2594
Phone: (303)691-3694 **Fax:** (303)691-5983
Email: office@nanonline.org
Website: http://www.NANonline.org
Josette G. Harris, PhD, Exec. Dir.

Fnded: 1975. **Mem:** 3,024. **Desc:** Clinical neuropsychologists and others interested in brain-behavior relationships. Works to preserve and advance knowledge regarding the assessment and remediation of neuropsychological disorders. Promotes the development of neuropsychology as a science and profession; develops standards of practice and training guidelines for the field; fosters communication between members; represents the professional interests of members; serves as an information resource; facilitates the exchange of information among related organizations. Offers continuing education programs; conducts research. **Pub:** *Archives of Clinical Neuropsychology*, bimonthly. Journal. *Price:* Included in membership dues; $185/year for nonmember institutions. • *Bulletin of the National Academy of Neuropsychologists*, quarterly. Bulletin. *Price:* Included in membership dues. • Membership Directory, biennial.

★ 4568 ★ National Academy of Opticianry (NAO)

8401 Corporate Dr No. 605
Landover, MD 20785
Phone: (301)577-4828 **Free:** 800-229-4828
Fax: (301)577-3880
Email: info@nao.org
Website: http://www.nao.org
Jim Iciek, Jr., Exec. Dir.

Fnded: 1973. **Mem:** 5,000. **Desc:** Offers review courses for national certification and state licensure examinations to members. Maintains speakers' bureau and Career Progression Program. **Pub:** *Academy Newsletter*, quarterly. Newsletter. • *Exam Review for Ophthalmic Dispensing*. • *Ophthalmic Dispensing Review Book*. Book. • *Optical Math Review*. • Brochure. • Videos.

★ 4569 ★ National Academy of Surgery (Academie nationale de chirurgie)

15, rue de l'Ecole de Medecine
F-75006 Paris, France
Phone: 33 1 43540232 **Fax:** 33 1 43293444
Email: ac.chirurgie@bhdc.jussieu.fr
Website: http://www.bium.univ-paris5.fr/acad-chirurgie

Fnded: 1731. **Mem:** 500. **Desc:** Promotes research and progress in surgery. **Pub:** *Annales de Chirurgie*, monthly. Journal.

★ 4570 ★ National Academy for Teaching and Learning About Aging

University of North Texas
PO Box 310919
Denton, TX 76203-0919
Phone: (940)565-3450 **Fax:** (940)565-3141
Email: couper.natla@snet.net
Website: http://www.unt.edu/natla
Donna Couper, PhD, Contact

Fnded: 1983. **Mem:** 250. **Desc:** Professionals in gerontology, education, health care, and other fields interested in developing aging education and intergenerational programming. Seeks to dispel myths about aging and old age; encourages communication among generations and works to create a social environment where people of all ages can live together. Serves as a clearinghouse of information on issues of aging and intergenerational programs; provides consultation and presentation services to individuals or groups that wish to develop aging education programs. Maintains resources for aging education and intergenerational programming. **Pub:** *AgeShare*. • *Schools in an Aging Society*. Six interrelated curriculum guides which provide education, for, with, and about older adults. *Price:* $55. • Teaching about Aging: Enriching Lives across the Lifespan (published by the National Retired Teachers Association; free & available from NRTA/AARP). **Frmly:** Center for Understanding Aging; (1996) Center for Understanding Aging.

★ 4571 ★ National Accessible Apartment Clearinghouse (NAAC)

201 N Union St., No. 200
Alexandria, VA 22314
Free: 800-421-1221 **Fax:** (703)518-6191
Email: clearinghouse@naahq.org
Website: http://www.forrent.com/naac/

Desc: Dedicated to providing an effective means to connect individuals with disabilities with apartments designed for an individual's particular needs.

★ 4572 ★ National Accreditation Council for Agencies Serving the Blind and Visually Impaired (NAC)

16920 Detroit Ave., No. 100
Lakewood, OH 44107
Phone: (216)258-3333 **Fax:** (216)258-2222
Email: shevgedeos@nacasb.org
Steven K. Hegedeos, Exec. Dir.

Fnded: 1966. **Mem:** 48. **Desc:** The only organization in the United States that exclusively accredits schools, agencies and programs serving people who are blind or visually impaired. Formed in 1966 with the broad-based support of national organizations in the field of blindness, many state and local organizations, and the U.S. Department of Health, Education and Welfare.

Influences special schools and agencies that serve people who are blind or visually impaired to meet established standards that promote effective, sound, and publicly accountable education and rehabilitation programs. "Accreditation is especially important in this field because so few agencies deliver these specialized services. In most cases, needed services for the blind or visually impaired are available from only one school or agency. As a result, the dynamic of competition is not present as a motivation for continued improvement, and it is difficult for funders or consumers to reach independent judgments as to the quality of the school or agency serving their community". **Pub:** *The Standard-Bearer*, annual. • Annual Report. • Also publishes self-study and evaluation guides, incorporating standards for management and services of agencies and schools for people who are blind and visually handicapped; publications are available in print, braille, and recorded editions. **Frmly:** (2003) National Accreditation Council for Agencies Serving the Blind and Visually Handicapped.

★ 4573 ★ National Accrediting Agency for Clinical Laboratory Sciences (NAACLS)

8410 W Bryn Mawr Ave., Ste. 670
Chicago, IL 60631
Phone: (773)714-8880 **Fax:** (773)714-8886
Email: info@naacls.org
Website: http://www.naacls.org
Olive Kimball, PhD, CEO

Fnded: 1973. **Mem:** 695. **Desc:** Independently accredits academic programs in hospitals, colleges, and universities for the following health professional classifications: Clinical Laboratory Scientist/Medical Technologist, Clinical Laboratory Technician/Medical laboratory Technician, Histologic Technician, Histotechnologist, Pathologists' Assistant. Independently approves academic programs in hospitals and colleges for the following: Cytogenetic Technologist, Phlebotomist, Clinical Assistant. Establishes standards for quality educational programs; determines if hospitals and colleges are maintaining standards through self-study and on-site visits. Provides workshops for program officials on self-study and accreditation. **Pub:** *Guide to Accreditation*. • *NAACLS News*, quarterly. Newsletter. Includes news related to allied health professions and listing of position vacancies. *Price:* Free to members and accredited program officials; $15/year for non-members. • *NAACLS Program Approval Guide*. • *National Accrediting Agency for Clinical Laboratory Sciences–Annual Report*. Annual Report. • *National Accrediting Agency for Clinical Laboratory Sciences–Essentials*. **Frmly:** (1973) Board of Schools of the ASCP.

★ 4574 ★ National Acupuncture Detoxification Association (NADA)

PO Box 1927
Vancouver, WA 98668-1927
Phone: (360)254-0186 **Fax:** (360)260-8620
Email: nadaclear@aol.com
Website: http://www.acudetox.com
Jay Renaud, MPA, Office Mgr.

Fnded: 1985. **Mem:** 1,010. **Nat'l Groups:** 1. **State Groups:** 2. **Desc:** Works to promote the use of acupuncture in the treatment of addictions. Provides training and educational materials. **Pub:** *Guidepoints: Acupuncture in Recovery*, monthly. Newsletter. *Price:* $185/year.

★ 4575 ★ National Adrenal Diseases Foundation (NADF)

505 Northern Blvd.
Great Neck, NY 11021
Phone: (516)487-4992
Email: nadfmail@aol.com
Website: http://www.medhelp.org/www/nadf.htm
Erin A. Foley, MPH, Pres.

Fnded: 1985. **Mem:** 1,300. **Local Groups:** 19. **Desc:** Individuals with adrenal diseases, especially Addison's disease, and their families; physicians. Seeks to provide a national selfhelp network for educational and emotional support for patients and their families. **Pub:** *NADF News*, quarterly. Newsletter. *Price:* $25/year. • Also publishes educational materials. **Frmly:** (1991) National Addison's Disease Foundation.

★ 4576 ★ National Adult Day Services Association

c/o National Council on the Aging
409 3rd St. SW, No. 200
Washington, DC 20024
Phone: (202)479-1200 **Free:** 800-424-9046
Fax: (202)479-0735
Email: info@ncoa.org
Website: http://www.nadsa.org
Constance Todd, Dir.

Fnded: 1979. **Mem:** 1,200. **Reg. Groups:** 10. **Desc:** Adult daycare practitioners; health and social service planners; individuals involved in planning and providing services for older persons. (Daycare centers offer services in a group setting ranging from active rehabilitation to social and health care.) Promotes and enhances adult daycare programs; provides services and activities for disabled older persons on a long-term basis; provides training and technical assistance and consultation services for daycare personnel; organizes funding; develops standards and guidelines for adult daycare programs; encourages adult daycare centers to participate in local area health planning activities to heighten the effectiveness of adult daycare. Plans and conducts training events for annual meeting and related conferences; maintains annotated bibliography; lobbies for approved public policy positions; surveys state adult daycare regulations and legislation. **Pub:** *Developing Adult Day Care: An Approach to Maintaining Independence for Impaired Older Persons*. • *NCOA Networks*, bimonthly. Newsletter. Reports on adult day care and other aging issues with a focus on public policy. *Price:* Free, for members only. • *Standards for Adult Day Care*.

★ 4577 ★ National Advisory Service for Parents of Children with Stomas (NASPCS)

c/o John Malcolm, Pres.
51 Anderson Dr.
Valley View Park
Darvel KA17 ODE, United Kingdom
Phone: 44 1560 322024
Email: john@stoma.freeserve.co.uk
Website: http://www.naspcs.co.uk

Fnded: 1988. **Mem:** 650. **Nat'l Groups:** 1. **Lang(s):** English. **Desc:** Parents of children suffering from serious bladder and bowel disorders. Provides an information service for parents on the practical day-to-day management of all aspects of coping with a child who has undergone a colostomy, ileostomy, or urostomy and provides advice on the incontinence often encountered with bowel and bladder problems. **Pub:** *My Child has Hirschspungs Disease*. Booklet. • *Our Special Children*. Booklet. **Frmly:** National Association for Support of Parents with Children with Stomas.

★ 4578 ★ National AIDS Committee - Germany (Nationaler AIDS-Beirat — NAB)

Federal Ministry for Health
D-53108 Bonn, Germany
Phone: 49 1888 4413210 **Fax:** 49 1888 4414932
Email: miesala@bmg.bund.de

Fnded: 1987. **Mem:** 27. **Lang(s):** German. Does not correspond in English. **Desc:** Organizations and individual experts interested in preventing the spread of HIV/AIDS. Counsels German government on AIDS related matters. **Pub:** *Voten des Nationalen AIDS-Beirates - 1987-1997*. Brochure.

★ 4579 ★ National AIDS Committee - Mexico (CONASIDA) (Centro Nacional para la Prevencion y Control del VIH/SIDA)

Calz. de Tlalfan 4585, 20. piso
Col. Toriello Guerra
14050 Mexico City, DF, Mexico
Phone: 52 5 55284848 **Fax:** 52 5 5284220
Email: conasida@prodigy.net.mx
Website: http://www.ssa.gob.mx/conasida

Fnded: 1986. **Mem:** 143. **State Groups:** 31. **Lang(s):** English, Spanish. **Desc:** Individual interested in preventing the spread of HIV/AIDS in Mexico. Offers public education programs on the transmission and effects of the disease. Campaigns to raise awareness and fund research. **Pub:** *Guia de Atencion Domiciliaria*, periodic. Booklet. Information for patients, consultants and hospitals on HIV/AIDS. • *Guia de Atencion Psicologica*. • *Guia para la Atencion Medica de Pacientes con Infeccion por VIH/SIDA en Consulta Externa y Hospitales*. • *Guias para Enfermeras*.

★ 4580 ★ National AIDS Committee - Seychelles

Ministry of Health
PO Box 52
Victoria, Seychelles
Phone: 248 388000 **Fax:** 248 224792
Email: aids@moh.gov.se

Fnded: 1987. **Mem:** 7. **Desc:** Promotes the study of AIDS.

★ 4581 ★ National AIDS Fund

1030 15th St. NW, Ste. 860
Washington, DC 20005-2208
Phone: (202)408-4848 **Free:** 800-234-AIDS
Fax: (202)408-1818
Email: info@aidsfund.org
Website: http://www.aidsfund.org
Candy Ferree, CEO

Fnded: 1988. **Mem:** 200. **State Groups:** 27. **Desc:** Promotes leadership and generates resources for effective community responses to HIV/AIDS. **Pub:** *News from the National AIDS Fund*, quarterly. Newsletter. • AIDS-in the workplace publications list available. **Frmly:** (1996) Rational Community AIDS Partnership.

★ 4582 ★ National AIDS Trust

New City Cloisters
188/196 Old St.
London EC1V 9FR, United Kingdom
Phone: 44 207 8146767 **Fax:** 44 207 2160111
Email: info@nat.org.uk
Website: http://www.nat.org.uk

Fnded: 1987. **Nat'l Groups:** 2. **Lang(s):** English. **Desc:** Individuals and organizations in the United Kingdom interested in preventing the spread of HIV/AIDS. Conducts educational programs, fundraising, policy work, employers initiatives, research, lobbying, and parliamentary liaison. **Pub:** *Impact*, 10/year. Magazine. Research reports.

★ 4583 ★ National Alliance for Autism Research (NAAR)

99 Wall St., Research Park
Princeton, NJ 08540
Phone: (609)430-9160 **Free:** 888-777-NAAR
Fax: (609)430-9163
Email: naar@naar.org
Website: http://www.naar.org
Glenn R. Tringali, COO

Fnded: 1994. **Desc:** Dedicated to finding the causes, prevention, effective treatment and, ultimately, cure of the autism spectrum disorders. **Pub:** *NAARATIVE*, 3/year. Newsletter. Includes autism research articles.

★ 4584 ★ National Alliance of Blind Students (NABS)
c/o American Council of the Blind
1155 15th St. NW, Ste. 1004
Washington, DC 20005
Phone: (202)467-5081 **Free:** 800-424-8666
Fax: (202)467-5085
Email: jsimeone1@sattbi.com
Website: http://www.acb.org/affiliates/
Jonathan Simeone, Pres.

Fnded: 1974. **Mem:** 150. **State Groups:** 8. **Desc:** Postsecondary students in academic, vocational, trade, and professional programs as well as disabled student service personnel. Aims to educate agencies, governments, institutions, and the public dealing with blind students as to their needs and educational pursuits in accredited postsecondary educational programs. Acts to protect rights and interests of blind students. Participates in annual National Student Seminar at the national convention of the American Council of the Blind. **Pub:** *Student Advocate*, quarterly. Newsletter. *Price:* Free to members.

★ 4585 ★ National Alliance of Breast Cancer Organizations (NABCO)
9 E 37th St., 10th Fl.
New York, NY 10016
Phone: (212)889-0606 **Free:** 888-80-NABCO
Fax: (212)689-1213
Email: NABCOinfo@aol.com
Website: http://www.nabco.org
Amy Langer, Exec. Dir.

Fnded: 1986. **Desc:** The National Alliance of Breast Cancer Organization (NABCO) is the leading non-profit information and education resource on breast cancer in the U.S. NABCO provides information to medical professionals and their organizations and to patients and their families, and advocates for beneficial regulatory change and legislation. With public and corporate partners, NABCO has collaborated on programs that have reached a national audience, heightening public awareness and connecting women with needed services. Services are free of charge. **Pub:** *NABCO News*, quarterly. Newsletter. Monitors developments relating to breast cancer. *Price:* Included in membership dues. • *NABCO's Breast Cancer Resource List*, annual. Contains information on materials and organizations that provide information about breast cancer. *Price:* Included in membership dues.

★ 4586 ★ National Alliance for Infusion Therapy (NAIT)
1001 Pennsylvania Ave. NW, 6th Fl.
Washington, DC 20004-2582
Phone: (202)347-0066 **Fax:** (202)624-7222
Email: aparver@pgsm.com
Alan K. Parver, Contact

Fnded: 1991. **Mem:** 20. **Desc:** National health care providers and manufacturers. Promotes the appropriate use of infusion therapies (parenteral or enteral administration of drugs or nutrients) at home or in other alternate-site settings. Seeks to raise awareness of infusion therapies through educational and research programs. Works to influence public policy and private payer advocacy of infusion therapy. Establishes and disseminates guidelines for quality patient care. **Pub:** *Infusion News*, bimonthly. Newsletter. *Price:* Free to members.

★ 4587 ★ National Alliance for the Mentally Ill (NAMI)
Colonial Place Three
2107 Wilson Blvd., Ste. 300
Arlington, VA 22201-3042
Phone: (703)524-7600 **Free:** 888-999-NAMI
Fax: (703)524-9094
Email: dana@nami.org
Website: http://www.nami.org
Dana L. Lebowitz, Mgr. Info. &Svc. Ctr.

Fnded: 1979. **Mem:** 220,000. **State Groups:** 52. **Local Groups:** 1200. **Desc:** Nations leading organization dedicated to improving the lives of children and adults with severe mental illness through support, education, research, and advocacy. Focus includes schizophrenia, bipolar disorder, major depression, and anxiety disorder. **Pub:** *Because Children Grow Up*, quarterly. Newsletter. • *NAMI Advocate*, quarterly. Magazine. *Price:* Included in membership dues. • *Nami-E-News*, Daily to weekly. Provides legislative policy updates online. • *Stigmabuster Alerts*, monthly. Report. Reports and recommends actions against prejudice and discrimination involving mental illness. • Handbooks. • Brochures.

★ 4588 ★ National Alliance of Methadone Advocates (NAMA)
435 2nd Ave.
New York, NY 10010
Phone: (212)595-6262 **Fax:** (212)595-6262
Email: nama4u@mail-x-change.com
Website: http://www.methadone.org/
Joycelyn Woods, Pres.

Fnded: 1988. **Mem:** 15,000. **Nat'l Groups:** 5. **Reg. Groups:** 20. **State Groups:** 10. **Local Groups:** 27. **Desc:** Methadone maintenance patients and supporters of methadone maintenance treatment. Promotes quality methadone maintenance treatment as the most effective modality for the treatment of opiate addiction. **Pub:** *Manual Series - Starting A Methadone Advocacy Group*. Manuals. *Price:* $10. • *NAMA Advocate*, quarterly. Newsletter. *Price:* $25/year, U.S.; $40 international. • Educational Series - 2.00 each.

★ 4589 ★ National Alliance for Research on Schizophrenia and Depression (NARSAD)
60 Cutter Mill Rd., Ste. 404
Great Neck, NY 11021
Phone: (516)829-0091 **Free:** 800-829-8289
Fax: (516)487-6930
Email: info@narsad.org
Website: http://www.narsad.org/
Constance Lieber, Pres.

Fnded: 1986. **Desc:** Raises funds for research on schizophrenia, depression, and other mental illnesses. **Pub:** *NARSAD Research*, quarterly. Newsletter. Highlights current scientific research. *Price:* Contribution.

★ 4590 ★ National Alliance of Senior Citizens (NASC)
2525 Wilson Blvd.
Arlington, VA 22201
Fax: (703)528-4380
Peter J. Luciano, CEO

Fnded: 1974. **Mem:** 117,000. **Desc:** Persons advocating the advancement of senior Americans through sound fiscal policy and through belief in the American system of individuality and personal freedom. Purpose is to inform the membership and the American public of the needs of senior citizens and of the programs and policies being carried out by the government and other specified groups. Represents the views of senior Americans before Congress and state legislatures. Maintains Golden Age Hall of Fame honoring individuals for outstanding service to the senior community. Conducts educational program; compiles statistics. Project "Life with Dignity: Compassionate Care for the Dying" helps to improve quality of life for people with terminal illness. Advocates living will and patients rights. **Pub:** *Senior Guardian*, bimonthly.

★ 4591 ★ National Alliance of State and Territorial AIDS Directors
444 N Capitol St. NW, Ste. 339
Washington, DC 20001
Phone: (202)434-8090 **Fax:** (202)434-8092
Email: jscofield@nastad.org
Website: http://www.nastad.org
Julie M. Scofield, Exec. Dir.

Fnded: 1992. **Mem:** 59. **State Groups:** 59. **Desc:** State and territorial directors of public state health HIV/AIDS programs and services. Dedicated to reducing the incidence of HIV infection in the U.S. and territories, providing comprehensive, compassionate, and quality care to all persons living with HIV/AIDS, and the development of responsible and compassionate public policies. **Pub:** *HIV Prevention Bulletin*, monthly. Newsletter.

★ 4592 ★ National Alopecia Areata Foundation (NAAF)
PO Box 150760
San Rafael, CA 94915-0760
Phone: (415)472-3780 **Fax:** (415)472-5343
Email: info@naaf.org
Website: http://www.naaf.org
Vicki Kalabokes, CEO

Fnded: 1981. **Mem:** 56,000. **Nat'l Groups:** 65. **Reg. Groups:** 4. **State Groups:** 6. **Local Groups:** 2. **Desc:** Individuals concerned about alopecia areata, a disease causing partial scalp hair loss, total scalp hair loss (alopecia totalis), or total loss of body hair (alopecia universalis); cause and cure are unknown and the course of the disease is unpredictable. Objectives are to: develop public awareness of the disease; provide a support network; raise funds for research; keep patients medically informed with explanations about AA and the latest treatments. Maintains medical advisory board; operates information booth at meetings of the American Academy of Dermatology. **Pub:** *National Alopecia Areata Foundation Newsletter*, quarterly. Newsletter. Covers treatment, research, and developments. Includes wig and cosmetic tips. *Price:* Included with donation of $35 or more. • Also publishes medical description of AA and assorted brochures.

★ 4593 ★ National AMBUCS
3315 N Main St.
High Point, NC 27265
Phone: (336)869-2166 **Fax:** (336)887-8451
Email: ambucs@ambucs.com
Website: http://www.ambucs.com
Tom Fender, Pres.

Fnded: 1927. **Mem:** 5,600. **Reg. Groups:** 6. **Local Groups:** 145. **Desc:** Dedicated to creating opportunities for independence for people with disabilities. Performs community service; provides physically challenged children with tricycles that can be operated by hand, foot or both: operates the Living Endowment Fund. **Pub:** *AMBUCS*, quarterly. Magazine. **Frmly:** American Business Clubs Spastic Paralysis Fund.

★ 4594 ★ National Amputation Foundation (NAF)
40 Church St.
Malverne, NY 11565
Phone: (516)887-3600 **Fax:** (516)887-3667
Email: amps76@aol.com
Website: http://www.nationalamputation.org
Donald A. Sioss, Exec. Sec.

Fnded: 1919. **Mem:** 2,500. **Desc:** Veterans with service-connected amputation. Assists all amputees, including nonveterans, in employment, social, and mental rehabilitation. Provides services, including legal counsel, vocational guidance and placement, social activities, liaison with other groups, and psychological aid. Sponsors Amp-to-Amp program arranging for amputees who have returned to a normal life to visit new amputees. **Pub:** *The Amp*, bimonthly. Newsletter.

★ 4595 ★ National Amputee Golf Association (NAGA)
11 Walnut Hill Rd.
Amherst, NH 03031-1713
Phone: (603)672-6444 **Free:** 800-633-6242
Fax: (603)672-2987
Email: info@nagagolf.org
Website: http://www.nagagolf.org
Bob Wilson, Dir.

Fnded: 1955. **Mem:** 2,400. **Reg. Groups:** 4. **Desc:** Individuals who have lost a hand, foot, or a combination thereof at a major joint. Purpose is to promote the mental and physical rehabilitation of amputees through the sport of golf. Conducts first swing program for therapists. Organizes local, regional, national, and international tournaments. Compiles statistics. **Pub:**

Amputee Golfer Magazine, annual. Magazine. *Price:* Included in membership dues. • Newsletter, semiannual, spring and fall. *Price:* Included in membership dues.

★ 4596 ★ National Ankylosing Spondylitis Society (NASS)
PO Box 179
Mayfield TN20 6ZL, United Kingdom
Phone: 44 1435 873527 **Fax:** 44 1435 873027
Email: nass@nass.co.uk
Website: http://www.nass.co.uk

Fnded: 1976. **Mem:** 8,000. **Reg. Groups:** 115. **Lang(s):** English. **Desc:** Promotes patient education in the medical and social aspects of the condition. Provides support through local UK groups for supervised physiotherapy one evening per week.

★ 4597 ★ National Aphasia Association (NAA)
29 John St., Rm. 1103
New York, NY 10038
Phone: (212)267-2814 **Free:** 800-922-4622
Fax: (212)267-2812
Email: naa@aphasia.org
Website: http://www.aphasia.org
Penny Montgomery-West, Response Dir.

Fnded: 1987. **Desc:** Works to promote the care, rehabilitation and quality of life of individuals with aphasia, a speech and language disorder caused by stroke, head trauma or other neurological conditions. Conducts public and professional education programs, facilitates the development of community programs to meet the needs of people with aphasia and their families; provides referrals to professionals. **Pub:** *Aphasia Community Group Manual.* Manual. Contains information to aid in the establishment of new support groups. *Price:* $30. • *Listing of Aphasia Community Groups.* Directory. *Price:* $2.75/copy. • *Newsletter of the National Aphasia Association*, semiannual. Newsletter. *Price:* $1. • *Videotape of 3 Community Groups.* Video. *Price:* $10.

★ 4598 ★ National Arab American Medical Association (NAAMA)
801 S Adams Rd., Ste. 208
Birmingham, MI 48009-7018
Phone: (248)646-3661 **Fax:** (248)646-0617
Email: naama@naama.com
Website: http://www.naama.com
Ellen R. Potter, Exec. Dir.

Fnded: 1974. **Mem:** 2,000. **State Groups:** 26. **Desc:** Medical professionals of Arab descent. Fosters exchange of scientific information. Encourages continuing education for members. Provides financial and technical support for medical students and institutions in the United States and in Arab countries. Offers medical assistance to needy individuals of Arab descent. **Pub:** *Al Hakeem*, quarterly. Newsletter. Contains medical and cultural articles. *Price:* Included in membership dues; $12/year. **Frmly:** (1997) Arab American Medical Association.

★ 4599 ★ National Arthritis Foundation
336 Smith St., Ste. 6-302
New Bridge Centre
Singapore 050336, Singapore
Phone: 65 2279726 **Fax:** 65 2270257
Email: nafsin@pacific.net.sg

Fnded: 1984. **Desc:** Aims to improve quality of life for arthritis suffers. Offers educational programs. Conducts research; disseminates information. **Pub:** Newsletter, periodic.

★ 4600 ★ National Arthritis and Musculoskeletal and Skin Disease Information Clearinghouse
c/o National Institute of Arthritis & Musculoskeletal & Skin Diseases
National Institutes of Health
1 AMS Cir.
Bethesda, MD 20892-3675
Phone: (301)495-4484 **Free:** 877-226-4267
Fax: (301)718-6366
Email: niamsinfo@mail.nih.gov
Website: http://www.niams.nih.gov

Desc: Provides information and resources on arthritis, musculoskeletal diseases, such as fibromyalgia, and skin diseases.

★ 4601 ★ National Asian Pacific American Families Against Substance Abuse (NAPAFASA)
340 E Second St., Ste. 409
Los Angeles, CA 90012
Phone: (213)625-5795 **Fax:** (213)625-5796
Email: jmori@aars-inc.org
Website: http://www.napafasa.org
Jeff Mori, Chm.

Fnded: 1988. **Nat'l Groups:** 200. **Desc:** Members include AAPI and human service organizations. Works to involve service providers, families, and youth to reach API communities in the promotion of health, social justice and the reduction of substance abuse and related problems. Special projects offer organizations technical assistance, training, program planning and clinical training.

★ 4602 ★ National Asian Pacific Center on Aging (NAPCA)
PO Box 21668
Seattle, WA 98101
Phone: (206)624-1221 **Fax:** (206)624-1023
Email: napca@napca.org
Website: http://www.napca.org/
Clayton Fong, Exec. Dir.

Fnded: 1979. **Reg. Groups:** 4. **Desc:** Goals are to: ensure and improve the delivery of health and social services to elderly Pacific/Asians; increase the capabilities of community-based services by expanding their information and technical base; include Pacific/Asians in planning and organizational activities, thus maintaining a strong link between the center and the community. Provides technical assistance to the generic service delivery system on program development and organizational capacity building and training. Compiles statistics. **Pub:** *Asian Pacific Affairs*, bimonthly. Newsletter. • *Demographic & Socio-Economic Characteristics of Elderly Asian & Pacific Island Americans.* • *Directory of Pacific/Asian Media Sources.* Directory. • *Pacific/Asian Elderly Bibliography.* Directory. • *Registry of Services for Pacific/Asian Elderly*, biennial. Directory. **Frmly:** (1993) National Pacific/Asian Resource Center on Aging.

★ 4603 ★ National Asian Women's Health Organization (NAWHO)
250 Montgomery St., Ste. 900
San Francisco, CA 94104
Phone: (415)989-9747 **Fax:** (415)989-9758
Email: nawho@nawho.org
Website: http://www.nawho.org
Karen Lim, Exec. Dir.

Fnded: 1993. **Desc:** Asian American women. Promotes increased awareness of the unique health needs of Asian American women among health care professionals and the public. Serves as a clearinghouse on Asian American women's health issues; conducts advocacy campaigns; compiles statistics.

★ 4604 ★ National Association of Addiction Treatment Providers (NAATP)
313 E Liberty St., Ste. 129
Lancaster, PA 17603-2748
Phone: (717)392-8480 **Fax:** (717)392-8481
Email: rhunsicker@naatp.org
Website: http://www.naatp.org
Ronald J. Hunsicker, Pres. /CEO

Fnded: 1978. **Mem:** 210. **State Groups:** 12. **Desc:** Corporate and private institutional alcohol and/or drug dependency treatment facilities. Promotes awareness of chemical dependency as a treatable disease; advocates high standards of health care in substance abuse treatment facilities. Encourages member education. Maintains contact with U.S. Congress and state and local governments. Serves in an advisory capacity to the Joint Commission on Accreditation of Healthcare Organizations and to the Commission on Accreditation of Rehabilitation Facilities. Compiles statistics on chemical dependency treatment and recovery. **Pub:** *NAATP Visions*, monthly. Newsletter. *Price:* Free. For members only. **Frmly:** (1987) National Association of Alcoholism Treatment Programs.

★ 4605 ★ National Association for Adults with Special Learning Needs (NAASLN)
c/o CEA
4380 Forbes Blvd.
Lanham, MD 20706
Free: 800-496-9222
Email: rcooper6@aol.com
Website: http://www.naasln.org/
Richard Cooper, Contact

Fnded: 1989. **Mem:** 350. **Desc:** Works to organize and promote a coalition of individuals interested in educating adults with special learning needs. Fosters development and implementation of educational programs for adults. Promotes unification of adult education professionals. Encourages research and dissemination of information on adult education. Acts as a forum for the exchange of information on adult education. Seeks to unify adults with special learning needs. Bestows annual NAASLN Distinguished Services Award.

★ 4606 ★ National Association for the Advancement of Psychoanalysis (NAAP)
80 8th Ave., Ste. 1501
New York, NY 10011-1501
Phone: (212)741-0515 **Fax:** (212)366-4347
Email: naap72@aol.com
Website: http://www.naap.org
Margery Quackenbush, Admin.

Fnded: 1972. **Mem:** 1,700. **Desc:** Psychoanalytic organizations and individual psychoanalysts from a variety of schools of psychoanalytic thought united for the advancement of psychoanalysis as a profession. Establishes standards for psychoanalytic training and works to improve its quality. Sets standards for certification of individual psychoanalysts; registers those who have met its training standards. **Pub:** *NAAP News*, quarterly. Covers institute, committee, and membership activities. Includes legislative news, calendar of events, and obituaries. *Price:* Included in membership dues; $12/year for nonmembers. • *Registry of Psychoanalysts*, annual. Directory. Lists qualified psychoanalysts and candidates-in-training. Includes list of member organizations and geographic index. *Price:* $15/copy. **Frmly:** (2000) National Association for the Advancement of Psychoanalysis and the American Accreditation in Psychoanalysis.

★ 4607 ★ National Association of Advisors for the Health Professions (NAAHP)
PO Box 1518
Champaign, IL 61824-1518
Phone: (217)355-0063 **Fax:** (217)355-1287
Email: staff@naahp.org
Website: http://www.naahp.org
Susan Maxwell, Exec. Dir.

Fnded: 1974. **Mem:** 1,275. **Reg. Groups:** 4. **Desc:** College and university faculty who advise and counsel students on health careers. Seeks to improve and preserve advisement at all educational levels of the health professions. Fosters and coordinates communication among the health professions and advisers. Marshalls resources; provides services concerning health professions advisement. Goals include: informed counseling for students seeking careers in the health professions; proper preparation of student evaluations for the professional schools; participation of advisers in curriculum development; improved communication between secondary and undergraduate institutions; coordination of record keeping and information exchange among undergraduate schools and local, state, and regional preprofessional programs. Makes available Advisor's Supplementary Student Evaluation Tool software program; conducts surveys. **Pub:** *Directory of the National Association of Advisors for the Health Professions*, annual. Directory. Includes health professional school announcements and order forms. *Price:* $25/issue. • *The Medical School Interview.* • *National Association of Advisors for the Health Professions–The Advisor*, quarterly. Focuses on manpower statistics, financial aid, admission procedures, curriculum, advising, recruitment, counseling practice, and ethics. *Price:* $70/year. • *Strategy for Success: A Handbook for Prehealth Students.* Handbook. • *Write for Success.* • Audiotapes. • Videos.

★ 4608 ★ National Association of Advisory Officers for Special Educational Needs

Princes St.
Tunbridge Wells TN2 4SL, United Kingdom
Phone: 44 1892 534034 **Fax:** 44 1799 521257
Email: diana.robinson@btclick.com

Desc: Advisory officers for special education. **Frmly:** (2000) National Association of Advisor Officers for Special Education.

★ 4609 ★ National Association of Air Medical Communication Specialists (NAAMCS)

PO Box 28
Otis Orchards, WA 99027-0028
Free: 877-396-2227
Email: shellsholl@aol.com
Website: http://www.naacs.org
Allan Adler, Pres.

Fnded: 1989. **Mem:** 300. **Desc:** Air medical communications specialists. Promotes professional advancement of members. Represents members at the national level; formulates standards of ethics and practice in air medical communications; sponsors educational and training programs. **Pub:** *NAACS Newsletter*, quarterly. Newsletter. • *NAACS Training Manual.* Manual.

★ 4610 ★ National Association of Alcohol and Drug Abuse Counsellors

122a Wilton Rd.
London SW1V 1JZ, United Kingdom
Phone: 44 870 7636139
Email: office@naadac.org.uk
Website: http://www.naadac.org.uk

Fnded: 1984. **Mem:** 160. **Desc:** Individual counsellors dedicated to the development of the professional specialism of alcoholism and drug abuse counselling as a means of securing the provision of quality care to those who experience primary and secondary addiction problems, their families and. dependants and others significant to them. Promotes recognition of the qualified alcoholism and drug abuse counsellor as a health care professional; fosters interaction and exchange of knowledge and experience between counsellor associations; advocates on a national level for alcoholism and drug abuse counsellors on issues affecting the profession; promotes a code of ethics. **Pub:** *NAADAC News*, quarterly. Newsletter.

★ 4611 ★ National Association on Alcohol, Drugs and Disability (NAADD)

2165 Bunker Hill Dr.
San Mateo, CA 94402-3801
Phone: (650)578-8047 **Fax:** (650)286-9205
Email: jdem@aimnet.com
Website: http://www.naadd.org/
John deMiranda, Exec. Dir.

Desc: Promotes awareness and education about substance abuse among people with co-existing disabilities; aims to create public awareness of issues related to alcoholism, drug addition, and substance abuse faced by persons with co-existing disabilities; provides a peer approach to enhance access to services, information, education and prevention through collaborative efforts of individuals and organizations. Sponsors the California Technology Assistance & Training Project. **Pub:** *The NAADD Report: The Newsletter on Alcohol, Drugs and Disability*, annual. Newsletter.

★ 4612 ★ National Association of Alternative Medicines (NAAM)

PO Box 35215
Chicago, IL 60707-0215
Phone: (708)453-0080 **Fax:** (708)453-0083
Email: naam@rentamark.com
Website: http://www.rentamark.com/naam/
L. Stollen, Contact

Fnded: 1975. **Mem:** 65,532. **Nat'l Groups:** 1. **Desc:** Practitioners of alternative medical specialties. Seeks to increase members' public visibility and professional influence. Provides member education; also provides trademark licensing and product and service endorsement services to support members' activities. A major platform for professional advancement and knowledge. **Pub:** *NAAM Journal*, monthly. Journal. • Journal, monthly. Invites authors to submit articles in Word format via email. *Price:* for members. **AKA:** (2000) American Alternative Medicine Association.

★ 4613 ★ National Association of Anorexia Nervosa and Associated Disorders (ANAD)

Box 7
Highland Park, IL 60035
Phone: (847)831-3438 **Fax:** (847)433-4632
Email: anad20@aol.com
Website: http://www.anad.org
Vivian Hanson Meehan, RN, Pres. /Founder

Fnded: 1976. **Nat'l Groups:** 350. **Desc:** Anorexics and bulimics, their families, health professionals, and others interested in the problems of anorexia nervosa and bulimia. Maintains chapters in 45 states, Canada, South Africa, Ghana, France, Italy, Puerto Rico, Argentina, England, Slovenia, Ireland, Switzerland, Colombia, Spain and Germany. Aims to: seek a better understanding of, prevent, and cure anorexia nervosa and associated eating disorders; educate the public and health professionals on illnesses relating to eating disorders and methods of treatment. Encourages and promotes research on the cause of eating disorders, methods of prevention, types of treatment and their effectiveness, and basic facts about victims. Acts as a resource center, compiling and providing information about eating disorders. Serves as an advocacy agency for those concerned with eating disorders. Works to end insurance discrimination against sufferers of eating disorders. Fights against the production, marketing, and distribution of dangerous diet aids and the use of misleading advertisements. Encourages and cosponsors local and regional meetings. Maintains speakers' bureau; provides children's services; compiles statistics. Conducts referral service, surveys, education, and early detection programs. Organizes selfhelp groups. **Pub:** *Working Together*, quarterly. Newsletter. *Price:* Included in membership dues. **Frmly:** (1980) Anorexia Nervosa and Associated Disorders.

★ 4614 ★ National Association of Area Agencies on Aging (NAAAA)

927 15th St., 6th Fl.
Washington, DC 20005
Phone: (202)296-8130 **Fax:** (202)296-8134
Email: info@n4a.org
Website: http://www.n4a.org
Sandy Markwood, CEO

Fnded: 1975. **Mem:** 665. **Desc:** Members are Area Agencies on Aging, established under the provisions of the Older Americans Act of 1965; also offers corporate and cooperating memberships. Promotes the achievement of a reasonable and realistic national policy on aging; assists the process of partnership and regular communication within a national network on aging. Acts as advocate for the needs of older persons at the national level. Maintains communication among members to enable an effective response to federal legislation and regulations. Disseminates information to the federal government, the private sector, and the public. Provides general administrative, training, and technical assistance to area agencies. **Pub:** *In Step with N4A*, monthly. Newsletter. • *National Directory for Eldercare Information and Referral*, biennial. Manuals. Contains listings of all area agencies throughout the US. *Price:* $50.

★ 4615 ★ National Association of Athletes Against Drugs (NAAAD)

2481 Pacific Ave., Ste. C
Long Beach, CA 90806-2953
Phone: (562)989-9692 **Fax:** (562)426-9863
Email: educat2100@aol.com
Elliott Smith, Chm.

Fnded: 1992. **Mem:** 1,293. **Reg. Groups:** 3. **Desc:** Professional athletes in motor sports. Promotes use of the fame enjoyed by racing drivers to deter youth from substance abuse. Seeks to increase participation by African-Americans in professional motor sports. Conducts educational programs; participates in charitable activities; makes available children's services; compiles statistics; maintains speakers' bureau. **Pub:** *The Informer*, periodic. Newsletter. *Price:* for members.

★ 4616 ★ National Association for Biomedical Research (NABR)

818 Connecticut Ave. NW, Ste. 200
Washington, DC 20006
Phone: (202)857-0540 **Fax:** (202)659-1902
Email: info@nabr.org
Website: http://www.nabr.org
Ms. Mary F. Hanley, Exec. VP

Fnded: 1979. **Mem:** 400. **Desc:** Universities, medical and veterinary schools, teaching hospitals, professional societies, voluntary health agencies, pharmaceutical companies and other research-related firms that use laboratory animals for biomedical research, education, and testing. Monitors and, when appropriate, attempts to influence legislation and regulations on behalf of members who are dependent on animals for biomedical research, education, and testing. **Pub:** *NABR Alert*, 6-10/year. Newsletter. Covers regulatory and legislative action related to the use of animals in biomedical research, research, and testing. *Price:* Included in membership dues. • *NABR Update*, 48/year. Bulletin. Covers national, state, and local regulatory and legislative activities affecting biomedical research. *Price:* Included in membership dues. • *National Association for BioMedical Research.* Annual Report. Describes the previous year's activities. *Price:* Included in membership dues.

★ 4617 ★ National Association of Boards of Examiners of Long Term Care Administrators (NABE)

1444 I St. NW, Ste. 700
Washington, DC 20005-2210
Phone: (202)712-9040 **Fax:** (202)216-9646
Email: nab@bostromdc.com
Website: http://www.nabweb.org
Randy Lindner, Exec. Dir.

Fnded: 1972. **Mem:** 550. **Desc:** State boards responsible for licensing nursing homes administrators. Produces exam to test the competence of nursing home adminstrators; operates continuing education review service; disseminates information and educational materials on nursing home administration. **Pub:** *NAB Study Guide: How To Prepare For the Nursing Home Administrators Examination.* The third edition. *Price:* $65.00. • *RC/AL Study Guide: How to Prepare for the Residential Care/Assisted Living Administrators Examination*, annual. *Price:* $34. **Frmly:** National Association of Boards of Examiners of Nursing Home Administrators.

★ 4618 ★ National Association of Boards of Pharmacy (NABP)

700 Busse Hwy.
Park Ridge, IL 60068

Phone: (847)698-6227 **Fax:** (847)698-0124
Email: custserv@nabp.net
Website: http://www.nabp.net
Carmen A. Catizone, Exec. Dir. /Sec.

Fnded: 1904. **Mem:** 68. **Desc:** Pharmacy boards of several states, District of Columbia, Puerto Rico, Virgin Islands, several Canadian provinces, the states of Victoria, Australia, and New South Wales, the Pharmaceutical Society of New Zealand, and the South African Pharmacy Council. Provides for interstate reciprocity in pharmaceutic licensure based upon a uniform minimum standard of pharmaceutic education and uniform legislation; improves the standards of pharmaceutical education licensure and practice. Provides legislative information; sponsors uniform licensure examination; also provides information on accredited school and college requirements. Maintains pharmacy and drug law statistics. **Pub:** *Annual Meeting Proceedings*, annual. Proceedings. • *NABP Newsletter*, 10/year. Newsletter. Reports on regulation and licensure in the pharmacy profession. Contains information on NABP competency assessment programs. *Price:* $35/year. • *The NAPLEX Candidate's Review Guide*, annual. • *State Board Newsletters*, quarterly. Newsletter. Covers 34 states. • *Survey of Pharmacy Law*, annual. Survey. • Surveys. • Also publishes periodically updated guides and examination manuals.

★ 4619 ★ National Association of Child Care Professionals

PO Box 90723
Austin, TX 78709
Free: 800-537-1118 **Fax:** (512)301-5080
Email: admin@naccp.org
Website: http://www.naccp.org
Sherry Workman, Exec. Dir.

Fnded: 1984. **Mem:** 2,662. **State Groups:** 4. **Desc:** Child care supervisors and individuals involved in decision making at a child care facility. Offers networking opportunities and support services to child care professionals. Dedicated to the professional development of child care directors. Conducts educational programs. **Pub:** *Caring for Your Children*, quarterly. Newsletter. Contains information for parents. *Price:* Free. For members only; $39 nonmembers. • *Professional Connections*, quarterly. Newsletter. Contains management information for directors. • *Team Work*, quarterly. Newsletter. Directed toward staff members. • Directory.Contains contact information for other child care professionals. • Management Tools of the Trade-Personnel resource management forms specific to child care industry.

★ 4620 ★ National Association of Child Care Resource and Referral Agencies (NACCRRA)

1319 F St. NW, Ste. 500
Washington, DC 20004-1106
Phone: (202)393-5501 **Fax:** (202)393-1109
Email: info@naccrra.org
Website: http://www.naccrra.org
Yasmina Vinci, Exec. Dir.

Fnded: 1987. **Mem:** 750. **Reg. Groups:** 8. **State Groups:** 32. **Local Groups:** 600. **Desc:** Network of community-based child care resource and referral programs that promote a diverse, high quality child care system with parental choice that is accessible to all families. National leadership to build such a system; promotes growth and development of quality resource and referral services.

★ 4621 ★ National Association of Childbearing Centers (NACC)

3123 Gottschall Rd.
Perkiomenville, PA 18074
Phone: (215)234-8068 **Fax:** (215)234-8829
Email: reachnacc@birthcenters.org
Website: http://www.birthcenters.org
Kate Bauer, Exec. Dir.

Fnded: 1983. **Mem:** 600. **Reg. Groups:** 6. **State Groups:** 2. **Desc:** Working on public and policy levels in government, industry and the health professions, NACC is dedicated to developing quality, holistic services for childbearing families that promote self-reliance and confidence in birth and parenting. Collects and disseminates information on birth centers. Sets national standards for birth center operation, promotes state regulation for licensure, and national accreditation by the Commission for the Accreditation of Birth Centers. Provides a Parent Information Service for consumers looking for birth centers. Provides information on birth center. **Pub:** *Birth Center Information Packet*. Articles. Covers growth and development, regulation, costs, reimbursement, research, and selected issues of NACC News. *Price:* $30. • *Continuous Quality Improvement Manual*. Manual. Contains forms and instructions for implementing a continuous quality improvement/risk management program in birth centers. *Price:* $100 for members; $150 for nonmembers. • *Marketing the Birth Center*. • *NACC Membership Directory*, annual. Membership Directory. *Price:* Included in membership dues. • *NACC News*, 3/year. • *NACC Uniform Data Set*. *Price:* $299 members; $599 nonmembers. • *National Birth Center Study*. Reprint. *Price:* $1. • *Sample Birth Center Policy and Procedure Manual*. Manual. Contains sample policies and procedures of an accredited birth center. Includes diskettes for customization. *Price:* $200 members; $300 nonmembers. • *Standards for Birth Centers*. *Price:* $15 for members; $30 for non-members. • *Survey Report of Birth Center Experience*. *Price:* $10 members; $20 nonmembers. • *"The Birth Center" Brochure*. Brochure. Contains information describing freestanding birth centers. Designed for public education and promotion of the concept of birth centers. *Price:* $49/100 brochures. • *"The Birth Center" Video*. Video. Designed to increase public awareness of the presence of birth centers. *Price:* $39.95.

★ 4622 ★ National Association for Children of Alcoholics (NACoA)

11426 Rockville Pike, St. 100
Rockville, MD 20852
Phone: (301)468-0985 **Free:** 888-554-2627
Fax: (301)468-0987
Email: nacoa@nacoa.org
Website: http://www.nacoa.org
Sis Wenger, Exec. Dir.

Fnded: 1983. **Mem:** 4,000. **Desc:** Authors, educators, physicians, psychologists, therapists, and children of alcoholics. Supports and serves as a resource for individuals of all age groups who are COAs. Objectives are to increase public and professional awareness and recognition of the special needs of children of alcoholics; to provide leadership in public policy at the national, state, and local level; to act as an informational and educational resource to academic and other community systems; to create networks that facilitate the exchange of information and resources; to initiate and advance professional knowledge and understanding; to advocate for accessible programs and services. Compiles statistics; conducts educational programs. **Pub:** *Children of Alcoholics: Selected Readings, Vol. II*. Book. • *It's Elementary: Meeting the Needs of High Risk Youth in the School Setting*. Booklet. • *NACoA Network*, bimonthly. Newsletter. *Price:* $20. • *Poor Jennifer: She's Always Losing Her Hat*. Video. • Also makes available posters, videos, booklets, brochures.

★ 4623 ★ National Association of Children's Hospitals and Related Institutions (NACHRI)

401 Wythe St.
Alexandria, VA 22314
Phone: (703)684-1355 **Fax:** (703)684-1589
Website: http://www.childrenshospitals.net
Lawrence A. McAndrews, Pres. /CEO

Fnded: 1968. **Mem:** 149. **Desc:** Children's hospitals and related institutions whose programs are clinical (as opposed to social or custodial). Purposes are: to promote the quality of child health care through the dissemination of information and the promotion of research and education programs related to such care; to participate in related charitable, scientific, and educational endeavors. Conducts surveys and research; disseminates information; maintains computerized services. Compiles statistics. **Pub:** *Childrens Hospitals Today*, quarterly. Magazine.

★ 4624 ★ National Association of Clinical Nurse Specialists (NACNS)

3969 Green St.
Harrisburg, PA 17110
Phone: (717)234-6799 **Fax:** (717)234-6798
Email: info@nacns.org
Website: http://www.nacns.org
Christine Carson Filipovich, Exec. Dir.

Fnded: 1995. **Mem:** 1,200. **Reg. Groups:** 11. **Desc:** Clinical Nurse Specialists. **Pub:** *Statement on Clinical Nurse Specialist Practice and Education*. Handbook. *Price:* $15/copy for members; $25/copy for nonmembers.

★ 4625 ★ National Association of Cognitive-Behavioral Therapists (NACBT)

PO Box 2195
Weirton, WV 26062
Phone: (304)723-3982 **Free:** 800-853-1135
Fax: (304)723-3982
Email: nacbt@nacbt.org
Website: http://www.nacbt.org/
Aldo R. Pucci, Pres.

Fnded: 1995. **Desc:** Promotes and supports the teaching and practice of cognitive-behavior psychotherapy and to support those professionals and students seeking to practice it; sets standards for credentialing.

★ 4626 ★ National Association of Colitis and Crohn's Disease (NACC)

4 Beaumont House
Sutton Rd.
Saint Albans AL1 5HH, United Kingdom
Phone: 44 1727 830038 **Fax:** 44 1727 862550
Email: nacc@nacc.org.uk
Website: http://www.nacc.org.uk

Fnded: 1979. **Mem:** 30,000. **Reg. Groups:** 70. **Lang(s):** English. **Desc:** Patients, relatives, health professionals, and anyone interested in colitis and Crohn's disease. Provides support and information for patients and families living with these conditions. **Pub:** Newsletter, quarterly.

★ 4627 ★ National Association of Community Health Centers (NACHC)

1330 New Hampshire Ave. NW, Ste. 122
Washington, DC 20036
Phone: (301)347-0400
Email: contact@nachc.com
Website: http://www.nachc.com
Tom Van Coverden, Pres. /CEO

Fnded: 1970. **Mem:** 950. **Desc:** Advocacy organization of ambulatory healthcare centers, administrators, clinicians, and consumers. Works to assure the continued growth and development of community-based healthcare delivery programs for medically underserved populations by providing technical assistance and education and training opportunities for health center staff and board members. Disseminates information and research data and provides representation in legislative and professional arenas. Sponsors educational institutes, workshops, and seminars throughout the year. **Pub:** *NACHC Link*. Newsletter. *Price:* Included in membership dues. • *The Vanguard*, quarterly. Newsletter. • *Washington Update*, monthly. Newsletter. **Frmly:** National Association of Directors and Administrators; (1977) National Association of Neighborhood Health Centers.

★ 4628 ★ National Association for Continence

PO Box 8310
Spartanburg, SC 29305-8310
Phone: (864)579-7900 **Free:** 800-BLA-DDER
Fax: (864)579-7902
Email: memberservices@nafc.org

Website: http://www.nafc.org
Nancy Muller, Exec. Dir.

Fnded: 1982. **Mem:** 140,000. **Nat'l Groups:** 1. **Desc:** Works to help individuals who have bladder control problems. Acts as a clearinghouse of information involving incontinence and assistive devices for consumers and their families as well as medical, nursing, and social service organizations. **Pub:** *Quality Care*, quarterly. Newsletter. *Price:* $25/year. • *Resource Guide-Continence Products and Services.* **Frmly:** Help for Incontinent People.

★ 4629 ★ National Association of Counsellors, Hypnotherapists and Psychotherapists

PO Box 719
Cambridge CB5 0NX, United Kingdom
Phone: 44 163 8741363 **Fax:** 44 163 8744190
Email: mail@nachp.org
Website: http://www.nachp.org

Desc: Aims to maintain a register of qualified therapists which is available to members of the public seeking treatment.

★ 4630 ★ National Association of County Aging Programs

440 1st St. NW
Washington, DC 20001
Phone: (202)942-4260 **Fax:** (202)942-4281
Email: msanz@naco.org
Sandra Reinsel-Markwood, Staff Liaison

Fnded: 1978. **Desc:** Affiliated with the National Association of Counties. Assists counties in their plans for providing services to the aging of the community.

★ 4631 ★ National Association of County Behavioral Health Directors (NACBHD)

1555 Connecticut Ave. NW, Ste. 200
Washington, DC 20036
Phone: (202)234-7543 **Free:** 800-228-6905
Fax: (202)462-9043
Email: lauren@nacbhd.org
Website: http://www.nacbhd.org
Lauren Wolfe, MS, Dep. Exec. Dir.

Fnded: 1996. **Mem:** 325. **Desc:** County/local behavioral health authorities responsible for the planning and delivery of mental health, developmental disabilities and substance abuse services and the state associations representing their interests. Promotes excellence in the delivery of county/local behavioral health services. **Pub:** *NACBHD Bulletin*, bimonthly. Newsletter. Contains policy information, articles of interest on local programs, association announcements, and job bank. *Price:* for members.

★ 4632 ★ National Association of County and City Health Officials (NACCHO)

1100 17th St. NW 2nd Fl.
Washington, DC 20036-4631
Phone: (202)783-5550 **Fax:** (202)783-1583
Email: info@naccho.org
Website: http://www.naccho.org
Debbie Mitchell, Exec. Dir.

Fnded: 1965. **Mem:** 1,000. **Desc:** County and city (local) health officials. Purposes are to stimulate and contribute to the improvement of local health programs and public health practices throughout the U.S.; disseminate information on local health programs and practices; participate in the formulation of the policies of the National Association of Counties. Is developing self-assessment instrument for use by local health officials. Operates Primary Care Project which helps to strengthen the link between local health departments and community health centers. Provides educational workshops for local health officials. **Pub:** *Membership Monthly*, monthly. Information guide for members. *Price:* Included in membership dues. • *NACCHO News*, bimonthly. *Price:* Included in membership dues. • Annual Report. **Frmly:** National Association of County Health Officials; (1975) National Association of County Health Officers.

★ 4633 ★ National Association of County Health Facility Administrators (NACHFA)

c/o National Association of Counties
440 First St., NW
Washington, DC 20001
Phone: (202)393-6226 **Fax:** (202)393-2630
Website: http://www.naco.org
Frank Colb, Staff Liaison

Fnded: 1977. **Mem:** 250. **Desc:** Administrators of freestanding and hospital-based long-term care facilities owned and operated by county governments or city-county consolidations; elected local officials. Promotes interests of county long-term care facilities; offers guidance in relevant legislative and regulatory areas. Provides technical assistance; conducts training workshops. Compiles statistics on public policy changes, such as changes in the Medicaid program, which affect long-term care facilities.

★ 4634 ★ National Association of the Deaf (NAD)

814 Thayer Ave., Ste. 250
Silver Spring, MD 20910-4500
Phone: (301)587-1788 **Fax:** (301)587-1791
Email: nadinfo@nad.org
Website: http://www.nad.org
Nancy J. Bloch, Exec. Dir.

Fnded: 1880. **Mem:** 22,000. **State Groups:** 51. **Desc:** Safeguards accessibility and civil rights of America's deaf population in areas of education, employment, healthcare, and telecommunications. **Pub:** *NADmag*, bimonthly. Magazine. • Also publishes catalog and textbooks on American Sign Language and other systems of manual communication.

★ 4635 ★ National Association of the Deaf in Iceland (Felag Heyrnarlausra)

Laugavegi 103
IS-105 Reykjavik, Iceland
Phone: 354 5613560 **Fax:** 354 5513567
Email: deaf@deaf.is
Website: http://www.deaf.is

Fnded: 1960. **Mem:** 200. **State Groups:** 1. **Lang(s):** English, Icelandic, Norwegian, Spanish, Swedish. **Desc:** People with hearing impairments, their families, and health care and speech and hearing professionals. Works to improve the quality of life of people with impaired hearing. Works to insure that the legal and economic rights of people with hearing impairments are respected. Conducts research and educational programs on sign language and other means of nonverbal communication. Serves as a liaison with other national and international associations with similar aims. Assists members in obtaining assistive technologies including text telephones, alarm services, and TTD messages. **Pub:** *Doff-laoio*, 3/year. Magazine. • *Doff-postur*, monthly. Newsletter. News regarding the deaf community in Iceland and abroad. • *TDD*, monthly. Magazine. News regarding the deaf community in Iceland and abroad. • *TTP*, 3/year. Newsletter.

★ 4636 ★ National Association for Deaf People (NADP)

35 N Frederick St.
Dublin 1, Ireland
Phone: 353 1 8723800 **Fax:** 353 1 8723816
Email: nad@iol.ie
Website: http://www.nadp.ie

Fnded: 1963. **Reg. Groups:** 8. **Lang(s):** English, Irish. **Desc:** Individuals and organizations. Seeks to improve the quality of life of people with hearing impairments; promotes full recognition of the rights of people with hearing loss. Makes available support and services; conducts educational and advocacy campaigns. Offers a job coaching service; operates Family Resource Centre; conducts sign language classes. **Pub:** *Link*, quarterly. Magazine. Contains information on deaf culture issues plus editorial.

★ 4637 ★ National Association of Deafened People

PO Box 50
Amersham HP6 6XB, United Kingdom
Phone: 44 1494 724830 **Fax:** 44 1494 431932
Email: enquiries@nadp.org.uk
Website: http://www.nadp.org.uk

Fnded: 1984. **Mem:** 500. **Nat'l Groups:** 1. **Reg. Groups:** 6. **Desc:** People with acquired profound hearing loss and professionals associated with them. Aims to work for improvements in the quality of life of deafened people, by providing a support service of information and advice and promoting an improvement in education, training and rehabilitation opportunities available. It also aims to increase public awareness of the needs and problems of deafened people, and to support research. **Pub:** *An Introduction to Cochlear Implants.* Booklet. • *Information Booklet.* • *Network*, quarterly. Newsletter.

★ 4638 ★ National Association of Dental Assistants (NADA)

900 S Washington St., No. G-13
Falls Church, VA 22046
Phone: (703)237-8616 **Fax:** (703)533-1153
R. Ludeman, Dir.

Fnded: 1974. **Mem:** 6,000. **Desc:** Professional dental auxiliaries. Seeks to: bring added stature and purpose to the profession through continuing education; make available to dental assistants the special benefits normally limited to members of specialized professional and fraternal groups. **Pub:** *Communication in the Workplace.* • *Dental Assistant Salary Survey*, biennial. Survey. • *The Explorer*, 11/year. Newsletter. Includes job exchange. *Price:* Included in membership dues; $20/year for nonmembers. • *Infection Control.* • *Mercury Poisoning.* • *Radiology.*

★ 4639 ★ National Association of Dental Laboratories (NADL)

1530 Metropolitan Blvd.
Tallahassee, FL 32308
Phone: (850)222-0053 **Free:** 800-950-1150
Fax: (850)222-0053
Email: nadl@nadl.org
Website: http://www.nadl.org
Bennett E. Napier, CAE, Exec. Dir.

Fnded: 1951. **Mem:** 2,900. **State Groups:** 45. **Desc:** Represents 2900 commercial dental laboratories, manufacturers/suppliers and educators serving the dental profession. Develops criteria for ethical dental laboratories. Offers business and personal insurance programs, Hazardous Materials Training Program, and an infectious disease prevention training program, business management and technical education programs. Compiles statistics; maintains speakers' bureau and museum; conducts educational and charitable programs. **Pub:** *The Journal of Dental Technology*, 10/year. Magazine. *Price:* $40 for members; $50 for members outside U.S. • *Leadership Newsletter*, periodic. Newsletter. • *Managing for Profit.* Book. • *NADL*, quarterly. Newsletter. *Price:* for members. • *Who's Who in the Dental Laboratory Industry*, annual. Directory. • Also publishes standardized accounting system and makes available videotapes. **Frmly:** National Association of Certified Dental Laboratories.

★ 4640 ★ National Association of Dental Plans (NADP)

8111 Lyndon B. Johnson Fwy., Ste. 935
Dallas, TX 75251-1347
Phone: (972)458-6998 **Fax:** (972)458-2258
Email: info@nadp.org
Website: http://www.nadp.org
Evelyn F. Ireland, CAE, Exec. Dir./Pres.

Fnded: 1989. **Mem:** 100. **Desc:** Dental HMO, PPO's and dental referral plans with Associate members that provide dental indemnity and dental practice management companies. Strives to improve consumer access to affordable quality dental care. **Pub:** *Data Reports*, quarterly. Reports.

★ 4641 ★ National Association of Directors of Nursing Administration in Long Term Care (NADONA/LTC)
10101 Alliance Rd., No. 140
Cincinnati, OH 45242
Phone: (513)791-3679 **Free:** 800-222-0539
Fax: (513)791-3699
Email: info@nadona.org
Website: http://www.nadona.org
Joan C. Warden-Saunders, R.N., Exec. Dir. & Founder

Fnded: 1986. **Mem:** 4,600. **Reg. Groups:** 5. **State Groups:** 35. **Desc:** Directors, assistant directors, and former directors of nursing in long term care. Goals are: to create and establish an acceptable ethical standard for practices in long term care nursing administration and to promote and encourage research in the profession; to develop and provide a consistent program of education and certification for the positions of director, associate director, and assistant director; to promote a positive image of the long term health care industry. Encourages members to share concerns and experiences; sponsors research programs. Advocates legislation pertaining to the practice of professional nursing. Maintains speakers' bureau. nursing. Maintains speakers' bureau. **Pub:** *The Director*, quarterly. Journal. Includes research, clinical papers and news items. *Price:* Included in membership dues.

★ 4642 ★ National Association of Disability Evaluating Professionals (NADEP)
PO Box 35407
Richmond, VA 23235
Phone: (804)378-8809
Email: mayrehab@aol.com
Website: http://www.nadep.com
Dr. Virgil R. May, III, Exec. Dir.

Fnded: 1984. **Mem:** 1,000. **Nat'l Groups:** 1. **Desc:** Lawyers, doctors, psychologists, employers, and others interested or involved in disability claims process, evaluation, and case management. Provides a forum for the exchange of information. Serves as a training center which prepares health professionals to qualify for the Certified Disability Examiner credential offered by the Commission on Disability Examiner Certification. **Pub:** *Disability Evaluation and Rehabilitation Review*, quarterly. Newsletter. *Price:* Included in membership. • *NADEP Guide to Functional Capacity Evaluation with Department Rating Applications Textbook.* Book. *Price:* $140 for nonmembers; $120 for members. **Frmly:** (1991) International Health Consultants.

★ 4643 ★ National Association of Disability Examiners (NADE)
PO Box 7886
Madison, WI 53707
Phone: (608)266-7604 **Free:** 800-443-9359
Fax: (608)266-8297
Email: theresa.klubertanz@ssa.gov
Website: http://www.nade.org/
Terri Klubertanz, Actg. Pres.

Fnded: 1963. **Mem:** 2,373. **Reg. Groups:** 7. **Local Groups:** 56. **Desc:** Disability claims examiners, attorneys, and physicians involved in determining the eligibility of applicants for social security benefits based on disability. Purpose is to foster, promote, and participate in activities designed to improve the documentation of applications for disability insurance benefits and the evaluation of medical and/or vocational information obtained in connection with such applications. Provides for the exchange of technical information, ideas, and philosophies. **Pub:** *NADE Advocate*, bimonthly. Newsletter. Includes listings of newly-certified examiners. *Price:* Included in membership dues. • *Nationwide Report*, quarterly. • Directory, annual.

★ 4644 ★ National Association for Drama Therapy (NADT)
733 15th St. NW, Ste. 330
Washington, DC 20005
Phone: (202)966-7409 **Fax:** (202)638-7895
Email: nadt@dmg-dc.com
Website: http://www.nadt.org
Rod Daniel, Contact

Fnded: 1979. **Mem:** 425. **Reg. Groups:** 2. **Desc:** Drama therapists (those trained in the therapeutic applications of creative drama and theatre) and others interested in the field of drama therapy, including those in the psychotherapy, rehabilitation, and education professions. (The association defines drama therapy as the intentional use of drama and theatrical processes to achieve the therapeutic goals of symptom relief, emotional and physical integration, and personal growth. It is used with individuals, groups, and families to maintain health and to treat emotional disorders, learning difficulties, geriatric problems, and social maladjustments.) Purposes are to: develop criteria and standards of training for drama therapists; maintain a system of registration and peer review; encourage research and development of professional training opportunities in drama therapy; represent the interests of members to legislative and regulatory agencies regarding the inclusion of drama therapy in mental health and education bills, state job lines, and insurance policies. Sponsors educational events; maintains speakers' bureau. **Pub:** *Dramascope*, semiannual. Newsletter. Includes book reviews, calendar of events, employment listings, descriptions of treatment programs and methods, and commentaries and reports. *Price:* Included in membership dues. • *Membership List/Registry*, annual. • *Proceedings of Annual Conference*, annual. Proceedings. • Bibliography. • Monographs. • Survey. • Also publishes information on workshops and courses in drama therapy.

★ 4645 ★ National Association on Drug Abuse Problems (NADAP)
355 Lexington Ave.
New York, NY 10017
Phone: (212)986-1170 **Fax:** (212)697-2939
Email: info@NADAP.com
Website: http://www.nadap.org
John Darin, Pres.

Fnded: 1971. **Desc:** Sponsored by business and labor organizations. Serves as an information clearinghouse and referral bureau for corporations and local communities interested in prevention of substance abuse and treatment of substance abusers. Provides: resources to local communities seeking to combat drug and alcohol abuse; corporate services for employers interested in creating a drug-free workplace. Community education and development services include: development of drug and alcohol awareness presentations for community organizations; identification of local substance abuse treatment resources; consultation on development of local prevention, treatment, and vocational programs. Corporate services include: provision of drug and alcohol information seminars in the workplace and through union organizations; assistance in formulation of company drug and alcohol policies; aid in the development and implementation of employee assistance programs; training of supervisors; assistance for companies and labor unions wishing to make full use of local treatment agency networks. Makes available vocational education services including training in job hunting, job interview workshops, training programs for substance abuse treatment professionals, and individual consultations for recovering substance abusers seeking to return to the job market. Provides placement services; has conducted surveys on the employability of rehabilitated drug users and found that former addicts perform comparably with others hired for similar jobs. Operates Neighborhood Prevention Network, through which local communities develop parent support groups and youth peer leadership groups dedicated to combatting drug and alcohol abuse. NPN provides substance abuse prevention and early intervention services for children and youth and ongoing training and materials dealing with specific issues in urban substance abuse. Maintains speakers' bureau. **Pub:** *Conference Proceedings*, biennial. Proceedings. • *NADAP News/Report*, quarterly. Newsletter. Covers current issues in the field of substance abuse. *Price:* Free. • Reports.

★ 4646 ★ National Association for the Dually Diagnosed (NADD)
132 Fair St.
Kingston, NY 12401
Phone: (845)331-4336 **Free:** 800-331-5362
Fax: (845)331-4569
Email: rfletcher@thenadd.org
Website: http://www.thenadd.org
Dr. Robert J. Fletcher, Founder/Exec. Dir.

Fnded: 1983. **Mem:** 1,500. **State Groups:** 6. **Desc:** Promotes understanding of and services for individuals with developmental disabilities and mental health needs. **Pub:** Books. • Audiotapes.

★ 4647 ★ National Association of Emergency Medical Technicians (NAEMT)
408 Monroe St.
Clinton, MS 39056-4210
Phone: (601)924-7744 **Free:** 800-34-NAEMT
Fax: (601)924-7325
Email: president@naemt.org
Website: http://www.naemt.org
Nathan Williams, Pres.

Fnded: 1975. **Mem:** 5,000. **State Groups:** 24. **Desc:** Nationally registered or state certified emergency medical technicians (EMTs) and EMT-paramedics. Promotes the professional status of EMTs and national acceptance of a uniform standard of recognition for their skills; encourages constant upgrading of these skills and EMT qualifications and educational requirements; engages in scientific research related to the care and transportation of the sick and injured; supports the establishment of emergency medical services systems. Sponsors insurance, credit card, and member loan programs. Maintains placement services. **Pub:** *NAEMT News*, bimonthly. Newsletter. *Price:* Free. For members only.

★ 4648 ★ National Association of EMS Educators (NAEMSE)
c/o J. Freel
700 N Bell Ave., Ste. 260
Carnegie, PA 15106-4310
Phone: (412)429-9550 **Fax:** (412)429-9554
Email: naemse@naemse.org
Website: http://www.naemse.org
Joann Freel, Exec. Dir.

Fnded: 1996. **Mem:** 2,038. **Desc:** Promotes EMS education, develops and delivers educational resources, and advocates research and life long learning. **Pub:** *Domain3*, quarterly. Journal. Features teaching tips, current research, an educator's toolbox. *Price:* included in membership dues. • *Educator Update*, bimonthly. Magazine.

★ 4649 ★ National Association of EMS Physicians (NAEMSP)
PO Box 15945-281
Lenexa, KS 66285-5945
Phone: (913)492-5858 **Free:** 800-228-3677
Fax: (913)541-0156
Email: info-naemsp@goamp.com
Website: http://www.naemsp.org
Dede Gish-Panjada, MBA, Exec. Dir.

Fnded: 1983. **Mem:** 1,480. **Desc:** Medical directors responsible for emergency medical services (EMS) programs throughout the United States; other physicians and nonphysicians dedicated to out-of-hospital emergency care. (Most physicians within this organization are medically-legally responsible for the provision of out-of-hospital emergency care.) Strives to foster excellence and provide medical leadership so that all individuals and communities receive quality out-of-hospital emergency medical services. Works to develop guidelines and strategies to reduce and prevent discomfort, disability, and death in the community; define roles, responsiblities, authority, and accountability of EMS physicians; promote communication and cooperation among EMS professionals; define the unique body of medical knowledge of prehospital and disaster medicine; promote cost-effective programs and interventions that optimize patient outcomes; advocate or initiate public policy for optimal emergency medical care; encourage and support quality EMS research. Provides forums for definition and debate of EMS issues. Encourages and promotes career development, career longevity, and professional well-being of EMS professionals. Defines and promotes ethical principles in the delivery of out-of-hospital emergency care. **Pub:** *EMS Medical Directors' Handbook.* Handbook. • *NAEMSP Newsletter*, bimonthly. Newsletter. • *Prehospital Emergency Care*, quarterly. Journal. • *Prehospital Systems and Medical Oversight.* Book. • *Quality Management in Prehospital Care.* Book.

★ 4650 ★ National Association of Federal Veterinarians (NAFV)

1101 Vermont Ave. NW, Ste. 710
Washington, DC 20005-6308
Phone: (202)289-6334 **Fax:** (202)842-4360
Email: dboyle@nafv.org
Website: http://users.erols.com/nafv/
Dr. Joe Yearous, Pres.

Fnded: 1918. **Mem:** 1,600. **State Groups:** 30. **Desc:** Professional society of veterinarians employed by the U.S. Government. Maintains speakers' bureau. **Pub:** *Federal Veterinarian*, monthly. Newsletter. Includes abstracts, obituaries, federal regulatory and legislative news, and association news. *Price:* Included in membership dues; $40/year for nonmembers. • *National Association of Federal Veterinarians–Directory*, annual. Directory. *Price:* $4 for members only. **Frmly:** Bureau of Animal Industry Veterinarians; (1943) National Association of Bureau of Animal Industry Veterinarians.

★ 4651 ★ National Association of First Responders (AAFAR-NAFR)

5334 Armadillo Ave.
Orange Beach, AL 36561-4211
Phone: (251)981-3383
Henry Weir, Jr., Pres.

Fnded: 1984. **Mem:** 3,755. **Nat'l Groups:** 417. **Reg. Groups:** 80. **State Groups:** 112. **Local Groups:** 220. **Desc:** Emergency medical responders who have had 40 hours of training. (EMRs, or first responders, arrive on the scene of a medical emergency and administer assistance prior to the arrival of paramedics or emergency medical technicians.) Provides a forum for exchange of ideas and medical information among EMRs. Offers a national certification program for first responders and educational and research programs. Maintains placement services and speakers' bureau. **Pub:** *National EMR Responder*, monthly. Newsletter. *Price:* Included in membership dues. **Frmly:** (1989) American Association of First Responders.

★ 4652 ★ National Association of Future Doctors of Audiology (NAFDA)

c/o Elizabeth Hoehl
University of Louisville
School of Medicine
Myers Hall
129 E Broadway
Louisville, KY 40202
Phone: (502)852-2620 **Fax:** (502)852-0865
Email: nafda@nafda.org
Website: http://www.nafda.org/
Elizabeth Hoehl, Pres.

Fnded: 1998. **Desc:** Audiology students. Provides forum on national, state and regional issues of concern to the AuD student, including opportunity to travel internationally to offer audiologic healthcare to underprivileged nations.

★ 4653 ★ National Association of General Practitioner Veterinarians (Bundesverband Praktischer Tierarzte — BPT)

Hahnstr. 70
D-60528 Frankfurt am Main, Germany
Phone: 49 69 6698180 **Fax:** 49 69 6668170
Email: bpt-ev@t-online.de
Website: http://www.tieraerzteverband.de

Fnded: 1951. **Mem:** 6,500. **Desc:** Veterinarians in Germany. Represents the professional, economic, and social interests of members. Advocates for animal health and welfare.

★ 4654 ★ National Association of Healthcare Access Management (NAHAM)

2025 M St. NW, Ste. 800
Washington, DC 20036
Phone: (202)367-1125 **Fax:** (202)367-2125
Email: info@naham.org
Website: http://www.naham.org
Steven Kemp, Exec. Dir.

Fnded: 1974. **Mem:** 1,100. **Reg. Groups:** 6. **Desc:** Healthcare access managers united to improve patient care and community relations. Promotes professional recognition and provides educational resources for the healthcare patient access field. Serves as a central source of technical information on changes and trends in healthcare that affect patient access services. Advocates progressive changes in healthcare practices; provides information on admissions and registration procedures. **Pub:** *Connections*, bimonthly. Newsletter. Contains list of employment opportunities. *Price:* Included in membership dues; $75/year for nonmembers. • *The NAHAM Management Journal*, quarterly. Journal. Contains reports on trends affecting admissions, patient registration, and patient access; includes descriptions of techniques, systems, and services. *Price:* Included in membership dues; $90/year for nonmembers. • *National Association of Healthcare Access Management–Membership Directory*, annual. Membership Directory. *Price:* for members only. **Frmly:** (1990) National Association of Hospital Admitting Managers.

★ 4655 ★ National Association for Healthcare Quality (NAHQ)

4700 W Lake Ave.
Glenview, IL 60025-1485
Phone: (847)375-4720 **Free:** 800-966-9392
Fax: 877-218-7939
Email: dsimmons@nahq.com
Website: http://www.nahq.org
Diane K. Simmons, Exec. Dir.

Fnded: 1976. **Mem:** 5,200. **State Groups:** 47. **Desc:** Healthcare professionals in quality assessment and improvement, utilization and risk management, case management, infection control, managed care, nursing, and medical records. Objectives are: to encourage, develop, and provide continuing education for all persons involved in health care quality; to give the patient primary consideration in all actions affecting his or her health and welfare; to promote the sharing of knowledge and encourage a high degree of professional ethics in health care quality. Offers accredited certification in the field of healthcare quality, utilization, and risk management. Facilitates communication and cooperation among members, medical staff, and health care government agencies. Conducts educational seminars and conferences. **Pub:** *Journal for Healthcare Quality*, bimonthly. Journal. *Price:* $125/year. • *NAHQ Guide to Quality Management.* • *NAHQ News*, quarterly. Newsletter. **Frmly:** (1979) National Association of Utilization Review Coordinators; (1991) National Association of Quality Assurance Professionals.

★ 4656 ★ National Association for Healthcare Recruitment (NAHCR)

307 Park Lake Cir.
Orlando, FL 32803
Phone: (407)843-6981 **Fax:** (407)423-4648
Email: ruthw@fha.org
Website: http://www.nahcr.com
Ruth Welke, Project Mgr. /Editor

Fnded: 1975. **Mem:** 1,000. **Reg. Groups:** 57. **Local Groups:** 50. **Desc:** Individuals employed directly by hospitals and other health care organizations which are involved in the practice of professional health care recruitment. Promotes sound principles of professional health care recruitment. Provides financial assistance to aid members in planning and implementing regional educational programs. Offers technical assistance and consultation services. Compiles statistics. **Pub:** *NAHCR Directions*, bimonthly. *Price:* $200/year. • *Recruiter Handbook.* Handbook. • *Trends Survey*, annual. Survey. • *Who's Who in Recruitment and Resources*, annual. **Frmly:** National Association of Nurse Recruiters; (1987) National Association of Healthcare Recruiters.

★ 4657 ★ National Association of Health Data Organizations (NAHDO)

375 Chipeta Way, Ste. A
Salt Lake City, UT 84108
Phone: (801)587-9104 **Fax:** (801)587-9125
Email: nahdoinfo@nahdo.org
Website: http://www.nahdo.org
Denise Love, Exec. Dir.

Fnded: 1986. **Mem:** 112. **Desc:** Members include state, federal, nonprofit and private health data organizations, employee benefits consultants, professional review organizations, data analysis firms, software vendors, and health services consultants, health care researchers, third-party payers, hospital associations, managed care organizations. Seeks to improve health care through the collection, dissemination, and application of health care data. Promotes public availability of and access to health data; supports use of health care data to guide formulation of health policy, purchasing, and establishment of needed health services. Sponsors educational programs, workshops, & seminars. Conducts surveys and comparative studies; maintains speakers' bureau. **Pub:** *Inventory of Statewide Hospital Discharge Data Activities.* Manual. *Price:* $225. • *NAHDO Annual Report*, annual. Annual Report. *Price:* Free.

★ 4658 ★ National Association for Health and Fitness

401 W Michigan St.
Indianapolis, IN 46202-3233
Phone: (317)955-0957 **Fax:** (317)634-7817
Email: info@physicalfitness.org
Website: http://www.physicalfitness.org
Jim Whitehead, Exec. Dir.

Fnded: 1979. **Mem:** 200. **Reg. Groups:** 4. **State Groups:** 40. **Desc:** State governor's fitness councils. Works with state government to establish and maintain governor's councils on physical fitness and health. Seeks to promote the quality of life for individuals in the U.S. through physical fitness, sports, and healthy lifestyles. **Pub:** *NAGCPFS*, quarterly. Newsletter. *Price:* Free. **Frmly:** (2000) National Association of Governor's Councils on Physical Fitness and Sport.

★ 4659 ★ National Association of Health Services Executives (NAHSE)

8630 Fenton St., No. 126
Silver Spring, MD 20910
Phone: (202)628-3953
Email: nationalHQ@nahse.org
Dr. Sandra Gould, PhD, Pres.

Fnded: 1968. **Mem:** 500. **Reg. Groups:** 16. **Local Groups:** 7. **Desc:** Black health care executive managers, planners, educators, advocates, providers, organizers, researchers, and consumers participating in academic ventures, educational forums, seminars, workshops, systems design, legislation, and other activities. Conducts National Work-Study Program and sponsors educational programs. **Pub:** *NAHSE Notes*, quarterly. Newsletter. *Price:* Free.

★ 4660 ★ National Association of Health Unit Coordinators (NAHUC)

1947 Madron Rd.
Rockford, IL 61107-1716
Phone: (815)633-4351 **Free:** 888-22-NAHUC
Fax: (815)633-4438
Email: office@nahuc.org
Website: http://www.nahuc.org
Faylua Core, Pres.

Fnded: 1980. **Mem:** 1,700. **Reg. Groups:** 9. **Local Groups:** 30. **Desc:** Coordinators of nonclinical nursing unit activities; educators, supervisors, students, and graduates in the field. Promotes the professional practice of unit coordinating. Has established standards of practice defining the role and responsibilities of health unit coordinators in the nonclinical area of health care and ensuring delivery of quality patient care. Works to establish certification guidelines for individual practitioners with a goal of national certification. Seeks recognition of the change in job title from clerk to that of coordinator, which the group believes better describes the nature of the position. Promotes continuing education and research; endeavors to develop accreditation of educational programs and standards of education for job entry. Provides vocational information to prospective students in the field; recruits students into the profession. Represents members' interests before allied health professionals, educational institutions, governmental bodies, and the community. Sponsors regional workshops, seminars, and other educational programs; compiles statistics. Maintains certification board and speakers' bureau; offers annual national certification exam and annual educational conference. **Pub:** *Information Booklet*, annual. Booklet. *Price:* $2. • *National Association of Health Unit Coordinators–Coordinator*, quarterly. Newsletter. *Price:* Included in membership dues; $15/year for nonmembers. • *National Association of Health Unit Coordinators - Education Program Procedure Guide*. Booklet. Provides information to assist in the development or evaluation of a formal educational program. *Price:* $30 for members; $50 for nonmembers. • *National Association of Health Unit Coordinators–Membership Directory*, annual. Membership Directory. *Price:* $5 for members only. • *Question & Answer Brochures*. Brochures. **Frmly:** (1990) National Association of Health Unit Clerks-Coordinators.

★ 4661 ★ National Association of Healthcare Consultants

1255 23rd St. NW
Washington, DC 20037-1174
Phone: (202)452-8282 **Free:** 800-313-6242
Fax: (202)833-3636
Email: consultants@healthcon.org
Website: http://www.healthcon.org
Melissa Forburger, Exec. Dir.

Fnded: 1994. **Mem:** 350. **Nat'l Groups:** 1. **Desc:** Consultants who "provide ethical, confidential, and professional advice to the healthcare industry." Promotes professional development of members; works to improve the standard of health care consulting services. Facilitates exchange of information among members; conducts educational and training programs; encourages members to attain Certified Healthcare Business Consultant (CHBC) status. Compiles statistics; makes available legal and marketing advice; provides group purchasing discount programs to members; maintains speakers' bureau. **Pub:** *Update*, periodic. Newsletter. *Price:* Not for sale. • Newsletter, periodic.

★ 4662 ★ National Association of Hispanic Nurses (NAHN)

1501 Sixteenth St. NW
Washington, DC 20036
Phone: (202)387-2477 **Fax:** (202)483-7183
Email: thehispanicnurses@earthlink.net
Website: http://www.thehispanicnurses.org/
Nilda Peragallo, Pres.

Fnded: 1976. **Mem:** 1,000. **Nat'l Groups:** 1. **State Groups:** 10. **Local Groups:** 24. **Desc:** Nurses on all educational levels, from all Hispanic subgroups; non-Hispanic nurses concerned about the health delivery needs of the Hispanic community; nursing students. Serves the nursing and health care delivery needs of the Hispanic community and the professional needs of Hispanic nurses. Provides a forum in which Hispanic nurses can analyze, research, and evaluate the health care needs of the Hispanic community. Disseminates findings of that research to local, state, and federal agencies so as to affect policy-making and resource allocation. Aims to ensure that Hispanic nurses have equal access to educational, professional, and economic opportunities. Identifies Hispanic nurses throughout the nation to determine the size of the work force available to provide culturally sensitive nursing care to Hispanics. **Pub:** *First National Hispanic Nurse Symposium Proceedings: Recruitment, Retention, Career Mobility - Strategy for Change*. Proceedings. • *Hispanic Nurse*, quarterly. *Price:* $15. **Frmly:** (1979) National Association of Spanish Speaking-Spanish Surnamed Nurses.

★ 4663 ★ National Association for Holistic Aromatherapy

4509 Interlake Ave., N, No. 233
Seattle, WA 98103
Phone: (206)547-2164 **Free:** 888-ASK-NAHA
Fax: (206)547-2680
Email: info@naha.org
Website: http://www.naha.org/
Jade Shutes, Pres.

Fnded: 1990. **Mem:** 1,600. **Nat'l Groups:** 7. **Reg. Groups:** 30. **Desc:** Seeks to establish and promote the art and science of aromatherapy as a health care alternative. Works to elevate and maintain high standards of aromatherapy eduction. Works to raise public awareness of the benefits of aromatherapy. Fosters communication and exchange among members. Offers educational programs. Maintains speakers' bureau. **Pub:** *Aromatherapy Journal*, quarterly. Newsletter. *Price:* $35/year. • *Membership and Practitioner Directory*, annual.

★ 4664 ★ National Association for Home Care (NAHC)

228 7th St. SE
Washington, DC 20003
Phone: (202)547-7424 **Fax:** (202)547-3540
Email: exec@nahc.org
Website: http://www.nahc.org
Val J. Halamandaris, Pres.

Fnded: 1982. **Mem:** 6,000. **Desc:** Providers of home health care, hospice, and homemaker-home health aide services; interested individuals and organizations. Develops and promotes high standards of patient care in home care services. Seeks to affect legislative and regulatory processes concerning home care services; gathers and disseminates home care industry data; develops public relations strategies; works to increase political visibility of home care services. Interprets home care services to governmental and private sector bodies affecting the delivery and financing of such services. Provides legal and accounting consulting services; conducts market research and compiles statistics. Offers members insurance discounts. Sponsors educational programs for organizations and individuals concerned with home care services. **Pub:** *Caring*, monthly. Magazine. *Price:* Included in membership dues; $45/year in U.S.; $65/year outside U.S. • *Homecare News*, monthly. Tabloid covering association news; serves as an information exchange between state associations and providers/suppliers to the industry. *Price:* Included in membership dues; $18/year for nonmembers. • *Hospice Forum*, biweekly. Newsletter. Covers legislative and research news. *Price:* Included in membership dues; $105/year for nonmembers. • *NAHC Report*, weekly. Newsletter. Covers legislative and regulatory issues related to the home health care industry. Contains employment opportunity listings. *Price:* Included in membership dues; $325/year for nonmembers. • *National Home Care and Hospice Directory*, annual. Directory.

★ 4665 ★ National Association of Hospital Hospitality Houses (NAHHH)

PO Box 18087
Asheville, NC 28814-0087
Phone: (828)253-1188 **Free:** 800-542-9730
Fax: (828)253-8082
Email: helpinghomes@nahhh.org
Website: http://www.nahhh.org
Celena E. Grey, Exec. Dir.

Fnded: 1986. **Mem:** 175. **Reg. Groups:** 10. **Desc:** Hospitals, hospital hospitality houses (HHH), charitable foundations, and interested individuals. (Hospital hospitality houses are temporary residential facilities for patients and their families.) Provides assistance to members and offers information and guidance to those who wish to establish an HHH. Conducts educational programs; operates resource center and speakers' bureau; compiles statistics. **Pub:** *Inside Hospitality*, quarterly. Newsletter. *Price:* Free. • *National Association of Hospitality Houses: Home Away From Home*. Brochure. Sent to members, hospitals, and healthcare agencies.

★ 4666 ★ National Association for Human Development (NAHD)

1424 16th St. NW, Ste. 102
PO Box 100
Washington, DC 20036
Phone: (202)328-2191 **Fax:** (202)265-6682
Email: info@voladv.org
Anne Radd, Exec. VP

Fnded: 1974. **Desc:** Seeks to help people establish and maintain physical and emotional health and vigor. Operates model demonstration projects and evaluation, research and training programs; conducts multimedia community awareness activities; sponsors "Active People Over 60" campaign. Provides specialized education in motivational communications; develops and implements employment training programs. Develops drug prevention educational programs, activities, and materials for minority populations; advocates on behalf of troubled children and youth. Offers resource development and technical assistance to other organizations. **Pub:** *Digest*, quarterly. • Booklets. • Manuals. • Also publishes evaluation sheets and audiovisual and media-oriented materials.

★ 4667 ★ National Association of Inpatient Physicians (NAIP)

190 N Independence Mall W
Philadelphia, PA 19106-1572
Phone: (215)351-2740 **Free:** 800-843-3360
Fax: (215)351-2536
Email: wellikson@mail.acponline.org
Website: http://www.naiponline.org
Laurence Wellikson, MD, Exec. Dir.

Desc: Promotes excellence and efficiency in clinical care; advances the practice of inpatient medicine. **Pub:** *The Hospitalist*. Newsletter. Forum for exchange of clinical and practice news. *Price:* included in membership dues.

★ 4668 ★ National Association of Laryngectomy Clubs

6 Rickett St., Ground Fl.
Fulham
London SW6 1RU, United Kingdom
Phone: 44 207 3819993 **Fax:** 44 207 3810025

Fnded: 1976. **Mem:** 4,000. **Nat'l Groups:** 95. **Desc:** Promotes the welfare of laryngectomees by providing literature to them, their friends and their families and also the relevant professionals. Membership is via a club only. **Pub:** Annual Report, annual. • Newsletter, quarterly. Also publishes emergency resuscitation video and audiotape.

★ 4669 ★ National Association of Lesbian/Gay Addiction Professionals (NALGAP)

901 N Washington St., No. 600
Alexandria, VA 22314
Phone: (703)465-0539 **Fax:** (703)741-6989
Email: clineal@nalgap.org
Website: http://www.nalgap.org
Rodger L. Beatty, PhD, Pres.

Fnded: 1979. **Mem:** 95. **Nat'l Groups:** 1. **Desc:** Doctors, nurses, social workers, psychologists, certified counselors, and other professionals who work with gay, lesbian, transgendered, and bisexual alcoholics and addicts; drug, alcohol, and gay agencies, organizations, and institutes. Provides a network for support and communication among professionals working with chemically dependent gay, lesbian, and bisexual people. Seeks to educate members of organizations and agencies about gay, lesbian, and bisexual people and addiction; assure that workshops, seminars, conferences, and publications that deal with addiction address the special needs and problems of gay, lesbian, and bisexual people and their families; coordinates services provided by educators and training personnel who are available to help others in the addiction field to better serve gay and lesbian clients. Acts as a clearinghouse for resource and research information in the field of addiction as it pertains to homosexuality; provides referral information about gay, lesbian, and bisexual groups of Alcoholics Anonymous World Services; develops and distributes a list of resource facilities for gay, lesbian, and bisexual alcoholics, addicts and their family and friends. Maintains a training and speakers' bureau. **Pub:** *The NALGAP Annotated Bibliography: Alcoholism, Substance Abuse, and Lesbians/Gay Men.* Book. • *NALGAP Newsletter*, periodic. Newsletter. *Price:* For members only. • *NALGAP Reporter*, semiannual. Newsletter. Includes book reviews. • *National Directory of Facilities and Services for Lesbian and Gay Alcoholics*, periodic. Directory. • Monographs. **Frmly:** (1984) National Association of Gay Alcoholism Professionals; (1997) National Association of Lesbian/Gay Alcoholism Professionals.

★ 4670 ★ National Association of Local Boards of Health (NALBOH)

c/o Marie Fallon
1840 E Gypsy Ln.
Bowling Green, OH 43402
Phone: (419)353-7714 **Fax:** (419)352-6278
Email: nalboh@nalboh.org
Website: http://www.nalboh.org
Warren Jensen, Chm.

Fnded: 1992. **Mem:** 800. **State Groups:** 10. **Desc:** Represents the interests of local boards of health throughout the United States and relates their concerns to individuals responsible for developing public health policy at the national level. Offers educational programs and speakers' bureau. **Pub:** *NewsBrief*, quarterly. Newsletter.

★ 4671 ★ National Association of Managed Care Physicians (NAMCP)

4435 Waterfront Dr., Ste. 101
Glen Allen, VA 23060
Phone: (804)527-1905 **Free:** 800-722-0376
Fax: (804)747-5316
Email: info@namcp.com
Website: http://www.namcp.com
W.C. Williams, III,MD, Exec. VP

Fnded: 1991. **Mem:** 8,000. **Desc:** Licensed physicians and allied health professionals working in managed health care programs; medical residents and students interested in managed health care; corporations or agencies providing services or goods to the industry; interested others. Enhances the ability of practicing physicians to proactively participate within the managed health care arena through research, communication, and education. Provides a forum for members to communicate their concerns about the changing health care environment, integrate into managed health care delivery systems, and assure continuous improvement in the quality of health care services provided. Develops practice criteria, quality assurance measures, and appropriate utilization management criteria. Offers educational programs; maintains speakers' bureau and placement services; conducts research programs; developing informational clearinghouse. **Pub:** *Managed Care Medicine*, bimonthly. Journal. *Price:* $95. • *NAMCP Guide to Managed Care.* Monograph. • *Profiles*, quarterly. Newsletter.

★ 4672 ★ National Association of Medicaid Directors (NASMD)

810 1st St. NE, Ste. 500
Washington, DC 20002-4267
Phone: (202)682-0100 **Fax:** (202)289-6555
Email: jrichardson@aphsa.org
Website: http://www.nasmd.org

Mem: 54. **Desc:** Directors and senior staff of state and territorial medical assistance programs. Promotes effective Medicaid policy and program administration; works with the federal government on issues through technical advisory groups. Conducts forums on policy and technical issues. **Pub:** *MMI Bulletin*, monthly. Newsletter. Summary of legal decisions, legislation, regulations, waivers relating to Medicaid program. *Price:* $90/year. **Frmly:** (1995) State Medicaid Directors Association.

★ 4673 ★ National Association of Medical Examiners (NAME)

1402 S Grand Blvd.
Saint Louis, MO 63104
Phone: (314)577-8298 **Fax:** (314)268-5971
Email: settledd@slu.edu
Website: http://www.thename.org
Denise Settlemoir, Exec. Dir.

Fnded: 1966. **Mem:** 950. **Desc:** Medical examiners, pathologists, and other licensed physicians who have responsibilities in connection with the official investigation of sudden, suspicious, and violent deaths. Attempts to establish greater understanding and support for the medical examiner system among the public, government officials, and the medical and legal professions. Has established standards for inspection and accreditation of a modern medico-legal investigative system. **Pub:** *American Journal of Forensic Medicine and Pathology*, quarterly. Journal.

★ 4674 ★ National Association of Medical Minority Educators (NAMME)

c/o Iral D. Porter
Health Careers Pathways Program
University of Kansas Medical Center
3007 Student Center Bldg, 39th & Rainbow
Kansas City, KS 66103
Phone: (212)843-3701 **Fax:** (212)650-3925
Email: premed@premed.edu
Website: http://www.namme-hpe.org
Ms. Iral D. Porter, M.B.A., Membership Chairperson

Fnded: 1975. **Mem:** 200. **Reg. Groups:** 4. **Desc:** Educators, administrators, and practitioners of medicine, osteopathic medicine, dentistry, veterinary medicine, optometry, podiatry, public health, and allied health. Promotes the increase of medical minority personnel; admissions of minority students to health professionals schools; retention and graduation of minority students in health profession schools; recruitment and development of minority faculty administrators and managerial personnel in the health professions; delivery of quality health care for minority populations; and recruitment, retention, and development of minority students in pre-health profession programs. Sponsors workshops for high school counselors and junior high and high school science teachers; provides training for minority affairs workers and officers. Offers annual student development sessions and recruitment fairs. Conducts research programs and systematic studies. **Pub:** *Financing Your Medical Education*, annual. Book. • *James Stills Quarterly - NAMME Edition*, quarterly. Newsletter.

★ 4675 ★ National Association Medical Staff Services (NAMSS)

PO Box 140647
Austin, TX 78714-0647
Phone: (512)454-7928 **Fax:** (512)454-3036
Email: namss@namss.org
Sandra Young-Mattson, CMSC, CPCS, Pres.

Fnded: 1971. **Mem:** 4,000. **Reg. Groups:** 5. **State Groups:** 48. **Local Groups:** 32. **Desc:** Individuals involved in the management and administration of healthcare provider services. Seeks to: enhance the knowledge and experience of medical staff services professionals; promote the certification of those involved in the profession. **Pub:** *Credentialing and Medical Staff Law.* • *Guidebook: Developing a Policy and Procedure Manual.* Manual. • *Medical Staff Leadership Orientation Manual.* • *NAMSS Membership Roster*, annual. Membership Directory. • *Synergy*, bimonthly. Magazine. *Price:* Included in membership dues; $65/year for nonmembers.

★ 4676 ★ National Association for Mental After-care in Residential Care Homes

Silverwells House
1 Old Mill Rd.
Bothwell
Glasgow G71 8AY, United Kingdom
Phone: 44 1698 852771 **Fax:** 44 1698 854712
Website: http://www.march.org.uk

Lang(s): English. **Desc:** Promotes services for people with mental health problems. Provides help and advice.

★ 4677 ★ National Association of Multicultural Rehabilitation Concerns (NAMRC)

c/o National Rehabilitation Association
633 S Washington St.
Alexandria, VA 22314
Phone: (703)836-0850 **Fax:** (703)836-0848
Email: info@nationalrehab.org
Website: http://www.nationalrehab.org/website/divs/namrc.html

Desc: Rehabilitation professionals, human services providers, educators, researchers, students, and other individuals with an interest in rehabilitation and people with disabilities. Promotes increased awareness of the barriers created by cultural insensitivity; seeks to ensure availability and quality of rehabilitation services to people of all cultural and ethnic backgrounds. Conducts continuing education courses and certification programs for rehabilitation professionals; supports legislation that encourages multiculturalism in American society and benefits people with disabilities. **Pub:** *Cultural Network Newsletter*, periodic. Newsletter.

★ 4678 ★ National Association of Neonatal Nurses (NANN)

4700 W Lake Ave.
Glenview, IL 60025-1485
Phone: (847)375-3660 **Free:** 800-451-3795
Fax: 888-477-6266
Email: info@nann.org
Website: http://www.nann.org
Brandon Dybala, Admin.

Fnded: 1984. **Mem:** 11,500. **Reg. Groups:** 60. **Desc:** Nurses currently working in neonatal intensive care units. Promotes professional development of members. Provides educational and networking opportunities. Disseminates legislative information. **Pub:** *Central Lines*, quarterly. Newsletter. • *Position Statements.* • *Practice Guidelines.* • *Technical Bulletins.*

★ 4679 ★ National Association of Nephrology Technicians/Technologists (NANT)

PO Box 2307
Dayton, OH 45401-2307
Phone: (937)586-3705 **Free:** 877-607-NANT
Fax: (937)586-3699
Email: nant@nant.melnet.com
Website: http://www.dialysistech.org
Francine W. Rickenbach, CAE

Fnded: 1983. **Mem:** 1,200. **State Groups:** 22. **Desc:** Nephrology technicians and technologists. Promotes the recognition, job security, and employment opportunities of nephrology technicians and technologists. Sets forth standards for the dialysis industry; educates dialysis practitioners; promotes research; disseminates new ideas; addresses technician and technologist practice issues. **Pub:** *A Manual on Water Treatment for Hemodialysis.* Book. Discusses each component of a hemodialysis water treatment system. *Price:* $20 for members; $40 for nonmembers. • *Dialysis Technology, Third Edition. Price:* $45 member; $60 nonmember. • *Nant News*, bimonthly. Newsletter. • *Study Guide for Technologists, Second Edition. Price:*

$20 member; $30 nonmember. **Frmly:** (1994) National Association of Nephrology Technologists.

★ 4680 ★ National Association of Nigerian Nurses and Midwives

PMB 3857
Lagos, Nigeria
Phone: 234 1 932173

Fnded: 1978. **Mem:** 7,100.

★ 4681 ★ National Association of Nurse Massage Therapists (NANMT)

2203 Woodridge Ct.
Grand Island, NE 68801
Free: 800-262-4017
Email: simpson@nebi.com
Website: http://www.nanmt.org
Cam Spencer, Pres.

Fnded: 1987. **Mem:** 187. **Desc:** Nurses and other healthcare professionals who practice massage therapy. Promotes the integration of massage and other therapeutic forms of bodywork into existing healthcare practice. Promotes Nurse Massage Therapists as specialists within the nursing profession. Establishes standards of professional practice and criteria for national certification of Nurse Massage Therapists. Educates the medical community and the general public about bodywork therapies. Monitors legislation. **Pub:** *NANMT Membership Directory*, annual. Membership Directory. *Price:* Included in membership dues. • *Nurse's Touch*, quarterly. Magazine. *Price:* Included in membership dues; $20/year for institutions.

★ 4682 ★ National Association of Nurse Practitioners in Women's Health (NPWH)

503 Capitol Ct. NE, Suite 300
Washington, DC 20002
Phone: (202)543-9693 **Fax:** (202)543-9858
Email: info@npwh.org
Website: http://www.npwh.org
Susan Wysocki, Pres.

Fnded: 1980. **Mem:** 2,834. **Desc:** Nurse practitioners involved in women's healthcare. Advocates quality healthcare to be inclusive of an individual's physical, emotional, and spiritual needs. Promotes women as decision-makers for their own healthcare. Encourages nurses to participate in continuing education programs. Disseminates information. **Pub:** *The Monthly Cycle*, monthly. Newsletter. *Price:* Available to members only. **Frmly:** (2001) National Association of Nurse Practitioners in Reproductive Health.

★ 4683 ★ National Association of Nutrition and Aging Services Programs (NANASP)

1101 Vermont Ave., Ste. 1001
Washington, DC 20005
Phone: (202)682-6899 **Fax:** (202)682-3984
Website: http://www.nanasp.org/

Desc: Dedicated to supporting a broad, comprehensive range of nutrition and other support services for the aging living in community dwellings; helps shape national policy; provides training for service providers; advocates on behalf of senior citizens.

★ 4684 ★ National Association of Optometrists and Opticians (NAOO)

PO Box 459
Marblehead, OH 43440
Phone: (419)798-2031 **Fax:** (419)798-8548
Email: fdrozak@cros.net
Franklin D. Rozak, Sec. /Treas.

Fnded: 1960. **Mem:** 13,225. **Desc:** Licensed optometrists, opticians, and corporations. Conducts public affairs programs of mutual importance to members; serves as an organizational center for special purpose programs; acts as a clearinghouse for information affecting the retail optical industry. **Frmly:** National Optical Association.

★ 4685 ★ National Association of Orthopaedic Nurses (NAON)

401 N Michigan Ave., Ste. 2200
Chicago, IL 60611
Free: 800-289-6266 **Fax:** (312)527-6658
Email: naon@sba.com
Website: http://www.orthonurse.org/
Marie Bass, Exec. Dir.

Fnded: 1980. **Mem:** 8,300. **Local Groups:** 154. **Desc:** Registered, licensed practical, or licensed vocational nurses involved or knowledgeable in orthopedic nursing. Enhances the personal and professional growth of orthopedic nurses through continuing education programs. Promotes research development and advances in orthopedic nursing; promotes an awareness of patients' rights. Stresses the concept of man's physical, psychological, social, emotional, and spiritual needs in the development of patient care plans. Maintains liaison with and serves as resource to hospitals, universities, industries, and government agencies. Operates special interest groups. Sponsors workshops; maintains speakers' bureau; offers research grants. Makes available audiovisual presentation. **Pub:** *News*, bimonthly. • *Orthopaedic Nursing*, bimonthly. Journal. • Bibliographies. • Monographs. • Proceedings.

★ 4686 ★ National Association of Orthopaedic Technologists (NAOT)

2950 Buskirk Ave., Ste. 170
Walnut Creek, CA 94596
Phone: (925)472-5822 **Fax:** (925)472-5901
Email: naot@hp-assoc.com
Website: http://naot.org
Kent Lindeman, Exec. Dir.

Fnded: 1982. **Mem:** 1,100. **Reg. Groups:** 4. **Local Groups:** 23. **Desc:** Allied health assistants working with orthopedic patients. Promotes continued professional education of members and other orthopedic health care providers; administers certification examination. Seeks to enhance public understanding of orthopedics. Conducts seminars; compiles statistics. **Pub:** *OnLine: Advancements in Orthopaedic Technology*, bimonthly. Newsletter. Includes orthopaedic articles, meeting updates, and technology tips.

★ 4687 ★ National Association of Ovulation Method Instructors UK

Oakfield
Wineham Lane
Bolney
Haywards Heath RH17 5SD, United Kingdom
Phone: 44 1444 881744 **Fax:** 44 1444 881744
Website: http://www.woomb.org

Fnded: 1977. **Lang(s):** English. **Desc:** Provides information on the Billings Ovulation Method of natural family planning; provides training for instructors. **Pub:** *Resource List*.

★ 4688 ★ National Association for Parents of the Visually Impaired (NAPVI)

PO Box 317
Watertown, MA 02471
Phone: (617)972-7441 **Free:** 800-562-6265
Fax: (617)972-7444
Email: napvi@perkins.pvt.k12.ma.us
Website: http://www.spedex.com/napvi
Susan LaVenture, Exec. Dir.

Fnded: 1980. **Mem:** 2,000. **Reg. Groups:** 7. **State Groups:** 16. **Desc:** Parents and families of visually impaired children; community groups and agencies; interested individuals. Goals are to provide support for members and to promote public understanding of the needs and rights of the visually impaired child. Seeks to address parental needs for: emotional support; information about care, education, and treatment for their children; aid in establishing local, state, and regional groups; quality services for blind and impaired children; communication of their expertise and expectations with other parents and federal, state, and local service agencies; assurance that their children are accepted by society. Conducts workshops for parents. Conducts research programs. **Pub:** *Awareness*, quarterly. Newsletter. *Price:* Included in membership dues. • *How to Pack 'Em In: A Guide to Planning Workshops.* • *Mainstreaming Your Visually Impaired Child: Legislative Handbook for Parents.* Handbook. • *Parents to the Rescue.* Book. • *Preschool Learning Activities for the Visually Impaired Child: A Guide for Parents.* Book. • *Take Charge!: A Resource Guide for Parents of the Visually Impaired.* • *Your Child's Information Journal.* • Audiotapes. • Brochures. • Reprints. • Videos.

★ 4689 ★ National Association of Pediatric Nurse Practitioners (NAPNAP)

20 Brace Rd., Ste. 200
Cherry Hill, NJ 08034
Phone: (856)857-9700 **Fax:** (856)857-1600
Email: info@napnap.org
Website: http://www.napnap.org
Cathy Van Horn, Off. Mgr.

Fnded: 1973. **Mem:** 6,700. **State Groups:** 51. **Desc:** Pediatric, school, and family nurse practitioners and interested persons. Seeks to improve the quality of infant, child, and adolescent health care by making health care services accessible and providing a forum for continuing education of members. Facilitates and supports legislation designed to promote the role of pediatric nurse practitioners; promotes salary ranges commensurate with practitioners' responsibilities; facilitates exchange of information between prospective employers and job seekers in the field. Supports research programs; compiles statistics. **Pub:** *Journal of Pediatric Health Care*, bimonthly. Journal. Includes annual index, book reviews, legislative news, literature abstracts, multi-media reviews, and product news. *Price:* $55/year for individuals; $104/year for institutions; $28/year for students. • *Pediatric Nurse Practitioner*, bimonthly. Newsletter. Contains calendar of events and legislative news. *Price:* Free to members. • Brochures.

★ 4690 ★ National Association of People With AIDS (NAPWA)

1413 K St. NW, Ste. 700
Washington, DC 20005
Phone: (202)898-0414 **Fax:** (202)898-0435
Email: napwa@napwa.org
Website: http://www.napwa.org
Terje Anderson, Exec. Dir.

Fnded: 1987. **Desc:** Serves as the collective voice and national consumer health education and advocacy resource for all people living with HIV disease in the United States, and those who care for us NAPWA advocates on behalf of all people living with HIV and AIDS in order to end the epidemic and the human suffering caused by HIV/AIDS. **Pub:** *Active Voice*, quarterly. Provides information about healthcare and advocacy issues. *Price:* Free. • *An Ounce of Prevention.* Informs family members and caregivers about the prevention of further HIV infection. • *Facts About AIDS.* Provides an introduction of HIV and related issues. • *Living with HIV.* Provides information on resources for treatment and offers prevention against further infection. • *Medical Alert*, quarterly. Identifies new approaches to treating HIV/AIDS, explains what new drugs are being tested and how they work, and provides treatment strategies. *Price:* Free.

★ 4691 ★ National Association of the Physically Handicapped (NAPH)

1375 Dewitt Dr.
Akron, OH 44313
Free: 800-743-5008
Email: trumanjm@aol.com
Website: http://www.naph.net
Jerry Snyder, Pres.

Fnded: 1958. **Mem:** 700. **Nat'l Groups:** 1. **State Groups:** 1. **Local Groups:** 13. **Desc:** Physically handicapped persons; associate members are nonhandicapped. Seeks to advance the social, economic, and physical welfare of the physically handicapped. Promotes involvement of the physically handicapped in the planning and administration of all programs in their interest. Sponsors fundraising activities. **Pub:** *NAPH National Newsletter*, quarterly. Newsletter. *Price:* included in membership dues; $12/year for nonmembers. • Brochure.

★ 4692 ★ National Association of Physician Nurses (NAPN)

900 S Washington St., No. G-13
Falls Church, VA 22046
Phone: (703)237-8616 **Fax:** (703)533-1153
Susan Young, Dir.

Fnded: 1973. **Mem:** 3,000. **Desc:** Physicians' nurses united to bring added stature and purpose to their profession and to create for themselves the benefits normally limited to members of specialized professional and fraternal groups. **Pub:** *The Nightingale*, monthly. Newsletter. *Price:* $30/year included in membership dues; $15/year for nonmembers. • *Salary Survey Report*, biennial. Report. • Also publishes special reports.

★ 4693 ★ National Association of Physician Recruiters (NAPR)

PO Box 150127
Altamonte Springs, FL 32715-0127
Phone: (407)774-7880 **Free:** 800-726-5613
Fax: (407)774-6440
Email: kmg-assn@worldnet.att.net
Website: http://www.napr.org
Bill Kautter, CAE, Exec. VP

Fnded: 1983. **Mem:** 300. **Desc:** Physician search firms (companies that recruit resident physicians or practicing physicians to fill positions nationwide). Promotes a positive public image of physician recruiting services. Seeks to establish accreditation standards for the field. Provides marketing services to the physician recruiting industry. Maintains speakers' bureau. Sponsors educational programs and seminars. Compiles statistics. **Pub:** *NAPA Business Report (Newsletter)*, annual, Client Brochure. Brochures. *Price:* $.75. • *NAPR Business Report*, quarterly. Newsletter.

★ 4694 ★ National Association of Physicians for the Environment (NAPE)

1643 Prince St.
Alexandria, VA 22314-2818
Phone: (301)571-9791 **Fax:** (301)530-8910
Email: nape@napenet.org
John T. Grupenhoff, PhD, Exec. VP

Fnded: 1993. **Mem:** 34. **Desc:** Physicians, medical and environmental organizations, and coporations. Promotes improved understanding of the impacts of environmental pollutants on the organs, systems, and disease processes of the human body. Strives to enlist physicians in the campaign to protect biological diversity; encourages institution of more stringent pollution control programs. Works to involve the medical professions in pollution control. Conducts educational programs for physicians. **Pub:** *NAPE Fact Sheet*. Brochure. • Annual Report. • Newsletter, periodic.

★ 4695 ★ National Association for Poetry Therapy (NAPT)

12950 NW 5th St.
Pembroke Pines, FL 33028
Free: (866)844-6278
Email: napt@dmg-dc.com
Website: http://www.poetrytherapy.org
Marge Silberling, Pres.

Fnded: 1981. **Mem:** 380. **Reg. Groups:** 16. **Desc:** Psychiatrists, psychologists, social workers, teachers, nurses, librarians, occupational therapists, paraprofessionals, ministers, counselors, recreation and rehabilitation specialists, and poets and professors of English and psychology. Objective is to promulgate the principles and techniques of poetry therapy for healing and personal growth. (Poetry therapy is used with patients in a variety of mental states ranging from "normal neurosis" to acute psychosis, as well as the physically handicapped and the learning disabled. Methods of using poetry for therapy vary and include reading poems and encouraging clients to write their own poetry. The general purpose is to lead the person into talking or writing about himself or herself and bringing out emotions not previously shown or discussed). Sponsors two degrees in the field of poetry therapy: Certified Poetry Therapist (CPT) and Registered Poetry Therapist (RPT). **Pub:** *Journal of Poetry Therapy*, quarterly. Magazine. *Price:* Included in membership dues. • *NAPT Museletter*, 3/year. Includes training and conference information. *Price:* included in membership dues; $15/year for nonmembers. • *Trainee's and Trainer's Guide*. *Price:* $20. **Frmly:** World Poetry Therapy Association; (1981) Association for Poetry Therapy.

★ 4696 ★ National Association of Postpartum Care Services

c/o Peter Neuberg
800 Detroit St.
Denver, CO 80206
Free: 800-45-DOULA **Fax:** (303)321-4058
Email: doulacare@aol.com
Website: http://www.napcs.org/
Peter Neuberg, Contact

Desc: Provides care services for women suffering from postpartum depression.

★ 4697 ★ National Association for Practical Nurse Education and Service (NAPNES)

8607 Second Ave., Ste. 404-A
Silver Spring, MD 20910-2745
Phone: (301)588-2491 **Fax:** (301)588-2839
Email: napnes@bellatlantic.net
Helen M. Larsen, Exec. Dir.

Fnded: 1941. **Mem:** 30,000. **State Groups:** 20. **Desc:** Licensed practical/vocational nurses, registered nurses, physicians, hospital and nursing home administrators, and interested others. Provides consultation service to advise schools wishing to develop a practical/vocational nursing program on facilities, equipment, policies, curriculum, and staffing. Promotes recruitment of students through preparation and distribution of recruitment materials. Sponsors seminars for directors and instructors in schools of practical/vocational nursing and continuing education programs for LPNs/LVNs; approves continuing education programs and awards contact hours; holds national certification courses in post licensure specialities such as pharmacology, long term care and gerontics. **Pub:** *Journal of Practical Nursing*, quarterly. Journal. Contains news of association activities, nursing law, and pending legislation affecting the nursing profession. *Price:* Included in membership dues; $15/year for nonmembers; $30/year for nonmembers outside the U.S. • *NAPNES Forum*, 8/year. Journal. Supplement to the *Journal of Practical Nusing*. • Also publishes brochures, pamphlets, and reprints.

★ 4698 ★ National Association of Pregnancy Massage Therapy (NAPMT)

1007 MoPac Cir., Ste. 202
Austin, TX 78746
Free: 888-451-4945
Email: napmt@texas.net
Carroll Patterson, Pres.

Desc: Works to provide therapeutic bodywork focusing on the special needs of pregnant women during pregnancy, birth and post-partum. **Pub:** *NAPMT Newsletter*. Newsletter.

★ 4699 ★ National Association for Premenstrual Syndrome

41 Old Rd.
East Peckham
Kent TN12 5AP, United Kingdom
Phone: 44 870 7772178 **Fax:** 44 870 7772177
Email: contact@pms.org.uk
Website: http://www.pms.org.uk

Fnded: 1983. **Mem:** 1,000. **Reg. Groups:** 8. **Desc:** Provides help, information and support to PMS sufferers and their families; promotes a better understanding of PMS and its treatment by the medical profession. **Pub:** *NAPS News*, monthly. Newsletter.

★ 4700 ★ National Association of Primary Care

Lettsom House
11 Chandos St.
Cavendish Sq.
London W1G 9DP, United Kingdom
Phone: 44 207 6367228 **Fax:** 44 171 6361601
Email: napc@primarycare.co.uk
Website: http://www.primarycare.co.uk

Fnded: 1991. **Mem:** 1,000. **Desc:** GP fundholding practices in England, Scotland, Wales & N Ireland. Aims to: promote good communication amongst fundholding practices; develop and extend the scope of services to patients offered by fundholding practices; encourage education research for and within fundholding practices; maintain and promote the highest ethical standards on the part of practitioners in fundholding practices; encourage the creation of new fundholding practices. **Frmly:** (2000) National Association of Fundholding Practices.

★ 4701 ★ National Association of Private Ambulance Services

21 Bassenhally Rd.
Whittlesey
Peterborough PE7 1RN, United Kingdom
Phone: 44 1733 350916 **Free:** 44 8000929112
Fax: 44 1733 350916
Email: napas@ambulanceservices.co.uk
Website: http://www.ambulanceservices.co.uk

Fnded: 1992. **Mem:** 47. **Reg. Groups:** 41. **Desc:** Provides self-regulation for private and professional ambulance service throughout the U.K and Ireland.

★ 4702 ★ National Association of Professional Geriatric Care Managers (PGCM)

1604 N Country Club Rd.
Tucson, AZ 85716-3102
Phone: (520)881-8008 **Fax:** (520)325-7925
Email: info@caremanager.org
Website: http://www.caremanager.org
Laury Adsit Gelardi, Exec. Dir.

Fnded: 1984. **Mem:** 1,700. **Reg. Groups:** 1. **State Groups:** 11. **Desc:** Promotes quality services and care for elderly citizens. Provides referral service and distributes information to individuals interested in geriatric care management. Maintains referral network. **Pub:** *GCM Journal*, quarterly. Journal. *Price:* $95/year. • *Inside GCM*, quarterly. Newsletter. • Membership Directory, annual. **Frmly:** National Association of Private Geriatric Care Managers.

★ 4703 ★ National Association of Professionals in Women's Health (NAPWH)

300 W Adams St., Ste.328
Chicago, IL 60606-5107

Desc: Health care professionals from a broad range of disciplines with a common interest in improving health outcomes for women. Seeks to "promote excellence and provide leadership, resources, and collegial support to all professionals who influence, develop, and champion quality health care programs for women." Works with community organizations to increase awareness of health care issues among women; sponsors continuing professional development courses for members; designs and implements community education programs.

★ 4704 ★ National Association of Protection and Advocacy Systems (NAPAS)

900 2nd St. NE, Ste. 211
Washington, DC 20002
Phone: (202)408-9514 **Fax:** (202)408-9520
Email: info@napas.org
Website: http://www.napas.org/
Curtis L. Decker, Exec. Dir.

Fnded: 1978. **Mem:** 96. **Reg. Groups:** 5. **State Groups:** 96. **Desc:** Executive directors and designees of state or territorial Developmental Disability, Mentally Ill Protection and Advocacy Systems, and Client Assistance Programs. Furthers the human, civil, and legal rights of persons with disabilities; advances the interests of protection and advocacy systems; facilitates coordination and mutual support among such systems and enhance their capacity to provide optimal services. Offers professional training; collects data. **Pub:** *NAPAS Newsletter*, periodic. Newsletter. • *State Protection and Advocacy Agencies*, annual. Directory. • Manuals. • Reports.

★ 4705 ★ National Association for Proton Therapy

1301 Highland Dr.
Silver Spring, MD 20910
Phone: (301)913-9360 **Fax:** (301)913-0372
Email: lenarzt@compuserve.com
Website: http://proton-therapy.org
Leonard Arzt, Contact

Fnded: 1989. **Mem:** 3. **Desc:** Oncologists and other health care professionals with an interest in the treatment of cancer. Promotes use of proton therapy to treat cancer patients. Conducts research and educational programs; gathers and disseminates information. **Pub:** *Proton News*, periodic. Newsletter.

★ 4706 ★ National Association for Pseudoxanthoma Elasticum (NAPE)

8764 Manchester Rd., Ste. 200
Saint Louis, MO 63144
Phone: (314)962-0100 **Fax:** (314)962-0100
Website: http://www.pxenape.org
Frances Benham, PhD, Board Chair

Fnded: 1989. **Mem:** 625. **Nat'l Groups:** 1. **Desc:** People who have Pseudoxanthoma Elasticum (PXE), as well as interested others(Pseudoxanthoma elasticum is a rare connective tissue disorder that can affect eyes, skin, and organs). Provides educational information about PXE. Compiles statistics. Serves to unite PXE patients with professionals who treat the disease and others who have the disease. Maintains database of patients with PXE. **Pub:** *PXE Awareness*, quarterly. Newsletter. Current treatment, research and legislative information. *Price:* $3/printed copy; $5/taped copy. **Frmly:** (1999) NAPE, Inc.

★ 4707 ★ National Association of Psychiatric Health Systems (NAPHS)

325 7th St., NW, Suite 625
Washington, DC 20004-2802
Phone: (202)393-6700 **Fax:** (202)783-6041
Email: naphs@naphs.org
Website: http://www.naphs.org
Mark Covall, Exec. Dir.

Fnded: 1933. **Mem:** 292. **Desc:** Advocates for behavoiral health. Represents provider systems that are committed to the delivery of responsive, accountable, and clinically effective preventing treatment, and care for children, adolescents, and adults with mental and substance use disorders. **Frmly:** (1993) National Association of Private Psychiatric Hospitals.

★ 4708 ★ National Association of Psychiatric Treatment Centers for Children (NAPTCC)

1025 Connecticut Ave. NW, Ste. 1012
Washington, DC 20036
Phone: (202)857-9735 **Fax:** (202)362-5145
Email: naptcc@aol.com
Joy Midman, Exec. Dir.

Fnded: 1983. **Mem:** 80. **Desc:** Treatment centers and programs for children and adolescents with or at risk of serious emotional or behavioral disorders, providing a full array of mental health and related services including residential treatment, partial hospitalization, outpatient treatment, therapeutic foster care, group homes, independent living programs, in-home treatment, intensive case management, and accredited education, special education, and alternative education programs. **Pub:** *Friday Facts*, weekly. • *Member Facilities*, annual. Directory. • Brochures.Contains informational material.

★ 4709 ★ National Association for Public Health Statistics and Information Systems (NAPHSIS)

801 Roeder Rd., Ste. 650
Silver Spring, MD 20910
Phone: (301)563-6001 **Fax:** (301)563-6012
Email: hq@naphsis.org
Website: http://www.NAPHSIS.org
Robert S. Bolan, Interim Dir.

Fnded: 1933. **Mem:** 300. **Desc:** Advocates, creates, and maintains comprehensive public health information systems that integrate vital records registration, public health statistics, and other health information. **Pub:** *The Journal*, bimonthly. Journal.

★ 4710 ★ National Association of Public Hospitals and Health Systems (NAPH)

1301 Pennsylvania Ave., NW, Ste. 950
Washington, DC 20004
Phone: (202)585-0100 **Fax:** (202)585-0101
Email: naph@naph.org
Website: http://www.naph.org
Christine Capito Burch, Exec. Dir.

Fnded: 1980. **Mem:** 70. **Desc:** Urban public hospitals. Promotes the development of federal, state, and local legislative and policy agendas for members. **Pub:** *Safety Net*, quarterly. • Newsletter, periodic. **Frmly:** (1998) National Association of Public Hospitals.

★ 4711 ★ National Association of Registered Nurses (NARN)

11512 Allecingie Pky., Ste. B
Richmond, VA 23235
Phone: (804)794-6513 **Free:** 800-383-9826
Fax: (804)379-7698
Email: fdebondt@aol.com
Website: http://www.associationsusa.org
Francis R. deBondt, PhD, Admin.

Fnded: 1979. **Mem:** 250. **Desc:** Nurses' associations. Seeks to offer nurses the opportunity to plan and create a financially sound future through financial management programs. Provides financial products, consultation, and services including Individual Retirement Accounts, full investment services, and group life insurance. Conducts educational programs. **Pub:** Brochures, periodic. • Newsletter, periodic.

★ 4712 ★ National Association of Rehabilitation Instructors (NARI)

c/o Nancy Marie-Luce
2939 Johnson Rd. SW
Huntsville, AL 35805-5844
Free: 800-671-6837 **Fax:** (205)533-1464
Julie Brock, Contact

Mem: 87. **State Groups:** 50. **Desc:** Objective is to promote rehabilitation of all persons with disabilities. Acts as a medium through which rehabilitation instructors can coordinate their efforts with other instructors, facilities, workshops, individuals, and organizations serving persons with disabilities. Conducts training workshops at the state level. **Pub:** *NARI Newsletter*, 3/year. Bulletin.

★ 4713 ★ National Association of Rehabilitation Professionals in the Private Sector (NARPPS)

3540 Soquel Ave., Ste. A
Santa Cruz, CA 95062-1776
Phone: (831)662-0310 **Free:** 800-240-9059
Fax: (831)662-8487
Email: gzimmermann@rehabpro.org
Website: http://www.rehabpro.com
Glenn Zimmermann, Exec. Dir.

Fnded: 1977. **Mem:** 3,300. **State Groups:** 36. **Desc:** Private rehabilitation companies, insurance companies, rehabilitation nurses, and rehabilitation professionals in the private sector. Seeks to promote the field of private rehabilitation and to provide for information exchange on rehabilitation issues and techniques. **Pub:** *NARPPS Journal*, quarterly. Journal. Includes book reviews and case studies. *Price:* Included in membership dues; $60/year for nonmembers; $35/year for libraries and schools. • *NARPPS National Directory*, annual. Directory. Contains membership listings by state; includes member name and advertisers indexes. *Price:* Included in membership dues; $50/copy for nonmembers. • *Rehabilitation Professional*, bimonthly. Newsletter.

★ 4714 ★ National Association of Rehabilitation Providers and Agencies

11250 Roger Bacon Dr., Ste. 8
Reston, VA 20190-5202
Phone: (703)437-4377 **Fax:** (703)435-4390
Email: nara@naranet.org
Website: http://www.naranet.org
Rick Guggolz, Exec. Dir.

Fnded: 1978. **Mem:** 100. **Desc:** Members are rehabilitation companies servicing patients (including Medicare recipients) with physical therapy, occupational therapy and speech pathology services in outpatient and long-term care settings. Associate members are rehabilitation vendors. **Pub:** *NARA News*, quarterly. Newsletter. Provides legislative news for rehabilitation companies; contains articles on Medicare, business management, etc. *Price:* included in membership dues.

★ 4715 ★ National Association of Rehabilitation Support Staff (NARSS)

c/o National Rehabilitation Association
633 S Washington St.
Alexandria, VA 22314
Phone: (703)836-0850 **Fax:** (703)836-0848
Email: info@nationalrehab.org
Website: http://www.nationalrehab.org/website/divs/narss.html

Desc: Office support staff in a rehabilitation setting. Promotes professional advancement of members; seeks to insure more effective rehabilitation services for people with disabilities. Conducts advocacy activities on behalf of people with disabilities; sponsors training courses for rehabiltation support staff; provides support and services to organizations representing people with disabilities. **Pub:** *NARSS Newsletter*, periodic. Newsletter.

★ 4716 ★ National Association for the Research and Therapy of Homosexuality (NARTH)

16633 Ventura Blvd., Ste. 1340
Encino, CA 91436
Phone: (818)789-4440 **Fax:** (818)786-6452
Email: narth4@earthlink.com
Website: http://www.narth.com
Joseph Nicolosi, PhD, Pres.

Fnded: 1992. **Mem:** 1,000. **Desc:** Mental health care providers, religious leaders, educators, and other individuals with an interest in the study of homosexuality. "NARTH investigates the causes and treatment of homosexuality, conducts research and educational programs, and maintains referral service for individuals seeking therapy to overcome homosexuality". **Pub:** *Collected Conference Papers*, annual. Proceedings. *Price:* $15. • *NARTH Bulletin*, 3/year. Magazine.

Price: $5. • *NARTH's "Understanding Homosexuality"*. Booklet. **Frmly:** (2003) National Association for the Research and Treatment of Homosexuality.

★ 4717 ★ National Association of Residents and Interns (NARI)

350 Fairway Dr., Ste. 200
Deerfield Beach, FL 33441-1834
Phone: (954)571-1877 **Free:** 800-221-2168
Fax: (954)571-8582
Email: membership@assnservices.com
Website: http://www.nari-assn.com
Joseph P. Santoli, Jr., Manager, Membership Services

Fnded: 1959. **Mem:** 40,000. **Desc:** Medical and dental students, interns, residents, and fellows. Contributes to the economic welfare of members through unsecured loan plans, affordable group insurance, group purchase discounts, and continuing medical education programs. **Pub:** *Association's Digest*, semiannual. Newsletter. Provides information on financial and business interests, industry news and member benefits. *Price:* Free for members.

★ 4718 ★ National Association for Rural Mental Health (NARMH)

1756 74th Ave. S, Ste. 101
Saint Cloud, MN 56301
Phone: (320)202-1820 **Free:** 800-809-5879
Fax: (320)202-1833
Email: narmh@facts.ksu.edu
Website: http://www.narmh.org
Donald Sawyer, Pres.

Fnded: 1977. **Mem:** 500. **Desc:** Mental health practitioners and administrators and others dedicated to improving mental health services in rural areas. Promotes effective rural mental health services. Promotes the use of services by rural community dwellers. **Pub:** *Rural Mental Health*, quarterly. Newsletter.

★ 4719 ★ National Association of School Nurses (NASN)

1416 Park St., Ste. A
Castle Rock, CO 80109
Phone: (303)663-2329 **Free:** (866)627-6767
Fax: (303)663-0403
Email: nasn@nasn.org
Website: http://www.nasn.org
Judith Robinson, Exec. Dir.

Fnded: 1969. **Mem:** 11,000. **State Groups:** 47. **Desc:** Improves health and educational success of children and youth by developing and providing leadership to advance school nursing practice. **Pub:** *Journal of School Nursing*, bimonthly. Magazine. Includes book reviews, resources, education topics and legislative updates. *Price:* included in membership dues; $70/year. • *NASNewsletter*, bimonthly. Newsletter. *Price:* Included in membership dues. • *Postural Screening*. *Price:* $7 members; $11 nonmembers. • *Scope and Standards of Professional School Nursing Practice*. *Price:* $10 members; $15 nonmembers. • *Vision Screening Guidelines for School Nurses*. *Price:* $7 members; $11 nonmembers. • Offers various guides, brochures, manuals, and other publications. **Frmly:** (1977) Department of School Nurses/NEA.

★ 4720 ★ National Association of School Psychologists (NASP)

4340 East West Hwy., Ste. 402
Bethesda, MD 20814
Phone: (301)657-0270 **Fax:** (301)657-0275
Email: cente@nasponline.org
Website: http://www.nasponline.org
Susan Gorin, Exec. Dir.

Fnded: 1969. **Mem:** 23,000. **Reg. Groups:** 5. **State Groups:** 51. **Desc:** School psychologists. Serves the mental health and educational needs of all children and youth. Encourages and provides opportunities for professional growth of individual members. Informs the public on the services and practice of school psychology, and advances the standards of the profession. Operates national school psychologist certification system. Sponsors children's services. **Pub:** *Communique Newspaper*, 8/year. Newspaper. • *School Psychology Review*, quarterly. Journal. • Catalog.Lists publications. • Monographs. • Reports.

★ 4721 ★ National Association of Senior Companion Project Directors (NASCPD)

c/o Lynne Brown-Zounes
Community Teamwork, Inc.
167 Dutton St.
Lowell, MA 01852
Phone: (978)459-0551
Email: brown@comteam.org
Website: http://www.nascpd.org/
Dwight Rasmussen, Contact

Fnded: 1978. **Mem:** 187. **Reg. Groups:** 5. **Desc:** Project directors from the Corp. for National Service's Senior Companion Program. Works to address the needs of SCP. Provides opportunities for expression and education for and by SCP project directors. Fosters communication between project directors, organizations, and agencies serving the SCP and the Corp. for National Service offices. Encourages the support and exchange of services among programs benefiting the aging. Seeks to prevent duplication and maximize the quality and level of services. Expands and promotes opportunities for senior companions worldwide. Assists in preserving government funding for SCP projects; works for increased stipends for volunteers. Works with Washington representatives on behalf of legislative changes affecting Corp. for National Service's and the SCP. Offers professional training and development. Conducts surveys. Operates speakers' bureau; compiles statistics. **Pub:** *NASCPD Newsletter*, periodic. Newsletter.

★ 4722 ★ National Association of Service Providers in Private Rehabilitation (NASPPR)

c/o National Rehabilitation Association
633 S Washington St.
Alexandria, VA 22314
Phone: (703)836-0850 **Fax:** (703)836-0848
Email: info@nationalrehab.org
Website: http://www.nationalrehab.org/website/divs/nasppr.html

Desc: Rehabilitation nurses and counselors, physical therapists, job placement professionals, and other individuals with an interest in the rehabilitation and employment of people with disabilities. Seeks to improve practice and outcomes in both the medical and placement phases of the rehabilitation process. Serves as a forum for the exchange of information among rehabilitation professionals; facilitates cooperation among members; sponsors educational and training programs.

★ 4723 ★ National Association of Seventh-Day Adventist Dentists (NASDAD)

c/o Judson Klooster
PO Box 101
Loma Linda, CA 92354
Phone: (909)558-8187 **Fax:** (909)558-0209
Email: nasdad@sd.llu.edu
Judson Klooster, Exec. Dir.

Fnded: 1944. **Mem:** 600. **Reg. Groups:** 11. **Desc:** Promotes the interests and businesses of dentists who are Seventh Day Adventists. **Pub:** *News*, quarterly. • *SDA Dentist*, annual.

★ 4724 ★ National Association for Sick Child Daycare (NASCD)

c/o Hugs & Kisses
1716 5 Ave. N
Birmingham, AL 35203
Phone: (205)324-8447 **Fax:** (205)324-8050
Email: jackiestewart@nascd.com
Website: http://www.nascd.com
Stewart Jacklyn, President

Fnded: 1979. **Mem:** 75. **Desc:** Works to promote the establishment of sick child daycare programs nationwide. Conducts educational programs; compiles statistics. **Pub:** *Survey of Sick Child Care Facilities*, quarterly. Newsletter. *Price:* $50 facility; $260 directory; $75 conference synopsis. • Brochure.

★ 4725 ★ National Association of Societies for the Care of the Handicapped (NASCOH)

PO Box UA 504
Union Ave.
Harare, Zimbabwe
Phone: 263 4 724678 **Fax:** 263 4 724678
Email: nascoh@zol.co.zw
Website: http://www.geocities.com/nascoh

Fnded: 1969. **Mem:** 52. **Desc:** Offers social and medical services to physically handicapped individuals. Conducts educational and informational programs. Acts as an advocate for the rights of the disabled. Co-ordinates the activities of societies working with and for people with disabilities. **Pub:** *NASCOH News*, quarterly. Magazine.

★ 4726 ★ National Association for Special Educational Needs (NASEN)

Nasen House
4/5 Amber Business Village
Amber Close
Amington
Tamworth B77 4RP, United Kingdom
Phone: 44 1827 311500 **Fax:** 44 1827 313005
Email: welcome@nasen.org.uk
Website: http://www.nasen.org.uk

Fnded: 1992. **Mem:** 11,300. **Reg. Groups:** 50. **Desc:** Mainly teachers and other practitioners in special education, also lectures in further and higher education, LEA staff, HMI and those from the caring professions. Promotes the development of children and young people with special educational needs, wherever they are located, and supports those who work with them. Details of course, conferences, and publications may be obtained. **Pub:** *British Journal of Special Education and Support for Learning*, quarterly. Journal. • *British Journal of Visual Impairment*. Journal. • *Journal of Research in Special Educational Needs*. Journal. • *Speciall*, 3/year. Magazine.

★ 4727 ★ National Association of Specialist Obstetricians and Gynaecologists (NASOG)

c/o Dr. Trevor Mudge
57 Anzac Way, Ste. 20
Ashford, SA 5035, Australia
Phone: 61 8 3710332 **Fax:** 61 8 3710479
Website: http://www.midcoast.com.au/prof/medical/assoc/nasog.html

Desc: Represents the industrial interests of the obstetricians and gynaecologists of Australia.

★ 4728 ★ National Association of State Alcohol and Drug Abuse Directors (NASADAD)

808 17th St. NW, Ste. 410
Washington, DC 20006
Phone: (202)293-0090 **Fax:** (202)293-1250
Email: dcoffice@nasadad.org
Website: http://www.nasadad.org
Lewis E. Gallant, PhD, Exec. Dir.

Fnded: 1971. **Mem:** 56. **Desc:** Purposes are: to represent the interests of state alcohol and drug abuse directors and their agencies before Congress and federal agencies; to foster development of comprehensive alcohol and drug abuse programs on state resources/services, alcohol and drug issues related to AIDS, drunk driving, and criminal justice activities in each state. Operates Project for Addiction Counselor Training, AIDS Policy Project, Criminal Justice Programs, Methadone Treatment Quality Assurance System project, and the National Prevention Network (NPN). Serves as an information clearinghouse. Conducts seminars on current and emerging alcohol and drug abuse issues. **Pub:** *Directory of State Alcohol and Drug Abuse Directors*, monthly. Directory. • *Special Report*. *Price:* $80/year. • *State Alcohol and*

Drug Abuse Profile, annual. Report. Provides data on state fiscal resources, services to clients, drug trends, model products, and special needs. *Price:* $45. • *State Resource and Services Related to Alcohol and Drug Problems*, annual. • *State Substance Abuse Quarterly*, quarterly. Newsletter. Covers significant national and state development. *Price:* $80. • *Treatment Works*. **Frmly:** (1978) National Association of State Drug Abuse Program Coordinators.

★ 4729 ★ National Association of State EMS Directors (NASEMSD)

111 Park Pl.
Falls Church, VA 22046-4513
Phone: (703)538-1799 **Fax:** (703)241-5603
Email: info@nasemsd.org
Website: http://www.nasemsd.org
Elizabeth B. Armstrong, CAE, Exec. Dir.

Fnded: 1981. **Mem:** 56. **Reg. Groups:** 4. **Desc:** Provides vision and leadership in the development and improvement of EMS systems and national EMS policy. **Pub:** *EMS Office, Structure, and Functioning*. *Price:* $35. • *EMT Certification, Licensing, and Reciprocity Requirements*. *Price:* $25. • *Training and Certification of EMS Personnel*. *Price:* $50. • *Trauma Center Designation Survey*. Survey. *Price:* $28.

★ 4730 ★ National Association of State Medicaid Directors (NASMD)

810 1st St. NE, Ste. 500
Washington, DC 20002
Phone: (202)682-0100 **Fax:** (202)682-3706
Lee Partridge, Dir.

Fnded: 1979. **Desc:** Representatives of state Medicaid agencies. Promotes effective and efficient management of federal and state health care programs. Facilitates communication and cooperation between state and federal Medicaid authorities; serves as a clearinghouse on Medicaid benefits.

★ 4731 ★ National Association of State Mental Health Program Directors (NASMHPD)

66 Canal Center Plz., Ste. 302
Alexandria, VA 22314
Phone: (703)739-9333 **Fax:** (703)548-9517
Website: http://www.nasmhpd.org
Dr. Robert W. Glover, Exec. Dir.

Fnded: 1963. **Mem:** 55. **Desc:** State commissioners and directors in charge of the state mental health agencies; associate members are assistant commissioners for children and youth, older persons, legal services, forensic services, and adult services. Promotes cooperation of state government agencies in delivery of services to people with severe mental illnesses; fosters the exchange of scientific and programmatic information in the administration of public mental health programs including treatment programs, community and hospital care of persons with mental illness, mental retardation, or substance abuse disorders. Monitors state and federal and congressional activities; gathers and analyzes information on organization, structure, funding, and programming of state government mental health programs. Operates under a cooperative agreement with the National Governors' Association (see separate entry).

★ 4732 ★ National Association of State School Nurse Consultants (NASSNC)

PO Box 708
Kent, OH 44240-0708

Desc: Registered nurses employed by state departments of education or health. Promotes development of standards of practice among school nurse consultants; facilitates continuing professional advancement of members. Serves as a forum for the exchange of information among members and between members and related professionals; promotes and supports research activities; formulates nursing standards; sponsors educational programs.

★ 4733 ★ National Association of State Units on Aging (NASUA)

1201 15th St. NW, No. 300
Washington, DC 20005
Phone: (202)898-2578 **Fax:** (202)898-2583
Email: info@nasua.org
Website: http://www.nasua.org/
Daniel A. Quirk, PhD, Exec. Dir.

Fnded: 1964. **Mem:** 57. **Desc:** Public interest organization that provides information, technical assistance, and professional development support to State Units on Aging. (A state unit is an agency of state government designated by the governor and state legislature to administer the Older Americans Act and to serve as a focal point for all matters relating to older people.) Serves as organized channel for officially designated state leadership in aging to exchange information and mutual experiences, and to join together for appropriate action on behalf of the elderly. Services include: information on federal policy and program developments in aging; training and technical assistance on a wide range of program and management issues; liaison with organizations representing the public and private sectors. **Pub:** *Directory of State Units on Aging*, periodic. Directory. • Books. • Manuals. • Reports. • Also publishes materials on aging policy and programs, policy briefs, legislative updates, and technical assistance documents.

★ 4734 ★ National Association of Substance Abuse Trainers and Educators (NASATE)

1521 Hillary St.
New Orleans, LA 70118
Phone: (504)286-5234
Dr. Tom Lief, Chairperson

Fnded: 1982. **Mem:** 100. **Reg. Groups:** 2. **Desc:** Accredited colleges and universities offering 12 or more course credit hours in the field of substance abuse. Goal is to provide a network for exchange on courses, student population, degreed and nondegreed programs, and graduate study in chemical dependency training. Acts as a clearinghouse for students interested in substance abuse training programs; assists universities with the development of such programs. Provides for the exchange of information among universities concerning certificates, continuing education units, degrees, and opportunities for transfer and enrollment in undergraduate, graduate, and professional schools. Examines the educational and training needs of students and their career mobility as substance abuse practitioners. **Pub:** *Annual Directory*. Directory.

★ 4735 ★ National Association of Supervisors and Administrators of Health Occupations Education (NASAHOE)

c/o Jo Ann Wakelyn
Virginia Department of Education
PO Box 2120
Richmond, VA 23218-2021
Phone: (804)225-2842 **Fax:** (804)371-2456
Email: jwakelyn@pen.k12.va.us
Website: http://www.pen.k12.va.us
Jo Ann Wakelyn, Pres.

Mem: 35. **Desc:** State administrators and local supervisors of health occupations education. Acts as resource sharing group, particularly in the area of curriculum development. Seeks to develop shared resources for recruitment. **Pub:** *NASAHOE News*, quarterly. Newsletter. **Frmly:** (1988) National Association for State Administrators of Health Occupations Education.

★ 4736 ★ National Association for the Support of Long Term Care (NASL)

1321 Duke St., Ste. 304
Alexandria, VA 22314
Phone: (703)549-8500 **Fax:** (703)549-8342
Email: member@nasl.org
Website: http://www.nasl.org
Peter Clendenin, Exec. VP.

Fnded: 1989. **Desc:** Long term care executives and businesses. Dedicated to providing a national communication forum and legislative and regulatory representation for the long term care industry.

★ 4737 ★ National Association of Swimming Clubs for the Handicapped

c/o The Willows
Mayles Lane
Wickham
Hampshire PO17 5ND, United Kingdom
Phone: 44 1329 833689

Fnded: 1966. **Mem:** 12,120. **Desc:** All ages with any disabilities. Aims to encourage disabled youngsters and adults to participate in swimming. Registered charity organization 247772.

★ 4738 ★ National Association of Theatre Nurses

Daisy Ayris House
6 Grove Park Ct.
Harrogate HG1 4DP, United Kingdom
Phone: 44 1423 508079 **Fax:** 44 1423 531613
Email: hq@natn.org.uk
Website: http://www.natn.org.uk

Fnded: 1964. **Mem:** 8,000. **Reg. Groups:** 47. **Desc:** Operating theatre nurses. Workshops and study days are organized locally and nationally throughout the year. **Pub:** *British Journal of Perioperitive Nurses*, monthly. Journal.

★ 4739 ★ National Association of Traveling Nurses (NATN)

PO Box 35215
Chicago, IL 60707-0215
Phone: (708)453-0080 **Fax:** (708)453-0083
Email: natn@rentamark.com
Website: http://www.travelingnurse.org
L. David Stoller, Chm.

Fnded: 1990. **Mem:** 78,,951. **Nat'l Groups:** 1. **Desc:** Members of the medical profession. Provides travel information. Provides information to nurses, health care professionals on traveling assignments and job placement opportunities. Offers substantial discounts for members at major hotels, resorts, and car rental agencies. Provides members with complete list of approved travel industry suppliers, including travel agents, vendors, airlines, cruise ship companies, and hotels. **Pub:** *Journal of Traveling Nurses*, quarterly. Journal. Online journal. *Price:* for members. • *National Online*. Newsletter. National invites authors to submit articles in "WORD" format via email for publication in the national online journal.

★ 4740 ★ National Association of VA Physicians and Dentists (NAVAPD)

11 Canal Centre Plz., Ste. 110
Alexandria, VA 22314-1595
Phone: (703)548-0280 **Fax:** (703)683-7939
Email: navapd@dgsys.com
Website: http://www.navapd.org
Robert M. Conroy, Pres.

Fnded: 1975. **Mem:** 2,000. **Desc:** Physicians and dentists at Department of Veterans Affairs Medical Centers. Purpose is to strengthen and improve the quality of care and conditions at VA health care facilities. Works to assure that veterans receive quality care. **Pub:** *NAVAPD News*, bimonthly. Newsletter. *Price:* Included in membership. • *NAVAPD Notes*, bimonthly.

★ 4741 ★ National Association of Vascular Access Networks (NAVAN)

11441 S State St., Ste. A, No. 113
Draper, UT 84020-9131
Phone: (801)576-1824 **Free:** 888-576-2826
Fax: (801)553-9137
Email: info@navannet.org
Website: http://www.navannet.org
Mary Lea Nations, Exec. Dir.

Fnded: 1988. **Mem:** 1,100. **Local Groups:** 10. **Desc:** Physicians, pharmacists, nurses, and manufacturers involved in the care and management of patients with vascular access devices. Seeks to advance the effectiveness of vascular access devices; promotes professional development of members. Serves as a network linking members; conducts educational programs. **Pub:** *JVAD*, periodic. Journal.

★ 4742 ★ National Association for Veterinary Acupuncture (NAVA)

951 W Bastanchury Rd.
Fullerton, CA 92835
Phone: (714)871-3000 **Fax:** (714)278-9335
Email: drdick@e-vet.com
Richard S. Glassberg, D.V.M., Pres.

Fnded: 1973. **Mem:** 60. **Desc:** Veterinarians, medical doctors, acupuncturists, and interested laymen. Purpose is to educate veterinarians and laymen in the field of veterinary acupuncture and to translate material into English. Conducts seminars; maintains speakers' bureau. **Pub:** *Compendium of Human and Veterinary Acupuncture.* • *Equine Acupuncture.*

★ 4743 ★ National Association of Veterinary Technicians in America (NAVTA)

PO Box 224
Battle Ground, IN 47920
Phone: (765)742-2216
Email: navta@navta.net
Website: http://www.navta.net/
Lisa Chase, Pres.

Desc: Committed to career growth and the advancement of the veterinary technology profession.

★ 4744 ★ National Association of Vision Professionals (NAVP)

c/o Prevention of Blindness Soc.
1775 Church St. NW
Washington, DC 20036
Phone: (202)234-1010 **Fax:** (202)234-1020
Email: mail@youreyes.org
Website: http://members.tripod.com/charlie216/
Michele Hartlove, Exec. Sec.

Fnded: 1976. **Mem:** 200. **Desc:** Individuals responsible for or connected with vision conservation and eye health programs in public or private agencies and institutions. Serves as a forum for ideas and programs, cooperates with other agencies, and promotes professional standards. Certifies vision screening personnel. **Pub:** *National Association of Vision Professionals–Newsletter*, quarterly. Newsletter. *Price:* Included in membership dues. **Frmly:** (1986) National Association of Vision Program Consultants.

★ 4745 ★ National Association for Visually Handicapped (NAVH)

22 W 21st St.
New York, NY 10010
Phone: (212)889-3141 **Fax:** (212)727-2931
Email: staff@navh.org
Website: http://www.navh.org
Dr. Lorraine Marchi, Founder/CEO

Fnded: 1954. **Mem:** 7,530. **Reg. Groups:** 2. **Desc:** Individuals, clubs, organizations, and foundations support NAVH's work in publishing and distributing large-print informational literature for the partially seeing. Acts as information clearinghouse regarding all public and private services available to the partially seeing. Offers guidance and counseling to parents of partially seeing children and to partially seeing adults. Educates the public and the professional community about the needs of the partially seeing. **Pub:** *About Children's Eyes.* Large print only. *Price:* Free. • *It's All Right to Be Angry.* • *Knitting Instructions.* • *Large Print Loan Library Catalog*, biennial. Catalog. Lists books in large print commercial publishers available from NAVH. • *National Association for Visually Handicapped–Bulletin: Annual Program Report*, annual. Newsletter. Reports on association activities and programs. Includes obituaries. • *NAVH Update*, quarterly. Newsletter. Provides updates on issues and devices for the visually handicapped. • *Visual Aids & Information Materials.* Catalog. Features visual aids available from NAVH. • Also publishes (in English, Russian, Spanish, and some Mandarin Chinese) pamphlets, guides, booklets, and manuals on eye diseases and services for visually impaired; also books on tape. **Frmly:** (1972) National Aid to Visually Handicapped.

★ 4746 ★ National Association of Women Pharmacists (NAWP)

c/o Office Manager
Royal Pharmaceutical Society of Great Britain
1 Lambeth High St.
London SE1 7JN, United Kingdom
Email: enquiries@nawp.org.uk
Website: http://www.nawp.org.uk

Fnded: 1905. **Mem:** 300. **Reg. Groups:** 3. **Local Groups:** 4. **Lang(s):** English. **Desc:** Women pharmacists. Promotes the careers of women in pharmacy and the role of women pharmacists in public life. Encourages continuing education and career development for women pharmacists. Maintains communication with pharmacists who have left the Register of the Royal Pharmaceutical Society of Great Britain (RPSGB) during a career break. Works with other women's organizations. Conducts courses and lectures, provides mentoring for members. **Pub:** *Careers in Pharmacy.* Book. • *NAWP*, 3/year. Newsletter.

★ 4747 ★ National Ataxia Foundation (NAF)

2600 Fernbrook Ln. N, No. 119
Minneapolis, MN 55447
Phone: (763)553-0020 **Fax:** (763)553-0167
Email: naf@mail.ataxia.org
Website: http://www.ataxia.org
Donna Gruetzmacher, Exec. Dir.

Fnded: 1957. **Mem:** 2,000. **Local Groups:** 58. **Desc:** Membership is open to any individual who wishes to contribute to the eradication of ataxia (a genetic disease characterized by the degeneration of the nerves of the spinal cord and the cerebellum, causing a loss of coordination and disturbance in gait and related conditions such as peroneal muscular atrophy, hereditary spastic paraplegia, and hereditary tremor. Ataxia may be inherited as a recessive or dominant trait and may strike persons from a very early age up to and even beyond 50 years of age. Ataxia is very similar to multiple sclerosis; however, multiple sclerosis is not inherited and has a different origin.) Objectives are: to make an early diagnosis of ataxia by locating all potential victims and encouraging them to have an examination; to educate the public and the helping professions about ataxia; to initiate basic research and coordinate efforts of worldwide research centers. Emphasis is on locating and understanding the genes responsible. Provides services and information to ataxia victims and their families. **Pub:** *Generations*, quarterly. Newsletter. Includes foundation news, calendar of events, and research updates. *Price:* Free to members and those who suffer from ataxia. • *Together - There is Hope.* Video. • Brochures. • Also publishes Together. . .(video) and brochures.

★ 4748 ★ National Attention Deficit Disorder Association (National ADDA)

1788 Second St., Ste. 200
Highland Park, IL 60035
Phone: (847)432-2332 **Fax:** (847)432-5874
Email: mail@add.org
Website: http://www.add.org
Nancy Ratey, Pres.

Fnded: 1989. **Desc:** Seeks to: promote a greater public awareness of the multiple needs of individuals with ADD and their families; address their educational, psychological, and social needs; encourage more responsiveness with regard to ADD in the academic and health care communities. Maintains database of support groups throughout the country. **Pub:** *Addalog.* Catalog. Lists books, brochures, monographs, and other materials available for purchasing. • *Focus.* Newsletter. • Monographs. • Pamphlets. **Frmly:** (1992) Attention-Deficit Disorder Association.

★ 4749 ★ National Autism Society of Sweden (Riksfoereningen Autism — RFA)

Hantverkargatan 87
S-112 38 Stockholm, Sweden
Phone: 46 8 7020580 **Fax:** 46 8 6440288
Email: info@autism.se
Website: http://w3.khurit.com/rfa/rfa/omsseng.asp

Fnded: 1973. **Mem:** 7,200. **Local Groups:** 25. **Desc:** Represents individuals with autism spectrum disorders and other disorders where autism is of frequent occurrence, including Fragile X, Tuberous Sclerosis, Rett Syndrome, and their relatives and professionals. **Pub:** *Ogonblick*, quarterly. Magazine. • Videos.

★ 4750 ★ National Beep Baseball Association (NBBA)

5568 Boulder-Crest St.
Columbus, OH 43235
Phone: (614)442-1444
Email: nbbasec@cs.com
Website: http://www.nbba.org
Jeana Weigand, Sec.

Fnded: 1975. **Mem:** 500. **Local Groups:** 20. **Desc:** Blind and visually impaired athletes, sighted volunteers, and others interested in participating in beep baseball. (Beep baseball uses a ball and two bases which emit sounds. Once the batter hits the ball, he or she must get to whichever base buzzes before one of the six other players fields the ball. The pitcher and catcher are sighted volunteers.) Promotes the development of amateur beep baseball and other recreational and competitive programs for the blind and visually impaired; holds tournaments. Sponsors speakers' bureau; conducts research programs. **Pub:** *Beep Baseball In A Nutshell*, annual. Bulletin. Features a brief description explaining the game and rules. *Price:* Free. • *History of NBBA.* Bulletin. • *NBBA Newsletter*, quarterly. Newsletter. Includes score statistics, tournament information and rule changes. *Price:* Included in membership dues.

★ 4751 ★ National Black Alcoholism and Addiction Council

1522 K St. NW, No. 450
Washington, DC 20005-1259
Phone: (202)296-2696 **Fax:** (315)798-8736
Email: nbacinc@earthlink.net
Website: http://www.nbacinc.org
Dr. John Robertson, Exec. Dir.

Fnded: 1978. **Mem:** 1,050. **Desc:** Individuals concerned about alcoholism among black Americans. Works to support and initiate activities that will improve alcoholism treatment services and lead to the prevention of alcoholism in the black community. Provides training on how to treat black alcoholics from a cultural perspective. Bestows political and service awards. Maintains biographical archives. Compiles statistics concerning alcoholism among blacks. **Pub:** *Model for Working With Children of Alcoholic and Drug Addicted Parents.* • *National News and Views*, semiannual. • *Treatment of Black Alcoholics.* **Frmly:** (1998) National Black Alcoholism Council.

★ 4752 ★ National Black Association for Speech-Language and Hearing (NBASLH)

PO Box 959
Athens, OH 45701
Phone: (740)594-4989 **Fax:** (740)594-6229
Email: nbaslh2@aol.com
Website: http://www.utexas.edu/coc/csd/multicultural/network/resource/nbaslh/nbaslh1.htm
Janice M. Wright, Exec. Dir.

Fnded: 1978. **Mem:** 500. **Desc:** Professionals and other individuals concerned with communicatively handicapped blacks. Strongly encourages the recruitment and training of black professionals to work with individuals suffering from speech, language, and hearing problems; maintains that conditions such as race, socioeconomic class, and cultural differences must be taken into account in order to understand and sensitively study the communicative process, and to treat communicative disorders. Supports related research; solicits, and provides, financial support for the training of black students in speech-language pathology and audiology. Disseminates information. **Pub:** *Echo*, quarterly. Newsletter. *Price:* $7.

★ 4753 ★ National Black Deaf Advocates (NBDA)

PO Box 305288
Charlotte Amalie, VI 00803
Phone: (340)774-5899 **Fax:** (340)774-8350
Email: rubytim@viaccess.net
Website: http://www.nbda.org/
Gwendolyn T. Powell, Pres.

Fnded: 1982. **Local Groups:** 20. **Desc:** Advocates for the rights of African-American deaf and hearing impared people. Seeks to promote the well-being, culture and empowerment of African-Americans who are deaf or hard of hearing. Conducts educational outreach programs; offers leadership training and training for interpreters and transliterators of color. Sponsors the Miss NBDA Pageant. **Pub:** *NBDA Network*, quarterly. Newsletter.

★ 4754 ★ National Black Leadership Initiative on Cancer (NBLIC)

PO Box 34828
Las Vegas, NV 89133
Phone: (702)655-3752 **Fax:** (702)655-3762
Email: dot.blic@yahoo.com
Dorothy M. Johnson, Chair

Fnded: 1994. **Mem:** 36. **Reg. Groups:** 44. **State Groups:** 1. **Local Groups:** 1. **Desc:** African-Americans and health care professionals concerned with the prevention, diagnosis, and treatment of people with cancer, particularly those of African-American descent. Seeks to facilitate "closing the gap in cancer incidence and mortality and increasing survival from cancer" by increasing awareness among African-AMRs of cancer and its prevention and treatment. Conducts educational programs to develop volunteer leaders in African-American communities, with emphasis on increasing understanding of breast, colorectal, and prostate cancer and the role played by diet in their prevention. **Pub:** Newsletter, monthly.

★ 4755 ★ National Black Nurses Association (NBNA)

8630 Fenton St., Ste. 330
Silver Spring, MD 20910
Phone: (301)589-3200 **Fax:** (301)589-3223
Email: nbna@erols.com
Website: http://www.nbna.org/
Millicent Gorham, Exec. Dir.

Fnded: 1971. **Mem:** 5,000. **Nat'l Groups:** 78. **Desc:** Registered nurses, licensed practical nurses, licensed vocational nurses, and student nurses. Functions as a professional support group and as an advocacy group for the black community and their health care. Recruits and assists blacks interested in pursuing nursing as a career. Presents scholarships to student nurses, including the Dr. Lauranne Sams Scholarship. Compiles statistics; maintains biographical archives. **Pub:** *Journal of Black Nurses Association*, semiannual. Journal. *Price:* Included in membership dues. • *National Black Nurses Association–Book of Reports*, annual. *Price:* available to members only. • *National Black Nurses Association–Proceedings*, periodic. • *NBNA Newsletter*, quarterly. Newsletter. Includes calendar of events, research updates, scholarships, grants, and fellowships. *Price:* Included in membership dues. • Annual Report.

★ 4756 ★ National Black Women's Health Project (NBWHP)

600 Pennsylvania Ave. SE, Ste. 310
Washington, DC 20003
Phone: (202)548-4000 **Fax:** (202)543-9743
Email: nbwhp@nbwhp.org
Website: http://www.BlackWomensHealth.org
Lorraine Cole, PhD, Pres.

Fnded: 1981. **Reg. Groups:** 5. **State Groups:** 26. **Local Groups:** 150. **Desc:** Provides education, advocacy, research and leadership development focusing on health issues that disproportionately affect black women across lifespan, devoted solely to the health of black women. groups. Also notes that black infant mortality is twice that of whites and that black women are often victims of family violence. Offers seminars outlining demographic information, chronic conditions, the need for health information and access to services, and possible methods of improving the health status of black women. Sponsors Center for Black Women's Wellness. Maintains library, database, and speakers' bureau. Conducts gender and race specific health research programs. Plans to: establish black women's wellness centers; develop Empowerment Through Wellness curriculum. **Pub:** *Body and Soul: A Black Women's Guide to Health and Well-Being.* • *It's Ok to Peek.* Video. • *It's Up to Us.* Video. • *Let Me Know What's Going On? My Body, My Self, My Life.* Video. • *On Becoming a Woman: Mothers and Daughters Talking Together.* Video. • *Our Bodies, Our Voices, Our Choices: A Black Women's Primer on Reproductive Health and Rights.* • Also publishes conference reports, brochures, and health fact sheets. Makes available educational films. **Frmly:** (1984) Black Women's Health Project.

★ 4757 ★ National Blood Foundation (NBF)

8101 Glenbrook Rd.
Bethesda, MD 20814-2749
Phone: (301)215-6552 **Fax:** (301)907-6895
Email: nbf@aabb.org
Website: http://www.aabb.org

Fnded: 1983. **Desc:** Promotes the safety and adequacy of America's blood supply by supporting research and education for blood banking and transfusion medicine.

★ 4758 ★ National Blood Transfusion Service

PO Box A101
Avondale
Harare, Zimbabwe
Phone: 263 4 707801 **Fax:** 263 4 707820
Email: lloyd@healthnet.zw

Fnded: 1986. **Desc:** Promotes the availability of blood supplies for tranfusions in Zimbabwe. Disseminates information. **Pub:** *Annual Report.* • Booklet. AIDS awareness and giving blood.

★ 4759 ★ National Board for Certification of Dental Laboratories (CDL)

1530 Metropolitan Blvd.
Tallahassee, FL 32308
Phone: (850)205-5626 **Free:** 800-950-1150
Fax: (850)222-0053
Email: nadl@nadl.org
Website: http://www.nadl.org/html/cdl.html
Bennett E. Napier, Exec. Dir.

Fnded: 1979. **Mem:** 600. **Desc:** Certified dental laboratories, including commercial, private, and dental or dental technology schools. Purpose is the certification and recognition of dental laboratories that demonstrate and document compliance with standards set by the industry for laboratory facilities, technical resources, safety, prevention of cross-contamination, and competence of personnel. **Pub:** *Certified Mail*, periodic. Newsletter. • Directory, semiannual.

★ 4760 ★ National Board for Certification in Dental Technology

c/o National Association of Dental Laboratories
1530 Metropoliton
Tallahassee, FL 32308
Phone: (850)205-5626 **Free:** 800-950-1150
Fax: (850)222-0053
Email: nadl@nadl.org
Website: http://www.nadl.org
Richard Harrell, Chm.

Fnded: 1958. **Mem:** 10,000. **Desc:** Certifies dental technicians with formal education in dental technology and a minimum of three years' experience who have passed written and practical exams administered by the NBC. Provides continuing education to certificants and recognizes competent dental technicians. Also certifies dental laboratories that meet published standards for personnel, facility and infection control practice. **Pub:** *Who's Who in the Dental Laboratory Industry*, annual. Directory. Online directory published in conjunction with the National Association of Dental Laboratories. *Price:* Free.

★ 4761 ★ National Board for Certification in Occupational Therapy (NBCOT)

The Eugene B. Casey Bldg. 800 S Frederick Ave. Ste 200
Gaithersburg, MD 20877-4150
Phone: (301)990-7979 **Fax:** (301)869-8492
Email: info@nbcot.org
Website: http://www.nbcot.org
Paul Grace, Exec. Dir.

Fnded: 1986. **Desc:** Participants are occupational therapists and occupational therapy assistants. Administers certification program and maintains certification records of certificants; operates disciplinary mechanisms. **Pub:** *Report to the Profession*, 2/yr.Newsletters. • Brochures. • Reports. **Frmly:** (1996) AOTCB; (1998) American Occupational Therapy Certification Board.

★ 4762 ★ National Board for Certification of Orthopaedic Technologists (NBCOT)

PMB No. 166
4736 Onondaga Blvd.
Syracuse, NY 13219
Free: (866)466-2268 **Fax:** (315)476-8840
Email: gonbcot@aol.com
Website: http://www.nbcot.net
Jeffrey Virgo, Chairman

Fnded: 1983. **Mem:** 1,500. **Desc:** Offers National Certification in Orthopaedic Technology to those Orthopaedic Technologists that have met the standards set forth by the NBCOT; allows re-certification by retesting or by obtaining Continuing Education Units. **Pub:** *Role Delineation.* Study guide for the Orthopaedic Technologist exam and the Orthopaedic Technologist-Surgery Certified exam.

★ 4763 ★ National Board for Certified Clinical Hypnotherapists (NBCCH)

1110 Fidler Ln., Ste. L1
Silver Spring, MD 20910
Phone: (301)608-0123 **Free:** 800-449-8144
Fax: (301)588-9535
Email: nbcch@natboard.com
Website: http://www.natboard.com/

Fnded: 1991. **Desc:** Dedicated to professionalizing the mental health specialty/sub-specialty of hypnotherapy, including addictions, counselors, marriage and family therapists, mental health counselors, pastoral counselors, psychiatric nurse, physicians, psychiatrists, psychologists, school counselors, and social workers; promotes standards for certification; sponsors educational activities; promotes public and professional awareness; sponsors scientific investigation into the uses of hypnotherapy. **Pub:** *Interlink.* Newsletter.

★ 4764 ★ National Board of Chiropractic Examiners (NBCE)

901 54th Ave.
Greeley, CO 80634
Phone: (970)356-9100 **Fax:** (970)356-6134
Email: nbce@nbce.org
Website: http://www.nbce.org
Horace C. Elliott, Exec. Dir.

Fnded: 1963. **Desc:** Develops, administers and scores examinations taken by applicants for chiropractic licensure by experienced practitioners seeking reciprocity, endorsement or relicensure. **Pub:** *NBCE Journal*. Journal.

★ 4765 ★ National Board of Examiners in Optometry
4340 E West Hwy., Ste. 1010
Bethesda, MD 20814
Phone: (301)652-5192 **Free:** 800-969-EXAM
Fax: (301)907-0013
Email: nbeo@optometry.org
Website: http://www.optometry.org
Dr. Norman E. Wallis, Exec. Dir.

Fnded: 1951. **Desc:** Administers entry-level criterion-referenced credentialing examinations to students and graduates of accredited schools and colleges of optometry for use by individual state licensing boards. Provides other evaluation, assessment, and survey services to the profession. **Pub:** *Candidates Guide*, annual. • *Test Points*, 3/year. Newsletter. • Annual Report. • Manuals.

★ 4766 ★ National Board of Forensic Chiropractors (NBOFC)
601 S Mill St.
PO Box 356
Manning, SC 29102
Phone: (803)435-5078 **Free:** 800-692-2256
Fax: (803)435-8096
Email: omyback@gte.net
Website: http://www.forensicexaminers.org/
Dr. Preston B. Fitzgerald, Sr., Contact

Fnded: 1996. **Desc:** Training association of examiners, scientists and professionals dedicated to orderly analysis, investigation and examination to obtain the truth, then provide expert opinion. **Pub:** Newsletter.

★ 4767 ★ National Board of Medical Examiners (NBME)
3750 Market St.
Philadelphia, PA 19104-3190
Phone: (215)590-9500 **Fax:** (215)590-9555
Email: webmail@nbme.org
Website: http://www.nbme.org
Donald E. Melnick, MD, Pres.

Fnded: 1915. **Mem:** 75. **Desc:** Purposes are: to prepare and administer qualifying examinations either independently or in conjunction with other organizations, of such high quality that legal agencies governing the practice of medicine within each state may, in their discretion, grant a license without further examination for those who have successfully completed such examinations; to cooperate with and, where appropriate, to make its specialized services available to the examining boards of the states, specialty boards, and other organizations concerned with the education and qualification of personnel in the fields of health; to assist medical schools, hospitals and related organizations and institutions in evaluation of the effectiveness of their educational programs; to initiate, develop, and participate in research designed to evaluate the effectiveness of educational programs and techniques, and to assess ever more precisely the knowledge, competence, and qualification of professionals in public health care; to provide educational opportunities for professional personnel in the methods, techniques, and values of testing methods related to knowledge and competence in the broad field of medicine. **Pub:** *National Board Examiner*, quarterly. Newsletter. Reports on new medical evaluation programs and new directions in the research and development of examinations. *Price:* Free. • Annual Report. • Also publishes information bulletins and policy statements.

★ 4768 ★ National Board of Naturopathic Examiners (NBNE)
PO Box 78600
North Capitol Station
Washington, DC 20013-8600
Dr. George A. Freibott, Trustee

Fnded: 1919. **Mem:** 5,000. **Nat'l Groups:** 1. **Reg. Groups:** 8. **State Groups:** 50. **Local Groups:** 2. **Desc:** Naturopathic physicians. Acts as a national testing association/board for diplomate status in naturopathy. Compiles statistics. Conducts research, educational, and charitable programs. Maintains speakers' bureau. **Pub:** *NBNE Newsletter*, quarterly. Newsletter. *Price:* $5/each.

★ 4769 ★ National Board for Nursing, Midwifery and Health Visiting for Northern Ireland
Centre House
79 Chichester St.
Belfast BT1 4JE, United Kingdom
Phone: 44 28 9023 8152 **Fax:** 44 28 9033 3298
Email: enquiries@nbni.n-i.nhs.uk

Fnded: 1979. **Mem:** 9. **Lang(s):** English. **Desc:** Non-executive members appointed by the Head of Department of Health and Social Services for Northern Ireland, executive members ie the Chief Executive, and Director of Finance & Administration of the National Board. The majority of members are registered nurses, midwives or health visitors. To approve institutions in relation to provision of training courses for nurses, midwives and health visitors which meet Central Council standards; to collaborate with Council in the promotion of improved training methods; and such other functions as the Head of the Department of Health may by order prescribe. **Pub:** Annual Report, annual. • Papers.

★ 4770 ★ National Board of Osteopathic Medical Examiners (NBOME)
8765 W Higgins Rd., Ste. 200
Chicago, IL 60631
Phone: (773)714-0622 **Fax:** (773)714-0631
Email: admin@nbome.org
Website: http://www.nbome.org
Joseph F. Smoley, PhD, Exec. Dir.

Fnded: 1935. **Mem:** 12. **Desc:** Examining and evaluating board to investigate the qualifications of, and administer examinations and grant diplomate status to osteopathic physicians. **Pub:** *Information Bulletin*, annual. Bulletin. **Frmly:** (1986) National Board of Examiners for Osteopathic Physicians and Surgeons.

★ 4771 ★ National Board of Podiatric Medical Examiners (NBPME)
PO Box 510
Bellefonte, PA 16823
Phone: (814)357-0487 **Fax:** (814)357-0581
Email: nbpmeofc@aol.com
Charles W. Gibley, Exec. Dir.

Fnded: 1956. **Mem:** 12. **Desc:** Professional podiatrists. Purpose is to prepare and administer examinations for podiatry students seeking state licensure. Monitors test validity and reliability. **Pub:** Annual Report. • Bulletin, annual. • Membership Directory, annual. **Frmly:** (1985) National Board of Podiatry Examiners.

★ 4772 ★ National Board for Respiratory Care (NBRC)
8310 Nieman Rd.
Lenexa, KS 66214-1579
Phone: (913)599-4200 **Fax:** (913)541-0156
Email: mthomas@goAMP.com
Website: http://www.nbrc.org
Melanie Thomas, Mgr. Candidate Services

Fnded: 1960. **Mem:** 16,000. **Desc:** Offers credentialing examinations for respiratory therapists, respiratory therapy technicians, pulmonary technologists, and perinatal/pediatric respiratory care specialists. **Pub:** Directory, annual. • Newsletter, bimonthly. **Frmly:** (1974) American Registry of Inhalation Therapists; (1982) National Board for Respiratory Therapy.

★ 4773 ★ National Brachial Plexus-Erb's Palsy Association
PO Box 23
Larsen, WI 54947-0023
Phone: (920)836-3843
Email: erbspalsy@usa.net
Website: http://www.nbpepa.org/
Brenda Copeland-Moore, Contact

Fnded: 1995. **Mem:** 1,000. **Desc:** Serves as a resource, information, and support center for the disease Brachial Plexus-Erb's Palsy. **Pub:** *BPI News*, quarterly. Newsletter.

★ 4774 ★ National Braille Association (NBA)
3 Townline Cir.
Rochester, NY 14623-2513
Phone: (585)427-8260 **Fax:** (585)427-0263
Email: nbaoffice@compuserve.com
Website: http://nationalbraille.org
Angela Coffaro, Exec. Dir.

Fnded: 1945. **Mem:** 1,500. **Desc:** Provides continuing education to those who prepare braille, and provides braille materials to persons who are visually impaired. Cooperates with other organizations in developing and expanding use of advanced braille codes; offers training workshops for transcribers and tactile illustrators. NBA Braille Book Bank maintains over 2000 titles and 500 standard technical tables in braille for immediate duplication; offers a transcribing service for braille readers. **Pub:** *Braille Technical Table Catalog*, periodic. Catalog. Contains technical tables in the NBA collection. Covers the fields of mathematics, statistics, chemistry, physics, computer science, and business. *Price:* Free. • *National Braille Association–Bulletin*, quarterly. Newsletter. Features articles of interest to members and persons working in the field of services to the visually impaired. Contains calendar of events. *Price:* Included in membership dues; $40/year for nonmembers in U.S.; $50/year outside U.S. • *National Braille Association–General Interest Catalog*, periodic. Catalog. Topics include work, recreation, and daily living. Directory of titles available in braille from NBA collection. Available in print and braille. *Price:* Free. • *National Braille Association–Music Catalog*, periodic. Catalog. Directory of music titles available in braille from NBA collection. Available in print and braille. *Price:* Free. • *National Braille Association–Textbook Catalog*, periodic. Catalog. Directory of titles of braille books from NBA collection of college-level and technical materials. Available in print and braille. *Price:* Free. • *NBA Publications*. Manuals. Cover tape recording, tactile graphics, mathematics and science brail le, textbook format braille, computer-assisted transcription, and large type. **Frmly:** (1964) National Braille Club.

★ 4775 ★ National Braille Press (NBP)
88 St. Stephen St.
Boston, MA 02115
Phone: (617)266-6160 **Free:** 888-965-8965
Fax: (617)437-0456
Email: orders@nbp.org
Website: http://www.nbp.org
William M. Raeder, Pres.

Fnded: 1927. **Desc:** Publishes books and magazines in braille, including booklets on computers, self-help, and children's books (also in print). Supported by private gifts and legacies. Sponsors Children's Braille Book Club, offering monthly selections of print-braille books. **Pub:** *National Braille Press Release*, semiannual. Newsletter. • *Our Special*, bimonthly. • *Syndicated Columnists Weekly*.

★ 4776 ★ National Brain Tumor Foundation (NBTF)
414 13th St., Ste. 700
Oakland, CA 94612-2603
Phone: (510)839-9777 **Free:** 800-934-CURE
Email: nbtf@braintumor.org
Website: http://www.braintumor.org
Janis Brewer, Exec. Dir.

Fnded: 1981. **Desc:** Medical researchers, doctors, brain tumor patients, and relatives working together to improve the quality of life for brain tumor patients and their families and find a cure through research. Raises funds for brain tumor research; offers patient services such as educational materials, a toll-free brain tumor information line, a quarterly newsletter, information about support groups and patient networks, and national and regional conferences. **Pub:** *Brain Tumors: A Guide.* Booklet. Contains information on brain tumors. *Price:* 1st copy free; $6 each additional copy. • *SEARCH*, quarterly. Newsletter. Informs readers of advances in treatment and psychosocial support. • Pamphlets. **Frmly:** (1989) Friends of Brain Tumor Research.

★ 4777 ★ National Breast Cancer Centre (NBCC)
Locked Bag 16
Camperdown, NSW 1450, Australia
Phone: 61 2 90363030 **Fax:** 61 2 90363077
Email: directorate@nbcc.org.au
Website: http://www.nbcc.org.au/default.htm

Fnded: 1995. **Desc:** Women, health professionals, cancer organizations, researchers and governments working to improve breast cancer outcomes for women.

★ 4778 ★ National Breast Cancer Coalition (NBCC)
1707 L St. NW, Ste. 1060
Washington, DC 20036
Phone: (202)296-7477 **Free:** 800-622-2838
Fax: (202)265-6854
Email: info@natlbcc.org
Website: http://www.stopbreastcancer.org
Fran Visco, Pres.

Fnded: 1991. **Mem:** 60,000. **Desc:** Promotes research into the cause of, optimal treatments and cure for breast cancer, aims to improve coordination and distribution of research funds and recruitment and training of scientists; strives to improve access to breast cancer screening, diagnosis, treatment and care for all women, particularly the underserved and uninsured, through legislation and change in regulation and delivery of breast health care; dedicated to increasing involvement and influence of those living with breast cancer in the areas of legislation, regulatory processes and all aspects of clinical trial design, including access to clinical trials. advocacy activities; formulated national action plan on breast cancer, to which the Clinton Administration committed in 1993. Operates: Aspen Project, which brings together industrial, scientific, governmental, and consumer representatives to develop innovative approaches to the prevention and treatment of breast cancer; Project LEAD, which trains grass roots advocates to influence public policies affecting people with breast cancer; Clinical Trials Project, which trains NBCC members to collaborate with scientific and industrial organizations to expedite clinical trials of breast cancer drugs and treatments. **Pub:** *Call to Action*, quarterly. Newsletter. *Price:* included in membership dues.

★ 4779 ★ National Burn Victim Foundation (NBVF)
PO Box 409
Basking Ridge, NJ 07920
Phone: (908)953-9091 **Fax:** (908)953-9099
Email: natlbvf@nac.net
Harry J. Gaynor, Exec. Dir.

Fnded: 1974. **Nat'l Groups:** 1. **Reg. Groups:** 2. **State Groups:** 1. **Desc:** Supporters are physicians specializing in burn treatment and care, fire services prevention personnel, nurses, communications experts, health and chemical industry representatives, and others interested in burn treatment and care. Maintains 24-hour emergency burn referral service. Conducts medical emergency burn care seminars and workshops for physicians, nurses, EMTs, and emergency rescue personnel. Operates Medical Disaster Response System, which utilizes private helicopters for transporting medical teams to disaster sites where large numbers of survivors have been tramatized. Collects burn data from New Jersey hospitals daily. Program currently provides direct professional services in New Jersey and information and referral services nationally. Offers consultation and evaluation services to the Division of Youth and Family Services and law enforcement agencies in cases involving suspected child abuse or neglect by burning. Presents burn awareness and prevention programs to schools, civic organizations, and day-care centers. Maintains speakers' bureau; conducts specialized education, children's services, and research programs; compiles statistics. **Pub:** *Burn Awareness.* Pamphlets. • *Child Abuse? Think Again.* Video. *Price:* $125. • *Disaster Medical Response.* Video. *Price:* $29.95. • *General Burn Awareness.* Video. • *Training Professionals - Child Abuse/Neglect Investigation.* Video. • Also publishes The Use of Forensics in the Investgation of Burn Injuries.

★ 4780 ★ National Business Coalition on Health
1015 18th St. NW, Ste. 730
Washington, DC 20036-5214
Phone: (202)775-9300 **Fax:** (202)775-1569
Email: mcornejo@nbch.org
Website: http://www.nbch.org
Greg Lehman, Pres. /CEO

Fnded: 1992. **Mem:** 80. **Desc:** Employer-led coalitions that group-purchase health care benefits for employees and measure and improve health care quality.

★ 4781 ★ National Cancer Center (NCC)
88 Sunnyside Blvd., Ste. 307
Plainview, NY 11803
Phone: (516)349-0610 **Fax:** (516)349-1755
Email: info@nationalcancercenter.org
Regina English, Exec. Dir.

Fnded: 1953. **Desc:** Supports cancer research and educational programs. Concentrates on cytology, immunology, detection, and prevention of cancer, and on invention and perfection of new methods and instruments for early diagnosis of cancer. **Frmly:** (1954) Eugene L. Garey Cancer Foundation; (1965) Cancer Cytology Foundation of America; (1986) National Cancer Cytology Center.

★ 4782 ★ National Cancer Institute of Canada (NCIC) (Institut National du Cancer du Canada — INCC)
10 Alcorn Ave., Ste. 200
Toronto, ON, Canada M4V 3B1
Phone: (416)961-7223 **Fax:** (416)961-7327
Email: ncic@cancer.ca
Website: http://www.ncic.cancer.ca

Fnded: 1947. **Mem:** 20. **Lang(s):** English, French. **Desc:** Coordinates and correlates the efforts of individuals and organized bodies with the goal of reducing the morbidity and mortality of cancer. This role is fulfilled through the support of clinical and laboratory-based research activities and research personnel. **Pub:** *Breast Cancer Bulletin*, semiannual. Newsletter. • *Canadian Cancer Statistics*, annual. • *Scientific Report*, annual. • *UPDATE*, quarterly. Newsletter. • Annual Report, annual.

★ 4783 ★ National Cancer Registrars Association (NCRA)
1310 Braddock Place, Ste. 102
Alexandria, VA 22314
Phone: (703)299-6640 **Fax:** (703)299-6620
Email: info@ncra-usa.org
Website: http://www.ncra-usa.org
Lori Swain, Exec. Dir.

Fnded: 1974. **Mem:** 2,500. **Desc:** Persons involved in central, state, regional, and hospital-based tumor registries including physicians, hospital administrators, and health care planners who maintain ongoing records of the cancer patient's history, diagnosis, therapy, and outcome. Purposes are to: promote research and education in tumor registry administration and practice; improve service to cancer patients; establish standards of education and provide a standardized course of study for tumor registrars; raise the level of knowledge and performance of tumor registrars through continuing education; disseminate information regarding current activities, research, and trends in the cancer field; initiate and/or participate in programs to improve and standardize the compiling of tumor - related information; interact with professional and governmental organizations that use data derived from tumor registries. Has conducted national educational programs including: coding and tumor registry workshops; symposia on head and neck tumors, lymphatic and hematopoietic neoplasms, and non-Hodgkin's lymphoma; tumor registry training program and seminars. Sponsors registry management training program at the University of Pittsburgh School of Health Related Professions to instruct tumor registrars. Offers certification examinations for tumor registrars; provides continuing education program to help members maintain certification; offers educational assistance for new registrars. **Pub:** *Connection*, quarterly. Newsletter. • *National Cancer Registrars Association–Membership Roster*, annual. *Price:* Included in membership dues. • *National Cancer Registrars Association–Proceedings/Annual Report*, annual. *Price:* Included in membership dues. • *National Cancer Registrars Association–The Journal of Registry Management.* Journal. Includes book reviews, peer reviewed scientific articles and lists of employment opportunities. *Price:* Included in membership dues; $40/year for nonmembers; $55/year for international subscriptions. • Surveys.Contains information on compensation. • Also publishes educational materials. **Frmly:** National Tumor Registrars Association.

★ 4784 ★ National Captioning Institute (NCI)
1900 Gallows Rd., Ste. 3000
Vienna, VA 22182
Phone: (703)917-7600 **Fax:** (703)917-9853
Email: koconnor@ncicap.org
Website: http://www.ncicap.org
Jack Gates, Pres. /COO

Fnded: 1979. **Desc:** Purpose is to caption television programs for the deaf and hard-of-hearing on behalf of public and commercial television broadcasters, cable-casters, and the home video industry. Makes available captioning services, making use of a "closed captioning" system that allows coded captions not visible on a normal television set to be decoded and made visible by the use of a special adapter which may be attached to a television set.

★ 4785 ★ National Care Homes Association
45/49 Leather Ln.
4th Fl.
London EC1N 7TJ, United Kingdom
Phone: 44 20 78317090 **Fax:** 44 20 78317040
Email: ncha@btclick.com

Fnded: 1981. **Mem:** 3,000. **Lang(s):** English. **Desc:** Independent sector care and nursing homes. Serves as a trade association representing members' interests. **Pub:** *Newsletter*, monthly. Newsletter.

★ 4786 ★ National Catholic AIDS Network (NCAN)
PO Box 960
Occidental, CA 95465
Phone: (707)874-3031 **Fax:** (707)874-1433
Email: info@ncan.org
Website: http://www.ncan.org
Fr. Rodney DeMartini, Exec. Dir.

Fnded: 1989. **Mem:** 4,500. **Reg. Groups:** 5. **Desc:** Provides support and exchange of information among Roman Catholic HIV/AIDS service workers and pastoral ministers. Disseminates educational materials on HIV/AIDS. **Pub:** *Connections*, quarterly. Newsletter. *Price:* Membership benefit.

★ 4787 ★ National Catholic Council on Alcoholism and Related Drug Problems (NCCA)
PO Box 248
Lafayette, IN 47902-0248
Phone: (765)420-0129 **Fax:** (765)420-0189

Email: inquiry@nccatoday.org
Website: http://www.nccatoday.org
Thomas A. Russell, Exec. Dir.

Fnded: 1949. **Mem:** 300. **Desc:** Promotes adequate treatment for all clergy and religious men and women suffering from alcoholism and drug dependency through consultation and supportive services. Cooperates with treatment programs for the spiritual, physical, and mental rehabilitation of alcoholics and drug dependent persons, especially with Alcoholics Anonymous World Services. Promotes pastoral ministry to alcoholics and their families. Educates Catholics, especially priests and religious men and women in pastoral ministries, on alcohol and alcohol problems as well as the use and abuse of alcohol and drugs. Sponsors workshops; conducts alcohol and drug abuse education programs in houses of formation and seminaries. Maintains speakers' bureau. **Pub:** *Alcoholism A Source Book for the Priest-Reprint of 1960 edition in 1998.* Book. • *The Best of the Blue Book Vol. II 1960-1997 published 1999.* Book. • *The Blue Book*, annual. Book. Proceedings of annual symposium. *Price:* $15 donation. • *NCCA Today*, quarterly. Newsletter. **Frmly:** National Clergy Conference on Alcoholism; (1988) National Clergy Council on Alcoholism and Related Drug Problems.

★ 4788 ★ National Catholic Pharmacists Guild of the United States (NCPG)

1012 Surrey Hills Dr.
Saint Louis, MO 63117-1438
Phone: (314)645-0085
John Paul Winkelmann, Exec. Dir. & Co-Pres.

Fnded: 1962. **Mem:** 400. **Nat'l Groups:** 1. **Desc:** Catholic pharmacists, pharmacy graduates, students, and pharmacy technicians. Upholds the principles of the Catholic faith and all laws of church and country, especially those pertaining to the practice of pharmacy; assists ecclesiastical authorities in the diffusion of Catholic pharmacy ethics; promotes donations of funds and supplies to the needy; opposes the sale of pornographic literature, especially that which is being sold in pharmacies; fosters solidarity and goodwill among all pharmacists. Provides pharmaceuticals and funds for people worldwide. **Pub:** *The Catholic Pharmacist*, quarterly. Journal. Includes obituaries, membership and professional news, new member listings, and book reports as well as other reports and issues. *Price:* Included in membership dues; $20/year for members only.

★ 4789 ★ National Caucus and Center on Black Aged (NCBA)

1220 L St. NW, Ste. 800
Washington, DC 20005
Phone: (202)637-8400 **Fax:** (202)347-0895
Email: info@ncba-aged.org
Website: http://www.ncba-aged.org
Karyne J. Conley, Pres. /CEO

Fnded: 1970. **Mem:** 3,000. **Local Groups:** 45. **Desc:** Seeks to improve living conditions for low-income elderly Americans, particularly blacks. Advocates changes in federal and state laws in improving the economic, health, and social status of low-income senior citizens. Promotes community awareness of problems and issues effecting low-income aging population. Operates an employment program involving 2000 older persons in 14 states. Sponsors, owns, and manages rental housing for the elderly. Conducts training and intern programs in nursing home administration, long-term care, housing management, and commercial property maintenance. **Pub:** *Golden Page*, quarterly. Newsletter. Reports developments concerning elderly blacks; includes association news and legislative update. *Price:* Included in membership dues. • Bulletin.

★ 4790 ★ National Center for American Indian and Alaska Native Mental Health Research (NCAIANMHR)

UCHSC Psychiatry Department
Nighthorse Campbell Native Health Bldg.
PO Box 6508, Mail Stop F800
Aurora, CO 80045-0508
Phone: (303)724-1414 **Free:** 800-820-9299
Fax: (303)724-1474
Email: billie.greene@uchsc.edu
Website: http://www.uchsc.edu/ai/ncaianmhr/journal/jover2.htm
Billie K. Greene, Journal Mgr.

Fnded: 1987. **Mem:** 41. **Desc:** Faculty, staff, and research associates in the mental health field. Conducts and supports research on management, prevention, and investigation of mental illness among Native Americans and Alaska Natives. Assists organizations in conducting and implementing mental health research. Disseminates information and statistics to public. **Pub:** *Behavioral Health Issues Among American Indians and Alaska Natives: Explorations on the Frontiers of the Biobehavioral Sciences.* Monograph. *Price:* $20. • *Calling From the Rim: Suicidal Behavior Among American Indian and Alaska Native Adolescents.* Monograph. *Price:* $20. • *Journal of the National Center for American Indian and Alaska Native Mental Health Research*, 3/year. Journal. Includes empirical research, case studies, unpublished dissertations, and articles on behavioral and social health sciences. *Price:* Free on-line. • *Mental Health Programs for American Indians: Their Logic, Structure and Function.* Monograph. *Price:* $20. • *New Directions in Prevention Among American Indian and Alaska Native Communities.* Monograph. *Price:* $14.95. • *The People Who Give More: Health and Mental Health Among the Contemporary Puyallup Indian Tribal Community.* Monograph. *Price:* $20.

★ 4791 ★ National Center for Complementary and Alternative Medicine (NCCAM)

PO Box 7923
Gaithersburg, MD 20898-7923
Phone: (301)519-3153 **Free:** 888-644-6226
Fax: (866)464-3616
Email: info@nccam.nih.gov
Website: http://nccam.nih.gov/
Stephen E. Straus, MD, Dir.

Fnded: 1992. **Desc:** Committed to exploring complementary and alternative healing practices, including but not limited to acupuncture, herbs, homeopathy, therapeutic massage, and traditional oriental medicine; trains CAM researchers; conducts biomedical research; disseminates information. Programs focus on evaluating the safety and efficacy of natural products, supporting pharmacological studies to determine potential interactive effects with standard treatment medications, evaluates CAM practices such as acupuncture and chiropractic. Acts as the NCCAM Clearinghouse. **Pub:** *Complementary & Alternative Medicine at the NIH*, quarterly. Newsletter. Features CAM updates, NIH research news, and information from the NCCAM. *Price:* Free.

★ 4792 ★ National Center for Disability Services (NCDS)

201 I.U. Willets Rd.
Albertson, NY 11507
Phone: (516)465-1470 **Fax:** (516)746-3298
Email: ecortez@ncds.org
Website: http://www.ncds.org
Edmund L. Cortez, Pres.

Fnded: 1952. **Desc:** Serves as a center providing educational, vocational, rehabilitation, and research opportunities for persons with disabilities. Work is conducted through the following: Abilities Health and Rehabilitation Services, a New York state licensed diagnostic and treatment center which offers comprehensive outpatient programs in physical therapy, occupational therapy, speech therapy, and psychological services; Career and Employment Institute, which evaluates, trains, and counsels more than 600 adults with disabilities each year, with the goal of productive competitive employment; Henry Viscardi School, which conducts early childhood, elementary, and secondary programs, as well as adult and continuing education programs; Research and Training Institute, which conducts research on the education, employment, and career development of persons with disabilities, and holds seminars and workshops for rehabilitation services professionals. Maintains library and speakers' bureau; compiles statistics; offers placement service; conducts research and educational programs. **Frmly:** (1991) Human Resources Center.

★ 4793 ★ National Center for Education in Maternal and Child Health (NCEMCH)

Georgetown University
PO Box 571272
Washington, DC 20057-1272
Phone: (202)784-9770
Email: info@ncemch.org
Website: http://www.ncemch.org
Rochelle Mayer, PhD, Contact

Fnded: 1982. **Desc:** Multidisciplinary staff in such diverse fields as pediatrics, public health, law, public policy, social work, psychology, behavioral health, nutrition, nursing, child development, education, communications, library science, and systems technology. Work with a broad range of public and private organizations to develop comprehensive program initiatives to advance the health of children and families.

★ 4794 ★ National Center for Environmental Health Strategies (NCEHS)

c/o Mary Lamielle, Dir.
1100 Rural Ave.
Voorhees, NJ 08043
Phone: (856)429-5358
Email: ncehs@ncehs.org
Website: http://www.ncehs.org/
Mary Lamielle, Dir. & Pres.

Fnded: 1986. **Mem:** 2,000. **Desc:** Persons with environmental illnesses, including those with chemical sensitivity disorders; medical, legal, and scientific professionals; government agencies; environmentalists; interested others. Promotes public awareness of health problems caused by chemical and environmental pollutants, focusing on chemical sensitivity disorders. Testifies before government agencies on behalf of persons with such health problems. Encourages the development and implementation of programs and policies aimed at assisting victims of pollutants and preventing future public health problems. Conducts educational programs and research. Gathers information and compiles statistics on indoor and outdoor pollutants, less-toxic products, pesticides, natural foods, and environmental disabilities, including alternative employment, workplace accommodations, social security disability and workmen's compensation, and housing. Maintains speakers' bureau. Provides advocacy and technical, referral, and children's services. Acts as a clearinghouse. **Pub:** *Chemical Sensitivity: A Report to the New Jersey Department of Health.* • *The Delicate Balance*, quarterly. Newsletter. Covers issues related to indoor contaminants, outdoor toxins, legislative and policy updates, research summaries, information on consumer products. *Price:* Included in membership dues; $15/year for nonmembers. • Also publishes reports, bibliographies, information packets, and books. **Frmly:** (1989) Environmental Health Association of New Jersey.

★ 4795 ★ National Center for FarmWorker Health

1770 FM 967
Buda, TX 78610
Phone: (512)312-2700 **Free:** 800-531-5120
Fax: (512)312-2600
Email: info@ncfh.org
Website: http://www.ncfh.org
E. Roberta Ryder, Chief Exec. Officer

Fnded: 1975. **Desc:** Seeks to make quality primary health care accessible to migrant and seasonal farm workers. Supports the establishment of a national network of migrant health centers through the production, processing, and distribution of information, including information on health problems specific to or more prevalent in the migrant community. Works to provide technical assistance for health development and research. Develops collaborative working relationship between agencies serving migrant farmworkers. Maintains job/resume bank, biographical archives, and library. Bestows awards; operates placement service; compiles statistics. biographical archives, library, and speakers' bureau. Bestows awards; operates placement service; compiles statistics. **Pub:** *Migrant Health Newsline*, bimonthly. Newsletter. Includes clinical supplement. • *Migrant Health Referral Directory*, annual. Directory. • *Migrant Health Resource Catalog.* Catalogs. • Books. • Directory. • Videos. **Frmly:** (1989) National Migrant Referral Project.

★ 4796 ★ National Center for Health Education (NCHE)

375 Hudson St.
New York, NY 10014
Phone: (212)463-4050 **Free:** 800-551-3488
Fax: (212)463-4060
Email: nche@nche.org
Website: http://www.nche.org
Lynne Whitt, Exec. VP

Fnded: 1975. **Desc:** Professionals promoting health education in schools, communities, and family settings. Aims to "extend the reach and power of education for health." Advocates health education and health promotion; builds coalitions of private and public sector groups; documents, develops, and disseminates model programs. Develops and manages Growing Healthy, a comprehensive school health education curriculum for kindergarten through grade six and "Starting Healthy" pre-kindergarten curriculum. **Pub:** *Growing Healthy (K-6).* Book. Contains school health education. • *Starting Healthy (Pre-K).* Book. Contains school health education.

★ 4797 ★ National Center for Homeopathy (NCH)

801 N Fairfax St., Ste. 306
Alexandria, VA 22314
Phone: (703)548-7790 **Free:** 877-624-0613
Fax: (703)548-7792
Email: info@homeopathic.org
Website: http://www.homeopathic.org
Sharon Stevenson, Exec., Contact

Fnded: 1974. **Mem:** 6,000. **Desc:** Comprises: National Center for Instruction in Homeopathy and Homeotherapeutics, and Homeopathic Information Service. Purposes are: to promote the art of healing according to the natural laws of cure from a strictly homeopathic standpoint; to facilitate the study of homeopathy by the medical and allied health professions; to implement the study of homeopathic philosophy and principles among laypersons; to fund scientific research in the field. Sponsors introductory courses in homeopathy to licensed health care practitioners and laypersons; maintains speakers' bureau and library. **Pub:** *Homeopathy Today*, monthly. Newsletter. Covers membership activities. Includes calendar of events, employment opportunity and new member listings, and book reviews. *Price:* $55 in U.S.; $75 outside U.S. • *Membership Directory & Homeopathic Resource Guide*, biennial. Directory. *Price:* $10. • Brochures. • Pamphlets. • Reprints. • Also distributes Homeopathic Household Kit.

★ 4798 ★ National Center for Neurogenic Communication Disorders (NCNCD)

University of Arizona
PO Box 210071
Tucson, AZ 85721-0071
Phone: (520)621-1472
Website: http://cnet.shs.arizona.edu/

Desc: Promotes research into speech and language disorders caused by diseases of the nervous system, with special interest in American Indian and Hispanic cultures.

★ 4799 ★ National Center for Post Traumatic Stress Disorder

VA Palo Alto Health Care System
795 Willow Rd. (352E117)
Menlo Park, CA 94025
Website: http://www.ncptsd.org/
Matthew J. Friedman, MD,PhD, Exec. Dir.

Desc: Promotes studies on the effects of psychological trauma. **Pub:** *NCP Clinical Quarterly*, quarterly. Provides an overview of the major clinical, theoretical and programmatic developments in the field of PTSD. • *PTSD Research Quarterly*, quarterly.

★ 4800 ★ National Center for Stuttering (NCS)

200 E 33rd St.
New York, NY 10016
Phone: (212)532-1460 **Free:** 800-221-2483
Fax: (212)683-1372
Email: martin.schwartz@nyu.edu
Website: http://www.stuttering.com
Martin F. Schwartz, Exec. Dir.

Fnded: 1974. **Desc:** Furnishes information to parents of children who stutter. Provides treatment for children and adults who stutter and training on the latest practices and theories for speech pathologists. **Pub:** *Annual Review of Published Literature.* • *Stutter No More.* Book. • Newsletter, quarterly. **Frmly:** Center for Speech Pathology.

★ 4801 ★ National Center for Therapeutic Riding (NCTR)

3600 Dustin Rd.
Burtonsville, MD 20866
Phone: (301)421-0380 **Fax:** (301)421-0384
Email: nctriding@aol.com
Website: http://www.nctrriding.org
Robyn Douglas-Watts, Exec. Dir.

Fnded: 1973. **Desc:** Nonprofit center that provides specialized horseback riding lessons to students with disabilities and other individuals from the Washington, DC area. Using the horse as a motivator, classes focus on teaching techniques for the physically handicapped, emotionally disturbed, learning disabled, or mentally retarded person. **Pub:** *NCTR Horsemanship Manual.* Manual. **Frmly:** (1980) Rock Creek Park Horse Centre.

★ 4802 ★ National Center for Voice and Speech (NCVS)

PO Box 642
Louisville, CO 80027
Free: 888-606-5788
Website: http://www.ncvs.org/more/

Fnded: 1990. **Desc:** Works to prevent, diagnose, treat voice and speech disorders through understanding underlying processes, including molecular, neurophysiologic, biomechanic, aerodynamic, acoustic.

★ 4803 ★ National Center for Youth with Disabilities

University of Minnesota - Box 721
420 Delaware St. SE
Minneapolis, MN 55455-0392
Phone: (612)625-3087 **Fax:** (612)626-2134
Nancy Okinow, MSW, Exec. Dir.

Fnded: 1985. **Desc:** Information and resource center that strives to raise awareness of the needs of adolescents with chronic illnesses and disabilities. Develops activities and programs. **Pub:** *Connections.* Newspaper. Highlights critical issues relating to youth with chronic illnesses and disabilities. Provides a forum for the exchange of information. • *Cydline Reviews.* • *Teenagers at Risk.* • Bulletins.

★ 4804 ★ National Certification Board of Pediatric Nurse Practitioners and Nurses (NCBPNP/N)

800 S Frederick Ave., Ste. 104
Gaithersburg, MD 20877-4151
Phone: (301)330-2921 **Free:** 888-641-2767
Fax: (301)330-1504
Email: info@pnpcert.org
Website: http://www.pnpcert.org
Janet S. Wyatt, Ph.D., CPNP, Exec. Dir.

Fnded: 1976. **Mem:** 12,000. **Desc:** Provides national and international pediatric nursing certification, exams, and continuing education programs. Credentials offered in Certified Pediatric Nurse Practitioner (CPNP) and Certified Pediatric Nurse (CPN). **Frmly:** (1989) National Board of Pediatric Nurse Practitioners and Associates.

★ 4805 ★ National Certification Board for Therapeutic Massage and Bodywork (NCBTMB)

c/o Christine D. Niero
8201 Greensboro Dr., Ste. 300
Mc Lean, VA 22102
Phone: (703)610-9015 **Free:** 800-296-0664
Fax: (703)610-9005
Email: info@ncbtmb.com
Website: http://www.ncbtmb.com/
Christine D. Niero, PhD, Exec. Dir.

Desc: Massage and bodywork practitioners. Formed to set standards of ethical and professional practice through a credible credentialing program.

★ 4806 ★ National Certification Commission for Acupuncture and Oriental Medicine (NCCAOM)

11 Canal Center Plaza, Ste. 300
Alexandria, VA 22314
Phone: (703)548-9004 **Fax:** (703)548-9079
Email: info@nccaom.org
Website: http://www.nccaom.org
Debra Persinger, PhD, Contact

Fnded: 1982. **Mem:** 13,000. **Desc:** National certification agency for practitioners of acupuncture, Chinese herbology, and Asian bodywork therapy in the United States. Establishes and maintains standards of competence for the safe and effective practice of Oriental medicine; to evaluate an applicant's qualifications in relation to these established standards through the administration of national board examinations; to certify practitioners who meet these standards. Acts as consultant to state agencies in regulation, certification, and licensing of the practice of acupuncture and Oriental medicine. of acupuncture and Oriental medicine. of acupuncture and Oriental medicine. **Pub:** *The Diplomate*, periodic. Newsletter. • *NCCAOM Directory of Diplomates*, annual. Directory. **Frmly:** (1997) National Commission for the Certification of Acupuncturists; (1998) National Commission for the Certification of Acupuncture and Oriental Medicine.

★ 4807 ★ National Certification Corp. for the Obstetric, Gynecologic and Neonatal Nursing Specialties (NCC)

645 N Michigan Ave., Ste. 900
Chicago, IL 60611
Phone: (312)951-0207
Website: http://www.nccnet.org
Betty Burns, CAE, Exec. Dir.

Fnded: 1975. **Mem:** 55,000. **Desc:** Promotes quality nursing care by encouraging nurses to demonstrate special knowledge by participating in a voluntary national certification program for obstetric/gynecologic nurse practitioners, inpatient obstetric nurses, neonatal intensive care nurses, neonatal nurse practitioners, low-risk neonatal nurses, electronic fetal monitoring, breastfeeding, menopause, and maternal newborn nurses. **Pub:** *NCC News*, periodic. Newsletter. • *Self Assessment Program.* Brochure. **Frmly:** (1991) NAACOG Certification Corporation.

★ 4808 ★ National Certification Council for Activity Professionals (NCCAP)

PO Box 62589
Virginia Beach, VA 23466
Phone: (757)552-0653
Email: info@nccap.org

Website: http://www.nccap.org

Desc: Activity professionals. Serves as a credentialing body setting standards and criteria to ensure that those served have optimal life experiences. Member of the National Registry of Certified Activity Professionals. **Pub:** Newsletter, quarterly.

★ 4809 ★ National Cervical Cancer Coalition (NCCC)

16501 Sherman Way, Ste. 110
Van Nuys, CA 91406
Phone: (818)909-3849 **Free:** 800-685-5531
Fax: (818)909-3849
Email: info@nccc-online.org
Website: http://www.nccc-online.org/
Alan Kaye, Exec. Dir.

Fnded: 1995. **Desc:** Grass roots campaign educating the public about cervical cancer prevention, outreach, screening, treatment, follow-up.

★ 4810 ★ National CFIDS Foundation

103 Althea Rd.
Needham, MA 02492
Phone: (781)449-3535 **Fax:** (781)449-8606
Email: info@ncf-net.com
Website: http://www.ncf-net.org
Gail R. Kansky, Pres.

Fnded: 1997. **Mem:** 4,000. **Desc:** Provides education, advocacy and fundraising for research. **Pub:** *The National Forum*, quarterly. Journal. *Price:* included in membership dues.

★ 4811 ★ National Child Care Association (NCCA)

1016 Rosser St.
Conyers, GA 30012
Free: 800-543-7161 **Fax:** (770)388-7772
Website: http://www.nccanet.org
Lynn L. White, Exec. Dir.

Fnded: 1987. **Mem:** 7,000. **State Groups:** 25. **Desc:** Works to promote and safeguard the interest of quality child care in the United States. Focuses on licensed, private providers of child care and preschool services. Conducts lobbying activities; offers casualty insurance programs; conducts educational and research programs; provides networking opportunities. **Pub:** *National Focus*, quarterly. Newsletter. • *Professional Development Video Series.* Videos.

★ 4812 ★ National Child Day Care Association (NCDCA)

1501 Benning Rd. NE
Washington, DC 20002-4599
Phone: (202)397-3800 **Fax:** (202)399-2666
Email: hardmont@aol.com
Website: http://www.nccfd.org
Travis Hardmon, Exec. Dir.

Desc: A local, nonprofit group that seeks to provide quality child care services for the Washington, DC area.

★ 4813 ★ National Childminding Association (NCMA)

8 Masons Hill
Bromley BR2 9EY, United Kingdom
Phone: 44 208 4646164 **Fax:** 44 208 2906834
Email: info@ncma.org.uk
Website: http://www.ncma.org.uk

Fnded: 1977. **Mem:** 50,000. **Local Groups:** 1000. **Lang(s):** English. **Desc:** Child care professionals, parents, and interested individuals. Promotes quality day care, recreation, and education for young children and seeks to advance the education of child care professionals. Offers seminars; conducts research. **Pub:** *Who Minds?*, quarterly. Magazine. • Pamphlets, periodic.

★ 4814 ★ National Children's Eye Care Foundation (NCECF)

c/o American Association for Pediatric Ophthalmology and Strabismus
PO Box 193832
San Francisco, CA 94119-3832
Phone: (415)561-8505 **Fax:** (415)561-8531
Email: aapos@aao.org
Website: http://med-aapos.bu.edu
Denise De Losada Wilson, Admin.

Fnded: 1970. **Desc:** Seeks to optimize the quality of life of infants, children, and families by fostering normal development and protection of vision through promoting programs of prevention, detection, treatment, research and education. **Pub:** Annual Report, annual. • Brochures. **Frmly:** (1982) Children's Eye Care Foundation.

★ 4815 ★ National Chronic Care Consortium (NCCC)

8100 26th Ave. S, Ste. 120
Bloomington, MN 55425
Phone: (952)858-8999
Website: http://www.nccconline.org

Desc: Nonprofit plans and providers. Aims to develop real-world solutions in chronic illness care. Serves as an operational laboratory for members in developing innovative care programs and as a national resource center.

★ 4816 ★ National Chronic Fatigue Syndrome and Fibromyalgia Association (NCFSFA)

PO Box 18426
Kansas City, MO 64133
Phone: (816)313-2000 **Fax:** (816)524-6782
Email: information@ncfsfa.org
Website: http://www.ncfsfa.org
Orvalene Prewitt, Contact

Fnded: 1985. **Mem:** 2,000. **Reg. Groups:** 2. **State Groups:** 14. **Local Groups:** 400. **Desc:** Individuals suffering from chronic fatigue syndrome and Fibromyalgia health care professionals. Chronic fatigue syndrome, also known as Chronic Epstein-Barr Virus syndrome, is characterized by persistent, recurring feelings of general weakness; other symptoms include sore throat, unexplained muscle pain, new headaches, devastating fatigue, impaired memory or concentration, tender lymph nodes, unrefreshing sleep and post-exertion malaise. Fibromyalgia is characterized as pain, generally felt all over, and can be compounded by fatigue, sleep disturbances, changes in mood, headaches and gastro-intestinal problems. Sponsors educational programs. Maintains speakers' bureau. **Pub:** *A Guide for Physicians When Considering a Diagnosis of Chronic Fatigue Syndrom in Children.* Brochure. • *A School's Guide for Students with CFS.* • *CFS: Addressing the Realities of a Chronic Illness.* Video. Includes educational information. • *CFS and School Success.* Brochure. • *CFS in the Workplace.* Brochure. • *CFS: Thief of Vitality.* Brochure. • *Chronic Fatigue Syndrome.* Bibliography. • *Coping Skills.* Brochure. • *Heart of America News*, quarterly. Newsletter. *Price:* Free for members. • *How to be a Phone Contact Packet.* • *How to Start a Support Group Packet.* • *Neuro-Psychological Rehabilitation Techniques.* Brochure. • *Patient Information Packet.* • *Physician Information Packet.* • *Social Security Disability Benefits.* Brochure. • *Understanding the Emotions Surrounding CFS.* Brochure. **Frmly:** (1985) National Chronic Epstein-Barr Virus Association; (1993) National Chronic Fatigue Syndrome Association.

★ 4817 ★ National Clearinghouse for Alcohol and Drug Information (NCADI)

PO Box 2345
Rockville, MD 20847-2345
Phone: (301)468-2600 **Free:** 800-729-6686
Fax: (301)468-6433
Email: info@health.org
Website: http://www.health.org/

Desc: Provides current information and materials concerning substance abuse. **Pub:** *Fact Sheets.* • Brochures.

★ 4818 ★ National Coalition of Abortion Providers (NCAP)

c/o Ron Fitzsimmons
908 King St., Ste. 400W
Alexandria, VA 22314-3097
Phone: (703)684-0055 **Fax:** (703)684-5051
Email: ron@ncap.com
Website: http://www.ncap.com
Ron Fitzsimmons, Exec. Dir.

Desc: Abortion providers.

★ 4819 ★ National Coalition for Adult Immunization (NCAI)

4733 Bethesda Ave., Ste. 750
Bethesda, MD 20814-5228
Phone: (301)656-0003 **Fax:** (301)907-0878
Email: ncai@nfid.org
Website: http://www.nfid.org/ncai
David A. Neumann, PhD, Dir.

Fnded: 1988. **Mem:** 126. **Desc:** Medical associations, advocacy groups, vaccine manufacturers and government health agencies. Dedicated to promoting adolescent and adult immunization and to raise immunization levels in high-risk and other target groups. Promotes and supports National Adult Immunization Awareness Week and the objectives of the U.S. Healthy People 2010 initiative. Educates physicians and public on vaccines for diptheria, hepatitis A and B, influenza, measles, mumps, pneumococcal pneumonia, rubella (German measles), tetanus, and chickenpox. **Pub:** *National Adult Immunization Awareness Week Campaign Kit*, annual. Fact sheets on vaccine-preventable diseases of adults and adolescents. • *Resource Guide for Adolescent and Adult Immunization*, semiannual.

★ 4820 ★ National Coalition for Campus Children's Centers

119 Schindler Education Center
University of Northern Iowa
Cedar Falls, IA 50614-0605
Phone: (319)273-3113 **Free:** 800-813-8207
Fax: (319)273-3109
Email: ncccc@uni.edu
Website: http://www.campuschildren.org
Bridget Shultz, Coord.

Fnded: 1980. **Mem:** 550. **Reg. Groups:** 4. **Desc:** Promotes child care centers on college campuses and provides information on organizing and operating these centers. Believes that campus child care programs should be an integral part of higher education systems and should provide safe and healthy environments for children, developmentally sound educational programs, and services to both parents and campus programs. **Pub:** Bibliographies. • Books. • Brochure. • Newsletter, 3/year. • Also compiles list of campus child care centers. **Frmly:** (1997) National Coalition for Campus Child Care; (1998) National Coalition for Children's Centers.

★ 4821 ★ National Coalition for Cancer Research (NCCR)

2300 N St. NW
Washington, DC 20004
Phone: (202)544-1880 **Fax:** (202)543-2565
Email: md@capitolassociates.com
Website: http://www.cancercoalition.org/
Carolyn B. Aldige, Pres.

Fnded: 1986. **Mem:** 19. **Desc:** Lay and professional organizations committed to the eradication of cancer. Dedicated to strengthening the National Cancer Program through public education and communication about the value of cancer research, treatment, and prevention.

★ 4822 ★ National Coalition for Cancer Survivorship (NCCS)
1010 Wayne Ave., Ste. 770
Silver Spring, MD 20910-5600
Phone: (301)650-9127 **Free:** 877-622-7937
Fax: (301)565-9670
Email: info@canceradvocacy.org
Website: http://www.canceradvocacy.org
Ellen Stovall, Pres. /CEO

Fnded: 1986. **Mem:** 2,500. **Reg. Groups:** 7. **Desc:** Ensures quality of cancer care for all Americans. Provides leadership and education, supports research, promotes responsible advocacy. helping survivors deal with life after cancer is diagnosed. Operates speakers' bureau. **Pub:** *Charting the Journey: An Almanac of Resources for Cancer Survivors*. Book. • *NCCS Networker*, quarterly. Newsletter. News and articles on cancer survivorship, interviews, and reviews. *Price:* included in membership dues. • *Survivors*. Book. • *Teamwork: The Cancer Patient's Guide to Talking With Your Doctor*. Booklet. • *What Cancer Survivors Need to Know About Health Insurance*. Booklet. • Also publishes many booklets on cancer-related topics.

★ 4823 ★ National Coalition of Creative Arts Therapy Associations (NCCATA)
c/o AMTA
8455 Colesville Rd., Ste. 1000
Silver Spring, MD 20910
Email: mb33@nyu.edu
Website: http://www.ncata.com
Miriam Roskin Berger, Chair

Fnded: 1979. **Mem:** 8,000. **Nat'l Groups:** 6. **Desc:** Creative arts therapists. Promotes therapeutic and rehabilitative uses of the arts in medicine, mental health, special education, and forensic and social services; coordinates member associations' activities and efforts in meeting common objectives while supporting and advancing each group's discipline. Works to: represent members' interests in legislative activities; define joint positions on public policy issues; facilitate communication among members; initiate educational and research programs. Compiles statistics. **Frmly:** (2002) National Coalition of Arts Therapy Associations.

★ 4824 ★ National Coalition on Health Care
1200 G St., NW, Ste. 750
Washington, DC 20005
Phone: (202)638-7151 **Fax:** (202)638-7166
Email: info@nchc.org
Website: http://www.nchc.org

Fnded: 1990. **Mem:** 100000,000. **Reg. Groups:** 96. **Desc:** Large and small businesses, labor unions, consumer groups, religious groups, and primary care providers. United to achieve better, more affordable healthcare for all Americans.

★ 4825 ★ National Coalition of Mental Health Professionals and Consumers
PO Box 438
Commack, NY 11725
Phone: (631)424-5232 **Free:** 888-729-6662
Fax: (516)549-3942
Email: ncmhpc@aol.com
Website: http://www.nomanagedcare.org/
Deborah Peel, MD, Pres.

Desc: Mental health professionals, consumers and consumer advocates. Works to address the negative impact of managed care on patients and professionals in mental health care; promotes pro-patient, pro-quality alternatives that preserve a patient's right to choice, privacy, and control over treatment, expose abuses in managed care, and bring about regulation of the managed care industry. **Pub:** *Consumer Protection Manual*. Manual. • Newsletter.

★ 4826 ★ National Coalition of Psychiatrists Against Motorcoach Therapy (NCPAMT)
c/o Dr. Anne Rose
4909 Briarwood Ave., No. 7
Royal Oak, MI 48073-1318
Jonathon Steele, PhD, Exec. Dir.

Fnded: 1985. **Mem:** 430. **Desc:** Psychiatrists, psychotherapists, psychologists, social workers, counselors, and mental health officials. Objective is to stop the practice of "Motorcoach Therapy," described by the coalition as the "escalating and unethical practice of procuring one-way bus fares for habitual and undesirable mental health patients" upon their release from local mental health facilities. Provides for information exchange; has launched an awareness campaign targeted primarily at mental health officials.

★ 4827 ★ National Coalition for Research in Neurological Disorders (NCR)
1250 24th St. NW, Ste. 300
Washington, DC 20037
Phone: (202)293-5453 **Fax:** (202)466-0585
Email: info@brainnet.org
Website: http://www.brainnet.org
Dominick P. Purpura, MD, Chair

Fnded: 1952. **Mem:** 57. **Desc:** Represents voluntary health agencies and professional societies concerned with obtaining funds for neurological research. Seeks to stimulate public information regarding the field of neurological disorders. Lobbies for increased funding for training and research in neurological disorders. **Pub:** *NCR News*, quarterly. **Frmly:** National Committee for Research in Neurological Disorders; (1988) National Committee for Research in Neruological and Communicative Disorders; (1989) National Coalition for Research in Neurological and Communicative Disorders.

★ 4828 ★ National Coalition on Rural Aging (NCRA)
409 3rd St. SW, No. 200
Washington, DC 20024
Phone: (202)479-1200 **Fax:** (202)479-0735
Email: info@ncoa.org
Website: http://www.ncoa.org/content.cfm?sectionID=40
Kristin Duke, Chairperson

Fnded: 1978. **Mem:** 500. **Desc:** Planners and providers of services for the aging, academicians and students, and others interested in issues related to older persons living in rural areas. Purposes are to develop social and public policies related to the needs and interests of rural older adults; to improve and increase services to rural older adults by working with national organizations and government agencies at all levels; to provide guidance to supportive organizations and communities; to encourage action on legislative, public policy, and service delivery issues. Disseminates information and promotes research and demonstration projects on the aging in rural America. Conducts training for individuals working with rural older adults, emphasizing the cultural mores of rural America and the methods of service provision which have proven adaptable to rural areas. Provides technical assistance and consultation significant to rural program planning and implementation. **Frmly:** (1999) National Center on Rural Aging.

★ 4829 ★ National College of Hypnosis and Psychotherapy
12 Cross St.
Nelson BB9 7EN, United Kingdom
Phone: 44 1282 699378 **Fax:** 44 1282 698633
Email: hypnosis_nchp@compuserve.com
Website: http://www.hypnotherapyuk.net

Fnded: 1977. **Mem:** 200. **Desc:** Mature students seeking a reputable, externally accredited (by the British Accreditation Council) training with a view to running their own practices, for interest or to augment their existing professional skills. Concerned with training in hypnotherapy/psychotherapy/counselling on part-time basis to appropriate, suitably motivated, mature students in London, Liverpool, Glasgow, and Northern Ireland. Courses are held at regular intervals throughout the year. Member of United Kingdom Council for Psychotherapy and European Association for Hypnopsychotherapy. Higher Education. Courses are held at regular intervals throughout the year. Member of United Kingdom Council for Psychotherapy.

★ 4830 ★ National Collegiate EMS Foundation (NCEMSF)
PO Box 113
Delmar, NY 12054-0113
Phone: (208)728-7342 **Fax:** (208)728-7352
Email: info@ncemsf.org
Website: http://www.ncemsf.org/
George J. Koenig, Pres.

Fnded: 1993. **Mem:** 500. **Reg. Groups:** 12. **Local Groups:** 150. **Desc:** Committed to the advancement of existing emergency response groups, assists in development of new response groups on college and university campuses. **Pub:** *Campus EMS Directory*, semiannual. Directory. Listing of campus EMS organizations. • *NCEMSF Newsletter*, quarterly. Newsletter. Contains information for and about campus-based EMS.

★ 4831 ★ National Commission on Correctional Health Care (NCCHC)
1300 W Belmont Ave.
Chicago, IL 60657
Phone: (773)880-1460 **Fax:** (773)880-2424
Email: ncchc@ncchc.org
Website: http://www.ncchc.org
Edward A. Harrison, Pres.

Fnded: 1983. **Mem:** 35. **Desc:** Professional organizations in the fields of medical and health care. Works to improve the quality of and set standards for medical care in correctional institutions in the U.S. including prisons, jails, and detention and juvenile facilities. Acts as an accrediting body for such facilities; develops training programs and conducts seminars; provides technical assistance; organizes special task forces on issues such as suicide and AIDS; annually bestows Award of Merit for achievement in the field of correctional health care. Compiles statistics; conducts research; disseminates information. **Pub:** *CorrectCare*, quarterly. Newspaper. • *Correctional Health Care: Guidelines for the Management of an Adequated Delivery System*. Manuals. • *Journal of Correctional Health Care*, semiannual. Journal. Contains articles on correctional health care topics including law, medicine, and ethics. *Price:* $30/year for individuals; $65/year for institutions. • Films. • Monographs. • Proceedings.

★ 4832 ★ National Commission on Human Life, Reproduction and Rhythm (NCHLRR)
PO Box 101501
Pittsburgh, PA 15237
Phone: (724)444-8013 **Fax:** (412)369-4550
Dr. Brain W. Donnelly, MD, Sec. -Treas.

Fnded: 1967. **Mem:** 25. **Desc:** Physicians united to strengthen the family unit and support traditional concepts of marriage, sex, and life. Encourages physicians to place more emphasis on personal attention to patients and less emphasis on the prescribing of medication; promotes pro-life values. Conducts scientific meetings dealing with subjects including: the role of the mother, particularly during her child's first three years; sex education; natural family planning; obstetric delivery; breastfeeding; abortion. Sponsors public meetings. **Pub:** *Child and Family*, quarterly. Journal. Contains scientific and philosophical articles in support of the traditional family. Consists primarily of reprinted material. *Price:* $12/year; $16/year outside U.S. • Also publishes reprint booklets.

★ 4833 ★ National Committee for Medical Research Ethics (NEM)
(Den Nasjonale Forskningsetiske Komite for Medisin — NEM)
c/o Prof. Georg Hoyer
University of Tromso
Tromso, Norway
Phone: 47 77644829 **Fax:** 47 77644831
Email: georg.hoyer@ism.uit.no
Website: http://www.etikkom.no

Fnded: 1990. **Mem:** 12. **Reg. Groups:** 5. **Lang(s):** English, Norwegian. **Desc:** Health care professionals, attorneys, ethicists, and others with an interest in ethical aspects of medical research. Promotes increased awareness of ethical issues within the medical research industry; conducts continuing professional education and public education programs.

★ 4834 ★ National Committee for the Prevention of Alcoholism and Drug Dependency (NCPADD)
c/o Thomas R. Neslund
12501 Old Columbia Pike
Silver Spring, MD 20904-6600
Phone: (301)680-6719 **Fax:** (301)680-6707
Email: 74617.1663@compuserve.com
Website: http://www.health20-20.org
Dr. Peter N. Landless, Exec. Dir.

Fnded: 1950. **Mem:** 50. **Nat'l Groups:** 60. **Reg. Groups:** 60. **Desc:** Health officials, physicians, educators, social workers, youth leaders, clergymen, temperance leaders, businessmen, judges, and others. To further the study of the effects of alcohol and other drugs on the physical, mental and moral powers of the individual citizen and on the social, economic, political, and religious life of the nation. Fosters nationwide educational program through films, lectures, forums, radio, and television programs. **Pub:** *ICPA Reporter*, quarterly. Bulletin. Describes worldwide activities of ICPA and local communities. *Price:* included in membership dues. **Frmly:** National Committee for the Prevention of Alcoholism.

★ 4835 ★ National Committee for the Prevention of Elder Abuse (NCPEA)
c/o Bob Blancato
1101 Vermont Ave., NW, Ste. 1001
Washington, DC 20002
Phone: (202)682-4140 **Fax:** (202)682-3984
Email: ncpea@erols.com
Website: http://www.preventelderabuse.org
Bob Blancato, Pres.

Fnded: 1987. **Mem:** 450. **State Groups:** 3. **Local Groups:** 10. **Desc:** Established to promote a greater understanding of the problem and the development of services to protect older persons and disabled adults in order to reduce the likelihood of their abuse and neglect. Performs research, advocacy, public awareness, and training services. **Pub:** *Journal of Elder Abuse & Neglect*, quarterly. Journal. • *nexus*, 3/year. • Membership Directory.

★ 4836 ★ National Committee for Quality Assurance (NCQA)
2000 L St., NW, Ste. 500
Washington, DC 20036
Phone: (202)955-3500 **Free:** 888-275-7585
Fax: (202)955-3599
Website: http://www.ncqa.org
Margaret E. O'Kane, Pres.

Fnded: 1979. **Desc:** Board of Directors representing employers, consumer and labor representatives, health plans, quality experts, regulators and representatives from organized medicine. mission: To improve the quality of health care delivered everywhere. Accredits quality assurance programs in prepaid managed health care organizations. Develops and coordinates programs for assessing the quality of care and service in the managed health care industry. Conducts research; holds training and educational seminars; operates speakers' bureau. **Pub:** *Health Plan Employer Data and Information Set*, annual. Handbook. • *Quality Matters*, 3/year. Newsletter. Discusses quality-related activities in the managed care industry and at NCQA. *Price:* $90/year.

★ 4837 ★ National Committee for Quality Health Care (NCQHC)
1100 Connecticut Ave. NW, Ste. 545
Washington, DC 20036
Phone: (202)331-7535 **Fax:** (202)331-7532
Email: ncqhc@erols.com
Website: http://www.ncqhc.org/
Catherine E. McDermott, Pres.

Fnded: 1978. **Mem:** 151. **Desc:** Coalition of health care professionals and organizations principally involved in the health care industry; includes hospitals, physicians, health maintenance organizations, nursing homes, manufacturers of health care equipment, investment bankers, architects, contractors, and accountants. Works to maintain and strengthen quality health care in the U.S. **Pub:** *An American Health Strategy: Ensuring the Availability of Quality Health Care.* • *Critical Condition: America's Health Care in Jeopardy.* • *Quality Bulletin*, bimonthly. Bulletin. • *Quality Outlook*, bimonthly. • Pamphlets. • Papers. **Frmly:** National Committee on Hospital Capital Expenditures.

★ 4838 ★ National Committee on the Treatment of Intractable Pain (NCTIP)
c/o Wayne Coy, Jr.
Cohn and Marks
1920 N St. NW, Ste. 300
Washington, DC 20036
Phone: (202)452-4836 **Fax:** (202)293-4827
Wayne Coy, Jr., Pres.

Fnded: 1977. **Mem:** 3,500. **Desc:** Individuals promoting education and research into more effective methods of pain prevention and control with the coordinated help of professionals in the medical, legal, bioethical, psychological, and religious fields. Endorses the British hospice concept of care of the dying, which allows the dying person to remain among family, friends, community, and skilled professionals and provides constant, effective medical and psychological support for pain control. Advocates legalization of heroin for medical purposes. Plans to sponsor speakers' bureau. **Pub:** *Newsletter of the National Committee on the Treatment of Intractable Pain*, annual. Newsletter. Covers concern generated by the use of medication to relieve intractable pain caused by cancer, specifically the effort to legalize heroin. *Price:* Free. • Monographs. • Reports. **Frmly:** (1977) American Intractable Pain Foundation.

★ 4839 ★ National Comprehensive Cancer Network (NCCN)
50 Huntington Pike, Ste. 200
Rockledge, PA 19046
Phone: (215)728-4788 **Free:** 888-909-6226
Fax: (215)728-3877
Email: information@nccn.org
Website: http://www.nccn.org
Kim Schwalje, Contact

Fnded: 1995. **Mem:** 19. **Desc:** Established to provide cancer care to the greatest number of patients in need; to advance cancer prevention, screening, diagnosis and treatment through excellence in basic and clinical research; to enhance the effectiveness and efficiency of cancer care delivery through the ongoing collection, synthesis and analysis of outcomes data. **Pub:** *The Complete Library of Practice Guidelines in Oncology.*

★ 4840 ★ National Conference of Local Environmental Health Administrators (NCLEHA)
c/o University of Washington
Department of Environmental Health
PO Box 357234
Seattle, WA 98195-7234
Phone: (206)616-2097 **Fax:** (206)543-8123
Email: ctreser@u.washington.edu
Website: http://depts.washington.edu/clehaweb/
Elwin Coll, Sec.

Fnded: 1939. **Mem:** 220. **Desc:** Professional environmental health personnel engaged in or officially concerned with municipal (city, county, or district) environmental health administration or teaching of environmental health. Promotes improvement and greater use of science and practice of environmental health in community life. **Pub:** Newsletter, quarterly. **Frmly:** (1969) Conference of Municipal Public Health Engineers; (1981) Conference of Local Environmental Health Administrators.

★ 4841 ★ National Contact Lens Examiners (NCLE)
6506 Loisdale Rd., Ste.209
Springfield, VA 22150-1815
Phone: (703)719-5800 **Free:** 800-296-1379
Fax: (703)719-9144
Email: mail@abo-ncle.org
Website: http://www.abo.org
Patricia M. Tolar, Chair

Fnded: 1979. **Mem:** 9,000. **Desc:** National certifying agency promoting continued development of opticians and technicians as contact lens fitters by formulating standards and procedures for determination of entry-level competency. Assists in the continuation, development, administration, and monitoring of a national Contact Lens Registry Examination (CLRE), which verifies entry-level competency of contact lens fitters. Issues certificates. Activities include: maintaining records of those certified in contact lens fitting; encouraging state occupational licensing and credentialing agencies to use the CLRE for licensure purposes; identifying contact lens dispensing education needs as a result of findings of examination programs; disseminating information to sponsors of contact lens continuing education programs.

★ 4842 ★ National Council on the Aging (NCOA)
409 3rd St. SW, 2nd Fl.
Washington, DC 20024
Phone: (202)479-1200 **Free:** 800-424-9046
Fax: (202)479-0735
Email: info@ncoa.org
Website: http://www.ncoa.org
Dr. James Firman, Pres. and CEO

Fnded: 1950. **Mem:** 7,500. **Desc:** Individuals and organizations who work on behalf of older Americans, including individuals in business and industry, organized labor, and the health professions; social workers, librarians, the clergy, and educators; housing, research, and government agencies; state and local agencies on the aging. Cooperates with other organizations to promote concern for older people and develop methods and resources for meeting their needs. Provides a national information and consultation center; holds conferences and workshops. Operates Family Friends Program, which recruits and trains older volunteers to work with families with chronically ill or disabled children. Conducts research and demonstration programs on issues important to older people such as: training and placement of older workers; economic security; services for the frail elderly living in their own homes; access to health and social services; increasing opportunities for socialization and participation in artistic, cultural, and educational programs and services; corporate programs; senior centers. Maintains the National Association of Older Worker Employment Services, Health Promotion Institute, National Center on Rural Aging, National Adult Day Services Association, National Institute on Community-Based Long-Term Care, National Institute of Senior Centers, National Institute of Senior Housing, National Interfaith Coalition on Aging, and National Institute on Financial Issues and Services for Elders. **Pub:** *Abstracts in Social Gerontology: Current Literature on Aging*, quarterly. Journal. Features books, reports, and articles on a variety of aging issues. Includes author and subject index. *Price:* Free to members. • *Innovations in Aging*, quarterly. Magazine. Covers issues and developments in the field of aging. *Price:* available to members only. • Books. • Brochures. • Pamphlets. **Frmly:** (1960)

National Committee on Aging of National Social Welfare Assembly.

★ 4843 ★ National Council on Alcoholism and Drug Dependence (NCADD)
20 Exchange Pl., Ste. 2902
New York, NY 10005-3201
Phone: (212)269-7797 **Free:** 800-622-2255
Fax: (212)269-7510
Email: national@ncadd.org
Website: http://www.ncadd.org
Stacia Murphy, Pres.

Fnded: 1944. **State Groups:** 11. **Local Groups:** 90. **Desc:** Works for the prevention and treatment of alcoholism and other drug dependence through programs of public education, information, and public policy advocacy. Sponsors National Alcohol Awareness Month each April. **Pub:** *NCADD Amethyst*, quarterly. Newsletter. *Price:* $50. • *NCADD Washington Report*, monthly. Newsletter. Newsletter reporting on washington issues related to alcolholism/drug dependence. *Price:* $97/year; $174/2 years; $259/3 years. • *Resource and Referral Guide*, annual. • *What Are the Signs of Alcoholism?*. • *What Can You Do About Someone Else's Drinking?*. • *Whos' Got the Power? You...or Drugs?*. Pamphlets. • Annual Report. **Frmly:** (1949) National Committee for Education on Alcoholism; (1955) National Committee on Alcoholism; (1990) National Council on Alcoholism.

★ 4844 ★ National Council for the Blind of Ireland (NCBI)
Whitworth Rd.
Druncomdra 9, Dublin, Ireland
Phone: 353 1 8307033 **Fax:** 353 1 8307787
Email: info@ncbi.ie
Website: http://www.ncbi.ie

Fnded: 1931. **Mem:** 6,500. **Nat'l Groups:** 1. **Reg. Groups:** 7. **Lang(s):** English, Irish. **Desc:** Individuals and organizations. Seeks to improve the quality of life of people with visual impairments; promotes increased independence for people with impaired vision. Makes available support and services; conducts educational and advocacy campaigns. **Pub:** *NCBI News*, bimonthly. Magazine. Also available in Braille.

★ 4845 ★ National Council for Community Behavioral Healthcare
12300 Twinbrook Pkwy., Ste. 320
Rockville, MD 20852
Phone: (301)984-6200 **Fax:** (301)881-7159
Email: charlesr@nccbh.org
Website: http://www.nccbh.org
Charles G. Ray, Pres.

Fnded: 1969. **Mem:** 900. **State Groups:** 38. **Desc:** Conducts educational programs. Maintains speakers' bureau **Pub:** *National Council News*, monthly. Newsletter. **Frmly:** (1997) National Council on Community Mental Health Centers; (1999) National Community Mental Healthcare Council.

★ 4846 ★ National Council of Disabled Peoples International in Pakistan (NCDPIP)
c/o Saluhuddin Malik
34 Sadar Bazar
Ghulam Mohammed Abad
Faisalabad, Pakistan
Phone: 92 41 680434 **Fax:** 92 41 695094
Email: dpipak@fsd.comsats.net.pk

Fnded: 1982. **Mem:** 125. **Nat'l Groups:** 1. **Reg. Groups:** 4. **Lang(s):** English, Urdu. **Desc:** Mentally and physically handicapped individuals, their families, and other supporters. Works for equality in participation and opportunity for the disabled. Acts as an umbrella organization registered with the Social Welfare Dept. for guidance and counseling to the provincial chapters for education and rehabilitation of disabled person in need throughout the country.

★ 4847 ★ National Council of Disabled Persons of Zimbabwe (NCDPZ)
PO Box 1952
Bulawayo, Zimbabwe
Phone: 263 9 214426 **Fax:** 263 9 208023
Email: ncd@telconet.co.za

Fnded: 1975. **Mem:** 500,000. **Reg. Groups:** 50. **Local Groups:** 71. **Lang(s):** English. **Desc:** Encourages unity of disabled persons in Zimbabwe. Promotes the interests of the disabled. Disseminates information. Continues to lobby for the implementation of our 1992 Disability Act, which our organization championed. **Pub:** *Disability Rights Up*, quarterly. Magazine. • *Program Report*, monthly. • Newsletter.

★ 4848 ★ National Council for Hospice and Specialist Palliative Care Services
34-44 Britannia St.
London WC1X 9JG, United Kingdom
Phone: 44 207 5208299 **Fax:** 44 207 5208298
Email: enquiries@hospice-spc-council.org.uk
Website: http://www.hospice-spc-council.org.uk

Fnded: 1991. **Mem:** 35. **Reg. Groups:** 15. **Desc:** Members are nominated by national charities and professional organisations or elected by regional hospice and palliative care units. To represent the views and interests of hospice and palliative care services to ministers, civil servants, MPs, the media and statutory and other agencies. To provide advice to hospice and specialist palliative care services in their relations with health authorities, local authorities and other agencies. **Pub:** *Information Exchange*, quarterly. Newsletter. • Papers.

★ 4849 ★ National Council on Independent Living (NCIL)
1916 Wilson Blvd., Ste. 209
Arlington, VA 22201
Phone: (703)525-3406 **Fax:** (703)525-3409
Email: ncil@ncil.org
Website: http://www.ncil.org
Anne-Marie Hughey, Exec. Dir.

Fnded: 1982. **Mem:** 380. **Local Groups:** 80. **Desc:** Independent living centers, organizations that provide support to independent living centers, and individuals. (Independent living centers offer programs to assist disabled individuals, including help in locating housing and finding appropriate personal care assistance, peer counseling, and independent living skills training.) Encourages the integration of people with disabilities into society; promotes independent lifestyles and decision-making for people with disabilities; works to strengthen independent living centers. Offers technical assistance and encourages cooperation among independent living centers. Seeks to develop leadership skills among people with disabilities; works to increase public awareness of the rights and needs of disabled individuals. Provides information and referral service; sponsors Peer Technical Assistance Network. Maintains speakers' bureau and placement service. **Pub:** *NCIL Newsletter*, quarterly. Newsletter. • *President's Bulletin*, monthly. Bulletin. **Frmly:** (1985) National Coalition of Independent Living Programs.

★ 4850 ★ National Council on Intellectual Disability (NCID)
PO Box 771
Mawson, ACT 2607, Australia
Phone: 61 6 62964400 **Fax:** 61 2 62964488
Email: ncid@dice.org.au
Website: http://www.dice.org.au

Fnded: 1953. **Mem:** 400. **Lang(s):** English. **Desc:** Organizations in Australia representing 25,000 individuals involved in the study of or the provision of services to individuals with intellectual disabilities. Works to: ensure that the best services are provided to the intellectually disabled and their families; eliminate discrimination against and establish equality for the developmentally disabled. Acts as a liaison between member organizations and government authorities; lobbies public officials. Seeks the establishment of free public education in adapted environments when necessary, the provision of free health care, the establishment of freedom in the choice of an occupation, the granting of voting rights, and the equal participation by intellectually disabled in poli cy development and management of related service organizations. Monitors and proposes modifications to relevant legislation. Works for the establishment of regional authorities on intellectual disability which will monitor research on intellectual disability and services for the intellectually disabled. Sponsors training programs and seminars; offers courses. **Frmly:** (1957) Australian Council of Organizations for Subnormal Children; (1971) Australian Council for the Mentally Retarded; (1984) Australian Association for the Mentally Retarded; (1988) AAMR - National Association on Intellectual Disability.

★ 4851 ★ National Council of Maori Nurses (Te Kaunihera O Nga Neehi Maori O Aotearoa)
Herne Bay 300
Richmond Rd., Grey Lynn
PO Box 46018
Auckland, New Zealand
Phone: 64 9 3603149 **Fax:** 64 9 3602180
Email: national.council@xtra.co.nz
Website: http://www.healthsite.co.nz/hauora_maori/ncmn

Local Groups: 6. **Lang(s):** English. **Desc:** Nurses of Maori descent. Promotes continuing professional development and advancement of members; works to ensure accessibility of health care to Maori people; conducts educational and training programs.

★ 4852 ★ National Council on Patient Information and Education (NCPIE)
4915 Saint Elmo Ave., Ste. 505
Bethesda, MD 20814-6082
Phone: (301)656-8565 **Fax:** (301)656-4464
Email: ncpie@erols.com
Website: http://www.talkaboutrx.org
Linda Golodner, Chair

Fnded: 1982. **Mem:** 160. **Desc:** Health care professional organizations, pharmaceutical manufacturing organizations, federal agencies, voluntary health agencies, and consumer groups. Increases the availability of information and improves the dialogue between consumers and health care providers about prescription medicines; increases professional awareness of the need to give adequate information on prescription therapy; expands consumers' participation with health professionals on matters of drug therapy. Communicates with health care providers on the importance of giving consumers oral and written information on prescription medicines and encourages consumers to ask questions about medicines and explain factors that may affect their ability to follow prescriptions. **Pub:** *A Parents Guide to Medicine Use By Children*. Brochure. • *The Active Consumer: Getting the Most from Your Medicines*. Brochure. • *Get the Answers*. Brochure. • *Guidelines for Improving Prescription Medicine Use Among Children and Teenagers*. Report. • *Medicine: Before You Take It, Talk About It*. Brochure. • *Medicines: What Every Woman Should Know*. Brochure. • *NCPIE News*, quarterly. Newsletter. • *Talk About Prescriptions: Month Planning Kit*, annual.

★ 4853 ★ National Council on Rehabilitation Education (NCRE)
c/o Charles Arokiasamy, Rh.D.
Rehabilitation Counseling Program
School of Education and Human Development
California State University - Fresno
5005 N Maple Ave., M.S 3
Fresno, CA 93740-8025
Phone: (559)278-0325 **Fax:** (559)278-0098
Email: charlesa@csufresno.edu
Website: http://www.rehabeducators.org/
Charles Arokiasamy, Admin. Sec.

Fnded: 1961. **Mem:** 540. **Nat'l Groups:** 1. **Reg. Groups:** 10. **Desc:** Academic institutions and organizations; professional educators, researchers, and students. Goals are to: assist in the documentation of the effect of education in improving services to persons with disability; determine the skills and training necessary for effective rehabilitation services; develop role models, standards, and uniform licensure and certification requirements for rehabilitation personnel; interact with consumers and public and private sector policy makers. Disseminates information and provides forum for discussion. Sponsors specialized education and placement service. Compiles statistics. Works closely with agencies and associations serving persons with disabilities. **Pub:** *NCRE Newsletter*, quarterly. Newsletter. Features member news. • *Rehabilitation Education*, quarterly. Journal. *Price:* $90/year for institutions. • Membership Directory, annual. *Price:* $25. • Monographs. • Report, quarterly. **Frmly:** (1976) Council of Rehabilitation Counselor Educators.

★ 4854 ★ National Council for Reliable Health Information (NCRHI)

PO Box 1747
Allentown, PA 18105
Phone: (610)437-1795
Email: sbinfo@quackwatch.com
Website: http://www.quackwatch.org
Dr. Stephen Barrett, Pres.

Fnded: 1977. **Mem:** 1,200. **Reg. Groups:** 13. **State Groups:** 12. **Local Groups:** 1. **Desc:** Health professionals, researchers, legal professionals, and other interested individuals. Seeks to educate the public on fraud and quackery in health care; offers advice to consumers; provides witnesses for health fraud trials; assists law enforcement officials with health fraud cases. Sponsors speakers' bureau and research programs. Offers aid to victims in the form of legal screening free of charge. **Pub:** *Available Resource Materials*. Pamphlet. Lists available materials by category. • *Join in Combatting Health Fraud, Misinformation, and Quackery*. Pamphlet. • *National Council Against Health Fraud Newsletter*, bimonthly. Newsletter. *Price:* Included in membership dues; $15/year for nonmember subs; $18/year for library subs. • *NCAHF Bulletin Board*, bimonthly. Bulletin. *Price:* available to members only. • *Recommended Consumer Protection Publications*, bimonthly. Pamphlet. • Reports. • Also publishes position statement on various topics. **AKA:** (2003) Quackwatch. **Frmly:** California Council Against Health Fraud; (1998) National Council Against Health Fraud.

★ 4855 ★ National Council of State Boards of Nursing (NCSBN)

111 E Wacker Dr., Ste. 2900
Chicago, IL 60601
Phone: (312)525-3600 **Free:** (866)293-9600
Fax: (312)279-1032
Email: info@ncsbn.org
Website: http://www.ncsbn.org
Kathy Apple, Exec. Dir.

Fnded: 1978. **Mem:** 61. **Desc:** State boards of nursing. Assists member boards in administering the National Council Licensure Examinations for Registered Nurses and Practical Nurses and works to insure relevancy of the exams to current nursing practice. Aids boards in the collection and analysis of information pertaining to the licensure and discipline of nurses. Provides consultative services, conducts research, develops model nursing legislation and administrative regulations, and sponsors educational programs. **Pub:** *Council Connector*, monthly. Newsletter. Newsletter for member boards. • *NCLEX Exam Test Plans*, annual. Booklets. Educational booklets. • Also publishes research results and monographs.

★ 4856 ★ National Council of State Emergency Medical Services Training Coordinators (NCSEMSTC)

111 Park Pl.
Falls Church, VA 22046
Phone: (703)538-1794 **Fax:** (703)241-5603
Email: ncsemstc@aol.com
Website: http://www.ncsemstc.org
Heidi Cooper, Assoc. Exec. Dir.

Fnded: 1977. **Mem:** 60. **Reg. Groups:** 9. **Desc:** Individuals employed by state-level emergency medical services agencies who are responsible for coordination or supervision of EMS training programs. Promotes the responsible movement of emergency medical technicians (EMTs) throughout the nation through standardization of policies related, but not limited to, curriculum, certification, recertification, revocation, and reciprocity; seeks to further develop the public recognition and trust of the emergency medical technician as a health care professional. **Pub:** *Membership List*, annual. Membership Directory.

★ 4857 ★ National Council of State Pharmacy Association Executives (NCSPAE)

c/o Rebecca Snead
Virginia Pharmacists Association
5501 Patterson Ave., No. 200
Richmond, VA 23226
Phone: (804)285-4145 **Fax:** (804)285-4227
Email: becky@vapharmacy.org
Website: http://www.ncspae.org
Jo An Condie, Pres.

Fnded: 1927. **Mem:** 52. **State Groups:** 52. **Desc:** Professional society of the executive officers of state pharmacy associations. **Frmly:** (1964) National Conference of State Pharmaceutical Association Secretaries; (1992) National Council of State Pharmaceutical Association.

★ 4858 ★ National Council for Therapeutic Recreation Certification (NCTRC)

7 Elmwood Dr.
New City, NY 10956
Phone: (845)639-1439 **Fax:** (845)639-1471
Email: nctrc@nctrc.org
Website: http://www.nctrc.org
Bob Riley, PhD, Exec. Dir.

Fnded: 1981. **Mem:** 17,170. **Desc:** Objectives are to: establish standards for certification and recertification of individuals who work in the therapeutic recreation field; grant recognition to individuals who voluntarily apply and meet established standards; monitor adherence to standards by certified personnel. **Pub:** *National Council for Therapeutic Recreation Certification: Certification Standards*. Book. • *NCTRC Newsletter*, semiannual. Newsletter.

★ 4859 ★ National Council of Voluntary Child Care Organisations

Unit 4, Pride Court
80-82 White Lion St.
London N1 9PF, United Kingdom
Phone: 44 20 78333319 **Fax:** 44 20 78338637
Email: office@ncvcco.org
Website: http://www.ncvcco.org

Fnded: 1942. **Mem:** 108. **Reg. Groups:** 8. **Lang(s):** English. **Desc:** Voluntary organisations providing child care or supporting child care work throughout England. Aims to be an independent, identifiable member-led organisation maintaining the distinctive voice of voluntary child care; promotes and sustains the voluntary sector's contribution to the provision of services for children and families. **Pub:** *Magnet*, monthly. Bulletin. • *Outlook*, quarterly. Newsletter.

★ 4860 ★ National Council on Women's Health

1300 York Ave.
PO Box 52
New York, NY 10021
Phone: (212)746-6967 **Fax:** (212)746-8691
Email: sdb2002@mail.med.cornell.edu
Website: http://www.ncwh.org
Roberta G. Rubin, MD, Pres.

Fnded: 1979. **Mem:** 500. **Desc:** Working partnership of health professionals and consumers whose mission is to educate the public and policy-makers on women's health issues and empower women to make informed healthcare choices. Open to everyone concerned with futhering the goals of the Council, fostering better quality health care, increased availability of information to patients, and improving doctor-patient relationship. The goals of the organization are accomplished through a variety of educational efforts including forums and conferences for the general public, publications for professionals and the public, and networking with a wide range of organizations concerned with women's health. **Pub:** Newsletter, quarterly.

★ 4861 ★ National CPA Health Care Advisors Association (HCAA)

111 E Wacker Dr., Ste. 990
Chicago, IL 60601
Free: 800-869-0491 **Fax:** (312)729-9800
Email: info@hcaa.com
Website: http://www.hcaa.com
Lisa Bruno, Exec. Dir.

Fnded: 1992. **Mem:** 47. **Desc:** Certified public accountant (CPA) firms providing financial and consulting services to health care professionals. Seeks to enhance members' ability to serve the health care industry. Facilitates resource sharing and the establishment of joint ventures among members; provides marketing services to members; conducts industry surveys; sponsors continuing professional development and training courses. **Pub:** *Practice Management Advisor*, quarterly. Newsletter. A customizable newsletter for clients of members.

★ 4862 ★ National Credentialing Agency for Laboratory Personnel (NCA)

PO Box 15945-289
Lenexa, KS 66285
Phone: (913)438-5110 **Fax:** (913)599-5340
Email: nca-info@goamp.com
Website: http://www.nca-info.org
Kathryn Sudduth, Sec. -Treas.

Fnded: 1977. **Mem:** 65,000. **Desc:** Persons who direct, educate, supervise, or practice in clinical laboratory science. To assure the public and employers of the competence of clinical laboratory personnel; to provide a mechanism for individuals demonstrating competency in the field to achieve career mobility. Develops and administers competency-based examinations for certification of clinical laboratory personnel; provides for periodic recertification by examination or through documentation of continuing education. Compiles statistics. **Pub:** *Clipboard*, semiannual. Newsletter. **Frmly:** (2001) National Certification Agency for Medical Lab Personnel.

★ 4863 ★ National Cristina Foundation (NCF)

500 W Putnam Ave.
Greenwich, CT 06830
Phone: (203)863-9100 **Fax:** (203)863-9230
Email: ncf@cristina.org
Website: http://www.cristina.org
Yvette Marrin, PhD, Pres.

Fnded: 1985. **Desc:** Looks for donations of commercially obsolete computer equipment, software, and audio/visual equipment from the business community, the government sector, and the public; redistributes this technology to partner organizations that maintain programs for persons with special needs, such as the disabled, the disadvantaged, and students at risk of school failure. Conducts public awareness campaigns; accepts donations through an online donor form. **Pub:** *Cristina Connections*. Magazine.

★ 4864 ★ National Cued Speech Association/Deaf Children's Literacy Project (NCSA)

23970 Hermitage Rd.
Cleveland, OH 44122-4008
Phone: (216)292-6213 **Free:** 800-459-3529
Email: cuedspdisc@aol.com
Website: http://www.cuedspeech.org
Pamela Beck, Mgr., NCSA Information Service

Fnded: 1982. **Mem:** 500. **Reg. Groups:** 2. **State Groups:** 8. **Desc:** Promotes and supports the effective use of Cued Speech for communication, language acquisition, and literacy. Provides information, referral and support for persons with language, hearing, speech, and learning needs. Sponsors instructional programs, exhibits, and family learning vacations. **Pub:** *Cued Speech Journal*, periodic. Journal. Covers various aspects of Cued Speech. *Price:* Included in membership dues; $10/year for nonmembers. • *On Cue*, quarterly. Newsletter. Contains calendar of events and regional reports. *Price:* Included in membership dues; $25/year for nonmembers.

★ 4865 ★ National Deaf Children's Society

15 Dufferin St.
London EC1Y 8UR, United Kingdom
Phone: 44 20 74908656 **Fax:** 44 20 72515020
Email: ndcs@ndcs.org.uk
Website: http://www.ndcs.org.uk

Fnded: 1944. **Mem:** 9,000. **Reg. Groups:** 12. **Local Groups:** 120. **Lang(s):** English. **Desc:** Supports families and young deaf people, chiefly through providing information and advice on education, state benefits, audiology and equipment. **Pub:** *Communication Tips and Terms*. Pamphlet. • *TALK*, quarterly. Magazine. • Annual Report, annual.

★ 4866 ★ National Deaf Education Network and Clearinghouse

800 Florida Ave., NE
Washington, DC 20002
Phone: (202)651-5051 **Fax:** (202)651-5054
Email: clearinghouse.infotogo@gallaudet.edu
Website: http://clerccenter.gallaudet.edu
Anita Glibert, Information Specialist

Desc: Information dissemination at the Gallaudet University Laurent Clerc National Deaf Education Center on diverse topics related to deaf and hard of hearing children, ages birth to 21 years old. **Pub:** *Odyssey Magazine*. Magazine. Reports on Clerc Center projects and contains peer-reviewed articles from contributors. *Price:* for members. • *World Around You*. Magazine. Provides motivation for independent and assisted reading, creative writing, and drawing for deaf and hard of hearing teens. *Price:* for members.

★ 4867 ★ National Dental Assistants Association (NDA)

3517 16th St. NW
Washington, DC 20010
Phone: (202)588-1697 **Fax:** (202)588-1244
Email: admin@ndaonline.org
Website: http://www.ndaonline.org
Dr. Romell J. Madison, Pres.

Mem: 500. **Desc:** An auxiliary of the National Dental Association. Works to encourage education and certification among dental assistants. Conducts clinics and workshops to further the education of members. Bestows annual Humanitarian Award; offers scholarships. **Pub:** *NDAA Journal*, annual. Journal.

★ 4868 ★ National Dental Association (NDA)

3517 16th St., NW
Washington, DC 20010
Phone: (202)588-1697 **Fax:** (202)588-1244
Email: admin@ndaonline.org
Website: http://www.ndaonline.org
Dr. Romell J. Madison, Pres.

Fnded: 1913. **Mem:** 7,000. **Reg. Groups:** 6. **State Groups:** 15. **Local Groups:** 48. **Desc:** Professional society for dentists. Aims to provide quality dental care to the unserved and underserved public and promote knowledge of the art and science of dentistry. Advocates the inclusion of dental care services in health care programs on local, state, and national levels. Fosters the integration of minority dental health care providers in the profession, and promotes dentistry as a viable career for minorities through support programs. Conducts research programs. Group is distinct from the former name of the American Dental Association. **Pub:** *Flossline*, bimonthly. Contains educational news. *Price:* Included in membership dues. • *NDA Journal*, quarterly. Journal. **Frmly:** (1932) Interstate Dental Association.

★ 4869 ★ National Dental EDI Council

2020 W Indian School, Ste. B-31
Phoenix, AZ 85015-5042
Phone: (602)266-7740 **Fax:** (602)277-6798
Email: ndedic@ndedic.org
Website: http://www.ndedic.org/

Desc: Works to unite all stakeholders in the promotion of electronic connectivity in the dental benefits industry, providing a forum for Electronic Data Interchange.

★ 4870 ★ National Dental Hygienists' Association (NDHA)

c/o Barbara Seldon, Trustee
28315 Kalong Cir. W
Southfield, MI 48034
Email: ndha@aol.com
Website: http://www.ndaonline.org/auxillary.htm
Diane Lane-Tyson, Pres.

Fnded: 1932. **Mem:** 100. **State Groups:** 10. **Desc:** Minority dental hygienists. To cultivate and promote the art and science of dental hygiene and to enhance the professional image of dental hygienists. Attempts to meet the needs of society through educational, political, and social activities while giving the minority dental hygienist a voice in shaping the profession. Encourages cooperation and mutual support among minority professionals. Seeks to increase opportunities for continuing education and employment in the field of dental hygiene. Works to improve individual and community dental health. Sponsors annual seminar, fundraising events, and scholarship programs; participates in career orientation programs; counsels and assists students applying for or enrolled in dental hygiene programs. Maintains liaison with American Dental Hygienists' Association. **Pub:** *The Lore*, quarterly. Newsletter. Information relative to NDHA and Dental Hygene Activities.

★ 4871 ★ National Denturist Association (NDA)

138 Winn Rd.
Falmouth, ME 04105
Phone: (207)642-6814 **Fax:** (207)781-2575
Email: wandaa@tscnet.com
Website: http://www.nationaldenturist.com/
Dr. Austin Carbone, Pres.

Fnded: 1975. **Mem:** 350. **Reg. Groups:** 8. **State Groups:** 22. **Desc:** Denturists and other dental professionals. Promotes recognition and authorization of the profession of denturism. Conducts research regarding law pertaining to the dental profession and to the profession and practice of denturism. Offers seminars for continuing education requirements. Compiles statistics. Provides political action counseling and organizing guidance. **Pub:** *NDA Denturist News*, quarterly. Newsletter. Contains educational and business management articles and political reports. Includes new product information and legal news. *Price:* Included in membership or free upon request.

★ 4872 ★ National Diabetes Information Clearing House (NDIC)

1 Information Way
Bethesda, MD 20892-3560
Phone: (301)654-3327 **Free:** 800-860-8747
Fax: (301)907-8906
Email: ndic@info.niddk.nih.gov
Website: http://www.niddk.nih.gov/health/diabetes/ndic.htm

Fnded: 1978. **Desc:** Works to increase knowledge and understanding about diabetes among patients, health care professions, general public. **Pub:** Booklets.Contain information on all aspects of diabetes. • Brochures.Contain information on all aspects of diabetes.

★ 4873 ★ National Digestive Diseases Information Clearinghouse (NDDIC)

2 Information Way
Bethesda, MD 20892-3570
Phone: (301)654-3810 **Free:** 800-891-5389
Fax: (301)907-8906
Email: nddic@info.niddk.nih.gov
Website: http://www.niddk.nih.gov
Kathy Kranzfelder, Dir.

Fnded: 1980. **Desc:** An information and referral service of the National Institute of Diabetes and Digestive and Kidney Diseases. Serves as a central information resource on the prevention and management of digestive diseases. Responds to written inquiries, develops and distributes publications about digestive diseases, and provides referrals to digestive disease organizations, including support groups. Maintains a database of patient and professional education materials, from which literature searches are generated. Provides bulk orders of publications to health and information professionals planning patient health education programs. **Pub:** *Age Page: Constipation.* • *Cirrhosis of the Liver.* • *Constipation.* • *Crohn's Disease.* • *Digestive Diseases Statistics.* • *Diverticulosis and Diverticulitis.* • *Facts and Fallacies About Digestive Diseases.* • *Gallstones.* • *Gas in the Digestive Tract.* • *Gastroesophageal Reflux Disease (Hiatal Hernia and Heartburn).* • *Harmful Effects of Medicines on the Adult Digestive System.* • *Hemorrhoids.* • *Irritable Bowel Syndrome.* • *Lactose Intolerance.* • *Pancreatitis.* • *Smoking and Your Digestive System.* • *Stomach and Duodenal Ulcers.* • *Ulcerative Colitis.* • *Your Digestive System and How it Works.* **AKA:** Digestive Diseases Clearinghouse. **Frmly:** (1985) National Digestive Diseases Education and Information Clearinghouse.

★ 4874 ★ National Disability Sports Alliance (NDSA)

25 W Independence Way
Kingston, RI 02881-1124
Phone: (401)792-7130 **Fax:** (401)792-7132
Email: info@ndsaonline.org
Website: http://www.ndsaonline.org
Jerry McCole, Exec. Dir.

Fnded: 1986. **Mem:** 3,000. **Nat'l Groups:** 1. **Reg. Groups:** 30. **State Groups:** 15. **Local Groups:** 100. **Desc:** Athletes with cerebral palsy, athletic officials including coaches and administrators, health care professionals, and other interested individuals. Seeks to offer competitive athletic opportunities for athletes with cerebral palsy or traumatic brain injury and stroke survivors; provides support and training assistance to athletes with varying degrees of disability. Organizes multi-sport competitions at the local, regional, national, and international levels; maintains 8-level classification system to ensure that competition is based on the functional level of participants rather than their neurological capability. Selects athletes to represent the U.S. in the Paralympic Games and other international competitions. Provides referral service to assist members in obtaining support for local sports programs; develops fundraising programs. Operates Youth Sports Program, which provides guidelines and assistance to young people with special needs who wish to learn a sport. Conducts educational clinics and seminars. Compiles statistics; maintains speakers' bureau and library. Plans to make available to members liability insurance and reduced rates on special sports equipment. **Pub:** *NDSA Classification and Rules Manual.* • *Update*, quarterly. Newsletter. **Frmly:** (2002) United States Cerebral Palsy Athletic Association.

★ 4875 ★ National Eating Disorder Information Centre (NEDIC)

College Wing, 1-211
200 Elizabeth St.
Toronto, ON, Canada M5G 2C4
Phone: (416)340-4156 **Free:** (866)633-4220
Fax: (416)340-4736
Email: nedic@uhn.on.ca

Fnded: 1985. **Lang(s):** English. **Desc:** Provides information and resources on causes, symptoms of, and therapeutic and health care treatments for eating disorders and the preoccupation with food and weight. Aims to raise awareness on eating disorders through conducting lectures and workshops. Sponsors Eating Disorder Awareness Week in Canada and publishes bulletins. **Pub:** Bulletin, 5/year. Provides information and resources on range of topics related to food and weight preoccupation.

★ 4876 ★ National Eating Disorders Association

603 Stewart St., Ste. 803
Seattle, WA 98101
Phone: (206)382-3587 **Fax:** (206)829-8501
Email: info@nationaleatingdisorders.org
Website: http://www.nationaleatingdisorders.org

Fnded: 2001. **Desc:** Formed to provide educational programming, prevention efforts, research, advocacy, treatment and outreach for those suffering from eating disorders such an anorexia and bulimia. Sponsors National Eating Disorders Awareness Week, in its 14th year, celebrated in fifty states. Distributes educational brochures, sponsors a Prevention Puppet Project designed to teach elementary school children about health self-esteem and body image. Created the GO GIRLS! program, designed to help high school girls learn more about body image and the role that the media plays in the way the feel about themselves and their bodies. Runs a national media advocacy campaign. **Pub:** *A Guide to the Primary Prevention of Eating Disorders*. Brochure. *Price:* $20 per 100. **Frmly:** (1980) Anorexia Nervosa Aid Society; (1983) American Anorexia Nervosa Association.

★ 4877 ★ National Eczema Association for Science and Education

4460 Redwood Hwy., Ste. 16-D
San Rafael, CA 94903-1953
Phone: (415)499-3474 **Free:** 800-818-7546
Fax: (415)472-5345
Email: info@nationaleczema.org
Website: http://www.nationaleczema.org
Robert O. McAlister, Exec. Dir.

Fnded: 1988. **Mem:** 10,000. **Desc:** Works to raise awareness of the inflammatory condition of the skin called eczema. Provides patient & provider education materials. Supports research. **Pub:** *The Advocate*, quarterly. Newsletter. Contains eczema related news & letters from patients and family members. *Price:* Donations accepted. • Brochures. • Videos. **Frmly:** (1997) Eczema Association for Science and Education.

★ 4878 ★ National Eczema Society (NES)

Hill House
Highgate Hill
London N19 5NA, United Kingdom
Phone: 44 207 2813553 **Fax:** 44 207 2816395
Email: helpline@excema.org
Website: http://www.eczema.org/

Fnded: 1975. **Mem:** 12,000. **Lang(s):** English. **Desc:** People with eczema, dermatitis, and sensitive skin. Seeks to improve the quality of life of people with eczema; promotes advancement of the diagnosis and treatment of eczema and related disorders. Provides information and support to those affected by the condtion. Conducts information days to raise public awareness of eczema; raises funds to support dermatological research; represents the interests of people with eczema before pertinent government agencies and health care organizations. **Pub:** *Exchange*, quarterly. Journal.

★ 4879 ★ National Education for Assistance Dog Services (NEADS)

PO Box 213
West Boylston, MA 01583
Phone: (978)422-9064 **Fax:** (978)422-3255
Email: info@neads.org
Website: http://www.neads.org
Sheila O'Brien, Exec. Dir.

Fnded: 1976. **Mem:** 6,000. **Reg. Groups:** 21. **State Groups:** 5. **Desc:** Interested individuals, clubs, and organizations. Trains dogs to alert deaf or hearing impaired individuals to specific sounds of the environment; also trains dogs to help disabled individuals. After extensive screening, dogs are trained by a professional staff for three to five months, learning: basic obedience; how to respond to household and other sounds including alarm clocks, door bells, smoke alarms, telephone, babies' crying, kettle whistles, oven timer, car horns, and sirens; how to perform assistance tasks such as pulling wheelchairs, using light switches, and retrieving articles from the floor or high shelves. Maintains speakers' bureau. **Pub:** *Hearing Ear Dogs: A Sound Relationship*. Brochure. • *Help Make a Miracle–Participate in Our Puppy Program*. Brochure. • *NEADS Newsletter*, quarterly. Newsletter. • *Service Dogs - Trained to Help the Physically Disabled*. Brochure. • *Sound Friendships - The Story of Willa and Her Hearing Ear Dog*. Book. • *Special Dogs for Special People*. Brochure. **Frmly:** New England Assistance Dog Service; (1989) Hearing Ear Dog Program; (1992) New England Assistance Dog Program.

★ 4880 ★ National Emergency Equipment Dealers Association (NEEDA)

c/o Kenton H. Pattie
8421 Frost Way
Annandale, VA 22003
Phone: (703)280-4622 **Fax:** (703)280-0942
Email: kentonp1@aol.com
Website: http://www.needa.org
Pattie H. Kenton, Exec. Dir.

Fnded: 1996. **Mem:** 88. **Desc:** Dealers and services of fire, rescue, and emergency medical service vehicles, supplies and equipment. Preserves and strengthens the free market systems for dealers through advocacy, information and training. **Pub:** *NEEDA Newsletter*, monthly. Newsletter. Appears daily on Web site. *Price:* $100 per year.

★ 4881 ★ National Emergency Medicine Association (NEMA)

306 W Joppa Rd.
Baltimore, MD 21204-4048
Phone: (410)494-0300 **Free:** 800-332-NEMA
Fax: (410)494-0725
Email: info@nmahealth.org
Website: http://www.nemahealth.org
Howard H. Farrington, Pres.

Fnded: 1982. **Mem:** 5,000. **Desc:** Seeks to prevent trauma and improve emergency medical care nationwide. Concerned with: promoting lifestyles that reduce the likelihood of trauma; educating the public on how to help a trauma victim before emergency personnel arrive; ensuring that trained emergency personnel have the necessary resources to effectively do their jobs; promoting effective treatment and care of trauma victims at hospitals and trauma centers; ensuring the availability of proper services and facilities to the recovering trauma victim. Provides The Heart of the Matter, an educational radio program, to more than 250 radio stations nationwide. Maintains speakers' bureau; offers grants; provides direct-mail program focusing on heart disease prevention. **Pub:** *A Guide to the Emergency Room*. • *Heart of the Matter*. • *Heartlines*, quarterly. Newsletter. • *How to Survive Trauma*.

★ 4882 ★ National Emergency Number Association (NENA)

422 Beecher Rd.
Columbus, OH 43230-1797
Free: 800-332-3911 **Fax:** (614)933-0911
Email: jgoerke@austin.rr.com
Website: http://www.nena9-1-1.org/
James D. Goerke, Interm Exec. Dir.

Fnded: 1982. **Mem:** 7,500. **Local Groups:** 46. **Desc:** Fosters the technical advancement, availability, and implementation of a universal emergency telephone number system. Promotes research, planning, training, and education. **Pub:** *Connections*, quarterly. Newsletter. Devoted to regional information. • *NENA News*, quarterly. Magazine. Covers many issues of the association.

★ 4883 ★ National EMS Pilots Association (NEMSPA)

526 King St., Ste. 415
Alexandria, VA 22314-3143
Phone: (703)836-8930 **Fax:** (703)836-8920
Email: dmancuso@aams.org
Website: http://www.nemspa.org

Fnded: 1988. **Mem:** 250. **Desc:** Pilots in the air medical industry and interested individuals. Works to help the air medical industry prosper safely and enhance the delivery of health care. Facilitates the exchange of information; evaluates new equipment; conducts educational programs; monitors governmental organizations; supports research; offers legal assistance. **Pub:** *Air Medical Journal*, bimonthly. Magazine. • *AirNet*, quarterly. Newsletter.

★ 4884 ★ National Endometriosis Society

Ste. 50
Westminster Place Gardens
1-7 Artillery Row
London SW1P 1RL, United Kingdom
Phone: 44 207 222 2781 **Fax:** 44 207 222 2786
Email: nes@endo.org.uk
Website: http://www.endo.org.uk

Fnded: 1982. **Mem:** 3,500. **Reg. Groups:** 60. **Lang(s):** English. **Desc:** Women with personal experience of endometriosis and clinicians. Funds research into endometriosis and raises public awareness of it among medical professionals and the public. **Pub:** *Endolink*, quarterly. Newsletter.

★ 4885 ★ National Environmental Health Association (NEHA)

720 S Colorado Blvd., Ste. 970, S Tower
Denver, CO 80246-1925
Phone: (303)756-9090 **Fax:** (303)691-9490
Email: staff@neha.org
Website: http://www.neha.org
Nelson E. Fabian, Exec. Dir. & CEO

Fnded: 1937. **Mem:** 5,100. **Nat'l Groups:** 3. **Reg. Groups:** 10. **State Groups:** 50. **Local Groups:** 3. **Desc:** Represents all professionals in environmental health and protection, including Registered Sanitarians, Registered Environmental Health Specialists, Registered Environmental Technicians, Certified Environmental Health Technicians, Registered Hazardous Substances Professionals and Registered Hazardous Substances Specialists. NEHA's mission is to advance the environmental health and protection profession for the purpose of providing a healthful environment for all. Educational materials, publications, credentials and meetings are available to NEHA members and non-member professionals who strive to improve the environment. **Pub:** *Food Environment News Digest*, 3/year. Magazine. Contains information relevant to food professionals. *Price:* $10 members; $17 non-members. • *Journal of Environmental Health*, 10/year. Journal. *Price:* $90. • *National Environmental Health Association–Membership Directory*, annual. Membership Directory. **Frmly:** (1937) California Association of Sanitarians; (1970) National Association of Sanitarians.

★ 4886 ★ National Episcopal AIDS Coalition (NEAC)

520 Clinton Ave.
Brooklyn, NY 11238
Phone: (718)857-9445 **Free:** 800-588-6628
Fax: (718)638-3039
Email: neac@neac.org
Website: http://www.neac.org
Richard F. Brewer, Admin.

Fnded: 1988. **Mem:** 1,400. **Desc:** Works to educate all Episcopalians about HIV/AIDS issues. Advocates for the physical, emotional and spiritual health of and the pastoral care for HIV/AIDS infected people. Develops support networks and communities. **Pub:** *Neaction*, quarterly. Newsletter.

★ 4887 ★ National Eye Care Project (NECP)

c/o American Academy of Opthalmology
PO Box 7424
San Francisco, CA 94142-7424
Phone: (415)561-8520 **Free:** 800-222-3937
Email: gnyman-york@aao.org
Gail Nyman-York, Public Svc. Mgr.

Fnded: 1986. **Desc:** Ophthalmologists dedicated to ensuring eye care for the elderly, particularly those who are economically disadvantaged. Provides medical and surgical eye care to individuals 65 and over who normally would not have access or the means to consult an ophthalmologist. Disseminates information on participating physicians and eye diseases. Offers referral services. A project of the Foundation of the American Academy of Ophthalmology. Publishes a fact sheet and information packet.

★ 4888 ★ National Eye Research Foundation (NERF)

c/o Andrew Kim
910 Skokie Blvd., No. 207A
Northbrook, IL 60062
Phone: (847)564-4652 **Free:** 800-621-2258
Fax: (847)564-0807
Email: nerf@eyemac.com
Website: http://www.nerf.org
Andrew K. Kin, Exec. Dir.

Fnded: 1955. **Mem:** 300. **Desc:** Persons with graduate degrees in the eye professions; persons without graduate degrees but employed in the field of eye care; others participating in the work of the foundation for charitable or public welfare purposes. Works to sponsor research and education relating to the eye and contact lenses and to promote interprofessional relations for better eye care. Serves as public information center for questions on eye care. Supports Vision Foundation for Blind Youth. Conducts research and certification program. **Pub:** *Contacto*, quarterly. Journal. *Price:* Included in membership dues; $85/year for nonmembers. • *The Pinnacle*, monthly. Newsletter.

★ 4889 ★ National Families in Action (NFIA)

Century Plaza II
2957 Clairmont Rd., Ste.150
Atlanta, GA 30329-1647
Phone: (404)248-9676 **Fax:** (404)248-1312
Email: nfia@nationalfamilies.org
Website: http://www.nationalfamilies.org
Sue Rusche, Chm. /Pres. /CEO

Fnded: 1977. **Desc:** Parents and other adults concerned about preventing drug abuse. Seeks to: educate parents, children, and the community about the use of drugs; counteract social pressures that condone and promote drug use; stop drug use. Worked for passage of statewide drug paraphernalia statutes. Collects and disseminates information about the effects of drugs. Maintains Drug Information Center, which contains more than 500,000 documents, studies, books, brochures, and films and videos relating to drug abuse. Operates after-school program for parents and youth. **Pub:** *Crack Update*. Brochure. Describes the effects of this highly addictive form of cocaine. *Price:* $35/100. • *False Messengers: How Addictive Drugs Change the Brain*. • *Guide to the Legalization Movement and How You Can Stop It*. Book. *Price:* $10. • *12 Reasons Not to Legalize Drugs*. *Price:* $15/100. • *12 Tips for Helping Your Children Stay Drug-Free*. *Price:* $15/100. • *You Have the Right to Know Curriculum Series*. Books. *Price:* $10/each. • Also publishes Inhalant Update. **Frmly:** (1982) DeKalb Families in Action; (1983) Families in Action; (1984) Families in Action Drug Information Center; (1990) Families in Action National Drug Information Center.

★ 4890 ★ National Family Association for Deaf-Blind

111 Middle Neck Rd.
Sands Point, NY 11050
Phone: (516)944-8900 **Free:** 800-255-0411
Fax: (516)944-7302
Email: nfadb@aol.com
Website: http://www.nfadb.org
Sheri Stanger, Pres.

Desc: Organization founded on the belief that individuals who are deaf-blind are valued members of society and are entitled to the same opportunities and choices as other members of the community. Runs a large national network of families who focus on issues surrounding deaf-blindness. Advocates for all persons who are deaf-blind of any chronological age and cognitive ability; supports national policy to benefit people who are deaf-blind; encourages the founding and strengthening of family organizations in each state dedicated to assisting families of persons who are deaf-blind; shares information related to deaf-blindness and provides resources and referrals; collaborates with professionals who work with persons who are deaf-blind.

★ 4891 ★ National Family Caregivers Association (NFCA)

10400 Connecticut Ave., Ste. 500
Kensington, MD 20895-3944
Phone: (301)942-6430 **Free:** 800-896-3650
Fax: (301)942-2302
Email: info@nfcacares.org
Website: http://www.nfcacares.org
Suzanne Geffen Mintz, Pres.

Fnded: 1992. **Mem:** 10,000. **Desc:** Individual caregivers, family friends, professionals, affiliated organizations, healthcare providers. Works to meet the needs of family caregivers and improve the caregiver's quality of life. Offers educational materials for caregivers and health professionals; advocates for respite assistance and other resources for caregivers. Provides information and referrals. **Pub:** *Love, Honor, Value*, quarterly. Newsletter. *Price:* Free with membership. • *Take Care!*, quarterly. Newsletter. *Price:* Free with membership. • Brochure. • The Resourceful Caregiver

★ 4892 ★ National Family Partnership (NFP)

c/o Informed Families Education Center
2490 Coral Way, Ste. 501
Miami, FL 33145
Phone: (305)856-4886 **Free:** 800-705-8997
Fax: (305)856-4815
Email: mosendorf@informedfamilies.org
Website: http://www.nfp.org
Peggy B. Sapp, Pres.

Fnded: 1980. **Mem:** 65. **Reg. Groups:** 32. **State Groups:** 22. **Desc:** Provides services, resources, and drug prevention programs for local parent and youth groups across the country. Sponsors Annual Red Ribbon Celebration in October; serves as a clearinghouse for state and federal legislation. **Pub:** *NFP Update*, quarterly. Newsletter. *Price:* $25/year for individuals; $100/year for groups. • Manuals. **Frmly:** National Federation of Parents for Drug-Free Youth.

★ 4893 ★ National Family Planning and Reproductive Health Association (NFPRHA)

1627 K St. NW, 12th Fl.
Washington, DC 20006
Phone: (202)293-3114 **Fax:** (202)293-1990
Email: info@nfprha.org
Website: http://www.nfprha.org
Judith M. DeSarno, Pres.

Fnded: 1971. **Mem:** 1,000. **Desc:** Hospitals, state and city departments of health, health care providers, private nonprofit clinics, and consumers concerned with the maintenance and improvement of family planning and reproductive health services. Serves as a national communications network and advocacy organization. Maintains contact with Congress and government agencies in order to monitor government policy and regulations. **Pub:** *NFPRHA Quart.*, quarterly. • *NFPRHA Report*. Reports on public policy affecting family planning and reproductive health. *Price:* included in membership dues; $200 for nonmembers. • Also publishes professional papers and educational materials. **Frmly:** (1979) National Family Planning Forum.

★ 4894 ★ National Federation of Access Centres

SW Regional Access Centre
disability Assist Service
University of Plymouth
Drake Circus
Plymouth PL4 8AA, United Kingdom
Phone: 44 1752 232696 **Fax:** 44 1752 232279
Email: m.m.kemp@plymouth.ac.uk
Website: http://www.nfac.org.uk

Lang(s): English. **Desc:** Provides clients with disabilities with an opportunity to evaluate a range of enabling technologies relevant to their learning, teaching, or other daily communication needs.

★ 4895 ★ National Federation of Arch Clubs (NFAC)

74 Meadow Grove
Dublin 16, Ireland
Phone: 353 1 2951081 **Fax:** 353 1 2963049

Lang(s): English, Irish. **Desc:** Individuals and organizations. Seeks to improve the quality of life of people with learning disablities and their families. Makes available recreational facilities for people with learning disabilities.

★ 4896 ★ National Federation for Biblio/ Poetry Therapy (NFBPT)

c/o Sherry Reiter
1904 E 1st St.
Brooklyn, NY 11223
Phone: (718)998-4572
Email: sreiter@erols.com
Sherry Reiter, Exec. Dir.

Fnded: 1983. **Mem:** 10. **Desc:** Establishes standards for individuals, organizations, and institutions engaged in the training of biblio/poetry therapists or the practice of biblio/poetry therapy as a profession. (Biblio/poetry therapy uses literature or poetry to help patients "respond to an emotional impact which can then be integrated in self-awareness and self-understanding.") A credentialing committee grants certification and the most advanced level, registration as a poetry therapist.

★ 4897 ★ National Federation of the Blind (NFB)

1800 Johnson St.
Baltimore, MD 21230
Phone: (410)659-9314 **Fax:** (410)685-5653
Email: nfb@nfb.org
Website: http://www.nfb.org
Marc Maurer, Pres.

Fnded: 1940. **Mem:** 50,000. **State Groups:** 52. **Local Groups:** 700. **Desc:** Federation of state (50 plus Washington, DC and Puerto Rico) and local (700) organizations representing over 50,000 blind people. Seeks the complete equality and integration of the blind into society. Monitors all legislation affecting the blind; evaluates present programs for the blind; stimulates and assists in promoting needed services. Supports and conducts scholarly research and publication of results. Works to improve policies toward the blind in such places as the U.S. Office of Personnel Management. Sponsors National White Cane Week annually for fundraising and educational purposes. Distributes information. Maintains National Blindness Information Center. **Pub:** *Braille Monitor*, monthly. Reports on action by the NFB on current legislative issues, legal cases, and social concerns affecting the blind; gives news of aids and appliances. *Price:* Included in membership dues; Available to nonmembers by donation. • *Future Reflections*, quarterly. Magazine. Offers guidance in the day-to-day aspects of raising a blind child. Includes literature reviews, calendar of events, and new product list. *Price:* Included in membership dues; $15/year for nonmembers. • *If Blindness Comes*. Book. General information book, includes answers to common questions about blindness. • *The Kernel Books*. Book. Series of books written by the blind. • *Voice of the Diabetic*, quarterly. Personal stories and practical guidance from blind diabetics and medical professionals; medical news; resource column; recipe corner. *Price:* Included in membership dues. • Brochures. • Pamphlets.

★ 4898 ★ National Federation of Licensed Practical Nurses (NFLPN)

605 Poole Dr.
Garner, NC 27529
Phone: (919)779-0046 **Fax:** (919)779-5642
Email: cbarbour@mgmt4u.com
Website: http://www.nflpn.org
Charlene Barbour, Exec. Dir.

Fnded: 1949. **Mem:** 5,000. **State Groups:** 22. **Desc:** Federation of state associations of licensed practical and vocational nurses. Aims to: preserve and foster the ideal of comprehensive nursing care for the ill and aged; improve standards of practice; secure recognition and effective utilization of LPNs; further continued improvement in the education of LPNs. Acts as clearinghouse for information on practical nursing and cooperates with other groups concerned with better patient care. Maintains loan program. **Pub:** *Licensed Practical Nurse*, quarterly. Journal. Includes state and legislative news and list of new members. *Price:* Included in membership dues. • *LPN*, quarterly. Magazine.

★ 4899 ★ National Federation of Opticiany Schools (NFOS)

c/o Randall L. Smith
9604 Escada Ct.
Chesterfield, VA 23832
Phone: (804)790-0026 **Fax:** (804)790-0026
Email: rlsmitl@jsr.cc.va.us
Website: http://www.nfos.org/
Randall L. Smith, Pres.

Desc: Promotes formal opticianry education offered by accredited educational institutions. Strives to develop formal education programs in identified areas of need; upgrade standards of opticianry education; facilitate exchange of teaching methods; achieve uniformity of formal education in opticianry; and assist national opticianry organizations.

★ 4900 ★ National Federation of Spiritual Healers

Old Manor Farm Studio
Church St.
Sunbury-On-Thames TW16 6RG, United Kingdom
Phone: 44 8451 232777 **Fax:** 44 1932 779648
Email: office@nfsh.org.uk
Website: http://www.nfsh.org.uk

Desc: Spiritual Healers. **Pub:** *Healing Today*, quarterly. Magazine.

★ 4901 ★ National Fibromyalgia Research Association (FNRA)

PO Box 500
Salem, OR 97308
Website: http://www.nfra.net/

Fnded: 1992. **Desc:** Dedicated to education, treatment and finding a cure for fibromyalgia. Produces a Fibromyalgia Awareness Pin to raise public awareness and research dollars.

★ 4902 ★ National Flight Paramedics Association (NFPA)

383 F St.
Salt Lake City, UT 84103
Free: 800-381-NFPA **Fax:** (801)534-0434
Email: jpburkejr@aol.com
Website: http://www.nfpa.rotor.com
Pat Petersen, Account Exec.

Fnded: 1986. **Mem:** 850. **State Groups:** 2. **Desc:** Flight paramedics. Promotes education, professionalism, and communication within the emergency medical service community. **Pub:** *Air Medical Journal*, semimonthly. Journal. *Price:* included in membership dues. • *Flight Paramedic News*, quarterly. Newsletter. *Price:* included in membership dues.

★ 4903 ★ National Foundation for Cancer Research (NFCR)

4600 W West Hwy., Ste. 525
Bethesda, MD 20814
Phone: (301)654-1250 **Free:** 800-321-2873
Fax: (301)654-5824
Email: fcsjr@nfcr.org
Website: http://www.researchforacure.com/site/PageServer
Franklin C. Salisbury, Jr., Pres.

Fnded: 1974. **Desc:** Purpose is to conduct basic scientific research and scientific investigation of the structure and function of normal and abnormal cells. This research is based on the belief that cancer is a disturbance of normal cellular function at the submolecular level. Funds 40 laboratories in the U.S. and 7 other countries. **Pub:** *National Cancer Bulletin*, periodic. Newsletter. *Price:* Free to donors. • Also publishes booklets and papers. **Frmly:** (1975) Bethesda National Foundation of Massachusetts.

★ 4904 ★ National Foundation for the Chemically Hypersensitive (NFCH)

4407 Swinson Rd.
Rhodes, MI 48652
Phone: (989)689-6369 **Fax:** (989)689-6877
Email: fred-nelson@mcsrelief.com
Website: http://www.mcsrelief.com
Fred Nelson, Dir.

Fnded: 1986. **Mem:** 16,000. **Reg. Groups:** 40. **State Groups:** 40. **Desc:** Individuals suffering from chemical hypersensitivity, their families, and friends; health care professionals; interested others. Promotes public awareness of chemical hypersensitivity disorders, such as multiple chemical sensitivities, environmental illness, food intolerance, total allergy syndrome, candida, and chronic fatigue. Disseminates information on symptoms of chemical hypersensitivity and the potential sources of exposure to the toxic substances that can result in hypersensitivity. Facilitates networking among those afflicted with chemical hypersensitivity. Compiles case histories and statistics; conducts research and educational programs; operates health care and legal referral services. Provides assistance in handling Social Security and worker's compensation claims and locating low-cost housing resources. Maintains speakers' bureau.

★ 4905 ★ National Foundation of Dentistry for the Handicapped (NFDH)

1800 15th St., Unit 100
Denver, CO 80202
Phone: (303)534-5360 **Fax:** (303)534-5290
Email: fleviton@nfdh.org
Larry Coffee, D.D.S., Pres.

Fnded: 1974. **State Groups:** 29. **Desc:** Promotes preventive dentistry for handicapped individuals in order to reduce dental disease. Sponsors Campaign of Concern and Donated Dental Services program, which enlists the cooperation of members of the dental profession, special education personnel, disabled individuals and their parents, counselors, and civic organizations in helping developmentally disabled people enjoy good dental health. These programs currently serves 23,841 people in 29 states. Conducts preventive health education through in-service training for members of participating special education schools, sheltered workshops, day centers, and group/nursing homes; teaches handicapped individuals how to maintain their own oral hygiene and provides them with dental supplies; evaluates the oral health status of each participant; suggests dentists who will accept handicapped patients if such a referral is desired. Sponsors Donated Dental Services Programs, which match indigent, elderly, and handicapped individuals with volunteer dentists. Operates a portable dental treatment system for the homebound, nursing home residents, and the developmentally disabled that is currently in use in Denver, CO, Newark, NJ, and Chicago, IL; has assisted in developing similar programs in Detroit, MI and Houston, TX. **Pub:** *Guidelines for Dental Programs in Institutions for Developmentally Disabled Persons*. • *Guidelines for Using Fluorides Among Handicapped Persons*. • *Special Smiles*, periodic. • Annual Report. • Also distributes audiovisual and written materials on dentistry for the handicapped.

★ 4906 ★ National Foundation for Depressive Illness (NAFDI)

PO Box 2257
New York, NY 10116
Phone: (212)696-1088 **Free:** 800-239-1265
Fax: (212)696-0563
Website: http://www.depression.org
Amy Russell, Administrator

Fnded: 1983. **Desc:** Provides public and professional education and information on recent medical advances in affective mood disorders. Conducts seminars on affective disorders, pharmaceutical development, and disease-related loss of productivity. Maintains speakers' bureau. Provides support group and referral services to appropriate doctors. **Pub:** *NAFDI News*, quarterly. Newsletter. • *Now We Can Treat the Illness Called Depression*. • Brochures.

★ 4907 ★ National Foundation for Ectodermal Dysplasias (NFED)

410 E Main
Box 114
Mascoutah, IL 62258
Phone: (618)566-2020 **Fax:** (618)566-4718
Email: info@nfed.org
Website: http://www.nfed.org
Mary Kaye Richter, Exec. Dir.

Fnded: 1981. **Mem:** 3,000. **Desc:** Families of ectodermal dysplasia patients and the medical community. (Ectodermal dysplasia is a genetic birth defect usually resulting in an abnormal development of the outer layer of cells in the embryo. The disorder may be characterized by absent or poorly functioning sweat glands, sparse hair follicles, abnormal hair texture, absence of hair and skin oils, disfigured finger and toe nails, hearing or sight deficiencies, abnormalities of the limbs and cleft palate. With proper medical care, ED patients can live fairly normal lives.) Locates patients and provides them with support and information. Assists the medical community in acquiring the necessary information for treating an ED patient, locates treatment facilities and provides referral services. Makes funds available to qualified applicants for dental and other necessary care. Conducts educational meetings and assists with research projects. Provides children's services; compiles statistics. Supports researchers financially and through access to patients when approved. **Pub:** *A Multi-Syndrome Guide to ED*. Booklet. • *A Skin Guide to Ectodermal Dysplasia*. Booklet. • *Dental Guide to the Ectodermal Dysplasia*. Booklet. • *The EDucator*, bimonthly. Newsletter. *Price:* $25/year. • *Evan's New Teeth*. Booklet. Booklet for children. • *Eye, Ear, Nose and Throat Guide to the Ectodermal Dysplasias*. Booklet. • *Family Guide to the Ectodermal Dysplasias*. Booklet.

★ 4908 ★ National Foundation for Facial Reconstruction (NFFR)

317 E 34th St., Rm. 901
New York, NY 10016
Phone: (212)263-6656 **Fax:** (212)263-7534
Email: info@nffr.org
Website: http://www.nffr.org
Whitney Burnett, Exec. Dir.

Fnded: 1951. **Desc:** Assists individuals with a craniofacial deformity. Supports the treatment and rehabilitation efforts of the Institute of Reconstructive Plastic Surgery at New York University Medical center. Assists in patient care, research, the training and education of personnel engaged in reconstructive plastic surgery, conducts public education campaigns that promote national awareness of the problems of facial deformities and available treatment methods, and initiates and stimulates research. **Pub:** *NFFR Newsletter*, annual. Newsletter. Reports on the rehabilitation of individuals with facial disfigurement. Includes case histories and research updates. *Price:* Free. • *Out of the Shadows. . .Into a Bright New Future.* Brochure. • Proceedings. **Frmly:** (1986) Society for the Rehabilitation of the Facially Disfigured.

★ 4909 ★ National Foundation for Infectious Diseases (NFID)
4733 Bethesda Ave., Ste. 750
Bethesda, MD 20814
Phone: (301)656-0003 **Fax:** (301)907-0878
Email: info@nfid.org
Website: http://www.nfid.org
Susan J. Rehm, MD, Pres.

Fnded: 1973. **Desc:** Supports research into the causes and cures of infectious diseases; assists in the education of both professionals and the public in infectious diseases. Conducts programs in prevention of infectious diseases. **Pub:** *Coccidiomycosis and Host-Fungus Interplay.* Proceedings. • *Double Helix,* quarterly. Newsletter. Reports on public welfare and support of research, education, and prevention of infectious disease. Monitors legislation. *Price:* Free. • *National Foundation for Infectious Diseases–Annual Report.* Annual Report. • *Recognition and Management of Nursing Home Infections.*

★ 4910 ★ National Foundation for Jewish Genetic Diseases (NFJGD)
250 Park Ave., Ste. 1000
New York, NY 10177
Phone: (212)371-1030 **Fax:** (212)319-5808
Website: http://www.nfjgd.org
George Crohn, Pres.

Fnded: 1974. **Desc:** Individuals concerned with the eradication of the seven known genetic diseases that affect children of predominantly Ashkenazi Jewish heritage. (These diseases include Gaucher's disease, Dystonia, Dysautonomia, Tay-Sachs, Bloom's Syndrome, Niemann-Pick, and Mucolipidosis IV.) Seeks to accomplish its goal by establishing carrier identification tests, providing genetic counseling which includes prenatal testing procedures, and conducting a nationwide education campaign to inform the public that these diseases exist and attack without warning. Supports basic medical research in the prevention and cure of these diseases. Acts as referral agency. Has sponsored symposia on chromosome breakage and neoplasia, Gaucher's disease, and cellular molecular biology of neuronal development. **Pub:** Books. • Brochures.

★ 4911 ★ National Foundation for Transplants (NFT)
1102 Brookfield, Ste. 200
Memphis, TN 38119
Phone: (901)684-1697 **Free:** 800-489-3863
Fax: (901)684-1128
Email: jhill@transplants.org
Website: http://www.transplants.org
Gary McMahan, Dir.

Fnded: 1983. **Desc:** Works to guide and assist fundraising for transplant patients and their families. Offers grants for smaller emergency transplants and medication needs. Provides financial support and advocacy. **Frmly:** (1999) Organ Transplant Fund.

★ 4912 ★ National Fragile X Foundation (NFXF)
PO Box 190488
San Francisco, CA 94119
Phone: (925)938-9300 **Free:** 800-688-8765
Fax: (925)938-9315
Email: natlfx@fragilex.org
Website: http://www.fragilex.org
Robert Miller, Exec. Dir.

Fnded: 1984. **Mem:** 2,000. **State Groups:** 80. **Desc:** Fragile X patients and their families; other individuals and institutions interested in the syndrome including health care professionals, special education teachers, genetics centers, hospitals, and libraries. (Fragile X syndrome is an X-linked genetic condition which causes varying degrees of mental retardation in affected males, and can cause mental retardation or psychological disorders in carrying females. FXS can be diagnosed by a DNA analysis test.) Seeks to increase awareness of the causes and treatment of FXS among members and the public. Works to stimulate research into the causes and treatment of the syndrome. Supports and provides assistance and advice to parents of children with FXS. Conducts research and educational programs. **Pub:** *Boys with Fragile X Syndrome.* Book. • *Children With Fragile X Syndrome: A Parents Guide.* Book. • *Educational Inclusion, A Mother's Perspective.* Video. • *Faces of Fragile X.* Video. • *Females & Fragile X.* Video. • *Fragile Handle with Care.* Book. • *Fragile X Syndrome and Hand Book For Parents and Professionals.* Booklets. • *Fragile X Syndrome: Diagnosis, Treatment & Research.* Book. • *Fragile X Syndrome The Basics.* Brochure. • *Medication Guide.* Book. • *National Fragile X Foundation Newsletter,* quarterly. Newsletter. • Also publishes family and professional information packets.

★ 4913 ★ National Gaucher Foundation (NGF)
5410 Edson Ln., Ste. 260
Rockville, MD 20852
Phone: (301)816-1515 **Free:** 800-GAU-CHER
Fax: (301)816-1516
Email: ngf@gaucherdisease.org
Website: http://www.gaucherdisease.org
Rhonda P. Buyers, Exec. Dir.

Fnded: 1984. **Mem:** 1,000. **Reg. Groups:** 2. **Local Groups:** 2. **Desc:** Persons with Gaucher Disease; interested medical professionals and individuals. Gaucher Disease, one of the most common inherited metabolic disorders, is caused by an enzyme deficiency which renders the body unable to break down and dispose of complex lipids (fat-like substances). These lipids accumulate in the spleen, liver, and bone marrow, causing enlargement of the organs and intermittent pain of varying severity. Gaucher is treatable through enzyme replacement therapy. (The disease is named for Phillippe C.E. Gaucher, a French physician who described it in 1882.) One in 14 Jews of E. European descent is a carrier and one in 450 has Gaucher Disease. Sponsors direct funding of and support for research and clinical programs at medical centers in the U.S. and abroad to develop a cure and/or treatment for Gaucher Disease. Seeks to help persons with the disorder by providing them the opportunity to share experiences and feelings on a confidential, personal basis. Disseminates technical and nontechnical information concerning the disease. Advocates increased screening for carriers and availability of prenatal diagnosis for families at risk. **Pub:** *Gaucher Disease Newsletter,* quarterly. Newsletter. Includes index, reprints of recent literature, legislative reports, and medical questions and answers. *Price:* $35/year.

★ 4914 ★ National Gerontological Nursing Association
7794 Grow Dr.
Pensacola, FL 32514
Phone: (850)473-1174 **Free:** 800-723-0560
Fax: (850)484-8762
Email: ngna@puetzamc.com
Website: http://www.ngna.org
Belinda E. Puetz, RN,PHD, Contact

Fnded: 1984. **Mem:** 1,400. **Local Groups:** 17. **Desc:** Gerontological nurses. Seeks to effectively improve the care and well-being of older adults. Provides a forum in which gerontological nursing issues are identified and explored. Develops and supports educational programs for nurses, health providers, and the general public. Disseminates information. **Pub:** *Geriatric Nursing,* bimonthly. Journal. • *SIGN,* bimonthly. Newsletter.

★ 4915 ★ National Guideline Clearinghouse (NGC)
c/o Vivian Coates, Proj.Dir.
ECRI
5200 Butler Pke.
Plymouth Meeting, PA 19462
Email: info@guideline.gov
Website: http://www.guideline.gov
Vivian Coates, Proj. Dir.

Desc: Provides physicians, nurses, health professionals, healthcare providers, health plans, integrated delivery systems, purchasers detailed information on clinical practice guidelines. **Pub:** Bibliographies.Covering development methodology, implementation, use.

★ 4916 ★ National Guild of Hypnotists (NGH)
PO Box 308
Merrimack, NH 03054-0308
Phone: (603)429-9438 **Fax:** (603)424-8066
Email: ngh@ngh.net
Website: http://www.ngh.net
Dr. Dwight F. Damon, Pres.

Fnded: 1951. **Mem:** 7,000. **State Groups:** 65. **Desc:** Certified and registered hypnotherapists, demonstrational (stage) hypnotists, and interested individuals. Objective is to unite all persons sharing a professional interest in hypnotism. Seeks to: establish standards for professional conduct; increase members' knowledge in there respective areas of specialization; improve members' professional skills to enhance the quality of services provided to clients; register individuals as hypnotherapists; encourage educational programs to further the knowledge and understanding of hypnosis; promote the acceptance of hypnosis; stimulate scientific research in the field and dissemination of results; cooperate with other professional societies that share mutual goals, ethics, and interests; provide members with group benefits; improve members' individual skills in the marketing of their services and management of their practices. Offers ongoing educational seminars and workshops, and certification program. Compiles statistics; conducts research programs. Operates speakers' bureau. Maintains hall of fame. Publishes Journal of Hypnotism and Hypno-Gram-quarterlies for members. Hypnosis Today-A hypnosis magazine for the general public. **Pub:** *Hypno-Gram,* quarterly. Newsletter. *Price:* included in membership dues. • *Hypnosis Today,* annual. Magazine. *Price:* $3.95. • *The Journal of Hypnotism,* quarterly. Magazine. *Price:* Included in membership dues. • *NGH Video Rental Library.* Videos. *Price:* for members. • Audiotapes. • Books.

★ 4917 ★ National Headache Foundation (NHF)
820 N Orleans, Ste. 217
Chicago, IL 60610
Free: 888-NHF-5552 **Fax:** (773)525-7357
Email: info@headaches.org
Website: http://www.headaches.org
Seymore Diamond, MD, Exec. Dir.

Fnded: 1970. **Mem:** 20,000. **Desc:** Headache sufferers, physicians, health care professionals. Serves as an information resource to headache sufferers, their families, and the physicians who treat them. Promotes research into potential headache causes and treatments. Educates the public to the fact that headaches are a legitimate biological disease and sufferers need understanding and continuity of care. Disseminates free information on headache causes and treatments. Funds research. Operates network of local support groups. **Pub:** *About Headaches.* Pamphlet. • *The Headache Handbook.* Brochure. • *How to Talk to Your Healthcare Provider About Headaches.* Brochure. • *NHF Head Lines,* bimonthly. Newsletter. Includes information on headache causes and treatments, foundation news, book reviews, research reports, support group updates, and reader Q&A. *Price:* Included in membership dues. • Headache: A Guide to Prevention & Treatment/A Patient's Guide to Migraine Prevention & Treatment/Headache Q & A. **Frmly:** (1986) National Migraine Foundation.

★ 4918 ★ National Health Association (NHA)

PO Box 30630
Tampa, FL 33630
Phone: (813)855-6607 **Fax:** (813)855-8052
Email: info@healthscience.org
Website: http://www.healthscience.org
Lynn Grudnik, Exec. Dir.

Fnded: 1948. **Mem:** 4,000. **Desc:** Public health education organization dedicated to teaching and preserving a tradition of health freedom and independence. Promotes health maintenance through natural means such as natural foods, fresh air, pure water, sunshine, fasting, exercise, and rest. Emphasizes a lifestyle that encourages people to maximize their health by living in harmony with their physiological needs. Operates Natural Hygiene Press; maintains Herbert Shelton Library on fasting, natural hygiene, and related subjects. **Pub:** *Health Science*, quarterly. Journal. *Price:* Included in membership dues. • Also publishes and distributes books and tapes. **Frmly:** American Physiological and Natural Hygiene Society; (2003) American Natural Hygiene Society.

★ 4919 ★ National Health Care Anti-Fraud Association (NHCAA)

1255 23rd St. NW, Ste. 200
Washington, DC 20037
Phone: (202)659-5955 **Fax:** (202)785-6764
Email: fraud@nhcaa.org
Website: http://www.nhcaa.org
William J. Mahon, Pres.

Fnded: 1985. **Mem:** 900. **Desc:** Network of private insurance companies and public and private agencies that work against health insurance fraud. **Pub:** *NHCAA Network*, quarterly. Newsletter. • Also plans to make available educational materials.

★ 4920 ★ National Health Care for the Homeless Council (NHCHC)

HCH Clinicians' Network
PO Box 60427
Nashville, TN 37206-0427
Phone: (615)226-2292 **Fax:** (615)226-1656
Email: council@nhchc.org
Website: http://www.nhchc.org
Mr. John Lozier, Exec. Dir.

Mem: 455. **Desc:** Agencies (35) and clinicians (425) with an interest in providing health care services to the homeless. Promotes increased availability of primary health care services to homeless people; seeks to prevent homelessness. Works to reform the U.S. health care system to best serve the needs of the homeless and indigent; cooperates with other organizations and agencies working to eradicate homelessness. Facilitates networking, information sharing, and peer support among members; conducts educational programs. **Pub:** *HCH Mobilizer*. Newspaper. *Price:* $15. • *Healing Hands*. Newsletter. *Price:* $25.

★ 4921 ★ National Health Council (NHC)

1730 M St. NW, Ste. 500
Washington, DC 20036
Phone: (202)785-3910 **Fax:** (202)785-5923
Email: info@nhcouncil.org
Website: http://www.nhcouncil.org
Myrl Weinberg, Pres.

Fnded: 1920. **Mem:** 115. **Desc:** National membership association of voluntary and professional societies in the health field; national organizations and business groups with strong health interests. Seeks to improve the health of patients, particularly those with chronic diseases, through conferences, publications, policy briefings and special projects. Distributes printed material on health careers and related subjects. Promotes standardization of financial reporting for voluntary health groups. **Pub:** *Council Currents*, bimonthly. Books. *Price:* Free. • *Directory of Health Groups in Washington*. Directory. • *Guide to America's Voluntary Health Agencies*. Directory. • *Standards of Accounting and Reporting for Voluntary Health and Welfare Organizations (The Black Book)*. Book. • *300 Ways to Put Your Talent to Work in the Health Field*. Book.

★ 4922 ★ National Health Federation (NHF)

PO Box 688
Monrovia, CA 91017
Phone: (626)357-2181 **Fax:** (626)303-0642
Email: info@thenhf.com
Website: http://www.nationalhealthfederation.org
Wes Dumond, CSR, Cust. Svcs. Rep.

Fnded: 1955. **Mem:** 6,000. **Local Groups:** 123. **Desc:** Persons interested in individual freedom of choice in matters relating to health. Represents belief "that organized medicine, the pharmaceutical industry, and other special interests have been responsible for many laws, rules, and regulations which very often better serve the interests of these groups than the interests of the American public." Seeks to serve as a "watch dog" and to institute corrective measures through investigation, education, legislation, and coordination of organizations with similar purposes. Supports research in areas such as laetrile testing; supports numerous educational foundation programs. Conducts lobbying activities. **Pub:** *Health Freedom News*, bimonthly. Magazine. *Price:* $3.95.

★ 4923 ★ National Health and Medical Research Council (NHMRC)

GPO Box 9848
Canberra, ACT 2601, Australia
Phone: 61 2 62899184 **Fax:** 61 2 62899197
Email: exec.sec@nhmrc.gov.au

Fnded: 1936. **Mem:** 30. **Lang(s):** English. **Desc:** Representatives from state and territory health authorities, professional and scientific colleges and associations, unions, universities, industry, business and consumer groups, welfare organizations, and the commonwealth administration. Evaluates reports from committees, expert panels, working parties and disseminates results. **Pub:** *Annual Report of NHMRC*, annual. Report. Contains research results.

★ 4924 ★ National Health Policy Forum (NHPF)

2131 K St. NW, Ste. 500
Washington, DC 20037
Phone: (202)872-1390 **Fax:** (202)862-9837
Email: nhpf@gwu.edu
Website: http://www.nhpf.org
Judith Miller Jones, Dir.

Fnded: 1971. **Desc:** Nonpartisan education program serving primarily senior federal legislative and regulatory health staff but also addressing the interests of state officials and their Washington representatives. Seeks to foster more informed government decision making. Helps decision makers forge the personal acquaintances and understanding necessary for cooperation among government agencies and between government and the private sector. Provides technical assistance to staff and grantees of its sponsoring foundations and corporate contributors. **Pub:** *Background Papers*. Papers. • *Issue Briefs*, 25-30/year. • *Site Visit Reports*. Reports.

★ 4925 ★ National Healthcare Cost & Quality Association (NHCQA)

11313 Weddington St.
North Hollywood, CA 91601
Phone: (818)761-6546 **Free:** 888-761-3600
Fax: (818)761-5568
Email: info@nhcqa.org

Desc: Dedicated to understanding cost and quality issues in the delivery of healthcare. **Pub:** *Real Healthcare*, semiannual. Magazine. *Price:* included in membership dues.

★ 4926 ★ National Healthy Mothers, Healthy Babies Coalition

121 N Washington St., Ste. 300
Alexandria, VA 22314
Phone: (703)836-6110 **Fax:** (703)836-3470
Email: info@hmhb.org
Website: http://www.hmhb.org
George Guido, Chm.

Fnded: 1981. **Mem:** 110. **Nat'l Groups:** 110. **State Groups:** 21. **Local Groups:** 30. **Desc:** Coalition of national and state organizations concerned with maternal and child health. Serves as a network through which members share ideas and information regarding issues such as prenatal care, nutrition for pregnant women, and infant mortality. **Pub:** *Healthy Mothers, Healthy Babies Newsletter*, quarterly. Newsletter. *Price:* Free. • *IEAC News*, quarterly. Newsletter. *Price:* Free. • *Power News*, quarterly. *Price:* Free. **Frmly:** (1999) Healthy Mothers, Healthy Babies.

★ 4927 ★ National Hearing Conservation Association (NHCA)

9101 Kenyon Ave., Ste. 3000
Denver, CO 80237
Phone: (303)224-9022 **Fax:** (303)770-1812
Email: nhca@gwami.com
Website: http://www.hearingconservation.org
Karen Wojdyla, Exec. Dir.

Fnded: 1977. **Mem:** 500. **Desc:** Individuals holding advanced academic degrees in a discipline involving hearing and hearing loss; professional service organizations engaged in industrial hearing conservation programs; companies that manufacture or sell occupational noise or hearing loss products. Promotes hearing conservation in all sectors of society. Encourages education and standards development among members and industrial groups; monitors legislation and regulatory activities related to hearing conservation. **Pub:** *NHCA Membership Directory*, annual. Membership Directory. Arranged alphabetically, geographically, and by member category. Includes consumer guide. *Price:* Included in membership dues; $25 per issue. • *Resources in Hearing Conservation*, annual. Compilation of references and films listed in previous "Spectrum" issues. *Price:* Included in membership dues; $20/issue. • *Spectrum*, quarterly. Newsletter. Provides information on technology, research, practice, and federal and state legal and regulatory activities. Includes book reviews. *Price:* Included in membership dues; $10/issue; $20 for supplements.

★ 4928 ★ National Heart Council (NHC)

306 W Joppa Rd.
Baltimore, MD 21204
Phone: (410)494-0300 **Fax:** (410)494-0725
Email: info@nemahealth.org
Website: http://www.nemahealth.org/heartcouncil.html
Howard H. Farrington, Pres.

Fnded: 1982. **Desc:** A project of the National Emergency Medicine Association. Seeks to further advances made in the field of emergency medicine, particularly as related to heart trauma. Awards grants to organizations and individuals for the purpose of conducting research, meetings, or other activities that gather and disseminate information on traumatic medicine, particularly cardiac disorders. **Pub:** *Heart Research Newsletter*, quarterly. Newsletter. • Also publishes guides, reports, and brochures; plans to produce videotapes on first aid for household accidents, heart attacks, and choking. **Frmly:** (1994) National Heart Research.

★ 4929 ★ National Heart Savers Association (NHSA)

9140 W Dodge Rd.
Omaha, NE 68114
Phone: (402)398-1993 **Fax:** (402)398-1994
Email: nhsa@aol.com
Website: http://www.heartsavers.org
Phil Sokolof, Pres.

Fnded: 1985. **Desc:** Promotes cardiac health care by informing the public of the dangers of a high-cholesterol diet. Conducts public cholesterol screening program; secured congressional designation of September as National Cholesterol Education Month. Has been successful in persuading major food processing and fast food restaurants companies to stop using palm and coconut oil, lard, and beef tallow, which are high in saturated fats, as ingredients in prepared foods. Promotes nutrition education in public schools and lobbies for more healthful school lunches. **Pub:** Books. • Pamphlets.

★ 4930 ★ National Hemophilia Foundation (NHF)

116 West 32nd St., 11th floor
New York, NY 10001
Phone: (212)328-3700 **Free:** 800-42-HANDI
Fax: (212)328-3777
Email: info@hemophilia.org
Website: http://www.hemophilia.org
Mark Skinner, Pres.

Fnded: 1948. **Mem:** 1,500. **Local Groups:** 48. **Desc:** Voluntary health organization consisting of individuals with hemophilia, their families, medical and paramedical professionals, and other interested persons. (Hemophilia is a hereditary disease in which blood clotting is abnormally delayed.) Supports research through postgraduate fellowship program; disseminates literature for the public and medical and paramedical personnel. Conducts educational programs. Operates information center to provide research assistance, referrals, and comprehensive resources on hemophilia, HIV/AIDS, and related topics. Chapters help in blood recruitment drives and referral services for patients and sponsor summer camps for young people with hemophilia. Maintains library. **Pub:** *Directory of Hemophilia Treatment Centers*, periodic. Directory. **Frmly:** (1956) Hemophilia Foundation.

★ 4931 ★ National Hepatitis C Coalition (NHCC)

PO Box 5058
Hemet, CA 92544
Phone: (909)658-4414
Email: support@nationalhepatitis-c.org
Website: http://nationalhepatitis-c.org/

Fnded: 1997. **Desc:** Works as hepatitis C support system; provides education and support through online communications, Hepatitis C Hotline, and grassroots operations across the country. Promotes awareness and research for effective treatments, cures, and vaccines.

★ 4932 ★ National Hispanic Council on Aging (NHCoA)

2713 Ontario Rd. NW
Washington, DC 20009
Phone: (202)265-1288 **Fax:** (202)745-2522
Email: nhcoa@nhcoa.org
Website: http://www.nhcoa.org
Marta Sotomayor, PhD, Pres.

Fnded: 1980. **Mem:** 50,000. **Nat'l Groups:** 25. **Reg. Groups:** 4. **State Groups:** 38. **Local Groups:** 20. **Desc:** Individuals and groups who work in administrative, planning, direct services, research, or educational areas who have a concern for the Hispanic elderly. Fosters the well-being of the Hispanic elderly through research, policy analysis, demonstration projects, development of educational resources, and training. Compiles research data and provides a network for organizations and community groups interested in the Hispanic elderly. Maintains speakers' bureau. **Pub:** *The Hispanic Elderly: A Cultural Signature, Latino Elderly: Issues and Solutions for 20th Centry Triple Jeopardy: Aged, Hispanic Women*, quarterly. Book. *Price:* $18.45 portage per book. • *Hispanic Elderly: Issues and Solutions for the 21st Century*. Book. • *Noticias on Hispanic Elderly Issues*, quarterly. Newsletter. Publicizes the activities of NHCoA. Includes calendar of events, legislative news, and notices of publications available. *Price:* $25/year. • *Triple Jeopardy: Hispanic Older Women*. Book.

★ 4933 ★ National Hispanic Medical Association

c/o Elena Rios, MD
1411 K St. NW, Ste. 200
Washington, DC 20005
Phone: (202)628-5895 **Fax:** (202)628-5898
Email: nhma@nhmamd.net
Website: http://home.earthlink.net/~nhma
Elena Rios, MD, Contact

Fnded: 1994. **Desc:** Hispanic physicians. Works to improve health care for Hispanics and underserved populations. Promotes Hispanic health policy issues in relevant forums. Conducts continuing education programs.

★ 4934 ★ National Hormone and Pituitary Program (NHPP)

Harbor - UCLA Medical Ctr.
1000 W Carson St.
Torrance, CA 90509
Phone: (310)222-3537 **Fax:** (310)222-3432
Email: parlow@humc.edu
Website: http://www.humc.edu/hormones
Dr. A.F. Parlow, Scientific Officer

Fnded: 1963. **Desc:** The agency collects human pituitary glands obtained through autopsies and extracts from them human growth hormone (hGH), human follicle stimulating hormone (hFSH), human luteinizing hormone (hLH), human adrenocorticotrophic hormone (ACTH), human thyroid stimulating hormone (hTSH), human prolactin, and beta-lipotropin. These and similar hormones of rat, ovine, bovine, porcine, and monkey origin are distributed to doctors in research centers for research in endocrinology. Promotes basic studies with all pituitary hormones and seeks to make these available to investigators. **Frmly:** (1983) National Pituitary Agency.

★ 4935 ★ National Hospice and Palliative Care Organization

1700 Diagonal Rd., Ste. 625
Alexandria, VA 22314-2848
Phone: (703)837-1500 **Free:** 800-658-8898
Fax: (703)837-1233
Email: nhpco_info@nhpco.org
Website: http://www.nhpco.org
Karen A. Davie, Pres.

Fnded: 1978. **Mem:** 5,000. **State Groups:** 48. **Local Groups:** 2400. **Desc:** Hospice organizations and individuals interested in the promotion of the hospice concept and program of care. (Hospice is a concept of caring for the terminally ill and their families which enables the patient to live as fully as possible, makes the entire family the unit of care, and centers the caring process in the home whenever appropriate. Inpatient facilities are available for those unable to be cared for at home.) Promotes standards of care in program planning and implementation; monitors health care legislation and regulation relevant to hospice care. Sponsors professional liaison and peer group networking. Collects data for the purpose of demonstrating definitive national trends in the hospice movement; encourages recognized medical and other health teaching institutions to provide instruction in hospice care of terminally ill patients and their families. Compiles statistics. Conducts educational and training programs in numerous aspects of hospice care for administrators and care-givers. Maintains nonlending library of hospice-related books. Operates helpline to assist public in identifying hospice programs in their area. **Frmly:** (2000) National Hospice Organization.

★ 4936 ★ National Hydrocephalus Foundation (NHF)

12413 Centralia
Lakewood, CA 90715-1623
Phone: (562)402-3523 **Fax:** (562)924-6666
Email: debbifields@nhfonline.org
Website: http://www.nhfonline.org/page2.html
Debbi Fields, Exec. Dir.

Fnded: 1980. **Mem:** 350. **Reg. Groups:** 1. **Local Groups:** 1. **Desc:** Works to assemble, disseminate, and research information about hydrocephalus, its treatments and outcomes, to families in need. **Pub:** *Life-Line*, quarterly. Newsletter. Contains current medical information, feature story on individual with hydrocephalus, Internet references, and more. *Price:* included in membership dues. • *Living with Hydrocephalus-Adult Guide*.

★ 4937 ★ National Hypertension Association (NHA)

324 E 30th St.
New York, NY 10016
Phone: (212)889-3557 **Fax:** (212)447-7032
Website: http://www.nathypertension.org
William M. Manger, MD, Chm.

Fnded: 1977. **Desc:** Physicians, medical researchers, and business professionals dedicated to the prevention of the complications of hypertension. Seeks to combat hypertension by developing, directing, and implementing effective programs to educate physicians and the public about the severe, life-threatening dangers of this health disorder. Conducts research on the cause of hypertension through basic laboratory studies. Provides the public with basic information on hypertension; conducts hypertension and hypercholesterol detection programs. Offers medical consulting to those found to have high blood pressure or hypercholesterolemia. Develops educational materials and participates in radio and television programs. **Pub:** *Clinical and Experimental Pheochromocytoma*. Book. • *High Blood Pressure and What You Can Do About It*, annual. Pamphlet. *Price:* $1. • *News Report*, annual. Newsletter. • *100 Questions and Answers About Hypertension*. Book. *Price:* $14.95. • Also publishes medical journal periodicals.

★ 4938 ★ National Immunotherapy Cancer Research Foundation

PO Box 1027
Flemington, NJ 08822
Phone: (908)806-4300 **Fax:** (908)806-3548
Dale A. Facchina, Pres. & CEO

Fnded: 1990. **Desc:** Promotes the use of immune system stimulation including vaccines, biological response modifiers, and other immuno-augmentative treatments as a cure for cancer. Raises funds for immunotherapy and immunology research in the prevention and treatment of cancer.

★ 4939 ★ National Indian Council on Aging (NICOA)

10501 Montgomery Blvd. NE, Ste. 210
Albuquerque, NM 87111
Phone: (505)292-2001 **Fax:** (505)292-1922
Email: info@nicoa.org
Website: http://www.nicoa.org
Dave Baldridge, Exec. Dir.

Fnded: 1976. **Mem:** 1,037. **Desc:** Native American/Alaska Native populations. The National Indian Council on Aging seeks to bring about improved comprehensive services to the American Indian and Alaska Native elderly. Objectives include: interaction with service provider agencies and advocacy organizations in the aging network, disseminate information to Indian communities and provide technical assistance and training opportunities to organizations. Research activities performed, as well as acting as a clearinghouse for current issues affecting the American Indian and Alaska Native elderly. **Pub:** *Elder Voices*, quarterly. Newsletter. *Price:* $5 for nonmembers. • *Mapping Indian Elders*. Reports. *Price:* $25. • Monographs. • Proceedings.

★ 4940 ★ National Industries for the Blind (NIB)

1901 N Beauregard St., Ste. 200
Alexandria, VA 22311-1727
Phone: (703)998-0770 **Fax:** (703)998-8268
Email: info@nib.org
Website: http://www.nib.org
Allan J. Clelland, Chm.

Fnded: 1938. **Mem:** 123. **Desc:** Association of agencies employing blind persons who undertake the production of certain goods and services for the federal government under the Javits-Wagner-O'Day Act. Offers gainful employment in these industries, located in 38 states, Puerto Rico, and the District of Columbia for those blind or multidisabled blind persons who are able and willing to work. Researches and recommends new products, prices, and price revisions to the Committee for Purchase From People Who Are Blind or Severely Disabled; allocates federal work orders among these agencies. Devises quality control systems; provides management and engineering services to increase plant efficiency and broaden opportunities for blind persons; assists the industries in procurement of raw materials. Marketing Division offers marketing, subcontracting, and industrial engineering expertise; Division of Rehabilitation Services works to establish evaluation and training programs to make possible the greater employment of multidisabled blind persons; Government Business Division deals with federal government contract administration, quality control, and pricing. Compiles statistics. **Pub:** *Opportunity*, quarterly. Magazine. Covers news and feature articles on agencies for the blind; describes industries, agencies, and projects that employ blind workers. • *60 Years of Success*, annual. Annual Report. • Report.

★ 4941 ★ National Information Center for Children and Youth with Disabilities (NICHCY)

PO Box 1492
Washington, DC 20013-1492
Phone: (202)884-8200 **Free:** 800-695-0285
Fax: (202)884-8441
Email: nichcy@aed.org
Website: http://www.nichcy.org
Suzanne Ripley, Dir.

Fnded: 1970. **Desc:** Provides information to assist parents, educators, care-givers, advocates, and others in helping children and youth with disabilities participate as fully possible in school, at home, and in the community. Provides personal responses to specific questions, referrals to other organizations/sources of help, prepared information packets, and technical assistance to parent and professional groups. **Pub:** *Disability Fact Sheet*, annual. • *News Digest*, periodic. Newsletter. Addresses current issues affecting individuals concerned with handicapped children and youth with disabilities. *Price:* Free. • *Parent Guide*. • *State Resource Sheet*, annual. • *Transition Summary*. • Booklets. • Papers. **Frmly:** National Information Center for the Handicapped; National Special Education Information Center; (1982) Parents Campaign for Handicapped Children and Youth; (1987) National Information Center for Handicapped Children and Youth; (1991) National Information Center for Children and Youth with Handicaps.

★ 4942 ★ National Inhalant Prevention Coalition (NIPC)

2904 Kerbey Ln.
Austin, TX 78703
Phone: (512)480-8953 **Free:** 800-269-4237
Fax: (512)477-3932
Email: nipc@io.com
Website: http://www.inhalants.org/

Fnded: 1992. **Desc:** Promotes awareness and prevention of the use of inhalants as dangerous drugs. **Pub:** *ViewPoint*, quarterly. Newsletter. Contains latest research findings.

★ 4943 ★ National Institute on Aging (NIA)

Bldg. 31, Rm. 5C27
31 Center Dr., MSC 2292
Bethesda, MD 20892
Phone: (301)496-1752
Website: http://www.nia.nih.gov/
Dr. Richard J. Hodes, Dir.

Desc: Promotes understanding of the nature of aging and to extend the healthy, active years of life.

★ 4944 ★ National Institute of Arthritis and Musculoskeletal and Skin Diseases Information Clearinghouse

c/o National Institutes of Health
1 AMS Cir.
Bethesda, MD 20892-3675
Phone: (301)495-4484 **Free:** 877-226-4267
Fax: (301)718-6366
Email: niamsinfo@mail.nih.gov
Website: http://www.niams.nih.gov

Desc: Collects, publishes, and disseminates professional and public educational materials for persons concerned with arthritis and musculoskeletal and skin diseases. **Pub:** Reports. **Frmly:** (1999) National Arthritis and Musculoskeletal and Skin Diseases Information Clearinghouse (NAMSIC).

★ 4945 ★ National Institute of Child Health and Human Development (NICHD)

Bldg. 31, Rm. 2A32, MSC 2425
31 Center Dr.
Bethesda, MD 20892-2425
Free: 800-370-2943
Email: nichdclearinghouse@mail.nih.gov
Website: http://www.nichd.nih.gov/about/mission.htm

Desc: Promotes research on the reproductive, neurobiological, developmental, behavioral processes determining and maintaining health of children, adults, families and populations.

★ 4946 ★ National Institute for Clinical Application of Behavioral Medicine (NICABM)

PO Box 523
Mansfield Center, CT 06250
Phone: (860)456-1153 **Free:** 800-743-2226
Fax: (860)423-4512
Email: info@nicabm.com
Website: http://www.nicabm.com
Ruth M. Buczynski, PhD, Pres.

Fnded: 1988. **Desc:** Works to provide information to behavioral health professionals. Conducts educational programs. **Pub:** Newsletter, quarterly.

★ 4947 ★ National Institute on Community-Based Long-Term Care (NICLC)

c/o National Council on the Aging
409 3rd St. SW
Washington, DC 20024
Phone: (202)479-1200 **Fax:** (202)479-0735
Email: info@ncoa.org
Website: http://www.ncoa.org/content.cfm?sectionID=42
Carol McClendon, Contact

Fnded: 1984. **Mem:** 1,100. **Desc:** A unit of the National Council on the Aging. Seeks to promote a comprehensive long-term care system that will integrate home-and community-based services, enabling older adults to live in their own homes as long as it is medically, socially, and economically feasible. Serves as information clearinghouse for long-term care professionals. Advocates public policies that support home and community-based services. Maintains speakers' bureau; offers educational sessions; compiles statistics. **Pub:** *Care Management Standards*. Book. • *NCOA Networks*, bimonthly. Newsletter. • *Perspective on Aging*, periodic. Journal. Provides information on aging issues.

★ 4948 ★ National Institute on Deafness and Other Communication Disorders Information Clearinghouse

1 Communication Ave.
Bethesda, MD 20892-3456
Free: 800-241-1044 **Fax:** (301)770-8977
Email: nidcdinfo@nidcd.nih.gov
Website: http://www.nidcd.nih.gov
Dr. Marin Allen, Project Officer

Fnded: 1988. **Desc:** Disseminates information on biomedical and behavioral research in human communication. **Pub:** *Information Resources for Human Communication Disorders*, annual. Directory. Encourages networking among those with an interest in deafness and communication disorders. *Price:* Single copies free. • *NIDCD Information Clearinghouse*. Newsletter. • *NIDCD Publications List*, annual. Pamphlet. **Frmly:** (1998) National Committee in Deafness and Other Communication Disorders.

★ 4949 ★ National Institute of Dental and Craniofacial Research (NIDCR)

45 Center Dr., MSC-6400
Bethesda, MD 20892-6400
Phone: (301)496-4261 **Fax:** (301)496-9988
Email: nidcrinfo@mail.nih.gov
Website: http://www.nidcr.nih.gov/
Lawrence Tabak, DDS, Dir.

Desc: Promotes general health by improving oral, dental and craniofacial health.

★ 4950 ★ National Institute on Drug Abuse (NIDA)

c/o National Institutes of Health
6001 Executive Blvd., Rm. 5213
Bethesda, MD 20892-9561
Phone: (301)443-1124
Website: http://www.drugabuse.gov/AboutNIDA.html
Dr. Glen R. Hanson, Actg. Dir.

Desc: Promotes research into the prevention and treatment of drug abuse. **Pub:** Reports.

★ 4951 ★ National Institute of Electromedical Information (NIEI)

PO Box 4633
Bay Terrace, NY 11360-4633
Phone: (718)849-8700 **Fax:** (718)225-1041
Email: sniei@aol.com
Stanley H. Kornhauser, PhD, Pres.

Fnded: 1984. **Mem:** 1,494. **Desc:** Health care practitioners, medical educators, research scientists, and electromedical device manufacturers. Disseminates information on research, case histories, new and proposed theories, and clinical applications of electromedicine to professionals, laypersons, federal agencies, U.S. industry, and universities. (Electromedicine deals with the application of diagnostic, monitoring and prosthetic electromedical devices used in research and clinical settings as well as the application of therapeutic electric currents in the prevention and treatment of diseases.) Supports the development of programs and materials for the preparation of those studying electromedicine; fosters the establishment of programs and creation of partnerships that provide resource-sharing networks and professional linkage among clinicians, researchers, colleges and universities, health care institutions, electromedical equipment manufacturers, and other scientific and educational organizations. Encourages exchange of information through an interdisciplinary forum between researchers and clinicians and advises and coordinates matters of mutual interest between members and other organizations. Enhances the career awareness of secondary or post-secondary students in the emerging fields of electromedical technology. Funds, when available, research and educational projects. Reviews standards and certification systems for determining the efficacy of electromedical devices. Offers seminars and tutorials. Maintains consulting service and speakers' bureau; compiles statistics. **Pub:** *American Journal of Electromedicine (AJE) included in Medical Electronics*, Temporarily Suspended. Journal. Includes case studies, original research documentation, interviews on state-of-the-art topics in electromedicine and product reports. • *National Institute of Electromedical Information–Membership Directory*, annual. Membership Directory. *Price:* Included in membership dues. • Books. • Bulletin, periodic. • Proceedings, periodic. • Also publishes book reviews and educational materials.

★ 4952 ★ National Institute of Hypertension Studies - Institute of Hypertension School of Research (NIHS)
PO Box 02006
Detroit, MI 48202
Fax: (313)872-0505
Dr. H. R. Lockett, Exec. Dir.

Fnded: 1975. **Desc:** Purposes are: to help find causes of and to help prevent essential hypertension; to educate people concerning essential hypertension; to diagnose, counsel, and refer afflicted individuals for treatment and follow-up activities; to conduct research on hypertension and to extend that research into the areas of crime and drug addiction and psychosocial and occupational stress. Sponsors hypertension detection clinics. Offers youth leadership courses. Compiles statistics and disseminates educational materials. Conducts research programs on psychosocial and occupational stress which offer diplomas to those completing the programs; survey project with Pharmaceutical Research and Manufacturers of America; also conducts research on drugs and hypertension. **Pub:** *IHS 1992 Report*, annual. Research report on causes of essential hypertension. • *OHRST Assessment Report Series*, annual. • *Pharmaceutical Research and Manufacturers of America.* • Magazine, periodic. **Frmly:** (1971) Institute of Hypertension Studies; (1981) Institute of Hypertension Studies - Institute of Hypertension School of Research.

★ 4953 ★ National Institute for Jewish Hospice (NIJH)
444 San Vincente Blvd.
Los Angeles, CA 90048
Phone: (323)467-7423 **Free:** 800-446-4448
Shirley Lamm, Exec. Dir.

Fnded: 1985. **Mem:** 50,000. **Desc:** Individuals, business firms, and organizations concerned about terminally ill Jewish people. Serves as a resource center that seeks to help terminal patients and their families deal with their grief by providing information on traditional Jewish views on death, dying, and managing the loss of a loved one. Offers guidance and training to patients and interested hospice personnel, health care professionals, clergy, and family members who work with terminally ill Jewish people. Maintains speakers' bureau; conducts research programs. Jewish living will, booklets and tapes are available. Accreditation is given by training onsite at hospices. **Pub:** *At Bedside.* • *Caring for the Jewish Terminally Ill.* • *For Families of the Jewish Terminally Ill.* • *Hemlock Is Poison for Society.* • *How to Console.* • *Introduction to Jewish Hospice.* • *The Jewish Living Will.* • *The Jewish Orphaned Adult.* • *Realities of the Dying.* • *Self-Healing and Hospice Care.* • *The Spiritual Component Cannot Be Ignored.* • *Strategies for Jewish Care.* • *The Undying Hope.*

★ 4954 ★ National Institute of Medical Herbalists
56 Longbrook St.
Exeter EX4 6AH, United Kingdom
Phone: 44 1392 426022 **Fax:** 44 1392 498963
Email: nimh@ukexeter.freeserve.co.uk
Website: http://www.nimh.org.uk

Fnded: 1864. **Mem:** 625. **Desc:** Practitioners of herbal medicine. **Pub:** *European Journal of Herbal Medicine*, 3/year. Journal. • *Register of Members.* Directory.

★ 4955 ★ National Institute of Mental Health (NIMH)
6001 Executive Blvd., Rm. 8184
MSC 9663
Bethesda, MD 20892-9663
Phone: (301)443-4513 **Fax:** (301)443-4279
Email: nimhinfo@nih.gov
Website: http://www.nimh.nih.gov

Desc: Conducts and supports mental health research and distribution information to the public.

★ 4956 ★ National Institute of Neurological Disorders and Stroke (NINDS)
Financial Management Branch
Bldg. 31, Rm. 8A34
31 Center Dr.
Bethesda, MD 20892-2350
Phone: (301)496-4927
Email: giftfunds@ninds.nih.gov
Website: http://www.ninds.nih.gov/about_ninds/mission.htm

Desc: Works to identify the causes and to prevent, diagnose and treat neurological disorders and stroke.

★ 4957 ★ National Institute of Nutrition (NIN)
408 Queen St., 3rd Fl.
Ottawa, ON, Canada K1R 5A7
Phone: (613)235-3355 **Fax:** (613)235-7032
Email: nin@nin.ca
Website: http://www.nin.ca

Fnded: 1983. **Lang(s):** English, French. **Desc:** Promotes the nutritional health of Canadians through research and education. Moves the nutrition agenda forward by encouraging exchange on key public policy issues. Conducts research that supports decision making across many sectors. **Pub:** *Healthy Bites*, quarterly. • *NIN Review*, annual. Report. • *Rapport*, quarterly. Newsletter. • Annual Report, annual.

★ 4958 ★ National Institute for Rehabilitation Engineering (NIRE)
PO Box 1088
Hewitt, NJ 07421
Phone: (973)853-6585 **Free:** 800-736-2216
Fax: (973)832-2894
Email: nire@theoffice.net
Website: http://www.theoffice.net/nire
Donald Selwyn, Exec. VP

Fnded: 1967. **Desc:** Multidisciplinary research, training, and service organization providing custom-designed and custom-made tools and devices, along with intensive personal task-performance and driver training, to aid the handicapped person in becoming more self-sufficient and independent. Often an organization of "last resort" for permanently, severely, or multihandicapped persons, the NIRE is staffed by electronics engineers, physicists, psychologists, optometrists, and other volunteers who work as a team with the handicapped person. These specialists review the handicapped person's abilities, disabilities, and task-performance goals and are thus able to help advise, plan, and implement programs to increase the person's abilities to perform desired tasks, using a combination of methods involving different practitioners and disciplines. Staff members also adapt, modify, and construct equipment specially suited to the individual client's need. No handicapped person is denied the institute's services due to an inability to pay, and fees for others are based on each person's income and means. Conducts occasional seminars for the handicapped and for professionals serving the handicapped. Provides speakers and seminar participants for other agencies' programs. Compiles statistics. **Pub:** *Rehabilitation Newsletter*, quarterly. Newsletter. Features announcements of upcoming seminars. *Price:* Included in membership dues.

★ 4959 ★ National Institute of Senior Centers (NISC)
c/o National Council on the Aging
409 3rd St. SW, No. 200
Washington, DC 20024
Phone: (202)479-1200 **Free:** 800-424-9046
Fax: (202)479-0735
Email: info@ncoa.org
Website: http://www.ncoa.org/content.cfm?sectionID=44
Constance Todd, Dir.

Fnded: 1970. **Mem:** 3,000. **Desc:** Individuals or organizations who are affiliated with senior centers at the local, state, or national level. (Senior centers are places where senior citizens can go for services, recreation, and information on topics such as nutrition, employment, and housing.) Assists senior centers, organizations, and communities in developing new centers and upgrading existing operations. Promotes professionalism within the senior center field and develops standards for senior centers nationwide. Maintains advocacy and public policy positions for senior centers; provides management training for persons working with senior centers. **Pub:** *NCOA Network*, bimonthly. Newspaper. Reports on senior citizen centers, including legislative updates, program and funding information, and current issues. *Price:* Free, for members only. • *Senior Center Operation: A Guide to Organization and Management.* • *Senior Center Standards.*

★ 4960 ★ National Institute of Transplantation (NIT)
2200 W 3rd St., Ste. 100
Los Angeles, CA 90057
Phone: (213)413-2779 **Fax:** (213)484-6652
Email: nit@transplantation.com
Website: http://www.transplantation.com
James Cicciarelli, PhD, Co-Dir.

Desc: Works to advance the science and art of organ transplantation. **Pub:** *NIT Newsletter*, semiannual. Newsletter.

★ 4961 ★ National Interfaith Coalition on Aging (NICA)
300 D St. SW, Ste. 801
Washington, DC 20024
Phone: (202)479-6655 **Free:** 800-424-9046
Fax: (202)479-0735
Email: rita.chow@ncoa.org
Website: http://www.ncoa.org/content.cfm?sectionID=41
Rita Chow, Dir.

Fnded: 1972. **Mem:** 300. **Desc:** Shares administrative capabilities and resources with National Council on the Aging. Religious and secular organizations and individuals concerned with the U.S. religious community's response to the problems of aging, and about the spiritual well-being of the elderly. Promotes communication and cooperative effort among religious organizations and individuals concerned about older people; assists churches and synagogues that attempt to respond to the needs of the elderly; identifies and supports programs and services for the elderly that are best implemented by religious organizations; facilitates continued participation in community affairs by the elderly. Serves as a resource and gerontological training agency for clergy and religious workers. **Pub:** *Journal of Religious Gerontology*, quarterly. Journal. Contains articles about developments in religious gerontology and religious concerns of aging. Includes book reviews and research reports. *Price:* $40/year.

★ 4962 ★ National Jewish Medical and Research Center
1400 Jackson St.
Denver, CO 80206
Phone: (303)388-4461 **Free:** 800-222-LUNG
Fax: (303)270-2165
Email: lungline@njc.org
Website: http://www.njc.org
Lynn Taussig, Pres.

Fnded: 1899. **Desc:** Devoted to treatment, research, and education in chronic respiratory diseases and immunological disorders such as asthma, tuberculosis, cystic fibrosis, chronic bronchitis, emphysema, interstitial lung disease, and systemic lupus erythematosus. Accepts non-sectarian patients of all ages. Disseminates information to the public. Maintains research library of 15,000 volumes. **Pub:** *Lung Line Letter*, quarterly. Newsletter. *Price:* Free. • *National Jewish Medical and Research Center–Annual Report. Price:* Free. • *National Jewish Medical and Research Center–Medical Scientific Update*, monthly. Newsletter. *Price:* Free. • *New Directions*, quarterly. Newsletter. Updates the center's research programs. *Price:* Free. **Frmly:** (1978) National Jewish Hospital/National

Asthma Center; (1998) National Jewish Center for Immunology and Respiratory Medicine.

★ 4963 ★ National Kidney Foundation (NKF)

30 E 33rd St., Ste. 1100
New York, NY 10016
Phone: (212)889-2210 **Free:** 800-622-9010
Fax: (212)779-0068
Email: info@kidney.org
Website: http://www.kidney.org
John Davis, Chief Exec. Officer

Fnded: 1950. **Local Groups:** 200. **Desc:** Supports research, patient services, professional and public education, organ and tissue donor program, and community service. Affiliates conduct community and patient services including: drug banks; transportation; early screening; patient seminars. Sponsors symposium for health care professionals. Maintains speakers' bureau and biographical archives; compiles statistics. **Pub:** *Advances in Renal Replacement Therapy*, quarterly. Journal. • *American Journal of Kidney Diseases*, monthly. Journal. Covers research in kidney and urinary tract diseases. Includes annual index and conference reports. *Price:* Included in membership dues. • *CNNT Newsletter*, quarterly. Newsletter. Contains employment opportunity listings and regional news. *Price:* Included in membership dues. • *CNSW Newsletter*, quarterly. Newsletter. Includes calendar of events, information on current literature, employment opportunities, and legislative and regional reports. *Price:* Included in membership dues. • *CRN News and Briefs*, quarterly. Newsletter. Contains employment opportunity listings, legislative news, and research reports. *Price:* Included in membership dues. • *Journal of Nephrology Social Work*, annual. Journal. • *Journal of Renal Nutrition*, quarterly. Journal. • *National Kidney Foundation–Clinical Nephrology Meetings Proceedings Book*. **Frmly:** (1958) National Nephrosis Foundation; (1964) National Kidney Disease Foundation.

★ 4964 ★ National Kidney and Urologic Diseases Information Clearinghouse (NKUDIC)

3 Information Way
Bethesda, MD 20892-3580
Phone: (301)654-4415 **Free:** 800-891-5390
Fax: (301)907-8906
Email: nkudic@info.niddk.nih.gov
Website: http://www.niddk.nih.gov

Fnded: 1987. **Desc:** An information and referral service of the National Institute of Diabetes and Digestive Kidney Diseases. Responds to written inquiries, develops and distributes publications about kidney and urologic diseases, and provides referrals to kidney and urologic organizations, including support groups. Maintains a database of patient and professional educational materials and performs searches. Provides bulk orders of publications to health and information professionals planning patient health education programs. Established by the National Institutes of Health. **Pub:** *Research Updates in Kidney and Urologic Health*, semiannual. Newsletter. • Booklets. • Directories. • Also publishes a variety of patient education materials including fact sheets and literature searches from the Combined Health Information Database (CHID).

★ 4965 ★ National Latina Health Organization (NLHO)

PO Box 7567
Oakland, CA 94601
Phone: (510)534-1362 **Fax:** (510)534-1364
Website: http://www.latinahealth.org/
Luz Alvarez Martinez, Exec. Dir.

Fnded: 1986. **Desc:** Puerto Rican, Chicana, Mexican, Cuban, Caribbean and South and Central American women. Works to increase awareness of health issues among Latin American women. Works to achieve bilingual access to quality health care and self-empowerment of Latinas through culturally sensitive educational programs, health advocacy, outreach, research, and the development of public policy. Cooperates with other organizations to defend reproductive rights, affordable birth control, sex education, prenatal care, and freedom from sterilization abuse. Offers technical training for community health facilitators. Organizes forums. **Pub:** Newsletter, periodic. Includes Latina health issues, legislation affecting Latinas, and calendar of events and activities on health and reproductive rights.

★ 4966 ★ National League of the Blind and Disabled (NLBD)

21 Hill St.
Dublin 1, Ireland

Fnded: 1893. **Mem:** 2,371. **Reg. Groups:** 3. **State Groups:** 4. **Local Groups:** 50. **Desc:** Blind, partially sighted and seeing disabled people 16 years of age and over. Represents, negotiates, campaigns for provisions of equality of resources and services for people with disabilities in education, rehabilitation, training, employment and benefits by the State and local authorities. **Pub:** *Advocate*, quarterly. Magazine.

★ 4967 ★ National League of the Blind of Ireland (NLBI)

21 Hillstreet
Dublin 1, Ireland
Phone: 353 1 8742792 **Fax:** 353 1 8787139

Fnded: 1898. **Mem:** 150. **Nat'l Groups:** 1. **Lang(s):** English. **Desc:** A self-administered organization of blind individuals in the Republic of Ireland. Conducts advocacy activities, negotiating with local authorities and utility companies for better services for blind people. Offers income support programs to provide financial assistance with optical, medical, dental, clothing, and educational expenses. Advises members on their rights regarding entitlement programs; offers free legal aid. Organizes hospital visitations and sporting and social events including debates and lectures.

★ 4968 ★ National League for Nursing (NLN)

61 Broadway 33rd Fl.
New York, NY 10006-2701
Phone: (212)363-5555 **Free:** 800-669-1656
Fax: (212)812-0393
Email: rcorcor@nln.org
Website: http://www.nln.org
Ruth Corcoran, EdD RN, CEO

Fnded: 1893. **Mem:** 12,300. **State Groups:** 33. **Desc:** Champions the pursuit of quality nursing education. A professional association of nursing faculty, education agencies, healthcare agencies, allied/public agencies, and public members whose mission is to advance quality nursing education that prepares the nursing workforce to meet the needs of diverse populations in an ever-changing health care environment. Serves as the primary source of information about every type of nursing education, from the LVN and LPN to the EDD and PHD. There are 33 affiliated constituent leagues that provide a local forum for members. The National League for Nursing Accrediting Commission is an independent corporate affiliate of the NLN, responsible for providing accreditation services to all levels of nursing education. NLN's bimonthly update is available free of charge on the website and by email. **Pub:** *Nursing Data Review*, annual. Book. Contains tables and graphs of data. • *Nursing Education Perspectives*, bimonthly. Journal. Contains news, legislative updates, education, service analyses, and editorials. • *State Approved Schools of Nursing - LPN*, annual. • *State Approved Schools of Nursing - RN*, annual. • Books.Covers education, leadership, nursing history, culture and diversity, theory development, and professional issues.

★ 4969 ★ National Lymphedema Network

1611 Telegraph Ave., Ste. 1111
Oakland, CA 94612-2138
Phone: 800-541-3259 **Fax:** (510)208-3110
Email: nln@lymphnet.org
Website: http://www.lymphnet.org
Saskia R.J. Thiadens, R.N., Exec. Dir.

Fnded: 1988. **Mem:** 2,800. **Desc:** Persons with lymphedema and their families, health care professionals. Provides education and support to patients, health care professionals and the general public by disseminating information on the prevention and management of primary and secondary lymphedema. Also support research into the causes and possible alternative treatments for this often incapacitating condition. Offers referral service to medical facilities, helps locate support groups and sponsors research and educational programs. **Pub:** *NLN Newsletter*, quarterly. Newsletter. Features cutting-edge medical articles, features, and resource listings. • *Resource Guide*. Contains list of treatment centers, health care professionals and sup pliers, Support Groups, PenPals, and updates on professional training courses.

★ 4970 ★ National Marfan Foundation (NMF)

22 Manhasset Ave.
Port Washington, NY 11050-2023
Phone: (516)883-8712 **Free:** 800-862-7326
Fax: (516)883-8040
Email: support@marfan.org
Website: http://www.marfan.org
Karen Wolk, CSW, Dir. Support Svcs.

Fnded: 1981. **Mem:** 25,000. **State Groups:** 15. **Local Groups:** 60. **Desc:** Persons affected with the Marfan syndrome and related connective tissue disorders; families of affected persons; genetic counselors; cardiologists, ophthalmologists, orthopedists, and other medical professionals. (Marfan syndrome is a heritable disorder of the connective tissue affecting the skeleton, lungs, eyes, heart, and blood vessels.) Objectives are to: disseminate accurate and timely information on Marfan syndrome; act as support network and provide a means for patients and relatives to share experiences; improve medical care. Supports and fosters research. **Pub:** *Cardiac Concerns, Ocular Concerns, Pediatric Concerns, Orthopedic Concerns*. Brochures. Overview of related disorders, physical activity guidelines. • *Connective Issues*, quarterly. Newsletter. Includes research reports, chapter news, and legislative reports. *Price:* Included in membership dues. • *How Do Your Genes Fit?*. Video. Explains about genetic disorders, especially, Marfan Syndrome. Contains information for middle school students, families and support groups. • *The Marfan Syndrome*. Booklet. • *The Marfan Syndrome: A Booklet for Teachers*. Booklet. • *The Marfan Syndrome: A Booklet for Teenagers*. Booklet.

★ 4971 ★ National Marrow Donor Program (NMDP)

3001 Broadway NE, Ste. 500
Minneapolis, MN 55413-1753
Phone: (612)627-5800 **Free:** 800-627-7692
Fax: (612)627-8125
Website: http://www.marrow.org
Jeffrey W. Chell, MD, CEO

Fnded: 1986. **Mem:** 468. **Desc:** Facilitates unrelated donor stem cell transplants for patients with life-threatening blood diseases who do not have matching donors in their families. Facilitates more than 150 transplants each month. Provides a single point of access for all sources of blood stem cells used in transplantation: marrow, peripheral blood, and umbilical cord blood. The Registry is able to search its own database and provides physicians with information on multiple stem cell sources for life-saving transplants. Since 1987, the NMDP has recruited a diverse Registry of approximately four million potential volunteer marrow and blood stem cell donors, provided transplants to more than 15,000 patients, developed education and recruitment initiatives to increase the diversity of the Registry, increased the number of minority patients receiving transplants each year, developed patient advocacy services, established a system of listing cord blood units within its own national Registry. Materials are available free of charge for both potential donors and patients. There is access to interpreters in over 141 languages for these materials. **Pub:** *Living*

Gift of Life. Brochure. • *Marrow Messenger*, annual. • *Medical Professionals' Guide to Unrelated Marrow Transplantation*. • *The Missing Piece*, annual. Brochure. • Brochures. **Frmly:** National Bone Marrow Donor Registry.

★ 4972 ★ National Mastitis Council (NMC)

2820 Walton Commons West, Ste. 131
Madison, WI 53711
Phone: (608)663-1255 **Fax:** (608)663-1249
Email: nmc@nmconline.org
Website: http://www.nmconline.org
Anne Saeman, Exec. Dir.

Fnded: 1961. **Mem:** 2,000. **Desc:** Seeks to resolve the problem of bovine mastitis (inflammation of the udder) by developing and distributing factual information on mastitis control and encouraging mastitis research. Conducts research and education programs. Helps organize and coordinate the activities of state councils. **Pub:** *National Mastitis Council–Annual Meeting Proceedings*. Proceedings. Contains papers on topics related to the production of high quality milk and the prevention of mastitis. *Price:* Included in membership dues; $15 to nonmembers. • *Udder Topics*, bimonthly. Newsletter. For people working in the dairy industry concerned with milk production. Covers topics related to the production of high quality milk. *Price:* Included in membership dues. • Also publishes books, brochures, flyers, and monographs.

★ 4973 ★ National Maternal and Child Health Clearinghouse (NMCHC)

c/o Health Resources and Services Admin.
U.S. Department of Health and Human Services
Parklawn Bldg.
5600 Fishers Ln.
Rockville, MD 20857
Phone: (301)443-2170
Email: ask@hrsa.gov
Website: http://www.ask.hrsa.gov/
Kristin C. Moyer, Project Dir.

Fnded: 1983. **Desc:** Federal, state, and local agencies; voluntary organizations; health professionals; consumers. Collects, and disseminates information on maternal and child health, including perinatal health; prenatal care; infant, child, and adolescent health; immunization; newborn screening; oral health; emergency medical services for children; health and safety in child care; lead poisoning prevention; violence and injury prevention; children with special health needs; family support and family-centered care; maternal and child health programs and services; human genetics, nutrition, and pregnancy care. Human Services, Health Resources and Services Administration, and Maternal and Child Health Bureau. **Pub:** *Maternal and Child Health Publicaitons Catalog*, annual. Catalog. Lists approximatley 350 volumes and ordering information. *Price:* Free. • *Maternal and Child Health Thesaurus, Second Edition*. • *Reaching Out: A Directory of National Organizations Related to Maternal and Child Health*. Directories. • *The Surgeon General's Workshop on Self-Help and Public Health*. Proceedings. • Approximately 350 active volumes; most written for professionals.

★ 4974 ★ National Meals on Wheels Foundation

PO Box 1727
Iowa City, IA 52244
Phone: (319)354-0862 **Fax:** (319)354-0845
Email: info@nationalmealsonwheels.org
Website: http://www.nationalmealsonwheels.org/
Connie Benton Wolfe, Exec. Dir.

Fnded: 1977. **Mem:** 1,000. **Desc:** Grants-making organization. **Pub:** *Collection of Innovative Models*. • *Monthly Membership Updates*, monthly. • *NANASP News*, quarterly. Newsletter. Contains legislative and membership updates, and new product information. *Price:* Included in membership dues. • *National Standards for Congregate Meals*. • *National Standards for Home-Delivered Meals*. • *Preparing Nutrition Programs for the Nineties*. • *Special Bulletins*, monthly. Bulletin. • *Special Report to Members*, quarterly. Newsletter. *Price:* Included in membership dues. • Annual Report, annual. **Frmly:** (1978) National Association of Title Seven Directors.

★ 4975 ★ National Medic-Card Systems (NMCS)

1070 Commerce St., Ste. D
San Marcos, CA 92069
Phone: (760)744-1560 **Fax:** (760)744-1569
Email: mikeb@bhprint.com
Michael C. Barksdale, Sales Mgr.

Fnded: 1978. **Desc:** Produces wallet-size medical cards that have five sections, fold into the size of a credit card, and describe individuals' medical conditions in detail. **Frmly:** (1986) National Medic-Card Society.

★ 4976 ★ National Medical Association (NMA)

1012 10th St. NW
Washington, DC 20001
Phone: (202)204-1223 **Fax:** (202)371-1162
Email: brainhardt@nmanet.org
Website: http://www.nmanet.org
Patricia Norman, Contact

Fnded: 1895. **Mem:** 4,000. **Reg. Groups:** 6. **State Groups:** 42. **Local Groups:** 93. **Desc:** Professional society of minority physicians. **Pub:** *Journal of the National Medical Association*, monthly. Journal. Contains scientific articles. *Price:* $35. • *NMA News*, quarterly. Newsletter. Contains medical and NMA news targeted to members.

★ 4977 ★ National Medical Fellowships (NMF)

5 Handover Sq., 15th Fl.
New York, NY 10004
Phone: (212)483-8880 **Fax:** (212)483-8897
Email: info@nmfonline.org
Website: http://www.nmfonline.org
Vivian Fox, Pres. /CEO

Fnded: 1946. **Reg. Groups:** 2. **Desc:** Promotes education of minority students in medicine. Provides need-based scholarships, special merit awards, and leadership opportunities to medical students of African American, Native American, Mexican American and mainland Puerto Rican heritage. **Pub:** *NMF Update*, quarterly. • Newsletter. • Annual Report. **Frmly:** (1952) Provident Medical Associates.

★ 4978 ★ National MedPeds Residents' Association (NMPRA)

c/o Renee Gaines
Department of Internal Medicine
1542 Tulane Ave., Rm. 447
New Orleans, LA 70112
Fax: (270)596-5951
Email: nmpra@medpeds.org
Website: http://www.medpeds.org/
David Kendrick, MD, Pres.

Fnded: 1967. **Mem:** 400. **Desc:** Promotes the practice of MedPeds, combined internal medicine and pediatrics; educates and serves MedPeds residency and serves as a resource for medical students interested in MedPeds. **Pub:** *MedPeds News*, quarterly. Newsletter. Serves as catalyst to increase communication between residents and residency programs in the combined field of medicine-pediatrics. *Price:* included in membership dues.

★ 4979 ★ National Mental Health Association (NMHA)

2001 N Beauregard St., 12th Fl.
Alexandria, VA 22311
Phone: (703)684-7722 **Free:** 800-969-NMHA
Fax: (703)684-5968
Email: infoctr@nmha.org
Website: http://www.nmha.org
Michael Faenza, CEO/Pres.

Fnded: 1909. **Mem:** 416,000. **Reg. Groups:** 340. **Desc:** Addresses all aspects of mental health and mental illness and is dedicated to improving mental health, preventing mental disorders, and achieving victory over mental illnesses. NMHA, in partnership with more than 340 affiliates across the country, accomplishes its mission through advocacy, public education, research, and service. **Pub:** *The ADA and People with Mental Illness: An Employer's Manual*. Book. A guide to accommodations for people w/mental & emotional disorders. *Price:* $40. • *Aiding People in Conflict: A Guide for Law Enforcement*. • *The Bell*, 12/year. Newsletter includes association news, calendar of events, legislative news, mental health/health trends and research news. **Frmly:** National Association for Mental Health; (1980) Mental Health Association.

★ 4980 ★ National Mental Health Consumers' Self-Help Clearinghouse (NMHCSHC)

1211 Chestnut St., Ste. 1207
Philadelphia, PA 19107
Phone: (215)751-1810 **Free:** 800-553-4KEY
Fax: (215)636-6312
Email: info@mhselfhelp.org
Website: http://www.mhselfhelp.org
Joseph Rogers, Exec. Dir.

Fnded: 1985. **Desc:** Serves mental health consumers/ex-patients and consumer/ex-patients, self-help groups, and consumer-run services. Provides technical assistance in the development of self-help projects, including advocacy groups, support groups, consumer-run services and self-advocacy efforts. Offers informational referrals, written material, and consulting services. **Pub:** *Advocacy and Recovery Using the Internet*. • *Art and Science of Writing Proposals That Win*. • *Consumer-Run Businesses and Services*. • *Consumer-Run Drop-In Centers*. • *Fighting Stigma*. • *History of the Consumer Movement*. • *Organizing and Operating a Speakers Bureau*. • *Raising Money for a Self-Help/Advocacy Group*. • *Self-Advocacy*. • *Serving on Boards and Committees*. • *Starting a Self-Help/Advocacy Group*. • *Systems Advocacy*.

★ 4981 ★ National Minority AIDS Council (NMAC)

1931 13th St. NW
Washington, DC 20009
Phone: (202)483-6622 **Fax:** (202)483-1135
Email: info@nmac.org
Website: http://www.nmac.org
Paul A. Kawata, Exec. Dir.

Fnded: 1986. **Mem:** 480. **Reg. Groups:** 2. **State Groups:** 20. **Local Groups:** 160. **Desc:** Public health departments and AIDS service organizations. Serves as a clearinghouse of information on AIDS as it affects minority communities in the U.S. Facilitates discussion among national minority organizations about AIDS. Maintains Project Health, Education, and AIDS Leadership, which provides computer usage, strategic planning, financial management, and volunteer program development assistance to AIDS service organizations, and Project Volunteer Information, Technical Assistance, and Leadership, which provides technical assistance in volunteer program development and maintenance. Conducts training conferences. Offers educational and research programs; compiles statistics. Maintains speakers' bureau. **Pub:** *Computer Technical Assistance Manual*. • *Leadership Reprint Series*, quarterly. Includes information on strategies for addressing HIV/AIDS and scientific updates. • *Legislative Update*, bimonthly. • *NMAC HEALer*, bimonthly. Includes updates on projects, community needs, and statistics. • *NMAC Update*, bimonthly. Newsletter. Includes association information and coverage of HIV/AIDS issues. • *Technical Assistance Manual for Volunteer Program Development*. • *Technical Assistance Newsletter*, bimonthly. Newsletter.

★ 4982 ★ National Minority Health Association (NMHA)
10 E Baltimore St., Ste. 1404
Baltimore, MD 21202
Free: (866)347-9959 **Fax:** (410)347-1542
Dr. David Dalton, Chm.

Fnded: 1987. **Mem:** 53,000. **Reg. Groups:** 5. **State Groups:** 27. **Local Groups:** 7. **Desc:** Health care providers and associations, consumers, executives and administrators, educators, pharmaceutical and health insurance companies, and other corporations with an interest in health care. Seeks to identify and focus attention on the health needs of minorities. Promotes: more effective research in minority health issues; better training of health care practitioners; development of programs that encourage minorities to pursue careers in the health care industry and educate minority communities on the importance of good health. Initiates discussions with professional health organizations, academic institutions, state and federal governments, and health departments to develop strategies to improve the quality and availability of health care, health delivery systems, and health professionals to minority communities. Maintains speakers' bureau, conducts research and educational programs; sponsors children's programs; complies statistics. **Pub:** *The National Minority Health Association News*, quarterly.

★ 4983 ★ National MPS Society
45 Packard Dr.
Bangor, ME 04401
Phone: (207)947-1445 **Fax:** (207)990-3074
Email: info@mpssociety.org
Website: http://www.mpssociety.org
Barbara Wedehase, Exec. Dir.

Fnded: 1974. **Mem:** 800. **Reg. Groups:** 9. **Desc:** Professionals and families devoted to educating the public and discovering and aiding families of MPS and ML children. Mucopolysaccharidoses (MPS) and mucolipidoses (ML) are extremely rare hereditary diseases caused by particular enzyme deficiencies and range in severity from strictly bone and joint involvement to massive complications in all organ systems. Helps to facilitate diagnosis and treatment through referrals to doctors and hospitals. Maintains parent referral service to direct families with newly diagnosed MPS and ML children to other members. **Pub:** *Courage*, quarterly. Newsletter. • *Ethan's Feeling Switch*. Book. *Price:* $5. • *Hunter*. Booklet. *Price:* $1. • *Hurler*. Booklet. *Price:* $1. • *I-Cell*. Booklet. • *Management Anesthesia*. Booklet. • *Management of MPS & ML*. Booklet. • *Maroteaux-Lamy*. Booklet. *Price:* $1. • *Morquio*. Booklet. *Price:* $1. • *Sanfilippo*. Booklet. • *Sly*. Booklet. **Frmly:** (1975) Parents for MPS; (1985) MPS Society.

★ 4984 ★ National Multiple Sclerosis Society (NMSS)
733 3rd Ave.
New York, NY 10017
Phone: (212)986-3240 **Free:** 800-FIGHT-MS
Fax: (212)986-7981
Email: info@nmss.org
Website: http://www.nmss.org
Michael J. Duggan, Pres.

Fnded: 1946. **Mem:** 470,000. **State Groups:** 93. **Desc:** Stimulates, supports, and coordinates research into the cause, treatment, and cure of multiple sclerosis; provides services for persons with MS and related diseases and their families; aids in establishing MS clinics and therapy centers. Conducts Creative Will, biennial competition for artists with MS. Maintains numerous committees including international and research and medical programs, and services. Maintains speakers' bureau; compiles statistics. **Pub:** *Inside MS*, 4/year. Magazine. Contains book reviews, research updates, legislative updates, and annual report. *Price:* Included in membership dues. **Frmly:** (1947) Association for Advancementof Research on Multiple Sclerosis.

★ 4985 ★ National Native American AIDS Prevention Center
436-14th St., Ste. 1020
Oakland, CA 94610
Phone: (510)444-2051 **Fax:** (510)444-1593
Email: information@nnaapc.org
Website: http://www.nnaapc.org
Michael Bird, Exec. Dir.

Fnded: 1987. **Desc:** Network of concerned Native people. Works to stop the spread of HIV and related diseases, including sexually transmitted disease and tuberculosis, among American Indians, Alaska Natives, and Native Hawaiians by improving their health status through empowerment and self determination. Serves as a resource to Native communities and to support community efforts by providing education and information services, thereby ehancing the physical, spiritual, and economic health of Native people. Sponsors educational programs. Maintains speakers' bureau. Compiles statistics. **Pub:** *Season*, annual. Journal. **Frmly:** (1998) National Indian AIDS Hotline.

★ 4986 ★ National Native American EMS Association (NNAEMSA)
c/o Chebon Tiger, Exec.Dir.
1701 S Mays, Ste. J
PO Box 197
Round Rock, TX 78664
Email: nnaemsa@earthlink.net
Website: http://heds.org/nnaemsa.htm
Chebon Tiger, Exec. Dir.

Desc: Represents and promotes first responders, emergency medical technicians, emergency nurses, and emergency physicians of Native American descent. **Pub:** *NNAEMSA News*. • Reports.

★ 4987 ★ National Necrotizing Fasciitis Foundation
c/o Donna Batdorff
2731 Porter SW
Grand Rapids, MI 49509-2140
Phone: (616)261-2538 **Fax:** (616)261-2539
Email: dbatdorff@nnff.org
Website: http://www.nnff.org
Donna Batdorff, Contact

Fnded: 1997. **Desc:** Strives to educate and offer support to those affected by necrotizing fasciitis (flesh eating bacteria).

★ 4988 ★ National Network for the Disabled
c/o Linda Walls
PO Box 3574
Gardena, CA 90247-7274
Phone: (310)638-5717 **Fax:** (310)638-5986
Linda Walls, Founder-Pres.

Fnded: 1980. **Mem:** 11,000. **Desc:** Provides support, companionship, and networking opportunities for elderly individuals and parents of disabled children. Conducts research. Sponsors education on such topics as assertiveness, resources, and medical options. Provides transportation and emergency services, including a food program through which meals are delivered to homes. Conducts special events for parents and children, including picnics and field trips; special programs on nutrition and accessible travel with groups. **Pub:** Brochure, monthly. • Newsletter, monthly. **Frmly:** Parent Networking Program.

★ 4989 ★ National Network for Youth (NNY)
1319 F St. NW, 4th Fl.
Washington, DC 20004
Phone: (202)783-7949 **Fax:** (202)783-7955
Email: nnymail@nn4youth.org
Website: http://www.nn4youth.org
Gretchen Noll, Exec. Dir.

Fnded: 1974. **Mem:** 850. **Reg. Groups:** 10. **State Groups:** 35. **Local Groups:** 400. **Desc:** Works to ensure that young people can be safe and grow up to lead healthy and productive lives. engages in public education efforts, promotes youth/adult partnerships, and strives to strengthen staff and community-based organization capacity to provide effective programs and services to youth in high-risk situations. Training and technical assistance is provided in a variety of areas including professional development of youth workers, youth leadership, peer education, HIV/AIDS and substance abuse prevention, grant writing, and community and youth development. The National Network for Youth is a sponsoring member of the Council on Accreditation of Services for Families and Children. **Pub:** *CYD Journal*, quarterly. Journal. Serves as an international voice to promote a holistic view of youth and community development. *Price:* $29. • *Doing What We Do Best: Guide to Replication of an Independent Living Project*. Outlines ways to develop a successful independent living program; includes project definition, implementation procedures, local reports, resources. *Price:* $3 for members; $4 for nonmembers. • *Helping Them Do Their Best: Guide to Using Volunteers in Runaway Centers*. Describes the benefits and essential components of a successful volunteer program; includes volunteer profile and innovative program models. *Price:* $3 for members; $4 for nonmembers. • *Network News*, quarterly. Provides updates on youth issues from a national perspective; features columns written by youth, an issues forum, legislative updates, and resources. *Price:* Free to members; $30/year for nonmembers. • *Policy Reporter*, quarterly. Newsletter. Reports on and analyzes current legislation, federal policy, and court decisions that impact services to youth. *Price:* Included in membership dues; $30/year for nonmembers. • Newsletters.Two newsletters emailed to members. *Price:* For members. **AKA:** National Network.

★ 4990 ★ National Neurofibromatosis Foundation (NNFF)
95 Pine St., 16th Fl.
New York, NY 10005
Phone: (212)344-6633 **Free:** 800-323-7938
Fax: (212)747-0004
Email: nnff@nf.org
Website: http://www.nf.org/
W. John Radziejewski, Dir. of Pub. Ed.

Fnded: 1978. **Mem:** 1,700. **State Groups:** 37. **Desc:** The leading resource on neurofibromatosis, a genetic disorder that causes tumors to grow along nerves throughout the body. Provides direct services to children and adults with NF, as well as information and resources to the public and medical professionals via a toll-free number and a website. **Pub:** *Neurofibromatosis News*, quarterly. Newsletter. *Price:* Free for members.

★ 4991 ★ National Neurotrauma Society
c/o Linda Garcia
PO Box 143060
Gainesville, FL 32608
Phone: (352)271-1169 **Fax:** (352)271-3060
Email: lindahou@aol.com
Website: http://www.neurotrauma.org
Linda Garcia, Contact

Mem: 500. **Desc:** Conducts scientific research in neurotrauma field.

★ 4992 ★ National Niemann Pick Disease Foundation (NPD)
c/o Barb Vorpahl
415 Madison Ave.
PO Box 49
Fort Atkinson, WI 53538
Phone: (920)563-0930 **Free:** 877-287-3672
Fax: (920)563-0931
Email: webmaster@nnpdf.org
Website: http://www.nnpdf.org
Barb Vorpahl, Chm.

Fnded: 1992. **Mem:** 4,500. **Desc:** Parents, medical and educational professionals, and friends. Works to promote medical research on Niemann-Pick Disease (NPD), a disorder which prevents metabolizing of the sphingomyelin lipid or cholesterol. Provides medical and educational information; offers support to families of children with NPD; facilitates genetic counseling for parents; supports legislation that affects patients and families with NPD; sponsors medical research. **Pub:** *Niemann-Pick Newsletter*, quarterly. Newsletter. *Price:* Free. • Directory.

★ 4993 ★ National Nurses Association of Kenya (NNAK)
PO Box 49422
Nairobi, Kenya
Phone: 254 20 229083 **Fax:** 254 20 335438

Fnded: 1958. **Local Groups:** 19. **Lang(s):** English. **Desc:** Nurses in Kenya. Promotes primary health care; facilitates exchange and cooperation between members; upholds ethics of the profession and encourages high standards. Represents members' interests before the government; provides help for members in times of difficulty; offers scholarships and operates trust fund. Operates foster child program. Works in conjunction with the National Council of Women in Kenya. Conducts workshops and seminars. **Pub:** *Kenya Nurses Newsletter*, quarterly. Newsletter. • *Kenya Nursing Journal*, semiannual. Journal.

★ 4994 ★ National Nursing Staff Development Organization
7794 Grow Dr.
Pensacola, FL 32514
Phone: (850)474-0995 **Free:** 800-489-1995
Fax: (850)484-8762
Email: nnsdo@puetzamc.com
Website: http://www.nnsdo.org
Belinda E. Puetz, PhD, Exec. Dir.

Fnded: 1989. **Mem:** 1,995. **Nat'l Groups:** 38. **Desc:** Advances the specialty practice of staff development for the enhancement of quality healthcare outcomes. Staff development, as a specialty of nursing practice, is defined by standards, based on research critical to quality patient and organizational outcomes. Provides a forum for networking among staff development educators. **Pub:** *Journal for Nurses in Staff Development*, periodic. Journal. • *Trendlines*, bimonthly. Newsletter.

★ 4995 ★ National Nutrition Foundation
c/o Merrilynne Hayes, Natl.Exec.Off.
PO Box 16
Upper Pakenham, VIC 3810, Australia
Phone: 61 3 59427421 **Fax:** 61 3 59427588
Email: m.hayes@nutritionaustralia.org
Website: http://www.nutritionaustralia.org/

Fnded: 1979. **Desc:** Promotes optimal health through food variety and physical activity to individuals living in Australia.

★ 4996 ★ National Optometric Association (NOA)
3723 Main St.
PO Box F
East Chicago, IN 46312
Phone: (219)398-1832 **Free:** 877-394-2020
Fax: (219)398-1077
Email: marshall@indiana.edu
Website: http://www.natoptassoc.org
Edward France, Jr., Pres.

Fnded: 1969. **Mem:** 450. **Nat'l Groups:** 1. **Reg. Groups:** 5. **Desc:** Optometrists dedicated to increasing awareness of the status of eye/vision health in the minority community and the national community at-large; and strives to make known the impact of the eye/vision dysfunction on the effectiveness and productivity of citizens and the academic proficiency of students. Conducts national minority recruiting programs, job placement, assistance programs for graduates, practitioners, and optometric organizations, and the promotion of delivery of care. Maintains speakers' bureau. Offers specialized education program. **Pub:** *NOA Newsletter*, semiannual. Newsletter. *Price:* Free.

★ 4997 ★ National Optometry Association (NOA)
PO Box 35215
Chicago, IL 60707-0215
Phone: (708)453-0080 **Fax:** (708)453-0083
Email: noa@rentamark.com
Website: http://www.rentamark.com/noa/

Fnded: 1975. **Mem:** 68,786. **Desc:** Optometrists. Seeks to increase members' public visibility and professional influence. Provides members with further education and recommends books to help the profession. Provides benefits. **Pub:** *NOA-E Journal*, monthly. Journal.

★ 4998 ★ National Oral Health Information Clearinghouse (NOHIC)
1 NOHIC Way
Bethesda, MD 20892-3500
Phone: (301)402-7364 **Fax:** (301)907-8830
Email: nohic@nidcr.nih.gov
Website: http://www.nohic.nidcr.nih.gov
Patricia Sheridan, Project Officer

Fnded: 1994. **Desc:** Serves as resource for patients, health professionals, and the public seeking information on the oral health of special care patients, including people with genetic or systemic disorders that compromise oral health, people whose medical treatment causes oral problems, and people with mental or physical disabilities that make good oral hygiene practices difficult. Collects and maintains an online database on oral health and special care issues. **Pub:** *Chemotherapy and Your Mouth*. Brochure. *Price:* Free. • *Diabetes and Periodontal Disease: A Guide for Patients*. Brochure. *Price:* Free. • *Radiation Treatment and Your Mouth*, annual. Brochure. *Price:* Free. • *Temporomandibular Disorders*. Brochure. *Price:* Free. • Also distributes other publications on special care topics, oral health care, oral cancer, smokeless tobacco, dry mouth, and oral complications of cancer treatment.

★ 4999 ★ National Organization on Adolescent Pregnancy, Parenting and Prevention (NOAPP)
2401 Pennsylvania Ave. NW, Ste. 350
Washington, DC 20037
Phone: (202)293-8370 **Fax:** (202)293-8805
Email: noappp@noappp.org
Website: http://www.noappp.org
A. Charlene Leach, Exec. Dir.

Fnded: 1979. **Mem:** 2,000. **Desc:** Professionals, policy makers, community and state leaders, and other concerned individuals and organizations. Promotes comprehensive and coordinated services designed for the prevention and resolution of problems associated with adolescent pregnancy, parenthood and prevention. Supports families in expanding their capability of nurturing children and setting standards that encourage their healthy development through loving, stable relationships. Programs include: providing advocacy services at local, state, and national levels for adolescent pregnancy issues; sharing information and promoting public awareness; conducting conferences, training institutes and workshops to encourage the establishment of effective programs; coalition building assistance. **Pub:** *NOAPPP Network Newsletter*, quarterly. Newsletter. Contains resource and research reviews, state highlights, legislative focus, and successful program models. **Frmly:** (1993) National Organization of Adolescent Pregnancy and Parenting.

★ 5000 ★ National Organization for Albinism and Hypopigmentation (NOAH)
PO Box 959
East Hampstead, NH 03826-0959
Free: 800-473-2310 **Fax:** (603)887-6049
Email: noah@albinism.org
Website: http://www.albinism.org
Michael McGowan, Pres.

Fnded: 1982. **Mem:** 1,000. **Reg. Groups:** 40. **State Groups:** 21. **Desc:** Individuals with albinism and their families; health care professionals; others interested in learning more about albinism. (Albinism is an inherited metabolic disorder that results in reduced pigment in the hair, eyes, and/or skin of those it affects; people with albinism also have impaired eye function including decreased visual acuity, involuntary eye movements, and increased sensitivity to light.) Seeks to educate teachers, health care professionals, and the public about albinism. Provides support to individuals with albinism and their families. Encourages research on the cause, results, and management of the disorder. **Pub:** *NOAH Information Bulletin*, periodic. Bulletin. Provides information on various aspects of albinism. • *NOAH News*, semiannual. • *The Student with Albinism in the Regular Classroom*. Book.

★ 5001 ★ National Organization for Associate Degree Nursing (N-OADN)
c/o Sharon L. Bernier
Montgomery College
7600 Takoma Ave.
Takoma Park, MD 20912
Phone: (301)650-1355 **Fax:** (301)650-1346
Email: sbernier@aol.com
Website: http://www.noadn.org
Sharon L. Bernier, Pres.

Fnded: 1986. **Mem:** 750. **State Groups:** 10. **Desc:** Individuals interested in retaining current competency level examinations and endorsement of RN licensure from state to state for associate degree nursing graduates. Represents and advances the status of associate degree nursing education and practice. Provides networking among members to facilitate the exchange of legislative information and support. Offers clearinghouse for interpretation of legal issues and liability insurance. **Pub:** *NOADN Newsletter*, quarterly. • Newsletter, quarterly. Includes national and state association news, activities, and information. • Also issues position papers. **Frmly:** (1986) National Organization for Advancement of Associate Degree Nursing.

★ 5002 ★ National Organization for Competency Assurance (NOCA)
2025 M St. NW, Ste. 800
Washington, DC 20036
Phone: (202)367-1165 **Fax:** (202)367-2165
Email: info@noca.org
Website: http://www.noca.org
Wade Delk, Exec. Dir.

Fnded: 1977. **Mem:** 300. **Desc:** Organizations conducting certification programs for occupations and professionals and trade associations representing these professionals. Seeks to increase public awareness, understanding, and acceptance of private sector credentialing as an alternative to licensure; promotes nonlicensed but certified practitioners as a means to achieving high quality and cost containment. **Pub:** *NOCA News*, quarterly. Newsletter. *Price:* $95/year. **Frmly:** (1989) National Commission for Health Certifying Agencies.

★ 5003 ★ National Organization on Disability (NOD)
910 16th St. NW, Ste. 600
Washington, DC 20006
Phone: (202)293-5960 **Fax:** (202)293-7999
Email: ability@nod.org
Website: http://www.nod.org
Brewster Thackeray, Dir. Communications

Fnded: 1982. **State Groups:** 50. **Local Groups:** 120. **Desc:** Works to promote the full and equal participation of people with disabilities in all aspects of life.

★ 5004 ★ National Organization of Life and Health Insurance Guaranty Associations (NOLHGA)
13873 Park Center Rd., Ste. 329
Herndon, VA 20171
Website: http://www.nolhga.com

Mem: 52. **Desc:** Promotes the life and health insurance guaranty industry.

★ 5005 ★ National Organization of Nurse Practitioners Faculties
1522 K St. NW, Ste. 702
Washington, DC 20005
Phone: (202)289-8044 **Fax:** (202)289-8046
Email: nonpf@nonpf.org
Website: http://www.nonpf.com
Kathryn Werner, MPA, Exec. Dir.
Fnded: 1981. **Mem:** 1,000. **Desc:** Works to promote public health by developing and implementing nurse practitioner education. Disseminates research related to nurse practitioner education; provides a forum for the exchange of information; works to influence policy affecting nurse practitioners; and develops national guidelins and criteria for nurse practitioner educational programs. **Pub:** *National Directory of NP Programs*, biennial. Directory. • *NONPF Quarterly Newsletter*, quarterly. Newsletter. • Brochure.

★ 5006 ★ National Organization for Rare Disorders (NORD)
PO Box 1968
Danbury, CT 06813-1968
Phone: (203)744-0100 **Free:** 800-999-6673
Fax: (203)798-2291
Email: orphan@rarediseases.org
Website: http://www.rarediseases.org
Susan Olivo, Admin. Assistant
Fnded: 1983. **Mem:** 65,000. **Nat'l Groups:** 130. **Desc:** Doctors, professionals, academics, voluntary health organizations, and individuals interested in rare disorders. Serves as a clearinghouse for information concerning rare disorders. Objectives are: to monitor the Orphan Drug Act; to link individuals with rare disorders together for mutual support; to stimulate research on rare diseases; to foster communication among voluntary agencies, health-related industries, and government bodies. (Orphan drugs are used in the treatment of rare disorders. Since their use is not widespread, most drug companies cannot expect to profit from the development and manufacture of these drugs. The Orphan Drug Act gives financial assistance and tax incentives to drug companies that develop these drugs.) Provides information on rare disorders and referrals to organizations. **Pub:** *NORD On-Line Bulletin*, monthly. Newsletter. Updating service for voluntary health agency members on legislation and other issues related to orphan drugs and diseases. Includes meeting schedule. *Price:* Included in membership dues, for organizations. • *NORD Resource Guide.* An alphabetical listing of national support groups and foundations that service the needs of people with rare disorders and disabilities. • *Orphan Disease Update*, 3/year. Newsletter. For individual members updating information on orphan diseases and orphan drug research; discusses legislative issues related to health. *Price:* Included in membership dues. • *Physician Guide to Rare Diseases.* Book.

★ 5007 ★ National Osteoporosis Foundation (NOF)
1232 22nd St., NW
Washington, DC 20037-1292
Phone: (202)223-2226 **Fax:** (202)223-2237
Email: nofmail@nof.org
Website: http://www.nof.org
Judith Cranford, Exec. Dir.
Fnded: 1984. **Mem:** 300,000. **Desc:** A national voluntary health organization dedicated to reducing the widespread prevalence of osteoporosis. (Osteoporosis is an excessive loss of bone tissue which often results in fractures of the hip, spine, and wrist.) Seeks to: increase public awareness and knowledge about osteoporosis; provide information about osteoporosis to sufferers and their families; educate physicians and allied health professionals; advocate for increased governmental support for research on osteoporosis; and support basic biomedical, epidemiological, clinical, behavioral, and social research and research training. Sponsors Research Grant Award program; conducts public and professional education programs. **Pub:** *Boning Up on Osteoporosis. Price:* $3 each; $2.75/101 or more. • *Facts About Osteoporosis, Arthritis and Osteoarthritis. Price:* $.30 each; $.25/500 copies or more. • *Falls and Related Fractures. Price:* $.75 each; $.70/500 or more. • *How Strong Are Your Bones*, periodic. *Price:* $.70 each; $.60/500 or more. • *Living with Osteoporosis. Price:* $.35 each; $.30/500 copies or more. • *Medications and Bone Loss. Price:* $.75 each; $.70/500 or more. • *Osteoporosis Education Kit. Price:* $65 each. • *Osteoporosis Report*, quarterly. Newsletter. Includes current medical journal references and listing of consumer publications and recent articles related to the subject of osteoporosis. *Price:* Included in membership dues. • *Stand Up to Osteoporosis. Price:* $.45 each; $.40/500 copies or more. **Frmly:** (1985) The Osteoporosis Foundation.

★ 5008 ★ National Osteoporosis Society
Camerton
Bath BA2 0PJ, United Kingdom
Phone: 44 1761 471771 **Fax:** 44 1761 471104
Email: info@nos.org.uk
Website: http://www.nos.org.uk
Fnded: 1986. **Mem:** 27,000. **Local Groups:** 130. **Desc:** National charity dedicated to improving the diagnosis, prevention, and treatment of osteoporosis. Works with health care professionals to facilitate greater understanding of the needs of individuals with the disease. Offers support to people with osteoporosis and their families through a range of detailed information booklets, a national telephone helpline and a network of regional support groups throughout the UK. Raises funds for research to increase understanding of the disease and improve treatment options and patient care. Raises awareness of the disease and campaigns to promote bone health.

★ 5009 ★ National Ovarian Cancer Association (NOCA)
27 Park Rd.
Toronto, ON, Canada M4W 2N2
Phone: (416)962-2700 **Free:** 877-413-7970
Fax: (416)962-2701
Email: noca@ovariancanada.org
Website: http://www.ovariancanada.org/
Desc: Committed to overcoming ovarian cancer, supports women and families living with the disease, promotes awareness to the public and health care professions, funds research to develop reliable early detection techniques, improved treatments and a cure.

★ 5010 ★ National Ovarian Cancer Coalition (NOCC)
500 NE Spanish River Blvd., Ste. 14
Boca Raton, FL 33431
Phone: (561)393-0005 **Free:** 888-OVA-RIAN
Fax: (561)393-7275
Email: noccnat@ovarian.org
Website: http://www.ovarian.org
Fnded: 1996. **Mem:** 16,000. **State Groups:** 25. **Desc:** Individuals with ovarian cancer and their families; health care professionals treating people with ovarian cancer. Seeks to advance the prevention, diagnosis, and treatment of ovarian cancer. Serves as a clearinghouse on ovarian cancer; provides support and services to members; conducts educational programs.

★ 5011 ★ National PACE Association (NPA)
801 N Fairfax St., Ste. 309
Alexandria, VA 22314
Phone: (703)535-1565 **Fax:** (703)535-1566
Email: info@npaonline.org
Website: http://www.npaonline.org
Desc: Promotes the availability of healthcare services to older adults through the Program of All-inclusive Care for the Elderly (PACE) and similar care models.

★ 5012 ★ National Parent Network on Disabilities (NPND)
6613 Church St., No. 100
Douglasville, GA 30134-1809
Email: npnd@mindspring.com
Desc: Families caring for people with special health care needs and developmental disabilities. Dedicated to empowering parents. Sponsors relays, leadership exchanges, weekly newsletter, legislative updates. **Pub:** *Friday Facts*, weekly. Newsletter.

★ 5013 ★ National Parkinson Foundation (NPF)
1501 NW 9th Ave.
Bob Hope Parkinson's Research Center
Miami, FL 33136-1494
Phone: (305)547-6666 **Free:** 800-327-4545
Fax: (305)548-4403
Email: mailbox@parkinson.org
Website: http://www.parkinson.org
Herbert C. Zemel, Pres.
Fnded: 1957. **Desc:** Doctors, nurses, scientists, pharmacologists, and therapists who research, diagnose, and treat Parkinsonism. Supports basic and clinical research for Parkinsonism and related neurological disorders and provides physical, speech, and occupational therapy. NPF is associated with the University of Miami School of Medicine, and supports the National Parkinson Institute, which provides diagnosis, treatment, care, and rehabilitation. Conducts educational programs. Distributes literature to medical libraries, nurses training schools, health clinics, physicians, and patients. Sponsors regional patient self-support groups where problems are discussed and experiences are exchanged under guidance of physicians, social workers, and psychologists. Maintains offices at 122 E. 42nd St., New York, NY 10017 and 4929 Wilshire Blvd., Los Angeles, CA 90010. **Pub:** *How to Start and Run a Support Group.* • *Membership List*, periodic. • *The Parkinson Handbook.* • *Parkinson Report*, quarterly. Newsletter. Contains research reports. *Price:* Included in membership dues; Available free of charge to others upon request. • Also publishes other books and brochures.

★ 5014 ★ National Pediatric and Family HIV Resource Center (NPHRC)
University of Medicine & Dentistry of New Jersey
30 Bergen St., ADMC No. 4
Newark, NJ 07103
Phone: (973)972-0410 **Free:** 800-362-0071
Fax: (973)972-0399
Email: ortegaes@umdnj.edu
Website: http://www.thebody.com/nphrc/nphrcpage.html
Fnded: 1990. **Desc:** Provides education, consultation, technical assistance and training for health and social service professionals caring for children, adolescents, and families with HIV and AIDS.

★ 5015 ★ National Pediatrics AIDS Network
c/o Gary Gale, Dir.
PO Box 1032
Boulder, CO 80306
Free: 800-646-1001
Email: gary@npan.org
Website: http://www.npan.org/
Gary Gale, Dir.
Desc: Works as a resource for children and adolescents with HIV/AIDS around the world.

★ 5016 ★ National Pediculosis Association (NPA)
50 Kearney Rd.
Needham, MA 02494
Phone: (781)449-6487 **Free:** 800-446-4NPA
Fax: (781)449-8129
Email: npa@headlice.org
Website: http://www.headlice.org
Deborah Z. Altschuler, Pres.
Fnded: 1983. **Desc:** Parents, physicians, school nurses, and individuals representing hospitals and county health departments. Works to eliminate the incidence, particularly among children, of pediculosis (head lice). Conducts public education campaign to make pediculosis control a public health priority; acts

as consumer advocate to ensure the quality and safety of products for treating pediculosis and scabies; encourages scientific research to discover methods of treatment that minimize the use of pesticides, which may harm pregnant and nursing women as well as infants and children. Disseminates information on identifying, treating, and preventing pediculosis, with emphasis on finding and removing nits (louse eggs) in the hair. Provides consultations to schools, camps, and other organizations. Maintains speakers' bureau and creates exhibits for professional meetings and conferences. Operates lending library of audiovisual aids; makes available other educational tools including posters and pamphlets. Sponsors National Pediculosis Prevention Month in September. Sponsors scientific advisory board of experts in such fields as entomology, dermatology, toxicology, pediatrics, parasitology, and pharmacology. **Pub:** *Keep Your Wits Not Your Nits.* • *Latest Greatest Coloring Book About Lice.*

★ 5017 ★ National Pensioners and Senior Citizens Federation (NPSCF)
3033 Lakeshore Blvd. W
Toronto, ON, Canada M8V 1K5
Phone: (416)251-7042
Email: helen.decoste@ns.sympatico.co

Fnded: 1945. **Nat'l Groups:** 750. **Lang(s):** English, French. **Desc:** Senior citizens' and pensioners' clubs. Seeks to stimulate public interest in the welfare of older Canadians. Provides services to improve the quality of life of senior citizens, including counselling and education. **Pub:** *National News*, quarterly. Newsletter. Seniors issues. • Brochure. • Papers.

★ 5018 ★ National Perinatal Association (NPA)
3500 E Fletcher Ave., Ste. 205
Tampa, FL 33613
Phone: (813)971-1008 **Free:** 888-971-3295
Fax: (813)971-9306
Email: npa@nationalperinatal.org
Website: http://www.nationalperinatal.org
Shelia S. Sorkin, Exec. Dir.

Fnded: 1976. **Mem:** 1,500. **Nat'l Groups:** 20. **Reg. Groups:** 1. **State Groups:** 27. **Desc:** Organizations and individuals interested in perinatal health care. Purpose is to promote improved patient care, education, research, advocacy and delivery systems for perinatal health. **Pub:** *Journal of Perinatology*, bimonthly. Journal. Examines all facets of perinatology/neonatology from a variety of perspectives. *Price:* Included in membership dues; $40/year for nonmembers. • *National Perinatal Association Bulletin*, quarterly. Newsletter. Includes article reviews and legislative news. *Price:* Included in membership dues. • Proceedings.

★ 5019 ★ National Perinatal Information Center
144 Wayland Ave., Ste. 300
Providence, RI 02906
Phone: (401)274-0650 **Fax:** (401)455-0377
Email: npic@npic.org
Website: http://www.npic.org
David E. Gagnon, MPH, Pres.

Fnded: 1985. **Mem:** 2,000. **Desc:** Gathers extensive patient data on hospital stays. Serves as perinatal research center for Maternal and Child Health Clearinghouse. Provides educational and research programs. Maintains speakers' bureau Performs children's services. **Pub:** *NPIC Newsletter*, quarterly. Contains articles on NPIC research. *Price:* included in membership dues. • Brochure, annual. • Directory.

★ 5020 ★ National Pharmaceutical Association (NPhA)
107 Kilmayne Dr., Ste. C
Cary, NC 27511
Free: 800-944-NPHA **Fax:** (919)469-5870
Email: npha@npha.net
Website: http://www.npha.net/
Lori Woodson, Pres.

Fnded: 1947. **Mem:** 2,235. **Desc:** State and local associations of professional minority pharmacists. To provide a means whereby members may "contribute to their common improvement, share their experiences, and contribute to the public good." **Pub:** *Journal of the NPhA*, quarterly. Journal. *Price:* $20/year for individuals (U.S.); $35/year for institutions (U.S.); $30/year for individuals (outside U.S.); $45/year for institutions (outside U.S.).

★ 5021 ★ National Phlebotomy Association (NPA)
1901 Brightseat Rd.
Landover, MD 20785
Phone: (301)386-4200 **Fax:** (301)386-4203
Email: naltphle@aol.com
Diane Crawford, CEO

Fnded: 1978. **Mem:** 12,000. **Reg. Groups:** 10. **Desc:** Offers educational programs for phlebotomists; to accredit phlebotomy programs; to give national certification examinations in phlebotomy at the request of approved program. (Phlebotomy is the collection of a blood specimen for analysis in the treatment of disease.) Conducts regional workshops and educational programs. Compiles statistics. **Pub:** *National Phlebotomy Association Certified Phlebotomists Registry*, periodic. • *Self Study Modules in Phlebotomy.*

★ 5022 ★ National Phobics Society
Zion Centre
339 Stretford Rd.
Hulme
Manchester M15 4ZY, United Kingdom
Phone: 44 870 7700456 **Fax:** 44 161 2279862
Email: natphob.soc@good.co.uk
Website: http://www.phobics-society.org.uk

Fnded: 1970. **Mem:** 6,000. **Desc:** Provides information, support, and advice to anyone affected by anxiety disorders, including panic attacks, OCD, BDD, agoraphobia, social phobia, and PTSD. **Pub:** *Don't Panic*, quarterly. Newsletter.

★ 5023 ★ National Physician's Association (NPA)
PO Box 35215
Chicago, IL 60707-0215
Phone: (708)453-0080 **Fax:** (708)453-0083
Email: npa@rentamark.com
Website: http://www.rentamark.com/npa/
L. Stollen, Contact

Fnded: 1975. **Nat'l Groups:** 1. **Desc:** Physicians. Seeks to increase members' public visibility and professional influence. Provides trademark licensing and product and service endorsement services to support members' activities. A platform for doctors to find new patients and receive information about the latest healthcare "breakthroughs", and receive advice on healthcare matters. **Pub:** *National Physicians Journal*, quarterly. Journal. NPA invites authors to submit articles in Word format via email for publication. *Price:* for members.

★ 5024 ★ National Podiatric Medical Association (NPMA)
c/o Raymond E. Lee, D.P.M.
1706 E 87th St.
Chicago, IL 60617
Phone: (773)374-1616 **Fax:** (773)374-5860
Email: npmadebby1@aol.com
Dr. Johndelle Jenkins, D.P.M., Contact

Fnded: 1971. **Mem:** 200. **Desc:** Minority podiatrists, predominately black. Promotes the science and art of podiatry. Seeks to: improve public health; raise the standards of the podiatric profession and education; stimulate a favorable relationship between all podiatrists; nurture growth and diffusion of podiatric information; stimulate public education concerning public health and features of podiatric medicine. Sponsors proposal of podiatric laws; works to eliminate religious and racial discrimination and segregation in American medical institutions. **Pub:** *Annual Seminar Ad Book.* • *National Podiatric Medical Association–Newsletter*, annual. Newsletter. Includes calendar of events and news from student-affiliated associations. *Price:* Included in membership dues. **Frmly:** (1987) National Podiatry Association.

★ 5025 ★ National Potter Syndrome Support Group
c/o Delores Schlegel
8221 Twp. Rd. 323
Holmesville, OH 44633
Phone: (330)279-4374
Email: potters_syndrome@mailcity.com
Website: http://www.geocities.com/potters_syndrome
Delores Schlegel, Contact

Fnded: 1995. **Mem:** 105. **Desc:** Supports and disseminates information to families affected with Potter Syndrome. **Pub:** *National Patter Syndrome Support Group Newsletter*, biennial. Newsletter.

★ 5026 ★ National Pressure Ulcer Advisory Panel (NPUAP)
11250 Roger Bacon Dr., Ste. 8
Reston, VA 20190-5202
Phone: (703)464-4849 **Fax:** (703)435-4390
Email: rguggolz@drohanmgmt.com
Website: http://www.npuap.org
Rick Guggolz, Exec. Dir.

Fnded: 1987. **Desc:** Dedicated to the prevention and management of pressure ulcers. Acts as information resource for health care professionals, government, public and health care agencies. Promotes research and legislative action. **Pub:** Newsletter, quarterly.

★ 5027 ★ National Prevention Network (NPN)
808 17th St. NW, Ste. 410
Washington, DC 20006
Phone: (202)293-0090 **Fax:** (202)293-1250
Email: dcoffice@nasadad.org
Website: http://www.nasadad.org
Alan Moghul, PhD, Dir., Prevention Svcs.

Fnded: 1982. **Mem:** 61. **Reg. Groups:** 5. **State Groups:** 50. **Desc:** Officials of state alcohol and drug agencies. Works to enhance national, state, and local programs for drug and alcohol abuse prevention; serves as a network among state agency personnel and other prevention professionals to assist in the development of effective and innovative substance abuse prevention strategies; seeks to establish guidelines for quality service. Collects and disseminates information and statistics on prevention services, programs, trends, activities, and issues. Provides consultation on technical matters; conducts research. **Pub:** *NPN Membership List*, quarterly.

★ 5028 ★ National Prison Hospice Association (NPHA)
PO Box 3769
Boulder, CO 80307
Phone: (303)544-5923 **Fax:** (303)444-2824
Email: npha@npha.org
Website: http://www.npha.org/
Fleet Maull, Founder/Dir.

Fnded: 1991. **Reg. Groups:** 4. **Desc:** Promotes hospice care for terminally ill inmates and those facing the prospect of dying in prison. Hospice is a comfort-oriented care that allows seriously ill and dying patients to die with dignity and humanity with as little pain as possible. **Pub:** *NPHA News*, annual. Newsletter. *Price:* Free.

★ 5029 ★ National Psoriasis Foundation/USA (NPF)
6600 SW 92nd Ave., Ste. 300
Portland, OR 97223
Phone: (503)244-7404 **Free:** 800-723-9166
Fax: (503)245-0626
Email: getinfo@npfusa.org
Website: http://www.psoriasis.org

Fnded: 1968. **Desc:** People who have psoriasis and psoriatic arthritis, their family members, friends, physicians, nurses, researchers and corporations. Untied to improve the quality of life for people who have psoriasis and psoriatic arthritis to educate the public about psoriasis and to support research. **Pub:** *Psoriasis Forum*. Newsletter. Features reports on new and updated psoriasis treatments, new drug approvals, and insurance problems.

★ 5030 ★ National Psychological Association for Psychoanalysis (NPAP)

150 W 13th St.
New York, NY 10011
Phone: (212)924-7440 **Fax:** (212)989-7543
Email: info@npap.org
Website: http://www.npap.org
Jeffrey Werden, Pres.

Fnded: 1948. **Mem:** 365. **Desc:** Professional society for practicing psychoanalysts. Conducts training program leading to certification in psychoanalysis. Offers information and private referral service for the public. Operates speakers' bureau. **Pub:** *National Psychological Association for Psychoanalysis–Bulletin*, biennial. Bulletin. *Price:* Free. • *National Psychological Association for Psychoanalysis–News and Reviews*, semiannual. *Price:* Included in membership dues. • *Psychoanalytic Review*, bimonthly. Journal. Includes book reviews.

★ 5031 ★ National Rare Blood Club (NRBC)

Associated Health Foundation
99 Madison Ave.
New York, NY 10016
Phone: (212)889-8245 **Free:** 800-772-8668
Fax: (212)448-1811
Edward Birnbaum, Pres.

Fnded: 1978. **Mem:** 16,000. **Desc:** Persons ages 18-65 with rare blood types who are physically able to donate blood. Operates as a voluntary community service with no fees or dues involved.

★ 5032 ★ National Register of Health Service Providers in Psychology

1120 G St., NW, Ste. 330
Washington, DC 20005
Phone: (202)783-7663
Email: judy@nationalregister.org
Website: http://www.nationalregister.org
Judy E. Hall, PhD, Exec. Off.

Fnded: 1974. **Mem:** 14,000. **Desc:** Licensed psychologists. Goal is to contribute to the continuous improvement of health services to the public by developing, reviewing and disseminating standards for evaluating credentials, disseminating information, conducting ethics programs, and evaluating education programs. Developed the subsidiary, HSP Verified, to develop electronic solutions for providing credentialing services. **Pub:** *The Register Report*, 3/year. Magazine.

★ 5033 ★ National Register of Hypnotherapists and Psychotherapists

12 Cross St.
Nelson BB9 7EN, United Kingdom
Phone: 44 1282 716839 **Fax:** 44 1282 698633
Email: nrhp@btconnect.com
Website: http://www.nrhp.co.uk

Fnded: 1985. **Mem:** 390. **Desc:** Therapists who have graduated from the National College of Hypnosis and Psychotherapy or equivalent trainings. Promotes and protects the professional status, standards, ethics and interest of its members and also promotes the interests of those members of the public who seek professional help, and for whom it provides a nationwide referral service. Member of the United Kingdom Council for Psychotherapy. **Pub:** *Directory of Practitioners*, annual. Directory. Contains a listing of qualified hypno-psychotherapists in UK. • *Information Leaflet*. • *Reports and Statistical Analyses of Membership*. Report.

★ 5034 ★ National Register of Personal Trainers (NRPT)

16 Borough High St.
London SE1 9QG, United Kingdom
Phone: 44 20 74079223 **Fax:** 44 20 74079225
Email: info@nrpt.co.uk
Website: http://www.nrpt.co.uk

Fnded: 1992. **Mem:** 1,000. **Desc:** Qualified fitness instructors available for one to one personal training throughout the UK. Representative and advisory body for personal fitness trainers in UK. Acts as a referral service for the general public when looking for a personal trainer; provides networking and secures the best possible services and products for personal trainers to enhance their professionalism. **Pub:** *One to One*, bimonthly. Newsletter. **Frmly:** (2001) National Register of Personal Fitness Trainers.

★ 5035 ★ National Registry of Certified Chemists (NRCC)

927 S Walter Reed Dr., No. 11
Arlington, VA 22204
Phone: (703)979-9001
Email: nrcc6@aol.com
Website: http://www.nrcc6.org
Gilbert E. Smith, PhD, Exec. Dir.

Fnded: 1967. **Mem:** 500. **Desc:** Certification programs for chemical hygiene officers, clinical chemists, clinical chemistry technologists, environmental analytical chemists, environmental analytical technicians, and toxicological chemists based on education, experience, and examination. **Pub:** Directory, annual. **Frmly:** (2001) National Registry in Clinical Chemistry.

★ 5036 ★ National Registry of Emergency Medical Technicians (NREMT)

Rocco V. Morando Bldg.
6610 Busch Blvd.
PO Box 29233
Columbus, OH 43229
Phone: (614)888-4484 **Fax:** (614)888-8920
Email: nremtwebofc@attmail.com
Website: http://www.nremt.org
Howard A. Werman, MD, Chairman

Fnded: 1970. **Mem:** 170,000. **Desc:** Promotes the improved delivery of emergency medical services by: assisting in the development and evaluation of educational programs to train emergency medical technicians; establishing qualifications for eligibility to apply for registration; preparing and conducting examinations designed to assure the competency of emergency medical technicians and paramedics; establishing a system for biennial registration; establishing procedures for revocation of certificates of registration for cause; maintaining a directory of registered emergency medical technicians. **Pub:** Newsletter, quarterly. **Frmly:** (1973) Registry of Emergency Medical Technicians - Ambulance.

★ 5037 ★ National Rehabilitation Administration Association (NRAA)

c/o National Rehabilitation Association
633 S Washington St.
Alexandria, VA 22314
Phone: (703)836-0850 **Fax:** (703)836-0848
Email: info@nationalrehab.org
Website: http://www.nationalrehab.org

Desc: Nonprofit rehabilitation instructors, state agency vocational rehabilitation instructors, and private instructors. Promotes continuing professional development of members. Conducts professional training sessions. **Pub:** *Journal of Rehabilitation Administration*, periodic. Journal. • *NRAA Newsletter*, periodic. Newsletter.

★ 5038 ★ National Rehabilitation Association (NRA)

633 S Washington St.
Alexandria, VA 22314
Phone: (703)836-0850 **Fax:** (703)836-0848
Email: info@nationalrehab.org
Website: http://www.nationalrehab.org/website/index.html

Fnded: 1925. **Mem:** 9,000. **Nat'l Groups:** 9. **Reg. Groups:** 7. **State Groups:** 52. **Desc:** Providing opportunities through knowledge and diversity for professionals in the fields of rehabilitation of people with disabilities. **Pub:** *Contemporary Rehab*, bimonthly. Newsletter. Includes calendar of events, listing of employment opportunities, chapter news, human interest stories, and practice information. *Price:* Included in membership dues. • *Journal of Rehabilitation*, quarterly. Journal. Includes articles on rehabilitation research and new technology. Also includes book reviews and annual index. *Price:* Included in membership dues; $65/year for nonmembers. • *Report of the Annual Mary E. Switzer Memorial Seminar*. Monographs. *Price:* $15/monograph.

★ 5039 ★ National Rehabilitation Counseling Association (NRCA)

8807 Sudley Rd., Ste. 102
Manassas, VA 20110-4719
Phone: (703)361-2077 **Fax:** (703)361-2489
Email: nrcaoffice@aol.com
Website: http://nrca-net.org/
Dr. Betty Hedgeman, Admin.

Fnded: 1958. **Mem:** 2,500. **Desc:** A division of the National Rehabilitation Association. Professional and student rehabilitation counselors. Works to expand the role of counselors in the rehabilitation process and seeks to advance members' professional development. Supports legislation favoring the profession. **Pub:** *Journal of Applied Rehabilitation Counseling*, quarterly. Journal. Includes research information and literature and book reviews. *Price:* Included in membership dues; $15 for nonmembers; $30 for institutions. • *With One Voice*, quarterly. Newsletter. Membership activities newsletter; includes legislative news and listing of employment opportunities. *Price:* Included in membership dues.

★ 5040 ★ National Rehabilitation Information Center (NARIC)

4200 Forbes Blvd., Ste. 202
Lanham, MD 20706
Phone: (301)459-5900 **Free:** 800-346-2742
Fax: (301)459-4263
Email: naricinfo@heitechservices.com
Website: http://www.naric.com
Mark X. Odum, Dir.

Fnded: 1977. **Desc:** Purpose is to improve delivery of information to the rehabilitation community. Disseminates the findings of programs funded by the National Institute on Disability and Rehabilitation Research; prepares custom bibliographies; helps locate answers to reference questions; searches for relevant materials in other commercially available databases. **Pub:** *NIDRR Program Directory*, annual. *Price:* $5. • *REHABDATA Thesaurus*. *Price:* $25. • Directory, annual. Available online only.

★ 5041 ★ National Remotivation Therapy Organization (NRTO)

103 McDonald St.
West Nanticoke, PA 18634
Phone: (570)735-7079
Website: http://www.remotivation.fws1.com
James Siberski, Exec. Dir.

Fnded: 1971. **Mem:** 412. **State Groups:** 5. **Desc:** Certified remotivation therapists organized to provide a forum for the discussion of ideas and information related to the field. Remotivation therapy involves the use of small group sessions to stimulate and revitalize individuals who have experienced a decline in interest in their surroundings, themselves, and other people. Conducts discussions of methods that allow patients an opportunity for verbal expression, renewal of listening skills, and resocialization. **Pub:** *NRTO Newsletter*, quarterly. Newsletter. *Price:* $20/year. • *Remotivation Therapy Information*. Brochure. • *Remotivator*, quarterly. Newsletter. **AKA:** National Remotivation Technique Organization.

★ 5042 ★ National Renal Administrators Association (NRAA)
1904 Naomi Pl.
Prescott, AZ 86303-5061
Phone: (928)717-2772 **Fax:** (928)441-3857
Email: nraa@nraa.org
Website: http://www.nraa.org
Michael Paget, Exec. Dir.

Fnded: 1977. **Mem:** 700. **Desc:** Administrative personnel involved with dialysis programs for patients suffering from kidney failure. Provides a vehicle for the development of educational and informational services for members. Maintains contact with health care facilities and government agencies. Operates placement service; compiles statistics; conducts political action committee. **Pub:** *Presidents Letter*, monthly. Newsletter. *Price:* Free to members; $10 nonmembers.

★ 5043 ★ National Resident Matching Program (NRMP)
2501 N St. NW, Ste. 1
Washington, DC 20037-1127
Phone: (202)828-0677 **Fax:** (202)828-1121
Email: nrmp@aamc.org
Website: http://www.aamc.org/nrmp
Robert L. Beran, PhD, Exec. Dir.

Fnded: 1951. **Desc:** National clearinghouse for matching the preferences of medical school graduates for medical residencies in the U.S. with the hospitals' choices of applicants. Runs matches for 17 medical sub-specialty fellowships. **Pub:** *NRMP Data*, annual. Booklet. *Price:* $35. **Frmly:** (1953) National InterAssociation Committee on Internships; (1968) National Intern Matching Program; (1978) National Intern and Resident Matching Program.

★ 5044 ★ National Resource Center for Health and Safety in Child Care (NRCHSCC)
c/o UCHSC at Fitzsimons
Campus Mail Stop F 541
PO Box 6508
Aurora, CO 80045-0508
Phone: (303)724-0665 **Free:** 800-598-KIDS
Fax: (303)724-0960
Email: natl.child.res.ctr.@uchsc.edu
Website: http://nrc.uchsc.edu
Marilyn J. Krajicek, RN, Dir.

Fnded: 1992. **State Groups:** 50. **Desc:** Seeks to enhance the quality of child care by supporting state and local health departments, child care regulatory agencies, child care providers, and parents in their effort to promote health and safety in child care. Provides information services and training and technical assistance. **Pub:** Bibliographies. • Brochure.

★ 5045 ★ National Restaurant Association Quality Assurance Study Group
c/o National Restaurant Association
1200 17th St. NW
Washington, DC 20036
Phone: (202)331-5900 **Free:** 800-424-5156
Fax: (202)331-2429
Email: ga@lists.restaurant.org
Website: http://www.restaurant.org/ga/index.cfm
Rosemary Y. Curtis, Admin. Asst.

Mem: 208. **Desc:** Professional quality assurance and quality control personnel sanitarians from the National Restaurant Association working in foodservice facilities. Provides members with the opportunity to share common goals, concerns, ideas, and problems. Conducts research and educational programs and semiannual study group meeting.

★ 5046 ★ National Reye's Syndrome Foundation (NRSF)
426 N Lewis
PO Box 829
Bryan, OH 43506
Phone: (419)636-2679 **Free:** 800-233-7393
Fax: (419)636-9897
Email: nrsf@reyessyndrome.org
Susan Landversicht, Dir. of Dev.

Fnded: 1974. **Mem:** 5,000. **Reg. Groups:** 6. **State Groups:** 47. **Local Groups:** 148. **Desc:** Families of children who have had Reye's Syndrome; doctors, scientists, nurses, and other health professionals and concerned individuals. (Reye's Syndrome is a disease affecting the liver and brain. Cause and cure unknown, its mortality rate is over 57 percent. Death may occur within a few hours after onset.) Aims to disseminate information to the public and the medical community and to raise and provide funds for research into the cause, treatment, cure, and prevention of the disease through research grants to individual scientists. Gives support and guidance to families experiencing Reye's Syndrome; assists federal and state agencies in obtaining data on Reye's cases; encourages governmental funding of research. Promotes service through a resource clearinghouse, support groups, and referral services. Promotes awareness via lay-oriented literature, information services, professional training, lay/professional slide presentations, and emergency room posters. Sponsors National Reye's Syndrome Month in September. Compiles statistics; maintains speakers' bureau. **Pub:** *National Reye's Syndrome Foundation–In the News*, semiannual. Newsletter. *Price:* Included in membership dues.

★ 5047 ★ National Rosacea Society
800 S Northwest Hwy., Ste. 200
Barrington, IL 60010
Free: 800-NO-BLUSH **Fax:** (847)382-5567
Email: rosaceas@aol.com
Website: http://www.rosacea.org
Day Olney, Contact

Fnded: 1997. **Desc:** Mission is to improve the lives of people with rosacea by raising awareness, providing public health information and supporting research on this widespread but little-known disorder. **Pub:** *Rosacea Review*, 3-4/year. Newsletter.

★ 5048 ★ National RSD Assistance Center
PO Box 1261
Knightdale, NC 27545
Email: rsdac@bellsouth.net
Website: http://www.rsdac.org/

Fnded: 1999. **Desc:** Individuals suffering from Reflex Sympathetic Dystrophy. Offers assistance for medications and utilities treatment, as well as food or utility bills if needed. Provides other contact resources for further assistance. Collects and disseminates information about the disease. RSD is a medical condition resulting from an injury to a nerve or soft tissue (e.g., broken bone, or even a sliver) that does not heal properly.

★ 5049 ★ National Runaway Switchboard (NRS)
3080 N Lincoln Ave.
Chicago, IL 60657
Free: 800-621-4000 **Fax:** (773)929-5150
Email: info@nrscrisisline.org
Website: http://www.nrscrisisline.org
Gordon Vance, Prog. Dir.

Fnded: 1974. **Reg. Groups:** 140. **Desc:** A 24-hour, toll-free national switchboard for runaways, families of runaways, and other troubled youth. Provides names and phone numbers of centers for shelter and other social services across the country, including counseling centers, referral lines, drug treatment facilities, and family planning services. Offers to relay messages between young people and their families if desired; can also set up conferences calls between youths and parents or agencies. The caller's confidentiality is maintained. Maintains speakers' bureau. Funded in part by the Family and Youth Services Bureau of the U.S. Department of Health and Human Services. Also provides free Bus ride home for qualified runaways. Access to AT&T Language Line. **Pub:** *FrontLine*, quarterly. Newsletter. Contains statistical data and reports on activities. *Price:* Free.

★ 5050 ★ National Rural Health Association (NRHA)
1 W Armour Blvd., Ste. 203
Kansas City, MO 64111
Phone: (816)756-3140 **Fax:** (816)756-3144
Email: mail@nrharural.org
Website: http://www.nrharural.org
Rob McVay, Contact

Fnded: 1978. **Mem:** 2,000. **Desc:** Administrators, physicians, nurses, physician assistants, health planners, academicians, and others interested or involved in rural health care. Creates a better understanding of health care problems unique to rural areas; utilizes a collective approach in finding positive solutions; articulates and represents the health care needs of rural America; supplies current information to rural health care providers; serves as a liaison between rural health care programs throughout the country. Offers continuing education credits for medical, dental, nursing, and management courses. **Pub:** *Journal of Rural Health*, quarterly. Journal. Includes rural health research, book reviews, abstracts of published research, and research reviews. *Price:* Included in membership dues; $50 for nonmembers; $125 for institutions. • Also publishes many other resources.

★ 5051 ★ National Rural Recruitment and Retention Network (3R Net)
2536 Kendall Ave.
Madison, WI 53705
Phone: (715)295-0742 **Free:** 800-787-2512
Fax: (715)343-8244
Email: info@3rnet.org
Website: http://www.3rnet.org/

State Groups: 45. **Desc:** 45 member state organizations. Strives to assist health professionals locate practice sites in rural areas throughout the United States.

★ 5052 ★ National School-Age Care Alliance (NSACA)
1137 Washington St.
Boston, MA 02124
Phone: (617)298-5012 **Fax:** (617)298-5022
Email: staff@nsaca.org
Website: http://www.nsaca.org
Mark Carter, Exec. Dir.

Fnded: 1981. **Mem:** 8,000. **Reg. Groups:** 5. **Local Groups:** 35. **Desc:** Professional providers of day care services for school age children outside of school hours. Seeks to advance the profession of school-age child care. Provides support and services to members including coalition building, networking, and group rates for video licensing. **Pub:** *Caring, Stimulating, Responsive*. Brochure. • *NSACA News*, quarterly. Newsletter.

★ 5053 ★ National Scoliosis Foundation (NSF)
5 Cabot Pl.
Stoughton, MA 02072-4624
Phone: (781)341-6333 **Free:** 800-673-6922
Fax: (781)341-8333
Email: NSF@scoliosis.org
Website: http://www.scoliosis.org

Fnded: 1976. **Mem:** 25,000. **State Groups:** 3. **Desc:** Supporters are businesses, organizations, and individuals concerned with the early detection and prevention of progressing scoliosis, kyphosis, and structural lordosis. Purposes are to promote programs and activities leading to the elimination of the crippling effects of scoliosis and to educate the public about all abnormal spinal curvatures. Assists local groups in identifying available medical resources and personnel to help conduct volunteer screening programs; encourages legislation requiring scoliosis screening for each student in the 5th through 10th grades throughout the U.S. Maintains resource center for individuals or schools seeking information on abnormal spinal curvatures; provides information on how to promote and assist in spinal screening programs; sponsors multimedia educational exhibits and programs for adults and children. Maintains speakers' bureau. **Pub:** *Spinal Connection*, biennial. Newsletter. Membership activities newsletter. *Price:* Free. • Booklets. • Brochures. • Manuals. • Also publishes resource lists and produces school audiovisual materials.

★ 5054 ★ National Senior Citizens Law Center (NSCLC)

1101 14th St. NW, Ste. 400
Washington, DC 20005
Phone: (202)289-6976 **Fax:** (202)289-7224
Email: nsclc@nsclc.org
Website: http://www.nsclc.org
Edward King, Exec. Dir.

Fnded: 1972. **Desc:** Legal services support center specializing in the legal problems of the elderly poor. Acts as advocate on behalf of elderly, poor clients in litigation and administrative affairs. Sponsors conferences and workshops on areas of the law affecting the elderly. **Pub:** *Nursing Home Law Letter*, quarterly. • *Washington Weekly*, weekly. Newsletter. • Also publishes handbooks, guides, and testimonies.

★ 5055 ★ National Service Dog Center (NSDC)

c/o Delta Society
580 Naches Ave. SW, No. 101
Renton, WA 98055
Phone: (425)226-7357 **Fax:** (425)235-1076
Email: info@deltasociety.org
Website: http://www.deltasociety.org
Nancy Kedward, Contact

Fnded: 1977. **Desc:** A joint program of the American Humane Association and the Delta Society. Provides a national service dog education, advocacy and referral service. Promotes the health benefits of service animals for people with disabilities. **Pub:** *Alert*, bimonthly. Newsletter. Reports on service animals and issues of concern to those who want information about service animals. • *Service Animal Resource Directory*, annual. Directory. Lists service dog training programs and information about selecting a supplier that best meets consumer's needs. • *Service Dogs Welcome!*. Video. **Frmly:** (1983) Hearing Dog Program; (1987) Hearing Dog Project; (1989) National Center for Hearing Dog Information; (1993) Hearing Dog Resource Center.

★ 5056 ★ National SIDS/Infant Death Resource Center (NSIDRC)

2070 Chain Bridge, Ste. 450
Vienna, VA 22182-2536
Phone: (703)821-8955 **Free:** (866)866-7437
Fax: (703)821-2098
Email: sids@circlesolutions.com
Website: http://www.sidscenter.org
Olivia Cowdrill, Proj. Dir.

Fnded: 1980. **Desc:** Funded by Maternal and Child Health Bureau, Health Resources and Services Administration, U.S. Department of Health and Human Services, National SIDS/Infant Death Resource Center. Provides resources, referrals, and technical assistance to SIDS families, public health and other professionals, and the general public. **Pub:** *Fact Sheets*. • *Information Exchange*, periodic. Newsletter. Includes list of resources, calendar of events, and national, state and legislative news. • *Table of SIDS Deaths and Mortality Rates*, annual. • Bibliographies, annual. Research bibliographies. • Also publishes fact sheets and educational publications. **Frmly:** (1991) National Sudden Infant Death Syndrome Clearinghouse.

★ 5057 ★ National Sjogren's Syndrome Association (NSSA)

PO Box 22066
Beachwood, OH 44122-0066
Phone: (216)292-3866 **Free:** 800-395-6772
Fax: (216)292-4955
Email: nickofohio@aol.com
Website: http://www.sjogrenssyndrome.org/
Barbara Henry, Exec. Dir.

Fnded: 1990. **Mem:** 4,500. **Desc:** Promotes public awareness of Sjogren's Syndrome; encourages research into the cause and cure of the disorder. (Sjogren's Syndrome is an autoimmune disorder characterized by dryness of all mucous membranes resulting from deficient secretion of the glands. Approximately 50% of Sjogren's Syndrome patients also have rheumatoid arthritis.) Sponsors chapters and offers information to the medical community. Conducts educational and research programs; maintains speakers' bureau. **Pub:** *Learning to Live with Sjogren's Syndrome*. Video. *Price:* $25. • *Patient Education Series*, quarterly. • *Sjogren's Digest*, quarterly. Newsletter. *Price:* Included in membership dues.

★ 5058 ★ National Sleep Foundation

1522 K St., NW, Ste. 510
Washington, DC 20005
Phone: (202)347-3471 **Fax:** (202)347-3472
Email: nsf@sleepfoundation.org
Website: http://www.sleepfoundation.org
James K. Walsh, PhD, Pres.

Fnded: 1990. **Desc:** Works to improve the quality of life of people suffering from sleep disorders and to prevent accidents related to sleep disorders. (Sleep disorders include: insomnia, narcolepsy, sleep apnea syndrome, sudden infant death syndrome, stroke, epilepsy, and other disorders of sleep and daytime alertness.) Educates health care professionals and the public about the existance and treatment of sleep disorders. Promotes the development of patient services, community resources, and support groups for individuals affected by sleep disorders. Sponsors educational and research programs. **Pub:** *Sleepmatters*. Magazine. • Brochures.

★ 5059 ★ National Society for Epilepsy

Chesham Ln.
Chalfont St. Peter
Gerrards Cross SL9 0RJ, United Kingdom
Phone: 44 1494 601300 **Fax:** 44 1494 871927
Website: http://www.epilepsynse.org.uk

Fnded: 1892. **Mem:** 2,000. **Desc:** Individuals with an interest in epilepsy who wish to support epilepsy education and research. Provides assessment, treatment, rehabilitation, long term and respite care for adults with epilepsy. The education department provides support and information, produces educational resources and runs conferences and seminars. Coordinates a national network of trained volunteers offering information services. **Pub:** *Epilepsy Review*, 3/year. Magazine.

★ 5060 ★ National Society of Genetic Counselors (NSGC)

c/o Bea Leopold
233 Canterbury Dr.
Wallingford, PA 19086-6617
Phone: (610)872-7608 **Fax:** (610)872-1192
Email: fyi@nsgc.org
Website: http://www.nsgc.org
Bea Leopold, Exec. Dir.

Fnded: 1979. **Mem:** 2,000. **Reg. Groups:** 6. **Desc:** The leaing voice, authority and advocate for the genetic counseling profession. **Pub:** *Journal of Genetic Counseling*, bimonthly. Journal. • *Perspectives in Genetic Counseling*, quarterly. Newsletter. • Also publishes high school and college level career packets.

★ 5061 ★ National Society for Histotechnology (NSH)

4201 Northview Dr., Ste. 502
Bowie, MD 20716-2604
Phone: (301)262-6221 **Fax:** (301)262-9188
Email: histo@nsh.org
Website: http://www.nsh.org
Lena Spencer, Pres.

Fnded: 1973. **Mem:** 4,800. **Reg. Groups:** 9. **State Groups:** 42. **Desc:** Histology laboratory technicians, pathologists, laboratory equipment manufacturers' representatives, and interested individuals. Encourages the professional growth and advancement of histoprofessionals and promotes the exchange of ideas and knowledge significant to histotechnology. Assists in the establishment and mutual understanding of related societies. Provides continuing education training courses. Investigates health hazards in the laboratory; ensures the safety of the laboratory; and participates in formulating federal laboratory regulations. **Pub:** *Journal of Histotechnology*, quarterly. Journal. Topics include anatomy, pathology, enzyme histochemistry, special stains, immunohistochemistry, cytology, and electron microscopy. *Price:* Included in membership dues; $70/year for nonmembers; $100/year for nonmembers outside U.S. • *NSH In Action*, quarterly. Annual Report. *Price:* for members. • *NSH in Action*, quarterly. Newsletter. • Booklets.Pertains to careers. • Also publishes training aids.

★ 5062 ★ National Society for Research into Allergy

PO Box 45
Hinckley LE10 0SZ, United Kingdom
Phone: 44 1455 250715 **Fax:** 44 1455 851546
Email: nsra.allergy@virgin.net

Fnded: 1980. **Mem:** 1,000. **Desc:** Main aim is to educate the populace on the devastating effects of allergy/intolerance and to see effective treatment in all teaching hospitals. Offers elimination diet and recipe books as well as councelling, advice, etc. on all types of allergy/intolerance/hyperventilation and the tests and treatments for same.

★ 5063 ★ National Spasmodic Dysphonia Association (NSDA)

1 E Wacker Dr., Ste. 2430
Chicago, IL 60601-1905
Free: 800-795-6732 **Fax:** (312)803-0138
Email: nsda@dysphonia.org
Website: http://www.dystonia.org/
Robert O. McAlister, PhD, Exec. Dir.

Fnded: 1990. **Mem:** 8,200. **Nat'l Groups:** 45. **Desc:** Individuals diagnosed with spasmodic dysphonia; doctors and scientists providing treatment and conducting research on the disease; interested others. Promotes public awareness of spasmodic dysphonia and the care, welfare, and rehabilitation of those with the disease. (Spasmodic dysphonia is a neurological movement disorder affecting muscular control of the vocal cords, often resulting in an abnormally raspy, breathy, or choppy speech pattern.) Makes information on the disease available to patients, their families, and the public. Encourages research to uncover the causes and treatments of spasmodic dysphonia; offers referral information on specialists administering the botulinum toxin presently used in many cases to temporarily treat the disease. Assists in the formation of local support groups to assist patients. **Pub:** *NSDA Newsletter*, biennial. Newsletter.

★ 5064 ★ National Spasmodic Torticollis Association (NSTA)

9920 Talbert Ave., Ste. 233
Fountain Valley, CA 92708
Phone: (714)378-7837 **Free:** 800-HUR-TFUL
Fax: (714)378-7830
Email: nstamail@aol.com
Website: http://www.torticollis.org
Bob Farmer, Pres.

Fnded: 1980. **Mem:** 3,400. **Reg. Groups:** 85. **Local Groups:** 48. **Desc:** Persons afflicted with spasmodic torticollis (ST), a syndrome in which the muscles on one side of the neck contract and pull the head to the side, sometimes pushing the chin up or down. ST usually occurs in adults and can sometimes be treated successfully with medication and physical therapy. Educates the public on ST so that persons with early symptoms know to seek proper medical help from a neurologist or neurosurgeon. Provides forum for discussion among ST sufferers and their families in order to share information and experiences and diminish feelings of alienation and self-consciousness. **Pub:**

NSTA News Magazine, quarterly. Magazine. Includes medical advisor's column. *Price:* Included in membership dues. • *P.T. In-Home Videotape*. Video. *Price:* $24 for members. • *Physicians Referral Directory*, annual. Directory. Lists neurologists who treat spasmodic torticollis. *Price:* Free. • *Relaxation/Affirmation Audiotape*. Audiotape. *Price:* $5.95. • *Series of "Helpful Hints" Letters*. • *What is NSTA?*. • Also publishes fact sheet. **Frmly:** Project S.T.

★ 5065 ★ National Special Needs Network Foundation (NSNNF)

c/o Jeffrey H. Minde
4613 N University Dr., No. 242
Coral Springs, FL 33067
Phone: (954)345-6465 **Fax:** (954)345-6465
Email: jhmnetwork@myacc.net
Website: http://www.nsnn.com/
Jeffrey H. Minde, Pres.

Desc: Special needs professionals. Dedicated to providing the finest and most complete special needs support services in America, including individuals and families with developmental and acquired disabilities, mental illnesses, and chronic medical conditions. **Frmly:** (2003) National Special Needs Network.

★ 5066 ★ National Spinal Cord Injury Association (NSCIA)

6701 Democracy Blvd., Ste. 300-9
Bethesda, MD 20817
Phone: (301)588-6959 **Free:** 800-962-9629
Fax: (301)588-9414
Email: nscia2@aol.com
Website: http://www.spinalcord.org
Marcie Roth, Exec. Dir.

Fnded: 1948. **Mem:** 150,000. **Local Groups:** 50. **Desc:** Seeks to inform and educate the medical and allied professions, persons with spinal cord injury or disease, their families, and the public on spinal cord injury. Provides information, referral and resource services to individuals with spinal cord injuries and diseases and their families to maximize quality of life. Also offers activities in public and professional prevention and education programs and services. Conducts recreation, advocacy, support group, and peer counseling programs through national network of chapters and support groups. referral service. **Pub:** *Spinal Cord Injury Life*, quarterly. Journal. Provides news and articles concerning persons with spinal cord injuries caused by trauma or disease. Includes book reviews. *Price:* Included in membership dues; $40/year subscription. • Also publishes fact sheets on research, sexuality and other topics. **Frmly:** National Spinal Cord Injury Foundation; (1979) National Paraplegia Foundation.

★ 5067 ★ National Stigma Clearinghouse

245 8th Ave., No. 213
New York, NY 10011
Phone: (212)255-4411
Email: stigmanet@webtv.net
Website: http://community-1.webtv.net/stigmanet/AbouttheNational/

Desc: Works to end exploitation of mental illness, encourage balanced portrayals of people with psychiatric vulnerabilities, promotes accuracy in using medical terms.

★ 5068 ★ National Stroke Association (NSA)

9707 E Easter Ln.
Englewood, CO 80112
Phone: (303)649-9299 **Free:** 800-STR-OKES
Fax: (303)649-1328
Email: info@stroke.org
Website: http://www.stroke.org
Andrew J. Beck, Sec.

Fnded: 1984. **Mem:** 7,500. **State Groups:** 16. **Local Groups:** 1200. **Desc:** Stroke survivors and their families; health care professionals and institutions; the lay community. Seeks to reduce the incidence and impact of stroke by promoting research, educating the public, and providing a network for stroke survivors and concerned persons. Serves as an information referral clearinghouse on stroke; makes available educational materials on stroke prevention, treatment, rehabilitation, resocialization, and research. Offers guidance in the development of stroke support groups and clubs. Maintains speakers' bureau and Stroke Information and Referral Center; compiles statistics. Conducts educational symposiums/meetings. **Pub:** *Be Stroke Smart*, bimonthly. Magazine. *Price:* Free. • *Hope: the Stroke Recovery Guide*. Book. • *Journal of Stroke and Cerebravascular Diseases*, quarterly. Journal. *Price:* $129/year for individual; $204/year for institution. • *State Listing of Stroke Clubs*, periodic. Directory. • *Stroke: Clinical Updates*, bimonthly. Newsletter. Professional newsletter with available slides. *Price:* Free with professional membership.

★ 5069 ★ National Student Nurses' Association (NSNA)

45 Main St., Ste. 606
Brooklyn, NY 11201
Phone: (718)210-0705 **Fax:** (718)210-0710
Email: nsna@nsna.org
Website: http://www.nsna.org
Diane J. Mancino, Ed.D., RN CAE, Exec. Dir.

Fnded: 1952. **Mem:** 31,000. **State Groups:** 48. **Local Groups:** 500. **Desc:** Students enrolled in state-approved schools for the preparation of registered nurses. Seeks to aid in the development of the individual nursing student and to urge students of nursing, as future leaders and health professionals, to be aware of and to contribute to improving the health care of all people. Encourages programs and activities in state groups concerning nursing, health, and the community. Provides assistance for state board review, as well as materials for preparation for state RN licensing examination. Cooperates with nursing organizations in recruitment of nurses and in professional, community, and civic programs. Sponsors Foundation of the National Student Nurses' Association in memory of Frances Tompkins to award scholarships to student nurses. **Pub:** *Dean's Notes*, 5/year. • *Imprint*, 5/year. Magazine. Features issues and trends of concern to nursing students. *Price:* included in membership dues; $5/single copy. • *NSNA News*, 2/year. Newsletter.

★ 5070 ★ National Student Speech Language Hearing Association (NSSLHA)

10801 Rockville Pike
Rockville, MD 20852
Phone: (301)897-5700 **Free:** 800-498-2071
Fax: (301)571-0481
Email: nsslha@asha.org
Website: http://www.nsslha.org
Dawn D. Dickerson, Dir. Of Operations

Fnded: 1972. **Mem:** 16,000. **Local Groups:** 285. **Desc:** Preprofessional organization for undergraduate and graduate students in speech-language pathology, speech and hearing sciences, and audiology. **Pub:** *Contemporary Issues in Communication Science and Disorders*, semiannual. Journal. *Price:* Included in membership dues; $20. **Frmly:** National Student Speech and Hearing Association.

★ 5071 ★ National Stuttering Association (NSP)

4071 E La Palma Ave., Ste. A
Anaheim, CA 92807
Phone: (714)630-7600 **Free:** 800-364-1677
Fax: (714)630-7707
Email: nsastutter@aol.com
Website: http://www.nsastutter.org
Annie Bradberry, Exec. Dir.

Fnded: 1977. **Mem:** 4,000. **Local Groups:** 79. **Desc:** Selfhelp organization of people who stutter, parents of children who stutter, and speech pathologists. Seeks to provide a safe, supportive environment for stutterers and their families through chapter meetings, special programs, workshops, tape series, and selfhelp groups. Concentrates on issues such as improving self-image and assuming personal responsibility rather than focusing on speech fluency. Educates the public about stuttering and functions as a referral service for those seeking professional help. (Does not provide speech therapy or trained therapists.) Offers consulting in program development and technical assistance to school districts, speech clinics, hospitals, rehabilitation centers, and other agencies involved in speech services. Advises members on how to be wise consumers of speech and related therapies. Maintains speakers' bureau. **Pub:** *Letting Go, Care*, monthly. Publication for parents. • *Letting Go, Stutter Buddies*. Audiotapes. Publication for children. • Audiotapes. • Brochures. • Pamphlets.

★ 5072 ★ National Subacute Care Association (NSCA)

1960 Gallows Rd., Ste. 210
Vienna, VA 22182
Phone: (703)790-8989 **Fax:** (703)790-8485
Email: info@nsca.net
Sanford. J. Hill, Exec. Dir.

Fnded: 1995. **Mem:** 1,500. **Desc:** Hospitals, nursing facilities, professionals and suppliers. Works to serve and represent the subacute and transitional healthcare industry. Provides information on subacute healthcare; promotes high level of ethics; develops standards. **Pub:** *NSCA News*, quarterly. Newsletter. • *Subacute Care*, quarterly. Journal. • Also issues InfoFaxes and Government Affairs Updates.

★ 5073 ★ National Surgical Assistant Association (NSAA)

740 B2 E Flynn Ln.
Phoenix, AZ 85014
Free: 888-633-0479 **Fax:** (602)212-9692
Email: nsaa@namgmt.com
Website: http://www.nsaa.net
Eugene Smith, Pres.

Fnded: 1983. **Mem:** 650. **Desc:** Professional surgical assistants throughout the United States. Provides standard guidelines and regulations. Establishes rules for those who practice and function as surgical assistants. Examines, reviews, and certifies the training, duration, experience, skills, and knowledge of its members. **Pub:** *CSA Node*, quarterly. Newsletter. Provides articles on latest surgical techniques and trends in the operating room. • Membership Directory.

★ 5074 ★ National Tay-Sachs and Allied Diseases Association (NTSAD)

2001 Beacon St., Ste. 204
Brighton, MA 02135
Phone: (617)277-4463 **Free:** 800-906-8723
Fax: (617)277-0134
Email: ntsad-boston@att.net
Website: http://www.ntsad.org
Jayne C. Gershkowitz, Exec. Dir.

Fnded: 1956. **Mem:** 400. **Reg. Groups:** 4. **Desc:** Supports educational, prevention, family service, and research programs concerning Tay-Sachs and allied degenerative lysosomal and leukodystrophy and neurological diseases occurring in infants, children, and adults. Provides educational literature on Tay-Sachs and allied diseases; serves as a referral agency for the layperson and professional on all aspects of Tay-Sachs and related diseases; promotes mass screening programs and appropriate legislation locally and nationally. Sponsors International Laboratory Quality Control and Reference Sample Center for TSD laboratories. Offers support groups and services for parents of children with Tay-Sachs and related diseases, grandparents and extended family members. Compiles statistics; operates speakers' bureau. **Pub:** *Breakthrough*, semiannual. Newsletter. • *Home Care Manual*. Manual. *Price:* $3 includes shipping and handling. • *Lay-Onset Tay-Sachs*. Information sheet. *Price:* Free. • *Lifeline*, quarterly. Newsletter. Distributed to affected families only. • *National Tay-Sachs and Allied Diseases Association–Breakthrough*, semiannual. Newsletter. • *What Every Family Should Know*, annual. Manual. *Price:* $4. • *What Is Canavan Disease?*. *Price:* 25 cents each, after 10. • *What Is Tay-Sachs Disease?*. *Price:* 25 cents each, after 10. • Also makes available brochures and educational materials. **Frmly:** (1966) National Tay-Sachs Association.

★ 5075 ★ National Therapeutic Recreation Society (NTRS)
22377 Belmont Ridge Rd.
Ashburn, VA 20148-4501
Phone: (703)858-0784 **Free:** 800-626-6772
Fax: (703)858-0794
Email: ntrsnrpa@aol.com
Website: http://www.nrpa.org/branches/ntrs.htm
Susan Potts, MS, Therapeutic Rec. Coord.

Fnded: 1966. **Mem:** 2,000. **Desc:** Professionals, educators, and students involved in the provision of therapeutic recreation services for persons with disabilities in clinical and residential facilities and in the community. Offers technical assistance services to agencies, institutions, and individuals. **Pub:** *Parks and Recreation*, monthly. Magazine. *Price:* Included in membership dues. • *Philosophy of Therapeutic Recreation: Ideas and Issues.* • *Preparing for a Career in Therapeutic Recreation.* • *Therapeutic Recreation Journal*, quarterly. Journal. Research journal. *Price:* $28 for members domestic; $34 for members foreign; $66 for nonmembers domestic; $72 for nonmembers foreign.

★ 5076 ★ National Transplant Society (NTS)
853 Sanders Rd., Ste. 314
Northbrook, IL 60062
Phone: (847)283-9333 **Fax:** (847)792-4108
Email: nts@organdonor.org

Desc: Advocates for issues relating to organ and tissue donation and transplantation. Seeks to enhance the availability of organs and human tissue for medical transplants. Maintains registry of donors; supports research.

★ 5077 ★ National Tuberculosis Controllers Association
2951 Flowers Rd. S, Ste. 102
Atlanta, GA 30341-4000
Phone: (770)455-0801 **Free:** 888-455-0801
Fax: (770)455-4221
Email: ntca@ntca-tb.org
Website: http://www.ntca-tb.org
Walter Q. Page, Exec. Dir.

Fnded: 1995. **Mem:** 459. **Desc:** Seeks to provide a collective voice for TB controllers to advance and advocate for tuberculosis control and elimination activities in the U.S. Advocates for policies and laws to advance tuberculosis control and elimination at the sate, local, and territorial levels. **Pub:** *The Red Snapper Review*, quarterly. Newsletter. Contains organizational and scientific news. *Price:* included in membership dues.

★ 5078 ★ National Union of Disabled Persons of Uganda (NUDPU)
PO Box 8567
Kampala, Uganda
Phone: 256 41 540179 **Fax:** 256 41 540178
Email: nudipu@starcom.co.ug

Fnded: 1987. **Mem:** 56. **Nat'l Groups:** 8. **Reg. Groups:** 48. **Lang(s):** English. **Desc:** People with disabilities and their families; health care personnel and other people working with individuals with disabilities. Seeks to improve the quality of life of people with disabilities; promotes advancement of assistive technologies and therapeutic methods. Provides support and services to people with disabilities and their families; conducts lobbying and advocacy activities; sponsors training programs. **Pub:** *NUDPU News*, semiannual. Newsletter. Bulletin containing information on disability activities in Uganda.

★ 5079 ★ National Upper Cervical Chiropractic Association (NUCCA)
c/o Lesley Louvar
2608 W Kenosha St., No. 224
Broken Arrow, OK 74012
Phone: (918)748-1900 **Fax:** (918)748-1900
Email: execdir@nucca.com
Website: http://www.nucca.org
Dr. Robert Goodman, Pres.

Fnded: 1966. **Mem:** 200. **Desc:** Promotes chiropractic, especially the NUCCA technique; seeks to improve the art of chiropractic; promotes education; sponsors studies.

★ 5080 ★ National Vaccine Information Center
421-E Church St.
Vienna, VA 22180
Phone: (703)938-3783 **Free:** 800-909-SHOT
Fax: (703)938-5768
Email: info@909shot.com
Website: http://www.909shot.com
Kathryn Williams, Contact

Fnded: 1982. **Mem:** 40,000. **Desc:** Parents of children who have had reactions to or been injured by vaccines; individuals interested in working to reform the vaccine system. Disseminates information concerning vaccines to parents and doctors in order to assure safer administration of vaccines. Promotes the development of safer vaccines. Refers parents of vaccine-injured children to doctors, lawyers, and other parents for support services. Maintains speakers' bureau; compiles statistics. **Pub:** *The Compensation System and How It Works.* • *Law Firm Directory.* Directory. • *The Vaccine Reaction*, quarterly. **AKA:** Dissatisfied Parents Together.

★ 5081 ★ National Vitiligo Foundation
611 S Fleishel Ave.
Tyler, TX 75701
Phone: (903)531-0074 **Fax:** (903)525-1234
Email: vtiligo@ballistic.com
Website: http://www.vitiligofoundation.org
James J. Nordlund, MD, Contact

Fnded: 1985. **Mem:** 25,000. **Reg. Groups:** 11. **Desc:** Doctors and patients; contributors and supporters. Provides information and counseling to vitiligo patients and their families. (Vitiligo is a skin disease which destroys pigment cells causing smooth, white-colored patches of skin.) Seeks to increase awareness and concern for the vitiligo patient. Raises funds for scientific and clinical research on the cause, treatment, and cure of vitiligo. **Pub:** *Handbook for Patients.* • *Handbook for Physicians.* • *Handbook for Schools.* • *Vitiligo*, semiannual. Newsletter. • Brochures.

★ 5082 ★ National Vulvodynia Association
PO Box 4491
Silver Spring, MD 20914-4491
Phone: (301)299-0775 **Fax:** (301)299-3999
Email: mate@nva.org
Website: http://www.nva.org
Phyllis Mate, Pres.

Fnded: 1994. **Mem:** 2,500. **Nat'l Groups:** 80. **Desc:** Strives to improve the lives of individuals affected by Vulvodynia, a spectrum of chronic vulvar pain disorders. **Pub:** *NVA News*, 3/year. Newsletter. *Price:* $40 included with donation, back issues available.

★ 5083 ★ National Wellness Institute
PO Box 827
Stevens Point, WI 54481-0827
Phone: (715)342-2969 **Free:** 800-243-8674
Fax: (715)342-2979
Email: nwi@nationalwellness.org
Website: http://www.nationalwellness.org
Anne Helmke, Dir. Member Services

Fnded: 1977. **Mem:** 1,800. **Desc:** Purposes are to provide national leadership in the wellness movement; to assist professionals working in health and wellness promotion in all types of settings; and organizations with planning, development, implementation, and evaluation of wellness programs; and to assist in the development of high quality wellness products and services. Acts as clearinghouse on wellness information. Provides consultations; offers professional development conferences. Sponsors National Wellness Association. **Pub:** *American Journal of Health Promotion*, bimonthly. Journal. • *Health Issues Update/Resource News*, bimonthly. Newsletter. An E-newsletter. *Price:* Included in membership dues. • *Health Promotion Practitioner*, bimonthly. Newsletter. An E-newsletter. • *Testwell Assessment Series.* • *Wellness Management*, quarterly. Newsletter. An e-newsletter. *Price:* Included in membership dues. • *Wellness Resource Directory*. Directory. • Brochures.

★ 5084 ★ National Wheelchair Basketball Association (NWBA)
c/o Roger Davis
710 Queensbury Loop
Winter Garden, FL 34787
Phone: (407)654-4315 **Fax:** (407)654-4315
Email: president@nwba.org
Website: http://www.nwba.org/
Harry Vines, Pres.

Fnded: 1949. **Mem:** 185. **Desc:** Wheelchair basketball teams comprised of individuals with severe permanent physical disabilities of the lower extremities. Seeks to provide opportunities on a national basis for the physically disabled to participate in the sport of wheelchair basketball, with its adjunct psychological, social, and emotional benefits, and to maintain a high level of competition through continuing refinement and standardization of playing rules and officiating. Sponsors sectional and regional tournaments leading up to the National Wheelchair Basketball Tournament. Maintains hall of fame; compiles statistics; participates in charitable activities. **Pub:** *National Wheelchair Basketball Tournament Program*, annual. • *Rules and Case Book*, annual. • *Standings and Statistics*, 10/year. • Directory, annual. Conference officers, team representatives names & addresses. • Newsletter, 12/year.

★ 5085 ★ National Wheelchair Softball Association (NWSA)
1616 Todd Ct.
Hastings, MN 55033
Phone: (612)437-1792 **Fax:** (612)437-3889
Email: ecmjon@mediaone.net
Jon Speake, Commissioner

Fnded: 1976. **Mem:** 24. **Desc:** Teams that are active in wheelchair softball competitions. Acts as governing agency for the promotion, interpretation, standardization, and continued growth of wheelchair softball. Coordinates efforts of member teams and encourages formation of new teams; protects the interests of members and enforces existing rules and regulations established by member teams. Conducts seminars on wheelchair softball and wheelchair sports; sponsors tournaments. Maintains hall of fame and compiles statistics.

★ 5086 ★ National Women's Health Network (NWHN)
514 10th St. NW, Ste. 400
Washington, DC 20004
Phone: (202)347-1140 **Fax:** (202)347-1168
Website: http://www.womenshealthnetwork.org
Cynthia Pearson, Exec. Dir.

Fnded: 1975. **Mem:** 8,000. **Desc:** An advocacy organization giving women a greater voice in the health care system in the United States. It is the only such membership organization and has a 28-year history of accomplishments on behalf of all women. Provides women with unbiased health information through its clearinghouse. Also monitors federal legislation to ensure that women's needs are not overlooked. **Pub:** *National Women's Health Network–Network News*, bimonthly. Newsletter. Keeps readers informed about the important developments in women's health, provides ways to improve one's health, recommends books. *Price:* Included in membership dues. • Also publishes health information packets, booklets, and brochures.

★ 5087 ★ National Women's Health Resource Center (NWHRC)

120 Albany St., Ste. 820
New Brunswick, NJ 08901
Phone: (732)828-8575 **Free:** 877-986-9472
Fax: (732)249-4671
Email: info@healthywomen.org
Website: http://www.healthywomen.org/
Amy R. Niles, Exec. Dir.

Fnded: 1988. **Desc:** Disseminates information about women's health. Serves as the national clearinghouse for women's health information. Provides comprehensive, unbiased health information. **Pub:** *National Women's Health Report*, bimonthly. Newsletter. Information on current women's health issues. *Price:* $30 for individuals; $80 for organizations and institutions.

★ 5088 ★ National Youth Sports Safety Foundation (NYSSF)

1 Beacon St., Ste. 3333
Boston, MA 02108
Phone: (617)367-6677 **Fax:** (617)722-9999
Email: nyssf@aol.com
Website: http://www.nyssf.org
Michelle Klein, Exec. Dir.

Fnded: 1989. **Desc:** Works to promote the safety and well-being of children and adolescents participating in sports. Strives to reduce the number and severity of injuries youth sustain in sports and fitness activities. Sponsors educational programs. Maintains speakers' bureau. **Pub:** *Sidelines*, quarterly. Newsletter. *Price:* included in membership dues; $9.5/year. • *Yearbook of Youth Sports Safety*. **Frmly:** National Youth Sports Foundation for the Prevention of Athletic Inuries.

★ 5089 ★ Native American Cancer Research (NACR)

c/o Linda Burhansstipanov
3022 S Nova Rd
Pine, CO 80470-7830
Phone: (303)838-9359 **Fax:** (303)838-7629
Website: http://members.aol.com/natamcan/
Linda Burhansstipanov, Pres. /Exec. Dir.

Fnded: 1999. **Desc:** Strives to reduce Native American cancer incidence and mortality, and to increase survival from cancer among Native Americans; implements cancer primary prevention, secondary prevention, risk reduction, screening (early detection), education, training, research, diagnoses, control, treatment, support, quality of life, and/or studies of cancer among Native Americans. **Pub:** *Native American Cancer Research Program Newsletter*, 3/year. Newsletter. Informs native and non-natives of Native American cancer prevention and control.

★ 5090 ★ Native American Women's Health Education Resource Center

PO Box 572
Lake Andes, SD 57356-0572
Phone: (605)487-7072 **Fax:** (605)487-7964
Email: nativewoman@igc.apc.org
Website: http://www.nativeshop.org/nawherc.html

Desc: Individuals and organizations interested in the health status of Native American women. Promotes improved health and access to health services for Native American women. Works to redress Eurocentrism in American society. Gathers and disseminates information on women's health and related topics. Conducts educational programs. **Pub:** Newsletter, periodic.

★ 5091 ★ Nature of Wellness

PO Box 10400
Glendale, CA 91209-3400
Phone: (818)790-6384 **Fax:** (818)790-9660
Email: supress@earthlink.net
Website: http://home.earthlink.net/~supress/

Desc: Seeks to inform the public about medical and scientific invalidity of animal experimentation and testing; investigates the impact of reliance by the medical/pharmaceutical/petrochemical industry on animal experimentation (in biomedical research) and animal testing (to assess the safety of drugs, pesticides and other chemicals) has on the health care system, environment and economy.

★ 5092 ★ NCCLS

940 W Valley Rd., Ste. 1400
Wayne, PA 19087-1898
Phone: (610)688-0100 **Fax:** (610)688-0700
Email: info@nccls.org
Website: http://www.nccls.org
John V. Bergen, PhD, Exec. Dir.

Fnded: 1968. **Mem:** 2,100. **Desc:** Government agencies, professional societies, clinical laboratories, and industrial firms with interests in medical testing. Purposes are to promote the development of national and international standards for medical testing and to provide a consensus mechanism for defining and resolving problems that influence the quality and cost of healthcare work performed. **Pub:** *Member/Volunteer Directory*. Directory. Information on NCCLS programs, projects, committees, members, volunteers, and staff. *Price:* Included in membership dues. • *NCCLS Update*, monthly. Newsletter. Includes new member information and meeting calendar. *Price:* Free. • Reports. • Videos. • Also publishes standards and guidelines and documents. **Frmly:** (1994) National Committee for Clinical Laboratory Standards; (1997) NCCLS: The Clinical Laboratory Standards Organization; (2000) National Committee for Clinical Laboratory Standards.

★ 5093 ★ NEA Health Information Network (NEA HIN)

1201 16th St., NW, Ste. 521
Washington, DC 20036
Phone: (202)822-7570 **Free:** 800-718-8387
Fax: (202)822-7775
Email: info@neahin.org
Website: http://www.neahin.org

Fnded: 1987. **Desc:** Dedicated to improve health, safety, and student achievement by providing school employees with vital, effective and timely health information. **Frmly:** (2001) Health Information Network.

★ 5094 ★ Nederlandse Federatie van Ouders van Dove Kinderen

c/o Els van der Zee
PO Box 754
NL-3500 AT Utrecht, Netherlands
Phone: 31 30 2900360
Email: fodok@wxs.nl
Website: http://www.fodok.nl

Mem: 9. **Lang(s):** Dutch. **Desc:** Organizations of parents of deaf children. Addresses the concerns of parents with deaf children; disseminates information.

★ 5095 ★ Neonatal Society

Academic Division of Child Health
School of Human Development
University Hospital
Nottingham NG7 2UH, United Kingdom
Phone: 44 115 9709257 **Fax:** 44 115 9709382

Fnded: 1959.

★ 5096 ★ Netherlands Association for Library, Information and Knowledge Professionals

Plompetorengracht 11
NL-3512 CA Utrecht, Netherlands
Phone: 31 30 2311263 **Fax:** 31 30 2311830
Email: nvbinfo@wxs.nl
Website: http://www.nvb-online.nl/contact.html?pagina=45

Fnded: 1912. **Mem:** 3,200. **Desc:** Represents and promotes library, information and knowledge professionals in the Netherlands. **Pub:** Newsletter, monthly.

★ 5097 ★ Netherlands Dietetic Association (NVD) (Nederlandse Vereniging van Dietisten)

Postbus 341
NL-5340 AH Oss, Netherlands
Phone: 31 412 624543 **Fax:** 31 412 637736
Email: bureau@nvdietist.nl
Website: http://www.nvdietist.nl

Fnded: 1941. **Mem:** 2,500. **Desc:** Strives to maintain high professional standards for dieticians working in the Netherlands. Represents members interests. Offers postgraduate training courses. **Pub:** *Dutch Journal for Dietitians*, periodic. Journal. • Brochures.

★ 5098 ★ Netherlands Institute for Care and Welfare

Catharijnesingel 47
Postbus 19152
NL-3501 DD Utrecht, Netherlands
Phone: 31 30 2306311 **Fax:** 31 30 2319641
Email: infolijn@nizw.nl
Website: http://www.nizw.nl

Lang(s): Dutch, English, French, German. **Desc:** Health professionals and institutions providing care to people with disabilities. Promotes an improved quality of life for people with disabilities. Represents members' interests; conducts research and educational programs.

★ 5099 ★ Netherlands Society of Cardiology (NSC) (Nederlandse Vereniging voor Cardiologie — NVVC)

PO Box 19192
NL-3501 DD Utrecht, Netherlands
Phone: 31 30 2345000 **Fax:** 31 30 2345002
Email: bureau@nvvc.nl
Website: http://www.cardiologie.nl

Fnded: 1934. **Mem:** 1,000. **Desc:** Promotes the profession of cardiology, cardiological research, and cardiac care in the Netherlands. Defends the professional interests of members. **Pub:** *Netherlands Heart Journal*, monthly. Journal. **Frmly:** (1999) Dutch Society of Cardiology.

★ 5100 ★ Netherlands Society for Dermatology and Venereology (Nederlandse Vereniging voor Dermatologie en Venereologie — NVDV)

c/o Dr. J.C.J.M. Veraart
Postbus 8552
NL-3503 RN Utrecht, Netherlands
Phone: 31 30 2474695 **Fax:** 31 30 2474439
Email: nvdv@vvaa.nl

Fnded: 1896. **Mem:** 500. **Desc:** Physicians and interested individuals. Promotes the study of dermatology and venereal infection and treatment. **Pub:** *Nederlands Tydschrift Voor Dermatologie en Veneredogie*, 8/year. Magazine. **Frmly:** (1999) Dutch Association for Dermatology and Venereology.

★ 5101 ★ Netherlands Society for Endocrinology (Nederlandse Vereniging voor Endocrinologie — NVE)

c/o D. Braat
Department of Gynaecology and Obstetrics
St. Radboudziekenhuis
Geert Grooteplein Zuid 14
NL-6500 HB Nijmegen, Netherlands
Phone: 31 24 3613932 **Fax:** 31 24 3541194

Fnded: 1947. **Mem:** 500. **Desc:** Fosters research and clinical practice in endocrinology.

★ 5102 ★ Netherlands Society of Gerontology
PO Box 222
NL-3500 AE Utrecht, Netherlands
Phone: 31 30 2769960 **Fax:** 31 30 2762880
Email: nig@nig.nl
Desc: Promotes gerontological research, training in the field of aging, and interests of gerontological organizations in international affairs.

★ 5103 ★ Netherlands Society of Tropical Medicine (Societe Nederlandaise de Medecine Tropicale)
c/o Nadamo Bos
PO Box 244
NL-3970 AE Driebergen Rijsenburg, Netherlands
Phone: 31 343 517126 **Fax:** 31 343 517126
Email: nadamo@worldaccess.nl
Website: http://www.rstmh.org/Netherlands.html
Fnded: 1907. **Mem:** 950. **Desc:** Physicians, nurses, midwives, social scientists, biologists, public relations officers, economists, and others working in the field of tropical medicine. Promotes research education and practice of tropical medicine and other related sciences. Areas of interest include: health care in developing countries, tropical surgery, topical pediatrics, maternal health and family planning. Collaborates with national and international organizations concerned with tropical health care. **Pub:** *Medicus Tropicus*, bimonthly. Magazine. • *Tropical Medicine and International Health*, monthly. Journal.

★ 5104 ★ Network Against Coercive Psychiatry (NACP)
172 W 79th St., No. 2E
New York, NY 10024
Phone: (212)560-7288 **Fax:** (212)799-9026
Email: seth17279@aol.com
Dr. Seth Farber, PhD, Contact
Fnded: 1989. **Desc:** Comprised of psychotherapists including psychiatrists, survivors of psychiatric incarceration, scholars and other concerned citizens. Promotes the idea of mental illness as a misleading and degrading metaphor. Works towards the possible development of a social movement against the mental health system.

★ 5105 ★ Network for Continuing Medical Education (NCME)
One Harmon Plaza
Secaucus, NJ 07094
Phone: (201)867-3550 **Free:** 800-223-0433
Fax: (201)867-2491
Website: http://www.ncme.com
Paul Gersh, Pres.
Fnded: 1965. **Mem:** 800. **Desc:** Hospitals that subscribe to receive NCME services. Produces and distributes monthly course package including videotape, posters, program brochure, and workbook to members. Course packages cover the full spectrum of medical topics and are designed to provide category 1 continuing medical education credit to physicians. **Pub:** *Video Journal Dermatology*, quarterly. • *Video Journal Oncology*, quarterly.

★ 5106 ★ Neuro-Developmental Treatment Association (NDTA)
1540 S Coast Hwy., Ste. 203
Laguna Beach, CA 92651
Free: 800-869-9295 **Fax:** (949)376-3456
Email: membership@ndta.org
Website: http://www.ndta.org
Brad Lund, Principal Dir.
Fnded: 1967. **Mem:** 3,800. **Reg. Groups:** 14. **Desc:** Physical and occupational therapists, speech pathologists, special educators, physicians, parents, and others interested in neurodevelopmental treatment. (NDT is a form of therapy for individuals who suffer from central nervous system disorders resulting in abnormal movement. Treatment attempts to initiate or refine normal stages and processes in the development of movement.) Informs members of new developments in the field and with ideas that will eventually improve functional independence. Locates articles related to NDT. Regional groups maintain libraries. **Pub:** *NDTA Network*, bimonthly. Newsletter. *Price:* for members. **Frmly:** International Bobath Alumni Association.

★ 5107 ★ Neurofibromatosis (NF)
9320 Annapolis Rd., Ste. 300
Lanham, MD 20706-3123
Phone: (301)918-4600 **Free:** 800-942-6825
Fax: (301)918-0009
Email: info@nfinc.org
Website: http://www.nfinc.org
Brenda Duffy, Pres.
Fnded: 1988. **Reg. Groups:** 9. **Desc:** Organizations providing support for individuals with neurofibromatosis (NF) and their families, physicians, and other health care providers. (NF is a genetic neurological disorder that can cause tumors to form on nerves and is linked to learning disabilities, hearing loss, vision impairment, epilepsy, and cancer.) Increases public awareness of NF through information dissemination; informs federal, state, and local legislators of the needs of NF families. Promotes, supports, and funds medical, clinical, educational, and sociological research that addresses the need to diagnose, treat, cure, and prevent NF. Identifies local NF support and peer counseling groups; offers referrals to medical resources and scientifically-evaluated research. Participates in networking of voluntary health organizations. **Pub:** *Neurofibromatosis Ink*, semiannual. Newsletter. Includes research summaries, reports, chapter news, and symposia information, bibliography, fundraising activities. • *Understanding Neurofibromatosis: An Introduction for Patients and Parents.* Booklets. *Price:* $3 for each multiple copy.

★ 5108 ★ Neurofibromatosis Association
82 London Rd.
Kingston Upon Thames KT2 6PX, United Kingdom
Phone: 44 208 5471636 **Fax:** 44 208 9745601
Email: nfa@zetnet.co.uk
Website: http://www.nfa.zetnet.co.uk
Fnded: 1981. **Mem:** 1,870. **Reg. Groups:** 36. **Desc:** Seeks to establish and maintain a network of family support workers who are able to support and offer practical help and advice to those affected by Neurofibromatosis and their families. Neurofibromatosis is a genetic disorder of the nerve tissue, the characteristics of which include six or more coffee colored marks on the skin in the first two years of life and nodules on or just below the surface of the skin, or tumors on both acoustical nerves. Fosters research; disseminates information. **Pub:** Newsletter, quarterly. • Annual Report.

★ 5109 ★ Neurofibromatosis Association of Ireland (NAI)
Carmichael Center
North Brunswick St.
Dublin 7, Ireland
Phone: 353 1 8726338 **Fax:** 353 1 8735737
Email: nfaireland@eircom.net
Website: http://www.nfaireland.ie
Fnded: 1985. **Mem:** 480. **Reg. Groups:** 3. **Lang(s):** English, Irish. **Desc:** Individuals and organizations. Seeks to improve the quality of life of people with neurofibromatosis and their families; promotes increased awareness of neurofibromatosis among health care providers and the public. Makes available support and services; conducts educational and advocacy campaigns; sponsors research. **Pub:** *Neuro News*, bimonthly. Newsletter.

★ 5110 ★ Neurologiskt Handikappades Riksforbund
c/o Monika Paulin
Box 32 84
S-103 65 Stockholm, Sweden
Phone: 46 8 6777010 **Fax:** 46 8 241315
Email: nhr@nhr.se
Website: http://www.nhr.se
Fnded: 1957. **Reg. Groups:** 119. **Desc:** Persons with neurological disabilities. Seeks to improve the quality of life for persons with multiple sclerosis and their families.

★ 5111 ★ Neuromuscular Diseases Association of Romania
Institute of Neurology
C.P. 44-12
R-75128 Bucharest, Romania
Phone: 40 1 3306273 **Fax:** 40 1 3213964
Email: ahnrom@inext.ro
Website: http://www.alsmndalliance.org/directory/romania.html
Desc: Promotes interest in neuromuscular diseases research among medical and scientific communities and the public in Romania. Disseminates information about the diseases.

★ 5112 ★ Neuropathy Association
Lincoln Bldg.
60 E 42nd St., Ste. 942
New York, NY 10165
Phone: (212)692-0662 **Free:** 800-247-6968
Fax: (212)692-0668
Email: info@neuropahty.org
Website: http://www.neuropathy.org
Catherine Law, CFO
Fnded: 1995. **Mem:** 50,000. **Local Groups:** 200. **Desc:** Offers support to persons suffering from disorders affecting the peripheral nerves; provides patient support and education, advocates for patients' interests, promotes research into the causes and cure for peripheral neuropathies. **Pub:** *A Guide to the Peripheral Neuropathies.* Booklet. • *Exercising with Neuropathy.* Booklet. • *Explaining Peripheral Neuropathy.* Booklet. • *Neuropathy News.* Newsletter.

★ 5113 ★ Neurosurgical Society of Australasia
College of Surgeons Gardens
240 Spring St.
Melbourne, VIC 3000, Australia
Phone: 61 3 92491294 **Fax:** 61 3 92491240
Email: college.nsa@surgeons.org
Website: http://www.nsa.on.net
Fnded: 1940.

★ 5114 ★ Neutropenia Support Association
905 Corydon
PO Box 243
Winnipeg, MB, Canada R3M 3S7
Phone: (204)489-8454 **Free:** 800-6-NEUTRO
Fax: (204)589-8454
Email: stevensl@neutropenia.ca
Website: http://www.neutropenia.ca/
Fnded: 1989. **Desc:** Works to increase awareness and understanding of neutropenia, a blood disorder, and other rare diseases. Promotes development and/or study of treatments, drug strategies, guidelines, drug approval, long term safety surveillance, sensitivity to chemotherapy drugs needed prior to transplantation, and genetics. Provides patient advocacy.

★ 5115 ★ Nevus Network
c/o The Congenital Nevus Support Group
PO Box 305
West Salem, OH 44287
Phone: (419)853-4525
Email: info@nevusnetwork.org
Website: http://www.nevusnetwork.org
BJ Bett, Co-Founder
Fnded: 1983. **Mem:** 900. **Reg. Groups:** 6. **Desc:** Works to support people with a large congenital nevus (large brown birth marks). Offers pen pals and information. **Pub:** *Nevus Network News*, periodic. Newsletter. *Price:* None. • Brochure.

★ 5116 ★ New England Gerontological Association (NEGA)
1 Cutts Rd.
Durham, NH 03824-3102
Phone: (603)868-5757
Email: genetsr@attbi.com
Website: http://www.negaonline.org
Dr. Eugene E. Tillock, Exec. Dir.

Fnded: 1958. **Mem:** 125. **Reg. Groups:** 1. **Desc:** Promotes the study of the aging process. Conducts educational programs in aging, health service administration and long-term care administration. **Pub:** *Gerontology Topics*, quarterly. Newsletter.

★ 5117 ★ New Hope Foundation
51 Throckmorton St.
Freehold, NJ 07728
Phone: (732)308-0113 **Fax:** (732)308-0115
Website: http://www.newhopefoundation.org
Alicia Goodhue, Contact

Desc: Private citizens, businesses, and organizations. Strives to serve those in need of treatment of alcoholism, drug addition, and gambling. Offers both inpatient and outpatient services.

★ 5118 ★ New Zealand Association of Gerontology
Auckland Hospital
Private Bag 92024
Auckland, New Zealand
Phone: 64 9 3074949 **Fax:** 64 9 3754344
Email: apoulter@adhb.govt.nz

Fnded: 1981. **Mem:** 400. **Nat'l Groups:** 1. **Reg. Groups:** 4. **Local Groups:** 4. **Desc:** Gerontologists in New Zealand. Studies ageing in all aspects. Encourages training for individuals caring for older people. Promotes gerontological research. **Pub:** *NZAG Newsletter*, quarterly. Newsletter. Includes information, feedback, and upcoming events.

★ 5119 ★ New Zealand Association of Optometrists
PO Box 1978
Wellington, New Zealand
Phone: 64 4 4732322 **Fax:** 64 4 4732328
Email: info@nzao.co.nz
Website: http://www.nzao.co.nz

Fnded: 1930. **Mem:** 800. **Reg. Groups:** 8. **Desc:** Optometrists in New Zealand. Seeks to ensure high standards of ethics and practice in optometry.

★ 5120 ★ New Zealand Association for the Scientific Study of Mental Deficiency (NZASSMD)
PO Box 19099
Wellington, New Zealand
Phone: 64 6 8774296
Email: mgahreus@xtra.co.uz

Fnded: 1980. **Lang(s):** English. **Desc:** Promotes research on intellectual disability. Unites professionals working in the field and facilitates data exchange; disseminates information. Establishes standards for practice and ethics. Monitors relevant legislation. **Pub:** *Australia and New Zealand Journal of Developmental Disability*, periodic. • Magazine, periodic.

★ 5121 ★ New Zealand Childcare Association (Te Tari Puna Ora o Aotearoa)
PO Box 11-863
Manners St.
Wellington, New Zealand
Phone: 64 4 4734672 **Fax:** 64 4 4737295
Email: rose.cole@nzchildcare.ac.nz
Website: http://www.nzchildcare.ac.nz

Fnded: 1963. **Mem:** 1,000. **Reg. Groups:** 17. **Desc:** Promotes and supports accessibility to quality child care in New Zealand. **Pub:** *Itirearea*, semimonthly. Newsletter. Also publishes texts concerned with parent education, student texts, and general information on childcare.

★ 5122 ★ New Zealand College of Midwives
PO Box 21-106
376 Manchester St.
Christchurch, New Zealand
Phone: 64 3 3772732 **Fax:** 64 3 3775662
Email: nzcom@nzcom.org.nz
Website: http://www.midwife.org.nz

Fnded: 1990. **Mem:** 2,000. **Reg. Groups:** 10. **Lang(s):** English. **Desc:** Midwives, consumer groups, and interested individuals. Promotes midwifery services and education, and represents the interests of midwives to governmental bodies and the public. Prescribes and monitors standards for the practice and education of midwifery. Acts as a consultant for governmental agencies; engages in the negotiation of government funding for community and independent midwifery services. Offers courses jointly with colleges and universities. **Pub:** *New Zealand College of Midwives*, semiannual. Journal. Contains articles on midwifery. • *New Zealand College of Midwives Midwifery News*, quarterly. Newsletter.

★ 5123 ★ New Zealand Continence Association (NZCA)
c/o Jill Brown, Sec.
41 Pembroke St.
Hamilton, New Zealand
Email: jill@continence.org.nz
Website: http://www.continence.org.nz/content.php

Desc: Provides services to people with continence problems, caregivers, health professionals, and general public, provides information and education on continence topics.

★ 5124 ★ New Zealand Dental Association (NZDA)
PO Box 28084
Auckland 5, New Zealand
Phone: 64 9 5242778 **Fax:** 64 9 5205256
Email: nzdainfo@nzda.org.nz
Website: http://www.nzda.org.nz

Fnded: 1905. **Mem:** 1,500. **Local Groups:** 15. **Lang(s):** English. **Desc:** Registered dental practitioners in New Zealand. Promotes improved dental health through the increased availability of dental and allied services. Collects and disseminates data on topics including AIDS, infection control, and oral health costs. **Pub:** *Membership Booklet of the New Zealand Dental Association*, annual. Directory. • *New Zealand Dental Journal*, quarterly. Journal. • *NZDA News*, bimonthly. Newsletter.

★ 5125 ★ New Zealand Dental Therapists Association
c/o Kathryn Holdaway
203 Lovedale Rd.
Hastings
Hawkes Bay, New Zealand
Phone: 64 6 8787504 **Fax:** 64 6 8787504
Email: nzdta@nzdta.co.nz
Website: http://www.nzdta.co.nz

Fnded: 1921. **Mem:** 460. **Nat'l Groups:** 1. **Reg. Groups:** 4. **Local Groups:** 18. **Lang(s):** English. **Desc:** Women dental therapists of New Zealand. Promotes the professional interests of members. Works to ensure the provision of dental services to children and adults in New Zealand. Establishes industry standards. **Pub:** *Dental Therapist Journal*, annual. Journal.

★ 5126 ★ New Zealand Dietetic Association (NZDA)
PO Box 5065
Wellington, New Zealand
Phone: 64 4 4733061 **Fax:** 64 4 4733062
Email: nzda@dietitians.org.nz
Website: http://www.dietitians.org.nz

Fnded: 1943. **Mem:** 500. **Reg. Groups:** 7. **Desc:** Enhances the profile of the dietetic profession; provides comment and information on key health and nutrition issues to government and the media; supports and strengthens the professional performance of members. **Pub:** *Journal of New Zealand Dietetic Association*, semiannual. Journal.

★ 5127 ★ New Zealand Endometriosis Foundation
PO Box 1683
Palmerston North 5301, New Zealand
Phone: 64 6 3592613 **Fax:** 64 6 3592613
Email: nzendo@xtra.co.nz
Website: http://www.nzendo.co.nz

Fnded: 1986. **Mem:** 500. **Local Groups:** 16. **Lang(s):** English. **Desc:** Offers education, information and support for girls and women with endometriosis and others interested in the disease. The Foundation fosters research and works with gynecologists and other health professionals in New Zealand and around the world. **Pub:** Newsletter, quarterly.

★ 5128 ★ New Zealand Genetical Society
Private Bag
Christchurch, New Zealand
Phone: 64 3 252511 **Fax:** 64 3 252074
Fnded: 1949.

★ 5129 ★ New Zealand Institute of Medical Radiation Technology (NZIMRT)
c/o Dave Morris, Gen.Sec.
PO Box 25668
St. Heliers
Auckland, New Zealand
Website: http://www.nzimrt.co.nz/mportal.aspx

Desc: Represents medical radiation technologists and radiation therapists in New Zealand.

★ 5130 ★ New Zealand Medical Association (NZMA)
26 The Terrace
PO Box 156
Wellington, New Zealand
Phone: 64 4 4724741 **Fax:** 64 4 4710838
Email: nzma@nzma.org.nz
Website: http://www.nzma.org.nz

Fnded: 1886. **Desc:** Members come from all disciplines within the medical profession. Aims to provide advocacy on behalf of doctors and their patients. Provides support and services to members and their practices.

★ 5131 ★ New Zealand Nurses Organization (NZNO)
PO Box 2128
Wellington, New Zealand
Phone: 64 4 9316747 **Fax:** 64 4 3829993
Email: nurses@nzno.org.nz
Website: http://www.nzno.org.nz

Fnded: 1909. **Mem:** 31,000. **Reg. Groups:** 11. **Desc:** Nurses, nurses' aids and medical radiation technologist. Represents and promotes nurses' interests and concerns on health issues through participation in health and social policy development. Conducts research on health issues. Offers health education programs. **Pub:** *New Zealand Nursing Journal*, 11/year. Journal.

★ 5132 ★ New Zealand Pain Society (NZPS)
PO Box 5303
Wellington, New Zealand
Phone: 64 4 4995957 **Fax:** 64 4 4995953
Email: info@nzps.org.nz
Website: http://www.nzps.org.nz

Fnded: 1983. **Mem:** 280. **Lang(s):** English. **Desc:** Health professionals and scientists interested in pain research and management. Works to improve the management of pain. Encourages research into pain mechanisms and pain syndromes; recommends the adoption of a uniform classification, nomenclature, and definition of pain and pain syndromes; advises national and regional agencies on standards relating to the use of drugs, appliances, and procedures in the therapy of pain; promotes education and training in pain management; facilitates information dissemination. Conducts lectures and workshops. **Pub:** *Directory*, annual. Directory. • *Ngau Mamae*, quarterly. Newsletter.

★ 5133 ★ New Zealand Private Hospitals Association (NZPHA)

PO Box 12 481
Wellington 6015, New Zealand
Phone: 64 4 4733159 **Fax:** 64 4 4733554
Email: lesley@nzpha.org.nz
Website: http://www.nzpha.org.nz

Fnded: 1946. **Lang(s):** English. **Desc:** Private hospitals in New Zealand. Represents, protects, and advocates the interests of its members and their associated services.

★ 5134 ★ New Zealand Psychological Society (NZPsS)

PO Box 4092
Wellington, New Zealand
Phone: 64 4 4734884 **Fax:** 64 4 4734889
Email: office@psychology.org.nz
Website: http://www.psychology.org.nz

Fnded: 1967. **Mem:** 700. **Reg. Groups:** 8. **Local Groups:** 8. **Lang(s):** English. **Desc:** Professional association for psychologists and interested individuals. Promotes psychology as a science. Represents interests of professional psychologists; provides services to members. Publishes "New Zealand Journal of Psychology." **Pub:** *AGM Agenda*, annual. Annual Report. • *Connections*, monthly. Newsletter. • *New Zealand Journal of Psychology*, semiannual. Journal. Two issues per volume. • *NZPSS Bulletin*, quarterly. Bulletin. • *Practice Issues for Clinical and Applied Psychologists in New Zealand*. Book. • *The Practice of Psychology & the Law: A Handbook*. Handbook.

★ 5135 ★ New Zealand Society for Music Therapy (NZSMT)

47 The Crows Nest
Whitby
Porirua 6006, New Zealand
Phone: 64 4 2347192 **Fax:** 64 4 2347191
Email: lewishome@xtra.co.nz
Website: http://www.nzsme.org.nz/therapy.html

Fnded: 1974. **Mem:** 150. **Reg. Groups:** 4. **Local Groups:** 4. **Lang(s):** English. **Desc:** Music therapy professionals. Promotes the therapeutic use of music as an educational tool for the intellectually and physically disabled, rehabilitation patients, and special education students. Initiates discussions with government departments concerning professional training courses and job establishment for music therapists. Encourages hospitals and community groups to consider employment of music therapists. Offers training courses; local branches conduct workshops and provide speakers. **Pub:** *Journal*, annual. Journal. • *MusT*, periodic. Newsletter.

★ 5136 ★ New Zealand Veterinary Association (NZVA)

PO Box 11-212
Manners St.
Wellington, New Zealand
Phone: 64 4 4710484 **Fax:** 64 4 4710494
Email: nzva@vets.org.nz
Website: http://www.vets.org.nz

Fnded: 1923. **Mem:** 1,500. **Reg. Groups:** 14. **Local Groups:** 15. **Lang(s):** English. **Desc:** Promotes excellence in the veterinary profession through service to its members. **Pub:** *New Zealand Veterinary Journal*, bimonthly. Journal. • *New Zealand Vetscript*, monthly.

★ 5137 ★ NHS Consultants Association

Hill House
Banbury
Oxon OX17 1QH, United Kingdom
Phone: 44 1295 750407 **Fax:** 44 1295 750407
Email: nhsca@pop3.poptel.org.uk
Website: http://www.nhsca.org.uk

Fnded: 1976. **Mem:** 600. **Desc:** Senior doctors committed to the NHS and the basic principles on which it was founded. Acts as a pressure group lobbying politicians and others concerned with health. **Pub:** Reports. **Frmly:** (2001) National Health Service Consultants Association.

★ 5138 ★ NIDCD - National Temporal Bone, Hearing and Balance Pathology Resource Registry (NTBR)

Massachusetts Eye and Ear Infirmary
243 Charles St.
Boston, MA 02114-3096
Phone: (617)573-3711 **Free:** 800-822-1327
Fax: (617)573-3838
Email: tbregistry@meei.harvard.edu
Website: http://www.tbregistry.org
Dr. Joseph B. Nadol, Jr., Contact

Fnded: 1960. **Reg. Groups:** 25. **Desc:** Promotes research of hearing and balance disorders through the study of the temporal bone and related brain structures. Encourages individuals with hearing or balance disorders to bequeath their temporal bones to scientific research. Serves as a clearinghouse for information on temporal bone research. Develops strategies to conserve human temporal bone collections. Maintains a nationwide network to retrieve donated temporal bone and brain tissue. **Pub:** *The Gift of Hearing, That Others May Hear*. Brochures. • *The Registry*, semiannual. Newsletter. Includes information about temporal bone research and donations. *Price:* Free. **Frmly:** (1992) National Temporal Bone Banks Program of The DRF; (1997) National Temporal Bone Registry; (1999) National Temporal Bone, Hearing and Balance Pathology Registry; (2003) National Temporal Bone, Hearing and Balance Pathology Resource Registry.

★ 5139 ★ Nightingale Research Foundation (NRF)

c/o Dr. Byron Hyde, Chair
121 Iona St.
Ottawa, ON, Canada K1Y 3M1
Fax: (613)523-1958
Email: nightingale@nightingale.ca
Website: http://www.nightingale.ca

Fnded: 1988. **Mem:** 8,000. **Lang(s):** English, French. **Desc:** Individuals with Myalgic Encephalomyelitis (Chronic Fatigue Syndrome); health care providers and medical researchers with an interest in non-HIV acquired immune deficiency syndromes. Seeks to advance scientific knowledge of the causes of non-HIV immune deficiency syndromes, and to develop more effective treatments for these diseases. Conducts research and educational programs for the public, health care professionals, and medical researchers; sponsors fundraising activities. **Pub:** *Nightingale*, annual. Newsletter. • Booklets. • Brochure.

★ 5140 ★ NIPPA-The Early Years Organisation (NIPPA)

6c Wildflower Way
Apollo Rd.
Belfast, United Kingdom
Phone: 44 2890 662825 **Fax:** 44 2890 381270
Email: mail@nippa.org

Fnded: 1965. **Mem:** 960. **Local Groups:** 19. **Lang(s):** English, Irish. **Desc:** Promotes the availability of child care facilities for women with children under 5 years of age. Fosters children's educational and physical development. **Pub:** *NIPPA Network*, quarterly. Newsletter. • Annual Report. • Books.

★ 5141 ★ NISH

2235 Cedar Ln.
Vienna, VA 22182-5200
Phone: (703)560-6800 **Fax:** (703)698-0124
Email: info@nish.org
Website: http://www.nish.org
Bob Chamberlin, Pres.

Fnded: 1974. **Mem:** 550. **Reg. Groups:** 6. **Desc:** Provides employment opportunities for people with severe disabilities under the Javits-Wagner O'Day Act. Promotes their placement into competitive industry. Conducts research and development to identify to the government commodities and services which are feasible for production and/or performance by work centers. (Work centers are nonprofit agencies that provide rehabilitative, training, and vocational services for persons with severe disabilities.) Provides training and technical assistance in the form of industrial engineering, production planning, quality control, inventory management, cost analysis, procurement, and contract administration. Acts as a liaison between work centers and the federal government. **Pub:** *NISH News*, monthly. Newsletter. Reports on work centers employing persons with severe disabilities, and legislation and regulations affecting these centers. *Price:* Free to participants of the J-W O'Day Program. • Annual Report. *Price:* Free. • Brochure. **Frmly:** (1991) National Industries for the Severely Handicapped.

★ 5142 ★ Nordic Aerobiological Society

Alvdalen
S-186 60 Vallentuna, Sweden
Phone: 46 8 51235500 **Fax:** 46 51235500
Email: mvp@innocent.com
Website: http://user.tninet.se/~cap624e

Fnded: 1977. **Desc:** Supports development of aerobiology and improves international cooperation, especially in Scandinavia.

★ 5143 ★ Nordic Association for Andrology (NAFA)

c/o Anders Bjartell
Department of Urology
Malmo University Hospital
S-205 02 Malmo, Sweden
Phone: 46 40331000 **Fax:** 40 40337352
Email: anders.bjartell@kir.mas.lu.se
Website: http://www.ki.se/org/nafa/

Desc: Membership is for all physicians and researchers interested in Andrology. Provides a meeting place for Nordic researchers and physicians interested in Andrology. Activities include annual meetings, and courses.

★ 5144 ★ Nordic Association for Clinical Sexology

Gronhojgardsvej 147
DK-2630 Taastrup, Denmark
Phone: 45 43996619 **Fax:** 45 43996619
Email: dacs@klinisksexologi.dk
Website: http://www.seksologinenseura.net

Fnded: 1979. **Lang(s):** Danish, English. **Desc:** promotes scientific exchange and practical collaboration in sexology between Denmark, Finland, Iceland, Norway, Estonia and Sweden; creates and promotes sexological knowledge and information.

★ 5145 ★ Nordic Association for Psychiatric Epidemiology (NAPE)

c/o Kristinn Tomasson
Bildshofoa 16
IS-110 Reykjavik, Iceland
Phone: 354 5504650

Fnded: 1997. **Desc:** Professionals within psychiatric epidemiology research. Promotes research within psychiatric epidemiology; recruits and supervises young researchers; aims to expand collaboration between Nordic and global countries; disseminates research results.

★ 5146 ★ Nordic Audiological Society (Nordisk Audiologisk Selskab — NAS)

Frankrigsgade 4
DK-2300 Copenhagen S, Denmark

Email: nasbc@vip.cybercity.dk
Website: http://www.nas.dk

Fnded: 1960.

★ 5147 ★ Nordic Cooperation on Disability (Nordiska Samarbetsorganet for Handikappfragor — NSH)

Box 510
S-162 15 Vallingby, Sweden
Phone: 46 8 6201890 **Fax:** 46 8 7392400
Email: nsh@nsh.se
Website: http://www.nsh.se

Fnded: 1980. **Mem:** 5. **Lang(s):** Danish, English, Finnish, Norwegian, Swedish. **Desc:** Governmental organization for Denmark, Finland, Iceland, Norway, and Sweden. Initiates, organizes, and expedites cooperation among Nordic countries on efforts concerning disability and rehabilitation.

★ 5148 ★ Nordic Council for Alcohol and Drug Research (NCADR) (Nordiska Namnden for Alkohol- och Drogforskning — NAD)

Annegatan 29 A 23
FIN-00100 Helsinki 10, Finland
Phone: 358 9 6948082 **Fax:** 358 9 6949081
Email: nads@kaapeli.fi
Website: http://www.kaapeli.fi/nad

Fnded: 1978. **Mem:** 5. **Lang(s):** Danish, Norwegian, Swedish. **Desc:** Researchers from Denmark, Finland, Iceland, Norway, and Sweden. Coordinates alcohol and drug research within Scandinavia; initiates new research projects. Organizes seminars. Disseminates information. **Pub:** Book, 0-4/year.

★ 5149 ★ Nordic Cystic Fibrosis Association

PO Box 1827
S-751 48 Uppsala, Sweden
Phone: 46 18151622
Email: info@rfcf.se

Fnded: 1982.

★ 5150 ★ Nordic Eating Disorders Society

PO Box 1613
S-701 16 Orebro, Sweden

★ 5151 ★ Nordic Environmental Mutagen Society (NordEMS)

POB 4404 Torshov
N-0403 Oslo, Norway

Fnded: 1980. **Desc:** Promotes research into genotoxic effects of environmental chemicals in the nordic countries.

★ 5152 ★ Nordic Federation of Heart and Lung Associations (NHL) (Nordiska Hjart and Lungsjukas Forbund)

Kampementsgatan 14
S-115 38 Stockholm, Sweden
Phone: 46 8 6626882
Email: info@heartlung.org
Website: http://www.heartlung.org

Fnded: 1948. **Mem:** 150,000. **Reg. Groups:** 126. **Lang(s):** Danish, Finnish, Icelandic, Norwegian, Swedish. **Desc:** Lung and heart disease specialists in 5 countries. Addresses medical issues in the context of social welfare. Engages in political activities; operates vocational and training centers. **Pub:** *BM-Bladet*, monthly. • *Silmu*, monthly. • *Status*, monthly. • *Trygd og Arbeid*, monthly.

★ 5153 ★ Nordic Federation for Medical Education

Co. Eivind Drange
Svingen 20A
N-5162 Laksevag, Norway
Phone: 47 51518648 **Fax:** 47 92050629
Email: drei@sir.no
Website: http://www.nfmu.org/

Fnded: 1966.

★ 5154 ★ Nordic Federation of Societies of Obstetrics and Gynecology (Nordisk Forening for Obstetrik och Gynekologi)

c/o Dr. Satu Suhonen, Sec.
Helsinki University Central Hospital
Women's Hospital
PO Box 610
FIN-00029 Helsinki, Finland
Email: satu.suhonen@hus.fi
Website: http://www.nfog.org

Fnded: 1933. **Mem:** 4,000. **Nat'l Groups:** 5. **Lang(s):** Swedish. **Desc:** Gynecologists and obstetricians from five Nordic countries. Conducts education programs; sponsors competitions and holds Nordic Congress for Obstetricians and Gynecologists every other year. **Pub:** *Acta Obstetrica Gynecologicia Scandinavica*, 10/year. Journal. Includes supplements. • *Bulletin*, quarterly. Newsletter. **Frmly:** Scandinavian Association of Obstetrics and Gynecology; (1999) Federation of Scandinavian Societies of Obstetrics and Gynecology.

★ 5155 ★ Nordic Gerontological Federation (NGF)

Ullevaal Hospital
N-0407 Oslo, Norway
Email: toril.utne@nordemens.no
Website: http://www.geronord.no

Fnded: 1973. **Desc:** Promotes gerontological research, development and education in the Nordic countries.

★ 5156 ★ Nordic Institute for Advanced Training in Occupational Health (NIATOH) (Nordisk Arbetsmiljoutbildning)

Topeliuksenkatu 41a A
FIN-00250 Helsinki, Finland
Phone: 358 9 47471 **Fax:** 358 9 47472497
Email: niva@ttl.fi
Website: http://www.niva.org

Fnded: 1982. **Lang(s):** Danish, English, Finnish, Norwegian, Swedish. **Desc:** Occupational health service personnel, doctoral students, and researchers. Provides courses in occupational health and working life questions. **Pub:** Catalog, annual. **Frmly:** (1989) Nordic Institute of Advanced Occupational Environment Studies.

★ 5157 ★ Nordic Medical Society of Paraplegia

Spinali's SCI Research Unit, Karolinska Hospital
S- 17176 Stockholm, Sweden
Phone: 46 8 51770050 **Fax:** 46 8 51770077

Fnded: 1987. **Desc:** Supports education and research into spinal cord lesion.

★ 5158 ★ Nordic Neurological Association

Umea University of Hospital
S-901 85 Umea, Sweden
Phone: 46 90 7851931

Fnded: 1922. **Desc:** Supports research and development of neurology in Scandinavian countries.

★ 5159 ★ Nordic Orthopedic Federation (Nordisk Ortopedisk Forening — NOF)

Umea University Hospital
S-901 85 Umea, Sweden
Email: olle.svensson@orthop.umu.se
Website: http://www.norf.org

Fnded: 1919. **Mem:** 2,500. **Nat'l Groups:** 5. **State Groups:** 5. **Desc:** Fosters orthopedic surgery within Nordic countries.

★ 5160 ★ Nordic Paediatric Federation (Nordisk Paediatrisk Forening)

Vestfold Central Hospital
N-3116 Tonsberg, Norway
Phone: 47 33342000

Fnded: 1916. **Desc:** Supports collaboration between Nordic paediatricians; concentrates on educational and organizational issues and other tasks of importance for Nordic paediatricians.

★ 5161 ★ Nordic Psychoanalytical Association

Industrigt 46
N-0357 Oslo, Norway
Phone: 47 22604692

★ 5162 ★ Nordic Radiologic Society (Nordisk Forening for Medisinsk Radiologi — NFMR)

University Hospital Malmo
S-20502 Malmo, Sweden
Phone: 46 40 331541 **Fax:** 46 40 969977
Email: olle.ekberg@rontgen.mas.lu.se

Fnded: 1919.

★ 5163 ★ Nordic Society for Disaster Medicine (Dordisk Ka)

c/o Knut-Ole Sundnes, Chair
N-2026 Skjetten, Norway
Phone: 47 63 849843
Email: kalle@wallman.nu

Fnded: 1991. **Desc:** Dedicated to improving medical disaster relief.

★ 5164 ★ Nordic Society for Psychosocial Oncology (Nordisk Forening for Psykosocial Onkologi — NFPO)

Trondheim Univ. Hospital, Department of Oncology
N-7006 Trondheim, Norway
Phone: 47 73997830 **Fax:** 47 73997821

Fnded: 1990. **Desc:** Promotes communication on research into psychosocial aspects in cancer patients.

★ 5165 ★ Nordic Society for Research in Brain Ageing (NorAge)

Norwegian Centre for Dementic Research
N-3170 Sem, Norway
Phone: 47 33341956 **Fax:** 47 33332153
Email: ainfinn-eek@nordemens.no

Fnded: 1991. **Desc:** Fosters the research in the brain's aging and its diseases.

★ 5166 ★ Nordic Society for Veterinary Pathology

Bulowsvej 17
DK-1870 Frederiksberg, Denmark
Phone: 45 35283105 **Fax:** 45 35283111
Email: helj@kvl.dk

Fnded: 1977. **Mem:** 40. **Nat'l Groups:** 5.

★ 5167 ★ Nordic Spine Deformity Society

Arhus University Hospital
DK-8000 Arhus, Denmark
Phone: 45 89493333 **Fax:** 45 89494120
Email: estender@dadlnet.dk

Fnded: 1974. **Desc:** Fosters research and treatment of scoliosis and all diseases of the back that may lead to spinal deformity.

★ 5168 ★ Nordic Telemedicine Association (NTA)
c/o Siri Birgitte Uldal
National Centre for Telemedicine
University Hospital of Tromso
PO Box 35
N-9038 Tromso, Norway
Phone: 47 77 75 41 49 **Fax:** 47 77 75 40 99
Email: tmasbu@rito.no
Website: http://www.nordictelemed.org
Fnded: 1999. **Desc:** Telemedicine organizations. Strives to strengthen and expand telemedicine activities; promotes collaboration with telemedicine groups worldwide.

★ 5169 ★ North American Association of Central Cancer Registries (NAACCR)
2121 W White Oaks Dr., Ste. C
Springfield, IL 62704
Phone: (217)698-0800 **Fax:** (217)698-0188
Email: info@naaccr.org
Website: http://www.naaccr.org
Fnded: 1987. **Mem:** 141. **Desc:** Cancer registries, government agencies, professional associations, and private groups interested in enhancing the quality and use of cancer registry data. Seeks to advance the use of cancer registration techniques in cancer control and epidemiological research, public health programs, and patient care. **Pub:** *NAACCR Narrative*, quarterly. Newsletter. **AKA:** NAACCR.

★ 5170 ★ North American Association of Urgent Care Medicine (NAFAC)
18870 Rutledge Rd.
Wayzata, MN 55391
Phone: (612)868-8417 **Fax:** (952)476-0646
Email: health1@aol.com
Website: http://www.nafac.com
William H. Wenmark, Pres.
Fnded: 1981. **Mem:** 500. **Desc:** Governing body for urgent care in North America. Representatives of hospital, corporate, and independently owned ambulatory urgent care centers. Seeks to: establish operational standards for such centers; in order for members to provide lower cost and more convenient outpatient urgent medical care; make the public aware of the concept of ambulatory urgent care centers and their usefulness in problem-based and episodic care. Cooperates with medical organizations; conducts public relations activities and studies on the industry as well as education programs and business support services. **Pub:** *Factor Studies*, triennial. Reports. National Research on Industry. **Frmly:** (1981) National Association of Centers for Urgent Treatment; (1984) National Association of Freestanding Emergency Centers; (2000) National Association for Ambulatrory Care Medicine; (2002) North American Association of Urgent Care Medicine; (2003) North American Association for Ambulatory Urgent Care.

★ 5171 ★ North American Brain Tumor Coalition (NABTC)
c/o Bennett, Turner & Coleman, LLP
1900 K St. NW, Ste. 750
Washington, DC 20006
Email: membership@nabraintumor.org
Website: http://www.nabraintumor.org
Fnded: 1991. **Desc:** Dedicated to eradicating brain tumors; promotes awareness, research, access to specialized care and other issues affecting brain tumor patients. Sponsors Brain Tumor Action Week in U.S., Brain Tumor Action Month, Canada.

★ 5172 ★ North American Clinical Dermatologic Society (NACDS)
c/o Mark Allen Crowe, MD
12613 133rd Ave E
Puyallup, WA 98374
Phone: (253)841-2453 **Fax:** (253)840-5519
Email: mcrowe@thedermdoc.com
Website: http://www.nacds.com
Mark Allen Crowe, MD, Sec. Gen.
Fnded: 1959. **Mem:** 210. **Desc:** Dermatologists practicing primarily in the U.S. and Canada and leaders of dermatology throughout the world. Promotes the interchange of information and research. **Pub:** *Program*, annual.

★ 5173 ★ North American College of Botanical Medicine
1116 Park Ave. SW
Albuquerque, NM 87102-2941
Phone: (505)873-8107 **Fax:** (505)873-4530
Email: phyto@swcp.com
Website: http://www.swcp.com/botanicalmedicine
Dick Brillault, Board Pres.
Fnded: 1996. **Desc:** Dedicated to providing herbal education by training herbalists and providing information for health care professionals and the community.

★ 5174 ★ North American Hyperthermia Society
820 Jorie Blvd.
Oak Brook, IL 60523
Phone: (630)571-2904 **Fax:** (630)571-7837
Website: http://www.thermaltherapy.org
Fnded: 1986. **Desc:** Promotes researchers in the field of thermal therapy; seeks to advance communication between theoreticians, experimentalists, and clinical practitioners; aims to increase understanding and use of hyperthermia; disseminates research findings. **Pub:** *International Journal of Hyperthermia*, bimonthly. Journal. Features research and clinical studies and trials on hyperthermia. *Price:* $905 for institutions; $548 for institutions.

★ 5175 ★ North American Menopause Society (NAMS)
PO Box 94527
Cleveland, OH 44101
Phone: (440)442-7550 **Fax:** (440)442-2660
Email: info@menopause.org
Website: http://www.menopause.org
Wulf H. Utian, MD,PhD, Exec. Dir.
Fnded: 1989. **Mem:** 2,500. **Desc:** Physicians, scientists, research and clinical personnel, and other health care professionals are active members; student or physicians serving residencies or fellowships are associate members. Promotes understanding of menopause in women. Advances the exchange of research plans and experience between members. Offers educational programs. **Pub:** *Flashes*, 3/year. Newsletter. *Price:* included in membership dues. • *Menopause Management*, bimonthly. A review publication. *Price:* included in membership dues. • *Menopause: The Journal of the North American Menopause Society*, bimonthly. Journal. *Price:* included in membership dues.

★ 5176 ★ North American Neuro-Ophthalmology Society (NANOS)
324 N Main St.
West Hartford, CT 06117-2507
Phone: (860)586-7507 **Fax:** (860)586-7550
Email: ctubby@nanosweb.org
Website: http://www.nanosweb.org
Cheryl-Ann Tubby, Admin. Dir.
Fnded: 1975. **Mem:** 400. **Nat'l Groups:** 1. **Desc:** Ophthalmologists and neurologists. Seeks to promote the field of neuro-ophthalmology. Supports education; encourages research; promotes clinical expertise. **Pub:** *Journal of Neuro-Ophthalmology*, quarterly. Journal.

★ 5177 ★ North American Neuromodulation Society
6287 Chesshire Ln. N
Osseo, MN 55311-4245
Phone: (763)559-4108 **Fax:** (763)559-4161
Email: american@neuromodulation.org
Website: http://www.neuromodulation.org/
Samuel J. Hassenbusch, MD, Pres.
Desc: Dedicated to advancing the field of neuromodulation therapies through clinical research, education and print material within the U.S.; aims to increase avenues of development for members through professional networking systems, ongoing communication and other opportunities. **Pub:** *Economic Newsletter*. Newsletter. Contains topics such as coding, reimbursement rates (RVU), payor coverage, and hospital topics. • *Neuromodulation*, quarterly. Journal. **Frmly:** (1994) American Neuromodulation Society.

★ 5178 ★ North American Primary Care Research Group (NAPCRG)
11400 Tomahawk Creek Pky.
Leawood, KS 66211-2672
Phone: (913)906-6000 **Free:** 800-274-2237
Fax: (913)906-6096
Email: napcrg@stfm.org
Website: http://www.napcrg.org
Roger Sherwood, Exec. Dir.
Fnded: 1972. **Mem:** 730. **Desc:** Physicians and other individuals interested in primary care research. (Primary care is the type of medicine practiced by physicians who do not require patient referrals from other physicians.) Promotes research on primary care topics. Maintains 11 special interest groups including: Ambulatory Sentinel Practice; Clinical Decision Making; Health Status Group. Disseminates information and serves as a forum for exchange of ideas on research projects. Maintains speakers' bureau. **Pub:** *Glossary of Primary Care Terms*. • *Process Classification for Family Care*. • Newsletter, quarterly. • Proceedings. • Reports.

★ 5179 ★ North American Registry of Midwives (NARM)
5257 Rosestone Dr.
Lilburn, GA 30047
Free: 888-842-4784
Website: http://www.narm.org
Debbie Pulley, Contact
Desc: Promotes the profession of Midwife; provides certification process that recognizes multiple routes of entry into midwifery and includes verification of knowledge and skills. **Pub:** *Certified Professional Midwives*. Brochure. • *North America Registry of Midwives News*. Newsletter.

★ 5180 ★ North American Riding for the Handicapped Association (NARHA)
PO Box 33150
Denver, CO 80233
Phone: (303)452-1212 **Free:** 800-369-7433
Fax: (303)252-4610
Email: narha@narha.org
Website: http://www.narha.org
William J. Scebbi, Exec. Dir.
Fnded: 1969. **Mem:** 3,700. **Reg. Groups:** 11. **Local Groups:** 500. **Desc:** Individuals and riding centers. Provides therapeutic riding for individuals with disabilities with good safety and proper care; offers appropriate training and certification for instructors working with the disabled. Provides educational programs. **Pub:** *AHA News*, 3/year. Newsletter. • *CAN Hoofbeats*, 3/year. Newsletter. • *EFMHA News*, 3/year. Newsletter. • *NARHA Guide*, annual. Directory. *Price:* Included in membership dues. • *NARHA News*, 8/year. *Price:* Included in membership. • *NARHA Strides*, quarterly. Magazine. *Price:* Included in membership.

★ 5181 ★ North American Skull Base Society (NASBS)
c/o Lawrence H. Leong
4815 Rugby Ave., Ste. 203
Bethesda, MD 20814
Phone: (301)654-6802 **Fax:** (301)718-8692
Email: info@nasbs.org
Website: http://www.nabss.org
Lawrence H. Leong, Exec. Dir.
Fnded: 1989. **Mem:** 500. **Desc:** Neurosurgeons, otolaryngologists, and others with an interest in dis-

eases associated with the skull base. Promotes advancement of medical practice relating to diseases of the skull base. Conducts continuing professional education programs. **Pub:** *Skull Base*, quarterly. Journal.

★ 5182 ★ North American Society of Adlerian Psychology (NASAP)
50 Northeast Dr.
Hershey, PA 17033
Phone: (717)579-8795 **Fax:** (717)533-8616
Email: nasap@msn.com
Website: http://www.alfredadler.org/
Becky LaFountain, Exec. Dir.

Fnded: 1951. **Mem:** 750. **Local Groups:** 20. **Desc:** Psychiatrists, psychologists, educators, social workers, clergy, and others interested in promoting the knowledge, training, and teaching of individual psychology, developed by the Austrian psychiatrist Alfred Adler (1870-1937). Encourages development of professional workers and groups in individual psychology; establishes standards for professional activities of members. Conducts research in child behavior and psychology, counseling, psychotherapy, group therapy, and treatment of the mentally ill. Sponsors training institutes and summer school program. Promotes establishment of family education associations and parent study groups. **Pub:** *Alfred Adler: As We Remember Him*. Book. • *An Adlerian Resource Book*. • *Journal of Individual Psychology*, quarterly. Journal. • *Membership List*, biennial. • *North American Society of Adlerian Psychology–Newsletter*, bimonthly. Newsletter. Includes calendar of events. *Price:* Included in membership dues; $20/year for nonmembers. **Frmly:** (1977) American Society of Alderian Psychology.

★ 5183 ★ North American Society for Cardiac Imaging (NASCI)
930 Edgecliff Way
Redwood City, CA 94061
Phone: (650)216-6621 **Fax:** (650)556-1678
Email: info@nasci.org
Website: http://www.nasci.org
Joan Oefner, CAE, Exec. Dir.

Fnded: 1973. **Mem:** 350. **Desc:** Approved individuals engaged in the practice and advancement of cardiac and vascular imaging are active members; medical students, other individuals, and corporations with an interest in cardiac imaging are sponsors. Seeks to advance the practice of cardiac imaging and to develop improved medical imaging technologies. Serves as a forum for the exchange of information among individuals and corporations with an interest in cardiac imaging; sponsors educational programs; maintains NASCI Research and Education Fund. **Pub:** *International Journal of Cardiovascular Imaging*, bimonthly. Journal. *Price:* included in membership dues. • *NASCI Membership Directory*, annual. Directory.

★ 5184 ★ North American Society for Dialysis and Transplantation (NASDT)
c/o Dr. Wadi Suki
6550 Fannin, Ste. 1273
Houston, TX 77030
Fax: (713)790-5053
Website: http://www.asts.org/ethics.cfm
Dr. Wadi Suki, Sec. -Treas.

Fnded: 1981. **Mem:** 200. **Desc:** Professionals active in the area of teaching, manufacturing, and administration in the fields of nephrology and transplantation including nephrologists, transplant surgeons and physicians, registered nurses, dialysis nurses, and transplant coordinators. Promotes education and research and disseminates current knowledge and technology in the field of kidney dialysis and transplantation.

★ 5185 ★ North American Society of Homeopaths (NASH)
1122 E Pike St., No. 1122
Seattle, WA 98122
Phone: (206)720-7000 **Fax:** (208)248-1942
Email: nashinfo@aol.com
Website: http://www.homeopathy.org/

Desc: Professional practitioners. Dedicated to the development and maintenance of homeopathic practice standards in North America. Strives to develop and support a qualified and certified homeopathic profession, distinct from, and in cooperation with other medical professionals; promotes individual's rights to receive homeopathic care. Provides certification and maintains register of those certified. Promotes public awareness of homeopathy. **Pub:** *The American Homeopath*. Journal. • *NASH News*. Newsletter.

★ 5186 ★ North American Society of Pacing and Electrophysiology/Heart Rhythm Association (NASPE)
Six Strathmore Rd.
Natick, MA 01760-2499
Phone: (508)647-0100 **Fax:** (508)647-0124
Email: info@naspe.org
Website: http://www.naspe.org
James H. Youngblood, CEO

Fnded: 1979. **Mem:** 3,200. **Desc:** Physicians, scientists, and allied professionals throughout the world dedicated to the study and management or cardiac arrhythmias; to improve the care of patients by promoting research, education and training, and providing leadership towards optimal health care policies and standards. **Pub:** *Journal of Cardiovascular Electrophysiology*, monthly. Journal. • *NASPE News*, 5/year. Newsletter. Covers membership activities. Includes calendar of events and information updates. • *North American Society of Pacing and Electrophysiology Annual Scientific Session Program*. • *PACE: The Journal of Pacing and Clinical Electrophysiology*, monthly. Journal. • Brochure. • Membership Directory, annual. Includes geographic index. **Frmly:** (2003) North American Society of Pacing and Electrophysiology.

★ 5187 ★ North American Society for Pediatric Gastroenterology, Hepatology and Nutrition (NASPGHAN)
PO Box 6
Flourtown, PA 19031
Phone: (215)233-0808 **Fax:** (215)233-3939
Email: naspghan@naspghan.org
Website: http://www.naspghan.org
Margaret Stallings, Exec. Dir.

Fnded: 1970. **Mem:** 1,000. **Desc:** Mission is to be a world leader in advancing the science and clinical practice of Pediatric Gastroenterology, Hepatology and Nutrition in health and disease. Strives to improve the care of infants, children and adolescents with digestive disorders by promoting advances in clinical care, research and education. Pediatric gastroenterologists specialize in the care of children with chronic abdominal pain, diarrhea, constipation, vomiting, bleeding from the GI tract, inflammatory bowel disease, liver diseases, diseases of the pancreas, poor weight gain and nutritional problems. Objectives include: improving the digestive health and nutrition of children worldwide and particularly in North America; fostering dialogue and research on pertinent issues that impact the pediatric gastroenterology patient and their family; providing opportunities for clinicians and researchers to gain knowledge of the scientific advances in the field; and disseminating scientific information in order to improve clinical outcomes and advance the practice of the field. **Pub:** *NASPGN Membership Directory*, annual. Membership Directory. • *Newsletter of the NASPGN*, 4-6/year. Newsletter. **Frmly:** (1988) North American Society for Pediatric Gastroenterology.

★ 5188 ★ North American Society for the Psychology of Sport and Physical Activity (NASPSPA)
c/o Gabriele Wulf
University of Nevada, Las Vegas
Department of Kinesiology
4505 Maryland Pkwy.
Las Vegas, NV 89154-3034
Phone: (702)895-0938 **Fax:** (702)895-1500
Email: gabriele.wulf@ccmail.nevada.edu
Website: http://www.naspspa.org
Gabriele Wulf, PhD, Sec. -Treas.

Fnded: 1966. **Mem:** 450. **Desc:** Kinesiologists, psychologists and physical educators. Promotes scientific research and relations within the behavioral sciences with an application to sport psychology, motor learning, control, and development through meetings, investigations, and other activities.

★ 5189 ★ North American Spine Society (NASS)
22 Calendar Ct., 2nd Fl.
La Grange, IL 60525
Phone: (708)588-8080 **Free:** 877-SPI-NEDR
Fax: (708)588-1080
Email: info@spine.org
Website: http://www.spine.org
Eric J. Muehlbauer, CAE, Exec. Dir.

Fnded: 1985. **Mem:** 3,400. **Desc:** Organization of physicians, osteopaths, orthopedists, neurosurgeons, physiatrists, radiologists, and other professionals that advances quality spine care through education, research and advocacy. Works to improve the quality of scientific practice in spinal disorders; exchange ideas and disseminate scientific information about clinical techniques; investigate and propagate methods by which malfunction of the spine can be corrected. Makes inquiries into practice characteristics, language usage and terminology, and treatment methods. **Pub:** *Common Coding Scenarios for Comprehensive Spine Care*, annual. Book. *Price:* Available for purchase. • *Contemporary Concepts in Spine Care*, bimonthly. Paper. • *Phase III Clinical Guidelines on Herniated Discs & Unremitting Low Back Pain*. Book. • *The Spine Journal*, bimonthly. Journal. Contains news on association activities, peer-reviewed research topics. *Price:* included in membership dues. • *Spine Line*, bimonthly. Magazine. Contains news on association activities, peer-reviewed research topics. *Price:* included in membership dues.

★ 5190 ★ North American Transplant Coordinators Organization (NATCO)
PO Box 15384
Lenexa, KS 66285-5384
Phone: (913)492-3600 **Fax:** (913)599-5340
Email: natco-info@goamp.com
Website: http://www.natco1.org
Deidre Gish-Panjada, Exec. Dir.

Fnded: 1979. **Mem:** 1,800. **Desc:** Nurses and allied health professionals working with organ recipients and those working to obtain and distribute human organs and tissues to waiting victims of end-stage organ failure. Seeks to influence increased procurement and use of transplantable organs and tissues under the direction of individuals and institutions responsible for the employment of members. Disseminates information to members, medical personnel, technicians, and the public regarding the benefits of organ transplantation, new techniques in organ procurement, advancements in immunology and preservation, transplant surgery, and other aspects of organ transplantation. Promotes and supports training and development programs for new transplant coordinators. Sponsors seminars, workshops, and annual training course on procurement for transplant coordinators. Offers job referral information. **Pub:** *NATCO–InTouch*, bimonthly. Newsletter. Includes calendar of events, employment opportunity listings, legislative updates, and conference reports. *Price:* Included in membership dues. • *North American Transplant Coordinators Organization–Membership Directory*, annual. Directory. *Price:* Included in membership dues. • *Progress in Transplantation*, QRT. Journal. Includes clinical articles addressing transplantation issues. *Price:* included in membership dues.

★ 5191 ★ Northern Ireland Association for Mental Health
80 University St.
Beacon House
Belfast BT7 1HE, United Kingdom
Phone: 44 28 90328474 **Fax:** 44 28 90232940

Fnded: 1959. **Mem:** 280. **Local Groups:** 32. **Desc:** Promotes dignity, choice, integration and participation for those with mental health needs living in the community. Aims to offer services of the highest standard to people with mental health needs; inform and educate the public about mental health; and press for high standards in the provision of mental health services. **Pub:** *Mental Health Matters*, quarterly.

★ 5192 ★ Northern Ireland Chest Heart and Stroke Association
21 Dublin Rd.
Belfast BT2 7HB, United Kingdom
Phone: 44 28 90320184 **Fax:** 44 28 90333487
Website: http://www.nichsa.com

Fnded: 1946. **Reg. Groups:** 16. **Lang(s):** English. **Desc:** Promotes the prevention of, and alleviate the suffering resulting from chest, heart, and stroke illnesses in Northern Ireland. Supports rehabilitation facilities; offers subsidized vacations for families affected by these diseases; provides nebulizers for asthmatic children and adults; provides help and advice; provides grants for people with low incomes; funds research.

★ 5193 ★ Norwegian Acupuncture Association (NFKA)
(Norsk Forening for Klassisk Akupunktur)
St. Olavsgt. 12
N-0165 Oslo, Norway
Phone: 47 22 988144 **Fax:** 47 22 361853
Email: nfka@akupunktur.no
Website: http://www.akupunktur.no

Fnded: 1978. **Mem:** 250. **Nat'l Groups:** 1. **Lang(s):** English, Norwegian. **Desc:** Doctors, nurses, dentists, and physiotherapists; students. Encourages the practice of acupuncture in Norway. Operates training institute for members. Conducts educational programs. **Pub:** *DE Qi-Tidsskrift for Kinesisk Medisin*, 3/year. Journal. Includes information on acupuncture and Chinese medicine. • Brochure, periodic.

★ 5194 ★ Norwegian Bardet-Biedl Syndrome Association (NLMBBSA)
(Interesseforeningen fur LMBB i Norge)
PO Box 4568
Torshov
N-0404 Oslo, Norway
Phone: 47 91564113
Email: be-bro@online.no

Fnded: 1984. **Mem:** 90. **Lang(s):** English, French, German. **Desc:** Persons with Laurence-Moon-Bardet-Biedl syndrome and their families. (LMBB is a genetic disorder; symptoms include retinitis pigmentosa, hypogenitalism, polydactyly, and obesity.) Offers assistance to children with LMBB and their parents as well as adults with LMBB, especially those newly diagnosed. **Frmly:** (1998) Norwegian LMBB's Syndrome Association.

★ 5195 ★ Norwegian Cystic Fibrosis Association (NCFA)
(Norsk Forening for Cystisk Fibrose — NFCF)
Postboks 4568
Torshov
N-0404 Oslo, Norway
Phone: 47 88004108 **Fax:** 47 22799199
Email: cfblad@folio.no
Website: http://www.cfnorge.no

Fnded: 1976. **Mem:** 798. **Nat'l Groups:** 1. **Reg. Groups:** 4. **Lang(s):** English, Norwegian. **Desc:** Persons with cystic fibrosis and interested individuals. Promotes improvements in the methods of care for persons with cystic fibrosis. Disseminates information; coordinates clinical research. **Pub:** *Nordic Cystic Fibrosis Magazine*, quarterly. Magazine.

★ 5196 ★ Norwegian Dental Association (Den Norske Tannlegeforening — NTF)
Postboks 3063, Elisenberg
N-0207 Oslo, Norway
Phone: 47 22547400 **Fax:** 47 22551109
Fnded: 1884.

★ 5197 ★ Norwegian Diabetes Association (NDF)
(Norges Diabetesforbund)
Postboks 6442
Etterstad
N-0605 Oslo, Norway
Phone: 47 23 051800 **Fax:** 47 23 051801
Email: norges.diabetesforbund@diabetes.no
Website: http://www.diabetes.no

Fnded: 1948. **Mem:** 34,000. **Nat'l Groups:** 5. **Reg. Groups:** 19. **Local Groups:** 150. **Lang(s):** English. **Desc:** Diabetics and their families; health personnel. Acts as support group. Disseminates information on availability of insulin, diabetes products, and health care. Lobbies the government to incorporate diabetes treatment into national health care plans and to provide free insulin, syringes, and urine and blood glucose strips. Provides research and medical services. Offers educational courses; conducts camps; maintains youth club. **Pub:** *Diabetes*, bimonthly. Magazine. Features educational material. Includes Annual medical supplement. • Booklets.

★ 5198 ★ Norwegian Dietetics Association
(Norsk Forening for Ernaering og Dietetikk)
Postboks 9202
Gronland
N-0134 Oslo, Norway
Phone: 47 21013600 **Fax:** 47 21013660
Email: nfed@kfo.no
Website: http://www.nfed.no

Fnded: 1948. **Mem:** 1,450. **Local Groups:** 18. **Lang(s):** Norwegian. **Desc:** Professional dietitians. Promotes advancement in the study and application of dietetics; advises government agencies and the public regarding a healthy diet. Conducts research and educational programs. **Pub:** *Kigkkenskriveren/Kjohhenskriveren*, 8/year. Magazine.

★ 5199 ★ Norwegian Dyslexia Association (NDA)
(Dysleksiforbundet i Norge — DIN)
Postboks 8731 Youngstorget
N-0028 Oslo, Norway
Phone: 47 22474450 **Fax:** 47 22429554
Email: post@dysleksiforbundet.no
Website: http://www.dysleksiforbundet.no

Fnded: 1976. **Mem:** 5,000. **Local Groups:** 40. **Lang(s):** English, Norwegian. **Desc:** Individuals with dyslexia and their parents; organizations. Acts as a support group. **Pub:** *Dyslektikeren*, bimonthly.

★ 5200 ★ Norwegian Epilepsy Association (NEA)
(Norsk Epilepsiforbund — NEF)
Storgaten 39
N-0192 Oslo, Norway
Phone: 47 23 353100 **Fax:** 47 23 353101
Email: nef@epilepsi.no
Website: http://www.epilepsi.no

Fnded: 1974. **Mem:** 3,800. **Reg. Groups:** 7. **Local Groups:** 39. **Lang(s):** English, Norwegian. **Desc:** Disseminates information to individuals with epilepsy and their families, health care centers, hospitals, and schools. Collaborates with related groups. **Pub:** *The Epilepsy Handbook*. Handbook. • *Epilepsy News*, quarterly. Magazine. Also publishes brochures (in Norwegian).

★ 5201 ★ Norwegian Federation of Organisations of Disabled People (NFODP)
(Funksjonshemmeds Fellesorganisasjon — FFO)
Sandakerveien 99
PO Box 4568
Nydalen
N-0404 Oslo, Norway
Phone: 47 2 2799100 **Fax:** 47 2 2799198
Email: info@ffo.no
Website: http://www.ffo.no

Fnded: 1950. **Mem:** 64. **Reg. Groups:** 19. **Local Groups:** 60. **Lang(s):** Norwegian. **Desc:** Organizations of disabled persons representing 260,000 individuals in Norway. Works for social integration and equality for disabled people; cooperates with the Norwegian Agency for International Development to ensure that aid also reaches the disabled. Serves as liaison between members and government; maintains contact with similar organizations abroad. **Pub:** *FFO's Ukeseddel*, weekly. Newsletter. • *Funksjonshemmedi I Europa*. Also issues press releases. **Frmly:** Norwegian League of Handicap Organizations.

★ 5202 ★ Norwegian Fibromyalgia Patients' Association (NFP)
(Norges Fibromyalgi Forbund — NFF)
Sollivn. 55
N-1366 Lysaker, Norway
Phone: 47 67583067 **Fax:** 47 67583158
Email: adm@fibromyalgi.no
Website: http://www.fibromyalgi.no

Fnded: 1985. **Mem:** 7,000. **Local Groups:** 67. **Lang(s):** English, Norwegian. **Desc:** Persons in Norway suffering from fibrositis or fibromyalgia (rheumatic disorders involving fibrous tissues). Funds research into the cause and cure of fibrositis or fibromyalgia. Promotes understanding of the disease; disseminates information. Conducts educational programs. **Pub:** *Fibromyalgi*, quarterly. Magazine.

★ 5203 ★ Norwegian Gerontological Society
Norwegian Centre for Dementia Research
Ullevaal Hospital, KGR
N-0407 Oslo, Norway
Phone: 47 22 117728 **Fax:** 47 23 016161
Email: toril.utne@nordemens.no

Desc: Promotes gerontological research, training in the field of aging, and interests of gerontological organizations in international affairs.

★ 5204 ★ Norwegian Immune Deficiency Foundation (NIDF)
(Norsk Immunsviktforening — NI)
c/o Eva Brox
Borgundveien 478
N-6015 Alesund, Norway
Phone: 47 70 146565 **Fax:** 47 70 146566
Email: evabrox@online.no
Website: http://immunsvikt.no

Fnded: 1983. **Mem:** 280. **Nat'l Groups:** 1. **Lang(s):** Norwegian. **Desc:** Persons with primary immunological disorders and their families; private companies. Acts as support group. Disseminates information. **Pub:** *Antibody deficiency*. Book. • *Immunsvikt hos Voksne og Barn*, periodic. • *Primary Antibody Deficiency and Self-Administration Home Therapy with s.c. immunoglobulin.*. Video. • *Subcut immunoglobulin therapy*. Video.

★ 5205 ★ Norwegian Multiple Sclerosis Society (NMSS)
(Multipel Sklerose Forbundet i Norge — MSFN)
Sorkedalsveien 3
N-0369 Oslo, Norway
Phone: 47 22 963580 **Fax:** 47 22 567695
Email: epost@ms.no
Website: http://www.ms.no

Fnded: 1966. **Mem:** 6,000. **Reg. Groups:** 37. **Local Groups:** 53. **Lang(s):** English. **Desc:** Promotes interest in multiple sclerosis research among medical and scientific communities and the public in Norway. Facilitates exchange of information among members. **Pub:** *Jeg har fatt MS*. Book. • *MS-bladet*, 5/year. Magazine. • *MS - En veiledning for helsepersonell*. Books. • *MS-En veiledning for pasienter og parorende*. Book. • Pamphlets.

★ 5206 ★ Norwegian Neuroscience Society (NNS)
c/o Terje Sagvolden, Pres.
Department of Physiology
University of Oslo
PO Box 1103 Blindern
N-0317 Oslo, Norway
Phone: 47 22851286 **Fax:** 47 22851249
Email: terje.sagvolden@basalmed.uio.no
Website: http://folk.uio.no/terjesa/nns/
Fnded: 1998. **Desc:** Promotes information exchange between European neuroscientists; provides educational courses.

★ 5207 ★ Norwegian Nurses Association (Norsk Sykepleierforbund — NSF)
Postboks 456, Sentrum
Oslo, Norway
Phone: 47 22 043304 **Fax:** 47 22 043240
Email: norsk.sykepleierforbund@nosf.no
Website: http://www.sykepleierforbundet.no
Fnded: 1912. **Mem:** 61,000.

★ 5208 ★ Norwegian Osteogenesis Imperfecta Foundation (NFOI) (Norsk Forening for Osteogenesis Imperfecta)
Postboks 4568
Nydalen
N-0404 Oslo, Norway
Phone: 47 22799100 **Fax:** 47 22799198
Email: nfei@c2i.net
Website: http://home.c2i.net/nfoi/
Fnded: 1979. **Mem:** 460. **Reg. Groups:** 2. **Lang(s):** English. **Desc:** Persons with OI and others interested in OI. (OI is a hereditary disease that causes various symptoms such as brittle bones, loose joints, short stature, poor teeth, and bad hearing.) NFOI is connected to a competence center: Trenings-OG Raadgivningssenteret (TRS) at Sunnaas Hospital. The center provides advice on different issues concerning OI. NFOI is also member of OI-NORDEN (Nordic Organization) and OIFE (European Foundation). **Pub:** *OI-NYTT*, quarterly. Journal. Also publishes brochures and pamphlets.

★ 5209 ★ Norwegian Ostomy Association (Norsk Forening for Stomi-og Reservoaropererte)
Postboks 5327
Majorstua
N-0304 Oslo, Norway
Phone: 47 22593000 **Fax:** 47 22853696
Email: norilco@kreft.no
Website: http://www.kreft.no//forkreftpasienter/pasientforeninger/norilco
Fnded: 1971. **Mem:** 6,000. **Local Groups:** 22. **Lang(s):** English, Norwegian. **Desc:** Individuals representing the interests of ostomy patients. Promotes information exchange among members. Works to improve quality of health care before and after surgery. **Pub:** *NORILCO-NYTT*, bimonthly. Magazine.

★ 5210 ★ Norwegian Parkinson Association (NPA) (Norges Parkinsonforbund — NPF)
Schweigaardsgt 34, F.2
N-0191 Oslo, Norway
Phone: 47 22 175861 **Fax:** 47 22 175862
Email: parkinson@cai.net
Website: http://www.parkinson.no
Fnded: 1984. **Mem:** 4,600. **Nat'l Groups:** 1. **Reg. Groups:** 17. **Local Groups:** 15. **Lang(s):** English. **Desc:** Parkinson patients and their relatives. Teaches patients about their disease and how to deal with the related problems. Represents members' interests in matters of social and health politics. Supports research efforts; conducts educational seminars. Offers lectures. **Pub:** *Parkinsonposten*, quarterly. Newsletter.

★ 5211 ★ Norwegian Physiotherapist Association (Norske Fysioterapeuters Forbund — NFF)
Postboks 7009, Majorstua
N-0306 Oslo, Norway
Phone: 47 22933050 **Fax:** 47 22565825
Email: Fysioterapi@online.no
Fnded: 1936.

★ 5212 ★ Norwegian Psychological Association
PO Box 8733
Youngstorget
N-0028 Oslo, Norway
Phone: 47 23103130 **Fax:** 47 22424292
Email: npfpost@psytol.no
Website: http://www.psykol.no
Fnded: 1994. **Mem:** 4,200. **Desc:** Professional association and union for psychologists.

★ 5213 ★ Norwegian Society for Biomedical Engineering (Medisinsk teknisk forening — MTF)
Postboks 287
N-2803 Gjovik, Norway
Phone: 47 72419677 **Fax:** 47 72410089

★ 5214 ★ Norwegian Society of Cardiology
Ostadalsveien 12B
N-0753 Oslo, Norway
Phone: 47 22507855 **Fax:** 47 22521658
Email: ncs@hjerte.org
Website: http://www.hjerte.org
Mem: 206. **Desc:** Promotes the study of cardiology in Norway. **Pub:** Journal, quarterly.

★ 5215 ★ Norwegian Society for Hematology (Norsk selskap for hematologi)
Hematologisk avdeling, Ulleval sykehus
N-0407 Oslo, Norway
Phone: 47 22119240 **Fax:** 47 22119181
Email: jonmagnus.tangen@ulleval.no
Fnded: 1987.

★ 5216 ★ Norwegian Society of Medical Physics (Norsk Forening for Medisinsk Fysikk — NFMF)
Radiofysisk avdeling, Haukeland Sykehus
N-5021 Bergen, Norway
Phone: 47 55972057 **Fax:** 47 55972046
Email: rhaf@haukeland.no

★ 5217 ★ Norwegian Society of Pharmacology and Toxicology (Norsk Selskap for Farmakologi og Toksikologi — NSFT)
Department of Pharmacotherapy
Ullevel Hospital
University of Oslo
PO Box 1065
N-0316 Blindern, Norway
Phone: 47 22 119000 **Fax:** 47 22 119013
Email: oyvind.melien@c2i.net
Website: http://www.farmakoterapi.uio.no/nsft
Mem: 426. **Desc:** Promotes pharmacology and toxicology in Norway.

★ 5218 ★ Norwegian Veterinary Association (DNV) (Norske Veterinarforening — DNV)
Postboks 6781
St Olavs pl
N-0130 Oslo, Norway
Phone: 47 22 994600 **Fax:** 47 22 994601
Email: dnv@vetnett.no
Website: http://www.vetnett.no
Fnded: 1888. **Mem:** 2,175. **Nat'l Groups:** 5. **Local Groups:** 15. **Lang(s):** English, Norwegian. **Desc:** Promotes the advancement of veterinary science in Norway. Sponsors educational and research programs. Compiles statistics; conducts charitable projects. **Pub:** *Norsk Veterinartidsskrift*, monthly. Journal.

★ 5219 ★ Novartis Foundation for Gerontological Research (NFGR)
Lichtstrasse
CH-4002 Basel, Switzerland
Phone: 41 61 3247353 **Fax:** 41 61 3244294
Website: http://www.mixer.fr/clients/pharma/novanfgr/
Fnded: 1986. **Desc:** Supports research for programs aimed at improving quality of life for elderly people. Promotes education and training for health care providers and the public.

★ 5220 ★ NRH Center for Health and Disability Research (CHDR)
1016 16th St. NW, Ste. 400
Washington, DC 20036
Phone: (202)466-1900 **Fax:** (202)466-1911
Website: http://www.nrhchdr.org
Susan E. Palsbo, PhD, Dir.
Fnded: 1985. **Desc:** Provides health and disability research.

★ 5221 ★ NSF International
PO BOX 130140
Ann Arbor, MI 48113-0140
Phone: (734)769-8010 **Free:** 877-867-3435
Fax: (734)769-0109
Email: info@nsf.org
Website: http://www.nsf.org
Fnded: 1944. **Desc:** Specializes in the areas of public health and environmental quality focusing on water quality, food safety, indoor air health and the environment. Develops standards, operates product certification and listings programs for products that meet or exceed public health safety standards. Maintains a worldwide network of auditors who conduct unannounced inspections of manufacturer facilities to ensure compliance and to protect the integrity of the NSF Certification Mark. Provides special research and testing services to industry, government, and foundations. **Pub:** *Bottled Water and Packaged Ice*, periodic. • *Class II Biohazard Cabinetry*, periodic. Book. • *Drinking Water Additives-Health Effects*, periodic. • *Drinking Water Treatment Units and Related Products, Components, and Materials*, periodic. • *Environmental Management Systems Standards and Guidance Documents*. • *Food Equipment and Related Products, Components, and Materials*, periodic. • *Plastics Piping Components and Related Materials*, periodic. • *Swimming Pools, Spas, and Hot Tubs*, periodic. • *Wastewater Treatment Units and Related Products and Components*, periodic. • Also publishes educational material. **Frmly:** (1993) National Sanitation Foundation.

★ 5222 ★ Nuclear Medicine Technology Certification Board (NMTCB)
2970 Clairmont Rd., Ste. 935
Atlanta, GA 30329
Phone: (404)315-1739 **Fax:** (404)315-6502
Email: board@nmtcb.org

Website: http://www.nmtcb.org
Bhaskar R. Dawadi, PhD, Exec. Dir.

Fnded: 1977. **Mem:** 19,500. **Desc:** Purposes are to provide for the certification of nuclear medical technologists and to develop, assess, and administer an examination relevant to nuclear medicine technology. Compiles statistics. **Pub:** *NMTCB Examination Report*, annual. *Price:* Free. • *NMTCB News*, semiannual. *Price:* Free to members. • Brochures.

★ 5223 ★ Nurse Healers Professional Associates International (NH-PAI)

3760 Highland Dr., No. 429
Salt Lake City, UT 84106
Phone: (801)273-3399 **Fax:** (509)693-3537
Email: nh-pai@therapeutic-touch.org
Website: http://www.therapeutic-touch.org
Rebecca M. Good, MA, RN, LPC, Coor.

Fnded: 1977. **Mem:** 700. **Desc:** Official organization for Therapeutic Touch (TT). Healthcare professionals and lay persons united to promote a holistic approach to healing and health maintenance and nontraditional healing methods. Disseminates information on therapeutic touch. Maintains speakers' bureau; conducts research and educational programs for Therapeutic Touch. Sets standards and scope of practice for TT and recognition program for Qualified Therapeutic Touch teachers and practitioners. **Pub:** *Cooperative Connection*, quarterly. Newsletter. Cooperative connection newsletter of the Nurse Healers Professonal Associate International, Inc (NH-PAI). *Price:* $20/year in U.S.; $28/year outside U.S. **Frmly:** (2002) Nurse Healers Professional Associates.

★ 5224 ★ Nurses Educational Funds (NEF)

304 Park Ave. S, No. 11F
New York, NY 10010-4301
Phone: (212)399-1428 **Fax:** (212)581-2368
Email: bbnef@aol.com
Barbara Butler, Exec. Dir.

Fnded: 1954. **Mem:** 30. **Desc:** Seeks to establish, maintain, and administer funds to provide financial assistance to registered nurses studying for advanced degrees; masters/doctoral level only formulate policies for the administration of such funds; collect and manage all funds contributed to it. Masters study must be full-time only GRE/or MAT scores are required. **Pub:** *Nurses Educational Funds Annual Report*, annual. Annual Report. Includes NEF activity highlights and financial summary for the fiscal year. *Price:* Available to members and donors only. **Frmly:** (1954) Isabel Hampton Robb Memorial Fund.

★ 5225 ★ Nurses' House

2113 Western Ave., Ste. 2
Guilderland, NY 12084-9559
Phone: (518)456-7858 **Fax:** (518)452-3760
Email: mail@nurseshouse.org
Website: http://www.nurseshouse.org
Susan Fraley, Exec. Dir.

Fnded: 1925. **Mem:** 1,100. **Reg. Groups:** 6. **Desc:** Registered nurses and interested individuals united to assist registered nurses in financial and other crises. Provides short-term financial aid for shelter, food, and utilities until nurses obtain entitlements or jobs. Offers counseling and referrals. Encourages homebound or retired nurses through a volunteer corps. **Pub:** *Appeal*, annual. Newsletter. • *The Dolphin*, semiannual. Newsletter. • Also publishes promotional flyer.

★ 5226 ★ Nurses Organization of Veterans Affairs (NOVA)

1726 M St. NW, Ste. 1101
Washington, DC 20036
Phone: (202)296-0888 **Fax:** (202)833-1577
Email: nova@vanurse.org
Website: http://www.vanurse.org
Deborah Beck, Exec. Dir.

Fnded: 1980. **Mem:** 3,200. **Reg. Groups:** 99. **Desc:** Voluntary, nonprofit professional society of Department of Veterans Affairs registered nurses. Objective is to provide VA nurses with the opportunity to preserve and improve quality care and professionalism through legislative influence. Conducts seminars, and educational programs. **Pub:** *News From NOVA*, quarterly. Newsletter. *Price:* $40/year for nonmembers. • Also publishes Legislatively Speakings. **Frmly:** (1989) Nurses Organization of the Veterans Administration.

★ 5227 ★ Nursing Association

159 Royal Rd.
Beau Bassin, Mauritius
Phone: 230 4645850
Fnded: 1955. **Mem:** 2,040.

★ 5228 ★ Nursing Touch and Massage Therapy Association International (NTMTAI)

1438 Shortcut, Ste. E
Slidell, LA 70458
Phone: (985)893-8002 **Fax:** (504)892-3493
Email: ntmta@aol.com

Desc: Massage therapists. Seeks to advance the study and practice of therapeutic massage. Conducts research, educational, and promotional activities.

★ 5229 ★ Nutrition Foundation of the Philippines (NFP)

107 E Rodriguez, Sr. Blvd.
Quezon City, Metro Manila 1102, Philippines
Phone: 63 2 7121474 **Fax:** 63 2 7113980

Fnded: 1959. **Mem:** 350. **Lang(s):** English. **Desc:** Nutritionists, educators, medical doctors, scientists, midwives, and food companies in the Philippines. Promotes public awareness and practice of sound nutritional principles. Conducts nutrition education campaigns primarily directed toward those most vulnerable to malnutrition. Trains individuals to participate in community nutrition programs and offers continuing educational opportunities for health care professionals. Provides technical assistance to public and private agencies working to improve nutrition in the Philippines, consulting services for program planning and implementation, and diet counseling program. Undertakes nutrition research and aids institutions conducting studies in the field; offers reference service. Operates speakers' bureau and placement and children's services. **Pub:** *Bulletin of the NFP*, bimonthly. Newsletter. Current trends in foods, nutrition, and dietetics. • *Low-Fat, Low-Cholesterol Cookbook*. Book. • *Monograp Series*. Book. Kitchen tested recipes for preschoolers.

★ 5230 ★ Nutrition Institute of America (NIA)

1524 Crystal St.
Kansas City, MO 64126
Phone: (816)241-8315 **Fax:** (816)231-6423
George Coulas, Pres.

Fnded: 1974. **Mem:** 6. **Desc:** Sponsors original research in nutrition and other areas that may affect our physical and emotional well-being. Sponsors lectures, symposia, adult education programs, and special tutor programs in nutrition; maintains extensive research library; compiles statistics. Presently inactive.

★ 5231 ★ Nutrition for Optimal Health Association (NOHA)

PO Box 380
Winnetka, IL 60093
Phone: (847)604-3258
Email: nohainfo@aol.com
Website: http://www.nutrition4health.org
Neil Levin, Pres.

Fnded: 1972. **Mem:** 300. **Desc:** Physicians and others interested in making informed health decisions through better nutrition. Promotes good nutrition as a means of achieving and maintaining optimal health; advances and disseminates scientifically based information on the practical application of sound nutritional principles to daily living. Offers cooking classes and workshops; conducts nutrition education programs and seminars. Maintains speakers' bureau. **Pub:** *Enjoy Nutritious Variety*, quarterly. Newsletter. • *NOHA News*, quarterly. Newsletter. Includes association news, book reviews and articles by members of NOHA's Professional Advisory Board. *Price:* Included in membership dues; $8/year for nonmembers. • Membership Directory, annual.

★ 5232 ★ Nutrition Society (NS)

10 Cambridge Ct.
210 Shepherds Bush Rd.
London W6 7NJ, United Kingdom
Phone: 44 20 76020228 **Fax:** 44 20 76021756
Email: office@nutsoc.org.uk
Website: http://www.nutsoc.org.uk

Fnded: 1941. **Mem:** 2,200. **Reg. Groups:** 2. **Lang(s):** English. **Desc:** Persons involved in nutrition research or in health maintenance organized to promote the scientific study of nutrition. Maintains special regional groups; disseminates information via journals. **Pub:** *British Journal of Nutrition*, monthly. Journal. • *Gazette*, periodic. Magazine. • *Nutrition Research Reviews*. Report. • *Proceedings of the Nutrition Society*, 3/year. Proceedings. • *Public Health Nutrition*, bimonthly. Journal.

★ 5233 ★ Nutrition Society of Australia (NSA)

PO Box 949
Kent Town, SA 5071, Australia
Phone: 61 8 83631307 **Fax:** 61 8 83631604
Email: info@nsa.asn.au
Website: http://www.nsa.asn.au/

Desc: Promotes the science of nutrition. Members include human nutritionists and dietitians, medical practitioners and nurses, agricultural scientists and veterinarians, food scientists, teachers and students.

★ 5234 ★ Nutrition Society of New Zealand

PO Box 56
Dunedin, New Zealand

★ 5235 ★ Nutrition Society of Southern Africa

PO Box 1697
Brits 0250, Republic of South Africa
Phone: 27 12 5214259 **Fax:** 27 12 5213510
Fnded: 1957.

★ 5236 ★ Obsessive-Compulsive Anonymous (OCA)

PO Box 215
New Hyde Park, NY 11040
Phone: (516)739-0662 **Fax:** (212)768-4679
Website: http://www.hometown.aol.com/west24th
Roy C., Contact

Fnded: 1988. **Mem:** 1,000. **Nat'l Groups:** 70. **Reg. Groups:** 70. **Desc:** Individuals suffering from obsessive-compulsive disorders. (OCD is characterized by recurrent unpleasant thoughts and/or repetitive, irrational mannerisms the sufferer feels compelled to perform.) Follows the 12-step method originated by Alcoholics Anonymous World Services to assist members in their recovery. **Pub:** *Obsessive Compulsive Anonymous Second Edition - 1999*. Book. *Price:* $19.00. • *Obsessive Compulsive Disorder: A Survival Guide for Family and Friends. Price:* $9.95.

★ 5237 ★ Obsessive-Compulsive Foundation (OCF)

337 Notch Hill Rd.
North Branford, CT 06471
Phone: (203)315-2190 **Fax:** (203)315-2196
Email: info@ocfoundation.org
Website: http://www.ocfoundation.org
Janet S. Emmerman, Pres.

Fnded: 1986. **Mem:** 11,000. **State Groups:** 9. **Desc:** Individuals with obsessive-compulsive disorders and their families and friends; professionals involved in the treatment of OCD. (OCD is often chronic and characterized by recurrent unpleasant thoughts and/or repetitive behaviors that the person feels driven to perform. Individuals with OCD realize their obsessions and compulsions are irrational or excessive, yet find they have no control over them. Individuals with OCD often become demoralized, depressed, and anxious.) Seeks to control and find a cure for OCD while improving the welfare of its individuals with OCD. Disseminates information on OCD and possible new therapies. Offers educational programs for professionals and the public. Assists with fundraising and forming local support groups; fosters communication between members. Funds research into causes and treatments. **Pub:** *Kidscope*, semiannual. Newsletter. For children and teens with OCD. • *OCD*. Brochure. • *OCD Newsletter*, bimonthly. Newsletter. • Also produces educational materials. **Frmly:** (1988) Obsessive Compulsive Disorder Foundation.

★ 5238 ★ Obstetrical and Gynaecological Society of Hong Kong

Duke of Windsor Social Service Bldg., 4/F
15 Hennessy Rd.
Hong Kong, People's Republic of China
Phone: 852 25278898 **Fax:** 852 28650345
Email: sysin@netvigator.com
Website: http://www.medicine.org.hk/ogshk/home.htm

Fnded: 1961. **Mem:** 330. **Lang(s):** Chinese, English. **Desc:** Obstetricians and gynecologists; medical students with an interest in the field. Seeks to advance the study and practice of obstetrics and gynecology. Conducts continuing professional development courses for members. **Pub:** *Hong Kong Journal of Gynecology, Obstetrics & Midwifery*, periodic. Journal.

★ 5239 ★ Obstetrical and Gynaecological Society of Malaysia

Plaza Mont' Kiara, Ste. C-07-02
No. 2 Jalan 1/70C, Mont' Kiara
50480 Kuala Lumpur, Malaysia
Phone: 60 3 62013009 **Fax:** 60 3 62017009
Email: ogsm@po.jaring.my
Website: http://www.ogsm.org.my/

Desc: Promotes the development of science and assist scientific research in all fields related to obstetrics and gynecology.

★ 5240 ★ Obstetrical and Gynaecological Society of Singapore

Women's Tower, Unit 8K38, Level 8
KK Women's & Children's Hospital
100 Bukit Timah Rd.
Singapore 229899, Singapore
Phone: 65 2951383 **Fax:** 65 2991969
Email: ogss@pacific.net.sg
Website: http://home1.pacific.net.sg/~ogss/

Desc: Works to promote and maintain high standard in obstetrics and gynaecology in Singapore. **Pub:** Papers.

★ 5241 ★ Obstetrician Family Center of Reproductive Health (Centro Obstetrico Familiar Salud Reproductiva — COF-Ecuado)

Pasaje Trivino E4-261
AV. 12, de Octubre
Apartado 17-12434 CCNU
Pichincha
Quito, Ecuador
Phone: 593 2 226515 **Fax:** 593 2 2901854
Email: direject@cofqsld.org.ec

Fnded: 1984. **Mem:** 79. **Nat'l Groups:** 6. **Reg. Groups:** 6. **Local Groups:** 6. **Lang(s):** Spanish. **Desc:** Works to increase public awareness of all aspects of sexuality and family life. Conducts educational and orientational programs for adolescents and parents on family planning, reproduction, sexuality, and family issues. Trains health care workers and family planning service providers. Investigates relevant topics and disseminates information. **Pub:** *Informe Annual del Adolescente*, annual. • *Manual del Adolescente*. • *Manual Metodos Anticonceptivos*. Manual. **Frmly:** Centro Obstetrico Familiar COF.

★ 5242 ★ Occupational and Environmental Diseases Association (OEDA)

PO Box 26
Enfield
Middlesex EN1 2NT, United Kingdom
Phone: 44 208 3608490
Website: http://www.oeda.demon.co.uk

Fnded: 1995. **Desc:** Asbestos is still responsible for much of our work. **Frmly:** (1978) Society for the Prevention of Asbestosis and Industrial Diseases.

★ 5243 ★ Occupational and Environmental Medical Association of Canada (OEMAC)

1147 Lawson Rd.
London, ON, Canada W6G 5K1
Phone: (519)439-7970 **Fax:** (519)439-8840
Email: oemac@emac.org
Website: http://www.oemac.org

Fnded: 1985. **Mem:** 350. **Lang(s):** English, French. **Desc:** Health care professionals with an active interest in occupational and environmental medicine. Promotes improved standards of education and practice in the field. Serves as a unified voice for Canadian occupational and environmental medicine; acts as a forum for exchange of scientific and professional information. Conducts continuing professional education programs. **Pub:** *Liaison*, quarterly. Newsletter. Contains information about the association's activities. • Directory, annual.

★ 5244 ★ ODPHP National Health Information Center (NHIC)

PO Box 1133
Washington, DC 20013-1133
Phone: (301)565-4167 **Free:** 800-336-4797
Fax: (301)984-4256
Email: info@nhic.org
Website: http://www.health.gov/nhic

Fnded: 1979. **Desc:** A health information referral service which links consumers and health professionals who have health questions with organizations best able to provide answers. Funded by the Office of Disease Prevention and Health Promotion, Public Health Service, U.S. Department of Health and Human Services. Maintains an online directory of more than 1800 health-related organizations that can provide health information. These include Federal and State agencies, voluntary associations, self-help and support groups, trade associations and professional societies. Prints directories and resource guides on a variety of health topics. **Pub:** *National Health Observances Planner*, annual. • *Prevention Report*, quarterly. Newsletter. **Frmly:** (1986) National Health Information Clearinghouse; (1987) ODPHP Health Information Center.

★ 5245 ★ Office of Health Economics

12 Whitehall
London SW1A 2DY, United Kingdom
Phone: 44 207 9309203 **Fax:** 44 207 7471419
Email: ohegeneral@ohe.org
Website: http://www.ohe.org

Fnded: 1962. **Desc:** Undertakes research on the economic aspects of medical care, with particular reference to the pharmaceutical industry. **Pub:** Papers.

★ 5246 ★ Ohashi Institute (OI)

147 W 25th St., 8th Fl.
New York, NY 10001-7205
Phone: (646)486-1187 **Free:** 800-810-4190
Fax: (646)486-1409
Email: ohashiinst@aol.com
Website: http://www.ohashi.com/institut.html
Wataru Ohashi, Dir.

Fnded: 1974. **Nat'l Groups:** 30. **State Groups:** 4. **Desc:** Dedicated to the promotion and teaching of the Oriental healing arts, specifically Ohashiatsu - a method of bodywork that elevates traditional Japanese shiatsu to a more complete experience of self-development and healing to promote health of body, mind and spirit. Program focuses on expanding awareness of self and others through the use of exercise, meditation and touch techniques based on Oriental healing philosophies. Courses for both laypeople and professionals in beginning, intermediate, advanced and post-graduate Ohashiatsu are offered. Instructor certification program available. Operates programs in the United States, South America and Europe. **Pub:** *Ohashiatsu News*. Newsletter. **Frmly:** (1983) Shiatsu Education Center of America.

★ 5247 ★ Oil Companies' European Organization for Environmental and Health Protection (CONCAWE)

Boulevard du Souverain 165
B-1160 Brussels, Belgium
Phone: 32 2 5669160 **Fax:** 32 2 5669181
Email: annemie.hermans@concawe.be
Website: http://www.concawe.be

Fnded: 1963. **Mem:** 34. **Lang(s):** English. **Desc:** Oil refining companies. Encourages the study of environmental and health issues that relate to the processing of crude oil and petroleum products; seeks to improve the understanding of environmental and health-related issues among authorities, users, and those involved in the industry. Examines topics such as emissions, labeling of petroleum products, and lead in gasoline. **Pub:** *CONCAWE Report*, periodic. **Frmly:** Study Group for Conservation of Clean Air and Water in Western Europe.

★ 5248 ★ Old Lesbians Organizing for Change (OLOC)

PO Box 980422
Houston, TX 77098
Email: info@oloc.org
Website: http://www.oloc.org
Arden Eversmeyer, Contact

Fnded: 1989. **Mem:** 1,000. **Desc:** Lesbians 60 years or older. Serves as a network to reduce ageism. Exchanges information on diversity of races, ethnicities, class backgrounds, and histories of members. Develops and disseminates educational materials on ageism and how to combat discrimination. **Pub:** *Facilitator's Handbook: Confronting Ageism for Lesbians 60 and Over*. Book. *Price:* $25. **AKA:** Old Lesbians Organizing.

★ 5249 ★ Oley Foundation for Home Parenteral and Enteral Nutrition

214 Hun Memorial, A-28
Albany Medical Center
Albany, NY 12208
Phone: (518)262-5079 **Free:** 800-776-OLEY
Fax: (518)262-5528
Email: bishopj@mail.amc.edu
Website: http://www.oley.org
Joan Bishop, Exec. Dir.

Fnded: 1983. **Mem:** 6,000. **Nat'l Groups:** 72. **Desc:** The Oley Foundation, a national non-profit organization, provides information and psycho-social support for home nutrition support patients, their families, caregivers and professionals. Programs include: bimonthly newsletter, national network of volunteers providing patient support, annual summer conference, regional meetings, toll-free patient-to-patient networking and information clearinghouse. Visit www.oley.org and/or call (800) 776-6539 for additional information. Seeks to enrich and enhance the lives of those requiring home nutrition support through an outreach system of patient volunteers, educational meetings and clearinghouse activities. **Pub:** *LifelineLetter*, bimonthly. Newsletter. *Price:* included in membership dues; $40/year for others. • Brochures.

★ 5250 ★ Ollier's/Maffucci Self-Help Group
PO Box 1533
Venice, FL 34284-1533
Phone: (941)496-9343 **Fax:** (941)496-9343
Email: olliers@aol.com
Website: http://www.ollier-maffucci.org
Bonnie Schmid-Hatch, Pres. /Founder

Fnded: 1987. **Mem:** 500. **Nat'l Groups:** 5. **State Groups:** 1. **Local Groups:** 1. **Desc:** Self-help group for persons with Ollier's disease, Maffacci and MHE or any diseases with enchodromas. (Ollier's disease is a rare, nongenetic bone disorder.) Aims to find as many patients as possible to support research program objectives. **Pub:** *Olliers News*, quarterly. Newsletter. *Price:* Donations. **Frmly:** (1998) Ollier's Disease Seflf-Help Group.

★ 5251 ★ Omicron Kappa Upsilon (OKU)
University of Nebraska Medical Center
College of Dentistry
40th & Holdgege St.
Lincoln, NE 68583-0740
Phone: (402)472-1339 **Fax:** (402)472-5290
Email: j.delahanty@umdnj.edu
Website: http://www.oku.org
Jan John, Corr. Sec.

Fnded: 1914. **Mem:** 17,500. **Desc:** Honorary society of men and women in the field of dentistry. **Pub:** Bulletin, annual.

★ 5252 ★ Oncology Nursing Society (ONS)
125 Enterprise Dr.
Pittsburgh, PA 15275
Phone: (412)859-6100 **Free:** (866)257-4ONS
Fax: 877-369-5497
Email: onsonline@ons.org
Website: http://www.ons.org
Pearl Moore, RN, CEO

Fnded: 1975. **Mem:** 30,000. **Local Groups:** 215. **Desc:** Registered nurses and other health care professionals with an interest in oncology. Seeks to: promote high professional standards in oncology nursing; provide a network for the exchange of information, resources, and peer support; encourage nurses to specialize in oncology; promote and develop educational programs in oncology nursing extending through the graduate level; identify, encourage, and foster nursing research in improving the quality of patient care. Conducts instructional and abstract sessions. Compiles statistics. **Pub:** *Clinical Journal of Oncology Nursing*, bimonthly. Journal. *Price:* $95/year. • *Oncology Nursing Forum*, bimonthly. Journal. Contains advertisers' index, calendar of events, information on new products, employment opportunity listings, chapter directory, and promotion news. *Price:* $115 for one-year subscription; $215 for two-year subscription; $95/year for institutions. • *ONS News*, monthly. Newsletter. Contains Washington, DC, news, calendar of events, employment opportunity listings, member news, and chapter news. *Price:* Included in membership dues.

★ 5253 ★ One-Arm Dove Hunt Association (OADH)
Box 582
Olney, TX 76374
Email: 1armjack@brazosnet.com
Jack R. Northrup, Co-Founder

Fnded: 1972. **Mem:** 550. **Desc:** Hand or arm amputees who enjoy the sport of shotgun shooting; interested nonamputees. Works to help amputees accept their handicap and to provide fellowship and shooting competitions. Activities include dove hunts, One-Arm Tales, One-Arm Talent, pool Tournament, golf tournament, horseshoe tournament, and dove dinner. **Pub:** Newsletter, annual.

★ 5254 ★ The One Shoe Crew (TOSC)
9328 Aizenberg Cir.
Elk Grove, CA 95624
Phone: (916)685-8746 **Fax:** (916)685-8746
Janice Piercy, Mgr.

Fnded: 1986. **Mem:** 2,500. **Desc:** Service for adults or teens whose feet have stopped growing. Finds cost-sharing partners for people who wear only one shoe or those who wear shoes of different sizes on each foot. (Clients include individuals with mismatched feet, amputees, people wearing a brace on one foot, and anyone with a one-sided foot problem who still wears one regular shoe.) Matches shoe size, width, needs, preferences, and approximate age of clients seeking partners. Many thousands of new, unused shoes and over 3,000 pairs of mismatched shoes (same shoe, different size) are available free to clients; shipping must be prepaid. Clients indicate the general shoe style they prefer. All services are free for U.S. Veterans.

★ 5255 ★ Operation Eyesight Universal (OEU)
4 Parkdale Cres. NW
Calgary, AB, Canada T2N 3T8
Phone: (403)283-6323 **Free:** 800-585-8265
Fax: (403)270-1899
Email: oeuca@giftofsight.com
Website: http://www.giftofsight.com

Fnded: 1963. **Mem:** 15,000. **Reg. Groups:** 3. **Lang(s):** English. **Desc:** Individuals, firms, churches, schools, service clubs, and other organizations united to promote sight restoration and blindness prevention through programs in developing countries. Provides medical, educational, assistance to needy individuals. Assists in the establishment of: special programs to combat blindness due to malnutrition; eye care hospitals; eye care departments in health care institutions; rural mobile eye programs. Works with local blindness prevention societies. Operates training programs. **Pub:** *Gift of Sight*, quarterly. Newsletter.

★ 5256 ★ Operation Rainbow
PO Box 571017
Houston, TX 77257-1017
Phone: (713)960-7800 **Fax:** (713)960-7803
Email: billmagee@operationrainbow.org
Website: http://www.operationrainbow.org
Bill Magee, Pres. /CEO

Fnded: 1978. **Desc:** Provides free reconstructive surgery for children in medically under-served countries and throughout the United States.

★ 5257 ★ Operation Smile International - Vietnam (OSIV)
2nd Fl., 63 Ly Thai To
Hanoi, Vietnam
Phone: 84 4 9348754 **Fax:** 84 4 9349024
Email: operationsmilevietnam@yahoo.com
Website: http://www.operationsmile.org

Lang(s): English, French, Vietnamese. **Desc:** Reconstructive surgeons and other health care professionals. Seeks to increase the availability of cosmetic and reconstructive surgery among impoverished children. Performs free reconstructive surgery on needy children; conducts training programs for surgeons; distributes medical equipment and supplies to indigenous health care centers.

★ 5258 ★ Ophthalmic Photographers' Society (OPS)
c/o Barbara McCalley
1869 W Ranch Rd.
Nixa, MO 65714-9230
Phone: (417)725-0181 **Free:** 800-403-1677
Fax: (417)724-8450
Email: opsmember@aol.com
Website: http://www.opsweb.org
Paul Montague, CRA, Contact

Fnded: 1969. **Mem:** 1,200. **Reg. Groups:** 3. **Desc:** Ophthalmologists, pathologists, medical and ophthalmic photographers, nurses, ophthalmic assistants, technicians, technologists, researchers, and engineers; organizations and individuals who are actively involved with ophthalmology or ophthalmic photography. Objective is to encourage the highest quality of ophthalmic photography and to promote development of new and improved techniques and equipment. (Ophthalmic photography involves photography of the eye for documentation and diagnostic purposes.) Provides continuing education and technical information. Serves as a forum for the discussion of ophthalmic photography. Provides testing, and subsequent certification as Certified Retinal Angiographer in performance of ophthalmic photography. **Pub:** *Journal of Ophthalmic Photography*, semiannual. Journal. *Price:* $26 US; $31 International. • *OPS Directory*, annual. Directory. • *OPS Newsletter*, bimonthly. Newsletter.

★ 5259 ★ Ophthalmological Society of the Republic of China
1 Chang-Teh St
Taipei 100, Taiwan
Fax: 886 2 3832310

Fnded: 1959.

★ 5260 ★ Opportunity Plus
PO Box 35481
Charlotte, NC 28235
Phone: (704)519-0600 **Fax:** (704)519-0699
Email: info@opportunity-plus.org
Website: http://www.opportunity-plus.org

Fnded: 1979. **Reg. Groups:** 5. **Desc:** Works with the physically disabled community by providing the opportunity to be independent through mentoring, training, and employment programs, and by educating the community at large through information, referral, and networking. **Pub:** *Mentor Newsletter*, quarterly. Newsletter. Includes client updates, resources, and legislative updates. **AKA:** (2002) Learning How. **Frmly:** (1987) Handicapped Organized Women; (1988) HOW.

★ 5261 ★ Optician Association
Alexanderstr. 25A
D-40210 Dusseldorf, Germany
Phone: 49 211 1863235 **Fax:** 49 211 86323535
Email: info@zva.de
Website: http://www.zva.de

Fnded: 1951. **Mem:** 7,500. **Desc:** Supports and represents the interests of opticians in Germany.

★ 5262 ★ Opticians Association of America (OAA)
PO Box 6600
Springfield, VA 22150-6600
Phone: (703)916-8856 **Free:** 800-443-8997
Fax: (703)916-7966
Email: oaa@opticians.org
Website: http://www.opticians.org
Earl M. Cleveland, Pres.

Fnded: 1926. **Mem:** 10,000. **State Groups:** 48. **Desc:** Retail dispensing opticians who fill prescriptions for glasses or contact lenses written by a vision care specialist. Works to advance the science of ophthalmic optics. Conducts research and educational programs. Maintains museum and speakers' bureau. Compiles statistics. **Pub:** *American Optician*, quarterly. Magazine. Contains calendar of events and research reports. *Price:* Included in membership dues. **Frmly:** (1972) Guild of Prescription Opticians of America.

★ 5263 ★ Option Institute and Fellowship (OIF)
2080 S Undermountain Rd.
Sheffield, MA 01257-9643
Phone: (413)229-2100 **Free:** 800-714-2779
Fax: (413)229-8931
Email: correspondence@option.org
Website: http://www.option.org
Barry N. Kaufman, Founder

Fnded: 1983. **Desc:** Provides individuals, couples, families, businesses and groups empowering personal growth programs and seminars using life-changing, experiential learning techniques that can greatly improve relationships, career, health and quality of life. Option Process counseling sessions with Certified

Option Process Mentors/Counselors are offered. **Pub:** *A Miracle to Believe In.* Book. • *A Sacred Dying.* Book. • *Giant Steps.* Book. • *Happiness Is a Choice.* Book. • *Out-Smarting Your Karma.* Book. • *Power Dialogues.* Book. • *Son-Rise: The Miracle Continues.* Book. • *To Love Is To Be Happy With.* Book.

★ 5264 ★ Optometric Extension Program Foundation (OEPF)
1921 E Carnegie, Ste. 3L
Santa Ana, CA 92705-5510
Phone: (949)250-8070 **Fax:** (949)250-8157
Email: smc.oep@att.net
Website: http://www.healthy.net/oep
Joseph B. Sullivan, OD, Pres.

Fnded: 1928. **Mem:** 4,000. **Desc:** Registered optometrists and optometric assistants enrolled for continuing education courses. Maintains speakers' bureau. Sponsors educational programs. **Pub:** *Journal of Behavioral Optometry*, bimonthly. Journal. Includes professional articles, calendar of events, and current affairs. *Price:* $65/year. • *Optometric Extension Program Foundation–Curriculum II*, annual. Text of 6-8 courses covering various optometry subjects. Includes literature and research reviews and annual index. *Price:* $350. • *Reference Directory*, biennial. Directory.

★ 5265 ★ Optometric Historical Society (OHS)
243 N Lindbergh Blvd.
Saint Louis, MO 63141
Phone: (314)991-4100 **Free:** 800-365-2219
Fax: (314)991-4101
Email: mdjones-od@phd.aol.org
Dr. Michael Johns, Exec. Dir.

Fnded: 1969. **Desc:** Optometrists and other individuals or groups interested in optometry, optics, and related disciplines. Purposes are to encourage the collection and preservation of materials relating to the history of optometry and to assist in the care of archives of optometric interest. **Pub:** Newsletter, quarterly.

★ 5266 ★ Optometrists Association Australia
204 Drummond St.
PO Box 185
Carlton South, VIC 3053, Australia
Phone: 61 3 96636833 **Fax:** 61 3 96637478
Email: oaanat@optometrists.asn.au
Website: http://www.optometrists.asn.au

State Groups: 6. **Lang(s):** English. **Desc:** Optometrists. Seeks to advance the profession of optometry; promotes ongoing professional development of members. Represents members' interests before government agencies and other organizations; provides resources to assist optometric practices. Makes available to the public information and services.

★ 5267 ★ Oral Health America
410 N Michigan Ave., Ste. 352
Chicago, IL 60611-4211
Phone: (312)836-9900 **Free:** 800-523-3438
Fax: (312)836-9986
Email: liz@oralhealthamerica.org
Website: http://www.oralhealthamerica.org
Robert J. Klaus, Pres. & CEO

Fnded: 1955. **Desc:** Funds dental education, research, and service programs. Operates speakers' bureau. **Pub:** *Advocate*, quarterly. Newsletters. • *Programs and Priorities*, periodic. • Annual Report. **Frmly:** (1963) Fund for Dental Education; (1973) American Fund for Dental Education; (1998) American Fund for Dental Health.

★ 5268 ★ Oral Hearing-Impaired Section (OHIS)
3417 Volta Pl. NW
Washington, DC 20007
Phone: (202)337-5220 **Fax:** (202)337-8314
Email: info@agbell.org
Website: http://www.agbell.org/sections/dhhs/
K. Todd Houston, PhD, Exec. Dir.

Fnded: 1964. **Mem:** 345. **Local Groups:** 3. **Desc:** Section of the Alexander Graham Bell Association for the Deaf. Persons who are deaf or hard of hearing predominantly use speech and lipreading work. Encourages deaf young people and their families to use speech, lipreading, and residual hearing. Participates in regional, national, and international conferences on deafness. Appears on television and radio programs to demonstrate communications skills. Seeks to dispel outmoded conceptions about deafness. Supports: richer educational opportunities for the hearing impaired; workshops and outings for deaf or hard of hearing children and their families and teachers; scholarship funds for qualified students with hearing impairments; improved methods for developing better speech, voice, lipreading, and auditory training techniques. **Pub:** *Valta Voices OHIS Section*, bimonthly. Magazine. **Frmly:** (1988) Oral Deaf Adults Section.

★ 5269 ★ ORBIS International
520 8th Ave, 11th Fl.
New York, NY 10018
Phone: (646)674-5500 **Free:** 800-ORBIS-US
Fax: (646)674-5599
Email: executive@ny.orbis.org
Website: http://www.orbis.org
Kathy Spahn, Pres. and Exec. Dir.

Fnded: 1973. **Desc:** Dedicated to saving sight and eliminating avoidable blindness worldwide. Responds to the needs of developing nations, where ninety percent of blind people live, with hands-on training for eye care professionals, public education about blindness, and technical assistance to improve access to quality ophthalmic services. Has the world's only flying eye hospital, a DC-10 that has been converted into a state-of-the-art medical facility, and flies to developing countries to provide intensive, comprehensive eye care training. Has long-term country programs in Bangladesh, China, Ethiopia, India and Vietnam. **Pub:** *ORBIS Observer*, quarterly. Newsletter. *Price:* Free. • *ORBIS Observer - Hong Kong.* Newsletter. • *ORBIS Observer - U.K.*. Newsletter. **Frmly:** Project Orbis.

★ 5270 ★ Ordre des Docteurs Veterinaires du Senegal
BP 139
Dakar, Senegal
Phone: 221 8322441 **Fax:** 221 8322441
Email: odvs@primature.sn

Fnded: 1993. **Mem:** 245. **Desc:** Veterinarians working to improve animal health and welfare in Senegal.

★ 5271 ★ Organic Acidemia Association (OAA)
c/o Kathy Stagni
13210 35th Ave N
Plymouth, MN 55441-2227
Phone: (763)559-1797 **Fax:** (763)694-0017
Email: oaanews@aol.com
Website: http://www.oaanews.org
Kathy Stagni, Exec. Dir.

Fnded: 1982. **Mem:** 800. **Desc:** Dietitians, researchers, and geneticists; clinics; parents and relatives of children suffering from organic acidemia disorders. (Organic acidemia is a class of genetic metabolic disorders that lead to cellular enzyme deficiencies and require restricted diets.) Fosters communication among parents and professionals; acts as support group. **Pub:** *Organic Acidemia Association Newsletter*, 3/year. Newsletter. *Price:* $25/year domestic; $35/year international.

★ 5272 ★ Organic Living Association
St. Mary's Villa
Hanley Swan
Worcester WR8 0EA, United Kingdom
Fax: 44 1684 310703

Fnded: 1971. **Mem:** 200. **Nat'l Groups:** 1. **Desc:** Aims to integrate the production and consumption of vegetables, fruit, cereals and dairy produce grown on healthy, naturally fertilized soil. Promotes human health by whatever humane means may be necessary; promotes establishment of ecological, self-reliant, self-sufficient villages. Disseminates knowledge of alternatives to allopathic medicine. **Pub:** Newsletter, bimonthly.

★ 5273 ★ Organisation Gestosis - Society for the Study of Pathophysiology of Pregnancy (OG) (Geburtshilfe und Gynakologie FMH)
Geburtshilfe und Gynakologie FMH
Gerbergasse 14
CH-4051 Basel, Switzerland
Phone: 41 61 2615555 **Fax:** 41 61 2615934

Fnded: 1969. **Mem:** 4,500. **Reg. Groups:** 11. **Lang(s):** English, German. **Desc:** Obstetricians, gynecologists, neonatologists, nephrologists, epidemiologists, pathologists, geneticists, immunologists, physiologists, and health officials in 75 countries in the field of EPH-Gestosis. EPH-Gestosis is a term adopted by the society to describe a malady that may occur during pregnancy wherein a woman exhibits excessive accumulation of body water, protein in the urine, and/or abnormal elevation of blood pressure; EPH is derived from the terms for 3 conditions: edema, proteinuria, and hypertension; gestosis is derived from the word gestation and the suffix -osis which means disturbance. The condition is prevalent in socioeconomically depressed areas where poor hygiene and malnutrition aggravate the effects of inadeq uate prenatal care. The society reports that EPH-Gestosis occurs in 10% of world population births, is responsible for as much as 50% of perinatal/fetal death, and is the cause of up to 33% of maternal mortality. Objectives are to: disseminate information to medical and lay personnel and the public; foster research, preventive health care, and therapy; internationalize nomenclature, classification, and definitions in the field of EPH-Gestosis for diagnosis, therapy, and comparative techniques; standardize methods of investigation; serve as documentation center; foster exchange of scientists. Conducts discussion groups and study groups on topics such as edema, proteinuria, cytology, serumprotein, and hypertension. Suggests alterations of definitions of EPH-Gestosis as offered by International Classification of Diseases of the World Health Organization. Makes recommendations for the most modern and successful measures of prevention and treatment of EPH-Gestosis. Collects and publishes papers submitted by researchers worldwide. Sponsors symposia and workshops; conducts surveys. worldwide. Sponsors symposia and workshops; conducts surveys. **Pub:** *Instruction Bulletin*, periodic. Bulletin. • *International Journal of Feto-Maternal Medicine*, periodic. Journal. • *OG News*, periodic. • Proceedings.

★ 5274 ★ Organization of European Cancer Institutes (OECI)
3, rue du Conseil-General
CH-1205 Geneva, Switzerland
Phone: 41 22 8091811 **Fax:** 41 22 8091810
Email: info@oeci.org
Website: http://www.oeci.org

Fnded: 1979. **Desc:** Enhances and promotes collaboration between cancer institutes in Europe.

★ 5275 ★ Organization for Nutrition Education (ONE)
c/o Shawna Berenbaum
College of Pharmacy and Nutrition
University of Saskatchewan
110 Science Place
Saskatoon, SK, Canada S7N 5C9
Phone: (306)966-5836 **Fax:** (306)966-6377
Email: berenbaum@sask.usask.ca
Website: http://www.stfx.ca/academic/human-nutrition/organization/main.html

Fnded: 1980. **Mem:** 200. **Lang(s):** English, French. **Desc:** Nutrition professionals and organizations and other individuals and corporations with an interest in nutrition and related fields. **Pub:** *National Membership*

Roster, annual. Directory. • *O.N.E. Annual Report*, annual. • *O.N.E. Bulletin*, 3/year. Newsletter. • *O.N.E. Report*. Annual Report.

★ 5276 ★ Organization for Safety and Asepsis Procedures (OSAP)
PO Box 6297
Annapolis, MD 21401
Phone: (410)571-0003 **Free:** 800-298-6727
Fax: (410)571-0028
Email: osap@clark.net
Website: http://www.osap.org

Fnded: 1984. **Desc:** Academicians, health care practitioners and dental industry representatives. Works to maximize problem solving of difficult dental infection control issues. **Pub:** Newsletter, quarterly. *Price:* included in membership dues.

★ 5277 ★ Organization of Teratology Information Services
1501 N Campbell
Arizona Poison and Drug Information Center, Rm. 1156
Tucson, AZ 85724
Phone: (520)626-3410 **Free:** 888-285-3410
Fax: (520)626-5115
Email: bdefects@ucsd.edu
Website: http://www.otispregnancy.org
Dee Quinn, Pres.

Fnded: 1990. **Mem:** 60. **State Groups:** 23. **Desc:** Provides information on teratology. Teratology is the study of agents used during pregnancy and their potential effects on the developing baby. **Pub:** *Fact Sheets*, annual. Report. Sixteen different fact sheets available on website.

★ 5278 ★ Orthodontic Education and Research Foundation (OERF)
3320 Rutger St.
Saint Louis, MO 63104-1008
Phone: (314)577-8189 **Fax:** (314)268-5673
Joe Mellion, Exec. Dir.

Fnded: 1957. **Mem:** 500. **Desc:** Orthodontists. Promotes research; conducts continuing education programs, seminars, and clinical and professional training. **Pub:** *OERF Journal*, annual. Proceedings. Includes new members listing. *Price:* Included in membership dues. • *OERF Newsletter*, annual. Newsletter.

★ 5279 ★ Orthodox Christian Association of Medicine, Psychology and Religion (OCAMPR)
PO Box 958
Cambridge, MA 02238
Phone: (617)868-6557 **Fax:** (617)495-7728
John T. Chirban, PhD, Pres.

Fnded: 1986. **Mem:** 2. **Desc:** Professionals in medicine, psychology, and religion. Facilitates interdisciplinary programs and community understanding of Orthodox Christianity concerning interdisciplinary studies. Encourages Christian fellowship among professionals. Sponsors charitable activities. Operates research center. **Pub:** *Conference Proceedings*, annual. Proceedings. Contains formal papers and reports of ethical, medical, and religious issues. • *Membership Directory*, periodic. Directory. Contains listing of Orthodox Health Professionals. *Price:* $2.50. • *Synergia*, quarterly. Newsletter.

★ 5280 ★ Orthopaedic Research Society (ORS)
c/o Brenda Welborn
6300 N River Rd., No. 727
Rosemont, IL 60018-4226
Phone: (847)384-4242 **Fax:** (847)823-4921
Email: welborn@aaos.org
Website: http://www.ors.org
Brenda Welborn, Exec. Dir.

Fnded: 1854. **Mem:** 1,700. **Desc:** Orthopaedic surgeons, physical and biological scientists, engineers, and other investigators. Seeks to promote research in orthopaedic surgery and musculoskeletal diseases. Provides educational activities; disseminates knowledge in these fields. **Pub:** *Journal of Orthopaedic Research*, semiannual. Journal. *Price:* included in membership dues. • Newsletter, semiannual. *Price:* included in membership dues.

★ 5281 ★ Orthopaedic Section, American Physical Therapy Association
2920 E Ave. S, Ste. 200
La Crosse, WI 54601
Phone: (608)788-3982 **Free:** 800-444-3982
Fax: (608)788-3965
Email: tdeflorian@orthopt.org
Website: http://www.orthopt.org
Terri DeFlorian, Exec. Dir.

Fnded: 1974. **Mem:** 13,000. **Desc:** Orthopaedic physical therapists and physical therapist assistants who belong to the American Physical Therapy Association; physical therapy educators and students. Supports the continued growth of the physical therapy profession through education and research; promotes development of a standard certification procedure for the field. Seeks to assure the quality of physical therapy curricula at both the undergraduate and postgraduate levels. Facilitates communication among orthopedic physical therapists and other health care professionals. Gathers and disseminates information on the care of musculoskeletal disorders. Provides access to a network of orthopaedic study groups. **Pub:** *Journal of Orthopaedic and Sports Physical Therapy*, monthly. Journal. • *Orthopaedic Physical Therapy Practice*, quarterly. • *Orthopaedic Section of the American Physical Therapy Association*. Newsletter. Describes orthopaedic physical therapy and what the section is all about.

★ 5282 ★ Orthopaedic Trauma Association (OTA)
6300 N River Rd., Ste. 727
Rosemont, IL 60018-4226
Phone: (847)698-1631 **Free:** 800-346-2267
Fax: (847)823-0536
Email: franzon@aaos.org
Website: http://www.ota.org
Nancy E. Franzon, Exec. Dir.

Fnded: 1983. **Mem:** 450. **Desc:** Physicians and other health care professionals with an interest in orthopedic trauma. Seeks to advance research and education in the practice of orthopedics; promotes development of improved orthopedic trauma treatment techniques; works to educate the public regarding safety issues in motor vehicle accidents. Serves as a clearinghouse on orthopedic trauma; conducts continuing professional development courses. **Pub:** *Fracture Lines*, periodic. Newsletter. *Price:* For members only. • *Journal of Orthopaedic Trauma*, periodic. Journal. • Abstracts of lectures given at annual meeting in JBJS and on-line.

★ 5283 ★ Orthopaedics Overseas (OO)
PO Box 65157
Washington, DC 20035-5157
Phone: (202)296-0928 **Fax:** (202)296-8018
Email: info@hvousa.org
Website: http://www.hvousa.org
Nancy Kelly, Exec. Dir.

Fnded: 1959. **Mem:** 775. **Desc:** Orthopedic surgeons interested in volunteering as consultants in developing countries. Trains physicians in developing countries in diagnostic, conservative, and operative management techniques. Addresses chronic and acute orthopedic problems and crippling diseases such as polio and arthritis. Operates programs in Cambodia, Bhutan, Nepal, Malawi, Kenya, St. Lucia, South Africa, Uganda, Vietnam, and Ethiopia. Formerly a project of CARE, the group is a division of Health Volunteers Overseas. HVO also sponsors Anesthesia Overseas, Dentistry Overseas, Nursing Overseas, Oral and Maxillofacial Surgery Overseas, and Pediatrics Overseas, Internal Medicine Overseas, Nurse Anesthesia Overseas, and Physical Therapy Overseas.

★ 5284 ★ Orthopedic Foundation for Animals (OFA)
2300 Nifong Blvd.
Columbia, MO 65201-3856
Phone: (573)442-0418 **Fax:** (573)875-5073
Email: ofa@offa.org
Website: http://www.offa.org
Dr. G.G. Keller, Project Dir.

Fnded: 1967. **Desc:** National and local dog clubs and individual breeders. Acts as a clearinghouse for information on orthopedic diseases of animals, particularly hip dysplasia in dogs (a hereditary condition resulting in abnormal development of the hip joints). Is attempting to develop a national control program through monitoring animals and conducting selective breeding and research. Conducts educational seminars; compiles statistics; sponsors a national referral service for animal breeders. Maintains library of all breed canine pelvic radiographs. **Pub:** *Proceedings of Canine Hip Dysplasia Symposium and Workshop*.

★ 5285 ★ Orthopedic Research Society (ORS)
6300 N River Rd., Ste. 727
Rosemont, IL 60018-4226
Phone: (847)698-1625 **Fax:** (847)823-4921
Email: ors@aaos.org
Website: http://www.ors.org
Brenda Welborn, Exec. Dir.

Fnded: 1954. **Mem:** 1,870. **Desc:** Orthopedic surgeons and other investigators who are elected as active members on the basis of previous scientific activity, continued participation in the field of research, and accomplishments in orthopedic surgery. Promotes orthopedic research and provides a meeting place for presentation and discussion of orthopedic research activities. **Pub:** *Journal of Orthopedic Research*, quarterly. Published for Musculoskeletal investigators. *Price:* $164 in U.S.; $190 elsewhere. • *Transactions of Annual Meeting*. Proceedings. *Price:* $45.

★ 5286 ★ Orthoptic and Binocular Vision Association (OBVA)
48 Church St.
Tamworth B79 7DE, United Kingdom
Phone: 44 1827 61600
Email: d.b.stidwill@aston.ac.uk

Fnded: 1958. **Mem:** 150. **Nat'l Groups:** 1. **Lang(s):** English. **Desc:** Optometrists are full members; optometry students and other health care professionals are associate members. Promotes orthoptic and vision training among health care professionals. Conducts educational programs in orthoptics and binocular vision. **Pub:** *OBVA Newsletter*, quarterly. Newsletter. Contains abstracts, cases, and comment.

★ 5287 ★ OsteoArthritis Research Society International (OARSI)
2025 M St., Ste.800
Washington, DC 20036
Phone: (202)367-1177 **Fax:** (202)367-2177
Email: oarsi@orsi.org
Website: http://www.oarsi.org

Desc: Researchers and health care professionals with an interest in osteoarthritis. Seeks to promote and encourage fundamental and applied research on osteoarthritis and its treatment. Gathers and disseminates information on osteoarthritis and related research; sponsors educational programs. **Pub:** *Membership Directory*, annual. Directory. • *OA Today*, quarterly. Newsletter. • *Osteoarthritis and Cartilage*, bimonthly. Journal.

★ 5288 ★ Osteogenesis Imperfecta Foundation (OIF)
804 W Diamond Ave., Ste. 210
Gaithersburg, MD 20878
Phone: (301)947-0083 **Free:** 800-981-2663
Fax: (301)947-0456
Email: bonelink@oif.org
Website: http://www.oif.org
Ms. Mary Beth Huber, Information & Resource Dir.

Fnded: 1970. **Mem:** 4,500. **State Groups:** 43. **Desc:** Osteogenesis Imperfecta Foundation, Inc. is a voluntary national health organization dedicated to helping people cope with osteogenesis imperfecta. The mission of the OI Foundation is to improve the quality of life for individuals affected by OI through education, awareness, mutual support and research into the treatment and potential cure of the disorder. Information is provided to individuals who have OI and their families, medical professionals and other members of the community. Resources and programs include a quarterly newsletter, a physician information service, written literature, informative videos, national conferences and local support groups. Compiles statistics. support groups. Compiles statistics. **Pub:** *Caring for Infants and Children with Osteogenesis Imperfecta.* Brochure. • *Going Places.* Video. • *Growing Up With OI: A Guide for Children.* Book. • *Growing Up With OI: A Guide for Families & Caregivers.* Book. • *Managing Osteogenesis Imperfecta: A Medical Manual.* Book. *Price:* $28.50. • *Osteogenesis Imperfecta: A Guide for Medical Professionals, Individuals, Families Affected by OI.* Brochure. • *Osteogenesis Imperfecta Foundation–Breakthrough*, quarterly. Newsletter. Contains medical reports, foundation news, and activities. *Price:* Free to members; $12/year for nonmembers. • *Plan for Success.* Video. • *Plan for Success: An Education's Guide to Students with Osteogenesis Imperfecta.* Brochure. • *Therapeutic Strategies for OI: A Guide for Physical Therapists and Occupational Therapists.* Brochure. • *You Are Not Alone.* Videos. *Price:* $7.50. • Also publishes other medical and general literature.

★ 5289 ★ Osteoporosis Society of Canada (La Societe de l'Osteoporose du Canada)
33 Laird Dr.
Toronto, ON, Canada M4G 3S9
Phone: (416)696-2663 **Free:** 800-463-6842
Fax: (416)696-2673
Email: osc@osteoporosis.ca
Website: http://www.osteoporosis.ca

Fnded: 1982. **Reg. Groups:** 13. **Lang(s):** English, French. **Desc:** Individuals and organizations interested in the prevention, diagnosis, and treatment of osteoporosis. Supports research programs that seek to improve the quality of life for women with osteoporosis. Promotes education about osteoporosis among professional health practitioners. Disseminates informational materials to individuals with osteoporosis, physicians, and the public. Offers audio visual programs; participates in public forums. **Pub:** *Osteoblast*, quarterly. Newsletter. A donor newsletter. • *Osteoporosis Update*, quarterly. Newsletter.

★ 5290 ★ Osterreichische Gesellschaft fur Familienplanung (OGF)
Ignaz-Semmelweis-Frauenklinik
Bastiengasse 36-38
A-1180 Vienna, Austria
Phone: 43 4 76153903
Email: office@oegf.at
Website: http://www.oegf.at

Fnded: 1966. **Mem:** 107. **Lang(s):** German. **Desc:** Works to improve the quality of life for individuals living in Austria by promoting family planning and responsible parenthood. Works to reduce the number of unwanted pregnancies and abortions and stop the spread of sexually transmitted diseases, especially AIDS. Provides programs in family planning, sex education, and health. Provides contraceptive services. Advocates for international aspects of reproductive and sexual health and rights among politicians and government officials. **Pub:** *Newsletter OEGF*, semiannual. Newsletter.

★ 5291 ★ Osterreichische Multiple Sklerose Gesellschaft
c/o Universitatsklinik f.
Neurologie
Waehringer Guertel 18-20
A-1090 Vienna, Austria
Phone: 43 1 404003121 **Fax:** 43 1 404003141
Email: msgs@akh-wien.ac.at

Fnded: 1965. **Reg. Groups:** 25. **Desc:** MS patients, families and professionals. Seeks to improve the quality of life for persons with multiple sclerosis and their families.

★ 5292 ★ Osterreichisches Nationalkomitee der FDI
c/o Bundeskurie Zahnarzte der Osterreichischen Arztekammer
Weihburggasse 9/3/22
A-1011 Vienna, Austria
Phone: 43 1 512512662 **Fax:** 43 1 512512667
Email: w.doneus@lion.cc

Desc: Represents the dental profession in Austria.

★ 5293 ★ Ostomy Association of China (OAC)
c/o Dr. Yu De-Hong MD, Pres.
174 Chang Hai Rd.
Shanghai 200433, People's Republic of China
Phone: 86 21 25070965 **Fax:** 86 21 65492727

Fnded: 1988. **Mem:** 400. **Nat'l Groups:** 1. **Reg. Groups:** 22. **Local Groups:** 23. **Lang(s):** English. **Desc:** Doctors, stoma nurses, and ostomates. Promotes the care of ostomates in China. Offers medical and practical advice and provides a way for ostomates to exchange information about their experiences. Operates the Ostomy Museum of China in Shanghai. **Pub:** *Friend of Ostomates*, monthly. • *From Anti Cancer*, bimonthly. Newspaper.

★ 5294 ★ Our Youths Foundation (OYF) (Fundacion Nuestros Jovenes — FNJ)
Baron de Carondelet 641 Y Villaengua
Quito, Ecuador
Phone: 593 2 247250 **Fax:** 593 2 443964
Email: fnjovenes@lettera.net
Website: http://www.fundacionnuestrosjovenes.org.ec

Fnded: 1982. **Mem:** 400. **Lang(s):** English, French, German, Spanish. **Desc:** Works to provide assistance to young substance abusers in Ecuador. Conducts drug awareness programs and offers medical and psychological assistance for young abusers. Investigates the extent and severity of illicit drug use in Ecuador and disseminates information to increase public awareness of the causes and effects of drug trafficking; VIH-SIDA prevention in high-risk groups and other health and educational projects. **Pub:** *Sin Limites*, bimonthly. Magazine. Contains analysis of adolescents' problems and prevention.

★ 5295 ★ Outpatient Intravenous Infusion Therapy Association (OPIVITA)
6240 Tacoma Mall Blvd., No. 104
Tacoma, WA 98409-6819
Phone: (253)627-1850 **Fax:** (253)274-0877
Email: opivita1@aol.com

Desc: Strives to educate physicians and their team members in the provision of safe and effective outpatient parenteral infusion therapy (OPAT).

★ 5296 ★ Outpatient Ophthalmic Surgery Society (OOSS)
793 A. Foothill Blvd., pmb 119
San Luis Obispo, CA 93405
Phone: 877-220-3585 **Fax:** 877-220-2793
Email: info@ooss.org
Website: http://www.ooss.org
Karen S. Morgan, Admin. Dir.

Fnded: 1981. **Mem:** 700. **Desc:** Ophthalmic surgeons. Purpose is to gather and share information about outpatient eye surgery in order to promote high-quality, low-cost patient care. **Pub:** *Dollars and Disease: The True Cost of Cataracts.* • Journal, annual. • Newsletter, quarterly. • Also publishes books; produces videotapes.

★ 5297 ★ Ovarian Cancer National Alliance
910 17th St. NW, Ste. 413
Washington, DC 20006
Phone: (202)331-1332 **Fax:** (202)331-2292
Email: ocna@ovariancancer.org
Website: http://www.ovariancancer.org/
Ann Kolker, Contact

Fnded: 1997. **Desc:** Works to promote knowledge about breast cancer and works toward a cure.

★ 5298 ★ Overcoming Mobility Barriers International (OMBI)
1022 S 41st St.
Omaha, NE 68105-8108
Phone: (402)342-5731 **Fax:** (402)342-5731
Kay E. Neil, Exec. Dir.

Fnded: 1979. **Mem:** 104. **Desc:** Government officials, service consumers and providers, and other persons interested in removing mobility barriers for elderly, handicapped, and disadvantaged persons. Advises and works in conjunction with other groups and government agencies to establish safety standards for special equipment used in retrofitting vehicles and works to retrain drivers in the use of nonconventional driving controls. Addresses such problems as possible allocation of fuel to social service agencies and others working in nontransit areas. **Pub:** *A Positive Approach*, quarterly. Newsletter. Includes calendar of events. *Price:* Included in membership dues.

★ 5299 ★ Ovulation Method Research and Reference Centre of Australia
27 Alexandra Pde.
North Fitzroy, VIC 3068, Australia
Phone: 61 3 94811722 **Fax:** 61 3 94824208
Website: http://www.billings-ovulation-method.org.au/index.shtml

Desc: Promotes the Billing Ovulation Method that teaches a woman to interpret natural signs of fertility through all life stages.

★ 5300 ★ Oxalosis and Hyperoxaluria Foundation (OHF)
5727 Westcliffe Dr.
Saint Louis, MO 63129
Phone: (618)281-9450 **Free:** 888-721-2432
Fax: (618)281-9452
Email: bdjrk@aol.com
Website: http://www.ohf.org
Brett Rosen, Pres.

Fnded: 1989. **Mem:** 900. **Desc:** Individuals affected by oxalosis and hyperoxaluria; health care professionals. Hyperoxaluria is a metabolic disease affecting the kidneys. Oxalosis occurs when calcium crystals have deposited elsewhere in the body, often the eyes, bones, and joints. Provides support services and information regarding the conditions and their affects. Encourages research. Operates referral service. **Pub:** *In Touch*, 3/year. Newsletter. • *Understanding Hyperoxaluria and Oxalosis.* Brochure.

★ 5301 ★ P.R.I.D.E. Foundation - Promote Real Independence for the Disabled and Elderly (P.R.I.D.E.)
391 Long Hill Rd.
Box 1293
Groton, CT 06340-1293
Phone: (860)445-1448 **Free:** 800-332-9122
Fax: (860)445-1448
Email: dresspride@aol.com
Website: http://www.sewtiqueonline.com
Evelyn S. Kennedy, Exec. Dir.

Fnded: 1978. **Desc:** Provides rehabilitation assistance for the handicapped and elderly in the areas of home management, independent dressing, and personal grooming. Designs and develops special garments that will help the handicapped feel more comfortable and dress independently; designs assistive devices for use in the kitchen, bedroom, and bathroom. Provides discussion leaders for community outreach and assistance to health agencies, social service groups, and volunteer organizations. Conducts workshops and educational forums for rehabilitation centers, educational institutions, and community agencies. Sponsored Project Pride, an in-class training program providing physically and mentally handicapped individuals with entry-level occupational skills in the sewing field. Conducts public exhibitions and demonstrations of clothing and adaptive devices. **Pub:** *Children's Fashions and Special Needs.* Paper. • *Dressing With Pride.* Book. • *Fashion and Clothing Accessibility.* Book. • *Resources and Clothing for Special Needs.* • *Scoliosis and Fashion.* Paper.

★ 5302 ★ Pacific Dermatologic Association (PDA)
2950 Buskirk Ave., Ste. 170
Walnut Creek, CA 94597
Phone: (925)472-5910
Email: alkayne@washington.edu
Website: http://www.pacificderm.org
Dr. David Taylor, Pres.

Fnded: 1948. **Mem:** 1,200. **Reg. Groups:** 1. **Desc:** Dermatologists united to provide opportunities for exchange of information and advancement of knowledge of dermatology and syphilology among physicians within the Pacific Rim. Conducts specialized education programs; sponsors competitions. **Pub:** *Transactions*, annual. • Membership Directory, triennial.

★ 5303 ★ Paget Foundation for Paget's Disease of Bone and Related Disorders (PDF)
120 Wall St., Ste. 1602
New York, NY 10005-4001
Phone: (212)509-5335 **Free:** 800-23-PAGET
Fax: (212)509-8492
Email: pagetfdn@aol.com
Website: http://www.paget.org
Charlene Waldman, Exec. Dir.

Fnded: 1978. **Desc:** Patients and their families and friends; physicians; paramedical professionals interested in improving health care of persons suffering from Paget's disease, a chronic disorder which may result in enlarged, deformed, and fragile bones in one or more regions of the skeleton, fibrous dysplasia, and primary hyperparathyroidism (PHPT). Also addresses related bone disorders such as fibrous dysplasia and both breast, prostate cancer hetastatic to bone. Conducts educational programs for patients, health care professionals, and the public; provides patient assistance and research advocacy; maintains referral service for patients seeking physicians who specialize in treating Paget's disease and PHPT. **Pub:** *Q+A.* Brochures. Ongoing series. • *Update*, 3/year. Newsletter. *Price:* Free. **Frmly:** (1992) Paget's Disease Foundation.

★ 5304 ★ Pain Management and Sclerotherapy
303 S Ingram Ct.
Middletown, DE 19709-7935
Phone: (302)996-0300 **Free:** 800-471-6114
Fax: (302)996-5300
Linda Pavina, Exec. Sec.

Fnded: 1938. **Mem:** 145. **Nat'l Groups:** 1. **Desc:** Dedicated to improving the practice of and disseminating knowledge about sclerotherapy. (The academy defines sclerotherapy as the stimulation of the formation of fibrous-connective tissues by the body, in a specific location, by the specific application of a sclerosing modality.) The most frequently used modality is the injection of certain medications, known as sclerosants. Primary studies involve the treatment of: unstable joints, venous abnormalities, and tendenoosseous points of hyper-irritability. Supports research program; maintains speakers' bureau. **Pub:** *Get the Point*, semiannual. Newsletter. Reports on the results of studies; evaluates differing sclerotherapeutic treatments. *Price:* Included in membership dues. • Directory, periodic. **Frmly:** (1956) American Osteopathic Academy of Sclerotherapy; (1959) American Academy of Sclerotherapy.

★ 5305 ★ Pain Society
21 Portland Pl.
London W1B 1PY, United Kingdom
Phone: 44 20 76318870 **Fax:** 44 20 73232015
Email: info@painsociety.org
Website: http://www.painsociety.org

Fnded: 1967. **Mem:** 1,400. **Desc:** Professional body representing healthcare professionals working in chronic and acute pain. Aims to relieve the suffering of pain by the promotion of education, training and research. Supplies general information and a list of pain clinics by county. **Pub:** *Pain Society Newsletter*, quarterly. Newsletter.

★ 5306 ★ Pakistan Kidney Patient Association
c/o Col. Shamim Ahmed Javed
Commercial Area Chaklala III
Rawalpindi, Pakistan
Phone: 92 51 5598789
Email: info@kidneypatients.org
Website: http://www.kidneypatients.org

Desc: Kidney patients, social workers, physicians, and other interested individuals working to provide low cost or free medical assistance to patients of kidney disease. Promotes awareness of kidney disease among the general public. Operates free clinics, laboratories and dialysis centers. **Pub:** Pamphlet, periodic.

★ 5307 ★ Pakistan Pharmacological Society
c/o Prof. S.M. Yousuf
664 Sector 46 G-9/1
Islamabad, Pakistan
Phone: 92 91 51255463

Mem: 225. **Desc:** Promotes pharmacology in Pakistan.

★ 5308 ★ Pakistan Voluntary Health and Nutrition Association (PVHNA)
9C, 18th Commercial St.
Karachi 29, Pakistan
Phone: 92 21 446709 **Fax:** 92 21 437653

Fnded: 1979. **Mem:** 30. **Lang(s):** English, Urdu. **Desc:** Seeks to improve public health in Pakistan. Promotes education in nutrition and family planning. Provides family planning organizations with training manuals. Conducts training programs in: water sanitation, child care, health care, and vocational education. Offers immunization services.

★ 5309 ★ Pan-African Association of Neurological Sciences (PAANS) (Association Pan-Africaine des Sciences Neurologiques — PAANS)
PO Box 20413
Nairobi, Kenya
Phone: 254 20 722487 **Fax:** 254 20 725776
Email: ruberti@africaonline.co.ke
Website: http://www.paans.nu.ac.za/

Fnded: 1972. **Mem:** 250. **Lang(s):** English, French. **Desc:** African neurologists specializing in neurosurgery, neuroradiology, neuropathology, neurophysiology, neurobiochemistry, and other branches of neuroscience; non-African neurologists maintaining connections with Africa. Furthers neurological sciences and encourages the exchange of ideas and information among neurologists in Africa and worldwide. Strives to acquaint the public and interested laymen with current developments in neuroscience. Conducts epidemiological research. **Pub:** *African Journal of Neurological Sciences*, semiannual. Journal. Contains information on neurology, neurosurgery, and neurosciencec. • *Pan African Association of Neurological Sciences Rules.*

★ 5310 ★ Pan-African Association of Plastic and Reconstructive Surgeons (PAPRS)
PO Box 3072-Halfway House
Johannesburg 1685, Republic of South Africa
Phone: 27 11 3101724 **Fax:** 27 11 3101861
Email: lamonta@iafrica.com

Fnded: 1996. **Mem:** 17. **State Groups:** 17. **Desc:** Encourages friendship between plastic surgeons in Africa. Seeks to improve the co-operation between the various countries on the continent and form a channel of communication with other international organizations.

★ 5311 ★ Pan American Association of Anatomy
912 Fairview Ave.
Bowling Green, OH 43402-1721
Fax: (419)383-3066
Email: baptista@paanatomy.org
Website: http://paanatomy.org
Dr. Carlos A. C. Baptista, Contact

Fnded: 1966. **Desc:** Anatomists. Seeks to stimulate the development and promotion of the Morphological Sciences on the American Continent. Facilitates scientific exchange and friendship among members. **Pub:** Newsletter.

★ 5312 ★ Pan-American League of Associations for Rhuematology (PANLAR)
c/o Dr. Abraham Garcia-Kutzbach
Clinicas Hospital Herrera Llerandi Norte
6a Avenida 7-55, Zona 10
Ala Norte 2o Piso
Guatemala City, Guatemala
Phone: 502 3343859 **Fax:** 502 3343859
Email: agarciak@ufm.edu.gt

Fnded: 1942. **Mem:** 10,000. **Reg. Groups:** 22. **Lang(s):** English, French, Portuguese, Spanish. **Desc:** Physicians and other professionals devoted to the prevention and treatment of rheumatic diseases. Seeks to educate health professionals. Conducts biomedical and epidemiological research. Offers assistance in the coordination of national, professional, and social agencies. Makes available professional publications. **Pub:** *PANLAR Bulletin*, biennial. Bulletin. **Frmly:** (2000) Pan American League Against Rhuematism.

★ 5313 ★ Pan American Sanitary Bureau
525 23rd St. NW
Washington, DC 20037
Phone: (202)974-3000 **Fax:** (202)974-3663
Website: http://www.paho.org/

Desc: Dedicated to improving and maintaining a healthy environment for people of the Americas; aims to develop a course to sustainable human development. Works as the Secretariat of the Pan American Health Organization.

★ 5314 ★ Panamanian Association for Planned Parenthood (Asociacion Panamena para el Planeamiento de la Familia — APLAFA)
Apartado Postal 4637
Panama City 5, Panama
Phone: 507 3170431 **Fax:** 507 2362979
Email: aplafa@orbi.net

Fnded: 1965. **Mem:** 100. **Reg. Groups:** 7. **Desc:** Fosters family values that include responsible parenting; educates the public about birth control options; conducts programs on health, children's concerns, and women in development.

★ 5315 ★ Pan-American Allergy Society (PAAS)
PO Box 947
Fredericksburg, TX 78624
Phone: (830)997-9853 **Fax:** (830)997-8625

Email: paas@ctesc.net
Website: http://www.paas.org
Ann Brey, Exec. Sec.

Fnded: 1956. **Mem:** 400. **Desc:** Physicians who include allergy diagnosis and management in their practice. Purpose is to serve as a forum for physicians who actively participate in the diagnosis and treatment of allergic disorders. Seeks to provide a means of social communication among members, thereby promoting interspecialty cooperation and an increase in individual excellence. Sponsors continuing medical education programs annually. **Pub:** *Pan American Allergy Society Report*, semiannual. Newsletter. • Membership Directory, biennial. **Frmly:** (1976) Gulf Coast Allergy Study Group.

★ 5316 ★ Pan-American Association of Ophthalmology (PAAO)

1301 S Bowen Rd., Ste. 365
Arlington, TX 76013
Phone: (817)265-2831 **Fax:** (817)275-3961
Email: info@paao.org
Website: http://www.paao.org
Dr. Rubens Belfort, Jr., Pres.

Fnded: 1939. **Mem:** 14,000. **Desc:** Ophthalmologists throughout the Western Hemisphere. Seeks to improve the treatment of eye diseases and prevention of blindness in the Americas through the exchange of ideas and treatments. **Pub:** *Noticiero*, quarterly. • *Pan-American Association of Ophthalmology-The Pan American*, semiannual. Newsletter. Includes obituaries and conference calendar. *Price:* Free.

★ 5317 ★ Panamerican Federation of Associations of Medical Schools (Federacion Panamericana de Asociaciones de Facultades y Escuelas de Medicina — FEPAFEM)

Apdo 60411
Caracas 1060, Venezuela
Phone: 58 212 936271 **Fax:** 58 212 936346

Fnded: 1962.

★ 5318 ★ Pan American Health Organization (PAHO)

525 23rd St. NW
Washington, DC 20037
Phone: (202)974-3000 **Fax:** (202)974-3663
Email: webmaster@paho.org
Website: http://www.paho.org
Dr. Bryna Brennan, Dir., Public Information

Fnded: 1902. **Mem:** 41. **Desc:** Governments of Western Hemisphere nations united to improve physical and mental health in the Americas. Coordinates regional activities combating disease including exchange of statistical and epidemiological information, development of local health services, and organization of disease control and eradication programs. Encourages development in health systems and technology; provides consulting services; conducts educational courses on public health topics including environmental health, food and nutrition, and tropical diseases. Has established Emergency Preparedness and Disaster Relief Coordination Program in order to increase the ability of health institutions to effectively handle emergencies. Operates the Natural Disaster Relief Voluntary Fund to support disaster relief activities. Maintains the Pan American Sanitary Bureau, the regional office for the Americas of the World Health Organization. Develops health documentaries and coordinates teleconferences. **Pub:** *Disaster Preparedness in the Americas*, quarterly. Newsletter. PAHO Emergency Preparedness and Disaster Relief Coordination Program. Covers disaster preparedness, mitigation, and management. *Price:* Free. • *EPI Newsletter*, bimonthly. Newsletter. Provides information on immunization programs in the Americas. Covers new technologies available for the execution of programs. *Price:* Distributed free to health workers. • *Epidemiological Bulletin*, bimonthly. Bulletin. Disseminates epidemiological information regarding communicable and noncommunicable diseases of public health importance. *Price:* Free. • *Health in the Americas*, quadrennial. • *Revista Panamericana de Salud Publica/Pan American Journal of Public Health*, monthly. Journal. Serves as a reference source regarding health problems in the Americas and progress made toward solutions. Includes book reviews and results. *Price:* $75/year. • Manuals. • Monographs. • Reports. • Also publishes scientific books and technical paper.

★ 5319 ★ Pan American Medical Association (PAMA)

c/o William E. Sorrel, M.D. Pres.
263 W End Ave., Ste. 1A
New York, NY 10023
William E. Sorrel, M.D., PhD, Pres.

Fnded: 1925. **Mem:** 6,000. **Nat'l Groups:** 58. **Desc:** Fosters the exchange of medical information and research results among physicians in Western Hemisphere countries. **Pub:** *Journal of the Pan American Medical Association*, biennial. Journal. *Price:* Free. For members only. **AKA:** Associacion Medica Pan Americana.

★ 5320 ★ Panamerican Society of Phlebology and Lymphology (Sociedad Panamericana de Flebologia y Linfologia)

Avellaneda 198
1642 San Isidro, Argentina
Phone: 54 11 47873606 **Fax:** 54 11 47873606
Email: cesanchez@intramed.net.ar

Fnded: 1978. **Desc:** Promotes exchange of scientific knowledge through congresses, meetings and workshops.

★ 5321 ★ Pancyprian Dental Association (PDA)

14 Thason
Rita Ct., 5th Fl.
Off. 501
Nicosia, Cyprus
Phone: 357 2 316812 **Fax:** 357 2 316937

Fnded: 1968. **Mem:** 440. **Local Groups:** 4. **Lang(s):** English, Greek. **Desc:** Dentists concerned with the dental health of the Cyprian populace. Conducts educational and public service programs. **Pub:** *Dental Tribune*, quarterly. Magazine.

★ 5322 ★ Pancyprian Veterinary Association

PO Box 25284
Nicosia 1308, Cyprus
Phone: 357 2 2420791 **Fax:** 357 2 2496625

Fnded: 1978. **Mem:** 150. **Desc:** Veterinarians working to improve animal health and welfare in Cyprus.

★ 5323 ★ Panhellenic Association of Opticians and Optometrists

49 Menadrou St., 4th Fl,
GR-10437 Athens, Greece
Phone: 30 1 5232616 **Fax:** 30 1 5232664

Fnded: 1926. **Mem:** 700. **Desc:** Opticians and optometrists. Promotes members' interests. Conducts training courses.

★ 5324 ★ Panhellenic Association of Pharmacists (PEF)

Korizi 6
Makrigianni
GR-117 43 Athens, Greece
Phone: 30 1 9227182 **Fax:** 30 1 9232964
Email: pepharm@otenet.gr

Fnded: 1929. **Mem:** 300. **Lang(s):** English, German, Greek. **Desc:** Pharmacists working in universities, hospitals, industries, marketing, national drug organizations, or in private and state jobs. Represents the interests of pharmacists. Seeks to improve the level of pharmaceutical science. Sponsors seminars. **Pub:** *Pharmakeutika Chronika*, quarterly. Magazine. Features professional and scientific articles. Also publishes abstracts of congresses and seminars.

★ 5325 ★ Papua New Guinea Veterinary Association

PO Box 741
Port Moresby, Papua New Guinea
Phone: 675 3259977 **Fax:** 675 3259310
Email: pngnaqs@dg.com.pg

Fnded: 1975. **Mem:** 10. **Desc:** Veterinarians working to improve animal health and welfare.

★ 5326 ★ Parenteral and Enteral Nutrition Society of Asia (PENSA)

4th Fl., Department of Nutrition Bldg.
Siriraj Hospital
Plannok Rd.
Bankoknoi
Bangkok 10700, Thailand
Phone: 66 2 4197740 **Fax:** 66 2 4129841
Email: secretary@pensa.org
Website: http://www.pensa.org

Fnded: 1995. **Desc:** Promotes research and development in nutritional support in Asian countries; improves the awareness of physicians of the importance of nutritional support in hospitalized patients.

★ 5327 ★ Parenteral Society

99 Ermin St.
Stratton St. Margaret
Swindon SN3 4NL, United Kingdom
Phone: 44 1793 824254 **Fax:** 44 1793 832551
Email: secretary@parenteral.demon.org.uk
Website: http://www.parenteral.org.uk

Fnded: 1981. **Mem:** 1,250. **Desc:** Fosters the advancement in the interests of public health, the practice and science of parenteral therapy and to preserve and improve the integrity and standards of the parenteral industry.

★ 5328 ★ Parents Active for Vision Education (PAVE)

4135 54th Pl.
San Diego, CA 92105-2303
Phone: (619)287-0081 **Free:** 800-PAVE-988
Fax: (619)287-0084
Email: info@pavevision.org
Website: http://www.pave-eye.com/vision

Fnded: 1988. **Local Groups:** 1. **Desc:** Parents and teachers with children in their homes and classrooms who suffer or have suffered from the effects of undiagnosed vision problems. Works to raise public awareness of learning related vision problems. Supports the development of comprehensive learning related vision screenings, vision education, and vision hygiene programs in schools and communities. Maintains speakers' bureau **Pub:** *The Hidden Disability: Undetected Vision Problems*. Pamphlet. *Price:* $23.50 100 copies, includes shipping and handling. • *Pavestones*, semiannual. Newsletter. *Price:* Free. • *Some Heroes Are Small*. Book. *Price:* $3.50 plus shipping and handling. • *Vision Alert: 20/20 is NOT Enough*. Video. *Price:* $40.

★ 5329 ★ Parents' and Carers' Association for the People With Down Syndrome

Kilinskiego str. 2
PL-90-145 Lodz, Poland
Phone: 48 42 6307348 **Fax:** 48 42 6565650
Email: mmalkusm@interia.pl

Fnded: 1990. **Mem:** 168. **Desc:** Provides support to people with Down's Syndrome, and their families.

★ 5330 ★ Parents of Galactosemic Children (PGC)

885 Del Sol St.
Sparks, NV 89436
Phone: (775)626-0885
Email: mesameadow@aol.com

Website: http://www.galactosemia.org
Evelyn A. Rice, Pres.

Fnded: 1985. **Mem:** 1,200. **Nat'l Groups:** 1. **Desc:** Parents of children born with galactosemia. (Children with galactosemia are missing an enzyme in all body cells that breaks galactose into gulcose, possibly causing jaundice, an enlarged liver, cataracts, kidney failure, and brain damage.) Works to obtain financial support for galactosemia research professionals. Offers support, educational programs, and other information to galactosemic families and interested professionals. Seeks ways for children and adults with galactosemia to live their lives to their fullest potential. **Pub:** Newsletter, semiannual.

★ 5331 ★ Parents and Professionals and Autism Northern Ireland (PAPA)

Donald House
Knockbracken Healthcare Park
Saintfield Rd.
Belfast BT8 8BH, United Kingdom
Phone: 44 28 90401729 **Fax:** 44 28 90403467
Email: info@autismni.org
Website: http://www.autismni.org

Fnded: 1989. **Mem:** 400. **Local Groups:** 14. **Lang(s):** English. **Desc:** Established by parents of autistic children and professionals that are concerned with autism in Northern Ireland. Seeks to ensure that people within the autistic spectrum and their caregivers have access to appropriate services, enabling people with autism to be valued members of their community. Provides resources, information, and advice on autism; encourages research and training; works in partnership with a range of voluntary, private, and statutory agencies; works to increase public awareness of autism. **Pub:** *Contact*, quarterly. Newsletter.

★ 5332 ★ Parents' Section of the Alexander Graham Bell Association for the Deaf (PS)

c/o Alexander Graham Bell Association for the Deaf
3417 Volta Pl. NW
Washington, DC 20007
Phone: (202)337-5220 **Fax:** (202)337-8314
Email: info@agbell.org
Website: http://www.agbell.org/sections.cfm
K. Todd Houston, Exec. Dir.

Fnded: 1958. **Mem:** 2,400. **Local Groups:** 28. **Desc:** Parents of hearing impaired children and individuals concerned with educational, social, psychological, and vocational needs of hearing impaired children. Encourages and supports parent group action and programs on behalf of hearing impaired children; works for auditory/oral teaching of children who are hearing impaired. Also publishes material concerning the problems of deaf children. **Frmly:** (1989) International Parents' Organization.

★ 5333 ★ Parents at Work (PAW)

1-3 Berry St.
London EC1V 0AA, United Kingdom
Phone: 44 20 72537243 **Fax:** 44 20 72536253
Email: info@parentsatwork.org.uk
Website: http://www.parentsatwork.org.uk

Fnded: 1985. **Mem:** 1,500. **Lang(s):** English. **Desc:** Campaign to improve quality of life for all working parents and their children. Lobbies employers and policy makers for improvement of childcare facilities. Provides working parents with childcare information. **Pub:** *Balanced Lives*, quarterly. Newsletter. • *Waving Not Drowning.* Newsletter. Features information for parents of disabled children who work or want to work. **Frmly:** (1994) Working Mothers Association.

★ 5334 ★ Parker Chiropractic Resource Foundation (PCRF)

2500 Walnut Hill Ln.
Dallas, TX 75229-5609
Chance Parker, Pres.

Fnded: 1951. **Mem:** 30,000. **Desc:** Doctors of chiropractic. Seeks to keep the chiropractic profession abreast of new developments, practices, and procedures concerning the administration of health care. **Pub:** *Share*, monthly. Magazine. **Frmly:** (1987) Parker Chiropractic Research Foundation.

★ 5335 ★ Parkinson Society of Canada (Societe Parkinson Canada)

4211 Yonge St., Ste. 316
Toronto, ON, Canada M2P 2A9
Phone: (416)227-9700 **Free:** 800-565-3000
Fax: (416)227-9600
Email: general.info@parkinson.ca
Website: http://www.parkinson.ca

Fnded: 1965. **Mem:** 16,000. **Reg. Groups:** 5. **Local Groups:** 100. **Lang(s):** English, French. **Desc:** Provides services to people with Parkinson's or related disorders, their families, and interested health care professionals. Seeks to publicize the nature and availability of treatment and assistance programs available to people with Parkinson's. Promotes research into the cause and cure of Parkinson's. Conducts fundraising activities; maintains support groups; makes available referral services. Sponsors research and educational programs. **Pub:** *Parkinson Post*, quarterly. Magazine. Current information on Parkinson's and Parkinson Society of Canada.

★ 5336 ★ Parkinson's Association of Ireland

Carmichael Centre
N Brunswick St.
Dublin, Ireland
Phone: 353 1 8722234 **Fax:** 353 1 8735737

Lang(s): English. **Desc:** Seeks to provide comfort and assistance to those living with Parkinson's Disease in Ireland.

★ 5337 ★ Parkinson's Disease Foundation (PDF)

710 West 168th St.
3rd Fl.
New York, NY 10032
Phone: (212)923-4700 **Free:** 800-457-6676
Fax: (212)923-4778
Email: info@pdf.org
Website: http://www.pdf.org/
Dr. Lewis P. Rowland, Pres.

Fnded: 1957. **Mem:** 95,000. **Local Groups:** 500. **Desc:** Raises funds for support of scientific research into causes, prevention, and cure of Parkinson's disease. Supports its own laboratories for research in Parkinsonism. Prepares and distributes information on patient care and rehabilitation including list of clinics where treatment is available, and a list of patient selfhelp groups. Supports a brain bank to permit anatomical and chemical studies. Sponsors scientific symposia. Offers patient and family counseling and advocacy services. Maintains research advisory board. Sponsors summer fellowship program for medical students and undergraduate. **Pub:** *Exercises for the Parkinson Patient and Hints for Daily Living.* • *Health Care Manual for the Professional Team. Price:* $10. • *Information Packet.* Booklets. *Price:* Free. • *PDF Newsletter*, 3-4/year. Newsletter. Covers developments in Parkinson's disease research, hints for daily living, and advice to health care professionals. Includes case studies. *Price:* Free. • *Progress, Promise, and Hope: The Parkinson Patient at Home.* • Brochures. **Frmly:** (1999) United Parkinson Foundation.

★ 5338 ★ Parkinson's Disease Society of the United Kingdom

215 Vauxhall Bridge Rd.
London SV1W 1EJ, United Kingdom
Phone: 44 20 79318080 **Fax:** 44 20 72339908
Email: enquiries@parkinsons.org.uk
Website: http://www.parkinsons.org.uk

Fnded: 1969. **Mem:** 27,000. **Reg. Groups:** 288. **Local Groups:** 250. **Desc:** Promotes awareness of Parkinson's disease.

★ 5339 ★ Partially Sighted Society (PSS)

9 Plato Pl.
72-74 St. Dionis Rd.
London SW6 4TU, United Kingdom
Phone: 44 1302 323132 **Fax:** 44 171 3170289

Fnded: 1973. **Mem:** 2,000. **Local Groups:** 20. **Desc:** Strives to improve social, medical, and domestic services available to the visually impaired in the United Kingdom and to increase educational and employment opportunities. Offers information and advice; provides visual aids and special printing and enlargement services. Operates 3 sight centers that offer vision assessment and training services. Arranges conferences, exhibitions, and displays. **Pub:** *Oculus*, quarterly. Newsletter. In large print. • Brochures, periodic. • Catalog, periodic.

★ 5340 ★ Partnership for a Drug Free America (DFA)

405 Lexington Ave., Ste. 1601
New York, NY 10174
Phone: (212)922-1560 **Free:** 888-575-3115
Fax: (212)922-1570
Email: bob_caruso@drugfree.org
Website: http://www.drugfreeamerica.org
Bob Caruso, Contact

Fnded: 1986. **Mem:** 2,500. **Desc:** A coalition of individuals and organizations representing the advertising, production, and communications industries. Seeks to utilize the creative skills of members to change social attitudes towards illegal drugs. Believes that drug abuse is a major crisis affecting American families and work environments. Works to evoke a social revulsion to what the group views as current public acceptance and complacency toward illegal drugs. Focuses on advertising strategies that will "unsell" illegal drugs, "de-normalize" drug usage in the U.S., and reinforce positive factors of life without drugs. Creates advertising campaigns targeted toward preteens, teenagers, young adults, and "influencers" (peers, parents, health care professionals, teachers, and opinion leaders). Is currently running media anti-drug advertisements, including an advertisement depicting an egg being fried as an analogy to the effects of drugs on the human brain. Conducts research evaluation program to assess attitudinal changes of targeted groups toward illegal drugs, monitor usage trends, and evaluate the effectiveness of these advertisments. **Pub:** *Partnership for a Drug-Free America Newsletter*, quarterly. Newsletter. • Bulletin, periodic. **Frmly:** (1990) Media-Advertising Partnership for a Drug-Free America.

★ 5341 ★ Partnership for Patient Safety (P4PS)

c/o Martin Hatlie
1 W Superior St., Ste. 2410
Chicago, IL 60610
Phone: (312)274-9695 **Fax:** (312)274-9696
Email: info@p4ps.com
Website: http://www.p4ps.org
Martin Hatlie, Pres.

Fnded: 2000. **Desc:** People and organizations involved in health care. Dedicated to reducing the harm caused by healthcare errors.

★ 5342 ★ Pathfinder International (PI)

9 Galen St., Ste. 217
Watertown, MA 02472
Phone: (617)924-7200 **Fax:** (617)924-3833
Email: information@pathfind.org
Website: http://www.pathfind.org
Frances K. Moseley, VP Resource Development

Fnded: 1957. **Desc:** Established to find, demonstrate, and promote new and more efficient family planning programs in developing countries. Objectives are to introduce and expand the availability of effective family planning services; improve the welfare of families in developing countries; assist developing countries in implementing population policies favorable to national development. Conducts activities with a concern for upholding human rights, enhancing the status and role of women, and respecting the views of family planning clients. **Pub:** *Pathways*, semiannual. Newsletter. Provides information on programs and updates on services. • Annual Report, annual. **AKA:** PF.

★ 5343 ★ Pathfinder International - Brazil (PI)

Praca 15 de Novembro, 13
Edificio Bouzas Salas 202/207
Terrerio de Jesus- Centro
40025-010 Salvador, Bahia, Brazil
Phone: 55 71 3210791
Email: claudari@pathfind.org
Website: http://www.pathfind.org

Lang(s): Portuguese, Spanish. **Desc:** Makes available low- and no-cost family planning services to the needy. Promotes population control through educational programs involving youth; trains indigenous people to sustain family planning services in their local areas.

★ 5344 ★ Pathological Society of Great Britain and Ireland

2 Carlton House Terrace
London SW1Y 5AF, United Kingdom
Phone: 44 20 79761260 **Fax:** 44 20 79761267
Email: administrator@pathsoc.org.uk
Website: http://www.pathsoc.org.uk

Fnded: 1906. **Mem:** 1,100. **Desc:** Those engaged in research or teaching in connection with pathology or allied science. Holds one scientific meetings each year. **Pub:** *Journal of Pathology*, monthly. Journal.

★ 5345 ★ Patient Advocates for Advanced Cancer Treatment (PAACT)

1143 Parmelee NW
PO Box 141695
Grand Rapids, MI 49504
Phone: (616)453-1477 **Fax:** (616)453-1846
Email: paact@paactusa.org
Website: http://www.paactusa.org

Fnded: 1984. **Mem:** 36,000. **Desc:** Prostate cancer patients and physicians. Engages in advocacy activities. Provides educational materials to those with prostate cancer. Conducts protocol studies and research. **Pub:** *Cancer Communication*, quarterly. Newsletter. • *Prostate Cancer Report*. Report.

★ 5346 ★ Paws With a Cause (PWC)

4646 S Division
Wayland, MI 49348
Phone: (616)877-7297 **Free:** 800-253-PAWS
Fax: (616)877-0248
Email: paws@ionline.com
Website: http://www.pawswithacause.org
A.J. Springstead Sapp, CEO

Fnded: 1979. **Mem:** 526. **Nat'l Groups:** 38. **Reg. Groups:** 2. **Desc:** Trains Assistance Dogs nationally for people with disabilities and provides lifetime team support which encourages independence. Promotes awareness through education. **Pub:** *Dogs for Dignity*, quarterly. Newsletter. *Price:* included in membership dues. • *The Story of Trapper*. Book. A children's story about the life of a service dog who changes the life of a family. **Frmly:** (1988) Ears for the Deaf.

★ 5347 ★ Pax Natura Society for Rehabilitation of the Deaf (PNSRD)

11460 60th Ave. NW
Edmonton, AB, Canada T6H 1J5
Phone: (780)435-7788 **Fax:** (780)435-7788

Fnded: 1975. **Mem:** 100. **Lang(s):** English, French. **Desc:** Individuals working to rehabilitate people with hearing impairment. Seeks to insure availability of social and health care services to people with hearing impairment throughout Canada. Sponsors supported living, educational, and rehabilitative services to people with impaired hearing. Conducts training programs for health care and social workers treating people with hearing impairments. Maintains summer camp and family retreat programs; undertakes fundraising activities. **Pub:** Annual Report, annual.

★ 5348 ★ Pediatric/Adolescent Gastroesophageal Reflux Association (PAGER)

PO Box 1153
Germantown, MD 20875-1153
Phone: (301)601-9541
Email: gergroup@aol.com
Website: http://www.reflux.org
Beth Anderson, Exec. Dir.

Fnded: 1992. **Mem:** 2,000. **Desc:** Provides information and support to parents, patients and doctors about Gastroesophageal Reflux. **Pub:** *Reflux Digest*, quarterly. Newsletter. Included research updates, practical information, family stories. *Price:* included in membership dues.

★ 5349 ★ Pediatric AIDS Foundation

2950 31st St., No. 125
Santa Monica, CA 90405
Phone: (310)314-1459 **Free:** 888-499-HOPE
Fax: (310)314-1469
Email: info@pedAIDS.org
Website: http://www.pedaids.org
Kate Carr, CEO & Pres.

Fnded: 1988. **Desc:** Confronts medical problems unique to children infected with HIV/AIDS, and focuses on finding medical answers that will bring hope. Identifies and funds critically needed pediatric AIDS research worldwide. Provides funds to hospitals around the country which serve children with HIV/AIDS through an Emergency Assistance Program. Encourages students to enter the field of pediatric AIDS through a Student Intern Award Program. Develops and distributes national Parent Education Program for parents of elementary and pre-school age children. **Pub:** Annual Report.

★ 5350 ★ Pediatric Brain Tumor Foundation of the United States (PBTFUS)

302 Ridgefield Ct.
Asheville, NC 28806
Phone: (828)665-6891 **Free:** 800-253-6530
Fax: (828)665-6894
Email: pbtfus@pbtfus.org
Website: http://www.pbtfus.org
Mike Traynor, Pres.

Fnded: 1991. **Desc:** Seeks to find the cause and cure of brain tumors in children. Supports medical research; promotes public awareness of the disease; aids in early detection and treatment of childhood brain tumors. **Pub:** *International Neuro-Oncology Journal*. Journal.

★ 5351 ★ Pediatric Digestion and Motility Disorders Society (PEDS)

PO Box 1360
Buffalo, NY 14203-1360
Phone: (716)852-2857
Email: pedskids@aol.com
Website: http://www.pedsgi.org

Desc: Volunteers. Work towards finding cures. Host events to fund research. Promote public awareness.

★ 5352 ★ Pediatric Endocrinology Nursing Society (PENS)

PO Box 2933
Gaithersburg, MD 20886-2933
Website: http://www.pens.org

Fnded: 1986. **Mem:** 325. **Desc:** Pediatric endocrine nurses. Promotes professional responsibility, accountability, ethics and respect; dedicated to the advancement of the art and science of pediatric endocrine nursing; establishes and maintains standards of practice; enhances nursing research, clinical expertise and recognition of excellence in nursing. **Pub:** *PENS Manual*. Manual. Contains individual chapters authored by nurses in the field of pediatric endocrinology. • *PENS Reporter*, quarterly. Newsletter. Includes society news, committee reports, deadlines, articles with focus on endocrine disorders and nursing research, lay organization information. *Price:* included in membership dues.

★ 5353 ★ Pediatric Orthopaedic Society of North America (POSNA)

6300 N River Rd., Ste. 727
Rosemont, IL 60018-4226
Phone: (847)698-1692 **Fax:** (847)823-0536
Email: goldberg@aaos.org
Website: http://www.posna.org
Sharon Goldberg, Exec. Dir.

Fnded: 1983. **Mem:** 800. **Desc:** Pediatric orthopedic surgeons. Purpose is to provide continuing education to members. Conducts tutorial programs. **Pub:** *Newsletter*, quarterly. Bulletin. *Price:* available to members only. • Membership Directory, annual.

★ 5354 ★ Pediatric Pharmacy Advocacy Group (PPAG)

9866 W Victoria Dr.
Littleton, CO 80128
Phone: (720)981-7356 **Fax:** (720)981-7357
Email: hankw@ppag.org
Website: http://www.ppag.org

Desc: Dedicated to safe and effective medication use to improve the lives of children by being a primary resource for drug therapy.

★ 5355 ★ People Against Cancer (PAC)

604 East St.
PO Box 10
Otho, IA 50569-0010
Phone: (515)972-4444 **Fax:** (515)972-4415
Email: info@peopleagainstcancer.com
Website: http://www.peopleagainstcancer.com
Frank D. Wiewel, Contact

Fnded: 1985. **Mem:** 2,000. **Desc:** Promotes research into alternative cancer therapy and prevention. Conducts educational, charitable, and research programs. **Pub:** *Options*, quarterly. Newsletter. • Bulletin. • Directory.

★ 5356 ★ People Against Impaired Driving (PAID)

c/o Kevin Catholic Jr/Sr High School
No. 107, 10005-84 St.
Edmonton, AB, Canada T5J 0H1
Phone: (403)462-2426 **Fax:** (403)462-2596

Fnded: 1982. **Mem:** 300. **Lang(s):** English, French. **Desc:** Volunteers opposed to impaired driving. Seeks to erradicate drunken and impaired driving; works to strengthen impaired driving statutes and improve their enforcement. Provides support and services to victims of impaired drivers and their families. Lobbies government agencies for more punitive measures against repeat impaired driving offenders. Conducts educational campaigns to raise public awareness of impaired driving and its effects; maintains speakers' bureau. **Pub:** *People Against Impaired Driving*. Brochure. • Newsletter, periodic.

★ 5357 ★ People-Animals-Love (PAL)

3201 New Mexico Ave. NW, Ste. 350
Washington, DC 20016
Phone: (202)895-1395 **Fax:** (202)274-1995
Email: palemail@aol.com
Website: http://www.peopleanimalslove.com
Susan L. Wellman, Exec. Dir.

Fnded: 1981. **Desc:** Purpose is to improve the quality of life of the elderly, the widowed, and the institutionalized by providing them with visits from pets and trained volunteers. Has initiated programs in nursing homes, prisons, hospices, and hospitals. Preliminary studies suggest that: pets may positively affect a person's blood pressure and general well-being; prisoners with pets often require less disciplinary action and medical attention; pets help lessen loneliness, hopelessness, and boredom; and that animals may be used effectively to reach at-risk children. Conducts summer P.A.L. camp to acquaint urban children with animals. Also visits inner city schools with farm animal program. Conducts P.A.L. Club, an after-school program targeting at-risk youth. **Pub:** *PAL Newsletter*, quarterly. Newsletter. • Brochure.

★ 5358 ★ People-to-People Health Foundation (HOPE)

Project HOPE Health Sciences
Educ. Center
225 Carter Hall Ln.
Millwood, VA 22646
Phone: (540)837-2100 **Free:** 800-544-HOPE
Fax: (540)837-1813
Email: webmaster@projecthope.org
Website: http://www.projecthope.org
Dr. John Howe, Pres. &CEO

Fnded: 1958. **Desc:** Promotes better world health and understanding through the training of medical, nursing, dental, and allied health personnel in developing areas of the world. Operates the Center for Health Affairs, which provides research and policy analysis to help develop solutions to problems in worldwide health systems. Develops programs which include the use of volunteer doctors, nurses, and allied health professionals to teach modern techniques in health sciences education, health services delivery systems, health facilities management, and health-related humanitarian assistance. Programs are currently operating in 37 countries, located in Africa, Asia, Eastern Europe, and North, Central, and South America. **Pub:** *Health Affairs*, quarterly. Journal. Covers domestic and international health policies; annual and five-year indexes available. *Price:* $45/year for individuals; $75/year for institutions. • *HOPE News*, quarterly. Newsletter. Covers Project HOPE's international and domestic programs. Includes calendar of events and news of fundraising activities. *Price:* Free. • Annual Report. **AKA:** Project HOPE.

★ 5359 ★ People's Medical Society (PMS)

PO Box 868
Allentown, PA 18105
Phone: (610)770-1670 **Free:** 800-624-8773
Fax: (610)770-0607
Email: mad1@peoplesmed.org
Website: http://www.peoplesmed.org
Pamela Maraldo, Chair

Fnded: 1982. **Mem:** 80,000. **Desc:** Promotes citizen involvement in the cost, quality, and management of the American health care system. Seeks to: train and encourage individuals to study local health care systems, practitioners, and institutions and promote preventive health care and medical cost control by these groups; address major policy issues and control health costs; encourage more preventive practice and research; promote self-care and alternative health care procedures; launch an information campaign to assist individuals in maintaining personal health and to prepare them for appointments with medical professionals. **Pub:** *Allergies: Questions You Have...Answers You Need.* • *Alzheimer's and Dementia: Questions You Have...Answers You Need.* • *Arthritis: Questions You Have, Answers You Need.* • *Asthma: Questions You Have, Answers You Need.* • *Breathe Better, Feel Better.* • *The Consumer's Medical Desk Reference.* • *Depression: Questions You Have, Answers You Need.* • *Headaches: 47 Ways to Stop the Pain.* • *Hearing Loss: Questions, You Have, Answers You Need.* • *Long-Term Care and Alternatives.* • *Medicare Made Easy.* • *Medicine on Trial.* • *Misdiagnosis: Woman as a Disease.* • *Natural Recipes for the Good Life.* • *150 Ways to Be a Savvy Medical Consumer.* • *People's Medical Society Newsletter*, bimonthly. Newsletter. Includes membership activities information. *Price:* Included in membership dues. • *Prostate: Questions You Have...Answers You Need.* • *77 Ways to Beat Colds and Flu.* • *So You're Going to be a Mother.* • *Tai Chi Made Easy.* • *Take This Book to the Gynecologist With You.* • *Take This Book to the Hospital With You.* • *28 Days to a Better Body.* • *Vitamins & Minerals: Questions You Have, Answers You Need.* • *Your Complete Medical Record.* • Bibliographies. • Bulletins.

★ 5360 ★ Perceptions, Inc. (PI)

1400 Broadway 5th Fl.
New York, NY 10018
Phone: (212)944-7717 **Fax:** (212)719-5609
Website: http://www.perceptions-inc.com/
Rene Nieva, Pres.

Fnded: 1978. **Desc:** Parents, professionals, schools, and libraries are subscribers. Publishes a newsletter that serves as an information source for parents wishing to develop expertise in meeting the educational, social, and emotional needs of their learning-disabled children. Holds seminars and workshops for parents and professionals. Maintains speakers' bureau. **Pub:** *Annual Index*. Directory. • Manual.Provides instructions on clothing and grooming.

★ 5361 ★ Perinatal Society of New Zealand (PSNZ)

c/o Women & Children's Health
Waikato Hospital
Private Bag 3200
Hamilton, New Zealand
Phone: 64 7 8398860 **Fax:** 64 7 8398724
Email: harrisde@walkatodhb.govt.nz

Fnded: 1979. **Mem:** 120. **Local Groups:** 12. **Lang(s):** English. **Desc:** Pediatricians, obstetricians, neo-natal and obstetric nurses, scientists, dietitians, radiologists, physiotherapists and other paediatric specialists and midwives in New Zealand. Aims to foster continued improvement in the standards of perinatal medicine and nursing. Works to increase public understanding of the activities in and the objectives of perinatology. Sponsors continuing education programs in perinatology. Promotes collaboration and open discussion among members. **Frmly:** (1990) New Zealand Perinatal Society.

★ 5362 ★ Periodic Paralysis Association (PPA)

1024 Royal Oaks Dr., Ste. 620
Monrovia, CA 91016
Phone: (626)303-3244 **Fax:** (626)337-1966
Email: info@periodicparalysis.org
Website: http://www.periodicparalysis.org
Patrick E. Cochran, Pres.

Fnded: 1997. **Desc:** Offers information, support to those inflicted with periodic paralysis and brings awareness to the public of this disorder.

★ 5363 ★ Peruvian Heart Association (PHA)

100 S Greenleaf Ave.
Gurnee, IL 60031-3378
Phone: (847)249-2111 **Free:** 800-367-7378
Fax: (847)249-2772
Email: milalatin@aol.com
Luis Vasquez, MD, Intl. Dir.

Fnded: 1967. **Mem:** 400. **Reg. Groups:** 6. **Desc:** Peruvian physicians, nurses, and other health care professionals specializing in cardiology who are devoted to research, training, teaching, and patient care. Offers continuing education courses for Peruvian physicians, enabling them to fulfill coursework required by Peruvian law for continuance of medical practice. Provides community health care information to residents of Lima, Peru concerning heart attacks, high blood pressure, cholesterol, diabetes, diet, and exercise. Conducts programs in conjunction with the American College of Cardiology and the American Heart Association, providing printed information and speakers on health care. Also provides information to U.S. doctors who wish to study and assist with Peruvian health care.

★ 5364 ★ Pharmaceutical Group of the European Union

159, rue Belliard
B-1040 Brussels, Belgium
Phone: 32 2 2380818 **Fax:** 32 2 2380819
Email: pharmacy@pgeu.org
Website: http://www.pgeu.org

Fnded: 1959. **Mem:** 25. **Lang(s):** English, French. **Desc:** International association representing community pharmacists. **Pub:** *Annual Reports*, annual. **Frmly:** Pharmaceutical Group of the European Community.

★ 5365 ★ Pharmaceutical Society of Denmark (Danmarks Farmaceutiske Selskab)

Universitetsparken 2
DK-2100 Copenhagen, Denmark
Phone: 45 31370850

Fnded: 1912.

★ 5366 ★ Pharmaceutical Society of Ghana (PSGh)

PO Box 2133
Accra, Ghana
Phone: 233 21 228341 **Fax:** 233 21 239583
Email: psgh@ighmail.com

Fnded: 1935. **Mem:** 1,200. **Lang(s):** English. **Desc:** Registered pharmacists in Ghana. Promotes and protects pharmacy and pharmacists and safeguards the interests and concerns of government and the public regarding pharmaceutical and related affairs. Encourages and regulates the education and training of pharmacists. **Pub:** *Ghana Pharmaceutical Journal*. Journal.

★ 5367 ★ Pharmaceutical Society of Japan (Nippon Yakugaku-Kai)

12-15, Shibuya 2-chome, Shibuya-ku
Tokyo, Japan
Phone: 81 3 34063321 **Fax:** 81 3 3481835
Email: koho_win@pharm.or.jp

Fnded: 1899.

★ 5368 ★ Pharmaceutical Society of Northern Ireland

73 University St.
Belfast BT7 1HL, United Kingdom
Phone: 44 2890 326927 **Fax:** 44 2890 439919
Email: chief.exec@psni.org.uk

Fnded: 1925. **Mem:** 1,707. **Desc:** Registered pharmacists. Acts as a professional and registration body for pharmacists and pharmacies in Northern Ireland.

★ 5369 ★ Pharmaceutical Society of Singapore (PSS)

Alumni Medical Centre
2 College Rd.
Singapore 169850, Singapore
Phone: 65 62211136 **Fax:** 65 62230969
Email: admin@pss.org.sg

Fnded: 1967. **Mem:** 1,026. **Lang(s):** English. **Desc:** Seeks to maximize the contribution of pharmacists to health care by enforcing a code of ethics, cooperating with other organizations, and providing educational programs. Sponsors competitions. **Pub:** *Singapore Pharmaceutical Bulletin*, quarterly. Bulletin. **Frmly:** (1967) Malayan Pharmaceutical Association.

★ 5370 ★ Pharmaceutical Society of South Africa (PSSA)

26 Juta St.
PO Box 31360
Braamfontein 2017, Republic of South Africa
Phone: 27 11 4423601 **Fax:** 27 11 4423601

Fnded: 1946. **Mem:** 5,500. **Lang(s):** Afrikaans, English. **Desc:** Registered pharmacists. Promotes high standards of ethics and practice in pharmacy. Conducts continuing professional education courses; facilitates communication among members; maintains museum. **Pub:** *South Africa Pharmaceutical Journal*, monthly. Journal.

★ 5371 ★ Pharmacological Society of Canada (PSC) (Societe de Pharmacologie du Canada — SPC)

Department of Physiology & Pharmacology
M223 Medical Sciences Bldg.
University of Western Ontario
London, ON, Canada N6A 5C1
Email: jane.rylett@med.uwo.ca
Website: http://www.physpharm.med.uwo.ca/psc/

Fnded: 1974. **Mem:** 300. **Desc:** Promotes research and education in pharmacology.

★ 5372 ★ Pharmacological Society of Canada (PSC) (Societe de Pharmacologie du Canada)

c/o Dr. Jana Sawynok, Pres.
Department of Pharmacology
Sir Charles Tupper Medical Bldg.
Dalhousie University
Halifax, NS, Canada B3H 4H7
Phone: (902)494-2596 **Fax:** (902)494-1388
Email: jana.sawynok@dal.ca
Website: http://www.pharmtox.med.uwo.ca/psc/

Mem: 326. **Desc:** Promotes pharmacology in Canada.

★ 5373 ★ Pharmacological Society in Taiwan

c/o Dr. Mao-Hsiung Yen
Department of Pharmacology
National Defense Medical Center
PO Box 90048-504, Neihu
Taipei 114, Taiwan
Phone: 886 2 87921704 **Fax:** 886 2 87921704
Email: mhyen@ndmctsgh.edu.tw

Mem: 270. **Desc:** Promotes pharmacology in Taiwan.

★ 5374 ★ Pharmacological and Therapeutic Society of Thailand

c/o Prof. S. Chompootaweep
Department of Pharmacology
Faculty of Medicine
Chulalongkorn University
Bangkok 10330, Thailand
Phone: 66 2 2511965 **Fax:** 66 2 2524963
Email: fmedsch@md2.md.chula.ac.th

Mem: 340. **Desc:** Promotes pharmacology in Thailand.

★ 5375 ★ Phi Alpha Sigma

313 S 10th St.
Philadelphia, PA 19107
Phone: (215)625-2650
Email: jrj002@jefferson.edu
Website: http://www.phialphasigma.org
Dr. Thomas Griffin, Pres.

Fnded: 1886. **Mem:** 120. **Nat'l Groups:** 1. **Reg. Groups:** 1. **State Groups:** 1. **Local Groups:** 1. **Desc:** Professional fraternity - medicine. **Pub:** *Bubbling Rales*, annual. Newsletter. *Price:* Free to alumni.

★ 5376 ★ Phi Chi Medical Fraternity (PCMF)

2039 Ridgeview Dr.
Floyds Knobs, IN 47119
Phone: (812)948-0581 **Free:** 800-800-7442
Fax: (812)941-8850
Email: phichi@phi-chi.org
Website: http://www.phi-chi.org
Daniel H. Cannon, MD, Chm., Exec. Trustees

Fnded: 1889. **Mem:** 40,818. **Local Groups:** 12. **Desc:** Professional fraternity - medicine. Maintains Phi Chi Welfare Association, which accepts voluntary contributions to a student loan fund and other services. **Pub:** *Constitution and Statutes.* • *Officers' Manual.* Manual. • *PC Chronicles*, semiannual. Magazine. Provides chapter news and information. *Price:* Included in membership dues. • *Phi Chi Directory.* Directory. • *Phi Chi History, 1889-1989.* • *Phi Chi Songs.* **Frmly:** (1989) Phi Chi.

★ 5377 ★ Phi Delta Epsilon Medical Fraternity

2228 E Solano Dr.
Phoenix, AZ 85016
Free: 800-347-3713 **Fax:** (602)956-3983
Email: phide@phide.org
Website: http://www.phide.org
George Craft, MD, Exec. Dir.

Fnded: 1904. **Mem:** 25,000. **Local Groups:** 41. **Desc:** Professional fraternity - medicine. **Pub:** *Phi Delta Epsilon News and Scientific Journal*, quarterly. Journal.

★ 5378 ★ Phi Lambda Kappa Medical Fraternity

3060 Bristol Rd., No. 239
Bensalem, PA 19020
Phone: (215)741-3978
Eleanor G. Halprin, Exec. Sec.

Fnded: 1907. **Mem:** 4,800. **Reg. Groups:** 17. **Local Groups:** 20. **Desc:** Professional fraternity - medicine. **Pub:** *Quarterly.*

★ 5379 ★ Phi Rho Sigma Medical Society

PO Box 90264
Indianapolis, IN 46290
Phone: (317)334-8720 **Fax:** (317)334-8721
Email: hrodenbe@iupui.edu
Harriet Rodenberg, Central Office Admin.

Fnded: 1890. **Mem:** 31,260. **Reg. Groups:** 13. **State Groups:** 12. **Desc:** Professional society - medicine. **Pub:** *Journal of Phi Rho Sigma*, quarterly. Journal. *Price:* Free. For members only.

★ 5380 ★ Phi Zeta

c/o Dr. Robert McClure
University of Missouri
Department of Veterinary Biomedical Sciences
101 Bingham Rd.
Columbia, MO 65203-3577
Phone: (314)449-4497
Email: mcclurerc@hotmail.com
Robert McClure, Sec. -Treas.

Fnded: 1925. **Local Groups:** 27. **Desc:** Honor society for veterinary medicine.

★ 5381 ★ Philippine Association of Gerontology

4th St. BBB Marulas
Valenzuela City, Philippines
Phone: 63 2 2916801 **Fax:** 63 2 29167113
Email: fgc@pacific.net.ph
Website: http://www.sfu.ca/iag/

Fnded: 1999. **Mem:** 65. **Nat'l Groups:** 1. **Lang(s):** English, Tagalog. **Desc:** Seeks to improve the welfare of senior citizens. Supports and encourages research in gerontology. Fosters communication and exchange of knowledge and experiences among members. **Pub:** Magazine. • Newsletter.

★ 5382 ★ Philippine Diabetes Association (PDA)

Unit 25, Facilities Center
548 Shaw Blvd.
Mandaluyong City 1501, Philippines
Phone: 531 1278 **Fax:** 531 1278
Email: secretariat@diabetesphil.org
Website: http://www.diabetesphil.org

Desc: Aims to improve quality of life for people with diabetes. Seeks to eliminate occurrence of diabetes in the Philippines.

★ 5383 ★ Philippine National AIDS Council

3F, Bldg. 12, Department of Health
Sta. Cruz
Manila, Philippines
Phone: 63 2 7430512 **Fax:** 63 2 7430512
Email: naspcp@doh.gov.ph
Website: http://www.doh.gov.ph/aids/

Fnded: 1988. **Reg. Groups:** 16. **Lang(s):** English. **Desc:** Provides AIDS information and education; offers AIDS counseling training. Implements programs for the management and care of HIV-infected individuals and persons with AIDS. Conducts research; compiles statistics. Maintains speakers' bureau; serves as a clearinghouse on AIDS and other sexually transmitted diseases; provides laboratory services. **Pub:** *Monthly Update*, quarterly. Newsletter. **Frmly:** (1998) National AIDS/STD Prevention and Control Program.

★ 5384 ★ Philippine Society of Anesthesiologists (PSA)

PMA Bldg.
North Ave., Rm. 102
Diliman
Quezon City, Metro Manila 1000, Philippines
Phone: 63 2 9295852
Email: psa@i-manila.com.ph
Website: http://www.psa-ph.org/

Desc: Anesthesiologists committed to safe and quality anesthesia care. Provides education programs.

★ 5385 ★ Philippine Society of Experimental and Clinical Pharmacology

c/o Dr. Cleotilde H. How
Department of Pharmacology
College of Medicine
University of the Philippines Manila
547 Pedro Gil St.
Manila 1000, Philippines
Phone: 63 2 5264248 **Fax:** 63 2 5218251
Email: pharmafaculty@hotmail.com

Mem: 202. **Desc:** Promotes experimental and clinical pharmacology in the Philippines.

★ 5386 ★ Philippine Urological Association (PUA)

PCS Bldg., 3rd Fl.
992 EDSA
Quezon City, Metro Manila 1105, Philippines
Fax: 63 2 9295501
Email: info@puanet.org
Website: http://www.puanet.org/

Fnded: 1957. **Mem:** 179. **Desc:** Promotes advancement of the art and science of urology in the Philippines.

★ 5387 ★ Phlebology Society of America (PSA)

c/o Denise M. Rossignol, Exec. Dir.
5 Daremy Ct.
Nesconset, NY 11767-1547
Phone: (631)366-1429 **Fax:** (631)366-3609
Email: denisemrossignol@cs.com
Dr. John B. Chang, Bd. Chm.

Fnded: 1962. **Mem:** 300. **Desc:** Physicians and scientists with an interest in phlebitis and other diseases of the vascular system. Seeks to advance the diagnosis and treatment of peripheral vascular disease. Serves as a certifying board for professional phlebologists; functions as a clearinghouse on phlebology; facilitates exchange of information among members. Conducts educational programs. **Pub:** *International Journal of Angiology*, quarterly. Journal.

★ 5388 ★ Phoenix House of New York

164 W 74th St.
New York, NY 10023
Phone: (212)595-5810 **Fax:** (212)496-6035
Email: phcomm@phoenixhouse.org

Website: http://www.phoenixhouse.org
Mitchell S. Rosenthal, MD, Pres.

Fnded: 1967. **Mem:** 760. **Desc:** Provides drug abuse treatment, vocational and educational services through individual, group and family counseling, and self help rehabilitation programs. Operates 20 facilities for adolescents and adults in New York, New Jersey and California and Texas. Operates extensive range of drug-free treatment programs including: Phoenix Academy (Board of Education certified, residential high school for adolescents); Step One (Board of Education certified day-school); IMPACT (outpatient intervention for teenagers and their parents); long-term residential treatment for adults; short-term outpatient and in-patient adult drug treatment. Also operates programs geared to specific populations, such as PORTAL program for homeless mothers and their children living in shelter accommodation; prison-based and community aftercare programs for male and female criminal offenders. Phoenix House Drug Education and Prevention Unit conducts adult and adolescent drug education workshops in public and private schools, corporations and other workplaces. **Pub:** *Phoenix House News*, quarterly. Newsletter. *Price:* Free. • Brochures. • Newsletter, quarterly. • Pamphlets. • Annual Report. **Frmly:** (2000) Phoenix House Foundation.

★ 5389 ★ Phoenix Society for Burn Survivors (PSBS)

2153 Wealthy St. SE, No. 215
East Grand Rapids, MI 49506
Phone: (616)458-2773 **Free:** 800-888-2876
Fax: (616)458-2831
Email: info@phoenix-society.org
Website: http://www.phoenix-society.org
Amy Acton, RN, Exec. Dir.

Fnded: 1977. **Mem:** 7,500. **Local Groups:** 340. **Desc:** Selfhelp service organization for burn survivors and their families. Works to ease the psychosocial adjustment of severely burned and disfigured persons during and after hospitalization so they may return to normal and satisfactory lives within their communities. Former burn survivors work as volunteers on a one-to-one basis with other burn survivors and their families. Offers a training program for volunteers; seeks to educate the public about the nature and problems of disfigurement; discourages concealment of disfigurement, which the society believes compounds the difficulty of adjustment; conducts research on psychological ramifications of burn disfigurement and disseminates information on burns and trauma and their treatment. Conducts school programs for burned children returning to classes. Maintains speakers' bureau and contains books on burn recovery, films, and videocassettes. **Pub:** *Audiovisual Materials on Burns, Disfigurement, and Related Subjects*, annual. List of audiovisual materials; includes educational and inspirational materials on coping with burns and disfigurement. *Price:* $10. • *Bibliographic References–Burns in Children*, annual. Bibliography. Lists reading material for the education and inspiration of parents, siblings, and professionals involved wiht burned children. *Price:* $5. • *Coping Strategies for Burn Survivors and Their Families.* • *Guidelines for Burn Volunteers.* • *Phoenix Society Newsletter*, quarterly. Newsletter. Provides news items on burn prevention, cosmetology for burn survivors, and other topics of interest; includes member news and book reviews. *Price:* Included in membership dues; $4/year for nonmembers; $10 outside U.S. **Frmly:** (1991) Phoenix Center.

★ 5390 ★ Phone-TTY

1246 Rte. 46 West
Parsippany, NJ 07054
Phone: (973)299-6627 **Fax:** (973)299-7768
Email: phonetty@aol.com
Website: http://www.phone-tty.com/
Anna M. Terrazzino, Exec. Dir.

Fnded: 1969. **Mem:** 20. **Desc:** Seeks to develop and promote better communication for the deaf using an ordinary telephone and current technology. Installs computerized phone-teletype equipment in the homes of individuals who are deaf, enabling these individuals to communicate with local police, hospitals, answering services, and news services, as well as members of the deaf community who have a PHONE-TTY in their homes. Researches, designs, manufactures, and distributes other communication devices for the deaf. Solicits grants and donations.

★ 5391 ★ Physically Handicapped Welfare Association

Joseph d'Argent Aven
Rose Hill, Mauritius
Phone: 230 4644845 **Fax:** 230 4650549

Fnded: 1960. **Mem:** 150. **Desc:** Aims to improve the lives of physically challenged people in Mauritius. Operates rehabilitation center. **Frmly:** (1981) Cripple Welfare Association.

★ 5392 ★ Physician Insurers Association of America (PIAA)

2275 Research Blvd., Ste. 250
Rockville, MD 20850
Phone: (301)947-9000 **Fax:** (301)947-9090
Email: ahorwich@thepiaa.org
Website: http://www.thepiaa.org
Ann Hokwich, Dir. of Admn. Services

Fnded: 1977. **Mem:** 60. **Desc:** Physician liability insurance companies, including domestic physician and dental liability insurers, international affiliates, and reinsurers. Seeks to further the best interests of member companies in areas related to physician liability insurance. Focuses on the availability and affordability of professional liability insurance and the effective delivery of quality healthcare. Conducts research and educational programs; monitors and advocates for legislation. **Pub:** *The Physician Insurer*, quarterly. Magazine. *Price:* $45/year. • *PIAA Membership Directory*, annual. Membership Directory. • Also publishes studies of major liability concerns in the insurance industry, including issues related to treatment of breast, lung, and colon cancer; medication errors; and laparoscopy procedures.

★ 5393 ★ Physicians Association for Anthroposophical Medicine (PAAM)

1923 Geddes Ave.
Ann Arbor, MI 48104
Fax: (734)662-1727
Email: paam@anthroposophy.org
Website: http://www.paam.net
Christian Wessling, MD, Pres.

Fnded: 1982. **Mem:** 70. **Nat'l Groups:** 1. **Desc:** Physicians promoting the use and learning of anthroposophical medicine. Sponsors educational programs. **Pub:** *Directory of Physicians*, biennial. Directory. *Price:* Free. • *PAAM Newsletter*, biennial. Newsletter.

★ 5394 ★ Physicians Committee for Responsible Medicine (PCRM)

5100 Wisconsin Ave., Ste. 400
Washington, DC 20016
Phone: (202)686-2210 **Fax:** (202)686-2216
Email: pcrm@pcrm.org
Website: http://www.pcrm.org
Neal D. Barnard, MD, Pres.

Fnded: 1985. **Mem:** 110,000. **Desc:** Physicians, scientists, healthcare professionals, and interested others. Increases public awareness about the importance of preventive medicine and nutrition, and raises scientific and ethical questions pertaining to the use of humans and animals in medical research. Supports research into U.S. agricultural and public health policies. Promotes the New Four Food Groups, a no-cholesterol, low-fat alternative to U.S.D.A. dietary recommendations. Maintains the Gold Plan program which includes information on low-fat, cholesterol-free entrees and nutrition for institutional food services. Offers fact sheets on nutrition, preventive medicine, and non-animal research topics. Maintains speakers' bureau. **Pub:** *Alternatives in Medical Education.* • *Best in the World (Cookbook)*. Book. • *Eat Right, Live Longer.* • *Food for Life.* • *Foods That Fight Pain.* • *Good Medicine*, quarterly. Magazine. Provides information about preventive medicine, nutrition, public health policy, medical/nutrition research updates, and AIDS research. *Price:* Included in membership dues. • *The Power of Your Plate.* • Brochures. • Also publishes fact sheets.

★ 5395 ★ Physiological Society of New Zealand (PSNZ)

c/o Assoc.Prof. Simon Malpas
Department of Physiology
University of Auckland
PO Box 92019
Auckland, New Zealand
Fax: 64 9 3737499
Email: s.malpas@auckland.ac.nz

Fnded: 1972. **Mem:** 180. **Lang(s):** English. **Desc:** Physiological scientists in New Zealand. Seeks to enhance the quality of physiological and related research in New Zealand by establishing links with similar societies throughout the world, enhancing the effectiveness of all levels of education in the teaching of physiological, biological and related sciences, and by acting as a national body to provide advice and information to the government and the community. Provides career advice and fosters career opportunities for graduate and postgraduate students.

★ 5396 ★ Pierre Fauchard Academy (PFA)

c/o Dr. Richard Kozal
PO Box 80330
Las Vegas, NV 89180-0330
Phone: (702)651-5013 **Free:** 800-232-0099
Fax: (702)651-5537
Email: rkozal@aol.com
Website: http://www.fauchard.org
Dr. Richard A. Kozal, Sec. -Treas.

Fnded: 1936. **Mem:** 6,000. **Reg. Groups:** 10. **State Groups:** 50. **Local Groups:** 5. **Desc:** Dentists "of high standards and leadership" who are nominated to the academy by state or section chairmen. Objectives are to educate dentists by providing literature on developments and opinions in dentistry; promote continuing education for all members of the dental profession; facilitate the exchange of knowledge among dentists; foster contact between dentistry leaders and those who seek advice on scientific, technical, or economic subjects; encourage advancement of professional and scientific standards; further the improvement of oral health of the public through prevention, therapy, and restoration; emphasize professional responsibility to the public. Sponsors annual Memorial Lecture honoring a past leader of dentistry. The academy is named for Pierre Fauchard (1678-1761), a French dentist who pioneered modern dental practice and dental education. **Pub:** *Dental Abstracts*, quarterly. *Price:* $25/year. • *Dental World*, bimonthly. Newsletter. Includes member news, meeting announcements, abstracts, book reviews, and editorials. • *Leadership Manual of the PFA.* Manual. • *Legacy, The Dental Profession.* Book. • *The Life and Times of Pierre Fauchard.* Book. • Membership Directory.

★ 5397 ★ Pill Addicts Anonymous (PAA)

PO Box 13738
Reading, PA 19612-3738

Fnded: 1979. **Mem:** 100. **State Groups:** 2. **Local Groups:** 2. **Desc:** Individuals who wish to recover from pill and drug addiction. Provides support through group sessions. **Pub:** Pamphlets.*Price:* Free.

★ 5398 ★ Pills Anonymous (PA)

PO Box 772
Bronx, NY 10451
Phone: (212)874-0700
Website: http://www.pillsanonymous.com

Fnded: 1975. **Local Groups:** 3. **Desc:** Persons addicted to drugs including tranquilizers, stimulants, analgesics, sedatives, cocaine, and marijuana. Purpose is to apply the Alcoholics Anonymous World Services' 12-step approach to persons dependent on addictive drugs. Provides emotional support to members, many of whom became addicted after using the drugs for legitimate reasons (for example, to alleviate the chronic pain of migraine headaches or arthritis) and teaches them methods of coping with pain that do not require drugs. **Frmly:** (1984) Pills Anonymous; (1992) Drugs Anonymous.

★ 5399 ★ Pilot Dogs (PD)
625 W Town St.
Columbus, OH 43215
Phone: (614)221-6367 **Fax:** (614)221-1577
Website: http://www.pilotdogs.org/
J. Jay Gray, Exec. Dir.

Fnded: 1950. **Mem:** 20,841. **Desc:** Provides guide dogs and training for the blind. **Pub:** *Pilot Light*, quarterly.

★ 5400 ★ Pioneer Total Abstinence Association
27 Upper Sherrard St.
Dublin 1, Ireland
Phone: 353 1 8749464 **Fax:** 353 1 8748485
Email: pioneer@s-j.ie
Website: http://www.pioneertotal.ie

Fnded: 1898. **Mem:** 500,000. **Nat'l Groups:** 6. **Reg. Groups:** 122. **Local Groups:** 1100. **Desc:** Promotes sobriety, principally by prayer and consecrated abstinence from alcohol of members. Encourages members to engage in good works. **Pub:** *Pioneer*, monthly. Magazine. Contains information on religion, general topics and youth.

★ 5401 ★ Pituitary Network Association (PNA)
PO Box 1958
Thousand Oaks, CA 91358
Phone: (805)499-9973 **Fax:** (805)480-0633
Email: pna@pituitary.org
Website: http://www.pituitary.org
Robert Knutzen, Chm.

Fnded: 1993. **Mem:** 5,000. **Nat'l Groups:** 4. **Reg. Groups:** 8. **State Groups:** 4. **Desc:** Patients supplying information to other patients, families and health care professionals. Publishes books and news magazines on pituitary issues. **Pub:** *Pituitary Patient Resource Guide*, biennial. Book. Reference guide for pituitary patients, their families, physicians, and all health care providers. *Price:* $39.95 for members; $49.95 for nonmembers. • *PNA Newsletter*, bimonthly. Newsletter. **Frmly:** (1993) PTNA; (2002) Pituitary Tumor Network Association.

★ 5402 ★ Planned Parenthood Association of Sierra Leone (PPASL)
45 Adelaide St.
PO Box 1094
Freetown, Sierra Leone
Phone: 232 22 22774 **Fax:** 232 22 22774
Email: ppasl@sierratel.sl
Website: http://www.ippf.org/regions/africa

Fnded: 1959. **Mem:** 750. **Lang(s):** English. **Desc:** Works to enhance the standard of living for individuals living in Sierra Leone by promoting family planning. Advocates family planning as a basic human right. Attempts to stop the spread of sexually transmitted diseases, especially AIDS. Offers programs in sex education, family planning, and health. Provides contraceptive and health care services. **Pub:** *PPASL News Letter*, semiannual. Newsletter. • Annual Report. • Reports. From baseline studies.

★ 5403 ★ Planned Parenthood Association of South Africa (PPASA)
172 Oxford Rd.
PO Box 1023
Saxonwold 2132, Republic of South Africa
Phone: 27 11 8801162 **Fax:** 27 11 8801191
Email: ppasa@ppasa.org.za
Website: http://www.ppasa.org.za

Fnded: 1930. **Mem:** 180. **Reg. Groups:** 5. **Lang(s):** Afrikaans, English, Sotho, Tswana, Xhosa, Zulu. **Desc:** Encourages family planning activities in South Africa and promotes family planning as a basic human right. Works to: improve maternal and child health; reduce the incidence of unwanted pregnancy and abortion; address issues related to adolescent sexuality and teen pregnancy; increase public knowledge of the prevention of AIDS and other sexually transmitted diseases; increase societal awareness of the relationship between population growth, natural resource consumption, and the conservation of the environment. Coordinates information, education, and training programs on sexual responsibility and reproductive health. Conducts research. **Pub:** *Aids Scan*, quarterly. Also publishes *Responsible Teenage Sexuality* (book).

★ 5404 ★ Planned Parenthood Association of Thailand (PPAT)
8 Soi Vibhavadi-Rangsit 44
Vibhavadi-Rangsit Rd.
Lad-Yao, Chatuchak
Bangkok 10900, Thailand
Phone: 66 2 9412320 **Fax:** 66 2 9412338
Email: ppat@samart.co.th
Website: http://www.ippf.org/regions/eseaor

Fnded: 1970. **Mem:** 655. **Lang(s):** Thai. **Desc:** Works to improve the quality of life for people living in Thailand by promoting responsible parenthood and family planning. Attempts to reduce the number of unwanted pregnancies and abortions. Offers programs in sex education, family planning, and health. Provides contraceptive and health care services. Conducts research. **Pub:** *PPAT News/Sarn Samphan Newsletter*, bimonthly. Newsletter. Explains PPAT activities.

★ 5405 ★ Planned Parenthood Federation of America (PPFA)
810 7th Ave.
New York, NY 10019
Phone: (212)541-7800 **Fax:** (212)245-1845
Email: communications@ppfa.org
Website: http://www.plannedparenthood.org/
Gloria Feldt, Pres.

Fnded: 1916. **Reg. Groups:** 169. **Desc:** Organizations providing leadership in making effective means of voluntary fertility regulation, including contraception, abortion, sterilization, and infertility services, available and fully accessible to all as a central element of reproductive health; stimulating and sponsoring relevant biomedical, socioeconomic, and demographic research; developing appropriate information, education, and training programs to increase knowledge about human reproduction and sexuality. Supports and assists efforts to achieve similar goals worldwide. Operates more than 900 centers that provide medically supervised reproductive health services and educational programs. **Pub:** Annual Report. • Books. • Pamphlets. **AKA:** Planned Parenthood; Planned Parenthood/World Population. **Frmly:** (1939) American Birth Control League.

★ 5406 ★ Planned Parenthood Federation of America - International
Asia & Pacific Regional Office
37 Petchburi Rd., Soi 15
Bangkok 10400, Thailand
Phone: 66 2 2548955 **Fax:** 66 2 2548956
Email: apro@ppfa.org
Website: http://www.plannedparenthood.org

Lang(s): English, Thai. **Desc:** Health care professionals, family planning and population organizations, and other interested individuals. Promotes increased availability of family planning services. Conducts educational programs to raise public awareness of population issues and family planning services; provides support and assistance to reproductive health and family planning clinics.

★ 5407 ★ Planned Parenthood Federation of Canada (PPFC) (Federation pour le planning des naissances du Canada — FPNC)
1 Nicholas St., Ste. 430
Ottawa, ON, Canada K1N 7B7
Phone: (613)241-4474 **Fax:** (613)241-7550
Email: admin@ppfc.ca
Website: http://www.ppfc.ca

Fnded: 1964. **Mem:** 26. **State Groups:** 6. **Local Groups:** 63. **Lang(s):** English, French. **Desc:** Promotes family planning and responsible parenthood. Encourages public awareness of contraceptive methods and the need for family planning. Works to reduce the number of unwanted pregnancies and abortions. Sponsors programs in family planning, sex education, and sexually transmitted diseases, especially AIDS. Provides contraceptive services. Acts as an advocate for family planning issues on a national level. Conducts research. **Pub:** *Beyond the Basics: A Sourcebook for Sexual and Reproductive Health Education.* Book. • *Youth Talk Back: Sex, Sexuality and Media Literacy.* Book. High school textbook that explores sociological issues related to sex, sexuality in the context of media literacy.

★ 5408 ★ Planned Parenthood Federation - Korea (PPFK)
121-146 Dangsandong 6-GA
Youngdeungpo-Ku
Seoul 150-650, Republic of Korea
Phone: 82 2 6348211 **Fax:** 82 2 4678217
Email: ppkf@unitel.co.kr

Fnded: 1961. **Local Groups:** 12. **Lang(s):** English, Korean. **Desc:** Family planning professionals in the Republic of Korea. Seeks to enhance the quality of life of Koreans by promoting family planning and improving maternal and infant health care. Encourages "culturally, economically, and socially healthy" families. Conducts educational programs for military personnel, industrial workers, students, and other groups; disseminates family planning information through mass media. Operates clinics, audio visual materials development center, and 10 sections. **Pub:** *Happy Home*, monthly. Magazine. • *PPFK Annual Report.*

★ 5409 ★ Planned Parenthood Federation of Nigeria (PPFN)
224 Ikorodu Rd.
Shamolu Layout, Palm Grove
PMB 12657
Lagos, Lagos, Nigeria
Phone: 234 1 820945 **Fax:** 234 1 7595580
Email: ppfn@rcl.nig.com
Website: http://www.ippf.org

Fnded: 1964. **Mem:** 3,000. **Nat'l Groups:** 1. **State Groups:** 30. **Local Groups:** 80. **Lang(s):** English. **Desc:** Works to improve the quality of life for individuals living in Nigeria by promoting responsible parenthood and family planning. Advocates family planning as a basic human right. Attempts to stop the spread of AIDS and other sexually transmitted diseases. Offers programs in sex education, family planning, and health. Provides contraceptive and health care services. **Pub:** *Planned News*, semiannual. Newsletter. **Frmly:** (1979) Family Planning Council of Nigeria.

★ 5410 ★ Plastic Surgery Administrative Association (PSAA)
4900 B S 31st St.
Arlington, VA 22206-1656
Phone: (703)931-4520
Email: psaa@mindspring.com
Website: http://www.plasticadmin.org/

Fnded: 1975. **Desc:** Plastic surgery administrators in all practices areas, including solo, group, academic, and surgi-center environments. Promotes the professional development of managers of plastic surgery practices; provides resources in order to achieve competency and efficiency; advocates for members on issues that affect the delivery of plastic surgery care; provides platform for networking. **Pub:** *Administrator*

Review, quarterly. Educational publication that informs members of new product information, clinical and administrative updates, and organization activities. *Price:* included in membership dues. • Newsletter, quarterly. Contains educational information.

★ 5411 ★ Plastic Surgery Educational Foundation (PSEF)
444 E Algonquin Rd.
Arlington Heights, IL 60005
Phone: (847)228-9900 **Free:** 888-4-PLASTIC
Fax: (847)228-9131
Email: memserv@plasticsurgery.org
Website: http://www.plasticsurgery.org
Paul Pomerantz, CAE, Exec. Dir.

Fnded: 1948. **Mem:** 4,500. **Desc:** Plastic and reconstructive surgeons. Purpose is to identify and respond to the educational needs of members and their patients. Sponsors regional and national demonstrations, lectures, educational seminars, symposia, and workshops focusing on plastic surgery techniques and procedures. Conducts annual in-service and self-assessment examinations dealing with topics such as aesthetic and breast surgery, hand and extremities, integument, maxillofacial surgery, and pediatric plastic surgery. Administers Visiting Professors Program; compiles statistics; sponsors charitable programs. **Pub:** *Plastic and Reconstructive Surgery*. Journal. • *Plastic Surgery News*. • Booklets. **Frmly:** (1981) Education Foundation of American Society of Plastic and Reconstructive Surgeons.

★ 5412 ★ Plastic Surgery Research Council (PSRC)
45 Lyme Rd., Ste. 304
Hanover, NH 03755
Phone: (603)643-2325 **Fax:** (603)643-1444
Email: psrc@sover.net
Website: http://www.ps-rc.org
Catherine B. Foss, Exec. Dir.

Fnded: 1955. **Mem:** 586. **Desc:** To foster fundamental research in the fields of plastic and reconstructive surgery. **Pub:** *Meeting Abstracts*, annual.

★ 5413 ★ Play Therapy International (PTI)
Fern Hill Centre, Fern Hill
Fairwarp
Uckfield TN22 3BU, United Kingdom
Phone: 44 1825 712360 **Fax:** 44 1825 713679
Email: ptiorg@aol.com
Website: http://www.playtherapy.org/

Fnded: 1996. **Mem:** 1,200. **Lang(s):** English, French. **Desc:** Professional child psychotherapists and play therapists, students, and other individuals with an interest in child psychology. Promotes advancement in the teaching, theory, and practice of play therapy and child psychotherapy. Conducts examinations and bestows certification to child psychotherapists and play therapists; makes available continuing professional advancement programs to members. Serves as a clearinghouse on play therapy; represents members within the psychological community and before public bodies. Sponsors research; provides children's services; maintains speakers' bureau. **Pub:** *Play News*, quarterly. Newsletter. • *World of Children*, semiannual. Journal.

★ 5414 ★ Polio Fellowship of Ireland (PFI)
Park House Vocational and Residential Training Center
Stillorgan Grove
Dublin, Ireland
Phone: 353 1 2888366 **Fax:** 353 1 2836128
Email: parkhouse@rehab.ie
Website: http://www.irishhealth.com/psg/polio.html

Fnded: 1949. **Lang(s):** English, Irish. **Desc:** Seeks to improve the quality of life of people who have physical disabilities, including polio, and mental health learning difficulties. Provides day activities, training, and residential accommodation.

★ 5415 ★ Polio Society (PS)
4200 Wisconsin Ave. NW, PMB 106-273
Washington, DC 20016
Phone: (301)897-8180 **Fax:** (202)466-1911
Becky Evans, Contact

Fnded: 1984. **Mem:** 3,500. **Local Groups:** 3. **Desc:** Polio survivors and health care professionals interested in the long-term health of patients who have had the disease. Gathers and disseminates information on post-polio syndrome. (PPS is a condition in which polio survivors suffer unaccustomed fatigue, joint and muscle pain, weakening or loss of muscle function, and respiratory problems.) Acts as liaison between members and medical facilities; maintains outreach program and referral service; sponsors support groups. Advocates on issues of disability and benefits. **Pub:** *Options*, quarterly. Newsletter. • Brochures.Informational brochures. • Also publishes information packets. **Frmly:** Post-Polio League for Information and Outreach.

★ 5416 ★ Polish Alzheimer's Association (PAA)
Ul. Hoza 54/1
PL-00-682 Warsaw, Poland
Phone: 48 22 6221122 **Fax:** 48 22 6221122
Email: alzheimer_pl@hotmail.com
Website: http://www.alzheimer.pl

Fnded: 1992. **Mem:** 500. **Nat'l Groups:** 1. **Local Groups:** 24. **Lang(s):** English, Polish. **Desc:** Individuals and organizations. Seeks to improve the quality of life of people with Alzheimer's disease and their families. Makes available support and services; facilitates research on Alzheimer's disease and related disorders; conducts educational programs. **Pub:** *Blizej Alzheimera*, quarterly. Newsletter. Contains information for the caregiver.

★ 5417 ★ Polish Anatomical Society (PAS) (Polskie Towarzystwo Anatomiczne — PTA)
Department of Anatomy
University School of Medical Sciences
6 Swiecicki St.
PL-60 781 Poznan, Poland
Phone: 48 61 8699181 **Fax:** 48 61 8658985
Email: wwozniak@usoms.poznan.pl

Fnded: 1926. **Mem:** 500. **Local Groups:** 12. **Lang(s):** English, French, German. **Desc:** Encourages scientific activities dealing with the morphological sciences, including anatomy, cell biology, embryology, histochemistry, histology, and zoology. Promotes modernization of educational methods. Conducts research. **Pub:** *Advances in Cell Biology*, quarterly. • *Folia Morphologica*, quarterly. **Frmly:** Polish Anatomical and Zoological Society.

★ 5418 ★ Polish Association of People Suffering From Epilepsy (PAPSE)
Fabryczna Str. 57
PL-15-482 Bialystok, Poland
Phone: 48 85 6754420 **Fax:** 48 85 6754420

Fnded: 1985. **Mem:** 400,000. **Reg. Groups:** 6. **Lang(s):** English, Polish. **Desc:** Nongovernmental organizations, foundations, funds, and individuals with an interest in people with epilepsy. Promotes an improved quality of life for people with epilepsy. Represents the rights and interests of people with epilepsy before government agencies; makes available international exchange program; identifies and seeks to acquire and distribute emerging technologies and equipment for the diagnosis and treatment of epilepsy. **Pub:** *Padaezki - Pytania I Odpowiedzi*. Book.

★ 5419 ★ Polish Cardiac Society
ul. Niemodlinska 33
PL-04-635 Warsaw, Poland
Phone: 48 22 8156553 **Fax:** 48 22 6133806
Email: drozdz@ptkardio.pl
Website: http://www.ptkardio.pl

Fnded: 1954. **Mem:** 2,300. **Nat'l Groups:** 13. **Reg. Groups:** 17. **Desc:** Promotes the study of cardiology in Poland. **Pub:** *Folia Cardiologica*. Journal. • *Polish Heart Journal*. Journal.

★ 5420 ★ Polish Medical Association (Polski Towarzystwo Lekarskie)
Al. Ujazdowskie St. 24
PL-00-478 Warsaw, Poland
Phone: 48 26 288699 **Fax:** 48 26 288699

Fnded: 1820. **Mem:** 30,000. **Reg. Groups:** 50. **Local Groups:** 284. **Lang(s):** Polish. **Desc:** Aims to maintain high professional and ethical standards in the medical profession. **Pub:** *Polski Tygodnik Lekavski also cited as: Polish Medical Weekly*, weekly. Magazine. • *Przeylad Lekavski also cited as: Medical Review.* • *Wiadomoici Leharshie also cited as: News for Physicians.*

★ 5421 ★ Polish Paediatric Pathology Society (Polski Towarzystwo Patologii Dzieciecej)
Aleja Dzieci Polskich 20
PL-04736 Warsaw, Poland
Phone: 48 22 8151971 **Fax:** 48 22 8151971
Email: ptpd@cxd.wow.pl

Fnded: 1996. **Mem:** 50. **Nat'l Groups:** 1. **Lang(s):** English, Polish. **Desc:** Pediatric pathologists. Seeks to advance the science and practice of pediatric pathology. Facilitates integration of scientific developments in the field; conducts continuing medical education programs. **Pub:** *Annals of Diagnostic Paediatric Pathology*, quarterly. Journal.

★ 5422 ★ Polish Pharmacological Society (Polskie Towarzystwo Farmakologiczne)
c/o Prof. Henryk I. Trzeciak
Department of Pharmacology
Silesian Medical University
18 Medykow St.
PL-40-752 Katowice-Ligota, Poland
Phone: 48 32 523835 **Fax:** 48 32 523835
Email: phacom@promarcos.com.pl

Mem: 462. **Desc:** Promotes pharmacology in Poland.

★ 5423 ★ Polish Society of Gerontology
Medical Academy
Department Gerontology
Ul. Kilinskiego 1
PL-15-230 Bialystok, Poland
Phone: 48 85 7422021 **Fax:** 48 85 7422539
Email: geronto@amb.ac.bialystok.pl

Desc: Promotes gerontological research, training in the field of aging, and interests of gerontological organizations in international affairs.

★ 5424 ★ Polish Society for Immunology (PSI) (Polskie Towarzystwo Immunologii Doswiadczalnej i Klinicznej)
Institute of Human Genetics
Polish Academy of Sciences
Strzeszynska 32
60-479 Poznan, Poland
Phone: 48 61 8233011 **Fax:** 48 61 8233235
Email: kurpimac@man.poznan.pl

Fnded: 1969. **Mem:** 547. **Local Groups:** 10. **Lang(s):** English, Polish. **Desc:** Researchers. Encourages, coordinates, and supervises immunological research activities in Poland. Assists instruction at universities and medical centers. Disseminates scientific information. Conducts educational and research programs. **Pub:** *Bulletin*, periodic. Bulletin. • *Central European Journal of Immunology*, quarterly.

★ 5425 ★ Polish Society of Veterinary Science (PSVS)
(Polskie Towarzystwo Nauk Weterynaryjnych)
Faculty of Veterinary Medicine in Warsaw
ul. Grochowska 272
PL-03-849 Warsaw, Poland
Phone: 48 22 8103397 **Fax:** 48 22 8103397
Email: ptnw@vetclub.pl
Website: http://www.vetcentrum.pl/ptnw

Fnded: 1952. **Mem:** 2,400. **Nat'l Groups:** 12. **Reg. Groups:** 17. **Lang(s):** English, Polish. **Desc:** Veterinarians in Poland. Promotes excellence in veterinary medicine. Maintains museum. **Pub:** *Medycyna Weterynaryjna*, monthly. Journal. Also publishes periodic congress and conference materials of divisions.

★ 5426 ★ Politzer Society - International Society for Otological Surgery
c/o Dr. O. Nuri Ozgirgin
Department of Otolaryngology
Baskent University Hospital
Bahcelievler
TR-06490 Ankara, Turkey
Phone: 90 312 2238534 **Fax:** 90 312 2157597
Email: ozgirgin@politzersociety.org
Website: http://www.politzersociety.org

Fnded: 1971. **Mem:** 300. **Desc:** Medical professionals involved in the science and practice of surgery and rehabilitation of diseases and disorders of the ear. Disseminates information. Conducts training programs.

★ 5427 ★ Polskie Towarzystwo Stwardnienia Rozsianego
c/o Hotel Marriott
Al Jerozolimskie 65/79
PL-00-697 Warsaw, Poland
Phone: 48 22 630 7220 **Fax:** 48 22 630 7220
Email: rgptsr@plearn.edu.pl

Desc: MS patients, families and professionals. Seeks to improve the quality of life for persons with multiple sclerosis and their families.

★ 5428 ★ Polycystic Ovarian Syndrome Association
PO Box 80517
Portland, OR 97280
Phone: (856)218-4815 **Free:** 877-775-PCOS
Fax: (413)751-4866
Email: info@pcosupport.org
Website: http://www.pcosupport.org
Kristin Rencher, Exec. Dir.

Fnded: 1997. **Mem:** 2,500. **Nat'l Groups:** 1. **Local Groups:** 12. **Desc:** Chapters worldwide provide support, education and advocacy for women suffering from polycystic ovary syndrome (PCOS). Host educational events combining lectures with support sessions. Advocate for women with PCOS in the media and medical community by attending and speaking at professional meetings as well as hosting exhibit booths. **Pub:** *PCOS Bulletin*, quarterly. Newsletter. *Price:* included in membership dues. • *PCOS Record*, monthly. Newsletter.

★ 5429 ★ Population and Community Development Association (PDA)
6 Sukhumvit Rd., SOI-12
Klongtoey
Bangkok 10110, Thailand
Phone: 66 2 2294611 **Fax:** 66 2 2294632
Email: pda@pda.or.th
Website: http://www.pda.or.th

Fnded: 1974. **Mem:** 483. **Local Groups:** 16. **Lang(s):** English, Thai. **Desc:** Seeks to improve the quality of life and increase economic levels in rural areas of Thailand. Coordinates development projects focusing on family planning, primary health care, and rural development. Offers training courses on the management of community-based development programs; conducts population research; educates communities on AIDS prevention. Worked to popularize birth control practices through socially entertaining programs such as condom-blowing contests and the Cops and Rubbers Project. Over the past 15 years Thailand's population growth has been cut in half through these types of programs. **Pub:** *From Condoms to Cabbages*. Book. An authorized biography of Mechai Viravaidya. • *PDA*, 3/year. Newsletter. • *Strategies to Strengthen NGO Capacity in Resource Mobilization through Business Activities*. UNAIDS best practice collection. • *TBIRD: News*, 3/year. Newsletter. Features TBIRD project activities.

★ 5430 ★ Portuguesa Multiple Sclerosis Society (SPEM)
(Sociedade Portuguesa de Esclerose Multipla)
Rua Tomas Alcaide 63C
P-1900-822 Lisbon, Portugal
Phone: 351 21 8394720 **Fax:** 351 21 8394729
Email: spem@spem.org
Website: http://www.spem.org

Fnded: 1984. **Mem:** 1,450. **Reg. Groups:** 9. **Lang(s):** English, French. **Desc:** MS patients, families and professionals. Seeks to improve the quality of life for persons with multiple sclerosis and their families. **Pub:** *Boletin Lsclerose Multipla*, quarterly. Magazine.

★ 5431 ★ Portuguese Society of Cardiology
Campo Grande 28-13
P-1700-093 Lisbon, Portugal
Phone: 351 21 7970685 **Fax:** 351 21 7931095
Email: secretariado@mail.spc.pt
Website: http://www.spc.pt

Fnded: 1949. **Mem:** 573. **Desc:** Promotes the study of cardiology in Portugal, including coronary heart disease prevention in clinical practice, and cardiovascular prevention in the elderly. **Pub:** *Boletim da Sociedade Portuguesa de Cardiologia*, monthly. Newsletter. • *Portuguese Journal of Cardiology*, monthly.

★ 5432 ★ Portuguese Society of Pharmacology
(Sociedade Portuguesa de Farmacologia)
c/o Dr. Ana M. Sebastiao
Laboratorio Neurosciencias
Faculdade Medicina de Lisboa
Av. Prof. Egas Moniz
P-1649-028 Lisbon, Portugal
Phone: 351 21 7936787 **Fax:** 351 21 7936787
Email: anaseb@neurosciencias.pt

Mem: 109. **Desc:** Promotes pharmacology in Portugal.

★ 5433 ★ Portuguese Society of Stomatology and Dental Medicine (PSSDM)
(Sociedade Portugesa de Estomatolgia Emedicina Dentaria — SPEMD)
Rua Prof. Fernando de Fonseca, 10A
Esc. 7
P-1600-618 Lisbon, Portugal
Phone: 351 217 520056 **Fax:** 351 217 520057
Email: mail@spemd.pt
Website: http://www.spemd.pt

Fnded: 1919. **Mem:** 2,200. **Local Groups:** 3. **Lang(s):** English, Portuguese. **Desc:** Stomatologists, dentists, and oral and maxillofacial surgeons in Portugal. Promotes research in all disciplines of oral medicine. Sponsors community dental hygiene programs. Establishes standards and qualifications for oral medicine specialists. Represents' members interests; operates legal defense fund for members. Monitors the manufacture of dental materials in Portugal. Promotes continuing education programs for members. **Pub:** *Revista Portugese de Estomatologia e Cirurgia Maxilofacial*, quarterly. Journal. Journal of dentistry and maxillofacial surgery. • *Stoma*, quarterly.

★ 5434 ★ Positively Women
347-349 City Rd.
London EC1V 1LR, United Kingdom
Phone: 44 20 77130444 **Fax:** 44 20 77131020
Email: info@positivelywomen.org.uk
Website: http://www.positivelywomen.org.uk/

Fnded: 1987. **Reg. Groups:** 1. **Lang(s):** English, French, Luganda, Swahili. **Desc:** Offers peer support and self-help services to women with HIV and/or AIDs and their children. Provides information; maintains a resource facility. **Pub:** *Positively Women Newsletter*, bimonthly. Newsletter.

★ 5435 ★ Postgraduate Center for Mental Health (PCMH)
c/o Vocational Services Department
344 W 36th St.
New York, NY 10018
Phone: (212)560-6720 **Fax:** (212)563-1291
Email: pcmhvoc@bigfoot.com
Website: http://www.webstrats.com/pcmhvoc.htm
Dr. Jacob Barak, Pres. & CEO

Fnded: 1945. **Desc:** Provides: therapy for individuals, groups, couples, and families; training; psychiatric day and evening care program; community services and public educational programs. Conducts research. Maintains: social rehabilitation clinic; child/adolescent and family clinic; adult clinic; employee support service; group residence for the mentally ill preparing for independent living. Training opportunities include: Adult Fellowship, Advanced Training for Social Workers, Child and Adolescent Counseling, Family Therapy, Group Therapy, Pastoral Counseling, Psychology Internship, and Social Work Internship. Offers mental health and organizational consultation to industry and government agencies. Maintains six residential facilities (supported housing) for homeless mentally ill. Oversees distribution of funds for programs providing housing and supportive services to people with HIV/AIDS. **Pub:** *Psychoanalysis and Psychotherapy*, semiannual. Journal. Includes professional book reviews and author and title indexes. *Price:* $37.50/year. **Frmly:** Institute for Research in Psychotherapy; (1962) Postgraduate Center for Psychotherapy.

★ 5436 ★ Postpartum Adjustment Services - Canada (PASS-CAN)
Unit 3 460 Woody Rd.
PO Box 7282, Sta. Main
Oakville, ON, Canada L6K 3T6
Phone: (905)844-9009 **Free:** 800-897-6660
Fax: (905)844-5973
Email: info@passcan.ca

Fnded: 1972. **Mem:** 500. **Lang(s):** English, French. **Desc:** Health care and mental health professionals; parents of preschool children. Seeks to "ease the transition to parenthood for families of infants or preschoolers" and to "reduce the stigma of postpartum depression or anxiety." Serves as the national clearinghouse on postpartum depression. Conducts advocacy, networking, and educational activities; maintains discussion and support groups for mothers experiencing postpartum anxiety or depression. Participates in charitable activities; maintains speakers' bureau. **Pub:** *ComPass*, periodic. Newsletter. • *Passwords*, periodic. Newsletter. • *Ups and Downs - A New Mother's Guide*. Booklet.

★ 5437 ★ Postpartum Support International (PSI)
c/o Laurence Kruckman
Indiana-University of Pennsylvania
Department of Anthropology
Indiana, PA 15705
Phone: (724)357-3935 **Fax:** (724)357-7637
Email: kruckman@iup.edu
Website: http://www.postpartum.net/
Laurence Kruckman, PhD, Pres. Elect

Fnded: 1987. **Desc:** Promotes international awareness, prevention and treatment of mental health issues related to childbearing. **Pub:** *PSI News*, quarterly. Newsletter.

★ 5438 ★ Potency Restored
8630 Fenton St., Ste. 218
Silver Spring, MD 20910
Phone: (301)588-5777 **Free:** 800-588-4170
Fax: (301)588-6220
Email: info@dr-giulio-scarzella.com
Website: http://www.dr-giulio-scarzella.com/impotence.html
Giulio I. Scarzella, MD, Exec. Dir.

Fnded: 1981. **Mem:** 90. **Desc:** Impotent men who have undergone inflatable penile implant (prosthetic) surgery or are considering the operation; partners of impotent men. Provides mutual help, understanding, and emotional support. Encourages members to become informed spokepersons in the field of impotence; presents scientific programs. Plans to start other groups around the country. **Pub:** Newsletter, monthly. **Frmly:** (1982) Impotence Anonymous.

★ 5439 ★ Practical Allergy Research Foundation (PARF)
1421 Colvin Blvd.
Buffalo, NY 14223
Phone: (716)875-0398 **Free:** 888-895-7277
Fax: (716)875-5399
Website: http://www.drrapp.com
Dr. Doris J. Rapp, MD, Pres.

Desc: Seeks to enhance public awareness of allergies, their symptoms, and remedies; fosters research in allergy. Produces and distributes teaching aids; participates in allergy teaching programs and seminars worldwide. Maintains speakers' bureau. **Pub:** *Allergies and the Hyperactive Child.* Book. • *Allergies and Your Family.* Book. • *Allergies Do Alter Activities and Behavior.* Video. • *Environmentally Sick Schools.* Video. • *The Impossible Child.* Book. • *Impossible Child or Allergic Child?.* Video. • *Is This Your Child?.* Book. • *Is This Your Child's World?.* Book. • *Recognize and Manage Your Allergies.* Book. • *Why An Environmentally Clean Classroom?.* Video. • *Why Some Children Can't Learn or Behave.* Video. • Audiotapes. • Catalog.

★ 5440 ★ Prader-Willi Foundation
267 Oxford St.
Rochester, NY 14607
Phone: (716)442-1655 **Free:** 800-442-1655
Fax: (716)271-2782
Email: alliance@proder-willi.org
Sheldon L. Tarakan, Pres.

Fnded: 1994. **Desc:** Devoted to serving individuals with Prader-Willi Syndrome. Provides information on subjects related to Prader-Willi Syndrome. Finances related projects such as residential development, family support, behavioral research, and awareness. Works with other Prader-Willi organizations. **Pub:** *Moris A. Angulo, MD Prader-Willi Syndrom: A Guide for Families & Others.* • *News & Notes,* quarterly. Newsletter. *Price:* Free.

★ 5441 ★ Prader-Willi Syndrome Association (U.S.A.) (PWSAUSA)
5700 Midnight Pass Rd., Ste. 6
Sarasota, FL 34242
Phone: (941)312-0400 **Free:** 800-926-4797
Fax: (941)312-0142
Email: national@pwsausa.org
Website: http://www.pwsausa.org
Janalee Heinemann, Exec. Dir.

Fnded: 1975. **Mem:** 3,000. **Nat'l Groups:** 1. **State Groups:** 34. **Desc:** Parents, physicians, educators, dieticians, group homes, and others interested in the Prader-Willi Syndrome, the most common known genetic cause of morbid obesity in children. (The significant manifestations of the syndrome are obesity, short stature, lack of muscle tone, hypogonadism, and central nervous system performance dysfunction.) Works to provide a forum for communication about the syndrome, particularly the means to cope with it; to promote research and the establishment of treatment facilities. **Pub:** *Gathered View,* bimonthly. Newsletter. Provides information on education, learning problems, and new resources for individuals with PWS. Includes book reviews and research updates. *Price:* Included in membership dues. • *Management of Prader-Willi Syndrome.* Book. • Handbooks.For parents. • Also publishes information packets and produces videos. **Frmly:** (1977) Prader-Willi Syndrome Parents and Friends; (1992) Prader-Willi Syndrome Association; (1998) Prader-Willi Syndrome Association U.S.A; (2002) PWSA USA.

★ 5442 ★ Pre-Eclampsia Society
c/o Dawn James
Rhianfa, Carmel
Caernarfon LL54 7RL, United Kingdom
Phone: 44 1286 882685
Email: dawnjames@clara.co.uk
Website: http://www.dawnjames.clara.net

Fnded: 1981. **Mem:** 500. **Desc:** Provides self help and support groups for those suffering or having suffered from pre-eclampsia.

★ 5443 ★ Pre-Retirement Association (PRA)
9 Chesham Rd.
Surrey
Guildford GU1 3LS, United Kingdom
Phone: 44 1483 301170 **Fax:** 44 1483 300981
Email: info@pra.uk.com
Website: http://www.pra.uk.com

Fnded: 1964. **Mem:** 404. **Local Groups:** 11. **Desc:** People with associated interests in a personal or professional capacity and companies willing to be associated with the development of retirement/redundancy advice/mid life planning. Promoting awareness of the needs of all those preparing for retirement. It provides education, planning and support services that relate to the successful management of transitional changes from an increasing diversity of employment patterns. Runs a course leading to a certificate in pre-retirement education with life planning. **Pub:** *PRA Resources Unit News,* quarterly. Newsletter. • *Preparation for Retirement: The Employer's Guide.* • *Your Retirement,* annual. Features basic information for retirees. **Frmly:** (2001) Pre-Retirement Association of Great Britain and Northern Ireland.

★ 5444 ★ Premenstrual Society
PO Box 429
Addlestone KT15 1DZ, United Kingdom
Phone: 44 1932 872560

Fnded: 1986. **Mem:** 500. **Reg. Groups:** 10. **Lang(s):** English. **Desc:** Seeks to provide advice and support for sufferers of premenstrual syndrome (PMS). Provides support for local groups and professionals in the field. **Pub:** *Premsol Newsletter,* semiannual. Newsletter.

★ 5445 ★ Premier Advocacy
444 N Capitol St. NW, Ste. 625
Washington, DC 20001-1511
Phone: (202)393-0860 **Fax:** (202)393-0864
Website: http://my.premierinc.com/frames/index.jsp?pagelocation=/all/advocacy/
Herb Kuhn, Corporate VP

Fnded: 1984. **Mem:** 40. **Desc:** Nonprofit multi-hospital systems. Sponsors educational programs for corporate officers and trustees of multi-hospital systems. Monitors, investigates, and develops policy positions on developments in the health care field. **Frmly:** Association AMHS Institute; (1988) American Healthcare Institute; (1998) AMHS Institute; (1999) Premier.

★ 5446 ★ Prescription Foot Orthotic Laboratory Association (PFOLA)
c/o Jay Skoog, Exec.Dir.
36 S Last Chance Gulch, Ste. A
Helena, MT 59601
Free: 800-347-6585 **Fax:** (406)443-4614
Email: jskoog@rmsmanagement.com
Website: http://www.nvo.com/pfola
Jay Skoog, Exec. Dir.

Fnded: 1990. **Mem:** 45. **Desc:** Works to promote and improve the efficacy of custom, prescription foot orthoses. **Pub:** Newsletters.*Price:* included in membership dues.

★ 5447 ★ Prevent Blindness America
500 E Remington Rd.
Schaumburg, IL 60173-5611
Phone: (847)843-2020 **Free:** 800-331-2020
Fax: (847)843-8458
Email: info@preventblindness.org
Website: http://www.preventblindness.org
Hugh R. Parry, Pres. /CEO

Fnded: 1908. **Nat'l Groups:** 1. **State Groups:** 22. **Local Groups:** 22. **Desc:** Charitable organization committed to preventing blindness and preserving sight through nationwide comprehensive programs of public and professional education, research, industrial, and community services. Services include promotion and support of local glaucoma screening programs, preschool vision testing, industrial eye safety, and collection of statistical and other data on nature and extent of causes of blindness and defective vision. Operates a toll-free information center dealing with eye health and safety topics. Through the Fight for Sight Research Division, the organization awards student fellowships, postdoctoral awards and grants in aid for medical research. Sponsors Wise Owl Program to promote widespread use of safety eyewear for various activities and occupations. Compiles statistics. **Pub:** *Prevent Blindness America–Annual Report,* annual. Magazine. Covers highlights and accomplishments of the previous fiscal year. Includes financial statements. *Price:* Free. • *Prevent Blindness News,* 3/year. Newsletter on eye health and safety. *Price:* $15/year. **Frmly:** (1915) National Committee for the Prevention of Blindness; (1928) National Society for the Prevention of Blindness; (1978) National Society to Prevent Blindness.

★ 5448 ★ Preventive Cardiovascular Nurses Association (PCNA)
613 Williamson St., Ste. 205
Madison, WI 53703
Phone: (608)250-2440 **Fax:** (608)250-2410
Email: info@pcna.net
Website: http://www.pcna.net
Sue Koob, Exec. Dir.

Fnded: 1991. **Mem:** 1,600. **Reg. Groups:** 16. **Desc:** Works to develop and promote the role of nurses in managing of patients with cardiovascular disease. Defines a certification process; disseminates information to increase consumer awareness; funds a training grant; seeks to have preventive cardiology designated a nursing specialty. **Pub:** *Prevention: PCNA Perspectives,* quarterly. Newsletter. • Membership Directory. **Frmly:** (2001) Lipid Nurse Task Force.

★ 5449 ★ Price-Pottenger Nutrition Foundation (PPNF)
7890 Broadway
Lemon Grove, CA 91945
Phone: (619)462-7600 **Free:** 800-366-3748
Fax: (619)433-3136
Email: info@price-pottenger.org
Website: http://www.price-pottenger.org
Ed Bennet, BS, Pres.

Fnded: 1952. **Mem:** 2,000. **Desc:** Seeks to increase awareness of natural health, organic gardening, nutrition and ecology. Disseminates information to the medical and dental professions, as well as to the public, through publications, seminars, classes, study groups, and scientific exhibits. Stresses the benefits of chemically-untreated "whole" foods. Named in honor of Weston A. Price, DDS and Francis M. Pottenger, Jr., M.D., known for their work in nutrition research. **Pub:** *Nutrition and Physical Degeneration.* Book. • *Pottenger's Cats: A Study in Nutrition.* Book. • *PPNF Health Journal: Health and Healing Wisdom,* quarterly. Journal. Contains articles on health, book reviews, recipes, and a calendar. *Price:* $35/yr; $100/yr for professional. **Frmly:** (1954) Santa Barbara Medical

Research Foundation; (1965) Weston A. Price Memorial Foundation; (1973) Price-Pottenger Foundation.

★ 5450 ★ PRIDE Youth Programs (PYP)
4684 Evergreen Dr.
Newaygo, MI 49337
Phone: (231)652-4400 **Free:** 800-668-9277
Fax: (231)652-2461
Email: prideyouth@ncats.net
Website: http://www.prideyouthprograms.org
Jay DeWispelaere, Pres. /CEO

Fnded: 1977. **Desc:** Parents, youth groups, educators, law enforcement officials, community groups, and corporations. Promotes drug abuse prevention through education. Provides current research information on drug abuse and facilitates the organization of parent peer groups, parent-school teams, and community action groups to reduce adolescent drug abuse. Gathers and disseminates information on the latest medical and scientific findings on the effects of drugs on youth, current patterns of drug and alcohol use among youth, social and cultural pressures that encourage youth to use drugs, and institutional and legal efforts being made to prevent drug abuse, reduce drug supplies, and prosecute drug traffickers. Conducts the PRIDE Community Action Plan to assist communities in establishing an effective drug abuse program and the PRIDE's Parent Training Program to assist concerned parents. Offers America's PRIDE, ClubPRIDE, and PRIDE Junior youth programs. Develops workplace drug training programs for corporations. Sponsors the annual PRIDE World Drug Conference, which seeks to bring parents, youth, and the public into contact with scientists, physicians, and policymakers dealing with adolescent drug abuse; also sponsors a series of one-day conferences for local community teams who are trained to return to their neighborhoods to organize workshops. Operates speakers' bureau; conducts educational programs and children's services; compiles statistics. Maintains library. **Pub:** *PRIDE Quarterly*. Newsletter. Discusses the legal, pharmacological, psychological, social, cultural, and physiological effects of adolescent drug use. Includes overviews. *Price:* $25/year. • Also publishes books and pamphlets. **AKA:** National Parents' Resource Institute for Drug Education. **Frmly:** (1982) Parent Resources and Information on Drug Education.

★ 5451 ★ Primary Immunodeficiency Association
Alliance House
12 Caxton St.
London SW1H 0QS, United Kingdom
Phone: 44 20 79767640 **Fax:** 44 20 79767641
Email: info@pia.org.uk
Website: http://www.pia.org.uk

Desc: Immunologists, physicians, and others working to raise awareness of immunodeficiency. Conducts research; disseminates information. **Pub:** *Primary Immunodeficiency Disease*. Booklet.

★ 5452 ★ Private Practice Section/ American Physical Therapy Association (PPS)
1710 Rhode Island NW, 8th Fl.
Washington, DC 20036
Phone: (202)457-1115 **Fax:** (202)457-9191
Email: info@ppsapta.org
Website: http://www.ppsapta.org
Stephen E. Anderson, Pres.

Fnded: 1955. **Mem:** 3,500. **Desc:** Physical therapists who are members of the American Physical Therapy Association and who are in private practice. Purposes are: to provide physical therapists with information on establishing and managing a private practice; to promote high standards of private practice physical therapy; to represent private practitioners before governmental and professional agencies; to disseminate information relating to private practice. Monitors federal and state legislation. Holds forums and seminars. Bestows Robert G. Dicus Award to recognize individuals for achievement in and commitment to the private practice of physical therapy. **Pub:** *An Employers Guide to Obtaining Physical Therapy Services*. • *How to Start a PT Private Practice*. • *IMPACT*, monthly. Magazine. Covers practice management, marketing, clinical developments, legislative and regulatory news, and research and professional issues. • *Private Practice Section Membership Directory*, annual. Membership Directory. Arranged alphabetically and geographically. Includes meeting schedule. *Price:* Included in membership dues; $300 for nonmembers. • *Private Practice Valuation Primer - How to Value a Practice for Sale or Purchase*. • *Twenty Questions About Private Practice*. Pamphlet. • Also makes available blood borne pathogen kit.

★ 5453 ★ Pro-Choice Public Education Project (PEP)
PO Box 3952
New York, NY 10163
Fax: (212)977-4578
Email: pep@protectchoice.org
Website: http://www.protectchoice.org/index.html

Desc: Seeks to educate young women about reproductive freedom and choice.

★ 5454 ★ Pro Familia: Deutsche Gesellschaft fur Familienplanung, Sexualpadagogik und Sexualberatung
Stresemannallee 3
D-60596 Frankfurt am Main, Germany
Phone: 49 69 639002 **Fax:** 49 69 639852
Email: info@profamilia.de
Website: http://www.profamilia.de

Fnded: 1952. **Mem:** 5,800. **Nat'l Groups:** 1. **Reg. Groups:** 16. **Local Groups:** 150. **Lang(s):** German. **Desc:** Promotes family planning as a basic human right. Works to reduce the number of unwanted pregnancies and abortions. Attempts to stop the spread of AIDS and other sexually transmitted diseases through education and contraceptive services. Sponsors programs in family planning, sex education, and health. Conducts research.

★ 5455 ★ Pro Familia Hungarian Scientific Society (HSSFWW)
Keleti Karoly utca 5-7
H-1024 Budapest, Hungary
Phone: 36 61 3456722 **Fax:** 36 61 3456678
Email: mcsnt@doki.net
Website: http://www.szexinfo.hu

Fnded: 1975. **Mem:** 900. **Lang(s):** English, French, Hungarian. **Desc:** Advocates family planning as a basic human right. Encourages public awareness of family planning and responsible parenthood. Works to reduce the number of unwanted pregnancies and abortions. Offers programs in sex education, family planning, and health care.

★ 5456 ★ Professional Association of German Internists (Berufsverband Deutscher Internisten)
Schone Aussicht 5
D-65193 Wiesbaden, Germany
Phone: 49 611 181330 **Fax:** 49 611 1813350
Email: info@bdi.de
Website: http://www.bdi.de

Fnded: 1959. **Mem:** 28,500. **Reg. Groups:** 23. **Local Groups:** 77. **Lang(s):** English, French. **Desc:** Protects and represents the interests of internal medicine specialists in Germany. Promotes continuing education. **Pub:** *BDI - Aktuell*, monthly. Newsletter. • *Der Internist*, monthly. Magazine.

★ 5457 ★ Professional Association of Health Care Office Management (PAHCOM)
461 E Ten Mile Rd.
Pensacola, FL 32534
Phone: (850)474-9460 **Free:** 800-451-9311
Fax: (850)474-6352
Email: pahcom@pahcom.com
Website: http://www.pahcom.com
Rose Chambers, Contact

Fnded: 1988. **Mem:** 3,200. **Nat'l Groups:** 1. **Local Groups:** 40. **Desc:** Office managers of group and solo medical practices. Operates certification program for health care office managers. **Pub:** *Compliance Program Guide*. Manual. • *Medical Law & Ethics*. Manual. • *Medical Office Management*, bimonthly. Newsletter. Provides current event information. *Price:* Free. For members only. • *Personnel Management*. Manual. • *Practice Enhancement*. Manual. • *Revenue Management*. Manual. **Frmly:** (2001) Professional Association of Health Care Office Managers.

★ 5458 ★ Professional Association of Nursery Nurses (PANN)
c/o Professional Association Teachers
2 St. James' Ct.
Friar Gate
Derby DE1 1BT, United Kingdom
Phone: 44 1332 372337 **Fax:** 44 1332 290310
Email: pann@pat.org.uk
Website: http://www.pat.org.uk

Fnded: 1982. **Mem:** 5,000. **Local Groups:** 11. **Lang(s):** English. **Desc:** Qualified and experienced child care practitioners within education, social services, the health service, the private sector (including nannies). Represents the interests of qualified and student nursery nurses, nannies, and other child care workers throughout the UK. Promotes professionalism at all times. **Pub:** *All You Need to Know About Working as a Nanny*. Information packet. • *Professionalism in Practice*, quarterly. Journal. Also publishes booklets, fact sheets, and information packs.

★ 5459 ★ Professional Board for Radiography and Clinical Technology
533 Vermeulen St.
Arcadia
PO Box 205
Pretoria 0083, Republic of South Africa
Phone: 27 12 3286680 **Fax:** 27 12 3285120
Email: daniek@hpcsa.co.za

Fnded: 1974. **Mem:** 3,997. **Lang(s):** Afrikaans, English. **Desc:** Works to maintain professional standards of education and conduct of radiographers; strives to prevent the admission of unqualified individuals into the radiography profession. Cooperates with the Health Professions Council of South Africa in approving training courses in radiography. Investigates reports of unprofessional conduct. Represents interests of the public. Disseminates information; compiles statistics. **Pub:** *HPCSA Bulletin*, quarterly. Bulletin. • *Technical Journal*, periodic. Journal. **Frmly:** (2000) Professional Board for Radiography.

★ 5460 ★ Professional Midwives Association of Germany (Bund Freiberuflicher Hebammen Deutschlands eV)
Am Alten Nordkanal 10
D-41748 Viersen, Germany
Phone: 49 69 79534971 **Fax:** 49 69 79534972
Email: geschaeftsstelle@bfhd.de
Website: http://www.bfhd.de

Fnded: 1984. **Mem:** 800. **Reg. Groups:** 12. **Lang(s):** English, Spanish. **Desc:** Represents the interests of self-employed midwives. Informs and contributes to the health education of the population. Promotes continuing education for midwives in the interests of mother and child. **Pub:** *Hebammen Info*, semimonthly. Newsletter. Contains articles about midwifery.

★ 5461 ★ Project Concern Hong Kong
Shop 105, Lei Cheng Uk Shopping Arcade
Lei Cheng Uk Estate
Hong Kong, People's Republic of China
Phone: 852 27769081 **Fax:** 852 27769083
Email: medcare@projectconcern.org.hk

Fnded: 1961. **Mem:** 12. **Nat'l Groups:** 35. **Local Groups:** 10. **Lang(s):** Chinese, English. **Desc:** National affiliate of the international organization. Health care practitioners and other interested individuals. Seeks to reduce morbidity and mortality, particularly among women and children. Establishes and operates medical and dental clinics and provides social services in economically disadvantaged areas. Sponsors charitable activities. **Pub:** *Project Concern Hong Kong Annual Report*, annual. Annual Report.

★ 5462 ★ Project Concern International (PCI)
3550 Afton Rd.
San Diego, CA 92123
Phone: (858)279-9690 **Free:** 877-PCI-HOPE
Fax: (858)694-0294
Email: postmaster@projectconcern.org
Website: http://www.projectconcern.org

Fnded: 1961. **Desc:** Works with communities worldwide to ensure low-cost, basic health care for those most in need, particularly mothers and children. Provides education, training, and medical assistance to safeguard the world's impoverished children. Works with volunteers to prepare local communities to care for their own children with long-term, self-sustaining projects. Maintains programs in Bolivia, Guatemala, El Salvador, Ghana, Honduras, Mexico, Nicaragua, India, Indonesia, Romania, Zambia and the United States. **Pub:** *Concern News*, quarterly. Newsletter. Includes news about the organization, special events and donors. *Price:* Free. • *Project Concern International–Annual Report*. Annual Report. Contains financial statements. *Price:* Free. **Frmly:** (1978) Project Concern, Inc.

★ 5463 ★ Project HOPE
255 Carter Hall Ln.
Millwood, VA 22646
Phone: (540)837-2100 **Fax:** (540)837-1813
Email: webmaster@projecthope.org
Website: http://www.projecthope.org/

Desc: Peacetime hospital ship conducting land-based medical training and health care education programs to advance healthcare globally.

★ 5464 ★ Project Inform (PI)
205 13th St., Ste. 2001
San Francisco, CA 94103
Phone: (415)558-8669 **Free:** 800-822-7422
Fax: (415)558-0684
Email: web@projectinform.org
Website: http://www.projectinform.org
Ellen La Pointe, Exec. Dir.

Fnded: 1985. **Mem:** 70,000. **Desc:** Information clearinghouse and hot line providing updated information on drug treatments for persons with AIDS or the Human Immunodeficiency Virus. Also provides information on organizations through which the drug treatments can be obtained. Works to speed up research process and focus on promising new treatments. **Pub:** *PI Perspective*, quarterly. Journal. Contains treatment information and focuses on advocacy issues. *Price:* Free. • Also publishes information packet and fact sheets on treatments and standards of care.

★ 5465 ★ Project Magic (PM)
Kansas Rehabilitation Hospital
1504 SW 8 St.
Topeka, KS 66606
Phone: (913)235-6600 **Free:** 888-221-8199
Website: http://www.dcopperfield.com
Julie DeJean, Dir.

Fnded: 1982. **Desc:** Provides information and facilitates communication between magicians, occupational therapists, and patients with physical, psychosocial, and developmental disabilities. Created by television magician David Copperfield, the project works to rehabilitate patients by teaching them magic tricks instead of, or in addition to, traditional therapy techniques. Seeks to motivate patients to develop new skills and improve their self-image by demonstrating magical tricks. Tricks such as sleight-of-hand teach physical dexterity and mental puzzles help people to improve memory, concentration, and the ability to think sequentially. Provides interested magicians and occupational therapists with information and written material on the therapeutic value of magic for disabled persons. Sponsors educational seminars and workshops for rehabilitation facilities and health professionals. **Pub:** *David Copperfield's Project Magic Booklet*, periodic.

★ 5466 ★ Project Renewal
200 Varick St., 9th Fl.
New York, NY 10014
Phone: (212)620-0340 **Fax:** (212)243-4868
Website: http://www.projectrenewal.org
Mr. Christie Williams, Dir. Development

Fnded: 1967. **Desc:** Provides care for homeless adults in New York City. Funded by the New York City Department of Mental Health, Mental Retardation and Alcoholism Services, the U.S. Department of Housing and Urban Development, the New York State Office of Mental Health, the New York City Department of Homeless Services, the New York City Human Resources Administrative Divison of AIDS Service, the New York State Office of Alcoholism and Substance Abuse Services, private individuals, and corporations and foundations. Main components of the program are: a 48 bed alcohol detoxification facility for homeless male alcoholics; a 150 person alcoholism outpatient clinic for sober homeless alcoholics; a 20 person, year-long program offering therapy and work rehabilitation for homeless alcoholics and other substance abusers; Midtown Outreach Program, which sends medical and outreach teams to homeless people on the streets and in shelters. Offers training, job placement, and permanent supported housing. **Frmly:** (1995) Manhattan Bowery Corporation.

★ 5467 ★ Prosthetics Outreach Foundation (POF)
726 Broadway, Ste. 306
Seattle, WA 98122-4311
Phone: (206)726-1636 **Fax:** (206)726-1637
Email: pofsea@pofsea.org
Website: http://www.pofsea.org
Winfried Danke, Exec. Dir.

Fnded: 1989. **Desc:** Committed to sharing clinical and technical experience and expertise from working more than a decade in prosthetics. Seeks to help the developing world to walk again through the fitting of quality prostheses at low or no cost to amputees in need. **Pub:** Newsletter, annual. *Price:* Free. **Frmly:** (1993) Prosthetics Research Foundation.

★ 5468 ★ Prosthodontics Society of South Africa (PROSSA)
Private Bag X1
Houghton 2041, Republic of South Africa
Phone: 27 11 4845258 **Fax:** 27 11 6425718

Fnded: 1970. **Mem:** 250.

★ 5469 ★ Protein Foods and Nutrition Development Association of India (PFNDAI)
Mahalaxmi Chambers
22 Bhulabhai Desai Rd.
Bombay 400 026, Maharashtra, India
Phone: 91 22 24928858 **Fax:** 91 22 4938998
Email: pfndai@vsnl.com
Website: http://www.pfndai.com

Fnded: 1968. **Mem:** 78. **Nat'l Groups:** 48. **Reg. Groups:** 1. **State Groups:** 7. **Local Groups:** 2. **Lang(s):** English. **Desc:** Indian food industries. Collects, analyzes, and disseminates information on nutrition and food science and technology. Promotes balanced nutrition; identifies nutrient needs and food preferences through surveys; offers consultive services to national and international agencies for the development of low-cost nutritional supplements; offers project consultive services to the food industry. Assists government agencies in formulating food standards, regulations, and legislation; compiles statistics. Provides job placement assistance for food scientists. Conducts research. **Pub:** *Pfndai Bulletin*, monthly. Bulletin. Contains news items connected with food science and nutrition. • Papers. Contains research reports and proceedings. • Videos.

★ 5470 ★ Protestant Guild for Human Services (PGHS)
411 Waverley Oaks Rd., Ste. 104
Waltham, MA 02452-8405
Phone: (781)893-6000 **Fax:** (781)893-1171
Email: admin@protestantguild.org
Website: http://www.protestantguild.org
Edmund T. Hagerty, Exec. Dir.

Fnded: 1945. **Local Groups:** 2. **Desc:** Non-sectarian organization with a volunteer board and highly-trained professional staff dedicated to serving individuals with special needs. Provides a wide spectrum of services to children, adolescents and young adults with a variety of developmental disabilities. **Pub:** *Annual Report*, annual. • *PGHS News*, semiannual. Newsletter. **Frmly:** Protestant Guild for the Blind.

★ 5471 ★ Psi Beta
1027 Westbridge Ln.
Chattanooga, TN 37405
Phone: (423)265-6555 **Free:** 888-PSI-BETA
Fax: (423)265-0033
Email: carol@psibeta.org
Website: http://www.psibeta.org
Carol Tracy, Exec. Dir.

Fnded: 1981. **Mem:** 17,000. **Nat'l Groups:** 1. **Reg. Groups:** 5. **Local Groups:** 160. **Desc:** Honor society - community, and junior college psychology students. Participates in psychology conventions. Provides means for contact with professors in students' areas of interest. Conducts educational programs and sponsors national awards. Promotes excellence in scholarship, leadership, research and community service. **Pub:** *Psi Beta Chapter Handbook*, annual. Handbook. *Price:* $16/copy. • *Psi Beta Newsletter*, 3/year. Newsletter. *Price:* Included in membership fee; $7.50/year for nonmembers.

★ 5472 ★ Psi Chi, National Honor Society in Psychology
PO Box 709
825 Vine St.
Chattanooga, TN 37401-0709
Phone: (423)756-2044 **Fax:** (423)265-1529
Email: psichi@psichi.org
Website: http://www.psichi.org
Kay Wilson, Exec. Officer

Fnded: 1929. **Mem:** 420,000. **Reg. Groups:** 7. **Local Groups:** 1010. **Desc:** Honor society - men and women, psychology. **Pub:** *Chapter Handbook*, annual. Manual. • *Eye on Psi Chi*, quarterly. Magazine. *Price:* Included in membership dues. • *Psi Chi Journal of Undergraduate Research*, quarterly. Journal.

★ 5473 ★ Psoriasis Association
7 Milton St.
Northampton NN2 7JG, United Kingdom
Phone: 44 1604 711129 **Fax:** 44 1604 792894
Website: http://www.timewarp.demon.co.uk/psoriasis.html

Fnded: 1968. **Desc:** Provides up to date information and promotes self-help and support to people with psoriasis; works to raise standards of patient care and improves education about psoriasis with the public and healthcare professionals.

★ 5474 ★ Psoriasis Association - Australia (PA)
16 Musgrave St.
Kirra, QLD 4225, Australia
Phone: 61 7 55991166 **Fax:** 61 7 55991166
Email: info@psoriasus.org.au
Website: http://www.psoriasis.org.au

Fnded: 1983. **Mem:** 4,000. **Lang(s):** English. **Desc:** People with psoriasis. Seeks to improve the quality of life of people with psoriasis. Serves as a clearinghouse on psoriasis and its treatment; sponsors fundraising activities; makes available counseling services; maintains support group network for people with psoriasis. **Pub:** *Members' Circular*, bimonthly. Newsletter.

★ 5475 ★ Psoriasis Association of New Zealand (PANZI)
PO Box 44-007
Lower Hutt
Lower Hutt 6315, New Zealand
Phone: 64 4 5687139 **Fax:** 64 4 5650422
Email: psoriasis@xtra.co.nz
Website: http://www.everybody.co.nz/support/psoriasis.html

Fnded: 1994. **Mem:** 400. **Reg. Groups:** 4. **Lang(s):** English. **Desc:** People with psoriasis. Seeks to improve the quality of life of people with psoriasis; promotes improved understanding of psoriasis and its treatment. Serves as a clearinghouse on psoriasis; assists people with psoriasis in locating support groups and services; sponsors educational programs for health care providers and the public. Holds two yearly national psoriasis awareness campaigns. **Pub:** *Psoriasis Association of New Zealand*. Brochure.

★ 5476 ★ Psoriasis Research Institute (PRI)
PO Box 208
Palo Alto, CA 94302-0208
Fax: (650)326-1262
Email: emf.pri@aol.com
Eugene M. Farber, MD, Pres.

Fnded: 1979. **Mem:** 15. **Desc:** Creates projects for the study, diagnosis, treatment, and eventual cure of psoriasis. Collects and disseminates information about psoriasis in an effort to advance the science of dermatology. Maintains Psoriasis Medical Center, which offers advanced therapeutic programs and equipment to treat all aspects of the disease. Offers counseling and biofeedback stress control for patients. Compiles statistics; conducts epidemiological study of psoriasis patients. Sponsors monthly selfhelp workshop for psoriasis patients utilizing audiovisual presentations, written materials, and discussions. **Pub:** *Conquering Psoriasis*. *Price:* $15 per copy. • *Psoriasis Medical Center*. Brochure. • *Psoriasis Newsletter*, 3/year. Newsletter. Contains innovative concepts in the treatment of psoriasis. *Price:* Free. • *Psoriasis Research Institute*. Pamphlet. • Also publishes research papers. **Frmly:** (1983) International Psoriasis Research Foundation.

★ 5477 ★ Psoriatric Arthropathy Alliance (PAA)
PO Box 111
Saint Albans AL2 3JQ, United Kingdom
Phone: 44 870 7703212 **Fax:** 44 870 7703212
Email: info@paalliance.org
Website: http://www.paalliance.org

Fnded: 1993. **Lang(s):** English. **Desc:** Individuals with psoriatic arthritis and its associated skin disorder, psoriasis. Seeks to "protect, serve, and respect the interests and rights of people who have or might become susceptible to psoriatic arthritis." Conducts educational programs to raise public awareness of psoriatic arthritis and related disorders; provides support and assistance to people with psoriatic arthritis and their families; sponsors advocacy programs benefiting members. **Pub:** *Psoriatic Care Fact File*. • *Skin 'N' Bones Connection*, semiannual. Pamphlets.

★ 5478 ★ PSRC of America
200 Madison Ave., Ste. 2108
New York, NY 10016
Phone: (212)686-9147 **Fax:** (212)779-9307
Email: cwielk@psrc-of-america.org
Website: http://www.psrc-of-america.org
Carol A. Wielk, Exec. Dir.

Fnded: 1977. **Desc:** Physicians, nurses, health care administrators, and consumers. Monitors the quality, appropriateness, and cost of health care given to patients in hospitals, ambulatory clinics, nursing facilities, and physicians' offices. Carries out work on behalf of managed care companies, health care institutions and facilities, insurance carriers and governmental entities. **Pub:** *Informational Health Care Bulletin*, periodic. **Frmly:** (1999) Professional Standards Review Council of America.

★ 5479 ★ Psychiatric Nurses Association of Ireland
2 Gardiner Pl.
Dublin 1, Ireland
Phone: 353 1 8746793 **Fax:** 353 1 8740315

Fnded: 1971. **Mem:** 4,700. **Reg. Groups:** 7. **Local Groups:** 32. **Desc:** Psychiatric nurses in Ireland. Seeks to advance the study and practice of psychiatric nursing. Encourages professional advancement for psychiatric nurses. Liaises with the Department of Health, Department of Environment, Health Boards, and Hospitals. **Pub:** *Psychiatric Nursing*, 3/year. Journal.

★ 5480 ★ Psychiatric Rehabilitation Services (PRS)
500 W Annandale Rd.
Falls Church, VA 22046
Phone: (703)536-9000 **Fax:** (703)533-9858
Email: pstilton@prsinc.org
Website: http://www.prsinc.org

Fnded: 1963. **Desc:** Working to help people with serious mental illness develop the skills and resources to recover and live satisfying and more self-sufficient lives in the community.

★ 5481 ★ Psychoanalytic Research Society
c/o Joseph Turkel
6 W 77th St., Ste. 1B
New York, NY 10024
Phone: (212)787-4092
Email: joeturkel@aol.com
Website: http://www.columbia.edu/~hc137/prs/
Harold Cook, Pres.

Desc: Promotes psychoanalytic research of an empirical, theoretical and clinical nature, including the planning and conducting of psychoanalytic research and dissemination of findings. **Pub:** *Bulletin of the Psychoanalytic Research Society*. Bulletin.

★ 5482 ★ Psychohistory Forum (PF)
627 Dakota Trail
Franklin Lakes, NJ 07417
Phone: (201)891-7486
Email: pelovitz@aol.com
Website: http://cliospsyche.org
Paul H. Elovitz, PhD, Dir.

Fnded: 1983. **Mem:** 100. **Desc:** Psychologists, psychiatrists, Psychotherapists, social workers, historians, psychohistorians, and laypeople having a scholarly interest in the integration of depth psychology and history. (Psychohistory is the study of psychobiography, group process, the mechanisms of defense, the history of childhood, creativity, dreams, and the difference between stated intention and actual behavior). Seeks to further psychohistory through the exchange of information. Conducts bimonthly workshops on topics related to psychohistory and training seminars on dream analysis, innovation, teaching, and methodology. Aids individuals in psychohistorical research. Holds lecture series. lecture series. lecture series. **Pub:** *Clio's Psyche: Understanding the Why of Culture Current Events, History and Society*, quarterly. Journal. *Price:* included in membership dues; $25 for nonmembers in U.S.; $35 for nonmembers outside U.S.; $48 for nonmembers in U.S. for 2 years. • *Immigrant Experience: Personal Narrative and Psychological Analysis*. Monograph. *Price:* $58 for nonmembers outside U.S. for 2 years.

★ 5483 ★ Psychological Society Ireland
CX House
2A Corn Exchange Pl.
Poolbeg St.
Dublin 2, Ireland
Phone: 353 1 6717122 **Fax:** 353 1 6717048
Email: psihq@eircom.net
Website: http://www.psihq.org

Fnded: 1970. **Mem:** 1,600. **Desc:** Strives to advance psychology as a pure and applied science. Maintains a code of ethics and standards of conduct. Provides professional diploma schemes.

★ 5484 ★ Psychological Society of South Africa (PsySSA)
POB 66083
Broadway 2020, Republic of South Africa
Phone: 27 11 6169373 **Fax:** 27 11 6169377
Email: psyssa@psyssa.com
Website: http://www.psyssa.com

Fnded: 1994. **Mem:** 2,500. **Reg. Groups:** 5. **Desc:** Promotes the common interests of members nationally and internationally while advances psychology as a science, profession and as a means of promoting well being. **Pub:** *South African Journal of Psychology*, quarterly. Journal.

★ 5485 ★ Psychology of Religion
c/o Nancy S. Thurston
Department of Psychology
George Fox University
414 N Meridian St.
Newberg, OR 97132-2697
Fax: (503)538-8383
Dr. Nancy Thurston, Sec.

Fnded: 1948. **Mem:** 1,350. **Desc:** A division of the American Psychological Association. Seeks to encourage and accelerate research, theory, and practice in the psychology of religion and related areas. Facilitates the dissemination of data on religious and allied issues and on the integration of these data with current psychological research, theory, and practice. **Pub:** *Psychology of Religion–Newsletter*, quarterly. Newsletter. Contains articles, interviews, book reviews, and announcements focusing on psychology and religion. *Price:* Free to members; $5/year to nonmembers. **Frmly:** (1971) American Catholic Psychological Association; (1993) Psychologists Interested in Religious Issues.

★ 5486 ★ Psychology Society (PS)
100 Beekman St.
New York, NY 10038-1810
Phone: (212)285-1872
Dr. Pierre C. Haber, Exec. Dir.

Fnded: 1960. **Mem:** 4,600. **Reg. Groups:** 5. **Local Groups:** 4. **Desc:** Professional membership is limited to psychologists who have a doctorate and are certified/licensed as such in the state where they practice. Associate membership is intended for teachers and researchers as well as persons who will attain professional status shortly. Seeks to further the use of psychology in therapy, family and social problems, behavior modification, and treatment of drug abusers and prisoners. Encourages the use of psychology in the solution of social and political conflicts. Operates an information bureau to answer inquiries of authors and media. Sponsors biennial overseas trip to enable members and their spouses to observe other programs and institutions. Collaborates with other associations. Evaluates programs in the use of psychology. Recommends legislation; appears in court cases where issues of mental health occur as expert and impartial witness. **Pub:** *PS Newsletter*, monthly. Newsletter. Includes book reviews, calendar of events, and research updates. *Price:* Included in membership dues. • *PS Quarterly*. Journal. *Price:* Included in membership dues. • *Psychology Society–Membership List*, biennial. Membership Directory.

★ 5487 ★ Psychometric Society (PS)
c/o Dr. Terry Ackerman
UNCG
207 Curry Bldg.
Greensboro, NC 27402-6171
Phone: (336)334-3474 **Fax:** (336)334-4120
Email: taackerm@uncg.edu
Website: http://www.psychometricsociety.org/
Dr. Terry Ackerman, Sec.

Fnded: 1935. **Mem:** 2,200. **Desc:** Persons interested in development of quantitative models for psychological phenomena and quantitative methodology in the social and behavioral sciences. **Pub:** *Psychometrika*, quarterly. Journal. Covers statistical models of psychological phenomena. Includes book and software reviews. *Price:* included in membership dues; $100 for organizations and nonmembers.

★ 5488 ★ Psychonomic Society (PS)
1710 Fortview Rd.
Austin, TX 78704
Phone: (512)462-2442 **Fax:** (512)462-1101
Email: cinnamon@psychonomic.org
Website: http://www.psychonomic.org
Robert F. Lorch, Jr., Sec. -Treas.

Fnded: 1959. **Mem:** 2,500. **Desc:** Persons qualified to conduct and supervise scientific research in psychology or allied sciences; members must hold a Ph.D. degree or its equivalent and must have published significant research other than the doctoral dissertation. Promotes the communication of scientific research in psychology and allied sciences. **Pub:** *Animal Learning and Behavior*, quarterly. Journal. Covers animal learning, motivation, emotion, and behavior, including classical and operant conditioning, sensory effects, and imprinting. *Price:* $36/year for individuals; $78/year for institutions. • *Behavior Research Methods, Instruments, and Computers*, quarterly. Journal. Contains articles in the areas of methods, techniques, and instrumentation of research in experimental psychology. *Price:* $46/year for individuals; $99/year for institutions. • *Cognitive, Affective, & Behavioral Neuroscience*, quarterly. Journal. • *Memory and Cognition*, bimonthly. Journal. Covers human memory and learning, conceptual processes, thinking, decision making, and skilled performance. *Price:* $50/year for individuals; $107/year for institutions. • *Perception and Psychophysics*, monthly. Journal. Provides articles on sensory processes, perception, and psychophysics, including reports of experimental investigations. *Price:* $68/year for individuals; $149/year for institutions. • *Program of the Annual Meeting of the Psychonomic Society*. Schedule and abstracts. *Price:* Included in membership dues; $7/copy to nonmembers in North America; $8.50/copy to nonmembers outside North America. • *Psychobiology*, quarterly. Journal. Encompasses all of the allied fields of the neurosciences relating directly to behavior; includes experimental, review, and theoretical papers. *Price:* $36/year for individuals; $73/year for institutions. • *Psychonomic Bulletin and Review*, quarterly. Journal. Contains short reports and full length review articles covering all areas of experimental psychology. *Price:* $42/year for individuals; $89/year for institutions.

★ 5489 ★ Psychotherapy Network
7705 13th St. NW
Washington, DC 20012
Phone: (202)829-2452 **Fax:** (202)726-7983
Email: info@psychnetworker.org
Website: http://www.psychotherapynetworker.org
Richard Simon, Dir.

Fnded: 1976. **Mem:** 65,000. **Desc:** Promotes the exchange of ideas and information among psychotherapists. **Pub:** *Psychotherapy Networker*, bimonthly. Magazine. Contains case studies, calendar of events, listing of employment opportunities, and book and movie reviews. *Price:* $24/year for individuals; $30 outside U.S. **Frmly:** (2003) Family Therapy Network.

★ 5490 ★ Public Citizen Health Research Group (PCHRG)
1600 20th St. NW
Washington, DC 20009
Phone: (202)588-1000 **Fax:** (202)588-7796
Email: member@citizen.org
Website: http://www.citizen.org/hrg
Joan Claybrook, Pres.

Fnded: 1971. **Desc:** Works on issues of health care delivery, workplace safety and health, drug regulation, food additives, medical device safety, and environmental influences on health. Petitions or sues federal agencies on consumers' behalf, testifies before Congress on health matters, and monitors the enforcement of health and safety legislation. Publicizes important health findings; makes available to the public a broad spectrum of research and consumer action materials in the form of books and reports. **Pub:** *Health Letter*, monthly. Newsletter. Consumer newsletter reporting on health and health policy issues. *Price:* $18/year. • *Health Research Group List of Publications*, annual. • *Worst Pills, Best Pills News*, monthly. Newsletter. Consumer newsletter reporting an drug safety issues. *Price:* $20/year.

★ 5491 ★ Public Health Association
58 Langdale Rd.
Manchester M14 5PN, United Kingdom
Email: info@dukpha.org.uk

Fnded: 1989. **Mem:** 1,000. **Reg. Groups:** 4. **State Groups:** 3. **Desc:** Aims to promote public health, by bringing people together across UK, especially tackling inequalities.

★ 5492 ★ Public Health Association of Australia (PHAA)
PO Box 319
Curtin, ACT 2605, Australia
Phone: 61 2 62852373 **Fax:** 61 2 62825438
Email: phaa@phaa.net.au
Website: http://www.phaa.net.au

Fnded: 1990. **Mem:** 1,800. **State Groups:** 7. **Lang(s):** English. **Desc:** Individuals, corporations, government agencies, and community-based organizations from more than 40 public health related disciplines. Provides a forum for the exchange of ideas, knowledge, and information on public health. Advocates for public health policy, development, research, and training. **Pub:** *Australian and New Zealand Journal of Public Health*, bimonthly. Journal.

★ 5493 ★ Public Health Committee of the Council of Europe
Council of Europe
F-67075 Strasbourg Cedex, France
Phone: 33 3 88412000 **Fax:** 33 3 88412745
Email: infopoint@coe.int
Website: http://www.coe.int/T/E/Social_Cohesion/soc-sp/

Desc: A steering committee of the Council of Europe. Representatives of national ministries of health. Coordinates activities of the committees of experts assembled by CE under the Partial Agreement in the Social and Pubic Health Field. The goal of the Agreement is to assist in the development of uniform legislation in participating countries in the areas of public health and consumer protection.

★ 5494 ★ Public Health Foundation (PHF)
1220 L St. NW, Ste. 350
Washington, DC 20005
Phone: (202)898-5600 **Fax:** (202)898-5609
Email: info@phf.org
Website: http://www.phf.org/
Ronald Bialek, MPP, Pres.

Fnded: 1970. **Desc:** Dedicated to achieving healthy communities through research, training, and technical assistance. **Pub:** *PHF E-News*. Newsletter. Promotes projects, products and plans. *Price:* Free.

★ 5495 ★ Puerto Rico Association of Pediatric Surgeons
PO Box 10426
Caparra Hts. Station
San Juan, PR 00922-0426
Phone: (787)777-3535 **Fax:** (787)720-6103
Email: titolugo@coqui.net
Website: http://home.coqui.net/titolugo/praps.htm

Fnded: 1997. **Desc:** General pediatric surgeons. Strives to improve the care of newborns, infants, children, adolescent and young adults with surgically related diseases. Provides educational forum, research and teaching of surgery, consults and recommends programs and policy statements.

★ 5496 ★ Puerto Rico Society of Microbiologists (PRSM)
PO Box 360175
San Juan, PR 00936-0175
Phone: (787)751-3057 **Fax:** (787)759-8559
Email: prsm40@hotmail.com
Website: http://www.asmusa.org/branch/brpr/objsmpr1b.htm

Fnded: 1957. **Desc:** Professionals in the field of microbiology. Aims to promote scientific interest in microbiology and to aid in the development and progress of professionals in the field. Organizes conferences, workshops, symposiums and conventions, sponsors student chapters. **Pub:** *PRSM-News*. Bulletin.

★ 5497 ★ Pull-thru Network (PTN)
2312 Savoy St.
Hoover, AL 35226-1528
Phone: (205)978-2930
Email: info@pullthrough.org
Website: http://www.pullthrough.org/
Bonnie McElroy, Pres.

Fnded: 1988. **Mem:** 550. **Desc:** Families, individuals, and professionals dedicated to children born with congenital defects of the lower intestine. Provides support to parents of children who've had or will have a "pull-through" type of surgery to correct a congenital defect such as imperforate anus, or Hirschsprung's disease, or any other conditions which may require an ostomy or cause bladder or bowel incontinence. Conducts educational programs. Affiliated with the United Ostomy Association. **Pub:** *Pull-Thru Network News*, quarterly. Newsletter.

★ 5498 ★ Pulmonary Hypertension Association (PHA)
850 Sligo Ave., No. 800
Silver Spring, MD 20910
Phone: 800-748-7274 **Fax:** (301)565-3994
Email: pha@phassociation.org
Website: http://www.phassociation.org
Rino Aldrighetti, Exec. Dir.

Fnded: 1990. **Mem:** 4,500. **Local Groups:** 100. **Desc:** Patients with pulmonary hypertension (PH) and primary pulmonary hypertension (PPH); families and physicians of patients; researchers. Provides fellowship and educational support for members and the public on PH and PPH, including current research and findings, early detection, resource organizations, organ transplantation, and support networks. Conducts support group meetings. Funds medical research **Pub:** *Advances in Pulmonary Hypertension*, quarterly. Journal. Medical journal. *Price:* Free. • *Pathlight*, quarterly. Newsletter. *Price:* $25 included in membership dues. • *Patients Guide to Pulmonary Hypertension, 2nd Ed.*, semiannual. Book. *Price:* $25; included in membership dues. • *Persistent Voices*, semiannual. Newsletter. Electronic newsletter. *Price:* Free; included in membership dues. • *PHA News*, biweekly. Newsletter. Electronic newsletter. *Price:* Free. **Frmly:** (1998) United Patients Association for Pulmonary Hypertension.

★ 5499 ★ Purine Research Society
c/o Tahma Metz
5424 Beech Ave.
Bethesda, MD 20814-1730
Phone: (301)530-0354 **Fax:** (301)564-9597
Email: purine@erols.com
Website: http://www2.dgsys.com/~purine/
Tahma Metz, Exec. Dir.

Fnded: 1986. **Desc:** Dedicated to funding research and treatment of diseases resulting from errors in purine metabolism, specifically purine autism, the largest single subgroup of autism. As with other metabolic diseases, purine disorders are caused by a defective gene that results in the production of an enzyme with too little or too much catalytic activity. Purine metabolic diseases include gout, Lesch-Nyhan syndrome, purine autism, ADA deficiency and others. We are supporting research to find the defective enzyme(s) responsible for purine overproduction in purine autism, particularly, and to find effective screening and treatment methods, including newborn screening, so that symptoms will never occur. **Pub:** Brochure. *Price:* Free. • Bulletin. **Frmly:** (1995) Purine 24, Inc.

★ 5500 ★ PXE International
c/o Sharon F. Terry
23 Mountain St.
Sharon, MA 02067-2234
Phone: (781)784-3817 **Fax:** (781)784-6672
Email: pxe@pxe.org
Website: http://www.pxe.org
Sharon F. Terry, Exec. Dir.

Fnded: 1995. **Mem:** 4,000. **Nat'l Groups:** 22. **Reg. Groups:** 20. **Desc:** Dedicated to supporting those affected by Pseudoxanthomas elasticum (PXE) and to research into its causes, treatments, and cure. (Pseudoxanthomas elasticum is a heritable connective tissue disorder causing calcification of connective tissue, potentially affecting the skin, arteries, gastrointestinal tissue, and the retina.) Provides information and support to patients, their families, and clinicians on diagnosis, effects, and treatment. Through a consortium of researchers worldwide, supports research by providing to researchers monetary grants and samples from its confidential Blood and Tissue Bank. Initiates and conducts epidemiological studies and other research. **Pub:** *MemberGram*, quarterly. Newsletter. Contains information on PXE; patient group and organization activities; research updates; profiles of patients, volunteers, and researchers. • Bulletin, periodic.

★ 5501 ★ Qualified Private Medical Practitioners and Hospitals' Association (QPMPA)
Floor V
Vallamattam Estate
Ravipuram, M.G. Rd.
Kochi 682 035, India
Phone: 91 484 2442121 **Fax:** 91 484 444344
Website: http://www.qpmpa.com

Fnded: 1972. **Mem:** 1,564. **Desc:** Promotes the private medical practitioners profession and hospitals industry.

★ 5502 ★ Quit
Ground Fl.
211 Old St.
London EC1V 9NR, United Kingdom
Phone: 44 207 2511551 **Fax:** 44 207 2511661
Email: info@quit.org.uk
Website: http://www.quit.org.uk

Fnded: 1926. **Lang(s):** Kurdish, Turkish. **Desc:** Offers information, advice and support to people who want to stop smoking. **Pub:** Brochures. Leaflets to help smokers quit.

★ 5503 ★ R. A. Bloch Cancer Foundation
4400 Main St., Ste. 500
Kansas City, MO 64111
Phone: (816)932-8453 **Free:** 800-433-0464
Fax: (816)931-7486
Email: hotline@hrbloch.com
Website: http://www.blochcancer.org
Donna O'Connor, Contact

Fnded: 1980. **Desc:** Sponsors the Cancer Hot Line, a support group that matches cancer patients with volunteers who are survivors of the same type of cancer. Also offers resource information and provides the book "Fighting Cancer" free of charge to anyone dealing with cancer. **Pub:** *Cancer. . .There's Hope.* Book. • *Cancer Hot Line News*, quarterly. • *Fighting Cancer.* Book. • *Guide for Cancer Supporters.* Book. **Frmly:** (1989) Cancer Connection.

★ 5504 ★ Rabbinic Center for Research and Counseling (RCRC)
128 E Dudley Ave.
Westfield, NJ 07090
Phone: (908)233-0419 **Fax:** (908)233-6459
Email: ihf@rcrconline.org
Website: http://www.rcrconline.org
Rabbi Irwin H. Fishbein, Dir.

Fnded: 1970. **Desc:** Individuals interested in the marriage relationship and marriage counseling with special emphasis on interfaith marriage. Purpose is to provide courses, workshops and counseling for intermarried couples, and to establish and operate outpatient clinics for treatment of emotional and mental disabilities by the application of both psychotherapeutic knowledge and religious guidance. Conducts research; maintains list of rabbis who officiate at interfaith marriages; distributes literature.

★ 5505 ★ The Radiance Technique International Association
PO Box 40570
Saint Petersburg, FL 33743
Phone: (727)347-2106 **Fax:** (727)347-2106
Email: trtia@aol.com
Website: http://www.trtia.org
Shoshanna Shay, Dir. Office Services

Fnded: 1980. **Desc:** Protects and preserves the science known as The Radiance Technique, an Authentic Reiki "science of universal energy which harmonizes and aligns the mind-body-spirit dynamic." Provides a network for those interested in The Radiance Technique. Maintains speakers' bureau. Compiles statistics and conducts research on the effectiveness of The Radiance Technique. Creates and promotes Radiant Peace Projects and sponsors the International Day of Radiant Peace on June 22 every year. **Pub:** *TRTIA Journal*, 3/year. Newsletter. *Price:* Included in membership dues. **Frmly:** (1980) American Reiki Association; (1987) American-International Reiki Association; (1997) Radiance Technique Association International; (1998) Radiance Technique and Peace Association International.

★ 5506 ★ Radiation Therapy Oncology Group (RTOG)
1101 Market St., 14th Fl.
Philadelphia, PA 19107
Phone: (215)574-3189 **Free:** 800-277-5463
Fax: (215)923-1737
Email: tmckeough@phila.acr.org
Website: http://www.rtog.org
Tim McKeough, Admin.

Fnded: 1971. **Mem:** 290. **Desc:** Clinical radiation therapy investigative centers united to conduct cooperative clinical trials and studies to improve the care of patients with cancer. Maintains 50 committees. **Pub:** *RTOG Report.* Reprint.

★ 5507 ★ Radical Caucus in Psychiatry (RCP)
c/o Carl Cohen, M.D.
SUNY Downstate Med. Center
Box 1203
450 Clarkson Ave.
Brooklyn, NY 11203
Phone: (718)270-2907 **Fax:** (718)287-0337
Email: cohen_c@hscbklyn.edu
Carl Cohen, MD, Coord.

Fnded: 1969. **Mem:** 75. **Desc:** Members of the American Psychiatric Association and individuals interested in mental health issues who take a politically progressive stand in psychiatry. Objective is to examine the socioeconomic and sociopolitical aspects of mental health issues from a left-oriented perspective. Areas of study have included a critical analysis of biological psychiatry, patient rights, and psychiatric treatment of mental patients in Latin America. Presents research findings to professionals and laypersons. Maintains speakers' bureau. **Pub:** Newsletter, annual.

★ 5508 ★ Radical Psychology Network (RadPsyNet)
c/o Colleen Loomis
VA/Stanford School of Medicine
VA Palo Alto Health Care System
Menlo Park Division
795 Willow Rd.
Menlo Park, CA 94025
Phone: (650)493-5000
Email: colleenloomis@yahoo.com
Website: http://www.radpsynet.org/
Colleen Loomis, Coord.

Fnded: 1993. **Mem:** 322. **Nat'l Groups:** 34. **Desc:** Strives to bring about social justice and create a society better able to meet human needs. **Pub:** *RadPsyNews.* Newsletter. • Papers.

★ 5509 ★ Radiological Society of North America (RSNA)
820 Jorie Blvd.
Oak Brook, IL 60523-2251
Phone: (630)571-2670 **Fax:** (630)571-7837
Email: informat@rsna.org
Website: http://www.rsna.org
Lise Steg Swanson, Account Exec.

Fnded: 1915. **Mem:** 35,000. **Desc:** Radiologists and scientists in fields closely related to radiology. Promotes study and practical application of radiology, radium, electricity, and other branches of physics related to medical science. **Pub:** *Radiographics*, bimonthly. Features pictorial presentations of selected scientific exhibits from the society's annual meeting. Includes case studies. • *Radiology*, monthly. Journal. Covers diagnostic radiology, neuroradiology, nuclear medicine, pediatric radiology, therapeutic radiology, cardiovascular radiology, and ultrasound. • *RSNA Educational Materials*, annual. Catalog. Lists video/slide set series for CME credits. • Membership Directory, annual. **Frmly:** (1918) Western Roentgen Society.

★ 5510 ★ Radiology Business Management Association (RBMA)
65 Enterprise
Aliso Viejo, CA 92656
Phone: 888-224-RBMA **Fax:** (949)330-6461
Email: info@rbma.org
Website: http://www.rbma.org
Sharon Urch, Exec. Dir.

Fnded: 1968. **Mem:** 1,600. **Reg. Groups:** 4. **State Groups:** 50. **Local Groups:** 10. **Desc:** Business managers for private radiology groups; corporate members include: vendors of equipment, services, or supplies. Purposes are to improve business administration of radiologists' practices to better serve patients and the medical profession; and to provide opportunities for professional development and recognition. Offers extensive educational and networking opportunities and informal placement service. Maintains information services emphasizing those aspects unique to the business of radiology. **Pub:** *Radiology Business Management Association–Bulletin*, bimonthly. Newsletter. Covers organizational topics, industry trends, and legislative developments affecting the private practice of radiology; includes annual index. *Price:* Included in membership dues; $100/year for nonmembers. • *Radiology Business Management Association–HIPAA Bulletin*, monthly. Bulletin. A radiology resource for education, implementation and compliance. • *Radiology Business Management Association–Membership Directory*, annual. Membership Directory. **Frmly:** (1990) Radiologists Business Managers Association.

★ 5511 ★ Radix Institute (RI)
3212 Monte Vista, NE
Albuquerque, NM 87106-2120
Free: 888-777-2349
Email: information@radix.org
Website: http://www.radix.org
Dale Cummings, Dir.

Fnded: 1963. **Mem:** 60. **Desc:** Educational and scientific organization dedicated to studying the creative process in nature as described by Wilhelm Reich. Reich, a psychoanalyst who began his work with Sigmund Freud, discovered and described the existence of the "muscular armor," or how blocked emotion is held in the chronic patterns of tension in the body. The Radix flow is experienced as feeling or emotion and is expressed in spontaneous movements of the body. Offers classes, workshops, and individual sessions in "Education in Feeling." Conducts teacher training and programs for professionals and research on the nature of the Radix. training and programs for professionals and research on the nature of the Radix. **Pub:** *List of Radix Teachers Worldwide*, annual. *Price:* Free. • *The Radix Journal*, biennial. Journal. *Price:* $26/year. • *Radix Newsletter*, 3/year. Newsletter. • Also publishes books and a newsletter. **Frmly:** Interscience Research Institute.

★ 5512 ★ Rainbow Celebration of Hope Network
16507 Parkridge Ct.
Houston, TX 77053
Phone: (713)326-8571
Email: rainchope@aol.com
Shelia Robey-Bailey, Contact

Fnded: 1999. **Mem:** 10. **Desc:** Provides spiritual and educational resources for individuals on dialysis; also provides means of support. **Pub:** Newsletter, annual. Covers past and future events and organizations.

★ 5513 ★ Rational Recovery Systems (RRS)
PO Box 800
Lotus, CA 95651
Phone: (530)621-2667 **Free:** 800-303-CURE
Fax: (530)622-4296
Email: rr@rational.org
Website: http://www.rational.org
Jack Trimpey, Pres.

Fnded: 1986. **Desc:** Rational Recovery means self-recovery from substance addiction through planned abstinence. Leads to complete abstinence from substance abuse using Addictive Voice Recognition Technique (AVRT). **Pub:** *AVRT Live (Addictive Voice Recognition Technique)*. Videos. Complete 12-video VHS set. *Price:* $749. • *Exploring AVRT*. Audiotapes. *Price:* $50. • *Greater Expectations*. Video. *Price:* $89.95. • *Journal of Rational Recovery*, quarterly. Journal. Contains articles by recovered addicts of alcohol, drugs, and eating disorders and others. *Price:* $36/year. • *Rational Recovery/The New Cure for Substance Addiction. Price:* $14.95. • *The Small Book: A Revolutionary Alternative for Overcoming Alcohol and Drug Dependence. Price:* $14.95. • *Taming the Feast Beast. Price:* $14.95. • *There's Nothing Wrong With You*. Video. *Price:* $89.95.

★ 5514 ★ Ray of Hope (ROH)
PO Box 2323
Iowa City, IA 52244
Phone: (319)337-9890 **Fax:** (319)337-9890
Email: rayofhopeinc@juno.com
E. Betsy Ross, Exec. Dir.

Fnded: 1977. **Mem:** 25. **Nat'l Groups:** 10. **Reg. Groups:** 13. **State Groups:** 2. **Local Groups:** 1. **Desc:** Selfhelp organization offering support for coping with sucide, loss, and grief. Organizes suicide survivor support groups. Offers training courses and consultation on bereavement and suicide postvention. Telephone counseling (pre-arranged). **Pub:** *After Suicide: A Unique Grief Process*. Booklet. *Price:* $5.95 plus $1.50 first book, and .25 each addition. • *Life After Suicide: A Ray of Hope for Those Left Behind*. Book. Guide for suicide survivor's bereavement process. *Price:* $27.95 plus $3 postage and .50 each additional book. • *Survivorship After Suicide*. Video. *Price:* $75 postage included.

★ 5515 ★ Raynaud's and Scleroderma Association (RSAT)
112 Crewe Rd.
Alsager
Cheshire ST7 2JA, United Kingdom
Phone: 44 1270 872776 **Fax:** 44 1270 883556
Email: info@raynauds.org.uk
Website: http://www.raynauds.demon.co.uk

Fnded: 1982. **Mem:** 8,000. **Nat'l Groups:** 1. **Reg. Groups:** 4. **Lang(s):** English. **Desc:** Individuals afflicted with Raynaud's Disease or scleroderma; concerned medical professionals. Raynaud's Disease is marked by interruption of blood flow to the extremities, primarily the toes and fingers but can include the ears and nose, due to spasmodic contraction of small blood vessels; in severe cases this phenomenon is often noted in individual suffering from scleroderma, which affects the blood vessels, immune system and connective tissue. Encourages better communication among doctors and patients and provides mutual support among those with the condition. Strives to heighten public awareness on Raynaud's Disease and scleroderma. Conducts fundraising activities to help finance research. **Pub:** *Raynaud's Association Newsletter*, quarterly. Newsletter. • Books, periodic. • Handbooks, periodic. **Frmly:** (1990) Raynaud's Association Trust.

★ 5516 ★ Re-Solv, the Society for the Prevention of Solvent and Volatile Substance Abuse (RS)
30A High St.
Stone ST15 8AW, United Kingdom
Phone: 44 1785 817885 **Fax:** 44 1785 813205
Email: information@re-solv.org
Website: http://www.re-solv.org

Fnded: 1984. **Mem:** 300. **Lang(s):** English. **Desc:** Promotes increased awareness on the part of parents, local authorities, retailers, and law enforcement officials of the problem of the "sniffing" of solvents and volatile substances. Acts as an information clearinghouse on solvent abuse. Liaises with other agencies, the Home Office, and other government bodies in the dissemination of information. Supports legislation that seeks to control solvent abuse. Provides videos and other materials for use in primary and secondary schools and by parents, teachers, doctors, social workers, retailers, and law enforcement personnel. doctors, social workers, retailers, and law enforcement personnel. doctors, social workers, retailers, and law enforcement personnel. **Pub:** *The Adolescent Epidemic*. Video. • *Chicken!*. Video. Video for young people; presents the story of how substance abuse affects the lives of young people and their families. • *Guide for the Carer*. Book.

★ 5517 ★ REACH: Association for Children with Hand or Arm Deficiency
PO Box 54
Helston
Cornwall TR13 8WD, United Kingdom
Phone: 44 845 1306225 **Fax:** 44 872 262098
Email: reach@reach.org.uk
Website: http://www.reach.org.uk

Fnded: 1978. **Mem:** 1,200. **Desc:** Aims to offer support to families of children with upper limb deficiency.

★ 5518 ★ Reach Ireland (RI)
Fair Stream
Hedge Rd.
Garristown
Dublin, Ireland
Phone: 353 1 8354953 **Fax:** 353 1 8427788
Email: reachorg@aol.com
Website: http://www.reach.org.uk

Fnded: 1990. **Mem:** 230. **Nat'l Groups:** 1. **Lang(s):** English, Irish. **Desc:** Individuals and organizations. Seeks to improve the quality of life of children with limb deficiencies and their families. Makes available support and services; conducts educational and advocacy campaigns. **Pub:** *Within Reach*, quarterly. Magazine.

★ 5519 ★ Reach Out for Youth with Ileitis and Colitis
84 Northgate Cir.
Melville, NY 11747-3042
Phone: (631)293-3102 **Fax:** (631)293-3103
Email: reachoutforyouth@reachoutforyouth.org
Website: http://www.reachoutforyouth.org
Susan Spellman, Exec. Dir.

Fnded: 1979. **Desc:** Works to provide support groups for families whose children have Inflammatory Bowel Disease (IBD). Provides educational and emotional support to patients and families; conducts fund-raising events; promotes research into the cause and treatment of IBD. **Pub:** *The Inner Circle*, quarterly. Newsletter. *Price:* Free. • *The Inside Story*. Brochure.

★ 5520 ★ Reach to Recovery
c/o American Cancer Society
1599 Clifton Rd.
PO Box 102454
Atlanta, GA 30368-2454
Free: 800-ACS-2345 **Fax:** (404)982-3691
Website: http://www.cancer.org/eprise/main/docroot/shr/content/shr_2.1_x_reach_to_recovery?sitearea=shr
Ena Wanless, Mgr. Breast Cancer Programs

Fnded: 1952. **Desc:** A peer support program for people with a personal concern about breast cancer; sponsored by the American Cancer Society. Trained volunteers provide support and information for people and help them meet the physical, emotional and cosmetic needs related to their disease and its treatment. Patient and volunteer may meet face to face or by telephone. Volunteers are able to provide support and up-to-date information, including literature for spouses, partners, children, other loved ones, and friends. **Pub:** *Reach to Recovery Program*. Brochure.

★ 5521 ★ Reclamation Inc.
2502 Waterford Dr.
San Antonio, TX 78217
Phone: (210)822-3569
Don H. Culwell, Dir.

Fnded: 1974. **Mem:** 20. **Local Groups:** 1. **Desc:** Former mental patients; interested others. Seeks to eliminate the stigma of mental illness and reclaim members' "human dignity." Serves as a voice for mental health patients in consumer, social, and political affairs. Helps members to live outside a hospital setting by providing assistance in the areas of resocialization, employment, and housing. Monitors media coverage; encourages "positive" presentations of mental health patients and increased coverage of mental health community service projects and events. **Pub:** *Positive Visibility*, quarterly. Newsletter. *Price:* included in membership dues.

★ 5522 ★ Recording for the Blind and Dyslexic (RFB)
20 Roszel Rd.
Princeton, NJ 08540
Phone: (609)452-0606 **Free:** 800-803-7201
Fax: (609)987-8116
Email: info@rfbd.org
Website: http://www.rfbd.org

Fnded: 1948. **Mem:** 40,000. **Reg. Groups:** 31. **Desc:** Provides library services, computerized books, books on audiotape, and other educational materials free of charge to individuals who are unable to read standard print because of a visual, physical, or perceptual disability. Materials are produced by 4800 volunteers at 31 recording studios throughout the U.S. Titles recorded supplement, but do not duplicate, those of the Library of Congress Talking Book program. **Pub:** *Disk Catalog*, quarterly. *Price:* $16/year. • *Recorded Catalog*, quarterly. *Price:* $16/year. • *Recording for the Blind–Annual Report*, annual. Annual Report. Includes financial statements for the fiscal year as well as highlights from the previous year. *Price:* Free. • *Recording for the Blind–Catalog Supplement*, periodic. • *RFB and D Impact*, quarterly. Newsletter. For donors, agencies, and schools serving the blind and print-disabled. *Price:* Free. **Frmly:** (1951) National Committee for Recording for the Blind; (2000) Recording for the Blind.

★ 5523 ★ Recovered Alcoholic Clergy Association (RACA)

Emmanuel Episcopal Church
498 Prince Ave.
Athens, GA 30601
Phone: (706)543-1294 **Fax:** (706)208-3790
Email: petercourtney@charter.net
Peter Courtney, Dir.

Fnded: 1968. **Mem:** 350. **Nat'l Groups:** 2. **Local Groups:** 100. **Desc:** Clergy in the Episcopal church orders and persons attending or teaching at Episcopal seminaries who have drinking problems. Recommends alcohol addiction treatment centers for members; trains individuals involved in confronting persons with drinking problems. Seeks to provide moral support to members; provides guidance to the families and/or colleagues of problem drinkers; maintains speakers' bureau. **Pub:** *No foolin*, monthly. Newsletter. • *RACA Directory*, annual. Directory. • Pamphlets.

★ 5524 ★ Recovered Medical Equipment for the Developing World (REMEDY)

c/o Darryl Rotman Kuperstock
333 Cedar St., 3-TMP
PO Box 208051
New Haven, CT 06520-8051
Phone: (203)737-5356 **Fax:** (203)785-6664
Email: remedy@yale.edu
Website: http://www.remedyinc.org/
Darryl Rotman Kuperstock, Exec. Dir.

Fnded: 1991. **Mem:** 300. **Desc:** Dedicated to achieving safe, efficient, and cost effective methods for recovering opened, but unused materials from hospital operating rooms. Provides teaching problem solving, and networking assistance. Sponsors the Agencies for International Relief E-mail (AIRE-mail) program that works to quickly fulfill the needs of urgent situations and special circumstances. **Pub:** *Remedy Newsletter*, semiannual. Newsletter. *Price:* Free.

★ 5525 ★ Recovery Inc.

802 N Dearborn St.
Chicago, IL 60610
Phone: (312)337-5661 **Fax:** (312)337-5756
Email: inquiries@recovery-inc.org
Website: http://www.recovery-inc.org
Shirley Sachs, Exec. Dir.

Fnded: 1937. **Mem:** 10,000. **Local Groups:** 800. **Desc:** Community mental health organization offering a self-help method developed by the neuropsychiatrist Dr. Abraham A. Low at the Psychiatric Institute of the University of Illinois Medical School. (The Recovery method is a system of techniques for controlling temperamental behavior and changing attitudes toward nervous symptoms and fears.) **Pub:** *Recovery Reporter*, bimonthly. Newsletter. *Price:* Included in membership dues. • *Recovery, Inc. Reports*. Newsletter. For professionals. • *Recovery, The Association of Nervous and Former Mental Patients–Directory*, annual. Directory. Lists the location and time of group meetings in the United States, Canada, and abroad. *Price:* $3 available to members only. **AKA:** Recovery, Inc., The Association of Nervous and Former Mental Patients.

★ 5526 ★ Recovery Ministries

876 Market Way
Clarkston, GA 30021
Phone: (516)997-0476
Virginia M. King, Exec. Dir.

Fnded: 1982. **Mem:** 600. **Desc:** A network of individuals, parishes, and Episcopal church diocesan committees addressing the issue of alcohol and drug use and addiction. Seeks to involve the Episcopal church in alcohol and other drug addiction issues. Serves as a resource clearinghouse. Sponsors annual Alcohol-Drug Awareness Sunday to provide information to congregations. **Pub:** *Alcohol-Drug Awareness Sunday Information Packet*, annual. Educational material. *Price:* $6. • *The NECAD News*, quarterly. *Price:* available to members only. • Brochures. • Newsletter. **Frmly:** (1997) National Episcopal Coalition on Alcohol and Drugs.

★ 5527 ★ Reflex Sympathetic Dystrophy Association of America (RSDSA)

PO Box 502
Milford, CT 06460
Phone: (203)877-3790 **Free:** 877-662-7737
Fax: (203)882-8362
Email: jwbroatch@aol.com
Website: http://www.rsds.org
James Broatch, MSW, Exec. Dir.

Fnded: 1984. **Mem:** 4,784. **Local Groups:** 100. **Desc:** People with Reflex Sympathetic Dystrophy Syndrome, also known as Complex Regional Pain Syndrome Type I and Type II; health care professionals treating RSDS patients. (RSDS is a disorder of the autonomic nervous system whose onset is usually preceded by a minor trauma such as a muscle sprain; symptoms of RSDS include severe pain, loss of muscle motion and use, swelling, skin and nail changes, and softening of the bones in affected areas.) Promotes increased awareness of RSDS among health care professionals and the public; conducts media campaigns; maintains national network of physicians involved in RSDS treatment and research. Encourages and supports RSDS research; has a national data bank for the coordination of RSDS research and treatment information. Aids in the formation of support groups for people with RSDS; develops in-service programs and seminars for use at hospitals and educational institutions. Makes available referral services. Conducts educational programs; maintains speakers' bureau; compiles statistics, funds research, has published clinical practice guidelines for diagnosis, treatment, and management of RSDS/CRPS. **Pub:** *Clinical Practice Guidelines for Diagnosis, Treatment, and Management of RSD/CRPS*. • *RSDSA Review*, quarterly. Newsletter. *Price:* Included in membership dues. • Also publishes fact sheets. **Frmly:** (1998) Reflex Sympathetic Dystrophy Association.

★ 5528 ★ Reflexology Association of America (RAA)

4012 Rainbow, Ste. K-PMB No. 585
Las Vegas, NV 89103-2059
Phone: (508)364-4234
Website: http://www.reflexology-usa.org/

Fnded: 1995. **Mem:** 500. **State Groups:** 20. **Desc:** Promotes the art of reflexology to promote physiological changes in the body. **Pub:** *Reflexology Across America*, quarterly. Newsletter. Disseminates information about reflexology. *Price:* included in membership dues.

★ 5529 ★ Reflexology Association of Australia (RAA)

PO Box 366
Cammeray, NSW 2062, Australia
Phone: 61 3 98994760
Email: seville@impaq.com.au

Desc: Promotes awareness and understanding of reflexology within the community; works to maintain high standard of professional practice; provide information and resources on matters pertaining to reflexology; provide ongoing professional development and support to members.

★ 5530 ★ Reflexology Association of Canada (RAC)

PO Box 83008
Edmonton, AB, Canada T5T 6S1
Phone: (780)443-4246 **Free:** 877-RAC-FEET
Fax: (780)444-6882
Email: memberserv@reflexologycanada.ca
Website: http://reflexologycanada.ca

Fnded: 1976. **Mem:** 3,000. **Desc:** Dedicated to training, educational standards and information dissemination to promote reflexology.

★ 5531 ★ Registered Nursing Home Association

15 Highfield Rd.
Edgbastion
Birmingham B15 3DU, United Kingdom
Phone: 44 121 4542511 **Fax:** 44 121 4540932
Email: rnhaho@aol.com
Website: http://www.rnha.co.uk

Fnded: 1968. **Mem:** 1,600. **Reg. Groups:** 33. **Desc:** Nursing Home Owners. **Pub:** *Nursing Home News*, monthly. Journal. • *RNHA Reference Book*, annual. Book. A reference book on nursing homes in U.K.

★ 5532 ★ Registry of Interpreters for the Deaf (RID)

333 Commerce St.
Alexandria, VA 22314
Phone: (703)838-0030 **Fax:** (703)838-0454
Email: admin@rid.org
Website: http://www.rid.org
Clay Nettles, Exec. Dir.

Fnded: 1964. **Mem:** 9,300. **Reg. Groups:** 5. **State Groups:** 58. **Desc:** Advocates sign language and oral interpreters. programs. Maintains 34 committees. Compiles statistics. **Pub:** *Registry of Interpreters for the Deaf–Proceedings of National Conventions*, biennial. Proceedings. *Price:* $11.95/copy. • *Views*, monthly. • Also publishes texts and other materials on interpretation, transliteration, and translation. **Frmly:** National Registry of Professional Interpreters and Translators for the Deaf.

★ 5533 ★ Regulatory Affairs Professionals Society (RAPS)

11300 Rockville Pike, Ste. 1000
Rockville, MD 20852
Phone: (301)770-2920 **Fax:** (301)770-2924
Email: raps@raps.org
Website: http://www.raps.org
Sherry Keramidas, PhD, Exec. Dir.

Fnded: 1976. **Mem:** 8,200. **Desc:** Represents the regulatory affairs profession and the individuals who are part of this dynamic field. RAPS members are the health regulatory leaders of today and tomorrow in areas such as medical devices, pharmaceuticals, biologics, biotechnology, and in vitro diagnostics. **Pub:** *Regulatory Affairs Focus*, monthly. Magazine. *Price:* included in membership dues; $120 for nonmembers.

★ 5534 ★ Rehabilitation Accreditation Commission (CARF)

4891 E Grant Rd.
Tucson, AZ 85712
Phone: (520)325-1044 **Fax:** (520)318-1129
Website: http://www.carf.org/

Fnded: 1966. **Desc:** Accrediting body promoting quality, value and optimal outcomes of services through consultative accreditation process centering on enhancing lives of those receiving services.

★ 5535 ★ Rehabilitation Engineering and Assistive Technology Society of North America (RESNA)

1700 N Moore St., Ste. 1540
Arlington, VA 22209-1903
Phone: (703)524-6686 **Fax:** (703)524-6630
Email: info@resna.org

Website: http://www.resna.org/
Larry Pencak, Exec. Dir.

Fnded: 1980. **Mem:** 1,250. **Desc:** Rehabilitation professionals, providers, and consumers. An interdisciplinary association for the advancement of rehabilitation and assistive technologies. Objectives are to improve the quality of life for disabled persons through the application of science and technology; influence policy relating to delivery of technology to disabled persons. Is concerned with the design and development of rehabilitation devices and the modification of housing and transportation systems. **Pub:** *Assistive Technology*, semiannual. Journal. • *Assistive Technology Sourcebook. Price:* $30. • *Augmentative Communication: Finding a Voice.* Video. Contains information on augmentative and alternative communication systems for funding sources and case managers. *Price:* $30. • *Backs: Correction or Accommodation.* Video. Contains information about static and adjustable back supports for funding sources and case managers. *Price:* $30. • *Communication: The Key to Teamwork.* Video. Includes explanations of assistive technology by rehabilitation experts for funding sources and case managers. *Price:* $30. • *Manual Mobility: Finding the Right Wheels.* Video. Contains information about rigid, folding, and lightweight wheelchairs for funding sources and case managers. *Price:* $30. • *RESNA News*, quarterly. • *Understanding the Technology When Selecting Wheelchairs. Price:* $10. • Brochures. • Manuals. • Membership Directory, annual. • Monographs. • Proceedings, annual. • Reports. • Also publishes an education series. **Frmly:** (1988) RESNA: Association for the Advancement of Rehabilitation Technology.

★ 5536 ★ Rehabilitation International (RI)
25 E 21st St.
New York, NY 10010
Phone: (212)420-1500 **Fax:** (212)505-0871
Email: rehabintl@rehab-international.org
Website: http://www.rehab-international.org/
Lex Frieden, Pres.

Fnded: 1922. **Mem:** 150. **Desc:** Organizations in 90 countries conducting programs for the rehabilitation of people with physical and mental disabilities. Disseminates information on every phase of disability prevention and rehabilitation. Assists experts in planning work or study programs outside their own countries; aids in practical development of national rehabilitation programs. **Pub:** *International Journal of Rehabilitation Research*, quarterly. Journal. • *International Rehabilitation Review*, triennial. Newsletter. Provides coverage of United Nations agencies, discusses the elimination of architectural and environmental barriers for the disabled. *Price:* $30/year. • *One-In-Ten*, quarterly. Newsletter. • *Proceedings of World Congress*, quadrennial. • *Rehabilitation*, semiannual. • Directory, annual. • Also publishes booklets and papers. **Frmly:** (1939) International Society for Crippled Children; (1960) International Society for the Welfare of Cripples; (1976) International Society for Rehabilitation of the Disabled.

★ 5537 ★ Rehabilitation Technology Association
West Virginia Rehabilitation Research and Training Center
PO Box 1004 Barron Dr.
Institute, WV 25112-1004
Phone: (304)766-2680
Email: rta@rtce.icdi.wvu.edu
Website: http://www.icdi.wvu.edu
Betty Tyler, Coor.

Fnded: 1982. **Mem:** 1,000. **Desc:** Individuals involved in the rehabilitation field. Uses technology to enhance performance in their jobs. **Pub:** *RTA Online Newsletter*, quarterly. Newsletter. Contains articles on rehabilitation and information technologies. *Price:* Free.

★ 5538 ★ Reiki Alliance
PO Box 41
Cataldo, ID 83810
Phone: (208)783-3535 **Fax:** (208)783-4848
Email: info@reikialliance.com
Website: http://www.reikialliance.com
Marvin Kelsey, Exec. Dir.

Fnded: 1983. **Mem:** 750. **Desc:** Teachers of Reiki, the Usui System of Reiki Healing. Supports teachers of the Usui System Of Reiki Healing in 40 countries. Promotes exchange among teachers and students; provides member referrals; supports workshops for additional teacher training. Sponsors annual Global Gathering. **Pub:** *Reiki Alliance Membership Newsletter*, 3/year. Newsletter. *Price:* Included in membership dues. • *Student Book.* Book.

★ 5539 ★ Relatives and Residents Association
5 Tavistock Place
London WC1H 9SN, United Kingdom
Phone: 44 20 76924302 **Fax:** 44 20 79166093
Email: relres@totalise.co.uk

Fnded: 1992. **Mem:** 2,500. **Nat'l Groups:** 2. **Local Groups:** 30. **Lang(s):** English. **Desc:** Provides advice and support to relatives and friends of older people in residential care homes, nursing homes and long stay hospitals. Also offers training to homes in order to promote good practice through involvement of relatives. **Pub:** *The Relatives & Residents Association*, 3/year. Newsletter. Contains news and updates nationally and within the organization.

★ 5540 ★ Remedios AIDS Foundation
1066 Remedios St.
Malate
Manila 1004, Philippines
Phone: 63 2 5240924 **Fax:** 63 2 5223431
Email: raf@phil.gn.apc.org

Fnded: 1991. **Mem:** 100. **Reg. Groups:** 4. **Lang(s):** English, Tagalog. **Desc:** Provides quality reproductive health information and services to targetted communities. Programs include counseling, resource center, Information Education Communicates materials, the Youth Zone, Clinica Remedios, support services, networking and advocacy. **Pub:** *Remedios Newsletter*, quarterly. Newsletter. • *Sourcebook on HIV/AIDS-STD Counseling.* Book.

★ 5541 ★ Remembering ADAM
PO Box 665
Hastings, PA 16646
Free: 877-767-2326
Email: adam51988@aol.com
Website: http://www.rememberingadam.com
Deborah A. Fowler, Contact

Fnded: 1999. **Mem:** 16. **Desc:** Volunteers. Provide speakers for events. Promote drug use awareness.

★ 5542 ★ Renal Association
Triangle House
Broomhill Rd.
London SW18 4XH, United Kingdom
Phone: 44 208 8752413 **Fax:** 44 208 8752434
Email: renal@immunology.org
Website: http://www.renal.org/

Fnded: 1950. **Desc:** Works as the professional body for nephrologists in the United Kingdom; promotes development of renal services within the U.K, including prevention and treatment of renal disorders.

★ 5543 ★ Renal Pathology Society (RPS)
c/o Guillermo Herrera
Department of Pathology
LSUMC Shreveport
1501 Kings Hwy
Shreveport, LA 71130-3932
Phone: (318)675-5878 **Fax:** (318)675-7662
Email: gherre@lsuhsc.edu
Website: http://www.renalpathsoc.org
Dr. Guillermo A. Herrerame, Sec. -Treas.

Fnded: 1993. **Mem:** 236. **Desc:** Works to spread and increase knowledge of pathology of the kidney and seeks to develop renal pathology as a subspecialty. Conducts research and educational programs. **Pub:** Directory. • Bulletin.

★ 5544 ★ Renal Physicians Association (RPA)
1700 Rockville Pke., Ste. 220
Rockville, MD 20852
Phone: (301)468-3515 **Fax:** (301)468-3511
Email: rpa@renalmd.org
Website: http://www.renalmd.org/
Dale Singer, Exec. Dir.

Fnded: 1973. **Mem:** 2,200. **Desc:** Physicians specializing in the treatment of renal (kidney) diseases. Promotes optimal care and high standards of treatment for patients. Serves as a national representative for physicians engaged in the study and management of patients with kidney and related disorders; specifically, expresses the concerns and needs of renal physicians to congressional and governmental agencies legislating, executing, and regulating the federal End Stage Renal Disease Program. Provides resources for the development of national policies concerning kidney disease such as ESRD legislative and network activities, federal funding for related research, and studies relative to treatment procedures and clinical practices. Conducts educational programs. Membership is open to practice managers who are responsible for billing and coding in nephrologists' offices. **Pub:** *RPA News*, bimonthly. Newsletter. *Price:* Included in membership dues.

★ 5545 ★ Reproductive Health Association of Cambodia
c/o Dr. Ouk Vong Vathiny
House No. 6, Rd. 150
Sangvat Veal Vong Khan 7 Makara
Phnom Penh, Cambodia
Phone: 855 23 982120 **Fax:** 855 23 885093
Email: vathiny@rhac.org.kh

Fnded: 1996. **Desc:** Represents reproductive health professionals in Cambodia.

★ 5546 ★ Reproductive Toxicology Center (RTC)
7831 Woodmont Ave., Ste. 375
Bethesda, MD 20814
Phone: (301)514-3081 **Fax:** (425)740-7498
Email: reprotox@reprotox.org
Website: http://reprotox.org
Anthony R. Scialli, MD, Dir.

Fnded: 1981. **Desc:** Works to gather and disseminate information on the effects of the chemical and physical environment on human fertility, pregnancy, and fetal development. Provides subscribers with information from the most relevant articles in the field.

★ 5547 ★ Republic of China Society of Cardiology (ROCSOC)
No. 8, Sect. 3, Ting-Chow Rd.
Taipei 100, Taiwan
Phone: 886 2 3687720 **Fax:** 886 2 3687926
Fnded: 1960.

★ 5548 ★ Research! America
1101 King St. No. 520
Alexandria, VA 22314-2944
Phone: (703)739-2577 **Free:** 800-366-CURE
Fax: (703)739-2372
Email: info@researchamerica.org
Website: http://www.researchamerica.org
Mary Woolley, Pres. & CEO

Fnded: 1989. **Mem:** 450. **Desc:** Academia, voluntary health organizations, professional and scientific societies, hospitals and independent research institutes, businesses and industries, and foundations and philanthropists. Works to increase public awareness of the benefits of medical and health research and to make medical and health research, including prevention research, a higher national priority. Seeks to stimulate interest in medical research careers. Appeals to institutions and the government to provide essential funding for medical and health research. Engages in multimedia communications programs and serves as a clearinghouse and source of information to members, the media, the general public, and elected officials including public opinion data we commission. Conducts public opinion polls and outreach programs; provides a unified link between citizens and local, state, and national opinion leaders and decision makers. **Pub:** *Membership Matters*, monthly. Newsletter. *Price:* Included in membership dues.

★ 5549 ★ Research Center Against Meningitis and Schistosomiasis (Centre de Recherches sur les Meningites et les Schistosomiases)

Boite Postale 10887
Niamey, Niger
Phone: 227 752045 **Fax:** 227 753180
Email: cermes@ird.ne
Website: http://www.mpl.ird.fr/cermes

Fnded: 1978. **Lang(s):** English, French. **Desc:** Health care professionals and researchers. Promotes development of improved diagnostic techniques and treatments for meningitis and schistosomiasis. Conducts research; gathers and disseminates information; makes available health services.

★ 5550 ★ Research and Education on Impaired Driving (REID)

c/o St. Kevin Catholic Jr/Sr High School
No. 107, 10005-84 St.
Edmonton, AB, Canada T5J 0H1
Phone: (403)462-2426 **Fax:** (403)462-2596

Fnded: 1982. **Mem:** 300. **Lang(s):** English, French. **Desc:** Volunteers opposed to drunk and impaired driving. Promotes increased public awareness of the dangers of impaired driving; seeks to improve enforcement of laws prohibiting drunken and impaired driving. Conducts educational programs; sponsors research; maintains speakers' bureau.

★ 5551 ★ Research to Prevent Blindness (RPB)

645 Madison Ave.
New York, NY 10022-1010
Phone: (212)752-4333 **Free:** 800-621-0026
Fax: (212)688-6231
Email: info@rpbusa.org
Website: http://www.rpbusa.org/hc2/index.asp
James V. Romano, PhD, COO

Fnded: 1960. **Desc:** National voluntary health foundation supported by foundations, corporations, and voluntary gifts and bequests from individuals. Established to stimulate basic and applied research into the causes, prevention, and treatment of blinding eye diseases. Grants funds for equipment, eye research professorships with up to 7 year salary support, assistance in financing construction campaigns for eye research laboratory facilities, and travel expenses for international scholars for short-term collaborative research in the U.S. Through seminars and other means, encourages communication among scientists, practicing ophthalmologists, and the public. Maintains scientific advisory panel. **Pub:** *Eye Research News Briefs*, annual. Newsletter. Contain reports on latest developments in eye research. *Price:* Free. • *Eye Research Seminar Papers*, biennial. Papers. • *Research to Prevent Blindness–Annual Report.* Contains information on RPB's activities in support of scientific research into the causes, treatment, and prevention of blindness. *Price:* Free.

★ 5552 ★ Research Society on Alcoholism (RSA)

4314 Medical Pkwy., No. 12
Austin, TX 78756-3332
Phone: (512)454-0022 **Fax:** (512)454-0812
Email: debbyrsa@bga.com
Website: http://www.RSOA.org
Debra Sharp, Exec. Dir.

Fnded: 1976. **Mem:** 1,400. **Desc:** Scientists who hold an M.D. or Ph.D. degree and others actively engaged in research on alcoholism and alcohol-related problems; doctoral students; professionals in related fields who are interested in supporting alcohol research. Purposes are to: serve as a forum for researchers working in the field; aid and further the application of research to problems related to alcoholism; disseminate scientific information; protect the rights of researchers and human research subjects; assess research priorities; enlighten the public about problems of alcoholism. Provides opportunities for communication and discussion among scientists, clinicians, and lay workers in alcoholism research, diagnosis, and treatment. Conducts lectures. **Pub:** *Alcoholism: Clinical and Experimental Research*, monthly. Journal. Includes book reviews and research reports. *Price:* $105 members; $145 members, foreign; $318 nonmembers. • *Recent Developments in Alcoholism*, annual. Monograph. *Price:* $382 Canada and Mexico; $406 nonmembers, foreign. • *RSA Directory*, periodic. Directory. *Price:* available to members only; available to members only.

★ 5553 ★ Research and Training Center on Independent Living (RTCIL)

University of Kansas
4089 Dole
RTC on Independent Living
1000 Sunnyside Ave.
Lawrence, KS 66045
Phone: (785)864-4095 **Fax:** (785)864-5063
Email: rtcil@ku.edu
Website: http://www.rtcil.org
Dr. James Budde, Dir.

Fnded: 1980. **Mem:** 180. **Desc:** U.S. independent living centers helping individuals with severe disabilities lead independent lives. Works to: identify attributes of successful self-help support groups; develop and test instruments to assess social support levels within self-help support groups; implement and evaluate intervention strategies for accurate and positive portrayals of people with disabilities by the media; deter unlawful parking in handicapped-designated parking spaces and enhance public awareness of issues related to disability and independent living; establish accreditation standards to evaluate ILC programs, services, and management. Has developed: Personal Attendant Care Management Training model in seven states to increase the ability of consumers to manage attendants an d reduce management problems and institutionalization; program to assist ILC consumers in identifying personal goals and initiating behavioral changes to attain them. Provides direct training and technical assistance to individuals, ILCs, state agencies, and consumers' groups; university courses, and presentations. Places an emphasis on the needs of underserved populations, including the mentally ill, patients with brain injuries, minorities, the elderly, and persons living in rural areas. **Pub:** *Catalogue of Publications*, annual. Lists publications available from the center; includes abstracts. • *Guidelines for Reporting and Writing About People with Disabilities.* • Manuals. • Monographs.

★ 5554 ★ Residency Review Committee for Emergency Medicine (RRCEM)

515 N State St., Ste. 2000
Chicago, IL 60610
Phone: (312)464-5404 **Fax:** (312)464-4098
Website: http://www.acgme.org
Dr. Larry Sulton, Dir.

Fnded: 1982. **Mem:** 12. **Desc:** Representatives from the American College of Emergency Physicians, the American Board of Emergency Medicine, Council on Medical Education of the American Medical Association, and the Emergency Medicine Residents' Association. Accredits residency training programs in emergency medicine. **Pub:** *Directory of Graduate Medical Education Programs*, annual. Directory.

★ 5555 ★ Resolve, The National Infertility Association

1310 Broadway
Somerville, MA 02144-1779
Phone: (617)623-1156 **Free:** 888-623-0744
Fax: (617)623-0252
Email: info@resolve.org
Website: http://www.resolve.org
Joan Bowen, Exec. Dir.

Fnded: 1974. **Mem:** 15,000. **Local Groups:** 56. **Desc:** Persons with problems of infertility and associated professionals who work with infertile couples such as adoption workers, physicians, and counselors. Seeks to provide "timely, compassionate support and information to people who are experiencing infertility, and to increase awareness of infertility issues." Offers information, referral, and support to persons with problems of infertility; conducts issue advocacy and public education programs. **Pub:** *Resolve National Newsletter*, quarterly. Newsletter. Provides information on medical, emotional, and legislative issues, and upcoming conferences. Includes book reviews, research reports, and letters. *Price:* Included in membership dues; $4/issue for nonmembers. • *Resolving Infertility.* Book. • Bibliography. • Brochure. • Also publishes fact sheets and briefs. **Frmly:** (1999) RESOLVE.

★ 5556 ★ Respiratory Nursing Society (RNS)

c/o NYSNA
11 Cornell Rd.
Latham, NY 12110
Phone: (518)782-9400
Email: rns@nysna.org
Website: http://www.respiratorynursingsociety.org/
Donna Wilson, Pres.

Fnded: 1990. **Mem:** 400. **Local Groups:** 2. **Desc:** Nurses who care for clients with pulmonary dysfunction, and who are interested in the promotion of pulmonary health. Fosters the personal and professional development of respiratory nurses, and quality care of their clients. Provides educational opportunities and promotes research in the field. **Pub:** *Respiratory Exchange*, quarterly. Newsletter.

★ 5557 ★ Responsible Hospitality Institute (RHI)

World Trade Center
1250 Sixth Ave., Ste. 217
San Diego, CA 92101
Phone: (619)234-0007 **Fax:** (619)234-0319
Email: jim@hospitalityweb.org
Website: http://www.hospitalityweb.org/rhi
Jim Peters, Pres.

Fnded: 1983. **Mem:** 300. **Local Groups:** 1. **Desc:** Individuals from the U.S., Canada, New Zealand, and Australia concerned with: accessibility of restaurants and other hospitality businesses to disabled persons; responsible operation of establishments selling alcoholic beverages. Presently Inactive. **Pub:** *Hospitality Insighter*, monthly. Newsletter. *Price:* $60. • *Networker.* **Frmly:** Intermission.

★ 5558 ★ Restless Legs Syndrome Foundation (RLS)

819 2nd St. SW
Rochester, MN 55902
Phone: (507)287-6465 **Free:** 877-463-6757
Fax: (507)287-6312
Email: rlsfoundation@rls.org
Website: http://www.rls.org
Georgianna Bell, Exec. Dir.

Fnded: 1990. **Mem:** 12,000. **Desc:** Sufferers of restless leg syndrome and other interested people. Supports research of effective treatments and a cure. Acts as and develops support groups for sufferers and their friends and families. Educates physicians, patients and the public to increase awareness. **Pub:** *Night Walkers*, quarterly. Newsletter. Includes information on research, support groups, and news. *Price:* $25/year for members.

★ 5559 ★ Restricted Growth Association
PO Box 4744
Dorchester DT2 9FA, United Kingdom
Phone: 44 1308 898445
Email: rga1@talk21.com
Website: http://www.rgaonline.org.uk

Fnded: 1970. **Mem:** 700. **Lang(s):** English. **Desc:** Open to persons with restricted growth, families with a child with restricted growth, health professionals, and other interested persons. Aims to help reduce the distress and disadvantages of persons of restricted growth by trying to reduce social barriers, improve the quality of life and enhance their role in society. Offers counseling training, family support, medical information and other practical help. Regional coordinators. **Pub:** *RGA Information Magazine*, semiannual. Magazine. • *RGA News*, quarterly. Newsletter. • *Walking Through Leaves: Autobiography of William Shakespeare.*

★ 5560 ★ Rethink
30 Tabernacle St.
London EC2A 4DD, United Kingdom
Phone: 44 20 73309100 **Fax:** 44 20 73309102
Email: info@rethink.org
Website: http://www.rethink.org

Fnded: 1972. **Mem:** 7,102. **Reg. Groups:** 8. **Local Groups:** 150. **Desc:** Exists to improve the lives of everyone affected by schizophrenia and other severe mental illnesses by providing quality support, services, and information and by influencing local, regional, and national policies. **Pub:** *A Meeting Of Minds - A Positive Response To Mental Disorder.* Video. Features the perspectives of schizophrenia sufferers, their careers, CPNs, social workers, and police officers. • *Cognitive Therapy.* Report. Covers a complimentary form of treatment. • *Does Severe Mental Illness Run In Families?.* • *Finding The Right Medication.* Handbook. A guide to drugs available to treat schizophrenia. • *500 Million More - Where and Why it is Needed.* Report. Highlights the underfunding of community care for people with a severe mental illness. • *Is Cost A Factor.* Survey. • *One in Ten.* Report. Covers suicide and other unnatural deaths involving people with schizophrenia. • *Schizophrenia.* Pamphlet. Covers the causes and symptoms of schizophrenia, including treatment. • *Schizophrenia And Research - UK.* Report. • *Schizophrenia - Notes for Relatives and Friends.* Pamphlet. • *The Silent Partners - The Needs and Experiences of People Who Care For People With A Severe Mental Illness.* Reprint. • *What is Schizophrenia?.* **Frmly:** (2002) National Schizophrenia Fellowship.

★ 5561 ★ Retinitis Pigmentosa International (RPI)
PO Box 900
Woodland Hills, CA 91365
Phone: (818)992-0500 **Free:** 800-FIGHT-RP
Fax: (818)992-3265
Email: info@rpinternational.org
Website: http://www.rpinternational.org
Helen Harris, Pres.

Fnded: 1972. **Mem:** 30,000. **State Groups:** 4. **Local Groups:** 1. **Desc:** Seeks to raise funds to support research and provide human service programs to assist the visually impaired. Offers charitable services. Maintains research programs. Also describes motion picture and television programs for the blind. Produces annual television special "The Eyes of Christmas" with celebrity memories and a motion picture described for the blind and vision impaired. **Pub:** *Nightlighter, Sound Bites*, annual. Newsletter.

★ 5562 ★ Retinoblastoma Society (RS)
St. Bartholomew's Hospital
London EC1A 7BE, United Kingdom
Phone: 44 207 6003309 **Fax:** 44 207 6008579
Email: rbinfo@rbsociety.org.uk
Website: http://www.rbsociety.org.uk

Fnded: 1986. **Mem:** 750. **Lang(s):** English. **Desc:** Children with retinoblastoma (eye cancer) and their families; other interested individuals. Seeks to improve the quality of life of people with eye cancer; promotes advancement in the prevention, diagnosis, and treatment of retinoblastoma. Provides support for people with retinoblastoma and their families; promotes awareness with health professionals; fundraising activities to support eye cancer research. **Pub:** *ORBS*, 3/year. Newsletter.

★ 5563 ★ Retirement Income Association
PO Box 21957
Santa Barbara, CA 93121-1957
James J. Maher, Pres.

Fnded: 1994. **Mem:** 250,000. **Desc:** Acts as a liaison between retired consumers and service and product providers. Offers access to insurance packages and health-related products and services. **Pub:** *Retirement Income Newsletter*, bimonthly. Newsletter. *Price:* $12.95. • *Retirement Today*, bimonthly. Newsletter. *Price:* $12.95/year.

★ 5564 ★ Retirement Research Foundation (RRF)
8765 W Higgins Rd., Ste. 430
Chicago, IL 60681-4170
Phone: (773)714-8080 **Fax:** (773)714-8089
Email: info@rrf.org
Website: http://www.rrf.org
Edward J. Kelly, Chm.

Desc: Works to promote aging and retirement issues. Supports efforts that improve care for the aging, and enable older adults to live at home or in residential settings that facilitate independent living.

★ 5565 ★ RGK Foundation
1301 W 25th St., Ste. 300
Austin, TX 78705-4236
Phone: (512)474-9298 **Fax:** (512)474-7281
Website: http://www.rgkfoundation.org
Gregory A. Kozmetsky, Pres.

Desc: Works to promote medical research.

★ 5566 ★ Richmond Fellowship of Austria (RFA)
Society for Mental Health
Hoffmanngasse 12
A-9020 Klagenfurt, Austria
Phone: 43 463 55112 **Fax:** 43 463 501256
Email: kuna.pmk@carinthia.com

Fnded: 1979. **Mem:** 400. **Nat'l Groups:** 2. **Lang(s):** English, Slovene. **Desc:** Community mental health services. Seeks to insure ethical and efficient administration of community mental health care programs and institutions. Conducts training programs for community mental health personnel; participates in charitable activities. **Pub:** *Pro Mente Kaouten*, quarterly. Newsletter.

★ 5567 ★ Richmond Fellowship International (RFI)
16 Europoint
5-11 Lavington St.
London SE1 0NZ, United Kingdom
Phone: 44 20 79456187 **Fax:** 44 20 79456190
Email: rfi.uk@virgin.net
Website: http://www.rfinternational.org

Fnded: 1981. **Mem:** 18. **Nat'l Groups:** 26. **Reg. Groups:** 1. **State Groups:** 6. **Lang(s):** English, French, Spanish. **Desc:** Promotes the establishment and operation of halfway houses and day centers for abused children, former psychiatric patients and recovering drug addicts. Organizes mental health training programs for social workers, psychologists, psychotherapists, and psychiatric nurses. Supports development of community based psychosocial rehabilitation services and service user advocacy. **Pub:** *Annual Report.* • Newsletter, periodic.

★ 5568 ★ Riding for the Disabled Association - Ireland (RDAI)
c/o Rathlinn
Templecarrig Lower
Delgany, Wicklow, Ireland
Phone: 353 1 2876498 **Fax:** 353 1 2876503

Fnded: 1969. **Mem:** 85. **Nat'l Groups:** 85. **Lang(s):** English, Irish. **Desc:** Equestrian coaches and enthusiasts. Promotes increased participation in equestrian activities among people with disabilities. Sponsors horseback riding programs for people with disabilities.

★ 5569 ★ Roger Wyburn-Mason and Jack M. Blount Foundation for the Eradication of Rheumatoid Disease (RDF)
7376 Walker Rd.
Fairview, TN 37062-8141
Phone: (615)799-1002 **Fax:** (615)799-1002
Email: admin@arthritistrust.org
Website: http://www.arthritistrust.org
Perry A. Chapdelaine, Exec. Dir. & Sec.

Fnded: 1982. **Mem:** 30,000. **Nat'l Groups:** 2. **Desc:** Seeks to eradicate rheumatoid disease and related arthritis. Where funds are available, performs or supports research. Provides physician list recommends publications primarily to show various causes of arthritis and treatments that must be explored to achieve wellness. Does not seek to over-emphasize a particular treatment program, but encourages removing burdens that stress the immune system, thus permitting the body to recover. These burdens may include, but may not be limited to, proper nutrition, candidiasis, food allergies, microorganism infections, foci or infection from root canals or extracted teeth, intestinal tract, or mercury poisoning from amalgams or other forms of dental metals, plus storage of herbicides and pesticides in fatty (lipids) parts of cells. **Pub:** *Arthritis.* Book. • *Arthritis: Little Known Treatments.* Book. Contains a collection of alternative, complementary, and holistic treatments. *Price:* 5. • *Away with Arthritis.* Book. *Price:* $15 15. • *The Causation of Rheumatoid Disease and Many Human Cancers – A New Concept in Medicine.* Pamphlet. *Price:* $10. • Also publishes several journals, papers, and articles on topics related to arthritis. **AKA:** Rheumatoid Disease Foundation; The Arthritis Trust of America.

★ 5570 ★ Rolf Institute (RI)
205 Canyon Blvd., Ste. 200
Boulder, CO 80302
Phone: (303)449-5903 **Free:** 800-530-8875
Fax: (303)449-5978
Email: info@rolf.org
Website: http://www.rolf.org
Lorraine Lombard, Contact

Fnded: 1971. **Mem:** 1,010. **Reg. Groups:** 14. **Desc:** Purposes are to: train and certify Rolfers and Movement Practitioners; serve the professional needs of members; inform the public about the benefits of Rolfing and Rolfing Movement Integration. (Rolfing is a technique devised by Dr. Ida P. Rolf, an American biochemist, for reordering the body to bring its major segments toward a vertical alignment.) Conducts research activities; maintains speakers' bureau. **Pub:** *Expressive Movement.* • *Healing Through Touch.* • *Ida Rolf Talks.* • *The Power of Balance.* • *Rolf Lines*, quarterly. *Price:* Only available to members of the Rolf Institute. • *Rolfing.* • *Rolfing and Physical Reality.* • *The Rolfing Experience.* • *Rolfing Stories of Personal Empowerment.* • Books. • Films. • Pamphlets. • Reprints. • Videos. **Frmly:** (1975) Ida P. Rolf Foundation for Structural Integration.

★ 5571 ★ Romanian Alzheimer Society
Bd. Mihail Kogalniceanu 95A
Sc. A. Et. 1, Ap. 8, Sector 5
R-70603 Bucharest, Romania
Phone: 40 21 6863470 **Fax:** 40 21 3348940
Email: alzsocro@fx.ro

Fnded: 1992. **Mem:** 250. **Lang(s):** English. **Desc:** Family caregivers, medical professionals, and volunteers involved with and concerned for people affected with dementia, including Alzheimer's disease. Works to support the elderly affected with mental disorders, particularly Alzheimer patients and their families.

★ 5572 ★ Romanian Association of Gerontology and Geriatrics
9 Caldarusani St.
Sector 1
R-78178 Bucharest, Romania
Phone: 40 1 6665050 **Fax:** 40 1 2231480

Desc: Promotes gerontological research, training in the field of aging, and interests of gerontological organizations in international affairs.

★ 5573 ★ Romanian Society of Cardiology (SRC) (Societatea de Cardiologie — SC)
Cardiology Department, Fundeni Hospital
258 Fundeni Way
R-72435 Bucharest, Romania
Phone: 40 21 2402224 **Fax:** 40 21 2402224
Email: rscardio@rscardio.com
Website: http://www.rscardio.ro

Fnded: 1947. **Mem:** 250. **Nat'l Groups:** 3. **Lang(s):** English, Romanian. **Desc:** Cardiologists. Promotes investigation into cardiovascular diseases. Areas of research include: clinical physiopathology; epidemiology; physiopathology; prophylaxy; therapeutics. Maintains educational programs. **Pub:** *Romanian Heart Journal*, quarterly. **Frmly:** (1991) Society of Cardiology.

★ 5574 ★ Rose Kushner Breast Cancer Advisory Center (RKBCAC)
PO Box 757
Palos Verdes Estates, CA 90274
Phone: (310)897-3445 **Fax:** (310)897-3444
Email: lkkushner@yahoo.com
Website: http://www.rkbcac.org/
Harvey D. Kushner, Ed.

Fnded: 1975. **Desc:** Information service for people, mostly women concerned about or with breast cancer. Provides information to public, patients and physicians concerning current knowledge about breast cancer detection, diagnosis, treatment and follow-up. **Pub:** *If You've Thought About Breast Cancer by Rose Kushner*, biennial. Booklet. *Price:* Free. **Frmly:** Breast Cancer Advisory Center; (1991) Women's Breast Cancer Advisory Center; (1991) Women's Breast Cancer Advisory Center.

★ 5575 ★ Royal Academy of Medicine in Ireland (RAMI)
6 Kildare St.
Dublin 2, Ireland
Phone: 353 1 6767650 **Fax:** 353 1 6611684
Email: secretary@rami.ie
Website: http://www.iformix.com

Fnded: 1882. **Mem:** 2,000. **Lang(s):** English. **Desc:** Physicians, medical researchers, and other scientists with an interest in medicine. Seeks to advance medical study, teaching, and practice. Serves as a forum for the exchange of information among members; sponsors research and educational programs. **Pub:** *Irish Journal of Medical Science*, quarterly. Journal. Medical journal.

★ 5576 ★ Royal Academy of Veterinary Sciences of Spain (Real Academia de Ciencias Veterinarias de Espana)
c/Maestro Ripoll, 8
E-28006 Madrid, Spain
Phone: 34 913943867 **Fax:** 34 913943864
Fnded: 1975.

★ 5577 ★ Royal Association for Deaf People (RAD)
Walsingham Rd.
Colchester CO2 7BP, United Kingdom
Phone: 44 1206 509509 **Fax:** 44 1206 769755
Email: tom.fenton@royaldeaf.org.uk

Fnded: 1841. **Desc:** Meets the needs of profoundly deaf people. **Frmly:** (2001) Royal Association in Aid of Deaf People.

★ 5578 ★ Royal Association for Disability and Rehabilitation (RADAR)
12 City Forum
250 City Rd.
London EC1V 8AF, United Kingdom
Phone: 44 20 72503222 **Fax:** 44 20 72500212
Email: radar@radar.org.uk
Website: http://www.radar.org.uk

Fnded: 1977. **Mem:** 500. **Desc:** Represents the rights and interests of disabled individuals in the United Kingdom. Strives to improve educational, health, and social services for disabled people and stresses their full integration and participation in community life. Seeks to eliminate barriers that impose restrictions on disabled people. Provides advice. UK Secretariat of Rehabilitation International. **Pub:** *Holiday Guides*, annual. • Bulletin, monthly. • Pamphlets.

★ 5579 ★ Royal Australasian College of Dental Surgeons
64 Castlereagh St.
Sydney, NSW 2000, Australia
Phone: 61 2 92323800 **Fax:** 61 2 92218108
Email: registrar@racds.org
Website: http://www.racds.org

Fnded: 1965. **Mem:** 1,400. **Nat'l Groups:** 5. **Reg. Groups:** 9. **State Groups:** 5. **Lang(s):** English. **Desc:** Dental surgeons. Promotes continuing professional development of members. Serves as a clearinghouse on dental surgical techniques and technologies; conducts educational programs for dental surgeons. Assists in the formulation of standards for dental surgical training and practice. Maintains museum. **Pub:** *Annals*, semiannual. Journal. • *College News*, periodic. Newsletter. • *Lecture Notes in Anatomy*, semiannual. • *Lecture Notes in Histology.* • *Lecture Notes in Microbiology.* • *Lecture Notes in Pathology.* • *Lecture Notes in Physiology.* • *Yearbook*, annual. Annual Report.

★ 5580 ★ Royal Australasian College of Physicians - Australia (RACP)
145 Macquarie St.
Sydney, NSW 2000, Australia
Phone: 61 2 92565444 **Fax:** 61 2 92523310
Email: racp@racp.edu.au
Website: http://www.racp.edu.au/
Fnded: 1938.

★ 5581 ★ Royal Australasian College of Surgeons (RACS)
Spring St.
Melbourne, VIC 3000, Australia
Phone: 61 3 92491200 **Fax:** 61 3 92491219
Fnded: 1927.

★ 5582 ★ Royal Australian College of Ophthalmologists
27 Commonwealth St.
Sydney, NSW 2010, Australia
Phone: 61 2 92677006 **Fax:** 61 2 92676534
Email: racosec@medeserv.cem.au
Fnded: 1969.

★ 5583 ★ Royal Australian and New Zealand College of Obstetricians and Gynaecologists (RANZCOG)
254-260 Albert St.
East Melbourne, VIC 3002, Australia
Phone: 61 3 94171699 **Fax:** 61 3 94190672
Email: ranzcog@ranzcog.edu.au
Website: http://www.ranzcog.edu.au/Open/College/college-main.htm

Fnded: 1978. **Desc:** Strives for excellence in health care delivery to women.

★ 5584 ★ Royal Australian and New Zealand College of Psychiatrists (RANZCP)
390 La Trobe St.
Melbourne, VIC 3000, Australia
Phone: 61 3 96400646 **Fax:** 61 3 96425652
Email: ranzcp@ranzcp.org
Website: http://www.ranzcp.org

Fnded: 1963. **Pub:** *Australian and New Zealand Journal of Psychiatry*, bimonthly. Journal. • *Australian Psychiatry*, quarterly. Magazine.

★ 5585 ★ Royal Australian and New Zealand College of Radiologists
51 Druitt St., Level 9
Sydney, NSW 2000, Australia
Phone: 61 2 92689777 **Fax:** 61 2 92689799
Email: ranzcr@ranzcr.edu.au
Website: http://www.racr.edu.au
Fnded: 1935.

★ 5586 ★ Royal College of Anaesthetists
48-49 Russell Sq.
London WC1B 4JY, United Kingdom
Phone: 44 20 78131900 **Fax:** 44 20 78131876
Email: info@rcoa.ac.uk
Website: http://www.rcoa.ac.uk
Fnded: 1988.

★ 5587 ★ Royal College of Dentists of Canada (RCDC) (College Royal des Chirugiends Dentistes du Canada)
5075 Yonge St., Ste. 405
Toronto, ON, Canada M2N 6C6
Phone: (416)512-6571 **Fax:** (416)512-6468
Email: office@rcdc.ca
Website: http://www.rcdc.ca/

Fnded: 1965. **Desc:** Promotes high standards of specialization in dental professions; provides licensing examinations.

★ 5588 ★ Royal College of General Practitioners
14 Princes Gate
Hyde Pk.
London SW7 1PU, United Kingdom
Phone: 44 207 5813232 **Fax:** 44 207 2253047
Email: info@rcgp.org.uk
Website: http://www.rcgp.org.uk

Fnded: 1952. **Mem:** 18,400. **Desc:** General practitioners. Responsible for the promotion of high quality general practice through education, research and standard setting. **Pub:** *British Journal of General Practice*, monthly. Journal.

★ 5589 ★ Royal College of Midwives
15 Mansfield St.
London W1G 9NH, United Kingdom
Phone: 44 20 73123535 **Fax:** 44 20 73123536
Email: info@rcm.org.uk
Website: http://www.rcm.org.uk/

Fnded: 1881. **Mem:** 36,000. **Nat'l Groups:** 4. **Local Groups:** 230. **Lang(s):** English. **Desc:** Promotes the practice of midwifery, and works to maintain high standards in the field. Provides educational programs to midwives in the areas of maternity, child care, and personal development. Represents worker rights of midwives to national legal and political authorities. Encourages and supports research. **Pub:** *Midwives.* Magazine. • *RCM Midwives Journal*, monthly. Journal.

★ 5590 ★ Royal College of Nursing
20 Cavendish Sq.
London W1G 0RN, United Kingdom
Phone: 44 207 4093333 **Fax:** 44 207 6473425
Email: webteam@rcn.org.uk
Website: http://www.rcn.org.uk
Fnded: 1916. **Mem:** 310,000. **Desc:** Nurses, midwives and health visitors. Represents nurses working at all levels of responsibility and in a wide variety of settings, from the NHS to the independent sector and from local government to private industry. **Pub:** *Nursing Standard*, weekly. Journal.

★ 5591 ★ Royal College of Nursing - Australia
1 Napier Close
Deakin, VIC 2600, Australia
Phone: 61 2 62825633 **Fax:** 61 2 62823565
Email: Canberra@rcna.org.au
Website: http://www.rcna.org.au
Fnded: 1949. **Mem:** 10,000. **Nat'l Groups:** 13. **Reg. Groups:** 2. **State Groups:** 8. **Desc:** Provides continuing professional development, policy analysis and development, advocacy and scholarship administration in the field of nursing. **Pub:** *Collegian*, quarterly. Journal.

★ 5592 ★ Royal College of Obstetricians and Gynaecologists - United Kingdom
27 Sussex Pl.
Regent's Park
London NW1 4RG, United Kingdom
Fax: 44 207 7230575
Email: pbarnett@rcog.org.uk
Website: http://www.rcog.org.uk
Fnded: 1929. **Mem:** 10,324. **Desc:** Obstetricians and gynecologists, having completed a period of training recognised by the College and passed all components of the MRCOG examination. The encouragement of the study and the improvement of the practice of obstetrics and gynaecology. This is achieved by running examinations, postgraduate meetings, publications, committees and working parties. **Pub:** *British Journal of Obstetrics and Gynaecology*, monthly. Journal. • *Journal for Continuing Professional Development from the Royal College of Obstetricians and Gynaecologists*. Journal. • *The Obstetrician and Gynaecologist*, quarterly.

★ 5593 ★ Royal College of Ophthalmologists
17 Cornwall Terr.
London NW1 4QW, United Kingdom
Phone: 44 207 9350702 **Fax:** 44 207 9359838
Email: margaret@rcophth.ac.uk
Website: http://www.rcophth.ac.uk
Fnded: 1988. **Mem:** 3,027. **Desc:** Medical Practitioners (ophthalmologists). **Pub:** *EYE*, bimonthly. Journal.

★ 5594 ★ Royal College of Paediatrics and Child Health
50 Hallam St.
London W1W 6DE, United Kingdom
Phone: 44 207 3075600 **Fax:** 44 207 3075601
Email: enquiries@rcpch.ac.uk
Website: http://www.rcpch.ac.uk
Fnded: 1928. **Mem:** 6,500. **Desc:** Consultant paediatricians, community child health doctors, trainee paediatricians, research workers, general practitioners and other medical specialists who work with children. Aims to advance the understanding, treatment and prevention of disease in childhood, to further the study of child health and to promote excellence in paediatric practice. **Pub:** *Archives of Disease in Children*, monthly. Journal. • *College Newsletter*, quarterly. Newsletter. **Frmly:** (1996) British Paediatric Association.

★ 5595 ★ Royal College of Pathologists of Australasia
Durham Hall
207 Albion St.
Surry Hills, NSW 2010, Australia
Phone: 61 2 83565858 **Fax:** 61 2 83565828
Email: rcpa@rcpa.edu.au
Website: http://www.rcpa.edu.au/
Fnded: 1956.

★ 5596 ★ Royal College of Pathologists - United Kingdom
2 Carlton House Terrace
London SW1Y 5AF, United Kingdom
Phone: 44 20 74516700 **Fax:** 44 20 74516701
Email: info@rcpath.org
Website: http://www.rcpath.org
Fnded: 1962. **Mem:** 7,500. **Lang(s):** English. **Desc:** Postgraduate medical and scientific graduates who have successfully completed all or part of the college's examinations following a specified period of approved training, or elected under specified college ordinances. Advances the science and practice of pathology, furthers public education, promotes study and research work in pathology and related subjects and publishes the results of such study and research. **Pub:** *College Bulletin*, quarterly. Journal. • *Manpower and Management Policy Documents*. • *Training and Examination Guidelines*. • Reports.

★ 5597 ★ Royal College of Physicians (RCP)
11 St. Andrew's Pl.
Regent's Park
London NW1 4LE, United Kingdom
Phone: 44 20 79351174 **Fax:** 44 20 74867038
Email: linda.cuthbertson@rcplondon.ac.uk
Website: http://www.rcplondon.ac.uk
Fnded: 1518. **Mem:** 17,500. **Reg. Groups:** 9. **Lang(s):** English. **Desc:** Individuals in 64 countries. Responsible for the postgraduate education and training of physicians in England, Wales, and Northern Ireland. Committed to maintaining the highest standards of medical practice. Advises the government, public, and members of the profession on health and medical issues. Conducts educational and training programs; organizes examinations; operates clinical effectiveness unit. **Pub:** *Annual Report*. • *College List*, annual. • *Working Party Reports*. • Journal, bimonthly.

★ 5598 ★ Royal College of Physicians of Edinburgh (RCPE)
9 Queen St
Edinburgh EH2 1JQ, United Kingdom
Phone: 44 131 2257324 **Fax:** 44 131 2203939
Email: president@rcpe.ac.uk
Website: http://www.rcpe.ac.uk
Fnded: 1681.

★ 5599 ★ Royal College of Physicians of Ireland
6 Kildare St.
Dublin 2, Ireland
Phone: 353 1 6616677 **Fax:** 353 1 6762920
Email: info@rcpi.ie
Website: http://www.rcpi.ie
Fnded: 1654. **Mem:** 4,500. **Desc:** Makes available post graduate medical education and training.

★ 5600 ★ Royal College of Physicians and Surgeons of Canada (RCPSC)
774 Echo Dr.
Ottawa, ON, Canada K1S 5N8
Phone: (613)730-8177 **Free:** 800-668-3740
Fax: (613)730-8830
Email: info@rcpsc.edu
Website: http://rcpsc.medical.org
Fnded: 1929. **Mem:** 33,178. **Lang(s):** English, French. **Desc:** Medical fellows (22,339); surgical fellows (10,839). Founded by the Canadian Medical Association. Prescribes requirements of specialty training in 58 medical, laboratory, and surgical specialties and subspecialties. Accredits specialty residency programs in Canada, judges the acceptability of residency education, and conducts the certifying examinations. Also assists its members (fellows) to maintain their specialty competence through continuing medical education and the maintenance of Certification Program. Intervenes in matters involving health and public policy and biomedical ethics; it is not a licensing or disciplinary body. **Pub:** *Annals RCPSC*, 8/year. Journal. Peer reviewed scientific articles.

★ 5601 ★ Royal College of Physicians and Surgeons of Glasgow
232-242 St. Vincent St.
Glasgow G2 5RJ, United Kingdom
Phone: 44 141 2216072 **Fax:** 44 141 2211804
Website: http://www.rcpsglasg.ac.uk
Fnded: 1599. **Mem:** 7,060. **Desc:** Physicians, surgeons, and dentists. Conducts educational and training programs. **Pub:** Annual Report.

★ 5602 ★ Royal College of Physicians and Surgeons of the United States of America (RCPS)
485 Allard Rd.
PO Box 24224
Grosse Pointe, MI 48236
Phone: (313)882-0641 **Fax:** (313)882-0979
Website: http://www.rcpsus.com
Martin Savitz, MD, Exec. Dir.
Fnded: 1984. **Mem:** 2,500. **Nat'l Groups:** 32. **Reg. Groups:** 30. **State Groups:** 4. **Local Groups:** 28. **Desc:** Physicians and allied health professionals interested in tropical medicine. Provides postgraduate continuing medical education; confers certificates and diplomas. Maintains speakers' bureau and hall of fame and provides placement services. Conducts research and educational programs; compiles statistics. **Pub:** *Bare Facts for Practicing Doctors*, semiannual. Magazine. Provides clinical info to doctors in tropical countries. • *Journal of the Royal College of Physicians and Surgeons*, semiannual. Journal. Focuses on continuing medical education and certificate/diploma award. *Price:* $50 for members; $75 for nonmembers; $110 institutions. • *JRCP&S*, periodic. Newsletter. • *Proceedings of the Royal College of Physicians and Surgeons*, semiannual. *Price:* $100.

★ 5603 ★ Royal College of Psychiatrists
17 Belgrave Sq.
London SW1X 8PG, United Kingdom
Phone: 44 20 72352351 **Fax:** 44 20 72451231
Email: rcpsych@rcpsych.ac.uk
Website: http://www.rcpsych.ac.uk
Fnded: 1971. **Mem:** 10,000. **Desc:** Psychiatrists. **Pub:** *British Journal of Psychiatry, Psychiatric Bulletin*, monthly. Journal.

★ 5604 ★ Royal College of Radiologists - United Kingdom (RCR)
38 Portland Pl.
London W1B 1JQ, United Kingdom
Phone: 44 207 6364432 **Fax:** 44 207 3233100
Email: enquiries@rcr.ac.uk
Fnded: 1939. **Mem:** 5,679. **Lang(s):** English. **Desc:** Diagnostic and interventional radiologists, nuclear medicine specialists, oncologists, radiotherapists, and ultrasound specialists. Works to advance the science and practice of radiological technology. Offers courses to further the education of practitioners. Establishes qualifications and examinations for fellowships and diplomas. **Pub:** *Clinical Oncology*, bimonthly. Journal. • *Clinical Radiology*, monthly. Journal. • *Members' Handbook*, biennial. Handbook. • *Newsletter*, quarterly. Newsletter. **Frmly:** (1975) Faculty of Radiologists.

★ 5605 ★ Royal College of Speech and Language Therapists
2 White Hart Yard
London SE1 1NX, United Kingdom
Phone: 44 207 3781200 **Fax:** 44 207 4037254
Email: postmaster@rcslt.org
Website: http://www.rcslt.org

Fnded: 1945. **Mem:** 8,500. **Lang(s):** English. **Desc:** Speech and language therapists, including practising members, non-practising and retired members. All members have a certificate to practise (or its equivalent) issued by the college. Supports qualified speech and language therapists working for the relief of disorders of communication among both adults and children and the accreditation of courses leading to qualification as a speech and language therapist. Careers information available on request. **Pub:** *Bulletin*, monthly. Magazine. Contains clinical articles, news, book reviews, and letters. • *Bulletin Supplement.* • *International Journal of Language and Communication Disorders*, quarterly. Journal. **Frmly:** (1995) College of Speech Therapists; (1997) College of Speech and Language Therapists.

★ 5606 ★ Royal College of Surgeons of Edinburgh
Nicolson St.
Edinburgh EH8 9DW, United Kingdom
Phone: 44 131 5271600 **Fax:** 44 131 5576406
Email: mail@rcsed.ac.uk
Website: http://www.rcsed.ac.uk

Fnded: 1505. **Desc:** Promotes the education, training and examination, the raising of standards in surgical practice.

★ 5607 ★ Royal College of Surgeons of England (RCS Eng)
35/43 Lincoln's Inn Fields
London WC2A 3PE, United Kingdom
Phone: 44 20 74053474 **Fax:** 44 20 78319438
Email: external@rcseng.ac.uk
Website: http://www.rcseng.ac.uk

Fnded: 1800. **Mem:** 15,000. **Lang(s):** English. **Desc:** Surgeons and dental surgeons in the United Kingdom. Aims to promote and encourage the study and practice of surgery as an art and a science. Maintains professional standards through examinations; establishes criteria for the qualification of consultant and dental surgeons in the National Health Service; advises government and other professional bodies on surgical matters; conducts research. Offers postgraduate courses in surgery and related subjects; sponsors seminars and workshops. Operates the Hunterian Museum. **Pub:** *Annals of the Royal College of Surgeons of England*, bimonthly. Report.

★ 5608 ★ Royal College of Surgeons in Ireland (RCSI)
123 Saint Stephen's Green
Dublin 2, Ireland
Phone: 353 1 4022100 **Fax:** 353 1 4022460
Website: http://www.rcsi.ie

Fnded: 1784.

★ 5609 ★ Royal College of Veterinary Surgeons
Belgravia House
62-64 Horseferry Rd.
London SW1P 2AF, United Kingdom
Phone: 44 207 2222001 **Fax:** 44 207 2222004
Email: admin@rcvs.org.uk
Website: http://www.rcvs.org.uk

Fnded: 1844. **Mem:** 21,200. **Lang(s):** Dutch, French, German. **Desc:** Graduates possessing a veterinary degree, registerable with the RCVS who intend to practice in the UK. Statutory body governing the veterinary profession in the UK. Responsible for quality of veterinary undergraduate education at the UK veterinary schools, provision of membership examination, and discipline of members. Establishment of certificate and diploma examinations. **Pub:** *Directory of Veterinary Practices*, annual. Directory. Lists all U.K. veterinary practices. • *Guide to Professional Conduct*, 3/year. • *RCVS Annual Report*, annual. Annual Report. • *RCVS News*, quarterly. • *RCVS Register and Directories*, annual. Directory.

★ 5610 ★ Royal Environmental Health Institute of Scotland
3 Manor Place
Edinburgh EH3 7DH, United Kingdom
Phone: 44 131 2256999 **Fax:** 44 131 2253993
Email: rehis@rehis.org.uk
Website: http://www.royal-environmental-health.org.uk

Fnded: 1983. **Mem:** 1,100. **Reg. Groups:** 2. **Desc:** Persons interested or engaged in any aspect of environmental health. **Pub:** *Environmental Health Scotland*, quarterly. Journal. Environmental Health Scotland.

★ 5611 ★ Royal Institute for Deaf and Blind Children (RIDBC)
361-365 North Rocks Rd.
North Rocks, NSW 2151, Australia
Phone: 61 2 98711233 **Fax:** 61 2 98712196
Email: online@ridbc.org.au
Website: http://www.ridbc.org.au

Fnded: 1860. **Lang(s):** English. **Desc:** Strives to provide the best education possible for children with vision and/or hearing disabilities so that they may achieve their full potential in life. Advances and disseminates knowledge in this field.

★ 5612 ★ Royal Institute of Public Health
28 Portland Place
London W1B 1DE, United Kingdom
Phone: 44 207 5802731 **Fax:** 44 207 5806157
Email: marketing@riph.org.uk
Website: http://www.riph.org.uk

Fnded: 1856. **Mem:** 1,700. **Nat'l Groups:** 12. **Lang(s):** English. **Desc:** Medical practitioners, dental practitioners, and environmental health officers from 19 countries. Seeks to advance public health and integrated health services. Provides a forum for information exchange among specialists. Reviews existing methodologies and proposes new practices. Serves as an advisory body to governmental and other organizations. Assists in developing continuing professional training for specialists in public health and preventive medicine. Conducts research. **Pub:** *Health & Hygiene*, quarterly. Journal. Features articles on health hygiene. • *Public Health*, bimonthly. Journal. Contains articles submitted on public health matters worldwide. **Frmly:** Society of Public Health; (1856) Society of Medical Officers of Health; (1973) Society of Community Medicine; (2002) Royal Institute of Health and Hygiene and Society of Public Health.

★ 5613 ★ Royal Medical Society
Student Centre
5/5 Bristol Sq.
Edinburgh EH8 9AL, United Kingdom
Phone 44 131 6502672 **Fax:** 44 131 6502672
Email: royalmedsoc@btinternet.com
Website: http://www.royalmedical.co.uk

Fnded: 1737. **Mem:** 2,500. **Desc:** Mainly medical students. Fellows and Life Members are medical graduates. An educational charity for medical students, run by medical students. **Pub:** *Res Medica*, periodic.

★ 5614 ★ Royal National Institute of the Blind England (RNIB)
105 Judd St.
London WC1H 9NE, United Kingdom
Phone: 44 207 3881266 **Fax:** 44 207 3882034
Email: helpline@rnib.org.uk
Website: http://www.rnib.org.uk

Fnded: 1868. **Reg. Groups:** 10. **Local Groups:** 40. **Lang(s):** English. **Desc:** "Wants a world in which blind and partially sighted people enjoy the same rights, freedoms, and responsibilities and quality of life as people who are fully sighted." Mission is to challenge blindness. Challenges the disabling effects of blindness by providing services to help people determine their own lives. Challenges society's actions, attitudes, and assumptions. Works to dismantle barriers that are put into the path of the blind and partially sighted people. Works to prevent, cure, and alleviate blindness. **Pub:** *Publications Catalogue.*

★ 5615 ★ Royal National Institute for Deaf People
19-23 Featherstone St.
London EC1Y 8SL, United Kingdom
Phone: 44 20 72968000 **Fax:** 44 207 2968199
Email: informationline@rnid.org.uk
Website: http://www.rnid.org.uk

Fnded: 1911. **Mem:** 25,455. **Reg. Groups:** 5. **Lang(s):** English. **Desc:** Individual registered members. Provides the following quality services for the deaf, deaf blind and hard of hearing people: information, residential care, training (deaf awareness), specialist telephone services (Typetalk), assistive devices for sale from Sound Advantage, and Communication Support Units. All services are accessed through Regional offices, except Typetalk and Sound Advantage. **Pub:** *One In Seven*, bimonthly. Magazine. News and news relating to deaf & hard of hearing people. Various leaflets and factsheets.

★ 5616 ★ Royal Pharmaceutical Society of Great Britain (RPSGB)
1 Lambeth High St.
London SE1 7JN, United Kingdom
Phone: 44 207 7359141 **Fax:** 44 207 7357629
Email: enquiries@rpsgb.org.uk
Website: http://www.rpsgb.org.uk

Fnded: 1841. **Mem:** 40,000. **Lang(s):** English. **Desc** Pharmacists. Professional, statutory and regulatory body for practicing pharmacists in Great Britain. **Pub:** *The Extra Pharmacopeia*, triennial. Book. • *Martindale Online Newsletter*, periodic. Newsletter. • *Martindale Online User Guide.* Handbook. • *Martindale Thesaurus.* Book.

★ 5617 ★ Royal Society of Medicine
1 Wimpole St.
London W1G 0AE, United Kingdom
Phone: 44 207 2902900 **Fax:** 44 207 2902992
Email: joanna.rose@rsm.ac.uk
Website: http://www.rsm.ac.uk

Fnded: 1805. **Mem:** 18,000. **Desc:** Doctors, dentists, vets and lay members with interest in medicine. **Pub:** *The AIDS Letter*, bimonthly. • *International Journal of STD and AIDS*, bimonthly. Journal. • *Journal of Medical Biography*, quarterly. Journal. • *Journal of Royal Society of Medicine*, monthly. Journal. • *Journal of Telemedicine and Telecare*, quarterly. Journal. • *Tropical Doctor*, quarterly.

★ 5618 ★ Royal Society of Medicine Foundation (RSMF)
207 E Westminster Rd. Ste. 201
Lake Forest, IL 60045
Phone: (847)234-6382 **Fax:** (847)234-6511
Email: RSMFIL@aol.com
Website: http://www.rsm.ac.uk
Dr. Richard S. Wilbur, Pres.

Fnded: 1967. **Mem:** 3,500. **Desc:** Serves as a forum for the discussion of topics relevant to the medical community in the U.S. and the United Kingdom. Sponsors conference series and exchange programs in conjunction with the Royal Society of Medicine. **Pub:** *Digest*, quarterly.

★ 5619 ★ Royal Society for the Promotion of Health
38A St. George's Dr.
London SW1V 4BH, United Kingdom
Phone: 44 207 6300121 **Fax:** 44 207 9766847
Email: rshealth@rshealth.org.uk

Website: http://www.rsph.org

Fnded: 1876. **Mem:** 6,000. **Desc:** Members are drawn from a wide variety of professions and occupations with an interest in improving the health of the population. They range from architects and engineers, the health related profession, to food scientists and caterers. Aims to improve the quality and dignity of human life worldwide and to promote the continuous improvement of health and safety through education communication and the encouragement of scientific research. **Pub:** *JRSH*, quarterly. Journal. **Frmly:** (1999) Royal Society of Health.

★ 5620 ★ Royal Society of Tropical Medicine and Hygiene (RSTMH)

Manson House
26 Portland Pl.
London W1B 1EY, United Kingdom
Phone: 44 207 5802127 **Fax:** 44 207 4361389
Email: mail@rstmh.org
Website: http://www.rstmh.org/

Fnded: 1907. **Mem:** 3,000. **Lang(s):** English. **Desc:** Medical and veterinary practititioners, scientists, and interested others representing 88 countries. Promotes health and seeks to advance the study, control, and prevention of tropical diseases in humans and animals. Encourages information exchange and facilitates discussion. **Pub:** *Bulletin of Tropical Medicine & International Health.* • *Transactions of the Royal Society of Tropical Medicine and Hygiene*, bimonthly. Journal. • *Yearbook of the Royal Society of Tropical Medicine and Hygiene.*

★ 5621 ★ Royal Surgical Aid Society

47 Great Russell St.
London WC1B 3PB, United Kingdom
Phone: 44 20 76374577 **Fax:** 44 20 73236878
Email: enquiries@agecare.org.uk
Website: http://www.agecare.org.uk

Fnded: 1862. **Mem:** 17. **Desc:** Seeks to improve the care and well being of older people who are physically frail or suffering from dementia, through a combination of continuous development of good practice in it's own homes, seeking pre-eminence in education and training, supporting research and innovation, providing awards for excellence, and continuing in the exchange of knowledge and ideas.

★ 5622 ★ RSDHope Group (RSDS)

PO Box 875
Harrison, ME 04040
Website: http://www.rsdhope.org/

Desc: Patients suffering from Reflex Sympathetic Dystrophy Syndrome, Chronic Pain, their parents and friends. Dedicated to increasing the awareness of Reflex Sympathetic Dystrophy Syndrome (RSDS), chronic pain. **Pub:** Newsletter.

★ 5623 ★ Rubinstein-Taybi Parent Group U.S.A. (RTSPG)

PO Box 146
Smith Center, KS 66967
Free: 888-447-2989
Website: http://www.rubinstein-taybi.org

Fnded: 1984. **Mem:** 380. **Desc:** Families with children diagnosed with Rubinstein-Taybi Syndrome. Provides information and support. **Pub:** *Rubinstein-Taybi Syndrome.* Brochure. **AKA:** RTS Parent Group U.S.A.

★ 5624 ★ Rural Institute

52 Corbin Hall
University of Montana
Missoula, MT 59812
Phone: (406)243-5467 **Free:** 800-732-0323
Fax: (406)243-4730
Email: muarid@selway.umt.edu
Website: http://ruralinstitute.umt.edu/

Desc: Devoted to supporting the independence, productivity, and inclusion into the community of persons with developmental disabilities and their families.

★ 5625 ★ Russian Chiropractic Association (RCA)

2 Leontivski Pereolo, 3rd entrance
Moscow, Russia
Phone: 7 503 2349656 **Fax:** 7 95 9520983
Email: spine@redline.ru
Website: http://www.sport-dc.com/rca.html

Fnded: 1992. **Desc:** Committed to the advancement of the Chiropractic profession in Russia.

★ 5626 ★ Russian Family Planning Association

18/20 Vadkovsky Per.
101479 Moscow, Russia
Phone: 7 95 9731559 **Fax:** 7 95 9731917
Email: info@family-planning.ru
Website: http://www.family-planning.ru

Fnded: 1991. **Mem:** 4,000. **Lang(s):** Russian. **Desc:** Advocates family planning and responsible parenthood as a basic human right and as a means to enhance the quality of life. Works to reduce the number of unwanted pregnancies and abortions. Attempts to stop the spread of AIDS and other sexually transmitted diseases. Offers programs in sex education, family planning, and health. Provides contraceptive and health care services. Conducts research. **Pub:** *Family Planning*, quarterly. Magazine. Provides information on family planning, contraception, and sex education. Also publishes books, brochures, booklets, and posters.

★ 5627 ★ Russian Scientific Society of Pharmacology (RSSP)

Institute of Pharmacology
Baltiskaya Str. 8
125315 Moscow, Russia
Phone: 7 95 1511881 **Fax:** 7 95 1511261
Email: root@pharm3.partners.bio.msu.ru

Mem: 295. **Desc:** Promotes pharmacology in Russia.

★ 5628 ★ Ruth Jackson Orthopaedic Society (RJOS)

c/o Mary Gebhardt
6300 N River Rd., Ste. 727
Rosemont, IL 60018
Phone: (847)698-1637 **Fax:** (847)823-0536
Email: gebhardt@aaos.org
Website: http://www.rjos.org
Mary Gebhardt, Contact

Fnded: 1983. **Mem:** 469. **Desc:** Women orthopaedic surgeons, residents, fellows, and medical students. Seeks to advance the science of orthopaedic surgery and to provide support for women orthopaedic surgeons. Named for practicing orthopaedic surgeon Dr. Ruth Jackson (1902-94), the first woman certified by the American Board of Orthopaedic Surgery and the first female member of the American Academy of Orthopaedic Surgeons. Conducts educational programs; operates placement service and speakers' bureau, holds biennial meeting, sponsors mentoring program, offers traveling fellowship and resident research award. **Pub:** *Membership List*, periodic. Newsletter. *Price:* $150. • *Ruth Jackson Society Newsletter*, semiannual. Newsletter. Includes articles on international members and careers and personal life; also contains calendar of events, upcoming meetings and courses. *Price:* Free for members only.

★ 5629 ★ S.A.F.E. Alternatives

c/o Linden Oaks Hospital
801 S Washington St.
Naperville, IL 60540
Phone: (630)305-5500 **Free:** 800-DONT-CUT
Website: http://www.safe-alternatives.com

Fnded: 1984. **Local Groups:** 1. **Desc:** Professional group assisting self-injurious individuals in the treatment of their addictive behavior patterns. Maintains speakers' bureau; compiles statistics. **Pub:** *Bodily Harm.* Book. *Price:* $14.95. **Frmly:** (1987) Self-Mutilators Support Group; (2003) SAFE - Self Abuse Finally Ends.

★ 5630 ★ Sacro Occipital Research Society International (SORSI)

PO Box 6067
Leawood, KS 66206
Free: 888-245-1011 **Fax:** (913)341-7685
Email: cbinyon@kc.rr.com

Fnded: 1958. **Desc:** Chiropractors in 6 countries. Promotes exchange and cooperation; conducts research; provides specialized education. **Frmly:** (1978) Sacro Occipital Research Society.

★ 5631 ★ Safety Assessment Federation

Nutmeg House
60 Gainsford St. Butlers
Butlers Wharf
London SE1 2NY, United Kingdom
Phone: 44 20 74030987 **Fax:** 44 20 74030137
Email: info@safed.co.uk
Website: http://www.safed.co.uk

Fnded: 1995. **Mem:** 17. **Desc:** Represents the interests of companies that undertake the independent safety inspection and certification of machinery plant and equipment. **Pub:** *Fact sheets.*

★ 5632 ★ St. Lucia Planned Parenthood Association (SLPPA)

83 Chaussee Rd.
Castries, St. Lucia
Phone: (758)452-4335 **Fax:** (758)453-7284
Email: parenthood@candw.lc
Website: http://www.ippfwhr.org/

Fnded: 1967. **Mem:** 6. **Lang(s):** English. **Desc:** Encourages responsible parenthood and family planning as a means to improve quality of life for people in St. Lucia. Advocates family planning as a basic human right. Provides health care and contraceptive services. Conducts research.

★ 5633 ★ Salvadoran Demographic Association (SDA) (Asociacion Demografica Salvadorena — ADS)

Edificio Profamilia
25 Av. Norte No. 583
Apartado Postal 1338
San Salvador, El Salvador
Phone: 503 2250588 **Fax:** 503 2250879
Email: info@ads.org.sv
Website: http://www.ads.org.sv

Fnded: 1962. **Mem:** 220. **Lang(s):** Spanish. **Desc:** Promotes responsible parenthood and family planning. Encourages public knowledge of contraception, family planning, AIDS, and other sexually transmitted diseases. Promotes family planning as a basic human right. Sponsors educational programs on family planning for teens and adults. **Pub:** *Anniversary Magazine*, annual. Magazine. Provides summary of covering and institutional goals. • *Informative News - Carta Informativa*, quarterly. • *Memoria de Labores*, annual. Annual Report. • *National Family Health Survey*, quinquennial.

★ 5634 ★ Samaritans - England

The Upper Mill
Kingston Rd.
Ewell KT17 2AF, United Kingdom
Phone: 44 20 83948300 **Fax:** 44 20 83948301
Email: admin@samaritans.org
Website: http://www.samaritans.org

Fnded: 1953. **Mem:** 18,300. **Local Groups:** 203. **Desc:** A nationwide charity providing confidential, emotional support to anyone in crisis, 24 hours a day, 365 days a year. Not a religious or political organization. **Pub:** *Educational Materials*, periodic. • *Samaritan News*, quarterly. • Books, periodic. • Videos, periodic.

★ 5635 ★ Samaritans - Western Australia

60 Bagot Rd.
Subiaco, WA 6008, Australia
Phone: 61 8 93815555 **Fax:** 61 9 3882368
Email: samarita@starwon.com.au

Website: http://www.thesamaritans.org.au

Fnded: 1967. **Mem:** 90. **Nat'l Groups:** 3. **Reg. Groups:** 3. **State Groups:** 2. **Local Groups:** 1. **Lang(s):** Chinese, English, German, Indonesian. **Desc:** National branch of Befrienders International Samaritans Worldwide. Offers supportive listening, usually by phone for suicidal and/or despairing people, and education for young persons who have attempted suicide and their families. Provides support and information services to health care professionals. **Pub:** *Directory of Youth Services*, annual. Directory. • *Information Handbook for Youth at Risk.* • *Survivor's Kit.* • *Teen Suicide Guidelines for Parents.* **Frmly:** (1998) Samaritan Befrienders.

★ 5636 ★ San Francisco AIDS Foundation (SFAF)

995 Market St. 200
San Francisco, CA 94103
Phone: (415)487-3000 **Free:** 800-367-AIDS
Fax: (415)487-3009
Email: feedback@staf.org
Website: http://www.sfaf.org
Pat Christen, Exec. Dir.

Fnded: 1982. **Desc:** Regional organization whose goals are to educate the public on the prevention of AIDS and to make various social service programs accessible to people with AIDS. Provides community forums; develops and distributes educational materials. Provides assistance to people with AIDS in obtaining emergency housing, social security and veterans' benefits, medical and insurance benefits, and legal referral services. Works with legislators, corporations, public health coalitions, activists, and the media to advance public health policy and improve media coverage. Maintains speakers' bureau. **Pub:** *Bulletin of Experimental Treatments for AIDS*, quarterly. Bulletin. Covers AIDS-related diseases, research, care, treatment, and clinical trials. *Price:* Free for individuals; Free for institutions. • Booklets. • Brochures. • Videos. • Also distributes AIDS educational materials. **Frmly:** AIDS/Kaposi's Sarcoma Research and Education Foundation.

★ 5637 ★ Sarcoma Alliance

775 E Blithedale, No. 334
Mill Valley, CA 94941
Phone: (415)381-7236
Email: ruth@sarcomaalliance.com
Website: http://www.sarcomaalliance.com
Suzanne Leider, Pres.

Fnded: 1999. **Desc:** Committed to guide, educate and support adults with sarcomas and their family, friends and caregivers.

★ 5638 ★ Sargent Cancer Care for Children (SCCC)

Mercantile Chambers
5th Fl, 53 Bothwell St.
Glasgow G2 6TS, United Kingdom
Phone: 44 1415 725700 **Fax:** 44 1415 725701
Website: http://www.sargent.org/

Fnded: 1969. **Lang(s):** English. **Desc:** Provides care for children and young adults experiencing cancer and their families; works closely within the hospital multidisciplinary team. The Malcolm Sargent House, Prestwick, provides supported short breaks for families year round. **Pub:** Brochures. • Annual Report.

★ 5639 ★ Scandinavian Association for Digestive Endoscopy (SADE)

Rikshospitalet Univ. Hospital
N-0027 Oslo, Norway
Phone: 47 22867612 **Fax:** 47 22867611
Email: larsaa@ioks.uio.no

★ 5640 ★ Scandinavian Association for Gastrointestinal Motility

c/o Einar Bjornsson
Department of Medicine II
Sahlgren's Hospital
S-413 45 Goteborg, Sweden
Email: einar.bjornsson@medicine.gu.sef

Fnded: 1987. **Desc:** Seeks to increase scientific knowledge of gastrointestinal motility and neurogastroenterology. Works to improve diagnosis and treatment of motility disturbances. **Pub:** Newsletter, periodic.

★ 5641 ★ Scandinavian Association of Plastic Surgeons (SAPS) (Nordisk Plastikkirurgisk Forening — NPF)

c/o Dr. Mikael Relander
Bokbackgranden 4B
FIN-20900 Turku, Finland
Phone: 358 2 2581560 **Fax:** 358 2 6102984
Email: mihael.relander@pp-timnet.fi

Fnded: 1951. **Mem:** 238. **Lang(s):** Danish, Finnish, Icelandic, Norwegian, Swedish. **Desc:** Plastic surgeons in 5 countries. Promotes the advancement of plastic surgery. Keeps members informed of developments in plastic surgery. Sponsors courses. **Pub:** *List of Members*, periodic. • *Scandinavian Journal of Plastic and Reconstructive Surgery and Hand Surgery*, quarterly. Journal.

★ 5642 ★ Scandinavian Association for Thoracic Surgery (SATS) (Nordisk Thoraxkirurgisk Forening — NTF)

c/o Prof. Hostrup Nielsen, MD
Department of Cardio-Thoracic Surgery
Skejby University Hospital
Brendstrupgaardsvej
DK-8200 Arhus N, Denmark
Phone: 45 89 495410 **Fax:** 45 89 496005
Email: phn@sks.aaa.dk
Website: http://www.scandinavian-ats.org

Fnded: 1949. **Mem:** 250. **Lang(s):** English. **Desc:** Scandinavian thoracic and cardiovascular surgeons. Conducts graduate lectures and presentations of scientific papers. **Frmly:** Scandinavian Association for Thoracic and Cardiovascular Surgery.

★ 5643 ★ Scandinavian Association of Urology (SAU) (Nordisk Urologisk Forening — NUF)

Rikshospitalet
Kir avd A
N-0027 Oslo A, Norway
Email: alxsch@online.no

Fnded: 1957. **Mem:** 750. **Lang(s):** Danish, English, Finnish, Icelandic, Norwegian, Swedish. **Desc:** Scandinavian physicians specializing in urology or having an interest in the field. Maintains international working groups. **Pub:** *NUF-Bulletinen*, semiannual. • *Scandinavian Journal of Urology and Nephrology*, quarterly.

★ 5644 ★ Scandinavian Association for Vascular Surgery (SAVS)

Karlskrona Hospital
S-371 85 Karlskrona, Sweden
Phone: 46 455 89500 **Fax:** 46 455 89487
Email: thomas.troeng@ltblekinge.se

Fnded: 1996.

★ 5645 ★ Scandinavian Fellowship for Oral Pathology and Oral Medicine (Skandinavisk Forening for Oral Patologi och Oral Medicin — SFOPOM)

c/o Ake Larsson, Sec.
Centre for Oral Health Sciences
S-214 21 Malmo, Sweden
Phone: 46 40 6658585 **Fax:** 46 40 6658585
Email: ake.larsson@od.mah.se

Fnded: 1971. **Desc:** Seeks to improve professional standards in oral pathology in Scandinavia.

★ 5646 ★ Scandinavian Institute of Dental Materials (Nordisk Institut for Odontologisk MaterialprEovning — NIOM)

PO Box 70
N-1305 Haslum, Norway
Phone: 47 67512200 **Fax:** 47 67591530
Email: niom@niom.no
Website: http://www.niom.no

★ 5647 ★ Scandinavian Neurological Association (SNA) (Nordisk Neurologisk Forening — NNF)

Department of Neurology
University of Helsinki
FIN-00290 Helsinki, Finland
Phone: 358 9 4712261 **Fax:** 358 9 4714009
Email: jorma.palo@helsinki.fi

Fnded: 1922. **Mem:** 5. **Lang(s):** Danish, English, Finnish, Icelandic, Norwegian, Swedish. **Desc:** Scandinavian national societies representing 900 neurologists and other specialists with an interest in neuroscience. Promotes neurological research and cooperation among Scandinavian neurologists. Provides educational counseling. **Pub:** *Congress Abstracts*, biennial. Proceedings.

★ 5648 ★ Scandinavian Neurosurgical Society (SNS) (Nordisk Neurokirurgisk Forening — NNF)

Institute of Clinical Neuroscience
Department of Neurosurgery
Karolinska Hospital
Box 30
S-171 76 Stockholm, Sweden
Phone: 46 8 51770000
Email: tiitmathiesen@neuro.ks.se

Fnded: 1945. **Mem:** 160. **Lang(s):** English. **Desc:** Scandinavian neurosurgeons and neurosurgical residents; practicing neurosurgeons outside of Scandinavia. Works to facilitate collaboration among Scandinavian neurosurgeons.

★ 5649 ★ Scandinavian Orthopaedic Association

Karolinska Sjukhuset
S-104 01 Stockholm, Sweden

★ 5650 ★ Scandinavian Society of Cataract and Refractive Surgery

c/o Magnus Otto
Department of Ophthalmology
Central Hospital
S-65185 Karlstad, Sweden
Phone: 46 54 524339 **Fax:** 46 54 152983
Email: ingrid.floren@oft.lu.se

Desc: Strives to advance scientific knowledge in the field of intraocular lens implantation and the practice of refractive surgery.

★ 5651 ★ Scandinavian Society for Cell Toxicology (SSCT)

Department of Biology
Abo University, Biocity
FIN-20520 Artellerigatan, Finland
Phone: 358 2 2154065 **Fax:** 358 2 2154748
Email: ichristi@abo.fi
Website: http://www.SSCT.net

Fnded: 1983. **Mem:** 75. **Nat'l Groups:** 4. **Desc:** Encourages communication among in vitro toxicologists, furthers the development of in vitro toxicology in the Nordic countries. **Pub:** *Workshop proceedings*, annual. Proceedings.

★ 5652 ★ Scandinavian Society of Clinical Physiology and Nuclear Medicine

S-221 85 Lund, Sweden

Fnded: 1981. Desc: Fosters nuclear and clinical physiological methods and thinking; encourages communication between Scandinavian countries.

★ 5653 ★ Scandinavian Society for Genito-Urinary Medicine (SSGM)
Univ. Hospital
N-7006 Trondheim, Norway
Phone: 47 0798000 **Fax:** 47 07997602

Fnded: 1982. **Desc:** Enhances research into the epidemiology of sexually transmitted diseases.

★ 5654 ★ Scandinavian Society for Head and Neck Oncology
Head and Neck Surgery, Haukeland University Hospital
N-5021 Bergen, Norway
Phone: 47 55972670 **Fax:** 47 55974956
Email: jan.olofsson@haukeland.no

Fnded: 1987. **Mem:** 200. **Pub:** *Abstracts.* Abstracts from annual meetings published in Clinical Otolaryngology.

★ 5655 ★ Scandinavian Society for the History of Medicine (Nordisk Medicinhistorisk Forening)
Ostra Hamngatan 11
S-411 10 Goteborg, Sweden

★ 5656 ★ Scandinavian Society for Immunology
Stockholm University
S-106 91 Stockholm, Sweden
Phone: 46 8 164164

Fnded: 1970. **Desc:** Promotes knowledge of immunology within the Scandinavian countries.

★ 5657 ★ Scandinavian Society for Laser Therapy
Lund University
S-22185 Lund, Sweden

★ 5658 ★ Scandinavian Society for Military Medicine
Swedish Defence Force
S-107 85 Stockholm, Sweden

Fnded: 1925.

★ 5659 ★ Scandinavian Society for Parasitology
c/o Dr. Charlotte Maddox-Hyttel
DVI; Bulowsvej 27
DK-1790 Copenhagen V, Denmark
Phone: 45 35300213 **Fax:** 45 35300181
Email: cmh@vetinst.dk
Website: http://www.hi.is/pub/ssp/

Fnded: 1967. **Mem:** 160. **Lang(s):** English. **Desc:** Researchers within the field of parasitology, biology, epidemiology, treatment, etc. **Pub:** *Bulletin of the Scandinavian Society for Parasitology*, semiannual. Journal.

★ 5660 ★ Scandinavian Society for Phlebology
Department of Surgery, Lund University
S- 221 85 Lund, Sweden

★ 5661 ★ Scandinavian Society for Prosthetic Dentistry (SSPD)
c/o Cecilia Christersson, Sec.
Odontologiska Fakulteten
Malmo Hogskola
Tandvardshogskolan
S-205 06 Malmo, Sweden
Phone: 46 40 6657000 **Fax:** 46 40 925359
Email: cecilia.christersson@od.mah.se
Website: http://www.odont.uio.no/prosthodont/sspd.html

Fnded: 1972.

★ 5662 ★ Scandinavian Society for Research in CardioThoracic Surgery (SSRCTS)
c/o J. Michael Hasenkam
Department of Cardiothoracic and Vascular Surgery
Skyjby Sygehus
Aarhus University Hospital
DK-8200 Arhus N, Denmark
Phone: 45 89 495480 **Fax:** 45 89 496016
Email: hasenkam@iekf.au.dk
Website: http://www.ssrcts.org

Fnded: 1990. **Mem:** 100. **Lang(s):** English. **Desc:** Cardiothoracic surgeons, students, and researchers. Provides a forum for young researchers to present their work.

★ 5663 ★ Scandinavian Society for the Study of Diabetes (SSSD)
PO Box 571
S-751 23 Uppsala, Sweden
Phone: 46 18 4714396

Fnded: 1965.

★ 5664 ★ Scandinavian Society for Surgery of the Hand (Skandinavisk Handkirurgiska Foreningen)
Lund University Hospital
S-205 02 Malmo, Sweden
Fax: 46 40928855

Fnded: 1951.

★ 5665 ★ Scandinavian Work Group on Reconstructive Microsurgery
Department of Plastic Surgery
Herlev Hospital
University of Copenhagen
DK-2730 Herlev, Denmark
Phone: 45 44535300 **Fax:** 45 44535332

★ 5666 ★ Schizophrenia Association of Great Britain
International Schizophrenia Centre
Bryn Hyfryd, The Crescent
Bangor LL57 2AG, United Kingdom
Phone: 44 1248 354048 **Fax:** 44 1248 353659
Email: info@sagb.co.uk
Website: http://www.sagb.co.uk

Fnded: 1970. **Mem:** 3,000. **Desc:** Provides information about schizophrenia for patients and families to increase understanding of the illness. **Pub:** Newsletter, semiannual. Contains articles on recent findings in Schizophrenia including nutritional aspects.

★ 5667 ★ Schizophrenia Ireland (SI)
38 Blessington St.
Dublin 7, Ireland
Phone: 353 1 8601620 **Fax:** 353 1 8601602
Email: info@sirl.ie
Website: http://www.sirl.ie

Lang(s): English, Irish. **Desc:** Individuals and organizations. Seeks to improve the quality of life of people with schizophrenia and their families. Makes available support and services; conducts educational and advocacy campaigns.

★ 5668 ★ Schizophrenia Society of Canada (Societe canadienne de schizophrenie)
50 Acadia Ave., St. 205
Markham, ON, Canada L3R 0B3
Phone: (905)415-2007 **Free:** 888-772-4673
Fax: (905)415-2337
Email: info@schizophrenia.ca
Website: http://www.schizophrenia.ca/

Fnded: 1979. **Reg. Groups:** 100. **Local Groups:** 10. **Desc:** Support group providing understanding of schizophrenia; disseminates information concerning the latest developments in schizophrenia research and treatment and society activities; advocates for legislation and improvements in services. Provides public awareness and education programs, family support, fundraising, or administration at various levels. **Pub:** *SSC Bulletin.* Bulletin. • Annual Report.

★ 5669 ★ Schizophrenics Anonymous (SA)
c/o National Schizophrenia Foundation
403 Seymour Ave., Ste. 202
Lansing, MI 48933
Phone: (517)485-7168 **Free:** 800-482-9534
Email: inquiries@nsfoundation.org
Website: http://www.sanonymous.org/
Eric Hufnagel, Pres. /CEO

Fnded: 1967. **Mem:** 100. **Desc:** Self-help organization. Groups are comprised of diagnosed schizophrenics who meet to share experiences, strengths, and hopes in an effort to help each other cope with common problems and recover from the disease; rehabilitation program follows the 12 principles of Alcoholics Anonymous World Services. Discussion topics include: symptoms and how to deal with them; the need to be responsible even though one is ill; overcoming guilt related to the illness. Each of the local groups attempts to recruit a volunteer mental health consultant from the area. The volunteer aids in program development and group discussion. **Pub:** Newsletter, semiannual. Provides health information. *Price:* $20. • Also distributes guidelines for establishing SA groups.

★ 5670 ★ Schweizerische Berufsverband fur Augenoptik und Optometrie (SBAO)
Sonnmattrain 7
CH-6043 Adligenswil, Switzerland
Phone: 41 41 3720682 **Fax:** 41 41 3720683
Email: sbao@datacomm.ch
Website: http://www.sbao.ch

Fnded: 1980. **Mem:** 740. **Lang(s):** English, French, German, Italian. **Desc:** Optometrists. Seeks to improve standards of optometric study, teaching, and practice. Conducts continuing professional development courses for members.

★ 5671 ★ Schweizerische Multiple Sklerose Gesellschaft
c/o Pascal Couchepin
Brinerstrasse 1
Postfach
CH-8036 Zurich, Switzerland
Phone: 41 1 466 6999 **Fax:** 41 1 466 6990
Email: info@multiplesklero.se.ch

Fnded: 1959. **Reg. Groups:** 39. **Desc:** MS patients, families and professionals. Seeks to improve the quality of life for persons with multiple sclerosis and their families.

★ 5672 ★ Scientific Society of Anaesthesiologists in Bulgaria
St. G. Sofiski 1
BG-1431 Sofia, Bulgaria
Phone: 359 2 521046 **Fax:** 359 2 548038
Email: tempus@ns.medfac.acad.bg

Fnded: 1970. **Mem:** 800. **Reg. Groups:** 2. **State Groups:** 5. **Desc:** Fosters research in anaesthesiology.

★ 5673 ★ Scientific Society of Forensic Meidlogy and Gastrointestinal Endoscopy
c/o Bulgarian Association of Surgeons and Gastroenterologists
5th City Clinical Hospital
Clinic of Internal Medicine

Stoletov 67-A
BG-1233 Sofia, Bulgaria
Phone: 359 2 9268105 **Fax:** 359 2 325141
Email: mechkov@techno-link.com

Fnded: 1973. **Mem:** 200. **Nat'l Groups:** 2. **Reg. Groups:** 1. **Lang(s):** English, French. **Desc:** Fosters research in hepatology, gastroenterology and gastrointestinal endoscopy. **Pub:** *Bulgarian Journal of Hepatogastroenterology*, quarterly. **Frmly:** Bulgarian Gastro-Surgical Club; Bulgarian Association of Surgeons and Gastroenterologists.

★ 5674 ★ Scientific Society of Nutrition and Dietetics

Department of hygiene, ecology and occupat. diseases
15 boul. D.Nestorov
BG-1431 Sofia, Bulgaria
Phone: 359 2 5940611 **Fax:** 359 2 595106
Email: galinapopova@dir.bg

Fnded: 1986. **Mem:** 101. **Lang(s):** English, Russian. **Desc:** Fosters research in apiotherapy.

★ 5675 ★ Scientific Society of Stomatology

Katedra po Protetichna Stomatologia
Department of Prosthetic Dentistry
1 G.Sofiiski str.
BG-1431 Sofia, Bulgaria
Phone: 359 2 542669 **Fax:** 359 2 9520559
Email: mitredoc@dentist.bg

Fnded: 1952. **Mem:** 104. **Nat'l Groups:** 1. **Reg. Groups:** 2. **State Groups:** 2. **Local Groups:** 15. **Lang(s):** English. **Desc:** Fosters research in all diseases of the mouth. **Pub:** *Stomatologia - Sofia BG*, semiannual. Journal.

★ 5676 ★ Scleroderma Foundation (SF)

12 Kent Way, Ste. 101
Byfield, MA 01922
Phone: (978)463-5843 **Free:** 800-722-4673
Fax: (978)463-5809
Email: sfinfo@sclerdoma.org
Website: http://www.scleroderma.org
Elaine Furst, Chm.

Fnded: 1983. **Mem:** 16,000. **Reg. Groups:** 75. **Desc:** Scleroderma organizations. Promotes medical research to find a cure for scleroderma, a chronic systemic disease affecting all organs resulting from uncontrolled growth of connective tissue. Seeks to foster an understanding of the disease through media and outreach programs; raises funds. Provides patients with educational materials and referrals to local organizations and medical specialists. Offers encouragement and consultation services towards the formation and development of local support groups. Acts as a clearinghouse for information about scleroderma research, drugs, and therapies. Conducts accredited programs for professionals. Maintains speakers' bureau; compiles statistics. Funds one million dollars a year in new research. **Pub:** *About Scleroderma*. Brochure. • *Helpful Hints for Living with Scleroderma*. • *Newsline*, quarterly. *Price:* Included in membership. • *Understanding and Managing Scleroderma*. Booklet. **Frmly:** (1984) International Scleroderma Federation; (1998) Scleroderma Federation.

★ 5677 ★ Scleroderma Research Foundation (SRF)

2320 Bath St., Ste. 315
Santa Barbara, CA 93105
Phone: (805)563-9133 **Free:** 800-441-CURE
Fax: (805)563-2402
Email: srfcure@srfcure.org
Website: http://www.srfcure.org/
Luke Evnin, Chm.

Fnded: 1978. **Reg. Groups:** 1. **Desc:** Seeks to find a cure for scleroderma, a life-threatening and degenerative illness. Funds and facilitates research and public awareness. **Pub:** *Scleroderma Handbook & Resource Guide*. Handbook. • *Scleroderma Research Foundation Newsletter*, semiannual. Newsletter. *Price:* Included in membership dues.

★ 5678 ★ Scleroderma Support Group (SSG)

224 Thompson St., No. 198
Hendersonville, NC 28792-2806
Phone: (401)781-5013
Email: seleroderma@hotmail.com
Website: http://www.angelfire.com/ri/scleroderma
Clara K. Ihlbrock, Pres.

Fnded: 1989. **Mem:** 1,000. **Nat'l Groups:** 1. **State Groups:** 2. **Desc:** Scleroderma patients and interested individuals. Serves as a support group for patients; provides information; raises funds for research; holds medical meetings and rap sessions.

★ 5679 ★ Scoliosis Association (SAI)

PO Box 811705
Boca Raton, FL 33481-1705
Phone: (561)994-4435 **Free:** 800-800-0669
Fax: (561)994-2455
Email: normlipin@aol.com
Website: http://www.scoliosis-assoc.org
Stanley Sacks, CEO

Fnded: 1976. **Mem:** 5,000. **Local Groups:** 52. **Desc:** Individuals or families involved or interested in scoliosis (lateral or sidewards curvature of the spine). Educates the public about scoliosis and other spinal deviations. Encourages and supports spinal screening programs in schools throughout the U.S. and Canada. Sponsors the formation of scoliosis chapters throughout the country which serve as support groups for the scoliosis patient and his or her family. Aids the patient in attaining a positive social and emotional adjustment during treatment of scoliosis. Plans to compile statistics; works with researchers in scoliosis. Raises funds for scoliosis research. Has sponsored scoliosis spinal conferences with several hospitals and leading spinal orthopaedists. **Pub:** *Backtalk*, periodic. Newsletter. Contains research and chapter news, article reprints, book reviews, and listings of publications. *Price:* $30 for individuals outside the U.S.; $40 for institutions; $40. • *Scoliosis, An Adult Perspective*. Video. *Price:* $19.95. • Bibliography.Lists books, articles, pamphlets, and papers on scoliosis. *Price:* $6 for part one; $3 for part two; $8 for parts one and two. • Brochure. • Also issues posters.

★ 5680 ★ Scoliosis Association (SAUK)

2 Ivebury Ct.
323-327 Latimer Rd.
London W10 6RA, United Kingdom
Phone: 44 20 89645343 **Fax:** 44 20 89645343
Email: sauk@sauk.org.uk
Website: http://www.sauk.org.uk

Fnded: 1981. **Mem:** 3,000. **Local Groups:** 29. **Lang(s):** English. **Desc:** Individuals affected by scoliosis; their parents and families. Seeks to increase knowledge and understanding of scoliosis (a lateral curvature of the spine) and emphasize the importance of early detection. Encourages contact between members; disseminates information to members and the public. **Pub:** *A Twist of Fate*. The psychological problems of coping with Scoliosis - especially for young people. • *Newsletter*, 2/year. Newsletter. • *Newsletter Index*. Lists and cross-references SAUK's newsletters. • *Schools Fact Sheet*. Contains information on scoliosis for parents of school-age children. • *Scoliosis: An Information Booklet*. Booklet.

★ 5681 ★ Scoliosis Research Society (SRS)

611 E Wells St.
Milwaukee, WI 53202
Phone: (414)289-9107 **Fax:** (414)276-3349
Email: jschaper@execinc.com
Website: http://www.srs.org
Tressa Goulding, Exec. Dir.

Fnded: 1966. **Mem:** 800. **Desc:** Orthopedic surgeons and physicians. Furthers research and education in spinal deformities, particularly scoliosis, a twisting of the spine to one side. Most cases are of unknown cause, though scoliosis can result from a birth defect, polio, or spinal injury and usually develops in children during the growth spurt between ages ten and 15. Early detection followed with use of a brace and exercise can halt the curvature and prevent deformity.

★ 5682 ★ Scope

6 Market Rd.
London N7 9PW, United Kingdom
Phone: 44 20 76197100
Email: cphelpline@scope.org.uk
Website: http://www.scope.org.uk

Lang(s): English. **Desc:** People with cerebral palsy, their families, and carers in England and Wales. Promotes equality for disabled people. Provides residential, job help, and education services for people with cerebral palsy; carries out research into issues affecting disabled people. **Pub:** *Disability Now*, monthly. Newspaper.

★ 5683 ★ Scottish Association of Health Councils

24 A Palmerston Place
Edinburgh EH12 5AL, United Kingdom
Phone: 44 131 2204101 **Fax:** 44 131 2204108
Email: admin1@sahc.sol.co.uk
Website: http://www.show.scot.nhs.uk/sahc

Fnded: 1977. **Mem:** 15. **Desc:** Membership is open to all 15 health councils in Scotland. Provides information, training resources and development of public participation to all health related matters. The organization is the focal point between Local Health Councils, the Scottish Executive and Health Department and other national organizations, SAHC is voluntary and funded by LHC's subscriptions. **Pub:** Papers.

★ 5684 ★ Scottish Association for Mental Health

Cumbrae House
15 Carlton Ct.
Glasgow G5 9JP, United Kingdom
Phone: 44 141 5687000 **Fax:** 44 141 5687001
Email: enquire@samh.org.uk
Website: http://www.samh.org.uk

Fnded: 1923. **Mem:** 239. **Local Groups:** 23. **Desc:** Health Boards, Regional Councils, District Councils, Psychiatric Hospitals, local and regional voluntary organisations, Trade Unions, Professional Bodies Universities, individuals, local associations for mental health. Campaigns for better hospital and community services; seeks to increase understanding of mental distress; provides direct services to people who have suffered from mental health problems, namely supported accommodation and training for employment on projects all over Scotland. Information, training and a development consultancy are also offered to local groups, professionals and affiliated local mental health associations. **Pub:** *Mental Health Matters*, quarterly. Newsletter.

★ 5685 ★ Scottish Childminding Association

7 Melville Terr., Ste. 3
Stirling FK8 2ND, United Kingdom
Phone: 44 1786 445377 **Fax:** 44 1786 449062
Website: http://www.childminding.org/

Desc: Promotes childminding as a quality childcare service. Works to inform childminders, parents, employers, local authorities and central government about good practice in childminding and ways to attain this.

★ 5686 ★ Scottish Committee of Optometrists

7 Queens Bldgs.
Queensferry Rd.
Rosyth
Fife
Saint Andrews KY11 2RA, United Kingdom
Phone: 44 383 419444 **Fax:** 44 383 416778

Email: secretarysco@aol.com

Fnded: 1935. **Mem:** 760. **Lang(s):** English. **Desc:** All optometrists in Scotland. Represents interests of independent optometrists in Scotland. **Pub:** *Look North*, bimonthly. Newsletter.

★ 5687 ★ Scottish Council on Deafness (SCoD)

Clerwood House
96 Clermiston Rd.
Edinburgh EH12 6UT, United Kingdom
Phone: 44 131 3146075 **Fax:** 44 131 3146077
Email: admin@scod.org.uk
Website: http://www.scod.org.uk/

Desc: Committed to addressing the needs of deaf, deafened, deafblind and hard of hearing individuals, their families and caregivers, and the professionals working with them. Works to improve the quality of life for all deaf people in Scotland.

★ 5688 ★ Scottish Council on Human Bioethics (SCHB)

200 Bath St.
Glasgow G2 4HG, United Kingdom
Phone: 44 7092 365757 **Fax:** 44 7092 365765
Email: secretary@schb.org.uk
Website: http://www.schb.org.uk/

Fnded: 1997. **Desc:** Doctors, lawyers, psychologists, ethicists and other professionals from disciplines associated with medical ethics whose principles are set out in the United Nations Universal Declaration of Human Rights. Works to collect and evaluate evidence and information relating to ethical issues to inform public debate; assist legislators, fellow professionals and other interested parties with ethical analysis and comment on issues; respond appropriately to the media.

★ 5689 ★ Scottish Council for Postgraduate Medical and Dental Education (SCPMDE)

Hanover Bldg., 2nd Fl.
66 Rose St.
Edinburgh EH2 2NN, United Kingdom
Phone: 44 131 2254365 **Fax:** 44 131 2255891
Email: enquiries@scpmde.scot.nhs.uk
Website: http://www.show.scot.nhs.uk/scpmde/

Desc: Directs, supports and commissions postgraduate studies in medical and dental education for approximately 4,700 doctors, dentists and clinical psychologists.

★ 5690 ★ Scottish Institute of Reflexology (SIR)

110 Easterhouse Rd., Flat ½
Glasgow G34 9RG, United Kingdom
Phone: 44 141 7730018
Email: mmreflex@aol.com
Website: http://www.scottishreflexology.org

Fnded: 1987. **Mem:** 430. **Desc:** Works to promote, monitor and maintain professional standards among reflexologists; aims to advance acceptance of reflexology as an alternative treatment; provides training courses.

★ 5691 ★ Scottish Motor Neurone Disease Association

76 Firhill Rd.
Glasgow G20 7BA, United Kingdom
Phone: 44 141 9451077 **Fax:** 44 141 9452578
Email: info@scotmnd.sol.co.uk
Website: http://www.scotmnd.org.uk

Fnded: 1981. **Mem:** 500. **Lang(s):** English. **Desc:** Promotes interest in motor neurone disease (MND) research among medical and scientific communities and the public in Scotland. Offers care and support services to MND patients in Scotland, and their families. Offers an information centre, equipment loan centre, organizes study days for health professionals. **Pub:** *Aware*, 3/year. Newsletter.

★ 5692 ★ Scottish National Blood Transfusion Association (SNBTA)

2 Otterburn Park
Edinburgh EH14 1JX, United Kingdom
Phone: 44 131 4437636

Fnded: 1940. **Mem:** 250,000. **Lang(s):** English. **Desc:** Blood donors. Promotes donation of blood; seeks to insure a reliable and safe supply of blood and plasma for use in medical transfusions. Represents the interests of blood and bone marrow donors before medical organizations and government agencies; provides support and assistance to the Scottish National Blood Transfusion Service; consults with medical organizations to improve blood donation and transfusion techniques. Maintains speakers' bureau. **Pub:** *Annual Report and Statement of Accounts*, annual. Annual Report.

★ 5693 ★ Scottish National Federation for the Welfare of the Blind

Balmashanner Rise
Forfar
Angus DD8 1PD, United Kingdom

Fnded: 1917. **Mem:** 63. **Lang(s):** English. **Desc:** Parent body for numerous charities and local authorities in Scotland concerned with the welfare of blind and partially sighted people. Provides information on social work, education, and employment services. **Pub:** Annual Report.

★ 5694 ★ Scottish Out of School Care Network (SOSCN)

6th Fl., Fleming House
134 Renfrew St.
Glasgow G3 6ST, United Kingdom
Phone: 44 141 3311301 **Fax:** 44 141 3321206
Email: info@soscn.org
Website: http://www.soscn.org

Fnded: 1991. **Mem:** 400. **Nat'l Groups:** 1. **Reg. Groups:** 30. **Local Groups:** 800. **Lang(s):** English. **Desc:** Organizations and agencies engaged in out-of-school child care. Promotes increased availability of affordable, quality child care. Establishes partnerships among members and between members and other organizations pursuing similar goals. Works to increase awareness of child care issues. Conducts research; makes available information about children's services; compiles statistics. **Pub:** *Connections*, quarterly. Newsletter.

★ 5695 ★ Scottish Pensions Association (SPA)

207 Pleasance
Edinburgh EH8 9RU, United Kingdom
Phone: 44 131 6678504
Email: websterspa@aol.com

Fnded: 1937. **Mem:** 10,000. **Reg. Groups:** 3. **Local Groups:** 90. **Lang(s):** English. **Desc:** Pensioners and those interested in issues affecting older peoples' lives, rights, and welfare. Aims to improve the quality of life for older people and urges that the State Pension should rise annually in line with prices or average earnings. Provides opportunities for members to gain a voice on the key issues affecting older people.

★ 5696 ★ Scottish Pharmaceutical Federation

135 Wellington St.
Glasgow G2 2XD, United Kingdom
Phone: 44 141 2211235 **Fax:** 44 141 2265047
Email: spf@npanet.co.uk
Website: http://www.npa.co.uk

Fnded: 1919. **Mem:** 1,050. **Desc:** Independent retail pharmacists in Scotland. Provides legal representation, general insurance, professional indemnity cover, staff training, clearing house and information services for Scotland. **Pub:** Newsletter, periodic.

★ 5697 ★ Scottish Pharmaceutical General Council

42 Queen St.
Edinburgh EH2 3NH, United Kingdom
Phone: 44 131 4677766 **Fax:** 44 131 4677767
Email: enquiries@spgc.org.uk
Website: http://www.spgc.org.uk

Fnded: 1913. **Desc:** Body recognised by Secretary of State for Scotland as representing the interests of the general body of chemist contractors in Scotland. Concerned with all NHS matters which affect retail pharmacy in Scotland.

★ 5698 ★ Scottish Society for Autism

Hilton House
Alloa Business Park
Whins Rd.
Alloa FK10 3SA, United Kingdom
Phone: 44 1259 720044 **Fax:** 44 1259 720051
Email: liddell@autism-in-scotland.org.uk
Website: http://www.autism-in-scotland.org.uk

Mem: 600. **Local Groups:** 8. **Lang(s):** English. **Desc:** Families affected by autism, Asperger syndrome, or related communication disorders, as well as professionals and caregivers in the field. Works to deliver a comprehensive range of expertise in care, support, and education for people with autism, their families, and caregivers in Scotland. Operates community houses, respite care centers, and schools; provides family support visits and other community support services.

★ 5699 ★ Scottish Society of the History of Medicine

Red Gable
Penhead
Saint Andrews KY16 8PB, United Kingdom

Fnded: 1948. **Mem:** 200. **Desc:** Aims to further the general history of medicine with particular attention to Scottish medicine. **Pub:** *Report of Proceedings*, semiannual. Proceedings.

★ 5700 ★ Scottish Spina Bifida Association (SSBA)

190 Queensferry Rd.
Edinburgh EH4 2BW, United Kingdom
Phone: 44 131 3320743 **Fax:** 44 131 3433651
Email: gail@ssba.org.uk
Website: http://www.ssba.org.uk

Fnded: 1965. **Mem:** 3,000. **Reg. Groups:** 5. **Local Groups:** 4. **Desc:** Seeks to increase public awareness and understanding of individuals with Spina Bifida/Hydrocephalus and allied disorders. Aims to secure provision for their special needs and those of their families.

★ 5701 ★ Scottish Sports Association for Disabled People

Fife Sports Institute
Viewfield Rd.
Glenrothes KY6 2RB, United Kingdom
Phone: 44 1592 415700 **Fax:** 44 1592 415710

Desc: Promotes sports for the disabled in Scotland.

★ 5702 ★ SEAMEO Regional Centre for Medical Microbiology, Parasitology and Entomology (SEAMEO TRO)

c/o Institute of Medical Research
Jalan Pahang
50588 Kuala Lumpur, Malaysia
Phone: 60 3 26988876 **Fax:** 60 3 26939335
Email: seameo@imr.gov.my

Fnded: 1970. **Desc:** A project of the Southeast Asian Ministers of Education Organization. Works to improve medical education and related programs in southeast Asia. Encourages study and research in the field. Conducts training programs and 2 graduate programs in medical microbiology and parasitology/entomology.

★ 5703 ★ SEAMEO Regional Centre for Public Health
c/o College of Public Health
625 Pedro Gil St.
Ermita
Manila, Philippines
Phone: 63 2 5242703 **Fax:** 63 2 5211394
Email: vchan@cph.upm.edu.ph

Fnded: 1927. **Mem:** 59. **Desc:** A project of the Southeast Asian Ministers of Education Organization. Encourages excellence in public health education programs in southeast Asia. Conducts training programs.

★ 5704 ★ Section for Long Term Care and Rehabilitation
c/o American Hospital Association
1 N Franklin St.
Chicago, IL 60606
Phone: (312)422-3302 **Fax:** (312)422-4590
Email: ssonik@aha.org
Website: http://www.aha.org
Susanne Sonik, Dir.

Fnded: 1984. **Mem:** 2,600. **Desc:** Functions as part of the American Hospital Association. Promotes understanding of the health and continuing care needs of persons of all ages and issues pertinent to health care provider organizations. Seeks to improve continuity of care between acute, pre- and post-acute, and long-term services; supports efforts to improve health care delivery to chronically ill, elderly and disabled. research.

★ 5705 ★ Section for Metropolitan Hospitals (SMH)
c/o American Hospital Association
1 N Franklin, Ste. 27
Chicago, IL 60606
Phone: (312)422-3000 **Fax:** (312)422-4583
Email: jsupplitt@aha.org
Website: http://www.hospitalconnect.com/aha
John T. Supplitt, Dir.

Fnded: 1984. **Mem:** 1,365. **Desc:** Institutional members of the American Hospital Association that are located within a metropolitan statistical area and/or provide a significant proportion of Medicare, Medicaid, and uncompensated care; participate in undergraduate and/or graduate medical education programs and research; provide high volumes of ambulatory care; offer specialized services; and are involved in professional and paraprofessional education and training programs. Represents views of members to the AHA and assists in the development and implementation of policies and programs to promote recognition, support, and growth for its members within the health care field. Serves as clearinghouse for metropolitan hospital delivery, finance, governance, management, and organizational issues. Compiles statistics; maintains databases; conducts forums.

★ 5706 ★ Section for Psychiatric and Substance Abuse Services (SPSPAS)
c/o American Hospital Association
One N Franklin
Chicago, IL 60606
Phone: (312)422-3000 **Free:** 800-242-4890
Fax: (312)422-4796
Email: hromero@aha.org
Website: http://www.aha.org/memberrelations/psas.org
Gary A. Mecklenburg, Pres.

Fnded: 1969. **Mem:** 3,000. **Desc:** Institutional members, both general hospitals and freestanding specialty hospitals, of the American Hospital Association who provide psychiatric, substance abuse, clinical psychology, and other behavioral health services. Assists the AHA in development and implementation of policies and programs to promote improvement of and advocacy for the nation's behavioral health care providers. Active in formulating and commenting on federal legislation and regulations relating to psychiatric and substance abuse services. Develops and maintains liaison relationships with key organizations important to behavioral health providers. **Frmly:** (1972) Psychiatric Hospital Section; (1984) Psychiatric Services Section; (1991) Special Constituency Section for Mental Health and Psychiatric Services; (1997) Special Constituency Section for Psychiatric and Substance Abuse Services.

★ 5707 ★ Secular Organizations for Sobriety (SOS)
4773 Hollywood Blvd.
Hollywood, CA 90027
Phone: (323)666-4295 **Fax:** (323)666-4271
Email: sos@CFIWest.org
Website: http://cfiwest.org/sos
James R. Christopher, Founder

Fnded: 1986. **Mem:** 20,000. **Desc:** Recovering alcoholics and drug addicts; families and friends of alcoholics or drug addicts. Serves as a support system free of any religious or spiritual undercurrent; believes sobriety is a process of personal responsibility. Espouses "a healthy skepticism" and encourages self-reliance and free thought. Maintains speakers' bureau. Compiles statistics. **Pub:** *Save Our Selves*, quarterly. Newsletter.

★ 5708 ★ The Seeing Eye
PO Box 375
Morristown, NJ 07963-0375
Phone: (973)539-4425 **Fax:** (973)539-0922
Website: http://www.seeingeye.org
Kenneth Rosenthal, Pres.

Fnded: 1929. **Nat'l Groups:** 1. **Desc:** Seeks to enhance the independence, dignity, and self-confidence of blind and visually impaired persons; provides assistance to graduates and their seeing-eyed dogs; educates the public in consideration of public policy. **Pub:** *The Seeing Eye Guide*, quarterly. Annual Report.

★ 5709 ★ Selective Mutism Foundation
c/o Sue Newman
PO Box 1198
Medford, NY 11763
Email: consultsn@aol.com
Website: http://selectivemutismfoundation.org/
Sue Newman, Co-Founder & Dir.

Fnded: 1991. **Mem:** 3,000. **Desc:** Individuals and families affected by selective mutism, an inherited anxiety disorder in which children with normal language skills or deficient language skills are unable to speak in school or other social situations. SM is often mistaken for normal shyness, and may go undetected for as long as two years. Promotes awareness and understanding of this condition. Encourages research and treatment. Maintains speakers' bureau. **Pub:** *Selective Mutism, A Silent Cry for Help*. Brochure. *Price:* Free. **Frmly:** (1993) Foundation for Elective Mutism, Inc.

★ 5710 ★ Self-Help Association for the Electrically Sensitive (Selbsthilfeverein fuer Elektrosensible)
Gesundheitshaus
Dachauerstr. 90
D-80335 Munich, Germany
Phone: 49 89 23337501

Fnded: 1989. **Mem:** 230. **Lang(s):** German. **Desc:** Individuals suffering from electrical hypersensitivity in Germany (electrical hypersensitivity is brought on from overexposure to electrical and magnetic fields emitted by appliances, particularly television sets, computers and mobile phones). Supports afflicted individuals and works to stop the spread of these conditions; works to insure recognition of these maladies by insurance companies and government agencies; promotes research into the causes and cure of electrical hypersensitivity.

★ 5711 ★ Self Help for Hard of Hearing People (SHHH)
7910 Woodmont Ave., Ste. 1200
Bethesda, MD 20814
Phone: (301)657-2248 **Fax:** (301)913-9413
Email: national@shhh.org
Website: http://www.shhh.org
Kathryn Stephens, Interim Exec. Dir.

Fnded: 1979. **Mem:** 12,000. **Reg. Groups:** 10. **State Groups:** 250. **Desc:** Devoted to the welfare and interests of those who cannot hear well, their relatives and friends. Strives to improve quality of hard of hearing people's lives through education, advocacy and self help. **Pub:** *Hearing Loss: The Journal of Self Help for Hard at Hearing People*, bimonthly. Magazine. Contains articles by hearing health professionals and personal narratives by people with hearing loss. Contains information on resources. • *Hospitality for Guests with Hearing Loss: A Guide for Hotel/Motel Compliance with the Americans with Disabilities Act.* • *Operation SHHH: Noise Abuse Prevention Posters.* • *Our Forgotten Children: Hard-of-Hearing Pupils in the Schools.* • *SHHH News*, quarterly. Newsletter. • *Telephone Strategies: A Technical and Practical Guide for Hard of Hearing People.* • Brochures. • Offers various publications on hearing loss, products, and related subjects. **AKA:** SHHH.

★ 5712 ★ Seniors Coalition (TSC)
9001 Braddock Rd., Ste. 200
Springfield, VA 22151
Phone: (703)239-1960 **Fax:** (703)239-1985
Email: tsc@senior.org
Website: http://www.senior.org
Mary Martin, Exec. Dir.

Fnded: 1989. **Desc:** Represents the interests and concerns of America's senior citizens at state and federal levels. **Pub:** *The Advocate*, quarterly. Magazine.

★ 5713 ★ SENSE
11-13 Clifton Terrace
Finsbury Park
London N4 3SR, United Kingdom
Phone: 44 20 72727774 **Fax:** 44 20 72726012
Email: enquiries@sense.org.uk
Website: http://www.sense.org.uk

Fnded: 1955. **Mem:** 650. **Reg. Groups:** 14. **Lang(s):** Welsh. **Desc:** Families, professionals and interested individuals. To provide services for deafblind people, their families, carers and the professionals with whom they work. Campaigns for legislative support for deafblind people. **Pub:** *Publications list.* • *Talking Sense*, 3/year. Magazine. For parents and professionals in the deafblind field. • Books. **Frmly:** (2001) National Deafblind and Rubella Association.

★ 5714 ★ Sequella Global Tuberculosis Foundation
c/o Carol A. Nacy
9610 Medical Center Dr., Ste. 220
Rockville, MD 20850
Phone: (301)762-3100 **Fax:** (301)762-2122
Email: information@sequellafoundation.org
Website: http://www.sequellafoundation.org
Carol A. Nacy, PhD, Pres.

Fnded: 1977. **Desc:** Researchers. Established as a resource for the Tuberculosis Research Community to help identify and develop concepts and tools for controlling the global epidemic.

★ 5715 ★ Serendipity Association
c/o Dr. Doug Henstreet
4614 Edgeware Rd., No. 4
San Diego, CA 92116-4760
Phone: (619)284-2468 **Fax:** (619)284-2468
Email: serendipityasn@yahoo.com
Dr. Doug Hemstreet, Chair

Fnded: 1973. **Desc:** Individuals and professionals interested in or working with holistic health care, world peace, and concepts involved with a "How to Make the World Work Project." Proposes reinventing our world to create a happy, healthy home for humanity, so that "all children everywhere are loved, housed, and well fed." Works to: reform educational system based on "correcting 14 vested Interest Distortions"; stop "government lies, deceit, and cover-ups in health, agriculture, education, defense, and waste." Promotes herbs, natural healing systems, and energy medicine for healing problems such as cancer and AIDS. Supports scientific research in the field of holistic medicine. Sponsors speakers, workshops, and training programs. Offers consulting services on designing and starting Holistic Health Centers and for government and corporations on reducing health care costs. **Pub:** *Serendipity News*, semiannual. Newsletter. *Price:* Included in membership dues. • Also publishes library information packages ($45). **Frmly:** (1999) Serendipity Association for Research and Implementation of Holistic Health and World Peace; (2003) Serendipity Association and How to Make the World Work Project.

★ 5716 ★ Seventh-Day Adventist Dietetic Association (SDADA)
6100 Leoni Rd.
Box 400
Grizzly Flats, CA 95636-0400
Phone: (916)782-5200 **Fax:** (916)782-5458
Email: rubyh@rsvl.ah.com
Fnded: 1956. **Mem:** 505. **Desc:** Seventh-Day Adventist registered dietitians; dietitians working in Seventh-Day Adventist institutions. Strives to motivate members to attain high professional standards and to actively promote Seventh-Day Adventist health principles. Provides resources and guidance concerning vegetarian lifestyles to dietitians. Disseminates nutrition information. **Pub:** *Diet Manual*. Includes vegetarian options. *Price:* $54.95. • *SDADA News*, quarterly. *Price:* available to members only. • *Seventh-Day Adventist Dietetic Association Diet Manual.* • *The Vegetarian Advantage.* Brochure.

★ 5717 ★ Sex Information and Education Council of Canada (SIECC)
850 Coxwell Ave.
Toronto, ON, Canada M4C 5R1
Phone: (416)466-5304 **Fax:** (416)778-0785
Email: sieccan@web.net
Website: http://www.sieccan.org
Fnded: 1964. **Mem:** 800. **Lang(s):** English, French. **Desc:** Individuals and organizations in fields including sex education, counselling, reproductive health and medicine, and rehabilitation and therapy. Fosters public and professional education about human sexuality. Facilitates networking among members. Maintains information service and speakers' bureau; conducts research programs; sponsors educational programs. **Pub:** *The Canadian Journal of Human Sexuality*, quarterly. Journal. • *SIECCAN Newsletter*, 2-3/year. Newsletter.

★ 5718 ★ Sexuality Information and Education Council of the U.S. (SIECUS)
130 W 42nd St., Ste. 350
New York, NY 10036-7802
Phone: (212)819-9770 **Fax:** (212)819-9776
Email: siecus@siecus.org
Website: http://www.siecus.org/
Tamara Krenin, Pres.
Fnded: 1964. **Desc:** Promotes education about sexuality. Advocates "the rght of individuals to make responsible sexual choices". Disseminates information. **Pub:** *Fact Sheets*. • *SIECUS Report*. Journal. • Manuals. • Pamphlets. • Booklets. • Bibliographies. • Also publishes guidelines for comprehensive sexuality education and position statement. Publications catalog available on request. **Frmly:** (1998) Sex Information and Education Council of the U.S.

★ 5719 ★ Sexually Transmitted Diseases Society of Southern Africa
PO Box 1038
Johannesburg 2000, Republic of South Africa
Fnded: 1983.

★ 5720 ★ Sexually Transmitted Infections Prevention Committee (STIPC)
Genitourinary Clinic
Boffa Hospital
Floriana MSD 05, Malta
Phone: 356 322306 **Fax:** 356 319243
Email: Philip.carabot@gov.mt
Fnded: 1986. **Mem:** 5. **Lang(s):** English. **Desc:** Makes recommendations for national AIDS and other sexually transmitted diseases policy formulation; advises Director General of Health, Malta. **Frmly:** (1999) National Committee for AIDS Prevention and Control.

★ 5721 ★ Share and Care Cockayne Syndrome Network
c/o Shirley Rodriguez
PO Box 570618
Dallas, TX 75357
Phone: (972)613-4590 **Fax:** (972)613-4590
Email: j93082@aol.com
Website: http://www.cockayne-syndrome.org
Shirley Rodriguez, contact
Fnded: 1993. **Mem:** 1,500. **Desc:** Professionals and families. Works to provide information on Cockayne Syndrome, a rare form of dwarfism, to help parents and doctors to make informed decisions in the care of these children. Provides support for families; encourages research. **Pub:** *Newsletter*, quarterly. Brochure. Research updates and articles on individual children.

★ 5722 ★ Shiatsu Therapists Alliance (STA)
1054 Centre St., Ste. 431
Thornhill, ON, Canada L4J 8E5
Phone: (416)579-5373
Email: shiatsutherapistsalliance@yahoo.ca
Desc: Works to inform and protect the public in matters regarding Shiatsu therapy; provides referrals to registered therapists; promotes ethical Shiatsu practice. Maintains speakers bureau. **Pub:** Newsletter.

★ 5723 ★ Shingles Support Society
c/o Marian Nicholson, Dir.
41 North Rd.
London N7 9DP, United Kingdom
Phone: 44 20 76079661
Email: marian@herpes.org.uk
Website: http://www.herpes.org.uk
Fnded: 1985. **Lang(s):** English. **Desc:** Individuals suffering from post-herpetic neuralgia and their families. Offers advice on self-help for post-herpetic neuralgia which can follow shingles. Provides information for primary care doctors by a consultant neurologist regarding drug treatment with dosage information.

★ 5724 ★ Shriners Hospitals for Children
2900 Rocky Point Dr.
Tampa, FL 33607-1460
Phone: (813)281-0300 **Free:** 800-237-5055
Website: http://www.shrinershq.org/hospitals/index.html
John D. Vermaas, Chm.
Fnded: 1922. **Mem:** 22. **Desc:** SHC operated orthopedic hospitals (19) and burn hospitals (4) founded by and affiliated with the Imperial Council of the Ancient Arabic Order of the Nobles of the Mystic Shrine for North America. Provides no-cost orthopedic and burn care to children under 18 years of age. Maintains the Shriners Hospitals for Children Endowment Fund. Conducts research; compiles statistics. **Pub:** *Between Us*, 3/year. Magazine. *Price:* Free. • *Imperial Council of the Ancient Arabic Order of the Nobles of the Mystic Shrine for North America.* • Booklet. • Brochures. • Pamphlets. • Also publishes fact sheets.

★ 5725 ★ Shwachman-Diamond Syndrome International
PMB 162
5195 Hampsted Village Center Way
New Albany, OH 43054-8331
Free: 877-737-4685 **Fax:** (614)939-0752
Email: 4sskids@shwachman-diamond.org
Website: http://www.shwachman-diamond.org/
Fnded: 1994. **Desc:** Provides emotional support to patients and their families; educates the medical community and general public about Schwachman-Diamond Syndrome; encourages training of and research by medical professionals; advocates support of research; links families through exchange of experience and ideas; disseminates current medical information; supports an International Patient Registry/Database. **Pub:** Newsletter.

★ 5726 ★ Siblings for Significant Change (SSC)
350 5th Ave., Ste.627
New York, NY 10118
Phone: (212)420-0776 **Free:** 800-841-8251
Fax: (212)643-1244
Email: gerriscfu@aol.com
Website: http://www.specialcitizens.com
Gerri Zatlow, Dir.
Fnded: 1982. **Mem:** 75. **Desc:** Siblings of disabled individuals; parents, educators, social workers, medical professionals, and researchers interested in siblings of disabled individuals. Provides peer support, legal assistance, and psychological counseling to siblings of the handicapped. Coordinates social activities for families with handicapped members and works on projects and audiovisual programs designed to increase national awareness of the difficulties faced by families of disabled individuals. Maintains speakers' bureau. Division of Special Citizens Futures Unlimited, a New York state organization that offers ongoing programs for autistic and autistic-like adults. **Pub:** *Directory of Sibling Related Services*. Directory. • Journal, semiannual. • Newsletter, periodic.

★ 5727 ★ Sickle Cell Disease Association of America (SCDAA)
200 Corporate Pointe, Ste. 495
Culver City, CA 90230-8727
Phone: (310)216-6363 **Free:** 800-421-8453
Fax: (310)215-3722
Email: scdaa@sicklecelldisease.org
Lynda King Anderson, Pres. /COO
Fnded: 1971. **Mem:** 65. **Local Groups:** 86. **Desc:** Community groups involved in sickle cell anemia programs throughout the U.S. (Sickle cell anemia is an inherited blood disease that primarily affects black people and is a major health problem within the black community.) Purposes are to: provide leadership on a national level in order to create awareness in all circles of the negative impact of sickle cell anemia on the health and economic, social, and educational well-being of the individual and his/her family and to create awareness of the requirements for resolution; prepare and distribute substantive educational materials; develop and promote implementation of service program standards that will be in the best interest of the affected population; provide ongoing technical assistance to interested groups; encourage adequate support for research. Resources include: counselor training; workshops and seminars; blood banks; screening and testing; tutorial services; camps for children with sickle cell disease; vocational rehabilitation; scholarships. Operates Charles F. Whitten Sickle Cell Summer Research Apprenticeships, Roland J. Nyman Research Fund, and Rick Berry Fund. **Pub:** *Comprehensive Guide to Sickle Cell Disease & SCDAA Services.* • *HELP, A Guide to Sickle Cell Disease Programs and Services*, periodic. • *SCD Parent/Teacher Guide.* • *Sickle Cell Disease Association of America Newsletter*, quarterly. Newsletter. *Price:* Free. • *Sickle Cell Disease Association of America Viewpoint*, periodic. • *Sickle Cell Disease Fact Brochures.* • Brochures. • Pamphlets. **Frmly:** National Association for Sickle Cell Disease.

★ 5728 ★ Sidelines National High-Risk Pregnancy Support Network
PO Box 1808
Laguna Beach, CA 92652

Phone: (949)497-2265 **Free:** 888-447-4754
Fax: (949)497-5598
Email: sidelines@sidelines.org
Website: http://www.sidelines.org
Candace Hurley, Exec. Dir.

Fnded: 1992. **Mem:** 20,000. **Reg. Groups:** 32. **Desc:** Former high-risk mothers dedicated to supporting women and their families experiencing a complicated or high-risk pregnancy. A pregnancy is termed "complicated" when the life or health of the mother and/or baby may be at risk. Committed to helping women overcome the risks of preterm birth, low birthweight, and other serious consequences of high risk pregnancies. Operates the One-On-One program where a mother and her family are paired with a trained "Phone Friend" who has previously been through a complicated pregnancy. Offers prenatal care information and grief and loss counseling. Provides the families with resources and referrals to local businesses, agencies, and services that can assist them. **Pub:** *Left Side Lines*, annual. Magazine. *Price:* $3.50 for hospitals, physicians and patients. • *Sidelines Parent Pack.* Book. *Price:* $15. • *That's What Friends Are For.* Guide for helping the bedresting mom and her family. • *When Pregnancy Isn't Perfect. Price:* $12. **Frmly:** (2002) Sidelines National Support Network.

★ 5729 ★ Sidran Traumatic Stress Foundation

200 E Joppa Rd., Ste. 207
Baltimore, MD 21286
Phone: (410)825-8888 **Fax:** (410)337-0747
Email: sidran@sidran.org
Website: http://www.sidran.org
Esther Giller, Pres. & Dir.

Fnded: 1986. **Desc:** Supports people with trauma-generated psychological disorders. Educates trauma survivors, their support people and caregivers through the development of programs, projects, and publications. Provides advocacy services; maintains speakers' bureau; information clearinghouse; professional training. **Pub:** *Sidran Bookshelf on Trauma and Dissociation*, annual. Catalog. • *Training Materials.* • *Workbooks.* • Books.Books for professional and lay audiences about the mental health effects of extremely traumatic experiences. **Frmly:** (2000) Sidran Foundation and Press.

★ 5730 ★ Sight Savers International - East, Central and Southern Africa Region

Mai Mahiu Rd., off Langata Rd.
Nairobi West
PO Box 34690
GPO
Nairobi, Kenya
Phone: 254 20 505750 **Fax:** 254 20 505548
Email: info@sightsavers.or.ke

Fnded: 1949. **Desc:** Promotes programs for the blind and visually impaired in Kenya, Uganda, Tanzania, Malawi, Zimbabwe. Fosters public awareness. Programmes in eye care, education and rehabilitation for the blind and visually impaired. **Pub:** *Horizons*, quarterly. Update on SSI activities worldwide. • *Xerophthaimia Bulletin*, periodic. Bulletin.

★ 5731 ★ Sight Savers International - England

Grosvenor Hall
Bolnore Rd.
Haywards Heath RH16 4BX, United Kingdom
Phone: 44 1444 446600 **Fax:** 44 1444 446688
Email: information@sightsavers.org

Fnded: 1950. **Mem:** 30. **Lang(s):** English. **Desc:** Works to prevent and cure blindness and also to provide education and rehabilitation for blind people in economically developing countries. Concentrates on comprehensive eye services which link the sectors together. Cooperates with indigenous government agencies and local leadership to develop and implement vision care programs. Conducts leadership development and educational programs to make projects sustainable using local resources and expertise. **Pub:** *Sight Savers News*, 3/year. Newsletter. Donor newsletter.

★ 5732 ★ Sigma Phi Alpha

University of Texas, Health Science Center
Houston, Dental B
PO Box 20068
Houston, TX 77225
Phone: (713)500-4085
Patricia Campbell, Treas.

Fnded: 1958. **Mem:** 9,000. **Local Groups:** 163. **Desc:** Honorary society, dental hygiene. **Pub:** *Sigma Phi Alpha*, annual. Newsletter. **AKA:** National Dental Hygiene Honor Society.

★ 5733 ★ Sigma Theta Tau International (STTI)

550 W North St.
Indianapolis, IN 46202
Phone: (317)634-8171 **Free:** 888-634-7575
Fax: (317)634-8188
Email: stti@stti.iupui.edu
Website: http://www.nursingsociety.org
Nancy Dickenson-Hazard, CEO

Fnded: 1922. **Mem:** 120,000. **Local Groups:** 406. **Desc:** One of the largest and most prestigious nursing organizations in the world. Committed to fostering nursing excellence, scholarship and leadership to improve health care worldwide, its members promote research-based practice by making resources available to all interested people and institutions. Sigma Theta Tau International is comprised of chapter honor societies that are located on more than 500 colleges and university campuses in all 50 states, Puerto Rico, Canada, South Korea, Taiwan, Australia, Pakistan, Brazil, Netherlands, and Hong Kong. Members are active in 94 countries and territories. **Pub:** *Directory of Nurse Researchers.* Directory. *Price:* $60 print; $25 compact disc. • *Journal of Nursing Scholarship*, quarterly. Journal. Includes manuscripts, books reviews, and opinion pieces. *Price:* $34/year; $56/2 years. • *The Online Journal of Knowledge Synthesis for Nursing (Full-Text Electronic Journal).* Journal. *Price:* $90/year for members; $105/year for non-members; $75/year for small institution; $350/year for large institution. • *Reflections on Nursing Leadership*, quarterly. Magazine. Includes President's message, executive update, inside the society, feature articles, people and announcements. *Price:* $20/2years. **Frmly:** (1985) Sigma Theta Tau.

★ 5734 ★ Sigmund Freud Archives (SFA)

c/o Harold P. Blum, M.D.
23 The Hemlocks
Roslyn, NY 11576
Phone: (516)621-6850 **Fax:** (516)621-3014
Email: haroldpblum@cs.com
Harold P. Blum, MD, Exec. Dir.

Fnded: 1951. **Mem:** 18. **Desc:** Psychoanalysts interested in the preservation and collection of scientific and personal writings of Sigmund Freud (1856-1939), Austrian neurologist and founder of psychoanalysis. Assists in research on Freud's life and work and the evolution of psychoanalytic thought; collects and classifies all documents, papers, publications, personal correspondence, and historical data written by, to, and on Freud.

★ 5735 ★ Signing Exact English Center for the Advancement of Deaf Children (SEE Center)

PO Box 1181
Los Alamitos, CA 90720
Phone: (562)430-1467 **Fax:** (562)795-6614
Email: seecenter@seecenter.org
Website: http://www.seecenter.org
Esther Zawolkow, Contact

Fnded: 1984. **Desc:** Working to promote early identification and intervention, to develop understanding of principles of Signing, to provide information to parents on deafness and related topics and to foster the positive development of self concept in the deaf child. Conducts workshops, and sign skills evaluations. Provides introductory information.

★ 5736 ★ Simon Foundation for Continence (SFC)

Box 835
Wilmette, IL 60091
Phone: (847)864-3913 **Free:** 800-23-SIMON
Fax: (847)864-9758
Email: simoninfo@simonfoundation.org
Website: http://www.simonfoundation.org
Cheryle B. Gartley, Pres.

Fnded: 1983. **Mem:** 140,000. **Desc:** Persons with urinary and bowel incontinence; family members, doctors, medical personnel, and others concerned with the condition. Seeks to educate the public on urinary and bowel problems, to provide information to persons with incontinence, and to remove the stigma attached to the condition. Acts as support group. Organizes "I Will Manage" selfhelp groups. Conducts research on the number of people who have the problems, and the types and causes of incontinence; compiles statistics. Maintains speakers' bureau. **Pub:** *A Time for Action.* Video. • *The Choice Is Yours.* Video. • *The Informer: Helping People with Incontinence*, quarterly. Newsletter. *Price:* Included in membership dues. • *Managing Incontinence: A Guide to Living with the Loss of Bladder Control.* Book. • *The Solution Starts with You.* Video. **Frmly:** Simon Foundation.

★ 5737 ★ Singapore Association for Counselling (SAC)

c/o Singapore Professional Centre
People's Association
Youth Block, Rm. 4
9 Stadium Link
Singapore 397750, Singapore
Phone: 65 3482586 **Fax:** 65 4409450
Website: http://www.spc.org.sg/member/sach1.htm

Desc: Counselors, social workers, psychologists, and others active in the profession of counseling. Encourages high standards of professional ethics, competence, conduct, educational qualifications, and achievement. Promotes research in counseling.

★ 5738 ★ Singapore Association for the Deaf

227 Mountbatten Rd.
Singapore 397998, Singapore
Phone: 65 63448274 **Fax:** 65 63457706
Email: aa@sadeaf.org.sg
Website: http://www.sadeaf.org.sg

Fnded: 1955. **Mem:** 5,252. **Desc:** Works to improve the quality of life for people with impaired hearing. Conducts educational programs. **Pub:** *Signal*, 3/year. Newsletter. Contains articles, news and announcements.

★ 5739 ★ Singapore Association for Mental Health (SAMH)

Block 69 Lorong 4
Toa Payho, Ste. 01-365
Singapore 310069, Singapore
Phone: 65 2553222 **Fax:** 65 2526834

Desc: Promotes services for the social and mental well-being of people in Singapore. Works to improve the care and rehabilitation of the mentally ill and emotionally disturbed.

★ 5740 ★ Singapore Dental Association (SDA)

2 College Rd.
Singapore 169850, Singapore
Phone: 65 62202588 **Fax:** 65 62247967
Email: admin@sda.org.sg
Website: http://www.sda.org.sg

Desc: Promotes the art and science of dentistry. Represents the interests of the dental profession. Upholds high ethical standards and professional conduct. Encourages study and research in the field of dental science and related subjects.

★ 5741 ★ Singapore Medical Association (SMA)
Alumni Medical Centre
2 College Rd., Level 2
Singapore 169850, Singapore
Phone: 65 62231264 **Fax:** 65 62247827
Email: sma@sma.org.sg
Website: http://www.sma.org.sg

Fnded: 1959. **Mem:** 3,200. **Lang(s):** English. **Desc:** Promotes medicine and allied sciences in Singapore. Maintains the honour and interests of the medical profession. Represents the medical profession before government and other organizations. Maintains standards of medical ethics and conduct. Provides a forum for social, cultural, and professional contact among members. Organizes public health educational programs; offers CPR training; administers a training programme for health care assistants. **Pub:** *Singapore Medical Association*, monthly. Newsletter. News article, classified ads. • *Singapore Medical Journal*, monthly. Journal. Includes scientific papers.

★ 5742 ★ Singapore Planned Parenthood Association (SPPA)
Blk. 3A Holland Close
No. 01-55
Singapore 272003, Singapore
Phone: 65 67758981 **Fax:** 65 67768296
Email: sppassn@singnet.com.sg
Website: http://www.sppa.org.sg

Fnded: 1949. **Mem:** 107. **Lang(s):** English. **Desc:** Promotes family planning as a basic human right and as a means to improve the quality of life for people living in Singapore. Works to reduce the number of unwanted pregnancies and abortions. Offers programs in sex education, family planning, and health. Provides contraceptive services. Acts as an advocate for family planning on a national level. **Pub:** *Monthly News Bulletin*, bimonthly. Bulletin. • Annual Report, annual. **Frmly:** (1986) Family Planning Association of Singapore.

★ 5743 ★ Singapore Psychiatric Association (SPA)
PO Box 177
Hougang Central Post Office
Singapore 915306, Singapore

Desc: Psychiatrists in Singapore. Fosters high standards. Promotes continuing education of members.

★ 5744 ★ Singapore Psychological Society (SPS)
PO Box 192
Newton Post Office
Singapore 912207, Singapore
Email: spsys@angelfire.com
Website: http://www.angelfire.com/sc2/sps/

Fnded: 1979. **Lang(s):** English. **Desc:** Psychologists, professors, and students. Promotes the advancement of psychology as a science and as a profession in Singapore.

★ 5745 ★ Singapore Radiological Society (SRS)
Outram Rd.
Singapore 169608, Singapore
Phone: 65 2223322 **Fax:** 65 2221720
Website: http://www.srs.org.sg

Desc: Promotes continuing medical education.

★ 5746 ★ Singapore Veterinary Association (SVA)
c/o Agri-Food and Veterinary Authority
5 Maxwell Rd., Ste. 18-00
Tower Block, MND Complex
Singapore 069110, Singapore
Phone: 65 2270670 **Fax:** 65 62206068
Email: sva@sva.org.sg
Website: http://www.sva.org.sg

Desc: Represents interests of veterinary surgeons and the veterinary profession in Singapore. Liaises with government agencies regarding veterinary science.

★ 5747 ★ Sister Kenny Rehabilitation Services (SKRS)
800 E 28th St.
Minneapolis, MN 55407
Phone: (612)863-4457 **Fax:** (612)863-2591
Mark Dixon, Exec. Dir.

Fnded: 1942. **Desc:** To investigate, evaluate, promote, and support projects in rehabilitation and provide rehabilitative patient care. (Named for Elizabeth Kenny, 1886-1952, an Australian nurse who developed a method for treating poliomyelitis with thermal compresses and physical therapy.) Compiles statistics on research activities and patient care activities. Specializes in the treatment of acutely and chronically disabled patients. A large number of patients are stroke victims, spinal cord-injured, or brain-damaged. Rehabilitation services are also used by patients with arthritis, cerebral palsy, Parkinson's disease, polio residuals, or other neuromuscular disorders or musculoskeletal injuries. Offers professional education programs to instruct medical and allied health profession als in the most recent and most relevant rehabilitation practices. Teaches rehabilitation personnel nursing skills needed to fulfill the special requirements of chronically ill and physically disabled people. **Frmly:** (1965) Sister Kenny Foundation; (1976) American Rehabilitation Foundation; (2002) Sister Kenny Institute.

★ 5748 ★ Sisters Network
8787 Woodway Dr., Ste. 4206
Houston, TX 77063
Phone: (713)781-0255 **Free:** (866)781-1808
Fax: (713)780-8998
Email: sisnet4@aol.com
Website: http://sistersnetworkinc.org
Karen E. Jackson, Contact

Fnded: 1994. **Mem:** 3,000. **Desc:** National African-American breast cancer survivorship organization. Promotes improved breast health among African-American women; seeks to reduced the incidence of breast cancer. Gathers and disseminates information on breast cancer prevention and self detection; provides emotional and psychological support to African-American women with breast cancer; supports breast cancer research initiatives and advocacy training. **Pub:** Newsletter, periodic.

★ 5749 ★ Sjogren's Syndrome Foundation (SSF)
8120 Woodmont Ave., No. 530
Bethesda, MD 20814
Phone: (301)718-0300 **Free:** 800-475-6473
Fax: (301)718-0322
Email: ssf@sjogrens.org
Website: http://www.sjogrens.com
Suzanne Stone, Exec. Dir.

Fnded: 1983. **Mem:** 8,700. **Local Groups:** 80. **Desc:** Individuals who have Sjogren's Syndrome, xerostomia (dry mouth), or keratoconjunctivitis sicca (dry eyes); specialists, internists, immunologists, rheumatologists, otolaryngologists, opthalmologists, gynecologists, gastroenterologists, pulmonologists, dermatologists, neurologists, urologists, pharmaceutical companies, and dentists. (Sjogren's Syndrome is a disorder marked by dryness of all mucous membranes, resulting from deficient secretion of the glands, particularly the lacrimal and salivary glands, those of the upper respiratory tract, the sweat glands, and the vaginal area. Approximately 50% of Sjogren's Syndrome patients also have rheumatoid arthritis, lupus, or scleroderma.) Objectives are to increase public awareness and medical knowledge about Sjogren's Syndrome, educate patients and their families, and allow patients to share information on coping with the syndrome. Supports research. Sponsors support groups with meetings in which doctors speak on aspects of the syndrome. Compiles statistics. **Pub:** *Moisture Seekers Newsletter*, monthly. Newsletter. Covers information on new products, treatments, and developments, status of research, and discussion by specialists. *Price:* Included in membership dues. • *The New Sjogren's Syndrome Handbook.* • Articles. • Brochure. **Frmly:** (1985) Moisture Seekers.

★ 5750 ★ Ski for Light
1455 W Lake St.
Minneapolis, MN 55408
Phone: (612)827-3232 **Fax:** (612)779-0211
Email: info@sfl.org
Website: http://www.sfl.org
Nancy McKinney, Pres.

Fnded: 1975. **Nat'l Groups:** 1. **Reg. Groups:** 10. **Desc:** Dedicated to encouraging and assisting interested groups in conducting cross-country skiing programs and other health sports activities for visually impaired and other physically disabled people. Brings together disabled and nondisabled people from throughout the U.S., Canada, Norway, and other countries. The group is modeled after the Knight's Race (Ridderrennet) in Norway, which has been held annually since 1964 with international participation. Sponsors physically demanding health sports events throughout the year in North America including the Ski for Light International Program. Maintains speakers' bureau. Maintains speakers' bureau. **Pub:** *SFL Bulletin*, quarterly. Bulletin. Contains organizational news. *Price:* Free. • *Ski for Light Even Journal.* Journal. **Frmly:** (1980) Ski for Light; (1983) HEALTHsports, Inc.

★ 5751 ★ Skin Cancer Foundation (SCF)
245 5th Ave., Ste. 1403
New York, NY 10016
Phone: (212)725-5176 **Free:** 800-SKIN-490
Fax: (212)725-5751
Email: info@skincancer.org
Website: http://www.skincancer.org
Perry Robins, MD, Pres.

Fnded: 1977. **Desc:** Sponsors medical symposia and public education programs on the prevention and early recognition of skin cancer. Grants its Seal of Recommendation to sunscreen products that meet the criteria and standards established by the SCF as effective aids in the prevention of sun-induced damage to the skin. **Pub:** *Flash!.* Newsletter. *Price:* $5.00. • *Melanoma Letter*, quarterly. Newsletter. Contains articles and commentary on advances in the prevention and treatment of skin cancer. *Price:* $25/year (minimum donation). • *Play it Safe in the Sun.* Book. *Price:* $9.95. • *Skin Cancer Foundation Journal*, annual. Journal. Contains short articles on the prevention, early detection, and treatment of skin cancer. Includes publications list. *Price:* $8/copy. • *Sun and Skin News*, quarterly. Newsletter. Provides practical advice on the prevention, treatment, and early detection of skin cancer. Includes research updates. *Price:* $25/year (minimum donation). • *Sun Sense: A Complete Guide.* Book. *Price:* $14.95. • *Understanding Melanoma, What you need to know.* Book. *Price:* $14.95. • *Worldwide Melanoma Update.* Newsletter. *Price:* $6. • Also publishes posters, charts, sun protection guidelines, slide sets, audiovisuals, CD-rom manuals and brochures. **Frmly:** (1978) National Skin Cancer Foundation.

★ 5752 ★ Sleep Research Society (SRS)
1 Westbrook Corp. Ctr., Ste. 920
Westchester, IL 60154
Phone: (708)942-1093 **Fax:** (708)942-0943
Email: iyore@aasmnet.org
Website: http://www.sleepresearchsociety.org
Ruth Benca, PhD, Pres.

Fnded: 1961. **Mem:** 850. **Desc:** Physiologists, psychologists, and physicians with research interests in the study of sleep. Disseminates scientific papers on the physiological and psychological aspects of sleep. Facilitates communication among research workers in this field, but does not sponsor research investigations on its own. **Pub:** *Sleep*, 9/year. Journal. Includes book reviews and bibliography of recent literature. *Price:*

included in membership dues; $129/year for nonmembers, US funds; $185/year to institutions, US funds; $159/year for nonmembers - foreign. • *Sleep Research Society–Sleep Research*, annual. Monograph. Series containing author and keyword-in-context index. *Price:* $220/year to institutions - foreign; Included in membership dues. **Frmly:** (1983) Association for the Psychophysiological Study of Sleep.

★ 5753 ★ Slovak Chamber of Dentists
Fibichova 14
SK-821 05 Bratislava, Slovakia
Phone: 421 2 43410517 **Fax:** 421 2 43413198
Email: skzl@skzl.sk
Website: http://www.skzl.sk

Fnded: 1992. **Mem:** 2,768. **Reg. Groups:** 38. **Desc:** Represents the dental profession in Slovakia. **Pub:** *Stomatolog*, monthly. Magazine. • *Zubny Lekar*. Journal.

★ 5754 ★ Slovak Family Planning Association (SSPRVR)
Ruzinovska 1
SK-82102 Bratislava, Slovakia
Phone: 421 7 43423880 **Fax:** 421 7 43423880
Email: sspprv@nextra.sk
Website: http://www.rodicovstvo.sk

Fnded: 1990. **Mem:** 310. **Lang(s):** English, Slovak. **Desc:** National branch of the International Planned Parenthood Federation. Promotes family planning and facilitates access to reproductive health services; works to ensure responsible parenthood. Conducts educational programs on population control, family planning, parenthood, and reproductive health. Operates family planning center. **Pub:** *Empatia*, quarterly. Journal.

★ 5755 ★ Slovak Multiple Sclerosis Society (Slovensky zvaz Sclerosis Mulitplex)
c/o Milan Surgos
Culenova 12
917 01 Trnava, Slovakia
Phone: 421 33 5513 009 **Fax:** 421 33 5344 581
Email: msinslovakia@pobox.sk
Website: http://web.stonline.sk/szsm

Fnded: 1990. **Mem:** 530. **Reg. Groups:** 16. **Desc:** MS patients, families and professionals. Seeks to improve the quality of life for persons with multiple sclerosis and their families.

★ 5756 ★ Slovak Pharmacological Society
c/o Prof. Pavel Svec
Department of Pharmacology & Toxicology
Faculty of Pharmacy
Comenius University
ul. Odbojarov 10
832 32 Bratislava, Slovakia
Phone: 421 7 60651 **Fax:** 421 7 55572065
Email: psvec@fpharm.uniba.sk
Website: http://fafstw.fpharm.uniba.sk/~SPhaS/

Mem: 245. **Desc:** Promotes pharmacology in Slovakia.

★ 5757 ★ Slovak Society of Biomedical Engineering and Medical Informatics (SBMI)
c/o Dr. Milan Tysler
Institute of Measurement Science
Slovak Academy of Science
Dubravska cesta 9
842 19 Bratislava, Slovakia
Phone: 421 2 54775950 **Fax:** 421 2 54775943
Email: umertysl@savba.sk

Desc: Promotes biomedical engineering and medical informatics; provides methodological and technical assistance for health care organizations in planning and implementing new information and medical technology.

★ 5758 ★ Slovak Society of Cardiology
Slovak Institute of Cardiovascular Diseases
Pod Krasnou horkou 1
SK-83348 Bratislava 37, Slovakia
Phone: 421 1 59320223 **Fax:** 421 1 59320223
Email: ssc@susch.sk
Website: http://www.cardiology.sk

Lang(s): English, Slovak. **Desc:** Cardiologists and other health care professionals with an interest in the human heart and its diseases. Seeks to enhance the professional standing and skill of members; represents members' interests before government agencies and the public.

★ 5759 ★ Slovak Society of Gerontology and Geriatrics (SSGG)
c/o Zoltan Mikes
Department of Geriatrics
Faculty of Medicine
Dumbierska 3
SK-831 01 Bratislava, Slovakia
Phone: 421 7 59545232 **Fax:** 421 7 59546263
Email: mikes@fmed.uniba.sk

Fnded: 1995. **Lang(s):** English, Slovak. **Desc:** Health care professionals and other individuals with an interest in the well-being of the elderly. Promotes delivery of improved health and social services to older people. Encourages professional advancement of health care practitioners. Makes available preventive and primary health care services; conducts research; maintains Geriatric Center.

★ 5760 ★ Slovak Society of Pediatrics
c/o Children's Hospital
1 Children's Clinic
Limbova 1
SK-833 40 Bratislava, Slovakia
Phone: 421 2 54774511 **Fax:** 421 2 54774511
Email: benedek@fmed.uniba.sk

Mem: 2,000. **Lang(s):** English, Slovak. **Desc:** Pediatricians and other health care professionals with an interest in child health. Promotes proper pediatric medical care; represents members' interests. **Pub:** *Detsky Lekar*, quarterly. Journal. Contains information regarding pediatric problems of primary care.

★ 5761 ★ Slovak Society of Physiology and Pathology of Respiration
c/o Dept. of Pathophysiology, Jes. Med. Fac.
Comenius University
26 Sklabinska str.
SK-037 53 Martin, Slovakia
Phone: 421 43 4238213 **Fax:** 421 43 4134807
Email: tatar@jfmed.uniba.sk

Fnded: 1968. **Mem:** 160. **Lang(s):** English, Slovak. **Desc:** Health care professionals treating respiratory ailments. Researchers in the field of respiratory (Experimental and Clinical Physiology and Pathophysiology of Respiration). Promotes professional advancement of members; represents members' interests. **Pub:** *Bulletin of the SSPPR*, 3/year. Newsletter.

★ 5762 ★ Slovenian Dental Association (SDA)
Komenskega 4
SLO-1000 Ljubljana, Slovenia
Phone: 386 1 2317868 **Fax:** 386 1 2301955
Email: katarina.jovanovic@quest.ames.si

Fnded: 1945. **Mem:** 350. **State Groups:** 1. **Lang(s):** English, German. **Desc:** Dentists and others interested in promoting and maintaining good dental health. Conducts educational programs; makes available children's services. **Pub:** *Informator*, periodic. Bulletin.

★ 5763 ★ Slovenian Pharmacological Society (Slovensko Drustvo Farmakologov — SFD)
Department of Pharmacology
Faculty of Medicine
Korytkova 2
SLO-1100 Ljubljana, Slovenia
Phone: 386 1 5437330 **Fax:** 386 1 5437331
Email: sfd@mf.uni-lj.si

Mem: 45. **Desc:** Promotes pharmacology in Slovenia.

★ 5764 ★ Slovenian Society of Cardiology
University Medical Centre
Clinic of Cardiology
Zaloska 7
SLO-1000 Ljubljana, Slovenia
Phone: 386 1 5222934 **Fax:** 386 1 5224599
Email: mfkenda@mf.uni.lj.si

Mem: 141. **Desc:** Promotes the study of cardiology in Slovenia. **Pub:** *Newsletter of the Slovenian Society of Cardiology*, semiannual.

★ 5765 ★ SMART Recovery
7537 Mentor Ave., Ste. 306
Mentor, OH 44060
Phone: (440)951-5357 **Fax:** (440)951-5358
Email: srmail1@aol.com
Website: http://www.smartrecovery.org/

Desc: Recovered, recovering, never addicted individuals committed to abstinence from addictive behavior, including alcohol, other substances, activities.

★ 5766 ★ SMARTRISK
790 Bay St., Ste. 401
Toronto, ON, Canada M5G 1N8
Phone: (416)977-7350 **Fax:** (416)596-2700
Email: info@smartrisk.ca
Website: http://www.smartrisk.ca

Fnded: 1992. **Lang(s):** English, French. **Desc:** Works to reduce the number of injuries in Canada. Sponsors campaigns to raise public awareness of preventable causes of injury in all aspects of daily life. **Pub:** *Heads Up*, monthly. Newsletter. Contains details on injury prevention, awareness and initiatives. **Frmly:** (2001) Canadian Injury Prevention Foundation.

★ 5767 ★ SmokeFree Educational Services
PO Box 905
New York, NY 10274-0905
Phone: (212)912-0960 **Fax:** (212)488-8911
Email: smokefree@usa.net
Website: http://www.smokefree.org
Joseph Cherner, Pres.

Fnded: 1987. **Mem:** 100,000. **Desc:** Mission statement is "to win the right to live and work in a smokefree environment, and to educate people about the unhealthy and socially undesirable consequences of tobacco addiction." Works for: more education for people on the consequences of tobacco addiction; tobacco-free schools; larger health warnings on cigarette ads and cigarette packs; health warnings on cigarettes sold to less developed countries; ending tobacco sponsorship of youth oriented events; eliminating cigarette vending machines; and 100% smokefree public places. **Pub:** *SmokeFree Air*, quarterly. Newsletter. *Price:* Included in membership dues. **AKA:** Smokefree America.

★ 5768 ★ Smokenders
901 NW 133rd St. A
Vancouver, WA 98665-6445
Free: 800-828-4357 **Fax:** (360)546-2518
Email: kwillcuts@smokenders.com
Website: http://www.smokenders.com
Kay Willcuts, VP

Desc: Teaches smokers to quit smoking through seminars or self-help kits.

★ 5769 ★ Social Psychiatry Research Institute (SPRI)
150 E 69th St., Ste. 2H
New York, NY 10021

Phone: (212)628-4800 **Fax:** (212)249-8546
Ari Kiev, MD, JD, Pres.
Fnded: 1970. **Desc:** Promotes, supports, and conducts, in and outside the U.S., research in the fields of mental health and psychiatry; to assemble data and findings for mental health and psychiatry. Is presently conducting double-blind psychopharmacological studies of antidepressant and antianxiety medications with volunteers. Has supported several suicide prevention and drug abuse projects. Has developed a 15-week home-study program on panic and agoraphobia.

★ 5770 ★ Social/Vocational Rehabilitation Clinic (SVRC)
c/o Post-Graduate Center West
344 W 36th St.
New York, NY 10018
Phone: (212)97‑-3200 **Fax:** (212)244-2034
Michelle Sternchos, Contact
Fnded: 1959. **Desc:** Clinic employing a comprehensive therapeutic clinical program for psychiatric outpatients. Aims at reducing hospital admissions and creating a therapeutic and social experience resulting in independent living, improved interpersonal relationships, and productivity in the work field. Offers a program of "therapeutic groups of creative, recreational, experiential, and work activities." Provides individual counseling, activity and therapy, and medication therapy; offers placement service; operates case management services. Sponsors vocational activities, family therapy, internship program, and community outreach activities. Functions as a psychotherapeutic service of the Postgraduate Center for Mental Health. **Frmly:** The Living Room; (1975) Social Rehabilitation Clinic; (1977) Psychiatric Day and Evening Clinic; (1988) Social Rehabilitation Clinic.

★ 5771 ★ Social Workers in the Field of Learning Disability
c/o Irish Association of Social Workers
IASW Offices
114/116 Pearse St.
Dublin 2, Ireland
Phone: 353 1 6774838 **Fax:** 353 1 6715734
Email: iasw@iol.ie
Website: http://iasw.eire.org
Fnded: 1972. **Mem:** 53. **Reg. Groups:** 4. **Lang(s):** English, Irish. **Desc:** Social workers working with people with learning disabilities. Seeks to improve the quality of life of people with learning disabilities; works to insure respect for the human rights of people with learning disabilities. Serves as a forum for the exchange of information among members; assists public agencies in devising public policies impacting people with learning disabilities.

★ 5772 ★ Sociedad de Anestesiologia de Chile
Av Providencia, 1476 4, Apto. 405, Castilla 195
Santiago, Chile
Phone: 56 2 2357564 **Fax:** 56 2 2357564
Email: sach@entelchile.net
Fnded: 1946.

★ 5773 ★ Sociedad Argentina de Ciencias Neurologicas, Psiquitricas y Neuroquirzrgicas
Santa Fe 1171
1059 Buenos Aires, Argentina
Phone: 54 1 411633
Fnded: 1920.

★ 5774 ★ Sociedad Argentina de Patologia
Santa Fe 1171
1059 Buenos Aires, Argentina
Phone: 54 1 411633
Fnded: 1933.

★ 5775 ★ Sociedad Chilena de Endocrinologia y Metabolismo
Bernarda Morin 488, Segundo Piso
Providencia
Santiago, Chile
Phone: 56 2 3412909 **Fax:** 56 2 3412909
Email: sochem@entelchile.net
Website: http://www.chillan.udec.cl/sochem
Fnded: 1958. **Mem:** 208. **Lang(s):** English, Spanish. **Pub:** *Boletin Endocrinoticias*, quarterly. Newsletter.

★ 5776 ★ Sociedad Chilena de Gastroenterologia
Trovador 4280 of 909
Santiago, Chile
Phone: 56 2 3425004 **Fax:** 56 2 3425005
Email: schgastr@netline.cl
Fnded: 1938.

★ 5777 ★ Sociedad Chilena de Hematologia
Casilla 166, Correo 55
Santiago, Chile
Phone: 56 2 3413113 **Fax:** 56 2 2693394
Fnded: 1943.

★ 5778 ★ Sociedad Chilena de Urologia
Esmeralda 678
Santiago, Chile
Phone: 56 2 6642469
Email: luicoz@entelchile.net
Fnded: 1935.

★ 5779 ★ Sociedad Espanola de Diabetes
Santa Isabel 51
E-28012 Madrid, Spain
Phone: 34 914682940 **Fax:** 34 915396306
Fnded: 1954.

★ 5780 ★ Sociedad Espanola de Geriatria y Gerontologia
Principe de Vergara, 57-59-1
E-28006 Madrid, Spain
Phone: 34 91 4111707 **Fax:** 34 91 5647944
Email: segg@segg.org
Website: http://www.segg.es
Fnded: 1948. **Mem:** 2,230. **Reg. Groups:** 15. **Lang(s):** Spanish. **Desc:** Promotes geriatric and gerontological research, training in the field of aging, and interests of gerontological organizations in international affairs. **Pub:** *Revista Espanola de Geriatria & Geratologia*. Journal.

★ 5781 ★ Sociedad de Farmacologia de Chile
Casilla 70000, Correo 7
Santiago, Chile
Phone: 56 2 776560 **Fax:** 56 2 2225515
Fnded: 1979.

★ 5782 ★ Sociedad de Genetica de Chile
Casilla 70061, Correo 7
Santiago, Chile
Phone: 56 2 776560
Email: rgalleg@udec.cl
Fnded: 1964.

★ 5783 ★ Sociedad Mexicana de Ingenieria Biomedica
Queretaro 210, 2 piso, Col Roma
06700 Mexico City, Mexico
Phone: 52 55744505 **Fax:** 52 55743928
Email: informacion@somib.org.mx
Fnded: 1978.

★ 5784 ★ Sociedad Mexicana de Pediatria
Tehuantepec 86-503, Col. Roma Sur
06760 Mexico City, Mexico
Phone: 52 55648371 **Fax:** 52 55647739
Fnded: 1930.

★ 5785 ★ Sociedad de Obstetricia y Ginecologia de Venezuela
Apdo 20081
Caracas 1020, Venezuela

★ 5786 ★ Sociedad de Psiquiatria del Uruguay
Bul Artigas 1521, SMU
Montevideo, Uruguay
Phone: 598 2 4014701 **Fax:** 598 2 4020272
Email: spu@mednet.org.uy
Website: http://www.chasque.apc.org/spu
Desc: Aims to develop the scientific analyses of theoretical and practical aspects of psychiatry.

★ 5787 ★ Sociedad Venezolana de Cardiologia (SVC)
Torre del Colegio, Piso 2, Oficina B-1
Caracas, Venezuela
Phone: 58 2 9766650 **Fax:** 58 2 9760846
Email: info@cardioven.org

★ 5788 ★ Sociedad Venezolana de Cirugia
Av Jose Maria Vargas, Urb. Santa Fe
Caracas 1080, Venezuela
Fnded: 1945.

★ 5789 ★ Sociedad Venezolana de Hematologia
San Jose
Caracas, Venezuela

★ 5790 ★ Sociedad Venezolana de Historia de la Medicina
Bolsa a San Francisco
Caracas 101, Venezuela

★ 5791 ★ Sociedad Venezolana de Medicina del Trabajo y Deportes
Los Caobos
Caracas, Venezuela

★ 5792 ★ Sociedad Venezolana de Oftalmologia
Av. Principal de los Ruices
Centro Empresarial de Los Ruices, piso 5, of. 507
Caracas 1050, Venezuela
Phone: 58 2 2398127
Email: svo@reacciun.ve
Website: http://www.svo.org.ve
Fnded: 1953.

★ 5793 ★ Sociedad Venezolana de Psiquiatria y Neurologia
Apdo 3380
Caracas, Venezuela

★ 5794 ★ Sociedad Venezolana de Puericultura y Pediatria
Edificio La Linea
Caracas 105, Venezuela

★ 5795 ★ Sociedad Venezolana de Radiologia
Av Andres Bello
Caracas, Venezuela

★ 5796 ★ Sociedade Brasileira de Engenharia Biomedica (SBEB)
Caixa Postal 68.510, Centro de Tecnologia - COPPE/UFRJ
21945-970 Rio de Janeiro, RJ, Brazil
Email: sbeb@peb.ufrj.br
Website: http://www.peb.ufrj.br/~sbeb

★ 5797 ★ Sociedade Portuguesa de Geriatria e Gerontologia
Av. Joao XXI 64-3 DT
P-1000 Lisbon, Portugal
Phone: 351 217951153 **Fax:** 351 217951118
Email: prismedica@prismedica.pt
Desc: Promotes gerontological research, training in the field of aging, and interests of gerontological organizations in international affairs.

★ 5798 ★ Societa Italiana di Colon-Proctologia (SICP)
Via Pierluigi da Palestrina, 63
I-00193 Rome, Italy
Phone: 39 06 3225056 **Fax:** 39 06 3613698
Fnded: 1993.

★ 5799 ★ Societa Italiana di Dermatologia Chirurgica
Largo Gemelli, 1
I-00168 Rome, Italy
Phone: 39 06 30154470

★ 5800 ★ Societa Italiana di Dermatologia e Venereologia (SIDEV)
Viale Benedetto XV, 7
I-16132 Genoa, Italy
Phone: 39 0103538416 **Fax:** 39 0103538401
Fnded: 1885.

★ 5801 ★ Societa Italiana di Endocrinologia (SIE)
Via Francesco Sforza, 35
I-20122 Milan, Italy
Phone: 39 0255631 **Fax:** 39 0255195438
Fnded: 1951.

★ 5802 ★ Societa Italiana di Endocrinologia e Diabetologia Pediatrica (SIEDP)
Largo del Pozzo, 71
I-41100 Modena, Italy
Phone: 39 059424572 **Fax:** 39 059424583
Email: berna@unimo.it

★ 5803 ★ Societa Italiana di Ginecologia ed Ostetricia (SIGO)
Via dei Soldati, 25
I-00186 Rome, Italy
Phone: 39 06 6875119 **Fax:** 39 06 6868142
Fnded: 1892.

★ 5804 ★ Societa Italiana di Medicina Generale (SIMG)
Via il Prato, 66
I-50123 Florence, Italy
Phone: 39 055284030 **Fax:** 39 055284038
Fnded: 1982.

★ 5805 ★ Societa Italiana di Medicina Perinatale (SIMP)
I-43100 Parma, Italy
Phone: 39 0521290453

★ 5806 ★ Societa Italiana di Medicina Respiratoria (SIMER)
Via Giovanni da Procida, 7/D
I-00162 Rome, Italy
Phone: 39 06 44240683

★ 5807 ★ Societa Italiana di Neurofisiologia Clinica
Via Sergio Pansini, 5
I-80131 Naples, Italy
Phone: 39 0817463793 **Fax:** 39 0815469861
Fnded: 1949.

★ 5808 ★ Societa Italiana di Oncologia Ginecologica (SIOG)
Via dei Soldati, 25
I-00186 Rome, Italy
Phone: 39 06 6875119 **Fax:** 39 06 6868142
Fnded: 1977.

★ 5809 ★ Societa Italiana di Patologia
Via L. Mangiagalli, 31
I-20133 Milan, Italy
Phone: 39 0270600515
Fnded: 1948.

★ 5810 ★ Societa Italiana di Pediatria (SIP)
Via Forli, 23
I-00161 Rome, Italy
Phone: 39 06 4403900 **Fax:** 39 06 44250889
Fnded: 1898.

★ 5811 ★ Societa Italiana di Psichiatria (SIP)
Via Tiburtina Valeria, 188
I-00191 Guidonia Montecelio, Italy
Phone: 39 07 74353876
Fnded: 1872.

★ 5812 ★ Societa Italiana di Psicologia (SIPs.)
Via Tagliamento, 76
I-00198 Rome, Italy
Phone: 39 06 8845136
Email: sipsit@tin.it

★ 5813 ★ Societa Italiana di Reumatologia (SIR)
Via G. Donizetti, 7
I-53100 Siena, Italy
Phone: 39 0577283322
Fnded: 1950.

★ 5814 ★ Societa Italiana di Urologia Pediatrica (SIUP)
Viale Ridolfi
I-36100 Venice, Italy
Fnded: 1982.

★ 5815 ★ Societa Medica Italiana di Paraplegia (SOMIPAR)
Corso Corsica, 17
I-10134 Turin, Italy
Phone: 39 011610780
Fnded: 1986.

★ 5816 ★ Societas Gerontological Fennica
Haartmannink 4
FIN-00290 Helsinki, Finland
Phone: 358 9 4712222 **Fax:** 358 9 4714013
Email: kaisu.pitkala@sll.fimnet.fi
Desc: Promotes gerontological research, training in the field of aging, and interests of gerontological organizations in international affairs.

★ 5817 ★ Societatea de Educatie Contraceptiva si Sexuala (SECS)
Calea 13 Septembrie 85
B1.77c, sc1, et8, ap75, Sector 5
R-76100 Bucharest, Romania
Phone: 40 1 41011081 **Fax:** 40 1 4101097
Email: secs@starnets.ro
Fnded: 1990. **Mem:** 1,027. **Reg. Groups:** 32. **Lang(s):** Romanian. **Desc:** Works to improve the quality of life for individuals living in Romania by promoting responsible parenthood and family planning. Attempts to reduce the number of unwanted pregnancies and abortions. Offers programs in family planning, sex education, and health. Acts as an advocate for family planning on a national level. **Pub:** *Newsletter*, quarterly. Newsletter.

★ 5818 ★ Societe Francaise d'Anesthesie et de Reanimation (SFAR)
74, rue Raynouard
F-75016 Paris, France
Phone: 33 1 45258225 **Fax:** 33 1 40503522
Email: sfar@invivo.edu
Website: http://www.sfar.org
Fnded: 1936. **Mem:** 4,125. **Lang(s):** French. Does not correspond in English. **Desc:** Anesthesiologists; interested others in France. Promotes scientific research and high standards of practice in the field. **Pub:** *Annales Francaises d'Anesthesie et de Reanimation*, monthly. Journal. • *Conferences d'Actuausation - Congres.*

★ 5819 ★ Societe Francaise d'Angeiologie (SFA)
145, rue de la Pompe
F-75116 Paris, France
Phone: 33 1 47551433 **Fax:** 33 1 47272147
Email: micazang@noos.fr
Fnded: 1947. **Mem:** 400. **Lang(s):** English, French. **Desc:** Individuals in France interested in angiology (the study of blood vessels and lymphatics). **Pub:** *Angeiologie*, bimonthly. Journal.

★ 5820 ★ Societe Internationale d'Urologie (SIU)
PO Box 55 Place du Parc
Montreal, QC, Canada H2X 4A3
Phone: (514)843-2865 **Fax:** (514)843-2844
Email: siu.elhilali@muhc.mcgill.ca
Website: http://www.siu-urology.org/
Fnded: 1907. **Mem:** 4,570. **Desc:** Represents and promotes urological societies globally.

★ 5821 ★ Societe Logique (SL)
3250 Saint Joseph Blvd. E
Montreal, QC, Canada H1Y 3G2
Phone: (514)522-8284 **Fax:** (514)522-2659
Email: info@societelogique.org
Fnded: 1981. **Mem:** 50. **Lang(s):** English, French. **Desc:** Architects interested in barrier-free design. Promotes erection of buildings accessible to people with physical disabilities. Serves as a clearinghouse on barrier-free architecture; provides consulting services to members; conducts educational programs; maintains speakers' bureau.

★ 5822 ★ Society for Academic Emergency Medicine (SAEM)
901 N Washington Ave.
Lansing, MI 48906-5137
Phone: (517)485-5484 **Fax:** (517)485-0801
Email: saem@saem.org
Website: http://www.saem.org
Roger J. Lewis, MD, Pres.
Fnded: 1989. **Mem:** 5,000. **Desc:** Physicians teaching emergency medicine, emergency medicine residents,

and nonphysicians teaching emergency care. Purposes are: to educate teachers of emergency medicine and encourage its development as an academic discipline; to apply sound educational principles, thus improving the quality of teaching in the field; to promote research in educational methods and clinical procedures. Provides a forum for the exchange of ideas and information. Promotes improved emergency patient care through more direct involvement of teachers and consumers in the needs assessment, planning, and implementation of projects and programs. Sponsors educational workshops; conducts lectures. **Pub:** *Academic Emergency Medicine*, monthly. Journal. • *SAEM Newsletter*, bimonthly. Newsletter. Promotes research and education in emergency medicine. *Price:* Included in membership dues.

★ 5823 ★ Society of Academic and Research Surgery
Royal College of Surgeons of England
35-43 Lincoln's Inn Fields
London WC2A 3PE, United Kingdom
Phone: 44 20 78696640 **Fax:** 44 20 78696644
Email: smitchell@rcseng.ac.uk
Website: http://www.surgicalresearchsociety.org.uk

Mem: 547. **Desc:** Surgeons. To provide for the interchange of information about research related to surgery and surgical disease. **Pub:** *British Journal of Surgery*. Journal.

★ 5824 ★ Society for Accessible Travel for the Handicapped (SATH)
347 5th Ave., Ste. 610
New York, NY 10016
Phone: (212)447-7284 **Fax:** (212)725-8253
Email: sathtravel@aol.com
Website: http://www.sath.org
Laurel VanHorn, Exec. Dir.

Fnded: 1976. **Mem:** 2,500. **Desc:** Travel professionals, consumers with disabilities, other individuals and corporations supporting this mission. Strives to raise awareness of needs of all travelers with disabilities, remove physical and attitudinal barriers to free access and expand travel opportunities in the United States and abroad. Operates speaker's bureau. library. Compiles statistics on the potential travel market of various handicapped groups and their locations. **Pub:** *Open World*, quarterly. Magazine. Contains articles on travel and related matters of interest to all handicapped persons. *Price:* Included in membership dues; $13/year plus shipping and handling; $24/2 years plus shipping and handling; $30/3 years plus shipping and handling. • *The Travel Related Industries Accessibility Guide, 1996*. • Information sheets on matter related to travel. The travel related Industries Accessibility Guide.

★ 5825 ★ Society for Accessible Travel and Hospitality (SATH)
347 5th Ave., Ste. 610
New York, NY 10016
Phone: (212)447-7284 **Fax:** (212)725-8253
Website: http://www.sath.org
Laurel Van Horn, Exec. Dir.

Fnded: 1976. **Desc:** Promotes awareness, respect and accessibility for disabled and mature travelers and employment for disabled in tourism industries. **Pub:** *Open World*. Magazine.

★ 5826 ★ Society for Adolescent Medicine (SAM)
1916 NW Copper Oaks Circle
Blue Springs, MO 64015
Fax: (816)224-8009
Email: cirwin@itsa.ucsf.edu
Website: http://www.adolescenthealth.org
Charles E. Irwin, Jr., Pres.

Fnded: 1968. **Mem:** 1,300. **Reg. Groups:** 18. **Desc:** Physicians, psychologists, social workers, psychiatrists, nurses, and other health care professionals. Goals are: to improve the quality of health care for adolescents; to encourage the investigation of normal growth and development during adolescence and of those diseases that affect adolescents; to stimulate the creation of health services for adolescents; to increase communication among health care professionals who care for adolescents; to foster and improve the quality of training of those individuals providing health care to adolescents. Seeks to: offer opportunities for discussion of teaching, research, and other common problems, through which coordinated efforts can be made toward their solution; publish and disseminate information related to adolescent medicine; identify, investigate, and list opportunities for careers in adolescent medicine; help plan and coordinate professional educational programs in the health care of the adolescent. Conducts research programs. **Pub:** *Journal of Adolescent Health*, monthly. Journal. Peer-reviewed scientific journal of articles on study results of the anthropology, biochemistry, endocrinology, physiology and psychology. *Price:* Included in membership dues; $199/year for nonmembers; $475/year for institutions.

★ 5827 ★ Society for the Advancement of Anaesthesia in Dentistry (SAAD)
53 Wimpole St.
London W10 8YH, United Kingdom
Phone: 44 207 9351656 **Fax:** 44 1246 208729
Email: saaduk@freeuk.com
Website: http://www.saaduk.org

Fnded: 1957. **Mem:** 2,100. **Desc:** Dentists and physicians interested in dental anesthesia. Seeks to advance pain and anxiety control in dentistry. Offers courses on intravenous techniques and relative analgesia. **Pub:** *Dental Sedation and Anaesthesia*. Book. • *SAAD Digest*, quarterly.

★ 5828 ★ Society of Air Force Clinical Surgeons
839 W Lincoln Ave., No. 716
Woodland, CA 95695
Phone: (530)661-0352 **Fax:** (530)661-0352
Email: rosepreuit@aol.com
Website: http://www.atech.org/SAFCS/about/history.htm
Rose A. Thomas, Exec. Dir.

Fnded: 1958. **Mem:** 640. **Desc:** Air Force Clinical Surgeons. Promotes excellence in surgery within the Air Force, serves as a forum for the presentation of scientific papers, fosters esprit de corps, and promulgates military surgical objectives.

★ 5829 ★ Society of Air Force Physicians (SAFP)
HQ AFMOA/SGOC
Bolling Air Force Base
110 Luke Ave., Ste. 400
Washington, DC 20332-7050
Phone: (202)767-4073 **Fax:** (202)404-7366
Jim Cox, Contact

Fnded: 1958. **Mem:** 300. **Desc:** Air Force internists, family practitioners, and specialists in emergency medicine, dermatology, allergy/immunology, and neurology. Objectives are to foster advancement of the art and science of medicine in the Air Force; encourage clinical and laboratory investigation; disseminate information.

★ 5830 ★ Society for Ambulatory Anesthesia (SAMBA)
520 N Northwest Hwy.
Park Ridge, IL 60068-2573
Phone: (847)825-5586 **Fax:** (847)825-5658
Email: samba@asahq.org
Website: http://www.sambahq.org/

Fnded: 1985. **Mem:** 2,000. **Desc:** Works to advance the study and growth of ambulatory anesthesia. Encourages high ethical and professional standards. Supports research, education and scientific progress in ambulatory anesthesia. **Pub:** *Anesthesia & Analgesia*. Journal. *Price:* $85/year.

★ 5831 ★ Society of American Gastrointestinal Endoscopic Surgeons (SAGES)
2716 Ocean Park Blvd., Ste. 3000
Santa Monica, CA 90405
Phone: (310)314-2404 **Fax:** (310)314-2585
Email: sagesweb@sages.org
Website: http://www.sages.org
Sallie Matthews, Exec. Dir.

Fnded: 1980. **Mem:** 4,300. **Desc:** Surgeons who perform gastrointestinal endoscopy and laparoscopy. Promotes the concepts of gastrointestinal endoscopy as an integral part of surgery and encourages academic, clinical, and research achievements in the field. Establishes standards of training and practice and guidelines for privileging. Provides a forum for the exchange of ideas on gastrointestinal endoscopy and related sciences. Conducts scientific studies. Offers Corporate Council membership that facilitates communication between the corporate sector and surgeons. **Pub:** *Surgical Endoscopy*, monthly. Journal. Contains information on Surgical Endoscopy. *Price:* $135/year. • Also publishes numerous guidelines on Gastrointestinal Endoscopic Surgery, privileging and standards of practice.

★ 5832 ★ Society of Anaesthesiologist of the Republic of China (SAROC)
271 Roosevelt Rd., Section 3
Taipei 10764, Taiwan
Phone: 886 2 3633912 **Fax:** 886 2 3633912
Email: saroc@tpts5.seed.net.tw
Fnded: 1956.

★ 5833 ★ Society of Andrology
Strada di Fiume, 447
I-34149 Cattinara, Italy
Phone: 39 0403994575 **Fax:** 39 0403994895
Fnded: 1976.

★ 5834 ★ Society of Andrology - India (SAI)
c/o Prof. P.R.K. Reddy
School of Life Sciences
University of Hyderabad
Hyderabad 60046, India
Phone: 91 40 23010223 **Fax:** 91 40 3010120
Email: prkra@uohyd.ernet.in
Website: http://andrology.tripod.com/

Fnded: 1988. **Desc:** Promotes research and teaching in the science of andology dealing with male reproduction.

★ 5835 ★ Society of Apothecaries of London
Apothecaries Hall
Black Friars Ln.
London EC4V 6EJ, United Kingdom
Phone: 44 207 2361189 **Fax:** 44 207 3293177
Email: clerk@apothecaries.org
Website: http://www.apothecaries.org

Fnded: 1617. **Mem:** 1,700. **Desc:** Members of the medical profession. Functions as City of London Livery Company and medical examining body.

★ 5836 ★ Society of Army Physician Assistants (SAPA)
6762 Candlewood Dr.
Fort Myers, FL 33919
Phone: (239)482-2162 **Fax:** (239)482-2162
Email: hal.slusher@juno.com
Website: http://www.sapa.org/
Harold E. Slusher, PAC, Exec. Dir.

Fnded: 1976. **Mem:** 1,000. **Desc:** Represents and supports the U.S. Army Physician Assistant, including, former, active, retired, reserve and National Guard PA's. Aims to provide a forum for discussion, representation with the AAPA; provides low cost continuing medical education (CME) to members and the PA profession. **Pub:** Newsletter, bimonthly. *Price:* included in membership dues. • Membership Directory. *Price:* included in membership dues.

★ 5837 ★ Society for Assisted Reproductive Technology (SART)
c/o American Society for Reproductive Medicine
1209 Montgomery Ave.
Birmingham, AL 35216-2809
Phone: (205)978-5000 **Fax:** (205)978-5015
Email: jzeitz@asrm.org
Website: http://www.sart.org
Joyce Zeitz, Exec. Admin.

Fnded: 1987. **Mem:** 370. **Desc:** Institutions conducting assisted reproductive procedures. Works to extend knowledge of human in vitro fertilization techniques. Conducts educational programs; gathers and disseminates information and outcome statistics on art.

★ 5838 ★ Society for the Autistically Handicapped (SFTAH)
199-205 Blandford Ave.
Kettering NN16 9AT, United Kingdom
Phone: 44 1536 523274 **Fax:** 44 1536 523274
Email: autism@rmplc.co.uk
Website: http://www.autismuk.com

Desc: Seeks to increase awareness of autism. Works to improve quality of life for people with autism. **Pub:** Newsletter, quarterly.

★ 5839 ★ Society for Basic Urologic Research (SBUR)
Department of Urology, 3125 RCP
University of Iowa
200 Hawkins Dr.
Iowa City, IA 52242-1099
Phone: (319)356-4275 **Fax:** (319)335-6971
Email: linda-buckner@uiowa.edu
Website: http://www.sbur.org/aboutus.asp

Fnded: disc. **Mem:** ussion, of. **Nat'l Groups:** liaiso. **Reg. Groups:** ollabo. **State Groups:** s amon. **Local Groups:** r scie. **Desc:** Molecular biologists, immunologists, epidemiologists, biochemists and clinical urologic scientists. Provides a forum for the presentation and discussion of urology; promotes collaborative investigations among member scientists; serves as a liaison between member scientists and funding agencies, industry representatives and academic institutions.

★ 5840 ★ Society of Behavioral Medicine (SBM)
7600 Terrace Ave., Ste. 203
Middleton, WI 53562
Phone: (608)827-7267 **Fax:** (608)831-5485
Email: sbm@tmahq.com
Website: http://www.sbmweb.org
Beth Klipping, Exec. Dir.

Fnded: 1978. **Mem:** 2,300. **Desc:** Behavioral and biomedical researchers and clinicians studying health promotion and disease prevention, with primary focus on the interactions between health and behavior. Seeks to function as a forum for the exchange of ideas and information between health care providers and basic scientists and medical researchers. Gathers and disseminates information to members and the public; conducts educational programs for health care professionals; works to integrate behavioral and biomedical research. **Pub:** *Annals of Behavioral Medicine*, quarterly. Journal. Features comprehensive area reviews of topics affecting biobehavioral research and practice; also contains abstracts of recent articles in the field. *Price:* $145 in US; $175 foreign. • *Annual Meeting Proceedings*. Proceedings. Supplement to *Annals of Behavioral Medicine*. • *Education and Training Directory*. Directory. *Price:* Directory is available on website. • *SBM Outlook*, quarterly. Newsletter. • Membership Directory, biennial. Directory is available only on website.

★ 5841 ★ Society for Behavioral Neuroendocrinology (SBN)
University of Virginia
Department of Biology
Gilmer Hall
Charlottesville, VA 22903
Website: http://www.sbn.org
Michael Baum, Pres.

Desc: Promotes the field of neuroendocrinology. **Pub:** *Hormones and Behavior*. Journal. *Price:* Electronic version included in membership dues; $75 paper version; $50 paper version for student members.

★ 5842 ★ Society of Biological Psychiatry (SBP)
Mayo Clinic of Jacksonville, Research-Birdsall 310
4500 San Pablo Rd.
Jacksonville, FL 32224
Phone: (904)953-2842 **Fax:** (904)953-7117
Email: peterson.maggie@mayo.edu
Website: http://www.sobp.org
Maggie Peterson, Mgr.

Fnded: 1945. **Mem:** 950. **Desc:** International professional society of psychiatrists, neurologists, neurosurgeons, pharmacologists, neuropharmacologists, physiologists, psychologists, and physicians in related biological studies. Studies the neuronal basis of human behavior and the biological basis of psychiatry. Compiles statistics. **Pub:** *Biological Psychiatry*, bimonthly. • *Membership Roster*, annual. Membership Directory.

★ 5843 ★ Society of British Neurological Surgeons (SBNS)
35-43 Lincoln's Inn Fields
London WC2A 3PE, United Kingdom
Fax: 44 161 2764567
Website: http://www.sbns.org
Fnded: 1926.

★ 5844 ★ Society for Cardiac Angiography and Interventions (SCA&I)
9111 Old Georgetown Rd.
Bethesda, MD 20814
Phone: (301)581-3450 **Free:** 800-992-7224
Fax: (301)581-3408
Email: info@scai.org
Website: http://www.scai.org
Norm Linsky, Exec. Dir.

Fnded: 1978. **Mem:** 2,000. **Desc:** Angiographers united to foster excellence in the field of cardiac catheterization, especially coronary arteriography and interventional angiography. (Angiography involves injecting substances opaque to radiation into blood vessels so that diagnostic X-rays of those blood vessels may be made.) Conducts clinical research. **Pub:** *Catheterization and Cardiovascular Interventions*, monthly. Journal. • *News Highlights*, quarterly. Newsletter. Includes calender of events and committee reports. *Price:* Free.

★ 5845 ★ Society for Cardiological Science and Technology
British Cardiac Society
9 Fitzroy Sq.
London W1P 5AH, United Kingdom
Phone: 44 20 73833887
Email: graham.tate@leedsth.nhs.uk
Website: http://www.scst.org.uk

Fnded: 1948. **Mem:** 1,000. **Reg. Groups:** 3. **Desc:** Persons whom the Council of the Society consider to be qualified to practice cardiography, technical cardiology and allied subjects. Aims to advance for the public benefit the science and practice of cardiography, technical cardiology and allied subjects by the promotion of improved standards of education and training and of research work therein and by making the results of such study and research available to practitioners and the general public. **Pub:** *SCST Update*, monthly.

★ 5846 ★ Society of Cardiothoracic Surgeons of Great Britain and Ireland
35-43 Lincoln's Inn Fields
London WC2A 3PE, United Kingdom
Phone: 44 207 8696893 **Fax:** 44 207 8696890
Email: sctsadmin@scts.org
Website: http://www.scts.org

Fnded: 1933. **Mem:** 561. **Desc:** Cardiac and thoracic surgeons. Concerned with the study of cardiothoracic disease. **Pub:** Bulletin, semiannual.

★ 5847 ★ Society of Cardiovascular Anesthesiologists (SCA)
2209 Dickens Rd.
PO Box 11086
Richmond, VA 23230-1086
Phone: (804)282-0084 **Fax:** (804)282-0090
Email: sca@societyhq.com
Website: http://www.scahq.org
Heather A. Spiess, Chief Staff Exec.

Fnded: 1977. **Mem:** 7,000. **Desc:** Anesthesiologists who specialize in cardiovascular surgical conditions. Purpose is to further medical education of cardiovascular anesthesiologists. Establishes goals and objectives for education of trainees in cardiovascular anesthesia; promotes personnel exchange between the U.S. and other countries; reviews related literature; maintains workshops; conducts research competitions. Sponsors Anesthesia Grand Rounds: Case Presentations as a section of the annual meeting. **Pub:** *Anesthesia and Analgesia*, monthly. Journal. • *Society of Cardiovascular Anesthesiologists–Newsletter*, bimonthly. Newsletter. Contains discussions of major issues within the cardiovascular anesthesiology field and reviews of related literature being published. *Price:* Included in membership dues. • Also publishes monographs.

★ 5848 ★ Society for Cardiovascular Magnetic Resonance (SCMR)
c/o Tom Sims
19 Mantua Rd.
Mount Royal, NJ 08061
Phone: (856)423-8955 **Fax:** (856)423-3420
Email: hq@scmr.org
Website: http://www.scmr.org
Tom Sims, Exec. Dir.

Fnded: 1994. **Mem:** 1,100. **Desc:** Physicians and scientists with an interest in cardiovascular magnetic resonance imaging are members; physiciansin-training and doctoral candidates with an interest in the field are associates; medical technologists with at least two years of experience in cardiovascular magnetic resonance are technologist members; nonscientific professionals employed by companies engaged in magnetic resonance imaging are industrial members. Seeks to advance the practice of cardiovascular magnetic resonance; works to improve study and teaching in the field. Facilitates exchange of information among members and between members and physicians and scientists working in related fields. Conducts educational programs in the application of magnetic resonance imaging to cardiovascular conditions. Serves as a clearinghouse on cardiovascular magnetic resonance imaging; sets equipment standards; conducts multicenter trials to develop cardiovascular magnetic resonance imaging methods, clinical applications, and practice standards. **Pub:** *Journal for Cardiovascular Magnetic Resonance*, quarterly. Journal.

★ 5849 ★ Society for Cardiovascular Pathology (SCVP)
c/o William C. Quist, MD
PO Box 1112
Brookline, MA 02446
Phone: (617)667-5742 **Fax:** (617)975-5620
Website: http://scvp.net
William C. Quist, MD, Treas.

Fnded: 1985. **Mem:** 200. **Desc:** Authorities in the field of cardiovascular pathology. Seeks to advance the study of cardiovascular disorders. **Pub:** *Cardiovascular Pathology*, bimonthly. Journal. Supports the scholarly activities of the SCVP.

★ 5850 ★ Society of Chairmen of Academic Radiology Departments (SCARD)
c/o Lise Steg Swanson
820 Jorie Blvd.
Oak Brook, IL 60523
Phone: (630)368-3731 **Fax:** (630)571-7837
Email: scard@rsna.org
Website: http://www.aur.org/scard/
Lise Steg Swanson, Acct. Exec.

Desc: Radiology department chairpersons. Dedicated to the advancement of the art and science of radiology; promotes medical education, research and patient care, the development of methods of teaching in radiology; provides a forum for problem solving and mutual interests.

★ 5851 ★ Society for Chaos Theory in Psychology and Life Sciences
Arizona State University, Dept. of Industrial Engineering
PO Box 875906
Tempe, AZ 85287-5906
Email: kevin.dooley@asu.edu
Website: http://www.societyforchaostheory.org
Kevin Dooley, Pres.

Fnded: 1991. **Mem:** 300. **Desc:** Researchers, theoriticians, and practitioners. Examines the application of "dynamical systems theory, far-from-equilibrium thermodynamics, self-organization, neural nets, evolutionary computation, fractals, cellular automata, related forms of chaos, catastrophes, bifurcations, nonlinear dynamics, and complexity theories to psychology and the life sciences." **Pub:** Newsletter. • Books. • Journal.

★ 5852 ★ Society of Chiropodists and Podiatrists
1 Fellmongers Path, Tower Bridge Rd.
London SE1 3LY, United Kingdom
Phone: 44 207 2348620 **Fax:** 44 207 2348621
Email: enq@scpod.org
Website: http://www.feetforlife.org

Fnded: 1945. **Mem:** 7,800. **Lang(s):** English. **Desc:** State registered chiropodists. The principal activities are to fulfill both a pre-registration and post-registration education function, to act as a trade union for its members employed in the National Health Service, to monitor the professional and ethical conduct and standards of its members, to publish professional journals, and to fulfil a public relations role. **Pub:** *The Journal of British Podiatric Medicine*, quarterly. Journal. Features articles on podiatric research. • *Podiatry Now*, monthly. Journal.

★ 5853 ★ Society of Chiropractic Orthospinology
8520 Hospital Dr.
Douglasville, GA 30134
Phone: (770)517-9921
Email: webmaster@orthospinology.org
Website: http://www.orthospinology.org/
Dr. Kirk Eriksen, Pres.

Desc: Doctors, student doctors, and patients. Promotes the Chiropractic approach for a healthy lifestyle, aims to increase understanding of the Orthospinology method. **Pub:** *Patient Brochure*. Brochure. *Price:* $2/psh, $10.

★ 5854 ★ Society for Clinical and Experimental Hypnosis (SCEH)
PO Box 642114
Pullman, WA 99164-2114
Phone: (509)335-7504 **Fax:** (509)335-2097
Email: sceh@wsu.edu
Website: http://sunsite.utk.edu/IJCEH/scehframe.htm
Jen Raupp, Exec. Dir.

Fnded: 1949. **Mem:** 950. **Desc:** United States constituent society of the International Society of Hypnosis. Professional society of physicians, dentists, doctoral level psychologists, and certain psychiatric social workers interested in research in hypnosis and its boundary areas as well as the therapeutic use of hypnosis in clinical practice. Encourages cooperation among professional and scientific disciplines in use of hypnosis; promotes educational standards; conducts introductory and advanced workshops and continuing education seminars in therapeutic hypnosis. Offers continuing education seminars in New York City and San Francisco, CA. **Pub:** *Focus*, quarterly. Newsletter. Contains research and clinical notes, society news, book reviews, and obituaries. *Price:* $11/year. • *International Journal of Clinical and Experimental Hypnosis*, quarterly. Journal. Contains book reviews, statistics, and research and clinical reports. *Price:* Included in membership dues; $49/year for nonmembers. • Membership Directory, periodic.

★ 5855 ★ Society for Clinical and Medical Hair Removal (SCME)
7600 Terrace Ave., Ste. 203
Middleton, WI 53562
Phone: (608)831-8009 **Fax:** (608)831-5485
Email: scme@eesgroupinc.com
Website: http://www.scmhr.org
Lisia Cooley-Walch, Pres.

Fnded: 1985. **Mem:** 1,000. **Reg. Groups:** 10. **Desc:** Professional society of electrologists (persons engaged in the removal of superfluous hair by galvanic blend or short wave methods for cosmetic and medical purposes). Conducts continuing education and leadership development seminars. **Pub:** *Perspectives*, periodic. • *SCME Directory of Membership*, annual. Membership Directory. • *SCME Newsletter*, quarterly. Newsletter. **Frmly:** (2002) Society of Clinical and Medical Electrologists.

★ 5856 ★ Society for Clinical Trials (SCT)
600 Wyndhurst Ave.
Baltimore, MD 21210
Phone: (410)433-4722 **Fax:** (410)435-8631
Email: sctbalt@aol.com
Website: http://www.sctweb.org
Mary C. Burke, Contact

Fnded: 1978. **Mem:** 1,450. **Desc:** Persons with training and expertise in behavioral science, bioethics, biostatistics, computer science, dentistry, epidemiology, law, management, medicine, nursing, and pharmacology. To promote the development and dissemination of knowledge about the design and conduct of clinical trials and other research employing similar methods. **Pub:** *Controlled Clinical Trials*, bimonthly. Journal.

★ 5857 ★ Society for Clinical Vascular Surgery
13 Elm St.
Manchester, MA 01944-1314
Website: http://www.vascsurg.org/doc/Jvonliebig.html

Fnded: 1969. **Desc:** Academic and community vascular surgeons. Promotes vascular surgery in the U.S.

★ 5858 ★ Society for Colposcopy and Cervical Pathology of Singapore (SCCPS)
c/o KK Women's & Children's Hospital
Unit 8K38 Women's Tower Level 8
100 Bukit Timah Rd.
Singapore 229899, Singapore
Phone: 65 62951383 **Fax:** 65 62991969
Website: http://www.sccps.org/

Desc: Promotes education and dissemination of knowledge through the use of colposcopy, pathology, cytology, cytogenetics, endocrinology, epidemiology and basic research relevant to understanding the physiology, pathogenesis, prevention, diagnosis and management of disease processes of premalignant and early malignancy of female lower genital tract, including the uterine cavity.

★ 5859 ★ Society for Companion Animal Studies (SCAS)
The Blue Cross
Shilton Rd.
Burford OX18 4PF, United Kingdom
Phone: 44 1993 825597 **Fax:** 44 1993 825598
Email: info@scas.org.uk
Website: http://www.scas.org.uk

Fnded: 1979. **Mem:** 350. **Nat'l Groups:** 1. **Lang(s):** English. **Desc:** Academics, physicians, psychologists, veterinarians, and laypersons in 13 countries interested in the study of the relationship between people and companion animals. Examines the effects animals have on the emotional and physical well being of individuals. Studies and disseminates results on the benefits companion animals bring to the clients of health and social care professionals. Conducts surveys and research projects. **Pub:** *Death of an Animal Friend*. Booklet. • *Guidelines for the Introduction of Pets in Nursing Homes and Other Institutions*. • *Issues in Research in Companion Animal Studies*. Report. • *Journal of Society for Companion Animal Studies*, quarterly. Journal. • *Pet Loss and Support for Bereaved Pet Owners*. Report. • *Pets, Health and Quality of Life for Older People*. • *When a Pet Dies*. Manual.

★ 5860 ★ Society of Computed Body Tomography and Magnetic Resonance (SCBT/MR)
c/o Matrix Meetings Inc
PO Box 1026
Rochester, MN 55903-1026
Phone: (507)288-5620 **Fax:** (507)288-0014
Email: matrixmeetings@charter.net
Website: http://www.scbtmr.org
Paul M. Silverman, MD, Pres.

Fnded: 1977. **Mem:** 100. **Desc:** Radiologists. Provides continuing medical educational courses on computed tomography and magnetic resonance imaging of the body. Course syllabus. **Frmly:** (1991) Society of Computed Body Tomography.

★ 5861 ★ Society for Computer Applications in Radiology (SCAR)
10105 Cottesmore Ct.
Great Falls, VA 22066-3540
Phone: (703)757-0054 **Fax:** (703)757-0454
Email: info@scarnet.org
Website: http://www.scarnet.org
Anna Marie Mason, Exec. Dir.

Fnded: 1980. **Mem:** 2,000. **Desc:** Individuals, corporations, and health facilities with an interest in medical imaging organized to promote and advance through study research, design and testing, the development and application of advanced technology information systems that will improve the delivery of medical imaging services. **Pub:** *Journal of Digital Imaging*, quarterly. Journal. • *SCAR News*, quarterly. Newsletter. • *SCAR University Primer 4: Electronic Reporting in the Digital Medical Enterprise*. • *SCAR University Primer 1: Security Issues in the Digital Medical Enterprise*. • *SCAR University Primer 3: QA: Meeting the Challenge of the Digital Medical Enterprise*. • *SCAR University Primer 2: Achiving Issues in the Digital Medical Enterprise*. • *Understanding Image Compression*. Handbook. • *Understanding Teleradiology*. Handbook.

★ 5862 ★ Society of Computing and Technology in Anaesthesia (SCATA)
c/o Associates of Anaesthesia
21 Portland Pl.
London W1B 1PY, United Kingdom
Website: http://www.scata.org.uk

Fnded: 1990. **Mem:** 340. **Desc:** Anesthesiology associations in Europe concerned with coding, standards for medical devices, and development of medical information technology. **Pub:** *SAN*. Newsletter.

★ 5863 ★ Society of Critical Care Medicine (SCCM)
701 Lee St., Ste. 200
Des Plaines, IL 60016
Phone: (847)827-6869 **Fax:** (847)827-6886
Email: info@sccm.org
Website: http://www.sccm.org
David Julian Martin, CEO/Exec. VP

Fnded: 1970. **Mem:** 9,100. **Reg. Groups:** 14. **Desc:** Physicians, nurses, scientists, technicians, respiratory therapists, engineers, pharmacists, and physicians assistants involved in the field of critical care medicine. Purposes are: to improve care for acute life-threatening illnesses and injuries; to promote development of optimal care facilities; to guarantee high educational standards in critical care medicine. SCCM has initiated self-assessment testing program in an effort to establish core curriculum and assist physicians in self-evaluation. SCCM established American College of Critical Care Medicine in 1988. **Pub:** *Critical Care Medicine*, monthly. Journal. *Price:* $130 for nonmembers. • *Educational and Scientific Symposium Syllabus*, annual. Proceedings. Compilation of proceedings of annual meeting. • *FORUM*, quarterly. Newsletter. Membership newsletter. • *New Horizons: The Science and Practice of Acute Medicine*, quarterly, February, May, August, November. Journal. *Price:* $105 for nonmembers.

★ 5864 ★ Society of Dermatology Physician Assistants (SDPA)
6218 E 78th Pl.
Tulsa, OK 74136
Phone: (918)523-1992 **Fax:** (918)523-1920
Email: monroejo@swbell.net
Website: http://www.pacifier.com/~jomonroe
Mary Monroe, Exec. Sec.

Fnded: 1993. **Mem:** 800. **Nat'l Groups:** 1. **Desc:** Physician assistants who are employed in or have an interest in the practice of dermatology. Seeks to advance the practice of dermatology physician assistants supervised by dermatologists; promotes continuing professional development of members. Acts as liaison between members and the American Academy of Dermatology; educates physicians and the public regarding the role of members in the practice of dermatology; assists in the training of dermatology physician assistants and students. Maintains writers' bureau. **Pub:** Newsletter, periodic. *Price:* for members only. **AKA:** (1995) Physician Assistants in Dermatology.

★ 5865 ★ Society of the Destitute Aged
PO Box DH 53
Egypt Lines
Highfield, Zimbabwe
Phone: 263 884525

Fnded: 1968. **Mem:** 50. **Desc:** Aims to improve living conditions for elderly destitute people in Zimbabwe. Conducts community sponsorship programs.

★ 5866 ★ Society for Developmental and Behavioral Pediatrics (SDBP)
c/o Noreen M. Spota
19 Station Ln.
Philadelphia, PA 19118-2939
Phone: (215)242-3378 **Fax:** (215)248-1981
Email: admin@sdbp.org
Website: http://www.sdbp.org
Noreen M. Spota, Admin. Dir.

Fnded: 1982. **Mem:** 750. **Reg. Groups:** 2. **State Groups:** 2. **Desc:** Pediatricians, child psychologists, and other allied health care professionals. Seeks to improve the health care of infants, children, and adolescents by promoting research, teaching, and clinical care in the area of developmental-behavioral pediatrics. **Pub:** *Journal of Developmental and Behavioral Pediatrics*, bimonthly. Journal. Includes original scientific articles, book and journal article reviews, commentaries, and letters to the editor. *Price:* Included in membership dues; $238/year for nonmembers. **Frmly:** Society for Behavioral Pediatrics.

★ 5867 ★ Society of Diagnostic Medical Sonography (SDMS)
2745 N Dallas Pky., No. 350
Plano, TX 75093-4706
Phone: (214)473-8057 **Fax:** (214)473-8563
Email: alysdale@sdms.org
Website: http://www.sdms.org
Amy Lysdale, Graphic Design and Communications Mgr.

Fnded: 1970. **Mem:** 13,500. **Reg. Groups:** 7. **State Groups:** 50. **Local Groups:** 40. **Desc:** Works to advance and educate its members and the medical community in the science of diagnostic medical sonography, to advance the science of ultrasound technology and to establish and maintain high standards of education and training. **Pub:** *Journal of Diagnostic Medical Sonography*, bimonthly. Journal. • *National Certification Examination Rewiew.* • *News Wave*, quarterly. • *SDMS Annual Conference Videotapes.* Videos. • *Sonography Benchmark Survey Annual Income.* Survey. • Books. **Frmly:** (1980) American Society of Ultrasound Technical Specialists.

★ 5868 ★ Society for Disability Studies
c/o Carol J. Gill, PhD
University of Illinois at Chicago, MC626
Department of Disability and Human Development
1640 W Roosevelt Rd., No. 236
Chicago, IL 60608-6904
Phone: (312)996-4664 **Fax:** (312)996-7743
Email: cg16@uic.edu
Website: http://www.uic.edu/orgs/sds/
Carol J. Gill, PhD, Exec. Officer

Fnded: 1986. **Mem:** 300. **Desc:** Social scientists and scholars studying the problems of disabled people in society. Strives to develop theoretical and practical knowledge about disability and promotes equal participation in society for individuals with disabilities. **Pub:** *Annual Proceedings*, annual. *Price:* $25.

★ 5869 ★ Society for Ear, Nose, and Throat Advances in Children (SENTAC)
c/o Sally R. Shott, MD, Sec.
Cincinnati Children's Hospital Medical Center
3333 Burnet Ave., ML 2018
Cincinnati, OH 45229-3039
Phone: (513)636-4355 **Fax:** (513)636-8133
Email: sally.shott@cchmc.org
Website: http://www.sentac.org
Sally R. Shott, MD, Sec.

Fnded: 1973. **Mem:** 350. **Desc:** Otolaryngologists, pediatricians, audiologists, speech pathologists, and related professionals. Works to evaluate the science and practice of medicine, surgery, and rehabilitation as related to diseases and disorders of the ear, nose, and throat in infants and children; to improve quality of care; to promote and coordinate research; to foster scientific exchange and coordination among professionals from related disciplines. Sponsors lectures and symposia. Provides forum for interchange of information on practice and research. **Pub:** *Directory and Meeting Abstracts*, annual. Directory. • Brochure.

★ 5870 ★ Society for Education in Anesthesia (SEA)
520 N NE Hwy.
Park Ridge, IL 60068-2573
Phone: (847)825-5568 **Fax:** (847)825-5658
Email: sea@asahq.org
Website: http://www.seahq.org
Stewart Hinckley, Exec. Dir.

Fnded: 1984. **Desc:** Anesthesiology educators. Committed to improve skills in anesthesia education. Offers an online discussion forum. **Pub:** *Journal of Education in Perioperative Medicine*, quarterly. Journal. Provides educationally important material to perioperative physicians.

★ 5871 ★ Society for Education on Contraception and Sexuality (SECS)
str. Paleolagu 4, PO 20
R-70273 Bucharest, Romania
Phone: 40 1 3126693 **Fax:** 40 1 3127088
Fnded: 1990. **Lang(s):** English, Romanian. **Desc:** Family planning organizations and health care personnel. Promotes universal access to family planning services. Serves as liaison linking members with government agencies responsible for public reproductive health and population programs; conducts continuing professional education courses for health care practitioners.

★ 5872 ★ Society of Emergency Medicine Physician Assistants (SEMPA)
950 N Washington St.
Alexandria, VA 22314-1552
Phone: (703)519-7334 **Fax:** (703)684-1924
Email: info@sempa.org
Website: http://www.sempa.org
Tom Moreno, Exec. Dir.

Fnded: 1990. **Mem:** 700. **Nat'l Groups:** 1. **Reg. Groups:** 6. **Desc:** Works to collect demographic data to share with the PA profession and other agencies; strives to devise a more standardized approach to credentialing the development and granting of clinical privileges. Seeks to enhance the EM PAs ability to provide the best quality patient care. **Pub:** *SEMPA News*, quarterly. Newsletter.

★ 5873 ★ Society for Endocrinology
17/18 The Courtyard
Woodlands
Bradley Stoke
Bristol BS32 4NQ, United Kingdom
Phone: 44 1454 642200 **Fax:** 44 1454 642222
Email: info@endocrinology.org
Website: http://www.endocrinology.org

Fnded: 1939. **Mem:** 2,000. **Desc:** Clinicians and scientists working within the field of hormones and hormone related disease. Undertakes scientific/medical publishing, conferences (including commercial exhibitions) and training courses. **Pub:** *Endocrine-Related Cancer*, quarterly. Journal. • *European Journal of Endocrinology*, monthly. Journal. • *Journal of Endocrinology*, monthly. Journal. • *Journal of Molecular Endocrinology*, bimonthly. Journal.

★ 5874 ★ Society for Endocrinology, Metabolism and Diabetes of South Africa (SEMDSA)
c/o Ms. Shelly Harris
PO Box 783155
Sandton 2146
Johannesburg, Republic of South Africa
Phone: 27 11 8070794 **Fax:** 27 11 8077989
Email: rsh@novonordisk.com
Website: http://www.diabetesafrica.com/idfmembers.html

Desc: Represents people with diabetes, endocrine and metabolic disorders. Promotes research and support of those with diabetes, endocrine and metabolic disorders in South Africa.

★ 5875 ★ Society of Environmental Toxicology and Chemistry (SETAC)
1010 N 12th Ave.
Pensacola, FL 32501-3367
Phone: (850)469-1500 **Fax:** (850)469-9778
Email: setac@setac.org
Website: http://www.setac.org
Jeffery A. Foran, Pres.

Fnded: 1979. **Mem:** 5,000. **Reg. Groups:** 16. **Desc:** Professionals in the fields of chemistry, toxicology, biology, and ecology; atmospheric, health, and earth sciences; and environmental engineering. Promotes the use of multidisciplinary approaches to examine the impacts of chemicals and technology on the environment. Strives to balance the interests of academia, business, and government. Conducts workshops and symposia on research topics of interest to members. **Pub:** *Environmental Toxicology and Chemistry*, monthly. Journal. Contains peer-reviewed research papers. *Price:* included in membership dues; $640 for institutions. • *Life-Cycle Assessment Data Quality: A*

Conceptual Framework. Report. • *Radiotelemetry Applications for Wildlife Toxicology Field Studies*. • *SETAC News*, bimonthly. Newsletter. Highlights environmental topics, SETAC activities, employment activities, and meetings of interest. • Membership Directory, annual. Lists addresses and specialties of members. *Price:* available to members only. • Publishes various technical and informal reports.

★ 5876 ★ Society for Epidemiologic Research (SER)
c/o Joseph L. Lyon
Department of Family & Preventive Medicine
50 N Medical Dr., 1C26
Salt Lake City, UT 84132
Phone: (801)581-7234 **Fax:** (801)585-9805
Email: jlyon@dfpm.utah.edu
Website: http://www.epiresearch.org/
Dr. Joseph L. Lyon, Sec. -Treas.

Fnded: 1967. **Mem:** 3,000. **Desc:** Epidemiologists, researchers, public health administrators, educators, mathematicians, statisticians, and others interested in epidemiological research. To stimulate scientific interest in and promote the exchange of information about epidemiological research. **Pub:** *American Journal of Epidemiology*, bimonthly. Journal. Includes research reports and reviews, computer programs for epidemiologists, and annual meeting abstracts. *Price:* $190/year. • *Society for Epidemiologic Research–Membership Directory*, every 3-5 years. Membership Directory. • *Society for Epidemiologic Research–Newsletter*, semiannual. Newsletter.

★ 5877 ★ Society of European Sonographers (SEUS)
36 Portland Pl.
London W1N 3DG, United Kingdom
Phone: 44 20 78157911 **Fax:** 44 20 78158099
Email: chudlet@sbu.ac.uk

★ 5878 ★ Society for Excellence in Eyecare
4400 Jenifer St., NW, Ste. 230
Washington, DC 20015
Phone: (202)244-7334 **Fax:** (202)362-4730
Email: peter@see.anasmm.com
Website: http://www.excellenteyesurgery.com
Peter Anas, Exec. Dir.

Fnded: 1989. **Mem:** 100. **Desc:** Seeks excellence in eye surgery and peri-operative care and is committed that patients with ocular problems are afforded safe, high quality and cost-effective care of the eye. Endeavors to seek education, training and advocacy, those policies, procedures and technologies that promote patient access to vision restoring treatment.

★ 5879 ★ Society for the Exploration of Psychotherapy Integration (SEPI)
134 Wooleys Ln.
Great Neck, NY 11023
Phone: (516)877-4803 **Fax:** (516)877-4805
Email: stricker@adelphi.edu
Website: http://www.cyberpsych.org/sepi/
Dr. George Stricker, Treas.

Fnded: 1984. **Mem:** 750. **Reg. Groups:** 15. **Desc:** Mental health professionals interested in the integration of theories and methods of psychotherapy. Encourages communication among members. Promotes collaborative work among psychotherapists who adhere to different theories and methods. **Pub:** *Journal of Psychotherapy Integration*, quarterly. Journal. Contains professional articles and book reviews.

★ 5880 ★ Society of Eye Surgeons (SES)
7801 Norfolk Ave.
Bethesda, MD 20814
Fax: (301)986-1876
Email: ief@iefusa.org
Website: http://www.iefusa.org
Kelvin Baervldd, Public Affairs Officer

Fnded: 1969. **Mem:** 1,000. **Desc:** Ophthamologists promoting the science of ophthalmic surgery worldwide. Supports the blindness prevention efforts of the International Eye Foundation. Provides educational, training, and eye care services by sponsoring teaching teams and professors to visit countries worldwide; fosters social exchange among physicians and scientists in the field of ophthalmology. **Pub:** *Eye to Eye*, semiannual. Newsletter. Provides program news.

★ 5881 ★ Society for Fermentation and Bioengineering Japan (Nihon Seibutsu-kogaku Kai)
2-1 Yamadaoka, Suita
Osaka 565, Japan
Phone: 81 6 8762731 **Fax:** 81 6 8792034
Fnded: 1923.

★ 5882 ★ Society for Fetal Urology
c/o Kris Evavold
5445 Meridian Mark Rd., No. 420
Atlanta, GA 30342
Phone: (404)252-5206
Website: http://www.fetalurology.org
Andrew J. Kirsch, MD, Sec. Treas.

Desc: Physicians committed to fetal and perinatal care. Seeks to improve the care of patients with fetal or perinatal urologic problems, especially hydronephrosis. Promotes communication between specialists; supports research; provides consultation. **Pub:** Newsletter, semiannual.

★ 5883 ★ Society of Gastroenterology Nurses and Associates (SGNA)
401 N Michigan Ave.
Chicago, IL 60611-4267
Phone: (312)321-5165 **Free:** 800-245-7462
Fax: (312)527-6658
Email: sgna@sba.com
Website: http://www.sgna.org
Mary Beth Hepp, Exec. Dir.

Fnded: 1974. **Mem:** 6,000. **Reg. Groups:** 60. **Desc:** To unite personnel engaged in the field of gastroenterology/endoscopy in order to promote the highest professional standards for gastroenterology nurses and associates. Conducts national and regional educational courses and research programs. Cooperates with other professional associations, hospitals, universities, industries, technical societies, research organizations, and governmental agencies. **Pub:** *Gastroenterology Nursing*, bimonthly. Includes subject and author indexes, book reviews, new product information. *Price:* $52/year for individuals; $80/year for institutions; $25/year for students; $15/copy. • *Gastroenterology Nursing - A Core Curriculum*. • *Job Description Handbook*. • *Manual of Gastrointestinal Procedures*. • *Pediatric Supplement*. • *Pulmonary Supplement*. • *SGNA News*, bimonthly. Newsletter. Contains regional directory, regional news, and articles on research and finance. *Price:* Free to members. **Frmly:** (1989) Society of Gastrointestinal Assistants.

★ 5884 ★ Society of Gastronintestinal Radiologists (SGR)
c/o International Meeting Managers, Inc.
4550 Post Oak Place, Ste. 342
Houston, TX 77027
Phone: (713)965-0566 **Fax:** (713)960-0488
Email: administration@sgr.org
Website: http://www.sgr.org/sgr_main.htm
Eric vanSonnenberg, MD, Pres.

Fnded: 1971. **Desc:** Strive to furnish leadership and foster advances in diagnostic, interventional, gastrointestinal and abdominal radiology; work to exchange knowledge pertaining to research practice and education in gastrointestinal and abdominal radiology. Annual lecture in memory of Walter B. Cannon, the pioneer physiologist who initiated gastrointestinal radiology and an annual postgraduate course in gastrointestinal radiology.

★ 5885 ★ Society of General Internal Medicine (SGIM)
2501 M St. NW, Ste. 575
Washington, DC 20037-1126
Phone: (202)887-5150 **Free:** 800-822-3060
Fax: (202)887-5405
Email: karlsond@sgim.org
Website: http://www.sgim.org
David Karlson, PhD, Exec. Dir.

Fnded: 1978. **Mem:** 3,000. **Reg. Groups:** 8. **Desc:** Physicians combining clinical practice with research. Promotes improved patient care, research, and teaching in primary care and general internal medicine. Sponsors research and educational programs. **Pub:** *Directory of Primary Care Internal Medicine Residency Programs and Fellowship Training Programs*, annual. Directory. Descriptiojns of 146 primary care general internal medicine programs. Lists 60 fellowship programs in general internal medicine. • *Journal of General Internal Medicine*, monthly. Journal. • *SGIM Forum*, monthly. Newsletter. **Frmly:** (1987) Society for Research and Education in Primary Care Internal Medicine.

★ 5886 ★ Society of Geriatric Cardiology (SGC)
Heart House
9111 Old Georgetown Rd.
Bethesda, MD 20814
Phone: (301)581-3449 **Fax:** (301)581-3408
Email: rpallott@sgcard.org
Website: http://www.sgcard.org
Rose Pallotta, Mgr.

Fnded: 1986. **Mem:** 500. **Desc:** Geriatric cardiologists and physicians in related fields are fellows; medical practitioners certified in specialties other than geriatrics or cardiologists are members; other individuals with an interest in geriatric cardiology are nonphysician members. Works to improve the clinical and therapeutic management of older individuals with cardiovascular disease; encourages use of preventive measures to avert the onset of cardiovascular aging and disease. Promotes more effective public policy and education regarding cardiac health. Conducts educational programs for physicians, other health care professionals, and the public. Supports research into cardiovascular aging and diseases relevant to older people. Serves as a clearinghouse on geriatric cardiology. Sponsors competitions. **Pub:** *American Journal of Geriatric Cardiology*, bimonthly. Journal. • *News Brief*, 3/year. Newsletter. **Frmly:** (1999) Council on Geriatric Cardiology.

★ 5887 ★ Society of Gerontology of the Republic Serbia
Gerontolosko Drustvo Srbije
Krfska 7
YU-11000 Belgrade, Serbia
Phone: 381 11 415734 **Fax:** 381 11 415734
Email: gerontolog@yahoo.com
Website: http://www.gds.org.yu

Fnded: 1973. **Mem:** 210. **Nat'l Groups:** 1. **Local Groups:** 8. **Lang(s):** English. **Desc:** Individuals who professionally deal with the problems of the aged and aging and their social, medical, legal, sociological, psychological, sociopolitical, economic, and other aspects. Seeks to improve gerontological theory and practice and to contribute to the implementation of the gerontological knowledge in the humanization of living conditions of the aged and aging. **Pub:** *Gerontology*, annual. Journal.

★ 5888 ★ Society of Government Service Urologists
7027 Weathered Post
PO Box 681965
San Antonio, TX 78268
Phone: (210)681-0587 **Fax:** (210)680-7725
Email: sgsu@txdirect.net
Website: http://www.txdirect.net/~sgsu
Preston Littrell, Admin.

Fnded: 1952. **Mem:** 731. **Desc:** Urologists. Promotes exchange of information on advancements in urological research. **Pub:** *SGSU*, quarterly. Newsletter. *Price:* Free.

★ 5889 ★ Society of Graduate Surgeons (SGS)
4929 Wilshire Blvd., No. 428
Los Angeles, CA 90010
Phone: (323)937-5514 **Fax:** (323)937-0959
C. James Dowden, Exec. Dir.

Fnded: 1950. **Mem:** 375. **Desc:** Surgeons who have completed general surgery residencies at USC-LA County Medical Center. Conducts post-graduate educational programs for members and surgeons.

★ 5890 ★ Society for Gynecologic Investigation (SGI)
409 12th St. SW
Washington, DC 20024-2188
Phone: (202)863-2544 **Fax:** (202)863-0739
Email: sgiava@aol.com
Website: http://sgionline.org/
Ava A. Tayman, Exec. Dir.

Fnded: 1953. **Mem:** 963. **Desc:** Present and former faculty members of institutions interested or engaged in fundamental gynecologic research. Purpose is to stimulate, encourage, assist, and conduct gynecologic research. **Pub:** *Journal of the Society for Gynecologic Investigation*, bimonthly. Journal. Published by Elsevier Sciences.

★ 5891 ★ Society of Gynecologic Oncologists (SGO)
401 N Michigan Ave.
Chicago, IL 60611
Phone: (312)644-6610 **Fax:** (312)527-6640
Email: sgo@sba.com
Website: http://www.sgo.org
M. Eileen Widner, Exec. Dir.

Fnded: 1969. **Mem:** 772. **Desc:** Purposes are to: improve the care of patients with gynecological cancer; encourage research in gynecologic oncology; advance knowledge in the field; upgrade standards of practice. Evaluates and seeks to address the trends in gynecologic oncology; assesses the future of the field.

★ 5892 ★ Society of Gynecologic Oncologists of Canada (GOC)
c/o Elizabeth Waite
780 Promenade Echo Dr.
Ottawa, ON, Canada K1S 5N8
Phone: (613)730-4192 **Free:** 800-561-2416
Fax: (613)730-4314
Email: ewaite@sogc.com
Website: http://www.g-o-c.org/

Fnded: 1980. **Desc:** Seeks to improve the care of women with gynecologic cancer; raise standards of practice and encourage research in gynecologic oncology; disseminates knowledge to practitioners, patients and public on gynecologic cancer, and cooperates with other organizations in women's health care, oncology, and related fields. Maintains speakers' bureau. **Pub:** Newsletter.

★ 5893 ★ Society of Health and Beauty Therapists
77 New Bond St
London W1Y 9DB, United Kingdom
Phone: 44 20 74933321

Fnded: 1962.

★ 5894 ★ Society of Health Education and Health Promotion Specialists (SHEPS)
c/o Sheffield Health
64 Terregles Ave.
Glasgow G41 4LX, United Kingdom
Phone: 44 114 2711305 **Fax:** 44 114 2711318
Email: frances.cunning@sheffield-ha.nhs.uk
Website: http://www.hj-web.co.uk/sheps/

Fnded: 1980. **Mem:** 500. **Reg. Groups:** 10. **Lang(s):** English. **Desc:** Provides a voice for health promotion theory and practice within the broader context of public health. **Frmly:** (2001) Society of Health Education and Promotion Specialists.

★ 5895 ★ Society for Health and Human Values (SHHV)
4700 W Lake Ave.
Glenview, IL 60025
Email: shhv@aol.com
George K. Degnon, Exec. Officer

Fnded: 1969. **Mem:** 900. **Desc:** Educators in the health professions united to develop new understandings, concepts, and programs in the area of human values and medicine with special emphasis on the education of health professionals. Conducts programs at national association meetings. Acts as resource service for educational institutions. **Pub:** *Advance Directives in Medicine*. Book. • *Literature and Medicine: A Claim for a Discipline*. Book. • *The Meaning of AIDS: Implications for Medical Science, Clinical Practice and Public Health Policy*. Book. • *Medicine & Religion: Strategies of Care*. Book. • *Ministers in Medical Education*. Book. • *Nurshing the Humanities in Medicine: Interactions with the Social Sciences*. Book. • *Of Value*, quarterly. • *The Visual Arts and Medical Education*. Book.

★ 5896 ★ Society for Healthcare Consumer Advocacy of the American Hospital Association (SHCA)
One North Franklin
Chicago, IL 60606
Phone: (312)422-3851 **Fax:** (312)422-4575
Email: shca@aha.org
Website: http://www.shca-aha.org
Glen Brown, Exec. Dir.

Fnded: 1972. **Mem:** 960. **State Groups:** 31. **Desc:** To advance the development of effective patient representative and advocacy programs in health care institutions. Conducts seminars and workshops. **Pub:** *In The Name of the Patient: Consumer Advocacy in Healthcare*. Book. *Price:* $35 for members; $45 for nonmembers. • *Membership Roster*, annual. **Frmly:** (1981) Society of Patient Representatives; (1988) National Society of Patient Representatives of the American Hospital Association; (1998) National Society of Patient Representation and Consumer Affairs of the American Hospital Association.

★ 5897 ★ Society for Healthcare Epidemiology of America (SHEA)
19 Mantua Rd.
Mount Royal, NJ 08061
Phone: (856)423-0087 **Fax:** (856)423-3420
Email: sheahq@talley.com
Website: http://www.shea-online.org
Michael L. Tapper, Pres.

Fnded: 1981. **Mem:** 1,100. **Desc:** Fosters the development and application of the science of healthcare epidemiology, broadly defined as any activity designed to study and/or improve outcomes in any type of healthcare institution or setting. **Pub:** *Infection Control and Hospital Epidemiology*, monthly. Journal. **Frmly:** Society of Hospital Epidemiologists of America; (2000) Society of Healthcare Epidemiologists of America.

★ 5898 ★ Society for Healthcare Strategy and Market Development of the American Hospital Association
1 N Franklin, 31st Fl.
Chicago, IL 60606
Phone: (312)422-3888 **Fax:** (312)422-4579
Email: stratsoc@aha.org
Website: http://www.stratsociety.org
Marty Campanello, Pres.

Fnded: 1996. **Mem:** 4,000. **Local Groups:** 57. **Desc:** Persons in hospitals, health systems and networks, managed care plans, ambulatory care and physician groups who are engaged in strategic planning, business development, marketing, or public relations activities. **Pub:** *Directory of Health Care Strategic Management and Communications Consultants*, annual. Directory. *Price:* Free to members; $40/copy for nonmembers. • *Membership Directory Society for Healthcare Strategy and Market Development*, annual. Membership Directory. *Price:* Included in membership dues. • *Spectrum*, bimonthly. Tabloid; includes calendar of events. *Price:* Included in membership dues. **Frmly:** (1984) American Society for Hospital Public Relations; (1990) American Society for Hospital Marketing and Public Relations; (1998) American Society for Healthcare Marketing and Public Relations.

★ 5899 ★ Society for Helping People with Autism (SPOSA)
Spolocnost na pomoc osobam s autizmom
PO Box 8
CS-841 02 Bratislava, Czech Republic
Fax: 42 7 54411774
Email: sposa@pobox.sk
Website: http://www.sposa.sk/page2.html

Fnded: 1994. **Desc:** Works to improve the quality of life for persons with autism and their families to ensure dignity within the community.

★ 5900 ★ Society for Hematopathology (SH)
3643 Walton Way Ext.
Augusta, GA 30909
Phone: (706)733-7550 **Fax:** (706)733-8033
Email: sh@uscap.org
Website: http://www.dartmouth.edu/~nlevy/wwwx.html
Carolyn Lane, Coord.

Fnded: 1981. **Mem:** 500. **Desc:** Physicians; doctors of science, osteopathy, veterinary medicine, and dental surgery. Promotes exchange of information and encourages clinical, morphologic, and functional investigation of the hematopoietic (pertaining to the formation of blood cells) and lymphoreticular (regarding reticuloendothelial cells of the lymph glands) systems. **Pub:** Newsletter.

★ 5901 ★ Society of Homeopaths
4a Artizan Rd.
Northampton NN1 4HU, United Kingdom
Phone: 44 1604 621400 **Fax:** 44 1604 622622
Email: info@homeopathy-soh.org
Website: http://www.homeopathy-soh.org

Fnded: 1978. **Mem:** 2,706. **Desc:** Professional homeopaths on the Society's register. Aims to develop and maintain high standards for the practise of homeopathy and to promote public awareness of homeopathy. It also supports the establishment of education and training in homeopathy. **Pub:** *The Homoeopath Journal*, quarterly. Journal. • *Register of Professional Homoeopaths*, semiannual. • Newsletter, quarterly.

★ 5902 ★ Society of Homes for the Handicapped (SHH)
G/F 2A Po On Rd.
Cronin Garden
Shamshuipo
Hong Kong, People's Republic of China
Phone: 852 227454214 **Fax:** 852 227864097
Email: fhs@fuhong.org

Fnded: 1977. **Mem:** 210. **Lang(s):** English. **Desc:** Works to integrate mentally and physically disabled individuals, as well as those who have recovered from mental illnesses, into Hong Kong society. Instructs family members on care for the disabled; operates residential homes and day care centers. Conducts courses for handicapped individuals; trains volunteers to work with the disabled. Provides vocational assessment and employment opportunities for the disabled. Offers social work services to families with disabled members. Organizes community educational programs for a better understanding and positive attitude towards persons with disabilities. **Pub:** *SHH Annual Report*, annual. Annual Report. • *SHH NEWS*, quarterly. Newsletter. SHH News and activities.

★ 5903 ★ Society for Human Ecology (SHE)
c/o Melville Cote
College of the Atlantic
105 Eden St.
Bar Harbor, ME 04609
Phone: (207)288-5015 **Fax:** (207)288-4126
Email: inquiry@ecology.coa.edu
Website: http://www.coa.edu
Katona Steven, Pres.

Fnded: 1981. **Mem:** 150. **Desc:** Educators, health practitioners, scientists, and other professionals in 30 countries studying human ecology and its applications. Focuses attention on the consequences of human action on manufactured, natural, and social environments. Promotes interdisciplinary collaboration; facilitates the exchange of information; identifies problems and recommends solutions from an ecological perspective. Conducts workshops and symposia. Participates in human ecology consortium. Organization is distinct from the International Organization for Human Ecology, formerly known as the Society for Human Ecology. **Pub:** *Human Ecology: A Gathering of Perspectives*. Proceedings. Proceedings from SHE's First International Conference, held in 1985. • *Human Ecology and Decision Making: An International and Interdisciplinary Collaboration*. • *Human Ecology Bulletin*, semiannual. • *Human Ecology–Coming of Age: An International Overview*. Proceedings. Proceedings of the symposium organized at the International Congress of Ecology in 1990. • *Human Ecology: Crossing Boundaries*. Selected papers from the 6th conference of SHE. • *Human Ecology: Research and Applications*. Proceedings. Proceedings from SHE's Second International Conference, held in 1988. • *Human Ecology: Steps to the Future*. Proceedings. Proceedings from SHE's Third International Conference. • *Human Ecology: Strategies for the Future*. Selected papers from the 4th conference of the SHE, held in 1990. • *International Directory of Human Ecologists*, periodic. Directory. Lists over 700 human ecologists worldwide, with descriptions of their work, research, and activities; includes addresses and phone numbers. • Brochure.

★ 5904 ★ Society for Industrial and Organizational Psychology (SIOP)
PO Box 87
Bowling Green, OH 43402-0087
Phone: (419)353-0032 **Fax:** (419)352-2645
Email: siop@siop.org
Website: http://www.siop.org
Michael J. Burke, Pres.

Fnded: 1982. **Mem:** 6,000. **Nat'l Groups:** 1. **Desc:** Dedicated to promoting human welfare through various applications of psychology to all types of organizations providing goods and services. **Pub:** *The Industrial-Organizational Psychologist (TIP)*, quarterly. Newsletter. Contains information about Society activities and articles of interest to those in the field. *Price:* included in membership dues, or for a small charge to others.

★ 5905 ★ Society of Infectious Diseases Pharmacists (SIDP)
502 E 11th St., Ste. 400
Austin, TX 78701-2656
Phone: (512)708-0611 **Fax:** (512)708-0627
Email: sidp@aams-texas.com
Website: http://www.sidp.org/
Charles H. Ballow, FCCP, Pres.

Desc: Pharmacists with a primary interest and practice in infectious diseases pharmacotherapy, and who have spent at least two years performing pharmacotherpeutic research are active members; pharmacists and other individuals not meeting the requirements for active membership, but who share an interest in infectious diseases pharmacotherapy, are associate members. Seesk to advance the study and practice of infectious diseases pharmacotherapy, and to enhance the professional status of members. Serves as a forum for discussion and exchange of information among members. Encourages pharmacotherapeutic research. **Pub:** *News Update*, monthly. Newsletter. • *SIDP*, 3/year. Newsletter.

★ 5906 ★ Society of Interventional Radiology (SIR)
10201 Lee Hwy., Ste. 500
Fairfax, VA 22030
Phone: (703)691-1805 **Free:** 800-488-7284
Fax: (703)691-1855
Email: info@sirweb.org
Website: http://www.sirweb.org
Pete Lauer, Exec. Dir.

Fnded: 1973. **Mem:** 4,000. **Desc:** Physicians who are leaders in the field of interventional radiology. Facilitates exchange of new ideas and techniques and provides educational courses for all physicians working in the field. Conducts annual postgraduate course. Conducts Interventional Radiology Political Action. **Pub:** *Directory of Angiography and Interventional Radiology Fellowship Programs*. Directory. • *Journal of Vascular and Interventional Radiology*, bimonthly. Journal. • *SIR Membership Directory*, annual. Membership Directory. • *SIR Newsletter*, bimonthly. Newsletter. **Frmly:** (2003) Society of Cardiovascular and Interventional Radiology.

★ 5907 ★ Society of Invasive Cardiovascular Professionals (SICP)
PO Box 61606
Virginia Beach, VA 23466
Phone: (757)497-3694 **Free:** 800-237-7285
Fax: (757)497-0010
Email: director@sicp.com
Website: http://www.sicp.com
Roger Siegfried, Pres.

Fnded: 1992. **Mem:** 700. **Desc:** Cardiac catheterization laboratory personnel. Supports the highest quality of patient care. Serves as a forum for exchange of information among members. Defines core curricula for cardiovascular professionals; makes available educational opportunities to members; establishes standards of ethics and practice for the field. Facilitates cardiovascular research. **Pub:** *Cath-Lab Digest*, monthly. Journal. *Price:* Free with membership. • *Journal of Invasive Cardiology*, monthly. Journal.

★ 5908 ★ Society for Investigative Dermatology (SID)
c/o Angela Welsh
820 W Superior Ave., Ste. 340
Cleveland, OH 44113-1800
Phone: (216)579-9300 **Fax:** (216)579-9333
Email: sid@sidnet.org
Website: http://www.sidnet.org
Angela Welsh, Admin. Dir.

Fnded: 1937. **Mem:** 2,300. **Desc:** Professional society promoting research in dermatology and allied subjects. **Pub:** *Journal of Investigative Dermatology*, monthly. Journal.

★ 5909 ★ Society of Japanese Virologists (Nippon Uirusu Gakkai)
5-16-9 Honkomagome, Bunkyo-ku
Tokyo, Japan
Fnded: 1953.

★ 5910 ★ Society of Laparoendoscopic Surgeons (SLS)
7330 SW 62nd Pl., Ste. 410
Miami, FL 33143-4825
Phone: (305)665-9959 **Free:** 800-446-2659
Fax: (305)667-4123
Email: info@sls.org
Website: http://www.sls.org
Paul A. Wetter, MD, Contact

Fnded: 1990. **Mem:** 6,700. **Desc:** Laparoscopic and endoscopic surgeons from all specialties and other health care professionals. Promotes improvement in laparoscopic and endoscopic surgical techniques; facilitates professional growth of members. Conducts educational programs. **Pub:** *Journal of the Society of Laparoendoscopic Surgeons*, quarterly. Journal. This is a multi-disciplinary journal of laparoscopy, endoscopy and minimally invasive surgery. *Price:* $250 in U.S. • *Laparoscopy and SLS Report*, semiannual. Newsletter. Membership newsletter. *Price:* $85.

★ 5911 ★ Society for Leukocyte Biology (SLB)
9650 Rockville Pike
Bethesda, MD 20814
Phone: (301)634-7810 **Free:** 800-433-2732
Fax: (301)634-7813
Email: slb@faseb.org
Website: http://www.leukocytebiology.org
Debbie Weinstein, PhD, Exec. Mgr.

Fnded: 1954. **Mem:** 1,025. **Desc:** Persons holding M.D. and/or Ph.D. degrees who conduct research with universities; private, industrial, and government institutes; hospital clinics; members of the pharmaceutical industry. Facilitates the association of persons studying the reticuloendothelial system; fosters research in the field. (The reticuloendothelial system comprises all the cells of the blood and body tissues, including macrophages, lymphocytes, and granulocytes. It is involved in the immune response and in inflammation and functions in host defense against such problems as malignancies, infection, and environmental pathogens.) Sponsors workshop on macrophage methodology. **Pub:** *Directory and Constitution*, annual. Directory. • *Journal of Leukocyte Biology*, monthly. Journal. • Books. • Newsletter, quarterly. **Frmly:** (1988) Reticuloendothelial Society.

★ 5912 ★ Society for Light Treatment and Biological Rhythms (SLTBR)
PO Box 591687
San Francisco, CA 94159-1687
Phone: (415)876-0716 **Fax:** (415)751-2758
Email: sltbrinfo@aol.com
Website: http://www.sltbr.org
Kathleen Matikonis, Exec. Dir.

Fnded: 1988. **Mem:** 400. **Desc:** Fosters research, professional development, and clinical applications in the fields of light therapy and biological rhythms.

★ 5913 ★ Society for Maternal Fetal Medicine (SMFM)
409 12th St. SW
Washington, DC 20024-2188
Phone: (202)863-2476 **Fax:** (202)554-1132
Email: info@smfm.org
Website: http://www.smfm.org
Patricia Stahr, Exec. Dir.

Fnded: 1977. **Mem:** 1,900. **Desc:** Obstetricians specializing in maternal-fetal medicine. Works to improve perinatal care through promotion and expansion of education in obstetrical perinatology. Provides a forum for exchange between members. **Pub:** *American Journal of Obstetrics and Gynecology*, periodic. Journal. **Frmly:** (1999) Society of Perinatal Obstetricians.

★ 5914 ★ Society of Medical Administrators (SMA)
c/o Medical Council of Canada
PO Box 82234 Station
Ottawa, ON, Canada K1G 3H7
Phone: (613)521-8787 **Fax:** (613)521-8831
Website: http://www.mcc.ca

Fnded: 1920. **Mem:** 50. **Lang(s):** English. **Desc:** Medical doctors in hospital or health care administration. Discusses issues concerning health care administration. **Pub:** Directory, annual. Also publishes minutes of the Annual Meeting. **Frmly:** (1951) Medical Superintendents Club.

★ 5915 ★ Society of Medical Consultants to the Armed Forces (SMCAF)
5 Southern Way
Fredericksburg, VA 22406
Phone: (301)295-9822 **Fax:** (301)295-3627

Email: jhutton@usuhs.mil
Fred A. Cecere, MD, Sec. -Treas.

Fnded: 1945. **Mem:** 1,000. **Desc:** Professional society of physicians and surgeons who have been in active military service and who have acted as consultants to the Surgeons General of the Army, Navy, or Air Force. To preserve and encourage the association of civilian consultants and military medical personnel and to assist in the development and maintenance of the highest standards of medical practice in the Armed Forces. **Pub:** *Roster*, every 2-3 years. • Newsletter, 3/year. **Frmly:** Society of U.S. Medical Consultants in World War II.

★ 5916 ★ Society for Medical Decision Making (SMDM)

1211 Locus St.
Philadelphia, PA 19107
Phone: (215)545-7697 **Fax:** (215)545-8107
Email: smdm-office@lists.smdm.org
Website: http://www.smdm.org
Daniel E. Reichard, Admin. Dir.

Fnded: 1979. **Mem:** 1,000. **Desc:** Individuals with an interest in "developing rational and systematic approaches" to medical decision making, including educators, clinicians, managers, and policy makers. Promotes improvement in all aspects of medical decision making. Evaluates decision making applications and disseminates conclusions. Facilitates multidisciplinary scholarship and research; conducts continuing professional education programs. **Pub:** *Medical Decision Making*, bimonthly. Journal. • Newsletter, semiannual.

★ 5917 ★ Society of Medical-Dental Management Consultants (SMD)

3646 E Ray Rd., B16-45
Phoenix, AZ 85044
Free: 800-826-2264 **Fax:** (602)759-3530
Email: chuck@smdmc.org
Website: http://www.smdmc.org
Charles R. Wold, CPA, Exec. Sec.

Fnded: 1968. **Mem:** 60. **State Groups:** 50. **Desc:** Professional medical and/or dental management consultants associated for educational and information sharing purposes. Objectives are to: advance the profession; share management techniques; improve individual skills; provide clients with competent and capable business management. Provides information on insurance and income tax. Conducts surveys; compiles statistics. **Pub:** *Membership Roster*, annual. Membership Directory. • *SMD Statistics.* • *Society of Medical-Dental Management Consultants–Newsletter*, monthly. Newsletter. *Price:* Included in membership dues. • Bulletin.

★ 5918 ★ Society of Medical Laboratory Technologists of South Africa (SMLTSA)
(Vereniging van Geneeskundige Laboratorium Tegnoloe van Suid-Afrika — VGLTSA)

PO Box 6014
Roggebaai 8012, Republic of South Africa
Phone: 27 21 4194857 **Fax:** 27 21 4212566
Email: smltsa@iafrica.com
Website: http://www.smltsa.org.za

Fnded: 1951. **Mem:** 1,700. **Local Groups:** 15. **Lang(s):** Afrikaans, English. **Desc:** Medical technologists, students, and interested persons organized to promote the medical technology profession. Works to: establish standards of practice; influence public policy; provide a forum for the exchange of ideas. Acts as an advisory and consulting body. Represents the profession before certifying, educational, employment, and registering authorities. Sponsors activities that advance scientific knowledge and encourage original work. **Pub:** *Constitution of the Society of Medical Laboratory Technologists of South Africa*. Book. • *Medical Technology*, semiannual. Journal. • *Medical Technology News*, periodic. Newspaper. • Newsletter.

★ 5919 ★ Society for Medicinal Plant Research
(Gesellschaft fur Arzneipflanzenforschung — GA)

c/o Dr. Renate Seitz
Emmeringerstr. 11
D-82275 Emmering, Germany
Phone: 49 8141 672749 **Fax:** 49 8141 673749
Email: ga-secretary@t-online.de
Website: http://www.ga-online.org

Fnded: 1953. **Mem:** 1,076. **Nat'l Groups:** 72. **Lang(s):** English, German. **Desc:** Scientists in 70 countries who promote medicinal plant research. Organized to serve as an international focal point for such interests as pharmacognosy, pharmacology, phytochemistry, plant biochemistry and physiology, chemistry of natural products; plant cell culture and application of medicinal plants in medicine. Acts as liaison with governments, pharmacopoeia commissions, and international health organizations on matters pertaining to the medicinal plant field. Serves as forum for international exchange of information on the different aspects of medicinal plant research. **Pub:** *Newsletter*, semiannual. Newsletter. Includes news of the society and congress announcements. • *Planta Medica*, monthly. Journal. **Frmly:** (1970) German Society for Medicinal Plant Research.

★ 5920 ★ Society for Medicine and Law in Israel

PO Box 6451
IL-31063 Haifa, Israel
Phone: 972 4 8375219 **Fax:** 972 4 8381587
Email: acarmi@research.haifa.ac.il

Fnded: 1972. **Mem:** 1,600. **Lang(s):** English. **Desc:** Promotes the advancement of medicine and law in Israel. **Pub:** *Refuah Umishpat*, semiannual. Journal.

★ 5921 ★ Society for Medicines Research (SMR)

c/o Ms. Lilian Attar
Triangle House
Broomhill Rd.
London SW18 4HX, United Kingdom
Phone: 44 208 8752431 **Fax:** 44 208 8752434
Email: secretariat@socmr.org
Website: http://www.socmr.org

Fnded: 1966. **Mem:** 526. **Lang(s):** English. **Desc:** Researchers at academic institutions and in the pharmaceutical industry; other concerned individuals. Promotes advancement in the field of medicinal education and research in order to provide the public with proper information on drug usage for relief of sickness. **Pub:** *Proceedings*, periodic. • Newsletter, 3-4/year. **Frmly:** (1994) Society for Drug Research.

★ 5922 ★ Society for Menstrual Cycle Research (SMCR)

10559 N 104th Pl.
Scottsdale, AZ 85258
Phone: (480)451-9731 **Fax:** (480)451-9731
Email: maryannafriederich@msn.com
Website: http://www.pop.psu.edu/smcr
Mary Anna Friederich, MD, Sec. -Treas.

Fnded: 1979. **Mem:** 100. **Desc:** Physicians, nurses, endocrinologists, geneticists, physiologists, psychologists, sociologists, researchers, educators, students, and others interested in the health needs of women as related to the menstrual cycle. Goals are: to identify research priorities, recommend research strategies, and promote interdisciplinary research on the menstrual cycle; to establish a communication network for facilitating interdisciplinary dialogue on menstrual cycle events; to disseminate information and promote discussion of issues among public groups. **Pub:** *Changing Perspectives on Menopause*. Book. • *Culture, Society and Menstruation*. Book. • *Membership Roster*, annual. Membership Directory. • *Menarche: The Transition from Girl to Woman.* Book. • *The Menstrual Cycle, Volume 1: A Synthesis of Interdisciplinary Research.* • *The Menstrual Cycle, Volume 2: Research and Implications for Women's Health.* • *Menstrual Health in Women's Lives.* • *Menstruation, Health, and Illness.* • *Mind-Body Rhythmicity, A Menstrual Cycle Prospective.* Book. • *Proceedings 8th Conference Society for Menstrual Cycle Research.* Proceedings. • Newsletter, quarterly.

★ 5923 ★ Society of Military Orthopaedic Surgeons (SOMOS)

810 North St.
Belgium, WI 53004-9531
Phone: (262)285-4280 **Fax:** (262)285-4231
Email: yolich@email.msn.com
Website: http://www.somos.org/
Ellen M. Yolich, Exec. Sec.

Fnded: 1958. **Mem:** 750. **Desc:** Orthopedic surgeons who have served in the active or reserve military. Objectives are to: stimulate scholarly contribution by military medical residents; act as clearinghouse; provide opportunities for consultation with and contributions of surgeons who are retired from the military; further the continuing education of orthopedic surgeons and residents. Presents scientific papers at annual meeting.

★ 5924 ★ Society of Military Otolaryngologists - Head and Neck Surgeons (SMO-HNS)

c/o Sue Pearce
9231 Shawdow Lawn Circle
Converse, TX 78109
Phone: (210)945-9006 **Fax:** (210)945-9024
Email: spearce@worldnet.att.net
Sue Pearce, Admn. Sec.

Fnded: 1952. **Mem:** 320. **Nat'l Groups:** 1. **Desc:** Otolaryngologists, head and neck surgeons and residents in training of the U.S. Army, Air Force, Navy, and former active duty members. Purposes are to further the social and professional contacts of military otolaryngologists and to advance the science and art of the field. **Frmly:** (1952) Society of Military Otolaryngologists.

★ 5925 ★ Society for Mucopolysaccharide Diseases (MPS)

46 Woodside Rd.
Amersham HP6 6RU, United Kingdom
Phone: 44 1494 434156 **Fax:** 44 1494 434252
Email: mps@mpssociety.co.uk
Website: http://www.mpssociety.co.uk

Fnded: 1982. **Mem:** 1,000. **Nat'l Groups:** 24. **Reg. Groups:** 12. **Lang(s):** English, French, German. **Desc:** Acts as a support group for individuals and their families worldwide afflicted with Mucopolysaccharide and related diseases. (MPS diseases, known individually as Hurler, Scheie, Hunter, Sanfilippo, Morquio, Maroteaux-Lamy, and Sly, and associated diseases called mucolipidosis, Fucosidosis, Mannosidosis, Fabry and Sialic Acid Disease, are genetic diseases. Children born with MPS are unable to produce certain enzymes necessary for appropriate metabolism to take place; consequently complex sugars become stored in connective tissues, causing progressive damage, including physical and mental handicaps. In many cases, MPS patients die before reaching adulthood.) Encourages public awareness of MPS diseases and the international transmission of medical knowledge and techniques. Raises funds to further MPS research and arranges for MPS families to assist in research such as carrier testing and biochemical diagnosis. Accepts donations to provide individual advocacy for MPS families. Sponsors research program on the natural history of MPS and the psychosocial problems of MPS children. **Pub:** *Conference Reports*, annual. Report. • *21 Years of Bone Marrow Transplant*, annual. Report. • Newsletter, quarterly.

★ 5926 ★ Society for Mucosal Immunology

4350 E West Hwy., Ste. 401
Bethesda, MD 20814-4411
Phone: (301)718-6516 **Fax:** (301)656-0989
Email: smi@paimgmt.com

Website: http://www.socmucimm.org
Peter Ernst, Contact

Fnded: 1987. **Mem:** 700. **Nat'l Groups:** 37. **Desc:** Clinician-scientists and basic scientists comprised of immunologists, physicians, dentists, veterinarians, biochemists and others interested in the immunology of the gastrointestinal, respiratory and urogential tracts, as well as the eye. Formed to advance research and education related to the field of mucosal immunology. **Pub:** *Mucosal Immunology Update*. *Price:* included in membership dues.

★ 5927 ★ Society of Multivariate Experimental Psychology (SMEP)

PO Box 400400
Charlottesville, VA 22904-4400
Phone: (804)924-3374
Email: maccallum.l@osu.edu
Website: http://www.smep.org/
Joe Rodgers, Sec. -Treas.

Fnded: 1960. **Mem:** 65. **Desc:** Psychologists interested in the branch of experimental psychology that centers on multivariate designs and associated special forms of analysis. Promotes substantive research and scientific discovery to develop mathematical/statistical models leading to their evaluation and integration into the development of psychological theory. **Pub:** *Multivariate Behavioral Research*, quarterly.

★ 5928 ★ Society for Multivariate Experimental Psychology

The Mere
Upton Park, United Kingdom

★ 5929 ★ Society for Muscular Dystrophy Information International (SMDI)

PO Box 479
Bridgewater, NS, Canada B4V 2X6
Phone: (902)685-3961 **Fax:** (902)685-3962
Email: smdi_intl@tallships.ca
Website: http://www.auracom.com/~smdi/index.html

Fnded: 1983. **Desc:** Dedicated to providing support and non-technical information for those concerned with muscular dystrophy or the allied disorders/disabilities, also referred to as neuromuscular disorders (NMDs). **Pub:** *Access-Able Information*, semiannual. Newsletter. Disability resource publication. • *SMDI International Newsletter*, semiannual. Newsletter. Features helpful information and topics regarding the disorders and disabilities, including organizations for these disorders located worldwide.

★ 5930 ★ Society for Neonatology and Paediatric Intensive Care (Gesellschaft fur Neonatologie und Padiatrische Intensivmedizin — GNPI)

Zentrum for Kinderheilkunde und Jugendmedizin
Justus-Liebig-Universitat
Feulgenstr. 12
D-35392 Giessen, Germany
Phone: 49 641 9943410 **Fax:** 49 641 9943419
Email: ludwig.gortner@paediat.med.uni-giessen.de
Website: http://www.gnpi.de

★ 5931 ★ Society of Neurological Surgeons (SNS)

200 1st St. SW
Rochester, MN 55905
Phone: (507)284-2254 **Fax:** (507)284-5206
Email: ras5@mailhub.cc.colmbia.edu
Website: http://www.societyns.org
David Piepgras, MD, Sec.

Fnded: 1920. **Mem:** 344. **Desc:** Neurological surgeons interested in and contributing to education.

★ 5932 ★ Society of Neurosurgical Anesthesia and Critical Care (SNACC)

PO Box 11086
Richmond, VA 23230-1086
Phone: (804)673-9037 **Fax:** (804)282-0090
Email: snacc@societyhq.com
Website: http://www.snacc.org/
Tod B. Sloan, MD, Pres.

Fnded: 1973. **Mem:** 500. **Desc:** Neurosurgeons and anesthesiologists interested in the care of patients with neurological disorders. Sponsors continuing medical education and research concerning the care of neurosurgical patients. **Pub:** *Annual Summary of Society Meeting Proceedings*, annual. Proceedings. • *Society Membership*, annual. • Newsletter, 3-4/year.

★ 5933 ★ Society of Nuclear Medicine (SNM)

1850 Samuel Morse Dr.
Reston, VA 20190-5316
Phone: (703)708-9000 **Fax:** (703)708-9020
Email: vpappas@snm.org
Website: http://www.snm.org
Virginia M. Pappas, Exec. Dir.

Fnded: 1954. **Mem:** 14,000. **Reg. Groups:** 15. **Desc:** Professional society of physicians, physicists, chemists, radiopharmacists, nuclear medicine technologists, and others interested in nuclear medicine, nuclear magnetic resonance, and the use of radioactive isotopes in clinical practice, research, and teaching. Disseminates information concerning the utilization of nuclear phenomena in the diagnosis and treatment of disease. Oversees the Technologist Section of the Society of Nuclear Medicine. **Pub:** *The Journal of Nuclear Medicine*, monthly. Journal. Includes advertisers' index, case reports, technical notes, book reviews, calendar of events and information on new products. *Price:* Included in membership dues; $120/year for nonmembers; $130/year for nonmembers in Canada and Mexico; $160/year for nonmembers outside North America. • *Journal of Nuclear Medicine Technology*, quarterly. Journal. Includes teaching editorials, commentaries, continuing education, and technologist news. Contains advertisers' index and calendar of events. *Price:* Included in membership dues; $70/year for nonmembers; $75/year for nonmembers in Canada and Mexico; $80/year for nonmembers outside North America. • *Society of Nuclear Medicine Membership Directory*, semiannual. Directory. Arranged geographically and alphabetically. *Price:* Included in membership dues; $100/issue for nonmembers. • Also publishes other books and patient pamphlets; produces audiovisual materials.

★ 5934 ★ Society of Nuclear Medicine Technologist Section

1850 Samuel Morse Dr.
Reston, VA 20190
Phone: (703)708-9000 **Fax:** (703)708-9015
Email: vpappas@snm.org
Website: http://www.snm.org/about/new_tech_1.html
Virginia Pappas, Exec. Dir.

Fnded: 1970. **Mem:** 7,000. **Reg. Groups:** 15. **Desc:** Members of the Society of Nuclear Medicine who have received formal training in nuclear medicine technology. Purposes are to: promote the continued development and improvement of nuclear medicine technology; enhance the development of nuclear medicine technologists; stimulate continuing education; develop a forum for the exchange of ideas and information. Serves as the central source of information for those interested and involved in the field of nuclear medicine technology. Represents the field in areas of licensure, accreditation, and certification. Sponsors training sessions. Conducts surveys; compiles statistics. **Pub:** *Journal of Nuclear Medicine Technology*, quarterly. Journal. *Price:* Included in membership dues. • Books. • Membership Directory, biennial. • Videos. **Frmly:** (2003) Technologist Section of the Society of Nuclear Medicine.

★ 5935 ★ Society of Nursery Nursing (SNN)

40 Archdale Rd.
East Dulwich
London SE22 9HJ, United Kingdom
Phone: 44 208 6930555 **Fax:** 44 208 6930555
Email: snn@totalise.co.uk

Fnded: 1991. **Mem:** 1,500. **Reg. Groups:** 5. **Local Groups:** 3. **Lang(s):** English. **Desc:** Nursing managers, nursing administrators and nurses, nursery teachers, school nurses, nannies, and other workers and employers with an interest in the education, health and welfare of children from birth to five years of age. Seeks to establish professional standards and a uniform code of ethics within the field; works to enhance the professional standing of members. Gathers and disseminates information to inform legislative debate concerning child health issues. Conducts examinations and educational programs and maintains speakers' bureau. **Pub:** *Nursery Nursing Administrator*, quarterly. Newsletter. **Frmly:** (2000) Society of Nursery Nursing Administrators.

★ 5936 ★ Society for Nutrition Education (SNE)

9202 N Meridian, Ste. 200
Indianapolis, IN 46260
Phone: (317)571-5618 **Fax:** (317)571-5603
Email: info@sne.org
Website: http://www.sne.org
Mary Ann Passi, CAE, Exec. Dir.

Fnded: 1967. **Mem:** 1,200. **Reg. Groups:** 15. **Desc:** Nutrition educators from the fields of dietetics, public health, home economics, medicine, industry, and education (elementary, secondary, college, university, and consumer affairs). Vision of SNE is healthy people in healthy communities. **Pub:** *Journal of Nutrition Education*, bimonthly. Journal. For educators, practitioners, and researchers on nutrition education. Includes book reviews and employment opportunity listings. *Price:* Included in membership dues; $119/year for individuals; $170/year for institutions; $60/year for individuals in training. • Also publishes journal supplements.

★ 5937 ★ Society for Obstetric Anesthesia and Perinatology (SOAP)

1910 Byrd Ave., Ste. 100
PO Box 11086
Richmond, VA 23230-1086
Phone: (804)282-5051 **Fax:** (804)282-0090
Email: soap@societyhq.com
Website: http://www.soap.org
Joy L. Hawkins, MD, Pres.

Fnded: 1969. **Mem:** 1,000. **Desc:** Physicians and scientists interested in perinatal health care. Purpose is to improve the health care of pregnant women and their unborn children. Conducts specialized education programs; compiles statistics. **Pub:** *Society for Obstetric Anesthesia and Perinatology Newsletter*, quarterly. Newsletter. *Price:* Included in membership dues.

★ 5938 ★ Society of Obstetricians and Gynaecologists of Canada

780 Echo Dr.
Ottawa, ON, Canada K1S 5R7
Phone: (613)730-4192 **Free:** 800-561-2416
Fax: (613)730-4314
Email: edore@sogc.com
Website: http://sogc.medical.org/corp/index_e.shtml

Fnded: 1944. **Lang(s):** English, French. **Desc:** Devoted to the medical specialty of obstetrics and gynaecology; promotes women's health through leadership, collaboration, education, research and advocacy.

★ 5939 ★ Society for Occlusal Studies (SOS)

c/o Dr. Bernard Williams
4601 W 109th St. Ste. 225
Overland Park, KS 66211-1314
Fax: (816)941-4832
Dr. Bernard Williams, Pres.

Fnded: 1964. **Mem:** 800. **Local Groups:** 95. **Desc:** Dentists and laboratory technicians who have completed the society's continuing education course in occlusion (bringing opposing surfaces of the teeth of the two jaws into contact). Promotes effective occlusal treatment. Conducts Principles of Occlusion Seminar,

Advanced Restorative Seminar, laboratory technician program, and practice management program. **Pub:** *Roster*, annual. • *SOS Newsletter*, quarterly. Newsletter. Covers developments in the treatment and diagnosis of temporomandibular joint dysfunction and principles of occlusion instrumentation. *Price:* Included in membership dues.

★ 5940 ★ Society for Occupational and Environmental Health (SOEH)
6728 Old McLean Village Dr.
Mc Lean, VA 22101
Phone: (703)556-9222 **Fax:** (703)556-8729
Email: soeh@degnon.org
Website: http://www.soeh.org
Ana Maria Osorio, MD, Pres.

Fnded: 1972. **Mem:** 350. **Desc:** Scientists, academicians, and industry and labor representatives. Seeks to improve the quality of both working and living places by operating as a neutral forum for conferences involving all aspects of occupational health. Focuses public attention on scientific, social, and regulatory problems; studies specific categories of hazards, methods for assessment of health effects, and diseases associated with particular jobs. Identifies hazards in the occupational and general environment and proposes actions to reduce their danger. **Pub:** *Archives of Environmental Health*. Journal. *Price:* Included in membership dues. • *Society for Occupational and Environmental Health–Bulletin*, quarterly. Newsletter. *Price:* Free, for members only.

★ 5941 ★ Society of Occupational Medicine
6 St. Andrew's Pl.
Regent's Park
London NW1 4LB, United Kingdom
Phone: 44 207 4862641 **Fax:** 44 207 4860028
Email: admin@som.org.uk
Website: http://www.som.org.uk/

Fnded: 1935. **Mem:** 2,000. **Desc:** Doctors working in occupational medicine. Many of the members have specialist qualifications in occupational medicine but others may be family practitioners connected with or holding part-time appointments in the specialty. Concerned with protecting the health of people at work and the prevention and management of occupational diseases and injuries. Seeks to interest and inform members through publications and scientific meetings, organised regionally and nationally. Stimulates research and education in occupational medicine and actively liaises with professional organisations relevant to occupational health. **Pub:** *Newsletter Periodical*, quarterly. Newsletter. • *Occupational Medicine Journal*, 8/year. Journal. • Papers.

★ 5942 ★ Society of Otorhinolaryngology and Head/Neck Nurses (SOHN)
116 Canal St., Ste. A
New Smyrna Beach, FL 32168
Phone: (904)428-1695 **Fax:** (904)423-7566
Email: info@sohnnurse.com
Website: http://www.sohnnurse.com/
Sandra L. Schwartz, R.N., Exec. Dir.

Fnded: 1976. **Mem:** 1,200. **Local Groups:** 15. **Desc:** Registered nurses specializing in otorhinolaryngology (the study of the ear, nose, and throat) and the head and neck. Seeks to: promote awareness of professional techniques and new developments in the field; enhance professional standards; create a channel for the exchange of ideas, concerns, and information; develop interaction with similar groups. Offers programs and seminars that have been approved for continuing education credits by the American Nurses' Association. **Pub:** *ORL-Head and Neck Nursing*, quarterly. Includes book reviews and current trends in nursing. *Price:* Included in membership dues; $30/year for nonmembers. • *Society of Otorhinolaryngology and Head-Neck Nurses–Update*, quarterly. Newsletter. Includes employment opportunity listings. *Price:* Included in membership dues.

★ 5943 ★ Society for Pediatric Anesthesia
1910 Byrd Ave., Ste. 100
PO Box 11086
Richmond, VA 23230-1086
Phone: (804)282-9780 **Fax:** (804)282-0090
Email: spa@societyhq.com
Website: http://WWW.pedsanesthesia.org
Steven C. Hall, Pres.

Desc: Working to foster quality anesthesia and perioperative care, and to alleviate pain in children

★ 5944 ★ Society for Pediatric Dermatology (SPD)
c/o Pat Fraser, Admin.
5422 N Bernard
Chicago, IL 60625
Phone: (773)583-9780 **Fax:** (773)583-9765
Email: patrici107@aol.com
Website: http://www.pedsderm.net
Pat Fraser, Admin.

Fnded: 1975. **Mem:** 500. **Desc:** Pediatricians, dermatologists, pediatric or dermatologic house officers, manufacturers of children's skin products, and researchers in biomedicine with studies in pediatric dermatology. Conducts research programs. **Pub:** *Society for Pediatric Dermatology–Newsletter*, quarterly. Newsletter. Reviews current publications in the field of pediatric dermatology; includes reviews in the areas of allergy and immunology, genetics and syndromes. *Price:* Included in membership dues.

★ 5945 ★ Society of Pediatric Nurses (SPN)
7794 Grow Dr.
Pensacola, FL 32514
Phone: (850)494-9467 **Free:** 800-723-2902
Fax: (850)484-8762
Email: spn@puetzamc.com
Website: http://www.pedsnurses.org
Belinda E. Puetz, PhD RN, Contact

Fnded: 1990. **Mem:** 1,550. **Nat'l Groups:** 30. **Desc:** Registered pediatric nurses are regular members; nursing students and other professionals with an interest in pediatric nursing are associate members. Promotes quality health and nursing care of children. Conducts advocacy campaigns to improve access to affordable care for children; works to advance techniques of pediatric nursing and health care. Sponsors research and educational programs for members; formulates standards of practice and ethics; fosters collaboration between members and other health care professionals, child health care advocates, and related organizations. **Pub:** *Journal of Pediatric Nursing*, bimonthly. Journal. • *SPN News*, bimonthly. Newsletter.

★ 5946 ★ Society for Pediatric Pathology
c/o United States & Canadian Academy of Pathology
3643 Walton Way Extension
Augusta, GA 30909
Phone: (706)364-3375 **Fax:** (706)733-8033
Email: spp@uscap.org
Website: http://path.upmc.edu/spp/
Ronald Jaffe, Pres.

Mem: 520. **Desc:** Pediatric pathologists. Seeks to advance the science and practice of pediatric pathology. Facilities integration of scientific developments in the field; conducts continuing medical education programs. **Pub:** *Pediatric & Developmental Pathology*, bimonthly. Journal.

★ 5947 ★ Society for Pediatric Psychology (SPP)
PO Box 170231
Atlanta, GA 30317
Email: gaylward@swimed.edu
Website: http://www.apa.org/divisions/div54/
Anthony Spirito, PhD, Pres.

Fnded: 1968. **Mem:** 995. **Desc:** A section of the American Psychological Association. Psychologists working in children's hospitals, developmental clinics, and pediatric and medical group practices. Fosters the development of theory, research, training, and professional practice in pediatric psychology and the application of psychology to medical and psychological problems of children, youths, and their families. Supports legislation benefiting children's health and welfare. Sponsors colloquia and symposia; provides speakers. **Pub:** *Journal of Pediatric Psychology*, quarterly. Journal. Includes research reports, literature and book reviews, case studies, graphs, tables, charts, and society meeting minutes. *Price:* Included in membership dues; $50 for nonmembers. • *Progress Notes, Newsletter of the Society for Pediatric Psychology*, 3/year. Newsletter. Contains research articles on pediatric psychology. Includes abstracts of published literature, society news, and lists of employment opportunities. *Price:* Included in membership dues.

★ 5948 ★ Society for Pediatric Radiology (SPR)
4550 Post Oak Pl., Ste. 342
Houston, TX 77027
Phone: (713)965-0566 **Fax:** (713)960-0488
Email: spr@meetingmanagers.com
Website: http://www.pedrad.org
Jennifer K. Boylan, Exec. Dir.

Fnded: 1958. **Mem:** 800. **Desc:** Physicians working in the field of pediatric radiology. Seeks to advance knowledge in pediatric imaging and improve medical care of infants and children. **Pub:** Membership Directory, annual.

★ 5949 ★ Society for Pediatric Research (SPR)
3400 Research Forest Dr., Ste. B7
The Woodlands, TX 77381
Phone: (281)419-0052 **Fax:** (281)419-0082
Email: info@aps-spr.org
Website: http://www.aps-spr.org
Debbie Anagnostelis, Exec. Dir.

Fnded: 1929. **Mem:** 2,500. **Desc:** Physicians and scientists under age 50 who are engaged in research in diseases of infancy and childhood; those over age 50 are senior members. **Pub:** *Pediatric Research*, monthly. Journal. Includes calendar of events, and abstracts. *Price:* $110/year.

★ 5950 ★ Society for Pediatric Urology (SPU)
Section of Urology, MC 4056
University of Chicago
5844 S Maryland Ave.
Chicago, IL 60637
Phone: (773)702-6150 **Fax:** (773)702-8702
Stephen Koff, Pres.

Fnded: 1941. **Mem:** 300. **Local Groups:** 45. **Desc:** Medical doctors who are specialists in urology (relating to the genito-urinary tract in health and disease) and who have a special interest in the field of childhood urological problems. Seeks to encourage the study, improve the practice, elevate the standards, and further the advancement of pediatric urology. Conducts educational programs. **Pub:** *Dialogues in Pediatric Urology*, monthly. Magazine. *Price:* $32. • *Pedictric Urology*, monthly. Newsletter. *Price:* Included in membership dues. • Audiotapes. • Books. • Pamphlets. • Videos.

★ 5951 ★ Society for Personality Assessment (SPA)
6109 H Arlington Blvd.
Falls Church, VA 22044
Phone: (703)534-4772 **Fax:** (703)534-6905
Email: officeSPA@aol.com
Website: http://www.personality.org
Dr. Stephen Finn, Pres.

Fnded: 1938. **Mem:** 3,000. **Desc:** Psychologists, behavioral scientists, anthropologists, and psychiatrists. Promotes the study, research, development, and application of personality assessment. **Pub:** *Journal of Personality Assessment*, 6/year. Journal. Includes book reviews, case reports, and annual directory. *Price:* Included in membership dues; $70/year for nonmembers; $270/year for institutions. • *SPA Exchange*, semiannual. Newsletter. **Frmly:** (1938) Rorschach Research Exchange; (1958) Society for Projective Techniques and Rorschach Institute; (1970) Society for Projective Techniques and Personality Assessment.

★ 5952 ★ Society for Personality and Social Psychology (SPSP)

c/o Gina Reisinger
University of Rochester
Department of Psychology
Rochester, NY 14627
Phone: (716)275-8724
Email: spsp@scp.rochester.edu
Website: http://www.spsp.org/
Claude Steele, Pres.

Fnded: 1974. **Mem:** 3,000. **Desc:** Social and personality psychologists. Conducts and disseminates research on social and personality psychology. Sponsors SPSP Diversity Programs. **Pub:** *Personality and Social Psychology Review*, quarterly. Journal. Contains original theoretical papers and conceptual review articles in personality and social psychology. *Price:* $126; included in membership dues; $50 for individuals; $170 for institutions. • *Personalty and Social Psychology Bulletin*, monthly. Journal. Contains original empirical papers in all areas of personality and social psychology. *Price:* $575 for regular institution; $50 for single issues, regular institution; $102; $11 for single issues.

★ 5953 ★ Society for Physician Assistants in Pediatrics (SPAP)

950 N Washington St.
Alexandria, VA 22314-1552
Free: 800-596-4398 **Fax:** (703)684-1924
Email: jrv1007@aol.com
Website: http://www.geocities.com/spap_peds1
Tom Moreno, Membership Coor.

Fnded: 1994. **Mem:** 250. **Desc:** Designed to gather and disseminate information affecting the practice of pediatric physician assistants, collect demographic data to share within the profession or with other organizations, assist in developing guidelines for physician assistant utilization in clinical settings, and to enhance the relationship with the American Academy of Pediatrics. **Pub:** *Physician Assistants in Pediatrics*, quarterly. Newsletter. *Price:* included in membership dues.

★ 5954 ★ Society of Physiologists, Biochemists and Pharmacologists

Department of Biochemistry, University
Pretoria 0002, Republic of South Africa

★ 5955 ★ Society for Police and Criminal Psychology

c/o A. Steven Dietz
City of Austin
8409 Ganttcrest Dr.
Austin, TX 78749
Phone: (512)530-8211
Email: steven.dietz@ci.austin.tx.us
Website: http://cep.jmu.edu/spcp/
A. Steven Dietz, Pres.

Desc: Promotes the scientific study of the criminal justice system, focusing on law enforcement, the judicial, and the corrections elements in criminal justice. Research includes the full range of human behaviors, motivations, and actions within the criminal justice system, along with causation of crime, victimization, and organizational influences. **Pub:** *Journal of Police and Criminal Psychology*, semiannual, spring and fall. Journal. Contains information on issues relevant to practitioners and academicians in the field of criminal justice. *Price:* included in membership dues.

★ 5956 ★ Society of Practising Veterinary Surgeons

2 The Old Gunroom
Blagdon Estate
Seaton Burn
Newcastle upon Tyne NE13 6DB, United Kingdom
Phone: 44 1670 789054 **Fax:** 44 1670 789359
Email: office@spvs.rog.uk
Website: http://www.spvs.org.uk

Desc: Represents the interests of veterinary surgeons.

★ 5957 ★ Society for Prevention of Infertility (SPI)

877 Park Ave.
New York, NY 10021
Phone: (212)288-3737 **Free:** 888-373-2229
Fax: (212)744-6536
Email: frfbaby@msn.com
Website: http://www.frfbaby.com
Masood A. Khatamee, Exec. Dir.

Fnded: 1990. **Mem:** 500. **Reg. Groups:** 100. **Desc:** Physicians specializing in obstetrics and gynecology; scientists representing public and private teaching hospitals, medical school faculties, and university research departments; practitioners who work with infertile men and women. Objectives are to: study sexually transmitted infectious diseases (STDs) and their effects on human fertility; reduce the incidence of infection and the possibility of resulting infertility. Coordinates and encourages research that can lead to successful forms of treatment and control of STDs, thus enhancing the opportunities for childless couples to achieve intrauterine pregnancies and bear healthy children. Encourages the exchange of information among those involved in research on and treatment of STDs. Designs educational and informational strategies intended for the prevention of infertility. **Frmly:** (1991) International Society of Infectious Diseases and Human Infertility.

★ 5958 ★ Society for Prevention Research (SPR)

1300 I St. NW, Ste. 250 West
Washington, DC 20005
Phone: (202)216-9670 **Fax:** (202)216-9671
Email: info@preventionresearch.org
Website: http://www.preventionresearch.org
Jennifer Lewis, Admin. Dir.

Fnded: 1992. **Mem:** 500. **Desc:** Scientists, practitioners, advocates, administrators, and policy makers concerned with the prevention of social, physical and mental health problems and the promotion of health, safety and well-being. Promotes the advancement of science-based prevention programs and policies through empirical research. Facilitates communication and cooperation among prevention interventionists working in fields that include etiology, epidemiology, and the social sciences. **Pub:** *Prevention Science*, quarterly. Journal.

★ 5959 ★ Society of Professors of Child and Adolescent Psychiatry (SPCAP)

3615 Wisconsin Ave. NW
Washington, DC 20016-3007
Phone: (202)966-7300 **Fax:** (202)966-2891
Email: mgomez@aacap.org
Matthew Gomez, Admin. Mgr.

Fnded: 1969. **Mem:** 150. **Desc:** Division directors from university psychiatric departments who meet annually to discuss issues in child and adolescent psychiatry. **Pub:** *SPCAP Membership Directory*, annual. Directory. **Frmly:** (1987) Society of Professors of Child Psychiatry.

★ 5960 ★ Society for Progressive Supranuclear Palsy (SPSP)

1838 Greene Tree Rd., Ste. 515
Baltimore, MD 21208
Phone: (410)486-3330 **Free:** 800-457-4777
Fax: (410)486-4283
Email: spsp@psp.org
Website: http://www.psp.org
Jackie J. Allison, Asst. Dir.

Fnded: 1990. **Nat'l Groups:** 1. **State Groups:** 60. **Desc:** Works to provide help and support to persons with progressive supranuclear palsy (PSP), a degenerative brain disorder. Sponsors medical research; educates physicians, persons with PSP and their families on the disease and care; provides advocacy and support, support groups, symposiums and videos. **Pub:** *The PSP Advocate*, quarterly. Newsletter.

★ 5961 ★ Society for the Psychological Study of Lesbian, Gay and Bisexual Issues (SPSLGBI)

c/o American Psychological Association
750 First St. NE
Washington, DC 20002
Phone: (202)336-6041 **Free:** 800-374-2721
Fax: (202)336-6040
Email: mdelong@apa.org
Website: http://www.apa.org/divisions/div44
James Fitzgerald, PhD, Pres.

Fnded: 1984. **Mem:** 1,600. **Nat'l Groups:** 1. **Desc:** Psychologists, graduate students in psychology, and others interested in the psychological study of lesbian, gay, and bisexual issues and the delivery of affirmative mental health services to gay, lesbian, and bisexual individuals. Promotes scholarship in the study of psychology as it relates to bisexual, gay, and lesbian issues; provides training for psychologists in the field. Cooperates with other groups sharing similar goals, including other divisions of the American Psychological Association. Conducts scholarly programs. **Pub:** *Division 44 Newsletter*, 3/year. Newsletter. • *Psychological Book Series on Lesbian and Gay Issues*, annual. *Price:* Included in membership dues. **Frmly:** (1998) Society for the Psychological Study of Lesbian and Gay Issues.

★ 5962 ★ Society for the Psychological Study of Social Issues (SPSSI)

208 I St. NE
Washington, DC 20002
Phone: (202)223-5100 **Fax:** (202)223-5555
Email: spssi@spssi.org
Website: http://www.spssi.org
Shari Miles, PhD, Exec. Dir.

Fnded: 1936. **Mem:** 2,600. **Desc:** Psychologists, sociologists, anthropologists, psychiatrists, political scientists, and social workers. Works to: obtain and disseminate to the public scientific knowledge about social change and other social processes; promote psychological research on significant theoretical and practical questions of social issues; encourage application of findings to problems of society. **Pub:** *Analyses of Social Issues & Public Policy (ASAP)*, quarterly. Journal. *Price:* included in membership dues; $55 for nonmembers. • *Journal of Social Issues (JSI)*, quarterly. Journal. *Price:* included in membership dues; $55 for nonmembers. • *Social Psychological Applications to Social Issues*, 3/year. Books. • *SPSSI Newsletter*, 3/year. Newsletter.

★ 5963 ★ Society for Psychophysiological Research (SPR)

1010 Vermont Ave., Ste. 1100
Washington, DC 20005
Phone: (202)393-4810 **Fax:** (202)783-2083
Email: spr@aps.washington.dc.us
Website: http://www.wlu.edu/~spr

Fnded: 1960. **Mem:** 906. **Desc:** Research group comprising representatives from psychology, psychiatry, physiology, medicine, and biomedical engineering concerned with the interrelationship between behavioral and biological processes. Conducts research including the evaluation of biofeedback in the treatment of disease states. Maintains historical archives. Conducts workshops. **Pub:** *Psychophysiology*, bimonthly.

★ 5964 ★ Society of Psychosomatic Obstetrics and Gynaecology, Brazil
c/o Dr. Alexandre Faisal Cury, Pres.
Faculdade Ciencias Medicas da Santa Casa SP
Rua Conego Eugenio Leite, 253
Jd. Paulistano
05414-010 Sao Paulo, SP, Brazil
Phone: 55 11 30313743 **Fax:** 55 11 36838196
Email: faisal@hcnet.usp.br
Website: http://www.ispog.org
Desc: Promotes the study of psychobiological and psychosocial, ethical and cross-cultural problems in the fields of obstetrics and gynaecology, women's health and reproductive health; facilitates the dissemination of new information in these fields. **Pub:** *Journal of Psychosomatic Obstetrics and Gynecology*. Journal.

★ 5965 ★ Society for Psychosomatic Research
Horseferry Rd.
London SW1P 2AP, United Kingdom
Fnded: 1955.

★ 5966 ★ Society for Psychotherapy Research (SPR)
308 Moore Bldg.
University Park, PA 16802
Phone: (814)863-1754 **Fax:** (814)863-7002
Email: naspr@psu.edu
Website: http://www.psychotherapyresearch.org/
Louis G. Castonguay, PhD, Pres., N. Amer. Chap.
Mem: 1,000. **Reg. Groups:** 4. **Desc:** Committed to the scientific study of psychotherapy. **Pub:** Newsletter.

★ 5967 ★ Society for Public Health Education (SOPHE)
750 First St. NE, Ste. 910
Washington, DC 20002-4242
Phone: (202)408-9804 **Fax:** (202)408-9815
Email: info@sophe.org
Website: http://www.sophe.org
Elaine Auld, Exec. Dir.
Fnded: 1950. **Mem:** 2,200. **Local Groups:** 23. **Desc:** Researchers and practitioners in health education/health promotion concerned with individual and population health problems. Seeks to promote, encourage, and contribute to the advancement of health of all people by encouraging research, improving health practices, elevating standards of achievement in public health education, and advocating for public health policies. **Pub:** *Health Education & Behavior*, bimonthly. Journal. Research and practice in social/behavioral sciences and health education. *Price:* Included in membership. • *Health Promotion Practice*, quarterly. Journal. Contains information on health promotion/health education policy, applications, practice. *Price:* included in membership dues. • *News and Views*, bimonthly. Newsletter. • *SOPHE Membership Directory & Buyer's Guide*. Membership Directory. **Frmly:** Society of Public Health Educators.

★ 5968 ★ Society for Radiation Oncology Administrators (SROA)
PO Box 51687
Albuquerque, NM 87181-1687
Free: (866)458-7762 **Fax:** (505)298-5063
Email: sroa@asrt.org
Website: http://www.sroa.org/
Robyn Blatter, Sec.
Fnded: 1984. **Mem:** 500. **Desc:** Individuals with managerial responsibilities in radiation oncology at the executive, divisional, or departmental level, and whose functions include personnel, budget, and development of operational procedures and guidelines for therapeutic radiology departments. Strives to improve the administration of the business and nonmedical management aspects of therapeutic radiology, to promote the field of therapeutic radiology administration, to provide a forum for communication among members, and to disseminate information among members. Maintains speakers' bureau; offers placement service. **Pub:** *SROA Membership Directory*, annual. Membership Directory. *Price:* Included in membership dues. • *SROA Newsletter*, quarterly. Newsletter. Includes calendar of events and employment listings. *Price:* Included in membership dues; $50 for non-members in U.S.; $60 for non-members outside U.S. **Frmly:** (1985) Radiation Oncology Administrators.

★ 5969 ★ Society of Radiographers of South Africa (SORSA) (Vereniging van Radiograwe van Suid-Afrika — VRSA)
PO Box 6014
Cape Town 8012, Republic of South Africa
Phone: 27 21 4194857 **Fax:** 27 21 212566
Email: smltsa@iafrica.com
Fnded: 1951. **Mem:** 1,500. **Lang(s):** English. **Desc:** Radiographers in South Africa. Strives for the establishment and maintenance of professional standards in the training and practice of radiography. Cooperates with governmental bodies in order to improve working conditions, salaries, and benefits. Represents members' interests nationally and internationally. Communicates with relevant authorities on educational and employment matters. Maintains liaisons with similar national and international organizations. Sponsors seminars and workshops. **Pub:** *The South African Radiographer*, 3/year. Journal. • Newsletter, quarterly.

★ 5970 ★ Society of Radiologists in Ultrasound (SRU)
44211 Slatestone Ct.
Leesburg, VA 20176-5109
Phone: (703)858-9210 **Fax:** (703)729-4839
Email: info@sru.org
Website: http://www.sru.org
Carol B. Benson, MD, Pres.
Fnded: 1975. **Desc:** Board certified and Board eligible radiologists interested in ultrasound imaging. Promotes the interests of radiologists in ultrasound. Funds research; educates non-physician health care professionals. **Pub:** *Managing Ultrasound Benefits*. Newsletter. Contains the latest ultrasound techniques and examinations. • Newsletter, 3/year.

★ 5971 ★ Society of Remedial Gymnasts and Recreational Therapies (SRG)
Cardiff University Hospital of Wales
Cardiff, United Kingdom
Fnded: 1946.

★ 5972 ★ Society for Reproductive Endocrinology and Infertility
c/o American Society for Reproductive Medicine
1209 Montgomery Hwy.
Birmingham, AL 35216-2809
Phone: (205)978-5000 **Fax:** (205)978-5005
Email: apitman@asrm.org
Website: http://www.socrei.org
Angelia Pitman, Admin.
Fnded: 1984. **Mem:** 810. **Desc:** Medical doctors with American Board of Obstetrics and Gynecology subspecialty certification as reproductive endocrinologists. Works to extend knowledge of human reproduction and endocrinology; makes available to members continuing education programs. Conducts seminars. **Pub:** *SREI Feedback*, quarterly. Newsletter. Includes Information for members on SREI activities. *Price:* included in membership dues.

★ 5973 ★ Society of Reproductive Surgeons (SRS)
1209 Montgomery Hwy.
Birmingham, AL 35216-2809
Phone: (205)978-5000 **Fax:** (205)978-5005
Email: cfinch@asrm.org
Website: http://www.reprodsurgery.org
Fnded: 1984. **Mem:** 450. **Desc:** Reproductive surgeons. Gathers and disseminates information on reproductive surgery; conducts continuing education programs for members. Makes available referrals list. **Pub:** *SRS Newsletter*, semiannual. Newsletter.

★ 5974 ★ Society for Research into Hydrocephalus and Spina Bifida (SRHSB)
c/o Dr. Terry Cubitt
Alton Health Centre
Alton GU34 2QX, United Kingdom
Phone: 44 1420 542542 **Fax:** 44 1420 549466
Email: srhsb@doctors.org.uk
Website: http://www.srhsb.org
Fnded: 1957. **Mem:** 284. **Lang(s):** English. **Desc:** Nursing, psychology, social work, scientific, and medical professionals from 29 countries with a common interest in hydrocephalus (an abnormal accumulation of fluid in the cranium) and spina bifida (a defect in the closing of the bony spinal canal). Object is to advance education and research on hydrocephalus and spina bifida. Brings together members to aid them in their endeavors to prevent, cure, and alleviate the conditions. **Pub:** *European Journal of Pediatric Surgery*, annual. Journal.

★ 5975 ★ Society of Rural Physicians of Canada (SRPC)
RR 5
Shawville, QC, Canada J0X 2Y0
Phone: (819)647-3971 **Free:** 877-276-1949
Fax: (819)647-3971
Email: admin@srpc.ca
Website: http://www.srpc.ca
Fnded: 1992. **Mem:** 1,200. **Reg. Groups:** 5. **Lang(s):** English, French. **Desc:** Physicians practicing in rural areas of Canada. Promotes delivery of health care services to individuals in remote areas nationwide. Seeks to ensure suitable working conditions for members. Sponsors annual continuing professional development course. Develops model policies for regulation and delivery of health care in rural areas; encourages medical research; provides support and services to members and to communities seeking to improve their health care resources; plans to establish a library. Offers free membership to students, residents, and honourary members. **Pub:** *Canadian Journal of Rural Medicine*, periodic. Newsletter.

★ 5976 ★ Society for a Science of Clinical Psychology
c/o Raymond P. Lorion
University of Pennsylvania
Graduate School of Education
Psychology in Education Division
3700 Walnut St.
Philadelphia, PA 19104-6216
Phone: (215)898-7367 **Fax:** (215)573-2115
Email: lorion@gse.upenn.edu
Website: http://pantheon.yale.edu/~tat22/
Thomas D. Borkovec, PhD, Pres.
Fnded: 1966. **Desc:** Promotes the integration of the scientist and the practitioner in training, research and applied undertakings in the field of clinical psychology.

★ 5977 ★ Society for the Scientific Study of Sexuality (SSSS)
c/o David L. Fleming
PO Box 416
Allentown, PA 18105
Phone: (610)530-2483 **Fax:** (610)530-2485
Email: thesociety@inetmail.att.net
Website: http://www.sexscience.org
David L. Fleming, Exec. Dir.
Fnded: 1957. **Mem:** 1,200. **Reg. Groups:** 3. **State Groups:** 4. **Desc:** Dedicated to advancing knowledge of sexuality. Support for research, and an interdisciplinary network of collaborating scholars. **Pub:** *Annual Review of Sex Research*, annual. Contains review articles on selected topics in the field of sexology. *Price:* $83/volume, agency; $56/volume, individual. • *Journal of Sex Research*, quarterly. Journal. Contains book reviews and case studies. *Price:* Included in

membership dues; $110/year for nonmembers; $160/year for libraries. • *Society for the Scientific Study of Sex–Membership Handbook/Directory.* Membership Directory. *Price:* available to members only. • *Society for the Scientific Study of Sex–Newsletter*, quarterly. Newsletter. Includes calendar of events. *Price:* Included in membership dues; $20/year for nonmembers. • Also publishes research and clinical material. **Frmly:** (1998) Society for the Scientific Study of Sex.

★ 5978 ★ Society for Sex Therapy and Research (SSTAR)
409 12th St. SW
PO Box 96920
Washington, DC 20090
Phone: (202)863-1645
Email: mbrooks@acog.org
Website: http://www.sstarnet.org/
Michelle Brooks-Hunter, Adminstrator

Fnded: 1974. **Mem:** 200. **Desc:** Professionals in social work, nursing, physiology, gynecology, urology, internal medicine, primate research, psychiatry, and psychology who have clinical or research interests in human sexual concerns. Seeks to facilitate communications among clinicians who treat problems of sexual identity, sexual function, and reproductive life. Provides a forum for exchange of ideas between researchers and patient care providers. **Pub:** Membership Directory, biennial. • Newsletter, 3-4/year. **Frmly:** (1979) Eastern Academy of Sexual Therapy.

★ 5979 ★ Society of Skeletal Radiology (SSR)
820 Jorie Blvd.
Oak Brook, IL 60523
Phone: (630)590-7714 **Fax:** (630)571-7837
Email: ssr@rsna.org
Website: http://www.skeletalrad.org
Dr. Arthur A. De Smet, MD, Pres.

Fnded: 1978. **Mem:** 270. **Desc:** Practicing radiologists. Represents the subspecialty of musculoskeletal radiology.

★ 5980 ★ Society for Social Medicine
c/o Ms. Angela Rowe
Population Health Group
School of Medicine, Health, Policy & Practice
University of East Angela
Norwich NR4 7TJ, United Kingdom
Phone: 44 20 76791732 **Fax:** 44 20 78130280
Email: a.rowe@uea.ac.uk
Website: http://www.socsocmed.org.uk/

Fnded: 1957.

★ 5981 ★ Society of Sports Therapists
c/o Graham N. Smith
45c Carrick St.
Glasgow G2 8PJ, United Kingdom
Phone: 44 141 2213660 **Fax:** 44 141 2211525
Email: admin@society-of-sports-therapists.org
Website: http://www.society-of-sports-therapists.org

Fnded: 1990. **Mem:** 1,500. **Desc:** Open to anyone over the age of 18 years who has successfully completed a course in sports therapy and satisfies the criteria for membership of the Society. Aims to provide a professional body for sports therapists which will educate, monitor and legislate on all matters pertaining to sports therapy.

★ 5982 ★ Society for the Study of Addiction to Alcohol and Other Drugs (SSA)
c/o Alex Schardy, Membership Admin.
4 Windsor Walk
London SE5 8AF, United Kingdom
Phone: 44 20 78480841 **Fax:** 44 20 77035787
Email: membership@addiction-ssa.org
Website: http://www.addiction-ssa.org

Fnded: 1884. **Mem:** 410. **Reg. Groups:** 1. **Lang(s):** English. **Desc:** Medical and allied health professionals seeking to stimulate scientific study of alcohol and drug addiction. Conducts research and educational programs. **Pub:** *Addiction*, monthly. Journal. • Monographs.

★ 5983 ★ Society for the Study of Inborn Errors of Metabolism (SSIEM)
c/o Department of Child Health
University Hospital of Wales
Heath Park
Cardiff
South Glamorgan S1O 2TH, United Kingdom
Phone: 44 29 2074 6322 **Fax:** 44 29 2074 6322
Email: graham.shortland@uhw-tr.wales.nhs.uk
Website: http://www.ssiem.org.uk

Fnded: 1962. **Mem:** 1,000. **Lang(s):** English. **Desc:** Biochemists, dietitians, pediatricians, pathologists, geneticists, and interested individuals in 41 countries. Purpose is to foster study of inherited metabolic disease diagnosis and treatment. Promotes exchange of ideas through meetings and publications. **Pub:** *Journal of Inherited Metabolic Diseases*, quarterly. Journal. • *Membership Handbook*, periodic. • Pamphlets. • Proceedings.

★ 5984 ★ Society for the Study of Normal Psychology
151 Talgarth Rd.
London W14, United Kingdom
Phone: 44 20 87489338 **Fax:** 44 20 85630551
Email: colethouse@clara.net
Website: http://www.studysociety.net

Mem: 270. **Nat'l Groups:** 8. **Reg. Groups:** 10. **Local Groups:** 3. **Pub:** *Contact*, 3/year. Newsletter. • Books.

★ 5985 ★ Society for the Study of Reproduction (SSR)
1619 Monroe St.
Madison, WI 53711-2063
Phone: (608)256-2777 **Fax:** (608)256-4610
Email: ssr@ssr.org
Website: http://www.ssr.org
P. Landis Keyes, Pres.

Fnded: 1967. **Mem:** 2,780. **Desc:** Researchers in obstetrics and gynecology, urology, zoology, animal husbandry, and physiology; clinicians in human and veterinary medicine. Purposes are to promote the study of reproduction by fostering interdisciplinary communication within the science. **Pub:** *Biology of Reproduction*, monthly, plus one supplement per year. Journal. Includes peer-reviewed scientific research in the field of reproductive biology. *Price:* $525 U.S.; $575 non U.S. • *Biology of Reproduction Monograph Series 1: Equine Reproduction VI.* Monograph.

★ 5986 ★ Society for Surgery of the Alimentary Tract (SSAT)
13 Elm St.
Manchester, MA 01944
Phone: (978)526-8330 **Fax:** (978)526-4018
Email: ssat@prri.com
Website: http://www.ssat.com
Robert P. Jones, Jr., Exec. Dir.

Fnded: 1960. **Mem:** 2,500. **Desc:** Licensed physicians with an interest in surgical aspects of digestive diseases. Seeks to advance the study, teaching, and practice of surgery of the alimentary tract; promotes continuing professional development of members. Serves as a forum for the discussion of new alimentary surgical techniques; encourages training opportunities and funding for alimentary surgical research. **Pub:** *Journal of Gastrointestinal Surgery*, bimonthly. Journal. • *Patient Care Guidelines.* Handbook.

★ 5987 ★ Society of Surgical Oncology (SSO)
c/o Rick Slawny
85 W Algonquin Rd., Ste. 550
Arlington Heights, IL 60005
Phone: (847)427-1400 **Fax:** (847)427-1294
Website: http://www.surgonc.org/
Rick Slawny, Exec. Dir.

Fnded: 1940. **Mem:** 1,700. **Desc:** Physicians and scientists working in the field of cancer. **Pub:** *Annals of Surgical Oncology*, 10/year. Journal. Includes proceedings of the society's annual scientific sessions. **Frmly:** (1974) James Ewing Society.

★ 5988 ★ Society of Teachers of the Alexander Technique (STAT)
Linton House, 1st Fl.
39-51 Highgate Rd.
London NW5 1RS, United Kingdom
Phone: 44 20 72843338 **Fax:** 44 20 74825434
Email: info@stat.org.uk
Website: http://www.stat.org.uk

Fnded: 1958. **Mem:** 1,864. **Nat'l Groups:** 1. **Lang(s):** English. **Desc:** Teachers (1130), students (242) and others (492) in 24 countries. Works to maintain professional standards and gain wider recognition of the Alexander Technique (a means of posture reeducation). Encourages research and communication among members. **Pub:** *Alexander Journal*, periodic. Journal. • *List of Teachers*, triennial. Directory. • *STATNEWS*, 3/year. Newsletter.

★ 5989 ★ Society of Teachers of Family Medicine (STFM)
11400 Tomahawk Creek Pkwy., Ste. 540
Leawood, KS 66211
Phone: (913)906-6000 **Free:** 800-274-2237
Fax: (913)906-6096
Email: admstaff@stfm.org
Website: http://www.stfm.org
Roger A. Sherwood, CAE, Exec. Dir.

Fnded: 1967. **Mem:** 5,000. **Desc:** Physicians involved in teaching or promoting family medicine; individuals in related fields. Organized to promote public welfare by maintaining and improving standards and practices of medical service, especially in the field of family medicine. Promotes these objectives by: supporting and expressing the tenets of family medicine as an academic discipline; maintaining and continually improving the quality of instructional and scientific skills and knowledge in the field of family medicine; providing a forum for the interchange of experience and ideas among its members and other interested persons; and encouraging research and teaching in family medicine. medicine. medicine. **Pub:** *Family Medicine*, monthly. Journal. Includes annual index, book reviews, and employment opportunities. *Price:* Included in membership dues; $12.50/copy for nonmembers; $88/year for individual nonmembers; $120/year for institutions. • *STFM Membership Directory*, annual. Membership Directory. • *STFM Messenger*, bimonthly. Newsletter. Covers general information related to family medicine issues. Includes research and education columns. *Price:* Included in membership dues. • Monographs.

★ 5990 ★ Society of Teachers of Speech and Drama
73 Berry Hill Rd.
Mansfield NG18 4RU, United Kingdom
Phone: 44 1623 627636
Email: ann.p.jones@btinternet.com
Website: http://www.stsd.org.uk

Fnded: 1908. **Mem:** 755. **Nat'l Groups:** 32. **Desc:** Members are involved in all branches of speech and drama work schools, colleges of further education and universities. They work in the professional and amateur theatre as producers, directors and coaches. Some are involved with the disabled whilst. others teach communication and presentation skills in the business world. The Society aims to uphold a high standard of teaching and support those working in the field. Each region has a representative who is responsible for promoting the work of the Society. A Conference is held in London in February and during August in another region. **Pub:** *Speech and Drama*, semiannual. Magazine. Contains articles on various subjects related to speech and drama. • Newsletter, 3/year, for members.

★ 5991 ★ Society for Theriogenology (ST)
PO Box 3007
Montgomery, AL 36109
Phone: (334)395-4666 **Fax:** (334)270-3399
Email: info@therio.org
Website: http://www.therio.org
Gary Althouse, Pres.

Fnded: 1954. **Mem:** 2,508. **Desc:** Veterinarians united to promote the practice of qualified veterinarians examining animals for breeding soundness; to facilitate these procedures by standardization of the criteria used by veterinarians; to assemble and evaluate the measurements of breeding soundness from literature and from unbiased records accumulated from all sources and distribute this information to all members. (Theriogenology is a branch of veterinary medicine that deals with reproduction, veterinary obstetrics, gynecology, and seminology.) Distributes morphology stain for use in making breeding soundness evaluations and standard forms for use in recording such evaluations. Maintains speakers' bureau. **Pub:** *Proceedings of Annual Meeting*, annual. *Price:* $50. • Newsletter, bimonthly. **Frmly:** (1975) American Veterinary Society for the Study of Breeding Soundness.

★ 5992 ★ Society of Thoracic and Cardiovascular Surgeons of Great Britain and Ireland
Walsgrave Hospital
Conventry CV2 2DX, United Kingdom
Phone: 44 24 76538936 **Fax:** 44 24 76538829

Fnded: 1933.

★ 5993 ★ Society of Thoracic Radiology (STR)
1711 Walden Ln. SW
Rochester, MN 55902
Phone: (507)288-5620 **Fax:** (507)288-0014
Email: str@thoracicrad.org
Website: http://www.thoracicrad.org
Robert D. Traver, Pres.

Fnded: 1983. **Mem:** 200. **Desc:** Radiologists. Provides for continuing medical education.

★ 5994 ★ Society of Thoracic Surgeons (STS)
633 N St. Clair St., No. 2320
Chicago, IL 60611
Phone: (312)202-5800 **Fax:** (312)202-5801
Email: sts@sts.org
Website: http://www.sts.org
Robert A. Wynbrandt, Exec. Dir.

Fnded: 1964. **Mem:** 4,700. **Desc:** Surgeons who confine their practice to the field of thoracic-cardiovascular surgery. Objectives are: to improve the quality and practice of thoracic and cardiovascular surgery as a specialty; to strengthen and establish basic standards in training programs; to encourage clinical and basic research; to promote the professional development of those surgeons specializing in the field; to represent and sponsor those surgeons who have recently entered the field. Conducts annual postgraduate program and three-day scientific session. **Pub:** *Annals of Thoracic Surgery*, monthly.

★ 5995 ★ Society of Toxicologic Pathology (STP)
1767 Business Center Dr., Ste. 302
Reston, VA 20190
Phone: (703)438-7508 **Fax:** (703)438-7508
Email: stp@toxpath.org
Website: http://www.toxpath.org
Clarissa Wilson, Exec. Dir.

Fnded: 1971. **Mem:** 700. **Reg. Groups:** 5. **Desc:** Promotes the advancement of the Individuals interested in toxicology and toxicologic pathology from industry, academic institutions, and government. **Pub:** *STP Newsletter*, quarterly. Newsletter. *Price:* available to members only. • *Toxicologic Pathology*, bimonthly. Journal. *Price:* $175/year for individuals in the U.S.; $195/year for individuals outside the U.S.; $195/year for institutions in the U.S.; $215/year for institutions outside the U.S. **Frmly:** (2003) Society of Toxicologic Pathologists.

★ 5996 ★ Society of Trauma Nurses (STN)
PMB 300
223 N Guadalupe
Santa Fe, NM 87501
Phone: (505)983-4923 **Fax:** (505)983-5109
Email: stn@traumanursesoc.org
Website: http://www.traumanursesoc.org
Beverlee Anderson, Exec. Dir.

Fnded: 1989. **Mem:** 650. **Nat'l Groups:** 1. **Reg. Groups:** 7. **Desc:** Nurses involved in all facets of trauma care. Seeks to communicate trauma nursing information and recognize excellence and innovation in trauma nursing. Addresses legislative issues; assists in the development of standards. Facilitates research. **Pub:** *Journal of Trauma Nursing*, quarterly. Journal. *Price:* Included in membership dues; $70/year for nonmembers; $85 outside U.S.

★ 5997 ★ Society for Treatment of Autism (STA)
404 94th Ave. SE
Calgary, AB, Canada T2J 0E8
Phone: (403)253-2291 **Free:** 888-301-2872
Email: atsc@autism.ca

Fnded: 1973. **Desc:** Provides educational and treatment programs for person with Autism and their families. Liaises with other community organizations.

★ 5998 ★ Society for the Treatment and Study of Stress
c/o J. Pierre Hogue, Pres.
125, av Pagnuelo
Montreal, QC, Canada
Phone: (514)277-8696 **Fax:** (514)875-0077
Email: age@cam.org

Desc: Promotes the study and treatment of stress.

★ 5999 ★ Society for Ultrastructural Pathology
c/o Joseph M. Harb, PhD
14655 East View Ct.
Brookfield, WI 53005
Phone: (414)781-6703
Email: khewanl@zappa.ultrakohl.com
Website: http://sup.ultrakohl.com/
Joseph Harb, PhD, Treas.

Fnded: 1986. **Mem:** 185. **Desc:** Promotes the art and science of diagnostic electron microscopy. Fosters the application of electron microscopy in the diagnosis and research of human diseases. Also provides an opportunity for the exchange of information, particularly ultrastructural and immunohistochemical, relevant to diagnostic pathology. Relevance of molecular pathology techniques to tumor pathology is also a focus. **Pub:** *Organelles in Tumor Diagnosis: An Ultrastructural Atlas*. Book. Atlas designed to identify diagnostic cell structures and tumors through the use of electron microscopy. *Price:* $39.50. • *Ultrastructural Pathology with Related Surgical and Molecular Pathology*, bimonthly. Journal. *Price:* $292.

★ 6000 ★ Society of United States Air Force Flight Surgeons
PO Box 35387
Brooks City-Base, TX 78235-0387
Phone: (210)536-2844 **Fax:** (210)536-2017
Email: michael.laughrey@brooks.af.mil
Website: http://www.sousaffs.org
Major Michael Laughrey, Exec. Officer

Fnded: 1960. **Mem:** 500. **Desc:** Flight surgeons who are members of the Aerospace Medical Association and who are currently serving on active duty with or have retired from the United States Air Force, or are serving in the Air Force Reserve or Air National Guard. Fosters advancement of aerospace medicine throughout the Air Force and encourages the clinical, laboratory, flight line, and in-flight investigation of medical problems in Air Force flying, missile, and space operations. **Pub:** *Aircraft Mishap Investigation Handbook*. Handbook. • *Flight Surgeon's Checklist*. Book. • *Flightlines*, quarterly. Newsletter. *Price:* Included in membership dues; $15/year for nonmembers.

★ 6001 ★ Society of U.S. Naval Flight Surgeons (SUSNFS)
PO Box 33008
Pensacola, FL 32508-3008
Phone: (850)452-2257
Email: dckleinberg@nomi.med.navy.mil
Website: http://www.aerospacemed.org

Fnded: 1976. **Desc:** Committed to advancement of the science, art, and practice of aerospace medicine and mission of the U.S. Navy.

★ 6002 ★ Society of University Otolaryngologists - Head and Neck Surgeons (SUO-HNS)
c/o Marvin Fried
USC School of Medicine
Department of Otolarynology
1200 N State St.
Box 795
Los Angeles, CA 90033
Phone: (323)226-7315 **Fax:** (323)226-2780
Donna Hoffman, M.A., Exec. Dir.

Fnded: 1964. **Mem:** 500. **Desc:** Otolaryngologists affiliated with universities through an approved residency training program, faculty appointment, or teaching or research position. Promotes the advancement of the art and science of otolaryngology by the development and improvement of undergraduate and graduate teaching programs. Encourages basic research and clinical investigation as an integral part of university training programs. Sponsors annual course; maintains society records. **Pub:** Directory, annual. **Frmly:** (1983) Society of University Olodaryngologists.

★ 6003 ★ Society of Urologic Nurses and Associates (SUNA)
c/o Richard P. Grimes
E Holly Ave.
PO Box 56
Pitman, NJ 08071-0056
Phone: (856)256-2335 **Free:** 888-827-7862
Fax: (856)589-7463
Email: suna@ajj.com
Website: http://www.suna.org
Richard P. Grimes, Exec. Dir.

Fnded: 1972. **Mem:** 2,800. **Reg. Groups:** 4. **Local Groups:** 30. **Desc:** Nurses and other health care providers working in the field of urology. Promotes excellence in urological education; establishes standards of care for urology patients. Conducts educational programs; holds examinations and bestows professional certification; facilitates communication among members. **Pub:** *Uro-Gram*, bimonthly. Newsletter.

★ 6004 ★ Society for Vascular Medicine and Biology (SVMB)
13 Elm St.
Manchester, MA 01944
Phone: (978)526-8330 **Fax:** (978)526-4018
Email: svmb@prri.com
Website: http://www.svmb.org
Dr. Judith Regensteiner, PhD, Chm.

Fnded: 1989. **Mem:** 270. **Desc:** Individuals with a professional interest in vascular medicine, surgery, or nursing are members; individuals in approved training programs are associates; individuals who have demonstrated leadership in vascular medicine teaching, practice, or research are fellows. Promotes advancement in the disciplines of vascular medicine and vascular biology. Provides consultation and advice to educational institutions, government agencies, and health care policy makers. Facilitates formation of vascular medicine training programs; promotes establishment of Centers of Excellence for the diagnosis and treatment of vascular diseases. Promulgates standards for postgraduate continuing medical education curricula. **Pub:** *Vascular Medicine*, quarterly. Journal. • *Vascular Medicine Directory*, periodic. Directory.

★ 6005 ★ Society for Vascular Nursing (SVN)
7794 Grow Dr.
Pensacola, FL 32514
Phone: (850)474-6963 **Free:** 888-536-4SVN
Fax: (850)484-8762
Email: svn@puetzamc.com
Website: http://www.svnnet.org
Belinda Puetz, PhD, RN , Exec. Dir.

Fnded: 1982. **Mem:** 700. **Local Groups:** 16. **Desc:** Nurses and other health care professionals interested in providing comprehensive care for persons with vascular disease. Seeks to educate public about prevention of PVD. Provides educational programs; conducts research. **Pub:** *Journal of Vascular Nursing*, quarterly. Journal. *Price:* Included in membership dues. • Also publishes patient educational materials. **Frmly:** (1992) Society for Peripheral Vascular Nursing.

★ 6006 ★ Society for Vascular Surgery (SVS)
13 Elm St.
Manchester, MA 01944
Phone: (978)526-8330 **Fax:** (978)526-4018
Email: svs@prri.com
Website: http://www.vascularweb.org
David M. Cloud, Exec. Dir.

Fnded: 1945. **Mem:** 594. **Desc:** Professional society of board-certified surgeons interested in promoting the study of and research in the circulatory system. **Pub:** *Journal of Vascular Surgery*, monthly.

★ 6007 ★ Society for Vascular Ultrasound (SVU)
4601 Presidents Dr., Ste. 260
Lanham, MD 20706-4831
Phone: (301)459-7550 **Free:** 800-788-8346
Fax: (301)459-5651
Email: info@svunet.org
Website: http://www.svunet.org
Steve Haracznak, Exec. Dir.

Fnded: 1977. **Mem:** 3,800. **Reg. Groups:** 20. **State Groups:** 5. **Local Groups:** 25. **Desc:** Vascular technologists and others in the field of noninvasive vascular technology. (Noninvasive vascular technology is a highly technical and specialized method of monitoring the blood flow in arms and legs and veins and arteries away from the heart in order to better diagnose disease and blood clots.) Seeks to establish an information clearinghouse providing reference and assistance in matters relating to noninvasive vascular technology; facilitate cooperation among noninvasive vascular facilities and other health professions; provide continuing education for individuals in the field; represents members on various regulatory issues. **Pub:** *Glossary of Terms*. Contains terms used in the vascular ultrasound profession. *Price:* $10 for members; $20 for nonmembers. • *Journal for Vascular Ultrasound*, quarterly. Journal. *Price:* Included in membership dues; $80/year for nonmembers; $105/year (outside the U.S. and Canada). • *Medicare Compliance Manual*. Handbook. *Price:* $250 for members; $350 for nonmembers. • *Patient Education Pamphlets*. Pamphlets. Covers peripheral arterial, venous, and cerebrovascular diseases. • *Referenced Study Outline*. *Price:* $10 for members; $15 for nonmembers. • *Spectrum*, bimonthly. Newsletter. *Price:* Included in membership dues; $50/year for nonmembers in the U.S. and Canada; $55/year overseas. • *Vascular Registry Review*. Two-volume (three-ring binder) set. *Price:* $75 for members; $100 for nonmembers. • Brochures. • Videos. • Also publishes information kits. **Frmly:** (1988) Society of Non-Invasive Vascular Technology; (2002) Society of Vascular Technology.

★ 6008 ★ Society for Veterinary Epidemiology and Preventive Medicine (SVEPM)
Epidemiology Department
Veterinary Laboratory Agency Weybridge
New Haw KT25 3NB, United Kingdom
Fnded: 1982.

★ 6009 ★ Society of Women in Urology
c/o Wendy J. Weiser
1111 N Plaza Dr., Ste. 550
Schaumburg, IL 60173-4946
Phone: (847)517-7225 **Fax:** (847)517-7229
Email: swiu@wjweiser.com
Wendy Weiser, Contact

Fnded: 1991. **Mem:** 260. **Desc:** Women working in the field of urology. **Pub:** *SWIU News*. Newsletter.

★ 6010 ★ Society for Women's Health Research
1828 L St. NW, Ste. 625
Washington, DC 20036
Phone: (202)223-8224 **Fax:** (202)833-3472
Email: info@womenshealth.org
Website: http://www.womens-health.org
Phyllis Greenberger, MSW, Exec. Dir.

Fnded: 1990. **Desc:** Seeks to improve the health of women by promoting equity in research. Advocates policies which promotes the inclusion of women in clinical trials; informs government agencies and private industry of issues affecting women's health and sex-based biology; educates women consumers on conditions that affect women; promotes funding for women's health research. **Pub:** *Journal of Women's Health*, 10/year. Journal. **Frmly:** (2001) Society for the Advancement of Womens Health Research.

★ 6011 ★ Solomon Islands Planned Parenthood Association (SIPPA)
PO Box 554
Lombi Cress
Honiara, Solomon Islands
Phone: 677 22991 **Fax:** 677 23653

Fnded: 1981. **Mem:** 9. **Lang(s):** English. **Desc:** Advocates family planning as a basic human right and as a means to enhance the standard of living for individuals living in the Solomon Islands. Work to stop the spread of sexually transmitted diseases such as AIDS. Offers programs in sex education, family planning, and health. Provides contraceptive services. Conducts research. **Pub:** Video.

★ 6012 ★ Sotos Syndrome Support Association (SSSA)
Three Danada Sq. E, PO Box 235
Wheaton, IL 60187
Email: sssa@well.com
Website: http://www.well.com/user/sssa
Eileen Thomas, Contact

Fnded: 1984. **Mem:** 125. **Desc:** Health care professionals and families of children with Sotos Syndrome. (Sotos Syndrome, also known as Cerebral Giantism, is a genetic disorder resulting in exceptional and rapid growth in the first five years, mental retardation, and speech and coordination impairments.) Purposes are to disseminate information to families of children diagnosed with Sotos Syndrome, form support groups, and provide referral and networking services. **Pub:** *SSSA Notes*, quarterly. Newsletter. Includes question and answer section, doctor's column, news updates, and comments from parents. *Price:* Included in membership dues. • Brochure. • Also publishes guidebook.

★ 6013 ★ South African Association of Paediatric Surgeons (SAAPS) (Suid-Afrikaanse Vereniging van Kinderchirurge — SAVK)
c/o Prof. H. Rode
Department of Paediatric Surgery
Red Cross War Memorial Children's Hospital
Rondebosch 7700, Republic of South Africa
Phone: 27 21 6585339 **Fax:** 27 21 6856632
Email: hrode@ich.uct.ac.za

Fnded: 1975. **Mem:** 50. **Nat'l Groups:** 1. **Reg. Groups:** 1. **Lang(s):** Afrikaans, English. **Desc:** Pediatric surgeons in South Africa. Promotes research, training, and clinical services in pediatric surgery. Grants postgraduate fellowships. Conducts educational programs; compiles statistics. **Pub:** *South African Medical Journal*, monthly. Journal.

★ 6014 ★ South African Association of Physicists in Medicine and Biology
PO Box 395
Pretoria 0001, Republic of South Africa
Fnded: 1960.

★ 6015 ★ South African Dental Association (SADA)
Private Bag 1
Houghton
Gauteng 2041, Republic of South Africa
Phone: 27 11 4845288 **Fax:** 27 11 6425718
Email: info@sada.co.za
Website: http://www.sadanet.co.za/

Fnded: 1922. **Mem:** 3,195. **Nat'l Groups:** 1. **Reg. Groups:** 11. **State Groups:** 11. **Lang(s):** Afrikaans, English. **Desc:** Practicing and retired dentists. Represents the dental profession in South Africa. Promotes research and investigation into dentistry and allied sciences. Sponsors National Dental Health Week in South Africa. **Pub:** *South African Dental Journal*, 10/year. Journal. Includes original scientific articles and general dental material. **Frmly:** (1998) Dental Association of South Africa.

★ 6016 ★ South African Diabetes Association (SADA) (Suid-Afrikaanse Diabetesberniging — SADV)
PO Box 604
Fontaine Bleau 2032, Republic of South Africa
Phone: 27 11 7884595 **Fax:** 27 11 4475100
Email: dfocus@worldonline.co.za

Fnded: 1969. **Mem:** 6,000. **Local Groups:** 9. **Lang(s):** Afrikaans, English. **Desc:** Individuals concerned with diabetes and associated diseases. Develops educational methods designed to give diabetics a better understanding and control of their disease. Promotes advancements in medical research and service to improve standards of treatment. Fosters exchange of information among members. Disseminates data on diabetes to increase public awareness of the disease; seeks to protect diabetics against discrimination due to their disease. Conducts research. Arranges social events and educational guidance for diabetics; organizes lectures. **Pub:** *Diabetes Focus*, quarterly. • *Sada News*, semiannual. Also publishes educational leaflets.

★ 6017 ★ South African Dietetics and Home Economics Association
PO Box 3046
Stellenbosch 7600, Republic of South Africa
Fnded: 1953.

★ 6018 ★ South African Genetics Society
Department of Genetics
Stellenbosch 7600, Republic of South Africa
Phone: 27 21 8084443 **Fax:** 27 21 8084336
Email: lw@maties.sun.ac.za
Fnded: 1956.

★ 6019 ★ South African Institute for Medical Research
PO Box 1038
Johannesburg 2000, Republic of South Africa
Phone: 27 11 7250511

★ 6020 ★ South African Medical Association (SAMA)
PO Box 74789
Lynnwood Ridge
Pretoria 0040, Republic of South Africa
Phone: 27 12 4812000 **Fax:** 27 12 4812100
Email: members@samedical.org
Website: http://www.samedical.org

Fnded: 1927. **Mem:** 12,000. **Reg. Groups:** 20. **Lang(s):** Afrikaans, English. **Desc:** Registered medical doctors and residents. Represents and protects interests of the medical profession in South Africa and promotes the medical and allied sciences. Makes representations on health policy and medico-political and social issues; advises members on matters affecting medical practice. Operates charitable program for dependents of deceased colleagues; awards loans to medical students. Holds symposia and clinical meetings; offers medical refresher courses. Bestows awards. **Pub:** *South African Journal of Continuing Medical Education*, monthly. Journal. • *South African Medical Journal*, biweekly. Journal. Also publishes booklets and brochures. **Frmly:** (2002) Medical Association of South Africa.

★ 6021 ★ South African Medical Research Council
PO Box 19070
Tygerberg 7505, Republic of South Africa
Phone: 27 21 9380911 **Fax:** 27 21 9380200
Email: lgething@eagle.mrc.ac.za

Fnded: 1969.

★ 6022 ★ South African National Multiple Sclerosis Society
295 Villiers Rd
Walmer 6070, Republic of South Africa
Phone: 27 41 512900 **Fax:** 27 41 515705

Fnded: 1963.

★ 6023 ★ South African National Tuberculosis Association (SANTA)
621 Leisk House, Corner Bree and Rissik Sts
Johannesburg 2001, Republic of South Africa
Phone: 27 11 3369636 **Fax:** 27 11 3339057
Email: santatb@iafrica.com

Fnded: 1947.

★ 6024 ★ South African Optometric Association (SAOA)
PO Box 2925
Halfway House 1685, Republic of South Africa
Phone: 27 11 8054517 **Fax:** 27 11 8053882
Email: pro@saoa.co.za
Website: http://www.saoa.co.za

Fnded: 1924.

★ 6025 ★ South African Orthopaedic Association (SAOA)
(Suid-Afrikaanse Ortopediese Vereniging — SAOV)
PO Box 12918
Brandhof 9324, Republic of South Africa
Phone: 27 51 4303280 **Fax:** 27 51 4303284
Email: saoa@megaweb.co.za
Website: http://www.saoa.org.za/

Fnded: 1942. **Mem:** 850. **Lang(s):** Afrikaans, English. **Desc:** Works to advance the science and art of orthopedic surgery and to protect the professional, financial, and educational interests of members. Provides orthopedic services to neighboring regions without orthopedic facilities. Promotes research in the field. **Pub:** *Journal of Bone and Joint Surgery*, monthly. Journal. • *Membership Directory*, annual. Directory. • *SA Orthopaedic Bulletin*, quarterly. Bulletin.

★ 6026 ★ South African Pharmacology Society (SAPS)
c/o SA ICSU Secretariat
Foundation for Research Development
PO Box 2600
Pretoria 0001, Republic of South Africa
Phone: 27 12 4814110 **Fax:** 27 12 4814007
Email: icsu@frd.ac.za

Fnded: 1966. **Mem:** 265. **Desc:** Pharmacists; pharmacologists; physicians; chemical pathologists; psychiatrists; analytical chemists; statisticians. Promotes work in pharmacology and related fields. **Pub:** Newsletter, biennial.

★ 6027 ★ South African Rheumatism and Arthritis Association
4 Park Ln, Parktown
Johannesburg 2001, Republic of South Africa

★ 6028 ★ South African Society of Anaesthesists (SASA)
Cargo corner Seventh Av, Ste. 101
Rosebank 2196, Republic of South Africa

★ 6029 ★ South African Society of Otorhinolaryngology
532 Louis Leipoldt Medical Centre
Bellville 7530, Republic of South Africa

★ 6030 ★ South African Society of Physiotherapy
PO Box 92125
Norwood 2117, Republic of South Africa
Phone: 27 11 4851467 **Fax:** 27 11 4851613
Email: ceo@saphysio.co.za
Website: http://www.physiosa.org.za

Fnded: 1925.

★ 6031 ★ South African Speech and Hearing Association
PO Box 31782
Braamfontein 2017, Republic of South Africa
Phone: 27 11 394011

Fnded: 1946.

★ 6032 ★ South African Veterinary Association
PO Box 25033
Monument Park
Pretoria, Republic of South Africa
Phone: 27 12 3461150 **Fax:** 27 12 3462929
Email: vethouse@sova.co.za

Fnded: 1920. **Desc:** Promotes veterinary services in South Africa.

★ 6033 ★ South American Commission for the Control of Foot-and-Mouth Disease
(Centro Panamericano de Fiebre)
Av. Presidente Kennedy, 7778
25040-000 Sao Bento, RJ, Brazil
Phone: 55 21 36619000 **Fax:** 55 21 36619001
Email: e-mail@panaftosa.ops-oms.org
Website: http://www.panaftosa.org.br

Fnded: 1973.

★ 6034 ★ South Pacific Underwater Medicine Society (SPUMS)
Australian and New Zealand College of Anaesthetists
630 St. Kilda Rd.
Melbourne, VIC 3004, Australia
Phone: 61 7 40550310 **Fax:** 61 7 40521583
Email: stevegoble@bigpond.com.au
Website: http://www.spums.org.au

Fnded: 1971. **Mem:** 1,000. **Lang(s):** English. **Desc:** Physicians and interested individuals in 10 countries. Serves to promote diving and hyperbaric medicines. **Pub:** *South Pacific Underwater Medicine Society Journal*, quarterly. Journal.

★ 6035 ★ Southern Africa AIDS Information Dissemation Service
Morkel House
17 Beveridge Rd.
PO Box A-509, Avondale
Harare, Zimbabwe
Phone: 263 4 336193 **Fax:** 263 4 336195
Email: info@safaids.org.zw
Website: http://www.safaids.org.zw

Fnded: 1994. **Lang(s):** English. **Desc:** Social welfare and health care organizations. Promotes increased awareness of AIDS and HIV and their prevention; seeks to improve the quality of life of people with AIDS and their families. Serves as a clearinghouse on AIDS and HIV. **Frmly:** (2000) Southern Africa Federation for AIDS.

★ 6036 ★ Southern Africa Cardiac Society
107 Chelmsford
Durban 4001, Republic of South Africa

★ 6037 ★ Southern Africa Federation of the Disabled (SAFOD)
19, Lobengula St.
PO Box 2247
Bulawayo, Zimbabwe
Phone: 263 9 69356 **Fax:** 263 9 74398
Email: safod@telconet.co.zw

Fnded: 1986. **Mem:** 10. **Lang(s):** English. **Desc:** Seeks to defend the rights of disabled people. Provides a forum for discussion among disabled persons. **Pub:** *Disability Frontline & CBR News*, quarterly. Newsletter. Includes focusing on disability issues and activities within the region.

★ 6038 ★ Southern African Association for Learning and Educational Difficulties (SAALED)
PO Box 2404
Clareinch 7740, Republic of South Africa
Phone: 27 21 7626306 **Fax:** 27 21 7626306
Email: info@saaled.org.za
Website: http://www.saaled.org.za

Fnded: 1973. **Mem:** 300. **Reg. Groups:** 4. **Local Groups:** 5. **Lang(s):** Afrikaans, English. **Desc:** Education professionals, associates, and parents. Works to influence official policy and improve educational facilities and practices for anyone with learning difficulties. Promotes interdisciplinary and interracial cooperation. Conducts community projects and charitable programs. **Pub:** *SAALED Newsletter*, semiannual. Newsletter. **Frmly:** (1992) Southern African Association for Learning and Educational Disabilities.

★ 6039 ★ Southern African Network of AIDS Service Organizations
PO Box 6690
Harare, Zimbabwe
Phone: 263 4 745748
Email: sanaso@mango.zw

Fnded: 1991. **Mem:** 1,100. **Nat'l Groups:** 145. **Reg. Groups:** 1. **State Groups:** 10. **Local Groups:** 44. **Lang(s):** English, Portuguese. **Desc:** Social service organizations working with NGO's and community based organizations working on HIV/AIDS in Southern Africa and with people living with HIV/AIDS in Southern Africa. Promotes increased access to information among people with AIDS; encourages coordination of members' activities. Serves as a clearinghouse on HIV and AIDS and their prevention; conducts advocacy lobbying programs to promote adequate resources and create supportive environments for an appropriate and effective response to HIV/AIDS. **Pub:** *SANASO Newsletter*, quarterly. Newsletter.

★ 6040 ★ Southern African Society of Human Genetics
PO Box 2034
Pretoria 0001, Republic of South Africa
Phone: 27 12 3192626 **Fax:** 27 12 3232788
Email: ehoney@medic.up.ac.za

Desc: Promotes clinical and laboratory service doing research and care for the genetic community.

★ 6041 ★ Sozialverband Vdk Deutschland
WurzerstraBe 4a
D-53175 Bonn, Germany
Phone: 49 228 820930 **Fax:** 49 228 8209343
Email: kontakt@vdk.de
Website: http://www.vdk.de

Fnded: 1950. **Mem:** 1100,000. **Reg. Groups:** 14. **Lang(s):** English, French, German. **Desc:** Victims of accidents and violence, elderly citizens, pensioners, mentally disabled individuals, victims of war or military service, and their dependents. Provides legal representation, accident and death insurance, and convalescent care; works to achieve social and vocational integration. Organizes recreational activities for members including: cultural events, parties, and travel excursions. Conducts public sensitization campaigns. Lobbying at national and European level. **Pub:** *Behinderte und Arbeitswelt.* • *Sozialrecht & Praxis*, periodic. Journal. Developments in social legislation and policy. • *Vdk Zeitung*, monthly. Journal. **Frmly:** German Organization of Victime of War and Military Service, Disabled People and Pensioners.

★ 6042 ★ Spanish Alpha 1 Association
Camino el Pato, 1
Bateria Colorada
E-11130 Cadiz, Spain
Phone: 34 956 537186
Email: alpha1info@arrakis.es
Website: http://www.alfa1.org

Fnded: 1999. **Desc:** Offers support and education for the Spanish speaking Alpha 1-Antitrypsin Deficiency patients and their families. Distributes Spanish educational materials. Works to increase awareness of Alpha 1-Antitrypsin Deficiency and the importance of early detection and treatment.

★ 6043 ★ Spanish ALS Association (ADELA) (Association Espanola de Esclerosis Lateral Amiotrofica)
Hierbabuena 12, local, bajo dcha.
E-28039 Madrid, Spain
Phone: 34 91 3113530 **Fax:** 34 91 4593926
Email: adela@adelaweb.com
Website: http://www.adelaweb.com

Fnded: 1990. **Mem:** 1,500. **Nat'l Groups:** 1. **State Groups:** 10. **Local Groups:** 20. **Lang(s):** Spanish. **Desc:** Promotes interest in amyotrophic lateral sclerosis or ALS (also called Lou Gehrig's disease) research among medical and scientific communities and the public in Spain. Offers support services to ALS sufferers and their families. Disseminates information about the disease. **Pub:** *Adela Informa*, quarterly. Bulletin. Contains general information about ALS. • *Adela Informa, Suplemento Cientifico.*

★ 6044 ★ Spanish Association for Parents with Autistic Children (Asociacion de Padres de Ninos Autistas — APNA)
Calle Navaleno, 9
E-28033 Madrid, Spain
Phone: 34 91 7662222 **Fax:** 34 91 7670038
Website: http://www.apna.es/mipagpre.html

Fnded: 1976. **Desc:** Families with autistic people addressing the needs of autistic people and their families. Provides diagnostic services, coordinates care services for outpatients, carries out services for technical, administration, and legal assessment for families with autistic people, periodically organizes "Parents Schools", organizes annual training courses.

★ 6045 ★ Spanish Association of Pharmacology (Sociedad Espanola de Farmacologia — SEF)
Bailen 20 4o 2a
E-08010 Barcelona, Spain
Phone: 34 93 2471273 **Fax:** 34 93 2471273
Email: socesfar@ctv.es

Mem: 683. **Desc:** Promotes pharmacology in Spain.

★ 6046 ★ Spanish Confederation of Family Alzheimer Associations (Confederacion Espanola de Familiares de Enfermos de Alzheimer y Otras Demencias — CEAFA)
Avenida Pio XII No 31 entreplanta of. 5
E-31008 Pamplona, Spain
Phone: 34 902 174517 **Fax:** 34 948 265739
Email: alzheimer@cin.es
Website: http://www.ceafa.org

Fnded: 1990. **Mem:** 40,000. **Lang(s):** English, Spanish. **Desc:** Individuals and organizations. Seeks to improve the quality of life of people with Alzheimer's disease and their families. Makes available support and services; facilitates research on Alzheimer's disease and related disorders; conducts educational programs. **Pub:** *En Mente*, quarterly. Newsletter. Contains information about activities.

★ 6047 ★ Spanish Confederation of Medical and Technical Advisers Associations (SCMTAA) (Confederacion Espanola de Asociaciones de Informadores Tecnicos Sanitarios — CEATIMEF)
Calle Mauricio Legendre, 2-3-I
E-28046 Madrid, Spain
Phone: 34 956 010025 **Fax:** 34 956 226919
Email: ceatimef-presidencia@ono.com
Website: http://www.ceatimef.com

Fnded: 1977. **Mem:** 12,000. **Reg. Groups:** 34. **Lang(s):** Spanish. **Desc:** Medical advisers. Promotes professional advancement of members. Represents members' interests before industrial organizations, government agencies, and the public.

★ 6048 ★ Spanish Society of Anatomy (Sociedad Anatomica Espanola)
c/o Prof. Javier Fonolla, Sec.
Dpto. Ciencias Morfologicas I
Fac. Medicina, Universidad Compultense
Ciudad Universitaria
E-28040 Madrid, Spain
Phone: 34 91 3941374 **Fax:** 34 91 3941374
Email: secant1@med.ucm.es
Website: http://www.med.ub.es/sae

Fnded: 1966. **Mem:** 300. **Desc:** Promotes development and advancement in anatomy and related sciences through research and education.

★ 6049 ★ Spanish Society of Cardiology
Nuestra Senora de Guadalupe, 5-7
28028 Madrid, Spain
Phone: 34 91 7242370 **Fax:** 34 91 7242371
Email: sec@secardiologia.es
Website: http://www.secardiologia.es

Mem: 2,179. **Desc:** Promotes the study of cardiology in Spain. **Pub:** Journal. • Newsletter.

★ 6050 ★ Spanish Society of Plastic, Reconstructive and Aesthetic Surgery (Sociedad Espanola de Cirugia Plastica, Reparadora y Estetica — SECPRE)
Villanueva 11, 3 planta
E-28001 Madrid, Spain
Phone: 34 915765995 **Fax:** 34 914315153
Email: info@secpre.org
Website: http://www.secpre.org/

Fnded: 1956.

★ 6051 ★ Spanish Society of Psychosomatic Obstetrics and Gynaecology
c/o Dr. Jesus Florido Navio
C/Lebrija. Urb Vista Real 13
E-18011 Granada, Spain
Email: jflorido@ugr.es
Website: http://www.ispog.org

Desc: Promotes the study of psychobiological and psychosocial, ethical and cross-cultural problems in the fields of obstetrics and gynaecology, women's health and reproductive health; facilitates the dissemination of new information in these fields. **Pub:** *Journal of Psychosomatic Obstetrics and Gynecology.* Journal.

★ 6052 ★ Speak Easy (SE)
95 Evergreen Ave.
Saint John's, NB, Canada E2N 1H4
Phone: (506)696-6799 **Fax:** (506)696-6799
Email: info@speakeasycanada.com
Website: http://www.speakeasycanada.com

Fnded: 1984. **Mem:** 1,000. **Lang(s):** English. **Desc:** People who stutter, parents of children who stutter, and health professionals with an interest in speech. Promotes public awareness of stuttering. Provides support and assistance to members; conducts educational programs; sponsors charitable initiatives. **Pub:** *Speaking Out*, monthly. Newsletter. • Brochure, periodic.

★ 6053 ★ Speak Easy International Foundation (SEIF)
233 Concord Dr.
Paramus, NJ 07652
Phone: (201)262-0895 **Fax:** (201)262-0895
Email: bob-antoinette@worldnet.att.net
Antoinette Gathman, Exec. Dir.

Fnded: 1977. **State Groups:** 8. **Local Groups:** 1. **Desc:** Support group and information source for individuals with a speech dysfluency (stuttering). Seeks to instill confidence in stutterers and reinforce fluency in their speech. Educates public, families, and friends on the problems of speech dysfluent individuals. **Pub:** *Speak Easy Newsletter*, quarterly. Newsletter. Contains activities of selfhelp groups, research reports on stuttering; convention schedules. *Price:* $25/year. • *Why Can't We Talk.* Video. Theatre-piece on stuttering. ng. *Price:* $129.95 institution; $25 individuals.

★ 6054 ★ Speakability
1 Royal St.
London SE1 7LL, United Kingdom
Phone: 44 207 2619572 **Fax:** 44 207 9289542
Email: speakability@speakability.org.uk
Website: http://www.speakability.org.uk

Fnded: 1980. **Mem:** 1,500. **Lang(s):** English. **Desc:** People with dysphasia (acquired language disorder), their friends and families, professionals working in the field. Works to raise awareness and understanding of dysphasia, offers help and advice through booklets and telephone helpline, membership scheme and newsletter, lectures and conferences. Professional backup and advocacy. Presses for improved provision of services; local branches, and self help groups are being developed across the country. **Pub:** *Dysphasia Matters: A Medical Teaching Pack.* Includes video and lecture packs. • *How to Help.* Booklets. • *Speaking Up*, quarterly. Newsletter. • *Talking About Dysphasia.* Audiotapes. **Frmly:** (2001) Action for Dysphasic Adults.

★ 6055 ★ Special Care Dentistry
211 E Chicago Ave., 5th Fl.
Chicago, IL 60611-9361
Phone: (312)440-2660 **Fax:** (312)440-2824
Email: specialcaredent@yahoo.com
James J. Balija, CAE, Exec. Dir.

Fnded: 1987. **Mem:** 1,600. **Nat'l Groups:** 3. **Desc:** Dentists, hygienists, and lay public interested in special care dentistry. Seeks to improve the quality of oral health for persons with special needs; offers fellowships in hospital care dentistry, geriatric care dentistry, and disability care dentistry. Conducts educational programs. **Pub:** *Oral Facial Emergencies.* Book. • *Oral Medicine in Hospital Practice.* Book. • *Special Care in Dentistry*, bimonthly. Journal. Features information of practice and patient care, trends, policy changes, and calendar of events. **Frmly:** (2001) Federation of Special Care Organizations in Dentistry.

★ 6056 ★ Special Olympics (SOI)
1325 G St., NW, Ste. 500
Washington, DC 20005
Phone: (202)628-3630 **Free:** 800-700-8585
Fax: (202)824-0200
Email: info@specialolympics.org
Website: http://www.specialolympics.org/
Timothy P. Shriver, Pres. and CEO

Fnded: 1968. **Mem:** 1200,000. **Desc:** International year-round program of sports training and competition for individuals with mental retardation. More than one million athletes in over 150 countries train and compete in 26 Olympic-type summer and winter sports. Founded in 1968 by Eunice Kennedy Shriver, Special Olympics provides people with mental retardation continuing opportunities to develop fitness, demonstrate courage, and experience joy as they participate in the sharing of gifts and friendship with other athletes, their families and the community. There is no cost to participate. **Pub:** *Spirit*, quarterly. Magazine. • *Update*, monthly. • Also publishes informational brochures, guides, instructional manual, and list of state programs.

★ 6057 ★ Special Olympics Albania
c/o Koco Gaba
RR Mine Peza
Pall 254/1/9
SHK 1/9
Tirana, Albania
Phone: 355 42 33946 **Fax:** 355 42 40964
Email: sabian@icc.al.eu.org

Desc: Offers support and training for disabled individuals in Albania who wish to participate in athletic competitions.

★ 6058 ★ Special Olympics Andorra
c/o Carolina Serra, Nat'l Dir.
Escola Meritxell dels Barrers 10
Santa Coloma, Andorra
Phone: 376 821731 **Fax:** 376 860540
Email: eensdm@mypic.ad

Desc: Offers support and training for disabled individuals in Andorra who wish to participate in athletic competitions.

★ 6059 ★ Special Olympics Argentina
c/o Pia Soldatti, Pres.
Nueva Olimpiada Especiales Argentina
Almirante Onofre Betbeder
1428 Capital Federal
1252 Buenos Aires, Argentina
Phone: 54 11 48960186 **Fax:** 54 11 48961413
Email: info@olimpiadaespecial.org.ar
Website: http://www.olimpiadaespecial.org.ar

Desc: Offers support and training for disabled individuals in Argentina who wish to participate in athletic competitions.

★ 6060 ★ Special Olympics Armenia
c/o Mr. Gavrush Mnatsakanyan, Pres.
43/65 Horenatsi St.
375018 Yerevan, Armenia
Phone: 374 1 576967 **Fax:** 374 1 541511
Email: arm_spolympics@mail.com

Desc: Offers support and training for disabled individuals participating in athletic competitions.

★ 6061 ★ Special Olympics Australia
c/o Rex Langthorne
PO Box 712
Glebe, NSW 2037, Australia
Phone: 61 2 95526188 **Fax:** 61 2 95523848
Email: rlangthorne@dsr.nsw.gov.au
Website: http://www.specialolympics.com.au/

Desc: Offers support and training for disabled individuals in Australia who wish to participate in athletic competitions.

★ 6062 ★ Special Olympics Austria
c/o Marc Angelini
Coburgstrasse 52
Postfach 15
A-8970 Schladming, Austria
Phone: 43 36 8723358 **Fax:** 43 36 8723859
Email: soo-schladming@specialolympics.at

Desc: Offers support and training for disabled individuals in Austria who wish to participate in athletic competitions.

★ 6063 ★ Special Olympics Azerbaijan
c/o Mr. Shahin Aliyev, Pres.
20 Bul-bul ave., 4th Fl, Rm. 12
370014 Baku, Azerbaijan
Phone: 994 12 983860 **Fax:** 994 12 985525
Email: azspecialolympics@mailru.com

Desc: Offers support and training for disabled individuals participating in athletic competitions.

★ 6064 ★ Special Olympics Bangladesh
c/o Lutful Hai, Exec.Dir.
Sharif Mansion, 4th Fl.
56-57 Motijheel C/A
GPO Box 829
Dhaka 1000, Bangladesh
Phone: 880 2 9553383 **Fax:** 880 2 8912085
Email: sobangla@bdmail.com

Desc: Offers support and training for disabled individuals in Bangladesh who wish to participate in athletic competitions.

★ 6065 ★ Special Olympics Belarus
c/o Mr. Valentin Shukh, Pres.
L. Libknehta, 68-906
220036 Minsk, Belarus
Phone: 375 172 862573 **Fax:** 375 172 862573
Email: olcom@user.unibel.by

Desc: Offers support and training for disabled individuals participating in athletic competitions.

★ 6066 ★ Special Olympics Benin
c/o Marie Jeanne Dagnon-Yalo
01 BP 3596 RP
Cotonou, Benin
Phone: 229 310383 **Fax:** 229 310383

Desc: Offers support and training for disabled individuals in Benin who wish to participate in athletic competitions.

★ 6067 ★ Special Olympics Bolivia
c/o Henry Jordan
Calle Mexico Coliseo Cerrado
3 er piso
Miaflores
La Paz, Bolivia
Phone: 591 2 227808
Email: apjordan@ceibo.entelnet.com.bo

Desc: Offers support and training for disabled individuals in Bolivia who wish to participate in athletic competitions.

★ 6068 ★ Special Olympics Bosnia and Herzegovina
c/o Ministry of Social Policy
A.B. Slimica 4
Sarajevo, Bosnia-Hercegovina
Phone: 387 71616433 **Fax:** 387 71648828

Desc: Offers support and training for disabled individuals in Bosnia & Herzegovina who wish to participate in athletic competitions.

★ 6069 ★ Special Olympics Botswana
c/o Botswana Council for the Disabled
Private Bag 459
Gaborone, Botswana
Phone: 267 373599 **Fax:** 267 311784
Email: bcd@info.bw

Desc: Offers support and training for disabled individuals in Botswana who wish to participate in athletic competitions.

★ 6070 ★ Special Olympics Bulgaria
c/o Nikolay Dagorov
57, Milin Kamak St., Fl. 4
BG-1421 Sofia, Bulgaria
Phone: 359 2 9633904 **Fax:** 359 2 387592
Email: law-kd@aster.net

Desc: Offers support and training for disabled individuals in Bulgaria who wish to participate in athletic competitions.

★ 6071 ★ Special Olympics Burkina Faso
c/o Alexandre Yougbare
BP 4411
Ouagadougou 01, Burkina Faso
Phone: 226 314978 **Fax:** 226 305370
Email: manou_ilboudo@yahoo.fr

Desc: Offers support and training for disabled individuals in Burkina Faso who wish to participate in athletic competitions.

★ 6072 ★ Special Olympics Cameroon
c/o Mbarga Panda Simon
PO Box 6991
Yaounde, Cameroon
Phone: 237 216650 **Fax:** 237 221873

Desc: Offers support and training for disabled individuals in Cameroon who wish to participate in athletic competitions.

★ 6073 ★ Special Olympics Canada
60 St. Clair Ave. W, Ste. 700
Toronto, ON, Canada M4T 2N5
Phone: (416)927-9050 **Free:** 877-291-7404
Fax: (416)927-8475
Email: info@specialolympics.ca
Website: http://www.cso.on.ca

Fnded: 1969. **Mem:** 30. **Lang(s):** English, French. **Desc:** Provides sport training and competition for people with a mental disability at local, provincial, national and international levels. Conducts research, provides coach training. **Pub:** *Canadian Special Olympics.* Brochure. • *Canadian Special Olympics National Office Bulletin*, semiannual. Newsletter. • *Canadian Special Olympics National Team.* Brochure.

★ 6074 ★ Special Olympics Chad
c/o Doubrain Ngabaye
BP 4196
N'Djamena, Chad
Phone: 235 516047 **Fax:** 235 521429

Desc: Offers support and training for disabled individuals in Chad who wish to participate in athletic competitions.

★ 6075 ★ Special Olympics China
c/o Yong Zhi Jun
44 Beichizi St.
Dongcheng District
Beijing 100006, People's Republic of China
Phone: 86 10 65139719 **Fax:** 86 10 65139722
Email: sochina@adpf.org.cn

Desc: Offers support and training for disabled individuals in China who wish to participate in athletic competitions.

★ 6076 ★ Special Olympics Colombia
c/o D. Alejandro Escallon
Carrera 13-A, No. 8734
Bogota, D.E., Colombia
Phone: 57 1 2182122 **Fax:** 57 1 2566775
Email: aescallo@elsitio.net.co

Fnded: 1975. **Mem:** 40. **Nat'l Groups:** 1. **Reg. Groups:** 14. **Lang(s):** Spanish. **Desc:** Offers support and training for disabled individuals in Colombia who wish to participate in athletic competitions. **Pub:** *Siempre Adelante*, quarterly. Magazine.

★ 6077 ★ Special Olympics Costa Rica
c/o Carlos Valverde
San Francisco de Dos Rios, de Productos de Concreto
San Jose 1000, Costa Rica
Phone: 506 2268135 **Fax:** 506 2273101
Email: sciefs@racsa.co.cr
Website: http://www.specialolympics.org

Desc: Offers support and training for disabled individuals in Costa Rica who wish to participate in athletic competitions.

★ 6078 ★ Special Olympics Croatia
c/o Verica Paulic
Trg Sportova 11, Rm. 30A
10000 Zagreb, Croatia
Phone: 355 1 6612200 **Fax:** 385 1 3091119
Email: igor.paulic@zg.tel.hr

Desc: Offers support and training for disabled individuals in Croatia who wish to participate in athletic competitions.

★ 6079 ★ Special Olympics Cuba
17 y 0 Vedado
Havana, Cuba
Phone: 53 7 8322452 **Fax:** 53 7 8553105
Email: tchkout@rimed.cu

Desc: Offers support and training for disabled individuals in Cuba who wish to participate in athletic competitions.

★ 6080 ★ Special Olympics Cyprus
c/o Andreas Hadjivasiliou
20 Ionos St. Engomini
PO Box 23931
Nicosia 1687, Cyprus
Phone: 357 22 662984 **Fax:** 357 22 664986
Email: megalemo@cytanet.com.cy

Desc: Offers support and training for disabled individuals in Cyprus who wish to participate in athletic competitions.

★ 6081 ★ Special Olympics Czech Republic
c/o Martina Stredova
Ricni 6
CS-11800 Prague, Czech Republic
Phone: 42 2 57313008 **Fax:** 42 2 57313008
Email: vstreda@subterra.cz

Desc: Offers support and training for disabled individuals in Czech Republic who wish to participate in athletic competitions.

★ 6082 ★ Special Olympics Denmark
c/o Dansk Handicap, Idraets-Forbund
Idraettens Hus-Brondby Stadion 20
DK-2605 Brondby, Denmark
Phone: 45 43262626 **Fax:** 45 43262470
Email: handicapidraet@dhif.dk

Desc: Offers support and training for disabled individuals in Denmark who wish to participate in athletic competitions.

★ 6083 ★ Special Olympics Dominican Republic
c/o Vicenta Peignand
Apartado de Coreos 1054
Santo Domingo, Dominican Republic
Phone: (809)688-6444 **Fax:** (809)688-1566
Email: dirladr@tricom.net

Desc: Offers support and training for disabled individuals in Dominican Republic who wish to participate in athletic competitions.

★ 6084 ★ Special Olympics Ecuador
c/o Hector Cueva Jimenez
Calle Berlin 158 y Ave. 9 de Octubre
Oficina 014 - 1er piso
Quito, Ecuador
Phone: 593 2 2508327 **Fax:** 593 2 2546567
Email: olimpesp@uio.satnet.net

Desc: Offers support and training for disabled individuals in Ecuador who wish to participate in athletic competitions.

★ 6085 ★ Special Olympics El Salvador
c/o Hector Hugo Matasol
Palacio de los Deportes
Indes 2o Nivel, Salon 3
San Salvador, El Salvador
Phone: 503 2711208 **Fax:** 503 2713374
Email: olimpiadases@vianet.com.sv

Desc: Offers support and training for disabled individuals in El Salvador who wish to participate in athletic competitions.

★ 6086 ★ Special Olympics Estonia
c/o Toomas Hendrick lives
Amrop International
Kaupmehe 8
EE-10114 Tallinn, Estonia
Phone: 372 2 6403155 **Fax:** 372 2 6558361
Email: meeli.hunt@amrop.com

Desc: Offers support and training for disabled individuals in Estonia who wish to participate in athletic competitions.

★ 6087 ★ Special Olympics Finland
c/o Finnish Sports Federation for Persons with Intellectual Disabilities
Radiokatu 20, 5.KRS
SF-00093 Slu, Finland
Phone: 358 9 8776868 **Fax:** 358 9 8776869
Email: eija.kangas-virtanen@sklu.org

Desc: Offers support and training for intellectually disabled individuals in Finland who wish to participate in sports.

★ 6088 ★ Special Olympics France
c/o Bruno Grob
182 rue Raymond Losserand
F-75014 Paris, France
Phone: 33 1 44126011 **Fax:** 33 1 44126019

Desc: Offers support and training for disabled individuals in France who wish to participate in athletic competitions.

★ 6089 ★ Special Olympics Gabon
c/o Daoveda Leocadie
BP 18349
Libreville, Gabon
Phone: 241 244980 **Fax:** 241 705658

Desc: Offers support and training for disabled individuals in Gabon who wish to participate in athletic competitions.

★ 6090 ★ Special Olympics Gambia
c/o Alieu Y. Cham
PO Box 2554
Serekunda, Gambia
Phone: 220 228601 **Fax:** 220 227861
Email: acham.baes@ganet.gm

Desc: Offers support and training for disabled individuals in Gambia who wish to participate in athletic competitions.

★ 6091 ★ Special Olympics Georgia
c/o Rcheulishrili Vaxtang
Apart 49, Chavchardnadze
380072 Tbilisi, Georgia
Phone: 995 32 331827 **Fax:** 995 32 970076
Email: ketosi@mailexcite.com

Desc: Offers support and training for disabled individuals in Georgia who wish to participate in athletic competitions.

★ 6092 ★ Special Olympics Germany
c/o Institut fur Sportwissenschaften der Universitat
Judenbuhl Western Euroweg, 11
D-97082 Wurzburg, Germany
Phone: 49 931 86010 **Fax:** 49 931 84390
Email: special_olympics@mail.uni-wuerzburg.de

Desc: Offers support and training for disabled individuals in Germany who wish to participate in athletic competitions.

★ 6093 ★ Special Olympics Ghana
c/o National Sports Council
PO Box 1272
Accra, Ghana
Phone: 233 21 674369 **Fax:** 233 21 662281
Email: soghana80@hotmail.com

Fnded: 1979. **Mem:** 15. **Nat'l Groups:** 1. **Reg. Groups:** 10. **Local Groups:** 11. **Desc:** Offers support and training for disabled individuals in Ghana who wish to participate in athletic competitions.

★ 6094 ★ Special Olympics Greece
c/o Epirotiki Bldg.
87 Akti Miaouli
GR-185 38 Piraeus, Greece
Phone: 30 1 6068956 **Fax:** 30 1 6068955
Email: spolimpicsgr@mail.com

Desc: Offers support and training for disabled individuals in Greece who wish to participate in athletic competitions.

★ 6095 ★ Special Olympics Honduras (Olimpiadas Especiales de Hondras)
c/o Ana de Galeano
Estadio de Beisbol
Complejo Deportivo Jose Simon Azcona
Tegucigalpa, Honduras
Phone: 504 2356405 **Fax:** 504 2356405
Email: oliesphonduras@sigmanet.hn

Desc: Offers support and training for disabled individuals in Honduras who wish to participate in athletic competitions.

★ 6096 ★ Special Olympics Hungary (Magyar Specialis Olimpia Eyesulet)
c/o Janos Wisinger
Istvanmezei ut. 1-3
H-1146 Budapest, Hungary
Phone: 36 1 2522236 **Fax:** 36 1 9995563
Email: hunolimp@nograd.net

Desc: Offers support and training for disabled individuals in Hungary who wish to participate in athletic competitions.

★ 6097 ★ Special Olympics Iceland
c/o Sveinn Aki Ludviksson
Ithrottamidstodin Laugardal
IS-104 Reykjavik, Iceland
Phone: 354 5144080 **Fax:** 354 5144081
Email: if@isisport.is
Website: http://isisport.is/if

Desc: Offers support and training for disabled individuals in Iceland who wish to participate in athletic competitions.

★ 6098 ★ Special Olympics India
c/o J.A. Benji Benjamin
106 Church St.
Lingarajapuram
St. Thomas Town
Bangalore 560 084, India
Phone: 91 80 25461379 **Fax:** 91 80 5478382
Email: benji_sivus@usa.net
Desc: Offers support and training for disabled individuals in India who wish to participate in athletic competitions.

★ 6099 ★ Special Olympics Ireland (SOI)
Park House, 4th Fl.
North Cicular Rd.
Dublin 7, Ireland
Phone: 353 1 8823972 **Fax:** 353 1 8688250
Email: info@specialolympics.ie
Website: http://www.specialolympics.ie
Fnded: 1978. **Mem:** 12,000. **Reg. Groups:** 4. **Lang(s):** English. **Desc:** Provides individuals with a learning difficulty with year-round opportunities to train for, and participate in, athletic competitions. Makes available coaches and training facilities for Special Olympics Athletes; administers and provides officials for local and national Special Olympics competitions. Participates in quadrennial International Special Olympics Games. **Pub:** *S.O. Alive*, 3/year, always spring, autumn, and Christmas. Newsletter.

★ 6100 ★ Special Olympics Italy
c/o Alessandro Palazzotti
via di Decima 40
I-00144 Rome, Italy
Phone: 39 06 52246486 **Fax:** 39 06 52246835
Email: soi@specialolympics.it
Website: http://www.specialolympics.it
Fnded: 2000. **Mem:** 15. **Desc:** Offers support and training for disabled individuals in Italy who wish to participate in athletic competitions.

★ 6101 ★ Special Olympics Japan
c/o Fukujiro Shiroki
Viale Bld. 3F
1-24 Kamitori-cho
Kumamoto 860-0845, Japan
Phone: 81 96 3524000 **Fax:** 81 96 3521820
Email: so-jpn@fa2.so-net.ne.jp
Website: http://www.specialolympics-nippon.gr.jp/
Desc: Offers support and training for disabled individuals in Japan who wish to participate in athletic competitions.

★ 6102 ★ Special Olympics Kazakhstan
Furmanova Str. 50, of. 412
480004 Alma-Ata, Kazakhstan
Phone: 7 3272 332979 **Fax:** 7 3272 332979
Email: specialkaz@asdc.kz
Fnded: 1991. **Mem:** 6,500. **Nat'l Groups:** 1. **Reg. Groups:** 14. **State Groups:** 1. **Local Groups:** 73. **Lang(s):** Russian. **Desc:** Individuals and organizations. Promotes the Special Olympics in Kazakhstan. Works to advance the social rehabilitation of people with mental retardation. **Pub:** *The Target*, quarterly. Newsletter.

★ 6103 ★ Special Olympics Kenya
c/o Joe N. Mutua
PO Box 70483
Nairobi, Kenya
Phone: 254 20 725836 **Fax:** 254 20 336885
Email: kitololo@africaonline.co.ke
Desc: Offers support and training for disabled individuals in Kenya who wish to participate in athletic competitions.

★ 6104 ★ Special Olympics Korea
c/o Jung-Hoon Lee
288-1 Hagye-Dong
Nowon-gu
Seoul 139-231, Republic of Korea
Phone: 82 2 9727630 **Fax:** 82 2 9784287
Email: hoon6910@chollian.net
Desc: Offers support and training for disabled individuals in Korea who wish to participate in athletic competitions.

★ 6105 ★ Special Olympics Latvia
c/o Dzidra Kupca
A. Briana St-8
LV-1001 Riga, Latvia
Phone: 371 2 7375587 **Fax:** 371 2 7376759
Email: dekko@inbox.lv
Fnded: 1998. **Mem:** 170. **Nat'l Groups:** 1. **Reg. Groups:** 5. **Lang(s):** English, Russian. **Desc:** Offers support and training for disabled individuals in Latvia who wish to participate in athletic competitions.

★ 6106 ★ Special Olympics Lesotho
c/o Lesotho Society of Mentally Handicapped Persons
Private Bag A-62
Lesotho Flour Mills
Maseru 100, Lesotho
Phone: 266 321292 **Fax:** 266 840504
Email: malebabo@yahoo.com
Website: http://www.specialolympics.org
Desc: Offers support and training for disabled individuals in Lesotho who wish to participate in athletic competitions.

★ 6107 ★ Special Olympics Malawi
c/o Sports Council Malawi
Box 452
Blantyre, Malawi
Phone: 265 675084 **Fax:** 265 675110
Email: mmathias@malawi.net
Desc: Offers support and training for disabled individuals in Malawi who wish to participate in athletic competitions.

★ 6108 ★ Special Olympics Malta
c/o Paul Micallef
New York Bldg., Ste. 9
Qawra Rd.
Qawra, Malta
Phone: 356 570326 **Fax:** 356 570326
Email: paul@novanet.net.mt
Desc: Offers support and training for disabled individuals in Malta who wish to participate in athletic competitions.

★ 6109 ★ Special Olympics Moldova
c/o Nicolai Barbieru
ul. Pushkina, 26
277024 Kishinev, Moldova
Phone: 373 2 244479 **Fax:** 373 2 227707
Desc: Offers support and training for disabled individuals in Moldova who wish to participate in athletic competitions.

★ 6110 ★ Special Olympics Nepal
c/o Dr. Jyoti Sherchan
Kamalpokhari
PO Box 12189
Kathmandu, Nepal
Phone: 977 1 424736 **Fax:** 977 1 425774
Email: sonepal@ccsl.com.np
Desc: Offers support and training for disabled individuals in Nepal who wish to participate in athletic competitions.

★ 6111 ★ Special Olympics Netherlands
c/o Netherlands Sports Federation for Citizens with Intellectual Handicaps
Regulierenring 2b
Postbus 200
NL-3980 Bunnik, Netherlands
Phone: 31 30 6597310 **Fax:** 31 30 6597373
Email: info@specialolympics.nl
Website: http://www.specialolympics.nl
Desc: Offers support and training for people with an intellectual disability in the Netherlands who wish to participate in athletic competitions.

★ 6112 ★ Special Olympics Norway
c/o IPU-Utvalget
Serviceboks 1, Ulleval I Stadion
N-0840 Oslo, Norway
Phone: 47 21029000 **Fax:** 47 21029481
Email: goril.hansen@nif.idrett.no
Desc: Offers support and training for disabled individuals in Norway who wish to participate in athletic competitions.

★ 6113 ★ Special Olympics Pakistan
c/o Parveen Ali
Defence Housing Society, Phase II
7-B 4th Central Ln.
Karachi, Pakistan
Phone: 92 21 5887260 **Fax:** 92 21 7725753
Email: pali@alephx.org
Desc: Offers support and training for disabled individuals in Pakistan who wish to participate in athletic competitions.

★ 6114 ★ Special Olympics Panama (Olimpiadas Especiales de Panama)
c/o Yolanda Eleta de Varela
Apartado Postal 394
Ancon
Panama City, Panama
Phone: 507 2288224
Email: olimesp@sinfo.net
Desc: Offers support and training for disabled individuals in Panama who wish to participate in athletic competitions.

★ 6115 ★ Special Olympics Paraguay (Olimpiadas Especiales de Paraguay)
c/o Irma Cuevas de Cabezudo
Rca. de Colombia 1112
Asuncion, Paraguay
Phone: 595 21 491493 **Fax:** 595 21 494314
Email: cabezudo@rieder.net
Desc: Offers support and training for disabled individuals in Paraguay who wish to participate in athletic competitions.

★ 6116 ★ Special Olympics Peru (Olimpiadas Especiales de Peru)
c/o Aldo Barbieri
Ave. Prolongacion Ricardo
Palma 1391, LaAurora
Miraflores
Lima 18, Peru
Phone: 51 14 470780 **Fax:** 51 14 473360
Email: olimpiadasespecialesperu@ddm.com.pe
Desc: Offers support and training for disabled individuals in Peru who wish to participate in athletic competitions.

★ 6117 ★ Special Olympics Philippines
c/o Nicanor Jorge
4 Lands St., Vasra Village
Quezon City, Metro Manila, Philippines
Phone: 63 2 9288448 **Fax:** 63 2 9295707
Email: best@pacific.net.ph
Desc: Offers support and training for disabled individuals in Philippines who wish to participate in athletic competitions.

★ 6118 ★ Special Olympics Poland
c/o Katerina Niemczycka
ul. Wilcza 38a
PL-00-679 Warsaw, Poland
Phone: 48 2 26270758 **Fax:** 48 2 26218418

Email: ospbiuro@olimpiadyspecjalne.pl
Website: http://www.olimpiadyspecjalne.pl

Fnded: 1985. **Mem:** 3,600. **Reg. Groups:** 18. **Local Groups:** 400. **Desc:** Offers support and training for disabled individuals in Poland who wish to participate in athletic competitions. **Pub:** *Jezyk*, quarterly. Bulletin. • *Tecza (Rainbow)*, biennial.

★ 6119 ★ Special Olympics Portugal
c/o Liga Portuguesa dos Deficientes Motores
Rua do Sitio do Casalinho da Ajuda
1349-011 Lisbon, Portugal
Phone: 351 21 3636174 **Fax:** 351 21 3648639
Email: lj.lpdm.crs@mail.telepac.pt

Desc: Offers support and training for disabled individuals in Portugal who wish to participate in athletic competitions.

★ 6120 ★ Special Olympics Romania
c/o Federatia Romana a Sportului Pentru Handicapati
Ministerul Tineretului si Sportului
str. Vasile Conte, n. 16
Sector 2
R-70139 Bucharest, Romania
Phone: 40 1 2122719
Email: maria_milea2000@k.ro

Desc: Offers support and training for disabled individuals in Romania who wish to participate in athletic competitions.

★ 6121 ★ Special Olympics Russia
c/o Dr. Andrei Pavlov, Pres.
15, Sadovniki Str.
115487 Moscow, Russia
Phone: 7 95 1120047 **Fax:** 7 95 1125430
Email: spolrussia@email.ru
Website: http://specialolympics.euro.ru

Fnded: 1999. **Mem:** 21,000. **Nat'l Groups:** 1. **Reg. Groups:** 30. **Desc:** Offers support and training for individuals with mental retardation participating in athletic competitions.

★ 6122 ★ Special Olympics Sabah
PO Box 10462
Kota Kinabalu
88805 Sabah, Malaysia
Phone: 60 88 223221 **Fax:** 60 88 244672
Email: so.sabah@org.my
Website: http://specialolympics.sabah.org.my

Fnded: 1998. **Mem:** 120. **State Groups:** 4. **Local Groups:** 10. **Desc:** Offers support and training for intellectually disabled individuals in Malaysia who wish to participate in athletic training and competitions.

★ 6123 ★ Special Olympics Singapore
c/o Robin Chua
Blk. 2, No. 01-65, St. George's Rd.
Singapore 322-002, Singapore
Phone: 65 2933182 **Fax:** 65 2938497
Email: sosinga@mbox4.singnet.com.sg

Desc: Offers support and training for disabled individuals in Singapore who wish to participate in athletic competitions.

★ 6124 ★ Special Olympics Slovakia
c/o Eva Lysicanova
Lamacska cesta 3
84104 Bratislava 4, Slovakia
Phone: 421 2 59418641 **Fax:** 421 2 59418641
Email: shso@ba.psg.sk
Website: http://www.shso.sk

Desc: Offers support and training for disabled individuals in Slovakia who wish to participate in athletic competitions.

★ 6125 ★ Special Olympics Slovenia
c/o Marijan Lacen
Samova 9/2o
SLO-1000 Ljubljana, Slovenia
Phone: 386 61 613617 **Fax:** 386 61 1362406
Email: info@zveza-sozitje.si

Desc: Offers support and training for disabled individuals in Slovenia who wish to participate in athletic competitions.

★ 6126 ★ Special Olympics South Africa
c/o Dr. Francois Jacobsz
Halfway House
PO Box 3818
Gauteng 1685, Republic of South Africa
Phone: 27 11 8055969 **Fax:** 27 11 8058081
Email: sosa@iafrica.com

Desc: Offers support and training for disabled individuals in South Africa who wish to participate in athletic competitions.

★ 6127 ★ Special Olympics Spain
c/o Francesc Martinez de Foix
Sant Antoni Maria Claret, 24, 40 piso
E-08037 Barcelona, Spain
Phone: 34 93 4572298 **Fax:** 34 93 4572793
Email: specialolympics@dyr.es
Website: http://www.dyr.es/org/specialolympics

Desc: Offers support and training for disabled individuals in Spain who wish to participate in athletic competitions.

★ 6128 ★ Special Olympics Sweden
c/o Victor Wahlstrom
Graddvagen 12
S-640 45 Kvicksund, Sweden
Phone: 46 278 626064 **Fax:** 46 278 24456
Email: peter_bjork@telia.com

Desc: Offers support and training for disabled individuals in Sweden who wish to participate in athletic competitions.

★ 6129 ★ Special Olympics Switzerland
Route u Petit-Moncor 17/19
Case postale 788
CH-1701 Fribourg, Switzerland
Phone: 41 26 4020045 **Fax:** 41 26 4020046
Email: specialolympics@compuserve.com
Website: http://www.specialolympics.ch

Desc: Offers support and training for disabled individuals in Switzerland who wish to participate in athletic competitions.

★ 6130 ★ Special Olympics Tajikistan
c/o Ms. Dilbar Sharipova .
Shotimura St.53 Apt. 4
Rudaki St. 21/6
734001 Dushanbe, Tajikistan
Phone: 992 372 213704 **Fax:** 992 372 213704
Email: sot@tojikistom.com

Desc: Offers support and training for disabled individuals participating in athletic competitions.

★ 6131 ★ Special Olympics Tanzania
c/o Claude Njimba
PO Box 1949
Dar es Salaam, United Republic of Tanzania
Phone: 255 51 183082 **Fax:** 255 51 112054

Desc: Offers support and training for disabled individuals in Tanzania who wish to participate in athletic competitions.

★ 6132 ★ Special Olympics Thailand
c/o Rachaniwan Bulakul
339 Soi Pipat, Silom Rd.
Bangrak
Bangkok 10500, Thailand
Phone: 66 2 2666708 **Fax:** 66 2 2381149
Email: sothai@inet.co.th

Fnded: 1987. **Mem:** 54. **Nat'l Groups:** 1. **Reg. Groups:** 4. **Desc:** Offers support and training for disabled individuals in Thailand who wish to participate in athletic competitions.

★ 6133 ★ Special Olympics Turkmenistan
c/o Mr. Bairam Seitlikov, Chair
PO Box 191
Krugozoi Main Post Office
744000 Ashgabat, Turkmenistan
Email: adji@online.tm

Fnded: 1990. **Mem:** 2,045. **Nat'l Groups:** 1. **Reg. Groups:** 5. **Lang(s):** English. **Desc:** Offers support and training for disabled individuals participating in athletic competitions.

★ 6134 ★ Special Olympics Uganda
c/o Edward Babumba
PO Box 5444
Kampala, Uganda
Phone: 256 41 267640 **Fax:** 256 41 345047
Email: souline@swiftuganda.com

Fnded: 1992. **Local Groups:** 45. **Desc:** Offers support and training for disabled individuals in Uganda who wish to participate in athletic competitions. **Pub:** *The Brave*, quarterly.

★ 6135 ★ Special Olympics Ukraine
c/o Mr. Konstantyn Slynavchuk, Pres.
20/6 Serpova St.
115-03115 Kiev, Ukraine
Phone: 380 44 444145 **Fax:** 380 44 4448200

Desc: Offers support and training for disabled individuals participating in athletic competitions.

★ 6136 ★ Special Olympics Uruguay (Olimpiadas Especiales de Uruguay)
c/o Alcides Abarno
Av. Brasil 2377, Depto. 1001
Montevideo, Uruguay
Phone: 598 2 7071007 **Fax:** 598 2 9021126

Desc: Offers support and training for disabled individuals in Uruguay who wish to participate in athletic competitions.

★ 6137 ★ Special Olympics Uzbekistan
c/o Mr. Adisman Dmitriv
Furkata Stl, Apt. 321
Tchilazarskij Rayon
700027 Tashkent, Uzbekistan
Phone: 998 712 1326279 **Fax:** 998 712 1391097
Email: nslavnova@uz.peacecorps.gov

Fnded: 2002. **Mem:** 2. **Reg. Groups:** 5. **State Groups:** 15. **Lang(s):** English, Russian. **Desc:** Offers support and training for disabled individuals participating in athletic competitions.

★ 6138 ★ Special Olympics Venezuela (Olimpiadas Especiales de Venezuela)
c/o Evelyn Guiralt
Residence Sans Souci, Edificio El Aman
Piso 12, Apart. 122
Avenida Solano Lopez Chacaito
Caracas 1050, Venezuela
Phone: 58 2 2618530 **Fax:** 58 2 9528390

Desc: Offers support and training for disabled individuals in Venezuela who wish to participate in athletic competitions.

★ 6139 ★ Special Olympics Zambia
c/o Jumali Nkhama
PO Box 31202
Lusaka, Zambia
Phone: 260 1 281529 **Fax:** 260 1 223645

Desc: Offers support and training for disabled individuals in Zambia who wish to participate in athletic competitions.

★ 6140 ★ Special Olympics Zimbabwe
c/o Bonny Woodman
Greendale
PO Box GD 143
Harare, Zimbabwe
Phone: 263 4 499701 **Fax:** 263 4 499701
Email: sozim@id.co.zw

Desc: Offers support and training for disabled individuals in Zimbabwe who wish to participate in athletic competitions.

★ 6141 ★ Special Recreation for disABLED International (SRDI)
701 Oaknoll Dr.
Iowa City, IA 52246-5168
Phone: (319)466-3192
Email: john-nesbitt@uiowa.edu
Website: http://www.jccniowa.org/~recdsabl
John A. Nesbitt, EdD, Pres. /CEO

Fnded: 1978. **Desc:** Seeks to serve and advocate special and therapeutic play and recreation for infants, children, youth, adults, and seniors throughout the world. Services include advisory and consultation, awards, employment information, professional education, public education, publishing, research, resource information and referral, technical assistance on programs and management methods, and an international library. Does international service work to: collect and disseminate international information on special recreation services for disabled persons, special recreation programs, and personnel training; conduct, provide, and support international exchange of technical, professional, and general information on special recreation for the disabled; cooperate with both governmental and voluntary organizations on national and international levels. Offers career guidance and placement service. Maintains speakers' bureau; compiles statistics. **Pub:** *Camping/Outdoor Recreation, National Institute on Camping for DisABLED.* Monograph. • *Community-Based Special Recreation, National Institute on New Models of Community-Based Special Recreation for DisABLED.* Monograph. • *Deaf-Blind, National Institute on Play and Recreation for Deaf-Blind.* Monograph. • *Health-PE-Recreation, World Seminar on Special Recreation, World Congress of the International Council on Health, Physical Education, Recreation and Dance.* Monograph. • *Mental Health, World Seminar on Special Recreation, World Congress of the World Federation for Mental Health, Manila, Philippines.* Monograph. **Frmly:** (1998) Special Recreation for Disabled.

★ 6142 ★ Speech Pathology Australia
2nd Floor, 11-19 Bank Place
Melbourne, VIC 3000, Australia
Phone: 61 3 96424899 **Fax:** 61 3 96424922
Email: office@speechpathologyaustralia.org.au
Website: http://www.speechpathologyaustralia.org.au

Fnded: 1949. **Mem:** 3,400. **Lang(s):** English. **Desc:** Speech pathologists working in private practice, hospitals, rehabilitation centers, education centers, and with agencies for specific disabilities. Represents and promotes the professional interests of speech pathologists in Australia. Lobbies government on behalf of members and their clients for improved services and facilities; works with the media to provide information on communication disorders; and sets professional standards for its members.

★ 6143 ★ Spina Bifida Association of America (SBAA)
4590 MacArthur Blvd. NW, Ste. 250
Washington, DC 20007-4226
Phone: (202)944-3285 **Free:** 800-621-3141
Fax: (202)944-3295
Email: sbaa@sbaa.org
Website: http://www.sbaa.org
Cindy Brownstein, CEO

Fnded: 1972. **Mem:** 6,000. **Local Groups:** 75. **Desc:** Individuals with spina bifida; their parents, relatives, and friends; concerned professionals. (Spina bifida, or "open spine," is the second most common disabling birth defect and results in muscle weakness or paralysis and incontinence. Its cause is unknown and there is no complete cure.) Purposes are to: develop an information service of materials relating to spina bifida; conduct research into the causes of the birth defect; improve vocational training of individuals with spina bifida; monitor development of legislation applying to disabled persons. Promotes public awareness and action through national media; provides referral services; participates in appropriate legislative activities; holds seminars on scientific, social, medical, and educational programs. Provides training of competent personnel to aid in the treatment, care, education, adjustment, and rehabilitation of individuals with spina bifida. **Pub:** *Insights*, bimonthly. Booklets. • *Spina Bifida Insights*, bimonthly. Newsletter. Reports on the developments in medicine, education, and legislation affecting the problems and needs of persons with spina bifida. *Price:* Included in membership dues; $25/year for nonmembers; $40/year for professionals; $50/year outside U.S. • Pamphlets. • Reports.

★ 6144 ★ Spina Bifida and Hydrocephalus Association of Canada (SBHAC)
977-167 Lombard Ave.
Winnipeg, MB, Canada R3B 0V6
Phone: (204)925-3650 **Free:** 800-565-9488
Fax: (204)925-3654
Email: spinab@mts.net
Website: http://www.sbhac.ca/

Fnded: 1981. **Mem:** 1,000. **Reg. Groups:** 12. **Lang(s):** English, French. **Desc:** Dedicated to improving the quality of life for all individuals with Spina Bifida and/or Hydrocephalus and their families; promotes awareness, education, and research. **Pub:** *Update*, 3/year. Newsletter. Provides up-to-date Canadian issues.

★ 6145 ★ Spinal Cord Society (SCS)
19051 County Hwy. 1
Fergus Falls, MN 56537-7609
Phone: (218)739-5252 **Fax:** (218)739-5262
Website: http://members.aol.com/scsweb/
Dr. Chase E. Carson, Pres.

Fnded: 1978. **Mem:** 9,000. **Local Groups:** 170. **Desc:** Spinal cord injury victims and their friends and families; physicians, nurses, physical and rehabilitation therapists, and other medical professionals. Purposes are to promote research and increase public awareness concerning the potential for a cure of paralysis due to spinal cord injury. Focuses on the cure rather than rehabilitation for paralysis due to spinal injury. Promotes funding of reversal-oriented pure and applied medical research; encourages establishment of spinal injury centers in conjunction with existing hospitals and medical centers; maintains data bank of chronic spinal cord injury case histories, continuously monitored and upgraded for improving treatment, guiding research, and screening patients for referral to other physician s or to a spinal injury center. Through concentration on research, data, and treatment, seeks to provide a base of information, statistical analysis, and experience, with accelerated progress and minimal duplication of effort. Maintains medical center in Minneapolis, MN that applies state-of-art treatment to paralysis victims. **Pub:** *Spinal Cord Society Newsletter*, monthly. Newsletter. Includes convention news, letters, and information on services. *Price:* $30/year.

★ 6146 ★ Spinal Injuries Action Association (SIAA)
76 James St. Lane
London N10 3DF, United Kingdom

Fnded: 1993. **Mem:** 1,200. **Nat'l Groups:** 1. **Lang(s):** English, Irish. **Desc:** Individuals and organizations. Seeks to improve the quality of life of people with spinal injuries and their families. Makes available support and services; conducts educational and advocacy campaigns. **Pub:** *Spinal News*, quarterly. Newsletter.

★ 6147 ★ Spinal Injuries Association (SIA)
76 St. James's Ln.
London N10 3DF, United Kingdom
Phone: 44 20 84442121 **Fax:** 44 20 84443761
Email: sia@spinal.co.uk
Website: http://www.spinal.co.uk

Fnded: 1974. **Mem:** 6,500. **Local Groups:** 10. **Lang(s):** English. **Desc:** National organisation for individuals with spinal cord injuries. Provides assistance through: an information service that answers member queries on all aspects of daily living including specialist holiday and travel information; a personal assistance service which provides short term, emergency cover; a solicitors referral scheme, a counseling service; publications and bi-monthly newsletter. **Pub:** *Sexuality Booklets.* Booklets. Covers sexuality, including heterosexual men, heterosexual women, gay men, and lesbians. • *Spinal Cord Injuries: Guidance for General Practitioners.*

★ 6148 ★ Spine Society of Europe (SSE)
Seefeldstr 16
CH-8610 Uster, Switzerland
Phone: 41 1 9941404 **Fax:** 41 1 9941403
Email: schild@active.ch
Website: http://www.eurospine.org

Fnded: 1998. **Desc:** Promotes research, prevention and treatment of spine diseases and related problems.

★ 6149 ★ Spondylitis Association of America (SAA)
PO Box 5872
Sherman Oaks, CA 91413
Phone: (818)981-1616 **Free:** 800-777-8189
Email: info@spondylitis.org
Website: http://www.spondylitis.org
Jane Bruckel, Exec. Dir.

Fnded: 1983. **Mem:** 4,000. **Desc:** Individuals affected by Ankylosing Spondylitis, psoriatic spondylitis, spondylitis associated with inflammatory bowel/Crohn's disease, undifferentiated spondyloarthropathy, and Reiter's Syndrome; and their families and friends; health care professionals; scientific researchers. (Ankylosing Spondylitis is a chronic condition most often affecting those between 17-40 years of age and characterized by pain or stiffness in the back. Although the cause and cure are not known, the condition may be managed through a program of medicines, posture awareness, and regular, therapeutic exercise; it is believed to be a hereditary condition.) Disseminates information; promotes public awareness and research; conducts educational programs; sponsors national support groups. **Pub:** *A Family of Related Diseases.* Booklet. • *Back in Action.* Videos. • *Guidebook for Patients.* • *Juvenile AS.* Booklet. • *Physical Therapy Exercises.* Audiotapes. • *Spondylitis Plus*, bimonthly. Newsletter. Includes information on treatment, research, and coping with the condition. *Price:* Included in membership dues. • *Straight Talk on Spondylitis.* Book. • *The Water Workout.* Video. **Frmly:** (1993) Ankylosing Spondylitis Association.

★ 6150 ★ Sports Medicine New Zealand (SMNZ)
PO Box 6398
Dunedin, New Zealand
Phone: 64 3 4777887 **Fax:** 64 3 4777882

★ 6151 ★ Standing Committee of the Hospitals of the European Union (HOPE)
35 Kapucijnenvoer
B-3000 Leuven, Belgium
Phone: 32 16 336902 **Fax:** 32 16 336906
Email: sg@hope.be
Website: http://www.hope.be

Fnded: 1966. **Mem:** 22. **Lang(s):** English, French, German. **Desc:** Works to develop the range and continuing improvement of services provided by hospitals. Gathers and disseminates information. **Pub:**

Hospital Healthcare Europe, annual. Book. Official HOPE reference book.

★ 6152 ★ Standing Committee of the International Congress on Animal Reproduction (ICAR)
(Comite Permanent International du Congres de Physiologie et Pathologie de la Reproduction Animale)
Gunn Bldg., Rm. 346
Faculty of Veterinary Science
University of Sydney
Sydney, NSW 2006, Australia
Phone: 61 2 93513363 **Fax:** 61 2 93513957
Email: garethe@vetsci.usyd.edu.au

Fnded: 1948. **Lang(s):** English. **Desc:** Veterinarians and agricultural scientists with an interest in the reproduction of farm animals and wildlife. Seeks to develop new breeding and animal husbandry techniques to insure efficient propagation of livestock and conservation of wildlife. **Pub:** *ICAR Conference Proceedings*, quarterly.

★ 6153 ★ Standing Liaison Committee of EU Speech and Language Therapists and Logopedists
(Comite Permanent de Liaison des Orthophonistes-Logopedes de l'UE — CPLOL)
2, rue des Deux Gares
F-75010 Paris, France
Phone: 33 1 40356375 **Fax:** 33 1 40374142
Email: info@cplol.org
Website: http://www.cplol.org

Fnded: 1988. **Mem:** 21. **Desc:** Speech and language therapists in the European Union. Promotes high standards of conduct for members; equivalence of qualifications; harmonization of legislation relating to the profession and of initial training; exchange of scientific knowledge and research in the fields of logopedics.

★ 6154 ★ STEPS: Association for People with Lower Limb Abnormalities
c/o Ms. Sue Banton
Lower Ground Floor, Lymm Court
11 Eagle Brow
Lymm WA13 0LP, United Kingdom
Phone: 44 671 7170044 **Fax:** 44 671 7170045
Email: info@steps-charity.org.uk
Website: http://www.steps-charity.org.uk

Fnded: 1980. **Mem:** 2,000. **Reg. Groups:** 15. **Desc:** Provides information and support for families of children with lower limb abnormalities. Objectives are to put families in touch with one another, develops a network of local contacts providing support, help and advise and to gather and exchange information with parents and health professionals.

★ 6155 ★ Sterilized Suture Manufacturers' Association (SSMA)
Vauxhall Industrial Estate
Ruabon Rd.
Clwyd LL14 6HA, United Kingdom
Phone: 44 1978 823664 **Fax:** 44 1978 810669

Fnded: 1945. **Mem:** 4.

★ 6156 ★ Stickler Involved People (SIP)
15 Angelina Dr.
Augusta, KS 67010
Phone: (316)775-2993
Email: sip@stickler.org
Website: http://sticklers.org/sip/
Pat Houchin, Coord.

Fnded: 1995. **Desc:** Dedicated to early diagnosis and treatment of Stickler Syndrome; provides support, medical information and offers ways in which to cope. **Pub:** *Stickler - The Elusive Syndrome*, quarterly. Book. *Price:* $29. • Newsletter, quarterly. *Price:* included in membership dues.

★ 6157 ★ Stomatological Society of Greece
17 Kallirroes St.
GR-117 43 Athens, Greece
Phone: 30 210 9214325 **Fax:** 30 210 9214204
Email: stomsoc@otenet.gr
Website: http://www.mednet.gr/stomsoc

Fnded: 1937. **Mem:** 600. **Lang(s):** English, Greek. **Desc:** Dentists. Promotes dentistry in Greece. Provides members with the latest technological information. **Pub:** *Stomatologia*, quarterly. Journal. Includes English summaries.

★ 6158 ★ Stop Teen-Age Addiction to Tobacco (STAT)
360 Huntington Ave., Cushing 241
Boston, MA 02115-5005
Phone: (617)373-7828 **Fax:** (617)369-0130
Email: stat@exit3.com
Website: http://www.smokefreeair.org/Org/Orgdet.cfm?ID=2559
Judy Sopenski, Dir.

Fnded: 1985. **Desc:** Devoted to reducing the use of tobacco by children and teens through grassroots community projects, policy research, public education, advocacy, communication and counter-advertising. Trains and educates professionals, practitioners, citizen activists and policy-makers on research and activities in tobacco addiction, youth access and prevention. Offers a range of educational courses and consulting services under contract with private and public organizations around the country. **Pub:** *Community Organizer's Manual*. • *60 Years of Deception: An Analysis and Compilation of Cigarette Advertising From 1925-1985*. • *Tobacco-Free Youth*. Catalog.

★ 6159 ★ StopSIDS.org
1673 Rte. 9, Ste. 2
Clifton Park, NY 12065
Free: 888-521-9499
Email: info@stopsids.org
Website: http://www.stopsids.org/
Dr. Tracey Mulhall, Co-Founder

Fnded: 2000. **Desc:** Committed to research and education in order to end sudden infant death syndrome (SIDS) and other infant deaths; promotes health in babies and children through chiropractic-atlas correction and other healthy lifestyle choices. **Pub:** *The Best-Kept Secret to Raising a Healthy Child...and the Possible Prevention of Sudden Infant Death Syndrome (SIDS)*. Book.

★ 6160 ★ Stratis Health
2901 Metro Dr., Ste. 400
Bloomington, MN 55425
Phone: (952)853-8523 **Free:** 800-444-3423
Fax: (612)853-8503
Email: info@stratishealth.org
Website: http://www.stratishealth.org
Jennifer Lundblad, VP

Fnded: 1971. **Mem:** 3,500. **Desc:** Physicians interested in ensuring the availabilty of quality health care at reasonable costs. Evaluates health care services at hospitals, retirement homes, and other facilities. Develops health care standards for hospitals and offers consultation services to operators of health care facilities to improve efficiency in services. Conducts research and development on latest treatments and medical technologies. Tests new medical technologies.

★ 6161 ★ Stress and Anxiety Research Society (STAR)
c/o Krys Kaniasty, Dept. of Psychology
Indiana University of Pennsylvania
Indiana, PA 15705
Phone: (724)357-5559 **Fax:** (724)357-2214
Email: hodapp@psych.uni-frankfurt.de
Website: http://www.star-society.org/
Dr. Volker Hodapp, Pres.

Fnded: 1980. **Desc:** Researchers sharing an interest in problems of stress, coping, and anxiety. Promotes international and multidisciplinary analysis of stress and related topics. Serves as a forum for exchange of scientific information regarding stress; gathers and disseminates stress research results; facilitates cooperative research among members. **Pub:** *Anxiety, Stress and Coping*, annual. Journal. Contains reprints of research reports, theoretical papers, and interpretive literature reviews; includes case studies and other correspondence. • *STAR Newsletter*, semiannual. Newsletter.

★ 6162 ★ Stroke Association
240 City Rd.
London EC1V 2PR, United Kingdom
Phone: 44 20 75660300 **Fax:** 44 20 74902686
Website: http://www.stroke.org.uk

Fnded: 1899.

★ 6163 ★ Stroke Clubs, International (SCI)
805 12th St.
Galveston, TX 77550
Phone: (409)762-1022
Email: strokeclub@aol.com
Ellis Williamson, CPA, Pres.

Fnded: 1968. **Mem:** 12,000. **Desc:** Active members are stroke victims; associate members are individuals interested in the problems of stroke victims. To unite stroke victims for the purpose of aiding each other; to instruct them and their families regarding the nature of stroke and the means for overcoming the resulting handicaps; to aid them in finding employment; and to give the stroke victim hope and encouragement. At monthly meetings, qualified speakers discuss the medical aspects of strokes and member stroke victims discuss their progress and problems. Maintains list of over 1,000 clubs throughout the U.S. **Pub:** *Stroke Club International Bulletin*, annual. Bulletin. Includes book and cassette recommendations. **Frmly:** (1973) The Stroke Club; (1978) Stroke Club of America.

★ 6164 ★ Stroke Network
PO Box 492
Abingdon, MD 21009
Website: http://www.strokenetwork.org

Desc: Stroke survivors and caregivers. Promotes stroke awareness, provides support to stroke survivors, offers information for those suffering physical problems such as Central Pain and emotional scars. Offers Web Casts, private chat rooms, bookstore. **Pub:** Newsletter, monthly.

★ 6165 ★ Stroke Society of Australasia (SSA)
Level 11, 167 Queen St.
Melbourne, VIC 3000, Australia
Phone: 61 3 96701000
Email: admin@strokesociety.com.au

Fnded: 1989.

★ 6166 ★ Student American Veterinary Medical Association (SAVMA)
c/o AVMA
1931 N Meacham Rd., Ste. 100
Schaumburg, IL 60173
Free: 800-248-2862
Website: http://www.avma.org/savma/about.htm

Fnded: 1969. **Mem:** 8,000. **Reg. Groups:** 28. **Desc:** Seeks to advance science and art of veterinary medicine, including its relationship to agriculture and public health. **Pub:** *INTERVET*, quarterly. Journal.

★ 6167 ★ Student National Medical Association (SNMA)
5113 Georgia Ave. NW
Washington, DC 20011
Phone: (202)882-2881 **Fax:** (202)882-2886
Email: snmamain@msn.com
Website: http://www.snma.org
Annette McLane, Exec. Dir.

Fnded: 1964. **Mem:** 5,000. **Reg. Groups:** 10. **Local Groups:** 155. **Desc:** Medical students, residents, and undergraduates of color. Seeks to help students in recruitment, admission, and retention in medical school and publishes information on problems and achievement in this area. Conducts annual research forum and community service projects. **Pub:** *Journal of the Student National Medical Association*, quarterly. Journal. • *SNMA News*, quarterly.

★ 6168 ★ Student Osteopathic Medical Association (SOMA)

142 E Ontario St.
Chicago, IL 60611
Free: 800-621-1772
Email: webmaster@studentdo.com
Website: http://www.studentdo.com/

Fnded: 1970. **Mem:** 6,000. **Desc:** Seeks to improve the quality of healthcare delivery; contributes to the education of osteopathic medical students, aims to improve awareness of osteopathic medicine, and establish communication between healthcare professionals. **Pub:** *Student DOctor*. Magazine. *Price:* included in membership dues.

★ 6169 ★ Sturge-Weber Foundation (SWF)

PO Box 418
Mount Freedom, NJ 07970
Phone: (973)895-4445 **Free:** 800-627-5482
Fax: (973)895-4846
Email: swf@sturge-weber.com
Website: http://www.sturge-weber.com
Joseph G. Morelli, MD, Chm.

Fnded: 1986. **Mem:** 1,500. **Reg. Groups:** 21. **Desc:** Persons with Sturge-Weber syndrome and their families; concerned professionals and supporters. Serves as an information clearinghouse on Sturge-Weber syndrome, port-wine stains, and Klippel-Trenaunay Weber syndrome. (Sturge-Weber syndrome is a congenital neurological disorder characterized by facial port-wine stains, seizures, glaucoma, and loss of motor control, accompanied in rare cases by internal organ irregularities.) Disseminates information; offers support to afflicted persons. Maintains speakers' bureau; compiles statistics. Funds research. **Pub:** *Branching Out Newsletter*, quarterly. Newsletter. *Price:* $30/year; $40/year outside U.S. • Brochures.

★ 6170 ★ Stuttering Foundation of America (SFA)

3100 Walnut Grove Rd., Ste. 603
PO Box 11749
Memphis, TN 38111-0749
Phone: (901)452-7343 **Free:** 800-992-9392
Fax: (901)452-3931
Email: stutter@stutteringhelp.org
Website: http://www.stutteringhelp.org
Jane Fraser, Pres.

Fnded: 1947. **Desc:** Provides comprehensive materials, including videotapes, books and brochures, on stuttering to both the public and professionals. Seeks to bring together speech pathologists concerned with the prevention and treatment of stuttering. Provides referrals to speech-language pathologists specializing in stuttering. Provides support for research into the causes of stuttering. **Pub:** *Advice to Those Who Stutter*. Book. • *The Child Who Stutters: To the Health Care Provider*. • *The Child Who Stutters: To the Pediatrician, 2nd Ed.*. • *Do You Stutter: A Guide for Teens, 3rd Ed.*. • *If Your Child Stutters: A Guide for Parents, 5th Ed.*. • *The School-Age Child Who Stutters: Working Effectively with Attitudes and Emotions*. • *Self Therapy for the Stutterer, 10th Ed.*. • *SFA Newsletter*, quarterly. Newsletter. Contains SFA activities and information on stuttering. *Price:* Free. • *Sometimes I Just Stutter*. • *Stuttering and Your Child: Questions and Answers, 3rd Ed.*. **Frmly:** (1991) Speech Foundation of America.

★ 6171 ★ Sudden Arrythmia Death Syndromes Foundation (SADS)

508 E S Temple, Ste. 20
Salt Lake City, UT 84102-1013
Phone: (801)531-0937 **Free:** 800-STO-PSAD
Fax: (801)531-0945
Email: sads@sads.org
Website: http://www.sads.org
Alice Lara, Exec. Dir.

Fnded: 1991. **Mem:** 29,000. **Reg. Groups:** 4. **Desc:** Seeks to identify, help diagnose and help treat children and young adults who are genetically predisposed to sudden death by cardia arrhythmias. Supports patients, families and physicians dealing with Long QT Syndrome (LQTS) and other sudden death syndromes; educates medical personnel and the public about cardiac arrhythmias; supports genetic research; links individuals with similar concerns for support; establishes support groups. **Pub:** *Acquired Long QT Syndrome*. Brochure. • *Inherited Long QT Syndrome*. Brochure. • Newsletter, triennial.

★ 6172 ★ Sudden Infant Death Syndrome (SIDS) Alliance (SIDSA)

1314 Bedford Ave., Ste. 210
Baltimore, MD 21208
Phone: (410)653-8226 **Free:** 800-221-SIDS
Fax: (410)653-8709
Email: info@sidsalliance.org
Website: http://www.sidsalliance.org/
Judith S. Jacobson, Exec. VP

Fnded: 1991. **Local Groups:** 50. **Desc:** Unites concerned citizens, health professionals, and parents who have lost a child to sudden infant death syndrome (SIDS), a condition commonly known as "crib death" that accounts for about 6000 infant deaths annually in the United States. (Deaths of this type usually occur at night and during the cold weather months among apparently healthy infants generally under 6 months of age.) Although the common causes and methods of prevention have yet to be determined, recent research findings suggest an increased risk of SIDS for infants sleeping on the stomach, sleeping on soft bedding, exposed to smoke, or overheated. Serves as a central source of medical and scientific information about SIDS. Works to eliminate SIDS through research; Assists bereaved parents who have lost a child to SIDS; seeks to make the public aware of SIDS and related issues. **Pub:** *Synopsis*, periodic. Newsletter.

★ 6173 ★ Sufi Psychology Association (SPA)

PO Box 2221
Davis, CA 95617-2221

Fnded: NNfo. **Mem:** unding ,pro. **Desc:** Psychologists, psychotherapists, psychiatrists and researchers. Promotes Sufi Psychology. **Pub:** *SPA Journal*, semiannual. Journal.

★ 6174 ★ Suicide Information and Education Centre (SIEC)

1202 Centre St. SE, Ste. 320
Calgary, AB, Canada T2G 5A5
Phone: (403)245-3900 **Fax:** (403)245-0299
Email: siec@suicideinfo.ca
Website: http://www.suicideinfo.ca

Fnded: 1982. **Lang(s):** English. **Desc:** Information center whose users include researchers, educators, students, health care professionals, social service agencies, librarians, and the general public. Obtains and provides access to a comprehensive collection of more than 27,000 English language documents on suicide and suicidal behaviors. Provides information to all professions and public on specific topics such as adolescent suicide and bereavement. **Pub:** *Counselling the Bereaved: Caregiver Handbook*. Booklets. • *Reach Out With Hope*. Videos. • *SIEC Alert*, bimonthly. Bulletin. Provides information highlights on topics related to suicidal behaviors. • *Suicide Attempts*. Pamphlets. • *Suicide in Canada: Facing the Facts*. Pamphlet. • *Youth Suicide and You*. Booklet.

★ 6175 ★ Support Dogs (SD)

9510 Page Ave.
Saint Louis, MO 63132
Phone: (314)423-1988 **Fax:** (314)423-5564
Email: sdi@supportdogs.org
Website: http://www.supportdogs.org
Joan Pace, Exec. Dir.

Fnded: 1981. **Mem:** 15,000. **Desc:** Helps people with special needs achieve greater independence and improve the quality of their lives by providing them with professionally trained dogs. Breeding program produces Golden Retrievers, Labradors, German Shepherds, and selected crossbreeds. Dogs are prematched and custom trained for each individual and assist their owners with tasks such as: opening mall and house doors; pulling wheelchairs long distances and up ramps; loading wheelchairs into vehicles; retreiving a dropped or distant object; bringing the phone and operating an emergency assistance switch; rising to high counters to assist with business transactions. **Pub:** *Support Dog News*, quarterly. Newsletter. Contains education about service dogs. *Price:* Free. **Frmly:** Support Dogs for the Handicapped.

★ 6176 ★ Support Organization for Trisomy 18/13 (SOFT 18/13)

c/o Barb VanHerreweghe
2982 S Union St.
Rochester, NY 14624
Phone: (716)594-4621 **Free:** 800-716-SOFT
Fax: (716)594-1957
Email: barbsoft@aol.com
Website: http://www.trisomy.org
Barb VanHerreweghe, Contact

Fnded: 1979. **Mem:** 2,100. **Nat'l Groups:** 1. **State Groups:** 50. **Local Groups:** 1. **Desc:** Families, friends, and professionals involved with children born with Trisomy 18 or Trisomy 13. (Trisomy 18 and 13 are genetic disorders in which there are three no. 18 or no. 13 chromosomes rather than the usual two. The disorders are characterized by mental retardation, neurological problems, and respiratory and circulatory deficiencies, and occur in approximately 1000 births per year in the U.S.) Offers support, understanding, and encouragement to families of affected individuals. Provides the public with information on these conditions and birth defects in general. Makes available to families and professionals a file of medical information. Representatives participate in workshops, seminars, lectures, and group studies at universities and hospitals. Conducts surveys and compiles statistics about medical treatment and problems. Maintains speakers' bureau and placement service. **Pub:** *Care of Infant & Child with T18 & T13*. *Price:* $10.95. • *Soft Notes*, bimonthly. • *The SOFT Touch*, 6/yr. Newsletter. Includes reader's forum and chapter news. *Price:* included in membership dues; $25. • *Trisomy 18 - A Book for Families*. *Price:* $10.95. • *Trisomy 13 - A Guidebook for Families*. *Price:* $10.95. • Brochures.

★ 6177 ★ Surfer's Medical Association

PO Box 1210
Aptos, CA 95001
Phone: (831)684-0916 **Fax:** (831)684-0916
Email: smacentral@aol.com
Website: http://www.damoon.net/sma/
Paula Smith, Exec. Dir.

Fnded: 1986. **Mem:** 1,000. **Reg. Groups:** 2. **Desc:** Surfer-health professionals and surfers interested in the health and medical aspects of surfing. Works to educate surfers and medical practitioners on the unique health problems of surfers. Represents the sport of surfing in the fields of medicine and science and also works to preserve the environment of beaches and oceans. Established the first international network of surfing health professionals. Sponsors members' research in this field. **Pub:** *Collected Surf Works*, 1-2/year. Book. Three volume set of articles and information on surfing and health. • *Surfing Medicine*. Journal. Contains original articles, research reports, conference updates, etc.

★ 6178 ★ Surgical Association of the Republic of China
Department of Surgery, National Taiwan University Hospital
Taipei, Taiwan
Phone: 886 2 7642409 **Fax:** 886 2 7656630
Fnded: 1967.

★ 6179 ★ Surgical Dressings Manufacturers' Association (SDMA)
c/o Q.M.S.
70 Egremont Rd.
Milnrow
Rochdale OL16 4ES, United Kingdom
Phone: 44 1706 41035 **Fax:** 44 1706 41035
Fnded: 1936.

★ 6180 ★ Surgical Eye Expeditions International (SEE Int'l)
27 C-2 E De La Guerra St.
Santa Barbara, CA 93101
Phone: (805)963-3303 **Free:** 800-20T-0SEE
Fax: (805)965-3564
Email: seeintl@seeintl.org
Website: http://www.seeintl.org
Steve Roth, Exec. Dir.
Fnded: 1974. **Mem:** 756. **Desc:** Provides free sight-restoring surgery to indigent and disadvantaged blind individuals in the United States and throughout the developing world. Recruits volunteer opthalmologists, nurses, and technicians. Conducts charitable and educational programs. Provides children's services. Organizes ophthalmic skills exchange. **Pub:** *SEE Vision*, quarterly. Newsletter. Provides recap of programs for professional members. • Annual Report.

★ 6181 ★ Surgical Research Society of Southern Africa (SRSSA) (Chirurgiese Navorsingsvereniging van Suide Afrika — CNSA)
Department of Surgery, 9th Fl.
Medical School, Wits University
7 York Rd.
Parktown 2193, Republic of South Africa
Phone: 27 12 5214153 **Fax:** 27 11 4842717
Email: surgres@chiron.wits.ac.za
Fnded: 1972. **Mem:** 270. **Local Groups:** 5. **Lang(s):** Afrikaans, English. **Desc:** Surgeons and surgeons in training. Promotes research, particularly among younger members, in clinical and experimental surgery. Sets surgical research standards. Provides funding to surgery departments of South African universities; offers grants and scholarships; sponsors competitions. **Pub:** *Abstracts of Society Meeting*, annual. • *South Africa Journal of Surgery*, periodic.

★ 6182 ★ Susan G. Komen Breast Cancer Foundation (SGKF)
5005 LBJ, Ste. 250
Dallas, TX 75244
Phone: (972)855-1600 **Free:** 800-IM-AWARE
Fax: (972)855-1605
Email: helpline@komen.org
Website: http://www.komen.org
Susan Braun, CEO/Pres.
Fnded: 1982. **Mem:** 75,000. **Nat'l Groups:** 118. **Desc:** Breast cancer patients, health care professionals, and other interested individuals. Works to: increase the recovery and survival rates of breast cancer patients; heighten public awareness of the risks of breast cancer and the need for early detection. Establishes breast screening and training in self-examination procedures; provides funding through grants for research and screening programs. Sponsors educational programs. Bestows awards; sponsors competitions; maintains speakers' bureau. **Pub:** *Frontline*, quarterly. Newsletter. Highlights current breast cancer issues and Komen events. *Price:* Free. **Frmly:** (1989) Susan G. Komen Foundation.

★ 6183 ★ Swedish Association of Dietitians (SAD) (Svensk Dietistforening — SD)
St. Eriksgatan 26
Box 12069
S-102 22 Stockholm, Sweden
Phone: 46 8 59899102 **Fax:** 46 8 59899055
Email: info@dietisten.com
Website: http://www.dietisten.com
Fnded: 1921. **Mem:** 1,200. **Local Groups:** 20. **Lang(s):** English. **Desc:** Promotes professional, economical and social interests for the members; promotes development of dietetic profession; promotes training, education and work of dietitians; promotes international, professional contacts. **Pub:** *Dietisten*, bimonthly. Journal. A journal of dietetics and catering.

★ 6184 ★ Swedish Association for the Electrosensitive
Box 6023
S-102 31 Stockholm, Sweden
Fax: 46 8 7128948
Email: info@feb.se
Website: http://www.feb.se
Fnded: 1987. **Mem:** 2,000. **Lang(s):** English, Swedish. **Desc:** Individuals suffering from electrical oversensitivity or electrical hypersensitivity in Sweden (electrical oversensitivity and hypersensitivity are brought on from overexposure to electrical and magnetic fields emitted by appliances, particularly television sets and video display terminals). Supports afflicted individuals and works to stop the spread of these conditions; works to insure recognition of these maladies by insurance companies and government agencies; promotes research into the causes and cure of electrical over- and hypersensitivity. Organizes grass roots groups. **Pub:** *Ljusglimten*, quarterly. Magazine. **Frmly:** (1998) Swedish Association for the Electrically and VDT Injured.

★ 6185 ★ Swedish Association of Neurologically Disabled (Neurologiskt Handikappades Riksforbund — NHR)
Box 3284
S-103 65 Stockholm, Sweden
Phone: 46 8 6777010 **Fax:** 46 8 241315
Email: nhr@nhr.se
Website: http://www.nhr.se
Fnded: 1957. **Mem:** 15,500. **Reg. Groups:** 26. **Local Groups:** 90. **Desc:** Promotes the interests of disabled individuals affected by neurological diseases living in Sweden. Works to offer support services. **Pub:** *Handikapp-Reflex*, bimonthly.

★ 6186 ★ Swedish Association of Occupational Therapists (SAOT) (Forbundet Sveriges Arbetsterapeuter — FSA)
Planiavagen 13
Box 760
S-131 24 Nacka, Sweden
Phone: 46 8 4662440 **Fax:** 46 8 4662424
Email: fsa@akademikerhuset.se
Website: http://www.fsa.akademikerhuset.se
Fnded: 1979. **Mem:** 9,136. **Reg. Groups:** 31. **Lang(s):** English, Swedish. **Desc:** Union of occupational therapists in Sweden. Compiles statistics; conducts research and educational programs; negotiates working conditions and wages. **Pub:** *Arbetsterapeuten*, monthly. Journal. Contains information about occupational therapy and employment listings. • *Arbetsterapeuten Publicerar Sig.* • *FOU-Rapporter*, semiannual.

★ 6187 ★ Swedish Association of Registered Physiotherapists (Legitimerade Sjukgymnasters Riksforbund — LSR)
Vasagatan 48
Box 3196
S-103 63 Stockholm, Sweden
Phone: 46 8 56706100 **Fax:** 46 8 56706199
Email: kansli@lsr.se
Website: http://www.sjukgymnastforbundet.se
Fnded: 1943. **Mem:** 11,000. **Lang(s):** English, Swedish. **Desc:** Union of physical therapists in Sweden. Sponsors educational programs; compiles statistics. **Pub:** *Nordisk Fysioterapi*, quarterly. Journal. • *Sjukgymnasten*, monthly. Magazine.

★ 6188 ★ Swedish Association for Sexuality Education (RFSU) (Riksforbundet for Sexuell Upplysning)
PO Box 121 28
SE-102 24 Stockholm, Sweden
Phone: 46 8 6920700 **Fax:** 46 8 6530823
Email: info@rfsu.se
Website: http://www.rfsu.se
Fnded: 1933. **Mem:** 620. **Lang(s):** Swedish. **Desc:** Promotes sexual and reproductive health as a basic human right. Works to reduce the number of unwanted pregnancies and abortions. Attempts to stop the spread of HIV/AIDS and other sexually transmitted infections. Offers programs in sexuality, sexual and reproductive health. Provides contraceptive and health care services. Conducts research. **Pub:** *Ottar*, quarterly. Magazine.

★ 6189 ★ Swedish Dental Association (SDA) (Sveriges Tandlakarforbund — STF)
PO Box 1217
S-111 82 Stockholm, Sweden
Phone: 46 8 6661500 **Fax:** 46 8 6625842
Email: info@tandlabarforbundet.se
Website: http://www.tandlakarforbundet.se/eng
Fnded: 1908. **Mem:** 9,000. **Lang(s):** English, Swedish. **Desc:** Union of dentists in Sweden. Offers over 200 continuing dental education courses annually. **Pub:** *Swedish Dental Journal*, bimonthly. Journal. • *Tandlakartidningen*, 18/year. Journal.

★ 6190 ★ Swedish Dental Trade Association (Foreningen Svensk Dentalhandel — FSD)
Box 22307
S-104 22 Stockholm, Sweden
Phone: 46 8 50893800 **Fax:** 46 8 50893801
Email: fsd@branschkansliet.se
Website: http://www.dentalhandel.se
Fnded: 1989. **Mem:** 60. **Lang(s):** English, Swedish. **Desc:** Companies manufacturing dental equipment and supplies. Establishes international standards and technical harmonization for dental equipment. Represents members' interests before government bodies, international agencies, and the public. Maintains liaison with organizations representing dentists, dental technicians, and dental supply dealers and distributors. Compiles statistics.

★ 6191 ★ Swedish Gerontological Society (SGS)
c/o Marianne Winqvist
Department of Sociology
PO Box 821
S-751 08 Uppsala, Sweden
Phone: 46 18 4711484
Email: marianne.winqvist@soc.uu.se
Website: http://www.dfr.se/sgs
Fnded: 1998. **Desc:** Devoted to the promotion of research on the elderly and aging; aims to further the field of gerontology in the community, including fields of community medicine, history, nursing, pedagogy, political science, psychology, social policy, social psychology, social work and sociology.

★ 6192 ★ Swedish Hemophilia Society (FBIS)
Box 55507
S-102 04 Stockholm, Sweden
Phone: 46 8 54640510 **Fax:** 46 8 54640514
Email: info@tbis.se
Website: http://www.fbis.se/eng.asp

Fnded: 1964. **Mem:** 1,325. **Nat'l Groups:** 1. **Reg. Groups:** 8. **Lang(s):** English, Swedish. **Desc:** Individuals with hemophilia and their families; health care professionals and other individuals providing support to people with hemophilia. Seeks to improve the quality of life of people with hemophilia; works to advance the treatment of hemophilia and related disorders. Facilitates communication and cooperation among members; sponsors educational programs.

★ 6193 ★ Swedish Medical Association (Sveriges Laekarfoerbund)
c/o Dr.Anders Milton
Villagatan 5
PO Box 5610
S-114 86 Stockholm, Sweden
Phone: 46 8 7903300 **Fax:** 46 8 205718
Email: info@slf.se
Website: http://www.ronden.se/slf

Fnded: 1903. **Mem:** 36,500. **Reg. Groups:** 28. **Desc:** Union of physicians in Sweden. Advocates collective negotiations on physicians' employment conditions, health policy, and medical education issues. Maintains professional and specialist groups. **Pub:** *Laekartidningen*, weekly. Journal.

★ 6194 ★ Swedish National Association of the Deaf (SDR)
Magnus Ladulasgatan 63, 4 tr.
S-118 27 Stockholm, Sweden
Phone: 46 8 4421461 **Fax:** 46 8 4421499
Email: sdr@sdrf.se
Website: http://www.sdrf.se/sdr

Fnded: 1922. **Mem:** 6,000. **Nat'l Groups:** 1. **Reg. Groups:** 3. **State Groups:** 1. **Local Groups:** 48. **Lang(s):** English, Swedish. **Desc:** Deaf people, their families, and health care and speech and hearing professionals. Works to improve the quality of life of people with impaired hearing. Works to insure that the legal and economic rights of people with hearing impairments are respected. Conducts research and educational programs on sign language and other means of nonverbal communication. Serves as a liaison with other national and international associations with similar aims. Assists members in obtaining assistive technologies including text telephones, alarm services, and TTD messages. **Pub:** *Dovtidningen*, monthly. Magazine.

★ 6195 ★ Swedish Occupational Therapy Association
c/o Foundation for Scandinavian Journal of Occupational Therapy
Planiavagen 13, Box 760
S-131 24 Nacka, Sweden
Phone: 46 8 4662440 **Fax:** 46 8 4662424
Email: fsa@akademikerhusef.se
Website: http://www.tandfo.co.uk/journals/archive/socctoc.html

Fnded: 1993. **Mem:** 5. **Lang(s):** Swedish. **Desc:** Promotes scientific research by means of publishing activities within the area of occupational therapy. **Pub:** *Scandinavian Journal of Occupational Therapy*, quarterly. Journal.

★ 6196 ★ Swedish Psychoanalytical Society (Svenska Psykoanalytiska Foreningen)
Vasterlanggatan 60
S-111 29 Stockholm, Sweden
Phone: 46 8 108095 **Fax:** 46 8 108095
Email: spaf@spaf.a.se
Website: http://www.spaf.a.se

Fnded: 1934. **Desc:** Helps with referrals for psychoanalysis and psychotherapy; pursues research projects related to psychoanalysis, and arranges lectures for the public on psychoanalytic topics.

★ 6197 ★ Swedish Psychological Association (SPA) (Sveriges Psykologforbund — SPF)
Box 3287
S-103 65 Stockholm, Sweden
Phone: 46 8 56706400 **Fax:** 46 8 56706499
Website: http://www.psykologforbundet.se

Fnded: 1955. **Mem:** 7,500. **Desc:** Union of psychologists in Sweden.

★ 6198 ★ Swedish Society for Anaesthesia and Intensive Care (Svensk Forening for Anestesi och Intensivvard — SAFI)
Linkoping University Hospital
S-581 85 Linkoping, Sweden
Fax: 46 013 222836
Fnded: 1946.

★ 6199 ★ Swedish Society of Cardiology (Svenska Cardiologforeningens)
Karolinska Hospital
Department of Cardiology
S-171 76 Stockholm, Sweden
Phone: 46 8 51779286 **Fax:** 46 8 333962
Email: anders.waldenstrom@medicin.umu.se
Website: http://www.svls.se/sektioner/ca

Mem: 1,171. **Desc:** Promotes the study of cardiology in Sweden.

★ 6200 ★ Swedish Society for Dermatology and Venereology
c/o Dr. Desiree Wiegleb Edstrom, MD
Department of Dermatology
Karolinska Hospital
SE-171 76 Stockholm, Sweden
Phone: 46 8 51777852 **Fax:** 46 8 51777851
Email: desiree.edstrom@ks.se
Website: http://www.svls.se/sektioner/ssdv/

Fnded: 1901. **Mem:** 450. **Lang(s):** English. **Desc:** Dermatologists in Sweden. Represents members' interests. **Pub:** *Forum for Nordic Dermatu-Venereology*, quarterly. Newsletter.

★ 6201 ★ Swedish Society for Geriatric Medicine and Gerontology
c/o Dr. Gunnar Akner
Nutrition and Pharmacotherapy Unit A1:05
Department of Geriatric Medicine
Karolinska Hospital
Karolinska Institute
S-17176 Stockholm, Sweden
Phone: 46 8 6510129 **Fax:** 46 8 6511441
Email: gunnar.akner@chello.se
Website: http://www.svls.se/sektioner/age/

Fnded: 1999. **Mem:** 625. **Lang(s):** English. **Desc:** Geriatricians, physicians, nurses, and paramedics. Supports the development of Swedish geriatric medicine and gerontology. Formulates the core curriculum for specialist training in geriatric medicine and serves as a center for international cooperation regarding scientific and educational matters.

★ 6202 ★ Swedish Society for Pharmacology, Clinical Pharmacology and Therapeutics
c/o Prof. Paul Hjemdahl
Department of Clinical Pharmacology
Karolinska Hospital
SE-171 76 Stockholm, Sweden
Phone: 46 8 51775293 **Fax:** 46 8 308592
Email: paul.hjemdahl@ks.se

Mem: 320. **Desc:** Promotes pharmacology and clinical pharmacology and therapeutics in Sweden.

★ 6203 ★ Swedish Society of Psychosomatic Obstetrics and Gynaecology
Department of Obstetrics & Gynecology
University Hospital of Norrland
S-901 85 Umea, Sweden
Phone: 46 90 133071
Email: ann.lalos@obstgyn.umu.se
Website: http://www.ispog.org

Desc: Promotes the study of psychobiological and psychosocial, ethical and cross-cultural problems in the fields of obstetrics and gynaecology, women's health and reproductive health; facilitates the dissemination of new information in these fields. **Pub:** *Journal of Psychosomatic Obstetrics and Gynecology*. Journal.

★ 6204 ★ Swedish Society for Research on Ageing
Vasa Hospital
S-441 33 Goteborg, Sweden

Desc: Promotes gerontological research, training in the field of aging, and interests of gerontological organizations in international affairs.

★ 6205 ★ Swedish Surgical Society (Svensk Kirurgisk Forening — SKF)
Kirurgiska Kliniken, Akademiska Sjukhuset
S-751 85 Uppsala, Sweden
Phone: 46 8 7292000
Fnded: 1905.

★ 6206 ★ Swedish Veterinary Association (Sveriges Veterinarforbund — SVF)
Box 12709
S-112 94 Stockholm, Sweden
Phone: 46 8 54555820 **Fax:** 46 8 54555839
Email: office@svf.se
Website: http://www.svf.se

Fnded: 1860. **Mem:** 2,400. **Lang(s):** English, Swedish. **Desc:** Swedish veterinarians. Functions as a trade union and professional organization. Conducts continuing education courses for members. **Pub:** *Svensk Veterinartidning - SVT*, 15/year. Journal.

★ 6207 ★ Swimming/Natation Canada
2197 Riverside Dr., Ste. 700
Ottawa, ON, Canada K1H 7X3
Phone: (613)260-1348 **Fax:** (613)260-0804
Email: natloffice@swimming.ca
Website: http://www.swimming.ca

Fnded: 1909. **Mem:** 83,604. **Lang(s):** English, French. **Desc:** Promotes swimming as a recreational and competitive activity for Canadians, including persons with a disability. Conducts educational and training programs; sponsors competitions. Seeks to provide opportunities for every individual in the sport to reach his/her maximum potential in fitness and excellence. **Frmly:** Canadian Wheelchair Swimming Association.

★ 6208 ★ Swiss Association of Logopedics (SALCD)
Feldeggstrasse 69
CH-8008 Zurich, Switzerland
Phone: 41 1 3882690 **Fax:** 41 1 3882695
Email: sekr@salogopaedie.ch
Website: http://www.salogopaedie.ch

Fnded: 1942. **Mem:** 1,250. **State Groups:** 1250. **Lang(s):** English, French, German, Italian. **Desc:** Speech and hearing professionals and other individuals in related fields. Seeks to advance the study, understanding, and treatment of communications disorders. Conducts research and educational programs. **Pub:** *Mitglieder - Bulletin*, quarterly. Bulletin.

★ 6209 ★ Swiss Association for Nutrition (Schweizerische Vereinigung fur Ernahrung — SVE)
Effingerstr. 2
Postfach 8333
CH-3001 Bern, Switzerland
Phone: 41 31 3850000 **Fax:** 41 31 3850005
Email: info@sve.org
Website: http://www.sve.org

Fnded: 1965. **Desc:** Promotes the exchange of experience between the research sector and the people confronted with practical aspects of nutrition; aims to increase the knowledge of nutrition.

★ 6210 ★ Swiss Dietetic Association (Schweizerischer Verband Diplomierter Ernanrungsberaterinnen — SVDE/ASDD)
Geschaftsstelle
Martigny - Platz
Bahnhofsdr. 7B
CH-6210 Sursee, Switzerland
Phone: 41 41 9260727 **Fax:** 41 41 9260299
Email: service@svde-asdd.ch
Website: http://www.sverb-asdd.ch

Fnded: 1942. **Mem:** 850. **Reg. Groups:** 8. **Desc:** Professional dietitians. Promotes advancement in the study and application of dietetics; advises government agencies and the public regarding a healthy diet. Conducts research and educational programs. **Pub:** *Ernahrungs Info*, bimonthly. Magazine.

★ 6211 ★ Swiss Foundation for Sexual and Reproductive Health
9, avenue de Beaulieu
case postale 313
CH-1000 Lausanne 9, Switzerland
Phone: 41 21 6612233 **Fax:** 41 21 6612234
Email: info@plan-s.ch
Website: http://www.plan-s.ch

Fnded: 1993. **Mem:** 200. **Lang(s):** French, German. **Desc:** Promotes family planning and responsible parenthood as a means to improve the quality of life for individuals in Switzerland. Advocates family planning as a basic human right. Works to reduce the number of unwanted pregnancies and abortions. Coordinates members' activities; conducts research.

★ 6212 ★ Swiss Hospital Association (SHA) (H Die Spitaler der Schweiz)
POB
Lorrainestrasse 4A
CH-3013 Bern, Switzerland
Phone: 41 31 3351111 **Fax:** 41 31 3351170
Email: geschaeftsstelle@hplus.ch

Fnded: 1930. **Mem:** 729. **Lang(s):** English, French, German. **Desc:** Safeguards, promotes, and represents the political, economic, and legal interests of public and private hospitals, clinics, and nursing homes. Serves as a liaison between health care authorities, health insurers and facilities. Plays an active role in defining medical, economic, social, and educations politics within the Swiss system of public health. Develops guidelines for compiling medical and administrative statistics, quality management, performance assessment, and controlling. Operates a publishing house and two education centers. **Pub:** *List of Members*, periodic. • *Medizinische Gesamtstatistik der Schweizer Spitaler*. • *Schweizer Spital*, monthly.

★ 6213 ★ Swiss Institute for Experimental Cancer Research (Institut Suisse de Recherche Experimentale sur le Cancer — ISREC)
155 Chemin des Boveresses
CH-1066 Epalinges-Lausane, Switzerland
Phone: 41 21 6925858 **Fax:** 41 21 6526933
Email: relations.publiques@isrec.unil.ch
Website: http://www-isrec.unil.ch

Fnded: 1964.

★ 6214 ★ Swiss Society of Cardiology
Schwarztorstrasse 18
CH-3007 Bern, Switzerland
Phone: 41 31 3888090 **Fax:** 41 31 3888098
Email: info@swisscardio.com
Website: http://www.swisscardio.com

Fnded: 1949. **Mem:** 520. **Desc:** Promotes the study of cardiology in Switzerland, including heart failure and pacemakers. **Pub:** *Kardiovaskulare Medizin/Medecine Cardiovasculare*, 8/year. Journal. • Newsletter, 3/year.

★ 6215 ★ Swiss Society of Dermatology and Venereology (Schweizerische Gesellschaft fur Dermatologie und Venerologie)
Herman-Greulich-Str 70
CH-8004 Zurich, Switzerland
Phone: 41 1 2988921

★ 6216 ★ Swiss Society of Gerontology (Schweizerische Gesellschaft fur Gerontologie — SGG)
Spital Bern Ziegler, Postfach
CH-3001 Bern, Switzerland
Phone: 41 31 9707798 **Fax:** 41 31 9707767
Email: info@sgg-ssg.ch
Website: http://www.sgg-ssg.ch

Fnded: 1953. **Desc:** Organizes regular scientific conferences and post-graduate education and interdisciplinary collaboration in research and practical work.

★ 6217 ★ Swiss Society for Health Policy (Schweizerische Gesellschaft fur Gesundheitspolitik — SGGP)
Haldenweg 10 A
CH-3074 Muri, Switzerland
Phone: 41 31 9526655 **Fax:** 41 31 9526800
Email: info@sggp.ch
Website: http://www.sggp.ch

Fnded: 1976.

★ 6218 ★ Swiss Society of Pharmacology and Toxicology (Societe Suisse de Pharmacologie et de Toxicologie)
c/o Prof. Karl G. Hofbauer
Biozentrum
Abteilung Pharmakologie
Klingelbergstrase 70
CH-4056 Basel, Switzerland
Phone: 41 61 2671645 **Fax:** 41 61 2672208
Email: karl.hofbauer@unibas.ch

Mem: 350. **Desc:** Promotes pharmacology and toxicology in Switzerland.

★ 6219 ★ Swiss Society of Psychosomatic Obstetrics and Gynaecology
c/o Dr. Noemi Deslex-Zaiontz
Weisse Gasse 3
CH-4051 Basel, Switzerland
Fax: 41 61 2612576
Email: deslex@balcab.ch
Website: http://www.ispog.org

Desc: Promotes the study of psychobiological and psychosocial, ethical and cross-cultural problems in the fields of obstetrics and gynaecology, women's health and reproductive health; facilitates the dissemination of new information in these fields. **Pub:** *Journal of Psychosomatic Obstetrics and Gynecology*. Journal.

★ 6220 ★ Swiss Society of Radiobiology and Medical Physics (Schweizerische Gesellschaft fur Strahlenbiologie und Medizinische Physik — SGSMP)
Abt fur Medizinische Strahlenphysik
Hallerhaus
Inselspital/ Universitat
CH-3010 Bern, Switzerland
Phone: 41 31 6328429 **Fax:** 41 31 6322676
Email: charlotte.lichtsteiner@insel.ch
Website: http://www.sgsmp.ch

Fnded: 1976. **Mem:** 210.

★ 6221 ★ Swiss Tropical Institute (STI) (Bureau Appui Sante Environnement — BASE)
Socinstrasse 57
Postfach
CH-4002 Basel, Switzerland
Phone: 41 61 2848111 **Fax:** 41 61 2718654
Website: http://www.sti.ch/

Fnded: 1987. **Lang(s):** French. **Desc:** Swiss organizations and government agencies concerned with international development and relief operations. Promotes improved health and quality of life in Chad. Seeks to develop local administrative capacities to ensure sustained economic and social development. Facilitates cooperation among development agencies; works to increase awareness of development issues among people in developing areas. Makes available health care services; conducts training courses to enable local communities to maintain autonomous primary health care facilities. Monitors environmental impact of development programs.

★ 6222 ★ Systematics Association
c/o Dr. Zofia Lawrence
CABI Bioscience UK Centre
Bakeham Lane
Egham TW20 9TY, United Kingdom
Phone: 44 1491 829080 **Fax:** 44 1491 829100
Email: z.lawrence@.cabi.org
Website: http://www.systass.org

Fnded: 1937. **Mem:** 600. **Desc:** Aims to provide a forum for discussing systematic problems and integrated new information from genetics, ecology and other specific fields into concepts and activities. **Pub:** Newsletter, quarterly. Contains association news and events.

★ 6223 ★ Taiwan Motor Neuron Disease Association
Neurological Service
Veterans General Hospital
201 Shih-pai Rd., Sec. 11
Taipei 11217, Taiwan
Phone: 886 2 28743815 **Fax:** 886 2 28743814
Email: mnda2874@ms39.hinet.net

Fnded: 1996. **Desc:** Individuals in Taiwan affected by neuromuscular diseases. Provides a forum for support and exchange of information. Works to raise awareness of the benefits of home care. **Pub:** Magazine, semiannual.

★ 6224 ★ Taiwan Pediatric Association (TPA)
10-1F, No. 69, Hang-Chow S Rd
Sec. 1
Taipei 10022, Taiwan
Phone: 886 2 23516446 **Fax:** 886 2 23516448
Email: pediatr@pediatr.org.tw

Fnded: 1960. **Mem:** 2,600. **Lang(s):** Chinese, English. **Desc:** Pediatricians and others working in the field of pediatric medicine in 6 countries. Promotes the health and welfare of infants, children, and adolescents. Encourages research and teaching in the field; sponsors educational and scientific programs. Facilitates information exchange. **Pub:** *Acta Paediatrica Sinica*, bimonthly. Journal. • *Members' Directory*, triennial. • *Supplement*, semiannual. For the purpose of continuing medical education. **Frmly:** (2000) Chinese Taipei Pediatric Association.

★ 6225 ★ Talking Newspaper Association of the United Kingdom
10 Browning Rd.
Heathfield TN21 8DB, United Kingdom
Phone: 44 1435 866102 **Fax:** 44 1435 865422
Email: info@tnauk.org.uk
Website: http://www.tnauk.org.uk

Fnded: 1974. **Mem:** 18,000. **Local Groups:** 430. **Lang(s):** English. **Desc:** Records newspapers and magazine on audio tape, computer disk, or CD-ROM for visually impaired persons. **Pub:** *Talking Newspaper News*, quarterly. Magazine.

★ 6226 ★ Tanzania Diabetes Association
c/o Dr. Kaushik L. Ramaiya
PO Box 65201
Muhimbili
Dar es Salaam, United Republic of Tanzania
Phone: 255 22 2114991 **Fax:** 255 22 2113459
Email: diabetes@cats-net.com
Website: http://www.diabetesafrica.com/idfmembers.html

Desc: Represents people with diabetes. Promotes research and support of those with diabetes in Tanzania.

★ 6227 ★ Tanzania Society for the Blind
PO Box 2254
Dar es Salaam, United Republic of Tanzania
Phone: 255 51 460858 **Fax:** 255 51 460857

Desc: Seeks to meet the special needs of the visually-impaired in Tanzania. Offers educational, training, and rehabilitation programs.

★ 6228 ★ Tanzania Veterinary Association
Sokoine University of Agriculture
PO Box 3174
Morogoro, United Republic of Tanzania
Phone: 255 23 2604647 **Fax:** 255 23 2604647
Email: deanfrm@suanet.ac.tz

Desc: Promotes veterinary sciences in Tanzania.

★ 6229 ★ TASH (TASH)
29 W Susquehanna Ave., Ste. 210
Baltimore, MD 21204
Phone: (410)828-8274 **Fax:** (410)828-6706
Email: nweiss@tash.org
Website: http://www.tash.org
Donna Gilles, Pres.

Fnded: 1973. **Mem:** 6,300. **Reg. Groups:** 2. **State Groups:** 35. **Desc:** Teachers, therapists, parents, administrators, university faculty, lawyers, and advocates involved in all areas of service to people with severe disabilities. Seeks to ensure an autonomous, dignified lifestyle for all people with severe disabilities; advocates quality education, from birth through adulthood, for disabled individuals. Disseminates updated information on solutions to problems, research findings, trends, and practices relevant to people with severe disabilities. Provides information and referral service. **Pub:** *JASH*, quarterly. Journal. *Price:* Included in membership dues. • *TASH Connections*, monthly. Magazine. **Frmly:** (1984) The Association for the Severely Handicapped; (2000) Association for Persons with Severe Handicaps.

★ 6230 ★ TDI
8630 Fenton St., Ste. 604
Silver Spring, MD 20910-3803
Phone: (301)589-3006 **Fax:** (301)589-3797
Email: ExecDir@tdi-online.org
Website: http://www.tdi-online.org
Claude Stout, Exec. Dir.

Fnded: 1968. **Mem:** 55,000. **Desc:** Hearing impaired individuals and their families, and organizations participating in telecommunications over regular telephone lines through special equipment. Promotes equal access to telecommunications and media for individuals who are deaf, late-deafened, hard of hearing, or deaf-blind. Strives to constantly improve technology and accessibility for all who rely on visual telecommunications. Advocate for standards and compatibility for all telecommunication devices. Promotes closed captioning on television, cable, and the Internet. Seeks to extend the installation of text telephones (TTYs) in public buildings, railroads, airlines, bus terminals, and other places where they can be of service to the hearing impaired. Sells International TTY Logo Decals to the public. **Pub:** *Emergency Acess Evaluation Kit.* Manual. Contains emergency personnel training for use of TTY's and dealing with deaf and hard of hearing callers. *Price:* $35. • *GA-SK Newsletter*, quarterly. Newsletter. • *National Directory of TTY Numbers*, annual. Directory. • *Using Your TTY/TDD Videotape. Price:* $34.95. **Frmly:** (1980) Teletypewriters for the Deaf; (2000) Telecommunications for the Deaf, Inc.

★ 6231 ★ Teens Teaching AIDS Prevention (TEENS TAP)
3030 Walnut
Kansas City, MO 64108
Phone: (816)561-8784 **Free:** 800-234-8336
Fax: (816)531-7199
Elizabeth Spaur, Youth Outreach Coor.

Fnded: 1987. **Mem:** 300. **Desc:** Sponsored by the Good Samaritan Project. Provides teenagers with information on AIDS through peer counseling. Also provides information to interested adults. Maintains speakers' bureau for schools and youth groups. Provides companions for children and teens with AIDS and their families. Makes available training and technical guidance to groups interested in organizing teen peer education programs. **Pub:** Brochures. • Manuals.

★ 6232 ★ Tel-Med
24769 Redlands Blvd., Ste. L
Loma Linda, CA 92354
Phone: (909)478-0330 **Fax:** (909)478-3312
Email: telmed@ix.netcom.com
Website: http://www.tel-med.com
Michael Carpenter, CFO

Fnded: 1971. **Mem:** 200. **Desc:** Hospitals, medical societies, universities, medical centers, public libraries, and other organizations offering the Tel-Med program. Tel-Med is a library of three to five minute recorded health related messages created to be played over the telephone for public use, free of charge. Provides messages to communities; local libraries are established where individuals from the community can call to listen to messages. Operates as an information service intended to educate and assist in recognizing early signs of illness and is not designed to diagnose or treat medical problems. Scripts are written by medical professionals and examined by a team of physicians; messages are reviewed at least annually. Offers services and information on a wide range of medical subjects including alcoholism, arthritis, bee stings, cancer, diabetes, drug abuse, influenza, medical costs, mental health, nutrition, parenting, sex education, smoking, vasectomies, and vaginitis. **Pub:** *Tel-Med Newsletter*, quarterly. Newsletter. • Annual Report, annual. • Brochures. • Also publishes tape listings and literature on implementation of the Tel-Med program.

★ 6233 ★ Tenovus - Scotland (TS)
234 St. Vincent St.
Glasgow G2 5RJ, United Kingdom
Phone: 44 141 2216268 **Fax:** 44 1292 311433
Email: gen.sec@talk21.com
Website: http://www.tenovus-scotland.org.uk

Fnded: 1967. **Reg. Groups:** 4. **Local Groups:** 1. **Lang(s):** English. **Desc:** Individuals and organizations. Promotes advancement of medical research projects undertaken by Scottish hospitals and university medical schools. Provides financial support and other assistance to medical research programs. Conducts fundraising activities. **Pub:** Newsletter, semiannual. • Brochure.

★ 6234 ★ Terry Fox Foundation (TFF)
789 Don Mills Rd., Ste. 802
Toronto, ON, Canada M3C 1T5
Phone: (416)962-7866 **Free:** 888-962-5677
Fax: (416)924-6597
Email: national@terryfoxrun.org
Website: http://www.terryfoxrun.org

Fnded: 1981. **Lang(s):** English, French. **Desc:** Individuals and organizations. Seeks to "maintain the vision and principles of Terry Fox;" promotes and supports research into the causes and treatment of cancer. Conducts fundraising activities benefiting cancer research. **Pub:** Newsletter, periodic. • Brochure.

★ 6235 ★ Thai Psychological Association
Phayathai Rd., Pathumwan
Bangkok 10330, Thailand
Phone: 66 2 1899235 **Fax:** 66 2 189923
Email: mkakanan@chula.ac.th

★ 6236 ★ Thalidomide Society
c/o Ms. Vivien Kerr
19 Central Ave.
Middlesex
Pinner HA5 5BT, United Kingdom
Phone: 44 20 88685309 **Fax:** 44 20 88685309
Email: info@thalsoc.demon.co.uk

Fnded: 1962. **Mem:** 330. **Desc:** Provides support, advice and information to thalidomide and similarly disabled people living in the U.K.

★ 6237 ★ THEO BC
100-112 E 3rd Ave.
Vancouver, BC, Canada V5T 1C8
Phone: (604)872-0770 **Fax:** (604)873-1758
Email: tcostello@theobc.org
Website: http://www.theobc.org

Fnded: 1976. **Mem:** 36. **Lang(s):** English, French. **Desc:** Individuals working with people with psychiatric, emotional, and social disabilities. Seeks to improve the quality of life of people with emotional and psychiatric disabilities. Conducts vocational and educational programs to enable people with emotional and psychiatric disabilities to join the mainstream of society; sponsors charitable activities. **Pub:** Newsletter, periodic. • Bulletin, periodic. • Brochure. **Frmly:** (2000) Arbutus Vocational Society.

★ 6238 ★ Therapeutic Communities of America (TCA)
1601 Connecticut Ave. NW, Ste. 803
Washington, DC 20009
Phone: (202)296-3503 **Fax:** (202)518-5475
Email: tcanet@erols.org
Linda Hay Crawford, Exec. Dir.

Fnded: 1975. **Mem:** 100. **Desc:** Treatment and rehabilitation substance abuse programs in the U.S. and Canada. Therapeutic community (TC) programs blend primary care, counseling and social services with resocialization, milieu therapy, behavior modification, progression through a hierarchy of occupational training and responsibility with the TC, and community reentry. May include outpatient, day treatment, aftercare services, and prevention, as well as programs for individuals involved with the juvenile and criminal justice systems. Works with, and for, clients, their families, and their employers. Interacts with health agencies, federal and state governments, law enforcement, the judiciary, community organizations, business, labor, and media. Provides leadership for national and international conferences. Maintains staff code of ethics and offers counselor certification program. **Pub:** *Data Bank Updates*, periodic. • *Legislative Updates*, periodic. • Monographs. • Newsletter, bimonthly. • Proceedings.

★ 6239 ★ Therapy Dogs International (TDI)
88 Bartley Rd.
Flanders, NJ 07836
Phone: (973)252-9800 **Fax:** (973)252-7171

Email: tdi@gti.net
Website: http://www.tdi-dog.org
Ursula Kempe, CEO

Fnded: 1976. **Mem:** 7,000. **Reg. Groups:** 32. **Desc:** Dedicated to the regulation, testing, selection, and registration of qualified dogs and handlers for the purpose of visitations to hospitals, nursing homes, and other institutions where therapy dogs are needed. **Pub:** *Therapy Dogs International*, 3/year. Newsletter. *Price:* included in membership dues. • Brochures.

★ 6240 ★ Think First Foundation: National Injury Prevention Program

5550 Meadowbrook Dr., Ste. 110
Rolling Meadows, IL 60008
Phone: (847)290-8600 **Free:** 800-844-6556
Fax: (847)290-9005
Email: thinkfirst@thinkfirst.org
Website: http://www.thinkfirst.org
Michael S. Turner, Chm.

Fnded: 1986. **State Groups:** 20. **Local Groups:** 200. **Desc:** Works to educate young people about personal vulnerability and the consequences of risk taking behavior. Our goal is to prevent permanent brain, spinal cord, and other traumatic injuries. Conducts school-based educational programs, reinforcement activities, general public education and public policy initiatives. **Pub:** *Prevention Pages*, quarterly. Newsletter. • *Think First for Kids Curriculum Packet*. Instructional materials for children in grads 1-3. *Price:* $249. **Frmly:** (2000) Think First Foundation: National Injury Prevention Programs.

★ 6241 ★ Think Twice Global Vaccine Institute

PO Box 9638
Santa Fe, NM 87504
Phone: (505)983-1856
Email: global@thinktwice.com
Website: http://thinktwice.com/
Nathan Wright, Contact

Fnded: 1996. **Desc:** Provides parents and concerned individuals with educational resources to make informed vaccine decisions. **Pub:** *Vaccines: Are They Really Safe and Effective?*.

★ 6242 ★ Thyroid Eye Disease (TED)

Solstice
Sea Rd.
Winchelsea Beach
Winchelsea TN36 4LH, United Kingdom
Phone: 44 179 7222338
Email: tedassn@eclipse.co.uk

Fnded: 1989. **Mem:** 700. **Lang(s):** English. **Desc:** Endocrinologists, ophthalmologists, radiologists, and other health care professionals; people with thyroid eye disease and their families. Seeks to advance the diagnosis and treatment of thyroid eye disease. Promotes increased awareness of thyroid eye disease in the medical community. Provides information, care, and support to people with thyroid eye disease; provides financial assistance to thyroid eye disease research. Maintains medical helpline. **Pub:** Newsletter, quarterly. • Bulletin, periodic.

★ 6243 ★ Thyroid Foundation of America

410 Stuart St.
Boston, MA 02116
Phone: (617)534-1500 **Free:** 800-832-8321
Fax: (617)726-4136
Email: info@allthyroid.org
Website: http://www.allthyroid.org
Dr. Lawrence C. Wood, Pres.

Fnded: 1985. **Mem:** 4,500. **Reg. Groups:** 1. **State Groups:** 2. **Local Groups:** 1. **Desc:** Individuals with thyroid conditions; health professionals. Provides education and support for thyroid patients and health professionals; promotes public awareness of thyroid problems. Conducts educational programs. Operates referral service. **Pub:** *The Bridge*, quarterly. Newsletter. Reports on current research, articles of interest to individuals with thyroid disorders. *Price:* Included in membership dues. • Brochures.

★ 6244 ★ Thyroid Society for Education and Research

7515 S Main St., Ste. 545
Houston, TX 77030
Phone: (713)799-9909 **Free:** 800-849-7643
Email: help@the-thyroid-society.org
Website: http://www.neosoft.com/~thyroid/thyroid.html
Dr. Mario Maldonado, MD, Medical Dir.

Desc: Promotes public awareness about thyroid disease. Provides patient education materials. **Pub:** *Could It Be My Thyroid?*. Book. Contains reference information for thyroid patients. *Price:* $22.

★ 6245 ★ Tissue Banks International (TBI)

815 Park Ave.
Baltimore, MD 21201-4887
Phone: (410)783-0183 **Free:** 800-756-4824
Fax: (410)454-4457
Email: tbi@tbionline.org
Website: http://www.tbionline.org
Gerald Cole, Pres. /CEO

Fnded: 1962. **Mem:** 76. **Desc:** A non-profit network of medical eye and tissue banks. Provides eye tissue for sight-restoring corneal transplant surgery. Also distributes bone, skin, and other soft tissues. Assists members with operational areas. Provides grants for research into the causes and cures of blindness. Distributes information on eye, tissue, and organ donation. Conducts educational and charitable programs. **Pub:** Brochure.

★ 6246 ★ TMJ Association (TMJA)

PO Box 26770
Milwaukee, WI 53226
Phone: (414)259-3223 **Fax:** (414)259-8112
Email: info@tmj.org
Website: http://www.tmj.org
Terrie Cowley, Pres.

Fnded: 1986. **Desc:** Provides updated information on temporomandibular problems; serves as a support network to patients; educated health care professionals, policymakers, research investigators and the general public about TMJ diseases and disorders; advocated in the public and private sectors for quality research that will yield evidence-based treatments and prevention of TMJ diseases and disorders; communicates with members of Congress, government agencies, and other in a position to set agendas to ensure ongoing research on TMJ diseases and disorders. **Pub:** *TMJ Communique*, annual. Newsletter. Provides news and updates. • *TMJ Science*, annual. Journal. Contains meeting summary and recommendations.

★ 6247 ★ Tokyo Institute of Psychiatry (TIP)

2-1-8 Kamikitazawa
Setagaya-ku
Tokyo 156-8585, Japan
Phone: 81 3 33045701 **Fax:** 81 3 33298035
Email: webmaster@prit.go.jp
Website: http://www.prit.go.jp/

Fnded: 1973. **Desc:** Conducts research into the causes, pathophysiology, treatments, and prevention of mental disorders, including psychosociocultural psychiatry and biological psychiatry; seeks to maintain and improve mental health.

★ 6248 ★ Tonga Family Planning Association (TFPA)

PO Box 1142
Nuku'alofa, Tonga
Phone: 676 21209 **Fax:** 676 23766
Email: fpatonga@kailanet.to

Lang(s): English, Tongan. **Desc:** Advocates family planning and responsible parenthood as a means to enhance the quality of life for individuals living in Tonga. Promotes family planning as a basic human right. Works to stop the spread of AIDS and other sexually transmitted diseases. Offers programs in sex education, family planning, and health. Provides contraceptive and health care services. Conducts research.

★ 6249 ★ Touch for Health Kinesiology Association

408 N Main St., Ste. 202
PO Box 392
New Carlisle, OH 45344-0392
Phone: (937)845-3404 **Free:** 800-466-8342
Fax: (937)845-3909
Email: admin@tfha.org
Website: http://www.tfhka.org
Gloria Godsey, Exec. Dir.

Fnded: 1974. **Mem:** 1,500. **Desc:** International network of independent instructors comprising laypersons, medical doctors, chiropractors, osteopaths, nurses, teachers, physical therapists, massage therapists, and other professionals. Promotes techniques for restoring natural energies and improving postural balance through muscle testing using applied kinesiology and acupressure points to improve muscle function and balance the body's energy. Stimulates trained professionals to utilize natural health care research techniques with laypeople and their associates, and disseminates information on research plans, methodology, and results of self-development programs in health care, both mental and physical. Increases the level of professional confidence and keeps interested instructors, trainers, laypeople, and those in the health care profession regularly and reliably informed on development in natural health care. Conducts research projects on Touch for Health methods and results. **Pub:** *Annual Meeting Journal*, annual. Journal. Compilation of papers presented at the annual meeting. *Price:* $30. • *Keeping in Touch*, quarterly. Newsletter. Includes coverage of research developments, book reviews, calendar of events tips for professionals, anecdotal reports, news of upcoming events. *Price:* $250 full page; $150 1/2 page; $75 1/4 page; $35 business card. • *Touch for Health Association Directory*, annual. Membership Directory. *Price:* $125 full page; $75 1/2 page; $50 1/4 page; $35 business card. • *Touch for Health Book*. Book. Reference manual. *Price:* $27.95. • *Touch for Health Folios*. *Price:* $24.95 full size; $19.95 pocket size. • *Touch for Health in Practice*, monthly. Newsletter. *Price:* Included w/ professional membership. • *Touch for Health Reference Chart*. *Price:* $34.95. **Frmly:** (1990) Touch for Health Foundation; (1993) Touch for Health Association of America; (1998) Touch for Health Association.

★ 6250 ★ Tourette Syndrome Association (TSA)

42-40 Bell Blvd.
Bayside, NY 11361-2820
Phone: (718)224-2999 **Fax:** (718)279-9596
Email: ts@tsa-usa.com
Website: http://www.tsa-usa.org/
Fred Cook, VP

Fnded: 1972. **Mem:** 30,000. **Reg. Groups:** 5. **State Groups:** 50. **Local Groups:** 300. **Desc:** People with Tourette Syndrome (TS) and their families and friends; physicians, nurses, teachers, psychologists, social workers, and other professionals; organizations such as mental health agencies. (TS is characterized by involuntary muscular movements and utterances of sounds or words, and is often undiagnosed or misdiagnosed.) Develops and disseminates educational materials to families, professionals, and agencies involved in health care, education, and governments. Schedules meetings and seminars for professionals and families to explore the latest information on TS. Stimulates support for research into the nature and causes of the disorder. Apprises members of rights, services, and benefits provided by the government and other organizations. Provides lists of doctors experienced in treating the disorder. Operates support groups and other services to help persons with TS and their families. Maintains sources for advocacy referral services in the areas of education, employment, and housing. **Pub:** *Leadership Bulletins*, 4/year. Bulletin. *Price:* Free. • *Medical Letter: Summary of the Recent Literature*, annual. • *Tourette Syndrome Association Newsletter*, quarterly. Newsletter. Includes book reviews. *Price:* Included in membership dues. **Frmly:** Gilles de la Tourette Syndrome Association.

★ 6251 ★ Tourette Syndrome (UK) Association
PO Box 26149
Dunfermline KY12 8YU, United Kingdom
Phone: 44 1383 629600 **Fax:** 44 1383 629609
Email: enquiries@tsa.org.uk

Fnded: 1981. **Mem:** 995. **Desc:** Dedicated to providing support, education, and public awareness to the neurological disorder Gilles de la Tourette Syndrome; promotes medical research into Tourette Syndome.

★ 6252 ★ Toxoplasmosis Trust (TTT)
Edgebrook House
13 E Feltes Ave.
Edinburgh EH4, United Kingdom
Phone: 44 131 3325589
Email: info@toxo.org.uk

Fnded: 1989. **Mem:** 5,000. **Lang(s):** English. **Desc:** Aims to raise awareness of toxoplasmosis among health professionals and the general public. (Toxoplasmosis is a parasitic infection, which, if caught during pregnancy, can cause damage to the unborn baby.) Provides information and support to those affected by or concerned about taxoplasmosis. **Pub:** *Toxoplasmosis and Lambing: How to Avoid an Unnecessary Risk.* • *Toxoplasmosis in Pregnancy: Avoid Unnecessary Risk.* • *Toxoplasmosis: Information for People with HIV and AIDS.* • *Toxoplasmosis: The Facts.* Videos. • *The Toxoplasmosis Trust Trust Update*, periodic. Magazine. • *Toxopliasmosis & Your Pet Cat.* • Newsletter, semiannual. • Reports. • Papers.

★ 6253 ★ Transcultural Nursing Society (TCNS)
c/o Donna Barnes
Madonna University, College of Nursing
36600 Schoolcraft Rd.
Livonia, MI 48150
Phone: (734)432-5470 **Free:** 888-432-5470
Fax: (734)432-5463
Email: barnestcn@juno.com
Website: http://www.tcns.org
Donna Barnes, Exec. Asst.

Fnded: 1974. **Mem:** 400. **Nat'l Groups:** 1. **Desc:** Nurses interested in advancing transcultural nursing in education and practice. Seeks to discuss health care of diverse cultures, disseminate transcultural nursing knowledge, improve and maintain quality healthcare, and promote transcultural nursing policies, practices, and leadership skills. Supports and conducts research; provides consultation services. **Pub:** *Journal of Transcultural Nursing*, quarterly. Journal. *Price:* included in membership dues.

★ 6254 ★ Transplant Recipients International Organization (TRIO)
2117 L St. NW, Ste. 353
Washington, DC 20037-1524
Phone: (202)293-0980 **Free:** 800-TRIO-386
Fax: (703)820-3948
Email: triointt@saol.com
Website: http://www.trioweb.org
Elizabeth Rubin, Pres.

Fnded: 1987. **Mem:** 3,500. **Nat'l Groups:** 1. **Reg. Groups:** 6. **Desc:** Transplant candidates, recipients, family members, donor families, and medical personnel. Provides support and medical information to patients and their families. Conducts educational programs. **Pub:** *TRIO Lifelines*, bimonthly. Newsletter. Includes chapter activities and current transplantation news. *Price:* included in membership dues.

★ 6255 ★ Transplantation Society (TS)
Central Business Office
205 Viger Ave. W, Ste. 201
Montreal, QC, Canada H2Z 1G2
Phone: (514)874-1998 **Fax:** (514)874-1580
Email: info@transplantation-soc.org
Website: http://www.transplantation-soc.org

Fnded: 1966. **Mem:** 3,000. **Lang(s):** English. **Desc:** Physicians and scientists who have made significant contributions to the advancement of knowledge in transplantation biology and medicine. Purpose is to further information in the general area of transplantation biology and medicine, with related interests in cancer immunology and host responses to infectious microorganisms. **Pub:** *Transplantation Proceedings*, bimonthly. Proceedings.

★ 6256 ★ Trauma Foundation at San Francisco General Hospital
c/o Andrew McGuire
Bldg. 1, Rm. 300
San Francisco, CA 94110
Phone: (415)821-8209 **Fax:** (415)282-2563
Email: tf@tf.org
Website: http://www.tf.org/
Andrew McGuire, Exec. Dir.

Fnded: 1973. **Desc:** Dedicated to improving the lives of survivors of traumatic injuries and injury prevention issues and policies, including fire safe cigarettes, automobile safety, gun control and alcohol policy. **Pub:** Videos.

★ 6257 ★ Treacher Collins Foundation (TCF)
PO Box 683
Norwich, VT 05055-0683
Phone: (802)649-3050 **Free:** 800-TCF-2055
Email: hopecharkins@hotmail.com
Website: http://www.treachercollinsfnd.org
Hope Charkins, M.S.W., Exec. Dir.

Fnded: 1988. **Desc:** Families, individuals, and professionals interested in developing and sharing knowledge about Treacher Collins Syndrome and related conditions. (Treacher Collins Syndrome, also known as Franceschetti-Klein Syndrome, is a rare genetic condition involving underdevelopment of the structures of the head and face.) Promotes research to improve the quality of life of individuals with Treacher Collins Syndrome. Provides networking and support. Operates referral and resource listing service. **Pub:** *Adults with Treacher Collins Syndrome Talk About Their Lives.* Video. • *American Resource List.* • *First Things First: Early Issues for Children with Treacher Collins Syndrome.* Video. • *Genetic Update: Treacher Collins Syndrome.* Offers information about the discovery of the gene which causes Treacher Collins; diagnostic and pre-natal testing; and TCF position on the discovery. • *The Genetics of Treacher Collins Syndrome.* Video. • *Parents Talk About Treacher Collins Syndrome.* Video. • *The Psycho/Social Implications of Treacher Collins Syndrome.* Video. • *Rare Should Not Mean Alone.* Video. Covers Treacher Collins syndrome and the services of the foundation. • *The Surgical Creation of an Ear.* Video. • *Terminology List.* • *Treacher Collins Syndrome - An Overview.* Booklet. • *Treacher Collins Syndrome: Nutrition, Feeding, and Eating.* Booklet. • Newsletter, annual. *Price:* Donations accepted. • Pamphlet. • Also publishes a networking list. **Frmly:** Treacher Collins Family Network.

★ 6258 ★ Treatment Action Group (TAG)
611 Broadway, Ste. 612
New York, NY 10012
Phone: (212)253-7922 **Fax:** (212)253-7923
Email: tag-nyc@msn.com
Website: http://www.treatmentactiongroup.org
William Berger, Admin. Dir.

Fnded: 1992. **Mem:** 50. **Desc:** Individuals who are HIV positive and individuals interested in AIDS treatment research. Promotes AIDS research; advocates for research and treatment. Conducts educational programs. **Pub:** *Tagline*, monthly. Newsletter. Features AIDS research and policy. *Price:* $30/year. • Also publishes various reports on AIDS research and treatments.

★ 6259 ★ Triangle Club
2030 P St. NW
Washington, DC 20035
Phone: (202)659-8641
Website: http://www.triangleclub.org

Fnded: 1980. **Mem:** 1,000. **Desc:** Regular groups of Alcoholics Anonymous World Services specifically composed of gays and lesbians. Purpose is to serve the gay and lesbian members of AA and to provide advice and support to other members of AA. Works for unity and service with AA for the betterment of the gay and lesbian members and AA; advocates freedom in communication as an important aid to recovery. Provides alcoholism professionals with information about gay and lesbian AA groups for use in counseling lesbian and gay alcoholics. Assists in the exchange of recorded tapes of lesbian and gay AA speakers. **Pub:** *World Directory of Gay/Lesbian Groups of Alcoholics Anonymous*, annual. Directory. • Newsletter, 4/year. • Also publishes calendar of events and pamphlet. **Frmly:** International Advisory Council for Homosexual Men and Women in Alcoholics Anonymous.

★ 6260 ★ Trigeminal Neuralgia Association (TNA)
2801 SW Archer Rd., Ste. C
Gainesville, FL 32608
Phone: (352)376-9955 **Fax:** (352)376-8688
Email: tnnational@tna-support.org
Website: http://www.tna-support.org
Claire W. Patterson, Pres.

Fnded: 1990. **Mem:** 20,000. **Nat'l Groups:** 3. **Local Groups:** 50. **Desc:** Individuals with trigeminal neuralgia, a neurological disorder characterized by sudden attacks of pain along the distribution of one or more branches of the trigeminal nerve in the face and head, and related facial pain conditions. Works to increase public and professional awareness and understanding of the disorder. Provides a forum for discussion among individuals with trigeminal neuralgia in order to share information and experiences and offer support to patients and their families. Offers physician referrals. Conducts educational programs. **Pub:** *Striking Back.* Book. Comprehensive guide for the layperson about TN. *Price:* $14 plus shipping. • *TNAlert*, quarterly. Newsletter. *Price:* Free. • *Trigeminal Neuralgia - An Overview for Patients and Their Families.*

★ 6261 ★ Trinity Medical Center
2701 17th St.
Rock Island, IL 61201-5393
Phone: (309)779-5000 **Fax:** (309)779-2303
Website: http://www.trinityqc.com
William Leaver, Pres.

Mem: 110. **Desc:** Hospitals sponsored by a Lutheran church or bearing the title Lutheran. Offers periodic grants for the advancement of health care chaplaincy programs. **Pub:** *Lutheran Health Resources Directory*, periodic. Directory. • Newsletter, quarterly.

★ 6262 ★ TRIPOD
1727 W Burbank Blvd.
Burbank, CA 91506-1312
Phone: (818)972-2080 **Fax:** (818)972-2090
Email: info@tripod.org
Website: http://www.tripod.org
Christopher W. Opie, Exec. Dir.

Fnded: 1983. **Desc:** Established a private/public partnership with Burbank Unified School District to assist individuals who are deaf or hard of hearing. Offers educational programs. **Pub:** *Language Says It All.* Videos. • *We Can Do Anything.* Video.

★ 6263 ★ Tropical Health and Education Trust (THET)
24 Eversholt St.
London NW1 1AD, United Kingdom

Phone: 44 20 76798127 **Fax:** 44 20 76798190
Email: vpthet1@aol.com
Website: http://www.thet.org

Fnded: 1989. **Lang(s):** English. **Desc:** Medical training institutions specializing in tropical medicine. Seeks to advance the study, teaching, and practice of tropical medicine. Serves as a liaison linking medical education institutions in Europe and the developing world; sponsors research and educational programs. **Pub:** *THET Annual Review*, annual. Annual Report. Contains review of previous year's activities.

★ 6264 ★ Tuberous Sclerosis Alliance (TSAlliance)

801 Roeder Rd., Ste. 750
Silver Spring, MD 20910
Phone: (301)562-9890 **Free:** 800-225-6872
Fax: (301)562-9870
Email: mleongini@tsalliance.org
Website: http://www.tsalliance.org
Michael Coburn, Pres. /CEO

Fnded: 1974. **Mem:** 8,000. **Nat'l Groups:** 1. **Desc:** Encourages and provides grants for research into the diagnosis, cause, management, and cure of tuberous sclerosis. (Tuberous sclerosis is a genetic disease characterized by one or more of the following: epileptic seizures, mental retardation, behavioral problems, non-malignant tumors, or skin lesions.) Provides support to families affected by the disease through a nationwide network of volunteer area representatives and the distribution of informational packets. Conducts educational programs for medical and allied professionals. **Pub:** *Perspective*, quarterly. Newsletter. Contains research articles, resources for patients and parents, legislative news. *Price:* Available to members. • Also publishes brochures, fact sheets, patient journal, Life Stages Guide. **Frmly:** (2001) National Tuberous Sclerosis Association.

★ 6265 ★ Tuberous Sclerosis Association

c/o Mrs. Janet Medcalf
PO Box 9644
Bromsgrove B61 0FP, United Kingdom
Phone: 44 1527 871898 **Fax:** 44 1527 579452
Email: support@tuberous-sclerosis.org
Website: http://www.tuberous-sclerosis.org

Fnded: 1977. **Mem:** 1,450. **Desc:** Supports families and individuals affected by tuberous sclerosis. Raises awareness of the condition and to educate professionals, sufferers and the general public.

★ 6266 ★ Tunisian Society of Cardiology and Cardiovascular Surgery

BP 30
El Omrane
TN-1005 Tunis, Tunisia
Phone: 216 71 563181 **Fax:** 216 71 563181
Website: http://www.escardio.org/society/natsoc/tunisia.htm

Mem: 96. **Desc:** Promotes the study of cardiology in Tunisia.

★ 6267 ★ Turkish Association of Orthopaedics and Traumatology (TAOT) (Turk Ortopedi ve Travmatoloji Dernegi — TOTD)

I.U. Istanbul Tip Fakultesi
Ortopedi ve Travmatoloji
Anabilim Dali
Capa
TR-34390 Istanbul, Turkey
Phone: 90 212 5241053 **Fax:** 90 212 6352835
Email: info@aott.org.tr

Fnded: 1939. **Mem:** 1,300. **Lang(s):** English, Turkish. **Desc:** Medical professionals specializing in orthopedics and trauma care. Conducts seminars on orthopedic surgery. Offers postgraduate educational courses; conducts research. **Pub:** *Acta Orthopaedica et Traumatologica Turcica*, 5/year. Journal. Includes abstracts in English. • Books.

★ 6268 ★ Turkish Dental Association (TDA)

Ziya Gokalp Cad No. 37/11
Kyzylay
Ankara, Turkey
Phone: 90 312 4359394 **Fax:** 90 312 4302959
Website: http://www.tdb.org.tr/english.html

Desc: Works to improve dental health in Turkey. Fosters continuing education programs for dentists and other oral health caregivers.

★ 6269 ★ Turkish Neuroscience Society

Ege University School of Medicine
Department of Physiology
TR-35100 Ismir, Turkey
Phone: 90 232 3882868 **Fax:** 90 232 3746597
Email: nhariri@alpha.med.ege.edu.tr
Website: http://med.ege.edu.tr/~tns/

Desc: Promotes research and study in the field of Neuroscience. Conducts educational programs.

★ 6270 ★ Turkish Pharmacological Society (TPS)

c/o Prof. Meral Tuncer
Department of Pharmacology
Faculty of Medicine
Hacettepe University
Sihhiye
TR-06100 Ankara, Turkey
Phone: 90 312 3245468 **Fax:** 90 312 3105312
Email: mtuncer@hacettepe.edu.tr
Website: http://www.tfd.org.tr

Mem: 490. **Desc:** Promotes pharmacology in Turkey.

★ 6271 ★ Turkish Psychological Association (TPA)

Mesrutiyet Cad. 22/12
Kizilay
TR-06640 Ankara, Turkey
Phone: 90 312 4256765 **Fax:** 90 312 4174059
Email: bilgi@psikolog.org.tr
Website: http://www.psikolog.org.tr

Fnded: 1976. **Mem:** 1,600. **Reg. Groups:** 3. **Lang(s):** English, Turkish. **Desc:** Psychologists and psychology faculty. Represents the science and the profession of psychology in Turkey. **Pub:** *Turk Psikoloji Dergisi (Turkish Journal of Psychology)*. Journal. Includes empirical articles, review papers, and articles concerning national policies for psychologists.

★ 6272 ★ Turkish Society of Cardiology (TSC) (Turk Kardiyoloji Dernegi — TKD)

Darulaceze cad. Funye sok.
Eksioglu Is Merbezi, 9/2
Okmeydani
TR-80270 Istanbul, Turkey
Phone: 90 212 2211730 **Fax:** 90 212 2211754
Email: tkd@ixir.com
Website: http://www.tkd.org.tr

Fnded: 1963. **Mem:** 1,080. **Nat'l Groups:** 9. **Lang(s):** English, Turkish. **Desc:** Cardiologists and specialists in related fields. Promotes increased public and professional awareness of cardiovascular diseases. Encourages and funds cardiological research; gathers and disseminates information to members. Offers postgraduate course in cardiology. Conducts survey on heart disease and risk factors. **Pub:** *Archives of the Turkish Society of Cardiology*, monthly. Journal. Contains research work, reviews, and case reports. English summaries available. • *Congress Supplement for Abstracts*, annual. • Directory, biennial.

★ 6273 ★ Turkiye Multipl Skleroz Dernegi

c/o Sule Ozkaner
Buyukdere Caddesi
Hukukcular Sitesi No. 24/21
Mecidiyekoy
Istanbul, Turkey
Phone: 90 212 275 2296 **Fax:** 90 212 265 9420

Fnded: 1989. **Mem:** 750. **Reg. Groups:** 5. **Desc:** MS patients, families and professionals. Seeks to improve the quality of life for persons with multiple sclerosis and their families.

★ 6274 ★ Turner Syndrome Society of the U.S. (TSS US)

14450 T. C. Jester, Ste. 260
Houston, TX 77014
Phone: (832)249-9988 **Free:** 800-365-9944
Fax: (832)249-9987
Email: tssus@turnersyndrome.org
Website: http://www.turnersyndrome.org
Merriott J. Terry, National Exec. Dir.

Fnded: 1987. **Mem:** 7,000. **Local Groups:** 36. **Desc:** Persons suffering from Turner syndrome; families of persons with the syndrome; health care professionals. TS is a genetic disorder affecting females, causing short stature and cardiac, kidney and spatial motor perception problems. TS can result in infertility and incomplete sexual maturation. Seeks to increase public awareness of the medical and sociopsychological effects TS has on patients. Maintains speakers' bureau. **Pub:** *Turner Syndrome*. Brochure. • *Turner Syndrome: A Guide for Families*. Booklet. • Videos. • Newsletter, quarterly. Online.

★ 6275 ★ Turner's Syndrome Society (TSS)

21 Blackthorn Ave.
Toronto, ON, Canada M6N 3H4
Phone: (416)781-2086 **Free:** 800-465-6744
Fax: (416)781-7245
Email: tssincan@web.net
Website: http://www.turnersyndrome.ca

Fnded: 1983. **Mem:** 500. **Lang(s):** English, French. **Desc:** Individuals with Turner's Syndrome (a chromosomal disorder affecting women), their families, and health care professionals and organizations with an interest in the disorder. Promotes an improved quality of life for people with Turner's Syndrome; seeks to advance research into living with Turner's Syndrome. **Pub:** *Turner's Syndrome News*, quarterly. Newsletter.

★ 6276 ★ Uganda Association for the Mentally Handicapped (UAMH)

5 Kms. Bombo Rd. Off 200 m. Kawaala Rd.
PO Box 9177
Kampala, Uganda
Phone: 256 41 566404 **Fax:** 256 41 566404

Fnded: 1983. **Mem:** 548. **Nat'l Groups:** 1. **Reg. Groups:** 4. **Local Groups:** 18. **Lang(s):** English, Luganda, Swahili. **Desc:** Provides for the education and care of mentally handicapped individuals in Uganda. Seeks to increase public awareness of the needs of the mentally handicapped. Offers programs to increase self-help, leisure, and communication skills. Conducts research and periodic courses, seminars, and workshops; offers children's services. Organizes competitions including the Special Olympics and Very Special Arts. Operates placement service. Maintains vocational training and respite care programs. **Pub:** *Information to Africa Network - FEPAPHAM*, quarterly. • *Parent-to-Parent Help: Contact Service*, annual. **Frmly:** (1999) Inclusion Uganda.

★ 6277 ★ Uganda Diabetes Association

PO Box 16602
Wandegeya
Kampala, Uganda
Fax: 256 41 532591
Website: http://www.diabetesafrica.com/idfmembers.html

Desc: Represents people with diabetes. Promotes research and support of those with diabetes in Uganda.

★ 6278 ★ UK Public Health Association (UKPHA)
Holborn Gate, 7th Fl.
330 High Holborn
London WC1A 7BA, United Kingdom
Phone: 44 8700 101932 **Fax:** 44 207 4000122
Email: info@ukpha.org.uk
Website: http://www.ukpha.org.uk/

Desc: Committed to promoting the development of public health policy at all levels of government, across all sectors, and to support those working in public health both professionally or in a voluntary capacity. **Pub:** Newsletter.

★ 6279 ★ UK Sports Association for People with Learning Disability
Ground Fl.
Leroy House
436 Essex Rd.
London N1 3QP, United Kingdom
Phone: 44 207 3541030 **Fax:** 44 20 735425930
Email: office@uksapld.freeserve.co.uk

Fnded: 1980. **Reg. Groups:** 4. **Desc:** Develops lins with governing bodies of sports. Supports regional associations in developing sporting and recreational opportunities for people with learning disabilities. **Pub:** *Bulletin*, quarterly. Newsletter. Features information on sport and learning disability.

★ 6280 ★ Ukrainian Gerontology and Geriatrics Society (UGGS)
Vyshgorodskaya St. 67
254114 Kiev, Ukraine
Phone: 380 44 4304068 **Fax:** 380 44 4329956
Email: admin@geront.kiev.ua

Fnded: 1965. **Mem:** 500. **Reg. Groups:** 10. **Lang(s):** English, Russian, Ukrainian. **Desc:** Health care professionals treating the elderly; scientists and clinicians with an interest in the aging process and diseases of the aged. Promotes gerontological research and increased availability of gerontological care; facilitates training of gerontology specialists. Represents the interests of gerontologists and gerontological organizations. **Pub:** *Problems of Aging & Longevity*, quarterly. Journal. Contains biology of aging, clinical gerontology and geriatrics, social gerontology and gerohygiene. **Frmly:** (1963) Gerontological & Geriatric Society of the USSR.

★ 6281 ★ Ukrainian Medical Association of North America (UMANA)
2247 W Chicago Ave., 2nd Fl.
Chicago, IL 60622
Phone: (773)278-6262 **Free:** 888-RXUMANA
Fax: (773)278-6962
Email: info@umana.org
Website: http://www.umana.org
George Hrycelak, Exec. Dir.

Fnded: 1950. **Mem:** 1,000. **Nat'l Groups:** 1. **Reg. Groups:** 19. **Local Groups:** 1. **Desc:** Physicians, surgeons, dentists, and persons in related professions who are of Ukrainian descent. Provides assistance to members; sponsors lectures. Maintains placement service, museum, biographical and medical archives, and library of 1800 medical books and journals in Ukrainian. **Pub:** *Journal of the Ukrainian Medical Association of North America (JUMANA)*, quarterly. Journal. Contains medical research articles and news. *Price:* Free to members; $10 otherwise. • *Newsletter to Membership*, quarterly. Newsletter. • *Umana News.* **Frmly:** American Ukrainian Medical Society.

★ 6282 ★ Ukrainian Society of Cardiology
Institute of Cardiology
5 Narodnoje Opolchenje St.
252151 Kiev, Ukraine
Phone: 380 44 2776622 **Fax:** 380 44 2774209
Email: alex@cardio.pp.kiev.ua
Website: http://www.rql.kiev.ua/cardio_j

Mem: 91. **Desc:** Promotes the study of cardiology in Ukraine. **Pub:** *Ukrainian Journal of Cardiology*, bimonthly.

★ 6283 ★ Ulster Cancer Foundation (UCF)
40-42 Eglantine Ave.
Belfast BT9 6DX, United Kingdom
Phone: 44 28 90663281 **Fax:** 44 28 90660081
Email: info@ulstercancer.org
Website: http://www.ulstercancer.org

Fnded: 1970. **Local Groups:** 60. **Lang(s):** English. **Desc:** Encourages and facilitates research on cancer and its prevention and early diagnosis. Seeks to help patients and their families cope with cancer. Works for new and better treatments for cancer, helps people reduce their risk of developing the disease. Conducts educational programs including clinics and training sessions for health care professionals; makes available children's services; sponsors competitions and bestows awards. Compiles statistics. **Pub:** *Cancer Control in Practice*. Book. A training and resource park for practice nurses. • *Cancer Education and Care in the Workplace*. Book. • *Environmental Health Perspectives on Cancer.* • *Focus on Cancer in Schools.* • *Smoking Matters for Young People.*

★ 6284 ★ UNAIDS - Joint United Nations Programme on HIV/AIDS
20, avenue Appia
CH-1211 Geneva 27, Switzerland
Phone: 41 22 7913666 **Fax:** 41 22 7914187
Email: unaids@unaids.org
Website: http://www.unaids.org

Fnded: 1995. **Lang(s):** English, French, German, Italian. **Desc:** Health care personnel and other individuals and organizations interested in stopping the global AIDS epidemic. Seeks to reduce the suffering of people with HIV and AIDS; works to "counter the impact of the pandemic on individuals, communities, and societies." Conducts educational programs in areas including AIDS prevention and treatment; makes available health and social services to people with HIV and AIDS.

★ 6285 ★ Undersea and Hyperbaric Medical Society (UHMS)
10531 Metropolitan Ave.
Kensington, MD 20895
Phone: (301)942-2980 **Fax:** (301)942-7804
Email: uhms@uhms.org
Website: http://www.uhms.org
Donald R. Chandler, Exec. Dir.

Fnded: 1967. **Mem:** 2,500. **Reg. Groups:** 4. **Desc:** Diving physiologists, physicians, biologists, and bioengineers with subsea or hyperbaric interests. Seeks to: develop and advance undersea and hyperbaric medicine and its supporting sciences; provide channels of scientific communication among researchers dedicated to the safe penetration of the oceans by man; disseminate information on diving problems. Conducts courses on diving medicine for physicians. **Pub:** *Case Histories of Diving and Hyperbaric Accidents.* • *Directory of Hyperbaric Chambers.* • *Diving Accident Management.* • *Diving Physiology in Plain English.* • *Fitness to Dive.* • *Flying After Diving.* • *Handbook and Membership Directory*, biennial. Directory. • *Hyperbaric Oxygen Therapy: A Committee Report.* • *Journal: Undersea & Hyperbaric Medicine*, quarterly. Journal. *Price:* $85. • *Key Documents of the Biomedical Aspects of Deep Diving.* • *Near Drowning.* • *Pressure*, bimonthly. Newsletter. Includes book reviews and obituaries. *Price:* $30/year. • *Treatment of Decompression Illness.* • *Underwater and Hyperbaric Medicine: Abstracts from the Literature*, bimonthly. *Price:* $100. • *Women in Diving.* • Are Asmatics Fit to Dive **Frmly:** (1986) Undersea Medical Society.

★ 6286 ★ Uniformed Services Academy of Family Physicians (USAFP)
2301 N Parham Rd., Ste. 4
Richmond, VA 23229
Phone: (804)968-4436 **Fax:** (804)968-4418
Email: fpnet@msn.com
Website: http://www.usafp.org/
Christy Duncan, Asst. Exec. Dir.

Fnded: 1973. **Mem:** 2,000. **Desc:** Family physicians, teachers of family medicine, medical students, and residents in the armed services, public health service, or Indian health service. Sponsors continuing education program. Sponsors educational programs.

★ 6287 ★ Union of American Physicians and Dentists (UAPD)
1330 Broadway, Ste. 730
Oakland, CA 94612
Phone: (510)839-0193 **Free:** 800-622-0909
Fax: (510)763-8756
Email: uapd@uapd.com
Website: http://www.uapd.com
Gary Robinson, Exec. Dir.

Fnded: 1972. **Mem:** 10,000. **Nat'l Groups:** 1. **Reg. Groups:** 1. **State Groups:** 1. **Local Groups:** 3. **Desc:** Independent national labor organization made up of self-employed medical doctors and dentists as well as those employed by hospitals, teaching institutions, counties, and municipalities. Seeks to: provide optimum medical care for the people; ensure quality facilities for the provision of medical care; enable physicians to give of themselves, unhindered by extraneous forces, for the welfare of their patients; ensure reasonable compensation for physicians commensurate with their training, skill, and the responsibility they bear for the life and health of their fellow human beings. **Pub:** *UAPD Report*, monthly. Newsletter. *Price:* Free with membership. • Also publishes materials on socioeconomic issues. **Frmly:** Union of American Physicians and Dentists.

★ 6288 ★ Union of the Deaf in Bulgaria
12-14 Denkooglu St.
BG-1000 Sofia, Bulgaria
Phone: 359 2 9804778 **Fax:** 359 2 9801696
Email: sgb@i-n.net

Fnded: 1934. **Mem:** 8,800. **Desc:** Promotes and protects members' cultural, educational, and social interests. **Pub:** *Tishina*, semimonthly. Newspaper. Reflects the problems of the deaf in Bulgaria and worldwide.

★ 6289 ★ Union of Disabled People in Bulgaria
Ghristo Belchev 21
BG-1000 Sofia, Bulgaria
Phone: 359 2 819016 **Fax:** 359 2 807601

Fnded: 1989. **Mem:** 30,000. **Desc:** Defends the interests of disabled persons. **Pub:** *Bulletin*, monthly. • *Kurazh*, periodic.

★ 6290 ★ Union of Estonian Emergency Medical Services (Eesti Kiirabi Liit)
Riia 18
EE-51010 Tartu, Estonia
Phone: 372 7 408804 **Fax:** 372 7 408809
Email: ekliit@pb.uninet.ee
Website: http://www.kiirabi.ee

Fnded: 1992. **Mem:** 1,118. **Reg. Groups:** 50. **Lang(s):** Estonian. **Desc:** Organizations and individuals providing emergency medical services; members of other medical specialty associations. Assists members in clarifying their rights and responsibilities under the present Estonian healthcare system. Represents the interests of EMS providers. Participates in training for EMS providers. Certifies emergency healthcare providers. Provides first aid training to the public. **Frmly:** Estonian First Medical Aid Association.

★ 6291 ★ Union of Estonian Psychologists (Eesti Psunholologide Liit)
PO Box 572
EE-11002 Tallinn, Estonia

Phone: 372 6 409476 **Fax:** 372 6 409475
Email: tniit@tpu.ee

Fnded: 1988. **Mem:** 73. **Desc:** Seeks to advance psychological science and practice in Estonia. **Pub:** Newsletter, periodic.

★ 6292 ★ Union of Middle Eastern and Mediterranean Pediatric Societies (UMEMPS) (Union des Societes de Pediatrie du Moyen-Orient et de la Mediterranee — USPMOM)

c/o Prof. T. Thomaidis
Milioni 6
GR-106 73 Athens, Greece
Phone: 30 1 3615168 **Fax:** 30 1 3615168

Fnded: 1966. **Mem:** 23. **Nat'l Groups:** 26. **Reg. Groups:** 1. **Lang(s):** English, French. **Desc:** National societies of pediatricians and pediatric surgeons.

★ 6293 ★ Union of Veterinarians in Bulgaria

15A P. Slaveikov Ave.
BG-1606 Sofia, Bulgaria
Phone: 359 2 513243 **Fax:** 359 2 542925

Fnded: 1893. **Mem:** 2,500. **Reg. Groups:** 36. **Local Groups:** 56. **Lang(s):** Bulgarian, English, Russian. **Desc:** Promotes and protects members' interests. **Pub:** *Veterinarna Zbirka*, monthly. Journal.

★ 6294 ★ Unione Nazionale Industrie Dentarie Italiane (UNDI)

Via Tamburini 2
I-20123 Milan, Italy
Phone: 39 02 7006121 **Fax:** 39 02 70006546
Email: foreignoffice@unidi.it

Fnded: 1969. **Mem:** 132. **Lang(s):** Dutch, English, French, German, Italian, Portuguese, Spanish. **Desc:** Companies manufacturing dental equipment and supplies. Establishes international standards and technical harmonization for dental equipment. Represents members' interests before government bodies, international agencies, and the public. Maintains liaison with organizations representing dentists, dental technicians, and dental supply dealers and distributors. Compiles statistics. **Pub:** *Unidipress*, bimonthly. Magazine.

★ 6295 ★ United Amputee Services Association

c/o Jim Moore, Dir.
PO Box 4277
Winter Park, FL 32793
Phone: (407)678-2920 **Fax:** (407)678-2203
Email: unitedamp@aol.com
Website: http://www.oandp.com/resources/organizations/uasa/index.htm
Kathy Hogan, Office Mgr.

Fnded: 1980. **Mem:** 400. **Desc:** Provides support and education to amputees and their families. **Pub:** *A Survivor's Guide for the Recent Amputee*. Booklet. Provides pertinent information regarding amputation. *Price:* $5 shipping and handling. • *Amputee Review*, quarterly. Newsletter. *Price:* included in membership dues.

★ 6296 ★ United Cerebral Palsy Associations (UCP)

1660 L St. NW, Ste. 700
Washington, DC 20036
Phone: (202)776-0406 **Free:** 800-USA-5UCP
Fax: (202)776-0414
Email: national@ucp.org
Website: http://www.ucp.org
E. Hal Nolan, Pres.

Fnded: 1949. **Mem:** 110. **Desc:** Voluntary national federation of state and local affiliates aiding persons with cerebral palsy and other disabilities, and their families. Goals are to prevent cerebral palsy, minimize its effects, and improve the quality of life for persons with cerebral palsy and other disabilities, and their families. Supports research and traineeships for medical and allied personnel; sponsors professional and public education in the prevention and management of cerebral palsy; cooperates with governmental and other agencies concerned with the welfare of persons with disabilities; acts as an advocate on the federal, state, and local levels for the civil rights of people with cerebral palsy and other disabilities, and their families. Establishes standards and promotes national accreditation of UCP affiliates; undertakes demonstration projects to establish models of exemplary community services for persons with cerebral palsy and other disabilities. Services provided by local and state affiliates include: medical, therapeutic, and social services for people with cerebral palsy and individuals with similar service needs; career development training; special education programs; recreational opportunities for children and adults; early intervention and assistive technology programs; family counseling services for parents of children with disabilities; personal assistance services; accessible and supported housing facilities where people with disabilities may live independently. **Pub:** *UCP Is Us*, bimonthly. Newsletter. Internal newsletter. • *Washington Watch*, biweekly. Newsletter. Electronic Newsletter. **Frmly:** (1949) National Foundation for Cerebral Palsy.

★ 6297 ★ United Cerebral Palsy Research and Educational Foundation (UCPREF)

1660 L St. NW, Ste. 700
Washington, DC 20036-5602
Phone: (202)776-0406 **Free:** 800-USA-5UCP
Fax: (202)776-0414
Email: national@ucp.org
Website: http://www.ucp.org
Pat Sandusky, Exec. Dir.

Fnded: 1955. **Desc:** Sponsors research directly related to the prevention of cerebral palsy and to improvement in the quality of life of persons with cerebral palsy and related developmental disorders. **Pub:** *Research Fact Sheets*, monthly. • Also publishes medical directors' reports and a foundation brochure.

★ 6298 ★ United European Gastroenterology Federation (UEGF)

c/o Prof. Juan R. Malagelada
Hospital General Vall d'Hebron
Pg. Val d'Hebron, 119-129
E-08035 Barcelona, Spain
Phone: 34 93 4281883 **Fax:** 34 93 2096205
Email: ega_uegf@ega.it
Website: http://www.uegf.org

Fnded: 1988. **Desc:** Promotes exchange of information in the field of gastroenterology.

★ 6299 ★ United Kingdom Council for Psychotherapy

167-169 Great Portland St.
London W1N 5PF, United Kingdom
Phone: 44 20 74363002 **Fax:** 44 20 74363013
Email: ukcp@psychotherapy.org.uk
Website: http://www.psychotherapy.org.uk

Fnded: 1989. **Mem:** 79. **Desc:** Psychotherapy organisations. The protection of the public by the promotion of appropriate standards for training, research, education and the practice of psychotherapy and by the dissemination of information. The publication of a register of psychotherapists. Liaison with Government and the European Commission as necessary. **Pub:** *Directory of Member Organisations*, annual. Directory. • *National Register of Psychotherapists*, annual.

★ 6300 ★ United Kingdom Home Care Association

42B Banstead Rd.
Carshalton Beeches SM5 3NW, United Kingdom
Phone: 44 20 82881551 **Fax:** 44 20 82881550
Email: enquiries@ukhca.co.uk
Website: http://www.ukhca.co.uk

Fnded: 1988. **Mem:** 1,300. **Lang(s):** English. **Desc:** Represents independent home care organizations providing home care and nursing care to people in their own homes. Identifies and promotes the highest standards of home care. **Pub:** *Home Care Workers Handbook*. Handbook. • *The Homecarer*, bimonthly. Newsletter.

★ 6301 ★ United Leukodystrophy Foundation (ULF)

2304 Highland Dr.
Sycamore, IL 60178
Phone: (815)895-3211 **Free:** 800-728-5483
Fax: (815)895-2432
Email: ulf@tbcnet.com
Website: http://www.ulf.org
Ron Brazeal, Exec. Dir.

Fnded: 1982. **Mem:** 12,000. **Desc:** Leukodystrophy patients, their families, and medical care professionals. (Leukodystrophy refers to a group of disorders which affect the brain, spinal cord, and peripheral nerves by damaging the insulating sheath around nerve strands, interfering with the flow of electrical impulses.) Provides information on leukodystrophy to patients, their families, and the general public; assists in identifying sources of medical care, social services, and counseling; coordinates a communication network among affected families. Promotes and supports research into the causes, treatment, and prevention of white matter disorders. Coordinates cooperation between donor and government agencies, scientific programs, and the private sector. Conducts educational and research programs. Offers second opinion program for those with undiagnosed white matter disorders. **Pub:** *The Facts About Leukodystrophy*. Brochures. • *ULF News*, quarterly. Newsletter. *Price:* Included in membership dues. • *What to Expect When the Diagnosis is a Neurodegenerative Disease*. Booklet.

★ 6302 ★ United Methodist Association of Health and Welfare Ministries (UMA)

601 W Riverview Ave.
Dayton, OH 45406-5543
Phone: (937)227-9494 **Free:** 800-411-9901
Fax: (937)222-7364
Email: nterry@umassociation.org
Website: http://www.umassociation.org
Mr. Dean W. Pulliam, CAE, CEO/Pres.

Fnded: 1940. **Mem:** 400. **Desc:** Membership association for 400 United Methodist related hospitals, retirement homes, community based ministries, youth and family service organizations, children's homes, churches, and individuals. Offers communications and church relations guidance. Provides leadership development training for health and human service professionals in United Methodist related organizations and agencies. Develops ethical and theological statements on institutional care. Operates Educational Assessment Guidelines Leading Toward Excellence (EAGLE), a self-assessment and peer review accreditation program. Operates a Field Consultation Program; members may access skilled professionals to assist with governance questions. Offers audiovisual services to members. Administers the Order of Good Shepherds program designed to recognize ministry in the workplace by employees at member organizations. Maintains speakers' bureau; compiles statistics. **Pub:** *Articles depicting innovative ministries by member organizations*, quarterly. Magazine. Professional journal related to operation of United Methodist related institutional ministries. *Price:* $40/year member; $60/year nonmember. • *Children, Youth, & Family Services Section Salary & Benefit Study*. • *National Directory of all United Methodist Related Health and Welfare Ministries*, annual. *Price:* $17/year for members; $27/year for nonmembers. • *Older Adult Ministries Section Salary & Benefit Study*. • *The UMA Journal*, quarterly. Magazine. Depicts innovative ministries by member organizations. **Frmly:** (1968) Board of Hospitals and Homes of The Methodist Church; (1972) Division of Health and Welfare Ministries of The United Methodist Church; (1983) National Association of Health and Welfare Ministries of The United Methodist Church.

★ 6303 ★ United Mitochondrial Disease Foundation (UMDF)

8085 Saltsburg Rd., Ste. 201
Pittsburgh, PA 15239
Phone: (412)793-8077 **Fax:** (412)793-6477
Email: info@umdf.org
Website: http://www.umdf.org
Antoinette Renda Beasley, Fin. Svcs. Coord.

Fnded: 1995. **Mem:** 3,000. **Nat'l Groups:** 1. **Reg. Groups:** 20. **State Groups:** 1. **Local Groups:** 1. **Desc:** Patients, parents or guardians, friends, relatives, medical professionals, hospitals, and other organizations. Promotes research for cures and treatments of mitochondrial disease; provides support to patients and families. Patient registry database includes information from symptoms and treatment to diagnostic methods and specific disorders. **Pub:** Newsletter, 3/year. *Price:* included in membership dues.

★ 6304 ★ United Network for Organ Sharing (UNOS)

PO Box 2484
Richmond, VA 23218-2484
Phone: (804)327-1432 **Free:** 888-TX1-NF01
Fax: (804)323-7343
Email: editor@unos.org
Website: http://www.unos.org
Jeremiah G. Turcotte, MD, Pres.

Fnded: 1984. **Mem:** 434. **Reg. Groups:** 11. **Desc:** Transplant and organ procurement centers, tissue-typing labs, and health care professionals engaged in organ transplant operations. Administers the National Organ Procurement and Transplantation Network and the U.S. Scientific Registry for Organ Transplantation, as mandated by law under contract with the U.S. Department of Health and Human Services. Maintains national waiting list for transplant candidates. Operates the Organ Center, which matches patients in need of transplants with donated organs. Formulates and implements national policies on equitable access and organ allocation and organ procurement standards. Conducts professional education courses for transplant personnel. Maintains and publicizes national statistics on organ donation and transplantation. **Pub:** *UNOS Update*, monthly. Magazine. *Price:* Free to domestic subscribers. **AKA:** UNOS.

★ 6305 ★ United Ostomy Association (UOA)

19772 MacArthur Blvd., Ste. 200
Irvine, CA 92612-2405
Free: 800-826-0826 **Fax:** (949)660-9262
Email: director@uoa.org
Website: http://www.uoa.org
Nancy Italia, Exec. Dir.

Fnded: 1962. **Mem:** 26,000. **Reg. Groups:** 12. **Local Groups:** 500. **Desc:** Individuals who have lost the normal function of their bowel or bladder necessitating colostomy, ileostomy, ileal conduit, or ureterostomy surgery, known as ostomy. Aids in rehabilitation of these persons through mutual aid, moral support, and exchange of practical information in managing the stoma and its necessary prosthetic appliances; sponsors visiting program allowing patients to ask non-medical questions of individuals who have experienced a similar condition. Works to educate the public as to the nature of ostomy, with a view to ending job and insurance discrimination. Encourages research on management of ostomy and prosthetic equipment and appliances; also encourages study of the costs for rehabilitating ostomy patients. Prepares exhibits for medical conventions. Maintains speakers' bureau; compiles statistics. **Pub:** *Ostomy Quarterly*. Magazine. Contains information on ostomy management, human interest stories, organizational news, nutrition tips, and ostomy and alternate procedures. • *Patient Care Manual*. Manual. Provides comprehensive information for all major ostomy and alternati e procedures.

★ 6306 ★ United Seniors Association (USA)

3900 Jermantown Rd., Ste. 450
Fairfax, VA 22030-4900
Phone: (703)359-6500 **Free:** 800-8US-AUSA
Fax: (703)359-6510
Email: usa@unitedseniors.org
Website: http://www.unitedseniors.org
Charles W. Jarvis, Chm. /Ch. Exec.

Fnded: 1991. **Mem:** 550,000. **Nat'l Groups:** 1. **Desc:** Seeks to educate and mobilize senior citizens about Social Security, Medicare, taxes, and other related issues. **Pub:** *The Senior American*, 4/year. Newsletter. *Price:* included in membership dues.

★ 6307 ★ United Seniors Health Cooperative

409 Third St. SW, Ste. 200
Washington, DC 20024
Phone: (202)479-6973 **Free:** 800-637-2604
Fax: (202)479-6660
Email: ushc@unitedseniorhealth.org
Website: http://www.unitedseniorshealth.org
Ann Werner, Pres. & CEO

Fnded: 1984. **Mem:** 10,000. **Desc:** The elderly, their families, and interested others. Assists elderly persons in independent living, health and insurance issues. Provides information resources for professionals serving seniors. **Pub:** *Dictionary of Eldercare Terminology*. • *United Seniors Health Report*, periodic. Newsletter. Provides information on important topics for seniors. *Price:* $15.

★ 6308 ★ United States Animal Health Association (USAHA)

PO Box K227
8100 Three Chopt Rd., Ste. 203
Richmond, VA 23288
Phone: (804)285-3210 **Fax:** (804)285-3367
Email: usaha@usaha.org
Website: http://www.usaha.org
Linda B. Ragland, Contact

Fnded: 1897. **Mem:** 1,100. **Reg. Groups:** 4. **Desc:** Veterinarians, livestock producers, and transportation and livestock companies concerned with the improvement of the health of livestock and poultry through disease control and eradication. **Pub:** *Foreign Animal Diseases Diagnosis and Control*, quarterly. Newsletter. • *Proceedings*, annual. *Price:* $30. **Frmly:** Association of State Sanitary Boards; United States Livestock Sanitary Association.

★ 6309 ★ U.S. Association for Blind Athletes (USABA)

33 N Institute St.
Colorado Springs, CO 80903
Phone: (719)630-0422 **Fax:** (719)630-0616
Email: usaba@usa.net
Website: http://www.usaba.org/
Dr. Charly Huebner, Exec. Dir.

Fnded: 1976. **Mem:** 3,000. **Nat'l Groups:** 1. **Reg. Groups:** 4. **State Groups:** 49. **Desc:** Visually impaired athletes; fully sighted physical educators, coaches, and special education teachers; interested volunteers. Aims to develop individual independence through sports opportunities and athletic competition. Promotes sports for the legally blind and visually impaired, organizes regional, national, and international competitions; works with other international organizations to promote goodwill and independence through friendly competition. Sports contested include alpine skiing, goalball, gymnastics, judo, Nordic skiing, powerlifting, speed skating, 5-side football, swimming, tandem cycling, track and field and wrestling. Sponsors coaches' training seminars, panel discussions, and training groups. Offers children's services; compiles statistics. **Pub:** *Directory of Organization Representatives*, quarterly. Directory. • *USABA Agenda*, monthly. Includes information on upcoming events. • *Vision*, quarterly. Magazine. Includes results of competitions and calender of events. *Price:* Included in membership dues. • Also publishes programs and grant proposals.

★ 6310 ★ United States Blind Golfers' Association (USBGA)

3094 Shamrock St. N
Tallahassee, FL 32308-2735
Phone: (850)893-4511 **Fax:** (850)893-4511
Email: jvbaker@mindspring.com
Website: http://www.blindgolf.com
Bob Andrews, Pres.

Fnded: 1953. **Mem:** 145. **Desc:** Blind and vision impaired golfers who compete for a national championship and U.S. Open, and various other tournaments around the country and internationally. Tournaments raise funds for various blind charities. Blind Junior Golf Program. **Pub:** *The Midnight Golfer*, semiannual. Newsletter. Includes information on blind golf; some international coverage. *Price:* Free. • Also provides learning packets and information on blind golf.

★ 6311 ★ United States and Canadian Academy of Pathology

3643 Walton Way Extension
Augusta, GA 30909
Phone: (706)733-7550 **Fax:** (706)733-8033
Email: iap@uscap.org
Website: http://www.uscap.org
Fred Silva, MD, Sec. -Treas.

Fnded: 1906. **Mem:** 8,200. **Desc:** Works for the advancement of pathology teaching, practice, and research. Disseminates information to members. Sponsors educational programs to serve the needs of pathologists of various levels of experience. Presents Maude Abbott Lectureship to a recognized and respected person in contemporary pathology. **Pub:** *Laboratory Investigation*, monthly. Journal. Focuses on significant advances in research dealing with human and experimental diseases. *Price:* Free to members. • *Modern Pathology*, bimonthly. Journal. Concentrates on the practice of diagnostic human pathology. *Price:* Free to members.

★ 6312 ★ U.S. Deaf Cycling Association (USDCA)

247 Jack London Ct.
Pittsburg, CA 94565-3661
Phone: (925)473-1943
Email: skedsmo@earthlink.net
Website: http://home.earthlink.net/~skedsmo/usdca.htm
Bobby Skedsmo, Sec.

Fnded: 1975. **Mem:** 29. **Reg. Groups:** 2. **Desc:** Promotes recreational and competitive cycling among the deaf and hearing impaired in the U.S. Conducts educational programs; sponsors competitions. **Pub:** *Breakaway*, 3/year. Newsletter. Features club activities and special features. *Price:* $1.

★ 6313 ★ United States Deaf Ski and Snowboard Association (USDSSA)

c/o Robert Lewis
9408 Inglewood Ct.
Frederick, MD 21701-7688
Fax: (410)279-4063
Email: rlewis@usdssa.org
Website: http://www.usdssa.org/
Robert Lewis, Pres.

Fnded: 1968. **Mem:** 350. **Reg. Groups:** 8. **Desc:** Promotes recreational and competitive skiing among the deaf and hearing impaired in the U.S. Provides deaf skiers with benefits, activities, and opportunities that will increase their enjoyment of the sport. Encourages ski racing among the deaf and sponsors national and regional races for deaf skiers, including the U.S.A. National Deaf Alpine and Nordic Ski Championships. Assists in the selection, organization, and training of the United States Deaf Ski Teams for international competition such as the World Winter Games for the Deaf. Presents awards; maintains hall of fame; offers children's services. **Pub:** Newsletter, 3/year. *Price:* available to members only.

★ 6314 ★ U.S. Flag Football of the Deaf
PO Box 230853
Centreville, VA 20120
Email: commissioner@usffd.org
Website: http://www.usffd.org/
Alex Calogar, Commissioner

Fnded: 1984. **Desc:** Hearing-impaired individuals. Organizes flag football games to be played every year across the nation. Compiles statistics and maintains hall of fame. **Pub:** *National Sports Organization - AAAD*, bimonthly. Newsletter.

★ 6315 ★ U.S.-Mexico Border Health Association (USMBHA)
5400 Suncrest Dr., Ste. C-5
El Paso, TX 79912-5615
Phone: (915)833-6450 **Fax:** (915)833-7840
Email: mail@usmbha.org
Website: http://www.usmbha.org
Dr. Alfonso Ruiz, Exec. Dir.

Fnded: 1943. **Mem:** 500. **Desc:** Physicians, public health administrators, nurses, sanitary engineers, veterinarians, scientists, laboratory workers, and other health officers from the 4 American and 6 Mexican states bordering the two countries. Seeks to make easier and more efficient the improvement of public health along both sides of the border; provides for exchange of experiences, discussion of mutual problems in human and animal diseases, and development of personal and professional contacts necessary for carrying out health projects. Sponsors seminars and workshops covering topics such as: food handling; rabies; tuberculosis; epidemiological principles; sexually transmitted diseases. Compiles statistics. **Pub:** *Journal of Border Health*, quarterly. Journal. Contains articles on U.S.-Mexico border health issues. *Price:* $5/issue. • *Report of Activities*, annual. • *U.S.-Mexico Border Health Association–News/Noticias*, quarterly. **Frmly:** (1975) United States-Mexico Border Health Association.

★ 6316 ★ United States Pharmacopeia
12601 Twinbrook Pky.
Rockville, MD 20852
Phone: (301)881-0666 **Free:** 800-822-8772
Fax: (301)816-8299
Email: webmaster@usp.org
Website: http://www.usp.org
Roger L. Williams, MD, Exec. VP & CEO

Fnded: 1820. **Mem:** 500. **Desc:** Dedicated to promoting the public health by establishing and disseminating officially recognized standards of quality and authoritative information for the use of medicines and other health care technologies by health professionals, patients and consumers. Also helps to monitor quality and prevent medication errors through national reporting programs. Achieves its goals through the contributions of volunteers representing pharmacy, medicine, and other health care professions, as well as science, academia, the US government, the pharmaceutical industry, and consumer organizations. **Pub:** *Pharmacopeial Forum*, bimonthly. Journal. • *Proceedings of Quinquennial Meetings*. • *The United States Pharmacopeia and the National Formulary*, annual. Includes semiannual supplement. • *USAN and USP Dictionary of Drug Names*, annual. **Frmly:** U.S. Pharmacopeial Convention.

★ 6317 ★ United States Sports Massage Federation (USMF)
2156 Newport Blvd.
Costa Mesa, CA 92627-1710
Phone: (949)642-0735 **Fax:** (949)642-1729
Email: doctorh@aimt-inc-smti.com
Website: http://www.aimt-inc-smti.com
M. K. Hungerford, PhD, Dir.

Fnded: 1989. **Mem:** 17. **Desc:** Sports massage therapists. Facilitates exchange of techniques and ideas among members. Promotes more widespread use of massage therapy by U.S. professional sports teams.

★ 6318 ★ University of Colorado Health Sciences Center Alumni Association
4200 E 9th Ave., A080
Denver, CO 80262
Phone: (303)315-8832 **Free:** 877-HSC-ALUM
Fax: (303)315-5398
Email: hscalumni@cufund.colorado.edu
Website: http://www.uchsc.edu/alumni/

Desc: Alumni association for the University of Colorado Health Sciences Center.

★ 6319 ★ University of Colorado School of Dentistry Alumni Association (SODAA)
c/o UCHSC Alumni Association
4200 E 9th Ave., A080
Denver, CO 80262
Email: randy.kluender@uchsc.edu
Website: http://www.uchsc.edu/sd/sd/alumni.html
Dr. Randy Kluender, Assoc. Dean

Mem: 1,130. **Desc:** Alumni association for University of Colorado Health Sciences Center, School of Dentistry.

★ 6320 ★ Upledger Institute (UI)
11211 Prosperity Farms Rd., Ste. D-325
Palm Beach Gardens, FL 33410
Phone: (561)622-4771 **Free:** 800-233-5880
Fax: (561)622-4771
Email: upledger@upledger.com
Website: http://www.upledger.com
John Matthew Upledger, CEO

Fnded: 1985. **Desc:** Promotes complementary health care; provides educational and training courses to osteopathic physicians, medical doctors, dentists, nurses, doctors of Chiropractic, doctors of Oriental medicine, naturopathic physicians, psychiatric specialists, psychologists, physical therapists, occupational therapists, speech therapists, massage therapists, acupuncturists, and other professional bodyworkers. Maintains speakers bureau. **Pub:** *UI Date*, semiannual. Newsletter. • *UptaDate*, annual. Newsletter.

★ 6321 ★ Urological Society of Australasia
Eastpoint, Ste. 512
180 Ocean St.
Edgecliff, NSW 2027, Australia
Phone: 61 2 93628644 **Fax:** 61 2 93621433
Email: secretary@urosoc.org.au
Website: http://www.urosoc.org.au/

Desc: Through the Royal Australasian College of Surgeons, the association is responsible for surgical standards and training; encourages research and liaison for fellowship as part of a 4-year structured training program.

★ 6322 ★ Urological Society of India (USI)
c/o Prof. Narmada P. Gupta, Hon.Sec.
Department of Urology
All India Institute of Medical Sciences
New Delhi 110 029, India
Phone: 91 11 26504884 **Fax:** 91 11 6527070
Email: npgupta@usi.org

Fnded: 1961. **Reg. Groups:** 4. **Desc:** Promotes the urological medical specialties in India. **Pub:** *Indian Journal of Urology*, semiannual. Journal. • Newsletter, quarterly.

★ 6323 ★ Urostomy Association of Great Britain and Ireland
c/o Angela Cooke
Buckland
Beaumont Park
Dunbar CM3 4DE, United Kingdom
Phone: 44 1245 224294 **Fax:** 44 1245 227569
Email: ua@centraloffice.fsnet.co.uk
Website: http://www.uagbi.org/

Fnded: 1971. **Desc:** Works to assist people who will undergo or have undergone surgery which results in a urinary diversion; assists caregivers in the rehabilitation process for the ostomate; improve quality of life for urostomates and their caregivers; undertakes research to enhance life for members.

★ 6324 ★ Uruguayan Association of the Analytical Psychotherapy (Asociacion Uruguaya de Psicoterapia Psicoanalitica — AUDEPP)
Canelones 2208
11200 Montevideo, Uruguay
Phone: 598 2 4084985 **Fax:** 598 2 4022066
Email: contacto@audepp.org
Website: http://www.audepp.org/

Mem: 400. **Desc:** Promotes research and development of the theoretical and technical aspects of psychoanalysis and psychotherapy.

★ 6325 ★ Uruguayan Society of Psychosomatic Obstetrics and Gynaecology
c/o Prof. Denise Defey
Department of Medical Psychology
School of Medicine
University of Uruguay
Av. Brazil 2359
11300 Montevideo, Uruguay
Phone: 598 2 7078718 **Fax:** 598 2 7078718
Email: agora@chasque.apc.org
Website: http://www.ispog.org

Desc: Promotes the study of psychobiological and psychosocial, ethical and cross-cultural problems in the fields of obstetrics and gynaecology, women's health and reproductive health; facilitates the dissemination of new information in these fields. **Pub:** *Journal of Psychosomatic Obstetrics and Gynecology*. Journal.

★ 6326 ★ USA Deaf Sports Federation (USADSF)
c/o Bobbie Beth Scoggins
911 Tierra Linda Dr.
Frankfort, KY 40601-4633
Fax: (502)695-2783
Email: homeoffice@usadsf.org
Website: http://www.usadsf.org
Bobbie Beth Scoggins, Pres.

Fnded: 1945. **Mem:** 4,000. **Nat'l Groups:** 20. **Reg. Groups:** 8. **State Groups:** 50. **Local Groups:** 200. **Desc:** Provides year-round training to athletes and coordinates athletic competition in a variety of sports at the state, regional, national, and international level. **Pub:** *Deaf Sports Review*, annual. Magazine. • *USADSF Bulletin*, quarterly. Bulletin. **Frmly:** (1999) American Athletic Association for the Deaf.

★ 6327 ★ USBloodDonors.org
c/o Pat Boone Foundation
9220 Sunset Blvd., Ste. 310
Los Angeles, CA 90069
Email: feedback@usblooddonors.org
Website: http://usblooddonors.org
Tami Reber, Contact

Desc: Establishes and maintains national register so blood, organ, tissue and other life-giving services can be donated.

★ 6328 ★ Vaccine and Infectious Disease Organization (VIDO)
120 Veterinary Rd.
University of Saskatchewan
Saskatoon, SK, Canada S7N 5E3
Phone: (306)966-7465 **Fax:** (306)966-7478
Email: info@vido.org
Website: http://www.usask.ca/vido/

Fnded: 1975. **Lang(s):** English, French. **Desc:** Promotes animal health through diagnosis and prevention of production-limiting diseases. Conducts research focusing on development of new vaccines to better treat infectious diseases and the discovery and application of biotechnologies. Serves as a clearinghouse on commercial veterinary diagnosis and treatment techniques; makes available laboratory and field study services. Makes available educational and extension services. **Pub:** Brochures. **Frmly:** (2003) Veterinary Infectious Disease Organization.

★ 6329 ★ Velo-Cardio-Facial Syndrome (VCFS)
c/o Dr. Robert J. Shprintzen
Upstate Medical University
University Hospital
708 Jacobsen Hall (CDU)
750 E Adams St.
Syracuse, NY 13210
Phone: (315)464-6590 **Fax:** (315)464-6593
Email: info@vcfsef.org
Website: http://www.vcfsef.org
Dr. Robert J. Shprintzen, Exec. Dir.

Mem: 1,300. **Desc:** Committed to educating the lay and professional public, offers family programs, provides parent-to-parent networking; promotes the diagnosis and treatment of individuals with VCF; distributes educational materials about Velo-Cardio-Facial (also known as Shprintzen Syndrome, DiGeorge Sequence, and Catch 22); and distributes questionnaire regarding the medical diagnosis and management of individuals with this disorder. **Pub:** Newsletter, periodic.

★ 6330 ★ Venezuelan Society of Pharmacology (Sociedad Venezolana de Farmacologia)
c/o Dr. Manuel Velasco
PO Box 76.333
El Marques
Caracas 1070-A, Venezuela
Phone: 58 2 125619871 **Fax:** 58 2 123214385
Email: veloscom@cantv.net

Mem: 125. **Desc:** Promotes pharmacology in Venezuela.

★ 6331 ★ Verbond der Vlaamse Tandartsen
Vrijheidslaan 61
B-1081 Brussels, Belgium
Phone: 32 2 4130013 **Fax:** 32 2 4148727
Email: verbond@vvt.be
Website: http://www.tandarts.be

Fnded: 1987. **Mem:** 3,300. **Desc:** Provides professional and scientific support to Belgian dentists and dental activities, focusing on Dutch speaking dentists.

★ 6332 ★ Vereniging Spierziekten Nederland
Lt. Gen. van Heutszlaan 6
NL-3743 JN Baarn, Netherlands
Phone: 31 35 5480480 **Fax:** 31 35 5480499
Email: vsn@vsn.nl
Website: http://www.vsn.nl

Fnded: 1967. **Mem:** 8,500. **Desc:** Works as a support group for individuals suffering from neuromuscular diseases, among others amyotrophic lateral sclerosis or ALS (also known as Lou Gehrig's Disease) and muscular dystrophy (e.g., Duchenne Musc. Dyst.) in the Netherlands. Strives to: heighten public awareness and understanding of the diseases; encourage research among medical and scientific communities; and improve the rehabilitation and professional care for the patients.

★ 6333 ★ Veris Research Information Service
5325 S 9th Ave.
La Grange, IL 60525-3602
Phone: (952)927-7104 **Free:** 800-554-1708
Fax: (952)927-6406
Email: slandvik@aol.com
Website: http://www.veris-online.org
Sharon Landvik, Exec. Officer

Desc: Acts as an information clearinghouse on antioxidants, including vitamin E, caroteroids, alpha-lipoic acid, and botanicals for health care professionals, researchers, and nutrition and health communicators. **Pub:** *VERIS*, quarterly. Fact sheets reporting on current research. • Also publishes research summaries. **Frmly:** (1998) Vitamin E Research and Information Service.

★ 6334 ★ Vestibular Disorders Association (VEDA)
PO Box 4467
Portland, OR 97208-4467
Phone: (503)229-7705 **Free:** 800-837-8428
Fax: (503)229-8064
Email: veda@vestibular.org
Website: http://www.vestibular.org
Connie Pilcher, Outreach Coord.

Fnded: 1983. **Mem:** 4,000. **Local Groups:** 115. **Desc:** Individuals suffering from vestibular disorders, their families and friends, and health care professionals. (Vestibular disorders are characterized by persistent dizziness or vertigo which often indicates a problem in the inner ear.) Provides support services including information and referrals; encourages public education about vestibular disorders and their effects. **Pub:** *Balancing Act, 2nd Ed.*. Book. *Price:* $15. • *BPPV: What You Need to Know.* Book. *Price:* $24.95 softbound; $34.95 hardbound. • *Getting Better.* Video. Closed caption VHS tape. *Price:* $25. • *Managing Your Symptoms.* Videos. Closed caption VHS tape. *Price:* $25. • *Meniere's Disease: What You Need to Know.* Book. *Price:* $24.95 softbound; $34.95 hardbound. • *On the Level*, quarterly. Newsletter. Includes coping tips, health-related items, reviews, and association news. *Price:* Included in membership dues. • *Stories and Strategies: Coping with Vestibular Disorders.* Booklet. • *VEDA Low-Salt Cookbook.* Book. *Price:* $17. • Audiotapes. • Bibliographies. • Pamphlets. • Reports. **Frmly:** (1989) Dizziness and Balance Disorders Association.

★ 6335 ★ Veterinarian Association for the Attention of Exotic and Wild Animals (Asociacion Veterinaria papa la Atencion de la Fauna Exotica y Salvaje)
Facultat de Veterinaria
Universitat Autonoma de Barcelona
E-08193 Bellaterra, Spain
Phone: 34 93 5812107 **Fax:** 34 93 5812006
Email: avafes@uab.es
Website: http://tau.uab.es/associacions/avafes/

Fnded: 1989. **Desc:** Advises individuals, ecological groups, and rescue centers on wild animal health. Fosters wildlife conservation.

★ 6336 ★ Veterinary Association of Malaysia
59 Jalan Sultan Azian Shah
31400 Ipoh, Malaysia
Phone: 60 5 5473507 **Fax:** 60 5 5473509
Email: vamsec@jphvri.po.my

★ 6337 ★ Veterinary Cancer Society (VCS)
PO Box 1763
Spring Valley, CA 91979-1763
Phone: (619)474-8929 **Fax:** (619)474-8947
Email: vcs@cox.net
Website: http://www.vetcancersociety.org
Dr. Barbara McGehee, Exec. Dir.

Fnded: 1974. **Mem:** 800. **Desc:** Veterinarians and others who have an interest in cancer in animals. Goals are to: achieve and maintain high standards of diagnosis, treatment, and prevention of animal cancers; advance interdisciplinary research in neoplastic diseases of animals; collect and disseminate information about animal tumors; conduct and evaluate studies, including cooperative clinical trials, of animal neoplasms. **Pub:** *VCS Newsletter*, quarterly. Newsletter. • Directory, periodic.

★ 6338 ★ Veterinary Council
53 Lansdowne Rd.
Dublin 4, Ireland
Phone: 353 1 6684402 **Fax:** 353 1 6604373
Fnded: 1931.

★ 6339 ★ Veterinary History Society
c/o The Royal Veterinary College
Royal College St.
London NW1 0TU, United Kingdom
Website: http://www.rvc.ac.uk/Guests/VetHistSoc/vhs.htm

Fnded: 1962. **Desc:** Veterinarians and other interested individuals. Fosters all aspects of veterinary history. **Pub:** *Veterinary History*, semiannual. Journal.

★ 6340 ★ Veterinary Hospital Managers Association (VHMA)
48 Howard St.
Albany, NY 12207
Phone: (518)433-8911 **Fax:** (518)463-8656
Email: vhma@caphill.com
Website: http://www.vhma.org
Christine M. Quinn, Exec. Dir.

Fnded: 1981. **Desc:** Individuals involved in veterinary practice management. Seeks to advance the study, teaching, and practice of veterinary practice management. Serves as a forum for the exchange of information among members; sponsors continuing professional development courses; formulates standards of ethics and practice for veterinary medical managers.

★ 6341 ★ Veterinary Orthopedic Society (VOS)
PO Box 313
Newmarket, NH 03857-0313
Phone: (603)659-7989 **Fax:** (603)659-7989
Email: vosclarkmt@aol.com
Website: http://www.landscapesearch.com
Mary Tuson Clark, Exec. Sec.

Fnded: 1972. **Mem:** 600. **Desc:** Veterinarians interested in orthopedic surgery. Promotes education and research in veterinary orthopedic surgery. Provides a forum for the exchange of ideas among veterinarians in academia, research, and practice. **Pub:** *Membership List*, periodic. Journal. • *VOS Newsletter*, annual. Newsletter. *Price:* Included in membership dues.

★ 6342 ★ VHA
220 E Las Colinas Blvd.
Irving, TX 75039-5500
Free: 877-847-1450 **Fax:** (972)830-0332
Email: feedback@vha.com
Website: http://www.vhahealthfoundation.org
Susan Crampton, Chm. /Pres.

Fnded: 1977. **Mem:** 2,150. **Reg. Groups:** 22. **Desc:** Health care alliance that represents 1,600 healthcare organizations nationwide, offering its members programs and services to help them improve their operational and clinical efficiency as well as community health. **Pub:** *Alliance*, monthly. Newsletter. Publication about VHA programs, And services and member activities. *Price:* available to members only. • Annual Report, annual. **Frmly:** (1995) Voluntary Hospitals of America.

★ 6343 ★ VHL Family Alliance (VHLFA)
171 Clinton Rd.
Brookline, MA 02445
Phone: (617)277-5667 **Free:** 800-767-4VHL
Fax: (617)734-8233
Email: info@vhl.org
Website: http://www.vhl.org
Joyce Graff, Chair

Fnded: 1993. **Mem:** 14,000. **Nat'l Groups:** 11. **State Groups:** 29. **Desc:** Patients affected by Von Hippel-Lindau Disease; their families; medical professionals;

interested others. Von Hippel-Lindau Disease is a genetic disorder involving abnormal growth forming "knots" of blood vessels in the retina, brain, or spinal cord areas. These knots are hemangiomas, a kind of tumor. Promotes education of the medical community, patients, and the general public about the disease. Provides an international support network to families affected by VHL. Conducts research and educational programs; funds research on VHL; maintains speakers' bureau. **Pub:** *VHL Family Forum*, quarterly. Newsletter. Contains the latest information on VHL, research into the disease, and support network information. *Price:* Included in membership. • *VHL Patient Handbook*. Booklet. • *What is VHL?*. Brochures. *Price:* $2 for 25. • *Your Family Health Tree*. Booklet. **AKA:** Von Hippel-Lindau Family Alliance.

★ 6344 ★ Victims of Asbestos and Industrial Disease (VAID)

547 Victoria Ave.
Windsor, ON, Canada N9A 4N1
Phone: (519)973-4800 **Free:** 800-565-3185
Fax: (519)973-1906

Fnded: 1986. **Mem:** 500. **Lang(s):** English, French. **Desc:** Individuals with asbestos-related illness and other industrial diseases. Promotes improved quality of life for members. Makes available medical, social, and legal services to victims of asbestos-related diseases and other industrial illnesses.

★ 6345 ★ Vietnam Assistance for the Handicapped - Ho Chi Minh City (VNAH)

27 Dang Tat St., Dist. I
Ho Chi Minh City, Vietnam
Phone: 84 8 8480330 **Fax:** 84 8 8480512
Email: vnah2@hem.vnn.vn
Website: http://vnah-hev.org

Fnded: 1992. **Lang(s):** English, Vietnamese. **Desc:** Organizations and individuals concerned about the status of people with disabilities. Seeks to fully integrate people with disabilities into economic and social life. Provides support and rehabilitation services to people with disabilities and their families.

★ 6346 ★ Vietnamese Medical Association of the U.S.A.

c/o B.S. NguyenleHieu, M.D.
Shelton Medical Clinic
302 C St.
PO Box 476
Shelton, NE 68876
Phone: (308)647-6828 **Fax:** (308)647-5219
B.S. Nguyenlehieu, MD, Contact

Fnded: 1989. **Mem:** 498. **Nat'l Groups:** 1. **State Groups:** 10. **Desc:** Vietnamese-American medical professionals. Promotes mutual support and fellowship among its members, while fostering and maintaining medical ethics. Assures the provision of equal educational and professional opportunities for its members and the welfare of the general Vietnamese community. Supports and assists the Vietnamese victims of the Vietnamese communist regime.

★ 6347 ★ Vision Australia Foundation

Brighton Centre
7 Mair St.
PO Box 123
Brighton, VIC 3186, Australia
Phone: 61 3 95995000 **Fax:** 61 3 95984240
Email: brighton@visionaustralia.org.au
Website: http://www.visionaustralia.org.au

Lang(s): English. **Desc:** Blind and vision impaired people in Australia. Provides assistance to members so that they may go on living lives they value.

★ 6348 ★ Vision Community Services - A Division of the Massachusetts Association for the Blind (VCS)

23A Elm St.
Watertown, MA 02472-2821
Phone: (617)926-4232 **Free:** 800-852-3029
Fax: (617)926-1412
Email: fweisse@mablind.org
Website: http://www.mablind.org
Fran Weisse, Dir. /Info. Svcs.

Fnded: 1903. **State Groups:** 3. **Desc:** Serves individuals who are newly blind or partially sighted, and those with progressive eye disease, as well as individuals who are blind. Provides information and referral services, individualized advocacy, self-help support groups, buddy telephone network, special services for elders, community volunteer services, recording studio, braille program, Newsline Boston, and a store of assistive devices. **Pub:** *VCS Resource List*, biennial. Catalog. In large print. Lists print, large print, cassette, disc, and braille brochures, pamphlets, fact sheets, and catalogs. Also available on cassette. *Price:* Free. • *VCS Resource Update*, bimonthly. Newsletter. In large print. Describes services and adaptive equipment for visually impaired individuals. Also available on cassette. *Price:* Free. **Frmly:** (2001) Vision Community Services.

★ 6349 ★ Visiting Nurse Associations of America (VNAA)

99 Summer St., Ste. 1700
Boston, MA 02110
Phone: (617)737-3200 **Free:** 800-426-2547
Fax: (617)737-1144
Email: vnaa@vnaa.org
Website: http://www.vnaa.org
Carolyn S. Markey, Pres. /CEO

Fnded: 1982. **Mem:** 210. **Desc:** Voluntary, nonprofit home health care agencies. Develops competitive strength among community-based nonprofit visiting nurse organizations; works to strengthen business resources and economic programs through contracting, marketing, governmental affairs and publications. **Pub:** *Nursing Procedure Manual*, monthly. Manual. *Price:* Free for members' CEOs. • *VNAA Spectrum*, monthly. *Price:* Free for members' CEOs. **Frmly:** (1985) American Affiliation of Visiting Nurses Associations and Services.

★ 6350 ★ Visually Impaired Data Processors International (VIDPI)

c/o American Council of the Blind
1155 15th St. NW, Ste. 1004
Washington, DC 20005
Phone: (202)467-5081 **Free:** 800-424-8666
Email: rrrogers@one.net
Website: http://www.acb.org/vidpi/
Robert R. Rogers, Pres.

Fnded: 1970. **Mem:** 75. **Desc:** Visually impaired electronic data processing employees; those seeking employment; employers, instructors, manufacturers, and students in the electronic data processing field. Advocates high standards in training visually impaired students. Seeks to increase employment opportunities; encourages the exchange of work technique ideas and the development of new equipment. Works with agencies to increase the availability of braille and recorded materials. Supports a speakers' bureau. **Pub:** *Views*, quarterly.

★ 6351 ★ Visually Impaired Veterans of America (VIVA)

c/o American Council of the Blind
1155 15th St. NW, Ste. 1004
Washington, DC 20005
Phone: (202)467-5081 **Free:** 800-424-8666
Email: rrrogers@one.net
Website: http://www.acb.org/vidpi/
David Dowland, Pres.

Fnded: 1975. **Mem:** 117. **Desc:** Veterans of the armed forces of the U.S. who have blindness or visual impairment. Purposes are: to maintain and foster the well-being and rehabilitation of all visually impaired veterans; to preserve the legal rights of all visually impaired veterans on the local, state, and national levels; to maintain, promote, and foster the social, economic, and cultural level of these veterans and to promote opportunities to increase their knowledge of educational, professional, and rehabilitation standards and methods. Seeks to acquire, preserve, and disseminate information relative to the functions and accomplishments of visually impaired veterans. Encourages research and development of new products for the blind. Maintains speakers' bureau; offers specialized education program. **Pub:** *VIVA Membership List*, annual. Membership Directory. Includes newsletter. • *VIVA Viewpoints*, quarterly. Newsletter. For blind veterans. *Price:* Included in membership dues.

★ 6352 ★ Vitamin Society of Japan (Nippon Bitamin Gakkai)

Yoshida, Sakyo-ku
Kyoto, Japan
Phone: 81 75 7510314

Fnded: 1947.

★ 6353 ★ Vocational Evaluation and Work Adjustment Association (VEWAA)

PO Box 26273
Colorado Springs, CO 80936
Phone: (719)638-4787 **Fax:** (719)638-6153
Email: info@vewaa.org
Website: http://www.vewaa.org
Robin Cook, Pres.

Fnded: 1967. **Mem:** 100. **Nat'l Groups:** 2. **Reg. Groups:** 7. **Desc:** Specialists in vocational evaluation and work adjustment whose goals are to improve and advance the field and to promote high ethical practices through training and research. Conducts educational programs at state, regional, and national levels. Works with other organizations to develop a certification program for vocational evaluators and work adjustment personnel. Keeps legislators informed of the needs of persons with disabilities; promotes adequate funding of state and federal programs benefiting persons with disabilities. Disseminates employment information to members. **Pub:** Bulletin, quarterly. • Newsletter, quarterly. • National Directory of Vocational Evaluation and Assessment Professionals.

★ 6354 ★ Voice Foundation (VF)

1721 Pine St.
Philadelphia, PA 19103
Phone: (215)735-7999 **Fax:** (215)735-9293
Email: voicefound@onrampcom.com
Website: http://www.voicefoundation.org
Robert T. Sataloff, Chm.

Fnded: 1969. **Mem:** 450. **Desc:** Sponsors research and education on the causes, prevention, and treatment of voice disorders. Sponsors educational programs. Holds fundraising events. **Pub:** *Journal of Voice*, quarterly. Journal. *Price:* $99/year for individuals; $126/year for individuals outside U.S.; $98/year for libraries/institutions; $112/year for libraries/institutions outside U.S. • *Voice Foundation Newsletter*, 3-4/year. Newsletter. *Price:* Included in membership dues. • Videos.

★ 6355 ★ Voluntary Euthanasia Society (VES)

13 Prince of Wales Ter.
London W8 5PG, United Kingdom
Phone: 44 20 79378721 **Fax:** 44 20 73762648
Email: info@ves.org.uk
Website: http://www.ves.org.uk/

Fnded: 1935. **Desc:** Doctors, lawyers and clergymen dedicated to legalizing euthanasia for competent adults suffering from terminal illnesses wanting to die.

★ 6356 ★ Voluntary Protection Programs Participants' Association (VPPPA)

7600 E Leesburg Pike, Ste. 440
Falls Church, VA 22043
Phone: (703)761-1146 **Fax:** (703)761-1148
Email: administration@vpppa.org
Website: http://www.vpppa.org

Mem: 450. **Desc:** Companies participating in voluntary protection programs and other workplace environmental protection, health, and safety programs. Promotes cooperation between labor, management, and government agencies to insure safe and environmentally sustainable workplaces. Works closely with federal environmental and safety agencies to develop and implement cooperative programs; provides information on environmental health and workplace safety to congressional committees considering legislation.

★ 6357 ★ Volunteer Trustees of Not-for-Profit Hospitals
818 18th St. NW, Ste. 900
Washington, DC 20006
Phone: (202)659-0338 **Fax:** (202)659-0116
Email: vt@sprintmail.com
Website: http://www.volunteertrustees.org
Linda B. Miller, Pres.

Fnded: 1980. **Mem:** 150. **State Groups:** 45. **Desc:** Representatives of 155 not-for-profit hospitals and their voluntary governing boards. Objectives are to: provide a trustee voice in policy-making and legislative activities; develop a communications network among trustees in order to provide the highest quality medical care at the lowest possible price; provide educational services to hospital governing boards; facilitate accurate portrayal of not-for-profit hospitals in the media and Congress. Areas of concern include: Medicare; controlling hospital costs; strategic planning for the not-for-profit hospital community. Compiles information on governing boards. Conducts roundtables.

★ 6358 ★ VSA arts
1300 Connecticut Ave. NW, 700
Washington, DC 20036
Phone: (202)628-2800 **Free:** 800-933-VSA1
Fax: (202)737-0725
Email: info@vsarts.org
Website: http://www.vsarts.org
Johanna Bentwood, Information Specialist

Fnded: 1974. **Nat'l Groups:** 87. **State Groups:** 47. **Desc:** An international Organization that promotes educational and lifelong learning opportunities through the arts for people of all abilities. Ambassador Jean Kennedy Smith founded the Organization in 1974 as an affiliate of The John F. Kennedy Center for the Performing Arts based on the concept that "the arts belong to all of us, and that everyone without exception must have equal opportunity to participate in, learn from, and enjoy the arts". The United States Congress has designated VSA arts as the coordinating Organization for arts programming for children and youth with disabilities. The Organization's educational programs use alternative curricula and teaching strategies designed to promote optimal learning experiences in a fully inclusive environment, providing youth and adults with an artistic means of self-expression, creating self-confidence and teaching marketable skills while fostering communication and independence. Offers comprehensive programs in literary, performing, and visual arts, in collaboration with local educational agencies, cultural institutions, institutions of higher education, arts agencies, disability Associations, and health and rehabilitation Organizations in 49 states and DC, and in more than 60 countries worldwide. Programs have served over 5 million people. **Pub:** *The Creative Spirit*, quarterly. Newsletter. • Also publishes manuals and guides and makes available videotapes. **Frmly:** (2000) Very Special Arts.

★ 6359 ★ Vulval Pain Society
PO Box 514
Slough SL1 2BP, United Kingdom
Website: http://www.vul-pain.dircon.co.uk

Fnded: 1996. **Mem:** 500. **Local Groups:** 2. **Desc:** Provides information and support to women who suffer from Vulval pain and discomfort.

★ 6360 ★ Vulvar Pain Foundation
PO Drawer 177
Graham, NC 27253
Phone: (336)226-0704 **Fax:** (336)226-8518
Website: http://www.vulvarpainfoundation.org

Fnded: 1992. **Mem:** 7,000. **Reg. Groups:** 17. **Desc:** Women who have vulvar pain and related disorders (fibromyalgia, interstitial cystitis, irritable bowel), family members, and interested health care professionals. Educates patients, physicians, and the public about successful treatment and current research. Identifies interested health care professionals, promotes scientific research, coordinates support networks and groups. **Pub:** *The Low Oxalate Cookbook*. Book. Contains dietary guidelines, recipes, and other related information. *Price:* $30. • *VPF*. Brochure. Describes the purposes, activities, and membership benefits of the foundation. *Price:* Free. • *The Vulvar Pain Newsletter*. Newsletter. **AKA:** The VP Foundation.

★ 6361 ★ W.M. Keck Foundation
550 S Hope St., Ste. 2500
Los Angeles, CA 90071
Phone: (213)680-3833
Website: http://www.wmkeck.org
Robert A. Day, Pres.

Fnded: 1954. **Desc:** Works to support medical research, science, and engineering.

★ 6362 ★ Wegener's Granulomatosis Association
PO Box 28660
Kansas City, MO 64188-8660
Phone: (816)436-8211 **Free:** 800-277-9474
Fax: (816)436-8211
Email: wga@wgassociation.org
Website: http://wgassociation.org
Joyce Kullman, Exec. Dir.

Fnded: 1986. **Mem:** 5,000. **Local Groups:** 50. **Desc:** Seeks to raise public awareness of Wegener's Granulomatosis. Alleviates the isolation of having the disease. Wegener's Granulomatosis is an uncommon life threatening disease, a form of vasculitis and an autoimmune disease. Disseminates information. **Pub:** *Wegener's Granulomatosis Support Group, Inc. International*, bimonthly. Newsletter. **Frmly:** (1999) Wegener's Granulomatosis Support Group; (2003) Wegener's Granulomatosis Support Group International.

★ 6363 ★ Weight Watchers International (WWI)
175 Crossways Park West
Woodbury, NY 11797-2055
Phone: (516)390-1632 **Fax:** (516)390-1795
Email: media@weightwatchers.com
Website: http://www.weightwatchers.com
Linda Huett, Pres. /CEO/Dir.

Fnded: 1963. **Desc:** The Weight Watchers Program includes a balanced diet, exercise and behavior modification. At weekly meetings, Weight Watchers members learn how to modify their current eating and exercise habits. Operates centers worldwide.

★ 6364 ★ Well Spouse Foundation (WSF)
63 W Main St., Ste. H
Freehold, NJ 07728
Free: 800-838-0879 **Fax:** (732)577-8644
Email: info@wellspouse.org
Website: http://www.wellspouse.org
Marty Beilin, Pres.

Fnded: 1988. **Mem:** 3,000. **Nat'l Groups:** 50. **Desc:** Husbands, wives, and partners of chronically ill patients. An emotional support network functioning to raise public consciousness about and advocate for the caregivers and families of the chronically ill. Establishes local support groups and supplies information and materials. Compiles statistics; conducts educational programs. **Pub:** *Mainstay*, quarterly. Newsletter. Contains membership news and information, advocacy issues, and helpful hints. *Price:* Included in membership dues. **Frmly:** National Well Spouse Foundation.

★ 6365 ★ Wellness Associates
PO Box 8422
Asheville, NC 28814
Phone: (828)251-5594
Email: info@thewellspring.com
Website: http://www.thewellspring.com
John W. Travis, MD, Dir.

Fnded: 1975. **Desc:** Provides high quality resource materials for lifestyle improvement integrating the major components of wellness: self-responsibility, stress management, nutrition, and physical awareness. Expands wellness education into the fields of emotional and psychological health. Recognizes spiritual growth and the search for meaning to be essential elements in the experience of wellness. Offers wellness publications and resources for helping professionals to assist them in realizing the principles of wellness in their own lives and to help their clients experience their own capacity for good health and wellbeing. Provides consultation for wellness centers, individuals, universities, agencies, hospitals, and government groups. **Pub:** *A Change of Heart: The Global Wellness Inventory*. Book. *Price:* $8. • *Simply Well: Choices for a Healthy Life*. Book. *Price:* $9.95. • *Wellness for Helping Professionals*. Book. *Price:* $39. • *Wellness Index*. Booklet. *Price:* $4.95. • *Wellness Inventory*. Booklet. *Price:* $2.95. • *Wellness Workbook*. Book. *Price:* $19.95. **Frmly:** (1979) Wellness Resource Center.

★ 6366 ★ Wellness Center (AWCI)
c/o UC Davis Medical Centre
2315 Stockton Blvd.
Sacramento, CA 95817
Phone: (916)734-9797
Email: ken.adams@ucdmc.ucdavis.edu
Website: http://wellness.ucdavis.edu/
Joseph Silva, CEO

Fnded: 1979. **Mem:** 1,500. **Desc:** Individuals concerned with wellness and preventive health care; firms, institutions, and organizations with wellness centers or employee assistance programs. Educates health practitioners and the public on methods of developing healthier lifestyles through the prevention and treatment of degenerative diseases and other health disorders. Provides professional training workshops in wellness counseling, an approach that integrates many scientific and medical disciplines, to assist members with problems related to weight control, stress, alcoholism, personal relationships, drug addiction, and other physical, mental, or social problems. Conducts individual and group counseling sessions and support groups. Provides speakers on topics such as wellness, lifestyle changes, longevity, diseases and alternative therapies. **Pub:** *Bibliographical Essay*, periodic. • *Directory of Members*, annual. Membership Directory. • *Life-Style for Wellness*, quarterly. Journal. Includes research reports, book reviews, and listings of employment opportunities. *Price:* $50/year. • *Mailing List*, periodic.

★ 6367 ★ Wellness Councils of America
9802 Nicholas St., Ste. 315
Omaha, NE 68114
Phone: (402)827-3590 **Fax:** (402)827-3594
Email: wellworkplace@welcoa.org
Website: http://www.welcoa.org
David Hunnicutt, Pres.

Fnded: 1988. **Mem:** 500. **Reg. Groups:** 10. **Desc:** Conducts health education at the workplace. Offers advisory services; maintains educational programs. **Pub:** *The Well Workplace*, monthly. Newsletter.

★ 6368 ★ Wellness International
5800 Democracy Dr.
Plano, TX 75024
Phone: (972)312-1100 **Fax:** (972)943-5260
Email: webmaster@winltd.com
Website: http://web.winltd.com
Susan Shapiro, Contact

Desc: Promotes application of the precepts of health maintenance organizations to public health problems in developing areas. Provides technical assistance to health services operating in developing regions.

★ 6369 ★ Wellstart International
PO Box 80877
San Diego, CA 92138-0877
Phone: (619)295-5192 **Fax:** (619)574-8159
Email: info@wellstart.org
Website: http://www.wellstart.org
Audrey Naylor, CEO

Desc: Seeks to advance the knowledge, skills, and ability of breastfeeding to health care providers in order to promote, protect, and support infant and maternal health and nutrition from conception through the completion of weaning.

★ 6370 ★ West African Society for Pharmacology (WASP) (Societe Ouest Africaine de Pharmacologie — SOAP)
c/o Prof. Charles O. Wambebe
Department of Pharmacology & Toxicology
National Institute for Pharmaceutical Research & Development
Idu Industrial Area
PMB 21
Abuja, Nigeria
Phone: 234 9 5231062 **Fax:** 234 9 5231043
Email: wambebe@niprd.anpa.net.ng

Mem: 350. **Desc:** Promotes pharmacology in West Africa.

★ 6371 ★ Western Pacific Society of Chemotherapy (WPSC)
PO Box 645
30770 Ipoh, Malaysia
Phone: 60 5 3131270 **Fax:** 60 5 3129127
Email: vkelim@pc.jaring.my

Fnded: 1986. **Desc:** Furthers knowledge in the field of microbial diseases.

★ 6372 ★ Western Surgical Association (WSA)
c/o Richard C. Thirlby, MD
Virginia Mason Medical Clinic
1100 Ninth Ave., C6-GSUR
Seattle, WA 98111
Phone: (206)223-6636 **Free:** 800-354-9527
Fax: (206)625-7245
Email: Richard.Thirlby@vmmc.org
Website: http://www.westernsurg.org
Dr. Richard Thirlby, MD, Sec.

Fnded: 1891. **Mem:** 700. **Desc:** Surgeons who have contributed to surgical education and advancement. Objectives are: to cultivate, promote, and diffuse knowledge of the art and science of surgery; to sponsor and maintain the highest standards of practice; to deliver the best possible care to all people. **Pub:** *Western Surgical Association Newsletter*, quarterly. Newsletter. Includes information on new members and information on upcoming meetings. *Price:* Free. • *Western Surgical Association Program*, annual. Book. Contains abstracts of papers to be presented at annual meeting, also includes transactions.

★ 6373 ★ Western Veterinary Conference (WVC)
2425 E Oquendo Rd.
Las Vegas, NV 89120-2406
Phone: (702)739-6698 **Fax:** (702)739-6420
Email: info@westernveterinary.org
Website: http://www.wvc.org
Dr. Steven Crane, Exec. Dir.

Fnded: 1928. **Mem:** 4,500. **Desc:** International veterinarians attending annual conference. Provides practical continuing education for veterinarians and technicians. Topics of study at conference include small and large animal medicine and surgery, general medicine, emergency clinic operation, radiographic and clinical pathologic methods, and current research. Autotutorial programs are available. **Frmly:** (1986) Intermountain Veterinary Medical Association.

★ 6374 ★ Weston A. Price Foundation
PMB 106-380
4200 Wisconsin Ave., NW
Washington, DC 20016
Phone: (202)333-4325 **Fax:** (202)333-0002
Email: westonaprice@msn.com
Website: http://www.westonaprice.org
Sally Fallon, Pres.

Fnded: 1999. **Mem:** 2,600. **Local Groups:** 130. **Desc:** Seeks to disseminate the research of Dr. Weston Price and restore nutrient-dense foods to the human diet through education, research, and activism. **Pub:** *Wise Traditions in Food, Farming, and the Healing Arts*, quarterly. Journal. Contains information on worldwide dietary, agricultural, and medical traditions. *Price:* included in membership dues.

★ 6375 ★ Wheelchair Motorcycle Association (WMA)
101 Torrey St.
Brockton, MA 02301
Phone: (508)583-8614
Dr. Eli Factor, Pres.

Fnded: 1975. **Mem:** 1,000. **Local Groups:** 1. **Desc:** Handicapped persons confined to wheelchairs interested in rediscovering the outdoors; institutional and individual supporters. Researches, develops, and tests off-road vehicles for quadriplegics and other severely handicapped persons. Has audiovisual program showing the use of cycles by the handicapped. **Pub:** *Climb for Independence*, quarterly. Newsletter. *Price:* Included in membership dues.

★ 6376 ★ Wheelchair Sports, USA (WSUSA)
3595 E Fountain Blvd., Ste. L-1
Colorado Springs, CO 80910
Phone: (719)574-1150 **Fax:** (719)574-9840
Email: wsusa@aol.com
Mar Porter, Off. Admin.

Fnded: 1958. **Mem:** 2,000. **Reg. Groups:** 14. **Desc:** Men and women athletes with significant permanent neuromuscular-skeletal disability (spinal cord disorder, poliomyelitis, or amputation) who compete in various amateur sports events in wheelchairs. Members compete in regional events and in the annual National Wheelchair Games, which include competitions in track and field (including pentathlon), swimming, archery, shooting, fencing, table tennis, weightlifting, basketball, and rugby. Compiles statistics; maintains hall of fame and speakers' bureau. competition. Compiles statistics; maintains hall of fame and speakers' bureau. competition. Compiles statistics; maintains hall of fame and speakers' bureau. **Pub:** *Constitution and By-Laws*, biennial. Newsletter. *Price:* $10 for 4 issues; $17 for 8 issues. • *WSUSA Newsletter*, quarterly. Newsletter. *Price:* $10/year. • Also publishes rule books. **Frmly:** (1994) National Wheelchair Athletic Association.

★ 6377 ★ Wilderness Medical Society (WMS)
3595 E Fountain Blvd., Ste. A1
Colorado Springs, CO 80910
Phone: (719)572-9255 **Fax:** (719)572-1514
Email: wms@wms.org
Website: http://www.wms.org
David Just, Exec. Dir.

Fnded: 1983. **Mem:** 4,200. **Desc:** Regular membership for persons with advanced degrees in the biomedical or life sciences with an interest in the medical, behavioral, and life sciences aspects of wilderness environments. Objectives are to promote research and educational activities that increase scientific knowledge about human activities in wilderness environments; stimulate interest and research in health consequences of wilderness activities; serve as central information source. Areas of interest include treatment of accident victims and victims of bites and stings, exotic infectious diseases and toxic plants, desert survival, avalanche control, and search and rescue. **Pub:** *Wilderness and Environmental Medicine*, quarterly. Journal. • *Wilderness Medicine Letter*, quarterly. Newsletter. *Price:* Included in membership dues.

★ 6378 ★ William Glasser Institute
22024 Lassen St., No. 118
Chatsworth, CA 91311
Phone: (818)700-8000 **Free:** 800-899-0688
Fax: (818)700-0555
Email: wginst@wglasser.com
Website: http://www.wglasser.com
William Glasser, MD, Pres.

Fnded: 1967. **Reg. Groups:** 9. **Desc:** Teaches Reality Therapy, Choice Theory, and Lead Management concepts to those who wish to use the knowledge in various working environments. **Pub:** *Journal of Reality Therapy*, semiannual. Journal. • Newsletter, 3/year. **Frmly:** Institute for Reality Therapy; (1998) Institute for Control Therapy, Reality Therapy, and Quality Management.

★ 6379 ★ William H. Donner Foundation
500 Fifth Ave., Ste. 1230
New York, NY 10110-0180
Phone: (212)719-9290 **Fax:** (212)302-8734
Website: http://www.donner.org

Fnded: 1961. **Desc:** Strives to fund thoughtful and creative medical-related projects.

★ 6380 ★ Williams Syndrome Association (WSA)
PO Box 297
Clawson, MI 48017-0297
Phone: (248)244-2229 **Fax:** (248)244-2230
Email: tmonkaba@aol.com
Website: http://www.williams-syndrome.org
Terry Monkaba, Exec. Dir.

Fnded: 1983. **Mem:** 8,000. **Reg. Groups:** 11. **State Groups:** 50. **Desc:** Individuals with Williams Syndrome and their families; medical and health care professionals; educators. (Williams Syndrome is characterized by similar facial features, low birth weight, heart disorders, hearing sensitivity, talkative personality, mild to severe learning disabilities, and developmental delays.) Provides support and assistance to families with a WS child. Conducts networking in the medical, scientific, educational, and professional communities for referral and study of newly-diagnosed WS individuals. Encourages medical behavior and supports research into all aspects of the syndrome. Compiles statistics. **Pub:** *Ben's Big Decision*. Book. Storybook and tape. *Price:* $19.95. • *Facts Brochure*. Brochures. *Price:* Free. • *Information for Teachers*. Handbook. For parents and professionals. *Price:* $7. • *The Promenade: A Story about Adolescents with Williams Syndrome*. Provides testing and evaluations for WSA. *Price:* $15; $4 for parents and professors. • *Williams Syndrome Association National Newsletter*, 4/year. Newsletter. Includes research updates and parent and professional forums. *Price:* $20/year.

★ 6381 ★ Wilson's Disease Association (WDA)
4 Navaho Dr.
Brookfield, CT 06804
Phone: (330)264-1450 **Free:** 800-399-0266
Fax: (509)757-6418
Email: wilsondiseaseassoc@yahoo.com
Website: http://www.wilsonsdisease.org
Kimberly F. Symonds, Exec. Dir.

Fnded: 1979. **Mem:** 1,000. **Nat'l Groups:** 1. **Local Groups:** 2. **Desc:** Patients of Wilson's disease relatives and friends of patients; physicians and other health care professionals. (Wilson's disease, named for S.A.K. Wilson, a pioneer in the study of the disease, is a genetic nervous disorder in which excessive amounts of copper collect in the liver, brain, and kidneys.) Purpose is to promote and sponsor research regarding the cause, treatment, cure, and prevention of Wilson's and related diseases. Stresses the importance of public awareness, early diagnosis, and treatment. Provides financial aid and moral support to needy individuals and organizations sharing the association's goals; serves as liaison among members and cooperating organizations. Collects and disseminates information to members and the public concerning developments, current research, and legislation in the field; acts as clearinghouse. **Pub:** *The Copper Connection*, quarterly. Newsletter. Includes research reports, member profiles, and book reviews. *Price:* included in membership dues. • *Wilson's Disease Association–Membership Directory*, annual. Membership Directory. *Price:* Included in membership dues. • *Wilson's Disease: Questions & Answers*. Brochures. • Also publishes many other brochures on various aspects of Wilson's disease.

★ 6382 ★ Winged Fellowship Trust
Angel House
20-32 Pentonville Rd.
London N1 9XD, United Kingdom
Phone: 44 207 8332594 **Fax:** 44 207 2780370
Email: admin@wft.org.uk
Website: http://www.wft.org.uk

Fnded: 1963. **Reg. Groups:** 5. **Lang(s):** English. **Desc:** Volunteers required to provide respite care for physically disabled persons in England. Organizes holidays for disabled individuals at five regional centers operated by the Trust. **Pub:** *Volunteer Information Brochure*, annual. Brochure. Includes descriptions of facilities and application form.

★ 6383 ★ Woman To Woman
c/o Dr. Lucie A. DiMaggio
1807 Elmwood Ave., Ste. 165
Buffalo, NY 14207-2434
Email: info@womantowomanvideos.org
Dr. Lucie A. DiMaggio, Founder

Desc: Provides videos and resource guides for newly diagnosed breast-cancer patients. Offers education, support and comfort. **Pub:** *NWL*. • Videos.

★ 6384 ★ Woman to Woman Support Network
Airport Plz., Unit 5
1341 W Main Rd.
Middletown, RI 02842
Phone: (401)841-9211
Email: jmartellino@cox.net
Website: http://www.thombs.com/woman2woman/

Desc: Provides free support and referals to women experiencing a problem pregnancy.

★ 6385 ★ Women in Endocrinology (WE)
c/o Ursula Kaiser, MD
Endocrine-Hypertension Division
Brigham and Women's Hospital
221 Longwood Ave.
Boston, MA 02115
Phone: (617)732-5768 **Fax:** (617)732-5764
Email: ukaiser@partners.org
Website: http://www.women-in-endo.org
Ursula Kaiser, MD, Sec. -Treas.

Desc: Women employed in the field of endocrinology; female endocrinology students and residents. Promotes "professional development and advancement of women in the field of endocrinology." Facilitates exchange of information among members; conducts educational programs.

★ 6386 ★ Women in Managed Care (WMC)
4435 Waterfront Dr., Ste. 101
PO Box 6026
Glen Allen, VA 23058-6026
Phone: (804)527-1905 **Fax:** (804)747-5316
Email: info@wimc.org
Website: http://www.wimc.org
Sloane Reed, Exec. Dir.

Fnded: 1996. **Mem:** 1,000. **Desc:** Women working for managed care health services providers. Promotes professional advancement of members. Conducts research and educational programs. **Pub:** *Women in Managed Care*, monthly. Newsletter.

★ 6387 ★ Women Organized to Respond to Life-Threatening Diseases (WORLD)
414 13th St., 2nd Fl.
Oakland, CA 94612-2603
Phone: (510)986-0340 **Fax:** (510)986-0341
Email: info@womenhiv.org
Website: http://www.womenhiv.org/
Rebecca Denison, Founder

Fnded: 1991. **Mem:** 12,000. **Desc:** An empowerment organization by and for women infected or affected by the HIV virus. Offers support and information to women who have AIDS and HIV. Offers retreats and educational classes. Maintains speakers bureau. **Pub:** *WORLD*, monthly. Newsletter. Personal testimonies of infected women; medical and political information. Easy-to-understand women specific HIV/AIDS treatment. **AKA:** WORLD.

★ 6388 ★ Women for Sobriety (WFS)
PO Box 618
Quakertown, PA 18951
Phone: (215)536-8026 **Fax:** (215)538-9026
Email: newlife@nni.com
Website: http://www.womenforsobriety.org
Becky Fenner, Dir.

Fnded: 1975. **Mem:** 5,000. **Nat'l Groups:** 200. **Desc:** Self-help groups of women alcoholics who use a program "based on abstinence, comprised of Thirteen Acceptance Statements that, when accepted and used, will provide each woman with a new way of life through a new way of thinking. Starts with coping first but then moves on to overcoming and a whole change in the approach to each day." Recognizes differences between male and female alcoholics in the method of successful recovery. Small groups organize and meet independently. Maintains speakers' bureau. **Pub:** *Sobering Thoughts*, monthly. Newsletter. Contains calendar of events, research updates, membership articles, and news on WFS meetings. *Price:* $14.95/year. • Also publishes tapes, workbooks, booklets, and videos.

★ 6389 ★ Women With Disabilities - Australia
PO Box 605
Rosny Park, TAS 7018, Australia
Phone: 61 3 62448288 **Fax:** 61 3 62448255
Email: wwda@ozemail.com.au
Website: http://www.wwda.org.au

Fnded: 1995. **Mem:** 1,700. **Nat'l Groups:** 1. **State Groups:** 7. **Desc:** Works for equality in participation and opportunity for disabled women. **Pub:** *WWDA News*, quarterly. Newsletter. Reports and information resources.

★ 6390 ★ Women's Association for Natural Medicinal Therapy
Private Mail Bag
Suva, Fiji
Phone: 679 315021 **Fax:** 679 315021
Email: wainimate@is.com.fj

Fnded: 1995. **Mem:** 30. **Lang(s):** English. **Desc:** Women practitioners of traditional medicine in Fiji, the Cook Islands, Naura, Kiribati, Tonga, Vanuatu, Papua New Guinea, the Solomon Islands, and Tahiti. Encourages: conservation of medicinal plants and their habitats; dissemination of information on traditional healing practices; communication among members; establishment of national traditional medicine associations.

★ 6391 ★ Women's Auxiliary of the ICA (WAICA)
1110 N Glebe Rd., Ste. 1000
Arlington, VA 22201
Phone: (703)528-5000 **Free:** 800-423-4690
Fax: (703)528-5023
Email: chiro@chiropractic.org
Website: http://www.chiropractic.org
Dr. DeeDee Humber, Pres.

Fnded: 1951. **Mem:** 500. **Desc:** Women chiropractors; wives, daughters, and mothers of chiropractors who are members of the International Chiropractors Association. Promotes and educates the public about chiropractice. Grants scholarships to chiropractic students. Supports charitable programs. **Pub:** *Membership Roster*, biennial. Membership Directory. • Newsletter, quarterly.

★ 6392 ★ Women's Dermatologic Society (WDS)
74 New Montgomery St., Ste. 230
San Francisco, CA 94105
Phone: (415)927-5727 **Fax:** (415)927-5726
Email: estreu@aad.org
Website: http://www.womensderm.org
Kerry Parker, CAE, Contact

Desc: Dermatology professionals promoting women in dermatology. Conducts mentoring program; provides networking opportunities **Pub:** Newsletter, quarterly.

★ 6393 ★ Women's Drug Research Project (WDR)
c/o Beth G. Reed
University of Michigan
School of Social Work
1065 Frieze Bldg.
Ann Arbor, MI 48109-1285
Phone: (734)763-5958
Beth G. Reed, Coord.

Fnded: 1973. **Desc:** Has investigated differences in the needs and problems of men and women entering drug abuse treatment programs. Studied two outpatient methadone programs and two residential therapeutic communities, which were established to gather new information about women addicts, their needs, and possible methods for meeting those needs. Also collected data from 20 programs in five cities for studies on treatment organization and psychosocial characteristics of addicts.

★ 6394 ★ Women's Health
52 Featherstone St.
London EC1Y 8RT, United Kingdom
Phone: 44 20 72516333 **Fax:** 44 20 72504152
Email: womenshealth@pop3.poptel.org.uk
Website: http://www.womenshealthlondon.org.uk

Fnded: 1982. **Mem:** 250. **Lang(s):** English. **Desc:** Women's health information organization in the UK. Works to empower women to make informed decisions about health and reproductive issues. Promotes a pro-choice perspective on women's health issues, including abortion. Informs women of their reproductive rights; provides information about women's health issues. Develops and promotes a feminist perspective of women's health and reproductive rights. **Pub:** *Women's Health*, quarterly. Newsletter. Covers information about women's health and reproductive issues. • Newsletter, quarterly. Focuses on a different health aspect each issue.

★ 6395 ★ Women's Health and Economic Development Association (WHEDA)
3B Ekpo Obot St.
PO Box 2665
Uyo, Nigeria
Phone: 234 85 203944
Email: wheda@fordwa.linkserve.com

Fnded: 1988. **Mem:** 18,000. **Nat'l Groups:** 4. **State Groups:** 20. **Local Groups:** 180. **Lang(s):** English. **Desc:** Works to prevent health problems of women in rural Nigerian communities. Provides education and counseling on nutritional and family planning issues. Encourages economic independence for women through supportive programs and activities. **Pub:** Articles. In newspapers and magazines. **Frmly:** (1988) Rural Women Health Association.

★ 6396 ★ Women's Healthcare Educational Network (WHEN)
9 Jackson St.
Tiffin, OH 44883
Free: 800-991-8877 **Fax:** (419)443-0785

Email: usainfo@whenusa.org
Sarah Hanna, Member Services Coor.

Fnded: 1990. **Mem:** 80. **Desc:** Network of businesses that specialize in serving the post-mastectomy woman. Strives to improve the manner in which external breast forms and their related products are provided. **Pub:** *One Voice*, quarterly. Newsletter. Contains information on breast cancer and other industry specific information. *Price:* included in membership dues; $10/year for non-members.

★ 6397 ★ Women's International Public Health Network (WIPHN)

7100 Oak Forest Ln.
Bethesda, MD 20817
Phone: (301)469-9210 **Fax:** (301)469-8423
Email: wiphn@erols.com
Dr. Naomi Baumslag, Pres.

Fnded: 1987. **Mem:** 12,500. **Desc:** Individuals and organizations with an interest in women's health issues. Promotes adoption of public health policies and programs providing greater access to health care for women. Conducts educational programs. **Pub:** *WIPHN News*, 3/year. Newsletter. *Price:* $35 for individuals; $50/yr for organizations.

★ 6398 ★ WOOMB Philippines

PO Box 191EA
Ermita, Metro Manila 1045, Philippines
Phone: 63 46 5400675

Fnded: 1994. **Mem:** 50. **Desc:** Advocates family planning and responsible parenthood as a basic human right and as a means to enhance the quality of life. Disseminates information on the Billings Ovulation Method of natural family planning.

★ 6399 ★ WOOMB Tanzania

c/o Sec., Tanzania Family Strengthening Association
PO Box 1003
Ndanda
Mtwara, United Republic of Tanzania

Desc: Advocates family planning and responsible parenthood as a basic human right and as a means to enhance the quality of life.

★ 6400 ★ Workgroup for Electronic Data Interchange (WEDI)

12020 Sunrise Valley Dr., Ste 100
Reston, VA 20191
Phone: (703)391-2716 **Fax:** (703)391-2759
Email: webmaster@wedi.org
Website: http://www.wedi.org
James A. Schuping, Contact

Desc: Promotes Electronic Commerce in the Health Care Industry.

★ 6401 ★ Working Group on Health and Development Issues (DEAG) (Werkgroep Medische Ontwikkelingssamenwerking — WEMOS)

Postbus 1693
NL-1000 BR Amsterdam, Netherlands
Phone: 31 20 4688388 **Fax:** 31 20 4686008
Email: wemos@wemos.nl
Website: http://www.wemos.nl

Fnded: 1980. **Mem:** 10. **Lang(s):** Dutch, English. **Desc:** Aims to improve health in developing countries through influencing international policy. **Pub:** *Exposed Deadly Exports: The Story of European Community Exports of Banned or Withdrawn Drugs to the Third World*. Book. • Books.

★ 6402 ★ World Allergy Organization (WAO)

611 E Wells St.
Milwaukee, WI 53202
Phone: (414)276-1791 **Fax:** (414)276-3349
Email: info@worldallergy.org
Website: http://www.worldallergy.org/
Denise Lemke, Exec. Dir.

Fnded: 1951. **Mem:** 38,000. **Nat'l Groups:** 52. **Reg. Groups:** 4. **Desc:** Umbrella organization for 56 international allergy associations representing 38,000 health professionals. **Pub:** *Allergy and Clinical Immunology International*, bimonthly. Journal. Includes research updates. *Price:* $44/year for members; $68/year for nonmembers. **Frmly:** (1980) International Association of Allergology; (2002) International Association of Allergology and Clinical Immunology.

★ 6403 ★ World Alliance of Neuromuscular Disorder Associations (WANDA)

GPO Box 414
Adelaide, SA 5001, Australia
Phone: 61 8 82345266 **Fax:** 61 8 82345866
Email: info@mdasa.org.au

Fnded: 1990. **Mem:** 65. **Nat'l Groups:** 65. **Reg. Groups:** 7.

★ 6404 ★ World Apheresis Association (WAA)

1, av Claude Vellefaux
F-75475 Paris, France
Phone: 33 1 42499210 **Fax:** 33 1 42409314
Email: ets-bussel@chu-stlouis.fr

★ 6405 ★ World Association for the Advancement of Veterinary Parasitology (WAAVP)

PO Box 8
North Aurora, IL 60542
Phone: (630)844-9676 **Fax:** (630)892-0818
Email: isvma@aol.com
Ann R. Donoghue, DVM, Sec. -Treas.

Fnded: 1963. **Mem:** 560. **Desc:** Veterinarians and other scientists in 60 countries interested in veterinary parasitology. Objectives are to encourage research in veterinary parasitology, to promote the exchange of information and material between organizations and individuals, and to organize meetings for the study of parasites of veterinary importance. Maintains scientific committees. **Pub:** *Membership Directory*, annual. Membership Directory. • *Newsletter*, 3/year. Newsletter. • *Proceedings of Scientific Conferences*, biennial. • *Statutes - List of Members*, biennial. **AKA:** Association Mondiale pour l'Advancement de Parasitologie Veterinaire.

★ 6406 ★ World Association for Bronchology

5-7 Shin Ogawa-machi, Sinjuku-ku
Tokyo 162, Japan
Phone: 81 3 32691865 **Fax:** 81 3 32691865

★ 6407 ★ World Association for Buiatrics (WAB) (Welt-Gesellschaft fur Buiatrik)

c/o Dr. O. Szenci, Sec.
Faculty of Veterinary Science
Szent Istvan University
PO Box 2
H-1400 Budapest, Hungary
Phone: 36 29 521301 **Fax:** 36 29 521303
Email: oszenci@univet.hu
Website: http://www.ulg.ac.be/fmv/wab.htm

Fnded: 1962. **Mem:** 10,000. **Lang(s):** English, French, German, Spanish. **Desc:** Veterinarians, practitioners, and scientists working with cattle in 48 countries. Seeks to study the diseases of cattle, including diagnosis, treatment, and prevention, and factors influencing cattle production. **Pub:** *Congress Reports*, biennial. • Newsletter, quarterly.

★ 6408 ★ World Association for Dynamic Psychiatry (WADP)

c/o Maria Ammon
Dynamic-Psychiatric Clinic
Geiselgasteigstrasse 203
Menterschwaige
D-81545 Munich, Germany
Phone: 49 89 6427230 **Fax:** 49 89 64272395

Fnded: 1980. **Mem:** 500. **Nat'l Groups:** 22. **Lang(s):** English, German. **Desc:** Disseminates the theory and practice of dynamic psychiatry developed at Gunter Ammon's Berlin School of Dynamic Psychiatry. Fosters and creates opportunities for dynamic psychiatry study in universities and other institutions. Promotes continuous advanced training in dynamic psychiatry for better patient care and improvement of public health. Conducts research into disease prevention, therapeutic method efficiency, and education standards; disseminates results. **Pub:** *Dynamische Psychiatrie/Dynamic Psychiatry*, bimonthly. • *WADP*, semiannual. Newsletter.

★ 6409 ★ World Association for Infant Mental Health (WAIMH)

Kellogg Center, Rm. 4
East Lansing, MI 48824-1022
Phone: (517)432-3793 **Fax:** (517)432-3694
Email: waimh@msu.edu
Website: http://www.msu.edu/user/waimh
Hiram E. Fitzgerald, Exec. Dir.

Fnded: 1992. **Mem:** 850. **Reg. Groups:** 19. **Desc:** Child development specialists, child psychiatrists, child psychoanalysts, infant care workers, linguists, nurses, obstetricians, pediatricians, psychologists, and social workers. Works to further research and understanding of mental development and disorders in children from conception through age 3. Promotes studies on the conditions affecting the mental health of infants, their parents, and other caregivers; explores mental development during infancy and its subsequent effects on psychopathological development. Advocates international multidisciplinary discussions of research and intervention in infant psychiatry within the framework of the total life cycle. Facilitates communication and exchange of information and theories; fosters discussion of questions, problems, and issues in infant mental health. **Pub:** *Infant Mental Health Journal*, bimonthly. Journal. *Price:* $45 for members; $58 for members outside the U.S.; $75 for USA non members. • *The Signal*, quarterly. Newsletter. *Price:* $99 for Non members outside the USA.

★ 6410 ★ World Association of Perinatal Medicine

Augustenburger Platz 1
D-13353 Berlin, Germany
Phone: 49 30 45064072 **Fax:** 49 30 45064901
Email: joachim.dudenhausen@charite.de

★ 6411 ★ World Association of Psychoanalysis (Association Mondiale de Psychanalyse — AMP)

5 rue de Lille
F-75007 Paris, France
Phone: 33 1 45485672 **Fax:** 33 1 45487938
Email: wapol@wapol.org
Website: http://www.wapol.org/

Fnded: 1992. **Mem:** 1,800. **Lang(s):** English, French. **Desc:** Mental health care professionals. Promotes advancement in psychoanalytical scholarship and practice. Serves as a clearinghouse on psychoanalysis and its applications; conducts research and educational programs.

★ 6412 ★ World Association of Sarcoidosis and Other Granulomatous Disorders (WASOG)

Via Juvara 9
20129 Milan, Italy
Phone: 39 02 2666906
Email: rizzatog@tin.it

Website: http://www.pinali.unipd.it/sarcoid

Fnded: 1958. **Mem:** 300. **Lang(s):** English. **Desc:** Physicians in 40 countries. Promotes and sponsors research and clinical activities on sarcoidosis concerning damage to the brain, eyes, heart, lungs, and skin. (Sarcoidosis is characterized by inflammation of the lungs, eyes, skin, and other tissue and results in immunological upset; its cause is unknown.) Maintains speakers' bureau and hall of fame. **Pub:** *Sarcoidosis*, semiannual. • *Transactions of the World Congress on Sarcoidosis*, biennial. **Frmly:** (1987) International Committee of Sarcoidosis.

★ 6413 ★ World Association for Social Psychiatry (WASP)

656 Romero Canyon Rd.
Santa Barbara, CA 93108
Phone: (805)969-1376 **Fax:** (805)969-1376
John L. Carleton, MD, Honorary Pres.

Fnded: 1964. **Mem:** 3,000. **Reg. Groups:** 26. **Desc:** Professionals, contributors, and interested individuals active in allied fields of social psychiatry including anthropology, social work, nursing, or occupational therapy. Objectives are to: study the nature of man and his surrounding culture; research methods to prevent and treat internal changes and behavioral disorders; advance the physical, social, and philosophic well-being of mankind. Fosters collaboration among members and distributes theoretical and practical information. Conducts workshops and demonstrations of rehabilitation centers. **Pub:** *French Journal of Social Psychiatry*, quarterly. Journal. • *International Journal of Social Psychiatry*, quarterly. Journal. • *World Journal of Social Psychiatry*, quarterly. Journal. **Frmly:** (1978) International Association for Social Psychiatry.

★ 6414 ★ World Association of Societies of Pathology and Laboratory Medicine

WASP Administrative Office
c/o Japanese Society of Laboratory Medicine
5F Takahashi Bldg., 1-7-1
Sarugakucho Chiyoda-ku
Tokyo 101-0064, Japan
Phone: 81 3 32950351 **Fax:** 81 3 32950352
Email: waspalm@jscp.org
Website: http://www.waspalm.org

Fnded: 1947. **Mem:** 23. **Lang(s):** English. **Desc:** National societies of laboratory medicine in 15 countries united to foster cooperation between members and improve standards in laboratory medicine. Maintains a variety of committees and educational programs. **Frmly:** (1969) International Society of Clinical Pathology.

★ 6415 ★ World Association of Veterinary Anatomists (WAVA)

Department of Veterinary Anatomy & Embryology
University of Antwerp
Universiteitspein 1
B-2610 Wilrijk, Belgium
Phone: 32 3 8202432 **Fax:** 32 3 8202433
Email: weyns@ruca.ua.ac.be
Website: http://vetanem.ruca.ua.ac.be/

Fnded: 1957. **Mem:** 350. **Reg. Groups:** 8. **Lang(s):** English, French, German, Spanish. **Desc:** Veterinarians and other professionals teaching and researching at veterinary institutions. Promotes the study and teaching of domestic animal anatomy. Seeks to establish a uniform nomenclature. Maintains International Committee on Veterinary Anatomical Nomenclature. **Pub:** *Anatomia, Histologia, Embryologia (Zentralblatt for Veterinarmedizin, Section C)*, quarterly. Journal. • *Nomina Anatomica Veterinaria - Nomina Histologica - Nomina Embryologica*. Book. • *WAVA-News*, annual.

★ 6416 ★ World Association of Veterinary Laboratory Diagnosticians (WAVLD)

PO Drawer 3040
College Station, TX 77841-3040
Phone: (979)845-3414 **Free:** 888-646-5623
Fax: (979)845-1794
Email: keugster@tvmdl.edu
A. K. Eugster, Sec. Treas.

Fnded: 1977. **Mem:** 650. **Nat'l Groups:** 5. **Desc:** Individuals in 30 countries engaged in laboratory diagnosis of animal diseases. Coordinates activities of regulatory, research, and service laboratories. Maintains guidelines for personnel qualifications and facility standards. Establishes uniform laboratory methods and seeks to improve and develop existing diagnostic techniques. Disseminates information; maintains speakers' bureau. **Pub:** *Symposium Proceedings*, triennial. Proceedings.

★ 6417 ★ World Association of Veterinary Microbiologists, Immunologists, and Specialists in Infectious Diseases (WAVMI) (Association Mondiale des Veterinaires Microbiologistes, Immunologistes et Specialistes des Maladies Infectieuses — AMVMI)

7, ave. du General de Gaulle
F-94704 Maisons-Alfort Cedex, France
Phone: 33 1 43967021 **Fax:** 33 1 43967022

Fnded: 1968. **Lang(s):** English, French. **Desc:** Facilitates international exchange among veterinary microbiologists, immunologists, and specialists in infectious diseases. Sponsors international course in animal immunology; conducts symposia. **Pub:** *Comparative Immunology, Microbiology and Infectious Diseases*, quarterly.

★ 6418 ★ World Association of Veterinary Pathologists (WAVP)

Ecole Nationale Veterinaire
F-94704 Maisons-Alfort, France
Phone: 33 1 43967109 **Fax:** 33 1 43967112
Email: parodi@net-alfort.fr

Fnded: 1952. **Desc:** Promotes the study of pathomorphology and pathophysiology of animal diseases and their pathogenesis.

★ 6419 ★ World Association of Wildlife Veterinarians (WAWV)

c/o Institute of Zoology
Regents Park
London NW1 4RY, United Kingdom
Phone: 44 171 4496668 **Fax:** 44 171 5861457
Email: t.sainsbury@ioz.ac.uk
Website: http://wildvet.home.netcom.com/home.html

Fnded: 1990. **Desc:** Coordinates and exchanges information on wildlife; promotes international meetings and seminars.

★ 6420 ★ World Autism Organisation (WAO)

Ronda del carril, 83
E-08530 Barcelona, Spain
Fax: 34 93 8605360
Email: contact@worldautism.org
Website: http://worldautism.org

Fnded: 1998. **Desc:** Seeks to increase awareness of autism; promotes development of improved diagnosis and treatment of people with autism. Works to enhance quality of life of people with autism.

★ 6421 ★ World Blind Union (WBU)

Jose Ortega y Gassett 22-24, 4
E-28006 Madrid, Spain
Phone: 34 91 5894533 **Fax:** 34 91 5894749
Email: umc@once.es
Website: http://umc.once.es

Fnded: 1984. **Mem:** 155. **Reg. Groups:** 7. **Lang(s):** English, French, Spanish. **Desc:** National associations of the blind and international agencies for the blind. Fosters international cooperation among organizations working for the welfare of the blind and the prevention of blindness in 155 countries. Encourages creation and development of national organizations of and for the blind; seeks to provide necessary technical and material aid to such groups. Provides guidance in fields of education, rehabilitation, vocational training, and employment. Works toward the introduction and improvement of minimum standards for the welfare of the blind worldwide. Encourages and conducts studies in the field of service to the blind and the prevention of blindness. Collects and disseminates information on the conditions of the blind in different coutries; informs members of social and legislative matters relating to blindness and its prevention. Maintains relations with numerous United Nations agencies including the World Health Organization, the International Council on Disability, and the International Agency for the Prevention of Blindness; sponsors the International Council for the Education of the Visually Impaired. **Pub:** *General Assembly Proceedings*, periodic. • *Review of the European Blind*, semiannual. • *The World Blind*, biennial. Magazine. Also available in braille and on casette.

★ 6422 ★ World Cancer Research Fund (WCRF)

105 Park St.
London W1Y 3FB, United Kingdom
Phone: 44 20 73434200 **Fax:** 44 20 73434201

Fnded: 1990. **Desc:** Promotes research into cancer prevention.

★ 6423 ★ World Chiropractic Alliance (WCA)

2950 N Dobson Rd., Ste. 1
Chandler, AZ 85224
Free: 800-347-1011 **Fax:** (480)732-9313
Website: http://www.worldchiropracticalliance.org/

Fnded: 1989. **Desc:** Dedicated to protecting and strengthening chiropractic around the world. **Pub:** *Position papers*. Papers. • Books.

★ 6424 ★ World Confederation for Physical Therapy (WCPT) (Confederation Mondiale pour la Therapie Physique)

46-48 Grosvenor Gardens
London SW1W 0EB, United Kingdom
Phone: 44 207 8819234 **Fax:** 44 207 8819239
Email: info@wcpt.org
Website: http://www.wcpt.org

Fnded: 1951. **Mem:** 83. **Nat'l Groups:** 65. **Reg. Groups:** 5. **Desc:** Confederation of 83 national associations representing physical therapists around the world supported mainly by subscriptions from its member organizations. Works to improve global health by: representing physical therapy and physical therapists internationally, collaborating with international and national organisations, encouraging high standards of physical therapy research, education and practice, and supporting communications of WCPT. **Pub:** *Annual Report*. • *Key Notes: Opinion Papers on a Variety of Professional Matters*, periodic. Reports. • *WCPT News*, semiannual. Newsletter. • Books, periodic.

★ 6425 ★ World Council of Coloproctology (WCCP)

Prince of Wales Private Hospital
Barker St.
Randwick, NSW 2031, Australia
Phone: 61 2 96504222 **Fax:** 61 2 96504924
Email: new@bigpond.net.au

Fnded: 1990. **Nat'l Groups:** 60. **Reg. Groups:** 5.

★ 6426 ★ World Council of Enterostomal Therapists (WCET)

PO Box 48099
60 Dundas St. E
Mississauga, ON, Canada L5A 4G8
Phone: (905)848-9400 **Fax:** (905)848-9413
Email: info@wcetn.org
Website: http://www.wcetn.org

Desc: Individuals engaged in caring for people with stomas, draining wounds, fistulae, incontinence management problems, and potential or actual tissue trauma. **Pub:** *WCET Journal*, periodic. Journal.

★ 6427 ★ World Council of Optometry (WCO)

c/o Anthony F Di Stefano OD
8360 Old York Rd.
Elkins Park, PA 19027
Phone: (215)780-1320 **Fax:** (215)780-1325
Email: wco@pco.edu
Website: http://www.worldoptometry.org/
Anthony F. Di Stefano, Exec. Dir.

Fnded: 1927. **Mem:** 84. **Nat'l Groups:** 54. **Reg. Groups:** 3. **Desc:** National optical and optometric organizations in 60 countries. Promotes optometry and vision care worldwide. Works to develop optometry through education, legal and legislative advice, discussion with authorities, and support of similar associations. Is concerned with protecting optometry from what the league sees as proposed restrictive legislation, and apathy toward the profession. Establishes educational standards; offers evaluation program for schools and colleges of optometry; provides consulting services. **Pub:** *International Country Contact Register*, periodic. • *Interoptics*, quarterly. Newsletter. • *Members Journals*, periodic. • *Optometric Mailing Directory*, periodic. Directory. Lists information on optometric organizations. • *Publications List*, periodic. • *Register of Schools and Colleges of Optometry*, periodic. • Brochure, periodic.

★ 6428 ★ World Federation of Acupuncture-Moxibustion Societies (WFAS)

18 Beixincang
Beijing 100700, People's Republic of China
Phone: 86 10 64063648 **Fax:** 86 10 64013968

Desc: Promotes cooperation among acupuncture-moxibustion groups; develops the science of acupuncture-moxibustion.

★ 6429 ★ World Federation of Catholic Medical Associations (FIAMC) (Federation Internationale des Associations Medicales Catholiques — FIAMC)

Palazzo San Calisto
V-00120 Vatican City, Vatican City
Phone: 39 6 69887372 **Fax:** 39 6 69887372
Email: fiamc.va@virgilio.it
Website: http://www.fiamc.org

Fnded: 1950. **Mem:** 52. **Nat'l Groups:** 64. **Reg. Groups:** 5. **Lang(s):** English, French. **Desc:** National associations and guilds of Catholic physicians. Seeks to: coordinate the efforts of Catholic medical associations worldwide; promote Christian principles throughout the medical profession; discuss and find new ethical approaches to biotechnological problems. Encourages the development of Catholic medical associations globally to assist in the moral, spiritual, and technical advancement of the Catholic physician; participates in the development of the medical profession. Maintains speakers' bureau. **Pub:** *Catholic Medical Quarterly*, quarterly. • *Decisions*, 3/year. Newsletter. • *Linacre Bulletin*, quarterly. • Journal, quarterly.

★ 6430 ★ World Federation of Chiropractic (WFC)

3080 Yonge St., Ste. 5065
Toronto, ON, Canada M4N 3N1
Phone: (416)484-9978 **Fax:** (416)484-9665
Email: info@wfc.org
Website: http://www.wfc.org

Fnded: 1988. **Mem:** 78. **Lang(s):** French, Spanish. **Desc:** Chiropractors, colleges, corporations, and national associations of chiropractors in over 78 countries. Represents the chiropractic profession internationally. Provides information and assistance in the fields of chiropractic and world health. Promotes uniformly high standards of chiropractic education, research, and practice. **Pub:** Membership Directory.

★ 6431 ★ World Federation of the Deaf (WFD)

PO Box 65
SF-00401 Helsinki, Finland
Fax: 358 9 5803572
Email: info@wfdnews.org
Website: http://www.wfdnews.org

Fnded: 1951. **Mem:** 123. **Nat'l Groups:** 124. **Reg. Groups:** 8. **Lang(s):** English. **Desc:** Ordinary members are National associations of the deaf that are legally constituted and represent in the widest sense the deaf in their country; other members are national or international associations, societies, and bodies for and of the deaf; health, educational, social, and similar establishments that accept the aims of the federation; professionals interested in deafness and related subjects; persons performing special tasks connected with the aims of the federation; parents and friends of the deaf. Represents the worldwide deaf community in international forums such as the United Nations. Makes policy statements and recommendations. Coordinates research and other projects with the deaf community; conducts surveys. Has established a network of experts on deafness and related issues. Promotes the use of national sign language as the first language of deaf people. **Pub:** *WFD News*, 3/year. Journal. • *WFD Survey of Deaf People in the Developing World*. Report.

★ 6432 ★ World Federation of Doctors Who Respect Human Life (United States Section) (WFDRHL)

PO Box 101501
Pittsburgh, PA 15237
Phone: (724)444-8045 **Fax:** (724)444-8013
Dr. Brain Donnelly, Sec. -Treas.

Fnded: 1976. **Mem:** 1,400. **Desc:** Physicians united to restore the "traditional Hippocratic medical position" through firm opposition to abortion, suicide, and direct euthanasia. Sponsors educational programs and seminars. Presently inactive. **Pub:** *Primum Non Nocere*, quarterly. Newsletter.

★ 6433 ★ World Federation of Hemophilia (WFH) (Federation Mondiale de l'Hemophilie — FMH)

1425 Rene-Levesque West
Ste. 1010
Montreal, QC, Canada H3G 1T7
Phone: (514)875-7944 **Fax:** (514)875-8916
Email: wfh@wfh.org
Website: http://wfh.org

Fnded: 1963. **Mem:** 1,000. **Nat'l Groups:** 88. **Reg. Groups:** 3. **Lang(s):** French, Spanish. **Desc:** Representatives of national hemophilia committees or societies. Assists individuals with hemophilia and persons with related disorders. Aims to stimulate interest in the development and improvement of diagnosis, treatment, rehabilitation, education, and research in hemophilia. Serves as a coordinating body to develop the collection, distribution and exchange of useful information and to make relevant investigations throughout the world. Encourages the establishment and development of other hemophilia organizations. Compiles statistics. **Pub:** *Hemophilia World*, quarterly. Newsletter. • *Information Update*, periodic. Bulletin.

★ 6434 ★ World Federation for Medical Education (WFME) (Federation Mondiale pour l'Enseignement Medical — FMEM)

Univ. of Copenhagen
Faculty of Health Sciences
Blegdamsvej 3
DK-2200 Copenhagen N, Denmark
Phone: 45 35327103 **Fax:** 45 35327070
Email: wfme@wfme.org
Website: http://www.sund.ku.dk/wfme/

Fnded: 1972. **Reg. Groups:** 6. **Lang(s):** English. **Desc:** Regional medical associations and associations of medical schools. Promotes the integrated study of medical education worldwide. Evaluates the effectiveness of medical education in meeting the needs of contemporary society. Acts as international representative of medical education before the World Health Organization, UNICEF, UNESCO, United Nations Development Programme, and the World Bank. **Pub:** *Report of the World Conference on Medical Education, Edinburgh, 1988/Proceedings of the World Summit on Medical Education, Edinburgh, 1994*. Report. • *Report of the World Summit on Medical Education, Edinburgh, 1994*. Report.

★ 6435 ★ World Federation for Mental Health (WFMH)

PO Box 16810
Alexandria, VA 22302-0810
Phone: (703)838-7543 **Fax:** (703)519-7648
Email: wfmh@erols.com
Website: http://www.wfmh.org
Preston Garrison, CEO

Fnded: 1948. **Mem:** 1,112. **Reg. Groups:** 9. **Desc:** Associations and individuals dedicated to achieving the highest level of public mental health. Objectives include charitable, scientific, literary, and educational activities in the field of mental health. Organizes training programs. Sponsors World Mental Health Day. **Pub:** Newsletter, quarterly. *Price:* Free to members. **Frmly:** (1948) International Committee for Mental Hygiene.

★ 6436 ★ World Federation of Neurology (WFN)

12 Chandos St.
London W1G 9DR, United Kingdom
Phone: 44 207 3234011 **Fax:** 44 207 3234012
Email: kimurakyoto@aol.com

Fnded: 1955. **Mem:** 23,000. **Nat'l Groups:** 86. **Reg. Groups:** 6. **Lang(s):** English. **Desc:** Neurologists and neuroscientists dedicated to improving the care of neurological patients and to preventing diseases of the nervous system. Disseminates information in the field of neurology. Organizes research groups on disease topics; compiles statistics. Maintains speakers' bureau. Conducts educational and research programs. **Pub:** *Journal of Neurological Sciences*, bimonthly. Contains research papers. • *World Neurology*, quarterly.

★ 6437 ★ World Federation of Neurosurgical Societies (WFNS)

c/o Dr. Edward Laws
University of Virginia Health Systems
Department of Neuro-Societies
PO Box 800212
Charlottesville, VA 22908
Phone: (434)924-2650 **Free:** 800-650-2650
Fax: (434)924-5894
Website: http://www.wfns.org
Dr. Edward Laws, Pres.

Fnded: 1957. **Mem:** 64. **Reg. Groups:** 5. **Desc:** National neurosurgical societies representing approximately 17,400 neurosurgeons. Works for the advancement of neurological surgery. **Pub:** *Critical Reviews in Neurosurgery*. Journal. • *Federation News*, quarterly. Newsletter. *Price:* $75. • *Proceedings of International Congress*, quadrennial. Proceedings. • *World Directory*, periodic. Directory.

★ 6438 ★ World Federation of Occupational Therapists (WFOT) (Federation Mondiale des Ergotherapeutes)

c/o WFOT Secretariat
PO Box 30
Forrestfield, WA 6058, Australia
Fax: 61 8 94539746
Email: wfot@multiline.com.au
Website: http://www.wfot.org.au

Fnded: 1952. **Mem:** 55. **Lang(s):** English. **Desc:** Membership is comprised of 55 countries which have Occupational Therapy Associations with approved constitutions and educational programmes; associate members, which are countries with approved constitutions; and individual members, who are qualified occupational therapists. Objectives are to: promote the occupational therapy profession; provide for exchange of information and publications; encourage international cooperation; establish standards of education for occupational therapists; maintain professional ethics; facilitate international exchange and placement of therapists and students. Promotes research; assists developing countries in formulating education programs for occupational therapists. **Pub:** *A Chronicle of the World Federation of Occupational Therapists.* • *WFOT Bulletin*, semiannual. Journal. • Bibliographies, periodic. Contains information on standards and requirements. • Manuals, periodic. Contains information on study courses. • Pamphlets, periodic. Contains information on standards and requirements.

★ 6439 ★ World Federation of Orthodontists (WFO)

401 N Lindbergh Blvd.
Saint Louis, MO 63141-7816
Phone: (314)993-1700 **Fax:** (314)993-5208
Email: wfo@wfo.org
Website: http://www.wfo.org/index.html
Lorraine DuPont, Exec. Sec.

Fnded: 1995. **Mem:** 6,448. **Desc:** Orthodontic specialists. Encourages high standards in orthodontics and promotes research in the field. **Pub:** *WFO Gazette*, semiannual. Newspaper. *Price:* included in membership dues.

★ 6440 ★ World Federation of Public Health Associations (WFPHA)

c/o Amer. Public Health Assn.
800 I St. NW
Washington, DC 20001-3710
Phone: (202)777-2486 **Fax:** (202)777-2534
Email: allen.jones@apha.org
Website: http://www.wfpha.org
George Benjamin, Exec. Dir.

Fnded: 1967. **Mem:** 64. **Nat'l Groups:** 64. **Reg. Groups:** 5. **Desc:** National public health associations united "to strengthen the public health profession and to improve community health throughout the world." Encourages formation of national public health associations. Organizes projects; conducts special studies; offers lectures; compiles reports; sponsors triennial world congress. **Pub:** *Reports of Triennial International Congresses*. Reports. • *WFPHA Report*, quarterly. Report.

★ 6441 ★ World Federation of Societies of Anaesthesiologists (WFSA) (Federation Mondiale des Societes d'Anesthesiologistes)

WFSA Office, Level 7
Imperial House, 15-19 Kingsway
London WC2B 6TH, United Kingdom
Phone: 44 20 78365652 **Fax:** 44 20 78365616
Email: info@wfsa-office.org
Website: http://www.anaesthesiologists.org

Fnded: 1955. **Mem:** 108. **Lang(s):** English, French, German, Spanish. **Desc:** Societies of anesthesiologists. Objectives are to: promote research in anesthesiology; disseminate scientific information; encourage the establishment of safety measures including equipment standardization; recommend suitable standards for training in anesthesiology. **Pub:** *WFSA Newsletter*, semiannual. Newsletter.

★ 6442 ★ World Federation of Surgical Oncology Societies (WFSOS)

1 Wimpole St.
London W1M 8AE, United Kingdom
Phone: 44 20 72902968 **Fax:** 44 20 72902989
Email: sarah.caruey@roysocmed.ac.uk

Desc: Promotes surgical oncology internationally; encourages and assists the formation of surgical oncology societies.

★ 6443 ★ World Federation for Ultrasound in Medicine and Biology

Dept. of Ultrasound, Herlev Hospital, University of Copenhag
DK-2730 Herlev, Denmark
Phone: 45 44884704 **Fax:** 45 44948009
Email: soha@herlevhosp.dk
Website: http://www.wfumb.org

Fnded: 1969. **Mem:** 50,000. **Reg. Groups:** 6. **Desc:** Promotes research in the field by international cooperation; disseminates scientific information on education programs internationally. **Pub:** *Ultrasound in Medicine and Biology*, monthly. Journal.

★ 6444 ★ World Forensic Psychiatry and Psychology Association (WFPPA)

Rue Franklin 140
1000 Brussels, Belgium
Fax: 32 2 7365176

★ 6445 ★ World Health Organization (WHO) (Organisation Mondiale de la Sante — OMS)

20, ave. Appia
CH-1211 Geneva 27, Switzerland
Phone: 41 22 7912111 **Fax:** 41 22 7913111
Email: info@who.int
Website: http://www.who.int

Fnded: 1948. **Mem:** 192. **Reg. Groups:** 6. **Lang(s):** Arabic, Chinese, English, French, Russian, Spanish. **Desc:** International health agency of the United Nations consisting of countries working toward the goal of "health for all," seeking to obtain the highest level of health care for all people. Believes health is a fundamental right of every human being without distinction of race, religion, political belief, economic situation, or social conditions and holds that all people deserve equal access to health services to enable them to lead socially and economically productive lives. Objectives are to: act as directing and coordinating authority on international health work; ensure valid and productive technical cooperation; promote research; prevent and combat diseases; generate and transfer information. Strives to eliminate poverty. Emphasizes the health needs of developing countries lacking resources and funds for modern medical technologies; works toward developing new techniques that will fulfill these needs by utilizing available resources, integrating educational, agricultural, town planning, and sanitation programs with health programs, combining peripheral health services and existing health systems, and applying appropriate technologies at reasonable costs. Establishes standards for food, biological, and pharmaceutical needs, develops standardized diagnostic procedures, and determines environmental health criteria. Promotes 8 elements of primary health care including: health education on prevention and cures; proper food supply and nutrition; adequate supply of safe water and sanitation; maternal and child health care; immunization; control of endemic diseases; and provisions of essential drugs. Acts as clearinghouse; coordinates activities with the United Nations on health and socioeconomic development; works with international nongovernmental organizations in the health sector. Supports International Agency for Research on Cancer. Maintains expert and scientific committees. **Pub:** *Bulletin of WHO*, bimonthly. Bulletin. • *International Digest of Health Legislation*, quarterly. • *World Health*, 10/year. Magazine. • *World Health Statistics Quarterly*. Includes summaries in Arabic, Chinese, Russian, and Spanish.

★ 6446 ★ World Health Organization - Regional Office for the Eastern Mediterranean (EMRO)

Abdul Razzak Al Sanhouri St.
PO Box 7608
Nasr City
Cairo 11371, Egypt
Phone: 20 2 6702535 **Fax:** 20 2 6702492
Email: postmaster@emro.who.int
Website: http://www.emro.who.int

Fnded: 1948. **Mem:** 22. **Lang(s):** Arabic, English, Farsi, French, Urdu. **Desc:** Regional office of the World Health Organization. Works to ensure that WHO programs effectively meet the particular public health needs of the Eastern Mediterranean; serves as a liaison between national and local public health agencies and the WHO. **Pub:** *Eastern Mediterranean Health Journal*, bimonthly. Journal. Contains information on public health and health systems research. Additional publications available on request.

★ 6447 ★ World Health Organization - Regional Office for Europe (EURO)

8 Scherfigsvej
DK-2100 Copenhagen O, Denmark
Phone: 45 39171717 **Fax:** 45 39171818
Email: webmaster@who.dk
Website: http://www.who.dk

Lang(s): Danish, English. **Desc:** Regional office of the World Health Organization. Works to ensure that WHO programs effectively meet the particular public health needs of Europe; serves as a liaison between national and local public health agencies and the WHO.

★ 6448 ★ World Health Organization - Regional Office for South-East Asia (SEARO)

World Health House
Indraprastha Estate
Mahatma Gandhi Rd.
New Delhi 110 002, Delhi, India
Phone: 91 11 23370804 **Fax:** 91 11 23379507
Email: pandeyh@whosea.org
Website: http://w3.whosea.org

Desc: Regional branch of the World Health Organization. Works to ensure that WHO programs effectively meet the particular public health needs of southeast Asia; serves as a liaison between national and local public health agencies and the WHO.

★ 6449 ★ World Health Organization - Regional Office for the Western Pacific (WPRO)

PO Box 2932
Manila 1000, Philippines
Phone: 63 2 5288001 **Fax:** 63 2 5211036
Email: postmaster@who.org.ph
Website: http://www.wpro.who.int

Desc: Regional branch of the World Health Organization. Works to ensure that WHO programs effectively meet the particular public health needs of the western Pacific; serves as a liaison between national and local public health agencies and the WHO.

★ 6450 ★ World Health Organization - Zimbabwe (WHOZ)

PO Box CY 348
Causeway
Harare, Zimbabwe
Phone: 263 4 253726 **Fax:** 263 4 253731
Email: regafro@afro.who.int
Website: http://www.afro.who.int

Lang(s): English. **Desc:** National branch of the international organization. Public health services and programs. Seeks to ensure that programs of the World Health Organization effectively meet the particular needs of people in Zimbabwe. Serves as a liaison between local public health programs and agencies and the WHO

★ 6451 ★ World Heart Federation

5, avenue du Mail
CH-1205 Geneva, Switzerland
Phone: 41 22 8070320 **Fax:** 41 22 8070339
Email: admin@worldheart.org
Website: http://www.worldheart.org

Fnded: 1978. **Mem:** 167. **Nat'l Groups:** 144. **Reg. Groups:** 8. **Lang(s):** English, French, German, Spanish. **Desc:** Promotes international study, prevention, and treatment of cardiovascular diseases; encourages, coordinates, and assists the development of educational and scientific programs focusing on cardiovascular problems. Seeks to help people achieve a longer and better life through prevention and control of heart disease and stroke, with a focus on low and middle income countries. **Pub:** *Heartbeat*, quarterly. **Frmly:** (1999) International Society and Federation of Cardiology.

★ 6452 ★ World Hypertension League

c/o Claude Lenfant, MD
9000 Rockville Pike, Bldg. 31, Rm. 5A-52
Bethesda, MD 20892-2486
Phone: (301)496-5166 **Fax:** (301)402-0818
Email: lenfantc@nhlbi.nih.gov
Website: http://www.mco.edu/org/whl/
Claude Lenfant, MD, Pres.

Nat'l Groups: 91. **Desc:** Federation of professional hypertension leagues, societies, and other national bodies. Liaises between member organizations; promotes internationally applicable methods and programs for hypertension control. **Pub:** Newsletter, bimonthly. Discusses the activities of member organizations and cardiovascular-related topics. • Yearbook, biennial. Summarizes the activities of the WHL and its member organizations over 2 years.

★ 6453 ★ World Institute on Disability (WID)

510 16th St., Ste. 100
Oakland, CA 94612
Phone: (510)763-4100 **Fax:** (510)208-9496
Email: webpoobah@wid.org
Website: http://www.wid.org
Stanley K. Yarnell, MD, Chm.

Fnded: 1983. **Desc:** International public policy center that conducts research on disability issues and overcoming obstacles to independent living for all people with disabilities. **Pub:** *An Independent Living Approach to Disability Policy Studies*. Report. *Price:* $17.50. • *The Cost of Program Models Providing Personal Assistance Services for Independent Living. Price:* $6. • *Ethical Issues in Disability and Rehabilitation: A Report on an International Conference*. Report. *Price:* $5. • *Executive Summary of Attending to America*. Video. *Price:* $5. • *Personal Assistance Service: People with Disabilities Forging Public Policy.*

★ 6454 ★ World Institute of Holistic Therapies

c/o Gabrielle Lesie
116 High St.
Ashland, OR 97520-0000
Phone: (541)552-9288 **Fax:** (541)552-9270
Email: admin@worldinstitute.net
Website: http://www.worldinstitute.net
Cheryl Rawson, Exec. Dir.

Fnded: 1997. **Mem:** 36. **Desc:** Seeks to implement a holistic approach for conscious living through education, research and service via a new understanding in consciousness, one which is reliant on the principle of self-responsibility. Implementation of this mission will be accomplished through the formation of partnerships with individuals and other organizations that work at the most advanced frontiers of education, research, healthcare and environmental health. Focused on creating a center of excellence for learning in areas that are key to our mission: experiential education, biological medicine, psychology of identity consciousness, and eco-development. By developing educational opportunities that promote a scientific understanding of the dynamic flow and interrelationship of all things, the institute desires to provide people with the tools to uplift their own lives, the lives of their families, the institutions that serve us, and by extension, the whole of humanity.

★ 6455 ★ World Medical Association (WMA) (Association Medicale Mondiale — AMM)

13 Ch. du Levant
BP 63
F-01212 Ferney-Voltaire, France
Phone: 33 450 407575 **Fax:** 33 450 405937
Email: wma@wma.net
Website: http://www.wma.net

Fnded: 1947. **Mem:** 78. **Reg. Groups:** 6. **Lang(s):** English, French, Spanish. **Desc:** Federation of national medical associations throughout the world. Goal is to achieve the highest international standards in medical education, medical science, medical ethics, and health care for people worldwide. Promotes closer ties and better communication among medical organizations and doctors of the world; studies professional problems in different countries. Represents and protects the rights and interests of physicians and people internationally. Encourages proper nutrition in developing countries; urges the teaching of human values in the practice of medicine. Seeks to improve maternal and child health care. Issues declarations on ethical topics including: abortion; AIDS; abuse of children and the elderly; euthanasia; genetic engineering; organ transplantation; the use and misuse of psychotropic drugs; torture; biomedical research on human subjects; medical care in rural areas; an international code of medical ethics; and rights of the patient. **Pub:** *World Medical Journal*, bimonthly. Journal. Contains medical and medico-political articles.

★ 6456 ★ World Medical Law Association

UZ-1K3, De Pintelaan 185
9000 Gent, Belgium
Phone: 32 9 2403859 **Fax:** 32 9 2404380

Fnded: 1967.

★ 6457 ★ World Medical Mission (WMM)

PO Box 3000
Boone, NC 28607
Phone: (828)262-1980 **Fax:** (704)266-1055
Email: jcastle@samaritan.org
Website: http://www.samaritan.org
W. Franklin Graham, III, Pres.

Fnded: 1977. **Desc:** Coordinates medical activities of the evangelical group Samaritan's Purse. Places Christian physicians who serve voluntarily in evangelical mission hospitals overseas and conducts emergency medical relief. Provides assistance in refurbishing and equipping mission hospitals and conducts training sessions. **Pub:** *On Call*, quarterly. • *The PaceMaker*, quarterly. • *World Medical Mission Newsletter*, 6/year. Newsletter. • Brochures.

★ 6458 ★ World Muscle Society (WMS)

c/o Haluk Topaloglu, Sec.
Department of Child Neurology
Hacettepe Children's Hospital
TR-06100 Ankara, Italy
Phone: 90 532 2341226 **Fax:** 90 312 4402034
Email: htopalog@hacettepe.edu.tr
Website: http://www.worldmusclesociety.org/

Fnded: 1995. **Desc:** Stimulates and disseminates knowledge in the field of neuromuscular disorders.

★ 6459 ★ World Organisation Ovulation Method Billings (WOOMB)

27 Alexandra Parade
North Fitzroy, VIC 3068, Australia
Phone: 61 3 94811722 **Fax:** 61 3 94824208
Email: billings@ozemail.com.au
Website: http://www.woomb.org

Desc: Works to research, study, and evaluate the female ovulation cycle and its direct relation to reproductive medicine. Disseminates information on natural family planning. **Pub:** Bulletin, quarterly.

★ 6460 ★ World Organization for Animal Health (OIE) (Office International des Epizooties)

12, rue de Prony
F-75017 Paris, France
Phone: 33 1 44151888 **Fax:** 33 1 42670987
Email: oie@oie.int
Website: http://www.oie.int

Fnded: 1924. **Mem:** 158. **Reg. Groups:** 5. **Lang(s):** English, French, Spanish. **Desc:** Veterinary services of national ministries of agriculture. Promotes and coordinates activities and research involving the epidemiology and control of contagious diseases in livestock. Collects and presents to governmental agencies data pertaining to epizootic diseases. Examines governmental agreements regarding animal health measures and assists in the supervision of their enforcement. Conducts specialized conferences and disease reporting seminars for chief veterinary officers and epidemiologists of member countries. Compiles statistics. WTO reference organization for animal health standards and world organization for animal health. Maintains documentation/information center. **Pub:** *International Animal Health Code*, annual. Includes recommendations for import/export of animals, animal products, diagnostic techniques, and vaccines. • *Manual of Standards for Diagnostic Tests and Vaccines*, periodic. Manual. Outlines standards for the surveillance and control of the most imortant animal diseases. • *World Animal Health*, annual.

★ 6461 ★ World Organization for Digestive Endoscopy (Organisation mondiale d'endoscopie digestive — OMED)

c/o Rikiya Fujita, Sec.
Cancer Institute Hospital
1-37-1 Kami-Ikebukuro
Toshima-ku
Tokyo 170-8455, Japan
Phone: 81 3 39180111 **Fax:** 81 3 53943828
Email: rikiya.fujita@jfcr.or.jp
Website: http://www.omed.org

Fnded: 1962. **Desc:** Promotes worldwide the study and advancement of gastrointestinal endoscopy; furthers the establishment of standards of practice and training in endoscopy.

★ 6462 ★ World Organization of Family Doctors

College of Medicine Bldg.
16 College Rd. 01-02
Singapore 169854, Singapore
Phone: 65 62242886 **Fax:** 65 63242029
Email: admin@wonca.com.sg
Website: http://www.globalfamilydoctor.com

Fnded: 1972. **Mem:** 56. **Reg. Groups:** 5. **Lang(s):** English, French, German, Spanish. **Desc:** Colleges, academies, or organizations in 53 countries concerned with the academic aspects of general family practice. Objectives are to: promote and maintain high standards of general family practice through education and research; foster worldwide communication and understanding among general practitioners; represent the academic and research activities of general practitioners to other worldwide bodies concerned with health or medical care. **Pub:** *The Family Doctor*, semiannual. Magazine. • *International Classification of Health Problems in Primary Care*. Book. • *Membership Directory*, annual. Directory. • *WONCA News*, bimonthly. **Frmly:** (1999) World Organization of National Colleges, Academies, and Academic Associations of General Practitioners/Family Physicians.

★ 6463 ★ World Organization of Gastroenterology (OMGE) (Organisation Mondiale de Gastroenterologie — OMGE)

Brunnsteinstrabe 10
D-81541 Munich, Germany
Phone: 49 89 41419240 **Fax:** 49 89 41419245
Email: omge@omge.org

Website: http://www.omge.org

Fnded: 1958. **Mem:** 75. **Reg. Groups:** 3. **Lang(s):** English, French, Spanish. **Desc:** National gastroenterology societies. Promotes research in the field of gastroenterology (the study of the diseases and pathology of the stomach and intestines). Fosters exchange of information among members. Compiles statistics. **Pub:** *Directory*, quadrennial. Directory. • *Nomenclature of Digestive Diseases.* • *OMGE Bulletin*, quadrennial. Bulletin. • *OMGE Newsletter*, annual. Newsletter. • *OMGE Statutes*, quadrennial.

★ 6464 ★ World Organization and Public Education Corp. of the National Association for the Advancement of Psychoanalysis

80 8th Ave., Ste. 1501
New York, NY 10011-5126
Phone: (212)741-0515 **Fax:** (212)366-4347
Email: naap72@aol.com
Website: http://www.naap.org
Margery Quackenbush, Admin.

Fnded: 1995. **Desc:** Works for public education for the National Association for the Advancement of Psychoanalysis. **Pub:** Brochure. **Frmly:** (2000) Public Education Corp. of the National Association for the Advancement of Psychoanalysis.

★ 6465 ★ World Organization for Specialized Studies on Diseases of the Esophagus (Organisation Mondiale d'Etudes Specialisees pour les Maladies de l'Oe hage)

c/o Robert Giuli, M.D.
Hopital Beaujon
2 blvd. Pershing
F-75017 Paris, France
Phone: 33 1 55379015 **Fax:** 33 1 55379040
Email: robert.giuli@oeso.org

Fnded: 1979. **Lang(s):** English, French. **Desc:** Thoracic and digestive surgeons, ear, nose, and throat specialists, intensive care specialists, pathologists, nutritionists, endoscopists, radio- and chemotherapists, and others who diagnose and treat patients suffering from cancer and other diseases of the esophagus. Acts as a forum for specialists to meet, study, and discuss the epidemiology, histological classification, and treatments of esophageal diseases. Conducts research programs. **Pub:** *Program of the International Polydisciplinary Congress*, periodic. **Frmly:** (2001) International Organization for Statistical Studies on Diseases of the Esophagus.

★ 6466 ★ World Parkinson Disease Association (WPDA)

via Zuretti, 35
I-20125 Milan, Italy
Phone: 39 0266713111 **Fax:** 39 026705283
Email: info@wpda.org
Website: http://www.wpda.org

Fnded: 1998.

★ 6467 ★ World Psychiatric Association (WPA)

c/o Mt. Sinai School of Medicine-CUNY
University of NY
Fifth Ave. & 100th St.
Box 1093
New York, NY 10029-6574
Phone: (718)334-5094 **Fax:** (718)334-5096
Email: wpa@dti.net
Website: http://www.wpanet.org
Prof. Juan E. Mezzich, Jr., Sec. Gen.

Fnded: 1950. **Mem:** 116. **Nat'l Groups:** 114. **Reg. Groups:** 18. **Desc:** Psychiatric societies and individuals in 90 countries. Objectives are: to promote international cooperation in the field of psychiatry; to advance inquiry into the etiology, pathology, and treatment of mental illness; to strengthen relations among psychiatrists working in various fields. Encourages the exchange of information concerning the medical problems of mental diseases; sponsors educational and research programs. Comprises 40 sections representing different specialties in psychiatry. **Pub:** *WPA News*, quarterly. Newsletter. *Price:* for members.

★ 6468 ★ World Rehabilitation Fund (WRF)

386 Park Ave. S, Ste. 500
New York, NY 10016
Phone: (212)725-7875 **Fax:** (212)725-8402
Email: wrfnewyork@msn.com
Website: http://www.worldrehabfund.org
Heather Burns Knierim, Pres.

Fnded: 1955. **Mem:** 19. **Desc:** Assist governmental and voluntary agencies in establishing, improving and expanding rehabilitation care services for persons with disabilities caused by landmines and other ordinance, national disasters and other causes. Provides technical assistance, training, medical equipment and supplies. Have offices in New York, Brussels, Beirut, Kampala, Guatemala City, Manila and Madras. Also have projects in Haiti and Pakistan.

★ 6469 ★ World Research Foundation (WRF)

41 Bell Rock Plz.
Sedona, AZ 86351
Phone: (928)284-3300 **Fax:** (928)284-3530
Email: info@wrf.org
Website: http://www.wrf.org
Laverne Boeckmann, Contact

Fnded: 1980. **Desc:** Informs the public of the latest developments in health and environmental issues. Provides health care professionals and the public with information on health tools and technologies currently available outside the U.S. but which have been overlooked or are unavailable in the U.S. Acts as a depository of public information. **Pub:** *World Research News*, quarterly. Newsletter. • Journal, quarterly. Contains traditional and nontraditional international health news. *Price:* $20. • Proceedings, annual. • Reports.

★ 6470 ★ World Small Animal Veterinary Association (WSAVA)

c/o David Wadsworth, Sec.
94 Norbreck Rd.
Lancashire
Blackpool FY5 1RP, United Kingdom
Phone: 44 253 823624 **Fax:** 44 253 857503
Website: http://www.wsava.org

Fnded: 1959. **Mem:** 39. **Desc:** WSAVA is an association of Veterinary associations, representing 47,000 individuals in 35 countries involved in practice, teaching, and research related to dogs, cats, caged birds, and other small animals. Primary purpose is to advance quality and availability of veterinary medicine and surgery relating to small animals. Encourages research; conducts surveys; sponsors meetings for studying conditions and matters affecting small animals; furthers international relationships between all veterinarians dealing with small animal health and welfare. **Pub:** *Journal of Small Animal Practice*, monthly. Journal. • *Proceedings of Congress*, annual. Papers.

★ 6471 ★ World Society for Stereotactic and Functional Neurosurgery (WSSFN)

c/o Andres Lozano, Sec.
University Health Network
Toronto Western Hospital Network
399 Bathurst St.
Toronto, ON, Canada M5T 2S8
Fax: (416)603-5298
Email: lozano@uhnres.utoronto.ca
Website: http://www.wssfn.org

Fnded: 1963.

★ 6472 ★ World Society for Stereotactic and Functional Neurosurgery (WSSFN)

c/o Massachusetts General Hospital
15 Parkman St., Ste. 331
Boston, MA 02114
Fax: (617)726-7546
Email: cosgrove@helix.mgh.harvard.edu
Website: http://www.wssfn.org/
Brian P. Brophy, Pres.

Fnded: 1963. **Mem:** 600. **Nat'l Groups:** 3. **Reg. Groups:** 4. **Desc:** Neurosurgeons and professors dedicated to the advancement of stereotactic studies and procedures. Original manuscripts submitted at meetings are published and used as reference books throughout the world. **Pub:** *Stereotactic and Functional Neurosurgery*, quarterly. Journal. • *Studies in Stereoencephalotomy*, quadrennial. **AKA:** World Stereotactic Society; WSSFN. **Frmly:** (1973) International Society for Research in Stereoencephalotomy.

★ 6473 ★ World Sports Medicine Association of Registered Therapists (WORLD SMAR)

206 Marine Ave.
PO Box 5642
Newport Beach, CA 92662
Phone: (626)574-1999 **Fax:** (626)574-1999
Email: americansportsmedicine@hotmail.com
Joe Borland, Contact

Fnded: 1993. **Mem:** 4,000. **Desc:** Sports medicine therapist, trainer, technician, and individuals involved in sports medicine and certified by any nationally recognized athletic trainers association. Establishes standards of competency for trainers, therapists, and sports medicine care providers that are recognized worldwide. **Pub:** *World Smart News.* • Brochure. *Price:* Free. • Bulletin, periodic. • Newsletter, quarterly. *Price:* Included in membership dues. **AKA:** World Smart.

★ 6474 ★ World Veterinary Association (WVA) (Welt-Tierarztegesellschaft)

Rosenlunds Alle 8
DK-2720 Vanlose, Denmark
Phone: 45 38710156 **Fax:** 45 38710322
Email: wva@ddd.dk
Website: http://www.worldvet.org

Fnded: 1959. **Mem:** 96. **Lang(s):** English, French, German, Spanish. **Desc:** Association of national (70), international (20), and commercial (4) organizations. Purposes are to: unify and promote the veterinary profession; encourages high standards of health and welfare in all species of animals; improve veterinary science through the exchange of information and education; establish uniform nomenclature. Sends volunteers to developing countries to assist in food production, processing and distribution, to teach basic techniques in disease control and eradication and to develop national veterinary services. **Pub:** *World Veterinary Directory*, periodic. Directory. • Bulletin, semiannual. • Membership Directory, annual.

★ 6475 ★ World Veterinary Poultry Association (WVPA) (Asociacion Mundial Veterinaria de Avicola — AMVA)

c/o Dr. U. Heffels-Redmann
Institut fur Geflugelkrankheiten
Justus-Liebig-Universitat Giessen
Frankfurter Str. 91
D-35392 Giessen, Germany
Phone: 49 641 9938452 **Fax:** 49 641 201548
Email: ursula.heffels-redmann@vetmed.uni-giessen.de
Website: http://www.wvpa.net

Fnded: 1959. **Mem:** 1,684. **Nat'l Groups:** 31. **Lang(s):** English, French, German. **Desc:** Veterinarians and other scientists in 56 countries engaged in practice, research, or education connected with avian pathology. Objectives are to: organize meetings for studying diseases and conditions; encourage research; promote the exchange of information and material for study between individuals and organizations; establish and maintain liaisons with other groups. Organizes avian medicine sections of the World Veterinary Congresses. **Pub:** *Aerosols*, annual. Newsletter. • *Avian Pathology*, bimonthly. Journal.

★ 6476 ★ Worldwide Aquatics Bodywork Association (WABA)
PO Box 889
Middletown, CA 95461
Phone: (707)987-3801 **Fax:** (707)987-9638
Email: info@waba.edu
Website: http://aspen.forest.net/waba/

Desc: Promotes the study, practice and teaching of Watsu and aquatic bodywork; maintains the Registry of the Worldwide Water Family.

★ 6477 ★ Wound, Ostomy and Continence Nurses Society: An Association of E.T. Nurses (WOCN)
4700 W Lake Ave.
Glenview, IL 60025
Phone: (847)375-6730 **Free:** 888-224-9626
Fax: (866)615-8560
Email: membership@wocn.org
Website: http://www.wocn.org
Dionne Wilson, Sr. Mgr.

Fnded: 1969. **Mem:** 4,000. **Nat'l Groups:** 10. **Reg. Groups:** 11. **Local Groups:** 20. **Desc:** Enterostomal therapy (ET) nurses, wound, ostomy and continence care nurses in 10 countries trained in WOCN accredited schools; individuals interested in objectives of the association who hold a valid license in medicine or nursing; health-related firms. Seeks to support ET, wound, ostomy, and continence, nurses by promoting educational, clinical, and research opportunities and to guide the delivery of expert health care to individuals with wounds, ostomies, and incontinence. **Pub:** *Guideline for Management of Wounds in Patients with Lower-Extremity Arterial Disease.* • *Journal of Wound, Ostomy and Continence Nursing*, bimonthly. Journal. • *Management of Urinary Incontinence.* Slides and handout. *Price:* $50 for members; $85 for nonmembers. • *Patient Information Data System. Price:* $95 for members; $125 for nonmembers. • *Professional Practice Manual.* Manual. *Price:* $85 for members; $125 for nonmembers. • *Standards of Care Guidelines for Management.* Booklets. • *WOCN News*, quarterly. Newsletter. • Membership Directory, annual. *Price:* $35 for members; $50 for nonmembers. • Fact Sheets and Position Statements N/C. **Frmly:** Wound, Ostomy and Continence Nurses Society, An Association of E.T. Nurses; (1993) International Association for Enterostomal Therapy.

★ 6478 ★ Xavier Society for the Blind (XSB)
154 E 23rd St.
New York, NY 10010
Phone: (212)473-7800
Rev. Alfred Caruana, S.J., Dir.

Fnded: 1900. **Mem:** 11,000. **Desc:** A center for publications, primarily Catholic, for the blind and visually handicapped, supported by charitable contributions. Transcribes numerous titles, including religious textbooks. Maintains a circulating library of books and other materials in Braille, large type, and on tape. Items are loaned by mail from catalogs of titles in each of 3 formats. Tapes are also circulated to the physically handicapped. **Pub:** *Catholic Review*, bimonthly. Magazine. Available in Braille, large print and on tape.

★ 6479 ★ Xi Psi Phi
c/o Dr. Keith W. Dickey
1623 Washington Ave., No. 300
Alton, IL 62002
Phone: (618)463-1889 **Fax:** (618)463-1882
Email: gobux@attbi.com
Website: http://www.xipsiphi.org
Dr. Keith W. Dickey, Sec. -Treas.

Fnded: 1889. **Mem:** 19,000. **Local Groups:** 22. **Desc:** Professional dental fraternity - dentistry. Maintains Hall of Fame. Conducts educational programs. **Pub:** *Quarterly*, quarterly. *Price:* $8.

★ 6480 ★ Y-ME National Breast Cancer Organization (Y-ME)
212 W Van Buren, Ste. 500
Chicago, IL 60607
Phone: (312)986-8338 **Free:** 800-221-2141
Fax: (312)294-8597
Email: mkirk@y-me.org
Website: http://www.y-me.org
Magaret C. Kirk, Chief Exec. Officer

Fnded: 1978. **Mem:** 15,000. **Nat'l Groups:** 25. **State Groups:** 23. **Local Groups:** 23. **Desc:** Purpose is to provide peer support, education and information to women who have or suspect they have breast cancer. Activities include presurgical counseling inservice programs for health professionals, hot line volunteer training, and technical assistance. Administers the Deborah David Dewar Fund, the Billie Klein Memorial Fund, Shellie Broutman Memorial, Eve & Susan Feldman Memorial and Mimi Kaplan Memorial. Provides a Latino program, teen breast health program, and adult workshops regarding mammography screening and breast self-exam. **Pub:** *A Women's Guide to Breast Cancer.* Brochure. • *Every Women's Guide to Breast Cancer. Price:* One copy is free. • *I Still Buy Green Bananas: Living with Hope...Breast Cancer.* Brochure. • *Just For Teens.* Brochure. • *When the Woman You Love Has Breast Cancer.* • *Y-ME Hotline*, bimonthly. Newsletter. • Breast Cancer Just for Teens!; A Woman's Guide to Breast Care. All brochures available in English and Spanish. **Frmly:** (1989) Y-Me Breast Cancer Support; (1994) Y-Me National Organization for Breast Cancer Information and Support.

★ 6481 ★ Yad Sarah
Yad Sarah House
Kiryat Weinberg
124 Herzl Blvd.
IL-956187 Jerusalem, Israel
Phone: 972 2 6444444 **Fax:** 972 2 6444423
Email: info@yadsarah.org.il
Website: http://www.yadsarah.org.il

Fnded: 1976. **Nat'l Groups:** 94. **Lang(s):** Arabic, Dutch, English, French, German, Hebrew, Portuguese, Russian, Spanish. **Desc:** Provides volunteer home care services and supplemental care for the handicapped, sick, and elderly in Israel so that they may live at home with their families without need for hospitalization or institutionalization. Lends medical equipment for no fee and assists disabled tourists. **Pub:** *Health News*, semiannual. Newsletter.

★ 6482 ★ Yemen Family Care Association (YFCA)
PO Box 795
Sana'a, Yemen
Phone: 967 1 288145 **Fax:** 967 1 270948
Email: yfca@y.net.ye

Fnded: 1976. **Mem:** 500. **Lang(s):** Arabic, English. **Desc:** Volunteer association which provides services for the mother, the child, and in the field of family planning, especially in poor under-served areas. Works to spread reproductive health culture within the society, especially among women and young people. In addition, the association works to increase the number of volunteers and to improve the quality of services and the expertise of staff and volunteers. **Pub:** *Al Osra*, bimonthly. Newsletter.

★ 6483 ★ Yes I Can Foundation for Exceptional Children
1110 N Glebe Rd., Ste. 300
Arlington, VA 22201-5704
Phone: (703)264-3660 **Free:** 800-224-6830
Fax: (703)264-9494
Email: yesican@cec.sped.org
Website: http://yesican.sped.org
Christine Mason, Acting Dir.

Fnded: 1922. **Mem:** 50,000. **State Groups:** 51. **Desc:** The Council for Exceptional Children. Advocates for quality education for all individuals with physical disabilities, multiple disabilities, and special health care needs served in schools, hospitals, or home settings. The council also advocates for gifted and talented children and youth. Operates the ERIC Clearinghouse on Disabilities and Gifted Education, and the National Clearinghouse for Professions in Special Education. Develops programs to help teachers, administrators, and related services professionals improve their practice. **Pub:** *DPHD Newsletter*, quarterly. Newsletter. Covers information regarding the education of individuals with physical disabilities and health impairments. *Price:* Included in membership dues. • *Exceptional Child Education Resources*, quarterly. Journal. Includes abstracts of book, nonprint media, and journal literature. • *Exceptional Children*, quarterly. Journal. Covers special education and research. *Price:* included in membership dues; $58/year for nonmembers. • *Teaching Exceptional Children*, bimonthly. Magazine. Includes classroom-oriented information about instructional methods, materials, and techniques for students of all ages with special needs. *Price:* included in membership dues; $58/year for nonmembers. • Audiotapes. • Books. • Films. • Videos. **Frmly:** (1968) Association of Educators for Homebound and Hospitalized Children; (1979) Division on Physically Handicapped, Homebound and Hospitalized; (1993) Division for Physically Handicapped; (2002) Foundation for Exceptional Children.

★ 6484 ★ Youth Development Coalition
3080 N Lincoln
Chicago, IL 60657
Free: 800-231-6946 **Fax:** (312)929-5150
Email: 1800hithome@horizonsd.org
Website: http://www.bakersfield.org/ydc
Nancy Eschbach, Contact

Desc: Provides assistance to youth and families in crisis situations.

★ 6485 ★ Yugoslav MND Association
c/o Dr. Zorica Stevic, MD, Ph.D., Assoc.Prof.
Institute of Neurology
Dr. Subtica br. 6
YU-11000 Belgrade, Serbia
Phone: 381 11 3614122 **Fax:** 381 11 684577
Email: zsmndyu@hotmail.com
Website: http://www.alsmndalliance.org/directory/yugoslavia.html

Fnded: 1977. **Desc:** Individuals in Yugoslavia affected by Motor Neruone Disease (MND), a muscle wasting condition. Participates in clinical trials of new medications. Provides a forum for support and exchange of information.

★ 6486 ★ Yugoslav Pharmacological Society (Farmakolosko Drustvo Jugoslavije)
c/o Prof. Ranka Samardzic
Department of Clinical Pharmacology
Pharmacology & Toxicology
PO Box 840
YU-11129 Belgrade, Serbia
Phone: 381 11 684479 **Fax:** 381 11 686025
Email: polovves@eunet.yu

Mem: 121. **Desc:** Promotes pharmacology in Serbia and Montenegro.

★ 6487 ★ Yugoslav Society of Cardiology
Institut of Cardiovascular Diseases
Clinic of Cardiology
Institutski put N4
YU-21204 Sremska Kamenica, Yugoslavia
Phone: 381 21 613286 **Fax:** 381 21 622881
Email: ukj@eunet.yu

Fnded: 1955. **Mem:** 330. **Desc:** Promotes the study of cardiology in Yugoslavia. **Pub:** *Cardiology*, quarterly. Journal. • *Hypertension*, quarterly. Journal.

★ 6488 ★ Zdruzenje Multiple Sklerose Slovenie (ZMSS)

c/o Alojz Jeselnik
Maroltova 14
SLO-1000 Ljubljana, Slovenia
Phone: 386 1 5687299 **Fax:** 386 1 5687287
Email: info@zdruzenje-ms.si
Website: http://www.zdruzenje-ms.si

Fnded: 1973. **Mem:** 1,593. **Reg. Groups:** 28. **Desc:** MS patients, families and professionals. Seeks to improve the quality of life for persons with multiple sclerosis and their families.

★ 6489 ★ Zero Balancing Association (ZBA)

801 W Main St., Ste. 202
Charlottesville, VA 22903
Phone: (434)244-2458 **Fax:** (434)244-2645
Email: info@zerobalancing.com
Website: http://www.zerobalancing.com
Cindi Pridgen, Exec. Dir.

Fnded: 1991. **Mem:** 500. **Desc:** Promotes the teaching and practice of Zero-Balancing, the hands-on body/mind system designed to align body energy with the body's physical structure; strives to relieve physical and mental symptoms and improve quality of life. Offers educational courses. **Pub:** *Interface*, quarterly. Newsletter. *Price:* Free for members.

★ 6490 ★ Zero to Three: National Center for Infants, Toddlers and Families

2000 M St. NW, Ste. 2000
Washington, DC 20036
Phone: (202)638-1144 **Free:** 800-899-4301
Fax: (202)638-0851
Website: http://www.zerotothree.org
Matthew E. Melmed, Exec. Dir.

Fnded: 1977. **Desc:** Professionals and researchers in the health care industry, policymakers, and parents working to improve the healthy physical, cognitive and social development of infants, toddlers, and their families. Members share their expertise about infants, toddlers, and their families. Sponsors training and technical assistance activities. **Pub:** *Zero to Three*, 6/year. Bulletin. Includes research and practice reports, book and video reviews, calendar of events, funding source information, and lists of training opportunities. *Price:* $60/year; $102/2 years; $144/3 years; Order in bulk for discounts. **Frmly:** (1992) National Center for Clinical Infant Programs; (2001) National Center for Infants, Toddlers and Families.

★ 6491 ★ Zimbabwe AIDS Network

PO Box CY 3006
Causeway
Harare, Zimbabwe
Phone: 263 4 700924 **Fax:** 263 4 700330
Email: zansec@zol.co.zw

Fnded: 1991. **Mem:** 150. **Nat'l Groups:** 150. **Lang(s):** English. **Desc:** Individuals and organizations working with people with HIV and AIDS. Seeks to increase public awareness of AIDS and its prevention; works to improve the quality of life of people with AIDS and their families. Serves as a clearinghouse on AIDS and HIV; provides support and services to people with AIDS. **Pub:** *The Web*, quarterly. Newsletter. Features national and regional news on HIV/AIDS.

★ 6492 ★ Zimbabwe Dental Association

PO Box 3303
Harare, Zimbabwe
Phone: 263 4 796389 **Fax:** 263 4 796389
Email: fmakoni@medsch.uz.ac.zw

Mem: 80. **Reg. Groups:** 2. **Lang(s):** English. **Desc:** Dentists and others working in the field of dentistry. Promotes dental health and the efficient practice of dentistry. Works to enhance the professional standing of members. **Pub:** Newsletter, periodic. **Frmly:** (2002) Dental Association of Zimbabwe.

★ 6493 ★ Zimbabwe Diabetic Association

c/o Mrs. N. Mujuru
Operational Office - Ward 3
Old Central Hospital
Parirenyatwa
PO Box 1797
Harare, Zimbabwe
Phone: 263 4 732089 **Fax:** 263 4 667488
Email: nmujuru@gta.gov.zw
Website: http://www.diabetesafrica.com/idfmembers.html

Desc: Represents people with diabetes. Promotes research and support of those with diabetes in Zimbabwe.

★ 6494 ★ Zimbabwe Medical Association

PO Box 3671
Harare, Zimbabwe
Phone: 263 4 720731

Lang(s): English. **Desc:** Registered medical doctors and residents. Represents and promotes the interests of the medical profession in Zimbabwe; promotes advancement in medicine and related sciences. Sponsors continuing professional education courses of members.

★ 6495 ★ Zimbabwe National Association for Mental Health (ZIMNAMH)

PO Box A 196
Avondale
Harare, Zimbabwe
Phone: 263 4 731272 **Fax:** 263 4 792946
Email: zimnamh@africaonline.co.zw

Fnded: 1981. **Mem:** 1,700. **Nat'l Groups:** 6. **Local Groups:** 250. **Desc:** Works to educate and rehabilitate the mentally ill. Informs the public about mental health issues. Promotes mental health for all throughout Zimbabwe. Contributes to increased awareness on the negative impact of child sexual abuse on children and to facilitate action to prevent and protect the child from all forms of sexual exploitation and sexual abuse. Promotes mental health for all through lobbying and advocacy and networks with other relevant stakeholders. **Pub:** *Zimnamh Newsletter*, quarterly. Newsletter. Containing information about mental health. • Pamphlets. Containing information about mental health. • Video.

★ 6496 ★ Zimbabwe National Family Planning Council (ZNFPC)

c/o Harare Hospital Grounds
Spilhaus Centre
Harare Hospital Grounds
CNR Highfield Rd., Swiss Way
PO Box 220, Southerton
Harare, Zimbabwe
Phone: 263 4 620281 **Fax:** 263 4 620280
Email: znfpc@ecoweb.co.zw

Fnded: 1957. **Lang(s):** English. **Desc:** Promotes family planning and responsible parenthood as a means to improve the quality of life for individuals living in Zimbabwe. Advocates family planning as a basic human right. Works to reduce the number of unwanted pregnancies and abortions. Offers programs in family planning, sex education and health. Provides contraceptive and health care services. Conducts research. **Pub:** *ZNFPC Newsletter*. Annual Report. Also publishes a variety of materials for the general public, clients, service providers, and policy makers. **Frmly:** (1985) Child Spacing and Fertility Association.

★ 6497 ★ Zimbabwe National Traditional Healers Association (ZINATHA)

PO Box 116
Reliance House
Corner of Takcawira and Speke Ave.
Harare, Zimbabwe
Phone: 263 4 751902

Fnded: 1980. **Mem:** 45,000. **Desc:** Promotes public awareness of alternative medicine. Coordinates actions of the Ministry of Health of Zimbabwe and traditional healers. Disseminates information. **Pub:** *ZINATHA*. Booklet.

★ 6498 ★ Zimbabwe Veterinary Association (ZVA)

PO Box CY 168
Causeway
Harare, Zimbabwe
Phone: 263 4 495859 **Fax:** 263 4 495859
Email: georgie@ecoweb.co.zw

Fnded: 1920. **Mem:** 180. **Local Groups:** 1. **Lang(s):** English. **Desc:** Veterinarians practicing in Zimbabwe. Encourages contact and information exchange among members. Conducts clinical meetings and seminars. **Pub:** *The Burdizzo*, quarterly. Newsletter. Contains news, letters, and association business. • *Zimbabwe Veterinary Journal*, semiannual. Journal. **Frmly:** (1980) Rhodesian Veterinary Association.

Chapter 2
State & Regional Organizations

This chapter lists the state and regional affiliates of 45 national organizations. Arrangement is alphabetical by subject categories, then by states, then by organization names. For additional information, consult the "User's Guide" located at the front of this directory.

Alzheimer's Disease

State chapters of the Alzheimer's Association are listed below. The national office is located at 919 N Michigan Ave., Ste. 1100, Chicago, Illinois 60611-1676. Additional information can be obtained by calling the national office at (800) 272-3900, or by consulting their web site at http://www.alz.org.

Arizona

★ 6499 ★ Alzheimer's Association
Desert Southwest Chapter
1028 E McDowell Rd.
Phoenix, AZ 85005
Phone: (602)528-0545 **Free:** 800-392-0022
Fax: (602)528-0546
Email: Scott.Gardner@alz.org
Website: http://www.alzaz.org
Scott Gardner, Exec Director
Remarks: Serves Arizona and Nevada.

California

★ 6500 ★ Alzheimer's Association
California Central Coast Chapter
2024 De La Vina, Ste. B
Santa Barbara, CA 93105
Phone: (805)563-0020 **Free:** 800-660-1993
Fax: (805)682-1811
Website: http://www.centralcoastz.org

★ 6501 ★ Alzheimer's Association
Los Angeles, Riverside, and San Bernardino Counties Chapter
5900 Wilshire Blvd., Ste. 1700
Los Angeles, CA 90036
Phone: (323)938-3379 **Free:** 800-660-1993
Fax: (323)938-1036
Website: http://www.alzla.org/

★ 6502 ★ Alzheimer's Association
Northern California and Northern Nevada Chapter
2065 W El Camino Real, Ste. C
Mountain View, CA 94040
Phone: (650)962-8111 **Free:** 800-660-1993
Fax: (650)962-9644
Website: http://www.alznorcal.org
Bill Fisher, EDIR, Contact

★ 6503 ★ Alzheimer's Association
Orange County Chapter
2540 N Santiago Blvd.
Orange, CA 92867
Phone: (714)283-1111 **Free:** 800-660-1993
Fax: (714)283-1240
Website: http://www.alzoc.org/

★ 6504 ★ Alzheimer's Association
San Diego Chapter
8514 Commerce Ave.
San Diego, CA 92121
Phone: (858)537-5040 **Free:** 800-660-1993
Fax: (858)537-5045
Email: info@sanalz.org
Website: http://www.sanalz.org

Colorado

★ 6505 ★ Alzheimer's Association
Rocky Mountain Chapter
789 Sherman St., Ste. 500
Denver, CO 80203
Phone: (303)813-1669 **Free:** 800-864-4404
Fax: (303)813-1670
Email: cheryl.dunaway@alz.org
Website: http://www.alzrockymtn.org
Linda Mitchell, Exec Director

★ 6506 ★ Alzheimer's Association
Rocky Mountain Chapter/Grand Junction Office
761 Rood Ave.
Grand Junction, CO 81501
Phone: (970)256-1274 **Free:** 800-864-4404
Fax: (970)243-6924
Email: maria.williams@alz.org
Website: http://www.alz.org

Connecticut

★ 6507 ★ Alzheimer's Association
Northern Connecticut Chapter
96 Oak St.
Hartford, CT 06106
Phone: (860)956-9560 **Free:** 800-356-5502
Fax: (860)956-9590
Website: http://www.alzct.org

★ 6508 ★ Alzheimer's Association
Southern Connecticut Chapter
2911 Dixwell Ave.
Hamden, CT 06518
Phone: (203)230-1777 **Fax:** (203)230-1712
Website: http://www.ctalz.org

Florida

★ 6509 ★ Alzheimer's Association
Central and North Florida Chapter
2010 Mizell Ave.
Winter Park, FL 32792
Phone: (407)629-1997 **Fax:** (407)629-2042
Email: annette.kelly@alz.org
Website: http://www.alzorlando.org/
Annette Kelly, Exec Director

★ 6510 ★ Alzheimer's Association
Florida Gulf Coast Chapter
9365 U.S. Hwy. 19 N, Ste. B
Pinellas Park, FL 33782
Phone: (727)578-2558 **Free:** 800-772-8672
Fax: (727)578-2286
Email: info@alz-tbc.org
Website: http://www.alz-tbc.org

★ 6511 ★ Alzheimer's Association
South Florida Chapter
1175 NE 125th St., Ste. 600
Miami, FL 33161
Phone: (305)891-6228 **Fax:** (305)892-0355

★ 6512 ★ Alzheimer's Association
Southeast Florida Chapter
8333 W McNab Rd., Ste. 210
Fort Lauderdale, FL 33321
Phone: (954)726-0002 **Free:** 800-861-7826
Fax: (954)726-0055
Website: http://www.alzsefc.org

Georgia

★ 6513 ★ Alzheimer's Association
Georgia Chapter
1925 Century Blvd., Ste. 10
Atlanta, GA 30345-3315
Phone: (404)728-1181 **Free:** 888-649-7800
Fax: (404)636-9768
Email: memoryga@bellsouth.net
Website: http://www.alzga.org
Jan Bequeath, Exec Director

Hawaii

★ 6514 ★ Alzheimer's Association
Aloha Chapter
1050 Ala Moana Blvd., Bldg. D
Honolulu, HI 96814
Phone: (808)591-2771 **Fax:** (808)591-9071

Illinois

★ 6515 ★ Alzheimer's Association
Central Illinois Chapter
606 W Glen Ave.
Peoria, IL 61614
Phone: (309)681-1100 **Free:** 800-681-1181
Fax: (309)681-1101
Email: marlene.rush@alz.org
Website: http://www.alzillinois.org/
Marlene Rush, Exec Director

★ 6516 ★ Alzheimer's Association
Greater Illinois Chapter
4709 Golf Rd., Ste. 1015
Skokie, IL 60076

Phone: (847)933-2413 **Free:** 800-272-3900
Fax: (847)933-2417
Website: http://www.alzheimers-illinois.org

Indiana

★ 6517 ★ Alzheimer's Association
Central Indiana Chapter
9135 N Meridian St., Ste. B-4
Indianapolis, IN 46260
Phone: (317)575-9620 **Free:** 888-575-9624
Fax: (317)582-0669
Email: Heather.Hershberger@alz.org
Website: http://www.standbyyou.org/
Heather Allen Hershberger, Exec Director

★ 6518 ★ Alzheimer's Association
Northern Indiana Chapter
108 N Main St., Ste. 707
South Bend, IN 46601
Phone: (574)232-4121 **Free:** 888-303-0180
Fax: (574)232-4235
Email: alznic@sbt.infi.net
Website: http://www.alz-nic.org/

Iowa

★ 6519 ★ Alzheimer's Association
Big Sioux Chapter
Mercy Medical Bldg.
522 4th St., Lower Level
PO Box 3716
Sioux City, IA 51101
Phone: (712)279-5802 **Free:** 800-426-6512
Fax: (712)277-8076
Email: help@alz-sioux.org
Website: http://www.alz-sioux.org
Remarks: Serves Iowa, Nebraska, and South Dakota.

★ 6520 ★ Alzheimer's Association
East Central Iowa Chapter
1642 42nd St. NE
Cedar Rapids, IA 52402
Phone: (319)294-9699 **Free:** 888-397-9635
Fax: (319)294-0068
Email: kelly.hauer@alz.org
Website: http://www.alzeci.org/

★ 6521 ★ Alzheimer's Association
Greater Iowa Chapter
Iowa Lutheran Hospital
700 E University, Level B
Des Moines, IA 50316
Phone: (515)263-2464 **Free:** 800-738-8071
Fax: (515)263-2466
Website: http://www.alz.org/greateriowa
Remarks: Serves Iowa and Illinois.

★ 6522 ★ Alzheimer's Association
Waterloo Branch Office
2101 Kimball Ave., Ste. 125
Waterloo, IA 50702
Phone: (319)272-2300 **Free:** 888-397-9635
Fax: (319)272-2109
Email: kristi.kajewski@alz.org
Website: http://www.alz.org

Kansas

★ 6523 ★ Alzheimer's Association
Heart of America Chapter
3846 W 75th St.
Prairie Village, KS 66208
Phone: (913)831-3888 **Free:** 800-733-1981
Fax: (913)831-1916
Email: kim.collins@alz.org
Website: http://www.alz.org/kcalz.org
Remarks: Serves Kansas and Missouri.

★ 6524 ★ Alzheimer's Association
Sunflower Chapter
347 S Laura
Wichita, KS 67211
Phone: (316)267-7333 **Free:** 877-267-7333
Fax: (316)267-6369
Website: http://www.alzheimerskansas.org

Kentucky

★ 6525 ★ Alzheimer's Association
Greater Kentucky and Southern Indiana Chapter
3703 Taylorsville Rd., Ste. 102
Louisville, KY 40220
Phone: (502)451-4266 **Free:** 800-221-1277
Fax: (502)456-2701
Website: http://www.alzinky.org/

Louisiana

★ 6526 ★ Alzheimer's Association
Greater New Orleans Chapter
1040 Calhoun St.
New Orleans, LA 70118
Phone: (504)895-6223 **Free:** 800-459-3528
Fax: (504)895-0493

★ 6527 ★ Alzheimer's Association
Northeast/Central Louisiana Chapter
PO Box 2471
Monroe, LA 71207
Phone: (318)322-2828 **Free:** 888-202-2828
Fax: (318)327-6301

Maine

★ 6528 ★ Alzheimer's Association
Maine Chapter
163 Lancaster St., Ste. 160B
Portland, ME 04101-2406
Phone: (207)772-0115 **Free:** 800-660-2871
Fax: (207)772-0354
Email: eleanor.goldberg@alz.org
Website: http://www.mainealz.org
Eleanor Goldberg, Exec Director

Maryland

★ 6529 ★ Alzheimer's Association
Greater Maryland Chapter
1850 York Rd., Ste. D
Lutherville Timonium, MD 21093
Phone: (410)561-9099 **Free:** 800-443-2273
Fax: (410)561-3433
Website: http://www.alzgmd.org

Massachusetts

★ 6530 ★ Alzheimer's Association
Massachusetts Chapter
36 Cameron Ave.
Cambridge, MA 02140
Phone: (617)868-6718 **Free:** 800-548-2111
Fax: (978)868-6720
Email: elaine.cohen@alz.org
Website: http://www.alzmass.org/
James Wessler, Exec Director
Alt. Contact: Spanish speaker's line: (617) 868-8599.

Michigan

★ 6531 ★ Alzheimer's Association
Greater Michigan Chapter
17220 W 12 Mile Rd., Ste. 100
Southfield, MI 48076
Phone: (248)557-8277 **Free:** 800-337-3827
Fax: (248)557-4642

★ 6532 ★ Alzheimer's Association
Michigan Great Lakes Chapter
107 Aprill Dr., Ste. 1
Ann Arbor, MI 48103
Phone: (734)677-3081 **Free:** 800-337-3827
Fax: (734)677-3091
Website: http://www.alzmigreatlakes.org

★ 6533 ★ Alzheimer's Association
North/West Michigan Chapter
225 W 30th St.
Holland, MI 49423
Phone: (616)392-8365 **Free:** 800-893-8365
Fax: (616)392-1712
Email: janet.magennis@alz.org
Website: http://www.nwmialz.org
Janet Magennis, Exec Director

Minnesota

★ 6534 ★ Alzheimer's Association
Minnesota-Dakotas Chapter
4550 W 77th St., Ste. 200
Minneapolis, MN 55435
Phone: (952)830-0512 **Free:** 800-232-0851
Fax: (952)830-0513
Email: john.kemp@alz.org
Website: http://www.alzmndak.org
John Kemp, Exec Director
Remarks: Serves Minnesota, North Dakota, and South Dakota.

Mississippi

★ 6535 ★ Alzheimer's Association
Mississippi Chapter
1900 Dunbarton Dr., Ste. I
Jackson, MS 39216
Phone: (601)987-0020 **Free:** 877-525-HELP
Fax: (601)987-9020

Missouri

★ 6536 ★ Alzheimer's Association
Mid-Missouri Chapter
1121 Business Loop 70 E, Ste. 2B
Columbia, MO 65201
Phone: (573)443-8665 **Free:** 800-693-8665
Fax: (573)499-9701
Email: penny.braun@alz.org
Website: http://www.alz.org/chapters/template/mid-mo/default.htm

★ 6537 ★ Alzheimer's Association
Saint Louis Chapter
9374 Olive Blvd.
Saint Louis, MO 63132
Phone: (314)432-3422 **Free:** 800-980-9080
Fax: (314)432-3824
Email: info@alzstl.org
Website: http://www.alzstl.org
Remarks: Also serves Illinois.

★ 6538 ★ Alzheimer's Association
Southwest Missouri Chapter
Glen Isle Ctr.
1500 S Glenstone
Springfield, MO 65804
Phone: (417)886-2199 **Free:** 800-487-0747
Fax: (417)886-0337
Website: http://www.alz-swmo.org/

Montana

★ 6539 ★ Alzheimer's Association
Montana Chapter
2900 12th Ave., Ste. 4E
Billings, MT 59101

Phone: (406)252-3053 **Fax:** (406)237-4285
Website: http://www.alz-mt.org

Nebraska

★ 6540 ★ Alzheimer's Association
Great Plains Chapter
5601 S 27th St., Ste. 201
Lincoln, NE 68512
Phone: (402)420-2540 **Free:** 888-487-2585
Fax: (402)420-2541
Website: http://www.alznebraska.org
Remarks: Serves Nebraska and Wyoming.

★ 6541 ★ Alzheimer's Association
Midlands Chapter
7101 Newport Ave., Ste. 305
Omaha, NE 68152
Phone: (402)572-3059 **Free:** 800-309-2112
Fax: (402)572-3038
Email: alz@infobridge.com
Website: http://www.omaha-cb-alz.org/
Connie Kudlacek, Exec Director
Remarks: Serves Iowa and eastern Nebraska.

New Jersey

★ 6542 ★ Alzheimer's Association
Greater New Jersey Chapter
400 Morris Ave., Ste. 251
Denville, NJ 07834
Phone: (973)586-4300 **Free:** 800-883-1180
Fax: (973)586-4342
Email: jean.gallo@alz.org
Website: http://www.alz.org/gnj

New Mexico

★ 6543 ★ Alzheimer's Association
New Mexico Chapter
8100 Mountain Rd. NE, Ste. 201
Albuquerque, NM 87110
Phone: (505)266-4473 **Free:** 800-777-8155
Fax: (505)266-0108
Email: info@nm-alzheimers.org
Website: http://www.nm-alzheimers.org/

New York

★ 6544 ★ Alzheimer's Association
Central New York Chapter
441 W Kirkpatrick St.
Syracuse, NY 13204-1361
Phone: (315)472-4201 **Free:** 800-339-4177
Fax: (315)472-4206
Website: http://www.alzcny.org

★ 6545 ★ Alzheimer's Association
Hudson Valley/Rockland/Westchester, NY Chapter
2 Jefferson Plaza, Ste. 203
Poughkeepsie, NY 12601
Phone: (845)471-2655 **Free:** 800-872-0994
Fax: (845)471-8960
Email: elaine.sproat@alz.org
Website: http://www.alz.org/midhudson/

★ 6546 ★ Alzheimer's Association
Long Island Chapter
3281 Veterans Memorial Hwy., Ste. E-13
Ronkonkoma, NY 11779
Phone: (631)580-5100 **Fax:** (631)580-3100
Website: http://www.alzheimersli.org
Fred M. Kadin, Exec Director

★ 6547 ★ Alzheimer's Association
New York City Chapter
360 Lexington Ave., 5th Fl.
New York, NY 10017
Phone: (212)983-0700 **Fax:** (212)697-6158
Email: Jed.Levine@alz.org
Website: http://www.alzheimernyc.org/

★ 6548 ★ Alzheimer's Association
Northeastern New York Chapter
85 Watervliet Ave.
Albany, NY 12206
Phone: (518)438-2217 **Free:** 800-303-2218
Fax: (518)438-2219
Email: alzneny@crisny.org
Website: http://www.alzneny.org/

★ 6549 ★ Alzheimer's Association
Rochester Chapter
435 E Henrietta Rd.
Rochester, NY 14620
Phone: (585)760-5400 **Free:** 800-724-0587
Fax: (585)760-5401
Email: alzroch@servtech.org
Website: http://www.alz-rochesterny.org

★ 6550 ★ Alzheimer's Association
Western New York Chapter
1284 French Rd.
Depew, NY 14043-4882
Phone: (716)656-8448 **Free:** 800-273-6737
Fax: (716)656-8525
Email: info@alzwny.org
Website: http://www.alzwny.org/

North Carolina

★ 6551 ★ Alzheimer's Association
Eastern North Carolina Chapter
400 Oberlin Rd., Ste. 208
Raleigh, NC 27605-1351
Phone: (919)832-3732 **Free:** 800-228-8738
Fax: (919)832-7989

★ 6552 ★ Alzheimer's Association
Western Carolina Chapter
3800 Shamrock Dr.
Charlotte, NC 28215
Phone: (704)532-7392 **Free:** 800-888-6671
Fax: (704)532-5421
Email: alz@perigree.net
Website: http://www.perigee.net/~alz/

Ohio

★ 6553 ★ Alzheimer's Association
Central Ohio Chapter
3380 Tremont Rd.
Columbus, OH 43221
Phone: (614)457-6003 **Free:** 800-735-6751
Fax: (614)457-6634
Email: cclark@alzheimerscentralohio.org
Website: http://www.alzheimerscentralohio.org/

★ 6554 ★ Alzheimer's Association
Cleveland Area Chapter
12200 Fairhill Rd.
Cleveland, OH 44120-1013
Phone: (216)721-8457 **Free:** 800-441-3322
Fax: (216)721-1629
Email: webinfo@alzclv.org
Website: http://www.alzclv.org/
Rimas J. Jasinevicius, Exec Director

★ 6555 ★ Alzheimer's Association
East Central Ohio Chapter
126 W Church St.
Newark, OH 43055
Phone: (740)345-5102 **Free:** 800-441-3322
Fax: (740)345-5099

★ 6556 ★ Alzheimer's Association
Greater Cincinnati Chapter
644 Linn St., Ste. 1026
Cincinnati, OH 45203
Phone: (513)721-4284 **Free:** 800-441-3322
Fax: (513)345-8446
Website: http://www.alz.org/grtrcinc
Remarks: Also serves Indiana and Kentucky.

★ 6557 ★ Alzheimer's Association
Greater East Ohio Area Chapter
1815 W Market St., Ste. 301
Akron, OH 44313
Phone: (330)864-5646 **Free:** 800-441-3322
Fax: (330)864-7336
Email: pamschuellerman@alz.org
Website: http://www.tricountyalz.org/
Pamela Schuellerman, Exec Director
Remarks: Also serves Pennsylvania.

★ 6558 ★ Alzheimer's Association
Miami Valley Chapter
The Laurelwood
3797 Summit Glen Dr., Ste. G100
Dayton, OH 45449
Phone: (937)291-3332 **Free:** 800-441-3322
Fax: (937)291-0463
Website: http://www.miamivalleycare.org/alzheimer

★ 6559 ★ Alzheimer's Association
Northwest Ohio Chapter
2500 N Reynolds Rd.
Toledo, OH 43615-2820
Phone: (419)537-1999 **Free:** 800-441-3322
Fax: (419)536-5591
Website: http://www.nwoalz.org

Oklahoma

★ 6560 ★ Alzheimer's Association
Oklahoma/Western Arkansas Chapter
6465 S Yale, Ste. 206
Tulsa, OK 74136-7810
Phone: (918)481-7741 **Free:** 800-493-1411
Fax: (918)481-7745
Website: http://www.alzokar.org

Oregon

★ 6561 ★ Alzheimer's Association
Oregon-Greater Idaho Chapter
1311 NW 21st Ave.
Portland, OR 97209
Phone: (503)413-7115 **Free:** 800-733-0402
Fax: (503)413-6909
Email: andi.miller@alz-or.org
Website: http://www.alz.org/oregon
Liz McKinney, Exec Director
Remarks: Also serves Washington.

Pennsylvania

★ 6562 ★ Alzheimer's Association
Delaware Valley Chapter
100 N 17th St., 2nd Fl.
Philadelphia, PA 19103
Phone: (215)561-2919 **Free:** 800-272-3900
Fax: (215)561-4663
Website: http://www.alz-delawarevalley.org
Remarks: Serves Delaware, New Jersey, and Pennsylvania.

★ 6563 ★ **Alzheimer's Association Greater Pennsylvania Chapter**
2001 N Front St., Ste. 321, Bldg. 2
Harrisburg, PA 17102
Phone: (717)232-3580 **Free:** 800-975-8848
Fax: (717)232-3609

Rhode Island

★ 6564 ★ **Alzheimer's Association Rhode Island Chapter**
245 Waterman St., Ste. 306
Providence, RI 02906
Phone: (401)421-0008 **Free:** 800-244-1428
Fax: (401)421-0115
Website: http://www.alz-ri.org

South Carolina

★ 6565 ★ **Alzheimer's Association Palmetto Chapter**
PO Box 7044
Columbia, SC 29202
Phone: (803)772-3346 **Free:** 800-636-3346
Fax: (803)772-3349
Email: paul.jeter@alz.org
Website: http://www.midnet.sc.edu/alz/alz.htm
Paul Jeter, Exec Director

★ 6566 ★ **Alzheimer's Association Upstate South Carolina Chapter**
521 N McDuffie St.
Anderson, SC 29621
Phone: (864)224-3045 **Free:** 800-273-2555
Fax: (864)225-1387
Email: alz@carol.net
Website: http://www.upstatescalz.org

Tennessee

★ 6567 ★ **Alzheimer's Association Eastern Tennessee Chapter**
Portland Bldg., Ste. H-102
2200 Sutherland Ave.
Knoxville, TN 37919
Phone: (865)544-6288 **Fax:** (865)544-6249
Email: corinne.patrick@alz.org
Website: http://www.tnalz.org

★ 6568 ★ **Alzheimer's Association Mid South Chapter**
4004 Hillsboro Rd., Ste. 219B
Nashville, TN 37215
Phone: (615)292-4938 **Fax:** (615)386-9768
Website: http://www.alztn.org
Remarks: Serves Alabama, Arkansas, and Tennessee.

★ 6569 ★ **Alzheimer's Association Northeast Tennessee Chapter**
207 N Boone St., Ste. 1500
Johnson City, TN 37604
Phone: (423)928-4080 **Fax:** (423)928-1152
Remarks: Also serves Virginia.

★ 6570 ★ **Alzheimer's Association Southeast Tennessee Chapter**
735 Broad St., Ste. 300
Chattanooga, TN 37402
Phone: (423)265-3600 **Free:** 800-616-1922
Fax: (423)265-3611

Texas

★ 6571 ★ **Alzheimer's Association Greater Austin Chapter**
3420 Executive Ctr. Dr., Ste. 301
Austin, TX 78731
Phone: (512)241-0420 **Free:** 800-367-2132
Fax: (512)241-0430
Email: alz@alz-austin.org
Website: http://www.alz-austin.org/
Gail Harmon, Exec Director

★ 6572 ★ **Alzheimer's Association Greater Dallas Chapter**
7610 N Stemmons Fwy., Ste. 600
Dallas, TX 75247-4228
Phone: (214)827-0062 **Free:** 800-515-8201
Fax: (214)827-2064
Email: dawn.mckinney@alz.org
Website: http://www.alzdallas.org/

★ 6573 ★ **Alzheimer's Association North Central Texas Chapter**
PO Box 9709
Fort Worth, TX 76147
Phone: (817)336-4949 **Free:** 800-471-4422
Fax: (817)336-4966
Email: theresa.hocker@alz.org
Website: http://www.alz.org/ncc
Theresa Hocker, Exec Director

★ 6574 ★ **Alzheimer's Association STAR Chapter**
4400 N Mesa, Ste. 9
El Paso, TX 79902
Phone: (915)544-1799 **Free:** 877-544-1799
Fax: (915)544-8746

Utah

★ 6575 ★ **Alzheimer's Association Utah Chapter**
1414 East 4500 South, Ste. 2
Salt Lake City, UT 84117
Phone: (801)274-1944 **Free:** 800-371-6694
Fax: (801)274-1226
Website: http://www.alzutah.org
Remarks: Also serves Idaho.

Vermont

★ 6576 ★ **Alzheimer's Association Vermont and New Hampshire Chapter**
PO Box 1139
Montpelier, VT 05601
Phone: (802)229-1022 **Free:** 800-698-1022
Fax: (802)229-5231
Email: susan.gordon@alz.org
Website: http://www.alz.org/vermont

Virginia

★ 6577 ★ **Alzheimer's Association Central and Western Virginia Chapter**
PO Box 4634
Charlottesville, VA 22905
Phone: (434)973-6122 **Free:** 888-809-7383
Fax: (434)973-4224
Email: kitter@cstone.net
Website: http://monticello.avenue.org/alzheimers/
Elizabeth Seabrook, Exec Director

★ 6578 ★ **Alzheimer's Association Greater Richmond Chapter**
4600 Cox Rd., Ste. 130
Glen Allen, VA 23060
Phone: (804)967-2580 **Free:** 800-598-4673
Fax: (804)967-2588
Email: sherry.peterson@alz.org
Website: http://www.richmondalzheimers.org/
Sherry E. Peterson, Exec Director

★ 6579 ★ **Alzheimer's Association National Capital Area Chapter**
11240 Waples Mill Rd., Ste. 402
Fairfax, VA 22030
Phone: (866)259-0042 **Free:** (866)259-0042
Fax: (703)359-4441
Website: http://www.alz-nca.org
Remarks: Serves Maryland, Virginia, and Washington DC.

★ 6580 ★ **Alzheimer's Association Southeastern Virginia Chapter**
20 Interstate Corporate Ctr., Ste. 233
Norfolk, VA 23502
Phone: (757)459-2405 **Free:** 800-755-1129
Fax: (757)461-7902
Website: http://www.alz.org/chapters/template/hamptrds/welcome.html

Washington

★ 6581 ★ **Alzheimer's Association Inland Northwest Chapter**
601 W Maxwell, No. 4
Spokane, WA 99201
Phone: (509)483-8456 **Free:** 800-256-6659
Fax: (509)483-6067
Website: http://www.inwalz.org
Remarks: Serves Idaho and Washington.

★ 6582 ★ **Alzheimer's Association Western and Central Washington State Chapter**
12721 30th Ave. NE, Ste. 101
Seattle, WA 98125
Phone: (206)363-5500 **Free:** 800-848-7097
Fax: (206)363-5700
Website: http://www.alzwa.org/

West Virginia

★ 6583 ★ **Alzheimer's Association West Virginia Chapter**
1111 Lee St. E
Charleston, WV 25301
Phone: (304)343-2717 **Free:** 800-491-2717
Fax: (304)343-2723
Website: http://wvalz.org
Remarks: Also serves Ohio and Virginia.

Wisconsin

★ 6584 ★ **Alzheimer's Association Greater Wisconsin Chapter**
2900 Curry Ln., Ste. A
Green Bay, WI 54311
Phone: (920)469-2110 **Free:** 800-360-2110
Fax: (920)469-2131
Remarks: Serves Minnesota and Wisconsin.

★ 6585 ★ **Alzheimer's Association South Central Wisconsin Chapter**
517 N Segoe Rd., Ste. 301
Madison, WI 53705
Phone: (608)232-3400 **Free:** 800-428-9280
Fax: (608)232-3407
Email: paul.rusk@alzwisc.org
Website: http://www.alzwisc.org/
Paul Rusk, Exec Director

★ 6586 ★ Alzheimer's Association Southeastern Wisconsin Chapter
6130 W National Ave., Ste. 200
Milwaukee, WI 53214
Phone: (414)479-8800 **Free:** 800-922-2413
Fax: (414)479-8819
Email: info@alzheimers-sewi.org
Website: http://www.alzheimers-sewi.org/
Sig Tomkalski, Exec Director

Amyotrophic Lateral Sclerosis

State chapters of the ALS Association are listed below. The national office is located at 27001 Agoura Rd., Ste. 150, Calabasas Hills, CA 91301-5104. Additional information can be obtained by calling the national office at (800) 782-4747, or by consulting their web site at http://www.alsa.org.

Arizona

★ 6587 ★ ALS Association Arizona Chapter
5040 E Shea Blvd., Ste. 151
Scottsdale, AZ 85254
Phone: (480)609-3888 **Fax:** (480)556-9927
Email: daniel@alsaz.org
Website: http://www.alsaz.org

California

★ 6588 ★ ALS Association Bay Area Chapter
140 Geary St., 4th Fl.
San Francisco, CA 94108-5611
Phone: (415)392-2572 **Fax:** (415)438-3972
Email: fightals@alsabayarea.org
Website: http://www.alsabayarea.org

★ 6589 ★ ALS Association Greater Los Angeles Chapter
PO Box 565
Agoura Hills, CA 91376
Phone: (818)865-8067 **Fax:** (818)865-8066
Email: ALSAGLAC@aol.com
Website: http://www.alsala.org

★ 6590 ★ ALS Association Greater Sacramento Chapter
2717 Cottage Way, Ste. 15
Sacramento, CA 95825
Phone: (916)979-9265 **Fax:** (916)979-9271
Email: lou@alssac.org
Website: http://www.alssac.org

★ 6591 ★ ALS Association Greater San Diego CIO
7925 Silverton, Ste. 506
San Diego, CA 92126-6350
Phone: (760)643-9293
Email: alsasd@email.com
Website: http://www.alsasd.com

★ 6592 ★ ALS Association Orange County Chapter
2230 W Chapman, No. 123
Orange, CA 92868
Phone: (714)938-1080 **Fax:** (714)938-1299
Email: information@alsaoc.org
Website: http://www.alsaoc.org
Cheryl Holt, Exec Director

Colorado

★ 6593 ★ ALS Association Rocky Mountain Chapter
PO Box 7964
Boulder, CO 80306
Phone: (720)890-8311 **Fax:** (970)532-1077
Email: sbaum@idcomm.com
Website: http://www.alsaco.org
Patti Abendroth, Exec Director

Connecticut

★ 6594 ★ ALS Association Connecticut Chapter
4 Oxford Rd.
Unit D1
Milford, CT 06460
Phone: (203)874-5050 **Fax:** (203)874-7070
Email: als.assoc@snet.net
Website: http://www.alsact.org
Bob O'Brien, Exec Director

Florida

★ 6595 ★ ALS Association Florida Chapter
5005 W Laurel St., Ste. 110
Tampa, FL 33607
Phone: (813)637-9000 **Free:** 888-257-1717
Fax: (813)637-9010
Email: office@als-florida.org
Website: http://www.als-florida.org

★ 6596 ★ ALS Association Florida Chapter East Coast Regional Office
1998 SW Taurus Ln.
Port Saint Lucie, FL 34984
Phone: (561)871-2453 **Fax:** (561)871-2223
Email: dotburk@aol.com
Website: http://www.alsa.org/serving/florida_goldcoast_chapter.cfm
Dottie Burkett, Exec Director

Indiana

★ 6597 ★ ALS Association Indiana Chapter
1980 E 116th St., Ste. 105
Carmel, IN 46032
Free: 888-508-3232
Email: alsa.in@juno.com
Brooke Billingsley, Exec Director

Kansas

★ 6598 ★ ALS Association Keith Worthington Chapter
8340 Mission Rd., Ste. B4
Prairie Village, KS 66206
Phone: (913)648-2062 **Free:** 800-878-2062
Fax: (913)642-2431
Email: bcooper@alsa-midwest.org
Website: http://www.alsa-midwest.org
Beckie Cooper, Exec Director

★ 6599 ★ ALS Association Keith Worthington Chapter Central/Western Kansas - Branch Office
5920 E Central, Ste. 102
Wichita, KS 67208
Phone: (316)612-0188 **Free:** 800-553-9056
Fax: (316)612-8768
Website: http://www.alsa-midwest.org

Kentucky

★ 6600 ★ ALS Association Kentucky CIO
PO Box 910130
Lexington, KY 40591-0130
Phone: (859)455-9859
Email: alsakentucky@msn.com
Website: http://www.alsakentucky.org

Maryland

★ 6601 ★ ALS Association National Capital Area Chapter
615 S Frederick Ave.
Ste. 308
Gaithersburg, MD 20877
Phone: (301)978-9855 **Fax:** (301)978-9854
Email: pfreiberg@alsa-ncac.org
Website: http://www.alsa-ncac.org
Remarks: This chapter serves Maryland, Washington, D.C., and Virginia.

Massachusetts

★ 6602 ★ ALS Association Massachusetts Chapter
75 McNeil Way
Ste. 201
Dedham, MA 02026
Phone: (781)326-8884 **Fax:** (781)326-4940
Email: customerservice@als-ma.org
Website: http://www.als-ma.org

★ 6603 ★ ALS Association Massachusetts Chapter - Wakefield Office
7 Lincoln St.
Wakefield, MA 01880
Free: 800-258-3323
Email: customerservice@als-ma.org
Website: http://www.als-ma.org
Donna Jordan, Exec Director

Michigan

★ 6604 ★ ALS Association ALS of Michigan, Inc.
21311 Civic Center Dr., Ste. 200
Southfield, MI 48076
Free: 800-882-5764 **Fax:** (248)354-6440
Email: alsofmi@alsofmi.org
Website: http://www.alsofmi.org

★ 6605 ★ ALS Association West Michigan Chapter
731 Front St. NW
Grand Rapids, MI 49504
Free: 800-387-7121 **Fax:** (616)459-4522
Email: alsawmc@aol.com
Website: http://www.alsa-westmichigan.org

Minnesota

★ 6606 ★ ALS Association Minnesota Chapter
333 N Washington Ave., Ste. 105
Minneapolis, MN 55401
Phone: (612)672-0484 **Free:** 888-672-0484
Fax: (612)672-9110
Email: info@alsmn.org
Website: http://www.alsmn.org
Marlin Possehl, Exec Director

Missouri

★ 6607 ★ ALS Association
Keith Worthington Chapter
Central Missouri - Branch Office
1447 F South Enterprise
Springfield, MO 65803
Phone: (417)886-5003 **Fax:** (417)886-5058
Website: http://www.alsa-midwest.org

★ 6608 ★ ALS Association
St. Louis Regional Chapter
5615 Pershing Ave., Ste. 20
Saint Louis, MO 63112
Phone: (314)534-0610 **Fax:** (314)361-3020
Email: info@alsastl.org
Website: http://www.alsa-stl.org

Nebraska

★ 6609 ★ ALS Association
Keith Worthington Chapter
Nebraska-Branch Office
10730 Pacific at Shaker Place
Ste. 228
Omaha, NE 68114
Phone: (402)991-8788 **Fax:** (402)991-3690
Email: rmiller@alsa-midwest.org
Website: http://www.alsa-midwest.org

Nevada

★ 6610 ★ ALS Association
Nevada Chapter
2101 S Jones, Ste. 120
Las Vegas, NV 89146
Phone: (702)248-4507 **Fax:** (702)248-8070
Email: alsanv@aol.com
Website: http://www.alsnevada.com

New Mexico

★ 6611 ★ ALS Association
New Mexico CIO
PO Box 16495
Albuquerque, NM 87191-6495
Phone: (505)323-6348
Email: cborgman@comcast.net
Website: http://www.alsa-nm.org

New York

★ 6612 ★ ALS Association
Greater New York Chapter
116 John St., Ste. 1304
New York, NY 10038
Free: 800-672-8857 **Fax:** (212)619-7409
Email: als@als-ny.org
Website: http://www.als-ny.org
Lauri Norvick, Exec Director

★ 6613 ★ ALS Association
Upstate New York CIO
PO Box 127
Elbridge, NY 13060
Phone: (315)253-9557
Email: donnalynn73@hotmail.com

North Carolina

★ 6614 ★ ALS Association
Jim "Catfish" Hunter Chapter
1425-113 Rock Quarry Rd.
Raleigh, NC 27610
Free: 877-568-4347 **Fax:** (919)844-4295
Email: jerry@catfishchapter.org
Website: http://www.catfishchapter.org/
Remarks: This chapter serves both North and South Carolina.

Ohio

★ 6615 ★ ALS Association
Northeast Ohio Chapter
2500 E 22nd St., Ste. 101
Cleveland, OH 44115
Phone: (216)592-2572 **Fax:** (216)592-2575
Email: mjarmst216@aol.com
Website: http://www.alsaohio.org
Judy Post, Administrator

★ 6616 ★ ALS Association
Western Ohio Chapter
1810 MacKenzie Dr.
Ste. 120
Columbus, OH 43220
Phone: (614)273-2572 **Fax:** (614)273-2573
Email: edalsawo@msn.com
Website: http://www.alsohio.org

Oregon

★ 6617 ★ ALS Association
Oregon and Southwest Washington CIO
3316 NE Clackamas
Portland, OR 97232
Phone: (503)238-5559 **Fax:** (503)977-4198
Email: cindyburdell@alsa-or.org
Website: http://www.alsa-or.org

Pennsylvania

★ 6618 ★ ALS Association
Greater Philadelphia Chapter
321 Norristown Rd., Ste. 260
Ambler, PA 19002
Phone: (215)643-5434 **Fax:** (215)643-9307
Email: alsassoc@alsphiladelphia.org
Website: http://www.alsphiladelphia.org
Mary Connell, President

★ 6619 ★ ALS Association
Western Pennsylvania Chapter
Landmarks Bldg.
One Station Square Dr., Ste. 550
Pittsburgh, PA 15219
Free: 800-967-9296 **Fax:** (412)471-2722
Email: info@alswp.org
Website: http://www.alswp.org

Rhode Island

★ 6620 ★ ALS Association
Rhode Island Chapter
1637 Warwick Ave.
Warwick, RI 02889
Phone: (401)732-1609 **Fax:** (401)732-2577
Email: alsarinf@aol.com
Website: http://www.alsari.org
Nancy Feroldi, Exec Director

Tennessee

★ 6621 ★ ALS Association
Central Tennessee Chapter
PO Box 190612
Nashville, TN 37219-0612
Phone: (615)255-4454
Email: alsa-central_tennessee@comcast.net

★ 6622 ★ ALS Association
Mid-South CIO
4746 Spottswood Ave., No. 192
Memphis, TN 38117
Phone: (901)351-3314
Email: awwalker45@aol.com
Remarks: This chapter serves western Tennessee, Mississippi, and Arkansas.

Texas

★ 6623 ★ ALS Association
North Texas Chapter
2100 Highway 360
Ste. 1900
Grand Prairie, TX 75050
Phone: (972)641-6200
Email: hope@alsanorthtexas.org
Website: http://www.alsanorthtexas.org
Remarks: The mission of the Dallas/Ft. Worth Chapter of the ALS Association is to help those living with ALS and their caregivers and to support research to find a cure. **Program(s):** Support groups, advocacy, education, and loaning of equipment and reading materials.

★ 6624 ★ ALS Association
South Texas Chapter
6800 Park Ten Blvd., Ste. 220N
San Antonio, TX 78213
Phone: (210)733-5204 **Fax:** (210)733-5206
Email: alsasotex@stic.net
Website: http://www.alsa-south-tx.org
April Coldsmith, Exec Director

★ 6625 ★ ALS Association
Southeast Texas CIO
3700 Wakeforest, No. 16
Houston, TX 77098
Phone: (713)526-7949 **Fax:** (713)533-9713
Email: markmiller@vippn.com
Remarks: This chapter serves Houston and the surrounding area.

Vermont

★ 6626 ★ ALS Association
Northern New England Chapter
80 Colchester Ave.
Burlington, VT 05401
Phone: (802)862-8882 **Fax:** (802)862-2138
Email: patriciakrusinski@msn.com
Remarks: This chapter serves Vermont, Hew Hampshire, and Maine.

Washington

★ 6627 ★ ALS Association
Evergreen Chapter
6627 S 191st Place
Ste. F-106
Kent, WA 98032
Phone: (425)656-1650 **Fax:** (425)656-1649
Email: info@alsa-ec.org
Website: http://www.alsa-ec.org

Wisconsin

★ 6628 ★ ALS Association
Southeast Wisconsin Chapter
2421 N Mayfair Rd., Ste. 212
Wauwatosa, WI 53226
Phone: (414)771-9400 **Fax:** (414)771-9503
Email: gehrigse@execpc.com
Website: http://www.se-wis-als.org

Arthritis

Listed below are chapters of the Arthritis Foundation, 1330 W Peachtree St., Atlanta, GA 30309, (800)283-7800, http://www.arthritis.org/.

Alabama

★ 6629 ★ Arthritis Foundation
Alabama Chapter
300 Vestavia Pkwy., Ste. 3500
Birmingham, AL 35216
Phone: (205)979-5700 **Free:** 800-879-7896
Fax: (205)979-4172
Email: info.al@arthritis.org
Website: http://www.arthritis.org/communities/chapters/Chapter.asp?Chapid=8
Dixie Kuykendall, President

Arizona

★ 6630 ★ Arthritis Foundation
Greater Southwest Chapter
1313 E Osborn Rd., Ste. 200
Phoenix, AZ 85014
Phone: (602)264-7679 **Free:** 800-477-7679
Fax: (602)264-0563
Email: info.caz@arthritis.org
Website: http://www.arthritis.org/communities/chapters/Chapter.asp?Chapid=64
Carol Chamberlin, President
Remarks: Serves Arizona, New Mexico, and El Paso, Texas.

Arkansas

★ 6631 ★ Arthritis Foundation
Arkansas Chapter
6213 Father Tribou St.
Little Rock, AR 72205
Phone: (501)664-7242 **Free:** 800-482-8858
Fax: (501)664-6588
Email: info.ar@arthritis.org
Website: http://www.arthritis.org/communities/chapters/Chapter.asp?Chapid=9
Diane Stephenson, President

California

★ 6632 ★ Arthritis Foundation
Northeastern California Chapter
3040 Explorer Dr., Ste. 1
Sacramento, CA 95827
Phone: (916)368-5599 **Free:** 800-571-3456
Fax: (916)368-5596
Email: info.neca@arthritis.org
Website: http://www.arthritis.org/communities/chapters/Chapter.asp?Chapid=35
Joan Stevie, President
Remarks: Also serves northern Nevada.

★ 6633 ★ Arthritis Foundation
Northern California Chapter
657 Mission St., Ste. 603
San Francisco, CA 94105-4120
Phone: (415)356-1230 **Free:** 800-464-6240
Fax: (415)356-1240
Email: info.nca@arthritis.org
Website: http://www.arthritis.org/communities/chapters/Chapter.asp?Chapid=33
Judith E. McAbee, President

★ 6634 ★ Arthritis Foundation
San Diego Area Chapter
9089 Clairemont Mesa Blvd., Ste. 104
San Diego, CA 92123-1288
Phone: (858)492-1090 **Free:** 800-422-8885
Fax: (858)492-9248
Email: info.sd@arthritis.org
Website: http://www.arthritis.org/communities/chapters/Chapter.asp?Chapid=50
Kathy Woodland, Director

★ 6635 ★ Arthritis Foundation
Southern California Chapter
4311 Wilshire Blvd., Ste. 530
Los Angeles, CA 90010-3775
Phone: (323)954-5750 **Free:** 800-954-2873
Fax: (323)954-5790
Email: info.sca@arthritis.org
Website: http://www.arthritis.org/communities/chapters/Chapter.asp?Chapid=49
Remarks: Also serves Hawaii and southern Nevada.

Colorado

★ 6636 ★ Arthritis Foundation
Rocky Mountain Chapter
2280 S Albion St.
Denver, CO 80222-4906
Phone: (303)756-8622 **Free:** 800-475-6447
Fax: (303)759-4349
Email: info.rm@arthritis.org
Website: http://www.arthritis.org/communities/chapters/Chapter.asp?Chapid=80
Ted Zerwin, President
Remarks: Serves Colorado and Wyoming.

Connecticut

★ 6637 ★ Arthritis Foundation
Southern New England Chapter
35 Cold Spring Rd., Ste. 411
Rocky Hill, CT 06067
Phone: (860)563-1177 **Free:** 800-541-8350
Fax: (860)563-6018
Email: info.sne@arthritis.org
Website: http://www.arthritis.org/communities/chapters/Chapter.asp?Chapid=66
Leslie Kotke, President
Remarks: Serves Connecticut and Rhode Island.

Delaware

★ 6638 ★ Arthritis Foundation
Delaware Chapter
100 W 10th St., Ste. 1105
Wilmington, DE 19801-1663
Phone: (302)777-1212 **Free:** 800-292-9599
Fax: (302)777-1841
Email: info.de@arthritis.org
Website: http://www.arthritis.org/communities/chapters/Chapter.asp?Chapid=15
Martha M. Buccino, President

District of Columbia

★ 6639 ★ Arthritis Foundation
Metropolitan Washington Chapter
4455 Connecticut Ave. NW, Ste. 300
Washington, DC 20008
Phone: (202)537-6800 **Fax:** (202)537-6859
Email: info.mwa@arthritis.org
Website: http://www.arthritis.org/communities/chapters/Chapter.asp?Chapid=32
Remarks: Serves Washington DC, Maryland, and Virginia.

Florida

★ 6640 ★ Arthritis Foundation
Florida Chapter
400 Hibiscus St., Ste. 200
West Palm Beach, FL 33401
Phone: (561)655-4970 **Free:** 800-672-0882
Fax: (561)655-2780
Email: info.fl@arthritis.org
Website: http://www.arthritis.org/communities/chapters/Chapter.asp?Chapid=61

Georgia

★ 6641 ★ Arthritis Foundation
Georgia Chapter
550 Pharr Rd., Ste. 550
Atlanta, GA 30305
Phone: (404)237-8771 **Free:** 800-933-7023
Fax: (404)237-8153
Email: info.ga@arthritis.org
Website: http://www.arthritis.org/communities/chapters/Chapter.asp?Chapid=19
Elizabeth A. Martin, President

Hawaii

★ 6642 ★ Arthritis Foundation
Soutbern California Chapter
Hawaii Office
615 Piikoi St., Ste. 1812
Honolulu, HI 96814
Phone: (808)596-2900 **Free:** 800-954-2873
Fax: (808)596-2904
Email: info.sca.hib@arthritis.org
Website: http://www.arthritis.org

Illinois

★ 6643 ★ Arthritis Foundation
Greater Chicago Chapter
303 E Wacker Dr., Ste. 300
Chicago, IL 60601-5206
Phone: (312)616-3470 **Free:** 800-735-0096
Fax: (312)616-9281
Email: info.gc@arthritis.org
Website: http://www.arthritis.org/communities/chapters/Chapter.asp?Chapid=11

★ 6644 ★ Arthritis Foundation
Greater Illinois Chapter
2621 N Knoxville Ave.
Peoria, IL 61604
Phone: (309)682-6600 **Free:** 800-795-9115
Fax: (309)682-6732
Email: info.gil@arthritis.org
Website: http://www.arthritis.org/communities/chapters/Chapter.asp?Chapid=20
Gary Dutro, President

Indiana

★ 6645 ★ Arthritis Foundation
Indiana Chapter
8660 Guion Rd.
Indianapolis, IN 46268
Phone: (317)879-0321 **Free:** 800-783-2342
Fax: (317)876-5608
Email: info.in@arthritis.org
Website: http://www.arthritis.org/communities/chapters/Chapter.asp?Chapid=22
Marva Cobb, President

Iowa

★ 6646 ★ Arthritis Foundation
Iowa Chapter
2600 72nd St., Ste. D
Des Moines, IA 50322-4724
Phone: (515)278-0636 **Free:** (866)378-0636
Fax: (515)278-2603
Email: info.ia@arthritis.org
Website: http://www.arthritis.org/communities/chapters/Chapter.asp?Chapid=21
Amy L. Selene, President

Remarks: Also serves Rock Island County, Illinois.

Kansas

★ 6647 ★ Arthritis Foundation
Kansas Chapter
1602 E Waterman
Wichita, KS 67211-1878
Phone: (316)263-0116 **Free:** 800-362-1108
Fax: (316)263-3260
Email: info.ks@arthritis.org
Website: http://www.arthritis.org/communities/chapters/Chapter.asp?Chapid=23
Doris E. Newman, President

Kentucky

★ 6648 ★ Arthritis Foundation
Kentucky Chapter
2908 Brownsboro Rd., Ste. 100
Louisville, KY 40206-3506
Phone: (502)585-1866 **Free:** 800-633-5335
Fax: (502)585-1657
Email: info.ky@arthritis.org
Website: http://www.arthritis.org/communities/chapters/Chapter.asp?Chapid=24
Cynthia A. Harbin, President
Remarks: Also serves southern Indiana.

Louisiana

★ 6649 ★ Arthritis Foundation
Louisiana Chapter
15254 Old Hammond Hwy., Ste. A4
Baton Rouge, LA 70816
Phone: (225)275-1119 **Free:** 800-673-7508
Fax: (225)275-1172
Email: info.la@arthritis.org
Website: http://www.arthritis.org/communities/chapters/Chapter.asp?Chapid=25
Debbie Goss, President

Maryland

★ 6650 ★ Arthritis Foundation
Maryland Chapter
1777 Reisterstown Rd., Ste. 150
Baltimore, MD 21208
Phone: (410)602-0160 **Free:** 800-365-3811
Fax: (410)602-0420
Email: info.md@arthritis.org
Website: http://www.arthritis.org/communities/chapters/Chapter.asp?Chapid=28
Jan Thompson, President
Remarks: Also serves eastern West Virginia.

Massachusetts

★ 6651 ★ Arthritis Foundation
Massachusetts Chapter
29 Crafts St., Ste. 450
Newton, MA 02458-1287
Phone: (617)244-1800 **Free:** 800-766-9449
Fax: (617)558-7686
Email: info.ma@arthritis.org
Website: http://www.arthritis.org/communities/chapters/Chapter.asp?Chapid=27
Joanne R. Donoghue, President

Michigan

★ 6652 ★ Arthritis Foundation
Michigan Chapter
17117 W 9 Mile Rd., Ste. 950
Southfield, MI 48075-4508
Phone: (248)424-9001 **Free:** 800-968-3030
Fax: (248)424-9005
Email: info.mi@arthritis.org
Website: http://www.arthritis.org/communities/chapters/Chapter.asp?Chapid=29
Michelle R.B. Glazier, President

Minnesota

★ 6653 ★ Arthritis Foundation
North Central Chapter
1902 Minnehaha Ave. W
Saint Paul, MN 55104
Phone: (651)644-4108 **Free:** 800-333-1380
Fax: (651)644-4219
Email: info.mn@arthritis.org
Website: http://www.arthritis.org/communities/chapters/Chapter.asp?Chapid=30
Remarks: Serves Minnesota, North Dakota, and South Dakota.

Mississippi

★ 6654 ★ Arthritis Foundation
Mississippi Chapter
350 N Mart Plaza
PO Box 9185
Jackson, MS 39286-9185
Phone: (601)362-6283 **Free:** 800-844-8400
Fax: (601)362-6469
Email: info.ms@arthritis.org
Website: http://www.arthritis.org/communities/chapters/Chapter.asp?Chapid=31
T.J. McSparrin, President

Missouri

★ 6655 ★ Arthritis Foundation
Eastern Missouri Chapter
8390 Delmar Blvd.
Saint Louis, MO 63124
Phone: (314)991-9333 **Free:** 800-406-2491
Fax: (314)991-4020
Email: info.emo@arthritis.org
Website: http://www.arthritis.org/communities/chapters/Chapter.asp?Chapid=16
Brenda Susan Van Slyck, President

★ 6656 ★ Arthritis Foundation
Western Missouri/Greater Kansas City Chapter
3420 Broadway, Ste. 105
Kansas City, MO 64111
Phone: (816)753-2220 **Free:** 888-719-5670
Fax: (816)753-2227
Email: info.wmo@arthritis.org
Website: http://www.arthritis.org/communities/chapters/Chapter.asp?Chapid=58
Brad Ziegler, President

Montana

★ 6657 ★ Arthritis Foundation
Rocky Mountain Chapter
Montana Branch
1643 Lewis Ave., Ste. 3
Billings, MT 59102-4151
Phone: (406)245-0231 **Free:** 888-245-0231
Fax: (406)245-0397
Email: info.rm.mb@arthritis.org
Website: http://www.arthritis.org

Nebraska

★ 6658 ★ Arthritis Foundation
Nebraska Chapter
7101 Newport Ave., Ste. 304
Omaha, NE 68152
Phone: (402)572-3040 **Free:** 800-642-5292
Fax: (402)572-3048
Email: info.ne@arthritis.org
Website: http://www.arthritis.org/communities/chapters/Chapter.asp?Chapid=34
Anne Hellbusch, Exec Director
Remarks: Also serves Iowa.

Nevada

★ 6659 ★ Arthritis Foundation
Southern California Chapter
Las Vegas Branch
2450 Chandler Ave., Ste. 17
Las Vegas, NV 89120-4059
Phone: (702)367-1626 **Free:** 800-954-2873
Fax: (702)367-6381
Email: info.sca.lvb@arthritis.org
Website: http://www.arthritis.org

New Hampshire

★ 6660 ★ Arthritis Foundation
Northern New England Chapter
New Hampshire Regional Office
6 Chenell Dr., Ste. 260
Concord, NH 03301
Phone: (603)224-9322 **Free:** 800-639-2113
Fax: (603)224-3778
Email: info.nne@arthritis.org
Website: http://www.arthritis.org

New Jersey

★ 6661 ★ Arthritis Foundation
New Jersey Chapter
200 Middlesex Tpke.
Iselin, NJ 08830
Phone: (732)283-4300 **Free:** 888-467-3112
Fax: (732)283-4633
Email: info.nj@arthritis.org
Website: http://www.arthritis.org/communities/chapters/Chapter.asp?Chapid=38
Dennis Hirschfelder, President

New York

★ 6662 ★ Arthritis Foundation
Central New York Chapter
5858 E Molloy Rd., Ste. 123
Syracuse, NY 13211
Phone: (315)455-8553 **Free:** 800-870-1771
Fax: (315)455-8714
Email: info.cny@arthritis.org
Website: http://www.arthritis.org/communities/chapters/Chapter.asp?Chapid=12

★ 6663 ★ Arthritis Foundation
Long Island Chapter
501 Walt Whitman Rd.
Melville, NY 11747
Phone: (631)427-8272 **Fax:** (631)427-3546
Email: info.li@arthritis.org
Website: http://www.arthritis.org/communities/chapters/Chapter.asp?Chapid=26
Patrick T. McAsey, President

★ 6664 ★ Arthritis Foundation
New York Chapter
122 E 42nd St., 18th Fl.
New York, NY 10168
Phone: (212)984-8700 **Fax:** (212)878-5960
Email: info.ny@arthritis.org
Website: http://www.arthritis.org/communities/chapters/Chapter.asp?Chapid=43

★ 6665 ★ Arthritis Foundation
Northeastern New York Chapter
1717 Central Ave., Ste. 105
Albany, NY 12205

Phone: (518)456-1203 **Free:** 800-420-5554
Fax: (518)869-3123
Email: rloy@arthritis.org
Website: http://www.arthritis.org/communities/chapters/Chapter.asp?Chapid=36
Ronald K. Loy, President

★ 6666 ★ Arthritis Foundation
Upstate New York Chapter
3300 Monroe Ave., Ste. 319
Rochester, NY 14618
Phone: (585)264-1480 **Fax:** (585)264-1517
Email: info.uny@arthritis.org
Website: http://www.arthritis.org/communities/chapters/Chapter.asp?Chapid=59
Carol Anne DeMoulin, President

North Carolina

★ 6667 ★ Arthritis Foundation
Carolinas Chapter
5019 Nations Crossing, Ste. 217
Charlotte, NC 28217
Phone: (704)529-5166 **Free:** 800-883-8806
Fax: (704)529-0626
Email: info.car@arthritis.org
Website: http://www.arthritis.org/communities/chapters/Chapter.asp?Chapid=54
Jim Batten, President
Remarks: Serves North Carolina and South Carolina.

Ohio

★ 6668 ★ Arthritis Foundation
Central Ohio Chapter
3740 Ridge Mill Dr.
Hilliard, OH 43026
Phone: (614)876-8200 **Free:** 888-382-4673
Fax: (614)876-8363
Email: info.coh@arthritis.org
Website: http://www.arthritis.org/communities/chapters/Chapter.asp?Chapid=13
Irene Baird, President

★ 6669 ★ Arthritis Foundation
Northeastern Ohio Chapter
Chagrin Plaza E, Ste. 210
23811 Chagrin Blvd.
Cleveland, OH 44122-5525
Phone: (216)831-7000 **Free:** 800-245-2275
Fax: (216)831-1764
Email: info.neoh@arthritis.org
Website: http://www.arthritis.org/communities/chapters/Chapter.asp?Chapid=37
Susan S. Loessin, President

★ 6670 ★ Arthritis Foundation
Northwestern Ohio Chapter
309 N Reynolds Rd., Ste. F
Toledo, OH 43615
Phone: (419)537-0888 **Free:** 800-551-PALS
Fax: (419)537-6553
Email: info.nwoh@arthritis.org
Website: http://www.arthritis.org/communities/chapters/Chapter.asp?Chapid=78
Cherie Chatreau-Grifo, Director

★ 6671 ★ Arthritis Foundation
Ohio River Valley Chapter
7811 Laurel Ave.
Cincinnati, OH 45243
Phone: (513)271-4545 **Free:** 800-383-6843
Fax: (513)271-4703
Email: info.orv@arthritis.org
Website: http://www.arthritis.org/communities/chapters/Chapter.asp?Chapid=65
Sidney Wittenberg, President
Remarks: Serves Kentucky, Ohio, and West Virginia.

Oklahoma

★ 6672 ★ Arthritis Foundation
Eastern Oklahoma Chapter
4520 S Harvard, Ste. 100
Tulsa, OK 74135-2932
Phone: (918)743-4526 **Free:** 800-400-4526
Fax: (918)743-6910
Email: info.eok@arthritis.org
Website: http://www.arthritis.org/communities/chapters/Chapter.asp?Chapid=17
Hope Sutherland, President

★ 6673 ★ Arthritis Foundation
Oklahoma Chapter
500 N Broadway, Ste. 200
Oklahoma City, OK 73102
Phone: (405)236-3399 **Free:** 800-627-5486
Fax: (405)236-3393
Email: info.ok@arthritis.org
Website: http://www.arthritis.org/communities/chapters/Chapter.asp?Chapid=44
Suzi White, President

Oregon

★ 6674 ★ Arthritis Foundation
Oregon Chapter
4412 SW Barbur Blvd., Ste. 220
Portland, OR 97239-4004
Phone: (503)222-7246 **Free:** 800-283-3004
Fax: (503)222-5542
Email: info.or@arthritis.org
Website: http://www.arthritis.org/communities/chapters/Chapter.asp?Chapid=45

Pennsylvania

★ 6675 ★ Arthritis Foundation
Central Pennsylvania Chapter
17 S 19th St.
PO Box 668
Camp Hill, PA 17011
Phone: (717)763-0900 **Free:** 800-776-0746
Fax: (717)763-0903
Email: info.cpa@arthritis.org
Website: http://www.arthritis.org/communities/chapters/Chapter.asp?Chapid=14

★ 6676 ★ Arthritis Foundation
Eastern Pennsylvania Chapter
219 N Broad St., 2nd Fl.
Philadelphia, PA 19107
Phone: (215)564-9800 **Free:** 800-355-9040
Fax: (215)564-6599
Email: info.epa@arthritis.org
Website: http://www.arthritis.org/communities/chapters/Chapter.asp?Chapid=18
Lyn Boocock-Taylor, President

★ 6677 ★ Arthritis Foundation
Western Pennsylvania Chapter
Warner Center, 5th Fl.
332 5th Ave.
Pittsburgh, PA 15222
Phone: (412)566-1645 **Free:** 800-522-9900
Fax: (412)391-1677
Email: info.wpa@arthritis.org
Website: http://www.arthritis.org/communities/chapters/Chapter.asp?Chapid=60
Jerry Ellis, President

Rhode Island

★ 6678 ★ Arthritis Foundation
Southern New England Chapter
Rhode Island Office
Airport Office Park
2348 Post Rd., Ste. 104
Warwick, RI 02886
Phone: (401)739-3773 **Fax:** (401)739-8990
Email: info.sne.rio@arthritis.org
Website: http://www.arthritis.org

South Carolina

★ 6679 ★ Arthritis Foundation
Carolinas Chapter
Coastal Region Office
1156 Bowman Rd., Ste. 225
Mount Pleasant, SC 29464
Phone: (843)416-1174 **Free:** 800-883-8806
Fax: (843)416-1173
Email: clebaron@arthritis.org
Website: http://www.arthritis.org

Tennessee

★ 6680 ★ Arthritis Foundation
Tennessee Chapter
1 Vantage Way, Ste. D-220
Nashville, TN 37228
Phone: (615)254-6795 **Free:** 800-454-4662
Fax: (615)254-8316
Email: info.tn@arthritis.org
Website: http://www.arthritis.org/communities/chapters/Chapter.asp?Chapid=53
Charles P. Taylor, President

Texas

★ 6681 ★ Arthritis Foundation
North Texas Chapter
2824 Swiss Ave.
Dallas, TX 75204
Phone: (214)826-4361 **Free:** 800-442-6653
Fax: (214)824-5842
Email: info.ntx@arthritis.org
Website: http://www.arthritis.org/communities/chapters/Chapter.asp?Chapid=40

★ 6682 ★ Arthritis Foundation
Northwest Texas Chapter
3001 W 5th St.
Fort Worth, TX 76107
Phone: (817)820-0635 **Free:** 800-283-7733
Fax: (817)820-0642
Email: info.nwtx@arthritis.org
Website: http://www.arthritis.org/communities/chapters/Chapter.asp?Chapid=42
Debra Phelan, President

★ 6683 ★ Arthritis Foundation
South Texas Chapter
3701 Kirby Dr., Ste. 1230
Houston, TX 77098
Phone: (713)529-0800 **Free:** 800-364-8000
Fax: (713)529-6622
Email: info.stx@arthritis.org
Website: http://www.arthritis.org/communities/chapters/Chapter.asp?Chapid=52

Utah

★ 6684 ★ Arthritis Foundation
Utah/Idaho Chapter
448 East 400 South, Ste. 103
Salt Lake City, UT 84111
Phone: (801)536-0990 **Free:** 800-444-4993
Fax: (801)536-0991
Email: info.utid@arthritis.org
Website: http://www.arthritis.org/communities/chapters/Chapter.asp?Chapid=62
Lisa B. Fall, President

Vermont

★ 6685 ★ Arthritis Foundation
Northern New England Chapter
257 S Union St.
Burlington, VT 05401
Phone: (802)864-4988 **Free:** 800-639-2113
Fax: (802)864-5339
Email: info.nne@arthritis.org
Website: http://www.arthritis.org/communities/chapters/Chapter.asp?Chapid=39
Remarks: Serves Maine, New Hampshire, and Vermont.

Virginia

★ 6686 ★ Arthritis Foundation
Virginia Chapter
3805 Cutshaw Ave., Ste. 200
Richmond, VA 23230
Phone: (804)359-1700 **Free:** 800-456-4687
Fax: (804)359-4900
Email: info.va@arthritis.org
Website: http://www.arthritis.org/communities/chapters/Chapter.asp?Chapid=55
C. Annie Magnant, President

Washington

★ 6687 ★ Arthritis Foundation
Washington/Alaska Chapter
3876 Bridge Way N, Ste. 300
Seattle, WA 98103
Phone: (206)547-2707 **Free:** 800-542-0295
Fax: (206)547-2805
Email: info.wa@arthritis.org
Website: http://www.arthritis.org/communities/chapters/Chapter.asp?Chapid=56
Karen Smith, President

Wisconsin

★ 6688 ★ Arthritis Foundation
Wisconsin Chapter
8556 W National Ave.
West Allis, WI 53227
Phone: (414)321-3933 **Free:** 800-242-9945
Fax: (414)321-0365
Email: info.wi@arthritis.org
Website: http://www.arthritis.org/communities/chapters/Chapter.asp?Chapid=57

Asthma & Allergies

State chapters of the Asthma and Allergy Foundation of America are listed below. The national office is located at 1233 Twentieth St. NW, Ste. 402, Washington, DC 20036. Additional information can be obtained by calling the national office at (800) 7-ASTHMA or by consulting their web site at http://www.aafa.org.

Alaska

★ 6689 ★ Asthma and Allergy Foundation of America
Alaska Chapter
PO Box 201927
Anchorage, AK 99520-1927
Phone: (907)696-4810
Email: aafaalaska@gci.net
Suzi Jackson, Exec Director

California

★ 6690 ★ Asthma and Allergy Foundation of America
Northern California Chapter
2269 Chestnut St., Ste. 481
San Francisco, CA 94123
Phone: (415)339-8880 **Fax:** (415)339-8881
Email: aafanorcal@yahoo.com
Ben Loewy, Exec Director

★ 6691 ★ Asthma and Allergy Foundation of America
Southern California Chapter
5900 Wilshire Blvd., Ste. 2330
Los Angeles, CA 90036
Phone: (323)937-7859 **Free:** 800-624-0044
Fax: (323)937-7815
Email: aafasocal@aol.com
Website: http://www.aafasocal.com
Francene Lifson, Exec Director

Florida

★ 6692 ★ Asthma and Allergy Foundation of America
Florida Chapter
11700 N 58th St., Ste. J
Tampa, FL 33617
Phone: (813)983-0244 **Fax:** (813)983-9057
Email: johnlittle@aafaflorida.org
Website: http://www.aafaflorida.org

Maryland

★ 6693 ★ Asthma and Allergy Foundation of America
Maryland-Greater Washington, D.C., Chapter
1777 Reisterstown Rd., Ste. 370
Baltimore, MD 21208
Phone: (410)653-2880 **Fax:** (410)653-9611
Email: info@aafa-md.org
Website: http://www.aafa-md.org
Linda R. Boyer, Exec Director

Massachusetts

★ 6694 ★ Asthma and Allergy Foundation of America
New England Chapter
220 Boylston St.
Chestnut Hill, MA 02467
Phone: (617)965-7771 **Fax:** (617)965-8886
Email: aafane@aol.com
Patricia Goldman, Exec Director

Michigan

★ 6695 ★ Asthma and Allergy Foundation of America
Michigan State Chapter
17520 W 12 Mile Rd., Ste. 102
Southfield, MI 48076-1943
Phone: (248)557-8050 **Free:** 888-444-0333
Fax: (248)557-8768
Email: aafamich@aol.com
Karen Katz, Exec Director

Missouri

★ 6696 ★ Asthma and Allergy Foundation of America
Greater Kansas City Chapter
9140 Ward Parkway, Ste. 120
Kansas City, MO 64114
Phone: (816)333-6608 **Free:** 888-542-8252
Fax: (816)333-6608
Email: infor@aafakc.org
Website: http://www.aafakc.org
Noel Albert, Exec Director

★ 6697 ★ Asthma and Allergy Foundation of America
Saint Louis Chapter
1500 S Big Bend, Ste. 1
Saint Louis, MO 63117
Phone: (314)645-2422 **Fax:** (314)645-2022
Email: aafa@mindspring.com
Website: http://postwebsites.com/stlouis/aafa
Patricia Williams, Exec Director

New Jersey

★ 6698 ★ Asthma and Allergy Foundation of America
Southeastern Pennsylvania Chapter
PO Box 115
32 Caspertown St.
Gibbstown, NJ 08027
Phone: (856)224-9547 **Fax:** (856)224-5893
Email: aafasepa@prodigy.net
Debi Maines, Exec Director

Oregon

★ 6699 ★ Asthma and Allergy Foundation of America
Oregon Chapter
14530 SW 144th Ave.
Tigard, OR 97224-1445
Phone: (503)579-8375
Email: hensches@teleport.com
Sandra L. Henschel, Exec Director

Texas

★ 6700 ★ Asthma and Allergy Foundation of America
North Texas Chapter
155 Southwood
Burleson, TX 76028
Phone: (817)483-8131 **Free:** 888-932-2232
Email: aafantx@hotmail.com
Website: http://www.aafa-ntx.org
Joan Hart, Exec Director

Washington

★ 6701 ★ Asthma and Allergy Foundation of America
Washington State Chapter
108 S Jackson St., Ste. 205
Seattle, WA 98104
Phone: (206)368-2866 **Free:** 800-778-2232
Fax: (206)368-2941
Email: aafawa@aafawa.org
Website: http://www.aafawa.org
Penny Nelson, Exec Director
Remarks: Based in Seattle. Serves the state of Washington.

Autism

State chapters of the Autism Society of America are listed below. The national office is located at 7910 Woodmont Ave., Ste. 300, Bethesda, MD 20814-3015. Additional information can be obtained by calling the national office at (800) 3-AUTISM, or by consulting their web site at http://www.autism-society.org/.

Alabama

★ 6702 ★ Autism Society of Alabama
771 2nd St.
Helena, AL 35080
Phone: (205)621-0548 **Free:** 877-428-8476
Fax: (205)681-1514
Email: director@autism-alabama.org
Website: http://www.autism-alabama.org

Arizona

★ 6703 ★ Autism Society of America Greater Phoenix Chapter
PO Box 10543
Phoenix, AZ 85064-0543
Phone: (480)940-1093
Website: http://aztec.asu.edu/phxautism/index.html

California

★ 6704 ★ Autism Society of America Inland Empire Chapter
PO Box 8932
Moreno Valley, CA 92552
Phone: (909)242-4413 **Free:** 800-328-8476
Fax: (909)242-4413
Email: dar4mar@aol.com
Website: http://www.inlandempireasa.org
Debbie Rosenbrook, President

★ 6705 ★ Autism Society of America San Diego County Chapter
PO Box 420908
San Diego, CA 92124
Phone: (619)298-1981 **Fax:** (619)278-0885
Email: info@sd-autism.org
Website: http://www.sd-autism.org
G. Fletcher, President

★ 6706 ★ Autism Society of Los Angeles United Autism Alliance
1612 W Olive Ave., Ste. 201
Burbank, CA 91506
Phone: (818)953-3855 **Fax:** (818)953-3850
Email: info@unitedautismalliance.org
Website: http://www.unitedautismalliance.org

Connecticut

★ 6707 ★ Autism Society of Connecticut
125 Harrington St.
Meriden, CT 06451
Phone: (203)235-7629
Email: ideasb@cshore.com
Website: http://www.autismsocietyofct.org

Delaware

★ 6708 ★ Autism Society of Delaware
PO Box 7336
Wilmington, DE 19803-0336
Phone: (302)777-7273
Email: DelAutism@aol.com
Website: http://www.wserv.com/delautism/
Artie Kempner, President

Florida

★ 6709 ★ Manasota Autism Society
PO Box 18934
Sarasota, FL 34276-1934
Phone: (941)328-0121 **Fax:** (941)328-0121
Email: mas@saraweb.com
Website: http://www.saraweb.com/MAS/

Kentucky

★ 6710 ★ Autism Society of Western Kentucky
PO Box 1647
Henderson, KY 42419-1647
Phone: (270)826-0510
Email: tawanda@dynasty.net
Website: http://www.kentucky-autism.org
Nancy Boyett, Contact

Michigan

★ 6711 ★ Autism Society of Michigan
6035 Executive Dr., Ste. 109
Lansing, MI 48911
Phone: (517)882-2800 **Free:** 800-223-6722
Fax: (517)882-2816
Email: miautism@aol.com
Website: http://www.autism-mi.org/
Chris Swartwout, President

Minnesota

★ 6712 ★ Twin Cities Autism Society
970 Raymond Ave., Ste. 101
Saint Paul, MN 55114-1146
Phone: (651)647-1083 **Fax:** (651)642-1230
Email: mpowell@goldengate.net
Website: http://www.tcas.org/

North Carolina

★ 6713 ★ Autism Society of North Carolina, Inc.
505 Oberlin Rd., Ste. 230
Raleigh, NC 27605-1345
Phone: (919)743-0204 **Free:** 800-442-2762
Fax: (919)743-0208
Email: jlawson@autismsociety-nc.org
Website: http://www.autismsociety-nc.org/

Ohio

★ 6714 ★ Autism Society of Greater Cincinnati
CCDD Bldg. E
3333 Burnet Ave., Rm. 4-32
Cincinnati, OH 45229
Phone: (513)636-7203 **Fax:** (513)636-2224
Email: asgc@fuse.net
Website: http://www.autismcincy.org/

Oregon

★ 6715 ★ Autism Society of Oregon
PO Box 13884
Salem, OR 97309
Phone: (503)234-5729 **Free:** 888-AUTISM-1
Fax: (503)363-9110
Email: aso@teleport.com
Website: http://www.autismoregon.com

Tennessee

★ 6716 ★ Autism Society of Middle Tennessee
480 Craighead St., Ste. 200
Nashville, TN 37204
Phone: (615)385-2077 **Fax:** (615)383-1176
Email: asmt@bellsouth.net
Website: http://www.autismmidtenn.org

Washington

★ 6717 ★ Autism Society of Washington
PO Box 310
East Olympia, WA 98540
Phone: (360)943-2205 **Fax:** (360)330-2240
Email: autismsociety@hotmail.com
Website: http://www.autismsocietyofwa.org
Kitsie Morris, Exec Director

Wisconsin

★ 6718 ★ Autism Society of Wisconsin
103 W College Ave., Ste. 601
Appleton, WI 54911-5744
Phone: (920)993-0279 **Free:** 888-4-AUTISM
Fax: (920)993-0279
Email: asw@asw4autism.org
Website: http://www.asw4autism.org/

Blind

The following are state affiliates of Prevent Blindness America, 500 E Remington Rd., Schaumburg, IL 60173, (800)331-2020, http://www.preventblindness.org/. For states that do not have affiliates listed, contact the national organization for help with inquiries.

Arizona

★ 6719 ★ Prevent Blindness America Arizona Division
240 W Osborn Rd., Ste. 232
Phoenix, AZ 85015
Phone: (602)636-1112
Email: pbaarizona1@prodigy.net

★ 6720 ★ Prevent Blindness America Arizona Division
240 W Osborn Rd., Ste. 232
Phoenix, AZ 85015
Phone: (602)636-1112
Email: info@pbaaz.org
Website: http://www.prevent-blindness.org/Phoenix/index.html

California

★ 6721 ★ Prevent Blindness America Northern California Affiliate
4200 California St., Ste. 101
San Francisco, CA 94118
Phone: (415)387-0934 **Free:** 800-338-3041
Email: PBNoCa@aol.com
Website: http://www.prevent-blindness.org/nca/

Connecticut

★ 6722 ★ Prevent Blindness America Connecticut Affiliate
984 Southford Rd.
Middletown, CT 06457
Phone: (860)347-2020 **Free:** 800-850-2020
Email: info@preventblindnessct.org
Website: http://www.prevent-blindness.org/ct/index.html

Florida

★ 6723 ★ Prevent Blindness America Florida Affiliate
3825 Henderson Blvd., Ste. 402
Tampa, FL 33629
Phone: (813)874-2020
Email: jtobin@preventblindnessfl.org
Website: http://www.prevent-blindness.org/florida

Georgia

★ 6724 ★ Prevent Blindness America
Georgia Affiliate
455 E Paces Ferry Rd., Ste. 222
Atlanta, GA 30305
Phone: (404)266-0071
Email: pbgeorgia@aol.com
Website: http://www.prevent-blindness.org/georgia

Illinois

★ 6725 ★ Prevent Blindness America
Illinois Division
39 S LaSalle St., Ste. 1224
Chicago, IL 60603
Phone: (312)346-9110 **Fax:** (312)346-9126
Email: jstolzenbach@pba-illinois.org

Indiana

★ 6726 ★ Prevent Blindness America
Indiana Affiliate
603 E Washington St., 5th Fl.
Indianapolis, IN 46204
Phone: (317)955-9580 **Free:** 800-232-2551
Email: jwagner@pbeye.org
Website: http://www.pbeye.org

Iowa

★ 6727 ★ Prevent Blindness America
Iowa Affiliate
1111 9th St., Ste. 250
Des Moines, IA 50314
Phone: (515)244-4341
Email: pbiowa@netins.net
Website: http://www.prevent-blindness.org/iowa

Kentucky

★ 6728 ★ Prevent Blindness America
Kentucky Division
117 Coral Ave.
Louisville, KY 40206
Phone: (502)895-8899 **Free:** 800-828-1179
Email: lrepperson@aol.com

Massachusetts

★ 6729 ★ Prevent Blindness America
Massachusetts Affiliate
100 Cummings Ctr., Ste. 330C
Beverly, MA 01915
Phone: (978)524-9500
Email: preventblind@aol.com
Website: http://www.prevent-blindness.org/MA/

Nebraska

★ 6730 ★ Prevent Blindness America
Nebraska Affiliate
7101 Newport Ave., Ste. 308
Omaha, NE 68152-2172
Phone: (402)572-3520 **Fax:** (402)572-3522
Email: preventblindnessnebraska@mb3.net
Website: http://www.prevent-blindness.org/ne/

New Jersey

★ 6731 ★ Prevent Blindness America
New Jersey Affiliate
2525 Rte. 130 S, Bldg. D
Cranbury, NJ 08512
Phone: (609)409-0770
Email: pblindness@aol.com
Website: http://www.preventblindnessnj.org

New York

★ 6732 ★ Fight For Sight, Inc.
381 Park Ave. S, Ste. 809
New York, NY 10016
Phone: (212)679-6060
Email: info@fightforsight.com
Website: http://www.fightforsight.com

★ 6733 ★ Prevent Blindness America
New York Division
375 Hudson St., 12th Fl.
New York, NY 10014-3660
Phone: (212)463-3682
Email: lbrenig@preventblindness.org
Website: http://www.preventblindness.org

North Carolina

★ 6734 ★ Prevent Blindness America
North Carolina Affiliate
3801 Lake Boone Trail, Ste. 410
Raleigh, NC 27607
Phone: (919)571-1014
Email: dmanley@pbnc.org
Website: http://www.prevent-blindness.org/nc/

Ohio

★ 6735 ★ Prevent Blindness America
Ohio Affiliate
1500 W 3rd Ave., Ste. 200
Columbus, OH 43212-2874
Phone: (614)464-2020
Email: preventblindnessohio@compuserve.com
Website: http://www.prevent-blindness.org/Ohio/

Oklahoma

★ 6736 ★ Prevent Blindness America
Oklahoma Affiliate
6 NE 63rd St., Ste. 150
Oklahoma City, OK 73105
Phone: (405)848-7123
Email: shan_pbo@swbell.net
Website: http://www.preventblindnessok.org

Tennessee

★ 6737 ★ Prevent Blindness America
Tennessee Affiliate
95 White Bridge Rd., Ste. 513
Nashville, TN 37205
Phone: (615)352-0450
Email: foryereyes@aol.com
Website: http://www.prevent-blindness.org/TN/

Texas

★ 6738 ★ Prevent Blindness America
Texas Affiliate
3211 W Dallas
Houston, TX 77019
Phone: (713)526-2559 **Free:** 888-987-4448
Email: pbtxhouston@compuserve.com
Website: http://www.prevent-blindness.org/TX/

Utah

★ 6739 ★ Prevent Blindness America
Utah Affiliate
661 South 200 East
Salt Lake City, UT 84111
Phone: (801)524-2020 **Free:** 800-675-5665
Email: preventblindness@uswest.net
Website: www.prevent-blindness.org/Utah

Virginia

★ 6740 ★ Prevent Blindness America
Virginia Affiliate
9840 Midlothian Turnpike, Ste. R
Richmond, VA 23235
Phone: (804)330-3195
Email: tim@pbv.org
Website: http://www.pbv.org

West Virginia

★ 6741 ★ Prevent Blindness America
West Virginia Division
729 9th Ave., No. 149
Huntington, WV 25701-2718
Phone: (304)529-1966 **Fax:** (304)525-4443
Email: prevent.blindness@verizon.net

Wisconsin

★ 6742 ★ Prevent Blindness America
Wisconsin Affiliate
759 N Milwaukee St.
Milwaukee, WI 53202
Phone: (414)765-0505
Email: info@preventblindnesswisconsin.org
Website: www.prevent-blindness.org/wi/

Cancer

Divisions of the American Cancer Society are listed below. The national office is located at 1599 Clifton Rd. NE, Atlanta, GA 30329, (800)ACS-2345, http://www.cancer.org/.

Alabama

★ 6743 ★ American Cancer Society
Baldwin County Office
26148 Capital Dr., Ste. F
Daphne, AL 36526
Phone: (251)621-7996 **Fax:** (251)447-0271

★ 6744 ★ American Cancer Society
Birmingham Branch
1100 Ireland Way, Ste. 201
Birmingham, AL 35205
Phone: (205)879-2242 **Fax:** (205)930-8895
Website: http://www2.cancer.org/state/al/index.html

★ 6745 ★ American Cancer Society
Dothan Office
2346 W Main St., Ste. 3
Dothan, AL 36303
Phone: (334)793-1012 **Fax:** (334)792-7278

★ 6746 ★ American Cancer Society
Florence Office
130 S Poplar St.
Florence, AL 35630
Phone: (256)767-0823 **Fax:** (256)767-0894

★ 6747 ★ American Cancer Society
Huntsville Office
2515-B Memorial Pkwy. SW
Huntsville, AL 35801
Phone: (256)536-1855 **Fax:** (256)534-0843

★ 6748 ★ American Cancer Society
Mobile Office
900 Western America Cir., Ste. 101
Mobile, AL 36609
Phone: (251)344-9856 **Fax:** (251)344-9882

★ 6749 ★ American Cancer Society
Montgomery Office
3054-C McGehee Rd.
Montgomery, AL 36111
Phone: (334)288-3432 **Fax:** (334)612-8181

★ 6750 ★ American Cancer Society
Tuscaloosa Office
2132 McFarland Blvd. E, Ste. C
Tuscaloosa, AL 35404
Phone: (205)758-0700 **Fax:** (205)758-0116

Alaska

★ 6751 ★ American Cancer Society
Anchorage Branch
1057 W Fireweed Ln., Ste. 204
Anchorage, AK 99503
Phone: (907)277-8696 **Free:** 800-478-9355
Fax: (907)263-2073
Email: cindy.emery@cancer.org
Website: http://www.cancer.org

Arizona

★ 6752 ★ American Cancer Society
Central Arizona Division
2929 E Thomas Rd.
Phoenix, AZ 85016-8034
Phone: (602)553-7129 **Fax:** (602)381-3096
Website: http://www2.cancer.org/state/az/index.html

★ 6753 ★ American Cancer Society
Northern Arizona Region
2724 E Lakin, Ste. 9
Flagstaff, AZ 86004
Phone: (928)526-3800 **Fax:** (928)526-5870

★ 6754 ★ American Cancer Society
Northwest Valley Office
12211 W Bell Rd., No. 102
Surprise, AZ 85374
Phone: (623)583-2828 **Fax:** (623)583-1163

★ 6755 ★ American Cancer Society
Rural Communities Region
2929 E Thomas Rd.
Phoenix, AZ 85016
Phone: (602)224-0524 **Fax:** (602)381-3096
Remarks: Serves Arizona, Nevada, and New Mexico.

★ 6756 ★ American Cancer Society
Southeastern Arizona Region
1636 N Swan, Ste. 151
Tucson, AZ 85712
Phone: (520)321-7989 **Fax:** (520)321-7988

★ 6757 ★ American Cancer Society
Western Yavapai and Mingus Verde Office
917 E Gurley St., Ste. 1B
Prescott, AZ 86301
Phone: (928)541-9270

Arkansas

★ 6758 ★ American Cancer Society
Arkansas Division
901 N University Ave.
Little Rock, AR 72207
Phone: (501)664-3480 **Fax:** (501)666-0068
Website: http://www2.cancer.org/state/ar/index.html

California

★ 6759 ★ American Cancer Society
Amador County Office
1765 Challenge Way, Ste. 115
Sacramento, CA 95815
Phone: (916)446-7933 **Fax:** (916)325-2351

★ 6760 ★ American Cancer Society
Antelope Valley-Eastern Sierra Unit
1043 W Ave. 4, Ste. B
Palmdale, CA 93551
Phone: (661)945-7585 **Fax:** (661)945-9039

★ 6761 ★ American Cancer Society
Auburn Unit
333 Sunrise Ave., Ste. 344
Roseville, CA 95661
Phone: (916)783-4181 **Fax:** (916)783-4175

★ 6762 ★ American Cancer Society
Bakersfield Unit
1523 California Ave.
Bakersfield, CA 93304
Phone: (661)327-2424 **Fax:** (661)327-2921

★ 6763 ★ American Cancer Society
Bishop Unit
c/o Antelope Valley-Eastern Sierra Unit
1043 W Ave. 4, Ste. B
Palmdale, CA 93551
Phone: (661)945-7585 **Fax:** (661)945-9039

★ 6764 ★ American Cancer Society
Border Regional Office
2655 Camino del Rio N, Ste. 100
San Diego, CA 92108
Phone: (619)299-4200 **Free:** 800-ACS-2345
Fax: (619)296-0928

★ 6765 ★ American Cancer Society
Brawley Regional Unit
Pioneers Memorial Hospital
207 W Legion Rd.
Brawley, CA 92227
Phone: (760)344-4195 **Fax:** (760)352-0316

★ 6766 ★ American Cancer Society
Central Alameda County Unit
1900 Mowry Ave., Ste. 405
Fremont, CA 94538
Phone: (510)742-8346 **Fax:** (510)742-8417

★ 6767 ★ American Cancer Society
Central Coast Counties Unit
1184 Monroe St., Stes. 1 & 2
Salinas, CA 93906
Phone: (831)442-2992 **Fax:** (831)442-2710

★ 6768 ★ American Cancer Society
Central Contra Costa County Unit
1885 Oak Park Blvd.
Pleasant Hill, CA
Phone: (925)934-7640 **Fax:** (925)934-5372

★ 6769 ★ American Cancer Society
Central Los Angeles Unit
3333 Wilshire Blvd., Ste. 900
Los Angeles, CA 90010
Phone: (213)386-6102 **Fax:** (213)480-0806

★ 6770 ★ American Cancer Society
Central Valley Regional Office
2222 W Shaw Ave., Ste. 201
Fresno, CA 93711
Phone: (559)451-0722 **Fax:** (559)451-0744
Email: mary.johnson@cancer.org
Website: http://www.cancer.org

★ 6771 ★ American Cancer Society
Central Ventura County Unit
250 W Citrus Grove, Ste. 200
Oxnard, CA 93030
Phone: (805)983-8864 **Fax:** (805)983-3751

★ 6772 ★ American Cancer Society
Corona/Norco Unit
1240 Palmyrita Ave., Ste. A
Riverside, CA 92507
Phone: (909)683-6415 **Fax:** (909)682-6804

★ 6773 ★ American Cancer Society
Desert Palms Unit
74-140 El Paseo, Ste.
Palm Desert, CA 92260
Phone: (760)568-2691 **Fax:** (760)341-8783

★ 6774 ★ American Cancer Society
Desert Sierra Regional Office
1240 Palmyrita Ave., Unit A
Riverside, CA 92507
Phone: (909)320-7142 **Free:** 800-ACS-2345
Fax: (909)682-6804

★ 6775 ★ American Cancer Society
Downey/Rio Hondo Unit
9901 Paramount Blvd., Ste. 245
Downey, CA 90240
Phone: (562)776-0201 **Fax:** (562)776-0373

★ 6776 ★ American Cancer Society
East Bay Regional Office
1700 Webster St.
Oakland, CA 94612
Phone: (510)452-5229 **Free:** 800-ACS-2345
Fax: (510)763-8826

★ 6777 ★ American Cancer Society
East Contra Costa County Unit
1885 Oak Park Blvd.
Pleasant Hill, CA 94523
Phone: (925)934-7640 **Fax:** (925)934-5372

★ 6778 ★ American Cancer Society
East Inland Valley Unit
8560 Vineyard Ave., Ste. 108
Rancho Cucamonga, CA 91730
Phone: (909)949-6115 **Fax:** (909)949-6813

★ 6779 ★ American Cancer Society
East San Gabriel Valley Unit
339 E Rowland St.
Covina, CA 91723
Phone: (626)966-9994 **Fax:** (626)966-8664

★ 6780 ★ American Cancer Society
El Dorado/Alpine Unit
333 Sunrise Ave., Ste. 344
Roseville, CA 95661
Phone: (916)783-4181 **Fax:** (916)783-4175

★ 6781 ★ American Cancer Society
Elk Grove/Laguna Unit
1765 Challenge Way, Ste. 115
Sacramento, CA 95815
Phone: (916)446-7933 **Fax:** (916)325-2351

★ 6782 ★ American Cancer Society
Fontana Unit
8560 Vineyard Ave., Ste. 108
Rancho Cucamonga, CA 91730
Phone: (909)949-6115 **Fax:** (909)949-6813

★ 6783 ★ American Cancer Society
Fresno County Unit
2222 W Shaw Ave., Ste. 201
Fresno, CA 93711
Phone: (559)451-0722 **Fax:** (559)451-0744

★ 6784 ★ American Cancer Society
Gold Coast Regional Office
426 E Barcellus, Ste. 304
Santa Maria, CA 93454
Phone: (805)925-8190 **Fax:** (805)925-1424

★ 6785 ★ American Cancer Society
Greater Conejo Valley Unit
50 W Hillcrest Dr., Ste. 208
Thousand Oaks, CA 91360
Phone: (805)497-0114 **Fax:** (805)497-9800

★ 6786 ★ American Cancer Society
Greater North Unit
Alton Deere Plaza
1940 E Deere Ave., Ste. 100
Santa Ana, CA 92705
Phone: (949)261-9446 **Fax:** (949)261-9419

★ 6787 ★ American Cancer Society
Greater Petaluma Area
400 N McDowell Blvd.
Petaluma, CA 94954
Phone: (707)766-8066 **Fax:** (707)545-3179

★ 6788 ★ American Cancer Society
Greater San Bernardino Area
1240 Palmyrita Ave., Ste. A
Riverside, CA 92507
Phone: (909)683-6415 **Fax:** (909)682-6804

★ 6789 ★ American Cancer Society
Greater Ventura Unit
3737 Telegraph Rd., Ste. D
Ventura, CA 93003
Phone: (805)644-6656 **Fax:** (805)644-6626

★ 6790 ★ American Cancer Society
High Desert Unit
14815 7th St.
Victorville, CA 92392
Phone: (760)245-2443

★ 6791 ★ American Cancer Society
Humboldt-Del Norte Counties Unit
2942 "F" St.
Eureka, CA 95501
Phone: (707)442-1436 **Fax:** (707)442-6427

★ 6792 ★ American Cancer Society
Imperial Central Unit
400 S 8th St.
El Centro, CA 92243
Phone: (760)352-6656 **Fax:** (760)352-0316

★ 6793 ★ American Cancer Society
Indian Wells Valley Unit
129 E Ridgecrest Blvd.
Ridgecrest, CA 93556
Phone: (760)371-1312 **Fax:** (760)371-2333

★ 6794 ★ American Cancer Society
Inland Mendocino Unit
497 Leslie St.
Ukiah, CA 95482
Phone: (707)462-7642 **Fax:** (707)462-0281

★ 6795 ★ American Cancer Society
Irvine Unit
Alton Deere Plaza
1940 E Deere Ave., Ste. 100
Santa Ana, CA 92705
Phone: (949)261-9446 **Fax:** (949)261-9419

★ 6796 ★ American Cancer Society
Kings County Unit
823 W Lacey Blvd.
Hanford, CA
Phone: (559)584-6691 **Fax:** (559)584-2815

★ 6797 ★ American Cancer Society
Lakeport Unit
1031 Jefferson St.
Napa, CA 94559
Phone: (707)255-5911 **Fax:** (707)255-3823

★ 6798 ★ American Cancer Society
Lodi Unit
207 E Alpine Ave.
Stockton, CA 95204
Phone: (209)941-2676 **Fax:** (209)941-2824

★ 6799 ★ American Cancer Society
Lompoc Valley Unit
604 E Ocean Ave.
Lompoc, CA 93436
Phone: (805)736-2610 **Fax:** (805)736-9413

★ 6800 ★ American Cancer Society
Long Beach-Harbor-Southeast Unit
936 Pine Ave.
Long Beach, CA 90813
Phone: (562)437-0791 **Fax:** (562)495-1782

★ 6801 ★ American Cancer Society
Los Angeles Coastal Cities, South Bay Branch
514 N Prospect Ave., Ste. 150
Redondo Beach, CA 90277
Phone: (310)937-2605 **Fax:** (310)937-2717

★ 6802 ★ American Cancer Society
Los Angeles Coastal Cities Unit
5731 W Slauson Ave., Ste. 200
Culver City, CA 90230
Phone: (310)348-0356 **Fax:** (310)645-1428

★ 6803 ★ American Cancer Society
Los Angeles Region
3333 Wilshire Blvd., Ste. 900
Los Angeles, CA 90010
Phone: (213)386-7660 **Fax:** (213)380-6286

★ 6804 ★ American Cancer Society
Los Banos Unit
PO Box 462
Los Banos, CA 93635
Phone: (209)827-4340 **Fax:** (209)722-6628

★ 6805 ★ American Cancer Society
Madera County Unit
425 N Gateway, Ste. C
Madera, CA 93637
Phone: (559)673-9425 **Fax:** (559)673-9432

★ 6806 ★ American Cancer Society
Marin County Unit
25 Bellam Blvd., Ste. 150
San Rafael, CA 94901
Phone: (415)454-8464 **Fax:** (415)456-1477

★ 6807 ★ American Cancer Society
Mendocino Coast Area
497 Leslie St.
Ukiah, CA 95482
Phone: (707)462-7642 **Fax:** (707)462-0281

★ 6808 ★ American Cancer Society
Merced/Mariposa County Unit
301 W 18th St., Ste. 101
Merced, CA 95340
Phone: (209)722-3341 **Fax:** (209)722-6628

★ 6809 ★ American Cancer Society
Mission Oaks Unit
274 Heather Ct.
Templeton, CA 93465
Phone: (805)238-9657 **Fax:** (805)434-3947

★ 6810 ★ American Cancer Society
Modoc County Unit
3290 Bechelli Ln.
Redding, CA 96002
Phone: (530)222-1058 **Fax:** (530)222-1409

★ 6811 ★ American Cancer Society
Mojave Valley Unit
1240 Palmyrita Ave., Ste. A
Riverside, CA 92507
Phone: (909)683-6415 **Fax:** (909)682-6804

★ 6812 ★ American Cancer Society
Morongo Basin Unit
56351 Twentynine Palms, Ste. B
Yucca Valley, CA 92284
Phone: (760)365-9828 **Fax:** (760)365-8317

★ 6813 ★ American Cancer Society
Mountain Valley Unit
2889 Cohasset Rd., Ste. 6
Chico, CA 95973
Phone: (530)342-4567 **Fax:** (530)345-5871

★ 6814 ★ American Cancer Society
Multi-Cities Unit
1240 Palmyrita Ave., Ste. A
Riverside, CA 92507
Phone: (909)683-6415 **Fax:** (909)682-6804

★ 6815 ★ American Cancer Society
Napa County Unit
1031 Jefferson St.
Napa, CA 94559
Phone: (707)255-5911 **Fax:** (707)255-3823

★ 6816 ★ American Cancer Society
Nevada City/Grass Valley Unit
618 5th St.
Marysville, CA 95901
Phone: (530)741-1366 **Fax:** (530)741-1383

★ 6817 ★ American Cancer Society
Newport-Mesa Unit
Alton Deere Plaza
1940 E Deere Ave., Ste. 100
Santa Ana, CA 92705
Phone: (949)261-9446 **Fax:** (949)261-9419

★ 6818 ★ American Cancer Society
North Coast Border Unit
1301 Northcrest Dr.
Crescent City, CA
Phone: (707)464-8277 **Fax:** (707)465-6710

★ 6819 ★ American Cancer Society
North State Unit
3290 Bechelli Ln.
Redding, CA 96002
Phone: (530)222-1058 **Fax:** (530)222-1409

★ 6820 ★ American Cancer Society
North Valley Region
1765 Challenge Way, Ste. 115
Sacramento, CA 95815
Phone: (916)446-7933 **Fax:** (916)325-4955

★ 6821 ★ American Cancer Society
Northern California Chinese Unit
39277 Liberty St., Ste. D-14
Fremont, CA 94538
Phone: (510)797-0600 **Fax:** (510)797-0698

★ 6822 ★ American Cancer Society
Orange County Regional Office
Alton Deere Plaza
1940 E Deere Ave., Ste. 100
Santa Ana, CA 92705
Phone: (949)261-9446 **Free:** 800-ACS-2345
Fax: (949)261-9419

★ 6823 ★ American Cancer Society
Palo Verde Valley Unit
74-140 El Paseo, Ste. 1
Palm Desert, CA 92260
Phone: (760)568-2691 **Fax:** (760)341-8783

★ 6824 ★ American Cancer Society
Perris Valley Unit
1240 Palmyrita Ave., Ste. A
Riverside, CA 92507
Phone: (909)683-6415 **Fax:** (909)682-6804

★ 6825 ★ American Cancer Society
Redlands/Yucaipa Unit
1240 Palmyrita Ave., Ste. A
Riverside, CA 92507
Phone: (909)683-6415 **Fax:** (909)682-6804

★ 6826 ★ American Cancer Society
Redwood Empire Region
c/o East Bay Region
1700 Webster St.
Oakland, CA 94612
Phone: (510)452-5229 **Fax:** (510)763-8826

★ 6827 ★ American Cancer Society
Riverside Unit
1240 Palmyrita Ave., Ste. A
Riverside, CA 92507
Phone: (909)683-6415 **Fax:** (909)682-6804

★ 6828 ★ American Cancer Society
Sacramento Unit
1765 Challenge Way, Ste. 115
Sacramento, CA 95815
Phone: (916)446-7933 **Fax:** (916)325-2351

★ 6829 ★ American Cancer Society
Saddleback Valley Unit
Alton Deere Plaza
1940 E Deere Ave., Ste. 100
Santa Ana, CA 92705
Phone: (949)261-9446 **Fax:** (949)261-9419

★ 6830 ★ American Cancer Society
San Diego County Unit
2655 Camino Del Rio N, Ste. 100
San Diego, CA 92108
Phone: (619)299-4200 **Fax:** (619)296-0928

★ 6831 ★ American Cancer Society
San Fernando Valley Unit
4940 Van Nuys Blvd., Ste. 301
Sherman Oaks, CA 91403
Phone: (818)905-7766 **Fax:** (818)905-9058

★ 6832 ★ American Cancer Society
San Francisco County Unit
235 Montgomery St., Ste. 320
San Francisco, CA 94104
Phone: (415)394-7100 **Free:** 800-ACS-2345
Fax: (415)394-7101

★ 6833 ★ American Cancer Society
San Gabriel Valley Unit
50 N Hill Ave., Ste. 200
Pasadena, CA 91106
Phone: (626)795-7774 **Fax:** (626)568-2888

★ 6834 ★ American Cancer Society
San Joaquin/Calaveras Unit
207 E Alpine Ave.
Stockton, CA 95204
Phone: (209)941-2676 **Fax:** (209)941-2824

★ 6835 ★ American Cancer Society
San Luis Obispo Unit
1428 Phillips Ln., Ste. 201
San Luis Obispo, CA 93401
Phone: (805)543-1481 **Fax:** (805)543-1515

★ 6836 ★ American Cancer Society
San Mateo County Unit
1650 S Amphlett Blvd., Ste. 110
San Mateo, CA 94402
Phone: (650)578-9902 **Fax:** (650)578-9940

★ 6837 ★ American Cancer Society
Santa Barbara Unit
1432 Chapala St.
Santa Barbara, CA 93101
Phone: (805)963-1576 **Fax:** (805)963-6093

★ 6838 ★ American Cancer Society
Santa Clara County Unit
1715 S Bascom Ave., Ste. 100
Campbell, CA 95008
Phone: (408)879-1032 **Fax:** (408)879-1031

★ 6839 ★ American Cancer Society
Santa Clarita Valley Unit
20655 Soledad Canyon Rd., Ste. 17
Santa Clarita, CA 91351
Phone: (661)298-0886 **Fax:** (661)298-0885

★ 6840 ★ American Cancer Society
Santa Cruz County Unit
Dominican Hospital Education Ctr.
1555 Soquel Dr.
Santa Cruz, CA 95065
Phone: (831)477-9523 **Fax:** (831)477-9506

★ 6841 ★ American Cancer Society
Santa Maria Valley Unit
220 S Palisade Dr., Ste. 103
Santa Maria, CA 93454
Phone: (805)922-2354 **Fax:** (805)928-6054

★ 6842 ★ American Cancer Society
Santa Rosa Unit
1451 Guerneville Rd., Ste. 220
Santa Rosa, CA 95403
Phone: (707)545-6720 **Fax:** (707)545-3179

★ 6843 ★ American Cancer Society
Sierra View Unit
456 W Putnam
Porterville, CA 93257
Phone: (559)782-7666

★ 6844 ★ American Cancer Society
Silicon Valley/Central Coast Regional Office
1715 S Bascom Ave., Ste. 100
Campbell, CA 95008
Phone: (408)879-1032 **Fax:** (408)879-1030

★ 6845 ★ American Cancer Society
Simi Valley Unit
1445 E Los Angeles Ave., Ste. 207
Simi Valley, CA 93065
Phone: (805)527-5360 **Fax:** (805)527-3357

★ 6846 ★ American Cancer Society
Siskiyou County Unit
3290 Bechelli Ln.
Redding, CA 96002
Phone: (530)222-1058 **Fax:** (530)222-1409

★ 6847 ★ American Cancer Society
Solano County Unit
1652 W Texas St., Ste. 110
Fairfield, CA 94533
Phone: (707)425-5006 **Fax:** (707)425-5639

★ 6848 ★ American Cancer Society
Sonoma Valley Area Office
400 N McDowell Blvd.
Petaluma, CA 94954
Phone: (707)766-8066 **Fax:** (707)545-3179

★ 6849 ★ American Cancer Society
South Central Los Angeles Unit
641 E El Segundo Blvd.
Los Angeles, CA 90059
Phone: (323)757-9992 **Fax:** (323)757-9995

★ 6850 ★ American Cancer Society
South Contra Costa County Unit
1885 Oak Park Blvd.
Pleasant Hill, CA 94523
Phone: (925)934-7640 **Fax:** (925)934-5372

★ 6851 ★ American Cancer Society
South Placer Unit
333 Sunrise Ave., Ste. 344
Roseville, CA 95661
Phone: (916)783-4181 **Fax:** (916)783-4175

★ 6852 ★ American Cancer Society
Stanislaus Unit
1604 Ford Ave., Ste. 8
Modesto, CA 95350
Phone: (209)524-7242 **Fax:** (209)524-7454

★ 6853 ★ American Cancer Society
Tehama County Unit
3290 Bechelli Ln.
Redding, CA 96002
Phone: (530)222-1058 **Fax:** (530)222-1409

★ 6854 ★ American Cancer Society
Temecula/Murrieta Unit
1240 Palmyrita Ave., Ste. A
Riverside, CA 92507
Phone: (909)683-6415 **Fax:** (909)682-6804

★ 6855 ★ American Cancer Society
Tri-Cities Unit
1900 Mowry Ave., Ste. 405
Fremont, CA 94538
Phone: (510)742-8346 **Fax:** (510)742-8417

★ 6856 ★ American Cancer Society
Tri-Valley Unit
7000 Village Pkwy., Ste. E
Dublin, CA 94568
Phone: (925)833-2784 **Fax:** (925)833-9137

★ 6857 ★ American Cancer Society
Tulare County Unit
211 N Encina
Visalia, CA
Phone: (559)734-1391 **Fax:** (559)734-0429

★ 6858 ★ American Cancer Society
Tuolumne County Unit
1604 Ford Ave., Ste. 8
Modesto, CA 95350
Phone: (209)524-7242 **Fax:** (209)524-7454

★ 6859 ★ American Cancer Society
Upper Napa Valley/Lake County Area Office
1031 Jefferson St.
Napa, CA 94559
Phone: (707)255-5911 **Fax:** (707)255-3823

★ 6860 ★ American Cancer Society
West Bay Regional Office
235 Montgomery St., Ste. 320
San Francisco, CA 94104
Phone: (415)394-7100 **Fax:** (415)394-7101

★ 6861 ★ American Cancer Society
West Contra Costa County Unit
2023 Vale Rd., Ste. 4
San Pablo, CA 94806
Phone: (510)236-6905 **Fax:** (510)236-6970

★ 6862 ★ American Cancer Society
West Inland Valley Unit
8560 Vineyard Ave., Ste. 108
Rancho Cucamonga, CA 91730
Phone: (909)949-6115 **Fax:** (909)949-6813

★ 6863 ★ American Cancer Society
West Unit
Alton Deere Plaza
1940 E Deere Ave., Ste. 100
Santa Ana, CA 92705
Phone: (949)261-9446 **Fax:** (949)261-9419

★ 6864 ★ American Cancer Society
Yolo County Unit
1765 Challenge Way, Ste. 115
Sacramento, CA 95815
Phone: (530)662-3464 **Fax:** (916)325-2351

★ 6865 ★ American Cancer Society
Yuba Sutter Colusa Unit
618 5th St.
Marysville, CA 95901
Phone: (530)741-1366 **Fax:** (530)741-1383

Colorado

★ 6866 ★ American Cancer Society
Boulder County Office
2130 Mountain View Ave., Ste. A
Longmont, CO 80501
Phone: (303)776-2689 **Fax:** (303)776-2875

★ 6867 ★ American Cancer Society
Colorado Springs Office
1445 N Union, Ste. B-100
Colorado Springs, CO 80909
Phone: (719)636-5101 **Fax:** (719)636-1480

★ 6868 ★ American Cancer Society
Grand Junction Office
2754 Compass Dr., Ste. 328
Grand Junction, CO 81506
Phone: (970)242-9593 **Fax:** (970)242-2283

★ 6869 ★ American Cancer Society
Larimer County Office
344 E Foothills Pkwy., Ste. 2E
Fort Collins, CO 80525
Phone: (970)226-0148 **Fax:** (970)223-6214

★ 6870 ★ American Cancer Society
Mile High Office
2253 S Oneida St.
Denver, CO 80224
Phone: (303)758-2030 **Free:** 800-882-9455
Fax: (303)759-1615

★ 6871 ★ American Cancer Society
Pueblo Office
720 N Main St., Ste. 418
Pueblo, CO 81003
Phone: (719)543-2824 **Fax:** (719)543-2877

★ 6872 ★ American Cancer Society
Southwest Colorado Office
3801 N Main Ave.
Durango, CO 81301
Phone: (970)247-0278 **Fax:** (970)247-4200

★ 6873 ★ American Cancer Society
Weld County Office
1020 9th Ave.
Greeley, CO 80631
Phone: (970)356-9727

Connecticut

★ 6874 ★ American Cancer Society
Rhode Island & Eastern Connecticut Division
Norwich Office
238 W Town St.
Norwich, CT 06360
Phone: (860)887-2547 **Fax:** (860)885-0820

★ 6875 ★ American Cancer Society
Southern New England Regional Office
Meriden Executive Pk.
538 Preston Ave.
Meriden, CT 06450
Phone: (203)379-4700 **Fax:** (203)379-5060

★ 6876 ★ American Cancer Society
Southwest New England Regional Office
372 Danbury Rd.
Wilton, CT 06897
Phone: (203)563-0740 **Fax:** (203)563-0738

Delaware

★ 6877 ★ American Cancer Society
New Castle Office
92 Read's Way, Ste. 205
New Castle, DE 19720
Phone: (302)324-4227 **Free:** 800-ACS-2345
Fax: (302)324-4233

District of Columbia

★ 6878 ★ American Cancer Society
District of Columbia Division
1875 Connecticut Ave. NW, Ste. 730
Washington, DC 20009
Phone: (202)483-2600 **Fax:** (202)483-1174

Florida

★ 6879 ★ American Cancer Society
Alachua Unit
2119 SW 16th St.
Gainesville, FL 32608
Phone: (352)376-6866 **Fax:** (352)336-3861

★ 6880 ★ American Cancer Society
Baker Office
1732 Kingsley Ave., Ste. 3
Orange Park, FL 32067
Phone: (904)264-6039 **Fax:** (904)264-6272

★ 6881 ★ American Cancer Society
Bartow Office
809 S Florida Ave.
Lakeland, FL 33801
Phone: (863)688-2326 **Fax:** (863)687-6939

★ 6882 ★ American Cancer Society
Bay Area Office
2012-A Lisenby Ave.
Panama City, FL 32405
Phone: (850)785-9205 **Fax:** (850)872-9431

★ 6883 ★ American Cancer Society
Big Bend Committee Office
241 John Knox Rd., Ste. 100
Tallahassee, FL 32308
Phone: (850)297-0588 **Fax:** (850)297-0592

★ 6884 ★ American Cancer Society
Brevard Area Office
4356-B Fortune Pl.
Melbourne, FL 32904
Phone: (321)723-7737 **Fax:** (321)723-3344

★ 6885 ★ American Cancer Society
Broward Office
3407 NW 9th Ave., Ste. 100
Fort Lauderdale, FL 33309
Phone: (954)564-0880 **Fax:** (954)561-8072

★ 6886 ★ American Cancer Society
Calhoun Office
2012-A Lisenby Ave.
Panama City, FL 32405
Phone: (850)785-9205 **Fax:** (850)872-9431

★ 6887 ★ American Cancer Society
Capital Area Office
241 John Knox Rd., Ste. 100
Tallahassee, FL 32308
Phone: (850)297-0588 **Fax:** (850)297-0592

★ 6888 ★ American Cancer Society
Charlotte Office
22107 Elmira Blvd.
Port Charlotte, FL 33952
Phone: (941)627-3000 **Fax:** (941)627-5229

★ 6889 ★ American Cancer Society
Citrus Unit
140 N Sportsman Pt.
Inverness, FL 34453
Phone: (352)637-5577 **Fax:** (352)637-2590

★ 6890 ★ American Cancer Society
Clay Unit
1732 Kingsley Ave., Ste. 3
Orange Park, FL 32073
Phone: (904)264-6039 **Fax:** (904)264-6272

★ 6891 ★ American Cancer Society
Collier Office
990 1st Ave. S, Ste. 200
Naples, FL 34102
Phone: (239)261-0337 **Fax:** (239)649-5571

★ 6892 ★ American Cancer Society
Dade Office
3901 NW 79th Ave., Ste. 224
Miami, FL 33166
Phone: (305)594-4363 **Fax:** (305)592-5140

★ 6893 ★ American Cancer Society
DeSoto Office
2100 S Tamiami Tr., Ste. A
Venice, FL 34293
Phone: (941)497-4309 **Fax:** (941)497-4752

★ 6894 ★ American Cancer Society
Duval Office
4030 Boulevard Center Dr.
Jacksonville, FL 32207
Phone: (904)398-0537 **Fax:** (904)396-0240

★ 6895 ★ American Cancer Society
East Polk Unit
192 Ave. D NW
Winter Haven, FL 33880
Phone: (863)294-0661 **Fax:** (863)293-3906

★ 6896 ★ American Cancer Society
East/Southeast Volusia Office
146 Orange Ave.
Daytona Beach, FL 32114
Phone: (386)253-1633 **Fax:** (386)253-1636

★ 6897 ★ American Cancer Society
Escambia Unit
701 E Cervantes St.
Pensacola, FL 32501
Phone: (850)438-4491 **Fax:** (850)433-5003

★ 6898 ★ American Cancer Society
First Coast Area Office
4030 Boulevard Center Dr.
Jacksonville, FL 32207
Phone: (904)398-0537 **Fax:** (904)396-0240

★ 6899 ★ American Cancer Society
Flagler Office
146 Orange Ave.
Daytona Beach, FL 32114
Phone: (386)439-3507 **Fax:** (386)253-1633

★ 6900 ★ American Cancer Society
Franklin Office
2012-A Lisenby Ave.
Panama City, FL 32405
Phone: (850)785-9205 **Fax:** (850)872-9431

★ 6901 ★ American Cancer Society
Gadsden/Chattahoochee Office
241 John Knox Rd., Ste. 100
Tallahassee, FL 32308
Phone: (850)297-0588 **Fax:** (850)297-0592

★ 6902 ★ American Cancer Society
Greater Tampa Office
1001 S MacDill Ave.
Tampa, FL 33629
Phone: (813)254-3630 **Free:** 800-ACS-2345
Fax: (813)349-4431
Website: http://www2.cancer.org/state/fl/index.htm

★ 6903 ★ American Cancer Society
Gulf Coast Area Office
701 E Cervantes St.
Pensacola, FL 32501
Phone: (850)438-4491 **Fax:** (850)438-9871

★ 6904 ★ American Cancer Society
Gulf Office
2012-A Lisenby Ave.
Panama City, FL 32405
Phone: (850)785-9205 **Fax:** (850)872-9431

★ 6905 ★ American Cancer Society
Hardee/Manatee/Highlands Unit
600 U.S. 301 Blvd. W, Ste. 136
Bradenton, FL 34205
Phone: (863)773-0333 **Fax:** (941)745-1760

★ 6906 ★ American Cancer Society
Hernando Office
8159 State Rd. 52
Hudson, FL 34667
Phone: (727)863-1019 **Fax:** (727)869-7228

★ 6907 ★ American Cancer Society
High-Five Unit
2119 SW 16th St.
Gainesville, FL 32608
Phone: (352)376-6866 **Fax:** (352)336-3861

★ 6908 ★ American Cancer Society
Holmes/Emerald Coast Office
4 Jackson St. NE
Fort Walton Beach, FL 32548
Phone: (850)244-3813 **Fax:** (850)664-5366

★ 6909 ★ American Cancer Society
Indian River Office
3375 20th St., Ste. 100
Vero Beach, FL 32960
Phone: (561)562-2272 **Fax:** (561)562-2666

★ 6910 ★ American Cancer Society
Jackson Office
2012-A Lisenby Ave.
Panama City, FL 32405
Phone: (850)785-9205 **Fax:** (850)872-9431

★ 6911 ★ American Cancer Society
Jacksonville Beaches/Ponte Vedra Office
2850 Isabella Blvd., Ste. 20
Jacksonville Beach, FL 32250
Phone: (904)249-0022 **Fax:** (904)270-0976

★ 6912 ★ American Cancer Society
Lake/Sumter Office
1411 E Main St., Ste. 3
Leesburg, FL 34748
Phone: (352)326-9599 **Fax:** (352)326-3855

★ 6913 ★ American Cancer Society
Lee/Cape Coral Office
4575 Via Royale, Ste. 110
Fort Myers, FL 33919
Phone: (239)936-1113 **Fax:** (239)936-3763

★ 6914 ★ American Cancer Society
Leon Office
241 John Knox Rd., Ste. 100
Tallahassee, FL 32308
Phone: (850)297-0588 **Fax:** (850)297-0592

★ 6915 ★ American Cancer Society
Liberty Office
2012-A Lisenby Ave.
Panama City, FL 32405
Phone: (850)785-9205 **Fax:** (850)872-9431

★ 6916 ★ American Cancer Society
Marco Island Office
917 N Collier Blvd.
Marco Island, FL 34145
Phone: (941)642-8800 **Fax:** (941)642-0027

★ 6917 ★ American Cancer Society
Marion Unit
2100 SE 17th St., Ste. 110
Ocala, FL 34471
Phone: (352)629-4727 **Fax:** (352)629-5107

★ 6918 ★ American Cancer Society
Martin Office
865 SE Monterey Commons Blvd.
Stuart, FL 34996
Phone: (772)287-7467 **Fax:** (772)287-7925

★ 6919 ★ American Cancer Society
Miami Beach/North Dade Office
3901 NW 79 Ave., Ste. 224
Miami, FL 33166
Phone: (305)594-4363 **Fax:** (305)947-8737

★ 6920 ★ American Cancer Society
Monroe/Keys Office
2502-B Roosevelt Blvd.
Key West, FL 33040
Phone: (305)292-2333 **Fax:** (305)294-3964

★ 6921 ★ American Cancer Society
Nassau Office
2850 Isabella Blvd., Ste. 20
Jacksonville Beach, FL 32250
Phone: (904)249-0022 **Fax:** (904)270-0976

★ 6922 ★ American Cancer Society
North Central Area Office
2119 SW 16th St.
Gainesville, FL 32608
Phone: (352)376-6866 **Fax:** (352)336-3861

★ 6923 ★ American Cancer Society
North Okaloosa Office
4 Jackson St. NE
Fort Walton Beach, FL 32548
Phone: (850)244-3813 **Fax:** (850)664-5366

★ 6924 ★ American Cancer Society
Okeechobee Office
3375 20th St., Ste. 100
Vero Beach, FL 32960
Phone: (561)562-2272 **Fax:** (561)562-2666

★ 6925 ★ American Cancer Society
Orlando Metro Office
1601 W Colonial Dr.
Orlando, FL 32804
Phone: (407)843-8680 **Fax:** (407)649-6502

★ 6926 ★ American Cancer Society
Osceola Unit
1601 W Colonial Dr.
Orlando, FL 32804
Phone: (407)843-8680 **Fax:** (407)423-2383

★ 6927 ★ American Cancer Society
Palm Beach Benefit Office
235 S County Rd., No. 20
Palm Beach, FL 33480
Phone: (561)655-3449 **Fax:** (561)655-3686

★ 6928 ★ American Cancer Society
Pasco Office
8159 State Rd. 52
Hudson, FL 34667
Phone: (727)863-1019 **Fax:** (727)869-7228

★ 6929 ★ American Cancer Society
Pinellas Office
4801 86th Ave. N
Pinellas Park, FL 33782
Phone: (727)546-9822 **Fax:** (727)545-3753

★ 6930 ★ American Cancer Society
Putnam Office
600 Zeigler Dr.
Palatka, FL 32177
Phone: (386)328-6224 **Fax:** (904)325-8086

★ 6931 ★ American Cancer Society
Saint Johns Office
2850 Isabella Blvd., Ste. 20
Jacksonville Beach, FL 32250
Phone: (904)249-0022 **Fax:** (904)270-0976

★ 6932 ★ American Cancer Society
Saint Lucie Office
3375 20th St., Ste. 100
Vero Beach, FL 32960
Phone: (561)562-2272 **Fax:** (561)562-2666

★ 6933 ★ American Cancer Society
Santa Rosa Unit
701 E Cervantes St.
Pensacola, FL 32501
Phone: (850)438-4491 **Fax:** (850)438-5003

★ 6934 ★ American Cancer Society
Sarasota Office
1750 17th St., Ste. A
Sarasota, FL 34234
Phone: (941)365-2858 **Fax:** (941)365-3256

★ 6935 ★ American Cancer Society
Seminole Unit
1601 W Colonial Dr.
Orlando, FL 32804
Phone: (407)843-8680 **Fax:** (407)649-6502

★ 6936 ★ American Cancer Society
South Palm Beach Office
3350 NW Boca Raton Blvd., Ste. A-34
Boca Raton, FL 33431
Phone: (561)394-7751 **Fax:** (561)394-7909

★ 6937 ★ American Cancer Society
South Sarasota Office
2100 S Tamiami Tr., Ste. A
Venice, FL 34293
Phone: (941)497-4309 **Fax:** (941)497-4752

★ 6938 ★ American Cancer Society
Suburban Hillsborough Unit
1462 Oakfield Dr.
Brandon, FL 33511
Phone: (813)685-0670 **Fax:** (813)689-1320

★ 6939 ★ American Cancer Society
Tri-City Office
22107 Elmira Blvd.
Port Charlotte, FL 33952
Phone: (941)627-3000 **Fax:** (941)627-5229

★ 6940 ★ American Cancer Society
Tri-County Office
2119 SW 16th St.
Gainesville, FL 32608
Phone: (352)376-6866 **Fax:** (352)336-3861

★ 6941 ★ American Cancer Society
Washington Office
2012-A Lisenby Ave.
Panama City, FL 32405
Phone: (850)785-9205 **Fax:** (850)872-9431

★ 6942 ★ American Cancer Society
West Palm Beach Office
5 Harvard Cir., Ste. 110
West Palm Beach, FL 33409
Phone: (561)616-9370 **Fax:** (561)616-9371

★ 6943 ★ American Cancer Society
West Polk Unit
809 S Florida Ave.
Lakeland, FL 33801
Phone: (863)688-2326 **Fax:** (863)687-6939

★ 6944 ★ American Cancer Society
West Volusia Office
218-A E New York Ave.
DeLand, FL 32724
Phone: (386)734-7836 **Fax:** (386)738-2215

Georgia

★ 6945 ★ American Cancer Society
Albany Office
323 Pine Ave.
Albany, GA 31701
Phone: 800-282-4914 **Fax:** (229)446-7709

★ 6946 ★ American Cancer Society
Athens Office
1060 Gaines School Rd., Ste. B-2
Athens, GA 30605
Phone: 800-282-4914 **Fax:** (706)549-2314

★ 6947 ★ American Cancer Society
Atlanta Office
2200 Century Pkwy., Ste. 950
Atlanta, GA 30345
Phone: (404)816-4994 **Fax:** (404)315-9348
Website: http://www2.cancer.org/state/ga/index.html

★ 6948 ★ American Cancer Society
Augusta Office
2623 Washington Rd., Bldg F, Ste. 104
Augusta, GA 30904
Phone: 800-282-4914 **Fax:** (706)731-0979

★ 6949 ★ American Cancer Society
Brunswick Office
2311 Heron St.
Brunswick, GA 31520
Phone: 800-282-4914 **Fax:** (912)262-0773

★ 6950 ★ American Cancer Society
Columbus Office
1233 12th St.
Columbus, GA 31902
Phone: 800-282-4914 **Fax:** (706)324-4749

★ 6951 ★ American Cancer Society
Dalton Office
300 W Emery St., Ste. 106
Dalton, GA 30720
Phone: 800-282-4914 **Fax:** (706)226-7531

★ 6952 ★ American Cancer Society
Fayetteville Office
135 Bradford Sq., Ste. B
Fayetteville, GA 30215
Phone: (404)816-4994 **Fax:** (770)460-1641

★ 6953 ★ American Cancer Society
Gainesville Office
2565 Thompson Bridge Rd, Ste. 114
Gainesville, GA 30501
Phone: (404)816-4994 **Fax:** (770)297-7418

★ 6954 ★ American Cancer Society
Gwinnett Office
6500 Sugarloaf Pkwy., Ste. 260
Duluth, GA 30097
Phone: (404)816-4994 **Fax:** (770)814-9517

★ 6955 ★ American Cancer Society
Macon Office
804 Cherry St., Ste. A
Macon, GA 31201
Phone: 800-282-4914 **Fax:** (478)741-5905

★ 6956 ★ American Cancer Society
Marietta Office
1825 Barrett Lakes Blvd., Ste. 280
Kennesaw, GA 30144
Phone: (404)816-4994 **Fax:** (770)429-9824

★ 6957 ★ American Cancer Society
Savannah Office
5102 Paulsen St., Bldg. 4
Savannah, GA 31405
Phone: 800-282-4914 **Fax:** (912)355-0955

★ 6958 ★ American Cancer Society
Statesboro Office
515 Denmark St., Ste. 500
Statesboro, GA 30458
Phone: 800-282-4914 **Fax:** (912)764-3089

★ 6959 ★ American Cancer Society
Waycross Office
406 Tebeau St.
Waycross, GA 31501
Phone: 800-282-4914 **Fax:** (912)283-9694

Guam

★ 6960 ★ American Cancer Society
Guam Unit
140 Aspinall St., Ste. 102
Agana, GU 96910
Phone: (671)477-9451 **Fax:** (671)477-9450

Hawaii

★ 6961 ★ American Cancer Society
Central/Leeward Unit
98-029 Hekaha St., Bldg 5, Ste. 6
Aiea, HI 96701
Phone: (808)486-8420 **Fax:** (808)935-9780

★ 6962 ★ American Cancer Society
East Hawaii Unit
614 Kilauea Ave., Ste. 2
Hilo, HI 96720
Phone: (808)935-9763 **Fax:** (808)935-9780

★ 6963 ★ American Cancer Society
Honolulu Office
2370 Nuuanu Ave.
Honolulu, HI 96817
Phone: (808)595-7544 **Free:** 800-ACS-2345
Fax: (808)595-7545
Website: http://www.hi-cancer.org

★ 6964 ★ American Cancer Society
Kauai Unit
3535 Kuhio Hwy.
Lihue, HI 96766
Phone: (808)245-2942 **Fax:** (808)245-2302

★ 6965 ★ American Cancer Society
Maui-Molokai-Lanai Unit
Cameron Ctr.
95 Mahalani St.
Wailuku, HI 96793
Phone: (808)244-5553 **Fax:** (808)244-6195

★ 6966 ★ American Cancer Society
Molokai Branch
PO Box 1618
Kaunakakai, HI 96748
Phone: (808)553-5154

★ 6967 ★ American Cancer Society
West Hawaii Unit
74-5588 R Pawai Pl.
Kailua Kona, HI 96740
Phone: (808)334-0442 **Fax:** (808)334-0443

★ 6968 ★ American Cancer Society
Windward Unit
130 Kailua Rd., Ste. 102B
Kailua, HI 96734
Phone: (808)262-5124 **Fax:** (808)262-4212

Idaho

★ 6969 ★ American Cancer Society
Eastern Idaho Office
900 E Harmony
Blackfoot, ID 83221
Phone: (208)785-2516 **Fax:** (208)785-6457

★ 6970 ★ American Cancer Society
Magic Valley Office
149 W 50 S
Rupert, ID 83350
Phone: (208)436-5238 **Fax:** (208)436-5267

★ 6971 ★ American Cancer Society
Northern Idaho Office
1602 Sherman Ave., Ste. 104
Coeur d'Alene, ID 83814
Phone: (208)667-9749 **Fax:** (208)765-5733

★ 6972 ★ American Cancer Society
Treasure Valley Office
2676 Vista Ave.
Boise, ID 83705
Phone: (208)343-4609 **Free:** 800-632-5934
Fax: (208)343-9922
Website: http://www2.cancer.org/state/id/index.html

Illinois

★ 6973 ★ American Cancer Society
Chicago Regional Office
77 E Monroe St., 12th Fl.
Chicago, IL 60603
Phone: (312)372-0471 **Free:** 800-227-2345
Fax: (312)372-0910
Website: http://www.il.cancer.org

★ 6974 ★ American Cancer Society
DuPage County Regional Office
999 Main St.
Glen Ellyn, IL 60137
Phone: (630)469-3011 **Free:** 800-ACS-2345
Fax: (630)469-3065
Email: shammes@cancer.org
Website: http://www.il.cancer.org/

★ 6975 ★ American Cancer Society
Eastern Illinois Office
2509 S Neil St.
Champaign, IL 61820
Phone: (217)356-9076 **Free:** 800-ACS-2345
Fax: (217)356-7721
Website: http://www.il.cancer.org/

★ 6976 ★ American Cancer Society
Fox Valley Regional Office
11 E Wilson St.
Batavia, IL 60510
Phone: (630)879-9009 **Free:** 800-ACS-2345
Fax: (630)879-9047
Website: http://www.il.cancer.org/

★ 6977 ★ American Cancer Society
Lake County Regional Office
777 Central Ave.
Highland Park, IL 60035
Phone: (847)432-0577 **Fax:** (847)432-0599

★ 6978 ★ American Cancer Society
Metro East Regional Office
118 S Seminary St.
Collinsville, IL 62234
Phone: (618)345-7911 **Fax:** (618)345-8320

★ 6979 ★ American Cancer Society
North Shore Illinois Office
820 Davis St., Ste. 340
Evanston, IL 60201
Phone: (847)328-5147 **Free:** 800-ACS-2345
Fax: (847)570-6043
Website: http://www.il.cancer.org

★ 6980 ★ American Cancer Society
Northern Illinois Regional Office
4312 E State St.
Rockford, IL 61108
Phone: (815)229-1287 **Free:** 800-ACS-2345
Fax: (815)229-1363
Website: http://il.cancer.org/

★ 6981 ★ American Cancer Society
Northwest Illinois Regional Office
3727 Blackhawk Rd.
Rock Island, IL 61201
Phone: (309)794-0601 **Free:** 800-ACS-2345
Fax: (309)793-3251
Website: http://www.il.cancer.org/

★ 6982 ★ American Cancer Society
Northwest Suburban Regional Office
100 W Palatine Rd., Ste. 150
Palatine, IL 60067
Phone: (847)358-3965 **Free:** 800-ACS-2345
Fax: (847)358-9218
Website: http://www.il.cancer.org/

★ 6983 ★ American Cancer Society
Prairie Land Regional Office
17060 Oak Park Ave.
Tinley Park, IL 60477
Phone: (708)633-7770 **Free:** 800-ACS-2345
Fax: (708)633-7773
Website: http://www.il.cancer.org/

★ 6984 ★ American Cancer Society
Riverside Regional Office
7234 W Ogden Ave., Ste. 3 S
Riverside, IL 60546
Phone: (708)484-8541 **Fax:** (708)484-3179

★ 6985 ★ American Cancer Society
Southern Regional Office
805 W DeYoung St., Ste. B
Marion, IL 62959
Phone: (618)998-9898 **Fax:** (618)997-8456

★ 6986 ★ American Cancer Society
West Central Regional Office
4234 N Knoxville Ave., Ste. B
Peoria, IL 61614
Phone: (309)688-3488 **Free:** 800-ACS-2345
Fax: (309)688-9493
Website: http://www.il.cancer.org/

★ 6987 ★ American Cancer Society
Western Illinois Regional Office
1305 Wabash
Springfield, IL 62704
Phone: (217)546-7586 **Free:** 800-ACS-2345
Fax: (217)546-7631
Website: http://www.il.cancer.org/

Indiana

★ 6988 ★ American Cancer Society
Central Indiana Area Service Center
6030 W 62nd St.
Indianapolis, IN 46278
Phone: (317)347-6670 **Free:** 800-233-6303
Fax: (317)347-6679
Denice Kallmyer, Exec Director

★ 6989 ★ American Cancer Society
Evansville Branch
1510 W Franklin St.
Evansville, IN 47710
Phone: (812)424-8281 **Free:** 800-227-2345
Fax: (812)424-1059
Gene Watson, Exec Director

★ 6990 ★ American Cancer Society
Indianapolis Office
6030 W 62nd St.
Indianapolis, IN 46278
Phone: (317)347-6670 **Fax:** (317)347-6679

★ 6991 ★ **American Cancer Society**
Lower Eastern Indiana Area Service Center
923 4th St.
PO Box 689
Columbus, IN 47201
Phone: (812)376-6781 **Fax:** (812)376-8031
Amy Eden, Exec Director

★ 6992 ★ **American Cancer Society**
Lower Eastern Indiana Area Service Center
Jenkins Hall
1401 Chester Blvd.
Richmond, IN 47374
Phone: (765)962-4180 **Fax:** (765)966-8023

★ 6993 ★ **American Cancer Society**
Mid-Indiana Area Service Center
2831 N Oakwood
Muncie, IN 47304-2254
Phone: (765)284-1696 **Fax:** (765)289-3254

★ 6994 ★ **American Cancer Society**
Mid-Indiana Area Service Center
707 W Historic 8th St.
Anderson, IN 46016
Phone: (765)642-6603 **Fax:** (765)642-6711
Gloria Collins, Contact

★ 6995 ★ **American Cancer Society**
Mid-Indiana Area Service Center
Kokomo Office
1150 S Dixon Rd.
Kokomo, IN 46902
Phone: (765)457-9173 **Fax:** (765)457-0595
Jim Seidel, Exec Director

★ 6996 ★ **American Cancer Society**
Mid-Indiana Area Service Center
Lafayette Office
401 S Earl St., Ste. 2C
Lafayette, IN 47904
Phone: (765)449-4799 **Fax:** (765)449-4065

★ 6997 ★ **American Cancer Society**
Mid-Indiana Area Service Center
Marion Office
1315 Gillespie St.
Marion, IN 46952
Phone: (765)668-7188 **Fax:** (265)668-7188

★ 6998 ★ **American Cancer Society**
Mid-Southwestern Area Service Center
318 Main St.
Vincennes, IN 47591
Phone: (812)886-9007 **Fax:** (812)886-9008

★ 6999 ★ **American Cancer Society**
Mid-Southwestern Indiana Area Service Center
1500 Meridian Rd.
Jasper, IN 47546
Phone: (812)482-7545 **Fax:** (812)482-6962
Christine Hopson, Exec Director

★ 7000 ★ **American Cancer Society**
North Central Indiana Area Service Center
535 W Edison, Unit 6
Mishawaka, IN 46545
Phone: (574)257-9789 **Fax:** (574)257-9790

★ 7001 ★ **American Cancer Society**
Northeast Indiana Area Service Center
2420 N Coliseum Blvd., Ste. 200
Fort Wayne, IN 46805
Phone: (219)471-3911 **Fax:** (219)483-5344
Peter Rinn, Exec Director

★ 7002 ★ **American Cancer Society**
Northwest Indiana Area Service Center
410 E Lincolnway
Valparaiso, IN 46383
Phone: (219)464-2895 **Fax:** (219)465-1044
Email: Judy.Rooney-Davis@cancer.org
Website: http://www.cancer.org
Judy Rooney-Davis, Exec Director

★ 7003 ★ **American Cancer Society**
Northwest Indiana Area Service Center
107 W 78th Pl.
Merrillville, IN 46410
Phone: (219)793-1030 **Fax:** (219)793-1033
Bill Lieber, Exec Director

★ 7004 ★ **American Cancer Society**
South Central Indiana Area Service Center
710 N Walnut St.
Bloomington, IN 47404
Phone: (812)336-8423 **Fax:** (812)339-9213
Email: jbretz@cancer.org
Website: http://www.cancer.org
Jim Bretz, Exec Director

★ 7005 ★ **American Cancer Society**
Southeast Indiana Area Service Center
230 Montgomery St., Ste. 105
Clarksville, IN 47129
Phone: (812)282-4266 **Free:** 800-227-2345
Fax: (812)282-5334
David Dougherty, Director

★ 7006 ★ **American Cancer Society**
Southwestern Indiana Area Service Center
1510 W Franklin St.
Evansville, IN 47710
Phone: (812)424-8281 **Fax:** (812)424-1059

★ 7007 ★ **American Cancer Society**
Wabash Valley Indiana Area Service Center
705 Putnam St.
Terre Haute, IN 47802
Phone: (812)232-2679 **Fax:** (812)232-2741
Julie Hansen, Exec Director

Iowa

★ 7008 ★ **American Cancer Society**
Burlington Office
1223 S Gear, Ste. 009
West Burlington, IA 52655
Phone: (319)752-4008 **Fax:** (319)752-6750

★ 7009 ★ **American Cancer Society**
Carroll Office
628 N Main St., Ste. 101
Carroll, IA 51401
Phone: (712)794-0100 **Fax:** (712)794-0101

★ 7010 ★ **American Cancer Society**
Cedar Rapids Office
4080 1st Ave. NE
Cedar Rapids, IA 52402
Phone: (319)365-5241 **Fax:** (319)365-1739

★ 7011 ★ **American Cancer Society**
Council Bluffs Office
2705 E Kanesville Blvd.
Council Bluffs, IA 51503
Phone: (712)323-6611 **Fax:** (712)323-7250

★ 7012 ★ **American Cancer Society**
Davenport Office
1351 W Central Park Ave., Ste. 1100
Davenport, IA 52804
Phone: (563)421-4227 **Fax:** (563)421-4229

★ 7013 ★ **American Cancer Society**
Des Moines Office
8364 Hickman, Ste. D
Des Moines, IA 50325
Phone: (515)253-0147 **Fax:** (515)253-0806

★ 7014 ★ **American Cancer Society**
Dubuque Office
367 Cedar Cross Rd.
Dubuque, IA 52003
Phone: (563)583-8249 **Fax:** (563)583-8240

★ 7015 ★ **American Cancer Society**
Fort Dodge Office
900 Central Ave., Ste. 21
Fort Dodge, IA 50501
Phone: (515)576-7078 **Fax:** (515)576-8353

★ 7016 ★ **American Cancer Society**
Iowa City Office
301 S Clinton St., 2nd Fl.
Iowa City, IA 52240
Phone: (319)337-8958 **Fax:** (319)337-8978

★ 7017 ★ **American Cancer Society**
Mason City Office
130 4th St. SW
Mason City, IA 50401
Phone: (641)422-9055 **Fax:** (641)422-9091

★ 7018 ★ **American Cancer Society**
Sioux City Office
Terra Ctr.
600 4th St., Ste. 229
Sioux City, IA 51101
Phone: (712)233-1148 **Fax:** (712)233-1507

★ 7019 ★ **American Cancer Society**
Storm Lake Office
541 Cayuga St.
Storm Lake, IA 50588
Phone: (712)732-9022 **Fax:** (712)732-9026

★ 7020 ★ **American Cancer Society**
Waterloo Office
200 E Ridgeway, Ste. 300
Waterloo, IA 50702
Phone: (319)272-2880 **Fax:** (319)272-2881

Kansas

★ 7021 ★ **American Cancer Society**
Kansas City Metro Office
6700 Antioch Rd., Ste. 100
Merriam, KS 66204-1200
Phone: (913)432-3277 **Free:** 800-ACS-2345
Fax: (913)432-1732
Website: http://www.cancer.org/state/heartland/

★ 7022 ★ **American Cancer Society**
Manhattan Office
3100 Heritage Ct., Ste. 80
Manhattan, KS 66503

Phone: (785)539-1547 **Free:** 800-359-1025
Fax: (785)539-1547
Website: http://www.cancer.org/state/heartland/index.html

★ 7023 ★ American Cancer Society
Southwest Kansas/Northwest Oklahoma Office
1712 32nd St.
Great Bend, KS 67530
Phone: (620)792-4994

★ 7024 ★ American Cancer Society
Topeka Office
1315 SW Arrowhead Rd.
Topeka, KS 66604
Phone: (785)273-4422 **Free:** 800-359-1025
Fax: (785)273-1503
Website: http://www.cancer.org/state/heartland/

★ 7025 ★ American Cancer Society
Wichita Office
435 S Broadway, Ste. 100
Wichita, KS 67202
Phone: (316)265-3400 **Free:** 800-478-4788
Fax: (316)265-3490
Website: http://www.cancer.org/state/heartland/

Kentucky

★ 7026 ★ American Cancer Society
Ashland Office
4338 13th St.
Ashland, KY 41102
Phone: (606)324-1819 **Fax:** (606)327-1744
Website: http://www2.cancer.org/state/ky/index.html

★ 7027 ★ American Cancer Society
Bowling Green Office
Greenwood Courtyard
2425 Scottsville Rd., Ste. 123
Bowling Green, KY 42104-4457
Phone: (270)782-3654 **Fax:** (270)846-0202
Website: http://www2.cancer.org/state/ky/

★ 7028 ★ American Cancer Society
Lexington Office
160 Moore Dr., Ste. 201
Lexington, KY 40503
Phone: (859)276-3223 **Fax:** (859)276-3056
Website: http://www2.cancer.org/state/ky/

★ 7029 ★ American Cancer Society
Louisville Area
Clark, Floyd Counties
701 W Muhammad Ali Blvd.
Louisville, KY 40203
Phone: (502)584-6782 **Free:** 800-ACS-2345
Fax: (502)584-8946

★ 7030 ★ American Cancer Society
Louisville Office
701 W Muhammad Ali Blvd.
Louisville, KY 40203
Phone: (502)584-6782 **Fax:** (502)584-6767
Website: http://www2.cancer.org/state/ky/index.html

★ 7031 ★ American Cancer Society
Northern Kentucky Office
Nicholas Center, Ste. A2
6612 Dixie Hwy.
Florence, KY 41042
Phone: (859)647-2200 **Fax:** (859)647-2246
Website: http://www2.cancer.org/state/ky/

★ 7032 ★ American Cancer Society
Owensboro Office
319 W 10th St.
Owensboro, KY 42301
Phone: (270)683-0425 **Fax:** (270)683-1471
Website: http://www2.cancer.org/state/ky/index.html

★ 7033 ★ American Cancer Society
Paducah Office
3140 Parisa Dr.
Paducah, KY 42003
Phone: (270)444-0375 **Free:** 800-ACS-2345
Fax: (270)444-0380

★ 7034 ★ American Cancer Society
Purchase District
3140 Parisa Dr.
Paducah, KY 42003
Phone: (502)444-0375 **Fax:** (502)444-0380
Website: http://www2.cancer.org/state/ky/index.html

★ 7035 ★ American Cancer Society
Somerset Kentucky Office
402 Coomer St.
Somerset, KY 42503
Phone: (606)679-6143 **Free:** 800-ACS-2345
Fax: (606)677-1943

Louisiana

★ 7036 ★ American Cancer Society
Alexandria Office
605C Medical Center Dr.
Alexandria, LA 71301
Phone: (318)445-4190 **Fax:** (318)445-5008

★ 7037 ★ American Cancer Society
Baton Rouge Office
4919 Jamestown Ave., Ste. 104
Baton Rouge, LA 70808
Phone: (225)927-0782 **Fax:** (225)927-0785

★ 7038 ★ American Cancer Society
Houma Office
614 Barrow St.
Houma, LA 70360
Phone: (985)851-7776 **Fax:** (985)851-5939

★ 7039 ★ American Cancer Society
Kenner Office
2200 Veterans Memorial Blvd., Ste. 214
Kenner, LA 70062
Phone: (504)469-0021 **Fax:** (504)469-0033
Website: http://www2.cancer.org/state/la/index.html

★ 7040 ★ American Cancer Society
Lafayette Office
1604 W Pinhook Rd., Ste. 182
Lafayette, LA 70508
Phone: (337)237-3736 **Fax:** (337)237-6907

★ 7041 ★ American Cancer Society
Lake Charles Office
1 Lakeshore Dr., Ste. 1585
Lake Charles, LA 70629
Phone: (337)433-5131 **Fax:** (337)439-9620

★ 7042 ★ American Cancer Society
Monroe Office
1761 N 19th St.
Monroe, LA 71201
Phone: (318)398-7248 **Fax:** (318)361-0718

★ 7043 ★ American Cancer Society
Shreveport Office
920 Pierremont Rd., Ste. 300
Shreveport, LA 71106
Phone: (318)227-8901 **Fax:** (318)865-4831

Maine

★ 7044 ★ American Cancer Society
Northeast New England Region
Topsham Office
1 Main St., Ste. 300
Topsham, ME 04086-1240
Phone: (207)373-3700 **Free:** 800-464-3102
Fax: (207)725-6680

Maryland

★ 7045 ★ American Cancer Society
Cumberland Office
111 S George St.
Cumberland, MD 21502
Phone: (301)722-2145 **Fax:** (301)724-6179

★ 7046 ★ American Cancer Society
Eldersburg Office
1393 Progress Way, Ste. 908
Eldersburg, MD 21784
Phone: (410)781-4316 **Fax:** (410)781-4317

★ 7047 ★ American Cancer Society
Gambrills Office
1041 Rte. 3 N, Bldg. A
Gambrills, MD 21054
Phone: (410)721-4304 **Fax:** (410)721-4307

★ 7048 ★ American Cancer Society
Hagerstown Office
1037 Haven Rd.
Hagerstown, MD 21742
Phone: (301)733-8272 **Fax:** (301)733-0285

★ 7049 ★ American Cancer Society
Salisbury Office
1138 Parsons Rd.
Salisbury, MD 21803
Phone: (410)749-1624 **Fax:** (410)860-0832

★ 7050 ★ American Cancer Society
Silver Spring Office
11331 Amherst Ave.
Silver Spring, MD 20902
Phone: (301)933-9350 **Fax:** (301)929-8243

★ 7051 ★ American Cancer Society
White Marsh Office
8219 Town Center Dr.
Baltimore, MD 21236
Phone: (410)931-6850 **Free:** 888-640-0427
Fax: (410)931-6875
Website: http://www.inet.net/imc/acsworking/md/index.shtml?md&total

Massachusetts

★ 7052 ★ American Cancer Society
Central New England Regional Office
Natick Business Park
6 Strathmore Rd.
Natick, MA 01760
Phone: (508)652-4300 **Fax:** (508)655-4907

★ 7053 ★ American Cancer Society
Massachusetts Bay Regional Office
25 Stuart St., 4th Fl.
Boston, MA 02116

Phone: (617)556-7400 **Fax:** (617)426-0383

★ 7054 ★ American Cancer Society
Midcoastal New England Region
Byfield Office
12 Kent Way, Ste. 209
Byfield, MA 01922
Phone: (978)462-0571 **Free:** 800-227-2345
Fax: (978)462-1566

★ 7055 ★ American Cancer Society
New England Division
30 Speen St.
Framingham, MA 01701
Free: 800-ACS-2345

★ 7056 ★ American Cancer Society
Southeast New England Regional Division
Brockton Office
1115 W Chestnut St., Ste. 301
Brockton, MA 02301
Phone: (508)584-9600 **Fax:** (508)584-9699

★ 7057 ★ American Cancer Society
Southeast New England Regional Office
1115 W Chestnut St.
Brockton, MA 02301
Phone: (508)584-9600 **Fax:** (508)584-9699

★ 7058 ★ American Cancer Society
Western New England Region
Pittsfield Office
39 Wahconah St., 2nd Fl.
Pittsfield, MA 01201
Phone: (413)734-6000 **Fax:** (413)445-0007

★ 7059 ★ American Cancer Society
Western New England Region
West Springfield Office
31 Capital Dr.
West Springfield, MA 01089
Phone: (413)734-6000 **Free:** 800-227-2345
Fax: (413)746-4099

Michigan

★ 7060 ★ American Cancer Society
Barry County Office
PO Box 509
Hastings, MI 49058
Phone: (616)945-4107

★ 7061 ★ American Cancer Society
Bay Area Service Center
1480 W Center Rd., Ste. 1
Essexville, MI 48732
Phone: (989)895-1730 **Free:** 800-728-2323
Fax: (989)895-1745
Website: http://www.gl.cancer.org
Linda Johnson, Exec Director

★ 7062 ★ American Cancer Society
Capital Area Service Center
1755 Abbey Rd.
East Lansing, MI 48823
Phone: (517)332-3300 **Fax:** (517)887-8152

★ 7063 ★ American Cancer Society
East Michigan Area Service Center
2353 S Linden Rd., Ste. B
Flint, MI 48532
Phone: (810)733-3702 **Fax:** (810)733-1480
Website: http://www.gl.cancer.org/
Becky Langtry, Exec Director

★ 7064 ★ American Cancer Society
Gladwin County Office
110 Ross St.
Beaverton, MI 48612
Phone: (989)895-1730 **Fax:** (989)435-8011

★ 7065 ★ American Cancer Society
Huron Valley Area Service Center
2010 Hogsback Rd., Ste. 6
Ann Arbor, MI 48105
Phone: (734)971-4300 **Fax:** (734)971-2818
Website: http://www.gl.cancer.org/
Amy Thompson-Boyk, Exec Director

★ 7066 ★ American Cancer Society
Ionia County Office
PO Box 45
Ionia, MI 48846
Phone: (866)364-6284

★ 7067 ★ American Cancer Society
Lakeshore Area Service Center
854 S Washington Ave., Ste. 410
Holland, MI 49423
Phone: (616)396-5576 **Fax:** (616)396-2673
Website: http://www.gl.cancer.org/
Jeff Compagner, Exec Director

★ 7068 ★ American Cancer Society
Livingston County Office
7208 W Grand River
Brighton, MI 48114
Phone: (810)225-8590 **Free:** (734)971-2818
Website: http://www.gl.cancer.org
Amy Thompson-Boyk, Exec Director

★ 7069 ★ American Cancer Society
Macomb Office
39425 Garfield, Ste. 24
Clinton Township, MI 48038
Phone: (586)263-8000 **Fax:** (586)263-5650
Website: http://www.gl.cancer.org/
Megan White, Exec Director

★ 7070 ★ American Cancer Society
Metro Detroit Area Service Center
18505 W 12 Mile Rd.
Southfield, MI 48076
Phone: (248)557-5353 **Free:** 800-227-2345
Fax: (248)557-6128
Megan White, Exec Director

★ 7071 ★ American Cancer Society
Montcalm County Office
PO Box 701
Greenville, MI 48838
Phone: (866)364-6284

★ 7072 ★ American Cancer Society
Muskegon Office
1383 E Laketon Ave.
Muskegon, MI 49442
Phone: (231)722-7407 **Fax:** (231)722-6267
Jeff Compagner, Director

★ 7073 ★ American Cancer Society
Northern Michigan Area Service Center
525 W 14th St., Ste. 5
Traverse City, MI 49684
Phone: (231)947-0860 **Free:** 800-723-0370
Fax: (231)947-0830
Website: http://www.gl.cancer.org/
Bob Burian, Exec Director

★ 7074 ★ American Cancer Society
South Central Michigan Service Center
715 W Michigan Ave.
Jackson, MI 49201
Phone: (517)787-0382 **Fax:** (517)787-1613
Email: sandysummerfelt@cancer.org
Website: http://www.gl.cancer.org/
Kathey Maitland, Exec Director

★ 7075 ★ American Cancer Society
Southwest Michigan Area Service Center
5110 Sprinkle Rd.
Portage, MI 49002
Phone: (616)349-8719 **Fax:** (616)349-0846

★ 7076 ★ American Cancer Society
Upper Peninsula Area Office
1400 S Carpenter Ave.
Iron Mountain, MI 49801
Phone: (906)776-2150 **Fax:** (906)776-2155

★ 7077 ★ American Cancer Society
West Michigan Area Service Center
400 Ann St. NW, Ste. 202
Grand Rapids, MI 49504
Phone: (616)364-6121 **Fax:** (616)364-6451
Website: http://www.gl.cancer.org/
Deb Sprague, Exec Director

Minnesota

★ 7078 ★ American Cancer Society
Bemidji Office
750 Paul Bunyan Dr. NW, Ste. 7
Bemidji, MN 56601
Phone: (218)444-2810 **Fax:** (218)444-2811

★ 7079 ★ American Cancer Society
Brainerd Office
17 Washington St., Ste. 2
Brainerd, MN 56401
Phone: (218)829-6212 **Fax:** (218)829-6258

★ 7080 ★ American Cancer Society
Duluth Office
130 W Superior St., LL2, Ste. 200
Duluth, MN 55802
Phone: (218)727-7439 **Free:** 800-582-5152
Fax: (218)727-8069
Website: http://www2.cancer.org/state/mw/

★ 7081 ★ American Cancer Society
Grand Rapids Office
Grand Rapids Community Cancer Center
2101 S Hwy. 169, Ste. 2
Grand Rapids, MN 55744
Phone: (218)326-4235 **Fax:** (218)326-5420

★ 7082 ★ American Cancer Society
Mankato Office
227 E Main, Ste. 110
Mankato, MN 56001
Phone: (507)345-1451 **Fax:** (507)345-3093

★ 7083 ★ American Cancer Society
Marshall Office
348 W Main St.
Marshall, MN 56258
Phone: (507)929-5000 **Fax:** (507)929-5005

★ 7084 ★ American Cancer Society
Minneapolis Office
3316 W 66th St.
Edina, MN 55435
Phone: (952)925-2772 **Free:** 800-582-5152
Fax: (952)925-6333

Website: http://www2.cancer.org/state/mn/

★ 7085 ★ American Cancer Society
Moorhead Office
1001 Center Ave., Ste. K
Moorhead, MN 56560
Phone: (218)233-6114 **Free:** 800-225-0289
Fax: (218)236-6307
Website: http://www2.cancer.org/state/mw/

★ 7086 ★ American Cancer Society
Rochester Office
882 7th St. NW
Rochester, MN 55901
Phone: (507)287-2044 **Free:** 800-582-5152
Fax: (507)287-2178
Website: http://www2.cancer.org/state/mw/

★ 7087 ★ American Cancer Society
Saint Cloud Office
3721 23rd St. S, Ste. 102
Saint Cloud, MN 56301
Phone: (320)255-0220 **Free:** 800-293-7028
Fax: (320)255-5517
Website: http://www2.cancer.org/state/mw/

★ 7088 ★ American Cancer Society
St. Paul Office
1096 Raymond Ave.
Saint Paul, MN 55108
Phone: (651)644-1224 **Free:** 800-349-0087
Fax: (651)644-2819

★ 7089 ★ American Cancer Society
Willmar Office
333 Litchfield Ave. SW
Willmar, MN 56201
Phone: (320)235-7237 **Fax:** (320)235-0796

Mississippi

★ 7090 ★ American Cancer Society
Gulfport Office
417 Security Sq.
Gulfport, MS 39507
Phone: (228)896-7024 **Fax:** (228)896-8620

★ 7091 ★ American Cancer Society
Hattiesburg Office
204 W Front St.
Hattiesburg, MS 39401
Phone: (601)545-7770 **Fax:** (601)545-7774

★ 7092 ★ American Cancer Society
Jackson Office
1380 Livingston Ln.
Jackson, MS 39213
Phone: (601)362-8874 **Free:** 800-227-2345
Fax: (601)362-8876
Website: http://www.cancer.org/ms.html

★ 7093 ★ American Cancer Society
Meridian Office
4825-A Poplar Springs Dr.
Meridian, MS 39305
Phone: (601)481-1712 **Fax:** (601)482-0258

Missouri

★ 7094 ★ American Cancer Society
Cape Girardeau Office
937 Broadway, Ste. 302
Cape Girardeau, MO 63701
Phone: (573)334-9197 **Fax:** (573)334-5115
Website: http://www.cancer.org/state/heartland/index.html

★ 7095 ★ American Cancer Society
Columbia Office
33 E Broadway, Ste. 100
Columbia, MO 65203
Phone: (573)443-1496 **Free:** 800-429-7753
Fax: (573)442-9955

★ 7096 ★ American Cancer Society
Hannibal Office
714 Broadway, Ste. 2
Hannibal, MO 63401
Phone: (573)221-4660 **Free:** 800-684-2733
Fax: (573)221-3326

★ 7097 ★ American Cancer Society
Heartland Division
1100 Pennsylvania Ave.
Kansas City, MO 64105
Free: 800-227-2345

★ 7098 ★ American Cancer Society
Jefferson City Office
2413 Hyde Park Rd.
Jefferson City, MO 65109
Phone: (573)635-4821 **Free:** 800-635-9194
Fax: (573)635-7821

★ 7099 ★ American Cancer Society
Joplin Office
2700 McClelland Blvd., Bldg. A, Ste. 110
Joplin, MO 64804
Phone: (417)624-6808 **Free:** 800-ACS-2345
Fax: (417)782-2348

★ 7100 ★ American Cancer Society
O Fallon Office
105 W Pitman
O Fallon, MO 63366
Phone: (636)379-8971 **Fax:** (636)379-8975

★ 7101 ★ American Cancer Society
Osage Beach Office
5740 Hwy. 54, Ste. 1002
Osage Beach, MO 65065
Phone: (573)302-7895 **Fax:** (573)317-1523

★ 7102 ★ American Cancer Society
St. Joseph Office
3931 Sherman Ave.
Saint Joseph, MO 64506
Phone: (816)233-2558 **Free:** 800-356-3161
Fax: (816)233-6952

★ 7103 ★ American Cancer Society
St. Louis Office
4207 Lindell Blvd.
Saint Louis, MO 63108
Phone: (314)286-8100 **Fax:** (314)286-8160
Email: june.shinners@cancer.org
Website: http://www.cancer.org

★ 7104 ★ American Cancer Society
Sikeston Office
201 N New Madrid St.
Sikeston, MO 63801
Phone: (573)471-1823 **Free:** 800-ACS-2345
Fax: (573)471-1372

★ 7105 ★ American Cancer Society
Springfield Office
3322 S Campbell, Ste. R
Springfield, MO 65807
Phone: (417)881-4668 **Fax:** (417)881-7955

★ 7106 ★ American Cancer Society
Trenton Office
406 E 9th St.
Trenton, MO 64683
Phone: (660)359-4484 **Fax:** (660)359-2115

Montana

★ 7107 ★ American Cancer Society
Billings Office
550 N 31st St., Ste. 103
Billings, MT 59101
Phone: (406)256-7150 **Free:** 800-252-5470
Fax: (406)256-7170

★ 7108 ★ American Cancer Society
Missoula Office
3550 Mullan Rd., Ste. 105
Missoula, MT 59808
Phone: (406)542-2191 **Fax:** (406)327-0146

Nebraska

★ 7109 ★ American Cancer Society
Kearney Office
3710 Central Ave.
Kearney, NE 68847
Phone: (308)237-7481 **Fax:** (308)236-2016

★ 7110 ★ American Cancer Society
Lincoln Office
5733 S 34th St., Ste. 500
Lincoln, NE 68516
Phone: (402)423-4888 **Free:** 877-232-4787
Fax: (402)423-4915

★ 7111 ★ American Cancer Society
Omaha Office
9850 Nicholas St., Ste. 200
Omaha, NE 68114
Phone: (402)393-5800 **Fax:** (402)393-7790

Nevada

★ 7112 ★ American Cancer Society
Greater Las Vegas Regional Office
1325 E Harmon Ave.
Las Vegas, NV 89119
Phone: (702)798-6877 **Free:** 800-ACS-2345
Fax: (702)798-0530

★ 7113 ★ American Cancer Society
Northern Nevada Regional Office
6490 S McCarran Blvd., Ste. 40
Reno, NV 89509
Phone: (775)329-0609 **Fax:** (775)329-8592

New Hampshire

★ 7114 ★ American Cancer Society
Midcoastal New England Regional Office
Bedford Office
Gail Singer Memorial Bldg.
360 State Rte. 101, Unit 8
Bedford, NH 03110
Phone: (603)472-8899 **Free:** 800-640-7101
Fax: (603)472-7093
Website: http://www.ne-cancer.org

New Jersey

★ 7115 ★ American Cancer Society
Central New Jersey Region
Fords Office
846 Main St.
Fords, NJ 08863

Phone: (732)738-6800 **Fax:** (732)738-8984

★ 7116 ★ American Cancer Society
Central New Jersey Region
Lawrenceville Office
3076 Princeton Pike
Lawrenceville, NJ 08648
Phone: (609)895-0101 **Fax:** (609)895-0944

★ 7117 ★ American Cancer Society
Jersey Shore Region
Shrewsbury Office
801 Broad St.
Shrewsbury, NJ 07702
Phone: (732)758-8220 **Fax:** (732)758-8225

★ 7118 ★ American Cancer Society
Jersey Shore Region
Toms River Office
1035 Hooper Ave.
Toms River, NJ 08753
Phone: (732)914-1000 **Fax:** (732)914-1004

★ 7119 ★ American Cancer Society
Metro New Jersey Region
Elizabeth Office
507 Westminster Ave.
Elizabeth, NJ 07208
Phone: (908)354-7373 **Fax:** (908)354-0284

★ 7120 ★ American Cancer Society
Metro New Jersey Region
Secaucus Office
150 Meadowlands Pkwy.
Secaucus, NJ 07094
Phone: (201)866-1020 **Fax:** (201)866-2401

★ 7121 ★ American Cancer Society
Metro New Jersey Region
West Orange Office
767 Northfield Ave.
West Orange, NJ 07052
Phone: (973)736-7770 **Fax:** (973)669-5817

★ 7122 ★ American Cancer Society
New Jersey Chinese Unit
Fords Office
846 Main St.
Fords, NJ 08863
Phone: (732)225-8588 **Fax:** (732)225-8589

★ 7123 ★ American Cancer Society
New Jersey Chinese Unit
Parsippany Office
669 Littleton Rd.
Parsippany, NJ 07054
Phone: (973)334-2249 **Fax:** (973)331-5944

★ 7124 ★ American Cancer Society
New Jersey Chinese Unit
Shrewsbury Office
801 Broad St.
Shrewsbury, NJ 07702
Phone: (732)224-8868 **Fax:** (732)224-8821

★ 7125 ★ American Cancer Society
Northern New Jersey Region
Hackensack Office
20 Mercer St.
Hackensack, NJ 07601
Phone: (201)343-2222 **Fax:** (201)343-1839

★ 7126 ★ American Cancer Society
Northern New Jersey Region
Wayne Office
468 Parish Dr., No. 6
Wayne, NJ 07470
Phone: (973)696-1885 **Fax:** (973)696-1916

★ 7127 ★ American Cancer Society
Northwest New Jersey Region
Flemington Office
84 Park Ave.
Flemington, NJ 08822
Phone: (908)782-6112 **Fax:** (908)782-3995

★ 7128 ★ American Cancer Society
Northwest New Jersey Region
Oxford Office
4 Opdyke's Ln.
Oxford, NJ 07863
Phone: (908)453-2103 **Fax:** (908)453-3724

★ 7129 ★ American Cancer Society
Northwest New Jersey Region
Parsippany Office
669 Littleton Rd.
Parsippany, NJ 07054
Phone: (973)331-9300 **Fax:** (973)331-9444

★ 7130 ★ American Cancer Society
Northwest New Jersey Region
Raritan Office
600 1st Ave.
Raritan, NJ 08869
Phone: (908)725-4664 **Fax:** (908)707-1858

★ 7131 ★ American Cancer Society
South Jersey Region
Absecon Office
626 N Shore Rd.
Absecon, NJ 08201
Phone: (609)645-7272 **Fax:** (609)641-9469

★ 7132 ★ American Cancer Society
South Jersey Region
Cape May Court House Office
Burdette Tomlin Memorial Hospital
2 Stone Harbor Blvd.
Cape May Court House, NJ 08210
Phone: (609)465-9587

★ 7133 ★ American Cancer Society
South Jersey Region
Cherry Hill Office
1851 Old Cuthbert Rd.
Cherry Hill, NJ 08034
Phone: (856)616-1650 **Fax:** (856)616-8449

★ 7134 ★ American Cancer Society
South Jersey Region
Vineland Office
1400 W Landis Ave.
Vineland, NJ 08360
Phone: (856)692-1364 **Fax:** (856)691-9130

New Mexico

★ 7135 ★ American Cancer Society
Albuquerque Regional Office
5800 Lomas Blvd. NE
Albuquerque, NM 87110-6539
Phone: (505)260-2105 **Free:** 800-ACS-2345
Fax: (505)266-9513
Website: http://www2.cancer.org/state/nm/index.html

★ 7136 ★ American Cancer Society
Clovis Office
PO Box 1856
Clovis, NM 88101
Phone: (505)762-5112 **Fax:** (505)742-1710

★ 7137 ★ American Cancer Society
Northern New Mexico Regional Office
531 Harkle Rd., Ste. B
Santa Fe, NM 87505
Phone: (505)988-5548 **Fax:** (505)986-1940

New York

★ 7138 ★ American Cancer Society
Brooklyn Regional Office
148 Pierrepont St.
Brooklyn, NY 11201
Phone: (718)237-7850 **Fax:** (718)852-9422

★ 7139 ★ American Cancer Society
Capital New York Region
Loudonville Office
260 Osborne Rd.
Loudonville, NY 12211
Phone: (518)438-7841 **Fax:** (518)438-9608

★ 7140 ★ American Cancer Society
Capital New York Region
Queensbury Office
Mt. Royal Plaza
959 State Rte. 9
Queensbury, NY 12804
Phone: (518)792-5358 **Fax:** (518)792-9204

★ 7141 ★ American Cancer Society
Central New York Region
East Syracuse Office
6725 Lyons St.
PO Box 7
East Syracuse, NY 13057
Phone: (315)437-7025 **Fax:** (315)437-8233
Website: http://www2.cancer.org/states/index.cfm?id=35

★ 7142 ★ American Cancer Society
Central New York Region
Malone Office
94 E Main St.
Malone, NY 12953
Phone: (518)483-3636 **Fax:** (518)483-3906

★ 7143 ★ American Cancer Society
Central New York Region
Utica Office
430 Court St., Ste. 205
Utica, NY 13502
Phone: (315)724-8125 **Fax:** (315)738-0517

★ 7144 ★ American Cancer Society
Hudson Valley Region
Kingston Office
95 Schwenk Dr.
Kingston, NY 12401
Phone: (845)331-8300 **Fax:** (845)331-4109

★ 7145 ★ American Cancer Society
Hudson Valley Region
Middletown Office
Wisner Professional Bldg.
419 E Main St.
Middletown, NY 10940
Phone: (845)343-5612 **Fax:** (845)343-8023

★ 7146 ★ American Cancer Society
Hudson Valley Region
Poughkeepsie Office
Vassar Brother's Hospital
45 Reade Pl.
Poughkeepsie, NY 12601
Phone: (845)452-2635 **Fax:** (845)452-8067

★ 7147 ★ American Cancer Society
Hudson Valley Region
Suffern Office
1 Executive Blvd., No. 206
Suffern, NY 10901
Phone: (845)368-1251 **Fax:** (845)368-1255

★ 7148 ★ American Cancer Society
Lakes Region Office
1400 Winton Rd. N
Rochester, NY 14609
Phone: (585)288-1950 **Fax:** (585)288-6467

★ 7149 ★ American Cancer Society
Manhattan/Bronx Regional Office
271 W 125th St., Ste. 210
New York, NY 10027
Phone: (212)663-8800 **Fax:** (212)663-8835

★ 7150 ★ American Cancer Society
Manhattan/Bronx Regional Office
19 W 56th St.
New York, NY 10019
Phone: (212)586-8700 **Fax:** (212)237-3855

★ 7151 ★ American Cancer Society
Nassau Regional Office
839 Stewart Ave.
Garden City, NY 11530
Phone: (516)229-4100 **Fax:** (516)229-4110

★ 7152 ★ American Cancer Society
New York Chinese Unit
Flushing Office
41-60 Main St., No. 206
Flushing, NY 11355
Phone: (718)886-8890 **Fax:** (718)886-8981

★ 7153 ★ American Cancer Society
Queens Regional Office
97-77 Queens Blvd., Ste. 1110
Rego Park, NY 11374
Phone: (718)263-2224 **Fax:** (718)261-0758

★ 7154 ★ American Cancer Society
Southern New York Region
Elmira Office
627 W Church St.
Elmira, NY 14905
Phone: (607)734-1552 **Fax:** (607)734-2435

★ 7155 ★ American Cancer Society
Southern New York Region
Endicott Office
31 Adams Ave.
Endicott, NY 13760
Phone: (607)786-7736 **Fax:** (607)785-6087

★ 7156 ★ American Cancer Society
Southern New York Region
Sidney Office
5 Oak Ave.
Sidney, NY 13838
Phone: (607)563-8462 **Fax:** (607)563-9044

★ 7157 ★ American Cancer Society
Staten Island Regional Office
58 New Dorp Plaza
Staten Island, NY 10306
Phone: (718)987-8871 **Fax:** (718)351-0361

★ 7158 ★ American Cancer Society
Suffolk Regional Office
20 Hampton Rd.
Southampton, NY 11968
Phone: (631)287-6277

★ 7159 ★ American Cancer Society
Suffolk Regional Office
75 Davids Dr.
Hauppauge, NY 11788
Phone: (631)436-7070 **Free:** 800-ACS-2345
Fax: (631)436-5380

★ 7160 ★ American Cancer Society
Westchester Regional Office
2 Lyon Pl.
White Plains, NY 10601
Phone: (914)949-4800 **Fax:** (914)949-8851

★ 7161 ★ American Cancer Society
Western New York Region
Amherst Office
101 John James Audubon Pkwy.
Amherst, NY 14228
Phone: (716)689-6981 **Fax:** (716)689-4923

★ 7162 ★ American Cancer Society
Western New York Region
Buffalo Office
1490 Jefferson Ave.
Buffalo, NY 14208
Phone: (716)882-6428 **Fax:** (716)885-4956

★ 7163 ★ American Cancer Society
Western New York Region
Jamestown Office
113 E 2nd St.
Jamestown, NY 14701
Phone: (716)487-1129 **Fax:** (716)661-3381

North Carolina

★ 7164 ★ American Cancer Society
Asheville Administrative Resource Center
120 Executive Park, Bldg. 1
Asheville, NC 28801
Phone: 800-282-4914 **Fax:** (828)252-8890

★ 7165 ★ American Cancer Society
Greenville Administrative Resource Center
930-B Wellness Dr.
Greenville, NC 27834
Phone: 800-282-4914 **Fax:** (252)695-0671

★ 7166 ★ American Cancer Society
Hope Lodge Office
930-A Wellness Dr.
Greenville, NC 27834
Phone: (252)816-4994 **Fax:** (252)695-6557

★ 7167 ★ American Cancer Society
Metrolina Administrative Resource Center
500 E Morehead St., Ste. 211
Charlotte, NC 28202
Phone: 800-282-4914 **Fax:** (704)376-0516

★ 7168 ★ American Cancer Society
Raleigh Administrative Resource Center
11 S Boylan Ave., Ste. 221
Raleigh, NC 27603
Phone: (919)834-8463 **Free:** 800-282-4914
Fax: (919)839-0551

★ 7169 ★ American Cancer Society
Triad Administrative Resource Center
4-A Oak Branch Dr.
Greensboro, NC 27407
Phone: 800-282-4914 **Fax:** (336)834-8777

★ 7170 ★ American Cancer Society
Wilmington Administrative Resource Center
3131 Wrightsville Ave.
Wilmington, NC 28403
Phone: 800-282-4914 **Fax:** (910)763-1936

North Dakota

★ 7171 ★ American Cancer Society
Bismarck Office
1102 S Washington St., Ste. 105
Bismarck, ND 58504
Phone: (701)224-9954 **Fax:** (701)250-9145

★ 7172 ★ American Cancer Society
Fargo Office
121 Roberts St.
Fargo, ND 58102
Phone: (701)232-1385 **Free:** 800-342-4535
Fax: (701)232-1109
Website: http://www.cancer.org/nd.html

★ 7173 ★ American Cancer Society
Grand Forks Office
1832 S Washington St.
Grand Forks, ND 58201
Phone: (701)792-3333 **Fax:** (701)792-3334

★ 7174 ★ American Cancer Society
Minot Office
600 22nd Ave. NW
Minot, ND 58701
Phone: (701)838-5550 **Fax:** (701)838-4710

Ohio

★ 7175 ★ American Cancer Society
Allen Area Office
616 S Collett St.
Lima, OH 45805
Phone: (419)225-8860 **Free:** 888-227-6446
Fax: (419)225-8862
Website: http://www.oh.cancer.org

★ 7176 ★ American Cancer Society
Clark/Miami Area Office
1130 Vester Ave.
Springfield, OH 45503
Phone: (937)399-0809 **Free:** 888-227-6446
Fax: (937)399-2060
Website: http://www.oh.cancer.org

★ 7177 ★ American Cancer Society
Cuyahoga County Office
10501 Euclid Ave.
Cleveland, OH 44106
Phone: (216)241-1177 **Free:** 888-227-6446
Fax: (216)241-0334
Website: http://www.oh.cancer.org

★ 7178 ★ American Cancer Society
Defiance Area Office
419 5th St., Ste. 2030
Defiance, OH 43512
Phone: (419)782-6866 **Free:** 888-227-6446
Fax: (419)782-4372
Website: http://www.oh.cancer.org

★ 7179 ★ American Cancer Society
Fairfield Area Office
151 Lake St.
Lancaster, OH 43130
Phone: (740)653-5632 **Free:** 888-227-6446
Fax: (740)653-5677
Website: http://www.oh.cancer.org

★ 7180 ★ American Cancer Society
Franklin County Office
870 Michigan Ave.
Columbus, OH 43215
Phone: (614)228-8466 **Free:** 888-227-6446
Fax: (614)228-4456
Website: http://www.oh.cancer.org

★ 7181 ★ American Cancer Society
Geauga Area Office
7861 Crile Rd.
Concord, OH 44077
Phone: (440)358-0864 **Free:** 888-227-6446
Fax: (440)358-9073
Website: http://www.oh.cancer.org

★ 7182 ★ American Cancer Society
Hamilton County Office
11117 Kenwood Rd.
Cincinnati, OH 45242
Phone: (513)891-1600 **Free:** 888-227-6446
Fax: (513)891-5583
Website: http://www.oh.cancer.org

★ 7183 ★ American Cancer Society
Hancock Office
110 S Main St.
Findlay, OH 45840
Phone: (419)423-0456 **Free:** 888-227-6446
Fax: (419)423-1120
Website: http://www.oh.cancer.org

★ 7184 ★ American Cancer Society
Lorain Area Office
43099 N Ridge Rd.
Elyria, OH 44035
Phone: (440)324-2211 **Free:** 888-227-6446
Fax: (440)324-4217
Website: http://www.oh.cancer.org

★ 7185 ★ American Cancer Society
Lucas County Office
135 Chesterfield Dr., No. 100
Maumee, OH 43537
Phone: (419)891-9200 **Free:** 888-227-6446
Fax: (419)891-9223
Website: http://www.oh.cancer.org

★ 7186 ★ American Cancer Society
Mahoning County Office
525 N Broad St.
Canfield, OH 44406
Phone: (330)533-0546 **Free:** 888-227-6446
Fax: (330)533-1678
Website: http://www.oh.cancer.org

★ 7187 ★ American Cancer Society
Marion Area Office
253 E Church St.
Marion, OH 43302
Phone: (740)387-3202 **Free:** 888-227-6446
Fax: (740)383-2988
Website: http://www.oh.cancer.org

★ 7188 ★ American Cancer Society
Mercer Area Office
105 S Walnut St.
Celina, OH 45822
Phone: 888-227-6446 **Fax:** (419)486-3490

★ 7189 ★ American Cancer Society
Montgomery Area Office
40 S Perry St., Ste. 120
Dayton, OH 45402
Phone: (937)223-8521 **Free:** 888-227-6446
Fax: (937)223-5435
Website: http://www.oh.cancer.org

★ 7190 ★ American Cancer Society
Muskingum Area Office
3612 Maple Ave.
Zanesville, OH 43702
Phone: (740)454-2589 **Free:** 888-227-6446
Fax: (740)374-5168
Website: http://www.oh.cancer.org

★ 7191 ★ American Cancer Society
Pickaway Area Office
469 E Ohio St.
PO Box 67
Circleville, OH 43113
Phone: 888-227-6446 **Fax:** (740)474-6078

★ 7192 ★ American Cancer Society
Ross Area Office
138 Marietta Rd., Ste. D
Chillicothe, OH 45601
Phone: (740)702-1160 **Free:** 888-227-6446
Fax: (740)702-1163
Website: http://www.oh.cancer.org

★ 7193 ★ American Cancer Society
Southwest Ohio Area Office
5378-A Cox Smith Rd.
Mason, OH 45040
Phone: 888-227-6446 **Fax:** (513)229-4994

★ 7194 ★ American Cancer Society
Stark Area Office
925 S Main St.
North Canton, OH 44720
Phone: (330)497-7100 **Free:** 888-227-6446
Fax: (330)966-0436
Website: http://www.oh.cancer.org

★ 7195 ★ American Cancer Society
Summit Area Office
1900 W Market St.
Akron, OH 44313
Phone: (330)865-1200 **Free:** 888-227-6446
Fax: (330)865-1205
Website: http://www.oh.cancer.org
Kathy Singer, Exec Director

★ 7196 ★ American Cancer Society
Trumbull Area Office
525 N Broad, Rte. 46
Canfield, OH 44406
Phone: 888-227-6446 **Fax:** (330)533-1678

★ 7197 ★ American Cancer Society
Tuscarawas Area Office
201A W Ohio Ave.
Dover, OH 44622
Phone: 888-227-6446 **Fax:** (330)602-5062

★ 7198 ★ American Cancer Society
Washington Area Office
215 Marion St.
Marietta, OH 45750
Phone: (740)374-5464 **Free:** 888-227-6446
Fax: (740)374-5464
Website: http://www.oh.cancer.org

★ 7199 ★ American Cancer Society
Wood Area Office
1045 N Main St., Ste. 8
Bowling Green, OH 43402
Phone: (419)353-5645 **Free:** 888-227-6446
Fax: (419)352-8041
Website: http://www.oh.cancer.org

Oklahoma

★ 7200 ★ American Cancer Society
Lawton Office
1305 W Gore Blvd., Ste. A
Lawton, OK 73501
Phone: (580)353-8145 **Fax:** (580)353-8146
Website: http://www.cancer.org/state/heartland/

★ 7201 ★ American Cancer Society
Norman Office
2420 Springer Dr., Ste. 205
Norman, OK 73069
Phone: (405)329-1332 **Free:** 888-320-3757
Fax: (405)329-1334
Email: amcgrew@cancer.org
Website: http://www.cancer.org/state/heartland/

★ 7202 ★ American Cancer Society
Oklahoma City Office
8400 Silver Crossing, Ste. H
Oklahoma City, OK 73132
Phone: (405)843-9888 **Free:** 800-733-9888
Fax: (405)848-0795
Website: http://www.cancer.org/state/heartland/

★ 7203 ★ American Cancer Society
Tulsa Office
5110 S Yale, Ste. 101
Tulsa, OK 74135
Phone: (918)743-6767 **Free:** 888-376-1725
Fax: (918)743-9655
Website: http://www.cancer.org/state/heartland

Oregon

★ 7204 ★ American Cancer Society
Eugene Office
2350 Oakmont Way, Ste. 200
Eugene, OR 97401
Phone: (541)484-2211 **Fax:** (541)687-9624

★ 7205 ★ American Cancer Society
Medford Office
31 W 6th
Medford, OR 97501
Phone: (541)779-6091 **Fax:** (541)779-1470

★ 7206 ★ American Cancer Society, Northwest Division
Portland Office
0330 SW Curry St.
Portland, OR 97201
Phone: (503)295-6422 **Free:** 800-577-6552
Fax: (503)228-1062

Pennsylvania

★ 7207 ★ American Cancer Society
Adams Office
424 E Middle St.
Gettysburg, PA 17325
Phone: (717)334-5352 **Fax:** (717)334-3974

★ 7208 ★ American Cancer Society
Bedford Office
322 S Juliana St., Ste. 8
Bedford, PA 15522
Phone: (814)623-8819 **Fax:** (814)623-6518

★ 7209 ★ American Cancer Society
Berks Office
498 Bellevue Ave.
Reading, PA 19605
Phone: (610)921-2328 **Fax:** (610)921-9521

★ 7210 ★ American Cancer Society
Blair Office
1004 N Juniata St.
Hollidaysburg, PA 16648
Phone: (814)695-9511 **Fax:** (814)695-8986

★ 7211 ★ American Cancer Society
Bux-Mont Office
High Point Professional Bldg.
700 Horizon Cir., Ste. 201
Chalfont, PA 18914
Phone: (215)712-3290 **Fax:** (215)712-3298

★ 7212 ★ American Cancer Society
Cambria Office
351 Budfield St.
Johnstown, PA 15904
Phone: (814)266-8744 **Fax:** (814)266-7754

★ 7213 ★ American Cancer Society
Cameron Office
135 W 4th St.
Emporium, PA 15834
Phone: (814)486-0911 **Fax:** (814)486-0825

★ 7214 ★ American Cancer Society
Capital Regional Office
3211 N Front St., Ste. 100
Harrisburg, PA 17110
Phone: (717)231-5780 **Fax:** (717)231-5784

★ 7215 ★ American Cancer Society
Carbon-Tamaqua Office
33 W Ridge St.
Lansford, PA 18232
Phone: (610)921-2328 **Fax:** (570)645-8845

★ 7216 ★ American Cancer Society
Centre Office
123 S Sparks St.
State College, PA 16801
Phone: (814)238-8908 **Fax:** (814)238-3236

★ 7217 ★ American Cancer Society
Chester County Office
428 Exton Commons
Exton, PA 19341
Phone: (610)363-6720

★ 7218 ★ American Cancer Society
Clarion Office
133B W Main St.
PO Box 408
Clarion, PA 16214
Phone: (814)226-7261 **Fax:** (814)226-8352

★ 7219 ★ American Cancer Society
Clearfield Office
119 E Market St.
Clearfield, PA 16830
Phone: (814)765-6988 **Fax:** (814)765-6744

★ 7220 ★ American Cancer Society
Corry Area Office
2 S Center St.
PO Box 103
Corry, PA 16407
Phone: (814)665-1691 **Fax:** (814)664-3851

★ 7221 ★ American Cancer Society
Crawford Office
464 Pine St.
Meadville, PA 16335
Phone: (814)337-8300 **Fax:** (814)337-8303

★ 7222 ★ American Cancer Society
Delaware County Office
600 N Jackson St., 2nd Fl.
Media, PA 19063
Phone: (610)565-1009 **Fax:** (610)892-9438

★ 7223 ★ American Cancer Society
DuBois Gateway Area Office
993 Beaver Dr.
Du Bois, PA 15801
Phone: (814)375-3548 **Fax:** (814)375-4430

★ 7224 ★ American Cancer Society
Elk Office
117 N Michael St.
Saint Marys, PA 15857
Phone: (814)834-9796 **Fax:** (814)834-7149

★ 7225 ★ American Cancer Society
Erie Office
2115 W 38th St.
Erie, PA 16508
Phone: (814)866-5077 **Fax:** (814)866-3890

★ 7226 ★ American Cancer Society
Franklin Office
452 E King St.
Chambersburg, PA 17201
Phone: (717)264-4412 **Fax:** (717)264-0765

★ 7227 ★ American Cancer Society
Fulton Office
452 E King St.
Chambersburg, PA 17201
Phone: (717)264-4412 **Fax:** (717)264-0765

★ 7228 ★ American Cancer Society
Hanover Office
1 Center Sq., Ste. 4
Hanover, PA 17331
Phone: (717)632-4918

★ 7229 ★ American Cancer Society
Huntingdon Office
RD 1, Box 33D
Huntingdon, PA 16652
Phone: (814)627-0083 **Fax:** (814)627-0089

★ 7230 ★ American Cancer Society
Jefferson Office
103 N Gilpin St.
Punxsutawney, PA 15767
Phone: (814)938-6460 **Fax:** (814)938-9437

★ 7231 ★ American Cancer Society
Lancaster Office
314 Good Dr.
Lancaster, PA 17603
Phone: (717)397-3744 **Fax:** (717)397-1526

★ 7232 ★ American Cancer Society
Lebanon Office
701 Cumberland St.
Lebanon, PA 17042
Phone: (717)273-4582 **Fax:** (717)273-3891

★ 7233 ★ American Cancer Society
Lehigh Valley Office
2121 City Line Rd.
Bethlehem, PA 18017
Phone: (610)921-2328 **Fax:** (610)882-5861

★ 7234 ★ American Cancer Society
McKean Office
121 Main St.
Bradford, PA 16701
Phone: (814)368-6183 **Fax:** (814)368-1174

★ 7235 ★ American Cancer Society
Mercer Office
19 Jefferson Ave.
Sharon, PA 16146
Phone: (724)346-3529 **Fax:** (724)346-1896

★ 7236 ★ American Cancer Society
Mifflin-Juniata Office
26 N Brown St.
Lewistown, PA 17044
Phone: (717)248-1421 **Fax:** (717)248-8015

★ 7237 ★ American Cancer Society
North Central Regional Office
1948 E 3rd St.
Williamsport, PA 17701
Phone: (570)326-4149 **Fax:** (570)326-7767

★ 7238 ★ American Cancer Society
Northeast Region
Greater Hazleton Unit
St. Gabriel House
132 S Wyoming St.
Hazleton, PA 18201
Phone: (570)459-1212 **Fax:** (570)454-2544

★ 7239 ★ American Cancer Society
Northeast Region
Monroe Unit
Business 209
RR 2, Box 2138
Stroudsburg, PA 18360
Phone: (570)421-7010 **Fax:** (570)421-8891

★ 7240 ★ American Cancer Society
Northeast Region
Susquehanna/Wyoming Unit
PO Box 4
Montrose, PA 18801
Phone: (570)278-1694 **Fax:** (570)278-2021

★ 7241 ★ American Cancer Society
Northeast Region
Wayne Unit
627 Main St., Lower Level
Honesdale, PA 18431
Phone: (570)253-3350 **Fax:** (570)253-9426

★ 7242 ★ American Cancer Society
Northeast Region
Wyoming Valley Unit
71 N Franklin St., Rm. 110
Wilkes Barre, PA 18701
Phone: (570)825-7763 **Fax:** (570)822-8673

★ 7243 ★ American Cancer Society
Northeast Region Office
Lackawanna Office
1101 Hill St.
Jessup, PA 18434
Phone: (570)383-4700 **Fax:** (570)383-4707

★ 7244 ★ American Cancer Society
Northeast Regional Office
Jessup Unit
1101 Hill St.
Jessup, PA 18434
Phone: (570)383-4700 **Fax:** (570)383-4707

★ 7245 ★ American Cancer Society
Northeast Regional Office
Pike Unit
110 W Harford St.
Milford, PA 18337
Phone: (570)296-7676

★ 7246 ★ American Cancer Society
Potter Office
538 E 2nd St., Rm. 1
Coudersport, PA 16915
Phone: (814)274-8330 **Fax:** (814)274-7724

★ 7247 ★ American Cancer Society
Schuylkill Office
512 N Centre St., Ste. 1-B
Pottsville, PA 17901
Phone: (610)921-2328 **Fax:** (570)622-8549

★ 7248 ★ American Cancer Society
Somerset Office
168 W Union St.
Somerset, PA 15501
Phone: (814)445-2584 **Fax:** (814)443-9585

★ 7249 ★ American Cancer Society
Southeast Philadelphia Regional Office
1626 Locust St.
Philadelphia, PA 19103
Phone: (215)985-5400 **Free:** 800-ACS-2345
Fax: (215)985-5406

★ 7250 ★ American Cancer Society
Southwest Region
Beaver Unit
320 Bilmar Dr.
Pittsburgh, PA 15205
Phone: (412)919-1100 **Free:** 888-227-5445
Fax: (412)919-1101

★ 7251 ★ American Cancer Society
Southwest Regional Office
320 Bilmar Dr.
Pittsburgh, PA 15205
Phone: (412)919-1100 **Fax:** (412)919-1101

★ 7252 ★ American Cancer Society
Venango-Forest Office
10 W Front St.
Oil City, PA 16301
Phone: (814)677-3077 **Fax:** (814)676-1995

★ 7253 ★ American Cancer Society
Warren Office
2 S State St.
North Warren, PA 16365
Phone: (814)723-5780 **Fax:** (814)723-0135

★ 7254 ★ American Cancer Society
York Office
924 N Colonial Ave.
York, PA 17403
Phone: (717)848-1841 **Fax:** (717)852-0919

Puerto Rico

★ 7255 ★ American Cancer Society
Puerto Rico Division
Arecibo Office
(Sociedad Americana del Cancer de Puerto Rico, Inc.)
URB Radioville
Calle No. 2, Casa No. 4
Arecibo, PR 00612
Phone: (787)879-0656 **Free:** 800-ACS-2345
Fax: (787)879-0656
Email: diananunzpr/acs/us@cancer.org
Website: http://www.cancer.org

★ 7256 ★ American Cancer Society
Puerto Rico Division
Caguas Office
(Sociedad Americana del Cancer de Puerto Rico, Inc.)
San Juan Bautista Medical Ctr.
Primer Piso Carr. 172
Caguas, PR 00725
Phone: (787)743-4040 **Fax:** (787)744-4336
Website: http://www@cancer.org

★ 7257 ★ American Cancer Society
Puerto Rico Division
Mayaguez Office
(Sociedad Americana del Cancer de Puerto Rico, Inc.)
Calle Prolongacion Vadi 203
Mayaguez, PR 00680
Phone: (787)833-3320 **Fax:** (787)833-3320

★ 7258 ★ American Cancer Society
Puerto Rico Division
Ponce Office
(Sociedad Americana del Cancer de Puerto Rico, Inc.)
716 Calle Ferrocarril
Ponce, PR 00717
Phone: (787)844-1037 **Fax:** (787)844-1037

Rhode Island

★ 7259 ★ American Cancer Society
Rhode Island Division
East Bay Unit
400 Main St.
Pawtucket, RI 02860-2996
Phone: (401)722-8480 **Free:** 800-364-5520
Fax: (401)727-9449
Website: http://www.ne-cancer.org

★ 7260 ★ American Cancer Society
Rhode Island & Eastern Connecticut Division
Providence Office
222 Richmond St., Ste. 200
Providence, RI 02903
Phone: (401)722-8480 **Fax:** (401)421-0535

South Carolina

★ 7261 ★ American Cancer Society
Aiken Office
115 Greenville St.
Aiken, SC 29801
Phone: 800-282-4914 **Fax:** (803)648-5094

★ 7262 ★ American Cancer Society
Central Midlands Office
Westpark Plaza
128 Stonemark Ln.
Columbia, SC 29210
Phone: (803)750-1693 **Free:** 800-282-4914
Fax: (803)750-4000
Website: http://www.cancer.org/state/sc/

★ 7263 ★ American Cancer Society
Charleston Office
5900 Core St., Ste. 504
North Charleston, SC 29406
Phone: 800-282-4914 **Fax:** (843)747-2761

★ 7264 ★ American Cancer Society
Greenville Office
154 Milestone Way
Greenville, SC 29615
Phone: 800-282-4914 **Fax:** (864)458-8454

★ 7265 ★ American Cancer Society
Greenwood Office
Hampton & Merriman
3 Village Square
Greenwood, SC 29648
Phone: 800-282-4914 **Fax:** (864)229-7653

★ 7266 ★ American Cancer Society
Hilton Head Office
15 Palmetto Business Park
Palmetto Bay Rd.
Hilton Head Island, SC 29928
Phone: 800-282-4914 **Fax:** (843)842-9898

★ 7267 ★ American Cancer Society
Myrtle Beach Office
950-48th Ave. N
Myrtle Beach, SC 29577
Phone: 800-282-4914 **Fax:** (843)213-0055

South Dakota

★ 7268 ★ American Cancer Society
Aberdeen Office
310 NW 8th Ave., Ste. 407
Aberdeen, SD 57401
Phone: (605)229-5906 **Fax:** (605)229-1019

★ 7269 ★ American Cancer Society
Mitchell Office
209 E 4th
Mitchell, SD 57301
Phone: (605)996-0121 **Fax:** (605)996-0204

★ 7270 ★ American Cancer Society
Pierre Office
221 S Central Ave.
Pierre, SD 57501
Phone: (605)224-7836 **Fax:** (605)224-7847

★ 7271 ★ American Cancer Society
Rapid City Office
2465 W Chicago St.
Rapid City, SD 57702
Phone: (605)342-7740 **Fax:** (605)399-2062

★ 7272 ★ American Cancer Society
Sioux Falls Office
4101 S Carnegie Pl.
Sioux Falls, SD 57106
Phone: (605)361-8277 **Free:** 800-660-7703
Fax: (605)361-8537
Website: http://www2.cancer.org/state/mw/

★ 7273 ★ American Cancer Society
Watertown Office
525 5th St. SE, Ste. 4
Watertown, SD 57201
Phone: (605)882-2957 **Fax:** (605)882-1701

Tennessee

★ 7274 ★ American Cancer Society
Chattanooga Office
850 Fort Wood St.
Chattanooga, TN 37403
Phone: (423)267-8613 **Fax:** (423)266-8494
Website: http://www2.cancer.org/state/tn/

★ 7275 ★ American Cancer Society
Jackson Office
2935 U.S. Hwy. 45 Bypass
Jackson, TN 38305
Phone: (731)664-4663 **Fax:** (731)664-7858

★ 7276 ★ American Cancer Society
Johnson City Office
508 Princeton Rd., Ste. 102
Johnson City, TN 37601
Phone: (423)926-2921 **Free:** 800-ACS-2345
Fax: (423)283-7112
Email: strivett@cancer.org
Website: http://www2.cancer.org/state/tn/

★ 7277 ★ American Cancer Society
Knoxville Office
871 Weisgarber Rd.
Knoxville, TN 37909
Phone: (865)584-1668 **Fax:** (865)584-1673
Website: http://www2.cancer.org/state/tn/

★ 7278 ★ American Cancer Society
Memphis Office
1378 Union Ave.
Memphis, TN 38104
Phone: (901)278-2000 **Free:** 800-227-2345
Fax: (901)278-2020

★ 7279 ★ American Cancer Society
Nashville Office
2000 Charlotte Ave.
Nashville, TN 37203
Phone: (615)327-0991 **Fax:** (615)327-4038
Website: http://www2.cancer.org/state/tn/

Texas

★ 7280 ★ American Cancer Society
Abilene Office
209 S Danville, Bldg. B, Ste. 107
Abilene, TX 79605
Phone: (915)692-6446 **Fax:** (915)691-9920
Website: http://www.acs-tx.org/Texas.nsf

★ 7281 ★ American Cancer Society
Amarillo Office
3915 Bell St.
Amarillo, TX 79109
Phone: (806)353-4306 **Fax:** (806)354-0668
Website: http://www.acs-tx.org/Texas.nsf

★ 7282 ★ American Cancer Society
Austin Office
2433 Ridgepoint Dr. B
Austin, TX 78754
Phone: (512)919-1870 **Fax:** (512)919-1846
Website: http://www.acs-tx.org/Texas.nsf

★ 7283 ★ American Cancer Society
Beaumont Office
755 S 11th St., Ste. 212
Beaumont, TX 77701-3723
Phone: (409)835-2138

★ 7284 ★ American Cancer Society
Bryan Office
3207 Briarcrest Dr.
Bryan, TX 77802
Phone: (979)776-1463 **Fax:** (979)774-0865

★ 7285 ★ American Cancer Society
Corpus Christi Office
4101 S Alameda
Corpus Christi, TX 78411
Phone: (361)857-0134 **Fax:** (361)854-3260

★ 7286 ★ American Cancer Society
Dallas Office
8900 Carpenter Fwy.
Dallas, TX 75247
Phone: (214)819-1200 **Fax:** (214)631-3869

★ 7287 ★ American Cancer Society
El Paso Office
909 E San Antonio
El Paso, TX 79901
Phone: (915)544-4425 **Fax:** (915)532-3748

★ 7288 ★ American Cancer Society
Fort Worth Office
3301 W Freeway
Fort Worth, TX 76107
Phone: (817)737-9990 **Fax:** (817)737-9977

★ 7289 ★ American Cancer Society
Houston Office
6301 Richmond
Houston, TX 77057
Phone: (713)266-2877 **Fax:** (713)266-4159

★ 7290 ★ American Cancer Society
Laredo Office
Plaza 3, Ste. 1
2329 E Saunders
Laredo, TX 78043
Phone: (956)723-7933 **Fax:** (956)723-6303

★ 7291 ★ American Cancer Society
Lubbock Office
3411 73rd St.
Lubbock, TX 79423
Phone: (806)792-7126 **Fax:** (806)793-0148

★ 7292 ★ American Cancer Society
Lufkin Office
4000 S Medford Dr., Ste. 17E
Lufkin, TX 75901
Phone: (936)634-2883 **Free:** 800-277-2345
Fax: (936)634-2792
Email: l.tullas@cancer.org
Website: http://www.cancer.org

★ 7293 ★ American Cancer Society
Midland Office
2304 W Wadley
Midland, TX 79705
Phone: (915)683-6374 **Fax:** (915)687-5360
Email: vhavins@cancer.org
Website: http://www.cancer.org

★ 7294 ★ American Cancer Society
Odessa Office
811 Central
Odessa, TX 79761
Phone: (915)334-6121 **Fax:** (915)334-7830

★ 7295 ★ American Cancer Society
Rio Grande Valley Office
5413 S McColl Rd.
Edinburg, TX 78539
Phone: (956)682-8320 **Free:** 800-227-2345
Fax: (956)682-8410

★ 7296 ★ American Cancer Society
San Angelo Office
3228 College Hills Blvd.
San Angelo, TX 76904
Phone: (915)944-2509 **Fax:** (915)949-4398

★ 7297 ★ American Cancer Society
San Antonio Office
8115 Datapoint Dr.
San Antonio, TX 78229
Phone: (210)614-4211 **Fax:** (210)615-7724

★ 7298 ★ American Cancer Society
Texarkana Office
5501 Plaza Dr.
Texarkana, TX 75503
Phone: (903)831-5422 **Fax:** (903)831-6521

★ 7299 ★ American Cancer Society
Texas City Office
9002 FM 1764
Texas City, TX 77591
Phone: (409)938-0672 **Fax:** (409)938-0007

★ 7300 ★ American Cancer Society
Tyler Office
1301 S Broadway
Tyler, TX 75701
Phone: (903)597-1348 **Free:** 800-ACS-2345
Fax: (903)531-2350

★ 7301 ★ American Cancer Society
Upper Valley Office
5413 S McColl Rd.
Edinburg, TX 78539
Phone: (956)682-8320 **Fax:** (956)682-8410

★ 7302 ★ American Cancer Society
Victoria Office
4401 Lilac
Victoria, TX 77901
Phone: (361)578-2849 **Free:** 800-ACS-2345
Fax: (361)578-8071
Website: http://www.acstx.org

★ 7303 ★ American Cancer Society
Waco Office
1311 New Rd.
Waco, TX 76710
Phone: (254)753-0806 **Free:** 800-227-2345
Fax: (254)753-0544
Email: jmadden@cancer.org
Website: http://www.cancer.org

★ 7304 ★ American Cancer Society
Wichita Falls Office
2304 Midwestern Pkwy., Ste. 206
Wichita Falls, TX 76308
Phone: (940)691-7201 **Free:** 800-227-2345
Fax: (940)696-0656

Email: mwaggone@cancer.org
Website: http://www.cancer.org

Utah

★ 7305 ★ American Cancer Society
Central Utah Office
819 Palisade Rd.
Sterling, UT 84665
Phone: (435)835-6351 **Fax:** (435)835-6350

★ 7306 ★ American Cancer Society
Greater Salt Lake Office
941 East 3300 South
Salt Lake City, UT 84106
Phone: (801)483-1500 **Fax:** (801)483-1558
Website: http://www2.cancer.org/state/ut/

★ 7307 ★ American Cancer Society
Ogden Office
2404 Washington Blvd., Ste. 218
Ogden, UT 84401
Phone: (801)393-8657 **Fax:** (801)393-2260

★ 7308 ★ American Cancer Society
Provo Office
286 South 600 East, Ste. A
Provo, UT 84606
Phone: (801)373-5886 **Fax:** (801)373-8220

★ 7309 ★ American Cancer Society
Southern Utah Office
592 N Mall Dr.
Saint George, UT 84790
Phone: (435)674-9707

Vermont

★ 7310 ★ American Cancer Society
Northwest New England Region
Montpelier Office
11 Loomis St.
Montpelier, VT 05602
Phone: (802)223-2348 **Fax:** (802)223-4818
Website: http://www.ne-cancer.org/

★ 7311 ★ American Cancer Society
Northwest New England Region
Rutland Office
734-9 US Rte. 4 E
Box H
Rutland, VT 05701
Phone: (802)775-0514 **Fax:** (802)773-8359

★ 7312 ★ American Cancer Society
Northwest New England Region
South Burlington Office
150 Kennedy Dr., Ste. 4
South Burlington, VT 05403
Phone: (802)658-0626

Virgin Islands

★ 7313 ★ American Cancer Society
Saint Croix Office
PO Box 6987
St. Croix, VI 00823
Phone: (340)778-2882 **Fax:** (340)778-2116

★ 7314 ★ American Cancer Society
Saint Thomas/Saint John Office
PO Box 10427
St. Thomas, VI 00801
Phone: (340)775-5373 **Fax:** (340)775-5373

Virginia

★ 7315 ★ American Cancer Society
Abingdon Office
205 W Main St., Ste. 23
Abingdon, VA 24210
Phone: (276)739-7780 **Fax:** (276)739-7781

★ 7316 ★ American Cancer Society
Charlottesville Office
3042-D Berkmar Dr.
Charlottesville, VA 22901
Phone: (434)978-7423 **Fax:** (434)978-1258

★ 7317 ★ American Cancer Society
Glen Allen Office
4240 Park Pl. Ct.
Glen Allen, VA 23060
Phone: (804)527-3700 **Fax:** (804)527-3700
Website: http://www.inet.net/imc/acsworking/va/

★ 7318 ★ American Cancer Society
Harrisonburg Office
1920 H Medical Ave.
Harrisonburg, VA 22801
Phone: (540)434-3360 **Fax:** (540)432-1621

★ 7319 ★ American Cancer Society
Lynchburg Office
2316 Atherholt Rd., Ste. 108
Lynchburg, VA 24501
Phone: (434)845-0973 **Fax:** (434)845-8719

★ 7320 ★ American Cancer Society
Martinsville Office
1079 Spruce St.
Martinsville, VA 24115
Phone: (276)638-8944 **Fax:** (276)638-3778

★ 7321 ★ American Cancer Society
Norfolk Office
2730 Ellsmere Ave.
Norfolk, VA 23513
Phone: (757)853-6638 **Fax:** (757)853-7006

★ 7322 ★ American Cancer Society
Peninsula Office
895 Middleground Blvd., Ste. 154
Newport News, VA 23606
Phone: (757)591-8330 **Fax:** (757)591-8328

★ 7323 ★ American Cancer Society
Roanoke Office
9 E Church Ave.
Roanoke, VA 24011
Phone: (540)344-8699 **Fax:** (540)345-2361

★ 7324 ★ American Cancer Society
Vienna Office
124 Park St. SE
Vienna, VA 22180
Phone: (703)938-5550 **Fax:** (703)938-6779

★ 7325 ★ American Cancer Society
Winchester Office
2654 Valley Ave., Ste. B
Winchester, VA 22601
Phone: (540)667-2315 **Fax:** (540)667-7798

Washington

★ 7326 ★ American Cancer Society
Everett Office
728 134th St. SW, Ste. 101
Everett, WA 98204
Phone: (425)741-8949 **Free:** 800-729-5588
Fax: (425)741-9638
Website: http://www2.cancer.org/states/index.cfm?id=50

★ 7327 ★ American Cancer Society
Kennewick Office
7325 W Deschutes Ave., Ste. A
Kennewick, WA 99336
Phone: (509)783-5108 **Fax:** (509)737-9702
Website: http://www2.cancer.org/states/index.cfm?id=50

★ 7328 ★ American Cancer Society
Spokane Office
1403 W Third
Spokane, WA 99204
Phone: (509)455-3440 **Free:** 800-227-2345
Fax: (509)455-3990

★ 7329 ★ American Cancer Society
Tacoma Office
1551 Broadway, Ste. 200
Tacoma, WA 98402
Phone: (253)272-5767 **Free:** 800-729-3880
Fax: (253)272-4485
Website: http://www2.cancer.org/states/index.cfm?id=50

West Virginia

★ 7330 ★ American Cancer Society
Bluefield Office
1808 Jefferson St.
Bluefield, WV 24701
Phone: (304)327-8770 **Fax:** (304)323-3161

★ 7331 ★ American Cancer Society
Charleston Office
301 RHL Blvd., Stes. 6 and 7
Charleston, WV 25309
Phone: (304)746-9950 **Free:** 800-288-3618
Fax: (304)746-9962

★ 7332 ★ American Cancer Society
Huntington Office
1336 Hal Greer Blvd.
Huntington, WV 25701
Phone: (304)523-7989 **Fax:** (304)523-7996

★ 7333 ★ American Cancer Society
Morgantown Office
300A Scott Ave.
Morgantown, WV 26505
Phone: (304)296-8155 **Fax:** (304)296-6172

★ 7334 ★ American Cancer Society
Parkersburg Office
3901 Briscoe Rd.
PO Box 4451
Parkersburg, WV 26104
Phone: (304)422-1472 **Fax:** (304)422-9569

Wisconsin

★ 7335 ★ American Cancer Society
Appleton Office
14 Tri Park Way, Bldg. 2
Appleton, WI 54914
Phone: (920)739-1201 **Fax:** (920)739-2442

★ 7336 ★ American Cancer Society
Eau Claire Office
2427 N Hillcrest Pkwy., Ste. 7
Altoona, WI 54720
Phone: (715)832-0181 **Fax:** (715)832-8570

★ 7337 ★ American Cancer Society
Franklin Office
9809 S Franklin Dr., Ste. 102
Franklin, WI 53132
Phone: (414)423-8570 **Fax:** (414)423-8538

★ 7338 ★ American Cancer Society
Green Bay Office
3311 S Packerland Dr.
De Pere, WI 54115
Phone: (920)338-1541 **Fax:** (920)338-1545

★ 7339 ★ American Cancer Society
La Crosse Office
1285 Rudy St., Ste. 103
Onalaska, WI 54650
Phone: (608)783-5000 **Fax:** (608)783-5005

★ 7340 ★ American Cancer Society
Madison Office
8317 Elderberry Rd.
Madison, WI 53717
Phone: (608)833-4555 **Fax:** (608)833-1195

★ 7341 ★ American Cancer Society
Pewaukee Office
N19 W24350 Riverwood Dr.
Waukesha, WI 53188
Phone: (262)523-5500 **Fax:** (262)523-9433
Website: http://www2.cancer.org/state/mw/

★ 7342 ★ American Cancer Society
Rhinelander Office
3716 Country Dr., Ste. 4
Rhinelander, WI 54501
Phone: (715)362-2400 **Fax:** (715)362-2433

★ 7343 ★ American Cancer Society
Sheboygan Office
515 Superior Ave.
Sheboygan, WI 53081
Phone: (920)457-5661 **Fax:** (920)457-8760

★ 7344 ★ American Cancer Society
Wausau Office
903 S 17th Ave., Ste. B
Wausau, WI 54401
Phone: (715)848-2881 **Fax:** (715)848-3797

★ 7345 ★ American Cancer Society
West Bend Office
237 N Main St.
West Bend, WI 53095
Phone: (262)338-4060 **Fax:** (262)338-3850

Wyoming

★ 7346 ★ American Cancer Society
Casper Office
152 N Durbin St., Ste. 312
Casper, WY 82601
Phone: (307)577-4892 **Fax:** (307)577-4892

★ 7347 ★ American Cancer Society
Cheyenne Office
4202 Ridge Rd.
Cheyenne, WY 82001
Phone: (307)638-3331 **Fax:** (307)638-1199
Website: http://www.cancer.org/state/wy/

★ 7348 ★ American Cancer Society
Green River Office
560 Uinta Dr., Ste. 3
Green River, WY 82935
Phone: (307)875-5020 **Fax:** (307)875-5024

★ 7349 ★ American Cancer Society
Northwest Wyoming Office
1411 E Fremont St.
Riverton, WY 82501
Phone: (307)857-3265 **Fax:** (307)857-3267

Cerebral Palsy

State chapters of the United Cerebral Palsy Association are listed below. The national office is located at 1660 L St. NW, Ste. 700, Washington, DC 20036. Additional informational can be obtained by calling the national office at (800) 872-5827, or by consulting their web site at http://www.ucpa.org/.

Alabama

★ 7350 ★ United Cerebral Palsy Association
Alabama Chapter
c/o East Central Alabama Chapter
301 EA. Darden Dr.
Box 694
Anniston, AL 36202
Phone: (256)237-8203 **Fax:** (256)235-2388
Email: ucpofeca@hiwaay.net

★ 7351 ★ United Cerebral Palsy Association
East Central Alabama Chapter
301 E A. Darden Dr.
Box 694
Anniston, AL 36202
Phone: (256)237-8203 **Fax:** (256)235-2388
Email: linda@ecaucp.org
Website: http://www.ecaucp.org

★ 7352 ★ United Cerebral Palsy Association
Greater Birmingham Chapter
120 Oslo Cir.
Birmingham, AL 35211
Phone: (205)944-3900 **Fax:** (205)944-3933
Email: lindab@ucpbham.com
Website: http://www.ucpbham.com

★ 7353 ★ United Cerebral Palsy Association
Huntsville and Tennessee Valley Chapter
2075 Max Luther Dr.
Huntsville, AL 35810
Phone: (256)852-5600 **Fax:** (256)852-6722
Email: therapy@ucphuntsville.org

★ 7354 ★ United Cerebral Palsy Association
Mobile Chapter
3058 Dauphin Sq. Connector
Mobile, AL 36607
Phone: (251)479-4900 **Fax:** (251)479-4998
Email: gharger1947@aol.com

★ 7355 ★ United Cerebral Palsy Association
Northwest Alabama Chapter
4212 Jackson Hwy.
Sheffield, AL 35660
Phone: (256)381-4310 **Fax:** (256)381-3478
Email: ucpofnwa@hiwaay.net

★ 7356 ★ United Cerebral Palsy Association
West Alabama Chapter
1100 UCP Pkwy.
Northport, AL 35476
Phone: (205)345-3031 **Fax:** (205)345-3035
Email: toniucpwa@comcast.net

Alaska

★ 7357 ★ United Cerebral Palsy Association
Alaska Chapter/PARENTS, Inc.
4743 Northern Lights Blvd.
Anchorage, AK 99508
Phone: (907)337-7678 **Fax:** (907)337-7671
Email: parents@parentsinc.org
Website: http://www.parentsinc.org

Arizona

★ 7358 ★ United Cerebral Palsy Association
Southern Arizona Chapter
3941 E 29th St., Ste. 601-604
Tucson, AZ 85711
Phone: (520)795-3108 **Fax:** (520)795-3196
Email: staff@ucpsa.org
Website: http://www.ucpsa.org

★ 7359 ★ United Cerebral Palsy Association of Central Arizona, Inc.
321 W Hatcher St., Ste. 102
Phoenix, AZ 85021
Phone: (602)943-5472 **Fax:** (602)943-4936
Email: info@ucpofaz.com
Website: http://www.ucpofaz.com

Arkansas

★ 7360 ★ United Cerebral Palsy Association
Central Arkansas Chapter
9720 N Rodney Parham Rd.
Little Rock, AR 72227
Phone: (501)224-6067 **Fax:** (501)227-5591
Email: info@ucpcark.org
Website: http://www.ucpcark.org

★ 7361 ★ United Cerebral Palsy Association
South Arkansas Chapter
714 W Grove
El Dorado, AR 71730
Phone: (870)863-8194 **Fax:** (870)881-4600

California

★ 7362 ★ United Cerebral Palsy Association
Central California Chapter
4224 N Cedar Ave.
Fresno, CA 93726-3700
Phone: (559)221-8272 **Fax:** (559)221-9347
Email: melishah@ccucp.org
Website: http://www.ccupc.org

★ 7363 ★ United Cerebral Palsy Association
Golden Gate Chapter
1970 Broadway, Ste. 600
Oakland, CA 94612
Phone: (510)832-7430 **Fax:** (510)839-1329
Email: info@ucpgg.org
Website: http://www.ucpgg.org

★ 7364 ★ United Cerebral Palsy Association
Greater Sacramento Chapter
191 Lathrop Way, Ste. N
Sacramento, CA 95815
Phone: (916)565-7700 **Fax:** (916)565-7773
Email: ucp@ucpsacto.org
Website: http://www.ucpsacto.org

★ 7365 ★ United Cerebral Palsy Association
Inland Empire Chapter
35325 Date Palm Dr., Ste. 136
Cathedral City, CA 92234
Phone: (760)321-8184 **Fax:** (760)321-8284
Email: ucpaie@aol.com

★ 7366 ★ United Cerebral Palsy Association
Los Angeles and Ventura Counties Chapter
6430 Independence Ave.
Woodland Hills, CA 91367
Phone: (818)782-2211 **Fax:** (818)909-9106
Email: ucpla@aol.com

★ 7367 ★ United Cerebral Palsy Association
North Bay Chapter
PO Box 7788
Santa Rosa, CA 95407-0788
Phone: (707)566-8647 **Fax:** (707)586-3279
Email: ucpnb@sonic.net

★ 7368 ★ United Cerebral Palsy Association
Orange County Chapter
3010 W Harvard St.
Santa Ana, CA 92704
Phone: (714)557-1291 **Fax:** (714)546-0943
Email: jminer@ucpaoc.org
Website: http://www.ucpaoc.org

★ 7369 ★ United Cerebral Palsy Association
San Diego County Chapter
8525 Gibbs Dr., Ste. 100
San Diego, CA 92123
Phone: (858)571-7803 **Fax:** (858)571-0919
Email: ucpsd@pacbell.net
Website: http://www.san.rr.com/ucpsd/

★ 7370 ★ United Cerebral Palsy Association
San Joaquin, Calaveras, and Amador Counties Chapter
333 W Benjamin Holt Dr., Ste. 1
Stockton, CA 95207
Phone: (209)956-0290 **Fax:** (209)956-0294
Email: jschumacher@ucpsj.org
Website: http://www.ucpsj.org

★ 7371 ★ United Cerebral Palsy Association
San Luis Obispo Chapter
3620 Sacramento Dr., Ste. 201-C
San Luis Obispo, CA 93401
Phone: (805)543-2039 **Fax:** (805)543-2045
Email: ucpslo@fix.net
Website: http://www.ucp-slo.org

★ 7372 ★ United Cerebral Palsy Association
Santa Barbara County Chapter
423 W Victoria St.
Santa Barbara, CA 93101
Phone: (805)966-1112 **Fax:** (805)962-7201
Email: ucpla@aol.com

★ 7373 ★ United Cerebral Palsy Association
Santa Clara and San Mateo Counties Chapter
480 San Antonio Rd., Ste. 215
Mountain View, CA 94040-1218
Phone: (650)917-6900 **Fax:** (650)948-8503
Email: ucp@ucpscsm.org
Website: http://www.ucpscsm.org

★ 7374 ★ United Cerebral Palsy Association
Stanislaus County Chapter
1213 13th St.
Modesto, CA 95354
Phone: (209)577-2122 **Fax:** (209)577-2392
Email: joanb30@hotmail.com

Connecticut

★ 7375 ★ United Cerebral Palsy Association
Eastern Connecticut Chapter
Shaw's Cove 6, Ste. 101
New London, CT 06320
Phone: (860)447-3889 **Fax:** (860)447-3789
Email: united.cerebra.palsy@snet.net

★ 7376 ★ United Cerebral Palsy Association
Greater Hartford Chapter
80 Whitney St.
Hartford, CT 06105
Phone: (860)236-6201 **Fax:** (860)236-6205
Email: ucpgh@netscape.net

★ 7377 ★ United Cerebral Palsy Association
Southern Connecticut Chapter
105C S Elm St.
Wallingford, CT 06492
Phone: (203)269-3511 **Fax:** (203)269-7411
Email: ucpasouthernct@yahoo.com

Delaware

★ 7378 ★ United Cerebral Palsy Association
Delaware Chapter
700A River Rd.
Wilmington, DE 19809-2746
Phone: (302)764-2400 **Fax:** (302)764-8713
Email: williammccool@juno.com

District of Columbia

★ 7379 ★ United Cerebral Palsy Association
Washington DC and Northern Virginia Chapter
3135 8th St. NE
Washington, DC 20017
Phone: (202)269-1500 **Fax:** (202)526-0519
Email: webmaster@ucpdc.org
Website: http://www.ucpdcnova.org

Florida

★ 7380 ★ United Cerebral Palsy Association
Child Development Centers
3305 S Orange Ave.
Orlando, FL 32806
Phone: (407)852-3300 **Fax:** (407)852-3301
Email: mbetts@ucpcdc.org
Website: http://www.ucpcdc.org

★ 7381 ★ United Cerebral Palsy Association
Kentucky Chapter
c/o Sunrise Group
9040 Sunset Dr.
Miami, FL 33173
Phone: (305)596-9040 **Fax:** (305)598-8240
Email: lleech@sunrisegroup.org
Website: http://www.sunrisegroup.org

★ 7382 ★ United Cerebral Palsy Association
North Florida Chapter/Tender Love and Care
1241-B East Ave.
Panama City, FL 32401
Phone: (850)769-7960 **Fax:** (850)769-1060
Email: kdrugachmc@aol.com

★ 7383 ★ United Cerebral Palsy Association
Northeast Florida Chapter
3311 Beach Blvd.
Jacksonville, FL 32207
Phone: (904)396-1462 **Fax:** (904)396-1199
Email: cpnefagency@hotmail.com

★ 7384 ★ United Cerebral Palsy Association
Northwest Florida Chapter
2912 N East St.
Pensacola, FL 32501-1324
Phone: (850)432-1596 **Fax:** (850)432-1930
Email: ucpnwfl@aol.com

★ 7385 ★ United Cerebral Palsy Association
Sarasota-Manatee Chapter
1090 S Tamiami Trail
Sarasota, FL 34236
Phone: (941)957-3599 **Fax:** (941)957-3499
Email: ucpsmi@gte.net

★ 7386 ★ United Cerebral Palsy Association
South Florida Chapter
1411 NW 14th Ave.
Miami, FL 33125
Phone: (305)325-1080 **Fax:** (305)325-1313
Email: info@ucpsouthflorida.org
Website: http://www.ucpsouthflorida.org

★ 7387 ★ United Cerebral Palsy Association
Tallahassee Chapter
1830 Buford Ct.
Tallahassee, FL 32308
Phone: (850)922-5630 **Fax:** (850)922-1258
Email: gator1@nettally.com
Website: http://www.nettally.com/ucp

★ 7388 ★ United Cerebral Palsy Association
Tampa Bay Chapter
2215 E Henry Ave.
Tampa, FL 33610
Phone: (813)239-1179 **Fax:** (813)237-3091
Email: kryals@ucptampa.org
Website: http://www.ucptampa.org

★ 7389 ★ United Cerebral Palsy Association of Florida, Inc.
1830 Buford Ct.
Tallahassee, FL 32308
Phone: (850)878-2141 **Fax:** (850)922-1258

Email: ucpadm@nettally.com

Georgia

★ 7390 ★ United Cerebral Palsy Association
Georgia Chapter
3300 Northeast Expy., Bldg. 9
Atlanta, GA 30341
Phone: (770)676-2000 **Fax:** (770)455-8040
Email: info@ucpga.org
Website: http://www.ucpga.org

Hawaii

★ 7391 ★ United Cerebral Palsy Association
Hawaii Chapter
414 Kuwili St., Ste. 105
Honolulu, HI 96817-5050
Phone: (808)532-6744 **Fax:** (808)532-6747
Email: ucpa@diverseabilities.org
Website: http://www.diverseabilities.org

Idaho

★ 7392 ★ United Cerebral Palsy Association
Idaho Chapter
5420 W Franklin Rd., Ste. A
Boise, ID 83705
Phone: (208)377-8070 **Fax:** (208)322-7133
Email: ucpidaho@aol.com

Illinois

★ 7393 ★ Easter Seals/United Cerebral Palsy Association
507 E Armstrong
Peoria, IL 61603
Phone: (309)686-1177 **Fax:** (309)686-2035
Email: sthompson@easterseals-ucp.org
Website: http://www.easterseals-ucp.org

★ 7394 ★ United Cerebral Palsy Association
East Central Illinois Chapter
2715 N 27th St.
Decatur, IL 62526-2126
Phone: (217)428-5033 **Fax:** (217)428-5094
Email: ucpeci@msn.com

★ 7395 ★ United Cerebral Palsy Association
Greater Chicago Chapter
160 N Wacker Dr.
Chicago, IL 60606
Phone: (312)368-0380 **Fax:** (312)368-0018
Email: pdulle@ucpnet.org
Website: http://www.ucpnet.org

★ 7396 ★ United Cerebral Palsy Association
Illinois Chapter
312 E Adams
Springfield, IL 62701
Phone: (217)528-9681 **Fax:** (217)528-9739
Email: ucpil@aol.com

★ 7397 ★ United Cerebral Palsy Association
Land of Lincoln Chapter
130 N 16th St.
Springfield, IL 62703
Phone: (217)525-6522 **Fax:** (217)525-9017
Email: ucpll@hotmail.com

★ 7398 ★ United Cerebral Palsy Association
Southern Illinois Chapter
9 Cusumano Professional Plaza Dr.
Mount Vernon, IL 62864
Phone: (618)244-2505 **Fax:** (618)244-3568
Email: ucpsi@onemain.com

★ 7399 ★ United Cerebral Palsy Association
Will County Chapter
311 S Reed St.
Joliet, IL 60436
Phone: (815)744-3500 **Fax:** (815)744-3504
Email: ucpwill@ucpwill.org
Website: http://www.ucpwill.org

Indiana

★ 7400 ★ United Cerebral Palsy Association
Greater Indiana Chapter
615 N Alabama St., Ste. 322
Indianapolis, IN 46204-1484
Phone: (317)632-3561 **Fax:** (317)632-3338
Email: donnar@ucpaindy.org

★ 7401 ★ United Cerebral Palsy Association
Wabash Valley Chapter
621 Poplar St.
Terre Haute, IN 47804
Phone: (812)232-6305 **Fax:** (812)234-3683
Email: ucp.wv@verizon.net

Kansas

★ 7402 ★ United Cerebral Palsy Association
Kansas Chapter
5111 E 21st St.
Wichita, KS 67208
Phone: (316)688-1888 **Fax:** (316)688-5687
Email: davej@cprf.org
Website: http://www.cprf.org

Louisiana

★ 7403 ★ United Cerebral Palsy Association
Baton Rouge Chapter
1805 College Dr.
Baton Rouge, LA 70808
Phone: (225)923-3420 **Fax:** (225)922-9316
Email: jketcham@ucpbr.org
Website: http://www.ucpbr.org

★ 7404 ★ United Cerebral Palsy Association
Greater New Orleans Chapter
1000 Leonidas St. and Leake Ave.
New Orleans, LA 70118
Phone: (504)865-0003 **Fax:** (504)865-0300
Email: info@ucpgno.com
Website: http://www.ucpgno.org

Maine

★ 7405 ★ United Cerebral Palsy Association
Northeastern Maine Chapter
700 Mt. Hope Ave., Ste. 320
Bangor, ME 04401
Phone: (207)941-2952 **Fax:** (207)941-2955
Email: ucp2@midmaine.com

Maryland

★ 7406 ★ United Cerebral Palsy Association
Central Maryland Chapter
1700 Reisterstown Rd., Ste. 226
Baltimore, MD 21208-2935
Phone: (410)484-4540 **Free:** 800-451-2452
Fax: (410)484-1807
Email: info@ucp-cm.org
Website: http://www.ucp-cm.org

★ 7407 ★ United Cerebral Palsy Association
Prince Georges and Montgomery Counties Chapter
3901 Woodhaven Ln.
Bowie, MD 20715
Phone: (301)262-4993 **Fax:** (301)262-4982
Email: ucppgmc@aol.com

★ 7408 ★ United Cerebral Palsy Association
Southern Maryland Chapter
211 Chinquapin Round Rd.
Annapolis, MD 21401
Phone: (410)280-2003 **Fax:** (410)269-5757
Email: ucpinfo@ucpsm.org
Website: http://www.ucpsm.org

Massachusetts

★ 7409 ★ United Cerebral Palsy Association
Berkshire County Chapter
141 North St.
Pittsfield, MA 01201
Phone: (413)442-1562 **Fax:** (413)499-4077
Email: ucp@netconnx.net

★ 7410 ★ United Cerebral Palsy Association
Metro Boston Chapter
71 Arsenal St.
Watertown, MA 02472
Phone: (617)926-5480 **Fax:** (617)926-3059
Email: ucpbost@aol.com

Michigan

★ 7411 ★ United Cerebral Palsy Association
Metropolitan Detroit Chapter
23077 Greenfield, Ste. 205
Southfield, MI 48075
Phone: (248)557-5070 **Fax:** (248)557-4456
Email: main@ucpdetroit.org
Website: http://www.ucpdetroit.org

★ 7412 ★ United Cerebral Palsy Association
Michigan Chapter
3401 E Saginaw, Ste. 216
Lansing, MI 48912
Phone: (517)203-1200 **Free:** 800-828-2714
Fax: (517)203-1203
Email: ucp@ucpmichigan.org
Website: http://www.ucpmichigan.org

Minnesota

★ 7413 ★ United Cerebral Palsy Association
Central Minnesota Chapter
510 25th Ave. N
Saint Cloud, MN 56303-3255
Phone: (320)253-0765 **Fax:** (320)253-6753
Email: info@ucpcentralmn.org

Website: http://www.ucpcentralmn.org

★ 7414 ★ United Cerebral Palsy Association
Minnesota Chapter
1821 University Ave. W, Ste. 219 S
Saint Paul, MN 55104-2892
Phone: (651)646-7588 Fax: (651)646-3045
Email: ucpmn@cpinternet.com

Missouri

★ 7415 ★ United Cerebral Palsy Association
Greater Kansas City Chapter
1044 Main St., Ste. 600
Kansas City, MO 64105
Phone: (816)531-4454 Fax: (816)531-3383
Email: bscott@ucpkc.org
Remarks: Also serves Kansas City, Kansas.

★ 7416 ★ United Cerebral Palsy Association
Greater Saint Louis Chapter
8645 Old Bonhomme Rd.
Saint Louis, MO 63132-3999
Phone: (314)994-1600 Fax: (314)994-0179
Email: forkoshr@ucpstl.org
Website: http://www.ucpstl.org

★ 7417 ★ United Cerebral Palsy Association
Missouri Chapter
8645 Old Bonhomme Rd.
Saint Louis, MO 63132-3999
Phone: (314)994-1600 Fax: (314)994-0179

★ 7418 ★ United Cerebral Palsy Association
Northwest Missouri Chapter
3303 Frederick Ave.
Saint Joseph, MO 64506
Phone: (816)364-3836 Fax: (816)390-8546
Email: ucpnwmo@ccp.com

Nebraska

★ 7419 ★ United Cerebral Palsy Association
Nebraska Chapter
7101 Newport Ave., Ste. 309
Omaha, NE 68152
Phone: (402)572-3686 Free: 800-729-2556
Fax: (402)572-3002
Email: ucpofne@aol.com

Nevada

★ 7420 ★ United Cerebral Palsy Association
Northern Nevada Chapter
4068 S McCarran Blvd., Ste. B
Reno, NV 89502-7532
Phone: (775)331-3323 Fax: (775)331-7913
Email: ucpnn@ucpnn.org
Website: http://www.ucpnn.org

New Jersey

★ 7421 ★ United Cerebral Palsy Association
Hudson County Chapter
8814 Kennedy Blvd.
North Bergen, NJ 07047
Phone: (201)662-0080 Fax: (201)861-4605
Email: hudsonucp@aol.com

★ 7422 ★ United Cerebral Palsy Association
Morris-Somerset Chapter
245 Main St., Ste. 113
Chester, NJ 07930
Phone: (908)879-2243 Fax: (908)879-8363
Email: info@ucpmsnj.com
Website: http://www.ucpmsnj.com

New York

★ 7423 ★ United Cerebral Palsy Association
Center for the Disabled
314 S Manning Blvd.
Albany, NY 12208
Phone: (518)437-5602 Fax: (518)437-5667
Email: krafchin@cftd.org
Website: http://www.cftd.org

★ 7424 ★ United Cerebral Palsy Association
Greater Suffolk Chapter
250 Marcus Blvd.
PO Box 18045
Hauppauge, NY 11788
Phone: (631)232-0011 Fax: (631)232-4422
Email: info@ucp-suffolk.org
Website: http://www.ucp-suffolk.org

★ 7425 ★ United Cerebral Palsy Association
Nassau County Chapter
380 Washington Ave.
Roosevelt, NY 11575
Phone: (516)378-2000 Fax: (516)378-0357
Email: info@ucpn.org
Website: http://www.ucpn.org

★ 7426 ★ United Cerebral Palsy Association
New York City Chapter
80 Maiden Ln., 8th Fl.
New York, NY 10038-4811
Phone: (212)683-6700 Fax: (212)685-8394
Email: info@ucpnyc.org
Website: http://www.ucpnyc.org

★ 7427 ★ United Cerebral Palsy Association
Western New York Chapter
7 Community Dr.
Buffalo, NY 14225
Phone: (716)505-5500 Fax: (716)894-8257
Email: info@ucpwny.org
Website: http://www.ucpwny.org

North Carolina

★ 7428 ★ United Cerebral Palsy Association
North Carolina Chapter
PO Box 27707
Raleigh, NC 27611-7707
Phone: (919)832-3787 Fax: (919)832-5928
Email: soneal@ucpnc.org
Website: http://www.ucpnc.com
Remarks: Also serves South Carolina.

Ohio

★ 7429 ★ United Cerebral Palsy Association
Central Ohio Chapter
440 Industrial Mile Rd.
Columbus, OH 43228-2411
Phone: (614)279-0109 Fax: (614)279-2527
Email: ucpoco@mindspring.com

★ 7430 ★ United Cerebral Palsy Association
Cincinnati Chapter
3601 Victory Pkwy.
Cincinnati, OH 45229
Phone: (513)221-4606 Fax: (513)872-5262
Email: ucpcrend@one.net
Remarks: Also serves Kentucky.

★ 7431 ★ United Cerebral Palsy Association
Greater Cleveland Chapter
10011 Euclid Ave.
Cleveland, OH 44106
Phone: (216)791-8363 Fax: (216)721-3372
Email: sdean@ucpcleveland.org
Website: http://www.ucpcleveland.org

Oklahoma

★ 7432 ★ United Cerebral Palsy Association
Oklahoma Chapter
5208 W Reno, Ste. 275
Oklahoma City, OK 73127
Phone: (405)917-7080 Fax: (405)917-7082
Email: oklahoma@ucpok.org
Website: http://www.ucpok.org

Oregon

★ 7433 ★ United Cerebral Palsy Association
Oregon and Southwest Washington Chapter
7830 SE Foster Rd.
Portland, OR 97206
Phone: (503)777-4166 Free: 800-473-4581
Fax: (503)771-8048
Email: ucpa@ucpaorwa.org
Website: http://www.ucpaorwa.org

Pennsylvania

★ 7434 ★ United Cerebral Palsy Association
Beaver, Butler and Lawrence Counties Chapter
114 Skyline Dr.
Butler, PA 16001
Phone: (724)283-3198 Fax: (724)283-5945
Email: ucpbbl@nauticom.net

★ 7435 ★ United Cerebral Palsy Association
Central Pennsylvania Chapter
44 S 38th St.
Camp Hill, PA 17011
Phone: (717)975-0611 Fax: (717)975-0839
Email: kidscenter@ucpcentralpa.org
Website: http://www.ucpcentralpa.org

★ 7436 ★ United Cerebral Palsy Association
MECA Chapter
3745 W 12th St.
Erie, PA 16505
Phone: (814)836-9113 Fax: (814)833-3919
Email: leaton@erie.net

★ 7437 ★ United Cerebral Palsy Association
Pennsylvania Chapter
1902 Market St.
Camp Hill, PA 17011
Phone: (717)761-6129 Fax: (717)761-2534
Email: info@ucpofpa.org

Website: http://www.ucpofpa.org

★ 7438 ★ United Cerebral Palsy Association
Philadelphia and Vicinity Chapter
102 E Mermaid Ln.
Philadelphia, PA 19118
Phone: (215)242-4200 **Fax:** (215)247-4229
Email: ucpkravitz@aol.com

★ 7439 ★ United Cerebral Palsy Association
Pittsburgh Chapter
4638 Centre Ave.
Pittsburgh, PA 15213
Phone: (412)683-7100 **Fax:** (412)683-4160
Email: info@ucppittsburgh.org
Website: http://trfn.clpgh.org/ucp/

★ 7440 ★ United Cerebral Palsy Association
South Central Pennsylvania Chapter
788 Cherrytree Ct.
Hanover, PA 17331
Phone: (717)632-5552 **Fax:** (717)632-2315
Email: sroberts@ucpsouthcentral.org

★ 7441 ★ United Cerebral Palsy Association
Southern Alleghenies Region Chapter
616 Somerset St.
Johnstown, PA 15901
Phone: (814)535-7708 **Fax:** (814)536-8833
Email: ucpsar@yahoo.com

★ 7442 ★ United Cerebral Palsy Association
Southwestern Pennsylvania Chapter
Washington Federal Sq.
190 N Main St., Ste. 306
Washington, PA 15301
Phone: (724)229-0851 **Fax:** (724)229-9252
Email: info@ucpswpa.org
Website: http://www.ucpswpa.org/
Remarks: Also serves West Virginia.

★ 7443 ★ United Cerebral Palsy Association
Western Pennsylvania Chapter
1 Corporate Cir., Ste. 2000
Greensburg, PA 15601
Phone: (724)832-8272 **Fax:** (724)837-8278
Email: gbg@ucpwpa.org
Website: http://www.ucpwpa.org

Rhode Island

★ 7444 ★ United Cerebral Palsy Association
Rhode Island Chapter
200 Main St., Ste. 210
PO Box 36
Pawtucket, RI 02862
Phone: (401)728-1800 **Fax:** (401)728-0182
Email: all@ucpri.org
Website: http://www.ucpri.org

Tennessee

★ 7445 ★ United Cerebral Palsy Association
Mid-South Chapter
4189 Leroy
Memphis, TN 38108
Phone: (901)761-4277 **Fax:** (901)761-7876
Email: ucp@ucpmemphis.org
Website: http://www.ucpmemphis.org

Remarks: Also serves Mississippi.

★ 7446 ★ United Cerebral Palsy Association
Middle Tennessee Chapter
209 10th Ave. S, Ste. 154
Nashville, TN 37203
Phone: (615)242-4091 **Fax:** (615)242-3582
Email: info@ucpnashville.org
Website: http://www.nashville.net/~ucp/index.html

Texas

★ 7447 ★ United Cerebral Palsy Association
Greater Houston Chapter
4500 Bissonnet, Ste. 340
Bellaire, TX 77401
Phone: (713)838-9050 **Fax:** (713)838-9098
Email: swaldner@ucphouston.org
Website: http://www.ucphouston.org

★ 7448 ★ United Cerebral Palsy Association
Metropolitan Dallas Chapter
8802 Harry Hines Blvd.
Dallas, TX 75235
Phone: (214)351-2500 **Free:** 800-999-1898
Fax: (214)351-2610
Email: eddyherrera@ucpdallas.org
Website: http://www.ucpdallas.org

★ 7449 ★ United Cerebral Palsy Association
Tarrant County Chapter
1555 Merrimac Cir., Ste. 102
Fort Worth, TX 76107
Phone: (817)332-7171 **Fax:** (817)332-7601
Email: info@ucptc.org
Website: http://www.ucptc.org

★ 7450 ★ United Cerebral Palsy Association
Texas Chapter
5555 N Lamar St., Ste. L139
Austin, TX 78751
Phone: (512)472-8696 **Free:** 800-798-1492
Fax: (512)472-8026
Email: ucptx@onr.com
Website: http://www.main.org/ucpa

Utah

★ 7451 ★ United Cerebral Palsy Association
Utah Chapter
3550 South 700 West
South Salt Lake, UT 84119
Phone: (801)266-1805 **Fax:** (801)266-2404
Email: shellyp@ucputah.org
Website: http://www.ucputah.org

Washington

★ 7452 ★ United Cerebral Palsy Association
South Puget Sound Chapter
6315 S 19th St., No. 25
Tacoma, WA 98466-6217
Phone: (253)565-1463 **Fax:** (253)565-0153
Email: info@ucp-sps.org
Website: http://www.ucp-sps.org

Wisconsin

★ 7453 ★ United Cerebral Palsy Association
Greater Dane County Chapter
1502 Greenway Cross
Madison, WI 53713
Phone: (608)273-4434 **Fax:** (608)273-3426
Email: ucpgdc@itis.com

★ 7454 ★ United Cerebral Palsy Association
North Central Wisconsin Chapter
740 N 3rd St.
Wausau, WI 54403
Phone: (715)842-8700 **Free:** 800-472-4408
Fax: (715)848-3511
Email: glamping@ucp-wausau.org
Website: http://www.ucp-wausau.org

★ 7455 ★ United Cerebral Palsy Association
Southeastern Wisconsin Chapter
7519 W Oklahoma Ave.
Milwaukee, WI 53219
Phone: (414)329-4500 **Free:** 888-482-7739
Fax: (414)329-4510
Email: ucpofsew@execpc.com
Website: http://www.ucp.org/ucp_local.cfm/155

★ 7456 ★ United Cerebral Palsy Association
West Central Wisconsin Chapter
206 Water St.
Eau Claire, WI 54703
Phone: (715)832-1782 **Fax:** (715)832-8203
Email: ucpwcw@aol.com

★ 7457 ★ United Cerebral Palsy Association
Wisconsin Chapter
206 Water St.
Eau Claire, WI 54703
Phone: (715)832-1782 **Free:** 800-261-1895
Fax: (715)832-8203
Email: ucpwcw@aol.com

Chronic Pain

State chapters of the American Pain Society are listed below. The national office is located at 4700 W Lake Ave., Glenview, IL 60025. Additional information can be obtained by calling the national office at (847) 375-4715, or by consulting their web site at http://www.ampainsoc.org/.

California

★ 7458 ★ American Pain Society
Western USA Pain Society
8700 Beverly Blvd.
Los Angeles, CA 90048
Phone: (310)855-8030 **Fax:** (310)659-3928
Website: Cedars-Sinai Comprehensive Cancer Center
Corinne Manetto, PhD, President

Illinois

★ 7459 ★ American Pain Society
Midwest Pain Society
4700 W Lake Ave.
Glenview, IL 60025
Phone: (847)375-4730 **Fax:** (847)375-4777

Email: jkokkines@amctec.com
Jim Kokkines, Contact

North Carolina

★ 7460 ★ American Pain Society
Southern Pain Society
PO Box 5033
Cary, NC 27512
Phone: (919)303-0045 **Fax:** (919)303-9666
Email: lori@southernpain.org
Website: http://www.southernpain.org
Lori H. Postal, Contact

Pennsylvania

★ 7461 ★ American Pain Society
Greater Philadelphia Pain Society
Park Towne Place, Ste. 108 N
2200 Ben Franklin Parkway
Philadelphia, PA 19130
Phone: (215)557-9705 **Fax:** (215)557-9683
Ed White, Contact

Virginia

★ 7462 ★ American Pain Society
Eastern Pain Association
PO Box 11086
Richmond, VA 23230-1086
Phone: (804)282-0063 **Fax:** (804)282-0090
Email: kay@societyhq.com
Kay Holmes, Contact

★ 7463 ★ American Pain Society
New England Pain Association
2209 Dickens Rd.
Richmond, VA 23230-1086
Phone: (804)282-4011 **Fax:** (804)282-0090
Email: nepa@societyhq.com
Website: http://www.ampainsoc.org/member/nepa/index.htm
Stewart Hinckley, Contact
Paul Arnstein, PhD, President

Crohn's & Colitis

State chapters of the Crohn's and Colitis Foundation of America are listed below. The national office is located at 386 Park Ave. S, 17th Fl., New York, NY 10016-8804. Additional information can be obtained by calling the national office at (800) 932-2423, or by consulting their web site at http://www.ccfa.org/.

Alabama

★ 7464 ★ Crohn's and Colitis Foundation of America
Alabama/Northwest Florida Chapter
244 Goodwin Crest Dr., Ste. 120
Birmingham, AL 35209
Phone: (205)941-9900 **Free:** 800-249-1993
Fax: (205)941-1411
Email: alabama@ccfa.org
Website: http://www.ccfa.org/chapters/alabama/
Pat Talty, Exec Director

Arizona

★ 7465 ★ Crohn's and Colitis Foundation of America
Arizona Chapter
1815 W Missouri Ave., Ste. 103
Phoenix, AZ 85015
Phone: (602)589-7233 **Free:** 800-582-7460
Fax: (602)589-0087
Website: http://www.ccfa.org/chapters/arizona/

California

★ 7466 ★ Crohn's and Colitis Foundation of America
Greater Los Angeles Chapter
3701 Wilshire Blvd., Ste. 1120
Los Angeles, CA 90010
Phone: (213)380-3800 **Fax:** (213)380-5593
Email: losangeles@ccfa.org
Website: http://www.ccfa.org/chapters/losangeles/
Hank Borenstein, Exec Director
Remarks: Also serves Hawaii.

★ 7467 ★ Crohn's and Colitis Foundation of America
Greater San Diego and Desert Area Chapter
2180 Garnet Ave., Ste. 3L
San Diego, CA 92109
Phone: (858)274-8898 **Fax:** (858)274-8896
Email: sandiego@ccfa.org
Website: http://www.ccfa.org/chapters/sandiego/
Pamela Meistrell, Exec Director

★ 7468 ★ Crohn's and Colitis Foundation of America
Long Beach Affiliate
Long Beach Memorial Medical Center
2801 Atlantic Ave., 5th Fl.
Long Beach, CA 90801-1428
Phone: (562)424-9000

★ 7469 ★ Crohn's and Colitis Foundation of America
Northern California Chapter
1730 S Amphlett Blvd., Ste. 230
San Mateo, CA 94402
Phone: (650)578-6590 **Free:** 800-241-0758
Fax: (650)578-6599
Email: ccfagba@pacbell.net
Website: http://www.ccfa.org/chapters/greaterbay/
Carol Gerstein, Exec Director
Frmly: Greater Bay Area Chapter.

★ 7470 ★ Crohn's and Colitis Foundation of America
Orange County Chapter
2030 E 4th St., Ste. 104
Santa Ana, CA 92705
Phone: (714)547-8500 **Fax:** (714)547-8585
Email: orangecounty@ccfa.org
Website: http://www.ccfa.org/chapters/orangecounty/
Kathy Castaneda, Exec Director

Colorado

★ 7471 ★ Crohn's and Colitis Foundation of America
Rocky Mountain Chapter
1777 S Bellaire St., Ste. 120
Denver, CO 80222
Phone: (303)639-9163 **Free:** (866)768-2232
Fax: (303)639-9166
Email: RockyMountain@ccfa.org
Website: http://www.ccfa.org/chapters/rockymountain/
Remarks: Serves Colorado, Nebraska, Utah, and Wyoming.

Connecticut

★ 7472 ★ Crohn's and Colitis Foundation of America
Central Connecticut Chapter
PO Box 185431
Hamden, CT 06518
Phone: (203)876-1693 **Fax:** (203)876-1693
Email: ctccfa@aol.com
Website: http://www.ccfa.org/chapters/centralct/

★ 7473 ★ Crohn's and Colitis Foundation of America
Northern Connecticut Affiliate
PO Box 370614
West Hartford, CT 06137-0614
Email: ccfanorthct@aol.com

Florida

★ 7474 ★ Crohn's and Colitis Foundation of America
Gold Coast/South Florida Chapter
8177 W Glades Rd., Ste. 216
Boca Raton, FL 33434
Phone: (561)218-2929 **Free:** 877-664-2929
Fax: (561)218-2240
Email: goldcoast@ccfa.org
Website: http://www.ccfa.org/chapters/goldcoast/

★ 7475 ★ Crohn's and Colitis Foundation of America
South Florida Chapter
1380 NE Miami Gardens Dr., Ste. 250
North Miami Beach, FL 33179
Phone: (305)354-2788 **Fax:** (305)354-7244
Email: southflorida@ccfa.org
Website: http://www.ccfa.org

Georgia

★ 7476 ★ Crohn's and Colitis Foundation of America
Georgia/Tennessee Chapter
2250 N Druid Hills Rd., Ste. 250
Atlanta, GA 30329
Phone: (404)982-0616 **Free:** 800-472-6795
Fax: (404)982-0656
Website: http://www.ccfa.org/chapters/georgia/
Marcia Greenburg, Exec Director

Illinois

★ 7477 ★ Crohn's and Colitis Foundation of America
Illinois/Carol Fisher Chapter
2250 E Devon Ave., Ste. 244
Des Plaines, IL 60018
Phone: (847)827-0404 **Free:** 800-886-6664
Fax: (847)827-6593
Website: http://www.ccfa.org/chapters/illinois/

Indiana

★ 7478 ★ Crohn's and Colitis Foundation of America
Indiana Chapter
931 E 86th St., Ste. 102
Indianapolis, IN 46240
Phone: (317)259-8071 **Free:** 800-332-6029
Fax: (317)259-8091
Website: http://www.ccfa.org/chapters/indiana/
Jan Koontz, Exec Director

Iowa

★ 7479 ★ Crohn's and Colitis Foundation of America
Eastern Iowa Affiliate
712 26th St. SE
Cedar Rapids, IA 52403-2917
Phone: (319)393-7876
Email: easterniowa@ccfa.org
Website: http://www.ccfa.org/chapters/easterniowa/
Allison Allen, Contact

★ 7480 ★ Crohn's and Colitis Foundation of America
Iowa State Chapter
PO Box 57562
Des Moines, IA 50322
Phone: (515)252-6179 **Fax:** (515)266-1512
Email: iowa@ccfa.org
Website: http://www.ccfa.org/chapters/iowa/

Kentucky

★ 7481 ★ Crohn's and Colitis Foundation of America
Kentucky Chapter
4801 Sherburn Ln., Ste. 201
Louisville, KY 40207
Phone: (502)893-3535 **Fax:** (502)893-3553
Email: kyccfai@aol.com
Website: http://www.ccfa.org/chapters/kentucky/
Remarks: Serves Kentucky and southern Indiana.

Louisiana

★ 7482 ★ Crohn's and Colitis Foundation of America
Louisiana Chapter
4141 Veterans Blvd., Ste. 336
Metairie, LA 70002
Phone: (504)888-1135 **Free:** 800-799-0157
Fax: (504)888-1132
Email: louisiana@ccfa.org
Website: http://www.ccfa.org/chapters/louisiana/
Dr. Robert Hammer, President

Maryland

★ 7483 ★ Crohn's and Colitis Foundation of America
Maryland/South Delaware Chapter
1107 Kenilworth Dr., Ste. 320
Baltimore, MD 21204
Phone: (410)825-5199 **Free:** 800-618-5583
Fax: (410)825-5431
Website: http://www.ccfa.org/chapters/md-southde/

Massachusetts

★ 7484 ★ Crohn's and Colitis Foundation of America
New England Chapter
280 Hillside Ave.
Needham, MA 02494
Phone: (781)449-0324 **Fax:** (781)449-0325
Email: ne@ccfa.org
Website: http://www.ccfa.org/chapters/ne/

Michigan

★ 7485 ★ Crohn's and Colitis Foundation of America
Michigan Chapter
31313 Northwestern Hwy., Ste. 209
Farmington Hills, MI 48334
Phone: (248)737-0900 **Fax:** (248)737-0904
Email: Miccfa@aol.com
Website: http://www.ccfa.org/chapters/michigan/
Bernie Riker, Exec Director

★ 7486 ★ Crohn's and Colitis Foundation of America
Western Michigan Office
125 Ottawa Ave. NW, Ste. 350
Grand Rapids, MI 49503
Phone: (616)774-0805 **Fax:** (616)774-4096
Email: westernmichigan@ccfa.org
Website: http://www.ccfa.org/chapters/westmich/
Pam Seymour, Contact

Minnesota

★ 7487 ★ Crohn's and Colitis Foundation of America
Minnesota/Dakotas Chapter
1885 University Ave. W, Ste. 355
Saint Paul, MN 55104
Phone: (651)917-2424 **Free:** 888-422-3266
Fax: (651)917-2425
Website: http://www.ccfa.org/chapters/minnesota/

Mississippi

★ 7488 ★ Crohn's and Colitis Foundation of America
Mississippi Affiliate
PO Box 631
Ridgeland, MS 39158
Phone: (601)605-1849
Email: mississippi@ccfa.org
Website: http://www.ccfa.org/chapters/mississippi/

Missouri

★ 7489 ★ Crohn's and Colitis Foundation of America
Gateway Chapter
8420 Delmar Ave., Ste. 500A
Saint Louis, MO 63124
Phone: (314)991-0220 **Free:** 800-783-8006
Fax: (314)991-8756
Website: http://www.ccfa.org/chapters/gateway/
Remarks: Serves Missouri, Kansas, southern Illinois, and northeast Arkansas.

New Jersey

★ 7490 ★ Crohn's and Colitis Foundation of America
New Jersey Chapter
45 Wilson Ave.
Manalapan, NJ 07726
Phone: (732)786-9960 **Fax:** (732)786-9964
Email: newjersey@ccfa.org
Website: http://www.ccfa.org/chapters/newjersey/
Rosemarie Golombos, Exec Director

New York

★ 7491 ★ Crohn's and Colitis Foundation of America
Central NY Affiliate
PO Box 47
Syracuse, NY 13206-0047
Free: 877-352-3621
Email: centralny@ccfa.org
Website: http://www.ccfa.org/chapters/centralny

★ 7492 ★ Crohn's and Colitis Foundation of America
Fairfield/Westchester Chapter
200 Bloomingdale Rd., 2nd Fl.
White Plains, NY 10605
Phone: (914)328-2874 **Fax:** (914)328-2946
Email: westfield@ccfa.org
Website: http://www.ccfa.org/chapters/westfield/
Renee Krutoff, Exec Director
Remarks: Serves Fairfield County, Connecticut, as well as Westchester, Putnam, Rockland, and Orange counties, New York.

★ 7493 ★ Crohn's and Colitis Foundation of America
Greater New York Chapter
386 Park Ave. S, 14th Fl.
New York, NY 10016-8804
Phone: (212)679-1570 **Fax:** (212)679-3567
Website: http://www.ccfa.org/chapters/newyork/

★ 7494 ★ Crohn's and Colitis Foundation of America
Long Island Chapter
585 Stewart Ave., Ste. 414
Garden City, NY 11530
Phone: (516)222-5530 **Fax:** (516)222-5535
Email: longisland@ccfa.org
Website: http://www.ccfa.org/chapters/longisland/

★ 7495 ★ Crohn's and Colitis Foundation of America
Rochester Chapter
1279 Chili Ave.
Rochester, NY 14624
Phone: (716)349-4144

★ 7496 ★ Crohn's and Colitis Foundation of America
Upstate/Northeastern New York Chapter
4 Normanskill Blvd.
Delmar, NY 12054
Phone: (518)439-0252
Email: capitalny@ccfa.org
Website: http://www.ccfa.org/chapters/capitalny/
Linda Winston, President

★ 7497 ★ Crohn's and Colitis Foundation of America
Western New York Chapter
PO Box 224
Williamsville, NY 14231-0224
Phone: (716)833-2870
Email: westernny@ccfa.org
Website: http://www.ccfa.org/chapters/westernny/

North Carolina

★ 7498 ★ Crohn's and Colitis Foundation of America
Carolinas Chapter
Charlotte Office
442 S Main St., Ste. 1
Davidson, NC 28036
Phone: (704)894-9751 **Free:** 888-455-3338
Fax: (704)894-9752
Email: northcarolina@ccfa.org
Website: http://www.ccfa.org

★ 7499 ★ Crohn's and Colitis Foundation of America
Carolinas Chapter
Columbia Office
134 McSwain Dr.
West Columbia, NC 29169
Phone: 888-455-3338 **Fax:** (704)894-9752
Email: carolinas@ccfa.org
Website: http://www.ccfa.org/chapters/scarolina/

★ 7500 ★ Crohn's and Colitis Foundation of America
Carolinas Chapter
Raleigh Office
8408 Glenwood Ave., Ste. H
Raleigh, NC 27612
Phone: (919)786-9852 **Free:** 800-360-1433
Fax: (919)786-9854
Email: raleigh@ccfa.org
Website: http://www.ccfa.org/chapters/northcarolina/

Ohio

★ 7501 ★ Crohn's and Colitis Foundation of America
Central Ohio Chapter
2021 E Dublin Granville Rd., Ste. 125
Columbus, OH 43229
Phone: (614)781-9970 **Free:** 800-625-5977
Fax: (614)781-9972
Email: centralohio@ccfa.org
Website: http://www.ccfa.org/chapters/centralohio/

★ 7502 ★ Crohn's and Colitis Foundation of America
Greater Cincinnati Chapter
2139 Auburn Ave.
Cincinnati, OH 45219
Phone: (513)585-1775 **Free:** 877-283-7513
Fax: (513)585-3071
Email: cincinnati@ccfa.org
Website: http://www.ccfa.org/chapters/cincinnati/
Andrea Sothfelder, Contact
Remarks: Also serves the greater Dayton area and northern Kentucky.

★ 7503 ★ Crohn's and Colitis Foundation of America
Northeast Ohio Chapter
23366 Commerce Park Rd., Ste. 210
Beachwood, OH 44122
Phone: (216)831-2692 **Fax:** (216)831-2792
Email: neohio@ccfa.org
Website: http://www.ccfa.org/chapters/neohio/

Oklahoma

★ 7504 ★ Crohn's and Colitis Foundation of America
Oklahoma Chapter
4504 E 67th St., Ste. 125
Tulsa, OK 74136
Phone: (918)523-8540 **Free:** 800-658-1533
Fax: (918)523-8560
Website: http://www.ccfa.org/chapters/oklahoma/

Pennsylvania

★ 7505 ★ Crohn's and Colitis Foundation of America
Philadelphia/Delaware Valley Chapter
367 E St. Rd.
Trevose, PA 19053
Phone: (215)396-9100 **Free:** 888-340-4744
Fax: (215)396-1170
Email: philadelphia@ccfa.org
Website: http://www.ccfa.org/chapters/philadelphia/

★ 7506 ★ Crohn's and Colitis Foundation of America
Western Pennsylvania/West Virginia Chapter
580 S Aiken Ave., Ste. 202
Pittsburgh, PA 15232
Phone: (412)687-9775 **Free:** 800-627-6467
Fax: (412)687-8544
Email: wpawv@ccfa.org
Website: http://www.ccfa.org/chapters/wpawv/

Puerto Rico

★ 7507 ★ Crohn's and Colitis Foundation of America
Puerto Rico Affiliate
56 Marbella St.
San Juan, PR 00907
Phone: (787)727-4481 **Fax:** (787)727-4481
Email: puertorico@ccfa.org
Website: http://www.ccfa.org/chapters/puertorico/

Texas

★ 7508 ★ Crohn's and Colitis Foundation of America
Houston Gulf Coast/South Texas Chapter
5120 Woodway, Ste. 8008
Houston, TX 77056
Phone: (713)572-2232 **Free:** 800-785-2232
Fax: (713)572-2433
Email: houston@ccfa.org
Website: http://www.ccfa.org/chapters/houston/
Monique Bossett, Exec Director

★ 7509 ★ Crohn's and Colitis Foundation of America
North Texas Chapter
9601 White Rock Trail, Ste. 102
Dallas, TX 75238
Phone: (972)243-8959 **Fax:** (972)243-8954
Email: grankin@coserv.net
Website: http://www.ccfa.org/chapters/ntexas/
Greg Rankin, Director

Virginia

★ 7510 ★ Crohn's and Colitis Foundation of America
Greater Washington DC/Virginia Chapter
901 King St., Ste 101
Alexandria, VA 22314
Phone: (703)739-2548 **Free:** 877-807-5271
Fax: (703)739-9657
Email: washingtondc@ccfa.org
Website: http://www.ccfa.org/chapters/washingtondc/

Washington

★ 7511 ★ Crohn's and Colitis Foundation of America
Northwest Chapter
320 Andover Park E, Ste. 270
Seattle, WA 98188
Phone: (206)574-0698 **Free:** 877-703-6900
Fax: (206)574-0869
Email: northwest@ccfa.org
Website: http://www.ccfa.org/chapters/northwest/
Remarks: Serves Alaska, Idaho, Montana, Oregon, and Washington.

Wisconsin

★ 7512 ★ Crohn's and Colitis Foundation of America
Wisconsin Chapter
2401 N Mayfair Rd., Ste. 19
Wauwatosa, WI 53226
Phone: (414)475-5520 **Free:** 877-586-5588
Fax: (414)475-5502
Email: wisconsin@ccfa.org
Website: http://www.ccfa.org/chapters/wisconsin/

Cystic Fibrosis

Listed below are chapters of the Cystic Fibrosis Foundation, 6931 Arlington Rd., Bethesda, MD 20814, (800)FIGHT-CF, http://www.cff.org/.

Alabama

★ 7513 ★ Cystic Fibrosis Foundation
Alabama Chapter
502 Montgomery Hwy., Ste. 101
Birmingham, AL 35216
Phone: (205)870-8565 **Free:** 800-523-2357
Email: alabama@cff.org
Website: http://www.cff.org
Kathleen Ash, Director

Arizona

★ 7514 ★ Cystic Fibrosis Foundation
Arizona Chapter
3800 N Central Ave. Ste 700
Phoenix, AZ 85012
Phone: (602)224-0068 **Fax:** (602)224-0432
Email: arizona@cff.org
Website: http://www.cff.org
Jan Lee Sproat, Director

Arkansas

★ 7515 ★ Cystic Fibrosis Foundation
Arkansas Chapter
1604 Merrill Dr. Ste. D
Little Rock, AR 72211
Phone: (501)224-5888 **Free:** 800-264-0030
Fax: (501)663-6711
Email: arkansas@cff.org
Website: http://www.cff.org
Gloria Redman, Director

California

★ 7516 ★ Cystic Fibrosis Foundation
Northern California Chapter
1939 Harrison St. Ste. 207
Oakland, CA 94612
Phone: (415)677-0155 **Fax:** (415)267-9695
Email: no-calif@cff.org
Website: http://www.cff.org

★ 7517 ★ Cystic Fibrosis Foundation
Southern California Chapter
9820 Willow Creek Rd., Ste. 245
San Diego, CA 92123
Phone: (858)578-2945 **Fax:** (858)578-2865
Email: san-diego@cff.org
Website: http://www.cff.org
Michele Mason, Director

★ 7518 ★ Cystic Fibrosis Foundation
Southern California Chapter—Los Angeles Office
1950 Santelle Blvd., Ste. 328
Los Angeles, CA 90025
Phone: (310)479-8585 **Fax:** (310)473-7307
Email: so-calif-la@cff.org
Website: http://www.cff.org
Katherine Caulfield, Director

★ 7519 ★ Cystic Fibrosis Foundation
Southern California / Utah Office
2150 Town Center Pl., Ste. 120
Anaheim, CA 92806
Phone: (714)938-1393 **Free:** 800-232-8731
Fax: (714)938-1462

Website: http://www.cff.org
Helen Johnson, Director

Colorado

★ 7520 ★ Cystic Fibrosis Foundation
Colorado Chapter
1755 Blake St.
Denver, CO 80202
Phone: (303)296-6610
Email: colorado@cff.org
Website: http://www.cff.org
Penny Barnow, Director

★ 7521 ★ Cystic Fibrosis Foundation
Colorado Chapter
Pikes Peak Office
118 N Tejon St., Ste. 200
Colorado Springs, CO 80903
Phone: (719)444-8966 **Fax:** (719)444-0926
Email: pikes-peak@cff.org
Website: http://www.cff.org
Barbara Furr-Cassidy, Director

Connecticut

★ 7522 ★ Cystic Fibrosis Foundation
Connecticut Chapter
185 Filas Dean Hwy.
Wethersfield, CT 06109
Phone: (860)257-6907 **Free:** 800-841-2828
Fax: (860)257-6903
Email: conn@cff.org
Website: http://www.cff.org
Rosemary Hoffmann, Director

Florida

★ 7523 ★ Cystic Fibrosis Foundation
Florida Chapter
2 Prospect Park Business Center
3443 NW 55th St., Bldg. 7
Fort Lauderdale, FL 33309
Phone: (954)739-5006 **Fax:** (954)739-2890
Email: florida@cff.org
Website: http://www.cff.org
Christina Landshut, Director

★ 7524 ★ Cystic Fibrosis Foundation
Florida Chapter
Tampa Regional Office
1315 S Howard Ave., Ste 102
Tampa, FL 33606
Phone: (813)258-0266 **Fax:** (813)258-3380
Email: tampa-fl@cff.org
Website: http://www.cff.org
Susan Baty, Director

★ 7525 ★ Cystic Fibrosis Foundation
Jacksonville Regional Office
2121 A Corporate Sq. Blvd, Ste. 170
Jacksonville, FL 32216
Phone: (904)724-0064 **Free:** 800-344-4823
Fax: (904)724-0280
Email: jax-fl@cff.org
Website: http://www.cff.org/jacksonville.htm
Claudia Werner, Director

★ 7526 ★ Cystic Fibrosis Foundation
Orlando Regional Office
1080 Woodcock Rd., Ste. 245
Orlando, FL 32803
Phone: (407)896-1113
Email: orlando-fl@cff.org
Website: http://www.cff.org
Suzanne Beranek, Director

★ 7527 ★ Cystic Fibrosis Foundation
Palm Beach Regional Office
2200 N Florida Mango Rd., Ste. 304
West Palm Beach, FL 33409
Phone: (561)683-9965
Email: palm-beach-fl@cff.org
Website: http://www.cff.org
Marie Cook, Director

Georgia

★ 7528 ★ Cystic Fibrosis Foundation
Georgia Chapter
2250 N Druid Hills Rd., Ste. 275
Atlanta, GA 30329
Phone: (404)325-6973 **Free:** 800-476-4483
Fax: (404)325-7921
Email: georgia@cff.org
Website: http://www.cff.org
Maureen A. Fraser, Director

Illinois

★ 7529 ★ Cystic Fibrosis Foundation
Greater Illinois Chapter
150 N Michigan Ave., Ste. 400
Chicago, IL 60601
Phone: (312)236-4491 **Free:** 800-824-5064
Fax: (312)236-2797
Email: illinois@cff.org
Website: http://www.cff.org
Ashton Chase, Director

Indiana

★ 7530 ★ Cystic Fibrosis Foundation
Indiana Chapter
1261 W 86th St., Ste. E2
Indianapolis, IN 46260
Phone: (317)202-9210 **Free:** 800-622-4826
Fax: (317)202-9215
Email: indiana@cff.org
Website: http://www.cff.org
Linda Moritz, Director

Iowa

★ 7531 ★ Cystic Fibrosis Foundation
Iowa Chapter
2600 72nd St., Ste. M
Des Moines, IA 50322
Phone: (515)252-1530 **Free:** 800-798-5151
Fax: (515)252-7684
Email: iowa@cff.org
Website: http://www.cff.org
Lisa Werner, Director

Kentucky

★ 7532 ★ Cystic Fibrosis Foundation
Kentucky / West Virginia Chapter
1941 Bishop Ln., Ste. 507
Louisville, KY 40218
Phone: (502)452-6353 **Free:** 800-526-8126
Fax: (502)456-2936
Email: kent-wv@cff.org
Website: http://www.cff.org
Mary Lee Stevens, Director
Program(s): Medical Education and Training Therapeutics Development Program.

Louisiana

★ 7533 ★ Cystic Fibrosis Foundation
Louisiana Chapter
4621 W Napoleon Ave., Ste. 207
Metairie, LA 70001
Phone: (504)455-5194 **Free:** 800-257-4166
Fax: (504)889-2592
Email: louisiana@cff.org
Website: http://www.cff.org
Renee Ganucheau, Director

★ 7534 ★ Cystic Fibrosis Foundation
Louisiana Chapter
Baton Rouge Regional Office
7354 Alberta Dr. Ste E
Baton Rouge, LA 70808
Phone: (225)769-9994 **Free:** 877-753-9990
Email: baton-rouge@cff.org
Website: http://www.cff.org
Nancy Wertz, Director

Maryland

★ 7535 ★ Cystic Fibrosis Foundation
Maryland Chapter
10616 Beaver Dam Rd., Ste. 6
Hunt Valley, MD 21030
Phone: (410)771-9000 **Free:** 800-731-2873
Email: maryland@cff.org
Website: http://www.cff.org
Josephine Schaeffer, Director

Massachusetts

★ 7536 ★ Cystic Fibrosis Foundation
Massachusetts/Rhode Island Chapter
220 N Main, Ste. 104
Natick, MA 01760
Phone: (508)655-6000 **Free:** 800-966-0444
Email: mass-ri@cff.org
Website: http://www.cff.org
Pamela Spitzer, Director

★ 7537 ★ Cystic Fibrosis Foundation
Rhode Island Chapter
220 N Main St., Ste. 104
Natick, MA 01760
Phone: (508)655-6000 **Free:** 800-966-0444
Email: mass-ri@cff.org
Website: http://www.cff.org
Pamela Spitzer, Director

Michigan

★ 7538 ★ Cystic Fibrosis Foundation
Ann Arbor Office
1100 N Main St.
Ann Arbor, MI 48104
Phone: (734)998-1234
Email: ann-arbor-mi@cff.org
Website: http://www.cff.org

★ 7539 ★ Cystic Fibrosis Foundation
Genesee Valley Regional Office
10775 S Saginaw, Ste. J
Grand Blanc, MI 48439
Phone: (810)603-3271 **Fax:** (810)603-3274
Email: geneseevalleyregional@cff.org
Website: http://www.cff.org
Kaygie Goggins, Director

★ 7540 ★ Cystic Fibrosis Foundation
Greater Michigan Chapter-Eastern Region
3064 Boardwalk
Saginaw, MI 48603
Phone: (989)790-2233 **Free:** 800-968-7169
Fax: (989)790-1050
Email: saginaw-mi@cff.org
Website: http://www.cff.org

★ 7541 ★ Cystic Fibrosis Foundation
Greater Michigan Chapter—Western Region
3835 28th St. SE, Ste. 105
Grand Rapids, MI 49512

Phone: (616)285-8140 **Free:** 800-968-1050
Fax: (616)285-4530
Email: grapids-mi@cff.org
Website: http://www.cff.org
Beth Heyboer, Director

★ 7542 ★ Cystic Fibrosis Foundation
Metro Detroit Chapter
2265 Livernois, Ste. 410
Troy, MI 48083
Phone: (248)269-8759 **Fax:** (248)362-2608
Email: detroit@cff.org
Website: http://www.cff.org
Patricia Lee, Director

Minnesota

★ 7543 ★ Cystic Fibrosis Foundation
Minnesota Chapter
1611 W County Rd. B, Ste. 221
Saint Paul, MN 55113
Phone: (651)631-3290 **Fax:** (651)631-3296
Email: minn@cff.org
Website: http://www.cff.org
Nancy L. Viking, Director
Remarks: Foundation raises money for research to find a cure for cystic fibrosis and to improve the quality of life for persons with the disease. **Program(s):** Gene Therapy; Clinical Research; Research and Development Program Centers; CFF-NIH Gene Therapy Centers; CF Care Centers.

Missouri

★ 7544 ★ Cystic Fibrosis Foundation
Gateway Chapter
200 S Hanley, Ste. 620
Saint Louis, MO 63105
Phone: (314)721-2490 **Free:** 800-727-1464
Fax: (314)721-2809
Email: gateway@cff.org
Website: http://www.cff.org/gateway.htm
Bert Merrell, Director

Nebraska

★ 7545 ★ Cystic Fibrosis Foundation
Nebraska Chapter
10838 Old Mill Rd., Ste. 6
Omaha, NE 68154
Phone: (402)330-6164
Email: nebraska@cff.org
Website: http://www.cff.org
Penny Biever, Director

New Hampshire

★ 7546 ★ Cystic Fibrosis Foundation
Northern New England Chapter
114 Perimeter Rd., Unit E
Nashua, NH 03063
Phone: (603)598-8191 **Free:** 800-757-0203
Fax: (603)598-8167
Email: no-new-eng@cff.org
Website: http://www.cff.org
Christopher Hendry, Director

New Mexico

★ 7547 ★ Cystic Fibrosis Foundation
New Mexico Chapter
4004 Carlisle NE, Ste. B
Albuquerque, NM 87107
Phone: (505)883-1455 **Fax:** (505)883-3998
Email: new-mexico@cff.org
Website: http://www.cff.org
Carolyn Jackson, Director

New York

★ 7548 ★ Cystic Fibrosis Foundation
Central New York Chapter
6700 Old Collamer Rd.
East Syracuse, NY 13057
Phone: (315)463-7965 **Free:** 800-962-6578
Fax: (315)463-8221
Email: central-ny@cff.org
Website: http://www.cff.org
Jennifer Janes, Director

★ 7549 ★ Cystic Fibrosis Foundation
Greater New York Chapter
60 E 42nd St., Ste. 1563
New York, NY 10165
Phone: (212)986-8783 **Fax:** (212)697-4282
Email: greater-ny@cff.org
Website: http://www.cff.org
Doris F. Tulcin, Exec Director

★ 7550 ★ Cystic Fibrosis Foundation
Greater New York Chapter
Long Island Office
420 Jericho Tpk., Ste. 320
Jericho, NY 11753
Phone: (516)827-1290 **Fax:** (516)827-1295
Email: long-island@cff.org
Website: http://www.cff.org
Yolan J. Wolf, Director

★ 7551 ★ Cystic Fibrosis Foundation
Northeastern New York Chapter
12 Avis Dr.
Latham, NY 12110
Phone: (518)783-7361 **Fax:** (518)783-7394
Email: ne-ny@cff.org
Website: http://www.cff.org
Linda Traylor, Director

★ 7552 ★ Cystic Fibrosis Foundation
Rochester Chapter
301 Exchange Blvd., Ste. 206
Rochester, NY 14608
Phone: (585)546-5890 **Fax:** (585)546-3903
Email: rochester-ny@cff.org
Website: http://www.cff.org
Kelly Hallenbeck, Director

North Carolina

★ 7553 ★ Cystic Fibrosis Foundation
Carolinas Chapter
1005 Bullard Ct., Ste. 105
Raleigh, NC 27615
Phone: (919)878-5040 **Free:** 800-822-9941
Fax: (919)878-5049
Email: carolinas@cff.org
Website: http://www.cff.org
Nancy Mallory, Director

★ 7554 ★ Cystic Fibrosis Foundation
Charlotte Office
1428 Orchard Lake Dr., No. B
Charlotte, NC 28270
Phone: (704)321-7852 **Free:** 800-336-0329
Fax: (704)321-7856
Email: charlotte-nc@cff.org
Website: http://www.cff.org
Janice Dumsha, Director

Ohio

★ 7555 ★ Cystic Fibrosis Foundation
Central Ohio Chapter
960 Kingsmill Pkwy., Ste. 101
Columbus, OH 43229
Phone: (614)846-2440 **Fax:** (614)846-2472
Email: central-oh@cff.org
Website: http://www.cff.org
Alyce Elbert, Director

★ 7556 ★ Cystic Fibrosis Foundation
Rainbow Chapter
2000 E 9th St., Ste. 420
Cleveland, OH 44115
Phone: (216)902-8140 **Free:** 800-368-2150
Email: rainbow@cff.org
Website: http://www.cff.org
Jennifer Basel, Director

Oklahoma

★ 7557 ★ Cystic Fibrosis Foundation
Sooner Chapter
2642 E 21st St., Ste. 100
Tulsa, OK 74114
Phone: (918)744-6354 **Free:** 800-814-5766
Email: sooner@cff.org
Website: http://www.cff.org
JoAnn Winn, Director

Oregon

★ 7558 ★ Cystic Fibrosis Foundation
Oregon / Idaho / Montana Chapter
5331 SW Macadam, Ste. 340
Portland, OR 97239
Phone: (503)226-3435 **Free:** 800-448-8404
Fax: (503)226-4165
Email: oregon@cff.org
Website: http://www.cff.org
Charlotte Governale, Director

Pennsylvania

★ 7559 ★ Cystic Fibrosis Foundation
Central Pennsylvania Chapter
55 S Progress Ave.
Harrisburg, PA 17109
Phone: (717)671-4000 **Free:** 800-671-2262
Fax: (717)671-4007
Email: central-pa@cff.org
Website: http://www.cff.org
Lisa Schlager, Director

★ 7560 ★ Cystic Fibrosis Foundation
Delaware Valley Chapter
2004 Sproul Rd., Ste. 208
Broomall, PA 19008
Phone: (610)325-6001 **Free:** 800-378-8423
Fax: (610)325-6588
Email: del-valley@cff.org
Website: http://www.cff.org
Susan Yannessa, Director

★ 7561 ★ Cystic Fibrosis Foundation
Northeastern Pennsylvania Chapter
1541 Alta Dr., Ste. 102
Whitehall, PA 18052
Phone: (610)820-0206 **Free:** 800-552-2199
Fax: (610)820-9367
Email: ne-pa@cff.org
Website: http://www.cff.org
Cynthia Phillips, Director
Program(s): Gene Therapy Studies.

★ 7562 ★ Cystic Fibrosis Foundation
Western Pennsylvania Chapter
810 River Ave., Ste. 100
Pittsburgh, PA 15212
Phone: (412)321-4422 **Free:** 800-562-5395
Fax: (412)321-9305
Email: west-pa@cff.org
Website: http://www.cff.org
Mary Pat Root Joseph, Director

Tennessee

★ 7563 ★ Cystic Fibrosis Foundation Tennessee Chapter
209 10th Ave S, Ste. 426
Nashville, TN 37203
Phone: (615)255-1167
Email: tenn@cff.org
Website: http://www.cff.org
Belinda Dinwiddie, Contact

★ 7564 ★ Cystic Fibrosis Foundation Tennessee Chapter Memphis Office
1028 Crest Haven, Ste. 203
Memphis, TN 38119
Phone: (901)818-9090
Email: memphis@cff.org
Website: http://www.cff.org
JoAnne Knox, Director

Texas

★ 7565 ★ Cystic Fibrosis Foundation Lone Star Chapter
8620 N New Braunsels, Ste. 110
San Antonio, TX 78217
Phone: (210)829-7267 **Fax:** (210)829-4204
Website: http://www.cff.org/
Beth Morgan, Director

★ 7566 ★ Cystic Fibrosis Foundation Northeast Texas Chapter
2929 Carlisle, Ste. 230
Dallas, TX 75204
Phone: (214)871-2222 **Fax:** (214)969-7439
Email: ne-texas@cff.org
Website: http://www.cff.org
Sila N. Foote, Contact

★ 7567 ★ Cystic Fibrosis Foundation Texas Gulf Coast Chapter
50 Briah Hollow Ln., Ste. 495 E
Houston, TX 77027
Phone: (713)621-0006 **Fax:** (713)621-2542
Email: texas-gulf@cff.org
Website: http://www.cff.org
Sissy Boyd, Director

Washington

★ 7568 ★ Cystic Fibrosis Foundation Washington/Alaska Chapter
100 W Harrison N Towers, Ste. 510
Seattle, WA 98119
Phone: (206)282-4770 **Free:** 800-647-7774
Email: washington@cff.org
Website: http://www.cff.org
Dottie Moore, Director

★ 7569 ★ Cystic Fibrosis Foundation Washington/Alaska Chapter
100 W Harrison N Towers, Ste. 510
Seattle, WA 98119
Phone: (206)282-4770 **Free:** 800-647-7774
Fax: (206)283-8359
Email: washington@cff.org
Website: http://www.cffwa.org/
Dottie Moore, Director

Wisconsin

★ 7570 ★ Cystic Fibrosis Foundation Wisconsin Chapter
2421 Mayfair Rd., Ste. 320
Milwaukee, WI 53226
Phone: (414)778-4820 **Free:** 800-472-7720
Fax: (414)778-4824
Email: wisconsin@cff.org
Website: http://www.cff.org
Lisa Weisman, Director

Dentistry

The following are constituent societies of the American Dental Association, 211 E Chicago Ave., Chicago, IL 60611, (312)440-2500, http://www.ada.org/.

Alabama

★ 7571 ★ Alabama Dental Association
836 Washington Ave.
Montgomery, AL 36104-3839
Phone: (334)265-1684 **Free:** 800-489-2532
Fax: (334)262-6218
Email: concactus@aldaonline.org
Website: http://www.aldaonline.org
Wayne McMahon, Exec Director
Wayne McMahan, Exec Director

Alaska

★ 7572 ★ Alaska Dental Society
9170 Jewel Lake Rd., Ste. 203
Anchorage, AK 99502-5381
Phone: (907)563-3003 **Fax:** (907)563-3009
Email: akdental@alaska.net
Website: http://www.akdental.org
Martha Reinbold, Exec Director

Arizona

★ 7573 ★ Arizona Dental Association
4131 N 36th St.
Phoenix, AZ 85018-4761
Phone: (602)957-4777 **Fax:** (602)957-1342
Email: azda@azda.org
Website: http://www.azda.org
Rick Murray, Exec Director
Greg McFarland, Exec Director

Arkansas

★ 7574 ★ Arkansas State Dental Association
2501 Crestwood Dr., Ste. 205
North Little Rock, AR 72116-7613
Phone: (501)771-7650 **Fax:** (501)771-1016
Email: asda@aristotle.net
Website: http://www.dental-asda.org
Billy Tarpley, Exec Director

California

★ 7575 ★ California Dental Association
1201 "K" St., 14th Fl.
Sacramento, CA 95814
Phone: (916)443-0505 **Free:** 800-736-8702
Fax: (916)443-2943
Email: info@cda.org
Website: http://www.cda.org
Dr. Dennis. Kalebjian, President
Timothy Comstock, Exec Director

Colorado

★ 7576 ★ Colorado Dental Association
3690 S Yosemite, Ste. 100
Denver, CO 80237-1808
Phone: (303)740-6900 **Fax:** (303)740-7989
Email: info@cdaonline.org
Website: http://www.cdaonline.org
Gary J. Cummins, Exec Director
Jim Towle, Exec Director

Connecticut

★ 7577 ★ Connecticut State Dental Association
62 Russ St.
Hartford, CT 06106-1522
Phone: (860)278-5550 **Fax:** (860)244-8287
Email: noel@csda.com
Website: http://www.csda.com
Noel Bishop, Exec Director

Delaware

★ 7578 ★ Delaware State Dental Society
Christiana Executive Campus
200 Continental Dr., Ste. 111
Newark, DE 19713
Phone: (302)368-7634 **Fax:** (302)368-7669
Email: dsds@delanet.com
Website: http://www.dedental.com
Betty Dencler, Exec Director
Margaret Novak, Exec Director

District of Columbia

★ 7579 ★ District of Columbia Dental Society
502 C St. NE
Washington, DC 20002-5810
Phone: (202)547-7613 **Fax:** (202)546-1482
Email: cbrown@cdental.org
Website: http://www.dcdental.org
C. Jay Brown, Exec Director

Florida

★ 7580 ★ Florida Dental Association
1111 E Tennessee St., Ste. 102
Tallahassee, FL 32308-6913
Phone: (850)681-3629 **Fax:** (850)561-0504
Email: dbuker@floridadental.org
Website: http://www.floridadental.org
Daniel J. Buker, Exec Director

Georgia

★ 7581 ★ Georgia Dental Association
Bldg. 17, Ste. 200
7000 Peachtree Dunwoody Rd. NE
Atlanta, GA 30328-1655
Phone: (404)636-7553 **Fax:** (404)633-3943
Email: phillips@gadental.org
Website: http://www.gadental.org
Martha Phillips, Exec Director

Hawaii

★ 7582 ★ Hawaii Dental Association
1345 S Beretania St., Ste. 301
Honolulu, HI 96814-1821
Phone: (808)593-7956 **Fax:** (808)593-7636
Email: hda@hawaiidentalassociation.net
Website: http://www.hawaiidentalassociation.net
Loren Liebling, Contact

Idaho

★ 7583 ★ Idaho State Dental Association
1220 W Hays St.
Boise, ID 83702-5315
Phone: (208)343-7543 **Fax:** (208)343-0775
Email: isda@mindspring.com
Website: http://www.isdaweb.com
A. Jerry Davis, Exec Director

Illinois

★ 7584 ★ Illinois State Dental Society
PO Box 376
Springfield, IL 62705
Phone: (217)525-1406 **Fax:** (217)525-8872
Email: rrechner@isds.org
Website: http://www.isds.org
Robert Rechner, Exec Director

Indiana

★ 7585 ★ Indiana Dental Association
PO Box 2467
Indianapolis, IN 46206-2467
Phone: (317)634-2610 **Fax:** (317)634-2612
Email: dbush@indental.org
Website: http://www.indental.org
Douglas M. Bush, Exec Director

Iowa

★ 7586 ★ Iowa Dental Association
505 5th Ave., Ste. 333
Des Moines, IA 50309-2379
Phone: (515)282-7250 **Fax:** (515)828-7256
Email: info@iowadental.org
Website: http://www.iowadental.org
Lawrence F. Carl, Exec Director
Robert W. Harpster, Contact

Kansas

★ 7587 ★ Kansas Dental Association
5200 SW Huntoon St.
Topeka, KS 66604-2398
Phone: (785)272-7360 **Fax:** (785)272-2301
Email: kevin@ksdental.org
Website: http://www.ksdental.org
Dr. Kevin J. Robertson, Exec Director

Kentucky

★ 7588 ★ Kentucky Dental Association
1940 Princeton Dr.
Louisville, KY 40205-1838
Phone: (502)459-5373 **Fax:** (502)458-5915
Email: porter_mike@msn.com
Website: http://www.kyda.org
Michael R. Porter, Exec Director

Louisiana

★ 7589 ★ Louisiana Dental Association
7833 Office Park Blvd.
Baton Rouge, LA 70809-7604
Phone: (225)926-1986 **Fax:** (225)926-1886
Email: info@ladental.org
Website: http://www.ladental.org
Dr. Mark S. Chaney, President
Ward Blackwell, Exec Director

Maine

★ 7590 ★ Maine Dental Association
PO Box 215
Manchester, ME 04351-0215
Phone: (207)622-7900 **Fax:** (207)622-6210
Email: info@medental.org
Website: http://www.medental.org
Frances Miliano, Exec Director

Maryland

★ 7591 ★ Maryland State Dental Association
6410 Dobbin Rd., Ste. F
Columbia, MD 21045-4774
Phone: (410)964-2880 **Free:** 800-766-2880
Fax: (410)964-0583
Email: elza@msda.com
Website: http://www.msda.com
David Williams, President
Elza Harrison, Exec Director

Massachusetts

★ 7592 ★ Massachusetts Dental Society
2 Willow St., Ste. 200
Southborough, MA 01745-1027
Phone: (508)480-9797 **Fax:** (508)480-0002
Email: madental@massdental.org
Website: http://www.massdental.org
Dr. Rene Bousquet, President
Dr. James B. Bramson, Exec Director

Michigan

★ 7593 ★ Michigan Dental Association
230 N Washington Sq., Ste. 208
Lansing, MI 48933-1312
Phone: (517)372-9070 **Fax:** (517)372-0008
Email: mda@michigandental.org
Website: http://www.michigandental.org
Gerri Cherney, Exec Director

Minnesota

★ 7594 ★ Minnesota Dental Association
2236 Marshall Ave.
Saint Paul, MN 55104-5758
Phone: (651)646-7454 **Fax:** (651)646-8246
Email: info@mndental.org
Website: http://www.mndental.org
Richard Diercks, Exec Director

Mississippi

★ 7595 ★ Mississippi Dental Association
2630 Ridgewood Rd.
Jackson, MS 39216-4903
Phone: (601)982-0442 **Fax:** (601)366-3050
Email: connie@msdental.org
Website: http://www.msdental.org
Connie Lane, Exec Director

Missouri

★ 7596 ★ Missouri Dental Association
230 W McCarty St.
PO Box 1707
Jefferson City, MO 65102-1707
Phone: (573)634-3436 **Fax:** (573)635-0764
Email: jake@modental.org
Website: http://www.modental.org
Dr. Jacob J. Lippert, Exec Director

Montana

★ 7597 ★ Montana Dental Association
17 ½ S Last Chance Gulch
Helena, MT 59601
Phone: (406)443-2061 **Fax:** (406)443-1546
Email: mda@mt.net
Website: http://www.mtdental.com
Mary McCue, Exec Director

Nevada

★ 7598 ★ Nevada Dental Association
6889 W Charleston Blvd., Ste. B
Las Vegas, NV 89117-1600
Phone: (702)255-4211 **Fax:** (702)255-3302
Email: nda@nvda.net
Website: http://www.nvda.org
Maury Astley, Exec Director

New Hampshire

★ 7599 ★ New Hampshire Dental Society
PO Box 2229
Concord, NH 03302-2229
Phone: (603)225-5961 **Fax:** (603)226-4880
Email: nhds@nhdental.com
Website: http://www.nhdental.com
Henry Dougherty, Exec Director

New Jersey

★ 7600 ★ New Jersey Dental Association
1 Dental Plaza
PO Box 6020
North Brunswick, NJ 08902-6020
Phone: (732)821-9400 **Fax:** (732)821-1082
Email: ddavis@njda.org
Website: http://www.njda.org
Ms. Ricky Dibofsky, Contact
Arthur Meisel, Exec Director

New Mexico

★ 7601 ★ New Mexico Dental Association
3736 Eubank Blvd. NE, Ste. D-2
Albuquerque, NM 87111-3556
Phone: (505)294-1368 **Fax:** (505)294-9958
Email: kcravens@nmdental.org
Website: http://www.newmexicodental.org
Kent Cravens, Exec Director
Rick Murray, Exec Director

New York

★ 7602 ★ New York State Dental Association
121 State St., 4th Fl.
Albany, NY 12207-1622
Phone: (518)465-0044 **Free:** 800-255-2100
Fax: (518)465-3219
Email: info@nysdental.org
Website: http://www.nysdental.org
Roy Lasky, Exec Director

North Carolina

★ 7603 ★ North Carolina Dental Society
PO Box 4099
Cary, NC 27519-4099
Phone: (919)677-1396 **Free:** 800-662-8754
Fax: (919)677-1397
Email: ncds@ncdental.org
Website: http://www.ncdental.org
Faye K. Marley, Contact

North Dakota

★ 7604 ★ North Dakota Dental Association
PO Box 1332
Bismarck, ND 58502-1332
Phone: (701)223-8870 **Fax:** (701)223-0855
Email: ndda@olsoncichy.com
Website: http://www.nddental.com
Joseph J. Cichy, Exec Director

Ohio

★ 7605 ★ Ohio Dental Association
1370 Dublin Rd.
Columbus, OH 43215-1009
Phone: (614)486-2700 **Fax:** (614)486-0381
Email: dentist@oda.org
Website: http://www.oda.org
David J. Owsiany, Exec Director
Nancy C. Quinn, Contact

Oklahoma

★ 7606 ★ Oklahoma Dental Association
629 NW Grand Blvd., Ste. A
Oklahoma City, OK 73118-6032
Phone: (405)848-8873 **Fax:** (405)848-8875
Email: odjessic@swbell.net
Website: http://www.okdentassoc.org
Stephen Glenn, Exec Director
Bob D. Berry, Exec Director

Oregon

★ 7607 ★ Oregon Dental Association
17898 SW McEwan Rd.
Portland, OR 97224-7798
Phone: (503)620-3230 **Fax:** (503)620-4169
Email: info@oregondental.org
Website: http://www.oregondental.org
William E. Zep, Exec Director
William E. Zepp, Exec Director

Pennsylvania

★ 7608 ★ Pennsylvania Dental Association
PO Box 3341
Harrisburg, PA 17105-3341
Phone: (717)234-5941 **Free:** 800-223-0016
Fax: (717)232-7169
Email: ckc@padental.org
Website: http://www.padental.org
Camille Kostelac-Cherry, Exec Director

Puerto Rico

★ 7609 ★ Colegio de Cirujanos Dentistas de Puerto Rico
Avenida Domenech 200
San Juan, PR 00918
Phone: (787)764-1969 **Fax:** (787)763-6335
Myrna Cruz-Garay, Exec Director

Rhode Island

★ 7610 ★ Rhode Island Dental Association
200 Centerville Rd.
Warwick, RI 02886-0204
Phone: (401)732-6833 **Fax:** (401)732-9351
Email: info@ridental.com
Website: http://www.ridental.com
Valerie Donnelly, Exec Director

South Carolina

★ 7611 ★ South Carolina Dental Association
120 Stonemark Ln.
Columbia, SC 29210-3841
Phone: (803)750-2277 **Fax:** (803)750-1644
Email: zomh@scda.org
Website: http://www.scda.org
Hal Zom, Exec Director
Hal Zorn, Exec Director

South Dakota

★ 7612 ★ South Dakota Dental Association
711 E Wells Ave., Ste. 240
PO Box 1194
Pierre, SD 57501-1194
Phone: (605)224-9133 **Fax:** (605)224-9168
Email: info@sddental.org
Website: http://www.sddental.org
Paul Knecht, Exec Director

Tennessee

★ 7613 ★ Tennessee Dental Association
2104 Sunset Pl.
PO Box 120188
Nashville, TN 37212-4917
Phone: (615)383-8962 **Fax:** (615)383-0214
Email: tda@tenndental.org
Website: http://www.tenndental.org
David S. Horvat, Exec Director

Texas

★ 7614 ★ Texas Dental Association
1946 S Interstate Hwy. 35, Ste. 400
Austin, TX 78704
Phone: (512)443-3675 **Fax:** (512)443-3031
Email: amsimmons@tda.org
Website: http://www.tda.org
Mary Kay Linn, Exec Director

Utah

★ 7615 ★ Utah Dental Association
1151 East 3900 South, Ste. B160
Salt Lake City, UT 84124-1216
Phone: (801)261-5315 **Fax:** (801)261-1235
Email: uda@uda.org
Monte Thompson, Exec Director

Vermont

★ 7616 ★ Vermont State Dental Society
100 Dorset St., Ste. 18
South Burlington, VT 05403-6241
Phone: (802)864-0115 **Fax:** (802)864-0116
Email: ptaylorvt@aol.com
Website: http://www.vsds.org
Peter Taylor, Exec Director

Virgin Islands

★ 7617 ★ Virgin Islands Dental Association
Medical Arts Complex, Ste. 10
St. Thomas, VI 00802
Phone: (340)777-5950 **Fax:** (340)775-4172
Email: jawdocvi@netscape.net
Dr. Horace Griffith, President

Virginia

★ 7618 ★ Virginia Dental Association
7525 Staples Mill Rd.
Richmond, VA 23228
Phone: (804)261-1610 **Fax:** (804)261-1660
Email: dickinson@vadental.org
Website: http://www.vadental.org
Dr. Terry D. Dickinson, Exec Director

Washington

★ 7619 ★ Washington State Dental Association
2033 6th Ave., Ste. 333
Seattle, WA 98121
Phone: (206)448-1914 **Fax:** (206)443-9266
Email: wsda@wsda.org
Website: http://www.wsda.org
Stephen A. Hardymon, Exec Director

West Virginia

★ 7620 ★ West Virginia Dental Association
2003 Quarrier St.
Charleston, WV 25311-2212
Phone: (304)344-5246 **Fax:** (304)344-5316
Email: wvrds@aol.com
Richard D. Stevens, Exec Director

Wisconsin

★ 7621 ★ Wisconsin Dental Association
111 E Wisconsin Ave., Ste. 1300
Milwaukee, WI 53202-4815
Phone: (414)276-4520 **Fax:** (414)276-8431
Email: dmcguire@wda.org
Website: http://www.wda.org
Dennis McGuire, Exec Director

Wyoming

★ 7622 ★ Wyoming Dental Association
502 S 4th St.
Laramie, WY 82070-3704
Phone: (307)755-4009 **Fax:** (307)745-8009
Email: keefeo2000@yahoo.com
Website: http://www.medicinebow.org/wyodental
Diane O'Keefe, Exec Director
Marvin Cronberg, Exec Director

Depression

State chapters of the Depression and Bipolar Support Alliance, formerly the National Depressive and Manic-Depressive Association, are listed below. The national office is located at 730 N Franklin St., Ste. 501, Chicago, Illinois 60610-7204. Additional information can be obtained by calling the national office at (800) 826-3632, or by consulting the web site at http://www.dbsalliance.org/.

Alabama

★ 7623 ★ Depression and Bipolar Support Alliance
Huntsville Chapter
PO Box 2933
Huntsville, AL 35804-2933
Phone: (256)536-3471
Email: dbsa_huntsville@yahoo.com
Website: http://www.geocities.com/dbsa_huntsville
Elayne Fountain, Contact

★ 7624 ★ Depression and Bipolar Support Alliance
Huntsville MDSG Chapter
660 Gallatin St.
Huntsville, AL 35801
Phone: (256)539-5419
Email: myra.yancey@mhcmc.org
Website: http://www.mhcmc.org/
Myrã Yancey, Contact

★ 7625 ★ Depression and Bipolar Support Alliance
Montgomery
Montgomery, AL
Phone: (334)230-9870
Email: dbsa_montgomery@bellsouth.net
Clairepatrese Sams Milligan, Contact

★ 7626 ★ Depression and Bipolar Support Alliance
Morgan County Chapter
PO Box 1502
Decatur, AL 35602-1502
Phone: (256)353-1160 **Fax:** (256)353-1163
Email: sue@mhainmc.org
Website: http://www.mhain.org/
Sue Brantley, Contact

★ 7627 ★ Depression and Bipolar Support Alliance
SOMI Bipolar Group
Mobile, AL
Phone: (251)340-6189
Eddy Jones, Contact

★ 7628 ★ Depression and Bipolar Support Alliance
Southeast Alabama Chapter
Dothan, AL
Phone: (334)794-7008
Robin Saliba, Contact

★ 7629 ★ Depression and Bipolar Support Alliance
Tuscaloosa Chapter
PO Box 1731
Tuscaloosa, AL 35403
Phone: (205)349-8791
Email: harley_1929@yahoo.com
Harley Sullivan, Contact

Arizona

★ 7630 ★ Depression and Bipolar Support Alliance
Bipolar Bears of Phoenix Chapter
936 W Impala Center
Mesa, AZ 85210
Phone: (480)838-3716 **Fax:** (480)994-4744
Email: bears@bipolarbears.org
Website: http://www.bipolarbears.org
Phil Sawyer, Contact

★ 7631 ★ Depression and Bipolar Support Alliance
Maricopa County Chapter
6411 E Thomas
Scottsdale, AZ 85251
Phone: (480)994-4407 **Fax:** (480)994-4744
Email: cnordyke@mhaarizona.org
Website: http://www.mhaaz.com
Cheryl Nordyke, Contact

Arkansas

★ 7632 ★ Depression and Bipolar Support Alliance
Arkansas Chapter
PO Box 94339
North Little Rock, AR 72190
Phone: (501)753-4767 **Fax:** (501)771-1226
Email: jerjun@juno.com
Jerry Quick, Contact

California

★ 7633 ★ Depression and Bipolar Support Alliance (DBSA)
Hemet, CA
Phone: (909)658-0181
Website: http://www.geocities.com/tdmda/hemetdbsa
Wesley Wilson, Contact

★ 7634 ★ Depression and Bipolar Support Alliance
Coachella Valley Chapter
100 S Sunrise Way, Box 357
Palm Springs, CA 92262-6737
Phone: (760)228-2824 **Fax:** (760)323-2404
Email: PalmSpringsDABA@yahoo.com
Mary Ritchie, Contact

★ 7635 ★ Depression and Bipolar Support Alliance (DBSA)
DBSA Napa
Napa, CA
Phone: (707)747-1989
Email: brennavarro9@aol.com
Brenda Navarro, Contact

★ 7636 ★ Depression and Bipolar Support Alliance (DBSA)
Depression Support/Visalia Chapter
11002 Ave. 352
Visalia, CA 93291
Phone: (559)733-7362 **Fax:** (559)733-7362
Email: rillmitch@thegrid.net
Dave Helling, Contact

★ 7637 ★ Depression and Bipolar Support Alliance (DBSA)
El Cajon
El Cajon, CA
Phone: (619)393-3568
Email: dbsa_el_cajon_owner@yahoogroups.com
Website: http://groups.yahoo.com/group/dmda_el_cajon/
Agnes Zsigovics, Contact

★ 7638 ★ Depression and Bipolar Support Alliance (DBSA)
Escondido Chapter
1540 E Valley Pkwy.
Escondido, CA 92027
Phone: (760)739-2971 **Free:** 800-336-2000
Fax: (760)735-9067
Email: kls5@pph.org
Website: http://www.pphs.org
Brian Heath, Contact

★ 7639 ★ Depression and Bipolar Support Alliance
Fontana/Upland Chapter
Fontana, CA
Phone: (909)947-1307 **Fax:** (909)947-4081
Samantha Johns, Contact

★ 7640 ★ Depression and Bipolar Support Alliance (DBSA)
Glendale Chapter
Glendale, CA
Phone: (323)662-5564
Email: getout@earthlink.net
Doris Outler, Contact

★ 7641 ★ Depression and Bipolar Support Alliance (DBSA)
Greater Long Beach Chapter
4634 Ostrom Ave.
Lakewood, CA 90713
Phone: (562)422-8891
Email: celtic1100@yahoo.com
Neil Young, Contact

★ 7642 ★ Depression and Bipolar Support Alliance
High Desert Chapter
20318 Thunderbird Rd., No. 2
Apple Valley, CA 92307
Phone: (760)946-0308
Email: galucla@aol.com
Gerri Logan, Contact

★ 7643 ★ Depression and Bipolar Support Alliance (DBSA)
Hillcrest UCSD
San Diego, CA 92128
Phone: (619)497-6664 **Fax:** (619)497-6696
Agnes Zsigovics, Contact

★ 7644 ★ Depression and Bipolar Support Alliance (DBSA)
Humboldt County
PO Box 7118
Eureka, CA 95502-7118
Phone: (707)839-4353
Email: les58paul@cs.com
Website: http://http://www.chargette.com/client/dmda/dmda.html
James Selle, Contact

★ 7645 ★ Depression and Bipolar Support Alliance
Indian Wells Valley Chapter
China Lake, CA
Phone: (760)377-3223
Email: ramer@ridgenet.net
Robert Millsop, Contact

★ 7646 ★ Depression and Bipolar Support Alliance (DBSA)
Inland Empire West
Ontario, CA
Phone: (909)947-1307 **Fax:** (909)947-4081
Email: dmjbf@aol.com
Samantha Johns, Contact

★ 7647 ★ Depression and Bipolar Support Alliance
La Jolla Chapter
8950 Villa La Jolla Dr., No. 2142
La Jolla, CA 92037
Phone: (858)535-4783 **Free:** 888-274-3637
Fax: (858)457-8527
Email: pmcgrath@ucsd.edu

★ 7648 ★ Depression and Bipolar Support Alliance
Los Angeles Chapter
PO Box 341201
Los Angeles, CA 90034-1201
Phone: (818)893-7363
Email: hankdor@aol.com
Doreen Scott, Contact

★ 7649 ★ Depression and Bipolar Support Alliance (DBSA)
Monterey Chapter
Monterey, CA
Phone: (831)646-8800 **Fax:** (831)657-0290
Email: jmpmiramar@yahoo.com
Website: http://www.dbsamonterey.com/
Rod Guthrie, Contact

★ 7650 ★ Depression and Bipolar Support Alliance (DBSA)
Mt. Shasta Chapter
PO Box 557
Mount Shasta, CA 96067
Phone: (530)918-7205 **Fax:** (530)926-2668
Kareen Thomas, Contact

★ 7651 ★ Depression and Bipolar Support Alliance (DBSA)
North County Young Warriors
Vista, CA
Phone: (760)860-2746
Email: ncyoungwarriors@aol.com
Kathy Bevilacqua, Contact

★ 7652 ★ Depression and Bipolar Support Alliance (DBSA)
Oceanside Chapter
Oceanside, CA
Phone: (760)597-9754
Email: dmdaca@aol.com
Robert D. Jones, Jr., Contact

★ 7653 ★ Depression and Bipolar Support Alliance
Orange County Chapter
PO Box 223
Tustin, CA 92781-0223
Phone: (714)744-8718
Email: gdierking@aol.com
Website: http://www.angelfire.com/ca/dmdaoc/index.html
Gloria Dierking, Contact

★ 7654 ★ Depression and Bipolar Support Alliance
Pasadena Chapter
Pasadena, CA
Phone: (626)446-0458
Jill Hall, Contact

★ 7655 ★ Depression and Bipolar Support Alliance
Riverside Chapter
16280 Whispering Spur
Riverside, CA 92504
Phone: (909)780-3366 **Fax:** (909)780-5758
Email: mddaofriv@ad.com
Website: http://www.geocities.com/mddariv/index.html

★ 7656 ★ Depression and Bipolar Support Alliance
Sacramento Chapter
2521 Key West Way
Sacramento, CA 95826
Phone: (916)684-1358 **Fax:** (916)363-3184
Email: marilynhillerman@yahoo.com
Marilyn Hillerman, Contact

★ 7657 ★ Depression and Bipolar Support Alliance (DBSA)
San Diego
San Diego, CA
Phone: (858)259-1391
Marilyn Hutson, Contact

★ 7658 ★ Depression and Bipolar Support Alliance
San Francisco Chapter
900 Hyde St., 3rd Fl.
San Francisco, CA 94109
Phone: (415)995-4792 **Fax:** (510)436-3144
Email: deborahmichelle@earthlink.net
Website: http://www.sfdmda.org
Deborah Sanders, Contact

★ 7659 ★ Depression and Bipolar Support Alliance
San Joaquin Chapter
PO Box 403
Lodi, CA 95241
Phone: (209)334-4642
Email: dmda_sanjoaquin@yahoo.com
Website: http://www.geocities.com/dmda_sanjoaquin
Glenda Lee, Contact

★ 7660 ★ Depression and Bipolar Support Alliance (DBSA)
San Mateo Co.
Belmont, CA
Phone: (650)595-5131
Ann Dinowitz, Contact

★ 7661 ★ Depression and Bipolar Support Alliance
Stanford Young Persons' Support Group
Stanford, CA
Phone: (650)245-1048
Email: dianaphrodite@yahoo.com
Diana Galbraith, Contact

★ 7662 ★ Depression and Bipolar Support Alliance
Stanislaus County Chapter
Modesto, CA
Phone: (209)544-8473 **Fax:** (209)869-1758
Email: dmda55@hotmail.com
Scott Hill, Contact

★ 7663 ★ Depression and Bipolar Support Alliance
Temecula Chapter
Temecula, CA
Phone: (909)926-8393
Email: threez@pe.net
Website: http://www.geocities.com/tdmda
Mark Monroe, Contact

★ 7664 ★ Depression and Bipolar Support Alliance
UCLA/West Los Angeles Chapter
300 Medical Plaza, 2nd Fl., Conf. Rm. 1
Los Angeles, CA 90095-8346
Phone: (310)466-9199
Email: jenniferhodges5683@hotmail.com
Jennifer Hodges, Contact

★ 7665 ★ Depression and Bipolar Support Alliance
Uplifters/Riverside Chapter
19880 Kirkpatrick Rd.
Perris, CA 92570
Phone: (909)780-0379 **Fax:** (909)780-5758
Email: arleekirk@juno.com
Arlie Kirkpatrick, Contact

★ 7666 ★ Depression and Bipolar Support Alliance (DBSA)
Visalia/Hanford Chapter
118 W Myrtle St.
Hanford, CA 93230
Phone: (559)585-1227
Irene Spindler, Contact

Colorado

★ 7667 ★ Depression and Bipolar Support Alliance (DBSA)
Aurora
Aurora, CO
Phone: (303)329-9894
Email: cstowell@juno.com
Alan Krasnow, Contact

★ 7668 ★ Depression and Bipolar Support Alliance (DBSA)
Colorado Springs/Initiatives Chapter
PO Box 366
Colorado Springs, CO 80901-0366
Phone: (719)477-1515 **Fax:** (719)477-1515
Email: dmdacolospgs@pcisys.net
Karen Fallahi, Contact

★ 7669 ★ Depression and Bipolar Support Alliance (DBSA)
Heritage Christian Center
Denver, CO 80220
Phone: (303)369-8514
Email: patbarry@copper.net
Patrick Berry, Contact

★ 7670 ★ Depression and Bipolar Support Alliance
North Star Chapter
Westminster, CO
Phone: (303)584-1957 **Fax:** (303)404-9264
Sharron Thomas, Contact

★ 7671 ★ Depression and Bipolar Support Alliance
Pueblo Chapter
1600 Grand Ave., No. 125
Pueblo, CO 81003
Phone: (719)583-9798 **Free:** 800-976-5929
Fax: (719)544-5708
Email: jackselway@puebloadvocacy.com
Website: http://www.puebloadvocacy.com/dmda
Jack Selway, Contact

★ 7672 ★ Depression and Bipolar Support Alliance
Southwest Chapter
455 S Lee St.
Lakewood, CO 80226
Phone: (303)331-2599 **Fax:** (303)830-8918
Joe Petrovich, Contact

★ 7673 ★ National Depressive and Manic-Depressive Association
Depression and Bipolar Support Alliance Boulder Chapter
Boulder, CO 80306-1343
Phone: (303)271-3533 **Fax:** (303)379-9786
Email: randalledwards99@hotmail.com
Randall Edwards, Contact

Connecticut

★ 7674 ★ Depression and Bipolar Support Alliance
Greenwich Chapter
c/o Greenwich Hospital
5 Perryridge Rd.
Greenwich, CT 06830
Phone: (203)975-2451 **Fax:** (203)863-4445
Email: fbtworld@aol.com
Website: http://www.greenhosp.org
Peter Flierl, Contact

★ 7675 ★ Depression and Bipolar Support Alliance (DBSA)
Middletown
Middletown, CT 06457
Phone: (860)346-0303

★ 7676 ★ Depression and Bipolar Support Alliance (DBSA)
Northwest Connecticut Chapter
Torrington, CT
Phone: (860)567-8928 **Fax:** (860)567-9007
Website: http://www.dbsanwct.tripod.com/
Doyle Finan, Contact

Delaware

★ 7677 ★ Depression and Bipolar Support Alliance
New Directions/Delaware Chapter
6 Hilton Rd.
Wilmington, DE 19810
Phone: (302)286-1161 **Fax:** (302)475-1574
Email: newdirectionsdelaware@yahoo.com
Website: http://www.newdirectionsdelaware.org
Dolores Grimes, Contact

District of Columbia

★ 7678 ★ Depression and Bipolar Support Alliance (DBSA)
Capital Area Chapter
Washington, DC
Phone: (301)279-0831
Email: cadma_99@yahoo.com
Alvin Martin, Contact

★ 7679 ★ **Depression and Bipolar Support Alliance**
Washington DC Chapter
Washington, DC 20016
Phone: (301)467-6717
Liz Engleman, Contact

Florida

★ 7680 ★ **Depression and Bipolar Support Alliance (DBSA)**
Broward County
Margrate, FL
Phone: (954)969-0291
Email: glennk@bellsouth.net
Website: http://www.bcdbsa.org
Glenn Krate, Contact

★ 7681 ★ **Depression and Bipolar Support Alliance**
Central Brevard Chapter
1407 N Lakemont Dr.
Cocoa, FL 32922
Phone: (321)632-9164
Email: cocoalocal@aol.com
Carolyn C. Hubbard, Contact

★ 7682 ★ **Depression and Bipolar Support Alliance (DBSA)**
Citrus County
Lecanto, FL
Phone: (352)341-1148
Email: korestis@tampabay.rr.com
Mary-Kelsey Orestis, Contact

★ 7683 ★ **Depression and Bipolar Support Alliance (DBSA)**
Collier County Chapter
1055 Rordon Ave.
Naples, FL 34103
Phone: (941)649-6241
Charis Nelson, Contact

★ 7684 ★ **Depression and Bipolar Support Alliance**
Depression/Bipolar Fellowship
919 SE 14th St.
Ocala, FL 34471-3917
Phone: (352)732-0879
Bob Rile, Contact

★ 7685 ★ **Depression and Bipolar Support Alliance (DBSA)**
Fort Meyers Chapter
1846 Braman Ave.
Fort Myers, FL 33901
Phone: (239)277-0778
Email: dbsaftmyersfl@aol.com
Anna Montoro, Contact

★ 7686 ★ **Depression and Bipolar Support Alliance**
Gainesville Chapter
PO Box 140604
Gainesville, FL 32614-0604
Phone: (352)335-0081
Sandy Wentworth, Contact

★ 7687 ★ **Depression and Bipolar Support Alliance (DBSA)**
Gold Coast Chapter
3501 Johnson St.
Hollywood, FL 33021
Phone: (954)923-0073 **Fax:** (954)985-6183
Email: surferchuck@msn.com
Website: http://www.goldcoastmda.com
Christine Ames, Contact

★ 7688 ★ **Depression and Bipolar Support Alliance (DBSA)**
Gold Coast (Women Only)
Tamarac, FL 33321-2901
Phone: (954)731-6228
Email: glennk@bellsouth.net
Website: http://www.bcdmda.org
Jann & Susan Krate, Contact
Crisis Phone(s): 24-hour line, (954) 463-0911.

★ 7689 ★ **Depression and Bipolar Support Alliance (DBSA)**
Greater Orlando
8638 Knotty Pine Ln.
Orlando, FL 32825
Phone: (407)277-7976 **Fax:** (407)468-6803
Email: themanicblues@cfl.rr.com
Marian Becker, Contact

★ 7690 ★ **Depression and Bipolar Support Alliance**
Hillsborough Chapter
Brandon, FL
Phone: (813)685-4818
Email: revrev@prodigy.net
Andrew Newelski, Contact

★ 7691 ★ **Depression and Bipolar Support Alliance**
Inverness Chapter
Inverness, FL
Phone: (352)341-5688
Email: korestis@tampabay.rr.net
Kelsey Orestis, Contact

★ 7692 ★ **Depression and Bipolar Support Alliance**
Jacksonville Beach Chapter
Jacksonville Beach, FL
Phone: (904)399-5468
Susan Seimer, Contact

★ 7693 ★ **Depression and Bipolar Support Alliance**
Jacksonville Beaches
Jacksonville, FL 32217
Phone: (904)241-4676 **Fax:** (904)448-8965
Email: dbsajax@dbsajax.com
Marcy Ashby, Contact

★ 7694 ★ **Depression and Bipolar Support Alliance (DBSA)**
Lakeland
Lakeland, FL
Phone: (863)431-2778
Adam O'Connor, Contact

★ 7695 ★ **Depression and Bipolar Support Alliance (DBSA)**
Libertyville
Libertyville, FL
Phone: (847)336-8346
John Philipp, Contact

★ 7696 ★ **Depression and Bipolar Support Alliance (DBSA)**
Naples Bipolar Group
Naples, FL
Phone: (239)643-6672
Email: microcmprt@earthlink.net
Steve Meek, Contact

★ 7697 ★ **Depression and Bipolar Support Alliance (DBSA)**
North Palm Beach County Chapter
18601 Misty Lake Dr.
Jupiter, FL 33458
Phone: (561)575-9787 **Fax:** (561)575-9787
Email: wsdgbp@aol.com
Joan Angle, Contact

★ 7698 ★ **Depression and Bipolar Support Alliance**
Palm Beaches Chapter
6347 Lacosta Dr., No. F
Boca Raton, FL 33433
Phone: (561)391-3401
Email: pbdmda@webtv.net
Harlan Friedman, Contact

★ 7699 ★ **Depression and Bipolar Support Alliance (DBSA)**
Pensacola Bipolar/Depression Support Group
Pensacola, FL
Phone: (850)291-9753
Email: jnwhite2001@yahoo.com
Jack White, Contact

★ 7700 ★ **Depression and Bipolar Support Alliance (DBSA)**
Pensacola Chapter
PO Box 2041
Pensacola, FL 32513-2041
Phone: (850)457-8456
Email: dmdapensacola@aol.com
Toni Beard, Contact

★ 7701 ★ **Depression and Bipolar Support Alliance**
Sarasota Chapter
5220 Ventura Ave.
Sarasota, FL 34235
Phone: (941)745-3518 **Fax:** (941)374-6235
Pat Schmidt, Contact

★ 7702 ★ **Depression and Bipolar Support Alliance (DBSA)**
South Brevard Chapter
Melbourne, FL 32901
Phone: (329)729-0888
Margaret Lee, Contact

★ 7703 ★ **Depression and Bipolar Support Alliance (DBSA)**
Suncoast Center Chapter
4024 Central Ave.
Saint Petersburg, FL 33711
Phone: (727)327-7656 **Fax:** (727)323-8978
Susan Rebillot, Contact

★ 7704 ★ **Depression and Bipolar Support Alliance (DBSA)**
Tallahassee Chapter
Tallahassee, FL 32303
Phone: (850)422-1675 **Fax:** (850)541-1941
Email: howard1861@earthlink.net
Sara Howard, Contact

★ 7705 ★ **Depression and Bipolar Support Alliance (DBSA)**
Tampa Bay Chapter
PO Box 340572
Tampa, FL 33694
Phone: (813)878-2906
Email: info@dbsatampabay.org
Website: http://www.tbstampabay.org
Neil Bush, Contact

★ 7706 ★ Depression and Bipolar Support Alliance (DBSA)
Volusia County
Daytona Beach, FL
Phone: (386)252-5785
Email: duboisjoanne@hotmail.com
Jack Paulden, Contact

★ 7707 ★ Depression and Bipolar Support Alliance (DBSA)
West Pasco Chapter
15012 Dennis Dr.
Port Richey, FL 34669
Phone: (727)819-9427 **Fax:** (727)819-9427
Bob Thompson, Contact

Georgia

★ 7708 ★ Depression and Bipolar Support Alliance (DBSA)
Greater Augusta Chapter
PO Box 1927
Augusta, GA 30903
Phone: (706)722-0010 **Fax:** (706)722-8819
Dan Cook, Contact

★ 7709 ★ Depression and Bipolar Support Alliance
Greater Savannah Chapter
455 Mall Blvd., No. 49
Savannah, GA 31406
Phone: (912)927-2064
John Ralston, Contact

★ 7710 ★ Depression and Bipolar Support Alliance (DBSA)
Jesup Chapter
1950 S Hwy. 301, No. 704
Jesup, GA 31546
Phone: (912)427-9281
Nina Howerton, Contact

★ 7711 ★ Depression and Bipolar Support Alliance (DBSA)
Metropolitan Atlanta Chapter
8198 Brookwood Valley Cir.
Atlanta, GA 30309
Phone: (404)355-8815
Email: info@atlantamoodsupport.com
Website: http://www.atlantamoodsupport.com
Stephen Propst, Contact

★ 7712 ★ Depression and Bipolar Support Alliance (DBSA)
Thomasville Chapter
PO Box 1378
Thomasville, GA 31799-1378
Phone: (229)227-9851
Email: ahansard@rose.net
Renee Hansard, Contact

Hawaii

★ 7713 ★ Depression and Bipolar Support Alliance
United Self Help Chapter
Honolulu, HI
Phone: (808)926-0466
Bud Bowles, Contact

Idaho

★ 7714 ★ Depression and Bipolar Support Alliance
New Beginnings Chapter
Idaho Falls, ID
Phone: (208)238-7073
Email: drmaddox670@aol.com
Debra Maddox, Contact

★ 7715 ★ Depression and Bipolar Support Alliance (DBSA)
North Idaho Chapter
Coeur d'Alene, ID
Phone: (208)666-3740 **Fax:** (208)666-2977
Rosemarie Olsen, Contact

★ 7716 ★ Depression and Bipolar Support Alliance
Saint Alphonsus Chapter
7470 Holbrook Ln., No. 112
Boise, ID 83704-5806
Phone: (208)658-9126
Fred Freeman, Contact

Illinois

★ 7717 ★ Depression and Bipolar Support Alliance (DBSA)
Alton/Godfrey
Godfrey, IL
Phone: (618)467-2179
Email: dougnjo@global.net
Website: http://www.webspawner.com/users/dbsaaltongodfrey/
Jolena Seibert, Contact

★ 7718 ★ Depression and Bipolar Support Alliance
Aurora Chapter
1N286 Woods Ave.
Wheaton, IL 60188
Phone: (630)653-3560
Email: sneezercat@aol.com
Thomas E. Johnson, Contact

★ 7719 ★ Depression and Bipolar Support Alliance
Belleville Chapter
St. Elizabeth's Hospital
211 S 3rd St.
Belleville, IL 62222
Phone: (618)234-2120 **Fax:** (618)222-4761
Richard Avdoian, Contact

★ 7720 ★ Depression and Bipolar Support Alliance
Berwyn Chapter
Berwyn, IL
Phone: (708)524-1794
Email: dmda_berwyn@yahoo.com
Pamela Strening, Contact

★ 7721 ★ Depression and Bipolar Support Alliance
Bloomington/Normal Chapter
710 E Front St.
Bloomington, IL 61701-5414
Phone: (309)821-1448
Email: seventenfronthouse@netscape.com
Kathy Brown, Contact

★ 7722 ★ Depression and Bipolar Support Alliance (DBSA)
DBSA West
Downers Grove, IL
Phone: (708)788-3858
Email: johnfrancis3@juno.com
John Wiley, Contact

★ 7723 ★ Depression and Bipolar Support Alliance
Fox Valley Chapter
2365 Coach and Surrey Lane
Aurora, IL 60506
Phone: (630)653-3560
Email: sneezercat@aol.com
Website: http://www.geocities.com/foxvalleydmda
Thomas E. Johnson, Contact

★ 7724 ★ Depression and Bipolar Support Alliance
Greater Chicago Area (DBSA)
4725 N Western Ave., No. 220
Chicago, IL 60625
Phone: (773)465-3280 **Fax:** (773)465-3385
Email: dmdamc@ameritech.net
Website: http://members.tripod.com/dmda-mc/index.htm
Chet Taranowski, Contact

★ 7725 ★ Depression and Bipolar Support Alliance (DBSA)
Gurnee Chapter
c/o Village Church of Gurnee
1319 N Hunt Club Rd.
Gurnee, IL 60031
Phone: (847)263-7079
Email: deniseanderson2@yahoo.com
Website: http://www.dmdagurnee.org
Denise Anderson, Contact

★ 7726 ★ Depression and Bipolar Support Alliance
Hinsdale Chapter
244 E Ogden, No. 114
Hinsdale, IL 60521
Phone: (708)788-3858
Kate Moran, Contact

★ 7727 ★ Depression and Bipolar Support Alliance
Illinois Valley Chapter
207 15th St.
Mendota, IL 61342-1311
Phone: (815)539-6432
Email: djmeyer@theramp.net
Doris J. Meyer, Contact
Frmly: Depressive and Manic-Depressive Association, Northern Illinois.

★ 7728 ★ Depression and Bipolar Support Alliance (DBSA)
Joliet Chapter
Joliet, IL
Phone: (815)773-7000
Lisa Mahaffey, Contact

★ 7729 ★ Depression and Bipolar Support Alliance
Libertyville Chapter
PO Box 8911
Waukegan, IL 60079-8911
Phone: (847)336-8346 **Fax:** (847)360-4296
John Philipp, Contact

★ 7730 ★ Depression and Bipolar Support Alliance (DBSA)
Mood Challenge Chapter
PO Box 6074
Peoria, IL 61601-6074
Phone: (309)686-4382
James B. Staley, Contact

★ 7731 ★ Depression and Bipolar Support Alliance (DBSA)
Mood Tides Chapter
Decatur, IL
Phone: (217)429-2132
Email: dbdevore@insightbb.com
Carolyn DeVore, Contact

★ 7732 ★ Depression and Bipolar Support Alliance (DBSA)
New Hope Elmhurst Chapter
PO Box 1332
Elmhurst, IL 60126
Phone: (630)415-3266
Pam Wagner, Contact

★ 7733 ★ Depression and Bipolar Support Alliance (DBSA)
North Shore Chapter
Kenilworth Union Church
211 Kenilworth Ave.
Kenilworth, IL 60043
Phone: (847)251-4272 **Fax:** (847)251-4289
Church Office Cobb, Contact

★ 7734 ★ Depression and Bipolar Support Alliance (DBSA)
Northwestern Medical Campus Chapter
675 N St. Clair, No. 20-250
Chicago, IL 60611
Phone: (312)695-3511
Email: vbrooks@nmff.org
Lindsay Sara, Contact

★ 7735 ★ Depression and Bipolar Support Alliance (DBSA)
South Suburban
Evergreen Park, IL
Phone: (708)424-3307
Jim Crofoot, Contact

★ 7736 ★ Depression and Bipolar Support Alliance (DBSA)
Urbana Champaign
4109 E Oaks Rd.
Urbana, IL 61802
Phone: (217)344-7901
Sten Johansen, Contact

Indiana

★ 7737 ★ Depression and Bipolar Support Alliance
BehaviorCorp
Carmel, IN
Phone: (317)587-0500 **Fax:** (317)574-1234
Email: lburch@behaviorcorp.org
Website: http://www.behaviorcorp.org
Larry L. Burch, Contact

★ 7738 ★ Depression and Bipolar Support Alliance
Central Indiana Chapter
Indianapolis, IN
Phone: (317)290-9686 **Fax:** (317)290-9685
Email: info@dmdacentralindiana.org
Website: http://www.dmdacentralindiana.org
Marchell K. Hunt, Contact

★ 7739 ★ Depression and Bipolar Support Alliance (DBSA)
Elkhart County Chapter
54470 Saddlebrook Crossing
Elkhart, IN 46514
Phone: (219)264-4053
Mary Kay Froschauer, Contact

★ 7740 ★ Depression and Bipolar Support Alliance
Four County Counseling Center
Logansport, IN
Phone: (219)722-5151 **Fax:** (219)722-9523
Email: ulrich@fourcounty.org
Website: http://www.fourcounty.org
Lawrence R. Ulrich, Contact

★ 7741 ★ Depression and Bipolar Support Alliance
Fulton County Chapter
321 E 8th St.
Rochester, IN 46975
Phone: (219)223-6870 **Fax:** (219)224-6870
Email: gsmokermhafc@rtcol.com
Ginelle Smoker, Contact

★ 7742 ★ Depression and Bipolar Support Alliance
Hamilton County Chapter
942 N 10th St.
Noblesville, IN 46060
Phone: (317)776-3455 **Fax:** (317)776-1155
Email: mhahc@juno.com
Kelli Spence, Contact

★ 7743 ★ Depression and Bipolar Support Alliance
Indiana Chapter
55 Monument Circle, No. 700
Indianapolis, IN 46204-2918
Phone: (317)686-0588 **Fax:** (317)638-3540
Email: mha@mentalhealthassociation.com
Website: http://www.mentalhealthassociation.com
Kevin Kilty, Contact

★ 7744 ★ Depression and Bipolar Support Alliance (DBSA)
Jefferson County
Madison, IN
Phone: (812)265-0045
Charles Morgan, Contact

★ 7745 ★ Depression and Bipolar Support Alliance (DBSA)
La Porte County
Michigan City, IN
Phone: (219)879-9173 **Fax:** (219)879-9173
Sharleen Stout, Contact

★ 7746 ★ Depression and Bipolar Support Alliance
North West Indiana Chapter
1083 N 475 E
Chesterton, IN 46304
Phone: (219)926-3424
Email: rkowal@netnitco.net
Ron Kowalski, Contact

★ 7747 ★ Depression and Bipolar Support Alliance (DBSA)
Northeast Indiana
Ashley, IN
Phone: (260)347-2291
Email: mmsmith@locl.net
Mary L. Smith, Contact

★ 7748 ★ Depression and Bipolar Support Alliance (DBSA)
Northeast Indiana
Corunna, IN
Phone: (260)347-2291
Email: mmsmith@locl.net
Mary L. Smith, Contact

★ 7749 ★ Depression and Bipolar Support Alliance
Northeastern Center, Inc.
220 S Main St.
PO Box 817
Kendallville, IN 46755
Phone: (219)347-2453 **Fax:** (219)347-2456
Email: necinfo@northeasterncenter.org
Website: http://www.northeasterncenter.org
Corey Walker, Contact

★ 7750 ★ Depression and Bipolar Support Alliance (DBSA)
SG Indianapolis Chapter
2506 Willowbrook Pkwy., No. 100
Indianapolis, IN 46205
Phone: (317)251-0005 **Fax:** (317)254-2800
Email: ksavoi@mcmha.org
Website: http://www.mcmha.org
Kim Savoie, Contact

★ 7751 ★ Depression and Bipolar Support Alliance (DBSA)
South West Indiana Chapter
123 NW 4th St., No. 614
Evansville, IN 47708
Phone: (812)426-2640 **Fax:** (812)426-7207
Email: vcmha@juno.com
Donna Carr, Contact

Iowa

★ 7752 ★ Depression and Bipolar Support Alliance (DBSA)
Des Moines Chapter
1120 E 6th St., No. 7
Des Moines, IA 50316
Phone: (515)244-9411
Email: ellieESP@aol.com
Ellie Philips, Contact

★ 7753 ★ Depression and Bipolar Support Alliance
Dubuque Mental Health Support Group
4950 Angel View Dr.
Dubuque, IA 52002
Phone: (563)556-2873
Email: pagronen1@mchsi.com
Penny Gronen, Contact

★ 7754 ★ Depression and Bipolar Support Alliance (DBSA)
Quad Cities Chapter
2720 Middle Rd.
Davenport, IA 52803
Phone: (319)355-3977
Email: dirko@netexpress.net
Kathy Kuhl, Contact

★ 7755 ★ Depression and Bipolar Support Alliance (DBSA)
SW Iowa
Atlantic, IA
Phone: (712)243-4650
Barry Buchanan, Contact

★ 7756 ★ Depression and Bipolar Support Alliance (DBSA)
Tri-State Consumers Group
PO Box 1917
Sioux City, IA 51102
Phone: (712)277-4687 **Fax:** (712)252-3871
Email: tristategroups@yahoo.com
Jamie Wilshire, Contact
Remarks: Serves Iowa and South Dakota.

★ 7757 ★ National Depressive and Manic-Depressive Association
Tri-State Consumers Group Chapter
4501 West St.
Sioux City, IA 51108
Phone: (712)277-4687
Denny Wilshire, Contact
Remarks: Serves Iowa and South Dakota.

Kansas

★ 7758 ★ Depression and Bipolar Support Alliance (DBSA)
Douglas County
Lawrence, KS
Phone: (785)842-0714
Email: charlier49@aol.com
Charlie Ross, Contact

★ 7759 ★ Depression and Bipolar Support Alliance (DBSA)
El Dorado Chapter
El Dorado, KS
Phone: (316)541-2935
Esther Fitzgerald, Contact

★ 7760 ★ Depression and Bipolar Support Alliance (DBSA)
Flint Hills Chapter (DMDSG)
2919 Northwood Dr.
Milford, KS 66514
Phone: (785)776-1332 **Fax:** (785)239-2251
Email: flinthillsdmda@hotmail.com
Website: http://www.flinthills.com/~bacon/DMDA
Jim Walker, Contact

★ 7761 ★ Depression and Bipolar Support Alliance (DBSA)
Kansas City Southside Chapter
2226 S 29th St.
Kansas City, KS 66106-5512
Phone: (913)384-0782
Email: babble@kc.rr.com
Website: http://www.depressionsupport.org
Janet Northcott, Contact

★ 7762 ★ Depression and Bipolar Support Alliance (DBSA)
Topeka Chapter
PO Box 4335
Topeka, KS 66604-0335
Phone: (785)272-1360 **Fax:** (785)272-1360
Email: ksbryce@aol.com
Bryce Miller, Contact

★ 7763 ★ Depression and Bipolar Support Alliance (DBSA)
Topeka Trinity Lutheran Church
Topeka, KS
Phone: (785)478-2211
Email: mmhood@cox.net
Mark Hood, Contact

★ 7764 ★ Depression and Bipolar Support Alliance
Wichita Chapter
1451 N Woodlawn
Wichita, KS 67208
Phone: (316)269-2534 **Fax:** (316)269-1409
Email: director30@hotmail.com
Barbara Andres, Contact

Kentucky

★ 7765 ★ Depression and Bipolar Support Alliance
Bluegrass Chapter
Frankfort, KY
Phone: (859)434-3399
Email: dthurberl@aol.com
Don Thurber, Contact

★ 7766 ★ Depression and Bipolar Support Alliance (DBSA)
Louisville Chapter
Louisville, KY
Phone: (502)595-8309 **Fax:** (502)587-8212
Email: mkuh144@msn.com
Michael Kuhl, Contact

★ 7767 ★ Depression and Bipolar Support Alliance
Western Kentucky Chapter
2544 Bittle Rd.
Owensboro, KY 42301
Phone: (270)683-3893
Clara Heintz, Contact

Louisiana

★ 7768 ★ Depression and Bipolar Support Alliance (DBSA)
New Orleans Chapter
1212 Melody Dr.
Metairie, LA 70002
Phone: (504)835-2413
Email: mzaeringer@aol.com
Website: http://www.dbsaneworleans.org
Marilyn Zaeringer, Contact

Maine

★ 7769 ★ Depression and Bipolar Support Alliance (DBSA)
Aces Chapter
2 Lyman Ave., No. 11
Saco, ME 04072-1954
Phone: (207)283-9375
Email: drmike@gwi.net
Dr. Michael Arenstam, Contact

★ 7770 ★ Depression and Bipolar Support Alliance (DBSA)
Falmouth (day meetings only)
Falmouth, ME
Phone: (207)878-8317 **Fax:** (207)878-8317
Email: khessl@maine.rr.com
Website: http://www.dbsafalmouth.rr.com
Kenneth Hess, Contact

★ 7771 ★ Depression and Bipolar Support Alliance (DBSA)
Portland Chapter
Portland, ME
Phone: (207)878-5131
Email: khess1@maine.rr.com
Jeffrey Irving, Contact

Manitoba

★ 7772 ★ Depression and Bipolar Support Alliance (DBSA)
South Central Counseling Consultants
Phone: (204)745-3350 **Fax:** (204)745-3394
Diane Findlay, Contact

★ 7773 ★ Mood Disorders Association of Manitoba, Inc. (DBSA)
4-1000 Notre Dame Ave.
Winnipeg, MB, Canada R3E 0N3
Phone: (204)786-0987 **Fax:** (204)786-1906
Email: sdmdm@depression.mb.ca
Website: http://www.depression.mb.ca

Maryland

★ 7774 ★ Depression and Bipolar Support Alliance (DBSA)
Capitol Area
Bethesda, MD
Phone: (301)279-0831
Email: cadma_99@yahoo.com
Alvin Martin, Contact

★ 7775 ★ Depression and Bipolar Support Alliance (DBSA)
Maryland Chapter
DRADA
600 N Wolfe St.
Baltimore, MD 21287-7381
Phone: (410)955-4647 **Fax:** (410)614-3241
Email: drada@jhmi.edu
Website: http://www.drada.org
Wendy Resnick, Contact

★ 7776 ★ Depression and Bipolar Support Alliance (DBSA)
PPD Moms (Postpartum/Related disorders only)
Rockville, MD
Phone: (301)467-6717
Email: pddmoms@fmhf.org
Website: http://www.fmhf.org

Massachusetts

★ 7777 ★ Depression and Bipolar Support Alliance (DBSA)
Attleboro Chapter
140 Park St.
Attleboro, MA 02703
Phone: (508)222-7525
Email: info@mddaboston.org
Website: http://www.mddaboston.org

★ 7778 ★ Depression and Bipolar Support Alliance (DBSA)
Boston Chapter
PO Box 102
Belmont, MA 02478
Phone: (617)855-2795 **Fax:** (617)855-3666
Email: info@mddaboston.org
Website: http://www.mddaboston.org
Everett Page, Contact

★ 7779 ★ Depression and Bipolar Support Alliance
Northeast Chapter
PO Box 2624
Worcester, MA 01653
Phone: (508)791-0060
Email: jeebee1952@msn.com
Jo-Ellen Stone, Contact

★ 7780 ★ Depression and Bipolar Support Alliance
Northern Worcester County Chapter
Leominster, MA
Phone: (978)874-2713
Eric Hawkins, Contact

★ 7781 ★ Depression and Bipolar Support Alliance (DBSA)
Westwood Lodge Hospital Chapter
45 Clapboardtree St.
Westwood, MA 02090
Phone: (781)431-9704
Email: jacqueline.swerling@cgey.com
Jacquie Swerling, Contact

Michigan

★ 7782 ★ Depression and Bipolar Support Alliance (DBSA)
Cadillac
Cadillac, MI
Phone: (231)775-5638 **Fax:** (231)775-6454
Email: jamesfitz@netonecom.net
Betty Clark, Contact

★ 7783 ★ Depression and Bipolar Support Alliance (DBSA)
Grand Rapids Chapter
858 Reynard St. SE
Grand Rapids, MI 49507
Phone: (616)246-0280
Tim Griffin, Contact

★ 7784 ★ Depression and Bipolar Support Alliance
Greater Flint Area/Rising Above Chapter
Lot 62 Merry Lane
Mount Morris, MI 48458-2426
Phone: (810)789-3609 **Fax:** (810)789-3609
Email: mvallet@gfn.org
Ellie M. Vallet, Contact

★ 7785 ★ Depression and Bipolar Support Alliance
Hillsdale & Jackson Counties Chapter
1200 N West Ave.
Jackson, MI 49202
Phone: (517)780-3384 **Fax:** (517)789-9981
Email: lesia.pikaart@lifewaysmco.com

★ 7786 ★ Depression and Bipolar Support Alliance (DBSA)
Kalamazoo
Portage, MI
Phone: (269)324-0049
Email: dbsa.kazoo@att.net
Website: http://home.att.net/~dbsa.kazoo
David Miner, Contact

★ 7787 ★ Depression and Bipolar Support Alliance (DBSA)
Metro Detroit
PO Box 32531
Detroit, MI 48232
Phone: (313)532-4217
Email: lifeinbalance@mdda-metro-detroit.org
Website: http://mdda-metro-detroit.org

★ 7788 ★ Depression and Bipolar Support Alliance (DBSA)
Metro Detroit
PO Box 132
Dearborn, MI 48121
Phone: (734)641-7994
Email: lifeinbalance@mdda-metro-detroit.org
Website: http://www.mdda-metro-detroit.org
Steve Wyatt, Contact

★ 7789 ★ Depression and Bipolar Support Alliance (DBSA)
Northeast Michigan Chapter
PO Box 715
Alpena, MI 49707
Phone: (989)354-4470
Email: nemdmda@northland.lib.mi.us
Marcelle Levitt, Contact

★ 7790 ★ Depression and Bipolar Support Alliance (DBSA)
Odyssey
Grand Haven, MI
Phone: (616)844-4172

★ 7791 ★ Depression and Bipolar Support Alliance
Traverse Bay Area/Suttons Bay Chapter
701 S Elmwood, No. 19
Traverse City, MI 49684
Phone: (231)342-3076
Jim Brubaker, Contact

★ 7792 ★ Depression and Bipolar Support Alliance (DBSA)
Tri-Cities
609 N Trumbull
Bay City, MI 48708
Phone: (989)662-7897
Email: richpe55@yahoo.com
Website: http://www.babha.org
Richard M. Philipp, Contact

Minnesota

★ 7793 ★ Depression and Bipolar Support Alliance (DBSA)
Golden Valley
Golden Valley, MN
Phone: (763)545-5659 **Fax:** (763)545-6953
Annette Langdon, Contact

★ 7794 ★ Depression and Bipolar Support Alliance
Help, Hope & Healing Chapter
Columbia Heights, MN
Phone: (763)571-6070
Joe Kunza, Contact

★ 7795 ★ Depression and Bipolar Support Alliance
Minnesota Chapter
2021 E Hennepin Ave., No. 412
Minneapolis, MN 55413
Phone: (612)379-7933 **Fax:** (612)331-1630
Email: dmdaminnesota@juno.com
Nikita Godette, Contact

Mississippi

★ 7796 ★ Depression and Bipolar Support Alliance (DBSA)
Coahoma County
Clarksdale, MS
Phone: (662)624-4636
Email: hardcore@gmt.net
Walter James Duncan, Jr., Contact

★ 7797 ★ Depression and Bipolar Support Alliance
Gulf Coast Chapter
4803 Harrison Cir.
Gulfport, MS 39507
Phone: (228)864-4579 **Free:** 800-584-6274
J. B. Morgan, Contact

★ 7798 ★ Depression and Bipolar Support Alliance (DBSA)
Jackson
Jackson, MS
Phone: (601)371-7529
Tommi Smith, Contact

★ 7799 ★ Depression and Bipolar Support Alliance (DBSA)
North Mississippi
Horn Lake, MS
Phone: (662)393-9998 **Fax:** (662)393-9988
Email: dbsanomiss@aol.com
Velma Creekmore, Contact

Missouri

★ 7800 ★ Depression and Bipolar Support Alliance (DBSA)
Greater Saint Louis Chapter
1905 S Grand Blvd.
Saint Louis, MO 63104
Phone: (314)776-3969 **Fax:** (314)776-7071
Email: dmdastl@aol.com
Helen Minth, Contact

★ 7801 ★ Depression and Bipolar Support Alliance (DBSA)
Joplin
Joplin, MO
Phone: (417)438-7173
Email: depressionfree@hotmail.com
Website: http://www.lifesupportministries.org
Ted Gillespie, Contact

★ 7802 ★ Depression and Bipolar Support Alliance (DBSA)
Kansas City Fairway Chapter
901 Tamoshanter
Kansas City, MO 64145
Phone: (816)942-5802 **Fax:** (913)281-3977
Email: tterwelp@worldnet.att.net
Tony Terwelp, Contact

★ 7803 ★ Depression and Bipolar Support Alliance
Southeast Missouri Chapter
PO Box 658
Cape Girardeau, MO 63702-0658
Phone: (573)332-0650 **Fax:** (573)334-4416
Kathryn Myers, Contact

Montana

★ 7804 ★ Depression and Bipolar Support Alliance
Cascade County Outreach Chapter
PO Box 3305
Great Falls, MT 59403
Phone: (406)453-7767 **Fax:** (406)453-7767
Rebecca L. Hewitt, Contact

Nebraska

★ 7805 ★ Depression and Bipolar Support Alliance (DBSA)
Greater Omaha Chapter
5157 Jackson St.
Omaha, NE 68106
Phone: (402)933-6326
Email: dmda@con.net
Website: http://www.geocities.com/dbsago
Bill Thielker, Contact

Nevada

★ 7806 ★ Depression and Bipolar Support Alliance (DBSA)
Southern Nevada
Las Vegas, NV
Phone: (702)257-6795

Email: dmdaofsn@yahoo.com
Cheryl Murphy, Contact

New Hampshire

★ 7807 ★ Depression and Bipolar Support Alliance (DBSA)
Nashua Chapter
PO Box 3761
Nashua, NH 03061
Phone: (603)930-5920
Email: winw@dmdanashua.org
Website: http://www.dmdanashua.org
Tom Doucedette, Contact

New Jersey

★ 7808 ★ Depression and Bipolar Support Alliance (DBSA)
Bergen County Recovery Group
PO Box 1296
Paramus, NJ 07653
Phone: (973)423-4394 **Fax:** (201)525-0844
Email: bergendmda@aol.com
Website: http://community.nj.cm/cc/dmda
Cecily Buck, Contact

★ 7809 ★ Depression and Bipolar Support Alliance (DBSA)
Colts Neck Chapter
East Brunswick, NJ
Phone: (732)919-7739
Email: antwon82763@aol.com
Website: http://community.nj.com/cc/dmdamon
Rick Allen, Contact

★ 7810 ★ Depression and Bipolar Support Alliance (DBSA)
Essex County Chapter
187 Bellevue Ave.
Montclair, NJ 07043
Phone: (973)744-5230
Email: margoatwell@msn.com
Website: http://community.nj.com/cc/dmda.essexcounty
Margo Atwell, Contact

★ 7811 ★ Depression and Bipolar Support Alliance (DBSA)
Middlesex County Chapter
61 Glenn Oaks Ct.
Old Bridge, NJ 08857
Phone: (732)735-8019 **Fax:** (732)679-6346
Email: ss_njdbsa@hotmail.com
Website: http://community.nj.com/cc/mcdmda
Sekhar Subramani, Contact

★ 7812 ★ Depression and Bipolar Support Alliance (DBSA)
Morristown Area
Chatham, NJ
Phone: (973)994-1143
Email: lsbl@panix.com
Website: http://community.nj.com/cc/lstnjdmdsg
Linda Boginsky, Contact

★ 7813 ★ Depression and Bipolar Support Alliance (DBSA)
Morristown/Madison
1 Stony Hill Pl.
Livingston, NJ 07039
Phone: (973)994-1143 **Free:** 800-367-6274
Email: LSB1@panix.com
Website: http://community.nj.com/cc/1stnjdmdsg
Linda Boginsky, Contact

★ 7814 ★ Depression and Bipolar Support Alliance (DBSA)
Sussex County Chapter
2 Smith St.
Newton, NJ 07860
Phone: (973)764-5013
Greg Ludwig, Contact

★ 7815 ★ Depression and Bipolar Support Alliance
Union County Chapter
99 Beauvoir Ave.
Summit, NJ 07901
Phone: (908)233-7074
Email: margoatwell@msn.com
Website: http://www.community.nj.com/cc/dmda.wes
Theldora Hawkins, Contact

New Mexico

★ 7816 ★ Depression and Bipolar Support Alliance (DBSA)
Albuquerque Chapter
PO Box 27619
Albuquerque, NM 87125-7619
Phone: (505)889-3632
Email: dmda4albq@yahoo.com
Leslie Kern, Contact

★ 7817 ★ Depression and Bipolar Support Alliance (DBSA)
Santa Fe
Santa Fe, NM
Phone: (505)954-4429
Email: nmsnowgoose@aol.com
Peggy Arogon, Contact

★ 7818 ★ Depression and Bipolar Support Alliance (DBSA)
Valencia County Chapter
Los Lunas, NM
Phone: (505)857-3647
Email: rdswift@wans.net
Rick Swift, Contact

New York

★ 7819 ★ Depression and Bipolar Support Alliance
Albany Chapter
Albany, NY 12202
Phone: (518)346-6800
Email: consumer@capital.net
Barbara Schumaker, Contact

★ 7820 ★ Depression and Bipolar Support Alliance (DBSA)
Binghamton Chapter
PO Box 1236
Binghamton, NY 13901
Phone: (607)778-2532
Jude Trepa, Contact

★ 7821 ★ Depression and Bipolar Support Alliance (DBSA)
Capitol District Mood Disorder Support Group
Albany, NY
Phone: (518)465-9413
Peter Berkery, Contact

★ 7822 ★ Depression and Bipolar Support Alliance
Dutchess County Chapter
510 Haight Ave.
Poughkeepsie, NY 12603
Phone: (914)473-2500 **Fax:** (914)473-4870
Email: mhadc@frontiernet.com
Website: http://www.mhadc.com

★ 7823 ★ Depression and Bipolar Support Alliance (DBSA)
Finger Lakes Chapter
375-377 W Church St.
Elmira, NY 14901
Phone: (607)734-4789
Email: contact@dbs-alliance-fingerlakes-mmi.org
Website: http://www.dbs-alliance-fingerlakes-mmi.org
George A. Griffith, Contact

★ 7824 ★ Depression and Bipolar Support Alliance (DBSA)
Ithaca Bipolar Explorers Club Chapter
1013 N Tioga St.
Ithaca, NY 14850
Phone: (607)255-7053 **Fax:** (607)255-5684
Email: cs19@cornell.edu
Carole Stone, Contact
Frmly: Depressive and Manic-Depressive Association, Ithaca Bipolar.

★ 7825 ★ Depression and Bipolar Support Alliance
Long Island Chapter
110 Grove St.
Merrick, NY 11566-2246
Phone: (516)379-1238

★ 7826 ★ Depression and Bipolar Support Alliance (DBSA)
MDSG New York Chapter
PO Box 30377
New York, NY 10011
Phone: (212)533-6374 **Fax:** (212)675-0218
Email: info@mdsg.org
Website: http://www.mdsg.org
Judy McEwen, Contact

★ 7827 ★ Depression and Bipolar Support Alliance (DBSA)
MFH
Gloversville, NY
Phone: (518)661-6507
Email: DBSAGville@aol.com
Kathy Austin, Contact

★ 7828 ★ Depression and Bipolar Support Alliance (DBSA)
Rochester Chapter
120 Holyoke St., No. 7
Rochester, NY 14615
Phone: (585)637-8868
Email: rochdmda@aol.com
Website: http://www.dbsaroch.org
Paul Schultz, Contact

★ 7829 ★ Depression and Bipolar Support Alliance
Westchester Chapter
White Plains Hospital Center
Davis Ave. at E Post Rd.
White Plains, NY 10601
Phone: (914)476-4720
Email: wcdmda@aol.com
Website: http://hometown.aol.com/wcdmda/index.html

North Carolina

★ 7830 ★ Depression and Bipolar Support Alliance
North Carolina Chapter
1046 Washington St.
Raleigh, NC 27605-1258

Phone: (919)821-4343 **Fax:** (919)821-4043
Email: ncdmda01@aol.com
Charles Hinton, Contact

North Dakota

★ 7831 ★ Depression and Bipolar Support Alliance
Fargo Chapter
124 8th St. N
Fargo, ND 58102
Phone: (701)237-5871 **Fax:** (701)237-0562
Email: mharrv@juno.com
Susan Helgeland, Contact

Ohio

★ 7832 ★ Depression and Bipolar Support Alliance (DBSA)
Toledo, OH
Phone: (866)553-3632 **Fax:** (419)255-4823
Email: dbsaohio@aol.com
Dorene Sherman, Contact

★ 7833 ★ Depression and Bipolar Support Alliance (DBSA)
Above the Moods Chapter
9299 State Rte. 66 N
Delphos, OH 45833
Phone: (419)692-2785
Irene Blockberger, Contact

★ 7834 ★ Depression and Bipolar Support Alliance (DBSA)
Akron Area
Akron General Medical Center
400 Wabash Ave.
Akron, OH 44307
Phone: (330)344-6475 **Fax:** (330)996-5802
Email: ccihlar@agmc.org
Website: http://www.agmc.org
Claudia Cihlar, RN, Contact

★ 7835 ★ Depression and Bipolar Support Alliance (DBSA)
Athens
PO Box 225
Athens, OH 45701
Phone: (740)594-0022 **Fax:** (740)594-0022
Email: dmdaathens@msn.com
Linda Bauer, Contact

★ 7836 ★ Depression and Bipolar Support Alliance (DBSA)
Bowling Green State University
Bowling Green, OH
Phone: (419)255-1459
Email: dbsabgsu@aol.com
Dorene Sherman, Contact

★ 7837 ★ Depression and Bipolar Support Alliance (DBSA)
Business and Professionals Group
Toledo, OH
Phone: (419)255-1459
Email: dmdato1@amplex.net
Dorene Sherman, Contact

★ 7838 ★ Depression and Bipolar Support Alliance
Cleveland Chapter
11501 Mayfield Rd., No. 100
Cleveland, OH 44106
Phone: (216)229-4841
J. Thomas Kalka, Contact

★ 7839 ★ Depression and Bipolar Support Alliance (DBSA)
Consumers Union of Lucas County
Toledo, OH
Phone: (419)242-1801
Email: dmdatol@amplex.net
Sandy Chambers, Contact

★ 7840 ★ Depression and Bipolar Support Alliance (DBSA)
Findlay
2330 S Main St.
Findlay, OH 45840
Phone: (419)422-9381
Email: bec1944@aol.com
Becky Hickle, Contact

★ 7841 ★ Depression and Bipolar Support Alliance (DBSA)
Four County
115 Deerfield Circle
Bryan, OH 43506
Phone: (419)636-2076 **Fax:** (419)267-3353
Email: gretick@bright.net
Caroline Gretick, Contact

★ 7842 ★ Depression and Bipolar Support Alliance (DBSA)
Greater Dayton
Dayton, OH
Phone: (937)781-9218
Email: dbsagreaterdayton@pop4.net
Vickie Snider, Contact

★ 7843 ★ Depression and Bipolar Support Alliance
Greater Toledo Chapter
961 S Reynolds Rd., No. 37
Toledo, OH 43615
Phone: (419)255-1459 **Fax:** (419)255-4823
Email: dmdatol@amplex.net
Dorene Sherman, Contact

★ 7844 ★ Depression and Bipolar Support Alliance (DBSA)
Medina
Human Services Bldg.
246 Northland Dr.
Medina, OH
Phone: (330)769-4884
Email: info@dbsamedina.org
Website: http://dbsamedina.org
Joan Rizzo, Contact

★ 7845 ★ Depression and Bipolar Support Alliance (DBSA)
Northwest Columbus
Columbus, OH
Phone: (614)792-9749
Email: wilks1953@cs.com
Mike Wilkinson, Contact

★ 7846 ★ Depression and Bipolar Support Alliance
Northwest Columbus Chapter
360 Meadow View Dr.
Powell, OH 43065
Phone: (740)548-6487
Email: dmdacolumbus@insight.rr.com
Barbara Ryan, Contact

★ 7847 ★ Depression and Bipolar Support Alliance (DBSA)
Oregon
Oregon, OH 43616
Phone: (419)255-1459
Email: margaretpaul212@yahoo.com
Dorene Sherman, Contact

★ 7848 ★ Depression and Bipolar Support Alliance (DBSA)
Swanton
Swanton, OH
Phone: (419)825-1745
Judy Alford, Contact

★ 7849 ★ Depression and Bipolar Support Alliance (DBSA)
Tiffin
Tiffin, OH
Phone: (419)448-5601
Email: zipp@acctiffin.com
Brenda Crosby, Contact

★ 7850 ★ Depression and Bipolar Support Alliance (DBSA)
Toledo Family Group
Toledo, OH
Phone: (419)255-1459
Email: dmdato1@amplex.net
Dorene Sherman, Contact

★ 7851 ★ Depression and Bipolar Support Alliance (DBSA)
Toledo Support Group
Toledo, OH
Phone: (419)255-1459
Email: dmdatol@amplex.net
Dorene Sherman, Contact

★ 7852 ★ Depression and Bipolar Support Alliance (DBSA)
Toledo Teen Group
Toledo, OH
Phone: (419)255-1459
Email: dmdato1@amplex.net
Dorene Sherman, Contact

★ 7853 ★ Depression and Bipolar Support Alliance (DBSA)
University of Toledo
Toledo, OH
Phone: (419)255-1459 **Fax:** (419)255-4823
Email: dbsaut@aol.com
Dorene Sherman, Contact

★ 7854 ★ Depression and Bipolar Support Alliance (DBSA)
Wayne County Chapter
Wooster, OH
Phone: (330)264-1590
Email: whudson54@aol.com
Walter Hudson, Contact

Oklahoma

★ 7855 ★ Depression and Bipolar Support Alliance (DBSA)
Oklahoma City, OK
Phone: (405)948-9300
Email: bth6800@aol.com
Bil Thomas, Contact

★ 7856 ★ Depression and Bipolar Support Alliance (DBSA)
Child Adolescents Group
Oklahoma City, OK
Phone: (405)634-4646
Email: bth6800@aol.com
Bil Thomas, Contact

★ 7857 ★ Depression and Bipolar Support Alliance (DBSA)
Community Counseling
Oklahoma City, OK

Phone: (405)235-3006
Roseanne Mann, Contact

★ 7858 ★ Depression and Bipolar Support Alliance
Edmond Chapter
Edmond, OK
Phone: (405)844-7967
Gerri Hames, Contact

★ 7859 ★ Depression and Bipolar Support Alliance (DBSA)
El Reno Chapter
El Reno, OK
Phone: (405)262-3909
Email: idbolain@hotmail.com
Larry Bolain, Contact

★ 7860 ★ Depression and Bipolar Support Alliance (DBSA)
GLBT
Oklahoma City, OK
Phone: (405)634-4646
Email: okglbtsupport@cox.net
Kane Watkins, Contact

★ 7861 ★ Depression and Bipolar Support Alliance (DBSA)
Jesus House
Okalahoma City, OK
Phone: (405)232-7164 **Fax:** (405)232-1369
Email: pnearder@yahoo.com
Pam Neader, Contact

★ 7862 ★ Depression and Bipolar Support Alliance (DBSA)
Midwest City Chapter
Midwest City, OK
Phone: (405)737-1923
Jackie Skaggs, Contact

★ 7863 ★ Depression and Bipolar Support Alliance (DBSA)
Norman Chapter
Norman, OK
Phone: (405)447-5819
Sharon Willis, Contact

★ 7864 ★ Depression and Bipolar Support Alliance (DBSA)
Northside Oklahoma City Chapter
14832 NW Expy.
Piedmont, OK 73078
Phone: (405)840-0607
Mary McCormick, Contact

★ 7865 ★ Depression and Bipolar Support Alliance
Oklahoma Chapter
5313 S May Ave.
Oklahoma City, OK 73119
Phone: (405)681-8073
Email: bth@aol.com
W. D. Thomas, Contact

★ 7866 ★ Depression and Bipolar Support Alliance (DBSA)
Southern Oklahoma
Ardmore, OK
Phone: (580)276-5834
Lisa Hays, Contact

★ 7867 ★ Depression and Bipolar Support Alliance (DBSA)
Southside Oklahoma City Chapter
Oklahoma City, OK
Phone: (405)755-8957
Warren Weaver, Contact

★ 7868 ★ Depression and Bipolar Support Alliance (DBSA)
Southwest Oklahoma Chapter
2328 NW 47th St.
Lawton, OK 73505
Phone: (580)695-1056
Email: johnwindham@yahoo.com
Website: http://www.lasillservices.com
John Windham, Contact

★ 7869 ★ Depression and Bipolar Support Alliance (DBSA)
Stillwater
Stillwater, OK
Phone: (405)372-2468
Email: fulgenzi@aol.com
Lawrence Fulgenzi, MD, Contact

★ 7870 ★ Depression and Bipolar Support Alliance (DBSA)
Tulsa
Tulsa, OK
Phone: (918)258-1684
Joyce Hill, Contact

★ 7871 ★ Depression and Bipolar Support Alliance (DBSA)
Yukon Chapter
Yukon, OK
Phone: (405)373-0059 **Fax:** (405)373-0059
Iva Cook, Contact

Ontario

★ 7872 ★ Mood Disorders Association of Ontario
40 Orchard View Blvd., Ste. 222
Toronto, ON, Canada M4R 1B9
Phone: (416)486-8046 **Fax:** (416)486-8127
Email: info@mooddisorders.on.ca
Website: http://www.mooddisorders.on.ca
Karen Liberman, Contact

Oregon

★ 7873 ★ Depression and Bipolar Support Alliance
Clackamas County Chapter
Oregon City, OR
Phone: (503)722-6500
Email: dmda_clackamas_county@hotmail.com
Casadi Marino, Contact

★ 7874 ★ Depression and Bipolar Support Alliance (DBSA)
Hillsboro
Portland, OR
Phone: (503)357-6331
Gen Horlacher, Contact

★ 7875 ★ Depression and Bipolar Support Alliance (DBSA)
Lane County Chapter
557 Fenster St.
Eugene, OR 97401
Phone: (541)935-2768
Email: hoya2112@aol.com
Sheila Brewster, Contact

★ 7876 ★ Depression and Bipolar Support Alliance (DBSA)
Moody Blues Stress Stop
Ashland, OR
Phone: (541)488-2130 **Fax:** (541)488-7417
Website: Http://www.ashlandhospital.org
Esther Nitzberg, Contact

★ 7877 ★ Depression and Bipolar Support Alliance (DBSA)
Portland Metro
Portland, OR
Phone: (503)245-2311
Glenda Watson, Contact

Pennsylvania

★ 7878 ★ Depression and Bipolar Support Alliance (DBSA)
Allegheny County Chapter
1945 5th Ave.
Pittsburgh, PA 15219
Phone: (412)391-3820 **Fax:** (412)391-3825
Email: jensings@earthlink.net
Delores Burgess, Contact

★ 7879 ★ Depression and Bipolar Support Alliance
Beaver County Chapter
219 3rd St.
Beaver, PA 15009
Phone: (724)775-9152 **Fax:** (724)775-9153
Email: svs2u@hotmail.com
Suzanne Vogel-Scibilia, MD, Contact

★ 7880 ★ Depression and Bipolar Support Alliance
Bipolar/Pottstown Chapter
Pottstown Memorial Medical Center
1600 E High St.
Pottstown, PA 19464
Phone: (610)327-7633 **Fax:** (610)327-7641
Linda W. Thompson, Contact

★ 7881 ★ Depression and Bipolar Support Alliance (DBSA)
Delaware County
Drexel Hill, PA
Phone: (610)544-0816 **Free:** 877-687-9552
Email: dmda562@msn.com
Joseph T. Bunting, Contact

★ 7882 ★ Depression and Bipolar Support Alliance
Delaware County Chapter
Upper Darby, PA
Phone: 877-687-9552 **Fax:** 877-687-9552
Email: dmda562@msn.com
Joseph T. Bunting, Contact

★ 7883 ★ Depression and Bipolar Support Alliance
Delaware Valley Chapter
PO Box 911
Bala Cynwyd, PA 19004-0901
Phone: (215)581-5438
Email: dmda562@msn.com
Ronald Berman, Contact

★ 7884 ★ Depression and Bipolar Support Alliance
Depressive & Manic Depressive Illness Support Group/WPIC
3811 O'Hara St.
Pittsburgh, PA 15213
Phone: (412)624-2211 **Fax:** (412)642-5734
Joan Buttenfield, RN, Contact

★ 7885 ★ Depression and Bipolar Support Alliance
Erie Chapter
1101 Peach St.
Erie, PA 16501
Phone: (814)452-4462 **Fax:** (814)456-6593
Email: shirleyf@surferie.net
Shirley Ruth French, Contact

★ 7886 ★ Depression and Bipolar Support Alliance (DBSA)
Friends for Friends Chapter
4641 Roosevelt Blvd.
Philadelphia, PA 19124-2399
Phone: (215)831-7809 **Fax:** (610)525-3832
Email: friendsforfriends@fbhs.org
Michael Solomon, Contact

★ 7887 ★ Depression and Bipolar Support Alliance (DBSA)
HUP Chapter
9639 James St.
Philadelphia, PA 19114
Phone: (215)552-8737
Email: hupdmda2dhazam@aol.com
Denis Hazam, Contact

★ 7888 ★ Depression and Bipolar Support Alliance
Lehigh Valley Chapter
2552 W South St.
Allentown, PA 18104
Phone: (610)252-2395
Email: info@dmda-lv.org
Website: http://www.dmda-lv.org
Regina Weppel, Contact

★ 7889 ★ Depression and Bipolar Support Alliance (DBSA)
Media
Media, PA
Phone: (610)892-0518
David Child, Contact

★ 7890 ★ Depression and Bipolar Support Alliance (DBSA)
New Directions Abington
Abington, PA
Phone: (215)886-8628
Email: compass123@comcast.net
Nick Breslin, Contact

★ 7891 ★ Depression and Bipolar Support Alliance
New Directions/Abington Chapter
PO Box 181
Hatboro, PA 19040
Phone: (215)887-4059
Email: boris@home.com
Amy Russell, Contact

★ 7892 ★ Depression and Bipolar Support Alliance (DBSA)
Pink & Blues (an LGBT group)
Mark Davis, PA
Phone: (215)546-0300
Email: Mark.Davis@phila.gov
Mark Davis, Contact

★ 7893 ★ Depression and Bipolar Support Alliance (DBSA)
Pocono Mountain Chapter
19 Crystal St.
East Stroudsburg, PA 18301
Phone: (570)420-1327 **Fax:** (570)424-6487
Email: lbutz@losch.net
Lisa Butz, Contact

★ 7894 ★ Depression and Bipolar Support Alliance (DBSA)
Reach Out Foundation
229 Plaza Blvd., No. 101
Morrisville, PA 19067
Phone: (215)428-0404
Email: rofbucks@aol.com
Kathleen Sharp, Contact

★ 7895 ★ Depression and Bipolar Support Alliance (DBSA)
Williamsport
Williamsport, PA
Phone: (570)971-2919
Email: jensings@earthlink.net
Jenna Melissas, Contact

Quebec

★ 7896 ★ Alliance for the Mentally Ill Quebec, Inc. (DBSA)
(Alliance pour les Malades Mentaux Inc.)
5253 Decarie, Ste. 150
Montreal, QC, Canada H3W 3C3
Phone: (514)486-1448 **Fax:** (514)486-6157
Email: amique@amiquebec.org
Website: http://www.amiquebec.org

Rhode Island

★ 7897 ★ Depression and Bipolar Support Alliance
Rhode Island Chapter
Providence, RI
Phone: (401)254-2573 **Fax:** (401)254-0609
Email: jmcnulty@nami.org
Jim McNulty, Contact

South Carolina

★ 7898 ★ Depression and Bipolar Support Alliance (DBSA)
Charleston Chapter
Charleston, SC
Phone: (843)723-2618
Email: manicgh@bellsouth.net
Website: http://www.justimage.net/darkhorse.htm
Melinda G. Harmon, Contact

★ 7899 ★ Depression and Bipolar Support Alliance (DBSA)
Greenwood
Greenwood, SC
Phone: (864)229-3570
Email: tjdorsey@emeraldis.com
Janet W. Dorsey, Contact

★ 7900 ★ Depression and Bipolar Support Alliance (DBSA)
South Carolina Chapter
Myrtle Beach, SC
Phone: (843)347-3035 **Fax:** (843)347-9379
Email: nscrauder@sc.rr.com
George Wright, Contact

★ 7901 ★ Depression and Bipolar Support Alliance
Ups & Downs
Greenville, SC
Phone: (864)455-3798 **Fax:** (864)455-4540
Robert Parker, Contact

Tennessee

★ 7902 ★ Depression and Bipolar Support Alliance (DBSA)
Madison Chapter
Madison, TN
Phone: (615)210-7656
Email: TeenaR@AOL.com
Teena Rodgers, Contact

★ 7903 ★ Depression and Bipolar Support Alliance (DBSA)
Memphis Chapter
Memphis, TN 38103
Phone: (901)384-3754
Email: dmda_memphis@yahoo.com
Kenneth Hetsel, Contact

★ 7904 ★ Depression and Bipolar Support Alliance
Nashville Centennial Chapter
Nashville, TN
Phone: (615)228-4810
Email: LizBeth782@aol.com
Elizabeth Reed, Contact

★ 7905 ★ Depression and Bipolar Support Alliance (DBSA)
Pendulum of Chattanooga
Chattanooga, TN
Phone: (423)698-2384 **Fax:** (423)698-6617
Email: coatsfh@aol.com
Marilou Coats, Contact

★ 7906 ★ Depression and Bipolar Support Alliance (DBSA)
Pendulum of Knoxville
Knoxville, TN
Phone: (865)545-7863
Laura Menefee-Green, Contact

★ 7907 ★ Depression and Bipolar Support Alliance (DBSA)
Two Rivers Chapter
Nashville, TN
Phone: (615)884-2160
Email: beckybarnett@tworivers.org
Becky Barrett, Contact

Texas

★ 7908 ★ Depression and Bipolar Support Alliance (DBSA)
Arlington
Arlington, TX
Phone: (817)416-1668

★ 7909 ★ Depression and Bipolar Support Alliance (DBSA)
Austin Chapter
Austin, TX 78701
Phone: (512)452-1771
Debbie Simms, Contact

★ 7910 ★ Depression and Bipolar Support Alliance
Bay Area Chapter
Friendswood, TX
Phone: (281)335-1000
Email: brew1@houston.rr.com
Paul Koll, Contact

★ 7911 ★ Depression and Bipolar Support Alliance (DBSA)
Brazos Valley Area Chapter
Bryan, TX

Phone: (979)268-2017
Email: kenwolman@msn.com
Jeff Tate, Contact

★ 7912 ★ Depression and Bipolar Support Alliance (DBSA)
Dallas Chapter
Dallas, TX
Phone: (817)654-7100
Carol King, Contact

★ 7913 ★ Depression and Bipolar Support Alliance
El Paso Chapter
El Paso, TX
Phone: (915)541-1400 **Fax:** (915)544-5992
Email: epdmda@aol.com
Website: http://www.epdmda.org
William E. Myers, Contact

★ 7914 ★ Depression and Bipolar Support Alliance (DBSA)
Ft. Worth and Tarrant Counties Chapter
Fort Worth, TX
Phone: (817)654-7100 **Fax:** (817)334-0025
Email: dbsa_fortworth_tc@yahoo.com
Molly Stegall, Contact

★ 7915 ★ Depression and Bipolar Support Alliance
Georgetown Chapter
Georgetown, TX
Phone: (512)863-5560
Anita Smith, Contact

★ 7916 ★ Depression and Bipolar Support Alliance (DBSA)
Grayson-Cook
Whitesboro, TX
Phone: (903)564-7112
Email: feelgoodtom@cox-internet.com
Website: http://www.gcdbsa.org
Thomas Evans, Contact

★ 7917 ★ Depression and Bipolar Support Alliance
Greater Austin Chapter
Austin, TX
Phone: (512)331-6866
Email: kjazz68-1999@yahoo.com
Karen Brown, Contact

★ 7918 ★ Depression and Bipolar Support Alliance
Houston and Harris County Chapter
Houston, TX
Phone: (713)528-1546 **Fax:** (281)514-2570
Email: jim.yeomans@compaq.com
Website: http://www.dmdahouston.org

★ 7919 ★ Depression and Bipolar Support Alliance (DBSA)
San Antonio Chapter
San Antonio, TX
Phone: (210)945-0698
Email: MVKSF@aol.com
Website: http://www.sadmda.org
Kathy Franklin, Contact

★ 7920 ★ Depression and Bipolar Support Alliance (DBSA)
San Marcos
San Marcos, TX
Phone: (512)754-9926 **Fax:** (512)396-5794
Email: dbsasm@yahoo.com
Charlotte Dallas, Contact

★ 7921 ★ Depression and Bipolar Support Alliance (DBSA)
Texas Chapter
Austin, TX
Phone: (512)478-2286 **Free:** 888-716-2807
Fax: (512)478-5223
Email: txdbsacoordinator@hotmail.com
Nancy Scholl, Contact

★ 7922 ★ Depression and Bipolar Support Alliance (DBSA)
Texas Panhandle
Amarillo, TX
Phone: (806)372-1023
Ardis Martin, Contact

★ 7923 ★ Depression and Bipolar Support Alliance
Tyler Chapter
Tyler, TX
Phone: (903)566-8401
Mary Mathison, Contact

Utah

★ 7924 ★ Depression and Bipolar Support Alliance
Uplift Chapter
444 W Stonehedge Dr., No. 8L
Salt Lake City, UT 84107
Phone: (801)264-8193
John Kreipl, Contact

Virginia

★ 7925 ★ Depression and Bipolar Support Alliance (DBSA)
Capitol Area
Arlington, VA
Phone: (301)279-0831
Email: cadma_99@yahoo.com
Alvin Martin, Contact

★ 7926 ★ Depression and Bipolar Support Alliance (DBSA)
Lynchburg Depressive Disorders Chapter
PO Box 216
Lynchburg, VA 24505
Phone: (804)237-5768 **Fax:** (434)237-6140
Email: lindaldda@aol.com
Linda Theisen, Contact

★ 7927 ★ Depression and Bipolar Support Alliance (DBSA)
Norfolk Chapter
6157 Westwood Terrace
Norfolk, VA 23508
Phone: (757)625-2275 **Fax:** (757)627-7199
Linda Matthews, Contact

★ 7928 ★ Depression and Bipolar Support Alliance (DBSA)
Portsmouth
Chesapeake, VA
Phone: (757)548-9323
Email: sredd@peoplec.com
Joy Redd, Contact

★ 7929 ★ Depression and Bipolar Support Alliance (DBSA)
Richmond Chapter
12189 Stokesley Ct.
Richmond, VA 23233
Phone: (804)748-0559 **Fax:** (804)360-8020
Ken Farmer, Contact

★ 7930 ★ Depression and Bipolar Support Alliance (DBSA)
Roanoke Anxiety & Depressive Disorders Chapter
2944 Lockridge Rd. SW
Roanoke, VA 24014
Phone: (540)344-0723 **Fax:** (540)344-1610
Susan Whately, Contact

★ 7931 ★ Depression and Bipolar Support Alliance (DBSA)
Shenwood
Woodstock, VA
Phone: (540)459-2916
Roy Sheetz, Contact

Washington

★ 7932 ★ Depression and Bipolar Support Alliance
Clark County Chapter
Vancouver, WA
Phone: (360)686-3496
Susan Plummer, Contact

★ 7933 ★ Depression and Bipolar Support Alliance (DBSA)
Eastside
Issaquah, WA
Phone: (425)391-3668
Email: Kathryn_clark@yahoo.com
Karoline Clark, Contact

★ 7934 ★ Depression and Bipolar Support Alliance
Greater Seattle Chapter
PO Box 22344
Seattle, WA 98122
Phone: (206)748-1577
Website: http://www.behavenet.com/seattledmda
Ken Clark, Contact

★ 7935 ★ Depression and Bipolar Support Alliance
Skagit Valley Chapter
Mount Vernon, WA
Phone: (360)424-8224
Email: oroboros@gte.net
Diana Dodds, Contact

★ 7936 ★ Depression and Bipolar Support Alliance (DBSA)
Tacoma Chapter
Hope for Depression and Bipolar Support Group
Tacoma, WA 98402
Phone: (253)565-9000
Email: laurie@tacid.org
Website: http://www.tacid.org
Laurie Teeter, Contact

★ 7937 ★ Depression and Bipolar Support Alliance
Tri-City Bi-Polar Support Group
35202 N Flagstone Dr.
Benton City, WA 99320
Phone: (509)946-9230
Email: cider_house_rules@yahoo.com

★ 7938 ★ Depression and Bipolar Support Alliance (DBSA)
Whatcom County Chapter
PO Box 4124
Bellingham, WA 98227
Phone: (360)392-4815 **Fax:** (360)733-2075
Email: raven98230@yahoo.com
Terri Danti, Contact

West Virginia

★ 7939 ★ Depression and Bipolar Support Alliance (DBSA)
Wheeling Chapter
Wheeling, WV
Phone: (304)242-0154
Email: stenger77@comcast.net
Penny Stenger, Contact

Wisconsin

★ 7940 ★ Depression and Bipolar Support Alliance (DBSA)
La Crosse Area Chapter
1515 State St.
La Crosse, WI 54601
Phone: (608)786-2360 **Fax:** (608)783-4996
Email: rpavenue@aol.com
Ray Pauloski, Contact

★ 7941 ★ Depression and Bipolar Support Alliance (DBSA)
Menomonee Falls Chapter
W167 N 8633 Jacobson Dr.
Menomonee Falls, WI 53051
Phone: (262)251-2697
Email: dbsasew@hotmail.com
Tom Malone, Contact

★ 7942 ★ Depression and Bipolar Support Alliance
Mood Disorders of Green Bay Chapter
N 8272 State Hwy. 55
Seymour, WI 54165
Phone: (920)833-6324
Deloris Clausen, Contact

★ 7943 ★ Depression and Bipolar Support Alliance (DBSA)
Ozaukee County Chapter
2141 N Briar Dr.
West Bend, WI 53095
Phone: (262)338-1614
Email: kkatty2@yahoo.com
Jane Kleinowski, Contact

★ 7944 ★ Depression and Bipolar Support Alliance (DBSA)
Southeastern Wisconsin Chapter
PO Box 510214
Milwaukee, WI 53202-0041
Phone: (414)964-2586
Email: dmdasewmilw@hotmail.com
Roseanne Schmidt, Contact

Wyoming

★ 7945 ★ Depression and Bipolar Support Alliance (DBSA)
Casper
Casper, WY
Phone: (307)259-1326
Allene Kilpatrick, Contact

Diabetes

State affiliates of the American Diabetes Association are listed below. The national service center is located at 1701 N Beauregard St., Alexandria, VA 22311, (800)DIABETES, http://www.diabetes.org/.

Alabama

★ 7946 ★ American Diabetes Association
200 Office Park Dr., Ste. 303
Birmingham, AL 35223
Phone: (205)870-5172 **Free:** 800-824-7891
Website: http://www.diabetes.org/adaal

Alaska

★ 7947 ★ American Diabetes Association
Alaska Area
801 W Fireweed, Ste. 103
Anchorage, AK 99503
Phone: (907)272-1424 **Free:** 800-DIABETES
Fax: (907)272-1428
Website: http://www.diabetes.org/adaak

Arizona

★ 7948 ★ American Diabetes Association
Arizona Affiliate
8125 N 23rd Ave., Ste. 222
Phoenix, AZ 85021-4961
Phone: (602)861-4731 **Free:** 800-342-2383
Fax: (602)995-1344
Website: http://www.diabetes.org/adaaz

Arkansas

★ 7949 ★ American Diabetes Association
Arkansas Affiliate
212 Natural Resources Dr.
Little Rock, AR 72205
Phone: (501)221-7444 **Free:** 888-DIABETES
Fax: (501)221-3138
Email: nbaxter@diabetes.org
Website: http://www.diabetes.org/adaar/

Connecticut

★ 7950 ★ American Diabetes Association
Connecticut Information Center
300 Research Pkwy.
Meriden, CT 06450
Phone: (203)639-0385 **Free:** 888-DIABETES
Website: http://www.diabetes.org/adact

Delaware

★ 7951 ★ American Diabetes Association
Delaware Information Center
Community Services Bldg.
100 W 10th St., Ste. 1002
Wilmington, DE 19801
Phone: (302)656-0030 **Fax:** (302)656-7331
Website: http://www.diabetes.org/main/application/commercewf

District of Columbia

★ 7952 ★ American Diabetes Association - Washington, D.C. Metro Area
1211 Connecticut Ave. NW, Ste. 204
Washington, DC 20036
Phone: (202)331-8303 **Free:** 800—DIABETES
Fax: (202)331-1402
Website: http://www.diabetes.org/adadc

Florida

★ 7953 ★ American Diabetes Association
Florida Information Center
1101 N Lake Destiny Rd., Ste. 415
Maitland, FL 32751
Phone: (407)660-1926 **Free:** 800-741-5698
Fax: (407)660-1080
Website: http://www.diabetes.org/adafl

Georgia

★ 7954 ★ American Diabetes Association
1 Corporate Sq., Ste. 120
Atlanta, GA 30329
Phone: (404)320-7100 **Free:** 800-342-2383
Fax: (404)320-0025
Website: http://www.diabetes.org/adaga

★ 7955 ★ American Diabetes Association
Greater Augusta, Georgia/Aiken, South Carolina Area
326 Greene St.
Augusta, GA 30901
Phone: (706)828-0420 **Free:** 800-433-7061
Website: http://www.diabetes.org

Idaho

★ 7956 ★ American Diabetes Association
1111 S Orchard, Ste. 234
Boise, ID 83705
Phone: (208)342-2774 **Free:** 888-DIABETES
Fax: (208)345-9334
Email: tsutton@diabetes.org
Website: http://www.diabetes.org/adaid
Remarks: Serving Southern Idaho.

Illinois

★ 7957 ★ American Diabetes Association
Greater Illinois Area
2580 Federal Dr., Ste. 403
Decatur, IL 62526
Phone: (217)875-9011 **Free:** 800-445-1667
Fax: (217)875-6849
Website: http://www.diabetes.org/adadil

Indiana

★ 7958 ★ American Diabetes Association
Indiana Information Center
7363 E 21st St.
Indianapolis, IN 46219
Phone: (317)352-9226 **Free:** 800-228-2897
Fax: (317)357-4288
Website: http://www.diabetes.org/adain

Iowa

★ 7959 ★ American Diabetes Association
Mid-American Region
6200 Aurora Ave., Ste. 504W
Des Moines, IA 50322
Phone: (515)276-2237 **Free:** 888-DIABETES
Fax: (515)276-2662
Website: http://www.diabetes.org
Remarks: Serving Iowa, Nebraska, and South Dakota.

Kansas

★ 7960 ★ American Diabetes Association
Kansas Area Office
837 S Hillside St.
Wichita, KS 67211-3005
Phone: (316)684-6091 **Free:** 800-676-4065
Website: http://www.diabetes.org/adaks

Kentucky

★ 7961 ★ American Diabetes Association
Kentucky Information Center
Watterson City Office Park
1941 Bishop Ln., Ste. 110
Louisville, KY 40218
Phone: (502)452-6072 **Free:** 888-DIABETES
Fax: (502)452-2705

Website: http://www.diabetes.org/adaky

Maine

★ 7962 ★ American Diabetes Association Maine Affiliate, Inc.
10 Bangor St., Ste. F
PO Box 2208
Augusta, ME 04330
Phone: (207)623-2232 **Free:** 800-870-8000
Website: http://www.diabetes.org/adame

Michigan

★ 7963 ★ American Diabetes Association Michigan Affiliate
30600 Telegraph Rd., Ste. 2255
Bingham Farms, MI 48025
Phone: (810)433-3830 **Free:** 800-525-9292
Website: http://www.diabetes.org/adami

Minnesota

★ 7964 ★ American Diabetes Association Minnesota Area, Great Lakes Region
715 Florida Ave. S, Ste. 307
Minneapolis, MN 55426
Phone: (763)593-5333 **Free:** 800-342-2383
Fax: (763)593-1520
Website: http://www.diabetes.org/adamn

Missouri

★ 7965 ★ American Diabetes Association Regional Office
1316 Parkade Blvd.
Columbia, MO 65203
Phone: (573)443-8611 **Free:** 800-404-2873
Fax: (314)875-2152
Email: pbixler@diabetes.org
Website: http://www.diabetes.org/missouri

Nevada

★ 7966 ★ American Diabetes Association Nevada Information Center
2785 E Desert Inn Rd., Ste. 140
Las Vegas, NV 89121
Phone: (702)369-9995 **Free:** 800-800-4232
Website: http://www.diabetes.org/adanv

New Hampshire

★ 7967 ★ American Diabetes Association New Hampshire Information Center
249 Canal St.
Manchester, NH 03101
Phone: (603)627-9579 **Free:** 888-DIA-BETES
Website: http://www.diabetes.org/adanh

New Jersey

★ 7968 ★ American Diabetes Association New Jersey Office
19 Schoolhouse Rd.
Somerset, NJ 08873-1235
Phone: (732)469-7979 **Free:** 888-DIABETES
Website: http://www.diabetes.org/adanj

New Mexico

★ 7969 ★ American Diabetes Association New Mexico Area Office
525 San Pedro NE, Ste. 101
Albuquerque, NM 87108
Phone: (505)266-5716 **Free:** 800-DIABETES
Fax: (505)268-4533
Website: http://www.diabetes.org/adanm

North Carolina

★ 7970 ★ American Diabetes Association North Carolina Information Center
2 Hanover Sq.
434 Fayetteville St. Mall, Ste. 1600
Raleigh, NC 27601
Phone: (919)743-5400 **Free:** 800-682-9692
Fax: (919)743-5430
Website: http://www.diabetes.org

North Dakota

★ 7971 ★ American Diabetes Association North Dakota/Northern Minnesota
315 N 4th St.
Grand Forks, ND 58203
Phone: (701)746-4427 **Free:** 800-666-6709
Fax: (701)746-9337
Email: ghand@diabetes.org
Website: http://www.diabetes.org

Ohio

★ 7972 ★ American Diabetes Association Central Ohio Area
937 N High St.
Worthington, OH 43085
Phone: (614)436-1917 **Free:** 888-DIABETES
Fax: (614)436-6351
Website: http://www.diabetes.org/

Oregon

★ 7973 ★ American Diabetes Association Oregon Information Center
380 SE Spokane St., Ste. 110
Portland, OR 97202
Phone: (503)736-2770 **Free:** 888-342-2383
Fax: (503)736-2774
Website: http://www.diabetes.org/adaor

South Carolina

★ 7974 ★ American Diabetes Association—South Carolina
2711 Middleburg Dr., Ste. 205
Kittrell Ctr.
Columbia, SC 29204
Phone: (803)799-4246 **Free:** 800-DIABETES
Fax: (803)799-5792
Email: lbundrick@diabetes.org
Website: http://www.diabetes.org/adasc

Tennessee

★ 7975 ★ American Diabetes Association Middle Tennessee Area
4205 Hillsboro Rd., Ste. 200
Nashville, TN 37215-3339
Phone: (615)298-3066 **Free:** 800-DIABETES
Fax: (615)292-5357
Website: http://www.diabetes.org/adatn

Texas

★ 7976 ★ American Diabetes Association Texas Information Center South Central Region
4425 W Airport Freeway, Ste. 130
Irving, TX 75062
Phone: (972)255-6900 **Fax:** (972)255-7900

Utah

★ 7977 ★ American Diabetes Association Serving Utah
250 E 300 S, Ste. 110
Salt Lake City, UT 84111
Phone: (801)363-3024 **Free:** 888-DIABETES
Email: gburns@diabetes.org
Website: http://www.diabetes.org/adaut

Vermont

★ 7978 ★ American Diabetes Association Vermont Information Center
77 Hegeman Dr.
Colchester, VT 05446
Phone: (802)654-7716 **Free:** 888-DIABETES
Fax: (802)654-7657
Email: tdanto@diabetes.org
Website: http://www.diabetes.org
Remarks: Serving Vermont.

Virginia

★ 7979 ★ American Diabetes Association National Office
1701 N Beauregard St.
Alexandria, VA 22311
Phone: (703)549-1500 **Free:** 800-232-3472
Fax: (703)836-7439
Email: customerservice@diabetes.org
Website: http://www.diabetes.org

West Virginia

★ 7980 ★ American Diabetes Association West Virginia Information Center
1221-A Ohio Ave.
Dunbar, WV 25064
Phone: (304)768-2596 **Free:** 800-DIABETES
Website: http://www.diabetes.org/adawv

Wisconsin

★ 7981 ★ American Diabetes Association Wisconsin Information Center
2323 N Mayfair Rd., No. 502
Wauwatosa, WI 53226
Phone: (414)778-5500 **Free:** 888-DIABETES
Website: http://www.diabetes.org/adawi

Wyoming

★ 7982 ★ American Diabetes Association Wyoming Area
330 S Center St.
Casper, WY 82601
Phone: (307)232-0322 **Free:** (866)877-4232
Fax: (307)232-0321
Email: nvreeland@diabetes.org
Website: http://www.diabetes.org

Dietetic Disorders

State chapters of the American Dietetic Association are listed below. The national office is located at 120 S Riverside Plaza, Ste. 2000, Chicago, IL 60606-6995. Additional information can be obtained by calling the national office at (312) 899-0040, or by consulting their web site at http://www.eatright.org/. Another source of information is the National Eating Disorders Association, at 603 Stewart St., Ste. 803, Seattle, WA 98101. Their phone number is (206) 382-3587, and their web site is http://www.nationaleatingdisorders.org/.

Alabama

★ 7983 ★ Alabama Dietetic Association
PO Box 11594
Montgomery, AL 36111-0594
Phone: (334)260-7970 **Fax:** (334)272-7128
Email: LV@gmsal.com
Website: http://www.eatrightalabama.org
Larry A. Vinson, Contact

Alaska

★ 7984 ★ Alaska Dietetic Association
PO Box 448
Girdwood, AK 99587-0448
Email: Aurbanus@provak.org
Website: http://www.eatrightalaska.org
Amy Urbanus, President

Arizona

★ 7985 ★ Arizona Dietetic Association
Document Development Services
PO Box 10344
Phoenix, AZ 85064
Phone: (602)955-4451 **Fax:** (602)957-4532
Email: azdietetic@aol.com
Website: http://www.eatrightarizona.org
Patty Williams, Exec Director

Arkansas

★ 7986 ★ Arkansas Dietetic Association
PO Box 55234
Little Rock, AR 72215-5234
Phone: (501)374-3300 **Fax:** (501)778-9050
Email: arda@up-link.net
Website: http://www.arkansaseatright.org/
Otty Newcomb, Contact

California

★ 7987 ★ California Dietetic Association
7740 Manchester Ave., Ste. 102
Playa del Rey, CA 90293-8499
Phone: (310)822-0177 **Fax:** (310)822-0177
Email: billkraus@dietitian.org
Website: http://www.dietitian.org/
Bill Kraus, MD, Contact

Colorado

★ 7988 ★ Colorado Dietetic Association
PO Box 1775
Estes Park, CO 80517
Phone: (970)577-8777 **Fax:** (970)577-0823
Email: codietassoc@aol.com
Website: http://www.eatrightcolorado.org/
Lorinda Sipe, Exec Director

Connecticut

★ 7989 ★ Connecticut Dietetic Association
138 Oakridge Rd.
Unionville, CT 06085
Phone: (860)673-2520 **Fax:** (860)673-6438
Email: cda@worldnett.att.net
Website: http://www.eatrightct.org
Vikki Allen, Contact

Delaware

★ 7990 ★ Delaware Dietetic Association
74-6A Abbey Lane
Newark, DE 19711
Phone: (302)831-8974
Email: jwalenta@christianacare.org
Website: http://www.dedietassn.org
Julie Walenta, President

District of Columbia

★ 7991 ★ District of Columbia Dietetic Association
DC Hospital Association
1250 I St. NW, Ste. 700
Washington, DC 20005-3922
Phone: (202)289-4215 **Fax:** (202)371-8151
Email: info@dcmada.org
Website: http://www.dcmada.org
Toni Brown, Contact

Florida

★ 7992 ★ Florida Dietetic Association
PO Box 12608
Tallahassee, FL 32317-2608
Phone: (850)386-8850 **Fax:** (850)386-7918
Email: DIETNUTR@aol.com
Website: http://www.eatrightflorida.org
Christine Stapell, MS, RD, Exec Director

Georgia

★ 7993 ★ Georgia Dietetic Association
1260 Winchester Pkwy., Ste. 205
Smyrna, GA 30080
Phone: (770)433-9044 **Fax:** (770)433-2907
Email: gdaexec@bellsouth.net
Website: http://www.gda-online.org
Christen Smith, Contact

Hawaii

★ 7994 ★ Hawaii Dietetic Association
98-945 Moanalua Rd., Apt. 905
Aiea, HI 96701-5044
Email: joann.Yasutake@kp.org
Website: http://www.nutritionhawaii.org
Jo Ann Yasutake, P, President

Idaho

★ 7995 ★ Idaho Dietetic Association
238 E 18th St.
Idaho Falls, ID 83404-6060
Email: metabolic@idahomed.com
Website: http://www.eatrightidaho.org
Becky Sulik, President

Illinois

★ 7996 ★ Illinois Dietetic Association
PO Box 234
Sparland, IL 61565
Phone: (309)274-9969 **Fax:** (309)274-9970
Email: tdmforida@yahoo.com
Website: http://www.eatrightillinois.org
Terri McBride, Exec Director

Indiana

★ 7997 ★ Indiana Dietetic Association
150 N Illinois St.
Elberfeld, IN 47613
Phone: (812)983-9911 **Fax:** (812)983-9911
Email: dsdenton90@aol.com
Website: http://www.dietetics.com/ida
Debra Denton, Contact

Iowa

★ 7998 ★ Iowa Dietetic Association
27924 Butler Center Rd.
Clarksville, IA 50619
Phone: (319)885-6557 **Fax:** (319)885-6558
Email: lursen@netins.net
Website: http://www.eatrightiowa.org
Monica Lursen, RD, Contact

Kansas

★ 7999 ★ Kansas Dietetic Association
3133 U Ave.
Dept. of Hotel, Restaurant, Institution Mgmt. and Dietetics
103 Justin Hall
Herington, KS 67449-5027
Email: eatrightks@tctelco.net
Website: http://www2.kumc.edu/sah/dietetics/kda/kdahome.htm
Diana Floyd, RD, President

Kentucky

★ 8000 ★ Kentucky Dietetic Association
PO Box 23555
Lexington, KY 40523-3555
Phone: (859)245-0717 **Fax:** (859)245-0717
Email: Adrienne@kyeatright.org
Website: http://www.kyeatright.org
Adrienne Grizzell, Contact

Louisiana

★ 8001 ★ Louisiana Dietetic Association
8550 United Plaza Blvd., Ste. 1001
Baton Rouge, LA 70809
Phone: (225)922-4570 **Fax:** (225)922-4611
Email: LDA@pncpa.com
Website: http://www.eatrightlda.org
Bland O'Connor, Exec Director

Maine

★ 8002 ★ Maine Dietetic Association
1174 North Rd.
North Yarmouth, ME 04097
Email: kinneye@mercyme.com
Website: http://www.eatrightmaine.org
Ellen Kinney, President

Maryland

★ 8003 ★ Maryland Dietetic Association
9107 Kilbride Rd..
Sparks Glencoe, MD 21152-9209
Email: hmullan@jhmi.edu
Website: http://www.eatwellmd.org
Hellen Mullan, President

Massachusetts

★ 8004 ★ Massachusetts Dietetic Association
326 Gloucester Hill Rd.
New Gloucester, MA 04260
Phone: (617)501-7083 **Fax:** (207)926-5735
Email: mdadirector@aol.com
Website: http://www.massnutrition.org
Carol Meerschaert, RD, Exec Director

Michigan

★ 8005 ★ Michigan Dietetic Association
Association Management Professionals, Inc.
3319 Greenfield Rd., No. 321
Dearborn, MI 48120
Phone: (313)271-7543 **Fax:** (313)271-1102
Email: ampteam@comcast.net
Website: http://www.eatrightmich.org
David Kasunic, CAE, Contact

Minnesota

★ 8006 ★ Minnesota Dietetic Association
1910 W County Rd., B Ste. 212
Saint Paul, MN 55113-5448
Phone: (651)628-9250 **Fax:** (651)628-0023
Email: mda@eatrightmn.org
Website: http://www.eatrightmn.org
D'ann Brosnahan, CAE, Contact

Mississippi

★ 8007 ★ Mississippi Dietetic Association
330 N Mart Plaza
Jackson, MS 39206
Phone: (601)981-0740 **Fax:** (601)362-9544
Email: msdietetic@yahoo.com
Website: http://www.eatrightmississippi.org
Gordon Haydel, Exec Director

Missouri

★ 8008 ★ Missouri Dietetic Association
PO Box 1225
Jefferson City, MO 65102-1225
Phone: (573)636-2822 **Fax:** (573)636-9749
Email: Broling@socket.net
Website: http://www.eatrightmissouri.org
Brenda Roling, Director

Montana

★ 8009 ★ Montana Dietetic Association
22 Willowbrook Ln.
Missoula, MT 59802-3334
Phone: (406)329-2673
Email: delguerra@saintpatrick.org
Laura Del Guerra, President

Nebraska

★ 8010 ★ Nebraska Dietetic Association
University of Nebraska, Lincoln
316G Leverton Hall, East Campus
Lincoln, NE 68583-0806
Email: bbenes1@unl.edu
Website: http://www.eatrightnebraska.org
Beverly Benes, President

Nevada

★ 8011 ★ Nevada Dietetic Association
8710 White Fir Dr.
Reno, NV 89523
Phone: (775)746-4774
Email: holzog@aol.com
Website: http://www.nevadard.org
Holly Herzog, RD, Contact

New Hampshire

★ 8012 ★ New Hampshire Dietetic Association
133 Hooper Hill Rd.
New Boston, NH 03070
Free: 800-926-6483
Email: barb@intern.my.com
Website: http://www.eatrightnh.org
Barbara Woodland, President

New Jersey

★ 8013 ★ New Jersey Dietetic Association
Professional Management Associates
203 Towne Centre Dr.
Hillsborough, NJ 08844
Phone: (908)359-1184 **Fax:** (908)359-7619
Email: mreardon@profmgmt.com
Website: http://www.eatrightnj.org
Marlene Reardon, Contact

New Mexico

★ 8014 ★ New Mexico Dietetic Association
309 Faculty Ln.
Corrales, NM 87048
Phone: (505)379-1461
Email: Jeanne.Collins@ish-inc.com
Jeanne Collins, President

New York

★ 8015 ★ New York State Dietetic Association
PO Box 30953
New York, NY 10011-0109
Phone: (212)691-7906 **Fax:** (212)741-9334
Email: fredtripp@prodigy.net
Website: http://www.eatrightny.org
Fred Tripp, MS, RD, Exec Director

North Carolina

★ 8016 ★ North Carolina Dietetic Association
1500 Sunday Dr., Ste. 102
Raleigh, NC 27607
Phone: (919)861-4529 **Free:** (866)562-3438
Fax: (919)787-4916
Email: Eheatherly@olsonmgmt.com
Website: http://www.eatrightnc.org
Erika Heatherly, Contact

North Dakota

★ 8017 ★ North Dakota Dietetic Association
2603 Olive St.
Grand Forks, ND 58201
Phone: (701)777-2539 **Fax:** (701)777-3268
Email: Sandy_Walen@mail.und.nodak.edu
Website: http://www.ndsu.nodak.edu/ndda
Sandy Walen, Contact

Ohio

★ 8018 ★ Ohio Dietetic Association
Blendonview Office Park
5008-05 Pine Creek Dr.
Westerville, OH 43081-4899
Phone: (614)895-1253 **Fax:** (614)895-3466
Email: oda@eatrightohio.org
Website: http://www.eatrightohio.org
Marlisa Bannister, Exec Director

Oklahoma

★ 8019 ★ Oklahoma Dietetic Association
125 HES
Stillwater, OK 74078-6116
Phone: (405)744-7469 **Free:** 877-OK-NUTRI
Fax: (405)744-6843
Email: o-d-a@okstate.edu
Website: http://www.oknutrition.org
Carol Beier, MS, RD, Exec Director

Oregon

★ 8020 ★ Oregon Dietetic Association
5811 SE Salmon St.
Portland, OR 97215-2738
Phone: (503)408-6448 **Fax:** (503)408-6448
Email: shelleyb@pop.nwlint.com
Website: http://www.eatrightoregon.org
Shelley Banfe, Contact

Pennsylvania

★ 8021 ★ Pennsylvania Dietetic Association
PO Box 60870
Harrisburg, PA 17106-0870
Phone: (717)236-1220 **Fax:** (717)233-2790
Email: mccann@epix.net
Website: http://www.eatrightpa.org
Colleen McCann, MPH,RD, Contact

Puerto Rico

★ 8022 ★ Puerto Rico Dietetic Association
PO Box 360915
San Juan, PR 00936-0915
Phone: (787)753-7144 **Fax:** (787)767-7880
Email: adapr@guajana.net
Minerva Martinez, Contact

Rhode Island

★ 8023 ★ Rhode Island Dietetic Association
PO Box 6892
Providence, RI 02904-6892
Phone: (401)729-4701
Website: http://www.eatrightri.org
Tricia Harrington, Contact

South Carolina

★ 8024 ★ South Carolina Dietetic Association
PO Box 1763
Columbia, SC 29202
Phone: (803)252-1087 **Fax:** (803)252-0589
Email: eatrightsc@capconsc.com
Website: http://www.eatrightsc.org
Kerin Duggins, Exec Director

South Dakota

★ 8025 ★ South Dakota Dietetic Association
25414 483rd Ave.
Garretson, SD 57030
Phone: (605)688-4039
Email: dawnrdc@msn.com
Website: http://www.sdaho.org/sddapage.htm
Dawn Conrad, RD, LN, Contact

Tennessee

★ 8026 ★ Tennessee Dietetic Association
2706 Greystone Rd.
Nashville, TN 37204
Phone: (615)463-7944 **Fax:** (615)297-9799
Email: allisona@juno.com
Website: http://www.eatright-tn.org
Nan Allison, RD,LDN, Contact

Texas

★ 8027 ★ Texas Dietetic Association
12300 Ford Rd., Suite 135
Dallas, TX 75234
Phone: (972)755-2530 **Fax:** (972)755-2530
Email: tda@challenge-management.com
Website: http://www.nutrition4texas.org
Gail Barron, CAE, Exec Director

Utah

★ 8028 ★ Utah Dietetic Association
1497 Sweetwater Ln.
Farmington, UT 84025-3074
Phone: (801)451-2221
Email: shortedmond@cs.com
Lynda Short, Contact

Vermont

★ 8029 ★ Vermont Dietetic Association
904 Elmore St.
Morrisville, VT 05661-8013
Phone: (802)888-5379 **Fax:** (802)847-3401
Email: helmwest@aol.com
Website: http://www.eatrightvt.org
Joan West, President

Virginia

★ 8030 ★ Virginia Dietetic Association
PO Box 439
Centreville, VA 20122
Phone: (703)815-8293 **Fax:** (703)815-8293
Email: vdahdqtrs@aol.com
Website: http://www.eatright-va.org
Jackie Darling, RD, Contact

Washington

★ 8031 ★ Washington State Dietetic Association
Apple A Day LLC
Seattle, WA 98146
Phone: (206)935-5104 **Fax:** (425)771-9588
Email: WSDA@quidnunc.net
Website: http://www.nutritionwsda.org
Barb Pyper, Contact

West Virginia

★ 8032 ★ West Virginia Dietetic Association
276 Richland Ave.
Morgantown, WV 26505-7310
Phone: (304)293-3402
Email: Bforbes3@wvu.edu
Website: http://www.wvda.org
Betty Forbes, President

Wisconsin

★ 8033 ★ Wisconsin Dietetic Association
1411 W Montgomery St.
Sparta, WI 54656-1003
Phone: (608)269-0042 **Free:** 888-232-8631
Fax: (608)269-0043
Email: wda@centurytel.net
Website: http://www.eatrightwisc.org
Lynn Lawler, RD, CD, Contact

Wyoming

★ 8034 ★ Wyoming Dietetic Association
Department of Family and Consumer Science
PO Box 3354
Laramie, WY 82071
Phone: (307)766-4145
Website: http://www.wyomingdieteticassociation.org
Cristin Stimpson, Contact

Disabilities

Listed below are intermediary affiliates of the National Easter Seal Society, 230 W Monroe St., Ste. 1800, Chicago, IL 60606, (312)726-6200, http://www.easter-seals.org/.

Alabama

★ 8035 ★ Easter Seals Alabama
6005-A E Shirley Ln.
Montgomery, AL 36117
Phone: (334)395-4489 **Free:** 800-388-7325
Fax: (334)395-4492
Email: bcaven@aleaster-seals.org
Website: http://www.al.easter-seals.org
Barry F. Cavan, President
Program(s): Easter Seal Rehabilitation Centers; Janice Capilouto Center for the Deaf; Easter Seal Opportunity Center; Camp Civitan; Camp ASCCA; Achievement Center; and support services.

★ 8036 ★ Easter Seals Birmingham Area
200 Beacon Pkwy. W
Birmingham, AL 35209
Phone: (205)942-6277 **Fax:** (205)945-4906
Email: jwebster@eastersealsbham.org
Johnny Webster, Exec Director
Program(s): Job training and employment services; school-aged children; and support services.

★ 8037 ★ Easter Seals Central Alabama
2125 E South Blvd.
Montgomery, AL 36116-2454
Phone: (334)288-0240 **Fax:** (334)288-7171
Email: easterseals@worldnet.att.net
Website: http://www.eastersealsmontgomery.com
Barry F. Cavan, President
Program(s): Continuing education; early intervention; job training and employment services; and medical rehabilitation and health services.

★ 8038 ★ Easter Seals West Alabama
1110 6th Ave. E
Tuscaloosa, AL 35401
Phone: (205)759-1211 **Fax:** (205)349-1162
Email: eswa@eastersealswestal.org
Website: http://www.easter-seals.org/tuscaloosa
Barry F. Cavan, President
Program(s): Job training and employment services; medical rehabilitation and health services; and support services.

★ 8039 ★ Goodwill Easter Seals of the Gulf Coast
2448 Gordon Smith Dr.
Mobile, AL 36617
Phone: (334)471-1581 **Free:** 800-411-0068
Fax: (334)476-4303
Email: frank@gesgc.org
Website: http://www.goodwill-easterseals.org
Barry F. Cavan, President
Program(s): Camping and recreation; early education and care; early intervention; job training and employment services; school-aged children; and support services.

Alaska

★ 8040 ★ Easter Seals Alaska
126 W 15th Ave.
Anchorage, AK 99501
Phone: (907)277-7325 **Fax:** (907)272-7325
Email: eseals@gci.net
Vilma Gutierrez-Osborne, CEO & Pres
Colette Michaelson, Contact
Program(s): Ketchikan Thrift Store; camping and recreation; continuing education; medical rehabilitation and health services; school-aged children; and support services.

Arizona

★ 8041 ★ Easter Seals Arizona
903 N 2nd St.
Phoenix, AZ 85004-1996
Phone: (602)252-6061 **Free:** 800-626-6061
Fax: (602)252-6065
Email: bpatchett@azseals.org
Website: http://www.azseals.org
Michael T. Fitzgerald, CEO & Pres
Program(s): Adult and senior services; camping and recreation; continuing education; early education and care; early intervention; job training and employment services; medical rehabilitation and health services; school-aged children; and support services.

★ 8042 ★ Easter Seals Arizona Tucson Office
5740 E 22nd St.
Tucson, AZ 85711
Phone: (520)745-5222 **Fax:** (520)745-9030
Michael T. Fitzgerald, President
Jim Neville, Mgr
Program(s): Camping and recreation; continuing education; early education and care; early intervention; job training and employment services; medical rehabilitation and health services; school-aged children; and support services.

★ 8043 ★ Easter Seals Arizona Yuma Office
661 E 32nd St., Ste. A
Yuma, AZ 85364
Phone: (520)726-6800 **Fax:** (520)726-1690
Email: azseals@msn.com
Michael T. Fitzgerald, CEO & Pres
Program(s): Continuing education; early education and care; early intervention; job training and employment services; medical rehabilitation and health services; and school-aged children.

Arkansas

★ 8044 ★ Easter Seals Arkansas
3920 Woodland Heights Rd.
Little Rock, AR 72212-2495
Phone: (501)227-3600 **Free:** 877-533-3600
Fax: (501)227-3658
Email: mail@ar.easter-seals.org
Website: http://www.arkeasterseals.org
Sharon Moone-Jochums, CEO & Pres
Program(s): Easter Seal Work Center; NISH Project; Butler House; Rehabilitation Center; camping and recreation; early education and care; early intervention; medical rehabilitation and health services; schoolaged children; and support services.

California

★ 8045 ★ Easter Seals Southern California Hollywood Office
6515 Sunset Blvd., 4th Fl.
Los Angeles, CA 90028
Phone: (323)462-2424 **Fax:** (323)462-1515
Email: sylvia.wolf@essc.org
Website: http://www.essc.org
Mark Whitley, Contact
Guadalupe Trevizo, Director

★ 8046 ★ Easter Seals Superior California Yuba City Center
144 Gibson Rd.
PO Box 266
Yuba City, CA 95992-0266
Phone: (916)673-4585 **Fax:** (916)673-4328
Email: info@easterseals.com
Website: http://www.easterseals.com
Gary Kasai, CEO & Pres

★ 8047 ★ Easter Seals Bay Area Contra Costa and Solano County Programs
1870 Arnold Industrial Pl., Ste. 1025
Concord, CA 94520
Phone: (510)689-1777 **Fax:** (510)689-2220
Email: sgerdtz@esba.org
Website: http://www.esba.org
Michael Pelfini, CEO & Pres
Program(s): Early intervention.

★ 8048 ★ Easter Seals Bay Area Tri-Valley Campus
7425 Larkdale Ave.
Dublin, CA 94568
Phone: (925)828-8857 **Fax:** (925)828-5245
Email: rhalog@esba.org
Website: http://www.esba.org
Dr. Michael Pelfini, CEO & Pres
Program(s): School-aged children.

★ 8049 ★ Easter Seals Central California
9010 Soquel Dr.
Aptos, CA 95003-4002
Phone: (831)684-2166 **Fax:** (831)685-6055
Email: dalvarez@es-cc.org
Website: http://www.es-cc.org
Bruce Hinman, CEO
Program(s): Camp Harmon; early education and care; early intervention; medical rehabilitation and health services; school-aged children; and support services.

★ 8050 ★ Easter Seals Central California Fresno Office
1685 E St., Ste. 101
Fresno, CA 93706
Phone: (559)264-7113 **Fax:** (559)264-8305
Email: twalker@theworks.com
Website: http://www.es-cc.org
Bruce Hinman, CEO
Ruth Hutchison, Vice President
Program(s): Early education and care; early intervention; medical rehabilitation and health services; school-aged children; and support services.

★ 8051 ★ Easter Seals Central California Marina Office
445 Reservation Rd., Ste. A
Marina, CA 93933-3301
Phone: (831)883-3010 **Fax:** (831)883-3013
Email: scook@earthlink.com
Website: http://www.es-cc.org
Bruce Hinman, CEO
Program(s): Camping and recreation; early education and care; medical rehabilitation and health services; residential and housing services; school-aged children; and support services.

★ 8052 ★ Easter Seals Northern California
1074 East Ave., Ste. A-1
Chico, CA 95973
Phone: (530)894-0205 **Fax:** (530)894-0206
Email: jschifferens@ca-no.easter-seals.org
Website: http://www.esncal.org
Jackie K. Reinhardt, CEO & Pres
John Schifferns, Mgr
Program(s): Adult and senior services; continuing education; early education and care; early intervention; medical rehabilitation and health services; school-aged children; and support services.

★ 8053 ★ Easter Seals Northern California
3289 Edgewood Rd.
Eureka, CA 95502-0109
Phone: (707)445-3106
Email: emorgan@northcoast.com
Website: http://www.esncal.org
Jackie K. Reinhardt, CEO & Pres
Eddie Morgan, Mgr
Program(s): Adult and senior services; camping and recreation; continuing education; early education and care; early intervention; medical rehabilitation and health services; school-aged children; and support services.

★ 8054 ★ Easter Seals Northern California Lakeport Office
501 B Main St.
Lakeport, CA 95453
Phone: (707)263-3949 **Fax:** (707)263-3985
Email: mborjon@ca-no.easter-seals.org
Website: http://www.esncal.org
Jackie K. Reinhardt, CEO & Pres
Program(s): Continuing education; early education and care; early intervention; medical rehabilitation and health services; school-aged children; and support services.

★ 8055 ★ Easter Seals Northern California Novato Office
20 Pimentel Ct., Ste. A1
Novato, CA 94949
Phone: (415)382-7450 **Fax:** (415)382-6052
Email: jreinhardt@ca-no.easter-seals.org
Website: http://www.esncal.org
Jackie K. Reinhardt, CEO & Pres
Program(s): Camping and recreation; continuing education; early education and care; early intervention; medical rehabilitation and health services; school-aged children; and support services.

★ 8056 ★ Easter Seals Northern California Rohnert Park Office
5440 State Farm Dr.
Rohnert Park, CA 94928
Phone: (707)584-1443 **Fax:** (707)584-3438
Email: skreuzer@ca-no.easter-seals.org
Website: http://www.esncal.org
Jackie K. Reinhardt, CEO & Pres
Susanne Kreuzer, Vice President
Program(s): Camping and recreation; continuing education; early education and care; early intervention; medical rehabilitation and health services; school-aged children; and support services.

★ 8057 ★ Easter Seals Southern California Alhambra Office
3055 W Valley Blvd.
Alhambra, CA 91803
Phone: (626)281-9404 **Fax:** (626)457-2868
Email: lupe.trevizoreinoso@essc.org
Website: http://www.essc.org
Guadalupe Trevizo, Director
Program(s): Adult and senior services; and support services.

★ 8058 ★ Easter Seals Southern California Escondido Office
1035 E Valley Pkwy.
Escondido, CA 92025
Phone: (760)737-3990 **Fax:** (760)432-8549
Email: debbie.ball@essc.org
Website: http://www.essc.org
Debbie Ball, Director
Program(s): Adult and senior services; camping and recreation; and medical rehabilitation and health services.

★ 8059 ★ Easter Seals Southern California Inland Counties Program
241 E 9th St.
San Bernardino, CA 92410-4408
Phone: (909)888-4125 **Fax:** (909)884-5741
Email: debbie.ball@essc.org
Website: http://www.essc.org
Mark Whitley, CEO
Debbie Davies, Director
Program(s): Adult and senior services; camping and recreation; school-aged children; and support services.

★ 8060 ★ Easter Seals Southern California Inland County Region Rancho Cucamonga Office
8560 Vinyard Ave., Ste. 201
Rancho Cucamonga, CA 91730
Phone: (909)481-5324 **Fax:** (909)481-5140
Email: debbie.ball@essc.org
Website: http://www.essc.org
Debbie Davies, Director
Program(s): Camping and recreation; school-aged children.

★ 8061 ★ Easter Seals Southern California Inland County Region Victorville Office
14360 St. Andrews Ave., No. 7
Victorville, CA 92392
Phone: (760)952-0018 **Fax:** (760)952-0059
Email: debbie.ball@essc.org
Website: http://www.essc.org
Debbie Davies, Director
Program(s): Adult and senior services; camping and recreation; school-aged children.

★ 8062 ★ Easter Seals Southern California Los Angeles Office
4727 Wilshire Blvd., Ste. 210
Los Angeles, CA 90010
Phone: (323)954-3770 **Fax:** (323)954-3775
Email: lupe.trevizoreinoso@essc.org
Website: http://www.essc.org
Guadalupe Trevizo, Director
Program(s): Adult and senior services.

★ 8063 ★ Easter Seals Southern California North-Central Los Angeles County Programs
315 Arden, Ste. 2
Glendale, CA 91203
Phone: (818)551-0128 **Fax:** (818)551-9846
Email: lupe.trevizoreinoso@essc.org
Website: http://www.essc.org
Guadalupe Trevizo, Director
Program(s): Adult and senior services.

★ 8064 ★ Easter Seals Southern California North Los Angeles County
1146 Commerce Center Dr.
Lancaster, CA 93534
Phone: (661)723-3414 **Fax:** (661)729-3318
Email: paula.pompa.craven@essc.org
Website: http://www.essc.org
Christine Edgeworth, Director
Program(s): Adult and senior services; job training and employment services; and support services.

★ 8065 ★ Easter Seals Southern California
North Los Angeles County Programs
25115 Ave. Stanford, Ste. B-122
Valencia, CA 91355
Phone: (661)257-8558 **Fax:** (661)257-8110
Email: christine.edgeworth@essc.org
Website: http://www.essc.org
Christine Edgeworth, Director
Program(s): Adult and senior services; camping and recreation; job training and employment services; school-aged children; and support services.

★ 8066 ★ Easter Seals Southern California
Orange County Programs
1661 N Raymond Ave., Ste. 100
Anaheim, CA 92801
Phone: (714)441-3070 **Fax:** (714)441-3477
Email: kathleen.kolenda@essc.org
Website: http://www.essc.org
Mark Whitley, CEO
Kathleen Kolenda, Director
Program(s): Adult and senior services; camping and recreation; medical rehabilitation and health services; and school-aged children.

★ 8067 ★ Easter Seals Southern California
Pasadena Office
100 N Hill Ave., Ste. 100
Pasadena, CA 91106
Phone: (626)793-7700 **Fax:** (626)793-8244
Mark Whitley, CEO
Guadalupe Trevizo, Director
Program(s): Adult and senior services.

★ 8068 ★ Easter Seals Southern California
Riverside
1450 University Ave., Ste. F2
Riverside, CA 92507
Phone: (909)248-4873 **Fax:** (909)248-4487
Email: debbie.ball@essc.org
Website: http://www.essc.org
Mark S. Whitley, CEO
Program(s): Adult and senior services.

★ 8069 ★ Easter Seals Southern California
Santa Ana Office
1801 E Edinger Ave., Ste. 190
Santa Ana, CA 92705-4734
Phone: (714)834-1111 **Fax:** (714)834-1128
Email: infor@essc.org
Website: http://www.essc.org
Mark Whitley, President
Program(s): Early education and care; and support services.

★ 8070 ★ Easter Seals Southern California
South San Diego County Programs
101 E 30th St., Unit C
National City, CA 91950
Phone: (619)336-0630 **Fax:** (619)336-0697
Email: debbie.ball@essc.org
Website: http://www.essc.org
Mark Whitley, CEO
Laura Orcutt, Director
Program(s): Adult and senior services; and camping and recreation.

★ 8071 ★ Easter Seals Southern California
Southwest Programs
Torrance Office
3625 Del Amo Blvd., Ste. 120
Torrance, CA 90503
Phone: (310)542-2148 **Fax:** (310)542-0048
Email: dee.prescott@essc.org
Website: http://www.essc.org
Mark S. Whitley, CEO & Pres
Dee Prescott, Director
Program(s): Adult and senior services; and school-aged children.

★ 8072 ★ Easter Seals Southern California
Van Nuys Office
16946 Sherman Way, Ste. 100
Van Nuys, CA 91406
Phone: (818)996-9902 **Fax:** (818)996-1606
Email: carlene.holden@essc.org
Website: http://www.essc.org
Christine Edgeworth, Director
Carlene Holden, Vice President
Program(s): Adult and senior services; and support services.

★ 8073 ★ Easter Seals Southern California
West Los Angeles County
6133 Bristol Pkwy., Ste. 200
Culver City, CA 90230
Phone: (310)641-4884 **Fax:** (310)641-4883
Email: dee.prescott@essc.org
Website: http://www.essc.org
Mark Whitley, CEO
Dee Prescott, Director
Program(s): Adult and senior services; and job training and employment services.

★ 8074 ★ Easter Seals Southern California
Whittier Office
13601 Whittier Blvd., Ste. 100
Whittier, CA 90605
Phone: (562)698-8229 **Fax:** (562)698-8499
Email: kathleen.kolenda@essc.org
Website: http://www.essc.org
Kathleen Kolenda, Director
Program(s): Adult and senior services.

★ 8075 ★ Easter Seals Superior California
3205 Hurley Way
Sacramento, CA 95864-3898
Phone: (916)485-6711 **Fax:** (916)485-2653
Email: info@eastersealsca.com
Website: http://www.eastersealsca.com
Gary Kasai, CEO & Pres
Program(s): Adult and senior services; early intervention; job training and employment services; medical rehabilitation and health services; and support services.

★ 8076 ★ Easter Seals Tri-Counties, California
4251 S Higuera St., Ste. 101
San Luis Obispo, CA 93401
Phone: (805)543-4122 **Fax:** (805)692-5330
Email: easter@fix.net
Janet Napier, Exec Director
Program(s): Early education and care; and support services.

★ 8077 ★ Easter Seals, Tri-Counties California
Ventura Office
10730 Henderson Rd.
Ventura, CA 93004-1898
Phone: (805)647-1141 **Fax:** (805)647-1148
Email: lholzinger@ca-tr.easter-seals.org
Website: http://www.ca-tr.easter-seals.org
Janet V. Napier, Exec Director
Program(s): Continuing education; early education and care; early intervention; medical rehabilitation and health services; school-aged children; and support services.

Colorado

★ 8078 ★ Easter Seals Colorado
5755 W Alameda Ave.
Lakewood, CO 80226-3500
Phone: (303)233-1666 **Free:** 800-875-4732
Fax: (303)233-1028
Email: escinfo@cess.org
Website: http://www.eastersealsco.org
Lynn Robinson, CEO & Pres
Program(s): Camping and recreation; medical rehabilitation and health services; and support services.

★ 8079 ★ Easter Seals Southern Colorado
310 E Abriendo Ave.
Pueblo, CO 81004
Phone: (719)265-2604 **Free:** 800-332-7019
Email: nwhittemore@ssfcu.org
Website: http://www.co-so.easter-seals.org
Nancy Whittemore, Director
Program(s): Camping and recreation; job training and employment services; and support services.

★ 8080 ★ Easter Seals Southern Colorado
Colorado Springs Office
225 S Academy Blvd., Ste. 104
Colorado Springs, CO 80910-2768
Phone: (719)574-9002 **Fax:** (719)574-1330
Email: jschmidt@easter-sealsessc.org
Website: http://www.co-so.easter-seals.org
John Schmidt, President
Program(s): Camping and recreation; medical rehabilitation and health services; school-aged children; and support services.

Connecticut

★ 8081 ★ Easter Seals
Greater Hartford Rehabilitation Center
100 Deerfield Rd.
Windsor, CT 06095-4207
Phone: (860)714-9500 **Fax:** (860)714-8979
Email: agouse@stfranciscare.org
Website: http://www.stfranciscare.org
Allen S. Gouse, PhD, Exec Director

★ 8082 ★ Easter Seals Connecticut
85 Jones St.
Hebron, CT 06248
Phone: (860)228-9438 **Free:** 800-874-7687
Fax: (860)228-9670
Email: johnq@eastersealsofct.org
Website: http://www.ct.easter-seals.org
John R. Quinn, President
Program(s): Camping and recreation; and support services.

★ 8083 ★ Easter Seals Norwalk
14 Strawberry Hill Ave.
Norwalk, CT 06855
Phone: (203)838-7231 **Fax:** (203)838-7283
Email: bto3norwalk@snet.net

Website: http://www.eastersealsofct.org
John R. Quinn, President
Program(s): Job training and employment services; school-aged children.

★ 8084 ★ Easter Seals Waterbury
22 Tompkins St.
Waterbury, CT 06708-1496
Phone: (203)754-5141 **Fax:** (203)757-1198
Email: rvitale@eswct.com
Website: http://www.eswct.com
Francis N. Deblasio, President
Program(s): Early education and care; early intervention; and medical rehabilitation and health services.

Delaware

★ 8085 ★ Easter Seals Delaware and Maryland's Eastern Shore
New Castle County
61 Corporate Circle
New Castle, DE 19720-2405
Phone: (302)324-4444 **Free:** 800-677-3800
Fax: (302)324-4441
Email: wja@nc.esdel.org
Website: http://www.de.easter-seals.org
Sandra J. Tuttle, President
William J. Adami, Vice President
Program(s): Adult and senior services; early intervention; job training and employment services; medical rehabilitation and health services; and support services.

District of Columbia

★ 8086 ★ Easter Seals Mid-Atlantic The Children's Center
2800 13th St. NW
Washington, DC 20009-5399
Phone: (202)387-4434 **Fax:** (202)462-7379
Email: shedgepeth@eseal.org
Website: http://www.eseal.org
Tracey Smith, Director
Sharon Hedgepeth, Director
Program(s): Continuing education; early education and care; early intervention; medical rehabilitation and health services; and support services.

Florida

★ 8087 ★ Easter Seals Broward County
6951 W Sunrise Blvd.
Plantation, FL 33313
Phone: (954)792-8772 **Fax:** (954)791-8275
Email: bdausman@esbc-fl.easter-seals.org
Rebecca C. Dausman, Exec Director
Program(s): Continuing education; early education and care; early intervention; job training and employment services; medical rehabilitation and health services; school-aged children; and support services.

★ 8088 ★ Easter Seals Florida
1040 Woodcock Rd., Ste. 215
Orlando, FL 32803
Phone: (407)896-7881 **Free:** 877-257-3257
Fax: (407)896-8422
Email: info@fl.easter-seals.org
Website: http://www.fl.easter-seals.org
Robert J. Griggs, President
Sue Ventura, Vice President

★ 8089 ★ Easter Seals Florida
1300 Executive Center Dr., Ste. 201
Tallahassee, FL 32301
Phone: (850)222-4606 **Fax:** (850)222-4615
Email: rgriggs@fl.easter-seals.org
Website: http://www.fl.easter-seals.org
Robert J. Griggs, CEO

★ 8090 ★ Easter Seals Florida Central Florida Region
1040 Woodcock Rd., Ste. 215
Orlando, FL 32803
Phone: (407)896-7881 **Fax:** (407)896-8422
Email: jnasser@fl.easter-seals.org
Website: http://www.fl.easter-seals.org
Robert J. Griggs, President

★ 8091 ★ Easter Seals Florida East Coast Region Melbourne Office
3661 S Babcock St.
Melbourne, FL 32901-8221
Phone: (321)723-4474 **Fax:** (321)676-3843
Email: gedwards@fl.easter-seals.org
Website: http://www.fl.easter-seals.org
Gail Edwards, Exec Director

★ 8092 ★ Easter Seals Florida Keys Region
5220 College Rd.
Key West, FL 33040
Phone: (305)294-1089 **Fax:** (305)296-1530
Email: mmurphy@fl.easter-seals.org
Website: http://www.fl.easter-seals.org
Bob Griggs, CEO & Pres
Jonathan Weinshank, Director
Program(s): Early education and care; early intervention; and medical rehabilitation and health services.

★ 8093 ★ Easter Seals Florida Palm Beach/Martin Region Martin County Regional Office
1700 SE Monterey Rd.
Stuart, FL 34996-4109
Phone: (561)286-4444 **Fax:** (561)286-4643
Email: kbarnes@fl.easter-seals.org
Website: http://www.fl.easter-seals.org
Kendra Barnes, Director

★ 8094 ★ Easter Seals Florida West Coast Region
7402 N 56th St., Ste. 906
Tampa, FL 33617
Phone: (813)988-7633 **Fax:** (813)914-0403
Email: garmstrong@fl.easter-seals.org
Website: http://www.fl.easter-seals.org
Robert J. Griggs, President
Gracy McLeary, Exec Director
Program(s): Early education and care; early intervention; medical rehabilitation and health services; and support services.

★ 8095 ★ Easter Seals Miami-Dade
1475 NW 14th Ave.
Miami, FL 33125-1692
Phone: (305)325-0470 **Fax:** (305)325-0578
Email: essdade@aol.com
Joan Bornstein, President

★ 8096 ★ Easter Seals North Florida
910 Myers Park Dr.
Tallahassee, FL 32301-4586
Phone: (850)222-4465 **Fax:** (850)222-4468
Email: enorthflorida@aol.com
Website: http://www.freenet.tlh.fl.us/EasterSeals/tallyes.htm
Christine Hall, President
Program(s): Early intervention; job training and employment services; and support services.

★ 8097 ★ Easter Seals Volusia and Flagler Counties Florida
1219 Dunn Ave.
Daytona Beach, FL 32120
Phone: (386)255-4568 **Free:** 877-255-4568
Fax: (386)258-7677
Email: info@fl.vf.easter-seals.org
Website: http://www.fl.vf.easter-seals.org
Lynn Sinnott, CEO & Pres
Program(s): Camping and recreation; continuing education; early education and care; early intervention; medical rehabilitation and health services; school-aged children; and support services.

Georgia

★ 8098 ★ Easter Seals East Georgia
1500 Wrightsboro Rd.
Augusta, GA 30904-2441
Phone: (706)667-9695 **Free:** (866)667-9695
Fax: (706)667-8831
Email: info@esega.org
Website: http://www.ga-ea.easter-seals.org
Sheila Thomas, Exec Director
Program(s): Job training and employment services; and support services.

★ 8099 ★ Easter Seals East Georgia
PO Box 1836
Thomson, GA 30824
Phone: (706)595-2212
Email: info@esega.org
Website: http://www.ga-ea.easter-seals.org
Sheila Thomas, Exec Director
Program(s): Job training and employment services.

★ 8100 ★ Easter Seals Middle Georgia
602 Kellam Rd.
Dublin, GA 31021
Phone: (478)275-8850 **Fax:** (478)275-8852
Email: ehooks@ga-mi.easterseals.org
Eloyce Hooks, Exec Director
Program(s): Job training and employment services; school-aged children; and support services.

★ 8101 ★ Easter Seals North Georgia
Prado North, Ste. 100
5600 Roswell Rd.
Atlanta, GA 30342
Phone: (404)943-1070 **Fax:** (404)943-0890
Email: info@ga-no.easter-seals.org
Website: http://www.ga-no.easter-seals.org
Donna Davidson, CEO & Pres

★ 8102 ★ Easter Seals Southern Georgia
1906 Palmyra Rd.
Albany, GA 31701-1598
Phone: (229)439-7061 **Free:** 800-365-4583
Fax: (229)435-6278
Email: benglish@swga-easterseals.org
Website: http://www.swga-easterseals.org
Beth English, Exec Director
Program(s): Adult and senior services; camping and recreation; early education and care; job training and employment services; residential and housing services; school-aged children; and support services.

★ 8103 ★ Easter Seals West Georgia
2515 Double Churches Rd.
Columbus, GA 31909
Phone: (706)660-1144 **Fax:** (706)660-1146
Email: easter-sealscolsga@mchsi.com
Barry F. Cavan, President
Sharon Borger, Exec Director
Program(s): Camping and recreation; early education and care; early intervention; job training and employment services; medical rehabilitation and health services; school-aged children; and support services.

Hawaii

★ 8104 ★ Easter Seals Hawaii
710 Green St.
Honolulu, HI 96813-2119
Phone: (808)536-1015 **Fax:** (808)536-3765
Email: info@eastersealshawaii.org

Website: http://www.eastersealshawaii.org
John F. Howell, CEO & Pres

Program(s): Adult and senior services; camping and recreation; continuing education; early education and care; early intervention; school-aged children; and support services.

Illinois

★ 8105 ★ Easter Seals Central Illinois
2715 N 27th St.
Decatur, IL 62526
Phone: (217)429-1052 **Free:** 800-500-7325
Fax: (217)423-7605
Email: jankel@easterseals-ci.org
Website: http://www.easterseals-ci.org
Janet Kelscheimer, President

Program(s): Camping and recreation; early education and care; early intervention; job training and employment services; medical rehabilitation and health services; school-aged children; and support services.

★ 8106 ★ Easter Seals of LaSalle and Bureau Counties
1013 Adams St.
Ottawa, IL 61350-4399
Phone: (815)434-0857 **Fax:** (815)434-2260
Leslie D. Ziel, Contact

Program(s): Camping and recreation; continuing education; early education and care; early intervention; medical rehabilitation and health services; school-aged children; and support services.

★ 8107 ★ Easter Seals Metro. Chicago
14 E Jackson Blvd., 9th Fl.
Chicago, IL 60604-2212
Phone: (312)939-5115 **Fax:** (312)939-0283
Email: essmc@eastersealchicago.org
Website: http://www.eastersealchicago.org
F. Timothy Muri, CEO & Pres

Program(s): Camping and recreation; medical rehabilitation and health services; and support services.

★ 8108 ★ Easter Seals Mid-Eastern Illinois
1137 E 5000 North Rd.
Bourbonnais, IL 60914
Phone: (815)932-0623 **Fax:** (815)932-2577
Email: eskkk@main.keynet.net
Website: http://www.easterseals-kankakee.org
Jackie Havener, Exec Director

Program(s): Camping and recreation; early education and care; early intervention; and medical rehabilitation and health services.

★ 8109 ★ Easter Seals Moline, Illinois
1504 13th Ave.
Moline, IL 61265-3196
Phone: (309)762-9552 **Fax:** (309)762-9610
George McDaniel, Exec Director

Program(s): Camping and recreation; and medical rehabilitation and health services.

★ 8110 ★ Easter Seals Southwestern Illinois
602 E 3rd St.
Alton, IL 62002
Phone: (618)462-7325 **Fax:** (618)462-8170
Website: http://www.mo.easter-seals.org
Craig A. Byrd, CEO & Pres

Program(s): Camping and recreation; and early education and care.

★ 8111 ★ Easter Seals Will-Grundy Counties
735 Essington, Ste. 103
Joliet, IL 60435-2830
Phone: (815)773-9362 **Fax:** (815)773-9365
Email: dcondotti@il-wg.easter-seals.org
Website: http://www.il-wg.easter-seals.org
Debra Condotti, President

Indiana

★ 8112 ★ Bridgepointe Goodwill Industries and Easter Seals, Inc.
1329 Applegate Ln.
Clarksville, IN 47129-9610
Phone: (812)283-7908 **Free:** 800-660-3355
Fax: (812)283-6248
Email: cmarshall@bridgepointe.org
Caren Marshall, Exec Director

Program(s): Camping and recreation; early education and care; early intervention; job training and employment services; medical rehabilitation and health services; school-aged children; and support services.

★ 8113 ★ Easter Seals ARC of Northeast Indiana
2542 Thompson Ave.
Fort Wayne, IN 46807
Phone: (260)456-4534 **Free:** 800-234-7811
Fax: (260)745-5200
Email: shinkle@arc-nei.org
Website: http://www.esarc.org
Steve Hinkle, CEO

Program(s): Camping and recreation; continuing education; early education and care.

★ 8114 ★ Easter Seals Committee Wayne & Union Counties
Centerville, IN 47330-0086
Phone: (317)855-2482 **Fax:** (317)855-2482
Email: easterseals@juno.com
Patricia Bowers, Exec Director

Program(s): Camping and recreation; school-aged children; and support services.

★ 8115 ★ Easter Seals Crossroads, Bartholomew County
4251 S 600 E
Columbus, IN 47203
Phone: (812)579-5790 **Fax:** (812)579-5790
Email: debbies@iquest.net
Deborah Siefker, Exec Director

Program(s): Camping, recreation, and support services.

Iowa

★ 8116 ★ Easter Seals Iowa
401 NE 66th Ave.
Des Moines, IA 50313
Phone: (515)289-1933 **Fax:** (515)289-1281
Email: info@eastersealsia.org
Donna Elbrecht, CEO & Pres

Program(s): Camping and recreation; early education and care; job training and employment services; medical rehabilitation and health services; school-aged children; and support services.

Kansas

★ 8117 ★ Easter Seals Kansas
3636 N Oliver
Wichita, KS 67220
Phone: (316)744-9291 **Fax:** (316)744-1428
Website: http://www.goodwilleastersealsks.org
Marie Mareda, President

Program(s): Job training and employment services; and support services.

Kentucky

★ 8118 ★ Easter Seals Kentucky
9810 Bluebrass Pkwy.
Louisville, KY 40299-1906
Phone: (502)584-9781 **Fax:** (502)589-2409
Email: bls@loueaster.org
Website: http://www.loueaster.org
Susan Eisenback, Exec Director

Program(s): Early intervention, medical rehabilitation, and health services.

★ 8119 ★ Easter Seals of Northern Kentucky
31 Spiral Dr.
Florence, KY 41042
Phone: (859)491-1171 **Fax:** (859)491-8132
Email: vickie@nkeaster.org
Margaret Baker-Wernersbach, Exec Director

Program(s): Medical rehabilitation and health services.

★ 8120 ★ Easter Seals West Kentucky
2229 Mildred St.
Paducah, KY 42001
Phone: (270)444-9687 **Free:** (866)673-3565
Fax: (270)444-0655
Email: info@ky-ws.easter-seals.org
Website: http://www.ky-ws.easter-seals.org
Kenneth R. Lucas, President

Program(s): Adult and senior services; continuing education; early education and care; early intervention; job training and employment services; medical rehabilitation and health services; school-aged children; and support services.

Louisiana

★ 8121 ★ Easter Seals Louisiana Covington Office
600 N Hwy. 190, Ste. 213
Covington, LA 70433
Phone: (504)892-7604 **Fax:** (504)892-5735
Email: escasmgt9@compsurf.com
Daniel H. Underwood, CEO

Program(s): Camping and recreation; early education and care; early intervention; medical rehabilitation and health services; school-aged children; and support services.

★ 8122 ★ Easter Seals Louisiana Monroe Office
1900 N 18th St., Ste. 203B
Monroe, LA 71201
Phone: (318)322-4788 **Fax:** (318)322-1549
Email: esldeltaproject@aol.com
Joan Oursler, Contact

Program(s): Camping and recreation; continuing education; early education and care; early intervention; medical rehabilitation and health services; school-aged children; and support services.

★ 8123 ★ Easter Seals Louisiana New Orleans Office
305 Baronne St., Ste. 400
New Orleans, LA 70112-1617
Phone: (504)523-7325 **Free:** 800-695-7325
Fax: (504)523-3465
Email: essla@aol.com
Daniel H. Underwood, CEO & Pres

Program(s): Camping and recreation; early education and care; early intervention; school-aged children; and support services.

★ 8124 ★ Easter Seals Louisiana Shreveport Office
900 Pierremont Rd., Ste. 220
PO Box 6105
Shreveport, LA 71106

Phone: (318)868-5840 **Fax:** (318)868-3612
Email: esshreveport@aol.com
Daniel H. Underwood, CEO & Pres
Gordon Grafton, Vice President
Program(s): Camping and recreation; early education and care; early intervention; medical rehabilitation and health services; school-aged children; and support services.

Maryland

★ 8125 ★ Easter Seals Mid-Atlantic
4041 Powder Mill Rd., Ste. 100
Beltsville, MD 20705
Phone: (301)931-8700 **Free:** 800-862-1377
Fax: (301)931-8690
Email: lreeves@eseal.org
Website: http://www.eseal.org
Lisa Reeves, CEO & Pres
Remarks: Serves Washington DC, Maryland, northern Virginia, south-central Pennsylvania, and eastern West Virginia.

★ 8126 ★ Easter Seals Salisbury
1915 N Salisbury Blvd.
Salisbury, MD 21801
Phone: (410)546-2894 **Fax:** (410)546-4913
Email: ncotter@gt.esdel.org
Website: http://www.de.easter-seals.org
Sandra J. Tuttle, President
Program(s): Early intervention, medical rehabilitation and health services, and support services.

Massachusetts

★ 8127 ★ Easter Seals Massachusetts
Denholm Bldg.
484 Main St.
Worcester, MA 01608-1817
Phone: (508)757-2756 **Free:** 800-244-2756
Fax: (508)831-9768
Email: maryd@eastersealsma.org
Website: http://www.eastersealsma.org
Kirk N. Joslin, CEO & Pres
Program(s): Camping and recreation; continuing education; early education and care; job training and employment services; medical rehabilitation and health services; school-aged children; and support services.

Michigan

★ 8128 ★ Easter Seals Southeastern Michigan
21111 Haggerty Rd.
Novi, MI 48375
Phone: (248)447-4711 **Fax:** (248)372-7472
John R. Cocciolone, CEO & Pres
Valerie Pearson, Director

★ 8129 ★ Easter Seals Genesee County
1420 W 3rd Ave.
Flint, MI 48504-4897
Phone: (810)238-0475 **Fax:** (810)238-9270
Email: eslily@intouchmi.com
Elliott C. Fauster, Exec Director
Program(s): Camping and recreation; medical rehabilitation and health services; school-aged children; and support services.

★ 8130 ★ Easter Seals Michigan
4065 Saladin Dr. SE
Grand Rapids, MI 49546-6299
Phone: (616)942-2081 **Free:** 800-292-2729
Fax: (616)942-5932
Email: essofmich@aol.com
Website: http://www.mi-ws.easter-seals.org
David Lankford, Contact
Kathy Hayden, Contact
Program(s): Adult and senior services; camping and recreation; early education and care; early intervention; job training and employment services; medical rehabilitation and health services; school-aged children; and support services.

★ 8131 ★ Easter Seals Michigan East Central Region
804 S Hamilton
Saginaw, MI 48602-1516
Phone: (517)797-0880 **Free:** 800-292-2729
Fax: (517)797-0888
Email: esofmi@aol.com
Website: http://www.mi-ws.easter-seals.org
Julie S. Dorsey, Director
Program(s): Adult and senior services; camping and recreation; early education and care; job training and employment services; medical rehabilitation and health services; school-aged children; and support services.

★ 8132 ★ Easter Seals Michigan Northwestern Region
109 S Union, Ste. 209
Traverse City, MI 49684
Phone: (231)941-1271 **Fax:** (231)941-1990
Email: essofmich@aol.com
Website: http://www.mi-ws.easter-seals.org
Robert Dean, CEO & Pres
Betty Reynolds-Maciejewski, Director
Program(s): Camping and recreation; continuing education; early education and care; early intervention; job training and employment services; medical rehabilitation and health services; school-aged children; and support services.

★ 8133 ★ Easter Seals Michigan Upper Peninsula Region
104 Coles Dr., Ste. A
Marquette, MI 49855-4059
Phone: (906)228-5816 **Free:** 800-292-2729
Fax: (906)228-6199
Email: esofupmich@aol.com
Karen Taylor, Director
Nancy A. Bell, Director
Program(s): Early education and care; medical rehabilitation and health services; school-aged children; and support services.

★ 8134 ★ Easter Seals Southeastern Michigan
22150 W 9 Mile Rd.
Southfield, MI 48034
Phone: (248)386-9600 **Free:** 800-757-3257
Fax: (248)386-9604
Email: jcocciolne@essmichigan.org
Website: http://www.essmichigan.org
Mr. John R. Cocciolone, CEO & Pres

Minnesota

★ 8135 ★ Easter Seals Minnesota Rochester Office
660 37th St. NW
Rochester, MN 55901
Phone: (507)287-8699 **Fax:** (507)281-3749
Michael Wirth-Davis, CEO & Pres

★ 8136 ★ Easter Seals Minnesota St. Paul Office
2543 Como Ave.
Saint Paul, MN 55108-1298
Phone: (651)646-2591 **Free:** 800-669-6719
Fax: (651)646-0302
Email: kmatter@goodwilleasterseals.org
Website: http://www.goodwilleasterseals.org
Michael Wirth-Davis, President
Program(s): Job training and employment services; and support services.

★ 8137 ★ Easter Seals Minnesota Waite Park Office
50 S 2nd St.
Waite Park, MN 56387
Phone: (320)654-9527 **Fax:** (320)654-9542
Michael Wirth-Davis, CEO & Pres
Program(s): Job training and employment services; and support services.

★ 8138 ★ Easter Seals Minnesota Willmar Office
2424 1st St. S
Willmar, MN 56201
Phone: (320)214-9238 **Fax:** (320)214-9140
Michael Wirth-Davis, CEO & Pres
Program(s): Job training and employment services; and support services.

Missouri

★ 8139 ★ Easter Seals Greater Kansas City
908 NE 116th Terrace
Kansas City, MO 64155
Phone: (816)734-7068 **Fax:** (816)734-7068
Email: kkroh@mo.easter-seals.org
Website: http://www.mo.easter-seals.org
Craig A Byrd, CEO & Pres
Program(s): Camping and recreation; early education and care; job training and employment services; medical rehabilitation and health services; school-aged children; and support services.

★ 8140 ★ Easter Seals Missouri
5025 Northrup Ave., Ste. 110
Saint Louis, MO 63110-2050
Phone: (314)664-5025 **Free:** 800-664-5025
Fax: (314)664-4838
Email: pat@easterseals-mo.org
Website: http://www.mo.easter-seals.org
Craig A. Byrd, CEO & Pres
Program(s): Support services.

★ 8141 ★ Easter Seals Southwest Missouri
2200 E Sunshine, Ste. 103
Springfield, MO 65804
Phone: (417)882-6500 **Fax:** (417)882-0230
Email: clawless@mo.easter-seals.org
Website: http://www.mo.easter-seals.org
Christine Lawless, Director
Program(s): Camping and recreation; early education and care; early intervention; school-aged children; and support services.

Montana

★ 8142 ★ Easter Seals Northern Rocky Mountains
4400 Central Ave.
Great Falls, MT 59405-1695
Phone: (406)761-3680 **Free:** 800-771-2153
Fax: (406)761-5110
Email: michelleb@esgw.org
Website: http://www.goodwill.org/localweb/greatfalls/
Michelle Belknap, CEO
Sally Cerny, President
Remarks: Serves Idaho, Montana, and Wyoming.

Nebraska

★ 8143 ★ Easter Seals Nebraska
2727 W 2nd, Ste. 471
Hastings, NE 68901
Phone: (402)462-3031 **Free:** 800-471-6425
Fax: (402)462-2040
Email: bkoehler@ne.easter-seals.org
Website: http://www.ne.easter-seals.org
Karen Ginder, President

Program(s): Job training and employment services.

Nevada

★ 8144 ★ Easter Seals Nevada
6100 Neil Rd., Ste. 201
Reno, NV 89511
Phone: (775)322-6555 **Fax:** (775)834-5933
Email: info@eastersealsnv.org
Donald Stromquist, President
Program(s): Adult and senior services; camping and recreation; job training and employment services; residential and housing services; school-aged children; and support services.

New Hampshire

★ 8145 ★ Easter Seals Lancaster
525 Prospect St.
Lancaster, NH 03584
Phone: (603)788-0911
Email: essofny@aol.com
Website: http://www.nh.easter-seals.org
Larry Gammon, CEO & Pres
Program(s): Residential and housing services; and school-aged children.

★ 8146 ★ Easter Seals New Hampshire
390 Union Ave.
Laconia, NH 03246
Phone: (603)524-8552 **Fax:** (603)524-8566
Email: essofny@aol.com
Website: http://www.nh.easter-seals.org
Larry Gammon, CEO & Pres
Program(s): Adult and senior services; and job training and employment services.

★ 8147 ★ Easter Seals New Hampshire Claremont Office
54 Pleasant St.
Claremont, NH 03743
Phone: (603)543-3795
Email: essofny@aol.com
Website: http://www.nh.easter-seals.org
Larry Gammon, CEO & Pres
Program(s): Job training and employment services.

★ 8148 ★ Easter Seals New Hampshire Concord Office
2 Industrial Dr.
Concord, NH 03301
Phone: (603)226-3791 **Fax:** (603)226-2540
Email: essofny@aol.com
Website: http://www.nh.easter-seals.org
Larry Gammon, CEO & Pres
Program(s): Adult and senior services; early education and care; early intervention; and support services.

★ 8149 ★ Easter Seals New Hampshire Derry Office
44 Birch St.
Derry, NH 03038
Phone: (603)432-1945 **Fax:** (603)434-2134
Email: essofny@aol.com
Website: http://www.nh.easter-seals.org
Larry Gammon, CEO & Pres
Program(s): Early intervention.

★ 8150 ★ Easter Seals New Hampshire Keene Office
12 Kingsbury St.
Keene, NH 03431
Phone: (603)355-1067 **Fax:** (603)358-3947
Email: essofny@aol.com
Website: http://www.nh.easter-seals.org
Larry Gammon, CEO & Pres
Program(s): Early education and care; job training and employment services; and school-aged children.

★ 8151 ★ Easter Seals New Hampshire Manchester Office
555 Auburn St.
Manchester, NH 03103
Phone: (603)623-8863 **Fax:** (603)621-3461
Email: mail@eseals.org
Website: http://www.nh.easter-seals.org
Larry Gammon, CEO & Pres
Christine McMahon, Contact
Program(s): Adult and senior services; camping and recreation; continuing education; early education and care; early intervention; job training and employment services; medical rehabilitation and health services; residential and housing services; school-aged children; and support services.

★ 8152 ★ Easter Seals New Hampshire Portsmouth Office
147 Congress St., Ste. A
Portsmouth, NH 03801
Phone: (603)431-7242 **Fax:** (603)427-2895
Email: essofny@aol.com
Website: http://www.nh.easter-seals.org
Larry Gammon, CEO & Pres
Program(s): Early education and care; job training and employment services; and school-aged children.

★ 8153 ★ Easter Seals Plymouth
1000 Texas Hill Rd.
Plymouth, NH 03264
Phone: (603)968-4467
Email: essofny@aol.com
Website: http://www.nh.easter-seals.org
Larry Gammon, CEO & Pres
Program(s): Residential and housing services.

★ 8154 ★ Easter Seals Rumney
1849 Rumney Rd.
Rumney, NH 03266
Phone: (603)786-2510
Email: essofny@aol.com
Website: http://www.nh.easter-seals.org
Larry Gammon, CEO & Pres
Program(s): Residential and housing services.

New Jersey

★ 8155 ★ Easter Seals New Jersey
1 Kimberly Rd.
East Brunswick, NJ 08816
Phone: (732)257-6662 **Free:** 800-468-0027
Fax: (732)257-7373
Email: mschneier@nj.easter-seals.org
Website: http://www.eastersealsnj.org
Brian J. Fitzgerald, CEO & Pres
Helen Drobnis, Director
Program(s): Adult and senior services; camping and recreation; job training and employment services; medical rehabilitation and health services; residential and housing services; and support services.

New Mexico

★ 8156 ★ Easter Seals New Mexico
2819 Richmond Dr. NE
Albuquerque, NM 87107-1918
Phone: (505)888-3811 **Free:** 800-279-5261
Fax: (505)888-0490
Email: esnm1@aol.com
Website: http://www.nm.easter-seals.org
Marlis Hadley, CEO & Pres
Program(s): Camping and recreation; continuing education; early education and care; school-aged children; and support services.

New York

★ 8157 ★ Easter Seals Monroe County
349 W Commercial St., Ste. 1350
East Rochester, NY 14445-2402
Phone: (585)264-9550 **Fax:** (585)264-9547
Email: fighttowin@aol.com
Website: http://www.eastersealsny.com
Larry Gammon, President
Program(s): Residential and housing services.

★ 8158 ★ Easter Seals New York Albany Office
230 Washington Ave. Ext.
Albany, NY 12203
Phone: (518)456-4880 **Free:** 800-727-8785
Fax: (518)456-5094
Email: fighttowin@aol.com
Website: http://www.eastersealsny.com
Larry Gammon, President
Ms. Chris McMahon, COO
Program(s): Camping and recreation; early education and care; medical rehabilitation and health services.

★ 8159 ★ Easter Seals New York New York City Chapter
300 Park Ave., 17th Fl.
New York, NY 10022
Phone: (212)572-6227 **Free:** 800-727-8785
Fax: (212)705-4210
Email: jkohomban@ny.easter-seals.org
Website: http://www.eastersealsny.com
Larry Gammon, President
Program(s): Camping and recreation; and support services.

North Carolina

★ 8160 ★ Easter Seals North Carolina
2315 Myron Dr.
Raleigh, NC 27607-3399
Free: 800-662-7119 **Fax:** (919)782-5486
Email: info@esnc.easter-seals.org
Website: http://www.nc.easter-seals.org
Adele R. Foschia, CEO
Program(s): Camping and recreation; continuing education; early education and care; early intervention; job training and employment services; medical rehabilitation and health services; school-aged children; and support services.

North Dakota

★ 8161 ★ Easter Seals/Goodwill North Dakota Fargo Office
15 S 21st St.
Fargo, ND 58103-9376
Phone: (701)237-9908
Gordon Hauge, CEO & Pres
Cindy Gabbert, Contact
Program(s): Continuing education; early education and care; early intervention; job training and employment services; medical rehabilitation and health services; school-aged children; and support services.

★ 8162 ★ Easter Seals/Goodwill North Dakota Mandan Office
211 Collins Ave.
Mandan, ND 58554-7206
Phone: (701)663-6828 **Fax:** (701)663-6859
Email: kodioak@btigate.com
Gordon Hauge, Contact
Cindy Sheldon, Contact
Program(s): Continuing education; early education and care; early intervention; job training and employment services; medical rehabilitation and health services; school-aged children; and support services.

★ 8163 ★ Easter Seals/Goodwill North Dakota
Minot Office
800 12th Ave. SW
Minot, ND 58702-1801
Phone: (701)838-0669 **Fax:** (701)838-5998
Gordon Hauge, CEO & Pres
Theresa Gochanour, Director
Program(s): Continuing education; early education and care; early intervention; job training and employment services; medical rehabilitation and health services; school-aged children; and support services.

★ 8164 ★ Easter Seals North Dakota
2125 Sims
Dickinson, ND 58601
Phone: (701)264-1060 **Free:** (866)895-1587
Fax: (701)264-1099
Email: kodiak@btigate.com
Gordon Hauge, CEO & Pres
Program(s): Continuing education; early education and care; early intervention; job training and employment services; school-aged children; and support services.

★ 8165 ★ Easter Seals North Dakota
Grand Forks Office
1811 DeMers Ave.
Grand Forks, ND 58208
Phone: (701)772-0704 **Fax:** (701)772-0336
Email: kodioak@btigate.com
Gordon Hauge, CEO & Pres
Laurie Forsberg, Contact
Program(s): Continuing education; early education and care; early intervention; job training and employment services; medical rehabilitation and health services; school-aged children; and support services.

★ 8166 ★ Easter Seals North Dakota
Jamestown Office
713 10th St. SE
Jamestown, ND 58402
Phone: (701)251-1446 **Fax:** (701)252-9527
Email: kodioak@btigate.com
Gordon Hauge, Contact
Rose Greer, Contact
Program(s): Continuing education; early education and care; early intervention; job training and employment services; medical rehabilitation and health services; school-aged children; and support services.

Ohio

★ 8167 ★ Easter Seals Central and Southeast Ohio, Inc.
Central Ohio Office
565 Children's Dr. W
Columbus, OH 43205-0166
Phone: (614)228-5523 **Free:** 800-860-5523
Fax: (614)228-8249
Email: kzuckerman@easterseals-cseohio.org
Website: http://www.oh-cn.easter-seals.org
Karin Zuckerman, CEO & Pres
Program(s): Adult and senior services; camping and recreation; early education and care; early intervention; medical rehabilitation and health services; and support services.

★ 8168 ★ Easter Seals Central and Southeast Ohio, Inc.
River Cities Office
609 Putnam St.
Marietta, OH 45750-0031
Phone: (740)374-8876 **Fax:** (740)374-4501
Website: http://www.oh-cn.easter-seals.org
Karin A. Zuckerman, CEO & Pres
Steve Parks, Mgr
Program(s): Camping and recreation; early intervention; medical rehabilitation and health services; schoolaged children; and support services.

★ 8169 ★ Easter Seals Central and Southeast Ohio, Inc.
Shawnee Regional Office
810 E Main St.
PO Box 354
Chillicothe, OH 45601
Phone: (740)773-1273 **Fax:** (740)773-0936
Email: abouilli@easterseals-cseohio.org
Website: http://www.oh-cn.easter-seals.org
Karin A. Zuckerman, President
Alexis Bouillon, Mgr
Program(s): Adult and senior services; camping and recreation; medical rehabilitation and health services; and support services.

★ 8170 ★ Easter Seals Northeast Ohio
Akron Office
3085 W Market St., Ste. 124
Akron, OH 44333-3363
Phone: (330)836-9741 **Fax:** (330)836-4967
Website: http://www.eastersealsneo.org
Sheila M. Dunn, CEO & Pres
Greg Tesniarz, Director
Program(s): Early education and care; early intervention; medical rehabilitation and health services; school-aged children; and support services.

★ 8171 ★ Easter Seals Northeast Ohio
Canton Office
3996 Fulton Dr. NW
Canton, OH 44718-3051
Phone: (330)649-9374 **Fax:** (330)649-9376
Email: linda@eastersealsneo.org
Website: http://www.eastersealsneo.org
Sheila M. Dunn, CEO & Pres
Greg Tesniarz, Director
Program(s): Camping and recreation; continuing education; early education and care; early intervention; medical rehabilitation and health services; and support services.

★ 8172 ★ Easter Seals Northeast Ohio
Cleveland Office
1929-A E Royalton Rd.
Cleveland, OH 44147
Phone: (440)838-0990 **Free:** 800-437-3288
Fax: (440)838-8440
Email: sdunn@eastersealsneo.org
Website: http://www.eastersealsneo.org
Sheila M. Dunn, CEO & Pres
Program(s): Camping and recreation; early education and care; early intervention; medical rehabilitation and health services; school-aged children; and support services.

★ 8173 ★ Easter Seals Northeast Ohio
Lakewood Office
14701 Detroit Ave., Ste. 252
Lakewood, OH 44107
Phone: (216)228-5170 **Fax:** (216)228-1018
Website: http://www.eastersealsneo.org
Sheila M. Dunn, CEO & Pres

★ 8174 ★ Easter Seals Northeast Ohio
University Heights Office
2175 Taylor
University Heights, OH 44118
Phone: 888-325-8532 **Fax:** (440)838-8440
Email: spowers@easter-sealsneo.org
Sheila M. Dunn, CEO

★ 8175 ★ Easter Seals Northeast Ohio
Willoughby Office
37415 Euclid Ave.
Willoughby, OH 44094
Phone: (440)953-2627 **Fax:** (440)953-2627
Website: http://www.eastersealsneo.org
Sheila M. Dunn, CEO & Pres
Program(s): Early intervention.

★ 8176 ★ Easter Seals Northwestern Ohio
Ashland Office
516 Claremont Ave.
Ashland, OH 44805
Phone: (419)281-5368 **Fax:** (419)289-8741
Email: jlambert@eastersealsnwohio.org
Website: http://www.eastersealsnwohio.org
Margaret Halter, Contact
Program(s): Adult and senior services; camping and recreation; early education and care; school-aged children; and support services.

★ 8177 ★ Easter Seals Northwestern Ohio
Fremont Office
309 Garrison St.
Fremont, OH 43420
Phone: (419)332-5921
Email: lgonzales@eastersealsnwohio.org
Website: http://www.eastersealsnwohio.org
Lori Gonzales, Contact
Program(s): Camping and recreation; continuing education; early education and care; early intervention; medical rehabilitation and health services; school-aged children; and support services.

★ 8178 ★ Easter Seals Northwestern Ohio
Lorain Office
1909 N Ridge Rd., Bldg. 6
Lorain, OH 44055-3344
Phone: (440)277-7337 **Fax:** (440)277-7339
Email: kwalter@eastersealsnwohio.org
Website: http://www.eastersealsnwohio.org
Kevin Walter, Exec Director
Program(s): Adult and senior services; camping and recreation; continuing education; early education and care; early intervention; medical rehabilitation and health services; school-aged children; and support services.

★ 8179 ★ Easter Seals Northwestern Ohio
Norwalk Office
226 State Rte. 61 E
Norwalk, OH 44857
Phone: (419)668-6791 **Fax:** (419)663-4529
Email: kwalter@eastersealsnwohio.org
Website: http://www.eastersealsnwohio.org
Philomena Fisher, Contact
Program(s): Adult and senior services; camping and recreation; continuing education; early education and care; school-aged children; and support services.

★ 8180 ★ Easter Seals Northwestern Ohio
Sandusky Office
Sandusky Plaza
1044 Cleveland Rd.
Sandusky, OH 44870
Phone: (419)626-8447 **Fax:** (419)627-9063
Website: http://www.eastersealsnwohio.org
Kevin Walter, Contact
Program(s): Camping and recreation; continuing education; early education and care; early intervention; medical rehabilitation and health services; school-aged children; and support services.

★ 8181 ★ Easter Seals Northwestern Ohio
Toledo Office
435 S Hawley St., Ste. A
Toledo, OH 43609
Phone: (419)241-2600 **Fax:** (419)241-5046
Email: kwalter@eastersealsnwohio.org
Website: http://www.eastersealsnwohio.org
Diana Harmon, Director
Lori Conti, Contact

Program(s): Camping and recreation; continuing education; early education and care; medical rehabilitation and health services; school-aged children; and support services.

★ 8182 ★ Easter Seals St. Clairsville
330 Fox-Shannon Pl.
Saint Clairsville, OH 43950
Phone: (740)695-5979 **Fax:** (740)695-6764
Email: mhon@wv.easter-seals.org
Website: http://www.wv.easter-seals.org
Martha Hon, CEO & Pres
Program(s): Early intervention; medical rehabilitation and health services; and school-aged children.

★ 8183 ★ Easter Seals Southwestern Ohio
Cincinnati Office
231 Clark Rd.
Cincinnati, OH 45215
Phone: (513)821-9890 **Free:** 800-288-1123
Fax: (513)821-9895
Email: twatson@oh-sw.easter-seals.org
Website: http://www.oh-sw.easter-seals.org
Tammy Watson, CEO & Pres
Program(s): Adult and senior services; continuing education; early education and care; early intervention; medical rehabilitation and health services; school-aged children; and support services.

★ 8184 ★ Easter Seals Trumbull County
155 S Park Ave.
Warren, OH 44481
Phone: (330)399-1001 **Fax:** (330)339-4001
Email: easterseals@cisnet.com
Website: http://www.oh-ya.easter-seals.org
Kenan J. Sklener, CEO
Program(s): Adult and senior services; early education and care; early intervention; medical rehabilitation and health services; and support services.

★ 8185 ★ Easter Seals West Central Ohio
Lima Office
3123 W Elm St.
Lima, OH 45805-2478
Phone: (419)222-7047 **Fax:** (419)222-9303
Email: k.oglesbee@goodwilldayton.org
Website: http://www.oh-wc.easter-seals.org
Amy Luttrell, President
Karen Oglesbee, Mgr
Program(s): Camping and recreation; early education and care; school-aged children; and support services.

★ 8186 ★ Easter Seals Youngstown Area
299 Edwards St.
Youngstown, OH 44502-1599
Phone: (330)743-1168 **Fax:** (330)743-1616
Email: eastersealsceo@cisnet.com
Website: http://www.oh-ya.easter-seals.org
Kenan J. Sklener, CEO
Program(s): Adult and senior services; early education and care; early intervention; medical rehabilitation and health services; school-aged children; and support services.

Oklahoma

★ 8187 ★ Easter Seals Oklahoma
Oklahoma City Office
2100 NW 63rd. St.
Oklahoma City, OK 73116
Phone: (405)848-2525 **Fax:** (405)842-9704
Email: easok@ilinkusa.net
Patricia Filer, CEO & Pres
Program(s): Adult and senior services; camping and recreation; early education and care; medical rehabilitation and health services; school-aged children; and support services.

★ 8188 ★ Easter Seals Oklahoma
Tulsa Office
2738 E 51st St., Ste. 130
Tulsa, OK 74105
Phone: (918)743-2311 **Fax:** (918)749-8510
Pat Filer, CEO & Pres
Program(s): Medical rehabilitation and health services.

Oregon

★ 8189 ★ Easter Seals
Medford Office
Medford, OR 97501
Phone: (541)842-2199 **Fax:** (541)842-2199
Email: medford@or.easter-seals.org
Website: http://www.or.easter-seals.org
Diane Mathews, Director
Program(s): Camping and recreation; school-aged children; and support services.

★ 8190 ★ Easter Seals Oregon
Eugene Center
3575 Donald St.
Eugene, OR 97405
Phone: (541)344-2247 **Free:** 800-244-5289
Fax: (541)344-7082
Email: eugene@or.easter-seals.org
Website: http://www.or.easter-seals.org
Jane Welch, Director
Program(s): Camping and recreation; continuing education; medical rehabilitation and health services; and support services.

★ 8191 ★ Easter Seals Oregon
Portland Office
5757 SW Macadam Ave.
Portland, OR 97201-3797
Phone: (503)228-5108 **Free:** 800-556-6020
Fax: (503)228-1352
Email: info@or.easter-seals.org
Website: http://www.or.easter-seals.org
Bob Baker, Vice President
Program(s): Camping and recreation; medical rehabilitation and health services; school-aged children; and support services.

Pennsylvania

★ 8192 ★ Easter Seals Central Pennsylvania
Altoona Office
501 Valley View Blvd.
Altoona, PA 16602
Phone: (814)941-1613 **Free:** 888-463-3039
Fax: (814)944-6500
Email: jhanlin@homenursingagency.com
Website: http://www.homenursingagency.com/eastseal.htm
Jeanne Hanlin, Contact
Program(s): Camping and recreation; continuing education; early education and care; early intervention; job training and employment services; medical rehabilitation and health services; school-aged children; and support services.

★ 8193 ★ Easter Seals Central Pennsylvania
State College Office
1300 S Allen St.
State College, PA 16801
Phone: (814)941-1613 **Free:** 888-463-3093
Fax: (814)238-3721
Email: bwallen@homenursingagency.com
Website: http://www.homenursingagency.com/eastseal.htm
Bill Wallen, Director
Carol McEwen, Director
Program(s): Camping and recreation; early education and care; and job training and employment services.

★ 8194 ★ Easter Seals Eastern Pennsylvania
1503 N Cedar Crest Blvd., Ste. 317
Allentown, PA 18104
Phone: (610)289-0114 **Fax:** (610)289-4282
Email: lindalm@easter-sealseasternpa.org
Website: http://www.easter-sealseasternpa.org
Linda LaMona, CEO & Pres

★ 8195 ★ Easter Seals Eastern Pennsylvania
Berks/Schuylkill Division
1040 Liggett Ave.
Reading, PA 19611
Phone: (610)775-1431 **Fax:** (610)796-1954
Email: essbks@voicenet.com
Website: http://www.easter-sealseasternpa.com
Linda LaMona, CEO & Pres
Program(s): Camping and recreation; early intervention; medical rehabilitation and health services; schoolaged children; and support services.

★ 8196 ★ Easter Seals Eastern Pennsylvania
Lehigh Valley Division
2200 Industrial Dr.
Bethlehem, PA 18017-2198
Phone: (610)866-8092 **Fax:** (610)866-3450
Website: http://www.easter-sealseasternpa.com
Barbara C. Carlson, Contact
Program(s): Camping and recreation; early education and care; early intervention; medical rehabilitation and health services; school-aged children; and support services.

★ 8197 ★ Easter Seals Eastern Pennsylvania
Lehighton Site
325 Alum St.
Lehighton, PA 18235
Phone: (610)379-9160 **Fax:** (610)379-9162
Website: http://www.easter-sealseasternpa.com
Linda LaMona, CEO & Pres
Program(s): Camping and recreation; early education and care; early intervention; medical rehabilitation and health services; and school-aged children.

★ 8198 ★ Easter Seals Eastern Pennsylvania
Pocono Division
109 Seven Bridge Rd.
East Stroudsburg, PA 18301-9100
Phone: (570)421-1254 **Fax:** (570)424-2346
Email: nancylt@easterseals-easternpa.org
Website: http://www.easterseals-easternpa.org
Linda LaMona, CEO & Pres
Program(s): Early intervention.

★ 8199 ★ Easter Seals Franklin and Adams Counties
34 Rd.side Ave.
Waynesboro, PA 17268
Phone: (717)762-5315 **Fax:** (717)762-0362
Email: easter-w@cvn.net
Robert S. Hoover, President
Program(s): Early education and care; early intervention; medical rehabilitation and health services; and support services.

★ 8200 ★ Easter Seals Franklin & Adams Counties
55 Hamilton Rd.
Chambersburg, PA 17201-6432
Phone: (717)264-7578 **Fax:** (717)264-1309
Email: easter-w@cvn.net

Website: http://www.gettysburg.edu/project/sl/health/easter.html
Robert S. Hoover, President
Program(s): Early education and care; early intervention; medical rehabilitation and health services; school-aged children; and support services.

★ 8201 ★ Easter Seals South Central Pennsylvania
York Office
2201 S Queen St.
York, PA 17402-4695
Phone: (717)741-3891 **Free:** 888-273-7351
Fax: (717)741-5359
Email: dnoel3@aol.com
Website: http://www.visiteasterseals.org
Debbie Noel, President

★ 8202 ★ Easter Seals Southeastern Pennsylvania
Bucks County Office
2400 Trenton Rd.
Levittown, PA 19056
Phone: (215)945-7200 **Fax:** (215)945-4073
Email: philaess@liberynet.org
Website: http://www.easterseals-sepa.org
Carl Webster, Exec Director
Program(s): Camping and recreation; continuing education; early education and care; early intervention; medical rehabilitation and health services; school-aged children; and support services.

★ 8203 ★ Easter Seals Southeastern Pennsylvania
Chester County Office
797 E Lancaster Ave., Ste. 2
Downingtown, PA 19335
Phone: (610)873-3990 **Fax:** (610)873-3992
Email: dkeiths@easterseals-sepa.org
Website: http://www.easterseals-sepa.org
Carl Webster, Exec Director
Program(s): Camping and recreation; continuing education; early education and care; early intervention; job training and employment services; medical rehabilitation and health services; school-aged children; and support services.

★ 8204 ★ Easter Seals Southeastern Pennsylvania
Delaware County Office
468 N Middletown Rd.
Media, PA 19063
Phone: (610)565-2353 **Fax:** (610)565-5256
Email: philaess@libertynet.org
Website: http://www.easterseals-sepa.org
Jan Wright, Director
Program(s): Camping and recreation; continuing education; early education and care; early intervention; medical rehabilitation and health services; and support services.

★ 8205 ★ Easter Seals Southeastern Pennsylvania
Montgomery County Office
1161 Forty Foot Rd.
Kulpsville, PA 19443
Phone: (215)368-7000 **Fax:** (215)368-1199
Email: philaess@libertynet.org
Website: http://www.easterseals-sepa.org
Carl Webster, Exec Director
Program(s): Camping and recreation; continuing education; early education and care; early intervention; medical rehabilitation and health services; school-aged children; and support services.

★ 8206 ★ Easter Seals Southeastern Pennsylvania
Philadelphia County Office
3975 Conshohocken Ave.
Philadelphia, PA 19131-5484
Phone: (215)879-1000 **Fax:** (215)879-8424
Email: philaess@libertynet.org
Mr. Carl Webster, CEO & Pres
John Podgajny, Director
Program(s): Camping and recreation; continuing education; early education and care; medical rehabilitation and health services; school-aged children; and support services.

★ 8207 ★ Easter Seals Western Pennsylvania
Cambria-Somerset Division
232 Walnut St.
Johnstown, PA 15901
Phone: (814)535-5508 **Fax:** (814)536-4943
Website: http://www.pa-ws.easter-seals.org
Lawrence P. Rager, Jr., CEO & Pres
Program(s): Early intervention; medical rehabilitation and health services; and support services.

★ 8208 ★ Easter Seals Western Pennsylvania
Cambria/Somerset Office
571 Main St.
Somerset, PA 15501
Phone: (814)445-4834
Website: http://www.pa-ws.easter-seals.org
Lawrence P. Rager, Jr., CEO & Pres
Program(s): Medical rehabilitation and health services.

★ 8209 ★ Easter Seals Western Pennsylvania
Clarion/Jefferson Division
103 N Gilpin St.
Punxsutawney, PA 15767
Phone: (814)938-6750 **Fax:** (814)938-9083
Website: http://www.pa-ws.easter-seals.org
Peg Swarm, Contact
Program(s): Early education and care; and job training and employment services.

★ 8210 ★ Easter Seals Western Pennsylvania
Fayette Division
141 Oakland Ave.
Uniontown, PA 15401
Phone: (724)437-4047 **Fax:** (724)437-5485
Lawrence P. Rager, Jr., CEO & Pres
Program(s): Camping and recreation; medical rehabilitation and health services; and support services.

★ 8211 ★ Easter Seals Western Pennsylvania
Fayette Division
c/o Greensboro Head Start
7 Glassworks Rd.
Greensboro, PA 15338
Phone: (724)437-4047 **Fax:** (724)437-5485
Website: http://www.pa-ws.easter-seals.org
Lawrence P. Rager, Jr., CEO & Pres
Program(s): Early education and care; and medical rehabilitation and health services.

★ 8212 ★ Easter Seals Western Pennsylvania
Pittsburgh Office
632 Fort Duquesne Blvd.
Pittsburgh, PA 15222
Phone: (412)281-7244 **Free:** 800-587-3257
Fax: (412)281-9333
Email: toutrich@pa-ws.easter-seals.org
Website: http://www.pa-ws.easter-seals.org
Lawrence P. Rager, Jr., CEO & Pres
Tina L. Outrich, Vice President
Program(s): Adult and senior services; continuing education; early education and care; job training and employment services; medical rehabilitation and health services; school-aged children; and support services.

★ 8213 ★ Easter Seals Western Pennsylvania
Venago Division
200 12th St.
Franklin, PA 16323-0231
Phone: (814)437-3071 **Fax:** (814)432-2269
Email: easterseals2@usachoice.net
Website: http://www.pa-ws.easter-seals.org
Lawrence P. Rager, Jr., CEO & Pres
Diana Griffith, Director
Program(s): Camping and recreation; early intervention; residential and housing services; and support services.

Puerto Rico

★ 8214 ★ Easter Seals Puerto Rico
Calle Universidad 500
Urbanizacion Perez Morris
Hato Rey
San Juan, PR 00918
Phone: (787)767-6710 **Fax:** (787)758-0950
Email: nmorales@serpr.org
Website: http://www.pr.easter-seals.org
Mrs. Nilda M. Morales, Exec Director
Program(s): Adult and senior services; camping and recreation; early intervention; and residential and housing services.

South Carolina

★ 8215 ★ Easter Seals South Carolina
Anderson County Office
1104 Ella St.
Anderson, SC 29621
Phone: (864)225-1371 **Fax:** (864)225-2943
Email: essand@carol.net
Website: http://www.sc.easter-seals.org
Cecilia Page, Contact
Program(s): Early education and care; and support services.

★ 8216 ★ Easter Seals South Carolina
Georgetown County Office
614 S Hazard St.
Georgetown, SC 29442
Phone: (843)546-2212 **Fax:** (843)545-5251
Email: eastergt@ftc.net
Website: http://www.sc.easter-seals.org
Richard S. Carter, CEO
Program(s): Support services.

★ 8217 ★ Easter Seals South Carolina
Greenville County Office
1122 Rutherford Rd.
Greenville, SC 29609
Phone: (864)232-4185 **Fax:** (864)232-8161
Website: http://www.sc.easter-seals.org
Richard S. Carter, CEO
Program(s): Support services.

★ 8218 ★ Easter Seals South Carolina
Greenwood County Office
118 W Alexander Ave.
Greenwood, SC 29648
Phone: (864)229-5428 **Fax:** (864)942-0553
Website: http://www.sc.easter-seals.org
Richard S. Carter, CEO
Program(s): Support services.

★ 8219 ★ Easter Seals South Carolina Pee Dee Office
119 S McQueen St.
Florence, SC 29501
Phone: (803)661-6909 **Fax:** (803)661-6905
Website: http://www.sc.easter-seals.org
Richard S. Carter, CEO
Remarks: Serves Darlington and Florence counties. **Program(s):** Job training, employment services, and support services.

★ 8220 ★ Easter Seals South Carolina Spartanburg County
1004 S Pine St.
Spartanburg, SC 29302
Phone: (864)582-8050 **Fax:** (864)582-1156
Website: http://www.sc.easter-seals.org
Connie Rollins, Director
Program(s): Support services.

★ 8221 ★ Easter Seals South Carolina State Headquarters
3020 Farrow Rd.
Columbia, SC 29203-7099
Phone: (803)256-0735 **Free:** 800-951-4090
Fax: (803)765-9765
Email: tskelton@eastersc.org
Website: http://www.sc.easter-seals.org
Richard S Carter, CEO
Program(s): Support services.

★ 8222 ★ Easter Seals South Carolina Trident Office
4500 Leeds Ave., Ste. 202B
Charleston, SC 29405
Phone: (843)308-7391 **Fax:** (843)308-7392
Email: eastersc@scsn.net
Website: http://www.sc.easter-seals.org
Robyn Linnen, Contact
Remarks: Serves Berkley, Charleston, and Dorchester counties. **Program(s):** Support services.

South Dakota

★ 8223 ★ Easter Seals South Dakota Eastern Regional Office
3801 S Western Ave., Ste. 106
Sioux Falls, SD 57105
Phone: (605)339-6969 **Fax:** (605)977-0640
Email: tanderson@sd.easter-seals.org
Website: http://www.essd.org
Ms. Pat Miller, CEO & Pres
Martin Hagemann, Contact
Program(s): Early education and care; school-aged children; and support services.

★ 8224 ★ Easter Seals South Dakota Pierre Office
1351 N Harrison Ave.
Pierre, SD 57501-2373
Phone: (605)224-5879 **Free:** 800-592-1852
Fax: (605)224-1033
Email: administrator@sd.easter-seals.org
Website: www.essd.org
Ms. Pat Miller, Contact
Program(s): Camping and recreation.

★ 8225 ★ Easter Seals South Dakota Western Regional Office
919 Main St., Ste. 203
Rapid City, SD 57702
Phone: (605)348-6459 **Fax:** (605)348-6459
Email: administrator@sd.easter-seals.org
Website: www.essd.org
Ms. Pat Miller, Contact
Ms. Lori Schreiner, Director
Program(s): Early education and care; school-aged children; and support services.

Tennessee

★ 8226 ★ Easter Seals Tennessee
2001 Woodmont Blvd.
Nashville, TN 37215
Phone: (615)292-6640 **Free:** 800-264-0078
Fax: (615)292-7206
Email: kroder@eastersealstn.com
Website: http://www.tn-easter-seals.org
Jayne Perkins, CEO & Pres
Ms. Kathleen Roder, Contact
Program(s): Continuing education; medical rehabilitation and health services; school-aged children; and support services.

Texas

★ 8227 ★ Easter Seals Central Texas
919 W 28-½ St.
Austin, TX 78705-3595
Phone: (512)478-2581 **Fax:** (512)476-1638
Email: smiller@eastersealstx.com
Website: http://www.eastersealstx.com
Sharon R. Miller, CEO & Pres
Program(s): Camping and recreation; early education and care; early intervention; job training and employment services; medical rehabilitation and health services; school-aged children; and support services.

★ 8228 ★ Easter Seals of Greater Dallas
3820 W Northwest Hwy., Ste. 100
Dallas, TX 75220
Phone: (972)394-8900 **Free:** 800-580-4718
Fax: (972)366-4209
Email: info@easterseals.com
Website: http://www.easterseals.com
Elizabeth Hart, CEO & Pres
Program(s): Medical rehabilitation and health services; and support services.

★ 8229 ★ Easter Seals Greater Northwest Texas
2100 Cicle Dr.
Fort Worth, TX 76119-8130
Phone: (817)536-8693 **Free:** 888-288-8324
Fax: (817)536-5214
Email: mail@easterseals-fw.org
Website: http://www.tx-nw.easter-seals.org
Ms. Francy Kragle, President
Program(s): Early intervention; medical rehabilitation and health services; and support services.

★ 8230 ★ Easter Seals Permian Basin
620 N Alleghany
Odessa, TX 79761
Phone: (915)332-8244 **Free:** 800-583-2404
Fax: (915)580-7428
Email: rehab@nwol.net
Tom Snoddy, Exec Director
Program(s): Early education and care; medical rehabilitation and health services; and support services.

★ 8231 ★ Easter Seals Rio Grande Valley Harlingen Office
1514 S 77 Sunshine Strip, Ste. 4
Harlingen, TX 78550
Phone: (956)423-9171 **Fax:** (956)423-7457
Email: prosenlund@easterseals-rgv.org
Website: http://www.easterseals-rgv.org
Deborah A. Paganelli, Exec Director
Program(s): Early intervention; medical rehabilitation and health services; and support services.

★ 8232 ★ Easter Seals Rio Grande Valley McAllen Office
1217 Houston St.
McAllen, TX 78501
Phone: (956)631-9171 **Free:** 800-728-5491
Fax: (956)631-7566
Email: prosenlund@easterseals-rgv.org
Website: http://www.easterseals-rgv.org
Deborah A. Paganelli, Exec Director
Program(s): Early education and care; early intervention; medical rehabilitation and health services; school-aged children; and support services.

★ 8233 ★ Easter Seals San Antonio
2203 Babcock Rd.
San Antonio, TX 78229-4498
Phone: (210)614-3911 **Fax:** (210)616-0443
Linda H. Tapia, Exec Director
Program(s): Medical rehabilitation and health services.

★ 8234 ★ Easter Seals Texarkana, Texas
1315 Walnut St.
Texarkana, TX 75501-4489
Phone: (903)794-2705 **Fax:** (903)793-1203
Email: temple@txk.com
Jerry Bedwell, President
Program(s): Adult and senior services; continuing education; early education and care; early intervention; medical rehabilitation and health services; school-aged children; and support services.

Utah

★ 8235 ★ Easter Seals Utah Salt Lake City Office
638 E Wilmington Ave.
Salt Lake City, UT 84106-1491
Phone: (801)486-3778 **Free:** 800-388-1991
Fax: (801)486-3123
Email: rstarley@eastersealsutah.org
Website: http://www.ut.easter-seals.org
Richard O. Starley, President
Program(s): Adult and senior services; camping and recreation; early education and care; job training and employment services; school-aged children; and support services.

Vermont

★ 8236 ★ Easter Seals Rutland
195 Stratton Rd.
Rutland, VT 05702
Phone: (802)775-4882
Email: mjohnso@eseals.org
Website: http://www.nh.easter-seals.org
Larry Gammon, CEO & Pres
Program(s): Residential and housing services; and school-aged children.

★ 8237 ★ Easter Seals Vermont
641 Comstock Rd., Ste. 1
Berlin, VT 05602
Phone: (802)223-4744 **Fax:** (802)229-0848
Email: mjohnso@eseals.org
Website: http://www.nh.easter-seals.org
Larry Gammon, CEO & Pres
Program(s): Early education and care; and school-aged children.

Virginia

★ 8238 ★ Easter Seals Central Virginia
9291 Laurel Grove Rd., Ste. 2
Mechanicsville, VA 23116-2969
Phone: (804)746-1007 **Fax:** (804)746-9214
Email: essoc@aol.com
Website: http://www.va.easter-seals.org
Edward J. Hamilton, President
Jewel Cooke, Director
Program(s): Adult and senior services; and support services.

★ 8239 ★ Easter Seals Northern Virginia
6319 Castle Pl., Ste. A
Falls Church, VA 22044-1907
Phone: (703)538-4480 **Fax:** (703)237-0249
Email: jcooke@va.easter-seals.org
Website: http://www.va.easter-seals.org
Edward J. Hamilton, PhD, CEO & Pres
Program(s): Camping, recreation, and support services.

★ 8240 ★ Easter Seals Virginia
201 E Main St.
Salem, VA 24153
Phone: (540)777-7325 **Free:** 800-365-1656
Fax: (540)777-2194
Email: info@va.easter-seals.org
Website: http://www.va.easter-seals.org
Edward J. Hamilton, PhD, CEO & Pres
Program(s): Early intervention and support services.

Washington

★ 8241 ★ Easter Seals Washington
1740 NE Riddell Rd., Ste. 315
Bremerton, WA 98310-3870
Phone: (360)373-2502 **Fax:** (360)373-5620
Email: spritchard@seals.org
Website: http://www.seals.org
Garry Wyckoff, CEO
Glenn LeDuc, Director
Program(s): Adult and senior services; job training and employment services.

★ 8242 ★ Easter Seals Washington State Office
521 2nd Ave. W
Seattle, WA 98119-5998
Phone: (206)281-5700 **Fax:** (206)281-5700
Email: esw@seals.org
Website: http://www.seals.org
Gary Wyckoff, Contact
Cathy Bisaillon, Vice President
Program(s): Adult and senior services; camping and recreation; continuing education; early education and care; early intervention; job training and employment services; medical rehabilitation and health services; school-aged children; and support services.

West Virginia

★ 8243 ★ Easter Seals West Virginia
1305 National Rd.
Wheeling, WV 26003-5780
Phone: (304)242-1390 **Free:** 800-677-1390
Fax: (304)243-5880
Email: mhon@wv-easter-seals.org
Website: http://www.wv.easter-seals.org
Martha Hon, CEO & Pres
Program(s): Camping and recreation; early education and care; early intervention; medical rehabilitation and health services; school-aged children; and support services.

Wisconsin

★ 8244 ★ Easter Seals Southeastern Wisconsin
3090 N 53rd St.
Milwaukee, WI 53210-1699
Phone: (414)449-4444 **Fax:** (414)449-4447
Email: tbiondo@wi-se.easter-seals.org
Website: http://www.wi-se.easter-seals.org
Tim Biondo, Exec Director
Program(s): Adult and senior services; camping and recreation; continuing education; early education and care; early intervention; medical rehabilitation and health services; school-aged children; and support services.

★ 8245 ★ Easter Seals Wisconsin
101 Nob Hill Rd., Ste. 301
Madison, WI 53713-3969
Phone: (608)277-8288 **Free:** 800-422-2324
Fax: (608)277-8333
Email: tpaprock@wi-easterseals.org
Website: www.wi-easterseals.org
Christine Fessler, CEO & Pres
Program(s): Camping and recreation; continuing education; early education and care; job training and employment services; school-aged children; and support services.

Domestic Violence

The following are state affiliates of the National Coalition Against Domestic Violence, PO Box 18749, Denver, CO 80218, (303)839-1852, http://www.ncadv.org/.

Alabama

★ 8246 ★ Alabama Coalition Against Domestic Violence
PO Box 4762
Montgomery, AL 36101
Free: 800-650-6522
Website: http://www.acadv.org

Alaska

★ 8247 ★ Alaska Network on Domestic Violence and Sexual Assault
130 Seward St., Rm. 209
Juneau, AK 99801
Phone: (907)586-3650 **Fax:** (907)463-4493
Website: http://www.andvsa.org

Arizona

★ 8248 ★ Arizona Coalition Against Domestic Violence
100 W Camelback Rd., Ste. 109
Phoenix, AZ 85013
Phone: (602)279-2900 **Fax:** (602)279-2980
Email: acadv@azcadv.org
Website: http://www.azacadv.org

Arkansas

★ 8249 ★ Arkansas Coalition Against Domestic Violence
1 Sheriff Ln., Ste. C
North Little Rock, AR 72114
Phone: (501)812-0571 **Fax:** (501)812-0578
Email: ssigmon@arkansas.net

California

★ 8250 ★ Coalition to End Domestic and Sexual Violence
2064 Eastman Ave., Ste. 104
Ventura, CA 93003
Phone: (805)654-8141 **Free:** 800-300-2181
Fax: (805)654-1264
Website: http://www.thecoalition.org/index.html
Crisis Phone(s): 24-hour hotline: (805) 656-1111.

★ 8251 ★ Statewide California Coalition for Battered Women
3711 Long Beach Blvd., Ste. 718
Long Beach, CA 90807
Phone: (562)981-1202 **Free:** 888-SCCBW-52
Fax: (562)981-3202
Email: sccbw@sccbw.org
Website: http://www.sccbw.org

Colorado

★ 8252 ★ Colorado Domestic Violence Coalition
PO Box 18902
Denver, CO 80218
Phone: (303)831-9632 **Free:** 888-778-7091
Fax: (303)832-7067
Email: ccadv@ix.netcom.com
Website: http://www.psynet.net/ccadv

Delaware

★ 8253 ★ Delaware Coalition Against Domestic Violence
PO Box 847
Wilmington, DE 19899
Phone: (302)658-2958 **Fax:** (302)658-5049
Crisis Phone(s): 24-hour bilingual line: (888) 522-2571.

District of Columbia

★ 8254 ★ District of Columbia Coalition Against Domestic Violence
513 U St., NW
Washington, DC 20001
Phone: (202)783-5332 **Fax:** (202)387-5684
Website: http://www.dccadv.org

★ 8255 ★ My Sister's Place
PO Box 29596
Washington, DC 20017
Phone: (202)529-5261
Crisis Phone(s): 24-hour hotline: (202) 529-5991.

Florida

★ 8256 ★ Florida Coalition Against Domestic Violence
308 E Park Ave.
Tallahassee, FL 32301
Phone: (850)425-2749 **Free:** 800-500-1119
Fax: (850)425-3091

Georgia

★ 8257 ★ Georgia Advocates for Battered Women and Children
250 Georgia Ave. SE, Ste. 308
Atlanta, GA 30312
Phone: (404)524-3847 **Free:** 800-334-2836
Fax: (404)524-5959

Hawaii

★ 8258 ★ Hawaii State Coalition Against Domestic Violence
716 Umi St., No. 210
Honolulu, HI 96819
Phone: (808)832-9316 **Fax:** (808)841-6028
Email: hscadv@pixi.com

Idaho

★ 8259 ★ Idaho Coalition Against Sexual and Domestic Violence
815 Park Blvd., Ste. 140
Boise, ID 83712
Phone: (208)384-0419 **Free:** 888-293-6118
Fax: (208)331-0687
Email: domvio@micron.net

Illinois

★ 8260 ★ Friends of Battered Women and Their Children
PO Box 5185
Evanston, IL 60204
Phone: (773)274-5232 **Fax:** (773)274-2214
Email: info@afriendsplace.org
Website: http://www.afriendsplace.org
Crisis Phone(s): (800) 603-HELP.

★ 8261 ★ Illinois Coalition Against Domestic Violence
801 S 11th St.
Springfield, IL 62703
Phone: (217)789-2830 **Fax:** (217)789-1939
Email: ilcadv@springnet1.com

★ 8262 ★ Life Span
PO Box 445
Des Plaines, IL 60016
Phone: (847)824-0382 **Fax:** (847)824-5311
Email: life-span@life-span.org
Website: http://www.life-span.org
Crisis Phone(s): 24-hour line: (847) 824-4454.

Indiana

★ 8263 ★ Indiana Coalition Against Domestic Violence
2511 E 46th St., Ste. 3
Indianapolis, IN 46205
Phone: (317)543-3908 **Free:** 800-332-7385
Fax: (317)377-7050
Website: http://www.violenceresource.org

Iowa

★ 8264 ★ Iowa Coalition Against Domestic Violence
2603 Bell Ave., Ste. 100
Des Moines, IA 50321
Phone: (515)244-8028 **Free:** 800-942-0333
Fax: (515)244-7417

Kansas

★ 8265 ★ Kansas Coalition Against Sexual and Domestic Violence
820 SE Quincy, Ste. 600
Topeka, KS 66612
Phone: (785)232-9784 **Fax:** (785)232-9937
Crisis Phone(s): state-wide hotline: (888) END-ABUSE.

Kentucky

★ 8266 ★ Kentucky Domestic Violence Association
PO Box 356
Frankfort, KY 40602
Phone: (502)875-4132 **Fax:** (502)875-4268

Louisiana

★ 8267 ★ Louisiana Coalition Against Domestic Violence
PO Box 77308
Baton Rouge, LA 70879-7308
Phone: (225)752-1296 **Fax:** (225)751-8927

Maine

★ 8268 ★ Maine Coalition to End Domestic Violence
128 Main St.
Bangor, ME 04401
Phone: (207)941-1194 **Fax:** (207)941-2327

Maryland

★ 8269 ★ Maryland Network Against Domestic Violence
6911 Laurel Bowie Rd., Ste. 309
Bowie, MD 20715
Phone: (301)352-4574 **Free:** 800-MD-HELPS
Fax: (301)809-0422

Massachusetts

★ 8270 ★ Massachusetts Coalition Against Sexual Assault and Domestic Violence
Jane Doe Inc.
14 Beacon St., Ste. 507
Boston, MA 02108
Phone: (617)248-0922 **Fax:** (617)248-0902
Website: http://www.besafe.org

Michigan

★ 8271 ★ Bay County Women's Center
PO Box 1458
Bay City, MI 48706
Phone: (517)686-4551 **Free:** 800-834-2098
Fax: (517)686-0906
Crisis Phone(s): 24-hour line: (517) 265-6776.

Minnesota

★ 8272 ★ Minnesota Coalition for Battered Women
450 N Syndicate St., Ste. 122
Saint Paul, MN 55104
Phone: (651)646-6177 **Fax:** (651)646-1527
Email: mcbw@pclink.com
Website: http://members.tripod.com/~DAWN-1/MCBW/index.html
Crisis Phone(s): (651) 646-0994.

Mississippi

★ 8273 ★ Mississippi State Coalition Against Domestic Violence
PO Box 4703
Jackson, MS 39296-4703
Phone: (601)981-9196 **Free:** 800-898-3234
Fax: (601)981-2501
Email: mcadv@misnet.com

Missouri

★ 8274 ★ Missouri Coalition Against Domestic Violence
415 E McCarty St.
Jefferson City, MO 65101
Phone: (573)634-4161 **Fax:** (573)636-3728

★ 8275 ★ Women's Support and Community Services
2838 Olive St.
Saint Louis, MO 63103
Phone: (314)531-9100
Crisis Phone(s): (314) 531-2003.

Montana

★ 8276 ★ Crisis Line
PO Box 6644
Great Falls, MT 59406
Phone: (406)453-HELP **Free:** 888-587-0199

★ 8277 ★ Montana Coalition Against Domestic and Sexual Violence
PO Box 633
Helena, MT 59624
Phone: (406)443-7794 **Fax:** (406)443-7818
Website: http://www.mt.net/~mcadsv

Nebraska

★ 8278 ★ Nebraska Domestic Violence and Sexual Assault Coalition
825 M St., Ste. 404
Lincoln, NE 68508-2253
Phone: (402)476-6256 **Free:** 800-876-6238
Fax: (402)476-6806
Website: http://www.ndvsac.org

Nevada

★ 8279 ★ Nevada Network Against Domestic Violence
100 W Grove, Ste. 315
Reno, NV 89509
Phone: (775)828-1115 **Free:** 800-500-1556
Fax: (775)828-9991

★ 8280 ★ SAFE House
18 Sunrise Dr., Ste. G-70
Henderson, NV 89014
Phone: (702)451-4203 **Fax:** (702)451-4302
Email: safe@intermind.net

New Hampshire

★ 8281 ★ New Hampshire Coalition Against Domestic and Sexual Violence
PO Box 353
Concord, NH 03302-0353
Phone: (603)224-8893 **Free:** 800-852-3388
Fax: (603)228-6096
Website: http://www.mhcadsv.org
Crisis Phone(s): outside of New Hampshire: (603) 225-9000.

New Jersey

★ 8282 ★ New Jersey Coalition for Battered Women
2620 Whitehorse/Hamilton Sq. Rd.
Trenton, NJ 08690
Phone: (609)584-8107 **Free:** 800-224-0211
Fax: (609)584-9750
Crisis Phone(s): For battered lesbians: (800) 224-0211.

★ 8283 ★ Strengthen Our Sisters
PO Box U
Hewitt, NJ 07421
Email: ssisters@warwick.net
Crisis Phone(s): 24-hour line: (973) 728-0007.

New Mexico

★ 8284 ★ New Mexico State Coalition Against Domestic Violence
PO Box 25266
Albuquerque, NM 87125
Phone: (505)246-9240 **Fax:** (505)246-9434
Email: nmcadv@nmcadv.org
Website: http://www.nmcadv.org/dv/

Alt. Contact: Legal helpline: (800) 773-3645.

New York

★ 8285 ★ New York State Coalition Against Domestic Violence
79 Central Ave.
Albany, NY 12206
Phone: (518)432-4864 **Free:** 800-942-6906
Fax: (518)463-3155

North Carolina

★ 8286 ★ North Carolina Coalition Against Domestic Violence
115 Market St.
Durham, NC 27701
Phone: (919)956-9124 **Fax:** (919)682-1449

North Dakota

★ 8287 ★ North Dakota Council on Abused Women's Services
State Networking Office
418 E Rosser Ave., Ste. 320
Bismarck, ND 58501
Phone: (701)255-6240 **Free:** 800-472-2911
Fax: (701)255-1904
Website: http://www.btigate.com/~endabuse

Ohio

★ 8288 ★ Ohio Domestic Violence Network
4041 N High St., Ste. 400
Columbus, OH 43214
Phone: (614)784-0023 **Free:** 800-934-9840
Fax: (614)784-0033
Website: http://www.ohiodvnetwork.org

Oklahoma

★ 8289 ★ Oklahoma Coalition Against Domestic Violence and Sexual Assault
2525 NW Expressway, Ste. 208
Oklahoma City, OK 73116
Phone: (405)848-1815 **Free:** 800-522-9054
Fax: (405)848-3469
Website: http://www.ocadvsa.org/

Oregon

★ 8290 ★ Oregon Coalition Against Domestic and Sexual Violence
520 NW Davis, Ste. 310
Portland, OR 97209
Phone: (503)223-7411 **Free:** 800-622-3782
Fax: (503)223-7490

Pennsylvania

★ 8291 ★ Laurel House
PO Box 764
Norristown, PA 19404
Phone: (610)275-4018
Email: LaurelHaus@aol.com
Website: http://www.libertynet.org/laurelh
Crisis Phone(s): (800) 642-3150.

★ 8292 ★ Pennsylvania Coalition Against Domestic Violence
National Resource Center on Domestic Violence
6440 Flank Dr., Ste. 1300
Harrisburg, PA 17112-2778
Phone: (717)545-6400 **Free:** 800-932-4632
Fax: (717)545-9456

★ 8293 ★ Pennsylvania Coalition Against Rape
125 N Enola Dr.
Enola, PA 17025
Phone: (717)728-9740 **Free:** 800-692-7445
Fax: (717)728-9781
Email: Stop@pcar.org
Website: http://www.pcar.org
Crisis Phone(s): (800) 692-7445.

★ 8294 ★ Women's Center of Montgomery County
101 Washington Ln., Ste. WC-1
Jenkintown, PA 19046
Website: http://www.wcmontco.org
Crisis Phone(s): 24-hour hotline: (800) 773-2424.

Rhode Island

★ 8295 ★ Rhode Island Council Against Domestic Violence
422 Post Rd., Ste. 202
Warwick, RI 02888
Phone: (401)467-9940 **Free:** 800-494-8100
Fax: (401)467-9943

South Carolina

★ 8296 ★ South Carolina Coalition Against Domestic Violence and Sexual Assault
PO Box 7776
Columbia, SC 29202-7776
Phone: (803)256-2900 **Free:** 800-260-9293
Fax: (803)256-1030

South Dakota

★ 8297 ★ South Dakota Coalition Against Domestic Violence and Sexual Assault
PO Box 141
Pierre, SD 57501
Phone: (605)945-0869 **Free:** 800-572-9196
Fax: (605)945-0870

Tennessee

★ 8298 ★ Tennessee Task Force Against Domestic Violence
PO Box 120972
Nashville, TN 37212
Phone: (615)386-9406 **Free:** 800-356-6767
Fax: (615)383-2967
Website: http://www.citysearch.com/nas/ttfadv

Texas

★ 8299 ★ Families in Crisis, Inc.
PO Box 25
Killeen, TX 76540
Phone: (254)634-1184 **Free:** 888-799-SAFE
Website: http://www.familiesincrisis.net

★ 8300 ★ Texas Council on Family Violence
PO Box 161810
Austin, TX 78716
Phone: (512)794-1133 **Free:** 800-525-1978
Fax: (512)794-1199
Website: http://www.ndvh.org

Utah

★ 8301 ★ Domestic Violence Advisory Council
120 North 200 West
Salt Lake City, UT 84103
Phone: (801)538-4100 **Free:** 800-897-LINK
Fax: (801)538-3993

Vermont

★ 8302 ★ Vermont Network Against Domestic Violence and Sexual Assault
PO Box 405
Montpelier, VT 05601
Phone: (802)223-1302 **Fax:** (802)223-6943
Email: vnadvsa@sover.net
Website: http://www.vnadvsa.together.com

Virginia

★ 8303 ★ Virginians Family Violence and Sexual Assault Hotline
2850 Sandy Bay Rd., Ste. 101
Williamsburg, VA 23185
Phone: (757)221-0990 **Free:** 800-838-VADV
Fax: (757)229-1553
Website: http://www.rtk.net/vadv/

Washington

★ 8304 ★ Washington State Coalition Against Domestic Violence
8645 Martin Way NE, Ste. 103
Lacey, WA 98516
Phone: (360)407-0756 **Fax:** (360)407-0761
Email: wscadv@cco.net

West Virginia

★ 8305 ★ West Virginia Coalition Against Domestic Violence
Elk Office Ctr.
4710 Chimney Dr., Ste. A
Charleston, WV 25302
Phone: (304)965-3552 **Fax:** (304)965-3572
Website: http://www.wvcadv.org

Wisconsin

★ 8306 ★ Manitowoc Domestic Violence Center
PO Box 1142
Manitowoc, WI 54220
Phone: (920)684-5770
Website: http://www.lakeshorebizdir.com/dvc.htm

★ 8307 ★ Wisconsin Coalition Against Domestic Violence
1400 E Washington Ave., Ste. 232
Madison, WI 53703
Phone: (608)255-0539 **Fax:** (608)255-3560

Wyoming

★ 8308 ★ Wyoming Coalition Against Domestic Violence and Sexual Assault
PO Box 236
Laramie, WY 82073
Phone: (307)755-5481 **Free:** 800-990-3877
Fax: (307)755-5482
Website: http://www.bcn.com/wcadvsa

Dyslexia

State chapters of the International Dyslexia Association are listed below. The national office is located at 8600 LaSalle Rd., Chester Bldg., Ste. 382, Baltimore, MD 21286-2044. Additional information can be obtained by calling the national office at

(800) ABCD-123, or by consulting their web site at http://www.interdys.org/.

Arizona

★ 8309 ★ International Dyslexia Association
Arizona Branch
PO Box 6284
Scottsdale, AZ 85261-6284
Phone: (480)941-0308
Website: http://www.dyslexia-az.org
Dawn Gutierrez, President
Remarks: Also serves parts of Nevada.

British Columbia

★ 8310 ★ International Dyslexia Association
British Columbia Branch
1260 Hornby St., Ste. 104
Vancouver, BC, Canada V6Z 1W2
Phone: (604)669-5811 **Fax:** (604)669-5161
Email: idabcb@infoserve.net
Fran Thompson, President
Remarks: Also serves Alberta, Northwest Territories, Saskatchewan, and Yukon Territory.

California

★ 8311 ★ International Dyslexia Association
Central California Branch
4594 Michigan Ave.
Fresno, CA 93703
Phone: (559)251-9385 **Fax:** (559)252-1216
Email: dyslexias@attbi.com
Website: http://communitycalendar.centralvalley.com/566
Joy Moody, President
Remarks: Also serves parts of Nevada.

★ 8312 ★ International Dyslexia Association
Inland Empire Branch
PO Box 6701
San Bernardino, CA 92412
Phone: (909)686-9837
Website: http://www.dyslexia-ca.org
Sandy Marzullo, President
Remarks: Also serves parts of Nevada.

★ 8313 ★ International Dyslexia Association
Los Angeles Branch
4379 Tujunga Blvd.
Studio City, CA 91604
Phone: (818)506-8866
Barbara Shaub, President

★ 8314 ★ International Dyslexia Association
Northern California Branch
PO Box 2618
Menlo Park, CA 94026
Phone: (650)328-7667 **Fax:** (650)325-3041
Email: cushen@itsa.ucsf.edu
Website: http://www.dyslexia-ncbida.org
Heidi Renner, President

★ 8315 ★ International Dyslexia Association
Orange County Branch
1801 E Parkcourt Pl., Bldg. D, Ste. 101
Santa Ana, CA 92701
Phone: (714)564-0777 **Fax:** (714)564-0770
Email: info@dyslexiaoc.org
Website: http://www.dyslexiaoc.org
Joanne Sellers, President

★ 8316 ★ International Dyslexia Association
San Diego Branch
2515 Camino del Rio Dr., Ste. 111
San Diego, CA 92108
Phone: (619)295-3722
Email: pph@tfb.com
Website: http://www.dyslexiasd.org
Jose Cruz, President

Colorado

★ 8317 ★ International Dyslexia Association
Rocky Mountain Branch
PO Box 3598
Boulder, CO 80307
Phone: (303)721-9425
Holly Graves, President
Remarks: Serves Colorado, Utah, and Wyoming.

Florida

★ 8318 ★ International Dyslexia Association
Florida Branch
4141 Bayshore Blvd., Ste. 1701
Tampa, FL 33611
Phone: (813)281-3148
Sylvia O. Richardson, President
Remarks: Also serves Puerto Rico.

Georgia

★ 8319 ★ International Dyslexia Association
Georgia Branch
1951 Greystone Rd. NW
Atlanta, GA 30318
Phone: (404)256-1232
Email: rdavis@schenck.org
Website: http://www.schenck.org
Rosalie Davis, President
Remarks: Also serves Alabama.

Hawaii

★ 8320 ★ International Dyslexia Association
Hawaii Branch
PO Box 61610
Honolulu, HI 96839-1610
Phone: (808)538-7007 **Fax:** (808)566-6837
Email: info@HIBIDA.org
Website: http://www.HIBIDA.org
Ron Yoshimoto, President
Remarks: Also serves American Samoa.

Illinois

★ 8321 ★ International Dyslexia Association
Illinois Branch
751 Roosevelt Rd., Ste. 301
Glen Ellyn, IL 60137
Phone: (630)469-6900 **Fax:** (630)469-6810
Email: ilbranch_ida@ameritech.net
Sue Grisko, President
Remarks: Also serves Missouri.

Indiana

★ 8322 ★ International Dyslexia Association
Indiana Branch
1100 W 42nd St., Ste. 385
Indianapolis, IN 46208
Phone: (317)926-1450 **Fax:** (317)927-9285
Email: inbofida@hotmail.com
Wayne LaMade, President

Iowa

★ 8323 ★ International Dyslexia Association
Iowa Branch
1030 5th Ave., Ste. 1450
Cedar Rapids, IA 52403
Phone: (319)551-2851 **Fax:** (319)365-1038
Email: sue_ida_ia@yahoo.com
Pat McGuire, President

Louisiana

★ 8324 ★ International Dyslexia Association
Louisiana Branch
410 N Hazel
Hammond, LA 70401
Phone: (504)876-0034 **Free:** 888-323-0332
Fax: (504)448-4423
Carolyn Blackwood, President
Remarks: Also serves Missouri.

Maryland

★ 8325 ★ International Dyslexia Association
Maryland Branch
PO Box 792
Brooklandville, MD 21022
Phone: (410)825-2881
Jean-Fryer Schedler, President

Massachusetts

★ 8326 ★ International Dyslexia Association
Massachusetts Branch
PO Box 662
Lincoln, MA 01773
Mary Ann Bonneau, President
Remarks: Serves Maine, New Hampshire, Vermont, Massachusetts, Rhode Island, Connecticut, and eastern Canada.

Michigan

★ 8327 ★ International Dyslexia Association
Michigan Branch
4050 Waverly Pl.
Ann Arbor, MI 48105
Phone: (734)663-9884
Email: postmaster@idamib.org
Website: http://www.idamib.org
Sally Burden, President

Minnesota

★ 8328 ★ International Dyslexia Association
Upper Midwest Branch
PMB 159
5021 Vernon Ave.
Minneapolis, MN 55436
Phone: (651)450-7589
Sarah Sevcik, President

Remarks: Also serves North Dakota, South Dakota, and Manitoba, Canada.

Missouri

★ 8329 ★ **International Dyslexia Association**
Kansas/Western Missouri Branch
7713 Quail Ridge Ct.
Parkville, MO 64152
Phone: (816)587-3240
Email: wolfden@jc.net
Lorrie Wolf, President
Remarks: Also serves Oklahoma.

Nebraska

★ 8330 ★ **International Dyslexia Association**
Nebraska Branch
6111 S 32nd St.
Lincoln, NE 68516
Phone: (402)434-6434
Email: gcarlson@lps.org
Website: http://www.lps.org
Gwelda Carlson, President

New Hampshire

★ 8331 ★ **International Dyslexia Association**
New Hampshire Branch
PO Box 3724
Concord, NH 03302
Phone: (603)229-7355
Mike Angwin, President

New Jersey

★ 8332 ★ **International Dyslexia Association**
New Jersey Branch
PO Box 32
Long Valley, NJ 07853
Phone: (908)879-0466 **Fax:** (908)879-0466
David Katz, President

New Mexico

★ 8333 ★ **International Dyslexia Association**
Southwest Branch
PO Box 25891
Albuquerque, NM 87125
Phone: (505)255-8234 **Fax:** (505)262-8547
Email: swida84@hotmail.com
Mary Gilroy, President

New York

★ 8334 ★ **International Dyslexia Association**
Buffalo Branch
c/o Gow School
Emory Rd.
South Wales, NY 14139
Phone: (716)687-2030
Email: bufida@gow.org
Kathy Rose, President
Remarks: Also serves Ontario, Canada.

★ 8335 ★ **International Dyslexia Association**
New York Branch
71 W 23rd St., Ste. 1527
New York, NY 10010
Phone: (212)691-1930 **Fax:** (212)633-1620
Email: info@nybida.org
Website: http://www.nybida.org
Judith R. Birsh, President

★ 8336 ★ **International Dyslexia Association**
Suffolk Branch
728 Route 25A
Northport, NY 11768
Phone: (631)423-7834 **Fax:** (631)423-7834
Email: ckent@optonline.net
Carol Kent, President

North Carolina

★ 8337 ★ **International Dyslexia Association**
North Carolina Branch
184-D2 Mountain Club Dr.
Vilas, NC 28692
Phone: (252)243-8843
Email: tommcd@boone.net
Tom McDonough, President

Ohio

★ 8338 ★ **International Dyslexia Association**
Central Ohio Branch
PO Box 16216
Columbus, OH 43216-6216
Phone: (614)899-5711
Email: abc@columbus.rr.com
Cameron James, President

★ 8339 ★ **International Dyslexia Association**
Northern Ohio Branch
34750 Ada Dr.
Solon, OH 44139-5808
Phone: (216)556-0883
Karen Lieberman, President

★ 8340 ★ **International Dyslexia Association**
Ohio Valley Branch
317 E 5th St.
Cincinnati, OH 45202
Phone: (513)651-4747
Carol Greiser, President
Remarks: Serves Ohio and Kentucky.

Oregon

★ 8341 ★ **International Dyslexia Association**
Oregon Branch
PO Box 3677
Portland, OR 97208-3677
Phone: (503)228-4455 **Free:** 800-530-2234
Fax: (503)228-3152
Email: orbida@aracnet.com
Website: http://www.aracnet.com/~orbida/
Betsy Ramsey, President

Pennsylvania

★ 8342 ★ **International Dyslexia Association**
Philadelphia Branch
PO Box 251
Bryn Mawr, PA 19010
Phone: (610)527-1548 **Fax:** (610)527-5011
Email: dyslexia@libertynet.org
Website: http://www.gpbida.org
Marianne Cook, President
Remarks: Also serves Delaware.

South Carolina

★ 8343 ★ **International Dyslexia Association**
South Carolina Branch
1500 Hallbrook Dr.
Columbia, SC 29209
Phone: (803)772-8065
Email: a.s.lawrence@worldnet.att.net
Amy Lawrence, President

Tennessee

★ 8344 ★ **International Dyslexia Association**
Tennessee Branch
6525 Brownlee Dr.
Nashville, TN 37205
Free: 877-TENN-IDA
Susan Smartt, President
Remarks: Also serves Kentucky.

Texas

★ 8345 ★ **International Dyslexia Association**
Austin Branch
Del Valle Junior High School
5500 Ross St.
Del Valle, TX 78617
Phone: (512)452-7658
Website: http://home.austin.rr.com/aabida/
Sharon Roberts, President

★ 8346 ★ **International Dyslexia Association**
Dallas Branch
13140 Coit Rd., Ste. 320
LB 120
Dallas, TX 75240
Phone: (972)233-9107 **Fax:** (972)490-4219
Leigh Miller, President
Remarks: Also serves Arkansas and Oklahoma.

★ 8347 ★ **International Dyslexia Association**
Houston Branch
PO Box 540504
Houston, TX 77254-0504
Phone: (713)529-1975
Email: cwills@briarwoodschool.org
Carole Wills, President

Virginia

★ 8348 ★ **International Dyslexia Association**
DC Capital Branch
4914 Reservoir Heights Ave.
Alexandria, VA 22311
Phone: (703)827-9019
Ruth Tifford, President
Remarks: Serves Washington DC and parts of Maryland, Virginia, and West Virginia.

★ 8349 ★ **International Dyslexia Association**
Virginia Branch
PO Box 23226
Richmond, VA 23226
Free: 800-988-8336
Email: vbida@hotmail.com
Rebecca Hurrell Aldred, President
Remarks: Also serves West Virginia.

Washington

★ 8350 ★ International Dyslexia Association
Washington State Branch
PO Box 7192
Seattle, WA 98133
Phone: (206)382-1020
Website: http://www.wabida.org
Pat Morton, President
Remarks: Also serves Alaska, Idaho, and Montana.

Wisconsin

★ 8351 ★ International Dyslexia Association
Wisconsin Branch
2002 N Cambridge Ave.
Milwaukee, WI 53202
Phone: (414)299-0551
Email: lorej@nconnect.net
Website: http://www.wis-dys.org
Jan Lorenzen, President

Epilepsy

The following are state affiliates of the Epilepsy Foundation of America, 4351 Garden City Dr., Landover, MD 20785, (800)EFA-1000, http://www.efa.org/.

Alabama

★ 8352 ★ Epilepsy Foundation of North and Central Alabama
701 37th St. S, Ste. 2
Birmingham, AL 35222-3222
Phone: (205)324-4222 **Free:** 800-950-6662
Website: http://www.epilepsyfoundation.org/ncalabama

★ 8353 ★ Epilepsy Foundation of South Alabama
951 Government St., Ste. 201
Mobile, AL 36604-2425
Phone: (251)432-0970 **Free:** 800-626-1582
Website: http://www.epilepsyfoundation.org/SouthAlabama

Arizona

★ 8354 ★ Epilepsy Foundation of Arizona
PO Box 25084
Phoenix, AZ 85002-5084
Phone: (602)406-3581 **Free:** 888-768-2690
Website: http://www.epilepsyfoundation.org/arizona

★ 8355 ★ Epilepsy Foundation of Arizona
PO Box 25084
Phoenix, AZ 85002-5084
Phone: (602)406-3581 **Free:** 888-768-2690
Website: http://www.epilepsyfoundation.org/arizona

California

★ 8356 ★ Epilepsy Foundation of Los Angeles, Orange, San Bernardino & Ventura Counties
5777 W Century Blvd.
Los Angeles, CA 90045-5600
Phone: (310)670-2870 **Free:** 800-564-0445
Website: http://www.epilepsy-socalif.org

★ 8357 ★ Epilepsy Foundation of Northern California
1624 Franklin St., Ste. 900
Oakland, CA 94612-2824
Phone: (510)893-6272 **Free:** 800-632-3532
Website: http://www.epilepsyfoundation.org/norcal

★ 8358 ★ Epilepsy Foundation of San Diego County
2055 El Cajon Blvd.
San Diego, CA 92104-1091
Phone: (619)296-0161 **Free:** 800-408-4322
Website: http://www.epilepsysandiego.org

Colorado

★ 8359 ★ Epilepsy Foundation of Colorado, Inc.
234 Columbine St., Ste. 333
Denver, CO 80206-4711
Phone: (303)377-9774 **Free:** 888-378-9779
Website: http://www.epilepsycolorado.org

Connecticut

★ 8360 ★ Epilepsy Foundation of Connecticut, Inc.
386 Main St.
Middletown, CT 06457-3360
Phone: (860)346-1924 **Free:** 800-899-3745
Website: http://www.epilepsyfoundation.org/connecticut

Delaware

★ 8361 ★ Epilepsy Foundation of Delaware
Tower Office Park
Newport, DE 19804-3167
Phone: (302)999-9313 **Free:** 800-422-3653
Website: http://www.epilepsyfoundation.org/delaware

Florida

★ 8362 ★ Epilepsy Foundation of Northeast Florida, Inc.
5209 San Jose Blvd., Ste. 101
Jacksonville, FL 32207-7663
Phone: (904)731-3752 **Free:** 888-897-8579
Website: http://www.efnef.org

★ 8363 ★ Epilepsy Foundation of South Florida, Inc.
Chase Federal Bldg., Ste. 700
7300 N Kendall Dr.
Miami, FL 33156-7840
Phone: (305)670-4949
Website: http://www.epilepsyofla.org

Georgia

★ 8364 ★ Epilepsy Foundation of Georgia
100 Edgewood Ave. NE, Ste. 1200
Atlanta, GA 30303-3069
Phone: (404)527-7155 **Free:** 800-527-7105
Website: http://www.epilepsyga.org/

Hawaii

★ 8365 ★ Epilepsy Foundation of Hawaii, Inc.
245 N Kukui St., Ste. 207
Honolulu, HI 96817-3921
Phone: (808)528-3058
Website: http://www.hawaiiepilepsy.com/efh

Idaho

★ 8366 ★ Epilepsy Foundation of Idaho
310 W Idaho St.
Boise, ID 83702-6039
Phone: (208)344-4340 **Free:** 800-237-6676
Website: http://www.epilepsyidaho.org

Illinois

★ 8367 ★ Epilepsy Foundation of Greater Chicago
20 E Jackson Blvd., 13th Fl.
Chicago, IL 60604-2200
Phone: (312)939-8622 **Free:** 800-273-6027
Website: http://www.epilepsyfoundation.org/chicago

★ 8368 ★ Epilepsy Foundation of North/Central Illinois
321 W State St., Ste. 208
Rockford, IL 61101-1119
Phone: (815)964-2689 **Free:** 800-221-2689
Website: http://www.epilepsyfoundation.org/ncillinois
Remarks: Also serves Iowa.

★ 8369 ★ Epilepsy Foundation of Southwestern Illinois
1931 W Main St.
Belleville, IL 62226-7479
Phone: (618)236-2181
Website: http://www.neuro.wustl.edu/easwi

Kentucky

★ 8370 ★ Epilepsy Foundation Kentuckiana
501 E Broadway, Ste. 110
Louisville, KY 40202-1797
Phone: (502)584-8817
Website: http://www.efky.org
Remarks: Serves Indiana and Kentucky.

Louisiana

★ 8371 ★ Epilepsy Foundation of Southeast Louisiana
3701 Canal St., Ste. H
New Orleans, LA 70119-6101
Phone: (504)486-6326 **Free:** 800-960-0587
Website: http://www.laepilepsy.org

Maryland

★ 8372 ★ Epilepsy Foundation of the Chesapeake Region
Hampton Plaza
300 E Joppa Rd., Ste. 1103
Towson, MD 21286-3012
Phone: (410)828-7700 **Free:** 800-492-2523
Website: http://www.abilitiesnetwork.org
Remarks: This affiliate serves Maryland, the District of Columbia, and Alexandria, Arlington, Fairfax, Falls Church, Loudoun, and Prince William counties in Virginia.

Massachusetts

★ 8373 ★ Epilepsy Foundation of Massachusetts and Rhode Island
540 Gallivan Blvd.
Boston, MA 02124-5401
Phone: (617)506-6041 **Free:** 888-576-9996
Website: http://www.epilepsyfoundation.org/massri

Michigan

★ 8374 ★ Epilepsy Foundation of Michigan
26211 Central Park Blvd., Ste. 100
Southfield, MI 48076-4154
Phone: (248)351-7979 **Free:** 800-377-6226
Website: http://www.epilepsyfoundation.org/michigan

★ 8375 ★ Epilepsy Foundation of Michigan
26211 Central Park Blvd., Ste. 100
Southfield, MI 48076-4154
Phone: (248)351-7979 **Free:** 800-377-6226
Website: http://www.epilepsyfoundation.org/michigan

Minnesota

★ 8376 ★ Epilepsy Foundation of Minnesota
2356 University Ave W, No. 405
Saint Paul, MN 55114-1850
Phone: (651)646-1771 **Free:** 800-779-0777
Website: http://www.efmn.org
Remarks: This affiliate also serves Barnes, Cass, Cavalier, Grand Forks, Griggs, Nelson, Pembina, Ramsey, Ransom, Richland, Sargent, Steele, and Walsh counties in North Dakota.

Mississippi

★ 8377 ★ Epilepsy Foundation of Mississippi
PO Box 16232
Jackson, MS 39236-6232
Phone: (601)362-2761 **Free:** 800-898-0291

Missouri

★ 8378 ★ Epilepsy Foundation of Kansas & Western Missouri
6550 Troost Ave., Ste. B
Kansas City, MO 64131-1266
Phone: (816)444-2800 **Free:** 800-972-5163
Website: http://www.efha.org

★ 8379 ★ Epilepsy Foundation of the Saint Louis Region
7100 Oakland Ave.
Saint Louis, MO 63117-1813
Phone: (314)645-6969 **Free:** 800-264-6970
Website: http://www.epilepsyfoundation.org/stlouis
Remarks: Also serves Illinois.

New Jersey

★ 8380 ★ Epilepsy Foundation of New Jersey
429 River View Plaza
Trenton, NJ 08611-3420
Phone: (609)392-4900 **Free:** 800-336-5843
Website: http://www.efnj.com

New York

★ 8381 ★ Epilepsy Foundation of Long Island, Inc.
506 Stewart Ave.
Garden City, NY 11530-4706
Phone: (516)739-7733 **Free:** 888-672-7154
Website: http://www.epilepsyfoundation.org/longislend

★ 8382 ★ Epilepsy Foundation of New York City
305 7th Ave., 12th Fl.
New York, NY 10001-6008
Phone: (212)633-2930
Website: http://www.epilepsyfoundation.org/nyc

★ 8383 ★ Epilepsy Foundation of Northeastern New York
3 Washington Sq.
Albany, NY 12205-5523
Phone: (518)456-7501 **Free:** 800-894-3223
Website: http://www.epilepsyfoundation.org/efneny

★ 8384 ★ Epilepsy Foundation of Rochester-Syracuse-Binghamton
1000 Elmwood Ave., Ste. 800
Rochester, NY 14620-3042
Phone: (716)442-4430 **Free:** 800-724-7930
Website: http://www.epilepsyfoundation.org/rochester

★ 8385 ★ Epilepsy Foundation of Southern New York, Inc.
1 Blue Hill Plaza, No. 1745
Pearl River, NY 10965-3104
Phone: (845)627-0627 **Free:** 800-640-0371
Website: http://www.epiinfo.org

North Carolina

★ 8386 ★ Epilepsy Foundation of North Carolina, Inc.
3001 Spring Forest Rd.
Raleigh, NC 27616-2817
Phone: (919)876-7788 **Free:** 800-451-0694
Website: http://www.supportnetworks.org/info/efnc.htm

Ohio

★ 8387 ★ Epilepsy Foundation of Central Ohio
454 E Main St., Ste. 250
Columbus, OH 43215-5354
Phone: (614)228-4401 **Free:** 800-878-3226
Website: http://www.epilepsy-ohio.org

★ 8388 ★ Epilepsy Foundation of Greater Cincinnati, Inc.
895 Central Ave., Ste. 550
Cincinnati, OH 45202-5757
Phone: (513)721-2905
Website: http://www.epilepsyfoundation.org/cincinnati
Remarks: This affiliate serves Clark and Floyd counties in Indiana as well as the majority of Kentucky.

★ 8389 ★ Epilepsy Foundation of Northeast Ohio
2800 Euclid Ave., Rm. 450
Cleveland, OH 44115-2418
Phone: (216)579-1330
Website: http://www.efneo.org

★ 8390 ★ Epilepsy Foundation of Northwest Ohio
1251 S Reynolds Rd., PMB 323
Toledo, OH 43615-3938
Phone: (419)351-7979 **Free:** 800-377-6226

★ 8391 ★ Epilepsy Foundation of Western Ohio
7523 Brandt Pike
Dayton, OH 45424-2337
Phone: (937)233-2500 **Free:** 800-360-3296
Website: http://www.epilepsyfoundation.org/western-ohio

Oregon

★ 8392 ★ Epilepsy Foundation of Oregon
619 SW 11th Ave., Ste. 225
Portland, OR 97205-2646
Phone: (503)228-7651 **Free:** 888-828-7651
Website: http://www.epilepsyfoundation.org/oregon
Remarks: This affiliate also serves Clark County in Washington.

Pennsylvania

★ 8393 ★ Epilepsy Foundation of Eastern Pennsylvania
7 Benjamin Franklin Pkwy.
Philadelphia, PA 19103-1208
Phone: (215)523-9180 **Free:** 800-887-7165
Website: http://www.efsepa.org

★ 8394 ★ Epilepsy Foundation of Western and Central Pennsylvania
Vocational Rehab Center
1323 Forbes Ave., No. 102
Pittsburgh, PA 15219-4725
Phone: (412)261-5880 **Free:** 800-361-5885
Website: http://www.efwp.org

Puerto Rico

★ 8395 ★ Sociedad Puertorriquena de Epilepsia
Hospital Ruiz Soler
Bayamon, PR 00959
Phone: (787)782-6200 **Fax:** (787)782-6262
Website: http://www.sociedadepilepsiapr.org

South Carolina

★ 8396 ★ Epilepsy Foundation of South Carolina
652 Bush River Rd., Ste. 211
Columbia, SC 29210-7537
Phone: (803)798-8502
Website: http://www.epilepsysc.org

Tennessee

★ 8397 ★ Epilepsy Foundation of East Tennessee
PO Box 3156
Knoxville, TN 37927-3156
Phone: (865)522-4991 **Free:** 800-522-4991
Website: http://www.efeasttn.org

★ 8398 ★ Epilepsy Foundation of Middle Tennessee
2002 Richard Jones Rd., Ste. C202
Nashville, TN 37215-2809
Phone: (615)269-7091 **Free:** 800-244-0768
Website: http://efmt.citysearch.com

★ 8399 ★ Epilepsy Foundation of Southeast Tennessee
744 McCallie Ave., Ste. 301
Chattanooga, TN 37403-2511
Phone: (423)756-1771
Website: http://www.epilepsy-setn.org
Remarks: This affiliate also serves Catoosa, Dade, and Walker counties in Georgia.

★ 8400 ★ Epilepsy Foundation of West Tennessee
70 Timber Creek Dr., No. 1
Cordova, TN 38018-4285
Phone: (901)624-7148
Remarks: This affiliate also serves DeSoto County, Mississippi.

Texas

★ 8401 ★ Epilepsy Foundation of Central and South Texas
10615 Perrin Beitel Rd., Ste. 602
San Antonio, TX 78217-3142
Phone: (210)653-5353 **Free:** 888-606-5353
Website: http://www.epilepsyfoundation.org/efcst

★ 8402 ★ Epilepsy Foundation of Greater North Texas
2906 Swiss Ave.
Dallas, TX 75204-5929
Phone: (214)823-8809 **Free:** 800-447-7778
Website: http://www.efgnt.org

★ 8403 ★ Epilepsy Foundation of Southeast Texas
2650 Fountain View Dr., Ste. 316
Houston, TX 77057-7619
Phone: (713)789-6295 **Free:** 888-548-9716
Website: http://www.epilepsyfoundation.org/setexas

Vermont

★ 8404 ★ Epilepsy Foundation of Vermont
PO Box 6292
Rutland, VT 05702-6292
Phone: (802)775-1686

Virginia

★ 8405 ★ Epilepsy Foundation of Virginia
UVA Health Services Ctr.
Charlottesville, VA 22908-0001
Phone: (434)924-8669
Website: http://www.efva.org/

Washington

★ 8406 ★ Epilepsy Foundation Washington
3800 Aurora Ave. N, No. 370
Seattle, WA 98103-8721
Phone: (206)547-4551 **Free:** 800-752-3509
Website: http://www.epilepsyfoundation.org/washington

Wisconsin

★ 8407 ★ Epilepsy Foundation of Central and Northeast Wisconsin
1004 1st St., Ste. 5
Stevens Point, WI 54481-2627
Phone: (715)341-5811 **Free:** 800-924-9932

★ 8408 ★ Epilepsy Foundation South Central Wisconsin
7617 Mineral Point Rd.
Madison, WI 53717-1623
Phone: (608)833-8888 **Free:** 800-657-4929
Website: http://www.epilepsyfoundation.org/socentralwisc

★ 8409 ★ Epilepsy Foundation of Southeast Wisconsin
735 N Water St., Ste. 701
Milwaukee, WI 53202-4104
Phone: (414)271-0110
Website: http://www.epilepsyfoundationsewi.org

★ 8410 ★ Epilepsy Foundation of Southern Wisconsin, Inc.
205 N Main St., Ste. 106
Janesville, WI 53545-3062
Phone: (608)755-1821 **Free:** 800-693-2287
Website: http://www.epilepsyfoundation.org/southwisc

★ 8411 ★ Epilepsy Foundation of Western Wisconsin
1812 Brackett Ave., Ste. 5
Eau Claire, WI 54701-4677
Phone: (715)834-4455 **Free:** 800-924-2105
Website: http://www.epilepsyfoundation.org/westernwisc

Health Care

The following are state affiliates of the American Health Care Association (1201 L St. NW, Washington, DC 20005, (202)842-4444, http://www.ahca.org/), a national organization representing long term health care facilities.

Alabama

★ 8412 ★ Alabama Nursing Home Association
4156 Carmichael Rd.
Montgomery, AL 36106
Phone: (334)271-6214 **Fax:** (334)244-6509
Email: anha@anha.org
Website: http://www.anha.org
Nancy Thomas, Contact

Alaska

★ 8413 ★ Alaska State Hospital and Nursing Home Association
426 Main St.
Juneau, AK 99801
Phone: (907)586-1790 **Fax:** (907)463-3573
Email: ldashnha@eagle.ptialaska.net
Website: http://www.ashnha.com
Linda Fink, Contact

Arizona

★ 8414 ★ Arizona Health Care Association
5020 N 8th Pl., Ste. A
Phoenix, AZ 85014
Phone: (602)265-5331 **Fax:** (602)265-4401
Email: azhca@goodnet.com
Website: http://www.azhca.org
Kathleen Collins Pagels, Contact

Arkansas

★ 8415 ★ Arkansas Health Care Association
1401 W Capitol, Ste. 180
Little Rock, AR 72201
Phone: (501)374-4422 **Fax:** (501)374-1077
Email: arkhca@aol.com
Website: http://arhealthcare.com
Randy Wyatt, Director

California

★ 8416 ★ California Association of Health Facilities
California Center for Assisted Living
PO Box 537004
2201 K St.
Sacramento, CA 95853
Phone: (916)441-6400 **Fax:** (916)441-6441
Email: gmacomber@cahf.mailport.com
Website: http://www.cahf.org
Peggy Goldstein, Contact

Colorado

★ 8417 ★ Colorado Health Care Association
225 E 16th Ave., Ste. 1100
Denver, CO 80203
Phone: (303)861-8228 **Fax:** (303)839-8068
Email: amiles@cohca.org
Website: http://www.cohca.org
Arlene Miles, Director

Connecticut

★ 8418 ★ Connecticut Association of Health Care Facilities
Connecticut Center for Assisted Living
99 E River Dr., 8th Fl.
East Hartford, CT 06108
Phone: (860)290-9424 **Fax:** (860)290-9478
Website: http://www.cahcf.org
Toni Fatone, Vice President

Delaware

★ 8419 ★ Delaware Health Care Facilities Association
726 Loveville Rd., Ste. 3000
Hockessin, DE 19707
Phone: (302)235-6895 **Fax:** (302)235-6899
Yrene E. Waldron, Director

District of Columbia

★ 8420 ★ District of Columbia Health Care Association
1250 H St. NW, Ste. 555
Washington, DC 20005
Phone: (202)393-5712 **Fax:** (202)393-7180
Email: dbeck@ppsv.com
David Beck, Director

Florida

★ 8421 ★ Florida Health Care Association
Florida Center for Assisted Living
307 W Park Ave.
Tallahassee, FL 32301
Phone: (850)224-3907 **Fax:** (850)681-2075
Email: wphelan@fhca.org
Website: http://www.fhca.org
William Phelan, Director

Georgia

★ 8422 ★ Georgia Nursing Home Association
160 Country Club Dr.
Stockbridge, GA 30281
Phone: (678)289-6555 **Fax:** (678)289-6400
Email: fwatson@gnha.org
Website: http://www.gnha.org/
Fred Watson, President

Hawaii

★ 8423 ★ Healthcare Association of Hawaii
932 Ward Ave., Ste. 430
Honolulu, HI 96814
Phone: (808)521-8961 **Fax:** (808)599-2879

Email: jwhite@hah.org
Website: http://www.hah.org
Terri J. Byers, Contact

Idaho

★ 8424 ★ Idaho Health Care Association
Idaho Center for Assisted Living
802 W Bannock, Ste. 304
PO Box 2623
Boise, ID 83701
Phone: (208)343-9735 **Fax:** (208)343-6891
Email: scott@ihca-net.org
Website: http://www.ihca-net.org
Robert Van de Merwe, Contact

Illinois

★ 8425 ★ Illinois Health Care Association
1029 S 4th St.
Springfield, IL 62703
Phone: (217)528-6455 **Fax:** (217)528-0452
Email: info@ihca.com
Website: http://www.ihca.com
William Kempiners, Director

Indiana

★ 8426 ★ Indiana Health Care Association
Indiana Center for Assisted Living
1 N Capitol, Ste. 1115
Indianapolis, IN 46204
Phone: (317)636-6406 **Fax:** (317)638-3749
Email: info@ihca.org
Website: http://www.ihca.org
Arthur L. Logsdon, J.D., President

Iowa

★ 8427 ★ Iowa Health Care Association
6750 Westown Pkwy., Ste. 100
West Des Moines, IA 50266
Phone: (515)327-5020 **Fax:** (515)327-5019
Email: promans@netins.net
Website: http://www.iowahealthcare.org
Steve Ackerson, Vice President

Kansas

★ 8428 ★ Kansas Health Care Association
221 SW 33rd St.
Topeka, KS 66611
Phone: (785)267-6003 **Fax:** (785)267-0833
Email: khca@cjnetworks.com
John Kiefhaber, Vice President

Kentucky

★ 8429 ★ Kentucky Association of Health Care Facilities
9403 Mill Brook Rd.
Louisville, KY 40223
Phone: (502)425-5000 **Fax:** (502)425-3431
Email: kyhealthcare@worldnet.att.net
Website: http://www.kahcf.org
Rich Miller, President

Maine

★ 8430 ★ Maine Health Care Association
317 State St.
Augusta, ME 04330
Phone: (207)623-1146 **Fax:** (207)623-4080
Website: http://www.mehca.org
Richard Erb, Contact

Maryland

★ 8431 ★ Health Facilities Association of Maryland
7060 Oakland Mills Rd., Ste. M
Columbia, MD 21046
Phone: (410)792-4390 **Fax:** (410)792-4617
Website: http://www.hfam.org/
Adele Wilzack, President

Massachusetts

★ 8432 ★ Massachusetts Extended Care Federation
2310 Washington St., Ste. 300
Newton Lower Falls, MA 02462
Phone: (617)558-0202 **Fax:** (617)558-3546
Website: http://www.mecf.org
Ned Morse, President

Michigan

★ 8433 ★ Health Care Association of Michigan
c/o Michigan Center for Assisted Living
PO Box 80050
Lansing, MI 48908
Phone: (517)627-1561 **Fax:** (517)627-3016
Website: http://www.hcam.org
Reginald Carter, Vice President

Minnesota

★ 8434 ★ Care Providers of Minnesota
2850 Metro Dr., Ste. 200
Bloomington, MN 55425
Phone: (952)854-2844 **Fax:** (952)854-6214
Email: rcarter@careproviders.org
Website: http://www.careproviders.org
Rick Carter, President

Mississippi

★ 8435 ★ Mississippi Health Care Association
114 Marketridge Dr.
Ridgeland, MS 39157
Phone: (601)956-3472 **Fax:** (601)977-0273
Website: http://www.mshca.org
Martha Carole Jones, Director

Missouri

★ 8436 ★ Missouri Health Care Association
236 Metro Dr.
Jefferson City, MO 65109
Phone: (573)893-2060 **Fax:** (573)893-5248
Earl Carlson, Director

Nebraska

★ 8437 ★ Nebraska Health Care Association
Nebraska Assisted Living Association
421 S 9th St., Ste. 137
Lincoln, NE 68508
Phone: (402)435-3551 **Fax:** (402)435-4829
Email: pats@nhca.org
Website: http://www.nhca.org
Patricia Snyder, Director

Nevada

★ 8438 ★ Nevada Health Care Association
4425 S Jones Blvd., Ste. 4
Las Vegas, NV 89103
Phone: (702)434-2273 **Fax:** (702)434-3974
Email: nevitc@msn.com
Charles Perry, Contact

New Hampshire

★ 8439 ★ New Hampshire Health Care Association
125 Airport Rd.
Concord, NH 03301
Phone: (603)226-4900 **Fax:** (603)226-3376
Website: http://www.nhhca.org
John Poirier, Director

New Jersey

★ 8440 ★ Health Care Association of New Jersey
2131 Rte. 33
Hamilton, NJ 08690
Phone: (609)890-8700 **Fax:** (609)584-1047
Email: raatnjahcf@aol.com
Website: http://www.hcanj.org
Paul Langevin, Contact

New Mexico

★ 8441 ★ New Mexico Health Care Association
New Mexico Center for Assisted Living
4411 McLeod NE, Ste. G
Albuquerque, NM 87109
Phone: (505)880-1088 **Fax:** (505)880-1157
Website: http://www.nmhca.org
Linda Sechovec, Director

New York

★ 8442 ★ New York State Health Facilities Association
33 Elk St., Ste. 300
Albany, NY 12207
Phone: (518)462-4800 **Fax:** (518)426-4051
Email: estafford@nyshfa.org
Website: http://www.nyshfa.org
Richard Herrick, Contact

North Carolina

★ 8443 ★ North Carolina Health Care Facilities Association
5109 Bur Oak Cir.
Raleigh, NC 27612
Phone: (919)782-3827 **Fax:** (919)787-8418
Email: nchcfa@nchcfa.net
Website: http://www.nchcfa.org
J. Craig Souza, President

North Dakota

★ 8444 ★ North Dakota Long Term Care Association
1900 N 11th St.
Bismarck, ND 58501
Phone: (701)222-0660 **Fax:** (701)223-0977
Email: ndltca@btigate.com
Website: http://www.ndltca.org
Shelly Peterson, President

Ohio

★ 8445 ★ Ohio Health Care Association
Ohio Centers for Assisted Living
55 Green Meadows Dr. S
Lewis Center, OH 43035
Phone: (614)436-4154 **Fax:** (614)436-0939
Email: scochran@ohca.org

Website: http://www.ohca.org
Peter van Runkle, Vice President

Oregon

★ 8446 ★ Oregon Health Care Association
Oregon Center for Assisted Living
8995 SW Miley Rd., Ste. 205
Wilsonville, OR 97070
Phone: (503)694-6580 **Fax:** (503)694-6587
Email: JCatOHCA@aol.com
Website: http://www.ohca.com
Jim Carlson, Director

Pennsylvania

★ 8447 ★ Pennsylvania Health Care Association
Center for Assisted Living Management
315 N 2nd St.
Harrisburg, PA 17101
Phone: (717)221-1800 **Fax:** (717)221-8690
Email: rmoran@phca.org
Website: http://www.phca.org
Alan Rosenbloom, Contact

Rhode Island

★ 8448 ★ Rhode Island Health Care Association
57 Kilvert St., Ste. 200
Warwick, RI 02886
Phone: (401)732-9333 **Fax:** (401)739-3103
Email: rihca@msn.com
Website: http://www.rihca.com
Alfred Santos, Vice President

South Carolina

★ 8449 ★ South Carolina Health Care Association
176 Laurelhurst Dr.
Columbia, SC 29210
Phone: (803)772-7511 **Fax:** (803)772-7943
Website: http://www.schca.org
J. Randall Lee, Vice President

South Dakota

★ 8450 ★ South Dakota Health Care Association
804 N Western Ave.
Sioux Falls, SD 57104
Phone: (605)339-2071 **Fax:** (605)339-1354
Email: sdhca@worldnet.att.net
Website: http://www.sdhca.org
Mark Deak, Director

Tennessee

★ 8451 ★ Tennessee Health Care Association
2809 Foster Ave.
PO Box 100129
Nashville, TN 37224
Phone: (615)834-6520 **Fax:** (615)834-2502
Website: http://www.thca.org
Richard Sadler, Director

Texas

★ 8452 ★ Texas Health Care Association
4214 Medical Pkwy., 3rd Fl.
Austin, TX 78756
Phone: (512)458-1257 **Fax:** (512)467-9575
Email: thca@jump.net
Website: http://www.txhca.org
Tim Graves, Director

Utah

★ 8453 ★ Utah Health Care Association
275 E South Temple, Ste. 200
Salt Lake City, UT 84111
Phone: (801)994-3990 **Fax:** (801)994-3994
Email: uhca@vii.com
Website: http://www.vii.com/~uhca/
Joan Gallegos, Director

Vermont

★ 8454 ★ Vermont Health Care Association
617 Comstock Rd., Ste. 8
Montpelier, VT 05602
Phone: (802)229-5700 **Fax:** (802)223-4826
Email: vhca@aol.com
Website: http://www.virtualvermont.com/healthcare/vhca
Mary Shriver, Director

Virginia

★ 8455 ★ Virginia Health Care Association
Virginia Center for Assisted Living
2112 W Laburnum Ave., Ste. 206
Richmond, VA 23227
Phone: (804)353-9101 **Fax:** (804)353-3098
Email: steve.morrisette@vhca.org
Website: http://www.vhca.org
Steve Morrisette, President

Washington

★ 8456 ★ Washington Health Care Association
2120 State St. NE, Ste. 102
Olympia, WA 98506
Phone: (360)352-3304 **Fax:** (360)754-2412
Email: jerryreilly@whca.org
Website: http://www.whca.org
Brendan Williams, Contact

West Virginia

★ 8457 ★ West Virginia Health Care Association
8 Capitol St., Ste. 700
Charleston, WV 25301
Phone: (304)346-4575 **Fax:** (304)342-0519
Email: wvhca@citynet.net
Website: http://www.wvhca.org
P. John Alfano, CEO

Wisconsin

★ 8458 ★ Wisconsin Health Care Association
121 S Pinckney St., Ste. 500
Madison, WI 53703
Phone: (608)257-0125 **Fax:** (608)257-0025
Website: http://www.whca.com
Thomas Moore, Director

Wyoming

★ 8459 ★ Wyoming Health Care Association
PO Box 2270
Cheyenne, WY 82003
Phone: (307)635-0178 **Fax:** (307)635-1911
Tom Jones, Contact

Heart

State affiliates of the American Heart Association are listed below. The Association's national center is located at 7272 Greenville Ave., Dallas, TX 75231, (800)AHA-USA1, http://www.americanheart.org/.

Alabama

★ 8460 ★ American Heart Association Southeast Affiliate Birmingham Chapter
1449 Medical Park Dr.
Birmingham, AL 35213
Phone: (205)510-1500 **Fax:** (205)510-1501
Website: http://www.americanheart.org/al

★ 8461 ★ American Heart Association Southeast Affiliate Dothan Chapter
1152 W Main St.
Dothan, AL 36301
Phone: (334)794-4570 **Fax:** (334)677-4488

★ 8462 ★ American Heart Association Southeast Affiliate Huntsville Chapter
605 Davis Cir., Bldg. 10, Ste. 26
Huntsville, AL 35801
Phone: (256)536-0400 **Fax:** (256)535-9631

★ 8463 ★ American Heart Association Southeast Affiliate Mobile Chapter
900 Western America Cir., Ste. 209
Mobile, AL 36609
Phone: (251)461-4000 **Fax:** (251)461-4001

★ 8464 ★ American Heart Association Southeast Affiliate Montgomery Chapter
448 S Lawrence St.
Montgomery, AL 36104
Phone: (334)832-4400 **Fax:** (334)832-4900

★ 8465 ★ American Heart Association Southeast Affiliate Sheffield Chapter
501 N Montgomery Ave., Rm. 305
Sheffield, AL 35660
Phone: (256)381-4042 **Fax:** (256)381-4092

★ 8466 ★ American Heart Association Southeast Affiliate Tuscaloosa Chapter
2901 7th St.
Tuscaloosa, AL 35401
Phone: (205)752-5521 **Fax:** (205)758-7775

Alaska

★ 8467 ★ American Heart Association Northwest Affiliate Anchorage Chapter
1057 W Fireweed Ln., Ste. 100
Anchorage, AK 99503
Phone: (907)263-2044 **Free:** 888-276-0858
Fax: (907)263-2045
Website: http://www.americanheart.org/ak
Craig Harpel, Vice President
Peggy Spittler, Director

Arizona

★ 8468 ★ American Heart Association
Desert/Mountain Affiliate
Phoenix Chapter
2929 S 48th St.
Tempe, AZ 85282
Phone: (602)414-5353 **Fax:** (602)414-5355

★ 8469 ★ American Heart Association
Desert/Mountain Affiliate
Tucson Chapter
5325 E Pima Rd.
Tucson, AZ 85712
Phone: (520)795-1403 **Fax:** (520)795-1426

★ 8470 ★ American Heart Association
Desert/Mountain Affiliate
Williams Chapter
117 W Rte. 66, Ste. 155
Williams, AZ 86046
Phone: (520)635-0368 **Fax:** (520)635-4800

Arkansas

★ 8471 ★ American Heart Association
Heartland Affiliate
Fayetteville Chapter
92 W Sunbridge
Fayetteville, AR 72703
Phone: (501)442-6540 **Fax:** (501)442-4580

★ 8472 ★ American Heart Association
Heartland Affiliate
Jonesboro Chapter
2512 S Culberhouse, Ste. E
Jonesboro, AR 72401
Phone: (870)931-3070 **Fax:** (870)930-9046

★ 8473 ★ American Heart Association
Heartland Affiliate
Little Rock Chapter
909 W 2nd St.
Little Rock, AR 72203
Phone: (501)375-9148 **Fax:** (501)375-9066
Website: http://www.americanheart.org/ar

California

★ 8474 ★ American Heart Association
Western States Affiliate
Bakersfield Division
404 Truxtun Ave.
Bakersfield, CA 93301
Phone: (661)327-1173 **Fax:** (661)323-6981
Website: http://www.heartsource.org

★ 8475 ★ American Heart Association
Western States Affiliate
Chico Division
1372 Longfellow Ave.
Chico, CA 95926
Phone: (530)342-4247 **Fax:** (530)345-4072
Website: http://www.heartsource.org

★ 8476 ★ American Heart Association
Western States Affiliate
East Bay Division
11200 Golf Links Rd.
Oakland, CA 94605
Phone: (510)632-9606 **Fax:** (510)635-5848
Website: http://www.heartsource.org

★ 8477 ★ American Heart Association
Western States Affiliate
Eureka Division
1400 N Dutton Ave., Ste. 20
Santa Rosa, CA 95401
Phone: (707)542-1992 **Fax:** (510)576-7377
Website: http://www.heartsource.org

★ 8478 ★ American Heart Association
Western States Affiliate
Fresno Division
1495 W Shaw Ave.
Fresno, CA 93711
Phone: (559)224-8215 **Fax:** (559)228-8115
Website: http://www.heartsource.org

★ 8479 ★ American Heart Association
Western States Affiliate
Inland Empire Division
1003 E Cooley Dr., Ste. 102
Colton, CA 92324
Phone: (909)424-1670 **Fax:** (909)825-2484
Website: http://www.heartsource.org

★ 8480 ★ American Heart Association
Western States Affiliate
Los Angeles County Division
1055 Wilshire Blvd., Ste. 900
Los Angeles, CA 90017
Phone: (213)580-1408 **Free:** 800-AHA-USA1
Fax: (213)580-1461
Email: caroll@heart.org
Website: http://www.heartsource.org
Carol Lugo, Exec Director

★ 8481 ★ American Heart Association
Western States Affiliate
Merced Division
PO Box 1325
Merced, CA 95341
Phone: (209)723-2974 **Fax:** (209)228-8115
Website: http://www.heartsource.org

★ 8482 ★ American Heart Association
Western States Affiliate
Monterey Peninsula Division
1514 Moffett St., Ste. A
Salinas, CA 93905
Phone: (831)757-6221 **Fax:** (831)757-6355
Website: http://www.heartsource.org

★ 8483 ★ American Heart Association
Western States Affiliate
North Bay Division
1400 N Dutton Ave., Ste. 20
Santa Rosa, CA 95401
Phone: (707)542-1992 **Fax:** (707)576-7377
Website: http://www.heartsource.org

★ 8484 ★ American Heart Association
Western States Affiliate
Orange County Division
4600 Campus Dr.
Irvine, CA 92612
Phone: (949)856-3555 **Fax:** (949)856-3364
Website: http://www.heartsource.org

★ 8485 ★ American Heart Association
Western States Affiliate
Palm Desert Division
74-020 Alessandro, Ste. A
Palm Desert, CA 92260
Phone: (760)346-8109 **Fax:** (760)773-0766
Website: http://www.heartsource.org

★ 8486 ★ American Heart Association
Western States Affiliate
Sacramento Division
2007 O St.
Sacramento, CA 95814
Phone: (916)446-6505 **Fax:** (916)443-2865
Website: http://www.heartsource.org

★ 8487 ★ American Heart Association
Western States Affiliate
Salinas Division
1514 Moffett St.
Salinas, CA 93905
Phone: (831)757-6221 **Fax:** (831)757-6355
Website: http://www.heartsource.org

★ 8488 ★ American Heart Association
Western States Affiliate
San Diego Division
3640 5th Ave.
San Diego, CA 92103
Phone: (619)291-7454 **Fax:** (619)291-9454
Website: http://www.heartsource.org

★ 8489 ★ American Heart Association
Western States Affiliate
San Francisco Division
120 Montgomery St., Ste. 1650
San Francisco, CA 94104
Phone: (415)433-2273 **Fax:** (415)228-8402
Email: howards@heart.org
Website: http://www.heartsource.org
Howard Shiflett, Exec Director

★ 8490 ★ American Heart Association
Western States Affiliate
San Joaquin County Division
1495 W Shaw Ave.
Fresno, CA 93711
Phone: (559)224-8215 **Fax:** (559)228-8115
Website: http://www.heartsource.org

★ 8491 ★ American Heart Association
Western States Affiliate
San Jose Division
1 Almaden Blvd., Ste. 500
San Jose, CA 95113
Phone: (408)977-4950 **Fax:** (408)977-4959
Website: http://www.heartsource.org

★ 8492 ★ American Heart Association
Western States Affiliate
San Luis Obispo Division
1371 Pacific St.
San Luis Obispo, CA 93401
Phone: (805)544-1505 **Fax:** (805)549-9627
Website: http://www.heartsource.org

★ 8493 ★ American Heart Association
Western States Affiliate
San Mateo Division
1710 Gilbreth Rd., Ste. 100
Burlingame, CA 94010
Phone: (650)259-6700 **Fax:** (650)259-6890
Website: http://www.heartsource.org

★ 8494 ★ American Heart Association
Western States Affiliate
Santa Barbara Division
212 W Figueroa St.
Santa Barbara, CA 93101
Phone: (805)963-8862 **Fax:** (805)963-8866
Website: http://www.heartsource.org

★ 8495 ★ American Heart Association
Western States Affiliate
Stockton Division
1212 W Robinhood Dr., Ste. 5-D
Stockton, CA 95207
Phone: (209)477-2683 **Fax:** (209)477-1271
Email: todd@heart.org
Website: http://www.heartsource.org
Tod Davis, Exec Director

★ 8496 ★ American Heart Association
Western States Affiliate
Ventura Division
333 Lantana St., Ste. 265
Camarillo, CA 93010
Phone: (805)445-7050 **Fax:** (805)445-9882
Email: kathys@heart.org
Website: http://www.heartsource.org
Kathy Shoemate, Exec Director
Remarks: Serves the cities of Ventura, Ojai, Oxnard, Port Hueneme, Camarillo, Somis, Moorpark, Simi Valley, Newbury Park, Thousand Oaks, Westlake Village, and Agoura.

Colorado

★ 8497 ★ American Heart Association
Desert/Mountain Affiliate
Boulder Chapter
3135 23rd St.
Boulder, CO 80304
Phone: (303)673-0292 **Fax:** (303)673-0249

★ 8498 ★ American Heart Association
Desert/Mountain Affiliate
Colorado Springs Chapter
415 N Tejon, Ste. 201
Colorado Springs, CO 80903
Phone: (719)635-7688 **Fax:** (719)635-3606

★ 8499 ★ American Heart Association
Desert/Mountain Affiliate
Denver Chapter
1280 S Parker Rd.
Denver, CO 80231
Phone: (303)369-5433 **Free:** 800-242-8721
Fax: (303)369-8087

★ 8500 ★ American Heart Association
Desert/Mountain Affiliate
Grand Junction Chapter
123 N 7th St.
Grand Junction, CO 81501
Phone: (970)241-4577 **Fax:** (970)241-4637

★ 8501 ★ American Heart Association
Desert/Mountain Affiliate
Pueblo Chapter
720 N Main St., Ste. 440
Pueblo, CO 81003
Phone: (719)583-9388 **Fax:** (719)583-4247

Connecticut

★ 8502 ★ American Heart Association
Connecticut Affiliate
5 Brookside Dr.
PO Box 5022
Wallingford, CT 06492
Phone: (203)294-0088 **Fax:** (203)294-3577
Website: http://www.americanheart.org/ct

Delaware

★ 8503 ★ American Heart Association
Pennsylvania-Delaware Affiliate
Kent County Chapter
1151 Walker Rd., Ste. 202
Dover, DE 19904
Phone: (302)734-9321 **Fax:** (302)734-5571

★ 8504 ★ American Heart Association
Pennsylvania-Delaware Affiliate
New Castle County Chapter
1096 Old Churchmans Rd.
Newark, DE 19713
Phone: (302)633-0200 **Fax:** (302)633-3964

★ 8505 ★ American Heart Association
Pennsylvania-Delaware Affiliate
Sussex County Chapter
Georgetown Professional Park, Ste. 201A
Georgetown, DE 19947
Phone: (302)856-7386 **Fax:** (302)856-2828

Florida

★ 8506 ★ American Heart Association
Boca Raton Chapter
500 NE Spanish River Blvd., Ste. 22
Boca Raton, FL 33431
Phone: (561)394-0170 **Fax:** (561)391-8669

★ 8507 ★ American Heart Association
Bonita Springs Chapter
28441 Bonita Crossings Blvd.
Bonita Springs, FL 34135
Phone: (941)498-9288 **Fax:** (941)498-9188

★ 8508 ★ American Heart Association
Ft. Lauderdale Chapter
1751 W Cypress Creek Rd.
Fort Lauderdale, FL 33309
Phone: (954)772-8100 **Fax:** (954)491-3511

★ 8509 ★ American Heart Association
Ft. Walton Beach Chapter
222 Hospital Dr. NE
Fort Walton Beach, FL 32548
Phone: (850)243-9715 **Fax:** (850)664-7976

★ 8510 ★ American Heart Association
Gainesville Chapter
210 NW 75th Dr., Ste. 1
Gainesville, FL 32607
Phone: (352)333-3244 **Fax:** (352)333-3254

★ 8511 ★ American Heart Association
Jacksonville Chapter
5851 St. Augustine Rd.
Jacksonville, FL 32207
Phone: (904)739-0197 **Fax:** (904)739-0012

★ 8512 ★ American Heart Association
Lakeland Chapter
1545 Lakeland Hills Blvd.
Lakeland, FL 33805
Phone: (863)686-8421 **Fax:** (863)683-4667

★ 8513 ★ American Heart Association
Melbourne Chapter
2800 Aurora Rd., Ste. I
Melbourne, FL 32935
Phone: (321)255-3557 **Fax:** (321)255-7810

★ 8514 ★ American Heart Association
Miami Chapter
2600 SW 3rd Ave., Ste. 900
Miami, FL 33129
Phone: (305)856-1449 **Fax:** (305)860-6780

★ 8515 ★ American Heart Association
New Port Richey Chapter
7137 Congress St.
PO Box 2251
New Port Richey, FL 34656-2251
Phone: (727)848-8924 **Fax:** (727)842-5931

★ 8516 ★ American Heart Association
Orlando Chapter
237 East Marks St.
Orlando, FL 32803
Phone: (407)843-1330 **Fax:** (407)423-9415

★ 8517 ★ American Heart Association
Ormond Beach Chapter
555 W Granada Blvd., Ste. A-1
Ormond Beach, FL 32174
Phone: (386)676-0001 **Fax:** (386)676-0204

★ 8518 ★ American Heart Association
Panama City Chapter
2697 Jenks Ave.
Panama City, FL 32405
Phone: (850)769-3070 **Fax:** (850)872-9133

★ 8519 ★ American Heart Association
Pensacola Chapter
4400 Bayou Blvd., Ste. 49-A
Pensacola, FL 32503
Phone: (850)473-0411 **Fax:** (850)473-2993

★ 8520 ★ American Heart Association
Saint Petersburg Chapter
9900 9th St. N
PO Box 21203
Saint Petersburg, FL 33742-1203
Phone: (727)570-8610 **Fax:** (727)570-8519
Website: http://www.americanheart.org/fl

★ 8521 ★ American Heart Association
Sarasota Chapter
2975 Bee Ridge Rd., Ste. B
Sarasota, FL 34239
Phone: (941)927-4997 **Fax:** (941)927-1427

★ 8522 ★ American Heart Association
Stuart Chapter
1111 S Federal Hwy., Ste. 110
Stuart, FL 34994
Phone: (561)286-1966 **Fax:** (561)220-2605

★ 8523 ★ American Heart Association
Tallahassee Chapter
1304 E 6th Ave.
Tallahassee, FL 32303
Phone: (850)878-3885 **Fax:** (850)942-2803

★ 8524 ★ American Heart Association
Tampa Chapter
1411 N Westshore Blvd., Ste. 216
Tampa, FL 33607
Phone: (813)289-6003 **Fax:** (813)289-4351

★ 8525 ★ American Heart Association
West Palm Beach Chapter
1301 S Olive Ave.
West Palm Beach, FL 33401
Phone: (561)655-8155 **Fax:** (561)832-6014

Georgia

★ 8526 ★ American Heart Association
Southeast Affiliate
Albany Chapter
1512 Gillionville Rd., Ste. 6
Albany, GA 31707
Phone: (912)883-5858 **Fax:** (912)883-5999

★ 8527 ★ American Heart Association
Southeast Affiliate
Athens Chapter
1353 Jennings Mill Rd., Ste. A
Bogart, GA 30622
Phone: (706)549-0939 **Fax:** (706)549-3141

★ 8528 ★ American Heart Association
Southeast Affiliate
Augusta Chapter
246 Davis Rd., Ste. E
Augusta, GA 30907
Phone: (706)855-5005 **Fax:** (706)855-5101

★ 8529 ★ American Heart Association
Southeast Affiliate
Brunswick Chapter
1614 Union St.
Brunswick, GA 31520
Phone: (912)264-5466 **Fax:** (912)264-1931

★ 8530 ★ American Heart Association
Southeast Affiliate
Columbus Chapter
1300 Wynnton Rd., Ste. 108
Columbus, GA 31906
Phone: (706)324-0173 **Fax:** (706)324-0174

★ 8531 ★ American Heart Association
Southeast Affiliate
Macon Chapter
3312 Northside Dr., Ste. 140-A
Macon, GA 31210
Phone: (478)405-3200 **Fax:** (478)405-3201

★ 8532 ★ American Heart Association
Southeast Affiliate
Marietta Chapter
1101 Northchase Pkwy., Ste. 1
Marietta, GA 30067
Phone: (678)385-2000 **Fax:** (678)385-2001
Website: http://www.americanheart.org/ga

★ 8533 ★ American Heart Association
Southeast Affiliate
Metro Atlanta Chapter
1101 Northchase Pkwy., Ste. 1
Marietta, GA 30067
Phone: (770)952-1316 **Fax:** (770)952-2208

★ 8534 ★ American Heart Association
Southeast Affiliate
Savannah Chapter
7505 Waters Ave., Ste. C7
Savannah, GA 31406
Phone: (912)355-0233 **Fax:** (912)355-0234

★ 8535 ★ American Heart Association
Southeast Affiliate
Valdosta Chapter
305 University Dr., Ste. 1
Valdosta, GA 31602
Phone: (229)247-1550 **Fax:** (229)241-8323

Hawaii

★ 8536 ★ American Heart Association
East Hawaii Chapter
400 Hualani St., Ste. 15
Hilo, HI 96720
Phone: (808)961-2825 **Fax:** (808)961-2827

★ 8537 ★ American Heart Association
Kauai Chapter
4303-C3 Rice St.
Lihue, HI 96766
Phone: (808)245-7311 **Fax:** (808)245-7311

★ 8538 ★ American Heart Association
Maui Chapter
J. Walter Cameron Center
95 Mahalani St., No. 13
Wailuku, HI 96793
Phone: (808)244-7185 **Fax:** (808)242-1857

★ 8539 ★ American Heart Association
Oahu Chapter
245 N Kukui St., Ste. 204
Honolulu, HI 96817
Phone: (808)538-7021

★ 8540 ★ American Heart Association
West Hawaii Chapter
74-5588 Pawai Pl., Bldg. H
Kailua Kona, HI 96740
Phone: (808)329-0783 **Fax:** (808)329-0784

Idaho

★ 8541 ★ American Heart Association
Northwest Affiliate
Greater Treasure Valley, Idaho/Oregon
270 S Orchard, Ste. B
Boise, ID 83705
Phone: (208)384-5066 **Free:** 800-589-4204
Fax: (208)336-5867
Email: jrobinso@heart.org
Website: http://www.americanheart.org/idmt
Mary T. MacConnell, Vice President
Julie Robinson, Director

Illinois

★ 8542 ★ American Heart Association
Midwest Affiliate
Chicago Chapter
208 S LaSalle St., Ste. 900
Chicago, IL 60604
Phone: (312)346-4675 **Fax:** (312)346-8236
Email: kwest2@heart.org
Website: http://www.americanheart.org/il/Chicago

★ 8543 ★ American Heart Association
Midwest Affiliate
Rockford Chapter
5192 Harrison Ave.
Rockford, IL 61108
Phone: (815)397-6112 **Free:** 800-694-8618
Fax: (815)397-5024

★ 8544 ★ American Heart Association
Midwest Affiliate
Springfield Chapter
2524 Farragut Dr., Ste. A
Springfield, IL 62704
Phone: (217)698-3838 **Free:** 800-252-8511
Fax: (217)698-4585
Website: http://www.americanheart.org/il

★ 8545 ★ American Heart Association
Midwest Affiliate
Westmont Chapter
801 N Cass Ave., Ste. 200
Westmont, IL 60559
Phone: (630)789-9222 **Fax:** (630)789-9235

Indiana

★ 8546 ★ American Heart Association
Midwest Affiliate
Evansville Chapter
233 SE 3rd St.
Evansville, IN 47713
Phone: (812)424-4464 **Free:** 800-966-7113
Fax: (812)424-4467

★ 8547 ★ American Heart Association
Midwest Affiliate
Indianapolis Chapter
8645 Guion Rd., Ste. H
PO Box 681550
Indianapolis, IN 46268
Phone: (317)876-4850 **Free:** 800-229-1503
Fax: (317)876-4859
Website: http://www.americanheart.org/in

★ 8548 ★ American Heart Association
Midwest Affiliate
Mishawaka Chapter
2410 N Grape Rd., Ste. 5A
Mishawaka, IN 46545
Phone: (219)258-4018 **Free:** 800-966-4572
Fax: (219)256-6687

Iowa

★ 8549 ★ American Heart Association
Heartland Affiliate
Cedar Rapids Chapter
3741 Center Point Rd. NE
Cedar Rapids, IA 52402
Phone: (319)378-1763

★ 8550 ★ American Heart Association
Heartland Affiliate
Council Bluffs Chapter
Edwards Professional Center
715 Harmony St., Ste. 101
Council Bluffs, IA 51503
Phone: (712)322-4755

★ 8551 ★ American Heart Association
Heartland Affiliate
Davenport Chapter
1606 Brady St., Ste. 213
Davenport, IA 52803
Phone: (563)323-4321

★ 8552 ★ American Heart Association
Heartland Affiliate
Des Moines Chapter
1111 9th St., Ste. 280
Des Moines, IA 50314
Phone: (515)244-3278 **Fax:** (515)244-5164
Website: http://www.americanheart.org/ia

★ 8553 ★ American Heart Association
Heartland Affiliate
Mason City Chapter
Westside Office Bldg.
1312-4th St. SW, No. 123
Mason City, IA 50401
Phone: (641)424-0256

★ 8554 ★ American Heart Association
Heartland Affiliate
Sioux City Chapter
Benson Bldg., Ste. 621
705 Douglas
Sioux City, IA 51101
Phone: (712)255-4798

★ 8555 ★ American Heart Association
Heartland Affiliate
Waterloo Chapter
1825 Logan Ave., No. 331
Waterloo, IA 50703
Phone: (641)235-3912

Kansas

★ 8556 ★ American Heart Association
Heartland Affiliate
Kansas City Chapter
6800 W 93rd St.
Overland Park, KS 66212
Phone: (913)648-6727 **Fax:** (913)648-0423

★ 8557 ★ American Heart Association
Heartland Affiliate
Topeka Chapter
5375 SW 7th St.
Topeka, KS 66606
Phone: (785)272-7056 **Free:** 800-284-3979
Fax: (785)272-2425
Email: mmclaugh@heart.org
Website: http://www.americanheart.org/ks

★ 8558 ★ American Heart Association
Heartland Affiliate
Wichita Chapter
2100 E Douglas
Wichita, KS 67214
Phone: (316)265-4238 **Fax:** (316)265-1390

Kentucky

★ 8559 ★ American Heart Association
Kentucky Affiliate
Central Kentucky Chapter
2201 Regency Rd., Ste. 401
Lexington, KY 40503-2339
Phone: (859)278-1632 **Fax:** (859)278-6236
Remarks: Serves Anderson, Bourbon, Clark, Fayette, Jessamine, Mercer, Scott, and Woodford counties.

★ 8560 ★ American Heart Association
Kentucky Affiliate
Eastern Kentucky Chapter
333 Guthrie St., Ste. 207
Louisville, KY 40202
Phone: (502)587-8641 **Free:** 800-AHA-USA1
Fax: (502)585-7001
Remarks: Serves Bullitt, Jefferson, Oldham and Shelby counties.

★ 8561 ★ American Heart Association
Kentucky Affiliate
Southcentral Kentucky Chapter
1212 Ashley Circle, Ste. 1
Bowling Green, KY 42104
Phone: 800-AHA-USA1 **Fax:** (270)842-8931

★ 8562 ★ American Heart Association
Kentucky Affiliate
Southwestern Kentucky Chapter
222 Kentucky Ave., Ste. 4
Paducah, KY 42003
Phone: 800-AHA-USA1 **Fax:** (270)442-3730

★ 8563 ★ American Heart Association
Kentucky Affiliate
Western Kentucky Chapter
318 St. Elizabeth St.
Owensboro, KY 42301
Phone: 800-AHA-USA1 **Fax:** (270)683-2149

Louisiana

★ 8564 ★ American Heart Association
Southeast Affiliate
Alexandria Chapter
2304 S MacArthur Dr., Ste. F
Alexandria, LA 71301
Phone: (318)443-7522 **Fax:** (318)443-2679

★ 8565 ★ American Heart Association
Southeast Affiliate
Baton Rouge Chapter
4962 Florida Blvd., Ste. 402
Baton Rouge, LA 70806
Phone: (225)248-7700 **Fax:** (225)248-7701

★ 8566 ★ American Heart Association
Southeast Affiliate
Houma Chapter
220 Progressive Blvd.
Houma, LA 70360
Phone: (985)851-3479 **Fax:** (985)580-2844

★ 8567 ★ American Heart Association
Southeast Affiliate
Lafayette Chapter
312 Guilbeau Rd., Ste. 6C
Lafayette, LA 70506
Phone: (337)988-2212 **Fax:** (337)988-2214

★ 8568 ★ American Heart Association
Southeast Affiliate
Lake Charles Chapter
1 Lakeside Plaza, Ste. 808
Lake Charles, LA 70601
Phone: (337)439-4050 **Fax:** (337)430-0305

★ 8569 ★ American Heart Association
Southeast Affiliate
New Orleans Chapter
105 Campus Dr. E
PO Box 159
Destrehan, LA 70047
Phone: (504)456-7224 **Free:** 800-242-8721
Fax: (985)764-8712
Website: http://www.americanheart.org/la

Maine

★ 8570 ★ American Heart Association
New England Affiliate
Maine Chapter
343 Gorham Rd.
South Portland, ME 04106
Phone: (207)879-5700 **Free:** 800-937-0944
Fax: (207)879-5918

Maryland

★ 8571 ★ American Heart Association
Baltimore Chapter
415 N Charles St.
Baltimore, MD 21201
Phone: (410)685-7074 **Free:** 800-242-8721
Fax: (410)539-5049
Website: http://www.americanheart.org/md

Massachusetts

★ 8572 ★ American Heart Association
New England Affiliate
Framingham Chapter
20 Speen St.
Framingham, MA 01701
Phone: (508)620-1700 **Free:** 800-662-1701
Fax: (508)620-6157
Email: webmaster@ahama.org
Website: http://www.americanheart.org/ma

★ 8573 ★ American Heart Association
New England Affiliate
South Yarmouth Chapter
2 White's Path
South Yarmouth, MA 02664
Phone: (508)760-6818 **Fax:** (508)760-6824

★ 8574 ★ American Heart Association
New England Affiliate
West Springfield Chapter
1111 Elm St., Ste. 9A
West Springfield, MA 01089
Phone: (413)827-0400 **Fax:** (413)827-9390

Michigan

★ 8575 ★ American Heart Association
Midwest Affiliate
Grand Rapids Chapter
The Lakeview Bldg.
3940 Peninsular Dr. SE, Ste. 180
Grand Rapids, MI 49546-6107
Phone: (616)285-1888 **Free:** 800-968-1040
Fax: (616)285-1895
Email: ahami.gr@greatid.com
Lisa Bennett, Vice President

★ 8576 ★ American Heart Association
Midwest Affiliate
Okemos Chapter
2140 University Park, Ste. 210
Okemos, MI 48864
Phone: (517)349-3102 **Fax:** (517)349-3240

★ 8577 ★ American Heart Association
Midwest Affiliate
Saginaw Chapter
3875 Bay Rd., Ste. 1-N
Saginaw, MI 48603
Phone: (989)792-6400 **Free:** 800-968-2422
Fax: (989)792-6556

★ 8578 ★ American Heart Association
Midwest Affiliate
Southfield Chapter
24445 Northwestern Hwy., Ste. 100
Southfield, MI 48075
Phone: (248)827-4214 **Fax:** (248)827-4234

Minnesota

★ 8579 ★ American Heart Association
Northland Affiliate
Central Minnesota Chapter
110 S 2nd St., Ste. 305
Waite Park, MN 56387-1367
Phone: (320)255-9930 **Fax:** (320)255-9808

★ 8580 ★ American Heart Association
Northland Affiliate
Duluth Chapter
401 W Michigan St.
Duluth, MN 55802
Phone: (218)727-7297 **Fax:** (218)727-0621

★ 8581 ★ American Heart Association
Northland Affiliate
Minneapolis Chapter
4701 W 77th St.
Minneapolis, MN 55435
Phone: (952)835-3300 **Fax:** (952)835-5828
Email: hmail@ahamn.attmail.com
Website: http://www.americanheart.org/mn

★ 8582 ★ American Heart Association
Northland Affiliate
Northwest Minnesota Chapter
220 W Washington
Fergus Falls, MN 56537
Phone: (218)739-3329 **Fax:** (218)739-3320

★ 8583 ★ American Heart Association
Northland Affiliate
Southeast Minnesota Chapter
1500 1st Ave. NE, Ste. 200
Rochester, MN 55906
Phone: (507)288-6749 **Fax:** (507)288-9287

★ 8584 ★ American Heart Association
Northland Affiliate
Southwest Minnesota Chapter
Northwestern Chapter Bldg., No. 205
209 S 2nd St.
Mankato, MN 56001
Phone: (507)345-8206 **Fax:** (507)345-8202

Mississippi

★ 8585 ★ American Heart Association
Southeast Affiliate
Biloxi Chapter
2320 14th St., Ste. 110
Gulfport, MS 39501
Phone: (228)864-1629 **Fax:** (228)864-4856

★ 8586 ★ American Heart Association
Southeast Affiliate
Greenwood Chapter
227 W Market, Ste. 8
Greenwood, MS 38930
Phone: (662)455-5877 **Fax:** (662)451-5810

★ 8587 ★ American Heart Association
Southeast Affiliate
Hattiesburg Chapter
609 Corinee St., Ste. B-1
Hattiesburg, MS 39401
Phone: (601)583-0108 **Fax:** (601)582-0496

★ 8588 ★ American Heart Association
Southeast Affiliate
Jackson Chapter
4830 McWillie Cir.
Jackson, MS 39206
Phone: (601)321-1200 **Fax:** (601)321-1201
Website: http://www.americanheart.org/ms
Teresa Humphrey, Director

Missouri

★ 8589 ★ American Heart Association
Heartland Affiliate
Columbia Office
2600 I-70 Dr. NW
Columbia, MO 65201
Phone: (573)446-3000 **Fax:** (573)445-6243
Email: hmail@ahamo.attmail.com
Website: http://www.americanheart.org/mo

★ 8590 ★ American Heart Association
Heartland Affiliate
Greater St. Louis Division
4643 Lindell Blvd.
Saint Louis, MO 63108
Phone: (314)367-3383 **Fax:** (314)367-8605
Email: hmail@ahamo.attmail.com
Website: http://www.americanheart.org/mo

★ 8591 ★ American Heart Association
Heartland Affiliate
Springfield Chapter
2446 E Madrid
Springfield, MO 65804
Phone: (417)881-1121 **Fax:** (417)881-8972

Montana

★ 8592 ★ American Heart Association of Idaho/Montana
Northwest Affiliate
Central Montana Chapter
600 Central Plaza, Ste. 304
Great Falls, MT 59401
Phone: (406)452-2362 **Free:** 800-592-7821
Fax: (406)452-0899
Email: aingerso@heart.org
Alice Ingersoll, Director

★ 8593 ★ American Heart Association of Idaho/Montana
Northwest Affiliate
Eastern Montana Chapter
2812 1st Ave. N, Rm. 216
Billings, MT 59101
Phone: (406)256-3855 **Fax:** (406)256-3728
Email: deckhard@heart.org
Dawn Eckhardt, Director

★ 8594 ★ American Heart Association of Idaho/Montana
Northwest Affiliate
Northwest Montana Chapter
PO Box 1236
Condon, MT 59826
Phone: (406)754-3015 **Fax:** (406)754-3015
Email: jwheeler@heart.org
Jabet Wheeler, Director

Nebraska

★ 8595 ★ American Heart Association
Heartland Affiliate
Lincoln Chapter
1550 S 70th St., Ste. 100
Lincoln, NE 68506
Phone: (402)489-5115 **Fax:** (402)489-6949
Website: http://www.americanheart.org/ne

★ 8596 ★ American Heart Association
Heartland Affiliate
Omaha Chapter
10100 J St., Ste. A
Omaha, NE 68127
Phone: (402)346-0771 **Fax:** (402)346-1717
Website: http://www.americanheart.org/ne

Nevada

★ 8597 ★ American Heart Association
Western States Affiliate
Clark County/Laughlin Division
6370 W Flamingo, Ste. 1
Las Vegas, NV 89103
Phone: (702)367-1366 **Fax:** (702)367-1975
Email: vickis@heart.org
Website: http://www.heartsource.org
Vicki K. Sylvia, Exec Director

★ 8598 ★ American Heart Association
Western States Affiliate
Reno Division
1281 Terminal Way, Ste. 111
Reno, NV 89502
Phone: (775)322-7065 **Fax:** (775)322-8959
Website: http://www.heartsource.org

New Hampshire

★ 8599 ★ American Heart Association
New England Affiliate
New Hampshire Chapter
20 Merrimack St., Ste. 1
Manchester, NH 03101
Phone: (603)669-5833 **Free:** 888-907-6933
Fax: (603)669-6745

New Jersey

★ 8600 ★ American Heart Association
Heritage Affiliate
Central New Jersey Chapter
2550 U.S. Hwy. 1
North Brunswick, NJ 08902
Phone: (732)821-2610 **Fax:** (732)821-2736
Website: http://www.americanheart.org/nj

★ 8601 ★ American Heart Association
Heritage Affiliate
Northern New Jersey Chapter
1 Bleeker St.
Millburn, NJ 07041
Phone: (973)376-3636 **Fax:** (973)912-9570

★ 8602 ★ American Heart Association
Heritage Affiliate
Southern New Jersey Chapter
600 S White Horse Pike
Audubon, NJ 08106
Phone: (856)546-5600 **Fax:** (856)546-0861

New Mexico

★ 8603 ★ American Heart Association
Desert/Mountain Affiliate
Albuquerque Chapter
6100 Pan American Fwy. NE, No. 345
Albuquerque, NM 87109
Phone: (505)823-8700 **Fax:** (505)823-8701

New York

★ 8604 ★ American Heart Association
Heritage Affiliate
Long Island Region
125 E Bethpage Rd.
Plainview, NY 11803
Phone: (516)777-8447 **Fax:** (516)370-1060

★ 8605 ★ American Heart Association
New York State Affiliate
Central Region
120 Lomond Ct.
Utica, NY 13502
Phone: (315)797-8906 **Fax:** (315)732-6563

★ 8606 ★ American Heart Association
New York State Affiliate
Dutchess County Region
301 Manchester Rd., Ste. 105
Poughkeepsie, NY 12603
Phone: (845)485-4703 **Fax:** (845)486-9950

★ 8607 ★ American Heart Association
New York State Affiliate
Genesee Valley Region
2113 Chili Ave.
Rochester, NY 14624
Phone: (716)426-4050 **Fax:** (716)426-1312

★ 8608 ★ American Heart Association
New York State Affiliate
Mid-State Region
59 Court St., 4th Fl.
Binghamton, NY 13903
Phone: (607)723-0208 **Fax:** (607)724-1875

★ 8609 ★ American Heart Association
New York State Affiliate
New York City Region
122 E 42nd St., 18th Fl.
New York, NY 10168
Phone: (212)878-5900 **Fax:** (212)878-5960
Email: ccendoma@heart.org
Website: http://www.americanheart.org/nyc

★ 8610 ★ American Heart Association
New York State Affiliate
Northeastern Region
440 New Karner Rd.
Albany, NY 12205
Phone: (518)869-1961 **Fax:** (518)869-8180

★ 8611 ★ American Heart Association
New York State Affiliate
Northern Region
PO Box 155
Watertown, NY 13601
Phone: (315)641-1000 **Fax:** (315)641-1098

★ 8612 ★ American Heart Association
New York State Affiliate
Orange-Rockland-Sullivan Regional Chapter
Good Samaritan Hospital
255 Lafayette Ave.
Suffern, NY 10901
Phone: (845)369-1320 **Fax:** (845)369-3801

★ 8613 ★ American Heart Association
New York State Affiliate
Southern Tier Region
PO Box 1461
Corning, NY 14830
Phone: (315)641-1000 **Fax:** (315)641-1098

★ 8614 ★ American Heart Association
New York State Affiliate
Upstate Region
5575 Thompson Rd.
Syracuse, NY 13214
Phone: (315)446-8334 **Fax:** (315)446-6986

★ 8615 ★ American Heart Association
New York State Affiliate
Westchester/Putnam Region
3020 Westchester Ave.
Purchase, NY 10577
Phone: (914)694-6464 **Fax:** (914)694-1285

★ 8616 ★ American Heart Association
New York State Affiliate
Western/Southwestern Region
25 Hazelwood Dr., Ste. 116
Amherst, NY 14228-2220
Phone: (716)564-1100 **Fax:** (716)564-1101

North Carolina

★ 8617 ★ American Heart Association
North Carolina Affiliate
Charlotte Chapter
1229 Greenwood Cliff, Ste. 109
Charlotte, NC 28204
Phone: (704)374-0632 **Fax:** (704)374-0634
Website: http://www.americanheart.org/nc

★ 8618 ★ American Heart Association
North Carolina Affiliate
Eastern North Carolina Chapter
3131 RDU Center Dr., Ste. 100
Morrisville, NC 27560
Phone: (919)463-8300 **Fax:** (919)463-8392

★ 8619 ★ American Heart Association
North Carolina Affiliate
Greater Greensboro Chapter
202 CentrePort Dr., No. 100
Greensboro, NC 27409
Phone: (336)668-0167 **Fax:** (336)668-8241

★ 8620 ★ American Heart Association
North Carolina Affiliate
Greenville Chapter
3015 S Memorial Dr., Ste. A
Greenville, NC 27834
Phone: (252)355-1112 **Fax:** (252)355-1375
Website: http://www.americanheart.org/nc

North Dakota

★ 8621 ★ American Heart Association
Northland Affiliate
Greater Fargo Area Chapter
712 51st SW St.
Fargo, ND 58103
Phone: (701)277-5029 **Fax:** (701)277-5029

★ 8622 ★ American Heart Association
Northland Affiliate
Jamestown Chapter
1005 12 Ave. SE
Jamestown, ND 58401
Phone: (701)252-5122 **Free:** 800-437-9710
Fax: (701)251-2092
Remarks: Serves eastern North Dakota and South Dakota.

★ 8623 ★ American Heart Association
Northland Affiliate
West North Dakota Chapter
1305 12 St. SW
Minot, ND 58701
Phone: (701)838-4635 **Free:** 800-437-9710
Fax: (701)838-4635

Ohio

★ 8624 ★ American Heart Association
Ohio Affiliate
Akron Metro Chapter
1236 Weathervane, Ste. 300C
Akron, OH 44313
Phone: (330)867-9987 **Fax:** (330)867-3460
Website: http://www.americanheart.org/oh

★ 8625 ★ American Heart Association
Ohio Affiliate
Cincinnati Metro Chapter
2936 Vernon Pl.
Cincinnati, OH 45219
Phone: (513)281-4048 **Fax:** (513)281-1433
Website: http://www.americanheart.org/oh
Amy Howe, Director

★ 8626 ★ American Heart Association
Ohio Affiliate
Cleveland Metro Chapter
1689 E 115th St.
Cleveland, OH 44106
Phone: (216)791-7500 **Fax:** (216)791-5202
Website: http://www.americanheart.org/oh

★ 8627 ★ American Heart Association
Ohio Affiliate
Columbus Metro
5455 N High St.
Columbus, OH 43214
Phone: (614)848-6676 **Free:** 800-282-0291
Fax: (614)848-4227
Remarks: Covering Franklin and Delaware counties.

★ 8628 ★ American Heart Association
Ohio Affiliate
Miami Valley Division
24 N Jefferson St., 3rd Fl.
Dayton, OH 45402
Phone: (937)224-3571 **Fax:** (937)224-0926
Website: http://www.americanheart.org/oh

★ 8629 ★ American Heart Association
Ohio Affiliate
Northwestern Ohio Chapter
5164 Monroe St., Ste. 201
Toledo, OH 43623
Free: 800-AHA-USA1 **Fax:** (419)841-8745
Website: http://www.americanheart.org/oh

★ 8630 ★ American Heart Association
Ohio Affiliate
Stark County Division
4916 Hills & Dales Rd.
Canton, OH 44708
Phone: (330)478-8383 **Fax:** (330)478-8681
Website: http://www.americanheart.org/oh

★ 8631 ★ American Heart Association
Ohio Affiliate
Youngstown Metro Chapter
840 Southwestern Run
Youngstown, OH 44514
Phone: (330)965-9230 **Fax:** (330)965-9233
Website: http://www.americanheart.org/oh

Oklahoma

★ 8632 ★ American Heart Association
Heartland Affiliate
Oklahoma City Chapter
5700 N Portland, Ste. 203
Oklahoma City, OK 73112
Phone: (405)942-2444 **Fax:** (405)942-6616
Website: http://www.americanheart.org/ok

★ 8633 ★ American Heart Association
Heartland Affiliate
Tulsa Chapter
2227 Skelly Dr., Ste. 100-S
Tulsa, OK 74105
Phone: (918)747-8254 **Free:** 888-242-0280
Fax: (918)745-2043

Oregon

★ 8634 ★ American Heart Association
Northwest Affiliate
Central Oregon Chapter
440 Charnelton St., No. 3
Eugene, OR 97401
Phone: (541)344-6345 **Fax:** (541)344-9289
Website: http://www.americanheart.org/or
Karen Young, Director

★ 8635 ★ American Heart Association
Northwest Affiliate
Portland/Southwest Washington Chapter
1425 NE Irving, No. 100
Portland, OR 97232
Phone: (503)233-0100 **Free:** 800-452-9445
Fax: (503)233-4464
Website: http://www.americanheart.org/or

★ 8636 ★ American Heart Association
Northwest Affiliate
Salem Chapter
PO Box 6015
Salem, OR 97304
Phone: (503)364-5400 **Fax:** (503)364-6200
Remarks: Serves Marion, Polk, and Yamhill counties.

★ 8637 ★ American Heart Association
Northwest Affiliate
Southern Oregon Chapter
10 Crater Lake Ave., Ste. 10
Medford, OR 97504
Phone: (541)799-2709 **Fax:** (541)734-3809
Website: http://www.americanheart.org/or
Janice Watson, Director

Pennsylvania

★ 8638 ★ American Heart Association
Pennsylvania-Delaware Affiliate
Altoona Chapter
Bldg. D, Ste. 101
501 Howard Ave.
Altoona, PA 16601
Phone: (814)949-3160 **Fax:** (814)949-0540

★ 8639 ★ American Heart Association
Pennsylvania-Delaware Affiliate
Berks Chapter
40 Berkshire Ct.
Wyomissing, PA 19610
Phone: (610)376-8001 **Fax:** (610)376-3008

★ 8640 ★ American Heart Association
Pennsylvania-Delaware Affiliate
Bethlehem Chapter
212 E Broad St.
Bethlehem, PA 18018
Phone: (610)867-0583 **Fax:** (610)867-7218

★ 8641 ★ American Heart Association
Pennsylvania-Delaware Affiliate
Capital Region Chapter
1517 Cedar Cliff Dr.
Camp Hill, PA 17001
Phone: (717)730-4080 **Fax:** (717)730-6725
Email: pda@heart.org

★ 8642 ★ American Heart Association
Pennsylvania-Delaware Affiliate
Chambersburg Chapter
225 E King St.
Chambersburg, PA 17201
Phone: (717)263-2870

★ 8643 ★ American Heart Association
Pennsylvania-Delaware Affiliate
Clearfield Chapter
440 Front St.
Clearfield, PA 16830
Phone: (814)765-7579

★ 8644 ★ American Heart Association
Pennsylvania-Delaware Affiliate
Conshohocken Chapter
625 W Ridge Pike, Bldg. A, Ste. 100
Conshohocken, PA 19428
Phone: (610)940-9540 **Fax:** (610)940-9541
Remarks: Covers Bucks, Chester, Delaware, Montgomery, and Philadelphia counties.

★ 8645 ★ American Heart Association
Pennsylvania-Delaware Affiliate
Erie Chapter
823 Filmore Ave.
Erie, PA 16505
Phone: (814)836-0013 **Fax:** (814)836-9213

★ 8646 ★ American Heart Association
Pennsylvania-Delaware Affiliate
Greensburg Chapter
615 S Main St.
Greensburg, PA 15601
Phone: (724)837-5468 **Fax:** (724)837-2037

★ 8647 ★ American Heart Association
Pennsylvania-Delaware Affiliate
Hermitage Chapter
59 N Crescent Dr.
Hermitage, PA 16148
Phone: (724)983-1055 **Fax:** (724)346-3706

★ 8648 ★ American Heart Association
Pennsylvania-Delaware Affiliate
Johnstown Chapter
400 Luray Ave.
Johnstown, PA 15904
Phone: (814)266-8905 **Fax:** (814)269-3134

★ 8649 ★ American Heart Association
Pennsylvania-Delaware Affiliate
Kulpmont Chapter
1020 Ash St.
Kulpmont, PA 17834
Phone: (570)373-1093

★ 8650 ★ American Heart Association
Pennsylvania-Delaware Affiliate
Lancaster Chapter
610 Community Way
Lancaster, PA 17603
Phone: (717)393-0725 **Free:** 800-264-2785
Fax: (717)393-0731

★ 8651 ★ American Heart Association
Pennsylvania-Delaware Affiliate
Lebanon Chapter
335 S 8th St.
Lebanon, PA 17042
Phone: (717)273-0463 **Fax:** (717)273-8616

★ 8652 ★ American Heart Association
Pennsylvania-Delaware Affiliate
Luzerne Chapter
71 N Franklin St.
Wilkes Barre, PA 18701
Phone: (570)822-6247 **Fax:** (570)823-9538

★ 8653 ★ American Heart Association
Pennsylvania-Delaware Affiliate
Pittsburgh Chapter
10 Duff Rd., Ste. 304
Pittsburgh, PA 15235
Phone: (412)243-5393 **Fax:** (412)243-5497

★ 8654 ★ American Heart Association
Pennsylvania-Delaware Affiliate
Scranton Chapter
730 Pittston Ave.
Scranton, PA 18505
Phone: (570)342-8374 **Fax:** (570)969-4122

★ 8655 ★ American Heart Association
Pennsylvania-Delaware Affiliate
Uniontown Chapter
7829 National Pike, Ste. 2
Uniontown, PA 15401
Phone: (724)437-2798 **Fax:** (724)437-5536

★ 8656 ★ American Heart Association
Pennsylvania-Delaware Affiliate
Venango/Clarion County Chapter
174 E Bissell Ave.
Oil City, PA 16301
Phone: (814)676-2445 **Fax:** (814)677-5469

★ 8657 ★ American Heart Association
Pennsylvania-Delaware Affiliate
Warren Chapter
185 Hospital Dr.
Warren, PA 16365
Phone: (814)723-4860 **Fax:** (814)723-4860

★ 8658 ★ American Heart Association
Pennsylvania-Delaware Affiliate
Williamsport Chapter
1704 Warren Ave.
Williamsport, PA 17701
Phone: (570)322-4733 **Fax:** (570)322-0435

★ 8659 ★ American Heart Association
Pennsylvania-Delaware Affiliate
York Chapter
Cape Horn Plaza, Ste. B2
2997 Cape Horn Rd.
Red Lion, PA 17356
Phone: (717)246-9661 **Fax:** (717)246-9578

Puerto Rico

★ 8660 ★ American Heart Association
San Juan Chapter
554 Cabo Alverio St.
San Juan, PR 00918
Phone: (787)751-6595 **Fax:** (787)250-0281

Rhode Island

★ 8661 ★ American Heart Association
Rhode Island Affiliate
275 Westminster St., Ste. 100
Providence, RI 02903
Phone: (401)274-4544 **Fax:** (401)274-3332
Website: http://www.americanheart.org/ri

South Carolina

★ 8662 ★ American Heart Association
South Carolina Affiliate
Charleston Chapter
409 King St., Ste. 300
Charleston, SC 29403
Phone: (843)853-1597 **Fax:** (843)853-2498
Website: http://www.americanheart.org/sc

★ 8663 ★ American Heart Association
South Carolina Affiliate
Columbia Chapter
400 Percival Rd.
PO Box 6604
Columbia, SC 29260

Phone: (803)738-9540 **Fax:** (803)787-0804
Website: http://www.americanheart.org/sc

★ 8664 ★ American Heart Association
South Carolina Affiliate
Florence Chapter
181 E Evans St., Ste. 204 BTC-009
Florence, SC 29506
Phone: (843)665-0985 **Fax:** (843)665-1855

★ 8665 ★ American Heart Association
South Carolina Affiliate
Myrtle Beach Chapter
1506 Gumm Plaza
Hwy. 501
Myrtle Beach, SC 29577
Phone: (843)626-3939 **Fax:** (843)626-2856

★ 8666 ★ American Heart Association
South Carolina Affiliate
Upstate South Carolina/Western North Carolina Chapter
310B Bennett Center Dr.
Greer, SC 29650
Phone: (864)801-9550 **Fax:** (864)801-3589

South Dakota

★ 8667 ★ American Heart Association
Northland Affiliate
Greater Sioux Falls Area Chapter
218 S Main Ave., Ste. 200
Sioux Falls, SD 57104
Phone: (605)743-5194 **Fax:** (605)743-5194

★ 8668 ★ American Heart Association
Northland Affiliate
West South Dakota Chapter
22161 New Underwood Rd.
New Underwood, SD 57761
Free: 800-437-9710

Tennessee

★ 8669 ★ American Heart Association
Southeast Affiliate
Chattanooga Chapter
519 E 4th St.
Chattanooga, TN 37403
Phone: (423)265-3466 **Fax:** (423)267-5508

★ 8670 ★ American Heart Association
Southeast Affiliate
Johnson City Chapter
208 Sunset Dr., Ste. 521
Johnson City, TN 37604
Phone: (423)282-5388

★ 8671 ★ American Heart Association
Southeast Affiliate
Knoxville Chapter
4708 Papermill Dr.
Knoxville, TN 37909
Phone: (865)588-7646 **Fax:** (865)584-4109

★ 8672 ★ American Heart Association
Southeast Affiliate
Memphis Chapter
11 S Orleans
Memphis, TN 38103
Phone: (901)572-4200 **Fax:** (901)572-4201

★ 8673 ★ American Heart Association
Southeast Affiliate
Nashville Chapter
1818 Patterson St.
Nashville, TN 37203
Phone: (615)340-4100 **Fax:** (615)340-4101
Website: http://www.americanheart.org/tn

Texas

★ 8674 ★ American Heart Association
Arkansas Affiliate
Texarkana Chapter
McKnight Center
4150 McKnight Rd.
Texarkana, TX 75503
Phone: (903)832-2477 **Fax:** (903)838-6006

★ 8675 ★ American Heart Association
Texas Affiliate
Abilene Chapter
149 N Willis, No. 10
Abilene, TX 79603
Phone: (915)627-0070 **Fax:** (915)627-0071

★ 8676 ★ American Heart Association
Texas Affiliate
Amarillo Chapter
6605 I-40 West, Bldg. A-6
Amarillo, TX 79106
Phone: (806)457-0090 **Fax:** (806)457-0099

★ 8677 ★ American Heart Association
Texas Affiliate
Austin Chapter
1700 Rutherford Ln.
Austin, TX 78754
Phone: (512)433-4000 **Fax:** (512)433-4200
Website: http://www.americanheart.org/tx

★ 8678 ★ American Heart Association
Texas Affiliate
Beaumont Chapter
5675 Eastex Fwy., Ste. 3
Beaumont, TX 77706
Phone: (409)980-8800 **Fax:** (409)980-8808

★ 8679 ★ American Heart Association
Texas Affiliate
Bryan Chapter
3833 S Texas Ave., No. 216
Bryan, TX 77802
Phone: (979)268-0068 **Fax:** (979)268-0070

★ 8680 ★ American Heart Association
Texas Affiliate
Corpus Christi Chapter
500 N Shoreline Blvd., Ste. 203 N
Corpus Christi, TX 78471
Phone: (361)692-0606 **Fax:** (361)692-0607

★ 8681 ★ American Heart Association
Texas Affiliate
Dallas Area Chapter
1615 Stemmons Fwy.
Dallas, TX 75207
Phone: (214)748-7212 **Fax:** (214)748-1307

★ 8682 ★ American Heart Association
Texas Affiliate
El Paso Chapter
233 Mesa Hills Dr.
El Paso, TX 79912
Phone: (915)833-1231 **Fax:** (915)581-0423

★ 8683 ★ American Heart Association
Texas Affiliate
Fort Worth Chapter
2401 Scott Ave.
Fort Worth, TX 76103
Phone: (817)315-5000 **Fax:** (817)315-5220

★ 8684 ★ American Heart Association
Texas Affiliate
Harlingen Chapter
712 Morgan Blvd., Ste. 102
Harlingen, TX 78550
Phone: (956)425-3924 **Fax:** (956)412-0139

★ 8685 ★ American Heart Association
Texas Affiliate
Houston Chapter
2626 S Loop W, Ste. 510
Houston, TX 77054
Phone: (713)610-5000 **Fax:** (713)610-5200

★ 8686 ★ American Heart Association
Texas Affiliate
Longview Chapter
1125 Judson Rd., No. 150
Longview, TX 75601
Phone: (903)323-8800 **Fax:** (903)323-8808

★ 8687 ★ American Heart Association
Texas Affiliate
Lubbock Chapter
4630 50th St., Ste. 400
Lubbock, TX 79414
Phone: (806)762-6599 **Fax:** (806)762-6598

★ 8688 ★ American Heart Association
Texas Affiliate
Midland Chapter
3205 W Cuthbert, A-8
Midland, TX 79701
Phone: (915)520-7041 **Fax:** (915)520-5714

★ 8689 ★ American Heart Association
Texas Affiliate
San Angelo Chapter
3135 Executive Dr.
San Angelo, TX 76904
Phone: (915)223-2345 **Fax:** (915)223-2211

★ 8690 ★ American Heart Association
Texas Affiliate
Tyler Chapter
5604 Old Bullard Rd., Ste. 106
Tyler, TX 75703
Phone: (903)324-1444 **Fax:** (903)324-1443

★ 8691 ★ American Heart Association
Texas Affiliate
Waco Chapter
6801 Sanger, Ste. 102
Waco, TX 76710
Phone: (254)299-0880 **Fax:** (254)299-0881

★ 8692 ★ American Heart Association
Texas Affiliate
Wichita Falls Chapter
811 6th St., Ste. 160
Wichita Falls, TX 76301
Phone: (940)397-0700 **Fax:** (940)397-0707

Utah

★ 8693 ★ American Heart Association
Western States Affiliate
Utah Chapter
1937 South 300 West, Ste. 120
Salt Lake City, UT 84115
Phone: (801)484-3838 **Fax:** (801)484-4448
Website: http://www.heartsource.org

Vermont

★ 8694 ★ American Heart Association
Vermont Affiliate
PO Box 485
434 Hurricane Ln.
Williston, VT 05495
Phone: (802)878-7700 **Free:** 800-639-6024
Fax: (802)878-7850

Virginia

★ 8695 ★ American Heart Association
Virginia Affiliate
Central Virginia Chapter
3025 Berkmar Dr.
Charlottesville, VA 22901
Phone: (434)973-5072 **Fax:** (434)973-1784

★ 8696 ★ American Heart Association
Virginia Affiliate
Greater Washington DC Regional Chapter
7203 Poplar St.
Annandale, VA 22003
Phone: (703)941-8500 **Fax:** (703)914-3795

★ 8697 ★ American Heart Association
Virginia Affiliate
Richmond Chapter
4217 Park Pl. Ct.
Glen Allen, VA 23060
Phone: (804)747-8334 **Fax:** (804)965-6421
Website: http://www.americanheart.org/va

★ 8698 ★ American Heart Association
Virginia Affiliate
Tidewater Chapter
360 Southport Cir., Ste. 104
Virginia Beach, VA 23452
Phone: (757)671-8636 **Fax:** (757)456-0486

★ 8699 ★ American Heart Association
Virginia Affiliate
Western Virginia Chapter
4504 Starkey Rd. SW, No. 115
Roanoke, VA 24014
Phone: (540)989-2810 **Fax:** (540)772-4243

Washington

★ 8700 ★ American Heart Association
Northwest Affiliate
Greater Pierce County Region
1101 S Fawcett, Ste. 100
Tacoma, WA 98402
Phone: (253)272-7854 **Fax:** (253)627-1035
Website: http://www.americanheart.org/wa

★ 8701 ★ American Heart Association
Northwest Affiliate
Greater Thurston County Chapter
505 4th Ave. W, Ste. D
Olympia, WA 98501
Phone: (360)236-8136 **Fax:** (360)236-8137

★ 8702 ★ American Heart Association
Northwest Affiliate
Inland Northwest Chapter
140 S Arthur Ave., Ste. 610
Spokane, WA 99202
Phone: (509)536-1500 **Free:** 800-536-1314
Fax: (509)536-1515
Website: http://www.americanheart.org/wa
Remarks: Also serves Idaho.

★ 8703 ★ American Heart Association
Northwest Affiliate
King County Chapter
155 NE 100th St., Ste. 306
Seattle, WA 98125
Phone: (206)525-7665 **Free:** 888-440-2328
Fax: (206)525-7645
Website: http://www.americanheart.org/wa

★ 8704 ★ American Heart Association
Northwest Affiliate
Tri-Cities Chapter
805 S Auburn
Kennewick, WA 99336
Phone: (509)582-9001 **Fax:** (509)582-6676
Remarks: Also serves north-central Oregon.

West Virginia

★ 8705 ★ American Heart Association
West Virginia Affiliate
Charleston Chapter
4510-C Pennsylvania Ave.
PO Box 12110
Charleston, WV 25302
Phone: (304)965-7998 **Fax:** (304)965-7992
Remarks: Also serves Ohio.

★ 8706 ★ American Heart Association
West Virginia Affiliate
Wheeling Chapter
McLain Bldg., Rm. 206
40 12th St.
Wheeling, WV 26003
Phone: (304)233-1525 **Fax:** (304)233-2075

Wisconsin

★ 8707 ★ American Heart Association
Northland Affiliate
Greater Milwaukee Chapter
795 N Van Buren St.
Milwaukee, WI 53202
Phone: (414)271-9999 **Free:** 800-242-8721
Fax: (414)271-3299
Email: ahawi@execpc.com
Website: http://www.americanheart.org/wi
Telecom. Serv: TDD: (414)271-0450.

★ 8708 ★ American Heart Association
Northland Affiliate
Northcentral Wisconsin Division
903 Grand Ave. C6
Rothschild, WI 54474
Phone: (715)359-4278 **Fax:** (715)359-7285

★ 8709 ★ American Heart Association
Northland Affiliate
Northeast Wisconsin Division
2149 Velp Ave.
Green Bay, WI 54303
Phone: (920)662-2268 **Fax:** (920)662-2273

★ 8710 ★ American Heart Association
Northland Affiliate
Northwest Wisconsin Division
800 Wisconsin St., Ste. 312
Eau Claire, WI 54703
Phone: (715)834-1108 **Fax:** (715)834-1401

★ 8711 ★ American Heart Association
Northland Affiliate
Southcentral Wisconsin Division
2850 Dairy Dr., Ste. 300
Madison, WI 53718
Phone: (608)221-8866 **Fax:** (608)221-9233

★ 8712 ★ American Heart Association
Northland Affiliate
Southwest Wisconsin Division
400 La Crosse St.
La Crosse, WI 54601
Phone: (608)784-4020 **Fax:** (608)782-8553

Hemophilia

The following are state affiliates of the National Hemophilia Foundation, 116 W 32nd St., 11th Fl., New York, NY 10001, (800)42-HANDI, http://www.hemophilia.org/.

Arizona

★ 8713 ★ Hemophilia Association, Inc.
4001 N 24th St.
Phoenix, AZ 85016
Phone: (602)955-3947 **Fax:** (602)955-1962
Email: mike@hemophiliaz.org
Website: http://www.hemophiliaz.org
Michael Rosenthal, Exec Director

Arkansas

★ 8714 ★ Hemophilia Foundation of Arkansas, Inc.
PO Box 1135
Greenbrier, AR 72058
Phone: (501)679-7300 **Free:** 800-484-9064
Laveane Lovelady, President
John Little, Vice President

California

★ 8715 ★ Central California Hemophilia Foundation
PO Box 163689
Sacramento, CA 95816
Phone: (916)448-0370 **Fax:** (916)489-1569
Email: hubbert@pacbell.net
Website: http://www.cchfsac.org
Sean Hubbert, President

★ 8716 ★ Hemophilia Association of San Diego
3570 Camino Del Rio N, Ste. 108
San Diego, CA 92108
Phone: (619)325-3570 **Fax:** (619)325-4350
Email: hemoofsd@aol.com
Website: http://www.hemophiliasd.org
Jessica Swann, Exec Director
Antonio Pascucci, President

★ 8717 ★ Hemophilia Foundation of Northern California
7700 Edgewater Dr., Ste. 710
Oakland, CA 94621
Phone: (510)568-6243 **Fax:** (510)568-6111
Email: consultvb@aol.com

Website: http://www.hfnconline.org
Val Bias, President

★ 8718 ★ Hemophilia Foundation of Southern California
33 S Catalina Ave., Ste. 102
Pasadena, CA 91106
Phone: (626)793-6192 **Free:** 800-371-4123
Fax: (626)796-5605
Email: hfsc@earthlink.net
Website: http://www.hemosocal.org
Rosemary Hutton, President

Colorado

★ 8719 ★ Hemophilia Society of Colorado
10020 E Girard Ave., Ste. 100
Denver, CO 80231
Phone: (303)750-6990 **Free:** 888-687-CLOT
Fax: (303)750-7035
Email: irarhojani@worldnett.att.net
Website: http://www.cohemo.org
Sherri Rhojani, President
Donna Reiner, President

Florida

★ 8720 ★ Hemophilia Foundation of Greater Florida
1350 N Orange Ave., Ste. 227
Winter Park, FL 32789
Phone: (407)629-0000 **Free:** 800-293-6527
Fax: (407)629-9600
Email: Hemofoundation@earthlink.net
Website: http://www.hemophiliaflorida.org
Fran Haynes, Exec Director
Barbara Burgeson, President

★ 8721 ★ National Hemophilia Foundation
Florida Chapter
17810 Littlewood Dr.
Spring Hill, FL 34610-7357
Phone: (727)856-7057 **Fax:** (727)856-2257
Email: dphilipsen@aol.com
Website: http://www.geocities.com/hotsprings/1809
Natalie Philipsen, Exec Director
Aleida Wiggins, President

Georgia

★ 8722 ★ Hemophilia of Georgia, Inc.
8800 Roswell Rd., Ste. 170
Atlanta, GA 30350
Phone: (770)518-8272 **Fax:** (770)518-3310
Email: mail@hog.org
Website: http://www.hog.org
Patricia Dominic, Exec Director
Hiram Allen, President

Hawaii

★ 8723 ★ Hemophilia Foundation of Hawaii
Kapiolani Medical Center
1164 Bishop St., Ste. 1501
Honolulu, HI 96813
Phone: (808)521-5483 **Fax:** (808)528-7430
Email: hemofdhi@pixi.com
Stanley Yates, President

Illinois

★ 8724 ★ Hemophilia Foundation of Illinois
332 S Michigan Ave., Ste. 1135
Chicago, IL 60604
Phone: (312)427-1495 **Fax:** (312)427-1602
Email: info@hemophiliaillinois.org
Website: http://www.hemophiliaillinois.org
Thomas Gauthier, Exec Director
Robert Robinson, President

Indiana

★ 8725 ★ Hemophilia of Indiana, Inc.
2216 E 44th St.
Indianapolis, IN 46205
Phone: (317)543-1299 **Fax:** (317)543-1291
Stephen Bassett, Exec Director
Othor Aldridge, President

Kentucky

★ 8726 ★ Kentucky Hemophilia Foundation, Inc.
Kosair Charities Center
982 Eastern Parkway
Louisville, KY 40217-1566
Phone: (502)634-8161 **Fax:** (502)634-9995
Email: kyhemo@bellsouth.net
Website: http://www.kyhemo.org
Ursela M. Lacer, Exec Director

Louisiana

★ 8727 ★ Louisiana Hemophilia Foundation
3636 S Sherwood Forest Blvd., Ste. 450
Baton Rouge, LA 70816-2285
Phone: (225)291-1675 **Fax:** (225)291-1679
Email: lahemophilia@etigers.net
Website: http://www.louisianahemophilia.org
Lori Keels, Exec Director
Howard Young, President

Massachusetts

★ 8728 ★ New England Hemophilia Association
180 Rustcraft Rd., Ste. 101
Dedham, MA 02026-4596
Phone: (781)326-7645 **Fax:** (781)329-5122
Email: neha@world.std.com
Catherine Cornell, Exec Director
Steve Jelinek, President

Michigan

★ 8729 ★ Hemophilia Foundation of Michigan
905 W Eisenhower Circle, Ste. 107
Ann Arbor, MI 48103
Phone: (734)332-4226 **Fax:** (734)332-4204
Email: harner@hfmich.org
Website: http://www.hfmich.org
Ivan C. Harner, Exec Director
Andrew Voegtle, President

Minnesota

★ 8730 ★ Hemophilia Foundation of Minnesota & the Dakotas
750 S Plaza Dr., Ste. 207
Mendota Heights, MN 55120
Phone: (651)406-8655 **Free:** 800-994-4363
Fax: (651)406-8656
Email: hfmd1@aol.com
Richard Baker, Exec Director
Shirley Wilson, Exec Director

Nebraska

★ 8731 ★ National Hemophilia Foundation
Nebraska Chapter
3610 Dodge St., No. 110-W
Omaha, NE 68131
Phone: (402)342-3329 **Fax:** (402)342-4329
Email: Mrye@hemophiliaone.com
Website: http://www.nebraskanhf.org
Matt Rye, President

Nevada

★ 8732 ★ Hemophilia Foundation of Nevada
PO Box 90158
Henderson, NV 89009
Phone: (702)564-4368 **Fax:** (702)564-2299
Email: hfnv@earthlink.net
Website: http://www.hemophilianevada.org
Brad Rassuchine, President
Renee Paper, Exec Director

New Mexico

★ 8733 ★ Sange de Oro, Inc.
Hemophilia Foundation of New Mexico
PO Box 7188
Albuquerque, NM 87194-7188
Phone: (505)341-9321
Email: Bjor@aol.com
Elisabeth Ortega Rangel, Exec Director

New York

★ 8734 ★ Bleeding Disorders Association of Northeastern New York
PO Box 3703
Albany, NY 12203
Phone: (518)782-9787 **Fax:** (518)782-9787
Email: hemovw@hotmail.com
Website: http://www.geocities.com/hotsprings/oasis/9190
Tom Brownell, President

★ 8735 ★ Hemophilia Center of Western New York, Inc.
462 Grider St.
Buffalo, NY 14215
Phone: (716)896-2470 **Fax:** (716)898-5537
Email: hemoctr@pce.net
Website: http://www.wnyhemophilia.com
Rosemary Holmberg, Exec Director
Thomas Long, President

★ 8736 ★ Mary M. Gooley Hemophilia Center, Inc.
1415 Portland Ave., Ste. 425
Rochester, NY 14621
Phone: (716)922-5700 **Fax:** (716)922-5775
Email: robert.fox@viahealth.org
Website: http://www.hemocenter.org
Robert Fox, Exec Director

North Carolina

★ 8737 ★ Hemophilia of North Carolina
2 Centerview Dr., Ste. 51
Greensboro, NC 27407
Free: 800-990-5557 **Fax:** (704)587-0815
Email: srfarr@worldnet.att.net
Jody Throckmorton, President

Ohio

★ 8738 ★ National Hemophilia Foundation
Central Ohio Chapter
670 Suntree Dr.
Worthington Highlands
Westerville, OH 43081-5013
Phone: (614)847-5634
Mike Capsel, President

★ 8739 ★ National Hemophilia Foundation
Greater Cincinnati/Northern Kentucky Chapter
1008 Marshall Ave., Ste. 3
Cincinnati, OH 45225
Phone: (513)961-4366 **Fax:** (513)871-6803
Email: ly113@aol.com
Linda Young, Exec Director

★ 8740 ★ Northern Ohio Hemophilia Foundation, Inc.
Independence Tower
5755 Granger Rd., Ste. 790
Cleveland, OH 44131
Phone: (216)739-1755 **Free:** 800-554-HEMO
Fax: (216)739-1758
Email: hemo@earthlink.net
Website: http://www.bleedingdisordersnorohio.org
Randi Paltrow, Exec Director

★ 8741 ★ Northwest Ohio Hemophilia Foundation
1 Stranahan Sq., Ste. 540
Toledo, OH 43604
Phone: (419)242-9587 **Fax:** (419)242-6316
Email: stephanieb@uhs-toledo.org
Website: http://www.uhs-toledo.org
Stephanie Branco, Director

★ 8742 ★ Southwestern Ohio Hemophilia Foundation
82 Elva Ct., Ste. B
Vandalia, OH 45377
Phone: (937)415-0644 **Fax:** (937)415-0604
Email: jlswohf@aol.com
Rita Falkenback, President

Oklahoma

★ 8743 ★ Oklahoma Hemophilia Foundation
1501 N Classen Blvd., Ste. B
Oklahoma City, OK 73106
Phone: (405)524-7069 **Free:** 800-735-3855
Fax: (405)524-7916
Email: mmorseohf@aol.com
Mike Morse, Exec Director

Pennsylvania

★ 8744 ★ National Hemophilia Foundation
Delaware Valley Chapter
222 S Easton Rd., Ste. 107
Glenside, PA 19038
Phone: (215)885-6500 **Fax:** (215)885-6074
Email: hemophilia@navpoint.com
Website: http://www.hemophiliasupport.org
Clifford Cohn, President

★ 8745 ★ National Hemophilia Foundation
Western Pennsylvania Chapter
532 S Aiken Ave., Ste. 102
Pittsburgh, PA 15232
Phone: (412)683-2231 **Fax:** (412)683-2568
Email: wpcnhf@pgh.net
Patricia Enright, Exec Director

Rhode Island

★ 8746 ★ Rhode Island Hemophilia Foundation
160 Plainfield St.
Providence, RI 02909
Phone: (401)944-6950 **Fax:** (401)944-4161
Emili Vaziri, President

South Carolina

★ 8747 ★ Hemophilia of South Carolina
PO Box 2386
Irmo, SC 29063
Free: 888-829-4849 **Fax:** 888-829-4849
Email: Factoreight@aol.com
Brandy Stewart, President

Tennessee

★ 8748 ★ Tennessee Hemophilia & Bleeding Disorders Foundation
7003 Chadwick Dr., Ste. 269
Brentwood, TN 37027
Phone: (615)373-0351 **Fax:** (615)373-4394
Email: thbdf@worldnet.att.net
Website: http://www.home.att.net/~thbdf
Sandy Jones, Contact

Texas

★ 8749 ★ National Hemophilia Foundation
Lone Star Chapter
16910 Shady Square Ct.
Houston, TX 77095
Phone: (281)861-6644 **Fax:** (281)861-6644
Debbie de la Riva, Exec Director

Utah

★ 8750 ★ Utah Hemophilia Foundation
880 E 3375 S
Salt Lake City, UT 84106
Phone: (801)484-0325 **Fax:** (801)484-4177
Email: soleil@hemophiliautah.org
Website: http://www.hemophiliautah.org
Susan Soleil, Exec Director

Virginia

★ 8751 ★ Hemophilia Association of the Capital Area
3251 Old Lee Hwy., Ste. 3
Fairfax, VA 22030-1504
Phone: (703)352-7641 **Fax:** (703)352-2145
Email: info@hacacares.org
Website: http://www.hacacares.org
Sandi Qualley, Exec Director

★ 8752 ★ National Hemophilia Foundation
United Virginia Chapter
9801 Husting Terrace
Chesterfield, VA 23832
Phone: (804)748-7896 **Fax:** (804)796-9043
Email: pader55@cs.com
Patricia DeRatto, Exec Director

Wisconsin

★ 8753 ★ Great Lakes Hemophilia Foundation
PO Box 704
Milwaukee, WI 53210-0704
Phone: (414)257-0200 **Free:** 888-797-4543
Fax: (414)257-1225
Email: Kmarquardt@glhf.org
Website: http://www.glhf.org
Kathleen M. Marquardt, Exec Director

Hospitals

Listed below are state hospital associations that are allied with the American Hospital Association, 1 N Franklin, Chicago, IL 60606, (312)422-3000, http://www.aha.org/.

Alabama

★ 8754 ★ Alabama Hospital Association
500 N East Blvd.
Montgomery, AL 36117
Phone: (334)272-8781 **Fax:** (334)270-9527
J. Michael Horsley, CEO & Pres

Alaska

★ 8755 ★ Alaska State Hospital and Nursing Home Association
426 Main St.
Juneau, AK 99801
Phone: (907)586-1790 **Fax:** (907)463-3573
Laraine Derr, CEO & Pres

Alberta

★ 8756 ★ Provincial Health Authorities of Alberta
44 Capital Blvd.
200/10044-108 St. NW
Edmonton, AB, Canada T5J 3S7
Phone: (780)426-8503 **Fax:** (780)424-4309
E. Michael Higgins, Exec Director

Arizona

★ 8757 ★ Arizona Hospital and Healthcare Association
2901 N Central Ave.
Phoenix, AZ 85012-2729
Phone: (602)445-4300 **Fax:** (602)445-4299
John R. Rivers, CEO & Pres

Arkansas

★ 8758 ★ Arkansas Hospital Association
419 Natural Resources Dr.
Little Rock, AR 72205-1539
Phone: (501)224-7878 **Fax:** (501)224-0519
James R. Teeter, CEO & Pres

California

★ 8759 ★ California Healthcare Association
1215 K St., Ste. 800
Sacramento, CA 95814
Phone: (916)552-7547 **Fax:** (916)552-7618
C. Duane Dauner, President
Alt. Contact: PO Box 1100, Sacramento, CA 95814.
Frmly: California Association of Hospitals and Health Systems.

★ 8760 ★ Healthcare Association of San Diego and Imperial Counties
707 Broadway, Ste. 905
San Diego, CA 92101-5391
Phone: (619)544-0777 **Fax:** (619)544-0888
Stephen A. Escoboza, CEO & Pres

★ 8761 ★ Healthcare Association of Southern California
515 S Figueroa St., Ste. 1300
Los Angeles, CA 90071-3322
Phone: (213)538-0700 **Fax:** (213)629-4272
James D. Barber, CEO & Pres

★ 8762 ★ Hospital Council of Northern and Central California
1215 K St., Ste. 730
Sacramento, CA 95814
Phone: (916)552-7608 **Fax:** (916)552-2618
Gregg Schnepple, CEO & Pres

Colorado

★ 8763 ★ Colorado Health and Hospital Association
7335 E Orchard Rd., Ste. 100
Greenwood Village, CO 80111
Phone: (720)489-1630 **Fax:** (720)489-9400
Larry Wall, President

Connecticut

★ 8764 ★ Connecticut Hospital Association
110 Barnes Rd.
PO Box 90
Wallingford, CT 06492-0090
Phone: (203)294-7200 **Fax:** (203)269-7713
Jennifer Jackson, President

Delaware

★ 8765 ★ Delaware Healthcare Association
1280 S Governors Ave.
Dover, DE 19904-4802
Phone: (302)674-2853 **Fax:** (302)734-2731
Joseph M. Letnaunchyn, President

District of Columbia

★ 8766 ★ District of Columbia Hospital Association
1250 Eye St. NW, Ste. 700
Washington, DC 20005-3930
Phone: (202)682-1581 **Fax:** (202)371-8151
Robert A. Malson, President

Florida

★ 8767 ★ Florida Hospital Association
307 Park Lake Cir.
PO Box 531107
Orlando, FL 32803-1107
Phone: (407)841-6230 **Fax:** (407)422-5948
Wayne NeSmith, President

★ 8768 ★ South Florida Hospital and Healthcare Association, Inc.
6363 Taft St., Ste. 200
Hollywood, FL 33024
Phone: (954)964-1660 **Fax:** (954)962-1260
Linda S. Quick, President

Georgia

★ 8769 ★ Georgia Hospital Association
1675 Terrell Mill Rd.
Marietta, GA 30067
Phone: (770)249-4500 **Fax:** (770)955-5801
Joseph A. Parker, President

Hawaii

★ 8770 ★ Healthcare Association of Hawaii
932 Ward Ave., Ste. 430
Honolulu, HI 96814-2126
Phone: (808)521-8961 **Fax:** (808)599-2879
Richard E. Meiers, CEO & Pres

Idaho

★ 8771 ★ Idaho Hospital Association
615 N 7th St.
Boise, ID 83701-1278
Phone: (208)338-5100 **Fax:** (208)338-7800
Steven A. Millard, President

Illinois

★ 8772 ★ Illinois Hospital Association
1151 E Warrenville Rd.
PO Box 3015
Naperville, IL 60566-7015
Phone: (630)505-7777 **Fax:** (630)505-4237
Kenneth C. Robbins, President

★ 8773 ★ Metropolitan Chicago Healthcare Council
222 S Riverside Plaza, 19th Fl.
Chicago, IL 60606
Phone: (312)906-6000 **Fax:** (312)993-0779
Earl C. Bird, CEO & Pres

Indiana

★ 8774 ★ Indiana Hospital and Health Association
1 American Sq.
PO Box 82063
Indianapolis, IN 46282
Phone: (317)633-4870 **Fax:** (317)633-4875
Kenneth G. Stella, President
Frmly: Indiana Hospital Association.

Iowa

★ 8775 ★ Iowa Hospital Association
100 E Grand Ave., Ste. 100
Des Moines, IA 50309
Phone: (515)288-1955 **Fax:** (515)283-9366
Kirk Norris, President
Frmly: Iowa Hospitals Association.

Kansas

★ 8776 ★ Kansas Hospital Association
215 SE 8th St.
Topeka, KS 66603
Phone: (785)233-7436 **Fax:** (785)233-6955
Donald A. Wilson, President
Alt. Contact: PO Box 2308, Topeka, KS 66601-2308.

Kentucky

★ 8777 ★ Kentucky Hospital Association An Association of Kentucky Hospitals and Health Systems
2501 Nelson Miller Pkwy.
PO Box 436629
Louisville, KY 40253-6629
Phone: (502)426-6220 **Fax:** (502)426-6226
Michael T. Rust, President

Louisiana

★ 8778 ★ Louisiana Hospital Association
9521 Brookline Ave.
Baton Rouge, LA 70809-1431
Phone: (225)928-0026 **Fax:** (225)923-1004
Lynn B. Nicholas, CEO & Pres
Alt. Contact: PO Box 80720, Baton Rouge, LA 70898-0720.

★ 8779 ★ Metropolitan Hospital Council of New Orleans
2450 Severn Ave., Ste. 210
Metairie, LA 70001
Phone: (504)837-1171 **Fax:** (504)837-1174
John J. Finn, PhD, President

Maine

★ 8780 ★ Maine Hospital Association
150 Capitol St.
Augusta, ME 04330
Phone: (207)622-4794 **Fax:** (207)622-3073
Steven R. Michaud, President

Maryland

★ 8781 ★ Healthcare Council of the National Capital Area
8201 Corporate Dr., Ste. 410
Landover, MD 20785-2229
Phone: (301)731-4700 **Fax:** (301)731-8286
Joseph P. Burns, CEO & Pres

★ 8782 ★ Maryland Hospital Association The Association of Maryland Hospitals & Health Systems
6820 Deerpath Rd.
Elkridge, MD 21075-6234
Phone: (410)379-6200 **Fax:** (410)379-8239
Calvin M. Pierson, President

Massachusetts

★ 8783 ★ Massachusetts Hospital Association
5 New England Executive Park
Burlington, MA 01803
Phone: (781)272-8000 **Fax:** (781)272-0466
Ronald M. Hollander, President

Michigan

★ 8784 ★ Healthcare Council of MidMichigan
3927 Beecher Rd.
Flint, MI 48532-3803
Phone: (810)766-8898 **Fax:** (810)762-4108
Bruce Trevithick, President

★ 8785 ★ Hospital Council of East Central Michigan
141 Harrow Ln., Ste. 11
Saginaw, MI 48603
Phone: (989)792-1725 **Fax:** (989)792-3099
Elizabeth S. Schnettler, President

★ 8786 ★ Michigan Health and Hospital Association
6215 W St. Joseph Hwy.
Lansing, MI 48917
Phone: (517)323-3443 **Fax:** (517)323-0946
Spencer C. Johnson, President

★ 8787 ★ North Central Council of the Michigan Hospital Association
616 Petoskey St., Ste. 208
Petoskey, MI 49770
Phone: (231)439-9812 **Fax:** (231)439-9813
Elizabeth Gertz, Exec Director

★ 8788 ★ Southeast Michigan Health and Hospital Council
24725 W 12 Mile Rd., Ste. 104A
Southfield, MI 48034
Phone: (248)358-2950 **Fax:** (248)358-1098
Donald P. Potter, President

★ 8789 ★ Southwestern Michigan Hospital Council
6215 W St. Joseph Hwy.
Lansing, MI 48917
Phone: (517)323-3443 **Fax:** (517)323-0946
Clark R. Ballard, President

Minnesota

★ 8790 ★ Minnesota Hospital and Healthcare Partnership
2550 University Ave. W, Ste. 350S
Saint Paul, MN 55114-1900
Phone: (651)641-1121 **Fax:** (651)659-1477
Bruce J. Rueben, President
Frmly: Minnesota Hospital Association.

Mississippi

★ 8791 ★ Mississippi Hospital Association
6425 Lakeover Rd.
PO Box 16444
Jackson, MS 39236-6444
Free: 800-289-8884 **Fax:** (601)368-3200
Sam W. Cameron, CEO & Pres

Missouri

★ 8792 ★ The Health Alliance of MidAmerica
10401 Holmes Rd., Ste. 280
Kansas City, MO 64131-3368
Phone: (816)941-3800 **Fax:** (816)941-0818
Michael R. Dunaway, Senior VP

★ 8793 ★ Missouri Hospital Association
PO Box 60
Jefferson City, MO 65102-0060
Phone: (573)893-3700 **Fax:** (573)893-2809
Marc D. Smith, President

Montana

★ 8794 ★ Montana Hospital Association
An Association of Montana Healthcare Providers
1720 9th Ave.
PO Box 5119
Helena, MT 59604
Phone: (406)442-1911 **Fax:** (406)443-3894
James F. Ahrens, President

Nebraska

★ 8795 ★ Nebraska Hospital Association
1640 L St., Ste. D
Lincoln, NE 68508
Phone: (402)458-4900 **Fax:** (402)475-4091
Laura J. Redoutey, President
Frmly: Nebraska Association of Hospitals and Health Systems.

Nevada

★ 8796 ★ Nevada Hospital Association
5250 Neil Rd., Ste. 302
Reno, NV 89502
Phone: (775)827-0184 **Fax:** (775)827-0190
Bill M. Welch, CEO & Pres
Frmly: Nevada Hospital Association.

New Brunswick

★ 8797 ★ New Brunswick Healthcare Association
861 Woodstock Rd.
Fredericton, NB, Canada E3B 7R7
Phone: (506)451-0750 **Fax:** (506)451-0760
Robert Simpson, Exec Director

New Hampshire

★ 8798 ★ New Hampshire Hospital Association
Foundation for Healthy Communities
125 Airport Rd.
Concord, NH 03301-7300
Phone: (603)225-0900 **Fax:** (603)225-4346
Michael J. Hill, President

New Jersey

★ 8799 ★ New Jersey Hospital Association
PO Box 1
760 Alexander Rd.
Princeton, NJ 08543-0001
Phone: (609)275-4000 **Fax:** (609)452-8097
Gary S. Carter, CEO & Pres

New Mexico

★ 8800 ★ New Mexico Hospitals and Health Systems Association
2121 Osuna Rd. NE
Albuquerque, NM 87113
Phone: (505)343-0010 **Fax:** (505)343-0012
Maureen L. Boshier, CEO & Pres

New York

★ 8801 ★ Greater New York Hospital Association, Subsidiaries, and Affiliates
555 W 57th St., 15th Flr.
New York, NY 10019
Phone: (212)246-7100 **Fax:** (212)262-6350
Kenneth E. Raske, President

★ 8802 ★ Healthcare Association of New York State
1 Empire Dr.
Rensselaer, NY 12144
Phone: (518)431-7600 **Fax:** (518)431-7915
Daniel Sisto, President

★ 8803 ★ Iroquois Healthcare Alliance
17 Halfmoon Executive Park Dr.
Clifton Park, NY 12065
Phone: (518)383-5060 **Fax:** (518)383-2616
Gary J. Fitzgerald, President
Alt. Contact: 5740 Commons Pk., E Syracuse, NY 13057; ph: 315445-1851, fax: 315445-2293.

★ 8804 ★ Nassau—Suffolk Hospital Council, Inc.
3001 Expressway Dr. N, Ste. 300
Islandia, NY 11749-5308
Phone: (631)435-3000 **Fax:** (631)435-2343
Kristina A. Krail, CEO

★ 8805 ★ Northern Metropolitan Hospital Association
400 Stony Brook Ct.
Newburgh, NY 12550
Phone: (845)562-7520 **Fax:** (845)562-0187
Arthur E. Weintraub, President

★ 8806 ★ Rochester Regional Healthcare Association
3445 Winton Pl.
Rochester, NY 14623
Phone: (716)273-8180 **Fax:** (716)273-8189
Robert M. Swinnerton, CEO & Pres

★ 8807 ★ Western New York Healthcare Association
1876 Niagara Falls Blvd.
Tonawanda, NY 14150-6439
Phone: (716)695-0843 **Fax:** (716)695-0073
William D. Pike, President

North Carolina

★ 8808 ★ North Carolina Hospital Association
An Association of Hospitals and Health Networks
PO Box 4449
Cary, NC 27519-4449
Phone: (919)677-2400 **Fax:** (919)677-4200
William A. Pully, President

North Dakota

★ 8809 ★ North Dakota Healthcare Association
3205 E Thayer Ave., NE Door
Bismarck, ND 58507-7340
Phone: (701)224-9732 **Fax:** (701)224-9529
Arnold R. Thomas, President
Frmly: North Dakota Hospital Association.

Nova Scotia

★ 8810 ★ Nova Scotia Association of Health Organizations
Bedford Professional Centre
2 Dartmouth Rd.
Bedford, NS, Canada B4A 2K7
Phone: (902)832-8500 **Fax:** (902)832-8505
Robert A. Cook, CEO & Pres

Ohio

★ 8811 ★ Akron Regional Hospital Association
190 Montrose W Ave., Ste. 201
Akron, OH 44321-2786
Phone: (330)668-6180 **Fax:** (330)668-2013
Marianne G. Lorini, President

★ 8812 ★ Center for Health Affairs
1226 Huron Rd. E
Cleveland, OH 44115

Phone: (216)696-6900 Fax: (216)696-1875
William T. Ryan, CEO & Pres

★ 8813 ★ Greater Cincinnati Health Council
2100 Sherman Ave., Ste. 100
Cincinnati, OH 45212-2775
Phone: (513)531-0200 Fax: (513)531-0278
Lynn R. Olman, President

★ 8814 ★ Greater Dayton Area Hospital Association
32 N Main St., Ste. 1441
Dayton, OH 45402
Phone: (937)228-1000 Fax: (937)228-1035
Joseph M. Krella, President

★ 8815 ★ Hospital Council of Northwest Ohio
3231 Central Park W Dr., Ste. 200
Toledo, OH 43617
Phone: (419)842-0800 Fax: (419)843-8889
W. Scott Fry, CEO & Pres

★ 8816 ★ Ohio Hospital Association The Association for Hospitals and Health Systems
155 E Broad St., 15th Fl.
Columbus, OH 43215
Phone: (614)221-7614 Fax: (614)221-4771
James R. Castle, CEO & Pres

Oklahoma

★ 8817 ★ Greater Oklahoma City Hospital Council
4000 Lincoln Blvd.
Oklahoma City, OK 73105
Phone: (405)359-5530 Fax: (405)359-5500
Jerry Maier, Chairman of the Board

★ 8818 ★ Oklahoma Hospital Association
4000 Lincoln Blvd.
Oklahoma City, OK 73105
Phone: (405)427-9537 Fax: (405)424-4507
Craig W. Jones, President

Ontario

★ 8819 ★ Catholic Health Association of Canada
1247 Kilborn Pl.
Ottawa, ON, Canada K1H 6K9
Phone: (613)731-7148 Fax: (613)731-7797
Richard Haughian, D.Th., President

★ 8820 ★ Ontario Hospital Association
200 Front St. W, Ste. 2800
Toronto, ON, Canada M5V 3L1
Phone: (416)205-1307 Fax: (416)205-1310
David MacKinnon, President

Oregon

★ 8821 ★ Oregon Association of Hospitals and Health Systems
Bldg. 2, Ste. 100
4000 Kruse Way Pl.
Lake Oswego, OR 97035-2543
Phone: (503)636-2204 Fax: (503)636-8310
Kenneth M. Rutledge, President

Pennsylvania

★ 8822 ★ Delaware Valley Healthcare Council of HAP
121 S Broad St., 20th Fl.
Philadelphia, PA 19107
Phone: (215)735-9695 Fax: (215)790-1267
Andrew B. Wigglesworth, President

★ 8823 ★ Hospital Council of Western Pennsylvania
500 Commonwealth Dr.
Warrendale, PA 15086
Phone: (724)772-7206 Fax: (724)772-8339
Ian G. Rawson, PhD, President

★ 8824 ★ Hospital and Healthsystem Association of Pennsylvania
4750 Lindle Rd.
PO Box 8600
Harrisburg, PA 17105-8600
Phone: (717)564-9200 Fax: (717)561-5334
Carolyn F. Scanlan, CEO & Pres
Frmly: Hospital Association of Pennsylvania.

Prince Edward Island

★ 8825 ★ Health Association of Prince Edward Island, Inc.
10 Pownal St.
Charlottetown, PE, Canada C1A 3V6
Phone: (902)368-3901 Fax: (902)368-3231
Ken Ezeard, President

Puerto Rico

★ 8826 ★ Puerto Rico Hospital Association
Villa Nevarez Professional Center, Officina 101-103
Centro Commercial Villa Nevarez
San Juan, PR 00927
Phone: (787)764-0290 Fax: (787)753-9748
Juan Rivera, Exec VP

Quebec

★ 8827 ★ Quebec Hospital Association
505 blvd. de Maisonneuve W, Ste. 400
Montreal, QC, Canada H3A 3C2
Phone: (514)282-4200 Fax: (514)282-4271
Daniel Adam, Exec VP

Rhode Island

★ 8828 ★ Hospital Association of Rhode Island
880 Butler Dr., Ste. 1
Providence, RI 02906
Phone: (401)274-4274 Fax: (401)274-1838
Edward Quinlan, President

Saskatchewan

★ 8829 ★ Saskatchewan Association of Health Organizations
1445 Park St.
Regina, SK, Canada S4N 4C5
Phone: (306)347-5500 Fax: (306)347-5500
Louise Simard, CEO & Pres

South Carolina

★ 8830 ★ South Carolina Hospital Association
101 Medical Circle
PO Box 6009
West Columbia, SC 29171-6009
Phone: (803)796-3080 Fax: (803)796-2938
Ken A. Shull, President

South Dakota

★ 8831 ★ South Dakota Association of Healthcare Organizations
3708 Brooks Pl.
Sioux Falls, SD 57106
Phone: (605)361-2281 Fax: (605)361-5175
David R. Hewett, CEO & Pres
Frmly: South Dakota Hospital Association.

Tennessee

★ 8832 ★ Tennessee Hospital Association
500 Interstate Blvd. S
Nashville, TN 37210
Phone: (615)256-8240 Fax: (615)242-4803
Craig A. Becker, President

Texas

★ 8833 ★ Dallas—Fort Worth Hospital Council
250 Decker Dr.
Irving, TX 75062
Phone: (972)719-4900 Fax: (972)719-4009
John C. Gavras, President

★ 8834 ★ Greater San Antonio Hospital Council
8620 N New Braunfels, Ste. 420
San Antonio, TX 78217
Phone: (210)820-3500 Fax: (210)820-3888
William Dean Rasco, CEO & Pres

★ 8835 ★ Texas Hospital Association
6225 US Hwy. 290 E
PO Box 15587
Austin, TX 78761-5587
Phone: (512)465-1000 Fax: (512)465-1090
Richard J. Bettis, CEO & Pres

Utah

★ 8836 ★ Utah Health Association Utah Hospital and Health Systems Association
2180 South 1300 East, Ste. 440
Salt Lake City, UT 84106-2843
Phone: (801)486-9915 Fax: (801)486-0882
Richard B. Kinnersley, President

Vermont

★ 8837 ★ Vermont Association of Hospitals and Health Systems
148 Main St.
Montpelier, VT 05602
Phone: (802)223-3461 Fax: (802)223-0364
Beatrice Grause, President
Frmly: Vermont Hospital Association.

Virginia

★ 8838 ★ Virginia Hospital and Healthcare Association
4200 Innslake Dr.
PO Box 31394
Richmond, VA 23294
Phone: (804)747-8600 Fax: (804)965-0475
Laurens Sartoris, President
Frmly: Virginia Hospital Association.

Washington

★ 8839 ★ Washington State Hospital Association
300 Elliott Ave. W, Ste. 300
Seattle, WA 98119-4118
Phone: (206)281-7211 **Fax:** (206)283-6122
Leo F. Greenawalt, CEO & Pres

West Virginia

★ 8840 ★ West Virginia Hospital Association
100 Association Dr.
Charleston, WV 25311-1571
Phone: (304)344-9744 **Fax:** (304)344-9745
Steven J. Summer, President

Wisconsin

★ 8841 ★ Wisconsin Health and Hospital Association
5721 Odana Rd.
Madison, WI 53719-1289
Phone: (608)274-1820 **Fax:** (608)274-8554
Stephen Brenton, President
Frmly: Wisconsin Hospital Association.

Wyoming

★ 8842 ★ Wyoming Hospital Association
PO Box 249
Cheyenne, WY 82003
Phone: (307)632-9344 **Fax:** (307)632-9347
Robert C. Kidd, II, President

Kidney

The following organizations are affiliates of the National Kidney Foundation, 30 E 33rd St., Ste. 1100, New York, NY 10016, (800)622-9010, http://www.kidney.org/.

Alabama

★ 8843 ★ National Kidney Foundation of Alabama, Inc.
562 Clay St.
PO Box 342
Montgomery, AL 36101
Phone: (334)265-1033 **Fax:** (334)264-6296
Email: nkfal@bellsouth.net
Website: http://www.nkfalabama.org

Arizona

★ 8844 ★ National Kidney Foundation of Arizona, Inc.
Arizona Kidney Foundation
4203 E Indian School Rd., Ste. 140
Phoenix, AZ 85018
Phone: (602)840-1644 **Fax:** (602)840-2360
Website: http://www.azkidney.org

Arkansas

★ 8845 ★ National Kidney Foundation of Arkansas, Inc.
1 Lile Ct., Ste. 201
PO Box 453
Little Rock, AR 72203
Phone: (501)664-4343 **Fax:** (501)664-7145
Email: nkfa@aristotle.net
Website: http://www.kidneyar.com

California

★ 8846 ★ National Kidney Foundation of Northern California, Inc.
11 Mission St., 3rd Fl.
San Francisco, CA 94105
Phone: (415)543-3303 **Fax:** (415)543-3331
Website: http://www.kidneynca.org

★ 8847 ★ National Kidney Foundation of Southern California, Inc.
5777 W Century Blvd., Ste. 1450
Los Angeles, CA 90045
Phone: (310)641-8152 **Free:** 800-747-5527
Fax: (310)641-5246
Email: jmartinez@kidneysocal.org
Website: http://www.kidneysocal.org

Colorado

★ 8848 ★ National Kidney Foundation of Colorado, Idaho, Montana, and Wyoming, Inc.
Cherry Creek Place III
3151 S Vaughn, Ste. 505
Aurora, CO 80014
Phone: (720)748-9991 **Fax:** (720)748-1273
Email: mlhanson@kidneycimw.org
Website: http://www.kidneycimw.org

Connecticut

★ 8849 ★ National Kidney Foundation of Connecticut, Inc.
920 Farmington Ave.
West Hartford, CT 06107
Phone: (860)232-6054 **Free:** 800-441-1280
Fax: (860)236-1367
Email: info@kidneyct.org
Website: http://www.kidneyct.org

District of Columbia

★ 8850 ★ National Kidney Foundation of the National Capital Area, Inc.
5335 Wisconsin Ave. NW, Ste. 300
Washington, DC 20015
Phone: (202)244-7900 **Fax:** (202)244-7405
Email: penglert@kidneywdc.org
Website: http://www.kidneywdc.org

Florida

★ 8851 ★ National Kidney Foundation of Florida, Inc.
Palmetto Bldg., No. 119
1040 Woodcock Rd.
Orlando, FL 32803
Phone: (407)894-7325 **Free:** 800-927-9659
Fax: (407)895-0051
Email: nkf@kidneyfla.org
Website: http://www.kidneyfla.org

Georgia

★ 8852 ★ National Kidney Foundation of Georgia, Inc.
2951 Flowers Rd. S, Ste. 221
Atlanta, GA 30341
Phone: (770)452-1539 **Free:** 800-633-2339
Fax: (770)452-7564
Email: cstarr@nkfg.org
Website: http://www.kidneyga.org

Hawaii

★ 8853 ★ National Kidney Foundation of Hawaii, Inc.
1314 S King St., No. 305
Honolulu, HI 96814
Phone: (808)593-1515 **Fax:** (808)593-8096
Email: stacey@kidneyhi.org
Website: http://www.kidneyhi.org

Illinois

★ 8854 ★ National Kidney Foundation of Illinois, Inc.
215 W Illinois, Ste. 1-C
Chicago, IL 60610
Phone: (312)321-1500 **Fax:** (312)321-1505
Email: kidney@nkfi.org
Website: http://www.nkfi.org/

Indiana

★ 8855 ★ National Kidney Foundation of Indiana, Inc.
911 E 86th St., No. 100
Indianapolis, IN 46240
Phone: (317)722-5640 **Free:** 800-382-9971
Fax: (317)722-5650
Email: NKFI@in.net
Website: http://www.kidneyindiana.org

Iowa

★ 8856 ★ National Kidney Foundation of Iowa, Inc.
c/o Mercy Medical Center
Mercy Medical Center
701 10th St. SE, No. 5618
Cedar Rapids, IA 52402
Phone: (319)369-4474 **Free:** 800-369-3619
Fax: (319)369-4419
Email: info@kidneyia.org
Website: http://www.kidneyia.org

Kansas

★ 8857 ★ National Kidney Foundation of Kansas and Western Missouri, Inc.
1900 W 47th Pl., Ste. 310
Westwood, KS 66205
Phone: (913)262-1551 **Free:** 800-444-8113
Fax: (913)722-4841
Email: info@kidneyksmo.org
Website: http://www.kidneyksmo.org

Kentucky

★ 8858 ★ National Kidney Foundation of Kentucky, Inc.
250 E Liberty St., No. 710
Louisville, KY 40202
Phone: (502)585-5433 **Fax:** (502)585-1445
Email: nkfk@nkfk.org
Website: http://www.nkfk.org

Louisiana

★ 8859 ★ National Kidney Foundation of Louisiana, Inc.
8200 Hampson, Ste. 425
New Orleans, LA 70118
Phone: (504)861-4500 **Free:** 800-462-3694
Fax: (504)861-1976
Email: kidneyla@gnofn.org
Website: http://www.kidneyla.org

Maine

★ 8860 ★ National Kidney Foundation of Maine, Inc.
630 Congress St.
PO Box 1134
Portland, ME 04104
Phone: (207)772-7270 **Free:** 800-639-7220
Fax: (207)772-4202
Website: http://www.kidney.me.org

Maryland

★ 8861 ★ National Kidney Foundation of Maryland, Inc.
1107 Kenilworth Dr., No. 202
Baltimore, MD 21204
Phone: (410)494-8545 **Free:** 800-671-5369
Fax: (410)494-8549
Website: http://www.kidneymd.org

Massachusetts

★ 8862 ★ National Kidney Foundation of Massachusetts, Rhode Island, New Hampshire, and Vermont, Inc.
129 Morgan Dr.
Norwood, MA 02062
Phone: (781)278-0222 **Fax:** (781)278-0333
Email: blinden@kidneyhealth.org
Website: http://www.kidneyhealth.org

Michigan

★ 8863 ★ National Kidney Foundation of Michigan, Inc.
1169 Oak Valley Dr.
Ann Arbor, MI 48108
Phone: (734)222-9800 **Free:** 800-482-1455
Fax: (734)222-9801
Email: kbergquist@nkfm.org
Website: http://www.nkfm.org

Minnesota

★ 8864 ★ National Kidney Foundation of Minnesota, Inc.
920 S 7th St.
Minneapolis, MN 55415
Phone: (612)337-7300 **Fax:** (612)904-4268
Remarks: Also serves North and South Dakota.

Mississippi

★ 8865 ★ National Kidney Foundation of Mississippi, Inc.
3000 Old Canton Rd., Ste. 100
PO Box 55802
Jackson, MS 39296
Phone: (601)981-3611 **Fax:** (601)981-3612
Email: gailgsweat@yahoo.com
Website: http://www.kidneyms.org

Missouri

★ 8866 ★ National Kidney Foundation of Eastern Missouri and Metro-East, Inc.
1423 Hanley Industrial Dr.
Saint Louis, MO 63144
Phone: (314)961-2828 **Free:** 800-489-9585
Fax: (314)961-0888
Email: mherrmann@nkfstl.com
Website: http://www.nkfstl.com

Nebraska

★ 8867 ★ National Kidney Foundation of Nebraska, Inc.
7101 Newport Ave., No. 301
Omaha, NE 68152
Phone: (402)572-3180 **Free:** 800-642-1255
Fax: (402)572-3211
Website: http://www.kidneyne.org

Nevada

★ 8868 ★ National Kidney Foundation of Nevada, Inc.
3050 E Desert Inn Rd., No. 121
Las Vegas, NV 89121
Phone: (702)735-9222 **Fax:** (702)735-9224
Email: nkfnv@aol.com
Website: http://vegasonline.com/NKF/NKFHP.htm

New Mexico

★ 8869 ★ National Kidney Foundation of New Mexico, Inc.
PO Box 14238
Albuquerque, NM 87191-4238
Phone: (505)293-5298
Email: connieqb@kidney-nm.org

New York

★ 8870 ★ National Kidney Foundation of Central New York, Inc.
731 James St., No. 200
Syracuse, NY 13203
Phone: (315)476-0311 **Free:** 877-854-3639
Fax: (315)476-3707
Email: NKF@CNYKidney.org
Website: http://www.cnykidney.org

★ 8871 ★ National Kidney Foundation of Greater New York, Inc.
30 E 33rd St.
New York, NY 10016
Phone: (212)889-2210 **Free:** 800-622-9010
Fax: (212)689-9261
Website: http://www.nkfofgreaterny.org
Frmly: National Kidney Foundation of New York /New Jersey, Inc.

★ 8872 ★ National Kidney Foundation of Northeast New York, Inc.
23 Computer Dr. E
Albany, NY 12205
Phone: (518)458-9697 **Free:** 800-999-9697
Fax: (518)458-9690
Email: nkfneny@crisny.org
Website: http://www.nkfneny.org

★ 8873 ★ National Kidney Foundation of Upstate New York, Inc.
3300 Monroe Ave., Ste. 100D
Rochester, NY 14618
Phone: (716)264-0420 **Free:** 800-724-9421
Fax: (716)264-0109
Email: nkfnyup@rochester.rr.com
Website: http://www.kidneynyup.org

★ 8874 ★ National Kidney Foundation of Western New York, Inc.
3871 Harlem Rd., No. 11
Buffalo, NY 14215
Phone: (716)835-1323 **Fax:** (716)835-2281
Email: nkfwny@hotmail.com
Website: http://www.nkfofwny.org

North Carolina

★ 8875 ★ National Kidney Foundation of North Carolina, Inc.
5950 Fairview Rd., No. 708
Charlotte, NC 28210
Phone: (704)552-1351 **Free:** 800-356-5362
Fax: (704)552-7870
Email: lskipper@nkfnc.org
Website: http://www.nkfnc.org

Ohio

★ 8876 ★ National Kidney Foundation of Ohio, Inc.
1373 Grandview Ave., No. 200
Columbus, OH 43212
Phone: (614)481-4030 **Fax:** (614)481-4038
Email: info@nkfofohio.org
Website: http://www.nkfofohio.org

Oklahoma

★ 8877 ★ National Kidney Foundation of Oklahoma, Inc.
3617 NW 58th St., No. 101
Oklahoma City, OK 73112
Phone: (405)947-6405 **Free:** 800-946-6405
Fax: (405)947-6463
Website: http://www.nkfo.org

Oregon

★ 8878 ★ National Kidney Foundation of Oregon and Washington, Inc.
1006 SE Grand Ave., Ste. 100
PO Box 15149
Portland, OR 97293-9149
Phone: (503)963-5364 **Free:** 888-3-KIDNEY
Fax: (503)238-1754
Email: help@kidneywa.org
Website: http://www.kidneyorwa.org

★ 8879 ★ National Kidney Foundation of Oregon and Washington, Inc. Medford Chapter
33 N Central Ave., No. 406
Medford, OR 97501
Phone: (541)773-8930 **Fax:** (541)773-8964
Email: medford@kidneyorwa.org
Website: http://www.kidneyorwa.org

Pennsylvania

★ 8880 ★ National Kidney Foundation of the Delaware Valley, Inc.
325 Chestnut St.
Philadelphia, PA 19106
Phone: (215)923-8611 **Fax:** (215)923-2199
Email: info@nkfdv.org
Website: http://www.nkfdv.org

★ 8881 ★ National Kidney Foundation of Western Pennsylvania, Inc.
555 Grant St., No. 380
Pittsburgh, PA 15219
Phone: (412)261-4115 **Fax:** (412)261-1405
Email: bonnieg@kidneywp.org
Website: http://www.kidneywp.org
Remarks: Also serves northern West Virginia.

South Carolina

★ 8882 ★ National Kidney Foundation of South Carolina, Inc.
5000 Thurmond Mall, Ste. 106
Columbia, SC 29201

Phone: (803)799-3870 **Free:** 800-488-2277
Fax: (803)799-3871
Email: bhughes@kidney-sc.org
Website: http://www.kidney-sc.org

South Dakota

★ 8883 ★ National Kidney Foundation of South Dakota, Inc.
400 S Sycamore, No. 104
Sioux Falls, SD 57110
Phone: (605)338-0518

Tennessee

★ 8884 ★ National Kidney Foundation of East Tennessee, Inc.
4450 Walker Blvd., No. 2
Knoxville, TN 37917
Phone: (865)688-5481 **Fax:** (865)688-0196
Email: helen@kidneyetn.org
Website: http://www.kidneyetn.org

★ 8885 ★ National Kidney Foundation of Middle Tennessee, Inc.
2120 Crestmoor Rd.
Nashville, TN 37215
Phone: (615)383-3887 **Fax:** (615)383-2647
Email: nkfmdtn@bellsouth.net
Website: http://www.nkfmdtn.org

★ 8886 ★ National Kidney Foundation of West Tennessee, Inc.
857 Mt. Moriah Rd., Ste. 201
Memphis, TN 38117
Phone: (901)683-6185 **Free:** 800-273-3869
Fax: (901)683-6189
Email: nkf@bellsouth.net

Texas

★ 8887 ★ National Kidney Foundation of North Texas, Inc.
3530 Forest Ln., Ste. 105
Dallas, TX 75234
Phone: (214)351-2393 **Free:** 877-543-6397
Fax: (214)351-3797
Email: info@nkft.org
Website: http://www.nkft.org

★ 8888 ★ National Kidney Foundation of South and Central Texas, Inc.
1919 Oakwell Farms Pkwy., Ste. 135
San Antonio, TX 78218
Phone: (210)829-1299 **Free:** 800-829-1299
Fax: (210)829-1248
Email: nkf@kidneytx.org
Website: http://www.kidneytx.org

★ 8889 ★ National Kidney Foundation of Southeast Texas, Inc.
2400 Augusta Dr., No. 252
Houston, TX 77057
Phone: (713)952-5499 **Free:** 800-961-5683
Fax: (713)952-5497
Website: http://nkfset.org

★ 8890 ★ National Kidney Foundation of the Texas Coastal Bend, Inc.
719 N Upper Broadway
PO Box 9172
Corpus Christi, TX 78469
Phone: (512)884-5892 **Fax:** (512)884-2332

★ 8891 ★ National Kidney Foundation of West Texas, Inc.
4601 50th St., Ste. 101
Lubbock, TX 79414
Phone: (806)799-7753 **Fax:** (806)799-0277
Email: nkfwt@nts-online.net
Website: http://www.nkfwt.org

Utah

★ 8892 ★ National Kidney Foundation of Utah, Inc.
Edgemont Professional Plaza
3707 N Canyon Rd., 1-D
Provo, UT 84604
Phone: (801)226-5111 **Fax:** (801)226-8278
Email: NKFU@KidneyUT.org
Website: http://www.KidneyUT.org

Virginia

★ 8893 ★ National Kidney Foundation of the Virginias, Inc.
2601 Willard Rd., Ste. 103
Richmond, VA 23294
Phone: (804)288-8342 **Free:** 888-543-6398
Fax: (804)282-7835
Email: randallm@kidneyva.org
Website: http://www.kidneyva.org

Washington

★ 8894 ★ National Kidney Foundation of Oregon and Washington, Inc.
2889 152nd Ave. NE, Ste. C
Redmond, WA 98052
Phone: (425)883-2869 **Free:** 888-4-KIDNEY
Fax: (425)883-3869
Email: help@kidneyorwa.org
Website: http://www.kidneyorwa.org

★ 8895 ★ National Kidney Foundation of Oregon and Washington, Inc. Yakima Chapter
32 N 3rd St., No. 412
Yakima, WA 98901
Phone: (509)452-2024 **Fax:** (509)225-6387
Email: yakima@kidneyorwa.org
Website: http://www.kidneyorwa.org

West Virginia

★ 8896 ★ National Kidney Foundation of Western Pennsylvania, Inc. Charleston Area Chapter
PO Box 2024
Charleston, WV 25327
Phone: (304)345-6998
Remarks: Also serves middle and southern West Virginia.

Wisconsin

★ 8897 ★ National Kidney Foundation of Wisconsin, Inc.
280 Regency Ct., No. 100
Brookfield, WI 53045
Phone: (262)821-0705 **Free:** 800-543-6393
Fax: (414)821-5641
Email: nkfw@kidneywi.org
Website: http://www.kidneywi.org

Learning Disabilities

Listed below are state offices of the Learning Disabilities Association of America, 4156 Library Rd., Pittsburgh, PA 15234-1349, (412)341-1515, http://www.ldanatl.org/.

Alabama

★ 8898 ★ Learning Disabilities Association of Alabama
PO Box 11588
Montgomery, AL 36111
Phone: (334)277-9151
Email: alabama@ldaal.org
Website: http://www.ldaal.org

Arizona

★ 8899 ★ Learning Disabilities Association of Arizona
13106 W Limewood Ave.
Sun City West, AZ 85375
Phone: (623)975-4551
Email: dcrawford_1@msn.com
Website: http://www.ldanatl.org/Affiliates/Az/welcome.htm

Arkansas

★ 8900 ★ Learning Disabilities Association of Arkansas
7509 Cantrell, Ste. 103C
Little Rock, AR 72207
Phone: (501)666-8777 **Fax:** (501)666-4070
Website: http://www.ldaarkansas.org

California

★ 8901 ★ Learning Disabilities Association of California
PO Box 601067
Sacramento, CA 95860-1067
Phone: (916)725-7881 **Free:** (866)532-6322
Fax: (916)725-8786
Email: office@ldaca.org
Website: http://www.ldaca.org

★ 8902 ★ Learning Disabilities Association San Diego
3550 Kearny Villa Rd., Ste. 222
San Diego, CA 92123
Phone: (858)467-9158 **Fax:** (858)467-1333
Website: http://www.LDASanDiego.org/

★ 8903 ★ Sacramento Learning Disabilities Association
PO Box 276645
Sacramento, CA 95827
Phone: (530)672-3145
Website: http://www.SacramentoLDA.org/

Colorado

★ 8904 ★ Learning Disabilities Association of Colorado
4500 E Iliff Ave.
Denver, CO 80222
Phone: (303)894-0992 **Fax:** (303)830-1645
Email: info@ldacolorado.com
Website: http://www.ldacolorado.com

Connecticut

★ 8905 ★ Learning Disabilities Association of Connecticut
999 Asylum Ave.
Hartford, CT 06105
Phone: (860)560-1711 **Fax:** (860)560-1750
Email: ldact@juno.com
Website: http://www.ldanatl.org/Affiliates/CT/LDAof-Connecticut.html

Florida

★ 8906 ★ Learning Disabilities Association of Florida
331 E Henry St.
Punta Gorda, FL 33950
Phone: (941)637-8957 **Fax:** (941)637-0617
Email: ldaf00@sunline.net
Website: http://www.ldafl.org/
Frmly: Florida ACLD.

Georgia

★ 8907 ★ Learning Disabilities Association of Georgia
PO Box 1337
Roswell, GA 30077
Phone: (678)461-4471 **Fax:** (678)461-4472
Email: services@ldag.org
Website: http://www.ldag.org/

Hawaii

★ 8908 ★ Learning Disabilities Association of Hawaii
200 N Vineyard Blvd., Ste. 310
Honolulu, HI 96817
Phone: (808)536-9684 **Free:** 800-533-9684
Fax: (808)537-6780
Email: ldah@gte.net
Website: http://www.ldanatl.org/Hawaii/ldah.html

Illinois

★ 8909 ★ Learning Disabilities Association of Illinois
10101 S Roberts Rd., Ste. 106
Palos Hills, IL 60465
Phone: (708)430-7532 **Fax:** (708)430-7592
Email: JanetLerner@juno.com
Website: http://www.ldanatl.org/Affiliates/IL/index.htm
Bev Johns, President

Indiana

★ 8910 ★ Learning Disabilities Association of Indiana
PO Box 20584
Indianapolis, IN 46220
Free: 800-284-2519
Email: bluhrig@inct.net
Website: http://www.inct.net/~bluhrig/

Kansas

★ 8911 ★ Learning Disabilities Association of Kansas
PO Box 4424
Topeka, KS 66604
Phone: (913)272-0033
Website: http://www.ldakansas.org/

Kentucky

★ 8912 ★ Learning Disabilities Association of Kentucky
2210 Goldsmith Lane, No. 222
Louisville, KY 40218
Phone: (502)473-1256 **Free:** 877-587-1256
Fax: (502)473-4695
Email: LDAofKY@aol.com
Website: http://www.ldaofky.org/

Maine

★ 8913 ★ Learning Disabilities Association of Maine
PO Box 67
Oakland, ME 04963
Phone: (207)465-7700 **Fax:** (207)873-4146
Email: ldame@ldame.org
Website: http://www.ldame.org/

Maryland

★ 8914 ★ Learning Disabilities Association of Maryland
PO Box 526
Bowie, MD 20718-0526
Free: 800-673-6777 **Fax:** (410)337-3702
Website: http://www.ldanatl.org/Affiliates/MD/md.htm

Massachusetts

★ 8915 ★ Learning Disabilities Association of Massachusetts
1275 Main St.
Waltham, MA 02451
Phone: (781)891-5009 **Fax:** (781)647-5141
Website: http://www.ldam.org/

Michigan

★ 8916 ★ Learning Disabilities Association of Michigan
200 Museum Dr., Ste. 101
Lansing, MI 48933
Phone: (517)485-8160

Mississippi

★ 8917 ★ Learning Disabilities Association of Mississippi
PO Box 4477
4080 Old Canton Rd.
Jackson, MS 39216
Phone: (601)362-1667 **Fax:** (601)362-9180
Email: ldams@bellsouth.net
Website: http://www.ldams.org

Missouri

★ 8918 ★ Learning Disabilities Association of Missouri
PO Box 3303
1942 E Meadowmere, No. 104
Springfield, MO 65808
Phone: (417)864-5110 **Fax:** (417)864-7290
Email: ldamo@cland.net
Website: http://www.ldamo.org

★ 8919 ★ Learning Disabilities Association of the Ozarks
PO Box 4362
Springfield, MO 65808
Phone: (417)882-2008
Website: http://www.ldaozarks.com/HOME_PAGEx.html

★ 8920 ★ St. Louis Learning Disabilities Association
10702 Manchester, Ste. 7
Saint Louis, MO 63122
Phone: (314)966-3088 **Fax:** (314)966-1806
Email: stloulda@mindspring.com
Website: http://www.ldastl.org/

Nebraska

★ 8921 ★ Learning Disabilities Association of Nebraska
PO Box 6464
Omaha, NE 68106

New Jersey

★ 8922 ★ Learning Disabilities Association of New Jersey
PO Box 401
Old Bridge, NJ 08857-0401
Phone: (732)360-0399

New Mexico

★ 8923 ★ Learning Disabilities Association of New Mexico
6301 Menaul Blvd. NE, No. 556
Albuquerque, NM 87110-3323
Phone: (505)821-2545
Email: bp@peavler.org
Website: http://www.vivanewmexico.com/nmlda/

New York

★ 8924 ★ Learning Disabilities Association of Central New York
722 W Manlius St.
East Syracuse, NY 13057
Phone: (315)432-0665 **Free:** 800-253-2269
Fax: (315)431-0606
Email: LDACNY@LDACNY.org
Website: http://www.ldacny.org

★ 8925 ★ Learning Disabilities Association of the Genesee Valley
339 East Ave.
Rochester, NY 14604
Phone: (716)263-3323
Website: http://www.ldagvi.org/

★ 8926 ★ Learning Disabilities Association of the Mohawk Valley
401 Columbia St.
Utica, NY 13502-3413
Phone: (315)797-1253 **Fax:** (315)797-4006
Website: http://www.ldalearningcenter.org/

★ 8927 ★ Learning Disabilities Association of Nassau and Suffolk
PO Box 461
Massapequa Park, NY 11762
Phone: (631)242-8943
Email: info@ldans.org
Website: http://www.ldans.org/

★ 8928 ★ Learning Disabilities Association of New York
27 W 20th St., Ste. 303
New York, NY 10011
Phone: (212)645-6730 **Fax:** (212)924-8896

★ 8929 ★ Learning Disabilities Association of New York City
27 W 20th St., Ste. 303
New York, NY 10011
Phone: (212)645-6730 **Fax:** (212)924-8896

Website: http://www.learningdisabilitynyc.org

★ 8930 ★ Learning Disabilities Association of New York City, Inc.
27 W 20th St., Ste. 303
New York, NY 10011
Phone: (212)645-6730 **Fax:** (212)924-8896
Email: helplineldanyc@earthlink.net

★ 8931 ★ Learning Disabilities Association of Western New York
2555 Elmwood Ave.
Kenmore, NY 14217
Phone: (716)874-7200 **Fax:** (716)874-7205
Email: LDAofWNY@aol.com
Website: http://members.aol.com/ldaofwny/home.html

North Carolina

★ 8932 ★ Learning Disabilities Association of North Carolina
PO Box 3542
Chapel Hill, NC 27515-3542
Phone: (919)493-5362 **Fax:** (919)489-0788
Email: ldanc@mindspring.com
Website: http://www.ldanc.org/

Oklahoma

★ 8933 ★ Learning Disabilities Association of Oklahoma
PO Box 1134
Jenks, OK 74037
Free: 800-532-6365
Email: ldao@fullnet.net

Pennsylvania

★ 8934 ★ Learning Disabilities Association of America
4156 Library Rd.
Pittsburgh, PA 15234-1349
Phone: (412)341-1515 **Fax:** (412)344-0224
Email: info@ldaamerica.org
Website: http://www.ldaamerica.org

★ 8935 ★ Learning Disabilities Association of Pennsylvania
Toomey Bldg., Box 208
Uwchland, PA 19480
Phone: (610)458-8193

★ 8936 ★ Learning Disabilities Association of Pennsylvania
Toomey Bldg., Box 208
Uwchland, PA 19480
Phone: (610)458-8193
Anna Mary McHugh, President
Lynn Reinhold, Vice President

Rhode Island

★ 8937 ★ Rhode Island Learning Disabilities Association
PO Box 8128
Cranston, RI 02920
Email: lindixx@email.com
Website: http://www.worldville.com/lifestyles/ldari/

South Dakota

★ 8938 ★ Learning Disabilities Association of South Dakota
PO Box 9760
Rapid City, SD 57709
Phone: (605)342-4320 **Free:** 888-388-5553

Email: dthom@rapidnet.com
Website: http://ldasd.rapidnet.com/

Texas

★ 8939 ★ Learning Disabilities Association of Texas
1011 W 31st St.
Austin, TX 78705
Phone: (512)458-8234 **Free:** 800-604-7500
Fax: (512)458-3826
Email: LDATexas@cs.com
Website: http://ourworld.compuserve.com/homepages/LDAT/

Utah

★ 8940 ★ Learning Disabilities Association of Utah
309 East 100 South, Ste. 2
PO Box 651052
Salt Lake City, UT 84165-1052
Phone: (801)363-6320 **Fax:** (801)363-6332
Email: LDAU@ldau.org
Website: http://www.ldau.org/

Vermont

★ 8941 ★ Learning Disabilities Association of Vermont
PO Box 1041
Manchester Center, VT 05255
Phone: (802)362-3127 **Fax:** (802)362-3128

Virginia

★ 8942 ★ Learning Disabilities Association of Virginia
Randolph Towers, No. 505
4100 N 9th St.
Arlington, VA 22203
Phone: (703)243-2614 **Fax:** (703)243-0894
Email: info@ldavirginia.org
Website: http://www.ldavirginia.org/index.html

Washington

★ 8943 ★ Learning Disabilities Association of Washington
7819 159th Pl., NE
Redmond, WA 98052
Phone: (425)882-0820 **Fax:** (425)861-4642
Email: info@ldawa.org
Website: http://www.ldawa.org

West Virginia

★ 8944 ★ West Virginia Learning Disabilities Association, Inc.
4726 Teays Valley Rd.
Scott Depot, WV 25560
Phone: (304)755-0347
Email: wvlda@hotmail.com
Frmly: Learning Disabilities Association of West Virginia.

Wisconsin

★ 8945 ★ Learning Disabilities Association of Wisconsin
1446 Baytree Ln.
Neenah, WI 54956
Phone: (920)720-5755 **Free:** 888-590-4141
Email: ldawisconsin@hotmail.com
Website: http://www.njsd.org/lda

Leukemia

State chapters of The Leukemia and Lymphoma Society are listed below. The national office is located at 1311 Mamaroneck Ave., White Plains, NY 10605. Additional information can be obtained by calling the national office at (800) 955-4LSA, or by consulting their web site at http://www.leukemia.org/.

Alabama

★ 8946 ★ The Leukemia and Lymphoma Society
Alabama Chapter
100 Chase Park S, Ste. 220
Birmingham, AL 35244
Phone: (205)989-0098 **Fax:** (205)989-0099
Valerie Hunton, Exec Director

Arizona

★ 8947 ★ The Leukemia and Lymphoma Society
Desert Mountain States Chapter
2990 E Northern Ave., Ste. E-100
Phoenix, AZ 85028
Phone: (602)788-8622 **Free:** 800-568-1372
Fax: (602)788-3455
Tim Metzer, Exec Director
Remarks: Serves Arizona, Utah, and western Texas.

California

★ 8948 ★ The Leukemia and Lymphoma Society
Greater Los Angeles Chapter
6033 W Century Blvd., Ste. 300
Los Angeles, CA 90045
Phone: (310)216-7600 **Fax:** (310)216-1500
Barbara Howell, Exec Director

★ 8949 ★ The Leukemia and Lymphoma Society
Greater Sacramento Area Chapter
3105 Fite Circle, Ste. 101
Sacramento, CA 95827
Phone: (916)369-7581 **Fax:** (916)369-0812
Tracy Newman, Exec Director
Remarks: Also serves much of Nevada.

★ 8950 ★ The Leukemia and Lymphoma Society
Northern California Chapter
1390 Market St., Ste. 1200
San Francisco, CA 94102
Phone: (415)625-1100 **Fax:** (415)625-1155

★ 8951 ★ The Leukemia and Lymphoma Society
San Diego/Hawaii Chapter
8575 Gibbs Dr., Ste. 262
San Diego, CA 92123
Phone: (858)277-1800 **Free:** 800-215-1098
Fax: (858)277-1748
Keith Turner, Exec Director
Alt. Contact: Hawaii Number: (808) 534-1222.

★ 8952 ★ The Leukemia and Lymphoma Society
Tri-County Chapter
2333 N Broadway, Ste. 320
Santa Ana, CA 92706
Phone: (714)881-0610 **Free:** 888-535-9300
Fax: (714)881-0616

Email: quinteroj@ca-tri.leukemia.org
Website: http://www.ca-tri.leukemia.org
Sam Thomas, Exec Director
Remarks: Also serves the Las Vegas, Nevada, area.

Colorado

★ 8953 ★ The Leukemia and Lymphoma Society
Rocky Mountain Chapter
5353 W Dartmouth Ave.
Denver, CO 80227
Phone: (303)984-2110 **Fax:** (303)984-2352
Remarks: Serves Colorado, Idaho, Montana, and Wyoming.

Connecticut

★ 8954 ★ The Leukemia and Lymphoma Society
Connecticut Chapter
300 Research Pkwy., Ste. 310
Meriden, CT 06450
Phone: (203)379-0445 **Free:** 888-282-9465
Fax: (203)379-0451
Elizabeth Garrigan, Exec Director

★ 8955 ★ The Leukemia and Lymphoma Society
Fairfield County Chapter
25 3rd St., 4th Fl.
Stamford, CT 06905
Phone: (203)967-8326 **Fax:** (203)325-8559
Email: fairfieldinfo@yahoo.com
Michael Angarola, Exec Director

Delaware

★ 8956 ★ The Leukemia and Lymphoma Society
Delaware Chapter
100 W 10 St., Ste. 209
Wilmington, DE 19801
Phone: (302)661-7300 **Free:** 800-220-1617
Fax: (302)661-0363

Florida

★ 8957 ★ The Leukemia and Lymphoma Society
Central Florida Chapter
3319 Maguire St., Ste. 101
Orlando, FL 32803
Phone: (407)898-0733 **Fax:** (407)896-8645
Tracy Tucker, Exec Director

★ 8958 ★ The Leukemia and Lymphoma Society
Northern Florida Chapter
9143 Phillips Hwy., Ste. 130
Jacksonville, FL 32256
Phone: (904)538-0721 **Free:** 800-868-0072
Fax: (904)538-9245
Eden Carr, Exec Director

★ 8959 ★ The Leukemia and Lymphoma Society
Palm Beach Area Chapter
4360 Northlake Blvd., Ste. 109
Palm Beach Gardens, FL 33410
Phone: (561)775-9954 **Free:** 888-478-8550
Fax: (561)775-0930
Email: McDonaldP@FL-wpb.leukemia.org
Website: http://www.FL-wpb.leukemia.org
Patricia McDonald, Exec Director

★ 8960 ★ The Leukemia and Lymphoma Society
Southern Florida Chapter
3325 Hollywood Blvd., Ste. 400
Hollywood, FL 33021
Phone: (954)961-3234 **Fax:** (954)961-7376
Email: silvermanb@fl-so.leukemia-lymphoma.org
Website: http://www.fl-so.leukemia-lymphoma.org
Barbara Silverman, Exec Director

★ 8961 ★ The Leukemia and Lymphoma Society
Suncoast Chapter
13907 N Dale Mabry Hwy., Ste. 101
Tampa, FL 33618
Phone: (813)963-6461 **Fax:** (813)963-1306
Anna Maria Gentile, Exec Director

Georgia

★ 8962 ★ The Leukemia and Lymphoma Society
Georgia Chapter
2625 Cumberland Pkwy, Ste. 205
Atlanta, GA 30339
Phone: (770)438-6006 **Free:** 800-399-7312
Fax: (770)438-6563
Laurie Papelian, Exec Director

Illinois

★ 8963 ★ The Leukemia and Lymphoma Society
Illinois Chapter
100 W Monroe Ave., Ste. 1610
Chicago, IL 60603
Phone: (312)726-0003 **Fax:** (312)726-4769
Lee J. Brown, Exec Director

Indiana

★ 8964 ★ The Leukemia and Lymphoma Society
Indiana Chapter
921 E 86th St., Ste. 205
Indianapolis, IN 46240
Phone: (317)726-2270 **Fax:** (317)726-2280
Dennis Norris, Exec Director

Iowa

★ 8965 ★ The Leukemia and Lymphoma Society
Iowa Chapter
8033 University Blvd., Ste. A
Des Moines, IA 50325
Phone: (515)270-6169 **Free:** 800-347-1074
Fax: (515)270-5392
Email: janna@crn.org
Website: http://www.crn.org
Janna LaCock, Exec Director

Kansas

★ 8966 ★ The Leukemia and Lymphoma Society
Kansas Chapter
555 N Woodlawn, Bldg. 1, Ste. 113
Wichita, KS 67208
Phone: (316)687-2222 **Free:** 800-779-2417
Fax: (316)687-1122
Email: kansas@ks.leukemia-lymphoma.org
Website: http://www.ks.leukemia-lymphoma.org

★ 8967 ★ The Leukemia and Lymphoma Society
Mid-America Chapter
Cloverleaf Bldg. 1, Ste. 202
6811 W 63rd St.
Shawnee Mission, KS 66202
Phone: (913)262-1515 **Free:** 800-256-1075
Fax: (913)262-2167
Email: janna@crn.org
Website: http://www.crn.org
Janna LaCock, Contact
Remarks: Serves western Missouri and eastern Kansas.

Kentucky

★ 8968 ★ The Leukemia and Lymphoma Society
Kentucky Chapter
710 W Main St., Ste. 201
Louisville, KY 40202
Phone: (502)584-8490 **Free:** 800-955-2566
Fax: (502)589-5316
Janelle Sumner, Exec Director

Louisiana

★ 8969 ★ The Leukemia and Lymphoma Society
Louisiana Chapter
3636 S I-10 Service Rd., Ste. 304
Metairie, LA 70001
Phone: (504)837-0945 **Free:** 888-290-0945
Fax: (504)837-9193
Susan Krilov, Exec Director

Maryland

★ 8970 ★ The Leukemia and Lymphoma Society
Maryland Chapter
Chester Bldg., Ste. 314
8600 La Salle Rd.
Baltimore, MD 21286
Phone: (410)825-2500 **Fax:** (410)825-2515
Website: http://www.mdleukemia.org
Sharon Yateman, Exec Director

Massachusetts

★ 8971 ★ The Leukemia and Lymphoma Society
Massachusetts Chapter
495 Old Connecticut Path, Ste. 220
Framingham, MA 01701
Phone: (508)879-5083 **Free:** 800-688-6572
Fax: (508)879-8163
Iris Gleason, Exec Director
Remarks: Serves Massachusetts, Maine, and New Hampshire.

Michigan

★ 8972 ★ The Leukemia and Lymphoma Society
Michigan Chapter
1421 E 12 Mile Rd., Bldg. A
Madison Heights, MI 48071
Phone: (248)582-2900 **Free:** 800-456-5413
Fax: (248)582-2925
Email: bizzisj@mi.leukemia-lymphoma.org
Website: http://www.mi.leukemia-lymphoma.org
Julia K. Bizzis, Exec Director

Minnesota

★ 8973 ★ The Leukemia and Lymphoma Society
Minnesota Chapter
5217 Wayzata Blvd., Ste. 221
Saint Louis Park, MN 55416
Phone: (952)545-3309 **Fax:** (952)545-5926
Murray Schmidt, Exec Director
Remarks: Serves Minnesota, North Dakota, and South Dakota.

Mississippi

★ 8974 ★ The Leukemia and Lymphoma Society
Mississippi Chapter
405 Fontaine Pl., Ste. 103
Ridgeland, MS 39157
Phone: (601)956-7447 **Free:** 877-538-5364
Fax: (601)956-6957
Julie Levanway, Exec Director

Missouri

★ 8975 ★ The Leukemia and Lymphoma Society
Gateway Chapter
77 W Port Plaza, Ste. 101
Saint Louis, MO 63146
Phone: (314)878-0780 **Free:** 800-264-2873
Fax: (314)878-4050
Judith Swiecicki, Exec Director
Remarks: Serves eastern Missouri and southern Illinois.

Nebraska

★ 8976 ★ The Leukemia and Lymphoma Society
Nebraska Chapter
2665 Farnam St.
Omaha, NE 68131
Phone: (402)344-2242 **Free:** 888-847-4974
Fax: (402)344-2422
Email: opbroekr@ne.leukemia.org
Website: http://www.ne.leukemia.org
Rosemary Opbroek, Exec Director

New Jersey

★ 8977 ★ The Leukemia and Lymphoma Society
Northern New Jersey Chapter
45 Springfield Ave.
Springfield, NJ 07081
Phone: (973)376-9559 **Fax:** (973)376-7072
Lorraine Seidel, Exec Director

★ 8978 ★ The Leukemia and Lymphoma Society
Southern New Jersey Chapter
216 Haddon Ave., Ste. 328
Westmont, NJ 08108
Phone: (856)869-0200 **Free:** 888-920-8557
Fax: (856)869-7383
Nanette Forte, Exec Director

New Mexico

★ 8979 ★ The Leukemia and Lymphoma Society
New Mexico Chapter
3150 Carlisle NE, Ste. 35
Albuquerque, NM 87110
Phone: (505)830-6040 **Free:** 888-286-7846
Fax: (505)830-6041
Cindi Ankiewicz, Exec Director
Remarks: Serves New Mexico and the Greater El Paso, Texas, area.

New York

★ 8980 ★ The Leukemia and Lymphoma Society
Central New York Chapter
Learbury Centre
401 N Salina St.
Syracuse, NY 13203
Phone: (315)471-1050 **Free:** 800-690-8944
Fax: (315)471-6434
Toni E. Bennett, Exec Director

★ 8981 ★ The Leukemia and Lymphoma Society
Long Island Chapter
555 Broad Hollow Rd., Ste. 403
Melville, NY 11747
Phone: (631)752-8500 **Fax:** (631)752-9066
Kerri Kaplan, Exec Director

★ 8982 ★ The Leukemia and Lymphoma Society
New York City Chapter
475 Park Ave. S, 21st Fl.
New York, NY 10016
Phone: (212)448-9206 **Fax:** (212)448-9214
Mary Kozik, Exec Director

★ 8983 ★ The Leukemia and Lymphoma Society
Westchester/Hudson Valley Chapter
1311 Mamaroneck Ave., Ste. 330
White Plains, NY 10605
Phone: (914)949-0084 **Fax:** (914)949-0391
Jean Montano, Exec Director

★ 8984 ★ The Leukemia and Lymphoma Society
Western New York/Finger Lakes Chapter
4053 Maple Rd., Ste. 110
Amherst, NY 14226
Phone: (716)635-9111 **Fax:** (716)837-0335
Nancy Hails, Exec Director

North Carolina

★ 8985 ★ The Leukemia and Lymphoma Society
North Carolina Chapter
5950 Fairview Rd., Ste. 250
Charlotte, NC 28210
Phone: (704)998-5012 **Free:** 800-888-9934
Fax: (704)998-5010
Selena Rogers, Exec Director

Ohio

★ 8986 ★ The Leukemia and Lymphoma Society
Central Ohio Chapter
2225 City Gate Dr., Ste. E
Columbus, OH 43219
Phone: (614)476-7194 **Free:** 800-686-2873
William Carnes, Exec Director

★ 8987 ★ The Leukemia and Lymphoma Society
Northern Ohio Chapter
902 Westpoint Pkwy., Ste. 300
Cleveland, OH 44145
Phone: (440)617-2873 **Fax:** (440)617-2879
Nathaniel A. Cross, Exec Director

★ 8988 ★ The Leukemia and Lymphoma Society
Southern Ohio Chapter
Fourth and Race Towers
105 W 4th St.
Cincinnati, OH 45202
Phone: (513)361-2100 **Fax:** (513)361-2109
Nancy Brinker, Exec Director

Oklahoma

★ 8989 ★ The Leukemia and Lymphoma Society
Oklahoma Chapter
3613 NW 56th St., Ste. 230
Oklahoma City, OK 73112
Phone: (405)943-8888 **Fax:** (405)945-8355
Email: odonnells@ok.leukemia-lymphoma.org
Website: http://www.ok.leukemia-lymphoma.org
Suzanne O'Donnell, Exec Director

Oregon

★ 8990 ★ The Leukemia and Lymphoma Society
Oregon Chapter
6501 SW Macadam Ave.
Portland, OR 97201
Phone: (503)245-9866 **Fax:** (503)245-9865
Gregory Knox, Exec Director

Pennsylvania

★ 8991 ★ The Leukemia and Lymphoma Society
Central Pennsylvania Chapter
800 Corporate Cir., Ste. 100
Harrisburg, PA 17110
Phone: (717)652-6520 **Free:** 800-822-2873
Fax: (717)652-8614

★ 8992 ★ The Leukemia and Lymphoma Society
Eastern Pennsylvania Chapter
2 International Plaza, Ste. 245
Philadelphia, PA 19113
Phone: (610)521-8274 **Fax:** (610)521-6132
Joanne Spink, Exec Director

★ 8993 ★ The Leukemia and Lymphoma Society
Western Pennsylvania and West Virginia Chapter
2 Gateway Ctr.
13 North
Pittsburgh, PA 15222
Phone: (412)395-2873 **Free:** 800-726-2873
Fax: (412)395-2888
George Omiros, Exec Director

Rhode Island

★ 8994 ★ The Leukemia and Lymphoma Society
Rhode Island Chapter
75 Sockanosset Crossroad, Ste. 206
Box 8099
Cranston, RI 02920
Phone: (401)943-8888 **Fax:** (401)943-1377
Lynn Aaronson, Exec Director

South Carolina

★ 8995 ★ The Leukemia and Lymphoma Society
South Carolina Chapter
1247 Lake Murray Blvd.
Irmo, SC 29063
Phone: (803)749-4299 **Fax:** (803)749-4088
Email: canningf@sc.leukemia-lymphoma.org
Website: http://www.sc.leukemia-lymphoma.org
Frank Canning, Exec Director

Tennessee

★ 8996 ★ The Leukemia and Lymphoma Society
Tennessee Chapter
446 Metroplex Dr., Ste. A-200
Nashville, TN 37211
Phone: (615)331-2980 **Free:** 800-332-2980
Fax: (615)331-2941
Email: llstennchap@netscape.net
Karen Rudzinski, Exec Director

Texas

★ 8997 ★ The Leukemia and Lymphoma Society
North Texas Chapter
12850 Spurling Dr., Ste. 220
Dallas, TX 75230
Phone: (972)239-0959 **Fax:** (972)239-0892
Richard Reader, Exec Director

★ 8998 ★ The Leukemia and Lymphoma Society
South/West Texas Chapter
950 Isom Rd., Ste. 104
San Antonio, TX 78216
Phone: (210)377-1775 **Free:** 800-683-2458
Fax: (210)344-3717
Cindy Atmar, Exec Director

★ 8999 ★ The Leukemia and Lymphoma Society
Texas Gulf Coast Chapter
5005 Mitchelldale, Ste. 115
Houston, TX 77092
Phone: (713)680-8088 **Fax:** (713)683-9504
Joan Jarrett, Exec Director

Virginia

★ 9000 ★ The Leukemia and Lymphoma Society
National Capital Area Chapter
5845 Richmond Hwy., Ste. 630
Alexandria, VA 22303
Phone: (703)960-1100 **Fax:** (703)960-0920
Email: samuelsc@dc-cap.leukemia-lymphoma.org
Website: http://www.tntdc.org
Darcy Valentine, Director
Remarks: Serves Washington DC, west-central Maryland, and northeastern Virginia.

★ 9001 ★ The Leukemia and Lymphoma Society
Virginia Chapter
2101 Executive Dr.
Tower Box 21
Hampton, VA 23666
Phone: (757)838-9351 **Free:** 800-866-4483
Fax: (757)827-7337
Diane Hagemann, Exec Director

Washington

★ 9002 ★ The Leukemia and Lymphoma Society
Washington and Alaska Chapter
530 Dexter Ave. N, Ste. 300
Seattle, WA 98109
Phone: (206)628-0777 **Free:** 888-345-4572
Fax: (206)292-9791
Email: WAChapter@wa.leukemia-lymphoma.org
Website: http://www.wa.leukemia-lymphoma.org
Kathryn Bennett, Exec Director

Wisconsin

★ 9003 ★ The Leukemia and Lymphoma Society
Wisconsin Chapter
1126 S 70th St., Ste. N405-A
Milwaukee, WI 53214
Phone: (414)256-4020 **Free:** 800-261-7399
Fax: (414)256-4025
Bede Barth, Exec Director

Liver Diseases

State chapters of the American Liver Foundation are listed below. The national office is located at 75 Maiden Lane, Ste. 603, New York, NY 10038. Additional information can be obtained by calling the national office at (800) GO-LIVER, or by consulting their web site at http://www.liverfoundation.org/.

Alabama

★ 9004 ★ American Liver Foundation
Alabama Chapter
617 Lorna Sq.
Birmingham, AL 35216
Phone: (205)822-1126 **Fax:** (205)824-2009
Email: paalliver@aol.com
Pamela Gallagher, Director

Arizona

★ 9005 ★ American Liver Foundation
Arizona Chapter
4545 E Shea Blvd., Ste. 164
Phoenix, AZ 85028
Phone: (602)953-1800 **Fax:** (602)953-1806
Email: alfofaz@qwest.net
Leanne Marco, Director

California

★ 9006 ★ American Liver Foundation
Greater Los Angeles Chapter
5777 Century Blvd., Ste. 865
Los Angeles, CA 90045
Phone: (310)670-4624 **Fax:** (310)670-4672
Email: dgracon@liver411.com
Website: http://www.liver411.com
Donna Gracon, Director

★ 9007 ★ American Liver Foundation
Northern California Chapter
870 Market St., Ste. 1046
San Francisco, CA 94102
Phone: (415)248-1060 **Free:** 800-292-9099
Fax: (415)248-1066
Email: info@liverlifeline.com
Website: http://www.liverlifeline.com
Linden Young, Director

★ 9008 ★ American Liver Foundation
San Diego Chapter
4452 Park Blvd., Ste. 102
San Diego, CA 92116
Phone: (619)291-5483 **Fax:** (619)295-7181
Email: alfsandiego@aol.com
Kristina Furrow, Director

Colorado

★ 9009 ★ American Liver Foundation
Rocky Mountain Chapter
3593 S Teller St., Ste. 403
Lakewood, CO 80235-2030
Phone: (303)988-4388 **Fax:** (303)988-4398
Email: rockymtnliver@qwest.com
Katherine Kinch, Director

Connecticut

★ 9010 ★ American Liver Foundation
Connecticut Chapter
110 Washington Ave, 3rd Fl.
North Haven, CT 06473
Phone: (203)234-6304 **Fax:** (203)234-6327
Email: info@ctalf.org
Website: http://www.ctalf.org
JoAnn Thompson, Director

District of Columbia

★ 9011 ★ American Liver Foundation
Greater Washington DC Chapter
1875 Eye St. NW, Ste. 1200
Washington, DC 20006
Phone: (202)872-6600 **Fax:** (202)872-6603
Email: alfdc@starpower.net
Website: http://www.liverdc.org
Yao P. Tyus, Director

Florida

★ 9012 ★ American Liver Foundation
Gulf Coast Chapter
101 American Center Place, Ste. 201
Tampa, FL 33619-4400
Phone: (813)740-0045 **Fax:** (813)740-2524
Email: alfgcc@aol.com
Maria Eddy, Director

Georgia

★ 9013 ★ American Liver Foundation
Georgia Chapter
1201 Clairmont Rd., Ste. 120
Decatur, GA 30030
Phone: (404)633-9169 **Free:** (866)-GA-LIVER
Fax: (404)633-8709
Email: alfga@mindspring.com
Charlotte Thompson, Director

Illinois

★ 9014 ★ American Liver Foundation
Illinois Chapter
27 E Monroe St., Ste. 700A
Chicago, IL 60603
Phone: (312)377-9030 **Fax:** (312)377-9035
Email: jackie@illinois-liver.org
Website: http://www.illinois-liver.org
Paul Ladniak, Contact

Massachusetts

★ 9015 ★ American Liver Foundation
New England Chapter
88 Winchester St.
Newton, MA 02461

Phone: (617)527-5600 **Free:** 800-298-6766
Fax: (617)527-5636
Email: info@liverfoundation-ne.org
Website: http://www.liverfoundation-ne.org
Judi Kaplan Elkin, Contact

Michigan

★ 9016 ★ American Liver Foundation
Michigan Chapter
31700 W 12 Mile Rd, Ste. 201
Farmington Hills, MI 48334
Phone: (248)489-5400 **Fax:** (248)489-0376
Email: miliver@coast.com
Ryan Ambrozaitis, Director

Minnesota

★ 9017 ★ American Liver Foundation
Minnesota Chapter
1500 McAndrews Rd. W, Ste. 214
Burnsville, MN 55337
Phone: (952)892-8441 **Fax:** (952)892-8442
Email: amlivermn@yahoo.com
Website: http://www.angelfire.com/mn2/amlivermn
Scott A. Suckow, Director
Remarks: Serves Minnesota and eastern North Dakota and South Dakota.

Missouri

★ 9018 ★ American Liver Foundation
Missouri Chapter
16 Hampton Village Plaza, Ste. 215
Saint Louis, MO 63109
Phone: (314)352-7377 **Free:** (866)455-4837
Fax: (314)352-7875
Email: alfmo@mcleodusa.net
Katherine Auble, Director
Remarks: Serves Missouri and southern Illinois.

New York

★ 9019 ★ American Liver Foundation
Greater New York Chapter
80 Wall St., Ste. 509
New York, NY 10005
Phone: (212)943-1059 **Free:** 877-307-7507
Fax: (212)943-1314
Email: nyliverfoundation@yahoo.com
Website: http://www.nyliverfoundation.com
Scott Suckow, Exec Director
Remarks: Also serves northeastern New Jersey.

★ 9020 ★ American Liver Foundation
Western New York Chapter
25 Canterbury Rd., Ste. 316
New York, NY 10025
Phone: (716)271-2859 **Fax:** (716)271-8642
Email: livrlady@aol.com
Nancy Koris, Director

North Carolina

★ 9021 ★ American Liver Foundation
North Carolina Triangle Chapter
PO Box 268
Morrisville, NC 27560
Phone: (919)481-3024 **Fax:** (919)481-9571
Email: ncalf@worldnet.att.net
Website: http://www.ntwrks.com/~tbordeaux/ncalf.htm
Larry Bordeaux, Director

Ohio

★ 9022 ★ American Liver Foundation
Northern Ohio Chapter
5755 Granger Rd., Ste. 335
Independence, OH 44131-1455
Phone: (216)635-2780 **Free:** (866)-OHIO-ALF
Fax: (216)635-2781
Email: morganalf@usalogin.net
Terri L. Manns, Director

Pennsylvania

★ 9023 ★ American Liver Foundation
Delaware Valley Chapter
111 Presidential Blvd., Ste. 214
Bala Cynwyd, PA 19004
Phone: (610)668-0152 **Fax:** (610)668-0155
Email: alfdelval@aol.com
Website: http://www.netaxs.com/~emagroup/alfdelva.htm
Peggy Gilbey McMackin, Director
Remarks: Serves Pennsylvania, Delaware, and souther New Jersey.

Tennessee

★ 9024 ★ American Liver Foundation
Mid-South Chapter
5583 Murray Rd., Ste. 205
Memphis, TN 38119
Phone: (901)766-7668 **Fax:** (901)766-2061
Email: midsouthalf@yahoo.com
Laura Jackson, Director

Texas

★ 9025 ★ American Liver Foundation
South Texas Chapter
2425 W Loop S, Ste. 660
Houston, TX 77027
Phone: (713)622-1318 **Fax:** (713)622-1376
Email: LiverSTX@aol.com
Patti Wittlif, Director

Washington

★ 9026 ★ American Liver Foundation
Pacific Northwest Chapter
2033 6th Ave., Ste. 260
Seattle, WA 98121
Phone: (206)443-3805 **Fax:** (206)443-1511
Email: pnwliver@uswest.net
Barbara Hernandez, Director

Wisconsin

★ 9027 ★ American Liver Foundation
Wisconsin Chapter
4929 N Lyndell Ave.
Glendale, WI 53217
Phone: (414)961-4936 **Fax:** (414)961-7288
Email: alfwisc@aol.com
Dee Eberle, Director

Lupus Erythematosus

The following are constituent chapters of the Lupus Foundation of America, 1300 Piccard Dr., Ste. 200, Rockville, MD 20850-4303, (301)670-9292, http://www.lupus.org/.

Alaska

★ 9028 ★ Lupus Foundation of America
Alaska Chapter
PO Box 240628
Anchorage, AK 99524-0268
Phone: (907)338-6332 **Free:** 800-307-5878
Email: LFA_Alaska@hotmail.com
Website: http://members.xoom.com/LFA_Alaska/index.html

Arkansas

★ 9029 ★ Lupus Foundation of America
Arkansas Chapter
220 Mockingbird
Hot Springs, AR 71913
Phone: (501)525-9380 **Free:** 800-294-8878
Email: lupusarkhs@cs.com

California

★ 9030 ★ Lupus Foundation of America
Northern California Chapter
2775 Cottage Way, Ste. 5
Sacramento, CA 95825
Phone: (916)973-0776
Email: saclupus@excite.com
Website: http://www.saclupus.org

★ 9031 ★ Lupus Foundation of America
San Diego Chapter
3914 Murphy Canyon Rd., Ste. A132
San Diego, CA 92123
Phone: (858)278-2788

Connecticut

★ 9032 ★ Lupus Foundation of America
Connecticut Chapter
97 South St., Ste. 110
West Hartford, CT 06110-1960
Phone: (860)953-0387
Email: CTLFA@aol.com
Website: http://www.lupusct.org

Delaware

★ 9033 ★ Lupus Foundation of America
Delaware Chapter
100 W 10th St., Ste. 1015
Wilmington, DE 19801
Phone: (302)622-8700 **Free:** 800-880-8686

Florida

★ 9034 ★ Lupus Foundation of America
Greater Florida Chapter
300 S Duncan Ave., Ste. 235-B
Clearwater, FL 33755
Phone: (727)447-7075 **Free:** 800-684-9276
Email: Greaterfla@aol.com
Website: http://www.lupusflorida.org

★ 9035 ★ Lupus Foundation of America
Northwest Florida Chapter
PO Box 17841
Pensacola, FL 32522-7841
Phone: (850)478-8107 **Free:** 800-458-8211
Email: info@lupus.pensacola.com
Website: http://www.lupus.pensacola.com

★ 9036 ★ Lupus Foundation of America
Southeast Florida Chapter
75 NE 6th Ave., Ste. 223
Delray Beach, FL 33483
Phone: (561)279-8606 **Free:** 800-339-0586

Email: lupusfl@bellsouth.net
Website: http://www.lupusfl.com

Georgia

★ 9037 ★ Lupus Foundation of America
Georgia Chapter
6425 Powers Ferry Rd. NW, Ste. 275
Atlanta, GA 30339-2920
Phone: (770)952-3891 **Free:** 800-800-4LFA
Email: lfagac@attglobal.net
Website: http://www.lfaga.org

Hawaii

★ 9038 ★ Hawaii Lupus Foundation
1200 College Walk, Ste. 114
Honolulu, HI 96817
Phone: (808)538-1522
Email: hlf@pixi.com

Indiana

★ 9039 ★ Lupus Foundation of America
Central Indiana Chapter
PO Box 51066
Indianapolis, IN 46251-1066
Phone: (317)858-9133
Email: lupuscentralin@cs.com

★ 9040 ★ Lupus Foundation of America
Northwest Indiana Chapter
PO Box 2763
Portage, IN 46368
Phone: (219)762-6575
Email: lupusnwichapter@aol.com

Iowa

★ 9041 ★ Lupus Foundation of America
Iowa Chapter
PO Box 13174
Des Moines, IA 50310-0174
Phone: (515)279-3048 **Free:** 888-279-3048
Email: LupusIAchapter@aol.com

Kansas

★ 9042 ★ Lupus Foundation of America
Kansas Chapter
PO Box 12204
Wichita, KS 67277-2204
Phone: (316)262-6180
Email: lupus@kansaslupus.org
Website: http://www.kansaslupus.org

Louisiana

★ 9043 ★ Louisiana Lupus Foundation
7732 Goodwood Blvd., Ste. L
Baton Rouge, LA 70806
Phone: (225)927-8052 **Free:** 888-60-LUPUS

Maryland

★ 9044 ★ Lupus Foundation of America
1300 Piccard Dr., Ste. 200
Rockville, MD 20850-4303
Phone: (301)670-9292 **Free:** 800-558-0121

Missouri

★ 9045 ★ Lupus Foundation of America
Kansas City Chapter
1012-A Main St.
Grandview, MO 64030
Phone: (816)761-0850
Email: lupuskcm@crn.org
Website: http://www.crn.org/lupus/

★ 9046 ★ Lupus Foundation of America
Missouri Chapter
8390 Delmar Blvd.
Saint Louis, MO 63124
Phone: (314)432-0008 **Free:** 800-958-7876
Email: information@lupusmo.org
Website: http://www.lupusmo.org

Nevada

★ 9047 ★ Lupus Foundation of America
Northern Nevada Chapter
1000 Bible Way, Ste. 69
Reno, NV 89502
Phone: (775)323-2444

★ 9048 ★ Lupus Foundation of America
Southern Nevada Chapter
PO Box 34645
Las Vegas, NV 89133-4645
Phone: (702)566-1425
Email: SNVLupus@aol.com

New Hampshire

★ 9049 ★ New Hampshire Lupus Foundation, Inc.
PO Box 5500
Manchester, NH 03108-5500
Phone: (603)424-0111
Email: Lupusnh@email.msn.com
Website: http://communities.msn.com/Lupusmemorabilia

New Jersey

★ 9050 ★ Lupus Foundation of America
New Jersey Chapter
PO Box 320
Elmwood Park, NJ 07407
Phone: (201)791-7868 **Free:** 800-322-5816
Email: NJ4lupus@aol.com

★ 9051 ★ Lupus Foundation of America
South Jersey Chapter
Business Executive Complexes
1873 Rte. 70 E, Ste. 110F
Cherry Hill, NJ 08003
Phone: (856)424-0255 **Free:** 877-475-8787
Email: lupssj@cs.com

New Mexico

★ 9052 ★ Lupus Foundation of America
New Mexico Chapter
2917 Carlisle Blvd. NE, Ste. 103
Albuquerque, NM 87110-2850
Phone: (505)881-9081
Email: lfanm@juno.com
Website: http://www.lupusnm.org

New York

★ 9053 ★ Lupus Foundation of America
Bronx Chapter
PO Box 1117
Bronx, NY 10462
Phone: (718)822-6542

★ 9054 ★ Lupus Foundation of America
Central New York Chapter
Pickard Office Bldg.
5858 E Molloy Rd., Ste. 173
Syracuse, NY 13211
Phone: (315)454-9886 **Fax:** (315)454-9887
Email: cnylupus@aol.com

★ 9055 ★ Lupus Foundation of America
Genesee Valley Chapter
500 Helendale Rd., Ste. 153
Rochester, NY 14609
Phone: (585)288-2910
Email: lupusgvc@frontiernet.net

★ 9056 ★ Lupus Foundation of America
Marguerite Curri Chapter
PO Box 139
Utica, NY 13503
Phone: (315)829-4272
Email: lupusmcurri@aol.com
Remarks: Serves the counties of Herkimer, Jefferson, Lewis, Madison, Oneida, Otsego and St. Lawrence.

★ 9057 ★ Lupus Foundation of America
Northeastern New York Chapter
790 Watervliet-Shaker Rd.
Latham, NY 12110
Phone: (518)786-9698 **Free:** 888-749-0100
Email: NENYLFA@aol.com
Website: http://nenylfa.tripod.com

North Carolina

★ 9058 ★ Lupus Foundation of America
Harnett County/Fayetteville/Raleigh Branch
PO Box 1622
Coats, NC 27521
Phone: (910)897-8917
Email: rbenson@intrastar.net
Website: http://www.ncneighbors.com/1090

★ 9059 ★ Lupus Foundation of America
Piedmont Chapter
1235-E East Blvd., No. 226
Charlotte, NC 28203
Phone: (704)375-8787
Email: lupuslinks@aol.com
Website: http://www.lupuslinks.org

★ 9060 ★ Lupus Foundation of America
Winston—Triad Lupus Chapter NCLF
2841 Foxwood Lane
Winston-Salem, NC 27103
Phone: (336)768-1493
Email: lfawinston-t.nclf@juno.com

Ohio

★ 9061 ★ Lupus Foundation of America
Akron Area Chapter
2769 Front St.
Cuyahoga Falls, OH 44221
Phone: (330)945-6767
Email: lupusakron@aol.com
Website: http://www.lupusohio.org

★ 9062 ★ Lupus Foundation of America
Columbus, Marcy Zitron Chapter
6161 Busch Blvd., Ste. 76
Columbus, OH 43229
Phone: (614)221-0811
Email: columbus@lupusohio.org
Website: http://www.lupusohio.org

★ 9063 ★ Lupus Foundation of America Greater Cleveland Chapter
12930 Chippewa Rd., Ste. 6
Rt. 82 at Riverview
Brecksville, OH 44141
Phone: (440)717-0183
Email: lupuscleveland@aol.com
Website: http://www.lupuscleveland.org

★ 9064 ★ Lupus Foundation of America Northwest Ohio Lupus Chapter
337 S Main St., Rm. 14
Findlay, OH 45840
Phone: (419)423-9313 **Free:** 888-33-LUPUS
Fax: (419)423-5959
Email: lupusnwo@juno.com
Website: http://www.lupusohio.org

Oklahoma

★ 9065 ★ Oklahoma Lupus Foundation
3131 N MacArthur, Ste. 106-B
Oklahoma City, OK 73122
Phone: (405)495-8787 **Free:** 800-725-6445
Email: oklupus@flash.net

Pennsylvania

★ 9066 ★ Lupus Foundation of America Southeastern Pennsylvania Chapter
25 Washington Ln., Ste. 39LL
Wyncote, PA 19095
Phone: (215)517-5070
Email: info@lupus-sepa.org
Website: http://www.lupus-sepa.org

★ 9067 ★ Lupus Foundation of Pennsylvania Erie Branch
3711 W 12th St., Unit 7
Erie, PA 16505
Phone: (814)838-0713 **Free:** 800-800-5776
Website: http://www.lupuspa.org

★ 9068 ★ Lupus Foundation of Pennsylvania Harrisburg Branch
5405 Jonestown Rd., Ste. 110
Harrisburg, PA 17112
Phone: (717)671-9515 **Free:** 888-215-8787
Fax: (717)671-9532
Email: cplclfa@aol.com
Website: http://www.lupuspa.org

★ 9069 ★ Lupus Foundation of Pennsylvania Pittsburgh Branch
Landmarks Bldg.
One Station Square Dr., Ste. 575
Pittsburgh, PA 15219
Phone: (412)261-5886 **Free:** 800-800-5776
Fax: (412)261-5365
Email: info@lupuspa.org
Website: http://www.lupuspa.org

★ 9070 ★ Lupus Foundation of Pennsylvania Pocono/Northeast Branch
Keystone College
One College Green
La Plume, PA 18440-0200
Phone: (570)945-5118 **Free:** 888-995-8787
Fax: (570)945-5119
Email: LUPUSNEPA@aol.com
Website: http://www.lupuspa.org

Rhode Island

★ 9071 ★ Lupus Foundation of America Rhode Island Chapter
8 Fallon Ave.
Providence, RI 02908
Phone: (401)421-7227

South Carolina

★ 9072 ★ Lupus Foundation of America South Carolina Chapter
PO Box 1427
Easley, SC 29641-1427
Phone: (864)269-2887 **Free:** 877-895-8787
Fax: (864)220-1009
Email: lupuslfasc@juno.com
Website: http://www.midnet.sc.edu/Lupus/Lupus.htm

Tennessee

★ 9073 ★ Lupus Foundation of America East Tennessee Chapter
10409 Lovell Center Dr.
Knoxville, TN 37922
Phone: (865)692-9825 **Free:** 888-59-LUPUS
Fax: (865)692-9826
Email: lupusTN1@aol.com

★ 9074 ★ Lupus Foundation of America Memphis Area Chapter
3181 Poplar Ave., Ste. 100
Memphis, TN 38111
Phone: (901)458-5302
Email: MemLupusFund@aol.com
Website: http://hometown.aol.com/tdhood69/myhomepage/business.html

★ 9075 ★ Lupus Foundation of America Nashville Area Chapter
4004 Hillsboro Rd., Ste. 223-B
Nashville, TN 37215
Phone: (615)298-2273
Email: lupustn@usit.com
Website: http://www.lupusnashville.org

Texas

★ 9076 ★ Lupus Foundation of America El Paso Area Branch
1401 Montana Ave., Ste. N
El Paso, TX 79902
Phone: (915)542-0330 **Fax:** (915)542-0012
Email: butterfly_hugs@cs.com

★ 9077 ★ Lupus Foundation of America North Texas Chapter
PO Box 810310
Dallas, TX 75381-0310
Phone: (972)345-4824 **Free:** 800-285-2369
Website: http://www.lupus-northtexas.org

★ 9078 ★ Lupus Foundation of America South Central Texas Chapter, Inc.
3308 Broadway, Stes. 209-210
San Antonio, TX 78209
Phone: (210)651-9480 **Free:** 800-809-3953
Email: lupustx@sbcglobal.net
Website: http://www.lupusstx.org

★ 9079 ★ Lupus Foundation of America Texas Gulf Coast Chapter
3730 Kirby Dr., Ste. 720
Houston, TX 77098
Phone: (713)529-0126 **Free:** 800-458-7870
Email: LFA@lupustexas.org
Website: http://www.lupustexas.org

★ 9080 ★ Lupus Foundation of America West Texas Chapter
1717 Ave. K, Ste. 224
Lubbock, TX 79401
Phone: (806)744-6666 **Free:** 800-580-5878
Email: lfawesttx@juno.com

Utah

★ 9081 ★ Lupus Foundation of America Utah Chapter, Inc.
455 E 500 S, Lower Level No. 2
Salt Lake City, UT 84111
Phone: (801)364-0366 **Free:** 800-657-6398
Email: LFAUtah1@mcleodusa.net
Website: http://lupuswest.topcities.com
Remarks: Also serves Idaho, Montana and Wyoming.

Vermont

★ 9082 ★ Lupus Foundation of America Vermont Chapter
PO Box 115
Waterbury, VT 05676
Phone: (802)244-5988
Email: LupusVT@aol.com

Virginia

★ 9083 ★ Lupus Foundation of America Eastern Virginia Chapter
Pembroke One
281 Independence Blvd., Ste. 434
Virginia Beach, VA 23462
Phone: (757)490-2793 **Fax:** (757)490-1086
Email: evalupus@yahoo.com

Washington

★ 9084 ★ Lupus Foundation of America Pacific Northwest Chapter
17962 Midvale Ave. N, Ste. 208
Shoreline, WA 98133
Phone: (206)546-6785 **Free:** 877-774-2992
Email: lupuspncwa@earthlink.net
Remarks: Serves Washington, Oregon and Idaho.

Wisconsin

★ 9085 ★ Lupus Foundation of America Wisconsin Chapter, Inc.
8544 W National Ave., Ste. 22-24
West Allis, WI 53227
Phone: (414)541-3033
Email: lupuswi@aol.com

Lyme Disease

State chapters of the Lyme Alliance are listed below. The national office is located at PO Box 454, Concord, MI 49237. Additional information can be obtained by calling the national office at (517) 563-3582, or by consulting their web site at http://www.lymealliance.org/.

California

★ 9086 ★ Lyme Disease Resource Center
PO Box 707
Weaverville, CA 96093
Email: info@lymedisease.org
Website: http://www.lymedisease.org/index.html
Nancy Brown, President

Connecticut

★ 9087 ★ Lyme Disease Foundation
1 Financial Plaza
Hartford, CT 06103-2601
Phone: (860)525-2000 **Free:** 800-886-5963
Fax: (860)525-8425
Email: Lymefnd@aol.com
Website: http://www.lyme.org

Massachusetts

★ 9088 ★ Massachusetts Lyme Disease Coalition
Cape Cod Lyme Disease Awareness Association
PO Box 1916
Mashpee, MA 02649
Phone: (508)563-7033
John Coughlan, President

Michigan

★ 9089 ★ Lyme Alliance, Inc.
PO Box 454
Concord, MI 49237
Phone: (517)563-3582 **Fax:** (517)524-7250
Email: barbfitz@concentric.net
Website: http://www.lymealliance.org

Minnesota

★ 9090 ★ Lyme Disease Coalition of Minnesota
902 Grandview Ave.
Duluth, MN 55812-1146
Phone: (218)728-3914
Email: lymenet_mn@yahoo.com
Website: http://www.freeyellow.com/members2/olivierlynn/page3.html
Tom Grier, President

New Jersey

★ 9091 ★ Lyme Disease Association
5019 Megill Rd.
Farmingdale, NJ 07727
Phone: (732)938-4834
Email: lymeliter@aol.com
Website: http://www.lymediseaseassociation.org
Pat Smith, President

Medicine

Listed below are state medical associations. The national organization is the American Medical Association, 515 N State St., Chicago, IL 60610, (312)464-5000, http://www.ama-assn.org/.

Alabama

★ 9092 ★ Medical Association of the State of Alabama
19 S Jackson St.
Montgomery, AL 36104
Phone: (334)954-2500 **Fax:** (334)269-5200
Email: cary@MASALINK.org
Website: http://www.MASALINK.org

Alaska

★ 9093 ★ Alaska State Medical Association
4107 Laurel St.
Anchorage, AK 99508
Phone: (907)562-0304 **Fax:** (907)561-2063
Email: ASMA@alaska.net
Website: http://www.akmed.org

Arizona

★ 9094 ★ Arizona Medical Association
810 W Bethany Home Rd.
Phoenix, AZ 85013
Phone: (602)246-8901 **Fax:** (602)242-6283
Website: http://www.azmedassn.org

Arkansas

★ 9095 ★ Arkansas Medical Society
PO Box 55088
Little Rock, AR 72215
Phone: (501)224-8967 **Fax:** (501)224-6489
Website: http://www.arkmed.org

California

★ 9096 ★ California Medical Association
PO Box 7690
San Francisco, CA 94120
Phone: (415)541-0900 **Fax:** (415)882-3349
Website: http://www.cmanet.org
Steve Thompson, Vice President

Colorado

★ 9097 ★ Colorado Medical Society
PO Box 17550
Denver, CO 80217-0550
Phone: (720)859-1001 **Fax:** (720)859-7509
Website: http://www.cms.org

Connecticut

★ 9098 ★ Connecticut State Medical Society
160 St. Ronan St.
New Haven, CT 06511
Phone: (203)865-0587 **Fax:** (203)865-4997
Website: http://www.csms.org

Delaware

★ 9099 ★ Medical Society of Delaware
131 Continental Dr., Ste. 405
Newark, DE 19713
Phone: (302)658-7596 **Fax:** (302)658-9669
Website: http://www.medsocdel.org

District of Columbia

★ 9100 ★ Medical Society of the District of Columbia
2175 K St. NW, Ste. 200
Washington, DC 20037
Phone: (202)466-1800 **Fax:** (202)452-1542
Website: http://www.msds.org

Florida

★ 9101 ★ Florida Medical Association
113 E College Ave.
PO Box 10269
Tallahassee, FL 32302
Phone: (850)224-6496 **Fax:** (850)222-8030
Website: http://www.fmaonline.org

Georgia

★ 9102 ★ Medical Association of Georgia
1330 W Peachtree St. NW, Ste. 500
Atlanta, GA 30309-2904
Phone: (404)876-7535 **Fax:** (404)881-5073
Website: http://www.mag.org
David A. Cook, Director

Hawaii

★ 9103 ★ Hawaii Medical Association
1360 S Beretania St., 2nd Fl.
Honolulu, HI 96814
Phone: (808)536-7702 **Fax:** (808)528-2376
Website: http://www.hma-assn.org

Idaho

★ 9104 ★ Idaho Medical Association
305 W Jefferson St.
Boise, ID 83701
Phone: (208)344-7888 **Fax:** (208)344-7903
Email: ima@micron.net
Website: http://www.idmed.org

Illinois

★ 9105 ★ Illinois State Medical Society
20 N Michigan Ave., Ste. 700
Chicago, IL 60602
Phone: (312)782-1654 **Fax:** (312)782-2023
Email: info@isms.org
Website: http://www.isms.org

Indiana

★ 9106 ★ Indiana State Medical Association
322 Canal Walk, Canal Level
Indianapolis, IN 46202
Phone: (317)261-2060 **Fax:** (317)261-2076
Website: http://www.ismanet.org

Iowa

★ 9107 ★ Iowa Medical Society
1001 Grand Ave.
West Des Moines, IA 50265
Phone: (515)223-1401 **Fax:** (515)223-0590
Website: http://www.iowamedical.org

Kansas

★ 9108 ★ Kansas Medical Society
623 SW 10th Ave.
Topeka, KS 66612
Phone: (785)235-2383 **Fax:** (785)235-5114
Email: ksmedsoc@inlandnet.net
Website: http://www.kmsonline.org

Kentucky

★ 9109 ★ Kentucky Medical Association
4965 U.S. Hwy. 42, Ste. 2000
Louisville, KY 40222
Phone: (502)426-6200 **Fax:** (502)426-6877
Website: http://www.kyma.org

Louisiana

★ 9110 ★ Louisiana State Medical Society
6767 Perkins Rd.
Baton Rouge, LA 70808
Phone: (225)763-8500 **Fax:** (225)763-6122
Website: http://www.lsms.org
Sharon Knight, JD, Director

Maine

★ 9111 ★ Maine Medical Association
PO Box 190
Manchester, ME 04351
Phone: (207)622-3374 **Fax:** (207)622-3332
Website: http://www.mainemed.com

Maryland

★ 9112 ★ Medical and Chirurgical Faculty of Maryland (MedChi)
Maryland State Medical Society
1211 Cathedral St.
Baltimore, MD 21201
Phone: (410)539-0872 **Fax:** (410)547-0915
Website: http://www.medchi.org

Massachusetts

★ 9113 ★ Massachusetts Medical Society
860 Winter St.
Waltham Woods Corporate Ctr.
Waltham, MA 02451-1423
Phone: (781)893-4610 **Fax:** (781)893-8009
Website: http://www.massmed.org

Michigan

★ 9114 ★ Michigan State Medical Society
120 W Saginaw
East Lansing, MI 48823
Phone: (517)337-1351 **Fax:** (517)337-2490
Website: http://www.msms.org

Minnesota

★ 9115 ★ Minnesota Medical Association
3433 Broadway St. NE, Ste. 300
Minneapolis, MN 55413-1761
Phone: (612)378-1875 **Fax:** (612)378-3875
Website: http://www.mnmed.org

Mississippi

★ 9116 ★ Mississippi State Medical Association
PO Box 2548
Ridgeland, MS 39158-2548
Phone: (601)853-6733 **Fax:** (601)853-6746
Website: http://www.msmaonline.com

Missouri

★ 9117 ★ Missouri Medical Association
113 Madison St.
PO Box 1028
Jefferson City, MO 65102
Phone: (573)636-5151 **Fax:** (573)636-8552
Website: http://www.msma.org

Montana

★ 9118 ★ Montana Medical Association
2021 11th Ave., Ste. 1
Helena, MT 59601
Phone: (406)443-4000 **Fax:** (406)443-4042
Website: http://www.mmaoffice.com

Nebraska

★ 9119 ★ Nebraska Medical Association
233 S 13th St., Ste. 1512
Lincoln, NE 68508
Phone: (402)474-4472 **Fax:** (402)474-2198
Email: nma@inetnebr.com
Website: http://www.nebmed.org

Nevada

★ 9120 ★ Nevada State Medical Association
3660 Baker Ln., Ste. 101
Reno, NV 89509
Phone: (702)825-6788 **Fax:** (702)825-3202
Email: nvstmeda@aol.com
Website: http://www.nsmadocs.org/index.html

New Hampshire

★ 9121 ★ New Hampshire Medical Society
7 N State St.
Concord, NH 03301
Phone: (603)224-1909 **Fax:** (603)226-2432
Website: http://www.nhms.org

New Jersey

★ 9122 ★ Medical Society of New Jersey
2 Princess Rd.
Lawrenceville, NJ 08648
Phone: (609)896-1766 **Fax:** (609)896-1368
Email: info@msnj.org
Website: http://www.msnj.org

New Mexico

★ 9123 ★ New Mexico Medical Society
7700 Jefferson NE, Ste. 400
Albuquerque, NM 87109
Phone: (505)828-0237 **Fax:** (505)828-0336
Email: nmms@nmms.org
Website: http://www.nmms.org/nmms/

New York

★ 9124 ★ Medical Society of the State of New York
420 Lakeville Rd.
Lake Success, NY 11042-5404
Phone: (516)488-6100 **Fax:** (516)488-1267
Website: http://www.mssny.org
Gerard L. Conway, Director

North Carolina

★ 9125 ★ North Carolina Medical Society
222 N Person St.
PO Box 27167
Raleigh, NC 27611
Phone: (919)833-3836 **Fax:** (919)833-2023
Website: http://www.ncmedsoc.org
Stephen W. Keene, Director

North Dakota

★ 9126 ★ North Dakota Medical Association
1025 3rd St. N
PO Box 1198
Bismarck, ND 58502-1198
Phone: (701)223-9475 **Fax:** (701)223-9476
Website: http://www.ndmed.com

Ohio

★ 9127 ★ Ohio State Medical Association
3401 Mill Run Dr.
Hilliard, OH 43026
Phone: (614)527-6762 **Fax:** (614)527-6763
Website: http://www.osma.org
Tim I. Maglione, Director

Oklahoma

★ 9128 ★ Oklahoma State Medical Association
601 NW Grand. Blvd.
Oklahoma City, OK 73118
Phone: (405)843-9571 **Fax:** (405)842-1834
Website: http://www.okmed.org

Oregon

★ 9129 ★ Oregon Medical Association
5210 SW Corbett St.
Portland, OR 97201
Phone: (503)226-1555 **Fax:** (503)241-7148
Website: http://www.ormedassoc.org
Scott C. R. Gallant, BA, Director

Pennsylvania

★ 9130 ★ Pennsylvania Medical Society
777 E Park Dr.
PO Box 8820
Harrisburg, PA 17105-8820
Phone: (717)558-7750 **Fax:** (717)558-7840
Website: http://www.pamedsoc.org

Puerto Rico

★ 9131 ★ Asociacion Medica de Puerto Rico
Ave. Fernandez Juncos No. 1305
Santurce, PR 00908
Phone: (787)721-6969 **Fax:** (787)722-1191
Website: http://www.asociacionmedicapr.com/index.htm
Alt. Contact: PO Box 9387, San Juan, PR 00908.

Rhode Island

★ 9132 ★ Rhode Island Medical Society
106 Francis St.
Providence, RI 02903
Phone: (401)331-3207 **Fax:** (401)751-8050
Email: RIMS@ids.net
Website: http://www.rimed.org

South Carolina

★ 9133 ★ South Carolina Medical Association
PO Box 11188
Columbia, SC 29211
Free: 800-327-1021 **Fax:** (803)772-6783
Website: http://www.scmanet.org
Jan McKellar, Director

South Dakota

★ 9134 ★ South Dakota State Medical Association
1323 S Minnesota Ave.
Sioux Falls, SD 57105
Phone: (605)336-1965 **Fax:** (605)336-0270
Website: http://www.usd.edu/med/sdsma

Tennessee

★ 9135 ★ Tennessee Medical Association
PO Box 120909
Nashville, TN 37212
Phone: (615)385-2100 **Fax:** (615)383-5918
Website: http://www.medwire.org/

Texas

★ 9136 ★ Texas Medical Association
401 W 15th St.
Austin, TX 78701-1680
Phone: (512)370-1300 **Fax:** (512)370-1693
Website: http://www.texmed.org

Utah

★ 9137 ★ Utah Medical Association
540 E 500 S
Salt Lake City, UT 84102
Phone: (801)355-7477 **Fax:** (801)532-1550
Website: http://www.utahmed.org
Val Bateman, Exec VP

Vermont

★ 9138 ★ Vermont Medical Society
PO Box 1457
Montpelier, VT 05601-1457
Phone: (802)223-7898 **Fax:** (802)223-1201
Website: http://www.vtmd.org

Virginia

★ 9139 ★ Medical Society of Virginia
4205 Dover Rd.
Richmond, VA 23221
Phone: (804)353-2721 **Fax:** (804)355-6189
Website: http://www.msv.org

Washington

★ 9140 ★ Washington State Medical Association
2033 6th Ave., Ste. 1100
Seattle, WA 98121
Phone: (206)441-9762 **Fax:** (206)441-5863
Website: http://www.wsma.org
Len Eddinger, Director

West Virginia

★ 9141 ★ West Virginia State Medical Association
4307 MacCorkle Ave. SE
PO Box 4106
Charleston, WV 25364
Phone: (304)925-0342 **Fax:** (304)925-0345
Website: http://www.wvsma.com

Wisconsin

★ 9142 ★ State Medical Society of Wisconsin
PO Box 1109
Madison, WI 53701
Phone: (608)257-6781 **Fax:** (608)283-5401
Website: http://www.wismed.org

Wyoming

★ 9143 ★ Wyoming Medical Society
1920 Evans Ave.
PO Box 4009
Cheyenne, WY 82003
Phone: (307)635-2424 **Fax:** (307)632-1973
Website: http://www.wyomed.org

Mental Health

Associations listed below are state affiliates of the National Mental Health Association, 2001 N. Beauregard St., 12th Fl., Alexandria, VA 22311, 800-969-NMHA, http://www.nmha.org/. Contact the national association for information on states not listed here.

Alabama

★ 9144 ★ National Mental Health Association in Etowah County
901 Goodyear Ave.
Gadsden, AL 35903
Phone: (256)492-3381 **Fax:** (256)494-5536
Email: mhaofet@internetpro.net
Cathy Spivey, Director

★ 9145 ★ National Mental Health Association in Madison County
701 Andrew Jackson Way
Huntsville, AL 35801
Phone: (256)536-9441 **Fax:** (256)534-7533
Email: director@mentalhealthalabama.org
Website: http://www.mentalhealthalabama.org
Sandra Moon, Director

★ 9146 ★ National Mental Health Association in Montgomery
1116 S Hull St.
Montgomery, AL 36104
Phone: (334)262-5500 **Fax:** (334)262-1576
Email: mhamontg@hiwaay.net
Darold Dunlavy, Exec Director

★ 9147 ★ National Mental Health Association in Morgan County
PO Box 1502
Decatur, AL 35602
Phone: (256)353-1160 **Fax:** (256)353-1163
Email: sue@mhainmc.org
Website: http://www.mhainmc.org
Sue Brantley, Director

★ 9148 ★ National Mental Health Association in Southwestern Alabama
PO Box 282
Montrose, AL 36559-0282
Phone: (334)626-9585
Email: mhaswa@msn.com

★ 9149 ★ National Mental Health Association in Tuscaloosa County
2123 9th St.
Tuscaloosa, AL 35401
Phone: (205)752-2689 **Fax:** (205)758-5773
Joan Brown, Director

Alaska

★ 9150 ★ National Mental Health Association in Alaska
4050 Lake Otis Pkwy., Ste. 204-A
Anchorage, AK 99508
Phone: (907)563-0880 **Fax:** (907)563-0881
Email: mhaa@alaska.net
Website: http://www.alaska.net/~mhaa/
Jan McGillivary, Director

Arizona

★ 9151 ★ National Mental Health Association of Arizona, Scottsdale
6411 E Thomas Rd.
Scottsdale, AZ 85251
Phone: (480)994-4407 **Fax:** (480)994-4744
Email: mhaaz@qwest.net
Website: http://www.mhaaz.com

★ 9152 ★ National Mental Health Association of Southern Arizona
1905 E 7th St., Bldg. 4
Tucson, AZ 85719
Phone: (520)882-4806 **Fax:** (520)882-0124
Email: mhatucson1@aol.com
Website: http://www.mhaaz.com
Cheryl Collier Becker, Director

Arkansas

★ 9153 ★ National Mental Health Association in Northwest Arkansas
PO Box 1993
Fayetteville, AR 72702-1993

California

★ 9154 ★ National Mental Health Association of Alameda County
1801 Adeline St., Rm. 203
Oakland, CA 94607
Phone: (510)835-5010 **Fax:** (510)835-9232
Email: mhaac@wenet.net
Website: http://www.mhaac.org

★ 9155 ★ National Mental Health Association of California
1127 11th St., Ste. 830
Sacramento, CA 95814
Phone: (916)557-1167 **Fax:** (916)447-2350
Email: rselix@mhac.org
Website: http://www.mhac.org
Rusty Selix, Director

★ 9156 ★ National Mental Health Association Los Angeles County
1336 Wilshire Blvd., 2nd Fl.
Los Angeles, CA 90017-1705
Phone: (213)413-1130 **Fax:** (213)413-1114
Email: rvanhorn@mhala.org
Website: http://www.mhala.org

★ 9157 ★ National Mental Health Association in Los Angeles County
1336 Wilshire Blvd., 2nd Fl.
Los Angeles, CA 90017
Phone: (213)413-1130 **Fax:** (213)413-1114
Email: mailbox@mhala.org
Website: http://www.mhala.org

★ 9158 ★ National Mental Health Association in Sacramento
9719 Lincoln Village Dr., St. 407
Sacramento, CA 95827
Phone: (916)366-4600 **Fax:** (916)855-5448
Email: information@mhasc.org
Website: http://www.mhasc.org

★ 9159 ★ National Mental Health Association in Sacramento
9719 Lincoln Village Dr., Ste. 407
Sacramento, CA 95827
Phone: (916)366-4600 **Fax:** (916)855-5448
Email: information@mhasc.org
Website: http://www.mhasc.org/open.htm

★ 9160 ★ National Mental Health Association in San Diego County
2047 El Cajun Blvd.
San Diego, CA 92104-1091
Phone: (619)543-0412 **Fax:** (619)543-0748
Email: mhasd@flash.net
Website: http://www.mhasd.org

★ 9161 ★ National Mental Health Association in San Diego County
2047 El Cajon Blvd.
San Diego, CA 92104
Phone: (619)543-0412 **Fax:** (619)543-0748
Email: mhasd@flash.net

★ 9162 ★ National Mental Health Association of San Francisco
1095 Market St., Ste. 408
San Francisco, CA 94103
Phone: (415)241-2926 **Fax:** (415)241-2928
Email: mhaofsf@aol.com

★ 9163 ★ National Mental Health Association of Santa Barbara
2017 Chapala St.
Santa Barbara, CA 93105
Phone: (805)569-1607 **Fax:** (805)682-0906
Email: sbmha@aol.com

★ 9164 ★ National Mental Health Association in Santa Barbara
2017 Chapala St.
Santa Barbara, CA 93105
Phone: (805)569-1607 **Fax:** (805)682-0906
Email: sbmha@aol.com
Annmarie Cameron, Exec Director

★ 9165 ★ Riverside Mental Health Advocacy Program
3634 Elizabeth St.
Riverside, CA 92506
Phone: (909)686-3706 **Fax:** (909)686-7267
Website: http://www.familyserviceriv.ca.com
Aggie Jenkins, President

Colorado

★ 9166 ★ National Mental Health Association of Colorado
6795 E Tennessee Ave., No. 425
Denver, CO 80224
Phone: (303)377-3040 **Free:** 800-456-3249
Fax: (303)377-4920
Email: jmrohner@mhacolorado.org
Website: http://www.mhacolorado.org
Victoria Simonsen, Director

★ 9167 ★ National Mental Health Association of El Paso County
12 N Meade Ave.
Colorado Springs, CO 80909
Phone: (719)633-4601 **Fax:** (719)633-0845
Email: mha@pppartnership.org
Website: http://www.pppartnership.org

★ 9168 ★ National Mental Health Association of the Midwest
PO Box 1468
Paonia, CO 81428
Phone: (970)527-4388 **Fax:** (970)527-6761
Email: rt.rt@juno.com

★ 9169 ★ National Mental Health Association of the Midwest
PO Box 1468
Paonia, CO 81428
Phone: (970)527-4388 **Fax:** (970)527-6761

★ 9170 ★ National Mental Health Association of Pueblo
PO Box 4623
Pueblo, CO 81003
Phone: (719)583-9798 **Fax:** (719)544-5708
Email: jackselway@puebloadvocacy.com
Website: http://www.puebloadvocacy.com

Connecticut

★ 9171 ★ National Mental Health Association of Connecticut
20-30 Beaver Rd.
Wethersfield, CT 06109
Phone: (860)529-1970 **Fax:** (860)529-6833
Email: webmaster@mhact.org
Website: http://www.mhact.org

Delaware

★ 9172 ★ National Mental Health Association in Delaware
812-D Philadelphia Pike
Wilmington, DE 19809
Phone: (302)765-9740 **Fax:** (302)765-9745
Email: dtreacy@dca.net
Website: http://www.mhainde.org

District of Columbia

★ 9173 ★ National Mental Health Association of Washington DC
1628 16th St. NW
Washington, DC 20009
Phone: (202)265-6363 **Fax:** (202)265-3265
Email: info@mhadc.org
Website: http://www.mhadc.org

Florida

★ 9174 ★ National Mental Health Association of Bay County
PO Box 2245
Panama City, FL 32402
Phone: (850)769-5441 **Fax:** (850)769-5528
Email: mhabay@knology.net

★ 9175 ★ National Mental Health Association of Broward County
7145 W Oakland Park Blvd.
Lauderhill, FL 33313
Phone: (954)746-2055 **Fax:** (954)746-6373
Email: mhaceo@aol.org
Website: http://www.mhabroward.org

★ 9176 ★ National Mental Health Association of Central Florida
608 Mariposa St.
Orlando, FL 32801
Phone: (407)843-1563 **Fax:** (407)843-4245
Email: mhacf@aol.com
Website: http://www.mhacf.com
Juanita Hernandez-Black, CEO & Pres

★ 9177 ★ National Mental Health Association of Collier County
2335 9th St. N, Ste. 404
Naples, FL 34103
Phone: (941)261-5405 **Fax:** (941)261-2931
Email: ccmha@mindspring.com
Website: http://www.ccmha.org

★ 9178 ★ National Mental Health Association of Greater Tampa Bay, Inc.
20505 U.S. Hwy. 19 N, Ste. 19
Clearwater, FL 33764
Phone: (727)669-1385 **Fax:** (727)669-1394
Email: mha@mha-tampabay.com
Website: http://www.mha-tampabay.com
Kelly Stuart Williams, CEO & Pres

★ 9179 ★ National Mental Health Association of Indian River County
2001 9th Ave., Ste. 301
Vero Beach, FL 32960
Phone: (561)569-9788 **Fax:** (561)569-2088

★ 9180 ★ National Mental Health Association in Northeast Florida, Inc.
4615 Phillips Hwy.
Jacksonville, FL 32207-2363
Phone: (904)399-5468 **Fax:** (904)399-3908
Email: mentalhealth@fcol.com
Website: http://www.mhajax.org
Claud Myers, CEO & Pres

★ 9181 ★ National Mental Health Association of Okaloosa and Walton Counties
PO Box 505
Fort Walton Beach, FL 32549
Phone: (850)244-1040 **Fax:** (850)244-2573
Email: mhaowfl@gnt.net
Website: http://www.mhaow.org
Program(s): Mental Health Education; 'Kids Link' Children's Mental Health Information and Referral Program; Mental Health Career Counseling; Domestic Violence Awareness.

★ 9182 ★ National Mental Health Association of Palm Beach County, Inc.
909 Fern St.
West Palm Beach, FL 33401
Phone: (561)832-3755 **Fax:** (561)832-3900
Email: info@mentalhealthpbc.com
Website: http://www.mentalhealthpbc.com

★ 9183 ★ National Mental Health Association of Palm Beach County, Inc.
909 Fern St.
West Palm Beach, FL 33401
Phone: (561)832-3755 **Fax:** (561)832-3990
Email: info@mentalhealthpbc.com
Website: http://www.mentalhealthpbc.com

★ 9184 ★ National Mental Health Association of Volusia and Flagler Counties
531 S Ridgewood Ave.
Daytona Beach, FL 32114-2554
Phone: (386)252-5785 **Fax:** (386)255-7560
Email: mhadbfl@bellsouth.net
Website: http://www.mhavolusia.org

★ 9185 ★ National Mental Health Association of West Florida, Inc.
840 W Lakeview Ave.
Pensacola, FL 32501
Phone: (850)438-9879 **Free:** 888-723-6544
Fax: (850)438-5901
Email: kgarber@mhawfl.org
Website: http://www.mhawfl.org
Karen Garber, CEO & Pres

Georgia

★ 9186 ★ National Mental Health Association of Clayton County
PO Box 524
Morrow, GA 30260-9998
Phone: (770)991-8509 **Fax:** (770)991-8507
Email: deborah_hanks@msn.com

★ 9187 ★ National Mental Health Association of Georgia
100 Edgewood Ave. NE, Ste. 502
Atlanta, GA 30303-3068
Phone: (404)527-7175 **Fax:** (404)527-7187
Email: executiveoffice@nmhag.org
Website: http://www.nmhag.org

★ 9188 ★ National Mental Health Association of Greater Augusta, Inc.
1720 Central Ave.
Augusta, GA 30904
Phone: (706)736-4339 **Fax:** (706)738-3548
Email: friendshipcenter@hotmail.com

★ 9189 ★ National Mental Health Association of Middle Flint
PO Box 1063
Oglethorpe, GA 31068
Phone: (478)472-4738

★ 9190 ★ National Mental Health Association of Newton County
PO Box 206
Covington, GA 30015-0206
Phone: (770)786-0807
Email: nccp@bellsouth.net

★ 9191 ★ National Mental Health Association of North Georgia Mountains
Stephens County Police Department
PO Box 579
Toccoa, GA 30577
Phone: (706)886-8655 **Fax:** (706)282-3316
Email: toccoagapd@alltel.net
Curtis Scott, President

★ 9192 ★ National Mental Health Association of Northeast Georgia
PO Box 6384
Athens, GA 30604
Phone: (706)549-7888 **Fax:** (706)549-1651
Email: mhanega@bellsouth.net

★ 9193 ★ National Mental Health Association of South Coastal Georgia
PO Box 189
Brunswick, GA 31521-0189
Phone: (912)638-2320 **Fax:** (912)638-1446
Email: mhaone@adelphia.org

★ 9194 ★ National Mental Health Association of Wayne County
PO Box 935
Jesup, GA 31598
Phone: (912)579-2205

Hawaii

★ 9195 ★ National Mental Health Association in Hawaii
200 N Vineyard Blvd., No. 300
Honolulu, HI 96817
Phone: (808)521-1846 **Fax:** (808)533-6995
Email: mha@i-one.com
Website: http://www.mhahawaii.org/

★ 9196 ★ National Mental Health Association in Hawaii County
HCR 1, Box 5822
Keaau, HI 96749
Phone: (808)965-6601 **Fax:** (808)966-9825
Email: grogan@ilhawaii.net
Website: http://mhahawaii.org

★ 9197 ★ National Mental Health Association in Kauai County
200 N Vineyard Blvd., No. 300
Honolulu, HI 96817
Phone: (808)521-1846
Website: http://www.mhahawaii.org

★ 9198 ★ National Mental Health Association in Maui County
95 Mahalani St.
Wailuku, HI 96793
Phone: (808)242-6461 **Fax:** (808)242-1857
Website: http://www.mhahawaii.org

Idaho

★ 9199 ★ National Mental Health Association of Idaho
PO Box 4725
Boise, ID 83711-4725
Phone: (208)893-9983 **Fax:** (208)327-0510
Email: kalek@juno.com

Illinois

★ 9200 ★ National Mental Health Association of DuPage County
188 W Randolph St., Ste. 2225
Chicago, IL 60601
Phone: (312)368-9070 **Fax:** (312)368-0283

★ 9201 ★ National Mental Health Association of Fayette County
2120 Lincoln St.
Evanston, IL 60201
Phone: (847)328-6198 **Fax:** (847)869-4701
Email: madel513653@aol.com

★ 9202 ★ National Mental Health Association in Illinois
188 W Randolph St., Ste. 2225
Chicago, IL 60601
Phone: (312)368-9070 **Fax:** (312)368-0283
Email: mhai@mhai.org
Website: http://www.mhai.org
Jan Holcomb, Director

★ 9203 ★ National Mental Health Association of Illinois Valley, Inc.
5407 N University
Peoria, IL 61614
Phone: (309)692-1766 **Fax:** (309)692-2966
Email: mhaiv@mhaiv.org
Website: http://www.mhaiv.org

★ 9204 ★ National Mental Health Association of Macon County, Inc.
1314 N Main
Decatur, IL 62526
Phone: (217)422-2988 **Fax:** (217)422-1108
Email: smartinmha@aol.com
Website: http://www.dps61.org

★ 9205 ★ National Mental Health Association in McLean County
PO Box 795
Bloomington, IL 61702-0795
Phone: (309)862-4408 **Fax:** (309)862-1542
Email: bisbeejk@aol.com

★ 9206 ★ National Mental Health Association of the North Shore
2120 Lincoln St.
Evanston, IL 60201-2282
Phone: (847)328-6198 **Fax:** (847)869-4701
Email: mhans@megsinet.net

★ 9207 ★ National Mental Health Association of the Rock River Valley
PO Box 4061
Rockford, IL 61110
Phone: (815)395-1839 **Fax:** (815)395-9117

★ 9208 ★ National Mental Health Association of Southwestern Illinois
PO Box 285
Edwardsville, IL 62025
Phone: (618)650-7216 **Fax:** (618)650-7216
Email: info@mhaswil.org

Indiana

★ 9209 ★ National Mental Health Association in Allen County
227 E Washington Blvd.
Fort Wayne, IN 46802
Phone: (219)422-6441 **Fax:** (219)423-3400

★ 9210 ★ National Mental Health Association in Blackford County
814 N Richmond
Hartford City, IN 47348
Phone: (765)348-7040 **Fax:** (765)348-7046
Email: dmitchell@towfin.com

★ 9211 ★ National Mental Health Association in Boone County
127 W Main St., Ste. 314
Lebanon, IN 46052
Phone: (765)482-3020 **Fax:** (765)482-9001
Email: mhabc@in-motion.net

★ 9212 ★ National Mental Health Association in Cass County
421 12th St.
Logansport, IN 46947
Phone: (219)722-3984

★ 9213 ★ National Mental Health Association in Clark County
6815 Hwy. 311
Sellersburg, IN 47172
Phone: (812)256-6291

★ 9214 ★ National Mental Health Association in Clay County
1211 E National Ave.
Brazil, IN 47834
Phone: (812)448-8801
Pat Heffner, Exec Director

★ 9215 ★ National Mental Health Association in Clinton County
51 W Clinton St., Ste. 101
Frankfort, IN 46041-1931
Phone: (765)659-3825

★ 9216 ★ National Mental Health Association in Daviess County
PO Box 183
Washington, IN 47501
Phone: (812)254-2423

★ 9217 ★ National Mental Health Association in Dearborn County
PO Box 354
Lawrenceburg, IN 47025
Phone: (812)577-5440

★ 9218 ★ National Mental Health Association in Dekalb County
902 Deer Ridge Crossing
Auburn, IN 46706
Phone: (219)925-2963 **Fax:** (219)925-1733
Cheryl Taylor, Exec Director

★ 9219 ★ National Mental Health Association in Delaware County
413 S Liberty St.
Muncie, IN 47305
Phone: (765)288-1924 **Fax:** (765)288-1956
Email: kwalkmhadc@aol.com
Vickie Strahan, Exec Director

★ 9220 ★ National Mental Health Association in Dubois County
PO Box 566
Jasper, IN 47547-0566
Phone: (812)482-3020
Leah Hayworth, President

★ 9221 ★ National Mental Health Association in Elkhart County
421 S 2nd St., Ste. 340
Elkhart, IN 46516
Phone: (219)295-8935 **Fax:** (219)295-1460
Email: mhaec@peoplepc.com

★ 9222 ★ National Mental Health Association in Floyd County
PO Box 63
New Albany, IN 47151
Phone: (812)941-0308

★ 9223 ★ National Mental Health Association in Franklin County
1216 N Main St.
PO Box 94
Brookville, IN 47012
Phone: (513)524-5371
Lisa Stiener, Exec Director

★ 9224 ★ National Mental Health Association in Fulton County
401 E 8th St., Ste. C
Rochester, IN 46975
Phone: (574)223-6870 **Fax:** (574)224-6870
Email: gsmokermhafc@rtcol.com
Genelle Smoker, Exec Director

★ 9225 ★ National Mental Health Association in Gibson
RR 3, Box 67
Owensville, IN 47665
Phone: (812)724-2141
Ruth Braselton, President

★ 9226 ★ National Mental Health Association in Greene County
RR 2, Box 132
Solsberry, IN 47459
Phone: (812)825-7108
Norman Sullivan, President

★ 9227 ★ National Mental Health Association in Hamilton County
942 N 10th St.
Noblesville, IN 46060
Phone: (317)776-3455 **Fax:** (317)776-3456

★ 9228 ★ National Mental Health Association in Hancock County
98 E North St.
Greenfield, IN 46140
Phone: (317)462-2877 **Fax:** (317)462-2877
Email: HCMHA98@aol.com
Ann Osborne, Exec Director

★ 9229 ★ National Mental Health Association in Hendricks County
6845 E U.S. 36, Ste. 880
Avon, IN 46123
Phone: (317)272-0027 **Fax:** (317)272-1176

★ 9230 ★ National Mental Health Association in Henry County
PO Box 449
New Castle, IN 47362
Phone: (765)529-4403 **Fax:** (765)593-2510

★ 9231 ★ National Mental Health Association in Howard County
507 N Webster St.
Kokomo, IN 46904-2221
Phone: (765)459-0309 **Fax:** (765)459-0300
Email: mhahowardco@aol.com
Jennifer Trobaugh, Exec Director

★ 9232 ★ National Mental Health Association in Indiana
55 Monument Cir., Ste. 455
Indianapolis, IN 46204
Phone: (317)638-3501 **Fax:** (317)638-3540
Email: MHAI@mentalhealthassociation.com
Website: http://www.mentalhealthassociation.com
Steve McCaffrey, President

★ 9233 ★ National Mental Health Association in Jackson County
PO Box 51
Seymour, IN 47274
Phone: (812)522-3480

★ 9234 ★ National Mental Health Association in Jay County
964 S Meridian St.
Portland, IN 47371
Phone: (219)726-8614
Sheron McClung, Exec Director

★ 9235 ★ National Mental Health Association in Johnson County
PO Box 748
Franklin, IN 46131
Phone: (317)535-6960

★ 9236 ★ National Mental Health Association in Knox County
PO Box 859
Vincennes, IN 47591
Phone: (812)895-1007 **Fax:** (812)885-2723

★ 9237 ★ National Mental Health Association in Kosciusko County
920 Fisher
PO Box 822
Warsaw, IN 46581
Phone: (219)269-2102 **Fax:** (219)269-3554
Email: mha@kconline.com
Sandra Frush, Exec Director

★ 9238 ★ National Mental Health Association in Lake County
9722 Parkway Dr.
Highland, IN 46322
Phone: (219)922-3822 **Fax:** (219)922-3825
Email: mhainlakecounty@yahoo.com

★ 9239 ★ National Mental Health Association in Lawrence County
RR 11, Box 23
Bedford, IN 47421
Phone: (812)275-3028

★ 9240 ★ National Mental Health Association in Marion County
2506 Willowbrook Pkwy., No. 100
Indianapolis, IN 46205-1542
Phone: (317)251-0005 **Fax:** (317)254-2800
Email: mtowell@mcmha.org
Marge Towell, Exec Director

★ 9241 ★ National Mental Health Association in Marshall County
401 W Jefferson St.
Plymouth, IN 46563
Phone: (219)935-5314

★ 9242 ★ National Mental Health Association in Monroe County
441 S College Ave.
Bloomington, IN 47403
Phone: (812)323-9720 **Fax:** (812)323-9132
Email: mha@bloomington.in.us
Elaine Moore, Exec Director

★ 9243 ★ National Mental Health Association in Morgan County
118 E Morgan St.
Martinsville, IN 46151
Phone: (765)342-1515
Email: mhamorg@scican.net

★ 9244 ★ National Mental Health Association in Parke County
RR 4, PO Box 250
Rockville, IN 47872
Phone: (765)245-2719

★ 9245 ★ National Mental Health Association in Perry County
PO Box 366
Tell City, IN 47586-0366
Phone: (812)547-7905 **Fax:** (812)547-5146
Email: wcwagner@psci.net

★ 9246 ★ National Mental Health Association in Porter County, Inc.
402 E Indiana Ave.
Valparaiso, IN 46383
Phone: (219)462-6267 **Fax:** (219)464-7483
Email: mha@netnitco.net
Margaret Stevens, Exec Director

★ 9247 ★ National Mental Health Association in Putnam County
10 ½ N Jackson St.
Greencastle, IN 46135
Phone: (765)653-3310 **Fax:** (765)653-2565
Email: mhapc2@ccrtc.com

★ 9248 ★ National Mental Health Association in Randolph County
430 S Meridian St.
Winchester, IN 47394
Phone: (765)932-2004

★ 9249 ★ National Mental Health Association in Rush County
Rush County Courthouse, 3rd Fl.
201 E 2nd St.
Rushville, IN 46173
Phone: (765)932-2004

★ 9250 ★ National Mental Health Association in St. Joseph County
211 W Madison St.
South Bend, IN 46601
Phone: (219)234-1049 **Fax:** (219)234-1040
Email: rjtraz@mindspring.com
Ryan J. Trzaskowski, Exec Director

★ 9251 ★ National Mental Health Association in Spencer County
HCR 68, Box 575
Saint Meinrad, IN 47577
Phone: (812)547-9630
Email: sschaefer@psci.net
Mary Posner, President

★ 9252 ★ National Mental Health Association in Steuben County
PO Box 372
Angola, IN 46703
Phone: (219)665-5981
Betty Bemesderfer, Exec Director

★ 9253 ★ National Mental Health Association in Tippecanoe County
915 Columbia St., Ste. 1
Lafayette, IN 47901-1476
Phone: (765)742-1800 **Fax:** (765)742-2085
Email: edir@dcwi.com
Website: http://dcwi.com/~mha/welcome.htm

★ 9254 ★ National Mental Health Association in Vanderburgh County
123 NW 4th St., Ste. 707
Evansville, IN 47708-1715
Phone: (812)426-2640 **Fax:** (812)426-7207
Email: vcmha@juno.com
Donna Carr, Exec Director

★ 9255 ★ National Mental Health Association in Vigo County
620 8th Ave.
Terre Haute, IN 47804
Phone: (812)232-5681 **Fax:** (812)234-2863
Email: mhavc@indy.net
Kathy Alexander, Exec Director

★ 9256 ★ National Mental Health Association in Wabash County
Box 310
North Manchester, IN 46962
Phone: (219)982-7766 **Fax:** (219)774-3432
Email: mamast@kconline.com
Mary Ann Mast, Exec Director

★ 9257 ★ National Mental Health Association in Wayne County
750 NW 13th St.
Richmond, IN 47374
Phone: (765)966-0221 **Fax:** (765)966-5915
Email: mha@infocom.com

★ 9258 ★ National Mental Health Association in Wells County
223 W Washington St.
Bluffton, IN 46714-2050
Phone: (219)824-1514

★ 9259 ★ National Mental Health Association in White County
Monticello Health Care
1120 N Main St.
Monticello, IN 47960
Phone: (219)583-9221
Pam Ashton, President

Iowa

★ 9260 ★ National Mental Health Association in Dubuque County
PO Box 283
Dubuque, IA 52004-0283
Phone: (563)582-2233 **Fax:** (319)584-0730
Email: dbqiamha@aol.com
Betty Allen, Secretary

★ 9261 ★ National Mental Health Association of Hamilton County
PO Box 334
Hamilton, IA 50116
Phone: (515)832-9620 **Fax:** (515)832-9591
Darren Helton, President

Kansas

★ 9262 ★ National Mental Health Association of the Heartland
739 Minnesota Ave.
Kansas City, KS 64101
Phone: (913)281-2221 **Fax:** (913)281-3977
Email: sdavis@mhah.org
Website: http://www.mhah.org
Frmly: Mental Health Association of the Heartland (Kansas).

★ 9263 ★ National Mental Health Association of Kansas
3745 SW Wanamaker Rd.
Topeka, KS 66610-1369
Phone: (785)252-8038 **Fax:** (985)233-5440
Email: asknbeg@terraworld.net
Gary W. Long, II, Director

★ 9264 ★ National Mental Health Association in Reno County
1520 N Plum
PO Box 2021
Hutchinson, KS 67504-2021
Phone: (316)663-7772 **Fax:** (316)665-4497
Email: mha_candace@yahoo.com

★ 9265 ★ National Mental Health Association of South Central Kansas
555 N Woodlawn, Ste. 3105
Wichita, KS 67208-4385
Phone: (316)685-1821 **Fax:** (316)685-0768
Email: rosemary@mhasck.org
Website: http://www.mhasck.org

Kentucky

★ 9266 ★ National Mental Health Association of Kentucky
120 Sears Ave., Ste. 213
Louisville, KY 40207
Phone: (502)893-0460 **Free:** 888-702-0463
Fax: (502)896-1306
Email: mhaky@kih.net
Website: http://www.mhaky.org
Sheriall Cunningham, Director

★ 9267 ★ National Mental Health Association of Northern Kentucky
605 Madison Ave.
Covington, KY 41011
Phone: (859)292-2487 **Fax:** (859)292-2485
Email: mhnky@aol.com
Website: http://members.aol.com/mhnky/mhnky.html

Louisiana

★ 9268 ★ National Mental Health Association in Caddo-Bossier
3825 Gilbert St., Ste. 209
Shreveport, LA 71104
Phone: (318)861-5971 **Fax:** (318)861-5972
Email: mhaincb@aol.com

★ 9269 ★ National Mental Health Association in Caldwell Parish
PO Box 136
Columbia, LA 71418
Phone: (318)649-5066
Email: hefnerp@aol.com

★ 9270 ★ National Mental Health Association in Catahoula Parish
403 Willow St.
Jonesville, LA 71343
Phone: (318)339-8562
Robbie M. Wilson, President

★ 9271 ★ National Mental Health Association in Franklin Parish
PO Box 128
Winnsboro, LA 71295
Phone: (318)435-3334
Drew Dunn, President

★ 9272 ★ National Mental Health Association in Louisiana
200 Lafayette St., Ste. 709
Baton Rouge, LA 70801
Phone: (225)343-1921 **Free:** 800-241-6425
Fax: (225)343-1983
Email: mhal15@aol.com

★ 9273 ★ National Mental Health Association in Metropolitan New Orleans
PO Box 850407
New Orleans, LA 70185
Phone: (504)897-1140 **Fax:** (504)897-2368
Email: mhamno@bellsouth.net

★ 9274 ★ National Mental Health Association in Red River County
Rte. 1, Box 274
Coushatta, LA 71019-7505
Phone: (318)932-5494
Betty Sullivan, President

★ 9275 ★ National Mental Health Association in Southwest Louisiana
PO Box 805
Lake Charles, LA 70602-0805
Phone: (337)582-1430 **Fax:** (337)582-1430
Email: melliott61@juno.com

★ 9276 ★ Tri Parish National Mental Health Association
PO Box 166
Jonesville, LA 71343
Phone: (318)339-8562

Maryland

★ 9277 ★ National Mental Health Association of Howard County
11702 Lightfall Ct.
Columbia, MD 21044
Phone: (410)995-3323 **Fax:** (410)997-4227
Donna Rawlings, Contact

★ 9278 ★ National Mental Health Association of the Lower Shore
PO Box 269
Snow Hill, MD 21863
Phone: (410)543-2057 **Fax:** (410)632-3224
Email: foxtrot@shore.intercom.net

★ 9279 ★ National Mental Health Association of Maryland
711 W 40th St., Ste. 460
Baltimore, MD 21211
Phone: (410)235-1178 **Fax:** (410)235-1180
Email: info@mhamd.org
Website: http://www.mhamd.org
Linda Raines, Director

★ 9280 ★ National Mental Health Association of Metropolitan Baltimore
711 W 40th St., Ste. 460
Baltimore, MD 21211
Phone: (410)235-1178 **Fax:** (410)235-1180
Email: mhaofmd@aol.com
Diane Cabot, Exec Director

★ 9281 ★ National Mental Health Association of Montgomery County
1000 Twinbrook Pkwy.
Rockville, MD 20851
Phone: (301)424-0656 **Fax:** (301)738-1030
Email: info@mhamc.org
Website: http://www.mhamc.org

★ 9282 ★ National Mental Health Association of Prince George's County
PO Box 89
Hyattsville, MD 20781
Phone: (301)699-2737 **Fax:** (301)699-2746
Website: http://www.mhapgc.freeservers.com

★ 9283 ★ National Mental Health Association of Southern Maryland
1170 Overlook Dr.
Accokeek, MD 20607-3516
Phone: (301)283-2410
Vivian Mills, President

★ 9284 ★ National Mental Health Association in Talbot County
108 Maryland Ave., Ste. 103
Easton, MD 21601
Phone: (410)822-0444 **Fax:** (410)820-7283
Email: bjadams@mhamdes.org
Website: http://www.mhamdes.org

★ 9285 ★ National Mental Health Association of Washington County
8162 Arcadia Ln.
Boonsboro, MD 21713
Phone: (301)739-4138
Sue Farrell, President

Michigan

★ 9286 ★ National Mental Health Association of Michigan
15920 W 12 Mile Rd.
Southfield, MI 48076
Phone: (248)557-6777 **Fax:** (248)557-5995
Email: mhamich@aol.com
Website: http://www.geocities.com/CapitolHill/Lobby/468

Mississippi

★ 9287 ★ National Mental Health Association of the Capitol Area
409 Briarwood Dr., Ste. 310
Jackson, MS 39206
Phone: (601)956-2800 **Fax:** (601)956-6380
Email: mhajxn@aol.com

★ 9288 ★ National Mental Health Association of Mississippi
PO Box 7329
Gulfport, MS 39506
Phone: (228)864-6274 **Fax:** (228)864-1310
Email: Keenminds@aol.com

Missouri

★ 9289 ★ National Mental Health Association of Greater Saint Louis
1905 S Grand Blvd.
Saint Louis, MO 63104
Phone: (314)773-1399 **Fax:** (314)773-5930
Email: mhagstl@aol.com
James House, II, CEO & Pres

★ 9290 ★ National Mental Health Association of the Heartland
739 Minnesota Ave.
Kansas City, MO 66101
Phone: (913)281-2221 **Fax:** (913)281-3977
Email: mevans@mhah.org
Website: http://www.mhah.org

Montana

★ 9291 ★ National Mental Health Association of Billings
3308 2nd Ave. N
PO Box 20891
Billings, MT 59104
Phone: (406)245-0697 **Fax:** (406)259-0624
Email: mhabillings@imt.net
Leanne Swanson, Exec Director

★ 9292 ★ National Mental Health Association of Daniels County
Box 746
Scobey, MT 59263
Phone: (406)487-2671
Esther Kramer, President

★ 9293 ★ National Mental Health Association of Great Falls
PO Box 2774
Great Falls, MT 59403
Phone: (406)268-6254

★ 9294 ★ National Mental Health Association of Montana
25 S Ewing, Ste. 200
Helena, MT 59601
Phone: (406)442-4276 **Fax:** (406)442-4986
Email: mham@in-tch.com
Website: http://www.mhamontana.org
Andrea Merrill, Director

★ 9295 ★ National Mental Health Association of Sheridan County
736 Shippe Canyon
Plentywood, MT 59254
Phone: (406)286-5625

★ 9296 ★ National Mental Health Association of Sweet Grass County
Box 372
Big Timber, MT 59011
Phone: (406)932-5594
Nora Hansen, President

Nebraska

★ 9297 ★ National Mental Health Association of Nebraska
PO Box 23001
Lincoln, NE 68504
Phone: (402)474-3183 **Fax:** (402)474-3274
Email: info@mha-ne.org
Website: http://www.mha-ne.org

New Jersey

★ 9298 ★ National Mental Health Association in Atlantic County
1147 N New Rd.
Absecon, NJ 08201
Phone: (609)272-1700 **Fax:** (609)484-0123
Email: mhaac@aol.com
Website: http://mhanj.org

★ 9299 ★ National Mental Health Association of Essex County
33 S Fullerton Ave.
Montclair, NJ 07042
Phone: (973)509-9777 **Fax:** (973)509-9888
Email: mhaecdavison@aol.com

★ 9300 ★ National Mental Health Association of Hudson County
3000 Kennedy Blvd., Ste. 305
Jersey City, NJ 07306
Phone: (201)653-4700 **Fax:** (201)653-4100
Email: mhahc@aol.com

★ 9301 ★ National Mental Health Association of Monmouth County
59 Broad St.
Eatontown, NJ 07724
Phone: (732)542-6422 **Fax:** (732)389-3163
Email: mhamonmouth@monmouth.com
Website: http://www.mentalhealthmonmouth.org

★ 9302 ★ National Mental Health Association of Morris County
28 Walnut St., Box 9
Madison, NJ 07940
Phone: (973)377-9280 **Fax:** (973)377-8608
Email: mhamc@aol.com

★ 9303 ★ National Mental Health Association of Morris County
28 Walnut St.
Box 9
Madison, NJ 07940
Phone: (973)377-9280 **Fax:** (973)377-8608
Email: mhamc@aol.com

★ 9304 ★ National Mental Health Association in New Jersey
88 Pompton Ave.
Verona, NJ 07044
Phone: (973)571-4100 **Free:** 800-367-8850
Fax: (973)857-1777
Email: info@mhanj.org
Website: http://www.mhanj.org

★ 9305 ★ National Mental Health Association of Ocean County
681 River Ave., Ste. 2J
Lakewood, NJ 08701
Phone: (732)905-1132 **Fax:** (732)905-0906
Email: mhaoc@aol.com

★ 9306 ★ National Mental Health Association in Passaic County
404 Clifton Ave.
Clifton, NJ 07011
Phone: (973)478-4444 **Fax:** (973)478-0941
Email: mhapc@aol.com
Joanne Green, Exec Director

★ 9307 ★ National Mental Health Association in Southwestern New Jersey
505 Cooper St.
Camden, NJ 08102
Phone: (856)966-6767 **Fax:** (856)541-3986
Email: mhaswnj2@aol.com

★ 9308 ★ National Mental Health Association of Union County
23 North Ave. E
Cranford, NJ 07016
Phone: (908)272-0300 **Fax:** (908)272-5696
Edmund Murphy, Exec Director

★ 9309 ★ Trenton Advocacy Association
121 Broad St., 2nd Fl.
Trenton, NJ 08628
Phone: (609)656-0110 **Fax:** (609)656-8078
Email: mhanjtrenton@aol.com

New Mexico

★ 9310 ★ National Mental Health Association in New Mexico
PO Box 1417
506 N Prince Dr.
Espanola, NM 87532
Phone: (505)753-4131 **Fax:** (505)382-4778
Email: mhanm@cybermesa.com

★ 9311 ★ National Mental Health Association in New Mexico
506 N Prince Dr.
PO Box 1417
Espanola, NM 87532
Phone: (505)753-4131
Email: mhanm@cybermesa.com
Deborah Fickling, Director

New York

★ 9312 ★ National Mental Health Association in Albany County
500 Central Ave.
Albany, NY 12206
Phone: (518)435-9931 **Fax:** (518)435-9937
Email: kimballm@crisny.org
Website: http://www.crisny.org
Michel Kimball, Exec Director

★ 9313 ★ National Mental Health Association in Allegany County
45 N Broad St.
Wellsville, NY 14895
Phone: (716)593-1991 **Fax:** (716)593-7104

★ 9314 ★ National Mental Health Association in Cattaraugus County, Inc.
129 N Union St.
PO Box 833
Olean, NY 14760
Phone: (716)372-0208 **Fax:** (716)372-0222

★ 9315 ★ National Mental Health Association in Cayuga County
PO Box 184
Cayuga, NY 13034
Phone: (315)258-9531 **Fax:** (315)258-3185
Email: arleenie@yahoo.com
Arleen Egry, President

★ 9316 ★ National Mental Health Association in Chautauqua County
413 Main St.
Jamestown, NY 14701
Phone: (716)487-0616 **Fax:** (716)483-3524
Email: chautmha@hotmail.com

★ 9317 ★ National Mental Health Association in Clinton County
159 Margaret St., Ste. 201
Plattsburgh, NY 12901
Phone: (518)563-8206 **Fax:** (518)563-9958
Email: hcook@bhsn.org
Website: http://www.bhsn.org

★ 9318 ★ National Mental Health Association of Columbia/Green Counties
713 Union St.
Hudson, NY 12534
Phone: (518)828-4619 **Fax:** (518)828-1196
Jeffrey Rovitz, Exec Director

★ 9319 ★ National Mental Health Association of Cortland County, Inc.
25 Clinton Ave.
PO Box 282
Cortland, NY 13045
Phone: (607)758-3107 **Fax:** (607)758-3107

★ 9320 ★ National Mental Health Association in Dutchess County
510 Haight Ave.
Poughkeepsie, NY 12603
Phone: (845)473-2500 **Fax:** (845)473-4870
Email: mhadc@hvc.rr.com
Website: http://www.mhadc.com

★ 9321 ★ National Mental Health Association of Erie County, Inc.
999 Delaware Ave.
Buffalo, NY 14209
Phone: (716)886-1242 **Fax:** (716)881-6428
Email: mhaec@localnet.com
Website: http://members.localnet.com/~mhaec

★ 9322 ★ National Mental Health Association in Essex County
RD 1, Box 1012
Westport, NY 12993-9702
Phone: (518)962-2077 **Free:** 800-440-8074
Fax: (518)962-8233
Email: mha@mhainessex.org

★ 9323 ★ National Mental Health Association in Franklin County
52 Broadway, Ste. 2B
Saranac Lake, NY 12983
Phone: (518)891-0504 **Free:** 800-776-9992
Fax: (518)891-6423
Email: mhafc@northnet.org

★ 9324 ★ National Mental Health Association in Fulton/Montgomery Counties
73 N Main St., Ste. 106
Gloversville, NY 12078
Phone: (518)725-2790 **Free:** 800-734-5864
Fax: (518)775-1076
Email: jcharney@mybizz.net
Website: http://www.mentalhealthassociation.org

★ 9325 ★ National Mental Health Association in Genessee County
25 Liberty St.
Batavia, NY 14020
Phone: (585)344-2611 **Fax:** (585)345-1418
Email: gencomha@2ki.net

★ 9326 ★ National Mental Health Association in Jefferson County
212 William St.
Watertown, NY 13601-2602
Phone: (315)788-0970 **Fax:** (315)788-8092
Email: mhajc@northnet.org
Roberta Hagerty, Contact

★ 9327 ★ National Mental Health Association of Nassau County, Inc.
186 Clinton St.
Hempstead, NY 11550
Phone: (516)489-2322 **Fax:** (516)489-2784
Email: mhanc@mhanc.org
Website: http://www.mhanc.org

★ 9328 ★ National Mental Health Association in New York City, Inc.
666 Broadway, Rm. 200
New York, NY 10012
Phone: (212)254-0333 **Fax:** (212)529-1959
Email: mhaofnyc@aol.com

★ 9329 ★ National Mental Health Association in New York State, Inc.
194 Washington Ave., Ste. 415
Albany, NY 12210
Phone: (518)434-0439 **Free:** 800-766-6177
Fax: (518)427-8676
Email: mhanys@mhanys.org
Website: http://www.mhanys.org/

★ 9330 ★ National Mental Health Association in Niagara County, Inc.
36 Pine St.
Lockport, NY 14094
Phone: (716)433-3780 **Fax:** (716)433-3847
Email: mhancny@aol.com
Website: http://www.mhanc.com

★ 9331 ★ National Mental Health Association of Onondaga County
3049 E Genesse St.
Syracuse, NY 13224
Phone: (315)445-5606 **Fax:** (315)445-1828
Email: fuscoaa@clrc.org
Website: http://www.mha-oc.org

★ 9332 ★ National Mental Health Association in Orange County
20 Walker St.
Goshen, NY 10924
Phone: (914)294-7411 **Free:** 800-832-1200
Fax: (914)294-7348
Email: mha@mhaorangeny.com
Website: http://www.mhaorangeny.com

★ 9333 ★ National Mental Health Association in Orleans County
113 E State St.
PO Box 269
Albion, NY 14411
Phone: (716)589-1158 **Fax:** (716)589-1158
Email: ritbo@aol.com

★ 9334 ★ National Mental Health Association of Oswego County
70 Bunner St.
Oswego, NY 13126-3703
Phone: (315)349-3533 **Fax:** (315)349-3533
Email: mhaosw@scsinter.net

★ 9335 ★ National Mental Health Association in Putnam County, Inc.
Brewster Town Ctr.
1620 Rte. 22
Brewster, NY 10509
Phone: (914)278-7600 **Fax:** (914)278-0600
Email: mhaputnm@bestweb.net
Website: http://www.bestweb.net/~mhaputnm/

★ 9336 ★ National Mental Health Association in Rochester/Monroe Counties, Inc.
339 East Ave., Ste. 201
Rochester, NY 14604
Phone: (585)325-3145 **Fax:** (585)325-3188
Email: pwoods@mharochester.org
Website: http://www.mharochester.org

★ 9337 ★ National Mental Health Association of Rockland County, Inc.
20 Squadron Blvd.
New City, NY 10956

Phone: (845)639-7400 **Fax:** (845)639-7419
Email: mharc@aol.com
Website: http://www.mharockland.org/

★ 9338 ★ National Mental Health Association in Schuyler County
106 Shannon St.
PO Box 141
Watkins Glen, NY 14891
Phone: (607)535-7426 **Fax:** (607)535-8284

★ 9339 ★ National Mental Health Association of the Southern Tier, Inc.
82 Oak St.
Binghamton, NY 13905
Phone: (607)771-8888 **Fax:** (607)771-8892
Email: mhaofst@tier.net
Website: http://www.tier.net/mhaofst
Casemiro Epe, Exec Director

★ 9340 ★ National Mental Health Association in Steuben County
115 Liberty
Bath, NY 14810
Phone: (607)776-6577 **Fax:** (607)776-7895

★ 9341 ★ National Mental Health Association in Suffolk County
199 N Wellwood Ave., Ste. 2
Lindenhurst, NY 11757
Phone: (631)226-3900 **Fax:** (631)225-1708
Email: louischerry@earthlink.net
Website: http://www.mhasuffolk.org

★ 9342 ★ National Mental Health Association in Tompkins County
518 W State St.
Ithaca, NY 14850
Phone: (607)273-9250 **Fax:** (607)272-5343
Email: info@mhaedu.org
Website: http://info.mhaedu.org

★ 9343 ★ National Mental Health Association in Ulster County
PO Box 2304
Kingston, NY 12402
Phone: (914)336-4747 **Fax:** (845)336-0192
Email: ependegar@mhainulster.com
Website: http://mhainulster.com

★ 9344 ★ National Mental Health Association in Warren/Washington
York Plaza
3043 State Route 4
Hudson Falls, NY 12839
Phone: (518)747-2284 **Fax:** (518)747-2253
Email: peter@wwamh.org
Website: http://www.wwamh.org

★ 9345 ★ National Mental Health Association of Westchester County, Inc.
2269 Saw Mill River Rd., Bldg. 1A
Elmsford, NY 10523
Phone: (914)345-5900 **Fax:** (914)347-8859
Email: help@mhawestchester.org
Website: http://www.mhawestchester.org

North Carolina

★ 9346 ★ National Mental Health Association in Beaufort County
4814 River Rd., Ste. 10
Washington, NC 27889
Phone: (252)946-9538
Email: nakreisher@aol.com

★ 9347 ★ National Mental Health Association in Burke County
PO Drawer 1266
Morganton, NC 28680
Phone: (828)439-4421 **Fax:** (828)439-4444

★ 9348 ★ National Mental Health Association in Caldwell County
247 Commercial St.
Lenoir, NC 28645
Phone: (828)757-5710 **Fax:** (828)757-5718
Email: weschester1@angelfire.com

★ 9349 ★ National Mental Health Association in Carteret County
PO Box 425
Swansboro, NC 28584
Phone: (252)393-2426 **Fax:** (252)745-2080
Email: patp@coastalnet.com

★ 9350 ★ National Mental Health Association in Cleveland County
201 W Marion St., Rm. 306
Shelby, NC 28150
Phone: (704)481-8637 **Fax:** (704)481-1960
Email: mha@cetlink.net

★ 9351 ★ National Mental Health Association in Columbus County
PO Box 534
Whiteville, NC 28472
Phone: (910)642-5168 **Fax:** (910)640-1010
Colene B. Stanley, President

★ 9352 ★ National Mental Health Association in Craven County
474 State Hwy. 306 S
Vanceboro, NC 28586
Phone: (252)745-4352

★ 9353 ★ National Mental Health Association in Cumberland County
310 Green St., Ste. 201-A
Fayetteville, NC 28302
Phone: (336)323-1954
Email: rmhacc@aol.com
Dana Covington, Contact

★ 9354 ★ National Mental Health Association in Davidson County
PO Box 1642
Lexington, NC 27293
Phone: (336)956-2952 **Fax:** (336)956-1647
Email: kaysaintsing@lexcominc.net

★ 9355 ★ National Mental Health Association in Forsyth County, Inc.
1 Brownsboro Plaza, Ste. 100
4265 Brownsboro Rd.
Winston-Salem, NC 27106
Phone: (336)759-9370 **Fax:** (336)759-3248
Email: andy@mha-fc.org
Website: http://www.mha-fc.org

★ 9356 ★ National Mental Health Association in Greensboro
1004 N Elm St.
Greensboro, NC 27401
Phone: (336)373-1402 **Fax:** (336)286-9642
Email: swalker@mhag.org
Website: http://www.greensboro.com/mha

★ 9357 ★ National Mental Health Association in High Point
910 Mill Ave.
PO Box 5693
High Point, NC 27260
Phone: (336)883-7480 **Fax:** (336)883-4013
Email: inncom@greensboro.com

★ 9358 ★ National Mental Health Association in Johnston County
26 Noble St.
Smithfield, NC 27577
Phone: (919)934-0311 **Fax:** (919)934-0311
Email: angelsamongus42@aol.com
Website: http://www.ncneighbors.com/1352/

★ 9359 ★ National Mental Health Association in McDowell
25 Academy St.
Marion, NC 28752
Phone: (828)652-3001 **Fax:** (828)652-1884
Email: tclontz@mcdowell.main.nc.us

★ 9360 ★ National Mental Health Association in Mecklenburg/Cabarrus Counties
3701 Latrobe Dr., Ste. 140
Charlotte, NC 28211
Phone: (704)365-3454 **Fax:** (704)365-9973
Email: mhameck@aol.com
Website: http://groups.gocarolinas.com/mhameck

★ 9361 ★ National Mental Health Association in Nash-Rocky Mount
PO Box 8773
Rocky Mount, NC 27804
Phone: (252)937-8820 **Fax:** (252)937-6702
Email: mhanrm@hotmail.com
Susan Smith, Director

★ 9362 ★ National Mental Health Association in New Hanover
301 N Front St., Ste. 4
PMD 265
Wilmington, NC 28401
Phone: (910)251-9005 **Fax:** (910)762-2265
Email: LauraWillisMHANC@aol.com

★ 9363 ★ National Mental Health Association in North Carolina
3820 Bland Rd.
Raleigh, NC 27609
Phone: (919)981-0740 **Fax:** (919)954-7238
Email: sgoff@mha-nc.org
Website: http://www.mha-nc.org

★ 9364 ★ National Mental Health Association in Onslow County
PO Box 425
Swansboro, NC 28584
Phone: (252)393-2426
Email: patp@coastalnet.com

★ 9365 ★ National Mental Health Association in Orange County
302 W Weaver St., Ste. F
PO Box 2253
Chapel Hill, NC 27515-2253
Phone: (919)942-8083 **Fax:** (919)688-4887
Email: mhaoc@intrex.net
Website: http://www.mhaoc.com
Megan L. Risley, Exec Director

★ 9366 ★ National Mental Health Association in Pamlico County
PO Box 425
Swansboro, NC 28584
Phone: (252)393-2426
Email: patp@coastalnet.com

★ 9367 ★ National Mental Health Association in Pitt County
101 W 14th St., Ste. 3
Greenville, NC 27835
Phone: (252)752-7448 **Fax:** (252)752-2729
Email: faeriename@aol.com

★ 9368 ★ National Mental Health Association in Randolph, Inc.
513-D White Oak St.
PO Box 4397
Asheboro, NC 27204-4397
Phone: (336)625-5551 **Fax:** (336)625-2331
Email: mharc@atomic.net

★ 9369 ★ National Mental Health Association of Rowan County
650 Statesville Blvd., Ste. 1
Salisbury, NC 28144
Phone: (704)636-9912 **Fax:** (704)639-0695
Website: http://www.dantana.com/mha

★ 9370 ★ National Mental Health Association in Rutherford County
286 Burch Hutchins Rd.
Forest City, NC 28043
Phone: (828)286-8884 **Fax:** (828)286-8330
Carolyn Osbourne, Exec Director

★ 9371 ★ National Mental Health Association in Stanly County
124 S 1st St.
PO Box 237
Albemarle, NC 28002
Phone: (704)982-7516 **Fax:** (704)982-7516
Email: lahnorwood@vnet.net
Linda Hoy, Exec Director

★ 9372 ★ National Mental Health Association of Stokes County
3868 Piney Mountain Rd.
Walnut Cove, NC 27052

★ 9373 ★ National Mental Health Association in Vance County
1221 Alpha St.
Henderson, NC 27536
Phone: (919)438-3412
Ralph Glover, President

★ 9374 ★ National Mental Health Association in Wake County
3820 Bland Rd.
Raleigh, NC 27609
Phone: (910)425-5971 **Fax:** (910)323-1954
Romaine Dougherty, Contact

★ 9375 ★ National Mental Health Association in Wayne County
719 E Ash St.
PO Box 1476
Goldsboro, NC 27534
Phone: (919)734-3530 **Fax:** (919)731-1186
Email: mhawc@esn.net
Website: http://www.ww2.esn.net/mhawc

★ 9376 ★ National Mental Health Association in Wilson County
509 W Nash St.
PO Box 652
Wilson, NC 27894
Phone: (252)242-2773 **Fax:** (252)237-6118
Email: mha_wc@bbnp.com
Rebecca R. Boyette, Exec Director

★ 9377 ★ National Mental Health Association in Yancey
PO Box 284
Burnsville, NC 28714
Phone: (828)682-7498

★ 9378 ★ Outreach and Prevention Services of Alamance, Inc.
711 Hermitage Rd.
Burlington, NC 27216
Phone: (336)438-2050 **Fax:** (336)438-2059
Email: hudsonjanA2@netscape.net

North Dakota

★ 9379 ★ Missouri Valley Mental Health Association
2817 Hawkens St., No. 4
Bismarck, ND 58503
Phone: (701)258-5169
Email: kipknaup@hotmail.com

★ 9380 ★ National Mental Health Association of the Lake Region
4746 76th Ave. NE
Devils Lake, ND 58301-9232
Phone: (701)662-8482
Grace Sharbono, President

★ 9381 ★ National Mental Health Association in North Dakota
1459 Interstate Loop
PO Box 4106
Bismarck, ND 58502-4106
Phone: (701)255-3692 **Free:** 800-472-2911
Fax: (701)255-2411
Email: director@mha-nd.org
Website: http://www.btigate.com/mhand

★ 9382 ★ National Mental Health Association of North Valley
136 Rolling Hills Circle
Grand Forks, ND 58201
Phone: (701)772-8792 **Fax:** (701)775-8645
Email: joschristy@juno.com
Website: http://www.btigate.com/~mhand
Jo Christenson, President

★ 9383 ★ National Mental Health Association in Souris Valley
1459 Interstate Loop
PO Box 160
Minot, ND 58702-0160
Phone: (701)255-3692 **Fax:** (701)255-2411
Email: mchand@btigate.com
Jennifer Bartsch, President

★ 9384 ★ National Mental Health Association of the South Central Region
2605 Circle Dr.
Jamestown, ND 58401-3924
Phone: (701)253-3842 **Fax:** (701)253-3204
Email: giedtd@state.nd.us
Nancy Schultz, President

★ 9385 ★ National Mental Health Association of South Valley
124 8th St. N
Fargo, ND 58102-4915
Phone: (701)237-5871 **Free:** 800-472-2911
Fax: (701)237-0562
Email: mharry@juno.com
Susan Helgeland, Exec Director

★ 9386 ★ National Mental Health Association of the Southwest
117 1st St. E
Dickinson, ND 58601
Phone: (701)227-7611 **Fax:** (701)227-7618
Email: 88buck@state.nd.us
Karen McConnell, President

★ 9387 ★ National Mental Health Association in the Tri-County Region
1402 9th Ave. W
Williston, ND 58801
Phone: (701)572-2651
Email: rhickok@dia.net
Rick Hickock, President

Ohio

★ 9388 ★ Mental Health Associations of Ohio
538 E Town St., Ste. D
Columbus, OH 43215
Phone: (614)221-1441 **Fax:** (614)221-1491
Email: mhafcoh@aol.com
Laura Moskow Sigal, Director

★ 9389 ★ National Mental Health Association of the Cincinnati Area, Inc.
2400 Reading Rd., Ste. 412
Cincinnati, OH 45202
Phone: (513)721-2910 **Fax:** (513)287-8544
Email: mhacincinnati@fuse.net
Website: http://www.mentalhealthassn.org

★ 9390 ★ National Mental Health Association of Franklin County
538 E Town St., Ste. D
Columbus, OH 43215
Phone: (614)221-1441 **Fax:** (614)221-1491
Email: mhafcoh@aol.com
Website: http://www.mhafc.org

★ 9391 ★ National Mental Health Association in Knox County
11 W Gambier St.
Mount Vernon, OH 43050-3301
Phone: (740)397-3088
Email: fladen4@yahoo.com

★ 9392 ★ National Mental Health Association in Licking County
65 Messimer Dr.
Newark, OH 43055
Phone: (740)522-1341 **Fax:** (740)522-4464
Email: mhalc@alink.com
Website: http://www.mhalc.org

★ 9393 ★ National Mental Health Association in Lucas County
1 Stranahan Sq., Ste. 540
Toledo, OH 43604-1900
Phone: (419)242-9587 **Fax:** (419)242-6316
Email: judyr@uhs-toledo.org
Website: http://www.uhs-toledo.org

★ 9394 ★ National Mental Health Association of Miami County
1100 Wayne St., Ste. 4002
Troy, OH 45373
Phone: (937)332-9293 **Fax:** (937)332-9293
Email: mhamc@mail2.wesnet.com
Website: http://www.mhamc.com

★ 9395 ★ National Mental Health Association of Ottawa County
1 Stranahan Sq., Ste. 540
Toledo, OH 43604-1900

Phone: (419)242-9587 **Fax:** (419)242-6316
Email: uhs@uhs-toledo.org
Website: http://www.uhs-toledo.org

★ 9396 ★ National Mental Health Association of Summit County
405 Tallmadge Rd.
Cuyahoga Falls, OH 44221
Phone: (330)923-0688 **Free:** 800-991-1311
Fax: (330)923-7573
Email: rlibertini@mhasc.net
Website: http://www.mentalhealthassociationofsummitcounty.org

★ 9397 ★ National Mental Health Association in Union County
131 N Main St.
Marysville, OH 43040
Phone: (937)642-0935 **Fax:** (937)644-9543
Email: paulus@netexp.net

Oklahoma

★ 9398 ★ National Mental Health Association in Tulsa
1870 S Boulder
Tulsa, OK 74119-5234
Phone: (918)585-1213 **Fax:** (918)585-1263
Email: mbrose@mhat.org
Website: http://www.mhat.org
Michael W. Brose, Exec Director

★ 9399 ★ National Mental Health Association in Tulsa
1870 S Boulder
Tulsa, OK 74119-5234
Phone: (918)585-1213 **Fax:** (918)585-1263
Email: mbrose@mhat.org
Website: http://www.mhat.org
Mike Brose, Exec Director

Oregon

★ 9400 ★ National Mental Health Association of Oregon
812 SW Washington St., Ste. 640
Portland, OR 97204
Phone: (503)227-8496 **Fax:** (503)227-8496
Email: beckie@quik.com

Pennsylvania

★ 9401 ★ The Advocacy Alliance, A National Mental Health Association
846 Jefferson Ave.
PO Box 1368
Scranton, PA 18501
Phone: (570)342-7762 **Fax:** (570)207-9194
Email: teo@theadvocacyalliance.org
Website: http://www.theadvocacyalliance.org

★ 9402 ★ National Mental Health Association of Adams County, Inc.
223 Baltimore St.
Gettysburg, PA 17325
Phone: (717)334-3139 **Fax:** (717)633-7104
Email: cmentzer@netrax.net

★ 9403 ★ National Mental Health Association of Allegheny County
1945 5th Ave.
Pittsburgh, PA 15219-5543
Phone: (412)391-3820 **Fax:** (412)391-3825
Email: mha@mhaac.net
Website: http://www.mhaac.net

★ 9404 ★ National Mental Health Association of the Capital Region
3 Crossgates Dr., Ste. 120
Mechanicsburg, PA 17055-2459
Phone: (717)796-0601 **Fax:** (717)796-0603
Email: astritemhacdp@paonline.com
Website: http://www.mentalhealthassoc.org

★ 9405 ★ National Mental Health Association of the Central Susquehanna Valley
37 Main St., Ste. 206
Bloomsburg, PA 17815
Phone: (570)784-9583 **Free:** 800-874-3220
Fax: (570)784-3220
Email: mhacsv@jlink.net

★ 9406 ★ National Mental Health Association in Cumberland, Dauphin & Perry
3 Crossgates Dr., Ste. 120
Mechanicsburg, PA 17055-2459
Phone: (717)796-0601 **Fax:** (717)796-0603
Email: johnc@mentalhealthassoc.org
Website: http://www.mentalhealthassoc.org/

★ 9407 ★ National Mental Health Association in Franklin/Fulton Counties
154 S 2nd St.
Chambersburg, PA 17201
Phone: (717)264-4301 **Fax:** (717)264-3591
Lisa Boice, Exec Director

★ 9408 ★ National Mental Health Association in Lancaster County
630 Janet Ave.
Lancaster, PA 17601
Phone: (717)397-7461 **Fax:** (717)397-2530
Email: mhalc@redrose.net
Mary Steffy, Director

★ 9409 ★ National Mental Health Association in Lebanon County
136 N 9th St.
Lebanon, PA 17046-4903
Phone: (717)273-5781 **Fax:** (717)273-6908
Email: mhaleb@lmf.net
Judith Feather, Director

★ 9410 ★ National Mental Health Association of Mercer County
19 N Water Ave.
Sharon, PA 16146-1343
Phone: (724)347-1303 **Fax:** (724)347-3199
Dr. James D. Robb, Director

★ 9411 ★ National Mental Health Association of Northwest Pennsylvania
1101 Peach St.
Erie, PA 16501-1812
Phone: (814)452-4462 **Fax:** (814)456-6593
Email: eccmhc@nc.inter.net

★ 9412 ★ National Mental Health Association in Pennsylvania
1414 N Cameron, Ste. C
Harrisburg, PA 17103
Phone: (717)236-8110 **Fax:** (717)236-0192
Email: swalther@paonline.com

★ 9413 ★ National Mental Health Association of Reading and Berks County
122 W Lancaster Ave., Ste. 207
Shillington, PA 19607-1348
Phone: (610)775-3000 **Fax:** (610)775-4000
Email: mharbc@ptd.net
Frmly: Berks County Mental Health Association.

★ 9414 ★ National Mental Health Association of Southeastern Pennsylvania
1211 Chestnut St., 11th Fl.
Philadelphia, PA 19107
Phone: (215)751-1800 **Fax:** (215)636-6300
Email: mha@mhasp.org
Website: http://www.mhasp.org

★ 9415 ★ National Mental Health Association in Westmoreland County
409 Coulter Ave., Ste. 4
Greensburg, PA 15601
Phone: (724)834-6351 **Fax:** (724)834-6352
Email: mhawc@westol.com
Website: http://www.westol.com/mhawc
Laura Hawkins, Director

★ 9416 ★ National Mental Health Association of York County
303 E Market St.
York, PA 17403-5614
Phone: (717)843-6973 **Fax:** (717)843-0185
Email: mentalhealth@mhay.org
Website: http://www.mhay.org
Kristin Keech, Director

Rhode Island

★ 9417 ★ National Mental Health Association of Rhode Island
Independence Sq.
500 Prospect St.
Pawtucket, RI 02860
Phone: (401)726-2285 **Fax:** (401)365-6170
Email: mmhari@mhari.org
Website: http://www.mhari.org

South Carolina

★ 9418 ★ National Mental Health Association in Abbeville County
761 Mt. Lebanon Rd.
Donalds, SC 29638
Phone: (864)379-2479

★ 9419 ★ National Mental Health Association in Aiken County
104 Florence St. SW
PO Box 1074
Aiken, SC 29801
Phone: (803)641-4164 **Fax:** (803)641-4166
Email: mhaac@duesouth.net
Website: http://www.mha-aikensc.org

★ 9420 ★ National Mental Health Association in Anderson County
PO Box 663
Anderson, SC 29622
Phone: (864)260-2221
Claudia Robinson, Contact

★ 9421 ★ National Mental Health Association in Bamberg County
PO Box 276
Denmark, SC 29042
Phone: (803)793-5786

★ 9422 ★ National Mental Health Association in Barnwell County
302 N Lartigue St.
Blackville, SC 29817
Phone: (803)284-3229

★ 9423 ★ National Mental Health Association in Beaufort/Jasper Counties
7 Office Park Dr., Ste. 228
PO Box 22538
Hilton Head Island, SC 29925
Phone: (843)842-5855 **Fax:** (843)842-5865

★ 9424 ★ National Mental Health Association in Calhoun County
Rte. 3, Box 504
Saint Matthews, SC 29135
Phone: (803)823-2612

★ 9425 ★ National Mental Health Association in Cherokee County
714 S Limestone St.
Gaffney, SC 29340
Phone: (803)489-8191
Shirley Tisdale, Contact

★ 9426 ★ National Mental Health Association in Chester County
PO Box 392
Chester, SC 29706
Phone: (803)385-2191

★ 9427 ★ National Mental Health Association in Claredon County
PO Box 278
Summerton, SC 29148
Phone: (803)485-2510

★ 9428 ★ National Mental Health Association in Colleton County
119 Charles St.
PO Box 1547
Walterboro, SC 29488
Phone: (843)549-1732 **Fax:** (843)549-2359

★ 9429 ★ National Mental Health Association in Darlington County
PO Box 131
Hartsville, SC 29551
Phone: (843)332-1481

★ 9430 ★ National Mental Health Association in Florence County
514-B S Dargen St.
Florence, SC 29506
Phone: (843)661-5407 **Fax:** (843)661-3859
Email: susanisrael@aol.com

★ 9431 ★ National Mental Health Association in Georgetown County
226 Queen St.
Georgetown, SC 29442
Phone: (843)527-6919 **Fax:** (843)527-2325
Email: jfenhagen@earthlink.net

★ 9432 ★ National Mental Health Association in Greenville County
301 University Ridge, Ste. 5600
Greenville, SC 29601-3675
Phone: (864)467-3344 **Fax:** (864)467-3547

★ 9433 ★ National Mental Health Association in Horey County
First Union Bank
2110 Oak St.
Myrtle Beach, SC 29577
Phone: (803)448-2688
Nick Sherfesee, President

★ 9434 ★ National Mental Health Association in Kershaw County
PO Box 586
Camden, SC 29020-2335
Phone: (803)432-7955 **Fax:** (803)425-0030
Email: whspence4@worldnet.att.net

★ 9435 ★ National Mental Health Association in Lancaster County
1769 Charles Ave.
Lancaster, SC 29720
Phone: (803)285-7471
Email: pbarry@gwm.sc.edu
Dr. Peter Barry, Contact

★ 9436 ★ National Mental Health Association in Laurens County
PO Box 81
Laurens, SC 29360
Phone: (864)984-1809

★ 9437 ★ National Mental Health Association in Lee County
261 Luckey Rd.
Bishopville, SC 29010
Phone: (803)428-5738

★ 9438 ★ National Mental Health Association in Marion County
3914 Elm Ct.
Mullins, SC 29574
Phone: (803)464-0630

★ 9439 ★ National Mental Health Association in Marlboro County
707 Crestview Dr.
Bennettsville, SC 29512
Phone: (803)479-4016
Beulah C. Black, President

★ 9440 ★ National Mental Health Association in McCormick County
PO Box 227
Mc Cormick, SC 29835
Phone: (803)391-2131

★ 9441 ★ National Mental Health Association in Mid-Carolina
PO Box 1657
Columbia, SC 29202-1657
Phone: (803)733-5425 **Fax:** (803)733-5427

★ 9442 ★ National Mental Health Association in Oconee County
PO Box 915
Walhalla, SC 29691
Phone: (864)638-3058

★ 9443 ★ National Mental Health Association in Orangeburg County
801 Shillings Bridge Rd.
Orangeburg, SC 29116
Phone: (803)533-0018 **Fax:** (803)516-0242
Brannon Underwood, Contact

★ 9444 ★ National Mental Health Association in Pickens County
3600 Pumkintown Hwy.
Pickens, SC 29671
Phone: (864)878-3974

★ 9445 ★ National Mental Health Association of the Piedmont
153 N Spring St.
Spartanburg, SC 29306
Phone: (864)582-3104 **Fax:** (864)582-3322

★ 9446 ★ National Mental Health Association in Saluda County
PO Box 191
Saluda, SC 29138
Phone: (803)356-9398

★ 9447 ★ National Mental Health Association in South Carolina
1823 Gadsden St.
Columbia, SC 29201
Phone: (803)779-5363 **Fax:** (803)779-0017
Email: mha@mha-sc.org
Website: http://www.mha-sc.org

★ 9448 ★ National Mental Health Association in Sumter County
c/o Sumter National Bank
PO Box 1629
Sumter, SC 29151
Phone: (803)755-7701
Lucy Thomas, President

★ 9449 ★ National Mental Health Association in York County
2778 Woodbridge Dr.
Fort Mill, SC 29715
Phone: (803)548-0952

Tennessee

★ 9450 ★ National Mental Health Association of Greater Knoxville
PO Box 52405
Knoxville, TN 37950-2405
Phone: (865)584-9125 **Fax:** (865)584-9125
Email: mhagk@lock-net.com
Website: http://www.korrnet.org/mha
Ben Harrington, Director

★ 9451 ★ National Mental Health Association of the Mid-South
200 Jefferson Ave., Ste. 1107
Memphis, TN 38103-2328
Phone: (901)323-0633 **Fax:** (901)323-0858
Email: mha@netten.net

★ 9452 ★ National Mental Health Association of Middle Tennessee
2416 21st Ave. S, Ste. 201
Nashville, TN 37212
Phone: (615)269-5355 **Fax:** (615)269-5413
Email: forinfo@mhamt.org
Website: http://www.ichope.com
Elizabeth Lentchner, Director

★ 9453 ★ National Mental Health Association of Tennessee
2416 21st Ave., Ste. 20
Nashville, TN 37212-5318
Phone: (615)242-7122 **Fax:** (615)242-9637
Email: anitab@mhatn.org
Website: http://www.mhatn.org

Texas

★ 9454 ★ National Mental Health Association in Abilene
PO Box 7282
Abilene, TX 79608
Phone: (915)673-2300 **Fax:** (915)673-2671
Email: mhaa@bitstreet.com
Website: http://www.abilenementalhealth.org

★ 9455 ★ National Mental Health Association in Beaumont/Jefferson Counties
670 N 7th St.
Beaumont, TX 77702-1741
Phone: (409)833-9657 **Fax:** (409)833-3522
Website: http://www.mentalhealthbeaumont.org
Pat Hays, President

★ 9456 ★ National Mental Health Association in Fort Bend County
10435 Greenbough Dr., Bldg. II, Ste. 200
Stafford, TX 77477
Phone: (281)261-1876 **Fax:** (281)261-1833
Email: mhafbc@wt.net
Website: http://www.mhafbc.org

★ 9457 ★ National Mental Health Association of Greater Dallas
624 N Good-Latimer Expy., Ste. 200
Dallas, TX 75204
Phone: (214)871-2420 **Fax:** (214)954-0611
Email: tsimmons@mhadallas.org
Website: http://www.mhadallas.org

★ 9458 ★ National Mental Health Association of Greater Houston
2211 Norfolk, Ste. 810
Houston, TX 77098
Phone: (713)523-8963 **Fax:** (713)522-0698
Email: bschwartz@mhahouston.org
Website: http://www.mhahouston.org
Program(s): Information and Referral Services, Advocacy, Self-Help Resource Center.

★ 9459 ★ National Mental Health Association in Greater San Antonio
8431 Fredricksburg Rd., Ste. 110
San Antonio, TX 78229
Phone: (210)614-7566 **Fax:** (210)614-7589
Email: mhasatx@axs4u.net

★ 9460 ★ National Mental Health Association in Tarrant County
3136 W 4th St.
Fort Worth, TX 76107-2113
Phone: (817)335-5405 **Fax:** (817)334-0025
Email: mhatc@mhatc.org
Lauralee Harris, President

★ 9461 ★ National Mental Health Association in Texas
8401 Shoal Creek Blvd.
Austin, TX 78757-7597
Phone: (512)454-3706 **Fax:** (512)454-3725
Email: mhainfo@mhatexas.org
Website: http://www.mhatexas.org
Clare Hudspeth, Exec Director

★ 9462 ★ National Mental Health Association in Texas
8401 Shoal Creek Blvd.
Austin, TX 78757-7597
Phone: (512)454-3706 **Fax:** (512)454-3725
Email: whatinfo@mhatexas.org
Website: http://www.mhatexas.org
Stella Mullins, President

★ 9463 ★ National Mental Health Association in Tyler
113 E Houston
Tyler, TX 75702
Phone: (903)592-0582 **Fax:** (903)592-7318
Tim King, President

Utah

★ 9464 ★ National Mental Health Association in Utah
1800 SW Temple, Ste. 503
Salt Lake City, UT 84115-3040
Phone: (801)596-3705 **Fax:** (801)596-3658
Email: mhaut@xmission.com
Website: http://www.xmission.com/~mhaut/index.htm

Vermont

★ 9465 ★ National Mental Health Association in Vermont
PO Box 165
Montpelier, VT 05601
Phone: (802)223-6263 **Fax:** (802)828-5252
Email: vamh1@aol.com
Website: http://www.vamh.org
Ken Libertoff, Director

Virginia

★ 9466 ★ National Mental Health Association of Augusta
Professional Bldg., Rm. 206
Staunton, VA 24401
Phone: (540)886-7181 **Fax:** (540)885-0640

★ 9467 ★ National Mental Health Association of Central Virginia
1010 Miller Park Sq.
Lynchburg, VA 24501
Phone: (804)847-9055 **Fax:** (804)847-3600
Email: mhacvexdir@aol.com

★ 9468 ★ National Mental Health Association of Charlottesville/Albemarle, Inc.
513 Stewart St., Ste. J
Charlottesville, VA 22902
Phone: (434)977-4673
Email: mha@avenue.org
Website: http://www.monticelloavenue.org

★ 9469 ★ National Mental Health Association in Chesterfield
PO Box 2188
Chesterfield, VA 23832
Phone: (804)748-7938
Email: kmorrow52@hotmail.com
Kenneth Marrow, President

★ 9470 ★ National Mental Health Association in Danville/Pittsylvania County
1225 W Main St.
PO Box 1106
Danville, VA 24543
Phone: (434)792-3700 **Fax:** (434)791-3187
Email: mha@gamewood.net
Website: http://pws.gamewood.net/~mha/

★ 9471 ★ National Mental Health Association of Fauquier County
PO Box 3549
Warrenton, VA 20188
Phone: (540)341-8732 **Fax:** 800-349-9057
Email: mhafc@mindspring.com
Website: http://www.fauquier-mha.org

★ 9472 ★ National Mental Health Association in Fredericksburg
2217 Princess Anne St., Ste. 219-1
Fredericksburg, VA 22401
Phone: (540)371-2704 **Free:** 800-684-6423
Fax: (540)372-3709
Email: mhaf@infi.net
Website: http://www.fls.infi.net/~mhaf

★ 9473 ★ National Mental Health Association in Halifax County
PO Box 329
South Boston, VA 24592
Phone: (804)572-3992 **Fax:** (804)572-8959
Irene Gravitt, Exec Director

★ 9474 ★ National Mental Health Association in Hanover
203 S Taylor St.
Ashland, VA 23005
Phone: (804)798-5902 **Fax:** (804)752-8373
Email: sunrisehse@aol.com
Website: http://www.hanovermentalhealth.org

★ 9475 ★ National Mental Health Association in Martinsville/Henry Counties
117 Broad St.
PO Box 582
Martinsville, VA 24114
Phone: (276)638-7801 **Fax:** (276)638-7960
Email: mha638@intelos.net
Website: http://intelos.net/mha638

★ 9476 ★ National Mental Health Association of New River Valley
303 Church St.
Blacksburg, VA 24060
Phone: (540)951-4990 **Fax:** (540)951-5015
Email: mhanry@bellatlantic.net
Website: http://donthide.org
Amy Forsyth-Stephens, Exec Director

★ 9477 ★ National Mental Health Association of Roanoke Valley
PO Box 592
Roanoke, VA 24004
Phone: (540)344-0931 **Fax:** (540)344-0932
Email: mharv@roanoke.infi.net

★ 9478 ★ National Mental Health Association of Rockbridge County
PO Box 1088
Lexington, VA 24450
Phone: (540)463-2911
Linda Munsey, Exec Director

★ 9479 ★ National Mental Health Association in South Hampton Roads
1513 E Sewells Point Rd.
Norfolk, VA 23502
Phone: (757)853-2606 **Fax:** (757)566-2013
Email: lhowards@aol.com

★ 9480 ★ National Mental Health Association of Virginia
503 E Main St., Ste. 707
Richmond, VA 23219
Phone: (804)225-5591 **Fax:** (804)225-5593
Email: vmfisher@hsc.vcu.edu
Website: http://www.mhav.org

★ 9481 ★ National Mental Health Association of Warren County
PO Box 358
Front Royal, VA 22630
Phone: (276)635-6223

★ 9482 ★ Peninsula Mental Health Association
2501 Washington Ave., 5th Fl.
Newport News, VA 23607
Phone: (757)245-0217 **Fax:** (757)245-5126
Bonnie Kelly, President

Washington

★ 9483 ★ National Mental Health Association of Washington
Washington Advocates for the Mentally Ill
802 NW 70th St.
Seattle, WA 98117
Phone: (206)789-7722 **Free:** 800-782-9264
Fax: (206)784-0957
Email: wami@wolfenet.com
Website: http://www.nami-wami.com
Eleanor Owen, Exec Director

West Virginia

★ 9484 ★ National Mental Health Association in the Greater Kanawha Valley, Inc.
1 United Way Sq.
Charleston, WV 25301-1098
Phone: (304)340-3512 **Fax:** (304)340-3508
Email: mha@wvinter.net
Ellen Ward, Director

★ 9485 ★ National Mental Health Association in Monongalia County
PO Box 1533
Morgantown, WV 26507
Phone: (304)292-0525
Penny Fletcher, Director

Wisconsin

★ 9486 ★ National Mental Health Association in Brown County
612 Skyline Blvd.
PO Box 1016
Green Bay, WI 54305
Phone: (920)468-6720
Barbara Bauer, President

★ 9487 ★ National Mental Health Association in Calumet County
W2643 St. Charles
Chilton, WI 53014
Phone: (920)849-1450 **Fax:** (920)894-2506
Email: wayne@tcei.com
Diane Kuckenbecker, President

★ 9488 ★ National Mental Health Association in Milwaukee County
734 N 4th St., No. 325
Milwaukee, WI 53203-2102
Phone: (414)276-3122 **Fax:** (414)276-3124
Email: mha@mhamilw.org
Website: http://www.mhamilw.org
Karen Robison, CEO & Pres

★ 9489 ★ National Mental Health Association in Sheboygan County
2020 Erie Ave.
Sheboygan, WI 53081
Phone: (920)458-3951 **Fax:** (920)458-3441
Email: mhasheb@bytehead.com
Beverly Randall, Director

Mental Retardation

Listed below are state offices of The Arc (1010 Wayne Ave., Ste. 650, Silver Spring, MD 20910; (301)565-3842, http://www.thearc.org/), a national organization on mental retardation.

Alabama

★ 9490 ★ The Arc of Alabama
300 S Hull St.
Montgomery, AL 36104
Phone: (334)262-7688
Website: http://www.arcalabama.org

★ 9491 ★ The Arc of Athens-Limestone
427 Rogers St.
Athens, AL 35611
Phone: (256)232-0366

★ 9492 ★ The Arc of Autauga and Western Elmore Counties
926 Selma Hwy.
Prattville, AL 36067
Phone: (334)365-4054

★ 9493 ★ The Arc of Baldwin County, Inc.
PO Box 400
Loxley, AL 36551
Phone: (334)964-4451

★ 9494 ★ The Arc of Blount County
615 Fairground Ave.
PO Box 210
Oneonta, AL 35121
Phone: (205)625-3552

★ 9495 ★ The Arc of Calhoun and Cleburne Counties
PO Box 1848
Anniston, AL 36202
Phone: (256)236-2857

★ 9496 ★ The Arc of Clarke County
PO Box 100
Jackson, AL 36545
Phone: (334)246-3000

★ 9497 ★ The Arc of Cullman County
95 County Rd. 1218
Vinemont, AL 35179
Phone: (205)739-1161

★ 9498 ★ The Arc of Dale County
717 W Main St.
Daleville, AL 36322
Phone: (334)255-3831

★ 9499 ★ The Arc of DeKalb County
201 Grand Ave. S
Fort Payne, AL 35967
Phone: (205)845-0165

★ 9500 ★ The Arc of Dothan/Houston Counties
7 Harrington Ln.
Dothan, AL 36305
Phone: (334)792-0002

★ 9501 ★ The Arc of Eastern Elmore County
PO Box 847
Wetumpka, AL 36092
Phone: (334)514-0708

★ 9502 ★ The Arc of Etowah County
PO Box 1172
Gadsden, AL 35902
Phone: (256)547-6800

★ 9503 ★ The Arc of Fayette/Lamar
1428 S Temple Ave.
Fayette, AL 35555
Phone: (205)932-8642

★ 9504 ★ The Arc of Franklin County
Red Bay, AL 35582
Phone: (256)356-8855

★ 9505 ★ The Arc of Geneva County
Rte. 1, Box 102
Coffee Springs, AL 36318

★ 9506 ★ The Arc of Jackson County
180 Mack Morris Dr.
Scottsboro, AL 35769
Phone: (256)259-1603

★ 9507 ★ The Arc of Jefferson County
215 21st Ave. S
Birmingham, AL 35205
Phone: (205)323-6383

★ 9508 ★ The Arc of Lawrence County
23343 State Hwy. 33
Courtland, AL 35618
Phone: (256)974-0496

★ 9509 ★ The Arc of Madison County
1100 Washington St.
Huntsville, AL 35801
Phone: (256)536-1035

★ 9510 ★ The Arc of Marshall County
5104 Porter Harvey Dr.
Guntersville, AL 35976
Phone: (256)582-5009

★ 9511 ★ The Arc of Montgomery
527 Buckingham Dr.
Montgomery, AL 36116
Phone: (334)281-6938
Website: http://www.mindspring.com/%7Emarc1
Lee Conner, Exec Director

★ 9512 ★ The Arc of Morgan County
401 14th St. SE, Bldg. 4E
Decatur, AL 35601
Phone: (256)355-6192

★ 9513 ★ The Arc of North Talladega County
PO Box 853
Talladega, AL 35160
Phone: (205)362-8064

★ 9514 ★ The Arc of Randolph County
PO Box 127
Roanoke, AL 36274
Phone: (334)863-8991

★ 9515 ★ The Arc of St. Clair County
282 Chula Vista Dr.
Pell City, AL 35125-6293
Phone: (205)884-2680

★ 9516 ★ The Arc of Shelby County
1960-H Chandalar Dr.
Pelham, AL 35124-4323
Phone: (205)664-9313

★ 9517 ★ The Arc of South Talladega County
PO Box 360
Sylacauga, AL 35150
Phone: (205)245-2323

★ 9518 ★ The Arc of The Chattahoochee Valley
PO Box 416
Valley, AL 36854
Phone: (205)644-2277

★ 9519 ★ The Arc of The Shoals
PO Box 501
Tuscumbia, AL 35674
Phone: (256)383-1472

★ 9520 ★ The Arc of Tuscaloosa County
PO Box 40246
Tuscaloosa, AL 35403
Phone: (205)556-4900
Email: bcarroll@dbtech.net
Website: http://www.dbtech.net/arc
Barbara Carroll, Exec Director

★ 9521 ★ The Arc of Walker County
910 Oak Hill Rd.
Jasper, AL 35504
Phone: (205)387-0562

★ 9522 ★ The Arc of Winston County
145 County Hwy. 76
Haleyville, AL 35565
Phone: (205)486-2178

★ 9523 ★ Mobile Association for Retarded Citizens, Inc. (MARC)
2424 Gordon Smith Dr.
Mobile, AL 36617
Phone: (251)479-7409 **Fax:** (251)473-7649
Email: jzoghby@mobilecan.org
Website: http://www.mobilearc.org
Jeffrey Zoghby, Exec Director

Alaska

★ 9524 ★ The Arc of Anchorage
2211 Arca Dr.
Anchorage, AK 99508
Phone: (907)277-6677
Website: http://www.arc-anchorage.org

Arizona

★ 9525 ★ The Arc of Arizona
5610 S Central Ave.
Phoenix, AZ 85040
Phone: (602)243-1787
Email: arcofarizona@aol.com
Website: http://www.arcarizona.org

★ 9526 ★ The Arc of Cottonwood
3165 Calle Del Montana
Sedona, AZ 86336

★ 9527 ★ The Arc of Douglas
PO Box 252
Douglas, AZ 85608
Phone: (520)364-7473

★ 9528 ★ The Arc of Gila County
PO Box 1262
Globe, AZ 85502
Phone: (520)425-6053

★ 9529 ★ The Arc of Graham County
PO Box 870
Safford, AZ 85548
Phone: (520)428-7968

★ 9530 ★ The Arc of Mesa
924 N Country Club
Mesa, AZ 85201
Phone: (602)969-3800

★ 9531 ★ The Arc of Mohave County
2090 Airway
Kingman, AZ 86401
Phone: (520)757-3988

★ 9532 ★ The Arc of Northeastern Pinal County
PO Box 535
Kearny, AZ 85237
Phone: (520)363-5581

★ 9533 ★ The Arc of the Prescott Area
PO Box 11784
Prescott, AZ 86301
Phone: (520)749-3197

★ 9534 ★ The Arc of Santa Cruz County
PO Box 972
Nogales, AZ 85628

★ 9535 ★ The Arc of Sierra Huachuca
120 N 6th St.
Sierra Vista, AZ 85635
Phone: (520)458-4611

★ 9536 ★ The Arc of Tempe
PO Box 26014
Tempe, AZ 85285-6014
Phone: (602)966-8536

★ 9537 ★ The Arc of Tucson, Inc.
PO Box 44324
Tucson, AZ 85733
Phone: (520)570-1295
Website: http://www.arcoftucson.org

★ 9538 ★ The Arc of Yuma County
256 S 2nd Ave., Ste. A
Yuma, AZ 85364
Phone: (928)783-1588

★ 9539 ★ Chandler/Gilbert Arc
3434 N San Marcos Pl.
Chandler, AZ 85224
Phone: (480)892-9422
Website: http://www.cgarc.org

★ 9540 ★ Early Intervention Infant Toddler Program, Inc.
413 E Florence Blvd.
Casa Grande, AZ 85222-4122
Phone: (520)836-7939

★ 9541 ★ Parents and Friends
3818 W Rose Ln.
Phoenix, AZ 85019

★ 9542 ★ The Peaks Arc
604 W Havasupai Rd.
Flagstaff, AZ 86001

Arkansas

★ 9543 ★ The Arc of Arkansas
2004 S Main St.
Little Rock, AR 72206-1597
Phone: (501)375-7770
Website: http://www.arcark.org

★ 9544 ★ The Arc of Nevada County
PO Box 480
Prescott, AR 71857
Phone: (870)887-6675

★ 9545 ★ The Arc of Randolph County
PO Box 425
Pocahontas, AR 72455-2114

★ 9546 ★ The Arc of Sebastian County
121 N 6th St.
Fort Smith, AR 72901
Phone: (501)783-5529

★ 9547 ★ The Arc of Sevier County
PO Box 246
De Queen, AR 71832
Phone: (870)642-6077

California

★ 9548 ★ Alpha Resource Center of Santa Barbara
4501 Cathedral Oaks Rd.
Santa Barbara, CA 93110
Phone: (805)683-2145

★ 9549 ★ The Arc of Alameda County
575 Independent Rd.
Oakland, CA 94621-3721
Phone: (510)639-4680
Website: http://www.arc-alameda.com

★ 9550 ★ The Arc of Amador and Calaveras Counties
75 Academy Dr.
Sutter Creek, CA 95685
Phone: (209)267-5978

★ 9551 ★ The Arc of Bakersfield
2240 S Union Ave.
Bakersfield, CA 93307
Phone: (661)834-2272
Website: http://www.barc-inc.org

★ 9552 ★ The Arc of Butte County
PO Box 3697
Chico, CA 95927-3697
Phone: (916)891-5866

★ 9553 ★ Arc California
1225 8th St., Ste. 590
Sacramento, CA 95814-2213
Phone: (916)552-6619
Email: arcgary@quiknet.com

★ 9554 ★ The Arc of El Dorado County
175 Placerville Dr., Ste. W
Placerville, CA 95667

★ 9555 ★ The Arc of Fresno
5755 E Fountain Way
Fresno, CA 93727
Phone: (559)291-0611
Website: http://www.arcfresno.org

★ 9556 ★ The Arc of Imperial Valley
502 E Main St.
PO Box 1828
El Centro, CA 92243
Phone: (760)352-0180
Email: arcinfo@arciv.org
Website: http://www.arciv.org

★ 9557 ★ The Arc of Orange County
225 W Carl Karcher Way
Anaheim, CA 92801
Phone: (714)744-5301

★ 9558 ★ The Arc of Riverside
8138 Mar Vista Ct.
Riverside, CA 92504
Phone: (909)688-5141
Email: ArcRiverCA@aol.com
Website: http://www.arcriversideca.org

★ 9559 ★ The Arc of the San Bernardino Area
796 E 6th St.
San Bernardino, CA 92410
Phone: (909)884-6484

★ 9560 ★ The Arc of San Diego
9575 Aero Dr.
San Diego, CA 92123
Email: info@arc-sd.com
Website: http://www.arc-sd.com

★ 9561 ★ The Arc of San Francisco
1500 Howard St.
San Francisco, CA 94103
Phone: (415)255-7200
Website: http://www.thearcsanfrancisco.org

★ 9562 ★ The Arc of Santa Maria Valley
PO Box 1037
Santa Maria, CA 93456
Phone: (805)922-7381
Email: kirkspry@vtc-sm.org
Website: http://www.vtc-sm.org

★ 9563 ★ The Arc of Solano
PO Box 4119
Vallejo, CA 94590
Phone: (707)552-2935

★ 9564 ★ The Arc of Sonoma County Advocacy Resource Center
PO Box 219
Santa Rosa, CA 95402
Phone: (707)578-5454

★ 9565 ★ The Arc of South Bay
1735 W Rosecrans Ave.
Gardena, CA 90249
Phone: (310)532-6333
Website: http://www.lafn.org/community/arcsobay

★ 9566 ★ The Arc of Southeast Los Angeles County
12049 S Woodruff Ave.
Downey, CA 90241-5669
Phone: (562)803-4606
Email: info@arcselac.org
Website: http://www.arcselac.org

★ 9567 ★ The Arc of Taft
204 Van Buren St.
Taft, CA 93268
Phone: (661)763-1532

★ 9568 ★ The Arc of Ventura County
5103 Walker St.
Ventura, CA 93003
Phone: (805)650-8611

★ 9569 ★ Casa De Esperanza
12000 Denholm Dr.
El Monte, CA 91732
Phone: (626)444-8943

★ 9570 ★ Contra Costa Association for Retarded Citizens
1340 Arnold Dr., Ste. 127
Martinez, CA 94553
Phone: (925)370-1818
Email: arcofcc@aol.com
Website: http://www.contracostaarc.com

★ 9571 ★ Life Options, Vocational and Resource Center (LOVARC)
123 N D St.
Lompoc, CA 93436-6911
Phone: (805)735-3428
Website: http://www.lovarc.com

★ 9572 ★ OPARC
8939 Vernon St., Ste. L
Montclair, CA 91763
Phone: (909)985-3116
Website: http://www.oparc.com

Colorado

★ 9573 ★ The Arc of Adams County
8805 Fox Dr., Ste. 100
Denver, CO 80260-6828
Phone: (303)428-0310

★ 9574 ★ The Arc of Arapahoe and Douglas Counties
7600 E Arapahoe Rd., No. 101
Englewood, CO 80112
Phone: (303)220-9228
Website: http://www.arc-arapahoe-douglas.org

★ 9575 ★ The Arc of Aurora
14111 E Alameda Ave.
Aurora, CO 80012-2509
Phone: (303)344-5390

★ 9576 ★ The Arc of Colorado
777 Grant St., Ste. 303
Denver, CO 80203
Phone: (303)864-9334

★ 9577 ★ The Arc of Colorado
777 Grant St., Ste. 303
Denver, CO 80203
Phone: (303)864-9334

★ 9578 ★ The Arc of Denver, Inc.
899 Logan St., No. 311
Denver, CO 80203
Phone: (303)831-7733

★ 9579 ★ The Arc in Jefferson County
8725 W 14th Ave., No. 100
Lakewood, CO 80215
Phone: (303)232-1338
Email: info@arcjc.org
Website: http://www.arcjc.org

★ 9580 ★ The Arc of Lake County
PO Box 317
Leadville, CO 80461
Phone: (719)486-3239

★ 9581 ★ The Arc of Mesa County
PO Box 2292
Grand Junction, CO 81501
Phone: (970)245-5775

★ 9582 ★ The Arc of the Pikes Peak Region
12 N Meade Ave.
Colorado Springs, CO 80909
Phone: (719)633-4601

★ 9583 ★ The Arc of Pueblo
2705 Vinewood
Pueblo, CO 81005
Phone: (719)545-5845
Website: http://www.arcofpueblo.org

★ 9584 ★ The Arc of Weld County
1025 9th Ave., Ste. 313
Greeley, CO 80631
Phone: (970)353-5219

★ 9585 ★ Association for Community Living in Boulder County, Inc.
6897 Paiute Ave., No. 6
Longmont, CO 80503
Phone: (303)652-3000
Email: info@aclboulder.org
Website: http://www.aclboulder.org

Connecticut

★ 9586 ★ The Arc of Connecticut
1030 New Britain Ave., Ste. 102
West Hartford, CT 06110
Phone: (860)953-8335

★ 9587 ★ The Arc of Greater Enfield
75 Hazard Ave., Unit E
Enfield, CT 06082
Phone: (860)763-5411

★ 9588 ★ The Arc of New London County
PO Box 361
Gales Ferry, CT 06335
Phone: (860)464-6302

★ 9589 ★ The Arc of Plainville
PO Box 12
Plainville, CT 06062
Phone: (860)747-1560

★ 9590 ★ The Arc of Quinebaug Valley
PO Box 398
Putnam, CT 06260
Phone: (860)928-1951

★ 9591 ★ The Arc of Southington, Inc.
201 W Main St.
Plantsville, CT 06479
Phone: (860)628-9220
Email: advocacy@arcsouthington.org
Website: http://www.arcsouthington.org

★ 9592 ★ The Arc of Waterbury
1929 E Main St.
Waterbury, CT 06705-1894
Phone: (203)575-0707

★ 9593 ★ Central Connecticut Arc, Inc.
1 Hartford Sq.
New Britain, CT 06052
Phone: (860)229-6665
Email: aruwet@ccarc.com

Website: http://www.ccarc.com
Anne L. Ruwet, Exec Director

★ 9594 ★ Farmington Valley Arc, Inc.
225 Commerce Dr.
PO Box 1099
Canton, CT 06019-1099
Phone: (860)693-6662
Email: favarh@connix.com
Website: http://www.connix.com/%7Efavarh

★ 9595 ★ Friends of New Milford, Inc.
283 Chestnutland Rd.
New Milford, CT 06776
Phone: (860)355-5343

★ 9596 ★ Litchfield County Association for Retarded Citizens, Inc. (LARC)
84-R Main St.
Torrington, CT 06790
Phone: (860)485-9364
Website: http://www.litchfieldarc.org

★ 9597 ★ Lower Valley Association for Retarded and Handicapped, Inc.
1 Hartford Ave.
Old Saybrook, CT 06475
Phone: (860)399-7431

★ 9598 ★ Marc Community Resources, Ltd.
12 Fairview St.
Portland, CT 06480
Phone: (860)342-0700

★ 9599 ★ MARC, Inc. of Manchester
376R W Middle Tpke.
Manchester, CT 06040
Phone: (860)645-5718
Email: lprytko@marcct.org
Website: http://www.marcct.org
Laurie Prytko, Exec Director

★ 9600 ★ The Meriden-Wallingford Society for the Handicapped, Inc.
223-226 Cook Ave.
Meriden, CT 06450
Phone: (860)237-9975

★ 9601 ★ Options Unlimited, Inc.
584 W Hill Rd.
Winsted, CT 06098
Phone: (860)738-1410

★ 9602 ★ Sarah, Inc.
246 Gooselane., Ste. 101
Guilford, CT 06437
Phone: (203)458-4040
Website: http://www.sarah-inc.org

★ 9603 ★ Sarah Seneca
11 Park Dr., Ste. 1
Branford, CT 06405
Phone: (203)315-3770

★ 9604 ★ Sarah Tuxis Residential Services, Inc.
45 Boston St.
Guilford, CT 06437
Phone: (203)458-8532
Email: Tuxis@cshore.com
Website: http://www.sarah-tuxis.org

★ 9605 ★ STAR, Inc.
182 Wolfpit Ave.
Norwalk, CT 06851
Phone: (203)846-9581

★ 9606 ★ Tri-County Arc
65 Route 66 E
Columbia, CT 06237
Phone: (860)228-2070

★ 9607 ★ WeCAHR
211 Main St.
Danbury, CT 06810
Phone: (203)792-3540

Delaware

★ 9608 ★ The Arc of Delaware
1016 Centre Rd., Ste. 1
Wilmington, DE 19805
Phone: (302)996-9400

District of Columbia

★ 9609 ★ District of Columbia Arc
900 Varnum St. NE
Washington, DC 20017
Phone: (202)636-2950

Florida

★ 9610 ★ The Arc of Alachua County, Inc.
3303 NW 83rd St.
Gainesville, FL 32606-6227
Phone: (352)334-4060
Email: dvanslooten@arcalachua.org
Website: http://www.arcalachua.org

★ 9611 ★ The Arc of Bradford County
PO Box 1026
Starke, FL 32091-1026
Phone: (904)964-7699

★ 9612 ★ The Arc of Brevard, Inc.
1694 Cedar St.
Rockledge, FL 32955
Phone: (407)690-3436
Email: fr4arc@arc-brevard.org
Website: http://www.arc-brevard.org

★ 9613 ★ The Arc of Charlotte County, Inc.
PO Box 3569
Port Charlotte, FL 33949
Phone: (941)627-8771
Email: cc_arc@geocities.com
Website: http://www.geocities.com/heartland/hills/4840/

★ 9614 ★ The Arc of Desoto
PO Box 787
Nocatee, FL 34268
Phone: (863)494-2328

★ 9615 ★ The Arc of Escambia County
3916 N 10th Ave.
Pensacola, FL 32503
Phone: (850)434-2638
Website: http://www.arc-escambia.org

★ 9616 ★ The Arc of Flagler
3510 S Ocean Shore Blvd.
Flagler Beach, FL 32136-4105

★ 9617 ★ Arc/Florida
411 E College Ave.
Tallahassee, FL 32301
Phone: (850)921-0460
Email: arcfl@supernet.net
Website: http://www.arcflorida.org

★ 9618 ★ The Arc of the Glades Area
4250 NW 16th St.
Belle Glade, FL 33430
Phone: (561)996-9583

★ 9619 ★ The Arc of the Gulf
303 Peters St.
Port Saint Joe, FL 32456
Phone: (904)229-6327

★ 9620 ★ The Arc of Indian River
1375 16th Ave.
Vero Beach, FL 32960
Phone: (561)562-6854

★ 9621 ★ The Arc of Jackson County
2944 Pennsylvania Ave., Ste. A
Marianna, FL 32448
Phone: (850)594-3901

★ 9622 ★ The Arc of Jacksonville
1050 N Davis St.
Jacksonville, FL 32209
Phone: (904)355-0155

★ 9623 ★ The Arc of the Keys, Inc.
PO Box 9285
Tavernier, FL 33070
Phone: (305)517-9508

★ 9624 ★ The Arc of Lee County
2570 Hanson St.
Fort Myers, FL 33901
Phone: (941)334-6285

★ 9625 ★ The Arc of Levy County
PO Box 86
Otter Creek, FL 32683
Phone: (352)486-4293

★ 9626 ★ The Arc of Madison-Jefferson
100 Commerce Dr.
PO Box 912
Madison, FL 32341
Phone: (850)973-4614

★ 9627 ★ The Arc of Marion County
2800 SE Maricamp Rd.
Ocala, FL 34471
Phone: (352)620-7460

★ 9628 ★ The Arc of Nassau County
PO Box 999
Yulee, FL 32097
Phone: (904)225-9355

★ 9629 ★ The Arc of Nature Coast
5283 Neff Lake Rd.
Brooksville, FL 34601
Phone: (352)544-2322
Email: thearc@thearc-naturecoast.org
Website: http://www.thearc-naturecoast.org

★ 9630 ★ The Arc of Palm Beach County
1201 Australian Ave.
Riviera Beach, FL 33404
Phone: (561)842-3213
Website: http://www.arcpbc.org

★ 9631 ★ The Arc of Putnam County, Inc.
1209 Westover Dr.
Palatka, FL 32177
Phone: (904)325-2249

★ 9632 ★ The Arc of the Ridge Area
120 E College Dr.
Avon Park, FL 33825
Phone: (863)452-1295

★ 9633 ★ The Arc of St. Johns County
2101 Arc Dr.
Saint Augustine, FL 32095
Phone: (904)824-7249 **Fax:** (904)824-8063
Website: http://www.arcsj.org

★ 9634 ★ The Arc of St. Lucie County, Inc.
PO Box 1016
Fort Pierce, FL 34954-1016
Phone: (561)465-5499

★ 9635 ★ The Arc of Santa Rosa
409 Dixie Rd.
Milton, FL 32570
Phone: (850)623-9320

★ 9636 ★ The Arc of South Florida
5555 Biscayne Blvd.
Miami, FL 33137-2656
Phone: (305)759-8500
Website: http://www.miamivr.com/arc

★ 9637 ★ The Arc of Taylor County
c/o Leon Advocacy and Resource Center
1589 Metropolitan Blvd.
Tallahassee, FL 32308
Phone: (850)422-0355
Email: larc@nettally.com
Website: http://www.leonarc.org

★ 9638 ★ The Arc of Volusia County
PO Box 9658
Daytona Beach, FL 32120
Phone: (904)274-4736

★ 9639 ★ The Arc of Walton County
1408 State Hwy. 83
PO Box 813
Defuniak Springs, FL 32435
Phone: (850)892-5013

★ 9640 ★ The Arc of Washington-Holmes Counties, Inc.
1335 South Blvd.
Chipley, FL 32428
Phone: (850)638-7517

★ 9641 ★ The Center for Independence, Inc.
5532 Auld Ln.
Holiday, FL 34690
Phone: (727)943-2019
Email: emile@marlowe.net
Website: http://www.thecenterforindependence.com
Frmly: The Association for Retarded Citizens/Pasco, Inc.

★ 9642 ★ Comprehensive Community Services, Inc.
511 Gold Kist Ave.
PO Drawer L
Live Oak, FL 32064
Phone: (904)362-7143

★ 9643 ★ Gadsden Association Rehabilitation Center
600 S Adams St.
Quincy, FL 32351
Phone: (850)627-9058

★ 9644 ★ Horizons of Okaloosa County, Inc.
PO Box 2350
Fort Walton Beach, FL 32549
Phone: (850)863-1530
Email: horizons@emeraldcoast.com
Website: http://www.horizons.nu

★ 9645 ★ Manosota Arc, Inc.
PO Box 9292
Bradenton, FL 34206-9292
Phone: (941)752-2976

★ 9646 ★ Osceola Association for Retarded Citizens
310 N Clyde Ave.
Kissimmee, FL 34741
Phone: (407)847-6016

★ 9647 ★ Pyramid, Inc.
345 S Magnolia Dr., Ste. B-11
Tallahassee, FL 32301
Phone: (850)671-1690

★ 9648 ★ Scarc
213 W McCollum Ave.
Bushnell, FL 33513
Phone: (352)793-5156

★ 9649 ★ Sunrise Arc of Lake County, Inc.
12340 County Rd. 44
Leesburg, FL 34788
Phone: (352)357-3486
Email: sunrisearc@aol.com
Website: http://www.sunrisearc.org

★ 9650 ★ UPARC
1501 N Belcher Rd., Ste. 249
Clearwater, FL 33765
Phone: (727)799-3330

Georgia

★ 9651 ★ The Arc of the Habersham Area
1068 Twin River Rd.
Demorest, GA 30535

★ 9652 ★ The Arc of Irwin County
PO Box 614
Ocilla, GA 31774

★ 9653 ★ The Arc of Macon
4664 Sheraton Dr.
Macon, GA 31210-1322
Phone: (912)477-7764

★ 9654 ★ The Arc of Newnan-Coweta
61 Hospital Rd.
Newnan, GA 30263
Phone: (770)253-1189

★ 9655 ★ The Arc of Stephens County
4331 Ledan
Gainesville, GA 30506

★ 9656 ★ The Arc of Walker County
PO Box 438
LaFayette, GA 30728
Phone: (706)638-1669

★ 9657 ★ The Coastal Arc
1211 Eisenhower Dr.
Savannah, GA 31416
Phone: (912)355-7633

★ 9658 ★ The Georgia Arc Network, Inc.
1996 Cliff Valley Way, Ste. 102
Atlanta, GA 30329
Phone: (404)634-5512
Email: Tomquery@worldnet.att.net
Website: http://www.arcga.org

★ 9659 ★ Hart County Association of Retarded Citizens, Inc.
PO Box 706
Hartwell, GA 30643

Hawaii

★ 9660 ★ The Arc in Hawaii
3989 Diamond Head Rd.
Honolulu, HI 96816-4413
Phone: (808)737-7995
Email: arc-hi@aloha.com

★ 9661 ★ The Arc of Hilo
1099 Waianuenue Ave.
Hilo, HI 96720
Phone: (808)935-7644

★ 9662 ★ The Arc of Kauai
3201 Akahi St.
Lihue, HI 96766
Phone: (808)245-4132

★ 9663 ★ The Arc of Kona
PO Box 127
Kealakekua, HI 96750
Phone: (808)323-2626

★ 9664 ★ The Arc of Maui
95 Mahalani St., Cameron Ctr.
Wailuku, HI 96793
Phone: (808)242-5781

Idaho

★ 9665 ★ The Arc of Eastern Idaho
PO Box 1545
Idaho Falls, ID 83403

★ 9666 ★ The Arc of Idaho, Inc.
PO Box 1016
Boise, ID 83701
Phone: (208)343-5583

Illinois

★ 9667 ★ Access Services of Northern Illinois
7399 Forest Hills Rd.
Loves Park, IL 61111
Phone: (815)282-8835
Email: info@AccessNI.com
Website: http://www.accessni.com

★ 9668 ★ Ada S. McKinley Community Services, Inc.
725 S Wells St.
Chicago, IL 60607

Phone: (312)554-0600

★ 9669 ★ Advocates Network of Kane and Kendall Counties
1736 W State St.
Geneva, IL 60134
Phone: (630)232-7661

★ 9670 ★ The Arc of Adams County
1824 Maine
Quincy, IL 62301
Phone: (217)224-8328

★ 9671 ★ The Arc of Glenkirk
3504 Commercial Ave.
Northbrook, IL 60062
Phone: (847)272-5111
Website: http://www.glenkirk.org

★ 9672 ★ The Arc of Illinois
1820 Ridge Rd., No. 300
Homewood, IL 60430
Phone: (708)206-1930
Email: tony@thearcofil.org
Website: http://www.thearcofil.org

★ 9673 ★ The Arc of Iroquois County
700 E Elm St.
Watseka, IL 60970
Phone: (815)432-6191
Email: info@thearcirq.org
Website: http://www.thearcirq.org

★ 9674 ★ The Arc of Lee County
500 Anchor Rd.
Dixon, IL 61021
Phone: (815)288-6691

★ 9675 ★ The Arc of McLean County MARC
1606 Hunt Dr.
Normal, IL 61761-2192
Phone: (309)451-8888 **Fax:** (309)451-8989
Website: http://www.marcofillinois.org

★ 9676 ★ The Arc of Park Lawn
10833 S Laporte Ave.
Oak Lawn, IL 60453
Phone: (708)425-3344

★ 9677 ★ The Arc of Rock Island County
4016 9th St.
Rock Island, IL 61201
Phone: (309)786-6474
Email: arcricIL@arcric.org
Website: http://www.arcric.org

★ 9678 ★ The Arc of Winnebago, Boone, and Ogle Counties
400 N 1st St.
Rockford, IL 61107-3978
Phone: (815)965-3455 **Fax:** (815)965-3673
Website: http://www.thearcofwinn-boone.org

★ 9679 ★ Aspire
9901 Derby Ln.
Westchester, IL 60154
Phone: (708)547-3550

★ 9680 ★ Association for the Developmentally Disabled in Woodford County
200 Moody St.
Eureka, IL 61530

★ 9681 ★ Association for Individual Development
309 W New Indian Trail Ct.
Aurora, IL 60506
Phone: (630)844-5040

★ 9682 ★ Bethphage
220 N LaFayette
Macomb, IL 61455
Phone: (309)837-5506

★ 9683 ★ Blue Island Citizens for Developmental Disabilities
2155 Broadway
Blue Island, IL 60406
Phone: (708)389-6578

★ 9684 ★ Chicago Association for Retarded Citizens (CARC)
8 S Michigan Ave., No. 1700
Chicago, IL 60603
Phone: (312)346-6230
Website: http://www.chgoarc.org

★ 9685 ★ Community Support Services, Inc.
7575 S Kostner
Chicago, IL 60652
Phone: (773)884-1000
Email: css@communitysupportservices.org
Website: http://www.communitysupportservices.org

★ 9686 ★ Community Support Services Inc.
9021 Ogden Ave.
Brookfield, IL 60513
Phone: (708)354-4547

★ 9687 ★ Futures Unlimited, Inc.
210 E Torrance Ave.
Pontiac, IL 61764
Phone: (815)842-1122

★ 9688 ★ Gateway Services, Inc.
406 S Gosse Blvd.
Princeton, IL 61356
Phone: (815)875-4548

★ 9689 ★ Helping Hand Rehabilitation Center
9649 W 55th St.
Countryside, IL 60525
Phone: (708)352-3580

★ 9690 ★ Kane Kendall Case Coordination Services
179 Oswalt Ave.
Batavia, IL 60510
Phone: (630)879-2277

★ 9691 ★ The Lambs Farm, Inc.
14245 W Rockland Rd.
Libertyville, IL 60048
Phone: (847)362-4636

★ 9692 ★ LARC, An Association for Retarded Citizens
19043 Wentworth Ave.
PO Box 77
Lansing, IL 60438
Phone: (708)474-1540 **Fax:** (708)474-1586
Email: LARCLansng@aol.com
Website: http://www.thetimesonline.com/org/larc/

★ 9693 ★ Malcolm Eaton Enterprises
570 W Lamm Rd.
Freeport, IL 61032
Phone: (815)235-7181

★ 9694 ★ Marklund
290 Town Center
Glendale Heights, IL 60139
Phone: (630)529-2018

★ 9695 ★ New Hope Association, Inc.
1624 E 154th St.
Dolton, IL 60419
Phone: (708)841-1071

★ 9696 ★ Oak-Leyden Developmental Services
411 W Chicago Ave.
Oak Park, IL 60302
Phone: (708)524-1050

★ 9697 ★ Occupational Development Center
1201 E Bell St., Ste. A
Bloomington, IL 61701
Phone: (309)820-0723

★ 9698 ★ Options and Advocacy for McHenry County
333 Commerce Dr., Ste. 800
Crystal Lake, IL 60014-3598
Phone: (815)477-4720

★ 9699 ★ Pathway Services Unlimited, Inc.
1201 S Main St.
PO Box 400
Jacksonville, IL 62651
Phone: (217)479-2300

★ 9700 ★ Peoria Association for Retarded Citizens, Inc.
PO Box 3418
Peoria, IL 61612
Phone: (309)691-3800
Email: peoriaarc@yahoo.com
Website: http://www.peoriaarc.org

★ 9701 ★ Seguin Retarded Citizens Association
6223 W Ogden Ave.
Berwyn, IL 60402
Phone: (708)788-5777

★ 9702 ★ Seguin Services, Inc.
3100 S Central Ave.
Cicero, IL 60804
Phone: (708)863-3803 **Fax:** (708)863-3863
Website: http://www.seguin.org

★ 9703 ★ South Chicago Parents and Friends of Retarded Children
10241 S Commercial Ave.
Chicago, IL 60617
Phone: (773)734-2222

★ 9704 ★ Southern Illinois Case Coordination Services, Inc.
519 S Locust
PO Box 588
Centralia, IL 62801
Phone: (618)532-4300

★ 9705 ★ SouthStar Services
1005 W End Ave.
Chicago Heights, IL 60411
Phone: (708)755-8030

★ 9706 ★ Springfield Association for Retarded Citizens (SPARC)
232 Bruns Ln.
Springfield, IL 62702
Phone: (217)793-2100
Email: inquire@springfieldsparc.org
Website: http://www.spfldsparc.org

★ 9707 ★ Suburban Access
925 W 175th St., 3rd Fl.
Homewood, IL 60430
Phone: (708)799-9190

★ 9708 ★ Trinity Services of Will County
100 N Gougar Rd.
Joliet, IL 60432
Phone: (815)485-6197

★ 9709 ★ Victor C. Neumann Association
5547 N Bavenswood
Chicago, IL 60640
Phone: (773)769-4313

★ 9710 ★ Western Illinois Service Coordination, Inc.
1117 E Jackson St.
Macomb, IL 61455
Phone: (309)833-1621

Indiana

★ 9711 ★ ADEC—Resources for Independence
PO Box 398
Bristol, IN 46507
Phone: (219)848-7451
Email: options@adecinc.com
Website: http://www.adecinc.com
Remarks: Serves Elkhart County.

★ 9712 ★ The Arc of Bartholomew County
PO Box 411
Columbus, IN 47202
Phone: (812)372-0610

★ 9713 ★ The Arc of Boone County
900 W Main
Lebanon, IN 46052
Phone: (765)482-6815
Email: bcarc@aol.com
Website: http://www.in-motion.net/~arc/

★ 9714 ★ The Arc of Brown County
PO Box 411
Columbus, IN 47202
Phone: (812)372-0610

★ 9715 ★ The Arc of Carroll County
35 N Washington St.
Delphi, IN 46923

★ 9716 ★ The Arc of Dearborn County
1030 Fairview
Lawrenceburg, IN 47025

★ 9717 ★ The Arc of Decatur County Inc.
PO Box 411
Columbus, IN 47202
Phone: (812)372-0610

★ 9718 ★ The Arc of Evansville
PO Box 4089
Evansville, IN 47724-0089
Phone: (812)428-4500
Website: http://www.evansvillearc.org

★ 9719 ★ The Arc of Hancock County
PO Box 93
Greenfield, IN 46140
Phone: (317)462-3727

★ 9720 ★ The Arc of Indiana
22 E Washington, Ste. 210
Indianapolis, IN 46204
Phone: (317)977-2375 **Free:** 800-382-9100
Fax: (317)977-2385
Email: arcin@in.net
Website: http://www.arcind.org

★ 9721 ★ The Arc of Jackson County, Inc.
PO Box 411
Columbus, IN 47202
Phone: (812)372-0610

★ 9722 ★ The Arc of Owen County
RR 7, Box 296
Spencer, IN 47460

★ 9723 ★ The Arc of Tippecanoe County
PO Box 6449
Lafayette, IN 47904
Phone: (765)423-5531

★ 9724 ★ The Arc of Vigo County
89 Cherry St.
Terre Haute, IN 47807
Phone: (812)232-4112

★ 9725 ★ Association for Retarded Citizens of Wabash County
PO Box 400
Wabash, IN 46992
Phone: (219)563-8411

★ 9726 ★ Benton County Association for Retarded Citizens
PO Box 12
Fowler, IN 47944

★ 9727 ★ Bi-County Services of Adams and Wells Counties
425 E Harrison Rd.
Bluffton, IN 46714
Phone: (219)824-1253
Email: info@adifferentlight.com
Website: http://www.bi-countyservices.com

★ 9728 ★ Blue River Services, Inc.
1365 Highway 135 NW
Corydon, IN 47112
Phone: (812)738-2408
Website: http://www.brsinc.org
Remarks: Serves Crawford, Harrison, and Washington counties.

★ 9729 ★ Carey Services, Inc.
2724 S Carey St.
Marion, IN 46953
Phone: (765)668-8961
Email: info@careyservices.com
Website: http://www.careyservices.com
Remarks: Serves Blackford and Grant counties.

★ 9730 ★ Clinton County Association for Retarded Citizens
5780 S County Rd. 250 E
Frankfort, IN 46041-8698
Phone: (765)659-6380

★ 9731 ★ Davies-Martin Rehabilitation Services
PO Box 249
Linton, IN 47441
Phone: (812)847-2231

★ 9732 ★ Dubois County Association for Retarded Citizens
1250 Justin St.
Jasper, IN 47546
Phone: (812)367-6111

★ 9733 ★ Easter Seals Arc of Northeast Indiana, Inc.
2542 Thompson Ave.
Fort Wayne, IN 46807
Phone: (219)456-4534
Website: http://www.esarc.org
Stephen L. Hinkle, President
Remarks: Serves Allen, Dekalb, Huntington and Steuben counties.

★ 9734 ★ Fountain County Association for Retarded Citizens
1500 E State Rd. 32
Veedersburg, IN 47987

★ 9735 ★ Green Acres Inc.
PO Box 1252
Richmond, IN 47375-1252
Phone: (765)966-0502
Email: wccrc@GACenter.org
Website: http://www.gacenter.org
Dan Stewart, CEO & Pres

★ 9736 ★ Greene County Area Rehabilitation Center
c/o Four Rivers Resource Services
PO Box 249
Linton, IN 47441
Phone: (812)847-2231
Email: fourrivers@frrs.org
Website: http://www.frrs.org

★ 9737 ★ Hopewell Center, Madison County
PO Box 3150
Anderson, IN 46018
Phone: (765)642-0201

★ 9738 ★ Jayland Association for Retarded Citizens
1104 S Massachusetts Ave.
Portland, IN 47371

★ 9739 ★ Jefferson Switzerland Association for Retarded Citizens
3355 N State Rte. 7
Madison, IN 47250

★ 9740 ★ Jennings County Association for Retarded Citizens
PO Box 411
Columbus, IN 47202
Phone: (812)372-0610

★ 9741 ★ Johnson County Association for Retarded Citizens
PO Box 216
Franklin, IN 46131
Phone: (317)738-5500

★ 9742 ★ Knox County Association for Retarded Citizens
2830 E ARC Ave.
Vincennes, IN 47591
Phone: (812)886-4312
Website: http://www.knoxcountyarc.com

★ 9743 ★ Lake County Association for the Retarded
2650 W 35th Ave.
Gary, IN 46408
Phone: (219)884-9441

★ 9744 ★ Landmark Services, Inc.
531 N Central Ave., Ste. 3
Connersville, IN 47331-2019
Phone: (765)825-3626

★ 9745 ★ Lawrence County Association for Retarded Citizens
PO Box 393
Bedford, IN 47421
Phone: (812)279-3229

★ 9746 ★ Marshall-Starke Development Center
1901 Pidco Dr.
Plymouth, IN 46563
Phone: (219)936-9400
Remarks: Serves Fulton, Marshall, and Starke counties.

★ 9747 ★ Noble Arc of Central Indiana
7701 E 21st St.
Indianapolis, IN 46219
Phone: (317)375-2700
Website: http://www.nobleofindiana.org
Remarks: Serves Hamilton, Howard, Marion, Shelby, and Tipton counties.

★ 9748 ★ Noble County Association for Retarded Citizens
506 S Orange St.
Albion, IN 46701
Phone: (219)636-2155

★ 9749 ★ Opportunity Enterprises, Porter County
PO Box 1206
Valparaiso, IN 46384
Phone: (219)464-9621

★ 9750 ★ Parke County Association for Retarded Citizens
PO Box 170
Rockville, IN 47872
Phone: (765)569-2076

★ 9751 ★ Passages, Inc.
PO Box 1005
Columbia City, IN 46725
Phone: (219)244-7688
Email: passages@whitleynet.org
Website: http://www.passagesinc.org

★ 9752 ★ Pike County Area Rehabilitation Center
PO Box 535
Petersburg, IN 47567
Phone: (812)354-6560

★ 9753 ★ Posey County Association for Retarded Citizens
609 Short St.
New Harmony, IN 47631

★ 9754 ★ Rush County Association for Retarded Citizens
814 W 11th St.
Rushville, IN 46173
Phone: (765)932-2961

★ 9755 ★ Spencer County Association for Retarded Citizens
PO Box 11
Dale, IN 47523
Website: http://www.spencercountyarc.org

★ 9756 ★ Stone Belt Arc, Inc.
2815 E 10th St.
Bloomington, IN 47408
Phone: (812)332-2168
Email: sbcarc@bloomington.in.us
Website: http://www.stonebelt.org
Remarks: Serves Monroe County.

★ 9757 ★ Sullivan County Area Rehabilitation Center
c/o Four Rivers Resource Services
PO Box 249
Linton, IN 47441
Phone: (812)847-2231
Email: fourrivers@frrs.org
Website: http://www.frrs.org

★ 9758 ★ Sycamore Services, Inc.
1001 Sycamore Ln.
PO Box 369
Danville, IN 46122
Phone: (317)745-4715 **Fax:** (317)745-8271
Email: info@sycamoreservices.com
Website: http://www.sycamoreservices.com
Remarks: Serves Hendricks County.

★ 9759 ★ Woodlawn Center of Cass and Pulaski Counties
1416 Woodlawn Ave.
Logansport, IN 46947
Phone: (219)753-4104

Iowa

★ 9760 ★ The Arc of Allamakee County
1270 Hwy. 9
Lansing, IA 52151

★ 9761 ★ The Arc of Appanoose County
700 N Main
Centerville, IA 52544

★ 9762 ★ The Arc of Black Hawk County
2518 Pleasant Dr.
Cedar Falls, IA 50613

★ 9763 ★ The Arc of Buchanan County
308 2nd St. SW
Independence, IA 50644
Phone: (319)334-2508

★ 9764 ★ The Arc of Cedar County
795 195th St.
Mechanicsville, IA 52306

★ 9765 ★ The Arc of Chickasaw County
1826 Jasper Ave.
New Hampton, IA 50659

★ 9766 ★ The Arc of Delaware County
1841 210th Ave.
Manchester, IA 52057

★ 9767 ★ The Arc of the Dubuque Area
3475 Windsor Ave.
Dubuque, IA 52001
Phone: (319)556-1785

★ 9768 ★ The Arc of East Central Iowa
214 1st St. SW
Cedar Rapids, IA 52404
Phone: (319)365-0487

★ 9769 ★ The Arc of Grundy County
105 Clark St.
Reinbeck, IA 50669

★ 9770 ★ The Arc of Hamilton County
702 Laura Ln.
Webster City, IA 50595

★ 9771 ★ The Arc of Hardin County
PO Box 336
Hubbard, IA 50122

★ 9772 ★ The Arc of Henry County
2444 Nebraska Ave.
New London, IA 52645

★ 9773 ★ The Arc of Iowa
715 E Locust
Des Moines, IA 50309-1915
Phone: (515)283-2358

★ 9774 ★ The Arc of Iowa County
503 Henry St.
Williamsburg, IA 52361

★ 9775 ★ The Arc of Jackson County
14065 407th Ave.
Bellevue, IA 52031

★ 9776 ★ The Arc of Jefferson and Nearby Counties
PO Box 71
Richland, IA 52585

★ 9777 ★ The Arc of Johnson County
1700 1st Ave., Ste. 16
Iowa City, IA 52240
Phone: (319)351-5017
Email: Arcofjc@mcleodusa.net
Website: http://www.jccn.iowa-city.ia.us/%7Ethearcjc/

★ 9778 ★ The Arc of Lee County
1102 Morgan
Keokuk, IA 52632

★ 9779 ★ The Arc of Lucas County
Rte. 1, Box 333
Chariton, IA 50049

★ 9780 ★ The Arc of Muscatine County
PO Box 251
Muscatine, IA 52761

★ 9781 ★ The Arc of North Central Iowa
Box 168
Mason City, IA 50402-0168

★ 9782 ★ The Arc of Sac County
2580 350th St.
PO Box 128
Wall Lake, IA 51466-0128

★ 9783 ★ The Arc of Scott County
729 21st St.
Bettendorf, IA 52722

★ 9784 ★ The Arc of Story County
PO Box 5004
Ames, IA 50010-5004
Phone: (515)232-9330

★ 9785 ★ The Arc of Tama County
231 W 3rd St.
Tama, IA 52339

★ 9786 ★ The Arc of Washington County
2240 Larch Ave.
Washington, IA 52353

★ 9787 ★ The Arc of Wayne County
PO Box 37
Promise City, IA 52583-0037

★ 9788 ★ The Arc of Winneshiek County
738 Ridge Rd.
Decorah, IA 52101

★ 9789 ★ The Arc of Woodbury County
3001 Malloy Rd.
Sioux City, IA 51103

Kansas

★ 9790 ★ The Arc of Anderson County
105 Park Plaza N, Apt. 9
Garnett, KS 66032

★ 9791 ★ The Arc of Atchison County
1201 S 7th
Atchison, KS 66002

★ 9792 ★ The Arc of Bourbon County
PO Box 802
Fort Scott, KS 66701

★ 9793 ★ The Arc of Butler County
2375 W Central Ave.
El Dorado, KS 67042-3208

★ 9794 ★ The Arc of Central Plains
Box 163
Hays, KS 67601
Phone: (785)628-6512

★ 9795 ★ The Arc of Cheyenne-Rawlins Counties
RR 1, Box 16B
Atwood, KS 67730

★ 9796 ★ The Arc of Cloud County
503 E 6th
Concordia, KS 66901

★ 9797 ★ The Arc of Douglas County
2518 Ridge Ct., Rm. 238
Lawrence, KS 66046
Phone: (785)749-0121
Email: thearcdc@grapevine.net
Website: http://www.grapevine.net/~thearcdc/

★ 9798 ★ The Arc of Leavenworth County
217A Delaware
Leavenworth, KS 66048
Phone: (913)651-6464

★ 9799 ★ The Arc of Marshall County
1150 11th Rd.
Marysville, KS 66508

★ 9800 ★ The Arc of Mitchell County
Rte. 1, Box 13
Beloit, KS 67420

★ 9801 ★ The Arc of Northwest Kansas
Rte. 2, Box 7
Norton, KS 67654

★ 9802 ★ The Arc of Russell County
647 E 5th St., No. 261
PO Box 371
Russell, KS 67665
Phone: (785)483-3742

★ 9803 ★ The Arc of Saline County
PO Box 362
Salina, KS 67401

★ 9804 ★ The Arc of Sedgwick County, Inc.
2919 W 2nd St.
Wichita, KS 67212
Phone: (316)943-1191
Website: http://www.arc-sedgwickcounty.org

★ 9805 ★ The Arc of Solomon Valley
507 S Madison
Plainville, KS 67663

★ 9806 ★ The Arc of Topeka
2701 Randolph
Topeka, KS 66611
Phone: (785)232-0597

★ 9807 ★ The Arc of Wabaunsee County
6 Cedar N
Eskridge, KS 66423

Kentucky

★ 9808 ★ The Arc of Barren County
PO Box 205
Glasgow, KY 42142
Phone: (270)651-3357

★ 9809 ★ The Arc of the Bluegrass, Inc.
898 Georgetown St.
Lexington, KY 40511
Phone: (859)233-1483 **Fax:** (859)231-9695
Email: ellerbrk@mis.net
Website: http://www.arcbluegrass.com

★ 9810 ★ The Arc of Kentucky
833 E Main St.
Frankfort, KY 40601
Phone: (502)875-5225
Website: http://www.arcofky.org

★ 9811 ★ The Arc of Lake Cumberland
PO Box 1377
Somerset, KY 42501

★ 9812 ★ The Arc of Logan County
443 Hopkinsville Rd.
Russellville, KY 42276

★ 9813 ★ The Arc of Madison County, Inc.
PO Box 161
Berea, KY 40403

★ 9814 ★ The Arc of Owensboro, Inc.
PO Box 1833
Owensboro, KY 42302
Phone: (502)685-2976

★ 9815 ★ Breckenridge County Educational Association for the Handicapped
Hardinsburg, KY 40143-9802

★ 9816 ★ Citizen Advocacy Program of Northern Kentucky
426 Hallam Ave.
Erlanger, KY 41018
Phone: (606)491-3344

★ 9817 ★ Frankfort Habilitation, Inc.
Rte. 7. U.S. Hwy. 127 S
Frankfort, KY 40601
Phone: (502)227-9529

★ 9818 ★ Hardin County Arc and Handicapped
PO Box 2013
Elizabethtown, KY 42702
Phone: (502)737-1140

★ 9819 ★ Hugh E. Sandefur Training Center
801 S Main St.
PO Box 714
Henderson, KY 42419-0714
Phone: (502)827-2401

★ 9820 ★ J. U. Kevil Foundation, Inc.
PO Box 345
Mayfield, KY 42066

★ 9821 ★ The Point/Arc of Northern Kentucky
104 Pike St.
Covington, KY 41011
Phone: (859)491-9191

Louisiana

★ 9822 ★ The Arc of Baton Rouge
8326 Kelwood Ave.
Baton Rouge, LA 70806
Phone: (225)927-0855 **Fax:** (225)924-3935
Website: http://www.arcbatonrouge.org

★ 9823 ★ The Arc of Beauregard
PO Box 13
Deridder, LA 70634
Phone: (337)462-2513

★ 9824 ★ The Arc of Caddo-Bossier
351 Jordan St.
Shreveport, LA 71101
Phone: (318)221-8392 **Fax:** (318)221-4262

Website: http://www.cbarc.org
Alt. Contact: Adult services can be contacted at 5320 Greenwood Rd., Shreveport, LA 71109; phone (318) 631-9501; fax (318) 631-9583.

★ 9825 ★ The Arc of Calcasieu
4100 J Bennett Johnston Ave.
Lake Charles, LA 70615
Phone: (337)433-3620
Email: hstroud@thecarc.com
Website: http://www.thecarc.com
Howard Stroud, Exec Director

★ 9826 ★ The Arc of DeSoto
1528 Old Jefferson Hwy.
PO Drawer 1238
Mansfield, LA 71052
Phone: (318)872-3255

★ 9827 ★ The Arc of Donaldsonville
PO Box 624
Donaldsonville, LA 70346
Phone: (504)473-4516

★ 9828 ★ The Arc of Evangeline
PO Box 677
Ville Platte, LA 70586
Phone: (318)363-5553

★ 9829 ★ The Arc of Greater New Orleans
5700 Loyola Ave.
New Orleans, LA 70115
Phone: (504)897-0134
Email: arcgnolee@juno.com
Website: http://www.arcgno.org

★ 9830 ★ The Arc of Iberia
PO Box 9610
New Iberia, LA 70562-9610
Phone: (318)364-7215

★ 9831 ★ The Arc of Iberville
PO Box 201
Plaquemine, LA 70765-0201
Phone: (225)687-4062

★ 9832 ★ The Arc of Jackson Parish
123 Gansville Rd.
Jonesboro, LA 71251

★ 9833 ★ The Arc of Lafayette
303 New Hope Rd.
Lafayette, LA 70506
Phone: (318)984-6110

★ 9834 ★ The Arc of Lafourche
PO Box 269
Thibodaux, LA 70302
Phone: (504)447-6214

★ 9835 ★ The Arc of Livingston
10494 Florida Blvd.
Walker, LA 70785
Phone: (504)664-7384

★ 9836 ★ The Arc of Louisiana
PO Box 65129
Baton Rouge, LA 70896-5129
Phone: (225)383-1033

★ 9837 ★ The Arc of Morehouse
10650 Lucy Hudson
Bastrop, LA 71220
Phone: (318)283-2338

★ 9838 ★ The Arc of North Webster
PO Box 351
Sarepta, LA 71071-0351
Phone: (318)847-4356

★ 9839 ★ The Arc of Rapides
3136 Cotton Wright Dr.
Alexandria, LA 71301
Phone: (318)445-5287

★ 9840 ★ The Arc of Sabine
545 W San Antonio
PO Box 1150
Many, LA 71449
Phone: (318)256-2025

★ 9841 ★ The Arc of St. Charles, Inc.
PO Box 455
Boutte, LA 70039-0455
Phone: (504)785-0971

★ 9842 ★ The Arc of St. James
Rte. 1, Box 924
Vacherie, LA 70090
Phone: (504)265-7910

★ 9843 ★ The Arc of St. John
101 Bamboo Rd.
Laplace, LA 70068
Phone: (504)652-8003

★ 9844 ★ The Arc of St. Martin
500 Lelia St.
PO Box 128
Saint Martinville, LA 70582
Phone: (337)394-4928

★ 9845 ★ The Arc of St. Mary
PO Box 3
Centerville, LA 70522
Phone: (318)836-9445

★ 9846 ★ The Arc of St. Tammany
1541 St. Ann Pl.
Slidell, LA 70460
Phone: (504)641-0197

★ 9847 ★ The Arc of Terrebonne
1 McCord Rd.
Houma, LA 70363
Phone: (504)876-4465
Email: TARC@cajun.net
Website: http://www.terrebonnearc.org

★ 9848 ★ The Arc of Vermilion
809 S Severin St.
Erath, LA 70533

★ 9849 ★ Assumption Arc
PO Drawer 1040
Napoleonville, LA 70390
Phone: (504)369-2907

★ 9850 ★ Community Opportunities of East Ascension
1122 SE Ascension Complex Blvd.
Gonzales, LA 70737
Phone: (225)621-2000 **Fax:** (225)621-2022
Email: jrr12@eatel.net
Website: http://www.homestead.com/coea
Mark Thomas, Exec Director

★ 9851 ★ Minden Association for Retarded Citizens
PO Box 423
Minden, LA 71058
Phone: (318)377-4774

★ 9852 ★ TARC
201 E Church St.
Hammond, LA 70401
Phone: (504)345-8811
Email: tarc@tarc-hammond.com
Website: http://www.tarc-hammond.com

Maine

★ 9853 ★ The Arc of Central Aroostook
26 Lombart St
PO Box 1245
Presque Isle, ME 04769
Phone: (207)764-0134

★ 9854 ★ The Arc of Green Valley
PO Box 127
Island Falls, ME 04747
Phone: (207)463-2156

★ 9855 ★ The Arc of Northern Aroostook
459 Main St.
Van Buren, ME 04785
Phone: (207)868-5203

★ 9856 ★ The Arc of Oxford County
85 Lincoln Ave.
Rumford, ME 04276
Phone: (207)369-0141

★ 9857 ★ The Arc of Sebasticook Farms
PO Box 65
Saint Albans, ME 04971
Phone: (207)938-4615

★ 9858 ★ The Arc/Waban Projects, Inc.
RR 1, Box 2405
Sanford, ME 04073
Phone: (207)324-7955

★ 9859 ★ Coastal Workshop
35 Limerock St.
PO Box 637
Camden, ME 04843
Phone: (207)236-6008

★ 9860 ★ Community Living Association
45 School St.
Houlton, ME 04730
Phone: (207)532-9446

★ 9861 ★ Community Partners, Inc.
PO Box 363
Biddeford, ME 04005
Phone: (207)282-7113

★ 9862 ★ Downeast Horizons, Inc.
RFD 1, Box 2042
Bar Harbor, ME 04609
Phone: (207)288-4234

★ 9863 ★ Independence Arc
PO Box 642
Brunswick, ME 04011
Phone: (207)725-4371

★ 9864 ★ Kathadin Friends Inc.
1024 Central St., Ste. A
Millinocket, ME 04462-2111

Phone: (207)723-9466

★ 9865 ★ Ken-A-Set Arc
PO Box 334
Waterville, ME 04903
Phone: (207)872-6484

★ 9866 ★ Landmark Human Resources
PO Box 178
Bridgton, ME 04009
Phone: (207)647-8396

★ 9867 ★ Life Enrichment Advancing People Inc.
36 ½ High St.
PO Box 979
Farmington, ME 04938
Phone: (207)778-3443

★ 9868 ★ Maine Independent Living Services Inc.
475 Western Ave., Ste. 13
Augusta, ME 04330
Phone: (207)326-1115

★ 9869 ★ Pathways, Inc. Arc
PO Box 1267
Auburn, ME 04210

★ 9870 ★ Work First Inc.
PO Box 86
Farmington, ME 04938
Phone: (207)778-3200

Maryland

★ 9871 ★ The Arc of Anne Arundel County, Inc.
931 Spa Rd.
Annapolis, MD 21401
Phone: (410)269-1883
Website: http://www.arcofannearundel.org
Kate Rollason, Exec Director

★ 9872 ★ The Arc of Baltimore
7215 York Rd.
Baltimore, MD 21212
Phone: (410)296-2272
Website: http://www.arcofbaltimore.org

★ 9873 ★ The Arc of Carroll County
180 Kriders Church Rd.
Westminster, MD 21158
Phone: (410)848-4124

★ 9874 ★ The Arc of Frederick County, Inc.
620-A Research Dr.
Frederick, MD 21703-8619
Phone: (301)693-0909 **Fax:** (301)695-6454
Email: info@arcfc.org
Website: http://www.arcfc.org

★ 9875 ★ The Arc of Howard County, Inc.
11735 Homewood Rd.
Ellicott City, MD 21042
Phone: (410)730-0638
Website: http://www.archoward.org

★ 9876 ★ The Arc of Maryland, Inc.
49 Old Solomon's Island Rd., Ste. 205
Annapolis, MD 21401
Phone: (410)571-9320 **Fax:** (410)974-6021
Email: info@thearcmd.org
Website: http://www.thearcmd.org

★ 9877 ★ The Arc of Montgomery County, Inc.
11600 Nebel St.
Rockville, MD 20852
Phone: (301)984-5777
Email: info@arcmontmd.org
Website: http://www.arcmontmd.org

★ 9878 ★ The Arc of the Northern Chesapeake Region
PO Box 610
Aberdeen, MD 21001
Phone: (410)836-7177
Website: http://www.arcncr.org

★ 9879 ★ The Arc of Prince George's County
1401 McCormick Dr.
Largo, MD 20774
Phone: (301)925-7050 **Fax:** (301)925-4387
Email: info@thearcofpgc.org
Website: http://www.thearcofpgc.org

★ 9880 ★ The Arc of Southern Maryland
PO Box 1860
Prince Frederick, MD 20678
Phone: (410)535-2413
Email: arcadmin@arcsomd.org
Website: http://www.arcsomd.org

★ 9881 ★ The Arc of Talbot County
PO Box 776
Easton, MD 21601
Phone: (410)820-5151

★ 9882 ★ The Arc of Washington County
820 Florida Ave.
Hagerstown, MD 21740
Phone: (301)733-3550

★ 9883 ★ The Arc of Worcester
PO Box 126
Newark, MD 21841
Phone: (410)632-2382

Massachusetts

★ 9884 ★ Advocacy Resource Center of Greater New Bedford
412 B County St.
New Bedford, MA 02740
Phone: (508)996-8551

★ 9885 ★ The Arc of the Brockton Area
1250 W Chestnut St.
Brockton, MA 02301
Phone: (508)583-8030

★ 9886 ★ The Arc of Cape Cod
PO Box 428
Hyannis, MA 02601
Phone: (508)790-3667

★ 9887 ★ The Arc of East Middlesex (EMARC)
20 Gould St.
Reading, MA 01867-2927
Phone: (781)245-5262
Email: info@theemarc.org
Website: http://www.theemarc.org
Jo Ann Simons, Exec Director

★ 9888 ★ The Arc of Greater Fall River
PO Box 1943
Fall River, MA 02722
Phone: (508)679-0001

★ 9889 ★ The Arc of Greater Lawrence
1 Parker St.
Lawrence, MA 01843
Phone: (978)975-8587
Website: http://www.classinc.org/arc_page.htm

★ 9890 ★ The Arc of Greater Plymouth
4 Main St.
Kingston, MA 02364
Phone: (781)585-1310
Website: http://www.thearcofgp.com

★ 9891 ★ The Arc of Greater Waltham
56 Chestnut St.
Waltham, MA 02453
Phone: (781)899-1344

★ 9892 ★ Arc Massachusetts
217 South St.
Waltham, MA 02453
Phone: (781)891-6270
Email: arcmass@gis.net
Website: http://www.arcmass.org

★ 9893 ★ The Arc of North Central, Inc.
564 Main St.
Fitchburg, MA 01420
Phone: (978)343-8852 **Fax:** (978)343-8852
Email: info@arcofnorthcentral.org
Website: http://arcofnorthcentral.org

★ 9894 ★ The Arc of Northern Bristol County
5 Bank St.
Attleboro, MA 02703
Phone: (508)226-1445
Website: http://www.arcnbc.org

★ 9895 ★ The Arc of Northern Essex
4 Summer St., Rm 6
Haverhill, MA 01830
Phone: (508)373-0552

★ 9896 ★ The Arc of South Norfolk County
789 Clapboardtree St.
Westwood, MA 02090
Phone: (617)762-4001
Website: http://www.sncarc.org

★ 9897 ★ The Arc of Southern Worcester County
14 Mechanic St.
Box 66
Southbridge, MA 01550
Phone: (508)764-4085

★ 9898 ★ Berkshire County Arc, Inc.
395 South St.
Pittsfield, MA 01201
Phone: (413)499-4241
Email: bcarc@netconnx.net
Website: http://www.bcarc.org

★ 9899 ★ Charles River Arc
49 E Militia Hits
Needham, MA 02492-0002
Phone: (781)444-4347 **Fax:** (781)444-5146
Email: familysupport@crarc.org
Website: http://www.crarc.org

★ 9900 ★ Greater Boston Arc
1505 Commonwealth Ave.
Boston, MA 02135-3605
Phone: (617)783-3900
Email: gbarc1@msn.com
Website: http://www.gbarc.org

★ 9901 ★ Minute Man Arc for Human Services, Inc.
1269 Main St.
West Concord, MA 01742
Phone: (978)371-1543 **Fax:** (978)287-0468
Email: MMAHS@aol.com
Website: http://www.minutemanarc.org

★ 9902 ★ North Shore Arc
64 Holten St.
Danvers, MA 01923
Phone: (978)762-4878

★ 9903 ★ South Shore ARC
371 River St.
North Weymouth, MA 02191
Phone: (781)335-3023
Email: info@southshorearc.org
Website: http://www.southshorearc.org

★ 9904 ★ The United Arc of Franklin and Hampshire Counties
111 Summer St.
Greenfield, MA 01301
Phone: (413)774-5558
Email: arc@crocker.com

Michigan

★ 9905 ★ The Arc of Allegan
219 Hubbard St.
Allegan, MI 49010
Phone: (616)673-8841

★ 9906 ★ The Arc of Arenac Area
PO Box 805
Standish, MI 48658

★ 9907 ★ The Arc of Arro/Berrien County
515 Ship St., Ste. 209
Saint Joseph, MI 49085
Phone: (616)429-8166

★ 9908 ★ The Arc of Bay County
709 Columbus Ave.
Bay City, MI 48708
Phone: (517)893-1346

★ 9909 ★ The Arc of Benzie County
11721 Maple Rd.
Beulah, MI 49617

★ 9910 ★ The Arc of Calhoun County
368 Capital Ave. NE
Battle Creek, MI 49017
Phone: (616)966-2575

★ 9911 ★ The Arc of Charlevoix-Emmet
6149 E Jordan Rd.
Ellsworth, MI 49729

★ 9912 ★ The Arc of Copper County
114 1st Centennial Heights
Calumet, MI 49913

★ 9913 ★ The Arc of Delta County
PO Box 651
Escanaba, MI 49829
Phone: (906)786-9212

★ 9914 ★ The Arc of Detroit
51 W Hancock
Detroit, MI 48201
Phone: (313)831-0202

★ 9915 ★ The Arc, Downriver
4212 13th St.
Wyandotte, MI 48192
Phone: (313)283-0710

★ 9916 ★ The Arc of Genesee County
G-5069 Van Slyke Rd.
Flint, MI 48507
Phone: (313)238-2140

★ 9917 ★ The Arc of Gogebic County
127 E Mary
PO Box 45
Bessemer, MI 49911

★ 9918 ★ The Arc of the Grand Traverse Area
PO Box 204
Traverse City, MI 49685-0204
Phone: (231)941-0560

★ 9919 ★ The Arc of Gratiot County
7205 N McClelland Rd.
Breckenridge, MI 48615-9504

★ 9920 ★ The Arc of Grosse Point/ Harper Woods
621 Washington
Grosse Pointe Park, MI 48230
Email: LKel584817@aol.com
Website: http://www.geocities.com/thearcgrossepointeharperwoods
Laura Kellett, Contact

★ 9921 ★ The Arc of Ionia County
5827 N Orleans Rd.
Orleans, MI 48865
Phone: (616)761-3151

★ 9922 ★ The Arc of Iosco
5589 Schaefer Rd.
Oscoda, MI 48750

★ 9923 ★ The Arc of Isabella
PO Box 171
Mount Pleasant, MI 48804
Phone: (517)772-8081

★ 9924 ★ The Arc of Kent County
1331 Lake Dr. SE, No. 2
Grand Rapids, MI 49506
Phone: (616)459-3339

★ 9925 ★ The Arc of Lenawee
PO Box 291
Adrian, MI 49221

★ 9926 ★ The Arc of Livingston
3075 E Grand River
Howell, MI 48843
Phone: (517)546-1228

★ 9927 ★ The Arc of Manistee
481 Bryant Ave.
Manistee, MI 49660

★ 9928 ★ The Arc Michigan
1325 S Washington Ave.
Lansing, MI 48910
Phone: (517)487-5426 **Free:** 800-292-7851
Fax: (517)487-0303
Website: http://www.arcmi.org
Eric Roberts, Exec Director

★ 9929 ★ The Arc of Midland
220 W Main St., No. 14
Midland, MI 48640
Phone: (989)631-4439 **Fax:** (989)832-5528
Email: arcadmin@thearcofmidland.org
Website: http://www.thearcofmidland.org

★ 9930 ★ The Arc of Monroe County
752 S Monroe St., Ste. B
Monroe, MI 48161-1453
Phone: (734)241-5881

★ 9931 ★ The Arc of Montcalm
PO Box 1011
Stanton, MI 48888

★ 9932 ★ The Arc of Muskegon
1145 E Wesley Ave.
Muskegon, MI 49442-2197
Phone: (231)777-2006
Email: arcmusk@i2k.com
Website: http://community.mlive.com/cc/arc-muskegon

★ 9933 ★ The Arc of Newaygo County
37 E Main St.
Fremont, MI 49412
Phone: (616)924-5840

★ 9934 ★ The Arc of Northwest Wayne County
26049 5 Mile Rd.
Redford, MI 48239
Phone: (313)532-7915 **Fax:** (313)532-7488
Email: ArcNW@aol.com
Website: http://comnet.org/arcnw

★ 9935 ★ The Arc of Oakland County
1641 W Big Beaver Rd.
Troy, MI 48084-3501
Phone: (248)816-1900
Email: tfk@thearcoakland.org
Website: http://www.thearcoakland.org
Thomas F. Kendziorski, Exec Director

★ 9936 ★ The Arc of Oceana
PO Box 121
Shelby, MI 49455

★ 9937 ★ The Arc of Ogemaw County
117 Somerset Terrace
Roscommon, MI 48653

★ 9938 ★ The Arc of St. Clair County
1033 26th St.
Port Huron, MI 48060
Phone: (313)982-3261

★ 9939 ★ The Arc of Sanilac
1155 Shabbona Rd.
Snover, MI 48472

★ 9940 ★ The Arc Services
310 Johnson St., Ste. 165
Saginaw, MI 48601
Phone: (517)752-6104

★ 9941 ★ The Arc Services of Macomb, Inc.
44050 N Gratiot Ave.
Clinton Township, MI 48036-1308
Phone: (810)469-1600
Email: arcmc@tir.com
Website: http://comnet.org/local/orgs/arc/index.html

★ 9942 ★ The Arc of Shiawassee
1905 W 21
Owosso, MI 48867
Phone: (517)723-7377
Email: arcshia@shianet.org
Website: http://www.angelfire.com/mi/arcshia

★ 9943 ★ The Arc of Tuscola County
2266 W Caro Rd.
Caro, MI 48723

★ 9944 ★ The Arc of Van Buren
65651 43 Hwy.
Bangor, MI 49013
Phone: (616)427-7247

★ 9945 ★ The Arc of Western Wayne County
2257 S Wayne Rd.
Westland, MI 48186
Phone: (734)729-9100 **Fax:** (734)729-9695
Email: thearcww@tir.com
Website: http://comnet.org/arcww

★ 9946 ★ The Association for Community Advocacy
1100 N Main St., No. 205
Ann Arbor, MI 48104
Phone: (734)662-1256

★ 9947 ★ Association for Macomb-Oakland Regional Center
8080 Huntington Ridge Ct.
Washington Township, MI 48094

★ 9948 ★ Community Advocates for Persons with Developmental Disabilities
814 S Westnedge
Kalamazoo, MI 49008-1162
Phone: (616)342-9801
Email: commadvoc@worldnet.att.net
Website: http://www.communityadvocates.org
George Martin, CEO & Pres

★ 9949 ★ Parents and Advocates for Wayne Community Services
28623 W Chicago
Livonia, MI 48150

★ 9950 ★ Tri-County Community Advocates for People with Developmental Disabilities, Inc.
921 N Washington Ave.
Lansing, MI 48906-5137
Phone: (517)484-3068

Minnesota

★ 9951 ★ The Arc of Alexandria
107 Donna Ave.
Alexandria, MN 56308
Phone: (320)762-2015

★ 9952 ★ The Arc of Anoka, Ramsey, and Suburban Counties
1526 E 122nd St.
Burnsville, MN 55337-6804
Phone: (952)890-3057

★ 9953 ★ The Arc of Blue Earth/Nicollet Counties
2113 Excalibur Rd.
North Mankato, MN 56003
Phone: (507)345-1542

★ 9954 ★ The Arc of Brown County
Box 641
New Ulm, MN 56073
Phone: (507)354-7445

★ 9955 ★ The Arc of Central Minnesota
6112 322nd St.
Saint Cloud, MN 56303
Phone: (320)240-9550

★ 9956 ★ The Arc of Clay County
Townsite Ctr., Rm. 141
810 4th Ave. S
Moorhead, MN 56560
Phone: (218)233-5949

★ 9957 ★ The Arc of Crow Wing County
2881 44th St. NW
Pine River, MN 56474
Phone: (218)587-5259

★ 9958 ★ The Arc of Fergus Falls
PO Box 1032
Fergus Falls, MN 56537

★ 9959 ★ The Arc of Freeborn County
407 E William St.
Albert Lea, MN 56007-2964
Phone: (507)377-3469

★ 9960 ★ The Arc of the Headwaters
522 Beltrami Ave., Ste. 108
Bemidji, MN 56601
Phone: (218)759-0097

★ 9961 ★ The Arc of Hennepin-Carver
4301 Hwy 7, No. 140
Minneapolis, MN 55416
Phone: (952)920-0855
Website: http://www.archennepincarver.org

★ 9962 ★ The Arc of Kandiyohi County
201 SW 4th St., No. 12
Willmar, MN 56201-0801
Phone: (320)231-1777

★ 9963 ★ The Arc of LeSueur County
812 Central Ave. S
New Prague, MN 56071

★ 9964 ★ Arc Minnesota
770 Transfer Rd., Ste. 26
Saint Paul, MN 55114-1422
Phone: (651)523-0823
Email: arcminn@mtn.org
Website: http://www.arcminnesota.com

★ 9965 ★ The Arc of Mower County
709 N Main St.
Austin, MN 55912
Phone: (507)433-8994

★ 9966 ★ The Arc of Norman County
209 Jamison Dr.
Ada, MN 56510

★ 9967 ★ The Arc of Northland
201 Ordean Bldg., Ste. 201
424 W Superior
Duluth, MN 55802
Phone: (218)726-4725

★ 9968 ★ The Arc of Range
309 7th St. S
Virginia, MN 55792
Phone: (218)741-2928

★ 9969 ★ The Arc of Rice County
12 6th St. NW
Faribault, MN 55021

★ 9970 ★ The Arc of St. Cloud
PO Box 251
Saint Cloud, MN 56302
Phone: (320)251-7272

★ 9971 ★ The Arc of Southeastern Minnesota
903 W Center, No. 140
Rochester, MN 55902
Phone: (507)287-2032

★ 9972 ★ The Arc of Southwestern Minnesota
1271 76th Ave.
Sherburn, MN 56171
Phone: (507)764-6894

★ 9973 ★ The Arc of Stevens County
Rte. 2, Box 200
Morris, MN 56267

★ 9974 ★ The Arc of Wadena County
513 2nd St. SW
Wadena, MN 56482

★ 9975 ★ The Arc of Waseca County
601 16th Ave. NE
Waseca, MN 56093
Phone: (612)758-2615

★ 9976 ★ The Arc of Western Stearns
34934 Queensfield Rd.
Sauk Centre, MN 56378

Mississippi

★ 9977 ★ The Arc of Adams County
PO Box 275
Natchez, MS 39121-0275
Phone: (601)442-2264

★ 9978 ★ The Arc of Biloxi
771 Water St.
Biloxi, MS 39530
Phone: (228)374-1200

★ 9979 ★ The Arc of Clay County
PO Box 613
West Point, MS 39773

★ 9980 ★ The Arc of Forrest County
PO Box 18800
Hattiesburg, MS 39404-8800

★ 9981 ★ The Arc of Itawamba County
Rte. 3, Box 184A
Fulton, MS 38843

★ 9982 ★ The Arc of Jones County
PO Box 1233
Laurel, MS 39441
Phone: (601)426-2944

★ 9983 ★ The Arc of Mississippi
7 Lakeland Cir., Ste. 600
Jackson, MS 39216
Phone: (601)982-1180
Website: http://www.arcms.org

★ 9984 ★ The Arc of Pearl River
PO Box 1816
Picayune, MS 39466

★ 9985 ★ The Arc of Tishomingo County
1133 County Rd. 992
Iuka, MS 38852
Phone: (662)423-4517

★ 9986 ★ The Arc of Warren County
100 Smokey Ln.
Vicksburg, MS 39180
Phone: (601)638-2761

★ 9987 ★ The Arc of Washington County
136 S Poplar St.
PO Box 1733
Greenville, MS 38702-1733
Phone: (662)332-3271

★ 9988 ★ The Arc of West Jackson County
1904 Government St.
Ocean Springs, MS 39564
Phone: (228)872-2939

★ 9989 ★ Gulf Coast Society for Retarded Citizens
PO Box 6651
Gulfport, MS 39506
Phone: (601)868-9755

★ 9990 ★ North Mississippi Special Needs Arc
403 S Commerce St.
Ripley, MS 38663
Phone: (662)837-9883

★ 9991 ★ Tri County Arc
PO Box 1084
Summit, MS 39666
Phone: (601)276-3603

Missouri

★ 9992 ★ The Arc of Clay and Platte Counties, Inc.
7400 C N Oak Traffic Way
Gladstone, MO 64118
Phone: (816)436-3009

★ 9993 ★ The Arc of Eastern Jackson County
704 E 121 St.
Kansas City, MO 64146

★ 9994 ★ The Arc of the Ozarks
1501 E Pythian
Springfield, MO 65802
Phone: (417)864-7887
Website: http://www.thearcoftheozarks.org

★ 9995 ★ The Arc of Stoddard County
PO Box 444
Dexter, MO 63841
Phone: (573)624-8525

★ 9996 ★ St. Louis Arc
1816 Lackland Hill Pkwy., No. 200
Saint Louis, MO 63146
Phone: (314)569-2211 **Fax:** (314)569-0778
Website: http://www.slarc.org

Montana

★ 9997 ★ Rocky Mountain Arc
207 S Montana St.
Butte, MT 59701

★ 9998 ★ Yellowstone Arc
602 18th St. W
Billings, MT 59102

Nebraska

★ 9999 ★ The Arc of Adams/Clay Counties
414 E 6th St.
Hastings, NE 68901
Phone: (402)463-5797

★ 10000 ★ The Arc of Buffalo County
2022 Ave. A, Ste. 17
Kearney, NE 68847
Phone: (308)237-4343

★ 10001 ★ The Arc of Butler County
328 S 4th St.
David City, NE 68632

★ 10002 ★ The Arc of Central Nebraska
720 W Stolley Park Rd.
Grand Island, NE 68801

★ 10003 ★ The Arc of Cheyenne County
1544 King
Sidney, NE 69162

★ 10004 ★ The Arc of Colfax County
935 Rd. 6
Schuyler, NE 68661-7160

★ 10005 ★ The Arc of Custer
PO Box 34
Broken Bow, NE 68822
Phone: (308)872-6067

★ 10006 ★ The Arc of Elkhorn Valley
800 Cornhusker Dr.
West Point, NE 68788

★ 10007 ★ The Arc of Hamilton/Merrick Counties
915 P St.
Aurora, NE 68818
Phone: (402)694-3519

★ 10008 ★ The Arc of Lincoln-Lancaster County
1101 Arapahoe, Ste. 5
Lincoln, NE 68502
Phone: (402)421-8866
Website: http://www.lincolnne.com/nonprofit.arc

★ 10009 ★ The Arc of Nebraska
1672 Van Dorn St.
Lincoln, NE 68502
Phone: (402)475-4407 **Free:** 800-666-7907
Website: http://www.arc-nebraska.org

★ 10010 ★ The Arc of Norfolk
PO Box 32
Norfolk, NE 68702
Phone: (402)379-1160

★ 10011 ★ The Arc, North Central
1310 Sheridan Pl.
Grand Island, NE 68803

★ 10012 ★ The Arc of Platte County
Rte. 2, Box 62
Genoa, NE 68640
Phone: (402)993-2489

★ 10013 ★ The Arc of Sarpy
3222 Chad St.
Bellevue, NE 68123
Phone: (402)291-8494

★ 10014 ★ The Arc of Saunders
1550 N Linder
Wahoo, NE 68066

★ 10015 ★ The Arc of Seward
255 N 7th
Staplehurst, NE 68439

★ 10016 ★ The Arc, South Central
11557 RD 740
Holdrege, NE 68949

★ 10017 ★ The Arc, Southeast
2423 R St.
Auburn, NE 68305

★ 10018 ★ The Arc, Southwest
RR3, Box 7621
Culbertson, NE 69024
Phone: (308)278-2788

★ 10019 ★ The Ollie Webb Center
1941 S 42nd St., Ste. 122
Omaha, NE 68105-2942
Phone: (402)346-5220

Nevada

★ 10020 ★ The Arc of Churchill County
PO Box 1641
Fallon, NV 89407
Phone: (775)423-4760

★ 10021 ★ The Arc of Ormsby
PO Box 491
Carson City, NV 89702
Phone: (702)882-8520

★ 10022 ★ The Arc of Washoe
790 Sutro St.
Reno, NV 89512
Phone: (775)333-9272

★ 10023 ★ Opportunity Village Arc
6300 W Oakey Blvd.
Las Vegas, NV 89146
Phone: (702)259-3707
Website: http://www.opportunityvillage.org

New Hampshire

★ 10024 ★ The Arc of Greater Manchester
PO Box 3363
Manchester, NH 03105-3363

★ 10025 ★ Concord Regional Arc, Inc.
PO Box 1173
Concord, NH 03302

★ 10026 ★ Salem Arc, Inc.
8 Centerville Dr.
Salem, NH 03079
Phone: (603)893-9889

New Jersey

★ 10027 ★ The Arc Ocean County Chapter
815 Cedar Bridge Ave.
Lakewood, NJ 08701
Phone: (732)363-3335

★ 10028 ★ The Arc Warren County Chapter
319 W Washington Ave.
Washington, NJ 07882
Phone: (908)689-7525

★ 10029 ★ The Arc of Atlantic County
101 Shore Rd.
Somers Point, NJ 08244
Phone: (609)926-0800

★ 10030 ★ The Arc of Bergen and Passaic Counties, Inc.
223 Moore St.
Hackensack, NJ 07601
Phone: (201)343-0322
Email: ArcBP@aol.com
Website: http://www.arcbergenpassaic.org

★ 10031 ★ The Arc of Burlington
1 Underwood Ct., Unit 2
Delran, NJ 08075
Phone: (856)764-9494
Email: info@arcofburlington.org
Website: http://www.arcofburlington.org

★ 10032 ★ The Arc of Camden
215 W White Horse Pike
Berlin, NJ 08009
Phone: (856)767-3650

★ 10033 ★ The Arc of Cape May County, Inc.
922 Rte. 47
PO Box 255
South Dennis, NJ 08245
Phone: (609)861-7100
Email: support@arcofcapemay.org
Website: http://www.arcofcapemay.org
Jean McCarthy, President

★ 10034 ★ The Arc of Cumberland
1680 W Sherman Ave.
Vineland, NJ 08360
Phone: (609)691-9138
Website: http://www.arccumberland.org

★ 10035 ★ The Arc of Essex
7 Regent St.
Livingston, NJ 07039
Phone: (973)535-1181
Website: http://www.arcessex.org

★ 10036 ★ The Arc of Gloucester
1555 Gateway Blvd.
Woodbury, NJ 08096
Phone: (856)848-8648

★ 10037 ★ The Arc of Hunterdon County
1322 State Route 31 N, Ste. 5
Annandale, NJ 08801
Phone: (908)730-7827
Website: http://www.archunterdon.org

★ 10038 ★ The Arc/Mercer, Inc.
231 Lawrenceville Rd.
Lawrenceville, NJ 08648
Phone: (609)278-1211
Email: arcmercer@aol.com
Website: http://www.arcmercer.org

★ 10039 ★ The Arc of Middlesex County
32 Ford Ave., 2nd Fl.
Milltown, NJ 08850
Phone: (732)247-8155
Email: arcmc@arc-middlesex.org
Website: http://www.arc-middlesex.org

★ 10040 ★ The Arc of Monmouth County
1158 Wayside Rd.
Tinton Falls, NJ 07712
Phone: (732)493-1919
Email: arcmon@superlink.net
Website: http://www.arcofmonmouth.org

★ 10041 ★ The Arc of Morris County
PO Box 123
Morris Plains, NJ 07950-0123
Phone: (973)326-9750

★ 10042 ★ The Arc of New Jersey
985 Livingston Ave.
North Brunswick, NJ 08902
Phone: (732)246-2525 **Fax:** (732)214-1834
Email: info@arcnj.org
Website: http://www.arcnj.org
Thomas Baffuto, Exec Director

★ 10043 ★ The Arc of Salem
150 Salem-Woodstown Rd.
PO Box 5
Salem, NJ 08079
Phone: (609)935-3600

★ 10044 ★ The Arc of Somerset County
141 S Main St.
Manville, NJ 08835
Phone: (908)725-8544
Email: ArcOffice@TheArcOfSomerset.org
Website: http://www.thearcofsomerset.org

★ 10045 ★ The Arc of Sussex
11 U.S. Rte. 206., Ste. 100
Augusta, NJ 07822
Phone: (973)383-7442
Website: http://www.scarc.org

★ 10046 ★ The Arc of Union County, Inc.
1225 South Ave.
Plainfield, NJ 07062
Phone: (908)754-5910
Email: info@arcunion.org
Website: http://www.arcunion.org

New Mexico

★ 10047 ★ The Arc of Artesia
1504 W Dallas Ave.
Artesia, NM 88210
Phone: (505)746-4811

★ 10048 ★ The Arc of Cibola County
1405 Dona
Grants, NM 87020

★ 10049 ★ The Arc of Curry County
2118 Carolina
Box 1835
Clovis, NM 88101

★ 10050 ★ The Arc of Las Cruces
2225 E Griggs Ave.
Las Cruces, NM 88001
Phone: (505)525-3811

★ 10051 ★ The Arc of Luna County
2020 S Columbus Rd.
Deming, NM 88030

★ 10052 ★ The Arc of New Mexico
3655 Carlisle NE
Albuquerque, NM 87110-5564
Phone: (505)883-4630 **Free:** 800-358-6493
Fax: (505)883-5564
Email: arcnm@arcnm.com
Website: http://www.arcnm.com

★ 10053 ★ The Arc of Otero County
873 Wright Ave.
Alamogordo, NM 88310
Phone: (505)437-0919

★ 10054 ★ The Arc of Roswell
712 N Lea
Roswell, NM 88201

★ 10055 ★ The Arc of Santa Fe
945 Vuelta del Sur
Santa Fe, NM 87505

★ 10056 ★ The Arc of Taos County
7421 NDCBU
Taos, NM 87571
Phone: (505)758-4274

★ 10057 ★ The Arc of Thriftown, Inc.
200 W Broadway
Farmington, NM 87401
Phone: (505)325-8998

★ 10058 ★ ARCA
11300 Lomas Blvd. NE
Albuquerque, NM 87112
Phone: (505)332-6700
Website: http://www.arc-a.org
Elaine Solimon, Exec Director

New York

★ 10059 ★ The Arc of Onondaga
600 S Wilbur Ave.
Syracuse, NY 13204
Phone: (315)476-7441
Email: tonipaglia@aol.com
Website: http://www.arcon.org
Toni Paglia, Contact

★ 10060 ★ The Arc of Ontario
3071 County Complex Dr.
Canandaigua, NY 14424
Phone: (716)394-7500
Email: contact@ontarioarc.org
Website: http://www.ontarioarc.org

★ 10061 ★ The Arc of Orleans County
PO Box 439
Albion, NY 14411-0439
Phone: (716)589-5516
Email: dcolquhoun@arcoforleans.com
Website: http://www.arcoforleans.org
Donald Colquhoun, Exec Director

★ 10062 ★ The Arc of Otsego County
35 Academy St.
PO Box 490
Oneonta, NY 13820
Phone: (607)432-8595

★ 10063 ★ The Arc of Schuyler County
203 12th St.
Watkins Glen, NY 14891
Phone: (607)535-6934
Email: manager@arcofschuyler.org
Website: http://www.schuylerarc.com

★ 10064 ★ The Arc of Seneca-Cayuga
1083 Waterloo Geneva Rd.
Waterloo, NY 13165
Phone: (315)539-5067
Email: mail@sencayarc.org
Website: http://www.sencayarc.org
Kevin M. Smith, Exec Director

★ 10065 ★ The Arc of Westchester
74 Westmoreland Ave.
White Plains, NY 10606
Phone: (914)428-8330
Website: http://www.westchesterarc.org

★ 10066 ★ Heritage Centers Erie County Chapter
101 Oak St.
Buffalo, NY 14203
Phone: (716)856-4201
Website: http://www.heritagecenters.org

★ 10067 ★ Herkimer Area Resource Center
333 S Main St.
PO Box 271
Herkimer, NY 13350
Phone: (315)866-8339

★ 10068 ★ Livingston-Wyoming Association for Retarded Citizens
18 Main St.
Mount Morris, NY 14510
Phone: (716)658-2828

★ 10069 ★ NYSArc
393 Delaware Ave.
Delmar, NY 12054
Phone: (518)439-8311 **Fax:** (518)439-1893
Email: nysarc@nysarc.org
Website: http://www.nysarc.org

★ 10070 ★ NYSARC, Inc. Chautauqua County Chapter
880 E 2nd St.
Jamestown, NY 14701
Phone: (716)483-2344

★ 10071 ★ NYSARC, Inc. Delaware County Chapter
RR 1, Box 67A
Walton, NY 13856
Phone: (607)865-7126

★ 10072 ★ NYSARC, Inc. Essex County Chapter
7 St. Patricks Pl.
Port Henry, NY 12974
Phone: (518)546-3381

★ 10073 ★ NYSARC, Inc. Franklin County Chapter
12 Mohawk St.
Tupper Lake, NY 12986
Phone: (518)359-3351

★ 10074 ★ NYSARC, Inc. Monroe County Chapter
1000 Elmwood Ave.
Rochester, NY 14620
Phone: (716)271-0660
Website: http://www.arcmonroe.org

★ 10075 ★ NYSARC, Inc. Montgomery County Chapter
Rte. 55
PO Box 639
Amsterdam, NY 12010
Phone: (518)842-5080

★ 10076 ★ NYSARC, Inc. Oneida-Lewis Chapter
245 Genesee St.
Utica, NY 13501
Phone: (315)738-1366
Website: http://www.thearcolc.org

★ 10077 ★ NYSARC, Inc. Steuben Chapter
6838 Industrial Park Rd.
Bath, NY 14810-8315
Phone: (607)776-4146
Email: steubenarc1@infoblvd.net
Website: http://www.steubenarc.com

★ 10078 ★ NYSARC, Inc. Yates County Chapter
235 North Ave.
Penn Yan, NY 14527
Phone: (315)536-7447

North Carolina

★ 10079 ★ The Arc of Alamance County, Inc.
PO Box 1275
Burlington, NC 27215
Phone: (336)438-2040
Email: thearcal@netpath.net
Website: http://www.netpath.net/%7Ethearcal/

★ 10080 ★ The Arc of Beaufort County Inc.
1534 W 5th St.
Washington, NC 27889
Phone: (252)946-0151

★ 10081 ★ The Arc of Brunswick County
PO Box 806
Supply, NC 28462

★ 10082 ★ The Arc of Buncombe County
PO Box 1365
Asheville, NC 28802
Phone: (704)253-1255

★ 10083 ★ The Arc of Cabarrus County
PO Box 1367
Concord, NC 28026-1367
Phone: (704)788-1616
Email: arccabarrus@ctc.net
Website: http://www.arcnc.org/cabarrus

★ 10084 ★ The Arc of Cherokee-Clay Inc.
PO Box 156
Murphy, NC 28906
Phone: (828)837-7874

★ 10085 ★ The Arc of Craven County
PO Box 12211
New Bern, NC 28562

★ 10086 ★ The Arc of Cumberland County
3623 Sycamore Dairy Rd.
Fayetteville, NC 28303
Phone: (910)867-2141
Email: ArcCumberland@aol.com
Website: http://www.disabilityresourcecenter.net

★ 10087 ★ The Arc of Davidson County
6 Vance Circle
Lexington, NC 27292
Phone: (704)246-2842

★ 10088 ★ The Arc of Durham County
3500 Westgate Dr., Ste 303
Durham, NC 27707
Phone: (919)493-8141
Email: thearcdc@mindspring.com
Website: http://www.arcnc.org/durham

★ 10089 ★ The Arc of Forsyth County
4265 Brownsboro Rd., Ste. 100
Winston-Salem, NC 27106-3425
Phone: (336)759-9619

★ 10090 ★ The Arc of Greensboro, Inc.
207-M S Westgate Dr.
Greensboro, NC 27407
Phone: (336)373-1076

★ 10091 ★ The Arc of Halifax County
PO Box 921
Littleton, NC 27850
Phone: (919)445-3378

★ 10092 ★ The Arc of Harnett County
PO Box 42
Buies Creek, NC 27506

★ 10093 ★ The Arc of Haywood County, Inc.
PO Box 832
Waynesville, NC 28786

★ 10094 ★ The Arc of High Point
153 E Bellevue Dr.
High Point, NC 27265
Phone: (336)883-0650
Website: http://www.arc-of-hp.com

★ 10095 ★ The Arc of Iredell County
328 Grant Rd.
Statesville, NC 28677
Phone: (704)873-2101

★ 10096 ★ The Arc of Jackson County
1262 Locust Creek Rd.
Sylva, NC 28779

★ 10097 ★ The Arc of Lee County
PO Box 4941
Sanford, NC 27331
Phone: (919)718-9122

★ 10098 ★ The Arc of Lenoir County
PO Box 1677
Kinston, NC 28503
Phone: (252)522-2814

★ 10099 ★ The Arc of Lincoln County
227 E Water St.
Lincolnton, NC 28092

★ 10100 ★ The Arc of Mecklenburg County, Inc.
5601 Executive Center Dr., No. 106
Charlotte, NC 28212
Phone: (704)535-4289
Website: http://www.homestead.com/arcmeck

★ 10101 ★ The Arc of Montgomery County
694 Horseshoe Bend Rd.
Troy, NC 27371
Phone: (910)428-4298

★ 10102 ★ The Arc of Moore County
PO Box 773
Southern Pines, NC 28387
Phone: 800-909-9272

★ 10103 ★ The Arc of North Carolina
4200 Six Forks Rd.
Raleigh, NC 27609
Phone: (919)782-4632 **Free:** 800-662-8706
Fax: (919)782-4634
Email: Rsewell108@aol.com
Website: http://www.arcnc.org

★ 10104 ★ The Arc of Onslow Advocacy for Special Needs
201 Taylor Notion Rd.
Cape Carteret, NC 28584
Phone: (252)393-4414

★ 10105 ★ The Arc of Orange County
PO Box 2594
Chapel Hill, NC 27515-2594
Phone: (919)942-5119
Website: http://www.arcoforange.org

★ 10106 ★ The Arc of Person County
PO Box 1182
Roxboro, NC 27573-1182

★ 10107 ★ The Arc of Pitt County
609-A Country Club Dr.
Greenville, NC 27834-6210
Phone: (919)756-1056

★ 10108 ★ The Arc of Robeson County
116 W 8th St.
Lumberton, NC 28359

★ 10109 ★ The Arc of Rockingham County
568 Glovenia St.
Eden, NC 27288

★ 10110 ★ The Arc of Rocky Mount
1230 Beal St.
Rocky Mount, NC 27804

★ 10111 ★ The Arc of Rowan County
1918 W Innes St.
Salisbury, NC 28144
Phone: (704)637-1521

★ 10112 ★ The Arc of Stanly County
PO Box 2448
Albemarle, NC 28002-2448
Phone: (704)983-3911
Website: http://www.arcofstanlync.org

★ 10113 ★ The Arc of Stokes County
221 Whispering Creek Dr.
King, NC 27021
Phone: (910)773-4166

★ 10114 ★ The Arc of Surry County
Rte. 1, Box 528
Dobson, NC 27017

★ 10115 ★ The Arc of Union County
102 E Franklin St.
Monroe, NC 28112
Phone: (704)283-1537

★ 10116 ★ The Arc of Vance County
2550 Flemingtown Rd.
Henderson, NC 27536

★ 10117 ★ The Arc of Wake County, Inc.
401 Oberlin Rd., Ste. 225
Raleigh, NC 27605
Phone: (919)832-2660

★ 10118 ★ The Arc of Wilson County
PO Box 3943
Wilson, NC 27895-3943
Phone: (252)237-8266

★ 10119 ★ The Arc of Yadkin County
PO Box 233
East Bend, NC 27018

★ 10120 ★ Columbus Arc, Inc.
777 Vinson Blvd.
Whiteville, NC 28472

★ 10121 ★ Davie County Arc, Inc.
PO Box 291
Mocksville, NC 27028

★ 10122 ★ Gaston County Arc, Inc.
200 E Franklin Blvd.
Gastonia, NC 28052
Phone: (704)861-1036

★ 10123 ★ Scotland County Association for Retarded Citizens
1028 Elizabeth Dr.
Laurinburg, NC 28352

North Dakota

★ 10124 ★ The Arc of Barnes County
141 2nd St. NE
Valley City, ND 58072

★ 10125 ★ The Arc of Bismarck
1211 Park Ave.
Bismarck, ND 58504
Phone: (701)222-1854

★ 10126 ★ The Arc of Cass County
2533 S University Dr.
PO Box 6461
Fargo, ND 58109-6461
Phone: (701)293-8191
Email: arccassnd@aol.com
Website: http://www.arccassnd.com

★ 10127 ★ The Arc of Little Missouri
608 1st St. NW
Bowman, ND 58623

★ 10128 ★ The Arc of North Dakota, Inc.
c/o The Arc, Upper Valley
PO Box 12420
Grand Forks, ND 58208-2420
Phone: (701)772-6191 **Free:** 877-250-2022

★ 10129 ★ The Arc of Stutsman County, Inc.
PO Box 1646
Jamestown, ND 58401

★ 10130 ★ The Arc, Upper Valley, Inc.
2500 Demers Ave.
PO Box 12420
Grand Forks, ND 58208-2420
Phone: (701)772-6191 **Free:** 877-250-2022
Website: http://www.thearcuppervalley.com

★ 10131 ★ Dickinson Area Arc, Inc.
PO Box 1421
Dickinson, ND 58601
Phone: (701)264-7828

Ohio

★ 10132 ★ The Arc of Allen County
546 S Collett
Lima, OH 45805
Phone: (419)225-6285

★ 10133 ★ The Arc of Ashtabula County
1120 Rte. 167
Jefferson, OH 44047

★ 10134 ★ The Arc of Auglaize County
428 W Haven Dr.
New Bremen, OH 45869
Phone: (419)629-2419

★ 10135 ★ The Arc of Butler County
5645 Liberty Fairfield Rd.
Hamilton, OH 45011
Phone: (513)863-3735

★ 10136 ★ The Arc of Clark County
PO Box 3011
Springfield, OH 45501
Phone: (513)323-3755

★ 10137 ★ The Arc of Clermont/Brown Counties
1075 Ohio Pike
Withamsville, OH 45245
Phone: (513)752-4330
Email: thearccb@aol.com
Website: http://www.thearc-cb.org

★ 10138 ★ The Arc of Erie County
The Kaleidoscope Ctr.
4405 Galloway Rd., No. 112
Sandusky, OH 44870
Phone: (419)625-9677
Email: arc@arcoferiecounty.linkohio.com
Website: http://arcoferiecounty.linkohio.com

★ 10139 ★ The Arc of Geauga, Inc.
12843 Opalocka
Chesterland, OH 44026

★ 10140 ★ The Arc of Hamilton County
1821 Summit Rd., No. 30
Cincinnati, OH 45237-2187
Phone: (513)821-2113

★ 10141 ★ The Arc of Knox County
600 N Fay St.
Mount Vernon, OH 43050

★ 10142 ★ The Arc of Licking County
175 S William St.
Newark, OH 43055
Phone: (740)345-9793

★ 10143 ★ The Arc of Lucas County
1 Stranahan Sq., No. 540
Toledo, OH 43604
Phone: (419)242-9587

★ 10144 ★ The Arc of Mercer County
372 E Main
PO Box 413
Saint Henry, OH 45883

★ 10145 ★ The Arc of Miami County
204 E Franklin St.
Troy, OH 45373
Phone: (513)339-6222

★ 10146 ★ The Arc of Ohio
1335 Dublin Rd., Ste. 205C
Columbus, OH 43212
Phone: (614)487-4720 **Free:** 800-875-2723
Fax: (614)487-4725
Email: TheArcOhio@aol.com
Website: http://www.thearcofohio.org
Gary Tonks, Exec Director

★ 10147 ★ The Arc of Ottawa County
1 Stranahan Sq., No. 540
Toledo, OH 43604-1900

★ 10148 ★ The Arc of Shelby County
PO Box 925
Sidney, OH 45365

★ 10149 ★ The Arc of Stark County
Belden Village Tower
4450 Belden Village St. NW, No. 503
Canton, OH 44718-2564
Phone: (330)492-5225

★ 10150 ★ The Arc of Summit and Portage Counties
90 N Prospect St.
Akron, OH 44304
Phone: (330)374-1594
Email: ArcSCPC@worldnet.att.net
Website: http://www.arcsummitportage.org

★ 10151 ★ The Arc of Warren County
3023 Ash Ct.
Mason, OH 45040
Phone: (513)763-2879

★ 10152 ★ The Arc of Washington County
PO Box 1003
Marietta, OH 45750

★ 10153 ★ The Arc of Wood County
PO Box 264
Bowling Green, OH 43402
Phone: (419)353-1099

★ 10154 ★ Center for Mental Retardation
1621 Euclid Ave., Ste. 802
Cleveland, OH 44115-2107
Phone: (216)621-4504

★ 10155 ★ Mahoning County Council for Retarded Citizens
3024 Center Rd., Rte. 224
Poland, OH 44514
Phone: (330)707-1134

★ 10156 ★ Society for the Handicapped of Medina County
4283 Paradise Rd.
Seville, OH 44273
Phone: (330)725-7041

Oklahoma

★ 10157 ★ The Arc of Edmond
PO Box 268
Edmond, OK 73083
Phone: (405)341-7132

★ 10158 ★ The Arc of Oklahoma
2442 N Walnut Ave., Ste. D
Oklahoma City, OK 73105
Phone: (405)528-1525

★ 10159 ★ Homelife Association
PO Box 35903
Tulsa, OK 74153-0903
Phone: (918)745-1114

★ 10160 ★ Tulsa Advocates for the Rights of Citizens with Developmental Disabilities
16 E 16th St., Ste. 405
Tulsa, OK 74119
Phone: (918)582-8272

Oregon

★ 10161 ★ The Arc of Benton County
Plaza 9 Shopping Ctr.
1885 NW 9th St.
Corvallis, OR 97330
Phone: (541)753-1711
Email: info@arcbenton.org
Website: http://www.arcbenton.org
Karin Frederick, Exec Director

★ 10162 ★ The Arc of Douglas County
PO Box 694
Roseburg, OR 97470
Phone: (541)672-5208

★ 10163 ★ The Arc of Eastern Oregon
PO Box 1393
Ontario, OR 97914
Phone: (541)889-2651

★ 10164 ★ The Arc of Jackson County
PO Box 1485
Medford, OR 97501
Phone: (541)779-4520

★ 10165 ★ The Arc of Josephine County
PO Box 54
Grants Pass, OR 97526
Phone: (541)479-0301

★ 10166 ★ The Arc of Lane County
2710 Taylor
Eugene, OR 97403
Phone: (541)343-5256
Website: http://www.arclane.org

★ 10167 ★ The Arc of Linn County
PO Box 577
Lebanon, OR 97355
Phone: (541)259-5528

★ 10168 ★ The Arc of Marion County
PO Box 12474
Salem, OR 97309
Phone: (503)581-3451

★ 10169 ★ The Arc of Multnomah County
619 SW 11th Ave., Ste. 234
Portland, OR 97205-2692
Phone: (503)223-7279
Website: http://www.thearcmult.org

★ 10170 ★ The Arc of Oregon
1745 State St.
Salem, OR 97301
Phone: (503)581-2726 **Free:** 877-581-2726
Fax: (503)363-7168
Email: arcoforg@CallAtg.com
Website: http://www.open.org/arcoforg

★ 10171 ★ The Arc of Polk
9990 Oak Hill Rd.
Independence, OR 97351

★ 10172 ★ The Arc of Tillamook County
2410 5th St.
PO Box 416
Tillamook, OR 97141

★ 10173 ★ The Arc of Umatilla County
215 W Orchard Ave.
Hermiston, OR 97838-1738
Phone: (541)567-7615

★ 10174 ★ The Arc of Washington County
PO Box 5778
Aloha, OR 97006-5778
Phone: (503)649-6110

★ 10175 ★ Central Oregon Arc, Inc.
2050 Bluebird Ln.
Bend, OR 97701

★ 10176 ★ Jackson County Family Consortium
2535 Griffin Creek Rd.
Medford, OR 97501-4219

★ 10177 ★ Residential Assistance Program
2050 NE Bluebird Ct.
Bend, OR 97701
Phone: (541)388-3060

★ 10178 ★ Share House, Inc.
3761 Kinciad St.
Eugene, OR 97405
Phone: (541)485-4330

★ 10179 ★ Specialized Housing, Inc.
5319 SW Westgate Dr., No. 124
Portland, OR 97221
Phone: (503)292-5066

Pennsylvania

★ 10180 ★ Achieva
711 Bingham St.
Pittsburgh, PA 15203
Phone: (412)995-5000 **Free:** 888-272-7229
Fax: (412)995-5001
Email: contact@achieva.info
Website: http://www.achieva.info
Frmly: Arc Allegheny.

★ 10181 ★ The Arc of Adams County
17 Rice Ave.
PO Box 551
Biglerville, PA 17307
Phone: (717)677-8487

★ 10182 ★ The Arc of Beaver County
Beaver Valley Professional Bldg., No. 103
1260 N Broadhead Rd.
Monaca, PA 15061
Phone: (724)775-1602

★ 10183 ★ The Arc of Berks County
1829 New Holland Rd., Ste. 9
Reading, PA 19607-2228
Phone: (610)603-0227

★ 10184 ★ The Arc of Blair County
431 Jackson Ave.
Altoona, PA 16602
Phone: (814)946-1011

★ 10185 ★ The Arc of Bucks County, Inc.
PO Box 755
Newtown, PA 18940-0755
Phone: (215)295-3848

★ 10186 ★ The Arc of Butler County
100 N Washington St.
Butler, PA 16001
Phone: (724)282-1500

★ 10187 ★ The Arc of Cambria County
960 Bedford St.
Johnstown, PA 15902
Phone: (814)535-1511

★ 10188 ★ The Arc of Centre County
1840 N Atherton St.
State College, PA 16803
Phone: (814)238-1444
Website: http://centreconnect.org/arc

★ 10189 ★ The Arc of Chester County
900 Lawrence Dr.
West Chester, PA 19380
Phone: (610)696-8090 **Fax:** (610)696-8300
Email: info@arcofchestercounty.org
Website: http://www.arcofchestercounty.org
Diane Carey, Exec Director

★ 10190 ★ The Arc of Crawford County
222 Chestnut St.
Meadville, PA 16335
Phone: (814)724-7346

★ 10191 ★ The Arc of Cumberland/Perry Counties
117 N Hanover St.
PO Box 386
Carlisle, PA 17013
Phone: (717)249-2611

★ 10192 ★ The Arc of Dauphin and Lebanon Counties
4309 Linglestown Rd., Ste. 114E
Harrisburg, PA 17112
Phone: (717)540-5800
Email: arcofdc@paonline.com
Website: http://www.arcofdc.org

★ 10193 ★ The Arc of Elk County
507 Arch St.
Saint Marys, PA 15857
Phone: (814)834-7851

★ 10194 ★ The Arc of Erie County
18 Hess Ave.
Erie, PA 16507
Phone: (814)452-4865

★ 10195 ★ The Arc of Fayette County
80 Old New Salem Rd.
Uniontown, PA 15401
Phone: (724)438-9042

★ 10196 ★ The Arc of Franklin/Fulton
Financial Trust Bldg., Ste. 218
Chambersburg, PA 17201
Phone: (717)264-4390

★ 10197 ★ The Arc of Indiana County
720 Church St.
Indiana, PA 15701
Phone: (724)349-8230

★ 10198 ★ The Arc of Jefferson County
RD 2, Box 513
Brockway, PA 15824

★ 10199 ★ The Arc of Juniata County
22 Cross St.
Mifflintown, PA 17059
Phone: (717)436-8827

★ 10200 ★ The Arc of Lackawanna County
115 Meadow Ave.
Scranton, PA 18508
Phone: (570)346-4010
Email: arclacka@intergrafix.net
Website: http://www.geocities.com/Heartland/Acres/6855/homepagearc.html

★ 10201 ★ The Arc of Lancaster County
630 Janet Ave.
Lancaster, PA 17601
Phone: (717)394-5251

★ 10202 ★ The Arc of Lehigh and Northampton Counties Inc.
1036 N Godfrey St.
Allentown, PA 18103
Phone: (610)434-8076
Email: thearc@ptd.net
Website: http://www.arcofl-n.org

★ 10203 ★ The Arc of Luzerne County
New Bridge Ctr.
480 Pierce St., Ste. 307
Kingston, PA 18704
Phone: (570)714-6320

★ 10204 ★ The Arc of Lycoming County
329 ½ Stanton St.
Williamsport, PA 17701
Phone: (570)326-6997

★ 10205 ★ The Arc of Mercer County
850 Hermitage Rd.
PO Box 1069
Hermitage, PA 16148
Phone: (724)981-2950
Email: shassel@mercerarc.org
Website: http://www.nauticom.net/www/mcar/

★ 10206 ★ The Arc of Montgomery County
Continental Plaza
1010 W 9th Ave.
King of Prussia, PA 19406
Phone: (610)265-4700
Email: owensmj@aol.com
Website: http://marcpa.org

★ 10207 ★ The Arc of Northumberland County
622 W Walnut St.
Shamokin, PA 17872
Phone: (570)648-2871

★ 10208 ★ The Arc—Pennsylvania
Bldg. No. 2, Ste. 221
2001 N Front St.
Harrisburg, PA 17102
Phone: (717)234-2621
Website: http://www.thearcpa.org

★ 10209 ★ The Arc of Philadelphia
2350 W Westmoreland St.
Philadelphia, PA 19140
Phone: (215)229-4550
Email: info@arcpddc.org
Website: http://www.arcpddc.org

★ 10210 ★ The Arc of Pike County
c/o Pike Area Agency on Aging
150 Pike County Blvd.
Hawley, PA 18428
Phone: (570)686-3656

★ 10211 ★ The Arc of Schuylkill County
143 Steins Rd.
Ashland, PA 17921

★ 10212 ★ The Arc of Warren/Forest Counties
PO Box 244
Warren, PA 16365
Phone: (814)723-8531

★ 10213 ★ The Arc of Washington County
PO Box 385
Meadow Lands, PA 15347
Phone: (724)222-6960
Website: http://www.thearcofwashpa.com

★ 10214 ★ The Arc of Wayne County
PO Box 1121
Honesdale, PA 18431

★ 10215 ★ The Arc of Westmoreland
Donohoe Rd.
RD 12, Box 227
Greensburg, PA 15601
Phone: (724)837-8159

★ 10216 ★ The Arc of Wyoming County
86 E Tioga St.
PO Box 338
Tunkhannock, PA 18657
Phone: (570)836-4001

★ 10217 ★ The Arc of York County
1803 Mount Rose Ave., Ste. C1
York, PA 17403
Phone: (717)846-6589

★ 10218 ★ Greene Arc, Inc.
RD 2, Box 107
Prosperity, PA 15329
Phone: (724)627-5511

★ 10219 ★ PARC
Armstrong County Chapter
309 Market St.
Kittanning, PA 16201
Phone: (724)545-3426

Rhode Island

★ 10220 ★ The Arc of Bristol County
PO Box 711
Bristol, RI 02809
Phone: (401)253-5900

★ 10221 ★ The Arc/Down Syndrome Society of Rhode Island
99 Bald Hill Rd.
Cranston, RI 02920
Phone: (401)463-5751

★ 10222 ★ The Arc of Greater Providence
220 Woonasquatucket Ave.
North Providence, RI 02911
Phone: (401)353-7000

★ 10223 ★ The Arc of Newport County
PO Box 4390
Middletown, RI 02842
Phone: (401)846-4600

★ 10224 ★ The Arc of Northern Rhode Island
320 Main St.
Woonsocket, RI 02895
Phone: (401)765-3700

★ 10225 ★ The Arc of South County
24 Salt Pond Rd., Bldg G3
Wakefield, RI 02879
Phone: (401)789-4386

★ 10226 ★ Cranston Arc, Inc.
905 Pontiac Ave.
Cranston, RI 02920
Phone: (401)941-1112
Website: http://www.cranstonarc.org

★ 10227 ★ Rhode Island Arc
99 Bald Hill Rd.
Cranston, RI 02920
Phone: (401)463-9191

★ 10228 ★ Rhode Island Arc
Blackstone Valley Chapter
115 Manton St.
Pawtucket, RI 02861
Phone: (401)727-0150
Email: contact@bvcriarc.org
Website: http://www.bvcriarc.org

★ 10229 ★ Rhode Island Arc
Kent County Chapter
3445 Post Rd.
Warwick, RI 02886
Phone: (401)739-2700
Website: http://www.kentcountyarc.org

★ 10230 ★ Rhode Island Arc
Westerly Chariho Chapter
93 Airport Rd.
Westerly, RI 02891
Phone: (401)596-2091
Email: info@oleancenter.org
Website: http://www.oleancenter.org

South Carolina

★ 10231 ★ The Arc of Anderson
1105 Hanover Rd.
Anderson, SC 29621

★ 10232 ★ The Arc of Cherokee County
PO Box 397
Gaffney, SC 29342

★ 10233 ★ The Arc of Horry County
PO Box 1628
250 Victory Ln.
Conway, SC 29526
Phone: (843)347-0261

★ 10234 ★ The Arc of the Midlands
PO Box 8707
Columbia, SC 29202
Phone: (803)935-5266

★ 10235 ★ The Arc of Pickens County
PO Box 1308
Easley, SC 29641
Phone: (864)859-5416

★ 10236 ★ The Arc of South Carolina
PO Box 8707
Columbia, SC 29202
Phone: (803)935-5266 **Free:** (866)300-9331
Email: TheARCSC@arcsc.org
Website: http://www.arcsc.org

South Dakota

★ 10237 ★ The Arc of Brown County
13084 385th Ave.
Aberdeen, SD 57401

★ 10238 ★ The Arc of Grant County
310 W 6th Ave.
Milbank, SD 57252

★ 10239 ★ The Arc of Kampeska
710 2nd St. NE
Watertown, SD 57201

★ 10240 ★ The Arc of Lake County
Box 450
Madison, SD 57042

★ 10241 ★ The Arc of Lyman-Brule
HCR 69, Box 42
Chamberlain, SD 57325

★ 10242 ★ The Arc of Mid-Dakota
RR 1, Box 215
Cavour, SD 57324

★ 10243 ★ The Arc of Oahe Chapter
PO Box 503
Pierre, SD 57501
Phone: (605)224-4501

★ 10244 ★ The Arc of South Dakota
708 SW 7th
PO Box 450
Pierre, SD 57501-0220
Phone: (605)224-8211

★ 10245 ★ East Central Arc
1800 Ohio Dr.
Brookings, SD 57006

★ 10246 ★ Sioux Arc
2308 S 1st Ave.
Sioux Falls, SD 57105

Tennessee

★ 10247 ★ Advocacy and Resources Corp.
453 Gould Dr.
Cookeville, TN 38506
Phone: (931)432-5981
Email: arc@arcdiversified.com
Website: http://www.arcdiversified.com
Frmly: The Arc of Putnam County.

★ 10248 ★ The Arc of Anderson County
PO Box 4823
Oak Ridge, TN 37831-4823
Phone: (865)481-0550

★ 10249 ★ The Arc of Claiborne County
Box 538
Tazewell, TN 37879
Phone: (423)626-6757

★ 10250 ★ The Arc of Coffee-Moore County
PO Box 1146
Tullahoma, TN 37388-1146
Phone: (931)759-4344

★ 10251 ★ The Arc of Cumberland County
PO Box 389
Crossville, TN 38557
Phone: (931)456-0206

★ 10252 ★ The Arc of Davidson County
1207 17th Ave. S, No. 100
Nashville, TN 37212
Phone: (615)321-5699

★ 10253 ★ The Arc of Hamblen County
PO Box 1793
Morristown, TN 37813
Phone: (423)581-1092

★ 10254 ★ The Arc of Hamilton County, Inc.
4613 Brainerd Rd.
Chattanooga, TN 37411
Phone: (423)624-6887
Email: arc@hamilton.theinbox.org
Website: http://www.geocities.com/localarc2001

★ 10255 ★ The Arc of Hickman County
571 Hurricane Branch Rd.
Pleasantville, TN 37147
Phone: (931)729-9625

★ 10256 ★ The Arc of Knox County
3000 N Central
Knoxville, TN 37914
Phone: (423)524-1311

★ 10257 ★ The Arc of Lincoln County
73 Prospect Rd.
Fayetteville, TN 37334
Phone: (931)433-7333

★ 10258 ★ The Arc of Marshall County
715 Fairlane Dr.
Lewisburg, TN 37091
Phone: (931)359-3125

★ 10259 ★ The Arc of Montgomery County
PO Box 2145
Clarksville, TN 37042
Phone: (931)905-0900

★ 10260 ★ The Arc of Obion County
4301 Mt. Zion Rd.
Union City, TN 38261
Phone: (901)885-5323

★ 10261 ★ The Arc of Sullivan County
400 Shelby St.
Box 100, People Pl.
Bristol, TN 37620
Phone: (423)652-1899

★ 10262 ★ The Arc of Tennessee
44 Vantage Way, Ste. 550
Nashville, TN 37228
Phone: (615)248-5878 **Free:** 800-835-7077
Email: arctn@worldnet.att.net
Website: http://www.thearctn.org

★ 10263 ★ The Arc of Warren County
71 Flood Rd.
Mc Minnville, TN 37110
Phone: (931)668-3710

★ 10264 ★ The Arc of Washington County
2700 S Roan St., Ste. 300B
Johnson City, TN 37601
Phone: (423)928-9362

★ 10265 ★ The Arc of Wayne County
RR 1, Box 282-D
Collinwood, TN 38450

★ 10266 ★ The Arc of Williamson County
129 W Fowlkes St., Ste. 151
Franklin, TN 37064
Phone: (615)790-5815

★ 10267 ★ Mid-South Arc
3485 Poplar Ave., No. 225
Memphis, TN 38111
Phone: (901)327-2473

Texas

★ 10268 ★ The Arc
PO Box 1484
Alvin, TX 77512
Phone: (281)388-1161

★ 10269 ★ The Arc of Anderson and Cherokee Counties
Rte. 8, Box 129
Jacksonville, TX 75766
Phone: (903)586-6150

★ 10270 ★ The Arc of the Bay Area
2704 Northern
League City, TX 77573
Phone: (281)484-7447

★ 10271 ★ The Arc of Baytown
5416 Shepard Rd.
PO Box 1085
Baytown, TX 77521

★ 10272 ★ The Arc of Bell County
PO Box 311
Temple, TX 76503

★ 10273 ★ The Arc of the Big Country
1021 Wolf Rd.
Abilene, TX 79602
Phone: (915)793-3500

★ 10274 ★ The Arc of Bluebonnet Circle
PO Box 1842
Brenham, TX 77833
Phone: (409)836-1002

★ 10275 ★ The Arc of Brown County
PO Box 1201
Brownwood, TX 76801
Phone: (915)543-5822

★ 10276 ★ The Arc of Bryan-College Station
2518 Dartmouth
College Station, TX 77840
Phone: (409)693-0812

★ 10277 ★ The Arc of Calhoun County
11 Pecan Dr.
Port Lavaca, TX 77979
Phone: (512)552-9403

★ 10278 ★ The Arc of the Capital Area
2818 San Gabriel
Austin, TX 78705
Phone: (512)476-7044 **Fax:** (512)476-9054
Email: info@arcofthecapitalarea.org
Website: http://www.arcofthecapitalarea.org

★ 10279 ★ The Arc of Cypress Creek
PO Box 11123
Spring, TX 77391-1123
Phone: (281)376-7072

★ 10280 ★ The Arc of Dallas
2114 Anson Rd.
Dallas, TX 75235
Phone: (214)634-9810
Email: info@arcdallas.org
Website: http://www.arcdallas.org

★ 10281 ★ The Arc of Denton County
PO Box 1279
Denton, TX 76202
Phone: (972)436-8471

★ 10282 ★ The Arc of East Texas
Rte. 9, Box 1900
Lufkin, TX 75901
Phone: (409)632-7944

★ 10283 ★ The Arc of Ector County
PO Box 13023
Odessa, TX 79768-3023
Phone: (915)362-2702

★ 10284 ★ The Arc of El Campo
PO Box 227
El Campo, TX 77437

★ 10285 ★ The Arc of Fort Bend County
3660 Glen Lakes Dr.
Missouri City, TX 77459
Phone: (281)499-2234
Website: http://www.arcoffortbend.org

★ 10286 ★ The Arc of Gillespie County
PO Box 770
Fredericksburg, TX 78624
Phone: (830)997-7163

★ 10287 ★ The Arc of Greater Corpus Christi
PO Box 72713
Corpus Christi, TX 78472-0713
Phone: (512)886-6900

★ 10288 ★ The Arc of Greater Houston
PO Box 924168
Houston, TX 77292-4168
Phone: (713)957-1600

★ 10289 ★ The Arc of Greater Tarrant County
259 Bailey Ave., Ste. A
Fort Worth, TX 76107
Phone: (817)877-1474

★ 10290 ★ The Arc of Gregg County
PO Box 522
Longview, TX 75606
Phone: (903)753-8773

★ 10291 ★ The Arc of Hopkins County
PO Box 1215
Sulphur Springs, TX 75482

★ 10292 ★ The Arc of Howard County
514 Westover Rd.
Big Spring, TX 79720
Phone: (915)264-5095

★ 10293 ★ The Arc of Hunt County
2603 Templeton St.
Greenville, TX 75401
Phone: (903)454-9170

★ 10294 ★ The Arc of Katy
PO Box 1106
Katy, TX 77492-1106

★ 10295 ★ The Arc of Kerrville
4800 Goat Creek Rd.
Kerrville, TX 78028

★ 10296 ★ The Arc of Madison-Leon County
Rte. 2, Box 162
Midway, TX 75852

★ 10297 ★ The Arc of Marshall
PO Box 24
Marshall, TX 75671

★ 10298 ★ The Arc of Matagorda County
4101 Holly Glen
Bay City, TX 77414
Phone: (409)245-6318

★ 10299 ★ The Arc of McLennan County
PO Box 3367
Waco, TX 76707
Phone: (254)756-7491

★ 10300 ★ The Arc of Midland
2701 N "A" St.
Midland, TX 79705
Phone: (915)498-8590
Email: brose@arcmidlandtx.org
Website: http://www.arcmidlandtx.org
Robert K. Rose, Exec Director

★ 10301 ★ The Arc of Milam
1705 Pakus St.
Rockdale, TX 76567

★ 10302 ★ The Arc of Northeast Tarrant County
PO Box 14455
Fort Worth, TX 76117
Phone: (817)834-7700

★ 10303 ★ The Arc of Panola County
102 N Shelby
Carthage, TX 75633
Phone: (903)693-4230

★ 10304 ★ The Arc of Plano
PO Box 260727
Plano, TX 75026
Phone: (972)682-9044

★ 10305 ★ The Arc of Potter and Randall Counties
202 S Louisiana
Amarillo, TX 79106
Phone: (806)372-5699

★ 10306 ★ The Arc of San Angelo
PO Box 1922
San Angelo, TX 76902
Phone: (915)655-3205

★ 10307 ★ The Arc of San Antonio
13430 West Ave.
San Antonio, TX 78216
Phone: (210)490-4300

★ 10308 ★ The Arc of Scurry County
PO Box 105
Snyder, TX 79550
Phone: (915)573-5610

★ 10309 ★ The Arc of Spring Branch/ Memorial
9524 Kempwood
Houston, TX 77080
Phone: (713)460-4274

★ 10310 ★ The Arc of Texas
1600 W 38th St., Ste. 200
Austin, TX 78731
Phone: (512)454-6694 **Free:** 800-252-9729
Fax: (512)454-4956
Email: secretary@thearcoftexas.org
Website: http://www.thearcoftexas.org

★ 10311 ★ The Arc of Texoma
223 N Walnut
Sherman, TX 75090
Phone: (903)892-6102

★ 10312 ★ The Arc of Tyler
810 Vine Heights
Tyler, TX 75701
Phone: (903)597-0995

★ 10313 ★ The Arc of Wharton
1017 ½ Alabama Rd.
Wharton, TX 77488
Phone: (409)282-9200

★ 10314 ★ The Arc of Wichita County
3307 Buchanan
Wichita Falls, TX 76308
Phone: (940)692-2303

Utah

★ 10315 ★ The Arc of Cache
426 East 500 South
River Heights, UT 84321

★ 10316 ★ The Arc of Davis County
811 South 500 West, No. 105
Bountiful, UT 84010

★ 10317 ★ The Arc of Morgan County
PO Box 597
Morgan, UT 84050

★ 10318 ★ The Arc of Salt Lake
2595 East 3300 South, Ste. 360
Salt Lake City, UT 84109
Phone: (801)412-3798

★ 10319 ★ The Arc of Utah
455 East 400 South, Ste. 202
Salt Lake City, UT 84111
Phone: (801)364-5060
Email: Arcutah@burgoyne.com

★ 10320 ★ The Arc of Utah County
687 West 1800 North
Provo, UT 84604

★ 10321 ★ The Arc of Washington County
334 W Tabernacle, Unit H
Saint George, UT 84770
Phone: (801)673-5251

Virginia

★ 10322 ★ The Arc of Augusta
1025 Fairfax Ave.
PO Box 102
Waynesboro, VA 22980
Phone: (540)943-1618

★ 10323 ★ The Arc of the Blue Ridge
PO Box 1401
Culpeper, VA 22701
Phone: (540)439-3505

★ 10324 ★ The Arc of Central Virginia
1508 Bedford Ave.
Lynchburg, VA 24504
Phone: (804)845-4071

★ 10325 ★ The Arc of the Eastern Shore
PO Box 626
Exmore, VA 23350
Phone: (757)442-3933

★ 10326 ★ The Arc of Greater Prince William/Insight, Inc.
13505 Hillendale Dr.
Woodbridge, VA 22193
Phone: (703)670-4800
Email: info@arcgpw.org
Website: http://www.arcgpw.org

★ 10327 ★ The Arc of Greater Williamsburg
202D Packets Ct.
Williamsburg, VA 23185
Phone: (757)229-3535

★ 10328 ★ The Arc of Halifax
PO Box 36
South Boston, VA 24592

★ 10329 ★ The Arc of Hanover County
PO Box 91
Ashland, VA 23005
Phone: (804)798-2400

★ 10330 ★ The Arc of Harrisonburg/ Rockingham County
1000 S High St.
Harrisonburg, VA 22801
Phone: (540)434-2469 **Fax:** (540)433-7759
Email: michaels@hrarc.org
Website: http://www.hrarc.org

★ 10331 ★ The Arc of Lenowisco
PO Box 1794
Gate City, VA 24251

★ 10332 ★ The Arc of Loudoun County (LARC)
PO Box 243
Leesburg, VA 20178
Phone: (703)777-1939
Website: http://www.loudoun-arc.org
Nancy Kysela, Director

★ 10333 ★ The Arc of Mecklenburg
515 N Lunenburg Ave.
South Hill, VA 23970

★ 10334 ★ The Arc of Northern Shenandoah Valley
PO Box 3263
Winchester, VA 22604
Phone: (540)665-0461

★ 10335 ★ The Arc of Northern Virginia
100 N Washington St., No. 234
Falls Church, VA 22046
Phone: (703)532-3214
Email: info@thearcofnova.org
Website: http://www.arcofnova.org

★ 10336 ★ The Arc of Petersburg
114 N Union St., Ste. B
PO Box 2085
Petersburg, VA 23804
Phone: (804)732-0685

★ 10337 ★ The Arc of the Piedmont
509 Park St.
Charlottesville, VA 22902
Phone: (434)977-4002 **Free:** 800-732-9507
Fax: (434)977-7964

Email: thearc@cstone.net
Website: http://www.avenue.org/arc

★ 10338 ★ The Arc of Rappahannock, Inc.
701 Westwood Office Park
Fredericksburg, VA 22401
Phone: (540)899-3789 Fax: (540)370-0179
Email: arc_r@msn.com
Website: http://www.arcvap.org

★ 10339 ★ The Arc of the Richmond Area
1901 Westwood Ave.
Richmond, VA 23227
Phone: (804)358-1874

★ 10340 ★ The Arc of Roanoke
3355 Shenandoan Ave. NW
PO Box 6220
Roanoke, VA 24017
Phone: (540)342-9624

★ 10341 ★ The Arc of Rockbridge
PO Box 657
Lexington, VA 24450
Phone: (540)348-5510

★ 10342 ★ The Arc of Smyth County
221 Look Ave.
Marion, VA 24354
Phone: (540)783-6801

★ 10343 ★ The Arc of Twin Galax County
PO Box 202
Woodlawn, VA 24381

★ 10344 ★ The Arc of Virginia
2025 E Main St., Ste. 120
Richmond, VA 23223
Phone: (804)649-8481 Fax: (804)649-3585
Email: tstokes@arcofva.org
Website: http://www.arcofva.org
Teja Stokes, Exec Director

★ 10345 ★ The Arc of the Virginia Peninsula
51 Battle Rd.
Hampton, VA 23666
Phone: (757)896-6461
Website: http://www.arcvap.org

★ 10346 ★ The Arc of Warren County
PO Box 1473
Front Royal, VA 22630-1473
Phone: (540)631-9092

★ 10347 ★ The Beach Arc
PO Box 8063
Virginia Beach, VA 23450
Phone: (757)340-5998
Website: http://groups.hamptonroads.com/BeachArc/

★ 10348 ★ Danville Association for Retarded Citizens, Inc.
7180 U.S. Hwy. N 29
Blairs, VA 24527
Phone: (804)836-3272

Washington

★ 10349 ★ The Arc of Clark County
9415 NE Fourth Plain Rd.
PO Box 2608
Vancouver, WA 98668-2608
Phone: (360)254-1562 Fax: (360)896-7382
Email: thearc@arcofclarkcounty.org
Website: http://www.arcofclarkcounty.org

★ 10350 ★ The Arc of Cowlitz Valley
1410 8th Ave., No. 15
Longview, WA 98632-3807
Phone: (360)425-5494
Website: http://www.cowlitzarc.org

★ 10351 ★ The Arc of King County
10550 Lake City Way NE, Ste. A
Seattle, WA 98125-7752
Phone: (206)364-6337
Email: inforef@arcofkingcounty.org
Website: http://www.arcofkingcounty.org

★ 10352 ★ The Arc of Kitsap and Jefferson Counties
3243 N Perry Ave.
Bremerton, WA 98310
Phone: (360)377-3473

★ 10353 ★ The Arc of the Olympic Peninsula
PO Box 2092
Port Angeles, WA 98362
Phone: (360)457-1301

★ 10354 ★ The Arc of Snohomish County
1615 California Ave.
Everett, WA 98201
Phone: (425)258-2459

★ 10355 ★ The Arc of Spokane
127 W Boone Ave.
Spokane, WA 99201
Phone: (509)328-6326
Website: http://www.arc-spokane.org

★ 10356 ★ The Arc of the Tri-Cities
761 Williams Blvd.
Richland, WA 99352
Phone: (509)946-5157

★ 10357 ★ The Arc of Washington State
1703 E State Ave. NE
Olympia, WA 98506
Phone: (360)357-5596 Free: 888-754-8798
Email: info@arcwa.org
Website: http://www.arcwa.org

★ 10358 ★ The Arc of Whatcom, Skagit, and Island Counties
1111 Cornwall, No. 205
Bellingham, WA 98225
Phone: (360)715-0170

West Virginia

★ 10359 ★ The Arc of Harrison County
PO Box 764
Clarksburg, WV 26301
Phone: (304)624-9114

★ 10360 ★ The Arc of Kanawha Putnam
1021 Quarrier St., Ste. 200
Charleston, WV 25301
Phone: (304)344-3403

★ 10361 ★ The Arc of Marion County
309 Cleveland Ave., Ste 101
Fairmont, WV 26554
Phone: (304)366-3213

★ 10362 ★ The Arc of Ohio County
439 Warwood Ave.
Wheeling, WV 26003
Phone: (304)277-1466

★ 10363 ★ The Arc of Wood County
521 Market St.
Box 17
Parkersburg, WV 26101
Phone: (304)422-3151 Fax: (304)422-1025
Email: arcwd@wirefire.com
Website: http://www.arcwd.org

★ 10364 ★ Bridges, Inc.
201 Walnut St., Ste. 207
Morgantown, WV 26505
Phone: (304)296-3092

Wisconsin

★ 10365 ★ The Arc of Barron County
103 E Sawyer St.
Rice Lake, WI 54868

★ 10366 ★ The Arc of Columbia County
711 E Cook St.
Portage, WI 53901
Phone: (608)742-9204

★ 10367 ★ The Arc Consumer Council
c/o Nan Upright-Sexton
7519 W Oklahoma Ave.
Milwaukee, WI 53219

★ 10368 ★ The Arc of Dane County
1320 Mendota St., Ste. 111A
Madison, WI 53714
Phone: (608)257-9738
Email: arcdane@chorus.net
Website: http://www.arcdanecounty.org
Ken Hobbs, Exec Director

★ 10369 ★ The Arc of Dunn County, Inc.
390 Red Cedar St., Ste. G
Menomonie, WI 54751-2265
Phone: (715)235-7373

★ 10370 ★ The Arc of Eau Claire
513 S Barstow St.
Eau Claire, WI 54701
Phone: (715)834-7204

★ 10371 ★ The Arc of Fond Du Lac County
500 N Park Ave.
Fond Du Lac, WI 54935
Phone: (920)923-3810

★ 10372 ★ The Arc of Juneau County
8978 County Rd. M
New Lisbon, WI 53950

★ 10373 ★ The Arc of Kenosha County, Inc.
c/o Kenosha Achievement Center
1218 79th St.
Kenosha, WI 53144

★ 10374 ★ The Arc of Langlade County
N2437 Sunnyside Rd.
Antigo, WI 54409
Phone: (715)627-7458

★ 10375 ★ The Arc of Lincoln County
11012 Koffke Dr.
Merrill, WI 54452
Phone: (715)453-4939

★ 10376 ★ The Arc of Marinette Area
2528 Gilbert St.
Marinette, WI 54143

★ 10377 ★ The Arc of Monroe County
509 Jefferson Ave.
Sparta, WI 54656-2118
Phone: (608)269-6157

★ 10378 ★ The Arc of Neenah-Menasha
375 Winnebago Ave.
Menasha, WI 54952
Phone: (920)725-0943

★ 10379 ★ The Arc of Outagamie County
633 W Wisconsin Ave.
Appleton, WI 54911
Phone: (920)731-9831

★ 10380 ★ The Arc of Ozaukee County
11649 N Lake Shore Dr.
Mequon, WI 53092
Website: http://www.ocarc.org

★ 10381 ★ The Arc of Racine County, Inc.
818 6th St.
Racine, WI 53403
Phone: (414)634-6303

★ 10382 ★ The Arc of Richland County
284425 Coop Wood Rd.
Richland Center, WI 53581

★ 10383 ★ The Arc of Washington County
916 Chestnut St.
West Bend, WI 53095

★ 10384 ★ The Arc of Waupaca County
45 20th St.
Clintonville, WI 54929

★ 10385 ★ The Arc of Western Racine County
26509 Ketterhagen Rd.
Burlington, WI 53105

★ 10386 ★ The Arc—Wisconsin
600 Williamson St.
Madison, WI 53703
Phone: (608)251-9272

★ 10387 ★ Green County Arc, Inc.
1615 22 ½ Ave.
Monroe, WI 53566

Wyoming

★ 10388 ★ The Arc, Diversified Services Inc.
PO Box EE
Torrington, WY 82240
Phone: (307)532-5911

★ 10389 ★ The Arc of Lander/Riverton
PO Box 213
Lander, WY 82520
Phone: (307)335-8801

★ 10390 ★ The Arc of Laramie County
PO Box 1812
Cheyenne, WY 82003
Phone: (307)632-1209
Website: http://www.arcoflaramiecounty.org

★ 10391 ★ The Arc, Magic City Enterprises Inc.
1780 Westland Rd.
Cheyenne, WY 82001
Phone: (307)637-8869

★ 10392 ★ The Arc of Natrona County
PO Box 393
Casper, WY 82602
Phone: (307)577-4913

★ 10393 ★ The Arc Regional Services
1150 N 3rd St.
Laramie, WY 82070
Phone: (307)742-6641

★ 10394 ★ The Arc of Sheridan County
PO Box 1028
Sheridan, WY 82801
Phone: (307)672-8665

★ 10395 ★ The Arc of Uinta and Lincoln Counties
528 Country Rd., Ste. 7
Evanston, WY 82930
Phone: (307)789-7679
Email: thearc@vcn.com
Website: http://www.geocities.com/thearcuinta/home.html
Cathy Frame, Exec Director

★ 10396 ★ The Arc of Weston County Children's Center
104 Stampede
Newcastle, WY 82701
Phone: (307)746-4560

★ 10397 ★ The Arc of Wyoming
318 W 'B' St.
PO Box 2161
Casper, WY 82602
Phone: (307)237-9110 **Free:** 800-801-0569
Fax: (307)577-4014
Email: arc-wy@home.com
Website: http://www.arcofwyoming.org

★ 10398 ★ Child Development Center
PO Box 7237
Sheridan, WY 82801
Phone: (307)672-6610

★ 10399 ★ Child Development Center of Natrona County
2020 E 12th St.
Casper, WY 82601
Phone: (307)235-5097

★ 10400 ★ Children's Resource Center/Special Touch Preschool Inc.
PO Box 1191
Powell, WY 82435
Phone: (307)754-2864

★ 10401 ★ The Learning Center
PO Box 342
Pinedale, WY 82941
Phone: (307)733-3791

★ 10402 ★ Lincoln-Uinta Child Development Association
PO Box 570
Mountain View, WY 82939
Phone: (307)782-6601

★ 10403 ★ Sweetwater County Child Development Center
821 Norton Ave.
Rock Springs, WY 82901
Phone: (307)352-6600

Multiple Sclerosis

State chapters of the Multiple Sclerosis Association of America (MSAA) and the National Multiple Sclerosis Society (NMSS) are listed below. The MSAA national office is located at 706 Haddonfield Rd., Cherry Hill, NJ 08002, 800-LEARN-MS, http://www.msaa.com/. Additional information can be obtained by contacting the NMSS national office at 733 Third Ave., New York, NY 10017, 800-FIGHT-MS, http://www.nationalmssociety.org.

Alabama

★ 10404 ★ National Multiple Sclerosis Society
Alabama Chapter
Birmingham, AL 35209
Phone: (205)879-8881 **Fax:** (205)879-8869
Email: alc@nmss.org
Website: http://www.alabamanmss.org
Tracy Smith, President

Alaska

★ 10405 ★ National Multiple Sclerosis Society
All America Chapter
Alaska Division
511 W 41st Ave., Ste. 101
Anchorage, AK 99503
Phone: (907)563-1115 **Fax:** (907)562-6673
Email: aka@nmss.org
Gary Wells, Contact

Arkansas

★ 10406 ★ Multiple Sclerosis Association of America
Mid-South Regional Office
107 Avonshire Terrace, Diamonhead
Hot Springs, AR 71913
Phone: (501)262-9380 **Free:** 877-MS-SOUTH
Fax: (501)262-9381
Email: midsouth@msaa.com
Website: http://www.msaa.com/regionms.htm
Adam Roberts, Director
Judith Harper-Bennie, Client Services Coordinator

★ 10407 ★ National Multiple Sclerosis Society
All America Chapter
Arkansas Division
Evergreen Pl.
1100 N University, Ste. 255
Little Rock, AR 72207
Phone: (501)663-6767 **Fax:** (501)666-4355
Email: marlene.vadjunec@nmss.org

Website: http://www.nmss.org
Marlene Vadjunec, Contact

California

★ 10408 ★ National Multiple Sclerosis Society
Channel Islands Chapter
14 W Valerio St.
Santa Barbara, CA 93101
Phone: (805)682-8783 **Fax:** (805)563-1489
Email: joan.young@cat.nmss.org
Website: http://www.nmssci.org
Joan Young, President

★ 10409 ★ National Multiple Sclerosis Society
Northern California Chapter
150 Grand Ave.
Oakland, CA 94612
Phone: (510)268-0572 **Free:** 800—FIGHT-MS
Fax: (510)268-0575
Email: info@msconnection.org
Website: http://www.msconnection.org
Julie Thomas, President

★ 10410 ★ National Multiple Sclerosis Society
Orange County Chapter
17500 Redhill Ave., Ste. 240
Irvine, CA 92614
Phone: (949)752-1680 **Fax:** (949)851-7739
Email: msinfo@cao.nmss.org
Website: http://www.nmssoc.org
Jamie MacDonald, President

★ 10411 ★ National Multiple Sclerosis Society
San Diego Chapter
8840 Complex Dr., Ste. 130
San Diego, CA 92123
Phone: (858)974-8640 **Fax:** (858)974-8646
Email: mssd@mssd.org
Website: http://www.mssd.org
Allan Shaw, President

★ 10412 ★ National Multiple Sclerosis Society
Silicon Valley Chapter
2589 Scott Blvd.
Santa Clara, CA 95050
Phone: (408)988-7557 **Fax:** (408)988-1816
Email: cau@nmss.org
Website: http://www.svcnmss.org
Carla Hines, President

★ 10413 ★ National Multiple Sclerosis Society
Southern California Chapter
2440 S Sepulveda Blvd., Ste. 115
Los Angeles, CA 90064
Phone: (310)479-4456 **Fax:** (310)479-4436
Email: leon.lebuffe@cal.nmss.org
Website: http://www.cal.nmss.org
Leon LeBuffe, President

Colorado

★ 10414 ★ National Multiple Sclerosis Society
Colorado Chapter
700 Broadway, Ste. 808
Denver, CO 80203-3442
Phone: (303)831-0700 **Free:** 800—FIGHT-MS
Fax: (303)831-8001
Email: general.information@coc.nmss.org
Website: http://www.fightmscolorado.org
Dianne Williams, President

Connecticut

★ 10415 ★ National Multiple Sclerosis Society
Greater Connecticut Chapter
705 N Mountain Rd.
Newington, CT 06111
Phone: (860)953-0601 **Fax:** (860)953-0602
Email: lgerrol@ctnmss.org
Lisa Gerrol, President

★ 10416 ★ National Multiple Sclerosis Society
Western Connecticut Chapter
1 Selleck St., Ste. 500
Norwalk, CT 06855
Phone: (203)838-1033 **Fax:** (203)831-2973
Email: bfaribanks@msswct.org
Website: http://www.msswct.org
M. Elizabeth Fairbanks, President

Delaware

★ 10417 ★ National Multiple Sclerosis Society
Delaware Chapter
2 Mill Rd., Ste. 106
Wilmington, DE 19806
Phone: (302)655-5610 **Fax:** (302)655-0993
Email: kate.cowperthwait@ded.nmss.org
Website: http://www.msdelaware.org/home/home.cfm
Kate Cowperthwait, President

District of Columbia

★ 10418 ★ National Multiple Sclerosis Society
National Capital Chapter
2021 K St., Ste. 715
Washington, DC 20006-1035
Phone: (202)296-5363 **Fax:** (202)296-3425
Email: info@MSandYou.org
Website: http://www.MSandYOU.org
Jeanne Oates Angulo, President

Florida

★ 10419 ★ National Multiple Sclerosis Society
Mid-Florida Chapter
3659 Maguire Blvd., Ste. 110
Orlando, FL 32803
Phone: (407)896-3873 **Fax:** (407)898-6736
Email: sylvia.navarro@flc.nmss.org
Tami Caesar, President

★ 10420 ★ National Multiple Sclerosis Society
North Florida Chapter
9550 Regency Sq. Blvd., Ste. 104
Jacksonville, FL 32225
Phone: (904)725-6800 **Fax:** (904)725-0500
Email: msnorfla@fln.nmss.org
Website: http://www.msnorthfl.org
Jennifer Lee, President

★ 10421 ★ National Multiple Sclerosis Society
South Florida Chapter
3201 W Commercial Blvd., Ste. 127
Fort Lauderdale, FL 33309
Phone: (305)599-0299 **Free:** 800—FIGHT-MS
Fax: (954)739-1398
Email: fls@nmss.org
Website: http://www.nmssfls.org
Karen Dresbach, President

Georgia

★ 10422 ★ National Multiple Sclerosis Society
Georgia Chapter
455 Abernathy Rd NE, Ste. 210
Atlanta, GA 30328
Phone: (404)256-9700 **Fax:** (404)351-4187
Email: mailbox@nmssga.org
Website: http://www.nmssga.org
Mary Creighton, President

Hawaii

★ 10423 ★ National Multiple Sclerosis Society
All America Chapter
Hawaii Division
418 Kuwili St., Ste. 105
Honolulu, HI 96817
Phone: (808)652-0811 **Fax:** (808)532-0814
Email: hih@nmss.org
Pam McElrath, President

Idaho

★ 10424 ★ National Multiple Sclerosis Society
All America Chapter
Idaho Division
1674 Hill Rd., Ste. 18
Boise, ID 83702
Phone: (208)388-1998 **Fax:** (208)388-1907
Email: idi@nmss.org
Blenda Davis, Contact

Illinois

★ 10425 ★ National Multiple Sclerosis Society
Greater Illinois Chapter
910 W Van Buren, 4th Fl.
Chicago, IL 60607
Phone: (312)421-4500 **Fax:** (312)421-4544
Email: cgic@msillinois.org
Steve Pratapas, President

Indiana

★ 10426 ★ National Multiple Sclerosis Society
Indiana State Chapter
7301 Georgetown Rd., Ste. 112
Indianapolis, IN 46268
Phone: (317)870-2500 **Fax:** (317)870-2520
Email: ini@nmss.org
Website: http://www.msindiana.org
Theresa Brun, President

Iowa

★ 10427 ★ National Multiple Sclerosis Society
Iowa Chapter
1300 50th St., Ste. 106
West Des Moines, IA 50266-5499
Phone: (515)270-6337 **Fax:** (515)270-0337
Email: iac@nmss.org
Website: http://www.ianmss.org
Brett Ridge, President

Kansas

★ 10428 ★ National Multiple Sclerosis Society
All America Chapter
South Central and Western Kansas Division
250 S Laura
Wichita, KS 67211
Phone: (316)264-1333 **Fax:** (316)264-5436
Email: kss@nmsskss.org
Pam McElrath, President

★ 10429 ★ National Multiple Sclerosis Society
Mid-America Chapter
PO Box 2292
Mission, KS 66201
Phone: (913)432-3926 **Fax:** (913)432-6912
Email: info@nmsskc.org
Scott Burnett, Chairman of the Board

Kentucky

★ 10430 ★ National Multiple Sclerosis Society
Kentucky Chapter
11700 Commonwealth Dr., Ste. 500
Louisville, KY 40299
Phone: (502)451-0014 **Free:** 800-873-6367
Fax: (502)451-9747
Email: cheryl.suhr@kyw.nmss.org
Website: http://www.kynmss.org
Cheryl Suhr, President

Louisiana

★ 10431 ★ National Multiple Sclerosis Society
Louisiana Chapter
3616 S I-10 Service Rd., Ste. 101
Metairie, LA 70001
Phone: (504)832-4013 **Free:** 800-346-7323
Fax: (504)831-7188
Email: karen.mcguire@lam.nmss.org
Karen McGuire, President

Maine

★ 10432 ★ National Multiple Sclerosis Society
Maine Chapter
PO Box 8730
Portland, ME 04104
Phone: (207)761-5815 **Fax:** (207)761-5817
Email: info@msmaine.org
Website: http://www.msmaine.org
Kris Dorer, President

Maryland

★ 10433 ★ National Multiple Sclerosis Society
Maryland Chapter
10946 Beaver Dam Rd., Ste. E
Hunt Valley, MD 21030
Phone: (410)527-1770 **Fax:** (410)527-9970
Email: info@nmss-md.org
Website: http://www.nmss-md.org
Rick Smith, President

Massachusetts

★ 10434 ★ National Multiple Sclerosis Society
Central New England Chapter
101A 1st Ave., Ste. 6
Waltham, MA 02451-1115
Phone: (781)890-4990 **Free:** 800-493-9255
Fax: (781)890-2089
Email: communications@mam.nmss.org
Website: http://www.msnewengland.org
Arlyn White, President

Michigan

★ 10435 ★ National Multiple Sclerosis Society
Michigan Chapter
21311 Civic Center Dr.
Southfield, MI 48076
Phone: (248)350-0020 **Fax:** (248)350-0029
Email: info@mig.nmss.org
Website: http://www.nmssmi.org
Patricia McDonald, President

Minnesota

★ 10436 ★ National Multiple Sclerosis Society
Minnesota Chapter
200 12th Ave. S
Minneapolis, MN 55415
Phone: (612)335-7900 **Fax:** (612)335-7997
Email: mnm@nmss.org
Website: http://www.mnms.org
Maureen Reeder, President

Mississippi

★ 10437 ★ National Multiple Sclerosis Society
All America Chapter
Mississippi Division
145 Executive Dr., Ste. 1
Madison, MS 39110
Phone: (601)856-7575 **Fax:** (601)856-7173
Email: info@msmnmss.org
Pam McElrath, President

Missouri

★ 10438 ★ National Multiple Sclerosis Society
Gateway Area Chapter
1867 Lackland Hill Pkwy.
Saint Louis, MO 63146
Phone: (314)781-9020 **Free:** 800—FIGHT-MS
Fax: (314)781-1440
Email: info@mos.nmss.org
Pat Knoerle-Jordan, President

Montana

★ 10439 ★ Multiple Sclerosis Association of America
NorthwWestern Regional Office
600 Central Ave., Ste. 13
Great Falls, MT 59401
Phone: (406)454-2758 **Free:** 800-565-6722
Fax: (406)454-2767
Email: northwest@msaa.com
Website: http://www.msaa.com
Sue Pencoske, Director

★ 10440 ★ National Multiple Sclerosis Society
All America Chapter
Montana Division
1629 Ave. D., Ste. 2-C
Billings, MT 59102
Phone: (406)252-9500 **Fax:** (406)252-5956
Email: mtt@nmss.org
Pam McElrath, President

Nebraska

★ 10441 ★ National Multiple Sclerosis Society
Nebraska Chapter
Community Health Plaza, Ste. 203
7101 Newport Ave.
Omaha, NE 68152
Phone: (402)572-3190 **Fax:** (402)572-3189
Email: nen@nmss.org
Pattie Gorham, President

Nevada

★ 10442 ★ National Multiple Sclerosis Society
Great Basin Sierra Chapter
1201 Terminal Way, Ste. 215
Reno, NV 89502
Phone: (775)329-7180 **Fax:** (775)329-7180
Email: nvn@nvn.nmss.org
Website: http://www.curems.org
Linda Lott, President

New Jersey

★ 10443 ★ Multiple Sclerosis Association of America
Northeastern Regional Office
706 Haddonfield Rd.
Cherry Hill, NJ 08002
Phone: (856)488-4500 **Free:** 800-532-7667
Fax: (856)488-8257
Email: sfreund@msaa.com
Website: http://www.msaa.com
Susan Freund, Director

★ 10444 ★ National Multiple Sclerosis Society
Greater North Jersey Chapter
1 Kalisa Way, Ste. 205
Paramus, NJ 07652
Phone: (201)967-5599 **Free:** 800-833-0087
Fax: (201)967-7085
Email: chapter@njb.nmss.org
Website: http://www.njbnmss.org
Joan Mistrough, President

★ 10445 ★ National Multiple Sclerosis Society
Mid-Jersey Chapter
246 Monmouth Rd.
Oakhurst, NJ 07755
Phone: (732)660-1005 **Fax:** (732)660-1338
Email: gail.svenciunas@njm.nmss.org
Michael Elkow, President

New Mexico

★ 10446 ★ National Multiple Sclerosis Society
All America Chapter
Rio Grande Division
2021 Girard SE, Ste. 201
Albuquerque, NM 87106
Phone: (505)244-0625 **Fax:** (505)244-0629
Email: nmx@nmss.org
Pam McElrath, President

New York

★ 10447 ★ National Multiple Sclerosis Society
Long Island Chapter
200 Parkway Dr. S
Hauppauge, NY 11788
Phone: (631)864-8337 **Free:** 800—FIGHT-MS
Fax: (631)864-8342

Email: jbiederman@nmssli.org
Johanna Biederman, CEO & Pres

★ 10448 ★ National Multiple Sclerosis Society
New York City Chapter
30 W 26th St., 9th Fl.
New York, NY 10010
Phone: (212)463-7787 **Fax:** (212)989-4362
Email: info@msnyc.org
Carol Kurzig, President

★ 10449 ★ National Multiple Sclerosis Society
Southern New York Chapter
2 Gannett Dr., Ste. LC
White Plains, NY 10604
Phone: (914)694-1655 **Fax:** (914)694-1656
Email: kathy.coulam@nyv.nmss.org
Website: http://www.fightms.org
Kathy Coulam, President

★ 10450 ★ National Multiple Sclerosis Society
Upstate New York Chapter
1650 South Ave., Ste. 100
Rochester, NY 14620-3901
Phone: (585)271-0801 **Free:** 877-869-6677
Fax: (585)442-2817
Email: chapter@msupstateny.org
James P. Ahearn, President

★ 10451 ★ National Multiple Sclerosis Society
Western New York/Northwestern Pennsylvania Chapter
4245 Union Rd., Ste. 108
Buffalo, NY 14225
Phone: (716)634-2261 **Fax:** (716)634-2979
Email: nyw@nmss.org
Arthur Cardella, President

North Carolina

★ 10452 ★ National Multiple Sclerosis Society
Central North Carolina Chapter
2211 W Meadowview Rd., Ste. 30
Greensboro, NC 27407
Phone: (336)299-4136 **Fax:** (336)855-3039
Email: ncc@nmss.org
Website: http://www.ncc.nmss.org
Elizabeth Green, President

★ 10453 ★ National Multiple Sclerosis Society
Eastern North Carolina Chapter
3101 Industrial Dr., Ste. 210
Raleigh, NC 27609
Phone: (919)834-0678 **Fax:** (919)834-9822
Email: nct@nmss.org
Website: http://www.encms.org
Robin Boettcher, President

★ 10454 ★ National Multiple Sclerosis Society
Mid-Atlantic Chapter
9844-C Southern Pines Blvd.
Charlotte, NC 28273
Phone: (704)525-2955 **Free:** 800-477-2955
Fax: (704)527-0406
Email: ncp@nmss.org
Website: http://www.ncp.nmss.org
Anne Marie McDermott, President

Ohio

★ 10455 ★ Multiple Sclerosis Association of America
Mid-Western Regional Office
1873 E Aurora Rd.
Twinsburg, OH 44087
Phone: (330)405-9055 **Free:** 800-589-7962
Fax: (330)405-9052
Email: midwest@msaa.com
Website: http://www.msaa.com/regionmw.htm
Renee Williams, Director

★ 10456 ★ National Multiple Sclerosis Society
Northwest Ohio Chapter
401 Tomahawk Dr.
Maumee, OH 43537
Phone: (419)897-9533 **Fax:** (419)897-9733
Email: oho@nmss.org
Website: http://www.oho.nmss.org
Jacque Pratt, President

★ 10457 ★ National Multiple Sclerosis Society
Ohio Buckeye Chapter
The Hanna Bldg., Ste. 333
1422 Euclid Ave.
Cleveland, OH 44115
Phone: (216)696-8220 **Free:** 800-667-7131
Fax: (216)696-2817
Email: oha@nmss.org
Website: http://www.nmssneo.org
Janet Kramer, President

★ 10458 ★ National Multiple Sclerosis Society
Ohio Valley Chapter
4460 Lake Forest Dr., Ste. 236
Cincinnati, OH 45242
Phone: (513)769-4400 **Fax:** (513)769-6019
Linda Stetson, President

Oklahoma

★ 10459 ★ National Multiple Sclerosis Society
Oklahoma Chapter
Bldg. 7, Ste. 103
4606 E 67th St.
Tulsa, OK 74136
Phone: (918)488-0882 **Fax:** (918)488-0913
Email: paula.cortner@oke.nmss.org
Website: http://www.oknmss.org
Paula Cortner, President

Oregon

★ 10460 ★ National Multiple Sclerosis Society
Oregon Chapter
1650 NW Naito Pkwy., Ste. 190
Portland, OR 97209
Phone: (503)223-9511 **Fax:** (503)223-2912
Email: info@orcnmss.org
Website: http://www.orcnmss.org
Carol Vogel Warner, President

Pennsylvania

★ 10461 ★ National Multiple Sclerosis Society
Allegheny District Chapter
1040 5th Ave., 2nd Fl.
Pittsburgh, PA 15219
Phone: (412)261-6347 **Fax:** (412)232-1461
Email: pax@nmss.org
Website: http://www.nmss-pgh.org
Colleen McGuire, President

★ 10462 ★ National Multiple Sclerosis Society
Central Pennsylvania Chapter
2209 Forest Hills Dr., Ste. 18
Harrisburg, PA 17112
Phone: (717)652-2108 **Fax:** (717)652-2590
Email: pac@nmss.org
Website: http://www.pac.nmss.org
Margie Adelmann, President

★ 10463 ★ National Multiple Sclerosis Society
Greater Delaware Valley Chapter
1 Reed St.
Philadelphia, PA 19147
Phone: (215)271-1500 **Fax:** (215)271-6122
Email: pae@nmss.org
Website: http://www.pae.nmss.org
Judith Cohen, President

Rhode Island

★ 10464 ★ National Multiple Sclerosis Society
Rhode Island Chapter
205 Hallene Rd., Ste. 209
Warwick, RI 02886
Phone: (401)738-8383 **Fax:** (401)738-8469
Email: ann.wood@nmss.org
Website: http://www.nmssri.org
Kathy Mechnig, President

South Carolina

★ 10465 ★ National Multiple Sclerosis Society
Mid-Atlantic Chapter
South Carolina Regional Office
2711 Middleburg Dr., Ste. 105
Columbia, SC 29204
Phone: (803)799-7848 **Free:** 800-922-7591
Fax: (803)765-2259

South Dakota

★ 10466 ★ National Multiple Sclerosis Society
Dakota Chapter
3800 W Technology Circle, Ste. 201
Sioux Falls, SD 57106
Phone: (605)336-7017 **Fax:** (605)336-8088
Email: dione.steuerwald@ndn.nmss.org
Website: http://www.msdakotachapter.org
Kathie Brown, President

Tennessee

★ 10467 ★ National Multiple Sclerosis Society
Mid South Chapter
4219 Hillsboro Rd., Ste. 306
Nashville, TN 37215
Phone: (615)269-9055 **Free:** 800-269-9055
Fax: (615)269-9470
Email: tns@nmss.org
Jim Ward, President

Texas

★ 10468 ★ National Multiple Sclerosis Society
All America Chapter
Panhandle Division
6222 Canyon Dr.
Amarillo, TX 79109
Phone: (806)468-7500 **Fax:** (806)468-8022
Email: info@nmsstxp.org
Pam McElrath, President

★ 10469 ★ National Multiple Sclerosis Society
All America Chapter
West Texas Division
1031 Andrews Hwy., Ste. 201
Midland, TX 79701
Phone: (915)522-2077 **Fax:** (915)694-7970
Email: txq@nmss.org
Pam McElrath, President

★ 10470 ★ National Multiple Sclerosis Society
Lonestar Chapter
8111 N Stadium Dr., Ste. 100
Houston, TX 77054
Phone: (713)526-8967 **Fax:** (713)394-7422
Email: txh@nmss.org
Website: http://www.nmsslonestar.org
Pat Bertotti, President

★ 10471 ★ National Multiple Sclerosis Society
North Central Texas Chapter
4086 Sandshell Dr.
Fort Worth, TX 76137
Phone: (817)306-7003 **Free:** 800—FIGHT-MS
Fax: (817)306-7055
Email: nms@nctms.org
Website: http://www.nctms.org
Evelyn Taylor, President

Utah

★ 10472 ★ National Multiple Sclerosis Society
Utah State Chapter
2995 S West Temple, Ste. C
Salt Lake City, UT 84115
Phone: (801)493-0113 **Free:** 800-527-8116
Fax: (801)493-0122
Email: info@fightmsutah.org
Tami Featherstone, President

Vermont

★ 10473 ★ National Multiple Sclerosis Society
All America Chapter
Vermont Division
100 Dorset St., Ste. 12
South Burlington, VT 05403
Phone: (802)862-0912 **Fax:** (802)864-6509
Email: vtn@nmss.org
Pam McElrath, President

Virginia

★ 10474 ★ National Multiple Sclerosis Society
Blue Ridge Chapter
1 Morton Dr., Ste. 106
Charlottesville, VA 22903
Phone: (434)971-8010 **Fax:** (434)979-4475
Email: vab@nmss.org
Website: http://www.vab.nmss.org
Faith Painter, President

★ 10475 ★ National Multiple Sclerosis Society
Central Virginia Chapter
2104 W Laburnum Ave., Ste. 102
Richmond, VA 23227
Phone: (804)353-5008 **Fax:** (804)353-5595
Email: melina.davis-martin@var.nmss.org
Website: http://nmss-cvc.communitypoint.org
Melina Davis-Martin, President

★ 10476 ★ National Multiple Sclerosis Society
Hampton Roads Chapter
405 S Parliament Dr., Ste. 105
Virginia Beach, VA 23462
Phone: (757)490-9627 **Fax:** (757)490-1617
Email: vax@nmss.org
Website: http://www.fightms.com
Sharon Grossman, President

Washington

★ 10477 ★ National Multiple Sclerosis Society
Greater Washington Chapter
192 Nickerson St., Ste. 100
Seattle, WA 98109
Phone: (206)284-4236 **Free:** 800-800-7047
Fax: (206)284-4972
Email: info@nmsswas.org
Patty Shepherd-Barnes, CEO & Pres

★ 10478 ★ National Multiple Sclerosis Society
Inland Northwest Chapter
818 E Sharp
Spokane, WA 99202
Phone: (509)482-2022 **Fax:** (509)483-1077
Email: wai@nmss.org
Website: http://www.omnicast.net/waims
Robert Hansen, President

West Virginia

★ 10479 ★ National Multiple Sclerosis Society
All America Chapter
West Virginia Division
111 Hale St.
Charleston, WV 25301
Phone: (304)343-5152 **Fax:** (304)343-5154
Email: information@ntlos.net
Pam McElrath, President

Wisconsin

★ 10480 ★ National Multiple Sclerosis Society
Wisconsin Chapter
Saratoga Dr., Ste. 1
Waukesha, WI 53186-0401
Phone: (262)547-8999 **Fax:** (262)547-4440
Email: info@wisms.org
Website: http://www.wisms.org
Colleen Kalt, CEO & Pres

Wyoming

★ 10481 ★ National Multiple Sclerosis Society
All America Chapter
Wyoming Division
400 E 1st St., Ste. 203
Casper, WY 82601
Phone: (307)234-2340 **Fax:** (307)234-4899
Email: nicholle.bridgmon@nmss.org
Pam McElrath, President

Myasthenia Gravis

State chapters of the Myasthenia Foundation are listed below. The national office is located at 5841 Cedar Lake Rd., Ste. 204, Minneapolis, MN 55416. Additional information can be obtained by calling the national office at (800) 541-5454, or by consulting their web site at http://www.myasthenia.org/.

Alabama

★ 10482 ★ Myasthenia Gravis Foundation of America
Alabama Chapter
200 Office Park Cir., Ste. 312
Birmingham, AL 35223
Phone: (205)868-1210 **Free:** (866)749-0844
Email: alchaptermgfa@aol.com

Arizona

★ 10483 ★ Myasthenia Gravis Foundation of America
Jim L. Walker, Arizona Chapter
935 E Main St., Ste. 206
Mesa, AZ 85203
Phone: (480)464-9648 **Fax:** (480)464-9754
Email: azmgfa@cox.net
Website: http://www.geocities.com/azmgfa
Trevor Lloyd, Chairman of the Board

Arkansas

★ 10484 ★ Myasthenia Gravis Foundation of America
Arkansas Chapter
PO Box 388
Mabelvale, AR 72103
Phone: (501)455-4448 **Fax:** (501)455-4055
Email: bktuck50@aol.com

Connecticut

★ 10485 ★ Myasthenia Gravis Foundation of America
Connecticut "Nutmeg" State Chapter
7 Dobson Dr.
East Hartford, CT 06118
Phone: (860)568-0657 **Free:** (866)329-8784
Email: RSpeaotMG@cs.com
Website: http://pages.cthome.net/ctnutmeg
Remarks: Serves Connecticut, Maine, Rhode Island, and Vermont.

Florida

★ 10486 ★ Myasthenia Gravis Foundation of America
East Central Florida Chapter
PO Box 623
Ormond Beach, FL 32175-0623
Phone: (386)672-2635 **Free:** 888-291-5067
Email: jimburkemgfa@cfl.rr.com
Website: http://www.myasthenia.org/chapters/E_Florida/

★ 10487 ★ Myasthenia Gravis Foundation of America
South Florida Gold Coast Chapter
2077 NE 21st Terr.
Jensen Beach, FL 34957
Phone: (727)334-9579
Email: lou_cor@bellsouth.net

★ 10488 ★ Myasthenia Gravis Foundation of America
West Central Florida Chapter
13540 Andova Dr.
Largo, FL 33774
Phone: (727)596-1491
Email: mpetersfl@aol.com

Georgia

★ 10489 ★ Myasthenia Gravis Foundation of America
Georgia State Chapter
PO Box 93604
Atlanta, GA 30318
Phone: (770)973-3269 **Free:** 800-743-4339
Fax: (770)319-3848
Email: gachapter_mgfa@hotmail.com
Website: http://members.tripod.com/~gcmgfa/
Remarks: Serves Georgia, Louisiana, Mississippi, and Tennessee.

Illinois

★ 10490 ★ Myasthenia Gravis Foundation of America
Illinois Chapter
2411 New St.
Blue Island, IL 60406
Phone: (708)385-3888 **Fax:** (708)385-0447
Email: myastheniaILL@aol.com
Website: http://www.myastheniagravis.org

Indiana

★ 10491 ★ Myasthenia Gravis Foundation of America
Greater Indianapolis Chapter
8922 Haverstick Rd.
Indianapolis, IN 46240
Phone: (317)846-1462
Email: spynke@aol.com

Kentucky

★ 10492 ★ Myasthenia Gravis Foundation of America
Kentucky Chapter
8510 Eastland Dr.
Spottsville, KY 42458
Phone: (270)826-1312
Email: heatherhagan@hotmail.com

Maryland

★ 10493 ★ Myasthenia Gravis Foundation of America
Maryland/DC/Delaware Chapter
PO Box 186
Pasadena, MD 21123-0186
Phone: (410)437-2881 **Free:** 800-803-5775
Email: maryland@myasthenia.org
Website: http://www.myasthenia.org/chapters/maryland

Massachusetts

★ 10494 ★ Myasthenia Gravis Foundation of America
Massachusetts/New Hampshire Chapter
PO Box 192
Shelburne Falls, MA 01370
Phone: (508)435-3808
Email: sba-mb@mindspring.com

Michigan

★ 10495 ★ Myasthenia Gravis Foundation of America
Detroit Chapter
17117 W 9 Mile Rd., Ste. 1745
Southfield, MI 48075
Phone: (248)423-9700 **Free:** 800-227-1763
Fax: (248)423-9705
Email: mgadetroit@mich.com
Website: http://www.mgadetroit.org

★ 10496 ★ Myasthenia Gravis Foundation of America
Great Lakes Chapter
2680 Horizon Dr. SE, Ste. C-9
Grand Rapids, MI 49546-7500
Phone: (616)956-0622 **Fax:** (616)956-9234
Email: office@greatlakesmgf.org
Website: http://www.greatlakesmgf.org

Minnesota

★ 10497 ★ Myasthenia Gravis Foundation of America
Minnesota Chapter
1001 S Lake Ave.
Duluth, MN 55802
Phone: (218)727-6064
Email: mgfamn@aol.com
Remarks: Serves Minnesota, Nebraska, North Dakota, and South Dakota.

Missouri

★ 10498 ★ Myasthenia Gravis Foundation of America
Greater Saint Louis Chapter
7514 Forrest View Dr.
Saint Louis, MO 63121
Phone: (314)382-7490
Email: MGFAStl@aol.com
Website: http://www.myathenia.org/chapters/St_Louis

New Jersey

★ 10499 ★ Myasthenia Gravis Foundation of America
Garden State Chapter
PO Box 4258
Wayne, NJ 07474
Phone: (973)628-6034 **Free:** 800-437-4949
Fax: (973)628-6035
Email: khaughey@mgnj.org
Website: http://www.mgnj.org

New Mexico

★ 10500 ★ Myasthenia Gravis Foundation of America
New Mexico Chapter
PO Box 26873
Albuquerque, NM 87125
Phone: (505)897-0932
Email: myasgrav@cybermesa.com
Website: http://www.myasthenia.org/chapters/New_Mexico
Remarks: Also serves Colorado.

New York

★ 10501 ★ Myasthenia Gravis Foundation of America
Metro New York Chapter
116 Goldie Ave.
North Bellmore, NY 11710
Phone: (631)409-8420 **Free:** 800-667-9807
Email: metronymgfa@yahoo.com
Website: http://mgfametrony.homestead.com/nymgmgfa.html

North Carolina

★ 10502 ★ Myasthenia Gravis Foundation of America
Carolinas Chapter
506 E Forest Hills Blvd.
Durham, NC 27707
Phone: (919)490-2937 **Free:** 800-842-8711
Fax: (919)489-7564
Email: carolinasmgfa@nc.rr.com
Remarks: Serves North Carolina and South Carolina.

Ohio

★ 10503 ★ Myasthenia Gravis Foundation of America
Mahoning-Shenango Valley Chapter
PO Box 282
Girard, OH 44420
Phone: (330)539-7582 **Fax:** (330)539-7582

★ 10504 ★ Myasthenia Gravis Foundation of America
Ohio Chapter
2907 Lincoln Way E, Unit B
Massillon, OH 44646
Phone: (330)834-9066
Email: ohiochaptermgf@nci2000.net
Website: http://ohiochaptermgf.org

Oklahoma

★ 10505 ★ Myasthenia Gravis Foundation of America
Oklahoma Chapter
6465 S Yale Ave., Ste. 623
Tulsa, OK 74136-7811
Phone: (918)494-4951
Email: okmgf@valornet.com
Website: http://www.myasthenia.org/chapters/oklahoma
Peggy Foust, Exec Director

Pennsylvania

★ 10506 ★ Myasthenia Gravis Foundation of America
Pennsylvania Chapter
2665 Pinewood Rd.
Lancaster, PA 17601
Phone: (866)7PA-MGFA
Email: pennamgfa@aol.com

Texas

★ 10507 ★ Myasthenia Gravis Foundation of America
Greater Dallas/Fort Worth Chapter
2022 Sage Valley Dr.
Richardson, TX 75080
Phone: (972)690-1302 **Fax:** (972)699-8698
Email: dfwmgf@hotmail.com

★ 10508 ★ Myasthenia Gravis Foundation of America
Greater South Texas Chapter
10592-A Fuqua St., Ste. 313
Houston, TX 77089-1402
Phone: (281)987-9393 **Fax:** (281)328-2430
Email: gowens@accesscomm.net

★ 10509 ★ Myasthenia Gravis Foundation of America
Northwest Texas Chapter
281 County Rd. 135
Ovalo, TX 79541
Phone: (915)554-7038 **Fax:** (915)554-7044
Email: nwtc@camalott.com

Utah

★ 10510 ★ Myasthenia Gravis Foundation of America
Utah State Intermountain Chapter
8717 South 910 East
Sandy, UT 84094
Phone: (801)816-2204

Virginia

★ 10511 ★ Myasthenia Gravis Foundation of America
Virginia Chapter
2304 Angus
Charlottesville, VA 22901
Phone: (434)295-9861 **Free:** 800-728-4405
Fax: (434)295-1909
Email: pma8n@cstone.net
Website: http://www.geocities.com/HotSprings/Spa/9948/
Remarks: Serves Virginia and West Virginia.

Washington

★ 10512 ★ Myasthenia Gravis Foundation of America
Pacific Northwest Chapter
18115 116th Ave. SE
Renton, WA 98058-6562
Phone: (425)235-1435 **Free:** 877-252-0677
Fax: (425)204-2070
Email: nwmg@cs.com
Remarks: Serves Alaska, Hawaii, Idaho, Montana, Nevada, Oregon, Washington, and Wyoming.

Wisconsin

★ 10513 ★ Myasthenia Gravis Foundation of America
Wisconsin Chapter
6644 W Revere Pl.
West Allis, WI 53219
Phone: (262)938-9800
Email: wiscmg@yahoo.com

Neurofibromatosis

State chapters of the National Neurofibromatosis Foundation are listed below. The national office is located at 95 Pine St., 16th Fl., New York, NY 10005. Additional information can be obtained by calling the national office at (800) 323-7938, or by consulting their web site at http://neurofibromatosis.org/.

California

★ 10514 ★ National Neurofibromatosis Foundation
California Chapter
2365 Westwood Blvd., Ste. 21
Los Angeles, CA 90064
Phone: (310)470-3888 **Free:** 888-314-6633
Fax: (310)441-1601
Email: NFCAL@aol.com
Website: http://www.neurofibromatosis.org/california
Stuart J. Rogoff, Vice President

Colorado

★ 10515 ★ National Neurofibromatosis Foundation
Colorado Chapter
11776 Glencoe St.
Thornton, CO 80233
Phone: (303)460-8313
Email: bkhnn1@aol.com
Website: http://www.neurofibromatosis.org/colorado
Kent Draper, President

Florida

★ 10516 ★ National Neurofibromatosis Foundation
Florida Chapter
735 36th Ave. N
Saint Petersburg, FL 33704
Free: 800-540-5721
Email: ssuzearle@aol.com
Website: http://www.neurofibromatosis.org/florida
Suzanne Earle, President

Georgia

★ 10517 ★ National Neurofibromatosis Foundation
Georgia Chapter
PO Box 1948
Hiram, GA 30141-1742
Phone: (770)445-4224
Email: ChikNMama1@aol.com
Rhonda Bridges, President

Illinois

★ 10518 ★ National Neurofibromatosis Foundation
Illinois Chapter
3224 Heather Glen Dr.
Aurora, IL 60504
Phone: (630)236-7356 **Free:** 800-500-6633
Email: donwojonf@aol.com
Website: http://www.neurofibromatosis.org/illinois
Don Wojtnyek, President

Iowa

★ 10519 ★ National Neurofibromatosis Foundation
Iowa Chapter
321 Glenview Dr.
Des Moines, IA 50312
Phone: (515)277-8494
Email: Drev@aol.com
Website: http://www.neurofibromatosis.org/iowa
Sheila Drevyanko, President

Louisiana

★ 10520 ★ National Neurofibromatosis Foundation
Louisiana Chapter
PO Box 499
Baton Rouge, LA 70821
Phone: (225)665-3547
Email: nflouisiana1@cox.net
Website: http://www.neurofibromatosis.org/louisiana
Debbie Bouy, President

Maryland

★ 10521 ★ National Neurofibromatosis Foundation
Mid-Atlantic Region Chapter
3357 Garrison Cir.
Abingdon, MD 21009
Phone: (410)887-5576
Email: NNFF@nf.org
Website: http://www.nf.org
Mike Daughaday, President

Massachusetts

★ 10522 ★ National Neurofibromatosis Foundation
Massachusetts Chapter
31 Springhill Ave.
Marlborough, MA 01752
Phone: (508)624-4533 **Free:** 888-585-5316
Fax: (508)624-7553
Email: nfma2000@aol.com
Website: http://www.neurofibromatosis.org/massachusetts
Matthew LaBarre, Vice President

Michigan

★ 10523 ★ National Neurofibromatosis Foundation
Michigan Chapter
6069 Brynthrop
Shelby Township, MI 48316
Phone: (810)731-7811
Email: hawkeyenf@aol.com
Website: http://www.neurofibromatosis.org/michigan
Peter Dingeman, President

Missouri

★ 10524 ★ National Neurofibromatosis Foundation
Missouri Chapter
1015 Locust St., Ste. 1032
Saint Louis, MO 63101
Phone: (314)436-6877 **Free:** 888-848-NNFF
Fax: (314)436-0524
Email: NFMissouri@aol.com
Website: http://www.neurofibromatosis.org/missouri
Rebecca Sastry, Exec Director

Nebraska

★ 10525 ★ National Neurofibromatosis Foundation
Northern Plains Chapter
PO Box 540843
Omaha, NE 68154-0843
Phone: (402)362-7279 **Free:** 877-449-7979
Email: NFNebraska@hotmail.com
Amy Hayes, President
Remarks: Serves Nebraska, North Dakota, and South Dakota.

New York

★ 10526 ★ National Neurofibromatosis Foundation
New York/New Jersey Chapter
95 Pine St., 16th Fl.
New York, NY 10005
Phone: (212)344-NNFF **Fax:** (212)747-0004
Website: http://www.neurofibromatosis.org/ny_nj
Pamela Linton, Exec Director

Oregon

★ 10527 ★ National Neurofibromatosis Foundation
Oregon Chapter
Patient Information and Support
1717 SW Park Ave., Apt. 1108
Portland, OR 97201
Phone: (503)412-6599
Email: walktours1@aol.com

Website: http://www.neurofibromatosis.org/oregon
Terri Wardell, Contact

South Carolina

★ 10528 ★ National Neurofibromatosis Foundation
South Carolina Chapter
PO Box 358
Cordova, SC 29039
Phone: (803)534-0962
Email: rudestu@bellsouth.net
Stu Wright, President

Tennessee

★ 10529 ★ National Neurofibromatosis Foundation
Tennessee Chapter
9025 Old Smyrna Rd.
Brentwood, TN 37027
Phone: (615)252-2360
Email: gbulso@bccb.com
Gino Bulso, President

Utah

★ 10530 ★ National Neurofibromatosis Foundation
Utah Chapter
1746 South 300 East
Kaysville, UT 84037
Phone: (801)451-0383 **Fax:** (801)968-0981
Email: bloomerjc@earthlink.net
Cherilyn Bloomer, President

Washington

★ 10531 ★ National Neurofibromatosis Foundation
Washington State Chapter
6628 212th St. SW, Ste. 100
Lynnwood, WA 98036
Phone: (425)672-9610 **Fax:** (425)672-9518
Email: NF@nnffwa.org
Website: http://www.neurofibromatosis.org/washington
Susan Blalock, Exec Director

Wisconsin

★ 10532 ★ National Neurofibromatosis Foundation
Wisconsin Chapter
Milwaukee, WI
Phone: (414)438-0985
Email: Epankownf@aol.com
Elaine Pankow, President

Wyoming

★ 10533 ★ National Neurofibromatosis Foundation
Wyoming Chapter
2434 Coulter Dr.
Casper, WY 82604
Phone: (307)473-7723
Email: n13good@aol.com
Norma Good, Contact

Nursing

The following state organizations are affiliates of the American Nurses Association, 600 Maryland Ave. SW, Ste. 100 West, Washington, DC 20024, (800)274-4ANA, http://www.nursingworld.org/.

Alabama

★ 10534 ★ Alabama State Nurses' Association
360 N Hull St.
Montgomery, AL 36104-3658
Phone: (334)262-8321 **Fax:** (334)262-8578
Email: alabamasna@mindspring.com
Website: http://www.nursingworld.org/snas/al
Karen L. Pakkala, RN, Exec Director

Alaska

★ 10535 ★ Alaska Nurses Association
2207 E Tudor Rd., Ste. 34
Anchorage, AK 99507-1069
Phone: (907)274-0827 **Fax:** (907)272-0292
Email: aknurse@aknurse.org
Website: http://www.aknurse.org
Camille Soleil, Exec Director

Arizona

★ 10536 ★ Arizona Nurses Association
1850 E Southern Ave., Ste. 1
Tempe, AZ 85282
Phone: (480)831-0404 **Fax:** (480)839-4780
Email: info@aznurse.org
Website: http://www.aznurse.org
Marla Weston, RN, MS, Exec Director

Arkansas

★ 10537 ★ Arkansas Nurses Association
804 N University
Little Rock, AR 72205
Phone: (501)664-5853 **Fax:** (501)664-5859
Email: arna@prodigy.net
Website: http://www.arna.org
David Eubanks, RN, Contact

California

★ 10538 ★ ANA/California
1121 L St., Ste. 409
Sacramento, CA 95814
Phone: (916)447-0225 **Fax:** (916)447-5568
Email: anacalif@pacbell.net
Website: http://www.anacalifornia.org
Tricia Hunter, RN, Contact

Colorado

★ 10539 ★ Colorado Nurses Association
950 S Cherry, Ste. 508
Denver, CO 80246
Phone: (303)757-7483 **Fax:** (303)758-0190
Email: cna@nurses-co.org
Website: http://www.nurses-co.org/cna
Linda Metzner, RN, JD, Exec Director

Connecticut

★ 10540 ★ Connecticut Nurses Association
Meritech Business Park
377 Research Pkwy., Ste. 2D
Meriden, CT 06450
Phone: (203)238-1207 **Fax:** (203)238-3437
Email: polly@ctnurses.org
Website: http://www.nursingworld.org/snas/ct
Polly T. Barey, MS, RN, Exec Director

Delaware

★ 10541 ★ Delaware Nurses Association
2644 Capitol Trail, Ste. 330
Newark, DE 19711
Phone: (302)368-2333 **Fax:** (302)366-1775
Email: delnurse@erols.com
Website: http://www.nursingworld.org/snas/de/
Ruth Bashford, MN, RN, Exec Director

District of Columbia

★ 10542 ★ American Nurses Association
600 Maryland Ave. SW, Ste. 100W
Washington, DC 20024-2571
Phone: (202)651-7000 **Free:** 800-274-4ANA
Fax: (202)651-7001
Email: lstierle@ana.org
Website: http://www.nursingworld.org/
Linda J. Stierle, MSN, CEO

★ 10543 ★ District of Columbia Nurses Association, Inc.
5100 Wisconsin Ave. NW, Ste. 306
Washington, DC 20016
Phone: (202)244-2705 **Fax:** (202)362-8285
Email: dcnurses1@aol.com
Website: http://dcnaonline.com
Tom Wachter, Contact

★ 10544 ★ Federal Nurses Association (FedNA)
600 Maryland Ave. SW, Ste. 100W
Washington, DC 20024
Phone: (202)651-7333 **Fax:** (202)651-7355
Email: FedNA@ana.org
Website: http://www.nursingworld.org/FedNA
Pamela C. Hagan, MSN, Contact

Florida

★ 10545 ★ Florida Nurses Association
PO Box 536985
Orlando, FL 32853-6985
Phone: (407)896-3261 **Fax:** (407)896-9042
Email: info@floridanurse.org
Website: http://www.floridanurse.org
Paula Massey, MN, RN, Exec Director

Georgia

★ 10546 ★ Georgia Nurses Association
3032 Briarcliff Rd. NE
Atlanta, GA 30329-2655
Phone: (404)325-5536 **Fax:** (404)325-0407
Email: gna-ceo@mindspring.com
Website: http://www.georgianurses.org
Deborah Hackman, CEO

Guam

★ 10547 ★ Guam Nurses Association
PO Box CG
Hagatna, GU 96932
Phone: (671)477-6877 **Fax:** (671)477-6877
Email: guamnurse@ite.net
Glynis S. Almonte, RN, Exec Director

Hawaii

★ 10548 ★ Hawaii Nurses Association
677 Ala Moana Blvd., Ste. 301
Honolulu, HI 96813
Phone: (808)531-1628 **Fax:** (808)524-2760
Email: nancy@hawaiinurses.org
Website: http://www.hawaiinurses.org
Nancy McGukin, Exec Director

Idaho

★ 10549 ★ Idaho Nurses Association
200 N 4th St., Ste. 20
Boise, ID 83702-6001
Phone: (208)345-0500 **Fax:** (208)385-0166
Email: idahonursesassn@hotmail.com
Website: http://www.nursingworld.org/snas/id
Judy Murray, PhD,RN, Exec Director

Illinois

★ 10550 ★ Illinois Nurses Association
105 W Adams St., Ste. 2101
Chicago, IL 60603
Phone: (312)419-2900 **Fax:** (312)419-2920
Email: cholmgren@illinoisnurses.com
Website: http://www.illinoisnurses.com
Cathy Holmgren, RN, Exec Director

Indiana

★ 10551 ★ Indiana State Nurses Association
2915 N High School Rd.
Indianapolis, IN 46224
Phone: (317)299-4575 **Fax:** (317)297-3525
Email: isnarn@prodigy.net
Website: http://www.indianurses.org
Ernest C. Klein, Jr., RN, Exec Director

Iowa

★ 10552 ★ Iowa Nurses Association
1501 42nd St., Ste. 471
West Des Moines, IA 50266
Phone: (515)225-0495 **Fax:** (515)225-2201
Email: iowanurses@aol.com
Website: http://www.iowanurses.org
Linda Goeldner, MA,CHE, Exec Director

Kansas

★ 10553 ★ Kansas State Nurses Association
1208 SW Tyler
Topeka, KS 66612-1735
Phone: (785)233-8638 **Fax:** (785)233-5222
Email: troberts@echo.sound.net
Website: http://www.nursingworld.org/snas/ks
Terri R. Roberts, JD, RN, Exec Director

Kentucky

★ 10554 ★ Kentucky Nurses Association
1400 S 1st St.
PO Box 2616
Louisville, KY 40201-2616
Phone: (502)637-2546 **Fax:** (502)637-8236
Email: mkeenan@kentucky-nurses.org
Website: http://www.kentucky-nurses.org
Maureen Keenen, JD, Contact

Louisiana

★ 10555 ★ Louisiana State Nurses Association
5700 Florida Blvd., Ste. 720
Baton Rouge, LA 70806
Phone: (225)201-0993 **Free:** 800-457-6378
Fax: (225)201-0971
Email: lsna@lsna.org
Website: http://www.lsna.org
Tawna Pounders, RN, Exec Director

Maine

★ 10556 ★ American Nurses Association-Maine (ANA-Maine)
PO Box 254
Auburn, ME 04212-0254
Phone: (207)667-0260
Email: josephn@acadia.net
Website: http://www.anamaine.org

Maryland

★ 10557 ★ Maryland Nurses Association
849 International Dr.
Airport Sq. 21, Ste. 255
Linthicum, MD 21090
Phone: (410)859-3000 **Fax:** (410)859-3001
Email: marylandnursesassociation@erols.com
Website: http://www.nursingworld.org/snas/md
Kathryn V. Hall, MS, RN, Exec Director

Massachusetts

★ 10558 ★ Massachusetts Association of Registered Nurses, Inc.
PO Box 70668
Quinsigamond Village Station
345 Greenwood St.
Worcester, MA 01607
Phone: (781)344-6926 **Fax:** (781)341-8495
Email: info@marnonline.org
Website: http://www.nursingworld.org/cmas/ma
Karen Daley, RN, President

Michigan

★ 10559 ★ Michigan Nurses Association
2310 Jolly Oak Rd.
Okemos, MI 48864-4599
Phone: (517)349-5640 **Fax:** (517)349-5818
Email: tom.renkes@minurses.org
Website: http://www.minurses.org
Tom Renkes, MS, RN, Exec Director

Minnesota

★ 10560 ★ Minnesota Nurses Association
1625 Energy Park Dr.
Saint Paul, MN 55108
Phone: (651)646-4807 **Free:** 800-536-4662
Fax: (651)647-5301
Email: emurphy@mnnurses.org
Website: http://www.mnnurses.org
Erin Murphy, RN, Exec Director

Mississippi

★ 10561 ★ Mississippi Nurses Association
31 Woodgreen Pl.
Madison, MS 39110
Phone: (601)898-0670 **Fax:** (601)898-0190
Email: mna@msnurses.org
Website: http://www.msnurses.org
Betty R. Dickson, Exec Director

Missouri

★ 10562 ★ Missouri Nurses Association
1904 Bubba Lane
PO Box 105228
Jefferson City, MO 65110-5228
Phone: (573)636-4623 **Free:** 888-662-MONA
Fax: (573)636-9576
Email: belinda@missourinurses.org
Website: http://www.missourinurses.org
Belinda Heimericks, RN, Exec Director

Montana

★ 10563 ★ Montana Nurses Association
104 Broadway, Ste. G-2
Helena, MT 59601
Phone: (406)442-6710 **Fax:** (406)442-1841
Email: info@mtnurses.org
Website: http://www.nursingworld.org/snas/mt/
Sami Butler, RN, Exec Director

Nebraska

★ 10564 ★ Nebraska Nurses Association
715 S 14th St.
Lincoln, NE 68508
Phone: (402)475-3859 **Fax:** (402)475-3961
Email: ne.nurses@prodigy.net
Website: http://www.nursingworld.org/snas/ne/index.htm
Chuck Stepanek, Exec Director

Nevada

★ 10565 ★ Nevada Nurses Association
PO Box 530399
Henderson, NV 89053-0399
Phone: (702)260-7886 **Fax:** (702)260-7052
Email: nvnurses@aol.com
Website: http://www.nvnurses.org
Richard Schlegel, CAE, Exec Director

New Hampshire

★ 10566 ★ New Hampshire Nurses Association
48 West St.
Concord, NH 03301-3595
Phone: (603)225-3783 **Fax:** (603)228-6672
Email: nh_nurses@compuserve.com
Website: http://www.nhnurses.myassociation.com
Robert Best, BSE, Exec Director

New Jersey

★ 10567 ★ New Jersey State Nurses Association
1479 Pennington Rd.
Trenton, NJ 08618-2661
Phone: (609)883-5335 **Fax:** (609)883-5343
Email: njsna@njsna.org
Website: http://www.njsna.org
Andrea Aughenbaugh, RN, CS, CEO

New Mexico

★ 10568 ★ New Mexico Nurses Association
PO Box 80300
Albuquerque, NM 87198
Phone: (505)268-7744 **Fax:** (505)268-7711
Email: nmnurses@hotmail.com
Website: http://www.nursingworld.org/snas/nm
Carrie Roberts, RN, Exec Director

New York

★ 10569 ★ New York State Nurses Association
11 Cornell Rd.
Latham, NY 12110
Phone: (518)782-9400 **Fax:** (518)782-9530
Email: martha.orr@nysna.org
Website: http://www.nysna.org
Martha L. Orr, MN, RN, Exec Director

North Carolina

★ 10570 ★ North Carolina Nurses Association
103 Enterprise St.
Box 12025
Raleigh, NC 27605
Phone: (919)821-4250 **Fax:** (919)829-5807
Email: rns@ncnurses.org
Website: http://www.ncnurses.org
Sindy Barker, CAE, Exec Director

North Dakota

★ 10571 ★ North Dakota Nurses Association
531 Airport Rd., Ste. D
Bismarck, ND 58504-6107
Phone: (701)223-1385 **Fax:** (701)223-0575
Email: ndna@prodigy.net
Sharon Moos, RN, Contact

Ohio

★ 10572 ★ Ohio Nurses Association
4000 E Main St.
Columbus, OH 43213-2983
Phone: (614)237-5414 **Fax:** (614)237-6081
Email: gharsheymeade@ohnurses.org
Website: http://www.ohnurses.org
Gingy Harshey-Meade, RN, CEO

Oklahoma

★ 10573 ★ Oklahoma Nurses Association
6414 N Santa Fe, Ste. A
Oklahoma City, OK 73116
Phone: (405)840-3476 **Fax:** (405)840-3013
Email: ona@oknurses.com
Website: http://www.oknurses.com
Jane Nelson, CAE, Exec Director

Oregon

★ 10574 ★ Oregon Nurses Association
9600 SW Oak, Ste. 550
Portland, OR 97223
Phone: (503)293-0011 **Fax:** (503)293-0013
Email: ona@oregonrn.org
Website: http://www.oregonrn.org
Susan E. King, MS, RN, Contact
Ken Fitzsimon, JD, Director

Pennsylvania

★ 10575 ★ Pennsylvania State Nurses Association
PO Box 68525
Harrisburg, PA 17106-8525
Phone: (717)657-1222 **Free:** 888-707-7762
Fax: (717)657-3796
Email: psna@psna.org
Website: http://www.psna.org
Michele P. Campbell, RN, Contact

Rhode Island

★ 10576 ★ Rhode Island State Nurses Association
550 S Water St., Unit 540B
Providence, RI 02903-4344
Phone: (401)421-9703 **Fax:** (401)421-6793
Email: risna@prodigy.net
Website: http://www.risnarn.org
Pamela L. McCue, MSN, Exec Director

South Carolina

★ 10577 ★ South Carolina Nurses Association
1821 Gadsden St.
Columbia, SC 29201
Phone: (803)252-4781 **Fax:** (803)779-3870
Email: scna@prodigy.net
Website: http://www.scnurses.org
Judith C. Thompson, Exec Director

South Dakota

★ 10578 ★ South Dakota Nurses Association
PO Box 1015
Pierre, SD 57501-1015
Phone: (605)945-4265 **Fax:** (605)945-4266
Email: sdnurse1@dtgnet.com
Website: http://www.nursingworld.org/snas/sd/
Ed Jacobson, Exec Director

Tennessee

★ 10579 ★ Tennessee Nurses Association
545 Mainstream Dr., Ste. 405
Nashville, TN 37228-1201
Phone: (615)254-0350 **Fax:** (615)254-0303
Email: lbrowntna@aol.com
Website: http://www.tnaonline.org
Louise Browning, CAE, Exec Director

Texas

★ 10580 ★ Texas Nurses Association
7600 Burnet Rd., Ste. 440
Austin, TX 78757-1292
Phone: (512)452-0645 **Fax:** (512)452-0648
Email: memberinfo@texasnurses.org
Website: http://www.texasnurses.org
Clair B. Jordan, RN, Exec Director

Utah

★ 10581 ★ Utah Nurses Association
3761 S 700 E, No. 201
Salt Lake City, UT 84106
Phone: (801)293-8351 **Free:** 800-236-1617
Fax: (801)293-8458
Email: una@xmission.com
Website: http://www.utahnurses.org
Bill Sartain, Exec Director

Vermont

★ 10582 ★ Vermont State Nurses Association
100 Dorset St., Ste. 13
South Burlington, VT 05403-6241
Phone: (802)651-8886 **Fax:** (802)651-8998
Email: vtnurse@prodigy.net
Website: http://www.nesna.org
Margaret M. Sharpe, RN, Exec Director

Virgin Islands

★ 10583 ★ Virgin Islands State Nurses Association
PO Box 583
Christiansted, VI 00821-0583
Phone: (809)773-1261
Email: vcgvina@viaccess.net
Verna Christian-Garcia, RN, Exec Director

Virginia

★ 10584 ★ Virginia Nurses Association
7113 Three Chopt Rd., Ste. 204
Richmond, VA 23226
Phone: (804)282-1808 **Fax:** (804)282-4916
Email: vnajmj@aol.com
Website: http://www.virginianurses.com
Jan Marshall Johnson, MS, RN, Exec Director

Washington

★ 10585 ★ Washington State Nurses Association
575 Andover Park W, Ste. 101
Seattle, WA 98188-3321
Phone: (206)575-7979 **Fax:** (206)575-1908
Email: wsna@wsna.org
Website: http://www.wsna.org
Judith A. Huntington, MN, RN, Exec Director

West Virginia

★ 10586 ★ West Virginia Nurses Association
100 Capitol St., Ste. 1009
PO 1946
Charleston, WV 25301
Phone: (304)342-1169 **Free:** 800-400-1226
Fax: (304)346-1861
Email: centraloffice@wvnurses.org
Website: http://www.wvnurses.org
Cheri Heflin, Exec Director

Wisconsin

★ 10587 ★ Wisconsin Nurses Association
6117 Monona Dr.
Madison, WI 53716
Phone: (608)221-0383 **Fax:** (608)221-2788
Email: wna@execpc.com
Website: http://www.wisconsinnurses.com
Gina Dennik-Champion, RN, Contact

Wyoming

★ 10588 ★ Wyoming Nurses Association
Majestic Bldg., Rm. 305
1603 Capitol Ave.
Cheyenne, WY 82001
Phone: (307)635-3955 **Fax:** (307)635-2173
Email: wyonurse@aol.com
Beverly McDermott, MS, RN, Exec Director

Optometry

The state optometric organizations listed below are affiliated with the American Optometric Association, 243 N Lindbergh Blvd., St. Louis, MO 63141, (314)991-4100, http://www.aoanet.org/.

Alabama

★ 10589 ★ Alabama Optometric Association, Inc.
400 S Union St., Ste. 435
Montgomery, AL 36104
Phone: (334)834-1057 **Fax:** (334)834-1691
Email: optometry@mindspring.com
Website: http://www.eyesite-aloa.org

Alaska

★ 10590 ★ Alaska Optometric Physicians Association
1689 C St., Ste. 222
Anchorage, AK 99501-5126
Phone: (907)770-3777 **Fax:** (907)272-7532
Email: akoa@alaska.com
Website: http://www.akoa.org

Alberta

★ 10591 ★ Alberta Association of Optometrists
10724-113 St.
Edmonton, AB, Canada T5H 3H8
Phone: (780)451-6824 **Fax:** (780)452-9918
Email: Psloan@optometrists.ab.ca
Website: http://www.optometrists.ab.ca

Arizona

★ 10592 ★ Arizona Optometric Association
1702 E Highland Ave., No. 213
Phoenix, AZ 85016
Phone: (602)279-0055 **Fax:** (602)264-6356
Email: Jane@azoa.org
Website: http://www.azoa.org

Arkansas

★ 10593 ★ Arkansas Optometric Association
441 S Victory St., Ste. 202
Little Rock, AR 72201
Phone: (501)661-7675 **Fax:** (501)661-1039
Email: aropt@swbell.net

★ 10594 ★ Southwest Council of Optometry
PO Box 1869
Alma, AR 72921
Phone: (501)632-2360 **Fax:** (501)632-4283
Email: swco@ipa.net

British Columbia

★ 10595 ★ British Columbia Association of Optometrists
No. 100-10751 Shellbridge Way
Richmond, BC, Canada V6X 2W8
Phone: (604)270-9909 **Fax:** (604)270-4950
Email: cwilliams@optometrists.bc.ca
Website: http://www.optometrists.bc.ca

California

★ 10596 ★ California Optometric Association
2415 K St.
Sacramento, CA 95816-5001
Phone: (916)441-3990 **Free:** 800-877-5738
Fax: (916)448-1423
Email: ELBrutvan@coavision.org
Website: http://www.coavision.org

Colorado

★ 10597 ★ Colorado Optometric Association, Inc.
1600 Broadway, Ste. 1320
Denver, CO 80202
Phone: (303)863-9778 **Fax:** (303)863-9775
Email: ghume@visioncare.org
Website: http://www.visioncare.org

Connecticut

★ 10598 ★ Connecticut Association of Optometrists
342 N Main St.
West Hartford, CT 06117-2507
Phone: (860)586-7508 **Fax:** (860)586-7550
Email: pberry@cao.org
Website: http://www.cao.org

Delaware

★ 10599 ★ Delaware Optometric Association, Inc.
PO Box 1009
Selbyville, DE 19975
Phone: (302)436-2020 **Fax:** (302)436-8846
Email: Jphilov@intercom.net

Florida

★ 10600 ★ Florida Optometric Association
PO Box 13429
Tallahassee, FL 32317
Phone: (850)877-4697 **Fax:** (850)878-0933
Email: Ken@floridaeyes.org
Website: http://www.floridaeyes.org

Georgia

★ 10601 ★ Georgia Optometric Association
1000 Corporate Ctr. Dr., No. 240
Morrow, GA 30260
Phone: (770)961-9866 **Fax:** (770)961-9965
Email: GBear79180@aol.com
Website: http://www.goaeyes.com

★ 10602 ★ Southern Council of Optometrists
4661 N Shallowford Rd.
Atlanta, GA 30338
Phone: (770)451-8206 **Fax:** (770)451-3156
Email: SJGSOCO@aol.com

Hawaii

★ 10603 ★ Hawaii Optometric Association
220 S King St., No. 801
Honolulu, HI 96813-4526
Phone: (808)537-5678 **Fax:** (808)537-1509
Email: Hoaopt@earthlink.net

Idaho

★ 10604 ★ Idaho Optometric Association, Inc.
25095 Homedale Rd.
Wilder, ID 83676-5811
Phone: (208)461-2000 **Fax:** (208)337-5613
Email: LEBenton@aol.com

Illinois

★ 10605 ★ Illinois Optometric Association
304 W Washington St.
Springfield, IL 62701
Phone: (217)525-8012 **Fax:** (217)525-8018
Email: ioa@ioaweb.org
Website: http://www.ioaweb.org

Indiana

★ 10606 ★ Indiana Optometric Association
201 N Illinois St., Ste. 1920
PO Box 44975
Indianapolis, IN 46244-0975
Phone: (317)237-3560 **Fax:** (317)237-3564
Email: rwuensc@attglobal.net
Website: http://www.ioa.org

Iowa

★ 10607 ★ Iowa Optometric Association
1454 30th St., Ste. 204
West Des Moines, IA 50266-1312
Phone: (515)222-5679 **Fax:** (515)222-9073
Email: IOAAED@aol.com
Website: http://www.iowaoptometry.org

Kansas

★ 10608 ★ Kansas Optometric Association
1266 SW Topeka Blvd.
Topeka, KS 66612
Phone: (785)232-0225 **Fax:** (785)232-6151
Email: Garykoa@cjnetworks.com

Kentucky

★ 10609 ★ Kentucky Optometric Association
PO Box 572
Frankfort, KY 40602
Phone: (502)875-3516 **Fax:** (502)875-3782
Email: Darleneeakin@kyeyes.org
Website: http://www.kyeyes.org

Louisiana

★ 10610 ★ Louisiana State Association of Optometrists
115-B N 13th St.
Oakdale, LA 71463
Phone: (318)335-0675 **Fax:** (318)335-0677
Email: LSAO@bellsouth.net

Maine

★ 10611 ★ Maine Optometric Association, Inc.
61A Pleasant Pond Lake
Litchfield, ME 04350
Phone: (207)582-9910 **Fax:** (207)582-1652
Email: nanmoa@aol.com
Website: http://www.MaineEyeDoctors.com

Manitoba

★ 10612 ★ Manitoba Association of Optometrists
200B-392 Academy Rd.
Winnipeg, MB, Canada R3N 0B8
Phone: (204)943-9811
Email: mboptom@aol.com

Maryland

★ 10613 ★ Maryland Optometric Association
720 Light St.
Baltimore, MD 21230
Phone: (410)727-7801 **Fax:** (410)752-8295
Email: moa@assnhqtrs.com
Website: http://www.marylandeyes.org

★ **10614** ★ **The Optometric Society of the District of Columbia**
7705 Cayuga Ave.
Bethesda, MD 20817
Phone: (301)229-4990

Massachusetts

★ **10615** ★ **Massachusetts Society of Optometrists, Inc.**
1071 Worcester Rd., No. 12
Framingham, MA 01701-5298
Phone: (508)875-7900 **Fax:** (508)875-0010
Email: Rich@massoptom.org
Website: http://www.massoptom.org

Michigan

★ **10616** ★ **Michigan Optometric Association**
530 W Ionia St., Ste. A
Lansing, MI 48933-1062
Phone: (517)482-0616 **Fax:** (517)482-1611
Email: mioptoassn@aol.com
Website: http://www.mioptassn.org

Minnesota

★ **10617** ★ **Minnesota Optometric Association, Inc.**
13355 10th Ave. N, Ste. 108
Minneapolis, MN 55441-5510
Phone: (763)765-2393 **Fax:** (763)765-2329
Email: Jim@mneyedocs.org
Website: http://www.mneyedocs.org

Mississippi

★ **10618** ★ **Mississippi Optometric Association, Inc.**
5420 I-55 N, Ste. D
Jackson, MS 39211
Phone: (601)956-7412 **Fax:** (601)956-7468
Email: MSOptometr@aol.com

Missouri

★ **10619** ★ **American Optometric Student Association**
243 N Lindbergh Blvd.
Saint Louis, MO 63141
Phone: (314)991-4100 **Fax:** (314)991-4101
Email: cmfrei@aol.com
Website: http://www.theaosa.org

★ **10620** ★ **Missouri Optometric Association, Inc.**
100 E High St., Ste. 301
Jefferson City, MO 65101-2960
Phone: (573)635-6151 **Fax:** (573)635-7989
Email: MOOPT@socket.net
Website: http://www.moeyecare.org

Montana

★ **10621** ★ **Armed Forces Optometric Association**
411 Sweetgrass Ct.
Great Falls, MT 59405
Phone: (406)452-5688 **Fax:** (406)452-5740
Email: execdir@afos2020.org
Website: http://www.afos2020.org

★ **10622** ★ **Montana Optometric Association, Inc.**
36 S Last Chance Gulch, Ste. A
Helena, MT 59601
Phone: (406)443-1160 **Fax:** (406)443-4614
Email: Suew@mteyes.com
Website: http://www.mteyes.com

Nebraska

★ **10623** ★ **Nebraska Optometric Association, Inc.**
PO Box 81706
Lincoln, NE 68501-1706
Phone: (402)474-7716 **Fax:** (402)476-6547
Email: noa@assocoffice.net
Website: http://www.noaonline.org

Nevada

★ **10624** ★ **Nevada Optometric Association, Inc.**
9101 W Sahara Ave., No. 105, PMB 172
Las Vegas, NV 89117-5772
Phone: (702)220-7444 **Fax:** (702)220-7444
Email: NOALV@aol.com
Website: http://www.nevadaoptometric.com

New Brunswick

★ **10625** ★ **New Brunswick Association of Optometrists**
364 York St., Ste. 230
Fredericton, NB, Canada E3B 3P7
Phone: (506)458-8759 **Fax:** (506)450-1271
Email: nbao@nbnet.nb.ca

New Hampshire

★ **10626** ★ **New Hampshire Optometric Association, Inc.**
767 Islington St., Ste. B
Portsmouth, NH 03801
Phone: (603)436-3717 **Fax:** (603)433-8815
Email: optometrist@attbi.com
Website: http://www.nhoptometry.org

New Jersey

★ **10627** ★ **New Jersey Optometric Association, Inc.**
20 Texas Ave.
Lawrenceville, NJ 08648
Phone: (609)671-0900 **Fax:** (609)671-1820
Email: njoa@aol.com
Website: http://www.eyecare.org

New Mexico

★ **10628** ★ **New Mexico Optometric Association, Inc.**
1008 Paseo del Pueblo Sur, PMB No. 241
Taos, NM 87571
Phone: (505)751-7242 **Fax:** (505)751-7243
Email: fleece@laplaza.org
Website: http://www.laplaza.org

New York

★ **10629** ★ **New York State Optometric Association, Inc.**
90 S Swan St.
Albany, NY 12210
Phone: (518)449-7300 **Free:** 800-231-9826
Fax: (518)432-5902
Email: NYSOA2020@aol.com
Website: http://www.nysoa.org

Newfoundland and Labrador

★ **10630** ★ **Newfoundland Association of Optometrists**
PO Box 2284, Stn. C
Saint John's, NL, Canada A1C 6E6
Phone: (709)739-8284 **Fax:** (709)739-8378
Email: nao@roadrunner.nf.net

North Carolina

★ **10631** ★ **North Carolina State Optometric Society, Inc.**
Box 1206
Wilson, NC 27894-1206
Phone: (252)237-6197 **Fax:** (252)237-9233
Email: nceyecare@aol.com
Website: http://www.nceyes.org

North Dakota

★ **10632** ★ **North Dakota Optometric Association, Inc.**
921 S 9th St.
Bismarck, ND 58504
Phone: (701)258-6766 **Fax:** (701)258-9005
Email: ndoa@btigate.com

Nova Scotia

★ **10633** ★ **Nova Scotia Association of Optometrists**
PO Box 21074
Cole Harbour RPO
Dartmouth, NS, Canada B2W 6B2
Phone: (902)435-2845 **Fax:** (902)435-2846
Email: nsao@accesswave.ca

Ohio

★ **10634** ★ **Ohio Optometric Association**
PO Box 6036
Worthington, OH 43085
Phone: (614)781-0708 **Fax:** (614)781-6521
Email: rcornett@ooa.org
Website: http://www.ooa.org

Oklahoma

★ **10635** ★ **Oklahoma Association of Optometric Physicians**
4545 N Lincoln Blvd., No. 105
Oklahoma City, OK 73105
Phone: (405)524-1075 **Fax:** (405)524-1077
Email: saundra@ix.netcom.com
Website: http://www.oaop.com

Ontario

★ **10636** ★ **Canadian Association of Optometrists**
234 Argyle Ave.
Ottawa, ON, Canada K2P 1B9
Phone: 888-263-4676 **Fax:** (613)235-2025
Email: gcampbell@opto.ca
Website: http://www.opto.ca

★ **10637** ★ **Ontario Association of Optometrists**
290 Lawrence Ave. W
Toronto, ON, Canada M5M 1B3
Phone: (416)256-4411 **Fax:** (416)256-9881
Email: master@optom.on.ca
Website: http://www.optom.on.ca

Oregon

★ 10638 ★ Oregon Optometric Physicians Association
4404 SE King Rd.
Milwaukie, OR 97222
Phone: (503)654-5036 **Free:** 800-922-2045
Fax: (503)659-4189
Email: Oopa@AssoMgt.com
Website: http://www.oregonoptometry.org

Pennsylvania

★ 10639 ★ Pennsylvania Optometric Association, Inc.
PO Box 3312
Harrisburg, PA 17105
Phone: (717)233-6455 **Fax:** (717)233-6833
Email: Charlie@poaeyes.org
Website: http://www.poaeyes.org

Prince Edward Island

★ 10640 ★ Prince Edward Island Association of Optometrists
216 Water St.
Summerside, PE, Canada C1N 1B3
Phone: (902)436-8549

Quebec

★ 10641 ★ Quebec Optometric Association
1265 Berri St., Ste. 740
Montreal, QC, Canada H2L 4X4
Phone: (514)288-6272
Email: aoq@login.net

Rhode Island

★ 10642 ★ Rhode Island Optometric Association
2484 Warwick Ave.
PMB 117
Warwick, RI 02889
Phone: (401)732-1752 **Fax:** (401)732-1771
Email: astanelun@aol.com
Website: http://www.rioa.org

Saskatchewan

★ 10643 ★ Saskatchewan Association of Optometrists
125-3rd Ave. S
Saskatoon, SK, Canada S7K 1L6
Phone: (306)652-2069
Email: saskop@sk.sympatico.ca

South Carolina

★ 10644 ★ South Carolina Optometric Association, Inc.
2730 Devine St.
Columbia, SC 29205
Phone: (803)799-6721 **Fax:** (803)799-2305
Email: optichk1@aol.com
Website: http://www.sc-eyecare.org

South Dakota

★ 10645 ★ South Dakota Optometric Society
PO Box 1173
Pierre, SD 57501
Phone: (605)224-8199 **Fax:** (605)224-6047
Email: Sdeyes3@home.com

Tennessee

★ 10646 ★ Tennessee Optometric Association, Inc.
2727 Branford Ave.
Nashville, TN 37204
Phone: (615)269-9092 **Fax:** (615)269-5986
Email: Garylodom@aol.com
Website: http://www.toaonline.org

Texas

★ 10647 ★ Texas Optometric Association, Inc.
1503 S I-35
Austin, TX 78741
Phone: (512)707-2020 **Fax:** (512)326-8504
Email: Spirit7651@aol.com
Website: http://www.texas.optometry.net

Utah

★ 10648 ★ Utah Optometric Association
230 W 200 S, Ste. 2110
Salt Lake City, UT 84101-3409
Phone: (801)364-9103 **Fax:** (801)364-9613
Email: uoa@xmission.com
Website: http://www.utaheyedoc.org

Vermont

★ 10649 ★ Vermont Optometric Association
PO Box 2027
120 Western Ave.
Brattleboro, VT 05303
Phone: (802)254-9012 **Fax:** (802)258-4705
Email: Dreye@together.net

Virginia

★ 10650 ★ Virginia Optometric Association
118 N 8th St.
Richmond, VA 23219-2305
Phone: (804)643-0309 **Fax:** (804)643-0311
Email: VOAEyeDocs@aol.com
Website: http://www.voanet.org

Washington

★ 10651 ★ Washington Association of Optometric Physicians
555-116th NE, No. 166
Bellevue, WA 98004-5205
Phone: (425)455-0874 **Fax:** (425)646-9646
Email: waop@eyes.org
Website: http://www.eyes.org

West Virginia

★ 10652 ★ The West Virginia Optometric Association, Inc.
815 Quarrier St., Ste. 345
Charleston, WV 25301-2616
Phone: (304)345-4710 **Fax:** (304)346-6416
Email: rprice0851@aol.com
Website: http://www.wvoa.com

Wisconsin

★ 10653 ★ Wisconsin Optometric Association, Inc.
5721 Odana Rd., Ste. 110
Madison, WI 53719
Phone: (608)274-4322 **Fax:** (608)274-8646
Email: Brownlowod@aol.com
Website: http://www.woa-eyes.org

Wyoming

★ 10654 ★ Wyoming Optometric Association
PO Box 3050
Cheyenne, WY 82003
Phone: (307)632-8819 **Fax:** (307)634-0804
Email: mgmtassn@aol.com
Website: http://www.optometry.wyoming.net

Osteopathic Medicine

Listed below are state divisional societies of the American Osteopathic Association, 142 E Ontario St., Chicago, IL 60611, (800)621-1773, http://www.aoa-net.org/.

Arizona

★ 10655 ★ Arizona Osteopathic Medical Association
5150 N 16th St., No. A122
Phoenix, AZ 85016
Phone: (602)266-6699 **Free:** 888-266-6699
Fax: (602)266-1393
Email: mweaver@az-osteo.org
Website: http://www.az-osteo.org
Amanda Weaver, MBA, Exec Director
David J. Wilson, DO, Vice President

Arkansas

★ 10656 ★ Arkansas Osteopathic Medical Association
412 Union Train Station
1400 West Markham
Little Rock, AR 72201
Phone: (501)374-8900 **Fax:** (501)374-8959
Email: osteomed@ipa.net
Website: http://www.arkosteomed.org
Ed Bullington, Exec Director
David Rowe, DO, Treasurer

California

★ 10657 ★ Osteopathic Physicians and Surgeons of California
1900 Point West Way, Ste. 188
Sacramento, CA 95815
Phone: (916)561-0724 **Fax:** (916)561-0728
Email: opsc@opsc.org
Website: www.opsc.org
Ken Young, CAE, Exec Director
Kevin M. Jenkins, DO, Vice President

Colorado

★ 10658 ★ Colorado Society of Osteopathic Medicine
650 S Cherry St., Ste. 440
Denver, CO 80246
Phone: (303)322-1752 **Fax:** (303)322-1956
Email: info@coloradodo.org
Website: http://www.coloradodo.org
Kathleen Brennan, Exec Director
Cynthia Egan, DO, Vice President

Delaware

★ 10659 ★ Delaware State Osteopathic Medical Society
PO Box 8177
Talleyville, DE 19803-8177
Phone: (302)764-1198 **Fax:** (302)764-1322
Email: dsoms@del.net

Website: http://www.deosteopathic.org
Christine Kelly, Contact
James Fierro, DO, Vice President

Florida

★ 10660 ★ Florida Osteopathic Medical Association
2007 Apalachee Pkwy.
Tallahassee, FL 32301
Phone: (850)878-7364 **Fax:** (850)942-7538
Email: admin@foma.org
Website: http://www.foma.org
Stephen R. Winn, Exec Director
Larry Mattingly, DO, Vice President

Georgia

★ 10661 ★ Georgia Osteopathic Medical Association
2160 Idlewood Rd.
Tucker, GA 30084-4815
Phone: (770)493-9278 **Fax:** (770)908-3210
Email: exdir@goma.org
Website: http://www.goma.org
Holly W. Barnwell, Exec Director
Ben Abraham, DO, Vice President

Idaho

★ 10662 ★ Idaho Osteopathic Medical Association
7685 Emerald
Boise, ID 83704
Phone: (208)376-2522 **Fax:** (208)375-5860
Ronald Higgenbotham, DO, Secretary

Illinois

★ 10663 ★ Illinois Osteopathic Medical Association
142 E Ontario
Chicago, IL 60611
Phone: (312)202-8179 **Free:** 800-621-1773
Fax: (312)202-8479
Email: ioms@ioms.org
Website: http://www.ioms.org
Michael Mallie, Exec Director

★ 10664 ★ New York State Osteopathic Medical Society, Inc.
142 E Ontario
Chicago, IL 60611
Phone: (312)202-8179 **Free:** 800-841-4131
Fax: (312)202-8224
Email: nysoms@nysoms.org
Website: http://www.nysoms.org
Michael Mallie, Exec Director

Indiana

★ 10665 ★ Indiana Osteopathic Association
3520 Guion Rd., Ste. 202
Indianapolis, IN 46222-1672
Phone: (317)926-3009 **Fax:** (317)926-3984
Email: mclaphan@aol.com
Website: http://www.inosteo.org
Michael H. Claphan, CAE, Exec Director

Iowa

★ 10666 ★ Iowa Osteopathic Medical Association
950 12th St.
Des Moines, IA 50309
Phone: (515)283-0002 **Fax:** (515)283-0355
Email: leah@ioma.org
Website: http://www.ioma.org
Norman Pawlewski, Exec Director

Kansas

★ 10667 ★ Kansas Association of Osteopathic Medicine
1260 SW Topeka Blvd.
Topeka, KS 66612
Phone: (785)234-5563 **Fax:** (785)234-5564
Email: kansasdo@aol.com
Charles Wheelen, Exec Director

Kentucky

★ 10668 ★ Kentucky Osteopathic Medical Association
1501 Twilight Tr.
Frankfort, KY 40601
Phone: (502)223-5322 **Fax:** (502)223-4937
Email: info@koma.org
Website: http://www.koma.org
Tom Underwood, Exec Director

Maine

★ 10669 ★ Maine Osteopathic Association
693 Western Ave., No. 1
Manchester, ME 04351
Phone: (207)623-1101 **Fax:** (207)623-4228
Email: info@mainedo.org
Website: http://www.mainedo.org
Kellie P. Miller, MS, Exec Director

Maryland

★ 10670 ★ Association of Military Osteopathic Physicians and Surgeons
1796 Severn Hills Lane
Severn, MD 21144-1061
Phone: (410)519-8217 **Fax:** (410)519-7657
Email: jyonts@amops.org
Website: http://www.amops.org
Jim Yonts, Exec Director

★ 10671 ★ Maryland Association of Osteopathic Physicians
3603 Southside Ave.
Phoenix, MD 21131
Phone: (410)683-8100 **Free:** 888-741-6267
Fax: (410)683-8200
Email: maops@maops.com
Darleen Won, Exec Director

Michigan

★ 10672 ★ Michigan Osteopathic Association
2445 Woodlake Cir.
Okemos, MI 48864-5941
Phone: (517)347-1555 **Fax:** (517)347-1556
Email: okemos@moa-do.com
Website: http://www.moa-do.com
Dennis M. Paradis, Exec Director

Mississippi

★ 10673 ★ Mississippi Osteopathic Medical Association
PO Box 16890
Jackson, MS 39236
Phone: (601)366-3105 **Free:** (866)423-6286
Fax: (601)366-2868
Email: info@moma-net.org
Website: http://www.moma-net.org
Jeffrey J. LeBoeuf, Exec Director

Montana

★ 10674 ★ Montana Osteopathic Association
224 W Main, No. 401
Lewistown, MT 59457
Phone: (406)538-7721 **Fax:** (406)538-5201
William J. Munro, DO, Exec Director

Nevada

★ 10675 ★ Nevada Osteopathic Medical Association
2920 N Green Valley Pkwy., No. 527
Henderson, NV 89014-0406
Phone: (702)434-7112 **Fax:** (702)434-7110
Email: nvoma@aol.com
Website: http://www.nevadaosteopathic.com
Denise Selleck-Davis, Exec Director

New Hampshire

★ 10676 ★ New Hampshire Osteopathic Association
7 N State St.
Concord, NH 03301
Phone: (603)224-1909
Joy Potter, Contact

New Jersey

★ 10677 ★ New Jersey Association of Osteopathic Physicians and Surgeons (NJAOPS)
1 Distribution Way, Ste. 201
Monmouth Junction, NJ 08852-3001
Phone: (732)940-9000 **Fax:** (732)940-8899
Email: njaops@njosteo.com
Website: http://www.njosteo.com
Frank Cagliari, Exec Director

North Dakota

★ 10678 ★ North Dakota State Osteopathic Association
1600 2nd Ave. SW, Ste. 120
Minot, ND 58701
Phone: (701)852-8798 **Free:** 800-437-4010
Fax: (701)837-5410
Website: http://www.nadk.net
Carmen Christianson Bell, MS, Exec Director

Ohio

★ 10679 ★ Ohio Osteopathic Association
53 W 3rd Ave.
PO Box 8130
Columbus, OH 43201-0130
Phone: (614)299-2107 **Fax:** (614)294-0457
Email: execdir@ooanet.org
Website: http://www.ooanet.org
Jon F. Wills, Exec Director

Oklahoma

★ 10680 ★ Oklahoma Osteopathic Association
4848 N Lincoln Blvd.
Oklahoma City, OK 73105-3335
Phone: (405)528-4848 **Free:** 800-522-8379
Fax: (405)528-6102
Email: lynette@okosteo.org
Website: http://www.okosteo.org
Lynette McClain, Exec Director

Oregon

★ 10681 ★ Osteopathic Physicians and Surgeons of Oregon
2121 SW Broadway, Ste. 300
Portland, OR 97201-3146
Phone: (503)222-2279 **Free:** 800-533-6776
Fax: (503)222-2392
Email: edied@opso.com
Website: http://www.opso.com
Jeff Heatherington, Exec Director

Pennsylvania

★ 10682 ★ Pennsylvania Osteopathic Medical Association
1330 Eisenhower Blvd.
Harrisburg, PA 17111-2395
Phone: (717)939-9318 **Free:** 800-544-POMA
Fax: (717)939-7255
Email: mlanni@poma.org
Website: http://www.poma.org
Mario E. J. Lanni, Exec Director

South Dakota

★ 10683 ★ South Dakota Osteopathic Association
MASSA—Berry Clinic
890 Lazelle St.
Sturgis, SD 57785
Phone: (605)347-3616 **Fax:** (605)347-4713
David Lauer, DO, Secretary

Tennessee

★ 10684 ★ Tennessee Osteopathic Medical Association
200 4th Ave. N, Ste. 900
Nashville, TN 37219
Phone: (615)242-3032 **Fax:** (615)254-7047
Email: dawalker@wmgt.org
Website: http://www.wmgt.org
DeeAnn Walker, Exec Director

Texas

★ 10685 ★ Texas Osteopathic Medical Association
1415 Lavaca St.
Austin, TX 78701-1634
Phone: (512)708-8662 **Free:** 800-444-8662
Fax: (512)708-1415
Email: terryb@txosteo.org
Website: http://www.txosteo.org/
Terry R. Boucher, MPH, Exec Director

Vermont

★ 10686 ★ Vermont State Association of Osteopathic Physicians and Surgeons, Inc.
72 Barre St.
Montpelier, VT 05602-3508
Phone: (802)229-9418 **Free:** 800-454-9663
Fax: (802)229-5619
Email: nocdos@shore.net
John M. Peterson, DO, Exec Director

Washington

★ 10687 ★ Washington Osteopathic Medical Association
PO Box 16486
Seattle, WA 98116
Phone: (206)937-5358 **Fax:** (206)933-6529
Email: kathie@woma.org
Website: http://www.woma.org
Kathleen S. Itter, Exec Director

West Virginia

★ 10688 ★ West Virginia Society of Osteopathic Medicine, Inc.
PO Box 5266
Charleston, WV 25361-0266
Phone: (304)345-9836 **Fax:** (304)345-9865
Email: wvdo@wvsominc.org
Website: http://www.wvsominc.org
Charlotte Cales Pulliam, Exec Director

Wisconsin

★ 10689 ★ Wisconsin Association of Osteopathic Physicians and Surgeons
34615 Rd. E
Oconomowoc, WI 53066-2543
Phone: (262)567-0520 **Fax:** (262)567-0520
Robert J. Finnegan, CAE, Exec Director

Parkinson's Disease

State chapters of the American Parkinson Disease Association are listed below. The national office is located at 1250 Hylan Blvd., Ste. 4B, Staten Island, NY 10305-1946. Additional information can be obtained by calling the national office at (800) 223-2732, or by consulting their web site at http://apdaparkinson.com/.

Alabama

★ 10690 ★ American Parkinson Disease Association
Birmingham Chapter
800 Jeffery Ln.
Birmingham, AL 35235
Phone: (205)833-4940
Email: Parkinson@pell.net
Paul E. Hayes, President

★ 10691 ★ American Parkinson Disease Association
North Alabama Chapter
1910 Crapemyrtle Green SE
Huntsville, AL 35802
Phone: (256)883-2835
Jean Smith, President

★ 10692 ★ American Parkinson Disease Association
Tuscaloosa Chapter
1515 19th Ave. E, Apt. 813
Tuscaloosa, AL 35404
Phone: (205)556-5327
Verna Patterson, President

Arizona

★ 10693 ★ American Parkinson Disease Association
Arizona Chapter
616 N Country Club Rd., Ste. C
Tucson, AZ 85716
Phone: (520)326-5400 **Free:** 800-541-4960
Email: holmes@u.arizona.edu
Bob Dolezal, President

Arkansas

★ 10694 ★ American Parkinson Disease Association
Arkansas Chapter
200 Scottwood
Hot Springs, AR 71901
Phone: (501)321-1539
Email: urmilgupta@aol.com
Urmil Gupta, President

California

★ 10695 ★ American Parkinson Disease Association
Greater Los Angeles Chapter
c/o First Charter Bank
9454 Wilshire Blvd.
Beverly Hills, CA 90212
Phone: (310)248-2109
Email: sblock@firstcharterbank.com
Steve Block, President

★ 10696 ★ American Parkinson Disease Association
San Diego Chapter
8555 Aero Dr., Ste. 205
San Diego, CA 92123-1745
Phone: (858)273-6763
Email: info@sd-pc.com
Website: http://www.sd-pc.com
William M. Stilwell, President

Connecticut

★ 10697 ★ American Parkinson Disease Association
Connecticut Chapter
27 Allendale Dr.
North Haven, CT 06473
Phone: (203)288-0546
Email: gladkt@hotmail.com
Website: http://www.ctapda.com
Gladys Tiedemann, President

Florida

★ 10698 ★ American Parkinson Disease Association
South Florida Chapter
10100 NW 2nd St.
Coral Springs, FL 33071
Phone: (954)786-2305
David Levy, President

★ 10699 ★ American Parkinson Disease Association
Sun Coast Parkinson Chapter
9937 87th St.
Largo, FL 33777
Phone: (727)391-8214
Email: vgbw@aol.com
Ginny Bernard, President

Georgia

★ 10700 ★ American Parkinson Disease Association
Atlanta Chapter
PO Box 49416
Atlanta, GA 30359
Phone: (770)979-3495
Email: bergatlapda@juno.com
Barbara Berger, RN, Contact

Idaho

★ 10701 ★ American Parkinson Disease Association
Middle Snake Idaho Chapter
5567 Willowlawn Way
Boise, ID 83714
Phone: (208)376-4401
Email: dojem@rmci.net
Don Mills, President

Illinois

★ 10702 ★ American Parkinson Disease Association
Midwest Chapter
2050 Pfingsten Rd., Ste. 127
Glenview, IL 60025
Phone: (847)724-7087
Email: cacapda@aol.com
Maxine Dust, President

Louisiana

★ 10703 ★ American Parkinson Disease Association
Bayou Chapter
PO Box 405
Thibodaux, LA 70302
Phone: (504)447-9043
Email: RWarch@mobiletel.com
Richard G. Weimer, President

Maine

★ 10704 ★ American Parkinson Disease Association
Maine State Chapter
107 Woodville Rd.
Falmouth, ME 04105
Phone: (207)781-3070
Email: cnbarker@maine.rr.com
Carl Barker, President

Maryland

★ 10705 ★ American Parkinson Disease Association
Anne Arundel County Chapter
PO Box 893
Severna Park, MD 21146
Phone: (410)729-3461
Tom Mislan, President

★ 10706 ★ American Parkinson Disease Association
Central Maryland Parkinson Outreach Chapter
PO Box 3153
Frederick, MD 21705
Phone: (301)682-9009
Email: bruff1terp@aol.com
Bill Ruff, President

★ 10707 ★ American Parkinson Disease Association
Delmarva Parkinson's Chapter/Support Group
4049 Oakland School Rd. at Trace Hollow Run
Salisbury, MD 21801
Phone: (410)543-0110
Email: johnston@intercom.net
Will Johnston, President

★ 10708 ★ American Parkinson Disease Association
Howard County Chapter
5625 Waterloo Rd.
Ellicott City, MD 21043
Phone: (410)465-2825 **Fax:** (410)465-2825
Email: pdmd@starpower.net
Website: http://www.apdaparkinson.com/howard_county.htm
Thomas Collins, President

★ 10709 ★ American Parkinson Disease Association
Western Maryland Chapter
13555 Donnybrook Dr.
Hagerstown, MD 21742
Phone: (301)790-2044
Email: nittanylion57@prodigy.net
Don and Pat Zilch, President
Peggy Barron, President

★ 10710 ★ American Parkinson Disease Association
Young Parkinson's Chapter of Maryland
601 N Caroline St., Ste. 5065
Baltimore, MD 21287-0875
Phone: (410)955-8795
Email: tcsc56@cs.com
Sandy Pollock, President

Massachusetts

★ 10711 ★ American Parkinson Disease Association
Massachusetts Chapter
203 Brimbal Ave.
Beverly, MA 01915
Phone: (978)922-1473
Email: apdafay@aol.com
Website: http://www.apdama.org
Fay Winson, President

Missouri

★ 10712 ★ American Parkinson Disease Association
Greater Saint Louis Chapter
660 S Euclid Ave.
Campus Box 8111
Saint Louis, MO 63110
Phone: (314)362-3299
Email: levins@neuro.wustl.edu
Website: http://www.geocities.com/parkinson_disease_saint_louis/
Joseph Marchbein, CPA, President

Montana

★ 10713 ★ American Parkinson Disease Association
Great Falls Chapter
2101 6th Ave. S
Great Falls, MT 59405
Phone: (406)761-6086
Ethel Stump, Contact

★ 10714 ★ American Parkinson Disease Association
Missoula Branch Chapter
2415 57th St.
Missoula, MT 59803
Phone: (406)251-5338
Email: mtcookies@msn.com
Carole Kamrath, President

Nebraska

★ 10715 ★ American Parkinson Disease Association
Nebraska Chapter
7701 Pacific St., Ste. 122
Omaha, NE 68114-5480
Phone: (402)397-2766
Sandy Woods-Kreifels, President

Nevada

★ 10716 ★ American Parkinson Disease Association
Southern Nevada Chapter
c/o University of Nevada School of Medicine
1707 W Charleston Blvd., Ste. 220
1001 Shadow Ln.
Las Vegas, NV 89102-2353
Phone: (702)464-3132
Julia Bernick, President

New Hampshire

★ 10717 ★ American Parkinson Disease Association
Granite State Chapter
61 Dublin Ave.
Nashua, NH 03063-2045
Phone: (603)889-3251
Email: gmchugh@ma.ultranet.com
George McHugh, President

New Jersey

★ 10718 ★ American Parkinson Disease Association
New Jersey Chapter
601 Hillside Ave.
Point Pleasant, NJ 08742
Phone: (732)714-0475
Email: hwl351@aol.com
Jack McMillian, Contact

New Mexico

★ 10719 ★ American Parkinson Disease Association
El Paso Chapter
112 Lisa
Box 107
Chaparral, NM 88021
Phone: (505)824-4306
Email: timotea@angelfire.com
Thomas Arellanes, President

★ 10720 ★ American Parkinson Disease Association
New Mexico Chapter
10817 Griffith Park NE
Albuquerque, NM 87123
Phone: (505)292-3844 **Free:** 800-278-5386
Email: tasec@cs.com
Bobby Dunagan, President

New York

★ 10721 ★ American Parkinson Disease Association
Faye Springer Memorial Rockaway Chapter
33 Point Breeze Ave.
Breezy Point, NY 11697
Marion Manley, President

★ 10722 ★ American Parkinson Disease Association
Nassau County Chapter
18 Wren Dr.
Woodbury, NY 11797
Phone: (516)798-8375
Sebastian Moschitto, President
Jim Hall, President

★ 10723 ★ American Parkinson Disease Association
New York Young Professionals Chapter
c/o Bear Stearns
383 Madison Ave., 5th Fl.
New York, NY 10179
Phone: (212)272-8280
Email: sschefrin@bear.com
Scott Schefrin, President

★ 10724 ★ American Parkinson Disease Association
Salvatore and Elena Esposito Chapter
18 St. Julian's Pl.
Staten Island, NY 10301
Phone: (718)727-2713
Email: winshear@pronetisp.net
Sophia Maestrone, President

★ 10725 ★ American Parkinson Disease Association
Southern Tier Chapter
PO Box 72
Binghamton, NY 13903
Phone: (607)723-7167
Winslow Shearman, Contact

★ 10726 ★ American Parkinson Disease Association
Suffolk County Chapter
c/o St. Catherine of Sienna Hospital
50 Rte. 25A
Smithtown, NY 11787
Phone: (631)862-3560
Email: newslady@obtonline.net
Website: http://www.suffolkapda.org/
Virginia Cravotta, President

North Carolina

★ 10727 ★ American Parkinson Disease Association
Asheville Chapter
C/O Robin Fox, R.N
Thomas Rehabilitation Hospital
68 Sweeton Creek Rd.
Asheville, NC 28803
Phone: (828)692-7623
Shirley Jankowski, Contact

Ohio

★ 10728 ★ American Parkinson Disease Association
Cincinnati Tri-State Chapter
125 W Galbraith Rd., Ste 218
Cincinnati, OH 45216
Phone: (513)984-1100 **Free:** 800-840-2732
Email: info@parkinsonswellness.org
Website: http://www.parkinsonswellness.org
Debbie Mills, President

Oklahoma

★ 10729 ★ American Parkinson Disease Association
Muskogee Area Chapter
9601 Taft Rd.
Muskogee, OK 74401
Phone: (918)687-4519
Roleen Bishop, President

★ 10730 ★ American Parkinson Disease Association
Oklahoma PD Chapter
19125 Park St.
Claremore, OK 74017
Phone: (918)341-5097
Dan Moore, President

★ 10731 ★ American Parkinson Disease Association
Owasso Area Chapter
12600 E 73rd St. N
Owasso, OK 74055
Phone: (918)834-2441
Donna Norris, President

★ 10732 ★ American Parkinson Disease Association
Ponca City Area Chapter
PO Box 743
Ponca City, OK 74602
Bill Hill, President

★ 10733 ★ American Parkinson Disease Association
Tulsa Area Chapter
PO Box 521165
Tulsa, OK 74152
Phone: (918)747-9320
Email: prairiec@swbell.net
Christine Kennedy, President

Pennsylvania

★ 10734 ★ American Parkinson Disease Association
Greater Delaware Valley Chapter
c/o APDA Information & Resource Center
Crozer-Chester Medical Center
1 Medical Center Blvd.
Upland, PA 19013
Phone: (610)447-2911
Robert Hurka, President

★ 10735 ★ American Parkinson Disease Association
J. Louis Blumberg Chapter
6700 Eastwood St.
Philadelphia, PA 19149
Phone: (215)342-6689
Belle Englander, President

★ 10736 ★ American Parkinson Disease Association
Pittsburgh Area Chapter
420 E North Ave., Ste. 206
Pittsburgh, PA 15212
Phone: (412)441-4100
Email: mallen@wpahs.org
Catherine Birk, MD, President

Rhode Island

★ 10737 ★ American Parkinson Disease Association
Rhode Island Chapter
PO Box 41659
Providence, RI 02940-1659
Phone: (401)823-5700 **Free:** 800-498-2732
Email: RIchapAPDA@aol.com
Website: http://www.parkinsondisease-rhodeisland.org
Athol Cochrane, President

Tennessee

★ 10738 ★ American Parkinson Disease Association
Middle Tennessee Chapter
c/o Information and Resource Center
2300 Patterson St.
Nashville, TN 37203
Phone: (615)329-9955
Email: asapmac@mindspring.com
Website: http://www.apdaparkinson.com/tn_chapter.htm
Meredith Car, President

Texas

★ 10739 ★ American Parkinson Disease Association
Central Texas Parkinson's Chapter
PO Box 153
Brownwood, TX 76804
Phone: (915)641-0020
Email: mamadunk@hotmail.com
Linda Duncan, President

★ 10740 ★ American Parkinson Disease Association
Hill Country Kerrville Chapter
145 Village Dr.
Kerrville, TX 78028
Phone: (830)895-2431
Email: beshaw@ktc.com
Fred Kleis, President

★ 10741 ★ American Parkinson Disease Association
Northeast Texas Chapter
1400 Preston Rd., Ste. 200
Plano, TX 75093
Phone: (214)345-4224
Email: bjwells@flash.net
Jerry Wells, Esq., President

★ 10742 ★ American Parkinson Disease Association
Parkinson's Caring, Sharing & Comparing Chapter of Central Texas
2809 Arroyo Ct. N
College Station, TX 77845
Phone: (979)696-6966
Email: b.erwin2@verizon.net
Bill Erwin, President

★ 10743 ★ American Parkinson Disease Association
San Antonio Chapter/Alamo Area Parkinson's Disease Support Group
8507 Chesam
San Antonio, TX 78250
Email: joanieduval@earthlink.net
Joan Duval, President

★ 10744 ★ American Parkinson Disease Association
West Texas Parkinsonism Society Chapter
5805 Duke Ave.
Lubbock, TX 79416
Phone: (806)793-3691
Steve Swain, President

Utah

★ 10745 ★ American Parkinson Disease Association
Northern Chapter of Utah
c/o APDA Information & Resource Center
University of Utah School of Medicine
Department of Neurology
50 N Medical Dr., Rm. 3R144
Salt Lake City, UT 84132
Phone: (801)585-2354
Email: mmkearns@worldnett.att.net
Miriam Kearns, President

Vermont

★ 10746 ★ American Parkinson Disease Association
Vermont Chapter
70 Hurdle Rd.
Moretown, VT 05660
Phone: (802)626-3707 **Free:** 888-763-3366
Email: advnture@sover.net
Bruce Talbot, President

Virginia

★ 10747 ★ American Parkinson Disease Association
Richmond Metro Chapter
PO Box 70283
Richmond, VA 23255
Phone: (804)740-6806
Email: Kathy_morton@wescanric.org
Kathy Morton, President

★ 10748 ★ American Parkinson Disease Association
Virginia Beach Chapter
Our Lady of Perpetual Help
4560 Princess Anne Rd.
Virginia Beach, VA 23462
Phone: (757)495-3062
Email: tcmedlc@tc.cc.va.us
Christine Medlin, Contact

Washington

★ 10749 ★ American Parkinson Disease Association
Washington State Chapter
PO Box 75169
Seattle, WA 98125-0169
Phone: (425)881-3116
Email: matulinde@aol.com
Maria Linde, President

West Virginia

★ 10750 ★ American Parkinson Disease Association
North Central West Virginia Chapter
107 C'Anna Sq.
Fairmont, WV 26554
Phone: (304)363-1028
Email: tracey_robertson@att.net
Tracey Robertson, President
Larry Policano, President

Wyoming

★ 10751 ★ American Parkinson Disease Association
Bighorn Basin Parkinson Chapter
PO Box 221
Powell, WY 82435
Phone: (307)754-2130
Dean Schultz, President

Pharmacy

Listed below are state pharmacy associations. The national organization is the National Council of State Pharmacy Association Executives, c/o Virginia Pharmacists Association, 5501 Patterson Ave., Ste. 200, Richmond, VA 23226, (804)285-4145, http://www.ncspae.org.

Alabama

★ 10752 ★ Alabama Pharmacy Association
1211 Carmichael Way
Montgomery, AL 36106-3672
Phone: (334)271-4222 **Fax:** (334)271-5423
Email: weley@aparx.org
Website: http://www.aparx.org
William Eley, II, Exec Director

Alaska

★ 10753 ★ Alaska Pharmaceutical Association
Box 10-1185
Anchorage, AK 99510-1185
Phone: (907)563-8880 **Fax:** (907)573-7880
Email: akphrmcy@alaska.net
Website: http://www.alaskapharmacy.org
Erin Byrne, Exec Director

Arizona

★ 10754 ★ Arizona Pharmacy Association
1845 E Southern Ave.
Tempe, AZ 85282-5831
Phone: (480)838-3385 **Fax:** (480)838-3557
Email: azpa@azpharmacy.org
Website: http://www.azpharmacy.org
Kathy Boyle, Exec Director

Arkansas

★ 10755 ★ Arkansas Pharmacists Association
417 S Victory
Little Rock, AR 72201
Phone: (501)372-5250 **Fax:** (501)372-0546
Email: rbeck@arpharmacists.org
Website: http://www.arpharmacists.org
Richard Beck, PD,CAE, CEO

California

★ 10756 ★ California Pharmacists Association
1112 I St., Ste. 300
Sacramento, CA 95814
Phone: (916)444-7811 **Fax:** (916)444-7929
Email: cmichelotti@cpha.com
Website: http://www.cpha.com
Carlo Michelotti, RPh, CEO

Colorado

★ 10757 ★ Colorado Pharmacists Society
5150 E Yale Cir., Ste. 304
Denver, CO 80222
Phone: (303)756-3069 **Fax:** (303)756-3649
Email: valkalnins@interfold.com
Website: http://www.coloradopharmacy.org
Val Kalnins, R.Ph., Exec Director

Connecticut

★ 10758 ★ Connecticut Pharmacists Association
35 Cold Spring Rd., Ste. 125
Rocky Hill, CT 06067
Phone: (860)563-4619 **Fax:** (860)257-8241
Email: marghiecpa@aol.com
Website: http://www.ctpharmacists.org
Marghie Giuliano, R.Ph., Exec VP

Delaware

★ 10759 ★ Delaware Pharmacists Society
PO Box 454
Smyrna, DE 19977-0454
Phone: (302)659-3088 **Fax:** (302)659-3089
Email: patsgrants@aol.com
Website: http://www.depharmacy.org
Pat Carroll-Grant, RPh, Exec Director

Florida

★ 10760 ★ Florida Pharmacy Association
610 N Adams St.
Tallahassee, FL 32301
Phone: (850)222-2400 **Fax:** (850)561-6758
Email: mjackson@pharmview.com
Website: http://www.pharmview.com
Michael Jackson, R.Ph., Exec VP

Georgia

★ 10761 ★ Georgia Pharmacy Association, Inc.
50 Lenox Pointe NE
Atlanta, GA 30324
Phone: (404)231-5074 **Fax:** (404)237-8435
Email: bharden@gpha.org
Website: http://www.gpha.org
Buddy Harden, Jr., R.Ph., Exec VP

Hawaii

★ 10762 ★ Hawaii Pharmacists Association
PO Box 22472
Honolulu, HI 96823-2472
Phone: (808)432-5536 **Fax:** (808)432-5535
Email: amtanigu@lava.net
Ronald Taniguchi, PharmD, Contact

Idaho

★ 10763 ★ Idaho State Pharmacy Association
PO Box 140117
305 W Jefferson St.
Boise, ID 83714-0117
Phone: (208)424-1107 **Fax:** (208)424-1102
Email: condie2@mindspring.com
Website: http://www.idahopharmacy.org
JoAn Condie, Exec Director

Illinois

★ 10764 ★ Illinois Pharmacists Association
204 W Cook St.
Springfield, IL 62704-2526
Phone: (217)522-7300 **Fax:** (217)522-7349
Email: terrim@ipha.org
Website: http://www.ipha.org
Terri McEntaffer, R.Ph., Exec Director

Indiana

★ 10765 ★ Indiana Pharmacists Alliance
729 N Pennsylvania St.
Indianapolis, IN 46204-1171
Phone: (317)634-4968 **Fax:** (317)632-1219
Email: ipalary@indianapharmacists.org
Website: http://www.indianapharmacists.org
Lawrence Sage, Exec VP
Frmly: Indiana Pharmacists Association.

Iowa

★ 10766 ★ Iowa Pharmacy Association
8515 Douglas Ave., Ste. 16
Des Moines, IA 50322
Phone: (515)270-0713 **Fax:** (515)270-2979
Email: ttemple@iarx.org
Website: http://www.iarx.org
Thomas Temple, R.Ph., CEO

Kansas

★ 10767 ★ Kansas Pharmacists Association
1020 SW Fairlawn Rd.
Topeka, KS 66604-2019
Phone: (785)228-2327 **Fax:** (785)228-9147
Email: bob@kansaspharmacy.org
Website: http://www.kansaspharmacy.org
Robert Williams, CAE, Exec Director

Kentucky

★ 10768 ★ Kentucky Pharmacists Association
1228 U.S. 127 S
Frankfort, KY 40601
Phone: (502)227-2303 **Fax:** (502)227-2258
Email: kyphassoc@aol.com
Mike Mayes, FACHE, Exec Director

Louisiana

★ 10769 ★ Louisiana Pharmacists Association
4744 Jamestown, Ste. 101
Baton Rouge, LA 70808
Phone: (225)926-2666 **Fax:** (225)926-1020
Email: lpa2000@tlxnet.net
Website: http://www.louisianapharmacists.org

Maine

★ 10770 ★ Maine Pharmacy Association
PMB 323
11 Bangor Mall Blvd., Ste. D
Bangor, ME 04401
Free: 800-639-1609 **Fax:** (207)989-6743
Email: mpa@mparx.com
Website: http://www.mainepharmacyassoc.com
Bob Morrisette, President

Maryland

★ 10771 ★ Maryland Pharmacists Association
650 W Lombard St.
Baltimore, MD 21201-1572
Phone: (410)727-0746 **Fax:** (410)727-2253
Email: mpha@erols.com
Website: http://www.rxstat.com/mpha/
Howard Schiff, Exec Director

★ 10772 ★ Washington, DC Pharmaceutical Association
908 Caddington Ave.
Silver Spring, MD 20901-1109
Phone: (301)593-3292 **Fax:** (301)593-7215
Email: midpharm@aol.com
Herb Kwash, Exec Director

Massachusetts

★ 10773 ★ Massachusetts Pharmacists Association
681 Main St., Ste. 3-32
Waltham, MA 02451
Phone: (781)736-0101 **Fax:** (781)736-0080
Email: carmelo@masspharmacists.org
Website: http://www.masspharmacists.org
Carmelo Cinquenonce, Exec VP

Michigan

★ 10774 ★ Michigan Pharmacists Association
815 N Washington Ave.
Lansing, MI 48906-5198
Phone: (517)484-1466 **Fax:** (517)484-4893
Email: larry@michiganpharmacists.org
Website: http://www.michiganpharmacists.org
Larry Wagenknecht, R.Ph., CEO

Minnesota

★ 10775 ★ Minnesota Pharmacists Association
1935 W County Rd. B-2
Roseville, MN 55113-2722
Phone: (651)697-1771 **Fax:** (651)697-1776
Email: julie@mpha.org
Website: http://www.mpha.org
Julie Johnson, R.Ph., Exec VP

Mississippi

★ 10776 ★ Mississippi Pharmacists Association
341 Edgewood Terrace Dr.
Jackson, MS 39206-6299
Phone: (601)981-0416 **Fax:** (601)981-0451
Email: mpha@bellsouth.net
S.E. "Bo" Dalton, R.Ph., Exec Director

Missouri

★ 10777 ★ Missouri Pharmacy Association
211 E Capitol Ave.
Jefferson City, MO 65101-3001
Phone: (573)636-7522 **Fax:** (573)636-7485
Email: jim@morx.com
Website: http://www.morx.com
Jim Frederich, R.Ph., Contact

Montana

★ 10778 ★ Montana Pharmacy Association
34 W 6th St., 1C
Helena, MT 59601
Phone: (406)449-3843 **Fax:** (406)443-1592
Email: jimesmith@qwest.net
Website: http://www.rxmt.org
Jim Smith, Exec Director

Nebraska

★ 10779 ★ Nebraska Pharmacists Association
6221 S 58th St., Ste. A
Lincoln, NE 68516
Phone: (402)420-1500 **Fax:** (402)420-1406
Email: gary@npharm.org
Website: http://www.npharm.org
Gary J. Cheloha, R.Ph., Exec VP

Nevada

★ 10780 ★ Nevada Pharmacy Alliance
PO Box 95277
Las Vegas, NV 89193
Phone: (702)433-7133 **Fax:** (702)435-2177
Email: nvphall@lvdi.net
Mary Grear, R.Ph., Exec VP

New Hampshire

★ 10781 ★ New Hampshire Pharmacists Association
2 Eagle Sq., Ste. 400
Concord, NH 03301-4956
Phone: (603)229-0292 **Fax:** (603)224-7769
Elizabeth Gower, RPh, Exec Director

New Jersey

★ 10782 ★ New Jersey Pharmacists Association
760 Alexander Rd.
PO Box 1
Princeton, NJ 08543-0001
Phone: (609)275-4246 **Fax:** (609)275-4066
Email: njpharm@aol.com
Website: http://www.njpha.com
Joe Morris, CEO

New Mexico

★ 10783 ★ New Mexico Pharmaceutical Association
4800 Zuni SE
Albuquerque, NM 87108
Phone: (505)265-8729 **Fax:** (505)255-8476
Email: d_tinker@nm-pharmacy.com
Website: http://www.NM-pharmacy.com
R. Dale Tinker, Exec Director

New York

★ 10784 ★ Pharmacists Society of the State of New York
201 Washington Ave. Ext.
Albany, NY 12203
Free: 800-632-8822 **Fax:** (518)464-0618
Email: craigb@pssny.org
Website: http://www.pssny.org
Craig Burridge, CAE, Exec Director
Frmly: Pharmaceutical Society of the State of New York.

North Carolina

★ 10785 ★ North Carolina Association of Pharmacists
109 Church St.
Chapel Hill, NC 27516
Phone: (919)962-2237 **Fax:** (919)968-9430
Email: fred@ncpharmacists.org
Website: http://www.ncpharmacists.org
Fred Eckel, R.Ph., Contact
Frmly: North Carolina Pharmaceutical Association.

North Dakota

★ 10786 ★ North Dakota Pharmaceutical Association
1906 E Broadway Ave.
Bismarck, ND 58501-4700
Phone: (701)258-4968 **Fax:** (701)258-9312
Email: ndpha@nodakpharmacy.com
Website: http://www.nodakpharmacy.com
Galen Jordre, R.Ph., Exec VP

Ohio

★ 10787 ★ Ohio Pharmacists Association
6037 Frantz Rd., Ste. 106
Dublin, OH 43017
Phone: (614)798-0037 **Fax:** (614)798-0978
Email: eboyd@ohiopharmacists.org
Website: http://www.ohiopharmacists.org
Ernest Boyd, PD,CAE, Exec Director

Oklahoma

★ 10788 ★ Oklahoma Pharmacists Association
Box 18731
45 NE 52nd St.
Oklahoma City, OK 73154
Phone: (405)528-3338 **Fax:** (405)528-1417
Email: pwoodward@opha.com
Website: http://www.opha.com
Phil Woodward, Exec Director
Frmly: Oklahoma Pharmaceutical Association.

Oregon

★ 10789 ★ Oregon State Pharmacists Association
29702-B SW Town Center Loop
Wilsonville, OR 97070
Phone: (503)582-9055 **Fax:** (503)582-9046
Email: tomh@oregonpharmacists.com
Website: http://www.oregonpharmacists.com
Tom Holt, Exec Director

Pennsylvania

★ 10790 ★ Pennsylvania Pharmacists Association
508 N 3rd St.
Harrisburg, PA 17101-1199
Phone: (717)234-6151 **Fax:** (717)236-1618
Email: ppa@papharmacists.com
Website: http://www.papharmacists.com
Carmen DiCello, R.Ph., Exec Director

Puerto Rico

★ 10791 ★ Colegio de Farmaceuticos de Puerto Rico
PO Box 360206
San Juan, PR 00936-0206
Phone: (787)753-7157 **Fax:** (787)759-9793
Email: cfpr2000@coqui.net
Milagros Morales, R.Ph., Exec Director

Rhode Island

★ 10792 ★ Rhode Island Pharmacists Association
500 Prospect St.
Pawtucket, RI 02860
Phone: (401)725-4141 **Fax:** (401)725-9960
Email: ripharm@aol.com
Website: http://www.ripharm.com

South Carolina

★ 10793 ★ South Carolina Pharmacy Association
1350 Browning Rd.
Columbia, SC 29210
Phone: (803)354-9977 **Fax:** (803)354-9207
Email: jbracewell@scpharmacyassociation.org
Website: http://www.scpharmacyassociation.org
Jim Bracewell, Exec VP

South Dakota

★ 10794 ★ South Dakota Pharmacists Association
514 W Elizabeth
Pierre, SD 57501-0518
Phone: (605)224-2338 **Fax:** (605)224-1280
Email: director2@sdpha.org
Website: http://www.sdpha.org
Bob Coolidge, Exec Director
Frmly: South Dakota Pharmaceutical Association.

Tennessee

★ 10795 ★ Tennessee Pharmacists Association
226 Capitol Blvd., Ste. 810
Nashville, TN 37219-1893
Phone: (615)256-3023 **Fax:** (615)255-3528
Email: bblack@tnpharm.org
Website: http://www.tnpharm.org
Baeteena Black, D.Ph., Exec Director

Texas

★ 10796 ★ Texas Pharmacy Association
PO Box 14709
Austin, TX 78761-4709
Phone: (512)836-8350 **Fax:** (512)836-0308
Email: jmartin@txpharmacy.com
Website: http://www.txpharmacy.com
Jim Martin, R.Ph., Exec Director

Utah

★ 10797 ★ Utah Pharmaceutical Association
1850 S Columbia Ln.
Orem, UT 84097-8036
Phone: (801)762-0452 **Fax:** (801)762-0454
Email: upha@upha.com
Website: http://www.upha.com
Reid L. Barker, Exec Director

Vermont

★ 10798 ★ Vermont Pharmacists Association
PO Box 790
Richmond, VT 05477-0790
Phone: (802)434-3001 **Fax:** (802)434-4803
Email: vpaorg@aol.com
Website: http://www.vtpharmacists.org
Fred Dobson, PhD, Exec Director

Virginia

★ 10799 ★ Virginia Pharmacists Association
5501 Patterson Ave., Ste. 200
Richmond, VA 23226
Phone: (804)285-4145 **Fax:** (804)285-4227
Email: rrsnead@erols.com
Website: http://pharmacy.su.edu/vpha
Rebecca Snead, R.Ph., Exec Director

Washington

★ 10800 ★ Washington State Pharmacists Association
1501 Taylor Ave. SW
Renton, WA 98055-3139
Phone: (425)228-7171 **Fax:** (425)277-3897
Email: rshafer@u.washington.edu
Website: http://www.pharmcare.org
Rod Shafer, R.Ph., CEO

West Virginia

★ 10801 ★ West Virginia Pharmacists Association
2003 Quarrier St.
Charleston, WV 25311-2212
Phone: (304)344-5302 **Fax:** (304)344-5316
Email: wvrds@aol.com
Richard Stevens, Exec Director

Wisconsin

★ 10802 ★ Pharmacy Society of Wisconsin
701 Heartland Tr.
Madison, WI 53717
Phone: (608)827-9200 **Fax:** (608)827-9292
Email: cdecker@pswi.org
Website: http://www.pswi.org
Christopher Decker, R.Ph., CEO
Frmly: Wisconsin Pharmacists Association.

Wyoming

★ 10803 ★ Wyoming Pharmacists Association
PO Box 2109
Glenrock, WY 82637
Phone: (307)436-8001 **Fax:** (307)436-8002
Email: wpha@juno.com
Website: http://www.wpha.net
Robert Smith, R.Ph., Exec Director

Physical Therapy

The following are state chapters of the American Physical Therapy Association, 1111 N Fairfax St., Alexandria, VA 22314-1488, (800)999-APTA, http://www.apta.org/.

Alabama

★ 10804 ★ American Physical Therapy Association
Alabama Chapter
323 De La Mare Ave.
Fairhope, AL 36532-2319
Phone: (251)990-9666 **Fax:** (251)990-8019
Email: rhonda@pradcom.com
Website: http://www.ptalabama.org
Rhonda Wilkinson, Contact
Karen Moore, Contact

Alaska

★ 10805 ★ American Physical Therapy Association
Alaska Chapter
8970 Northwood Park Cir.
Eagle River, AK 99577
Phone: (907)566-3749
Email: runwithstrength@gci.net
Bethany Lawso, Contact

Arizona

★ 10806 ★ American Physical Therapy Association
Arizona Chapter
4035 E Fanfol
Phoenix, AZ 85028
Phone: (602)569-9101 **Free:** 800-264-APTA
Fax: (602)996-3966
Email: info@azapta.org
Website: http://www.azapta.org
Pauline Wampler, Director

Arkansas

★ 10807 ★ American Physical Therapy Association
Arkansas Chapter
PO Box 2068
Conway, AR 72033-2068
Phone: (501)269-8247 **Fax:** (501)327-1370
Email: arpta@cyberback.com

Website: http://www.arpta.org
Lauren Maxwell, Director

California

★ 10808 ★ American Physical Therapy Association
California Chapter
2520 Venture Oaks Way, Ste. 150
Sacramento, CA 95833-4228
Phone: (916)929-2782 **Fax:** (916)646-5960
Email: pevans@ccapta.org
Website: http://www.ccapta.org
Patricia Evans, Contact

Colorado

★ 10809 ★ American Physical Therapy Association
Colorado Chapter
7853 E Arapahoe Ct., Ste. 2100
Englewood, CO 80112-1361
Phone: (303)694-4728 **Free:** 800-875-2782
Fax: (303)694-4869
Email: apta@assnoffice.com
Website: http://www.assnoffice.com/apta
Ellen Caruso, Exec Director

Connecticut

★ 10810 ★ American Physical Therapy Association
Connecticut Chapter
330 Main St., 3rd Fl.
Hartford, CT 06106-5408
Phone: (860)246-4414 **Fax:** (860)541-6484
Email: abrunetti@tcor.com
Website: http://www.ctpt.org
Allyson J. Brunetti, Contact

District of Columbia

★ 10811 ★ American Physical Therapy Association
District of Columbia Chapter
6981 32nd St. NW
Washington, DC 20015
Phone: (202)723-2819 **Fax:** (202)537-1388
Email: tmsgloria@aol.com
Gloria Rogers, President

Florida

★ 10812 ★ American Physical Therapy Association
Florida Chapter
1705 S Gadsden St.
Tallahassee, FL 32301
Phone: (850)222-1243 **Fax:** (850)224-5281
Email: ccrosby@fpta.org
Website: http://www.fpta.com
Craig Crosby, Director

Georgia

★ 10813 ★ American Physical Therapy Association
Georgia Chapter
1260 Winchester Pkwy., Ste. 205
Smyrna, GA 30080
Phone: (770)433-2418 **Fax:** (770)433-2907
Email: ptagexec@bellsouth.net
Website: http://www.ptagonline.org
Kathy Brooks, Director

Hawaii

★ 10814 ★ American Physical Therapy Association
Hawaii Chapter
1360 S Bertania St., Ste. 301
Honolulu, HI 96814-1514
Phone: (808)247-0105 **Fax:** (808)523-7809
Email: jgold@hillandknowlton.com
Website: http://www.hapta.org
Joanne Reid, PT, Contact

Idaho

★ 10815 ★ American Physical Therapy Association
Idaho Chapter
PO Box 1273
Boise, ID 83701-1273
Phone: (208)342-6647 **Fax:** (208)342-6647
Email: ipta@aol.com
Website: http://www.ptidaho.org
Jill Cooper, Director

Illinois

★ 10816 ★ American Physical Therapy Association
Illinois Chapter
1010 Jorie Blvd., Ste. 134
Oak Brook, IL 60523
Phone: (630)571-1400 **Free:** 800-552-4782
Fax: (630)571-1406
Email: staylor@ipta.org
Website: http://www.ipta.org
Stephanie Taylor, Contact

Indiana

★ 10817 ★ American Physical Therapy Association
Indiana Chapter
PO Box 26692
Indianapolis, IN 46226-0692
Phone: (317)823-3681 **Fax:** (317)823-3681
Email: schroeder@inapta.org
Website: http://www.inapta.org
Teresa Schroeder, Director

Iowa

★ 10818 ★ American Physical Therapy Association
Iowa Chapter
1228 8th St., Ste. 106
West Des Moines, IA 50265-2622
Phone: (515)222-9838 **Free:** 800-925-3064
Fax: (515)222-9839
Email: mail@iowaapta.org
Website: http://www.iowaapta.org
Michael C. Mandel, Director

Kansas

★ 10819 ★ American Physical Therapy Association
Kansas Chapter
214 SW 6th St., Ste. 300
Topeka, KS 66603-3719
Phone: (785)233-5400 **Fax:** (785)290-0476
Email: executivedirector@kpta.kscoxmail.com
Website: http://www.kpta.com
Brenda Straub, Contact

Kentucky

★ 10820 ★ American Physical Therapy Association
Kentucky Chapter
4010 Dupont Cir., Ste. 584
Louisville, KY 40207
Phone: (502)899-9341 **Fax:** (502)899-9342
Email: kpta@bluegrass.net
Website: http://www.KPTA.org
Maria Gray, Director

Louisiana

★ 10821 ★ American Physical Therapy Association
Louisiana Chapter
8550 United Plaza Blvd., Ste. 1001A
Baton Rouge, LA 70809-2256
Phone: (225)922-4614 **Fax:** (225)922-4611
Email: bconnor@pncpa.com
Website: http://www.lpta.org
Bland O'Connor, Director

Maine

★ 10822 ★ American Physical Therapy Association
Maine Chapter
PO Box 1783
Portland, ME 04104-1783
Phone: (207)799-1584 **Fax:** (207)799-1584
Email: jangeyer1@aol.com
Website: http://www.maineapta.org
Jan Geyer, Contact

Maryland

★ 10823 ★ American Physical Therapy Association
Maryland Chapter
PO Box 1099
Laurel, MD 20725-1099
Phone: (301)362-4290 **Free:** 800-306-5596
Fax: 800-675-9438
Email: aptamd@erols.com
Website: http://www.aptamd.org
Wayne Becraft, President

Massachusetts

★ 10824 ★ American Physical Therapy Association
Massachusetts Chapter
34 Atlantic St.
Gloucester, MA 01930-1625
Phone: (978)281-5393 **Fax:** (978)282-4384
Email: kag@shore.net
Website: http://aptaofma.org
Karen A. Gallagher, Director

Michigan

★ 10825 ★ American Physical Therapy Association
Michigan Chapter
PO Box 21236
Lansing, MI 48909-1236
Phone: (517)347-0880 **Free:** 800-242-8131
Fax: (517)347-4720
Email: mpta@mpta.org
Website: http://www.mpta.com
Terry Warren, Director

Minnesota

★ 10826 ★ American Physical Therapy Association
Minnesota Chapter
1711 W County Rd. B, Ste. 101 S
Roseville, MN 55113-4036
Phone: (651)635-0902 **Fax:** (651)635-0903
Email: mnapta@isd.net
Judy Hawley, Contact

Mississippi

★ 10827 ★ American Physical Therapy Association
Mississippi Chapter
921 N Congress St.
Jackson, MS 39202-2554
Phone: (601)354-3629 **Free:** 800-247-1106
Fax: (601)355-1506
Email: insightltd@msn.com
Deirdre McGowan, PhD, Director

Missouri

★ 10828 ★ American Physical Therapy Association
Missouri Chapter
205 E Capitol, Ste. 100
Jefferson City, MO 65101
Phone: (573)556-6730 **Free:** 888-222-6782
Fax: (573)556-6731
Email: mcapta@aol.com
Website: http://www.mopt.org
Debbie Stover, Director

Montana

★ 10829 ★ American Physical Therapy Association
Montana Chapter
PO Box 4553
Missoula, MT 59806-4553
Phone: (406)251-5232 **Fax:** (406)251-5270
Email: mapta@montana.com
Website: http://www.mapta.com
Robin Childers, Director

Nebraska

★ 10830 ★ American Physical Therapy Association
Nebraska Chapter
PO Box 540427
Omaha, NE 68154-0427
Phone: (402)491-3660 **Fax:** (402)431-1372
Email: npta@npta.org
Website: http://www.npta.org
Judy Kramolisch, Director

Nevada

★ 10831 ★ American Physical Therapy Association
Nevada Chapter
8665 W Flamingo Rd., Ste. 131
PMB 105
Las Vegas, NV 89147
Phone: (702)571-1535 **Fax:** (702)889-1674
Email: npta@infi.net
Website: http://www.nvapta.org
Carolyn Muse Grant, Contact

New Hampshire

★ 10832 ★ American Physical Therapy Association
New Hampshire Chapter
PO Box 978
Manchester, NH 03105-0978
Phone: (603)627-7970 **Fax:** (603)627-3970
Email: nhapta@xtdl.com
Website: http://www.nhapta.org
James H. Bradley, Director

New Jersey

★ 10833 ★ American Physical Therapy Association
New Jersey Chapter
1100 US Hwy. 130, Ste. 3
Robbinsville, NJ 08691-1108
Phone: (609)208-0200 **Fax:** (609)208-1000
Email: aptanj@aptanj.org
Website: http://www.aptanj.org
Judy Oiler, Director

New York

★ 10834 ★ American Physical Therapy Association
New York Chapter
5 Palisades Dr., Ste. 330
Albany, NY 12205
Phone: (518)459-4499 **Free:** 800-459-4489
Fax: (518)459-8953
Email: lesliew@nypta.org
Website: http://www.nypta.org
Leslie J. Wood, Director

North Carolina

★ 10835 ★ American Physical Therapy Association
North Carolina Chapter
316 W Millbrook Rd., Ste. 105
Raleigh, NC 27609
Phone: (919)841-0268 **Free:** 800-948-2672
Fax: (919)841-0269
Email: NCPTAHQ1@aol.com
Website: http://www.ncpt.org
Donna Willis, Contact

North Dakota

★ 10836 ★ American Physical Therapy Association
North Dakota Chapter
Department of Physical Therapy
University of North Dakota
Grand Forks, ND 58202-9037
Phone: (701)777-3873 **Fax:** (701)777-4199
Email: awhite@medicine.nodak.edu
Alyson White, Director

Ohio

★ 10837 ★ American Physical Therapy Association
Ohio Chapter
2066 W Henderson Rd., Ste. 202
Columbus, OH 43220-2452
Phone: (614)538-9612 **Fax:** (614)538-9614
Email: opt@ohiopt.org
Website: http://www.ohiopt.org
Nancy Garland, Contact

Oklahoma

★ 10838 ★ American Physical Therapy Association
Oklahoma Chapter
223 W Ridgewood
Shawnee, OK 74801
Phone: (405)275-7588 **Fax:** (405)275-7588
Email: JGSecret@aol.com
Joyce Gowin, CPS, Director

Oregon

★ 10839 ★ American Physical Therapy Association
Oregon Chapter
147 SE 102nd
Portland, OR 97216
Phone: (503)262-9247 **Free:** 877-492-4919
Fax: (503)253-9172
Email: opta@teleport.com
Website: http://www.opta.org
Sandra Fisher, CAE, Director

Pennsylvania

★ 10840 ★ American Physical Therapy Association
Pennsylvania Chapter
4701 Devonshire Rd., Ste. 106
Harrisburg, PA 17109
Phone: (717)541-9169 **Fax:** (717)541-9182
Email: PAPTASSN@aol.com
Website: http://www.ppta.org
Kim Annibali, Director

Puerto Rico

★ 10841 ★ American Physical Therapy Association
Puerto Rico Chapter
Prodriquez Olmo K-26
Arecibo, PR 00612
Phone: (787)854-3700 **Fax:** (787)817-6037
Email: damarisv@coqui.net
Damaris Vazquez, PT, President

Rhode Island

★ 10842 ★ American Physical Therapy Association
Rhode Island Chapter
PO Box 1409
Kingston, RI 02881-0492
Phone: (401)874-5391 **Fax:** (401)874-5630
Email: RIAPTA@email.com
Bruce Goodeluck, President

South Carolina

★ 10843 ★ American Physical Therapy Association
South Carolina Chapter
3650-A Center Cir.
Fort Mill, SC 29715
Phone: (803)802-5454 **Fax:** (815)371-1499
Email: executiveofficer@scapta.org
Website: http://www.scapta.org
Jane Boston, Exec Director

South Dakota

★ 10844 ★ American Physical Therapy Association
South Dakota Chapter
PO Box 88033
Sioux Falls, SD 57109-0033
Phone: (605)339-4839 **Fax:** (605)357-8780

Email: sodakpt@aol.com
Website: http://www.sdpta.org
Deby McCauley, Contact

Tennessee

★ 10845 ★ American Physical Therapy Association
Tennessee Chapter
PO Box 23071
Nashville, TN 37202
Phone: (615)269-5312 **Fax:** (615)297-5852
Email: tpta1@aol.com
Website: http://www.tptaonline.org
Debbie Lowenthal, Contact

Texas

★ 10846 ★ American Physical Therapy Association
New Mexico Chapter
5125 Highlands
McKinney, TX 75070
Email: hjhammonds@msn.com
Website: http://www.nmapta.org
Holly Hammonds, Director

★ 10847 ★ American Physical Therapy Association
Texas Chapter
400 W 15th St., Ste. 805
Austin, TX 78701-1647
Phone: (512)477-1818 **Fax:** (512)477-1434
Email: weitz@tpta.org
Website: http://www.tpta.org
Tim Weitz, Exec Director

Utah

★ 10848 ★ American Physical Therapy Association
Utah Chapter
2101 East 3870 South
Salt Lake City, UT 84109
Phone: (801)278-4016 **Fax:** (801)278-2752
Email: uapta@softsolutions.com
Diane Buma, Director

Vermont

★ 10849 ★ American Physical Therapy Association
Vermont Chapter
1878 Mountain Rd., Ste. 1
Stowe, VT 05672-4775
Phone: (802)253-2273 **Fax:** (802)253-7754
Email: psweat@zoo.uvm.edu
Philip L. Sweet, PT, President

Virginia

★ 10850 ★ American Physical Therapy Association
Virginia Chapter
1111 N Fairfax St.
Alexandria, VA 22314-1488
Free: 800-999-2782 **Fax:** (703)706-8575
Email: debbiekelly@apta.org
Website: http://www.vpta.org
Debbie Kelly, Director

Washington

★ 10851 ★ American Physical Therapy Association
Washington Chapter
208 NW Rogers
Olympia, WA 98502-4940
Phone: (360)352-7290 **Free:** 800-554-5569
Fax: (206)352-7298
Email: caryn.porter@ptwa.org
Website: http://www.ptwa.org
Caryn Porter, Director

West Virginia

★ 10852 ★ American Physical Therapy Association
West Virginia Chapter
2110 Kanawha Blvd. E, Ste. 220
Charleston, WV 25311
Phone: (304)345-6808 **Fax:** (304)344-4139
Email: jrm@wvapta.org
Website: http://www.movementscience.com/host_wvpta/
Nancy Tonkin, Contact

Wisconsin

★ 10853 ★ American Physical Therapy Association
Wisconsin Chapter
802 W Broadway, Ste. 208
Madison, WI 53713
Phone: (608)221-9191 **Fax:** (608)221-9697
Email: wpta@wpta.org
Website: http://www.wpta.org
Karen Oshman, Director

Wyoming

★ 10854 ★ American Physical Therapy Association
Wyoming Chapter
13475 Wisconsin
Casper, WY 82609
Phone: (307)235-3910
Email: kjbpt@touchtronics.net
Website: http://www.wypta.org
Kathy Brunken, PT, President

Respiratory Diseases

The associations listed below are constituents of the American Lung Association, 61 Broadway, 6th Fl., New York, NY 10019, 800-LUNG-USA, http://www.lungusa.org/.

Alabama

★ 10855 ★ American Lung Association of Alabama
3125 Independence Dr., Ste. 325
Birmingham, AL 35209
Phone: (205)933-8821 **Fax:** (205)930-1717
Email: aodom@alabamalung.org
Website: http://www.alabamalung.org

Alaska

★ 10856 ★ American Lung Association of Alaska
500 W International Airport Rd., Ste. 1
Anchorage, AK 99518
Phone: (907)276-5864 **Fax:** (907)565-5587
Email: christie@aklung.org
Website: http://www.aklung.org
Christie McIntire, Contact

Arizona

★ 10857 ★ American Lung Association of Arizona/New Mexico
102 W McDowell Rd.
Phoenix, AZ 85003-1299
Phone: (602)258-7505 **Free:** 800-LUNG-USA
Fax: (602)258-7507
Email: bpfeifer@lungaz.org
Website: http://www.lungaz.org

★ 10858 ★ American Lung Association of Arizona/New Mexico
Northern Arizona Branch
102 W McDowell Rd.
Phoenix, AZ 85003-1299
Phone: (602)258-7505 **Fax:** (602)258-7507
Email: cclees@lungaz.org
Website: http://www.lungaz.org

★ 10859 ★ American Lung Association of Arizona/New Mexico
Southern Arizona Branch
2819 E Broadway
Tucson, AZ 85716
Phone: (520)323-1812 **Fax:** (520)323-1816
Email: jjones@lungaz.org
Website: http://www.lungaz.org

Arkansas

★ 10860 ★ American Lung Association of Arkansas
211 Natural Resources Dr.
Little Rock, AR 72205-1539
Phone: (501)224-5864 **Fax:** (501)224-5645
Email: carogers@aristotle.net
Website: http://www.lungark.org

California

★ 10861 ★ American Lung Association of California
424 Pendleton Way
Oakland, CA 94621-2189
Phone: (510)638-LUNG **Fax:** (510)638-8984
Email: contact@californialung.org
Website: http://www.californialung.org
Ben Abate, PhD, President

★ 10862 ★ American Lung Association of California
Redwood Empire Branch
115 Talbot Ave.
Santa Rosa, CA 95404
Phone: (707)527-LUNG **Fax:** (707)542-6111
Email: lungassn@neteze.com

★ 10863 ★ American Lung Association of California
Superior Branch
1108 Sheridan Ave., Ste. B
Chico, CA 95926
Phone: (530)345-5864 **Fax:** (530)345-6035
Email: patty@alacsb.org
Website: http://www.lungusa.org/superiorbranch/index.html

★ 10864 ★ American Lung Association of Central California
4948 N Arthur
PO Box 9389
Fresno, CA 93794
Phone: (559)222-4800 **Fax:** (559)221-2081
Email: info@amerilungcencal.org
Website: http://www.amerilungcencal.org

★ 10865 ★ American Lung Association of the Central Coast
550 Camino El Estero, Ste. 100
Monterey, CA 93940-3231
Phone: (831)373-7306 **Free:** 800-LUNG-USA
Fax: (831)373-5530
Email: admin@alaccoast.org
Website: http://www.alacoast.org

★ 10866 ★ American Lung Association of the East Bay
295 27th St.
Oakland, CA 94612-3894
Phone: (510)893-5474 **Fax:** (510)893-9008
Email: eastbaylung@alac.org

★ 10867 ★ American Lung Association of the Inland Counties
441 Mac Kay Dr.
San Bernardino, CA 92408-3230
Phone: (909)884-5864 **Fax:** (909)884-6249
Email: lungassn@pe.net

★ 10868 ★ American Lung Association of Los Angeles County
5858 Wilshire Blvd., No. 300
PO Box 36926
Los Angeles, CA 90036-0926
Phone: (323)935-5864 **Fax:** (323)935-1873
Email: lalung@lalung.org
Website: http://www.lalung.org

★ 10869 ★ American Lung Association of Orange County
1570 E 17th St.
Santa Ana, CA 92705
Phone: (714)835-5864 **Fax:** (714)835-0169
Email: alaoc1@aol.com
Website: http://www.oclung.org

★ 10870 ★ American Lung Association of Sacramento-Emigrant Trails
909 12th St.
Sacramento, CA 95814-2997
Phone: (916)444-LUNG **Free:** 800-LUNG-USA
Fax: (916)444-6661
Email: staff@saclung.org
Website: http://www.saclung.org

★ 10871 ★ American Lung Association of San Diego & Imperial Counties
2750 4th Ave.
PO Box 3879
San Diego, CA 92163-1879
Phone: (619)297-3901 **Fax:** (619)297-8402
Email: info@lungsandiego.org
Website: http://www.lungsandiego.org

★ 10872 ★ American Lung Association of San Francisco and San Mateo Counties
2171 Junipero Serra Blvd., Ste. 720
Daly City, CA 94014-1980
Phone: (650)994-5864 **Fax:** (650)994-4601
Email: lung@alasfsm.org

★ 10873 ★ American Lung Association of Santa Barbara and Ventura Counties
1510 San Andres St.
Santa Barbara, CA 93101-4104
Phone: (805)963-1426 **Fax:** (805)962-2843
Email: dkweeks@aol.com

★ 10874 ★ American Lung Association of Santa Clara-San Benito Counties
1469 Park Ave.
San Jose, CA 95126-2530
Phone: (408)998-5864 **Fax:** (408)998-0578
Email: info@lungsrus.org
Website: http://www.lungsrus.org

Colorado

★ 10875 ★ American Lung Association of Colorado
1600 Race St.
Denver, CO 80206-1198
Phone: (303)388-4327 **Fax:** (303)377-1102
Email: sgoulding@alacolo.org
Website: http://www.alacolo.org

★ 10876 ★ American Lung Association of Colorado
Northern Region
2601 S Lemay, No. 7-117
Fort Collins, CO 80525
Phone: (970)223-6111 **Fax:** (970)223-6111
Email: johnalfredwolfe@attbi.com

★ 10877 ★ American Lung Association of Colorado
Pikes Peak Region
421 S Tejon, Ste. 100
Colorado Springs, CO 80903
Phone: (719)635-3891 **Fax:** (719)635-4057
Email: nutz@alacolo.org
Website: http://www.alacolo.org

★ 10878 ★ American Lung Association of Colorado
Southern Region
409 N Main St., Ste. 314
Pueblo, CO 81003
Phone: (719)296-8800 **Fax:** (719)296-8811
Email: jbeasley@alacolo.org
Website: http://www.alacolo.org

★ 10879 ★ American Lung Association of Colorado
Western Region
PO Box 3154
Grand Junction, CO 81502
Phone: (970)245-2120 **Fax:** (970)245-2288
Email: canderson@alacolo.org
Website: http://www.alacolo.org

Connecticut

★ 10880 ★ American Lung Association of Connecticut
45 Ash St.
East Hartford, CT 06108-3272
Phone: (860)289-5401 **Free:** 800-992-2263
Fax: (860)289-5405
Email: alaofct@alact.org
Website: http://www.alact.org

Delaware

★ 10881 ★ American Lung Association of Delaware
1021 Gilpin Ave., Ste. 202
Wilmington, DE 19806-3280
Phone: (302)655-7258 **Fax:** (302)655-8546
Website: http://www.alade.org

District of Columbia

★ 10882 ★ American Lung Association of the District of Columbia
475 H St. NW
Washington, DC 20001-2617
Phone: (202)682-5864 **Fax:** (202)682-5874
Email: info@aladc.org
Website: http://www.aladc.org

Florida

★ 10883 ★ American Lung Association of Central Florida
1333 W Colonial Dr.
Orlando, FL 32804-7133
Phone: (407)425-5864 **Fax:** (407)425-2876
Email: alacf@gdi.net

★ 10884 ★ American Lung Association of Florida
5526 Arlington Rd.
Jacksonville, FL 32211-5216
Phone: (904)743-2933 **Free:** 800-940-2933
Fax: (904)743-2916
Email: alaf@lungfla.org
Website: http://www.lungfla.org

★ 10885 ★ American Lung Association of Florida
Northwest Region
4300 Bayou Blvd., Ste. 2
Pensacola, FL 32503-2677
Phone: (850)478-5864 **Fax:** (850)474-6354
Email: alafnw@networktel.net

★ 10886 ★ American Lung Association of Florida
Spaceport Region
412 S Palmetto Ave.
Daytona Beach, FL 32114-4922
Phone: (386)255-6447 **Fax:** (386)253-2410
Email: alafsp@bellsouth.net

★ 10887 ★ American Lung Association of Gulfcoast Florida
110 Carillon Pkwy.
Saint Petersburg, FL 33716
Phone: (727)347-6133 **Free:** 800-771-5863
Fax: (727)345-0287
Email: alagf@alagf.org

★ 10888 ★ American Lung Association of South Florida, Inc.
2020 S Andrews Ave.
Fort Lauderdale, FL 33316-3430
Phone: (954)524-4657 **Fax:** (954)524-3162
Email: carolruggeri@sflung.org
Website: http://www.sflung.org

★ 10889 ★ American Lung Association of Southeast Florida
2701 N Australian Ave.
West Palm Beach, FL 33407-4526
Phone: (561)659-7644 **Fax:** (561)835-8967
Email: amlungsefl@inhaleexhale.org
Website: http://www.inhaleexhale.org

★ 10890 ★ American Lung Association of The Big Bend Region
539 Silver Slipper Ln., Ste. A
Tallahassee, FL 32303-4873
Phone: (850)386-2065 **Fax:** (850)422-1894
Email: alafbbr@earthlink.net

Georgia

★ 10891 ★ American Lung Association of Georgia
2452 Spring Rd.
Smyrna, GA 30080
Phone: (770)434-5864 **Free:** 800-LUNG-USA
Fax: (770)319-0349
Website: http://www.alaga.org

Hawaii

★ 10892 ★ American Lung Association of Hawaii
245 N Kukui St., Ste. 100
Honolulu, HI 96817
Phone: (808)537-5966 **Fax:** (808)537-5971
Website: http://www.ala-hawaii.org

Idaho

★ 10893 ★ American Lung Association of Idaho/Nevada
Boise Office
1111 S Orchard, Ste. 245
Boise, ID 83705-1966
Phone: (208)345-5864 **Fax:** (208)345-5896

Illinois

★ 10894 ★ American Lung Association of Illinois
3000 Kelly Ln.
Springfield, IL 62707
Phone: (217)787-5864 **Free:** 800-LUNG-USA
Fax: (217)787-5916
Email: info@lungil.org
Website: http://www.lungil.org
Harold Wimmer, CEO
Lori Younker, Mgr

★ 10895 ★ American Lung Association of Metropolitan Chicago
1440 W Washington Blvd.
Chicago, IL 60607
Phone: (312)243-2000 **Fax:** (312)243-3954
Website: http://www.lungchicago.org

Indiana

★ 10896 ★ American Lung Association of Indiana
9445 Delegates Row
Indianapolis, IN 46240
Phone: (317)573-3900 **Fax:** (317)573-3909
Email: info@lungin.org
Website: http://www.lungin.org

Iowa

★ 10897 ★ American Lung Association of Iowa
5601 Douglas Ave.
Des Moines, IA 50310-1800
Phone: (515)278-5864 **Fax:** (515)334-9564
Email: tammy@alaia.org
Website: http://www.alaia.org

Kansas

★ 10898 ★ American Lung Association of Kansas
4300 SW Drury Ln.
Topeka, KS 66604-2419
Phone: (785)272-9290 **Fax:** (785)272-9297
Website: http://www.kslung.org

Kentucky

★ 10899 ★ American Lung Association of Kentucky
4100 Churchman Ave.
PO Box 9067
Louisville, KY 40209-0067
Phone: (502)363-2652 **Fax:** (502)363-0222
Email: menisam@kylung.org
Website: http://www.kylung.org

Louisiana

★ 10900 ★ American Lung Association of Louisiana
2325 Severn Ave., Ste. 8
Metairie, LA 70001-6918
Phone: (504)828-5864 **Fax:** (504)828-5867
Email: bfont@bellsouth.net
Website: http://www.louisianalung.org

Maine

★ 10901 ★ American Lung Association of Maine
122 State St.
Augusta, ME 04330
Phone: (207)622-6394 **Fax:** (639)426-2919
Email: Cgagne@MaineLung.org
Website: http://www.mainelung.org

Maryland

★ 10902 ★ American Lung Association of Maryland
1840 York Rd., Ste. M
Timonium, MD 21093-5156
Phone: (410)560-2120 **Free:** 800-LUNG-USA
Fax: (410)560-0829
Email: info@marylandlung.org
Website: http://www.marylandlung.org

Massachusetts

★ 10903 ★ American Lung Association of Greater Norfolk County
25 Spring St.
Walpole, MA 02081-4302
Phone: (508)668-6729 **Fax:** (508)668-6796
Email: lungusa2@earthlink.net

★ 10904 ★ American Lung Association of Massachusetts
One Abbey Ln.
Middleboro, MA 02346-3230
Phone: (508)947-7204 **Fax:** (508)947-7208
Email: alam@gis.net
Carlos Alvarez, Exec Director

★ 10905 ★ American Lung Association of Middlesex County
5 Mountain Rd.
PO Box 265
Burlington, MA 01803
Phone: (781)272-2866 **Fax:** (781)273-2846
Email: alaofmc@aol.com
David Ales, Exec Director

★ 10906 ★ American Lung Association of Western Massachusetts
393 Maple St.
Springfield, MA 01105
Phone: (413)737-3506 **Fax:** (413)737-3511

Michigan

★ 10907 ★ American Lung Association of Michigan
25900 Greenfield, Ste. 401
Oak Park, MI 48237
Phone: (248)784-2000 **Free:** 800-543-LUNG
Fax: (248)784-2008
Email: alam@alam.org
Website: http://www.alam.org

★ 10908 ★ American Lung Association of Michigan
Capital Region
403 Seymour Ave.
Lansing, MI 48933-1179
Phone: (517)484-4541 **Free:** 800-678-5864
Fax: (517)484-2118
Email: smspringer@voyager.net

★ 10909 ★ American Lung Association of Michigan
Genesee Valley Region
519 S Saginaw, Ste. 312
Flint, MI 48502
Phone: (810)232-3177 **Fax:** (810)232-6257
Email: genesee@123.net

★ 10910 ★ American Lung Association of Michigan
Grand Valley and Southwest Regions
2815 Michigan St. NE, Ste. B
Grand Rapids, MI 49506
Phone: (616)942-0513 **Fax:** (616)942-0650
Email: grandvalleyalam@voyager.net

★ 10911 ★ American Lung Association of Michigan
Huron Valley Region
412 Huron St.
Ann Arbor, MI 48104
Phone: (734)994-0155 **Fax:** (734)327-2968
Email: huron@123.net

★ 10912 ★ American Lung Association of Michigan
Metro Detroit Region
25900 Greenfield, Ste. 401
Oak Park, MI 48237
Phone: (248)784-2000 **Fax:** (248)784-2008
Email: MBaumgartner@alam.org
Website: http://www.alam.org

★ 10913 ★ American Lung Association of Michigan
Northwest Region
153-½ E Front St., Ste. D
Traverse City, MI 49684-2508
Phone: (231)946-1344 **Fax:** (231)946-0150
Email: northw@northlink.net

★ 10914 ★ American Lung Association of Michigan
Upper Peninsula Region
227 W Washington St.
Marquette, MI 49855-4321
Phone: (906)228-9833 **Fax:** (906)228-3430
Email: cjmargrif@lushen.com

Minnesota

★ 10915 ★ American Lung Association of Minnesota
490 Concordia Ave.
Saint Paul, MN 55103-2441
Phone: (651)227-8014 **Fax:** (651)227-5459
Website: http://www.alamn.org

Mississippi

★ 10916 ★ American Lung Association of Mississippi
731 Pear Orchard Rd., Ste. 18
PO Box 2178
Ridgeland, MS 39158
Phone: (601)206-5810 **Free:** 800-586-4872
Fax: (601)206-5813
Email: ebarber@alams.org

Website: http://www.alams.org
Elizabeth Barber, Director

★ 10917 ★ American Lung Association of South Mississippi
PO Box 8911
Gulfport, MS 39506-8911
Fax: (228)896-2213
Email: mmcgahan@alams.org
Website: http://www.alams.org

Missouri

★ 10918 ★ American Lung Association of Eastern Missouri
1118 Hampton Ave.
Saint Louis, MO 63139-3196
Phone: (314)645-5505 **Fax:** (314)645-7128
Email: tyoung@alaem.org
Website: http://www.alaem.org

★ 10919 ★ American Lung Association of Western Missouri
2007 Broadway
Kansas City, MO 64108-2080
Phone: (816)842-5242 **Fax:** (816)842-5470
Email: kcmo@alawmo.com
Joe Gilman, Director

Montana

★ 10920 ★ American Lung Association of the Northern Rockies
825 Helena Ave.
Helena, MT 59601-3459
Phone: (406)442-6556 **Fax:** (406)442-2346
Email: ala-nr@ala-nr.org
Website: http://www.ala-nr.org
Remarks: Serves Montana and Wyoming.

Nebraska

★ 10921 ★ American Lung Association of Nebraska
Community Health Plaza
7101 Newport Ave., Ste. 303
Omaha, NE 68152
Phone: (402)572-3030 **Fax:** (402)572-3028
Email: ala@lungnebraska.org
Website: http://www.lungnebraska.org

Nevada

★ 10922 ★ American Lung Association of Idaho/Nevada
1091 Haskell St.
PO Box 7056
Reno, NV 89510-7056
Phone: (775)829-5864 **Fax:** (775)829-5850
Email: dszabo@lungs.org
Website: http://www.lungs.org

New Hampshire

★ 10923 ★ American Lung Association of New Hampshire
9 Cedarwood Dr., Ste. 12
Bedford, NH 03110
Phone: (603)669-2411 **Fax:** (603)645-6220
Email: info@nhlung.org
Website: http://www.nhlung.org

New Jersey

★ 10924 ★ American Lung Association of New Jersey
1600 Rte. 22 E
Union, NJ 07083-3407
Phone: (908)687-9340 **Fax:** (908)851-2625
Email: info.alanj@verizon.net

★ 10925 ★ American Lung Association of Northern New Jersey
333B Rte. 46 W, Ste. 205
Fairfield, NJ 07004
Phone: (973)227-7720 **Fax:** (973)227-3270

★ 10926 ★ American Lung Association of Southern New Jersey
109 S Main St., Ste. 18
Cranbury, NJ 08512
Phone: (609)918-0313 **Fax:** (609)918-0314

New Mexico

★ 10927 ★ American Lung Association of Arizona/New Mexico New Mexico Branch
216 Truman NE
Albuquerque, NM 87108
Phone: (505)265-0732 **Fax:** (505)260-1739
Email: joem@alanm.org
Website: http://www.alanm.org

New York

★ 10928 ★ American Lung Association of Central New York
1620 Burnet Ave.
Syracuse, NY 13206
Phone: (315)422-6142 **Fax:** (315)422-9710
Email: alaofcny@aol.com

★ 10929 ★ American Lung Association of the City of New York, Inc.
432 Park Ave. S, 8th Fl.
New York, NY 10016
Phone: (212)889-3370 **Fax:** (212)889-3375
Email: info@alany.org
Website: http://www.alany.org

★ 10930 ★ American Lung Association of the Finger Lakes Region
1595 Elmwood Ave.
Rochester, NY 14620
Phone: (716)442-4260 **Fax:** (716)442-4263
Email: aladeb@rochester.rr.com
Website: http://www.ggw.org/ala-fl/

★ 10931 ★ American Lung Association of the Hudson Valley
35 Orchard St.
White Plains, NY 10603-3397
Phone: (914)949-2150 **Fax:** (914)949-4765
Email: info@alahv.org
Website: http://www.alahv.org

★ 10932 ★ American Lung Association of Mid-New York
587 Main St., Ste. 109
New York Mills, NY 13417
Phone: (315)736-6099 **Fax:** (315)736-5976
Email: ALAMNY@aol.com
John Storey, Exec Director

★ 10933 ★ American Lung Association of Nassau Suffolk, New York
225 Wireless Blvd.
Hauppauge, NY 11788-3914
Phone: (631)231-5864 **Fax:** (631)231-5118
Email: postmaster@alans.org

★ 10934 ★ American Lung Association of New York State, Inc.
3 Winners Circle, Ste. 300
Albany, NY 12205-1187
Phone: (518)453-0172 **Fax:** (518)489-5864
Email: postmaster@alanys.org
Website: http://www.alanys.org

★ 10935 ★ American Lung Association of Northeastern New York
3 Winners Circle, Ste. 300
Albany, NY 12205
Phone: (518)459-4197 **Fax:** (518)489-5864
Email: postmaster@alaneny.org
Website: http://www.alaneny.org

★ 10936 ★ American Lung Association of Western New York
210 John Glenn Dr., No. 3
Buffalo, NY 14228
Phone: (716)691-5864 **Fax:** (716)691-5012
Email: cschweitzer@alawny.org
Website: http://www.alawny.org

North Carolina

★ 10937 ★ American Lung Association of North Carolina
1323 Capital Blvd., Ste. 102
PO Box 27985
Raleigh, NC 27611
Phone: (919)832-8326 **Free:** 800-892-5650
Fax: (919)856-8530
Email: swillcox@lungnc.org
Website: http://www.lungnc.org

North Dakota

★ 10938 ★ American Lung Association of North Dakota
212 N 2nd St.
PO Box 5004
Bismarck, ND 58502-5004
Phone: (701)223-5613 **Free:** 800-252-6325
Fax: (701)223-5727
Email: aland@gcentral.com
Susan Kahler, Exec Director

Ohio

★ 10939 ★ American Lung Association of Ohio, Columbus State Office
1950 Arlingate Ln.
Columbus, OH 43228-4102
Phone: (614)279-1700 **Fax:** (614)279-4940
Email: kelsey@ohiolung.org
Website: http://www.ohiolung.org

Oklahoma

★ 10940 ★ American Lung Association of Oklahoma
2805 E Skelly Dr., Ste. 806
Tulsa, OK 74105
Phone: (918)747-3441 **Fax:** (918)747-4629
Email: dakin@oklung.org
Website: http://www.oklung.org
Darla Akin, Contact

Oregon

★ 10941 ★ American Lung Association of Oregon
7420 SW Bridgeport Rd., Ste. 200
Portland, OR 97224
Phone: (503)924-4094 **Free:** 800-LUNG-USA
Fax: (503)924-4120
Email: admin@lungoregon.org
Website: http://www.lungoregon.org

Pennsylvania

★ 10942 ★ American Lung Association of Pennsylvania
6041 Linglestown Rd.
Harrisburg, PA 17112-1208
Phone: (717)541-5864 **Free:** 800-932-0903
Fax: (717)541-8828

Puerto Rico

★ 10943 ★ American Lung Association of Puerto Rico
395 Domenech Ave.
PO Box 195247
San Juan, PR 00919-5247
Phone: (787)765-5664 **Fax:** (787)765-5964
Email: info@pulmon.org
Website: http://www.pulmon.org
Yolanda Rosario, Director

Rhode Island

★ 10944 ★ American Lung Association of Rhode Island
298 W Exchange St.
Providence, RI 02903-3700
Phone: (401)421-6487 **Fax:** (401)331-5266
Email: alaofri@aol.com

South Carolina

★ 10945 ★ American Lung Association of South Carolina
1817 Gadsden St.
Columbia, SC 29201-2392
Phone: (803)779-5864 **Free:** 800-849-5864
Fax: (803)254-2711
Email: alasc@lungsc.org
Website: http://www.lungsc.org

★ 10946 ★ American Lung Association of South Carolina
Coastal Region
1941 Savage Rd., Ste. 200-A
Charleston, SC 29407-4789
Phone: (843)556-8451 **Fax:** (843)556-3332
Email: scatlin@lungsc.org
Website: http://www.lungsc.org
Sally Catlin, Director

★ 10947 ★ American Lung Association of South Carolina
Midlands Region
1817 Gadsden St.
Columbia, SC 29201-2392
Phone: (803)779-5864 **Fax:** (803)254-2711
Email: gsteele@lungsc.org
Website: http://www.lungsc.org
Gabrielle Steele, Director

★ 10948 ★ American Lung Association of South Carolina
Piedmont Region
84 Villa Rd., B-2
Greenville, SC 29615
Phone: (864)233-0517 **Fax:** (864)233-2124
Email: ckinghorn@lungsc.org
Website: http://www.lungsc.org
Cynthia Kinghorn, Director

South Dakota

★ 10949 ★ American Lung Association of South Dakota
1212 W Elkhorn, Ste. 1
Sioux Falls, SD 57104-0233
Phone: (605)336-7222 **Free:** 800-873-5864
Fax: (605)336-7227
Email: lung@americanlungsd.org
Website: http://www.recess.org/

Tennessee

★ 10950 ★ American Lung Association of Tennessee
One Vantage Way, Ste. C250
Nashville, TN 37228
Phone: (615)329-1151 **Free:** 800-432-5864
Fax: (615)329-1723
Email: alastaff@alatn.org
Website: http://www.alatn.org

Texas

★ 10951 ★ American Lung Association of Texas
5926 Balcones Dr., Ste. 100
PO Box 26460
Austin, TX 78755-0460
Phone: (512)467-6753 **Fax:** (512)467-7621
Email: alatexas@texaslung.org
Website: http://www.texaslung.org

★ 10952 ★ American Lung Association of Texas
Alamo and Southern Region
The Callaghan Bldg.
7475 Callaghan Rd., Ste. 203
San Antonio, TX 78229
Phone: (210)308-8978 **Fax:** (210)308-8992
Email: alasoutx@onr.com

★ 10953 ★ American Lung Association of Texas
Central Region
5926 Balcones Dr., Ste. 105
PO Box 26566
Austin, TX 78755-0566
Phone: (512)467-2534 **Fax:** (512)467-7539
Email: alacentx@onr.com
Website: http://www.texaslung.org

★ 10954 ★ American Lung Association of Texas
Dallas Region
8150 Brookriver Dr., S-102, LB-151
Dallas, TX 75247
Phone: (214)631-5864 **Fax:** (214)630-8092
Email: dallas@texaslung.org
Website: http://www.texaslung.org

★ 10955 ★ American Lung Association of Texas
Fort Worth Region
2630 W Freeway, Ste. 202
Fort Worth, TX 76102
Phone: (817)332-4549 **Fax:** (817)332-4961
Email: jaustin@texaslung.org
Website: http://www.texaslung.org

★ 10956 ★ American Lung Association of Texas
Houston and Southeast Region
2425 W Loop S, Ste. 330
PO Box 27396
Houston, TX 77227-7396
Phone: (713)629-1600 **Fax:** (713)629-5828

★ 10957 ★ American Lung Association of Texas
Rio Grande Valley Region
3827 N 10th St., No. 203
McAllen, TX 78501
Phone: (956)631-0514 **Fax:** (956)668-9615
Email: lrunnels@flash.net

★ 10958 ★ American Lung Association of Texas
Western Region
444 Executive Center Blvd., Ste. 206
El Paso, TX 79902
Phone: (915)532-6776 **Fax:** (915)532-7231
Email: westreg@flash.net

Utah

★ 10959 ★ American Lung Association of Utah
1930 South 1100 East
Salt Lake City, UT 84106-2317
Phone: (801)484-4456 **Fax:** (801)484-5461
Email: wldavis@utahlung.org

Vermont

★ 10960 ★ American Lung Association of Vermont
30 Farrell St.
South Burlington, VT 05403-6196
Phone: (802)863-6817 **Fax:** (802)863-6818
Email: info@vtlung.org
Sharon Wheelock, Contact

Virgin Islands

★ 10961 ★ American Lung Association of the Virgin Islands
PO Box 974
St. Thomas, VI 00804
Phone: (340)774-8620 **Fax:** (340)774-8620

Virginia

★ 10962 ★ American Lung Association of Virginia
9221 Forest Hill Ave.
Richmond, VA 23235
Phone: (804)267-1900 **Fax:** (804)267-5634
Email: resourcecenter@lungva.org

Washington

★ 10963 ★ American Lung Association of Washington
2625 3rd Ave.
Seattle, WA 98121
Phone: (206)441-5100 **Free:** 800-732-9339
Fax: (206)441-3277
Email: alaw@alaw.org
Website: http://www.alaw.org

West Virginia

★ 10964 ★ American Lung Association of West Virginia
415 Dickinson St.
PO Box 3980
Charleston, WV 25339-3980
Phone: (304)342-6600 **Fax:** (304)342-6096
Email: chantal@alawv.org
Website: http://www.alawv.org

Wisconsin

★ 10965 ★ American Lung Association of Wisconsin
13100 W Lisbon Rd., Ste. 700
Brookfield, WI 53005-2508
Phone: (262)703-4200 **Fax:** (262)781-5180
Email: amlung@lungwisconsin.org

Social Work

Listed below are chapters of the National Association of Social Workers, 750 1st St. NE, Ste. 700, Washington, DC 20002, (202)408-8600, http://www.naswdc.org/.

AE

★ 10966 ★ National Association of Social Workers
International Chapter
CMR 419 Box 1913
APO, AE 09102
Email: naswintl@aol.com
Website: http://www.naswintl.org

Alabama

★ 10967 ★ National Association of Social Workers
Alabama Chapter
Governors Park II
2921 Marti Ln., No. G
Montgomery, AL 36116
Phone: (334)288-2633 **Fax:** (334)288-1398
Email: naswal@earthlink.net

Alaska

★ 10968 ★ National Association of Social Workers
Alaska Chapter
4161 Patterson Circle
Anchorage, AK 99504-4680
Phone: (907)332-6279 **Fax:** (907)332-6270
Email: naswak@alaska.net
Website: http://www.naswak.org

Arizona

★ 10969 ★ National Association of Social Workers
Arizona Chapter
1050 E Southern Ave., Ste. F-5
Tempe, AZ 85282
Phone: (480)968-4595 **Fax:** (480)894-9726
Email: chapter@naswaz.com
Website: http://www.naswaz.com

Arkansas

★ 10970 ★ National Association of Social Workers
Arkansas Chapter
1123 S University 1010
Little Rock, AR 72204
Phone: (501)663-0658 **Free:** 800-797-6279
Fax: (501)663-6406
Email: naswar@cei.net
Website: http://www.naswar.org

California

★ 10971 ★ National Association of Social Workers
California Chapter
1016 23rd St.
Sacramento, CA 95816
Phone: (916)442-4565 **Free:** 800-538-2565
Fax: (916)442-2075
Email: naswca@naswca.org
Website: http://www.naswca.org

★ 10972 ★ National Association of Social Workers
California Chapter
Los Angeles Office
315 W 9th St., Ste. 321
Los Angeles, CA 90015
Phone: (213)452-0090 **Fax:** (213)452-0094
Email: membership@naswca.org
Website: http://www.naswca.org

Colorado

★ 10973 ★ National Association of Social Workers
Colorado Chapter
2345 S Federal Blvd., Ste. 200
Denver, CO 80219
Phone: (303)753-8890 **Free:** 800-595-NASW
Fax: (303)753-8891
Email: naswco@qwest.net
Website: http://www.naswco.org

Connecticut

★ 10974 ★ National Association of Social Workers
Connecticut Chapter
2139 Silas Deane Hwy., Ste. 205
Rocky Hill, CT 06067
Phone: (860)257-8066 **Fax:** (860)257-8074
Email: naswct@snet.net
Website: http://www.naswct.org

Delaware

★ 10975 ★ National Association of Social Workers
Delaware Chapter
3301 Green St.
Claymont, DE 19703
Phone: (302)792-0646 **Fax:** (302)792-0678
Email: naswde@dca.net
Website: http://www.geocities.com/HotSprings/6271/DENASW.html

District of Columbia

★ 10976 ★ National Association of Social Workers
DC Metro Washington Chapter
PO Box 75236
Washington, DC 20013
Phone: (202)371-8282 **Fax:** (202)371-6578
Email: office@naswmetro.org
Website: http://www.naswmetro.org

Florida

★ 10977 ★ National Association of Social Workers
Florida Chapter
345 S Magnolia Dr., Ste. 14-B
Tallahassee, FL 32301
Phone: (850)224-2400 **Free:** 800-352-6279
Fax: (850)561-6279
Email: naswfl@unr.net
Website: http://www.naswfl.org

Georgia

★ 10978 ★ National Association of Social Workers
Georgia Chapter
3070 Presidential Dr., Ste. 226
Atlanta, GA 30340
Phone: (770)234-0567 **Fax:** (770)234-0565
Email: naswga@mindspring.com
Website: http://www.naswga.org

Guam

★ 10979 ★ National Association of Social Workers
Guam Chapter
Rm. 205, HSS Bldg., UOG
PO Box 5176
UOG Station
Mangilao, GU 96923
Phone: (671)735-2877
Email: naswgu@netpci.com

Hawaii

★ 10980 ★ National Association of Social Workers
Hawaii Chapter
677 Ala Moana Blvd., No. 911
Honolulu, HI 96813
Phone: (808)521-1787 **Fax:** (808)521-3299
Email: info@naswhi.org
Website: http://www.naswhi.org

Idaho

★ 10981 ★ National Association of Social Workers
Idaho Chapter
PO Box 7393
Boise, ID 83707
Phone: (208)345-4060 **Fax:** (208)345-4062
Email: naswid@qwest.net
Website: http://www.naswid.20m.com

Illinois

★ 10982 ★ National Association of Social Workers
Illinois Chapter
180 N Michigan Ave., Ste. 400
Chicago, IL 60601
Phone: (312)236-8308 **Fax:** (312)236-6627
Email: office@naswil.org
Website: http://www.naswil.org

Indiana

★ 10983 ★ National Association of Social Workers
Indiana Chapter
1100 W 42nd St., Ste. 375
Indianapolis, IN 46208

Phone: (317)923-9878 **Fax:** (317)925-9364
Email: naswind@aol.com

Iowa

★ 10984 ★ National Association of Social Workers
Iowa Chapter
4211 Grand Ave., Level 3
Des Moines, IA 50312
Phone: (515)277-1117 **Fax:** (515)277-2277
Email: naswiowa@aol.com
Website: http://www.angelfire.com/ia2/nasw

Kansas

★ 10985 ★ National Association of Social Workers
Kansas Chapter
Jayhawk Towers
700 SW Jackson St., Ste. 801
Topeka, KS 66603-3740
Phone: (785)354-4804 **Fax:** (785)354-1456
Email: knasw@birch.net
Website: http://www.knasw.com

Kentucky

★ 10986 ★ National Association of Social Workers
Kentucky Chapter
310 St. Clair, Ste. 104
Frankfort, KY 40601
Phone: (502)223-0245 **Fax:** (502)223-0525
Email: naswky@dcr.net
Website: http://www.naswky.org

Louisiana

★ 10987 ★ National Association of Social Workers
Louisiana Chapter
700 N 10th St., Ste. 200
Baton Rouge, LA 70802
Phone: (225)346-1234 **Free:** 800-899-1984
Fax: (225)346-5035
Email: admin@naswla.org
Website: http://www.naswla.org

Maine

★ 10988 ★ National Association of Social Workers
Maine Chapter
222 Water St.
Hallowell, ME 04347-1397
Phone: (207)622-7592 **Fax:** (207)623-4860
Email: naswmaine@aol.com
Alt. Contact: PO Box 5065, Augusta, ME 04332.

Maryland

★ 10989 ★ National Association of Social Workers
Maryland Chapter
5710 Executive Dr., No. 105
Baltimore, MD 21228
Phone: (410)788-1066 **Fax:** (410)747-0635
Email: mdnasw@aol.com
Website: http://www.nasw-md.org

Massachusetts

★ 10990 ★ National Association of Social Workers
Massachusetts Chapter
14 Beacon St., No. 409
Boston, MA 02108
Phone: (617)227-9635 **Fax:** (617)227-9877
Email: chapter@naswma.org
Website: http://www.naswma.org

Michigan

★ 10991 ★ National Association of Social Workers
Michigan Chapter
741 N Cedar St., Ste. 100
Lansing, MI 48906
Phone: (517)487-1548 **Fax:** (517)487-0675
Email: office@nasw-michigan.org
Website: http://www.nasw-michigan.org

Minnesota

★ 10992 ★ National Association of Social Workers
Minnesota Chapter
1885 University Ave. W, Ste. 340
Saint Paul, MN 55104
Phone: (651)293-1935 **Fax:** (651)293-0952
Email: email@naswmn.org
Website: http://www.naswmn.org

Mississippi

★ 10993 ★ National Association of Social Workers
Mississippi Chapter
PO Box 4228
Jackson, MS 39216
Phone: (601)981-8359 **Free:** 800-543-7098
Fax: (601)981-6922
Email: naswms@aol.com
Website: http://members.aol.com/naswms

Missouri

★ 10994 ★ National Association of Social Workers
Missouri Chapter
Parkade Ctr., Ste. 138
601 Business Loop 70 W
Columbia, MO 65203
Phone: (573)874-6140 **Free:** 800-333-6279
Fax: (573)874-8738
Email: chapter@nasw-mo.org
Website: http://www.nasw-mo.org

Montana

★ 10995 ★ National Association of Social Workers
Montana Chapter
25 S Ewing St., Ste. 406
Helena, MT 59601
Phone: (406)449-6208 **Fax:** (406)449-2533
Email: naswmt@mt.net
Website: http://www.naswmt.com

Nebraska

★ 10996 ★ National Association of Social Workers
Nebraska Chapter
PO Box 83732
Lincoln, NE 68501
Phone: (402)477-7344 **Free:** 877-816-6279
Fax: (402)476-6547

Email: naswne@assocoffice.net
Website: http://www.naswne.org

Nevada

★ 10997 ★ National Association of Social Workers
Nevada Chapter
1555 E Flamingo Rd., Ste. 158
Las Vegas, NV 89119
Phone: (702)791-5872 **Fax:** (702)791-5873
Email: naswnv@worldnet.att.net
Website: http://www.nasw-nv.com

New Hampshire

★ 10998 ★ National Association of Social Workers
New Hampshire Chapter
c/o New Hampshire Association for the Blind
25 Walker St.
Concord, NH 03301
Phone: (603)226-7135 **Fax:** (603)228-3836
Email: naswnh@worldpath.net
Website: http://www.naswnh.org

New Jersey

★ 10999 ★ National Association of Social Workers
New Jersey Chapter
2 Quarterbridge Plaza
Hamilton, NJ 08619
Phone: (609)584-5686 **Fax:** (609)584-5681
Email: naswnj@aol.com
Website: http://www.naswnj.org

New Mexico

★ 11000 ★ National Association of Social Workers
New Mexico Chapter
1503 University Blvd. NE
Albuquerque, NM 87102
Phone: (505)247-2336 **Fax:** (505)243-0446
Email: nasw@qwest.net
Website: http://www.naswnm.org
Remarks: Send faxes "Attn: Dolores."

New York

★ 11001 ★ National Association of Social Workers
New York City Chapter
50 Broadway, 10th Fl.
New York, NY 10004
Phone: (212)668-0050 **Fax:** (212)668-0305
Email: schachter@naswnyc.org
Website: http://www.naswnyc.org/

★ 11002 ★ National Association of Social Workers
New York State Chapter
188 Washington Ave.
Albany, NY 12210
Phone: (518)463-4741 **Free:** 800-724-6279
Fax: (518)463-6446
Email: naswnys@aol.com
Website: http://www.naswnys.org

North Carolina

★ 11003 ★ National Association of Social Workers
North Carolina Chapter
PO Box 27582
Raleigh, NC 27611-7581
Phone: (919)828-9650 **Free:** 800-280-6207
Fax: (919)828-1341
Email: naswnc@aol.com
Website: http://www.naswnc.org

North Dakota

★ 11004 ★ National Association of Social Workers
North Dakota Chapter
PO Box 1775
Bismarck, ND 58502-1775
Phone: (701)223-4161 **Fax:** (701)224-9824
Email: naswnd@aptnd.com
Website: http://www.naswdakotas.com

Ohio

★ 11005 ★ National Association of Social Workers
Ohio Chapter
118 E Main St., Ste. 3 W
Columbus, OH 43215
Phone: (614)461-4484 **Fax:** (614)461-9793
Email: ohnasw@ameritech.net
Website: http://www.naswoh.org

Oklahoma

★ 11006 ★ National Association of Social Workers
Oklahoma Chapter
2801 N Lincoln Blvd.
Oklahoma City, OK 73105
Phone: (405)239-7017 **Fax:** (405)236-3638
Email: naswok@ionet.net
Website: http://www.ionet.net/~naswok/

Oregon

★ 11007 ★ National Association of Social Workers
Oregon Chapter
7688 SW Capitol Hwy.
Portland, OR 97219
Phone: (503)452-8420 **Fax:** (503)452-8506
Email: nasworegon@nasworegon.org
Website: http://www.nasworegon.org

Pennsylvania

★ 11008 ★ National Association of Social Workers
Pennsylvania Chapter
1337 N Front St.
Harrisburg, PA 17102
Phone: (717)232-4125 **Fax:** (717)232-4140
Email: exec@nasw-pa.org
Website: http://www.nasw-pa.org

Puerto Rico

★ 11009 ★ National Association of Social Workers
Puerto Rico Chapter
PO Box 192051
San Juan, PR 00919-2051
Phone: (787)758-3588 **Fax:** (787)281-8433

Rhode Island

★ 11010 ★ National Association of Social Workers
Rhode Island Chapter
260 W Exchange St., Ste. 306
Providence, RI 02903
Phone: (401)274-4940 **Fax:** (401)274-4941
Email: rinasw@aol.com

South Carolina

★ 11011 ★ National Association of Social Workers
South Carolina Chapter
PO Box 5008
Columbia, SC 29250
Phone: (803)256-8406 **Fax:** (803)254-4116
Email: scnasw@earthlink.net
Website: http://www.scnasw.org

South Dakota

★ 11012 ★ National Association of Social Workers
South Dakota Chapter
1000 N West Ave., No. 360
Spearfish, SD 57783
Phone: (605)339-9104 **Fax:** (605)339-9104
Email: naswsd@aptnd.com
Website: http://www.naswdakotas.com

Tennessee

★ 11013 ★ National Association of Social Workers
Tennessee Chapter
1808 W End Ave., Ste. 805
Nashville, TN 37203
Phone: (615)321-5095 **Fax:** (615)327-2676
Email: tnnasw@aol.com
Website: http://www.naswtn.com

Texas

★ 11014 ★ National Association of Social Workers
Texas Chapter
810 W 11th St.
Austin, TX 78701
Phone: (512)474-1454 **Free:** 800-888-6279
Fax: (512)474-1317
Email: naswtex@naswtx.org
Website: http://www.naswtx.org/

Utah

★ 11015 ★ National Association of Social Workers
Utah Chapter
University of Utah GSSW No. 229
395 S 1500 E
Salt Lake City, UT 84112-0260
Phone: (801)583-8855 **Fax:** (801)583-6218
Email: utnasw@aros.net
Website: http://www.utnasw.org/

Vermont

★ 11016 ★ National Association of Social Workers
Vermont Chapter
PO Box 1348
Montpelier, VT 05601
Phone: (802)223-1713 **Fax:** (802)223-1713
Email: naswvt@madriver.com
Website: http://www.naswvt.org

Virgin Islands

★ 11017 ★ National Association of Social Workers
Virgin Islands Chapter
Havensight Secretarial Services
2 Buccaneer Mall
St. Thomas, VI 00802
Phone: (340)776-3424 **Fax:** (340)777-8108

Virginia

★ 11018 ★ National Association of Social Workers
Virginia Chapter
1506 Staples Mill Rd.
Richmond, VA 23230
Phone: (804)204-1339 **Fax:** (804)204-1539
Email: naswva@naswva.com
Website: http://www.naswva.com

Washington

★ 11019 ★ National Association of Social Workers
Washington Chapter
8711 15th Ave. NW
Seattle, WA 98117
Phone: (206)706-7084 **Fax:** (206)706-7085
Email: admin@nasw-wa.org
Website: http://www.nasw-wa.org

West Virginia

★ 11020 ★ National Association of Social Workers
West Virginia Chapter
1608 Virginia St. E
Charleston, WV 25311
Phone: (304)345-6279 **Fax:** (304)343-3295
Email: mail@naswwv.org
Website: http://www.naswwv.org/

Wisconsin

★ 11021 ★ National Association of Social Workers
Wisconsin Chapter
16 N Carroll St., Ste. 220
Madison, WI 53703
Phone: (608)257-6334 **Free:** (866)462-7994
Fax: (608)257-8233
Email: naswwi@tds.net
Website: http://www.naswwi.org

Wyoming

★ 11022 ★ National Association of Social Workers
Wyoming Chapter
PO Box 701
Cheyenne, WY 82003
Phone: (307)634-2118 **Fax:** (307)778-9518
Email: wynasw@worldnet.att.net

Urological Diseases

State chapters of the American Urological Association are listed below. The national office is located at 1120 N Charles St., Baltimore, MD 21201. Additional information can be obtained by calling the national office at (410) 727-1100, or by consulting their web site at http://auanet.org/.

California

★ 11023 ★ American Urological Association
Western Section
1950 Old Tustin Ave.
Santa Ana, CA 92705
Phone: (714)550-9155 **Fax:** (714)550-9234
Email: urologyusa@aol.com
Website: http://www.urologyusa.com
Frank J. DeSantis, Exec Director
Remarks: The Western section comprises the states of Alaska, Arizona, California, Hawaii, Idaho, Montana, Nevada, Oregon, Utah, Washington and Wyoming; the Canadian provinces of Alberta, British Columbia and Saskatchewan; and the island possessions of the United States in the Pacific Ocean.

Illinois

★ 11024 ★ American Urological Association
North Central Section
1111 N Plaza Dr., Ste. 550
Schaumburg, IL 60173-4950
Phone: (847)517-1544 **Fax:** (847)517-7229
Email: ncs@wjweiser.com
Wendy Weiser, Exec Director
Remarks: Comprises the states of Illinois, Indiana, Iowa, Michigan, Minnesota, North Dakota, Ohio, South Dakota and Wisconsin.

★ 11025 ★ American Urological Association
South Central Section
1111 N Plaza Dr., Ste. 550
Schaumburg, IL 60173-4950
Phone: (847)605-0850 **Fax:** (847)517-7229
Email: scs@wjweiser.com
Wendy Weiser, Exec Director
Remarks: Comprises the states of Arkansas, Colorado, Kansas, Missouri, Nebraska, New Mexico, Oklahoma and Texas, in addition to Mexico, Belize and the Republics of Costa Rica, El Salvador, Honduras and Nicaragua.

★ 11026 ★ American Urological Association
Southeastern Section
1111 N Plaza Dr., Ste. 550
Schaumburg, IL 60173-4950
Phone: (847)969-0248 **Fax:** (847)517-7229
Email: ses@wjweiser.com
Website: http://www.sesaua.org
Wendy Weiser, Contact
Remarks: Comprises the states of Alabama, Florida, Georgia, Kentucky, Louisiana, Mississippi, North Carolina, South Carolina and Tennessee, in addition to Puerto Rico, the Virgin Islands and the Republic of Panama.

Massachusetts

★ 11027 ★ American Urological Association
Mid-Atlantic Section
13 Elm St.
Manchester, MA 01944-1314
Phone: (978)526-8330 **Fax:** (978)526-4018
Email: maaua@prri.com
Website: http://www.auanet.org/membership/sections/midatlantic/
Robert P. Jones, EdD, Exec Director
Remarks: Comprises the southern portion of the state of New Jersey and the eastern portion of the state of Pennsylvania. The states of Delaware, Maryland, Virginia and West Virginia are also included, as well as Washington, D.C.

★ 11028 ★ American Urological Association
New England Section
13 Elm St.
Manchester, MA 01944
Phone: (978)526-8330 **Fax:** (978)526-4018
Email: neaua@prri.com
Aurelie M. Alger, JD, Exec Director
Remarks: Comprises the states of Connecticut, Maine, Massachusetts, New Hampshire, Rhode Island and Vermont.

★ 11029 ★ American Urological Association
Northeastern Section
13 Elm St.
Manchester, MA 01944
Phone: (978)526-8330 **Fax:** (978)526-4018
Email: nsaua@prri.com
David Cloud, Exec Director
Remarks: Comprises the state of New York (except the southeastern portion) and the western portion of the state of Pennsylvania. The eastern portion of Canada, including the provinces of Ontario, Quebec, New Brunswick, Nova Scotia, Prince Edward Island, Newfoundland and Manitoba are also included.

New York

★ 11030 ★ American Urological Association
New York Section
1216 Fifth Ave., Rm. 554
New York, NY 10029
Phone: (212)722-4300 **Fax:** (212)722-1842
Email: auany@aol.com
Ida Flores, Exec Director
Remarks: Comprises the southeastern portion of the state of New York, including Long Island, and the northern portion of the state of New Jersey.

Veterinary Medicine

The following are state groups of the American Veterinary Medical Association, 1931 N Meacham Rd., Ste. 100, Schaumburg, IL 60173, (847)925-8070, http://www.avma.org/.

Alabama

★ 11031 ★ Alabama Veterinary Medical Association
PO Box 3514
Montgomery, AL 36109-0514
Phone: (334)261-3012 **Fax:** (334)261-3013
Email: franzc55@cs.com
Website: http://www.alvma.com
Charles F. Franz, DVM, Exec Director

Alaska

★ 11032 ★ Alaska State Veterinary Medical Association
PO Box 112269
Anchorage, AK 99511-2269
Phone: (907)344-7913 **Fax:** (907)349-1255
Dr. Paul Frederickson, Contact

Arizona

★ 11033 ★ Arizona Veterinary Medical Association
5502 N 19th Ave.
Phoenix, AZ 85015-7936
Phone: (602)242-7936 **Fax:** (602)249-3828
Email: ekane@azvma.org
Website: http://www.azvma.org
Emily Kane, Exec Director

Arkansas

★ 11034 ★ Arkansas Veterinary Medical Association
8 Shackleford Plaza, Ste. 208
Little Rock, AR 72211
Phone: (501)221-1477 **Fax:** (501)221-6691
Email: info@arkvetmed.org
Website: http://www.arkvetmed.org
Mr. Robert Blount, Exec Director

California

★ 11035 ★ California Veterinary Medical Association
1400 River Park Dr., Ste. 100
Sacramento, CA 95815-4505
Phone: (916)649-0599 **Fax:** (916)646-9156
Email: dschumacher@cvma.net
Website: http://www.cvma.net
Dr. Richard Schumacher, Exec Director

Colorado

★ 11036 ★ Colorado Veterinary Medical Association
Denver Area Veterinary Medical Society
789 Sherman St., Ste. 550
Denver, CO 80203
Phone: (303)318-0447 **Fax:** (303)318-0450
Email: info@colovma.com
Website: http://www.colovma.com
Ralph Johnson, Exec Director

Connecticut

★ 11037 ★ Connecticut Veterinary Medical Association
731 Hebron Ave.
Glastonbury, CT 06033
Phone: (860)659-9683 **Fax:** (860)657-8244
Email: connveterinary@aol.com
Website: http://www.ctvma.org
Simon Flynn, Exec Director

Delaware

★ 11038 ★ Delaware Veterinary Medical Association
937 Monroe Terrace
Dover, DE 19904
Phone: (302)674-8581 **Fax:** (302)674-8581
Email: appelplej@aol.com
Website: http://www.avma.org/statevma/devma
Lynn Appel, Exec Director

District of Columbia

★ 11039 ★ District of Columbia Veterinary Medical Association
2501 Que St. NW, No. 320
Washington, DC 20007
Phone: (301)734-5873 **Fax:** (301)734-4314
Website: http://www.avma.org/statevma/dcvma
Dr. Michele April, Contact

Florida

★ 11040 ★ Florida Veterinary Medical Association
7131 Lake Ellenor Dr.
Orlando, FL 32809-5738
Phone: (407)851-3862 **Fax:** (407)240-3710
Email: fvma@bellsouth.net

Website: http://www.fvma.org
Donald N. Schaefer, Exec Director

Georgia

★ 11041 ★ Georgia Veterinary Medical Association
2814 Spring Rd., Ste. 217
Atlanta, GA 30339
Phone: (678)309-9800 **Fax:** (678)309-3361
Email: gvma@mindspring.com
Website: http://www.gvma.net
Beth Monte, Exec Director

Hawaii

★ 11042 ★ Hawaii Veterinary Medical Association
4400 Kalanianaole Hwy., Ste. 6
Honolulu, HI 96821
Phone: (808)733-8828 **Fax:** (808)733-8829
Website: http://www.hawaiivetmed.org
Dr. Eric Ako, Exec VP

Idaho

★ 11043 ★ Idaho Veterinary Medical Association
PO Box 6573
Boise, ID 83707
Phone: (208)375-1551 **Fax:** (208)376-4430
Email: msvicki1@mindspring.com
Website: http://www.ivma.org
Vicki Smith, Exec Director

★ 11044 ★ Utah Veterinary Medical Association
PO Box 6573
Boise, ID 83707
Phone: (208)375-1551 **Fax:** (208)375-4430
Email: msvicki1@mindspring.com
Vicki Smith, Exec Director

★ 11045 ★ Wyoming Veterinary Medical Association
PO Box 6573
Boise, ID 83707
Phone: (208)375-1551 **Fax:** (208)376-4430
Email: msvicki1@mindspring.com
Website: http://www.wyvma.org
Vicki Smith, Exec Director

Illinois

★ 11046 ★ Illinois State Veterinary Medical Association
161 S Lincolnway, Ste. 302
North Aurora, IL 60542
Phone: (630)892-2321 **Fax:** (630)892-0818
Email: isvma@aol.com
Website: http://www.isvma.org
Eve C. Larocca, Exec Director

Indiana

★ 11047 ★ Indiana Veterinary Medical Association
309 W Washington St., Ste. 202
Indianapolis, IN 46204
Phone: (317)974-0888 **Fax:** (317)974-0985
Email: ivma@iquest.net
Website: http://www.invma.org
Lisa Perius, Exec Director

Iowa

★ 11048 ★ Iowa Veterinary Medical Association
5921 Fleur Dr.
Des Moines, IA 50321
Phone: (515)285-6701 **Fax:** (515)285-7809
Email: ivma@netins.net
Website: http://www.iowavma.org
Dave Furneaux, Exec Director

Kansas

★ 11049 ★ Kansas Veterinary Medical Association
816 SW Tyler, Ste. 200
Topeka, KS 66612-1635
Phone: (785)233-4141 **Fax:** (785)233-2534
Email: 74253.653@compuserve.com
Website: http://www.vet.ksu.edu/links/KVMA
Gary Reser, CAE, Exec VP

Kentucky

★ 11050 ★ Kentucky Veterinary Medical Association
PO Box 4067
Frankfort, KY 40604-4067
Phone: (502)226-5862 **Fax:** (502)226-6177
Email: kvma@aol.com
Website: http://www.avma.org/statevma/kyvma
Louise Cook, Exec Director

Louisiana

★ 11051 ★ Louisiana Veterinary Medical Association
8550 United Plaza Blvd., Ste. 1001
Baton Rouge, LA 70809
Phone: (225)928-5862 **Fax:** (225)922-4611
Email: lvma@pncpa.com
Website: http://www.lvma.org
Bland O'Connor, Exec Director

Maine

★ 11052 ★ Maine Veterinary Medical Association
PO Box 8
Rumford Center, ME 04278
Phone: (207)364-8660 **Fax:** (207)364-7209
Email: hersey@megalink.net
Website: http://www.avma.org/statevma/mevma
Dr. Charles Hersey, Exec Director

Maryland

★ 11053 ★ Maryland Veterinary Medical Association
5024 R Campbell Blvd.
Nottingham, MD 21236-5943
Free: 888-884-6882 **Fax:** (410)931-8111
Email: MDVMA@aol.com
Website: http://www.mdvma.org
Buzz Thomas, Exec Director

Massachusetts

★ 11054 ★ Massachusetts Veterinary Medical Association
169 Lakeside Ave.
Marlborough, MA 01752-4503
Phone: (508)460-9333 **Fax:** (508)460-9969
Email: staff@massvet.org
Website: http://www.ultranet.com/~massvet
Susan Weinstein, Exec Director

Michigan

★ 11055 ★ Michigan Veterinary Medical Association
2144 Commons Pkwy.
Okemos, MI 48864-3986
Phone: (517)347-4710 **Fax:** (517)347-4666
Email: prescott@michvma.org
Website: http://www.michvma.org
Dr. Peter A. Prescott, Exec Director

Minnesota

★ 11056 ★ Minnesota Veterinary Medical Association
393 N Dunlap St., Ste. 400
Saint Paul, MN 55104
Phone: (651)645-7533 **Fax:** (651)645-7539
Email: info@mvma.org
Website: http://www.mvma.org
Sharon Vangsness, CAE, Exec Director

Mississippi

★ 11057 ★ Mississippi Veterinary Medical Association
209 S Lafayette St.
Starkville, MS 39759
Phone: (662)324-9380 **Fax:** (662)324-9380
Email: msvma@futuresouth.com
Dr. Harvey F. McCrory, Contact

Missouri

★ 11058 ★ Missouri Veterinary Medical Association
2500 Country Club Dr.
Jefferson City, MO 65109
Phone: (573)636-8612 **Fax:** (573)659-7175
Email: movma@mchsi.com
Website: http://www.movma.org
Richard Antweiler, Exec Director

Montana

★ 11059 ★ Montana Veterinary Medical Association
PO Box 6322
Helena, MT 59604
Phone: (406)447-4259 **Fax:** (406)442-8018
Email: stuart@initco.net
Website: http://www.avma.org/statevma/mtvma
Stuart Doggett, Exec Director

Nebraska

★ 11060 ★ Nebraska Veterinary Medical Association
PO Box 2118
Hastings, NE 68902-2118
Phone: (402)463-4704 **Fax:** (402)463-5683
Email: gmo@inebraska.com
Website: http://www.nvma.org
Don Ellerbee, Exec Director

Nevada

★ 11061 ★ Nevada Veterinary Medical Association
PO Box 34420
Reno, NV 89533
Phone: (775)324-5344 **Fax:** (775)747-9170
Email: nvma@775.net
Website: http://www.aci.net/nvma
Michelle Wagner, Exec Director

New Hampshire

★ 11062 ★ New Hampshire Veterinary Medical Association
PO Box 616
Concord, NH 03302-0616
Phone: (603)224-2432 **Fax:** (603)225-0556
Email: nhvmaip@mediaone.net
JoAnn Poole, Exec Director

New Jersey

★ 11063 ★ New Jersey Veterinary Medical Association
66 Morris Ave., Ste. 2A
Springfield, NJ 07081
Phone: (973)379-1100 **Fax:** (973)379-6507
Email: rickaaamac@earthlink.com
Website: http://www.njvma.org
Richard Alampi, Exec Director

New Mexico

★ 11064 ★ New Mexico Veterinary Medical Association
3037 San Patricia NW
Albuquerque, NM 87107
Phone: (505)343-1691 **Fax:** (505)294-9958
Email: nmvma@earthlink.net
Website: http://home.earthlink.net/~nmvma/
Marjorie Nelson, Contact

New York

★ 11065 ★ New York City Veterinary Medical Association
331 W 57th St., S293
New York, NY 10019-3101
Phone: (212)246-0057 **Fax:** (212)586-3949
Email: VMANYC@aol.com
Effie Cooper, Contact

★ 11066 ★ New York State Veterinary Medical Society
9 Highland Ave.
Albany, NY 12205-5417
Phone: (518)437-0787 **Fax:** (518)437-0957
Email: INFO@NYSVMS.org
Website: http://www.nysvms.org
Julie Lawton, Exec Director
Frmly: New York State Veterinary Medical Association.

North Carolina

★ 11067 ★ North Carolina Veterinary Medical Association
138 Spring Ave.
Fuquay Varina, NC 27526
Phone: (919)557-9385 **Fax:** (919)557-9389
Email: mprasor@cs.com
Website: http://www.ncvma.org
Mollie Rasor, Exec Director

★ 11068 ★ South Carolina Association of Veterinarians
PO Box 505
Hwy 903/123
Maury, NC 28554
Phone: (252)747-8180 **Fax:** (252)747-4100
Email: vetmeeting@aol.com
Ralph Lee, Exec VP

North Dakota

★ 11069 ★ North Dakota Veterinary Medical Association
921 S 9th St.
Bismarck, ND 58504
Phone: (701)221-7740 **Fax:** (701)258-9005
Email: nkopp@btigate.com
Nancy Kopp, Contact

Ohio

★ 11070 ★ Ohio Veterinary Medical Association
3168 Riverside Dr.
Columbus, OH 43221
Phone: (614)486-7253 **Fax:** (614)486-1325
Email: ohiovma@ohiovma.org
Website: http://www.ohiovma.org
Jack Advent, CAE, Exec Director

Oklahoma

★ 11071 ★ Oklahoma Veterinary Medical Association
PO Box 14521
Oklahoma City, OK 73113
Phone: (405)478-1002 **Fax:** (405)478-7193
Email: okvma@compuserve.com
Website: http://www.okvma.org
Dr. Charles Helwig, Exec Director

Oregon

★ 11072 ★ Oregon Veterinary Medical Association
1880 Lancaster Dr. NE, Ste. 118
Salem, OR 97305
Phone: (503)399-0311 **Fax:** (503)363-4218
Email: ovma@teleport.com
Glenn M. Kolb, Exec Director

Pennsylvania

★ 11073 ★ Pennsylvania Veterinary Medical Association
PO Box 8820
Harrisburg, PA 17105-8820
Phone: (717)588-7841 **Free:** 888-550-7862
Fax: (717)558-7845
Email: pvma@pamedsoc.org
Website: http://www.pavma.org
Charlene Wandzilak, Exec Director

Puerto Rico

★ 11074 ★ Puerto Rico Veterinary Medical Association
352 Ave. San Claudio, Ste. 248
San Juan, PR 00926-4107
Phone: (787)283-2840 **Fax:** (787)761-3440
Email: cmvpr@prw.net
Sandra Sanchez, Contact

Rhode Island

★ 11075 ★ Rhode Island Veterinary Medical Association
PO Box 3
Cumberland, RI 02864
Free: 877-521-0103 **Fax:** (866)277-0238
Email: rivma@rivma.org
Website: http://www.rivma.org
Nancy Klaffky, Contact

South Dakota

★ 11076 ★ South Dakota Veterinary Medical Association
South Dakota VMA
Box 2175, SDU
Brookings, SD 57007-1396
Phone: (605)688-6649 **Fax:** (605)688-6003
Email: janice_kampmann@sdstate.edu
Dr. Daryl K. Thorpe, Exec Director

Tennessee

★ 11077 ★ Tennessee Veterinary Medical Association
200 4th Ave. N, Ste. 900
Nashville, TN 37219
Phone: (615)254-3687 **Fax:** (615)254-7047
Email: tvma@wmgt.org
Website: http://www.tvmanet.org
Dee Ann Walker, CAE, Exec Director

Texas

★ 11078 ★ Texas Veterinary Medical Association
6633 Hwy 290 E, Ste. 201
Austin, TX 78723
Phone: (512)452-4224 **Fax:** (512)452-6633
Email: tvma@tvma.org
Website: http://www.tvma.org
Dr. Elbert Hutchins, Exec Director

Vermont

★ 11079 ★ Vermont Veterinary Medical Association
2073 Spear St.
Charlotte, VT 05445
Phone: (802)425-3495 **Fax:** (802)425-3495
Email: vvma@together.net
Website: http://www.vtvets.org
Sue Moraska, Exec Director

Virginia

★ 11080 ★ Virginia Veterinary Medical Association
4001 Springfield Rd.
Glen Allen, VA 23060
Phone: (804)270-9013 **Fax:** (804)270-2160
Email: vavma@aol.com
Website: http://www.vvma.org
Robin R. Schmitz, Exec Director

Washington

★ 11081 ★ Washington State Veterinary Medical Association
PO Box 962
Bellevue, WA 98009-0962
Phone: (425)454-8381 **Fax:** (425)454-8382
Email: wsvma1@aol.com
Website: http://www.wsvma.org
Sandra J. Bertelsen, Exec VP

West Virginia

★ 11082 ★ West Virginia Veterinary Medical Association
35 Turner Rd.
Elkview, WV 25071
Phone: (304)965-3373
Website: http://www.avma.org/statevma/wvvma
Gail Jones, Contact

Wisconsin

★ 11083 ★ Wisconsin Veterinary Medical Association
301 N Broom St.
Madison, WI 53703
Phone: (608)257-3665 **Fax:** (608)257-8989
Email: wvma@wvma.org
Website: http://www.wvma.org
Leslie Grendahl, Exec Director

Chapter 3
Foundations & Other Funding Organizations

Entries listed below are arranged alphabetically by organization names within three categories: (1) Private Foundations, (2) Corporate Foundations, and (3) Other Funding Organizations. For additional information, consult the "User's Guide" located at the front of this directory.

Private Foundations

★ 11084 ★ A. E. Finley Foundation
PO Box 98266
Raleigh, NC 27624-8266
Phone: (919)782-0529 **Fax:** (919)235-3348
Website: http://www.aefinleyfoundation.org
Robert Brown, President

Fnded: 1957. **Philosophy:** The A. E. Finley foundation "contributes to and supports charitable, scientific, literary, religious, and educational organizations. It endeavors to contribute to soundly managed and operated qualifying organizations which fundamentally give service with a broad scope and impact, aid all kinds of people, and contribute materially to the general welfare." **Priorities:** *Arts & Humanities:* 4%. Supports art museums, theater, public broadcasting, and historic preservation. *Civic & Public Affairs:* 3%. Supports community foundations and clubs. *Education:* 60%. Funds colleges, universities, leadership training, schools and fellowships. *Environment:* 6%. Supports food distribution programs, senior services, Special Olympics, Young Men's Christian Association's, Young Women's Christian Association and United Way. *International:* 22%. Supports cancer, diabetes, respiratory, Alzheimers disease and hospitals. *Note:* Total contributions made in fiscal 1999. **Typ. Recipients:** Cancer, Children's Health/Hospitals, Hospices, Hospitals, Hospitals (University Affiliated), Medical Education, People with Disabilities, Respiratory, Single-Disease Health Associations, Substance Abuse. **Geo. Dist:** NC; NC, Triangle area; VA.

★ 11085 ★ A. J. Fletcher Foundation
PO Box 12800
Raleigh, NC 27605
Phone: (919)890-6081 **Fax:** (919)890-6279
Website: http://www.ajf.org
Thomas McGuire, Jr., Vice President & Executive Director

Fnded: 1961. **Philosophy:** Although the primary focus of the foundation has traditionally been on education, communications, and the arts, the foundation will also consider requests from agencies and organizations addressing a wide variety of social issues and charitable endeavors. The foundation has broadened its focus to include health and human services, illiteracy, public education, poverty programs, and statewide service organizations, and has provided seed money for new and emerging nonprofit organizations. In an effort to maintain long-term relationships with grantees, the foundation provides grants for technical assistance, management training, and other developmental programs that benefit an agency long after allocated funds are gone. It also encourages partnerships through seminars and conferences that offer information aimed at fostering financial stability. The foundation will share resources and knowledge in a statewide interactive network that includes other nonprofits and donor groups. **Priorities:** *Arts & Humanities:* 52%. Public television, historic preservation, music, and theater. *Civic & Public Affairs:* 5%. *Education:* About 19%. Primarily to colleges and universities in North Carolina. *Environment:* 22%. Emphasis on child welfare. *International:* 1%. *Note:* Total contributions made in fiscal 1999. **Typ. Recipients:** Children's Health/Hospitals, Eyes/Blindness, Family Planning, Health-General, Hospices, People with Disabilities, Public Health, Single-Disease Health Associations. **Geo. Dist:** NC.

★ 11086 ★ A. L. Mailman Family Foundation
707 Westchester Ave.
White Plains, NY 10604
Phone: (914)683-8089 **Fax:** (914)686-5519
Email: almf@mailman.org
Website: http://www.mailman.org
Ms. Luba Lynch, Executive Director

Fnded: 1980. **Philosophy:** "The A.L. Mailman Family Foundation's mission is to enhance the ability of families and communities to nurture their children. We believe that the most effective way to fulfill this mission is by focusing on early childhood." The foundation's program areas are: Early Care and Education, focusing on, "High quality programs and experiences for all children." Family Support, feared toward showing that, "All families have the tools to support their children." Moral Education & Social Responsibility, which aims to produce, "Children raised and educated to be caring adults." *A.L. Mailmain Family Foundation Mission and Program Areas.* **Priorities:** *Civic & Public Affairs:* 14%. Public policy groups, legal aid, and minority affairs. *Education:* 44%. Funds colleges, universities and preschool education. Grants focus on early child care. *Environment:* 33%. Child welfare and family services. *International:* 5%. Children's health and hospitals. *Note:* Total contributions made in 1999. **Typ. Recipients:** Alzheimers Disease, Cancer, Children's Health/Hospitals, Clinics/Medical Centers, Domestic Violence, Family Planning, Health Organizations, Medical Education, Mental Health, Nutrition, People with Disabilities, Prenatal Health Issues, Public Health, Research/Studies Institutes. **Geo. Dist:** nationally.

★ 11087 ★ A. Lindsay and Olive B. O'Connor Foundation
PO Box D
Hobart, NY 13788
Phone: (607)538-9248 **Fax:** (607)538-1650
Donald Bishop, II, President & Executive Director

Fnded: 1965. **Philosophy:** The foundation gives to a variety of causes that all serve to enhance the quality of life in rural, upstate New York. A majority of donations support organizations concerned with issues affecting civic and public affairs. Educational institutions and the arts also typically receive funding. **Priorities:** *Arts & Humanities:* 28%. Major support for museums. *Civic & Public Affairs:* 27%. Focus on community revitalization projects. *Education:* 5%. Funds education associations and colleges and universities. *Environment:* 3%. Supports family services. *International:* 19%. Primarily supports hospitals. *Note:* Total contributions made in 1999. **Typ. Recipients:** Emergency/Ambulance Services, Heart, Hospices, Hospitals, Medical Education, People with Disabilities, Single-Disease Health Associations. **Geo. Dist:** NY, Delaware County and contiguous rural counties in upstate New York.

★ 11088 ★ A. V. Hunter Trust, Inc.
650 S Cherry, Suite 535
Denver, CO 80246-1897
Phone: (303)399-5450 **Fax:** (303)399-5499
Website: http://www.avhuntertrust.org
Sharon Siddons, Executive Director & Secretary

Fnded: 1937. **Philosophy:** In distributing contributions, the trustees adhere to A. V. Hunter's will which states, "the trustees shall from time to time... use the net income from said trust and property included therein, in the aid, support, maintenance and assistance, by gift, donation, or otherwise as to them may seem advisable, of then existing, established non-sectarian, charitable institutions or projects or endeavors located in the State of Colorado...whose objects or purposes are to give aid, comfort, support or assistance to children, or aged persons or indigent adults." **Priorities:** *Civic & Public Affairs:* About 8%. Job resource centers, employment programs for women, and Native American affairs. *Education:* 16%. Outward Bound programs and adult learning. *Environment:* About 50%. Planned Parenthood, youth organizations, and volunteer programs. *International:* 18%. Hospice, health centers, and dentistry programs for the disadvantaged. *Note:* Total contributions made in 2001. **Typ. Recipients:** Adolescent Health Issues, Children's Health/Hospitals, Clinics/Medical Centers, Domestic Violence, Emergency/Ambulance Services, Family Planning, Health Organizations, Hospices, Hospitals, Hospitals (University Affiliated), Medical Rehabilitation, Multiple Sclerosis, Nursing Services, People with Disabilities, Prenatal Health Issues, Public Health, Research/Studies Institutes, Sexual Abuse, Single-Disease Health Associations, Substance Abuse. **Geo. Dist:** Denver, CO.

★ 11089 ★ Abbot and Dorothy H. Stevens Foundation
PO Box 111
North Andover, MA 01845
Phone: (978)688-7211 **Fax:** (978)686-1620
Elizabeth Beland, Administrator

Fnded: 1953. **Philosophy:** The purpose of the Abbot and Dorothy H. Stevens Foundation is to assist local charitable organizations. Grants are made across the major categories of support. Specific interests include the arts, law and justice, colleges, hospitals, churches, conservation/preservation, education, and social services. **Priorities:** *Arts & Humanities:* 28%. Supports museums, art centers, libraries, and performing arts. *Civic & Public Affairs:* 11%. Funds other philanthropic organizations. *Education:* 15%. Funds colleges, universities, and precollege education. *Environment:* 29%. Supports human services and summer youth programs. *International:* 8%. Gives to hospitals and health associations. *Note:* Total contributions made in 2000. **Typ. Recipients:** Cancer, Children's Health/Hospitals, Clinics/Medical Centers, Emergency/Ambulance Services, Health-General, Home-Care Services, Hospitals, Medical Research, Mental Health, Nursing

Services, People with Disabilities, People with Disabilities, Substance Abuse. **Geo. Dist:** MA, preference given to Merrimack Valley Area and greater Lawrence Area.

★ 11090 ★ Abell Foundation

111 South Calvert St., Suite 2300
Baltimore, MD 21202
Phone: (410)547-1300 **Fax:** (410)539-6579
Email: abell@abell.org
Website: http://www.abell.org
Robert Embry, Jr., President

Fnded: 1953. **Philosophy:** The foundation recognizes the "complex interdependent issues affecting the quality of life in Maryland." From this perspective, the foundation looks to "join others in seeking solutions to pervasive and stubborn social and economic problems, promote the development of fuller human potential and achievement of self-sufficiency through educational opportunities, and strengthen organizations to provide greater access and more effective services." Emphases include educational reform, job creation, tourism, strengthening families, reducing drug addiction, and alleviating hunger and homelessness. **Priorities:** *Arts & Humanities:* 7%. Museums, theater, music, dance, opera, and arts associations. *Civic & Public Affairs:* 10%. Primarily for economic development. *Education:* 31%. Public and private education. *Environment:* 40%. Child welfare, pregnancy prevention programs, food banks, shelters, youth organizations, job training, and community services. *International:* 9%. Public health concerns. *Note:* Total contributions made in 2000. **Typ. Recipients:** Clinics/Medical Centers, Domestic Violence, Eyes/Blindness, Family Planning, Health Organizations, Medical Education, Mental Health, Nutrition, People with Disabilities, Preventive Medicine/Wellness Organizations, Substance Abuse. **Geo. Dist:** Baltimore, MD.

★ 11091 ★ Abell-Hanger Foundation

PO Box 430
Midland, TX 79702
Phone: (915)684-6655 **Fax:** (915)684-4474
Email: ahf@abell-hanger.org
Website: http://www.abell-hanger.org
David Smith, Executive Director

Fnded: 1954. **Philosophy:** The foundation was created to carry on the philanthropic endeavors that Mr. Abell pursued during his professional and civic career. He once commented that "one likes to be successful, not just for the money, but because of what one can do for one's community, one's country, and for mankind. Business success provides the opportunity to do some of the things most of us dream about doing for our community and its various institutions, organizations, and agencies." Since its inception, the foundation has focused its funding on the arts, community and social services (especially for youth and the handicapped), health, social sciences, and higher education. **Priorities:** *Arts & Humanities:* 17%. Supports museums, libraries, and the Midland Odessa Symphony and Chorale. *Civic & Public Affairs:* 10%. Supports community development. *Education:* 38%. Supports schools, colleges and universities. *Environment:* 23%. Supports children's services, senior services, drug abuse centers, food banks and people with disabilities. *International:* 11%. Supports health sciences, hospitals, and disease and disorder centers and ambulance purchases. *Note:* Total contributions made in fiscal 2001. **Typ. Recipients:** AIDS/HIV, Alzheimers Disease, Cancer, Child Abuse, Children's Health/Hospitals, Domestic Violence, Emergency/Ambulance Services, Eyes/Blindness, Family Planning, Health Funds, Health Organizations, Hospices, Hospitals, Medical Education, Medical Rehabilitation, Medical Research, Medical Training, Multiple Sclerosis, Nursing Services, People with Disabilities, Public Health, Single-Disease Health Associations, Substance Abuse. **Geo. Dist:** TX.

★ 11092 ★ Abercrombie Foundation

PO Box 68
Versailles, KY 40383
Phone: (859)873-4477
John Backer, General Manager

Fnded: 1950. **Philosophy:** "The Board of Trustees of the Foundation has decided to give preference to grant requests from: institutions involved in the education of young people at the secondary and university levels, particularly private universities; organizations working to preserve our natural resources and beautify our environment in rural as well as urban areas; institutions and organizations that provide medical services, information and assistance to the community at large; institutions conducting medical research aimed at alleviating significant current health problems; institutions and organizations that aid children in physical or emotional distress; and institutions and organizations devoted to the education and prevention of substance abuse." **Priorities:** *Arts & Humanities:* 2%. Supports music conservancies. *Civic & Public Affairs:* 1%. *Education:* 68%. Colleges, universities, and family literacy programs received funding. *Environment:* 1%. Animal welfare, family services, and elder care received grants. *International:* 28%. Supports geriatric health and cancer research. *Note:* Total contributions made in 2001. **Typ. Recipients:** Cancer, Children's Health/Hospitals, Clinics/Medical Centers, Diabetes, Domestic Violence, Family Planning, Geriatric Health, Medical Education, Medical Research, Mental Health, People with Disabilities, Prenatal Health Issues, Research/Studies Institutes, Speech & Hearing, Substance Abuse. **Geo. Dist:** KY.

★ 11093 ★ Abney Foundation

100 Vine St.
Anderson, SC 29621
Phone: (864)964-9201 **Fax:** (864)964-9209
Email: info@abneyfoundation.org
Website: http://www.abneyfoundation.org
Carl Edwards, Executive Director

Fnded: 1957. **Philosophy:** The Abney Foundation primarily supports higher education in South Carolina. Interests include colleges, technical schools, and universities. The foundation also supports hospitals, hospices, homes, food distribution, youth organizations, and churches. **Priorities:** *Arts & Humanities:* 1%. Supports theater, music, arts funds. *Civic & Public Affairs:* 7%. Supports community affairs. *Education:* 79%.Supports colleges, universities and scholarship. *Environment:* 3%. Supports youth services, special olympics, meals on wheels, and the elderly Young Men's Christian Association. *International:* 4%. Supports hospices, health clinics, diabetes and medical research. *Note:* Total contributions made in 2000. **Typ. Recipients:** Cancer, Clinics/Medical Centers, Diabetes, Home-Care Services, Hospices, Hospitals, Medical Education, Medical Research. **Geo. Dist:** SC.

★ 11094 ★ Abraham and Sonia Rochlin Foundation

275 Hill St., Suite 250
Reno, NV 89501
Phone: (775)329-1611 **Fax:** (775)329-1983
Heide Rochlin, President

Fnded: 1969. **Philosophy:** The foundation primarily supports civic affairs with Jewish interests. Israeli endowment funds account for most of the giving. Other interests include Jewish religious organizations and universities. **Priorities:** *Arts & Humanities:* 1%. Public broadcasting. *Education:* 9%. Higher education. *International:* 7%. Medical research, cancer centers, geriatric health, and hospices. *Note:* Total contributions made in 2000. **Typ. Recipients:** Alzheimers Disease, Cancer, Clinics/Medical Centers, Hospices, Long-Term Care, Medical Research, Preventive Medicine/Wellness Organizations, Respiratory, Single-Disease Health Associations. **Geo. Dist:** internationally; CA; NV; NY.

★ 11095 ★ Achelis Foundation

767 3rd Ave., 4th Floor
New York, NY 10017-2023
Phone: (212)644-0322 **Fax:** (212)759-6510
Email: main@achelis-bodman-fnds.org
Website: http://www.fdcenter.org/grantmaker/achelis-bodman
Joseph Dolan, Secretary & Executive Director

Fnded: 1940. **Philosophy:** The foundation was created to distribute funds for "charitable, benevolent, educational, and religious uses and purposes." It largely supports youth, social-service agencies, educational institutions (especially school-reform and school-choice programs), major cultural programs, health (including medical research and rehabilitation programs.) Other interests include volunteerism, entrepreneurship, strengthening the two-parent family, fatherhood (and father absence), job training and placement into private-sector jobs, and economic development. Special consideratin is given to leadership development, parental involvement, consumer choice, economic empowerment, independent quality research, prevention and early intervention, advancing the state of art, self-help and self-reliance, innovations and new cost-saving approaches and improving the quality of urban life. The foundation also focuses on returning fathers to their families. Obtaining measurable outcomes of clients and program results in health and social-service agencies is also a goal of the foundation. **Priorities:** *Arts & Humanities:* 9%. Supports museums, dance, and music. *Civic & Public Affairs:* 25%. Including entrepreneurship and job placement. *Education:* 40%. Primary support for education and school reform. *Environment:* 13%. Emphasis on fatherhood, families, restoring marriage, youth, volunteerism, community, and society. *International:* 5%. Supports biomedical research, hospitals, and medical rehabilitation. *Note:* Total contributions made in 2001. **Typ. Recipients:** AIDS/HIV, Alzheimers Disease, Cancer, Children's Health/Hospitals, Clinics/Medical Centers, Domestic Violence, Emergency/Ambulance Services, Eyes/Blindness, Health Funds, Health Organizations, Health-General, Hospitals, Hospitals (University Affiliated), Medical Education, Medical Rehabilitation, Medical Research, Medical Training, Mental Health, Nursing Services, Outpatient Health Care, People with Disabilities, Public Health, Speech & Hearing, Substance Abuse, Transplant Networks/Donor Banks. **Geo. Dist:** New York, NY.

★ 11096 ★ Addison H. Gibson Foundation

One PPG Place, Suite 2230
Pittsburgh, PA 15222
Phone: (412)261-1611 **Fax:** (412)261-5733
Email: ldunbar@gibson-fnd.org
Website: http://www.gibson-fnd.org
Lynn Dunbar, Assistant Director

Fnded: 1936. **Philosophy:** The foundation's primary interests are health care and higher education. It continues the tradition established by its founder of providing direct assistance on behalf of self-supporting individuals in need of medical care for which they, and their families, cannot afford. The foundation also operates an education loan fund, providing funds at low interest to college and graduate students who have successfully completed one or more full years of their studies. **Priorities:** *Education:* 59%. Supports educational loans. *International:* 41%. Makes grants to medical providers on behalf of individuals who have correctable medical conditions. **Typ. Recipients:** Children's Health/Hospitals, Clinics/Medical Centers, Eyes/Blindness, Health Funds, Health Organizations, Hospitals, Medical Education, Medical Rehabilitation, Medical Research, People with Disabilities, Public Health. **Geo. Dist:** only western Pennsylvania.

★ 11097 ★ Adolph Coors Foundation

4100 East Mississippi Ave., Suite 1850
Denver, CO 80246
Phone: (303)388-1636 **Fax:** (303)388-1684
Salley Rippey, Executive Director

Fnded: 1975. **Philosophy:** The foundation traditionally has funded a variety of organizations. In the area of health, emphasis has been on programs that are preventive in nature and that can demonstrate a reduction in health-care costs. Educational grants usually are directed to private independent four-year colleges and universities that do not receive a significant amount of tax-derived funding. Preservation of historic sites and buildings is funded when there is evidence that a facility will be used by a variety of organizations. Limited grants are made to cultural organizations for capital or special projects. Human service funding targets organizations that help people become self-sufficient and realize their potential. Distribution of the funds from Adolph Coors, Jr.'s, bequest are confined to Colorado. Limited foundation grants for activities outside Colorado were made possible in 1977 with a bequest from the estate of Gertrude Steele Coors. Most of the foundation's activities outside Colorado are directed to institutions and programs that endeavor to preserve and promote traditional values and the principles of a free-market economy. The foundation does not act on behalf of the Adolph Coors Company; nor does it engage in activities for the benefit of the company, its employees, or its distributors. **Priorities:** *Arts & Humanities:* 9%. Funds orchestra and music associations. *Civic & Public Affairs:* 10%. Includes grants to cultural institutions. *Education:* About 30%. Primarily precollege and higher education. *Environment:* 37%. Supports youth activities, community and human services. *International:* 12%. *Note:* Total contributions made in fiscal 1999. **Typ. Recipients:** AIDS/HIV, Children's Health/Hospitals, Clinics/Medical Centers, Domestic Violence, Emergency/Ambulance Services, Health Organizations, Hospitals, Medical Rehabilitation, Medical Research, Mental Health, Nursing Services, People with Disabilities, Preventive Medicine/Wellness Organizations, Public Health, Sexual Abuse, Single-Disease Health Associations, Substance Abuse. **Geo. Dist:** CO.

★ 11098 ★ Adrian and Jessie Archbold Charitable Trust

401 East 60th St., Suite 36B
New York, NY 10022
Phone: (212)371-1152 **Fax:** (212)753-9327
Myra Mahon, Director

Fnded: 1976. **Philosophy:** The trust makes most of its grants in the areas of education, health, and civic affairs. Educational funding favors religious education, colleges and universities, private academies, and law. Health support includes single disease associations, medical centers, health foundations, and hospitals. In civic affairs, interests include foundations and fellowship centers. Other recipient areas also are supported. **Priorities:** *Arts & Humanities:* 12%. Gives to museums, libraries, dance, theater, and music. *Civic & Public Affairs:* 15%. Supports public policy, parks, community development, farms, memorials, and botanical gardens. *Education:* 49%. Supports colleges and universities, scholarships, and medical education. *Environment:* 8%. Supports drug abuse, athletics, and children's organizations. *International:* 7%. Funds hospitals, medical centers, and single-disease health associations. *Religion:* 2%. *Note:* Total contributions made in fiscal 2000. **Typ. Recipients:** AIDS/HIV, Cancer, Children's Health/Hospitals, Clinics/Medical Centers, Emergency/Ambulance Services, Family Planning, Health Funds, Health Organizations, Health-General, Hospitals, Hospitals (University Affiliated), Medical Education, Medical Rehabilitation, Medical Research, Mental Health, People with Disabilities, Prenatal Health Issues, Public Health, Single-Disease Health Associations, Substance Abuse. **Geo. Dist:** NY, eastern United States.

★ 11099 ★ Agnes M. Lindsay Trust

660 Chestnut St.
Manchester, NH 03104
Phone: (603)669-1366 **Fax:** (603)665-8114
Email: admin@lindsaytrust.org
Website: http://www.lindsaytrust.org
Susan Bouchard, Administrative Director

Fnded: 1939. **Philosophy:** The Agnes M. Lindsay Trust supports colleges, universities, and private secondary schools through scholarship funds. It makes grants for capital needs to certain elementary and secondary schools, especially those schools that serve a special need (for example, to blind, deaf, or learning disabled children). In addition, the foundation supports a number of social welfare organizations, many of which work with special needs populations, health projects, children's hospitals, homes, and youth organizations. **Priorities:** *Arts & Humanities:* 7%. Supports cultural art. *Civic & Public Affairs:* 1%. Supports community affairs. *Education:* 36%. Supports colleges, universities, other educational insitutions, and programs. *Environment:* 44%. Supports YMCA, youth services, and family services. *International:* 15%. Supports hospitals and visiting nurses. *Note:* Contributions were made in 1999. **Typ. Recipients:** AIDS/HIV, Cancer, Children's Health/Hospitals, Clinics/Medical Centers, Domestic Violence, Eyes/Blindness, Geriatric Health, Health Organizations, Heart, Hospices, Hospitals, Long-Term Care, Medical Education, Medical Rehabilitation, Mental Health, Nursing Services, Outpatient Health Care, People with Disabilities, Prenatal Health Issues, Substance Abuse. **Geo. Dist:** ME; MA; NH; VT.

★ 11100 ★ Ahmanson Foundation

9215 Wilshire Boulevard
Beverly Hills, CA 90210
Phone: (310)278-0770 **Fax:** (310)278-4581
Lee Walcott, Jr., Vice President & Managing Director

Fnded: 1952. **Philosophy:** "The Foundation concentrates its funding on cultural projects supporting the arts, education at the collegiate and precollegiate levels, medicine and delivery of health care services, specialized library collections, programs related to homelessness and low-income populations, preservation of the environment, and a wide range of human service projects. The vast majority of the Foundation's philanthropy is directed toward organizations and institutions based in and serving the greater Los Angeles community. "Simultaneously, the Foundation is particularly committed to the support of non-profit organizations and institutions which continually demonstrate sound fiscal management, responsibility to efficient operation, and program integrity. "Through such focused interests and a shared vision with the non-profit sector the Foundation endeavors to increase the quality of life in Southern California and to enhance its cultural legacy." **Priorities:** *Arts & Humanities:* 28%. Funds art museums, collections management, film, performing arts, children's arts programs, public broadcasting, libraries, and historical societies. *Civic & Public Affairs:* Less than 1%. Gives to housing programs, minority affairs, community foundations, and police associations. *Education:* 37%. Supports universities and secondary schools; primary education and literacy programs; and religious and humanities education. *Environment:* 7%. Gives to youth organizations, shelters, food banks, family service agencies, and child mentoring programs. *International:* 21%. Funds medical research, hospital equipment, hospitals, psychiatric services, clinics, and dementia care. *Note:* Total contributions made in fiscal 2000. **Typ. Recipients:** Adolescent Health Issues, AIDS/HIV, Alzheimers Disease, Cancer, Children's Health/Hospitals, Clinics/Medical Centers, Domestic Violence, Emergency/Ambulance Services, Eyes/Blindness, Family Planning, Health Funds, Health Organizations, Heart, Hospitals, Long-Term Care, Medical Education, Medical Research, Mental Health, Multiple Sclerosis, Nursing Services, Outpatient Health Care, People with Disabilities, Prenatal Health Issues, Public Health, Research/Studies Institutes, Single-Disease Health Associations, Speech & Hearing, Substance Abuse, Trauma Treatment.

★ 11101 ★ Alavi Foundation

500 Fifth Ave., Suite 3900
New York, NY 10110
Phone: (212)944-8333 **Fax:** (212)921-0325
Dr. Mohammad Geramian, President

Fnded: 1973. **Philosophy:** The foundation makes most of its grants in the areas of education, religion, and international organizations. Educational funding favors Muslim and Islamic education, universities, and private schools. Other support goes to major American universities. Religious interests include mosques, temples, and religious centers. **Priorities:** *Civic & Public Affairs:* 6%. Supports ethnic Islamic organizations. *Education:* 53%. Supports Islamic education, language schools, and colleges and universities. *Environment:* Less than 1%. *International:* Less than 1%. *Note:* Total contributions were made in fiscal 2001. **Typ. Recipients:** Arthritis, Cancer, Children's Health/Hospitals, Eyes/Blindness, Health Organizations, Heart, Hospitals, Medical Education, Multiple Sclerosis, People with Disabilities, Single-Disease Health Associations, Transplant Networks/Donor Banks. **Geo. Dist:** internationally; nationally.

★ 11102 ★ Albert A. List Foundation

1328 Broadway, Suite 524, PMB 117
New York, NY 10001-2121
Phone: (212)631-0065 **Fax:** 888-826-1402
Email: listdn@earthlink.net
Website: http://fdncenter.org/grantmaker/listfdn
Vikki List, President

Fnded: 1953. **Philosophy:** The foundation supports three general focus areas: Democracy and Citizen Participation, Freedom of Expression; and New Problems/New Solutions. The Democracy and Citizen Participation program supports campaign finance reform, voter education and participation, confrontation of anti-democratic objectives, and projects that provide or encourage alternative visions for justice and democracy. The Freedom of Expression program supports organizations that protect the right of inquiry and expression or support strategies to ensure those freedoms. The New Problems/New Solutions program is meant to support groups working for social change that seek to address new challenges. **Priorities:** *Arts & Humanities:* 21% Supports museums, art organizations, public broadcasting, and the performing arts. *Civic & Public Affairs:* 51%. Supports "Democracy and Citizen Participation," with grants funding public policy, civil rights, women's groups, legal and justice issues, minority affairs, and media watchdog groups. *Education:* 4%. Funds education initiatives. *Environment:* 6%. Primarily supports family planning. *Note:* Total contributions made in 2000. **Typ. Recipients:** Clinics/Medical Centers, Family Planning, Long-Term Care, Public Health. **Geo. Dist:** nationally and regionally.

★ 11103 ★ Albert and Ethel Herzstein Charitable Foundation

6131 Westview
Houston, TX 77055
Phone: (713)681-7868 **Fax:** (713)681-3652
Email: albertandethel@herzsteinfoundation.org
Website: http://www.herzsteinfoundation.org
L. Hajtman, President

Fnded: 1965. **Philosophy:** The foundation gives to a variety of organizations in several fields, but the majority of its donations support education, civic and community, human services and health. **Priorities:** *Arts & Humanities:* 6%. Supports theater, ballet, public broadcasting, and historic preservation. *Civic & Public Affairs:* 34%. Gives to community foundations and civic programs. *Education:* 45%. Supports colleges and universities, Junior Achievement, and academies. *Environment:* 15%. Supports family and youth services, human services, and healthcare. *Note:* Total contributions made in 2001. **Typ. Recipients:** Adolescent Health Issues, AIDS/HIV, Alzheimers Disease, Cancer, Children's Health/Hospitals, Clinics/Medical Centers, Diabetes, Emergency/Ambulance Services, Eyes/Blindness, Health Organizations, Health-General, Heart, Hospitals, Medical Education, Medical Research, Mental Health, Multiple Sclerosis, People with Disabilities, Prenatal Health Issues, Respiratory, Single-Disease Health Associations, Substance Abuse. **Geo. Dist:** Houston, TX.

★ 11104 ★ Albert Pick, Jr. Fund

30 North Michigan Ave., Suite 1002
Chicago, IL 60602
Phone: (312)236-1192
Email: info@albertpickjrfund.org
Website: http://www.albertpickjrfund.org
Cleopatra Alexander, Executive Director

Fnded: 1947. **Philosophy:** The Albert Pick, Jr. Fund makes grants across the major categories of support.

In health and human services interests include programs in wellness, community-based health-care delivery, youth, family planning, or geriatric services. Also included is mental health, physical rehabilitation, and crisis care services. Funding for the arts goes to a wide spectrum of organizations, including public broadcasting, festivals, museums, and the performing arts. Educational support includes early childhood education and at-risk intervention, universities, and post-secondary institutions. Civic and community funding supports neighborhood development, environmental affairs, human relations, and minority rights. **Priorities:** *Arts & Humanities:* 11%. Museums, arts festivals, opera, theater, and performing arts. *Civic & Public Affairs:* 29%. Public interest, housing, zoos, and foundations. *Education:* 26%. Educational programs, learning centers, literacy, career training, and schools. *Environment:* 19%. Youth and family concerns, YMCA/YWCA, shelters and senior services. *International:* 9%. Health centers, hospitals and hospice. *Note:* Total contributions made in 2000. **Typ. Recipients:** AIDS/HIV, Children's Health/Hospitals, Clinics/Medical Centers, Domestic Violence, Emergency/Ambulance Services, Family Planning, Health Organizations, Hospices, Hospitals, Long-Term Care, Medical Training, People with Disabilities, Prenatal Health Issues, Preventive Medicine/Wellness Organizations, Public Health, Sexual Abuse, Single-Disease Health Associations, Substance Abuse. **Geo. Dist:** Chicago, IL.

★ 11105 ★ Alex Hillman Family Foundation

630 Fifth Ave., Room 2604
New York, NY 10111
Phone: (212)265-3115 **Fax:** (212)765-3134
Rita Hillman, President

Fnded: 1966. **Philosophy:** The Alex Hillman Family Foundation makes most of its grants in the areas of arts and education. The foundation's major priority is funding the arts. Interests include museums, music academies, film, and public broadcasting. Educational funding supports nursing schools. **Priorities:** *Arts & Humanities:* 8%. Supports music, museum of art, public broadcasting and film and video. *Civic & Public Affairs:* 1%. *Education:* 49%. Supports medical education, nursing education, and universities. *International:* 6%. Supports hospital, health organizations, and cancer research. *Note:* Total contributions made in 2000. **Typ. Recipients:** Emergency/Ambulance Services, Health Organizations, Heart, Hospices, Hospitals, Medical Education, Nursing Services, People with Disabilities. **Geo. Dist:** New York, NY, metropolitan area.

★ 11106 ★ Alex and Marie Manoogian Foundation

21001 Van Born Rd.
Taylor, MI 48180
Phone: (313)274-8799
Eugene Gargaro, Jr., Secretary & Director

Fnded: 1942. **Philosophy:** The foundation is very active in the affairs of the Armenian community in the United States. Grants generally are made to Armenian social service organizations and Armenian religious and educational institutions. Funding also is directed to other institutions and organizations in higher and private secondary education, as well as arts organizations. **Priorities:** *Arts & Humanities:* Less then 1%. Supports cultural association. *Civic & Public Affairs:* Less than 1%. Funds ethnic groups. *Education:* Less than 1%. Funds colleges and universities. *International:* 3%. Funds a health center. *Note:* Total contributions made in 2000. **Typ. Recipients:** Cancer, Hospitals, Medical Education, People with Disabilities, Public Health, Substance Abuse. **Geo. Dist:** nationally.

★ 11107 ★ Alexander and Margaret Stewart Trust

Brawner Bldg., Suite 210
888 17th St. Northwest
Washington, DC 20006-3313
Phone: (202)785-9892 **Fax:** (202)785-0918
Doris Lustine, Executive Secretary

Fnded: 1951. **Philosophy:** "The Alexander and Margaret Stewart Trust makes grants to organizations, primarily in Washington, D.C., that provide care or treatment for those suffering from cancer or childhood afflictions." "Cancer: Under the will of Mary E. Stewart, the Trustees entertain grant applications for care and treatment of people afflicted with cancer. The Trust occasionally may fund the purchase of equipment used in cancer diagnosis and treatment. It rarely funds the education of students or doctors engaged in cancer research. The Trust is supporting research of emerging cancer therapies, but does not accept proposals for such research, working instead with experts to fund research at selected institutions." "Child Health: Under the will of Helen S. Devore, grants are made for the care of children who are physically or mentally ill or handicapped, and for research, education, or prevention of diseases common to early childhood. This includes societal behavioral patterns that have a negative impact on the welfare of children." "The Trustees welcome evidence that a requested program has ongoing community support and acceptance before funding is considered and will consider funding start-up costs (not 'planning' projects) for a new program with the intention that the donee organization will continue the program using alternate sources of funding. Programs aiding the economically deprived are favored." 1997 Application Guidelines **Priorities:** *Education:* 13%. Supports universitys. *Environment:* 6%. Supports community services organizations, family planning, child welfare, and people with disabilities. *International:* 81%. Supports trust solicited cancer research, cancer care, and hospices. **Typ. Recipients:** Cancer, Child Abuse, Children's Health/Hospitals, Clinics/Medical Centers, Eyes/Blindness, Family Planning, Health Organizations, Health-General, Hospices, Hospitals, Long-Term Care, Medical Education, Mental Health, Nursing Services, People with Disabilities, Prenatal Health Issues, Single-Disease Health Associations. **Geo. Dist:** Washington, DC, metropolitan area.

★ 11108 ★ Alfred I. duPont Foundation

4600 Touchton Rd. East, Bldg. 200, Suite 120
Jacksonville, FL 32246
Phone: (904)232-4123
Rosemary Wills, Director

Fnded: 1936. **Philosophy:** The Alfred I. duPont Foundation makes most of its grants in the areas of education, social services, and the arts. Educational funding favors medical and religious education and college funds. Social service funding favors homes, while the support for the arts focuses on galleries and preservation societies. The foundation will also support health services, civic affairs, and churches. **Priorities:** *Arts & Humanities:* 12%. Supports museums, historical preservation, and music. *Civic & Public Affairs:* 11%. Supports law and justice, gardens, and parks. *Education:* 42%. Supports education funds and associations, and colleges and universities. *Environment:* 11%. Supports homes, services for the elderly, and scouting. *International:* 16%. Supports medical research. *Note:* Total contributions made in 2001. **Typ. Recipients:** Alzheimers Disease, Arthritis, Children's Health/Hospitals, Clinics/Medical Centers, Emergency/Ambulance Services, Health Organizations, Hospices, Long-Term Care, Medical Education, Medical Rehabilitation, Multiple Sclerosis, Nursing Services, People with Disabilities, Public Health, Single-Disease Health Associations. **Geo. Dist:** southeastern United States; FL.

★ 11109 ★ Alfred Jurzykowski Foundation

15 East 65th St.
New York, NY 10021
Phone: (212)535-8930
Bluma Cohen, Executive Director & Vice President

Fnded: 1960. **Philosophy:** The foundation supports projects and programs in Poland and Brazil. Many types of U.S. tax-exempt organizations receive support. Interests include the disabled, child welfare, community service organizations, and family planning. **Priorities:** *Arts & Humanities:* 7%. Supports public libraries, theater, art museum, and orchestra society. *Civic & Public Affairs:* 6%. Support given to civic and public policy organizations. *Education:* 19%. Funds educational programs with an international focus. *Environment:* 10%. Funds youth programs, the homeless, Big Brothers and Big Sisters, and food for the poor. *Note:* Total contributions made in 2000. **Typ. Recipients:** AIDS/HIV, Cancer, Children's Health/Hospitals, Clinics/Medical Centers, Family Planning, Health Organizations, Home-Care Services, Hospices, Hospitals, Medical Education, People with Disabilities. **Geo. Dist:** New York, NY, metropolitan area.

★ 11110 ★ Alfred P. Sloan Foundation

630 Fifth Ave., Suite 2550
New York, NY 10111
Phone: (212)649-1649 **Fax:** (212)757-5117
Website: http://www.sloan.org
Ralph Gomory, President

Fnded: 1934. **Philosophy:** The foundation's main interests and programs are concentrated primarily in five categories: science and technology, including the areas of fellowships, direct support of research, and the history of science and technology; standard of living and economic performance, including the areas of industries, nonprofit sectors, the university as a system and the system of universities, assessment of government performance, and the family and the workplace; education and careers in science and technology, including the areas of careers, the scientific and technical work force, immigration of scientists and engineers, learning outside the classroom, public understanding of science and technology, underrepresented minorities, women, and retention; selected national issues; and civic projects. Science and Technology are major interests of the foundation. Programs include fellowships, direct support of research, and the history of science and technology. Sloan Research Fellowships are granted in the areas of economics, chemistry, mathematics, neuroscience, computer science, and physics. The fellowships are made to stimulate fundamental research by young scholars of outstanding promise at a time in their careers when other support may be difficult to secure. The foundation makes a number of grants that focus on molecular studies of evolution. Grants support research projects, scientific conferences, and workshops designed to introduce the study of evolution into the research agendas of molecular biologists. Postdoctoral fellowships are awarded to young scientists interested in developing the interdisciplinary skills necessary for conducting molecular research on evolution. Another program area is Education and Careers in Science and Technology. Programs in this area strengthen science and engineering education and increase interest in these fields. Issues of main concern include career choice, developing student interests, learning outside the classroom, and increasing public understanding. The foundation also funds programs that involve selected national issues. It attempts to contribute to other major national issues including drug abuse, energy and the environment, and traditional civic programs that benefit the city of New York. **Priorities:** *Arts & Humanities:* 16%. Funding is awarded to film institutes, public broadcasting, and theater. *Civic & Public Affairs:* 18%. Supports standard of living and economic performance, public policy centers, selected national issues, community foundations, and an aquarium. *Education:* 62%. Supports educational programs and institutions focused on careers in science and technology. Funds fellowships in chemistry, computer science, economics, mathematics, neuroscience, and physics. *Environment:* 3%. Supports research on the effects of women working in families. Also funds child advocacy and parenting programs. *Religion:* 1%. Contributes to marine science and other scientific research. Provides substantial support to the National Academy of Sciences. *Note:* Total contributions made in 2001. **Typ. Recipients:** AIDS/HIV, Domestic Violence, Health Policy/Cost Containment, Medical Education, Medical Research, Public Health, Research/Studies Institutes, Substance Abuse. **Geo. Dist:** nationally.

★ 11111 ★ Allegheny Foundation
One Oxford Center
301 Grant St., Suite 3900
Pittsburgh, PA 15219-6401
Phone: (412)392-2900
Website: http://www.scaife.com
Joanne Beyer, President

Fnded: 1953. **Philosophy:** The foundation reports that it "confines most of its grant awards to programs for historic preservation, civic development, education, youth development, and animal welfare." Although the foundation makes grants to local chapters of national organizations for programs which benefit the local economy, preference is shown for locally based and operated organizations and programs. **Priorities:** *Arts & Humanities:* 22%. Museums, theater, and historical societies. *Civic & Public Affairs:* 54%. Public policy, economic development, and community services. *Education:* 15%. Supports educational funds and associations. *Environment:* 15%. Youth organizations and animal welfare. *Note:* Total contributions made in 2001. **Typ. Recipients:** Cancer, Medical Education, People with Disabilities. **Geo. Dist:** PA, including western Pennsylvania.

★ 11112 ★ Alletta Morris McBean Charitable Trust
400 S El Camino Real, Suite 777
San Mateo, CA 94402
Phone: (650)558-8480 **Fax:** (650)558-8481
Email: mcbeancharitabletrust@att.net
Charlene Kleiner, Assistant Secretary

Fnded: 1986. **Philosophy:** The trustees give special attention to organizations whose charitable activities are focused on the City of Newport, Rhode Island, and Aquidneck Island, Rhode Island, and are designed to enhance the quality of life in and to perpetuate the history of the City of Newport and Aquidneck Island. **Priorities:** *Arts & Humanities:* 22%. Focuses funding on historic preservation projects. Also funds museums and libraries. *Civic & Public Affairs:* 3%. Funds community foundations and commissions, economic development, and aquariums. *Education:* 23%. Supports universities and public and private schools. *Environment:* 4%. Supports youth organizations, services for seniors, and humane societies. *International:* 27%. Funds donor banks, hospitals, and nursing services. *Note:* Total contributions made in 2000. **Typ. Recipients:** Emergency/Ambulance Services, Health-General, Home-Care Services, Hospices, Hospitals, Mental Health, Nursing Services. **Geo. Dist:** Aquidneck Island, RI; Newport, RI.

★ 11113 ★ Alsam Foundation
50 South LaSalle St., Suite L-5
Chicago, IL 60603-1006
Phone: (208)854-0414 **Fax:** (208)854-0415
George Moosman, President

Fnded: 1984. **Philosophy:** The foundation typically funds scholarship programs, religious concerns, arts organizations, health causes, and civic and community affairs projects. **Priorities:** *Arts & Humanities:* Less than 1%. Supports public broadcasting. *Education:* 59%. Supports scholarships, colleges and universities, and medical education. *Environment:* 1%. Funds youth organizations, animal protection, and child welfare. *International:* 35%. Funds clinics and medical research. *Note:* Total contributions made in fiscal 2001. **Typ. Recipients:** Arthritis, Cancer, Medical Education, Medical Research, Research/Studies Institutes, Single-Disease Health Associations. **Geo. Dist:** CO; UT.

★ 11114 ★ Altman Foundation
521 Fifth Ave., 35th Fl.
New York, NY 10175-3599
Phone: (212)682-0970
Karen Rosa, Vice President & Executive Director

Fnded: 1913. **Philosophy:** "In carrying out its mission, the Altman Foundation seeks to strengthen communities and enhance the well-being of all New Yorkers. The Foundation's grants support programs and institutions that enrich the quality of life within the five boroughs of New York City, with a particular interest in initiatives that help individuals, families and communities benefit from the services and opportunities that will enable them to achieve their full potential." 1997 Guidelines Brochure **Priorities:** *Arts & Humanities:* 14%. Programs that extend the benefit of the arts through established and meaningful organizations and institutions, including programs identifying and providing pre-professional-level training to youngsters in specific art disciplines. *Civic & Public Affairs:* 4%. Funds botanical gardens and community foundations. *Education:* 23%. Independent and non-public primary and secondary schools, colleges and universities with interest in scholarships and access programs for promising disadvantaged students. *Environment:* 20%. Social Welfare programs developing long-term solutions that strengthen communities. *International:* 21%. Voluntary hospitals, health centers and programs in the health field that focus on improving access to services and providing assistance to those in need of special care. *Religion:* 3%. Supports computer and math programs. *Note:* Total contributions were made in 2000. **Typ. Recipients:** AIDS/HIV, Cancer, Child Abuse, Children's Health/Hospitals, Clinics/Medical Centers, Domestic Violence, Emergency/Ambulance Services, Eyes/Blindness, Geriatric Health, Health Funds, Health Organizations, Health Policy/Cost Containment, Home-Care Services, Hospitals, Medical Education, Mental Health, Outpatient Health Care, People with Disabilities, Prenatal Health Issues, Preventive Medicine/Wellness Organizations, Public Health. **Geo. Dist:** NY, focusing on the five boroughs of New York City.

★ 11115 ★ Amateur Athletic Foundation of Los Angeles
2141 West Adams Boulevard
Los Angeles, CA 90018
Phone: (323)730-4600 **Fax:** (323)730-4637
Email: info@aafla.org
Website: http://www.aafla.org
Carmen Zimmerle, Executive Assistant

Fnded: 1984. **Philosophy:** The Amateur Athletic Foundation's mission is to promote and enhance youth sports in Southern California and to increase the knowledge of sports and its impact on people's lives. The Foundation grants awards to youth sports organizations within the eight southern most counties of CA and conducts youth sports and coaching education programs. The current objectives of the foundation's board of directors encourage grant making to organizations that provide ongoing, structured youth programs combining the essential elements of teaching, learning, and competition. **Priorities:** *Civic & Public Affairs:* 2%. Funds community center, community groups, and ethnic affairs. *Education:* 7%. Gives to colleges, universities, an education foundation, and school athletic programs. *Environment:* 91%. Funds youth athletic programs and equipment. *Note:* Total contributions made in 2000. **Typ. Recipients:** Children's Health/Hospitals, Clinics/Medical Centers, People with Disabilities. **Geo. Dist:** CA, Imperial County; CA, Los Angeles County; CA, Orange County; CA, Riverside County; CA, San Bernadino County; CA, San Diego County; CA, Santa Barbara County; CA, Ventura County.

★ 11116 ★ The Ambrose Monell Foundation
1 Rockefeller Plaza, Suite 301
New York, NY 10020
Phone: (212)586-0700 **Fax:** (212)245-1863
Email: info@monellvetlesen.org
Website: http://www.monellvetlesen.org/monell/default.htm
George Rowe, Jr., President

Fnded: 1952. **Philosophy:** The foundation was set up to help improve "the physical, mental, and moral condition of humanity throughout the world." It pursues this goal by supporting health, the arts, education, social services, science, and civic causes. **Priorities:** *Arts & Humanities:* 15%. Supports public broadcasting, opera, ballet, libraries, symphonies, and museums. *Civic & Public Affairs:* 13%. Public policy groups, a botanical garden, and legal aid causes. *Education:* 29%. Focus on higher education. *Environment:* Approx. 1%. *International:* 34%. Includes the highest grant to the Monell Ohem Senior Center in Philadelphia, PA. Also supports hospitals, medical research, and single-disease health associations. *Religion:* 6%. Supports an earth observatory and research. *Note:* Total contributions made in 2000. **Typ. Recipients:** AIDS/HIV, Alzheimers Disease, Arthritis, Cancer, Clinics/Medical Centers, Clinics/Medical Centers, Emergency/Ambulance Services, Eyes/Blindness, Geriatric Health, Health-General, Hospitals, Hospitals (University Affiliated), Medical Education, Medical Rehabilitation, Medical Research, Mental Health, Public Health, Research/Studies Institutes, Respiratory, Speech & Hearing. **Geo. Dist:** nationally; New York, NY, metropolitan area.

★ 11117 ★ Amelia Peabody Charitable Fund
1 Hollis St.
Wellesley, MA 02482-4631
Phone: (781)237-6468
Website: http://www.ameliapeabody.org
Margaret St. Clair, Trustee

Fnded: 1942. **Philosophy:** The purpose of the Amelia Peabody Charitable Fund is to assist local charitable and educational organizations, with emphasis on hospitals, cultural programs, education institutions, and conservation groups. **Priorities:** *Arts & Humanities:* 3%. Primary support for museums and libraries. *Civic & Public Affairs:* 12%. Supports public policy, job training, ethnic organizations, and community development. *Education:* 26%. Supports public and charter schools, learning centers, and special education. *Environment:* 48%. Supports YMCA, shelters, recreation, family services, and youth organizations. *International:* 7%. Focus is on hospitals, single-disease associations, pediatric health, and medical research. *Religion:* Less than 1%. *Note:* Total contributions made in 2000. **Typ. Recipients:** Alzheimers Disease, Arthritis, Cancer, Children's Health/Hospitals, Clinics/Medical Centers, Diabetes, Emergency/Ambulance Services, Eyes/Blindness, Family Planning, Geriatric Health, Health Organizations, Health-General, Heart, Home-Care Services, Hospitals, Long-Term Care, Medical Education, Medical Research, Medical Training, Nursing Services, People with Disabilities, Prenatal Health Issues, Public Health, Single-Disease Health Associations, Speech & Hearing, Substance Abuse. **Geo. Dist:** New England; Boston, MA, metropolitan area.

★ 11118 ★ Amelia Peabody Foundation
One Hollis St., Suite 215
Wellesley, MA 02482
Phone: (781)237-6468 **Fax:** (781)237-5014
Email: jsmith@ameliapeabody.org
Website: http://www.ameliapeabody.org
Margaret St. Clair, Co-Managing Trustee

Fnded: 1985. **Philosophy:** "The primary mission of the Amelia Peabody Foundation is to increase the number, range, and depth of positive learning experiences available to materially disadvantaged young people living in the cities and towns of Massachusetts." **Priorities:** *Arts & Humanities:* 1%. Supports museums and theaters. *Civic & Public Affairs:* 8%. Supports public policy, community foundations, towns and municipalities, and housing. *Education:* 36%. Supports arts/humanities education, legal education, schools, and universities. *Environment:* 30%. Supports Young Men's Christian AssociationA, youth programs, recreation/athletics, and emergency relief. *International:* 22%. Funds public health and medical centers. *Note:* Total contributions made in 2000. **Typ. Recipients:** Clinics/Medical Centers, Diabetes, Emergency/Ambulance Services, Health Organizations, Hospitals, Medical Education, Medical Research, People with Disabilities, Public Health, Single-Disease Health Associations, Substance Abuse. **Geo. Dist:** MA.

★ 11119 ★ American Foundation Corp.
720 National City Bank Bldg.
Cleveland, OH 44114
Phone: (216)241-6664 **Fax:** (216)241-6693
Barb Lattner, Treasurer

Fnded: 1974. **Philosophy:** The American Foundation Corporation makes most of its grants in the areas of civic affairs, education, the arts, and social services. In civic affairs, interests include an arboretum, conservation and environmental affairs, and wildlife resources. Educational funding favors private academies, colleges and universities, and technical education. Support for the arts goes to art associations and institutes, the performing arts, and museums. Social service funding includes child welfare, youth organizations, and animal protection. The foundation also supports other recipient areas. **Priorities:** *Arts & Humanities:* 30%. Major support for a library; also supports museums. *Civic & Public Affairs:* 12%. Supports parks, gardens, municipalities, neighborhood organizations, fire departments, and zoos. *Education:* 28%. Supports colleges, universities, secondary schools, and education organizations. *Environment:* 14%. Funds animal protection, women's organizations, camps, and family planning services. *International:* 10%. Supports hospitals, nursing, and clinics. *Note:* Total contributions made in 2000. **Typ. Recipients:** Cancer, Children's Health/Hospitals, Clinics/Medical Centers, Emergency/Ambulance Services, Family Planning, Heart, Hospices, Hospitals, Hospitals (University Affiliated), Long-Term Care, Medical Education, Medical Rehabilitation, Mental Health, Nursing Services, People with Disabilities. **Geo. Dist:** nationally; OH.

★ 11120 ★ Amon G. Carter Foundation
PO Box 1036
Fort Worth, TX 76101-1036
Phone: (817)332-2783 **Fax:** (817)332-2787
Email: jrobinson@agcf.org
Website: http://www.agcf.org
John Robinson, Grant Administrator-Exec. Vice Pres.

Fnded: 1945. **Philosophy:** The foundation supports visual and performing arts, education, health, and social services in Fort Worth and Tarrant County, Texas. Current board policy allocates half of annual grant funds to the Amon Carter Museum for general support and acquisitions. Remaining funds are used for the general grant program. Support for education includes primary and secondary education, both public and private. Grants are also made to colleges and universities located in Texas. Contributions in the health field are made to hospitals and to local and national single-disease health organizations. Social service grants emphasize programs that benefit youth, the aged, and the disabled. Recipients include a variety of youth organizations, recreation facilities, homes, and shelters. The foundation provides limited support to civic groups, including police and fire fighter associations, several Fort Worth parks and gardens, and the city zoo. **Priorities:** *Arts & Humanities:* 81%. Provides major support to the Amon Carter Museum of art; also supports performing arts centers, music, theater, and dance. *Civic & Public Affairs:* 4%. Gives to housing, urban development, and community foundations. *Education:* 8%. Funds private/parochial schools, colleges and universities, and scholarship funds. *Environment:* 3%. Supports Boys & Girls clubs, recreation programs, homeless, family services and the hungry. *International:* 3%. Supports hospitals, medical centers, medical research, blood centers, and nursing homes. *Note:* Total contributions made in 2000. **Typ. Recipients:** AIDS/HIV, Alzheimers Disease, Cancer, Children's Health/Hospitals, Clinics/Medical Centers, Diabetes, Emergency/Ambulance Services, Family Planning, Health Organizations, Health Policy/Cost Containment, Hospices, Hospitals, Hospitals (University Affiliated), Medical Education, Medical Rehabilitation, Medical Research, Mental Health, Nursing Services, People with Disabilities, Prenatal Health Issues, Public Health, Research/Studies Institutes, Respiratory, Single-Disease Health Associations, Substance Abuse, Transplant Networks/Donor Banks. **Geo. Dist:** Fort Worth, TX, including Tarrant County.

★ 11121 ★ Andersen Foundation
100 4th Ave., North
Bayport, MN 55003-1096
Phone: (651)642-5150 **Fax:** (651)430-5537
Mary Gillstrom, Assistant Secretary

Fnded: 1959. **Philosophy:** The foundation traditionally contributes a significant portion of its funding to education, with emphasis on assisting private colleges who do not accept state and federal funds and local medical projects. **Priorities:** *Civic & Public Affairs:* 4%. *Education:* 55%. Supports private colleges and universities. *Environment:* 9%. Supports scouts and youth and family services. *International:* 24%. Supports hospitals and medical centers. *Note:* Total contributions made in 2000. **Typ. Recipients:** Cancer, Children's Health/Hospitals, Clinics/Medical Centers, Domestic Violence, Emergency/Ambulance Services, Eyes/Blindness, Health Funds, Health Organizations, Heart, Hospices, Hospitals, Kidney, Medical Research, Mental Health, People with Disabilities, Research/Studies Institutes, Single-Disease Health Associations, Substance Abuse. **Geo. Dist:** nationally; MN.

★ 11122 ★ Andrew W. Mellon Foundation
140 East 62nd St.
New York, NY 10021
Phone: (212)838-8400 **Fax:** (212)888-4172
Website: http://www.mellon.org
Michele Warman, General Counsel & Secretary

Fnded: 1969. **Philosophy:** The purpose of the foundation is to "aid and promote such religious, charitable, scientific, literary, and educational purposes as may be in the furtherance of the public welfare or tend to promote the well-doing or well-being of mankind." The foundation currently makes grants on a selective basis in the areas of higher education; culture and the performing arts; population; conservation and the environment; and certain areas of public affairs. It has eliminated its support of public health care. The foundation's overriding interest continues to be in education and is strongly focused on higher education. It includes support for libraries, research institutes, and publishing endeavors that are a part of higher education. Grants to universities stress faculty development in several ways. The foundation makes grants to encourage outstanding minority students to pursue doctoral degrees in humanities. In addition, the foundation funds other new approaches to graduate education in the arts and sciences. In the field of conservation and the environment, the foundation supports research on issues relating to energy, natural resources including ground water and the oceans, global systems, and toxic waste. The foundation "looks for ways to fill gaps in the understanding of basic processes, to encourage good ideas, to provide bridging funds for good programs with temporary financial problems, and to encourage new lines of research." Institution-building and the training of young scientists are priorities. The foundation has a continuing interest in the field of population. It supports organizations that conduct research or provide technical assistance to family-planning programs. It also funds research on contraceptives. It would like to see more emphasis placed on the value of research as a guide to grant making. The foundation expects to continue funding for library automation projects, especially through consortia of libraries, publishers, and others concerned with scholarly communication. **Priorities:** *Arts & Humanities:* 16%. Funds museums, art conservation, the performing arts, libraries, dance, and arts festivals. *Civic & Public Affairs:* 1%. Population issues and public affairs programs receive funding. *Education:* 55%. Primarily supports institutions of higher learning and scholarship/fellowship programs. *Note:* Total contributions made in 2001. **Typ. Recipients:** Family Planning, Medical Education, Medical Research, Public Health. **Geo. Dist:** nationally.

★ 11123 ★ The Andy Warhol Foundation for the Visual Arts
65 Bleecker St., 7th Fl.
New York, NY 10012
Phone: (212)387-7555 **Fax:** (212)387-7560
Email: info@warholfoundation.org
Website: http://www.warholfoundation.org
Pamela Clapp, Program Director

Fnded: 1987. **Philosophy:** The foundation's mission is the "advancement of the visual arts." According to the foundation's statement of purpose, the visual arts include painting, sculpture, printmaking, photography, film, video, decorative arts, and art publishing. The foundation's objective is to "foster innovative expression and the creative process by encouraging and supporting cultural organizations that in turn, directly or indirectly, support artists and their work... The foundation is focused primarily on supporting work of a challenging and often experimental nature, while noting that the interpretation of those terms may vary from place to place and culture to culture." The foundation will only consider proposals from performing arts groups (dance, theater, and music groups) for specific aspects of their activity that incorporate the visual arts in their performances. Grants are awarded to curatorial programs at museums, artists' organizations, and other cultural organizations in the United States and abroad to assist in the innovative presentation of the visual arts with an emphasis on projects that cultivate new, expanded, and diverse audiences. Projects may include exhibitions, catalogs, audience development, and other organizational activities directly related to these areas. This category also supports the work of choreographers and performing artists where the visual arts are an inherent element of the production. The historic preservation program awards grants to organizations seeking to preserve and enhance historic buildings, districts, and landscapes, and to organizations seeking to increase public participation in the urban planning process. In addition to its grant making, the foundation has worked with the DIA Center for the Arts and the Carnegie Institute to establish the Andy Warhol Museum in Pittsburgh, PA–the artist's hometown. The foundation has provided the museum with art work and archival material for its permanent collection. The foundation has also supported the museum with grants. The foundation does not fund exhibitions or other activities relating to Andy Warhol's work. **Priorities:** *Arts & Humanities:* 100%. Supports visual arts, curatorial programs, and historic preservation and historic restoration. *Note:* Total contributions made in fiscal 2001. **Typ. Recipients:** AIDS/HIV. **Geo. Dist:** nationally.

★ 11124 ★ Animal Assistance Foundation
455 Sherman St., Suite 462
Denver, CO 80203
Phone: (303)744-4405 **Fax:** (303)744-7065
Email: info@aaf-fd.org
Website: http://www.aaf-fd.org
David Gies, Executive Director

Fnded: 1975. **Philosophy:** The Animal Assistance Foundation is a nonprofit organization dedicated to domestic pet population control and to the enhancement of animal welfare through charitable, scientific, and educational means. This will be accomplished by providing leadership on animal welfare issues, assuring the continuing operation of the Harrison Memorial Animal Hospital, contributing funds and other assistance to animal welfare organizations, and supporting veterinary, scientific, and social domestic pet research. **Priorities:** *Environment:* 100%. Provides support for pet population control, research, and humane education. All grants relate in some way to helping companion animals. *Note:* Total contributions made in fiscal 2001. **Typ. Recipients:** AIDS/HIV, Domestic Violence, Substance Abuse. **Geo. Dist:** CO.

★ 11125 ★ Ann Jackson Family Foundation
PO Box 5580
Santa Barbara, CA 93150
Phone: (805)969-2258 **Fax:** (805)969-0315

Fnded: 1978. **Philosophy:** The Ann Jackson Family Foundation gives to charities and services which "foster religious, charitable, educational, and scientific purposes and to organizations which promote the prevention of cruelty to children and animals." **Priorities:** *Arts & Humanities:* 16%. Historic preservation and art museums. *Civic & Public Affairs:* 13%. Botanic and zoological gardens, and community foundations. *Education:* 28%. Secondary schools. *Environment:* 28%. Youth and family services. *International:* 13%. A Mental health associations, hospitals, and health centers. *Note:* Total contributions made in fiscal 2001. **Typ. Recipients:** Cancer, Clinics/Medical Centers, Emergency/Ambulance Services, Eyes/Blindness, Family Planning, Family Planning, Geriatric Health, Health Organizations, Heart, Hospitals, Medical Rehabilitation, Medical Research, Mental Health, Multiple Sclerosis, Nursing Services, People with Disabilities, Prenatal Health Issues, Respiratory, Substance Abuse. **Geo. Dist:** Santa Barbara, CA, and surrounding areas.

★ 11126 ★ Annenberg Foundation

St. Davids Center, Suite A-200
150 Radnor-Chester Rd.
Saint Davids, PA 19087
Phone: (610)341-9066 **Fax:** (610)964-8688
Email: info@annenbergfoundation.org
Website: http://www.annenbergfoundation.org
Dr. Gail Levin, Executive Director

Fnded: 1989. **Philosophy:** The Annenberg Foundation believes that there is nothing more important than the quality of K-12 education in determining how productive and fulfilling the future will be for America's young people and for society as a whole. Through the Annenberg Challenge grant–its $500 million program in support of systemic public school reform–the foundation and its partner organizations and school districts work to promote school reform nationwide. The Challenge provides 18 matching grants for urban, rural, and arts-centered school reform programs, which are tailored to the needs of individual schools. Serving more than 1.3 million students in largely disadvantaged schools, the Challenge is the largest public/private partnership for school reform in the history of American public education. The Annenberg Foundation's investment in the Challenge program, which was first announced in December 1993, will conclude in 2002. (Additional details about the Challenge sites may be found on the Foundation's web page.) In addition to the Challenge, The Annenberg Foundation still focuses on primary and secondary education, but also has interests in the areas of arts and culture, health care, civic causes, and international institutions. **Priorities:** *Arts & Humanities:* 28%. Historical preservation, and public broadcasting. *Education:* 54%. K-12 education, including curriculum improvement, professional development, and arts education. Counseling and mentoring and parent education and involvement are also priorities. *Environment:* 2%. *International:* 16%. *Note:* Total contributions made in fiscal 2001. **Typ. Recipients:** Cancer, Children's Health/Hospitals, Clinics/Medical Centers, Emergency/Ambulance Services, Family Planning, Health Funds, Health Organizations, Hospitals, Medical Education, Medical Research, Mental Health, Nursing Services, People with Disabilities, Preventive Medicine/Wellness Organizations, Research/Studies Institutes, Substance Abuse. **Geo. Dist:** nationally.

★ 11127 ★ Annie E. Casey Foundation

Care of Office of the President
701 Saint Paul St.
Baltimore, MD 21202
Phone: (410)547-6600 **Fax:** (410)547-6624
Website: http://www.aecf.org

Fnded: 1948. **Philosophy:** "In general, the grant making of the Annie E. Casey Foundation is limited to initiatives that have significant potential to demonstrate innovative policy, service delivery, and community supports for children and families. The challenge of helping rebuild distressed communities is at the center of the Annie E. Casey Foundation's grantmaking plans for the next decade. Working with neighborhoods and state and local governments, the Foundation will provide significant grants and other forms of assistance to a limited number of sites in a long-term effort to strengthen the support services, social networks, physical infrastructure, employment, self-determination, and economic vitality of distressed communities. The Foundation's work is divided into three areas: 1. Improving Major Systems Serving Disadvantaged Children and Families 2. Transforming Neighborhoods 3. Promoting Accountability and Innovation." The Annie E. Casey Foundation web site: *Major Foundation Initiatives* **Priorities:** *Civic & Public Affairs:* 36%. Focus on Baltimore. *Education:* 6%. Public schools and education reform, emphasis on urban areas. *Environment:* 52%. Supports social services programs and the Casey family services program. *International:* 6%. Health care and mental health. *Note:* Total contributions made in 1999. **Typ. Recipients:** Children's Health/Hospitals, Clinics/Medical Centers, Clinics/Medical Centers, Family Planning, Health Organizations, Health Policy/Cost Containment, Hospitals, Medical Education, Mental Health, Nutrition, People with Disabilities, Prenatal Health Issues, Preventive Medicine/Wellness Organizations, Public Health, Substance Abuse. **Geo. Dist:** nationally.

★ 11128 ★ Anschutz Family Foundation

555 17th St., Suite 2400
Denver, CO 80202
Phone: (303)293-2338 **Fax:** (303)299-1235
Website: http://www.anschutzfamilyfoundation.org
Sue Anschutz-Rodgers, President & Executive Director

Fnded: 1982. **Philosophy:** " The Anschutz Family Foundation supports Colorado nonprofit organizations that assist people to help themselves while nurturing and preserving their self-respect. The Foundation encourages endeavors that strengthen families and communities and advance individuals to become productive and responsible citizens. There is a special interest in self-sufficiency, community development, and programs aimed at the economically disadvantaged, the young, the elderly, and the disabled. The Foundation is also dedicated to funding efforts in rural Colorado." 2001 Annual Report **Priorities:** *Arts & Humanities:* 8%. Supports arts outreach, the performing arts, and historical preservation. *Civic & Public Affairs:* 23%. Supports capacity building, community foundations, public policy, economic and community development, and self-sufficiency initiatives. *Education:* 4%. Supports educational foundations, literacy, public and charter schools, and colleges. *Environment:* 62%. Funds youth organizations, early childhood development, senior services, services for the disabled, homeless shelters, food programs, family services, crime prevention, women's issues, humane societies, and outdoor programs. *Note:* Total contributions made in fiscal 2001. **Typ. Recipients:** AIDS/HIV, Alzheimers Disease, Cancer, Children's Health/Hospitals, Clinics/Medical Centers, Domestic Violence, Emergency/Ambulance Services, Family Planning, Geriatric Health, Health Organizations, Heart, Home-Care Services, Hospices, Hospitals, Medical Rehabilitation, Medical Research, Mental Health, Multiple Sclerosis, Nursing Services, People with Disabilities, Preventive Medicine/Wellness Organizations, Public Health, Research/Studies Institutes, Single-Disease Health Associations, Substance Abuse, Trauma Treatment. **Geo. Dist:** CO.

★ 11129 ★ Applebaum Foundation

11111 Biscayne Blvd., Tower 3, Apt. 653
North Miami, FL 33181
Phone: (301)651-6478
Warren Weiss, Vice President

Fnded: 1949. **Philosophy:** The Applebaum Foundation makes most of its grants in the areas of education and religion. Educational funding favors specific departments at the University of Miami and educational institutions with Jewish curriculums. Religious funding favors Jewish organizations for Israeli relief and synagogues. The foundation also supports health services and some civic affairs. **Priorities:** *Arts & Humanities:* 1%. *Civic & Public Affairs:* 1%. *Education:* 65%. Primary support for the University of Miami and Jewish education. *Environment:* 1%. Gives to the United Way and to organizations dealing with the disabled. *International:* 9%. Emphasis on a university hospital; also supports medical research. *Note:* Total contributions made in fiscal 2001. **Typ. Recipients:** Cancer, Children's Health/Hospitals, Geriatric Health, Health Funds, Health Organizations, Health-General, Heart, Hospitals, Kidney, Medical Education, Medical Research, People with Disabilities, Public Health, Respiratory, Single-Disease Health Associations, Transplant Networks/Donor Banks. **Geo. Dist:** nationally; FL; NY.

★ 11130 ★ Arca Foundation

1308 19th St., NW
Washington, DC 20036
Phone: (202)822-9193 **Fax:** (202)785-1446
Email: grants@arcafoundation.org
Website: http://www.arcafoundation.org
Donna Edwards, Executive Director

Fnded: 1952. **Philosophy:** "The purpose of the foundation is to support not-for-profit organizations in the United States whose work encourages a more open foreign policy, based on respect for international law, human rights and the sovereignty of all nations. The foundation also supports projects concerned with domestic social change. In 1999, the Arca Foundation continued its focus on U.S. policy toward Cuba, building on a decade of experience in supporting citizen participation in policy debates and peaceful change in the hemisphere. Our grantmaking has emphasized issues and countries where a shift in U.S. policy or public opinion can make a significant, if not decisive difference. Arca's grantmaking in 1999 continued to emphasize the urgent need for campaign finance reform supporting educational efforts at the state and national level. Other domestic grants reflected the board's concern with the dramatic deterioration of conditions for working people in this country, and the need to build strong coalitions to level the playing field for everyone." 1999 Annual Report **Priorities:** *Civic & Public Affairs:* 19%. For issues concerning U.S. domestic policy, musgrove seminars, and campaign reform. *Environment:* 36%. Funds domestic social change. *Note:* Total contributions made in 1999. **Typ. Recipients:** Health Policy/Cost Containment, Substance Abuse. **Geo. Dist:** nationally.

★ 11131 ★ Arcadia Foundation

105 East Logan St.
Norristown, PA 19401-3060
Phone: (610)275-8460 **Fax:** (610)275-8460
Marilyn Steinbright, President

Fnded: 1964. **Philosophy:** The foundation generally supports art, civic, human service, health, and educational organizations working to improve the quality of life in Pennsylvania. **Priorities:** *Arts & Humanities:* 33%. Supports theater, public broadcasting, and music. *Civic & Public Affairs:* 3%. Urban affairs, organizations, and housing. *Education:* 34% Private and public education. *Environment:* 22%. Focus on community service organizations in eastern Pennsylvania. *International:* 4%. Supports hospitals, health associations, and pediatric health. *Note:* Total contributions made in fiscal 2001. **Typ. Recipients:** Arthritis, Children's Health/Hospitals, Clinics/Medical Centers, Diabetes, Emergency/Ambulance Services, Health Organizations, Hospices, Hospitals, Hospitals (University Affiliated), Long-Term Care, Medical Education, Mental Health, Nursing Services, People with Disabilities, Single-Disease Health Associations. **Geo. Dist:** PA, zip codes 18000 to 19800.

★ 11132 ★ Arcana Foundation

1156 15th St. Northwest, No. 605
Washington, DC 20005
Phone: (202)789-7280 **Fax:** (202)842-2297
Email: arcanajk@aol.com
Joan Kennan, Executive Director

Fnded: 1986. **Philosophy:** The foundation supports programs in Washington, DC, that work to alleviate poverty and enhance cultural activities. It also makes grants to organizations that Mr. and Mrs. von Hoffman have been actively involved with in the past. **Priorities:** *Arts & Humanities:* 21%. Supports libraries, art museums, music, and public broadcasting. *Civic & Public Affairs:* 11%. Support for community services and housing and employment programs. *Education:* 13%. Supports secondary education. *Environment:* 51%. Funding for the aged, child welfare, substance abuse rehabilitation, and the homeless. *International:* 1% *Note:* Total contributions made in fiscal 2001. **Typ. Recipients:** Children's Health/Hospitals, Clinics/Medical Centers, Diabetes, Domestic Violence, Family Planning, Geriatric Health, Health Organizations, Hospices, Long-Term Care, Medical Research, Mental Health, People with Disabilities, Prenatal Health Issues, Public Health, Substance Abuse. **Geo. Dist:** DC.

★ 11133 ★ Arie and Ida Crown Memorial

222 North LaSalle St., Suite 2000
Chicago, IL 60601
Phone: (312)236-6300 **Fax:** (312)984-1499
Email: aicm@crown-chicago.com
Susan Crown, President

Fnded: 1947. **Philosophy:** "The Arie and Ida Crown Memorial (AICM) supports projects that offer opportunities to the disadvantaged, strengthen the bond of families and improve the quality of people's lives. As a general rule, the Foundation funds programs that serve members of the Jewish community and residents of Chicago (Cook County)." "In the tradition of its founders, a core purpose of AICM is to bolster the Jewish community. Special emphasis is placed on programs offering assistance to the disenfranchised, promoting Jewish education, fortifying the family unit, strengthening Jewish culture and tradition, assisting in the resettlement efforts and promoting Jewish identity." 1996 Guidelines. **Priorities:** *Arts & Humanities:* 4%. Funds music, opera, arts institutes, museums, theater, and public broadcasting. *Civic & Public Affairs:* 18%. Funds public and foreign policy, parks, and zoos. *Education:* 29%. Supports education funds, religious education, and higher education. *Environment:* 12%. Funds family services, child welfare, and youth organizations. *International:* 11%. Medical centers and single-disease associations receive support. *Religion:* 4%. Supports science museums and planetariums. *Note:* Total contributions made in 2000. **Typ. Recipients:** Alzheimers Disease, Children's Health/Hospitals, Clinics/Medical Centers, Diabetes, Domestic Violence, Eyes/Blindness, Family Planning, Health Organizations, Health-General, Hospitals, Hospitals (University Affiliated), Medical Rehabilitation, Medical Research, Mental Health, People with Disabilities, Public Health, Single-Disease Health Associations, Substance Abuse. **Geo. Dist:** Chicago, IL, including Cook County.

★ 11134 ★ Arkell Hall Foundation

68 Front St.
PO Box 240
Canajoharie, NY 13317-0240
Phone: (518)673-5417 **Fax:** (518)673-5493
Joseph Santangelo, Vice President and Treasurer

Fnded: 1948. **Philosophy:** "The primary mission of the Arkell Hall Foundation is the operation and maintenance of a home for elderly persons. Funds which may become available above the needs of the Home may be distributed annually to organizations providing services within the Target Community." "The most important requirement is significant direct impact in the Western Montgomery County New York community. Projects or organizations not primarily serving the Target Community or with large service areas (such as national or regional) will not qualify for funding." 1997 Grant Program Guidelines **Priorities:** *Arts & Humanities:* 41%. Supports a library, art gallery, and the performing arts. *Civic & Public Affairs:* 5%. Supports community affairs. *Education:* 31%. Supports secondary and training schools, and colleges and universities. *Environment:* 11%. Supports youth services, animal affairs, and social services. *International:* 11%. Supports hospices, hospitals, and disease and disorder awareness programs. *Note:* Total contributions made in fiscal 2001. **Typ. Recipients:** Alzheimers Disease, Cancer, Children's Health/Hospitals, Clinics/Medical Centers, Diabetes, Domestic Violence, Emergency/Ambulance Services, Health Funds, Health Organizations, Health-General, Heart, Hospices, Hospitals, Long-Term Care, Medical Education, Medical Research, Nursing Services, Outpatient Health Care, People with Disabilities, Prenatal Health Issues, Single-Disease Health Associations, Substance Abuse. **Geo. Dist:** NY, Western Montgomery County.

★ 11135 ★ Arnold and Mabel Beckman Foundation

100 Academy Drive
Irvine, CA 92612
Phone: (949)721-2222 **Fax:** (949)721-2225
Email: jdorrance@beckman-foundation.com
Website: http://www.beckman-foundation.com
Jacqueline Dorrance, Executive Director

Fnded: 1977. **Philosophy:** "The Arnold and Mabel Beckman Foundation makes grants to nonprofit research institutions to promote research in chemistry and the life sciences, broadly interpreted, and particularly to foster the investigation of methods, instruments and materials that will open up new avenues of research in science. The Beckman Young Investigators Program is intended to provide research support to the most promising young faculty members in the early stages of academic careers in the chemical and life sciences." **Priorities:** *Education:* 18%. Supports educational scholarship. *Environment:* 9%. In support of Boy Scouts. *Religion:* 73%. Supports science centers, and organizations with science related interests. *Note:* Contributions made in fiscal 1999. **Typ. Recipients:** Clinics/Medical Centers, Eyes/Blindness, Medical Research, Research/Studies Institutes, Speech & Hearing. **Geo. Dist:** nationally.

★ 11136 ★ Arthur J. Schmitt Foundation

629 Green Bay Rd., Suite 1
Wilmette, IL 60091
Phone: (847)853-0231
John Donahue, Executive Director

Fnded: 1941. **Philosophy:** "Reflecting the strong sense of responsible stewardship to God evidenced in the life of Arthur J. Schmitt, the Arthur J. Schmitt Foundation commits itself to placing its resources toward fashioning a better and more humane world. To this end, and drawing from its founder's quest for leadership, the foundation pledges to support endeavors that will enable the development of human potential, especially in persons in whom notable promise of achievement is discerned. "In its activities, deliberations and decisions, the Arthur J. Schmitt Foundation is rooted in a spirit of Christian concern, with a special, but not exclusive, commitment to the Roman Catholic Tradition, in devotion to country, and in an informed awareness of present day world realities. The foundation realizes that in so doing, it exemplifies the central commitments of Arthur J. Schmitt. "Through this mission the foundation preserves the memory of its founder, Arthur J. Schimitt, and shares his story and his values with those who benefit from the foundation's resources." 1996 Brochure **Priorities:** *Arts & Humanities:* 1% *Education:* 65%. Supports Catholic educational institutions (49%); scholarships (12%). *Environment:* 28%. Community services, people with disabilities, youth organizations, and shelters. *International:* 1%. Supports home-care services. *Note:* Total contributions made in fiscal 2001. **Typ. Recipients:** AIDS/HIV, Health Funds, Home-Care Services, Home-Care Services, Hospitals, Long-Term Care, Medical Education, Mental Health, People with Disabilities, Research/Studies Institutes, Substance Abuse. **Geo. Dist:** Chicago, IL, metropolitan area.

★ 11137 ★ Arthur S. DeMoss Foundation

Phillips Point West Tower, Suite 1600
777 South Flagler Drive
West Palm Beach, FL 33401
Phone: (561)804-9020 **Fax:** (561)804-9025
Mrs. Arthur DeMoss, Contact

Fnded: 1955. **Philosophy:** The foundation's focus is conducting its own projects, staffed by its own people. Additionally, a few grants are awarded. Sponsored projects are Power for Living, a multi-national evangelical outreach, which promotes the free book, *Power for Living: Executive Ministries*, dedicated to "winning and discipling business and professional executives to Jesus Christ;" Life Action Ministries, which is concerned with "teaching Biblical principles regarding the building of Christian families and Christian homes;" and Rebirth of America, which promotes the free book of the same name, and is concerned with the departure of present day America from "our founding fathers' respect for God's moral law." Foundation grantmaking is restricted to Christian evangelical causes. **Priorities:** *Note:* Total contributions made in 1998. **Typ. Recipients:** Family Planning, Medical Rehabilitation, Medical Research. **Geo. Dist:** nationally and internationally.

★ 11138 ★ Arthur Vining Davis Foundations

225 Water St., Ste. 1510
Jacksonville, FL 32202-5185
Phone: (904)359-0670 **Fax:** (904)359-0675
Email: arthurvining@bellsouth.net
Website: http://www.jvm.com/davis/
Dr. Jonathan Howe, Executive Director

Fnded: 1952. **Philosophy:** Mr. Davis' philanthropic philosophy emphasized higher education and religious activities, with some attention to medicine. The foundations will continue their commitment to Mr. Davis' ideals, again concentrating their funding in the area of private higher education, and, to a lesser extent, to medicine, religion, public television, and secondary education. Grants in private higher education concentrate on institutions with outstanding records of teaching and learning in the liberal arts and sciences, and those with broadly acknowledged academic excellence, adequate financial resources, and a record of good trustee and alumni support. Grants generally range from $100,000 to $200,000 for projects proposed by the applicant college president with the goal of reinforcing institutional excellence. The trustees prefer to give grants in the medical field for programs that encourage caring attitudes in the delivery of health care. Projects should have the potential for widespread practical application and should be of interest to other groups. New ideas are encouraged, especially if they facilitate communications with patients by doctors, nurses, and other caregivers; ameliorate patient anxieties; and foster caring attitudes. Grants range from $50,000 to $200,000. The majority of grants in the field of religion are made to fully accredited by the Association of Theological Schools seminaries that prepare persons for ordained ministry. As with the higher education program, support generally goes to schools known for academic excellence and financial stability. Grants generally range from $75,000-$150,000 for projects proposed by the institutions president or Dean. Support for public television seeks to emphasize the Foundation's interest in education, including television for children. Grants ordinarily are made to provide partial support for a major series of educational programs. A series should be assured of national distribution through the public broadcasting system. Grants in secondary education will be made to professional development programs which strengthen teachers and teaching in high schools. Collaborative partnerships between faculties of colleges and high schools, or combined efforts involving reform organizations, colleges/universities, and high schools are encouraged. **Priorities:** *Arts & Humanities:* 12%. Supports public television specials and series. *Education:* 85%. Supports colleges and higher education. *International:* 1%. Supports health care demonstration project. *Note:* Total contributions made in 2001. **Typ. Recipients:** Cancer, Children's Health/Hospitals, Clinics/Medical Centers, Health Organizations, Health Policy/Cost Containment, Health-General, Hospices, Hospitals, Hospitals (University Affiliated), Medical Education, Medical Research, Mental Health, Research/Studies Institutes. **Geo. Dist:** nationally.

★ 11139 ★ Assisi Foundation of Memphis

PO Box 381437
Memphis, TN 38183
Phone: (901)684-1564 **Fax:** (901)684-1997
Barry Flynn, Executive Director

Fnded: 1994. **Priorities:** *Arts & Humanities:* 8%. Gives to libraries, museums, and public broadcasting. *Education:* 30%. Provides major support to the University of Tennessee; also funds public pre-college schools, literacy programs, colleges, and charter/private schools. *International:* 31%. Supports clinics, hospitals, pediatric health, medical research institutes, medical foundations, single-disease health associations, and hospice. *Note:* Total contributions made in 2000. **Typ. Recipients:** AIDS/HIV, Cancer, Children's Health/Hospitals, Clinics/Medical Centers, Health Organizations, Hospitals, Medical Research. **Geo. Dist:** TN.

★ 11140 ★ Atherton Family Foundation

900 Fort St. Mall, Suite 1300
Honolulu, HI 96813
Phone: (808)537-6333 **Fax:** (808)521-6286
Email: lschiff@hcf-hawaii.org
Lissa Schiff, Private Foundation Services Officer

Fnded: 1976. **Philosophy:** The foundation supports programs within a broad spectrum of activities, although funding is limited to organizations based in the state of Hawaii. Support of "educational programs, projects, and institutions... continue to have the highest priority, as do those with a religious nature." Organizations concerned with health and social services also are given careful attention. In reviewing proposals, the foundation's directors look for programs that seek to fulfill a "critical need in the community or provide a direct benefit to a group or class of people for the alleviation of a problem, or for the provision of an amenity that enhances life for the people in Hawaii." In addition, the directors have established a scholarship program as a memorial to Juliette M. Atherton. **Priorities:** *Arts & Humanities:* 19%. Supports visual arts, performing arts, folk arts, arts academies, and history and historic preservation. *Civic & Public Affairs:* 8%. *Education:* 42%. Supports Christian K-12 education, educational programs, universities, education councils, literacy, and scholarships. *Environment:* 22%. Supports youth and family services and United Way. *International:* 4%. Gives to hospice, cancer centers, disease and disorders programs, and hospitals. *Note:* Contributions were made in 2000. **Typ. Recipients:** Cancer, Children's Health/Hospitals, Clinics/Medical Centers, Domestic Violence, Emergency/Ambulance Services, Family Planning, Geriatric Health, Health Funds, Health Organizations, Hospices, Hospitals, Long-Term Care, Medical Education, Medical Rehabilitation, Medical Research, Medical Training, Mental Health, Nursing Services, People with Disabilities, Prenatal Health Issues, Substance Abuse. **Geo. Dist:** HI.

★ 11141 ★ Atkinson Foundation

1720 South Amphlett Blvd.
Suite 100
San Mateo, CA 94402
Phone: (650)357-1101 **Fax:** (650)357-1101
Email: atkinfdn@aol.com
Elizabeth Curtis, Administrator & Director

Fnded: 1939. **Philosophy:** "The Foundation hopes to provide opportunities for people to attain their highest potential in areas of spiritual, educational, social and economic life, to assist their efforts to become independent and self-sufficient and generally to improve the quality of their lives." The foundation gives primary consideration to "nonprofit organizations serving the residents of San Mateo County, California, through programs that benefit children, youth, families, immigrants, the elderly and the ill, the disadvantaged, needy and homeless, the mentally and physically disabled, and those suffering from drug, alcohol, or physical abuse"; schools and institutions of higher education serving the needs of students in San Mateo County; the United Methodist Church and other church-related organizations serving the spiritual, material or social welfare needs of residents of San Mateo County; selected support for other denominations, religious education and mission programs; "U.S. nonprofits providing assistance, support and training in Mexico, Central America or the Caribbean for the sustainable development of local water and food resources, for economic initiatives such as cooperative banks, agrobusinesses and microenterprise, and for programs such as sanitation, nutrition, health education, and family planning". Atkinson Foundation Grant Priorities and Restrictions. **Priorities:** *Arts & Humanities:* 9%. Funds librarys and history organizations. *Civic & Public Affairs:* 6% Supports community affairs, job training, workers' rights, nonprofit management, and housing. *Education:* 7%. Contributes to education programs in preschool, elementary, and secondary schools, community colleges, universities, adult and vocational schools and related organizations. *Environment:* 37%. Supports social service programs that benefit children and youth; families; immigrants and refugees; the elderly and ill; and the disadvantaged, needy, and homeless. *International:* 6%. Funds disease-specific organizations, children's health, and health education. *Note:* Total contributions made in 2001. **Typ. Recipients:** AIDS/HIV, Alzheimers Disease, Children's Health/Hospitals, Clinics/Medical Centers, Domestic Violence, Eyes/Blindness, Family Planning, Health-General, Heart, Hospitals, Medical Rehabilitation, Medical Research, Mental Health, People with Disabilities, Public Health, Substance Abuse. **Geo. Dist:** United States-based international organizations serving Latin America; United States-based international organizations serving the Caribbean; CA, San Mateo County.

★ 11142 ★ Atlantic Foundation

14 Fairgrounds Rd., Suite A
Hamilton, NJ 08619
Phone: (609)689-1040 **Fax:** (609)689-1059
J. Johnson, Jr., Chairman

Fnded: 1964. **Philosophy:** The Atlantic Foundation primarily funds organizations affiliated with science, specifically oceanography and marine science. The foundation's major recipient is the Harbor Branch Oceanographic Institute. Technical educational institutes also are funded on occasion. **Priorities:** *Arts & Humanities:* 70%. Funds sculpture and literary organizations. *Civic & Public Affairs:* 1%. *Environment:* Less than 1%. *Religion:* 27%. Emphasis is on the Harbor Branch Oceanographic Institution. *Note:* Total contributions made in 2000. **Typ. Recipients:** Substance Abuse. **Geo. Dist:** eastern United States.

★ 11143 ★ Atlantic Foundation of New York

125 Park Ave., 21st Floor
New York, NY 10017
Phone: (212)922-0350 **Fax:** (212)922-0360
Alan Ruby, Secretary & Treasurer

Fnded: 1990. **Priorities:** *Arts & Humanities:* 5%. Gives to libraries and public broadcasting. *Civic & Public Affairs:* 17%. Supports women's affairs, public policy organizations, nonprofit management, law and justice. *Education:* 58%. Supports colleges, universities, medical education, and various education programs. *Environment:* 20%. Supports child welfare, and family and senior services. *Note:* Total contributions made in 2000. **Typ. Recipients:** Adolescent Health Issues, Home-Care Services. **Geo. Dist:** nationally.

★ 11144 ★ Atran Foundation, Inc.

23-25 East 21st St., 3rd Floor
New York, NY 10010
Phone: (212)505-9677
Diane Fischer, Secretary

Fnded: 1945. **Philosophy:** The Atran Foundation makes most of its grants in support of Jewish religious organizations, education, and civic affairs. Educational support goes to Jewish universities, medical education, and social science education. In civic affairs, interests include women's affairs, business interests, and community affairs. The foundation supports other recipient areas on a limited basis. **Priorities:** *Arts & Humanities:* 6%. *Civic & Public Affairs:* 2%. *Education:* 37%. *International:* 1%. *Note:* Total contributions made in fiscal 2001. **Typ. Recipients:** Clinics/Medical Centers, Emergency/Ambulance Services, Geriatric Health, Hospitals, Hospitals (University Affiliated), Long-Term Care, Medical Education, Medical Research, People with Disabilities, Research/Studies Institutes. **Geo. Dist:** NY.

★ 11145 ★ Audrey and Sydney Irmas Charitable Foundation

16027 Ventura Blvd., Suite 601
Encino, CA 91436
Phone: (818)382-3313 **Fax:** (818)382-3315
Robert Irmas, Administrator Trustee

Fnded: 1986. **Philosophy:** The foundation distributes its giving evenly between Jewish religious organizations, civic affairs, the arts, and social services. The foundation also supports health services. **Priorities:** *Arts & Humanities:* 13%. Museums, opera, and photography. *Civic & Public Affairs:* 8%. Law and justice, affordable housing, and feminism studies. *Education:* 9%. *Environment:* 4%. *International:* 12%. *Note:* Total contributions made in 2000. **Typ. Recipients:** Adolescent Health Issues, AIDS/HIV, Cancer, Child Abuse, Children's Health/Hospitals, Clinics/Medical Centers, Diabetes, Eyes/Blindness, Health Organizations, Hospitals, Medical Education, Medical Research, Mental Health, Research/Studies Institutes, Single-Disease Health Associations, Substance Abuse, Transplant Networks/Donor Banks. **Geo. Dist:** Los Angeles, CA.

★ 11146 ★ Autry Foundation

4383 Colfax Ave.
Studio City, CA 91604
Phone: (818)752-7770 **Fax:** (818)752-7779
Jacqueline Autry, President

Fnded: 1974. **Philosophy:** The foundation's primary purpose is to support the Autry Museum of Western Heritage. The foundation also supports other arts organizations, health concerns, and educational organizations. **Priorities:** *Arts & Humanities:* 67%. Major support for the Autry Museum of Western Heritage; also funds other museums, film, and broadcasting. *Civic & Public Affairs:* 2%. *Education:* 12%. Supports higher education and pre-college projects. *Environment:* 15%. Funds youth organizations, family services, community programs, and recreation and athletics. *International:* 3%. *Note:* Total contributions made in 2000. **Typ. Recipients:** Alzheimers Disease, Cancer, Child Abuse, Children's Health/Hospitals, Clinics/Medical Centers, Diabetes, Domestic Violence, Eyes/Blindness, Health Organizations, Health-General, Heart, Hospices, Hospitals, Medical Research, People with Disabilities, Prenatal Health Issues, Public Health, Research/Studies Institutes, Respiratory, Single-Disease Health Associations, Speech & Hearing, Substance Abuse. **Geo. Dist:** CA, including southern California.

★ 11147 ★ B. B. Owen Trust

PO Box 830068
Richardson, TX 75083
Phone: (972)783-7170 **Fax:** (972)783-7175
Monty Jackson, Trustee

Fnded: 1974. **Philosophy:** The B. B. Owen Charitable Trust primarily contributes most of its grants to health care, specifically medical centers in Texas. Other areas of interest include food and clothing distribution, community centers, homes, religion, and civic affairs. **Priorities:** *Arts & Humanities:* 10%. Funds ballet. *Civic & Public Affairs:* 28%. City of McKinney parks, and local Texas government. *Education:* 6%. Supports the University of Dallas and Junior Achievement. *Environment:* 19%. Boys & Girls Clubs, YMCA, YWCA, childrens charities. *International:* About 16%. Supports pediatric health, hospitals, and health funds. *Note:* Total contributions made in fiscal 1999. **Typ. Recipients:** Cancer, Children's Health/Hospitals, Clinics/Medical Centers, Eyes/Blindness, Family Planning, Hospitals, Hospitals (University Affiliated), Kidney, Medical Education, Medical Research, Nursing Services, People with Disabilities, Preventive Medicine/Wellness Organizations, Single-Disease Health Associations, Substance Abuse. **Geo. Dist:** TX, Dallas.

★ 11148 ★ B. C. McCabe Foundation

8152 Painter Ave., Suite 201
Whittier, CA 90602
Phone: (562)696-1433 **Fax:** (562)698-5508
James Shepard, Trustee

Fnded: 1976. **Philosophy:** The foundation typically supports social service organizations, educational institutions, health concerns, and religious welfare causes within California. **Priorities:** *Arts & Humanities:* 5%. Art center. *Civic & Public Affairs:* 4%. Women's services. *Education:* 8%. Colleges. *Environment:* 56%. Youth guidance, clubs, and homes. *International:* 20%. Hospitals and health projects. *Note:* Total contributions made in 2000. **Typ. Recipients:** AIDS/HIV, Children's Health/Hospitals, Clinics/Medical Centers, Diabetes, Emergency/Ambulance Services, Health Organizations, Hospitals, Medical Education, Nursing Services, Nutrition, People with Disabilities, Substance Abuse, Trauma Treatment. **Geo. Dist:** CA.

★ 11149 ★ Ball Brothers Foundation

222 South Mulberry
PO Box 1408
Muncie, IN 47308
Phone: (765)741-5500 **Fax:** (765)741-5518
Email: ballfoundation@yahoo.com
Douglas Bakken, Executive Director

Fnded: 1926. **Philosophy:** "The Foundation was established 'to promote religious, educational or charitable purposes, or all of these, within the State of Indiana." "While Foundation grants support a wide range of Indiana institutions and organizations, the majority of funds have been distributed to Muncie and East Central Indiana." "The Foundation's goal has been to facilitate the building of community. Current areas of funding interest include higher education, K-12 public education, arts, humanities and cultural organizations and outdoor recreation programs, and youth services." "The Foundation, in partnership with other philanthropic entities across Indiana... (facilitates) programs dedicated to stimulating giving and volunteering and seeking ways to enrich and broaden the quality of life in the state." "The Foundation, since 1983, has been the primary funder of the Minnetrista Cultural Foundation, and operator of the Minnetrista Cultural Center, a 70,000 square foot community facility, opened in 1988." "During the past several years, the Foundation has been involved with area public schools in seeking ways to facilitate the introduction of computers and seeking ways to capitalize on the global network, namely (the) Internet." 1997 General Information. **Priorities:** *Arts & Humanities:* 72%. Supports musical performance, museums, libraries, and historical preservation; major grants to the Minnetrista Cultural Foundation and the Ball State University Art Museum. *Civic & Public Affairs:* 9%. Funds community development. *Education:* 10%. Substantial gifts went to Ball State University and local schools. *Environment:* 7%. Supports United Way, Young Men's Christian Association, scouting, and Special Olympics. *International:* 1%. Funds hospitals and preventive medical organizations. *Note:* Total contributions made in 2000. **Typ. Recipients:** AIDS/HIV, Children's Health/Hospitals, Diabetes, Health Organizations, Heart, Hospitals, Medical Rehabilitation, People with Disabilities, Preventive Medicine/Wellness Organizations, Public Health. **Geo. Dist:** IN, East Central Indiana; Muncie, IN.

★ 11150 ★ Banbury Fund Inc.

PO Box 5315, FDR St.
New York, NY 10150-5315
Phone: (212)888-3535

Fnded: 1946. **Philosophy:** The fund places an emphasis on educational institutions, environmental causes, civic affairs, and scientific and health care organizations. **Priorities:** *Arts & Humanities:* 5%. Performing arts, museums. *Civic & Public Affairs:* 5%. Supports civic and community development. *Education:* 47%. Supports educational programs, schools, and colleges and universities. *Environment:* 7%. Supports humane studies, United Way, and family and youth services. *International:* 13%. Supports hospices and disease and disorder awareness affairs. *Religion:* 4%. Supports Cold Spring Harbor Laboratory. *Note:* Total contributions made in 2000. **Typ. Recipients:** AIDS/HIV, Cancer, Clinics/Medical Centers, Emergency/Ambulance Services, Eyes/Blindness, Family Planning, Health Organizations, Hospices, Hospitals, Hospitals (University Affiliated), Medical Education, Public Health. **Geo. Dist:** NY.

★ 11151 ★ Barker Welfare Foundation

1007 Glen Cove Ave.
Glen Head, NY 11545
Phone: (516)759-5592 **Fax:** (516)759-5497
Email: barkersmd@aol.com
Sarane Ross, President & Director

Fnded: 1934. **Philosophy:** "The mission of the Barker Welfare Foundation is to make grants to qualified charitable organizations whose initiatives improve the quality of life, with an emphasis on strengthening youth and families and which reflect the philosophy of Catherine B. Hickox, the Founder." The Barker Welfare Foundation gives the majority of its support in the areas of social service and the arts. In the social service category, the foundation emphasizes youth, family services, community centers, and homes. In the arts, a majority of support goes to dance, historic preservation, libraries, museums, music, and theater. The foundation also gives some support to civic causes, health organizations, and educational institutions. In May 1994, the foundation changed its funding policy for the metropolitan Chicago, IL, area. The foundation will no longer accept unsolicited applications for grants; all grants made in that area will be foundation-initiated. **Priorities:** *Arts & Humanities:* 28%. Primary support for music, libraries, museums, opera, ballet, and public broadcasting. *Civic & Public Affairs:* 6%. Emphasis on neighborhood associations and foundations. *Environment:* 57%. Targets youth organizations, family services, child welfare, and people with disabilities. *Note:* Total contributions made in fiscal 2001. **Typ. Recipients:** Adolescent Health Issues, AIDS/HIV, Cancer, Child Abuse, Children's Health/Hospitals, Clinics/Medical Centers, Emergency/Ambulance Services, Family Planning, Heart, Home-Care Services, Hospitals, Long-Term Care, Medical Rehabilitation, Medical Training, Mental Health, Nursing Services, Nutrition, Outpatient Health Care, People with Disabilities, Prenatal Health Issues, Public Health, Substance Abuse. **Geo. Dist:** Chicago, IL; Michigan City, IN; New York, NY.

★ 11152 ★ Barra Foundation

8200 Flourtown Ave., Suite 12
Wyndmoor, DE 19038-7976
Phone: (215)233-5115 **Fax:** (215)836-1033
William Harral, III, President

Fnded: 1963. **Philosophy:** The Barra Foundation seeks to advance knowledge and education, particularly "in the fields of American art history and material culture from the colonial period to 1900." To this end, the foundation supports innovative pilot studies and projects not supported by other agencies or individuals. **Priorities:** *Arts & Humanities:* 66%. Funds museums, historical societies, libraries, public broadcasting, and arts associations. *Civic & Public Affairs:* 12%. Supports career and economic development organizations, zoos and community organizations. *Education:* 9%. Gives to higher education and summer youth education projects. *Environment:* 4%. Funds community services, youth organizations, and united funds. *International:* 6%. Supports medical centers and health associations. *Religion:* 2%. Supports the Academy of Natural Sciences of Philadelphia. *Note:* Total contributions made in 2000. **Typ. Recipients:** Alzheimers Disease, Cancer, Children's Health/Hospitals, Clinics/Medical Centers, Emergency/Ambulance Services, Family Planning, Health Organizations, Health-General, Home-Care Services, Hospices, Hospitals, Hospitals (University Affiliated), Long-Term Care, Medical Education, Medical Rehabilitation, Medical Research, People with Disabilities, Preventive Medicine/Wellness Organizations, Public Health, Single-Disease Health Associations. **Geo. Dist:** Philadelphia, PA.

★ 11153 ★ Bass Foundation

309 Main St.
Fort Worth, TX 76102
Phone: (817)336-0494 **Fax:** (817)332-2176
Email: fcabal@sidrichardson.org
Valleau Wilkie, Jr., Executive Director

Fnded: 1945. **Philosophy:** The Bass Foundation makes most of its grants in the areas of civic affairs, the arts, and education. Funding for civic affairs favors zoos and conservation efforts. The arts receive support in the areas of museums, the performing arts, and art councils. Educational funding favors universities, and private education. The foundation also supports medical centers, churches, and social services. **Priorities:** *Arts & Humanities:* 1%. Supports fine arts, arts groups, and an orchestra. *Civic & Public Affairs:* 83%. Supports volunteer services, Texas Wild exhibit, rural affiliate, and safety. *Education:* 5%. Supports private schools, higher education. *Environment:* About 1%. Funds United Way. *Note:* Total contributions made in 2001. **Typ. Recipients:** Children's Health/Hospitals, Emergency/Ambulance Services, Family Planning, Geriatric Health, Hospitals, Substance Abuse. **Geo. Dist:** Fort Worth, TX.

★ 11154 ★ Bat Hanadiv Foundation No. 3

2 Wall St., 13th Floor
New York, NY 10005
Phone: (212)732-3200 **Fax:** (212)732-3232
Jerome Caufield, Attorney

Fnded: 1981. **Philosophy:** The Bat Hanadiv Foundation No. 3 gives primarily to Jewish causes in Israel. The foundation's three main interests include educational institutions, civic groups, and the arts. In the area of education, grants fund universities and scientific education. **Priorities:** *Education:* 35%. Supports science education, Jewish studies, and special education. *Note:* Total contributions made in 2000. **Typ. Recipients:** Hospices, Hospitals, Substance Abuse.

★ 11155 ★ Baughman Foundation

PO Box 1356
Liberal, KS 67905-1356
Phone: (620)624-1371 **Fax:** (620)624-4177
Email: baughman@swko.net
Eugene Slaymaker, President

Fnded: 1958. **Philosophy:** The foundation gives to local municipalities and local organizations, primarily providing scholarships and capital or special project support. **Priorities:** *Arts & Humanities:* 16%. Gives to libraries, art/humanities councils, museums, historical societies, and public broadcasting. *Civic & Public Affairs:* 17%. Funds economic development, towns, fire and police departments, chambers of commerce, and parks. *Education:* 42%. Supports public schools, colleges and universities, economic education, 4-H, Junior Achievement, and scholarship funds. *Environment:* 22%. Supports athletics/recreation programs, youth activities, senior services, rape and domestic violence services, animal welfare organizations, and shelters. *International:* 3%. Hospitals, health foundations, and emergency medical services receive support. *Note:* Total contributions made in 2001. **Typ. Recipients:** Alzheimers Disease, Clinics/Medical Centers, Diabetes, Domestic Violence, Emergency/Ambulance Services, Health Organizations, Hospitals, People with Disabilities, Sexual Abuse, Single-Disease Health Associations, Substance Abuse. **Geo. Dist:** Liberal, KS.

★ 11156 ★ Beatrice P. Delany Charitable Trust

1211 Ave. of the Americas
New York, NY 10036
Phone: (212)789-5374
Mr. John Enteman, Administrator

Fnded: 1977. **Philosophy:** The trust traditionally supports programs and organizations in the areas of education, religion, civic groups, health, social services, and the arts. **Priorities:** *Arts & Humanities:* 11%. Supports music, with major support given to the Chicago Symphony Orchestra also funds opera, theater, and public broadcasting. *Civic & Public Affairs:* 14%. Major support given to the Devereux Foundation. Also supports botanical gardens & zoos. *Education:* 30%. Supports colleges and universities, religious education, medical education. *Environment:* 14%. Supports young men's christian association, United Way, child welfare, homes, and youth programs. *International:* 18%. Funds hospitals, medical centers, and disease and disorder concerns, hospice and cancer. *Note:* Total contributions made in fiscal 2000. **Typ. Recipients:** Cancer, Children's Health/Hospitals, Clinics/Medical Centers, Health-General, Hospitals, Medical Education, Medical Research, Mental Health, Multiple Sclerosis. **Geo. Dist:** nationally; Chicago, IL.

★ 11157 ★ Beazley Foundation

3720 Brighton St.
Portsmouth, VA 23707
Phone: (757)393-1605 **Fax:** (757)393-4708
Website: http://www.beazleyfoundation.org
Richard Bray, Jr., President

Fnded: 1948. **Philosophy:** "In keeping with the informal policy established by Mr. Beazely, the Trustees of the Beazely Foundation will award grants to organizations that are tax exempt under Section 501(c)(3) of the Internal Revenue Code and which are engaged in educational, charitable and religious activities." "Although there are no set distribution percentages for the three areas of giving, it is expected that the foundation will continue to emphasize grants to education with a smaller percentage going to charitable projects and a still smaller percentage to religious activities. The Foundation prefers, when making grants to religious activities, to gift ecumenical projects as opposed to grants to individual churches or denominations." "Geographically, the Foundation's goal is to grant the largest percentage of the funds during any one year to projects supporting the citizens of Portsmouth with a majority of the remaining funds to projects within the Tidewater Area preferably, but in the Commonwealth of Virginia at a minimum, with a very small percentage going to organizations outside the Commonwealth." **Typ. Recipients:** AIDS/HIV, Cancer, Child Abuse, Children's Health/Hospitals, Clinics/Medical Centers, Domestic Violence, Emergency/Ambulance Services, Geriatric Health, Health Organizations, Health-General, Hospitals, Hospitals (University Affiliated), Medical Education, Medical Rehabilitation, People with Disabilities, Public Health, Single-Disease Health Associations, Substance Abuse. **Geo. Dist:** Hampton Roads, VA area; Portsmouth, VA.

★ 11158 ★ Beinecke Foundation Inc.

8 Sound Shore Drive
Suite 120
Greenwich, CT 06830
Phone: (203)861-7311
John Robinson, President

Fnded: 1966. **Philosophy:** "The Beinecke Foundation, Inc. funds two types of programs: 1.Unsolicited projects reflecting an applicant's particular interests. 2.Projects reflecting an applicant's interest which are developed in response to a Foundation call for proposals." The foundation's interests include environmental affairs, higher education, New York City cultural institutions, and Protestant giving. **Priorities:** *Arts & Humanities:* 13%. Supports museums, historical societies, and art centers. *Civic & Public Affairs:* 30%. Supports botanical gardens. *Education:* 29%. Funds higher education. *Environment:* 7%. Funds youth clubs. *International:* 5%. Funds single-disease health associations. *Note:* Total contributions made in 2000. **Typ. Recipients:** Cancer, Children's Health/Hospitals, Emergency/Ambulance Services, Family Planning, Health Organizations, Hospitals, Medical Research, Research/Studies Institutes, Single-Disease Health Associations. **Geo. Dist:** CT; NY.

★ 11159 ★ Beirne Carter Foundation

1802 Bayberry Ct., No. 301
Richmond, VA 23226
Phone: (804)521-0272 **Fax:** (804)521-0274
Email: bcarterfn@aol.com
Website: http://www.bcarterfdn.org
Lucille Lindamood, Grant Administrator

Fnded: 1986. **Philosophy:** The foundation supports a variety of organizations that have direct impact on Virginia, from Richmond to southern Virginia. Organizations that typically receive support include environmental affairs, family services, the disadvantaged, rural arts, and history programs. **Priorities:** *Arts & Humanities:* 14%. Supports historic preservation, theater, libraries, museums, arts centers, and public broadcasting. *Civic & Public Affairs:* 7%. Contributes to urban renewal, transportation, community associations, parks, and aquariums. *Education:* 52%. Funds primary schools, parochial schools, colleges and universities. *Environment:* 18%. Focus on shelters, food distribution, youth organizations, child welfare, and family services. *International:* 7%. Gives to medical centers, nursing services, and pediatric health care. *Religion:* 1%. Funds a science museum. *Note:* Total contributions made in 2001. **Typ. Recipients:** AIDS/HIV, Arthritis, Cancer, Child Abuse, Children's Health/Hospitals, Clinics/Medical Centers, Domestic Violence, Emergency/Ambulance Services, Family Planning, Hospices, Hospitals, Hospitals (University Affiliated), Medical Education, Medical Research, Mental Health, Nursing Services, People with Disabilities, Preventive Medicine/Wellness Organizations, Public Health, Research/Studies Institutes, Respiratory, Single-Disease Health Associations, Transplant Networks/Donor Banks. **Geo. Dist:** VA.

★ 11160 ★ Ben B. Cheney Foundation

1201 Pacific Ave. South, Suite 1600
Tacoma, WA 98402
Phone: (253)572-2442 **Fax:** (253)572-2902
Mr. William Rieke, Executive Director

Fnded: 1955. **Philosophy:** The Ben B. Cheney Foundation "prefers to fund projects that develop new and innovative approaches to community problems, facilitate the improvement of services or programs, or invest in equipment and facilities that will have a lasting impact on community needs." Under its program guidelines, the foundation states that it seeks to disburse funds to civic projects, culture, charity, education, health, social services, youth, and the elderly. **Priorities:** *Arts & Humanities:* 24%. Focus is on museums, music, libraries, historical societies, and the performing arts. *Civic & Public Affairs:* 8%. Funds community development, housing, parks, and an aquarium. *Education:* 31%. Support for colleges, universities, and a scholarship program. *Environment:* 13%. Supports Young Men's Christian Association, food banks, and youth organizations. *International:* 15%. Supports hospitals and mental health. *Religion:* 2%. Funds science centers and science museums. *Note:* Total contributions made in 2000. **Typ. Recipients:** AIDS/HIV, Cancer, Children's Health/Hospitals, Clinics/Medical Centers, Domestic Violence, Emergency/Ambulance Services, Eyes/Blindness, Health Funds, Health Organizations, Heart, Hospitals, Long-Term Care, Medical Training, Mental Health, People with Disabilities, Single-Disease Health Associations, Speech & Hearing, Substance Abuse. **Geo. Dist:** CA, Del Norte, Humboldt, Lassen, Shasta, Siskiyou, and Trinity Counties in northern CA; CA, especially northern CA; OR, especially southwestern OR; WA, especially southwestern WA, Tacoma-Pierce County.

★ 11161 ★ Ben and Esther Rosenbloom Foundation

106 Old Court Rd., Suite 302
Baltimore, MD 21208
Phone: (410)653-0239
Howard Rosenbloom, Executive Director

Fnded: 1982. **Philosophy:** The foundation primarily gives to Jewish human service organizations. **Priorities:** *Arts & Humanities:* 1%. Supports music, art institutes, and museums. *Civic & Public Affairs:* 1%. Funds public policy organizations. *Environment:* 4%. Primarily united funds and community service organizations. *International:* 5%. Funds hospitals and single-disease health associations. *Note:* Total contributions made in 2000. **Typ. Recipients:** AIDS/HIV, Cancer, Domestic Violence, Emergency/Ambulance Services, Eyes/Blindness, Health Organizations, Heart, Hospitals, Kidney, Medical Rehabilitation, People with Disabilities, Single-Disease Health Associations. **Geo. Dist:** Baltimore, MD.

★ 11162 ★ Beneficia Foundation

1 Pitcairn Place, Suite 3000
Jenkintown, PA 19046-3593
Phone: (215)887-6700 **Fax:** (215)881-6092
Email: ak3371@pitcairn.com
Alisha King, Contact

Fnded: 1953. **Philosophy:** "Beneficia's mission is to enhance the quality of life through conservation of the environment and promotion of the arts. Beneficia favors programs which are innovative, catalytic, addressing unmet needs, and striving towards self-sustainability. Priorities for giving in the area of the environment include: inventory, protection and stewardship of high priority ecosystems (especially tropical and marine); creation of economic incentives for the conservation of biodiversity; and policy and legislation. Priorities for the giving in the area of the arts include: performing arts, especially classical music, theater and opera; and the visual arts with an emphasis on museums and art centers." **Priorities:** *Arts & Humanities:* 11%. Focus on performing arts, museums, and music. *Civic & Public Affairs:* 11%. Supports botanical gardens and zoological societies, and legal concerns. *Education:* 6%. Funds higher education. *Environment:* 4%. Violence prevention. *International:* About 1%. *Religion:* About 1%. Botanical research. *Note:* Total contributions made in 2001. **Typ. Recipients:** Cancer, Children's Health/Hospitals, Health-General, Medical Education, Nursing Services, Nutrition, People with Disabilities. **Geo. Dist:** no restrictions.

★ 11163 ★ Benjamin and Mary Siddons Measey Foundation

PO Box 258
Media, PA 19063
Phone: (610)566-5800 **Fax:** (610)566-8197
James Brennan, Member, Board of Managers

Fnded: 1958. **Philosophy:** The Benjamin and Mary Siddons Measey Foundation supports two areas of giving: education and health. Educational support favors universities and their medical schools. In health care, interests include university hospitals and health consortiums. **Priorities:** *Education:* 99%. Mainly supports medical education. *International:* Less than 1%. Supports a cancer center. *Note:* Total contributions made in 2000. **Typ. Recipients:** Cancer, Children's Health/Hospitals, Clinics/Medical Centers, Geriatric Health, Health Funds, Health Organizations, Hospitals, Hospitals (University Affiliated), Medical Education, Medical Research, Public Health. **Geo. Dist:** Philadelphia, PA.

★ 11164 ★ Benjamin and Roberta Russell Educational Foundation

PO Box 369
Alexander City, AL 35011-0272
Phone: (256)329-1320 **Fax:** (256)329-5346
James Nabors, Secretary & Treasurer

Fnded: 1944. **Philosophy:** The foundation's primary interest is education, with a focus on higher education. Support often goes to universities, community colleges, and private academies. The foundation also will contribute to hospitals, health relief agencies, single-disease associations, and children's welfare organizations. **Priorities:** *Arts & Humanities:* 8%. Supports libraries and the performing arts. *Civic & Public Affairs:* Less than 1%. Supports municipal projects. *Education:* 42%. Funds scholarships, colleges, universities, and secondary schools. *Environment:* 34%. Supports scouting and youth organizations, food and shelter, and humane societies. *International:* 16%. Supports single-disease health organizations, hospitals, health funds, and hospices. *Note:* Total contributions made in 2000. **Typ. Recipients:** Alzheimers Disease, Children's Health/Hospitals, Diabetes, Emergency/Ambulance Services, Hospices, Hospitals, Kidney, Multiple Sclerosis, Single-Disease Health Associations. **Geo. Dist:** Southeastern USA; AL.

★ 11165 ★ Benson and Edith Ford Fund

100 Renaissance Ctr., 34th Fl.
Detroit, MI 48243

Phone: (313)259-7777 **Fax:** (313)393-7579
David Hempstead, Secretary & Trustee

Fnded: 1943. **Philosophy:** The foundation makes grants in the areas of youth organizations and child welfare, hospitals, civic affairs, the arts, and education. A wide variety of grants are given in each of these areas. **Priorities:** *Arts & Humanities:* 45%. Funds support the fine arts, historical societies, the performing arts, and music; a major grant went to the Henry Ford Museum and Greenfield Village. *Civic & Public Affairs:* 6%. Supports the Detroit Zoological Society, a neighborhood club, and parks. *Education:* 5%. Supports private pre-college education, colleges and universities, and college funds. *Environment:* 13%. Gives to scouts, food banks, youth programs, homes, United Way, and animal protection. *International:* 8%. Supports hospitals, health centers, and single-disease health associations. *Religion:* 22%. Supports the Edison Institute and Woods Hole Oceanographic Institute. *Note:* Total contributions made in 2000. **Typ. Recipients:** Alzheimers Disease, Cancer, Children's Health/Hospitals, Clinics/Medical Centers, Emergency/Ambulance Services, Eyes/Blindness, Family Planning, Health Organizations, Hospitals, Long-Term Care, People with Disabilities, Preventive Medicine/Wellness Organizations, Public Health, Substance Abuse. **Geo. Dist:** MI, especially Detroit.

★ 11166 ★ Benwood Foundation

Suntrust Bank Bldg.
736 Market St., Suite 1600
Chattanooga, TN 37402
Phone: (423)267-4311 **Fax:** (615)267-9049
Email: benwoodfnd@benwood.org
Corinne Allen, Executive Director

Fnded: 1950. **Philosophy:** The purpose and activities of the foundation, as defined in its charter, cover a wide spectrum of philanthropy. Within this framework, the trustees have discretion to interpret the donor's philanthropic goals in accordance with today's needs. A broad range of organizations receive funding. The foundation contributes in six general areas: social services; health; the environment; education; the arts and humanities; and economic development. **Priorities:** *Arts & Humanities:* 13%. Gives to museums, historical societies, performing arts, public broadcasting, and art associations. *Civic & Public Affairs:* 17%. Funds urban and community affairs, zoos, public safety, and community foundations. *Education:* 28%. Primarily supports colleges and universities, public and private schools, and educational foundations. *Environment:* 13%. United funds, children's organizations, and athletics. *International:* 13%. Funds medical centers and health organizations. *Note:* Total contributions made in 2000. **Typ. Recipients:** Alzheimers Disease, Clinics/Medical Centers, Emergency/Ambulance Services, Health Organizations, Hospitals, Medical Education, Medical Research, Mental Health, People with Disabilities, Public Health, Research/Studies Institutes, Substance Abuse. **Geo. Dist:** Chattanooga, TN.

★ 11167 ★ Bernard McDonough Foundation

311 Fourth St.
Parkersburg, WV 26101
Phone: (304)424-6280 **Fax:** (304)424-6281
Email: jwakley@marmac.net
James Wakley, President & Director

Fnded: 1961. **Priorities:** *Arts & Humanities:* 9%. Supports libraries, museums, and performing arts. *Civic & Public Affairs:* 4%. Funds civic organizations, community foundations, and housing. *Education:* 38%. Colleges, universities, and public schools. *Environment:* 28%. Supports United Way, family causes, aging concerns, people with special needs and social services. *International:* 11%. Supports health, disease and disorder concerns. *Note:* Contributions were made in 2000. **Typ. Recipients:** Alzheimers Disease, Cancer, Cancer, Children's Health/Hospitals, Clinics/Medical Centers, Emergency/Ambulance Services, Health Organizations, Health-General, Heart, Hospices, Hospitals, Hospitals (University Affiliated), Medical Education, Mental Health, Multiple Sclerosis, People with Disabilities, Research/Studies Institutes. **Geo. Dist:** WV.

★ 11168 ★ Bernard Osher Foundation

909 Montgomery, No. 300
San Francisco, CA 94133
Phone: (415)861-5587 **Fax:** (415)677-5868
Email: nagle@osherfoundation.com
Patricia Tracy-Nagle, Executive Administrator & Secretary

Fnded: 1977. **Philosophy:** "The foundation's objective is to improve the quality of life for Bay Area residents through support of cultural and educational organizations and institutions...The foundation supports programs in these fields of interest: Arts and Humanities (programs which encourage artistic creativity in the visual and performing arts and promote scholarship in the literary arts); and Education (fellowships for colleges, universities, and conservatories for students of exceptional promise, with emphasis on graduate studies, and enrichment programs for schools, grades K-12)." **Priorities:** *Arts & Humanities:* 31%. Emphasis on music, museums, and performing arts. *Civic & Public Affairs:* 13%. Support festivals, zoos, and community foundations. *Education:* 39%. Primary support for the University of California, Berkeley. *Environment:* 5%. Youth organizations, family services, and united funds. *Religion:* 11%. Supports The Exploratorium, and California Academy of Sciences. *Note:* Total contributions made in 2000. **Typ. Recipients:** AIDS/HIV, Cancer, Diabetes, Family Planning, Health Organizations, Hospitals, Medical Education, Medical Research, Mental Health, People with Disabilities, Substance Abuse. **Geo. Dist:** CA, Alameda County; CA, San Francisco County.

★ 11169 ★ Bernice Barbour Foundation, Inc.

14434 Laurel Trail
Wellington, FL 33414-7648
Phone: (561)791-0861 **Fax:** (561)753-9153
Email: eve@bernicebarbour.org
Website: http://www.bernicebarbour.org
Eve Lloyd-Thompson, Secretary & Treasurer

Fnded: 1987. **Philosophy:** "The Bernice Barbour Foundation is a private charity established by the late Bernice Wall Barbour. It is a trust to be used for the preservation and care of animals, and prevention of cruelty to animals in the United States." Eve Lloyd Thompson, Treasurer and Secretary **Priorities:** *Civic & Public Affairs:* 2%. Supports zoos and aquariums. *Education:* 51%. Funds colleges and universities for veterinary science. *Environment:* 35%. Supports animal welfare organizations. *Religion:* 27%. Supports research and equipment at veterinary schools. *Note:* Total contributions made in 2001. **Typ. Recipients:** Clinics/Medical Centers, Emergency/Ambulance Services, Medical Education, Medical Rehabilitation, Medical Research, People with Disabilities. **Geo. Dist:** nationally.

★ 11170 ★ Bill and Melinda Gates Foundation

PO Box 23350
Seattle, WA 98102
Phone: (206)709-3140 **Fax:** (206)709-3280
Email: info@gatesfoundation.org
Website: http://www.gatesfoundation.org

Fnded: 1999. **Philosophy:** "The Bill & Melinda Gates Foundation places a major focus on helping to improve people's lives through health and learning. We will continue to look for strategic opportunities to extend the benefits of modern science and technology to people around the world, especially where poverty serves as an obstacle to participating in these benefits. As in the past, we will invest in partnerships with individuals and organizations that bring experience, expertise and commitment to their own efforts to help people through better health and learning. "In our home communities of the Pacific Northwest, we will support a broad range of projects and programs, with a special emphasis on vulnerable children and their families. "The challenges and problems of human existence are as daunting as ever. But the prospect of major gains in human well-being is historically unique. The Bill & Melinda Gates Foundation is animated by a vivid sense of the wonderful possibilities of the future and is grounded in a consciousness of the responsibility to ensure that our resources are used wisely and well." Letter About the Foundation by Founders Bill Gates III and Melinda Gates, and Co-Chairs William H. Gates, Sr., and Patty Stonesifer **Priorities:** *Arts & Humanities:* 5%. Supports libraries and efforts to enhance public access to information. *Civic & Public Affairs:* 2%. Gives to charitable organizations in Pacific Northwest communities. *Education:* 28%. Funds model schools and districts, professional development for instructors and administrators, and promotes higher education of minorities through the Gates Millenium Scholars Program. *International:* 48%. Supports work in the areas of Vaccine Preventable Diseases, Reproductive and Child Health, and Conditions Associated with Poverty. *Note:* Contributions analysis was provided by foundation and is based on grants awarded in 2000. **Typ. Recipients:** AIDS/HIV, Children's Health/Hospitals, Health Organizations, Health Policy/Cost Containment, Health-General, Medical Education, Medical Research, Public Health, Research/Studies Institutes. **Geo. Dist:** Pacific Northwest; internationally; nationally.

★ 11171 ★ Billy Rose Foundation

805 Third Ave., 23rd Floor
New York, NY 10022
Phone: (212)407-7745 **Fax:** (212)407-7799
Ms. Terri Mangino, Executive Director

Fnded: 1958. **Philosophy:** Of primary interest to the foundation is "making available to the American people works of genius in music, drama, painting, sculpture, all art forms." **Priorities:** *Arts & Humanities:* 41%. Supports arts organizations, music, theater, museums, film & video, ballet, opera, and libraries. *Civic & Public Affairs:* 2%. Funds botanical gardens, civic affairs, and public affairs. *Education:* 9%. Supports arts education, colleges, and universities. *International:* 4%. Supports corrective procedures and nursing services. *Note:* Total contributions made in 1998. **Typ. Recipients:** Cancer, Clinics/Medical Centers, Family Planning, Health Organizations, Hospitals, Medical Rehabilitation, Medical Research, Nursing Services, People with Disabilities, Single-Disease Health Associations, Transplant Networks/Donor Banks. **Geo. Dist:** New York, NY.

★ 11172 ★ Bingham Trust

PO Box 2004
New York, NY 10109
Patricia Davidson, Trustee

Fnded: 1934. **Philosophy:** Every five years, the trust shifts its primary focus to entirely new fields of interest. Funds available in the grant cycle beginning January 1, 1996, and ending December 31, 2000, have been entirely committed to four institutions providing transitional housing for certain psychiatric patients, four public middle schools to improve the schools' coordination with families and social services, two organizations developing and distributing contraceptives in underdeveloped countries, a program for the application of DNA technology in the fields of anthropology and archaeology, and a small number of minor grants selected by the trustees. The trust's fields of interest in the cycle starting January 1, 2001, will not be determined until the year 2000. **Priorities:** *Civic & Public Affairs:* 9%. Giving includes foundations, clubs and housing. *Education:* 22%. Funding to middle schools, universities, school for the deaf and other school programs. *Environment:* 22%. Supports United Way, shelters, child welfare, homes and human development services. *International:* 15%. Supports children's health, hospitals, health centers, and arthritis. *Note:* Totl contributions made in 2000. **Typ. Recipients:** Arthritis, Cancer, Children's Health/Hospitals, Clinics/Medical Centers, Eyes/Blindness, Health-General, Home-Care Services, Hospitals, Mental Health. **Geo. Dist:** nationwide.

★ 11173 ★ Blandin Foundation

100 North Pokegama Ave.
Grand Rapids, MN 55744
Phone: (218)326-0523 **Fax:** (218)327-1949
Email: bfinfo@blandinfoundation.org
Website: http://www.blandinfoundation.org
Linda Gibeau, Grants Manager

Fnded: 1941. **Philosophy:** "We strive to accomplish our mission of strengthening rural communities in Minnesota by partnering statewide with organizations on long-term projects, by making grants to selected communities to pursue action plans and by partnering with the Foundation's home community, the Grand Rapids area, to create an exemplary community. The Blandin Foundation focuses its grant funding *statewide* on several major goals to be able to best assist communities. The Foundation will fund a limited number of projects and programs in each focus area. The intent is to fund projects and programs in each focus area. The intent is to fund projects which have large enough scope to reach rural communities throughout Minnesota. Current focus areas include: Life-long Learning; Leadership; Diversity; (and) Economic Opportunity." Blandin Foundation Grant Guidelines. **Priorities:** *Arts & Humanities:* 5%. Provides major support to the Guthrie Theater; also funds museums, art associations, and public broadcasting. *Civic & Public Affairs:* 63%. Supports projects that promote economic opportunity/development, community safety, and community leadership training. Also legal aid organizations, municipalities, housing initiatives, and Native American affairs. *Education:* 14%. Funds public schools, colleges, and universities; also runs a scholarship program. *Environment:* 11%. Contributes to social and youth services, counseling, persons with disabilities, Young Men's Christian Association, recreation and athletic programs, and United Way. *International:* 6%. Supports health care centers, hospice, and nursing homes. *Note:* Contributions analysis reflects grants awarded in 2001. **Typ. Recipients:** Children's Health/Hospitals, Clinics/Medical Centers, Domestic Violence, Emergency/Ambulance Services, Health Organizations, Health Policy/Cost Containment, Hospices, Long-Term Care, Medical Education, Medical Research, Mental Health, Nursing Services, Outpatient Health Care, People with Disabilities, Public Health, Substance Abuse. **Geo. Dist:** MN.

★ 11174 ★ Blowitz-Ridgeway Foundation

One Northfield Plaza, Suite 528
570 Frontage Rd.
Northfield, IL 60093-1213
Phone: (847)446-1010
Tina Erickson, Administrator

Fnded: 1984. **Philosophy:** One of the primary funding areas of the foundation is "the support of non-profit agencies which provide health care to economically disadvantaged children and adolescents." Additional interests include child welfare, family services, and youth organizations. Priority is given to medical, psychiatric, psychological, and/or residential care, and research programs in medicine, psychology, social science, and education. **Priorities:** *Civic & Public Affairs:* 7%. Funds housing and job training. *Education:* 26%. Supports a high schools, arts education, and educational foundations. *Environment:* 29%. Supports homeless shelters, food distribution, family services, services for victims of violence, youth organizations, and early childhood development initiatives. *International:* 34%. Funds healthcare services and medical research. *Note:* Total contributions for fiscal 2002. **Typ. Recipients:** AIDS/HIV, Alzheimers Disease, Arthritis, Cancer, Child Abuse, Children's Health/Hospitals, Clinics/Medical Centers, Domestic Violence, Emergency/Ambulance Services, Eyes/Blindness, Family Planning, Health Organizations, Health-General, Health-General, Home-Care Services, Hospices, Hospitals, Hospitals (University Affiliated), Long-Term Care, Medical Rehabilitation, Medical Research, Mental Health, Nursing Services, Outpatient Health Care, People with Disabilities, Prenatal Health Issues, Public Health, Respiratory, Sexual Abuse, Single-Disease Health Associations, Speech & Hearing. **Geo. Dist:** IL.

★ 11175 ★ Blue Moon Fund

433 Park St.
Charlottesville, VA 22902-5178
Phone: (804)295-5160 **Fax:** (804)295-1648
Email: info@bluemoonfund.org
Website: http://www.wajones.org

Fnded: 1944. **Philosophy:** "Blue Moon Fund was established in April 2002 by Diane Edgerton Miller and Pat Jones Edgerton. Together they share more than 70 years of experience in philanthropy and dedication to preserving the sustainable quality of life on our planet. In 1944, Diane's grandfather and Pat's father, W. Alton Jones created a family foundation using his personal assets. His vision for the foundation was that it work for the "betterment of mankind." Over its 57 years, the Jones Foundation evolved from a general philanthropic foundation into a strategic, initiative-based international entity focusing on environmental sustainability and preventing nuclear war. In 2001, the Jones Foundation underwent a restructuring process from which emerged three new foundations, of which one is Blue Moon Fund. Blue Moon Fund is investigating work on "global sustainability" with a specific focus on human consumption, the natural world, and economic advancement. The fund's founders believe that the human and biologcal interdependency of our world necessitates a true understanding of how we are all connected. We share a world of rapidly diminishing resources, one in which our very existence and security depends upon nuturing and preserving our earth. Understanding the impact of the human imprint on our ecological systems is key to learning and developing the proper respect for the "vastness of our world." The founders hope to take blue moon fund to stratospheric heights with their passion and ideology." Blue Moon Fund website. **Priorities:** *Civic & Public Affairs:* 23%. Funds public policy institutes, peace organizations, sustainable economic development, and weapons control organizations. *Education:* 16%. Supports programs at colleges and universities. *Religion:* 3%. Funds science and research organizations. *Note:* Total contributions made in 2000. **Typ. Recipients:** Cancer, Children's Health/Hospitals, Medical Education, Mental Health, Respiratory, Substance Abuse. **Frmly:** W. Alton Jones Foundation.

★ 11176 ★ Blum-Kovler Foundation

919 North Michigan Ave., Suite 2800
Chicago, IL 60611
Phone: (312)664-5050 **Fax:** (312)664-8983

Fnded: 1957. **Philosophy:** The foundation gives to a wide variety of agencies in the arts, civic affairs, education, health, welfare, and religion categories. **Priorities:** *Arts & Humanities:* 15%. Funds museums, arts centers, arts associations, historical societies, and public broadcasting. *Civic & Public Affairs:* 34%. Funds community development and public policy. *Education:* 13%. Private secondary education and colleges and universities. *Environment:* 17%. Supports child welfare, community services, crime prevention, and people with disabilities. *International:* 17%. Focus on hospitals, medical research, diabetes, and children's health. *Note:* Total contributions made in 2002. **Typ. Recipients:** Cancer, Children's Health/Hospitals, Clinics/Medical Centers, Diabetes, Health Funds, Health Organizations, Hospices, Hospitals, Hospitals (University Affiliated), Medical Education, Medical Rehabilitation, Medical Research, Mental Health, People with Disabilities, Public Health, Research/Studies Institutes, Single-Disease Health Associations, Substance Abuse, Transplant Networks/Donor Banks. **Geo. Dist:** Washington, DC; Chicago, IL, metropolitan area; New York, NY.

★ 11177 ★ Blumenthal Foundation

PO Box 34689
Charlotte, NC 28234-4689
Phone: (704)377-6555 **Fax:** (704)377-9237
Website: http://www.blumenthalfoundation.org
Philip Blumenthal, Director

Fnded: 1953. **Philosophy:** According to the foundation's literature, it considers grant requests, primarily in the Charlotte/Mecklenburg Co. area of North Carolina, in several fields including the following: religious and interfaith groups, social services, education, the arts and humanities, health care, the environment, and Jewish institutions and philanthropies. The foundation provides grants for seed money, annual operating budgets, capital campaigns, conferences and seminars, special projects, and endowments. **Priorities:** *Arts & Humanities:* 6%. Supports a number of organizations dedicated to fine arts. *Civic & Public Affairs:* 2%. Supports zoological services, community concerns, and leadership organizations. *Education:* 13%. Local and statewide initiatives. *Environment:* 3%. Supports youth. *International:* About 1%. *Note:* Total contributions made in fiscal 2001. **Typ. Recipients:** Adolescent Health Issues, AIDS/HIV, Clinics/Medical Centers, Family Planning, Health Organizations, Hospitals, Mental Health, Single-Disease Health Associations, Substance Abuse. **Geo. Dist:** headquarters; Charlote, NC. **Frmly:** Blumenthal Foundation for Charity, Religion and Education.

★ 11178 ★ Bodman Foundation

767 Third Ave., 4th Floor
New York, NY 10017
Phone: (212)644-0322 **Fax:** (212)759-6510
Email: main@archelis-bodman-fnds.org
Website: http://www.fdncenter.org/grantmaker/archelis-bodman
Joseph Dolan, Secretary & Executive Director

Fnded: 1945. **Philosophy:** The foundation was set up to reflect the philanthropic interests of both Mr. and Mrs. Bodman, including religious, educational, and charitable organizations "for the moral, ethical, and physical well-being and progress of mankind." The foundation maintains a strong local orientation. The foundation has adopted a focus on putting responsible, full-time fathers back into two-parent intact families, as well as an emphasis on measurable outcomes of clients and program results in health and social-service agencies. Areas of interest include youth rehabilitation, biomedical research, child welfare, cultural institutions, health and hospitals, social services, education and job training, and job placement into private sector, prevention and early intervention, entrepreneurship, school reform and charter schools. **Priorities:** *Arts & Humanities:* 5%. Supports music, museums, and arts education. *Civic & Public Affairs:* 12%. Supports job training, public policy, botanical gardens, and family issues. *Education:* 38%. Primarily funds precollege education; also supports literacy and colleges and universities. *Environment:* 25%. Supports boys and girls clubs, volunteerism, substance abuse programs, family services, and youth programs. *International:* 6%. Supports biomedical research, hospitals, and single-disease research. *Religion:* 2%. Funds science councils. *Note:* Total contributions made in 2000. **Typ. Recipients:** Cancer, Child Abuse, Children's Health/Hospitals, Clinics/Medical Centers, Domestic Violence, Emergency/Ambulance Services, Eyes/Blindness, Health Funds, Health Organizations, Hospices, Hospitals, Medical Education, Medical Rehabilitation, Medical Research, Outpatient Health Care, People with Disabilities, Single-Disease Health Associations, Speech & Hearing, Substance Abuse, Transplant Networks/Donor Banks, Trauma Treatment. **Geo. Dist:** NJ, Northern New Jersey; New York, NY, metropolitan area.

★ 11179 ★ Boettcher Foundation

600 Seventeenth St., Suite 2210 South
Denver, CO 80202
Phone: (303)534-1937
Email: grants@boettcherfoundation.org
Website: http://www.boettcherfoundation.org
Timothy Schultz, President & Executive Director

Fnded: 1937. **Philosophy:** The foundation typically supports education, civic, health, cultural, and community groups. As education is a strong interest of the foundation, educational organizations consistently receive a large percentage of grants. In the area of civic and cultural programs, it emphasizes the economic development of Colorado communities through support of cultural and tourist attractions. In recent years, the foundation's health priorities have focused on programs enhancing cost containment efforts and preventative services, especially in rural areas of

Colorado. In 1998, the largest dollar amounts awarded were for capital projects, such as building or equipment needs. The grants most frequently, were in the form of challenges. **Priorities:** *Arts & Humanities:* 9%. Performing arts, museums, historical centers, and archeology. *Civic & Public Affairs:* 5%. Supports gardens and aquariums, with minor support for community development. *Education:* 44%. Universities and educational programs; scholarships. *Environment:* 29%. Youth and child services, food banks, rehabilitation, and the disabled. *International:* 13%. Hospitals and health institutes. *Note:* Total contributions were made in 2000. **Typ. Recipients:** AIDS/HIV, Alzheimers Disease, Children's Health/Hospitals, Clinics/Medical Centers, Domestic Violence, Emergency/Ambulance Services, Eyes/Blindness, Family Planning, Health-General, Hospices, Hospitals, Long-Term Care, Medical Education, Medical Rehabilitation, Mental Health, Multiple Sclerosis, People with Disabilities, Preventive Medicine/Wellness Organizations, Public Health, Sexual Abuse, Single-Disease Health Associations, Substance Abuse. **Geo. Dist:** Denver, CO.

★ 11180 ★ Booth-Bricker Fund

826 Union St., Suite 300
New Orleans, LA 70112
Phone: (504)581-2430 **Fax:** (504)566-4785
Gray Parker, Chairman

Fnded: 1976. **Philosophy:** The Booth-Bricker Fund supports a variety of local organizations, "and makes contributions for the purposes of promoting, developing, and fostering religious, charitable, scientific, literary, or educational programs." Educational support is provided to universities, day schools, and private schools. Health care favors both general care and specialty hospitals in New Orleans. Museums, theater, and public broadcasting are favored areas of support for the arts. The fund also gives to local church organizations and provides general support for social service organizations. **Priorities:** *Arts & Humanities:* 16%. Supports music and museums, historic preservation, and public broadcasting. *Civic & Public Affairs:* 8%. Funds civic groups and public policy organizations. *Education:* 45%. Funds colleges, universities, and pre-college religious education. *Environment:* 7%. Contributes to children's groups, united funds, and community service organizations. *International:* 3%. Gives to medical centers, hospitals, and health associations. *Note:* Total contributions made in 2001. **Typ. Recipients:** Children's Health/Hospitals, Clinics/Medical Centers, Eyes/Blindness, Health Organizations, Hospitals, Hospitals (University Affiliated), Long-Term Care, People with Disabilities, Public Health, Single-Disease Health Associations. **Geo. Dist:** LA, priority given to New Orleans.

★ 11181 ★ Booth Ferris Foundation

1211 Ave. of Americas
New York, NY 10036
Phone: (212)483-2323 **Fax:** (212)596-3712
Hildy Simmons, Co-Trustee

Fnded: 1957. **Philosophy:** The foundation's primary funding area is education, "especially theological, smaller colleges, and independent secondary schools." Social service and cultural activities in New York City receive a limited number of contributions. Civic, social service, education, and religious projects are funded, but to a lesser degree. Support usually goes to established organizations, particularly those in which the donors were interested during their lifetimes. **Priorities:** *Arts & Humanities:* 20%. Funds museums, theaters, historical societies, art funds, and the performing arts. *Civic & Public Affairs:* 29%. Supports community development, nonprofit management, housing, legal aid, and economic enterprise programs. *Education:* 27%. Primarily funds colleges and universities. *Environment:* 16%. Funds children's charities, camps and recreation programs, and community services. *Note:* Total contributions made in 2000. **Typ. Recipients:** Children's Health/Hospitals, Emergency/Ambulance Services, Eyes/Blindness, Family Planning, Health Organizations, Hospitals, Nutrition, People with Disabilities, Research/Studies Institutes, Substance Abuse. **Geo. Dist:** nationally; New York, NY, metropolitan area.

★ 11182 ★ The Bothin Foundation

Presidio Blvd., Suite 1016
PO Box 29906
San Francisco, CA 94129-0906
Phone: (415)561-6540 **Fax:** (415)561-6477
Website: http://www.pacificfoundationservices.com
Lyman Casey, Executive Director & Treasurer

Fnded: 1926. **Philosophy:** With limited funds available, "the foundation traditionally has supported charitable organizations promoting youth, the elderly, the environment, the disabled, health care, minorities, community social services and the arts. Grants for the arts are made only to those groups predominantly serving youth or with heavy emphasis on youth participation. As a rule, the foundation prefers to make grants for capital or building and equipment needs." Annual Report **Priorities:** *Arts & Humanities:* 7%. Funds music, festivals, and art museums. *Civic & Public Affairs:* 12%. Supports civic and public policy. *Education:* 10%. Funds precollege education and educational programs. *Environment:* 55%. Supports food banks, shelters, disabled-citizen concerns, and youth groups. *International:* 10%. Funds health services for disadvantaged youth and children, hospice, and AIDS awareness. *Note:* Total contributions made in 2001. **Typ. Recipients:** AIDS/HIV, Cancer, Clinics/Medical Centers, Domestic Violence, Emergency/Ambulance Services, Eyes/Blindness, Family Planning, Health Organizations, Home-Care Services, Hospices, Hospitals, Hospitals (University Affiliated), Kidney, Medical Rehabilitation, Mental Health, People with Disabilities, Prenatal Health Issues, Sexual Abuse, Speech & Hearing, Substance Abuse. **Geo. Dist:** San Francisco, CA, metropolitan area.

★ 11183 ★ Bradley-Turner Foundation

PO Box 140
Columbus, GA 31902
Phone: (706)571-6040 **Fax:** (706)571-3408
Tom Black, Administrator

Fnded: 1943. **Philosophy:** The foundation generally funds higher educational institutions, arts and cultural organizations, religious associations, and social services. **Priorities:** *Arts & Humanities:* 11%. Gives to museums, history museums, ballet, orchestras, and historic preservation. *Civic & Public Affairs:* 30%. Funds housing, cot foundations, community initiatives, job training and placement, fire departments, and civic clubs. *Education:* 39%. Supports colleges and universities, public and private schools, literacy programs, and education foundations. *Environment:* 8%. Funds youth programs, shelters, community services, United Way, and Young Men's Christian Association. *International:* 7%. Gives to hospitals, children's health, and single disease health associations. *Note:* Total contributions made in 2000. **Typ. Recipients:** Cancer, Child Abuse, Children's Health/Hospitals, Clinics/Medical Centers, Emergency/Ambulance Services, Health Organizations, Hospices, Hospitals, Hospitals (University Affiliated), Long-Term Care, Medical Education, Medical Rehabilitation, Medical Research, Outpatient Health Care, People with Disabilities, Single-Disease Health Associations. **Geo. Dist:** GA.

★ 11184 ★ Brady Family Foundation

3 Pond Rd.
Gloucester, MA 01930-1834
Phone: (978)283-5800
Patrick Brady, Trustee

Fnded: 1994. **Priorities:** *Arts & Humanities:* Less than 1%. *Civic & Public Affairs:* 99%. *Education:* Less than 1%. *Environment:* Less than 1%. *International:* 1%. *Note:* Total foundation contributions made in 2001. **Typ. Recipients:** Cancer, Children's Health/Hospitals, Medical Research, Multiple Sclerosis, Single-Disease Health Associations. **Geo. Dist:** MA; NY. **Frmly:** Cyrk International Foundation.

★ 11185 ★ Britton Fund

1422 Euclid Ave., Suite 1010
Cleveland, OH 44115-2078
Phone: (216)363-6489
Nick Valentino, Treasurer

Fnded: 1952. **Philosophy:** The fund generally supports medical organizations, community services, and educational institutions in the Cleveland, Ohio, area. **Priorities:** *Arts & Humanities:* 9%. Arts centers, music, historic preservation, community affiliate, and museums. *Civic & Public Affairs:* 14%. Supports women's affiliate, disaster relief, and vocational services. *Education:* 18%. Primarily for student aid. *Environment:* 24%. Food banks, shelters, family planning, community services, and YMCAs. *International:* 17%. Major grant to University Hospitals in Cleveland, Ohio. Also supports Alzheimer's research, medical rehabilitation, medical centers, and geriatric care. *Religion:* 17%. Funds museum. *Note:* Total contributions made in 2001. **Typ. Recipients:** Alzheimers Disease, Cancer, Children's Health/Hospitals, Clinics/Medical Centers, Domestic Violence, Emergency/Ambulance Services, Eyes/Blindness, Eyes/Blindness, Family Planning, Geriatric Health, Health Organizations, Hospitals, Hospitals (University Affiliated), Long-Term Care, Medical Education, Medical Rehabilitation, Medical Research, Mental Health, Multiple Sclerosis, Nursing Services, People with Disabilities, Sexual Abuse, Single-Disease Health Associations, Speech & Hearing. **Geo. Dist:** OH, Greater Cleveland including Cayahoga, Geauga, and lake counties.

★ 11186 ★ Brown Foundation

PO Box 130646
Houston, TX 77219-0646
Phone: (713)523-6867 **Fax:** (713)523-2917
Email: bfi@brownfoundation.org
Website: http://www.brownfoundation.org
Nancy Pittman, Executive Director

Fnded: 1951. **Philosophy:** Since its establishment, the foundation has supported a variety of organizations, mostly in the state of Texas. Major areas of giving include education, the arts and humanities, health and medicine, civic & public affairs and human services. In the field of education, the foundation focuses on searching out and supporting non-traditional and innovative approaches designed to improve public education at the primary and secondary levels. **Priorities:** *Arts & Humanities:* 33%. Funds art galleries, arts centers, museums, historical societies, film programs, and the peforming arts. Major support for the Smithsonian Institute. *Civic & Public Affairs:* 14%. Gives to community and neighborhood affairs, housing, parks, public policy, and environmental affairs. *Education:* 31%. Supports engineering education, colleges and universities, faculty endowments, public and private schools, and scholarships. *Environment:* 7%. Funds family services, services for the disabled, shelters, child welfare organizations, abuse prevention programs, rape crisis centers, the United Way, and youth organizations. *International:* (Medicine and Science) 15%. Supports children's health care, organ donation centers, cancer research, hospitals, clinics, drug abuse programs, and medical science and research. *Note:* Total contributions made in fiscal 2001. **Typ. Recipients:** Adolescent Health Issues, Alzheimers Disease, Cancer, Child Abuse, Children's Health/Hospitals, Clinics/Medical Centers, Domestic Violence, Family Planning, Health Organizations, Heart, Hospices, Hospitals, Medical Education, Medical Research, Mental Health, People with Disabilities, Research/Studies Institutes, Single-Disease Health Associations. **Geo. Dist:** TX, particularly Houston.

★ 11187 ★ Broyhill Family Foundation

PO Box 500
Golfview Park
Lenoir, NC 28645
Phone: (828)758-6100
Paul Broyhill, Chairman & Manager

Fnded: 1945. **Philosophy:** The Broyhill Family Foundation, formerly the Broyhill Foundation, originally was established to help needy individuals obtain a college education through loans. The foundation also funds civic organizations, community and human services, hospitals and health organizations, and the arts. Although the foundation no longer offers loans directly to students, it is funding a Special Investment Loan Program available through the College Foundation, which provides student aid. **Priorities:** *Arts & Humani-*

ties: 2%. Support given to art and culture. *Civic & Public Affairs:* 17%. Funds community and public affairs. *Education:* 43%. Emphasis on educational institutions and programs, including colleges and universities. *Environment:* 17%. Grants were made to social, family, and youth services. *International:* 14%. Hospices, disease and disorder concerns, single-disease organizations, hospitals, and AIDS causes receive support. *Note:* Total contributions made in 2001. **Typ. Recipients:** Children's Health/Hospitals, Clinics/Medical Centers, Emergency/Ambulance Services, Eyes/Blindness, Health Organizations, Health-General, Hospices, Hospitals, Medical Education, Medical Research, Mental Health, People with Disabilities, Preventive Medicine/Wellness Organizations, Public Health, Research/Studies Institutes, Substance Abuse. **Geo. Dist:** NC, preference to Cardwell County and surrounding areas.

★ 11188 ★ Bruce McMillan, Jr. Foundation

PO Box 9
Overton, TX 75684
Phone: (903)834-3148 **Fax:** (903)834-3947
Ralph Ward, Jr., President, Treasurer & Director

Fnded: 1951. **Philosophy:** The Bruce McMillan, Jr., Foundation supports the areas of education, religion, scientific, literary and charitable. Educational funding favors colleges and universities and agricultural programs. Scholarships are generally restricted to students from eight high schools in the Overton, TX, area. Health care support goes to cancer research, blood centers, and treatment centers. Religious support favors individual churches in the Overton, TX, area, and social services support includes youth organizations. **Priorities:** *Arts & Humanities:* 1%. For a museum. *Civic & Public Affairs:* 1%. *Education:* 68%. Supports educational endowments for secondary schools and colleges. *Environment:* 5%. Youth and family services programs. *International:* 6%. Health centers. *Note:* Total contributions made in fiscal 2001. **Typ. Recipients:** Cancer, Child Abuse, Children's Health/Hospitals, Domestic Violence, Emergency/Ambulance Services, Family Planning, Health Organizations, Heart, Heart, Prenatal Health Issues, Public Health, Sexual Abuse, Single-Disease Health Associations, Substance Abuse, Transplant Networks/Donor Banks. **Geo. Dist:** TX, emphasis on the Overton area.

★ 11189 ★ The Bryant Foundation

PO Box 1239
Stephens City, VA 22655-1239
Phone: (540)868-2183
Arthur Bryant, II, President & Treasurer

Fnded: 1949. **Philosophy:** The foundation primarily is interested in supporting education in Virginia. Most of the giving focuses, but is not limited to, higher education. Smaller grants are made to other major categories of support. Other interests include libraries, community endowments, health services, religion, and community centers. Many of the foundation's secondary interests support athletic or recreational projects. **Priorities:** *Arts & Humanities:* 22%. Funds historic preservation, cultural and history museums, and libraries. *Education:* 67%. Supports colleges, universities, and private pre-college schools. *Environment:* About 1%. Children's homes, community centers, and Young Men's Christian Association. *International:* 9%. Gives to hospitals, free clinics, health care foundations, cancer organizations, and the American Red Cross. *Note:* Total contributions made in 2000. **Typ. Recipients:** Cancer, Clinics/Medical Centers, Emergency/Ambulance Services, Health Organizations, Health Organizations, Health-General, Hospitals, Long-Term Care, Medical Rehabilitation, Medical Research, Prenatal Health Issues, Public Health, Respiratory, Single-Disease Health Associations. **Geo. Dist:** VA.

★ 11190 ★ Buchanan Family Foundation

222 East Wisconsin Ave.
Lake Forest, IL 60045
Phone: (847)234-0235
Huntington Eldridge, Jr., Treasurer

Fnded: 1967. **Philosophy:** The foundation generally supports hospitals and health organizations, cultural and environmental causes, and colleges and universities, all within the metropolitan Chicago, IL, area. **Priorities:** *Arts & Humanities:* 14%. Supports public broadcasting, festivals, libraries, historical society, music, and opera, symphony and theaters. *Civic & Public Affairs:* 12%. Supports aquarium, zoo, parks, and community foundations. *Education:* 22%. Supports colleges and universities, endowments and secondary schools. *Environment:* 14%. Supports community service organizations, scouts, YMCA and United Way. *International:* 23%. Supports hospitals and medical centers; research foundation. *Religion:* 4%. Funds planetarium, science museum. *Note:* Total contributions made in 2000. **Typ. Recipients:** Children's Health/Hospitals, Clinics/Medical Centers, Emergency/Ambulance Services, Family Planning, Health Organizations, Hospitals, Medical Rehabilitation, Medical Research, Nursing Services, Prenatal Health Issues, Single-Disease Health Associations. **Geo. Dist:** Chicago, IL.

★ 11191 ★ Buffett Foundation

1430 Kiewit Plaza
Omaha, NE 68131
Phone: (402)345-9168
Allen Greenberg, Executive Director & Secretary

Fnded: 1964. **Philosophy:** The Buffet Foundation makes most of its grants to social service organizations focusing on planned parenthood and international population growth. The foundation also sponsors several scholarships and an outstanding teacher award program (restricted to Omaha public school teachers only). **Priorities:** *Civic & Public Affairs:* 16%. Supports reproductive law and policy, and womens affairs. *Education:* 12%. Funds scholarships and fellowships for higher education. *Environment:* 15%. Major support is awarded to family planning services. Also supports United Way and youth programs. *International:* 33%. Supports medical research, reproductive health issues, and access to reproductive health care. *Note:* Total contributions made in fiscal 2001. **Typ. Recipients:** Clinics/Medical Centers, Family Planning, Health-General, Hospitals, Hospitals (University Affiliated), Medical Education, Medical Research, Public Health. **Geo. Dist:** no geographic restrictions.

★ 11192 ★ Bugher Foundation

600 5th Ave.
New York, NY 10020
Phone: (212)632-3000 **Fax:** (212)896-2580
Email: dau@daniel-adams.com
Don Adams, Trustee

Fnded: 1961. **Philosophy:** The foundation is dedicated to cardiovascular disease research. **Priorities:** *Education:* 23% Supports universities, schools, and medical edu. *International:* 77%. Supports American Heart Association, blood centers, and cardiovascular research. *Note:* Total contributions were made in fiscal 2000. **Typ. Recipients:** Cancer, Emergency/Ambulance Services, Heart, Medical Education, Medical Research, Single-Disease Health Associations, Transplant Networks/Donor Banks. **Geo. Dist:** nationally.

★ 11193 ★ Buhl Foundation (PA)

650 Smithfield St., Suite 2300
Pittsburgh, PA 15222
Phone: (412)566-2711 **Fax:** (412)566-2714
Email: buhl@buhlfoundation.org
Doreen Boyce, President

Fnded: 1927. **Philosophy:** The foundation's focus is on innovation, with emphasis on funding "opportunities with potential impact beyond the institution which has been funded." The foundation's concerns include "the developing and harnessing of new technologies to address the administration and purposes of organizations or processes of learning and teaching;...the investigation of problems with a view to generating creative solutions and cooperation among diverse disciplines or organizations;...(and) the generation and dissemination of new knowledge where that knowledge has the possibility of direct practical application." The foundation's board of managers designated that proposals with the following characteristics are of particular interest: educational programs; programs for young people; studies to produce practical applications which make a contribution to basic theory; attempts which relate specialists in a common approach to problems or which call for cooperative efforts among separate agencies; institutional, experimental, or demonstrational approaches to resolving problems when they are innovative; and previously supported and promising programs where time extension or new developments afford opportunity for enhancement of values. **Priorities:** *Arts & Humanities:* 18%. Funds the arts, theater, music, and libraries. *Civic & Public Affairs:* 10%. Funds community education and job training programs, community foundations, and leadership programs. *Education:* 42%. Funds colleges and universities, boards of education, and elementary education programs. *Environment:* 15%. Funds social services, rehabilitation centers, and the United Way. *Note:* Total contributions made in fiscal 2001. **Typ. Recipients:** Cancer, Child Abuse, Children's Health/Hospitals, Emergency/Ambulance Services, Health Organizations, Heart, Hospitals, Mental Health, Nursing Services, People with Disabilities, Sexual Abuse, Substance Abuse. **Geo. Dist:** Pittsburgh, PA, metropolitan area.

★ 11194 ★ Bullitt Foundation

1212 Minor Ave.
Seattle, WA 98101-2825
Phone: (206)343-0807 **Fax:** (206)343-0822
Email: info@bullitt.org
Website: http://www.bullitt.org
Marilyn Fike, Administrator

Fnded: 1952. **Philosophy:** The purpose of the Bullitt Foundation is to protect and restore the natural physical environment. During the past year the foundation has given grants solely to environmental causes. Gifts are confined to the Pacific Northwest. The foundation has seven specific priorities among environmental issues. *Energy and Climate Change.* "The foundation will promote a swift transition toward the efficient use of energy sources that are safe, sustainable, and environmentally attractive." *Forests and Land Ecosystems.* "The foundation seeks to maintain species endemic to the Northwest, and the ecosystems on which they depend, and to safeguard the beauty, natural wealth, and recreational activities of the region." *Growth Management and Transportation.* "The foundation supports efforts to promote land-use policies and practices that protect environmentally sensitive areas; accommodate agriculture, fisheries, and forestry; and promote communities in which residential, commercial, industrial, and civic functions are integrated." *Public Outreach, Education, and Capacity Building.* "The foundation supports projects that educate the public, promote stewardship, ensure adequate funding and support for quality environmental education in schools, and encourage more informed and active voters." *Rivers, Wetlands, and Estuaries.* "The foundation strives to protect aquatic resources, from the pure water of mountain streams to the productive richness of marine environments." *Sustainable Agriculture.* "The foundation supports efforts that preserve farmlands, conserve biodiversity, and foster sustainable agricultural policies and practices." *Toxic Substances, Mining, and Radioactive Waste.* "The foundation supports efforts to advance policies and practices that reduce toxic substance use, eliminate the release of toxic substances, reform destructive mining practices, and clean up areas already contaminated by toxic substances." The foundation will also consider environmental proposals that do not fall within the seven priority areas, but that do fall within its geographic area and overall mission. Bullitt Foundation Annual Report **Priorities:** *Civic & Public Affairs:* 4%. *Environment:* 2%. *Note:* Contributions made in fiscal 2000. **Typ. Recipients:** Preventive Medicine/Wellness Organizations. **Geo. Dist:** AK, Coastal Rainforests; ID; MT, Western part of state; OR; WA; BC.

★ 11195 ★ Bunbury Co., Inc.

2 Railroad Place
Hopewell, NJ 08525
Phone: (609)333-8800 **Fax:** (609)333-8900
Email: BunburyCo@aol.com
Website: http://www.bunburycompany.org
Samuel Lambert III, Treasurer

Fnded: 1952. **Philosophy:** "Through its grant making, Bunbury seeks to assist organizations working within a broad spectrum of philanthropic activities. Those organizations include, but are not limited to, those dealing with disadvantaged youth and families; ecology and the natural world, education in the broadest sense; and promotion of the arts." The Bunbury Company Application Guidelines **Priorities:** *Arts & Humanities:* 12%. Supports the performing arts, historical societies, and arts councils. *Civic & Public Affairs:* 26%. Supports community funds, fire departments, and trade organizations. *Education:* 38%. Supports colleges and universities, literacy, and education foundations. *Environment:* 14%. Supports family planning, family and youth services, and housing. *International:* 5%. Supports a medical center. *Note:* Total contributions made in 2001. **Typ. Recipients:** AIDS/HIV, Cancer, Children's Health/Hospitals, Clinics/Medical Centers, Domestic Violence, Emergency/Ambulance Services, Family Planning, Hospitals, Medical Research, Mental Health, Nursing Services, People with Disabilities, Public Health, Substance Abuse. **Geo. Dist:** NJ, Burlington County; NJ, Camden County; NJ, Hunterdon County; NJ, Middlesex County; NJ, Monmouth County; NJ, Ocean County; NJ, Somerset County; NJ, Mercer County.

★ 11196 ★ Bunker Foundation

PO Box 223609
Carmel, CA 93922
Phone: (650)740-3273
Susan Ingemason, President

Fnded: 1995. **Priorities:** *Arts & Humanities:* 3%. Supports public broadcasting and a museum. *Civic & Public Affairs:* 15%. Supports public policy and parks. *Education:* 21%. Supports public and private schools and higher education. *Environment:* 8%. Supports United Way, animal protection, and children's organizations. *International:* 50%. Supports medical research and hospitals and medical centers. *Note:* Total contributions made in fiscal 1998. **Typ. Recipients:** Cancer, Children's Health/Hospitals, Diabetes, Family Planning, Hospices, Hospitals (University Affiliated), Medical Research, Speech & Hearing. **Geo. Dist:** CA. **Frmly:** Susan Ingemason McNealy Foundation.

★ 11197 ★ Burdine Johnson Foundation

PO Box 1230
Buda, TX 78610-1230
Phone: (512)312-1336 **Fax:** (512)295-4773
Robert Giberson, Trustee

Fnded: 1960. **Philosophy:** The Burdine Johnson Foundation primarily supports religious, private, and secondary education. Other interests include the performing arts, family planning, and civic affairs. **Priorities:** *Arts & Humanities:* 21%. Supports foundation for performing arts and preservation associations. *Civic & Public Affairs:* 1%. *Education:* 69%. Supports public and private schools, religious education, and universities. *Environment:* 5%. Supports community center, seniors, and family planning. *International:* 1%. Supports children's hospitals and cancer centers. *Note:* Total contributions made in 2000. **Typ. Recipients:** Cancer, Children's Health/Hospitals, Domestic Violence, Emergency/Ambulance Services, Family Planning, Medical Education, Medical Research, Multiple Sclerosis, Sexual Abuse, Single-Disease Health Associations, Substance Abuse, Transplant Networks/Donor Banks. **Geo. Dist:** TX.

★ 11198 ★ The Burnett Foundation

801 Cherry St., Suite 1585
Unit 16
Fort Worth, TX 76102-6881
Phone: (817)877-3344 **Fax:** (817)338-0448
Thomas Beech, Executive Vice President

Fnded: 1978. **Philosophy:** The Burnett Foundation was founded in 1978 by Anne Burnett Tandy. Since its earliest days the Foundation's grants have reflected the philosophy and special genius of its founder. "Organization-Building grants that help nonprofit organizations become more effective, more responsive and more creative in carrying out their missions. In several instances, the Foundation's support has helped create new organizations. "Community-Building grants that help the citizens of a community capitalize and build on their community's strengths and develop strategies to deal with challenges and opportunities facing them. Most of the Foundation's Community-Building grants have targeted inner-city neighborhoods. "Grants have been made in the fields of arts and humanities, health, human services, community development and education. Historically, the Foundation has focused its energy and resources in Fort Worth, Texas and in the last few years also in Sante Fe, New Mexico." 1996 Annual Report **Priorities:** *Arts & Humanities:* 77%. Major support is given to museums, also supports music, opera, art festivals, ballet, and the performing arts. *Civic & Public Affairs:* 15%. Supports parks, housing, and community foundation. *Education:* 2%. Supports scholarship and universities. *Environment:* 5%. Supports United Way, food distribution, Young Women's Christian Association, youth programs, and counseling. *International:* 1%. Substance abuse and AIDS prevention. *Note:* Total contributions made in 2001. **Typ. Recipients:** AIDS/HIV, Alzheimers Disease, Cancer, Child Abuse, Children's Health/Hospitals, Clinics/Medical Centers, Domestic Violence, Emergency/Ambulance Services, Family Planning, Health Policy/Cost Containment, Hospitals, Medical Education, Medical Research, Mental Health, People with Disabilities, Prenatal Health Issues, Research/Studies Institutes, Sexual Abuse, Single-Disease Health Associations, Substance Abuse. **Geo. Dist:** occasionally grants are provided nationally, at the trustee's discretion; Santa Fe, NM; Ft. Worth, TX.

★ 11199 ★ Burton D. Morgan Foundation

PO Box 1500
Akron, OH 44309-1500
Phone: (330)258-6512 **Fax:** (330)258-6559
Website: http://www.bdmorganfdn.org
John Frank, President

Fnded: 1967. **Philosophy:** The Burton D. Morgan Foundation primarily supports education, including private Episcopal schools and universities. Other interests include churches, arts centers, art associations, and civic affairs in northeastern Ohio. The foundation's present areas of focus include programs to support the free/private enterprise system, economics, education, and mental health. **Priorities:** *Arts & Humanities:* 5%. Supports public broadcasting, music, and history. *Civic & Public Affairs:* 46%. Supports the EAA Aviation Foundation, community foundations, urban and economic development, philanthropic causes, and employment. *Education:* 28%. Focus on colleges and universities and education associations. *Environment:* 3%. Supports Young Men's Christian Association and general social services. *International:* 2%. Supports children's health and hospitals. *Note:* Total contributions made in 2000. **Typ. Recipients:** Children's Health/Hospitals, Domestic Violence, Emergency/Ambulance Services, Family Planning, Health Organizations, Heart, Hospices, Hospitals, Medical Education, Mental Health, Nursing Services, People with Disabilities, Public Health, Research/Studies Institutes, Substance Abuse. **Geo. Dist:** OH, Summit County.

★ 11200 ★ Burton G. Bettingen Corp.

9777 Wilshire Boulevard, Suite 615
Beverly Hills, CA 90212
Phone: (310)276-4115 **Fax:** (310)276-4693
Email: burtonbet@aol.com
Patricia Brown, Executive Director

Fnded: 1984. **Philosophy:** The current focus of the corporation is child welfare including assistance to child prostitutes, runaways, and abandoned children. The corporation has two separate giving funds: the Haven Fund is committed to supporting child welfare; the General Fund includes support for youth but also supports organizations in several fields including education, health, environment, and welfare. The corporation provides broad types of support including program, capital funds, research, and endowments. **Priorities:** *Arts & Humanities:* 3%. Supports museums and public television. *Civic & Public Affairs:* 10%. Supports community development and philanthropy concerns. *Education:* 14%. Supports educational programs, schools, colleges and universities. *Environment:* 33%. Supports youth services and social services. *International:* 30%. Supports health and medical centers, hospitals, disease and disorder concerns. *Note:* Contributions made in fiscal 1999. **Typ. Recipients:** AIDS/HIV, Alzheimers Disease, Cancer, Child Abuse, Children's Health/Hospitals, Emergency/Ambulance Services, Family Planning, Health Organizations, Health Policy/Cost Containment, Home-Care Services, Hospitals, Hospitals (University Affiliated), Long-Term Care, Medical Education, Medical Research, Mental Health, People with Disabilities, Preventive Medicine/Wellness Organizations, Research/Studies Institutes, Respiratory, Sexual Abuse, Single-Disease Health Associations, Substance Abuse. **Geo. Dist:** Los Angeles, CA.

★ 11201 ★ Bush Foundation

332 Minnesota St., E-900
Saint Paul, MN 55101
Phone: (651)227-0891 **Fax:** (651)297-6485
Email: info@bushfoundation.org
Website: http://www.bushfoundation.org
Anita Pampusch, President

Fnded: 1953. **Philosophy:** The foundation concentrates its grants in the areas of education, humanities and the arts, community and social welfare, health, and leadership development. The foundation is predominantly a regional giver, making grants primarily in Minnesota, North Dakota, and South Dakota. However, it operates two non-regional grant programs, offering matching grants to historically black private colleges and grants to accredited tribally controlled Indian colleges. The foundation's matching capital grants program and faculty development program for black private colleges is run in cooperation with the William and Flora Hewlett Foundation of Menlo Park, CA. Grants to education programs take the form of faculty development and matching capital grants for undergraduate colleges in Minnesota and the Dakotas; faculty development and matching capital grants to historically black private colleges; grants to encourage elementary and secondary school age girls and all minority students to pursue math and science education; faculty development grants to Indian colleges. In the area of health, the foundation supports programs to improve the quality, accessibility, and efficiency of health care services within its geographic region. Grants are concentrated on training programs for health professionals, efforts to improve access to health care in rural and under-served areas, and the promotion of minority career development in the health field. Human services funding supports programs for troubled and disadvantaged youth; emergency housing and employment counseling services for homeless women with children; programs to assist victims of domestic violence; and programs that provide rehabilitation services for developmentally disabled adults. Other interests include rural economic development, rural family assistance programs, and law and corrections. The Bush Medical Fellows Program seeks to develop physicians' potential for increased competence and leadership in clinical medicine, health care delivery, administration, and education. Miscellaneous grants are made to community foundations and such areas as public broadcasting and the environment. **Priorities:** *Arts & Humanities:* 10%. Focus on public broadcasting, museums, theaters, music, arts centers, and arts funds. *Education:* 39%. Emphasis on colleges and universities primarily in Minnesota, North Dakota, and South Dakota. Fellowships are also supported. *Environment:* 33%. Support for youth organizations, child welfare, immigrant programs, and family services. *International:* 1%. Funds hospitals and direct health care organizations. *Note:* Total contributions made in fiscal 2001. **Typ. Recipients:** AIDS/HIV, Children's Health/Hospitals, Clinics/Medical Centers,

Domestic Violence, Family Planning, Geriatric Health, Health Organizations, Health-General, Medical Education, Medical Rehabilitation, Medical Training, Mental Health, Nursing Services, People with Disabilities, Public Health, Research/Studies Institutes, Sexual Abuse, Substance Abuse. **Geo. Dist:** nationally; MN; ND; SD.

★ 11202 ★ Byrne Foundation
35 Rope Ferry Rd.
Hanover, NH 03755
Phone: (603)643-4555
Dorothy Byrne, President

Fnded: 1993. **Philosophy:** The foundation's primary interests include cancer research, Dartmouth College, and general philanthropy. **Priorities:** *Arts & Humanities:* 2%. Supports public broadcasting. *Civic & Public Affairs:* 4%. Supports community foundations, economic development. *Education:* 27%. Supports secondary schools, Dartmouth College. *Environment:* 6%. Funds community centers, youth programs, services for the elderly. *International:* 57%. Supports cancer research centers. *Note:* Total contributions made in 1998. **Typ. Recipients:** Cancer, Child Abuse, Children's Health/Hospitals, Clinics/Medical Centers, Emergency/Ambulance Services, Health Organizations, Hospices, Hospitals, Medical Rehabilitation, Medical Research, Multiple Sclerosis, People with Disabilities, Public Health, Respiratory, Substance Abuse. **Geo. Dist:** NH, Upper Valley Region; VT, Upper Valley Region.

★ 11203 ★ Cabot Family Charitable Trust
70 Federal St.
Boston, MA 02110
Phone: (617)451-1744
Ruth Scheer, Executive Director

Fnded: 1942. **Philosophy:** The trust supports colleges and universities, the arts, scientific organizations, and civic causes. Giving is generally limited to the greater Boston, Massachusetts, area. **Priorities:** *Arts & Humanities:* 40%. Supports orchestra, museums. *Civic & Public Affairs:* 10%. Supports libraries, community foundations. *Education:* 26%. Supports colleges and universities. *Environment:* 7%. Supports family services, YMCA, family planning. *Religion:* 10%. Supports scientific organization. *Note:* Total contributions made in 2001. **Typ. Recipients:** Children's Health/Hospitals, Clinics/Medical Centers, Family Planning, Health Organizations, Hospitals, Medical Education, Mental Health, People with Disabilities, Public Health. **Geo. Dist:** CA; MA.

★ 11204 ★ Caleb C. and Julia W. Dula Educational and Charitable Foundation
112 South Hanley Rd., 2nd Floor
Saint Louis, MO 63105-3418
Phone: (314)726-2800 **Fax:** (314)863-3821
James Mauze, General Counsel

Fnded: 1939. **Philosophy:** The foundation primarily supports the arts and civic affairs. Art funding favors libraries, symphonies, and historic preservation. Civic affairs support goes to foundations, zoos and botanical gardens, and environmental affairs. The foundation also makes contributions to education, hospitals and nursing services, and social services. **Priorities:** *Arts & Humanities:* 18%. Supports theaters, music, dance, and historical societies. *Civic & Public Affairs:* 21%. Botanical gardens, zoos, and foundations were funded. *Education:* 24%. Secondary schools and universities received grants. *Environment:* 19%. Supports people with disabilities, youth organizations, family services, and animal welfare. *International:* 13%. Funding went to hospitals and single-disease health associations. *Note:* Total contributions made in 2000. **Typ. Recipients:** Alzheimers Disease, Cancer, Children's Health/Hospitals, Clinics/Medical Centers, Diabetes, Emergency/Ambulance Services, Family Planning, Health Organizations, Hospitals, Medical Education, Nursing Services, People with Disabilities, Preventive Medicine/Wellness Organizations, Single-Disease Health Associations. **Geo. Dist:** MO; NY.

★ 11205 ★ The California Endowment
21650 Oxnard St.
Suite 1200
Woodland Hills, CA 91367
Phone: 800-449-4149 **Fax:** (818)703-4193
Email: questions@calendow.org
Website: http://www.calendow.org
Manny Padilla, Internal Communication Manager

Fnded: 1996. **Philosophy:** "The California Endowment supports a multicultural approach to health and has four strategic program areas: Access-to increase access for all Californians to health care; Cultural Competency-to develop a culturally competent health system; Work Force Diversity-to promote a diverse California workforce; Disparities in Health-to eliminate health disparities and promote improvements in health and well-being among at-risk populations. Additionally, we offer two responsive grantmaking programs: Communities First-responding to the needs of communities at the center of developing solutions for health-related issues; Local Opportunities Fund-providing communities with resources to address important health issues on a local, grassroots level." **Priorities:** *International:* 100%. Supports health services, public health institutes and foundations, clinics, hospitals, medical education, the uninsured and medically underserved. *Note:* Total contributions made in fiscal 2002. **Typ. Recipients:** Adolescent Health Issues, AIDS/HIV, Cancer, Child Abuse, Children's Health/Hospitals, Clinics/Medical Centers, Domestic Violence, Eyes/Blindness, Family Planning, Geriatric Health, Health Funds, Health Organizations, Health Policy/Cost Containment, Health-General, Hospitals, Medical Rehabilitation, Mental Health, Nutrition, People with Disabilities, Prenatal Health Issues, Public Health, Public Health, Research/Studies Institutes, Respiratory. **Geo. Dist:** CA.

★ 11206 ★ California Wellness Foundation
6320 Canoga Ave., Suite 1700
Woodland Hills, CA 91367
Phone: (818)593-6600 **Fax:** (818)593-6614
Email: tcwf@tcwf.org
Website: http://www.tcwf.org
Gary Yates, President & Chief Executive Officer

Fnded: 1991. **Typ. Recipients:** Children's Health/Hospitals, Clinics/Medical Centers, Family Planning, Geriatric Health, Health Organizations, Hospitals, Medical Education, Medical Research, Public Health, Trauma Treatment.

★ 11207 ★ Callaway Foundation, Inc.
209 Broome St.
PO Box 790
LaGrange, GA 30241
Phone: (706)884-7348 **Fax:** (706)884-0201
H. Speer Burdette, President

Fnded: 1943. **Philosophy:** The philosophy of the Callaway Foundation was initiated by Fuller E. Callaway, Sr., who had a profound interest in the "health, education, and welfare of the people in the community in which he lived and did business." The foundation is primarily intended for religious, charitable, and educational benefits to the people in Troup County and LaGrange, GA. The foundation prefers to provide capital funds for established and active community organizations, especially those that offer lasting benefit to the community. The foundation also supports organizations and projects considered worthy by others as evidenced by various sources of support. The board of trustees will consider matching funds for such groups and to qualifying churches within the city limits of LaGrange. **Priorities:** *Arts & Humanities:* 4%. Supports arts centers, museums, music, and the performing arts. *Civic & Public Affairs:* 27%. Funds municipalities and housing. *Education:* 42%. Focus on LaGrange College. *International:* 4%. Major support for West Georgia Health System. *Note:* Total contributions made in fiscal 2001. **Typ. Recipients:** AIDS/HIV, Alzheimers Disease, Cancer, Clinics/Medical Centers, Emergency/Ambulance Services, Eyes/Blindness, Family Planning, Health Organizations, Health Policy/Cost Containment, Heart, Hospitals, Long-Term Care, Medical Education, Medical Rehabilitation, People with Disabilities, Public Health, Single-Disease Health Associations, Substance Abuse, Transplant Networks/Donor Banks. **Geo. Dist:** LaGrange, GA, including Troup County.

★ 11208 ★ Cameron Baird Foundation
120 Delaware Ave., 6th Fl.
Buffalo, NY 14202
Phone: (716)845-6000
Brian Baird, Trustee

Fnded: 1960. **Philosophy:** The Cameron Baird Foundation makes most of its grants in the areas of the arts, civic affairs, and education. Arts funding favors musical performances in Buffalo, NY. Funding for civic affairs emphasizes the environment. Educational giving focuses on minority scholarships. The foundation funds a variety of other interests, such as family planning and youth organizations. **Priorities:** *Arts & Humanities:* 60%. Primary support for orchestras, arts institutes, opera, and arts associations. *Civic & Public Affairs:* 3%. Women's affairs and housing. *Education:* 6%. Supports private secondary schools and colleges. *Environment:* 12%. Funds family planning, youth organizations, child welfare, and community services. *International:* 1%. Hospitals, children's health, hospices, and single-disease health associations. *Note:* Total contributions were made in 2000. **Typ. Recipients:** Children's Health/Hospitals, Family Planning, Hospices, Multiple Sclerosis, People with Disabilities, Public Health. **Geo. Dist:** Buffalo, NY.

★ 11209 ★ Camille and Henry Dreyfus Foundation
555 Madison Ave., 20th Floor
New York, NY 10022-3301
Phone: (212)753-1760
Email: admin@dreyfus.org
Website: http://www.dreyfus.org
Dr. Mark Cardillo, Executive Director

Fnded: 1946. **Philosophy:** The foundation's goal is to "advance the science of chemistry, chemical engineering, and related sciences as a means of improving human relations and circumstances around the world." To reflect this philosophy, the foundation offers funding through seven programs: Camille Dreyfus Teacher-Scholar Awards, Henry Dreyfus Teacher-Scholar Awards, New Faculty Awards, Faculty Start-up Grants for Undergraduate Institutions, Scholar/Fellow Program for Undergraduate Institutions, Special Grant Program in the Chemical Sciences, and the Postdoctoral Program in Environmental Science. The Camille Dreyfus Teacher-Scholar Awards Program focuses primarily on individual research attainment and promise, with the expectation that the nominee will demonstrate a commitment to education as well; the Henry Dreyfus Teacher-Scholar Awards Program stresses teaching, mentorship, and the nominee's accomplishments as a role model for undergraduates planning careers in the chemical sciences. The Camille and Henry Dreyfus New Faculty Award Program offers starter grants in research for newly appointed faculty members at graduate institutions just prior to their first year of teaching. Candidates are nominated by their respective institutions, and each institution is limited to one nomination. The Camille and Henry Dreyfus Faculty Start-up Grants for Undergraduate Institutions began in 1993. The program aims to provide funding for new faculty members in the chemical sciences at the start of their research and teaching activities. An unrestricted grant of $12,500 is awarded in September of the year the new faculty member formally begins the first year appointment, in order to encourage new faculty to begin the teaching-research interplay as early as possible in their careers. The Special Grant Program in Chemical Sciences supports innovative ways to advance the chemical sciences, primarily by enhancement of academic curricula and of presentation of chemistry to the public. The Scholar/Fellow Program for Undergraduate Institutions aims to encourage teaching and research in undergraduate colleges. The program is designed to attract talented Ph.D. recipients to careers in undergraduate education and to recognize outstanding research accomplishments or potential among established undergraduate faculty. The Postdoctoral Program in Environmental Chemistry was established in 1996. This program encourages experts in the field of environmental science to submit proposals for the training of Ph.D. chemists and chemical engineers in research activities related to chemistry and the environment. This award is granted annually to five institutions and the total of the each grant is $90,0000. **Priorities:** *Education:* 100%. Support directed toward the chemical sciences. The foundation focuses its funding on established award programs in colleges and universities. *Note:* Total contributions made in 2000. **Typ. Recipients:** Emergency/Ambulance Services, Medical Research. **Geo. Dist:** nationally.

★ 11210 ★ Camp Younts Foundation

PO Box 813
Franklin, VA 23851
Phone: (757)562-3439 **Fax:** (757)569-7839
Bobby Worrell, Executive Director

Fnded: 1955. **Philosophy:** The foundation typically supports small colleges, private academies, and military institutes. Another priority is civic affairs, specifically, Southampton County, VA, and through the Elms Foundation. Other areas of support include churches, homes, and child welfare organizations. **Priorities:** *Arts & Humanities:* 10%. Funds museums and historical organisation. *Civic & Public Affairs:* 13%. Funds philanthropic organizations, botanical gardens and local historical society. *Education:* 65%. Higher education and seminars. *Environment:* 2%. People with disabilities and recreation and athletics. *International:* About 1%. Primarily supports the Southampton Memorial Hospital in addition to single disease associations. *Note:* Contributions were made in 2001. **Typ. Recipients:** Cancer, Geriatric Health, Hospitals, Medical Education, Nursing Services, People with Disabilities, Single-Disease Health Associations. **Geo. Dist:** southeastern states; VA.

★ 11211 ★ The Cannon Foundation, Inc.

57 Union St. South
PO Box 548
Concord, NC 28026-0548
Phone: (704)786-8216 **Fax:** (704)785-2052
Email: fdavis@cannonfoundationinc.org
Website: http://www.thecannonfoundationinc.org
Frank Davis, Executive Director

Fnded: 1943. **Philosophy:** The foundation is dedicated to carrying out the donor's "commitment to the people of Cabarrus County and the state of North Carolina through his philanthropy in health, education, and religion." **Priorities:** *Arts & Humanities:* 10%. Gives to museums and historic preservation. *Civic & Public Affairs:* 25%. Primary support for family services and youth organizations. *Education:* 23%. Funds colleges, universities, and elementary education. *International:* 36%. Supports hospitals, hospices, clinics, and health services. *Note:* Total contributions made in fiscal 1999. Percentages were provided by foundation and are approximate. **Typ. Recipients:** Adolescent Health Issues, AIDS/HIV, Children's Health/Hospitals, Clinics/Medical Centers, Domestic Violence, Emergency/Ambulance Services, Family Planning, Geriatric Health, Health Organizations, Health-General, Home-Care Services, Hospices, Hospitals, Nutrition, People with Disabilities, People with Disabilities, Prenatal Health Issues, Public Health, Research/Studies Institutes, Substance Abuse, Transplant Networks/Donor Banks. **Geo. Dist:** NC.

★ 11212 ★ Carl B. and Florence E. King Foundation

5956 Sherry Lane, Suite 620
Dallas, TX 75225
Phone: (214)750-1884 **Fax:** (214)750-1651

Fnded: 1966. **Philosophy:** "The Foundation contributes to a variety of concerns and organizations, including Goodwill Industries, the YMCA and YWCA, the Boy Scouts of America, and a wide range of Texas youth groups. Even before the value and popularity of academic scholarships became evident, the King Foundation was providing a number of deserving college students with financial assistance. That focus continues today." "The King Foundation also provides funds for the construction of schools, hospitals, and homes for the aged, handicapped, and indigent. Selected grants assist medical research organizations and other charitable or scientific associations. The Foundation makes contributions to educational institutions as well." The Carl B. and Florence E. King Foundation 1997 brochure and guidelines **Priorities:** *Arts & Humanities:* 14%. Public broadcasting, symphonies, and theater programs for young audiences. *Education:* About 34%. Focus on Texas universities, scholarships, 4-H programs, prep schools, and religious education. *Environment:* About 8% *International:* About 10%. Supports health organizations. *Note:* Total contributions made in 2000. **Typ. Recipients:** Cancer, Children's Health/Hospitals, Clinics/Medical Centers, Diabetes, Emergency/Ambulance Services, Eyes/Blindness, Family Planning, Health Funds, Health Organizations, Hospices, Hospitals, Medical Education, Medical Rehabilitation, Medical Research, Nursing Services, People with Disabilities, Prenatal Health Issues, Substance Abuse. **Geo. Dist:** Dallas, TX, including metropolitan area.

★ 11213 ★ Carl J. Herzog Foundation

321 Railroad Ave.
Greenwich, CT 06830
Phone: (203)629-2424 **Fax:** (203)629-2545
David Babson, Jr., Treasurer & Director

Fnded: 1952. **Philosophy:** The Carl J. Herzog Foundation is primarily interested in supporting medical research and dermatology. **Priorities:** *Civic & Public Affairs:* Less than 1%. Supports community foundations. *Education:* 19%. Supports higher education. *Environment:* 1%. YWCA's. *International:* 79%. Supports medical research in dermatology. *Note:* Total contributions made in 2001. **Typ. Recipients:** Cancer, Clinics/Medical Centers, Health Funds, Health Organizations, Health-General, Hospitals, Hospitals (University Affiliated), Medical Education, Medical Research, Research/Studies Institutes, Single-Disease Health Associations, Substance Abuse. **Geo. Dist:** nationally.

★ 11214 ★ The Carl and Lily Pforzheimer Foundation, Inc.

650 Madison Ave., 23rd Floor
New York, NY 10022
Phone: (212)223-6500 **Fax:** (212)223-2693
Mary Kitabjian, III, Executive Secretary

Fnded: 1942. **Philosophy:** Some of the major responsibilities of the foundation include the continuing publication of scholarly material directly related to the Carl H. Pforzheimer Collection of Shelley and His Circle, previously owned by the foundation and now located at the New York Public Library. It also supports scholarly works by leading university presses of books dealing with fields in which the foundation has a major interest, such as English and American literature. In general, the foundation provides limited support to ongoing programs in education, health care, the arts, and organizations with which the foundation is familiar. While the foundation does not make grants to individuals, it does donate to institutions that may sponsor individuals working in fields or on projects closely identified with the previously mentioned interests. **Priorities:** *Arts & Humanities:* 37%. Funds dance, theater, libraries, music, and cultural concerns. *Civic & Public Affairs:* 5%. Gives to community development, and civic groups. *Education:* 46%. Supports colleges and universities, literacy programs, and precollege education. *Environment:* 4%. Funds children's groups and community centers. *International:* 6%. Supports medical centers. *Religion:* 1%. *Note:* Total contributions made in 2000. **Typ. Recipients:** AIDS/HIV, Clinics/Medical Centers, Emergency/Ambulance Services, Eyes/Blindness, Hospitals, Nursing Services, People with Disabilities, Substance Abuse. **Geo. Dist:** nationally; New York, NY.

★ 11215 ★ Carnegie Corp. of New York

437 Madison Ave.
New York, NY 10022
Phone: (212)371-3200 **Fax:** (212)754-4073
Website: http://www.carnegie.org
Adam Liebling, Grants Associate

Fnded: 1938. **Philosophy:** The corporation's charter states that funds are to be used to promote "the advancement and diffusion of knowledge and understanding among the people of the United States." Its Charter was later amended to permit the use of funds for the same purposes in certain countries that are or were members of the British overseas Commonwealth. The corporation makes grants into the following program areas: education, international peace and security, international development, and democracy. A major goal of the education program's goal is rebuild the public confidence in education. To accomplish this goal the corporation will focus on early childhood education, urban school reform, and higher education. The International Peace and Security program builds on previous activities of the Corporation. The program will have three major focuses: non-proliferation of weapons, Russia and other Post Soviet States, and New Dimensions of Security. The International Development program will not accept unsolicited proposals until after October 1999. The following themes define the Program: strengthening African universities, enhancing women's opportunities in higher education and revitalizing public libraries. The corporation has devoted grants to improving the effectiveness of government, increasing public understanding of social issues, and encouraging active participation. **Priorities:** *Arts & Humanities:* 6%. Public Broadcasting Service. *Civic & Public Affairs:* 15%. Supports public policy and human rights programs; libraries. *Education:* 29%. Program development and improvement and science education. *Environment:* 22%. Supports national youth and adolescent programs. *Note:* Total contributions made in fiscal 1999. **Typ. Recipients:** Adolescent Health Issues, Child Abuse, Children's Health/Hospitals, Clinics/Medical Centers, Family Planning, Health Organizations, Health Policy/Cost Containment, Medical Education, Medical Research, Mental Health, Prenatal Health Issues, Public Health, Substance Abuse. **Geo. Dist:** internationally, especially to countries that are or have been members of the British commonwealth.

★ 11216 ★ Carolyn Foundation

901 Marquette Ave., Suite 2630
Minneapolis, MN 55402-3230
Phone: (612)596-3279 **Fax:** (612)338-2084
Email: berdahl.carolyn@winternet.com
Website: http://www.carolynfoundation.org
Rebecca Erdahl, Executive Director

Fnded: 1964. **Philosophy:** The Carolyn Foundation is interested principally in health and welfare, education, the arts, programs addressing social problems, and the environment. It is a regional foundation and limits funding to Minneapolis and St. Paul, MN, and New Haven, CT, and to some national environmental organizations with programs affecting these areas. **Priorities:** *Arts & Humanities:* 20%. Funds ballet, public broadcasting, music, and theater. *Civic & Public Affairs:* 15%. Supports community projects, housing, community development and women's affairs. *Education:* 15%. Gives to universities, prepatory schools, literacy and arts/ humanities education. *Environment:* 29%. Funds family welfare, family planning services, youth programs, and United Way. *International:* 5%. Supports cancer and general health. *Note:* Total contributions made in 2000. **Typ. Recipients:** Child Abuse, Children's Health/Hospitals, Clinics/Medical Centers, Domestic Violence, Emergency/Ambulance Services, Family Planning, Health Organizations, Hospitals, Medical Rehabilitation, Mental Health, Nursing Services, People with Disabilities, Research/Studies Institutes, Substance Abuse. **Geo. Dist:** New Haven, CT; Minneapolis-St. Paul, MN.

★ 11217 ★ Carrie Estelle Doheny Foundation Trust

707 Wilshire Boulevard, Suite 4960
Los Angeles, CA 90017
Phone: (213)488-1122 **Fax:** (213)488-1544
Email: doheny@dohenyfoundation.org
Website: http://www.dohenyfoundation.org
Shirley Bernard, Senior Grants Administrator

Fnded: 1948. **Philosophy:** The foundation was established "for the advancement of education, medicine, religion, science, the improvement of the health and welfare of infants, children, adults, families, the help and care of the sick, the aged and the incapacitated, and aid to the needy." The foundation supports a variety of local organizations, with emphasis on Roman Catholic groups, medical research, hospital care, education, child health and welfare, and assistance to the sick and needy. **Priorities:** *Education:* 28%. Supports higher and secondary educational institutions and programs. *Environment:* 6%. Supports family services. *International:* 27%. Funds hospitals, medical centers, and disease and disorder concerns. *Note:* Total contributions made in 2000. **Typ. Recipients:** Cancer, Children's Health/Hospitals, Clinics/Medical Centers, Domestic Violence, Emergency/Ambulance Services, Eyes/Blindness, Family Planning, Health Organizations, Heart, Hospitals, Long-Term Care, Medical Research, Medical Training, Nutrition, People with Disabilities, Prenatal Health Issues, Public Health, Research/Studies Institutes, Single-Disease Health Associations, Speech & Hearing. **Geo. Dist:** nationally.

★ 11218 ★ Carson Family Charitable Trust

c/o US Trust Co. New York
114 W 47th St., Tax Svcs.
New York, NY 10036
Phone: (212)852-3834 **Fax:** (212)852-1714
Russell Carson, Trustee

Fnded: 1991. **Priorities:** *Arts & Humanities:* 10%. Supports art museums and libraries. *Education:* 78%. Funds scholarships, private pre-college education, and colleges. *Environment:* 5%. Supports substance abuse prevention and Planned Parenthood. *International:* 7%. Supports medical research and hospitals. *Note:* Total contributions made in 1999. **Typ. Recipients:** Cancer, Clinics/Medical Centers, Emergency/Ambulance Services, Family Planning, Heart, Hospitals, Hospitals (University Affiliated), Single-Disease Health Associations, Substance Abuse. **Geo. Dist:** no restrictions.

★ 11219 ★ Carthage Foundation

One Oxford Centre
301 Grant St., Suite 3900
Pittsburgh, PA 15219-6401
Phone: (412)392-2900 **Fax:** (412)392-2922
Website: http://www.scaife.com/carthage.html
Michael Gleba, Treasurer

Fnded: 1964. **Philosophy:** The foundation's primary interests include national and international organizations that deal with public policy issues. **Priorities:** *Arts & Humanities:* 2%. Primary support for accuracy in media. *Civic & Public Affairs:* (Public Policy) 67%. Major grant to the Free Congress Research and Education Foundation. *Education:* 11%. Public policy education. *Environment:* 1%. Funds social services and substance abuse prevention. *International:* 1%. Supports the Institute for Health Freedom. *Note:* Total contributions made in 1998. **Typ. Recipients:** Domestic Violence, Health Policy/Cost Containment, Public Health, Substance Abuse. **Geo. Dist:** no restrictions.

★ 11220 ★ Castle Rock Foundation

4100 East Mississippi Ave., 1850
Denver, CO 80246
Phone: (303)388-1636 **Fax:** (303)388-1684
Email: generalinfo@castlerockfdn.org
Website: http://www.castlerockfoundation.org
Sally Rippey, Secretary

Fnded: 1993. **Philosophy:** "The mission of the Castle Rock Foundation is to: promote a better understanding of the free enterprise system; preserve the principles upon which our democracy was founded, to help ensure a limited role for government and the protection of individual rights as provided for in the Constitution; encourage personal responsibility and leadership; and to uphold traditional Judeo-Christian values." **Priorities:** *Arts & Humanities:* 7%. Supports museums and historical preservation. *Civic & Public Affairs:* 37%. Supports civic and public affairs, civil rights, and law and justice. *Education:* 18%. Supports educational institutions programs, leadership training, economics education, and colleges. *Environment:* 12%. Supports scouting, youth programs. *International:* 7%. *Note:* Total contributions were made in fiscal 2001. **Typ. Recipients:** Cancer, Clinics/Medical Centers, Health Policy/Cost Containment, Medical Research, Preventive Medicine/Wellness Organizations. **Geo. Dist:** nationally.

★ 11221 ★ Cecil B. Day Foundation

4725 Peachtree Corners Circle, Suite 300
Norcross, GA 30092
Phone: (770)446-1500 **Fax:** (770)446-2527
Edward White, Jr., President

Fnded: 1968. **Philosophy:** The primary purpose of the foundation is to "assist local churches in their Christian Mission of sharing the gospel of Jesus Christ in New England and the Atlanta, GA regions." The foundation hopes to function as a catalyst to bring the evangelical community closer together, and to fund institutions or ministers who lack denominational means of assistance. Priority is given to groups without other means of obtaining financial support. **Priorities:** *Civic & Public Affairs:* 7%. Gives to housing organizations and citizens' groups. *Education:* 4%. Contributes to learning centers, child development programs, and a nursing college. *Environment:* 6%. Supports youth programs and athletic programs. *International:* 1%. A home for cancer patients receives support. *Note:* Total contributions made in 2000. **Typ. Recipients:** AIDS/HIV, Cancer, Family Planning, Medical Education, Public Health. **Geo. Dist:** New England; Atlanta, GA, including statewide.

★ 11222 ★ Cele H. and William B. Rubin Family Fund

32 Monadnock Rd.
Wellesley Hills, MA 02481-1338
Phone: (781)235-4751 **Fax:** (781)235-4692
Ellen Gordon, President

Fnded: 1943. **Philosophy:** The Cele H. and William B. Rubin Family Fund gives across the major categories of support, but primarily focuses on civic affairs and higher education. Civic interests include economic development, housing programs, and zoos and parks. The foundation also supports women's affairs within these categories of support. **Priorities:** *Arts & Humanities:* 67%. Primary support goes to the Old Colony Charitable Fund. Also funds performing arts and libraries. *Civic & Public Affairs:* Less than 1%. Supports women's affairs, ethnic organizations, and other charitable organizations. *Education:* 25%. Colleges, universities, business schools, educational foundations, and private schools. *Environment:* 1%. Funds YMCAs, United Way, youth programs, and food banks. *International:* 4%. Supports single-disease societies and institutes. *Note:* Total contributions made in 2000. **Typ. Recipients:** Alzheimers Disease, Arthritis, Cancer, Clinics/Medical Centers, Diabetes, Health Organizations, Heart, Hospices, Hospitals, Kidney, Medical Education, Medical Rehabilitation, Medical Research, Multiple Sclerosis, People with Disabilities, Prenatal Health Issues, Public Health, Research/Studies Institutes, Single-Disease Health Associations. **Geo. Dist:** nationally.

★ 11223 ★ Champlin Foundation

300 Centerville Rd., Suite 300S
Warwick, RI 02886-0226
Phone: (401)736-0370 **Fax:** (401)736-7248
Email: champlinfdns@worldnet.att.net
Website: http://www.fndcenter.org/grantmaker/champlin
Keith Lang, Executive Director

Fnded: 1932. **Philosophy:** The aim of the foundations is to provide funds to Rhode Island organizations helping the broadest possible segment of the population. The foundations are interested in preserving land for recreation and open space. The foundations support land protection efforts in conjunction with the Nature Conservancy, the Rhode Island Department of Environmental Management, and the Audubon Society of Rhode Island. Although cultural projects involving libraries and library services receive considerable support, the foundations generally do not support the arts. Funding is offered instead to organizations with constituencies that are unable to provide monetary support. Some interest is shown for historic preservation efforts. The foundations have developed a scholarship program enabling Rhode Island public high school students to attend Brown University, and have recently instituted a program to fund equipment for Rhode Island public schools. They also have an interest in social service agencies, facilities for youth, hospitals, and health care agencies. **Priorities:** *Arts & Humanities:* 28%. Supports historic preservation, public libraries, museums, and public broadcasting. *Civic & Public Affairs:* 1%. Supports volunteer fire companies. *Education:* 13%. Majority of support to public elementary schools for educational equipment. *Environment:* 28%. Supports housing, family planning, substance abuse prevention, youth and fitness, and animal humane societies. *International:* 8%. Funds construction and mortgage costs for medical facilities. *Note:* Giving analysis provided by foundation. Total contributions made in 2000. **Typ. Recipients:** Clinics/Medical Centers, Emergency/Ambulance Services, Family Planning, Geriatric Health, Health Funds, Health Organizations, Health-General, Heart, Hospices, Hospitals, Long-Term Care, Medical Rehabilitation, Nursing Services, People with Disabilities, Prenatal Health Issues, Public Health, Transplant Networks/Donor Banks. **Geo. Dist:** Providence, RI.

★ 11224 ★ Charles A. Dana Foundation

745 Fifth Ave., Suite 900
New York, NY 10151
Phone: (212)223-4040 **Fax:** (212)317-8721
Email: danainfo@dana.org
Website: http://www.dana.org
William Safire, Chairman & Chief Executive Officer

Fnded: 1950. **Philosophy:** "The Dana Foundation, established in 1950 by industrialist, philanthropist, and legislator Charles A. Dana, is a private philanthropic foundation with principal interests in science, health, and education. The Foundation's curent areas of emphasis are in immunology and neuroscience research, and in K-12 education, particularly the training of arts educators." "SCI and Health Grants: For the decade of the 1990s, The Foundation focused on brain research. In 2001, interests expanded to include research in immunology. Grants in these areas are made principally through competitive Clinical Hypotheses Programs in Immuno-imaging, Neuroimmunology, Neuroimaging, and Brain-Cardiovascular system interactions. These competitive grant programs support pilot testing of experimental and innovative ideas that in immunology and neuroscience research have the potential of advancing clinical applications. The Foundation also supports an invitational program in which leading scientists are invited to compete for research grants designed to improve immune system responses to biological agents." "Education Grants: The Dana Foundation has supported advances in education throughout its history. The Foundation's current interest is focused primarily on professional development programs that foster improved teaching of the performing arts in public schools. Programs emphasize innovation training projects that are exported from, or imported to, New York City, Washington, DC, Los Angeles, and their surrounding areas... The Foundation's continuing interest in fostering innovations in K-12 Education is maintained through grant support for the Dana Center for Educational Innovation at the University of Texas in Austin." *The Dana Foundation 2001 Annual Report* **Priorities:** *Arts & Humanities:* 7%. Funds performing arts, art museums, and film. *Education:* 35%. Mainly funds college and university projects to support education of the public about the importance of brain research. *Environment:* Less than 1%. The New York Times 9/11 Neediest Fund received foundation support. *International:* 58%. Focus on immunology and brain diseases and disorders–long term, multifaceted support, and short-term, flexible support. *Note:* Total contributions made in 2001. **Typ. Recipients:** AIDS/HIV, Cancer, Children's Health/Hospitals, Clinics/Medical Centers, Emergency/Ambulance Services, Geriatric Health, Health Organizations, Health Policy/Cost Containment, Health-General, Heart, Hospitals, Medical Education, Medical Research, Medical Training, Mental Health, Multiple Sclerosis, People with Disabilities, Public Health, Single-Disease Health Associations, Speech & Hearing, Substance Abuse. **Geo. Dist:** nationally.

★ 11225 ★ Charles A. Frueauff Foundation

Three Financial Center
900 South Shackleford, Suite 300
Little Rock, AR 72211
Phone: (501)978-1078
Website: http://www.frueaufffoundation.com
Sue Frueauff, Secretary

Fnded: 1950. **Philosophy:** The Charles A. Frueauff Foundation's main areas of support are higher education, social services, health agencies and hospitals. The foundation reports that it is currently focusing on welfare reform and daycare. **Priorities:** *Education:* 41%. Supports scholarships at colleges and universities; also provides funds for capital expenditures, general operations, and special programs at educational institutions and for educational programs. *Environment:* 42%. Supports services for the handicapped, community services, and youth programs and services. *International:* 17%. Funds hospitals, hospices, single-disease health associations, and medical schools. *Note:* Total contributions made in 2001. **Typ. Recipients:** Children's Health/Hospitals, Clinics/Medical Centers, Emergency/Ambulance Services, Health Organizations, Hospices, Hospitals, Medical Education, Nursing Services, People with Disabilities, Public Health, Substance Abuse, Transplant Networks/Donor Banks. **Geo. Dist:** east of the Rocky Mountains.

★ 11226 ★ Charles Edison Fund

One Riverfront Plaza, 4th Floor
Newark, NJ 07102-5401
Phone: (973)648-0500 **Fax:** (973)648-0400
Email: alberta@charlesedisonfund.org
Website: http://www.charlesedisonfund.org
John Keegan, President & Chairman

Fnded: 1948. **Philosophy:** "The Charles Edison Fund is an endowed philanthropic institution dedicated to the support of worthwhile endeavors generally within the areas of medical research, science education and historic preservation. The fund is an extension of the benefactions and aspirations of its Founder, a man of discerning foresight, rare achievement and background." "In more recent years a pattern of giving has emerged within the Fund. Its contributions tend to be almost equally divided among medical research projects, science education and historic preservation. Additionally, but with some exceptions, institutions and organizations assisted are based principally in the New York-New Jersey Metropolitan area. This concentration of interest facilitates the efforts of the Trustees to evaluate the work of recipient groups, frequently accomplished by personal visitations." **Priorities:** *Arts & Humanities:* 56%. Primarily supports the Thomas Edison Preservation Society; also funds other historic preservation organizations and historic sites. *Civic & Public Affairs:* 6%. Gives to community foundations, leadership development programs, and philanthropic organizations. *Education:* 28%. Supports colleges, universities, private pre-college schools, scholarship funds, and science and medical education. *International:* 9%. Funds medical research and hospitals. *Note:* Total contributions made in 2000. **Typ. Recipients:** Arthritis, Cancer, Children's Health/Hospitals, Clinics/Medical Centers, Diabetes, Eyes/Blindness, Hospitals, Hospitals (University Affiliated), Medical Education, Medical Rehabilitation, Medical Research, Medical Training, Mental Health, People with Disabilities, Prenatal Health Issues, Single-Disease Health Associations, Speech & Hearing, Trauma Treatment. **Geo. Dist:** NJ, primarily metropolitan area; NY, primarily metropolitan area.

★ 11227 ★ Charles Engelhard Foundation

645 5th Ave.
New York, NY 10022
Phone: (212)935-2430 **Fax:** (212)935-2434
Mary Ogorzaly, Secretary

Fnded: 1949. **Philosophy:** The foundation gives to a variety of cultural, civic, and educational organizations. Less emphasis is placed on religion and social services. **Priorities:** *Arts & Humanities:* 27%. Funds libraries, art museums, literary art programs, dance, theater, opera, and music. *Civic & Public Affairs:* 4%. Gives to community foundations, ethnic affairs, public policy centers, and philanthropic organizations. *Education:* 31%. Primarily supports private and parochial secondary schools; also funds colleges and universities. *Environment:* 15%. Supports family programs, services for the disabled, and animal welfare organizations. *International:* 6%. Hospitals, nursing facilities, medical centers, and single-disease health associations receive support. *Note:* Total contributions made in 2000. **Typ. Recipients:** AIDS/HIV, Cancer, Children's Health/Hospitals, Clinics/Medical Centers, Family Planning, Health Organizations, Health-General, Home-Care Services, Hospices, Hospitals, Medical Education, Medical Research, People with Disabilities, Preventive Medicine/Wellness Organizations, Public Health, Single-Disease Health Associations, Substance Abuse. **Geo. Dist:** primarily the Northeastern United States.

★ 11228 ★ Charles G. Koch Charitable Foundation

655 15th St., Suite 445
Washington, DC 20005-2001
Phone: (202)393-2354 **Fax:** (202)393-2355
Email: email@cgkfoundation.org
Website: http://www.cgkfoundation.org
Kelly Young, Vice President

Fnded: 1981. **Philosophy:** "The Foundation's mission is to advance the well-being of humanity through the development of a free and civil society. To achieve this mission, we essentially fund research and education programs that examine the benefits of using market-process analysis to develop solutions to critical social problems. The Foundation elects to focus specifically on the following issues: environment, labor, legal, and fiscal." **Priorities:** *Arts & Humanities:* 2%. Supports the Kansas Cultural Trust. *Civic & Public Affairs:* 47%. Supports philanthropic causes, civic and community services, and legal affairs. *Education:* 49%. Supports education programs, schools, and universities. *Note:* Total contributions made in 2000. **Typ. Recipients:** Clinics/Medical Centers, Medical Research. **Geo. Dist:** nationally; KS; LA; MN; OK; TX.

★ 11229 ★ Charles H. Farnsworth Trust

PO Box 351, M-10
Boston, MA 02101
Phone: (617)664-3889
Marilyn Butler, Vice President

Fnded: 1930. **Philosophy:** The purpose of the Charles H. Farnsworth Trust "is to assist elderly persons to live in dignity and with independence. In describing the purpose of his legacy, Mr. Farnsworth made clear his interest in housing, particularly in affordable housing options providing support services to the elderly. Program interests include services to the elderly in their homes, such as health care, homemaker assistance, and nutritional support; collective and supportive housing and services; and research, planning, and communication to better inform individuals, institutions, and the community at large of ways to improve the quality and quantity of housing and support services for the elderly." 1998 Form 990 Supplement **Priorities:** *Arts & Humanities:* 4%. Supports community music centers. *Civic & Public Affairs:* 10%. Supports housing, legal aid, and community development. *Environment:* 53%. Gives to elderly causes and senior services. *International:* 33%. Funds visiting nurses associations and health services to the elderly. *Note:* Total contributions made in fiscal 2001. **Typ. Recipients:** Alzheimers Disease, Clinics/Medical Centers, Diabetes, Emergency/Ambulance Services, Eyes/Blindness, Geriatric Health, Health Funds, Health Organizations, Home-Care Services, Hospices, Hospitals, Hospitals (University Affiliated), Long-Term Care, Medical Research, Mental Health, Nursing Services, People with Disabilities, Prenatal Health Issues, Public Health, Speech & Hearing. **Geo. Dist:** MA.

★ 11230 ★ Charles H. Hood Foundation, Inc.

95 Berkeley St., Rm. 201
Boston, MA 02116
Phone: (617)695-9439 **Fax:** (617)423-4619
Raymond Considine, Secretary & Executive Director

Fnded: 1942. **Philosophy:** "The Charles H. Hood Foundation is interested in supporting projects concerned with child health in New England. Emphasis is on the initiation and furtherance of medical research which will help to diminish health problems affecting large numbers of children. The Foundation funds productive research efforts undertaken by junior faculty in medically oriented tax exempt institutions in the six New England states. It undertakes no research on its own. The intent of the award is to support initial independent investigations, provide the opportunity to demonstrate creativity, and assist in the transition to other sources of research funding." *Charles H. Hood Foundation Application Guidelines* **Priorities:** *International:* 100%. Support given to hospitals and medical centers. *Note:* Total contributions made in 2000. **Typ. Recipients:** Adolescent Health Issues, Cancer, Children's Health/Hospitals, Clinics/Medical Centers, Diabetes, Eyes/Blindness, Hospitals, Hospitals (University Affiliated), Medical Research, Medical Training, Nutrition, Prenatal Health Issues, Public Health. **Geo. Dist:** CT; ME; MA; NH; RI; VT.

★ 11231 ★ Charles H. Revson Foundation

55 East 59th St.
New York, NY 10022
Phone: (212)935-3340 **Fax:** (212)688-0633
Email: info@revsonfoundation.org
Website: http://www.revsonfoundation.org
Eli Evans, President

Fnded: 1956. **Philosophy:** The foundation has four principal areas of interest: urban affairs with an emphasis on New York City; education; biomedical research policy; and Jewish education and philanthropy. Related to each of these interests are concerns for governmental accountability, the development of public leadership, the changing role of women, and the impact of modern communications on education. Many of the foundation grants are public-policy-oriented. Funds most often go to universities, such as City College of New York, Columbia University, and New York University; legal services organizations, such as Legal Aid Society of New York; national advocacy organizations, such as NAACP, Legal Defense Fund, and Children's Defense Fund; and biomedical research institutions, such as the National Academy of Sciences and Memorial Sloan-Kettering. Numerous grants have been awarded to the Children's Television Workshop and the Educational Broadcasting Corporation, the majority for productions about Jewish-related subjects. **Priorities:** *Arts & Humanities:* 14%. Supports public broadcasting and major support for history regarding the Holocaust and Jewish heritage. *Civic & Public Affairs:* 42%. Support public policy, womens affairs, Law & Justice, community and welfare to work. *Education:* 16%. Major support is in the form f fellowship, also supports international studies, public education, and legal education. *Environment:* 3%. Supports food distribution and the homeless. *International:* 12%. Supports biomedical research and adolescent health issues. *Note:* Total contributions made in 1999. **Typ. Recipients:** AIDS/HIV, Cancer, Clinics/Medical Centers, Medical Education, Medical Research. **Geo. Dist:** internationally; nationally; New York, NY.

★ 11232 ★ Charles Hayden Foundation

130 Liberty St., Suite 2707
New York, NY 10006-1196
Phone: (212)785-3677 **Fax:** (212)785-3689
Website: http://www.fdncenter.org/grantsmaker/hayden
Kenneth Merin, President, Chief Executive Officer

Fnded: 1937. **Philosophy:** "The Charles Hayden Foundation seeks to promote the mental, moral, and physical development of school-aged youth in the New York and Boston metropolitan areas. Our focus is on those institutions and programs primarily serving youth most a risk of not reaching their full potential, especially youth in low-income communities. Priority is given to programs that intervene early in young people's lives and continuously provide opportunities and support over an extended period. The Foundation looks for the same attributes whether program or capital support is being sought." "Program support grants are focused on efforts to help youth develop the skills and knowledge needed to succeed in school and lay the foundations for satisfying and productive lives. Programs must have well-defined goals that are expected to be met in a specified time frame. Priority is given to: expanding community-based programs offering youth educational, social, recreational and career services (e.g. after school programs); and improving student achievement by strengthening K-12 education, especially elementary and middle school education, for youth in Boston and New York City and in nearby cities of Cambridge, Chelsea, Newark and Jersey City. Most public school support gets to charter schools for capital or for program purposes. K-12 support goes to efforts using independent school resources to expand opportunities for needy inner-city youth. The foundation also supports efforts to strengthen informal education enrichment programs offered outside of schools in institutions such as museums and zoos." "Capital support grants go for renovation, expansion, construction and acquisition of physical facilities and purchase and repair of non-expendable equipment. Emphasis is on assisting those organizations in need of physical facilities to improve the availability and quality of programs for young people. While we acknowledge the problem of deferred maintenance in youth-serving facilities, we will look carefully at the record of past attention to maintenance and an organization's long-term strategy for repair and renovation. Organizations eligible for capital grants include: youth-serving agencies and other community-based organizations whose facilities are largely used by and for youth development; non-public educational institutions serving needy students; charter schools that lack access to significant capital support from local public sources; children's museums, theaters and performing groups; and science and environmental centers with facilities used specifically for youth-oriented activities." 1996 Annual Report **Priorities:** *Arts & Humanities:* 7%. Funds libraries and children's museums. *Civic & Public Affairs:* 25%. Supports nonprofit management organizations, and civic ventures. *Education:* 17%. Supports after school and enrichment programs. *Environment:* 35%. Supports community service organizations, camps, community centers, scouts and at-risk youth programs. *Religion:* 10%. Funds the American Museum of Natural History. *Note:* Total contributions made in fiscal 2000. **Typ. Recipients:** AIDS/HIV, Family Planning, Hospitals, People with Disabilities, Research/Studies Institutes, Substance Abuse. **Geo. Dist:** Boston, MA, metropolitan area; New York, NY, metropolitan area.

★ 11233 ★ Charles J. Strosacker Foundation

PO Box 471
Midland, MI 48640-0471
Phone: (989)832-0066
Bobbie Arnold, Executive Vice President

Fnded: 1957. **Philosophy:** The foundation was established "to assist and benefit political subdivisions of the State of Michigan, and religious, charitable, benevolent, scientific, or educational organizations." **Priorities:** *Arts & Humanities:* 12%. Supports arts centers, museums, visual arts, and historic preservation. *Civic & Public Affairs:* 23%. General civic interests, largely in the Midland, MI, area, including community foundations, parks, and county fairs. *Education:* 25%. Universities, colleges, secondary schools, arts education, legal and medical education, and minority education are funded. *Environment:* 29%. Donates to American Red Cross, domestic violence council, united funds, family services, Young Men's Christian Association, and youth programs. *International:* 8%. Funds medical centers, AIDS organizations, and general health concerns. *Religion:* 3%. Supports the Michigan Molecular Institute. *Note:* Total contributions made in 2001. **Typ. Recipients:** AIDS/HIV, Clinics/Medical Centers, Domestic Violence, Emergency/Ambulance Services, Family Planning, Geriatric Health, Health Organizations, Health Policy/Cost Containment, Hospices, Hospitals, Medical Education, Mental Health, Nursing Services, Public Health, Substance Abuse, Transplant Networks/Donor Banks. **Geo. Dist:** Midland, MI, some statewide funding.

★ 11234 ★ Charles M. Bair Memorial Trust

PO Box 30678
Billings, MT 59115
Phone: (406)657-8083 **Fax:** (406)657-8034
Penny Doak, Vice President and Trust Officer

Fnded: 1978. **Philosophy:** The trust's priorities include hospitals and medical centers in Montana that were named in the original trust document, Christian Science churches, and scholarships to graduates of Harlowton and White Sulphur Springs high schools. High school graduates in Meagher and Wheatland counties also are supported. **Priorities:** *International:* 97%. Emphasis on hospitals and medical centers. **Typ. Recipients:** Clinics/Medical Centers, Hospitals. **Geo. Dist:** MT, Meagher County; MT, Wheatland County.

★ 11235 ★ Charles and M. R. Shapiro Foundation

200 North LaSalle St., Suite 2100
Chicago, IL 60601
Phone: (312)346-3100 **Fax:** (312)621-1750
Email: nshubert@muchlaw.com
Norman Shubert, President

Fnded: 1958. **Philosophy:** The Charles and M. R. Shapiro Foundation makes most of its grants to Jewish religious organizations. A secondary interest is Jewish education. Minor grants go to civic affairs, health, social services, and the arts. **Priorities:** *Arts & Humanities:* About 4%. *Civic & Public Affairs:* 3%. *Education:* 27%. Religious education, colleges and universities, and special education. *Environment:* 11%. Youth organizations, the elderly, and community services. *International:* 14%. Alzheimer's research, emergency health care, and cancer research. *Note:* Total contributions made in fiscal 1999. **Typ. Recipients:** Alzheimers Disease, Cancer, Clinics/Medical Centers, Emergency/Ambulance Services, Geriatric Health, Health-General, Hospices, Hospitals, Medical Research, Mental Health, Multiple Sclerosis, People with Disabilities, Single-Disease Health Associations. **Geo. Dist:** nationally; Chicago, IL.

★ 11236 ★ Charles Stewart Mott Foundation

Mott Foundation Bldg.
503 S Saginaw St., Suite 1200
Flint, MI 48502-1851
Phone: (810)238-5651 **Fax:** (810)766-1753
Email: info@mott.org
Website: http://www.mott.org

Fnded: 1926. **Philosophy:** Founder Charles Stewart Mott believed that "every person, always, is in a kind of informal partnership with his community. His own success is dependent to a large degree on that community, and the community, after all, is the sum total of the individuals who make it up." While this remains the guiding principle of the foundation, its grant making has been refined and broadened over time to reflect changing national and world conditions. Grant making is now organized in four programs: Civil Society, Environment, Flint Area, and Poverty. In addition, the foundation maintains the flexibility to investigate new opportunities through an Exploratory and Special Projects program. Fundamental to all grant making are certain values: learning how people can live together to create a sense of community, whether at the neighborhood level or as a global society; building strong communities through collaboration to provide a basis for positive change; nurturing strong, self-reliant individuals to ensure a well-functioning society; promoting the social, economic, and political empowerment of all individuals to preserve fundamental democratic principles and rights; encouraging responsible citizen participation to help foster social cohesion; developing leadership to build upon the needs and values of people and to inspire the aspirations and potential of others; and respecting the diversity of life to maintain a sustainable human and physical environment. In the final analysis, the mission of the Charles Stewart Mott Foundation is to support efforts that promote a just, equitable, and sustainable society. In the Environment giving area, the goal is "to support efforts of an engaged citizenry working to create accountable and responsive institutions, sound public policies, and appropriate models of development that protect the diversity and integrity of selected ecosystems in North America and around the world". In the Flint Area, the goal is "to foster a well-functioning, connected community that is capable of meeting the economic, social, and racial challenges ahead". Grantmaking is focused in four areas: Developing Public Capital, Creating National Models, Building Upon Legacy, and Effecting Public Policy. Poverty giving focuses on improving life outcomes for children, youth, and families in low-income communities. At its core, this program centers upon the importance of families and communities working together on behalf of children. Its areas of interest are the following: building communities to provide strong, safe environments that nurture and ensure growth opportunities for children, youth, and families; strengthening families so they can nurture children and youth and create strong communities; improving education to enable children, youth, and families to have access to paths out of poverty, and to serve as a resource to strengthen communities; and expanding economic opportunity to provide economic empowerment, job creation, and increased income to enable families to move out of poverty. **Priorities:** *Civic & Public Affairs:* 44%. *Education:* 21%. Funds public school systems, preschool and early childhood development. *Environment:* Less than 1%. Supports scouting and United Way. *Note:* Contributions made in 2000. **Typ. Recipients:** AIDS/HIV, Family Planning, Health Policy/Cost Containment, Home-Care Services, People with Disabilities, Public Health, Research/Studies Institutes, Substance Abuse. **Geo. Dist:** internationally; nationally; Flint, MI.

★ 11237 ★ Charlotte R. Schmidlapp Fund

Department 00864
Cincinnati, OH 45263
Phone: (513)579-6034 **Fax:** (513)534-0960
Lawra Baumann, Manager, Charitable Plan Giving Services

Fnded: 1907. **Philosophy:** The primary focus of the fund is to support programs aimed at helping young women establish themselves in life. The fund has begun a program of grants for women in the study of math and science. To help increase the number of role models for young women, grants are made to female teachers of math and science. The fund also supports critically needed day care for the children of female high school and college students. Although the challenges today are different from when Mr. Schmidlapp established the fund, it continues to help women in significant ways. **Priorities:** *Arts & Humanities:* 3%. Supports museums and art associations. *Civic & Public Affairs:* 16%. Funds urban and women's centers. *Education:* 19%. Focus on women's and children's education. *Environment:* 24%. Funds child welfare and youth organizations. *International:* 38%. Hospitals and pediatric health. *Note:* Total contributions made in fiscal 1998. **Typ. Recipients:** Cancer, Children's Health/Hospitals, Clinics/Medical Centers, Health Organizations, Health-General, Hospitals, Nursing Services, Prenatal Health Issues, Public Health. **Geo. Dist:** IN; KY; Cincinnati, OH.

★ 11238 ★ Chatlos Foundation

PO Box 915048
Longwood, FL 32791-5048
Phone: (407)862-5077
Website: http://www.chatlos.org
William Chatlos, President

Fnded: 1953. **Philosophy:** The Chatlos Foundation gives funding priority to Bible colleges, religious causes, medical issues, liberal arts colleges, and social concerns. The foundation prefers to provide program support. As a result, the foundation makes fewer grants to capital funds, conference expenses, administrative costs, multiyear grants or computer projects. **Priorities:** *Education:* 41%. Supports school, colleges, universities, scholarship, and religious education. *Environment:* 2%. Supports scouts, homeless/shelters, young men's christian association, substance abuse, the disabled and the aged, food distribution, and prison alternatives. *International:* 30%. Supports children's health, AIDS, and medical centers. *Note:* Total contributions made in 2000. **Typ. Recipients:** AIDS/HIV, Arthritis, Cancer, Children's Health/Hospitals, Clinics/Medical Centers, Emergency/Ambulance Services, Eyes/Blindness, Health Organizations, Heart, Hospitals, Hospitals (University Affiliated), Long-Term Care, Medical Education, Medical Research, Nursing Services, People with Disabilities, Public Health, Trauma Treatment. **Geo. Dist:** nationally.

★ 11239 ★ Chauncey and Marion Deering McCormick Foundation

410 North Michigan Ave., Room 590
Chicago, IL 60611
Phone: (312)644-6720 **Fax:** (312)644-7555
Lawson Whitesides, Jr., President

Fnded: 1957. **Philosophy:** The foundation primarily concentrates on local giving to organizations such as arts institutions, hospitals, universities, museums, wildlife conservation groups, private secondary schools, churches, and social services agencies. The foundation supports capital campaigns, art purchases, library funds, and building funds. **Priorities:** *Arts & Humanities:* 40%. Supports art institutes, libraries, museums, the theater, and the performing arts. *Civic & Public Affairs:* 2%. Supports animal services zoos. *Education:* 28%. Supports schools, colleges and universities. *Environment:* 7%. Supports child welfare, planned parenthood, and the United Way. *International:* 13%. Supports hospices, hospitals, and medical centers. *Note:* Total contributions made in fiscal 2001. **Typ. Recipients:** Cancer, Clinics/Medical Centers, Emergency/Ambulance Services, Family Planning, Health Organizations, Hospices, Hospitals, Hospitals (University Affiliated), Medical Education, Medical Rehabilitation, Medical Research, Mental Health, Single-Disease Health Associations. **Geo. Dist:** Chicago, IL, metropolitan area.

★ 11240 ★ Chichester duPont Foundation

3120 Kennett Pike
Wilmington, DE 19807
Phone: (302)658-5244 **Fax:** (302)658-5091
Gregory Fields, Secretary

Fnded: 1946. **Philosophy:** The foundation is primarily interested in supporting today's youth. Giving goes to social service organizations for the direct benefit of children. Most of the support is for operating budgets and capital campaigns. Another interest is education at the primary and secondary levels. Giving has been for endowment funds and youth recreation facilities in schools. The foundation also gives to civic affairs and organizations' building funds and operating budgets. The arts and health are minimally supported. **Priorities:** *Arts & Humanities:* 10%. Funds museums, historical societies, historic sites, and theater. *Civic & Public Affairs:* 2%. Gives to horicultural gardens and a sailing training program. *Education:* 9%. Funds a state university and public pre-college schools. *Environment:* 44%. Supports child and family services, community centers, senior services, animal welfare, family planning, and Young Men's Christian Association. *International:* 8%. Hospitals, cancer care, a dermatology association, cerebral palsy and a therapeutic riding program receive support. *Religion:* 1%. Contributes to a natural history museum. *Note:* Total contributions made in 2000. **Typ. Recipients:** Arthritis, Cancer, Child Abuse, Children's Health/Hospitals, Clinics/Medical Centers, Emergency/Ambulance Services, Family Planning, Health Organizations, Heart, Hospices, Hospitals, Long-Term Care, Medical Education, Medical Rehabilitation, Medical Research, Nursing Services, People with Disabilities, Preventive Medicine/Wellness Organizations, Public Health, Single-Disease Health Associations, Substance Abuse. **Geo. Dist:** mid-Atlantic United States; northeastern United States.

★ 11241 ★ Chiles Foundation

111 Southwest Fifth Ave., Suite 4050
Portland, OR 97204
Phone: (503)222-2143 **Fax:** (503)228-7079
Email: cf@qwest.net
Earle Chiles, President & Trustee

Fnded: 1941. **Philosophy:** "The foundation's principal purposes are to assist and support higher education, medical advancement, and arts and culture." **Priorities:** *Arts & Humanities:* 13%. Supports the performing arts, public broadcasting, art centers, and museums. *Civic & Public Affairs:* 2%. Supports community foundations, and national park. *Education:* 59%.Funds colleges, and universitys. *Environment:* Less than 1%. Supports youth organizations. *International:* 11%.Supports research programs. **Typ. Recipients:** Cancer, Clinics/Medical Centers, Emergency/Ambulance Services, Health Funds, Health Organizations, Heart, Hospitals, Medical Research, Multiple Sclerosis, Nursing Services, Prenatal Health Issues, Public Health, Single-Disease Health Associations. **Geo. Dist:** primarily Pacific Northwest.

★ 11242 ★ China Medical Board of New York

750 3rd Ave., 23rd Floor
New York, NY 10017-2701
Phone: (212)682-8000 **Fax:** (212)949-8726
Email: Rschwarz@chinamedicalboard.org
Dr. M. Schwarz, President

Fnded: 1928. **Philosophy:** The board's primary interest is supporting medical, nursing, and public health education and research. Contributions are made to eleven different countries and territories in East and Southeast Asia, as directed by its charter. "The Board is especially interested in grants to advance the recipient institution's pursuit of excellence and for the enhancement of the academic and professional content of medical, nursing, and public health education and training." The board also reports that it has a program for higher education in nursing. Categories of support programs include national fellowship grants, regional fellowship grants, research grants, education grants, and endowment grants. In addition, the Medical Education for Students in Rural Areas project enables students to receive basic medical science education at Chulalongkorn Faculty of Medicine in Bangkok and their clinical education in one of two provincial hospitals. **Priorities:** *Note:* Total contributions made in fiscal 2001. **Typ. Recipients:** Health Organizations, Medical Education, Medical Research. **Geo. Dist:** East and Southeast Asia.

★ 11243 ★ Chisholm Foundation

114 W 47th St.
New York, NY 10036-1532
Phone: 800-878-7878
Dennise Lopez, Contact

Fnded: 1960. **Philosophy:** The foundation typically supports secondary and higher education, public policy groups, the arts, and social services. **Priorities:** *Arts & Humanities:* 22%. Museums, arts institutes, theater, and opera received funding. *Civic & Public Affairs:* 7%. Supports public policy organizations, community affairs groups, and arboretums and gardens, and women's affairs. *Education:* 48%. Emphasis on Millsaps College; funds private schools and colleges and universities. *Environment:* 13%. Contributions go to family services, animal rescue, scouts, sexual violence centers, shelters, and United Way. *International:* 4%. Funds hospital and cancer centers. *Note:* Total contributions made in 2001 **Typ. Recipients:** AIDS/HIV, Cancer, Children's Health/Hospitals, Clinics/Medical Centers, Domestic Violence, Emergency/Ambulance Services, Geriatric Health, Health-General, Hospitals, Medical Education, People with Disabilities, Sexual Abuse, Single-Disease Health Associations, Transplant Networks/Donor Banks. **Geo. Dist:** DC; MS; New York, NY.

★ 11244 ★ Christ Is Our Salvation Foundation (CIOS)

PO Box 20815
Waco, TX 76702-0815
Phone: (254)752-5551 **Fax:** (254)752-4711
Paul Piper, Sr., Trustee

Fnded: 1952. **Philosophy:** The foundation primarily is interested in supporting Christian religious organizations. Churches, missions, conventions, and bible classes all are given support. Religious education is a secondary interest, along with support for civic affairs, social services, and the arts. **Priorities:** *Arts & Humanities:* 1%. *Civic & Public Affairs:* 3%. Supports community foundations. *Education:* 9%. Supports colleges and universities. *International:* 2%. Primarily supports hospitals. *Note:* Total contributions made in fiscal 2001. **Typ. Recipients:** Cancer, Children's Health/Hospitals, Clinics/Medical Centers, Health Organizations, Hospitals, People with Disabilities, Public Health, Substance Abuse. **Geo. Dist:** midwestern states; TX.

★ 11245 ★ Christian A. Johnson Endeavor Foundation

1060 Park Ave.
New York, NY 10128-1033
Phone: (212)534-6620 **Fax:** (212)410-0568
Email: clubin@cajef.org
Julie Kidd, President

Fnded: 1952. **Philosophy:** The foundation is primarily interested in supporting educational projects and educational outreach arts programs. It concentrates its giving on private institutions of higher learning at the baccalaureate level and on educational outreach programs of visual and performing arts organizations. The foundation also funds the Educational Leadership Program, which sponsors seminars and meetings for leaders in the education world. **Priorities:** *Arts & Humanities:* 10%. Funds museums, theater, music, and opera. *Civic & Public Affairs:* 2%. *Education:* 82%. Supports colleges, universities, and scholarship funds. *Environment:* 2%. Funds Boys' Harbor. *Note:* Total contributions made in fiscal 2001. **Typ. Recipients:** Eyes/Blindness, Heart, People with Disabilities. **Geo. Dist:** U.S. Eastern Region.

★ 11246 ★ Christopher Reynolds Foundation

267 5th Ave., Suite 1001
New York, NY 10016
Phone: (212)532-1606 **Fax:** (212)532-1403
Email: crfny@aol.com
Website: http://www.creynolds.org
Andrea Panaritis, Exec. Director, Secretary, & Treasurer

Fnded: 1952. **Philosophy:** The Christopher Reynolds Foundation makes most of its grants in the areas of international development, policy, and social science. Civic affairs contributions are a major priority, with interests in international policy and national security. Educational funding supports large universities with international studies programs. **Priorities:** *Note:* Total contributions made in fiscal 2001. **Typ. Recipients:** Clinics/Medical Centers, Medical Education, Mental Health, Public Health, Public Health, Speech & Hearing. **Geo. Dist:** U.S. organizations working in Indochina; MI; NY; OH.

★ 11247 ★ Christy-Houston Foundation

1296 Dow St.
Murfreesboro, TN 37130
Phone: (615)898-1140 **Fax:** (615)895-9524
Email: christy-houston@mindspring.com
Robert Mifflin, Executive Director

Fnded: 1987. **Philosophy:** The foundation is dedicated to the "improvement of the quality of life for the citizens and residents of Rutherford County, TN, with an emphasis on the promotion and enhancement of health care." The foundation has reported that it is placing a greater focus on social services in Rutherford County, TN, and that it plans in the future to fund a Boys and Girls Club, a YMCA, and a senior citizen's center. **Priorities:** *Arts & Humanities:* 1%. Supports museum. *Civic & Public Affairs:* 22%. Supports towns/ municipalities and parks. *Education:* 6%. Supports school, universities, and scholarship. *Environment:* 13%. Supports daycare, people with disabilities, and community service organizations. *International:* 58%. Funds nursing homes. *Note:* Total contributions made in fiscal 2001. **Typ. Recipients:** Clinics/Medical Centers, Domestic Violence, Emergency/Ambulance Services, Health Organizations, Heart, Hospices, Hospitals, Kidney, Medical Education, Public Health. **Geo. Dist:** Rutherford County, TN.

★ 11248 ★ Claneil Foundation

630 West Germantown Pike, Suite 400
Plymouth Meeting, PA 19462-1074
Phone: (610)828-6331 **Fax:** (610)828-6405
Cathy Weiss, Executive Director

Fnded: 1968. **Philosophy:** "The Claneil Foundation is interested in making a difference in the lives of individuals, families, organizations and communities. The Foundation supports nonprofit activities that fall within the following categories: The Arts and Humanities; Community Development; Education; The Built and Natural Environment; Health and Human Services". Claneil Foundation, Inc. Interim Guidelines. **Priorities:** *Arts & Humanities:* 11%. Primarily for historic preservation and museums. *Civic & Public Affairs:* 24%. Supports community foundations, women's affairs, Native American affairs, and economic development. *Education:* 9%. Gives to colleges and universities, faculty development, special education, and minority education. *Environment:* 12%. Supports community services, family services, and shelters. *International:* 25%. Funds trauma treatment, hospitals, prenatal care, pediatric and geriatric health, and long-term care. *Religion:* 4%. Gives to a science center. *Note:* Total contributions made in 2000. **Typ. Recipients:** AIDS/HIV, Alzheimers Disease, Cancer, Children's Health/Hospitals, Clinics/Medical Centers, Domestic Violence, Family Planning, Geriatric Health, Health Funds, Health Organizations, Home-Care Services, Hospitals, Long-Term Care, Medical Education, Medical Research, Mental Health, Prenatal Health Issues, Preventive Medicine/Wellness Organizations, Single-Disease Health Associations, Substance Abuse, Trauma Treatment. **Geo. Dist:** MA; PA; Philadelphia, PA, metro area.

★ 11249 ★ Clara Blackford Smith and W. Aubrey Smith Charitable Foundation

330 W Main St.
Denison, TX 75020
Phone: (903)415-2300
Linda Hunt, Board Member

Fnded: 1985. **Philosophy:** "The Clara Blackford Smith and W. Aubrey Smith Charitable Foundation was established under the will of Mrs. Smith and the funds are to be used exclusively for religious, charitable, educational, scientific and literary purposes. The Foundation is administered by NationsBank of Texas, N.A. The by-laws state the Foundation generally will limit support to non-profit organizations within the State of Texas, primarily in Grayson County." 1997 Grant Application Information Sheet **Priorities:** *Arts & Humanities:* 1%. Supports performing arts and museums. *Civic & Public Affairs:* 34%. Primarily for community organizations in the city of Denison. *Education:* 12%. Public education, colleges, universities, literacy, scholarship, student aid and minority education. *Environment:* 19%. Supports programs for athletics/recreation, camps, shelters, and United Way. *International:* 34%. Funds medical center, public health, and rehabilitation centers. *Note:* Total contributions made in fiscal 2000. **Typ. Recipients:** Cancer, Clinics/Medical Centers, Diabetes, Domestic Violence, Emergency/Ambulance Services, Geriatric Health, Health Funds, Health Organizations, Hospices, Hospitals, Medical Education, Medical Rehabilitation, Medical Research, Nursing Services, People with Disabilities, Public Health, Substance Abuse. **Geo. Dist:** TX, primarily Grayson County.

★ 11250 ★ Clara and Spencer Werner Foundation

711 South Main St.
PO Box 493
Paris, IL 61944
Phone: (217)466-1215 **Fax:** (217)466-1017
Email: cswernerf@tigerpaw.com
Jerry Klug, Chairman

Fnded: 1953. **Philosophy:** The foundation gives only to Lutheran organizations; its primary interest is religious education. **Priorities:** *Education:* 26%. Provides for scholarship fund and religious education. *Note:* Total contributions made in fiscal 2001. **Typ. Recipients:** Alzheimers Disease, Health Organizations. **Geo. Dist:** IL, including surrounding states.

★ 11251 ★ Clark Foundation (NY)

One Rockefeller Plaza, 31st Floor
New York, NY 10020-2102
Phone: (212)977-6900 **Fax:** (212)977-3424
Charles Hamilton, Executive Director

Fnded: 1931. **Philosophy:** The foundation continues to support the hospitals and the museums in Cooperstown, NY. Funding is also given for educational, youth, employment, and social service organizations. An important area of foundation activity is the scholarship program for students from the Cooperstown area. Students may attend any college of their choice. Funds are earmarked for each particular student and administered through the college. **Priorities:** *Arts & Humanities:* 6%. Funds opera, museums, and historical associations. *Civic & Public Affairs:* 22%. Supports community development, women's issues, housing, business issues, and employment services. *Education:* 21%. Supports scholarships, precollege and college education, and outward bound programs. *Environment:* 47%. Supports united funds, children's organizations, and family services. *International:* 2%. *Note:* Total contributions made in fiscal 2001. **Typ. Recipients:** AIDS/HIV, Cancer, Clinics/Medical Centers, Emergency/Ambulance Services, Family Planning, Health Funds, Health Organizations, Hospitals, Kidney, Medical Education, Medical Training, Mental Health, Outpatient Health Care, People with Disabilities, Substance Abuse. **Geo. Dist:** nationally; Cooperstown, NY; New York, NY.

★ 11252 ★ Clark-Winchcole Foundation

3 Bethesda Metro Center, Suite 550
Bethesda, MD 20814
Phone: (301)654-3607
Vincent Burke, President & Trustee

Fnded: 1964. **Philosophy:** The foundation gives to broad purposes in the Washington, DC, area, with emphasis on social services and the arts. **Priorities:** *Arts & Humanities:* 30%. Supports museums, performing arts, and historical preservation. *Education:* 27%. Student aid, secondary education, and literacy programs. *Environment:* About 13%. Funds social welfare and youth groups. *International:* About 13%. American Red Cross, hospitals, and health foundations. *Note:* Total contributions made in 1998. **Typ. Recipients:** Cancer, Children's Health/Hospitals, Clinics/Medical Centers, Emergency/Ambulance Services, Health Organizations, Hospices, Hospitals, Long-Term Care, Medical Rehabilitation, Mental Health, Nursing Services, People with Disabilities, Public Health, Research/Studies Institutes, Single-Disease Health Associations, Speech & Hearing, Substance Abuse. **Geo. Dist:** Washington, DC, including metropolitan area.

★ 11253 ★ Claude R. Lambe Charitable Foundation

655 15th St., Suite 445
Wichita, KS 67201
Phone: (316)828-5552
Kelly Young, Vice President

Fnded: 1982. **Philosophy:** The foundation favors research and study organizations, primarily those concerned with economics and public policy issues. **Priorities:** *Civic & Public Affairs:* 85%. Economic policy, free enterprise, and law and justice. *Education:* 6%. Primarily targeting colleges, universities and institutes that focus on social sciences. *Note:* Total contributions made in 2000. **Typ. Recipients:** Health Policy/Cost Containment.

★ 11254 ★ Claude Worthington Benedum Foundation

223 Fourth Ave., Suite 1400
Pittsburgh, PA 15222
Phone: (412)288-0360 **Fax:** (412)288-0366
Email: wpgetty@benedum.org
Website: http://www.fdncenter.org/grantmaker/benedum
William Getty, President & Trustee

Fnded: 1944. **Philosophy:** The foundation operates two grantmaking programs, one in West Virginia and one in the Pittsburgh Region. West Virginia Program: In education, the foundation wants to encourage public education reform with teachers and administrators; support a fundamental reform of teacher education; use the strengths of higher education to serve the needs of the state; and support measures that strengthen the state's independent colleges. In health, the foundation wants to reshape the rural health care delivery by fostering new and more effective systems of service; encourage community-based initiatives in disease prevention and health promotion; foster research and analysis of rural health policy; and support health education to restructure rural health care. In community improvement, the foundation wants to support programs that encourage, enable and empower local residents; understands that local action must include housing, recreation, leisure activities, libraries, small businesses and the arts; recognizes that adequate shelter is the first prerequisite for decent living and development of affordable housing must be a priority. In economic development, the foundation will work with intermediaries to develop alternate economic opportunities; encourages economic development strategies that build upon West Virginia's human, natural, physical, technological and other resources; and encourages the wise use of land and water resources for environmental responsibility and economic gain. In the arts, the foundation seeks to strengthen arts organizations that provide educational, social and economical renewal; believes the major art organizations benefit themselves, their regions and the state by improving their quality and their capacity to reach new audiences; and will work with intermediaries to provide technical assistance to large and small arts organizations. Pittsburgh Region Grants Program: In regional economic development the foundation wants to encourage development focusing on job creation; promote public-private sector collaborations; support initiatives of the Cultural District and its resident art organizations to strengthen their financial viability, improve programs and build new audiences; and provide on-going support to the United Way. **Priorities:** *Arts & Humanities:* 24%. Supports symphony, opera, and ballet. *Civic & Public Affairs:* 17%. Supports economic development and employment/job training. *Education:* 26%. Supports educational foundations, initiatives, programs, and institutions. *Environment:* 20%. Supports homes, family services, domestic violence prevention, and United Way. *International:* 6%. Supports health funds and organizations. *Note:* Total contributions made in 2000. **Typ. Recipients:** Children's Health/Hospitals, Clinics/Medical Centers, Diabetes, Domestic Violence, Emergency/ Ambulance Services, Health Organizations, Health Policy/Cost Containment, Hospitals, Medical Education, Nursing Services, Nutrition, People with Disabilities, Prenatal Health Issues, Preventive Medicine/ Wellness Organizations, Public Health, Research/ Studies Institutes. **Geo. Dist:** Pittsburgh, PA; WV.

★ 11255 ★ Clay Foundation

1426 Kanawha Boulevard, East
Charleston, WV 25301
Phone: (304)344-8656 **Fax:** (304)344-3805
Email: cfiwv@aol.com
Charles Avampato, President

Fnded: 1987. **Philosophy:** The Clay Foundation was established "to promote and enhance the quality of life of the citizens of West Virginia." The foundation's goal is to fund innovative projects or support services which best serve the residents of the state. Although the foundation considers requests from a broad range of organizations, it currently has a special interest in programs in the field of aging; health care research and education; vocational education programs; and services to disadvantaged youth and their families. **Priorities:** *Arts & Humanities:* 12%. Funds art center construction, opera, symphony and museum. *Civic & Public Affairs:* 7%. Supports economic development and community foundations. *Education:* 29%. Funds higher and pre-college education, after-school programs, and literacy. *Environment:* 48%. Provides funding for housing, United Way, recreation, and indigent families. *International:* 4%. *Note:* Total contributions made in 2001. **Typ. Recipients:** Children's Health/Hospitals, Clinics/Medical Centers, Health Organizations, Health Policy/Cost Containment, Hospices, Hospitals, Medical Education, Mental Health, People with Disabilities, Preventive Medicine/Wellness Organizations, Speech & Hearing. **Geo. Dist:** WV.

★ 11256 ★ Clayton Fund
600 Travis, 7th Fl.
Houston, TX 77002
Phone: (713)216-1453
William Askey, Contact

Fnded: 1989. **Philosophy:** The trust was created for charitable or educational purposes. These purposes include aid to the needy, especially children; the environment; family planning; education; agriculture; and arts and culture. **Priorities:** *Arts & Humanities:* 6%. Supports opera, theater, and music. *Civic & Public Affairs:* 5%. Urban/community affairs and clubs. *Education:* 39%. Medical education, colleges and universities, and minority education. *Environment:* 27%. Planned Parenthood, food banks, and youth organizations. *International:* 5%. Public health issues and children's health. *Note:* Total contributions made in 2000. **Typ. Recipients:** Cancer, Children's Health/Hospitals, Clinics/Medical Centers, Domestic Violence, Emergency/Ambulance Services, Family Planning, Family Planning, Health Organizations, Heart, Hospitals, Hospitals (University Affiliated), Medical Education, Medical Rehabilitation, Mental Health, People with Disabilities, Prenatal Health Issues, Public Health, Single-Disease Health Associations, Speech & Hearing, Transplant Networks/Donor Banks. **Geo. Dist:** nationally.

★ 11257 ★ Cleveland H. Dodge Foundation
670 West 247th St.
Bronx, NY 10471
Phone: (718)543-1220 **Fax:** (718)543-0737
Email: chdodgefdn@aol.com
Website: http://www.chdodgefoundation.org
Phyllis Criscuoli, Executive Director & Treasurer

Fnded: 1917. **Philosophy:** The foundation gives priority to organizations supported by the donor and members of his family that continue to perform effective services. In keeping with Cleveland Dodge's philanthropic beliefs, the foundation also funds "institutions aiming to build good moral character in youth without being narrowly sectarian or seeking to proselytize, including social agencies serving needy youth." **Priorities:** *Arts & Humanities:* 20%. Supports libraries and museums. *Civic & Public Affairs:* 20%. Funds parks and gardens. *Education:* 39%. Gives to higher education. *Environment:* 12%. Funds youth groups and community services. *Note:* Total contributions made in 1998. **Typ. Recipients:** Emergency/Ambulance Services, Family Planning, Health Organizations, Nursing Services, People with Disabilities, Public Health. **Geo. Dist:** Northeastern United States; AZ; NM; New York, NY, including metropolitan area.

★ 11258 ★ Clipper Ship Foundation
77 Summer St., 8th Floor
Boston, MA 02110
Phone: (617)426-7172 **Fax:** (617)426-5441
Email: philanthropy@grantsmanagement.com
Website: http://www.grantsmanagement.com
Anna Karlsson, Foundation Assistant

Fnded: 1979. **Philosophy:** The foundation's principal objective is to assist nonprofit, operating organizations serving the Boston community and help them broaden the scope of their activities and fulfill their goals. Special attention will be given to those organizations involved with "the homeless, the destitute, the handicapped, children and the aged, or supplying the special needs of minority, low-income individuals and families." Worldwide disaster relief is also an occasional concern of the foundation. **Priorities:** *Arts & Humanities:* 5%. Supports the performing arts. *Civic & Public Affairs:* 29%. Supports community affairs and economic development. *Education:* 15%. Funds education. *Environment:* 39%. Funds health and human services. Supports child welfare, people with disabilities, and emergency services. *International:* 4%. Supports health programs. *Note:* Total contributions made in fiscal 2000. **Typ. Recipients:** AIDS/HIV, Clinics/Medical Centers, Domestic Violence, Emergency/Ambulance Services, Eyes/Blindness, Family Planning, Hospices, Hospitals, Long-Term Care, Medical Rehabilitation, Mental Health, Nursing Services, People with Disabilities, Prenatal Health Issues, Preventive Medicine/Wellness Organizations, Public Health, Speech & Hearing, Substance Abuse. **Geo. Dist:** Boston, MA, within Route 128 area and cities of Brockton, MA.

★ 11259 ★ Clowes Fund
320 N Meridian, Suite 316
Indianapolis, IN 46204-1722
Phone: (317)833-0144 **Fax:** (317)833-0145
Email: staff@clowesfund.org
Website: http://www.clowesfund.org
Elizabeth Casselman, Exec. Dir.

Fnded: 1952. **Philosophy:** The fund typically supports higher educational institutions, the performing arts, and social services, primarily in Indiana and Massachusetts. **Priorities:** *Arts & Humanities:* 32%. Supports museums, the performing arts, cultural centers and theaters. *Civic & Public Affairs:* 6%. Funds housing, zoos and parks, and urban affairs. *Education:* 35%. Literacy, scholarships, and endowments. *Environment:* 11%. Supports youth organizations, child welfare, and substance abuse prevention. *International:* 2%. Health associations and funds, and hospitals. *Note:* Total contributions made in 1998. The fund typically does not support environmental causes, health, or religion. **Typ. Recipients:** Child Abuse, Children's Health/Hospitals, Clinics/Medical Centers, Diabetes, Domestic Violence, Family Planning, Health Funds, Health Organizations, Hospices, Hospitals, Hospitals (University Affiliated), Medical Education, Medical Research, Nursing Services, Outpatient Health Care, People with Disabilities, Respiratory, Substance Abuse. **Geo. Dist:** Indianapolis, IN; MA.

★ 11260 ★ Cockrell Foundation
1600 Smith, Suite 3900
Houston, TX 77002-7348
Phone: (713)209-7500 **Fax:** (713)209-7599
Email: mnw@cockrell.com
M. Williams, Executive Vice President

Fnded: 1966. **Philosophy:** The Cockrell Foundation is a family organization serving primarily the Houston area. The foundation is required by the last will and testament of Ernest Cockrell, Jr., to give one-half of annual funding to the University of Texas at Austin School of Engineering. It outlines no giving priorities for remaining funds and gives to a variety of areas. **Priorities:** *Arts & Humanities:* Less than 1%. Natural science and fine arts museums. *Civic & Public Affairs:* About 1%. Community Support. *Education:* 31%. Higher education and continuing education programs. *Environment:* 47%. Youth and human services. *International:* 19%. Supports hospitals, medical centers, and specified disease organizations. *Note:* Total contributions made in 2002. **Typ. Recipients:** Adolescent Health Issues, Alzheimers Disease, Cancer, Child Abuse, Children's Health/Hospitals, Clinics/Medical Centers, Diabetes, Emergency/Ambulance Services, Eyes/Blindness, Family Planning, Health Organizations, Heart, Hospices, Hospitals, Medical Education, Medical Research, Mental Health, People with Disabilities, Prenatal Health Issues, Single-Disease Health Associations, Speech & Hearing. **Geo. Dist:** Houston, TX.

★ 11261 ★ Coleman Foundation (IL)
575 West Madison St., Suite 4605
Chicago, IL 60661-2549
Phone: (312)902-7120 **Fax:** (312)902-7124
Email: Coleman@colemanfoundation.org
Website: http://www.colemanfoundation.org
Michael Hennessy, President

Fnded: 1953. **Philosophy:** The foundation traditionally supports secondary and higher educational institutions, hospitals, medical training, and health organizations concerned with a single disease. Community and youth-oriented human service organizations are also supported. Limited funding goes to civic and cultural organizations. Program areas funded by the foundation include entrepreneurship awareness education, cancer research in the Midwest, housing and education of the handicapped, and education. **Priorities:** *Arts & Humanities:* Less than 1%. *Civic & Public Affairs:* 14%. Supports community development, community foundations, and entrepreneurship. *Education:* 60%. Funds scholarship, universities and colleges, entrepreneurship, society, religious education, arts/humanities education, business education, medical education, and agricultural education. *Environment:* 3%. Supports community services, Big Brothers/Big Sisters, homes, food distribution, Young Men's Christian Association, and athletics/recreation. *International:* 23%. Supports medical centers, cancer, eyes/blindness, healthcare organizations, hospice, and hospitals. *Note:* Total contributions made in 2000. **Typ. Recipients:** AIDS/HIV, Cancer, Clinics/Medical Centers, Eyes/Blindness, Health Organizations, Hospices, Hospitals, Hospitals (University Affiliated), Medical Education, Medical Rehabilitation, Medical Research, People with Disabilities, Preventive Medicine/Wellness Organizations, Public Health, Research/Studies Institutes, Sexual Abuse, Single-Disease Health Associations. **Geo. Dist:** nationally; especially the midwest; Chicago, IL.

★ 11262 ★ Collins Foundation
1618 Southwest 1st Ave., Suite 505
Portland, OR 97201-5706
Phone: (503)227-7171 **Fax:** (503)295-3794
Email: information@collinsfoundation.org
Website: http://www.collinsfoundation.org
Dr. Jerry Hudson, Executive Vice President

Fnded: 1947. **Philosophy:** The foundation was established to use its funds for religious, charitable, and educational purposes within the state of Oregon. It is always open to new ideas and causes which it can support. It looks favorably on small, creative programs that can serve the community. **Priorities:** *Arts & Humanities:* 20%. Supports museums, performing arts, libraries, and public broadcasting. *Civic & Public Affairs:* 4%. Supports community affairs, an aquarium, and housing. *Education:* 30%. Supports higher education and educational programs. *Environment:* 14%. Supports YMCA, youth organizations, and human services. *International:* 10%. Supports hospitals, medical centers, community health, and single disease associations. *Religion:* 2%. Supports a science museum. *Note:* Contributions were made in 2002. **Typ. Recipients:** Alzheimers Disease, Cancer, Children's Health/Hospitals, Clinics/Medical Centers, Emergency/Ambulance Services, Family Planning, Health Funds, Health Organizations, Health Policy/Cost Containment, Heart, Hospices, Hospitals, Hospitals (University Affiliated), Medical Research, Mental Health, People with Disabilities, Prenatal Health Issues, Preventive Medicine/Wellness Organizations, Public Health, Research/Studies Institutes, Substance Abuse, Trauma Treatment. **Geo. Dist:** OR.

★ 11263 ★ Colorado Trust
1600 Sherman St.
Denver, CO 80203-1604
Phone: (303)837-1200 **Fax:** (303)839-9034
Email: rachel@coltrust.org
Website: http://www.coloradotrust.org
Christie McElhinney, Senior Communications Officer

Fnded: 1985. **Philosophy:** The mission of The Colorado Trust is to involve citizens in community change, develop human potential, and promote the health and well-being of the people of Colorado. To fulfill its mission, the foundation supports innovative projects, conducts studies, develops services, and provides education to produce long-lasting benefits. The Trust has developed these initiatives: *Community Action for Health Promotion Initiative (1995-2002)* Designed to increase local health-promotion activities in Colorado and to build the capacity of Colorado communities to identify and address preventable health problems, the initiative is a seven-year $5.2 million program. More than 50 communities in Colorado will receive funding, primarily for these subject areas: adolescent mental health, adolescent pregnancy, child abuse and neglect, chronic disease, congenital abnormalities and infant mortality, dental health, elderly mental health, injuries, low birth-weight, the effects of poverty on child health, reproductive health, substance abuse, tobacco use, and violence. *Volunteers for Rural Seniors Initiative* This six-year, $2.8 million initiative will support independent living projects for rural seniors by creating or expanding volunteer-based community service systems. To apply for a grant, Colorado communities must exist outside a metropolitan area and have a population of 25,000 or less. *Coalition for the Medically Underserved (1997 - 2000)* In 1997, a 35-member coalition, representing health-care providers and agencies, health insurance companies, businesses, and state and county governments began meeting to identify solutions for improving access to quality health care for the medically underserved in Colorado. The Colorado Trust has allocated $420,700 in grants to the coalition to continue its work to remove any substantial differences in access to quality health care and prevention programs among all people in Colorado by the year 2007. *Community Voices: Healthcare for the Underserved Initiative (1999-2003)* In partnership with the W.K.Kellogg Foundation, the Colorado Trust has awarded Denver Health Medical Center a $2.4 million grant over five years to improve access to health-care services for Denver's medically underserved population. Components of the Community Voices Initiative inlaid a targeted public outreach and awareness effort, the creation of a user-friendly system to ensure that eligible patients are enrolled in appropriate health insurance plans, and the provision of case management to help high-risk patients access appropriate medical care. **Priorities:** *Arts & Humanities:* 2%. *Civic & Public Affairs:* 1%. *Education:* 19%. Focus on health education at the university level. *Environment:* 27%. Funds youth initiatives, child care, family services, child development, substance abuse centers, and violence prevention. *International:* 51%. Supports medically underserved, children's immunization programs, hospice, hospitals, mental health centers, healthy communities, and local health promotion initiatives. *Note:* Total contributions made in 2000. **Typ. Recipients:** Adolescent Health Issues, AIDS/HIV, Children's Health/Hospitals, Clinics/Medical Centers, Domestic Violence, Emergency/Ambulance Services, Family Planning, Geriatric Health, Health Funds, Health Organizations, Health Policy/Cost Containment, Health-General, Hospices, Hospitals, Long-Term Care, Medical Education, Medical Research, Mental Health, Nursing Services, Nutrition, People with Disabilities, Prenatal Health Issues, Preventive Medicine/Wellness Organizations, Public Health, Sexual Abuse, Single-Disease Health Associations, Substance Abuse, Transplant Networks/Donor Banks. **Geo. Dist:** CO.

★ 11264 ★ Columbia Foundation

One Lombard St., Suite 305
San Francisco, CA 94111
Phone: (415)986-5179 **Fax:** (415)986-1732
Email: susan@columbia.org
Website: http://www.columbia.org
Susan Clark, Executive Director

Fnded: 1940. **Philosophy:** "While the foundation's broad philanthropic purpose has given it flexibility to respond to changing social conditions, it has nevertheless maintained its long-standing interest in world peace, human rights, the environment, cross-cultural and international understanding, the quality of urban life, and the arts." "Arts and Culture: institutional advancement of San Francisco's major arts organizations and the creation of art by individual artists or groups of artists engaged in a new collaboration or in community service through their art." "Environment: enhanced understanding and application of principles of sustainability according to which the future capacity of the earth to support life is preserved with a focus on non-polluting agriculture and the preservation and restoration of biological diversity and wild ecosystems including ancient forest, wetlands, and other endangered wilderness areas." "Human rights: work to stop the use of capital punishment, to advocate for the right to die with dignity, to normalize attitudes toward homosexuality and eradicate homophobia, the right to express convictions, to be free from discrimination, and the right of every person to physical and mental integrity." "Urban community: Promote the viability and quality of life over time without using up the natural processes and products on which life itself depends. In the context of sustainable urban community development, an integral part of this goal is community planning which fosters a healthy, mutually-reinforcing balance between ecological, economic, and social concerns." 1996 & 1997 Application, 1999 guidelines. "Priority is given to the following types of projects: those that promote social change rather than providing an ongoing service; venture funding for new ideas or for efforts to address controversial issues; programs in the early stages of development when the potential is high out funding is scarce; programs that promote the renewal or advancement of major community institutions of long-term interest to the foundation; and programs that educate and train community leaders in sustainability as a new governing principle for all community and economic development." **Priorities:** *Arts & Humanities:* 22%. Opera, orchestras, art exhibits. *Civic & Public Affairs:* 36%. Gay/Lesbian rights, violence prevention, urban community development. *Education:* 9%. University and bilingual programs. *Environment:* 2%. *International:* 1%. Supports single-disease health associations. *Note:* Total contributions made in fiscal 2001. **Typ. Recipients:** AIDS/HIV, Domestic Violence, Emergency/Ambulance Services, Health Funds, Health Policy/Cost Containment, Hospices, Long-Term Care, Medical Research, Nutrition, Preventive Medicine/Wellness Organizations, Public Health. **Geo. Dist:** CA, especially northern California; San Francisco, CA, including metropolitan area; London.

★ 11265 ★ The Commonwealth Fund

1 East 75th St.
New York, NY 10021-2692
Phone: (212)606-3858 **Fax:** (212)606-3500
Email: cmwf@cmwf.org
Website: http://www.cmwf.org
Andrea Landes, Director, Grants Management

Fnded: 1918. **Philosophy:** The fund's current giving is focused on four areas: improving insurance coverage and access to care, improving the quality of health care services, international health policy and practice, and improving New York City public spaces and services. Internationally, since 1925, the fund has also awarded Harkness Fellowships to enable citizens of the United Kingdom, Australia, and New Zealand to study and travel in the United States. In 1998, the fund announced two new programs: The Pediatric Developmental Service Program and the Health Care in New York City Program. **Priorities:** *Civic & Public Affairs:* 19%. Supports economic policy and public policy. *Education:* 34%. Supports medical education. *International:* 47%. Supports medical research, geriatric health, health policy public health and research institutes. *Note:* Total contributions made in 2001. **Typ. Recipients:** Adolescent Health Issues, Cancer, Children's Health/Hospitals, Clinics/Medical Centers, Diabetes, Domestic Violence, Family Planning, Geriatric Health, Health Funds, Health Organizations, Health Policy/Cost Containment, Health-General, Heart, Home-Care Services, Hospitals, Long-Term Care, Medical Education, Medical Research, Medical Training, Mental Health, Nursing Services, Prenatal Health Issues, Preventive Medicine/Wellness Organizations, Public Health, Research/Studies Institutes, Substance Abuse. **Geo. Dist:** nationally; some emphasis on New York City.

★ 11266 ★ Compton Foundation

535 Middlefield Rd., Suite 160
Menlo Park, CA 94025
Phone: (650)328-0101 **Fax:** (650)328-0171
Website: http://www.comptonfoundation.org
Edith Eddy, Executive Director

Fnded: 1973. **Philosophy:** "In a world in which most problems have become increasingly interrelated and universal in dimension, and where survival of human life under conditions worth living is in jeopardy, the Compton Foundation is concerned first and foremost with the prevention of war, and the amelioration of world conditions that tend to cause conflict. Primary among these conditions are the increasing pressures and destabilizing effects of excessive population growth, the alarming depletion and unequal distribution of the world's natural resources, the tenuous status of human rights, and the steady deterioration of the world's environment." The foundation categorizes these global human survival problems into the areas of Peace and World Order, Population, and the Environment. Other, more limited concerns of the foundation include Equal Educational Opportunity, Community Welfare and Social Justice, and Culture and the Arts. 1997 Policies and Guidelines **Priorities:** *Arts & Humanities:* 3%. Supports arts associations, museums, music, dance, and opera. *Civic & Public Affairs:* 24%. Supports public policy organizations. *Education:* 25%. Supports colleges and universities. *Environment:* 23%. Funds planned parenthood groups, child welfare, and youth organizations. *International:* 2%. Gives to health organizations. *Religion:* 3%. Supports research center. *Note:* Total contributions made in 2000. **Typ. Recipients:** AIDS/HIV, Family Planning, Health Organizations, Health Policy/Cost Containment, Medical Education, Public Health. **Geo. Dist:** internationally; nationally; San Francisco, CA, including Marin an Snata Clara Counties.

★ 11267 ★ Comstock Foundation

PO Box 2127
9th Fl.
Spokane, WA 99210-2127
Phone: (509)353-4156 **Fax:** (509)353-2278
Website: http://www.watrust.com

Fnded: 1950. **Philosophy:** The foundation carries out Josie Shadle's charitable interests in its current grants program. Almost all grants are made to organizations in Spokane, WA, for specific projects which serve the people of Spokane. Within those limits, the foundation is best characterized by the number and diversity of projects and organizations that it supports. The foundation prefers to make grants for capital projects rather than contribute to operating expenses. Capital grants vary from building and remodeling to providing needed office equipment, such as computers. In special circumstances, the trustees may choose to help a worthy organization with rent, mortgage payments, or other operating costs for short intervals. Whenever possible, the foundation prefers to join with other donors in funding a project, rather than assuming a major portion of the amount needed. **Priorities:** *Arts & Humanities:* 4%. *Civic & Public Affairs:* 1%. *Education:* About 45%. Mainly supports Gonzaga University. *Environment:* 42%. *International:* 8%. *Note:* Contributions made in 1997. **Typ. Recipients:** AIDS/HIV, Cancer, Children's Health/Hospitals, Clinics/Medical Centers, Eyes/Blindness, Health Organizations, Hospitals, Medical Education, Medical Rehabilitation, Multiple Sclerosis, Nursing Services, People with Disabilities, Prenatal Health Issues, Single-Disease Health Associations, Substance Abuse. **Geo. Dist:** Spokane, WA, including metropolitan area and Spokane County.

★ 11268 ★ Conn Memorial Foundation, Inc.

2910 West Bay to Bay Boulevard, Suite 200
Tampa, FL 33629
Phone: (813)282-4922 **Fax:** (813)221-7527

Email: maggie.osborn@connfoundation.com
Maggie Osborn, Director of Services

Fnded: 1954. **Philosophy:** The Foundation "exists for the purpose of providing leadership, direction and funding assistance to tax-exempt and nonprofit youth and family organizations." The Foundation's primary interests are children, youth, and family programs; education, human service, and emergency/disaster relief; and program capital support and agency expansion. The foundation reports that scholarship assistance will be made available to foundation funded agencies whose clients seek education beyond high school. **Priorities:** *Arts & Humanities:* 4%. *Civic & Public Affairs:* 8%. Urban community affairs, aquariums, and African American affairs. *Education:* 10%. *Environment:* 45%. Youth organizations, community service, and child abuse counseling programs. *International:* 2%. *Note:* Total contributions made in fiscal 2001. **Typ. Recipients:** AIDS/HIV, Cancer, Child Abuse, Children's Health/Hospitals, Clinics/Medical Centers, Health Organizations, People with Disabilities, Research/Studies Institutes, Substance Abuse. **Geo. Dist:** FL, Hillsborough and Pinellas counties.

★ 11269 ★ Connelly Foundation
One Tower Bridge, Suite 1450
West Conshohocken, PA 19428
Phone: (610)834-3222 **Fax:** (610)834-0866
Email: eawilcox@connellyfdn.org
Website: http://www.connellyfdn.org
E. Wilcox, Grants Administrator

Fnded: 1955. **Philosophy:** The Connelly Foundation is a private grantmaking organization whose mission is to enhance the quality of life in the Delaware Valley. **Priorities:** *Arts & Humanities:* 8%. Theaters, libraries, museums. *Civic & Public Affairs:* 7%. Rehabilitation for houses. *Education:* 57%. Largely Catholic universities and secondary schools. *Environment:* 11%. Homelessness, addiction, childcare. *International:* 11%. Children's Hospital, cancer therapy, equipment upgrades. *Religion:* 1%. Supports scientific centers and scientific research. *Note:* Total contributions made in 1998. **Typ. Recipients:** AIDS/HIV, Alzheimers Disease, Cancer, Child Abuse, Children's Health/Hospitals, Clinics/Medical Centers, Domestic Violence, Emergency/Ambulance Services, Family Planning, Geriatric Health, Health Funds, Health Organizations, Heart, Home-Care Services, Hospices, Hospitals, Hospitals (University Affiliated), Long-Term Care, Medical Education, Medical Rehabilitation, Medical Research, Nursing Services, Outpatient Health Care, People with Disabilities, Prenatal Health Issues, Preventive Medicine/Wellness Organizations, Public Health, Research/Studies Institutes, Substance Abuse, Transplant Networks/Donor Banks. **Geo. Dist:** Greater Delaware Valley Region; Philadelphia, PA.

★ 11270 ★ Conrad N. Hilton Foundation
100 West Liberty St., Suite 840
Reno, NV 89501
Phone: (775)323-4221 **Fax:** (775)323-4150
Email: cnhf@hiltonfoundation.org
Website: http://www.hiltonfoundation.org
Steven Hilton, President

Fnded: 1944. **Philosophy:** Conrad Hilton believed, "the practice of charity will bind us...in one great brotherhood. As the funds you will expend here come from many places in the world, so let there be no territorial, religious, or color restrictions on your benefactions, but beware of organized, professional charities with high-salaried executives and a heavy ratio of expenses. Be ever watchful for the opportunity to shelter little children with the umbrella of your charity; be generous to their schools, their hospitals and their places of worship. For, as they must bear the burdens of our mistakes, so are they in their innocence the repositories of our hopes for the upward progress of humanity. Give aid to their protectors and defenders, the Sisters, who devote their love and life's work for the good of mankind, for they appeal especially to me as being deserving of help from the foundation." 2000 Annual Report. The Foundation's mission is to alleviate human suffering. Directors select priority areas including blindness, early childhood development, domestic violence, homelessness, and substance abuse prevention and research. Programs include an international education program for multi-handicapped blind children, their parents, and professionals who work with them (Perkins School for the Blind); nationwide delivery of the Project ALERT curriculum to help middle school students resist drugs (BEST Foundation for a Drug Free Tomorrow); and a comprehensive disease prevention program in Ghana, West Africa, centered around sources of clean water (World Vision). The foundation reports that it has undertaken a global collaborative to control and eliminate trachoma in 10 to 12 countries in Africa and Asia through the Carter Center, World Vision, and Helen Keller International. The foundation is also seeking to improve care and services for infants and toddlers with disabilities through its Early Head Start and Migrant Head Start programs. **Priorities:** *Arts & Humanities:* Less than 1%. *Civic & Public Affairs:* 11%. *Education:* 13%. *Environment:* 25%. Supports drug abuse prevention and treatment, mental health, animal protection, at-risk youth, Big Brothers/Big Sisters, child welfare, domestic violence and child abuse prevention, family services, recreation and athletic organizations, United Way, and volunteer services. *International:* 28%. Supports blindness prevention and treatment, AIDS/HIV organizations, cancer centers, children's health, health organizations, hospitals, preventative medicine and wellness organizations, and single-disease health associations. *Religion:* Less than 1%. *Note:* Total contributions made in fiscal 2002. **Typ. Recipients:** Arthritis, Children's Health/Hospitals, Clinics/Medical Centers, Diabetes, Domestic Violence, Emergency/Ambulance Services, Eyes/Blindness, Family Planning, Geriatric Health, Health Organizations, Health-General, Heart, Hospices, Hospitals, Medical Research, Multiple Sclerosis, People with Disabilities, Public Health, Research/Studies Institutes, Single-Disease Health Associations, Substance Abuse, Transplant Networks/Donor Banks. **Geo. Dist:** internationally; nationally.

★ 11271 ★ Constantin Foundation
4809 Cole Ave., LB-127
Dallas, TX 75205-3578
Phone: (214)522-9300 **Fax:** (214)521-7025
Betty Hillin, Executive Director

Fnded: 1947. **Philosophy:** Traditionally, most grants have been awarded to private colleges, universities, and secondary schools. The remainder of funds have supported hospitals and medical centers, and social service organizations. **Priorities:** *Arts & Humanities:* 2%. Supports performing arts for youth. *Education:* 53%. Private schools and the University of Dallas. *Environment:* 41%. Supports shelters, volunteer centers and youth organizations. *International:* 4%. Supports the Arthritis Foundation. *Note:* Total contributions made in 1998. **Typ. Recipients:** Alzheimers Disease, Arthritis, Cancer, Child Abuse, Children's Health/Hospitals, Clinics/Medical Centers, Eyes/Blindness, Family Planning, Health Organizations, Hospitals, Hospitals (University Affiliated), Medical Research, Mental Health, People with Disabilities, Single-Disease Health Associations, Substance Abuse. **Geo. Dist:** TX, Dallas County; Dallas, TX, including metropolitan area.

★ 11272 ★ Cooke Foundation
1164 Bishop St., 8th Floor
Honolulu, HI 96813
Phone: (808)537-6333 **Fax:** (808)521-6286
Email: info@hcf-hawaii.org
Website: http://www.hcf-hawaii.org
Lisa Schiff, Grants Administrator

Fnded: 1920. **Philosophy:** "Grantmaking fields in the order of interest to the Trustees are arts, culture and humanities; human services; youth development; environment and species protection; health; community development; and education. Grants may be awarded for innovative programs, demonstration programs, and time-limited projects. The Trustees will consider matching other funds, and are particularly interested in helping organizations develop an expanded financial base or test new ways to generate revenue. Staff training and other activities to increase standards of performance and efficiency are considered. Joint project requests from two or more organizations seeking to explore and resolve community problems are of interest to the Trustees. Although most of the funding from the Foundation goes to O'ahu-based recipients, the Foundation is statewide in the scope of grantmaking." 2001 Annual Report **Priorities:** *Arts & Humanities:* 39%. Supports museums, historical and archeological projects, music, dance, public broadcasting, theater, arts centers, and arts education. *Civic & Public Affairs:* 5%. Supports community development and housing. *Education:* 22%. Supports public and private pre-college education, and universities. *Environment:* 21%. Supports family services, mental health, drug rehabilitation, youth causes, food banks, and community centers. *International:* 6%. Supports hospitals, health clinics, and single-disease associations. *Note:* Total contributions made in fiscal 2001. **Typ. Recipients:** AIDS/HIV, Alzheimers Disease, Cancer, Children's Health/Hospitals, Clinics/Medical Centers, Domestic Violence, Emergency/Ambulance Services, Family Planning, Health Organizations, Health Policy/Cost Containment, Health-General, Heart, Hospices, Hospices, Hospitals, Medical Research, Mental Health, People with Disabilities, Prenatal Health Issues, Public Health, Single-Disease Health Associations, Substance Abuse. **Geo. Dist:** HI, especially Oahu.

★ 11273 ★ Cooper Foundation
211 N 12th St., No. 304
Lincoln, NE 68508
Phone: (402)476-7571 **Fax:** (402)476-2356
Email: art@cooperfoundation.org
Website: http://www.cooperfoundation.org
E. Thompson, President

Fnded: 1934. **Priorities:** *Arts & Humanities:* 32%. Supports music, art centers, theater, and public broadcasting. *Education:* 39%. Supports schools and colleges. *Environment:* 14%. Supports child welfare, YWCA, and homes. *Note:* Total contributions made in 1999. **Typ. Recipients:** Cancer, Children's Health/Hospitals, Domestic Violence, Emergency/Ambulance Services, Hospitals, Kidney, Medical Education, People with Disabilities, Prenatal Health Issues, Public Health, Substance Abuse. **Geo. Dist:** Lincoln, NE, including Lancaster County.

★ 11274 ★ Corbett Foundation
127 West 9th St., Suite 3
Cincinnati, OH 45202
Phone: (513)241-3320 **Fax:** (513)723-4422
Karen McKim, Executive Director

Fnded: 1958. **Philosophy:** "Grants are generally restricted to the field of cultural arts and education and community projects; however, to the extent the funds are available, grants may be made for other purposes." In recent years, the foundation has made major grants to the University of Cincinnati College Conservatory of Music for capital improvements. **Priorities:** *Arts & Humanities:* 61%. Focus is primarily in the Cincinnati area. *Civic & Public Affairs:* 31%. Public policy. *Education:* 7%. Supports high school and performing arts. *Environment:* About 1%. Scouting. *International:* 2%. Hospital. *Note:* Total contributions made in fiscal 2002. **Typ. Recipients:** Alzheimers Disease, Nutrition, Preventive Medicine/Wellness Organizations, Substance Abuse. **Geo. Dist:** Cincinnati, OH.

★ 11275 ★ Corella and Bertram Bonner Foundation
10 Mercer St.
Princeton, NJ 08540
Phone: (609)924-6663 **Fax:** (609)683-4626
Email: wmeisel@bonner.org
Website: http://www.bonner.org
Wayne Meisel, President

Fnded: 1981. **Philosophy:** According to the foundation's literature, its purpose is to "help the person who is hurting." The foundation is primarily interested in directing financial assistance to the basic needs of food, education, and health care. Its goal is "to displace despair with opportunity. ... and it is the intent to develop partners in these programs to ensure the success of all resources invested in each grant." To meet this plan, the foundation focuses on several major areas: crisis ministry, education, medical services, aid to the handicapped, and general relief. The Crisis Ministry Program financially supports initiatives from food-banks and community-based religious organizations and coalitions that are directly involved in the feeding of the hungry. The focus of these initiatives is on religious community leadership against hunger and its underlying causes. In addition to its contributions to numerous food banks throughout the United States, the foundation also supports education. The Bonner Scholars Program supports academically qualified individuals that otherwise would not be able to attend college because of financial need. The foundation works closely with selected colleges to identify and support deserving students. In return, Bonner Scholars are expected to contribute to society by tutoring and mentoring others. The foundation will also consider requests from organizations serving those communities who are in need of emergency or continuing assistance. **Priorities:** *Civic & Public Affairs:* 4%. Supports People in Action. *Education:* 48%. Funds Learn and Serve America. *Environment:* 17%. Youth programs. *International:* 14%. Mayo Foundation. *Note:* Total contributions made in fiscal 2001. **Typ. Recipients:** Clinics/Medical Centers, Health Funds, Hospitals, Medical Research, Research/Studies Institutes. **Geo. Dist:** nationally; East Coast region.

★ 11276 ★ Courtney S. Turner Charitable Trust

1200 Main St., 14th Fl.
Kansas City, MO 64105
Phone: (816)979-7481 **Fax:** (816)691-7916
David Ross, Sr., Trust Officer

Fnded: 1986. **Philosophy:** The Courtney S. Turner Charitable Trust has two primary interests: education and the arts. Educational funding favors new programs in higher education. Funding for the arts emphasizes music, museums, and theater. Social services are a secondary interest, with minor support to youth organizations. **Priorities:** *Arts & Humanities:* 37%. Supports music, threatre, and public broadcasting. *Civic & Public Affairs:* 10%. Supports gardens. *Education:* 23%. Supports colleges and education funds. *Environment:* 10%. Supports YWCA, scouts, and a community center. *International:* 9%. Supports hospital foundation and a health center. *Religion:* 10%. Supports a science museum. *Note:* Total contributions made in 2000. **Typ. Recipients:** Children's Health/Hospitals, Clinics/Medical Centers, Domestic Violence, Health-General, Heart, Hospitals, Hospitals (University Affiliated), Multiple Sclerosis, Nursing Services, People with Disabilities, Public Health, Sexual Abuse, Substance Abuse. **Geo. Dist:** Atchison, MO; Kansas City, MO, metropolitan area.

★ 11277 ★ Cowles Charitable Trust

PO Box 219
Rumson, NJ 07760
Phone: (732)936-9826
Mary Croft, Secretary & Treasurer

Fnded: 1948. **Philosophy:** The Cowles Charitable Trust makes most of its grants in the areas of education, arts, health, and environment. Educational funding favors colleges and universities. Funding in the arts emphasizes museums, arts associations, arts centers, music, and theater groups. The trust also will fund civic groups, social services, and health organizations. **Priorities:** *Arts & Humanities:* 40%. Funds arts centers, museums, libraries, opera, and ballet. *Civic & Public Affairs:* 8%. Funds municipalities, parks, and housing. *Education:* 25%. Supports precollege and higher education. *Environment:* 18%. Supports family and children's services, United Way. *International:* 16%. Gives to medical centers and health associations. *Note:* Total contributions made in 2000. **Typ. Recipients:** AIDS/HIV, Cancer, Children's Health/Hospitals, Clinics/Medical Centers, Domestic Violence, Emergency/Ambulance Services, Family Planning, Health Organizations, Hospitals, Hospitals (University Affiliated), Medical Education, Medical Rehabilitation, Medical Research, Mental Health, People with Disabilities, Single-Disease Health Associations, Substance Abuse. **Geo. Dist:** nationally; FL; New York City, NY.

★ 11278 ★ Crescent Porter Hale Foundation

655 Redwood Highway, Suite 301
Mill Valley, CA 94941
Phone: (415)388-2333 **Fax:** (415)381-4799
Ulla Davis, Executive Director

Fnded: 1961. **Philosophy:** The foundation supports organizations devoted to education in the fields of art, music, elementary, secondary, and university education. "The foundation will consider other worthwhile programs which can be demonstrated as serving broad community purposes, leading toward the improvement of the quality of life. Agencies serving disadvantaged youth, the disabled, or the elderly are of particular interest to the foundation." "Emphasis is placed on organizations engaged in Catholic endeavors." **Priorities:** *Arts & Humanities:* 4%. Gives to dance, music, and an arts and crafts museum. *Civic & Public Affairs:* 6% Funds housing, community initiatives, parks, women's affairs, and employment training and placement. *Education:* 26%. Supports colleges, private secondary schools, and educational organizations for religious concerns. *Environment:* 25%. Funds youth and family services, community centers, violence prevention programs, food distribution, and shelters. *International:* 2%. Contributes to pediatric cancer programs and a hospital volunteer program. *Note:* Total contributions made in 2000. **Typ. Recipients:** AIDS/HIV, Arthritis, Cancer, Family Planning, Health Organizations, Hospices, Hospitals, Long-Term Care, Medical Education, Medical Research, Nursing Services, People with Disabilities, Research/Studies Institutes, Sexual Abuse, Single-Disease Health Associations, Substance Abuse. **Geo. Dist:** San Francisco, CA, Bay area.

★ 11279 ★ Crestlea Foundation

100 W 10th St., Suite 1109
Wilmington, DE 19801
Phone: (302)654-2477 **Fax:** (302)654-2323
Stephen Martinenza, Secretary & Treasurer

Fnded: 1955. **Philosophy:** The foundation has three main areas of interest, but does not limit giving to these areas specifically. Secondary and higher education are major interests, followed by support for libraries and museums in Pennsylvania and Delaware. The third main interest is youth activities and family planning. In addition, the foundation distributes the remainder of its support to community affairs, nature conservation, and churches. **Priorities:** *Arts & Humanities:* 29%. Arts funds, libraries, museums, music, and historic preservation. *Civic & Public Affairs:* 4%. Funds civic affairs, free enterprise, community foundations, and housing. *Education:* 25%. $2,000,000 grant to Pomfred School. Mainly precollege private education and computer equipment. Also supports religious education and literacy. *Environment:* 23%. United Way, day care programs, people with disabilities, scouts, senior services, and family planning services. *International:* 6%. Supports hospitals, hospice, and health organizations. *Note:* Total contributions made in 2001. **Typ. Recipients:** Alzheimers Disease, Cancer, Children's Health/Hospitals, Clinics/Medical Centers, Family Planning, Geriatric Health, Health Organizations, Hospices, Hospitals, Long-Term Care, Medical Education, People with Disabilities, Preventive Medicine/Wellness Organizations, Public Health, Single-Disease Health Associations. **Geo. Dist:** Wilmington, DE, including surrounding area.

★ 11280 ★ Crystal Trust

1088 Du Pont Bldg.
Wilmington, DE 19898
Phone: (302)651-0533
Stephen Doberstein, Director

Fnded: 1947. **Philosophy:** The trust has no specific mandate other than that of serving the Wilmington community. It supports a wide variety of causes. Emphasis is on gifts for capital and other one-time special purposes, and against gifts for continuing expenses of operations or deficits. **Priorities:** *Arts & Humanities:* 9%. Museums and historic preservation. *Civic & Public Affairs:* 5%. Primary support for the Delaware Department of State. *Education:* 56%. Includes a major grant to Wilmington College. *Environment:* 19%. Supports people with disabilities, family services, child welfare, youth organizations, and the aged. *International:* 6%. Health centers and single-disease health associations. *Note:* Total contributions made in 2000. **Typ. Recipients:** Cancer, Child Abuse, Clinics/Medical Centers, Domestic Violence, Family Planning, Geriatric Health, Health Funds, Health Organizations, Health-General, Hospices, Hospitals, Long-Term Care, Medical Education, Medical Research, Mental Health, People with Disabilities, Preventive Medicine/Wellness Organizations, Public Health, Single-Disease Health Associations. **Geo. Dist:** nationally.

★ 11281 ★ CTW Foundation, Inc.

PO Box 911
Wilmington, DE 19899-0911
Phone: (302)429-9425
Robert Tucker, President

Fnded: 1954. **Priorities:** *Arts & Humanities:* 16%. Supports art foundations, performing arts, and museums. *Education:* 22%. Supports universities, colleges, and schools. *Environment:* 55%. Supports domestic violence services and people with disabilities. *International:* 4%. Supports medical centers and single-disease health associations. *Note:* Total contributions made in 2000. **Typ. Recipients:** Cancer, Children's Health/Hospitals, Clinics/Medical Centers, Domestic Violence, Health Funds, Health Organizations, Hospices, Hospitals, Medical Education, Medical Rehabilitation, Medical Research, Medical Training, People with Disabilities, Preventive Medicine/Wellness Organizations, Public Health. **Geo. Dist:** nationally.

★ 11282 ★ The Cullen Foundation

601 Jefferson, Suite 4000
Houston, TX 77002
Phone: (713)651-8835 **Fax:** (713)651-2374
Website: http://www.cullenfdn.org
Alan Stewart, Executive Director

Fnded: 1947. **Philosophy:** The foundation supports a variety of educational and health institutions, social service programs, and arts groups. **Priorities:** *Arts & Humanities:* 16%. Funds music, museums, public broadcasting, ballet, and theater. *Civic & Public Affairs:* 4%. Funds housing programs, philanthropic organizations, and community development organizations. *Education:* 57%. Supports colleges and universities, private religious education, medical education, and public school reform. *Environment:* 13%. Contributes to the United Way, food banks, child welfare, camps and scouting, and substance abuse centers. *International:* 9%. Funds a heart institute and health care systems. *Religion:* 2%. Supports the Houston Museum of Natural Science. *Note:* Total contributions made in 2000. **Typ. Recipients:** AIDS/HIV, Alzheimers Disease, Cancer, Child Abuse, Children's Health/Hospitals, Clinics/Medical Centers, Emergency/Ambulance Services, Family Planning, Heart, Hospices, Hospitals, Medical Education, Medical Rehabilitation, Medical Research, Speech & Hearing, Substance Abuse. **Geo. Dist:** Houston, TX, including surrounding area.

★ 11283 ★ Cuneo Foundation

9101 Greenwood Ave., Suite 210
Niles, IL 60714
Phone: (847)296-3351 **Fax:** (847)296-3310
John Cuneo, Jr., President

Fnded: 1945. **Philosophy:** The two major priorities of the Cuneo Foundation are Catholic churches and social services. Catholic church funding favors churches in Chicago. Support for social services favors children's homes, youth organizations, and support for the needy. Nominal support goes to a number of educational institutions, including private schools, universities, and religious education. Health services, the arts, and civic affairs are lower priorities.

Priorities: *Arts & Humanities:* 1%. *Civic & Public Affairs:* 3%. *Education:* 18%. Supports parochial schools. *Environment:* 19%. Youth agencies, shelters and food banks are funded. *International:* 12%. Funds single-disease health associations. *Religion:* 1%. *Note:* Total contributions made in 1998. **Typ. Recipients:** Alzheimers Disease, Cancer, Children's Health/Hospitals, Geriatric Health, Health Funds, Heart, Hospices, Hospitals, Long-Term Care, Medical Education, Medical Research, People with Disabilities, Public Health, Single-Disease Health Associations. **Geo. Dist:** Chicago, IL, including metropolitan area.

★ 11284 ★ D and DF Foundation

1 Maritime Plz., Suite 1400
San Francisco, CA 94111
Phone: (415)427-2449 **Fax:** (415)288-0549
Donald Fisher, Trustee

Fnded: 1986. **Priorities:** *Arts & Humanities:* 4%. Funds museums, dance, and music. *Civic & Public Affairs:* 69%. Supports parks, community foundations, and clubs. *Education:* 19%. Supports pre-college education and universities. *Environment:* 6%. Supports United Way, social services agencies, children's organizations, and volunteer services. *International:* 2%. Supports medical research and women's health. *Note:* Total contributionss in fiscal 1999. **Typ. Recipients:** AIDS/HIV, Cancer, Clinics/Medical Centers, Health Funds, Health Organizations, Health-General, Hospitals, Medical Education, Medical Research, People with Disabilities. **Geo. Dist:** CA.

★ 11285 ★ Daisy Marquis Jones Foundation

1600 South Ave., Suite 250
Rochester, NY 14620
Phone: (585)461-4950 **Fax:** (585)955-4940
Email: mail@dmjf.org
Website: http://www.dmjf.org
Roger Gardner, President & Trustee

Fnded: 1968. **Philosophy:** The foundation considers itself "a citizen of the community and responds to special opportunities to improve local conditions and to help people solve their own problems." The foundation also encourages preventive programs and focuses on projects involving the disadvantaged. The foundation makes grants primarily to improve the quality of health care in Monroe and Yates counties. Other areas of support include community development, senior citizens, youth, men, women, and improving the administration of justice. The foundation "seeks to make the best use of its limited resources and, in keeping with the foundation's 'new directions,' will focus on primary prevention and advocacy issues. The foundation will continue to emphasize projects involving the disadvantaged." **Priorities:** *Arts & Humanities:* 3%. Supports arts councils, public broadcasting, historic preservation, performing arts, and theater. *Civic & Public Affairs:* 14%. Supports housing, community development, employment/job training, philanthropic organizations, women's affairs, law and justice, and botanical gardens/parks. *Education:* 16%. Supports preschools, minority education, and scholarship funds. *Environment:* 29%. Supports Young Men's Christian Association, Big Brothers/Big Sister, senior services, shelters for the homeless, food banks, United Way, and at-risk youth. *International:* 37%. Supports medical centers, children's health, hospice, health organizations, speech and training, AIDS, mental health, and cancer treatment. *Note:* Total contributions made in 2000. **Typ. Recipients:** Adolescent Health Issues, AIDS/HIV, Alzheimers Disease, Cancer, Children's Health/Hospitals, Clinics/Medical Centers, Domestic Violence, Emergency/Ambulance Services, Family Planning, Geriatric Health, Health Organizations, Hospices, Hospitals, Hospitals (University Affiliated), Long-Term Care, Medical Education, Medical Rehabilitation, Mental Health, Nursing Services, Nutrition, Outpatient Health Care, People with Disabilities, Prenatal Health Issues, Preventive Medicine/Wellness Organizations, Public Health, Research/Studies Institutes, Speech & Hearing, Substance Abuse. **Geo. Dist:** NY, Monroe County; NY, Yates County.

★ 11286 ★ Dale J. Bellamah Foundation

PO Box 676370
Rancho Santa Fe, CA 92067
Phone: (858)756-1154 **Fax:** (858)756-3856
Email: dwilson@mnttrust.com
Website: http://www.mnttrust.com
Frank Potenziani, Vice President & Director

Fnded: 1972. **Philosophy:** The foundation's interests include higher education scholarships, business school programs in international business and law in Eastern Europe, research in diabetes, hospitals, the U.S. Olympic Committee, youth programs, and care of the mentally retarded. **Priorities:** *Civic & Public Affairs:* 1%. Funds ethnic organization. *Education:* 66%. Primarily for scholarships and fellowships. *Environment:* 19%. Funds the U.S. Olympic Committee and training center and a youth organization. *International:* 13%. Supports the American Diabetes Association. *Note:* Total contributions made in 2000. **Typ. Recipients:** Arthritis, Cancer, Diabetes, Hospitals, Medical Education, People with Disabilities, Single-Disease Health Associations. **Geo. Dist:** NM.

★ 11287 ★ Dan Murphy Foundation

PO Box 711267
Los Angeles, CA 90071
Phone: (213)623-3120
Sir Daniel Donohue, President

Fnded: 1957. **Philosophy:** The Dan Murphy Foundation's primary concerns are the charities and activities of the Roman Catholic church, in the Archdiocese of Los Angeles. Organizations of interest include religious orders, higher education, high schools and elementary schools, social services (especially religious welfare), and medical institutions. **Priorities:** *Arts & Humanities:* 1%. *Education:* 23%. Funds Catholic colleges and schools, and religious education. *Environment:* 3%. *International:* 2%. *Religion:* Less than 1%. *Note:* Total contributions made in 2000. **Typ. Recipients:** Cancer, Children's Health/Hospitals, Clinics/Medical Centers, Emergency/Ambulance Services, Eyes/Blindness, Eyes/Blindness, Family Planning, Health Organizations, Hospices, Hospitals, Long-Term Care, Medical Education, Medical Rehabilitation, Medical Research, Mental Health, Nursing Services, People with Disabilities, Prenatal Health Issues, Substance Abuse. **Geo. Dist:** CA; Los Angeles, CA, metropolitan area.

★ 11288 ★ Dane G. Hansen Foundation

110 West Main St.
PO Box 187
Logan, KS 67646
Phone: (785)689-4832 **Fax:** (785)689-4833
Email: hansentr@ruraltel.net
Ross Beach, President & Trustee

Fnded: 1965. **Philosophy:** The foundation's mission is to "improve the quality of life for citizens of Kansas." Support is provided to a variety of organizations and programs in the arts, civic and public affairs, education, health, and social services. The foundation maintains an education scholarship program to aid students attending Kansas colleges and universities. The foundation also provides scholarships for vocational education and for theological and graduate studies. **Priorities:** *Arts & Humanities:* 4% Supports arts councils and libraries. *Civic & Public Affairs:* 34%. Funds improvements to city and public services. *Education:* 46%. Educational institutions and programs are funded. *Environment:* 8%. Funding went to youth causes, special needs children, and animal training concerns. *International:* 7%. Supports hospice, disease and disorder concerns, hospitals and medical centers. *Note:* Contributions were made in fiscal 2001. **Typ. Recipients:** Cancer, Children's Health/Hospitals, Clinics/Medical Centers, Emergency/Ambulance Services, Eyes/Blindness, Health Organizations, Health-General, Heart, Hospices, Hospitals, Long-Term Care, Medical Education, Medical Rehabilitation, Medical Research, People with Disabilities, Single-Disease Health Associations. **Geo. Dist:** KS, Northwestern part of state.

★ 11289 ★ Danforth Foundation

211 North Broadway, Suite 2390
Saint Louis, MO 63102
Phone: (314)588-1900 **Fax:** (314)588-0035
Dr. Bruce Anderson, President

Fnded: 1927. **Philosophy:** "The Danforth Foundation is a private, independent foundation whose mission is to help St. Louis become the leading region in America. Its goals are to do the follow: help established institutions become world class; help organizations which show great promise of making significant contributions to St. Louis; support creation, renovation, and enhancement of selected facilities; and support other projects which promise long-term contributions to the quality of life in the region." The Danforth Foundation also supports several of its own initiatives. Foundation and three partners: the National Governors Association, the National Conference of State Legislatures, and the Education Commission of the States. Its mission is to help stat and local government officials improve the well-being of high-risk children and their families. A ten-year initiative launched in 1992, the Policymakers Program has helped more than 300 government executives and legislators from 40 states revise ways in which social services are delivered to their residents. The Danforth Program for Successful Schools supported the work of 20 school teams in the states of Missouri, California, Ohio, and Florida in developing The Danforth Program for Teachers supported two initiatives designed to improve teaching and learning in the St. Louis metropolitan area: the Action Research Collaborative and the Professional Development Schools Collaborative. Funds for these initiatives were transferred to the St. Louis Regional Professional Development Center as of June 1, 1997. **Priorities:** *Civic & Public Affairs:* 34%. Supports towns/municipalities, policy making, community and economic development, community foundations, and nonprofit management. *Education:* 28%. Funds universities, early childhood development research and facilities, public school systems, and teacher training. *Environment:* 14%. Funds youth organizations, child care programs, violence prevention, Young Men's Christian Association, and the United Way. *Religion:* 19%. Supports the Plant Science Institute. *Note:* Total contributions made in fiscal 2001, excluding program-related investments. **Typ. Recipients:** Children's Health/Hospitals, Clinics/Medical Centers, Domestic Violence, Family Planning, Health Organizations, Hospitals, Mental Health, Research/Studies Institutes. **Geo. Dist:** Saint Louis, MO.

★ 11290 ★ Daniel Foundation of Alabama

820 Shades Creek Parkway, Suite 1200
Birmingham, AL 35209
Phone: (205)879-0902 **Fax:** (205)879-0906
S. Smith, Executive Director

Fnded: 1977. **Philosophy:** The concerns of the Daniel Foundation encompass a wide variety of educational, social service, cultural, and community interests in the state of Alabama, particularly in Birmingham. **Priorities:** *Arts & Humanities:* 13%. Gives to Birmingham performing arts groups, museums, and historical societies. *Civic & Public Affairs:* 22%. Funds housing, community foundations, and a botanical garden. *Education:* 50%. Primarily supports colleges, universities, and secondary schools. *Environment:* 6%. Supports youth groups, anti-substance abuse programs, the aged, and community services. *International:* 5%. Funds medical centers and children's hospital. *Religion:* 3%. Funds Discovery 2000. *Note:* Total contributions made in 2001. **Typ. Recipients:** AIDS/HIV, Cancer, Child Abuse, Children's Health/Hospitals, Clinics/Medical Centers, Eyes/Blindness, Health Organizations, Hospices, Hospitals, Long-Term Care, Medical Education, Medical Rehabilitation, Medical Research, Mental Health, Multiple Sclerosis, People with Disabilities, Public Health, Research/Studies Institutes, Single-Disease Health Associations, Substance Abuse. **Geo. Dist:** southeastern states; AL.

★ 11291 ★ Davee Foundation

225 W Wacker Dr., Suite 3000
Chicago, IL 60606

Phone: (312)201-2000
Ruth Davee, President

Fnded: 1964. **Priorities:** *Arts & Humanities:* 4%. Funds orchestras, dance, theater, opera, art museums, public broadcasting, literary arts, humanities associations, and libraries. *Civic & Public Affairs:* 2%. Gives to citizens/voters groups, public policy organizations, a zoo, women's affairs, urban renewal, and parks. *Education:* 91%. Provides major support to the Northwestern University Medical School; also funds other colleges and universities. *Environment:* Less than 1%. Family planning organizations, shelters, senior services, youth organizations, and veterans organizations receive foundation funds. *International:* 1%. Contributes to hospitals, a medical rehabilitation center, hospice, and single-disease health associations. *Note:* Total contributions made in 2000. **Typ. Recipients:** Alzheimers Disease, Cancer, Family Planning, Hospices, Hospitals, Hospitals (University Affiliated), Medical Education, Medical Rehabilitation, Medical Research, People with Disabilities. **Geo. Dist:** IL.

★ 11292 ★ Davenport-Hatch Foundation
1 East Ave.
Rochester, NY 14604
Phone: (716)238-3300
Bill McKee, Contact

Fnded: 1952. **Philosophy:** The foundation makes grants across the major categories of support. In the area of health care, interests include hospitals and single-disease health associations. Social services support goes to community service organizations, children and families, and youth organizations. Educational support includes scholarships and capital support, mostly to private schools. Art interests include history and music, and the remainder goes to civic affairs and religion. **Priorities:** *Arts & Humanities:* 5%. Supports philharmonic orchestras, museums, and performing arts. *Civic & Public Affairs:* 1%. Supports the Susan B. Anthony House. *Education:* 11%. Supports colleges, universities, and educational programs. *Environment:* 67%. Supports United Way, child welfare, and youth services. *International:* 12%. Supports hospitals, health services, the elderly, hearing and speech impaired, and disease and disorder concerns. *Religion:* 3%. Supports the Rochester Museum and Science Center. *Note:* Contributions were made in fiscal 2001. **Typ. Recipients:** AIDS/HIV, Alzheimers Disease, Cancer, Clinics/Medical Centers, Domestic Violence, Emergency/Ambulance Services, Family Planning, Geriatric Health, Health Organizations, Health-General, Heart, Home-Care Services, Hospices, Hospitals, Kidney, Long-Term Care, Medical Education, Medical Rehabilitation, Medical Research, Medical Training, Mental Health, Multiple Sclerosis, Nursing Services, People with Disabilities, Prenatal Health Issues, Public Health, Single-Disease Health Associations, Speech & Hearing, Substance Abuse, Trauma Treatment. **Geo. Dist:** Rochester, NY, including surrounding metropolitan area.

★ 11293 ★ David Geffen Foundation
PO Box 8509
Universal City, CA 91618-8509
Phone: (818)733-6300　**Fax:** (818)733-6129
David Geffen, Trustee

Fnded: 1986. **Priorities:** *Arts & Humanities:* 17%. Funds theater, music, art museums, art funds, and historic preservation. *Civic & Public Affairs:* 18%. Supports civil liberties, gay and lesbian causes, and legal defense organizations. *Education:* 18%. Primarily supports colleges and universities, with a focus on cinema and television education programs. *Environment:* 1%. Conributions to shelters, programs for the homeless, senior services, youth organizations, food distribution, and services for victims of domestic violence and rape. *International:* 31%. Gives to AIDS causes and research, hospitals, children's health concerns, free clinics, and single-disease health associations. *Note:* Total contributions made in 2000. **Typ. Recipients:** AIDS/HIV, Cancer, Children's Health/Hospitals, Clinics/Medical Centers, Diabetes, Emergency/Ambulance Services, Family Planning, Health Organizations, Health Policy/Cost Containment, Hospices, Hospitals, Medical Education, Medical Research, Public Health, Single-Disease Health Associations, Substance Abuse. **Geo. Dist:** CA; Washington, DC; NY.

★ 11294 ★ David, Helen, and Marian Woodward Fund-Atlanta
191 Peachtree St. NE
MC GA1102
Atlanta, GA 30303
Phone: (404)332-6677　**Fax:** (404)332-1389
Website: http://www.wachovia.com/corp_inst/charitable_services/
Bennie Boswell, Jr., Manager, Community Affairs

Fnded: 1975. **Philosophy:** The fund focuses its giving in the Atlanta, GA, area. Contributions reflect an emphasis on health care and education; social services, religious organizations, civic groups, and the arts also receive support from the fund. **Priorities:** *Arts & Humanities:* 16%. Supports historic preservation; music, and general architects. *Civic & Public Affairs:* 22%. Supports community foundations, clubs, parks, and ethnic organizations. *Education:* 39%. Primarily funding private precollege education. Also supports religious education. *Environment:* 12%. Supports scouting, young men's christian association and camps. *International:* 8% Supports medicine centers, alzheimers, and health organizations. *Note:* Total contributions made in fiscal 2001. **Typ. Recipients:** Child Abuse, Children's Health/Hospitals, Clinics/Medical Centers, Health Organizations, Health Policy/Cost Containment, Hospitals, Long-Term Care, People with Disabilities, Public Health, Single-Disease Health Associations, Substance Abuse. **Geo. Dist:** GA, emphasis on Atlanta and neighboring states.

★ 11295 ★ David and Lucile Packard Foundation
300 Second St., Suite 200
Los Altos, CA 94022
Phone: (650)948-7658　**Fax:** (650)948-5793
Website: http://www.packard.org
Richard Schlosberg, III, President & Trustee

Fnded: 1964. **Philosophy:** The foundation makes grants in the following categories: science; conservation; population; children, families, and communities; arts; and special areas that include organizational effectiveness and philanthropy. Current initiatives include childcare center technology and health-care access, quality, and insurance for low-income children; land, marine, and energy conservation will also receive support. **Priorities:** *Arts & Humanities:* 2%. Focus on cultural facilities, arts education, and institutional support. *Civic & Public Affairs:* 15%. Primarily funds organizations concerned with population issues, reproductive rights, and family planning. *Education:* 6%. Supports fellowships and research at colleges and universities. *Environment:* 46%. Supports programs for children, families, and communities that improve health and economic security; promote child and youth development; prevent domestic violence; and build community and national capacity. *International:* 24%. Focus is on children's health. *Religion:* 12%. Funds ocean science, interdisciplinary science, sustainability science, and underrepresented groups in the scientific community. Also provides fellowships for science and engineering. *Note:* Total contributions made in 2001. **Typ. Recipients:** Children's Health/Hospitals, Clinics/Medical Centers, Emergency/Ambulance Services, Family Planning, Health Organizations, Health Policy/Cost Containment, Health-General, Heart, Hospitals, Long-Term Care, Medical Education, Medical Research, Nursing Services, Nutrition, People with Disabilities, Prenatal Health Issues, Preventive Medicine/Wellness Organizations, Public Health, Research/Studies Institutes. **Geo. Dist:** internationally; nationally; CA, Monterey County; CA, San Mateo County; CA, Santa Clara County; CA, Santa Cruz County.

★ 11296 ★ David Rockefeller Fund
30 Rockefeller Plz., Rm. 5600
New York, NY 10112
Phone: (212)649-5600
Marnie Pillsbury, Executive Director

Fnded: 1989. **Priorities:** *Arts & Humanities:* 65%. Supports libraries, art and cultural museums, music festivals, historic preservation, public broadcasting, and orchestras. *Civic & Public Affairs:* 3%. Gives to state and national parks and fire departments. *Education:* 3%. Colleges, nursery schools, and an outward bound school receive support. *Environment:* 16%. Supports the United Way, scouts, child care, drug and alcohol abuse centers, Young Men's Christian Association, youth organizations, family services, and animal welfare. *International:* 8%. Funds hospitals, medical centers, community health programs, hospice, and nursing associations. *Religion:* 2%. Gives to genetics and biological laboratories, and a natural history museum. *Note:* Total contributions made in 2000. **Typ. Recipients:** Children's Health/Hospitals, Clinics/Medical Centers, Family Planning, Hospitals, Hospitals, Nursing Services, Prenatal Health Issues, Public Health. **Geo. Dist:** Seal Harbor, ME; Pocantico, NY.

★ 11297 ★ David Schwartz Foundation
630 Third Ave.
New York, NY 10017
Phone: (212)586-4225　**Fax:** (212)586-0649
Richard Schwartz, President

Fnded: 1945. **Philosophy:** The David Schwartz Foundation makes most of its grants to education and the arts. Funding supports universities, medical education, and private and day schools. Arts funding goes to the performing arts, historic preservation, and museums. Other areas of support include Jewish religious organizations, civic affairs, health, and social services. **Priorities:** *Arts & Humanities:* 18%. Supports arts funds, theater, museums, and music organizations. *Civic & Public Affairs:* 4%. Gives to playgrounds, civic organizations, women's affairs, and philanthropic organizations. *Education:* 67%. Focus on colleges, universities, and arts and medical education. *Environment:* Less than 1%. *International:* Less than 1%. *Note:* Total contributions made in fiscal 2001. **Typ. Recipients:** AIDS/HIV, Cancer, Children's Health/Hospitals, Clinics/Medical Centers, Family Planning, Hospitals, Medical Education, Medical Research, Public Health, Single-Disease Health Associations. **Geo. Dist:** New York, NY.

★ 11298 ★ de Kay Foundation
1211 Ave. of America
New York, NY 10036
Phone: (212)789-4151
Daniel Ordan, Contact

Fnded: 1967. **Philosophy:** The de Kay Foundation makes grants to a few organizations. One-third of contributions goes to St. Barnabas Hospital in New York. Another one-third of funds was split between the Federation for Protestant Welfare Agencies and the Community Service Society of New York. The remaining one-third funds the groups which enable elderly individuals (over age 65) in the Tri-State region to remain in their homes. Applications must be submitted through social service agencies. Individuals applying directly will be rejected. **Priorities:** *Environment:* 25%. Supports the Community Service Society of New York and the Federation of Protestant Welfare agencies. *International:* 50%. Supports St. Barnabas Hospital. *Note:* Total contributions made in fiscal 1999. **Typ. Recipients:** Hospitals. **Geo. Dist:** New York, NY.

★ 11299 ★ Dekko Foundation, Inc.
PO Box 548
1208 Lakeside Drive
Kendallville, IN 46755-0548
Phone: (219)347-1278　**Fax:** (219)347-7103
Email: dekko@dekkofoundation.org
Website: http://www.dekkofoundation.org

Fnded: 1981. **Philosophy:** The foundation provides grants to charitable organizations primarily in communities where Group Dekko had plants prior to 1992. Education receives the majority of the foundation's giving. The foundation's mission is "to foster economic freedom through education." Approximately 40-60% of all grants will be proactive. **Priorities:** *Civic & Public Affairs:* 33%. Supports community development. *Education:* 35%. Focus on primary education. *Environment:* 30%. Primarily for the foundation's Youth Initiative, empowering young people to serve their community, and Early Childhood Programs. *Religion:* 1%. *Note:* Total contributions made in fiscal 2000. **Typ. Recipients:** Domestic Violence, Emergency/Ambulance Services, People with Disabilities, Public Health. **Geo. Dist:** AL, Limestone County; IN, DeKalb County; IN, Kosciuszko County; IN, LaGrange County; IN, Noble County; IN, Steuben County; IN, Whitley County; IA, Clarke County; IA, Decatur County; IA, Lucas County; IA, Ringgold County; IA, Union County.

★ 11300 ★ Del E. Webb Foundation

PO Box 3350
101 Saguaro Drive
Wickenburg, AZ 85358
Phone: (520)684-7223 **Fax:** (520)684-5665
Robert Johnson, President & Director

Fnded: 1960. **Philosophy:** The foundation primarily applies its resources to preserve and enrich the benefits to be derived by residents of Arizona, Nevada, and California from improved and expanded medical services and medical research. *Del E. Webb Foundation Principles*. Traditional areas of support include health care, health facilities, medical education, and medical research. **Priorities:** *Arts & Humanities:* 1%. Funds a museum. *Civic & Public Affairs:* 13%. Supports community organizations, national parks, and housing. *Education:* 20%. Supports science and math education, universities, medical education, and private precollege education. *Environment:* 5%. Youth organizations, community service organizations, and programs for people with disabilities receive funding. *International:* 61%. Supports medical centers, cancer research, and public health issues. *Note:* Total contributions made in 2000. **Typ. Recipients:** Cancer, Child Abuse, Children's Health/Hospitals, Clinics/Medical Centers, Diabetes, Emergency/Ambulance Services, Eyes/Blindness, Geriatric Health, Health Funds, Health Organizations, Home-Care Services, Hospitals, Kidney, Long-Term Care, Medical Education, Medical Research, Medical Training, People with Disabilities, Prenatal Health Issues, Preventive Medicine/Wellness Organizations, Public Health, Public Health, Research/Studies Institutes, Single-Disease Health Associations, Speech & Hearing, Trauma Treatment. **Geo. Dist:** AZ; CA; NV.

★ 11301 ★ Dellora A. and Lester J. Norris Foundation

303 E Main St.
PO Box 4325
Saint Charles, IL 60174
Phone: (630)584-2500 **Fax:** (630)584-1020
Eugene Butler, Treasurer

Fnded: 1979. **Philosophy:** The foundation gives primarily to health institutions, especially hospitals; social service organizations, where the emphasis is on child welfare, family services, and youth organizations; and higher and secondary education. The foundation also provides funding to the arts, civic organizations, and churches. Funding is generally limited to organizations started by or supported by Mr. and Mrs. Norris during their lifetimes. **Priorities:** *Arts & Humanities:* 8%. Museums, libraries, opera, music, arts festivals, and historical societies. *Civic & Public Affairs:* 15%. Community foundations. *Education:* 38%. Supports pivate secondary education and colleges and universities. *Environment:* 8%. Youth organizations, family services, and child welfare. *International:* 22%. Focus on health funds, hospitals, and single-disease health associations. *Note:* Total contributions made in 2000. **Typ. Recipients:** AIDS/HIV, Cancer, Children's Health/Hospitals, Clinics/Medical Centers, Diabetes, Health Funds, Health Organizations, Heart, Hospices, Hospitals, Medical Rehabilitation, Medical Research, Mental Health, People with Disabilities, Public Health, Respiratory, Single-Disease Health Associations, Substance Abuse. **Geo. Dist:** nationally; CO; FL; IL.

★ 11302 ★ DeRoy Testamentary Foundation

26999 Central Park Boulevard, Suite 160N
Southfield, MI 48076
Phone: (248)827-0920 **Fax:** (248)827-0922
Email: DeRoyFdtn@aol.com
Julie Rodecker Holly, Vice President

Fnded: 1979. **Philosophy:** The foundation makes most of its grants in the areas of education, social services, the arts, and health care. Educational funding favors university English departments, arts and business education, scholarship funds, and drop-out programs. Funding for social service organizations favors animal protection, family services, homes for the aged, and community centers. The foundation also funds health foundations and hospitals. **Priorities:** *Arts & Humanities:* 29%. Supports museums, music and theater. *Civic & Public Affairs:* 15%. Funds women's programs, justice issues, and community programs. *Education:* 15%. Contributes to colleges, universities, and local schools. *Environment:* 24%. Supports a humane society, family services, and child welfare organizations. *International:* 17%. Funds hospitals, home care, and hospices. *Note:* Giving priorities provided by foundation in 2003. **Typ. Recipients:** Cancer, Children's Health/Hospitals, Clinics/Medical Centers, Domestic Violence, Emergency/Ambulance Services, Eyes/Blindness, Family Planning, Health Organizations, Hospices, Hospitals, Long-Term Care, Medical Education, Medical Rehabilitation, Medical Research, Mental Health, Nursing Services, People with Disabilities, Prenatal Health Issues, Public Health, Trauma Treatment. **Geo. Dist:** Metropolitan Detroit, MI.

★ 11303 ★ DeWitt Wallace-Reader's Digest Fund

2 Park Ave., 23rd Floor
New York, NY 10016
Phone: (212)251-9700 **Fax:** (212)679-6990
Email: wrdf@wallacefunds.org
Website: http://www.wallacefoundation.org
M. DeVita, President

Fnded: 1965. **Philosophy:** "To foster fundamental improvement in the quality of educational and career development opportunities for all school-age youth and to increase access to these improved services for young people in low-income communities." "These principles guide the translation of the mission of Dewitt Wallace-Readers Digest Fund into specific grantmaking across its program areas: education and career development are lifelong processes that are most effective when they involve active engagement in meaningful pursuits and build on the learner's strengths and current knowledge; education and career development occur in a wide range of settings, including schools, families, community institutions, and the work place; career development is a component of the education process that connects school to work and prepares young people for the productive adulthood; youth are best served when programs to educate and guide them are coordinated and complimentary; increasing young people's access to high quality services requires community institutions to be more inclusive in their outreach and more responsive to the diverse needs of today's youth; improving the quality of services for young people requires investments in the adults who work with and on behalf of youth in schools and community organizations; fundamental improvement in services for youth requires work on several levels of a problem at the same time, combining investments in direct service with complementary efforts to educate leaders in both the public and private sectors." **Priorities:** *Arts & Humanities:* 5%. *Civic & Public Affairs:* 10%. *Education:* 76%. *Environment:* 9%. Contributions through community based organizations. *Note:* Total contributions made in 2000. Percentages provided by foundation. **Typ. Recipients:** Clinics/Medical Centers, Hospitals, Medical Research, People with Disabilities, Research/Studies Institutes. **Geo. Dist:** nationally.

★ 11304 ★ Dibner Fund

PO Box 7575
Wilton, CT 06897
Phone: (203)761-9904 **Fax:** (203)761-9989
Email: Dibnerfund@worldnet.att.net
Marci Sternheim, Executive Director

Fnded: 1957. **Philosophy:** The mission of the Dibner Fund is to sustain, in select instances through long term support, institutions or organizations to which the donor was particularly committed, as well as others primarily involved with achieving better understanding of the history of science and technology with primary support of the Dibner Institute and Burndy Library in this field, located in Cambridge, MA. The Fund is uniquely characterized by its highly focused support of unsolicited and internally selected institutions and programs, mostly science driven. Examples of this are those that emphasize education and scholarship in the pure and applied sciences as well as others of special interest to the trustees; institutions, agencies and programs encouraging youth to pursue and sustain careers in science and technology; programs to encourage and assist foreign-born scientists and engineers who emigrate to the US; and other community, educational, health care, environmental and cultural agencies or institutions chosen by the board. In 1998, the Dibner Fund added one new category–peaceful coexistence–and expanded its humanitarian and environmental grantmaking areas. Humanitarian aid focuses on disaster relief and medical aid. Environmental grants focus on fresh water and rivers. The Dibner Fund **Priorities:** *Arts & Humanities:* 16%. Supports public broadcasting, libraries, museums, and history organizations. *Civic & Public Affairs:* 9%. Gives to parks, aquariums, and nonprofit management. *Education:* 12%. Supports colleges and universities and scholarship funds. *Environment:* 4%. Supports aid for people with disabilities and the United Way. *International:* 7%. Supports hospitals. *Religion:* 40%. Major funding goes to the Dibner Institute for the History of Science and Technology. Also funds science centers and scientific history. *Note:* Total contributions made in 2000. **Typ. Recipients:** Cancer, Children's Health/Hospitals, Diabetes, Emergency/Ambulance Services, Hospices, Hospitals, People with Disabilities, Single-Disease Health Associations. **Geo. Dist:** nationally and internationally.

★ 11305 ★ Dillon Foundation

PO Box 537
Sterling, IL 61081
Phone: (815)626-9000 **Fax:** (815)626-4000
Peter Dillon, President & Director

Fnded: 1953. **Philosophy:** The Dillon Foundation makes most of its grants in the area of civic affairs, especially in Sterling Township, IL. Educational institutions, including public schools and universities, are secondary interests. Minor support goes to other charitable recipient areas. **Priorities:** *Civic & Public Affairs:* 48%. Supports City of Sterling. *Education:* 26%. Supports elementary schools, universities, and college associations. *Environment:* 23%. Supports YMCA, senior services and United Way. *International:* 1%. Supports Cancer Center and hospice. *Note:* Total contributions made in 1998. **Typ. Recipients:** Cancer, Children's Health/Hospitals, Clinics/Medical Centers, Emergency/Ambulance Services, Family Planning, Health Organizations, Hospices, Hospitals, Medical Rehabilitation, Medical Research, People with Disabilities, Public Health, Research/Studies Institutes, Single-Disease Health Associations. **Geo. Dist:** Sterling, IL, including metropolitan area.

★ 11306 ★ Dr. C. C. and Mabel L. Criss Memorial Foundation

1700 Farnam St.
Omaha, NE 68102
Phone: (402)963-2155 **Fax:** (402)348-6666
James Strasheim, Trustee

Fnded: 1978. **Philosophy:** The foundation primarily supports organizations and institutions in Omaha, NE. Colleges and universities receive major contributions. Private secondary education is also a priority. Large grants usually support the construction and expansion of schools. Health care, research, and hospitals are supported. Local cultural associations and historical preservation organizations are of interest to the foundation. Community services also receive funding. **Priorities:** *Arts & Humanities:* 7%. Supports performing arts, university of Nebraska library, and museums. *Civic & Public Affairs:* Less than 1%. Funds Nebraska Station Bar Foundation. *Education:* 77%. Supports leadership training colleges and universities and religious education in Nebraska. *Environment:* 10%. Supports family services, the United Way, people with disabilities, scouts, and substance abuse and treatment. *International:* Less than 1%. Funds Children's Hospital and Alzheimer's Disease Association. *Note:* Contributions were made in fiscal 2002. **Typ. Recipients:** Alzheimers Disease, Children's Health/Hospitals, Heart, Hospices, Hospitals, Prenatal Health Issues. **Geo. Dist:** Omaha, NE.

★ 11307 ★ Dr. P. Phillips Foundation

PO Box 3753
Orlando, FL 32802
Phone: (407)422-6105 **Fax:** (407)422-4952
J. Hinson, President

Fnded: 1953. **Philosophy:** The foundation supports a wide variety of charitable organizations in Orange County, FL. Education, social services, the arts, and civic affairs are its main priorities. Social service funding favors child and youth development programs. The foundation supports all categories of the arts, including funds, museums, festivals, symphonies, theaters, and historical societies. Civic affairs in Orlando and Orange County, FL., are also a major interest. Other interests include educational funding for public schools, continuing education programs for youth in Central Florida, and science centers. **Priorities:** *Arts & Humanities:* 12%. *Civic & Public Affairs:* 1%. *Education:* 17%. Focus on primary and secondary education. *Environment:* 53%. Primarily for youth organizations and recreational activities. *International:* 16%. Emphasis on access to care, mental health services, and rehabilitation services. *Note:* Total contributions made in fiscal 2001. **Typ. Recipients:** AIDS/HIV, Alzheimers Disease, Cancer, Clinics/Medical Centers, Diabetes, Domestic Violence, Emergency/Ambulance Services, Eyes/Blindness, Health Organizations, Hospices, Mental Health, Multiple Sclerosis, People with Disabilities, Prenatal Health Issues, Public Health, Single-Disease Health Associations. **Geo. Dist:** FL, Orange County.

★ 11308 ★ Dr. Ralph and Marian Falk Medical Research Trust

231 South LaSalle St., Suite 0260
Chicago, IL 60697-0001
Phone: (312)828-2345 **Fax:** (312)987-0806
M. Ryan, Senior Vice President

Fnded: 1992. **Philosophy:** "The purpose of the research trust is to provide support for medical research in the areas of diseases for which no definite cure is known." Dr. Ralph and Marian Falk Medical Research Trust 1998 IRS Form 990 **Priorities:** *Education:* 46%. Supports universities and medical education. *International:* 54%. Supports medical centers and medical research. *Note:* Total contributions made in 2001. **Typ. Recipients:** Arthritis, Cancer, Children's Health/Hospitals, Clinics/Medical Centers, Hospitals, Hospitals (University Affiliated), Medical Education, Medical Rehabilitation, Medical Research, Prenatal Health Issues, Public Health, Research/Studies Institutes. **Geo. Dist:** nationally.

★ 11309 ★ Dr. Scholl Foundation

1033 Skokie Boulevard, Suite 230
Northbrook, IL 60062
Phone: (312)782-5210
Website: http://www.drschollfoundation.com
Pamela Scholl, President

Fnded: 1947. **Philosophy:** The foundation was established, as described in its charter, "for religious, charitable, scientific, literary, and educational purposes, and to do all things necessary or expedient to carry out the foregoing purposes. No part of the activities of the corporation shall be used for propaganda or otherwise to influence legislation." The foundation supports private education at all levels including elementary, secondary, and post-secondary schools; colleges and universities; and medical education. Support is also available for general charitable programs including grants to hospitals, programs for senior citizens, children, and the developmentally disabled. The foundation also shows an interest in civic, cultural, religious, and social welfare projects. **Priorities:** *Arts & Humanities:* 9%. Opera, public broadcasting, libraries, and historical preservation. *Civic & Public Affairs:* 4%. Funds horticultural societies, an aquarium, and employment initiatives. *Education:* 32%. Arts education, colleges and universities, schools, and science education. *Environment:* 12%. Supports sports programs, the disabled, and family services. *International:* 12%. Children's health, blindness, single-disease associations, and infant welfare. *Religion:* 9%. Science museums. *Note:* Total contributions made in 2000. **Typ. Recipients:** Cancer, Children's Health/Hospitals, Clinics/Medical Centers, Eyes/Blindness, Health Funds, Health Organizations, Heart, Hospices, Hospitals, Medical Education, Medical Research, People with Disabilities, Prenatal Health Issues, Research/Studies Institutes, Single-Disease Health Associations, Substance Abuse. **Geo. Dist:** nationally; IL.

★ 11310 ★ Dr. W. C. Swanson Family Foundation, Inc.

2955 Harrison Boulevard, Suite 201
Ogden, UT 84403
Phone: (801)392-0360 **Fax:** (801)392-0429
Cindy Purcell, President

Fnded: 1978. **Philosophy:** The stated purpose of the foundation is "for religious, charitable, literary, scientific, or educational purposes, or for the prevention of cruelty to children or animals." Although the foundation's purpose remains the same, the scope of the mission has broadened to include medical research and public information through the use of film and mass media. The foundation developed and sponsored a documentary entitled "A Story of Healing" which won the Academy Award for Documentary-Short Subject, March 1998. **Priorities:** *Arts & Humanities:* 12%. Support for museums, performing arts, arts centers, music, and dance. *Civic & Public Affairs:* 3%. Housing and local government. *Education:* 33%. Primary support for universities in Utah and primary and secondary education. *Environment:* 21%. Emphasis on child welfare, family services, and prevention of domestic violence. *International:* 10%. Focus on pediatric helath and health associations. *Religion:* 1%. Giving to dinosaur park and museum. *Note:* Total contributions made in 1998. **Typ. Recipients:** Cancer, Child Abuse, Children's Health/Hospitals, Domestic Violence, Emergency/Ambulance Services, Health Organizations, Health-General, Heart, Hospices, Hospitals, Medical Education, Medical Rehabilitation, People with Disabilities, Public Health, Sexual Abuse, Substance Abuse, Trauma Treatment. **Geo. Dist:** UT, primarily Northern Utah and Weber County; grants from the rest of Utah are next in priority, then regional requests, and lastly national and international.

★ 11311 ★ Dodge Jones Foundation and Subsidiary

PO Box 176
Abilene, TX 79604
Phone: (915)673-6429 **Fax:** (915)673-2028
Lawrence Gill, Grants Administrator

Fnded: 1954. **Philosophy:** The foundation focuses its activity in the areas of education, community services, health, civic affairs, historic preservation, and youth organizations. **Priorities:** *Arts & Humanities:* 53%. Supports libraries, public broadcasting, fine arts and museums. *Civic & Public Affairs:* 7%. Supports municipalities and community organizations. *Education:* 21%. Supports colleges, universities and private academies. *Environment:* 14%. Supports children's services, camps, YWCA, scouting and day care. *International:* 3%. Supports hospital and medical centers. *Note:* Total contributions made in 2000. **Typ. Recipients:** AIDS/HIV, Alzheimers Disease, Cancer, Children's Health/Hospitals, Clinics/Medical Centers, Emergency/Ambulance Services, Family Planning, Geriatric Health, Health Organizations, Health Policy/Cost Containment, Heart, Hospices, Hospitals, Medical Education, Medical Rehabilitation, Medical Research, Mental Health, People with Disabilities, Public Health, Speech & Hearing, Substance Abuse. **Geo. Dist:** TX.

★ 11312 ★ Dolan Children's Foundation

340 Crossways Park Dr.
Woodbury, NY 11797-0000
Phone: (516)803-9200
William Frewin, Jr., Vice President

Fnded: 1998. **Priorities:** *Arts & Humanities:* 2%. Supports arts league. *Education:* 94%. Private education. *Environment:* 2%. Supports family services and child welfare. *International:* Less than 1%. Primarily supports cystic fibrosis associations. *Note:* Total contributions made in 2001. **Typ. Recipients:** Single-Disease Health Associations.

★ 11313 ★ Dolan Family Foundation

340 Crossways Park Drive
Woodbury, NY 11797
Phone: (516)803-3890 **Fax:** (516)364-4592
Marianne Dolan-Weber, Chairman

Fnded: 1987. **Philosophy:** The foundation generally supports educational institutions and health and medical research organizations. **Priorities:** *Education:* About 55%. *Environment:* 8%. Community services. *International:* 27%. **Typ. Recipients:** Hospitals, Medical Research, People with Disabilities. **Geo. Dist:** nationally and internationally; NY.

★ 11314 ★ Don and Sybil Harrington Foundation

801 South Fillmore, Suite 700
Amarillo, TX 79101
Phone: (806)373-8353 **Fax:** (806)373-3656
Email: haf@aaf-hf.org
Website: http://www.aaf-hr.org
Jim Allison, Executive Director

Fnded: 1957. **Philosophy:** The foundation has a wide range of funding interests including health, human services, and education in the Panhandle area of Texas. **Priorities:** *Arts & Humanities:* 10%. Supports performing arts and historical societies. *Civic & Public Affairs:* 18%. Funds community organizations. *Education:* 7%. *Environment:* 32%. Supports United Way, scouts, and youth organizations. *International:* 26%. Funds medical centers and cancer research. *Religion:* 4%. Supports a discovery center. *Note:* Total contributions made in 2000. **Typ. Recipients:** Arthritis, Cancer, Children's Health/Hospitals, Clinics/Medical Centers, Domestic Violence, Emergency/Ambulance Services, Eyes/Blindness, Geriatric Health, Health Organizations, Hospices, Hospitals, Medical Education, Medical Rehabilitation, Medical Research, People with Disabilities. **Geo. Dist:** TX, 26 Northern Counties in Texas.

★ 11315 ★ Donald W. Reynolds Foundation

1701 Village Center Circle
Las Vegas, NV 89134
Phone: (702)804-6000 **Fax:** (702)804-6099
Email: generalquestions@dwrf.org
Website: http://www.dwreynolds.org
Karina Mayer, Administrative Officer

Fnded: 1954. **Philosophy:** The foundation's reports its current interests as follows. *National Programs* Aging and Quality of Life: "At present, this program focuses on strengthening the geriatric knowledge and skills of physicians who will care for the growing number of frail elders in the United States over the coming decades." Cadriovascular Clinical Research: "This program supports a limited number of centers in leading academic health centers that are devoted to fighting atherosclerotic heart disease through cutting edge research and training." *Capital Programs* Capital

Grants: "The Foundation makes capital grants in Arkansas, Nevada, and Oklahoma to qualified charitable organizations which demonstrate a sustainable program, exhibit an entrepreneurial spirit, and assist those served to be healthy, self-sufficient and productive members of the community. Grants are intended to have a major impact on the applicant, the clients served by that organization and the surrounding community. Applicants must serve a well-documented need in one or more of the following areas: arts and culture, civic and public affairs, education, health or human services." Community Services Centers Grants: "This program is designed to help privately supported, nonprofit organizations to join together to house their operations in a shared facility. Independent of each other, smaller organizations may not need or be able to afford to operate their own buildings. However, together, a group of organizations with compatible program goals, shared constituencies, or similar space and location needs could be logically co-located in one, larger facility. The desired result is that efficiencies derived from sharing common space and functions will improve nonprofit programs and that programmatic synergy created will benefit the people served." Donald W. Reynolds Foundation 2002 statement of priorities. **Priorities:** *Arts & Humanities:* 11%. Supports public broadcasting, ballet, historic preservation, museums, theater, and arts festivals. *Education:* 16%. Supports universities and colleges, medical education, literacy, legal education, and arts/humanities education. *Environment:* 17%. Supports United Way, youth programs, food distribution, senior services, special Olympics, Big Brothers/Big Sisters, and scouting. *International:* 21%. Supports cancer and heart research, medical centers, and children's health. *Note:* Total contributions made in fiscal 2001. **Typ. Recipients:** AIDS/HIV, Cancer, Clinics/Medical Centers, Emergency/Ambulance Services, Geriatric Health, Health Funds, Health Organizations, Heart, Hospices, Hospitals, Medical Education, People with Disabilities, Single-Disease Health Associations, Substance Abuse. **Geo. Dist:** nationally for aging and cardiovascular research programs; AR; NV; OK.

★ 11316 ★ Donnell B. and Elizabeth Dee Shaw Stewart Educational Foundation

c/o First Security Bank of Utah NA
PO Box 9936
Ogden, UT 84409
Phone: (801)626-9531
Mary Barker, Trustee

Fnded: 1977. **Typ. Recipients:** Children's Health/Hospitals, Emergency/Ambulance Services, Eyes/Blindness, Health Organizations, Heart, Hospices, Hospitals, People with Disabilities, Single-Disease Health Associations, Substance Abuse. **Geo. Dist:** Ogden, UT.

★ 11317 ★ Dora Roberts Foundation

PO Box 2050
Fort Worth, TX 76113
Phone: (817)884-4442 **Fax:** (817)884-4294
Rick Piersall, Senior Vice President, Bank One

Fnded: 1948. **Philosophy:** The Dora Roberts Foundation makes grants primarily to social services programs, including those for community centers, food and clothing, and the aged. Health support favors rehabilitation, hospitals, and medical centers. Educational interests include junior colleges, high schools, and foundations for education. The foundation also supports religious programs and civic affairs. **Priorities:** *Arts & Humanities:* 7%. Supports history and music. *Civic & Public Affairs:* 14%. Supports safety, clubs, festivals, towns/municipalities, and civic affairs. *Education:* 18%. Supports schools, universities, and colleges. *Environment:* 37%. Supports recreation/athletics, food distribution, animal protection, scouts, community centers, and United Way. *International:* 3%. Supports medical rehabilitation. *Note:* Total contributions made in fiscal 1999. **Typ. Recipients:** Cancer, Heart, Hospices, Hospitals, Medical Education, Medical Rehabilitation, Sexual Abuse. **Geo. Dist:** TX, Big Spring.

★ 11318 ★ Dorot Foundation

c/o Marks Paneth ET AL
622 Third Ave.
New York, NY 10017-6701
Phone: (212)503-8800
Email: info@dorot.org
Website: http://www.dorot.org
Prof. Ernest Frerichs, Executive Director

Fnded: 1958. **Philosophy:** The foundation is a major funder of colleges and universities in New England, Israel, and Canada. Other interests include funding for museums of interest to Israel or the Jewish faith, and other Jewish causes. **Priorities:** *Arts & Humanities:* 9%. Supports the Archives for Historical Documentation with primary support given to the New York Public Library. *Civic & Public Affairs:* 81%. Supports public and civic affairs. *Education:* Less than 1%. Supports universities, and educational programs. *Environment:* 3%. Supports the 92nd St. YM-YWHA and children's services. *Religion:* Less than 1%. *Note:* Contributions were made in fiscal 2002. **Typ. Recipients:** AIDS/HIV, Clinics/Medical Centers, Hospices, Medical Education, Medical Research, Medical Training, Mental Health, People with Disabilities, Public Health, Substance Abuse. **Geo. Dist:** U.S.-based affiliates of Israeli organizations; northeast United States.

★ 11319 ★ Dorothy U. Dalton Foundation

Greenleaf Trust Bldg.
490 W South St.
Kalamazoo, MI 49007
Phone: (616)388-9800 **Fax:** (616)388-9868
Ronald Kilgore, Secretary & Treasurer

Fnded: 1978. **Philosophy:** The Dorothy U. Dalton Foundation primarily supports social service organizations. The foundation supports the YMCA and YWCA, youth organizations, relief for the needy, and united funds. Secondary interests include museums, civic centers, and health clinics in Kalamazoo, MI. **Priorities:** *Arts & Humanities:* 55%. Generally in support of capital campaigns involving theater, the arts, festival, and symphonies. *Civic & Public Affairs:* 16%. Primary support for The Kalamazoo Foundation Center and housing resources. *Education:* 4%. Supports the American Red Cross Building Stronger campaign. *Environment:* 19%. Interests include the United Way, children's organizations, vacation camps, and junior achievement. *International:* 5%. Medical centers. *Note:* Total contributions made in fiscal 2001. **Typ. Recipients:** AIDS/HIV, Alzheimers Disease, Children's Health/Hospitals, Clinics/Medical Centers, Domestic Violence, Emergency/Ambulance Services, Family Planning, Geriatric Health, Health Organizations, Hospices, Hospitals, Long-Term Care, Mental Health, Nursing Services, Nutrition, Outpatient Health Care, People with Disabilities, Sexual Abuse, Speech & Hearing, Substance Abuse. **Geo. Dist:** MI, Kalamazoo County.

★ 11320 ★ Dorrance Family Foundation

7600 East Doubletree Ranch Rd. Suite 300
Scottsdale, AZ 85258
Phone: (480)367-7000
Carolyn O'Malley, Executive Director

Fnded: 1991. **Philosophy:** The foundation provides major support to the Arizona Science Center. Funding also goes to health organizations, arts associations, and community services primarily within Phoenix, AZ. **Priorities:** *Arts & Humanities:* 22%. Primarily for museums and symphonies. *Civic & Public Affairs:* 31%. Supports the Desert botanical gardens. *Education:* 38%. Private, precollege education, and student aid. *Environment:* 1%. Community centers, blind services, animal welfare, and youth organizations. *International:* 3%. Hospices, medical research, and children's health. *Religion:* 5%. Supports the Arizona Science Center. *Note:* Total contributions made in 2001. **Typ. Recipients:** AIDS/HIV, Arthritis, Cancer, Children's Health/Hospitals, Domestic Violence, Family Planning, Health Organizations, Heart, Hospices, Hospitals, Kidney, Medical Research, People with Disabilities, Public Health, Sexual Abuse, Substance Abuse. **Geo. Dist:** AZ.

★ 11321 ★ Dover Foundation

PO Box 208
Shelby, NC 28151
Phone: (704)487-8890 **Fax:** (704)482-6818
Email: doverfnd@shelby.net
Hoyt Bailey, President

Fnded: 1944. **Philosophy:** The Dover Foundation is primarily interested in supporting higher education in North Carolina, including scholarships. Secondary interests include religious organizations, medical foundations and hospitals, human services, arts and humanities, and youth organizations. **Priorities:** *Arts & Humanities:* 8%. Supports arts councils, museums, and public television. *Civic & Public Affairs:* 1%. Funds general civic concerns. *Education:* 28%. Supports higher education in North Carolina. *Environment:* 28%. Gives to homes and youth groups. *International:* 16%. Funds hospitals, hospices, health associations, and medical research. *Note:* Total contributions made in fiscal 2001. **Typ. Recipients:** Cancer, Child Abuse, Clinics/Medical Centers, Domestic Violence, Emergency/Ambulance Services, Family Planning, Geriatric Health, Health Funds, Health Organizations, Heart, Hospices, Hospitals, Kidney, Medical Education, Medical Research, Mental Health, Preventive Medicine/Wellness Organizations, Public Health, Research/Studies Institutes, Respiratory. **Geo. Dist:** NC.

★ 11322 ★ Drue Heinz Trust

PO Box 68
FDR Station
New York, NY 10150
Phone: (212)371-5757 **Fax:** (212)759-0479
Julia Shea, Foundation Manager

Fnded: 1954. **Philosophy:** The Drue Heinz Foundation is primarily interested in supporting the arts, including major support to the Carnegie Museum of Art. The foundation also supports arts associations, museums, libraries, and the performing arts. Other recipient areas are funded on a limited basis. **Priorities:** *Arts & Humanities:* 29%. Supports literary arts, museums, film, music, theater, and libraries. *Civic & Public Affairs:* 14%. Funds nonprofit management, philanthropic organizations, minority affairs, legal aid, and community associations. *Education:* 3%. Gives to arts education and literacy programs. *Environment:* 1%. Gives to shelters, seeing eye dog programs, and children's programs. *International:* Less than 1%. Contributes to hospitals, medical centers, and cancer research. *Note:* Total contributions made in 2001. **Typ. Recipients:** AIDS/HIV, Cancer, Children's Health/Hospitals, Clinics/Medical Centers, Emergency/Ambulance Services, Eyes/Blindness, Family Planning, Geriatric Health, Hospitals, Medical Education, Medical Rehabilitation, Medical Research, People with Disabilities, Single-Disease Health Associations. **Geo. Dist:** New York, NY.

★ 11323 ★ Duffield Family Foundation

2223 Santa Clara Ave., Ste. B
Alameda, CA 94501
Phone: (510)337-8989 **Fax:** (510)337-8988
Email: info@maddiesfund.org
Website: http://www.maddiesfund.org
Laurie Peek, Secretary

Fnded: 1995. **Philosophy:** The foundation primarily supports programs for domestic animal welfare that promote humane education, adoption and rescue, medical assistance and emergency care, quality of life, spaying and neutering, and human/animal interaction. **Priorities:** *Arts & Humanities:* 6%. A museum received funding. *Civic & Public Affairs:* 1%. Support went to the Oakland Zoo. *Education:* 1%. Gives to animal-related educational programs. *Environment:* 92%. Emphasis on humane societies and animal welfare causes. *Note:* Total contributions made in fiscal 1999. **Typ. Recipients:** Cancer, Child Abuse, Children's Health/Hospitals, Medical Education, People with Disabilities. **Geo. Dist:** CA.

★ 11324 ★ Duke Endowment

100 North Tryon St., Suite 3500
Charlotte, NC 28202-4012

Phone: (704)376-0291 **Fax:** (704)376-9336
Email: droberson@tde.org
Website: http://www.dukeendowment.org
David Roberson, Director, Communications

Fnded: 1924. **Philosophy:** Mr. Duke limited his benefaction to North Carolina and South Carolina. Pursuant to the terms of the trust indenture, funds are directed only to four educational institutions (Duke University, Davidson College, Furman University, and Johnson C. Smith University); nonprofit hospitals in North Carolina and South Carolina for operations, programs, and for improving and expanding facilities; nonprofit child care institutions in North Carolina and South Carolina; and the rural United Methodist Church and its pastors in North Carolina; and retired ministers who have served at least five years in an annual conference of the United Methodist Church in North Carolina, and their surviving dependents. The endowment currently addresses health issues that include health care financing, small and rural hospitals, access to primary care, community affiliations, children's health, and care of the indigent. In education, key issues include the problems of private colleges and universities such as endowments, faculty recruitment and retention, student financial aid, and physical plants. In the area of child care, a primary focus involves programs to reunite and strengthen families. Finally, grants to rural churches are centered around community needs, pastoral education, and the construction of churches. **Priorities:** *Education:* 43%. Specifically to four eligible religiously affiliated colleges and universities. *Environment:* 7%. Child care and child welfare programs. *International:* 34%. Hospitals in North and South Carolina. *Note:* Total contributions made in 1999. Analysis provided by foundation. **Typ. Recipients:** Adolescent Health Issues, AIDS/HIV, Alzheimers Disease, Cancer, Children's Health/Hospitals, Clinics/Medical Centers, Diabetes, Emergency/Ambulance Services, Family Planning, Geriatric Health, Health Organizations, Health Policy/Cost Containment, Health-General, Heart, Home-Care Services, Hospices, Hospitals, Hospitals (University Affiliated), Long-Term Care, Medical Education, Medical Rehabilitation, Medical Research, Medical Training, Nursing Services, Nutrition, Outpatient Health Care, People with Disabilities, Prenatal Health Issues, Preventive Medicine/Wellness Organizations, Public Health, Respiratory, Substance Abuse. **Geo. Dist:** NC; SC.

★ 11325 ★ Dumont Foundation

11500 Olympic Blvd., Suite 340
Los Angeles, CA 90064-1527
Phone: (310)478-2888 **Fax:** (310)312-1544
Email: s.ziegler@verizon.net
Frances Clarke, President

Fnded: 1967. **Priorities:** *Arts & Humanities:* 35%. Art institute. *Education:* 65%. Gives to Colleges and universities mainly for medical research. *Note:* Total contributions in 2001. **Typ. Recipients:** Alzheimers Disease, Arthritis, Children's Health/Hospitals, Clinics/Medical Centers, Eyes/Blindness, Heart, Hospitals, Medical Education, Medical Research. **Geo. Dist:** Los Angeles, CA.

★ 11326 ★ Dunspaugh-Dalton Foundation

1533 Sunset Drive, Suite 150
Coral Gables, FL 33143
Phone: (305)668-4192 **Fax:** (305)361-2818
William Lane, Jr., President

Fnded: 1963. **Philosophy:** The primary focus of the foundation's grantmaking is education. Other areas of interest include social services, health, and the arts. **Priorities:** *Arts & Humanities:* 7%. Focus on music, public broadcasting, and museums. *Civic & Public Affairs:* 14%. Funds botanical gardens, aquariums, and community associations. *Education:* 51%. Primarily for higher education. *Environment:* 18%. Funds youth concerns and United Way. *International:* 7%. Gives to hospitals, medical centers, hospices, and health associations. *Religion:* 1%. Funds science and space planetarium. *Note:* Total contributions made in 2001. **Typ. Recipients:** Alzheimers Disease, Cancer, Children's Health/Hospitals, Clinics/Medical Centers, Emergency/Ambulance Services, Family Planning, Geriatric Health, Health Organizations, Hospices, Hospitals, Hospitals (University Affiliated), Long-Term Care, Medical Education, Medical Rehabilitation, Medical Research, Mental Health, Nursing Services, People with Disabilities, Research/Studies Institutes, Single-Disease Health Associations, Speech & Hearing, Substance Abuse. **Geo. Dist:** nationally; CA; FL, Dade County; NC.

★ 11327 ★ Dyson Foundation

25 Halcyon Rd.
Millbrook, NY 12545-9611
Phone: (845)677-0644 **Fax:** (845)677-0650
Email: info@dyson.org
Website: http://www.dyson.org
Diana Gurieva, Executive Director

Fnded: 1957. **Philosophy:** Over the years, the foundation has made grants to a variety of organizations in the arts, higher education, medicine and health, and social services. However, with greater experience and an increasingly defined focus, the Foundation's current priorities for new grants are limited to the following areas: Funding Program in Health and Medicine, part of the Anne E. Dyson Community Pediatrics Training Initiative, which aims to develop pediatric professionals with greater skills and interest in community-based medicine, advocacy and the capacity to improve the health of children in their communities; Funding Program for the Mid-Hudson Valley of New York State, which seeks to improve and enhance the quality of life in the region by supporting social services, education, health, community development, and arts and cultural programs. The foundation will consider proposals in all these areas in Dutchess County, New York. Applicants from other areas considered to be part of the Mid-Hudson Valley (generally Putnam, Ulster, Greene, Columbia and Orange Counties) will be considered as long as the proposed program has a substantial impact on Dutchess County. Of special interest are projects focusing on economically disadvantaged children and youth, improving community healthcare services, strengthening the infrastructure of not-for-profit sector, and increasing philanthropy and charitable giving in the area; Legacy and Family Interest Grants are tied to the historic or current interests of members of the Dyson family and in all cases are initiated by the family directors; Directors' Discretionary Grants. **Priorities:** *Arts & Humanities:* 8%. Libraries, music programs, public radio, historic site, and dance theater. *Civic & Public Affairs:* 1%. Funds women's legal services. *Education:* 46%. Funds colleges, universities, and medical school. *Environment:* 9%. Youth organizations, Planned Parenthood organizations, and resource development for youth. *International:* 35%. Hospitals, health education, cancer institute, and medical centers. *Note:* Total contributions made in 2000. **Typ. Recipients:** AIDS/HIV, Cancer, Children's Health/Hospitals, Eyes/Blindness, Family Planning, Family Planning, Geriatric Health, Health Funds, Health Organizations, Hospitals, Medical Education, Medical Rehabilitation, Medical Research, People with Disabilities, Prenatal Health Issues, Public Health, Substance Abuse, Trauma Treatment. **Geo. Dist:** nationally; NY, Mid-Hudson Valley.

★ 11328 ★ E. J. Grassmann Trust

PO Box 4470
Warren, NJ 07059-0470
Phone: (908)753-2440 **Fax:** (908)753-9384
William Engel, Executive Director & Trustee

Fnded: 1979. **Philosophy:** The trust attempts to fund the types of organizations that Mr. Grassmann supported during his lifetime. Preferred organizations include local hospitals and health organizations; organizations engaged in ecological endeavors; educational institutions; and organizations that help the needy, particularly children. The trust's *Guidelines for Grants* indicate that, "Preference will be given to organizations with low administration expenses, that show efforts to encourage individuals to help themselves, and that make efforts to achieve a broad base of funding sources." **Priorities:** *Arts & Humanities:* 11%. Contributes to historical societies, performing arts organizations, museums and theaters. *Civic & Public Affairs:* 10%. Funds community development and planning, housing, and an arboretum. *Education:* 37% Supports colleges, academies and secondary schools. *Environment:* 9%. Funds children's and outreach services, Young Men's Christian Association, camps, and family planning services. *International:* 23%. Gives to hospitals, single-disease associations, and public health programs. *Note:* Total contributions made in 2001. **Typ. Recipients:** AIDS/HIV, Cancer, Children's Health/Hospitals, Clinics/Medical Centers, Emergency/Ambulance Services, Family Planning, Health Organizations, Health-General, Hospices, Hospitals, Medical Education, Medical Rehabilitation, Nursing Services, People with Disabilities, Public Health, Single-Disease Health Associations, Trauma Treatment. **Geo. Dist:** GA, middle Georgia; NJ, Union County and surounding area.

★ 11329 ★ E. K. and Lillian F. Bishop Foundation

701 5th Ave., Floor 47
Seattle, WA 98104
Phone: (520)749-2004 **Fax:** (520)749-2990
Email: thomas.nevers@azbar.org
Tom Nevers, Grants Manager

Fnded: 1971. **Philosophy:** "The E.K. and Lillian F. Bishop Foundation promotes the welfare of young people through grants to qualified organizations. The Foundation supports a wide range of charitable, cultural, educational and recreational programs. Inspirational experiences such as opportunities to explore the arts, to participate in sports and in wholesome group activities are considered to be of special importance. Some of the projects supported by the Foundation include a youth employment center, community cultural and athletic events, special medical equipment and treatment centers for young people. The Awards Committee looks for projects that focus on prevention of problems and those that seek innovative solutions to youth-oriented problems. Enlisting community support for a project is also encouraged." Foundation Guidelines. **Priorities:** *Arts & Humanities:* 4%. Funds cultural enrichment programs. *Civic & Public Affairs:* 12%. Supports employment assistance, city government, and fire departments. *Education:* 8%. Supports educational programs, colleges and universities. *Environment:* 70%. Funds social service organizations, youth activities, and athletics. *International:* 4%. Gives to hospitals and clinics. *Note:* Total contributions made in fiscal 2000. **Typ. Recipients:** Children's Health/Hospitals, Clinics/Medical Centers, Domestic Violence, Emergency/Ambulance Services, Eyes/Blindness, Family Planning, Health Funds, Heart, Hospitals, Medical Research, Nursing Services, Research/Studies Institutes, Single-Disease Health Associations, Substance Abuse, Trauma Treatment. **Geo. Dist:** WA; WA, Grays Harbor County.

★ 11330 ★ E. L. Cord Foundation

1 East 1st St., No. 901
Reno, NV 89501
Phone: (775)323-0373 **Fax:** (775)325-8523
William Bradley, Trustee

Fnded: 1962. **Philosophy:** "The E. L. Cord Foundation plans to focus its attention on its interests in the following general fields and activities connected or included therein, as recipients of grants. 1. Charitable 2. Scientific 3. Religious 4. Literacy and 5. Educational" 1997 Grant Policies and Procedures **Priorities:** *Arts & Humanities:* 36%. Supports art and automobile museums, public broadcasting, peforming arts, libraries, historical societies and historic preservation. *Civic & Public Affairs:* 8%. Gives to counties and municipalities, chambers of commerce, parks, legal aid, women's organizations, and Native American Affairs. *Education:* 33%. Funds colleges, universities, and public schools. *Environment:* 15%. Supports self-help programs, animal welfare organizations, senior services, food distribution, family services, and youth programs. *International:* 5%. Contributes to medical centers, hospitals, hospice, and cancer treatment centers. *Note:* Total contributions made in 2000. **Typ. Recipients:** Cancer, Children's Health/Hospitals, Clinics/Medical Centers, Diabetes, Domestic Violence, Emergency/Ambulance Services, Health-General, Hospices, Hospitals, Medical Education, Medical Research, People with Disabilities, Single-Disease Health Associations, Substance Abuse. **Geo. Dist:** NV, northern and rural counties.

★ 11331 ★ E. L. Wiegand Foundation
Wiegand Center
165 West Liberty St., Suite 200
Reno, NV 89501
Phone: (775)333-0310 **Fax:** (775)333-0314
Kristen Avansino, President & Executive Director

Fnded: 1982. **Philosophy:** The foundation funds "programs and projects...at educational institutions in the academic areas of science, business, fine arts, law and medicine; and...at health and medical research institutions in the areas of heart, eye, and cancer surgery, treatment, and research, with priority given to programs and projects that benefit children." To a lesser degree, the foundation considers applications from civic and community affairs organizations, public affairs institutions, and cultural institutions. The foundation shows a strong preference for organizations affiliated with the Roman Catholic Church. **Priorities:** *Arts & Humanities:* 12%. Supports libraries, arts foundations, museum, and ballet. *Civic & Public Affairs:* 12%. Supports employment/job training, community foundation, public policy, and law and justice. *Education:* 40%. Funds colleges, universities, science education, religious education, scholarship, and medical education. *Environment:* 8%. Supports athletics/recreation, scouts, and youth programs. *International:* 23%. Supports medical centers, hospital, heart, and home care services. *Religion:* 3%. Supports science museums. *Note:* Total contributions made in fiscal 1998. **Typ. Recipients:** Alzheimers Disease, Cancer, Children's Health/Hospitals, Clinics/Medical Centers, Diabetes, Health Organizations, Health-General, Heart, Hospitals, Long-Term Care, Medical Education, Medical Research, Nursing Services, People with Disabilities, Prenatal Health Issues, Public Health, Respiratory, Single-Disease Health Associations, Substance Abuse. **Geo. Dist:** AZ; CA, Northern California; Washington, DC; ID; NV; New York, NY; OR; UT; WA.

★ 11332 ★ E and M Charities
PO Box 209
Muscatine, IA 52761-0069
Phone: (563)264-8000
David Stanley, President

Fnded: 1979. **Philosophy:** E and M Charities makes most of its grants in the areas of education and social services. Educational funding favors tax service education, religious education, community colleges, and public school systems. Funding for social services goes to family services and marriage counseling, community centers, and youth organizations. Methodist religious organizations also receive support. Grants to other recipient areas are limited. **Priorities:** *Arts & Humanities:* 1%. Supports arts council and performing arts. *Civic & Public Affairs:* 40%. Legislative exchange programs, nonprofits, economy policy, and community foundations. *Education:* 4%. Supports public schools and colleges. *Environment:* 16%. Funds charitable organizations. *Note:* Contributions made in 2001. **Typ. Recipients:** Health Organizations, Respiratory. **Geo. Dist:** nationally.

★ 11333 ★ E. M. Lynn Foundation
2501 N Military Trl.
Boca Raton, FL 33431
Phone: (561)994-1900 **Fax:** (561)994-1910
Christine Lynn, Trustee

Fnded: 1977. **Philosophy:** The foundation generally supports a variety of charitable organizations; however, recent giving has been devoted to the Lynn University. **Priorities:** *Arts & Humanities:* 6%. Supports museums, music, theater. *Civic & Public Affairs:* About 8%. Supports philanthropic organizations and foundations. *Education:* 58%. Multiple grants to Lynn University. *Environment:* 3%. Funds youth groups and social services. *International:* About 25%. Gives to hospitals and single-disease health associations. *Note:* Total contributions made in fiscal 2000. **Typ. Recipients:** AIDS/HIV, Alzheimers Disease, Arthritis, Cancer, Clinics/Medical Centers, Diabetes, Emergency/Ambulance Services, Family Planning, Health Funds, Health-General, Heart, Hospices, Hospitals, Hospitals (University Affiliated), Kidney, Medical Education, Medical Research, People with Disabilities, Preventive Medicine/Wellness Organizations, Research/Studies Institutes, Respiratory, Single-Disease Health Associations, Substance Abuse, Transplant Networks/Donor Banks. **Geo. Dist:** FL, Southern Florida; NY; NC; PA; VA.

★ 11334 ★ E. Rhodes and Leona B. Carpenter Foundation
PO Box 58880
Philadelphia, PA 19102-8880
Phone: (215)963-5212
Joseph O'Connor, Jr., Contact

Fnded: 1975. **Philosophy:** While education traditionally receives the majority of funding and consideration from the foundation, the foundation maintains a giving pattern to a wide variety of organizations, generally located in the eastern part of the country but stretching to California. It considers requests from museums for the purchase, restoration, and conservation of Asian art and also considers proposals from organizations relating to education in the field of Asian art. The foundation also supports hospices and hospitals. The foundation has outlined a few proposal guidelines for organizations that include the following: public institutions which had direct relationships with Leona or Rhodes Carpenter during their lifetimes, public charities in support of graduate theological education, public charities where E. R. Carpenter Company has had a long-time manufacturing or business facilities including the Richmond, VA, area where requests are limited to the performing arts, museums for the purchase and restoration of Asian art, and organizations involved in providing hospice care. **Priorities:** *Arts & Humanities:* 39%. Supports arts centers, museums, libraries, ballet, music. *Civic & Public Affairs:* 1%. *Education:* 34%. Funds religious schools, secondary schools, nursing schools, and colleges and universities. *Environment:* 9%. Supports family centers, youth programs, shelters, food banks, and prevention of domestic/sexual abuse. *International:* 8%. Supports medical centers, hospices, and health clinics. *Religion:* 7%. Funds science museums. *Note:* Total contributions made in 2000. **Typ. Recipients:** AIDS/HIV, Cancer, Children's Health/Hospitals, Clinics/Medical Centers, Domestic Violence, Emergency/Ambulance Services, Family Planning, Health Organizations, Health Policy/Cost Containment, Hospices, Hospitals, Medical Education, Medical Rehabilitation, Nursing Services, People with Disabilities, Public Health, Research/Studies Institutes, Sexual Abuse, Single-Disease Health Associations, Substance Abuse. **Geo. Dist:** east of the Mississippi River; VA.

★ 11335 ★ Earhart Foundation
2200 Green Rd., Suite H
Ann Arbor, MI 48105
Phone: (734)761-8592 **Fax:** (734)761-2722
David Kennedy, President

Fnded: 1929. **Philosophy:** The foundation initially centered its grant making on charitable, religious, and educational purposes. Emphasis was also placed on the social sciences and the humanities. Currently, the foundation directs a majority of its funding to fellowship research grants to individuals from established institutions pursuing endeavors of their own choice. Designated graduate students, scholars, and research principals are considered for support. Three program areas have been established for awards: The H. B. Earhart Fellowships are awarded to graduate students ready to embark upon careers in college or university teaching or in research. Graduate students are nominated by faculty sponsors, and applications for this program are not accepted. The Fellowship Research Grants Program is open to individuals who have established themselves professionally and who are affiliated with educational or research institutions. The effort funded should lead to the advancement of knowledge through teaching, lecturing, and publication. Earhart Foundation grants are occasionally awarded to "publicly supported" educational and research organizations qualified for private foundation support. However, resources allotted to this program have been reduced as the foundation concentrates more funding on individual research grants. **Priorities:** *Civic & Public Affairs:* 18%. Funds economic research and public policy. *Education:* 80% Supports colleges, universities, and educational programs. About half of education spending goes to fellowships. *Environment:* 1%. *Note:* Total contributions made in 2000. **Typ. Recipients:** People with Disabilities.

★ 11336 ★ Earl C. Sams Foundation
101 N Shoreline Blvd., Suite 602
Corpus Christi, TX 78401
Phone: (361)888-6485 **Fax:** (361)884-4241
Bruce Hawn, President

Fnded: 1946. **Philosophy:** The Earl C. Sams Foundation, Inc., is a charitable foundation focusing primarily on south Texas area needs. The foundation's primary interests are educational, medical, social, youth, zoological, and environmental causes. **Priorities:** *Arts & Humanities:* 8%. Supports museums and dance, and music. *Civic & Public Affairs:* 36%. Funds zoological concerns, aquariums, and parks. *Education:* 11%. Gives to educational foundations, colleges, and elementary education. *Environment:* 23%. Funds youth organizations, united funds, and family and drug counseling. *International:* 7%. Supports hospitals, single-disease health associations, and medical rehabilitation. *Note:* Total contributions made in 2000. **Typ. Recipients:** AIDS/HIV, Alzheimers Disease, Arthritis, Cancer, Child Abuse, Children's Health/Hospitals, Diabetes, Emergency/Ambulance Services, Family Planning, Health-General, Heart, Kidney, Medical Education, Medical Rehabilitation, Medical Research, Mental Health, People with Disabilities, Substance Abuse. **Geo. Dist:** TX, Southern Texas.

★ 11337 ★ Eberly Foundation
PO Box 2023
Uniontown, PA 15401-1643
Phone: (724)438-3789
Website: http://www.psu.edu/
Robert Eberly, Sr., President

Fnded: 1963. **Priorities:** *Arts & Humanities:* 9%. Funds libraries, museums, public broadcasting, historic preservation, performance art. *Civic & Public Affairs:* 19%. Funds economic development, city services and projects, national parks. *Education:* 53%. Supports universities, school districts, secondary education. *Environment:* 1%. Funds shelters, family services, community centers. *International:* 18%. Funds hospitals, single-disease health organizations. *Note:* Total contributions made in 1999. **Typ. Recipients:** Children's Health/Hospitals, Clinics/Medical Centers, Emergency/Ambulance Services, Heart, Hospitals, Medical Education, People with Disabilities. **Geo. Dist:** PA.

★ 11338 ★ Eden Hall Foundation
600 Grant, Suite 3232
Pittsburgh, PA 15219
Phone: (412)642-6697 **Fax:** (412)642-6698
George Greer, Chairman

Fnded: 1984. **Philosophy:** The foundation has four primary areas of interest: "social welfare and the improvement of conditions of the poor and needy; educational programs dedicated to the advancement and dissemination of useful knowledge, and support and maintenance of private colleges, universities, and other educational institutions; the advancement of better health through support and maintenance of hospitals or organizations whose primary purpose is the prevention and alleviation of sickness and disease; and the advancement of good morals." **Priorities:** *Arts & Humanities:* 1%. Supports libraries, museums and theater. *Civic & Public Affairs:* 5%. Supports economic development, a zoological society and women's affairs. *Education:* 43%. Supports colleges, universities, schools, minority education and scholarships. *Environment:* 36%. Support family services, Big Brother/Big Sister, homes Young Men's Christian Association, and United Way. *International:* 9%. Supports children's health programs, hospital, and health care centers.

Note: Total contributions made in 2000. **Typ. Recipients:** AIDS/HIV, Arthritis, Cancer, Children's Health/Hospitals, Clinics/Medical Centers, Diabetes, Domestic Violence, Emergency/Ambulance Services, Family Planning, Health Funds, Health Organizations, Hospices, Hospitals, Kidney, Medical Education, Medical Rehabilitation, Mental Health, Multiple Sclerosis, Nursing Services, People with Disabilities, Prenatal Health Issues, Research/Studies Institutes, Single-Disease Health Associations, Substance Abuse. **Geo. Dist:** PA, primarily western area.

★ 11339 ★ Edgar and Elsa Prince Foundation

190 South River Ave.
Suite 300
Holland, MI 49423
Phone: (616)494-8143 **Fax:** (616)494-8110
Elsa Prince, President

Fnded: 1977. **Philosophy:** The foundation typically supports churches, ministries, religious social welfare organizations, and religiously affiliated schools. **Priorities:** *Arts & Humanities:* Less than 1%. *Civic & Public Affairs:* 4%. Supports community foundations, housing, and public policy. *Education:* 29%. Funds Christian schools and educational initiatives. *Environment:* 11%. Supports family services, youth organizations, and community services. *International:* 1%. Supports health services and single-disease associations. *Note:* Total contributions made in fiscal 2001. **Typ. Recipients:** Children's Health/Hospitals, Emergency/Ambulance Services, Family Planning, Heart, Hospices, Hospitals, Long-Term Care, Medical Rehabilitation, Medical Research, People with Disabilities, Prenatal Health Issues, Public Health, Single-Disease Health Associations, Trauma Treatment. **Geo. Dist:** MI.

★ 11340 ★ Edith L. Trees Charitable Trust

One PNC Plaza, 2nd Floor
249 Fifth Ave.
Pittsburgh, PA 15222
Phone: (412)762-3808
James Ferguson, III, Trust Officer

Fnded: 1976. **Philosophy:** The Edith L. Trees Charitable Trust provides support to organizations that serve mentally retarded children. Generally, the trust focuses its efforts in three categories–social services, education, and civic causes. The trust's social service funding supports Associations for Retarded Citizens (ARCs), community service organizations, and community centers. The trust's contributions to education fund schools and special/gifted education, and its civic funds support philanthropic organizations. **Priorities:** *Civic & Public Affairs:* 2%. Funds employment/job training services and community affairs. *Education:* 25%. Funds special education and vocational training for the mentally retarded and visually impaired; also funds autism research at universities. *Environment:* 55%. Supports services for disabled and mentally retarded children and adults; funds recreational activities and camps for physically and developmentally disabled youth. *International:* 14%. Supports children's hospital, rehabilitation centers, and single-disease health associations. *Note:* Total contributions made in 2000. **Typ. Recipients:** Children's Health/Hospitals, Clinics/Medical Centers, Eyes/Blindness, Health Organizations, Health Policy/Cost Containment, Health-General, Hospitals (University Affiliated), Medical Rehabilitation, Mental Health, People with Disabilities, Public Health, Single-Disease Health Associations. **Geo. Dist:** Pittsburgh, PA.

★ 11341 ★ Edmond de Rothschild Foundation

1585 Broadway
New York, NY 10036
Phone: (212)969-3250 **Fax:** (212)969-2900
Paul Epstein, Director

Fnded: 1963. **Philosophy:** The Edmond de Rothschild Foundation is primarily interested in funding organizations located in France and Israel. Major categories of contributions include educational institutions, health care, and the sciences. The foundation also will fund charitable organizations in the United States on a limited basis. **Priorities:** *Arts & Humanities:* 40%. Supports performing arts groups and museums. *Civic & Public Affairs:* 4%. Funds community organizations. *Education:* 16% Contributes to colleges and universities. *International:* 36% Funds medical centers and hospitals. *Note:* Total contributions made in fiscal 2001. **Typ. Recipients:** Cancer, Clinics/Medical Centers, Emergency/Ambulance Services, Geriatric Health, Heart, Hospitals, Medical Education, Multiple Sclerosis, Single-Disease Health Associations. **Geo. Dist:** New York, NY.

★ 11342 ★ Edna McConnell Clark Foundation

250 Park Ave., Suite 900
New York, NY 10177-0026
Phone: (212)551-9100 **Fax:** (212)986-4558
Email: info@emcf.org
Website: http://www.emcf.org
Nancy Roob, Vice President

Fnded: 1950. **Philosophy:** The Edna McConnell Clark Foundation is currently undergoing a transition in grantmaking. The Foundation's new grantmaking approach, referred to as Institution and Field Building (IFB), is designed to help, "...build the capacities of nonprofit organizations to achieve their own objectives through multi-year organizational development grants." In connection with this new approach to grantmaking, the Foundation has decided to focus solely on youth development organizations and programs. Foundation President Michael A. Bailin recently described the foundation's new direction. "Having decided to work exclusively in youth development with a focus on young people from low-income families, we understand the importance of articulating to others outside the Foundation what we hope to accomplish. While we are still working to clarify our objectives, here is what we can say right now. In broad strokes, we intend that as a result of participating in the programs our grantees provide outside of school time, children and young people aged 9 through 24 will *gain academic skills and perform better in school*, advancing more consistently from grade to grade. Older youth or young adults will be able to *find meaningful employment*, with opportunities for advancement. We also hope to see greater numbers of young people *more actively involved in the civic and cultural life of their communities*. Finally, we expect our gratees' program participants to *steer clear of harmful activities*, such as getting pregnant at too early an age, becoming mixed up in crime, or abusing drugs." *Edna McConnell Clark Foundation 2001 Annual Report* The foundation continues to maintain a Venture Fund to explore new areas for potential grantmaking and to support projects that are consistent with its mission but that fall outside or cut across its established program areas. **Priorities:** *Civic & Public Affairs:* 14%. Principally for the New York Neighborhoods Program. Also funds justice programs. *Education:* 18%. Funds student achievement initiatives. *Environment:* 58%. Primarily supports child welfare and youth development. *International:* 4%. Supports tropical disease research. *Note:* Total contributions made in fiscal 2001. **Typ. Recipients:** Child Abuse, Domestic Violence, Eyes/Blindness, Hospitals, Medical Research, Nursing Services, Substance Abuse. **Geo. Dist:** Northeast corridor (Boston to Washington, DC).

★ 11343 ★ Educational Foundation of America

35 Church Lane
Westport, CT 06880-3515
Phone: (203)226-6498 **Fax:** (203)227-0424
Email: efa@efaw.org
Website: http://www.efaw.org
Diane Allison, Executive Director

Fnded: 1959. **Philosophy:** In general, the foundation makes grants for specific projects in the areas of population issues, the arts, education, the environment, energy, Native American issues, and other interests including medicine and peace. The foundation has recently intensified its activity in population issues, with support for programs enhancing public awareness and parent education, increasing demographic studies, reproductive rights, and strengthening public policy interests. Other civic concerns focus on problems of energy use, conservation, and nonprofit management. Education funding has emphasized nursing programs, science and mathematical programs, special education studies, minority educational projects, international studies, and population and environmental programs. Arts funding has helped institutions and programs in visual arts, dance, music, and theater. **Priorities:** *Civic & Public Affairs:* 19%. Supports public policy, taxpayer and consumer associations, corporate responsibility programs, and economic policy. *Education:* 19%. Funds preschool, elementary and secondary education, colleges and universities. *Environment:* 5%. Funds child welfare organizations, family planning, and social service agencies. *International:* 4%. Community health programs, hospitals and medical centers, and single-disease health associations receive support. *Note:* Total contributions made in 2000. **Typ. Recipients:** Cancer, Children's Health/Hospitals, Clinics/Medical Centers, Family Planning, Geriatric Health, Medical Education, Medical Research, Prenatal Health Issues, Public Health, Substance Abuse. **Geo. Dist:** nationally.

★ 11344 ★ Edward C. Johnson Fund

82 Devonshire St., S3
Boston, MA 02109
Phone: (617)563-6806
Website: http://www.fidelityfoundation.org
Anne-Marie Soulliere, Foundation Director

Fnded: 1964. **Philosophy:** The Edward C. Johnson Fund has made grants to educational institutions, museums, historic preservation and other cultural organizations, for the protection and improvement of the environment, and to community organizations. Purposes include capital campaigns, program support, and special projects. **Priorities:** *Arts & Humanities:* 54%. Museums, historical societies, arts associations, music, and libraries, with major grants to Peabody Essex Museum and Museum of Fine Arts Boston. *Civic & Public Affairs:* 1%. Community projects, foundations, and clubs. *Education:* 10%. Secondary schools and universities, with major grants to Boston College and Garrison Forest School, and economic education. *Environment:* 2%. Supports athletics, Young Men's Christian Association, and homes. *International:* 17%. Hospitals and medical associations. *Religion:* 1%. Supports Bermuda Underwater Exploration Institute. *Note:* Total contributions made in 2000. **Typ. Recipients:** Alzheimers Disease, Cancer, Clinics/Medical Centers, Emergency/Ambulance Services, Eyes/Blindness, Health Organizations, Home-Care Services, Hospitals, Medical Education, Medical Research, Mental Health, Nursing Services, Preventive Medicine/Wellness Organizations, Single-Disease Health Associations. **Geo. Dist:** New England.

★ 11345 ★ Edward D. and Anna Mitchell Family Foundation

6310 San Vicente Boulevard, Suite 500
Los Angeles, CA 90048
Phone: (323)935-6222 **Fax:** (323)930-1361
Jonathan Mitchell, President

Fnded: 1953. **Philosophy:** The foundation's primary interest is Israel-related organizations and education. Other interests include medical research and education. **Priorities:** *Arts & Humanities:* 5%. Supports music, museums, and art centers. *Civic & Public Affairs:* 14%. Emphasis on a charitable trust and a community foundation. *Education:* 47%. Supports educational funds and programs. *Environment:* 5%. Supports united funds, shelters, family planning, and children's welfare programs. *International:* 13%. Focus on AIDS, Parkinsons disease research, hospitals, and health associations. *Note:* Total contributions made in 1998. **Typ. Recipients:** AIDS/HIV, Children's Health/Hospitals, Clinics/Medical Centers, Diabetes, Emergency/Ambulance Services, Family Planning, Health Organizations, Heart, Hospitals, Long-Term Care, Medical Education, Medical Research, Medical Training, People with Disabilities, Single-Disease Health

Associations. **Geo. Dist:** Los Angeles, CA; New York, NY.

★ 11346 ★ Edward E. Ford Foundation

1912 Sunderland Pl. NW
Washington, DC 20036-1608
Phone: (202)955-1028 **Fax:** (202)955-8097
Email: office@eeford.org
Website: http://www.eeford.org
Robert Hallett, Executive Director

Fnded: 1957. **Philosophy:** Although the charter is broad in its scope, the "major objective of the Foundation is to encourage and improve secondary education as provided by independent private schools in the United States." The foundation believes that the most significant impact stems from a narrow focus. The foundation's interest in education stems from Mr. Ford's notion that students who graduate from such institutions go on to become productive, motivated contributors to our society, and that schools provide a choice in education for both students and their parents. Since 1957, the board has given almost $52 million to a variety of issues affecting secondary private education without favoring any one type of school or project. In recent years, more funding has gone to co-educational schools and non-boarding institutions, and matching grants have been slightly more common than outright grants. Grants have been made for scholarships, professional development for teachers, summer workshops, buildings, curriculum, and computer education for faculty. Grants always are made to individual schools. Applicants must be members of the National Association of Independent Schools (NAIS). Presently, the board has an interest in supporting projects designed to benefit faculty in NAIS schools. The foundation also is interested in computer education and related technology for faculty. The foundation initiated a students grant program in 1993 for regional and state associations of NAIS. **Priorities:** *Education:* 100%. Supports faculty enrichment, capital and building projects, scholarships, and educational programs at private and parochial secondary schools. *Note:* Total contributions made in fiscal 2001. **Typ. Recipients:** Substance Abuse. **Geo. Dist:** nationally, including United States territories.

★ 11347 ★ Edward G. Schlieder Educational Foundation

313 Carondelet St., 1st Fl.
New Orleans, LA 70130
Phone: (504)533-5535 **Fax:** (504)533-3669
Pierre Lapeyre, Assistant Secretary

Fnded: 1945. **Philosophy:** The foundation primarily supports higher education in Louisiana. **Priorities:** *Education:* 100%. Supports schools, and colleges. *Note:* The foundation reports that 100% of grants are restricted exclusively to educational institutions within the State of Louisiana. While grants may from time to time be specifically designated for special programs or areas of the grantee institution, the foundation indicates that all contributions benefit educational concerns. Total contributions made in 2000. **Typ. Recipients:** Cancer, Children's Health/Hospitals, Health Organizations, Health Policy/Cost Containment, Hospitals (University Affiliated), Medical Education, Medical Research, Nutrition. **Geo. Dist:** LA, limited to educational institutions in Louisiana.

★ 11348 ★ Edward John Noble Foundation, Inc.

PO Box 954
383 Main St., Unit 2
Ridgefield, CT 06877
Phone: (203)438-5690
E.J. Smith, President

Fnded: 1940. **Philosophy:** The foundation's donor believed that grant making must be a working process and not merely a passive distribution of money; not simply to help others, but to enable others to help themselves. The foundation continues to devote its attention to the arts, education, and health, as Mr. Noble wanted, but is also interested in supporting conservation and preservation of the environment. In the arts, the foundation assists major cultural organizations in New York City and their educational programs. In higher education, the foundation encourages effective interdisciplinary programs of environmental studies. In secondary education, support is given to programs likely to improve educational opportunities for disadvantaged gifted and talented youth in New York City. The foundation supports several conservation projects on St. Catherine's Island and selected other programs which help preserve the natural environment. In the health field, the foundation primarily supports projects which show the greatest promise of stabilizing the population and providing effective population education. The foundation also considers proposals from established arts organizations interested in management training programs for interns. The foundation sees a developing role in intern programs for efficient administration of institutions and for training the arts managers of the future. **Priorities:** *Arts & Humanities:* 62%. Primary support for museums, performing arts, music, and opera. *Civic & Public Affairs:* 5%. *Education:* 10%. Colleges, universities, and secondary schools. *Environment:* Approx. 1%. Focus on family planning. *International:* Approx. 1%. Supports hospitals and medical centers. *Religion:* 8%. Support for a natural history museum. *Note:* Total contributions made in 2000. **Typ. Recipients:** Cancer, Clinics/Medical Centers, Family Planning, Health Organizations, Health-General, Hospitals, Medical Education, Medical Research, Medical Training, Trauma Treatment. **Geo. Dist:** GA, Georgia coast; New York, NY, metropolitan area.

★ 11349 ★ Edward Mallinckrodt, Jr. Foundation

1 N Jefferson
Saint Louis, MO 63103
Phone: (314)849-0464
Email: langenom@agedwards.com
Oliver Langenberg, Chairman

Fnded: 1953. **Philosophy:** "The basic aim of the Foundation is to dispense that amount required by law for the purpose of advancing knowledge in the various fields of clinical and laboratory research. It is further the general aim to confine contributions to those worthy projects that are in need of initial start-up funding to move the projects foward to the point of other independent support or to support highly promising young investigators at the time when start-up funds are limited and initial progress is dependent on additional funding." **Priorities:** *International:* 100%. Health care and research in major medical universities. *Note:* Total contributions made in 2001. **Typ. Recipients:** Cancer, Children's Health/Hospitals, Clinics/Medical Centers, Emergency/Ambulance Services, Kidney, Medical Research, Speech & Hearing. **Geo. Dist:** nationally.

★ 11350 ★ Edward S. Moore Foundation

47 Arch St.
Greenwich, CT 06830
Phone: (203)629-4591 **Fax:** (203)629-4594
John Cross, III, President

Fnded: 1957. **Philosophy:** The foundation distributes donations to a variety of organizations primarily in New York and Connecticut. The foundation typically supports educational institutions, the arts, hospitals and health organizations, and social services, particularly those organizations concerned with the welfare of young people. **Priorities:** *Arts & Humanities:* 16%. Museums, music programs, and historical societies. *Civic & Public Affairs:* 5%. Zoos and aquariums receive funding. *Education:* 21%. Colleges and universities, and mentoring programs. *Environment:* 32%. Primarily supports child welfare and family services organizations. *International:* 12%. Hospitals - mostly children's health concerns. *Note:* Total contributions made in 2000. **Typ. Recipients:** Children's Health/Hospitals, Clinics/Medical Centers, Domestic Violence, Health Organizations, Hospitals, Hospitals (University Affiliated), Medical Education, Medical Rehabilitation, Medical Research, Mental Health, People with Disabilities. **Geo. Dist:** CT; NY.

★ 11351 ★ Edward W. Hazen Foundation

309 Fifth Ave., Suite 200-3
New York, NY 10016
Phone: (212)889-3034 **Fax:** (212)889-3039
Email: hazen@hazenfoundation.org
Website: http://www.hazenfoundation.org
Barbara Taveras, President

Fnded: 1925. **Philosophy:** The Foundation seeks to "assist young people, particularly minorities and those disadvantaged by poverty, to achieve their full potential as individuals and as active participants in a democratic society. This goal remains faithful to Mr. Hazen's original intentions and values – values that honored individual achievement and civic participation." "The Edward W. Haze Foundation has two major grantmaking programs: Public Education and Youth Development. Recognizing that children are best considered within the context of family and community, and reflecting the Foundation's belief in the pivotal role that a strong public education system can play in helping youth fulfill their potential, the Foundation has designed its grantmaking strategy with the following goals in mind: effective schools for all students; and full partnership for parents and communities working to reform and restructure their school systems." To achieve these goals, the Foundation supports new or emerging Community and Parent Organizing initiatives which seek educational equity and improved student achievement; Educational Advocacy efforts which address issues of equity and accountability, including issue analysis, policy recommendations and community education; and Community-based programs which seek to strengthen the connections between schools, families and communities. The Foundation also focuses on youth organizing around concrete social issues. "By fostering new and increased roles for youth in communities and schools the Foundation seeks to contribute to the development of a new generation of grassroots leaders committed to improving conditions in their schools and communities. Toward this end, the Foundation supports new or emerging Leadership Development initiatives which provide advocacy and community organizing skills to middle and high school-age youth; Innovative programs of community based and youth-based organizations which wish to broaden their approach to youth development to include youth organizing around concrete social issues, public education in particular; and school-based programs of community-based and grassroots organizations which help middle and high school age youth develop the interest and skills necessary to become involved in meaningful social change efforts." 1996 Guidelines **Priorities:** *Civic & Public Affairs:* 59%. Supports public policy, law and justice, philanthropic organizations, economic policy, and women's issues. *Education:* 29%. Supports higher education, social sciences education, and education associations. *Environment:* 6%. Supports substance abuse, child welfare, and family services. *Note:* Total contributions made in 2001. **Typ. Recipients:** AIDS/HIV, Family Planning, Medical Research, Mental Health, Public Health, Sexual Abuse, Single-Disease Health Associations. **Geo. Dist:** nationally.

★ 11352 ★ Edwin Gould Foundation for Children

23 Gramercy Park South
New York, NY 10003
Phone: (212)982-5200 **Fax:** (212)982-6886
Email: bbelfer@egf-ny.org

Fnded: 1923. **Philosophy:** "The Foundation is dedicated to improving the educational, personal and professional opportunities of young people. Believing that organizations can achieve more together than they can alone, we collaborate with many other foundations, corporations, nonprofits and a variety of public entities. Through grants and in-kind support as well as leveraging financial and human resources, we nurture programs that we believe can be models of reform." "In Edward Gould's day children typically needed temporary homes, protection against TB, or summer camp opportunities. Today's children face different challenges, including family breakdown, overcrowded schools, a changing job market, a woeful lack of community programs and support systems, and powerful negative peer pressures. Perhaps the most alarming is the growth of what might be called a 'street culture' of drugs, violence, and gangs that confronts young people daily and forces them to make important choices too early and too often in their lives." "As a small foundation in what might be the most challenging urban settings, we have chosen to address these issues in two ways. First we concentrate on a small number of programs and support them over a sustained period. Secondly we have expanded the roles we play in addition to grantmaking. By housing several organizations in our building, we are building a partnership network that encourages the sharing of ideas and resources." Annual Report **Priorities:** *Civic & Public Affairs:* 16%. Supports aquariums, safety, and business/free enterprise. *Education:* 77%. Emphasis on the Edwin Gould Academy and a number of other educational associations. Supports scholarship funds. *Environment:* 5%. Youth programs. *Note:* Total contributions made in 2000. **Typ. Recipients:** Health Organizations, Medical Education. **Geo. Dist:** New York, NY.

★ 11353 ★ Edwin S. Webster Foundation

77 Summer St., Ste. 800
Boston, MA 02110
Phone: (617)426-7172 **Fax:** (617)426-5441
Email: mjenney@grantsmanagement.com
Website: http://www.grantsmanagement.com
Michelle Jenney, Foundation Assistant

Fnded: 1948. **Philosophy:** The Edwin S. Webster Foundation primarily supports "charitable organizations that are well known to the trustees, with emphasis on hospitals, medical research, education, youth agencies, cultural activities, and programs addressing the needs of minorities." **Priorities:** *Arts & Humanities:* 14%. Supports museums, theater and orchestras. *Civic & Public Affairs:* 8%. Supports gardens and a zoo. *Education:* 26%. Supports education associations, education funds, and public and private schools. *Environment:* 14%. Supports emergency relief, community services, youth services, and family services. *International:* 27%. Supports hospital and medical centers. *Religion:* 8%. Supports a science laboratory and a museum. *Note:* Total contributions made in 2000. **Typ. Recipients:** Cancer, Children's Health/Hospitals, Clinics/Medical Centers, Diabetes, Emergency/Ambulance Services, Eyes/Blindness, Family Planning, Family Planning, Health Organizations, Heart, Hospitals, Hospitals (University Affiliated), Medical Education, Medical Rehabilitation, Medical Research, Mental Health, People with Disabilities, Public Health, Single-Disease Health Associations, Substance Abuse, Trauma Treatment. **Geo. Dist:** New England.

★ 11354 ★ Edyth Bush Charitable Foundation, Inc.

199 East Welbourne Ave.
PO Box 1967
Winter Park, FL 32790-1967
Phone: 888-647-4322 **Fax:** (407)647-7716
Email: dhessler@edythbush.org
Website: http://www.edythbush.org
David Odahowski, President

Fnded: 1966. **Philosophy:** The foundation's original goal was to support charitable, religious, educational, and literary purposes; with special consideration to organizations that help underprivileged or needy people improve themselves or that relieve human suffering. The foundation adheres to the intent of Edyth Bush in its giving patterns, supporting organizations in the areas of education, human services, health, and the arts. Supported art organizations demonstrate nationally recognized quality; strong emphasis is placed on K-12 educational programs. nationally recognized quality; strong emphasis is placed on K-12 educational programs. **Priorities:** *Arts & Humanities:* 15%. Supports museums and the performing arts. *Civic & Public Affairs:* 20%. Funds community *Education:* 2%. Supports public education. *Environment:* 45%. Supports youth organizations, humane society, and community service organizations. *International:* 9%. Supports health care. **Typ. Recipients:** Alzheimers Disease, Cancer, Clinics/Medical Centers, Eyes/Blindness, Health Organizations, Hospitals, Mental Health, Nursing Services, People with Disabilities, Single-Disease Health Associations. **Geo. Dist:** FL, Lake County; FL, Orange County; FL, Osceola County; FL, Seminole County.

★ 11355 ★ Effie and Wofford Cain Foundation

4131 Spicewood Springs Rd., Suite A-1
Austin, TX 78759
Phone: (512)346-7490 **Fax:** (512)346-7491
Email: mbratz@cainfoundation.org
Mrs. Lynn Fowler, Exec. Director, Secretary & Treasurer

Fnded: 1952. **Philosophy:** The foundation traditionally focuses its support on educational institutions and programs, social service organizations, medical institutions, and medical research programs. **Priorities:** *Arts & Humanities:* 3%. Cultural institutions. *Civic & Public Affairs:* 3%. Public and community benefit. *Education:* 31%. Educational institutions. *Environment:* 4%. Human needs and services. *Religion:* Scientific and medical institutions. **Typ. Recipients:** Alzheimers Disease, Arthritis, Cancer, Child Abuse, Children's Health/Hospitals, Clinics/Medical Centers, Diabetes, Domestic Violence, Emergency/Ambulance Services, Health Organizations, Heart, Hospitals, Hospitals (University Affiliated), Medical Education, Medical Research, Medical Training, Mental Health, People with Disabilities, Public Health, Respiratory, Single-Disease Health Associations, Substance Abuse. **Geo. Dist:** TX.

★ 11356 ★ Eisenberg Foundation for Charities

2340 South Arlington Heights Rd., Suite 615
Arlington Heights, IL 60005
Phone: (847)981-0545 **Fax:** (847)981-0548
James Marousis, Treasurer & Director

Fnded: 1989. **Philosophy:** Foundation makes grants for "medicine and health, education, and physical, emotional and social assistance, primarily for the benefit of underprivileged youth and elderly." **Priorities:** *Civic & Public Affairs:* Less than 1%. *Education:* 8%. Supports universities, medical education, and education foundations. *Environment:* 10%. Supports senior services, youth programs, people with disabilities, homes and children's services. *International:* 69%. Supports medical centers, health care counsels, nursing homes health foundations and medical research. *Note:* Total contributions made in 2000. **Typ. Recipients:** AIDS/HIV, Alzheimers Disease, Cancer, Children's Health/Hospitals, Clinics/Medical Centers, Geriatric Health, Health Organizations, Health Policy/Cost Containment, Hospitals, Hospitals (University Affiliated), Long-Term Care, Medical Education, Medical Rehabilitation, Medical Research, Multiple Sclerosis, People with Disabilities, Prenatal Health Issues, Public Health, Research/Studies Institutes. **Geo. Dist:** IL, DuPage County; Chicago, IL, metropolitan area; Rochester, MN.

★ 11357 ★ El Pomar Foundation

10 Lake Circle
Colorado Springs, CO 80906
Phone: (719)633-7733 **Fax:** (719)577-5702
Email: grants@elpomar.org
Website: http://www.elpomar.org
William Hybl, Chairman & Chief Executive Officer

Fnded: 1937. **Philosophy:** In general, the foundation supports educational and health institutions; civic, community, and social services; and the arts in Colorado. The foundation places greater emphasis on civic, community, and emergency needs of the poor. The foundation also concentrates on programs designed to promote excellence in nonprofit organizations. **Priorities:** *Arts & Humanities:* 6%. Supports arts centers, performing arts, museums, historical societies, and public broadcasting. *Civic & Public Affairs:* 32%. Funds zoos, community foundations, parks, environmental affairs, botanical gardens, and women's affairs. *Education:* 27%. Supports minority education, leadership education, space science and economics education, literacy programs, and Colorado colleges. *Environment:* 23%. Gives to youth programs, Big Brothers/Big Sisters, child care, food distribution, safe houses/shelters, disaster relief, the United Way, and senior services. *International:* 7%. Funds hospitals, community health centers, hospice, dental and eye health, blood centers, and health foundations. *Note:* Total contributions made in 2001, excluding Awards for Excellence, Youth in Community Service, and In-kind support grants. **Typ. Recipients:** Alzheimers Disease, Arthritis, Cancer, Children's Health/Hospitals, Clinics/Medical Centers, Diabetes, Domestic Violence, Emergency/Ambulance Services, Eyes/Blindness, Health Organizations, Health-General, Hospices, Hospitals, Long-Term Care, Medical Rehabilitation, Medical Research, Mental Health, Nursing Services, People with Disabilities, Preventive Medicine/Wellness Organizations, Public Health, Substance Abuse, Transplant Networks/Donor Banks. **Geo. Dist:** CO.

★ 11358 ★ Eleanor and Edsel Ford Fund

100 Renaissance Ctr., Suite 3400
Detroit, MI 48243
Phone: (313)259-7777 **Fax:** (313)393-7579
David Hempstead, Secretary & Trustee

Fnded: 1944. **Philosophy:** Contributions are "committed pursuant to testamentary direction left by Eleanor Clay Ford." The purpose of the fund is to provide financial support to corporations, trusts, community chests, funds, or foundations, organized and operated solely for religious, charitable, scientific, literary or educational purposes, or for the prevention of cruelty to children or animals. **Priorities:** *Arts & Humanities:* 24%. Supports music and Arts Founders Society. *Education:* 43%. Supports arts/humanities education and schools. *International:* 21%. Funds support the Henry Ford Health System. *Religion:* 11%. Supports the Edison Institute. *Note:* Total contributions made in 2000. **Typ. Recipients:** Health Organizations, Hospitals, Public Health. **Geo. Dist:** Detroit, MI, including metropolitan area.

★ 11359 ★ Eleanor Naylor Dana Charitable Trust

375 Park Ave., Suite 3807
New York, NY 10152
Phone: (212)754-2890 **Fax:** (212)754-2892

Fnded: 1979. **Philosophy:** The trust gives funding priority in two areas: biomedical research, where it supports clinical investigation and "innovative projects designed to improve medical practice and prevent disease;" and the performing arts, "particularly those organizations which have an impact on the cultural climate of the nation." **Priorities:** *Arts & Humanities:* 42%. Supports performing arts. *Education:* 4%. Colleges and universities. *International:* 49%. Funds biomedical research, hospitals, and childrens health. *Note:* Total contributions made in fiscal 2000. **Typ. Recipients:** AIDS/HIV, Cancer, Children's Health/Hospitals, Clinics/Medical Centers, Diabetes, Eyes/Blindness, Family Planning, Heart, Hospitals, Hospitals (University Affiliated), Medical Education, Medical Research, Mental Health, Public Health, Transplant Networks/Donor Banks, Trauma Treatment. **Geo. Dist:** including the East Coast; New York, NY.

★ 11360 ★ Elinor Patterson Baker Foundation

10 Mason St.
Greenwich, CT 06830
Phone: (203)869-3000 **Fax:** (203)869-7412
Email: apanoli@bankofny.com
Anne Panoli, Foundation Administrator

Fnded: 1984. **Philosophy:** "The Elinor Patterson Baker Foundation makes grants for the general charitable purposes of organizations that fulfill the aims, principles, goals, and purposes of The Humane Society of the United States." **Priorities:** *Arts & Humanities:* 1%. *Civic & Public Affairs:* 1%. *Education:* 4%. *Environment:* 75%. Supports animal welfare organizations. *Note:* Total contributions made in fiscal 2000. **Typ. Recipients:** Clinics/Medical Centers, People with Disabilities. **Geo. Dist:** nationally and to U.S.-based international organizations.

★ 11361 ★ Elis Olsson Memorial Foundation
PO Box 151
West Point, VA 23181
Phone: (804)843-9066 **Fax:** (804)843-9068
Thelma Downey, Executive Director

Fnded: 1966. **Philosophy:** The foundation makes most of its grants to educational institutions. Interests include private high schools, seminaries, universities, medical colleges, and literacy institutes. Secondary interests include family services, historical preservation, and various other charitable organizations. **Priorities:** *Arts & Humanities:* 14%. Supports museums and historic preservation. *Civic & Public Affairs:* 16%. Supports a foundation. *Education:* 32%. Primarily supports schools in Virginia. *Environment:* 16%. Family services, youth organizations, and the disabled. *International:* 9%. Focus on medical education and health associations. *Religion:* 4%. For a science museum. *Note:* Total contributions made in 2000. **Typ. Recipients:** Alzheimers Disease, Cancer, Children's Health/Hospitals, Clinics/Medical Centers, Emergency/Ambulance Services, Health Funds, Health Organizations, Health-General, Heart, Hospices, Hospitals, Hospitals (University Affiliated), Long-Term Care, Medical Education, Medical Rehabilitation, Medical Research, People with Disabilities, Public Health, Research/Studies Institutes, Respiratory, Single-Disease Health Associations. **Geo. Dist:** VA.

★ 11362 ★ Elisabeth Severance Prentiss Foundation
PO Box 5756
Cleveland, OH 44101
Phone: (216)222-2736 **Fax:** (216)222-2410
Michael Gelland, Contact

Fnded: 1944. **Philosophy:** "The Elisabeth Severance Prentiss Foundation is a charitable trust dedicated to the support and advancement of health care services in the greater Cleveland community. The foundation awards monetary grants to qualifying institutions and agencies for medical research and programs designed to improve the method of health care services." The trust agreement's five objectives are to promote medical and surgical research; to promote public health; to aid hospitals and health institutions in Cuyahoga County, OH, with support for capital and operating expenses; to improve methods of hospital administration; and to promote equitable health care delivery and cost-containment programs. The foundation lacks the resources to provide continuous aid to organizations for operating expenses while at the same time funding new areas of need. Therefore, its primary objective at this time is to support new, essential services that are likely to become self-sustaining. **Priorities:** *Civic & Public Affairs:* Less than 1%. *Education:* 13%. Supports nursing programs and university hospital programs. *Environment:* 8%. Funds neighborhood family practice, Planned Parenthood, and family services. *International:* 78%. Supports health centers, clinics, and foundations, hospices, hospitals, American Red Cross, mental health, children's health, and cancer *Note:* Total contributions made in 2000. **Typ. Recipients:** Adolescent Health Issues, AIDS/HIV, Alzheimers Disease, Cancer, Children's Health/Hospitals, Clinics/Medical Centers, Emergency/Ambulance Services, Eyes/Blindness, Family Planning, Geriatric Health, Health Organizations, Health Policy/Cost Containment, Heart, Hospices, Hospitals, Hospitals (University Affiliated), Long-Term Care, Medical Education, Medical Rehabilitation, Medical Research, Medical Training, Mental Health, Multiple Sclerosis, Nursing Services, Outpatient Health Care, People with Disabilities, Public Health, Research/Studies Institutes, Sexual Abuse, Single-Disease Health Associations, Substance Abuse, Transplant Networks/Donor Banks. **Geo. Dist:** Cleveland, OH, metropolitan area.

★ 11363 ★ Elizabeth Morse Genius Charitable Trust
231 S Lasalle St.
Chicago, IL 60697
Phone: (312)828-5554 **Fax:** (312)987-0806
Charles Slamar, Jr., Trust Officer

Fnded: 1992. **Priorities:** *Arts & Humanities:* 11%. Supports performing arts, public broadcasting and local orchestras. *Civic & Public Affairs:* 20%. Supports community development and legal advocacy. *Education:* 4%. Supports educational insitutions. *Environment:* 44%. Supports social services, youth concerns and the homeless shelters. *International:* 19%. Supports hospitals and medical/wellness centers. *Note:* Contributions were made in fiscal 2001. **Typ. Recipients:** AIDS/HIV, Cancer, Child Abuse, Children's Health/Hospitals, Clinics/Medical Centers, Domestic Violence, Emergency/Ambulance Services, Hospitals, Long-Term Care, Mental Health, People with Disabilities, Public Health. **Geo. Dist:** Chicago, IL.

★ 11364 ★ Elizabeth Morse Genius Foundation
PO Box 40
Winter Park, FL 32790
Phone: (407)644-0555 **Fax:** (407)644-9504
Harold Ward, III, President & Trustee

Fnded: 1959. **Philosophy:** The foundation primarily supports education funds, education associations, and the arts. **Priorities:** *Arts & Humanities:* 27%. Supports arts funds, music, public broadcasting, historic preservation, and libraries. *Education:* 71%. Major support for an education fund and a college. *Environment:* Less than 1%. *Note:* Total contributions made in 2000. **Typ. Recipients:** Clinics/Medical Centers, Family Planning, Health Organizations, Hospitals. **Geo. Dist:** Winter Park, FL.

★ 11365 ★ Elizabeth and Stephen Bechtel Jr. Foundation
PO Box 193809
San Francisco, CA 94119-3809
Phone: (415)284-8572 **Fax:** (415)284-8571
Email: esb@fremontgroup.org
Mrs. Lauren Dachs, Executive Dir.

Fnded: 1957. **Philosophy:** The foundation has traditionally supported higher education organizations, environmental affairs, and cultural activities. Major support from the foundation has been pledged to the California Institute of Technology Campaign for Caltech, the University of California, and Stanford University. **Priorities:** *Arts & Humanities:* 9%. *Civic & Public Affairs:* 12%. *Education:* 60%. *Environment:* 7%. *International:* 5%. *Note:* Total contributions made in 2000. **Typ. Recipients:** Adolescent Health Issues, Cancer, Children's Health/Hospitals, Clinics/Medical Centers, Emergency/Ambulance Services, Eyes/Blindness, Health Organizations, Hospitals, Hospitals (University Affiliated), Long-Term Care, Medical Education, Medical Research, Multiple Sclerosis, Nutrition, People with Disabilities, Prenatal Health Issues, Research/Studies Institutes, Single-Disease Health Associations, Substance Abuse. **Geo. Dist:** San Francisco, CA, Bay area.

★ 11366 ★ Ella West Freeman Foundation
PO Box 13218
New Orleans, LA 70185-3218
Phone: (504)895-1988 **Fax:** (504)895-1988
Email: firstline@compuserve.com
Website: http://www.ellawest.org
Louis Freeman, Jr., Chairman

★ 11367 ★ Ellen Browning Scripps Foundation
6121 Terryhill Drive
La Jolla, CA 92037
Phone: 800-326-3776
Website: http://www.scrippsfoundation.org
E. Dawson, Sr. Vice President & Manager

Fnded: 1935. **Philosophy:** The Ellen Browning Scripps Foundation makes most of its grants in the areas of education, the arts, health, and civic affairs. Educational funding favors Scripps College and private schools. Funding for the arts goes to museums, libraries, and historic preservation. Health interests include research, medical centers, and hospitals. In civic affairs, interests include zoos, women's affairs, and the environment. The foundation also supports a variety of social service interests. **Priorities:** *Arts & Humanities:* About 18%. Museums, libraries, and opera. *Civic & Public Affairs:* About 15%. Primary support given to the San Diego Zoological Society. *Education:* About 23%. Colleges and private education. *Environment:* About 14%. Scouting and youth programs, Meals on Wheels, and services for the elderly. *International:* 20%. Hospices and hospitals. *Religion:* 5%. Natural history and maritime museums, aerospace, and oceanography studies. *Note:* Total contributions made in fiscal 1999. **Typ. Recipients:** Children's Health/Hospitals, Eyes/Blindness, Hospices, Hospitals, Medical Research, People with Disabilities, Research/Studies Institutes, Single-Disease Health Associations, Transplant Networks/Donor Banks. **Geo. Dist:** CA, San Diego County.

★ 11368 ★ Ellison Foundation
1 Memorial Drive
Cambridge, MA 02142-1300
Phone: (617)225-3830 **Fax:** (617)255-3801
Elton Drew, Trustee

Fnded: 1952. **Philosophy:** The foundation was formed for the purposes of disbursing funds solely and exclusively for religious, charitable, scientific, literary, or educational purposes, and for the prevention of cruelty to children or animals. Health care receives major support. **Priorities:** *Arts & Humanities:* 4%. Gives to historical societies, historic preservation/historic sites, art museums, and libraries. *Civic & Public Affairs:* 4%. Contributes to community foundations and an aquarium. *Education:* 16%. Funds colleges, scholarship funds, and secondary schools. *Environment:* 7%. Supports shelters and child welfare organizations. *International:* 65%. Supports hospitals, medical centers, cancer organizations, and visiting nurse programs, and eye and ear health. *Religion:* 1%. Funds a science museum and veterinary medicine research. *Note:* Total contributions made in 2000. **Typ. Recipients:** Cancer, Children's Health/Hospitals, Clinics/Medical Centers, Health Organizations, Hospitals, Hospitals (University Affiliated), Medical Education, Medical Rehabilitation, Nursing Services, People with Disabilities, Public Health, Speech & Hearing. **Geo. Dist:** nationally; MA, primarily.

★ 11369 ★ Ellwood Foundation
PO Box 550049
Houston, TX 77255
Phone: (713)785-5507 **Fax:** (713)780-8833
H. Hightower, Trustee

Fnded: 1958. **Philosophy:** The Ellwood Foundation primarily makes grants in the areas of health services and social services. Health support goes to medical research, mental health, hospitals, health foundations, single-disease associations, and health organizations. In social services, funding favors homes, child welfare, the disabled, and youth centers. Grants are made to other recipient areas on a limited basis. **Priorities:** *Arts & Humanities:* 5%. Supports the Institute of Texas Cultures. *Civic & Public Affairs:* 5%. *Education:* 17%. Supports educational programs and institutions. *Environment:* 17%. Supports children and youth services, drug and alcohol abuse assistance, and the disabled. *International:* 50%. Supports hospice, medical centers, hospitals, disease and disorder concerns. *Religion:* 3%. Supports the Institute of Molecular Studies. *Note:* Contributions were made in fiscal 2001. **Typ. Recipients:** Alzheimers Disease, Cancer, Child Abuse, Children's Health/Hospitals, Clinics/Medical Centers, Eyes/Blindness, Health Organizations, Heart, Hospices, Hospitals, Hospitals (University Affiliated), Long-Term Care, Medical Education, Medical Rehabilitation, Medical Research, Mental Health, People with Disabilities, People with Disabilities, Prenatal Health Issues, Public Health, Single-Disease Health Associations, Speech & Hearing, Substance Abuse. **Geo. Dist:** Houston, TX.

★ 11370 ★ Elmer and Mamdouha Bobst Foundation

Elmer Holmes Bobst Library
New York University
70 Washington Square St., Room 1209
New York, NY 10012-1091
Phone: (212)998-2440 **Fax:** (212)995-3679
Ms. Mamdouha Bobst, President

Fnded: 1968. **Philosophy:** The foundation's interests include support for the E. and M. Bobst Institute at the Richard Nixon Library, the promotion of health and cancer research, Islamic organizations in the United States and abroad, and youth and community service organizations. **Priorities:** *Civic & Public Affairs:* About 1%. Supports foreign policy. *Education:* 95%. Supports precollege education, colleges and universities. *Environment:* 3%. Supports animal welfare and youth services. *International:* 2%. Hospitals, health funds, and single-disease health associations. *Note:* Total contributions made in 2001. **Typ. Recipients:** AIDS/HIV, Arthritis, Cancer, Children's Health/Hospitals, Clinics/Medical Centers, Emergency/Ambulance Services, Health Funds, Health Organizations, Heart, Hospices, Hospitals, Hospitals (University Affiliated), Medical Education, Medical Research, Public Health, Single-Disease Health Associations, Transplant Networks/Donor Banks. **Geo. Dist:** New York, NY.

★ 11371 ★ Elsa U. Pardee Foundation

Box 2767
Midland, MI 48641-2767
Phone: (989)832-3691
Email: info@pardeefoundation.org
Website: http://www.pardeefoundation.org
Lucille Dougherty, Staff Assistant

Fnded: 1944. **Philosophy:** The purpose of the foundation is "to support research in the field of cancer, and to provide for others those advantages of knowledge and techniques still undiscovered in the treatment of cancer." Current foundation policy allocates one-third to cancer treatment, one-third to cancer research projects, and one-third to established cancer research institutes. Grants support hospitals, universities, and research institutes for projects to study control of, and cures for, cancer. Assistance with the cost of cancer treatment to families was also an area of interest to the founder, and her niece, Elsa G. Allen. Besides increasing its commitment to cancer research, the foundation also continues to fund high quality endeavors that have proven their significance. Each year the foundation devotes about one-third of funding to proposals recommended by its Medical Committee as innovative new projects. **Priorities:** *Education:* 5%. *International:* 100%. Supports cancer research. Approximately one-third goes to new research, one-third to ongoing programs, and about one-third for treatment costs for cancer victims. *Note:* Total contributions made in 2001. **Typ. Recipients:** Cancer, Clinics/Medical Centers, Hospitals, Medical Research, Transplant Networks/Donor Banks. **Geo. Dist:** nationally.

★ 11372 ★ Emma Eccles Jones Foundation

PO Box 45385
Salt Lake City, UT 84145
Phone: (801)532-1500
Clark Giles, Committee Member

Fnded: 1972. **Priorities:** *Arts & Humanities:* 43%. Supports dance, art programs, public broadcasting, theaters, libraries, opera, music, and museums. *Civic & Public Affairs:* 11%. Supports community foundations, and gardens. *Education:* 26%. Primarily supports colleges, and universitys. *Environment:* 20%. Supports animal protection, planned parenthood, scouts, and youth organizations. *Note:* Total contributions made in fiscal 1998. **Typ. Recipients:** Children's Health/Hospitals, Clinics/Medical Centers, Emergency/Ambulance Services, Family Planning, Hospitals (University Affiliated), Medical Education, Medical Research. **Geo. Dist:** UT.

★ 11373 ★ Engelberg Foundation

1050 N Lake Way
Palm Beach, FL 33480
Phone: (561)848-7089
Alfred Engelberg, Trustee

Fnded: 1991. **Priorities:** *Arts & Humanities:* 9%. Gives to art endowments and performing arts. *Education:* 32%. Focus on art and law education. *Environment:* 8%. Supports programs for the homeless and community service. *International:* 23%. Genetics, hospitals, Medicaid studies, and teen pregnancy prevention programs. *Religion:* 3%. Grants made to research. *Note:* Total contributions in fiscal 2001. **Typ. Recipients:** AIDS/HIV, Cancer, Children's Health/Hospitals, Clinics/Medical Centers, Family Planning, Health Organizations, Hospitals, Long-Term Care, Outpatient Health Care, Public Health. **Geo. Dist:** NY.

★ 11374 ★ English-Bonter-Mitchell Foundation

110 West Berry, 8th Floor
Fort Wayne, IN 46802
Phone: (260)461-6199 **Fax:** (260)461-6198
Michele Herald, Trust Officer

Fnded: 1972. **Philosophy:** The foundation's giving focuses on culture and youth programs. Support also is directed toward higher education, hospitals, churches and religious organizations, social services, and community development. **Priorities:** *Arts & Humanities:* 27%. Supports public broadcasting, arts funds, historical preservation, orchestra, music, and theater. *Civic & Public Affairs:* 6%. Supports parks and zoos. *Education:* 34%. Supports Junior Achievement, education associations, colleges, and universities. *Environment:* 28%. Supports Big Brothers/Big Sisters, scouting, the disabled, YMCA, and United Way. *International:* 4%. Supports hospital foundations, medical centers, and hospice. *Note:* Total contributions made in 2000. **Typ. Recipients:** Children's Health/Hospitals, Clinics/Medical Centers, Emergency/Ambulance Services, Health Funds, Health Organizations, Hospices, Hospitals, Medical Education, Medical Rehabilitation, Mental Health, People with Disabilities, Public Health, Single-Disease Health Associations, Substance Abuse. **Geo. Dist:** IN, primarily Fort Wayne.

★ 11375 ★ Enid and Crosby Kemper Foundation

PO Box 419692
Kansas City, MO 64141-6692
Phone: (816)860-7711 **Fax:** (816)860-5690
Website: http://www.umb.com
Steve Campbell, Trust Administrator

Fnded: 1972. **Philosophy:** The foundation traditionally has placed emphasis on higher and private secondary education and cultural programs, particularly museums and music. Significant support has also been extended to health and youth-related causes. **Priorities:** *Arts & Humanities:* 83%. Primarily to museums, historical societies, and music. *Civic & Public Affairs:* Less than 1%. *Religion:* 16%. Supports Science City. *Note:* Total contributions made in 2000. **Typ. Recipients:** Children's Health/Hospitals, Clinics/Medical Centers, Health Organizations, Hospitals, Kidney, Medical Research, People with Disabilities, Public Health, Single-Disease Health Associations, Speech & Hearing, Substance Abuse. **Geo. Dist:** Kansas City, MO, metropolitan area.

★ 11376 ★ Erik E. and Edith H. Bergstrom Foundation

PO Box 520
Palo Alto, CA 94302-0520
Phone: (650)323-0596 **Fax:** (650)324-4596
Erik Bergstrom, President and CEO

Fnded: 1981. **Philosophy:** "All women should have access to the education and means to limit their family size to the number of children they can financially and emotionally sustain. This foundation supports family planning programs because they promote health and well being not only for women, but also for their families and for the entire world." **Priorities:** *Civic & Public Affairs:* 4%. Public Policy. *Environment:* 23%. Planned parenthood services. *Note:* Total contributions made in fiscal 2000. **Typ. Recipients:** Family Planning, Health Organizations. **Geo. Dist:** U.S.-based organizations operating in Latin America.

★ 11377 ★ Essel Foundation

2500 Westchester Ave.
Purchase, NY 10577
Phone: (914)698-7133
Constance Lieber, President

Fnded: 1966. **Philosophy:** The Essel Foundation is primarily interested in supporting mental illness research. Regular contributions are made to support depression and schizophrenia treatment and research. Higher education is an additional area of interest. **Priorities:** *Arts & Humanities:* Less than 1%. Supports public radio. *Education:* 9%. Funds colleges and universities. *International:* 87%. Provides major support to the National Alliance for Research on Schizophrenia and Depression; also funds other mental health associations, research centers, and hospitals. *Note:* Total contributions made in fiscal 2000. **Typ. Recipients:** Cancer, Clinics/Medical Centers, Geriatric Health, Medical Research, Mental Health, Single-Disease Health Associations. **Geo. Dist:** New York, NY.

★ 11378 ★ Esther A. and Joseph Klingenstein Fund, Inc.

787 Seventh Ave., 6th Floor
New York, NY 10019-6016
Phone: (212)492-6181 **Fax:** (212)492-7007
John Klingenstein, President

Fnded: 1946. **Philosophy:** The Fund's major interests are in two program areas: neuroscience and independent secondary education. The primary focus of the neuroscience program is the annual fellowship awards to young investigators (up to ten a year) doing basic research in neuroscience, specifically related to the etiology of epilepsy. In independent secondary education, major support is for the development of faculty members and administrators through programs at the Klingenstein Center for Independent Education at Teachers College, Columbia University. Grants are also made to organizations concerned with the separation of church and state; animal-based research for the advancement of medicine; and prevention of teenage pregnancy. The directors continue to support institutions in which they are personally involved. **Priorities:** *Arts & Humanities:* About 15%. Museums and libraries. *Education:* 62%. Support independent secondary education and the Klingenstein Fellowships. *Environment:* 1%. Children's Aid Society. *International:* About 13%. Support for neuroscience/epilepsy research and animal-based medical research. *Religion:* Less than 1%. Cold Spring Harbor Laboratory Association. **Typ. Recipients:** Adolescent Health Issues, Cancer, Children's Health/Hospitals, Clinics/Medical Centers, Family Planning, Hospitals, Hospitals (University Affiliated), Medical Education, Medical Research, Mental Health, People with Disabilities, Preventive Medicine/Wellness Organizations, Public Health, Research/Studies Institutes, Single-Disease Health Associations. **Geo. Dist:** nationally.

★ 11379 ★ Ethel Wilson Bowles and Robert Bowles Memorial Fund

301 East Colorado Boulevard, Suite 900
Pasadena, CA 91101
Phone: (626)796-9123
Emrys Ross, Trustee

Fnded: 1974. **Philosophy:** The foundation funds medical research, medical schools, and hospitals in California. **Priorities:** *Education:* 46%. Supports medical schools and an institute of technology. *International:* 54%. Funds hospitals and medical centers. *Note:* Total contributions made in 2000. **Typ. Recipients:** Children's Health/Hospitals, Hospitals, Hospitals (University Affiliated), Medical Education, Medical Research, Single-Disease Health Associations. **Geo. Dist:** CA.

★ 11380 ★ Eugene and Agnes E. Meyer Foundation

1400 16th St. Northwest, Suite 360
Washington, DC 20036-2217
Phone: (202)483-8294 **Fax:** (202)328-6850
Website: http://www.meyerfoundation.org
Julie Rogers, President

Fnded: 1944. **Philosophy:** The foundation hopes to improve the quality of life in Washington D.C., by supporting community efforts and promoting community responsibility. The foundation takes an innovative and comprehensive approach to the problems and changing needs of the Washington metropolitan area. "We recognize that human needs in a large metropolitan area are always changing and our grant-making process was designed with flexibility in mind." Grants are awarded in six broad program areas: neighborhood development and housing; community service; arts and humanities; education; health and mental health; and law and justice. **Priorities:** *Arts & Humanities:* 32%. Theater, museums, dance, and music. *Civic & Public Affairs:* 27%. Community service grants, neighborhood development/housing, and law and justice programs. *Education:* 6%. Recording for blind and dyslexic, high schools, and multicultural career programs. *Environment:* 19%. *International:* 16%. Mental health services, AIDS, and drug/alcohol treatment programs. *Note:* Total contributions made in 2000. **Typ. Recipients:** AIDS/HIV, Children's Health/Hospitals, Clinics/Medical Centers, Domestic Violence, Family Planning, Health Organizations, Health-General, Hospices, Long-Term Care, Mental Health, People with Disabilities, Prenatal Health Issues, Public Health, Substance Abuse. **Geo. Dist:** Washington, DC, metropolitan area; MD, suburban Maryland; VA, Northern Virginia.

★ 11381 ★ Eugene B. Casey Foundation

800 South Frederick Ave.
Suite 100
Gaithersburg, MD 20877
Phone: (301)948-4595 **Fax:** (301)948-9159
Betty Brown-Casey, Chairman, President & Treasurer

Fnded: 1981. **Philosophy:** "Grants are primarily restricted to the Maryland and Washington, D.C., area in amounts sufficient to have an impact, and generally limited to the same charitable activities as in the foundation's past years." Major support goes to organizations directly affiliated with the foundation, including the Casey Family Foundation at Washington College and the Eugene B. Casey Center for Diagnostic Cardiolology. Other foundation interests include hospices, mental health, family services, shelters, arts for the disabled and youth, and Washington, D.C., area colleges and universities. **Priorities:** *Arts & Humanities:* 33%. Supports the performing arts and public broadcasting services. *Civic & Public Affairs:* 21%. Supports affordable housing, public policy, Native American affairs, and human rights. *Education:* 13%. Supports educational programs, preparatory schools, colleges and universities, arts & humanities education, literacy, and architects education. *Environment:* 2%. Supports youth services, the homeless, the elderly, battered women, and substance abuse. *International:* 31%. Supports hospices, hospitals, medical centers, medical research, and eyes/blindness. *Note:* Total contributions made in fiscal 2000. **Typ. Recipients:** Cancer, Child Abuse, Children's Health/Hospitals, Clinics/Medical Centers, Domestic Violence, Emergency/Ambulance Services, Eyes/Blindness, Family Planning, Health Funds, Health Organizations, Heart, Hospices, Hospitals, Hospitals (University Affiliated), Medical Education, Medical Research, Mental Health, Nutrition, People with Disabilities, Substance Abuse. **Geo. Dist:** Washington, DC, including metropolitan area.

★ 11382 ★ Eugene M. Lang Foundation

535 5th Ave., Suite 906
New York, NY 10017
Phone: (212)949-4100 **Fax:** (212)286-8964
Eugene Lang, Contact

Fnded: 1963. **Philosophy:** The foundation typically supports education, the arts, health, and civic causes. **Priorities:** *Arts & Humanities:* 4%. Supports opera, theater, music, libraries, museums, and arts festivals. *Civic & Public Affairs:* Less than 1%. *Education:* 57%. Emphasis on colleges and universities. *Environment:* Less than 1%. *International:* 31%. Focus on New York Hospital Medical Center and pediatric cancer research. *Religion:* About 6%. American Museum of Natural History. *Note:* Total contributions made in 2000. **Typ. Recipients:** AIDS/HIV, Cancer, Children's Health/Hospitals, Clinics/Medical Centers, Health Organizations, Hospitals, Medical Rehabilitation, Mental Health. **Geo. Dist:** internationally; nationally; New York, NY.

★ 11383 ★ The Eugene McDermott Foundation

3808 Euclid
Dallas, TX 75205
Phone: (214)521-2924
Mary Cook, President

Fnded: 1972. **Philosophy:** The foundation traditionally has supported medical facilities, science, schools, the arts, educational programs, and cultural organizations. **Priorities:** *Arts & Humanities:* 71%. Supports libraries, music, museums, theater, opera, and dance. *Civic & Public Affairs:* 2%. Urban affairs, zoos, and botanical gardens. *Education:* 23%. Funds colleges and universities, private schools, education funds, and arts education. *Environment:* 3%. Supports youth and senior organizations. *Note:* Total contributions made in fiscal 2000. **Typ. Recipients:** AIDS/HIV, Cancer, Child Abuse, Children's Health/Hospitals, Clinics/Medical Centers, Domestic Violence, Emergency/Ambulance Services, Family Planning, Hospitals, Hospitals (University Affiliated), Medical Education, People with Disabilities, Prenatal Health Issues, Preventive Medicine/Wellness Organizations, Public Health, Single-Disease Health Associations, Substance Abuse, Transplant Networks/Donor Banks. **Geo. Dist:** Dallas, TX.

★ 11384 ★ Eva L. and Joseph M. Bruening Foundation

1422 Euclid Ave., Suite 627
Cleveland, OH 44115-1901
Phone: (216)621-2632 **Fax:** (216)621-8198
Website: http://www.fmscleveland.com/bruening
Janet Narten, Executive Director

Fnded: 1988. **Philosophy:** The mission of the foundation is to enhance the quality of life in Cuyahoga County, OH. Priority is given to initiatives designed to educate youth, comfort the aged, and provide encouragement and support to the disabled and disadvantaged. The foundation supports practical programs that meet clearly defined community needs in a creative and efficient manner. The foundation welcomes grant requests for capital, start-up operations, and program support from tax-exempt, non-profit organizations whose goals and objectives match those of the foundation. **Priorities:** *Arts & Humanities:* (Arts/Culture) 5%. Supports dance, theater, historical societies, and cultural arts programs. *Civic & Public Affairs:* (Public/Society Benefit) 5%. Funds community programs, nonprofit management, and urban development. *Education:* 14%. Funds secondary schools, education programs, literacy programs, and colleges and universities. *Environment:* 50%. Supports community services, homes, senior and children's services, services for the homeless, food banks, domestic violence organizations, and crisis centers. *International:* 22%. Primarily funds clinics, pediatric/adolescent health and women's health. *Note:* Total contributions made in 2000. **Typ. Recipients:** Adolescent Health Issues, AIDS/HIV, Alzheimers Disease, Cancer, Children's Health/Hospitals, Clinics/Medical Centers, Domestic Violence, Emergency/Ambulance Services, Eyes/Blindness, Family Planning, Geriatric Health, Health Organizations, Hospices, Hospitals, Long-Term Care, Nursing Services, People with Disabilities, Prenatal Health Issues, Preventive Medicine/Wellness Organizations, Public Health, Research/Studies Institutes, Sexual Abuse, Single-Disease Health Associations, Speech & Hearing, Substance Abuse. **Geo. Dist:** OH, Cuyahoga County.

★ 11385 ★ Evan and Marion Helfaer Foundation

735 North Water St.
Milwaukee, WI 53202
Phone: (414)287-7184 **Fax:** (414)276-0172
Pat Denning, Co-Trustee & Administrator

Fnded: 1971. **Philosophy:** The foundation makes grants across the major categories of support. Educational funding favors universities, colleges, medical and engineering schools, and private high schools. Health service support goes to hospitals and cancer and blood centers. Funding for the arts includes performing arts, museums, and historic preservation. Social service interests include youth organizations, united funds, and community centers. The foundation will make grants to other recipient areas as well. **Priorities:** *Arts & Humanities:* 16%. Focus on museums, libraries, arts funds, theater, and music. *Civic & Public Affairs:* 34%. Funds stadiums and community projects. *Education:* 19%. Primary and secondary schools and colleges and universities are funded. *Environment:* 23%. Grants are made to youth organizations, united funds, child welfare, services. *International:* 3%. Support goes to a health education center and hospitals. *Note:* Total contributions made in fiscal 2001. **Typ. Recipients:** Cancer, Child Abuse, Children's Health/Hospitals, Clinics/Medical Centers, Geriatric Health, Health Organizations, Heart, Hospitals, Medical Education, Medical Research, Mental Health, Nursing Services, People with Disabilities, Public Health, Single-Disease Health Associations, Substance Abuse, Transplant Networks/Donor Banks. **Geo. Dist:** Milwaukee, WI.

★ 11386 ★ Evelyn and Walter Haas, Jr. Fund

One Market Landmark, Suite 400
San Francisco, CA 94105
Phone: (415)856-1400 **Fax:** (415)856-1500
Email: info@haasjr.org
Website: http://www.haasjr.org
Clayton Juan, Grants Administrator

Fnded: 1953. **Philosophy:** The Evelyn and Walter Haas, Jr. Fund was established to support cultural, educational, and human welfare programs that enrich the lives of residents of the San Francisco area. The 2000 program guidelines reflect the direction of the fund's future grantmaking. Currently, the fund's four program areas are "Strengthening Children, Youth, Families, and the Elderly; Strengthening Neighborhoods; Promoting Diversity and Inclusiveness; and Enhancing Nonprofit Leadership and Governance." "Strengthening Neighborhoods" focuses on efforts to stabilize and improve urban neighborhoods, with a particular emphasis on community development through programs that involve residents and promote leaders who can energize local improvements. In order to reweave community and home safety nets, especially in low-income neighborhoods, "Strengthening Children, Youth, Families, and the Elderly" supports programs that nurture the young to become healthy, productive, caring adults, and enhance elders' well-being and encourage their self-sufficiency. The fund helps ensure that youth have opportunities to enhance their personal development during nonschool hours through activities that include recreation, sports, education, and community service; develops and enhances community-based prevention programs that enable parents to play active roles in their children's development, and foster cooperation between home and school; supports school-linked and community-based approaches that coordinate and leverage resources to effect enduring, systemic improvements in services for healthy child and youth development; and enhances the quality of life for the elderly by strengthening a continuum of independent living services.

"Promoting Diversity and Inclusiveness" focuses on promoting a sense of community that respects and embraces diversity with particular interest in strategies designed to overcome barriers caused by racism, seism, and homophobia. Work is done in three arenas: building community; affirming pluralism; and fair and equitable treatment. "Enhancing Nonprofit Leadership and Governance" looks to enhance the effectiveness of local nonprofit groups working in the Fund's interest areas through leadership development, management and technical assistance, and public policy. **Priorities:** *Arts & Humanities:* 19%. Supports museums, music, theater, and public broadcasting. *Civic & Public Affairs:* 51%. Funds neighborhood and economic development, nonprofit administration, civil liberties, parks, and housing. *Education:* 7%. Supports universities, mentoring, educational funds, and secondary schools. *Environment:* 16%. Funds YMCA, children and youth programs, neighborhood centers, and food banks and shelters. *International:* 1%. *Note:* Total contributions made in 2000. **Typ. Recipients:** Alzheimers Disease, Child Abuse, Clinics/Medical Centers, Domestic Violence, Geriatric Health, Health Organizations, Home-Care Services, Hospices, Hospitals, Long-Term Care, Mental Health, Nursing Services, Nutrition, People with Disabilities, Research/Studies Institutes, Research/Studies Institutes. **Geo. Dist:** CA, Alameda County; CA, San Francisco County.

★ 11387 ★ Ewing Halsell Foundation

711 Navarro, Suite 537
San Antonio, TX 78205
Phone: (210)223-2649 **Fax:** (210)271-9089
Gilbert Denman, Jr., Trustee, Chairman of the Board

Fnded: 1957. **Philosophy:** The foundation requires that all contributions be made to help improve the quality of life for Texas citizens. "The foundation makes most of its grants in the San Antonio area and in those Southwestern parts of Texas where a large part of the income producing assets of the foundation are located, and where it can best evaluate needs for assistance." The foundation believes strongly in public involvement and fostering a wide range of philanthropic support. Therefore, matching funds are encouraged but not always required. The foundation may make a challenge grant to stimulate other financial participation. challenge grant to stimulate other financial participation. **Priorities:** *Arts & Humanities:* 51%. Supports public broadcasting, symphony and museum. *Civic & Public Affairs:* 5%. Supports community foundations, housing, zoos and parks. *Education:* 15%. Support public and private schools. *Environment:* 15%. Supports United Way, youth and family services. *International:* 8%. Supports medical research. *Note:* Total contributions made in fiscal 1999. **Typ. Recipients:** AIDS/HIV, Cancer, Children's Health/Hospitals, Clinics/Medical Centers, Domestic Violence, Emergency/Ambulance Services, Family Planning, Geriatric Health, Health Organizations, Heart, Hospitals, Medical Research, Nursing Services, People with Disabilities, Public Health, Single-Disease Health Associations, Substance Abuse. **Geo. Dist:** San Antonio, TX.

★ 11388 ★ Ewing Marion Kauffman Foundation

4801 Rockhill Rd.
Kansas City, MO 64110-2046
Phone: (816)932-1000 **Fax:** (816)932-1440
Email: info@emkf.org
Website: http://www.emkf.org
Sharon Cohen, Vice President

Fnded: 1966. **Philosophy:** "The Ewing Marion Kauffman Foundation is a private foundation that works toward the vision of self-sufficient people in healthy communities. Our mission is to research and identify unfulfilled needs of society and to develop, implement and/or fund breakthrough solutions that have a lasting impact and offer people a choice and hope for the future." "Focusing on youth Development and entrepreneurship, the Foundation works toward five outcomes. . .that comprise a strategic 'filter' through which we evaluate all funding opportunities: Children enter school prepared to succeed. Children and youth make a successful transition through childhood and adolescence to responsible adulthood. Youth and adults have the knowledge, skills and values to make entrepreneurship a choice for the future. Entrepreneurs have the knowledge, skills and values to accelerate job and wealth creation in America. Not-for-profit leaders have the entrepreneurial knowledge, skills and values to advance their organization's social missions." "Through partnerships, the Foundation believes it can most effectively support social and economic solutions that support children, their families and communities, and accelerate the development of entrepreneurship in America." **Priorities:** *Arts & Humanities:* 4%. Supports the city museum. *Civic & Public Affairs:* 60%. Funds public policy and entrepreneurial training institutes and education. *Education:* 27%. Funds higher education and educational development programs. *Environment:* 5%. Supports youth development group, including community and economic development centered around youth concerns. *International:* 4%. Supports a health center. *Note:* Total contributions made in 2000. **Typ. Recipients:** Clinics/Medical Centers, Health Policy/Cost Containment, Mental Health, Prenatal Health Issues, Substance Abuse. **Geo. Dist:** Kansas City, MO.

★ 11389 ★ F. B. Heron Foundation

100 Broadway, 17th Floor
New York, NY 10005
Phone: (212)404-1800 **Fax:** (212)404-1805
Website: http://www.heronfdn.org
Sharon King, President

Fnded: 1992. **Priorities:** *Civic & Public Affairs:* 79%. Funds housing, minority and urban affairs, economic development, and community foundations. *Education:* 9%. Supports educational funds and higher education. *Environment:* 10%. Supports shelters, food banks, and services for families and children. *Note:* Total contributions made in 2000. **Typ. Recipients:** AIDS/HIV, Domestic Violence, Emergency/Ambulance Services, Home-Care Services, Research/Studies Institutes, Substance Abuse.

★ 11390 ★ F. J. O'Neill Charitable Corp.

3550 Lander Rd.
Cleveland, OH 44124
Phone: (216)464-2121 **Fax:** (216)464-1517
Hugh O'Neill, President

Fnded: 1979. **Philosophy:** The corporation's main concerns are higher education and religion. Colleges and universities are funded primarily, as well as churches and religious organizations in Ohio. Of particular interest to the corporation are local concerns and self-help projects. "Applications to the Corporation are considered on their merits. Need and the good to be accomplished are prime considerations." **Priorities:** *Arts & Humanities:* 2%. Museums, historical societies, and theaters. *Civic & Public Affairs:* 12%. Foundations and housing. *Education:* 55%. Supports private precollege education. *Environment:* 8%. Gives to youth concerns, drug abuse programs, and united funds. *International:* 8%. Health care facilities. *Religion:* 4%. *Note:* Total contributions made in 2000. **Typ. Recipients:** Cancer, Children's Health/Hospitals, Clinics/Medical Centers, Emergency/Ambulance Services, Eyes/Blindness, Geriatric Health, Health Organizations, Health-General, Heart, Home-Care Services, Hospices, Hospitals, Long-Term Care, Medical Rehabilitation, Medical Research, Nursing Services, People with Disabilities, Public Health, Single-Disease Health Associations, Substance Abuse. **Geo. Dist:** OH, Eastern Ohio.

★ 11391 ★ F. M. Kirby Foundation

17 DeHart St.
PO Box 151
Morristown, NJ 07963-0151
Phone: (973)538-4800
Website: http://fdncenter.org/grantmaker/kirby/
S. Kirby, Executive Director

Fnded: 1931. **Philosophy:** The foundation provides funds to organizations in areas where family members live and work, and to organizations in which Fred M. Kirby, the original donor, had an interest. The foundation states its philosophy as follows: "A distinctive feature of American life, dating back to colonial times, is the remarkable richness and diversity of its voluntary, non-profit sector. Although government has become alarmingly involved in people's lives over the last few decades, we believe people should be encouraged to solve their own problems exclusive of government aid, and on the local level. Private philanthropy is there to help them." **Priorities:** *Arts & Humanities:* 16%. Provides funding to museums, performing arts, historical preservation, and theater. *Civic & Public Affairs:* 2%. Supports individual rights organizations, zoos, legal affairs, and population interests. *Education:* 51%. Funds colleges and universities and private schools. *Environment:* 4%. Funds the United Way, family planning and family services, youth organizations, and the prevention of domestic violence. *International:* 25%. Supports medical research, hospitals, single-disease health associations, and health funds. *Note:* Total contributions made in 2000. **Typ. Recipients:** AIDS/HIV, Alzheimers Disease, Arthritis, Cancer, Children's Health/Hospitals, Domestic Violence, Emergency/Ambulance Services, Eyes/Blindness, Family Planning, Geriatric Health, Health Funds, Health Organizations, Health-General, Heart, Hospices, Hospitals, Medical Education, Medical Rehabilitation, Medical Research, Nursing Services, People with Disabilities, Public Health, Respiratory, Single-Disease Health Associations, Substance Abuse, Transplant Networks/Donor Banks. **Geo. Dist:** some giving nationally; Morristown, NJ; Hillsborough, NC; Wilkes-Barre, PA.

★ 11392 ★ F. R. Bigelow Foundation

55 5th St. E, Suite 600
Saint Paul, MN 55101-1797
Phone: (651)224-5463 **Fax:** (651)224-8123
Email: inbox@saintpaulfoundation.org
Website: http://www.saintpaulfoundation.org
Paul Verret, President

Fnded: 1934. **Philosophy:** "The F.R. Bigelow Foundation is willing to consider grant applications from all properly qualified nonprofit corporations. Historically, the primary areas of interest have been education, social service, humanities and the arts. The Children, Families, and Community Initiative (CFCI) was established by the trustees in 1990 with a five-year grant of $2.5 million. The purpose of CFCI is to address the needs of children living in the Frogtown and Summit-University neighborhoods in the context of family and community. This program is overseen by an active, multi-cultural Steering Committee of persons who live and/or work in the two neighborhoods. In 1995, the Trustees authorized a second five-year grant of $2.5 million to continue the work of CFCI through the year 2000. In 1998 a majority of CFCI's efforts were devoted to improving the grantmaking process, strengthening internal operations and developing a long-range plan for beyond the year 2000. Over half of grant dollars were directed toward youth leadership, and academic development, collaboration between community-based organizations serving youth, after school and summer enrichment, community building, and neighborhood entrepreneurs." 1998 Annual Report **Priorities:** *Arts & Humanities:* 20%. Performing arts, museums, and historical societies. *Civic & Public Affairs:* 16% Crime prevention efforts, community foundations, and urban affairs. *Education:* 15%. Public education, universities, and lifelong learning support. *Environment:* 21%. Primarily supports youth and family programs. *International:* 2%. Support and expansion of health programs. *Religion:* 10%. Funds a science museum. *Note:* Total contributions made in 2000. **Typ. Recipients:** Alzheimers Disease, Cancer, Children's Health/Hospitals, Emergency/Ambulance Services, Family Planning, Health Organizations, Health-General, Hospices, Hospitals, Medical Rehabilitation, Mental Health, People with Disabilities, Preventive Medicine/Wellness Organizations, Public Health, Research/Studies Institutes, Single-Disease Health Associations, Substance Abuse. **Geo. Dist:** St. Paul, MN.

★ 11393 ★ Fan Fox and Leslie R. Samuels Foundation

350 Fifth Ave., Suite 4301
New York, NY 10118

Phone: (212)239-3030 **Fax:** (212)239-3039
Email: info@samuels.org
Website: http://www.samuels.org
Joseph Mitchell, President, Treasurer, and Director

Fnded: 1981. **Philosophy:** The foundation is generally interested in funding organizations in the metropolitan New York area dealing with the performing arts and health. In the performing arts, particular interests are music, especially opera, ballet, dance, theater and programs for young artists. Health-related grants are directed toward improving the delivery of health services to the people of New York City, particularly children and the elderly. **Priorities:** *Arts & Humanities:* 53%. Primarily supports performing arts, including theater, ballet, dance, and music. *Education:* 7%. Supports medical and arts education. *Environment:* 4%. Supports human service organizations. *International:* 36%. Funds hospitals and medical centers for the delivery of health services, home-care services, and geriatric health. *Note:* Total contributions made in fiscal 2001. **Typ. Recipients:** Adolescent Health Issues, AIDS/HIV, Alzheimers Disease, Cancer, Children's Health/Hospitals, Clinics/Medical Centers, Diabetes, Geriatric Health, Health Organizations, Health Policy/Cost Containment, Heart, Home-Care Services, Hospices, Hospitals, Long-Term Care, Medical Education, Medical Rehabilitation, Medical Research, Mental Health, Nursing Services, People with Disabilities, Prenatal Health Issues, Public Health, Research/Studies Institutes, Respiratory, Substance Abuse. **Geo. Dist:** New York, NY, metropolitan area.

★ 11394 ★ Fannie E. Rippel Foundation

180 Mt. Airy Rd., Suite 200
Basking Ridge, NJ 07920-2021
Phone: (908)766-0404
Email: rippel@gti.net
Website: http://www.fdncenter.org/grantmaker/rippel
Edward Probert, President & Chief Executive Officer

Fnded: 1953. **Philosophy:** The objectives of the Fannie E. Rippel Foundation were specified in the will of Julius S. Rippel and in the foundation's certificate of incorporation. These objectives are "to aid, assist, fund, equip, and provide for maintenance of corporations, institutions or associations, organizations or societies which are maintained for the relief and care of aged women; to provide and furnish funds for the erection of...hospitals; to provide and furnish funds for the equipment of...hospitals either in whole or in part; to aid or provide for the maintenance of hospitals in whole or in part; to provide and furnish funds for corporations, institutions and other organizations organized, maintained and existing for the purpose of treatment of and/or research concerning heart disease; to provide and furnish funds for corporations, institutions and other organizations organized, maintained and existing for the purpose of treatment of and/or research concerning cancer." Fannie E. Rippel Foundation Fiscal 2000 IRS Form 990 The foundation states that it is also interested in strategies to reach under-served rural and urban populations, women's health, prevention and strategies to change the behavior of populations including research and access to preventative care, humanistic medicine and mind-body-spirit connections as relating to the healing process. **Priorities:** *Arts & Humanities:* 3%. *Education:* 36%. *International:* 61%. *Note:* Total contributions made in fiscal 2000. **Typ. Recipients:** Cancer, Children's Health/Hospitals, Clinics/Medical Centers, Diabetes, Emergency/Ambulance Services, Eyes/Blindness, Geriatric Health, Health Organizations, Health-General, Heart, Hospitals, Hospitals (University Affiliated), Medical Education, Medical Rehabilitation, Medical Research, Public Health, Research/Studies Institutes. **Geo. Dist:** nationally; Middle Atlantic Seaboard.

★ 11395 ★ Faye McBeath Foundation

1020 North Broadway
Milwaukee, WI 53202
Phone: (414)272-6262 **Fax:** (414)272-6235
Email: info@fayemcbeath.org
Website: http://www.fayemcbeath.org
Sarah Dean, Executive Director

Fnded: 1964. **Philosophy:** Miss McBeath stipulated specific guidelines when she established the foundation. Under the terms of the trust, grants are made to organizations within the state of Wisconsin and for the following purposes: to promote research and education in the fields of medical science and public health; to provide medical, nursing, and hospital care for the sick and disabled; to promote child welfare; to promote research in civic and government affairs directed toward improved efficiency of local government; and to disseminate the results of the research. Miss McBeath said that "the foundation was to spend at least 20 percent of its disbursements each decade on each of the first four categories." Currently, the foundation directs special attention to projects consistent with the following priorities: *Welfare of Children:* Grants in this area help to strengthen the family, as the key factor in education, motivation, and development of children, including programs which improve parenting skills and reduce the incidence of child abuse and family violence; to enhance the development and school readiness of preschool children; to stress the development and well-being of children's creativity, imagination, and self-esteem, with emphasis on learning skills and development; to promote experiences which bring excitement and challenge to the learning process and to dramatize the rewards of educational success; to develop quality educational initiatives that prepare youth for employment; to enhance the quality of precollegiate education; and to address special youth problems, such as adolescent pregnancy, unemployment, and teen suicide. *Health Care and Education:* Funding is made to promote improvement in the health of high-risk populations, especially infants, the elderly, and the poor through projects designed to improve prenatal care, encourage healthy lifestyles, and prevent disease; to provide and expand alternatives to institutional and inpatient care; to facilitate access to comprehensive medical care for elderly, youth, minorities, and the indigent; to enhance the development of the Milwaukee Regional Center as a viable resource for the community and state; and to improve the capability of local universities and colleges to educate health-care providers. *Care of Elderly Persons:* Support is given to sustain older persons in their homes and neighborhoods by strengthening alternatives to institutional care, such as support services, special housing, and home care; to promote independence of older adults and activities for them in education, volunteer work, and employment; to stimulate social interaction between children, youth, and older adults; to strengthen the older person's family and informal support systems, such as respite care and friendly visitor programs; and to increase access to existing community services for isolated older adults. **Priorities:** *Arts & Humanities:* 8%. *Civic & Public Affairs:* 32%. *Education:* 10%. *Environment:* 32%. Supports child care, youth services, planned parenthood, Young Women's Christian Association, and the elderly. *International:* 12%. Funds hospitals, specialty clinics, and disease and disorder concerns. *Note:* Total contributions made in 2000. **Typ. Recipients:** AIDS/HIV, Alzheimers Disease, Child Abuse, Children's Health/Hospitals, Clinics/Medical Centers, Domestic Violence, Eyes/Blindness, Family Planning, Geriatric Health, Health Organizations, Health Policy/Cost Containment, Hospices, Hospitals, Long-Term Care, Medical Education, Medical Rehabilitation, Mental Health, Nursing Services, People with Disabilities, Public Health, Single-Disease Health Associations, Speech & Hearing, Substance Abuse, Transplant Networks/Donor Banks. **Geo. Dist:** WI, particularly the Milwaukee metropolitan area.

★ 11396 ★ Feldman Foundation

Box 1046
Dallas, TX 75221
Phone: (214)689-4337 **Fax:** (214)689-5886
Robert Feldman, Trustee

Fnded: 1964. **Philosophy:** Since its inception, the foundation has supported Jewish welfare agencies and organizations that show an interest in Israel. **Priorities:** *Education:* 14%. Includes colleges and universities. *Environment:* 1%. Supports senior citizens and United Way organizations. *Note:* Total contributions made in 2001. **Typ. Recipients:** Family Planning, Hospitals, Hospitals (University Affiliated), Long-Term Care, Medical Education, Medical Research, Preventive Medicine/Wellness Organizations, Single-Disease Health Associations. **Geo. Dist:** national organizations for support of Israel; TX.

★ 11397 ★ Field Foundation of Illinois

200 South Wacker Dr., Suite 3860
Chicago, IL 60606
Phone: (312)831-0910 **Fax:** (312)831-0961
Email: hlindsey@fieldfoundation.org
Handy Lindsey, Jr., President

Fnded: 1960. **Philosophy:** "The Field Foundation seeks to provide support for community, civic, and cultural organizations in the Chicago area, enabling both new and established programs to test innovations, to expand proven strengths, or to address specific, time-limited operational needs." **Priorities:** *Arts & Humanities:* 17%. Supports art institutes, galleries, and the opera. *Civic & Public Affairs:* 23%. Supports park development, housing, and community projects. *Education:* 21%. Supports literacy, public schools, and universities. *Environment:* 23%. Supports YMCA, youth services, Hull House, and homeless services. *International:* 20%. Supports HIV facility and health care programs. *Note:* Total contributions made in fiscal 2001. **Typ. Recipients:** AIDS/HIV, Children's Health/Hospitals, Clinics/Medical Centers, Domestic Violence, Emergency/Ambulance Services, Health Organizations, Heart, Hospitals, Hospitals (University Affiliated), Medical Education, Medical Rehabilitation, People with Disabilities, Prenatal Health Issues, Public Health, Sexual Abuse, Substance Abuse. **Geo. Dist:** Chicago, IL, including metropolitan area.

★ 11398 ★ Figtree Foundation

PO Box 130843
Birmingham, AL 35213
Phone: (205)879-0712 **Fax:** (205)879-6382
Jo Morrison, President

Fnded: 1986. **Philosophy:** The Figtree Foundation primarily supports religion, targeting a variety of Jewish causes. The foundation also focuses donations on education. Minor interests include civic affairs, health associations, social services, and the arts. **Priorities:** *Arts & Humanities:* 9%. Funds public broadcasting, libraries, and music. *Civic & Public Affairs:* 2%. Supports public policy and advocacy. *Education:* 13%. Primarily Jewish colleges and schools. *Environment:* 4%. Community support. *International:* 9%. Funds single-disease associations. *Note:* Total contributions made in 2000. **Typ. Recipients:** Cancer, Health-General, Hospices, Medical Rehabilitation, Medical Research, People with Disabilities, Single-Disease Health Associations, Substance Abuse. **Geo. Dist:** Birmingham, AL.

★ 11399 ★ First Fruit

14 Corporate Plz.
Newport Beach, CA 92660
Phone: (949)640-9090
Email: info@firstfruit.org
Website: http://www.firstfruit.org
Robert Martin, Executive Director

Fnded: 1976. **Philosophy:** The foundation's main interests are religion and education. Religious support varies from prison fellowships to a variety of religious affiliations and beliefs. Usually, religious gifts have international interests. Educational support is mainly centered on giving to seminaries with a worldwide scope. The foundation supports other areas of philanthropy only if it involves religious activities or international concerns. **Priorities:** *Education:* 2%. Religious education. *Note:* Total contributions made in 2001. **Typ. Recipients:** People with Disabilities. **Geo. Dist:** internationally.

★ 11400 ★ Flatley Foundation

50 Braintree Hill Office Park, Suite 400
Braintree, MA 02184-8754
Phone: (781)848-2000 **Fax:** (781)849-4400
Thomas Flatley, Trustee

Fnded: 1982. **Priorities:** *Civic & Public Affairs:* 36%. Major support for Fidelity Charitable Gift Fund. Also funds legal affairs, housing, and Irish American organizations. *Education:* 4%. Supports a scholarship fund and higher education. *Environment:* 1%. Supports United Way and human services. *International:* 2%. Funds hospitals and health centers. *Note:* Total contributions made in 2001. **Typ. Recipients:** Cancer, Diabetes, Emergency/Ambulance Services, Health Organizations, Hospitals, People with Disabilities, Prenatal Health Issues, Public Health, Substance Abuse. **Geo. Dist:** MA.

★ 11401 ★ Fleming Foundation

500 W 7th St., Suite 1007
Fort Worth, TX 76102-4732
Phone: (817)335-3741 **Fax:** (817)338-4844
G. Louden, CPA

Fnded: 1936. **Philosophy:** The goal of the foundation is to perpetuate Mr. Fleming's community and charitable interests, primarily focusing on educational institutions, the arts, and health services. The foundation also reports that it will no longer provide grants to religious organizations. **Priorities:** *Arts & Humanities:* 54%. Supports performing arts and music. *Education:* 5%. Supports private schools. *Environment:* 40%. Supports boys and girls clubs. *Note:* Total contributions made in 2001. **Typ. Recipients:** AIDS/HIV, Alzheimers Disease, Cancer, Children's Health/Hospitals, Clinics/Medical Centers, Eyes/Blindness, Family Planning, Health Organizations, Heart, Hospitals, Medical Rehabilitation, Mental Health, People with Disabilities, Research/Studies Institutes, Single-Disease Health Associations, Substance Abuse. **Geo. Dist:** Fort Worth, TX, including Tarrant County.

★ 11402 ★ Fletcher Jones Foundation

523 W Sixth St., Suite 301
Los Angeles, CA 90014
Phone: (213)943-4646 **Fax:** (213)943-4648
Email: chris@fletcherjonesfdn.org
Christine Sisley, Executive Director

Fnded: 1969. **Philosophy:** According to the foundation, "the trustees of the foundation give consideration to charitable, scientific, literary, and educational areas, plus a minor portion to general-purpose grants. However, from time to time, the trustees may give special emphasis to any one of the above-listed areas. At present, grants are given primarily to private colleges and universities, particularly those in California." The foundation's 1996 annual report stated: "Since the Foundation began making grants about 25 years ago, we have given special emphasis to the private colleges and universities in California. Earlier this year, the Trustees approved a change in that policy. You might call it a slight change. A majority of the Trustees, after considerable thought and discussion, became persuaded that some of our support for education at the college level should go to the public institutions and, in particular, to the University of California." **Priorities:** *Arts & Humanities:* 1%. Supports the performing arts, public broadcasting, museums, and libraries. *Civic & Public Affairs:* 1%. *Education:* 94%. Largely funds scholarships and fellowships at colleges and universities in California. *Environment:* 3%. Funds scouting, children's welfare, and people with disabilities. *International:* 1%. Supports health associations, hospitals, and speech & hearing. *Note:* Total contributions made in 2000. **Typ. Recipients:** Children's Health/Hospitals, Clinics/Medical Centers, Domestic Violence, Eyes/Blindness, Health Organizations, Health-General, Hospices, Hospitals, Medical Research, Nursing Services, People with Disabilities, Public Health, Research/Studies Institutes, Single-Disease Health Associations. **Geo. Dist:** CA.

★ 11403 ★ Flinn Foundation

1802 North Central Ave.
Phoenix, AZ 85004
Phone: (602)744-6800 **Fax:** (602)744-6815
Email: info@flinn.org
Website: http://www.flinn.org
John Murphy, Executive Director

Fnded: 1965. **Philosophy:** "The Flinn Foundation fulfills its mission to improve the quality of life primarily by serving as a resource for health and health care in Arizona. It takes a proactive approach to its grantmaking. Under this approach, the Foundation often formulates general concepts or program models designed to impact a specific need or problem, then solicits funding requests from organizations in specified fields of interest. Grant recipients are largely chosen through (1) a Request for Proposals (RFP) which is sent to a wide group of organizations believed to be eligible to apply for grant funds and identified as having an interest in the subject area targeted by the Foundation; or (2) an invited proposal process in which the Foundation invites one or more organizations to apply for funding for a specific activity or project." Flinn Foundation web site **Priorities:** *Arts & Humanities:* 26%. Supports symphony orchestras, theater, opera, dance, art museums, arts councils, and children's theater programs. *Civic & Public Affairs:* 3%. Gives to community foundations, community action, and nonprofit management programs. *Education:* 56%. Supports state universities and the Flinn Scholars program. *Environment:* 4%. Funds community services, child welfare organizations, and abuse/violence prevention. *International:* 11%. Supports pediatric health programs, hospitals, hospice, single-disease health associations, health care cost containment initiatives, health foundations, and mental health. *Note:* Total contributions made in 2000. **Typ. Recipients:** Adolescent Health Issues, AIDS/HIV, Alzheimers Disease, Child Abuse, Children's Health/Hospitals, Clinics/Medical Centers, Family Planning, Geriatric Health, Health Organizations, Health Policy/Cost Containment, Heart, Hospices, Hospitals, Medical Education, Medical Research, Medical Training, Nursing Services, People with Disabilities, Prenatal Health Issues, Public Health, Research/Studies Institutes, Sexual Abuse, Substance Abuse. **Geo. Dist:** AZ.

★ 11404 ★ The Florence Gould Foundation

80 Pine St., Ste. 1701
New York, NY 10005-1702
Phone: (212)701-3400 **Fax:** (212)269-5420
John Young, President

Fnded: 1957. **Philosophy:** The Florence J. Gould Foundation is primarily interested in promoting Franco-American friendship and understanding. **Priorities:** *Arts & Humanities:* 38%. Supports museums, libraries, opera, orchestra, and theater. *Civic & Public Affairs:* 2%. Supports gardens and parks. *Education:* 25%. Supports arts and humanities education, colleges, and universities. *Environment:* 2%. Funds human services. *Religion:* 3%. Supports marine biology. *Note:* Total contributions made in 1999. **Typ. Recipients:** AIDS/HIV, Alzheimers Disease, Children's Health/Hospitals, Clinics/Medical Centers, Geriatric Health, Medical Education, People with Disabilities. **Geo. Dist:** nationally.

★ 11405 ★ Florence V. Burden Foundation

10 East 53rd St., 32nd Floor
New York, NY 10022
Phone: (212)872-1150 **Fax:** (212)872-1149
Marjorie Lipkin, Executive Director

Fnded: 1967. **Philosophy:** The Burden Foundation's approach is not just to make grants, but to make productive grants. Initial grants are often applied research projects designed to advance knowledge and practice in the foundation's fields or to demonstrate that a significant advance is feasible. The foundation is interested in issues of broad national importance, looking for projects on the cutting edge of social innovation that will demonstrate new ways to solve basic or enduring problems. The foundation's overall theme is to strengthen families and communities. It has changed priorities replacing crime and justice with a focus on children while continuing its focus on the elderly with its aging program area. For aging, the foundation addresses the following: to support family caregivers, both those caring for frail elders as well as elders caring for grandchildren; and to benefit elders and children, families and communities through intergenerational programs. For children, the foundation addresses the following: to intervene early in children's lives, to build their self-esteem and socialization skills, and to prevent abuse and violence. The foundation will focus on children and youth up to 18 years of age. **Typ. Recipients:** AIDS/HIV, Alzheimers Disease, Child Abuse, Children's Health/Hospitals, Clinics/Medical Centers, Diabetes, Domestic Violence, Emergency/Ambulance Services, Eyes/Blindness, Family Planning, Geriatric Health, Health Organizations, Health-General, Hospices, Hospitals, Long-Term Care, People with Disabilities, Single-Disease Health Associations, Substance Abuse, Transplant Networks/Donor Banks. **Geo. Dist:** Northeast; NY.

★ 11406 ★ Foellinger Foundation

520 East Berry St.
Fort Wayne, IN 46802
Phone: (260)422-2900 **Fax:** (260)422-9436
Email: info@foelinger.org
Cheryl Taylor, President

Fnded: 1958. **Philosophy:** The Foundation has a broad range of interests that include Youth and Families, Education and the Arts, Community Development, and Human Services. "The Foundation's Board of Directors emphasizes grant making to support programs and projects that focus on young people and their families, especially the economically disadvantaged. The Foundation encourages applicant organizations to develop linkages with nonprofit agencies and governmental entities in order to more effectively deliver services. Because the Foundation's resources are limited, the Board seeks funding partnerships to provide the maximum leverage for grant effectiveness." The foundation prefers seeking worthy causes rather than merely responding to solicitations. **Priorities:** *Arts & Humanities:* 8%. Supports museums, theaters, and symphonies. *Civic & Public Affairs:* 11%. Funds parks, recreation projects, and community partnerships. *Education:* 48%. Supports universities and public schools. *Environment:* 18%. Supports the United Way, summer park programs, and youth organizations. *International:* 5%. Primary funding goes toward cancer care, health clinics, AIDs prevention and education. *Note:* Contributions made in fiscal 2001. **Typ. Recipients:** AIDS/HIV, Clinics/Medical Centers, Domestic Violence, Health Organizations, Medical Rehabilitation, People with Disabilities, Preventive Medicine/Wellness Organizations, Public Health, Substance Abuse. **Geo. Dist:** Fort Wayne, IN, including Allen County.

★ 11407 ★ Fondren Foundation

PO Box 2558
Houston, TX 77252-8037
Phone: (713)216-4513
Ms. Martie Herrick, Assistant Secretary-Treasurer

Fnded: 1948. **Philosophy:** Traditionally, the foundation has focused on education, including higher education and private schools, and health. Major past health recipients have been the Ella F. Fondren Building, a part of Methodist Hospital, as well as university and community hospitals. The foundation also has given generously to the social services, the arts and humanities, and civic and public affairs. **Priorities:** *Arts & Humanities:* 11%. Museums, libraries, historic preservation, performing arts, and music. *Civic & Public Affairs:* 8%. Primarily for a zoo and a park. *Education:* 35%. Supports private primary and secondary schools and colleges and universities. *Environment:* 29%. Provides funding primarily for child welfare and youth organizations. *International:* 14%. Supports children's health and cardiac research. *Religion:* 2%. Supports a health science center and a nature center. *Note:* Total contributions made in fiscal 2001. **Typ. Recipients:** AIDS/HIV, Alzheimers Disease, Cancer, Children's Health/Hospitals, Clinics/Medical Centers, Emergency/Ambulance Services, Family Planning, Geriatric Health, Heart, Hospices, Hospitals, Medical Education, Medical Rehabilitation, Medical Research, Mental Health, People with Disabilities, Prenatal Health Issues, Public Health, Research/Studies Institutes, Single-Disease Health Associations, Speech & Hearing,

Substance Abuse, Transplant Networks/Donor Banks. **Geo. Dist:** nationally; Houston, TX.

★ 11408 ★ Ford Family Foundation
1600 Northwest Stewart Parkway
Roseburg, OR 97470
Phone: (541)957-5574 **Fax:** (541)957-5720
Website: http://www.tfff.org
Norman Smith, President

Fnded: 1957. **Philosophy:** Through grantmaking and internal initiative development, the Ford Family Foundation endeavors to help individuals, through organized learning opportunities, to be contributing and successful citizens; and, to support nonprofit activities, agencies and projects, with particular emphasis on mid-size and small communities in the state of Oregon and Siskiyou County, California. (Form 990 1998 Grant guidelines) **Priorities:** *Arts & Humanities:* 6%. Funds music, libraries, and the performing arts. *Civic & Public Affairs:* 14%. Supports housing, parks and gardens, municipalities/towns, and community foundations. *Education:* 36%. Supports scholarships through the Ford Scholars Program (three scholarship programs in the state of Oregon and Siskiyou County, California.) Foundation also funds grants for technology, colleges, and local school districts. Interests include purchasing computer equipment, literacy projects, athletic programs, and counseling work. *Environment:* 22%. Supports services for the handicapped, youth programs, homes, Young Men's Christian Association, and food distribution programs. *International:* 9%. Supports children's hospitals, medical centers, emergency care, and single-disease associations. *Religion:* 5%. Funds science museums. *Note:* Total contributions made in fiscal 2001. **Typ. Recipients:** Adolescent Health Issues, Cancer, Child Abuse, Children's Health/Hospitals, Clinics/Medical Centers, Domestic Violence, Emergency/Ambulance Services, Health Organizations, Health-General, Hospices, Hospitals, Mental Health, People with Disabilities, Prenatal Health Issues, Substance Abuse. **Geo. Dist:** CA, Siskiyou County; OR, rural communities only with population of 30,000 or fewer people.

★ 11409 ★ Ford Foundation
320 East 43rd St.
New York, NY 10017
Phone: (212)573-5000 **Fax:** (212)351-3677
Email: office-communications@fordfound.org
Website: http://www.fordfound.org
Barron Tenny, Secretary

Fnded: 1936. **Philosophy:** "The Ford Foundation is a resource for innovative people and institutions worldwide. Our goals are to: strengthen democratic values; reduce poverty and injustice; promote international cooperation; and advance human achievement." Ford Foundation Annual Report 2001 Program activities are supported primarily within the following broad categories: Asset Building and Community Development; Education, Media, Arts, and Culture; and Peace and Social Justice. Within these three broad categories, the Foundation also funds projects using film, television, and radio to explore public policy issues and uses a limited portion of its capital funds to make program-related investments in enterprises that will advance philanthropic purposes. **Priorities:** *Arts & Humanities:* 5%. Media, Arts and Culture–public broadcasting; promoting a free and responsible news media; independent production of film, video, and radio programming; and strengthening art institutions. *Civic & Public Affairs:* 16%. Community Development, Resource Development and Economic Development–with a focus on development finance and economic security; workforce development; environment and development; and community development. *Education:* 39%. Education, Knowledge and Religion–supports education reform; higher education and scholarship; and religion, society and culture educational initiatives. Major emphasis on education research and reform K-12. Made a substantial, one-time commitment above routine budget levels to establish the Ford Foundation International Fellowships Program. *International:* 8%. Human Development and Reproductive Health–funds efforts in the areas of children, youth and families; and sexuality and reproductive health. *Note:* Total contributions made in fiscal 2001. **Typ. Recipients:** AIDS/HIV, Domestic Violence, Family Planning, Health Organizations, Medical Research, Nutrition, Public Health, Substance Abuse. **Geo. Dist:** internationally, especially Asia, Latin America, and Africa; nationally.

★ 11410 ★ Forest Foundation
820 A St., Suite 345
Tacoma, WA 98402
Phone: (253)627-1634 **Fax:** (253)627-6249
Frank Underwood, Executive Director

Fnded: 1962. **Philosophy:** The Forest Foundation is concerned primarily "with the growth and development of the individual because the individual is primary to solving societal problems and creatively enhancing the human condition. Its focus is on stimulating, encouraging, and supporting activities and programs of established, voluntary non-profit organizations that emphasize individual growth and responsibility." The foundation focuses on these specific program areas: community improvement; culture and the arts; education; the environment; and human services, which includes child welfare, day care, the disabled, drug rehabilitation, hunger/emergency shelter, senior adults, and youth. youth. **Priorities:** *Arts & Humanities:* 26%. Supports museums, theater, historical societies, music, and opera. *Civic & Public Affairs:* 32%. Housing, economic development, and community foundations. *Education:* 24%. Emphasis on secondary schools and education funds. *Environment:* 8%. Focus on child welfare, youth organizaions, and family services. *International:* 4%. Mental health and a blood services center. *Note:* Total contributions made in fiscal 2001. **Typ. Recipients:** AIDS/HIV, Cancer, Child Abuse, Clinics/Medical Centers, Domestic Violence, Emergency/Ambulance Services, Family Planning, Health Funds, Health Organizations, Hospitals, Medical Education, Medical Research, Mental Health, People with Disabilities, Public Health, Sexual Abuse, Single-Disease Health Associations, Transplant Networks/Donor Banks. **Geo. Dist:** WA, southwestern Washington; especially Pierce County.

★ 11411 ★ Forest Lawn Foundation
625 Fair Oaks Ave., Suite 360
South Pasadena, CA 91030
Phone: (626)441-6358 **Fax:** (626)441-3672
Email: ljb@forestlawnfoundation.org
Website: http://www.forestlawnfoundation.org
Linda Blinkenberg, Executive Director

Fnded: 1951. **Philosophy:** The foundation's interests are chiefly focused on social services around Los Angeles. Youth organizations, the Braille Institute, and services for the needy are generally funded. Recently, the foundation has focused more attention on education and youth prevention programs. Although the foundation has other interests, most of the giving goes to community interests and health, including hospitals and hospices. **Priorities:** *Arts & Humanities:* 1%. Gives to a library. *Education:* 14%. Funds Junior Achievement, the Braille Institute, colleges and universities and after-school programs. *Environment:* 68%. Supports Young Men's Christian Association, scouting, Boy and Girls Clubs, senior citizen programs, emergency relief, and food distribution programs. *International:* 15%. Supports the American Red Cross, medical centers, hospitals, and hospice. *Note:* Total contributions made in 2000. **Typ. Recipients:** Child Abuse, Children's Health/Hospitals, Clinics/Medical Centers, Emergency/Ambulance Services, Health Organizations, Heart, Home-Care Services, Hospices, Hospitals, Nursing Services, People with Disabilities, Prenatal Health Issues, Public Health, Single-Disease Health Associations, Substance Abuse. **Geo. Dist:** Los Angeles, CA, including Los Angeles County and Orange County.

★ 11412 ★ Forrest C. Lattner Foundation
777 East Atlantic Ave., Suite 317
Delray Beach, FL 33483
Phone: (561)278-3781
Susan Lloyd, President & Secretary

Fnded: 1982. **Philosophy:** The Forrest C. Lattner Foundation makes most of its grants in the areas of health care, civic affairs, and the arts. Health service funding favors hospitals, mental health, pediatrics, and single-disease associations. Civic affairs funding favors other philanthropic organizations, housing, and botanical gardens. Support for the arts focuses on art centers, museums, and public broadcasting. Minor support is given to education and social services. **Priorities:** *Arts & Humanities:* About 15%. Public television, theaters, and library associations. *Civic & Public Affairs:* About 4%. Housing and social services. *Education:* 13%. Secondary schools and colleges. *Environment:* About 26%. Supports youth organizations, the aged, guidance centers, and the prevention of domestic violence. *International:* 24%. Health clinics, health associations, and medical research. *Note:* Total contributions made in 2000. **Typ. Recipients:** AIDS/HIV, Alzheimers Disease, Cancer, Children's Health/Hospitals, Clinics/Medical Centers, Domestic Violence, Emergency/Ambulance Services, Eyes/Blindness, Family Planning, Health Funds, Health-General, Heart, Home-Care Services, Hospices, Hospitals, Medical Education, Medical Research, Mental Health, People with Disabilities, Public Health, Research/Studies Institutes, Single-Disease Health Associations, Substance Abuse, Trauma Treatment. **Geo. Dist:** midwest; FL.

★ 11413 ★ Foster Foundation
1929 43rd Ave. East, Suite 300
Seattle, WA 98112
Phone: (206)726-1815
Jill Goodsell, Administrator

Fnded: 1984. **Philosophy:** The foundation states that its purpose is to "enhance the quality of life in the Pacific Northwest and Alaska through the support of qualified needs in areas of cultural activities, education, social and community services, health and the environment." The Foster Foundation makes most of its grants in the areas of education, social services, and health. Education support favors the University of Washington and literacy institutes. Support for social services includes children's homes, united funds, youth organizations, and food banks. Health interests include hospitals, AIDS and cancer research, and nursing. The foundation makes grants in other areas of support as well. **Priorities:** *Arts & Humanities:* 8%. Funds Seattle arts organizations. *Education:* 32%. Primarily for private precollege education, literacy, and higher education. *Environment:* 34%. Supports community centers, youth groups, and homelessness. *International:* 14%. Gives to hospitals, medical centers, and cancer and AIDS research. *Note:* Total contributions made in 2001. **Typ. Recipients:** AIDS/HIV, Cancer, Children's Health/Hospitals, Clinics/Medical Centers, Emergency/Ambulance Services, Family Planning, Geriatric Health, Health Organizations, Hospices, Hospitals, Medical Research, Nursing Services, People with Disabilities, Public Health, Research/Studies Institutes, Respiratory, Single-Disease Health Associations. **Geo. Dist:** Seattle, WA.

★ 11414 ★ Foundation for Child Development
145 East 32nd St.
14th Floor
New York, NY 10016-6055
Phone: (212)213-8337 **Fax:** (212)213-5897
Email: inforequest@ffcd.org
Website: http://www.ffcd.org
Ruby Takanish, President

Fnded: 1900. **Philosophy:** The foundation is "dedicated to the principle that all families should have the social and material resources to raise their children to be healthy, educated, and productive members of their communities. The Foundation seeks to understand children, particularly the disadvantaged, and to promote their well-being. We believe that families, schools, nonprofit organizations, businesses, and government at all levels share complementary responsibilities in the critical task of raising new generations. "Seeking to achieve its goals, the Foundation supports: basic and policy-relevant research about the factors that promote and support the optimal development of children and adolescents; policy analysis, advocacy, services, and public education to enhance the discussion and adoption of social policies that support families in their important child-raising responsibilities; leadership development activities linked to the programmatic focus of the foundation. "The Foundation believes that by integrating these approaches, FCD will strengthen its effectiveness in achieving its mission." Foundation Mission Statement **Priorities:** *Civic & Public Affairs:* 39%. Supports public policy, philanthropic organizations, economic policy, urban and rural affairs. *Education:* 25%. Supports social science education, leadership training, preschool education, colleges and universities, and technical education. *Environment:* 13%. Supports day care, family services, and child welfare. *International:* 19%. Funds childrens health, and nutrition, and medical rehabilitation. *Religion:* 3%. Supports scientific centers and institution and scientific organizations. *Note:* Total contributions made in fiscal 2001. **Typ. Recipients:** Child Abuse, Children's Health/Hospitals, Domestic Violence, Family Planning, Geriatric Health, Health Funds, Hospitals, Medical Education, Medical Rehabilitation, Medical Research, Mental Health, Nutrition, People with Disabilities, Public Health, Research/ Studies Institutes. **Geo. Dist:** New York area.

★ 11415 ★ Foundation for Deep Ecology

1062 Fort Cronkhite
Sausalito, CA 94965
Phone: (415)229-9339 **Fax:** (415)229-9340
Email: info@deepecology.org
Website: http://www.deepecology.org
Jerry Mather, Megatechnology & Globalization Program

Fnded: 1991. **Philosophy:** The Foundation for Deep Ecology concentrates on supporting fundamental ecological issues with certain general goals: to articulate the root causes of today's problems; to support activism that reverses or quells the present drives of society; and to protect forest lands, habitats, and other places around the world. Grant making is divided into three broad categories: Wilderness and Biodiversity, which concerns itself with the decimation of the world's tropical and temperate forests, habitats and biodiversity; Sustainable Agriculture, which supports programs retarding or reversing the destruction of the world's forests and new thinking and alternative models for agriculture; and Megatechnology and Economic Globalization, which seeks proposals for effective analysis, organization, and action on issues related to the industrialization of agriculture and forestry. **Priorities:** *Civic & Public Affairs:* 3%. Supports public policy organizations and community foundations. *Religion:* Less than 1%. *Note:* Total contributions made in fiscal 2000. **Typ. Recipients:** Public Health. **Geo. Dist:** internationally; nationally.

★ 11416 ★ Foundation for Seacoast Health

100 Campus Dr., Suite 1
Portsmouth, NH 03801
Phone: (603)422-8200 **Fax:** (603)422-8207
Email: ffsh@communitycampus.org
Website: http://www.ffsh.org
Susan Bunting, President

Fnded: 1984. **Philosophy:** The Foundation for Seacoast Health supports Seacoast area nonprofit organizations and scholarships for students pursuing health-related fields of study. The foundation has recently shifted in hopes of "narrowing the funding focus and concentrating on fewer, more comprehensive programs, assisting the most successful foundation-funded programs in becoming financially independent; concentrating resources on improving health care delivery systems, rather than on particular services; and focusing on prevention rather than intervention through a gradual shift in funding from the elderly and adolescent populations to the earlier childhood years, focusing on the child's health in relation to the family unit." Although the foundation has concentrated on health care for the elderly and adolescents in the past, it feels that as a whole, health care funding should begin supporting programs aimed at young children in order to encourage a healthier population for the future. "The Foundation for Seacoast Health will continue to focus its resources on programs which have a prevention orientation and which address the systemic issues of health care access and utilization. Believing that the future of our community rests with our children, our top priority will be programs which promote the health of infants, children, and adolescents." Annual Report **Priorities:** *Civic & Public Affairs:* 1%. *Education:* 9%. For health-related scholarships. *Environment:* 12%. Supports Families First and community child care centers. *International:* 78%. Supports health-related initatives through major grants programs, including the infant/child/adolescent program, the health promotion program, the women's health initiative, medical financial assistance, and the discretionary fund. *Note:* Total contributions made in 2000. **Typ. Recipients:** Adolescent Health Issues, AIDS/HIV, Cancer, Cancer, Children's Health/Hospitals, Clinics/Medical Centers, Diabetes, Domestic Violence, Emergency/Ambulance Services, Family Planning, Geriatric Health, Health Funds, Health Organizations, Health Policy/Cost Containment, Health-General, Home-Care Services, Hospices, Hospitals, Medical Rehabilitation, Mental Health, Nursing Services, People with Disabilities, Prenatal Health Issues, Preventive Medicine/Wellness Organizations, Public Health, Sexual Abuse, Single-Disease Health Associations, Substance Abuse, Trauma Treatment. **Geo. Dist:** Eliot, ME; Kittery, ME; York, ME; Greenland, NH; New Castle, NH; Newington, NH; North Hampton, NH; Portsmouth, NH; Rye, NH.

★ 11417 ★ France-Merrick Foundation

The Exchange, Suite 118
1122 Kenilworth Drive
Towson, MD 21204
Phone: (410)832-5700 **Fax:** (410)832-5704
Robert Schaefer, Executive Director

Fnded: 1962. **Philosophy:** The foundation provides most of its support to civic and cultural activities, public education, private and higher education, historic preservation and conservation, and health and social services. **Priorities:** *Arts & Humanities:* 11%. Emphasis on historic preservation. *Civic & Public Affairs:* 19%. Supports foundations and community projects. *Education:* 38%. Primarily supports parochial/private elementary and secondary schools and colleges and universities. *Environment:* 18%. Support for the homeless, child welfare, family services, and united funds. *International:* 14%. *Note:* Total contributions made in fiscal 2001. **Typ. Recipients:** Cancer, Children's Health/Hospitals, Clinics/Medical Centers, Domestic Violence, Health Organizations, Health-General, Hospices, Hospitals, Hospitals (University Affiliated), Medical Education, People with Disabilities, Public Health. **Geo. Dist:** Baltimore, MD, within the metropolitan area.

★ 11418 ★ Frances and Benjamin Benenson Foundation

708 3rd Ave., 28th Floor
New York, NY 10017
Phone: (212)867-0990 **Fax:** (212)983-1952
Charles Benenson, President

Fnded: 1983. **Philosophy:** The foundation has two primary interests: the arts and education. Scholarships for minority students is the foundation's chief focus, and other funding for education emphasizes educational foundations and universities. Funding for the arts favors museums, the performing arts, and libraries. Secondary interests include religious organizations and social services. **Priorities:** *Arts & Humanities:* 24%. Supports museums, public libraries, modern art, and the performing arts. *Civic & Public Affairs:* 3%. Assists community development and urban affairs. *Education:* 24%. Supports educational programs, schools, colleges, and universities. *Environment:* 34%. Supports youth services, the United Way, and social services. *International:* 3%. Supports single-disease associations. *Note:* Contributions made in fiscal 2000. **Typ. Recipients:** AIDS/HIV, Cancer, Children's Health/Hospitals, Clinics/Medical Centers, Diabetes, Emergency/Ambulance Services, Family Planning, Health Organizations, Hospitals, People with Disabilities, Single-Disease Health Associations, Substance Abuse. **Geo. Dist:** New York, NY.

★ 11419 ★ The Frances L. and Edwin L. Cummings Memorial Fund

501 Fifth Ave., Suite 708
New York, NY 10017-6103
Phone: (212)286-1778 **Fax:** (212)682-9458
Elizabeth Costas, Administrative Director

Fnded: 1982. **Philosophy:** The Cummings Fund's philosophy is to assist organizations seeking to "benefit the health and well-being of mankind." The sole giving restriction is that the "cultural arts" may never be the recipient of foundation funds. The primary interest is in the piloting or expansion of new, innovative programs of organizations operating in, or within close proximity to, New York City. The Cummings Fund encourages smaller and lesser-known community-based organizations to submit grant requests which address the sometimes unique needs of that specific community. The fund has a particular interest in programs serving young people. The major fields of interest are as follows: social welfare, especially programs addressing child abuse homelessness, teenage pregnancy, parenting education, and youth employment and job training; education, with a focus on students from disadvantaged backgrounds, especially efforts to reform the public education system or programs that serve public school children; and health care, especially institutions and programs serving economically and socially disadvantaged populations. A minor area of interest is medical research, especially involving AIDS and cancer. **Priorities:** *Education:* 51%. Supports public education, especially programs serving minorities, the disadvantaged, and the physically and/or mentally disabled. *Environment:* 39%. Supports child abuse prevention, parent education, juvenile delinquency, teenage pregnancy programs, youth employment and job training. *International:* 9%. Funds institutions serving economically and socially disadvantaged populations; cancer, blindness, and AIDS research. *Note:* Total contributions made in fiscal 2002. **Typ. Recipients:** AIDS/HIV, Cancer, Child Abuse, Children's Health/Hospitals, Clinics/Medical Centers, Domestic Violence, Eyes/Blindness, Family Planning, Health Organizations, Home-Care Services, Hospitals, Medical Rehabilitation, Medical Research, Mental Health, Outpatient Health Care, People with Disabilities, Public Health, Substance Abuse. **Geo. Dist:** New York, NY, including surrounding area.

★ 11420 ★ Frances Wood Wilson Foundation, Inc.

250 East Ponce de Leon Ave., Suite 702
Decatur, GA 30030
Phone: (404)370-0035 **Fax:** (404)370-1624
W. Wingfield, President

Fnded: 1954. **Philosophy:** The foundation generally awards its grants to programs and institutions involved in child welfare, religious, civic, health, or educational activities in Georgia, except for programs carried on by Chestnut Hill Benevolent Association in Boston, MA. All grants are made to tax-exempt organizations. Scholarship awards are made to the respective educational institution, rather than to individual students. **Priorities:** *Arts & Humanities:* 8%. Supports historical societies, ballet, and arts centers. *Civic & Public Affairs:* 8%. Supports zoos and parks. *Education:* 32%. Emphasis on colleges and universities. *Environment:* 14%. Recreation and athletics, youth organizations, and child welfare. *International:* 11%. Children's health, hospitals, and cancer causes. *Religion:* 2%. Supports natural history museums. *Note:* Total contributions made in fiscal 2001. **Typ. Recipients:** Cancer, Child Abuse, Children's Health/Hospitals, Clinics/Medical Centers, Health Organizations, Health-General, Hospices, Hospitals, Medical Education, Medical Rehabilitation, Nursing Services, People with Disabilities, Single-Disease Health Associations. **Geo. Dist:** GA.

★ 11421 ★ Francis Families Foundation

800 West 47th St., Suite 717
Kansas City, MO 64112

Phone: (816)531-0077 Fax: (816)531-8810
Email: lyn@francisfoundation.org
Website: http://www.francisfoundation.org
Lyn Knox, Program Officer

Fnded: 1989. **Philosophy:** The foundation supports post doctoral medical fellowships in pulmonary research and anesthesiology, and educational and cultural institutions in the greater Kansas City metropolitan area. The foundation's fellowship program administrative office, located at the School of Public Health, Department of Environmental Health, Harvard University, is under the direction of Joseph D. Brain, Sc.D. Fellowship awards are made to institutions located throughout the United States and Canada. Grants are awarded to provide a stipend, including fringe benefits and travel expenses. Support for research project cost is not allowed. A fellow must have 75% of his or her time available for research. The foundation also supports educational, art, and cultural institutions in the greater Kansas City, MO, metropolitan area. Areas of interest include theater, art, music, dance, cultural endeavors, and education. Support may be ongoing or a one-time contributions and may include capital campaigns pledges or special projects. However, funding to capital campaigns is limited. The foundation has narrowed the focus in Kansas City to give primary consideration to early childhood development. **Priorities:** *Arts & Humanities:* 19%. Focus on art institutes, museums, and theater. *Civic & Public Affairs:* 46%. Primarily supports child and youth development and community foundations. *Education:* 4%. Supports schools and education centers, and provides fellowships. *Environment:* 11%. Supports youth programs, family services, and United Way. *International:* 19%. Supports hospitals and children's health. *Note:* Total contributions made in 2000. **Typ. Recipients:** Children's Health/Hospitals, Clinics/Medical Centers, Health Organizations, Hospitals, Hospitals (University Affiliated), Medical Education, Medical Research, Prenatal Health Issues, Public Health, Research/Studies Institutes, Respiratory, Single-Disease Health Associations. **Geo. Dist:** nationally; Kansas City, MO.

★ 11422 ★ Frank E. and Seba B. Payne Foundation

231 South LaSalle St.
Chicago, IL 60697
Phone: (312)828-1785 **Fax:** (312)828-0806
M. Ryan, Vice President, Bank of America

Fnded: 1962. **Philosophy:** Grants are made solely at the discretion of the trustees for any "religious, charitable, scientific, literary, or educational purposes, and in addition, for the prevention of cruelty to children or animals." **Priorities:** *Arts & Humanities:* 6%. Supports music, libraries, theaters and media. *Civic & Public Affairs:* Approx. 1%. Community projects. *Education:* 52%. Scholarships, secondary schools and colleges. *Environment:* 6%. Youth and community support. *International:* 32%. Hospitals and health centers. *Note:* Total contributions made in fiscal 2000. **Typ. Recipients:** AIDS/HIV, Children's Health/Hospitals, Clinics/Medical Centers, Domestic Violence, Emergency/Ambulance Services, Emergency/Ambulance Services, Eyes/Blindness, Family Planning, Hospitals, Nursing Services, People with Disabilities, Public Health, Single-Disease Health Associations, Speech & Hearing, Substance Abuse, Transplant Networks/Donor Banks. **Geo. Dist:** Chicago, IL; Bethlehem, PA.

★ 11423 ★ Frank Loomis Palmer Fund

777 Main St., CTEH 40222B
Hartford, CT 06115
Phone: (860)952-7405 **Fax:** (860)952-7395
Email: marjorie_alexandre_davis@fleet.com
Marjorie Davis, Vice President

Fnded: 1936. **Philosophy:** The Frank Loomis Palmer Fund distributes its income "to corporations, societies, institutions, and trusts located or operating in the city of New London, CT, which are devoted exclusively to religious, charitable, scientific, literary, historical, or educational purposes, including the encouragement of art. The Fund's purpose is to encourage new projects and to provide seed money rather than to supplement operating expenses; to disseminate the dollars to reach, aid, and assist the largest volume of people." **Priorities:** *Arts & Humanities:* 12%. Funds art centers, museums, and historical preservation. *Civic & Public Affairs:* 22%. Funds community development organizations. *Education:* 21%. Gives to primary and secondary education, and colleges and universities. *Environment:* 28%. Supports drug prevention programs and youth organizations. *International:* 8%. Funds hospitals, hospices, and health groups. *Religion:* 2%. Contributes to science centers and maritime societies. *Note:* Total contributions made in fiscal 1999. **Typ. Recipients:** AIDS/HIV, Children's Health/Hospitals, Domestic Violence, Emergency/Ambulance Services, Family Planning, Health Organizations, Hospices, Hospitals, Medical Rehabilitation, Mental Health, Nursing Services, People with Disabilities, Public Health, Single-Disease Health Associations, Substance Abuse. **Geo. Dist:** New London, CT.

★ 11424 ★ Frank Stanley Beveridge Foundation, Inc.

301 Northeast 51st St., Suite 1130
Boca Raton, FL 33431-4929
Phone: (561)241-8388 **Fax:** (561)241-8332
Email: administrator@beveridge.org
Website: http://www.beveridge.org
Philip Caswell, President

Fnded: 1947. **Philosophy:** The foundation was organized "to aid and provide for the benefit of such poor and needy persons...and to aid and provide for the advancement or promotion of science, learning, medicine, surgery, literature, music, art or human welfare." The foundation annually sets aside approximately one-third of funds for the general maintenance of Stanley Park in Westfield, MA, one-third for organizations in Hampden and Hampshire Counties, and one-third for nonprofits located in regions where Beveridge family members reside, namely the Tampa and Palm Beach, FL, areas. The foundation will consider grant proposals from the following institutional/program activity areas: animal welfare, arts and culture, civil rights, community improvement, conservation/environment, crime, disasters/safety, diseases/medical disciplines, medical research, education, employment, food and agriculture, general and rehabilitative health, housing, human services, mental health, crisis intervention, philanthropy/volunteerism, public affairs and society benefit, recreation, religion, science, social sciences, and youth development. **Priorities:** *Arts & Humanities:* 10%. Museums, public broadcasting, music, and libraries. *Civic & Public Affairs:* 6%. Primarily supporting the Stanley Park of Westfield; also funds community foundations. *Education:* 35%. Supports primary and secondary schools, colleges, and special education. *Environment:* 15%. Focus on youth organizations, people with disabilities, and animal welfare. *International:* 10%. Single-disease health associations and hospitals. *Note:* Total contributions made in 2001. **Typ. Recipients:** Cancer, Clinics/Medical Centers, Diabetes, Emergency/Ambulance Services, Eyes/Blindness, Geriatric Health, Health Organizations, Hospices, Hospitals, Medical Education, Mental Health, Nursing Services, People with Disabilities, Public Health, Research/Studies Institutes, Single-Disease Health Associations. **Geo. Dist:** CA, Orange County; FL, Boca Raton; HI, Kauai County; MA, Hampden County; MA, Hampshire County; NH; RI.

★ 11425 ★ Fred L. Emerson Foundation, Inc.

PO Box 276
Auburn, NY 13021
Phone: (315)253-9621 **Fax:** (315)253-5235
Ronald West, Executive Director & Secretary

Fnded: 1943. **Philosophy:** "Among the foundation's interests are education (primarily private higher education), hospitals and health programs, community agencies, churches, cultural institutions, youth and community service programs, and social welfare agencies." Fred L. Emerson Foundation 2000 IRS Form 990 Support to private colleges and universities is in the form of scholarship endowment and building funds. The foundation generally makes grants for annual campaigns, emergency funds, capital and building funds, equipment and materials, renovation projects, special endowments, research, scholarships, matching and challenge grants, and special local community projects. **Priorities:** *Arts & Humanities:* 16%. Funds museums, history organizations, public broadcasting, and performing arts. *Civic & Public Affairs:* 1%. Gives to local fire departments and public policy associations. *Education:* 63%. Supports private colleges and universities. *Environment:* 11%. Supports local children's athletic and recreation programs. *International:* 8%. Contributes to hospice, cancer centers, hospitals, ambulatory services, and a rehabilitation center. *Note:* Total contributions made in 2000. **Typ. Recipients:** Cancer, Emergency/Ambulance Services, Eyes/Blindness, Family Planning, Health Organizations, Health-General, Heart, Hospices, Hospitals, Long-Term Care, Medical Rehabilitation, Medical Research, People with Disabilities, Single-Disease Health Associations, Substance Abuse. **Geo. Dist:** NY, Cayuga County; NY, Upstate; Auburn, NY.

★ 11426 ★ Fred Maytag Family Foundation

PO Box 366
Newton, IA 50208
Phone: (641)791-1133
Ellen Bergeron, Foundation Administrator

Fnded: 1945. **Philosophy:** The foundation focuses its funding primarily on higher educational institutions, the arts, health and human service organizations, and civic groups. **Priorities:** *Arts & Humanities:* 14%. Primarily to arts organizations in Des Moines. *Civic & Public Affairs:* 17%. Emphasis on parks and clubs in Iowa. *Education:* 18%. Supports colleges and university foundations. *Environment:* 13%. Funds youth programs in Iowa. *International:* 4%. Mainly to health centers. *Note:* Total contributions made in 2000. **Typ. Recipients:** Cancer, Child Abuse, Children's Health/Hospitals, Clinics/Medical Centers, Emergency/Ambulance Services, Family Planning, Health Organizations, Heart, Hospices, Hospitals, Medical Education, Medical Rehabilitation, Medical Research, Mental Health, People with Disabilities, Single-Disease Health Associations, Substance Abuse. **Geo. Dist:** Des Moines, IA; Newton, IA.

★ 11427 ★ Frederick P. and Sandra P. Rose Foundation

200 Madison Ave., 5th Floor
New York, NY 10016
Phone: (212)210-6666
Sandra Rose, President & Director

Fnded: 1982. **Priorities:** *Arts & Humanities:* 27%. Funds libraries, art museums, and the performing arts. *Civic & Public Affairs:* 3%. Supports voters organizations, community parks, and public safety forces. *Education:* 10%. Gives to colleges, universities, and music education. *Environment:* Less than 1%. *International:* Less than 1%. *Religion:* 42%. Provides major support to the American Museum of Natural History. *Note:* Total contributions made in fiscal 2000. **Typ. Recipients:** Cancer, Children's Health/Hospitals, Clinics/Medical Centers, Health Organizations, Health-General, People with Disabilities, Single-Disease Health Associations. **Geo. Dist:** NY.

★ 11428 ★ Frederick S. Upton Foundation

100 Ridgeway
Saint Joseph, MI 49085
Phone: (616)982-1905 **Fax:** (616)982-0323
Email: supton@qtm.net
Stephen Upton, Trustee

Fnded: 1954. **Philosophy:** The foundation's primary purpose is local giving, with emphasis on higher education, religion, cultural programs, community funds, and youth organizations. **Priorities:** *Arts & Humanities:* 32%. Supports artists guilds, libraries, and symphonies. *Civic & Public Affairs:* 5%. Supports councils, community centers, and public safety. *Education:* 15%. Funds colleges. *Environment:* 22%. Supports United Funds, women's organizations, and family programs. *International:* 19%. Supports hospitals. *Note:* Total contributions made in 1999. **Typ. Recipients:** AIDS/HIV, Children's Health/Hospitals, Domestic Violence, Family Planning, Geriatric Health, Health Organizations, Hospitals, People with Disabilities, Public Health. **Geo. Dist:** IL; IN; MA; MI, Southwest Michigan; OH; PA; SC; WI.

★ 11429 ★ Freed Foundation

1025 Thomas Jefferson St. NW, Suite 308E
Washington, DC 20007
Phone: (202)337-5487
Elizabeth Freed, President

Fnded: 1954. **Philosophy:** The Freed Foundation is "interested in non-traditional learning environments, especially those which benefit children. Whether related to socio-economic issues, traumatic childhood experiences, absence of positive role models, or other influences, many children cannot be reached through mainstream educational settings and do not have access to appropriate alternatives. We hope to focus on educational grants in the areas on environmental awareness, artistic creativity, and/or cultural enrichment. We feel connected and interested in learning. Programs focused on enriching children's lives by improving self-esteem, mental health and overall well-being are top priorities. We sincerely hope to make a difference by investing our resources in this manner." President's Message, 1996 Annual Report **Priorities:** *Arts & Humanities:* 23%. Supports history, theater, and the performing arts. *Civic & Public Affairs:* 6%. Supports botanical gardens. *Education:* 46%. Supports minority education, Rutgers University, afterschool/enrichment programs, and literacy. *Environment:* 6%. Supports camps, youth programs, family services, and crime prevention. *International:* 14%. Supports prenatal health issues, eyes/blindness, and AIDS. *Note:* Total contributions made in 2000. **Typ. Recipients:** AIDS/HIV, Alzheimers Disease, Cancer, Child Abuse, Children's Health/Hospitals, Clinics/Medical Centers, Domestic Violence, Emergency/Ambulance Services, Eyes/Blindness, Family Planning, Health Policy/Cost Containment, Hospices, Hospitals, Medical Education, Medical Rehabilitation, Mental Health, Nutrition, People with Disabilities, Public Health, Research/Studies Institutes, Sexual Abuse, Single-Disease Health Associations, Substance Abuse. **Geo. Dist:** Washington, DC, including metropolitan area; NJ; NY.

★ 11430 ★ Friedman Family Foundation

PMB 719, 204 E 2nd Ave.
San Mateo, CA 94401
Phone: (650)342-8750 **Fax:** (650)342-8750
Email: fffdn@aol.com
Website: http://www.friedmanfoundation.org
Lisa Kawahara, Program Director

Fnded: 1964. **Priorities:** *Civic & Public Affairs:* 49%. Supports public policy organizations and community foundations. *Education:* 9%. Supports after school/enrichment programs and private schools. *Environment:* 18%. Supports youth programs, community service organizations, shelters/homeless and family services. *International:* 2%. Supports single-disease health associations, medical centers and health services. *Note:* Total contributions made in fiscal 2001. **Typ. Recipients:** AIDS/HIV, Child Abuse, Children's Health/Hospitals, Clinics/Medical Centers, Domestic Violence, Emergency/Ambulance Services, Health Organizations, Health Policy/Cost Containment, Heart, Hospitals, Medical Research, Mental Health, People with Disabilities, Public Health, Single-Disease Health Associations. **Geo. Dist:** San Francisco, CA, focus on Bay area.

★ 11431 ★ Frist Foundation

3319 West End Ave., Suite 900
Nashville, TN 37203-1076
Phone: (615)292-3868 **Fax:** (615)292-5843
Email: askfrist@fristfoundation.org
Website: http://www.fristfoundation.org
Peter Bird, Jr., Executive Director

Fnded: 1982. **Philosophy:** The Frist Foundation makes most of its grants in the areas of education, social services, and the arts. Most of its resources are funneled through its "initiatives", including: Youth Leadership and Service: supports a comprehensive effort to promote volunteerism among Nashville's youth and to identify and train young people for roles as community leaders. The initiative includes support for the Young Leaders Council; established in 1985, this program trains business people up to 39 years of age for board positions with nonprofit agencies. Through classroom sessions and through individual placements with agencies, participants are exposed to the challenges of the not-for-profit field ranging from fund-raising to legal responsibilities. The Frist Awards of Achievement: This competition, offered annually since 1985, provides unrestricted grants to Nashville organizations best exemplifying improvement and achievement in nonprofit management including innovation, productivity, and volunteer involvement. Unrestricted grants of $15,000 are awarded to the top agency in each of three categories. The program is a partnership with the Center for Nonprofit Management, and is administered by the CNM. Internship Grants Program: This program is designed to help organizations stretch their capabilities. The foundation offers grants to organizations to enable them to hire student interns to accomplish specific projects. The program is also aimed at introducing college students (graduate and undergraduate) to the nonprofit field while linking nonprofit organizations more closely to college campuses. Educator Awards: Administered by the PENCIL Foundation, enables Nashville area teachers to pursue self-designed programs of professional self-improvement. The program is also open to principals seeking to hone their management skills and knowledge. **Priorities:** *Arts & Humanities:* 20%. Major funding goes to the Frist Center for the Visual Arts; also funds art centers, music, theaters, museums, and ballet. *Civic & Public Affairs:* 25%. Primary support is for community affairs organizations. *Education:* 19%. Focus on the Center for Nonprofit Management and education associations and foundations. *Environment:* 16%. Supports health and human services organizations. *Note:* Total contributions made in 2001. **Typ. Recipients:** Child Abuse, Children's Health/Hospitals, Clinics/Medical Centers, Domestic Violence, Emergency/Ambulance Services, Family Planning, Health Funds, Health Organizations, Health Policy/Cost Containment, Medical Education, Medical Training, Mental Health, Nursing Services, People with Disabilities, Public Health, Sexual Abuse, Speech & Hearing, Substance Abuse. **Geo. Dist:** TN; Nashville, TN.

★ 11432 ★ Fritz B. Burns Foundation

4001 West Alemeda Ave., Suite 203
Burbank, CA 91505
Phone: (818)840-8802 **Fax:** (818)840-0468
Joseph Rawlinson, President

Fnded: 1955. **Philosophy:** The foundation emphasizes areas of funding established by the donor during his lifetime. The foundation offers "educational contributions with an emphasis on buildings, equipment, endowments, student scholarship and loan funds, and faculty fellowships." Hospitals, hospital equipment, and medical research also are supported. **Priorities:** *Arts & Humanities:* 1%. *Civic & Public Affairs:* 3%. *Education:* 56%. Supports colleges, universities, and precollege educational institutions. *Environment:* 3%. *International:* 23%. Primarily hospitals and medical centers. *Note:* Total contributions made in fiscal 2001. **Typ. Recipients:** Children's Health/Hospitals, Clinics/Medical Centers, Emergency/Ambulance Services, Family Planning, Health Organizations, Hospitals, Medical Research, Nursing Services, Nutrition, People with Disabilities, Prenatal Health Issues, Research/Studies Institutes, Single-Disease Health Associations. **Geo. Dist:** Los Angeles, CA, metropolitan area.

★ 11433 ★ Frost Foundation

511 Armijo, No. A
Santa Fe, NM 87501
Phone: (505)986-0208 **Fax:** (505)986-0430
Email: frost0729@aol.com
Website: http://www.frostfound.org
Mary Whited-Howell, President

Fnded: 1959. **Philosophy:** The focus of the Frost Foundation has expanded over the years to include health groups, social services, humanitarian needs, and the environment. The foundation focuses its charitable giving on three major program areas, namely social service and humanitarian needs, the environment, and education. Social service projects will include, but not be limited to, street and domestic violence, child abuse, specific public health issues such as alcohol and drug abuse, homelessness, and problems of the elderly. Regarding the environment, the foundation will consider programs in research, education, and action to conserve and protect the environment for the well-being and safety of plants, animals, and human beings. Education projects will stress new, innovative, creative, practical programs to address students' and society's needs today, and which will recognize the changing sociological structure and concerns. The foundation favors causes which address urgent and timely needs, utilize funds and personnel creatively and efficiently, promise new ideas for the benefit of humanity, and have far-reaching impact. **Priorities:** *Arts & Humanities:* About 6%. Supports museums, music, and Opera. *Civic & Public Affairs:* 10%. Supports programs that benefit the homeless, and also gives grants towards community projects and nonprofit management. *Education:* 15%. Supports programs that address students' and society's needs today, also those that address the changing sociological structure and concerns and also supports literacy. *Environment:* 35%. Animal protection, prevention of domestic violence and child abuse, early childhood and family support, United Way, Big Brothers/Big Sister, and family planning services. *International:* 18%. Public health issues, hospices, and emergency health organizations. *Note:* Total contributions made in 2000. **Typ. Recipients:** AIDS/HIV, Cancer, Children's Health/Hospitals, Clinics/Medical Centers, Domestic Violence, Emergency/Ambulance Services, Family Planning, Geriatric Health, Health-General, Hospices, Hospitals, Hospitals (University Affiliated), Medical Education, Medical Rehabilitation, Medical Research, Mental Health, Outpatient Health Care, People with Disabilities, Prenatal Health Issues, Public Health, Research/Studies Institutes, Sexual Abuse, Single-Disease Health Associations, Substance Abuse. **Geo. Dist:** LA; NM.

★ 11434 ★ Fuller E. Callaway Foundation

209 Broome St.
LaGrange, GA 30241
Phone: (706)884-7348 **Fax:** (706)884-0201
H. Burdette, General Manager, President & Treasurer

Fnded: 1917. **Philosophy:** The foundation traditionally devotes significant resources to nursing scholarships: the George E. Sims, Jr. Nursing Scholarship Program administered by West Georgia Health System, and two foundation-sponsored scholarship programs. The remainder goes to LaGrange area schools and LaGrange College, local community service organizations, and churches. **Priorities:** *Arts & Humanities:* Approx. 1%. *Civic & Public Affairs:* 83%. Supports urban and community affairs organizations in La Grange, Georgia. *Education:* 1%. Major support for scholarship programs. *Environment:* 15%. Focus on child welfare and community service organizations. *International:* Approx. 1%. *Note:* Total contributions made in 2001. **Typ. Recipients:** Arthritis, Cancer, Children's Health/Hospitals, Domestic Violence, Health Organizations, Heart, Hospitals, Medical Education, Multiple Sclerosis, Nursing Services, Respiratory, Single-Disease Health Associations. **Geo. Dist:** LaGrange, GA, including Troup County, GA.

★ 11435 ★ Fullerton Foundation

PO Box 2208
Gaffney, SC 29342-2208
Phone: (864)489-6678 **Fax:** (864)487-9946
Email: cjbonner@fullertonfoundation.org
Walter Cavell, Executive Director

Fnded: 1954. **Philosophy:** The Fullerton Foundation makes grants in the areas of education, health, and social services. All of the educational funding supports university-level medical training. Health care support goes to medical centers, hospitals, and health associations. Social service funding favors children's homes and community centers. **Priorities:** *Civic & Public Affairs:* 2%. Supports community foundation. *Education:* 56%. Supports medical education and scholarships. *Environment:* 11%. Supports children's organizations and services for the developmentally disabled. *International:* 28%. Funding goes primarily to university-affiliated hospitals. *Note:* Total contributions made in fiscal 2001. **Typ. Recipients:** Cancer, Children's Health/Hospitals, Clinics/Medical Centers, Emergency/Ambulance Services, Family Planning, Geriatric Health, Health Funds, Health Organizations, Health Policy/Cost Containment, Health-General, Hospitals, Hospitals (University Affiliated), Long-Term Care, Medical Education, Medical Research, Nursing Services, Nutrition, Outpatient Health Care, People with Disabilities, Prenatal Health Issues, Preventive Medicine/Wellness Organizations, Public Health, Research/Studies Institutes, Transplant Networks/Donor Banks, Trauma Treatment. **Geo. Dist:** NC; SC.

★ 11436 ★ Fund for New Jersey

94 Church St., Suite 303
New Brunswick, NJ 08901
Phone: (732)220-8656 **Fax:** (732)220-8654
Email: fundnj@worldnet.att.net
Website: http://www.fundfornj.org
Mark Murphy, Executive Director & Secretary

Fnded: 1969. **Philosophy:** The fund supports "organizations whose efforts have implications for future public policies in New Jersey, organizations that promote public discussion and awareness of New Jersey's neglected problems and that act to rectify them." Social and Economic Opportunity, Environment and Land Use, and Public Affairs in New Jersey are the three fund-designated giving categories. Grants are awarded to inform, demonstrate, publicize, educate, and organize, thus providing essential links for individuals to shape New Jersey's future. "The fund will favor approaches and projects that build consensus by bridging diverse communities and interests; promote prevention and early intervention to address problems, nurture and advance emerging leaders from diverse backgrounds who will bring new perspectives to our public policy debates; pursue the adoption of the 'best' practices and programs; increase the accountability of public institutions and purposes; impact the lives of inner-city residents, particularly youth; help build a sense of community and counteract fragmenting social polarization; prepare individuals, organizations, and communities to exercise authority over important aspects of their lives; demonstrate effective approaches to resolving problems and meeting community needs; and educate the public and governmental leaders on critical issues." "The Fund for New Jersey was a founding member of the Camden Development Collaborative which was created in 1995 to assist the residents of Camden in developing a sustainable economic and social environment for the growth of their children and families." 1996 Annual Report. **Priorities:** *Arts & Humanities:* 2%. *Civic & Public Affairs:* 21%. Support for organizations furthering public policy in New Jersey. *Education:* 46%. Support for college/university programs in public policy. *Environment:* 10%. Emphasis on social and economic opportunity. *International:* 3%. *Note:* Total contributions made in 2000. **Typ. Recipients:** AIDS/HIV, Child Abuse, Domestic Violence, Health Organizations, Hospitals, Medical Education, Prenatal Health Issues, Public Health, Substance Abuse. **Geo. Dist:** NJ.

★ 11437 ★ G. Harold and Leila Y. Mathers Charitable Foundation

118 N Bedford Rd., Suite 203
Mount Kisco, NY 10549-2555
Phone: (914)242-0465 **Fax:** (914)242-0665
Email: jhandleman@mathersfoundation.org
Website: http://www.mathersfoundation.org
James Handelman, Executive Director

Fnded: 1975. **Philosophy:** The foundation typically focuses its giving in the field of medical research performed at various hospitals, medical research institutes, and universities throughout the country. **Priorities:** *Arts & Humanities:* Less than 1%. *Civic & Public Affairs:* Less than 1%. *Education:* 67%. Supports colleges and universities and medical education. *Environment:* 1%. Supports family services. *International:* 32%. Supports hospital, single-disease associations, and biomedical research. *Note:* Total contributions made in 2000. **Typ. Recipients:** Cancer, Children's Health/Hospitals, Clinics/Medical Centers, Emergency/Ambulance Services, Health-General, Heart, Hospitals, Hospitals (University Affiliated), Medical Education, Medical Research, Public Health, Research/Studies Institutes, Single-Disease Health Associations. **Geo. Dist:** nationally.

★ 11438 ★ G. Unger Vetlesen Foundation

One Rockefeller Plaza
Suite 301
New York, NY 10020-2002
Phone: (212)586-0700 **Fax:** (212)245-1863
Email: info@monellvetlesen.org
Website: http://www.monellvetlesen.org
George Rowe, Jr., President & Director

Fnded: 1955. **Philosophy:** The foundation typically supports oceanographic and geological research at scientific institutes. **Priorities:** *Arts & Humanities:* Less than 1%. *Civic & Public Affairs:* 1%. Gives to a seaport museum. *Education:* 26%. Funds universities with a focus on oceanography and marine biology programs. *Religion:* 69%. Supports oceanographic institutes, observatories, and research in marine biology, oceanography, and climate/atmospheric change. *Note:* Total contributions made in 2000. **Typ. Recipients:** Medical Education, Medical Research. **Geo. Dist:** nationally; MA; NY.

★ 11439 ★ GAR Foundation

50 South Main St.
PO Box 1500
Akron, OH 44309-1500
Phone: (330)643-0201 **Fax:** (330)258-6559
Email: gar@bdblaw.com
Website: http://www.garfdn.org
Robert Briggs, Executive Director

Fnded: 1967. **Philosophy:** The foundation supports higher and secondary educational institutions. It also contributes to a variety of programs in the arts, including public broadcasting, music, performing arts, museums, and libraries. Religious organizations, civic groups, and social service agencies are funded on a lesser scale. **Priorities:** *Arts & Humanities:* 16%. Supports museums, theaters, public broadcasting, music, historical societies, and art centers. *Civic & Public Affairs:* 40%. Funds community foundations, zoos, public policy concerns, and community causes. *Education:* 16%. Colleges and universities, education funds, and secondary education receive support. *Environment:* 20%. Supports youth organizations, united funds, homes, people with disabilities, and prevention of domestic violence. *International:* 3%. *Religion:* 2%. *Note:* Total contributions made in 2000. **Typ. Recipients:** Alzheimers Disease, Cancer, Children's Health/Hospitals, Clinics/Medical Centers, Emergency/Ambulance Services, Eyes/Blindness, Family Planning, Health Funds, Health Organizations, Hospices, Hospitals, Medical Education, Mental Health, Multiple Sclerosis, Nursing Services, People with Disabilities, Prenatal Health Issues, Public Health, Substance Abuse. **Geo. Dist:** OH, Summit County and 5 surrounding counties.

★ 11440 ★ Gardner and Florence Call Cowles Foundation

715 Locust St.
Des Moines, IA 50309
Phone: (515)284-8117 **Fax:** (515)699-7035
Charles Edwards, President & Trustee

Fnded: 1934. **Philosophy:** The foundation's grantgiving activities are confined to Iowa. Grants are made primarily to four-year private colleges. The foundation also supports various cultural institutions and selected social agencies, and is planning to focus more on human services. **Priorities:** *Arts & Humanities:* 52%. Supports performing arts and art centers. *Civic & Public Affairs:* 15%. Funds community development and zoos. *Education:* 44%. Supports four-year private colleges and universities. *Environment:* 2%. Supports family planning and youth programs. *Religion:* 2%. Funds science center. *Note:* Total contributions made in 2001. **Typ. Recipients:** Family Planning. **Geo. Dist:** IA.

★ 11441 ★ Gates Family Foundation

3575 Cherry Creek North Drive, Suite 100
Denver, CO 80209
Phone: (303)722-1881 **Fax:** (303)316-3038
Email: info@gatesfamilyfoundation.org
Website: http://www.gatesfamilyfdn.org
Tom Kaesemeyer, Executive Director

Fnded: 1946. **Philosophy:** The Gates Foundation's purpose is to "enhance the quality of life of those who live and work in Colorado through activities that promote broad education, self-sufficiency, connection to nature, and cultural appreciation. In their grantmaking activities, the trustees are mindful that the free enterprise system provided the opportunity to create the wealth that makes the Foundation's work possible. Emphasis is placed on capital projects. Special attention is paid to the Denver metropolitan area." 2001 Annual Report Among the foundation's interests are improvement of the quality of life for Denver residents, including support of cultural activities, provision of better low-cost health care, preservation of parks and historic areas, support of conservation and outdoor recreation programs, and the growth and development of independent schools and colleges. In addition, the foundation supports greater cooperation between the public and private sectors; the development of leadership and managerial skills of elected officials and public sector managers; assessment of and means to address the problems faced by public education; and the development of nonacademic programs for young people, particularly those that encourage the development of character and leadership skills. The foundation continues its interest in organizations that promote free enterprise and constructive public policy dialogue. Programs of special interest to the trustees are occasionally initiated by the foundation. **Priorities:** *Arts & Humanities:* 23%. Funds theaters, museums, historic preservation, and public broadcasting. *Civic & Public Affairs:* 22%. Supports community organizations, foundations, urban issues, environmental organizations, and parks. *Education:* 33%. Supports universities, public K-12 schools, and charter schools. *Environment:* 22%. Funds youth services, human services, and recreation. *Note:* Total contributions made in 2001. **Typ. Recipients:** Child Abuse, Domestic Violence, Family Planning, Health Policy/Cost Containment, Health-General, Medical Rehabilitation, People with Disabilities, Substance Abuse. **Geo. Dist:** CO.

★ 11442 ★ Gebbie Foundation

110 W 3rd St., No. 308
Jamestown, NY 14701
Phone: (716)487-1062 **Fax:** (716)484-6401
Thomas Cardman, Executive Director

Fnded: 1964. **Philosophy:** The foundation's mission is "to support appropriate charitable and humanitarian programs to improve the quality of life, primarily in Chautauqua County." Traditionally, the foundation has supported the founder's specific interests and giving patterns. Major initiatives focus on children, youth, and education, "to provide opportunities to young children and families for growth and learning; to encourage them to become productive citizens; assist those interested in extending their education; and provide funding to enhance educational programs." The foundation also supports arts appreciation and participation, historical societies, and libraries. Human services programs that assist those who suffer from social, economic, or cultural deprivation are of particular interest to the foundation. The foundation provides assistance for community development issues, including the maintenance, preservation, and enhancement of economic, health, and environmental assets. 1997 Annual Report **Priorities:** *Arts & Humanities:* 12%. Theater, libraries, historical societies, ballet, and arts organizations. *Civic & Public Affairs:* 23%. Community development, assistance in bringing new business to the area, legal aid, civic centers, and neighborhood projects. *Education:* 7%. Scholarship funding, preschool education, colleges, environment education, and education reform. *Environment:* 45%. Local YWCA organizations, United Way, youth programs, daycare, family services, food banks, animal protection. *International:* 9%. Supports local hospitals, Chautauqua Health Network, hospice and cancer. *Note:* Total contributions made in fiscal 2001. **Typ. Recipients:** Alzheimers Disease, Cancer, Children's Health/Hospitals, Domestic Violence, Emergency/Ambulance Services, Health-General, Heart, Hospices, Hospitals, Medical Education, Medical Rehabilitation, Medical Research, Mental Health, Nursing Services, People with Disabilities, Prenatal Health Issues, Public Health, Research/Studies Institutes, Speech & Hearing, Substance Abuse. **Geo. Dist:** NY.

★ 11443 ★ General Service Foundation

557 N Mill St., Suite 201
Aspen, CO 81611
Phone: (970)920-6834 **Fax:** (970)920-4578
Email: info@generalservice.org
Website: http://www.generalservice.org
Carleen Indereiden, Grants Manager

Fnded: 1946. **Philosophy:** The current interests of the foundation are International Peace, Reproductive Health and Rights, and Western Water. Under the International Peace Program the foundation seeks to address the root causes of conflict and to promote peaceful and stable communities, primarily in Mexico, Central America, and the Caribbean. The foundation considers programs and projects which address the following issues, as well as their interrelationships: political rights and civil freedoms; economic, social and cultural rights; equitable solutions to the human impact of global competition on workers in the region; and fostering U.S. engagement in global and regional affairs, international institutions and a foreign policy that promotes a peaceful and equitable world. Funding is given principally for education and policy analysis and formation, rather than for research. The foundation also may make contributions to organizations working to accomplish the following objectives: develop leadership and participation in the non-governmental organization community; further communication and collaborative efforts among non-governmental organizations; and strengthen interregional organizations, both governmental and non-governmental. The Reproductive Health and Rights Program is dedicated to improving access to comprehensive reproductive health care, including abortion, for women and adolescents; and to supporting education efforts which increase awareness and action around issues of reproductive health, sexuality, and reproductive choices. In the U.S., funding focuses on surgical and medical abortion; family planning and contraception; and comprehensive sexuality education. In Mexico, funding is primarily aimed at advocating reproductive rights and access to comprehensive health care at the national level; and building decentralized capacity within the reproductive and sexual rights movement on the state level. The Western Water program is geared toward preserving and protecting water flows for aquatic and riparian ecosystems in the rivers of the American interior West. Target states are Idaho, Montana, Wyoming, Colorado, New Mexico, Utah, and Arizona. Although a wide range of activites are funded within this program, priority is given to organizations attempting to impact legal and/or policy changes. The foundation also maintains smaller giving programs for which recipients are preselected. The Discretionary Arts Program does not contribute through unsolicited proposals, but through a small discretionary program. The funds are distributed only at the request of the board of directors. The Education Program's mission is to fund educational projects within targeted communities as well as Native American youth education programs. Proposals in this program are considered only at the request and initiation of members of the Education Committee. **Priorities:** *Civic & Public Affairs:* 46%. Supports reproductive rights, Native American and human rights, and law and justice organizations. *Education:* 3%. Gives to institutions of higher education. *International:* 7%. Primary support for reproductive and women's health. *Note:* Total contributions made in 2001. **Typ. Recipients:** AIDS/HIV, Family Planning, Health-General, Medical Research, Public Health. **Geo. Dist:** nationally; the Caribbean.

★ 11444 ★ Generoso Pope Foundation

700 White Plains Rd., Suite 315
Scarsdale, NY 10583
Phone: (914)723-3044
Mr. Anthony Pope, President & Secretary

Fnded: 1947. **Philosophy:** The foundation reflects the personal philanthropic interests of the Pope family, especially their interest in Roman Catholic institutions and in organizations that study and record the experience of Italian immigrants in America. Many recipients are given funds annually. Other foundation interests include welfare funds, higher and secondary education, and hospitals. **Priorities:** *Arts & Humanities:* 2% supports museums, public radio, performing arts, journalism, and art. *Civic & Public Affairs:* 16% supports police benevolence and community services. *Education:* 33% supports colleges, universities, educational programs. *Environment:* 7%. Supports March of Dimes, Meals on Wheels, and battered women's services. *International:* 30%. Supports hospitals, medical centers, pediatric medicine, rehabilitation, disease and disorder concerns. *Note:* Contributions were made in 2000. **Typ. Recipients:** Children's Health/Hospitals, Clinics/Medical Centers, Diabetes, Domestic Violence, Eyes/Blindness, Geriatric Health, Health Funds, Health Organizations, Hospitals, Long-Term Care, Medical Education, Medical Rehabilitation, Medical Research, Mental Health, People with Disabilities, Prenatal Health Issues, Public Health, Single-Disease Health Associations. **Geo. Dist:** New York, NY, metropolitan area; limited support elsewhere. **Frmly:** Pope Foundation.

★ 11445 ★ George D. Smith Fund

805 Third Ave.
New York, NY 10022
Phone: (212)702-5801
Lawrence Milas, Vice President

Fnded: 1956. **Philosophy:** The George D. Smith Fund primarily supports health care services and medical research. Other interests include universities, civil rights, family planning, and public broadcasting. **Priorities:** *Arts & Humanities:* 12%. Funds public radio. *Education:* 43%. Supports universities and secondary public schools. *Environment:* 7%. Supports Planned Parenthood of America. *International:* 14%. Contributes to a medical center. *Note:* Total contributions made in 2001. **Typ. Recipients:** Clinics/Medical Centers, Family Planning, Health Funds, Health Organizations, Hospitals (University Affiliated), Medical Education. **Geo. Dist:** CA; NE; NY; UT.

★ 11446 ★ George F. Baker Trust

477 Madison Ave., Suite 1650
New York, NY 10022
Phone: (212)755-1890 **Fax:** (212)319-6316
Ms. Rocio Suarez, Executive Director

Fnded: 1937. **Philosophy:** Grants from the trust are for general charitable giving, largely to institutions in the New York area that have received continuous support over the years from the donor and his family. Special consideration is given to education, hospitals, social services, youth agencies, conservation, and historic preservation. **Priorities:** *Arts & Humanities:* 6%. Supports museums, school libraries, and cultural concerns. *Civic & Public Affairs:* 14%. *Education:* 44%. Supports secondary and preparatory schools, academies, colleges and universities. *Environment:* 5%. Supports youth services and neighborhood affairs. *International:* 10%. Supports medical centers, rehabilitation centers, and hospitals. *Religion:* 3%. *Note:* Contributions were made in 2000. **Typ. Recipients:** AIDS/HIV, Cancer, Children's Health/Hospitals, Clinics/Medical Centers, Diabetes, Emergency/Ambulance Services, Family Planning, Health-General, Heart, Hospitals, Hospitals (University Affiliated), Medical Education, Medical Rehabilitation, Medical Research, People with Disabilities, Prenatal Health Issues, Public Health, Substance Abuse. **Geo. Dist:** Nationally; New York, NY.

★ 11447 ★ George F. and Sybil H. Fuller Foundation

1B Central St.
Boylston, MA 01505
Phone: (508)869-6723 **Fax:** (508)869-2601
Russell Fuller, Chairman, Treasurer & Trustee

Fnded: 1955. **Philosophy:** The foundation generally supports higher educational organizations, cultural institutions, hospitals, historic preservation efforts, and social services. Within the past year, the foundation has placed more emphasis on community service organizations working to improve the quality of life in Massachusetts. **Priorities:** *Arts & Humanities:* 21%. Includes museums, historic preservation, music, and theater. *Civic & Public Affairs:* 25%. Supports Chambers of Commerce, community foundations, safety, and housing. *Education:* 26%. Funds primarily colleges and universities. *Environment:* 18%. Supports the Young Men's Christian Association, Young Women's Christian Association, homes, community centers, and United Way. *International:* 5%. Supports community health associations. *Note:* Total contributions made in 2000. **Typ. Recipients:** Children's Health/Hospitals, Clinics/Medical Centers, Diabetes, Emergency/Ambulance Services, Health Organizations, Health-General, Hospices, Hospitals, Medical Education, Medical Research, Nursing Services, People with Disabilities, Public Health, Single-Disease Health Associations, Substance Abuse. **Geo. Dist:** MA, Worcester County.

★ 11448 ★ George Foundation

Private Mail Box
310 Morton St. - Suite C
Richmond, TX 77469
Phone: (281)342-6109 **Fax:** (281)341-7635
Email: radamson@thegeorgefoundation.org
Website: http://www.thegeorgefoundation.org
Roland Adamson, Executive Director

Fnded: 1945. **Philosophy:** The George Foundation is "trust for religious, charitable, scientific, literary and/or educational purposes." The founders directed the trustees of their foundation to administer its funds "for the use and benefit of the people of Fort Bend County, primarily, yet (the Trustees) may extend the benefits thereof to the people of other counties in the State of Texas." **Priorities:** *Arts & Humanities:* 5%. Provides major funding to the Ft. Bend County Museum Association. *Civic & Public Affairs:* 1%. Funds community foundations and community festivals. *Education:* 76%. Supports universities, colleges, public schools, literacy programs, and scholarship funds. *Environment:* 7%. Supports the United Way, youth services, family planning, social services for women and children, and scouts. *International:* 9%. Supports

★ 11449 ★ George and Frances Ball Foundation

PO Box 1408
Muncie, IN 47308
Phone: (765)741-5500 **Fax:** (317)741-5518
Email: jjpcuis@iquest.net
Joyce Beck, Administrative Assistant

Fnded: 1937. **Philosophy:** The foundation supports higher education and the arts primarily in east central Indiana and the immediate surrounding area. Educational funding goes primarily to colleges and universities, with substantial funding to Ball State University in Muncie, IN. The foundation supports a variety of cultural organizations, especially the Minnetrista Cultural Foundation, also in Muncie. In addition, the foundation funds libraries and museums. Civic affairs and social services also are funded. **Priorities:** *Arts & Humanities:* 44%. *Civic & Public Affairs:* 8%. *Education:* 44%. *International:* 8%. *Note:* Historical percentages 1937-2001. **Typ. Recipients:** Children's Health/Hospitals, Emergency/Ambulance Services, Family Planning, Health Organizations, Hospitals, Medical Education, Medical Rehabilitation, Medical Research, People with Disabilities, Substance Abuse. **Geo. Dist:** IN, Delaware County; IN, East Central Indiana; Muncie, IN.

★ 11450 ★ George Frederick Jewett Foundation
Russ Bldg.
235 Montgomery St., Suite 612
San Francisco, CA 94104
Phone: (415)421-1351 **Fax:** (415)421-0721
Email: tfbjewettf@aol.com
Ann Gralnek, Senior Advisor

Fnded: 1957. **Philosophy:** "Following the death of Mary Cooper Jewett Gaiser in 1996, the trustees of the foundation determined to divide the foundation into separate philanthropic entities. During the reorganization and beginning with its 1998 grant cycle, there will be two separate funds within the George Frederick Jewett Foundation divided equally between the two entities. These funds will be directed by the two branches of the Jewett Family and will be known as Jewett Fund A and Jewett Fund B of the George Frederick Jewett Foundation." "The primary interests of the Jewett Fund A within the Foundation are: Arts and Culture, Education, and Environment (with particular emphasis on Land Conservation, Oceanographic Studies, and Population). Some consideration will also be given to Health/Social Services and Medical Research. The Jewett Fund A of the Foundation focuses its grants largely, although not exclusively, to San Francisco, California, and Spokane, Washington." "The priority interests of Jewett Fund B of the Foundation are: Education, Libraries, Music, Preservation, Protection of the Environment, including Population Issues, and Scientific Research. Jewett Fund B of the Foundation focuses its grants largely in geographic areas in which Trustees and family members have knowledge of particular needs." George Frederick Jewett Foundation 1997 Annual Report **Priorities:** *Arts & Humanities:* 18%. *Civic & Public Affairs:* 6%. Supports parks. *Education:* 28%. Supports colleges, universities and private schools. *Environment:* 12%. Supports family planning and community service organizations. *International:* 8%. Supports health clinic and research/studies institute. *Note:* Total contributions made in 2000. **Typ. Recipients:** Cancer, Clinics/Medical Centers, Diabetes, Emergency/Ambulance Services, Family Planning, Hospitals, Medical Education, Medical Rehabilitation, Nursing Services, People with Disabilities, Prenatal Health Issues, Public Health, Speech & Hearing, Substance Abuse. **Geo. Dist:** San Francisco, CA; WA, Eastern Washington; Spokane, WA.

★ 11451 ★ George Gund Foundation
45 Prospect Ave. West
1845 Guildhall Bldg.
Cleveland, OH 44115
Phone: (216)241-3114 **Fax:** (216)241-6560
Email: dabbott@gundfdn.org
Website: http://www.gundfdn.org
David Abbott, Executive Director

Fnded: 1952. **Philosophy:** The foundation's operations reflect George Gund's belief that creative solutions are needed to cure society's ills. This belief demands the seeking and fostering of innovative ideas to enhance people's understanding of their environment and increase their ability to cope with its ever-changing requirements. The foundation attempts this through its giving to education, human services, economic revitalization, arts, environmental quality, and civic affairs. Grantmaking for primary and secondary education focuses on improving educational programs for low-income and minority youth, especially in the Cleveland Public Schools. Emphasis is placed on projects in Cuyahoga County dealing with public school improvement, community and parental involvement, policy development, staff development, and program evaluation. Grantmaking in early childhood focuses on strengthening the child care system in Greater Cleveland as well as early intervention programs for disadvantaged preschoolers. In human services, the foundation supports programs within Cuyahoga County that enhance the welfare and stability of children and families and promote greater self-sufficiency for persons of low-income. Grantmaking in health focuses primarily on Greater Cleveland programs that seek to prevent infant mortality and improve community health. The foundation also supports national and local family planning and reproductive rights organizations, retinal degenerative disease research, local AIDS services and educational programs, and national AIDS policy formation. In environmental affairs, primary grantmaking in Greater Cleveland focuses on ecosystems, rivers and watersheds, parks, and open space, and efforts to encourage citizen awareness. Grantmaking in Ohio focuses on state-wide issues and organizations promoting improved public policy or providing coordination and support for local environmental groups. Local grantmaking in the Great Lakes basin emphasizes region-wide protection of environmental resources and strengthening the infrastructure of the environmental community, including programs that develop leadership and management capacity in nonprofit organizations. In civic affairs, the foundation focuses on public policy, increasing governmental effectiveness, and encouraging citizen participation in the Greater Cleveland area. Grantmaking also supports economic and community revitalization efforts at the local and state level, including the creation of jobs. **Priorities:** *Arts & Humanities:* 13%. Supports museums, music, ballet, public broadcasting, dance and theater. *Civic & Public Affairs:* 31%. Supports civil rights, law & justice, festivals, botanical gardens/parks, and public policy. *Education:* 27%. Supports universities, journalism/media education, scholarship, and leadership training. *Environment:* 7%. Supports United Way, family planning services, child welfare and camps. *International:* 11%. Supports AID/HIV, eyes/blindness, medical center. *Religion:* 6%. Supports science museums. *Note:* Total contributions made in 1998. **Typ. Recipients:** AIDS/HIV, Children's Health/Hospitals, Clinics/Medical Centers, Emergency/Ambulance Services, Eyes/Blindness, Family Planning, Hospitals, People with Disabilities, Single-Disease Health Associations. **Geo. Dist:** Cleveland, OH, including northeastern Ohio region.

★ 11452 ★ George H. Deuble Foundation
c/o DCC Corp.
5757 Mayfair Rd.
PO Box 2288
North Canton, OH 44720-1546
Phone: (330)828-9770
Andrew Deuble, Secretary & Trustee

Fnded: 1947. **Philosophy:** The foundation makes grants across the major categories of support. Social service support goes to family planning, child welfare, community centers, and employment. Support for education includes scholarships, universities, technical education, and funds. Health support includes brain research, nursing, and single-disease associations. Arts funding favors historic preservation and museums. The foundation also funds civic and religious causes. **Priorities:** *Arts & Humanities:* 26%. Restoration funds, museums, and arts institutes. *Civic & Public Affairs:* 2%. *Education:* About 16%. Primary schools and colleges and universities. *Environment:* 26%. United funds, youth organizations, the disabled, and YM-YWCAs. *International:* 26%. A medical foundation, hospitals, and medical research. *Note:* Total contributions made in 2001. **Typ. Recipients:** Health Funds, Heart, Hospitals, Medical Research.

★ 11453 ★ George Hoag Family Foundation
11340 West Olympic Blvd., Ste. 300
Los Angeles, CA 90064
Phone: (310)473-9050 **Fax:** (310)473-9091
Mr. Charles Smith, Secretary/Executive Director

Fnded: 1940. **Philosophy:** The foundation "primarily applies its resources to preserve and enrich the benefits to be derived by California residents, and principally those residing in Orange County, from improved and expanded medical services, opportunities for youth and other humanitarian or similar community projects." **Priorities:** *Arts & Humanities:* 4%. Supports a philharmonic society and ballet. *Civic & Public Affairs:* 14%. Funds community foundations and housing programs. *Education:* 4%. Funds a college foundation, academic decathalon, and other educational programs. *Environment:* 36%. Supports youth organizations and and food banks. *International:* 35%. Supports hospitals, clinics, and healthcare-related programs. *Note:* Total contributions made in 1998. **Typ. Recipients:** Adolescent Health Issues, AIDS/HIV, Alzheimers Disease, Cancer, Child Abuse, Children's Health/Hospitals, Clinics/Medical Centers, Diabetes, Domestic Violence, Emergency/Ambulance Services, Eyes/Blindness, Health Organizations, Health-General, Heart, Hospices, Hospitals, Medical Research, Outpatient Health Care, People with Disabilities, Prenatal Health Issues, Preventive Medicine/Wellness Organizations, Public Health, Research/Studies Institutes, Single-Disease Health Associations, Substance Abuse. **Geo. Dist:** CA, Orange County.

★ 11454 ★ George I. Alden Trust
370 Main St., 12th Fl.
Worcester, MA 01608
Phone: (508)798-8621 **Fax:** (508)791-6454
Email: trustees@aldentrust.org
Website: http://www.aldentrust.org
Susan Woodbury, III, Chairman

Fnded: 1912. **Philosophy:** The primary interest of the George I. Alden Trust is education. The focus is on higher education, although a few projects in secondary education are also supported. The trust has funded endowments for scholarship support for students, laboratory and other equipment purchases, and building programs. The trust favors educational institutions combining academic excellence with efficient and economically sound administration. **Priorities:** *Arts & Humanities:* 9%. Supports libraries. *Civic & Public Affairs:* 7%. Supports community foundations. *Education:* 69%. Supports college, universities, and literacy. *Environment:* 14%. Supports Young Men's Christian Association in Massachusetts. *Religion:* 1%. Funds science centers. **Typ. Recipients:** Clinics/Medical Centers, Emergency/Ambulance Services, Family Planning, Health Organizations, Medical Education, Medical Research. **Geo. Dist:** New England area; Worcester, MA.

★ 11455 ★ George Link, Jr. Foundation
1290 Ave. of the Americas, 5th Floor
New York, NY 10104
Phone: (201)846-8481
Michael Cantanzaro, Vice President & Director

Fnded: 1980. **Philosophy:** The foundation typically supports health organizations, educational institutions, religious causes, and social services. **Priorities:** *Arts & Humanities:* 3%. Museums and cultural centers. *Civic & Public Affairs:* 5%. Housing & Ethnic organizations, and safety. *Education:* 31%. Colleges and high schools. *Environment:* 14%. Community services, primarily organized by religious groups. *International:* 19%. Hospitals and medical centers. *Note:* Total contributions made in 1998. **Typ. Recipients:** Cancer, Children's Health/Hospitals, Clinics/Medical Centers, Health Funds, Health Organizations, Heart, Hospitals, Long-Term Care, Medical Education, Medical Rehabilitation, Medical Research, Mental Health, People with Disabilities, Public Health, Single-Disease Health Associations. **Geo. Dist:** Northeast; NJ; NY.

★ 11456 ★ George and Mary Josephine Hamman Foundation
3336 Richmond, Suite 310
Houston, TX 77098
Phone: (713)522-9891 **Fax:** (713)522-9693
Email: hammanfdn@aol.com
Website: http://www.hammanfoundation.org
E. Fritsche, Executive Director

Fnded: 1954. **Philosophy:** The foundation makes grants across the major categories of support. Health care interests include single-disease associations, hospices, health organizations, and hospitals. The arts are supported through funding to museums, the performing arts, ballet, and art centers. Educational funding favors private schools, education centers, special education schools for the deaf, colleges, and private universities. Social service interests include family planning, the homeless, homes, child welfare, and the disabled. Other interests include churches and religious groups. **Priorities:** *Arts & Humanities:* 20%. Focus on museums, music, and theater. *Civic & Public Affairs:* 11%. Support for a park, nature center, and community affairs organization. *Education:* 27%. Primarily to colleges and universities, primary and secondary schools, and scholarships. *Environment:* 14%. Family planning, child welfare, youth organizations, and the homeless. *International:* 19%. Supports single-disease health associations and hospitals. *Note:* Total contributions made in fiscal 1999. **Typ. Recipients:** Alzheimers Disease, Cancer, Children's Health/Hospitals, Clinics/Medical Centers, Domestic Violence, Emergency/Ambulance Services, Eyes/Blindness, Family Planning, Health Organizations, Heart, Hospices, Hospitals, Hospitals (University Affiliated), Medical Education, Medical Rehabilitation, Medical Research, Mental Health, People with Disabilities, Single-Disease Health Associations, Speech & Hearing, Substance Abuse. **Geo. Dist:** Houston, TX.

★ 11457 ★ George S. and Dolores Dore Eccles Foundation

Deseret Bldg.
79 South Main St., 12th Floor
Salt Lake City, UT 84111
Phone: (801)246-5336 **Fax:** (801)350-3510
Lisa Eccles, Executive Director

Fnded: 1958. **Philosophy:** "The George S. and Dolores Dore Eccles Foundation is dedicated to improving the welfare of mankind. It is a foundation which serves the Intermountain West with a particular focus on the State of Utah. The Foundation provides assistance to institutions and organizations with a history of achievement, effectiveness and good management. Moreover, the Foundation supports programs and projects which enrich the quality of life and learning and have the potential to make a significant difference in the community. The Foundation's fields of interest include the arts, community organizations, education and medicineical." **Priorities:** *Arts & Humanities:* 24%. Supports performing arts, and college campus libraries. *Civic & Public Affairs:* 4%. Supports community affairs. *Education:* 52%. Supports educational institutions and programs. *Environment:* 5%. Focus on children and youth services, and a domestic violence prevention facility. *International:* 2%. Supports health concerns. *Note:* Contributions were made in 2000. **Typ. Recipients:** Arthritis, Clinics/Medical Centers, Domestic Violence, Eyes/Blindness, Health Organizations, Hospices, Hospitals, Medical Education, Medical Research, Mental Health, Nursing Services, Outpatient Health Care, People with Disabilities, Preventive Medicine/Wellness Organizations, Public Health, Research/Studies Institutes, Single-Disease Health Associations, Speech & Hearing. **Geo. Dist:** preference for Intermountain area of United States; UT.

★ 11458 ★ George W. Brackenridge Foundation

711 Navarro St., Suite 535
San Antonio, TX 78205
Phone: (210)224-1011 **Fax:** (210)223-3657
Gilbert Denman, Jr., Trustee

Fnded: 1920. **Philosophy:** Foundation support goes to accredited Texas educational organizations for individual scholarhips, scholarship programs, and educational facilities and programs. The foundation also supports the arts and zoos. **Priorities:** *Arts & Humanities:* 11%. Supports museums, visual arts, and performing arts. *Civic & Public Affairs:* About 1%. *Education:* 86%. Supports educational programs, colleges, and universities. *Environment:* About 1%. *International:* 2%. Supports health centers. *Religion:* About 1%. Supports research. *Note:* Total contributions made in 2001. **Typ. Recipients:** Clinics/Medical Centers, Medical Education, Medical Training. **Geo. Dist:** TX.

★ 11459 ★ Geraldine R. Dodge Foundation

163 Madison Ave.
PO Box 1239
Morristown, NJ 07962-1239
Phone: (973)540-8442 **Fax:** (973)540-1211
Email: info@grdodge.org
Website: http://www.grdodge.org
David Grant, Executive Director

Fnded: 1974. **Philosophy:** "The foundation works in two ways: one, by responding to imaginative proposals that fall within the declared areas and which promise to have impact, to be replicable, and to effect systemic change; and two, by developing initiatives shaped by close listening to practitioners and resource people in areas where the concentration of funds is likely to improve the quality of life." "Expectations for every project go far beyond the transmittal of funds: they grow out of an extensive review process that continues. Further, we seek to collaborate with other funders, individual, foundation, and corporate, as well as select government units in areas of mutual interest. We often provide seed money that allows a project to take root and find other sources of funding, but we will also willingly follow other funders of successful innovations." "The Foundation seeks to be an enabler, backing persons and ideas and institutions who serve a purpose that transcends self-interest and may contribute to sustain human society and the environment that shelters it." The foundation has five major program areas that receive funding: education, the arts, local projects, the welfare of animals, and public issues. Precollegiate education in the northeastern United States is awarded funds to develop teachers and curriculums and to make good education more accessible. The arts in New Jersey are supported, encouraging art education, promoting the role of the individual artist, supporting public access to the arts, and encouraging stability and development of art institutions. Programs in Morris County, NJ are funded by the focus on local projects. The foundation supports animal welfare projects with national implications, and provides direct assistance to a local animal shelter assistance program. Humane treatment and species conservation are major interests of the foundation. National programs for the environment, including conservation, education, and pollution reduction, are the recipients of public issues funding, with the majority of support for efforts in New Jersey and the Northeast. **Priorities:** *Arts & Humanities:* 26%. Focus on literary arts, performing arts, museums, music, theater, and arts festivals. *Education:* 35%. Primarily for education reform, literacy, higher education, and public education. *Environment:* 16%. Supports family planning organizations, animal protection. *Note:* Total contributions made in 2000. **Typ. Recipients:** Domestic Violence, Family Planning, Medical Education, Medical Research. **Geo. Dist:** nationally; NJ.

★ 11460 ★ Gheens Foundation

One Riverfront Plaza, Suite 705
Louisville, KY 40202
Phone: (502)584-4650 **Fax:** (502)584-4652
Email: lindahw@aye.net
James Davis, Executive Director

Fnded: 1957. **Philosophy:** "The Gheens Foundation is one of the largest private foundations in Kentucky and the Trustees oversee the distribution of approximately $4 million each year. Most of the grants are made in the Louisville/New Orleans area and are used to support a wide range of endeavors at all levels, including education, economic development, medical, arts, social/health services, handicapped, mental health programs, etc." *The Gheens Foundation, Inc.: A Brief History* **Priorities:** *Arts & Humanities:* 3%. Primarily for historical societies, museums, and memorial landmarks. *Civic & Public Affairs:* 16%. Support for economic development projects in Louisville. *Education:* 42%. Colleges and universities, primary and secondary education, literacy programs, and education associations. *Environment:* 21%. Supports united funds, youth organizations, and family services. *International:* 7%. Supports medical centers. *Religion:* 2%. Gives to the Louisville Science Center. *Note:* Total contributions made in fiscal 2000. **Typ. Recipients:** Cancer, Children's Health/Hospitals, Clinics/Medical Centers, Diabetes, Eyes/Blindness, Family Planning, Geriatric Health, Health Organizations, Hospices, Hospitals, Hospitals (University Affiliated), Medical Education, Medical Rehabilitation, Medical Research, Mental Health, People with Disabilities, Preventive Medicine/Wellness Organizations, Public Health, Single-Disease Health Associations, Substance Abuse. **Geo. Dist:** Louisville, KY; LaFourche Parish, LA.

★ 11461 ★ Gilder Foundation

c/o Anchin, Block & Anchin, LLP
1375 Broadway
New York, NY 10018
Phone: (212)765-2500
Richard Gilder, Jr., President

Fnded: 1965. **Priorities:** *Arts & Humanities:* 67%. Supports museums, performing arts, music, libraries and historical societies. *Civic & Public Affairs:* 9%. Funding goes to anti-defamation, city parks, community foundations, and philanthropic organizations. *Education:* 21%. Universities, colleges, institutes, and schools receiving funding some applied to scholarship programs. *International:* 1%. *Note:* Total contributions made in 1999. **Typ. Recipients:** Clinics/Medical Centers, Family Planning, Health Organizations, Health-General, Hospitals, People with Disabilities, Public Health. **Geo. Dist:** New York, NY.

★ 11462 ★ Gladys Brooks Foundation

1055 Franklin Ave., Suite 102
Garden City, NY 11530
Phone: (516)746-6103 **Fax:** (516)877-1758
Website: http://www.gladysbrooksfoundation.org
Jessica Rutledge, Administrative Assistant

Fnded: 1981. **Philosophy:** The foundation was created "to provide for the intellectual, moral, and physical welfare of the people of this country by establishing and supporting non-profit libraries, educational institutions, hospitals, and clinics. The foundation will consider grant applications in the fields of libraries, education, hospitals, and clinics." Library grant applications will be considered for endowments, construction, and equipment. In education, grant applications will be considered generally for educational endowments to fund scholarships based solely on leadership and academic ability of the student; endowments to support salaries of educators who confine their activities primarily to classroom instruction in the liberal arts, mathematics, and the sciences during the academic year; and erection or endowment of buildings, wings, or additions thereto of buildings for educational purposes. Grant applications from hospitals and clinics will be considered generally where the proposal demonstrates one or more of the following: (a) a new health need; (b) an improvement in the quality of health care; or (c) reduced health costs with better patient outcomes. "No grant will be considered that is to support a laboratory research project." **Priorities:** *Arts & Humanities:* 8%. Supports museums, libraries and historic preservation. *Civic & Public Affairs:* 6%. Cathedral Community Cares. *Education:* 42%. Supports Colleges and universities, education foundations, tutoring programs, and schools. *Environment:* 11%. *International:* 28%. Supports hospitals. *Note:* Total contributions made in 2000. **Typ. Recipients:** Cancer, Children's Health/Hospitals, Clinics/Medical Centers, Emergency/Ambulance Services, Hospitals, Medical Education, Medical Research, Nursing Services, People with Disabilities, Research/Studies Institutes, Single-Disease Health Associations. **Geo. Dist:** CT; DE; DC; IN; ME; MD; MA; NH; NJ; NY; NC; OH; PA; RI; SC; VT; VA; WA; WV.

★ 11463 ★ Gladys and Roland Harriman Foundation

63 Wall St.
140 Broadway, 4th Floor
New York, NY 10005-1101
Phone: (212)493-8182 **Fax:** (212)493-5570
William Hibberd, Secretary

Fnded: 1966. **Philosophy:** The foundation generally gives a majority of funding to educational institutions, primarily to private secondary schools and colleges and universities. Hospitals and medical research organizations, as well as the arts, are also major beneficiaries. **Priorities:** *Arts & Humanities:* 32%. Supports museums, public broadcasting, performing arts, and libraries. *Civic & Public Affairs:* 1%. Funds community affairs and community development. *Education:* 23%. Supports secondary and preparatory schools, colleges, and universities. *Environment:* 13%. Supports child welfare and services for the elderly; major grant to Boys Club of New York. *International:* 20%. Supports the American Red Cross, medical centers, cancer centers, and hospitals. *Religion:* 6%. Supports the American Museum of Natural History. *Note:* Total contributions made in 2000. **Typ. Recipients:** Cancer, Child Abuse, Clinics/Medical Centers, Diabetes, Domestic Violence, Emergency/Ambulance Services, Family Planning, Geriatric Health, Health Organizations, Hospitals, Medical Education, Medical Research, Speech & Hearing, Substance Abuse. **Geo. Dist:** nationally; New York, NY.

★ 11464 ★ Gleason Foundation

1000 University Ave.
PO Box 22970
Rochester, NY 14692-2970
Phone: (585)241-4030 **Fax:** (585)241-4099
Email: susy.elniski@gleasonfoundation.org
Ralph Harper, Secretary, Treasurer

Fnded: 1959. **Philosophy:** The foundation focuses its interests on education, including secondary education and manufacturing/engineering, research, and technology. It also supports community funds, youth groups, social service agencies, public interest and civic affairs groups, and cultural activities. **Priorities:** *Arts & Humanities:* 7%. Supports museums, historical preservation, libraries, dance, and music. *Civic & Public Affairs:* 26%. Supports economic and public policy organizations, justice issues, women's organizations, and community foundations. *Education:* 40%. Supports private and charter schools, scholarship funds, and colleges and universities. *Environment:* 11%. Supports United Way, volunteer services, emergency relief, food banks, and community service organizations. *International:* 13%. Funds medical centers and emergency care. *Religion:* 1%. *Note:* Total contributions made in 2000. **Typ. Recipients:** Child Abuse, Children's Health/Hospitals, Clinics/Medical Centers, Domestic Violence, Emergency/Ambulance Services, Family Planning, Medical Rehabilitation, Medical Research, Nursing Services, Nutrition, People with Disabilities. **Geo. Dist:** Rochester, NY. **Frmly:** Gleason Memorial Fund.

★ 11465 ★ Golden Family Foundation

500 Fifth Ave., 50th Floor
New York, NY 10110
Phone: (212)391-8960
William Golden, President

Fnded: 1952. **Philosophy:** The Golden Family Foundation makes grants across the major categories of support. Most recently, large contributions were made to science and civic affairs. Other support goes to environmental affairs, Jewish religious organizations, higher education, health, the arts, and international organizations. **Priorities:** *Arts & Humanities:* 7%. Gives to museums, history, historic preservation, libraries, theater, and music. *Civic & Public Affairs:* 15%. Supports botanical gardens, community foundations, parks, and professional associations. *Education:* 14%. Primarily funds medical education, science/mathematics education, and universities. *International:* Less than 1%. Contributes to single-disease health associations and health foundations. *Religion:* 54%. Supports science museums and science laboratories. *Note:* Total contributions made in 2001. **Typ. Recipients:** Clinics/Medical Centers, Family Planning, Hospitals, Medical Education, Medical Rehabilitation, Medical Research, Research/Studies Institutes, Single-Disease Health Associations. **Geo. Dist:** some giving nationally; New York, NY, including metropolitan area.

★ 11466 ★ The Gordon Fund

125 Broad St.
New York, NY 10004-2498
Phone: (212)558-4000 **Fax:** (212)558-3064
Mary Roberts, Trustee

Fnded: 1985. **Philosophy:** The foundation makes grants across the major categories of support. The foundation's primary interest is education, with an emphasis on Harvard University and other colleges. Support for civic affairs includes environmental concerns and foreign relations. Health support favors public health and cancer research and treatment. Religious giving focuses on Catholic churches and organizations. Other support goes to social services and the arts. **Priorities:** *Arts & Humanities:* 9%. Funds museums, libraries, music, and literary arts. *Civic & Public Affairs:* 5%. Contributes to leadership development, public policy, parks, and nonprofit management. *Education:* 59%. Supports colleges, universities and private schools. *Environment:* 13%. Supports sports/recreation programs and community service organizations. *International:* 8%. Gives to hospitals, single-disease health associations, public health, and health and wellness projects. *Note:* Total contributions made in 2001. **Typ. Recipients:** Cancer, Emergency/Ambulance Services, Health-General, Hospitals, Medical Education, Medical Research, People with Disabilities, Research/Studies Institutes, Respiratory, Single-Disease Health Associations. **Geo. Dist:** CT; ME; MA; NH; NJ; NY; PA.

★ 11467 ★ Gordon and Mary Cain Foundation

8 Greenway Plaza, Suite 702
Houston, TX 77046
Phone: (713)960-9283 **Fax:** (713)877-8107
James Weaver, President

Fnded: 1988. **Philosophy:** The foundation makes grants across the major categories of support. Social service support goes to human services, homes, aid to the homeless, youth organizations, and united funds. Educational funding favors colleges and universities. Various programs also are supported in health care, science, the arts, and civic affairs. **Priorities:** *Arts & Humanities:* 8%. Supports theater, museums, music, and literary organizations. *Civic & Public Affairs:* 7%. Funds public policy, economic development, and gardens. *Education:* 57%. Supports secondary schools, medical schools, colleges and universities. *Environment:* 7%. Supports youth programs and services, and community centers. *International:* 12%. Funds cancer and heart institutes, hospitals, and research. *Religion:* 2%. Supports science museums and institutes. *Note:* Total contributions made in 2000. **Typ. Recipients:** AIDS/HIV, Cancer, Children's Health/Hospitals, Clinics/Medical Centers, Diabetes, Emergency/Ambulance Services, Eyes/Blindness, Family Planning, Health Policy/Cost Containment, Heart, Hospices, Hospitals, Medical Education, Medical Rehabilitation, Medical Research, Public Health, Single-Disease Health Associations, Substance Abuse. **Geo. Dist:** Houston, TX; Lake Wales, FL; Linville, NC.

★ 11468 ★ Gottesman Fund

1818 North St., NW, Suite 700
Washington, DC 20036
Phone: (202)785-2727 **Fax:** (202)331-9306
Milton Gottesman, Vice President

Fnded: 1965. **Philosophy:** The fund primarily supports the Jewish religion and higher education, including teaching and medicine. Other interests include organizations involved with Israel and civic foundations. **Priorities:** *Arts & Humanities:* Less than 1%. *Civic & Public Affairs:* 5%. Grants are made to community foundations and philanthropic organizations. *Education:* 48%. Jewish schools, universities, and day schools are funded. *Environment:* Less than 1%. *International:* Less than 1%. *Religion:* 14%. Supports natural history museums. *Note:* Total contributions made in fiscal 2001. **Typ. Recipients:** AIDS/HIV, Arthritis, Cancer, Children's Health/Hospitals, Clinics/Medical Centers, Clinics/Medical Centers, Family Planning, Health Organizations, Hospitals, Hospitals (University Affiliated), Medical Education, Medical Rehabilitation, Medical Research, People with Disabilities, Public Health, Single-Disease Health Associations. **Geo. Dist:** east of the Mississippi River; FL; NY.

★ 11469 ★ Grable Foundation

650 Smithfield St., Suite 240
Pittsburgh, PA 15222
Phone: (412)471-4550 **Fax:** (412)471-2267
Email: grable@grablefdn.org
Website: http://www.grablefdn.org
Susan Brownlee, Executive Director

Fnded: 1977. **Philosophy:** The foundation's mission is "to help children and youth to become independent, caring, contributing members of society by supporting programs critical to a child's successful development. In order of priority, The Grable Foundation will focus on: improving educational opportunities so that children can achieve their potential; supporting community efforts that create an environment in which children can succeed; strengthening families so they can serve as the core support of children and society." **Priorities:** *Arts & Humanities:* 6%. Supports arts museums, music, and theater. *Civic & Public Affairs:* 18%. Supports public policy and women's affairs. *Education:* 33%. Supports literacy, after school/enrichment programs, universities, and schools. *Environment:* 19%. Supports Young Men's Christian Association, youth organizations, United Way, camps, and day care. *International:* 16%. Supports substance rehabilitation, prenatal health issues, and health organizations. *Religion:* 5%. Funds science centers. *Note:* Total contributions made in 1998. **Typ. Recipients:** Children's Health/Hospitals, Family Planning, Health Organizations, Health-General, Hospitals, Mental Health, Prenatal Health Issues, Substance Abuse. **Geo. Dist:** PA, southwest region.

★ 11470 ★ Grace and Franklin Bernsen Foundation

15 West 6th St., Suite 1308
Tulsa, OK 74119-5407
Phone: (918)584-4711 **Fax:** (918)584-4713
Email: info@bernsen.org
Website: http://www.bernsen.org
Sandra Griffin, Administrator

Fnded: 1985. **Philosophy:** The foundation "provides grants in support of religious, charitable, scientific, literary or educational purposes, or for the prevention of cruelty to children." Arts funding favors ballet, art centers, museums, and performing arts. Educational funding goes to one university and to programs in Tulsa public schools. Health organizations, youth organizations, community centers, food banks, and the United Way are also supported. **Priorities:** *Arts & Humanities:* 12%. Supports museums, theater, dance, libraries, and historical societies. *Civic & Public Affairs:* 16%. Contributes to investment forums, zoos, and community funds. *Education:* 26%. Gives to colleges, universities, education foundations, public pre-college schools, and childhood development programs. *Environment:* 34%. Supports youth and family services, camps, crime prevention programs, shelters, child abuse prevention, and food and shelter programs. *International:* 2%. Funds hospice, infant medical care, and nursing services. *Religion:* 1%. Gives to an air and space museum. *Note:* Total contributions made in fiscal 2001. **Typ. Recipients:** Child Abuse, Children's Health/Hospitals, Clinics/Medical Centers, Domestic Violence, Emergency/Ambulance Services, Health Organizations, Heart, Hospices, Hospitals, Medical Education, Medical Rehabilitation, Medical Research, Mental Health, Multiple Sclerosis, Nursing Services, People with Disabilities, Prenatal Health Issues, Public Health, Respiratory, Sexual Abuse, Single-Disease Health Associations, Speech & Hearing, Substance Abuse. **Geo. Dist:** Tulsa, OK.

★ 11471 ★ Graham Foundation for Advanced Studies in the Fine Arts

4 West Burton Place
Chicago, IL 60610-1416
Phone: (312)787-4071
Email: info@grahamfoundation.org
Website: http://www.grahamfoundation.org
Richard Solomon, Director

Fnded: 1956. **Priorities:** *Arts & Humanities:* 57%. Supports historic preservation, architectural history, museums, and literature on architectural history and the built environment. *Civic & Public Affairs:* 6%. Funds urban and community planning. *Education:* 35%. Supports universities, scholarships, dissertation awards, and university presses. Focus is on education in architecture and history of the built environment. *Note:* Total contributions made in 2001. **Typ. Recipients:** Health Organizations. **Geo. Dist:** internationally; nationally.

★ 11472 ★ The Grainger Foundation
100 Grainger Parkway
Lake Forest, IL 60045-5201
Phone: (847)535-1000

Fnded: 1967. **Philosophy:** While the foundation's funding interests are broad, it places "emphasis on capital funds, and special program funds for higher education (colleges and universities), cultural and historical institutions (art, symphonies, and museums), hospitals, and human service organizations." **Priorities:** *Arts & Humanities:* 5%. Cultural and historical institutions and art museums. *Civic & Public Affairs:* Less than 1%. *Education:* 73%. Colleges and universities, and private secondary education; focus on science and technology education. *Environment:* 2%. Recreation/athletics, crime prevention, youth organizations, and human services. *International:* 19%. Supports hospitals. *Note:* Total contributions made in 2000. **Typ. Recipients:** Cancer, Children's Health/Hospitals, Clinics/Medical Centers, Health Organizations, Hospitals, Medical Education, Medical Research, Research/Studies Institutes, Substance Abuse. **Geo. Dist:** Chicago, IL, including metropolitan area.

★ 11473 ★ Grayce B. Kerr Fund
117 Bay St.
Easton, MD 21601
Phone: (410)822-6652 **Fax:** (410)822-4546
Email: gbkf@bluecrab.org
Heather Brady Masone, contact

Fnded: 1986. **Philosophy:** "The Grayce B. Kerr Fund, Inc., established in 1986, is a dynamic philanthropic foundation committed to enhancing the quality of life. The Fund awards grants that significantly impact and sustain long term change and growth in organizations and institutions. "Currently, the Fund's principal areas of interest include nurturing educational achievement and excellence, fostering life skills critical to self-sufficiency, and encouraging cultural growth. The Fund supports economic and other research activities directed toward improving the information base available for public policy-making. "Leadership effecting positive change in our community is a goal of Grayce B. Kerr Fund, Inc." Annual Report **Priorities:** *Arts & Humanities:* 12%. *Civic & Public Affairs:* 8%. *Education:* 48%. *Environment:* 5%. *International:* 13%. *Religion:* 14%. **Typ. Recipients:** Cancer, Children's Health/Hospitals, Family Planning, Hospices, Hospitals, Medical Research, Mental Health, Public Health.

★ 11474 ★ Green Fund
14 East 60th St., Suite 702
New York, NY 10022
Phone: (212)755-2445 **Fax:** (212)755-0021
Bruce Rosenblatt, Contact

Fnded: 1947. **Philosophy:** Because the fund initiates its grants program, it will not respond to solicitations. The fund concentrates its donations in the New York metropolitan area, providing general support for social service groups, especially to Jewish welfare organizations, health-related institutions, education, and the arts. **Priorities:** *Arts & Humanities:* 4%. Ballet, opera, music, libraries, public broadcasting, and theater. *Civic & Public Affairs:* 52%. Supports women's rights issues, parks/botanical gardens and housing. *Education:* 7%. Focus on colleges and universities, legal education. *Environment:* 2%. Supports homeless/shelters, family planning services, and child abuse. *International:* 1%. Hospitals, geriatric health, and cancer research are supported. *Note:* Total contributions made in fiscal 2001. **Typ. Recipients:** Cancer, Children's Health/Hospitals, Clinics/Medical Centers, Family Planning, Geriatric Health, Health Funds, Health Organizations, Hospices, Hospitals, Medical Education, Medical Rehabilitation, Medical Research, Nursing Services, People with Disabilities, Prenatal Health Issues, Single-Disease Health Associations. **Geo. Dist:** New York, NY.

★ 11475 ★ Greentree Foundation
400 Madison Ave., Suite 1001
New York, NY 10017
Phone: (212)888-7755 **Fax:** (212)888-1574
Email: rschaffer@greentreefdn.org
Richard Schaffer, President

Fnded: 1982. **Philosophy:** "The Greentree Foundation supports focused projects initiated by local community groups that provide clearly defined participatory roles for schools, parents, children, and community-based organizations. We seek to reduce educational deficiencies and lessen social and cultural tensions." 1997 Guidelines **Priorities:** *Arts & Humanities:* 9%. Supports museums, libraries, art centers and theater groups. *Civic & Public Affairs:* 9%. Funds community development/revitalization programs, botanical gardens, diversity programs, and neighborhood associations. *Education:* 53%. Supports colleges, universities, tutoring and after-school programs, arts education, and private pre-college schools. *Environment:* 18%. Supports youth programs, shelters, food distribution, and child and family services. *Note:* Total contributions made in 2000. **Typ. Recipients:** Child Abuse, Family Planning, Hospitals, Medical Education, Mental Health, Research/Studies Institutes. **Geo. Dist:** New York, NY, including metropolitan area.

★ 11476 ★ Greenwall Foundation
2 Park Ave., 24th Floor
New York, NY 10016-9301
Phone: (212)679-7266
Email: admin@greenwall.org
Website: http://www.greenwall.org
William Stubing, President

Fnded: 1949. **Philosophy:** The foundation primarily supports work in medical research, education, and the arts. Medical funding targets areas of special interest to the foundation including bioethics and basic research in insulin-dependent diabetes mellitus. Educational funding focuses on programs to improve the teaching of mathematics and natural sciences. In the arts, the foundation encourages requests from emerging artists and the development of new artistic work. **Priorities:** *Arts & Humanities:* 1%. Supports theater. *Civic & Public Affairs:* 10%. Supports parks/botanical gardens, towns/municipalities, and law & justice. *Education:* 72%. Supports public schools, educational programs, colleges, universities, and medical education. *International:* 10%. Gives to medical centers, hospitals, the Joslin Diabetes Center, and health organizations. *Religion:* 2%. Supports science academies. *Note:* Contributions were made in 2000. **Typ. Recipients:** Alzheimers Disease, Children's Health/Hospitals, Clinics/Medical Centers, Diabetes, Health Organizations, Health Policy/Cost Containment, Heart, Hospitals, Hospitals (University Affiliated), Long-Term Care, Medical Education, Medical Research, Public Health. **Geo. Dist:** NY.

★ 11477 ★ Gregg-Graniteville Foundation
PO Box 418
Graniteville, SC 29829
Phone: (803)663-7552 **Fax:** (803)663-6435
Patricia Knight, Secretary-Treasurer

Fnded: 1941. **Philosophy:** The purposes of the foundation are to make contributions or to render financial aid to the churches, schools, colleges, public libraries, and other educational and religious organizations located in Aiken County, SC, and Richmond County, GA; to provide scholarships or to finance other educational training; and to construct, own, operate, and maintain parks, gymnasiums, swimming pools, and other facilities for the benefit of the health and welfare of the people who work in the Graniteville, SC, area. **Priorities:** *Arts & Humanities:* 1%. Dance, music, and libraries. *Civic & Public Affairs:* 1%. Major support for the Gregg Park Civic Center. Also supports clubs. *Education:* 27%. Primarily for colleges and universities and religious education. *Environment:* 4%. Community service organizations, Special Olympics, and atheltics/recreation. *International:* 60%. Medical rehabilitation and single disease health associations. *Note:* Total contributions made in 2000. **Typ. Recipients:** Cancer, Diabetes, Domestic Violence, Emergency/Ambulance Services, Geriatric Health, Health Organizations, Hospitals, Hospitals (University Affiliated), Medical Rehabilitation, Mental Health, People with Disabilities, Research/Studies Institutes, Single-Disease Health Associations. **Geo. Dist:** GA, Richmond County; SC, Aiken County.

★ 11478 ★ Grousbeck Family Foundation
c/o Stanford University Graduate School of Business
Rm. L336
Stanford, CA 94305-5015
Phone: (650)723-0709
H. Grousbeck, President

Fnded: 1991. **Priorities:** *Arts & Humanities:* 6%. *Civic & Public Affairs:* 23%. Supports community organizations. *Education:* 57%. Supports special education colleges and universities. *Environment:* 4%. services, refugee assistance and homes. *Note:* Total contributions made in 1999. **Typ. Recipients:** Children's Health/Hospitals, Eyes/Blindness, Health Organizations, People with Disabilities, Public Health. **Geo. Dist:** nationally.

★ 11479 ★ Grover Hermann Foundation
1000 Hillgrove, Suite 200
Western Springs, IL 60558
Phone: (708)246-8331 **Fax:** (708)246-8319
Katheryn Rhoads, Executive Director

Fnded: 1955. **Philosophy:** The Grover Hermann Foundation funds education, health, community, public policy, and religious programs throughout the United States. In the category of education, higher education receives the greatest consideration, with preference for private rather than tax-supported institutions. Scholarships, fellowships, endowments, challenge grants, and capital grants are considered. Private colleges are strongly favored over tax-supported institutions. In the health category, the foundation considers grants for facilities, basic research, disease-specific organizations, and other health programs having demonstrable significance. Community grants are considered for local development, libraries, organizations for youth, the aged or disadvantaged, and other community-related activities. In the area of public policy, the foundation considers organizations dedicated to the strengthening and improvement of our governmental, economic and social systems and that recognize and promote the values of individual liberty, a strong work ethic, free-market competition and limited government. Religious grants favor established organizations and well-defined secular causes. **Priorities:** *Arts & Humanities:* 4%. Supports ballet and theater. *Civic & Public Affairs:* 70%. Supports public policy and community foundations. *Education:* 16%. Supports education associations, universities, and scholarship foundation. *Environment:* 3%. Supports youth organizations. *International:* 6%. Supports medical research. *Note:* Total contributions made in 2000. **Typ. Recipients:** Child Abuse, Children's Health/Hospitals, Domestic Violence, Emergency/Ambulance Services, Health Organizations, Health Policy/Cost Containment, Health-General, Hospices, Hospitals, Long-Term Care, Medical Education, Medical Rehabilitation, Medical Research, Mental Health, Nursing Services, People with Disabilities, Single-Disease Health Associations, Speech & Hearing. **Geo. Dist:** Chicago, IL.

★ 11480 ★ Grundy Foundation
680 Radcliffe St.
PO Box 701
Bristol, PA 19007
Phone: (215)788-5460 **Fax:** (215)788-0915
Roland Johnson, Executive Director

Fnded: 1961. **Philosophy:** According to the broad directive in Mr. Grundy's will, the foundation considers scientific, literary, educational, and charitable projects in the Commonwealth of Pennsylvania. The board of trustees has limited the foundation's work to Bucks County, primarily to the borough of Bristol. The foundation currently is involved in a variety of projects in support of Bristol's ongoing revitalization program. **Priorities:** *Arts & Humanities:* 46%. Supports historic preservation, museums, and the performing arts. *Civic & Public Affairs:* 5%. Funds economic development, urban affairs, and community associations. *Education:* 13%. Contributes to public education. *Environment:* 28%. Supports United Way, family services, senior services, youth programs, and disaster relief agencies. *International:* 4%. Gives to public health programs and single-disease health associations. *Note:* Total contributions made in 2001. **Typ. Recipients:** Cancer, Children's Health/Hospitals, Clinics/Medical Centers, Domestic Violence, Emergency/Ambulance Services, Family Planning, Health-General, Hospitals, Long-Term Care, Mental Health, People with Disabilities, Public Health, Respiratory, Sexual Abuse, Substance Abuse. **Geo. Dist:** Bristol, PA, and Bucks County.

★ 11481 ★ Gustavus and Louise Pfeiffer Research Foundation

89 Diamond Spring Rd., CN 3050
Denville, NJ 07834
Phone: (973)983-0480 **Fax:** (973)586-3456
Website: http://www.fdncenter.org/grantmaker/pfeiffer
Matthew Herold, Jr., Secretary

Fnded: 1942. **Philosophy:** Primary support goes to the advancement of medicine and pharmacy. The foundation generally limits biomedical research to breast, ovarian, and prostate cancer, predictive factors in cardiovascular disease, and gerontological immunology. **Priorities:** *Education:* 51%. Supports medical education. *International:* 49%. Supports medical research in the fields of breast, prostate, and ovarian cancer, and cardiovascular disease. *Note:* Total contributions made in 2001. **Typ. Recipients:** AIDS/HIV, Cancer, Children's Health/Hospitals, Clinics/Medical Centers, Diabetes, Geriatric Health, Health Policy/Cost Containment, Health-General, Heart, Hospitals, Hospitals (University Affiliated), Kidney, Medical Education, Medical Research, Public Health, Research/Studies Institutes, Single-Disease Health Associations. **Geo. Dist:** nationally.

★ 11482 ★ H. A. and Mary K. Chapman Charitable Trust

One Warren Place, Suite 1816
6100 South Yale Ave.
Tulsa, OK 74136
Phone: (918)496-7882 **Fax:** (918)496-7887
Donne Pitman, Trustee

Fnded: 1976. **Philosophy:** The bulk of funding goes to health and educational organizations. Most grants are to organizations in Oklahoma, primarily in the metropolitan Tulsa area. **Priorities:** *Arts & Humanities:* 3%. Supports ballet, museums, opera and theater. *Education:* 57%. Colleges, religion education, high schools and education funds. *Environment:* 22%. Supports youth and family services, YWCA, United Way, Goodwill Industries, and youth organizations. *International:* 18%. Hospitals and medical research. *Note:* Total contributions made in 1999. **Typ. Recipients:** Cancer, Child Abuse, Children's Health/Hospitals, Clinics/Medical Centers, Domestic Violence, Geriatric Health, Health Organizations, Health-General, Hospices, Hospitals, Medical Education, Medical Research, Mental Health, Nursing Services, People with Disabilities, Prenatal Health Issues, Public Health, Research/Studies Institutes, Respiratory, Single-Disease Health Associations, Speech & Hearing, Substance Abuse. **Geo. Dist:** Tulsa, OK.

★ 11483 ★ H. C. S. Foundation

1801 East 9th St., Suite 1035
Cleveland, OH 44114-3103
Phone: (216)781-3502 **Fax:** (216)781-3504
L. Hiltz, Trustee

Fnded: 1959. **Philosophy:** The foundation primarily supports education through capital grants. Other interests include the arts, health services, religion, and social services. **Priorities:** *Arts & Humanities:* 7%. Supports children's theater and public broadcasting. *Civic & Public Affairs:* 54%. Funds Renaissance Village, Cincinnati Zoo and Botanical Garden, community development, and legal concerns. *Education:* 7%. Supports universities. *Environment:* 6%. Funds human services and athletics. *International:* 18%. Supports medical centers, infant care, and hearing and speech centers. *Religion:* 2%. Funds a science center. *Note:* Total contributions made in 2000. **Typ. Recipients:** Cancer, Clinics/Medical Centers, Eyes/Blindness, Family Planning, Health Funds, Health Organizations, Heart, Hospitals, Long-Term Care, Medical Rehabilitation, People with Disabilities, Prenatal Health Issues, Speech & Hearing, Substance Abuse, Trauma Treatment. **Geo. Dist:** MD; Cincinnati, OH.

★ 11484 ★ H. Leslie Hoffman & Elaine S. Hoffman Foundation

225 South Lake Ave., Suite 1150
Pasadena, CA 91101
Phone: (626)793-0043 **Fax:** (626)793-0047
J. Popovich, Trustee

Fnded: 1952. **Philosophy:** The H. Leslie Hoffman and Elaine S. Hoffman Foundation's main focus is educational institutions in the Los Angeles, CA, area. The foundation also supports social service organizations, health concerns, and the arts. **Priorities:** *Arts & Humanities:* 9%. Contributes to museums, libraries, and performing arts organizations. *Civic & Public Affairs:* 4%. Gives to municipalities, community foundations, and legal aid programs. *Education:* 34%. Primarily supports colleges and universities. *Environment:* 33%. Supports YMCA, scouts, child welfare, family services, and a food bank. *International:* 15%. Funds single-disease health associations, pediatric health, medical research, and hospitals. *Note:* Total contributions made in 2001. **Typ. Recipients:** Arthritis, Arthritis, Cancer, Children's Health/Hospitals, Clinics/Medical Centers, Diabetes, Emergency/Ambulance Services, Eyes/Blindness, Health Organizations, Health-General, Heart, Hospices, Hospitals, Medical Education, Medical Research, People with Disabilities, Substance Abuse. **Geo. Dist:** Los Angeles, CA, metro area.

★ 11485 ★ H. N. and Frances C. Berger Foundation

PO Box 13390
Palm Desert, CA 92255-3390
Phone: (760)341-5293
Website: http://www.hnberger.org
Christopher McGuire, Vice President & Assistant Secretary

Fnded: 1994. **Priorities:** *Civic & Public Affairs:* 1%. *Education:* 59%. Supports colleges and universities, including some scholarship programs. *Environment:* 4%. Supports charities, Big Brothers/Big Sisters, and women's services. *International:* 29%. Funding goes to medical centers, rehabilitation services, medical research, and hospitals. *Note:* Total contributions made in 1999. **Typ. Recipients:** AIDS/HIV, Alzheimers Disease, Cancer, Clinics/Medical Centers, Domestic Violence, Health-General, Hospices, Hospitals, Medical Rehabilitation, Medical Research, People with Disabilities, Research/Studies Institutes. **Geo. Dist:** CA; KY.

★ 11486 ★ Hagedorn Fund

345 Park Ave., 8th Fl.
New York, NY 10021
Phone: (212)464-0134
Monica Neal, Vice President

Fnded: 1953. **Philosophy:** The Hagedorn Fund makes most of its grants in two areas: social services and health care. In social services, interests include children, religious charities, homes, and domestic violence. Health care support favors single-disease associations and hospitals. Other areas of interest include religious and legal education, community colleges, minority college funds, libraries, and civic affairs. **Priorities:** *Arts & Humanities:* 7%. Supports public broadcasting, music, libraries, historic preservation, and art societies. *Civic & Public Affairs:* 9%. Supports gardens, economic development, and parks. *Education:* 22%. Supports higher education, after school/enrichment programs, and education funds. *Environment:* 33%. Supports family planning, family services, youth programs, and child welfare. *International:* 11%. Supports hospitals, AIDS, and cancer research. *Note:* Total contributions made in 2001. **Typ. Recipients:** AIDS/HIV, Arthritis, Cancer, Children's Health/Hospitals, Clinics/Medical Centers, Diabetes, Emergency/Ambulance Services, Eyes/Blindness, Family Planning, Health Organizations, Health Policy/Cost Containment, Heart, Hospices, Hospitals, Medical Education, Medical Rehabilitation, Mental Health, Nursing Services, People with Disabilities, Respiratory. **Geo. Dist:** Cuyahoga County, OH.

★ 11487 ★ Hal and Charlie Peterson Foundation

PO Box 293870
Kerrville, TX 78029-3870
Phone: (830)896-2262 **Fax:** (830)896-2283
Email: hcpfn@ktc.com
John Mosty, Secretary-Treasurer

Fnded: 1990. **Philosophy:** The foundation generally supports educational institutions, the arts, and health-related causes. Funding is limited to Kerr and adjacent counties in Texas. **Priorities:** *Arts & Humanities:* 13%. Funds museums, theater, and historic preservation. *Civic & Public Affairs:* 8%. Supports municipalities, safety organizations, and housing. *Education:* 29%. Private and public education, medical education, and colleges and universities. *Environment:* 32%. Funds United Way, YMCAs, recreation and athletics, scouting, and people with disabilities. *International:* 9%. Support for hospitals, clinics, and single-disease associations. *Note:* Total contributions made in 2000. **Typ. Recipients:** Alzheimers Disease, Cancer, Clinics/Medical Centers, Emergency/Ambulance Services, Health-General, Hospices, Hospitals, Medical Education, Medical Rehabilitation, Nursing Services, People with Disabilities, Preventive Medicine/Wellness Organizations, Substance Abuse. **Geo. Dist:** TX, Kerr and adjacent counties.

★ 11488 ★ The Hall Family Foundation

PO Box 419580, Department 323
Kansas City, MO 64141-6580
Phone: (816)274-8515 **Fax:** (816)274-8547
William Hall, President

Fnded: 1993. **Philosophy:** "The Hall Family Foundation is a private philanthropic organization dedicated to enhancing the quality of human life. Programs that enrich the community, help people and promote excellence are considered to be of prime importance. The Foundation views its critical function as that of a catalyst. It seeks to be responsive to programs that are innovative, yet strive to create permanent solutions to community needs in the greater Kansas City area. The Hall Family Foundation concentrates its philanthropic efforts on five areas of interest in the greater Kansas City area: Education, in a continuing tradition of concern for youth, the Foundation has an interest in programs that enhance or promote excellence in elementary, secondary and higher education. Programs which address the educational needs of urban school children, and efforts and initiatives targeting systemic educational reform are a high priority; Children, Youth and Families, the Foundation has a strong interest in improving the lives of children, youth and families and values programs which help prevent family violence, improve child well-being, expand youth services and respond to families' physical and emotional health needs; the Arts, the Foundation considers programs which encourage excellence in the community's major performing and visual arts organizations and is interested in programs that enhance quality, strengthen management, broaden existing funding bases and increase audience development; Community Development, the Foundation is interested in programs and initiatives which help prevent or overcome blight and deterioration of the central city and its neighborhoods with redevelopment projects which help to stabilize these areas a high priority; Additional Interests; included in this category is Foundation support of community-wide efforts that seek to provide long-term solutions to local issues of high priority." **Priorities:** *Arts & Humanities:* 44%. Supports performing arts, art centers, and museums. *Civic & Public Affairs:* 10%. Supports community development initiatives. *Education:* 13%. Supports education centers, colleges and universities, and provides scholarships. *Environment:* 9%. Funds children, youth and family services. *International:* 5%. *Religion:* 10%. *Note:* Five-year summary of contributions supplied by foundation. **Typ. Recipients:** Child Abuse, Children's Health/Hospitals, Clinics/Medical Centers, Domestic Violence, Health Organizations, Health-General, Home-Care Services, Hospitals, Hospitals (University Affiliated), Medical Education, Medical Rehabilitation, Mental Health, Public Health, Sexual Abuse, Substance Abuse. **Geo. Dist:** Kansas City, MO, metropolitan area.

★ 11489 ★ Hall-Perrine Foundation

115 3rd St. Southeast, Suite 803
Cedar Rapids, IA 52401-1222
Phone: (319)362-9079 **Fax:** (319)362-7220
Jack Evans, President, Chief Executive Officer

Fnded: 1953. **Philosophy:** "The foundation is interested in assisting local tax-exempt public institutions and organizations dedicated to the solution of problems of people of all ages. The foundation has a particular interest in all areas of health care. It also has a concern for the advancement of education, seeks to support projects to resolve social problems, and is interested in the encouragement and maintenance of community cultural activities." **Priorities:** *Arts & Humanities:* Less than 1%. *Civic & Public Affairs:* 4%. Supports chambers of commerce, housing, and philanthropy. *Education:* 33%. Funds colleges and universities, Junior Achievement, and scholarship foundations. *Environment:* 63%. Supports United Way, scouting, youth organizations, and community centers. *International:* Less than 1%. *Religion:* Less than 1%. *Note:* Total contributions approved in 2000. **Typ. Recipients:** Clinics/Medical Centers, Domestic Violence, Emergency/Ambulance Services, Family Planning, Geriatric Health, Health Organizations, Heart, Hospitals, Hospitals, People with Disabilities, Substance Abuse. **Geo. Dist:** IA, Linn County; Cedar Rapids, IA.

★ 11490 ★ Harden Foundation

PO Box 779
Salinas, CA 93902-0779
Phone: (831)442-3005 **Fax:** (831)443-1429
Email: jgrainger@hardenfoundation.org
Website: http://www.hardenfoundation.org
Joseph Grainger, Executive Director

Fnded: 1963. **Philosophy:** "In general, the Foundation seeks to support not-for-profit organizations that will achieve all or some of the following objectives: improve the well-being of young people; strengthen the family; develop individual self-reliance and health; prevent inappropriate institutionalization of individuals; improve the quality of life through cultural activities; encourage more humane treatment of animals; eliminate duplication and improve coordination of social and community services." 1995-1996 Annual Report **Priorities:** *Arts & Humanities:* 11%. Supports libraries, music, and museum. *Civic & Public Affairs:* 8%. Supports legal aid, clubs, and inner-city developmemt. *Education:* 7%. Supports agriculture education, education funds. *Environment:* 58%. Supports Big Brothers/Big Sisters, scouts, Young Men's Christian Association, shelters/homelesss, at-risk youth, family services, counseling, and food distribution programs. *International:* 14%. Supports eyes/blindness, hospital, medical funds, AIDS/HIV, and home-care services. *Note:* Contributions made in fiscal 2001. **Typ. Recipients:** AIDS/HIV, Alzheimers Disease, Child Abuse, Children's Health/Hospitals, Clinics/Medical Centers, Domestic Violence, Emergency/Ambulance Services, Eyes/Blindness, Family Planning, Health Funds, Heart, Home-Care Services, Hospices, Hospitals, Long-Term Care, Medical Rehabilitation, Mental Health, Nursing Services, Nutrition, Outpatient Health Care, People with Disabilities, Prenatal Health Issues, Respiratory, Single-Disease Health Associations, Substance Abuse. **Geo. Dist:** CA, Monterey County; Salinas Valley, CA.

★ 11491 ★ Harkness Foundation for Dance

145 East 48th St., Suite 26C
New York, NY 10017-0025
Phone: (212)755-5540 **Fax:** (212)755-5542
Theodore Bartwink, Treasurer

Fnded: 1986. **Philosophy:** The Harkness Foundation for Dance focuses on funding for the performing arts, dance venues, and dance scholarships. Limited funding is also available for non-performing arts organizations, with some funding going to health and social service causes. **Priorities:** *Arts & Humanities:* 64%. Supports dance, theater, opera, cultural and performing arts centers, and arts associations. *Civic & Public Affairs:* Less than 1%. Gives to parks, career transition services for dancers, and legal aid for the arts. *Education:* 14%. Funds arts/humanities education, colleges, and universities. *Environment:* 11%. Supports social service agencies and Young Men's Christian Association. *International:* 11%. Contributes to joint health and dance medicine programs. *Note:* Total contributions made in 2001. **Typ. Recipients:** AIDS/HIV, Cancer, Hospitals. **Geo. Dist:** some giving nationally; New York, NY.

★ 11492 ★ Harold K. Hochschild Foundation

477 Madison Ave.
New York, NY 10022-5802
Phone: (212)371-2100 **Fax:** (212)759-2946
Adam Hochschild, Trustee

Fnded: 1980. **Philosophy:** The foundation primarily supports the arts, with emphasis on historic preservation, and museums. Civic affairs are a secondary interest, with support to human rights, public policy, and international trade affairs. Other support funds environmental affairs, health care, and social services. The foundation has begun to place a greater emphasis on civil liberties, arms control, and ecology. **Priorities:** *Arts & Humanities:* 60%. Major support to the Adirondack Historical Association of New York; also funds libraries and arts centers. *Civic & Public Affairs:* 22%. Funds public policy, civil rights, labor organizations, and safety. *Education:* 1%. *Environment:* Less than 1%. *International:* 2%. *Religion:* 1%. *Note:* Total contributions made in 2000. **Typ. Recipients:** Emergency/Ambulance Services, Family Planning, Health Organizations, Health Policy/Cost Containment, Home-Care Services, Nutrition, Public Health. **Geo. Dist:** internationally; nationally; NY.

★ 11493 ★ Harold K. L. Castle Foundation

146 Hekili St., Suite 203A
Kailua, HI 96734
Phone: (808)262-9413 **Fax:** (808)261-6918
Email: bradenkf@aloha.com
Website: http://www.castlefoundation.org
Katherine Braden, Vice President & Treasurer

Fnded: 1962. **Philosophy:** The foundation favors private education, the community, health and human services (especially youth), youth concerns, and the arts, in Hawaii. The foundation places more emphasis on programs that can effect true systemic change rather than programs which do not address the cause of the problem. The foundation's giving is becoming more proactive. The foundation is assisting the community to determine its goals and is providing program start-ups and seed money to help the community reach its goals. **Priorities:** *Arts & Humanities:* 8%. Supports museums, fine arts, the performing arts, and music. *Civic & Public Affairs:* 2%. Funds community and economic development, and legal affairs. *Education:* 69%. Funds public school governance reform, private school development, and science education. *Environment:* 11%. Emphasis on youth concerns, United Way, and community services. *International:* 6%. Supports medical centers, cancer research, and Easter Seals Society. *Note:* Total contributions made in 2000. **Typ. Recipients:** AIDS/HIV, Cancer, Child Abuse, Children's Health/Hospitals, Clinics/Medical Centers, Domestic Violence, Emergency/Ambulance Services, Health Organizations, Heart, Hospices, Hospitals, Medical Rehabilitation, Mental Health, People with Disabilities, Prenatal Health Issues, Single-Disease Health Associations, Substance Abuse. **Geo. Dist:** HI, focusing on Windward Oahu.

★ 11494 ★ Harold McAlister Charitable Foundation

4801 Wilshire Boulevard, Suite 232
Los Angeles, CA 90010
Phone: (323)937-0927 **Fax:** (323)937-4727

Fnded: 1959. **Philosophy:** Health services are a major interest of the foundation, although no specific health field is supported uniformly. Social services organizations also receive regular support, with primary interests in child welfare, animal protection, services for the disabled, and other community-support organizations. Higher education in California also is a major priority. **Priorities:** *Arts & Humanities:* 3%. *Civic & Public Affairs:* 8%. *Education:* 21%. Mainly supports colleges and universities. *Environment:* 6%. Focus on child welfare, youth organizations, family services, and animal protection. *International:* 60%. Supports hospitals, single-disease health associations, and children's health services. *Note:* Total contributions made in fiscal 2001. **Typ. Recipients:** Arthritis, Cancer, Children's Health/Hospitals, Clinics/Medical Centers, Emergency/Ambulance Services, Geriatric Health, Health Organizations, Heart, Hospitals, Kidney, Long-Term Care, Medical Research, Nutrition, People with Disabilities, Public Health, Research/Studies Institutes, Research/Studies Institutes, Respiratory, Sexual Abuse, Single-Disease Health Associations, Speech & Hearing, Substance Abuse. **Geo. Dist:** Los Angeles, CA.

★ 11495 ★ Harriet Ford Dickenson Foundation

3450 Park Ave.
New York, NY 10154
Phone: (212)464-1937 **Fax:** (212)464-1919
James Largey, Vice President

Fnded: 1958. **Priorities:** *Arts & Humanities:* 47%. Supports opera, museums, ballet, orchestras, libraries, public broadcasting, historic preservation, and music programs. *Civic & Public Affairs:* 11%. Funds botanical gardens, parks, civic groups, legal aid, affordable housing programs, and professional organizations. *Education:* 2%. Gives to colleges and universities. *Environment:* 15%. Supports the United Way, family planning organizations, youth groups, youth services, and camps and recreation programs. *International:* 10%. Hospitals and single-disease health associations receive support. *Note:* Total contributions made in 2000. **Typ. Recipients:** Family Planning, Hospitals, People with Disabilities. **Geo. Dist:** NY, Broome County.

★ 11496 ★ Harriett Ames Charitable Trust

1600 Market St., 29th Floor
Philadelphia, PA 19103
Phone: (215)585-4609 **Fax:** (215)585-5488
Email: lynn.brickman@hawthorn-pnc.net
Lynn Brickman, Administrator Officer

Fnded: 1952. **Philosophy:** The trust's primary funding interests include hospitals and organizations engaged in medical research, educational institutions, and Jewish welfare organizations. The trust also supports cultural and youth programs. **Priorities:** *Arts & Humanities:* 67%. Supports museums, film, visual arts, music, and arts funds. *Civic & Public Affairs:* 3%. *Education:* 22%. Funds precollege and higher education. *Environment:* 1%. *International:* 5%. Supports hospitals and medical centers. *Note:* Total contributions made in 2001. **Typ. Recipients:** Alzheimers Disease, Cancer, Clinics/Medical Centers, Diabetes, Eyes/Blindness, Geriatric Health, Health Funds, Health Organizations, Hospitals, Medical Education, Medical Research, Multiple Sclerosis, People with Disabilities, Research/Studies Institutes, Single-Disease Health Associations, Trauma Treatment. **Geo. Dist:** nationally; NY.

★ 11497 ★ Harris and Eliza Kempner Fund

2201 Market St., Suite 601
Galveston, TX 77550-1529
Phone: (409)762-1603 **Fax:** (409)762-5435
Email: information@kempnerfund.org
Website: http://kempnerfund.org
Elaine Perachio, Executive Director

Fnded: 1946. **Philosophy:** The Harris and Eliza Kempner Fund has established three priorities in the Galveston, TX, area which has traditionally received more than 80% of the fund's annual contributions. The fund intends to focus on the needs of children and youth including education, health care, and human services, as well as access to social and cultural enrichment. A second priority is addressing the need for affordable housing for low- to moderate-income families. Finally, economic development will receive particular attention in the coming years. Preference is given to seed money grants, operating funds, and small capital needs. In addition to its general grant program, the fund operates a matching gift program for family members and it began Program Related Investments in 1992. The fund made its first three Program-Related Investments in Galveston. Currently, there are nine volunteer members comprising the board of trustees. Seven are family members and two are non-family. The fund also has established three advisory committees, which review grant requests in education, the environment, or population control and third world development. For the student loans, the fund has narrowed its general application process to a program in which selected colleges recommend a specified number of needy upperclassmen. Historically, the fund provides support to a broad range of activities in the Galveston community. The arts and humanities, human services, and health care have all received substantial contributions. The Galveston County Jewish Welfare Association and the University of Texas Medical Branch (UTMB), which is also located in Galveston, have both received continuing support. UTMB has received more than $2.5 million from the fund over the years. Annually, the fund also provides support to the United Way of Galveston. **Priorities:** *Arts & Humanities:* 16%. Emphasis on opera, historical foundations, and arts centers. *Civic & Public Affairs:* 12%. Supports urban and community affairs projects. *Education:* 18%. Supports medical education, primary and secondary education, and scholarships. *Environment:* 30%. Focus on youth organizations, united funds, and family planning. *International:* 13%. Primary support for a university medical center. *Note:* Total contributions made in 2000. **Typ. Recipients:** Adolescent Health Issues, AIDS/HIV, Alzheimers Disease, Cancer, Child Abuse, Children's Health/Hospitals, Clinics/Medical Centers, Domestic Violence, Emergency/Ambulance Services, Family Planning, Health Organizations, Heart, Hospices, Medical Education, Mental Health, Nursing Services, People with Disabilities, Prenatal Health Issues, Research/Studies Institutes, Single-Disease Health Associations, Substance Abuse. **Geo. Dist:** TX, Galveston county.

★ 11498 ★ Harry A. and Margaret D. Towsley Foundation

140 Ashman St., PO Box 349
Midland, MI 48640
Phone: (989)837-1100 **Fax:** (989)837-3240
Lynn White, President

Fnded: 1959. **Philosophy:** The foundation generally focuses its philanthropic work on the problems and needs of private higher education and health education and services. In this area, the University of Michigan is a primary beneficiary of support. Cultural arts, religion, community services, and innovative projects also receive considerable funding. **Priorities:** *Arts & Humanities:* 13%. Museums, opera, summer festival, and theater. *Civic & Public Affairs:* 11%. Supports community foundations. *Education:* 30%. Mostly colleges and universities, schools, education foundations, and arts/humanities education. *Environment:* 20%. Supports children services, family services, food programs, emergency services, family planning services, and senior services. *International:* 10%. Hospices, health centers, AIDS funds, and hospitals. *Note:* Total contributions made in 2000. **Typ. Recipients:** AIDS/HIV, Alzheimers Disease, Cancer, Child Abuse, Children's Health/Hospitals, Clinics/Medical Centers, Emergency/Ambulance Services, Family Planning, Geriatric Health, Health Organizations, Health-General, Hospices, Hospitals, Medical Education, Medical Rehabilitation, Medical Research, Nursing Services, Public Health, Respiratory, Single-Disease Health Associations, Substance Abuse, Transplant Networks/Donor Banks. **Geo. Dist:** MI, especially Ann Arbor and Washtenaw County.

★ 11499 ★ Harry C. Moores Foundation

100 South 3rd St.
Columbus, OH 43215
Phone: (614)227-8884 **Fax:** (614)227-2390
Mary Cummins, Contact

Fnded: 1961. **Philosophy:** The Harry C. Moores Foundation is primarily interested in supporting social services, education, and health. Funding for social services favors food and clothing distribution, homes, and youth organizations. Education interests include universities, colleges, religious education, and minority education. Health funding goes to hospitals, health organizations, and single-disease associations. The foundation also supports the arts, civic affairs, and religion. **Priorities:** *Arts & Humanities:* 5%. Supports art and culture. *Civic & Public Affairs:* 15%. Supports community affairs. *Education:* 11%. Supports educational institutions and programs. *Environment:* 41%. Supports youth and family services, food banks, abuse and addiction programs. *International:* 16%. Supports health, disease and disorder concerns. *Religion:* 5%. Supports the Center for Science and Industry. *Note:* Contributions made in fiscal 1999. **Typ. Recipients:** AIDS/HIV, Alzheimers Disease, Arthritis, Cancer, Children's Health/Hospitals, Clinics/Medical Centers, Diabetes, Emergency/Ambulance Services, Eyes/Blindness, Family Planning, Health Funds, Health Organizations, Health Policy/Cost Containment, Heart, Hospitals, Long-Term Care, Mental Health, Multiple Sclerosis, People with Disabilities, Respiratory, Single-Disease Health Associations, Speech & Hearing, Substance Abuse. **Geo. Dist:** Columbus, OH, metropolitan area.

★ 11500 ★ Harry C. Trexler Trust

33 South 7th St., Suite 205
Allentown, PA 18101
Phone: (610)434-9645 **Fax:** (610)437-5721
Thomas Christman, Executive Director

Fnded: 1934. **Philosophy:** Following the wishes of the donors, the trustees look to fund organizations which are "of the most benefit to humanity" in Allentown or Lehigh County. Areas of funding are not rigid, but will continually change in response to the needs of the area. Present areas of concern are culture and parks, education, youth, the elderly, and the disadvantaged. **Priorities:** *Arts & Humanities:* 13%. Contributes to music groups, art associations, public libraries, museums, theater, and historic preservation. *Civic & Public Affairs:* 39%. Principally supports the City of Allentown, PA. Supports economic development, parks, safety, and housing. *Education:* 13%. Primarily funds colleges and art and religious education. Also supports literacy, scholarship, and arts/humanities education. *Environment:* 19%. Funds youth groups YMCAs, food distribution programs, people with disabilities, daycare, and homes. *International:* 7%. Supports indigent care and blood drives. *Religion:* 2%. Supports science centers. *Note:* Total contributions made in fiscal analysis for 2001 is approximate. **Typ. Recipients:** Children's Health/Hospitals, Clinics/Medical Centers, Emergency/Ambulance Services, Eyes/Blindness, Home-Care Services, Long-Term Care, Medical Rehabilitation, Nursing Services, People with Disabilities, Transplant Networks/Donor Banks. **Geo. Dist:** PA, Lehigh County.

★ 11501 ★ Harry Frank Guggenheim Foundation

527 Madison Ave., 15th Floor
New York, NY 10022-4304
Phone: (212)644-4907 **Fax:** (212)644-5110
Email: hfgacf@aol.com
Website: http://www.hfg.org
Karen Colvard, Program Officer

Fnded: 1929. **Philosophy:** "The Foundation welcomes proposals from any of the natural and social sciences and the humanities that promise to increase understanding of the causes, manifestations, and control of violence, aggression, and dominance. Highest priority is given to research that can increase understanding and amelioration of urgent problems of violence, aggression, and dominance in the modern world." "Particular questions that interest the Foundation concern violence, aggression, and dominance in relation to social change, the socialization of children, inter-group conflict, drug trafficking and use, family relationships, and investigations of the control of aggression and violence...Priority will also be given to areas and methodologies not receiving adequate attention and support from other funding sources." **Priorities:** *Civic & Public Affairs:* 5%. Funds nonprofit management organizations and foundations. *Education:* 63%. Supports natural and social science research at universities. *Environment:* 2%. Supports community organizations and United Way. *Religion:* 2%. Gives to the National Academy of Sciences. *Note:* Total contributions made in 2000. **Typ. Recipients:** Alzheimers Disease, Child Abuse, Children's Health/Hospitals, Eyes/Blindness, Health Funds, Hospitals, Kidney, Medical Education, Medical Research, People with Disabilities, Substance Abuse. **Geo. Dist:** nationally and internationally.

★ 11502 ★ Harry and Jeanette Weinberg Foundation

7 Park Center Court
Owings Mills, MD 21117-4200
Phone: (410)654-6900 **Fax:** (410)654-3943
Website: http://www.hjweinbergfoundation.org
Bernard Siegel, President & Director

Fnded: 1959. **Philosophy:** The foundation's current fields of interests are the aged, the homeless, and other disadvantaged groups. It supports building funds, capital campaigns, endowment funds, and special projects. **Priorities:** *Arts & Humanities:* Less than 1%. *Civic & Public Affairs:* 5%. Funds community foundations, housing, nonprofit management, police departments, and community development. *Education:* 4%. Primarily funds pre-college education/educational programs; provides some support to institutions of higher learning. *Environment:* 11%. Contributes to organizations serving youth, the elderly, and families. *International:* 20%. Supports hospitals, medical centers, and single-disease health associations. *Note:* Total contributions made in fiscal 2001. **Typ. Recipients:** Clinics/Medical Centers, Diabetes, Geriatric Health, Health Funds, Health Organizations, Heart, Hospitals, Long-Term Care, Medical Rehabilitation, Mental Health, Public Health. **Geo. Dist:** no restrictions.

★ 11503 ★ Harry and Maribel G. Blum Foundation

919 North Michigan Ave., Suite 2800
Chicago, IL 60611
Phone: (312)664-5050 **Fax:** (312)664-8983
H. Kovler, Vice President

Fnded: 1967. **Philosophy:** The foundation's primary interest is Jewish organizations, including religious and social service organizations. It also supports health care, child welfare, and educational institutions. **Priorities:** *Civic & Public Affairs:* 46%. Zoos, aquariums, parks. *Education:* 9%. Supports higher education. *Environment:* 6%. Youth and housing. *International:* 35%. Diabetes, hospitals. *Note:* Total contributions made in 2001. **Typ. Recipients:** Cancer, Children's Health/Hospitals, Clinics/Medical Centers, Diabetes, Health Organizations, Hospitals, Medical Education, Medical Rehabilitation, Medical Research, People with Disabilities, Prenatal Health Issues, Single-Disease Health Associations, Transplant Networks/Donor Banks. **Geo. Dist:** nationally; IL.

★ 11504 ★ Harry S. and Isabel C. Cameron Foundation
PO Box 2518
Houston, TX 77252-2518
Phone: (713)247-7865
Email: diane.guiberteau@bankofamerica.com
Diane Guiberteau, Administrator

Fnded: 1966. **Philosophy:** The foundation, following the interests of its donors, supports educational institutions in Texas. It also shows an interest in religious organizations and social service agencies. **Priorities:** *Arts & Humanities:* 9%. Major support for the Museum of Fine Arts in Houston. *Civic & Public Affairs:* 11%. Funds urban affairs projects. *Education:* 23%. Focus on Catholic secondary education and colleges and universities. *Environment:* 11%. Provides support for youth organizations, child welfare, United Way, and community services. *International:* 10%. Funds hospitals and single-disease health associations. *Note:* Total contributions made in fiscal 2000. **Typ. Recipients:** AIDS/HIV, Alzheimers Disease, Cancer, Children's Health/Hospitals, Clinics/Medical Centers, Emergency/Ambulance Services, Eyes/Blindness, Health Organizations, Hospices, Hospitals, Medical Education, Medical Rehabilitation, Mental Health, Nursing Services, People with Disabilities, Public Health, Single-Disease Health Associations, Substance Abuse. **Geo. Dist:** Houston, TX, including metropolitan area.

★ 11505 ★ Harry S. Moss Heart Trust
PO Box 831041
Bank of America, 19th Floor
Dallas, TX 75283-1041
Phone: (214)209-2005
Dan Kelly, Trust Officer & Vice President

Fnded: 1973. **Philosophy:** The trust provides funds for research, equipment, and buildings for the prevention and cure of heart disease, primarily in Dallas County, TX. **Priorities:** *Environment:* 2%. Supports a children's camp. *International:* 98%. Supports heart disease research. *Note:* Total contributions made in 2001. **Typ. Recipients:** Children's Health/Hospitals, Clinics/Medical Centers, Diabetes, Health Organizations, Heart, Hospitals, Hospitals (University Affiliated), Medical Education, Medical Research, Nursing Services, People with Disabilities, Single-Disease Health Associations. **Geo. Dist:** Dallas, TX.

★ 11506 ★ Hartford Courant Foundation
285 Broad St.
Hartford, CT 06115
Phone: (860)241-6472 **Fax:** (860)520-6988
Email: hcfoundation@courant.com
Website: http://www.hartfordcourantfoundation.org
Kate Miller, Executive Director

Fnded: 1950. **Philosophy:** "The Hartford Courant Foundation seeks to make a sustainable impact on the vitality of Connecticut's capital region by being a catalyst for hope, inspiration and creativity and by improving the lives of its people, especially its children." "The Foundation makes grants primarily in support of education, the arts, community development, health and social services, with an emphasis on programs benefiting children, youth and families. Grants in the area of the arts will be made only for outreach or education programs for children or families." Hartford Courant Foundation Guidelines. **Priorities:** *Arts & Humanities:* 20%. Supports public broadcasting, theater, museums, orchestras, and history organizations. *Civic & Public Affairs:* 30%. Funds community and economic development, law and justice organizations, housing programs, civic associations, women's affairs, ethnic organizations, and citizens organizations. *Education:* 15%. Supports literacy programs, colleges/universities, and tutorial and learning disabilities programs. A limited amount of funding supports preselected private/parochial secondary schools. *Environment:* 25%. Funds programs for children and for families in need such as Young Men's Christian Association and youth activities, parenting and counseling programs, and domestic abuse programs. *International:* 5%. Gives to health-related programs, health centers, and clinics. *Note:* Total contributions made in 2001. **Typ. Recipients:** AIDS/HIV, Child Abuse, Children's Health/Hospitals, Clinics/Medical Centers, Domestic Violence, Family Planning, Hospitals, Hospitals (University Affiliated), Medical Rehabilitation, Medical Research, Mental Health, Nursing Services, People with Disabilities, Prenatal Health Issues, Public Health, Substance Abuse. **Geo. Dist:** CT, Central Connecticut.

★ 11507 ★ Harvey and Bernice Jones Charitable Trust
922 E Emma Ave.
PO Box 2035
Springdale, AR 72765
Phone: (479)756-8090 **Fax:** (479)750-7444
Website: http://www.jonesnet.org
Bernice Jones, Director

Fnded: 1989. **Philosophy:** The trust concentrates its grant program on education, medical services, and religious organizations in Arkansas. The primary emphasis is on assisting organizations near Springdale, AR, where Bernice Jones lives. The trust concentrates on helping a few select organizations with ongoing support. **Priorities:** *Education:* 73%. Supports public schools and scholarships. *Environment:* 19%. Supports the Harvey and Bernice Jones Center for Families and athletics. *International:* 6%. Funds hospitals and children's health. *Note:* Contributions were made in fiscal 2000. **Typ. Recipients:** Children's Health/Hospitals, Clinics/Medical Centers, Eyes/Blindness, Health-General, Hospitals, Long-Term Care. **Geo. Dist:** AR, Northwest Arkansas.

★ 11508 ★ Harvey Randall Wickes Foundation
4800 Fashion Square Boulevard
472 Plaza North
Saginaw, MI 48604
Phone: (989)799-1850 **Fax:** (989)799-3327
Email: HRWICKES@concentric.net
James Finkbeiner, President

Fnded: 1945. **Philosophy:** In accordance with the donor's wishes, the main purpose of the foundation is to provide buildings and equipment to educational, health, and social service organizations in the Saginaw, MI, area. Support for the area's three hospitals is also given. The foundation also supports the United Way, and parks and recreation facilities in Saginaw Township. **Priorities:** *Arts & Humanities:* 18%. Supports theater, museums, and orchestra. *Civic & Public Affairs:* 37%. Supports zoos and community foundations. *Education:* 11%. Supports universities and private schools. *Environment:* 11%. Supports youth services, housing, crime prevention, and homes. *International:* 13%. Supports health organizations. *Note:* Total contributions made in 1998. **Typ. Recipients:** Cancer, Child Abuse, Clinics/Medical Centers, Emergency/Ambulance Services, Eyes/Blindness, Health Funds, Health Organizations, Hospitals, Medical Rehabilitation, People with Disabilities, Public Health, Substance Abuse. **Geo. Dist:** MI, Saginaw County.

★ 11509 ★ Hattie M. Strong Foundation
1620 Eye St. NW, Suite 700
Washington, DC 20006
Phone: (202)331-1619 **Fax:** (202)466-2894
Judith Cyphers, Secretary & Director of Grants

Fnded: 1928. **Philosophy:** The Hattie M. Strong Foundation primarily supports a loan program for American students in their last year of undergraduate or graduate school. The foundation also administers a grant program in support of education projects focusing on the Washington, DC, area. "The foundation considers innovative and effective programs that promote literacy, provide training and basic lifeskills development, and educational enrichment and remedial programs." **Priorities:** *Education:* In fiscal 2001, the foundation gave 100% of its funding to education. About 64% went to loans to college students, and 36% went to organizations in the Washington, DC, area that provide educational opportunities for at-risk youth and adults, tutoring, and afterschool programs. **Typ. Recipients:** Medical Rehabilitation, Research/Studies Institutes. **Geo. Dist:** nationally for student loan program; Washington, DC, metropolitan area for community education grant program.

★ 11510 ★ Hawn Foundation
5949 Sherry Lane, No. 775
Dallas, TX 75225-3553
Phone: (214)696-6595 **Fax:** (214)696-6596
Joe Hawn, Jr., President

Fnded: 1962. **Philosophy:** The Hawn Foundation primarily makes grants in the areas of education and health care. Educational funding favors universities, religious education, and minority education. In health care, interests include health and research foundations, nursing, single-disease associations, and hospitals. Other recipient areas include social services and the arts. **Priorities:** *Arts & Humanities:* 3%. Funds the Dallas Museum of Art and music. *Civic & Public Affairs:* 9%. Supports Salesmanship Club, housing. *Education:* 5%. Supports schools and universities. *Environment:* 5%. Youth and family services. *International:* 70%. Funds single-disease associations, hospitals, and medical centers. *Religion:* 1%. Funds museum. *Note:* Total contributions made in fiscal 2000. **Typ. Recipients:** Alzheimers Disease, Arthritis, Cancer, Child Abuse, Children's Health/Hospitals, Clinics/Medical Centers, Diabetes, Emergency/Ambulance Services, Eyes/Blindness, Health Funds, Health Organizations, Health-General, Heart, Hospitals, Hospitals (University Affiliated), Long-Term Care, Medical Rehabilitation, Medical Research, Mental Health, Multiple Sclerosis, Nursing Services, People with Disabilities, Public Health, Research/Studies Institutes, Respiratory, Single-Disease Health Associations, Substance Abuse. **Geo. Dist:** Dallas, TX.

★ 11511 ★ The Hearst Foundation, Inc.
888 7th Ave., 45th Floor
New York, NY 10106-0057
Phone: (212)586-5404 **Fax:** (212)586-1917
Email: hearst@fdn.org
Website: http://www.hearstfdn.org
Robert Frehse, Jr., Executive Director & Vice President

Fnded: 1945. **Philosophy:** "Within a general policy of assisting institutions to provide access and opportunity to underrepresented, low-income and minority populations, the Directors of the Hearst Foundations have established certain priorities. Education is among them. The Foundation's primary focus is support of undergraduate education through the establishment of endowed scholarships at private liberal arts colleges and universities. In addition, endowed scholarship support is provided for professional study in teaching, medicine, nursing, engineering, math, science, and the health care professions at the undergraduate and graduate levels. A limited number of proposals are also accepted from K-12 independent schools with outstanding academic programs, and demonstrated track records of outreach to economically disadvantaged students. In general, grants are not made to public schools. However, private organizations or coalitions seeking improvement of public education and broadening access to education will be considered. Another priority is health. The Foundation's interests in the health field seek to improve and increase health care, while facilitating wellness, prevention, and rehabilitation. Working largely through leading regional hospitals and medical centers, the Foundation support programs which increase access for underserved urban and rural populations. Areas of interest include perinatology and pediatrics, cancer, stroke, aging, women's health issues, and medical research. A third priority is social services. Preference is given to well-established, larger agencies, providing comprehensive services. Requests for technical assistance, management training, and leadership development, designed to help nonprofit agencies deliver services more efficiently and effectively are also considered. A fourth priority is culture. The Foundation's priority in the arts is to increase access and educational opportunities for diverse populations and underserved communities. The major portion of funds endow arts education and/or community outreach programs through major cultural institutions. Special attention is given to programs which enrich the lives of young people through exposure to the arts." 1997 Guidelines for Grant Applications. **Priorities:** *Arts & Humanities:* 39%. Supports theater, music, museums, dance, opera, libraries, and history. *Civic & Public Affairs:* 5%. Funds industrial development and leadership organizations. *Education:* 44%. Supports colleges and universities, science and mathematics education, religious education, scholarship funds, literacy, and schools. *Environment:* 2%. Supports Big Brothers/Big sister, family services, child care services, youth organizations, and community centers. *International:* 8%. Supports emergency services, hospitals, transplant networks/donor banks, cancer, medical research, and medical centers. *Note:* Total contributions made in 2000. **Typ. Recipients:** AIDS/HIV, Cancer, Children's Health/Hospitals, Clinics/Medical Centers, Emergency/Ambulance Services, Heart, Home-Care Services, Hospitals, Hospitals (University Affiliated), Medical Education, Medical Rehabilitation, Medical Research, Mental Health, Nursing Services, People with Disabilities, Prenatal Health Issues, Public Health, Research/Studies Institutes, Single-Disease Health Associations, Substance Abuse. **Geo. Dist:** nationally.

★ 11512 ★ Heckscher Foundation for Children

17 East 47th St.
New York, NY 10017
Phone: (212)371-7775 **Fax:** (212)371-7787
Virginia Sloane, President

Fnded: 1921. **Philosophy:** The foundation promotes the health and general welfare of children and makes grants in a number of different areas within this framework. The general welfare of children is interpreted broadly to include child care, recreation, and exposure of children to the arts. Needy and orphaned children are a special concern of the foundation, evidenced by support for adoption services, children's homes, distribution of clothing and other essentials for needy children, and the provision of gifts at Christmas. **Priorities:** *Arts & Humanities:* 16%. Supports music, historic preservation, dance, theater, and public broadcasting. *Civic & Public Affairs:* 12%. Funds community foundations, economic enterprise organizations, women's affairs, housing, and inner-city development. *Education:* 19%. Supports colleges, after-school programs, arts school, and a school for the deaf. *Environment:* 32%. Supports homes, shelter/homeless, youth organizations, community centers, camps, YMCAs, child and family services, and child welfare organizations. *International:* 11%. Gives to hospitals, medical centers, single-disease health associations, and children's health programs. *Note:* Total contributions made in 2000. **Typ. Recipients:** Adolescent Health Issues, AIDS/HIV, Cancer, Children's Health/Hospitals, Clinics/Medical Centers, Emergency/Ambulance Services, Family Planning, Health Organizations, Hospitals, Medical Education, Medical Rehabilitation, Medical Research, Mental Health, Nursing Services, People with Disabilities, Preventive Medicine/Wellness Organizations, Single-Disease Health Associations, Speech & Hearing, Substance Abuse, Transplant Networks/Donor Banks. **Geo. Dist:** New York, NY.

★ 11513 ★ Helen Brach Foundation

55 W Wacker Dr., Suite 701
Chicago, IL 60601
Phone: (312)372-4417 **Fax:** (312)372-0290
Toni Peville, Associate Director

Fnded: 1974. **Philosophy:** Helen Brach established her foundation to be used as the primary vehicle for her annual gifts to charity. The foundation's grants have not been limited to any single area, but "areas of interest, among others, have included efforts to save wildlife, curtail the abuse of children and animals, provide funding for education at the secondary and college level, funding for scientific and literary purposes, and help for those serving the physically and mentally disabled, the poor, the blind, the homeless, the teenaged unwed mother, and the elderly." **Priorities:** *Civic & Public Affairs:* 13%. Supports urban affairs and community foundations. *Education:* 21%. Supports secondary and preparatory schools, colleges, and universities. *Environment:* 31%. Supports child welfare, and social and adult services and churches. *International:* 8%. Supports health care and medical centers. *Note:* Total contributions made in fiscal 1999. **Typ. Recipients:** AIDS/HIV, Children's Health/Hospitals, Clinics/Medical Centers, Geriatric Health, Health Funds, Health Organizations, Hospices, Hospitals, Long-Term Care, Medical Rehabilitation, Medical Research, Mental Health, Nursing Services, Nutrition, People with Disabilities, Preventive Medicine/Wellness Organizations, Public Health, Trauma Treatment. **Geo. Dist:** nationally; IL.

★ 11514 ★ Helen Clay Frick Foundation

1 Mellon Center, Rm. 3825
PO Box 185
Pittsburgh, PA 15230
Phone: (412)234-5784 **Fax:** (412)234-1073
Email: robinson.bk@mellon.com
Barbara Robinson, Trust Administrator

Fnded: 1947. **Philosophy:** The major focus of the Frick Foundation has been on the fine arts, which stems from its founder's interest in art and the collection acquired by her father. Much of the annual funds go to the Frick Collection in New York City. Other areas of interest are the environment and education. **Priorities:** *Arts & Humanities:* 34%. Supports arts museums, historic preservation, and the performing arts. *Civic & Public Affairs:* 11%. Supports botanical gardens, clubs. *Education:* 9%. Funds medical education, religious education, and universities. *Environment:* 6%. Supports community service organizations, animal protection, and child welfare. *Religion:* 12%. Supports science museums, general-science, and science centers. *Note:* Total contributions made in 2000. **Typ. Recipients:** Hospitals, Medical Education. **Geo. Dist:** New York, NY; Pittsburgh, PA.

★ 11515 ★ Helen Hay Whitney Foundation

450 East 63rd St.
New York, NY 10021-7928
Phone: (212)751-8228 **Fax:** (212)688-6794
Email: hhwf@earthlink.net
Website: http://www.hhwf.org
Barbara Hugonnet, Administrative Director

Fnded: 1947. **Philosophy:** "The Helen Hay Whitney Foundation supports early postdoctoral training in all basic biomedical sciences. To attain its ultimate goal of increasing the number of imaginative, well-trained, and dedicated medical scientists, the foundation grants financial support of sufficient duration to help further the careers of young men and women engaged in biological or medical research." Residents of the United States, Canada, and Mexico, who hold M.D., Ph.D., or equivalent degrees are eligible to apply for fellowships for beginning postdoctoral training in biomedical research. Also eligible are nonresidents training in the United States. Fellowships are normally for three years, with awards of $25,000 the first year, $27,000 the second year, and $29,000 the third year, as well as an annual allowance of $2,000 to defray research expenses. **Priorities:** *Education:* 50%.Primary focus is on medical education grants and fellowships. *Environment:* 5%. Supports general human services. *International:* 45% Supports universities and institutes for medical research fellowships. *Note:* Total contributions made in fiscal 2000. **Typ. Recipients:** Cancer, Children's Health/Hospitals, Hospitals, Medical Education, Medical Research, Research/Studies Institutes. **Geo. Dist:** North America.

★ 11516 ★ Helen K. and Arthur E. Johnson Foundation

1700 Broadway, Suite 1100
Denver, CO 80290-1039
Phone: (303)861-4127 **Fax:** (303)861-0607
Website: http://www.johnsonfoundation.net
John Alexander, President & Executive Director

Fnded: 1948. **Philosophy:** The foundation supports a wide variety of creative efforts to solve human problems and to enrich the quality of life. It concentrates its efforts on health, education, youth, civic and cultural affairs, community and social services, and senior citizens. **Priorities:** *Arts & Humanities:* 9%. Supports opera, museum, music. *Civic & Public Affairs:* 11%. Supports community foundations, housing and botanical gardens/parks. *Education:* 22%. Funds student aid, scholarship, school, college, and universities. *Environment:* 22%. Supports senior services, Big Brothers/Big Sisters, shelters/homeless, United Way, scouts, emergency relief and people with disabilities. *International:* 28%. Supports eyes/blindness, respiratory, Alzheimers, hospice and children's hospital, and AIDS. *Religion:* 4%. Supports science museums. *Note:* Total contributions made in 2000. **Typ. Recipients:** AIDS/HIV, Alzheimers Disease, Cancer, Children's Health/Hospitals, Clinics/Medical Centers, Eyes/Blindness, Family Planning, Health Organizations, Health-General, Hospices, Hospitals, Long-Term Care, Medical Rehabilitation, Medical Research, Medical Training, Multiple Sclerosis, Nursing Services, People with Disabilities, Public Health, Research/Studies Institutes, Sexual Abuse, Single-Disease Health Associations, Speech & Hearing, Substance Abuse, Transplant Networks/Donor Banks. **Geo. Dist:** CO.

★ 11517 ★ Helena Rubinstein Foundation

477 Madison Ave., 7th Floor
New York, NY 10022-5802
Phone: (212)750-7310 **Fax:** (212)750-9798
Website: http://www.fdncenter.org/grantmaker/rubinstein
Diane Moss, President & Chief Executive Officer

Fnded: 1953. **Philosophy:** When she created the foundation, Ms. Rubinstein wanted to affirm a principle she often expressed, "My fortune comes from women and should benefit them and their children, to better their quality of life." The foundation has developed and broadened its original philanthropic concepts to meet the changing needs of society and continues to support an increasing number of innovative programs in education, the arts, arts-in-education, women's issues, and community services. In 1996, the foundation reported a plan to reduce annual grantmaking and long-term commitments in order to insure future economic stability. Along with this reduction in grantmaking was a commitment to a greater emphasis on school-to-work and welfare-to-work initiatives to prepare young people and poor people for productive futures. The foundation continues to stress the importance of higher education by funding scholarships and remains committed to art education. **Priorities:** *Arts & Humanities:* (Arts/Arts Education) 23%. Funds art museums, the opera, theater, ballet, children's museums, music, dance, and public broadcasting. *Civic & Public Affairs:* (Community Services) 38%. Supports community affairs, economic development, housing, job training programs, and public and women's affairs. *Education:* 34%. Gives to colleges, universities, and educational programs. *International:* 5%. Supports children's health, research, women's healthcare and aid to the homeless. *Note:* Total contribution made in fiscal 2001. **Typ. Recipients:** AIDS/HIV, Alzheimers Disease, Cancer, Children's Health/Hospitals, Clinics/Medical Centers, Eyes/Blindness, Family Planning, Geriatric Health, Health Organizations, Hospitals, Medical Education, Medical Rehabilitation, Medical Research, Medical Training, Nursing Services, Prenatal Health Issues, Preventive Medicine/Wellness Organizations, Public Health, Single-Disease Health Associations, Substance Abuse. **Geo. Dist:** New York, NY.

★ 11518 ★ Helene Fuld Health Trust

HSBC Bank USA
452 Fifth Ave., 17th Floor
New York, NY 10018
Phone: (212)525-2418
Email: marianne.caskran@us.hsbc.com
Website: http://www.fuldtrust.org
Marianne Caskran, Grants Administrator

Fnded: 1969. **Philosophy:** "The primary mission of the Helene Fuld Health Trust is to support and promote the health, welfare, and education of student nurses. The first priority of the Trust remains financial aid to nursing students. The Trust will seek opportunities to establish endowed scholarships at select nursing schools through an invitational process. Acknowledging the increased complexity of and sophisticated knowledge required for health care delivery, the Trust will give preference to programs that offer BSN degrees and higher. The trust will not accept unsolicited grant requests for financial aid. The trust will also award grants to leading nursing schools and other organizations which undertake innovative programs designed to develop and expand the professional and leadership skills of nursing students, faculty, and administration. Proposals for these grants will be by invitation only." Helene Fuld Health Trust Guidelines **Priorities:** *Education:* 100%. Primarily supports colleges and universities for nursing education. *Note:* Total contributions made in fiscal 2001. **Typ. Recipients:** Children's Health/Hospitals, Clinics/Medical Centers, Health Organizations, Health-General, Hospitals, Medical Education, Medical Research, Nursing Services. **Geo. Dist:** nationally.

★ 11519 ★ Helmerich Foundation

1579 East 21st St.
Tulsa, OK 74114
Phone: (918)742-5531
Walter Helmerich, III, Trustee

Fnded: 1965. **Philosophy:** The Helmerich Foundation makes grants to the arts, particularly to the performing arts in Tulsa, Oklahoma, religious organizations, and educational institutions and funds. Other areas of interest include civic concerns, social services, and health foundations and centers. The foundation prefers to make large grants that have an impact on projects. Therefore, other recipient areas are funded on a limited basis. **Priorities:** *Arts & Humanities:* 12%. Primarily for libraries, museums, music, and the performing arts. *Civic & Public Affairs:* 3%. Funds zoological park, community development. *Education:* 29%. Supports schools, education funds, universities. *Environment:* 24%. Funds community and family services and child welfare. *International:* 26%. Funds health centers and health foundations. *Note:* Total contributions made in fiscal 2001. **Typ. Recipients:** AIDS/HIV, Cancer, Children's Health/Hospitals, Clinics/Medical Centers, Diabetes, Domestic Violence, Emergency/Ambulance Services, Eyes/Blindness, Health Organizations, Hospices, Mental Health, Nursing Services, People with Disabilities, People with Disabilities, Public Health, Respiratory. **Geo. Dist:** Tulsa, OK.

★ 11520 ★ Henry Ford II Fund

100 Renaissance Center, 34th Floor
Detroit, MI 48243
Phone: (313)259-7777 **Fax:** (313)393-7579
David Hempstead, Secretary & Trustee

Fnded: 1953. **Philosophy:** The fund reports that "the purpose of each grant or contribution is to provide financial support to corporations, trusts, community chests, funds or foundations, organized and operated solely for religious, charitable, scientific, literary or educational purposes, or for the prevention of cruelty to children or animals." The awards "are generally limited to charitable organizations already favorably known to, and of interest to, the substantial contributors of the foundation." **Priorities:** *Arts & Humanities:* Less than 1%. Supports public broadcasting. *Civic & Public Affairs:* 21%. Supports community organisation and foundations. *Education:* 44%. Supports universities, colleges, education associations, and minority education. *Environment:* 9%. Supports the United Way, food banks, and child welfare. *International:* 14%. Supports children's hospitals. *Religion:* 6%. Funds the Edison Institute. *Note:* Total contributions made in 2000. **Typ. Recipients:** Children's Health/Hospitals, Emergency/Ambulance Services, Eyes/Blindness, Health Organizations, Hospitals, Medical Rehabilitation, Medical Research, People with Disabilities. **Geo. Dist:** Detroit, MI.

★ 11521 ★ Henry Luce Foundation

111 West 50th St., Suite 4601
New York, NY 10020-1202
Phone: (212)489-7700 **Fax:** (212)581-9541
Website: http://www.hluce.org
Michael Gilligan, President & Director

Fnded: 1936. **Philosophy:** "During the past two years, Public Policy projects have dealt with a range of topics, including citizenship, immigration policy, taxation, youth violence, the environment and the roll of the United Nations." "Grants made through the Higher Education category support special scholarly or educational initiatives that fall outside the guidelines for the foundation's other programs." "The Luce Scholars Program was created to enable young Americans to immerse themselves in Asian culture for a year. The Asia Foundation, the organization that administers the Asian aspects of the program, arranges professional placements for each scholar." "Every year, 67 American colleges and universities nominate candidates who have no formal study of Asia." "The Luce Fund for Asian Studies is a new $12 million initiative designed to strengthen the study of Asia at leading American liberal arts colleges." "The fund provides seed money for junior faculty positions and program development over a four-year period. Project grants support a range of concerns in the humanities and social sciences. Typically, these grants fund research and faculty development, cultural and scholarly exchange, language and library programs, and policy studies." "The foundation continues to bring attention to the cultural wealth of Asia through art exhibitions that highlight pioneering scholarship." "The Luce Foundation's program in Theology supports activities of faith and learning that strengthen the role of religion in daily life. For more than six decades, the Theology Program has emphasized theological education and scholarship, while also embracing projects that support churches and religious leadership. These activities reflect Henry R. Luce's intent to honor the work of his parents, who were Presbyterian missionary educators in China." "The Luce Fund in American Art funds scholarly exhibitions and publications and is open to all periods and genres of American art history." "Twenty-six dissertation awards for doctoral research in American art continue to assist the next generation of art historians specializing in this field. The primary program provides 10 full fellowships annually through an open national competition administered by the American Council of Learned Societies." "The foundation also makes grants for dissertation research to 30 invited schools that show a strong commitment to American art." "The Women in Science Program offers three categories of funding: undergraduate scholarships, graduate fellowships, and term support for tenure-track junior faculty appointments. The program seeks... to encourage women to enter, study, graduate and teach... in fields where there have been barriers to their advancement. These include physics, chemistry, biology, computer science, meteorology, engineering, and mathematics." 1998-1999 Biennial Report. **Priorities:** *Arts & Humanities:* 10%. Focus on museums. *Education:* 29%. Supports higher education. *Note:* Total contributions made in 1999. **Typ. Recipients:** Geriatric Health, Medical Education, Medical Education, Public Health. **Geo. Dist:** nationally; East and Southeast Asia.

★ 11522 ★ Henry and Lucy Moses Fund, Inc.

1301 Ave. of the Americas, 40th Fl.
New York, NY 10019-6076
Phone: (212)554-7800 **Fax:** (212)554-7700
Irving Sitnick, President & Director

Fnded: 1942. **Philosophy:** The foundation reflects the interests of Mr. and Mrs. Moses, now both deceased. Its major concerns are welfare activities, hospitals and health-related causes. Other areas which receive support are education, youth programs, social services, and music. **Priorities:** *Arts & Humanities:* 16%. *Civic & Public Affairs:* 18%. *Education:* 21%. Supports Columbia University and its trustees. *Environment:* 8%. *International:* 17%. *Note:* Contributions made in 2000. **Typ. Recipients:** Cancer, Clinics/Medical Centers, Family Planning, Health Organizations, Hospitals, Long-Term Care, Medical Education, Medical Research, Nursing Services, People with Disabilities, Single-Disease Health Associations. **Geo. Dist:** some funding nationally; New York, NY, metropolitan area.

★ 11523 ★ Henry and Marilyn Taub Foundation

354 Eisenhower Pkwy.
Livingston, NJ 07039
Phone: (201)287-2500 **Fax:** (201)287-2580
Fred Lafer, President & Treasurer

Fnded: 1967. **Philosophy:** The Henry and Marilyn Taub Foundation provides funds for Jewish religious organizations. The arts, civic affairs, health services and social services also are supported by the foundation, particularly when they are affiliated with the Jewish faith. **Priorities:** *Arts & Humanities:* 2%. Funds the performing arts. *Education:* 8%. Supports colleges and universities. *International:* 3%. Funds single-disease centers. *Note:* Total contributions made in 1998. **Typ. Recipients:** Cancer, Clinics/Medical Centers, Domestic Violence, Emergency/Ambulance Services, Eyes/Blindness, Hospitals, Hospitals, Medical Education, Medical Rehabilitation, Medical Research, People with Disabilities, Single-Disease Health Associations, Substance Abuse. **Geo. Dist:** Eastern United States; NJ; NY.

★ 11524 ★ Henry P. Kendall Foundation

176 Federal St.
Boston, MA 02110
Phone: (617)951-2525 **Fax:** (617)443-1977
Website: http://www.kendall.org
Theodore Smith, Executive Director

Fnded: 1957. **Philosophy:** The Foundation's interests have traditionally focused on protecting the planet's natural environment and reducing the threats of nuclear war and weapons proliferation. "At the stage of the Foundation's history it's program is focused almost entirely on the environment and actions needed to secure its physical, biological and aesthetic wealth for future generations." 1998 Annual Report. **Priorities:** *Arts & Humanities:* About 24%. Supports a historical society, educational and cultural programs for adults, and a major grant to the Kendall Whaling Museum ($717,355). *Civic & Public Affairs:* About 12%. Supports aquariums, wilderness and marine organizations and arms control. *Education:* 7%. Supports universities. *Religion:* About 5%. Funds the Franklin Institute. *Note:* Total contributions made in 2000. **Typ. Recipients:** Medical Education. **Geo. Dist:** New England and the Pacific Northwest; AK; maritime provinces; western Canada.

★ 11525 ★ Henry P. and Susan C. Crowell Trust

1800 Office Club Pointe, Suite 220
Colorado Springs, CO 80920
Phone: (719)272-8300 **Fax:** (719)272-8305
Email: crowellhp@aol.com
Website: http://www.crowellfoundation.org
John Bass, President & Secretary

Fnded: 1927. **Philosophy:** The mission of the trust "is limited to the teaching and active extension of the doctrines of evangelical Christianity through approved grants to qualified organizations." **Priorities:** *Arts & Humanities:* 1%. *Civic & Public Affairs:* 1%. *Education:* 8%. Mainly religious education. *Note:* Contributions made in 1998. **Typ. Recipients:** Clinics/Medical Centers, Hospitals. **Geo. Dist:** nationally.

★ 11526 ★ Herbert H. and Grace A. Dow Foundation

1018 West Main St.
Midland, MI 48640-4292
Phone: (989)631-3699 **Fax:** (989)631-0675
Email: info@hhdowfoundation.org
Website: http://www.hhdowfoundation.org
Margaret Riecker, President

Fnded: 1936. **Philosophy:** "The Herbert H. and Grace A. Dow Foundation, while limited in its grantmaking to organizations within Michigan, has charter goals to improve educational, religious, economic, and cultural lives of Michigan's people as those needs can be defined in a world which constantly presents new or different challenges and opportunities. The Foundation TrusteeS carefully consider proposals submitted, and look for programs where their contributions can be leveraged. Organizations requesting funding should be sure that they have planned for that programs future self sufficiency." The foundation tends "to support organizations that have clearly stated objectives, strong and purposeful management, and are publicly accountable; have needs which are not normally funded by government or public financing; are not hesitant to explore, initiate, volunteer, or execute, original ideas or concepts; are willing to collaborate with other persons or organizations to give synergy to a common objective or goal; and have purposes which tend to advance private enterprise and the preservation of a free, open, and self-resourceful society." 1999 Herbert H. and Grace A. Dow Foundation, Annual Report. **Priorities:** *Arts & Humanities:* 18%. Funds arts centers, museums, historic preservation, and libraries. *Civic & Public Affairs:* 8%. Gives to municipalities and community foundations. *Education:* 36%. Supports public and private pre-college schools, colleges, and universities. *Environment:* 23%. Supports the United Way, community centers, family and children's services, and services for the disabled. *International:* 4%. Funds medical centers, hospitals, and HIV/AIDS organizations. *Religion:* 6%. The Michigan Molecular Institute receives major support. *Note:* Total contributions made in 2001. **Typ. Recipients:** Children's Health/Hospitals, Clinics/Medical Centers, Emergency/Ambulance Services, Geriatric Health, Health Policy/Cost Containment, Hospitals, Medical Rehabilitation, People with Disabilities, Public Health, Substance Abuse. **Geo. Dist:** MI, statewide; Midland, MI.

★ 11527 ★ Herbst Foundation

30 Van Ness Ave., Suite 3600
San Francisco, CA 94102
Phone: (415)252-1220 **Fax:** (415)252-1205
Dwight Merriman, Jr., President

Fnded: 1961. **Philosophy:** The foundation's primary purpose is to provide capital support (bricks-and-mortar) to organizations in the city and county of San Francisco. Primary concerns include education and social services. **Priorities:** *Arts & Humanities:* 7%. Supports libraries, museums and music. *Civic & Public Affairs:* 1%. Supports philanthropic organizations and public policy. *Education:* 46%. Supports public and private education. *Environment:* 35%. Supports family services, counseling, people with disabilities, YMCA's, youth programs, and child welfare. *International:* 9%. Supports health associations, a blood center, and hospitals. *Note:* Total contributions made in fiscal 2001. **Typ. Recipients:** AIDS/HIV, Alzheimers Disease, Clinics/Medical Centers, Diabetes, Eyes/Blindness, Family Planning, Geriatric Health, Health Organizations, Hospitals, Medical Education, Medical Rehabilitation, Medical Research, People with Disabilities, Speech & Hearing, Transplant Networks/Donor Banks. **Geo. Dist:** nationally; CA, San Francisco County; San Francisco, CA.

★ 11528 ★ Herman Goldman Foundation

61 Broadway, 18th Floor
New York, NY 10006
Phone: (212)797-9090 **Fax:** (212)797-9162
Richard Baron, Executive Director

Fnded: 1943. **Philosophy:** From its founding in 1943 until Mr. Goldman's death in 1968, the foundation was modest in size. Through funds from Mr. Goldman's estate, the foundation's assets increased significantly and it established firm guidelines for the distribution of its resources. Those program guidelines emphasize education, social development and justice, health, and the arts. **Priorities:** *Arts & Humanities:* 11%. Supports museums, and performing and visual arts. *Civic & Public Affairs:* 14%. Philanthropic organizations are funded. *Education:* 17%. Funds universities, and educational institutions and programs. *Environment:* 24%. Emphasis is placed on family services. *International:* 16%. Priorities focus on hospitals, geriatric care, medical centers, and disease and disorder concerns. *Note:* Total contributions made in fiscal 2001. **Typ. Recipients:** AIDS/HIV, Cancer, Clinics/Medical Centers, Geriatric Health, Health Funds, Health Organizations, Hospitals, Hospitals (University Affiliated), Long-Term Care, Medical Education, Medical Research, Mental Health, Multiple Sclerosis, People with Disabilities, Prenatal Health Issues, Single-Disease Health Associations. **Geo. Dist:** New York, NY, including metropolitan area.

★ 11529 ★ Herman T. and Phenie R. Pott Foundation

PO Box 387
Saint Louis, MO 63166
Phone: (314)418-2643 **Fax:** (314)418-2349
James Collins, Executive Director

Fnded: 1963. **Philosophy:** The foundation makes most of its grants in the areas of social services and education. Social service funding favors shelters, family resource centers, children's services, and united funds. Funding in education emphasizes universities and college funds in St. Louis. The trust also will fund civic affairs, the St. Louis Mercantile Library, and health services. **Priorities:** *Arts & Humanities:* 10%. Supports a library, opera theater, and an arts council. *Civic & Public Affairs:* 4%. Botanical gardens, philanthropic organizations, and employment. *Education:* 13%. Gives to schools, colleges, and universities. *Environment:* 31%. Supports shelters, family resource centers, children's services, youth organizations, the United Way, shelters, Special Olympics and Big Brothers/Big Sisters. *International:* 18%. Pediatric health, mental health, and single-disease health associations. *Note:* Total contributions made in 2000. **Typ. Recipients:** Alzheimers Disease, Child Abuse, Children's Health/Hospitals, Diabetes, Domestic Violence, Emergency/Ambulance Services, Eyes/Blindness, Family Planning, Health Organizations, Heart, Hospitals, Medical Rehabilitation, Medical Research, Mental Health, Multiple Sclerosis, People with Disabilities, Preventive Medicine/Wellness Organizations, Respiratory, Single-Disease Health Associations. **Geo. Dist:** St. Louis, MO.

★ 11530 ★ Herrick Foundation

840 W Long Lake Rd., Suite 200
Troy, MI 48098
Phone: (248)267-3321 **Fax:** (248)879-2001
Kenneth Herrick, Chairman, President, and Treasurer

Fnded: 1949. **Philosophy:** The foundation traditionally supports colleges, universities, educational projects, churches, hospitals, health organizations, civic groups, social service agencies, cultural organizations, and scientific organizations primarily in Michigan. **Priorities:** *Arts & Humanities:* 7%. Supports libraries, public broadcasting, and museums. *Civic & Public Affairs:* 11%. Supports community foundations and fire departments. *Education:* 38%. Supports secondary education and colleges and universities. *Environment:* 12%. Primarily for youth organizations. *International:* 14%. Funds hospitals and health organizations. *Note:* Total contributions made in fiscal 2001. **Typ. Recipients:** Alzheimers Disease, Cancer, Children's Health/Hospitals, Clinics/Medical Centers, Diabetes, Emergency/Ambulance Services, Health Funds, Health Organizations, Health-General, Heart, Hospices, Hospitals, Hospitals (University Affiliated), Kidney, Long-Term Care, Medical Education, Medical Research, Nursing Services, People with Disabilities, Preventive Medicine/Wellness Organizations, Single-Disease Health Associations, Substance Abuse. **Geo. Dist:** MI, Primarily Michigan, occasionally Washington, D.C., Indiana, Mississippi, Ohio, Tennesse, Oklahoma and Wisconsin.

★ 11531 ★ Hess Foundation

1185 Ave. of the Americas
New York, NY 10036
Phone: (212)536-8421
Norma Hess, President

Fnded: 1954. **Philosophy:** The foundation concentrates its giving in the areas of higher and secondary education, hospitals, medical research, temples, and social services. **Priorities:** *Arts & Humanities:* 22%. Supports Lincoln Center, performing arts, museums, the opera, and libraries. *Civic & Public Affairs:* 2%. *Education:* 22%. Funds colleges, universities, educational programs, medical education, and arts and humanities education. *Environment:* 6%. Supports United Way, YMCA, services for the handicapped, meals on wheels, and recreation/athletics. *International:* 34%. Supports hospitals, medical centers, gay men's health, hospice, disease and disorder concerns, and children's health. *Religion:* 2%. *Note:* Total contributions made in fiscal 2000. **Typ. Recipients:** AIDS/HIV, Alzheimers Disease, Children's Health/Hospitals, Clinics/Medical Centers, Clinics/Medical Centers, Emergency/Ambulance Services, Health Organizations, Health-General, Hospices, Hospitals, Medical Education, People with Disabilities, Prenatal Health Issues, Single-Disease Health Associations. **Geo. Dist:** nationally; New York, NY; Paris.

★ 11532 ★ Hill Crest Foundation

PO Box 530507
Birmingham, AL 35253
Phone: (205)870-0400 **Fax:** (205)870-0484
Charles Terry, Sr., Chairman

Fnded: 1988. **Philosophy:** The Hill Crest Foundation is primarily engaged in making grants to programs in the field of mental health. In addition to the primary area of support, the officers have decided to support a wide variety of organizations in several fields including the arts, civic and public affairs, education, health care, religion, and social services. The foundation also supports charitable organizations with several grant types including capital, operating support, project, research, and a donation to a scholarship fund. The foundation's grant-making activity is concentrated in Jefferson County, AL, and the surrounding areas. Applications from out of state are given low priority. **Priorities:** *Arts & Humanities:* 6%. Supports museums and music. *Civic & Public Affairs:* 4%. *Education:* 37%. Primarily to colleges and universities, medical education, religious education, and Social science. *Environment:* 32%. Supports people with disabilities, YMCA/YWCA, youth programs. *International:* 14%. Funds research and specialized services. *Note:* Total contributions made in fiscal 2001. **Typ. Recipients:** AIDS/HIV, Alzheimers Disease, Cancer, Children's Health/Hospitals, Diabetes, Domestic Violence, Eyes/Blindness, Family Planning, Health Funds, Health Organizations, Hospitals, Hospitals (University Affiliated), Medical Education, Medical Rehabilitation, Mental Health, Nutrition, People with Disabilities, Prenatal Health Issues, Public Health, Respiratory, Single-Disease Health Associations, Substance Abuse, Trauma Treatment. **Geo. Dist:** Birmingham, AL, metropolitan area.

★ 11533 ★ Hillcrest Foundation

901 Main, 19th Floor
Dallas, TX 75202
Phone: (214)209-1965 **Fax:** (214)209-1940
Dan Kelly, Specialist

Fnded: 1959. **Philosophy:** The Hillcrest Foundation was created to help alleviate poverty problems, to aid the advancement of education, and to promote health care in Texas. The grant applicant must be a charitable organization located in Texas, with a purpose compatible with the principles of the foundation. **Priorities:** *Arts & Humanities:* 11%. Supports libraries museum, historical preservation, and film/video *Civic & Public Affairs:* 15%. Supports non-profit management arboretums/botanical gardens, transitional living, philanthropic organizations, and law and justice. *Education:* 32%. Supports religious education, education funds, afterschool programs, technical education, and science education, and student aid. *Environment:* 22%. Supports emergency relief, youth programs, homeless, food distribution, crime prevention, camps, homes, and substance abuse. *International:* 17%. Supports Alzheimers, gereatric health, hospital, hospice, medical centers, childrens health, hearing, and oral health. *Religion:* 3%. Supports scientific research, observatories, and scientific labs. *Note:* Total contributions made in 2000. **Typ. Recipients:** Alzheimers Disease, Arthritis, Cancer, Child Abuse, Children's Health/Hospitals, Clinics/Medical Centers, Diabetes, Domestic Violence, Emergency/Ambulance Services, Health Organizations, Heart, Hospitals, Long-Term Care, Medical Education, Medical Research, Mental Health, Nursing Services, Outpatient Health Care, People with Disabilities, Prenatal Health Issues, Public Health, Research/Studies Institutes, Respiratory, Single-Disease Health Associations, Substance Abuse. **Geo. Dist:** Dallas, TX.

★ 11534 ★ Hillman Foundation

2000 Grant Bldg.
Pittsburgh, PA 15219
Phone: (412)338-3466 **Fax:** (412)338-3463
Email: foundation@hillmanfo.com
Ronald Wertz, President

Fnded: 1951. **Philosophy:** The foundation allocates its resources primarily to programs designed to improve the quality of life in Pittsburgh and the southwestern Pennsylvania region. Funding is given to organizations in six program areas, including all levels of education, community and civic affairs, social services, cultural advancement and the arts, health and medicine, and youth and youth services. Over the next several years, the foundation intends to "maintain a contributions program of multiple interests based on the single principal of helping people and organizations to improve themselves and the surrounding region. The current policy of giving priority to requests submitted by qualified organizations located in the Pittsburgh and Southwestern Pennsylvania area will continue." **Priorities:** *Arts & Humanities:* 25%. Supports museums, art institutes and public broadcasting. *Civic & Public Affairs:* 16%. Supports economic development, zoos, urban and community affairs and public policy. *Education:* 26%. Private education and community colleges. *Environment:* 22%. Supports family services, United Way, YMCA's, youth programs, and child welfare. *International:* 8%. Supports a cancer center and United Cerebral Palsy. *Note:* Total contributions made in 2001. **Typ. Recipients:** AIDS/HIV, Cancer, Children's Health/Hospitals, Domestic Violence, Eyes/Blindness, Family Planning, Health Organizations, Long-Term Care, Medical Education, Medical Rehabilitation, Medical Research, Mental Health, Nursing Services, Outpatient Health Care, People with Disabilities, Research/Studies Institutes, Sexual Abuse, Single-Disease Health Associations, Speech & Hearing, Substance Abuse. **Geo. Dist:** PA, Southwestern part of state; Pittsburgh, PA.

★ 11535 ★ Hillsdale Fund

PO Box 20124
Greensboro, NC 27420
Phone: (336)274-5471
E. Doolan, Vice President

Fnded: 1963. **Philosophy:** The Hillsdale Fund makes most of its grants in the areas of civic affairs, education, and social services. Funding for civic affairs favors environmental affairs and community development programs. Educational funding emphasizes public education. Social services favor food and clothing distribution and other relief agencies. The arts are a secondary interest with support to public broadcasting and historical preservation. Health, religion, and other recipient areas are also supported. **Priorities:** *Arts & Humanities:* 6%. Supports historic preservation, theater, museums, and arts funds. *Civic & Public Affairs:* 28%. Emphasis is on parks, public policy organizations, community foundations, public safety, and economic development. *Education:* 12%. Supports secondary schools, colleges, and universities. *Environment:* 29%. Supports child welfare, youth organizations, food banks, United Way, and services for the aged. *International:* 9%. Supports rural health, pediatric health, hospice, and single-disease associations. *Religion:* 3%. *Note:* Total contributions made in 2000. **Typ. Recipients:** AIDS/HIV, Alzheimers Disease, Cancer, Children's Health/Hospitals, Emergency/Ambulance Services, Family Planning, Health Organizations, Health-General, Hospices, Hospitals, Multiple Sclerosis, People with Disabilities, Preventive Medicine/Wellness Organizations, Public Health, Single-Disease Health Associations, Substance Abuse. **Geo. Dist:** U.S. Eastern Region; NC.

★ 11536 ★ Hobby Family Foundation

2131 San Felipe
Houston, TX 77019-5620
Phone: (713)521-4694 **Fax:** (713)521-3950
Jennifer Cole, Secretary

Fnded: 1945. **Philosophy:** The foundation has shifted its funding toward local cultural and educational organizations in the Houston area. **Priorities:** *Arts & Humanities:* 51%. Supports museums and performing arts; includes major grant to the Houston Music Hall. *Civic & Public Affairs:* 34%. Major support for the Southwest Texas development Foundation. *Education:* 11%. *Environment:* 2%. *Note:* Contributions made in 1998. **Typ. Recipients:** AIDS/HIV, Alzheimers Disease, Cancer, Children's Health/Hospitals, Domestic Violence, Emergency/Ambulance Services, Eyes/Blindness, Family Planning, Health Funds, Health Organizations, Heart, Hospices, Hospitals, Mental Health, People with Disabilities, Single-Disease Health Associations. **Geo. Dist:** Houston, TX.

★ 11537 ★ Hoblitzelle Foundation

5956 Sherry Lane, Suite 901
Dallas, TX 75225-6522
Phone: (214)373-0462 **Fax:** (214)750-7412
Email: hoblitzelle@worldnet.att.net
Website: http://home.att.net/~hoblitzelle
Paul Harris, Executive Vice President

Fnded: 1942. **Philosophy:** The foundation supports educational, scientific, literary, and charitable organizations which "carry out the charitable and philanthropic purposes of the founders." The foundation seeks "to provide the basic tools for people to improve the quality of life in Texas." **Priorities:** *Arts & Humanities:* 13%. Supports arts museum, music, libraries, ballet, and theater. *Civic & Public Affairs:* 14%. Funds botanical gardens/parks, safety clubs, zoos, and women's affairs, and chambers of commerce. *Education:* 32%. Supports religious welfare organizations. *Environment:* 24%. Supports community centers, United Way, emergency relief, shelter/homeless, scouts, family services, food distribution and family planning services. *International:* 11%. Supports eye/blindness, heart associations, arthritis, oral health, and medical centers. *Religion:* 2%. Supports science centers and institutes. *Note:* Total contributions made in 2001. **Typ. Recipients:** AIDS/HIV, Alzheimers Disease, Cancer, Children's Health/Hospitals, Clinics/Medical Centers, Diabetes, Emergency/Ambulance Services, Eyes/Blindness, Family Planning, Health Funds, Health Organizations, Health-General, Hospices, Hospitals, Hospitals (University Affiliated), Long-Term Care, Medical Education, Medical Research, Medical Training, Multiple Sclerosis, Nursing Services, People with Disabilities, Prenatal Health Issues, Public Health, Single-Disease Health Associations, Substance Abuse, Transplant Networks/Donor Banks, Trauma Treatment. **Geo. Dist:** TX; Dallas, TX.

★ 11538 ★ Homeland Foundation (NY)

230 Park Ave.
PMB 359
New York, NY 10017
Fax: (212)949-0949
E. Lisk-Wyckoff, Jr., President

Fnded: 1938. **Philosophy:** "The Homeland Foundation has a threefold purpose: To maintain Wethersfield House, Wethersfield Gardens, and Wethersfield Stables in Amenia, NY, for the general public, and Wethersfield Farm for open space, scenic enjoyment, and for conservation purposes. To conduct and fund the cultural and intellectual activities of the Wethersfield Institute and of Homeland Foundation. To provide financial support to institutions and projects that foster the Roman Catholic Faith, and especially those that strengthen the unity of the Catholic community in the United States with the Holy See; educational initiatives geared to promote Christian culture as it is seen in the history of Western Europe; and projects that address questions touching Christian life, especially major questions of philosophy, theology, political science, and sociology." **Priorities:** *Arts & Humanities:* 14%. Funds libraries, museums, and music. *Civic & Public Affairs:* 2%. *Education:* 30%. Funds higher education, including religious education and scholarships. *Environment:* 13%. Contributes to shelters, volunteer services, and youth organizations. *International:* 2%. *Note:* Total contributions made in fiscal 2000. **Typ. Recipients:** Cancer, Clinics/Medical Centers, Emergency/Ambulance Services, Family Planning, Heart, Hospitals, Long-Term Care, Prenatal Health Issues. **Geo. Dist:** internationally; nationally; NY, metropolitan area.

★ 11539 ★ Homer and Martha Gudelsky Family Foundation

11900 Tech Rd.
Silver Spring, MD 20904
Phone: (301)622-0100 **Fax:** (301)622-3507
Medda Gudelsky, Secretary & Director

Fnded: 1968. **Philosophy:** The foundation's major interests are education and health care. Educational funding favors secondary and higher education in suburban Maryland. The foundation also has interests in the environment, arts, religious groups, and civic projects. **Priorities:** *Arts & Humanities:* 11%. Gives to theater, museums, and public broadcasting. *Civic & Public Affairs:* Less than 1%. A volunteer fire department receives support. *Education:* 29%. Funds institutions of higher learning and arts education. *Environment:* 3%. Supports substance abuse rehabilitation, children's services, and programs for people with disabilties. *International:* 12%. Contributes to hospitals and mobil medical services. *Note:* Total contributions made in 2001. **Typ. Recipients:** Cancer, Clinics/Medical Centers, Emergency/Ambulance Services, Hospitals, Long-Term Care, Medical Education, Research/Studies Institutes, Substance Abuse. **Geo. Dist:** Washington, DC; FL; MD.

★ 11540 ★ The Hoover Foundation

101 East Maple St.
North Canton, OH 44720
Fax: (216)497-5857
Lawrence Hoover, Chairman

Fnded: 1945. **Philosophy:** The Hoover Foundation makes most of its grants in the areas of education, civic affairs, social services, and the arts. Educational funding favors educational enhancement programs, colleges, private high schools, and technical education. Funding for civic affairs goes to municipalities, the environment, and consumer affairs. Social service support includes united funds, community centers, and animal protection. In the arts, interests include libraries, art institutes, historical preservation, and the performing arts. **Priorities:** *Arts & Humanities:* 35%. Supports libraries, museums, music, and the performing arts. *Civic & Public Affairs:* 6%. Supports employment/job training and a community foundation. *Education:* 17%. Supports religious education, education reform, colleges and public schools. *Environment:* 40%. Supports domestic violence/child abuse services, community centers, YMCA, United Way, and family planning services. *International:* 1%. Supports single-disease health associations, medical centers, and medical research. *Note:* Total contributions made in 2000. **Typ. Recipients:** Children's Health/Hospitals, Domestic Violence, Emergency/Ambulance Services, Eyes/Blindness, Family Planning, Health Funds, Health Organizations, Heart, Hospitals, Medical Research, Multiple Sclerosis, People with Disabilities, Respiratory, Substance Abuse, Transplant Networks/Donor Banks. **Geo. Dist:** OH, Stark County.

★ 11541 ★ Horace W. Goldsmith Foundation

375 Park Ave., Suite 1602
New York, NY 10152
Phone: (212)319-8700 **Fax:** (212)319-2881
Mr. James Slaughter, Chief Executive Officer & Director

Fnded: 1955. **Philosophy:** The foundation is interested in the support of higher education, the performing arts and cultural groups, and social welfare programs. Funding by the foundation is self-initiated. **Priorities:** *Arts & Humanities:* 27%. Funds museums, libraries, and the performing arts. *Civic & Public Affairs:* 4%. Contributes to housing, parks, botanical gardens, and community development. *Education:* 35%. Supports business education, legal education, colleges, and universities. *Environment:* 1%. Contributes to senior services, substance abuse treatment, and other human services. *International:* 14%. Supports medical centers and hospitals. *Religion:* 3%. Gives to science centers, science museums, and an academy of natural sciences. *Note:* Total contributions made in 2000. **Typ. Recipients:** AIDS/HIV, Cancer, Children's Health/Hospitals, Clinics/Medical Centers, Family Planning, Geriatric Health, Health Organizations, Heart, Hospitals, Hospitals (University Affiliated), Long-Term Care, Medical Education, Medical Rehabilitation, Medical Research, Nursing Services, People with Disabilities, Public Health, Research/Studies Institutes, Single-Disease Health Associations, Substance Abuse. **Geo. Dist:** New York, NY, including metropolitan area.

★ 11542 ★ Horizons Foundation

4020 E Madison St., Suite 322
Seattle, WA 98112
Phone: (206)323-8061
Ralph Hadac, Executive Director & Treasurer

Fnded: 1990. **Philosophy:** The foundation focuses on health organizations, environmental causes, and the arts in the Puget Sound area. **Priorities:** *Arts & Humanities:* 3%. Funds performing arts, museums, and outreach programs. *Civic & Public Affairs:* 17%. Contributes to public policy organizations, minority affairs, zoos, and philanthropic organizations. *Education:* 1%. Gives to a public university. *Environment:* 42%. Focus on teen pregnancy prevention, parenting skills, violence/sexual assault prevention, and youth and family services. *International:* 3%. Women's, children's, and community health organizations and mental health centers receive support. *Note:* Total contributions made in 2001. **Typ. Recipients:** Child Abuse, Children's Health/Hospitals, Clinics/Medical Centers, Domestic Violence, Family Planning, Family Planning, Health-General, Mental Health, Prenatal Health Issues, Sexual Abuse. **Geo. Dist:** WA, Puget Sound region.

★ 11543 ★ Houston Endowment

600 Travis, Suite 6400
Houston, TX 77002-3000
Phone: (713)238-8100 **Fax:** (713)238-8101
Email: sjohns@houstonendowment.org
Website: http://www.houstonendowment.org
H. Nelson, III, President

Fnded: 1937. **Philosophy:** The purpose of the endowment "is the support of any charitable, educational or religious undertaking." The directors place priority on organizations and programs serving the greater Houston area and the State of Texas. Support is given to a wide variety of charitable activities, including those in the areas of education, health, the arts, culture, civic, and human services. "While the Houston Endowment Inc. provides the funds for many scholarships, it does not provide scholarships to individuals on the basis of individual application to the foundation. The foundation's scholarships programs are administered in one of two ways. First, Houston Endowment Inc. funds the Jesse H. Jones and Mary Gibbs Jones High School Scholarship Program." Second, the Endowment provides funding for scholarships in various fields of study by making grants to selected colleges and universities. For a list of colleges and universities and their contact information, refer to the Endowment's website. **Priorities:** *Arts & Humanities:* 8%. Funds visual and performing arts. *Civic & Public Affairs:* 22%. Supports community enhancement initiatives, including community development, community education, housing, and parks and natural spaces. *Education:* 37%. Supports K-12 and higher education. *Environment:* 27%. Supports health and human services organizations, including services for the elderly and disabled. *International:* 6%. Funds medical facilities and research, and access to health care. *Note:* Total contributions made in 2000. **Typ. Recipients:** AIDS/HIV, Alzheimers Disease, Cancer, Child Abuse, Children's Health/Hospitals, Children's Health/Hospitals, Clinics/Medical Centers, Diabetes, Domestic Violence, Emergency/Ambulance Services, Family Planning, Geriatric Health, Health Organizations, Health Policy/Cost Containment, Heart, Hospices, Hospitals, Medical Education, Medical Rehabilitation, Medical Research, Medical Training, Mental Health, Nursing Services, Outpatient Health Care, People with Disabilities, Research/Studies Institutes, Single-Disease Health Associations, Substance Abuse, Transplant Networks/Donor Banks. **Geo. Dist:** TX, some statewide giving; Harris County, TX; Houston, TX.

★ 11544 ★ Howard Gilman Foundation

111 West 50th St.
New York, NY 10020
Phone: (212)307-1073 **Fax:** (212)262-4108
Website: http://www.howardgilman.org
Jennifer Amis, Program Administrator

Fnded: 1981. **Priorities:** *Arts & Humanities:* 49%. Supports dance, opera, music, museums, theater, fine arts, and photography. *Civic & Public Affairs:* 5%. Gives to municipalities and philanthropic organizations. *Education:* 22%. Funds medical schools, colleges, and universities. *Environment:* 1%. Contributes to animal welfare organizations and to children's and immigrant services. *International:* 11%. Medical centers and HIV/AIDS organizations receive support. *Religion:* Less than 1%. *Note:* Total contributions made in fiscal 2000. **Typ. Recipients:** AIDS/HIV, Children's Health/Hospitals, Clinics/Medical Centers, Health Organizations, Health-General, Heart, Hospitals, Hospitals (University Affiliated), Medical Education, Medical Research, Public Health, Single-Disease Health Associations. **Geo. Dist:** internationally; nationally; New York, NY.

★ 11545 ★ Howard Heinz Endowment

30 Dominion Tower
625 Liberty Ave.
Pittsburgh, PA 15222-3199
Phone: (412)281-5777 **Fax:** (412)281-5788
Email: info@heinz.org
Website: http://www.heinz.org
Maxwell King, Executive Director

Fnded: 1941. **Philosophy:** "Throughout their histories, the Howard and Vira I. Heinz Endowments have been privileged to enjoy a remarkable intimate relationship with the communities and organizations they serve. From this relationship continually emerges two of the Endowments' primary strengths: their sensitivity to the needs of their region, and their willingness to shoulder risks on its behalf. It has been characteristic of the Endowments to want to listen and respond personally to requests for help. We are neighbors, after all, not disinterested observers. For that reason, there has been a reluctance over the years to print formalized program guidelines, suggesting as they might an unfeeling institutionalization of process. We do not intend for that to happen. But we also appreciate how dramatically the philanthropic landscape has changed in recent years. With the demand for philanthropic resources increasing rapidly and with ever greater urgency, we must respond to the call from prospective grantseekers for guidance specificity and direction... The Endowments' present grantmaking reflects over half a century of applied values and experiential learning. Three signature themes emerge from this rich history: leadership, cooperation and enterprise. These themes will continue to guide us in the future." *A Message From the Executive Director* **Priorities:** *Arts & Humanities:* 25%. Supports history, museums, dance, arts festivals, public broadcasting, libraries, theater, music, and ballet. *Civic & Public Affairs:* 38%. Supports community foundations, economic development, public policy, public affairs, and botanical gardens. *Education:* 12%. Supports universities, leadership training, continuing education, schools, and literacy. *Environment:* 18%. Supports family services, youth programs, domestic violence and child abuse prevention, United Way, and food distribution programs. *International:* 4%. Supports hospitals, childrens health, and nutrition. *Religion:* 1%. *Note:* Total contributions made in 2000. **Typ. Recipients:** Child Abuse, Children's Health/Hospitals, Clinics/Medical Centers, Domestic Violence, Family Planning, Health Organizations, Health Policy/Cost Containment, Heart, Hospitals, Medical Education, Medical Rehabilitation, Medical Research, Mental Health, Nursing Services, Nutrition, Prenatal Health Issues, Preventive Medicine/Wellness Organizations, Public Health, Research/Studies Institutes, Substance Abuse. **Geo. Dist:** PA, Southwest Pennsylvania; Pittsburgh, PA.

★ 11546 ★ Howard Hughes Medical Institute

Office of Grants and Special Programs
4000 Jones Bridge Rd.
Chevy Chase, MD 20815-6789
Phone: (301)215-8500 **Fax:** (301)215-8888
Email: grantvpr@hhmi.org
Website: http://www.hhmi.org

Fnded: 1954. **Philosophy:** In late 2000, the Institute purchased a 281-acre site, just outside Washington, DC upon which it intends to develop a research campus for a cost of approx. $500 million. Disbursements for this new facility through 2002 were $68 million. The largest private initiative in U.S. history to enhance science education at all levels, the Institute disburses grants for preschool through postgraduate training. Through its grants program, the Institute also supports the research of outstanding biomedical scientists outside the United States and provides funding to help medical schools sustain their commitment to research. **Priorities:** *Education:* 100%. Supports scientific research training, science education, and research by scientists outside the United States. *Note:* Total contributions made in fiscal 2001. **Typ. Recipients:** Arthritis, Cancer, Hospitals (University Affiliated), Medical Education, Medical Research. **Geo. Dist:** internationally; nationally.

★ 11547 ★ HRK Foundation

345 Saint Peter St., Suite 1200
Saint Paul, MN 55102
Phone: (651)293-9001 **Fax:** (651)298-0551
Email: hrkfoundation@hrkgroup.com
Website: http://www.hrkfoundation.org
Kathleen Fluegel, Foundation Director

Fnded: 1962. **Philosophy:** "HRK Foundation is a family foundation defined and sustained by a sense of spirituality, creativity, and stewardship. Through quiet leadership and philanthropy, the Board seeks to promote healthy families and communities, to enhance the quality of and access to education, and to improve the fabric of our society." "The work of HRK Foundation will be carried out through a commitment to and support for: "The Arts: People and organizations that nourish the human spirit and encourage our connectedness. "Health: Programs that strengthen families and promote healthy lives for children and/or provide services for people affected by HIV/AIDS. "Community Building: Efforts which increase adequate and affordable housing; encourage responsible land use; promote conservation and preservation of community resources; advance the work of neighbors who reach across their differences for the common good. "Education: Educational approaches that promote holistic personal development–intellectual, social, emotional, and spiritual." HRK Foundation Grant Guidelines **Priorities:** *Arts & Humanities:* 37%. Supports people and organizations that nourish the human spirit and encourage our connectedness. Recipients include libraries, public radio, arts, the opera, and humanities council. *Civic & Public Affairs:* 21%. Funds community-building efforts which increase adequate and affordable housing, encourage responsible land use, promote conversation and preservation of community resources, and advance the work of neighbors who reach across their differences for the common good. *Education:* 28%. Supports educational approaches and institutions that promote holistic personal development-intellectual, social emotional, and spiritual. *International:* 14%. Supports programs that strengthen families and promote healthy lives for children, and/or provide services for people affected by HIV/AIDS. *Note:* Contributions were made in 2001. **Typ. Recipients:** AIDS/HIV, Children's Health/Hospitals, Clinics/

Medical Centers, Emergency/Ambulance Services, Family Planning, Health Funds, Health Organizations, Hospitals, Medical Education, Medical Rehabilitation, Mental Health, People with Disabilities, Public Health, Single-Disease Health Associations, Substance Abuse, Transplant Networks/Donor Banks. **Geo. Dist:** MN, Twin Cities metropolitan area; WI, St. Croix Valley and Ashland and Bayfield Counties. **Frmly:** Mary Anderson Foundation MAHADH Foundation MAHADH Foundation to HRK Foundation.

★ 11548 ★ Huber Foundation
PO Box 277
Rumson, NJ 07760
Phone: (732)933-7700
Lorraine Barnhart, Executive Director

Fnded: 1949. **Philosophy:** The foundation focuses its grant making on "the issues of Reproductive Freedom, Population Education, and Family Planning." The Huber Foundation 2000 Annual Report. **Priorities:** *Civic & Public Affairs:* 64%. Funds legal defense, women's rights, and reproductive rights groups. *Education:* 4%. College civil liberties programs. *Environment:* 23%. Family planning organizations. *Note:* Total contributions made in 2000. **Typ. Recipients:** Clinics/Medical Centers, Family Planning, Health Organizations, Hospitals, Public Health. **Geo. Dist:** nationally.

★ 11549 ★ Hudson-Webber Foundation
333 West Fort St., Suite 1310
Detroit, MI 48226
Phone: (313)963-7777 **Fax:** (313)963-2818
David Egner, President

Fnded: 1943. **Philosophy:** The Hudson-Webber Foundation's objective is "to improve the vitality and quality of life of the metropolitan Detroit community." The foundation has a particular interest in the revitalization of downtown Detroit and institutions and programs that directly benefit its citizens. The foundation concentrates its efforts and resources in five program areas: the Detroit Medical Center, economic development of southeastern Michigan (with emphasis on the creation of employment opportunities), Detroit physical revitalization, the arts, and crime abatement in Detroit. **Priorities:** *Arts & Humanities:* 14%. Supports historical preservation, art institutes, orchestra and opera. *Civic & Public Affairs:* 25%. Supports community foundations and job training. *Education:* 10%. Supports universities. *Environment:* 12%. Supports United Way, family services and youth programs. *International:* 30%. Supports hospital research and medical centers. *Religion:* 8%. Supports science center. *Note:* Total contributions made in 1998. **Typ. Recipients:** Cancer, Child Abuse, Children's Health/Hospitals, Clinics/Medical Centers, Domestic Violence, Family Planning, Health Organizations, Hospitals, Nursing Services, People with Disabilities, Prenatal Health Issues, Public Health, Substance Abuse, Transplant Networks/Donor Banks. **Geo. Dist:** MI, Oakland County; MI, Southeastern Michigan; MI, Wayne County; Detroit, MI.

★ 11550 ★ Hugh and Hazel Darling Foundation
520 S Grand Ave. 7th Floor
Los Angeles, CA 90071-2645
Phone: (213)683-5200 **Fax:** (213)627-7795
Email: rstack@dhrlaw.com
Richard Stack, Trustee

Fnded: 1988. **Philosophy:** The Hugh and Hazel Darling Foundation supports the advancement of education in California, with primary emphasis on legal education and education programs calculated to impart a better understanding and appreciation of our legal system through its support of educational institutions. Due to multi-year pledges, funds for new projects are limited. "We've made multi-year commitments to what we believe to be worthwhile projects, so that limits our ability to commit new funds," explained Richard L. Stack, trustee of the foundation. **Priorities:** *Arts & Humanities:* 1%. Supports public media. *Civic & Public Affairs:* 4%. Supports public law education. *Education:* 93%. Funds universities and colleges. *Environment:* 2%. Funds youth organizations and the blind. **Typ. Recipients:** People with Disabilities, Speech & Hearing. **Geo. Dist:** CA.

★ 11551 ★ Hugh I. Shott, Jr. Foundation
500 Federal St.
PO Box 1559
Bluefield, WV 24701
Phone: (304)325-8181 **Fax:** (304)325-3727
Richard Wilkinson, President

Fnded: 1985. **Philosophy:** The Hugh I. Shott, Jr. Foundation's mission is to "improve social and economic quality of life in the trade area of the Bluefield Daily Telegraph." 2001 application form. Educational funding supports college foundations and public school districts. Civic affairs interests include municipalities, community development, and business. **Priorities:** *Arts & Humanities:* 8%. Performing arts and historic preservation. *Civic & Public Affairs:* 47%. Community programs and foundations, parks and towns/municipalties. *Education:* 17%. College and university foundations mainly in Bluefield, VA. *Environment:* 25%. Supports health organizations and medical centers, sports, youth programs, volunteer projects, and United Way. *International:* 3%. *Note:* Total contributions made in 2000. **Typ. Recipients:** Clinics/Medical Centers, Emergency/Ambulance Services, Family Planning, Hospices, Hospitals, People with Disabilities, Public Health. **Geo. Dist:** VA, Southwest Virginia; WV, Southern West Virginia.

★ 11552 ★ Hugh J. Andersen Foundation
PO Box 204
Bayport, MN 55003-0204
Phone: (651)439-1557 **Fax:** (651)439-9480
Email: hjafdn@srinc.biz
Website: http://www.scenicriver.org
Katie Wood, Grants Consultant

Fnded: 1962. **Philosophy:** "The mission of the Hugh J. Andersen Foundation is to give back to our community through focused efforts that foster inclusivity, promote equality, and lead to increased human independence, self-sufficiency and dignity. To fulfill this mission, the Foundation acts as a grantmaker, innovator, and convenor." 2000 Hugh J. Andersen Foundation Annual Report The foundation places a high priority on organizations that benefit people in St. Croix Valley, which the board has defined as Washington County in Minnesota, and Pierce, Polk, and St. Croix counties in Wisconsin. Projects designed to benefit the people of St. Paul, MN, receive secondary consideration, as will projects serving other parts of Minnesota. Limited consideration will be given to organizations with a national or international scope. The foundation is particularly interested in direct services provided by programs that serve children and youth, especially those that provide personal development activities; that provide various social support services to the community at large; that are engaged in health-related services, other than hospitals and research facilities; and that provide educational opportunities and enrichment to the general community. Consideration will be given to battered women's shelters, special projects or programming in public schools, programs for the developmentally or physically disabled, programs for seniors, and public or civic projects and activities within the St. Croix Valley. **Priorities:** *Arts & Humanities:* 7%. Supports performing arts, theater and arts councils. *Civic & Public Affairs:* 2%. Funds nonprofit management. *Education:* 7%. Supports programs serving children and youth, including children's museums, minority education, and literacy initiatives. *Environment:* 57%. Supports housing, community development, youth groups and camps, women's and family services, support for victims of violence, and United Way. *International:* 20%. Funds health-related services that educate and improve community well-being. *Note:* Total contributions made in fiscal 2000. **Typ. Recipients:** AIDS/HIV, Cancer, Children's Health/Hospitals, Clinics/Medical Centers, Diabetes, Domestic Violence, Emergency/Ambulance Services, Family Planning, Health Organizations, Hospitals, Medical Rehabilitation, Medical Research, People with Disabilities, Sexual Abuse, Single-Disease Health Associations, Substance Abuse. **Geo. Dist:** MN, St. Paul (secondary focus); St. Croix Valley, MN, St. Croix Valley also covers WI; WI, Pierce County; WI, Polk County; WI, St. Croix County.

★ 11553 ★ Hugh Kaul Foundation Trust
PO Box 11426
Birmingham, AL 35202
Phone: (205)326-4696 **Fax:** (205)581-7433
Karla Gayle, Vice President & Trust Officer

Fnded: 1990. **Philosophy:** The trust is a private foundation which makes grants to charitable organizations in the Greater Birmingham metropolitan area, in Clay County, and in Coosa County of the state of Alabama. **Priorities:** *Arts & Humanities:* 13%. Funds museums, art councils, libraries, film, music, public broadcasting, and performing arts. *Civic & Public Affairs:* 19%. Funds community foundations, economic development, parks and botanical gardens, and civic groups. *Education:* 38%. Supports colleges, universities, precollege education, and education funds. *Environment:* 7%. Supports YMCA/YWCAs, children's groups, scouting, community centers, and elder concerns. *International:* 17%. Supports speech and hearing concerns and hospitals. *Note:* Total contributions were made in 2000. **Typ. Recipients:** Cancer, Children's Health/Hospitals, Eyes/Blindness, Family Planning, Hospitals, Medical Education, Medical Research, Mental Health, Public Health, Single-Disease Health Associations, Speech & Hearing, Substance Abuse. **Geo. Dist:** AL, Coosa County; AL, Jefferson County; Birmingham, AL, Clay County.

★ 11554 ★ Hugoton Foundation
900 Park Ave.
New York, NY 10021
Phone: (212)734-5447 **Fax:** (212)734-5448
Joan Stout, President

Fnded: 1981. **Philosophy:** The Hugoton Foundation makes most of its grants in the areas of health care and education. Funding for health care favors hospitals. Education support goes primarily to medical and nursing schools, colleges, and secondary education. The foundation also supports other recipient areas on a limited basis. **Priorities:** *Arts & Humanities:* Less than 1%. Gives to libraries. *Civic & Public Affairs:* Less than 1%. Contributes to the USO and a community fund. *Education:* 27%. Funds universities; parochial schools; and business, religious and nursing schools. *Environment:* 6%. Funds recreation/athletics, emergency relief, substance abuse centers, child welfare, and animal protection. *International:* 50%. Supports hospital, medical centers, blood banks, heart research, and nursing services. *Religion:* 3%. Gives to a natural history museum. *Note:* Total contributions made in 2001. **Typ. Recipients:** Alzheimers Disease, Cancer, Children's Health/Hospitals, Clinics/Medical Centers, Emergency/Ambulance Services, Eyes/Blindness, Geriatric Health, Health Organizations, Heart, Hospitals, Medical Education, Medical Rehabilitation, Medical Research, Mental Health, Mental Health, Nursing Services, People with Disabilities, Research/Studies Institutes, Respiratory, Single-Disease Health Associations, Transplant Networks/Donor Banks. **Geo. Dist:** Miami, FL; New York, NY.

★ 11555 ★ Hunt Alternatives Fund
500 E Eighth Ave.
Denver, CO 80203
Phone: (212)722-7606 **Fax:** (303)839-1013
Elsa Holguin, Executive Director

Fnded: 1981. **Philosophy:** Among other objectives, The Hunt Alternatives Fund aims to strengthen the role of women in society, accelerate systemic change, nurture coalitions in blighted neighborhoods, and cultivate the arts (when used as a catalyst for social progress). The Fund concentrates on grassroots efforts in prevention, advocacy and leadership development–particularly those that target the causes, rather than the symptoms. The Fund is especially interested in fostering the long-term viability of non-profit organizations by helping them identify new or increased sources of asistance and develop strategies for self-sufficiency. programs, the individual Leadership and Youth Leadership awards to recognize leadership by individuals in the community. **Priorities:** *Civic & Public Affairs:* 97%. Support a variety of civic causes through the Swanee Hunt Operating Fund. Also funds neighborhood development and women's affairs. *Environment:* 2%. With emphasis on children and families. *International:* 1%. *Note:* Total contributions made in fiscal 1998. **Typ. Recipients:** AIDS/HIV, Cancer, Child Abuse, Children's Health/Hospitals, Clinics/Medical Centers, Domestic Violence, Emergency/Ambulance Services, Family Planning, Health Organizations, Health-General, Medical Education, Mental Health, People with Disabilities, Prenatal Health Issues, Public Health, Respiratory, Sexual Abuse, Single-Disease Health Associations, Substance Abuse. **Geo. Dist:** Denver, CO, metropolitan area.

★ 11556 ★ Huston Foundation

1 Fayette St., Suite 190
Conshohocken, PA 19428-2064
Phone: (610)832-4949 **Fax:** (610)832-4960
Email: hustonfndn@aol.com
Susan Heilman, Executive Assistant

Fnded: 1957. **Philosophy:** "The main purpose of the Huston Foundation's contributions program is to lend financial assistance to help improve social, cultural, intellectual, and economic environments primarily within the continental United States and to Protestant Evangelical Christian organizations worldwide." Grants are divided between religious and secular segments and are primarily made in the categories of health, human services, education, civic affairs, the arts, and community development. The foundation reports that at least 51% of the funding each year supports Protestant Evangelical Christian organizations. **Priorities:** *Arts & Humanities:* 6%. Supports arts societies and theatres. *Civic & Public Affairs:* 8%. Supports philanthropic organizations and economic development. *Education:* 22%. Supports Private Christian education. *Environment:* 15%. Supports family services, YMCA's, youth programs, and child welfare. *International:* 1%. Supports ophthalmic research. *Note:* Total contributions made in 2000. **Typ. Recipients:** Child Abuse, Children's Health/Hospitals, Clinics/Medical Centers, Emergency/Ambulance Services, Eyes/Blindness, Family Planning, Health Organizations, Hospices, Hospitals, Medical Education, Medical Rehabilitation, Medical Research, Nursing Services, People with Disabilities, Public Health, Sexual Abuse, Single-Disease Health Associations. **Geo. Dist:** nationally; PA, Eastern Pennsylvania.

★ 11557 ★ Hyams Foundation

175 Federal St., 14th Floor
Boston, MA 02110
Phone: (617)426-5600 **Fax:** (617)426-5696
Email: info@hyamsfoundation.org
Website: http://www.hyamsfoundation.org
Elizabeth Smith, Executive Director

Fnded: 1921. **Philosophy:** The mission of the Hyams Foundation is to increase economic and social justice and power within low-income communities. The Hyams Foundation believes that investing in strategies that enable low-income people to increase their economic security, build wealth and become active participants in their communities will have the greatest social return in these times. The Foundation will carry out its mission by: supporting civic participation by low-income communities; promoting economic development that benefits low-income neighborhoods and their residents; and developing the talents and skills of low-income youth. The Foundation has chosen to focus on civic participation, economic development, and young people, believing that they present three key opportunities for change. Within each priority area, the Foundation will support strategies that reflect several key principles. They are: building capacity within low-income communities and neighborhoods, particularly in communities of color which are disproportionately low-income; connecting low-income communities and neighborhoods to one another and to the broader community at large; identifying and building on those assets and "anchor" institutions that are unique to individual low-income communities; emphasizing the leadership and direct participation of low-income individuals; promoting meaningful diversity and cross-cultural understanding in all communities and institutions; and encouraging comprehensive solutions to achieving economic and social justice while promoting collaboration and cooperation among individuals and organizations. **Priorities:** *Civic & Public Affairs:* 53%. Supports community development, public policy issues, housing, job training, legal aid, and urban affairs. *Education:* 18%. Funds adult education, literacy, and educational funds. *Environment:* 17%. Supports neighborhood centers, human services, child care, and senior services. *International:* 2%. *Note:* Total contributions made in 2000. **Typ. Recipients:** Adolescent Health Issues, AIDS/HIV, Children's Health/Hospitals, Clinics/Medical Centers, Domestic Violence, Family Planning, Health Funds, Health Organizations, Hospitals, Medical Research, Mental Health, Substance Abuse. **Geo. Dist:** Boston, MA; Chelsea, MA.

★ 11558 ★ Hyde and Watson Foundation

437 Southern Boulevard
Chatham, NJ 07928
Phone: (973)966-6024 **Fax:** (973)966-6404
Website: http://www.fdncenter.org/grantmaker/hydeandwatson
Hunter Corbin, President

Fnded: 1983. **Philosophy:** The foundation is primarily interested in the support of capital projects that are of lasting value and that will increase the quality, capacity, or efficiency of a grantee's program or services. Typical projects of interest include the purchase, relocation, renovation, or improvement of facilities; purchase of capital equipment; construction; development of materials; and certain areas of medical research. The foundation supports projects in the broad fields of education, health, social services, the arts and humanities, and religion. A substantial portion of the foundation's grant funds each year are allocated to projects for which the foundation's support makes a major contribution. foundation's support makes a major contribution. **Priorities:** *Arts & Humanities:* 5%. Supports public broadcasting, historic preservation, museums, music, theater, and art foundations. *Civic & Public Affairs:* 3%. Supports community foundations, job training, neighborhood development, and parks. *Education:* 39%. Supports private schools, universities, and educational programs. *Environment:* 35%. Supports family services, scouting, YMCA, and animal protection. *International:* 13%. Supports hospitals, hospice, single-disease associations, medical research, and children's health. *Note:* Total contributions made in 2000. **Typ. Recipients:** Adolescent Health Issues, Alzheimers Disease, Cancer, Children's Health/Hospitals, Clinics/Medical Centers, Domestic Violence, Emergency/Ambulance Services, Eyes/Blindness, Geriatric Health, Health Organizations, Health-General, Heart, Hospices, Hospitals, Hospitals (University Affiliated), Medical Education, Medical Rehabilitation, Medical Research, Nursing Services, People with Disabilities, Prenatal Health Issues, Public Health, Research/Studies Institutes, Respiratory, Single-Disease Health Associations, Speech & Hearing, Substance Abuse, Transplant Networks/Donor Banks, Trauma Treatment. **Geo. Dist:** NJ, Essex County; NJ, Morris County; NJ, Union County; New York, NY, metropolitan area.

★ 11559 ★ I. A. O'Shaughnessy Foundation

W-1271 First Bank Bldg.
332 Minnesota St.
Saint Paul, MN 55101
Phone: (651)222-2323 **Fax:** (651)222-6368
Email: iaoshaughnessyfd@qwest.net

Fnded: 1941. **Philosophy:** The foundation funds higher education, hospitals, youth organizations, community services, churches, the arts, and sciences. **Priorities:** *Arts & Humanities:* 4%. Supports art and music. *Civic & Public Affairs:* 5%. Funds community foundations. *Education:* 66%. Largely supports Catholic universities and secondary schools. *Environment:* 5%. Funds centers for families and children. *International:* 3%. Supports psychiatric treatment facilities, a therapeutic riding center, and other medical organizations. *Note:* Total contributions made 2001. **Typ. Recipients:** Alzheimers Disease, Cancer, Children's Health/Hospitals, Clinics/Medical Centers, Domestic Violence, Heart, Hospices, Hospitals, Medical Education, Medical Rehabilitation, People with Disabilities, Prenatal Health Issues. **Geo. Dist:** IL; KS; MN; TX.

★ 11560 ★ Independence Foundation

Offices at the Bellevue
200 South Broad St., Suite 1101
Philadelphia, PA 19102
Phone: (215)985-4009 **Fax:** (215)985-3989
Email: ssherman@independencefoundation.org
Website: http://www.independencefoundation.org
Susan Sherman, President

Fnded: 1932. **Philosophy:** "True to our charter, the current Directors continue to use and apply the property and the income therefrom, 'exclusively in such charitable, benevolent, scientific, and educational activities as will promote the well-being of mankind and the alleviation of human suffering.' (Charter)." "The interests of the Foundation concentrate on initiatives that demonstrate innovation and make a difference to residents of Philadelphia and the surrounding Pennsylvania counties. These include Nurse Managed Health Care, Culture and the Arts, Legal Aid, and Contemporary Social Problems." "The foundation supports initiatives in community-based and community focused nurse managed primary health care where services to people are not always available. The foundation is particularly interested in promoting wellness through comprehensive primary health care. This may include health promotion, disease prevention, family planning, early intervention and related supportive services that focus particularly on basic human needs of food and shelter. The foundation is also interested in efforts that address the challenge of balancing quality, access and cost in health care." 1996 Annual Report **Priorities:** *Arts & Humanities:* 30%. Funds museums, music associations, and art centers. *Civic & Public Affairs:* 15%. Supports ethnic associations, community councils, zoos, and legal concerns. *Education:* 10%. Supports colleges, particularly nursing and law programs. *Environment:* 15%. Funds health and human service programs, family planning, and associations for people with disabilities. *International:* 25%. Funds hospitals and community-based, nurse-managed healthcare projects. *Note:* Total contributions made in 2001. **Typ. Recipients:** AIDS/HIV, Children's Health/Hospitals, Clinics/Medical Centers, Domestic Violence, Emergency/Ambulance Services, Eyes/Blindness, Family Planning, Health Organizations, Health Policy/Cost Containment, Hospitals, Hospitals (University Affiliated), Medical Education, Medical Rehabilitation, Medical Research, Mental Health, Nursing Services, People with Disabilities, Prenatal Health Issues, Preventive Medicine/Wellness Organizations, Public Health. **Geo. Dist:** PA, Bucks County; PA, Chester County; PA, Delaware County; PA, Montgomery County; Philadelphia, PA, metropolitan area.

★ 11561 ★ International Foundation

170 Changebridge Rd.
Unit C5-4, Second Floor
Montville, NJ 07045
Phone: (973)227-6107 **Fax:** (973)227-6821
Dr. Edward Holmes, Grants Chairman

Fnded: 1948. **Philosophy:** "The International Foundation exists to help people of the developing world in their endeavors to solve some of their problems, to attain a better standard of living and to obtain a reasonable degree of self-sufficiency. "The Trustees of The International Foundation believe in granting support to those projects which have promise of successfully accomplishing stated objectives to meet defined specific needs. "The Trustees encourage proposals for the developing world which advance a stable social order, provide necessary services for its people, and encourage cultural and artistic endeavors that favor a rising quality of life. "Grants are made in five general areas: agriculture, health, education, social development, and environment. "Some aid to refugees and grants for population planning are also given." The International Foundation Brochure, 2000 **Priorities:** *Note:* Contributions made in 2000. **Typ. Recipients:** Children's Health/Hospitals, Clinics/Medical Centers, Emergency/Ambulance Services, Eyes/Blindness, Family Planning, Health Funds, Health Organizations, Health-General, Hospitals, Medical Rehabilitation, Medical Training, Nutrition, People with Disabilities, Public Health, Public Health, Single-Disease Health Associations. **Geo. Dist:** internationally.

★ 11562 ★ Ira W. DeCamp Foundation

Global FoundationS Group
60 Wall St., 36th Floor
New York, NY 10260
Phone: (212)483-2323 **Fax:** (212)648-5082
Lisa Philp, Vice President

Fnded: 1975. **Philosophy:** The chief purpose of the foundation is to support health care organizations, medical research, and medical education; social services, and workforce development. **Priorities:** *Arts & Humanities:* 2%. Primarily supports libraries. *Civic & Public Affairs:* 2%. Supports women's affairs and community development. *Education:* 44%. Emphasis on medical education. *Environment:* 8%. Supports child welfare, people with disabilities, youth organizations, and the homeless. *International:* 34%. Primary support for hospitals in New York City. *Religion:* 1%. Funds a laboratory. *Note:* Total contributions made in fiscal 2000. **Typ. Recipients:** AIDS/HIV, Alzheimers Disease, Cancer, Children's Health/Hospitals, Clinics/Medical Centers, Emergency/Ambulance Services, Eyes/Blindness, Geriatric Health, Health Funds, Health Organizations, Heart, Hospices, Hospitals, Hospitals (University Affiliated), Kidney, Long-Term Care, Medical Education, Medical Rehabilitation, Medical Research, Medical Training, Mental Health, Nursing Services, Outpatient Health Care, People with Disabilities, Public Health, Research/Studies Institutes, Single-Disease Health Associations, Speech & Hearing, Substance Abuse, Transplant Networks/Donor Banks. **Geo. Dist:** New York, NY, including the metropolitan area.

★ 11563 ★ Ireland Foundation

1422 Euclid Ave., Suite 1030
Cleveland, OH 44115-2004
Phone: (216)363-1033 **Fax:** (216)363-1038
Louise Humphrey, President & Trustee

Fnded: 1951. **Philosophy:** The fund generally supports private, secondary schools; the arts; and other philanthropic causes. A majority of funding is distributed within the state of Ohio, but some giving is national. **Priorities:** *Arts & Humanities:* 38%. Historic preservation, museums, and opera. *Civic & Public Affairs:* 3%. Primarily supporting the Archbold Foundation. *Education:* 11%. Supports private precollege education and colleges and universities. *Environment:* 4%. People with disabilities and united funds. *International:* 42%. Cancer research, hositals, and nursing services. *Religion:* 1%. Funds Tall Timers Research. *Note:* Total contributions made in 2000. **Typ. Recipients:** Cancer, Children's Health/Hospitals, Clinics/Medical Centers, Family Planning, Health Organizations, Hospitals, Hospitals (University Affiliated), Medical Education, Medical Rehabilitation, Medical Research, Nursing Services, People with Disabilities, Prenatal Health Issues. **Geo. Dist:** Cleveland, OH.

★ 11564 ★ Irene E. and George A. Davis Foundation

One Monarch Place, Suite 1450
Springfield, MA 01144
Phone: (413)734-8336 **Fax:** (413)734-7845
Email: info@davisfdn.org
Website: http://www.davisfdn.org
Mary Walachy, Executive Director

Fnded: 1970. **Philosophy:** The foundation focuses its grantmaking activities on the local Western Massachusetts community with an emphasis on higher education, religious organizations, and the fine arts. The foundation's literature states, "While the Foundation will entertain proposals form all interest areas, the Foundation seeks to support programs which will offer creative responses to the communities' most pressing needs and concerns, which are preventative and farsighted, and which reach a broad segment of the community." **Priorities:** *Arts & Humanities:* 11%. Supports museums, libraries, festivals, and the performing arts. *Civic & Public Affairs:* 6%. Supports community foundations, public policy, and a zoo. *Education:* 41%. Supports colleges and universities, music education, and private and public schools. *Environment:* 16%. Supports youth programs, Young Men's Christian AssociationA, services for the elderly, United Way, and animal protection. *International:* 7%. Supports community health organizations and hospitals. *Note:* Total contributions made in 2000. **Typ. Recipients:** AIDS/HIV, Children's Health/Hospitals, Clinics/Medical Centers, Domestic Violence, Emergency/Ambulance Services, Geriatric Health, Health Organizations, Hospitals, Mental Health, Nursing Services, People with Disabilities, Prenatal Health Issues, Public Health, Research/Studies Institutes, Single-Disease Health Associations. **Geo. Dist:** MA.

★ 11565 ★ Irene W. and C. B. Pennington Foundation

8550 United Plaza Blvd., Ste. 1001
Baton Rouge, LA 70809
Phone: (225)922-4600
William Hodgkins, Contact

Fnded: 1982. **Philosophy:** The foundation primarily favors social service organizations, with emphasis on youth organizations and community centers. In the past, large grants were given to universities in Louisiana. Minor grants are given to other recipient areas. **Priorities:** *Arts & Humanities:* 2%. Arts centers. *Civic & Public Affairs:* 18%. Foundations and community groups. *Education:* 19%. Gives to private precollege education. *Environment:* 28%. Funds youth groups and YMCAs. *International:* 17%. Support includes the Pennington Medical Foundation. *Religion:* 13%. *Note:* Total contributions made in 2000. **Typ. Recipients:** Cancer, Children's Health/Hospitals, Clinics/Medical Centers, Domestic Violence, Emergency/Ambulance Services, Emergency/Ambulance Services, Family Planning, Health-General, Hospices, Hospitals, Kidney, Medical Research, Mental Health, Nutrition, Public Health, Sexual Abuse, Substance Abuse. **Geo. Dist:** Baton Rouge, LA.

★ 11566 ★ Irvine Health Foundation

18301 Von Karman Ave., Suite 440
Irvine, CA 92612
Phone: (949)253-2959 **Fax:** (949)253-2962
Email: ebk@ihf.org
Website: http://www.ihf.org
Edward Kacic, President

Fnded: 1985. **Philosophy:** "The Irvine Health Foundation is a nonprofit grant-making foundation whose goal is to improve the health, consisting of physical, mental and emotional wellbeing, of the residents of Orange County, California. The foundation is focused on promoting health and wellness, ensuring the availability of accessible, quality, health-related services, working in the area of health policy and supporting research designed to develop new knowledge in areas related to health." **Priorities:** *Arts & Humanities:* 1%. *Civic & Public Affairs:* 13%. *Education:* 34%. *Environment:* 22%. Supports services for the homeless and child welfare. *International:* 12%. Supports women's health, medical research, and public health. *Note:* Total contributions made in fiscal 2001. **Typ. Recipients:** AIDS/HIV, Alzheimers Disease, Child Abuse, Children's Health/Hospitals, Clinics/Medical Centers, Domestic Violence, Emergency/Ambulance Services, Family Planning, Geriatric Health, Health Organizations, Health Policy/Cost Containment, Hospices, Hospitals, Medical Education, Medical Research, Mental Health, Multiple Sclerosis, Nursing Services, People with Disabilities, Prenatal Health Issues, Preventive Medicine/Wellness Organizations, Public Health, Respiratory, Sexual Abuse, Single-Disease Health Associations, Speech & Hearing, Substance Abuse. **Geo. Dist:** CA, Orange County.

★ 11567 ★ Irving Goldman Foundation

52 Vanderbilt Ave., 16th Floor
New York, NY 10017
Phone: (212)557-6700
Lloyd Goldman, President

Fnded: 1984. **Priorities:** *Arts & Humanities:* 4%. Gives to museums and film. *Education:* 55%. Supports universities, Hebrew schools, minority education, and the Educational Alliance. *Environment:* 3%. Focus is on child welfare. *International:* 7%. Contributes to women's health, breast cancer, diabetes, and hospitals. *Note:* Total contributions made in 2001. **Typ. Recipients:** Cancer, Children's Health/Hospitals, Diabetes, Geriatric Health, Hospitals, Hospitals (University Affiliated), Medical Research, Single-Disease Health Associations. **Geo. Dist:** NY.

★ 11568 ★ Irving I. Moskowitz Foundation

21500 S Pioneer
Hawaiian Gardens, CA 90716
Phone: (562)809-0186 **Fax:** (562)860-3436
Dr. Irving Moskowitz, President

Fnded: 1968. **Philosophy:** The foundation primarily supports organizations affiliated with the Jewish faith. **Priorities:** *Civic & Public Affairs:* 9%. Public policy concerns. *Education:* 1%. Supports a university. *Environment:* 13%. Youth organizations, food distribution, and community services. *International:* 19%. Supports a medical center. *Note:* Total contributions made in 2000. **Typ. Recipients:** Clinics/Medical Centers, Medical Rehabilitation, Mental Health, Single-Disease Health Associations. **Geo. Dist:** nationally.

★ 11569 ★ Irving S. Gilmore Foundation

136 East Michigan Ave., Suite 900
Kalamazoo, MI 49007
Phone: (269)342-6411 **Fax:** (269)342-6465
Email: fritz@isgilmorefoundation.org
Website: http://www.isgilmorefoundation.org
Frederick Freund, Executive Director

Fnded: 1972. **Philosophy:** "The mission of the Foundation is to support and enrich the cultural, social, and economic life of greater Kalamazoo." **Priorities:** *Arts & Humanities:* 26%. Supports arts councils, symphonies, community and professional theater, art museums, libraries, and historic preservation. *Civic & Public Affairs:* 7%. Funds community development initiatives, towns/municipalities, neighborhood associations, and housing. *Education:* 54%. Provides major support to Western Michigan University; also emphasises arts and business education and learning centers. *Environment:* 9%. Focus on community services, programs for the disabled, youth organizations, senior services, family services, and United Way. *International:* 3%. Hospitals, AIDS research and treatment, health care for pregnant mothers and newborns, clinics, and a hearing/speech center. *Note:* Total contributions made in 2000. **Typ. Recipients:** AIDS/HIV, Clinics/Medical Centers, Emergency/Ambulance Services, Eyes/Blindness, Family Planning, Medical Education, Nursing Services, People with Disabilities, Public Health, Single-Disease Health Associations, Speech & Hearing, Substance Abuse. **Geo. Dist:** Kalamazoo, MI, including greater metropolitan area.

★ 11570 ★ Island Foundation (MA)

589 Mill St.
Marion, MA 02738-1553
Phone: (508)748-2809 **Fax:** (508)748-0991
Email: islandfdn@earthlink.net
Julie Early, Executive Director

Fnded: 1979. **Philosophy:** "The Island Foundation welcomes proposals in three general categories: the environment, alternative education, and building the capacity of organizations in New Bedford, Massachusetts. Priorities within these areas are described below. Environment: The Island Foundation funds environmental projects within New England (primarily Maine, Massachusetts and Rhode Island) that are (1) regional or statewide collaborative initiatives that improve and/or protect coastal and freshwater resources; or (2) research projects to investigate the environmental impacts of toxic chemicals. In addition, the foundation supports right whale research, university-based ecological economics, and land conservation efforts in southeastern Massachusetts, although the Foundation is not requesting proposals on these topics at this time." "Building Capacity in New Bedford: With a focus on the city of New Bedford, Massachusetts, the Island Foundation seeks local nonprofits that enhance the quality of life of residents, encourage community involvement, and promote sustainable economic development within this city and the surrounding region." "Alternative Education: Through the Year 2001, the Island Foundation has committed its education resources to the *Personal Leadership Development for Making the Right Choices* program at Thompson Island Outward Bound Education Center, located on one of the Boston (Massachusetts) harbor islands...Given the multi-year contribution to the *Choices* program, the Island Foundation is not seeking alternative education proposals at this time." Island Foundation Guidelines **Priorities:** *Arts & Humanities:* 10%. Funds New Bedford museums. *Civic & Public Affairs:* 9%. Supports community foundations, zoos, and other civic organizations. *Education:* 33%. Supports one multiyear urban Outward Bound education program. *Environment:* 9%. Supports community centers and YMCA. *International:* 3%. Supports therapeutic center. *Note:* Total contributions made in 1999. **Typ. Recipients:** Adolescent Health Issues, AIDS/HIV, Domestic Violence, Family Planning, Kidney, Medical Rehabilitation, People with Disabilities, Substance Abuse. **Geo. Dist:** New Bedford, MA.

★ 11571 ★ Ittleson Foundation

15 East 67th St.
New York, NY 10021
Phone: (212)794-2008 **Fax:** (212)794-0351
Website: http://www.ittlesonfoundation.org
Anthony Wood, Executive Director

Fnded: 1932. **Philosophy:** The foundation currently is interested in programs which address issues associated with AIDS, mental health, and the environment. The foundation's literature states, "While our strategies change from year to year, our interest is in a sense constant. We want the United States to be a stronger and healthier country tomorrow than it is today. Our fields of interest by their very nature express benchmarks toward that goal. A democracy is only worthy of that name when it both forcefully and compassionately addresses the needs of the most sick (and) the most disturbed..." The foundation focuses on projects that address the consequences of AIDS on the mental health of people with the disease, their families, and caregivers. The foundation is also supportive of innovative prevention efforts, especially those that address the needs of youth. In environment, the foundation is interested in the education of a new generation of environmentalists, urban environmental issues, and efforts at resource protection. The foundation supports programs that provide new opportunities to recruit young people into the environmental studies field, and it seeks pilot projects that will test new approaches to solving environmental problems, and bring about changes through policy research or applied research, such as tests of innovative technology; analyses of regulations and laws; innovative recycling projects; and similar efforts. The foundation encourages projects that link formal professional competence with community-based efforts. The foundation promotes the well-being of mankind through support of mental health, psychiatric research, and behavioral science research. Since 1932, mental health has been the primary focus and will continue to be a strong interest. The foundation is especially interested in innovative projects that address underserved populations, such as the elderly, poor, and minorities. The foundation encourages projects that link formal professional competence to informal networks of support in order to make services available. The foundation is interested in providing seed money for the start-up of innovative programs that improve the social welfare of citizens. Preference is given to pilot projects, test and demonstration projects, and applied research of public policy. Projects should be of nationally scope or significance beyond the local area of implementation and should result in a product or outcome of some consequence in the real world. **Priorities:** *Education:* 26%. Supports universities, schools, and religious education. *Environment:* 4%. Supports food distribution, homes, shelter/homeless. *International:* 44%. Major supportis for AIDS/HIV. Also supports nursing services, and mental health. *Note:* Total contributions made in 2000. **Typ. Recipients:** AIDS/HIV, Cancer, Child Abuse, Children's Health/Hospitals, Emergency/Ambulance Services, Geriatric Health, Health Organizations, Hospitals, Medical Education, Medical Research, Mental Health, Nutrition, People with Disabilities, Prenatal Health Issues, Preventive Medicine/Wellness Organizations, Public Health, Research/Studies Institutes, Single-Disease Health Associations, Substance Abuse. **Geo. Dist:** nationally.

★ 11572 ★ J. Aron Charitable Foundation

126 East 56th St., Suite 2300
New York, NY 10022
Phone: (212)832-8352
Mr. Peter Aron, President & Executive Director

Fnded: 1934. **Philosophy:** The foundation generally supports arts and cultural programs, educational institutions, hospitals and health organizations, and social service agencies. **Priorities:** *Arts & Humanities:* 23%. Supports museums, with major funding to the South Street Seaport Museum; music, libraries, and historical preservation also receive funding. *Civic & Public Affairs:* 3%. Supports municipalities, ethnic organizations, and housing. *Education:* 23%. Funds colleges and universities, and private pre-college education. *Environment:* 9%. Supports the Phoenix House Development Fund, United Way, youth organizations, and shelters. *International:* 30%. Funds hospitals, medical centers, medical research, and single-disease associations. *Note:* Total contributions made in 1999. **Typ. Recipients:** Clinics/Medical Centers, Emergency/Ambulance Services, Eyes/Blindness, Family Planning, Geriatric Health, Hospitals, Hospitals (University Affiliated), Medical Education, Medical Research, Mental Health, People with Disabilities, Research/Studies Institutes, Respiratory, Single-Disease Health Associations, Single-Disease Health Associations, Substance Abuse. **Geo. Dist:** New Orleans, LA, including metropolitan area; New York, NY.

★ 11573 ★ J. Bulow Campbell Foundation

50 Hurt Plaza, Suite 850
Atlanta, GA 30303-2917
Phone: (404)658-9066 **Fax:** (404)659-4802
Betsy Hamilton, Associate Director

Fnded: 1940. **Philosophy:** The J. Bulow Campbell Foundation prefers to give grants to non-governmental organizations "having a program of acknowledged or potential excellence and giving evidence or promise of regional leadership." In considering grants for Presbyterian causes, the foundation follows Mr. Campbell's example "by identifying grant opportunities that are consistent with the purposes of the Southern Presbyterian Church." In considering grants to educational institutions, emphasis is placed on privately supported institutions noted for academic excellence, with priority given to "projects designed to improve the quality of intellectual performance, and the level of spiritual life." The foundation prefers to contribute to projects of a permanent nature or to capital funding rather than to underwrite current operating expenses or recurring programs. In some cases, an exception will be made for an important project which requires startup funds to ensure initial success. It would be expected that the program become self-sustaining after the initial period. In general, the foundation is very selective in its giving decisions. It prefers to give a smaller number of grants to important, well-planned projects rather than to provide assistance to a larger number of less significant projects. The foundation makes all grants without publicity. Although recipients may reveal that a grant has been received, the source must remain confidential. **Priorities:** *Arts & Humanities:* 3%. Gives to a historical society and a public library. *Civic & Public Affairs:* 24%. Funds Habitat for Humanity, citizen's groups, community foundations, and parks. *Education:* 47%. Supports religious education, private schools, colleges and universities. *Environment:* 7%. Funds scouting, Young Men's Christian Association, and a girls' ranch. *International:* 2%. Contributes to Easter Seals and a mental health foundation. *Note:* Total contributions made in 2000. **Typ. Recipients:** Cancer, Children's Health/Hospitals, Clinics/Medical Centers, Emergency/Ambulance Services, Health Organizations, Hospices, Hospitals, Long-Term Care, Medical Education, Medical Research, Mental Health, Nursing Services, People with Disabilities, Single-Disease Health Associations. **Geo. Dist:** AL; FL; Atlanta, GA, including surrounding area; NC; SC; TN.

★ 11574 ★ J. E. and L. E. Mabee Foundation, Inc.

401 South Boston Ave., Suite 3000
Tulsa, OK 74103-4017
Phone: (918)584-4286 **Fax:** (918)584-5540
John Conway, Jr., Vice Chairman, Secretary-Treasurer

Fnded: 1948. **Philosophy:** The general objectives of the foundation are to assist religious, charitable, and educational organizations. The foundation generally makes its largest grants in the area of education, specifically to construct and renovate facilities. Such capital grants are given to institutions of higher learning. Youth issues are also an important foundation focus. Grants in this area generally fund building programs. In the health field, the foundation funds capital projects for hospitals, health agencies, and institutions engaged in the discovery, treatment, and care of diseases. **Priorities:** *Arts & Humanities:* 7%. Funding for renovations at museums and other cultural institutions. *Civic & Public Affairs:* 3%. Contributes to Goodwill Industries and foundations. *Education:* 34%. Emphasis on college and university building funds. *Environment:* 26%. Primarily funds capital projects for youth organizations, shelters, and domestic violence centers. Provides program support to the United Way. *International:* 17%. Focus on capital campaigns at hospitals, medical centers, and health systems. *Note:* Total contributions made in fiscal 2001. **Typ. Recipients:** Alzheimers Disease, Cancer, Children's Health/Hospitals, Clinics/Medical Centers, Diabetes, Domestic Violence, Health Funds, Health Organizations, Health-General, Health-General, Heart, Hospices, Hospitals, Long-Term Care, Medical Education, Medical Rehabilitation, Medical Research, Mental Health, Nursing Services, People with Disabilities, Preventive Medicine/Wellness Organizations, Public Health, Research/Studies Institutes, Single-Disease Health Associations, Substance Abuse. **Geo. Dist:** AR; KS; MO; NM; OK; TX.

★ 11575 ★ J. E. and Z. B. Butler Foundation

825 3rd Ave.
New York, NY 10082
Leon Glaser, Section, Treasurer

Fnded: 1958. **Philosophy:** The foundation is committed to supporting social service, health, education, civic, religious, and environmental organizations. The foundation takes a special interest in Jewish causes. **Priorities:** *Civic & Public Affairs:* 29%. Supports community foundations and legal aid. *Education:* 8%. Supports universities and education organizations. *Environment:* 19%. Funds domestic violence, child abuse, battered women and family advocacy programs. *International:* 10%. Supports hospitals and medical centers. *Note:* Total contributions made in 2000. **Typ. Recipients:** AIDS/HIV, Alzheimers Disease, Cancer, Children's Health/Hospitals, Clinics/Medical Centers, Domestic Violence, Family Planning, Health Organizations, Home-Care Services, Hospitals, Long-Term Care, Nursing Services, People with Disabilities, Prenatal Health Issues, Single-Disease Health Associations, Substance Abuse. **Geo. Dist:** New York, NY.

★ 11576 ★ J. F. Maddox Foundation

PO Box 2588
Hobbs, NM 88241-2588
Phone: (505)393-6338 **Fax:** (505)397-7266
Email: bobreid@leaco.net
Robert Reid, Executive Director, Secretary

Fnded: 1963. **Philosophy:** "The mission of the J.F Maddox Foundation is to significantly improve the quality of life in southeastern New Mexico by investing in education, community development, and other social programs. The Foundation particularly supports initiatives driven by innovative leadership, designed for substantial impact, and committed to lasting value." *J. F Maddox Foundation Mission Statement* **Priorities:** *Arts & Humanities:* 2%. Supports music, public broadcasting, and museums. *Civic & Public Affairs:* 16%. Supports community foundations, law/justice, towns/municipalities, and foundations. *Education:* 68%. Supports schools, colleges, universities, scholarships, religious education, and public schools. *Environment:* 13%. Supports shelters, food distribution, counseling, United Way, and children's services. *International:* Less than 1%. *Note:* Total contributions made in 2000. **Typ. Recipients:** Alzheimers Disease, Cancer, Child Abuse, Diabetes, Domestic Violence, Emergency/Ambulance Services, Hospices, Hospitals, Hospitals (University Affiliated), Nutrition, People with Disabilities, Substance Abuse. **Geo. Dist:** NM, Southeast New Mexico; TX, West Texas.

★ 11577 ★ J. L. Bedsole Foundation

PO Box 1137
Mobile, AL 36633
Phone: (251)432-3369 **Fax:** (251)432-1134
Email: bedsole2@bellsouth.net
Mabel Ward, Executive Director

Fnded: 1949. **Priorities:** *Arts & Humanities:* 23%. Contributes to libraries, history organizations, opera, arts councils, and public broadcasting. *Civic & Public Affairs:* 24%. Focus on community redevelopment projects, chambers of commerce, and community foundations in the Mobile, AL, area. *Education:* 28%. Provides education support primarily in large gifts to private schools, state universities, and colleges. *Environment:* 5%. Supports Young Men's Christian Association, food banks, volunteer services, and substance abuse organizations. *International:* 7%. Supports hospitals, health foundations, and services for the developmentally disabled. *Religion:* 11%. Funds a science museum. *Note:* Total contributions made in 2000, excluding scholarships. **Typ. Recipients:** Children's Health/Hospitals, Clinics/Medical Centers, Eyes/Blindness, Health Organizations, Health-General, Hospitals, Medical Education, Mental Health, Outpatient Health Care, People with Disabilities, Public Health, Single-Disease Health Associations, Substance Abuse. **Geo. Dist:** AL, Southwest part of the state; Mobile, AL.

★ 11578 ★ J. M. Kaplan Fund

261 Madison Ave., 19th Floor
New York, NY 10016
Phone: (212)767-0630 **Fax:** (212)767-0639
Peter Davidson, Chairman

Fnded: 1945. **Philosophy:** "We maintain our belief that private foundations best serve the general interest when they act with a clear point of view and are willing to take chances so that fresh ideas in both the private and public realms can be safely tested. We believe that only by supporting the positive capacities and assets of individuals and organizations can needs be successfully identified and addressed. To these ends we are loyal to proven efforts and grantees with a track record, and at the same time take pleasure in helping new undertakings get off the ground. We seek to reinforce the honorable tradition of progressive social policy and enable talented people to make wonderful things happen - in city streets and neighborhoods, at the exhibition, in parks, on the printed page, in the classroom and field, and at the official hearing." 1996 Annual Report **Priorities:** *Arts & Humanities:* 22%. Supports libraries, museums, music, arts foundations, architecture and design. *Civic & Public Affairs:* 21%. Supports human rights, legal aid, community development, parks, and urban and rural restoration organizations. *Education:* 27%. Supports colleges, public and private schools, and literacy campaigns. *Environment:* 8%. Supports human needs, youth services, food banks, AIDS-related programs, and services for the homeless. *International:* 1%. *Note:* Total contributions made in 2000. **Typ. Recipients:** AIDS/HIV, Cancer, Children's Health/Hospitals, Family Planning, Health Organizations, Respiratory. **Geo. Dist:** New York, NY.

★ 11579 ★ J. M. McDonald Foundation

PO Box 3219
Evergreen, CO 80439
Phone: (303)674-9300 **Fax:** (303)674-9216
Donald McJunkin, President

Fnded: 1952. **Philosophy:** The foundation reflects Mr. McDonald's concerns in greater educational opportunity and educational institutions, the problems of the physically and mentally handicapped and the aged, and the potential for research to improve human conditions. The foundation supports established organizations. Colleges generally receive grants for facilities. The foundation makes grants to social service organizations and has a particular interest in child welfare and care of the aged and needy. The foundation also makes grants to hospitals for facilities. **Priorities:** *Arts & Humanities:* 23%. Supports public broadcasting and museums. *Civic & Public Affairs:* 4%. *Education:* 34%. Funds colleges and education associations. *Environment:* 28%. Supports youth groups and children's services. *International:* 9%. Supports outpatient health care. *Note:* Total contributions made in 2000. **Typ. Recipients:** Cancer, Child Abuse, Children's Health/Hospitals, Clinics/Medical Centers, Domestic Violence, Emergency/Ambulance Services, Family Planning, Geriatric Health, Health Organizations, Heart, Hospices, Hospitals, Medical Education, Medical Rehabilitation, Medical Research, Mental Health, Outpatient Health Care, People with Disabilities, Public Health, Research/Studies Institutes, Single-Disease Health Associations, Speech & Hearing, Substance Abuse. **Geo. Dist:** Northeast USA; primarily upstate NY.

★ 11580 ★ J. Paul Getty Trust

1200 Getty Center Dr., Suite 800
Los Angeles, CA 90049-1685
Phone: (310)440-7320 **Fax:** (310)440-7703
Email: enovotny@getty.edu
Website: http://www.getty.edu/grants

Fnded: 1953. **Philosophy:** "The Getty is an international cultural and philanthropic organization serving both general audiences and specialized professionals. We are a tax-benefited institution, educational in purpose and character, that focuses on the visual arts in all of their dimensions and their capacity to strengthen and to inspire aesthetic and humanistic values. The Getty makes a difference by weaving together the presentation, enjoyment, study, and conservation of the visual arts in order to increase the public's knowledge and sensitivity, expand its awareness and creativity, and sharpen its understanding and caring–all with the conviction that cultural enlightenment and community involvement in the arts can help lead to a more civilized society." *The J. Paul Getty Trust Report 1998-1999* The Getty Grant Program supports a wide range of projects undertaken by institutions and individuals throughout the world that promote research in the history of art, advancement of the understanding of art, and the conservation of cultural heritage. Projects are not restricted as to historical period or geographic location. In the area of scholarship, specific grant categories include grants for postdoctoral fellowships, collaborative research projects, multi-volume or series publications, research centers, curatorial research fellowships, archival projects, and reference works. In the area of conservation, grants support the treatment of works of art, research conservation surveys, conservation education and training, architectural conservation, and archaeological site management. Grants to museums support cataloguing of collections and the interpretation of permanent collections. Museums may also receive funding to assist with multi-volume or series publications and conservation projects. Grants are also occasionally awarded to national and international professional organizations with programs dedicated to scholarship, art museums, and conservation. Museums and visual arts organizations in Los Angeles County may receive funding for organizational assessments and electronic cataloguing of collections. A special initiative of the program is related to cultural diversity and includes internship grants to museums and visual arts organizations in the Los Angeles area, as well as other grants to increase cultural diversity within the professions related to the Grant Program's areas of interest. The J. Paul Getty Trust also makes grants to a small number of scholars and students through the programs of the Getty Research Institute for the History of Art and the Humanities, as well as the J. Paul Getty Museum. **Priorities:** *Arts & Humanities:* 73%. Supports art and architectural conservation, art museums and arts organizations. Also provides multicultural internships, postdoctoral fellowships, organizational assessments, and electronic cataloguing grants to arts organizations in the Los Angeles area. Supports national and international organizations that serve the fields of art, art scholarship, conservation, and museums. *Education:* 16%. Funds Education and Research Grants and Residential Scholar Programs that advance scholarship in art and architectural history. *Note:* Total contributions made in 2001. **Typ. Recipients:** Adolescent Health Issues, Health-General. **Geo. Dist:** internationally; nationally.

★ 11581 ★ J. Roderick MacArthur Foundation

9333 North Milwaukee Ave.
Niles, IL 60714
Phone: (847)966-0143 **Fax:** (847)581-8730
Marylou Bane, Administrator

Fnded: 1976. **Philosophy:** The foundation supports charitable organizations that protect human rights, civil liberties, social justice, and freedom of expression. **Priorities:** *Arts & Humanities:* 74%. Supports Harper's Magazine Foundation and a children's museum. *Civic & Public Affairs:* 5%. Supports public policy and initiatives to abolish the death penalty. *Education:* 5%. Funds media education and a school. *Environment:* 13%. Supports Vietnam Veterans of America Foundation. *Religion:* Less than 1%. *Note:* Total contributions made in 2000. **Typ. Recipients:** Home-Care Services, Substance Abuse. **Geo. Dist:** nationally.

★ 11582 ★ J. S. Bridwell Foundation

807 8th St., Suite 500
Wichita Falls, TX 76301-3365
Phone: (940)322-4436 **Fax:** (940)761-3365
Mac Cannedy, President

Fnded: 1949. **Philosophy:** The foundation has a broad range of interests that is limited only by its geographic priority of organizations or projects in Texas. Grants primarily are addressed to social services, but the foundation contributes to Southern Methodist University in Dallas, TX, for the Bridwell Library. The foundation has demonstrated a giving pattern of ongoing support to certain established charities, such as the Salvation Army, United Way, and Easter Seals. While the foundation gives to many organizations, it has shown a particular interest in organizations that address the concerns of disadvantaged youth, such as the Methodist Home in Waco, TX. address the concerns of disadvantaged youth, such as the Methodist Home in Waco, TX. **Priorities:** *Arts & Humanities:* 20%. Supports performing arts and museums. *Civic & Public Affairs:* 3%. Gives to volunteer fire departments, and community and public affairs groups. *Education:* 2%. Funds educational programs, with major support given to Midwestern State University. *Environment:* 13%. Emphasis on child and youth services, united funds, food banks, and senior citizen services. *International:* 60%. Rehabilitation centers, hospitals, hospices, and disease and disorder concerns received support. *Note:* Total contributions made in 1999. **Typ. Recipients:** Cancer, Children's Health/Hospitals, Clinics/Medical Centers, Emergency/Ambulance Services, Health Organizations, Heart, Hospices, Long-Term Care, Medical Rehabilitation, Medical Research, Medical Training, People with Disabilities, Single-Disease Health Associations, Substance Abuse. **Geo. Dist:** TX.

★ 11583 ★ J. W. Kieckhefer Foundation

PO Box 1151
Prescott, AZ 86302
Phone: (928)445-4010 **Fax:** (928)445-4012
Eugene Polk, Administrative Officer, Trustee

Fnded: 1953. **Philosophy:** The foundation is a general purpose charity which emphasizes social services. The foundation gives grants for annual campaigns, seed money, emergency funds, capital funds (including building funds, equipment, materials, and renovation), special endowments for chairs and lecture series, research-related programs, conferences and seminars, and general purposes. The foundation provides continuous support and gives both one-time and multiple-year grants. **Priorities:** *Arts & Humanities:* 15%. Supports museums, arts centers, and music. *Civic & Public Affairs:* 9%. Emphasis on housing, legal aid, and community development. *Education:* 8%. Universities, education associations, and secondary education. *Environment:* 39%. Primarily supports child welfare, the aged, and people with disabilities. *International:* 22%. Focus on hospitals and medical centers, medical research, and single-disease health associations. *Religion:* 6%. Funds science centers. *Note:* Total contributions made in 2000. **Typ. Recipients:** Alzheimers Disease, Cancer, Child Abuse, Children's Health/Hospitals, Clinics/Medical Centers, Domestic Violence, Eyes/Blindness, Family Planning, Geriatric Health, Health Funds, Health Organizations, Heart, Hospices, Hospitals, Kidney, Medical Education, Medical Rehabilitation, Medical Research, People with Disabilities, Prenatal Health Issues, Preventive Medicine/Wellness Organizations, Public Health, Research/Studies Institutes, Respiratory, Single-Disease Health Associations, Substance Abuse. **Geo. Dist:** nationally; AZ.

★ 11584 ★ J. Willard and Alice S. Marriott Foundation

PO Box 150
Washington, DC 20058
Phone: (301)380-2246 **Fax:** (301)380-8957
Email: bonnie.white@marriott.com
Bonnie White, Grant Manager

Fnded: 1966. **Philosophy:** The foundation primarily awards grants to local organizations. It also gives to a few general scholarship funds. The majority of funding, however, goes to previously supported organizations. **Priorities:** *Arts & Humanities:* 1%. Gives to arts centers, music, public broadcasting, and performing arts. *Civic & Public Affairs:* 1%. Funds trade associations, municipalities, and civic concerns. *Education:* 62%. Funds higher education and educational associations. *Environment:* 28%. Supports youth groups, united funds, human services organizations, and the disabled. *International:* 8%. Focus on health funds, hospitals, medical research, and single-disease health associations. *Note:* Total contributions made in 2000. **Typ. Recipients:** AIDS/HIV, Arthritis, Cancer, Children's Health/Hospitals, Clinics/Medical Centers, Emergency/Ambulance Services, Eyes/Blindness, Health Organizations, Heart, Hospitals, Hospitals (University Affiliated), Medical Education, Medical Research, Multiple Sclerosis, Nutrition, People with Disabilities, Prenatal Health Issues, Public Health, Research/Studies Institutes, Speech & Hearing, Substance Abuse, Trauma Treatment. **Geo. Dist:** nationally; Washington, DC, metropolitan area; MD; VA.

★ 11585 ★ Jack N. and Lilyan Mandel Foundation

2829 Euclid Ave.
Cleveland, OH 44115
Phone: (216)875-6500 **Fax:** (216)875-6580
Jack Mandel, Trustee

Fnded: 1963. **Priorities:** *Arts & Humanities:* Less than 1%. *Civic & Public Affairs:* 85%. Major support for Mandel Supporting Foundations. *Education:* 9%. *Environment:* Less than 1%. *International:* Less than 1%. *Note:* Total contributions made in 2000. **Typ. Recipients:** AIDS/HIV, Alzheimers Disease, Children's Health/Hospitals, Clinics/Medical Centers, Diabetes, Emergency/Ambulance Services, Eyes/Blindness, Geriatric Health, Heart, Multiple Sclerosis, People with Disabilities, Public Health, Single-Disease Health Associations. **Geo. Dist:** OH.

★ 11586 ★ Jackson Hole Preserve

30 Rockefeller Plaza, Room 5600
New York, NY 10112
Phone: (212)649-5819 **Fax:** (212)649-5829
Carmen Reyes, Jr., Treasurer

Fnded: 1940. **Philosophy:** The Jackson Hole Preserve supports organizations involved in the conservation and preservation of wildlife, nature, and land. Recently, the preserve made grants to historic preservation societies in New York. However, most of the funding usually goes to environmental affairs. "Our grant-making activities are directed toward information and action programs that increase public understanding of conservation issues and citizen participation in their resolution." **Priorities:** *Arts & Humanities:* 3%. Supports museum and historic preservation. *Civic & Public Affairs:* 3%. Supports civic planning. *Education:* 2%. Educational materials development. *Note:* Total contributions made in 2000. **Typ. Recipients:** Hospitals, Single-Disease Health Associations. **Geo. Dist:** NY, Hudson River Valley region; VT; WY.

★ 11587 ★ Jacob G. Schmidlapp Trust No. 1

Department 00864
Cincinnati, OH 45263
Phone: (513)579-6034 **Fax:** (513)744-6997
Lawra Baumann, Foundation Officer

Fnded: 1927. **Philosophy:** The Jacob G. Schmidlapp Trust No. 1 believes that funds should be used "for relief in sickness, suffering and distress, the care of young children, or the helpless and afflicted." To this purpose, the trust concentrates on social services, health facilities, and educational institutions that directly or indirectly benefit children, the sick, and the disadvantaged in the Cincinnati area. In the future, the trust expects to elicit proposals for programs which are especially effective in achieving the goals set by Mr. Schmidlapp while at the same time meeting the community needs of today. **Priorities:** *Arts & Humanities:* 10%. Gives to art and history museums, and public broadcasting. *Civic & Public Affairs:* 17%. Supports parks and arboretums, community foundations, urban leagues, and community associations. *Education:* 33%. Funds colleges and universities and primary and secondary education. *Environment:* 22%. Supports Young Men's Christian Association, scouts, child welfare, and the United Way. *International:* 13%. Gives to wellness programs, rehabilitation centers, hospice, and pediatric disease organizations. *Note:* Total contributions made in fiscal 2001. **Typ. Recipients:** Adolescent Health Issues, Arthritis, Cancer, Children's Health/Hospitals, Clinics/Medical Centers, Diabetes, Domestic Violence, Emergency/Ambulance Services, Family Planning, Geriatric Health, Health Funds, Health Organizations, Heart, Hospices, Hospitals, Long-Term Care, Medical Education, Medical Rehabilitation, Mental Health, Nursing Services, People with Disabilities, Prenatal Health Issues, Preventive Medicine/Wellness Organizations, Public Health, Single-Disease Health Associations, Speech & Hearing, Substance Abuse, Trauma Treatment. **Geo. Dist:** Cincinnati, OH, metropolitan area.

★ 11588 ★ Jacob and Hilda Blaustein Foundation

10 E Baltimore St., Suite 1101
Baltimore, MD 21202
Phone: (410)347-7201 **Fax:** (410)659-0552
Email: info@blaufund.org
Michael Hirschhorn, President

Fnded: 1957. **Philosophy:** Jewish identity and continuity, health, intergroup relations, and the arts are the foundation's four program areas. **Priorities:** *Arts & Humanities:* 4%. Supports public art organizations, historical organizations, educational broadcasting and libraries. *Civic & Public Affairs:* 10%. Supports the Ellis Island Foundation, rescue services, and civic foundations. *Education:* 20%. Supports education centers, universities, and religious education. *International:* 33%. Supports hospitals, medical centers, and single-disease health organizations. *Note:* Total contributions made in 1998. **Typ. Recipients:** Cancer, Children's Health/Hospitals, Clinics/Medical Centers, Emergency/Ambulance Services, Eyes/Blindness, Health Organizations, Health-General, Heart, Hospitals, Medical Education, Mental Health, People with Disabilities, Preventive Medicine/Wellness Organizations, Public Health, Single-Disease Health Associations, Transplant Networks/Donor Banks. **Geo. Dist:** Baltimore, MD.

★ 11589 ★ James G. Boswell Foundation

101 West Walnut St.
Pasadena, CA 91103-3642
Phone: (626)583-3002 **Fax:** (626)583-3090
Jim Henry, Executive Director

Fnded: 1947. **Philosophy:** The foundation generally supports agricultural education and general higher education. Health concerns, precollege private schools, cultural organizations, rural affairs groups, and youth organizations also receive minor support. **Priorities:** *Arts & Humanities:* 2%. Gives to a historical society. *Civic & Public Affairs:* 13%. Funds community foundations and law & justice organizations. *Education:* 67%. Supports educational programs and institutions, with an emphasis on agricultural education programs. *Environment:* 6%. Funds athletic programs, girl and boy scouts, 4-H, Young Men's Christian Association, and the United Way. *International:* 12%. Supports health centers and a cancer center. *Note:* Contributions were made in 2000. **Typ. Recipients:** Cancer, Clinics/Medical Centers, Health Organizations, Heart, Hospitals, Medical Education, Medical Research, People with Disabilities, Prenatal Health Issues, Public Health. **Geo. Dist:** CA.

★ 11590 ★ James Graham Brown Foundation, Inc.

4350 Brownsboro Rd.
Suite 200
Louisville, KY 40207
Phone: (502)896-2440 **Fax:** (502)896-1774
Email: mason@jgbf.org
Website: http://www.jgbf.org
Mason Rummel, Executive Director

Fnded: 1943. **Philosophy:** The mission of the foundation is to "foster the well-being, quality of life and image of Louisville and Kentucky." The primary categories of funding of the James Graham Brown Foundation, Inc. are education, civic, economic development, culture and humanities, human services, and health.The foundation tends to fund projects with an emphasis in bricks and mortar, renovation, equipment purchases,and pre-selected scholarship funds. The foundation also prefers to support organizations located in Kentucky. "Special projects for civic or economic development which have an explicit objective to improve the quality of life of Kentuckians and the image of Kentucky are of particular interest to the Foundation as well." James Graham Brown Foundation Program Guidelines and Application Procedures. **Priorities:** *Arts & Humanities:* 3%. Supports historic preservation and museums. *Civic & Public Affairs:* 29%. Supports industrial development, zoos, nonprofit management, economic development, and community foundations. *Education:* 49%. Funds colleges, universities and literacy organizations. *Environment:* 17%. Supports the United Way, volunteer services, youth services, scouting, and family services. *International:* 2%. Gives to hospitals, hospice, pediatric health, and single-disease health associations. *Note:* Total contributions made in 2001. **Typ. Recipients:** Arthritis, Cancer, Children's Health/Hospitals, Clinics/Medical Centers, Emergency/Ambulance Services, Eyes/Blindness, Family Planning, Geriatric Health, Health Organizations, Hospices, Hospitals, Medical Rehabilitation, Mental Health, Multiple Sclerosis, People with Disabilities, Prenatal Health Issues, Respiratory, Single-Disease Health Associations, Substance Abuse. **Geo. Dist:** KY.

★ 11591 ★ James H. Cummings Foundation

1807 Elmwood Ave., Rm. 112
Buffalo, NY 14207
Phone: (716)874-0040 **Fax:** (716)874-0040
William McFarland, Executive Director & Secretary

Fnded: 1962. **Philosophy:** The foundation was created "to further medical science, medical research, and medical education... to provide services for underprivileged boys and girls" and "to assist aged and infirm persons." Grants are generally for capital expenditures, in particular for the purchase of medical research equipment. The foundation prefers to support organizations that do not receive government funding. Priority is given to medical proposals. **Priorities:** *Arts & Humanities:* 1%. Music *Education:* 31%. Supports higher education. *Environment:* 14% Supports underprivileged children aged and infirm persons. *International:* 50%. Supports medical science, medical research, and medical education. *Note:* Total contributions made in fiscal 2001. **Typ. Recipients:** Cancer, Children's Health/Hospitals, Clinics/Medical Centers, Family Planning, Geriatric Health, Health Organizations, Health-General, Heart, Hospices, Hospitals, Medical Rehabilitation, Medical Rehabilitation, Medical Research, Medical Training, Nursing Services, People with Disabilities, Prenatal Health Issues, Public Health, Respiratory, Speech & Hearing, Substance Abuse. **Geo. Dist:** Buffalo, NY; Hendersonville, NC; Toronto, ON.

★ 11592 ★ The James Irvine Foundation

One Market, Steuart Tower, Suite 2500
San Francisco, CA 94105
Phone: (415)777-2244 **Fax:** (415)777-0869
Website: http://www.irvine.org
Ann Clarke, Director of Grants Administration

Fnded: 1937. **Philosophy:** "The James Irvine Foundation is a general purpose private foundation granting funds to support projects and programs for the benefit of California residents. The Foundation is dedicated to enhancing the social, economic, and physical quality of life throughout California and to enriching the state's intellectual and cultural environment." "The James Irvine Foundation: 2000 Summary Information for the Public" The Foundation's funding priorities are Arts; Children, Youth and Families; Civic Culture; Higher Education; Sustainable Communities; and Special Projects. improve the economic and social well-being of the disadvantaged and their communities, foster self-sufficiency, and assist the ethnic minorities to function more effectively as full participants in society To encourage communication, understanding, and cooperation among diverse cultural, ethnic, and socioeconomic groups To promote civic participation, social responsibility, public understanding of issues, and the development of sound public policy To enrich the quality and diversity of educational, cultural, health, and human service programs throughout the State. The Foundation makes grants in seven categorical areas: Arts; Children, Youth and Families; Civic Culture; Higher Education; Sustainable Communities; and Special Projects. **Priorities:** *Arts & Humanities:* 21%. Supports public broadcasting, museums, dance, and cultural centers. *Civic & Public Affairs:* 17%. Funds community foundations, community building, naturalization and civic participation in California's Central Valley, human and race relations, collaborative regional development, and state and local governance reform. *Education:* 35%. Focus on higher education and research studies. *Environment:* 14%. Supports programs for children, youth, and families. *International:* 7%. Funds rural health and public health clinics. *Note:* Total contributions made in 2000. **Typ. Recipients:** AIDS/HIV, Children's Health/Hospitals, Clinics/Medical Centers, Domestic Violence, Family Planning, Health Organizations, Health Policy/Cost Containment, Health-General, Hospitals, Hospitals (University Affiliated), Medical Research, Nursing Services, People with Disabilities, Prenatal Health Issues, Preventive Medicine/Wellness Organizations, Public Health, Research/Studies Institutes. **Geo. Dist:** CA.

★ 11593 ★ James L. Stamps Foundation

2000 E Fourth St., Suite 230
Santa Ana, CA 92705
Phone: (714)568-9740 **Fax:** (714)568-9754
Delores Boutault, Manager

Fnded: 1963. **Philosophy:** The Stamps Foundation primarily supports Christian religious organizations and Christian-based education. Churches, fellowships, and conferences along with seminaries and bible schools account for most of the foundation's interests. Support to social services is based on a religious outlook. **Priorities:** *Education:* 56%. Primary support for Christian colleges and universities and scholarships. *Environment:* 4%. Supports camps, seniorior citizen organizations and food banks. *Note:* Total contributions made in 2000. **Typ. Recipients:** Clinics/Medical Centers, Emergency/Ambulance Services, Public Health. **Geo. Dist:** CA, Southern California.

★ 11594 ★ James M. Johnston Trust for Charitable and Educational Purposes

2 Wisconsin Circle, Suite 600
Chevy Chase, MD 20815
Phone: (301)907-0135
Julia Sanders, Office Manager

Fnded: 1968. **Philosophy:** The trust, following the interests of its donor, concentrates its grant-making program on education, particularly at the University of North Carolina at Chapel Hill. Support is directed toward scholarship programs, nursing education, and faculty development. **Priorities:** *Civic & Public Affairs:* 2%. Supports a fire department. *Education:* 82%. Funds scholarships, colleges, universities, art education, secondary schools, and academies. *Environment:* 5%. Supports youth organizations, services for the disabled, and the scouts. *International:* 7%. Primary support for hospitals and children's health. *Note:* Total contributions made in 2000. **Typ. Recipients:** Cancer, Children's Health/Hospitals, Diabetes, Emergency/Ambulance Services, Heart, Hospices, Hospitals, Long-Term Care, Medical Education, Medical Rehabilitation, Medical Research, Medical Training, Mental Health, Nursing Services, People with Disabilities, Single-Disease Health Associations. **Geo. Dist:** Washington, DC; NC.

★ 11595 ★ James S. McDonnell Foundation

1034 South Brentwood Boulevard, Suite 1850
Saint Louis, MO 63117-1229
Phone: (314)721-1532 **Fax:** (314)721-7421
Email: info@jsmf.org
Website: http://www.jsmf.org
Dr. Susan Fitzpatrick, Program Officer

Fnded: 1950. **Philosophy:** "The foundation's primary program interests are in biomedical and behavioral sciences, with over 90% of its annual grant awards supporting basic and applied research. Support for research, however, is provided primarily through foundation-initiated programs. Foundation-initiated programs are managed by advisory boards which assist in developing program guidelines, issue requests for proposals (RFPs), review submitted proposals and conduct program evaluation. In this way, the foundation is able to benefit from expert advice, fund work in targeted areas of interest, assure program applicants adequate peer review, and make specific funding decisions based on the relative merits of all proposals elicited by an RFP. Current foundation-initiated programs include: The McDonnell-Pew Program in Cognitive Neuroscience; Molecular Medicine in Cancer Research; Cognitive Studies for Educational Practice; The Initiative to Support Collaborative Research in Eastern Europe; and Cognitive Rehabilitation. The foundation's commitment to these programs severely limits funds available for other investigator-initiated research." 1997 Foundation Policies and Application Guidelines **Priorities:** *Civic & Public Affairs:* 31%. JSM Charitable Trust. *Education:* 53%. Supports universities. *International:* 14%. Funds biomedical and behavioral sciences research, and medical centers. *Note:* Contributions were made in 2000. **Typ. Recipients:** Cancer, Children's Health/Hospitals, Clinics/Medical Centers, Eyes/Blindness, Health Organizations, Hospitals, Medical Education, Medical Rehabilitation, Medical Research, Mental Health, Research/Studies Institutes. **Geo. Dist:** internationally; nationally.

★ 11596 ★ Jane Coffin Childs Memorial Fund for Medical Research

333 Cedar St.
Rm. LW 300
New Haven, CT 06510
Phone: (203)785-4612 **Fax:** (203)785-3301
Email: jccfund@yale.edu
Website: http://www.jccfund.org
Kimberly Roberts, Administrative Director

Fnded: 1937. **Philosophy:** The fund traditionally has supported basic cancer research, rather than the investigation of the clinical aspects of the disease. Current funding is limited to post-doctoral fellowships for physicians and scientists. **Priorities:** *International:* 100%. Fellowships for cancer research. *Note:* Total contributions made in fiscal 2001. **Typ. Recipients:** Cancer, Children's Health/Hospitals, Clinics/Medical Centers, Health-General, Hospitals, Medical Education, Medical Research, Medical Training, Research/Studies Institutes. **Geo. Dist:** nationally and internationally.

★ 11597 ★ Janirve Foundation

One North Pack Square, Suite 416
Asheville, NC 28801
Phone: (828)258-1877 **Fax:** (828)258-1837
Charles Dyson, Chairman, Advisory Committee

Fnded: 1964. **Philosophy:** The foundation supports a wide range of charities with emphasis on social services, health, and education. Support also goes to the arts and humanities and environmental causes. The foundation "encourages the submission of proposals which set forth new or different and innovative approaches toward dealing with a problem affecting a significant sector of society." **Priorities:** *Arts & Humanities:* 7%. Supports symphonies, libraries, arts councils, and history. *Civic & Public Affairs:* 26%. Public policy, vocational services, community foundations, economic development, and housing receive support. *Education:* 13% Supports colleges and universities, schools, and literacy. *Environment:* 39%. Supports food banks, shelters, youth services, child abuse centers, Goodwill Industries, and Special Olympics. *International:* 4%. Funds hospitals, hospice, single-disease organizations, and drug rehabilitation. *Note:* Total contributions made in 2000. **Typ. Recipients:** Adolescent Health Issues, Alzheimers Disease, Cancer, Child Abuse, Children's Health/Hospitals, Clinics/Medical Centers, Domestic Violence, Emergency/Ambulance Services, Family Planning, Geriatric Health, Health Organizations, Health-General, Hospices, Hospitals, Long-Term Care, Medical Education, Medical Rehabilitation, People with Disabilities, Preventive Medicine/Wellness Organizations, Public Health, Single-Disease Health Associations, Transplant Networks/Donor Banks. **Geo. Dist:** Palm Beach, FL; West Palm Beach, FL; NC, Western North Carolina.

★ 11598 ★ Jay and Betty Van Andel Foundation

2905 Lucerne SE
Grand Rapids, MI 49546
Phone: (616)942-3267
Jay Van Andel, President

Fnded: 1963. **Philosophy:** The foundation has directed its philanthropy into four main categories–the arts, religious organizations, educational institutions, and civic groups. The foundation's contributions to the arts focus on museums, music, and opera in Grand Rapids, MI. The foundation's religious interests include Christian organizations and missions, churches, and religious welfare organizations. The foundation's educational funding supports religious educational organizations, scholarship funds, and colleges and universities. Its funding to civic groups includes conservative public policy think tanks and a zoological society. **Priorities:** *Arts & Humanities:* 2%. Gives to museums, opera, ballet, historical societies, and orchestras. *Civic & Public Affairs:* 5%. Funds zoos, community foundations, public policy organizations, and chambers of commerce. *Education:* 4%. Contributes to colleges, universiies, and Christian schools. *Environment:* 1%. Gives to community centers, the United

Way, YMCA, and human service agencies. *International:* 1%. Hospitals, health foundations, hospice programs, and neurological disease organizations receive support. *Religion:* 84%. Provides major support to the Van Andel Institute for scientific research and education; also funds the Creation Research Society. *Note:* Total contributions made in 2000. **Typ. Recipients:** Alzheimers Disease, Children's Health/Hospitals, Clinics/Medical Centers, Health Organizations, Health-General, Hospices, Hospitals, Long-Term Care, Medical Research, People with Disabilities, Public Health, Research/Studies Institutes. **Geo. Dist:** MI.

★ 11599 ★ The Jay and Rose Phillips Family Foundation

10 Second St. NE, Suite 200
Minneapolis, MN 55413
Phone: (612)623-1654 **Fax:** (612)623-1653
Email: phillipsfnd@phillipsfnd.org
Website: http://www.phillipsfnd.org
Patricia Cummings, Executive Director & Secretary

Fnded: 1944. **Philosophy:** "The mission of The Jay and Rose Phillips Family Foundation is to honor the legacy of its founders, Jay and Rose Phillips, by continuing the family tradition of sharing resources for the public good, while exercising leadership and flexibility in responding to emerging community needs." "Consistent with the legacy of grantmaking created by Jay and Rose Phillips, the Foundation makes grants selectively in the following areas: Human Services; Health; Education; Programs for people with disabilities; Programs to combat discrimination". "During times of severe economic hardship and financial distress, the Foundation's primary concern is in providing support for projects that address unmet human and social needs." Jay and Rose Phillips Family Foundation *Guidelines and Special Concerns for Grantmaking* **Priorities:** *Arts & Humanities:* 3%. Supports opera, music, theater, history, and public broadcasting. *Civic & Public Affairs:* (Public Policy) 12%. Supports womens affairs, housing, law & justice, native american affairs, civil rights and zoos. *Education:* 22%. Supports school, scholarship, religious education, universities minority education. *Environment:* 34%. Supports senior services, food distribution programs, United Way, young men's christian association, homes, family services, Young Women's Christian Association, scouts, and special olympics. *International:* 7%. Supports medical research hospital, and single-disease health associations. *Note:* Total contributions made in 2000. **Typ. Recipients:** AIDS/HIV, Cancer, Children's Health/Hospitals, Clinics/Medical Centers, Family Planning, Health Organizations, Health-General, Heart, Hospices, Hospitals, Long-Term Care, Medical Education, Medical Rehabilitation, Medical Research, Multiple Sclerosis, People with Disabilities, Prenatal Health Issues, Public Health, Research/Studies Institutes, Sexual Abuse, Single-Disease Health Associations. **Geo. Dist:** MN, seven-county metropolitan area of Minneapolis/St. Paul, MN.

★ 11600 ★ Jean and Louis Dreyfus Foundation

420 Lexington Ave., Suite 626
New York, NY 10170
Phone: (212)599-1931 **Fax:** (212)599-2956
Email: jldreyfusfdtn@hotmail.com
Edmee Firth, Executive Director

Fnded: 1978. **Philosophy:** "The mission of the Foundation is to enhance the quality of life of New Yorkers, particularly the aging and the disadvantaged. It disburses grants mostly in the greater New York City area and primarily in fields supportive of aging, arts-in-education, literacy, education and social services. The Foundation is committed to funding direct service organizations and those projects which will produce systemic change. To this end the Foundation supports pilot programs which can eventually be replicated or which will be funded by independent or government sources in the future. Occasionally organizations will be awarded grants to strengthen their infrastructure or for general operating support. The Foundation encourages matching funds from other charitable organizations, public financial drives, individuals, and government bodies." *The Jean & Louis Dreyfus Foundation, Inc. Annual Report 2001* **Priorities:** *Arts & Humanities:* 24%. Supports art museums, theater, music, arts education programs, and arts foundations. *Education:* 25%. Gives to universities, arts education, literacy programs, and after-school programs. *Environment:* 51%. Supports senior services, violence prevention, family planning, volunteer services, youth programs, ethnic and women's organizations, career development, and hospitals. *Note:* Total contributions made in 2001. **Typ. Recipients:** Adolescent Health Issues, AIDS/HIV, Alzheimers Disease, Cancer, Children's Health/Hospitals, Clinics/Medical Centers, Family Planning, Geriatric Health, Health Funds, Health Organizations, Health Policy/Cost Containment, Home-Care Services, Hospitals, Long-Term Care, Medical Education, Medical Training, Mental Health, Nursing Services, Nutrition, Prenatal Health Issues, Public Health, Substance Abuse. **Geo. Dist:** New York, NY.

★ 11601 ★ Jeffris Family Foundation

PO Box 650
Janesville, WI 53547-0650
Phone: (608)757-1039 **Fax:** (608)754-7248
Thomas Jeffris, President & Director

Fnded: 1977. **Philosophy:** The foundation typically supports historic preservation projects and community and urban affairs programs. **Priorities:** *Arts & Humanities:* 47%. Supports historic preservation and historical societies. *Civic & Public Affairs:* 53%. Municipalities are funded. *Note:* Total contributions made in 2000. **Typ. Recipients:** Emergency/Ambulance Services. **Geo. Dist:** WI.

★ 11602 ★ Jesse Philips Foundation

3870 Honey Hill Lane
Dayton, OH 45405
Phone: (937)496-1300
Caryl Philips, President

Fnded: 1960. **Philosophy:** The Jesse Philips Foundation makes grants across all major categories of support. The foundation's primary giving interests include social services, health, education, religion, the arts, science, and civic affairs. Religious funding favors Jewish organizations. **Priorities:** *Arts & Humanities:* 28%. Supports theater, ballet, arts centers, and historic preservation. *Civic & Public Affairs:* 3%. *Education:* 51%. Supports universities, scholarships, and general education. *Environment:* 8%. Supports scouting, animal protection, and family planning services. *International:* 4%. Funds medical centers. *Religion:* 1%. Supports science research and science institution. *Note:* Total contributions made in fiscal 2001. **Typ. Recipients:** AIDS/HIV, Cancer, Children's Health/Hospitals, Clinics/Medical Centers, Family Planning, Health Funds, Health Organizations, Hospitals, Medical Research, Mental Health, Respiratory, Single-Disease Health Associations, Transplant Networks/Donor Banks. **Geo. Dist:** OH, Montgomery County.

★ 11603 ★ Jesselson Foundation

450 Park Ave., Suite 2603
New York, NY 10022
Phone: (212)751-3666 **Fax:** (212)751-3377
Michael Jesselson, Vice President

Fnded: 1955. **Philosophy:** The foundation primarily supports Jewish causes, with interest shown for civic, social welfare, and educational organizations. **Priorities:** *Education:* 21%. Primarily for Jewish education. *Environment:* 3%. Emphasis on youth organizations. *International:* 2%. *Note:* Total contributions made in fiscal 2001. **Typ. Recipients:** Cancer, Children's Health/Hospitals, Clinics/Medical Centers, Diabetes, Heart, Hospitals, Long-Term Care, Medical Education, Medical Research, Single-Disease Health Associations. **Geo. Dist:** Nationwide.

★ 11604 ★ Jessie B. Cox Charitable Trust

Hemenway & Barnes
60 State St.
Boston, MA 02109-1899
Phone: (617)227-7940 **Fax:** (617)227-0781
Email: dso@hembar.com
Website: http://www.hembar.com/cox
Susan Fish, Grants Administrator

Fnded: 1982. **Philosophy:** "The purpose of the trust is to increase significantly the ability of New England non-profit organizations to carry out their stated missions in the fields of health, education, the environment, and the development of philanthropy in the community. "In the health field, the trust is particularly interested in supporting primary healthcare, and advocacy projects, and research that will have a positive effect on the prevention and treatment of illness and disability, particularly among children and youth; increased access to appropriate levels of care for New England's underserved populations; and delivery of health services to the poor. In the education area, the trust is particularly interested in supporting projects which will have a significant effect on the availability of academic resources, both traditional and innovative; increased access, incentives and opportunities for educational participation by underserved populations in New England; the availability of instruction and training in the visual and performing arts; and improved academic performance and achievement. "The trust is interested in supporting environmental projects which will have a positive impact on protection of critical natural resources; energy conservation; public awareness of the critical environmental issues facing the region; and protection of the public's health, especially in low-income and minority communities." In philanthropy, the trust seeks to "encourage the development and expansion of emerging community foundations, increase philanthropic resources in underserved areas, and provide modest support for certain special efforts of philanthropic donors." Jessie B. Cox Charitable Trust *Guidelines and Policies* **Priorities:** *Education:* 23%. Supports education associations and colleges and universities. *International:* 32%. Focus on health centers, public health, pediatric health, and single-disease health associations. *Note:* Total contributions made in 2001. **Typ. Recipients:** Adolescent Health Issues, AIDS/HIV, Children's Health/Hospitals, Diabetes, Family Planning, Health Organizations, Health Policy/Cost Containment, Health-General, Home-Care Services, Hospitals, Hospitals (University Affiliated), Medical Education, Medical Research, Mental Health, Nursing Services, Nutrition, People with Disabilities, Prenatal Health Issues, Preventive Medicine/Wellness Organizations, Public Health, Respiratory, Substance Abuse. **Geo. Dist:** New England.

★ 11605 ★ Jessie Ball duPont Fund

One Independent Dr., Suite 1400
Jacksonville, FL 32202-5011
Phone: (904)353-0890 **Fax:** (904)353-3870
Website: http://www.dupontfund.org
Sherry Magill, President

Fnded: 1976. **Philosophy:** In 1994, the foundation established the Jessie Ball duPont Fund Making a Difference Award, formerly the Turnaround Award. This award recognizes an individual who can make a difference or literally turn around an organization that meets a critical societal need. In 1991, the foundation launched several new programs. The trustees established the Jessie Ball duPont Fund Award to honor selected individuals at the Fund's eligible institutions. The honorees are chosen for their courage, integrity, creativity, perseverance, and compassion. Their life work focuses on promoting just relations and equality in their communities. The fund also began the Clergy Enrichment Fund, which is designed to respond to the needs of ordained clergy at the fund's eligible religious institutions and includes a sabbatical program and a professional development fund. A strong preference is given to clergy who serve at small, financially-assisted churches. Another program, the Nonprofit Initiative, is a program that addresses the needs of eligible non-profits with discretionary funds, technical assistance, and a leadership developmental institute. Both programs have their own set of application guidelines. In 1990, the fund launched the Jessie Ball duPont Fund Small Liberal Arts College Initiative. As part of the initiative, the fund has awarded over $3,000,000 to 37 eligible colleges, with an enrollment of fewer than 2,900 students each. In addition to the Small Liberal Arts College Initiative, the fund has application guidelines for a People-In-Need program and a Feasibility Grant program. Through grants to eligible institutions, the fund seeks to help solve the needs of today's society, especially in the South, and to anticipate emerging issues that may become major concerns in the future. The fund's objectives are to enable individuals to reach their full potential in today's society and to enable society to fulfill its obligation to its members; to support projects that are not adequately funded by other sources; and to assist and encourage eligible institutions to work with other organizations to address common problems and achieve common goals. In addition, the fund attempts to enable the eligible institutions to generate additional resources by attracting a broad constituency of donors and volunteer participation; and to preserve and use our historical heritage. **Priorities:** *Civic & Public Affairs:* 36% (Nonprofits). Funds nonprofit management, and broad-based community issues including community economic development and human services organizations. *Education:* 38%. Primarily supports colleges and universities. *Note:* Total contributions made in fiscal 2001. **Typ. Recipients:** AIDS/HIV, Alzheimers Disease, Cancer, Children's Health/Hospitals, Clinics/Medical Centers, Domestic Violence, Emergency/Ambulance Services, Eyes/Blindness, Health Organizations, Heart, Hospitals, Hospitals (University Affiliated), Long-Term Care, Medical Education, Mental Health, Nursing Services, People with Disabilities, Respiratory, Sexual Abuse, Single-Disease Health Associations, Speech & Hearing. **Geo. Dist:** southern states; DE, nationally; FL; VA.

★ 11606 ★ Jessie Smith Noyes Foundation, Inc.

150 Broadway, Suite 1915
New York, NY 10038-4499
Phone: (212)571-2300 **Fax:** (212)689-6549
Email: noyes@noyes.org
Website: http://www.noyes.org
Victor DeLuca, President

Fnded: 1947. **Philosophy:** The foundation is committed to "protecting and restoring Earth's natural systems and promoting a sustainable society by strengthening individuals, institutions and communities pledged to pursuing those goals." As opportunities and needs suggest new directions and areas of emphasis, the foundation continues to modify its program to assure its relevance to contemporary society and to a sustainable future. Currently, the foundation funds projects that promote environmentally sound approaches to development, and that address toxins, sustainable agriculture, reproductive rights, sustainable communities, New York metropolitan area environment, and related interests. The foundation's objective in its sustainable communities program is to promote communities that are environmentally sound, economically vital, and socially just. Priorities include supporting individuals and organizations in implementing programs that respect the interconnectedness of human and natural communities. The toxins program's objective is to reduce threats posed by toxins to the environment and human health. The reproductive rights program seeks to promote quality reproductive health care as a human right. Priorities are to broaden the base and agenda of the reproductive rights movement and to influence legislation, policy, and reform initiatives. Reproductive rights in the United States are a focus, especially programs assisting women of color. The foundation's Metro-New York program seeks to promotes an environmentally sound metropolitan New York through an active, informed, and empowered local citizenry. It accomplishes this objective by strengthening organizations working on environmental issues; by improving public policies and responsiveness of public agencies; and by developing effective coalitions and networks among different organizations, both within the environmental movement and between environmental groups and others. The sustainable agriculture program has the objective of helping to "build a system of food and fiber production that sustains the environment and benefits people." The priorities of this program are strengthening organizations working toward the objective, improving sustainable agriculture policies and practices, and demonstrating the benefits and feasibility of sustainable agriculture. In addition to the programs described above, the foundation makes annual membership contributions and grants to specific charities designated by Charles F. Noyes. Small programs addressing redefining fiduciary responsibility and environmental justice are also implemented by the foundation. Issues of social justice and the environment are a key consideration throughout the grant decision-making process. The foundation does not accept applications for discretionary grants. **Priorities:** *Civic & Public Affairs:* 10%. *Education:* 9%. *Environment:* 26%. Reproductive rights. *International:* 5%. *Note:* Total contributions made in 2000. In addition to its program grants, the foundation also makes annual contributions to pre-selected charities, discretionary grants, and membership contributions. **Typ. Recipients:** AIDS/HIV, Alzheimers Disease, Emergency/Ambulance Services, Family Planning, Health Organizations, Health Policy/Cost Containment, Hospitals, Medical Education, Medical Research, Public Health. **Geo. Dist:** nationally.

★ 11607 ★ Jewish Foundation for Education of Women

135 East 64th St.
New York, NY 10021
Phone: (212)288-3931 **Fax:** (212)288-5798
Website: http://www.jfew.org
Marge Goldwater, Executive Director

Fnded: 1984. **Philosophy:** The foundation was established to assist women in achieving their goals through higher education. The foundation is offering the following programs for the School Year 1999/2000: Scholarships for Emigres Training for Careers in Jewish Education. This program is open to emigres from the former Soviet Union who are pursuing careers in Jewish education. Candidates in Jewish education. Candidates in Jewish education, rabbinical and cantorial studies, and Jewish studies are invited to write the foundation for an application. Awards range from $10,000 to $20,000. Approximately seven scholarships will be awarded. Scholarships in the Health Professions. This program will provide scholarships to emigres from the former Soviet Union who are studying medicine, dentistry, nursing, pharmacy, occupational and physical therapy, and physician assistance. Typical awards are $5,000. Approximately 72 scholarships will be awarded. The foundation is offering additional scholarships through the colleges and universities designated below. These scholarships will be awarded through faculty recommendations; students cannot apply directly. CUNY Teacher Incentive Program: This program will provide stipends to CUNY graduates who are studying for a master's degree in education at CUNY and interested in pursuing a teaching career in the New York City public school system. Qualified students should contact the office of the Vice Chancellor for Academic Affairs at CUNY for further information ARTS Scholarships at The Juilliard School, Tisch School of the Arts at New York University, and the Manhattan School of Music: These scholarships are being offered to qualified students enrolled in their programs. Faculty members will select recipients. CUNY Dissertation Fellowships in the Humanities: A small number of fellowships will be awarded through the CUNY Graduate Center to qualified applicants. Barnard College Summer Internships: This program will support summer internships for qualified Barnard College students. Summer stipends are also available for qualified students in Barnard's Double Degree Program with the Jewish Theological Seminary. The foundation also offers scholarships for students of five New York City schools of social work. Faculty members make the decisions. Scholarships are also provided to disadvantaged teens through various social service groups. **Priorities:** *Education:* 100%. Supports higher education. *Note:* Total contributions made in fiscal 2001. **Typ. Recipients:** Medical Education. **Geo. Dist:** NY, five boroughs of New York.

★ 11608 ★ Jewish Healthcare Foundation

Center City Tower, Suite 2330
650 Smithfield St.
Pittsburgh, PA 15222
Phone: (412)261-1400 **Fax:** (412)232-6240
Email: info@jhf.org
Website: http://www.jhf.org
Karen Wolk-Feinstein, President

Fnded: 1991. **Philosophy:** "The Jewish Healthcare Foundation uses its resources to identify and support creative ideas and partnerships with the potential to make our region's health care system one of the best in the country. Our operating principles require that grants build upon proven techniques and the best information available. Funded programs should contribute to reshaping the system and lead to long-term solutions. While addressing ongoing concerns, the foundation will also address emerging health care concerns. The foundation views grants as investments that should strive to have a maximum impact on health status and systems by (1) changing health behaviors, (2) improving networks of care, or (3) generating good public programs. At the Jewish Healthcare Foundation we believe that connecting people with other skilled, informed and inventive people, provides the most direct route to the highest standards in health care. Jewish values compel us to connect system improvements to the Jewish and general communities and their institutions. By working to improve the physical and emotional health of individuals and communities, the JHF honors Jewish heritage and values. Our current agenda focuses on the following funding priorities: Financing Health: Insuring Quality–issues of insurance enrollment, entitlement, coverage and benefits affect access, quality, disease management and early detection. Advancing Health: Information Technology and Medical Research–quality in health care depends increasingly on the speed with which the health sector is transformed into an information driven industry. Integrating Health: Physician, Behavioral, Environmental and Public Health–integrating these elements will improve the health status of all Americans; integrating services for the frail and vulnerable across the continuum of acute rehabilitation, end-of-life, home based and residential services, will produce better outcomes." **Priorities:** *Arts & Humanities:* 3%. Supports public broadcasting. *Civic & Public Affairs:* 17%. Supports community foundations, law and justice organizations, job training, philanthropic organizations. *Education:* 19%. Supports universities, medical colleges, and religious education. *Environment:* 7%. Supports United Way, scouting, senior services, and Young Women's Christian AssociationAs. *International:* 31%. Supports hospitals, cancer research, AIDS organizations, respiratory health, and medical rehabilitation. *Note:* Total contributions made in 2000. **Typ. Recipients:** Adolescent Health Issues, AIDS/HIV, Alzheimers Disease, Cancer, Children's Health/Hospitals, Clinics/Medical Centers, Domestic Violence, Geriatric Health, Health Funds, Health Organizations, Health Policy/Cost Containment, Health-General, Health-General, Heart, Home-Care Services, Hospitals, Hospitals (University Affiliated), Kidney, Long-Term Care, Medical Education, Medical Research, Medical Training, Mental Health, Nursing Services, Nutrition, People with Disabilities, Prenatal Health Issues, Preventive Medicine/Wellness Organizations, Public Health, Single-Disease Health Associations, Substance Abuse, Transplant Networks/Donor Banks. **Geo. Dist:** PA, Western Pennsylvania.

★ 11609 ★ JM Foundation

60 East 42nd St., Room 1651
New York, NY 10165
Phone: (212)687-7735 **Fax:** (212)697-5495
Carl Helstrom, Associate Executive Director

Fnded: 1936. **Philosophy:** "The Foundation's primary goals include: Assisting people with disabilities to lead fulfilling, independent lives. Promoting prevention and patient-centered health care. Encouraging market-oriented public policy solutions. Enhancing America's unique system of free enterprise, entrepreneurship, and voluntarism. Strengthening American families and reinforcing the crucial role of parents. The Foundation sponsors a variety of special initiatives and organizations to achieve its aims." "The Board of Directors has established priorities in two general areas: health and rehabilitation and education and public policy research." 2001 Annual Report The JM Foundation is closely involved with the Philanthropy Roundtable, the State Policy Network, and the National Results Council. **Priorities:** *Civic & Public Affairs:* 42%. Supports public policy research, legal concerns, and urban affairs. *Education:* 16%. Funds education reform and research on educational policy. *Environment:* 23%. Supports people with disabilities, family services, and youth organizations. *International:* 12%. Supports medical research, medical centers, substance abuse rehabilitation, mental health, and medical rehabilitation. *Note:* Total contributions made in 2001. **Typ. Recipients:** Cancer, Children's Health/Hospitals, Clinics/Medical Centers, Eyes/Blindness, Family Planning, Geriatric Health, Health Organizations, Health Policy/Cost Containment, Heart, Hospitals, Medical Education, Medical Rehabilitation, Medical Research, People with Disabilities, Prenatal Health Issues, Preventive Medicine/Wellness Organizations, Public Health, Research/Studies Institutes, Single-Disease Health Associations, Speech & Hearing, Substance Abuse, Trauma Treatment.

★ 11610 ★ Joe C. Davis Foundation

908 Audubon Drive
Nashville, TN 37204
Phone: (615)297-1030 **Fax:** (615)463-2763
Email: bartonshan@home.com
Anne Fergerson, Administrative Assistant

Fnded: 1976. **Philosophy:** The Joe C. Davis Foundation supports health and education in the Nashville, TN, area. **Priorities:** *Arts & Humanities:* 12%. Funds a local public library. *Civic & Public Affairs:* 6%. *Education:* 33%. Supports secondary education and colleges and universities. *Environment:* 25%. Supports the YMCA in Nashville and other family and children's services. *International:* 24%. Funds a medical school. *Note:* Total contributions made in fiscal 2000. **Typ. Recipients:** Alzheimers Disease, Cancer, Children's Health/Hospitals, Clinics/Medical Centers, Diabetes, Health Organizations, Health Policy/Cost Containment, Hospices, Hospitals, Hospitals (University Affiliated), Medical Education, Medical Research, Public Health, Speech & Hearing, Substance Abuse. **Geo. Dist:** Nashville, TN, including metropolitan area.

★ 11611 ★ Joe and Emily Lowe Foundation

249 Royal Palm Way, Suite 502
Palm Beach, FL 33480
Fax: (561)655-7130
Ellen Liman, President

Fnded: 1949. **Philosophy:** The foundation funds a wide variety of causes in the arts, civic and public affairs, education, health, social services, and religion (emphasizing Jewish causes). **Priorities:** *Arts & Humanities:* 25%. Performing arts, public broadcasting, opera, theater, and ballet. *Civic & Public Affairs:* 6%. Supports legal centers. *Education:* 8%. Colleges and specialty schools. *Environment:* 12%. Youth and family projects. *International:* 20%. Hospitals and health centers. *Note:* Total contributions made in 1999. **Typ. Recipients:** Cancer, Children's Health/Hospitals, Clinics/Medical Centers, Emergency/Ambulance Services, Eyes/Blindness, Family Planning, Heart, Hospices, Hospitals, Kidney, Medical Education, Medical Rehabilitation, Mental Health, People with Disabilities, Single-Disease Health Associations, Substance Abuse. **Geo. Dist:** Palm Beach, FL; New York, NY, metropolitan area.

★ 11612 ★ John A. and Delia T. Robert Charitable Trust 2

PO Box 10247
Birmingham, AL 35202
S. Compere, Trust Officer

Fnded: 1995. **Priorities:** *Arts & Humanities:* 8%. Funds libraries. *Civic & Public Affairs:* 8%. Supports zoos. *Education:* 19%. Supports school and scholarship. *Environment:* 16%. *International:* 34%. *Note:* Total contributions made in 2001. **Typ. Recipients:** Child Abuse, Health Organizations, Hospitals, People with Disabilities, Public Health. **Geo. Dist:** Birmingham, AL.

★ 11613 ★ The John A. Hartford Foundation, Inc.

55 East 59th St., 16th Fl.
New York, NY 10022-1178
Phone: (212)832-7788 **Fax:** (212)593-4913
Email: mail@jhartfound.org
Website: http://www.jhartfound.org
James O'Sullivan, Grants Manager

Fnded: 1929. **Philosophy:** The John A. Hartford Foundation's primary program emphasis is its Aging and Health Program, which seeks to strengthen the capacity of the American health care system to meet the needs of an aging population. Giving is focused on increasing the capacities of academic geriatricians and health professionals and on integrating and improving services for the elderly. Examples of ongoing grant programs include: The Centers of Excellence program, in which selected academic medical centers use Foundation grants to strengthen recruitment to academic geriatric careers and provide training and research opportunities for faculty geriatricians, and, The Beeson Scholars career development awards, administered by the American Federation for Aging Research, to develop a new cadre of physician-scientists to be leaders in geriatric research and care. The program,"Improving Depression Care for Elders, seeks to assist the office-based primary care physician be developing, implementing and evaluating a disease management model for the care of depressed elders. The Social Work Initiative is broadly designed to improve social work practice with older adults through the development of better education and training programs, which builds on the Foundation's Geriatric Interdisciplinary Team Training and General Physician programs." The Social Work Initiative also parallels the Foundation's Academic Geriatrics and Nursing Institute. 1998 Annual Report. **Priorities:** *Education:* 53%. Supports universitys. *International:* 47%. Supports geriatric health. *Note:* Total contributions made in 2001. **Typ. Recipients:** Arthritis, Cancer, Clinics/Medical Centers, Geriatric Health, Health Funds, Health Organizations, Health Policy/Cost Containment, Health-General, Home-Care Services, Hospitals, Long-Term Care, Medical Education, Medical Rehabilitation, Medical Research, Medical Training, Mental Health, People with Disabilities, Public Health, Research/Studies Institutes. **Geo. Dist:** nationally.

★ 11614 ★ John Ben Snow Memorial Trust

Jefferson Tower
50 Presidential Plaza, Suite 106
Syracuse, NY 13202
Jonathan Snow, Trustee

Fnded: 1974. **Philosophy:** The John Ben Snow Memorial Trust makes most of its grants in the areas of education, civic affairs, and the arts. Educational funding favors universities and community colleges. Journalism is an area of focus. The arts are supported by grants to historic preservation, museums, and art centers. Grants also are made to other recipient areas, including disabled assistance organizations. **Priorities:** *Arts & Humanities:* 27%. Supports public broadcasting, art centers, and museums. *Civic & Public Affairs:* 17%. Funds community groups and municipalities. *Education:* 32%. Contributes to colleges, universities, law schools, and education associations. *Environment:* 17%. Funds youth groups. *International:* 5%. *Note:* Total contributions made in 2000. **Typ. Recipients:** Cancer, Clinics/Medical Centers, Family Planning, Geriatric Health, Health Funds, Hospices, Hospitals, Medical Education, Medical Research, People with Disabilities. **Geo. Dist:** Eastern USA; NY.

★ 11615 ★ John D. and Catherine T. MacArthur Foundation

140 South Dearborn St.
Chicago, IL 60603-5285
Phone: (312)726-8000 **Fax:** (312)920-6258
Email: 4answers@macfound.org
Website: http://www.macfound.org
Richard Kaplan, Assistant Vice President

Fnded: 1970. **Philosophy:** "The Foundation is dedicated to helping groups and individuals foster lasting improvements in the human condition. The foundation seeks the development of healthy individuals and effective communities; peace within and among nations; responsible choices about human reproduction; and a global ecosystem capable of supporting healthy human societies. The Foundation pursues this mission by supporting research, policy development, dissemination, education and training, and practice." The Foundation makes grants through two major integrated programs. The Program on Human and Community Development supports work in community development, the arts, economic opportunity, youth development, education, mental health, research and other areas. The Program on Global Security and Sustainability focuses upon issues of peace, population and the environment. The Foundation's special programs are the General Program, through which a number of special initiatives that promote excellence and diversity in the media, and the MacArthur Fellows Program. **Priorities:** *Civic & Public Affairs:* (Human and Community Development) 38%. Focus on economic opportunity, building community capacity, cross-cutting initiatives, and land grants/donations to Florida. Also supports youth development and population issues. *Education:* 7%. Provides fellowships through the MacArthur Fellows Program. *Note:* Total contributions made in 2000. **Typ. Recipients:** Clinics/Medical Centers, Family Planning, Geriatric Health, Health Organizations, Health Policy/Cost Containment, Medical Education, Medical Research, Mental Health, Preventive Medicine/Wellness Organizations, Public Health, Research/Studies Institutes. **Geo. Dist:** internationally; nationally; FL, Palm Beach County: human and community development grants; Chicago, IL, education reform grants; Chicago, IL, human and community development grants; global security and sustainability grants; global security and sustainability grants; global security and sustainability grants; global security and sustainability grants.

★ 11616 ★ John Edward Fowler Memorial Foundation

1725 K St. NW, Suite 1201
Washington, DC 20006
Phone: (202)728-9080 **Fax:** (202)728-9082
Website: http://fdncenter.org/grantmaker/fowler
Richard Lee, President

Fnded: 1964. **Philosophy:** The Fowler Foundation is interested in supporting "smaller, well managed, non-profit organizations that have innovative ideas about how to help people help themselves." Most grants are limited to grassroots programs in the Washington, DC, area. *John Edward Fowler Memorial Foundation 1999 Grants Report* **Priorities:** *Arts & Humanities:* 6% Supports Performing arts. *Civic & Public Affairs:* 1%. Primarily for employment and job training programs. *Education:* 17%. Funds after school programs for at-risk youth, and literacy programs. *Environment:* 56%. Primarily supports at-risk youth, shelters, and transitional housing. *International:* 3%. Funds pediatric and low-income health and clinics. *Note:* Total contributions made in 2001. **Typ. Recipients:** AIDS/HIV, Alzheimers Disease, Cancer, Children's Health/Hospitals, Clinics/Medical Centers, Domestic Violence, Emergency/Ambulance Services, Geriatric Health, Hospices, Hospitals, Hospitals (University Affiliated), Long-Term Care, Mental Health, Multiple Sclerosis, Outpatient Health Care, People with Disabilities, Prenatal Health Issues, Public Health. **Geo. Dist:** Washington, DC, including immediate metropolitan area.

★ 11617 ★ John Ernest Bamberger and Ruth Eleanor Bamberger Memorial Foundation

136 South Main St., Suite 418
Salt Lake City, UT 84101-1690
Phone: (801)364-2045 **Fax:** (801)322-5284
Eleanor Roser, Chairman

Fnded: 1947. **Philosophy:** The foundation provides support primarily for social services, education, including scholarships for undergraduate student nurses, health organizations, and civic causes. **Priorities:** *Arts & Humanities:* 3%. *Civic & Public Affairs:* 10%. Legal aid and Native American affairs. *Education:* 9%. Secondary education, scholarships, literacy, private education, and colleges and universities. *Environment:* 73%. Youth organizations, child welfare, and YMCAs. *International:* 3%. Public health, AIDS. *Note:* Total contributions made in 2000. **Typ. Recipients:** Alzheimers Disease, Cancer, Children's Health/Hospitals, Clinics/Medical Centers, Domestic Violence, Emergency/Ambulance Services, Eyes/Blindness, Family Planning, Health Organizations, Health-General, Hospices, Hospitals, Long-Term Care, Medical Education, Mental Health, Multiple Sclerosis, Nursing Services, People with Disabilities, Public Health, Respiratory, Sexual Abuse, Single-Disease Health Associations, Substance Abuse. **Geo. Dist:** Salt Lake City, UT.

★ 11618 ★ John G. and Marie Stella Kenedy Memorial Foundation

1700 Tower II
Corpus Christi, TX 78478
Phone: (361)887-6565 **Fax:** (361)887-6582
Email: kmf@kenedy.org
Judy Gilbreath, Office Manager & Grants Officer

Fnded: 1960. **Philosophy:** A majority of the foundation's funding supports dioceses and religious organizations in Texas. Educational institutions and social services also receive funding. **Priorities:** *Civic & Public Affairs:* About 4%. Housing. *Education:* 29%. Academic scholarships. *Environment:* 12%. Focus on people with disabilities, child welfare, youth organizations, and substance abuse prevention. *International:* 2%. *Note:* Total contributions made in fiscal 2001. **Typ. Recipients:** AIDS/HIV, Hospitals, People with Disabilities, Substance Abuse. **Geo. Dist:** TX.

★ 11619 ★ John H. and Wilhelmina D. Harland Charitable Foundation

2 Piedmont Center, Suite 106
Atlanta, GA 30305
Phone: (404)264-9912 **Fax:** (404)266-8834
Email: harland@randomc.com
John Conant, Secretary

Fnded: 1972. **Philosophy:** The foundation was established to provide ongoing support to organizations personally supported by the donors, as well as to fund other institutions of a similar nature. The Harlands had a particular interest "in causes that serve children and higher education." These remain primary concerns of the foundation, but consideration is given to grant requests that fall within the following categories: education, health, community services, children and youth services, cultural and religious organizations. The trustees have a particular interest in improved education for children and young people, opportunities for handicapped and disabled children, character development, and preparing youth for graduation from high school and productive employment. **Priorities:** *Arts & Humanities:* 18%. Funds arts centers, theaters, museums. *Civic & Public Affairs:* 6%. Supports housing, economic development, and legal affairs. *Education:* 11%. Supports pre-college education, literacy, and higher learning. *Environment:* 39%. Gives to youth programs, boys and girls clubs, and family services. *International:* 16%. Funds hospitals, health centers, and single-disease organizations. *Note:* Total contributions made in 2001. **Typ. Recipients:** Child Abuse, Children's Health/Hospitals, Clinics/Medical Centers, Domestic Violence, Emergency/Ambulance Services, Geriatric Health, Health Organizations, Hospitals, Long-Term Care, Medical Education, Medical Rehabilitation, Mental Health, Nutrition, People with Disabilities, Public Health, Research/Studies Institutes, Single-Disease Health Associations, Speech & Hearing, Substance Abuse. **Geo. Dist:** Atlanta, GA, metropolitan area.

★ 11620 ★ John Huntington Fund for Education

20620 North Park Boulevard, Suite 215
Cleveland, OH 44118
Phone: (216)321-7185 **Fax:** (216)932-0331
Ann Pinkerton, Treasurer

Fnded: 1954. **Philosophy:** The foundation was established to fund student scholarships in the areas of science, nursing, and technology. The foundation makes grants to universities, nursing schools, art institutes, and other scholarship programs in Ohio. **Priorities:** *Arts & Humanities:* 2%. Supports an art institute. *Education:* 96%. Supports educational programs and scholarships. *International:* 2%. Supports a hospital. *Note:* Total contributions made in 2001. **Typ. Recipients:** Hospitals (University Affiliated), Medical Education. **Geo. Dist:** Cuyahoga County, OH, Cuyahoga County.

★ 11621 ★ The John L. Weinberg Foundation

85 Broad St.
New York, NY 10004-2434
Phone: (212)902-6897 **Fax:** (212)888-7559
Email: john.l.weinberg@gs.com
John Weinberg, Trustee

Fnded: 1959. **Philosophy:** The John L. Weinberg Foundation primarily supports hospitals and university-level education. Other areas of interest include civic affairs, the arts, and social services. **Priorities:** *Arts & Humanities:* 37%. Supports libraries, museums, public broadcasting, and historic preservation. *Civic & Public Affairs:* 7%. Supports historic homes and parks. *Education:* 23%. Colleges and universities, minority education, private precollege education, arts and humanities education, and scholarship funds. *Environment:* 7%. Supports animal protection, food distribution programs, Young Men's Christian Association, United Way, and scouting. *International:* 19%. Supports hospital, medical centers, single disease health associations, and mental health. *Note:* Total contributions made in fiscal 2001. **Typ. Recipients:** AIDS/HIV, Cancer, Children's Health/Hospitals, Clinics/Medical Centers, Diabetes, Emergency/Ambulance Services, Geriatric Health, Health Funds, Hospitals, Medical Research, People with Disabilities, Single-Disease Health Associations, Substance Abuse. **Geo. Dist:** nationally; Greenwich, CT; New York, NY.

★ 11622 ★ John M. Hopwood Charitable Trust

PNC Bank
2 PNC Plaza, 25th Floor
620 Liberty Ave.
Pittsburgh, PA 15222-2705
Phone: (412)762-3502 **Fax:** (412)705-1043
Email: bruce.bickel@pncbank.com
Bruce Bickel, Senior Vice President and Manager

Fnded: 1948. **Philosophy:** Though the trust makes grants across the major categories of support, medical organizations its primary interest. In health services, interests include hospital foundations, health programs, and hospitals. Arts support favors museums, libraries, festivals, theater, and other performing arts. Support for education includes giving to colleges, universities, and private schools. Social service support goes to united funds, community centers, and community activities. The trust also places emphasis on environmental concerns. **Priorities:** *Arts & Humanities:* 4%. Supports performing arts, museums, art centers, and public broadcasting. *Civic & Public Affairs:* 12%. Gives to, civic leagues, economic development, and housing. *Education:* 33%. Contributes to colleges, universities, private schools, education funds, scholarships, and literacy. *Environment:* 14%. Funds youth groups, Young Men's Christian Association, Big Brothers/Big Sisters, scouts, drug awareness and United Way. *International:* 27%. Supports hospitals and hospital associated foundations, mental health and single disease health associations. *Note:* Total contributions made in 2000. **Typ. Recipients:** Cancer, Children's Health/Hospitals, Clinics/Medical Centers, Domestic Violence, Emergency/Ambulance Services, Health Organizations, Hospices, Hospitals, Kidney, Long-Term Care, Medical Education, Medical Rehabilitation, Mental Health, Multiple Sclerosis, Nursing Services, People with Disabilities, Public Health, Single-Disease Health Associations, Speech & Hearing, Substance Abuse. **Geo. Dist:** PA, Western part of state.

★ 11623 ★ John M. Olin Foundation

330 Madison Ave., 22nd Floor
New York, NY 10017
Phone: (212)661-2670 **Fax:** (212)661-5917
Website: http://www.jmof.org
James Piereson, Executive Director

Fnded: 1953. **Philosophy:** The general purpose of the foundation "is to provide support for projects that reflect or are intended to strengthen the economic, political, and cultural institutions upon which the American heritage of constitutional government and enterprise is based. The foundation also seeks to promote a general understanding of these institutions by encouraging the thoughtful study of the connections between economic and political freedoms, and the cultural heritage that sustains them." The foundation encourages research on the formulation, implementation, and evaluation of public policy in the social and economic fields. Foundation-sponsored projects in this area have included tax policy, monetary policy, welfare policy, and fiscal policy. The foundation supports projects that address the relationship between American institutions and the international context in which they operate. Foundation-sponsored projects in this area have included studies of national security affairs, strategic issues, American foreign policy, and the international economy. The foundation also seeks to promote understanding of the moral, cultural, and institutional foundations of free government. The foundation, therefore, has supported studies of the American Constitution, the operation of the American political institutions, and the moral and cultural principles underlying these institutions. The foundation seeks to deepen understanding of the American judicial system and to preserve the rule of law as the foundation of American constitutional government. Support has gone to public interest law and to studies related to the judicial system, jurisprudence, and the relationship between law and economics. In each of these four areas, the foundation attempts to advance its objectives through research, institutional support, fellowships, professorships, lectures, books, scholarly journals, conferences and seminars, and occasional radio and television programs. **Priorities:** *Civic & Public Affairs:* 25%. Supports civil rights and legal aid. *Education:* 73%. Supports education funds and programs. *Environment:* 2%. Primarily supports crime prevention. *Note:* Total contributions made in 2000. **Typ. Recipients:** Health Organizations, Health Policy/Cost Containment, Single-Disease Health Associations. **Geo. Dist:** internationally; nationally.

★ 11624 ★ John and Mary Franklin Foundation Inc.

NC1-002-11-18 Bank of America Plaza
Charlotte, NC 28255
Phone: (404)607-5209
Dr. Marilu McCarty, Executive Secretary

Fnded: 1955. **Philosophy:** In 1955, John Franklin wrote that the foundation was to be organized solely for charitable, religious, scientific, and educational purposes. He listed fifteen charities which he and his wife had supported in the preceding year as an indication of their personal preferences. These consisted of health care institutions and social service organizations, primarily for young people. Mr. Franklin also described his and his wife's charitable interests in the fields of science, religion, and education. In the field of science, they were particularly interested in medical research, and listed the Heart Fund, Cancer Fund, and March of Dimes as typical recipients. In education, their primary interest was in educating the disabled so that they might lead fuller lives, listing the Atlanta Speech School and the Muscular Dystrophy Fund as examples. While not specifying any religious charity by name, Mr. Franklin did state that appropriations should be made without respect to denomination, creed, or color and should be governed by the demands of the particular time. The foundation is managed by a nine-member board of trustees which has followed and expanded on the pattern of grants described by John Franklin. Grants generally are limited to the metropolitan Atlanta area, although special grants occasionally are made to institutions in other areas of Georgia and in adjoining states. **Priorities:** *Arts & Humanities:* 12%. Supports ballet, choir, historical preservation, and art centers. *Civic & Public Affairs:* 1%. Funds parks and botanical gardens. *Education:* 66%. Supports schools, colleges and universities, and scholarship funds. *Environment:* 11%. Supports youth organizations and United Way. *International:* 3%. Supports American Red Cross and children's health. *Religion:* 3%. *Note:* Total contributions made in 2001. **Typ. Recipients:** Cancer, Children's Health/Hospitals, Clinics/Medical Centers, Emergency/Ambulance Services, Family Planning, Geriatric Health, Health Policy/Cost Containment, Hospices, Hospitals, Long-Term Care, Medical Education, Medical Rehabilitation, Medical Research, Medical Training, Mental Health, People with Disabilities, Single-Disease Health Associations. **Geo. Dist:** Atlanta, GA, including metropolitan area.

★ 11625 ★ John McShain Charities

300 East Lancaster Ave., Suite 200
Wynnewood, PA 19096-2105
Fax: (215)564-2343
Mary McShain, President

Fnded: 1949. **Philosophy:** The foundation's purpose is to make donations primarily to education, as well as to benefit Roman Catholic churches, religious organizations, and welfare funds. The foundation has also supported music, community organizations, and hospitals. **Priorities:** *Arts & Humanities:* 1%. Supports museums, libraries and a fine arts committee. *Civic & Public Affairs:* 2%. Supports community foundations. *Education:* 72%. Emphasis on secondary and preparatory schools, colleges, and universities. *Environment:* 1%. Funds human services. *International:* 1%. Supports hospitals. *Note:* Total contributions made in fiscal 1999. **Typ. Recipients:** AIDS/HIV, Clinics/Medical Centers, Health Organizations, Hospitals, Long-Term Care, People with Disabilities. **Geo. Dist:** some grants nationally; Philadelphia, PA.

★ 11626 ★ John Merck Fund

11 Beacon St., Suite 1230
Boston, MA 02108
Phone: (617)723-2932 **Fax:** (617)523-6029
Email: info@jmfund.org
Ms. Ruth Hennig, Executive Director

Fnded: 1970. **Philosophy:** The fund makes grants in the following fields: developmental disabilities, to medical teaching hospitals for research in connection with developmental disabilities in children; the environment, to encourage preservation of productive farmland in Vermont, and to address global problems relating to climate change and the dangers of synthetic chemicals; reproductive health, to support access to women's reproductive health care in the U.S.; international human rights; and disarmament, for promoting nonproliferation of nuclear weapons; and job opportunities in the northeast U.S. "The Fund endeavors to assist outstanding individuals working on promising projects in organizations that may have difficulty attracting funds; favors grants for pilot projects that have potential for widespread application; supports advocacy, including litigation, to establish precedents the Fund considers to be in the public interest; concentrates on smaller organizations, including startups; favors matching grants." The foundation has recently begun to focus on economic opportunities and to support job creation projects. **Priorities:** *Civic & Public Affairs:* 37%. Supports law & justice, public policy, economic development, philanthropic organizations, rural affairs, womens affairs, and employment/job training. *Education:* 10%. Supports medical education, technical education, and universities. *Environment:* 3%. Supports family planning services. *International:* 5%. Supports medical research, reproductive health issues, and public health. *Note:* Total contributions made in 1998. **Typ. Recipients:** Adolescent Health Issues, Cancer, Children's Health/Hospitals, Emergency/Ambulance Services, Family Planning, Geriatric Health, Health Funds, Health Organizations, Health-General, Medical Education, Medical Research, Mental Health, People with Disabilities, Prenatal Health Issues, Public Health, Respiratory, Single-Disease Health Associations. **Geo. Dist:** nationally; VT.

★ 11627 ★ John P. McGovern Foundation

2211 Norfolk, Suite 900
Houston, TX 77098-4044
Phone: (713)524-5255 **Fax:** (713)661-3031
Dr. John McGovern, President

Fnded: 1961. **Philosophy:** The foundation primarily supports medical research organizations and medical funds, primarily in the area of the prevention of alcohol and substance abuse, with some focus on prevention of allergies. **Priorities:** *Arts & Humanities:* 9%. Supports libraries and museums. *Civic & Public Affairs:* 13%. Funds a foundation and community associations. *Education:* 45%. Supports universities and student exchange programs. *Environment:* 17%. Youth programs. *International:* 15%. Supports a medical institute and museum of health and medical science. *Note:* Total contributions made in 2001. **Typ. Recipients:** Cancer, Child Abuse, Children's Health/Hospitals, Clinics/Medical Centers, Domestic Violence, Eyes/Blindness, Health Funds, Health Organizations, Health-General, Heart, Hospitals, Medical Education, Medical Rehabilitation, Medical Research, Mental Health, Public Health, Research/Studies Institutes, Substance Abuse. **Geo. Dist:** some giving nationally; Houston, TX.

★ 11628 ★ John P. Murphy Foundation

Terminal Twr.
50 Public Sq., Ste. 924
Cleveland, OH 44113-2203
Phone: (216)623-4770 **Fax:** (216)623-4773
Mr. Allan Zambie, Executive Vice President

Fnded: 1960. **Philosophy:** The foundation's articles of incorporation state that the foundation will distribute its grants for "charitable, educational, scientific, literary, and religious purposes." Educational grants are usually made to colleges and universities. Artistic and cultural grants generally range from $1,000 to $50,000. Grants to social service organizations typically are below $5,000, and are given to a wide variety of needs. Community service grants also are given to numerous types of organizations. Most of the foundation's health grants are given to hospital building programs. **Priorities:** *Arts & Humanities:* 40%. Includes the highest grant of $5,000,000 to the University of Notre Dame law school. *Civic & Public Affairs:* 15%. Supports community affairs organizations. *Education:* 20%. Primarily supports colleges and universities and educational associations. *Environment:* 13%. United funds, food banks, child welfare, and YMCAs. *International:* 11%. Hospitals, nursing services, clinics, and medical rehabilitation. *Religion:* Approx. 1%. *Note:* Total contributions made in 2001. **Typ. Recipients:** Cancer, Children's Health/Hospitals, Clinics/Medical Centers, Family Planning, Health Funds, Health Organizations, Heart, Hospices, Hospitals, Hospitals (University Affiliated), Long-Term Care, Medical Education, Medical Rehabilitation, Medical Research, Mental Health, Nursing Services, People with Disabilities, Preventive Medicine/Wellness Organizations, Public Health, Sexual Abuse, Single-Disease Health Associations, Substance Abuse. **Geo. Dist:** Cleveland, OH, metropolitan area and adjacent counties in Northeastern Ohio.

★ 11629 ★ John R. McCune Charitable Trust

6 PPG Place
Pittsburgh, PA 15222
Phone: (412)644-7796 **Fax:** (412)644-8059
James Edwards, Executive Director

Fnded: 1972. **Philosophy:** The trust primarily provides grants to health-care institutions, institutions of secondary and higher education, and social service agencies. The trust does not make pledges beyond one year. The majority of the trust's grants are awarded to institutions or agencies located in western Pennsylvania. **Priorities:** *Arts & Humanities:* 4%. Supports music and museums. *Civic & Public Affairs:* 11%. Primarily for community foundations, neighborhood development, and training centers. *Education:* 42%. Supports colleges, universities, pre-college education, and scholarships. *Environment:* 16%. Funds children's centers, YMCAs, youth groups, animal protection senior concerns, and food banks. *International:* 18%. Gives to hospitals, health care centers, medical research, and Alzheimers. *Note:* Total contributions made in fiscal 2000. **Typ. Recipients:** Alzheimers Disease, Cancer, Child Abuse, Children's Health/Hospitals, Clinics/Medical Centers, Diabetes, Geriatric Health, Health Funds, Health Organizations, Hospitals, Medical Research, Mental Health, Multiple Sclerosis, People with Disabilities, Prenatal Health Issues, Public Health, Research/Studies Institutes, Single-Disease Health Associations, Substance Abuse, Transplant Networks/Donor Banks. **Geo. Dist:** Pittsburgh, PA, including western Pennsylvania.

★ 11630 ★ The John R. Oishei Foundation

One HSBC Center, Suite 3650
Buffalo, NY 14203-2805
Phone: (716)856-9490 **Fax:** (716)856-9493
Website: http://www.oisheifdt.org
Thomas Baker, Executive Director

Fnded: 1941. **Philosophy:** "The Foundation's mission is to act as a catalyst for change in the greater Buffalo community by supporting creative programs which attempt to advance the status quo, are strategically sound and are strongly focused on excellence. Its principal grant-making areas include medical research and care, education, cultural and social needs. The fundamental goal of the Foundation is to enhance the quality of life for members of the Buffalo community as well as to enhance the reputation of the city and the region." **Priorities:** *Arts & Humanities:* 18%. Supports theaters, libraries, music, galleries, and arts institutes. *Civic & Public Affairs:* 4%. Major support for the Erie County Bar Association. *Education:* 48%. Supports secondary schools, colleges and universities in Buffalo, NY. *Environment:* 6%. Supports charities, orphanages, youth activities, aid to children, aid to the underprivileged, counseling, and the elderly. *International:* 20%. Funds medical research, health systems, the Red Cross, and hospitals. *Note:* Total contributions made in 2000. **Typ. Recipients:** AIDS/HIV, Alzheimers Disease, Children's Health/Hospitals, Emergency/Ambulance Services, Geriatric Health, Health Organizations, Hospices, Hospitals, Long-Term Care, Medical Education, Medical Research, People with Disabilities, Substance Abuse. **Geo. Dist:** NY, Greater Western New York area; Buffalo, NY. **Frmly:** Julia R. and Estelle L. Foundation.

★ 11631 ★ John Randolph and Dora Haynes Foundation

888 West 6th St., Suite 1150
Los Angeles, CA 90017-2737
Phone: (213)623-9151 **Fax:** (213)623-3951
Email: info@haynesfoundation.org
Website: http://www.haynesfoundation.org
Diane Cornwell, Administrative Director

Fnded: 1926. **Philosophy:** "The Foundation attempts to reflect directly the interests of Dr. and Mrs. Haynes by focusing its resources on the fields which particularly concerned them. Accordingly, the Trustees of the Foundation support study and research in political science, economics, public policy, history, social psychology, and sociology, favoring projects with specific application to the Los Angeles area. By dissemination of the results of the research, and by other means, the Foundation seeks to improve public awareness and understanding of current issues." "Foundation also provides in the social sciences, undergraduate scholarships, graduate fellowships, and faculty research fellowships to selected colleges and universities in the greater Los Angeles area." 2000 Annual Report **Priorities:** *Arts & Humanities:* 14%. Supports historical societies, libraries, public broadcasting, and museums. *Civic & Public Affairs:* 21%. Supports philanthropy, private foundations, and political organizations. *Education:* 66%. Funds fellowships, internships, and scholarships to colleges and other educational institutions. *Note:* Total contributions made in fiscal 2001. **Typ. Recipients:** Children's Health/Hospitals, Geriatric Health, Health Policy/Cost Containment, Medical Education, Medical Research, Substance Abuse. **Geo. Dist:** Los Angeles, CA, metropolitan area.

★ 11632 ★ John S. Dunn Research Foundation

3355 West Alabama, Suite 720
Houston, TX 77098-1718
Phone: (713)626-0369 **Fax:** (713)626-3866
John Dunn, Jr., President

Fnded: 1985. **Philosophy:** The foundation typically funds organizations "whose primary efforts are medically related to educational and research activities." **Priorities:** *Civic & Public Affairs:* 2%. *Education:* 50%. Funds medical education and private schools. *Environment:* 4%. Supports medically-related social service concerns. *International:* 41%. Supports medical research, hospitals, clinics, and single-disease associations. *Note:* Total contributions made in 2000. **Typ. Recipients:** Alzheimers Disease, Cancer, Children's Health/Hospitals, Clinics/Medical Centers, Diabetes, Eyes/Blindness, Family Planning, Health Funds, Health Organizations, Heart, Hospices, Hospitals, Hospitals (University Affiliated), Medical Education, Medical Rehabilitation, Medical Research, People with Disabilities, Public Health, Respiratory, Single-Disease Health Associations, Speech & Hearing. **Geo. Dist:** TX.

★ 11633 ★ John S. and James L. Knight Foundation

Wachovia Financial Center, Suite 3300
200 Biscayne Boulevard
Miami, FL 33131
Phone: (305)908-2600 **Fax:** (305)908-2698
Email: publications@knightfdn.org
Website: http://www.knightfdn.org
Hodding Carter, III, President & Chief Executive Officer

Fnded: 1950. **Philosophy:** "To heighten the impact of our grant making, Knight Foundation's trustees have elected to focus on two signature programs, Journalism and Knight Community Partners, each with its own eligibility requirements. A third program, The National Venture Fund, supports innovative opportunities and initiatives at the national level that relate directly or indirectly to Knight's work in its 26 communities. In a rapidly changing world, the Foundation also remains flexible enough to respond to unique challenges, ideas and projects that lie beyond its identified program areas, yet would fulfill the broad vision of its founders." John S. and James L. Knight Foundation Statement of Purpose **Priorities:** *Arts & Humanities:* 15%. Supports museums, performing arts, libraries, literary arts, historic preservation, historical societies, and arts/humanities councils. *Civic & Public Affairs:* 36%. Funds professional journalism associations, organizations defending free press, public policy organizations, community foundations, community development programs, municipalities, housing, nonprofit management, and minority/women's affairs. *Education:* 29%. Supports the education of current and future journalists; also funds colleges and universities, literacy programs, and education reform. *Environment:* 12%. Emphasis on child and social welfare, homelessness, and disaster relief. Also funds the United Way. *International:* 1%. Contributes to the American Red Cross, mental health centers, hospice, hospitals, and medical centers. *Religion:* 2%. Funds a science museum. *Note:* Total contributions approved in 2001. **Typ. Recipients:** Cancer, Children's Health/Hospitals, Emergency/Ambulance Services, Health Organizations, Hospices, Hospitals, Medical Research, Mental Health, Prenatal Health Issues, Substance Abuse. **Geo. Dist:** nationally.

★ 11634 ★ John Simon Guggenheim Memorial Foundation

90 Park Ave.
New York, NY 10016
Phone: (212)687-4470 **Fax:** (212)697-3248
Email: fellowships@gf.org
Website: http://www.gf.org

Fnded: 1925. **Philosophy:** The foundation "offers fellowships to further the development of scholars and artists by assisting them to engage in research in any field of knowledge and creation in any of the arts, under the freest possible conditions and irrespective of race, color, or creed." The foundation offers fellowships through two annual competitions: one open to citizens and permanent residents of the United States and Canada, and the other open to citizens and permanent residents of Latin America and the Caribbean. **Priorities:** *Arts & Humanities:* Less than 1%. *Civic & Public Affairs:* 2%. Supports community development. *Education:* 96%. Supports fellowships at colleges and universities, faculty development, arts/humanities education, medical education, and technical education. *Note:* Contributions analysis represents total contributions in 2000. The foundation reports that percentages vary from year to year. **Typ. Recipients:** Medical Education, Medical Research. **Geo. Dist:** nationally; Latin America and the Caribbean.

★ 11635 ★ John Smith Charities

PO Box 608
Greenville, SC 29608
Fax: (864)271-5930
Bill Bridges, Administrator

Fnded: 1985. **Philosophy:** John Smith Charities primarily supports education and social services. Educational funding favors colleges, religious education, universities, and private education. Social service support goes to public housing, food distribution, family counseling, and youth camps. Other recipient areas are supported by the foundation are the arts, and health care. **Priorities:** *Arts & Humanities:* 8%. Funds performing arts, symphonies, public broadcasting, theaters, museums, and historical societies. *Civic & Public Affairs:* 38%. Supports community foundations, and women's affairs. *Education:* 37%. Includes a major grant to the South Carolina Governor's School for the Arts. *Environment:* 8%. Supports scouts and YMCA. *Note:* Total contributions made in fiscal 2001. **Typ. Recipients:** Cancer, Clinics/Medical Centers, Emergency/Ambulance Services, Health Organizations, Hospitals, Hospitals (University Affiliated), Long-Term Care, Medical Education, Mental Health, People with Disabilities, Single-Disease Health Associations. **Geo. Dist:** SC, Upstate South Carolina.

★ 11636 ★ John Stauffer Charitable Trust

301 North Lake Ave., 10th Floor
Pasadena, CA 91101-4108
Phone: (626)793-9400 **Fax:** (626)793-5900
Mr. H. Senecal, Trustee

Fnded: 1974. **Philosophy:** The trust is limited to supporting colleges, universities, and hospitals. Giving to colleges and universities emphasizes efforts to acquire and erect buildings and other facilities; obtain equipment, instruments, books, and furnishings; and provide scholarships, fellowships, and professorships that specifically target science and chemistry. Support to hospitals is more limited and goes toward acquiring land, erecting buildings and other facilities, and obtaining equipment, instruments, and furnishings. The trust prefers to give grants to institutions that maintain balanced operating budgets and avoid deficit financing. The trustees encourage the use of plaques to memorialize the name of John Stauffer. **Priorities:** *Education:* 75%. Primarily supports colleges and universities. *International:* 25%. Supports hospitals. *Note:* Total contributions made in fiscal 2001. **Typ. Recipients:** Cancer, Children's Health/Hospitals, Clinics/Medical Centers, Emergency/Ambulance Services, Family Planning, Health Organizations, Heart, Hospitals, Medical Rehabilitation, Medical Research, Mental Health, Outpatient Health Care, People with Disabilities, Public Health, Substance Abuse. **Geo. Dist:** CA.

★ 11637 ★ John Steele Zink Foundation

1259 East 26th St.
Tulsa, OK 74114
Phone: (918)749-8249
Jacqueline Zink, Trustee

Fnded: 1972. **Philosophy:** The John Steele Zink Foundation provides funding to various cultural programs, including museums, theater companies, dance, and music in the Tulsa area. It supports philanthropic organizations, educational funds, and local colleges. The foundation is committed to social service in its contributions to community and youth organizations, as well as to united funds. It also supports local churches. **Priorities:** *Arts & Humanities:* 23%. Mostly funding music programs and theater. *Civic & Public Affairs:* 26%. Foundation continuing support and operating funds. *Education:* 16% Colleges and universities in Tulsa OK. *Environment:* 14%. Scouting and youth programs, support groups and humane society. *International:* 17%. Single-disease health associations and emergency health projects. *Note:* Total contributions made in fiscal 2001. **Typ. Recipients:** AIDS/HIV, Child Abuse, Children's Health/Hospitals, Clinics/Medical Centers, Domestic Violence, Emergency/Ambulance Services, Family Planning, Health Organizations, Heart, Hospices, Hospitals, Mental Health, Multiple Sclerosis, People with Disabilities, Prenatal Health Issues, Sexual Abuse, Speech & Hearing, Substance Abuse. **Geo. Dist:** Tulsa, OK.

★ 11638 ★ John Templeton Foundation

5 Radnor Corporate Center, Suite 100
100 Matsonford Rd.
PO Box 8322
Radnor, PA 19087-8322
Phone: (610)687-8942 **Fax:** (610)687-8961
Email: info@templeton.org
Website: http://www.templeton.org

Fnded: 1988. **Philosophy:** The John Templeton Foundation was established in 1987 by renowned international investor, Sir John Templeton, to encourage a fresh appreciation of the critical importance, for all peoples and cultures, of the moral and spiritual dimensions of life. Through it's programs, the Foundations seeks to encourage the world to catch the vision of the tremendous possibilities for spiritual progress in an open and humble approach to life; encourage institutions of learning to incorporate training towards excellence in character in their efforts to prepare the next generation for service; to encourage growth in appreciating the potential of free societies; and to promote the understanding of the significant responsibilities associated with freedom in its several aspects, moral, spiritual, political and economic. "Website." **Typ. Recipients:** Cancer, Health Organizations, Health-General, Medical Research, Mental Health.

★ 11639 ★ John W. Anderson Foundation

402 Wall St.
Valparaiso, IN 46383
Phone: (219)462-4611
William Vinovich, Vice Chairman

Fnded: 1967. **Philosophy:** "The John W. Anderson Foundation was created in 1967 for the purpose of supporting such charitable, religious, scientific, literary or educational purposes within the United States as the Trustees, in their discretion, shall determine will best promote the mental, moral, intellectual and physical improvement, assistance and relief of inhabitants of the United States, of all races and creeds and particularly youth who reside in and near Lake and Porter Counties in Northwest Indiana." John W. Anderson Foundation 1999 Annual Report, Grant Application and Guidelines Brochure. **Priorities:** *Arts & Humanities:* 3%. Gives to music and public broadcasting. *Civic & Public Affairs:* 2%. Supports economic development. *Education:* 27%. Funds colleges and universities and education funds. *Environment:* 53%. Supports youth groups, united funds, and social services. *International:* 12%. Contributions go to medical research and health associations. *Note:* Total contributions were made in 2000. **Typ. Recipients:** Cancer, Children's Health/Hospitals, Clinics/Medical Centers, Emergency/Ambulance Services, Family Planning, Health Organizations, Heart, Hospices, Medical Education, Medical Rehabilitation, Mental Health, Nursing Services, People with Disabilities, Public Health, Research/Studies Institutes, Single-Disease Health Associations. **Geo. Dist:** IL, funds some organizations in Northeastern Illinois; IN.

★ 11640 ★ John W. and Effie E. Speas Memorial Trust

PO Box 419119
Kansas City, MO 64105
Phone: (816)979-7481 **Fax:** (816)979-7916
David Ross, Senior Vice President

Fnded: 1947. **Philosophy:** The Speas Memorial Trust supports a variety of health and social service organizations, with some focus on mental health and substance abuse programs. Recently, it has initiated services for the elderly in the Kansas City metropolitan area, with emphasis on helping the elderly to continue to reside in their own homes, and on providing respite care. The trust also contributes to university medical schools. **Priorities:** *Civic & Public Affairs:* 4%. Supports community foundations. *Education:* 28%. Supports healthcare programs at colleges and universities. *Environment:* 20%. Supports family services, United Way, and youth organizations. *International:* 39%. Funds hospitals, medical centers, and cancer research. *Note:* Total contributions made in 2000. **Typ. Recipients:** Alzheimers Disease, Cancer, Child Abuse, Children's Health/Hospitals, Clinics/Medical Centers, Emergency/Ambulance Services, Eyes/Blindness, Geriatric Health, Health Organizations, Health Policy/Cost Containment, Heart, Home-Care Services, Hospices, Hospitals, Hospitals (University Affiliated), Kidney, Long-Term Care, Medical Education, Medical Rehabilitation, Medical Research, Medical Training, Mental Health, Multiple Sclerosis, Nursing Services, Nutrition, People with Disabilities, Prenatal Health Issues, Preventive Medicine/Wellness Organizations, Public Health, Single-Disease Health Associations, Speech & Hearing, Substance Abuse, Transplant Networks/Donor Banks. **Geo. Dist:** KS, Johnson County; KS, Wyandotte County; MO, Cass County; MO, Clay County; MO, Jackson County; MO, Platte County.

★ 11641 ★ John Wesley and Anna Hodgin Hanes Foundation

100 North Main
PO Box 3099
Winston-Salem, NC 27150-7131
Phone: (336)732-5372 **Fax:** (336)732-6537
Linda Tilley, Relationship Manager

Fnded: 1947. **Philosophy:** The Trust Agreement for the foundation stated that "the income and principal of the Trust shall be used exclusively for such charitable, scientific, literary, or educational purposes...as a majority of the individual trustees...shall determine." The foundation has a primary interest in Winston-Salem and Forsyth county in North Carolina where it is located. "It has always been interested in improving the life of the citizens of North Carolina and will continue to support this interest with funding. However, it is a prime requirement of the foundation that organizations seeking funding show that the community in which the organization is located and the organization's trustees have given substantial financial support prior to consideration by the foundation." **Priorities:** *Arts & Humanities:* 13%. Supports music, performing arts, and libraries. *Civic & Public Affairs:* 10%. Supports economic development, housing, and philanthropic organizations. *Education:* 31%. Supports higher education, community college, technical college and other education. *Environment:* 36%. YMCA's, seniors, hunger programs, youth programs and child welfare. *International:* 4%. Supports hospitals and wellness programs. *Religion:* 1%. Supports a science center. *Note:* Total contributions made in 2001. **Typ. Recipients:** AIDS/HIV, Alzheimers Disease, Clinics/Medical Centers, Domestic Violence, Emergency/Ambulance Services, Eyes/Blindness, Family Planning, Health Funds, Hospices, Hospitals, Medical Education, Medical Rehabilitation, People with Disabilities, Public Health, Single-Disease Health Associations, Substance Abuse, Transplant Networks/Donor Banks. **Geo. Dist:** NC, Winston-Salem and Forsyth County area; Winston-Salem, NC.

★ 11642 ★ Jon and Karen Huntsman Foundation

500 Huntsman Way
Salt Lake City, UT 84108
Phone: (801)584-5700

Fnded: 1988. **Priorities:** *Arts & Humanities:* 4%. *Civic & Public Affairs:* Less than 1%. *Education:* 70%. Funds scholarships, law schools, colleges and universities. *Environment:* 16%. Supports athletics and human services. *International:* 8%. Focus is on single-disease associations. *Note:* Total contributions made in 1999. **Typ. Recipients:** Cancer, Children's Health/Hospitals, Domestic Violence, Emergency/Ambulance Services, Medical Research, People with Disabilities, Single-Disease Health Associations. **Geo. Dist:** UT.

★ 11643 ★ Joseph Alexander Foundation

400 Madison Ave., Suite 906
New York, NY 10017
Phone: (212)355-3688
Robert Weintraub, President & Director

Fnded: 1960. **Philosophy:** The Joseph Alexander Foundation makes most of its grants in the areas of health, education, and social services. Health funding favors cancer and AIDS research and treatment, hospitals, and geriatric care. Educational support primarily goes to Jewish universities, medical education, and legal education. In social services, interests include the aged, the disabled, homes for children, family services, and community centers. The foundation also makes grants to other recipient areas. **Priorities:** *Arts & Humanities:* 9%. Historic preservation, museums. *Civic & Public Affairs:* 5%. Supports community foundations *Education:* 30%. Funds colleges and universities, Jewish studies, and education associations. *International:* 26%. Supports medical research, hospitals, single-disease health associations, and geriatric health. *Note:* Total contributions made in fiscal 2001. **Typ. Recipients:** AIDS/HIV, Alzheimers Disease, Cancer, Children's Health/Hospitals, Clinics/Medical Centers, Diabetes, Emergency/Ambulance Services, Eyes/Blindness, Family Planning, Geriatric Health, Health Funds, Health Organizations, Hospices, Hospitals, Kidney, Long-Term Care, Medical Education, Medical Rehabilitation, Medical Research, Mental Health, Multiple Sclerosis, Nursing Services, People with Disabilities, Single-Disease Health Associations, Substance Abuse, Transplant Networks/Donor Banks, Trauma Treatment. **Geo. Dist:** nationally; New York, NY.

★ 11644 ★ Joseph B. Whitehead Foundation

50 Hurt Plaza, Suite 1200
Atlanta, GA 30303
Phone: (404)522-6755 **Fax:** (404)522-7026
Email: fdns@woodruff.org
Website: http://www.jbwhitehead.org
Charles McTier, President

Fnded: 1937. **Philosophy:** The foundation was established with a particular interest in benefiting children. Its primary areas of giving include human services, particularly for children and youth; elementary and secondary education; health care; economic development and civic affairs; literacy and vocational training; art and cultural activities; and environmental education. **Priorities:** *Civic & Public Affairs:* 6%. Funds community foundations and housing. *Education:* 15%. Supports general education programs, primary and secondary schools, higher education, and special education. *Environment:* 71%. Supports United Way, YMCA, child/youth welfare, housing and shelter, care of elderly, and the disabled. *International:* 3%. Focus is on hospitals and medical care, public and preventive health, and general health. *Note:* Total contributions made in 2000. **Typ. Recipients:** Alzheimers Disease, Arthritis, Cancer, Child Abuse, Children's Health/Hospitals, Clinics/Medical Centers, Domestic Violence, Family Planning, Health Organizations, Health Policy/Cost Containment, Health-General, Home-Care Services, Hospitals, Kidney, Medical Rehabilitation, Mental Health, Nursing Services, People with Disabilities, Prenatal Health Issues, Preventive Medicine/Wellness Organizations, Public Health, Respiratory, Single-Disease Health Associations, Substance Abuse, Trauma Treatment. **Geo. Dist:** Atlanta, GA, including metropolitan area.

★ 11645 ★ Joseph and Bessie Feinberg Foundation

505 North Lake Shore Drive
Suite 1005
Chicago, IL 60611
Reuben Feinberg, President

Fnded: 1969. **Philosophy:** A majority of the foundation's funding goes to higher education in support of universities and Jewish theological seminaries. Jewish religious organizations are also a major interest. The foundation supports other charitable recipient organizations with minor grants. **Priorities:** *Arts & Humanities:* 3%. Funds public broadcasting, art festivals, performing arts, museums, and historical societies. *Civic & Public Affairs:* 1%. Gives to legal aid organizations, community development, and public policy organizations. *Education:* 66%. Funds colleges, universities, Jewish studies and theology education. *Environment:* Less than 1%. Children's charities and refugee assistance programs receive support. *International:* 12%. Supports medical centers, the Gastro Intestinal Research Foundation, and other disease and disorder concerns. *Note:* Total contributions made in fiscal 2000. **Typ. Recipients:** Children's Health/Hospitals, Clinics/Medical Centers, Health Organizations, Heart, Hospitals, Kidney, Medical Education, Medical Research, Multiple Sclerosis, People with Disabilities, Single-Disease Health Associations. **Geo. Dist:** Chicago, IL; NY.

★ 11646 ★ Joseph Drown Foundation

1999 Ave. of the Stars, Suite 1930
Los Angeles, CA 90067
Phone: (310)277-4488 **Fax:** (310)277-4573
Email: staff@jdrown.org
Website: http://www.jdrown.org
Wendy Wachtell, Vice President, Program Director

Fnded: 1953. **Philosophy:** The foundation's focus remains education and medical research. In education, it funds loan programs in higher education and reform programs in K-12. Some funding is also available for scholarships. The focus on medical and scientific research remains broad, but no unsolicited grant requests in this area are accepted. The grant-making in community health and social services is geared towards improving life in the local community. The focus is on programs that deal with issues such as high drop-out rates, teen pregnancy, lack of sufficient health care, substance abuse, and violence. The funding in the arts and humanities is limited to outreach and education. **Priorities:** *Arts & Humanities:* 2%. Primarily supports outreach and art education programs. *Civic & Public Affairs:* 3%. Supports legal defense and feminist efforts. *Education:* 30%. Supports public and private education. *Environment:* 11%. Gives to child welfare, youth organizations, and senior services. *International:* 51%. Primary support for single-disease health associations, medical research, and hospitals. *Note:* Total contributions made in fiscal 2000. **Typ. Recipients:** Adolescent Health Issues, Alzheimers Disease, Arthritis, Cancer, Children's Health/Hospitals, Clinics/Medical Centers, Diabetes, Emergency/Ambulance Services, Eyes/Blindness, Family Planning, Geriatric Health, Health Organizations, Health-General, Heart, Hospitals (University Affiliated), Long-Term Care, Medical Education, Medical Research, Mental Health, Outpatient Health Care, People with Disabilities, Preventive Medicine/Wellness Organizations, Research/Studies Institutes, Single-Disease Health Associations, Speech & Hearing, Substance Abuse. **Geo. Dist:** CA.

★ 11647 ★ Joseph Meyerhoff Fund

25 S Charles St.
Baltimore, MD 21201
Phone: (410)727-3200 **Fax:** (410)727-3207
Email: tmr@magnajm.com
Ms. Terry Rubenstein, Vice President & Secretary

Fnded: 1953. **Philosophy:** The fund supports a wide variety of charitable organizations. Jewish organizations are favored. Peace initiatives and interests in Israel also are major interests. A range of educational support is also given by the fund. **Priorities:** *Arts & Humanities:* 14%. Funds the symphony orchestra, public broadcasting, libraries, performing arts and the B&O Railroad Museum. *Civic & Public Affairs:* 3%. Funds parks, civic and community affairs. *Education:* 5%. Funds colleges, universities, and educational programs. *Environment:* 9%. Funds community services. *International:* 8%. Funds the Sinai Hospital Department for Development. *Religion:* 2%. *Note:* Contributions were made in 2000. **Typ. Recipients:** Hospitals, Speech & Hearing. **Geo. Dist:** Baltimore, MD; New York, NY.

★ 11648 ★ Joseph P. Kennedy, Jr. Foundation

1325 G St., Northwest, Suite 500
Washington, DC 20005-4709
Phone: (202)393-1250 **Fax:** (202)824-0351
Email: sswenson@specialolympics.org
Website: http://www.jpkf.org
Lucille Zeph, Executive Director

Fnded: 1946. **Philosophy:** "The Joseph P. Kennedy, Jr. Foundation believes that persons with mental retardation have the ability to live, learn, work, recreate, and worship like everyone else. We recognize that people with mental retardation may need assistance to do these things." "We believe that families of people with mental retardation, especially families of children with mental retardation, benefit from support and information to successfully include their family member in the everyday activities of their community." The foundation maintains two firm objectives: to seek the prevention of mental retardation by identifying its causes and to improve the means by which society deals with its citizens with mental retardation. To accomplish these objectives, the foundation has traditionally used its funds and influence in those areas in which a "multiplier effect" could be achieved. This is accomplished in these ways: "1. Enhance the quality of life of persons with mental retardation and their families." "2. Provide seed funding to capitalize on Federal and/or State or Local spending on behalf of persons with mental retardation and their families by funding initiatives that evolve beyond where existing programs are going, and do not duplicate public efforts." "3. Increase professional and public awareness of the needs of persons with mental retardation and their families." "4. Work to reduce the incidence of mental retardation." The foundation supports a variety of demonstration programs in newly-defined areas in the field of mental retardation with the hope that the programs will be replicable on a wide scale to benefit persons with mental retardation and their families. Recent grants have supported projects relating to access to medical care and the use of drugs by pregnant teens. Reflecting a growing awareness of the importance of the ethical implications of mental retardation, the foundation also has funded major intellectual and training efforts in the broad area of bioethics. Another major area of concern is teen pregnancy. Because a significant cause of mental retardation is prematurity and low birth weight among the newborn babies of adolescents, the foundation developed a values-based curriculum, "A Community of Caring," for use in programs for pregnant teens in clinics, hospitals, agencies, or schools. The program is currently being implemented to address pregnancy prevention and examine other high-risk behavior by youth. Small one-time grants may be provided to civic and public affairs organizations each year. The foundation also reports that it is decreasing activity in the sciences and focusing more upon projects which help integrate persons with mental retardation into community life, as well as on projects which empower persons with mental retardation. Programs focusing on family support; health care and oral health; and self advocacy will be highlighted in future funding priorities. **Priorities:** *Arts & Humanities:* 13%. Museums. *Civic & Public Affairs:* 14%. Supports public policy groups that deal with the disabled. *Education:* 27%. Primarily for special education and job training projects. *Environment:* 19%. Focus on programs for people with disabilities. *International:* 18%. Supports hospitals, people with disabilities and health organizations. *Note:* Total contributions made in fiscal 2000. **Typ. Recipients:** Children's Health/Hospitals, Clinics/Medical Centers, Family Planning, Health Policy/Cost Containment, Hospitals, Medical Education, Medical Research, Medical Training, Mental Health, People with Disabilities, Prenatal Health Issues, Preventive Medicine/Wellness Organizations, Substance Abuse. **Geo. Dist:** nationally.

★ 11649 ★ Josiah Macy, Jr. Foundation

44 East 64th St.
New York, NY 10021
Phone: (212)486-2424 **Fax:** (212)644-0765
Website: http://www.josiahmacyfoundation.org/jmacy1.html
Martha Wolfgang, Vice President

Fnded: 1930. **Philosophy:** Traditionally, the Macy Foundation has focused on medicine and health. This stems from Mrs. Ladd's personal interest in these areas. Her instructions, intended to guide the foundation's giving, were concerned with "fundamental aspects of health, of sickness, and of methods for the relief of suffering." "Today the Foundation focuses support on issues that challenge the education of health professionals, such as the increasing need for teamwork, the provision of primary care in the changing environment of health-care management and delivery, and the increasing need for diversity of health-care professionals. In addition, some programs address the fundamental shifts in medical and other health professional education necessitated by the rapid rate of advance in such areas as human genetics." Two recent conferences sponsored by the Foundation focused on ways to improve working relationships between medicine and public health, and the growing challenge of health education posed by rapid advances in genetics. 1997 annual report **Priorities:** *Civic & Public Affairs:* 2%. Includes support for other foundations or community programs. *Education:* 57%. Includes support for colleges and universities. *International:* 29%. Includes support for medical training, nursing, health policy organizations, and health professionals training. *Religion:* 12%. Includes support for laboratories. *Note:* Total contributions made in fiscal 2001. **Typ. Recipients:** AIDS/HIV, Cancer, Children's Health/Hospitals, Clinics/Medical Centers, Family Planning, Health Funds, Health Organizations, Health Policy/Cost Containment, Health-General, Hospitals, Hospitals (University Affiliated), Medical Education, Medical Research, Medical Research, Medical Training, Nursing Services, Public Health, Single-Disease Health Associations, Substance Abuse. **Geo. Dist:** nationally.

★ 11650 ★ Josiah W. and Bessie H. Kline Foundation

515 S 29th St.
Harrisburg, PA 17104
Phone: (717)561-4373 **Fax:** (717)561-0826
John Obrock, Secretary

Fnded: 1952. **Philosophy:** The foundation makes most of its grants in the areas of education, health, and social services in south-central Pennsylvania. Educational funding supports various small colleges and universities in Pennsylvania. Health interests include medical centers, health foundations, and hospitals. Social service support goes to community centers, family services, and youth organizations. The foundation also makes grants to the arts and civic affairs in south-central Pennsylvania. **Priorities:** *Arts & Humanities:* 22%. Funds public broadcasting, theater, opera, and libraries. *Education:* 26%. Emphasis on Pennsylvania Colleges and Universities, minority education and public education. *Environment:* 45%. Primary support given to organizations such as United Way, the Pennsylvannia Special Olympics, organizations that support crippled children. food banks and scouting. *International:* 1%. Supports health associations. *Note:* Total contributions made in 2000. **Typ. Recipients:** Alzheimers Disease, Arthritis, Cancer, Children's Health/Hospitals, Clinics/Medical Centers, Diabetes, Emergency/Ambulance Services, Family Planning, Health Organizations, Health-General, Heart, Hospices, Hospitals, Kidney, Medical Rehabilitation, Medical Research, Mental Health, Multiple Sclerosis, Nursing Services, Outpatient Health Care, People with Disabilities, Public Health, Single-Disease Health Associations, Substance Abuse. **Geo. Dist:** PA.

★ 11651 ★ Joukowsky Family Foundation

410 Park Ave., Suite 1610
New York, NY 10022
Phone: (212)355-3151 **Fax:** (212)355-3147
Email: info@joukowsky.org
Website: http://www.joukowsky.org
Nina Joukowsky-Koprulu, Director & President

Fnded: 1981. **Philosophy:** The Joukowsky Family Foundation makes most of its grants in the area of education. Additional funding is available for civic affairs, the arts, health care, international affairs, religion, and social services. **Priorities:** *Arts & Humanities:* 6%. Historical associations and music. *Education:* 82%. Primary support for colleges and universities and preparatory schools. *Environment:* 5%. Supports united funds, family planning, child welfare, and the homeless. *Note:* Contributions made in fiscal 2001. **Typ. Recipients:** Diabetes, Domestic Violence, Family Planning, Hospices, Hospitals, Medical Education, Medical Rehabilitation, Medical Research, People with Disabilities, Single-Disease Health Associations. **Geo. Dist:** U.S. Northeast Region; internationally; nationally. **Frmly:** The Joukowsky Foundation.

★ 11652 ★ Joyce Foundation

3 First National Plaza
70 West Madison St., Suite 2750
Chicago, IL 60602
Phone: (312)782-2464 **Fax:** (312)782-4160
Email: info@joycefdn.org
Website: http://www.joycefdn.org
Ellen Alberding, President

Fnded: 1948. **Philosophy:** "The Joyce Foundation supports efforts to protect the natural environment of the Great Lakes, to reduce poverty and violence in the region, and to ensure that its people have access to good schools, decent jobs, and a diverse and thriving culture. We are especially interested in improving public policies, because public systems such as education and welfare directly affect the lives of so many people, and because public policiees help shape private sector decisions about jobs, the environment, and the health of our communities. To ensure that public policies truly reflect public rather than private interests, we support efforts to reform the system of financing election campaigns. Our current program areas are: Employment Program: improve public policies around welfare-to-work, problems of low-wage workers entering and moving up in the job market, helping the hard-to-employ gain job skills, improve job retention and stability, increase resources for and access to quality training and education programs that lead to higher-paying jobs; Environment: Greak Lakes water issues including water quality and water quantity, water infrastructure, climate change, and pros and cons of privatizing water systems, clean energy and transportation; Gun Violence: focuses on a public health approach to reducing gun injuries and deaths in the US, achieve comprehensive federal health and safety oversight of the firearms industry including both federal and Midwestern state policies; Money and Politics: judicial reform, public interest obligations of broadcasters, campaign finance reform especially in the Midwest, and Culture: increase participation of people of color in major cultural institutions, increase cultural programming in communities, including stabilizing culturally specific art groups, encourage major institutions to develop new work that is relevant to minority audiences. We focus our grantmaking on initiatives that promise to have an impact on the Great Lakes region, specifically the states of Illinois, Indiana, Iowa, Michigan, Minnesota, Ohio and Wisconsin. A limited number of environment grants are made to organizations in Canada. Education grantmaking focuses on public schools in Chicago, Cleveland and Milwaukee. Culture grants are restricted to the Chicago metropolitan area." Joyce Foundation 2000 Annual Report **Priorities:** *Arts & Humanities:* 2%. Supports museums, theater, and music organizations. *Civic & Public Affairs:* 28%. Funds employment, policies to prevent gun violence, and money and politics initiatives. *Education:* 25%. Supports organizations promoting education reform, minority education, and colleges and universities. *Environment:* 11%. Funds gun violence prevention programs. *Note:* Total contributions made in 2000. **Typ. Recipients:** Adolescent Health Issues, Emergency/Ambulance Services, Health Policy/Cost Containment, Medical Education, Public Health. **Geo. Dist:** IL; Chicago, IL; IN; IA; MI; MN; OH; WI.

★ 11653 ★ Joyce Mertz-Gilmore Foundation

218 East 18th St.
New York, NY 10003-3694
Phone: (212)475-1137 **Fax:** (212)777-5226
Email: info@mertzgilmore.org
Website: http://www.mertzgilmore.org
Jay Beckner, Executive Director

Fnded: 1959. **Philosophy:** "The Joyce Mertz-Gilmore Foundation has environment, human rights, peace and security, and New York City grantmaking programs. The Foundation prefers to make general support grants to organizations whose work closely parallels its interests. The Foundation also supports specific programs or projects when appropriate." Environment: "The Foundation supports organizations promoting increased energy efficiency and the development and use of renewable energy sources for the future. Key areas of interest include: promoting efficiency and renewables through revision of state and local utility regulations and sound national policies; increasing public awareness and interest in energy efficiency; and promoting renewable energy in developing countries." Human Rights: "The Foundation supports organizations which investigate and publicize human rights abuses, advocate non-political applications of international human rights law, encourage the free flow of information within and between countries or work to build the capacity of non-governmental human rights groups in developing countries, Central Europe and former Soviet republics. The Foundation supports policy efforts, advocacy and information dissemination related to the fair and humane treatment of the growing, worldwide refugee population. The Foundation also promotes development approaches which draws upon resources and knowledge of the refugees themselves, and empowers refugees to press for their own needs and rights. The Foundation supports national or regional efforts to protect and extend the rights of immigrants and refugees, and lesbian and gay men. The Foundation makes grants to groups which undertake advocacy and policy work, citizen awareness activities and/or litigation to establish clear precedents for protecting the civil rights of these groups. The Foundation supports voluntary sector capacity- and infrastructure-building in Central Europe and the former Soviet republics." New York City Human and Built Environment: "The Foundation supports HIV/AIDS public education and policy work with and emphasis on the involvement of underserved communities in the policy making process. The Foundation supports efforts to ensure that all New Yorkers have access to public parks, open space, waterfronts and green spaces in their neighborhoods, emphasizing the relationship between public spaces and community development and stabilization. The Foundation supports technical assistance providers working with community-based organizations. The Foundation supports organizations making small grants and/or providing technical assistance and training programs for local community leadership and resource development in underserved neighborhoods." **Priorities:** *Arts & Humanities:* 3%. New York City Dance. *Civic & Public Affairs:* 45%. Supports the New York City Human and Built Environment program, international human rights, immigrant, gay, and lesbian rights in the United States. *Education:* 1%. *Environment:* 2%. *Religion:* 1%. *Note:* Total contributions made in 2000. **Typ. Recipients:** AIDS/HIV, Hospitals (University Affiliated). **Geo. Dist:** internationally; nationally; New York, NY.

★ 11654 ★ Judd S. Alexander Foundation

PO Box 2137
Wausau, WI 54402-2137
Phone: (715)845-4556 **Fax:** (715)848-9336
Website: http://www.juddsalexanderfoundation.org
Gary Freels, President

Fnded: 1973. **Philosophy:** The Judd S. Alexander Foundation makes most of its grants in the areas of social services and civic affairs. Social service interests include youth organizations, recreation, and human development. In civic affairs, funding favors community philanthropic organizations, economic development, and municipalities. Other areas of interest include health care, the arts, and education. **Priorities:** *Arts & Humanities:* 2%. Performing arts, museums, and music. *Civic & Public Affairs:* 76%. Chambers of commerce, county services. *Education:* 13%. Precollege and college education. *Environment:* 9%. Big Brothers, children and youth services. *International:* Approx. 1%. *Note:* Total contributions made in fiscal 2001. **Typ. Recipients:** Cancer, Clinics/Medical Centers, Health Funds, Heart, Hospices, Hospitals, Medical Training, People with Disabilities, Public Health, Respiratory, Single-Disease Health Associations. **Geo. Dist:** programs that directly affect and benefit the residents of Marathon County.

★ 11655 ★ Judy and Michael Steinhardt Foundation

650 Madison Ave., 17th Floor
New York, NY 10022
Phone: (212)371-7300
Michael Steinhardt, Trustee

Fnded: 1986. **Priorities:** *Civic & Public Affairs:* 19%. Supports the Steinhardt Family Foundation and miscellaneous civic causes. *Education:* 15%. Funds colleges and universities. *Note:* Total contributions made in fiscal 2000. **Typ. Recipients:** Cancer, Children's Health/Hospitals, Clinics/Medical Centers, Family Planning, Health Organizations, Hospitals, Nutrition, People with Disabilities. **Geo. Dist:** NY.

★ 11656 ★ Julius Frankel Foundation

PO Box 755, Tax Div.
Chicago, IL 60690
Phone: (312)461-2655
John Georgas, Contact

Fnded: 1959. **Philosophy:** The foundation principally supports the arts, concentrating on music and dance; higher education; hospitals and health organizations; and social welfare groups. **Priorities:** *Arts & Humanities:* 32%. Supports museums, opera, symphonies, and ballet. *Civic & Public Affairs:* 3%. Funds youth job programs, housing programs, and community foundations. *Education:* 23%. Emphasis on schools and institutes. *Environment:* 13%. Grants are made to youth centers and programs, and family services. *International:* 24%. Supports hospitals, medical centers, and rehabilitation centers. *Religion:* 5%. Science museum. *Note:* Total contributions made in fiscal 2001. **Typ. Recipients:** Children's Health/Hospitals, Clinics/Medical Centers, Hospices, Hospitals, Hospitals (University Affiliated), Long-Term Care, Medical Education, Medical Rehabilitation, Medical Rehabilitation, Medical Research, People with Disabilities, Public Health, Speech & Hearing, Substance Abuse. **Geo. Dist:** IL.

★ 11657 ★ June Rockwell Levy Foundation

175 Federal St.
Boston, MA 02110
Phone: (617)482-5270
Jonathan Loring, President

Fnded: 1947. **Philosophy:** The June Rockwell Levy Foundation supports a variety of charitable organizations. Health care support favors general hospitals and medical foundations. Private education and colleges are favored for educational support. All areas of social services and civic affairs are supported by the foundation. The arts and international organizations receive minor support. **Priorities:** *Arts & Humanities:* 32%. Supports public libraries, repertory theater, museums, the philharmonic, and symphony orchestras. *Civic & Public Affairs:* 9%. Supports community and civic affairs. *Education:* 14%. Supports educational institutions, services, and programs. *Environment:* 18%. Supports family services, Planned Parenthood, United Way, animal shelters, and social services. *International:* 17%. Supports hospitals, rehabilitation centers, and disease and disorder concerns. *Note:* Contributions were made in 1998. **Typ. Recipients:** AIDS/HIV, Cancer, Children's Health/Hospitals, Clinics/Medical Centers, Diabetes, Domestic Violence, Emergency/Ambulance Services, Family Planning, Geriatric Health, Health Funds, Health Organizations, Home-Care Services, Hospices, Hospitals, Long-Term Care, Medical Education, Medical Education, Medical Rehabilitation, Medical Research, Mental Health, Nursing Services, People with Disabilities, Public Health, Sexual Abuse, Single-Disease Health Associations, Substance Abuse. **Geo. Dist:** MA; RI.

★ 11658 ★ Jurodin Fund

PO Box 4120
Greenwich, CT 06831
Fax: (203)531-1790
Irene Steiner, Secretary

Fnded: 1960. **Philosophy:** The Jurodin Fund primarily supports education and religious organizations. Education funding favors colleges and legal education. Jewish religious organizations are also a major priority. Secondary interests include medical centers, civic affairs, and the arts. **Priorities:** *Arts & Humanities:* Less than 1%. Contributes to museums, music, libraries, and public broadcasting. *Education:* 99%. Major grant to New York University; also funds other colleges and universities. *Environment:* Less than 1%. Supports United Way. *International:* Less than 1%. Funds hospitals, a cancer center, and a vision health organization. *Note:* Total contributions made in 2000. **Typ. Recipients:** Cancer, Clinics/Medical Centers, Emergency/Ambulance Services, Eyes/Blindness, Family Planning, Health Organizations, Hospitals, Medical Education, Medical Rehabilitation, Medical Research, Nursing Services, People with Disabilities, Single-Disease Health Associations. **Geo. Dist:** U.S. Northeast Region; New York, NY.

★ 11659 ★ Kansas Health Foundation

309 East Douglas
Wichita, KS 67202-3405
Phone: (316)262-7676 **Fax:** (316)262-2044
Email: nclaassen@khf.org
Website: http://www.kansashealth.org
Nancy Claassen, Grants Manager

Fnded: 1978. **Philosophy:** The Foundation has three program finding categories: Public Health, Leadership, and Children's Health. The Public Health mission is "to develop and support population-based health in Kansas so preventative measures are utilized to improve the health of Kansans." The Leadership mission is "to build the capacity of individuals to improve the health of all Kansans." The Children's Health mission is "to improve the health of Kansans by creating an environment that puts children first so they become caring, thinking and contributing adults." 2000 Annual Report. **Priorities:** *International:* 71%. Funds public health and childrens health. *Note:* Total contributions made in 2001. **Typ. Recipients:** Adolescent Health Issues, AIDS/HIV, Alzheimers Disease, Cancer, Child Abuse, Children's Health/Hospitals, Clinics/Medical Centers, Domestic Violence, Emergency/Ambulance Services, Geriatric Health, Health Organizations, Health Policy/Cost Containment, Health-General, Heart, Home-Care Services, Hospices, Hospitals, Hospitals (University

Affiliated), Medical Education, Medical Rehabilitation, Medical Research, Medical Training, Nursing Services, Nutrition, People with Disabilities, Prenatal Health Issues, Preventive Medicine/Wellness Organizations, Public Health, Research/Studies Institutes, Respiratory, Sexual Abuse, Substance Abuse. **Geo. Dist:** KS.

★ 11660 ★ Kaplen Foundation

PO Box 792
Tenafly, NJ 07670-0792
Phone: (201)227-0722
Wilson Kaplen, Trustee

Fnded: 1963. **Typ. Recipients:** Children's Health/Hospitals, Clinics/Medical Centers, Emergency/Ambulance Services, Hospitals, Medical Education, Medical Rehabilitation, Medical Research, Mental Health, People with Disabilities, Public Health, Single-Disease Health Associations, Substance Abuse. **Geo. Dist:** NJ.

★ 11661 ★ Kate B. Reynolds Charitable Trust

PO Box 3099
Winston-Salem, NC 27150-6732
Phone: (336)732-5252 **Fax:** (336)723-7765
Website: http://www.kbr.org
E. Cope, President

Fnded: 1947. **Philosophy:** Three-quarters of the total income from the trust is expended through the Health Care Division, which supports innovative health care programs throughout North Carolina, with the remaining 25% of contributions being disbursed through the Poor and Needy Division. Each division has its own advisory board to provide guidance on plans and priorities for the use of funds and to review and recommend approval of specific grant requests. The Health Care Division funds are used to encourage and support innovative programs that increase the availability of health services to under-served groups. This division also provides support for other types of health programs which have merit and which are related to the goal of the division. The Poor and Needy Division funds are used to support organizations which provide for basic needs, such as food, clothing, shelter, and health care. The division also funds efforts that seek to reduce reliance upon support services or that promote maximum levels of functioning for those with chronic problems, and supports other types of programs that have merit and are related to the goal of the division. **Priorities:** *Environment:* 25%. Funds programs that help the financially needy people of Winston-Salem and Forsyth counties. Trust's objectives are to provide for basic needs (food, clothing, shelter, and healthcare), to fund efforts that seek to reduce reliance upon support services, or that promote maximum levels of functioning for those with chronic problems. *International:* 75%. Funds programs that help improve the health of financially needy people in North Carolina. Trust's objectives are to increase the availability of health services to underserved groups, promote good health and prevent illness, and support well-conceived studies that clearly define health problems in North Carolina. *Note:* Total contributions made in fiscal 2001. **Typ. Recipients:** Adolescent Health Issues, AIDS/HIV, Alzheimers Disease, Cancer, Children's Health/Hospitals, Clinics/Medical Centers, Diabetes, Domestic Violence, Emergency/Ambulance Services, Family Planning, Geriatric Health, Health Organizations, Health Policy/Cost Containment, Health-General, Heart, Home-Care Services, Hospices, Hospitals, Long-Term Care, Medical Education, Medical Rehabilitation, Mental Health, Nursing Services, Outpatient Health Care, People with Disabilities, Prenatal Health Issues, Preventive Medicine/Wellness Organizations, Public Health, Single-Disease Health Associations, Speech & Hearing, Substance Abuse. **Geo. Dist:** NC, Forsyth County: grants for the poor and needy; NC, health care grants.

★ 11662 ★ Katherine Mabis McKenna Foundation

PO Box 185
Latrobe, PA 15650
Phone: (724)537-6900 **Fax:** (724)537-6906
Linda Boxx, Chairman

Fnded: 1969. **Philosophy:** The Katherine Mabis McKenna Foundation makes grants across the major categories of support. Grants are made primarily to the environment and youth services in western Pennsylvania. **Priorities:** *Arts & Humanities:* 13%. Supports museums, libraries and historical preservation. *Civic & Public Affairs:* 34%. Funds gardens, parks and community foundations. *Education:* 33%. Supports education foundation, local school districts, colleges and universities. *Environment:* 7%. Supports Big Brothers, Big Sisters, scouting and United Way. *Religion:* approx. 1%. Supports science center. *Note:* Contributions were made in 2000. **Typ. Recipients:** Arthritis, Cancer, Emergency/Ambulance Services, Hospitals, Medical Rehabilitation, People with Disabilities, Research/Studies Institutes, Single-Disease Health Associations. **Geo. Dist:** PA, Eastern Westmoreland County.

★ 11663 ★ Kelly Gene Cook, Sr. Charitable Foundation

278 Waterford Way
Montgomery, TX 77356
Phone: (936)449-6272
Email: pegpool@aol.com
Peggy Pool, President

Fnded: 1986. **Philosophy:** The foundation supports higher education, primarily through scholarship programs. Designated programs are coordinated through the financial aid offices at Millsaps College, the University of Mississippi, and Mississippi State University. Other contributions are made on a limited basis to other institutions. **Priorities:** *Civic & Public Affairs:* About 1%. *Education:* 67%. Supports educational institutions and programs including scholarships to colleges and universities. *Environment:* 27%. Supports youth and family services. *International:* 5%. Supports the Mental Health Association. *Note:* Total contributions made in 2001. **Typ. Recipients:** Domestic Violence, Medical Education, Medical Training, Mental Health, People with Disabilities, Substance Abuse. **Geo. Dist:** internationally; nationally; MS.

★ 11664 ★ Kelvin and Eleanor Smith Foundation

26380 Curtiss Wright Parkway, Suite 105
Cleveland, OH 44143
Phone: (216)289-5789 **Fax:** (216)289-5948
Carol Zett, Grants Manager

Fnded: 1955. **Philosophy:** "The Foundation's principal interests are in the fields of non-sectarian education, the free enterprise system, the performing and visual arts, health care, and other activities of the type supported by the United Way Services of Cleveland. Grants may be made in support of current operations or for special projects; grants for endowment are not made." **Priorities:** *Arts & Humanities:* 36%. Supports museums, public radio, theater, opera, and arts associations. *Civic & Public Affairs:* 35%. Funds botanical gardens, parks, orboretums, and career guidance. *Education:* 16%. Contributes to colleges, universities, arts/music education, and private pre-college schools. *Environment:* 4%. Supports child welfare, shelters, and animal welfare organizations. *International:* 7%. Gives to hospitals, hospice programs, clinics, and nursing homes. *Religion:* 2%. Science centers receive foundation funding. *Note:* Total contributions made in fiscal 2000. **Typ. Recipients:** Cancer, Children's Health/Hospitals, Clinics/Medical Centers, Eyes/Blindness, Family Planning, Health Organizations, Hospices, Hospitals (University Affiliated), Medical Education, Medical Rehabilitation, Mental Health, Nursing Services, People with Disabilities, Prenatal Health Issues, Speech & Hearing, Substance Abuse. **Geo. Dist:** Cleveland, OH, metropolitan area.

★ 11665 ★ Kenneth T. and Eileen L. Norris Foundation

11 Golden Shore, Suite 450
Long Beach, CA 90802
Phone: (562)435-8444 **Fax:** (562)436-0584
Email: gerringer@ktn.org
Website: http://www.norrisfoundation.org
Ronald Barnes, Executive Director & Trustee

Fnded: 1963. **Philosophy:** When the foundation was established in 1963, grants were focused in two areas: medicine and private education in Southern California. However, "Today's Norris Foundation continues to allocate large portions of its resources to medicine and education but encompasses a broader agenda–one that also includes community and youth programs, science and the arts. In each program area, the sure hand of Ken Norris has shaped the results, producing a pattern of giving designed to encourage, extend, reconfigure or transform projects originating from a diverse assortment of nonprofit recipients." Norris Foundation 1995-1996 Annual Report **Priorities:** *Arts & Humanities:* 13%. Funds theaters, libraries, and museums. *Civic & Public Affairs:* 3%. Supports Las Floristas. *Education:* 39%. Supports colleges and universities; emphasis on medical education. *Environment:* 4%. Emphasis on youth organizations. *International:* 39%. Primary support for the Norris Cancer Center, hospitals and medical centers, single-disease health associations, and pediatric health. *Religion:* 1%. Funds a natural history museum and college scientist achievement rewards. *Note:* Total contributions made in fiscal 1999. **Typ. Recipients:** AIDS/HIV, Alzheimers Disease, Cancer, Children's Health/Hospitals, Clinics/Medical Centers, Diabetes, Emergency/Ambulance Services, Eyes/Blindness, Family Planning, Health Organizations, Heart, Hospices, Hospitals, Kidney, Medical Education, Medical Rehabilitation, Medical Research, People with Disabilities, Research/Studies Institutes, Respiratory, Single-Disease Health Associations, Speech & Hearing, Substance Abuse, Trauma Treatment. **Geo. Dist:** CA, Los Angeles County area.

★ 11666 ★ Kentland Foundation

PO Box 879
Berryville, VA 22611-1082
Phone: (540)955-1268 **Fax:** (540)955-4942
Helene Walker, President

Fnded: 1966. **Philosophy:** The Kentland Foundation makes most of its grants to education and religion. Funding favors literacy, religious education, universities, and parochial education. Other significant interests include youth organizations, housing, churches, and health services. **Priorities:** *Civic & Public Affairs:* 1%. *Education:* 29%. Funds pre-college parochial education. *Environment:* 5%. Funds scouting. *International:* 5%. Gives to hospitals and hospice. *Note:* Contributions made in 2000. **Typ. Recipients:** Cancer, Children's Health/Hospitals, Clinics/Medical Centers, Domestic Violence, Emergency/Ambulance Services, Family Planning, Health Funds, Hospices, Hospitals, Long-Term Care, Medical Education, Medical Research, Nutrition, People with Disabilities, Prenatal Health Issues, Preventive Medicine/Wellness Organizations, Preventive Medicine/Wellness Organizations, Public Health, Research/Studies Institutes, Sexual Abuse. **Geo. Dist:** mid-Atlantic states.

★ 11667 ★ Kern Foundation Trust

50 S LsSalle St., L-5
Chicago, IL 60675
Phone: (312)630-6000 **Fax:** (312)444-4122
Email: dgr@ntrs.com
Dale Rudy, Contact

Fnded: 1959. **Philosophy:** The Kern Foundation Trust's aim is to support "the dissemination of the theosophical philosophy as broadly as possible, in a non-proselytizing, non-propagandizing manner." **Priorities:** *Education:* 5%. *Note:* Total contributions made in 1998. **Typ. Recipients:** People with Disabilities. **Geo. Dist:** CA; IL.

★ 11668 ★ Kerr Foundation, Inc.

12501 North May Ave.
Oklahoma City, OK 73120
Phone: (405)749-7991 **Fax:** (405)749-2877
Email: aholz@thekerrfoundation.org
Website: http://www.thekerrfoundation.org
Robert Kerr, Jr., Chairman of Board

Fnded: 1963. **Philosophy:** The foundation's main concern is to support organizations and institutions that provide new or enhanced opportunities to Oklahomans and the Southwest region, particularly the young. The stated areas of interest are "education, health, cultural development, and community service." **Priorities:** *Arts & Humanities:* 21%. Funds museums, art funds, and cultural and historic preservation. *Civic & Public Affairs:* 6%. Gives to public policy organizations and community groups. *Education:* 47%. Supports colleges, universities, education funds, and scholarships. *Environment:* 11%. Funds shelters, youth groups, and senior concerns. *International:* 6%. Contributes to health centers and associations. *Religion:* 6%. *Note:* Total contributions made in 2000. **Typ. Recipients:** Cancer, Children's Health/Hospitals, Clinics/Medical Centers, Domestic Violence, Emergency/Ambulance Services, Family Planning, Geriatric Health, Health Organizations, Health-General, Hospitals (University Affiliated), Medical Education, Mental Health, People with Disabilities, Prenatal Health Issues, Public Health, Single-Disease Health Associations, Substance Abuse. **Geo. Dist:** OK.

★ 11669 ★ Kettering Fund

1560 Kettering Tower
Dayton, OH 45423
Phone: (937)228-1021 **Fax:** (937)449-7239
Email: ketteringfund@aol.com
Judy Thompson, Executive Director

Fnded: 1958. **Philosophy:** The fund supports groups furthering "general philanthropy with an emphasis in higher education and cultural development." **Priorities:** *Arts & Humanities:* About 11%. Supports art museums and foundations and Carillon Historical Park. *Civic & Public Affairs:* 26%. Zoos and parks, urban affairs, and civic institutions. *Education:* 42%. Supports higher education. *Environment:* 7%. Focus is on youth activities. *International:* 10%. Supports single-disease health associations, and medical centers. *Religion:* Less than 1%. Funds National Aviation Hall of Fame. *Note:* Total contributions made in fiscal 2000. **Typ. Recipients:** Arthritis, Children's Health/Hospitals, Clinics/Medical Centers, Emergency/Ambulance Services, Family Planning, Health Organizations, Hospices, Hospitals, Long-Term Care, Medical Education, Nursing Services, People with Disabilities, Public Health, Transplant Networks/Donor Banks. **Geo. Dist:** OH, especially Dayton.

★ 11670 ★ Kiplinger Foundation

1729 H St., Northwest
Washington, DC 20006
Phone: (202)887-6559 **Fax:** (202)496-1817
Andrea Wilkes, Secretary

Fnded: 1948. **Philosophy:** The Kiplinger Foundation makes most of its grants in the areas of education, civic affairs, and the arts. Funding for education is primarily limited to matching gifts made by employees to educational institutions. There is no scholarship funding available. In civic affairs, interests include journalism centers and press associations. Funding for the arts goes to music schools, performing arts, museums, galleries, historic preservation, and theater. Grants also are made to other recipient areas such as welfare and social services, youth agencies, and health organizations on a more limited basis. **Priorities:** *Arts & Humanities:* 22%. Funds symphonies, historical societies, museums, opera, ballet, and arts centers. *Civic & Public Affairs:* 6%. Includes funding for the National Press Foundation. *Education:* 69%. Support mostly given in the form of matching gifts to universities, public and private secondary schools, and education committees. *Environment:* 2%. Supports the United Way, shelters, food banks, and community services. *International:* 1%. Supports health programs. *Note:* Total contributions made in 2000. **Typ. Recipients:** Cancer, Children's Health/Hospitals, Emergency/Ambulance Services, Family Planning, Health Organizations, Hospices, Hospitals, Medical Rehabilitation, Mental Health, Nursing Services, People with Disabilities, Public Health, Research/Studies Institutes, Sexual Abuse, Substance Abuse. **Geo. Dist:** Washington, DC, including metropolitan area.

★ 11671 ★ Kirkpatrick Foundation, Inc.

1200 NW 63rd, Suite 500
PO Box 268822
Oklahoma City, OK 73126-8822
Phone: (405)840-2882 **Fax:** (405)840-2946
Email: kfi@compuserve.com
Susan Shaw-McCalmont, Executive Director

Fnded: 1955. **Philosophy:** The Kirkpatrick Foundation makes most of its grants in the areas of civic affairs, the arts and cultural programs, education, and social services. Educational support mainly goes to precollegiate programs. In social services, interests include youth organizations, and child welfare. An emphasis is placed on sharing information between educational and social service organizations. **Priorities:** *Arts & Humanities:* 81%.Supports a variety of art organizations in Oklahoma City. *Education:* 22%. Primary support for arts education. *Religion:* Less than 1%. *Note:* Total contributions made in 2000 **Typ. Recipients:** Children's Health/Hospitals, Clinics/Medical Centers, Domestic Violence, Emergency/Ambulance Services, Family Planning, Heart, Hospitals, Medical Education, Medical Research, People with Disabilities, Public Health, Single-Disease Health Associations. **Geo. Dist:** Oklahoma City, OK, including metropolitan area. **Frmly:** Kirkpatrick Foundation.

★ 11672 ★ Knapp Foundation, Inc. (MD)

PO Box O
Saint Michaels, MD 21663
Phone: (410)745-5660
Antoinette Vojvoda, President

Fnded: 1929. **Philosophy:** The Knapp Foundation makes most of its grants in the areas of "wildlife conservation projects and college and university library projects. Several small contributions are disbursed each year that represent a predetermined group of organizations that the foundation has supported for fifty years or more." **Priorities:** *Arts & Humanities:* About 2%. Museums. *Civic & Public Affairs:* 8%. Primarily to aquariums and botanical gardens. *Education:* 17%. Supports colleges and universities. *Environment:* 3%. Primarily for youth organizations and the disabled. *International:* 1%. Supports the American Foundation for the Blind. *Religion:* 7%. Funds natural science museums. *Note:* Total contributions made in 1999. **Typ. Recipients:** Cancer, Children's Health/Hospitals, Emergency/Ambulance Services, Hospitals, Medical Education, People with Disabilities, Research/Studies Institutes, Single-Disease Health Associations. **Geo. Dist:** East-coast states.

★ 11673 ★ Koch Foundation, Inc.

2830 Northwest 41st St., Suite H
Gainesville, FL 32606
Phone: (352)373-7491 **Fax:** (352)337-1548
Michael Marconi, Executive Director

Fnded: 1979. **Philosophy:** "The Koch Foundation provides financial support for evangelization efforts to official Catholic organizations throughout the world that propagate the Roman Catholic faith. Grants are made for direct evangelization programs, education and spiritual formation of evangelists, resource-poor Catholic schools that are the principal means of evangelization in the community, a Catholic presence in the media, and capital expenditures; such as, construction and repair of churches or formation centers. In capital expenditures, priority is given to situations involving financially distressed, underdeveloped areas." *Women in Faith & Action: Koch Foundation, Inc. 2001 Annual Report* **Priorities:** *Arts & Humanities:* 6%. Funds Catholic mass media projects. *Education:* 4%. Supports Catholic schools. *Note:* Total contributions made in 2001. **Typ. Recipients:** Prenatal Health Issues. **Geo. Dist:** internationally; nationally.

★ 11674 ★ Kohlberg Foundation

111 Radio Cir.
Mount Kisco, NY 10549
Phone: (914)242-2388
Nancy White-McCabe, Executive Director

Fnded: 1989. **Priorities:** *Arts & Humanities:* 12%. Gives to performing arts organizations, art museums, libraries, history/preservation organizations, and film. *Civic & Public Affairs:* 37%. Supports grantmakers associations, consumer services, zoos, legal aid, fire departments, municipalities, and philanthropic organizations. *Education:* 2%. Contributes to public schools; art, sports, and environmental education; law schools, and education funds. *Environment:* 4%. Funds day care, sports and recreation programs, youth activities, and child and family services. *International:* 10%. Gives to cancer research organizations, cancer centers, single-disease health associations, pediatric health organizations, hospitals, ambulance services, and hospices. *Religion:* 24%. Supports biological and environmental research. *Note:* Total contributions made in 2001. **Typ. Recipients:** Cancer, Children's Health/Hospitals, Clinics/Medical Centers, Diabetes, Family Planning, Health-General, Hospitals, Mental Health, Research/Studies Institutes, Single-Disease Health Associations, Speech & Hearing. **Geo. Dist:** nationally.

★ 11675 ★ Kohler Foundation

725 Woodlake Rd., Suite X
Kohler, WI 53044
Phone: (920)458-1972 **Fax:** (920)458-4280
Email: terriyoho@kohler.com
Terri Yohoi, Executive Director

Fnded: 1940. **Philosophy:** The foundation makes grants primarily for education and cultural programs in Wisconsin. The foundation also funds a scholarship program for higher education of Sheboygan County, WI, residents studying the arts. **Priorities:** *Arts & Humanities:* 67%. Supports performing arts, art galleries, and cultural programs. *Civic & Public Affairs:* About 1%. Wade House. *Education:* 27%. Support for scholarships. Also funds colleges and universities, public schools, and enrichment programs. *Environment:* 3%. Family and community services. *International:* Less than 1%. Rehabilitation center of Sheboygan. *Note:* Total contributions made in 2000. **Typ. Recipients:** Child Abuse, Children's Health/Hospitals, Family Planning, Medical Education, Medical Rehabilitation, Nursing Services, People with Disabilities. **Geo. Dist:** CA; CO; IL; IN; MN; NJ; NY; NC; WI.

★ 11676 ★ Koret Foundation

33 New Montgomery St., Suite 1090
San Francisco, CA 94105-4509
Phone: (415)882-7740 **Fax:** (415)882-7775
Email: info@koretfoundation.org
Website: http://www.koretfoundation.org

Fnded: 1966. **Philosophy:** "The Koret Foundation is a Jewish-sponsored charitable trust that seeks to enhance the human spirit by furthering education, economic opportunity and community life in the San Francisco Bay Area and Israel. The Foundation's grant-making objectives are based on ethical values derived from Jewish traditions. The Koret Foundation was created by Joseph and Stephanie Koret, Jewish immigrants from Eastern Europe whose entrepreneurial vision and success provided the resources that have endowed the Koret Foundation's grant-making capabilities. "By enabling the organizations and institutions we support to advance economic opportunity, security and quality of life, the Koret Foundation strives to fulfill its missions to the communities we serve and to the citizens of those communities. "While the majority of funds granted annually by the Koret Foundation go to organizations with established records of successful service, an increasing portion of the Foundation's funding is dedicated to seeding and supporting new and innovative programs that hold the promise of being catalysts for positive change." The foundation's areas of interest include the Local and National Jewish Community with grants to Jewish communal organizations, care for elderly citizens, Jewish cultural identity, Jewish education, and emigre resettlement; the Israel/International Jewish Community with grants to economic reform and development, higher education, and emigre resettlement and career development; and the General Community with grants to cultural and community development, independent living for the elderly, public policy and economic development, youth employment, and higher education. **Priorities:** *Arts & Humanities:* 5%. Emphasis on museums, theater, and opera. *Civic & Public Affairs:* 14%. Primary support for the San Francisco Zoological Society and the Korean Center. *Education:* 14%. Focus on universities in California. *Environment:* 9%. United funds and food banks. *Note:* Total contributions made in 2000. **Typ. Recipients:** Emergency/Ambulance Services, Geriatric Health, Hospitals (University Affiliated), Long-Term Care, Medical Education, Research/Studies Institutes. **Geo. Dist:** San Francisco, CA, including Bay area.

★ 11677 ★ Kresge Foundation

3215 West Big Beaver Rd.
PO Box 3151
Troy, MI 48007-3151
Phone: (248)643-9630 **Fax:** (248)643-0588
Website: http://www.kresge.org
John Marshall, III, President & Chief Executive Officer

Fnded: 1924. **Philosophy:** "The Kresge Foundation, an independent private foundation, was created in 1924 by Sebastian S. Kresge 'to promote the well-being of mankind.' Through our grantmaking programs, we seek to strengthen the capacity of charitable organizations to provide effective programs of quality. Our geographic scope is national, and on occasion, international." "The Foundation's grants support a range of organizations reflecting almost the entire breadth of the nonprofit sector. This diverse group is responding to new challenges presented by their communities or sustaining activities that have demonstrated their effectiveness. We believe that a challenge grant toward an organization's capital project does more than just build a building or reward good programs. It presents an opportunity to build institutional capacity by helping an organization broaden and deepen its base of support from the private sector and by encouraging volunteer involvement in the fund-raising effort and beyond." "In December, 1998, The Kresge Foundation Trustees approved the Kresge HBCU Initiative, a five-year, $18 million program to support advancement efforts at historically Black colleges and universities...The ultimate goal of the Initiative is to strengthen HBCUs by increasing ongoing and additional funding sources available to them." 1998 Annual Report **Priorities:** *Arts & Humanities:* 18%. Supports theater, museums, music, libraries, and cultural activities. *Civic & Public Affairs:* 14%. Supports community foundations, economic development, and public affairs programs. *Education:* 25%. Higher education institutions and educational programs receive support. *Environment:* 24%. Supports YMCA, scouting, American Red Cross programs, United Way, and youth organizations. *International:* 4%. Supports hospitals, hospice, and healthcare programs. *Religion:* 1%. *Note:* Total contributions made in 2001. **Typ. Recipients:** AIDS/HIV, Alzheimers Disease, Cancer, Child Abuse, Children's Health/Hospitals, Clinics/Medical Centers, Diabetes, Domestic Violence, Emergency/Ambulance Services, Eyes/Blindness, Family Planning, Health Organizations, Hospices, Hospitals, Long-Term Care, Medical Education, Medical Rehabilitation, Medical Research, Mental Health, Nursing Services, Outpatient Health Care, People with Disabilities, Preventive Medicine/Wellness Organizations, Research/Studies Institutes, Sexual Abuse, Single-Disease Health Associations, Substance Abuse, Trauma Treatment. **Geo. Dist:** nationally.

★ 11678 ★ Kulas Foundation

50 Public Square, Suite 924
Cleveland, OH 44113-2203
Phone: (216)623-4770 **Fax:** (216)623-4773
Email: azambie@gateway.net
Nancy McCann, President

Fnded: 1938. **Philosophy:** Funding is provided to music programs at colleges and universities, art centers, and community organizations. The foundation identified three categories of grant recipients: musical, educational, and civic and charitable activities. The foundation has made several major grants to support research in the field of music therapy. **Priorities:** *Arts & Humanities:* 45%. Museums, performing arts, visual arts, and public broadcasting. *Civic & Public Affairs:* 2%. Community development projects. *Education:* 18%. Supports colleges and universities. *Environment:* 3%. Supports child welfare, counseling, and community service organizations. *International:* 9%. Medical centers. **Typ. Recipients:** Cancer, Children's Health/Hospitals, Clinics/Medical Centers, Eyes/Blindness, Health Organizations, Hospices, Hospitals, Hospitals (University Affiliated), Long-Term Care, Medical Education, Nursing Services. **Geo. Dist:** Cleveland, OH, including metropolitan area.

★ 11679 ★ L. E. Phillips Family Foundation

3925 N Hastings Way
Eau Claire, WI 54703
Phone: (715)839-2139 **Fax:** (715)839-2148
Website: http://www.goPresto.com
Mary Jo Cohen, President and Director

Fnded: 1943. **Philosophy:** The foundation supports organizations in Wisconsin. Funding has gone primarily to the Melvin S. Cohen Trust for the Minneapolis Federation for Jewish Service. The remainder of funding is disbursed among cultural organizations, educational institutions, health agencies, social service groups, and religious organizations. **Priorities:** *Arts & Humanities:* 3%. *Civic & Public Affairs:* 6%. Focus on the L.E. Phillips Career Development Center. *Education:* 4%. Supports colleges and universities. *Environment:* 3%. Youth organizations and religious welfare. *Note:* Total contributions made in fiscal 2001. **Typ. Recipients:** AIDS/HIV, Children's Health/Hospitals, Geriatric Health, Health Organizations, Health Policy/Cost Containment, Health-General, Heart, Hospitals, Hospitals (University Affiliated), Medical Education, Medical Education, Medical Rehabilitation, Medical Research, People with Disabilities, Public Health, Single-Disease Health Associations, Substance Abuse. **Geo. Dist:** WI, Chippewa County; WI, Eau Claire County; WI, Northwestern Wisconsin.

★ 11680 ★ L. G. Balfour Foundation

75 State St., 7th Floor
Mail Code: MABOFO7B
Boston, MA 02109
Phone: (617)346-2484 **Fax:** (617)346-2495
Kerry Sullivan, Director, Grants

Fnded: 1973. **Philosophy:** L. G. Balfour built his fortune through his long association with educational institutions. His foundation reflects this by giving primarily to programs designed to improve access to education for all potentially qualified students. The foundation funds various scholarship programs and is particularly interested in supporting programs designed to eliminate barriers to education for capable but financially needy students, especially minorities. The foundation concentrates on programs carried out by qualified charitable institutions in Massachusetts and the New England area. The foundation will consider proposals for any charitable purpose in Attleboro, MA, or the surrounding area. Primary consideration, however, will be given to the educational and medical needs of the community. In addition to the competitive grant programs described above, the foundation funds a scholarship program for L. G. Balfour Company employees and provides grants to specific educational, fraternal, and medical institutions named by L. G. Balfour before his death. **Priorities:** *Education:* 100%. Supports various programs for students in New England, especially minorities or youth with a financial need. **Typ. Recipients:** Hospitals. **Geo. Dist:** New England area; MA.

★ 11681 ★ L. K. Whittier Foundation

625 South Fair Oaks Ave., Suite 360
South Pasadena, CA 91030
Phone: (626)441-5188 **Fax:** (626)441-3672
Linda Blinkenberg, Secretary & Chief Financial Officer

Fnded: 1955. **Philosophy:** The foundation makes grants primarily in Southern California, specifically Los Angeles. The foundation assists in the establishment and development of innovative endeavors in the areas of health and medicine, the sciences, and education. **Priorities:** *Arts & Humanities:* 27%. Supports public broadcasting. *Education:* 16%. Supports technical education and general education. *Environment:* 12%. Supports camps and scouting. *International:* 45%. Funds children's health care. *Note:* Total contributions made in fiscal 2001. **Typ. Recipients:** Cancer, Children's Health/Hospitals, Clinics/Medical Centers, Eyes/Blindness, Family Planning, Geriatric Health, Health Organizations, Hospitals, Medical Education, Medical Research, People with Disabilities, Research/Studies Institutes, Single-Disease Health Associations. **Geo. Dist:** CA, Southern California, particularly Los Angeles.

★ 11682 ★ Laffey-McHugh Foundation

PO Box 2286
Wilmington, DE 19899
Phone: (302)654-1680 **Fax:** (302)654-1681
Arthur Connolly, Jr., President

Fnded: 1949. **Philosophy:** The foundation continues to reflect the interests of the original donors by supporting Roman Catholic churches and church-related institutions, including schools, child-welfare agencies, and religious-welfare groups. The foundation also makes grants to institutions of higher education, both sectarian and nonsectarian, and to local hospitals, cultural organizations, and nonsectarian-welfare agencies. **Priorities:** *Arts & Humanities:* About 5% Supports public broadcasting, libraries, museums, and the performing arts. *Civic & Public Affairs:* 7%. Community affairs and housing are funded. *Education:* 18%. Supports colleges, universities, religious schools, and educational programs. *Environment:* 25%. Family and childrens services and united funds. *International:* About 19%. Supports children's health, hospice, disease and disorder concerns. *Note:* Contributions were made in 2000. **Typ. Recipients:** Alzheimers Disease, Cancer, Child Abuse, Children's Health/Hospitals, Clinics/Medical Centers, Family Planning, Geriatric Health, Heart, Hospices, Hospitals, Long-Term Care, Nursing Services, Outpatient Health Care, People with Disabilities, Preventive Medicine/Wellness Organizations, Public Health, Single-Disease Health Associations, Substance Abuse. **Geo. Dist:** DE; NY; PA.

★ 11683 ★ Lakeside Foundation

50 Fremont St., Suite 3520
San Francisco, CA 94105
Phone: (925)284-8634 **Fax:** (925)284-8131
Paul Davies, Jr., Vice President, Secretary & Director

Fnded: 1953. **Priorities:** *Civic & Public Affairs:* 22%. Major grant to the Hoover Institution. *Education:* 44%. Funds schools, colleges, major grant to Samuel Merritt College. *Environment:* 2%. Funds social welfare foundations. *International:* 24%. Funds medical centers, single-disease health associations, hospitals. *Religion:* 5%. Funds science institutes and laboratories. *Note:* Total contributions made in 1999. **Typ. Recipients:** Arthritis, Cancer, Children's Health/Hospitals, Clinics/Medical Centers, Emergency/Ambulance Services, Hospitals, Medical Education, Medical Research, Nursing Services, People with Disabilities, Single-Disease Health Associations, Speech & Hearing, Transplant Networks/Donor Banks. **Geo. Dist:** San Francisco, CA, including metropolitan area.

★ 11684 ★ Lannan Foundation

313 Read St.
Santa Fe, NM 87501-2628
Phone: (505)986-8160 **Fax:** (505)986-8195
Email: jo@lannan.org
Website: http://www.lannan.org
Frank Lawler, Vice President

Fnded: 1950. **Philosophy:** The Foundation gives in the following areas: the arts, literature, indigenous communities and special project. "(The) art program is designed to further the careers of emerging and under-recognized artists, foster serious criticism and discussion of contemporary art, and to bring new, experimental and sometimes controversial works of arts to a wide audience." "(The literary program supports) the creation of literature written originally in the English language and to develop a wider audience for contemporary prose and poetry." The foundation gives out literary awards and grants. "(The indigenous communities program is) dedicated to benefiting rural Native Americans who suffer from racial and cultural discrimination, lack of education and economic opportunities, in adequate health care and widespread poverty." **Priorities:** *Arts & Humanities:* 26%. Focus on museums, literary arts, arts funds, and Native American arts/cultural organizations. *Civic & Public Affairs:* 43%. Funds organizations dealing with Native American issues and law/justice. *Education:* 27%. Supports institutions of higher education, with a focus on Native American colleges and universities. *Note:* Total contributions made in 2000. **Typ. Recipients:** Domestic Violence, Hospitals, Medical Rehabilitation.

★ 11685 ★ Lauder Foundation

767 5th Ave., 40th Fl.
New York, NY 10153
Phone: (212)572-4426
Barbara Capri, Administrator

Fnded: 1962. **Philosophy:** The foundation supports museums and the arts, education, Jewish organizations, medical research, social service agencies, and conservation groups. Some funding is given to public affairs organizations and hospitals. **Typ. Recipients:** Cancer, Clinics/Medical Centers, Eyes/Blindness, Health Funds, Heart, Hospices, Hospitals, Hospitals (University Affiliated), Medical Research, Multiple Sclerosis, People with Disabilities, Public Health, Research/Studies Institutes, Substance Abuse. **Geo. Dist:** New York, NY.

★ 11686 ★ Laura Moore Cunningham Foundation

PO Box 1157
Boise, ID 83701
Phone: (208)365-2512
Harry Bettis, President

Fnded: 1964. **Philosophy:** The Laura Moore Cunningham Foundation is primarily interested in providing business scholarships through educational institutions located in Idaho. The foundation also contributes to several Idaho hospitals. In addition, the foundation awards various smaller grants to support social services, civic organizations, and the arts. **Priorities:** *Arts & Humanities:* 11%. Funds public broadcasting, museums, and music. *Civic & Public Affairs:* 6%. Gives to economic development organizations, a fire department, community festivals, and ethnic affairs. *Education:* 59%. Primarily gives to colleges and universities for scholarship funding. *Environment:* 9%. Supports homes and programs for seniors, youth and family services, and emergency assistance. *International:* 1%. Supports medical centers and health services. *Note:* Total contributions made in fiscal 2001. **Typ. Recipients:** Child Abuse, Children's Health/Hospitals, Clinics/Medical Centers, Emergency/Ambulance Services, Family Planning, Health Organizations, Health-General, Heart, Hospices, Hospitals, Hospitals (University Affiliated), Long-Term Care, Medical Education, Nursing Services, People with Disabilities, Prenatal Health Issues, Single-Disease Health Associations. **Geo. Dist:** ID.

★ 11687 ★ Laurel Foundation

Two Gateway Center, Suite 1800
Pittsburgh, PA 15222
Phone: (412)765-2400 **Fax:** (412)765-2407
Donna Panazzi, Vice President

Fnded: 1951. **Philosophy:** The Laurel Foundation makes grants to organizations serving southwestern Pennsylvania. In civic affairs, interests include community development, libraries, museums, conservation, and natural resource management. Educational support favors literacy, traditional education centers, vocational training, and apprenticeship programs. Funding for social services goes to health and human services, population control, and youth organizations. The arts are supported by funding to theaters, the performing arts, and festivals. "In response to a considerable increase in grant requests, the Trustees have reviewed the Foundation's priorities and have identified specific goals and objectives with which to guide their deliberations. With an emphasis on outcomes and accountability, grants will focus on programs which offer long-term benefits for participants and the community. The Foundation favors programs that foster individual responsibility and self-sufficiency, exhibit a commitment to sound fiscal and program management, implement collaborative efforts to leverage resources and increase efficiency, and that demonstrate measurable outcomes through the application of conclusive evaluation procedures." 1997 Annual Report **Priorities:** *Arts & Humanities:* 28%. Theater, music, museums, and historic preservation. *Civic & Public Affairs:* 13%. Supports programs dealing with legal issues, community leadership, and the nonprofit sector. Some support given to community development and beautification projects as well. *Education:* 13%. Secondary and higher education. *Environment:* 11%. Animal welfare programs and youth and family services. *International:* 8%. Preventive medicine, and women's and children's health issues. *Note:* Total contributions made in 2000. **Typ. Recipients:** Alzheimers Disease, Children's Health/Hospitals, Clinics/Medical Centers, Emergency/Ambulance Services, Family Planning, Health Funds, Hospitals, Medical Education, Medical Research, Nursing Services, People with Disabilities, Public Health, Substance Abuse. **Geo. Dist:** Pittsburgh, PA, including southwestern PA.

★ 11688 ★ Lee and Ramona Bass Foundation

309 Main St.
Fort Worth, TX 76102
Phone: (817)336-0494 **Fax:** (817)332-2176
Website: http://www.sidrichardson.org/lrbf.htm
Valleau Wilkie, Jr., Executive Director

Fnded: 1993. **Philosophy:** The foundation typically considers funding in the following areas: schools, colleges, and universities within Texas, with emphasis placed upon faculty development and liberal arts programs; community programs and projects, particularly related to the arts and the environment, such as museums, zoos, and educational/research institutions; and national and regional conservation programs. **Priorities:** *Arts & Humanities:* 49%. Supports museums, symphony, fine arts. *Civic & Public Affairs:* 22%. Major support to Forth Worth Zoological Association. *Education:* About 3%. Universities, institutes, Episcopal school. *Environment:* About 2%. Texas A&M Kingsville. *International:* Less than 1%. *Note:* Total contributions made in 2000. **Typ. Recipients:** Children's Health/Hospitals, Medical Research. **Geo. Dist:** no restrictions.

★ 11689 ★ Leighton-Oare Foundation

211 West Washington Ave., Suite 2400
South Bend, IN 46601
Phone: (574)232-5977 **Fax:** (574)234-5967
Judd Leighton, Chairman

Fnded: 1955. **Philosophy:** The Leighton-Oare Foundation is primarily interested in health services, education, and the arts. Health service funding heavily favors health foundations. Educational funding favors colleges and universities. The arts are supported mainly through grants to music and a historical society. Minor interests include civic affairs, religion, and social services. **Priorities:** *Arts & Humanities:* Less than 1%. *Civic & Public Affairs:* 64%. Funds community foundations and civic projects. *Education:* 16%. Supports precollege and higher education, and legal education. *Environment:* Less than 1%. *International:* 20%. Supports the Memorial Health Foundation, arthritis, and medicine research. *Note:* Total contributions made in 2000. **Typ. Recipients:** Arthritis, Children's Health/Hospitals, Clinics/Medical Centers, Geriatric Health, Health Funds, Hospices, Hospitals, Medical Research, Medical Research, Multiple Sclerosis, Public Health, Research/Studies Institutes, Substance Abuse. **Geo. Dist:** IN.

★ 11690 ★ Leland Fikes Foundation

3050 Lincoln Plaza
500 North Akard, Suite 3050
Dallas, TX 75201-6696
Phone: (214)754-0144
Nancy Solana, Vice President & Secretary

Fnded: 1952. **Philosophy:** The Fikes Foundation offers support to a wide variety of cultural, civic, educational, health, scientific, and social service organizations. A preference is shown toward local projects and organizations. **Priorities:** *Arts & Humanities:* 7%. Supports cultural development, symphonies, museums, libraries, theater, and arts festivals. *Civic & Public Affairs:* 17%. Funds public policy, nonprofit management, housing concerns, zoos, and botanical gardens. *Education:* 25%. Focus on private schools, colleges and universities, and literacy. *Environment:* 19%. Supports youth organizations, family planning, community services, camps, food banks, and family services. *International:* 23%. Primary support for university hospitals. Also supports AIDS organizations, medical research, and mental health. *Religion:* 3%. Supports science centers. *Note:* Total contributions made in 2000. **Typ. Recipients:** AIDS/HIV, Cancer, Children's Health/Hospitals, Clinics/Medical Centers, Diabetes, Domestic Violence, Eyes/Blindness, Family Planning, Health Organizations, Heart, Hospitals, Hospitals (University Affiliated), Medical Education, Medical Research, Mental Health, Nursing Services, People with Disabilities, Prenatal Health Issues, Public Health, Single-Disease Health Associations, Substance Abuse, Transplant Networks/Donor Banks, Trauma Treatment. **Geo. Dist:** Dallas, TX.

★ 11691 ★ Leon Lowenstein Foundation

126 East 56th St., 28th Floor
New York, NY 10022
Phone: (212)319-0670 **Fax:** (212)319-0670
Robert Bendheim, President

Fnded: 1941. **Philosophy:** The foundation provides funding "to higher education and health for the benefit of New York City." **Priorities:** *Arts & Humanities:* About 4% supports performing arts, museums, libraries. *Civic & Public Affairs:* About 6%. Supports community and public affairs. *Education:* About 55%. Supports educational institutions and programs. *Environment:* 2%. Supports United way, social, children and family services. *International:* About 30%. Supports rehabilitation centers, hospitals, disease and disorder concerns. *Note:* Contributions were made in 2000. **Typ. Recipients:** Arthritis, Cancer, Children's Health/Hospitals, Clinics/Medical Centers, Emergency/Ambulance Services, Eyes/Blindness, Health Organizations, Hospitals, Medical Education, Medical Rehabilitation, Medical Research, Mental Health, Nursing Services, People with Disabilities, Single-Disease Health Associations, Substance Abuse. **Geo. Dist:** New York, NY, metropolitan area.

★ 11692 ★ Lettie Pate Evans Foundation, Inc.

50 Hurt Plaza, Suite 1200
Atlanta, GA 30303
Phone: (404)522-6755 **Fax:** (404)522-7026
Email: fdns@woodruff.org
Website: http://www.lpevans.org
Charles McTier, President

Fnded: 1945. **Philosophy:** The foundation's primary interests are education and the arts. **Priorities:** *Arts & Humanities:* 19%. Cultural organizations, historical preservation, museums, and performing arts. *Education:* 42%. Colleges and universities and religion education. *Environment:* 5%. Human Services. *International:* 38%. Children's health care. *Note:* Total contributions made in 2000. **Typ. Recipients:** Cancer, Health Organizations, Hospitals, Nursing Services, Public Health. **Geo. Dist:** GA, emphasis on Atlanta; VA.

★ 11693 ★ Lettie Pate Whitehead Foundation

50 Hurt Plaza, Suite 1200
Atlanta, GA 30303

Phone: (404)522-6755 **Fax:** (404)522-7026
Email: fdns@woodruff.org
Website: http://www.lpwhitehead.org
Charles McTier, President

Fnded: 1946. **Philosophy:** As specified under the will of Conkey Pate Whitehead, the foundation is limited to providing funds for needy female Christian students in Alabama, Florida, Georgia, Louisiana, Mississippi, North Carolina, South Carolina, Tennessee, and Virginia. Grants are made directly to institutions of higher education which, in turn, allocate scholarship funds to individual students. Scholarships are based on financial need. This educational program accounts for about 90% of giving. The remainder of support is given to homes for needy elderly Christian women. **Priorities:** *Civic & Public Affairs:* (Housing & Neighborhood Revitalization) About 13%. For the benefit of needy, elderly Christian women. *Education:* 87%. Scholarships for needy female Christian students in southern states. *Note:* Total contributions made in 2000. **Typ. Recipients:** Alzheimers Disease, Cancer, Clinics/Medical Centers, Geriatric Health, Home-Care Services, Hospices, Long-Term Care, Medical Education. **Geo. Dist:** AL; FL; GA; LA; MS; NC; SC; TN; VA.

★ 11694 ★ Lied Foundation Trust

3907 West Charleston Boulevard
Las Vegas, NV 89102
Phone: (702)878-1559 **Fax:** (702)878-6469
Christina Hixson, Trustee

Fnded: 1972. **Philosophy:** The Lied Foundation Trust traditionally funds three main areas: higher education, religious organizations, and youth organizations in Las Vegas. Major contributions are made to higher education, particularly to Kansas University, the Lied Institute for Real Estate Studies, and the University of Nevada. The Boys and Girls Club of Las Vegas is also a main interest. The foundation also funds other organizations primarily in the areas of social services and education. **Priorities:** *Arts & Humanities:* About 5%. Funds performing arts, public libraries, museums and dance theaters. *Civic & Public Affairs:* About 4%. Supports legal services and cities. *Education:* 61%. Provides scholarships; supports secondary education, and colleges and universities. *Environment:* 24%. Animal welfare and protection. *International:* 4%. Supports an ear institute. *Religion:* 2%. Funds science museums. *Note:* Total contributions made in 2000. **Typ. Recipients:** Health Organizations, Hospitals (University Affiliated), People with Disabilities, Research/Studies Institutes, Speech & Hearing, Speech & Hearing, Transplant Networks/Donor Banks. **Geo. Dist:** CA; IA; KS; NE; NV.

★ 11695 ★ Life Sciences Research Foundation

115 W University Parkway
Baltimore, MD 21210
Phone: (410)467-2597
Email: sdirenzo@molbio.princeton.edu
Susan DiRenzo, Assistant Director

Fnded: 1984. **Priorities:** *Education:* 100%. Awards postdoctoral research fellowships to graduates of graduate schools in the biological sciences for basic research in life sciences. The purpose of the grants is to train and support high quality young scientists in the very best research environments. *Note:* Total contributions made in 2001. **Typ. Recipients:** Cancer, Children's Health/Hospitals, Hospitals (University Affiliated), Medical Education, Medical Research, Research/Studies Institutes.

★ 11696 ★ Lillian B. Disney Foundation

c/o Motto, Kryla & Fisher
899 Adams St., Suite E
Saint Helena, CA 94574
Phone: (707)963-9222
Diane Miller, Secretary & Treasurer

Fnded: 1974. **Typ. Recipients:** Cancer, Clinics/Medical Centers, People with Disabilities. **Geo. Dist:** CA.

★ 11697 ★ Lilly Endowment

Program Office
2801 North Meridian St.
PO Box 88068
Indianapolis, IN 46208-0068
Phone: (317)924-5471 **Fax:** (317)926-4431
Website: http://www.lilly.com/about/community/foundation/endowment.html

Fnded: 1937. **Philosophy:** "We consider proposals in three program areas: community development, education, and religion. We are also interested in initiatives that benefit youth, that foster leadership education among nonprofit institutions, and that promote the causes of philanthropy and volunteerism." "Community Development: Our community development grantmaking focuses primarily on the quality of life in Indianapolis and Indiana, and we grant funds for human/social needs, central city and neighborhood revitalization, low-income housing, and arts and culture in Indianapolis. We also support amateur athletics and fitness organizations, facilities and programs that help advance the city's economic revitalization and community recreational opportunities. On a statewide level, we provide major support for the development of endowments of community foundations and the advancement of United Ways." "Education: Our educational grantmaking revolves primarily around our interest in improving education in Indiana, with special emphasis on higher education and on programs designed to increase the number of Indiana residents with bachelor's degrees. We support a number of invitational grant programs, many of which are aimed at Indiana's colleges' and universities' abilities to increase the state's educational attainment level. We also support on an invitational basis private historically black colleges and universities throughout the United States." "Religion: Our primary aim in this field is to deepen and enrich the religious lives of American Christians, principally by supporting efforts to encourage, support and educate a new generation of talented pastors and to strengthen current pastors in their capacities for excellence in ministry. We seek to help congregations be vibrant, healthy communities of faith, and we encourage efforts that make available and accessible the wisdom of the Christian tradition for contemporary life. We support seminaries, theological schools and other educational and religious institutions that share these aims. We also support projects that strengthen the contributions which religious ideas, practices, values, and institutions make to the common good of our society." "Besides grantmaking in our three principal areas of community development, education and religion, the Endowment also awards grants in support of youth development, leadership education, and fundraising and philanthropy." 2001 Annual Report **Priorities:** *Civic & Public Affairs:* (Community Development) 23%. Supports human and social services, neighborhood revitalization, housing, arts and culture, community foundations, athletics and recreation. Also funds youth development and fundraising and philanthropy. *Education:* 54%. Supports higher education in Indiana, and leadership education. *Note:* Total contributions made in 2001. **Typ. Recipients:** Emergency/Ambulance Services, Family Planning, Health Organizations, People with Disabilities, Substance Abuse. **Geo. Dist:** nationally; IN, statewide; Indianopolis, IN.

★ 11698 ★ Lincy Foundation

150 S Rodeo Dr., Suite 250
Beverly Hills, CA 90212
Phone: (310)271-3490 **Fax:** (310)271-3416
James Aljian, Chairman

Fnded: 1989. **Philosophy:** The Lincy Foundation is primarily interested in aiding Armenian interests through its support of the United Armenian Fund and other organizations. The foundation has also supported care for the elderly with two large grants going to homes for the aged in southern California. **Priorities:** *Arts & Humanities:* About 1%. Supports television stations. *Civic & Public Affairs:* 39%. Supports Armenian Organization, parks, youth assistance, Habitat for Humanity. *Education:* 40%. Supports schools and universities. *Environment:* About 11%. Youth, homes for the aged, United Way. *International:* About 7%. Single-disease research and hospitals. *Note:* Total contributions made in 2000. **Typ. Recipients:** AIDS/HIV, Arthritis, Cancer, Children's Health/Hospitals, Clinics/Medical Centers, Diabetes, Emergency/Ambulance Services, Eyes/Blindness, Geriatric Health, Health Funds, Health Organizations, Heart, Hospices, Hospitals, Hospitals (University Affiliated), Kidney, Long-Term Care, Medical Education, Medical Research, Mental Health, People with Disabilities, Prenatal Health Issues, Public Health, Sexual Abuse, Single-Disease Health Associations, Transplant Networks/Donor Banks. **Geo. Dist:** CA; DC; GA; KS; MA; MI; NV; NY; NC; PA; VA.

★ 11699 ★ Little Family Foundation

PO Box 185
Pittsburgh, PA 15230
Phone: (617)722-7772

Fnded: 1946. **Philosophy:** The Little Family Foundation's main emphasis is to promote quality education as a stepping stone to success in the business world. The foundation has established the Little Family Foundation Fellowship Awards in conjunction with the national office of Junior Achievement in Colorado Springs, CO. The foundation also supports arts organizations and conservation minded organizations. **Priorities:** *Arts & Humanities:* About 6%. Supports public broadcasting, museums, and music. *Civic & Public Affairs:* About 17%. Contributes to zoos and aquariums. *Education:* About 36%. Funds business and higher education. *Environment:* About 29%. Funds youth groups and united funds. *Religion:* About 3%. *Note:* Total contributions made in 2000. **Typ. Recipients:** AIDS/HIV, Cancer, Domestic Violence, Family Planning, Hospitals, Long-Term Care, Medical Rehabilitation, Medical Research, Nursing Services, People with Disabilities, Single-Disease Health Associations, Substance Abuse. **Geo. Dist:** nationally.

★ 11700 ★ Liz Claiborne and Art Ortenberg Foundation

650 5th Ave., 15th Floor
New York, NY 10019
Phone: (212)333-2536 **Fax:** (212)956-3531
Email: lcaof@fcc.net
Website: http://www.lcaof.org
James Murtaugh, Program Director

Fnded: 1984. **Philosophy:** Environmental concerns top the priority list of the Liz Claiborne and Art Ortenberg Foundation. Typically, the foundation chooses well-established programs with firm reputations, such as the Nature Conservancy, the World Wildlife Fund, and the New York Zoological Society-Wildlife Conservation International. The foundation's board of directors has identified two primary program interests for the future: mitigation of conflict between the land and resource use practices of rural communities and conservation of biological diversity; and, implementation of field-based scientific, technical, and practical training programs in conservation biology for local people. Typically, the foundation funds modest, carefully designed field projects, in which local communities have a substantial proprietary interest. The foundation also provides very limited funding for organizations concerned with health care, social services, education, and the arts. **Priorities:** *Arts & Humanities:* 2%. Supports historic preservation, theater, art museums, public radio, and Library of Congress. *Civic & Public Affairs:* 2%. Emphasis is on a botanical garden and public policy groups concerned with the protection of native lands. *Education:* 1%. Supports colleges and universities, and elementary schools. *Environment:* 1%. Youth and family services, community centers, United Way, and YWCA. *International:* 1%.Funds hospital, medical centers, and single-disease health associations. *Note:* Total contributions made in fiscal 2001. **Typ. Recipients:** AIDS/HIV, Emergency/Ambulance Services, Family Planning, Health Organizations, Hospitals, People with Disabilities, Single-Disease Health Associations. **Geo. Dist:** internationally especially undeveloped countries; Northern Rockies area and nationally.

★ 11701 ★ Lloyd A. Fry Foundation
120 S LaSalle St., Suite 1950
Chicago, IL 60603
Phone: (312)580-0310 **Fax:** (312)580-0980
Website: http://www.fryfoundation.org
Jill Darrow-Seltzer, Executive Director

Fnded: 1983. **Philosophy:** The foundation focuses its philanthropic efforts in the areas of education, health, civic affairs, social services, and the arts. In education, the foundation is receptive to efforts to improve Chicago inner-city education at the elementary and secondary levels. It works toward this goal through support of programs aimed at Chicago school reform, faculty development programs, and scholarship programs for minority students. The foundation also funds universities, cultural organizations, private agencies, and community groups that improve Chicago public education. Foundation giving in the arts also reflects a commitment to education through the support of arts outreach projects for inner-city students. Chicago's major cultural institutions and mid-sized arts organizations also receive support. In the area of health, the foundation continues to focus on health education and disease prevention among low-income and minority populations, as well as on efforts to improve health care for the medically indigent in Chicago. Improving health services for low-income children is a special emphasis in this area. Grants to civic and social service organizations reflect foundation interests in monitoring local government, studying the legal system, and providing legal services to needy individuals and organizations. Other concerns include job training and placement for minority youth and neighborhood economic development. **Priorities:** *Arts & Humanities:* 7%. Supports performing arts and public broadcasting. *Civic & Public Affairs:* 13%. Supports urban and community affairs, employment, legal issues, and zoos. *Education:* 31%. Supports private schools, educational foundations and initiatives, public and private colleges and universities. *Environment:* 24%. Supports youth programs, the homeless, community organizations, and family services. *International:* 5%. Supports medical centers and research. *Note:* Total contributions made in fiscal 2000. **Typ. Recipients:** AIDS/HIV, Child Abuse, Children's Health/Hospitals, Clinics/Medical Centers, Domestic Violence, Geriatric Health, Health Organizations, Health Policy/Cost Containment, Heart, Hospitals, Medical Rehabilitation, Mental Health, Nursing Services, People with Disabilities, Prenatal Health Issues, Public Health, Single-Disease Health Associations, Substance Abuse. **Geo. Dist:** Chicago, IL.

★ 11702 ★ Lois U. Horvitz Foundation
c/o Parkland Management Company
1001 Lakeside Ave., Suite 900
Cleveland, OH 44114-1151
Phone: (216)479-2200 **Fax:** (216)479-2222
Thomas Oden, Trustee

Fnded: 1988. **Philosophy:** "During 1998, the Foundation was reorganized into four separate foundations. They are the Lois U. Horvitz Foundation, the MJH Foundation, the PTS Foundation and the PAH Foundation ("H.R.H. Family Foundations"). The Harry R. Horvitz Scholarship Program is now funded by the H.R.H. Family Foundations, continuing the family's strong commitment to the communities in which the family had owned newspapers and to those newspapers' former employees. Each year the Foundation makes only a few significant grants in an effort to provide meaningful impact for an organization or a specific project. Grants may be considered for capital projects, endowments for specific purposes and for specific projects. These grants are not limited to any single purpose (i.e., education, health care, or social services)." Lois H. Horvitz Foundation 2001 Form 990. **Priorities:** *Arts & Humanities:* 33%. Supports an art museum. *Education:* 29%. Funds a scholarship fund and an independent college preparatory school. *Environment:* 11%. Supports children's services, substance abuse treatment, and a charity fund. *International:* 17%. Gives to a medical center and the Cleveland Clinic. *Religion:* 1%. A science center receives funding. *Note:* Total contributions made in fiscal 2001. **Typ. Recipients:** Clinics/Medical Centers, Domestic Violence, Hospices, Substance Abuse. **Geo. Dist:** preference is given where Horvitz family members reside. **Frmly:** H.R.H. Family Foundation.

★ 11703 ★ Lon V. Smith Foundation
9440 Santa Monica Boulevard, Suite 300
Beverly Hills, CA 90210-4614
Phone: (310)276-9306 **Fax:** (310)276-3824
Marguerite Murphy, Secretary & Treasurer

Fnded: 1952. **Philosophy:** The primary focus of the foundation is on social services in the Los Angeles area. A variety of organizations are supported, including services for the disabled, child welfare programs, youth organizations, family services, shelters, and homes. The foundation also is interested in supporting health services. A variety of health organizations are supported by the foundation, including hospitals, single-disease associations, family clinics, counseling, and pediatrics. **Priorities:** *Arts & Humanities:* 1%. Museums. *Civic & Public Affairs:* 11%. Family services, legal associations, and Habitat for Humanity. *Education:* 7%. Educational programs and schools. *Environment:* 37%. Family and youth services including Boy Scouts of America and shelters for abused women. *International:* 35%. Alzheimer's Association, children's health issues and medical centers are funded. *Note:* Total contributions made in 2000. **Typ. Recipients:** Alzheimers Disease, Cancer, Children's Health/Hospitals, Clinics/Medical Centers, Diabetes, Domestic Violence, Emergency/Ambulance Services, Geriatric Health, Health Organizations, Hospitals, Hospitals, Hospitals (University Affiliated), Long-Term Care, Medical Education, Medical Research, Nursing Services, Nutrition, Outpatient Health Care, People with Disabilities, Prenatal Health Issues, Preventive Medicine/Wellness Organizations, Public Health, Research/Studies Institutes, Single-Disease Health Associations, Speech & Hearing, Substance Abuse. **Geo. Dist:** Los Angeles, CA.

★ 11704 ★ Longleaf Foundation
6410 Poplar Ave., Suite 900
Memphis, TN 38119
Phone: (901)761-2474
Website: http://www.hecsoft.com/grants/Tennessee/The%20Longleaf%20Foundation
Joseph Ott, Secretary, Treasurer, Director & Manager

Fnded: 1995. **Priorities:** *Arts & Humanities:* 5%. *Civic & Public Affairs:* 1%. *Education:* 52%. *Environment:* 23%. *International:* 1%. *Note:* Total contributions made in 1998. **Typ. Recipients:** Clinics/Medical Centers, Family Planning, Home-Care Services. **Geo. Dist:** Memphis, TN.

★ 11705 ★ Longwood Foundation
100 West 10th St., Suite 1109
Wilmington, DE 19801
Phone: (302)654-2489 **Fax:** (302)654-2323
Peter Morrow, Executive Director

Fnded: 1937. **Philosophy:** One of the foundation's primary interests has been to support and develop Longwood Gardens, once the home of Pierre du Pont. It is among the finest horticultural gardens open to the public in America. The gardens cover 1,000 acres, and include a conservatory, an arboretum, flower gardens, an open air theater, illuminated fountains, greenhouses, and several other attractions. To a lesser extent, funds traditionally have been given to the Eleutherian Mills Historical Library, a research library which assembles and houses historical documents and records relating to the Brandywine Valley and its development. The foundation also has supported educational institutions for the construction of scientific, engineering training, and library facilities. Local conservation and horticultural groups, hospitals, and a variety of social service agencies have received substantial funding from the foundation. **Priorities:** *Arts & Humanities:* 8%. Funds archaeology and historic preservation, libraries, museums, arts centers, historical societies, and the performing arts. *Civic & Public Affairs:* 32%. Provides major support to Longwood Gardens; also supports other horticultural and botanical gardens, fire and police departments, and an urban league. *Education:* 34%. Grantmaking focuses on primary and secondary education. *Environment:* 7%. Emphasis on community services, youth organizations, child welfare, day care, united funds, the aged, and family services. *International:* 12%. Contributes to health systems, hospitals, hospice, and wellness programs. *Note:* Total contributions made in fiscal 2001. **Typ. Recipients:** AIDS/HIV, Cancer, Children's Health/Hospitals, Clinics/Medical Centers, Emergency/Ambulance Services, Family Planning, Geriatric Health, Health Organizations, Hospices, Hospitals, Long-Term Care, Medical Research, People with Disabilities, Preventive Medicine/Wellness Organizations, Public Health, Substance Abuse. **Geo. Dist:** DE; PA, Southern Chester County.

★ 11706 ★ Loren M. Berry Foundation
3055 Kettering Boulevard, Suite 418
Dayton, OH 45439
Phone: (937)293-0398
William Lincoln, Treasurer & Trustee

Fnded: 1960. **Philosophy:** The foundation supports a variety of youth organizations, social and family service organizations, and united funds. The foundation prioritizes higher education and educational foundations. Community affairs, the arts, and health concerns are also important. **Priorities:** *Arts & Humanities:* 11%. Funds art institutes, theater, historical preservation, and public broadcasting. *Civic & Public Affairs:* 8%. Supports public policy and economic development. *Education:* 28%. Supports higher education, education funds, schools, and scholarship programs. *Environment:* 11%. Grants awarded to Young Men's Christian Association, Planned Parenthood, and services for children and youth. *International:* 20%. Contributes to hospitals, disease and disorder concerns, the American Red Cross, and medical centers. *Religion:* 15%. Supports aviation museum. *Note:* Total contributions made in 2001. **Typ. Recipients:** Alzheimers Disease, Cancer, Children's Health/Hospitals, Clinics/Medical Centers, Domestic Violence, Emergency/Ambulance Services, Eyes/Blindness, Family Planning, Geriatric Health, Health Organizations, Heart, Hospices, Hospitals, Medical Rehabilitation, People with Disabilities, Single-Disease Health Associations, Transplant Networks/Donor Banks. **Geo. Dist:** Dayton, OH.

★ 11707 ★ Louis and Anne Abrons Foundation
437 Madison Ave.
New York, NY 10017
Phone: (212)756-3376 **Fax:** (212)832-6698
Richard Abrons, President

Fnded: 1950. **Philosophy:** The foundation focuses giving on social welfare organizations; civic and public affairs associations, including environmental causes; educational institutions; and Jewish organizations. **Priorities:** *Arts & Humanities:* 9%. Supports performing arts, museums, and public libraries. *Civic & Public Affairs:* 5%. Supports parks, ethnic organizations, and community and public affairs. *Education:* 18%. Supports colleges and universities, schools, minority education. *Environment:* 28%. Supports family services and neighborhood concerns, with major support given to the Henry Street Settlement. *International:* 11%. Supports hospitals, nursing, children's health, and single-disease health associations. *Note:* Total contributions made in 2000. **Typ. Recipients:** Cancer, Children's Health/Hospitals, Family Planning, Health Organizations, Hospitals, Medical Education, Medical Research, Mental Health, Nursing Services, Substance Abuse. **Geo. Dist:** New York, NY.

★ 11708 ★ Louis Calder Foundation
230 Park Ave., Room 1525
New York, NY 10169
Website: http://www.lcfnyc.org
Allison Sargent, Grant Program Manager

Fnded: 1951. **Philosophy:** Foundation grants reflect a high level of social awareness, with particular attention to the problems and needs of those in New York City. The current policy of the foundation is to concentrate "its grantmaking to organizations whose programs and projects are directed to improving the condition of the people of the City of New York. Current funding priorities are grants which support the efforts of community based organizations whose programs are designed to enhance the potential and increase the self sufficiency of New York City's disadvantaged children and youth and their families." **Priorities:** *Arts & Humanities:* 22%. Libraries, public broadcasting, museums, ballet, and music. *Civic & Public Affairs:* 5%. Support law & justice, botanical gardens, and housing. *Education:* 27%. Colleges and universities, private and public pre-college education, literacy, after school enrichment programs, leadership training, education reform, medical education, scholarships, and legal education. *Environment:* 33%. Youth organizations, programs for at-risk youth, family services and child welfare. *International:* 7%. Mainly hospitals. *Note:* Total contributions made in fiscal 2000. **Typ. Recipients:** Adolescent Health Issues, AIDS/HIV, Cancer, Children's Health/Hospitals, Health Organizations, Heart, Hospitals, People with Disabilities, Research/Studies Institutes. **Geo. Dist:** New York City.

★ 11709 ★ Louis and Harold Price Foundation

450 Park Ave., Suite 1102
New York, NY 10022-2605
Phone: (212)753-0240 **Fax:** (212)752-9338
Email: grantinquiry@pricefoundation.org
Website: http://www.pricefoundation.org
Rosemary Guidone, President

Fnded: 1951. **Philosophy:** The foundation supports a business institute, Jewish welfare funds, hospitals, community funds, and higher education, including scholarship funds. Grants also are given to youth agencies, camps for children, temple support, medical research, the arts, and services for the blind and other disabled persons. The foundation responds more favorably to proposals from organizations in California, Colorado and New York. **Priorities:** *Arts & Humanities:* 6%. *Civic & Public Affairs:* 13%. *Education:* 32%. Includes a large grant to the Price Institute for Entrepreneurial Studies. *Environment:* 11%. Supports community services, child welfare, and programs for the disabled. *International:* 35%. Funds hospitals, medical research, mental health, and single-disease health organizations. *Note:* Total contributions made in 2000. **Typ. Recipients:** AIDS/HIV, Alzheimers Disease, Alzheimers Disease, Arthritis, Cancer, Children's Health/Hospitals, Clinics/Medical Centers, Emergency/Ambulance Services, Eyes/Blindness, Health Funds, Health Organizations, Health-General, Heart, Hospitals, Kidney, Long-Term Care, Medical Rehabilitation, Medical Research, Mental Health, Multiple Sclerosis, Outpatient Health Care, People with Disabilities, Public Health, Research/Studies Institutes, Single-Disease Health Associations. **Geo. Dist:** Los Angeles, CA, including the metropolitan area; New York, NY, including the metropolitan area.

★ 11710 ★ Louis R. Lurie Foundation

555 California St., Suite 5100
San Francisco, CA 94104
Phone: (415)392-2470 **Fax:** (415)421-8669
Robert Lurie, President

Fnded: 1948. **Philosophy:** The foundation gives to a wide range of local interests in the San Francisco and Chicago areas. While there is no specific area of focus, the foundation does give substantially to organizations concerned with civic and community issues, the social sciences, education, the arts and humanities, and a variety of health issues. **Priorities:** *Arts & Humanities:* 10%. Supports museums, theater, performing arts, and cultural associations. *Civic & Public Affairs:* 4%. Funds housing and community affairs. *Education:* 17%. Preparatory schools, colleges, and educational programs receive grants. *Environment:* 15%. Family services, child welfare, and food banks receive support. *International:* 13%. Gives to hospitals, medical centers, rehabilitation institutes, elder care, and disease and disorder concerns. *Religion:* 3%. Funds a research center. *Note:* Total contributions made in 2000. **Typ. Recipients:** AIDS/HIV, Alzheimers Disease, Cancer, Child Abuse, Children's Health/Hospitals, Clinics/Medical Centers, Domestic Violence, Emergency/Ambulance Services, Family Planning, Geriatric Health, Health Funds, Health Organizations, Hospitals, Medical Education, Medical Rehabilitation, Medical Research, Mental Health, People with Disabilities, Prenatal Health Issues, Public Health, Research/Studies Institutes, Single-Disease Health Associations, Speech & Hearing, Substance Abuse. **Geo. Dist:** San Francisco, CA, metropolitan area; Chicago, IL.

★ 11711 ★ The Louis and Rachel Rudin Foundation, Inc.

345 Park Ave., 33rd Floor
New York, NY 10154
Phone: (212)407-2400 **Fax:** (212)407-2540
Robin Avram, Administrator

Fnded: 1968. **Philosophy:** The purpose of the foundation is to aid medical and nursing schools in the education and training of doctors and nurses. **Priorities:** *Education:* 100%. Supports medical education through scholarships. *Note:* Contribution made in fiscal 2000. **Typ. Recipients:** Alzheimers Disease, Cancer, Children's Health/Hospitals, Eyes/Blindness, Geriatric Health, Home-Care Services, Medical Education, Medical Training, Mental Health. **Geo. Dist:** NY.

★ 11712 ★ Louis and Sandra Berkman Foundation

PO Box 576
Steubenville, OH 43952
Phone: (740)283-3722 **Fax:** (740)283-1224
Linda Pinkle, Secretary

Fnded: 1952. **Philosophy:** The foundation primarily supports higher education. Minimal funding goes to health organizations and religious welfare causes. **Priorities:** *Arts & Humanities:* About 1%. *Civic & Public Affairs:* 17% *Education:* 59%. Colleges and universities, with major grants to Bethany College and Franciscan University. *Environment:* 2%. Youth programs. *International:* 3%. Medical centers, cancer research, and public health. *Note:* Total contributions made in 2001. **Typ. Recipients:** Cancer, Children's Health/Hospitals, Clinics/Medical Centers, Emergency/Ambulance Services, Eyes/Blindness, Family Planning, Health Organizations, Heart, Hospices, Hospitals, Medical Research, Prenatal Health Issues, Public Health, Single-Disease Health Associations, Transplant Networks/Donor Banks. **Geo. Dist:** MA; OH; PA.

★ 11713 ★ Louise H. and David S. Ingalls Foundation

20600 Chagrin Boulevard, Suite 430
Shaker Heights, OH 44122
Phone: (216)921-6000 **Fax:** (216)921-7709
Email: wwwatson@visnet.com
Jane Watson, Contact

Fnded: 1953. **Philosophy:** The foundation makes most of its grants in the areas of education, health, and the arts. Educational funding favors colleges and private secondary schools. Health care interests include hospital building campaigns, research, and pediatrics. Support for the arts goes to museums, art associations, and the performing arts. Secondary interests include youth organizations and civic affairs. **Priorities:** *Arts & Humanities:* 17%. Funds museums, music, arts festivals, historical societies, and performing arts. *Civic & Public Affairs:* 12%. Supports community foundations, botanical gardens, and clubs. *Education:* 27%. Supports pre-college and higher education. *Environment:* 4% Contributes to youth programs, family services, and community services. *Religion:* 28%. Supports museums. *Note:* Total contributions made in 2000. **Typ. Recipients:** Clinics/Medical Centers, Emergency/Ambulance Services, Eyes/Blindness, Family Planning, Health Organizations, Hospitals, Long-Term Care, Medical Education, Medical Rehabilitation, Nursing Services, People with Disabilities, Single-Disease Health Associations, Transplant Networks/Donor Banks. **Geo. Dist:** CT; NY; OH, Ohio, Connecticut, Virginia, and New York; VT.

★ 11714 ★ Louise Manoogian Simone Foundation

21001 Van Born Rd.
Taylor, MI 48180
Phone: (313)274-8799
Louise Simone, President & Director

Fnded: 1962. **Philosophy:** The Simone foundation's principal areas of interest are organizations supporting Armenian culture, religion, and education. The foundation also contributes to the arts, with emphasis on museums. **Priorities:** *Arts & Humanities:* 1%. Public broadcasting. *Civic & Public Affairs:* 1%. Civic concerns. *Education:* Less than 1%. *Environment:* Less than 1%. *Note:* Total contributions made in fiscal 2000. **Typ. Recipients:** Children's Health/Hospitals, Family Planning, Health-General, Public Health, Research/Studies Institutes. **Geo. Dist:** nationally, with an emphasis on the eastern states.

★ 11715 ★ Louise Taft Semple Foundation

425 Walnut St.
Cincinnati, OH 45202
Phone: (513)381-2838 **Fax:** (513)381-0205
Penny Freedman, Contact

Fnded: 1941. **Philosophy:** The Louise Taft Semple Foundation makes most of its grants in the areas of the arts, humanities, education, and social services. Social service funding favors united funds, homes, youth organizations, and community centers. Educational support goes to private and public school systems, university legal education, and religious learning. In the arts, support favors art funds, museums, and opera. **Priorities:** *Arts & Humanities:* 33%. Primary support for Aronoff Performing Arts Center, arts funds, ballet, music, opera, and public broadcasting. *Civic & Public Affairs:* 11%. Focus on a zoological society, women's affairs, legal aid, and towns/municipalities. *Education:* 29%. Support for primary and secondary education, faculty development, arts education, and schs. *Environment:* 20%. Supports United Way, YMCA, scouting, and youth programs. *International:* 6%. Supports children's health and speech & hearing. *Note:* Total contributions made in 2000. **Typ. Recipients:** Children's Health/Hospitals, Medical Rehabilitation, People with Disabilities, Preventive Medicine/Wellness Organizations, Speech & Hearing, Substance Abuse, Substance Abuse. **Geo. Dist:** OH, Hamilton County; Cincinnati, OH.

★ 11716 ★ Lowell Berry Foundation

3685 Mount Diablo, Suite 269
Lafayette, CA 94549
Phone: (925)284-4427 **Fax:** (925)284-4332
Debbie Coombe, Office Manager

Fnded: 1950. **Philosophy:** The primary objective of the foundation is to assist in strengthening Christian ministry at the local church level. Its second purpose is to assist local social service programs in California. The foundation has a large number of ongoing grant programs, and the number of new grants is restricted to programs in California's Contra Costa and northern Alameda counties. The foundation's recipients include evangelical Christian religious programs, higher education, religious welfare organizations, and family services. **Priorities:** *Civic & Public Affairs:* 1%. Funds community affairs and public policy. *Education:* 7%. Supports colleges and universities and education funds. *Environment:* 10%. Gives to youth organizations, animal protection groups, food banks, shelters, and athletic organizations. *International:* 1%. Supports health services and medical centers. *Religion:* 1%. Supports a science center. *Note:* Total contributions made in 2001. **Typ. Recipients:** Cancer, Child Abuse, Children's Health/Hospitals, Clinics/Medical Centers, Domestic Violence, Family Planning, Medical Rehabilitation, Medical Research, People with Disabilities, Public Health, Substance Abuse. **Geo. Dist:** CA, Contra Costa County; CA, Northern Alameda County.

★ 11717 ★ Loyola Foundation, Inc.

308 C St., Northeast
Washington, DC 20002

Phone: (202)546-9400
Albert McCarthy, III, Executive Director, Secretary

Fnded: 1957. **Philosophy:** The Loyola Foundation was established "to assist overseas Catholic mission activities. In the beginning we hoped to assist, in a very small and limited way, a vast area of the world." Over the last thirty years, the foundation has broadened its interests, but primarily supports four areas: vehicles; construction, renovation, and repairs; equipment and furnishings; and agricultural and water projects. The foundation funds basic, durable vehicles to missions that apply. It will not fund buses to be used by the local population or trucks for hauling equipment. Construction, renovation, and repair projects include schools, churches, and community centers. Grants for equipment have primarily been to church-run trade schools, health centers, religious educational projects, and self-help centers. Grants for furnishings include churches, rectories, convents, classrooms, and schools. Water projects include some well digging and storage tank construction. The foundation has supported missions around the world and often visits the locations it funds. The areas include Africa, the Middle East, Asia, the Caribbean, and Central and South America. **Priorities:** *Civic & Public Affairs:* 9%. Supports community and neighborhood development. *Education:* 11%. Religious schools and universities. *Environment:* 5%. Funds family and social services. *Note:* Total contributions made in fiscal 1999. **Typ. Recipients:** Cancer, Medical Education, Public Health, Substance Abuse. **Geo. Dist:** internationally.

★ 11718 ★ Lucius N. Littauer Foundation

60 East 42nd St., Suite 2910
New York, NY 10165
Phone: (212)697-2677
William Frost, President

Fnded: 1929. **Philosophy:** The primary focus of the foundation is to provide funds for scholars engaged in research in Jewish studies at the postdoctoral level. Other current areas of interest are medical research with an emphasis on medical ethics, and the environment. The foundation established the position of Littauer Hebraica Technical and Research Services Librarian in the Judaica Department of the Harvard College Library. In 1994, the foundation awarded a multi-year grant to Columbia University to establish the Lucius N. Littauer Foundation Professorship of Classical Jewish Civilization. Also, the foundation has founded and contributed to Judaic book funds at colleges and universities throughout the United States. Other current areas of interest are medical ethics and the environment. The foundation also supports some social welfare projects, including federated fund drives, Jewish welfare funds, and selected public interest groups. Some funding is available for health and environmental concerns. **Priorities:** *Arts & Humanities:* 3%. Support includes film, television, museums, libraries and archives, and the performing arts. *Civic & Public Affairs:* 5%. Supports public television specials and series. *Education:* 29%. Supports conferences, programs, and workshops held at colleges and universities, scholarships, and fellowships. *Environment:* 2%. Supports social welfare. *International:* 3%. Funds medical centers and hospitals. *Note:* Total contributions made in 2001. **Typ. Recipients:** Clinics/Medical Centers, Geriatric Health, Geriatric Health, Health Organizations, Health Policy/Cost Containment, Hospitals, Hospitals (University Affiliated), Medical Education, People with Disabilities. **Geo. Dist:** internationally; nationally; New York, NY.

★ 11719 ★ Lund Foundation

535 North Brand Boulevard, Suite 504
Glendale, CA 91203
Phone: (818)291-4000 **Fax:** (818)291-4004
Email: lundfaun@earthlink.net
Robert Wilson, Vice President & Secretary

Fnded: 1973. **Philosophy:** The foundation typically supports the arts, educational institutions, health oranizations, and social services in the greater Los Angeles area. **Priorities:** *Arts & Humanities:* About 3%. Museums, foundations, orchestras. *Civic & Public Affairs:* 8%. Community foundations. *Education:* About 9%. Primarily to colleges and educational foundations. *Environment:* 37%. Funds youth groups, community centers, and family services. *International:* About 42%. Hospitals, pediatric health, and single-disease health associations. *Note:* Total contributions made in 2000. **Typ. Recipients:** Arthritis, Cancer, Children's Health/Hospitals, Clinics/Medical Centers, Emergency/Ambulance Services, Hospitals, Medical Research, Mental Health, Multiple Sclerosis, People with Disabilities, Single-Disease Health Associations, Substance Abuse, Trauma Treatment. **Geo. Dist:** AZ; CA; FL; GA; MA; TX.

★ 11720 ★ Lynde and Harry Bradley Foundation

Attn: Michael W Grebe
PO Box 510860
Milwaukee, WI 53203-0153
Phone: (414)291-9915 **Fax:** (414)291-9991
Website: http://www.bradleyfdn.org

Fnded: 1942. **Philosophy:** The programs of the Lynde and Harry Bradley Foundation "support limited, competent government; a dynamic marketplace for economic, intellectual, and cultural activity; and a vigorous defense at home and abroad of American ideas and institutions." Funding is concentrated locally in cultural programs, education, social services, medical programs, health agencies, and public policy. National support goes toward research and education in domestic and international public policy. The foundation reports that projects that are likely to be supported will "generally share the following assumptions: That free men and women should be treated as self-governing, responsible citizens, not as victims or clients. They will aim to restore the intellectual and cultural legitimacy of citizenly common sense, the received wisdom of experience, everyday morality, and personal character, refurbishing their roles as reliable guideposts of everyday life. They will seek to reinvigorate and reempower the traditional, local institutions–families, schools, churches, and neighborhoods–that provide training in and room for the exercise of genuine citizenship, that pass on everyday morality to the next generation, and that cultivate personal character. They will encourage decentralization of power and accountability away from centralized, bureaucratic, national institutions back to the states, localities, and revitalized mediating structures where citizenship is more fully realized. In addition to these thematic considerations, eligible projects will exhibit these features: They may address any arena of public life-economics, politics, culture, or civil society-where citizenship as here understood is an important issue. It is important to note that our view of citizenship is not narrowly focused on voting and elections. They may address the problem of citizenship at home or abroad, where the fall of many (and the perpetuation of some) totalitarian regimes has made this particularly urgent. In light of our emphasis on decentralization, and considering the Foundation's deep roots in Milwaukee and Wisconsin-areas with proud traditions of innovation and experimentation in democratic citizenship–community and state projects will be of particular interest to us. Such projects will aim to improve the life of the community through increasing cultural and educational opportunities, grass-roots economic development, and effective and humane social and health services, reflecting where possible the Foundation's focus on the resuscitation of citizenship." *Report of the Lynde and Harry Bradley Foundation* **Priorities:** *Arts & Humanities:* 11%. Supports theaters, symphonies, and art museums. *Civic & Public Affairs:* 36%. Funds neighborhoods, policy research, and domestic policy programs. *Education:* 41%. Supports research projects, scholarship programs, school choice efforts, universities. *Environment:* 3%. Supports family services. *Note:* Total contributions made in 2001. **Typ. Recipients:** Children's Health/Hospitals, Clinics/Medical Centers, Health Policy/Cost Containment, Hospitals, Transplant Networks/Donor Banks. **Geo. Dist:** nationally; WI.

★ 11721 ★ Lyndhurst Foundation

517 East Fifth St.
Chattanooga, TN 37403-1826
Phone: (423)756-0767 **Fax:** (423)756-0770
Website: http://www.lyndhurstfoundation.org
Jack Murrah, President

Fnded: 1938. **Philosophy:** Through the end of the century, the foundation intends to focus upon a number of activities. In Chattanooga, the foundation will focus on: continued development of the Tennessee Riverpark; redevelopment of the Southside as a live-and-work urban neighborhood with a zero-emissions industrial park; facilitation of historic preservation; stimulation of downtown housing development; strengthening of the city's arts and cultural life; protection and enhancement of the community's natural environment; the reform of the community's elementary and secondary public schools; the continued development of improved housing opportunities for people of modest means; and innovations in social service programs that provide genuine progress against social problems and genuine enhancement of community strengths. In the South, the foundation will focus on: continued development of the Center for Documentary Studies at Duke University, a center supporting responsible involvement in the world by encouraging photographers, filmmakers, writers, scholars, teachers, and students to work by direct observation, to participate in the lives of individuals and communities, and to render these lives in works of artistic, literary, and social value; support of individuals providing significant contributions within various fields of interest (through the Lyndhurst Prize program); continued evolution of a significant education reform initiative in rural Alabama; and protection and enhancement of the natural environment of the Southern Appalachian region. Most of the foundation's grants are distributed solely at the foundation's initiative. This means that, in most categories, the foundation does not seek or fund uninvited requests. For instance, within the field of education, the foundation has made a commitment extending through the end of the century to support certain reform initiatives within the city of Chattanooga and in rural Alabama. Within two categories, however, the foundation is open to requests. These are in the fields of arts and culture within the Chattanooga area, and environmental improvement throughout the six-state region (Tennessee, North Carolina, South Carolina, Georgia, Alabama, and Mississippi) that defines the Southeast. Strong preference is given to programs that focus on the Southern Appalachian region. **Priorities:** *Arts & Humanities:* 56%. Theater, museums, documentary studies organization. *Civic & Public Affairs:* 19%. Includes organizations concerned with the revitalization of Chattanooga. *Education:* About 9%. Charter schools, universities, community foundations. *Environment:* 2%. Community services. *International:* less than 1%. Supports health centers. *Note:* Total contributions made in 2000. **Typ. Recipients:** Child Abuse, Clinics/Medical Centers, Mental Health, Sexual Abuse, Substance Abuse. **Geo. Dist:** Southeastern USA; Chattanooga, TN.

★ 11722 ★ Lynn R. and Karl E. Prickett Fund

PO Box 20124
Greensboro, NC 27420
Charles Cheek, Trustee

Fnded: 1964. **Philosophy:** The foundation generally supports civic affairs, social service groups, and education. Civic affairs funding favors civil rights, the environment, and municipalities. Funding for social services emphasizes community relations and planned parenthood. Educational funding favors funds, higher education, and political education. The arts and health care are also supported. **Priorities:** *Arts & Humanities:* 8%. Supports art institutes, and music. *Civic & Public Affairs:* 17%. Supports festivals, aquariums, community foundations, civil rights, and legal aid. *Education:* 16%. Mainly supports colleges and universities, education funds, and private secondary schools. *Environment:* 35%. Supports food distribution, youth organizations, and animal protection. *International:* 10%. Primarily supports single-disease health associations. *Religion:* 1%. Supports scientific organizations and research. *Note:* Total contributions made in 2000. **Typ. Recipients:** AIDS/HIV, Alzheimers Disease, Cancer, Children's Health/Hospitals,

Emergency/Ambulance Services, Eyes/Blindness, Family Planning, Geriatric Health, Health Organizations, Multiple Sclerosis, Single-Disease Health Associations, Substance Abuse. **Geo. Dist:** nationally.

★ 11723 ★ Lyon Foundation

PO Box 546
Bartlesville, OK 74005
Phone: (918)336-0066
James Connor, President

Fnded: 1975. **Philosophy:** Recent grants have been made primarily to social service organizations. The foundation favors community centers, youth organizations, and support for services for the disabled. Other recipient areas include health foundations, nutrition programs, and housing. In the past, contributions have been made across all major categories of support. **Priorities:** *Arts & Humanities:* 13%. Funds historical preservation. *Civic & Public Affairs:* 33%. Supports the City of Bartlesville, fire departments, and legal concerns. *Education:* 27%. Supports colleges, nursing scholarships, and community education. *Environment:* 23%. Supports Young Men's Christian Association, a community center, senior citizens organizations, alcohol and drug abuse prevention, and a local Pony League. *International:* 4%. Funds a hospital and family care. *Note:* Total contributions made in 2000. **Typ. Recipients:** Alzheimers Disease, Clinics/Medical Centers, Emergency/Ambulance Services, Geriatric Health, Health Organizations, Hospitals, Medical Education, Medical Rehabilitation, Mental Health, Nutrition, People with Disabilities, Public Health, Substance Abuse. **Geo. Dist:** Bartlesville, OK.

★ 11724 ★ M. B. and Edna Zale Foundation

3102 Maple Ave., Suite 225
Dallas, TX 75201-1233
Phone: (214)855-0627 **Fax:** (214)220-0633
Leonard Krasnow, President

Fnded: 1951. **Philosophy:** The foundation "honors the tradition of its founders through grants that stimulate change. To accomplish this mission, the Foundation acts as a catalyst for collaboration and makes grants in communities where the trustees live or have an interest." M. B. and Edna Zale Foundation 1996 Annual Report. **Priorities:** *Arts & Humanities:* 1%. subpanelports museums, history, theater, and opera. *Civic & Public Affairs:* 5%. Supports civil rights womens affairs, and clubs. *Education:* 10%. Supports colleges and universities, secondary schools, and literacy. *Environment:* 14%. Supports shelters, community services, child welfare, United Way, food distribution programs, family planning services, and people with disabilities. *International:* 15%. Hospital, geriatric health, and clinics. *Religion:* 1%. Supports a science center. *Note:* Total contributions made in 1999. **Typ. Recipients:** Cancer, Children's Health/Hospitals, Clinics/Medical Centers, Diabetes, Emergency/Ambulance Services, Geriatric Health, Health Organizations, Health-General, Heart, Hospitals, Hospitals (University Affiliated), Kidney, Long-Term Care, Medical Education, Mental Health, Nutrition, People with Disabilities, Speech & Hearing. **Geo. Dist:** preference is given to funding organizations in Florida, Georgia, New York, and Texas.

★ 11725 ★ M. D. Anderson Foundation

PO Box 2558
Houston, TX 77252-8037
Phone: (713)216-5348 **Fax:** (713)216-2119
Toloria Allen, Grants Administrator

Fnded: 1936. **Philosophy:** The foundation provides funding for the "improvement of working conditions among workers generally, as well as among particular classes of unskilled, skilled, and agricultural workers; to the establishment, support and maintenance of hospitals, homes and institutions for the care of the sick, the young, the aged, the incompetent and the helpless among the people; to the improvement of living conditions among people generally as well as in particular sections or localities; and to the promotion of health, science, education, and advancement and diffusion of knowledge and understanding among people." **Priorities:** *Arts & Humanities:* 11%. Supports museums and music. *Civic & Public Affairs:* 8%. Funds neighborhood development, legal organizations, and zoos. *Education:* 50%. Funds colleges, universities, education centers, and religious pre-college education. *Environment:* 10%. Supports shelters, services for people with disabilities, and youth organizations. *International:* 14%. Supports hospitals, medical centers, clinics, and nursing. *Religion:* 1%. *Note:* Total contributions made in 2000. **Typ. Recipients:** Adolescent Health Issues, Cancer, Child Abuse, Children's Health/Hospitals, Clinics/Medical Centers, Emergency/Ambulance Services, Eyes/Blindness, Family Planning, Geriatric Health, Health Organizations, Health Policy/Cost Containment, Heart, Hospices, Hospitals, Medical Education, Medical Rehabilitation, Medical Research, Mental Health, Nursing Services, People with Disabilities, Prenatal Health Issues, Public Health, Research/Studies Institutes, Single-Disease Health Associations, Substance Abuse, Transplant Networks/Donor Banks. **Geo. Dist:** TX, Harris County; Houston, TX, and metropolitan area.

★ 11726 ★ M. G. and Lillie A. Johnson Foundation

PO Box 2269
Victoria, TX 77902
Phone: (512)575-7970 **Fax:** (512)575-2264
Email: mgj@cox-internet.com
Robert Halepeska, Executive Vice President

Fnded: 1958. **Philosophy:** The foundation's stated priority is support for health and higher education institutions in the Gulf Coast area of Texas. Historically, all grants are made to qualifying entities located in the 13 county area lying between Wharton and San Patricio counties. **Priorities:** *Arts & Humanities:* 2%. Supports the performing arts and libraries. *Civic & Public Affairs:* 17%. Provides funding for municipalities, towns, fire departments, and public safety organizations to purchase medical and safety equipment. *Education:* 26%. Supports three area colleges. *Environment:* 28%. Contributes to youth groups, drug abuse programs, food banks, senior citizens, and children's homes. *International:* 27%. Awards grants to area hospitals for the purchase of equipment. *Note:* Total contributions made in fiscal 2002. Giving priorities were provided by the foundation. **Typ. Recipients:** Clinics/Medical Centers, Domestic Violence, Emergency/Ambulance Services, Eyes/Blindness, Health Funds, Heart, Hospices, Hospitals, Long-Term Care, Medical Education, Medical Rehabilitation, Mental Health, Nursing Services, Nutrition, People with Disabilities, Public Health, Research/Studies Institutes, Sexual Abuse, Substance Abuse, Transplant Networks/Donor Banks, Trauma Treatment. **Geo. Dist:** Gulf Coast between San Patricio and Wharton; TX.

★ 11727 ★ M. J. Murdock Charitable Trust

PO Box 1618
Vancouver, WA 98668
Phone: (360)694-8415 **Fax:** (360)694-1819
Website: http://www.murdock-trust.org
John Van Zytveld, Senior Program Director

Fnded: 1975. **Philosophy:** "The trust's mission is to enrich the quality of life in the Pacific Northwest by providing grants to organizations that seek to strengthen the region's educational and cultural base in creative and sustainable ways. Although the major funding interests are education and scientific research, grants are also given to a wide variety of organizations, including those that serve the arts, public affairs, health and medicine, human services, and people with disabilities." 1997 Guidelines The trust favors programs aimed at solutions for and the prevention of social problems, either through research or the application of existing knowledge and capabilities. Of major interest are projects which "expand man's knowledge of himself and his world; and which promote those values and activities of society leading to a happier, healthier, freer, and more productive life." The trust's primary function is to "provide 'up-front' or venture capital, along with that of other donors and the applicant's own resources. Funds are provided for the testing and validation of promising concepts, and in the launching of well thought-out programs which have the potential to thrive beyond the stage of initial funding." Science continues to be a major interest of the trust, reflecting Mr. Murdock's own scientific bent. The trust is taking an increasingly informed, active role in improving science and science education in the Pacific Northwest. It will explore additional pre-collegiate science possibilities that address the issue of the diminished supply of science educators and researchers, and will "seek to reinvigorate undergraduate science, and to support research and specialized science-education opportunities that address critical needs" of the region. **Priorities:** *Arts & Humanities:* 11%. Focus on historical societies, theater, and music. *Civic & Public Affairs:* 15%. *Education:* 44%. Interests include higher education, informal education at museums, research at major universities, and natural science research. *Environment:* 14%. Funds human service organizations. *International:* 5%. *Religion:* Approx. 1%. Supports scientific research. *Note:* Total contributions made in 2000. **Typ. Recipients:** Alzheimers Disease, Cancer, Children's Health/Hospitals, Clinics/Medical Centers, Emergency/Ambulance Services, Eyes/Blindness, Health Policy/Cost Containment, Hospitals, Hospitals (University Affiliated), Medical Education, Medical Rehabilitation, Medical Research, Mental Health, People with Disabilities, Preventive Medicine/Wellness Organizations, Public Health. **Geo. Dist:** Pacific Northwest USA; AK; ID; MT; OR; WA.

★ 11728 ★ M. R. Bauer Foundation

208 South LaSalle St., Suite 1750
Chicago, IL 60604-1188
Phone: (312)372-1947 **Fax:** (312)372-2389
Email: klawrence@LKsu.com
Kent Lawrence, President & Executive Director

Fnded: 1994. **Philosophy:** The foundation typically supports judicial system reform projects and programs reducing unwanted pregnancy. Colleges and universities, hospitals and health organizations, civic and public affairs causes, cultural concerns, and social welfare organizations also are supported. **Priorities:** *Arts & Humanities:* 1%. Museums, theater, music, arts associations, and arts festivals. *Civic & Public Affairs:* 18%. Primarily for judicial reform projects. *Education:* 3%. Colleges and universities, and medical education. *Environment:* 20%. Family planning, food and clothing distribution, youth organizations, and community services. *International:* 50%. Hospitals, medical centers, and single-disease health associations. *Note:* Total contributions made in 2001. **Typ. Recipients:** Adolescent Health Issues, Cancer, Children's Health/Hospitals, Clinics/Medical Centers, Emergency/Ambulance Services, Family Planning, Health Organizations, Hospitals, Long-Term Care, Medical Education, Medical Rehabilitation, Medical Research, Mental Health, Multiple Sclerosis, Prenatal Health Issues, Research/Studies Institutes, Single-Disease Health Associations. **Geo. Dist:** Chicago, IL.

★ 11729 ★ M. S. Doss Foundation, Inc.

PO Box 1677
Seminole, TX 79360-1677
Phone: (915)758-2770 **Fax:** (915)758-9591
Joe McGill, President

Fnded: 1984. **Philosophy:** The M. S. Doss Foundation primarily supports social service organizations. Recipients include children's homes and youth organizations. The foundation makes grants to other recipient areas, with an emphasis on building funds. **Priorities:** *Arts & Humanities:* 1%. Supports music. *Civic & Public Affairs:* 18%. Supports community affairs. *Education:* 3%. Supports educational institutions in Texas. *Environment:* 67% Supports youth services, food banks, senior services, and women's shelters. *International:* 6%. Supports the Cerebral Palsy Treatment Center and hospitals. *Note:* Contributions were made in 2002. **Typ. Recipients:** Child Abuse, Children's Health/Hospitals, Clinics/Medical Centers, Diabetes, Domestic Violence, Hospices, Hospitals, Medical Education, Medical Rehabilitation, People with Disabilities, Single-Disease Health Associations, Substance Abuse. **Geo. Dist:** NM, eastern New Mexico; TX, western Texas.

★ 11730 ★ Mabel Louise Riley Foundation

77 Summer St., 8th Floor
Boston, MA 02110
Phone: (617)399-1850 **Fax:** (617)399-1851
Email: rileyfoundation@kl.com
Website: http://www.agmconnect.org/riley1.html
Nancy Saunders, Administrative Manager

Fnded: 1972. **Philosophy:** The Mabel Louise Riley Foundation is a general purpose fund with the wide mission of "improving the quality of life for the people of Massachusetts, particularly in Boston." Miss Riley's wish that the trustees give "particular consideration to the needs of children and youth" is a factor in grant decisions. The foundation places an emphasis on education, and also supports youth and young adults through summer activity programs, arts for youth, and various human service programs. Comprehensive community development in low-income and minority neighborhoods is a priority that includes employment and job training, housing, historic preservation, urban affairs, and access to the arts for underserved populations. General city-wide attempts to enhance the quality of life in Boston, activities which have potential for lasting impact upon the Boston population, services to needy constituencies, and cultivation of potentially self-sufficient programs that may serve as models are also supported. **Priorities:** *Arts & Humanities:* 10%. Supports museums, libraries, music, and cultural and arts centers. *Civic & Public Affairs:* 34%. Supports community development, urban affairs, economic development, ethnic organizations, zoos and gardens, and housing. *Education:* 13%. Funds education associations, training organizations, charter schools, and higher education. *Environment:* 37%. Supports youth organizations, YMCA, human services, family and child welfare, and shelters. *International:* 3%. Community health centers and single-disease associations receive funding. *Note:* Total contributions made in 2000. **Typ. Recipients:** Clinics/Medical Centers, Diabetes, Emergency/Ambulance Services, Family Planning, Health Policy/Cost Containment, Long-Term Care, Medical Education, Mental Health, People with Disabilities, Prenatal Health Issues, Substance Abuse. **Geo. Dist:** Boston, MA.

★ 11731 ★ Maclellan Foundation

Provident Bldg., Suite 501
One Fountain Square
Chattanooga, TN 37402
Phone: (423)755-1366 **Fax:** (423)755-1640
Email: info@maclellanfdn.org
Website: http://www.maclellan.net
Hugh Maclellan, Jr., President, Treasurer & Trustee

Fnded: 1945. **Philosophy:** "The purpose of the Maclellan Foundation is to serve strategic international and national organizations committed to furthering the Kingdom of Christ and select local organizations, which foster the spiritual welfare of the community. We will serve by providing financial and leadership resources to extend the Kingdom of God in accordance with the Great Commission. The Maclellan Foundation sees as its primary strategies to play a key leadership role in aggressively leveraging its resources to complete the Great Commission in three areas. These three areas are being proactive in funding strategic, evangelical Christian organizations which are strategic, cost efficient, and have a big multiplying effect; strengthening strategic Christian organizations led by Godly leaders acting in a responsible, organizational manner; and encouraging other evangelical donors in their giving to such organizations." Maclellan Foundation Giving Guidelines **Priorities:** *Note:* Total contributions made in 2000. **Typ. Recipients:** Family Planning, Public Health, Substance Abuse. **Geo. Dist:** internationally; nationally; Chattanooga, TN.

★ 11732 ★ Malcolm Hewitt Wiener Foundation

1270 Ave. of the Americas
New York, NY 10020
Adelaide Lewis, Contact

Fnded: 1984. **Philosophy:** The Malcolm Hewitt Wiener Foundation makes grants across the major categories of support. In civic affairs, interests include world peace intitiatives, foreign relations, and economics. Arts funding favors art institutes, museums, historical preservation, and libraries. Social service primarily supports family services and family planning. Funding for education supports colleges and universities. Health care contributions include hospitals and health organizations. **Priorities:** *Arts & Humanities:* 26%. Supports ballet, orchestra, performing arts. *Civic & Public Affairs:* 10%. Supports parks, libraries, law and justice organizations. *Education:* 45%. Supports colleges and universities, arts and humanities education. *Environment:* 3%. Supports family planning. *International:* 7%. Supports New York Hospital-Cornell Medical Center. *Note:* Total contributions made in 2000. **Typ. Recipients:** AIDS/HIV, Children's Health/Hospitals, Clinics/Medical Centers, Emergency/Ambulance Services, Family Planning, Health Organizations, Health-General, Hospitals, Hospitals (University Affiliated), Medical Education, Medical Research, Nursing Services, People with Disabilities, Public Health, Single-Disease Health Associations, Transplant Networks/Donor Banks. **Geo. Dist:** nationally; New York, NY.

★ 11733 ★ Mamie McFaddin Ward Heritage Foundation

PO Box 3928
Beaumont, TX 77704-3928
Phone: (409)880-1426 **Fax:** (409)880-1437

Fnded: 1976. **Philosophy:** "The Foundation's primary purpose is to support the McFaddin-Ward House Museum, located in Beaumont, TX. The Foundation may also make grants to non-profit organizations in the local community for educational, cultural and charitable purposes." **Priorities:** *Arts & Humanities:* 39%. Supports historic preservation, museums, and theater. *Civic & Public Affairs:* 24%. Funds urban affairs and housing. *Education:* 10%. Supports private schools. *Environment:* 12%. Supports scouting and substance abuse treatment. *International:* 15%. Supports pediatric health, outreach programs, organ donation, and mental health. *Note:* Total contributions made in 2001. **Typ. Recipients:** Cancer, Children's Health/Hospitals, Clinics/Medical Centers, Emergency/Ambulance Services, Geriatric Health, Long-Term Care, Medical Rehabilitation, Medical Research, Mental Health, Nutrition, Substance Abuse. **Geo. Dist:** TX, Jefferson County.

★ 11734 ★ Mardag Foundation

600 5th St. Center
Saint Paul, MN 55101-1797
Phone: (651)224-5463 **Fax:** (651)224-8123
Email: inbox@mardag.org
Website: http://www.mardag.org/
Paul Verret, President

Fnded: 1969. **Philosophy:** "The Mardag Foundation is committed to making grants to qualified nonprofit organizations within the State of Minnesota that help to enhance and improve the quality of life. Our focus is on children, the elderly and other at-risk populations, education, and the arts. Where appropriate, the Foundation will be an active participant with others in grantmaking programs, and will be proactive in addressing issues as well as responsive to applications for grants." The foundation normally will: make grants for capital, program, or expansion projects of a time-limited nature; help meet start-up costs for promising new programs that demonstrate sound management and clear goals relevant to community needs; support established agencies seeking to expand their services or experiencing temporary financial difficulty; make some grants payable over a number years; provide funds to match resources or offer challenge grants; expect an indication of the general process that will be used to monitor or evaluate the impact or effect of the grants. In recent years, the foundation arranged a partnership with other private and public funders to address the critical needs in education and the problems of illiterate adults in Minnesota, and to achieve a better understanding of the needs of minority students. Included in the foundation's assistance is a three-year statewide program intended to help independent secondary schools improve their economic stability, and develop competitive curricula in an increasingly technological society. Funding for social service projects in Minnesota remains a priority as values, public funding, and local economics continue to change. In 1996, the foundation adopted a provisional policy outlining how it intends to address devolution and changes in public funding. 1996 Annual Report **Priorities:** *Arts & Humanities:* 11%. Arts centers, historical societies, music, and theaters. *Civic & Public Affairs:* 10%. Inner-city development. *Education:* 10%. Colleges and universities, minority education, and education associations. *Environment:* 66%. Child welfare, domestic violence, and family services. *International:* 3%. Public health. *Note:* Total contributions made in 1998. **Typ. Recipients:** Alzheimers Disease, Child Abuse, Domestic Violence, Emergency/Ambulance Services, Family Planning, Geriatric Health, Health Organizations, Hospices, Hospitals, Long-Term Care, Mental Health, People with Disabilities, Public Health, Sexual Abuse, Single-Disease Health Associations, Substance Abuse. **Geo. Dist:** MN.

★ 11735 ★ Margaret L. Wendt Foundation

40 Fountain Plaza, Suite 277
Buffalo, NY 14202-2220
Phone: (716)855-2146 **Fax:** (716)855-2149
Robert Kresse, Secretary & Trustee

Fnded: 1955. **Philosophy:** The foundation makes grants in the following designated areas: schools, religious organizations, hospitals and health organizations, youth programs, the arts, and social and community welfare organizations. **Priorities:** *Arts & Humanities:* 32%. Supports historical societies, theater, opera, and public broadcasting. *Civic & Public Affairs:* 5%. Funds urban programs, community services, and zoos. *Education:* 13%. Supports colleges and universities. *Environment:* 8%. Funds United Way, boys and girls clubs, camps, food and shelter, and family support programs. *International:* 8%. Nursing medical research, psychiatric care, medical centers, and children's hospitals. *Religion:* 1%. *Note:* Total contributions made in fiscal 2001. **Typ. Recipients:** AIDS/HIV, Alzheimers Disease, Children's Health/Hospitals, Clinics/Medical Centers, Emergency/Ambulance Services, Family Planning, Health Funds, Health Organizations, Heart, Home-Care Services, Hospices, Hospitals, Long-Term Care, Medical Education, Medical Research, Mental Health, Nursing Services, Outpatient Health Care, People with Disabilities, Research/Studies Institutes, Single-Disease Health Associations, Speech & Hearing, Substance Abuse. **Geo. Dist:** NY, Western New York state; Buffalo, NY.

★ 11736 ★ Margaret T. Morris Foundation

PO Box 592
Prescott, AZ 86302
Phone: (928)445-4010
Eugene Polk, Trustee

Fnded: 1967. **Philosophy:** The foundation supports all areas of philanthropy equally. Acceptable proposals have included arts associations, libraries, community development, support for educational programs at the primary and secondary levels, single-disease health organizations, hospitals, churches and religious community living, youth clubs, shelters, homes, and food and clothing distributors. **Priorities:** *Arts & Humanities:* 8%. Libraries, museums, performing arts and public broadcasting receive funding. *Civic & Public Affairs:* 14%. Supports community development and housing. *Education:* 26%. Emphasis on higher education. *Environment:* 17%. Supports services for youth, seniors, and programs for differently abled groups. *International:* 28%. Hospitals and health services are supported. *Note:* Total contributions made in 2000. **Typ. Recipients:** AIDS/HIV, Alzheimers Disease, Cancer, Children's Health/Hospitals, Clinics/Medical Centers, Emergency/Ambulance Services, Family Planning, Geriatric Health, Health Organizations, Health Policy/Cost Containment, Health-General, Home-Care Services, Hospices, Hospitals, Long-Term Care, Medical Education, Medical Research, Mental Health, People with Disabilities, Prenatal Health Issues, Preventive Medicine/Wellness Organizations, Public Health, Research/Studies Institutes, Single-Disease Health Associations. **Geo. Dist:** nationally.

★ 11737 ★ Marie H. Bechtel Charitable Remainder Uni-Trust

201 West 2nd St., Ste. 1000
Davenport, IA 52801
Phone: (563)328-3333 **Fax:** (563)328-3352
R. Bittner, Trustee

Fnded: 1978. **Philosophy:** The Marie H. Bechtel Charitable Remainder Uni-Trust was established with the purpose of serving the needs of the Scott County, IA, community. The trust has a broad range of interests that includes youth, education, public affairs, civic affairs, the arts, health, and social services. Both Harold and Marie Bechtel were lifetime residents of Scott County. Their primary purpose in establishing the trust was "to support all interests which serve to enhance the community, to restore its vitality, and to create meaningful education and employment today and in the future." Since Harold Bechtel's death in 1987, nearly all distributions have been to local organizations or Iowa educational institutions, but there have been several outside of Iowa. **Priorities:** *Arts & Humanities:* 10%. Supports libraries, arts museums, and a music festival. *Civic & Public Affairs:* 23%. Supports urban affairs and development, beautification foundation, and community support. *Education:* 36%. Supports universities, schools, colleges and business school. *Environment:* 21%. Supports Young Men's Christian Association, youth programs, and homes. *Religion:* 10%. Supports a Natural Science museum. *Note:* Total contributions made in 2001. **Typ. Recipients:** Cancer, Medical Education, Public Health. **Geo. Dist:** IA, Scott County.

★ 11738 ★ Marion I. and Henry J. Knott Foundation

3904 Hickory Ave.
Baltimore, MD 21211-1834
Phone: (410)235-7068 **Fax:** (410)889-2577
Email: knott@knottfoundation.org
Website: http://www.knottfoundation.org
M. Contori, Exec. Dir.

Fnded: 1986. **Philosophy:** The Marion I. and Henry J. Knott Foundation makes grants to "further Roman Catholic activities and other charitable, cultural, educational, health care, and human service activities." Program areas funded include arts and humanities, Catholic activities, education (limited to Catholic and non-sectarian private schools), health care, and social and human services. The foundation supports the following types of projects: capital/building campaigns, endowment funds (except for arts and humanities), new and/or ongoing programs, and operating expenses. **Priorities:** *Arts & Humanities:* 11%. Museums and arts centers, opera, and historical societies. *Civic & Public Affairs:* About 23%. Focus on urban affairs. *Education:* 31%. Primarily supports private primary and secondary education. *Environment:* About 24%. Supports shelters, food banks, counseling, and family services. *International:* About 2%. Supports health associations. *Note:* Total contributions made in 2000. **Typ. Recipients:** AIDS/HIV, Alzheimers Disease, Cancer, Children's Health/Hospitals, Clinics/Medical Centers, Eyes/Blindness, Health Funds, Health Organizations, Hospices, Medical Education, Medical Rehabilitation, Mental Health, Multiple Sclerosis, Nutrition, People with Disabilities, Prenatal Health Issues, Preventive Medicine/Wellness Organizations, Public Health, Single-Disease Health Associations, Substance Abuse, Trauma Treatment. **Geo. Dist:** CA; MD.

★ 11739 ★ Marion O. and Maximilian E. Hoffman Foundation

6000 Northern Blvd.
Muttontown, NY 11732
Phone: (516)624-4955
Ursula Niarakis, President

Fnded: 1984. **Philosophy:** The foundation makes most of its grants in the areas of environmental affairs, education, and the arts. Conservation causes receive major emphasis. Educational funding favors higher education, scholarships, and private schools. Funding for the arts emphasizes film, museums, and theater. Other support also goes to social services. **Priorities:** *Arts & Humanities:* 1%. *Environment:* 4%. *Note:* Total contributions made in fiscal 2001. **Typ. Recipients:** AIDS/HIV, Cancer, Clinics/Medical Centers, Health Organizations, Hospitals, Medical Research, People with Disabilities, Single-Disease Health Associations. **Geo. Dist:** New York, NY.

★ 11740 ★ Marmot Foundation

1100 N Market St.
Wilmington, DE 19890
Phone: (302)651-1000
Charles Gummey, Jr., Secretary (For Delaware Organizations)

Fnded: 1968. **Philosophy:** The foundation's primary focus is social service organizations, including united funds and community center support. Youth organizations are also a major priority. The trustees are also interested in education, from day schools to high schools to the university level. Health services are considered a secondary interest, with most support going directly to hospitals. **Priorities:** *Arts & Humanities:* Supports museums, arts and cultural programs, and libraries. *Civic & Public Affairs:* Supports housing and community development. *Education:* Funds secondary schools, colleges and universities, adult literacy, and reading. *Environment:* Supports United Way, children and family services, family planning, homeless shelters, and senior citizen services. *International:* Supports hospitals, hospice, healthcare, and health associations. **Typ. Recipients:** Arthritis, Cancer, Children's Health/Hospitals, Clinics/Medical Centers, Diabetes, Emergency/Ambulance Services, Eyes/Blindness, Family Planning, Health Funds, Health Organizations, Heart, Hospices, Hospitals, Hospitals (University Affiliated), Medical Education, Mental Health, Outpatient Health Care, People with Disabilities, Preventive Medicine/Wellness Organizations, Public Health, Research/Studies Institutes, Substance Abuse, Trauma Treatment. **Geo. Dist:** DE; FL.

★ 11741 ★ Marriner S. Eccles Foundation

P. O. Box 628
Salt Lake City, UT 84110-0628
Phone: (801)246-1436
Shannon Toronto, Executive Director

Fnded: 1973. **Philosophy:** The foundation's giving is restricted to private, nongovernmental charitable, scientific, and educational organizations located in Utah for the benefit of the citizens of that state. **Priorities:** *Arts & Humanities:* 17%. Supports performing arts, museums, and art centers. *Civic & Public Affairs:* 10%. *Education:* 34%. Funds colleges and universities. *Environment:* 26%. Includes issues related to teen pregnancy and substance abuse. *International:* 12%. Primarily to hospitals and single-disease health associations. *Note:* Total contributions made in fiscal 2001. **Typ. Recipients:** AIDS/HIV, Arthritis, Cancer, Children's Health/Hospitals, Clinics/Medical Centers, Diabetes, Emergency/Ambulance Services, Eyes/Blindness, Family Planning, Geriatric Health, Health Organizations, Health-General, Hospices, Hospitals, Medical Education, Mental Health, Nursing Services, People with Disabilities, Public Health, Respiratory, Single-Disease Health Associations, Substance Abuse. **Geo. Dist:** UT.

★ 11742 ★ Mars Foundation

6885 Elm St.
McLean, VA 22101
Phone: (703)821-4900 **Fax:** (703)448-9678
Susan Martin, Assistant Secretary

Fnded: 1956. **Philosophy:** Grants are generally awarded in the form of unrestricted general support. Though priority is given to programs for children and the environment, other grantees include: educational organizations; fine art associations; and public health organizations, including groups concerned with population problems and medical care and assistance. **Priorities:** *Arts & Humanities:* 12%. Supports the fine arts and historic preservation. *Civic & Public Affairs:* 6%. Urban and economic affairs. *Education:* About 36%. Supports elementary and secondary education and colleges and universities. *Environment:* 20%. Supports family planning organizations, child welfare, animal protection, shelters, and youth organizations. *International:* 7%. Primarily for single-disease health associations, hospitals, hospices, and medical training. *Note:* Total contributions made in 1998. **Typ. Recipients:** Cancer, Children's Health/Hospitals, Clinics/Medical Centers, Domestic Violence, Family Planning, Health Funds, Hospices, Medical Education, Medical Research, Nursing Services, People with Disabilities, People with Disabilities, Single-Disease Health Associations, Substance Abuse. **Geo. Dist:** nationally; Washington, DC, including metropolitan area.

★ 11743 ★ Marshall L. and Perrine D. McCune Charitable Foundation

345 E Alameda St.
Santa Fe, NM 87501-2229
Phone: (505)983-8300 **Fax:** (505)983-7887
Email: fsowers@swcp.com
Website: http://www.nmmccune.org
Frances Sowers, Associate Director

Fnded: 1988. **Typ. Recipients:** AIDS/HIV, Children's Health/Hospitals, Clinics/Medical Centers, Diabetes, Hospices, Hospitals, Nursing Services, Prenatal Health Issues, Preventive Medicine/Wellness Organizations, Public Health, Sexual Abuse. **Geo. Dist:** NM.

★ 11744 ★ Martha Holden Jennings Foundation

The Halle Bldg.
1228 Euclid Ave., Suite 710
Cleveland, OH 44115
Phone: (216)589-5700 **Fax:** (216)589-5730
Website: http://www.mhjf.org
William Hiller, Executive Director

Fnded: 1958. **Philosophy:** The foundation continues its mission to fund projects to "explore new frontiers in elementary and secondary public school education in Ohio and to promote more effective teaching in those schools." In seeking to improve the quality of primary and secondary education, the foundation has "invested heavily in major outreach areas. These include: early childhood education; urban schools; family involvement; improvements in math and science; ... assisting schools with technology; and partnerships involving universities and urban schools in Ohio." Grants also are aimed at programs to build a bridge of understanding and cooperation among colleges, universities, and public schools in order to achieve a higher quality of teaching and improved curricula and materials. The foundation itself administers several programs. These include a grants program for individual teachers and administrators to implement proposals or test new approaches to education designed by the recipients. The foundation also operates an educators' retreat to bring together public school educators, deans of colleges of education, and representatives of the Ohio Department of Education. Other programs offer workshops, lectures, and awards to develop needed skills, provide intellectual stimulation, and recognize outstanding teachers. **Priorities:** *Education:* 100% The Foundation reports its priorities are state initiatives, focusing on technology, and the master teachers program. The state initiatives program encompases three separate intiatives: parent involvement to improve student achievement by strengthening partnerships between families and schools; early childhood with a commitment to operate four Reggio Emilia preschools; and urban schools, with a focus on solving the problems of Large urban schools including early childhood education, prevention of disruptive and dangerous behavior, career planning and placement, assistance for "at-risk" students, intervention and accountability alliance, partnerships with parents and development for educators. The foundation's area of interest focusing on Technology includes programs such as training teachers in technology, software training, preparing high school students for high-tech careers and establishing a distance learning network. Each year the foundation also recognizes three Master Teachers from Ohio that are currently hosting the Jennings Scholar Lecture Series for the master teachers program. *Note:* Total contributions made in 1999. **Typ. Recipients:** Adolescent Health Issues, Heart, Mental Health, People with Disabilities, Preventive Medicine/Wellness Organizations, Substance Abuse. **Geo. Dist:** OH, Cuyahoga County.

★ 11745 ★ Martin Foundation

Castillo Square
5051 Castillo Drive, Suite 204
Naples, FL 34103
Gerladine Martin, President

Fnded: 1954. **Philosophy:** "Since its inception, the Martin Foundation has supported many worthy local civic projects and organizations, such as: the Public Library; YM-YWCA; Public Television; Park Development; Civic Plaza; Environmental Center; Midwest Museum of American Art; and the Elkhart County Community Foundation to mention a few." "In addition the Foundation has supported national and international organizations and projects including: University of California, Berkeley, graduate scholarship program; Field Museum of Natural History; Indiana University, South Bend for the endowed professorship in piano; Interlochen Center for the Arts; Massachusetts Institute of Technology for the Lee and Geraldine Martin Professorship in Environmental Studies and the Martin Fund; Nature Conservancy; Samaritan Institute, an international counseling network; and World Wildlife Fund." "The Foundation will continue to fund worthwhile local civic and community projects and has an interest in creative projects at the national level which attempt to address some of the world's challenging problems." 1996/1997 Guidelines and Annual Report **Priorities:** *Arts & Humanities:* 9%. Gives to arts centers, museums, and public broadcasting. *Civic & Public Affairs:* 8%. Funds women's issues, civil rights, and community foundations. *Education:* 58%. Contributes to higher education. Major grant to MIT. *Environment:* 7%. Primarily supports youth concerns, Young Men's Christian Association, and family planning services. *International:* 7%. Supports caregivers, health policy/cost containment, hospitals, and the Red Cross. *Note:* Total contributions made in fiscal 2001. **Typ. Recipients:** AIDS/HIV, Alzheimers Disease, Cancer, Child Abuse, Clinics/Medical Centers, Domestic Violence, Emergency/Ambulance Services, Family Planning, Health-General, Hospices, Hospitals, Medical Education, Medical Research, Medical Training, Mental Health, Nursing Services, People with Disabilities, Public Health, Single-Disease Health Associations, Substance Abuse. **Geo. Dist:** nationally.

★ 11746 ★ Marty and Dorothy Silverman Foundation

150 East 58th St., 29th Floor
New York, NY 10155
Fax: (212)755-1410
Lorin Silverman, Secretary-Treasurer

Fnded: 1986. **Philosophy:** The foundation provides grants to programs that address the needs of indigent senior citizens including nursing homes and hospitals. Additionally, grants may be made to other educational, scientific, cultural, and health and welfare agencies. **Priorities:** *Arts & Humanities:* 3%. Contributes to the performing arts, public broadcasting, and museums. *Civic & Public Affairs:* 19%. Funds legal aid, urban affairs, and housing organizations. *Education:* 4%. Gives to institutions of higher learning, with an emphasis on legal and medical education. *Environment:* 16%. Funds YMHA/YWHAs, senior services, and social service agencies. *International:* 36%. Supports hospitals, medical centers, health associations, and geriatric health concerns. *Note:* Total contributions made in fiscal 2000. **Typ. Recipients:** AIDS/HIV, Alzheimers Disease, Cancer, Child Abuse, Clinics/Medical Centers, Domestic Violence, Family Planning, Geriatric Health, Health Organizations, Health Policy/Cost Containment, Heart, Hospitals, Long-Term Care, Medical Education, Medical Research, Mental Health, Nursing Services, People with Disabilities, Public Health, Single-Disease Health Associations. **Geo. Dist:** New York, NY.

★ 11747 ★ Mary and Daniel Loughran Foundation

601 13th St. NW, Ste. 1000
Washington, DC 20005
Phone: (202)434-7005 **Fax:** (202)347-4866
F. Burke, Executive Director & Secretary

Fnded: 1967. **Philosophy:** The foundation primarily supports higher education in Washington, DC, and Virginia. The trustees also support agricultural education and schools for handicapped children. Youth organizations also are a primary focus, with emphasis on infant homes and maternity care. The foundation supports other charitable organizations in addition to its main interests. **Priorities:** *Arts & Humanities:* 15%. Museums and historic building preservation. *Civic & Public Affairs:* 2%. Legal aid. *Education:* 38%. Scholarship, educational instituitions. *Environment:* 24%. Youth organizations and community centers. *International:* 12%. Hospital support. *Note:* Total contributions made in fiscal 1999. **Typ. Recipients:** Adolescent Health Issues, Cancer, Children's Health/Hospitals, Clinics/Medical Centers, Emergency/Ambulance Services, Eyes/Blindness, Family Planning, Heart, Hospitals, Long-Term Care, Medical Education, Medical Rehabilitation, Medical Research, People with Disabilities, Prenatal Health Issues, Sexual Abuse, Single-Disease Health Associations. **Geo. Dist:** DC; MD; VA.

★ 11748 ★ Mary Duke Biddle Foundation

1044 West Forest Hills Boulevard
Durham, NC 27707
Phone: (919)493-5591 **Fax:** (919)489-0118
Dr. James Semans, Chairman

Fnded: 1956. **Philosophy:** Mrs. Biddle's interests are still reflected in the foundation's giving pattern. Major recipients include cultural organizations, educational institutions, and community groups. In addition, the foundation shows an interest in aiding the handicapped. The trust agreement establishing the foundation specified that at least one-half of the annual income must go to Duke University for religious, scientific, literary, medical research, or educational purposes. Traditionally, support is given to Duke Memorial United Methodist Church, Durham, NC; Christ Church United Methodist, New York, NY; and Irvington Presbyterian Church, Irvington-on-Hudson, NY. The foundation provides grants for new programs, commissioning new works of art, for feasibility studies, and to organizations that provide assistance to individuals. In addition, challenge grants, planning grants, and start-up grants are made. The trustees are involved in the investigation of proposals and are willing to consider innovative projects and new ventures, even if success cannot be certain. Funding usually takes the form of general, program, and fellowship funds. In the area of music and the cultural arts, the foundation gives grants to organizations that support individual artists. Grants to individuals, however, are not made. Education grants are given to a wide variety of educational efforts in North Carolina and New York. Grants for aid to communities also are made. **Priorities:** *Arts & Humanities:* 36%. Emphasis on the Duke University Institute of Art. Also supports opera, theater, music, libraries, artists guilds, and the performing arts. *Civic & Public Affairs:* 2%. Gives to parks, community foundations and organizations, civil rights and botanical gardens. *Education:* 50%. Primary support for Duke University programs. Also funds scholarship and literacy. *Environment:* 7%. Funds community outreach, family and youth services, Special Olympics and counseling. *International:* 4%. Duke University Medical Center, blindness/eyes, AIDs, and physical therapy. *Note:* Total contributions made in 2000. **Typ. Recipients:** AIDS/HIV, Cancer, Clinics/Medical Centers, Geriatric Health, Health Organizations, Health-General, Hospices, Hospitals (University Affiliated), Medical Education, Medical Rehabilitation, Mental Health, People with Disabilities. **Geo. Dist:** NY; NC.

★ 11749 ★ Mary Hillman Jennings Foundation

2203 Allegheny Tower
Pittsburgh, PA 15222
Phone: (412)434-5606 **Fax:** (412)434-5907
Paul Euwer, Jr., Executive Director

Fnded: 1968. **Philosophy:** The foundation's principal areas of interest are education, social services, and health. In addition, the foundation funds civic, arts, and religious organizations. **Priorities:** *Arts & Humanities:* 11%. Supports museums, ballet, theater, historical preservation, and libraries. *Civic & Public Affairs:* 2%. Supports community foundations, guild groups, and leadership initiatives. *Education:* 27%. Supports private precollege education, and colleges and universities. *Environment:* 9%. Supports community service organizations, YMCA, youth services, shelters, and food distribution. *International:* 45%. Supports medical centers, hospitals, and medical research. *Religion:* 1%. *Note:* Total contributions made in 2000. **Typ. Recipients:** Alzheimers Disease, Cancer, Children's Health/Hospitals, Clinics/Medical Centers, Diabetes, Domestic Violence, Emergency/Ambulance Services, Family Planning, Health Organizations, Hospices, Hospitals, Long-Term Care, Medical Rehabilitation, Medical Research, Nursing Services, Outpatient Health Care, People with Disabilities, Public Health, Sexual Abuse, Single-Disease Health Associations, Substance Abuse, Trauma Treatment. **Geo. Dist:** Pittsburgh, PA.

★ 11750 ★ Mary J. Hutchins Foundation

11 John St.
New York, NY 10038
Phone: (212)964-3859
Richard Mirabella, Treasurer

Fnded: 1935. **Philosophy:** The Mary J. Hutchins Foundation primarily supports health care and social service organizations. Health support goes to general and specialty nonprofit hospitals. Nursing also is supported. Social service support favors homes and shelters, charity and welfare organizations, and youth clubs. Civic affairs agencies are supported on a limited basis. The foundation also endeavors to provide aid to poor and needy adults regardless of race, creed, or nationality. **Priorities:** *Arts & Humanities:* 2%. Gives to a gallery showing benefiting AIDS. *Civic & Public Affairs:* 5%. Contributes to community foundations, nonprofit management organizations, and neighborhood associations. *Education:* 4%. Funds independent schools and a speech school. *Environment:* 39%. Contributes to youth activities, scouts, child welfare organizations, shelters, family planning services, family counseling, and United Way. *International:* 41%. Supports hospitals and medical centers, eye and ear health, mental health, and epilepsy and multiple sclerosis organizations. *Note:* Total contributions made in 2001. **Typ. Recipients:** Clinics/Medical Centers, Emergency/Ambulance Services, Eyes/Blindness, Family Planning, Hospices, Hospitals, Hospitals (University Affiliated), Medical Education, Medical Rehabilitation, Medical Research, Mental Health, Multiple Sclerosis, Nursing Services, People with Disabilities, Sexual Abuse, Single-Disease Health Associations. **Geo. Dist:** New York, NY, metro area.

★ 11751 ★ Mary Livingston Griggs and Mary Griggs Burke Foundation

55 East Fifth St.
1400 5th St.
Saint Paul, MN 55101-1792
Phone: (651)227-7683 **Fax:** (651)602-2670
Marvin Pertzik, Secretary & Treasurer

Fnded: 1966. **Philosophy:** The foundation supports the arts, and institutions or programs with a cultural, historical, or educational focus. The foundation has additional interests in social services and conservation, environmental, and beautification efforts. **Priorities:** *Arts & Humanities:* 57%. Supports museum, opera, ballet, libraries, dance, public broadcasting and ethnic/folk art. *Civic & Public Affairs:* 7%. Supports zoological societies botanical gardens and parks. *Education:* 5%. Supports arts/humanities education, minority education, and colleges. *Environment:* 13%. Supports homeless, family planning services, daycare, and United Way. *Religion:* 2%. Supports science museums. *Note:* Total contributions made in fiscal 2001. **Typ. Recipients:** AIDS/HIV, Clinics/Medical Centers, Family Planning, Heart, Hospitals, Medical Research. **Geo. Dist:** Minneapolis, MN; St. Paul, MN; New York, NY.

★ 11752 ★ Mary Moody Northen Foundation

PO Box 1300
Galveston, TX 77553
Phone: (409)765-9770 **Fax:** (409)762-7055
Betty Massey, Executive Director

Fnded: 1964. **Philosophy:** While the foundation supports charitable activities in Texas and Virginia, it primarily concentrates its charitable activities to two foundation-administered programs, including the restoration of the W. L. Moody, Jr., residence in Galveston, TX. The foundation will develop the residence as a house museum and research center dedicated to the Moody family and its role in the history of Galveston. The foundation also supports Mountain Lake Properties, which is comprised of 2,600 acres of mountain timberland, meadows, and a volcanic lake. The foundation will preserve and operate this property for the benefit of the public in the same manner as national and state forest properties. properties. **Priorities:** *Arts & Humanities:* 81%. Support for museums and historic preservation. *Education:* 7%. Supports higher education. *Note:* Total contributions made in fiscal 2000. **Typ. Recipients:** Cancer, Child Abuse, Mental Health, Single-Disease Health Associations. **Geo. Dist:** TX; VA.

★ 11753 ★ Mary Ranken Jordan and Ettie A. Jordan Charitable Foundation

1 US BankPlaza, Suite 3500
Saint Louis, MO 63101
Phone: (314)552-6000 **Fax:** (314)552-7000
Email: farnold@thompsoncoburn.com
Fred Arnold, Chairman, Advisory Committee

Fnded: 1958. **Philosophy:** The foundation makes most of its grants in the areas of education, the arts, and children's health and welfare. Educational support favors colleges, universities, special education for the disabled, private secondary education, and art education. Arts interests include the performing arts, museums, historical preservation, and libraries. In social services, support goes to homes, youth organizations, food and clothing distribution, united funds, and community centers. Other recipient areas are funded on a limited basis. **Priorities:** *Arts & Humanities:* 27%. Supports public television, the performing arts, art museums, opera, and theater. *Civic & Public Affairs:* 16%. Supports zoos, parks, botanical gardens, and employment/job training. *Education:* 24%. Mainly supports colleges and universities. *Environment:* 10%. Supports family programs, scouting, people with disabilities, and Young Men's Christian Association. *International:* 19%. Supports health centers, hospitals, and single-disease health organizations. *Religion:* 3%. Supports science academies. *Note:* Contributions were made in 2000. **Typ. Recipients:** Children's Health/Hospitals, Clinics/Medical Centers, Clinics/Medical Centers, Diabetes, Emergency/Ambulance Services, Hospitals, Medical Education, Mental Health, People with Disabilities, Respiratory. **Geo. Dist:** MO, emphasis on St. Louis area.

★ 11754 ★ Mary Reynolds Babcock Foundation

2920 Reynolda Rd.
Winston-Salem, NC 27106-5123
Phone: (336)748-9222 **Fax:** (336)777-0095
Email: info@mrbf.org
Website: http://www.mrbf.org
Gayle Williams, Executive Director

Fnded: 1953. **Philosophy:** The Babcock Foundation concentrates on assisting people in the South to build communities that nurture people, encourage enterprise, bridge differences, foster fairness, and promote civility. The foundation places special emphasis on strategies that increase communities' commitment, sense of responsibility, and capacity toward three ends: assuring the well-being of children, youth, and families;bridging the faultlines of race and class; and protecting and investing in human and natural resources for the long term. "In particular, we seek to have impact in areas where poverty prevails or race divides." The foundation will invest in organizations, individuals, and communities through three grantmaking programs: Organizational Development Program, for 75-100 local, statewide, and regional organizations over five years; Community Problem Solving, a program of intensive work with coalitions of organizations in 10-15 communities in the Southeast; and Grassroots Leadership Development. **Priorities:** *Arts & Humanities:* 17%. Supports historic preservation. *Civic & Public Affairs:* 69%. Primary support for economic development, nonprofit management, urban and community affairs, housing, employment and job training women's affairs and philanthropic. *Education:* 3%. Focus on education reform, colleges and universities, public education, and literacy. *Environment:* 6%. Supports community services, youth and family services, food banks and emergency relief. *International:* 1%. *Note:* Total contributions made in 2000. **Typ. Recipients:** Emergency/Ambulance Services, Family Planning, Health Organizations, Hospitals, Nutrition. **Geo. Dist:** Southeastern United States.

★ 11755 ★ Mary S. and David C. Corbin Foundation

910 Society Bldg.
Akron, OH 44308
Phone: (330)762-6427 **Fax:** (330)762-6428
Email: corbin@nls.net
James Hartenstein, Treasurer

Fnded: 1970. **Philosophy:** The foundation primarily supports higher education, health organizations, and civic affairs in the Akron, Ohio, area. **Priorities:** *Arts & Humanities:* 18%. Supports museums and historic preservation. *Civic & Public Affairs:* 24%. Supports botanical gardens, urban affairs, and economic development. *Education:* 18%. Major grant to the University of Akron. *Environment:* 30%. Youth organizations, family services, scouting, and YMCAs receive support. *International:* 5%. Funds hospitals, cardiac care, the American Red Cross, and Multiple Sclerosis. *Note:* Total contributions made in 2001. **Typ. Recipients:** Alzheimers Disease, Arthritis, Cancer, Cancer, Children's Health/Hospitals, Clinics/Medical Centers, Domestic Violence, Emergency/Ambulance Services, Health Organizations, Heart, Hospices, Hospitals, Long-Term Care, Mental Health, Multiple Sclerosis, Nursing Services, People with Disabilities, Prenatal Health Issues, Trauma Treatment. **Geo. Dist:** Akron, OH.

★ 11756 ★ Mary Stuart Rogers Foundation

PO Box 3153
Modesto, CA 95353
Phone: (626)523-6416 **Fax:** (626)523-2315

Fnded: 1985. **Priorities:** *Education:* 60%. Funds colleges, universities, schools, and religious education. *Environment:* 3%. Funds family services. *International:* 3%. Supports children's health. *Note:* Total contributions made in 2000. **Typ. Recipients:** Cancer, Children's Health/Hospitals, Diabetes, Domestic Violence, Eyes/Blindness, Health Organizations, Heart, Hospitals, Medical Research, People with Disabilities, Public Health, Single-Disease Health Associations. **Geo. Dist:** CA.

★ 11757 ★ Mary W. Harriman Foundation

63 Wall St., Suite 3101
New York, NY 10005
Phone: (212)493-8182 **Fax:** (212)493-5570
William Hibberd, Secretary

Fnded: 1925. **Philosophy:** Board and family members directly involved with the distribution of funds give to groups that provide "a solid philanthropic benefit to the New York area." **Priorities:** *Arts & Humanities:* 21%. Supports libraries, museums, public broadcasting, the performing arts, and ballet. *Civic & Public Affairs:* 15%. Supports urban development, parks, and botanical gardens. *Education:* 38%. Supports secondary and preparatory schools, colleges and universities, and minority education. *Environment:* 11%. Supports children services, disabled services, social services, and family planning services. *International:* 5%. Supports cancer centers, visiting nurse organizations. *Religion:* 1%. Supports the American Museum of Natural History. *Note:* Total contributions made in 2000. **Typ. Recipients:** AIDS/HIV, Cancer, Child Abuse, Children's Health/Hospitals, Emergency/Ambulance Services, Family Planning, Hospices, Hospitals, Medical Education, Medical Rehabilitation, Mental Health, Nursing Services, People with Disabilities. **Geo. Dist:** New York, NY, metropolitan area.

★ 11758 ★ Massey Charitable Trust

PO Box 1178
Coraopolis, PA 15108
Phone: (412)262-5992
Walter Carroll, Executive Director & Trustee

Fnded: 1968. **Philosophy:** The trust makes grants across the major categories of support. In education, funding favors colleges, minority education, and special education for the handicapped. Social service support goes to living services, family services, counseling, youth organizations, and food and clothing distribution. Health support favors single-disease associations, rehabilitation services, and specialty hospitals. In the arts, interests include opera, art centers, historic preservation, and public broadcasting. **Priorities:** *Arts & Humanities:* 19%. Supports symphonies, opera, museums, and arts centers. *Civic & Public Affairs:* 7%. Focus on the Pittsburgh Leadership Foundation, and community and public affairs. *Education:* 25%. Funds colleges, universities, and educational programs. *Environment:* 15%. Supports child and youth services, women's shelters, the disabled, elderly services, and planned parenthood. *International:* 18%. Supports hospitals, visiting nurse foundation, and disease and disorder concerns. *Note:* Total contributions made in 2000. **Typ. Recipients:** Alzheimers Disease, Arthritis, Cancer, Children's Health/Hospitals, Clinics/Medical Centers, Diabetes, Emergency/Ambulance Services, Eyes/Blindness, Family Planning, Health Funds, Health Organizations, Hospices, Hospitals, Hospitals (University Affiliated), Kidney, Long-Term Care, Medical Education, Medical Rehabilitation, Medical Research, Nursing Services, People with Disabilities, Public Health, Sexual Abuse, Single-Disease Health Associations, Substance Abuse. **Geo. Dist:** PA, emphasis on Southwest Pennsylvania; Pittsburgh, PA.

★ 11759 ★ Massey Foundation

Four N Fourth St. Suite 100
PO Box 26765
Richmond, VA 23219
Phone: (804)288-9500
William Massey, Jr., Director

Fnded: 1957. **Philosophy:** The foundation has traditionally directed its philanthropy to medical, civic, and education activities in the southeastern United States. The foundation's current interests include private and state colleges and universities, as well as selected secondary schools for capital and special needs. The foundation has traditionally given to educational projects in the Appalachian coal fields where the family originated. In addition to educational institutions, the foundation supports religious and charitable organizations. The foundation supports hospitals and selected health care facilities with both capital and program grants. Symphonies, museums, and special arts organizations receive consideration, particularly regional facilities open to the general public. **Priorities:** *Arts & Humanities:* 4%. Richmond Ballet, museums, music, theater and the Virginia Historical Society. *Civic & Public Affairs:* Less than 1%. Renaissance, philanthropy, and a botanical garden. *Education:* 86%. Mostly colleges and universities. Also supports engineering education, educational funds and technical institutes *Environment:* 5%. Supports a boys home, YMCA/YWCA, and scouting. *International:* Less than 1%. Hospitals and cancer research. *Religion:* 3%. Virginia Institute of Marine Science and a science museum. *Note:* Total contributions made in fiscal 2001. **Typ. Recipients:** Cancer, Emergency/Ambulance Services, Health Organizations, Hospitals, Hospitals (University Affiliated), Medical Education, Mental Health, Preventive Medicine/Wellness Organizations, Single-Disease Health Associations. **Geo. Dist:** KY; VA; WV.

★ 11760 ★ Mathile Family Foundation

6450 Sand Lake Rd., Suite 200
Dayton, OH 45414-2645
Phone: (937)264-4600 **Fax:** (937)264-4635
Kippy Ungerleider-King, Grant Associate

Fnded: 1987. **Priorities:** *Civic & Public Affairs:* 68%. Provides major support to the Downtown Dayton Renaissance Fund; also funds urban ars, community foundations, and community development. *Education:* 17%. Primarily supports Catholic colleges and college preparatory schools. *Environment:* 5%. Supports child welfare, food/clothing distribution, recreation programs, scouts, United Ways, and YMCA/YWCA. *International:* 3%. Funds a children's hospital and single-disease health associations. *Note:* Total contributions were made in fiscal 2000. **Typ. Recipients:** Cancer, Children's Health/Hospitals, Domestic Violence, Hospices, Long-Term Care, Single-Disease Health Associations. **Geo. Dist:** Dayton, OH, metropolitan area.

★ 11761 ★ Matilda R. Wilson Fund

100 Renaissance Center, 34th Floor
Detroit, MI 48243
Phone: (313)259-7777 **Fax:** (313)393-7579
George Miller, Jr., President

Fnded: 1954. **Philosophy:** The foundation generally contributes to Southeast Michigan organizations offering services in the following areas: the arts, youth services, education, health, and human services. **Priorities:** *Arts & Humanities:* 16%. Funds a historical society, opera, theater, and symphony orchestra, a library, and public broadcasting. *Civic & Public Affairs:* 14%. Major support for a zoological society. *Education:* 42%. Supports MI colleges and universities and minority education. *Environment:* 12%. Funds United Way, family services, food distribution, youth programs and shelters. *International:* 5%. Supports hospices, hospitals, and oral health. *Religion:* 5%. Supports the Detroit Science Center. *Note:* Total contributions made in 2000. **Typ. Recipients:** Children's Health/Hospitals, Clinics/Medical Centers, Emergency/Ambulance Services, Eyes/Blindness, Health Organizations, Hospices, Hospitals, Medical Education, People with Disabilities, Public Health, Research/Studies Institutes, Substance Abuse. **Geo. Dist:** nationally; MI.

★ 11762 ★ Maurice Amado Foundation

3940 Laurel Canyon Boulevard, Suite 809
Studio City, CA 91604
Phone: (818)980-9190 **Fax:** (818)980-9190
Website: http://www.mauriceamadofdn.org
Pam Kaizer, Executive Director

Fnded: 1961. **Philosophy:** The foundation supports activities that emphasize the Sephardic Jewish heritage, with special interest in cultural and educational projects. **Priorities:** *Arts & Humanities:* 12%. Museums, symphonies, opera, a film festival, history, and a library. *Education:* 17%. Funds a variety of educational institutions; also supports sephardic Jewish studies. **Typ. Recipients:** Cancer, Children's Health/Hospitals, Clinics/Medical Centers, Domestic Violence, Emergency/Ambulance Services, Geriatric Health, Health Organizations, Hospitals, Hospitals (University Affiliated), Long-Term Care, Medical Education. **Geo. Dist:** Los Angeles, CA; New York, NY.

★ 11763 ★ Max Factor Family Foundation

9777 Wilshire Boulevard, Suite 1011
Beverly Hills, CA 90212
Phone: (310)274-8193 **Fax:** (310)274-9058
Barbara Bentley, Trustee

Fnded: 1941. **Philosophy:** The foundation's primary concerns lie in geriatric health, research grants for doctors, scholarships for minorities in health-related fields, Jewish welfare organizations, and children's diseases. **Priorities:** *Education:* 5%. Gives to literacy programs and law schools. *Environment:* 18%. Funds support anti-violence programs, senior services, and children's concerns, including a $3,000 grant to Shoes that Fit in California. *International:* 44%. Supports medical centers and clinics. *Note:* Total contributions made in 2001. **Typ. Recipients:** Cancer, Children's Health/Hospitals, Clinics/Medical Centers, Diabetes, Domestic Violence, Emergency/Ambulance Services, Eyes/Blindness, Geriatric Health, Health Funds, Health Organizations, Health-General, Heart, Hospitals, Long-Term Care, Medical Education, Medical Research, Mental Health, People with Disabilities, Public Health, Single-Disease Health Associations, Speech & Hearing, Substance Abuse. **Geo. Dist** CA.

★ 11764 ★ Max H. Gluck Foundation

10375 Wilshire Boulevard, No. 2
Los Angeles, CA 90024-4728
Phone: (310)276-6962
Mrs. Camilla Kocol, Executive Director

Fnded: 1955. **Philosophy:** The foundation is devoted to supporting the arts through direct support of specific museums and opera companies or by supporting art education. While most of the interests lie in the arts, the foundation also supports children's services, especially day care, health, and public education in California's largest cities. **Priorities:** *Arts & Humanities:* 29%. Supports opera, art museums, children's museums and a literary project. *Civic & Public Affairs:* 7%. Gives to a zoo. *Education:* 32%. Funds universities and higher education in the arts and music. *Environment:* 7%. Funds senior services, Boys and Girls Clubs, and other social services. *Religion:* 25%. Supports natural history museums. *Note:* Total contributions made in fiscal 2001. **Typ. Recipients:** AIDS/HIV, Arthritis, Children's Health/Hospitals, Clinics/Medical Centers, Diabetes, Emergency/Ambulance Services, Family Planning, Hospitals, Medical Education, People with Disabilities, Prenatal Health Issues, Research/Studies Institutes, Single-Disease Health Associations. **Geo. Dist:** Los Angeles, CA, including metropolitan area; NY.

★ 11765 ★ Max Kade Foundation

450 Park Ave.
New York, NY 10022
Phone: (212)752-4693 **Fax:** (212)964-1549
Mr. Hans Hachmann, Contact

Fnded: 1944. **Philosophy:** The foundation's primary interest lies in higher education, particularly at the graduate and postdoctoral level. Grants are generally made to universities, colleges, and other educational and research institutions. The foundation seeks to promote international understanding and sharing of knowledge, through the exchange of young postdoctoral research scholars and visiting faculty members between U.S. and European universities. Research scholars are nominated by their home institutions. The foundation's major fields of interest are research and training in medicine or the natural and physical sciences (math, physics, chemistry, and biochemistry), and the study of foreign languages, literature, and culture. **Priorities:** *Education:* 93%. Funds colleges, universities, and educational programs. Focus is on medical research, chemistry and biochemistry, engineering, mathematics and physics, visiting faculty, study abroad, and Max Kade language centers. *International:* 7%. Funds postoctoral research exchange programs in hospitals, medical centers, and universities. *Note:* Total contributions made in 200. **Typ. Recipients:** Cancer, Children's Health/Hospitals, Clinics/Medical Centers, Diabetes, Eyes/Blindness, Geriatric Health, Heart, Hospitals, Medical Education, Medical Research, Medical Training, Nutrition, Research/Studies Institutes. **Geo. Dist:** nationally.

★ 11766 ★ Max and Victoria Dreyfus Foundation, Inc.

50 Main St., Suite 1000
White Plains, NY 10606
Phone: (914)682-2008
Lucy Gioia, Office Administrator

Fnded: 1965. **Philosophy:** The foundation supports a variety of organizations in the arts, education, social services, health, and civic areas. **Priorities:** *Arts & Humanities:* 12%. Supports arts societies and the performing arts. *Civic & Public Affairs:* 12%. Housing and community programs. *Education:* 32%. Educational programs and funds. *Environment:* 23%. Primarily youth programs. *International:* 12%. Medical research and health care programs. *Religion:* 2%. *Note:* Total contributions made in 2000. **Typ. Recipients:** AIDS/HIV, Cancer, Children's Health/Hospitals, Clinics/Medical Centers, Emergency/Ambulance Services, Eyes/Blindness, Family Planning, Health Organizations, Health Organizations, Health-General, Heart, Home-Care Services, Hospices, Hospitals, Hospitals (University Affiliated), Medical Education, Medical Rehabilitation, Medical Research, Mental Health, People with Disabilities, Sexual Abuse, Single-Disease Health Associations, Substance Abuse. **Geo. Dist:** nationally.

★ 11767 ★ Maximilian E. and Marion O. Hoffman Foundation

970 Farmington Ave., Suite 203
West Hartford, CT 06107
Phone: (860)521-2949 **Fax:** (860)561-5082
Doris Chaho, President

Fnded: 1986. **Philosophy:** The foundation primarily supports health care, public policy, and environmental concerns; however, education, social services, and the arts also receive support from the foundation. **Priorities:** *Arts & Humanities:* 12%. Supports orchestra, theater and public broadcasting. *Education:* 33%. Supports private education. *Environment:* 8%. Supports people with disabilities and shelters/homes. *International:* 12%. Supports hospital and medical centers. *Religion:* 1%. Supports science center. *Note:* Total contributions made in fiscal 2001. **Typ. Recipients:** Adolescent Health Issues, AIDS/HIV, Alzheimers Disease, Cancer, Child Abuse, Children's Health/Hospitals, Clinics/Medical Centers, Diabetes, Emergency/Ambulance Services, Geriatric Health, Health Organizations, Health-General, Heart, Home-Care Services, Hospitals, Hospitals (University Affiliated), Kidney, Medical Education, Medical Rehabilitation, Mental Health, Nursing Services, Nutrition, People with Disabilities, Prenatal Health Issues, Research/Studies Institutes, Respiratory, Single-Disease Health Associations, Substance Abuse. **Geo. Dist:** U.S. Northeastern Region.

★ 11768 ★ McBean Family Foundation

400 S El Camino Real, Suite 777
San Mateo, CA 94402
Phone: (650)558-8480 **Fax:** (650)558-8481
Email: mcbeanfamilyfoundation@att.net
Charlene Kleiner, Secretary

Fnded: 1955. **Philosophy:** The foundation provides support for health organizations, educational institutions, civic affairs, human services, and the arts. Funding is generally limited to the San Francisco area and Northern California. **Priorities:** *Arts & Humanities:* Less than 1%. *Civic & Public Affairs:* 30%. Supports civic and community organizations. *Education:* 14%. Funds schools and higher education. *International:* 30%. Supports health care, hospice, and human services for children and families. *Note:* Total contributions made in 2001. Analysis provided by the foundation. **Typ. Recipients:** AIDS/HIV, Alzheimers Disease, Cancer, Child Abuse, Clinics/Medical Centers, Eyes/Blindness, Health Organizations, Hospices, Hospitals, Long-Term Care, Medical Education, Medical Research, People with Disabilities, Prenatal Health Issues, Sexual Abuse, Speech & Hearing. **Geo. Dist:** CA, San Francisco Bay area.

★ 11769 ★ McCamish Foundation
3060 Peachtree Rd. Northwest, 19th Floor
Atlanta, GA 30305
Phone: (404)261-4418 **Fax:** (404)262-2681
Email: kreynolds@mccamishgroup.com
Roy Jones, Chief Operating Officer

Fnded: 1989. **Philosophy:** The McCamish Foundation's main concern is social services with multiple grants funding Noah's Ark, an animal protection agency. Other social service concerns include athletics, senior services, and disabled adults. Education also receives large support, including funding for Reinhart College, leadership training, and educational foundations. The foundation also supports religious organizations, public policy groups, and environmental concerns. **Priorities:** *Civic & Public Affairs:* 5%. Supports public policy research, business and legal concerns, and aquariums and botanical gardens. *Education:* 13%. Funds higher education and enrichment programs. *Environment:* 49%. Funds youth groups, services for the elderly, and religious welfare. *International:* 9%. Supports medical centers, rehabilitation, and single-disease associations. *Note:* Total contributions in 2000. **Typ. Recipients:** Alzheimers Disease, Arthritis, Cancer, Child Abuse, Children's Health/Hospitals, Clinics/Medical Centers, Domestic Violence, Emergency/Ambulance Services, Health-General, Heart, Hospitals, Medical Education, Medical Rehabilitation, People with Disabilities, Prenatal Health Issues, Preventive Medicine/Wellness Organizations, Public Health, Single-Disease Health Associations. **Geo. Dist:** Atlanta, GA.

★ 11770 ★ McCann Foundation
35 Market St.
Poughkeepsie, NY 12601
Phone: (245)452-3085 **Fax:** (245)452-3093
John Gartland, Jr., Trustee

Fnded: 1969. **Philosophy:** The McCann Foundation focuses on the needs of the Dutchess County, NY, community. The foundations awards grants to a number of educational, cultural, religious, social, and recreational organizations "to help them achieve their goals and better serve their communities." As a foundation, their role "is to seek and fund opportunities and projects that benefit the community and everyone who lives, works, studies and visits in Dutchess County." McCann Foundation Annual Report, 1996 During 1996, the foundation directly supported two major community projects. These included the conversion of a former IBM building into a new home for Our Lady of Lourdes High School, as well as a major multipurpose, sports facility expansion of The McCann Recreation Center at Marist College. **Priorities:** *Arts & Humanities:* 1%. Funds public broadcasting. *Civic & Public Affairs:* 3%. Supports public defense, botanical gardens, and community groups. *Education:* 61%. Includes a major grant to Marist College. *Environment:* 25%. Funds recreational activities and community services. *Note:* Total contributions made in 1999. **Typ. Recipients:** Cancer, Children's Health/Hospitals, Emergency/Ambulance Services, Hospices, Hospitals, People with Disabilities, Trauma Treatment. **Geo. Dist:** NY, Dutchess County; Poughkeepsie, NY.

★ 11771 ★ McCasland Foundation
PO Box 400
Duncan, OK 73534
Phone: (580)252-5580 **Fax:** (580)252-5791
Barbara Braught, Executive Director

Fnded: 1952. **Philosophy:** The foundation funds colleges and universities, mostly within Oklahoma, as well as arts organizations, community foundations, and social services agencies. **Priorities:** *Arts & Humanities:* 49%. Funds music, libraries, construction of a museum and statue, and historical societies. *Civic & Public Affairs:* 8%. Urban affairs. *Education:* 22%. Primarily funds colleges and universities. *Environment:* 12%. Supports united funds and youth groups. *International:* 3%. Pediatric health and health centers. *Religion:* 2%. Gives to science museums. *Note:* Total contributions made in 2000. **Typ. Recipients:** Alzheimers Disease, Cancer, Children's Health/Hospitals, Clinics/Medical Centers, Emergency/Ambulance Services, Health Organizations, Heart, Hospices, Hospitals, Long-Term Care, Medical Education, Medical Rehabilitation, Medical Research, People with Disabilities, Single-Disease Health Associations, Substance Abuse. **Geo. Dist:** OK, primarily Oklahoma.

★ 11772 ★ McConnell Foundation
PO Box 492050
Redding, CA 96049-2050
Phone: (530)226-6200 **Fax:** (530)226-6210
Email: info@mcconnellfoundation.org
Website: http://www.mcconnellfoundation.org
Lee Salter, President & Executive Director

Fnded: 1964. **Philosophy:** Currently, the foundation promotes innovative projects in Shasta and Siskiyou counties in California in the areas of arts and culture, community enrichment, designated special projects, education, environment, health care, recreation, and social services. Within these general giving areas, the foundation has four specific areas of interest including the following: environment, environmental education, and recreation; projects that benefit the working poor; projects for the larger good; and promotion of volunteerism. Support is limited to nonprofit, tax-exempt organizations, public education (high school and above), and governmental entities. **Priorities:** *Arts & Humanities:* 68%. Supports museums, public broadcasting, and libraries. *Civic & Public Affairs:* 8%. Funds community services and redevelopment, parks, women's affairs, and towns/municipalities. *Education:* 5%. Supports public education, scholarships, pre schools, and education foundations. *Environment:* 5%. Supports family planning services, family services, Young Men's Christian Association, United Way, and senior services. *International:* 13%. Funds hospitals, emergency care, and community health projects. *Note:* Total contributions in 2000. **Typ. Recipients:** Clinics/Medical Centers, Domestic Violence, Emergency/Ambulance Services, Family Planning, Hospices, Hospitals, Medical Rehabilitation, Medical Research, Medical Training, Nutrition, People with Disabilities, Public Health, Substance Abuse. **Geo. Dist:** CA, Shasta County; CA, Siskiyou County.

★ 11773 ★ McCune Foundation
750 Six PPG Place
Pittsburgh, PA 15222
Phone: (412)644-8779 **Fax:** (412)644-8059
Email: info@mccune.org
Website: http://www.mccune.org
Henry Beukema, Executive Director

Fnded: 1979. **Philosophy:** The McCune Foundation has a broad mission to support efforts which improve communities. The Distribution Committee emphasizes the following program areas: education, the humanities, human services, and civic affairs. The foundation recognizes the importance of community-based organizations that are working to remedy the effects of economic dislocation, while addressing future issues. With an awareness of limited resources in comparison to growing needs, the Foundation is particularly interested in innovative/collaborative approaches to address regional problems and priorities, primarily in Southwestern Pennsylvania. **Priorities:** *Arts & Humanities:* About 17%. Primary support for historic organizations, museums, and theater. *Civic & Public Affairs:* 20%. Funds economic and community development concerns. *Education:* 36%. Focus on colleges. *Environment:* 21%. Focus on services for families and children. *International:* 5%. Funds hospitals. *Religion:* 2%. *Note:* Total contributions made in fiscal 2000. **Typ. Recipients:** AIDS/HIV, Cancer, Children's Health/Hospitals, Clinics/Medical Centers, Domestic Violence, Geriatric Health, Health Funds, Health Organizations, Health Policy/Cost Containment, Hospices, Hospitals, Hospitals (University Affiliated), Medical Education, Medical Rehabilitation, Medical Research, Medical Training, Mental Health, Nursing Services, Nutrition, People with Disabilities, Prenatal Health Issues, Public Health, Single-Disease Health Associations, Substance Abuse. **Geo. Dist:** CT; NM; OK; PA, Southwestern Pennsylvania; Pittsburgh, PA.

★ 11774 ★ McGregor Fund
333 West Fort St., Suite 2090
Detroit, MI 48226-3134
Phone: (313)963-3495 **Fax:** (313)963-3512
Email: info@mcgregorfund.org
Website: http://www.mcgregorfund.org
C. Campbell, President & Assistant Secretary

Fnded: 1925. **Philosophy:** "Concern for the needs of the homeless and hungry remains a priority of the fund." In addition, "partnerships and cooperative endeavors which address the critical issues facing greater Detroit continue to be a key element." To these ends, the fund supports a broad range of civic, health, and human service programs in the Detroit area. It also has expanded its interest in the environment and in the arts and humanities. In keeping with Mr. McGregor's belief that education was an essential prerequisite to solving society's ills, the fund supports specific projects at independent elementary and secondary schools serving metropolitan Detroit, colleges and universities in the Detroit area, and Michigan's public research universities. Grants are also awarded under two special programs, one for elementary and secondary schools serving students from low-income families in Detroit and the other for private liberal arts colleges and universities in Michigan and Ohio. In addition to the general and special programs, six discretionary grants are awarded to educational institutions selected each year by the trustees. The McGregor Fund is a member of several national and statewide service organizations that promote the advancement of the nonprofit sector. The fund is no longer supporting national or local chapters of disease-specific organizations. **Priorities:** *Arts & Humanities:* 21%. Supports symphony orchestra hall, and the Museum of African American History. *Civic & Public Affairs:* 19%. Community affairs. *Education:* 22%. Supports public schools, colleges, universities, and educational programs. *Environment:* 28%. United Way, children's services, food for the needy, and shelters. *International:* 8%. Funds hospitals, AIDS awareness, and American Red Cross. *Religion:* 1%. *Note:* Contributions made in fiscal 2001. **Typ. Recipients:** AIDS/HIV, Children's Health/Hospitals, Emergency/Ambulance Services, Family Planning, Health Organizations, Hospitals, Long-Term Care, Mental Health, Nursing Services, People with Disabilities, Prenatal Health Issues, Substance Abuse. **Geo. Dist:** Detroit, MI, metropolitan area.

★ 11775 ★ McInerny Foundation
c/o Pacific Century Trust
PO Box 3170
Honolulu, HI 96802-3170
Phone: (808)538-4540 **Fax:** (808)538-4647

Fnded: 1937. **Philosophy:** The McInernys established the foundation "in order to promote the welfare of the people of the Hawaiian Islands." Under the terms of the deed of trust creating the foundation, the income is to be used for "charitable, scientific or educational purposes, or for the prevention of cruelty to children or animals." Use of this income is flexible, in order to meet changing conditions, and to "best serve the charitable requirements of the people of the Hawaiian Islands." Grants currently are made in five fields: education, social services, environment, culture and arts, and health and rehabilitation. **Priorities:** *Arts & Humanities:* 12%. Supports museums, arts education, literature, public broadcasting, and the performing arts. *Civic & Public Affairs:* 6%. Supports economic development, housing, legal aid, and community foundations. *Education:* 40%. Supports pre-school through higher education. *Environment:* 29%. Funds United Way, social service organizations, youth groups, and humane societies. *International:* 11%. Supports clinics, medical centers, and single-disease associations. *Note:* Total contributions made in fiscal 2000. **Typ. Recipients:** AIDS/HIV, Cancer, Children's Health/Hospitals, Clinics/Medical Centers, Domestic Violence, Emergency/Ambulance Services, Family Planning, Health Organizations, Home-Care Services, Hospices, Hospitals, Long-Term Care, Medical Education, Medical Rehabilitation, Mental Health, People with Disabilities, Prenatal Health Issues, Public Health,

Single-Disease Health Associations, Substance Abuse. **Geo. Dist:** HI.

★ 11776 ★ McIntosh Foundation

15840 Meadows Wood Dr.
Wellington, FL 33414-9026
Phone: (561)792-3763
Michael McIntosh, President & Director

Fnded: 1953. **Philosophy:** With the advent in the past few years of a large number of foundations with hundreds of millions of dollars in assets (and many with billions) almost all of whom are addressing a broad range of social issues, it seemed to make sense that a relatively small foundation like the McIntosh Foundation should think of narrowing its focus. "Accordingly, because of its long-term interest in Southeast Alaska dating back to the early 1970's, several years ago it decided to focus its modest resources on the environment and economic issues (timber, commercial fishing, tourism, etc.) affecting the Tongass National Forest. The Tongass, aside from being by far the U.S.'s largest National Forest, comprises 95% of the land area of the 50,000 square miles that is Southeast Alaska. It is also the last great remaining temperate rainforest on earth." 1999 Philosophy Statement. **Priorities:** *Arts & Humanities:* 1%. Supports historic preservation and libraries. *Civic & Public Affairs:* 5%. Supports legal concerns and community foundations. *Education:* 9% Funds higher education. *International:* Less than 1%. *Note:* Total contributions made in 2000. **Typ. Recipients:** Cancer, Clinics/Medical Centers, Geriatric Health, Health Organizations, Hospitals, Nursing Services, People with Disabilities, Single-Disease Health Associations. **Geo. Dist:** AK; AK, Tongass National Forest, Southeast Alaska.

★ 11777 ★ MCJ Foundation

310 South St.
PO Box 1975
Morristown, NJ 07962
Phone: (973)540-9020 **Fax:** (973)538-8175
Suzanne Spero, Vice President & Director

Fnded: 1983. **Philosophy:** "The MCJ Foundation was founded in the belief that the revitalization of our nation's inner-city neighborhoods through education, social services, economic opportunity and various collaborative efforts that involve the men and women from these communities is essential to ensure the uplifting of our nation's minorities and underprivileged children." "The Foundation currently focuses on programs that encourage and enable the development of mentoring relations, quality education, activities and job training for 'youth at risk,' entrepreneurial opportunities, affordable housing, community service activities, arts and cultural diversity, and health." **Priorities:** *Arts & Humanities:* 26%. Major support for the New Jersey Performing Arts Center; also funds theater, museums, film, and public broadcasting. *Civic & Public Affairs:* 24%. Supports job training, mentoring, and urban affairs organizations. *Education:* 20%. Funds colleges, universities, Junior Achievement, and primary and secondary schools. *Environment:* 27%. Focus on youth organizations and child welfare. *International:* 3%. Supports hospitals and single-disease associations. *Note:* Total contributions made in 2000. **Typ. Recipients:** Cancer, Children's Health/Hospitals, Clinics/Medical Centers, Family Planning, Health Funds, Health-General, Hospitals, Medical Research, People with Disabilities, Public Health, Substance Abuse. **Geo. Dist:** Newark, NJ; New York, NY.

★ 11778 ★ McKnight Foundation

710 Second St. South, Suite 400
Minneapolis, MN 55401
Phone: (612)333-4220 **Fax:** (612)332-3833
Email: info@mcknight.org
Website: http://www.mcknight.org
Richard Scott, Vice President Finance and Admin.

Fnded: 1953. **Philosophy:** "Our mission is to improve the quality of life for present and future generations and to seek paths to a more humane and secure world. We support efforts to strengthen communities, families, and individuals, particularly those in need. We contribute to the arts, encourage preservation of our natural environment, and promote research in selected fields. We continually explore innovative ideas to advance our goals in partnership with those we serve." "Making grants in the human services in seven-county Twin Cities metro area is the core of the foundation's work. It seeks to meet the needs of and empower people who are poor or disadvantaged; to identify effective long-term strategies to meet those needs; and to address the underlying problems of the community and the institutional causes of those problems. Within the human services area, the foundation is primarily supporting programs in the following areas: the development of children and young people; the linkage between housing and social services; family stability at a time of change in family structure; employment for people who are hard to employ; community development with an emphasis on enhancing the safety, livability and economic stability of neighborhoods; and greater public understanding of the needs of people confronting these challenges." The foundation has also shown recent interest in community improvement and economic development, affordable housing in the Twin Cities, public affairs, and international development issues (such as women's rights and health and human services). International grant making focuses on relieving the suffering of disadvantaged people in Africa and refugees in Southeast Asia, enhancing international stability with an emphasis on peacekeeping efforts, and improving the understanding of global issues in Minnesota and the upper Midwest. **Priorities:** *Arts & Humanities:* 14%. Supports arts councils, arts education and criticism, community arts, and dance/film/video. *Environment:* 68%. Supports programs providing services to those whose opportunities have been limited by poverty. Also provides program support to community improvement, housing, public affairs, and family loan programs. *Religion:* 5%. Research and applied science–includes plant and crop research. *Note:* Total contributions made in 2001. **Typ. Recipients:** Adolescent Health Issues, Child Abuse, Domestic Violence, Family Planning, Hospitals, Medical Rehabilitation, Medical Research, Medical Training, Mental Health, People with Disabilities, Sexual Abuse. **Geo. Dist:** environment grants are made within the ten states along the Mississippi River; some funding internationally; MN, emphasis on the Minneapolis-St. Paul metropolitan area.

★ 11779 ★ McLean Contributionship

945 Haverford Rd.
Bryn Mawr, PA 19010-3814
Phone: (610)527-6330 **Fax:** (610)527-9733
Website: http://fdncenter.org/grantmaker/mclean
Sandra McLean, Executive Director

Fnded: 1951. **Philosophy:** The trustees believe the resources of the Contributionship can be used most effectively by making a relatively limited number of grants for projects of long-term benefit rather than by underwriting continuing operating expenses. The trustees focus on capital projects, brick and mortar, and endowments, or will provide seed money for the understanding and preservation of the environment, education, medical purposes, scientific developments, and compassionate care of the elderly. **Priorities:** *Arts & Humanities:* 16%. Supports arts, cultural organizations, historical societies, museums, media, and performing arts. *Education:* 29%. Supports higher education, elementary and secondary education, continuing education, and libraries. *Environment:* 15%. Job training, food/nutrition, recreation, youth development, and United Way. *International:* 13%. Diseases (ALS), Health-general and rehabilitative: hospitals, nursing homes and Programs, rehab, and medical research. *Note:* Total contributions made in 2000. **Typ. Recipients:** AIDS/HIV, Cancer, Children's Health/Hospitals, Diabetes, Domestic Violence, Emergency/Ambulance Services, Eyes/Blindness, Family Planning, Geriatric Health, Health-General, Hospitals, Long-Term Care, Medical Education, Medical Rehabilitation, Medical Research, Mental Health, Nursing Services, People with Disabilities, Prenatal Health Issues, Public Health, Single-Disease Health Associations, Transplant Networks/Donor Banks. **Geo. Dist:** PA, primarily metropolitan Philadelphia.

★ 11780 ★ McMahon Foundation

PO Box 2156
Lawton, OK 73502
Phone: (580)355-4622 **Fax:** (580)357-3248
James Wood, Director

Fnded: 1940. **Philosophy:** The foundation makes grants primarily for education (including scholarship funds), the arts, youth, the handicapped, and community funds for local projects. Past contributions in Lawton went to an auditorium, a museum devoted to the history of the Great Plains, a city/county health center, a nursing home for the elderly, a mental health center, a public library, a recreational park, and a boys' club gymnasium. Support for other civic and arts organizations has been provided as well. **Priorities:** *Arts & Humanities:* 5%. Supports arts and humanities. *Civic & Public Affairs:* 41%. Supports community development. *Education:* 49%. Supports schools and universities. *Environment:* 3%. Funds the United Way and rehabilitation services. *Note:* Total contributions made in fiscal 1999. **Typ. Recipients:** Emergency/Ambulance Services, Hospices, Nursing Services, Substance Abuse. **Geo. Dist:** OK, Comanche County; OK, only Oklahoma; Lawton, OK.

★ 11781 ★ McMillen Foundation

6610 Mutual Drive
Fort Wayne, IN 46825
Phone: (260)484-8631 **Fax:** (260)483-0474
John McMillen, President

Fnded: 1947. **Philosophy:** The McMillen Foundation makes most of its grants in the areas of social services and education. Social service funding favors recreational support for the benefit of youth. Educational support is directed at health education and outreach programs. Minor grants are given to other recipient areas. **Priorities:** *Arts & Humanities:* 5%. Supports historic preservation and music. *Civic & Public Affairs:* 5%. Major support for the Headwater Park Commission. *Education:* 35%. Emphasis on an education fund and medical education. *Environment:* 52%. Primary support for a recreation association and a YWCA. *Religion:* 2%. Supports science centers. *Note:* Total contributions made in 1998. **Typ. Recipients:** AIDS/HIV, Clinics/Medical Centers, Domestic Violence, Family Planning, Geriatric Health, Health Organizations, Health-General, Hospices, People with Disabilities, Public Health, Sexual Abuse, Substance Abuse. **Geo. Dist:** IN, Allen County; Ft. Wayne, IN.

★ 11782 ★ The Meadows Foundation

3003 Swiss Ave.
Wilson Historic District
Dallas, TX 75204-6049
Phone: (214)826-9431 **Fax:** (214)827-7042
Website: http://www.mfi.org
Bruce Esterline, Vice President, Grants

Fnded: 1948. **Philosophy:** The Meadows Foundation looks for "imaginative, innovative ways to solve community problems; for projects leading to organizational self-sufficiency; for capital plans which will enable programs to flourish; and for ways to alleviate pain, to ameliorate social ills, and to promote better human relationships." The foundation continues its tradition of balanced giving in basic areas of human activity and need: the arts, social services, health, education, and civic programs. In 1978, the foundation funded the Algur H. Meadows Award for Excellence in the Arts, established by the Meadows School of the Arts at Southern Methodist University. The annual award of $50,000 is for exceptional achievement or distinguished service in the creative or performing arts. Other grants in arts and culture support various community and educational institutions, including gifts to museums and historic preservation projects. Human services grants support disaster relief, child care, dependency rehabilitation, handicapped, youth, and counseling programs. Educational grants include preschool through postgraduate levels, at both public and private institutions, and numerous community-based organizations. The foundation's Charitable Schools Program is geared toward encouraging and supporting youth volunteerism. Grants for health services are especially targeted towards disadvantaged or rural citizens. Civic and public affairs grants improve the built or natural environment. The foundation sponsors a program housing nonprofit agencies for creative resource sharing on several unique blocks of turn-of-the-century houses in Dallas. In recent years, there has been an increasing interest in public education, mental health/illness, and the environment. **Priorities:** *Arts & Humanities:* 25%. Focus on museums, fine arts, performing arts, and history and archaeology organizations. *Civic & Public Affairs:* 21%. Supports urban affairs, community and public development. Environmental research conservation organizations are also supported under this program area. *Education:* 15%. Supports institutions that implement programs in literacy, tutoring, drop-out recovery, teacher education, and reading readiness. *Environment:* 22%. Supports child development centers, youth organizations, senior services, crime prevention, domestic violence programs, homeless shelters, food banks, and community centers. *International:* 17%. Emphasis on hospitals, medical centers, mental health centers, single-disease health associations, and special cause centers that deal with abuse and rehabilitation. *Note:* Total contributions made in 2000. **Typ. Recipients:** AIDS/HIV, Alzheimers Disease, Cancer, Child Abuse, Children's Health/Hospitals, Clinics/Medical Centers, Diabetes, Domestic Violence, Emergency/Ambulance Services, Eyes/Blindness, Family Planning, Geriatric Health, Health Funds, Health Organizations, Health Policy/Cost Containment, Health-General, Heart, Home-Care Services, Hospices, Hospitals, Hospitals (University Affiliated), Kidney, Long-Term Care, Medical Education, Medical Training, Mental Health, Outpatient Health Care, People with Disabilities, Preventive Medicine/Wellness Organizations, Public Health, Single-Disease Health Associations, Speech & Hearing, Substance Abuse, Transplant Networks/Donor Banks. **Geo. Dist:** TX, emphasis on Dallas.

★ 11783 ★ Medina Foundation

801 2nd Ave., Floor 13
Seattle, WA 98104
Phone: (206)652-8783 **Fax:** (206)652-8791
Email: info@medinafoundation.org
Website: http://www.medinafoundation.org
Patricia McKay, Executive Director

Fnded: 1948. **Philosophy:** The purpose of the foundation is "to aid in improving the human condition in the greater Puget Sound community by fostering positive change and the growth and improvement of people." The foundation specifies four areas of interest: emergency food and shelter; the physically and mentally handicapped and their development; promotion of efficiency and effectiveness of charity-supported and governmental organizations within the foundation's interests; and private education (preschool through grade 12) programs to improve teachers' abilities, programs to improve leadership and development, projects fostering communications among various segments of the education community, and support of vocational schools and programs. **Priorities:** *Civic & Public Affairs:* 18%. Housing, community development, resource centers, clubs, and employment/job training. *Education:* 14%. Teacher development, alternative schools, vocational schools, and development of physically and mentally handicapped. *Environment:* 53%. Senior services, youth shelters, alcohol and drug abuse programs, parenting programs, and community services. *International:* 7%. Clinics and services for education and mental health. *Note:* Total contributions made in 2000. **Typ. Recipients:** Cancer, Children's Health/Hospitals, Clinics/Medical Centers, Domestic Violence, Emergency/Ambulance Services, Geriatric Health, Health Organizations, Hospitals, Medical Education, Medical Rehabilitation, Mental Health, People with Disabilities, Preventive Medicine/Wellness Organizations, Single-Disease Health Associations, Substance Abuse. **Geo. Dist:** WA, greater Puget Sound region.

★ 11784 ★ Merck Family Fund

303 Adams St.
Milton, MA 02186
Phone: (617)696-3580 **Fax:** (617)696-7262
Email: merck@merckff.org
Website: http://www.merckff.org
Jenny Russell, Executive Director

Fnded: 1954. **Philosophy:** The Merck Family Fund is dedicated to protecting the natural environment and addressing the root causes of problems faced by socially and economically disadvantaged people by working to build a sense of community in impoverished neighborhoods. The fund's environmental program focuses on protecting and restoring vital eastern United States ecosystems and promoting economic practices that will assure a sustainable environment for future generations. The fund's community-building program focuses on creating green and open space and meeting the needs of disadvantaged youth. **Priorities:** *Civic & Public Affairs:* 37%. Supports aquariums, gardens, parks, housing, economic development, and minority affairs. *Environment:* 5%. Supports youth and family centers and food banks. *Note:* Total contributions made in 2000. **Typ. Recipients:** Family Planning, Home-Care Services, Hospitals, Long-Term Care, People with Disabilities, Preventive Medicine/Wellness Organizations. **Geo. Dist:** nationally for the Sustainable Economics program; Northern forests, Southern Appalachians, and Southern Coastal Plain for the Eastern Ecosystems program; Boston, MA, community-building program; New York, NY, community-building program; Providence, RI, community-building program.

★ 11785 ★ Mericos Foundation

625 S Fair Oaks Ave., Suite 360
South Pasadena, CA 91030
Phone: (626)441-5188 **Fax:** (626)441-3672
Email: linda@sowest.net
Linda Blinkenberg, Secretary & Director

Fnded: 1980. **Philosophy:** Mericos Foundation makes grants across the major categories of support. Educational funding favors universities and public school systems. Education funding also supports science, math, and technology programs. Social services support includes family planning; child welfare; and youth development, citizenship, and responsibility. Arts interests include historic preservation, museums, and arts organizations. Health care support goes to critical health programs, nursing services, and hospices. In civic affairs, interests include the environment as well as zoos and botanical gardens. and technology. **Priorities:** *Arts & Humanities:* 4%. Historical Society and libraries. *Civic & Public Affairs:* 4%. Community affairs. *Education:* 61%. High schools, higher education, and scholarship endowments. *Environment:* 27%. Youth, senior and family program support. *International:* 3%. *Note:* Total contributions made in 2000. **Typ. Recipients:** Children's Health/Hospitals, Clinics/Medical Centers, Domestic Violence, Family Planning, Geriatric Health, Health-General, Heart, Hospices, Medical Research, Nursing Services, People with Disabilities. **Geo. Dist:** Santa Barbara, CA, including surrounding area.

★ 11786 ★ Mervin Bovaird Foundation

401 S Boston, Suite 3300
Tulsa, OK 74103-4070
Phone: (918)592-3300
Mr. R. Cooper, President & Trustee

Fnded: 1955. **Philosophy:** The purpose of the foundation, as stated in its articles of incorporation, is "to receive and administer funds for scientific, educational and charitable purposes, all for the public welfare." The foundation primarily supports scholarship programs at the University of Tulsa. Funding also is provided for social services, civic causes, and health organizations in the Tulsa, OK, area. **Priorities:** *Arts & Humanities:* 15%. Museums, music, ballet, and opera. *Civic & Public Affairs:* 9%. Primary support for a municipal park. *Education:* 18%. Supports educational concerns mostly in the form of scholarships to students from Tulsa attending the University of Tulsa. *Environment:* 31%. Primary support for family services, child welfare, and youth organizations. *International:* 19%. Hospitals, medical research, and single-disease health associations. *Note:* Total contributions made in 2001. **Typ. Recipients:** Arthritis, Cancer, Children's Health/Hospitals, Clinics/Medical Centers, Domestic Violence, Emergency/Ambulance Services, Family Planning, Family Planning, Health Organizations, Health Policy/Cost Containment, Heart, Hospices, Hospitals, Kidney, Long-Term Care, Medical Rehabilitation, Medical Research, Mental Health, Multiple Sclerosis, People with Disabilities, Prenatal Health Issues, Sexual Abuse, Single-Disease Health Associations, Speech & Hearing, Substance Abuse. **Geo. Dist:** Tulsa, OK, metropolitan area.

★ 11787 ★ Meyer Memorial Trust

425 NW 10th Ave., Suite 400
Portland, OR 97209
Phone: (503)228-5512
Email: mmt@mmt.org
Website: http://www.mmt.org
Doug Stamm, Executive Director

Fnded: 1982. **Philosophy:** Upon creation of the charitable trust, Mr. Meyer stated, "Realizing as I do the uncertainties of the future, I want my trustees to be able to exercise broad discretion in shaping and carrying out charitable programs which can be tailored to fit changing conditions and problems." The trust conducts three types of grant-making activities. General purpose grants are made within Oregon and Clark County, Washington to a broad range of causes, including culture and the arts, education, health, and social services. The trust operates a Small Grants Program, initiated in 1988, under which grants of $500 to $12,000 are awarded for small projects. These grants are limited to Oregon and Clark County, Washington. The trust also makes grants in Support for Teacher Initiatives, a special program initiated in 1994 which provides grants up to $2,000 to individual teachers and $7,000 to teams of teachers for projects that promise to stimulate and facilitate more effective learning by students in the classroom, and is also limited to Oregon and Clark County, Washington. **Priorities:** *Arts & Humanities:* 15%. Museums, symphonies, historic preservation, and cultural centers. *Education:* 16%. Science and math education, private pre-college education, and after school enrichment programs. *Environment:* 28%. Supports programs for workers with disabilities, at-risk family programs, child development services, and youth organizations. *International:* 9%. Mental health services, children's health, and medical centers. *Note:* Total contributions made in fiscal 2001. Contributions analysis was provided by foundation, and includes General Purpose, Small Grants, and support for teacher programs. **Typ. Recipients:** AIDS/HIV, Alzheimers Disease, Cancer, Child Abuse, Children's Health/Hospitals, Clinics/Medical Centers, Domestic Violence, Emergency/Ambulance Services, Family Planning, Geriatric Health, Health Organizations, Health Policy/Cost Containment, Heart, Hospices, Hospitals, Long-Term Care, Medical Education, Medical Rehabilitation, Medical Research, Medical Training, Mental Health, Nursing Services, People with Disabilities, Prenatal Health Issues, Public Health, Sexual Abuse, Single-Disease Health Associations, Substance Abuse. **Geo. Dist:** OR; WA, Clark County.

★ 11788 ★ Middendorf Foundation

2 East Read St.
Baltimore, MD 21202
Phone: (410)752-7088 **Fax:** (410)625-5728
E. Hathaway, President & Trustee

Fnded: 1953. **Philosophy:** The foundation's primary interest is supporting health care, specifically the establishment of health clinics. Arts funding favors historical preservation in Maryland. Civic affairs, the Boys Latin School in Baltimore, and family services also are supported. **Priorities:** *Arts & Humanities:* 28%. Restoration and endowments. *Civic & Public Affairs:* 8%. Supports parks, economic development, and community foundations. *Education:* 7%. Universities and secondary schools. *Environment:* 13%. Youth clubs, Special Olympics, and meals on wheels programs. *International:* 37%. Medical centers and health foundations. *Religion:* 3%. Science Center. *Note:* Total contributions made in fiscal 2001. **Typ. Recipients:** Cancer, Child Abuse, Clinics/Medical Centers, Emergency/Ambulance Services, Eyes/Blindness, Family Planning, Geriatric Health, Health Organizations,

Health-General, Hospices, Hospitals, Medical Education, Mental Health, People with Disabilities, Prenatal Health Issues, Preventive Medicine/Wellness Organizations, Public Health, Respiratory, Single-Disease Health Associations, Substance Abuse, Trauma Treatment. **Geo. Dist:** MD.

★ 11789 ★ Mildred H. McEvoy Foundation

370 Main St.
12th Floor
Worcester, MA 01608
Phone: (508)798-8621 **Fax:** (508)791-1201
Sumner Tilton, Jr., Trustee

Fnded: 1963. **Philosophy:** "The McEvoy Foundation provides grants to health, educational, cultural and human service organizations that are exempt under Section 501(c)(3) of the Internal Revenue Code and that are based in the Boothbay, Maine area. It supports requests to organizations which are providing solutions to or prevention of problems within the immediate community and which are receiving additional support from other funding sources." Mildred H. McEvoy Foundation Guidelines **Priorities:** *Arts & Humanities:* 45%. Multiple grants went to Grand Banks Schooner Museum Trust and the Boothbay Railway Village Museum; other museums and historical societies received support. *Civic & Public Affairs:* 11%. Supports community services and the horticultural society, and botanical gardens. *Education:* 17%. Supports secondary and preparatory schools, colleges, and universities. *Environment:* 8%. Supports Boothbay Region YMCA and child welfare. *International:* 13%. Supports health centers, hospitals, and biomedical research organizations. *Religion:* 5%. Supports the New England Science Center. *Note:* Total contributions made in 2000. **Typ. Recipients:** Cancer, Children's Health/Hospitals, Clinics/Medical Centers, Emergency/Ambulance Services, Family Planning, Hospitals, Hospitals (University Affiliated), Long-Term Care, Medical Education, Medical Research, Nursing Services, Public Health, Single-Disease Health Associations, Substance Abuse. **Geo. Dist:** Boothbay Harbor, ME.

★ 11790 ★ Milken Family Foundation

1250 4th St., 3rd Floor
Santa Monica, CA 90401-1353
Phone: (310)570-4800 **Fax:** (310)570-4801
Email: admin@mff.org
Website: http://www.mff.org
Richard Sandler, Executive Vice President

Fnded: 1982. **Philosophy:** "The purpose of the Milken Family foundaton is to discover and advance inventive and effective ways of helping people help themselves and those around them to lead productive and satisfying lives. The Foundation advances this mission primarily through its work in education and medicine." "In education, the Foundation is committed to: Strengthening the profession by recognizing and rewarding outstanding educators; by expanding their professional leadership and policy influence; and by encouraging talented young people to become educators. Stimulating creativity and productivity among educators and students of all ages–especially by using technology to improve learning and teaching. Fostering the involvement of both the family and the community in schools. Helping build vibrant communities–especially by involving young people who have special needs, or who live in neighborhoods considered disadvantaged, in school-based programs that contribute to the revitalization of their community and to the well-being of its residents." "In medicine, the Foundation is committed to: Advancing and supporting basic and applied medical research–especially in the areas of prostate cancer and epilepsy–and recognizing and rewarding outstanding scientists in these areas. Supporting basic health care programs to assure the well-being of community members of all ages." "A wealth of human potential is represented by individual people of all ages whose vision and purpose make them dynamic forces for change. The Foundation's mission is to help realize this potential by giving support that enables people to create and carry out effective, lasting solutions to the challenges facing our communities." 1997 Funding Guidelines **Priorities:** *Civic & Public Affairs:* 21%. Supports community affairs, urban league, and public policy, safety, and housing. *Education:* 62%. Supports educational programs and institutions, leadership training. *International:* 25%. Supports medical centers and disease and disorder concerns, hospice and childrens health. *Note:* Contributions were made in fiscal 1998. **Typ. Recipients:** AIDS/HIV, Cancer, Children's Health/Hospitals, Clinics/Medical Centers, Eyes/Blindness, Hospitals, Long-Term Care, Medical Research, People with Disabilities, Single-Disease Health Associations, Substance Abuse, Substance Abuse. **Geo. Dist:** CA.

★ 11791 ★ Millbrook Tribute Garden

PO Box AC
Millbrook, NY 12545
Phone: (845)677-6823
Kathy Shanks, Secretary

Fnded: 1943. **Philosophy:** The Millbrook Tribute Garden makes grants across the major categories of support. Educational support favors Millbrook's private schools. Religious support goes to individual churches and religious welfare. Health care interests include hospitals. **Priorities:** *Arts & Humanities:* 7%. Supports a library and the performing arts. *Civic & Public Affairs:* 8%. Supports community development, botanical gardens and a horticultural society. *Education:* 30%. Supports secondary and preparatory schools, colleges, and universities. *Environment:* 21%. Supports youth services, senior citizens services, volunteer services, and planned parenthood. *International:* 9%. Supports hospitals and centers for women with AIDS. *Note:* Total contributions made in fiscal 2001. **Typ. Recipients:** AIDS/HIV, Family Planning, Hospices, Hospitals, Medical Rehabilitation. **Geo. Dist:** Millbrook, NY, and vicinity.

★ 11792 ★ Minnie Stevens Piper Foundation

GPM South Tower, Suite 200
800 NW Loop 410
San Antonio, TX 78216-5699
Phone: (210)525-8494 **Fax:** (210)341-6627
Email: cotero@mspf.org
Website: http://www.mspf.org
Carlos Otero, Executive Director & Secretary

Fnded: 1950. **Philosophy:** "The foundation was formed to support charitable, scientific or educational undertakings by providing for or contributing toward the education of financially limited but worthy students; by assisting young men and women residents of Texas, attending or wishing to attend colleges and universities in the State of Texas, to complete their education and obtain degrees; by contributing to community chests, and supporting any other nonprofit organization or activity dedicated to the furtherance of the general welfare within the State of Texas." The following continuing programs are presently operated by the foundation: STUDENT LOAN PROGRAM: A revolving fund totaling $2,500,000 with loans limited to amounts repaid to the fund by former borrowers. A total of approximately $350,000 is available yearly. PIPER PROFESSORS PROGRAM: Ten awards of $2,500 each are made annually to professors for superior teaching at the college level. Selection is made on the basis of nominations submitted by each college or university in the State of Texas. STUDENT AID CENTER AND BEXAR COUNTY SCHOLARSHIP CLEARINGHOUSE: The Student Aid Center provides information through the Student Aid Library regarding college admissions, financial assistance, career planning, and international study to students, parents and counselors. The Bexar County Scholarship Clearing House serves as a liaison between applicants and scholarship donors. The purpose of the clearing house is to eliminate unnecessary duplication of work on the part of the counselors, students, donors, and parents; to broaden the scope of scholarship opportunities in this area; to expedite processing of scholarships to an earlier period of the senior year; and to standardize scholarship application forms. PIPER SCHOLARS PROGRAM: Four-year scholarships are awarded to academically promising and superior high school seniors in amounts sufficient for their needs to attend the college or university of their choice in the State of Texas. Applicants must be U.S. Citizens/Permanent Residents and Texas residents. Students selected and named Piper Scholars must maintain a "B" average throughout their undergraduate college career to remain in the program. **Priorities:** *Arts & Humanities:* 8%. Supports libraries, performing arts, public broadcasting and music. *Civic & Public Affairs:* Less than 1%. *Education:* 85%. Provides academic scholarships and awards. *Environment:* Less than 1%. *International:* 3%. Supports medical research and single-disease health associations. *Religion:* 1%. Supports a science academy. *Note:* Total contributions made in 2000. **Typ. Recipients:** Cancer, Domestic Violence, Eyes/Blindness, Health Organizations, Hospitals, Medical Education, Medical Research, Mental Health, People with Disabilities, Public Health, Substance Abuse. **Geo. Dist:** TX.

★ 11793 ★ Miriam and Peter Haas Fund

201 Filbert St., 5th Floor
San Francisco, CA 94133
Phone: (415)296-9249 **Fax:** (415)296-8842
Email: mphf@mphf.org
Cheryl Polk, Executive Director & Secretary

Fnded: 1982. **Philosophy:** "The Miriam and Peter Haas Fund, a private foundation located in San Francisco, was incorporated in 1982 and for the first ten years was administered by the trustees. In 1992, the Fund received a large bequest. With new resources, the trustees hired staff, established a more formalized structure and chose early childhood as their primary focus. Based upon research conducted in 1993 and 1994, foundation staff and trustees developed a grantmaking framework to be implemented in stages over several years. It is designed to support activities that provide San Francisco's young (ages 2-5), low-income children and their families with access to high-quality early childhood programs that are a part of a comprehensive, coordinated system. The Fund recognizes the importance of connecting the work of its direct service grants to the ongoing discussions of public policy and will seek specific opportunities to share and collaborate with organizations to improve early childhood settings. The Fund will also continue trustee-initiated grantmaking to arts, education, public affairs and health and human services organizations." "We believe that young children and their families must be able to access high quality early childhood programs which are affordable and part of a comprehensive, coordinated system. Working with others, in long term sustained effort, we believe this vision is attainable." "With this in mind, the Fund's Early Childhood program reflects a multi-level approach. Our strategic support of the field–in areas such as planning, policy, finance, leadership development and comprehensive services–will be complemented by efforts to meet the immediate needs of young children. By weaving these pieces together, we hope to provide thoughtful, responsive and comprehensive grantmaking." "It is our belief that high quality early childhood programs improve children's chances for success in school and life. The Model Centers Initiative is designed to improve the quality of early childhood programs by strengthening and enhancing organizational capacity, service delivery, family involvement, comprehensive services, curriculum, professional and leadership development, and other key components of selected centers over a multi-year period." *Miriam and Peter Haas Fund Statement About the Fund* **Priorities:** *Arts & Humanities:* 66%. Supports art museums, public broadcasting, theater, ballet, orchestras, libraries, and historic preservation. *Civic & Public Affairs:* 5%. Funds community foundations, housing, legal aid, and economic development. *Education:* 11%. Gives to colleges, universities, public schools, and preschools. *Environment:* 8%. Supports day care, community centers, child advocacy, family services, Young Men's Christian Association, and United Way. *International:* 2%. Contributes to pediatric health organizations, hospitals, free clinics, HIV/AIDS organizations, and single-disease health associations. *Note:* Total contributions made in 2000. **Typ. Recipients:** AIDS/HIV, Cancer, Children's Health/Hospitals, Clinics/Medical Centers, Domestic Violence, Family Planning, Hospitals, Long-Term Care, Medical Rehabilitation, Medical

Research, Mental Health, People with Disabilities, Public Health, Research/Studies Institutes, Substance Abuse. **Geo. Dist:** CA, San Francisco County.

★ 11794 ★ Monfort Family Foundation

PO Box 337300
Greeley, CO 80633
Phone: (970)454-1357 **Fax:** (970)454-2535
Dave Evans, Administrator

Fnded: 1970. **Philosophy:** The foundation primarily supports student programs at the university level. Other educational interests include technical training and support. "Funds are earmarked primarily for projects and/or groups promoting access to education, development of the arts and humanities, conducting scientific research into the causes and/or prevention of life-threatening diseases and the treatment thereof, and providing various forms of aid to the disadvantaged." **Priorities:** *Arts & Humanities:* 1%. *Civic & Public Affairs:* 8%. *Education:* 88%. Mainly scholarships for university students. *Environment:* 2%. Contributes mainly to boys and girls organizations. *International:* Less than 1%. Single-disease health organizations, children's hospitals, and medical centers. *Note:* Total contributions made in 2000. **Typ. Recipients:** AIDS/HIV, Arthritis, Cancer, Children's Health/Hospitals, Clinics/Medical Centers, Hospitals, Medical Rehabilitation, Multiple Sclerosis, People with Disabilities, Prenatal Health Issues, Public Health, Respiratory, Single-Disease Health Associations, Speech & Hearing, Substance Abuse, Trauma Treatment. **Geo. Dist:** CO, Northern Colorado.

★ 11795 ★ Monterey Fund

1 Metrotech Center N, 9th Fl.
Brooklyn, NY 11201
Phone: (347)643-4590 **Fax:** (347)643-4765
Gilbert Sherman, Contact

Fnded: 1967. **Typ. Recipients:** Cancer, Children's Health/Hospitals, Clinics/Medical Centers, Hospitals, Medical Education, People with Disabilities, Prenatal Health Issues, Public Health, Single-Disease Health Associations. **Geo. Dist:** New York, NY, metropolitan area.

★ 11796 ★ Montgomery Street Foundation

930 Montgomery St., Suite 1107
San Francisco, CA 94104
Fax: (415)398-0612
Carol Elliott, Secretary & Treasurer

Fnded: 1952. **Philosophy:** The foundation primarily supports colleges and universities with moderate grants. Grants to higher education focus on economic education and business schools. Civic interests include law and justice and better business. The foundation also supports a number of social service and health interests. **Priorities:** *Arts & Humanities:* 4% supports historic art, the opera and museum. *Civic & Public Affairs:* 11% supports public and civic affairs. *Education:* 16% supports colleges and universities. *Environment:* 9% supports planned parenthood, handicapped, child sexual abuse treatment, and treatment center for the blind. *International:* 50% supports children's health, and medical research. *Religion:* 7% supports scientific learning center and museum, and science institute. *Note:* Contributions were made in 1998. **Typ. Recipients:** Cancer, Child Abuse, Children's Health/Hospitals, Clinics/Medical Centers, Domestic Violence, Emergency/Ambulance Services, Family Planning, Geriatric Health, Health Funds, Health Organizations, Heart, Hospices, Hospitals, Long-Term Care, Medical Education, Medical Research, People with Disabilities, Public Health, Research/Studies Institutes, Single-Disease Health Associations, Substance Abuse. **Geo. Dist:** San Francisco, CA, metropolitan area.

★ 11797 ★ Moody Foundation

2302 Postoffice St., Suite 704
Galveston, TX 77550
Phone: (409)763-5333 **Fax:** (409)763-5564
Email: pmoore@moodyf.org
Website: http://www.moodyf.org
Peter Moore, Grants Director

Fnded: 1942. **Philosophy:** In recent years, much of the foundation's funding has supported foundation-initiated projects, primarily through the Transitional Learning Community, a comprehensive head-injury rehabilitation facility, and through Moody Gardens. The Gardens complex, located on Galveston Island, now includes a convention center, a swimming beach, 3-D I-MAX theater, visitors' center, equestrian arena for therapeutic horseback riding, a nine-story glass pyramid biome housing a tropical rainforest the Moody Hospitality Institute and a world class aquarium. The rainforest pyramid provides environmental education while complementing the Gardens' horticultural therapy program. The entire complex has been designed with special attention to the needs of persons with disabilities, both for recreation and employment. The foundation's remaining grants support a wide variety of programs benefiting the people of Texas (mainly in Galveston) in the areas of education, health, social service, law enforcement, civic and public affairs, performing arts and medical research. **Priorities:** *Arts & Humanities:* 1%. Gives to museums, a film festival, public broadcasting, and libraries. *Civic & Public Affairs:* 29%. Provides major funding for Moody Gardens, Inc., a complex in Galveston, TX including gardens, an aquarium, and a convention center. *Education:* 3%. Supports special education programs, Episcopal schools, colleges and universities. *Environment:* 2%. Funds services for the homeless and poor, family services, and animal welfare programs. *International:* 64%. Provides substantial support to the Transitional Learning Community, a residential rehabilitation and research facility for the treatment of traumatic brain injuries. Also contributes to nursing homes and to neurological research, post-trauma health, mental health, and physical therapy programs. *Note:* Total contributions made in 2000, excluding scholarships provided to individuals through the Moody Scholars Program. **Typ. Recipients:** AIDS/HIV, Cancer, Children's Health/Hospitals, Domestic Violence, Emergency/Ambulance Services, Eyes/Blindness, Family Planning, Geriatric Health, Health Organizations, Health Policy/Cost Containment, Heart, Hospices, Hospitals, Hospitals (University Affiliated), Kidney, Long-Term Care, Medical Education, Medical Rehabilitation, Medical Research, Mental Health, Nursing Services, People with Disabilities, Prenatal Health Issues, Respiratory, Single-Disease Health Associations, Speech & Hearing, Substance Abuse, Transplant Networks/Donor Banks. **Geo. Dist:** TX; Dallas, TX; Galveston, TX.

★ 11798 ★ Moriah Fund, Inc.

1 Farragut Square South
1634 I St. Northwest, Suite 1000
Washington, DC 20006
Phone: (202)783-8488 **Fax:** (202)783-8499
Email: jedwards@moriahfund.org
Janice Edwards, Grants Manager

Fnded: 1985. **Philosophy:** "The Moriah Fund was established in 1985; its philosophy of giving is rooted in fundamental Jewish values: a concern for the disadvantaged and an emphasis on self-help; a commitment to equity and justice; and a desire to improve the quality of life for Jews and non-Jews alike. In accordance with these values, the mission and operations of the Moriah Fund incorporate concern for the basic needs of all people-especially the most disadvantaged-and for the well-being and continuation of the Jewish people." "Moriah's grant making program seeks to promote pluralism and democracy, help disadvantaged people gain self-sufficiency and control over their lives, promote sustainable development, women's rights and reproductive health and protect and preserve the environment. Moriah supports programs that strengthen local involvement, leadership and institutional development. The Fund focuses on areas where private funding can make a difference, that is, areas that receive inadequate government funds, or that leverage public and private support through advocacy and the modeling of innovative programs." 1998 Annual Report **Priorities:** *Civic & Public Affairs:* 23%. Funds public policy, legal affairs, women's concerns, human rights, job training, and community development. *Education:* 2%. *Environment:* 7%. Supports family planning, childcare, food banks, and youth and family services. *International:* 7%. Funds mental health, women and children's health, and mental health care. *Note:* Total contributions made in 2000. **Typ. Recipients:** Adolescent Health Issues, Children's Health/Hospitals, Clinics/Medical Centers, Family Planning, Health Organizations, Health Policy/Cost Containment, Long-Term Care, Medical Training, Mental Health, People with Disabilities, Prenatal Health Issues, Public Health. **Geo. Dist:** internationally; emphasis on Latin America, particularly Guatemala; Washington, DC; MD; NY.

★ 11799 ★ Morris Goldseker Foundation of Maryland

1040 Park Ave., Suite 310
Baltimore, MD 21201
Phone: (410)837-5100 **Fax:** (410)837-7927
Email: sscott@goldsekerfoundation.org
Website: http://www.goldsekerfoundation.org
Sally Scott, Program Officer

Fnded: 1974. **Philosophy:** The foundation has established four program areas of interest: community affairs, education, human services, and neighborhood development. In all of these areas, highest priority is given to programs of direct service to disadvantaged people and programs that improve the quality of life, increase access and opportunity, promote self-reliance, encourage creativity, and represent the tradition of private voluntary action beyond peoples' own particular spheres of activity. Also of special interest are programs that strengthen institutions and systems of delivery; address long-term solutions to community problems; strengthen neighborhoods; strengthen the private nonprofit sector; attract other resources; and improve efficiency of operations. In 1996, the Foundation announced that funding to health interests would be discontinued, and that greater emphasis would be placed on public education. In 2000, the Foundation's Board of Trustees and its Selection Committee adopted a two-track approach to grantmaking. The approach designates priority areas that build on existing experience and investments, but also retains the ability to respond to new ideas and opportunities with established program areas. Between 2001-2003, and possibly beyond, most of the grantmaking funds will focus on the first-track priority areas. In these areas - community development, regionalism, and non-profit sector - the Foundation will be more directly engaged and active partner. The existing grantmaking policies apply to the priority areas. The second track focuses on the Foundation's established program areas - neighborhood development, community affairs, human services, and education. **Priorities:** *Arts & Humanities:* 6%. Supports historic preservation and libraries. *Civic & Public Affairs:* 58%. Supports planning and housing associations, neighborhood development, and community revitalization. *Education:* 23%. Funds colleges and universities, private schools, and scholarship funds. *Environment:* 4%. Funds human services programs, including youth and work programs and food banks. *International:* 1%. Supports a regional health network. *Note:* Total contributions made in 2000. **Typ. Recipients:** Child Abuse, Clinics/Medical Centers, Domestic Violence, Family Planning, Health Organizations, Medical Education, Mental Health, People with Disabilities, Research/Studies Institutes, Substance Abuse. **Geo. Dist:** Baltimore, MD.

★ 11800 ★ Morris and Gwendolyn Cafritz Foundation

1825 K St. Northwest, Suite 1400
Washington, DC 20006
Phone: (202)223-3100 **Fax:** (202)296-7567
Email: grantscoord@cafritzfoundation.org
Website: http://www.cafritzfoundation.org
Anne Allen, Executive Director

Fnded: 1948. **Philosophy:** The foundation has reflected the interests of its founders. The foundation's areas of concern have been the arts and humanities, education, community services, and health in Washington, DC. "The general policy is to concentrate grants to organizations, operating within the Washington metropolitan area, with projects of direct assistance to the District of Columbia." The foundation supports the arts and humanities, gives money for scholarships to local students, and supports education, local health, and community services. This emphasis on the Washington, DC, community is expected to continue. **Priorities:** *Arts & Humanities:* Supports music, theater, dance, libraries, ethnic and folk art, public broadcasting, and ballet. *Civic & Public Affairs:* Supports botanical gardens, parks, civil rights, municipalities, community foundation, housing, job training, legal aid, and ethnic organizations. *Education:* Funds public school, arts/humanities education, education reform, literacy science education, environmental education, and leadership training. *Environment:* Supports domestic violence, Big Brothers/Big Sisters, daycare, scouts, emergency relief, family services, youth organizations volunteer services, and shelters. *International:* Supports children's health, public health, and medical training. **Typ. Recipients:** Adolescent Health Issues, AIDS/HIV, Children's Health/Hospitals, Diabetes, Domestic Violence, Emergency/Ambulance Services, Family Planning, Geriatric Health, Health Organizations, Hospices, Hospitals, Long-Term Care, Medical Education, Medical Rehabilitation, Mental Health, Nursing Services, People with Disabilities, Prenatal Health Issues, Single-Disease Health Associations, Substance Abuse. **Geo. Dist:** Washington, DC, including metropolitan area.

★ 11801 ★ Morris Stulsaft Foundation

100 Bush St., Suite 825
San Francisco, CA 94104-2521
Phone: (415)986-7117 **Fax:** (415)986-2521
Email: stulsaft@aol.com
Website: http://www.stulsaft.org
Joseph Valentine, Executive Director

Fnded: 1953. **Philosophy:** The foundation, in accordance with its stated goal, is organized to aid and assist needy and deserving children. It has traditionally funded organizations in the broad categories of social services and recreation, education, health, and the arts. Social service funding includes support for child welfare (including adoption services and child abuse prevention); recreational activities (particularly for handicapped youth); traditional youth groups; religious welfare organizations; day care and children's centers; programs for disadvantaged and mentally and physically disabled youth; prevention of substance abuse; family planning and parental services; homes and shelters; job training; volunteer assistance; and immigrant services. In the area of education, interests include minority education; remedial education, tutoring, and drop-out prevention; vocational education; literacy; special education; and preschool, arts, and bilingual education. Health funding includes mental health and child development; pediatric nursing services and in-house care for sick children; respite care; hospitals; and single-disease health associations. Grants in the arts went to public broadcasting, museums, and the performing arts for programs which promote arts appreciation and involve youth (especially minority and low-income youth) in arts activities. **Priorities:** *Arts & Humanities:* 8%. Funds music, museums, and arts. *Civic & Public Affairs:* 10%. *Education:* 14%. Emphasis on primary and secondary education. *Environment:* 54%. Supports a wide variety of community and social welfare causes in the San Francisco Bay Area. *International:* 9%. Supports hospitals, medical clinics, pediatric health organizations. *Note:* Total contributions made in fiscal 2001. Percentages provided by foundation and include capital grant contributions. **Typ. Recipients:** Adolescent Health Issues, AIDS/HIV, Cancer, Child Abuse, Children's Health/Hospitals, Diabetes, Domestic Violence, Emergency/Ambulance Services, Eyes/Blindness, Family Planning, Heart, Hospitals, Medical Education, Medical Rehabilitation, Medical Research, Mental Health, Nursing Services, People with Disabilities, Prenatal Health Issues, Preventive Medicine/Wellness Organizations, Public Health, Research/Studies Institutes, Sexual Abuse, Single-Disease Health Associations, Speech & Hearing, Substance Abuse, Trauma Treatment. **Geo. Dist:** CA, Alameda County; CA, Contra Costa County; CA, Marin County; CA, San Francisco County; CA, San Mateo County; CA, Santa Clara County.

★ 11802 ★ Mr. and Mrs. Lyndon C. Whitaker Charitable Foundation

308 N 21st St., Suite 400
Saint Louis, MO 63103
Phone: (314)241-3452
Christy Gray, Executive Director

Fnded: 1975. **Philosophy:** "The Foundation funds organizations that promote, contribute, and further develop the cultural heritage and vitality of the St. Louis, MO community. It supports programs and organizations that preserve the natural and cultural heritage of parks and encourage the use of parks. The Foundation supports preventive and primary health care for those in need, and supports medical research that can improve the quality of life for all." **Priorities:** *Arts & Humanities:* 27%. Supports historical preservation, museums, theater, music, and art. *Civic & Public Affairs:* 37%. Supports parks, zoos, and gardens. *Education:* 22%. Supports public schools, and universities. *Environment:* 5%. Supports food distribution and youth programs. *International:* 9%. Supports single-disease health associations. *Note:* Total contributions made in fiscal 2001. **Typ. Recipients:** Alzheimers Disease, Cancer, Clinics/Medical Centers, Family Planning, Health-General, Hospices, Hospitals, Hospitals (University Affiliated), Medical Education, Medical Research, People with Disabilities, Public Health, Respiratory, Single-Disease Health Associations. **Geo. Dist:** St. Louis, MO, metropolitan area.

★ 11803 ★ Naomi and Nehemiah Cohen Foundation

PO Box 73708
Washington, DC 20056
Phone: (202)234-5454 **Fax:** (202)234-8797
Email: nncf@starpower.net
Allison McWilliams, Associate Director

Fnded: 1959. **Philosophy:** "The Naomi and Nehemiah Cohen Foundation provides funding to charitable and educational organziations that promote peaceful existence between Israel, Palestinians and the Arab States; provide human services and educational, cultural and economic opportunities to women, minorities, underserved communities and the Jewish community; protect women's rights, including freedom of reproductive choice; protect the environment; promote responsible government and social justice." *Naomi and Nehemiah Cohen Foundation Mission Statement* **Priorities:** *Arts & Humanities:* 2%. Theater, art galleries/museums, and public television. *Civic & Public Affairs:* 8%. Public policy, human rights, social justice, and economic development. *Education:* 7%. Scholarship funds, foundations, and policy studies. *Environment:* 16%. *International:* 16%. Medical centers, planned parenthood programs, and clinics. *Note:* Total contributions made in 2001. Analysis provided by foundation. **Typ. Recipients:** Arthritis, Cancer, Children's Health/Hospitals, Clinics/Medical Centers, Diabetes, Emergency/Ambulance Services, Eyes/Blindness, Family Planning, Health Organizations, Health-General, Heart, Hospices, Hospitals, Hospitals (University Affiliated), Long-Term Care, Medical Education, Mental Health, Prenatal Health Issues, Single-Disease Health Associations, Substance Abuse. **Geo. Dist:** Washington, DC.

★ 11804 ★ Nathan Cummings Foundation

475 10th Ave., 14th Floor
New York, NY 10018
Phone: (212)787-7300 **Fax:** (212)787-7377
Email: info@nathancummings.org
Website: http://www.nathancummings.org
Lance Lindblom, President

Fnded: 1949. **Philosophy:** "The Nathan Cummings Foundation is rooted in the Jewish tradition and committed to democratic values and social justice, including fairness, diversity, and community. We seek to build a socially and economically just society that values nature and protects the ecological balance for future generations; promotes humane health care; and fosters arts and culture that enriches communities. The core programs include arts and culture; the environment; health; interprogram initiatives for social and economic justice; and Jewish life. The goal of the Environment program is to, "facilitate environmental justice and environmentally sustainable communities by supporting the accountability of corporations, governments, and other institutions for their environmental practices." The goal of the Health program is to, "improve people's health and wellbeing, especially those who confront barriers due to low- to moderate-socioeconomic status, race, ethnicity, or gender; recognizing the link between physical health and the economic, social, environmental, psychological, and spiritual factors that affect individuals, families, and communities." The goal of the Jewish Life and Values program is to, "extend the presence and influence of the values of tolerance, social justice (*tzedec*) loving-kindness (*chesed*), mutual respect, and ethical behavior within the Jewish world both to enhance Jewish life and to assist in the promotion of a more just society." The goal of Contemplative Practice grants is to, "promote the development and dissemination of contemplative practice programs–from all traditions–which address the foundation's core values." The goal of Interprogram Initiatives for Social and Economic Justice is to, support social and economic justice, in order to encourage equitable and sustainable development that promotes democracy; as well as community, cultural, social, spiritual and individual wellbeing. Interprogram will advance this goal by supporting the exploration, development, and implementation of public policy, private efforts, and activities for institutional and systemic changes." The Nathan Cummings Foundation Program Guidelines. **Priorities:** *Arts & Humanities:* 26%. Supports community-based organizations and museum initiatives. *International:* 19%. Supports beginning of life and end of life health, and access to health services programs. *Note:* Total contributions made in 2001. **Typ. Recipients:** AIDS/HIV, Cancer, Children's Health/Hospitals, Clinics/Medical Centers, Family Planning, Geriatric Health, Health Funds, Health Organizations, Health Policy/Cost Containment, Health-General, Hospitals, Long-Term Care, Medical Education, Medical Research, Mental Health, People with Disabilities, Prenatal Health Issues, Preventive Medicine/Wellness Organizations, Public Health, Trauma Treatment. **Geo. Dist:** nationally.

★ 11805 ★ Needmor Fund

1840 Folsom St., Suite 110
Boulder, CO 80302
Phone: (303)449-5801
Website: http://www.fdncenter.org/grantmaker/needmor

Fnded: 1956. **Priorities:** *Civic & Public Affairs:* 58%. Supports employment, Gay/Lesbian issues, public policy. *Education:* 3%. Supports public education, education funds and religious education. *Environment:* 29%. Supports family planning, family services, scouting, and food distribution programs. *International:* 1%.Funds public health. *Note:* Total contributions made in 2000. **Typ. Recipients:** People with Disabilities, Public Health. **Geo. Dist:** nationally; Toledo, OH, and surrounding area.

★ 11806 ★ Nelda C. and H. J. Lutcher Stark Foundation

601 W Green Ave.
PO Box 909
Orange, TX 77631-0909
Phone: (409)883-3513 **Fax:** (409)883-3530
Website: http://www.starkfoundation.org
Sherrie Sheppard, Grants Administrator

Fnded: 1961. **Philosophy:** The foundation's primary purpose is the operation of the Stark Museum of Art, the Frances Ann Lutcher Theater for Performing Arts, the Miriam Lutcher Stark Contest in Reading and Declamation, the Shangri La Botanical Gardens and Nature Center, and the W. H. Stark House, the historic home of the Stark family. The foundation was established "to encourage, promote and assist education through grants and scholarships to educational institutions. The Foundation also seeks to enrich the lives of Southeast Texans through the arts; improve quality of life of Southeast Texas through support of medical research, services, and education; assist community organizations providing special services of need to individuals; and preservation of the heritage of Southeast Texas." 2001 Annual Report **Priorities:** *Arts & Humanities:* 3%. Supports historical societies, museums, opera, libraries, and art. *Civic & Public Affairs:* 4%. Funds housing, public safety, and fire prevention. *Education:* 47%. Supports scholarships, Junior Achievement, educational institutions and programs, and schools. *Environment:* 12%. Supports rehabilitation, youth services, and veterans. *International:* 32%. Supports hospices, medical centers, and retina and cancer research. *Note:* Contributions were made in 2001. **Typ. Recipients:** Cancer, Children's Health/Hospitals, Eyes/Blindness, Hospices, People with Disabilities, Single-Disease Health Associations, Transplant Networks/Donor Banks. **Geo. Dist:** LA, Southwest Louisiana; TX, Southeast Texas.

★ 11807 ★ Neva and Wesley West Foundation

PO Box 7
Houston, TX 77001-0007
Phone: (713)520-0400 **Fax:** (713)520-1131
Stuart Stedman, Trustee

Fnded: 1956. **Philosophy:** The Neva & Wesley West Foundation predominantly supports the arts. Other areas of interest include health and medical organizations, environmental issues, and educational concerns. Traditionally, donations are not granted outside Texas. **Priorities:** *Arts & Humanities:* 33%. Supports museums, opera, theater, symphony, ballet. *Civic & Public Affairs:* 1%. Supports gardens. *Education:* 14%. Supports schools, colleges. *Environment:* 1%. Supports homes, womens shelters, scouts. *International:* 12%. Supports medical research. *Note:* Total contributions made in 2000. **Typ. Recipients:** Children's Health/Hospitals, Emergency/Ambulance Services, Eyes/Blindness, Family Planning, Health Organizations, Hospitals, Medical Education, Medical Research, Mental Health, Prenatal Health Issues, Public Health, Speech & Hearing. **Geo. Dist:** Houston, TX.

★ 11808 ★ New-Land Foundation

1114 Ave. of the Americas, 46th Floor
New York, NY 10036-7798
Phone: (212)479-6162 **Fax:** (212)841-6275
Renee Schwartz, Secretary

Fnded: 1941. **Philosophy:** The foundation is currently interested in funding programs in the following areas: civil rights/justice, the environment (other than hazardous waste), population control, and peace and arms control. The foundation does not typically fund programs in medicine, religion, educational institutions, or general social programs, including conferences and symposiums. **Priorities:** *Civic & Public Affairs:* 23%. Supports public policy, community foundations, and law & justice. *Education:* 4%. Supports educational programs. *Environment:* 2%. Supports Planned Parenthood of New York and other family planning orgs. *Note:* Total contributions made in 2000. **Typ. Recipients:** Clinics/Medical Centers, Family Planning, Hospitals, Medical Education, Medical Research, Mental Health, Research/Studies Institutes. **Geo. Dist:** nationally.

★ 11809 ★ New World Foundation

666 West End Ave.
New York, NY 10025
Phone: (212)249-1023 **Fax:** (212)472-0508
Email: cgreer@newwf.org
Website: http://www.newwf.org
Mr. Colin Greer, President

Fnded: 1954. **Philosophy:** Due to the recent decrease in availability of federal funding, the New World Foundation has decided to provide support to community and public institutions. The foundation seeks to implement connections between activists and policymakers, and decrease future levels of poverty, homelessness, and chronic unemployment. Other interests are race, gender, and class issues as well as a variety of causes, largely progressive in nature. The foundation supports programs from the local to the national level. The following principal areas of giving are Equal Rights and Opportunities: those programs which promote participation of all groups in all aspects of American life; Education and Youth: those projects that use community resources to enhance the quality of public education; Public Health: programs to raise public and personal health standards, including health needs of the disadvantaged, as well as environmental and occupational health and safety; and Community Initiatives: those projects that encourage citizen efforts in equal justice and opportunity, improve quality of community life, enhance delivery systems, and meet local needs in a variety of other areas **Priorities:** *Civic & Public Affairs:* 19%. Primarily supports community institutions that promote equal opportunities and encourage citizens to participate in society. *Education:* 11%. Supports educational associations and literary assistance. *Environment:* 38%. Funds food banks and shelters. *Note:* Total contributions made in fiscal 2001. **Typ. Recipients:** Health Organizations, People with Disabilities. **Geo. Dist:** nationally.

★ 11810 ★ New York Foundation

350 Fifth Ave., Suite 2901
New York, NY 10118-2996
Phone: (212)594-8009
Website: http://www.nyf.org
Madeline Lee, Executive Director

Fnded: 1909. **Philosophy:** The foundation supports groups in New York City that are working on problems of urgent concern to disadvantaged communities and neighborhoods. The foundation is particularly interested in start-up grants to new, untested programs that have few other sources of support. The overarching goal of the foundation's grants program is empowerment of the people whose work the foundation supports. The foundation emphasizes activities that enable individuals and groups to become more effective participants in the political and policy-making process. It also emphasizes self-help programs that enable groups to help themselves. In a series of planning meetings, the board reaffirmed the foundation's strong interest in community organizing and advocacy by and on behalf of the populations of concern to the foundation. They also narrowed somewhat the conditions under which the foundation will consider support for direct service programs. Among applicants whose primary aim is direct service, preference will be given to organizations that look likely to move toward advocacy and organizing, and to programs created by newly emerging communities, where service provision is often only the first step to the development of a voice for the community. **Priorities:** *Civic & Public Affairs:* 59%. Focus on poor disadvantaged minorities of the New York City area. *Education:* 1%. Supports Barnard College. *Environment:* 34%. Funds services for disadvantaged groups; including human service organizations serving youth, families, and the elderly. *International:* 6%. Supports ministry and Audre Lorde Project. *Note:* Total contributions made in 2000. **Typ. Recipients:** Adolescent Health Issues, AIDS/HIV, Cancer, Domestic Violence, Geriatric Health, Health Organizations, Health Policy/Cost Containment, Heart, Hospitals, Hospitals (University Affiliated), Mental Health, Nutrition, Outpatient Health Care, People with Disabilities, Prenatal Health Issues, Preventive Medicine/Wellness Organizations, Public Health, Single-Disease Health Associations, Substance Abuse. **Geo. Dist:** New York, NY, metropolitan area.

★ 11811 ★ Nicholas H. Noyes, Jr. Memorial Foundation

1950 E Greyhound Pass, 18-356
Carmel, IN 46033-7730
Phone: (317)844-8009 **Fax:** (317)844-8099
Email: admin@noyesfoundation.org
Website: http://www.noyesfoundation.org
Nancy Ayres, President

Fnded: 1951. **Philosophy:** The foundation distributes its giving to a variety of interests. Educational funding favors secondary schools and private academies. Social service recipients include united funds, housing, work centers, and day care. Most of the support for the arts is centered on the performing arts in Indianapolis. Health care favors nursing and hospitals. Other interests include zoos, conservation, and religion. **Priorities:** *Arts & Humanities:* 22%. Funds museums, music, dance, and art centers. *Civic & Public Affairs:* 3%. Supports zoos and economic development. *Education:* 40%. Funds colleges, universities, precollege education, and education funds. *Environment:* 28%. Supports youth groups, childcare, united funds, and family services. *International:* 4%. Contributes to hospitals, rehabilitation, and medical centers. *Note:* Total contributions made in 2000. **Typ. Recipients:** Cancer, Children's Health/Hospitals, Clinics/Medical Centers, Diabetes, Emergency/Ambulance Services, Family Planning, Hospitals, Medical Rehabilitation, Medical Research, Nursing Services, People with Disabilities, Single-Disease Health Associations, Substance Abuse. **Geo. Dist:** Indianapolis, IN.

★ 11812 ★ Nina Mason Pulliam Charitable Trust

135 N Pennsylvania St., Suite 1200
Indianapolis, IN 46204-1956
Phone: (317)231-6075
Mary Price, Contact

Fnded: 1997. **Philosophy:** The Nina Pulliam Charitable Trust seeks to help people in need, especially women, children and families; to protect animals and nature; and to enrich community life in the metropolitan areas of Indianapolis and Phoenix. (2001 Form 990) **Priorities:** *Arts & Humanities:* 18%. Supports museums, theater, libraries, and music. *Civic & Public Affairs:* 51%. Supports zoological parks, national parks, community parks, housing, and women's issues. *Education:* 2%. Supports an education foundation. *Environment:* 21%. Supports domestic violence shelters, youth clubs and organizations, United Way, and recreation centers. *Religion:* 4%. Supports a science center. *Note:* Total contributions made in 2001. **Typ. Recipients:** People with Disabilities. **Geo. Dist:** AZ; IN.

★ 11813 ★ Nora Eccles Treadwell Foundation

241 Joaquin Ave.
San Leandro, CA 94577
Phone: (510)895-1032
Patricia Canepa, Chairman & Director

Fnded: 1962. **Philosophy:** The foundation's principal concerns are medical research, primarily in the areas of cardiovascular disease, diabetes, and arthritis. Currently, its major priority is the Nora Eccles Treadwell Cardiovascular Research and Training Institute at the University of Utah's Medical Center. **Priorities:** *International:* 100%. Supports medical research, primarily cardiovascular, arthritis, and diabetes. Major grant to the University of Utah. *Note:* Total contributions made in 2000. **Typ. Recipients:** Arthritis, Children's Health/Hospitals, Diabetes, Emergency/Ambulance Services, Family Planning, Health Funds, Health Organizations, Health-General, Heart, Hospitals, Hospitals (University Affiliated), Medical Education, Medical Research, Mental Health, People with Disabilities, Prenatal Health Issues, Single-Disease Health Associations. **Geo. Dist:** CA; UT.

★ 11814 ★ Norcross Wildlife Foundation

PO Box 269
Wales, MA 01081-0269
Phone: (212)362-4831 **Fax:** (212)362-4783
Website: http://www.norcrossws.org

Fnded: 1964. **Philosophy:** The foundation supports a variety of organizations, but environmental affairs remain the primary focus for its giving program. **Priorities:** *Arts & Humanities:* 1%. Primarily supports libraries. *Civic & Public Affairs:* 22%. Supports community affairs and municipalities. *Education:* 1%. Supports educational institutions. *Environment:* 8%. Supports people with disabilities, and social and youth services. *Religion:* 1%. Funds a natural history society. *Note:* Total contributions made in 2000. **Typ. Recipients:** AIDS/HIV, Children's Health/Hospitals, Clinics/Medical Centers, Emergency/Ambulance Services, Hospitals, Medical Education, People with Disabilities. **Geo. Dist:** nationally.

★ 11815 ★ Nord Family Foundation
347 Midway Boulevard, Suite 210
Elyria, OH 44035
Phone: (440)324-2822 **Fax:** (440)324-6427
Email: exedir@nordff.org
Website: http://www.nordff.org
Sharon White, Controller

Fnded: 1988. **Philosophy:** The trustees have clarified the foundation's grant-making priorities into the two themes of strengthening the family and strengthening the public service in all of its grant making, and also serve as a general purpose foundation in Lorain County, OH. The foundation has also established three specific priorities for action: improving the county's leadership, education, and physical appearance. An agenda entitled "Lorain County 2020" was recently published with input from the foundation and community leaders. The foundation reports that it is initiating a Grassroots Leadership Program and a Family Investment Fund. **Priorities:** *Arts & Humanities:* 23%. Supports historical associations, dance, theater, music and public broadcasting. *Civic & Public Affairs:* 17%. Focus is on urban affairs, housing, economic development, and job training. *Education:* 22%. Emphasis is on primary and secondary education, education associations, minority education, and scholarships. *Environment:* 25%. Interests include community service organizations, child welfare, family planning, food distribution programs, emergency relief, YMCA, and community centers. *International:* 7%. Supports community health, blood banks, single-disease associations, and medical rehabilitation. *Religion:* Less than 1%. *Note:* Total contributions made in 2000. **Typ. Recipients:** Adolescent Health Issues, Alzheimers Disease, Cancer, Child Abuse, Children's Health/Hospitals, Clinics/Medical Centers, Domestic Violence, Emergency/Ambulance Services, Eyes/Blindness, Family Planning, Health Organizations, Health-General, Mental Health, Nursing Services, People with Disabilities, Public Health, Sexual Abuse. **Geo. Dist:** Denver, CO; OH, Cuyahoga County area; OH, Lorain County area; Columbia, SC.

★ 11816 ★ Norman Foundation
147 East 48th St.
New York, NY 10017
Phone: (212)230-9830 **Fax:** (212)230-9849
Email: info@normanfdn.org
Website: http://www.normanfdn.org
June Makela, Program Director

Fnded: 1938. **Philosophy:** The foundation has identified three main areas of interest: economic justice, civil rights/individual liberties and environmental justice. "Economic justice grants are awarded to projects that seek to redress economic inequities or facilitate wider access to employment, education, housing and the like. Grants in the area of civil rights/individual liberties typically fund projects designed to combat systemic discrimination and violence directed against disenfranchised groups, such as racial minorities, women, gays and lesbians, and the disabled. Other grants have gone to projects addressing government and corporate abuses of power, particularly those that create threats to the environment, human health and safety." The foundation encourages cooperation between local groups at the grassroots level and national advocacy groups; a successful proposal would most likely combine a grassroots approach with a strong advocacy component. The foundation provides general support and project-oriented support and places great importance on diversity within organizations. The foundation has an interest in dealing directly in economic, "since the creation of decent, healthy jobs with fair incomes and benefits is not only a good in itself, it empowers people to achieve more" in the foundation's areas of interest. Also of particular interest are strategies on how to engage more Americans in their civic lives and to increase faith and involvement in community institutions. **Priorities:** *Civic & Public Affairs:* 71%. Supports general civil funding and the Welfare Rights Organizing Coalition in Seattle. *Education:* 3%. *Environment:* 9%. Supports youth programs. *International:* 2%. *Note:* Total contributions made in 1999. **Typ. Recipients:** AIDS/HIV, Children's Health/Hospitals, Domestic Violence, Family Planning, Health Policy/Cost Containment, Hospices, Medical Research, Mental Health, People with Disabilities, Public Health. **Geo. Dist:** nationally.

★ 11817 ★ Norman and Rosita Winston Foundation
1285 Ave. of the Americas
New York, NY 10019-6064
Phone: (212)373-3000 **Fax:** (212)373-2187
John O'Neil, Attorney

Fnded: 1954. **Philosophy:** The foundation focuses its funding on higher education, the arts, health and medical research, civic organizations, and social services. **Priorities:** *Arts & Humanities:* About 42%. Supports museums, performing arts, music, ballet, libraries, opera, and public broadcasting. *Civic & Public Affairs:* 3%. Urban affairs projects. *Education:* About 28%. Primary support for colleges, universities, and medical education. *Environment:* 2%. *International:* 9%. Focus on cancer research. *Religion:* 3%. *Note:* Total contributions made in 1996. **Typ. Recipients:** Cancer, Geriatric Health, Heart, Hospitals, Long-Term Care, Medical Education, Medical Research, Research/Studies Institutes, Sexual Abuse. **Geo. Dist:** NY.

★ 11818 ★ Northwest Area Foundation
60 Plato Boulevard East, Suite 400
Saint Paul, MN 55107
Phone: (651)224-9635 **Fax:** (651)225-7701
Email: info@nwaf.org
Website: http://www.nwaf.org
Karl Stauber, President

Fnded: 1934. **Philosophy:** The Northwest Area Foundation seeks to help communities most in need create positive futures - economically, ecologically, and socially. To implement the mission, the Foundation will help communities work toward a balanced system that will reduce poverty; stimulate economic growth; sustain the natural environment; and develop effective institutions, relationships, and individuals. One hundred percent of the Foundation's resources will be devoted to supporting its mission through three programs: Community Ventures: The Foundation will identify approximately 16 communities in which to work intensively. Its commitment to each community will be long-term, as much as 10 years or longer. Investments in these community partnerships will total approximately $150 million over the next decade. Community Connections: The Foundation also will make available an array of shorter-term services, programs, and small grants to an additional number of communities. These will be consistent with the Foundation's new mission. Investments in these activities will total approximately $25 million over the next decade. Community Horizons: Recognizing the dilemma of rural communities where both population and opportunity have been declining for decades, the Foundation will help selected communities develop and retain teams of leaders who can help chart the future. This program, which will be fully operating in three to five years, will total approximately $25 million over the next decade. **Typ. Recipients:** AIDS/HIV, Clinics/Medical Centers, Family Planning, Health Organizations, Health Policy/Cost Containment, Mental Health, Nursing Services, Outpatient Health Care. **Geo. Dist:** ID; IA; MN; MT; ND; OR; SD; WA.

★ 11819 ★ Oak Foundation U.S.A.
PriceWaterhouseCoopers LLP
333 Market St.
San Francisco, CA 94105
Phone: (415)498-7866
Alan Parker, Vice President & Director

Fnded: 1986. **Priorities:** *Arts & Humanities:* Less than 1%. *Civic & Public Affairs:* 22%. Supports housing, women's organizations, law and justice issues, civil rights, and an aquarium. *Education:* 4%. Supports enrichment programs. *Environment:* 3%. Supports community service organizations. *International:* 14%. Supports hospitals, healthcare, single-disease associations, and health institutes. *Religion:* 4%. Supports scientists' organizations. *Note:* Total contributions made in 2000. **Typ. Recipients:** AIDS/HIV, Cancer, Clinics/Medical Centers, Emergency/Ambulance Services, Hospitals, Medical Education, Medical Rehabilitation, Medical Research, Mental Health, People with Disabilities, Single-Disease Health Associations. **Geo. Dist:** CA.

★ 11820 ★ Oberkotter Foundation
1600 Market St., Suite 3600
Philadelphia, PA 19103
Phone: (215)751-2601 **Fax:** (215)751-2678
Email: George_Nofer@SHSL.com
George Nofer, Co-Trustee

Fnded: 1992. **Priorities:** *Education:* 67%. Funds schools for the deaf and medical schools. *International:* 33%. Supports hospitals, medical research, and hearing foundations. *Note:* Total contributions made in 2000. **Typ. Recipients:** Alzheimers Disease, Cancer, Children's Health/Hospitals, Clinics/Medical Centers, Diabetes, Health Organizations, Hospitals, Medical Education, Medical Research, People with Disabilities, Public Health, Research/Studies Institutes, Speech & Hearing.

★ 11821 ★ O'Donnell Foundation
100 Crescent Court, Suite 1660
Dallas, TX 75201
Phone: (214)871-5800 **Fax:** (214)855-8988
Carolyn Bacon, Executive Director

Fnded: 1957. **Philosophy:** The foundation's primary focus is on education, especially science and engineering. It also funds civic and public affairs organizations, medical centers, and the arts. **Priorities:** *Arts & Humanities:* Approx. 1%. Funds art museums. *Civic & Public Affairs:* Approx. 1%. Supports other foundations. *Education:* 98%. Supports public primary and secondary schools in Texas. Major building grant to University of Texas at Austin. *Environment:* Approx. 1%. Supports Life Sciences Research Foundation. *Note:* Total contributions made in fiscal 2000. **Typ. Recipients:** Clinics/Medical Centers, Hospitals (University Affiliated), Medical Education, Respiratory. **Geo. Dist:** TX.

★ 11822 ★ The Offield Family Foundation
400 North Michigan Ave., Room 407
Chicago, IL 60611
Phone: (312)467-5480 **Fax:** (312)467-0473
Marie Larson, Secretary

Fnded: 1953. **Philosophy:** The foundation supports a wide variety of charitable organizations. Most of the support goes to civic affairs, including conservation issues and women's affairs. Health is also a major priority, mainly supporting hospitals. Public broadcasting and family planning are consistently supported, while public education remains a minor interest. **Priorities:** *Arts & Humanities:* 20%. Cultural parks, arts centers, and public broadcasting. *Civic & Public Affairs:* 13%. Women's resources, clubs, and community foundations. *Education:* 3%. Public precollege education, colleges, and universities. *Environment:* 16%. Planned Parenthood, youth clubs, and food banks. *International:* 14%. Medical centers, burn centers, and hospitals. *Note:* Contributions made in fiscal 2000. **Typ. Recipients:** Cancer, Children's Health/Hospitals, Clinics/Medical Centers, Emergency/Ambulance Services, Family Planning, Health Funds, Health Organizations, Hospices, Hospitals, Hospitals (University Affiliated), Medical Education, Medical Research, People with Disabilities, Public Health, Substance Abuse, Transplant Networks/Donor Banks, Trauma Treatment. **Geo. Dist:** nationally.

★ 11823 ★ Ohrstrom Foundation
717 Fifth Ave.
New York, NY 10022
Phone: (212)759-5380 **Fax:** (212)486-0935
Ms. Dorothy Barry, Jr., Treasurer

Fnded: 1953. **Philosophy:** The Ohrstrom Foundation makes most of its grants in the areas of environmental affairs, education, arts/humanities, health/medical, community service, civil rights, and religion. In education, interests include technical training, universities, and private schools. **Priorities:** *Arts & Humanities:* 7%. focus on libraries and museums. *Civic & Public Affairs:* 36%. Supports ethnic and community organizations. *Education:* 22%. Funds secondary schools and colleges and universities. *Environment:* 13%. Supports substance abuse programs, animal protection, youth organizations, and community service organizations. *International:* 6%. Supports hospitals and single-disease health associations. *Note:* Total contributions made in fiscal 2001. **Typ. Recipients:** Arthritis, Cancer, Emergency/Ambulance Services, Health Organizations, Heart, Hospices, Hospitals, Medical Research, People with Disabilities, Research/Studies Institutes, Single-Disease Health Associations, Substance Abuse. **Geo. Dist:** nationally; VA.

★ 11824 ★ Olive B. Cole Foundation

6207 Constitution Drive
Fort Wayne, IN 46804
Phone: (260)436-2182 **Fax:** (260)432-3146
John Hogan, Executive Vice President & Treasurer

Fnded: 1954. **Philosophy:** The goal of the Cole Foundation is local giving, chiefly in the areas of education, community projects, and recreation. It strives to fund new organizations and maintain old recipients. **Priorities:** *Arts & Humanities:* 15%. Libraries, historical preservation, museums, music, and public broadcasting. *Civic & Public Affairs:* 3%. Parades/festivals, job training programs, community foundations, a zoo, and parks. *Education:* 48%. Education funds, precollege public education, and colleges and universities. *Environment:* 34%. People with disabilities, community centers, youth organizations, the elderly, and athletics. *Note:* Total contributions made in fiscal 2001. **Typ. Recipients:** AIDS/HIV, Alzheimers Disease, Cancer, Children's Health/Hospitals, Clinics/Medical Centers, Emergency/Ambulance Services, Health Organizations, Home-Care Services, Hospices, People with Disabilities, People with Disabilities, Trauma Treatment. **Geo. Dist:** IN, North Eastern Indiana, Noble, La Grange, De Kalb, and Steuben counties.

★ 11825 ★ Oliver S. and Jennie R. Donaldson Charitable Trust

New York, NY 10109-1910
Phone: (212)852-1000 **Fax:** (212)852-3377
Linda Franciscovich, Managing Director

Fnded: 1969. **Philosophy:** The foundation makes grants across the major categories of support. Most of the grants are made in the areas of education, health, civic affairs, and social services. Educational funding favors colleges and universities. Funding for health care goes to support cancer treatment and research at a number of facilities, hospitals, and health organizations. In civic affairs, interests primarily include conservation and preservation organizations. Social service funding supports community centers, homes, and animal protection organizations. **Priorities:** *Arts & Humanities:* 17%. Supports public libraries, cultural festival, museums. *Civic & Public Affairs:* 1%. Supports civic and community affairs. *Education:* 13%. Supports colleges, universities, and educational programs. *Environment:* 6%. Supports volunteer consulting, animal welfare, and youth services. *International:* 39%. Supports hospitals, children's health, cancer and heart research. *Religion:* 17%. Supports stem cell, dioxins, and cancer research. *Note:* Contributions were made in 2001. **Typ. Recipients:** Cancer, Child Abuse, Children's Health/Hospitals, Clinics/Medical Centers, Emergency/Ambulance Services, Health Organizations, Health-General, Heart, Hospitals, Medical Research, Mental Health, Nursing Services, People with Disabilities, Preventive Medicine/Wellness Organizations, Research/Studies Institutes, Single-Disease Health Associations. **Geo. Dist:** northeastern United States.

★ 11826 ★ Oppenstein Brothers Foundation

PO Box 13095
Kansas City, MO 64199-3095
Phone: (816)234-8671 **Fax:** (816)234-8690
Sheila Rice, Program Officer

Fnded: 1975. **Philosophy:** The Oppenstein Brothers Foundation was created by a bequest of Mr. Michael Oppenstein in order that the accumulated wealth of his brothers and himself might be used "for religious, charitable, scientific and educational purposes serving the public welfare..." The foundation's giving areas include social welfare, education (excluding scholarship assistance), arts (primarily educational programming for children), health (programs that promote wellness), and social services. **Priorities:** *Arts & Humanities:* 37%. Arts outreach, music, and ballet. *Civic & Public Affairs:* 7%. Housing and urban and community affairs. *Education:* 6%. Primary education and colleges and universities *Environment:* 26%. Primary support for child welfare, food banks, shelter, united funds, and youth organizations. *International:* 9%. Health centers and clinics and single-disease health associations. *Note:* Total contributions made in fiscal 1999. **Typ. Recipients:** AIDS/HIV, Alzheimers Disease, Cancer, Child Abuse, Children's Health/Hospitals, Clinics/Medical Centers, Domestic Violence, Emergency/Ambulance Services, Eyes/Blindness, Family Planning, Health Organizations, Heart, Hospices, Hospitals, Medical Rehabilitation, Mental Health, People with Disabilities, Prenatal Health Issues, Public Health, Sexual Abuse, Single-Disease Health Associations, Substance Abuse. **Geo. Dist:** Kansas City, MO, metropolitan area.

★ 11827 ★ Orchard Foundation

PO Box 2587
South Portland, ME 04116
Phone: (207)799-0686
Email: orchard@maine.rr.com
Website: http://www.orchardfoundation.org
M. Erlich, Trustee

Philosophy: Orchard Foundation funds organizations in three fields of interest: Environment; Children, Youth, and Families; and Campaign Finance Reform. Environment: The foundation focuses primarily on air quality, biodiversity, fresh and coastal waters, forests, toxic substances, and pollution prevention. Preference is given to legal, legislative, and administrative process advocacy projects. Children, Youth, and Families: Within this field of interest, the foundation funds projects in three categories. The category of Child & Family Advocacy focuses on projects that promote child welfare at local and state levels by addressing systemic issues as opposed to direct service projects. The area of Literacy supports programs that encourage or teach reading. Although family literacy projects are considered, the main focus is on children's literacy. Pregnancy Prevention focuses on programs that encourage middle and high school students to delay childbearing using either a direct service or a policy-oriented approach. Programs to be funded under this category should emphasize birth control skills. Campaign Finance Reform: The foundation supports statewide efforts to implement campaign finance reform, with preference given to organizations that have already researched their state's "money in politics" situation and are able to develop and advocate for the implementation of statewide reforms. Orchard Foundation Program Areas, 2001 **Priorities:** *Arts & Humanities:* 4%. Supports libraries, museums, and historical preservation. *Civic & Public Affairs:* 8%. Funds public policy initiatives. *Education:* 41%. Supports Boston-area higher education institutions, private secondary schools, and literacy projects. *Environment:* 10%. Interests include children, youth, and family welfare. *International:* 4%. Supports children's hospitals and clinics. *Note:* Total contributions in 2000. **Typ. Recipients:** AIDS/HIV, Alzheimers Disease, Arthritis, Child Abuse, Children's Health/Hospitals, Clinics/Medical Centers, Domestic Violence, Family Planning, Health Funds, Hospices, Hospitals, Medical Education, Medical Research, Multiple Sclerosis, Nursing Services, Outpatient Health Care, People with Disabilities. **Geo. Dist:** New England area; NY.

★ 11828 ★ Ordean Foundation

501 Ordean Bldg.
Duluth, MN 55802
Phone: (218)726-4785 **Fax:** (218)726-4848
Email: ordean@cpinternet.com
Stephen Mangan, Executive Director

Fnded: 1933. **Philosophy:** Through his will in 1926, Mr. Ordean directed the founding of "a corporation for the purpose of administering and furnishing relief and charity for the worthy poor...without discrimination as to age, sex, color, or religious inclination. Mr. Ordean also made sizeable bequests to the service of disabled and orphaned children, youth, disadvantaged women, the elderly and infirm." The foundation's mission concentrates on the funding of services and facilities for the needy, treatment of the chronically or temporarily mentally ill, the care and rehabilitation of the physically impaired, and the support of youth guidance programs. **Priorities:** *Arts & Humanities:* 4%. Funds children's museum. *Civic & Public Affairs:* 14%. Supports housing and economic development. *Education:* 12%. Funds colleges. *Environment:* 51%. Emphasis on youth organizations, food and clothing distributions, prevention of domestic violence, child welfare, community centers, and Young Men's Christian Association and Young Women's Christian Association. *International:* 11%. Funding for health centers and single disease health associations. *Note:* Total contributions made in 2000. **Typ. Recipients:** AIDS/HIV, Alzheimers Disease, Children's Health/Hospitals, Clinics/Medical Centers, Domestic Violence, Emergency/Ambulance Services, Family Planning, Health Organizations, Home-Care Services, Medical Education, Medical Rehabilitation, Mental Health, People with Disabilities, Prenatal Health Issues, Public Health, Single-Disease Health Associations, Substance Abuse. **Geo. Dist:** Duluth, MN, Hermantown, and Proctor areas.

★ 11829 ★ Orville D. and Ruth A. Merillat Foundation

1800 West U.S. 223
PO Box 1071
Adrian, MI 49221
Phone: (517)265-5425 **Fax:** (517)265-3041
Mr. John Thurman, Treasurer

Fnded: 1983. **Philosophy:** The foundation provides substantial support for a variety of preselected Christian causes. Educational interests include higher education, theological education, and religious schools. Among human services receiving support are Christian service groups, youth organizations, and child welfare and family service agencies. The foundation also supports conferences of churches, crusades, ministries, evangelical associations, and Bible distribution efforts. **Priorities:** *Arts & Humanities:* 2%. Opera and fine arts. *Civic & Public Affairs:* 7%. Public policy and community organizations. *Education:* 24%. Supports colleges and Christian schools. *Environment:* 19%. Family and youth councils and centers. *International:* 4%. Health centers. *Note:* Total contributions made in fiscal 2001. **Typ. Recipients:** Health Funds, Hospices. **Geo. Dist:** MI, particularly Adrian.

★ 11830 ★ Otto Bremer Foundation

445 Minnesota St., Suite 2000
Saint Paul, MN 55101-2107
Phone: (651)227-7621 **Fax:** (651)312-3665
Email: obf@bremer.com
Website: http://www.ottobremer.org
John Kostishack, Executive Director

Fnded: 1944. **Philosophy:** The Foundation is committed to playing a contributing role in strengthening nonprofits throughout its Service area. Foundation grants favor organizations located in communities serviced by Bremer Banks, which are located in Minnesota, North Dakota, Montana, and Wisconsin. Principal grant recipients within these rural communities are "agencies which address the needs of individuals affected by poverty; activities which address general community needs and encourage citizen participation; educational internships; promotion of individual and community health; and activities of religious organizations which address community needs." The foundation annually reevaluates priorities within these categories in order to remain responsive to the communities' needs. "The current focus areas are...working with nonprofit organizations to bring to communities...providing resources to assist beneficiaries in becoming self supporting organizations that have an impact on the future." Otto Bremer Foundation 1999 Annual Report. **Priorities:** *Note:* Total contributions made in 1999. **Typ. Recipients:** AIDS/HIV, Clinics/Medical Centers, Diabetes, Domestic Violence, Emergency/Ambulance Services, Geriatric Health, Health Organizations, Hospices, Hospitals, Medical Education, Mental Health, Nursing Services, Outpatient Health Care, People with Disabilities, Public Health, Substance Abuse. **Geo. Dist:** MN; MT; ND; WI.

★ 11831 ★ The Overbrook Foundation

122 East 42nd St., Suite 2500
New York, NY 10168-2500
Phone: (212)661-8710 **Fax:** (212)661-8664
Email: Sheila@overbrook.org
M. McGoldrick, Grants Manager

Fnded: 1948. **Philosophy:** The foundation reflects the interests of the descendants of Frank and Helen Altschul. Foundation support is often given on a continuing basis. Although the foundation makes some large grants, it prefers to make smaller grants to a variety of institutions. Many of the recipient organizations have a national or international orientation. Major interests of the foundation include Jewish welfare funds, higher and secondary education, hospitals, international relations, cultural programs, and community funds. funding focus. funding focus. **Priorities:** *Arts & Humanities:* 9% Supports libraries, museums, performing and visual art. *Civic & Public Affairs:* 37%. Supports community and public affairs. *Education:* 15%. Supports educational programs and institutions. *Environment:* 10%. Supports planned parenthood, handgun violence prevention, children's services, and recording services for the blind and dyslexic. *International:* 7%. Supports hospitals, mental health centers, medical centers, gay men's health, and medical research institutes. *Note:* Contributions were made in 2000. **Typ. Recipients:** AIDS/HIV, Emergency/Ambulance Services, Family Planning, Health Organizations, Hospices, Hospitals, Hospitals (University Affiliated), Medical Research, Mental Health, Nursing Services, People with Disabilities, Single-Disease Health Associations, Substance Abuse. **Geo. Dist:** nationally; CT; New York, NY, metropolitan area.

★ 11832 ★ Oxford Foundation

125D Lancaster Ave.
Strasburg, PA 17579
Phone: (717)687-9335 **Fax:** (717)687-9336
Email: pcalhoun@oxfordfoundation.org
Website: http://www.oxfordfoundation.org
Philip Calhoun, Executive Director

Fnded: 1947. **Philosophy:** The Oxford Foundation makes grants across the major categories of support. In education, interests include colleges, universities, public school districts, private education, medical training, and day schools. Health support goes to medical centers, health organizations, and Alzheimer's research. Social service support includes community centers, family services, shelters, and youth organizations. Funding for civic affairs favors foundations, agricultural support, and zoos. **Priorities:** *Arts & Humanities:* 6%. Supports historic preservation, music, museums, and the performing arts. *Civic & Public Affairs:* 18%. Supports fire fighters, gardens, public policy, research, planning, advocacy, and community and economic development. *Education:* 28%. Supports schools, educational foundations, and colleges and universities. *Environment:* 13%. Supports child welfare, youth development, people with disabilities, senior services, and community partnerships. *International:* 22%. Funds medical centers, community health programs, children's health care, and single-disease health associations. *Note:* Total contributions made in 2001. **Typ. Recipients:** Alzheimers Disease, Arthritis, Cancer, Children's Health/Hospitals, Clinics/Medical Centers, Diabetes, Domestic Violence, Emergency/Ambulance Services, Family Planning, Hospices, Hospitals, Hospitals (University Affiliated), Medical Education, Medical Research, Mental Health, Nursing Services, People with Disabilities, Prenatal Health Issues, Public Health, Sexual Abuse, Single-Disease Health Associations, Substance Abuse. **Geo. Dist:** PA.

★ 11833 ★ Park Foundation

PO Box 550
Ithaca, NY 14851
Phone: (607)272-9124 **Fax:** (607)272-6057
Mrs. Leslie Myers, Executive Director

Fnded: 1966. **Priorities:** *Arts & Humanities:* 21%. Provides major support to public broadcasting; also funds libraries and arts organizations. *Education:* 78%. Supports colleges and universities, with particular focus on funding projects and fellowships. *Note:* Total contributions made in 2000. **Typ. Recipients:** Cancer, Diabetes, Eyes/Blindness, Heart, Hospices, Hospitals, Medical Rehabilitation, Prenatal Health Issues. **Geo. Dist:** NY, Central New York.

★ 11834 ★ Patrick and Anna M. Cudahy Fund

1007 Church St., Suite 414
Evanston, IL 60201
Phone: (847)866-0760 **Fax:** (847)475-0679
Email: secretary@cudahyfund.org
Website: http://www.cudahyfund.org
Judith Borchers, Executive Director

Fnded: 1934. **Philosophy:** The fund supports a broad range of civic, educational, and social service programs, and organizations which are primarily located in the Milwaukee, Madison, and Chicago areas. Current interests include national programs dealing with the environment and other public interest issues, secondary and higher education, religious welfare, and civic and cultural affairs. The fund also supports international social welfare projects. **Priorities:** *Arts & Humanities:* 5%. Gives to museums, theater, libraries, and public broadcasting. *Civic & Public Affairs:* 12%. Funds housing, women's affairs, job training, public policy, and business associations. *Education:* 5%. Contributes largely to Catholic educational institutions and literacy programs. *Environment:* 34%. Supports child and family services, food distribution, programs for the homeless, senior services, and programs for the disabled. *International:* 6%. Gives to clinics, AIDS/HIV treatment centers, health care for the blind and deaf, and mental health programs. *Note:* Total contributions made in 2001. **Typ. Recipients:** Clinics/Medical Centers, Domestic Violence, Family Planning, Geriatric Health, Health Organizations, Long-Term Care, People with Disabilities, Preventive Medicine/Wellness Organizations, Public Health, Substance Abuse. **Geo. Dist:** internationally; nationally; Chicago, IL; WI.

★ 11835 ★ Patrick and Catherine Weldon Donaghue Medical Research Foundation

18 North Main
West Hartford, CT 06107-1919
Phone: (860)521-9011 **Fax:** (860)521-9018
Email: director@donaghue.org
Website: http://www.donaghue.org

Fnded: 1989. **Philosophy:** "The Donaghue Medical Research Foundation funds innovative basic biomedical, pre-clinical research, as well as epidemiological, community health and health services research in the areas of cancer, cardiovascular disease, mental health and neurodegenerative diseases." "The Donaghue Foundation, in seeking to promote knowledge of practical benefit to human life through research, conducts several initiatives in support of Connecticut-based health research and related work." "Research in Clinical and Community Health Issues is a funding initiative for biomedical, behavioral and other health-related research projects that address the major medical conditions and social problems influencing the health of individuals, groups, and communities. The Foundation is especially interested in clinical, epidemiological and health service research studies that focus on the development and evaluation of more effective methods for preventing, diagnosing and treating illnesses and conditions that have a major impact on the people of Connecticut." "The Donaghue Investigator Program is an initiative aimed at supporting particularly promising medical researchers holding faculty appointments at Connecticut institutions. The funding emphasis is on the investigator and his or her program of research rather than upon a specific study." "Practical Benefit Initiatives. In these areas the Foundation initiates research projects showing particular promise for producing practical benefit to human life. In areas the Foundation wishes to pursue, an interactive process between the Foundation and prospective investigators is used to develop projects for funding." The Patrick and Catherine Weldon Donaghue Medical Research Foundation 1998 Annual Report **Priorities:** *International:* 100%. The foundation funds individuals at health-research institutions. In 2001, the giving was distributed as follows: 20% for Research in Clinical and Community Health Issues; 56% for Practical Benefit Initiatives; and 24% for The Donaghue Investigator Program. **Typ. Recipients:** Cancer, Children's Health/Hospitals, Heart, Medical Education, Medical Research, People with Disabilities, Public Health. **Geo. Dist:** CT.

★ 11836 ★ Paul Ogle Foundation

Box 946
Jeffersonville, IN 47130
Phone: (812)282-7566 **Fax:** (812)284-5519
Email: rlanum@stites.com
Website: http://www.ogle-fdn.org
Robert Lanum, Chairman

Fnded: 1979. **Philosophy:** The Paul Ogle Foundation focuses on capital improvement projects and one-time projects that fall within the mission and current priorities of the foundation. Scholarship funding goes to colleges in Indiana and Kentucky. Social services, such as youth welfare organizations, are a priority. **Priorities:** *Arts & Humanities:* 9%. Supports historical societies, libraries, and arts funds. *Civic & Public Affairs:* 12%. Supports community foundations, urban parks, zoos, and municipalities. *Education:* 44%. Primarily gives to colleges, universities, and schools. *Environment:* 27%. Funds youth clubs, scouting, and the United Way. *International:* Less than 1%. Funds American Red Cross. *Religion:* 4%. Supports a science center. *Note:* Total contributions made in 2000. **Typ. Recipients:** Clinics/Medical Centers, Domestic Violence, Emergency/Ambulance Services, Heart, Medical Rehabilitation, People with Disabilities. **Geo. Dist:** IN, Clark County; IN, Floyd County; IN, Harrison County; IN, Scott County; IN, Switzerland County; IN, Washington County.

★ 11837 ★ Paul and Phyllis Fireman Charitable Foundation

1601 Forum Place, Suite 905
West Palm Beach, FL 33401
Phone: (561)684-1900 **Fax:** (561)684-2168
Phyllis Fireman, Trustee

Fnded: 1985. **Philosophy:** The foundation's major priority is funding civic affairs organizations, specifically anti-defamation leagues. The foundation is also interested in education and favors Jewish educational institutions, both at the university and secondary levels. Minor support also goes to social services, the arts, and religion. **Priorities:** *Arts & Humanities:* 4%. Gives to art and children's museums, libraries, and performing arts. *Civic & Public Affairs:* 69%. Supports ethnic organizations, diversity programs, civil rights, community foundations, housing programs, and law/justice organizations. *Education:* 6%. Funds colleges, universities, pre-college schools, and educational programs. *Environment:* 9%. Supports the United Way, shelters/homeless, food distribution, youth clubs, and family services. *International:* 6%. Supports hospitals, medical centers, free clinics, single-disease health associations, medical research, and an eating disorders center. *Note:* Total contributions made in 2000. **Typ. Recipients:** AIDS/HIV, Alzheimers Disease, Arthritis, Cancer, Children's Health/Hospitals, Clinics/Medical Centers, Domestic Violence, Emergency/Ambulance Services, Geriatric Health, Health Organizations, Health-General, Heart, Home-Care Services, Hospices, Hospitals, Medical Education, Medical Rehabilitation, Medical Research, Multiple Sclerosis, Nutrition, People with Disabilities, Preventive Medicine/

Wellness Organizations, Public Health, Single-Disease Health Associations, Transplant Networks/Donor Banks. **Geo. Dist:** New York, NY.

★ 11838 ★ Paul Stock Foundation

PO Box 2020
Cody, WY 82414-2020
Phone: (307)587-5275 **Fax:** (307)527-7897
Charles Kepler, President

Fnded: 1958. **Philosophy:** The foundation's primary mission is to provide student aid for Wyoming residents to pursue higher education. The foundation also focuses on youth agencies, arts groups, and community activities. **Priorities:** *Arts & Humanities:* 1%. Funds the Buffalo Bill Memorial Association. *Civic & Public Affairs:* 86%. Supports activities in the city of Cody, Wyoming. *Education:* 13%. Student aid, vocational/technical education, and a major endowment to the University of Wyoming. *Note:* Total contributions made in 1999. **Typ. Recipients:** Long-Term Care, Medical Rehabilitation, Research/Studies Institutes. **Geo. Dist:** WY.

★ 11839 ★ Pauline Allen Gill Foundation

5500 Preston Rd., Suite 215
Dallas, TX 75205
Phone: (214)521-7243 **Fax:** (214)521-7233
Nancy Seay, Vice President

Fnded: 1975. **Philosophy:** The foundation gives primarily to health care, educational institutions, and the arts. The foundation also supports social services, religion, civic affairs, and environmental concerns. **Priorities:** *Arts & Humanities:* 1%. Supports music and art museums. *Civic & Public Affairs:* 25%. Supports nonprofit management, housing and gardens and parks. *Education:* 19%. Supports private schools and literacy. *Environment:* 5%. Supports community centers, counseling, family services, and United Way. *International:* 27%. Supports medical centers, hospitals, and visiting nurses. *Note:* Total contributions made in 2000. **Typ. Recipients:** AIDS/HIV, Arthritis, Children's Health/Hospitals, Clinics/Medical Centers, Domestic Violence, Emergency/Ambulance Services, Eyes/Blindness, Family Planning, Health Organizations, Heart, Hospitals, Hospitals (University Affiliated), Kidney, Medical Education, Medical Research, Nursing Services, Nutrition, People with Disabilities, Public Health, Research/Studies Institutes, Single-Disease Health Associations, Substance Abuse, Trauma Treatment. **Geo. Dist:** Dallas, TX.

★ 11840 ★ Pearl M. and Julia J. Harmon Foundation

PO Box 52568
Tulsa, OK 74152-0568
Phone: (918)743-6191
Website: http://www.HarmonFoundation.com
George Hangs, Jr., Secretary & Treasurer

Fnded: 1962. **Philosophy:** The foundation supports a wide variety of causes, primarily in the Tulsa, OK, area. Major funding is directed to supporting the Harmon Science Center, an interactive science museum in Tulsa, OK. The foundation does not accept applications for outright grants, but rather directs the distribution of funds through interest-free or reduced-rate loans to charitable organizations. It does not restrict funding to set organizations and attempts to respond to the changing needs of the community. **Priorities:** *Arts & Humanities:* 18%. Funds opera, music, and libraries. *Civic & Public Affairs:* 1%. Supports towns/municipalities, safety. *Education:* 18%. Supports universities, education-general, and schools. *Environment:* 22%. Supports food distribution, senior services, and family planning services. *International:* 5%. Supports medical rehabilitation, home-care services, and emergency/ambulance services. *Note:* Total contributions made in 1999. **Typ. Recipients:** Clinics/Medical Centers, Domestic Violence, Emergency/Ambulance Services, Family Planning, Health Organizations, Health-General, Medical Rehabilitation, Mental Health, Nursing Services, People with Disabilities, Prenatal Health Issues, Research/Studies Institutes, Sexual Abuse, Substance Abuse. **Geo. Dist:** AR; KS; NM; Tulsa, OK; TX.

★ 11841 ★ Peery Foundation

2560 Mission College Boulevard, Suite 101
Santa Clara, CA 95054
Phone: (408)980-0130 **Fax:** (408)988-4893
Richard Peery, President

Fnded: 1977. **Philosophy:** Much of the foundation's support goes to the Church of Latter-day Saints. Other interests focus on youth organizations in a variety of areas, including the arts, scholarships, and social activities. **Priorities:** *Arts & Humanities:* 7%. Supports theater, symphony, historical societies, and arts associations. *Civic & Public Affairs:* 3%. Focus on community affairs. *Education:* 66%. Supports secondary education, colleges, and educational programs. *Environment:* 5%. Supports children and youth services, family services, and food banks. *International:* 17%. Primarily for children's health and single-disease health associations. *Note:* Total contributions made in fiscal 2000. **Typ. Recipients:** Arthritis, Cancer, Children's Health/Hospitals, Emergency/Ambulance Services, Hospices, Medical Research, People with Disabilities, Prenatal Health Issues, Respiratory, Sexual Abuse, Single-Disease Health Associations, Speech & Hearing. **Geo. Dist:** CA. **Frmly:** Richard T. Peery Foundation.

★ 11842 ★ Penzance Foundation

909 3rd Ave., 5st Floor
New York, NY 10022
Phone: (212)653-8802 **Fax:** (212)653-8803
John Emery, Vice President

Fnded: 1981. **Philosophy:** The foundation's giving program generally supports the preferences of Mrs. Clark, with the majority of funding going to educational institutions and social service organizations, principally to youth groups. Medical facilities are also beneficiaries of the foundation's grant-making program. **Priorities:** *Arts & Humanities:* 22%. Funds museums. *Education:* 48%. Funds colleges, universities, private precollege education, and educational associations. *Environment:* 6%. Funds family services and Boys and Girls clubs. *Note:* Total contributions made in fiscal 2001. **Typ. Recipients:** Family Planning, Health Organizations, Hospitals, Kidney, Medical Rehabilitation, Medical Research. **Geo. Dist:** MA; NY.

★ 11843 ★ Perkins-Prothro Foundation

2304 Midwestern Parkway, Suite 200
Wichita Falls, TX 76308
Phone: (940)691-7770 **Fax:** (940)691-6304
Joe Prothro, President

Fnded: 1967. **Philosophy:** The Perkins-Prothro Foundation makes endowments to several universities in Texas in support of higher education. Health services and religion are also of interest to the foundation. Other recipient areas include the arts and community services. **Priorities:** *Arts & Humanities:* 5%. *Civic & Public Affairs:* 9%. *Education:* 75%. Supports a humanities research center and colleges and universities. *Environment:* 6%. *International:* 2%. Hospitals and hospice programs. *Note:* Total contributions made in 2000. **Typ. Recipients:** Cancer, Children's Health/Hospitals, Clinics/Medical Centers, Emergency/Ambulance Services, Health Organizations, Health Policy/Cost Containment, Health-General, Heart, Hospices, Hospitals, Medical Rehabilitation, People with Disabilities, Prenatal Health Issues, Public Health, Single-Disease Health Associations, Substance Abuse. **Geo. Dist:** TX, central Texas area only.

★ 11844 ★ Perot Foundation

PO Box 269014
Plano, TX 75026
Phone: (972)535-1969 **Fax:** (972)535-1991
Carolyn Rathjen, Director

Fnded: 1969. **Philosophy:** The majority of contributions made by the Perot Foundation support higher education, especially medical education at Texas universities. The foundation also supports medical research, religious welfare organizations, and social services. Grants to other recipient areas are made on a limited basis. **Priorities:** *Arts & Humanities:* 8%. Funds music, museums, and opera. *Civic & Public Affairs:* 2%. *Education:* 20%. Emphasis on medical education and scholarship funding. *Environment:* 9%. Funds United Way, scouting, community services, and child welfare. *International:* 55%. Primary support for medical centers, research, nursing services, children's health, and single-disease health associations. *Religion:* Less than 1%. *Note:* Total contributions made in 2000. **Typ. Recipients:** AIDS/HIV, Alzheimers Disease, Cancer, Child Abuse, Children's Health/Hospitals, Emergency/Ambulance Services, Emergency/Ambulance Services, Family Planning, Health Organizations, Heart, Hospitals, Medical Education, Medical Research, Mental Health, Nursing Services, Nutrition, People with Disabilities, Prenatal Health Issues, Public Health, Single-Disease Health Associations, Substance Abuse. **Geo. Dist:** TX, emphasis on Dallas.

★ 11845 ★ Peter Kiewit Foundation

8805 Indian Hills Drive, Suite 225
Omaha, NE 68114
Phone: (402)344-7890 **Fax:** (402)344-8099
Lyn Ziegenbein, Executive Director

Fnded: 1980. **Philosophy:** The foundation makes charitable contributions in the designated areas of education, community development and service, culture, social welfare, health, and character building and physical improvement. The foundation also maintains a scholarship program for graduating high school seniors in the Omaha area. **Priorities:** *Arts & Humanities:* 9%. Funds public libraries, historic preservation, fine art museums, and performing arts. *Civic & Public Affairs:* 53%. Supports civic affairs, housing, municipalities, community foundations, police and fire departments, chambers of commerce, parks, playgrounds, and a zoo. *Education:* 24%. Funds colleges, universities, and educational foundations. *Environment:* 9%. Funds Young Men's Christian Association, United Way, scouts, Boys and Girls Clubs, sports/recreation programs, and child and family services. *International:* 5%. Supports community health programs, single-disease health associations, and hospitals. *Note:* Total contributions made in fiscal 2001. **Typ. Recipients:** AIDS/HIV, Cancer, Clinics/Medical Centers, Emergency/Ambulance Services, Family Planning, Health Organizations, Hospitals, Medical Rehabilitation, Nutrition, People with Disabilities, Trauma Treatment. **Geo. Dist:** Rancho Mirage, CA; IA, the portion of Iowa which is within a 100-mile radius of Omaha, NE; NE; Omaha, NE; Sheridan, WY.

★ 11846 ★ Pew Charitable Trusts

One Commerce Sq.
2005 Market St., Suite 1700
Philadelphia, PA 19103
Phone: (215)575-9050 **Fax:** (215)575-4939
Email: info@pewtrusts.com
Website: http://www.pewtrusts.com
Rebecca Rimel, President & CEO

Fnded: 1948. **Philosophy:** "The Pew Charitable Trusts support the work of nonprofit organizations in the fields of culture, education, the environment, health and human services, public policy, and religion. Through their grantmaking, the Trusts seek to encourage individual development and personal achievement, cross-disciplinary problem solving, and innovative, practical approaches to meeting the changing needs of a global community. The Trusts are based in Philadelphia and maintain a special commitment to the city and its neighboring region. The mission of the Culture program is to assure that the arts, in all their diversity, flourish in the United States, and to promote their increased integration into the fabric of American life. The Education program seeks to raise the performance of students at all levels of education, especially their capabilities to learn for understanding and to acquire the literacies they need for productive employment and effective citizenship in an increasingly complex society. The Education program's principal focus is on supporting the reform of the educational system, elementary school through university, in order to raise standards and improve student performance.

The mission of the Environment program is to promote policies and practices that protect the global atmosphere and preserve healthy forest and marine ecosystems. Much of the Environment program's grantmaking focuses on the development of special initiatives, the mobilization of strategic coalitions to pursue specific policy objectives, and the funding of clusters of projects whose goals reinforce or compliment each other. Because of the program's highly focused nature, the great majority of projects supported are initiated by program staff and/or developed in close collaboration with other foundations and environmental organizations. The Health and Human Services program is designed to promote the health and well-being of the American people and to strengthen disadvantaged communities. Nationally, the trusts give to biomedical research and training; and a public health initiative is being developed. In the Philadelphia area, the trusts support the Pew Fund for Health and Human Services in Philadelphia and the Fund for Urban Neighborhood Development. The mission of the Public Policy program is to create sustainable improvements to America's democratic life through promoting improvements in the conduct and financing of elections, research on the causes and consequences of declines in social trust, efforts to call Americans to re-engage in the civic life of their nation and communities, and increases in overall government performance. The Religion program seeks to advance a deeper understanding of religion's contributions to the ideas, beliefs, morals, and institutions that shape culture and society, and to help people of faith improve their efforts to make a greater contribution to contemporary public life. The Venture Fund is a unique tool for the Trusts, enabling us to explore opportunities that fall outside the clearly defined goals and objectives of the six program areas." **Priorities:** *Arts & Humanities:* 1%. *Civic & Public Affairs:* 9%. *Education:* 5%. Supports K-12 and higher education. *Environment:* 2%. *International:* 5%. Supports biomedical research, scientists, and science policies; also funds human services. *Religion:* 9%. *Note:* Total contributions made in 2001. **Typ. Recipients:** Adolescent Health Issues, AIDS/HIV, Cancer, Children's Health/Hospitals, Domestic Violence, Emergency/Ambulance Services, Family Planning, Geriatric Health, Health Organizations, Health Policy/Cost Containment, Home-Care Services, Medical Education, Nutrition, Prenatal Health Issues, Public Health, Substance Abuse. **Geo. Dist:** internationally; nationally; Philadelphia, PA.

★ 11847 ★ Pfaffinger Foundation

316 W Second St., Suite PH-C
Los Angeles, CA 90012
Phone: (213)680-7460 **Fax:** (213)680-7474
Mary Tower, President

Fnded: 1936. **Philosophy:** The foundation primarily assists employees, former employees, and surviving spouses of former employees of the Times Mirror Company, a publishing firm in Los Angeles. Limited support for charitable institutions in the greater Los Angeles area is given when funds are available. **Priorities:** *Civic & Public Affairs:* 83%. Major grant to California Community Foundation. *Environment:* 12%. Food banks, YMCAs, the United Way, youth, family, and senior citizen services. *International:* 4%. Focus on women's, children's, and geriatric health. *Note:* Total contributions made in 2000. **Typ. Recipients:** Alzheimers Disease, Child Abuse, Children's Health/Hospitals, Clinics/Medical Centers, Domestic Violence, Emergency/Ambulance Services, Family Planning, Geriatric Health, Health Organizations, Health Policy/Cost Containment, Hospitals, Mental Health, Public Health, Substance Abuse. **Geo. Dist:** CA, Southern California.

★ 11848 ★ Phil Hardin Foundation

PO Drawer 5533
Meridian, MS 39302-5533
Phone: (601)483-4282 **Fax:** (601)483-5665
Email: info@philhardin.org
Website: http://www.philhardin.org
C. Wacaster, Vice President

Fnded: 1964. **Philosophy:** "Our vision is to renew and rebuild communities and their economics by means of education. Our goals to guide efforts to accomplish this vision are: Goal 1: Strengthen the capacity of communities to nurture and educate young children. Goal 2: Strengthen the capacity of higher education institutions to renew communities and their economies. Goal 3: Strengthen the capacity of communities for locally initiated educational improvement and economic development. Goal 4: Strengthen policy and leadership at the local levels that support action and success in regard to the foundation's goals." **Priorities:** *Arts & Humanities:* 7%. Supports historic preservation, history, and museum. *Civic & Public Affairs:* 21%. Supports recently audited financial statement development. *Education:* 63%. Supports colleges, universities, faculty development, tutoring programs, and literacy. *Environment:* 4%. Supports family services. *International:* 1%. Supports speech/hearing. *Note:* Total contributions made in 1998. **Typ. Recipients:** Health Policy/Cost Containment, Hospitals (University Affiliated), Medical Rehabilitation, Medical Research, Outpatient Health Care, People with Disabilities, Speech & Hearing. **Geo. Dist:** nationally; MS.

★ 11849 ★ Philip L. Graham Fund

1150 15th St., Northwest
Washington, DC 20071
Phone: (202)334-6640 **Fax:** (202)334-4498
Email: plgfund@washpost.com
Candice Bryant, President

Fnded: 1963. **Philosophy:** "From its earliest days, the fund's dual mission has been first, to use its resources for the betterment of the Washington, DC, metropolitan area and second, to provide assistance to activities in the field of journalism and communications." Areas of funding priority reflect the interests of the late Mr. Graham and include: programs enriching the lives of children; projects aiding needy citizens in the community; cultural organizations, especially those promoting the visual or dramatic arts; programs improving pre-college public education; and journalism and communications organizations promoting minority interests and freedom of the press worldwide. **Priorities:** *Arts & Humanities:* 24%. Supports theater, multicultural performing arts, museums, libraries, and arts in education. *Civic & Public Affairs:* 8%. Funds minority and women's affairs, affordable housing, volunteerism, and environment. *Education:* 22%. Supports elementary, secondary, and higher education, early childhood, at-risk youth, and services for the learning disabled. *Environment:* 38%. Funds organizations that address mental health, abused women and children, hunger, shelters, hospitals, vocational training, family services, prenatal care, child care, youth, AIDS, literacy, blindness, and seniors. *International:* 5%. *Note:* Total contributions made in 2000. Also provides discretionary grants for shelter, food, and other assistance to the poor and homeless. **Typ. Recipients:** AIDS/HIV, Cancer, Children's Health/Hospitals, Clinics/Medical Centers, Diabetes, Domestic Violence, Emergency/Ambulance Services, Family Planning, Geriatric Health, Health Organizations, Heart, Home-Care Services, Hospices, Hospitals, Long-Term Care, Mental Health, Outpatient Health Care, People with Disabilities, Prenatal Health Issues, Public Health, Substance Abuse, Transplant Networks/Donor Banks. **Geo. Dist:** Washington, DC, including metropolitan area.

★ 11850 ★ Philip L. Van Every Foundation

PO Box 32368
Charlotte, NC 28232
Phone: (704)554-1421 **Fax:** (704)556-5636
Sean Jamison, Jr., Executive Director

Fnded: 1961. **Philosophy:** The foundation's primary interests are health-related organizations, social welfare causes, and civic concerns in North Carolina. **Priorities:** *Arts & Humanities:* 14%. Supports theater, public broadcasting, and music. *Civic & Public Affairs:* 13%. Supports community affairs. *Education:* 17%. Supports colleges and universities. *Environment:* 22%. Supports housing, homes, substance abuse services, and YWCA. *International:* 12%. Supports single-disease health associations. *Religion:* 2%. Supports scientific organizations. *Note:* Total contributions made in 2000. **Typ. Recipients:** AIDS/HIV, Arthritis, Cancer, Emergency/Ambulance Services, Health Organizations, Hospices, Hospitals, Medical Education, Medical Research, Multiple Sclerosis, Single-Disease Health Associations, Speech & Hearing, Substance Abuse, Trauma Treatment. **Geo. Dist:** NC.

★ 11851 ★ Philip M. McKenna Foundation

PO Box 186
Latrobe, PA 15650
Phone: (724)537-6901 **Fax:** (724)537-6906
T. Boxx, Chairman

Fnded: 1967. **Philosophy:** The Philip M. McKenna Foundation's "is to support the advancement of a free, prosperous, and well-ordered society based on traditional American civic principles, private enterprise, and the cultual heritage of western civilization. This purpose and public philosophy entails a core commitment to limited constitutional government, free market economics, and moral virtue. In conducting this mission, support is directed toward research and educational programs with a long-term focus, as well as public policy programs focused on more immediate concerns. The interests of the foundation also includes support the benefit of the community and scientific, educational, and charitable causes compatible with the foundations heritage and priorities." Mission statement. **Priorities:** *Civic & Public Affairs:* 54%. Supports public policy, legal concerns, and economics. *Education:* 38% Contributes to economic education at colleges and universities. *Environment:* 2%. Supports youth initiatives. *Religion:* 3%. Funds science museums. *Note:* Total contributions made in 2000. **Typ. Recipients:** Health Policy/Cost Containment, Hospitals, Research/Studies Institutes. **Geo. Dist:** nationally for public policy; PA, Southwestern Pennsylvania for community and civic programs.

★ 11852 ★ Pinewood Foundation

437 Madison Ave., 37th Fl.
New York, NY 10022
Fax: (212)812-4335
Celeste Bartos, President

Fnded: 1956. **Philosophy:** The foundation typically funds arts organizations, museums, and cultural programs, and also supports education organizations. **Priorities:** *Arts & Humanities:* 15%. Museums, film and public broadcasting. *Civic & Public Affairs:* 11%. Women's issues, human rights. *Education:* 34%. Colleges and universities. *Note:* Contributions made in fiscal 2000. **Typ. Recipients:** AIDS/HIV, Clinics/Medical Centers, Eyes/Blindness, Family Planning, Health Organizations, Hospices, Hospitals, Hospitals (University Affiliated), Medical Education, Medical Research, Multiple Sclerosis, Prenatal Health Issues, Public Health, Research/Studies Institutes, Single-Disease Health Associations. **Geo. Dist:** New York, NY.

★ 11853 ★ Pinkerton Foundation

630 Fifth Ave., Ste. 1755
New York, NY 10111
Phone: (212)332-3385 **Fax:** (212)332-3399
Website: http://www.fdncenter.org/grantmaker/pinkerton
Joan Colello, Executive Director & Secretary

Fnded: 1966. **Philosophy:** "The foundation's original mandate was to work to prevent and reduce the incidence of crime and juvenile delinquency and, in the early years, the foundation made grants to a wide range of programs supporting human services and education for the disadvantaged. Building on the original mandate and concerns of its founder, the foundation concentrates its current grant-making program on two segments of the population: first, economically disadvantaged children and youth and families at risk; and second, severely learning-disabled children and adults of borderline intelligence. Within these groups, the foundation seeks to support programs that develop individual competencies, instill values, and increase opportunities to participate in society. Of particular interest are projects that demonstrate promising new ideas for greater program effectiveness or that replicate projects that have proven effective elsewhere. The foundation supports community-based programs in New York City, with preference given to projects for children, youth, and families that intervene before a pattern of failure has been established. The foundation also occasionally supports research and demonstration projects in its principal program areas. While grants for direct service projects are usually limited to New York City, those with potential for national impact or replication may go beyond this geographic limitation." **Priorities:** *Arts & Humanities:* 3%. *Civic & Public Affairs:* 30%. Funds vocational initiatives and community development. *Education:* 15%. Supports programs for middle and schools. *Environment:* 45% Funds youth services and community centers. *Note:* Contributions made in 2000. **Typ. Recipients:** AIDS/HIV, Clinics/Medical Centers, Domestic Violence, Family Planning, Hospitals, Hospitals (University Affiliated), Nursing Services, Outpatient Health Care, People with Disabilities, Public Health, Research/Studies Institutes. **Geo. Dist:** New York City, NY.

★ 11854 ★ Plough Foundation

6410 Poplar Ave., Ste. 710
Memphis, TN 38119
Phone: (901)761-9180 **Fax:** (901)761-6186
Email: mail@plough.org
Rick Masson, Jr., Executive Director & Trustee

Fnded: 1960. **Philosophy:** The foundation supports reform of the public school system and homeless programs in Shelby County, TN. The foundation also plans to place more emphasis on crime prevention and law enforcement. In the area of social services, it has emphasized education reform, Jewish Federation, united funds, homeless projects, youth organizations, and issues related to crime prevention. The foundation's current special interests include: public education, specifically early intervention programs for children; families in crisis, preferably programs and ideas that take a realistic approach to the problems and offer avenues for the participants to become self-sufficient; youth programs, mainly programs that specifically address the needs of and opportunities for young people; stretching the nonprofit dollar, particularly programs and activities that demonstrate unique, innovative ways to maximize resources; homeless programs that are part of a comprehensive system; and crime, specifically programs addressing prevention and law enforcement. The foundation will no longer be making grants to schools of pharmacy. The foundation will, however, continue to make deferred payments to certain institutions. **Priorities:** *Arts & Humanities:* 19%. Ballet, music, arts associations. *Civic & Public Affairs:* 18%. Community affairs and public policy. *Education:* 9%. Public education and education reform. *Environment:* 12%. Family services, united funds, and youth organizations. *International:* 23%. Health centers and hospitals. *Note:* Total contributions made in 1998. **Typ. Recipients:** Cancer, Clinics/Medical Centers, Emergency/Ambulance Services, Hospitals, Medical Education, Mental Health, Outpatient Health Care, People with Disabilities, Single-Disease Health Associations, Substance Abuse. **Geo. Dist:** TN, primarily in Shelby County and Memphis.

★ 11855 ★ Polk Brothers Foundation, Inc.

20 West Kinzie Ave.
Suite 1110
Chicago, IL 60610
Phone: (312)527-4684 **Fax:** (312)527-4681
Email: info@polkbrosfdn.org
Website: http://www.polkbrosfdn.org
Nikki Stein, Executive Director

Fnded: 1957. **Philosophy:** "Founded in 1955, the Foundation remains a Chicago concern. Reflecting the underlying philosophy of the Polk Family, the Foundation supports programs that work directly with populations of need–particularly children. Grants are made for both new and ongoing initiatives in four program areas: social service, education, culture and health." "Since its start, the Foundation has focused on clearly defining its mission. By working with grantees to identify specific goals, develop strategies to reach those objectives and evaluating progress made, the Foundation continues to strive for success in its endeavor." "The goal of the Foundation's grantmaking is to improve the quality of life... (especially in the Chicago area)...with a particular focus on economically-disadvantaged children and youth. We believe that there are three elements that help us achieve that objective: assisting our grantees to enhance their programs; motivating them to increase the capacity of their organizations to implement their programs; and inspecting and improving our own grantmaking process to ensure it contributes to the first two components. We utilize evaluation as a meaningful way to inform all three elements." "When we look at a grant and the way the money is utilized, we really study three factors. First we consider the quality of the program. We ask ourselves if the idea makes sense and has a reasonable chance of making the impact desired. Equally important is the group's ability to attack the identified problem. Does it have a board and staff committed to the program, competent management and adequate fundraising capability?" "Finally, we analyze an agency's past performance, recognizing that circumstances may dictate the need for flexibility and adjustment and that progress, rather than instant results, may be a more reasonable measure of success during a given time frame. Our own objective then is to blend rigor and realism in developing and utilizing evaluation methods that are useful to grantees as well as to us." Polk Bros. 1995 Annual Report, *Evaluating for Impact* The foundation responds to requests from social service, cultural, educational, and health organizations that provide direct services in Chicago. The foundation has implemented the Full Service Schools Initiative. "The Initiative seeks to meet students' and families' needs for a wide range of educational, health, and social service programs through partnerships between schools and community organizations. By locating programs at schools, we can take advantage of excellent facilities that normally shut down at the end of the school day, while providing families much better access to a wide range of resources." 1996 Annual Report **Priorities:** *Arts & Humanities:* 23%. Supports art and culture. *Civic & Public Affairs:* 11%. Supports community and public affairs. *Education:* 25%. Supports educational institutions and programs. *Environment:* 18%. Supports youth, family, and social services. *International:* 5%. Supports health care centers and services. *Religion:* 2%. Supports museums of natural history, with the majority of support given to the Museum of Science and Industry. *Note:* Contributions were made in fiscal 2000. **Typ. Recipients:** AIDS/HIV, Child Abuse, Clinics/Medical Centers, Health Organizations, Hospitals, Medical Rehabilitation, Mental Health, Nursing Services, People with Disabilities, Prenatal Health Issues, Public Health, Substance Abuse. **Geo. Dist:** Chicago, IL.

★ 11856 ★ Powell Family Foundation

4350 Shawnee Mission Parkway, Suite 280
Fairway, KS 66205
Phone: (913)236-0003 **Fax:** (913)262-0058
Carrie Hoelscher, Secretary

Fnded: 1969. **Philosophy:** The foundation primarily serves the Kansas City area through grants in education, community support, religion, and youth programs. Camps are strongly supported, with funding allocated to resident and day camps both for facilities and camperships. Grants in education provide scholarships as well as support for innovative educational programs, including projects to use the arts and the outdoors to motivate students. In particular, the foundation supports the Powell Gardens near Lone Jack, MO, a complex established to encourage research and education in horticulture and natural resources. Grants to religious organizations are made primarily to Christian Science churches and religious welfare programs. Occasional grants may be awarded to other denominational groups that provide social services in the Kansas City community. **Priorities:** *Civic & Public Affairs:* About 94%. Supports the Powell Gardens and women's affairs. *Education:* 6%. *Note:* Total contributions made in 1998. **Typ. Recipients:** Cancer, Family Planning. **Geo. Dist:** Kansas City, MO, metropolitan area.

★ 11857 ★ Powell Foundation

2121 San Felipe, Suite 110
Houston, TX 77019
Phone: (713)523-7557 **Fax:** (713)523-7553
Email: info@powellfoundation.org
Website: http://www.powellfoundation.org
Nancy Powell Moore, Foundation Manager

Fnded: 1967. **Philosophy:** "The purpose of The Powell Foundation is to distribute funds for public charitable purposes, principally for the support, encouragement and assistance to education, health, conservation, and the arts with a direct impact within the Foundation's geographic zone of interest, i.e., principally, Harns, Travis, and Walker Counties, Texas." "The Powell Foundation's current emphasis is in the field of education in the broadest sense. Other areas of interest continue to be community service projects focused on the needs of children, the disadvantaged, the urban environment, and the visual and performing arts, especially in the Greater Houston area." Powell Foundation Guidelines. **Priorities:** *Arts & Humanities:* 14%. Supports the theater, museums, ballet, opera, symphony and art festivals. *Education:* 63%. Educational programs, schools, academies, colleges, and universities receive funding. *International:* 11%. Funds the American Red Cross, health associations, medical research, and Planned Parenthood. *Note:* Total contributions made in 2001. **Typ. Recipients:** Adolescent Health Issues, AIDS/HIV, Child Abuse, Clinics/Medical Centers, Emergency/Ambulance Services, Eyes/Blindness, Family Planning, Hospitals (University Affiliated), Mental Health, Public Health, Research/Studies Institutes, Single-Disease Health Associations, Speech & Hearing, Substance Abuse. **Geo. Dist:** TX, Harris County; TX, Travis County; TX, Walker County.

★ 11858 ★ Presbyterian Health Foundation

711 Stanton L. Young Blvd., Suite 604
Oklahoma City, OK 73104-5023
Phone: (405)271-8150 **Fax:** (405)271-2911
Jean Gumerson, President

Fnded: 1985. **Priorities:** *Education:* 19%. Supports universities and colleges, medical education, and scholarships. *Environment:* 2%. Supports United Way. *International:* 62%. Supports medical research and medical centers. *Note:* Total contributions made in fiscal 2000. **Typ. Recipients:** Cancer, Child Abuse, Children's Health/Hospitals, Clinics/Medical Centers, Eyes/Blindness, Health Organizations, Health-General, Hospitals (University Affiliated), Medical Education, Medical Research, Prenatal Health Issues, Public Health. **Geo. Dist:** OK.

★ 11859 ★ Priddy Foundation

807 8th St.
City National Bldg., Suite 1010
Wichita Falls, TX 76301
Phone: (940)723-8720 **Fax:** (940)723-8656
Email: info@priddyfdn.org
Website: http://www.priddyfdn.org
David Wolverton, President

Fnded: 1963. **Philosophy:** The foundation focuses giving on human services, education, the arts, and civic concerns in northern Texas. **Priorities:** *Arts & Humanities:* 1%. Supports theater and arts education. *Civic & Public Affairs:* 80%. Supports community foundations, housing, nonprofit management, womens affairs, and neighborhood groups. *Education:* 4%. Supports higher education. *Environment:* 10%. Supports relief agencies, child welfare, scouting, counseling, senior services, and meals on wheels program. *International:* 2%. Supports a health care center. *Note:* Total contributions made in 1999. **Typ. Recipients:** Alzheimers Disease, Clinics/Medical Centers, Emergency/Ambulance Services, Health Organizations, Hospices, Hospitals, Medical Education, Medical Rehabilitation, Mental Health, People with Disabilities,

Prenatal Health Issues. **Geo. Dist:** OK, Southern OK; TX, Northern Texas; Wichita Falls, TX.

★ 11860 ★ Pritzker Foundation

200 West Madison St., Suite 2500
Chicago, IL 60606
Phone: (312)750-8400 **Fax:** (312)750-8545
Thomas Pritzker, Vice President & Director

Fnded: 1944. **Philosophy:** The Pritzker Foundation supports Jewish organizations, the arts, health, education, and social services in the Chicago metropolitan area, by providing small grants, ranging from $25 to $1,000, to a large number of organizations. Significant grants are made to a limited number of recipients that include the Jewish United Fund, Crusade of Mercy, several Jewish organizations and synagogues, and programs in support of Israel. In addition, the foundation awards the annual Pritzker Architecture Prize of more than $100,000, administered through the Hyatt Foundation. **Priorities:** *Arts & Humanities:* 9%. Funds public libraries, children's museums, modern & contemporary art museums, the opera, theater, visual and performing arts. *Civic & Public Affairs:* 8%. Funds parks, community affairs, zoology, and aquariums. Also supports private foundations. *Education:* 73%. Supports secondary schools, colleges, universities, and educational programs. *Environment:* 1%. *International:* 2%. Supports medical centers, health centers, and single-disease associations. *Religion:* 4%. Supports science museums and planetariums. *Note:* Total contributions made in 2000. **Typ. Recipients:** Cancer, Children's Health/Hospitals, Clinics/Medical Centers, Domestic Violence, Eyes/Blindness, Family Planning, Health Organizations, Health-General, Hospitals, Medical Education, Medical Rehabilitation, Medical Research, Mental Health, People with Disabilities, Public Health, Research/Studies Institutes, Single-Disease Health Associations, Substance Abuse. **Geo. Dist:** Chicago, IL, metropolitan area.

★ 11861 ★ Prospect Hill Foundation

99 Park Ave., Suite 2220
New York, NY 10016-1601
Phone: (212)370-1165 **Fax:** (212)599-6282
Email: ashipley@prospecthill.org
Website: http://www.fdncenter.org/grantmaker/prospecthill
Constance Eiseman, Executive Director

Fnded: 1960. **Philosophy:** The areas for which the foundation is interested in receiving proposals are nuclear weapons control, environmental conservation, and family planning services in Latin America. The nuclear weapons control grants program seeks to improve communications, understanding, and a sense of mutual risk among leaders in the U.S. and the former Soviet Union; lead to commitments among world leaders to limit and reduce nuclear weapons arsenals; and implement strategies for limiting the proliferation of nuclear weapons, weapons development, and the capacity to manufacture nuclear weapons. The environmental conservation program is concerned with strategies for the preservation of public and private lands and strengthening public policies for environmental protection, water quality, and ecosystem protection in the northeastern U.S. The population program is concerned with programs in Latin America which encourage access to family planning services. Proposals from social services, arts, cultural, and educational institutions are accepted upon invitation only. **Priorities:** *Arts & Humanities:* 17%. Supports historic preservation, museums, music, dance, libraries, and theater. *Civic & Public Affairs:* 9%. Supports zoological societies, botanical gardens, conservancy, and population issues. *Education:* 40%. Supports colleges and preparatory schools. *Environment:* 7%. Focus on community service organizations. *International:* 1%. Supports hospitals. *Note:* Total contributions made in fiscal 2001. **Typ. Recipients:** Emergency/Ambulance Services, Family Planning, Heart, Hospitals, Prenatal Health Issues. **Geo. Dist:** nationally; NY.

★ 11862 ★ Public Welfare Foundation

1200 U St. NW
Washington, DC 20009
Phone: (202)965-1800 **Fax:** (202)265-8852
Website: http://www.publicwelfare.org
Larry Kressley, Executive Director

Fnded: 1947. **Philosophy:** "The Public Welfare Foundation is dedicated to supporting organizations that provide services to disadvantaged populations, and to those working for lasting improvements in the delivery of services that meet basic human needs. Our funding is focused in nine program areas: Criminal Justice, Human Rights and Global Security, Disadvantaged Elderly, Disadvantaged Youth, Environment, Health, Community Economic Development and Security, Population & Reproductive Health, and Community Support. The Foundation is willing to allocate seed money and to take risks to helping organizations with little else but dedication to a sound idea, a reasonable plan for carrying it out, and a strong base in and commitment to their communities. An important factor in the Foundation's grantmaking decisions is identifying specific, short-term financial needs our support would address. A grant should not create a long-term dependency or function simply as a contribution. An organization's ability to demonstrate community support, whether in the form of grants or in-kind contributions, is an additional factor. Our funding has no geographic restrictions. Grants outside the U.S. are generally made to organizations with offices both in the U.S. and in the region where the program is operating, although the foundation has increased its efforts to directly fund organizations in other countries. Regardless, the involvement of the local or regional community is always an important consideration." **Priorities:** *Civic & Public Affairs:* 21%. Supports community economic development and participation, grassroots organizations, low wage workers, technical assistance to grassroots organizations, advocacy and policy development. Also supports criminal justice, including alternatives to incarceration, institutional prevention, advocacy, and policy development. *Environment:* 17%. Funds programs for disadvantaged elderly and youth, welfare reform, family planning services, family services, daycare, and homeless services. *International:* 29%. Funds health advocacy, access and reform, preventive and primary services, hunger and nutrition, occupational health and safety, mental health advocacy and services. Supports reproductive rights, education, and health; health policy, health Funds, AIDS, and health reform. *Note:* Total contributions made in fiscal 2001. **Typ. Recipients:** Adolescent Health Issues, AIDS/HIV, Children's Health/Hospitals, Clinics/Medical Centers, Domestic Violence, Emergency/Ambulance Services, Family Planning, Geriatric Health, Health Organizations, Health Policy/Cost Containment, Health-General, Hospitals, Hospitals (University Affiliated), Medical Research, Mental Health, Nutrition, People with Disabilities, Prenatal Health Issues, Public Health. **Geo. Dist:** nationally.

★ 11863 ★ R. C. Baker Foundation

PO Box 6150
Orange, CA 92863-6150
Phone: (714)750-8987
Frank Scott, Chairman

Fnded: 1952. **Philosophy:** The foundation supports organizations and projects concerned with the arts, education, community services, health, and social services. **Priorities:** *Arts & Humanities:* 8%. Emphasis on museums, the performing arts, and public broadcasting. *Civic & Public Affairs:* 11%. Focus on legal aid, community services, and police officers associations. *Education:* 26%. Supports colleges and universities, education associations, and scholarship funds. *Environment:* 19%. Primary funding for youth organizations and child welfare. *International:* 33%. Primary support for hospitals and single-disease health associations. *Note:* Total contributions made in 2000. **Typ. Recipients:** Cancer, Children's Health/Hospitals, Clinics/Medical Centers, Domestic Violence, Emergency/Ambulance Services, Eyes/Blindness, Health Organizations, Hospitals, Medical Rehabilitation, Medical Research, Mental Health, Multiple Sclerosis, Nursing Services, People with Disabilities, Preventive Medicine/Wellness Organizations, Research/Studies Institutes, Single-Disease Health Associations, Speech & Hearing, Substance Abuse. **Geo. Dist:** western US.

★ 11864 ★ R. D. and Joan Dale Hubbard Foundation

PO Box 2498
Ruidoso, NM 88355-2498
Phone: (505)258-5919 **Fax:** (505)258-3749
James Stoddard, Executive Director

Fnded: 1986. **Philosophy:** "From its beginning, the Foundation adopted an entrepreneurial approach to philanthropy that reflects the spirit of (its founders). Both R.D. and Joan Dale Hubbard are Kansas natives and both were teachers in Kansas. They maintain strong ties to education and to the people in the West. ... Together the Hubbards established the Foundation's philanthropic trust, which centers around cultural, education and general benefit to mankind. The foundation's two major categories of support are the arts and humanities, and education." **Priorities:** *Arts & Humanities:* 23%. Supports museum, music, theater, and ballet. *Civic & Public Affairs:* 5%. Funds community foundations. *Education:* 58%. Funds scholarship, universities, colleges, and schools. *Environment:* 8%. Supports Big brothers/Big Sisters and special olympics. *International:* 6%. Supports medical centers, home-care services, hospital. *Note:* Total contributions made in 2000. **Typ. Recipients:** AIDS/HIV, Alzheimers Disease, Cancer, Children's Health/Hospitals, Clinics/Medical Centers, Domestic Violence, Heart, Home-Care Services, Medical Education, Medical Research, Medical Training, People with Disabilities, Single-Disease Health Associations. **Geo. Dist:** CA; IL; KS; NE; NM; OK; TX.

★ 11865 ★ R. J. McElroy Trust

500 KWWL Bldg.
Suite 318
Waterloo, IA 50703
Phone: (319)287-9102 **Fax:** (319)287-9105
Email: mcelroy@cedarnet.org
Website: http://www.cedarnet.org/mcelroy
Linda Klinger, Executive Director

Fnded: 1965. **Philosophy:** The R.J. McElroy Trust assists non-profit organizations which provide educational services to deserving youth, giving high priority to grants which provide seed money to programs rather than capital projects. **Priorities:** *Arts & Humanities:* 14%. Supports libraries, arts forums, theater, the symphony, and public broadcasting. *Civic & Public Affairs:* 18%. Supports community services, urban development, parks and botanical gardens. *Education:* 37%. Supports community schools, colleges, and universities, including scholarships and fellowships. Supports medicine education and science education. *Environment:* 23%. Supports youth and family services, Young Women's Christian Association's, Big Brothers/Big Sisters, community centers and camps. *International:* 6%. Supports hospitals, mental illness and respiratory *Note:* Total contributions made in 2000. **Typ. Recipients:** AIDS/HIV, Children's Health/Hospitals, Clinics/Medical Centers, Domestic Violence, Family Planning, Hospices, Hospitals, Medical Education, Medical Training, People with Disabilities, Prenatal Health Issues, Research/Studies Institutes, Substance Abuse. **Geo. Dist:** IA, Black Hawk County and rural counties in the Waterloo area; Waterloo, IA.

★ 11866 ★ R. K. Mellon Family Foundation

One Mellon Center
500 Grant St., Suite 4106
Pittsburgh, PA 15219-2502
Phone: (412)392-2800 **Fax:** (412)392-2849
Website: http://www.fdncenter.org/grantmaker/rkmellon
Michael Watson, Vice President

Fnded: 1978. **Philosophy:** The foundation's giving priorities are Southwestern Pennsylvania and Conservation. Southwestern Pennsylvania funding is focused on Regional Economic Development, Education, System Reform, and Families, Youth & Child Development. Conservation grants are provided for American Land Conservation, and to protect natural resources, contain sprawl, manage forests, and conserve land in the Pennsylvania Regional Focus area. Richard King Mellon Foundation Grant Application **Priorities:** *Arts & Humanities:* 28%. Focus on museums, historic preservation, and music. *Civic & Public Affairs:* 6%. Supports zoos and community services. *Education:* 31%. Primary support for colleges, universities, and private secondary schools. *Environment:* 13%. Community services and youth organizations. *International:* 8%. Hospitals and medical research. *Note:* Total contributions made in 2000. **Typ. Recipients:** AIDS/HIV, Cancer, Clinics/Medical Centers, Domestic Violence, Emergency/Ambulance Services, Health Funds, Health Organizations, Health-General, Hospitals, Hospitals (University Affiliated), Long-Term Care, Medical Education, Medical Rehabilitation, Medical Research, Medical Training, Mental Health, Nursing Services, People with Disabilities, Preventive Medicine/Wellness Organizations, Sexual Abuse, Single-Disease Health Associations, Substance Abuse, Transplant Networks/Donor Banks. **Geo. Dist:** PA, Western Pennsylvania; Pittsburgh, PA.

★ 11867 ★ Ralph E. Ogden Foundation

Pleasant Hill Rd.
PO Box 290
Mountainville, NY 10953
Phone: (845)534-3423 **Fax:** (845)534-5854
Georgene Zlock, Secretary

Fnded: 1947. **Philosophy:** The foundation's major priority is the arts, with large contributions to the Storm King Art Center, Mountainville, NY. All categories of the arts are supported. Other interests are minor, but include international organizations, education, health, and social services. **Priorities:** *Arts & Humanities:* 84%. Supports art galleries, art centers, museums, opera, and music. *Civic & Public Affairs:* 1% Supports community and civic affairs and public gardens and trails. *Education:* 3% Funds colleges, universities, and educational programs. *Environment:* 3%. Supports health-care and senior welfare. *International:* 1%. Supports hospital. *Note:* Contributions were made in 2000. **Typ. Recipients:** Clinics/Medical Centers, Health Organizations, Health Policy/Cost Containment, Hospices, Hospitals, Medical Education, Public Health, Substance Abuse. **Geo. Dist:** nationally; NY.

★ 11868 ★ Ralph M. Parsons Foundation

1055 Wilshire Boulevard, Suite 1701
Los Angeles, CA 90017
Phone: (213)482-3185 **Fax:** (213)482-8878
Email: hoppe@rmpf.org
Website: http://www.rmpf.org
Wendy Hoppe, Executive Director & Secretary

Fnded: 1961. **Philosophy:** "The Foundation is concerned with the encouragement and support of projects and programs deemed beneficial to humankind in several major areas of interest...The emphasis upon individual categories may vary from year to year, and exceptions to these guidelines may occur solely at the discretion of the Foundation." The foundation's primary areas of interest include the following: higher education, with emphasis on the fields of engineering, technology, and the sciences; social impact, focusing on assistance to socially or economically disadvantaged groups in society; civic and cultural affairs, with a preference for programs that enhance the cultural life of all people by providing opportunities for access to cultural experiences; civic grants are awarded to address significant concerns which arise in the community; health, with emphasis on services to disadvantaged elderly, families, and youth, through support of programs and medical equipment associated with these services; and special projects, providing giving flexibility through foundation-initiated grants for projects of interest to the Board that are related to the broad purposes of the foundation but fall outside its established areas of interest. **Priorities:** *Arts & Humanities:* About 27%. *Civic & Public Affairs:* 3%. *Education:* 23%. Primarily to colleges and universities for technical education. *Environment:* 37%. Senior services, youth organizations, and day care. *International:* 10%. Supports hospitals, medical research, cancer treatment, and children's health. *Note:* Total contributions made in 1998. **Typ. Recipients:** Adolescent Health Issues, AIDS/HIV, Alzheimers Disease, Cancer, Child Abuse, Children's Health/Hospitals, Clinics/Medical Centers, Domestic Violence, Eyes/Blindness, Family Planning, Geriatric Health, Health Organizations, Heart, Hospitals, Hospitals (University Affiliated), Long-Term Care, Medical Research, Mental Health, People with Disabilities, Prenatal Health Issues, Preventive Medicine/Wellness Organizations, Speech & Hearing, Substance Abuse, Trauma Treatment. **Geo. Dist:** CA, Los Angeles County.

★ 11869 ★ Ramapo Trust

126 East 56th St., 10th Floor
New York, NY 10022
Phone: (212)308-7355 **Fax:** (212)750-0132
Email: heathercarey@broodalefoundation.org
Website: http://www.brookdalefoundation.org
Stephen Schwartz, President

Fnded: 1973. **Philosophy:** The trust "is a charitable institution whose resources have centered on gerontology and geriatrics. The trust will consider innovative projects which serve the aging, or increase knowledge in the field of aging." The trust places emphasis on services for families of Alzheimer's disease patients and for grandparents and other kin raising grandchildren or other relatives children. **Priorities:** *Arts & Humanities:* 8%. Funds performing arts. *Civic & Public Affairs:* 3%. Supports community groups and legal aid. *Education:* 24%. Funds universities, schools, and research. *Environment:* 7%. Supports elder care, services for the disabled, and family services. *International:* 49%. Focus on geriatric medicine; supports medical centers, mental health, and cancer treatment. *Note:* Total contributions made in fiscal 2001. **Typ. Recipients:** Alzheimers Disease, Cancer, Clinics/Medical Centers, Domestic Violence, Geriatric Health, Health Funds, Health Organizations, Health-General, Heart, Hospitals, Hospitals (University Affiliated), Long-Term Care, Medical Education, Medical Research, Mental Health, Nursing Services, Public Health, Sexual Abuse, Substance Abuse. **Geo. Dist:** nationally.

★ 11870 ★ Randolph Foundation

255 East 49th St., Suite 23D
New York, NY 10017
Phone: (212)752-7148 **Fax:** (212)752-7316
Heather Higgins, Trustee

Fnded: 1990. **Philosophy:** "The Randolph Foundation will continue to focus on public policy issues, but from a slightly different perspective: we are particularly concerned with fostering those underlying values and attitudes that enable free-market and democratic systems to function and flourish. We believe those values are reflected in individual character, and are central to the institutional foundations of a free society; morality and public life, family and community, and competitive educational structures affecting the preservation and continuing development of American Civilization." "The Randolph Foundation has defined this program area under the broad heading of 'Cultural Values, Civic Virtues'. This would include reemphasizing such concepts as: obligations as well as rights; self-control as well as self-expression; personal ethics over legal obligations; responsibility as opposed to dependency; individual merit in contrast to group entitlement; reliance on the private sphere before government; and values that are superior, not relative." "Within this area, the Randolph Foundation is also interested in investing its limited resources to encourage new and worthwhile ideas, individuals, projects, and organizations. Solicitations for support which do not meet these criteria, however worthwhile, will almost certainly be declined." 1997 **Priorities:** *Arts & Humanities:* 8%. Supports the visual arts. *Civic & Public Affairs:* 64%. Primary support for public policy groups. *Education:* 25%. Focus on colleges, universities, and education associations. *International:* 3%. *Note:* Total contributions made in 2000. **Typ. Recipients:** AIDS/HIV, Cancer, Children's Health/Hospitals, Health Organizations, Medical Research, Outpatient Health Care. **Geo. Dist:** nationally.

★ 11871 ★ Raskob Foundation for Catholic Activities, Inc.

PO Box 4019
Wilmington, DE 19807
Phone: (302)655-4440 **Fax:** (302)655-3223
Website: http://www.rfca.org
Frederick Perella, Jr., Executive Vice President

Fnded: 1945. **Philosophy:** The foundation's purpose is to "engage in such exclusively religious, charitable, literary, and educational activities as will aid the Roman Catholic Church and institutions and organizations identified with it." In determining its own priorities, the foundation takes into account the priorities of the National Conference of Catholic Bishops. It also strives to help the church meet some of the major needs of priests and nuns, and the problems of immigrants and refugees. Toward this end, the foundation supports projects both within the United States and abroad. **Priorities:** *Arts & Humanities:* Approx. 1%. *Civic & Public Affairs:* 31%. Funds community leadership. *Education:* 12%. Supports Catholic schools and universities. *Environment:* 13%. Funds family services and youth ministry. *International:* 1%. *Religion:* 2%. *Note:* Total contributions made in 2000. **Typ. Recipients:** Adolescent Health Issues, AIDS/HIV, Children's Health/Hospitals, Clinics/Medical Centers, Domestic Violence, Family Planning, Health Organizations, Hospices, Hospitals, Medical Education, Medical Rehabilitation, Mental Health, Nursing Services, People with Disabilities, Preventive Medicine/Wellness Organizations, Public Health, Substance Abuse. **Geo. Dist:** internationally; nationally.

★ 11872 ★ Rauch Foundation

229 Seventh St., Suite 306
Garden City, NY 11530-5766
Phone: (516)873-9808 **Fax:** (516)873-0708
Email: info@rauchfoundation.org
Website: http://www.rauchfoundation.org
Nancy Douzinas, President

Fnded: 1961. **Philosophy:** "Today, the Foundation concentrates the majority of our grant making to benefit vulnerable young children and their families. The Foundation's mission in this area is to foster the development of programs and policies that promote, strengthen, and maintain the health and well-being of families and their children from conception through age six. Our program interests include family planning, prenatal care, parenting education, income security, family support, and early childhood education. The Foundation encourages proposals for projects that seek to: help families become more self-reliant and build family strengths; change program focus from the child alone to the family as a whole; assist families to remain intact and encourage more fathers to be strong partners in parenting and supporting their children; expand the availability of preventive services and shift existing services from remediation to prevention; extend the reach and effectiveness of current policies or programs; improve policies that impact programs; and streamline the delivery of services." "Environment: The foundation also has initiated two small grant programs in Nassau County and Maryland. The programs will evolve over the next few years, but are expected to focus on community-based efforts to preserve, protect, and clean up the environment. Performing Arts: A modest program is planned for support of music programs in Nassau County next year. The Foundation reported that it is not currently accepting unsolicited proposals in this areas." "Leadership: The Foundation Board will develop a small program focused on leadership over the next year. At this time, the Foundation is not accepting unsolicited proposals in this area." 1997 Guidelines Guidelines **Priorities:** *Arts & Humanities:* 6%. *Civic & Public Affairs:* 18%. Funds community affairs. *Education:* 11%. Supports schools, universities, and literacy programs. *Environment:* 40%. Supports planned parenthood, volunteerism, youth, and family services. *International:* About 2%. *Religion:* 4%. *Note:* Total contributions made in fiscal 2001. **Typ. Recipients:** Child Abuse, Family Planning, Health-General, Hospices, Nursing Services, People with Disabilities, Prenatal Health Issues, Public Health. **Geo. Dist:** MD, small environmental program in Maryland; NY, Nassau County.

★ 11873 ★ Ray C. Fish Foundation

2001 Kirby Dr., Suite 1005
Houston, TX 77019
Phone: (713)522-0741 **Fax:** (713)529-4033
Barbara Daniel, President

Fnded: 1957. **Philosophy:** "Under the charter of the Ray C. Fish Foundation, grants are made for the support, establishment, operation, or advancement of qualified educational, scientific, or other charitable organizations in the state of Texas." The foundation's first large grant, $5 million, was made in 1966 as seed money for the Texas Heart Institute. Other health interests include the American Heart Association, the Living Bank, and various Houston hospitals. Educational interests include colleges, universities, and schools located in Texas, especially those at which there are professorships, chairs, and endowed scholarship funds in the name of Mr. and Mrs. Fish. The foundation supports a broad range of community service programs and organizations. The foundation also supports various Houston museums and performing arts groups. **Priorities:** *Arts & Humanities:* 15%. Supports history, ballet, museum, music, libraries, and historic preservation. *Civic & Public Affairs:* 26%. Supports arboretums, urban affairs, public policy, parks, and nature centers. *Education:* 24%. Primarily funds colleges and universities, medical education, religious, education, and field specific education. *Environment:* 11%. Emphasis on youth organizations, community affairs, child welfare, food/clothing distribution, sexual abuse, and young men's christian association. *International:* 16%. Supports hospitals, single-disease health associations, and a medical rehabilitation center. *Note:* Total contributions made in fiscal 1999. **Typ. Recipients:** Alzheimers Disease, Cancer, Child Abuse, Clinics/Medical Centers, Emergency/Ambulance Services, Family Planning, Health Organizations, Heart, Hospices, Hospitals, Hospitals (University Affiliated), Kidney, Medical Education, Medical Rehabilitation, Medical Research, People with Disabilities, Research/Studies Institutes, Single-Disease Health Associations, Single-Disease Health Associations. **Geo. Dist:** Galveston, TX; Houston, TX, including metropolitan area; Kerrville, TX.

★ 11874 ★ Raymond John Wean Foundation

PO Box 760
Warren, OH 44482-0760
Phone: (330)394-5600 **Fax:** (330)394-5601
Email: RJWeanFdn@aol.com
Raymond Wean, Jr., Chairman

Fnded: 1949. **Philosophy:** Grants from the foundation primarily support people and communities within the geographic area served. The foundation rewards excellence in those communities and supports groups and projects that empower citizens to meet their full potential. Its main areas of interest include: education, community development, health, the arts, youth and family services, and personal development leading to employment. **Priorities:** *Arts & Humanities:* 17%. Supports art institutes, museums. *Civic & Public Affairs:* 10%. Supports gardens, libraries. *Education:* 60%. Supports public and private schools; colleges and universities, preschool. *Environment:* 3%. Supports camps, youth programs, family services. *International:* 4%. Supports hospitals, medical centers. *Religion:* 1%. Supports science museum. *Note:* Total contributions made in 1998. **Typ. Recipients:** Cancer, Children's Health/Hospitals, Clinics/Medical Centers, Family Planning, Health Organizations, Health Policy/Cost Containment, Hospices, Hospitals, Long-Term Care, Medical Education, Medical Rehabilitation, Medical Research, Mental Health, Nursing Services, People with Disabilities, Public Health, Single-Disease Health Associations, Substance Abuse. **Geo. Dist:** FL, Southeast Florida; OH, Northeast Ohio; PA, Southeast Pennsylvania.

★ 11875 ★ Reeves Foundation (OH)

PO Box 441
Dover, OH 44622-0441
Phone: (330)364-4660
Don Ulrich, Executive Director

Fnded: 1966. **Philosophy:** Foundation interests include hospitals, historic preservation, municipalities, and educational projects. The foundation will also fund other recipient areas. Priority is given to organizations benefiting Tuscarawas County, Ohio. **Priorities:** *Arts & Humanities:* 22%. Supports libraries, public broadcasting, and historic preservation. *Civic & Public Affairs:* 14%. Supports towns/municipalities, parks/gardens, safety, and community foundations. *Education:* 49%. Supports scholarships, educational funds, religious education, and schools. *Environment:* 3%. Supports counseling, family services, Young Men's Christian Association, and emergency relief. *International:* 9%. Supports hospital, cancer research, and health organizations. *Note:* Total contributions made in 2000. **Typ. Recipients:** Alzheimers Disease, Cancer, Children's Health/Hospitals, Clinics/Medical Centers, Emergency/Ambulance Services, Hospices, Hospitals, Hospitals, People with Disabilities, Public Health. **Geo. Dist:** OH, Tuscarawas County.

★ 11876 ★ Regenstein Foundation

8600 West Bryn Mawr Ave., Suite 705N
Chicago, IL 60631
Phone: (773)693-6464 **Fax:** (773)693-2480
Thomas Staszak, Acting Vice President

Fnded: 1950. **Philosophy:** The foundation's primary interests are in arts, music, education, and social services in the Chicago metropolitan area. **Priorities:** *Arts & Humanities:* 15%. Funds public broadcasting, art institutes, music, libraries, history, and opera. *Civic & Public Affairs:* 62%. Supports the Lincoln Park Zoo. *Environment:* 10%. Gives to youth groups, united funds, animal concerns, people with disabilities, food distribution, scouts, and child welfare. *International:* 13%. Funds hospitals. *Note:* Total contributions made in 2000. **Typ. Recipients:** Clinics/Medical Centers, Family Planning, Health Organizations, Heart, Hospitals, Medical Education, Medical Rehabilitation, Mental Health, Nursing Services, People with Disabilities, Prenatal Health Issues, Sexual Abuse, Transplant Networks/Donor Banks. **Geo. Dist:** Chicago, IL, metropolitan area.

★ 11877 ★ Reinberger Foundation

27600 Chagrin Boulevard
Cleveland, OH 44122
Phone: (216)292-2790 **Fax:** (216)292-4466
Robert Reinberger, Co-Director

Fnded: 1968. **Philosophy:** The foundation does not place any restrictions on the types of organizations which may request a grant; nor does it have a fixed pattern of giving. Priorities are apt to change from year to year. All giving, however, is limited strictly to the greater Cleveland and Columbus areas. The foundation prefers to provide funds for operating purposes and capital improvements. It usually does not provide seed money or fund new projects, preferring to help well-established, traditional organizations. **Priorities:** *Arts & Humanities:* 36%. Supports museums, music, performing arts, public broadcasting, and cultural affairs. *Civic & Public Affairs:* 11%. Supports zoos, botanical gardens, and community development. *Education:* 17%. Primary support for colleges and universities. Also funds schools and arts education. *Environment:* 12%. Supports children's services and senior citizens' community centers. *International:* 14%. Supports hospitals, clinics, children's health, and medical rehabilitation. *Religion:* 7%. Supports science museums and science centers. *Note:* Contributions were made in 2000. **Typ. Recipients:** Alzheimers Disease, Cancer, Children's Health/Hospitals, Clinics/Medical Centers, Family Planning, Health Organizations, Health-General, Hospitals, Hospitals (University Affiliated), Long-Term Care, Medical Education, Medical Rehabilitation, Medical Research, People with Disabilities, Public Health, Speech & Hearing. **Geo. Dist:** Cleveland, OH; Columbus, OH.

★ 11878 ★ Research Corp.

Science Advancement Program
101 North Wilmot Rd., Suite 250
Tucson, AZ 85711-3335
Phone: (520)571-1111 **Fax:** (520)571-1119
Email: awards@rescorp.org
Website: http://www.rescorp.org
Dr. Raymond Kellman, Vice President

Fnded: 1912. **Philosophy:** The support of scientific research and experimentation at scholarly institutions is the main activity of Research Corporation. All awards are made within academic settings and within the core physical sciences, chemistry, physics, and astronomy. The emphasis of the foundation has been on support of people and their programs rather than bricks and mortar or broad institutional initiatives. Another goal of Research Corporation is to encourage and support programs that include and motivate students. For instance, the Cottrell College Science Awards encourage research with undergraduates; equipment, summer stipends, and supplies are provided. The Cottrell Scholars Awards reward beginning faculty who wish to excel at both teaching and research; all awards are for $50,000, which can be used largely at the discretion of the scholar. A small group of undergraduate colleges, which have been conspicuously successful at producing science graduates, participate in the Department Development Program; the foundation invites proposals from promising candidates in undergraduate chemistry and physics departments that have the potential to join this group. Research Opportunity Awards are mid-career awards for tenured science faculty aimed at reestablishing vigorous research programs. "Research Corporation is open to opportunities within our fields of activity that fall outside the regular programs. Proposals for support of projects that will enhance science research or that bear on the infrastructure of science can be considered. Occasionally, proposals may also be encouraged for research projects that are exceedingly novel, that run counter to scientific paradigms and are unlikely to achieve support from more traditional sources. Because our resources are limited, only the most challenging and innovative proposals are likely to succeed." 1995 Award Programs Summary **Priorities:** *Education:* 99%. Supports academic science in two ways: by providing funding for original research in chemistry, physics, and astronomy; and by stressing undergraduate teaching and involvement of students in research: Cottrell College Science program to support projects at predominantly undergraduate institutions (44%); new Research Innovation Awards program (29%); Cottrell Scholars Awards for graduate faculty (12%); Partners in Science program (9%); general grants to research and science education(3%); remaining funds supported the Research Opportunity Awards (3%), given to mid-career scientists to further their research. *Note:* Total contributions made in 2000. **Typ. Recipients:** Diabetes, Health-General, Medical Education, Substance Abuse. **Geo. Dist:** nationally.

★ 11879 ★ Retirement Research Foundation

8765 West Higgins Rd., Suite 430
Chicago, IL 60631-4170
Phone: (773)714-8080 **Fax:** (773)714-8089
Email: info@rrf.org
Website: http://www.rrf.org
Marilyn Hennessy, President

Fnded: 1950. **Philosophy:** The foundation is particularly interested in innovative programs in aging that have the potential for national and regional impact. Funding interests fall into four areas: to improve the availability and quality of community-based and institutional long term care; to provide new and expanded opportunities for older adults to engage in meaningful roles in society such as employment and volunteerism that will strengthen community activities including advocacy, community leadership, community services, and intergenerational programs; to seek causes and solutions to significant problems of older adults through support of basic, applied, and policy research for which federal funding is not available; and to increase the number of professionals and para-professionals adequately prepared to serve the elderly population through support of selected education and training initiatives which enhance knowledge and skills of participants. The foundation currently operates the Congregational Connection Program (CCP) and the Organizational Capacity Building Program (OCB). **Priorities:** *Arts & Humanities:* Less than 1%. *Civic & Public Affairs:* 7%. Supports community foundations and legal aid. *Education:* 13%. Supports religious education, universities, fellowships, colleges, faculty development, literacy, and medical education. *Environment:* 21%. Supports senior services, community service organizations, shelters, and family services. *International:* 46%. Supports Alzheimers, medical research, geriatric health, public health, hospitals, health organizations, and hospices. *Note:* Total contributions made in 2000. **Typ. Recipients:** Alzheimers Disease, Alzheimers Disease, Cancer, Children's Health/Hospitals, Clinics/Medical Centers, Diabetes, Emergency/Ambulance Services, Family Planning, Geriatric Health, Health Organizations, Health Policy/Cost Containment, Heart, Home-Care Services, Hospices, Hospitals, Long-Term Care, Medical Education, Medical Research, Mental Health, Nursing Services, People with Disabilities, Preventive Medicine/Wellness Organizations, Public Health, Single-Disease Health Associations, Speech & Hearing, Transplant Networks/Donor Banks. **Geo. Dist:** nationally; Midwest: direct service projects; FL, direct service projects; Chicago, IL, metropolitan area.

★ 11880 ★ RGK Foundation

1301 West 25th St.
Suite 300
Austin, TX 78705-4236
Phone: (512)474-9298 **Fax:** (512)474-7281
Email: jhampton@rgkfoundation.org
Website: http://www.rgkfoundation.org
Gregory Kozmetsky, President, Chairman

Fnded: 1966. **Philosophy:** The Foundation's focus " includes three main component areas of Education, Community, and Medicine/Health. The Foundation's primary interests within Education include programs that focus on formal K-12 education (particularly mathematics, science, and reading), after-school tutoring and enrichment, integrating technology into curriculum, teacher development, and higher education. The Foundation is particularly interested in programs that raise literacy levels and programs that attract female and minority students into the fields of mathematics, science, and technology. Within Community, the Foundation supports a broad range of human services programs, youth development programs, community improvement programs, and cultural arts programs. Human service programs of current interest to the Foundation include early childhood development, parenting education, domestic violence, and child abuse prevention. The Foundation supports youth development programs that work to build character, leadership and social skills. The Foundation is interested in supporting community improvement projects that enhance nonprofit management and promote philanthropy and voluntarism. Cultural arts programs supported by the Foundation are typically educational outreach activities for youth. The Foundation's current interests in the area of Medicine/Health are programs that promote the health and well-being of children and families and, on a more limited basis, medical research programs." RGK Foundation website **Priorities:** *Arts & Humanities:* 5%. Supports public broadcasting, libraries, and museums. *Civic & Public Affairs:* 9%. Supports community organizations, leadership organizations, and women's affairs. *Education:* 58%. Funds schools and higher education, including medical schools. *Environment:* 22%. Funds community centers, youth and children's programs, shelters. *International:* 6%. Funds hospitals, health clinics, and medical research. *Note:* Total contributions made in 2000. **Typ. Recipients:** Arthritis, Cancer, Child Abuse, Children's Health/Hospitals, Clinics/Medical Centers, Diabetes, Domestic Violence, Eyes/Blindness, Geriatric Health, Health Organizations, Health Policy/Cost Containment, Heart, Hospices, Hospitals, Hospitals (University Affiliated), Kidney, Medical Education, Medical Education, Medical Research, Mental Health, Nursing Services, People with Disabilities, Prenatal Health Issues, Public Health, Research/Studies Institutes, Respiratory, Single-Disease Health Associations, Speech & Hearing, Substance Abuse, Transplant Networks/Donor Banks. **Geo. Dist:** nationally.

★ 11881 ★ Rhodebeck Charitable Trust

260 Madison Ave., 18th Floor
New York, NY 10167
Fax: (212)488-6260
Huyler Held, Trustee

Fnded: 1987. **Philosophy:** The Rhodebeck Charitable Trust makes most of its grants in the area of social services. Interests include homes, the homeless, food distribution, and children's services. **Priorities:** *Arts & Humanities:* 10%. *Civic & Public Affairs:* 72%. Legal defense funds, housing programs, jobs for youth, and community service organizations. *Environment:* 8%. Child welfare. *Note:* Total contributions made in fiscal 1999. **Typ. Recipients:** Alzheimers Disease, Child Abuse, Children's Health/Hospitals, Geriatric Health, Health Organizations, Home-Care Services, Mental Health, Nursing Services, Substance Abuse. **Geo. Dist:** New York, NY.

★ 11882 ★ Rice Foundation

8600 Gross Point Rd.
Skokie, IL 60077-2151
Phone: (847)581-9999
Peter Nolan, President

Fnded: 1947. **Philosophy:** The foundation generally supports civic organizations and social services in the Chicago metropolitan area. The arts have also been a funding focus. **Priorities:** *Arts & Humanities:* 3%. Supports performing arts and festivals. *Civic & Public Affairs:* 4%. Funds community foundations, zoos, botanical gardens, and arboretums. *Education:* 14%. Funds secondary educational institutions and education foundations. *Environment:* 30%. Supports child and youth services, a crime commission, developmental services, homes, and camps. *International:* 43%. Hospitals, wellness centers, and disease and disorder concerns. *Note:* Total contributions made in 2000. **Typ. Recipients:** Arthritis, Cancer, Children's Health/Hospitals, Clinics/Medical Centers, Geriatric Health, Health Organizations, Health-General, Home-Care Services, Hospitals, Hospitals (University Affiliated), Long-Term Care, Medical Education, Medical Rehabilitation, Mental Health, People with Disabilities, Prenatal Health Issues, Single-Disease Health Associations. **Geo. Dist:** Chicago, IL.

★ 11883 ★ Rich Foundation

11 Piedmont Center, Suite 204
Atlanta, GA 30305
Phone: (404)262-2266 **Fax:** (404)266-2123
Anne Berg, Grant Consultant

Fnded: 1942. **Philosophy:** The foundation typically supports human service organizations, health organizations, educational institutions, and the arts and humanities. Funding is limited to the metropolitan Atlanta area. **Priorities:** *Arts & Humanities:* 25%. Music, arts centers, theater, opera, and ballet. *Civic & Public Affairs:* 1%. Parks, botanical gardens, and urban affairs. *Education:* 12%. Colleges and universities, primary and secondary education, and education associations. *Environment:* 28%. Emphasis on united funds, family services, child welfare, youth organizations, religious welfare organizations, and the aged. *International:* 20%. Hospitals and medical centers, single-disease health associations, and pediatric health. *Note:* Total contributions made in fiscal 1999. **Typ. Recipients:** Cancer, Child Abuse, Children's Health/Hospitals, Emergency/Ambulance Services, Eyes/Blindness, Health Organizations, Heart, Hospitals, Medical Education, Medical Research, Mental Health, Nursing Services, People with Disabilities, Prenatal Health Issues, Single-Disease Health Associations. **Geo. Dist:** Atlanta, GA, metropolitan area.

★ 11884 ★ Richard and Helen DeVos Foundation

126 Ottowa Northwest, Suite 500
Grand Rapids, MI 49503
Phone: (616)454-4114 **Fax:** (616)454-0970
Email: virginiav@rdvcorp.com
Ginny Vander Hart, Foundation Director

Fnded: 1969. **Philosophy:** The foundation primarily funds religious programs and associations, as well as some churches. Education (largely religious) is also a major focus. **Priorities:** *Arts & Humanities:* 1%. Supports art museums, the library of Michigan, symphonies, and performing arts. *Civic & Public Affairs:* 13%. Supports City Vision, city gardens, and community action. *Education:* 39%. Supports colleges, universities, and educational services and programs. *Environment:* 7%. Supports youth services, family services, soup kitchens, and social services. *International:* 7%. Supports health services. *Note:* Contributions were made in 2000. **Typ. Recipients:** Clinics/Medical Centers, Emergency/Ambulance Services, Family Planning, Health Funds, Health Organizations, Health-General, Hospitals, Long-Term Care, Medical Research, People with Disabilities, Prenatal Health Issues, Public Health, Single-Disease Health Associations, Transplant Networks/Donor Banks. **Geo. Dist:** nationally; FL, including central Florida; Grand Rapids, MI.

★ 11885 ★ Richard and Jane Manoogian Foundation

21001 Van Born Rd.
Taylor, MI 48180
Phone: (313)274-8799
Richard Manoogian, President & Treasurer

Fnded: 1984. **Priorities:** *Arts & Humanities:* 34%. Supports museums, art institutes, and art space. *Civic & Public Affairs:* 7%. Funds a founders society, and housing. *Education:* 12%. Universities, colleges, creative studies, college funds, and schools receive funding. *Environment:* 2%. Funds mainly the United Way. *Note:* Total contributions made in 1999. **Typ. Recipients:** Cancer, Clinics/Medical Centers, Family Planning, Medical Research, People with Disabilities, Single-Disease Health Associations.

★ 11886 ★ Richard King Mellon Foundation

One Mellon Center
500 Grant St., Suite 4106
Pittsburgh, PA 15219-2502
Phone: (412)392-2800
Website: http://fdncenter.org/grantmaker/rkmellon/
Michael Watson, Vice President and Director

Fnded: 1947. **Philosophy:** The Foundation has two distinct areas of interest: programs that relate to regional economic development, education, system reform, regional conservation, system reform, and families/youth in Pittsburgh and Southwestern Pennsylvania; and the American Land Conservation Program, and conservation of natural areas on a national level. *Education:* Priority is given to for early childhood and preschool education as well as higher educational institutions. Aims to support charter, parochial, and independent schools; ensure the global competitiveness of U.S. institutions of higher learning; and strengthen workforce education. *Families and Youth:* Within this area, the goal is the aggressive pursuit of creative approaches to overcoming the many obstacles now facing disadvantaged families and children, especially through the expansion of successful model programs. The focus is on early childhood development, promotion of effective parenting, and strengthening of youth programs. *Regional Economic Development:* Support is available for community development, economic development, and employment development programs. The foundation looks for programs that stimulate downtown re-development; support development of new economy; aid in recruitment and retention of young talent; market the amenities and cultural attractions in Southwestern Pennsylvania; and enable the entire region to participate in improved economic status. *System Reform:* The goals of system reform grantmaking is to support efforts to redesign and improve human service delivery; enhance leadership in the nonprofit sector; establish standards and best practices for youth programs; and encourage organizational collaboration. *Conservation:* Continues to be the major focus. The foundation's American Land Conservation Program operates on a national level to acquire and preserve key tracts of land within the United States that are in danger of being lost to development. On a regional level, the foundation funds programs the preserve natural assets, acquire land and easements to preserve open space, clean up streams, contain sprawl, and education the public on environmental issues in Pennsylvania. *Richard King Mellon Foundation Funding Policy* **Priorities:** *Arts & Humanities:* 1%. Gives to various cultural organizations in the Pittsburgh area. *Civic & Public Affairs:* 16%. Funds economic development, community development, and civic organizations. *Education:* 10%. Contributes to colleges, universities, and public and private pre-college schools and academies. *Environment:* 6%. Funds programs and services for family, youth, and children; and supports human service agencies. *Note:* Total contributions made in 2000. **Typ. Recipients:** AIDS/HIV, Cancer, Children's Health/Hospitals, Clinics/Medical Centers, Domestic Violence, Emergency/Ambulance Services, Family Planning, Geriatric Health, Health Organizations, Health Policy/Cost Containment, Hospices, Hospitals, Long-Term Care, Medical Education, Medical Rehabilitation, Medical Research, Medical Training, Mental Health, Nursing Services, People with Disabilities, Prenatal Health Issues, Preventive Medicine/Wellness Organizations, Public Health, Research/Studies Institutes, Sexual Abuse, Single-Disease Health Associations, Substance Abuse. **Geo. Dist:** nationally for conservation programs; PA, Southwestern Pennsylvania; Pittsburgh, PA.

★ 11887 ★ Richard Lounsbery Foundation

51 East 63rd St. Suite 1
New York, NY 10021
Phone: (212)319-7033 **Fax:** (212)753-9286
Ms. Marta Norman, Executive Director

Fnded: 1959. **Philosophy:** The Richard Lounsbery Foundation makes most of its grants in the area of education. Educational funding favors higher education, with emphasis on scientific research at universities. Other interests include medical and scientific research, international concerns, civic and environmental causes, and the arts. **Priorities:** *Arts & Humanities:* About 15%. Supports museums and music. *Civic & Public Affairs:* About 9%. Supports institutes, foundations, legal aid. *Education:* About 46%. Colleges/Universities. *International:* About 5%. Cancer centers and research. *Religion:* About 20%. Scientific institutions. *Note:* Total contributions made in 2000. **Typ. Recipients:** AIDS/HIV, Cancer, Hospitals, Hospitals (University Affiliated), Medical Education, Medical Rehabilitation, Medical Research, Nutrition, People with Disabilities, Research/Studies Institutes, Respiratory, Single-Disease Health Associations. **Geo. Dist:** internationally; nationally; CA; CO; CT; DC; IL; KY; MA; NJ; NY; OH; PA; UT; VA; WA.

★ 11888 ★ Richard and Rhoda Goldman Fund

One Lombard St., Suite 303
San Francisco, CA 94111
Phone: (415)788-1090 **Fax:** (415)788-7890
Email: info@goldmanfund.org
Website: http://www.goldmanfund.org
Robert Gamble, Executive Director

Fnded: 1951. **Philosophy:** "The Richard & Rhoda Goldman Fund is a private foundation reflecting the founders' long-term commitment to support charitable organizations that enhance the quality of life, primarily in the Bay Area. The fund is interested in supporting programs that will have a positive impact in an array of fields including: the Environment, Population, Jewish Affairs, Children and Youth, Elderly, Social and Human Services, Health, Education, and the Arts." Richard and Rhoda Goldman Fund Program Priorities **Priorities:** *Arts & Humanities:* 4%. Gives to libraries, fine arts, museums, opera and ballet. *Civic & Public Affairs:* 15%. Funds public policy programs, law/justice organizations, and neighborhood development. *Education:* 11%. Primarily supports colleges and universities. *Environment:* 5%. Supports youth programs, violence prevention, and family planning. *International:* 2%. Gives to hospital and medical centers. *Note:* Total contributions made in 2000. **Typ. Recipients:** AIDS/HIV, Alzheimers Disease, Cancer, Child Abuse, Children's Health/Hospitals, Clinics/Medical Centers, Domestic Violence, Family Planning, Health Organizations, Health Policy/Cost Containment, Health-General, Heart, Hospices, Long-Term Care, Medical Research, Medical Training, Nursing Services, Public Health. **Geo. Dist:** San Francisco, CA, including metropolitan area.

★ 11889 ★ Richard S. Reynolds Foundation

1403 Pemberton Rd., Suite 102
Richmond, VA 23233
Phone: (804)740-7350 **Fax:** (804)740-7807
Victoria Pitrelli, Executive Director

Fnded: 1965. **Philosophy:** The foundation gives to a variety of groups mainly in the Richmond, VA, area. Education, arts and sciences, religion, and community service groups generally receive a majority of the foundation's giving. **Priorities:** *Arts & Humanities:* 27%. Giving to the performing arts and museums. *Civic & Public Affairs:* 10%. Primarily for housing and community programs. *Education:* 48%. Colleges, universities, and primary and secondary education. *Environment:* 20%. Emphasis on youth organizations and emergency shelters. *International:* 1%. Hospitals, medical research, and single-disease health asssociations. *Note:* Total contributions made in fiscal 2001. **Typ. Recipients:** Cancer, Children's Health/Hospitals, Clinics/Medical Centers, Emergency/Ambulance Services, Health Funds, Heart, Hospitals, Medical Education, Medical Rehabilitation, Medical Research, Mental Health, Multiple Sclerosis, People with Disabilities, Respiratory. **Geo. Dist:** VA, Central Virginia, particularly Richmond.

★ 11890 ★ Richard and Susan Smith Family Foundation

27 Boylston St.
Chestnut Hill, MA 02467-1719
Phone: (617)278-5220
Susan Smith, Trustee

Fnded: 1970. **Typ. Recipients:** Cancer, Children's Health/Hospitals, Health Organizations, Health-General, Hospices, Hospitals, Medical Rehabilitation, Medical Research, Prenatal Health Issues, Single-Disease Health Associations, Speech & Hearing. **Geo. Dist:** Boston, MA, metropolitan area.

★ 11891 ★ Rigler-Deutsch Foundation

PO Box 828
Burbank, CA 91503
Fax: (213)878-0329
James Rigler, Vice President

Fnded: 1966. **Philosophy:** The foundation primarily gives to arts and cultural orgainzations in New York, NY, and Los Angeles, CA. Since 1994 the foundation has contributed a majority of its funding towards the Classic Arts Showcase, which is a twenty-four hour a day classic arts network with an MTV style format. **Priorities:** *Arts & Humanities:* 48%. Primary support for opera, ballet, theaters, and music. *Civic & Public Affairs:* 2%. Civil rights and public policy. *Education:* 3%. Arts education. *Environment:* 5%. *International:* 1%. AIDS and mental health organizations. *Note:* Total contributions made in 2000. **Typ. Recipients:** AIDS/HIV, Cancer, Children's Health/Hospitals, Family Planning, Health Funds, Hospitals, Medical Research, Mental Health, Prenatal Health Issues, Speech & Hearing, Substance Abuse. **Geo. Dist:** Los Angeles, CA; New York, NY.

★ 11892 ★ Rita J. and Stanley H. Kaplan Foundation

866 United Nations Plaza, No. 306
New York, NY 10017
Phone: (212)688-1047 **Fax:** (212)688-6907
Email: rskfnd@aol.com
Nancy Greenblatt, Executive Director

Fnded: 1984. **Philosophy:** The foundation primarily supports the performing arts and Jewish museums. Other recipient areas include medical centers, Jewish religious organizations, and a variety of social services and civic affairs interests. **Priorities:** *Arts & Humanities:* 15%. Public broadcasting, opera, theater, and museums of fine art. *Civic & Public Affairs:* 13%. Community and urban affairs and clubs. *Education:* 33%. Funds primary and secondary schools with an emphasis on Jewish education. *Environment:* 1%. Supports youth programs. *International:* 20%. Primarily for medicine centers and medical research. *Note:* Total contributions made in 2000. **Typ. Recipients:** Adolescent Health Issues, AIDS/HIV, Cancer, Clinics/Medical Centers, Emergency/Ambulance Services, Family Planning, Health Funds, Health Organizations, Hospitals, Hospitals (University Affiliated), Medical Education, Medical Research, People with Disabilities, Preventive Medicine/Wellness Organizations, Public Health, Single-Disease Health Associations, Transplant Networks/Donor Banks. **Geo. Dist:** New York, NY.

★ 11893 ★ Robert G. Cabell III and Maude Morgan Cabell Foundation

PO Box 85678
Richmond, VA 23285-5678
Phone: (804)780-2000 **Fax:** (804)697-2989
John Werner, Executive Director

Fnded: 1957. **Philosophy:** The foundation makes grants across the major categories of support. In education, interests include colleges and universities. Social service support goes to shelters, food banks, senior centers, and youth organizations. Funding for the arts favors historic preservation. Grants also are made to other recipient areas. **Priorities:** *Arts & Humanities:* 29%. Supports museums, libraries, and historical societies. *Civic & Public Affairs:* 38%. Funds neighborhood revitalization, housing, women's affairs, and clubs. *Education:* 8%. Funds colleges and higher education. *Environment:* 12%. Supports the Young Men's Christian Association, family planning services, youth programs, food banks, and family services. *International:* 2%. Supports preventative healthcare. *Religion:* 5%. Suppports a science museum. *Note:* Total contributions made in 2000. **Typ. Recipients:** Alzheimers Disease, Arthritis, Child Abuse, Children's Health/Hospitals, Clinics/Medical Centers, Diabetes, Domestic Violence, Emergency/Ambulance Services, Family Planning, Geriatric Health, Health Organizations, Heart, Hospitals, People with Disabilities, Public Health, Research/Studies Institutes, Single-Disease Health Associations, Transplant Networks/Donor Banks. **Geo. Dist:** Richmond, VA.

★ 11894 ★ Robert J. Kleberg, Jr. and Helen C. Kleberg Foundation

700 North Saint Mary's St., Suite 1200
San Antonio, TX 78205
Phone: (210)271-3691 **Fax:** (210)271-9089
Robert Washington, Grants Coordinator

Fnded: 1950. **Philosophy:** The foundation's goal is to support organizations reflecting the interests of the late donors. The greatest emphasis has been on medical research. Other areas supported by the foundation include veterinary science, wildlife research and preservation, health services, higher education, community organizations, and the arts and humanities. **Priorities:** *Arts & Humanities:* 4%. Funds museums, libraries, performing arts, and music. *Civic & Public Affairs:* About 1%. Botanical gardens; resource center. *Education:* 55%. Colleges, universities, and secondary education. *Environment:* About 3%. Supports women's services, single-cause organizations. *International:* 33%. Primary support for medical research. *Religion:* Less than 1%. Nature and botanical support. *Note:* Total contributions made in 1998. **Typ. Recipients:** Alzheimers Disease, Cancer, Children's Health/Hospitals, Clinics/Medical Centers, Domestic Violence, Emergency/Ambulance Services, Eyes/Blindness, Family Planning, Health Organizations, Health-General, Heart, Hospitals, Kidney, Medical Education, Medical Rehabilitation, Medical Research, Nursing Services, People with Disabilities, Research/Studies Institutes, Respiratory, Speech & Hearing, Transplant Networks/Donor Banks, Trauma Treatment. **Geo. Dist:** nationally; TX.

★ 11895 ★ Robert Lehman Foundation
Kelley, Drye & Warren, LLP
101 Park Ave.
New York, NY 10178
Phone: (212)808-7946 **Fax:** (212)808-7897
Email: pguth@kelleydrye.com
Paul Guth, Secretary

Fnded: 1943. **Philosophy:** The primary purpose of the foundation is to maintain the Robert Lehman collection at the Metropolitan Museum of Art. The foundation also supports cultural programs and higher educational institutions, with emphasis on arts education. **Priorities:** *Arts & Humanities:* 73%. Supports museums, arts centers and galleries, and historical societies. Major grants to the Metropolitan Museum of Art and the Museum of Modern Art. *Civic & Public Affairs:* 1%. *Education:* 26%. Primarily supports art education. *Note:* Total contributions made in fiscal 2000. **Typ. Recipients:** AIDS/HIV, Cancer, Children's Health/Hospitals, Clinics/Medical Centers, Emergency/Ambulance Services, Home-Care Services, Hospitals, People with Disabilities. **Geo. Dist:** nationally, particularly the Northeast; New York, NY.

★ 11896 ★ Robert and Myra Kraft and J Hiatt Foundation, Inc.
1 Agrand St.
Worcester, MA 01607
Phone: (508)791-2301 **Fax:** (508)792-1578

Fnded: 1953. **Priorities:** *Education:* 100%. Supports higher education, with a focus on the Northeast. *Note:* Contributions were made in fiscal 1998. **Typ. Recipients:** Cancer, Hospitals, Medical Research. **Geo. Dist:** MA. **Frmly:** Jacob and Francis Hiatt Foundation.

★ 11897 ★ Robert R. McCormick Tribune Foundation
435 North Michigan Ave., Suite 770
Chicago, IL 60611
Phone: (312)222-3512 **Fax:** (312)222-3523
Email: rrmtf@tribune.com
Website: http://www.rrmtf.org

Fnded: 1990. **Philosophy:** "The Robert R. McCormick Tribune Foundation is dedicated to a democratic society and its quality of life. Its mission is to improve the social and economic environment; to encourage a free and responsible discussion of issues affecting the nation; to enhance the effectiveness of American education; and to stimulate responsible citizenship." The foundation seeks to fulfill its mission through four programs. The Communities program is designed to combine the efforts of the McCormick Tribune Foundation, Tribune Company units, and other organizations to directly impact local communities throughout the country. A complete listing of communities participating in this unique grantmaking program is available at the foundation's website. The Education program is designed focus on the quality of early childhood education; increase the number of accredited preschool programs; enhance the skills and recognition of preschool program directors and teachers; improve the early childhood education system; heighten public understanding of the importance of early childhood education. This program is in the Chicago area. The Journalism program is designed to ensure a viable future for journalism, through research, development and education; promote diversity of news staffing and content; encourage informed coverage of national security issues; and support freedom of expression. This program is nationwide. The Citizenship program is designed to promote patriotism and voluntarism. This program is in the Chicago area. The foundation continues to provide operating support to Cantigny, the former estate of Robert R. McCormick, which is operated as a park in Wheaton, IL. Also, in 1992, the foundation opened, operates, and supports the Cantigny First Division Museum to house and exhibit World War I antiques and memorabilia. **Priorities:** *Civic & Public Affairs:* 75%. Supports the Communities program, which functions through regional partners and which is engaged in stimulating charitable giving from the general public. *Note:* Total contributions made in 2000. **Typ. Recipients:** AIDS/HIV, Cancer, Children's Health/Hospitals, Clinics/Medical Centers, Domestic Violence, Emergency/Ambulance Services, Eyes/Blindness, Health Organizations, Heart, Hospices, Hospitals, Medical Education, Medical Rehabilitation, Medical Research, Mental Health, Multiple Sclerosis, Nursing Services, People with Disabilities, Prenatal Health Issues, Public Health, Respiratory, Single-Disease Health Associations, Substance Abuse. **Geo. Dist:** varies by program area; Chicago, IL, metropolitan area. **Frmly:** Robert R. McCormick Charitable Trust.

★ 11898 ★ Robert R. Meyer Foundation
PO Box 11426
Birmingham, AL 35202
Phone: (205)326-4696 **Fax:** (205)581-7433
Carla Gail, Vice President & Trustee

Fnded: 1949. **Philosophy:** The foundation provides a broad base of support to all types of charitable organizations in the Birmingham area. **Priorities:** *Arts & Humanities:* 14%. Gives to libraries and art festivals. *Civic & Public Affairs:* 9%. Funding includes community development. *Education:* 37%. Funds Alabama universities and colleges. *Environment:* 28%. Supports YMCAs, YWCAs, and youth groups. *International:* 9%. Supports single-health groups and community organizations. *Note:* Total contributions were made in 2000. **Typ. Recipients:** AIDS/HIV, Cancer, Clinics/Medical Centers, Domestic Violence, Eyes/Blindness, Family Planning, Health Organizations, Hospitals, Long-Term Care, Medical Education, Mental Health, Nursing Services, People with Disabilities, Public Health, Research/Studies Institutes, Speech & Hearing, Substance Abuse. **Geo. Dist:** Birmingham, AL, metropolitan area.

★ 11899 ★ Robert R. Young Foundation
680 Steamboat Rd.
Greenwich, CT 06830
Fax: (203)661-4247
David Wallace, President

Fnded: 1959. **Philosophy:** The foundation generally supports colleges and universities, hospitals, and social services in New York and New England. **Priorities:** *Arts & Humanities:* 1%. *Education:* 89%. Supports universities and local schools. *Environment:* 1%. Supports youth programs, youth services, and united way. *International:* 8%. Supports hospitals. *Note:* Total contributions made in 2000. **Typ. Recipients:** Arthritis, Cancer, Children's Health/Hospitals, Clinics/Medical Centers, Diabetes, Emergency/Ambulance Services, Family Planning, Heart, Hospices, Hospitals, Medical Research, Mental Health, Multiple Sclerosis, People with Disabilities, Single-Disease Health Associations, Substance Abuse. **Geo. Dist:** New England; NY.

★ 11900 ★ Robert Russell Memorial Foundation
1221 Brickell Ave., 21st Fl.
Miami, FL 33131
Phone: (305)579-0500 **Fax:** (305)961-5503
Norman Lipoff, Chairman & Trustee

Fnded: 1984. **Philosophy:** The foundation primarily supports Jewish organizations in Miami. It also supports educational institutions with Jewish or Middle Eastern studies and programs in Israel. **Priorities:** *Education:* 8%. Secondary higher education. *Environment:* 9%. United Way, scouting, and youth programs. *Note:* Contributions made in fiscal 2000. **Typ. Recipients:** Clinics/Medical Centers, Hospitals, Medical Education, Medical Training. **Geo. Dist:** nationally and internationally; FL, emphasis on Dade County.

★ 11901 ★ Robert S. and Grayce B. Kerr Foundation
PMB 25106
PO Box 20000
Jackson, WY 83001
Phone: (307)733-8829 **Fax:** (307)733-9702
Sarah Lacy, Administrative Assistant

Fnded: 1986. **Philosophy:** The foundation seeks to identify those people, programs, and policies which best address needs in the arts, education, and the environment (habitat preservation) within Oklahoma and Wyoming. Funding is limited to organizations that benefit these specified fields of interest and geographic affiliations. **Priorities:** *Arts & Humanities:* 46%. Emphasis on museums, public broadcasting, and historical societies. *Civic & Public Affairs:* 9%. Supports a community foundation. *Education:* 22%. Primarily for universities in Oklahoma. *Environment:* 6%. Supports child welfare, family services, and community services organizations. *International:* 6%. Supports medical centers and hospitals. *Note:* Total contributions made in 2000. **Typ. Recipients:** AIDS/HIV, Child Abuse, Clinics/Medical Centers, Domestic Violence, Emergency/Ambulance Services, Eyes/Blindness, Health Organizations, Hospices, Hospitals, Long-Term Care, Medical Education, Medical Rehabilitation, Medical Research, Nursing Services, People with Disabilities, Prenatal Health Issues, Substance Abuse. **Geo. Dist:** OH; OK; WY.

★ 11902 ★ Robert Sterling Clark Foundation
135 East 64th St.
New York, NY 10021
Phone: (212)288-8900 **Fax:** (212)288-1033
Ms. Margaret Ayers, Executive Director

Fnded: 1952. **Philosophy:** The foundation limits its funding to the three areas within its current concentration: strengthening cultural institutions in New York; improving the performance of public institutions in New York; and ensuring access to family planning services. While the foundation concentrates on cultural and public institutions in New York, the foundation reports that it, "will continue to support national organizations working in these areas to ensure that women have access to comprehensive reproductive health information and services. Funds will also be made available to organizations working in individual states to support the development of pro-choice coalitions to counteract local anti-choice initiatives." Robert Sterling Clark Foundation Fiscal 2000 IRS Form 990 **Priorities:** *Arts & Humanities:* 16%. Funds theater, music, dance, museums, and arts councils. *Civic & Public Affairs:* 51%. Supports public policy organizations, civil rights, women's affairs, reproductive rights, economic development, economic policy, job training, and botanical gardens/parks. *Education:* 2%. Gives to schools, educational/after-school programs, and education funds. *Environment:* 22%. Supports youth organizations, child welfare, family planning, and food distribution. *International:* 2%. Primarily supports women's/reproductive health organizations. *Religion:* 2%. Funds a science center. *Note:* Total contributions made in fiscal 2000. **Typ. Recipients:** Domestic Violence, Family Planning, Health Organizations, Health-General, Long-Term Care, Mental Health, Public Health. **Geo. Dist:** nationally; New York, NY.

★ 11903 ★ Robert Stewart and Helen Pfeiffer Odell Fund
420 Montgomery St., 7th Fl.
San Francisco, CA 94104
Phone: (415)396-3215 **Fax:** (415)834-0604
Gene Ranghiasci, Vice President

Fnded: 1967. **Philosophy:** The foundation makes most of its grants to benefit youth in California. The primary interest is social services, specifically child welfare programs and youth organizations. Other interests include funding for schools, health care, and the arts. **Priorities:** *Arts & Humanities:* 3%. Contributes to music and historical societies. *Civic & Public Affairs:* 8%. Funds housing, zoos, legal issues, and a festival. *Education:* 47%. Supports private precollege education and scholarship funds. *Environment:* 18%.

Funds youth groups and child welfare. *International:* 5%. Supports medical foundations. *Religion:* 1%. Funds exploratorium. *Note:* Total contributions made in 2000. **Typ. Recipients:** Children's Health/Hospitals, Clinics/Medical Centers, Eyes/Blindness, Health Organizations, Hospitals, Medical Rehabilitation, Medical Research, Mental Health, People with Disabilities, Public Health. **Geo. Dist:** CA, Northern California, with emphasis on San Francisco.

★ 11904 ★ Robert W. Wilson Foundation

520 83rd St., Suite 3R
Brooklyn, NY 11209
Phone: (718)748-6113
Robert Wilson, President

Fnded: 1992. **Priorities:** *Arts & Humanities:* 28%. Supports museums, libraries, music, dance, historic preservation, public broadcasting, and art foundations. *Civic & Public Affairs:* 32%. Funds gardens, justice organizations, public policy, and women's organizations. *Education:* 1%. *Environment:* 1%. *International:* 1%. Medical research and deafness research receive funding. *Note:* Total contributions made in 2000. **Typ. Recipients:** Arthritis, Clinics/Medical Centers, Emergency/Ambulance Services, Health-General, Medical Research, Mental Health, Multiple Sclerosis, People with Disabilities, Single-Disease Health Associations, Speech & Hearing, Substance Abuse. **Geo. Dist:** Washington, DC; Bronx, NY; New York, NY; Roseburg, OR; Arlington, VA.

★ 11905 ★ Robert W. Woodruff Foundation

50 Hurt Plz., Suite 1200
Atlanta, GA 30303
Phone: (404)522-6755 **Fax:** (404)522-7026
Email: fdns@woodruff.org
Website: http://www.woodruff.org
Charles McTier, President

Fnded: 1937. **Philosophy:** The foundation's principal giving interests include education, health care, human services, cultural and civic affairs, and the environment. Preference is given to one-time capital projects. Awards for basic operating expenses usually are avoided. **Priorities:** *Arts & Humanities:* Approx. 1%. Supports public broadcasting, performing arts, and library. *Civic & Public Affairs:* 7%. Supports legal services programs, community foundations, State of GA, Office of the Governor. *Education:* 18%. Supports colleges and universities, education foundations. *Environment:* 2%. Supports Boys and Girls Clubs, senior services, counseling service, and United Way. *International:* 56%. Supports the Robert W. Woodruff Health Sciences Center Fund. *Religion:* 5%. *Note:* Total contributions made in 2000. **Typ. Recipients:** Alzheimers Disease, Cancer, Children's Health/Hospitals, Emergency/Ambulance Services, Geriatric Health, Health Organizations, Health Policy/Cost Containment, Health-General, Hospices, Long-Term Care, Medical Education, Medical Rehabilitation, Medical Research, Mental Health, Nursing Services, Public Health, Trauma Treatment. **Geo. Dist:** Atlanta, GA, some statewide giving.

★ 11906 ★ Robert Wood Johnson Foundation

College Rd. East
PO Box 2316
Princeton, NJ 08543-2316
Phone: 888-631-9989 **Fax:** (609)987-8845
Email: rtoth@rwjf.org
Website: http://www.rwjf.org
Richard Toth, Director, Office of Proposal Management

Fnded: 1936. **Philosophy:** The foundation's four objectives are the following: to ensure that Americans of all ages have access to basic health care at reasonable cost; to improve care and support for people with chronic health conditions; to promote healthy communities and lifestyles; and to reduce the personal, social and economic harm caused by substance abuse of tobacco, alcohol and illicit drugs. The Substance Abuse Policy Research program helps identify, analyze, and evaluate public- and private-sector policies aimed at reducing the harm caused by abuse of tobacco, alcohol, illegal drugs, and combinations of the three. The foundation assists efforts to fund projects to improve access to care for people with the most serious geographic, cultural, financial, and other barriers to care; to make arrangements for health care more effective and affordable; and to help people maintain or more quickly regain their functional abilities for everyday life. The foundation directs its purpose to focusing upon improving health services; helping those groups most susceptible to disease; addressing individual health problems on a large scale; and promoting bold, creative approaches and solutions to health concerns. The foundation, therefore, explores and funds new areas of medical care concerned with infant, child, and adolescent welfare; chronic illness and disability, particularly among the elderly; AIDS concerns; substance abuse; mental illness; the organization and quality of health services; medical ethical issues; quality and availability of health professionals; and the problems arising from technological advances in medicine. Programs span the areas of education, social services, and civic affairs, yet all related to health interests. The foundation also makes funding available to support research, evaluation, and demonstration projects that will assess the impact of major changes in the financing and organization of health services on health-care costs, quality, and access to care. Additional funds are made available in an effort to strengthen the nation's nursing services, supporting projects that address nursing manpower and educational development. The Health Policy Fellowships Program develops the capacity of outstanding mid-career health professionals in academic and community-based settings to assume leadership roles in health policy and management. Health Tracking is a major initiative that examines and reports on our nation's changing health-care system and how these changes are affecting the American people; and pulls together insights from many foundation programs. **Priorities:** *Environment:* 21%. *International:* 75%. Supports programs that assure that all American have access to basic health care at reasonable cost, and those programs that improve the way services are organized and provided to people with chronic health conditions. *Note:* Contributions made in 2000. **Typ. Recipients:** Adolescent Health Issues, AIDS/HIV, Alzheimers Disease, Cancer, Children's Health/Hospitals, Clinics/Medical Centers, Family Planning, Geriatric Health, Health Funds, Health Organizations, Health Policy/Cost Containment, Health-General, Heart, Home-Care Services, Hospitals, Long-Term Care, Medical Education, Medical Training, Mental Health, Nursing Services, People with Disabilities, Prenatal Health Issues, Public Health, Research/Studies Institutes, Respiratory, Single-Disease Health Associations, Substance Abuse. **Geo. Dist:** nationally.

★ 11907 ★ Robert Z. Hawkins Foundation

One East Liberty St., Suite 509
Reno, NV 89501
Phone: (775)786-1105 **Fax:** (775)786-4886
Email: rzhawkins@aol.com
William Wallace, Chairman

Fnded: 1980. **Philosophy:** "Grants may be made to organizations operated exclusively for charitable, religious, educational, scientific or literary purposes, or for the prevention of cruelty to children or animals, which hold a letter from the Internal Revenue Service determining that the organization is a qualified Section 501 (c)(3) organization." "Grants may also be made to religious organizations, and to political subdivisions, if made exclusively for public purposes." **Priorities:** *Arts & Humanities:* 8%. Focus on public broadcasting, museums, music and opera. *Civic & Public Affairs:* 32%. Supports The City of Reno and county parks. *Education:* 20%. Supports colleges, universities, medical education, parochial education scholarships and engineering education. *Environment:* 29%. Supports youth organizations, animal welfare, substance abuse, United Way, emergency services and camps. *International:* 4%. Health funds, hospitals, mental illness. *Religion:* 1%. Funds scientific research. *Note:* Total contributions made in 2000. **Typ. Recipients:** Cancer, Children's Health/Hospitals, Diabetes, Domestic Violence, Emergency/Ambulance Services, Health Organizations, Hospitals, Long-Term Care, Medical Education, Mental Health, People with Disabilities, Public Health, Single-Disease Health Associations, Substance Abuse, Transplant Networks/Donor Banks. **Geo. Dist:** CA; NV, Northern Nevada; Reno, NV.

★ 11908 ★ Robertson Foundation

American Express TBS, Inc.
1185 Ave. of the Americas
New York, NY 10036
Phone: (212)372-1000
Julian Robertson, Jr., Trustee

Fnded: 1997. **Typ. Recipients:** Cancer, Clinics/Medical Centers.

★ 11909 ★ Rockefeller Brothers Fund, Inc.

437 Madison Ave., 37th Floor
New York, NY 10022-7001
Phone: (212)812-4200 **Fax:** (212)812-4299
Email: rock@rbf.org
Website: http://www.rbf.org
Benjamin Shute, Jr., Secretary

Fnded: 1940. **Philosophy:** "The fund seeks to achieve its major objective of improving the well-being of all people through support of efforts in the United States and abroad that contribute ideas, develop leaders, and encourage institutions in the transition to global interdependence and that counter world trends of resource depletion, militarization, protectionism, and isolation which now threaten to move humankind everywhere further away from cooperation, trade and economic growth, arms restraint, and conservation." In order to achieve these goals, the fund makes grants in four general areas. *Sustainable Development*: This program is designed to foster strategies to combat global warming and seeks to contribute to international cooperation on this issue, conserve terrestrial and marine biodiversity by protecting and restoring ecosystems and by fostering sustainable communities that pursue locally-appropriate development strategies. *Peace and Security*: The Fund seeks to contribute to encouraging broad public dialogue and debate on America's role in the world and on the values and principles that should shape it. *Democratic Practice*: This program seeks to identify and support new ways to foster civic engagement, including innovative models and programs that catalyze the civic energy of young people. *Health*: Charles E. Culpeper Human Advancement: This program funds human advancement and fulfillment of individual potential by supporting arts and culture, working to improve the quality of education, recognizing and encouraging individual leadership, and helping to mitigate the impact of health threats that undermine human advancement on a nation- or region-wide scale. The Fund also supports the Ramon Magsaysay Award Foundation, which grants the Ramon Magsaysay Awards, named after the former president of the Philippines, that were established by the trustees of the Fund in the late 1950s, and the Pocantico Programs which provide public access to the Pocantico Historic Area, the heart of the Rockefeller family estate in Westchester County, New York, and were established when the Fund leased the area from the National Trust for Historic Preservation in 1991. **Priorities:** *Arts & Humanities:* 12%. Funds the performing arts, visual and literary arts, and cultural and historic preservation. *Civic & Public Affairs:* 25%. Grants are given nationally and internationally to the Nonprofit Sector and to civic, community-based, neighborhood and public spaces programs in New York City. *Education:* 8%. Funds programs that enhance quality of the professionals in the education field and encourage people of color to enter the teaching profession. Also funds organizations/programs that provide quality early childhood education and care. *International:* 11%. Provides funding for biomedical research, health services research, the study of social and ethical issues in health and disease, and American medical education. *Note:* Total grant payments made in 2000. Excludes employee matching gifts, grant and program management expenses, and direct charitable activities relating to the Fund's fellowship and other programs. **Typ. Recipients:** Speech & Hearing. **Geo. Dist:** internationally; nationally; New York, NY.

★ 11910 ★ Rockefeller Family Fund
437 Madison Ave., 37th Floor
New York, NY 10022
Phone: (212)812-4252 **Fax:** (212)812-4299
Email: mmccarthy@rffund.org
Website: http://www.rffund.org
Mr. Lee Wasserman, Director

Fnded: 1967. **Philosophy:** The Rockefeller Family Fund makes grants in five program areas: Citizen Participation and Government Accountability, increasing voter participation and structural improvement to systems of government; Economic Justice for Women, enhancing the economic status of women by providing them with equitable employment opportunities and improving their work lives; The Environment, emphasizing the reduction of military pollution, the conservation of natural resources and the protection of health as affected by the environment; Institutional Responsiveness, supporting projects to influence public opinion and private institutions on issues of social concern; and Self-Sufficiency, which helps groups working within the fund's program areas to increase their income by obtaining funds from new sources or improving their ability to raise money from current sources. **Priorities:** *Civic & Public Affairs:* 68%. Program areas include citizen education and participation, economic justice for women, institutional responsiveness, and self-sufficiency. *Note:* Total contributions made in 2000. **Typ. Recipients:** Health Policy/Cost Containment, Health-General, People with Disabilities, Public Health. **Geo. Dist:** nationally; the fund does not generally consider projects which pertain to one city or state, unless the project could serve as a national model.

★ 11911 ★ Rockefeller Foundation
420 Fifth Ave.
New York, NY 10018-2702
Phone: (212)869-8500 **Fax:** (212)764-3468
Website: http://www.rockfound.org
Lynda Mullen, Secretary

Fnded: 1913. **Philosophy:** The foundation's stated mission when it was founded in 1913 was, "to promote the well-being of mankind throughout the world." It is dedicated to identifying and attacking the underlying causes of human suffering and need at their source. The foundation carries out its mission through grants and fellowships to individuals and institutions in the following areas: arts and humanities; equal opportunity; agricultural sciences; health sciences; population sciences; global environment; and special African initiatives, including female education. The balance of the foundation's programs support work in building democracy, international security, international philanthropy, and other special interests and initiatives. The foundation operates the Bellagio Study and Conference Center in northern Italy for international conferences and for residencies for artists, scholars and policymakers, and other professionals from around the world. **Priorities:** *Arts & Humanities:* 3%. Supports arts and humanities programs that help to understand and engage difference across changing societies. *Civic & Public Affairs:* About 21%. Equal opportunity to support diverse urban communities, including employment, good schools, freedom from discrimination, and full participation in the democratic process. *Education:* 18%. Supports educational programs, higher education, and school districts for reform policies. *Environment:* 2%. Population sciences, including family planning and reproductive health services. *International:* 19%. Focus on building human capacity for population-based health care in developing nations. *Religion:* 1%. Supports agricultural sciences to increase crop yields of smallholder farmers in developing countries profitably and without degrading natural resources. *Note:* Total contributions made in 2000. **Typ. Recipients:** AIDS/HIV, Family Planning, Health Organizations, Health-General, Medical Education, Medical Research, Medical Training, Public Health, Research/Studies Institutes. **Geo. Dist:** internationally; nationally.

★ 11912 ★ Rockwell Fund, Inc.
1330 Post Oak Boulevard, Suite 1825
Houston, TX 77056
Phone: (713)629-9022 **Fax:** (713)629-7702
Email: mvogt@rockfund.org
Website: http://www.rockfund.org
Martha Vogt, Senior Program Officer

Fnded: 1931. **Philosophy:** The fund supports a broad range of activities, with preference for causes in the Houston area. **Priorities:** *Arts & Humanities:* 9%. Supports museums and the theater. *Civic & Public Affairs:* 2%. Supports community services and environmental organizations. *Education:* 36%. Supports independent schools, colleges, and universities. *Environment:* 36%. Supports human services, youth services, and social services. *International:* 17%. Supports hospices, mental health centers, hospitals, and emergency care centers. *Note:* Total contributions made in 2001. **Typ. Recipients:** Adolescent Health Issues, AIDS/HIV, Cancer, Child Abuse, Children's Health/Hospitals, Clinics/Medical Centers, Emergency/Ambulance Services, Eyes/Blindness, Family Planning, Health Organizations, Heart, Hospices, Hospitals, Medical Rehabilitation, Medical Research, Mental Health, Nursing Services, People with Disabilities, Prenatal Health Issues, Public Health, Single-Disease Health Associations, Single-Disease Health Associations, Speech & Hearing, Substance Abuse, Transplant Networks/Donor Banks. **Geo. Dist:** Houston, TX, limited giving outside of the Houston area.

★ 11913 ★ Rollin M. Gerstacker Foundation
PO Box 1945
Midland, MI 48641-1945
Phone: (989)631-6097 **Fax:** (989)832-8842
Gail Lanphear, President

Fnded: 1957. **Philosophy:** The foundation adheres to Mrs. Gerstacker's belief "that it was the responsibility of private citizens to enrich their communities to the best of their abilities." In accordance with this philosophy, the foundation traditionally has given to homes for the elderly, colleges and universities, the Mid-Michigan Medical Center, research institutions, youth, and community services, particularly in Midland, MI. These areas of interest remain the focus of foundation giving. **Priorities:** *Arts & Humanities:* 9%. Supports music, museums, theater and historical associations. *Civic & Public Affairs:* 24%. Primarily funds public policy institutes, community foundations, municipalities, and housing. *Education:* 41%. Supports colleges, universities, and research institutes. *Environment:* 11%. Funds domestic violence prevention, youth organizations, United Way, and child welfare. *International:* 5%. Supports nursing, hospitals, mental health, and single-disease associations. *Religion:* 4%. Funds research institutions. *Note:* Total contributions made in 2001. **Typ. Recipients:** AIDS/HIV, Alzheimers Disease, Arthritis, Clinics/Medical Centers, Domestic Violence, Emergency/Ambulance Services, Eyes/Blindness, Geriatric Health, Hospitals, Medical Rehabilitation, Medical Research, Mental Health, Multiple Sclerosis, Nursing Services, People with Disabilities, Public Health, Research/Studies Institutes, Single-Disease Health Associations, Substance Abuse, Transplant Networks/Donor Banks. **Geo. Dist:** Midland, MI; Cleveland, OH.

★ 11914 ★ RosaMary Foundation
PO Box 13218
New Orleans, LA 70185-3218
Phone: (504)895-1984 **Fax:** (504)895-1988
Website: http://www.rosamary.org
Richard Freeman, Jr., Chairman

Fnded: 1939. **Philosophy:** "The Foundation supports grant seekers within the Greater New Orleans area. Highest priority is given to grants in the following categories: Education, with emphasis on private institutions; Human service organizations; Arts, both performing and applied; Community development activities; Governmental oversight activities." RosaMary Foundation Mission Statement. **Priorities:** *Arts & Humanities:* 22%. Includes museums, music, and arts associations. *Civic & Public Affairs:* 24%. Supports community improvement/development, public affairs concerns, and public protection. *Education:* 30%. Primarily for colleges and universities. *Environment:* 5%. Focus on youth development, housing/shelter, and other human service organizations. *International:* 2%. Emphasis on mental health and crisis intervention. *Note:* Total contributions made in 2002. **Typ. Recipients:** AIDS/HIV, Clinics/Medical Centers, Eyes/Blindness, Family Planning, Health Organizations, Hospitals, Medical Research, People with Disabilities, Research/Studies Institutes, Transplant Networks/Donor Banks. **Geo. Dist:** New Orleans, LA.

★ 11915 ★ Rosamond Gifford Charitable Corp.
518 James St., Suite 280
Syracuse, NY 13203
Phone: (315)474-2489 **Fax:** (315)475-4983
Email: kgoldfarb@giffordfd.org
Website: http://www.giffordfd.org
Kathryn Goldfarb, Executive Director

Fnded: 1954. **Philosophy:** "The Rosamund Gifford Charitable Corporation is a philanthropic foundation dedicated to the continuing stewardship of the funds entrusted to our care and committed to using our financial and human resources to build the capacity of individuals, institutions, and associations to enhance the economic vitality and the quality of life of the people of our community." *The Rosamund Gifford Charitable Corporation 1998 Annual Report* "In 1998, The Rosamund Gifford Charitable Corporation adopted a new strategic plan to guide us toward fulfillment of our mission. The continuing vision of the Gifford Foundation, which is reflected in that plan, is to be a proactive force to bring about a transformation in the philosophy and structures that serve the people, the associations and the institutions of our community. As a focus for changing structures, the Foundation will be convening leaders, building strategic partnerships with other funders, proactively seeking gift recipients and creating a public image as a respected facilitator and agent of community improvement." *The Rosamund Gifford Corporation 1998 Annual Report* **Priorities:** *Arts & Humanities:* 25%. Museums, music, and theaters. *Civic & Public Affairs:* 20%. Primarily for municipal services and housing. *Education:* 15%. Supports community schools, higher education, and literacy. *Environment:* 33%. Supports community services, youth programs, and the United Way. *International:* 4%. AIDS and American Lung Association. *Note:* Total contributions made in 2000. **Typ. Recipients:** Alzheimers Disease, Clinics/Medical Centers, Emergency/Ambulance Services, Family Planning, Health Organizations, Health-General, Heart, Hospices, Hospitals, Kidney, Long-Term Care, Medical Research, Mental Health, Nursing Services, People with Disabilities, Prenatal Health Issues, Public Health, Sexual Abuse, Single-Disease Health Associations, Substance Abuse. **Geo. Dist:** NY, Syracuse and Onondaga County.

★ 11916 ★ Rose E. Tucker Charitable Trust
900 Southwest Fifth Ave., 26th Floor
Portland, OR 97204
Phone: (503)224-3380 **Fax:** (503)220-2480
Email: tuckertrust@stoel.com
Terrence Pancoast, Trustee

Fnded: 1976. **Philosophy:** The trust makes most of its grants in the areas of social services, education, civic, and the environment. Social service support includes adult care, youth organizations, family planning, and food distribution. Educational funding favors grants, including capital projects and scholarships, to universities and colleges in Oregon. Funding for the arts supports museums, libraries, and the performing arts. **Priorities:** *Arts & Humanities:* 14%. Supports performing arts, museums, theaters, festivals, and historical societies. *Civic & Public Affairs:* 20%. Funds community organizations, policy institutes, and parks and zoos. *Education:* 25%. Funds colleges, universities, and schools. *Environment:* 19%. Funds Young Men's Christian Association, food banks, and youth programs. *International:* 9%. Supports medical aid.

Religion: 2%. Funds a science museum. *Note:* Total contributions made in fiscal 2001. **Typ. Recipients:** Alzheimers Disease, Clinics/Medical Centers, Emergency/Ambulance Services, Family Planning, Health Funds, Health Organizations, Health-General, Hospitals, Medical Rehabilitation, Mental Health, People with Disabilities, Prenatal Health Issues, Public Health, Single-Disease Health Associations, Substance Abuse. **Geo. Dist:** Portland, OR, metropolitan area; some statewide giving.

★ 11917 ★ Rose M. Badgeley Residuary Charitable Trust

140 Broadway, 11th Fl.
New York, NY 10005
Phone: 800-975-4722 **Fax:** (212)658-7790
Roberta Grossman, Vice President

Fnded: 1977. **Philosophy:** The trust supports non-profit organizations with religious, charitable, scientific, literary or educational purposes. **Priorities:** *Arts & Humanities:* 14%. Primarily funds music concerns. Also supports theater. *Civic & Public Affairs:* 4%. Focus on philanthropic organizations. *Education:* 19%. Funds private precollege education. *Environment:* 12%. Supports youth groups and services for the homeless. *International:* 34%. Supports hospitals, medical centers, and cancer research. *Note:* Total contributions made in fiscal 1999. **Typ. Recipients:** AIDS/HIV, Alzheimers Disease, Cancer, Children's Health/Hospitals, Clinics/Medical Centers, Emergency/Ambulance Services, Eyes/Blindness, Geriatric Health, Health Organizations, Heart, Hospitals, Hospitals (University Affiliated), Medical Rehabilitation, Medical Research, Mental Health, Nursing Services, People with Disabilities, Prenatal Health Issues, Single-Disease Health Associations, Substance Abuse, Transplant Networks/Donor Banks. **Geo. Dist:** NY. **Frmly:** Rose M. Badgeley Charitable Trust.

★ 11918 ★ Rosenberg Foundation

47 Kearny St., Suite 804
San Francisco, CA 94108
Phone: (415)421-6105 **Fax:** (415)421-0141
Email: rosenfdn@rosenbergfdn.org
Website: http://www.rosenbergfdn.org
Kirke Wilson, President, Secretary

Fnded: 1935. **Philosophy:** The Rosenberg Foundation currently has three program priorities: families in poverty in rural and urban areas in California, the changing population of California, and child support reform. Regarding the first priority, the foundation supports programs that reduce dependency, promote self-help, create access to the economic mainstream, or address the causes of poverty among children and families. Programs under the second priority receiving prime consideration will be those that promote the full social, economic, and cultural integration of immigrants and minorities into a pluralistic society. The Rosenberg Foundation is seeking projects which test new ideas and which show significant and permanent improvement in public social policy. Regarding the third priority, the foundation supports projects that are working to improve the child support system through advocacy and public education in the areas of paternity establishment, collection and distribution of support orders, and development of the national child support assurance program. **Priorities:** *Civic & Public Affairs:* 65%. Funds legal centers, public policy, employment, housing, and child support system reform. *Education:* 4%. Supports multicultural education. *Environment:* 29%. Supports programs that help to improve the situations of children and their families in poverty. *Note:* Total contributions made in 2000. **Typ. Recipients:** Health Policy/Cost Containment. **Geo. Dist:** CA, grantss are made outside California to operate productions in California and to national organizations benefiting Californians.

★ 11919 ★ Rosenstiel Foundation

575 Madison Ave., 11th Fl.
New York, NY 10022-2511
Phone: (212)940-8837 **Fax:** (212)940-6776
Maurice Greenbaum, Secretary & Treasurer

Fnded: 1950. **Philosophy:** The Rosenstiel Foundation primarily supports the arts, civic affairs, and health care. Arts funding favors museums, theater, and dance. Support for civic affairs goes to centers for Polish culture and other international affairs. Secondary interests include education with gifts to universities and science education. The foundation will also fund social service organizations. **Priorities:** *Arts & Humanities:* 24%. Funds museums, theaters, symphonies, opera, and arts associations. *Civic & Public Affairs:* 29%. Supports ethnic organizations and public policy associations. *Education:* 28%. Focus on private secondary education, universities, and education funds. *Environment:* 2%. *International:* 10%. Health associations, hospitals, hospices, medical research, and medical rehabilitation. *Note:* Total contributions made in 2000. **Typ. Recipients:** AIDS/HIV, Cancer, Children's Health/Hospitals, Clinics/Medical Centers, Eyes/Blindness, Health Organizations, Health-General, Heart, Hospices, Hospitals, Kidney, Medical Education, Medical Rehabilitation, Medical Research, Nursing Services, People with Disabilities, Public Health, Research/Studies Institutes, Single-Disease Health Associations, Substance Abuse. **Geo. Dist:** Eastern USA; New York, NY.

★ 11920 ★ Ross Family Charitable Foundation

c/o Starr & Co.
350 Park Ave., 9th Floor
New York, NY 10022
Phone: (212)759-6556
Courtney Ross, Trustee

Fnded: 1989. **Priorities:** *Arts & Humanities:* 1%. Gives to a sculpture garden, museums, and film preservation. *Civic & Public Affairs:* 2%. Police associations, community councils, and community foundations receive support. *Education:* 96%. Funds universities, colleges, scholarship funds, private schools, and film education programs. *International:* Less than 1%. Supports a cancer center and AIDS causes. *Note:* Total contributions made in 1999. **Typ. Recipients:** AIDS/HIV, Cancer, Children's Health/Hospitals, Hospitals, Medical Research, People with Disabilities, Research/Studies Institutes. **Geo. Dist:** NY.

★ 11921 ★ Ross Foundation

PO Box 335
Arkadelphia, AR 71923
Phone: (870)246-9881 **Fax:** (870)246-9674
Email: joenix@sbcglobal.net
Ross Whipple, President

Fnded: 1966. **Philosophy:** The Ross Foundation has two primary interests: promoting the economic, cultural, and educational interests of Arkadelphia and Clark County through various projects and programs, as well as promoting conservation and the management of natural resources. The foundation's funding is generated through the timber industry. Therefore, grants are made to support the environment and conservation. **Priorities:** *Arts & Humanities:* 2%. Arts center. *Education:* 34%. Colleges and universities, science/mathematical education, agricultural education, and environmental education. *Environment:* 18%. United Way, youth activities, and community service organizations. *International:* 35%. *Note:* Total contributions made in 2000. **Typ. Recipients:** AIDS/HIV, Child Abuse, Clinics/Medical Centers, Domestic Violence, Emergency/Ambulance Services, Hospitals, Public Health, Respiratory, Substance Abuse. **Geo. Dist:** AR, Arkadelphia County; AR, Clark County.

★ 11922 ★ Rowland Foundation

PO Box 13
Cambridge, MA 02238
Phone: (617)497-4634 **Fax:** (617)497-4627
Dr. Philip DuBois, President

Fnded: 1960. **Philosophy:** The foundation primarily funds "academic institutions, social welfare, hospitals, museums, conservation, historical associations, medical research, and the arts." **Priorities:** *Civic & Public Affairs:* 5%. Funds the Crotched Mountain Foundation. *Education:* 3%. Supports research at Harvard University. *Religion:* 92%. Major support is awarded to the Rowland Institute for Science. *Note:* Total contributions made in fiscal 2000. **Typ. Recipients:** Cancer, Children's Health/Hospitals, Eyes/Blindness, Family Planning, Health Funds, Health Organizations, Heart, Hospitals, Medical Education, Medical Rehabilitation, Medical Research, People with Disabilities, Single-Disease Health Associations. **Geo. Dist:** primarily New England.

★ 11923 ★ Roy A. Hunt Foundation

One Bigelow Square, Suite 630
Pittsburgh, PA 15219-3030
Phone: (412)281-8734 **Fax:** (412)255-0522
Website: http://www.rahuntfdn.org
Torrence Hunt, Jr., President & Trustee

Fnded: 1966. **Philosophy:** The foundation primarily supports the institutions in which the current trustees are interested. **Priorities:** *Arts & Humanities:* 17%. Contributes to arts centers, public broadcasting, historical societies, and the performing arts. *Civic & Public Affairs:* 15%. Funds cultural groups, public affairs, community organizations, and women's and minority groups. *Education:* 13%. Supports pre-college education, colleges, and universities. *Environment:* 21%. Funds United Way, community centers, services for the disadvantaged, and YMCAs. *International:* 10%. Funds hospitals and single-disease associations. *Religion:* Less than 1%. *Note:* Total contributions made in fiscal 2002. **Typ. Recipients:** AIDS/HIV, Alzheimers Disease, Cancer, Children's Health/Hospitals, Clinics/Medical Centers, Family Planning, Health Organizations, Hospitals, Medical Rehabilitation, Mental Health, Single-Disease Health Associations, Substance Abuse. **Geo. Dist:** limited national giving; Boston, MA; Pittsburgh, PA.

★ 11924 ★ Roy and Christine Sturgis Charitable and Educational Trust (TX)

PO Box 830241
Dallas, TX 75283-0241
Phone: (214)209-2422 **Fax:** (214)209-1997
Daniel Kelly, Trust Officer

Fnded: 1981. **Philosophy:** The trust's main priorities include education, the arts, health, and "the relief of human suffering." Youth and social services and science are also areas of interest. The trust is primarily interested in supplementing needs for capital requirements or special projects, research, and programs that have a measurable beginning and end. Endowments, start-up funds, and limited general operating expenses also are considered. Grants subject to matching requirements receive special consideration. **Priorities:** *Arts & Humanities:* 7%. Supports performing arts, museums, libraries, and historical commissions. *Civic & Public Affairs:* 8%. Funding for parks, zoos, clubs, and restoration. *Education:* 46%. Supports colleges, universities, and literacy. *Environment:* 24%. Funds social services, scouting, youth activities, Young Men's Christian Association camps, United Way, and senior citizens. *International:* 9%. Funds hospitals, health centers, nursing and blindness. *Religion:* 3%. Supports a science museum. *Note:* Total contributions made in fiscal 2000. **Typ. Recipients:** Adolescent Health Issues, Alzheimers Disease, Cancer, Children's Health/Hospitals, Clinics/Medical Centers, Diabetes, Domestic Violence, Eyes/Blindness, Health Organizations, Health-General, Heart, Hospices, Hospitals, Hospitals (University Affiliated), Kidney, Long-Term Care, Medical Education, Nursing Services, People with Disabilities, Single-Disease Health Associations, Substance Abuse, Transplant Networks/Donor Banks. **Geo. Dist:** AR; TX, Dallas County.

★ 11925 ★ Roy J. Carver Charitable Trust

202 Iowa Ave.
Muscatine, IA 52761-3733
Phone: (563)263-4010 **Fax:** (563)263-1547
Email: info@carvertrust.org
Website: http://www.carvertrust.org
Troy Ross, Executive Administrator

Fnded: 1982. **Philosophy:** Roy J. Carver's "commitment to helping young people through educational opportunities and to building a better world through medical and scientific research are cornerstones of the charitable trust. As a matter of policy, the trust favors grants that make its participation a vital factor in the success of the project. Such projects should promote the ethical, intellectual, and physical development of young men and women; establish, equip, or provide for the maintenance of institutions of learning; or contribute to the advancement of knowledge and its practical applications through medical and scientific research." Roy J. Carver Charitable Trust, *Grant Policies and Proposal Guidelines* **Priorities:** *Arts & Humanities:* 11%. Supports historical preservation, public broadcasting, museum. *Civic & Public Affairs:* 7%. Supports public libraries. *Education:* 41%. Public and private education. *Environment:* 5%. Provides resources for handicapped children and YMCA. *International:* 35%. Funds medical research. *Note:* Total contributions made in fiscal 2001. **Typ. Recipients:** AIDS/HIV, Alzheimers Disease, Cancer, Child Abuse, Children's Health/Hospitals, Domestic Violence, Emergency/Ambulance Services, Eyes/Blindness, Hospitals (University Affiliated), Medical Education, Medical Research, Nursing Services, People with Disabilities. **Geo. Dist:** organizations with which the founder had significant involvement; IA.

★ 11926 ★ Russell Family Foundation

4756 University Village Place, Suite 474
4756 University Village Place North East
Seattle, WA 98105
Phone: (206)568-4949
Dawn Vinberg, Program Manager

Fnded: 1995. **Priorities:** *Arts & Humanities:* 16%. Gives to art museums, public broadcasting, music, ballet, and arts councils. *Civic & Public Affairs:* 26%. Funds nonprofit management, community foundations, affordable housing, and professional associations. *Education:* 38%. Supports universities, private academies, a Christian school, and literacy/reading programs. *Note:* Total contributions made in 1999. **Typ. Recipients:** Mental Health. **Geo. Dist:** WA.

★ 11927 ★ Russell Sage Foundation

112 E 64th St.
New York, NY 10021
Phone: (212)750-6000 **Fax:** (212)371-4761
Email: info@rsage.org
Website: http://www.russellsage.org
Eric Wanner, President

Fnded: 1907. **Philosophy:** The Russell Sage Foundation functions as a research center, a funding source for various studies, a member of the nation's social science community, and a publisher. Over the years, the foundation has regularly sponsored innovative research in the social sciences, with emphasis on contemporary questions of social policy and scientific development. It also has directed a portion of its funds toward the needs of New York City and the surrounding vicinity. The foundation now dedicates itself exclusively to strengthening the methods, data, and theoretical core of the social sciences as a means of improving social policies. **Priorities:** *Civic & Public Affairs:* 30%. Supports economic policy, census studies, U.S. social policy, and immigration studies. *Education:* 61%. Funds programs in colleges and universities that focus on one or all of the following four areas: (1) research on the future of work, including the causes and consequences of the decline in demand for low-skill workers in advanced economies; (2) research on current U.S. immigration that focuses on the adaptation of the second generation to American society; (3) a joint program with the Andrew W. Mellon Foundation that supports research on curricula designed to foster active literacy among disadvantaged students; and (4) a program on the social psychology of cultural contact that focuses on improving relations between racial and ethnic groups in schools, workplaces, and neighborhood settings. *Environment:* 2%. *Note:* Total contributions made in fiscal 2000. **Typ. Recipients:** Health Policy/Cost Containment, Medical Education, Medical Research, Mental Health. **Geo. Dist:** nationally.

★ 11928 ★ Ruth and Vernon Taylor Foundation

518 17th St., Suite 1670
Denver, CO 80202
Phone: (303)893-5284 **Fax:** (303)893-8263
Friday Green, Trustee

Fnded: 1953. **Philosophy:** The foundation's charter decrees the areas of giving to be educational, religious, charitable, and scientific causes. Over the years, the foundation has expanded its interests to include the arts and humanities. **Priorities:** *Arts & Humanities:* 15%. Gives to museums, arts centers, and historic preservation. *Civic & Public Affairs:* 11%. Supports parks, zoos, and aquariums. *Education:* 16%. Primarily colleges and universities. *Environment:* 16%. Supports boys and girls clubs, respite care, and community associations. *International:* 7%. Funds biomedical and single-disease research. *Religion:* 3%. Funds aquariums. *Note:* Total contributions made in fiscal 2001. **Typ. Recipients:** Cancer, Child Abuse, Children's Health/Hospitals, Clinics/Medical Centers, Emergency/Ambulance Services, Family Planning, Health Funds, Health Organizations, Heart, Hospices, Hospitals, Medical Rehabilitation, Medical Research, People with Disabilities, Public Health, Research/Studies Institutes, Single-Disease Health Associations, Substance Abuse. **Geo. Dist:** nationally; Mid-Atlantic states; CO; IL; MT; TX; WY.

★ 11929 ★ S & G Foundation of Wyoming

No. 25185
PO Box 20,000
Jackson, WY 83001-7000
Phone: (914)351-2260
Gale Davis, Secretary & Treasurer

Fnded: 1998. **Priorities:** *Arts & Humanities:* Less than 1%. *Civic & Public Affairs:* 2%. Supports civic organizations and funds. *Education:* 93%. Supports higher education. Major grants to United World College and Colby College. *Environment:* Less than 1%. *Note:* Total contributions made in fiscal 2002. **Typ. Recipients:** People with Disabilities. **Geo. Dist:** nationally.

★ 11930 ★ S. H. Cowell Foundation

120 Montgomery St., Suite 2570
San Francisco, CA 94104
Phone: (415)397-0285 **Fax:** (415)986-6786
Website: http://www.shcowell.org
Susan Vandiver, Vice President Grants Programs

Fnded: 1955. **Philosophy:** The foundation supports a broad array of programs, and "is most interested in awarding grants to agencies which have clearly demonstrated community participation and support as well as evidence of private, non-governmental funding." The foundation's interests include aiding organizations concerned with the welfare of children and minorities; promoting the relative self-sufficiency of physically or mentally handicapped persons; providing general improvement in basic social programs in needy areas; assisting family planning organizations; supporting programs for the prevention of alcoholism; promoting job training programs; and providing for low-income housing. The foundation has recently begun placing greater emphasis on programs that offer affordable housing to the poor and programs that support public primary schools in high-density, low-income areas. It also focuses on the needs of Hispanics in California. Greater emphasis is being placed on serving the needs of children and families at risk in a comprehensive, coordinated way. The foundation's program in support of small arts organizations has been terminated. **Priorities:** *Arts & Humanities:* 1%. Supports the performing arts. *Civic & Public Affairs:* 41%. Funds housing and housing development, population concerns, and arms control. *Education:* 3%. Supports secondary schools and universities. *Environment:* 42%. Community programs, alcoholism, emergency relief, family planning, the United Way, and youth services. *International:* 6%. Funds health-care programs. *Note:* Total contributions made in 1998. **Typ. Recipients:** AIDS/HIV, Cancer, Child Abuse, Children's Health/Hospitals, Clinics/Medical Centers, Domestic Violence, Family Planning, Health Organizations, Medical Research, Nutrition, People with Disabilities, Public Health, Substance Abuse, Trauma Treatment. **Geo. Dist:** CA.

★ 11931 ★ S. H. and Helen R. Scheuer Family Foundation Inc.

350 Fifth Ave., Suite 1413
New York, NY 10118
Phone: (212)947-9009 **Fax:** (212)947-9770
Email: linda@61associates.com
Linda Ehrlich, Administrative Director

Fnded: 1943. **Philosophy:** The foundation gives most of its grants to local Jewish philanthropic, health, welfare, and higher education organizations; other support goes to arts and humanities, education, and social services. **Priorities:** *Arts & Humanities:* 13%. Funds archaeological research, opera, museums and theater. *Civic & Public Affairs:* 1%. *Education:* 30%. Funds colleges, universities, schools, and education funds. *Environment:* 2%. Includes YMHA/YWHAs. *International:* 2%. Supports medical centers, hospital funds and breast cancer research. *Note:* Total contributions made in fiscal 2000. **Typ. Recipients:** Clinics/Medical Centers, Domestic Violence, Family Planning, Geriatric Health, Hospitals, Medical Education, Mental Health, Nursing Services, People with Disabilities. **Geo. Dist:** New York, NY, metropolitan area.

★ 11932 ★ S. Mark Taper Foundation

12011 San Vicente Boulevard, Suite 400
Los Angeles, CA 90049-4986
Phone: (310)476-5413 **Fax:** (310)471-4993
Website: http://www.cerritos.edu/cerritos/development/funders_taper.html
Raymond Reisler, Executive Director

Fnded: 1989. **Priorities:** *Arts & Humanities:* 9%. Supports museums, historic preservation, theater, and music. *Civic & Public Affairs:* 12%. Supports community organizations and legal aid. *Environment:* 6%. Funds food banks and youth organizations. *International:* 69%. Supports hospitals, clinics, and single-disease health associations. Major grants to Cedars-Sinai Medical Center ($2,300,000) and National Institute of Transplantation ($1,265,000). *Note:* Total contributions made in 2001. **Typ. Recipients:** Child Abuse, Clinics/Medical Centers, Domestic Violence, Health Organizations, People with Disabilities, Prenatal Health Issues, Public Health, Sexual Abuse, Single-Disease Health Associations, Speech & Hearing, Substance Abuse, Transplant Networks/Donor Banks. **Geo. Dist:** CA.

★ 11933 ★ Sabbah Family Foundation

PO Box 19608
Greensboro, NC 27419-9608
Phone: (336)294-4494 **Fax:** (336)547-0840
Maurice Sabbah, President, Treasurer & Director

Fnded: 1987. **Priorities:** *Arts & Humanities:* Less than 1%. Funds art foundation. *Civic & Public Affairs:* 86%. Funds civic foundations. Major grant to Oklahoma Community Foundation ($18,000,000). *Education:* Less than 1%. Funds secondary and higher education. *Environment:* Less than 1%. Funds Young Men's Christian Association. *Note:* Total contributions made in fiscal 2000. **Typ. Recipients:** Cancer, Children's Health/Hospitals, Health-General, Hospices. **Geo. Dist:** Oklahoma City, OK.

★ 11934 ★ Sage Foundation

PO Box 1919
Brighton, MI 48116
Phone: (810)227-7660
Melissa Fadim, Chairman, President & Treasurer

Fnded: 1954. **Philosophy:** "In general, it is the objective of the Sage Foundation is to make grants and contributions that further charitable, religious, scientific, literary, and educational purposes. The Sage Foundation hopes and intends to accomplish these objectives through people and the actions of people." Sage Foundation 2001 Form 990. **Priorities:** *Arts & Humanities:* 52%. Supports music, arts institutes, music, and arts festivals. *Civic & Public Affairs:*

2%. *Education:* 6%. Emphasis on colleges and universities and secondary education. *Environment:* 6%. *International:* 26%. Focus on health funds and medical centers. *Note:* Total contributions made in 2000. **Typ. Recipients:** AIDS/HIV, Alzheimers Disease, Arthritis, Cancer, Children's Health/Hospitals, Clinics/Medical Centers, Domestic Violence, Emergency/Ambulance Services, Geriatric Health, Health Funds, Health Organizations, Heart, Hospices, Hospitals, Hospitals (University Affiliated), Long-Term Care, Medical Research, Mental Health, People with Disabilities, Public Health, Single-Disease Health Associations, Substance Abuse. **Geo. Dist:** nationally.

★ 11935 ★ St. Giles Foundation
420 Lexington Ave., Suite 2329
New York, NY 10170
Phone: (212)338-9001
Richard Arkwright, President

Fnded: 1979. **Philosophy:** The St. Giles Foundation has a special interest in medical science. It also funds hospitals and child services. **Priorities:** *Education:* 13%. Special education and student aid. *International:* 87%. Mainly supporting children's health, hospitals, and medical research. *Note:* Contributions made in fiscal 2001. **Typ. Recipients:** AIDS/HIV, Cancer, Children's Health/Hospitals, Clinics/Medical Centers, Health-General, Hospitals, Medical Education, Medical Rehabilitation, Medical Research, Mental Health, People with Disabilities, Prenatal Health Issues. **Geo. Dist:** NY.

★ 11936 ★ Samuel Freeman Charitable Trust
114 West 47th St.
New York, NY 10036-1532
Phone: (212)852-3629 **Fax:** (212)852-3377
Linda Franciscouicif, Contact

Fnded: 1981. **Philosophy:** The Samuel Freeman Charitable Trust makes grants across the major categories of support. Major interests include municipalities, colleges, cancer research, museums, and social services. **Priorities:** *Arts & Humanities:* 12%. Funds museums, theater, music, dance, libraries, and historic preservation. *Civic & Public Affairs:* 3%. Gives to aquariums, botanical gardens, philanthropic organizations, fire and police departments, and community action programs. *Education:* 44%. Supports colleges, universities, private/parochial schools, and education funds. *Environment:* 12%. Contributes to YMCA and animal welfare. *International:* 5%. Gives to hospitals, medical research, health foundations, cancer organizations and other single-disease health associations. *Religion:* 17%. Supports oceanography and biological research laboratories. *Note:* Total contributions made in 2000. **Typ. Recipients:** AIDS/HIV, Cancer, Clinics/Medical Centers, Diabetes, Eyes/Blindness, Family Planning, Health-General, Hospitals, Medical Education, Medical Research, Multiple Sclerosis, People with Disabilities, Single-Disease Health Associations, Substance Abuse. **Geo. Dist:** mid-Atlantic region.

★ 11937 ★ Samuel Goldwyn Foundation
9570 W Pico Blvd., Suite 400
Los Angeles, CA 90035
Phone: (310)473-7575 **Fax:** (310)860-3195
Meyer Gottlieb, Treasurer

Fnded: 1947. **Philosophy:** The foundation's trustees generally support all areas of philanthropy. In the past, large grants have been given to the arts. Libraries, theaters, museums, and public broadcasting have all received funding. Other interests include support for police academies, public education, the aged, child care, and a variety of health concerns. **Priorities:** *Arts & Humanities:* 46%. Supports museums, music, theater, film and video, dance, libraries, and public broadcasting. *Civic & Public Affairs:* 1%. Funds police, women's affairs, and foundations. *Education:* 24%. Contributes to pre-college schools, universities, centers for the learning disabled, and educational programs. *Environment:* 16%. Supports family planning services, youth organizations, homes, senior services, and disaster relief. *International:* 9%. Gives to clinics, hospitals, pediatric health, AIDS and cancer organizations, single-disease associations, and an eye institute. *Note:* Total contributions made in 2001. **Typ. Recipients:** AIDS/HIV, Cancer, Children's Health/Hospitals, Clinics/Medical Centers, Domestic Violence, Emergency/Ambulance Services, Eyes/Blindness, Family Planning, Health Funds, Health Organizations, Health-General, Heart, Hospitals, Long-Term Care, Mental Health, People with Disabilities, Research/Studies Institutes, Sexual Abuse, Single-Disease Health Associations, Speech & Hearing. **Geo. Dist:** nationally; Los Angeles, CA, metropolitan area; New York, NY, metropolitan area.

★ 11938 ★ Samuel I. Newhouse Foundation
335 Madison Ave., 9th Fl.
New York, NY 10017
Phone: (212)588-2200 **Fax:** (212)588-2222

Fnded: 1945. **Philosophy:** The foundation principally supports the arts, higher education, Jewish causes, and social services. **Priorities:** *Arts & Humanities:* 27%. Funds art centers, museums, libraries, and performing arts. *Civic & Public Affairs:* 17%. Supports towns and municipalities. *Education:* 21%. Supports higher education and scholarships. *Environment:* 9%. Primarily United Way. Also supports substance abuse and people with disabilities. *International:* 15%. Funds single-disease health associations, hospital, and medical research. *Note:* Total contributions made in fiscal 2001. **Typ. Recipients:** Cancer, Clinics/Medical Centers, Health Organizations, Heart, Hospitals, Medical Education, Medical Research, Mental Health, People with Disabilities, Single-Disease Health Associations, Substance Abuse. **Geo. Dist:** nationally; New York, NY.

★ 11939 ★ Samuel M. Soref and Helene K. Soref Foundation
50 S LaSalle St., Suite L-5
Chicago, IL 60675
Phone: (312)630-6000

Fnded: 1983. **Philosophy:** The foundation primarily grants major contributions to large, select Jewish organizations. **Priorities:** *Civic & Public Affairs:* 2%. Supports ethnic organizations. *Education:* 46%. Supports Jewish educational institutions and Judaic programs in non-Jewish schools, and universities. *Environment:* 9%. Suports homes, shelters, food banks, and senior services. *International:* 1%. *Note:* Total contributions made in 2000. **Typ. Recipients:** Children's Health/Hospitals, Emergency/Ambulance Services, Health Organizations, Hospitals, Long-Term Care, Medical Education, People with Disabilities, Speech & Hearing. **Geo. Dist:** CA; FL.

★ 11940 ★ Samuel N. and Mary Castle Foundation
The Pacific Garden Center, Makai Tower
733 Bishop St., Suite 1275
Honolulu, HI 96813
Phone: (808)522-1101 **Fax:** (808)522-1103
Email: acastle@aloha.net
Website: http://fdncenter.org/grantmaker/castle/
Alfred Castle, Executive Director

Fnded: 1925. **Philosophy:** The charter of the Samuel N. and Mary Castle Foundation reflects Mary Tenney Castle's desire "to support such charitable benevolence, religious and education purposes as the Trustees may from time to time decide." The foundation's purpose is "to make grants to appropriate charitable organizations primarily within the state of Hawaii." Through the years the foundation's interests have been primarily in the support of early education and care, private education, Protestant churches and arts and cultural organizations with ties to the Castle family. Mary Castle established the Henry and Dorothy Castle Memorial Fund in 1895, setting aside funds for the training and education of children. In 1953, the memorial became a funding source for organizations providing care and learning opportunities to young children. The foundation reports that projects targeting children (prenatal to age five) and their families are of priority interest. **Priorities:** *Arts & Humanities:* 14%. Funds music and theater focused on children, and public broadcasting. *Civic & Public Affairs:* 10%. Gives to community foundations and community development programs. *Education:* 56%. Primarily funds primary and preschool education; also supports some institutions of higher learning. *Environment:* 6%. Contributes to child welfare, family services, and youth activities. *International:* 1%. Public health organizations receive funding. *Note:* Total contributions made in 2001. **Typ. Recipients:** AIDS/HIV, Cancer, Children's Health/Hospitals, Emergency/Ambulance Services, Health Organizations, Hospices, Hospitals, Mental Health, People with Disabilities, Prenatal Health Issues, Respiratory, Speech & Hearing, Substance Abuse. **Geo. Dist:** HI.

★ 11941 ★ Samuel Roberts Noble Foundation
PO Box 2180
2510 Sam Noble Parkway
Ardmore, OK 73402
Phone: (580)223-5810 **Fax:** (580)221-6212
Email: macawley@noble.org
Website: http://www.noble.org
Michael Cawley, President & Trustee

Fnded: 1945. **Philosophy:** Because the trustees were given wide latitude in the activities that could be carried out, the foundation has been successful in adapting to the changing needs of society. By combining in-house research and traditional grant making, the foundation seeks to improve the quality of life in rural and urban communities. The foundation conducts research in the areas of plant biology research and agricultural research, consultation and demonstration. The plant biology division focuses on genetic engineering in plants. The agricultural division continues its interests in conservation, farming techniques, and agricultural economics. In addition to research, the division offers demonstration and consultation programs to regional farmers and ranchers. Although the foundation's main focus includes basic plant biology research and agricultural research, consultation, and demonstration, the foundation also awards grants in other areas when additional funds are available. Other areas of giving focus on capital funding for higher education, health research and delivery systems, and public affairs. Generally, these areas of giving remain geographically limited, with primary emphasis in Oklahoma. The foundation reports that in 1997 a new operating program in forage biotechnology was added to its in-house operations. 1997 Guidelines **Priorities:** *Arts & Humanities:* 4%. Supports historic preservation, music, museums, and art institutes. *Civic & Public Affairs:* 9%. Community affairs and public policy. *Education:* 54%. For research at colleges and universities, school building construction major grant to University of Oklahoma. *Environment:* 7%. Funds day care, Young Men's Christian Association. *International:* 22%. Health research and delivery systems. *Religion:* 1%. *Note:* About 70% of total giving supports organizations in Oklahoma. Total contributions made in fiscal 2000. **Typ. Recipients:** Cancer, Child Abuse, Children's Health/Hospitals, Clinics/Medical Centers, Diabetes, Domestic Violence, Emergency/Ambulance Services, Eyes/Blindness, Family Planning, Health Organizations, Health Policy/Cost Containment, Heart, Hospices, Hospitals, Medical Education, Medical Rehabilitation, Medical Research, Mental Health, Nursing Services, People with Disabilities, Preventive Medicine/Wellness Organizations, Public Health, Research/Studies Institutes, Single-Disease Health Associations, Substance Abuse, Transplant Networks/Donor Banks. **Geo. Dist:** Southwestern USA; OK.

★ 11942 ★ Samuel Rubin Foundation
777 United Nations Plaza, Suite 10D
New York, NY 10017
Phone: (212)697-8945 **Fax:** (212)682-0886
Website: http://www.samuelrubinfoundation.org
Cora Weiss, President

Fnded: 1949. **Philosophy:** The foundation's general purpose is to carry on the vision of its founder, Samuel Rubin, whose life was dedicated to the pursuit of peace and justice and the search for an equitable reallocation of the world's resources. The foundation believes that these objectives can be achieved only through the fullest implementation of social, economic, political, civil, and cultural rights for all people. **Priorities:** *Arts & Humanities:* 6%. Supports public broadcasting, cultural projects, and the performing arts. *Civic & Public Affairs:* 55%. Supports community affairs, economic projects, and peace and justice issues. *Education:* 8%. Supports schools, educational programs, and colleges. *International:* 1%. *Note:* Total contributions made in fiscal 2000. **Typ. Recipients:** Domestic Violence, Health-General, Hospitals, Medical Research. **Geo. Dist:** internationally; nationally.

★ 11943 ★ Samuel S. Fels Fund

1616 Walnut St., Suite 800
Philadelphia, PA 19103
Phone: (215)731-9455 **Fax:** (215)731-9457
Website: http://www.samfels.org
Helen Newbold, Executive Director

Fnded: 1935. **Philosophy:** "The general purpose of the Fund, as stated in the Charter, is to initiate and to assist any activities or projects of a scientific, educational or charitable nature which tend to improve human daily life and to bring to the average person greater health, happiness, and a fuller understanding of the meaning and purposes of life. To this end the Fund makes grants in the categories of Arts and Humanities, Education, Community Programs, and Health, all in the city of Philadelphia. The ideal proposal to Fels is one that addresses positive social change. We also mean to be useful to organizations at points of particular need such as expansion, experimentation, or reorganization or in times of particular need for advocacy. The Fund also runs an annual program, the Fels Internships in Community Service. Recent grantees are invited to submit descriptions of projects that could be done by graduate students over the course of ten weeks in the summer. Organizations whose projects are selected receive $6,000 to pay the graduate students, whom they select. The program is a way to draw talen to the not-for-profit sector and to carry out serious work on the community's behalf." *Samuel S. Fels Fund: A Report for the Year Ended December 31, 2001* **Priorities:** *Arts & Humanities:* 6%. Funds theater, ballet, fine arts, music, dance. *Civic & Public Affairs:* 54%. Supports botanical gardens/parks, ethnic organization, law and justice, women's affairs, and urban/community affairs. *Education:* 13%. Supports literacy, science/mathematics education, and legal education. *Environment:* 5%. Funds internships, free memberships. *International:* 12%. Gives to medical research, AIDS, prenatal health, issues, and clinics/medical centers. *Note:* Total contributions made in 2001. **Typ. Recipients:** Adolescent Health Issues, AIDS/HIV, Cancer, Child Abuse, Children's Health/Hospitals, Clinics/Medical Centers, Diabetes, Domestic Violence, Emergency/Ambulance Services, Family Planning, Health Organizations, Health Organizations, Home-Care Services, Hospitals, Long-Term Care, Nutrition, People with Disabilities, Prenatal Health Issues, Public Health. **Geo. Dist:** Philadelphia, PA.

★ 11944 ★ Sandra Atlas Bass and Edythe and Sol G. Atlas Fund

185 Great Neck Rd.
Great Neck, NY 11021
Phone: (516)487-9030 **Fax:** (516)466-6847
Sandra Bass, President

Fnded: 1962. **Philosophy:** The fund makes most of its grants in the areas of social services, health, and religion. Social service funding favors programs for the blind and disabled. Health support primarily funds single disease associations, while major support for religion goes to the United Jewish Federation Appeal. Other areas of interest include education, the arts, and international organizations. **Priorities:** *Civic & Public Affairs:* 2%. *Education:* 10%.Supports Veterinary Medical College and scholarships. *Environment:* 47%. Major support goes to animal rights, protection, and animal services. Also supports volunteer services. *International:* 21%. Supports single-disease associations, hospitals, and services for the blind. *Note:* Total contributions made in 2001. **Typ. Recipients:** Cancer, Children's Health/Hospitals, Diabetes, Emergency/Ambulance Services, Hospitals, Hospitals (University Affiliated), Kidney, Medical Education, Medical Research, Multiple Sclerosis, People with Disabilities, Respiratory, Single-Disease Health Associations, Trauma Treatment. **Geo. Dist:** Long Island, NY; New York, NY.

★ 11945 ★ Sapirstein-Stone-Weiss Foundation

One American Rd.
Cleveland, OH 44144
Phone: (216)252-7300 **Fax:** (216)252-6777
Gary Weiss, Vice President & Secretary

Fnded: 1952. **Philosophy:** The foundation is interested in supporting all major support categories for the Jewish faith. Social services, education, and religion are major priorities. Social service funding goes to Jewish community centers. Funding for education supports Jewish religious education and universities. **Priorities:** *Note:* Total contributions made in fiscal 2000. **Typ. Recipients:** Clinics/Medical Centers, Hospitals, Long-Term Care, People with Disabilities. **Geo. Dist:** Eastern USA.

★ 11946 ★ Sarah and Pauline Maier Foundation

PO Box 6190
Charleston, WV 25362
Phone: (304)343-2201 **Fax:** (304)343-2243
Email: edhmaier@genrlcorp.com
Edward Maier, President

Fnded: 1958. **Philosophy:** The foundation primarily supports higher education in West Virginia, including universities, colleges, legal education, and education funds. Other education related pursuits in Kanawha County, including the arts, a medical center, and civic affairs, are supported. The foundation awarded a 5 year grant of $3,000,000 to the Center for Arts and Sciences of West Virginia, Inc in 1996. **Priorities:** *Arts & Humanities:* 3%. Supports arts associations, theaters, and museums. *Civic & Public Affairs:* About 1%. *Education:* 96%. Supports West Virginia colleges. *International:* About 1%. Supports American Heart Association. *Note:* Total contributions made in fiscal 2000. **Typ. Recipients:** Clinics/Medical Centers, Heart, Medical Education. **Geo. Dist:** WV.

★ 11947 ★ Sarah Scaife Foundation

One Oxford Centre
301 Grant St., Suite 3900
Pittsburgh, PA 15219-6401
Phone: (412)392-2900
Website: http://www.scaife.com
Michael Gleba, Vice President, Programs

Fnded: 1941. **Philosophy:** The Sarah Scaife Foundation directs its resources primarily to the support of organizations involved in research, publications, and education concerning major domestic and international public policy issues. The foundation assists a variety of groups that provide decision makers and the general public with informed source material in a timely manner. **Priorities:** *Arts & Humanities:* 1%. Funds a historical society. *Civic & Public Affairs:* 62%. Supports public policy research and legal foundations. *Education:* 22%. Supports programs at colleges and universities, with a focus on domestic public policy and international studies. *Environment:* 1%. Funds Goodwill Industries. *International:* 2%. Funds a health policy institute. *Note:* Total contributions made in 1999. **Typ. Recipients:** Health Policy/Cost Containment, Medical Rehabilitation, People with Disabilities, Substance Abuse. **Geo. Dist:** nationally.

★ 11948 ★ Sarita Kenedy East Foundation Inc.

80 Pine St., Suite 1701
New York, NY 10005-1702
Phone: (212)701-3292
Margaret Devine, president

Fnded: 1962. **Philosophy:** The Sarita Kenedy East Foundation's major interest is supporting Roman Catholic churches, monasteries and religious organizations. Few grants are made outside the foundation's primary interest. **Priorities:** *Arts & Humanities:* 3%. Funds cultural and media initiatives. *Civic & Public Affairs:* 8%. Supports community initiatives. *Education:* 13%. Supports Catholic schools. *Environment:* 9%. Funds youth and family organizations. *International:* 18%. Supports medical services. *Note:* Total contributions made in 2001. **Typ. Recipients:** Cancer, Hospitals, Nursing Services, Outpatient Health Care, Public Health. **Geo. Dist:** nationally.

★ 11949 ★ Sarkeys Foundation

530 East Main St.
Norman, OK 73071
Phone: (405)364-3703 **Fax:** (405)364-8191
Website: http://www.sarkeys.org
Susan Frantz, Contact

Fnded: 1962. **Philosophy:** The foundation's mission is "to improve the quality of life in Oklahoma and the Southwest." Major areas of support include higher education, health care and medical research, and cultural and humanitarian programs of regional significance. **Priorities:** *Arts & Humanities:* 16%. Gives to arts associations, ballet libraries, theater, opera, historical societies, and museums. *Civic & Public Affairs:* 15%. Funds community foundations, citizens organizations, and botanical gardens. *Education:* 45%. Supports colleges and universities, literacy programs, and science, math, and arts education. *Environment:* 14%. Supports human services, community centers, at-risk youth, day care, domestic violence prevention, camps, and family services. *International:* 8%. Hospice and nursing care centers receive support. *Religion:* 2%. An aerospace science and technology center receives funding. *Note:* Total contributions made in 2001. **Typ. Recipients:** AIDS/HIV, Alzheimers Disease, Cancer, Child Abuse, Children's Health/Hospitals, Clinics/Medical Centers, Diabetes, Domestic Violence, Emergency/Ambulance Services, Eyes/Blindness, Family Planning, Health Organizations, Hospices, Hospitals, Medical Education, Medical Rehabilitation, Medical Research, Mental Health, People with Disabilities, Prenatal Health Issues, Public Health, Sexual Abuse, Single-Disease Health Associations, Speech & Hearing, Substance Abuse. **Geo. Dist:** OK.

★ 11950 ★ Scaife Family Foundation

One Oxford Centre
301 Grant St., Suite 3900
Pittsburgh, PA 15219-6401
Phone: (412)392-2900 **Fax:** (412)392-2922
Website: http://www.scaife.com/scaife.html
Joanne Beyer, Vice President, Secretary & Treasurer

Fnded: 1983. **Philosophy:** "The Scaife Family Foundation grant awards will support and develop programs that address the well-being of the family and traditional values. The Foundation will remain flexible in order to offer support in areas of importance as determined by the Trustees. Grant awards are not limited to a particular geographic area, but organizations and projects in the Pittsburgh and Western Pennsylvania area will be given special consideration." **Priorities:** *Arts & Humanities:* 12%. Major support for libraries and opera. *Civic & Public Affairs:* 27%. Supports employment, entrepreneurship, legal affairs issues, housing, economic development, and public policy groups. *Education:* 28%. Supports education funds, medical education, and universities. *Environment:* 21%. Supports family services, child welfare, United Way, youth organizations, and services for the disabled. *International:* 6%. Funds research, health foundations, hospitals, and single-disease associations. *Note:* Total contributions made in 1999. **Typ. Recipients:** Cancer, Child Abuse, Children's Health/Hospitals, Clinics/Medical Centers, Eyes/Blindness, Family Planning, Health Funds, Health Organizations, Hospices, Hospitals, Kidney, Medical Education, Medical Rehabilitation, Medical Research, Mental Health, Nursing Services, People with Disabilities, Prenatal Health Issues, Public Health, Single-Disease Health Associations, Speech & Hearing, Substance Abuse. **Geo. Dist:** nationally; PA, Western Pennsylvania; Pittsburgh, PA.

★ 11951 ★ Scherman Foundation
16 East 52nd St., Suite 601
New York, NY 10022-5306
Phone: (212)832-3086 **Fax:** (212)838-0154
Website: http://www.scherman.org
Sandra Silverman, President & Executive Director

Fnded: 1943. **Philosophy:** "The giving program of the Foundation emphasizes long-term general support, reflecting the Directors' commitment to sustained support for current grantees, and the belief that strong nonprofit leaders who are closest to the issues can best decide on the most effective use of grant funds. The main areas of interest of the Scherman Foundation are the environment, peace and security, reproductive rights, human rights and liberties, the arts, and social welfare. In the last two areas particularly, priority is given to organizations in New York City. The foundation emphasizes general support grants, as it is assumed that nonprofit organizations with strong leadership are better able than donors to decide on the most effective use of funds." **Priorities:** *Arts & Humanities:* 14%. Supports theaters, public broadcasting, dance, music, museum, opera, and arts festivals. *Civic & Public Affairs:* 17%. Funds public policy organizations in the fields Disarmament and Peace and Human Rights and Liberties. *Environment:* 49%. Under the category of Social Welfare, the foundation supports violence prevention, housing initiatives, youth organizations, and women's affairs. A major emphasis is reproductive rights and services. *Note:* Total contributions made in 2001. **Typ. Recipients:** AIDS/HIV, Domestic Violence, Family Planning, Family Planning, Health Organizations, Outpatient Health Care. **Geo. Dist:** New York, NY, emphasis on metropolitan New York City for the arts and social welfare.

★ 11952 ★ Schumann Fund for New Jersey
21 Van Vleck St.
Montclair, NJ 07042
Phone: (973)509-9883 **Fax:** (973)509-1149
Email: breisman@worldnet.att.net
Website: http://fdncenter.org/grantmaker/schumann/index.html
Barbara Reisman, Executive Director

Fnded: 1988. **Philosophy:** The Schumann Fund for New Jersey has established program priorities that fall into four broad categories to assist nonprofit organizations in New Jersey. The fund supports efforts to encourage academic and social success for young children, especially the urban poor, which enhance the potential for lifelong accomplishment through Early Childhood Development. The fund also supports the protection of natural resources and wildlife through sound land-use planning and balanced economic growth through its Environmental Protection grant program. Essex County, NJ, remains a priority as the fund supports local activities directed at solving community problems, with particular concern for families with young children, education, and social services. The fund also supports efforts to enhance the study, review, and public discussion of important policy issues facing New Jersey through its Public Policy program., particularly in the areas of school reform and educational innovation. Grant proposals that address the fund's priorities receive special consideration if they aim to permanently and positively change the way society deals with a problem, if the proposed project promises to become largely self-sufficient, and if the proposal indicates the recipient has invested a high level of time and/or money to the program. **Priorities:** *Civic & Public Affairs:* 36%. Supports philanthropic organizations, community foundations, urban/community affairs, law & justice, and public policy. *Environment:* 18%. Supports daycare, at-risk youth, family services, emergency services, and child welfare. *Note:* Total contributions made in 2000. **Typ. Recipients:** AIDS/HIV, Child Abuse, Diabetes, Family Planning, Health Organizations, Mental Health, Prenatal Health Issues, Public Health, Single-Disease Health Associations. **Geo. Dist:** NJ, Essex County.

★ 11953 ★ Schwartz Foundation
821 E Gate Dr.
Mount Laurel, NJ 08054
Bernard Schwartz, President

Fnded: 1983. **Philosophy:** The Schwartz Foundation is primarily interested in supporting Jewish religious organizations. **Priorities:** *Arts & Humanities:* 2%. Libraries and museums. *Civic & Public Affairs:* 86%. Community concerns and urban affairs. *Education:* 3%. Schools and a Hebrew academy. *Environment:* 2%. Crime prevention and youth services. *International:* 1%. *Note:* Total contributions made in fiscal 2001. **Typ. Recipients:** Alzheimers Disease, Geriatric Health, Multiple Sclerosis, People with Disabilities, Single-Disease Health Associations. **Geo. Dist:** PA, emphasis on Philadelphia.

★ 11954 ★ Scurlock Foundation
700 Louisiana, Suite 3920
Houston, TX 77002
Phone: (713)236-0550 **Fax:** (713)222-2419
Elizabeth Blanton Wareing, President

Fnded: 1954. **Priorities:** *Arts & Humanities:* 16%. Supports museums, opera, dance, fine arts, libraries, and theaters. *Civic & Public Affairs:* 23%. Funds zoos, parks, fire departments, and community organizations. *Education:* 47%. Supports colleges and universities, private secondary education, and special education. *International:* 7%. Supports hospitals, geriatric health, single-disease health associations, and cancer centers. *Note:* Total contributions made in 2000. **Typ. Recipients:** Cancer, Children's Health/Hospitals, Clinics/Medical Centers, Diabetes, Eyes/Blindness, Geriatric Health, Hospices, Hospitals, Hospitals (University Affiliated), Medical Education, Medical Research, Mental Health, Multiple Sclerosis, People with Disabilities, Public Health, Single-Disease Health Associations, Speech & Hearing. **Geo. Dist:** TX.

★ 11955 ★ Seabury Foundation
50 S LaSalle St.
Chicago, IL 60675
Phone: (312)630-6000
Tom Iskalis, Contact

Fnded: 1947. **Philosophy:** "The Seabury Foundation is a family foundation that funds projects in the areas of education, social services, health, conservation, and the arts in the city of Chicago. Particular emphasis is placed on programs that nurture strong family relationships, promote individual self-sufficiency, and encourage civic participation. The foundation seeks to improve access of all persons to the education, services, and resources that will support them in living secure, productive, and creative lives." **Priorities:** *Arts & Humanities:* 17%. Supports museums, historical society, theater, music, and art. *Civic & Public Affairs:* 14%. Supports neighborhoods, community affairs, and the Chicago Zoological Society. *Education:* 22%. Funds colleges, universities, educational services and programs. *Environment:* 27%. Girls Scouts of America, YMCA, youth and family services. *International:* 12%. Planned Parenthood, community health services, hospitals, hospice, and Down Syndrome National Association. *Note:* Total contributions made in 2000. **Typ. Recipients:** Adolescent Health Issues, Cancer, Children's Health/Hospitals, Clinics/Medical Centers, Domestic Violence, Emergency/Ambulance Services, Family Planning, Hospices, Hospitals, Medical Rehabilitation, Medical Research, Mental Health, Nursing Services, People with Disabilities, Prenatal Health Issues, Public Health, Single-Disease Health Associations. **Geo. Dist:** Chicago, IL, metropolitan area.

★ 11956 ★ The Seaver Institute
555 S Flower St. Suite 4580
Los Angeles, CA 90071
Phone: (213)673-2090 **Fax:** (213)673-2089
Email: seaverinstitute@aol.com
Victoria Seaver-Dean, President

Fnded: 1955. **Philosophy:** The Seaver Institute provides seed money to highly regarded organizations for particular projects which offer the potential for significant advancement in their fields. Although Science and Education have been the primary recipients of the Institute's benefactions, innovative projects in the Arts and Humanities are equally important. **Priorities:** *Arts & Humanities:* 6%. Funds museums and libraries. *Civic & Public Affairs:* 14%. Supports philanthropy. *Education:* 62%. Primary support for colleges and universities. *Environment:* 1%. *International:* Less than 1% *Religion:* 6%. Emphasis on the California Institute of Technology and the Woods Hole Oceanographic Institute. *Note:* Total contributions made in fiscal 2000. **Typ. Recipients:** Children's Health/Hospitals, Eyes/Blindness, Hospices, Hospitals, Medical Education, Medical Research, Research/Studies Institutes, Single-Disease Health Associations, Substance Abuse, Transplant Networks/Donor Banks. **Geo. Dist:** nationally.

★ 11957 ★ Second Foundation
1111 Superior Ave. Suite 1000
Cleveland, OH 44114-2507
Phone: (216)696-4200 **Fax:** (216)696-7303
Email: pranney@ssrl.com
Phillip Ranney, Secretary

Fnded: 1984. **Philosophy:** The Second Foundation makes most of its grants in the areas of higher education, projects related to the environment such as museums and libraries, and organizations located in Cuyahoga County previously supported by the foundation's founder. "Organizations promoting self-help by the recipients are looked upon favorably by the trustees." **Priorities:** *Arts & Humanities:* 15%. Supports libraries and museums. *Civic & Public Affairs:* 6%. Supports community development and a botanical garden. *Education:* 62%. Supports colleges and universities and scholarships. *Environment:* 6%. Supports Western Reserve Residences, senior citizen services, United Way. *International:* 6%. Funds elder care, hospice. *Religion:* 4. Supports science centers. *Note:* Total contributions made in 2000. **Typ. Recipients:** Child Abuse, Clinics/Medical Centers, Domestic Violence, Health Funds, Hospitals, Hospitals (University Affiliated), Research/Studies Institutes. **Geo. Dist:** OH, Cuyahoga County.

★ 11958 ★ Self Family Foundation
PO Box 1017
Greenwood, SC 29648-1017
Phone: (864)941-4011 **Fax:** (864)941-4091
Email: application@selffoundation.org
Website: http://www.selffoundation.org
Mamie Nicholson, Program Officer

Fnded: 1942. **Philosophy:** "Grantmaking is based on the belief that all communities have strengths as well as weaknesses, and that positive, long-term change occurs when a community's strengths serve as the basis for action. The Self Family Foundation will support organizations that help people rebuild their communities from the inside out by focusing on assets and mobilizing relationships between local institutions, businesses and residents. Primary geographic area of interest is Greenwood, South Carolina and surrounding counties. The Self Family Foundation will consider requests from other regions of South Carolina, if they have statewide impact. Primary grant target areas: Education–enhancing children's school readiness; working together with schools, families, youth-serving organizations and other community organizations to support the intellectual and social development of our young people. Health Care–individual and community wellness and prevention; revitalizing neighborhoods through collaboration with community organizations, businesses, public institutions and local residents. Secondary grant target areas: Arts, culture and history–increasing awareness of and access to activities specifically within Greenwood, South Carolina." *The Self Family Foundation Program Guidelines & Application Procedures* **Priorities:** *Arts & Humanities:* 3%. Supports arts councils, libraries, and opera. *Civic & Public Affairs:* 17%. Supports parks, inner-city development, community foundations, and Habitat for Humanity. *Education:* 42%. Supports local schools, literacy, colleges, universities, and enrichment programs. *Environment:* 30%. Supports United Way, domestic abuse, family services, animal protection, scouting, and camps. *International:* 8%. Supports children's health and hospice. *Note:* Total contributions made in 2000. **Typ. Recipients:** Adolescent Health Issues, Alzheimers Disease, Cancer, Child Abuse, Children's Health/Hospitals, Clinics/Medical Centers, Domestic Violence, Eyes/Blindness, Family Planning, Heart, Home-Care Services, Hospices, Hospitals, Medical Education, Medical Research, People with Disabilities, Research/Studies Institutes, Sexual Abuse. **Geo. Dist:** SC, emphasis on Greenwood area.

★ 11959 ★ Sequoia Foundation

PO Box 1278
Tacoma, WA 98401
Phone: (253)272-8336
Frank Underwood, Executive Director

Fnded: 1982. **Philosophy:** The current areas of geographic interest for conservation, environment, and social service grants are Mexico, Central America, the Himalayan Mountain region, and the Northwest United States. Grants are given in the foundation's program areas of conservation/environment and social services, where a component of the program is to generate or stabilize economic development. These program areas will tend to remain constant, but the geographic areas on which the foundation will focus its conservation and social service grants will change over time. Because the foundation intends to keep its programs flexible at all times, its focus will vary as conditions change and new needs arise. The Sequoia Foundation focuses its support on established organizations seeking to meet national and international needs rather than on local issues. **Priorities:** *Arts & Humanities:* 5%. Museums. *Civic & Public Affairs:* 1%. Chamber of Commerce. *Education:* 54%. Primary support for universities and preparatory schools. *Environment:* 37%. Focus on the New Horizon Foundation. *International:* 1%. *Note:* Total contributions made in fiscal 2001. **Typ. Recipients:** Family Planning, Health Organizations, Hospitals, Medical Education, Medical Rehabilitation, Mental Health, Public Health, Public Health. **Geo. Dist:** nationally, with emphasis on the Western and Northwestern USA; Seattle, WA; Tacoma, WA.

★ 11960 ★ Seth Sprague Educational and Charitable Foundation

114 W 47th St.
New York, NY 10036
Phone: (212)852-1000 **Fax:** (212)852-3377
Linda Franciscovich, Managing Director

Fnded: 1939. **Philosophy:** The foundation gives to a broad range of interests, with a focus on education, social services, community affairs, and health. **Priorities:** *Arts & Humanities:* 16%. Historic preservation, performing arts, and museums. *Civic & Public Affairs:* 12%. Employment and job training, botanical gardens, and community foundations. *Education:* 19%. Private precollege education, legal education, and colleges/universities. *Environment:* 19%. Substance abuse programs, youth organizations, and child welfare. *International:* 22%. Hospitals, AIDS/HIV, and medical centers. *Religion:* 7%. *Note:* Total contributions made in 2000. **Typ. Recipients:** AIDS/HIV, Arthritis, Cancer, Children's Health/Hospitals, Clinics/Medical Centers, Domestic Violence, Emergency/Ambulance Services, Family Planning, Geriatric Health, Health Funds, Health Organizations, Health-General, Hospices, Hospitals, Medical Education, Medical Rehabilitation, Medical Research, Medical Training, Mental Health, Nursing Services, People with Disabilities, Single-Disease Health Associations, Substance Abuse. **Geo. Dist:** nationally; MA; NY.

★ 11961 ★ Seymour H. Knox Foundation

1 HSBC Center Suite 3840
Buffalo, NY 14203
Phone: (716)854-6811 **Fax:** (716)856-0517
Email: kbojw@aol.com
James Wendel, Assistant Secretary & Assist. Treasurer

Fnded: 1945. **Philosophy:** The foundation lists the following giving areas: arts and music, universities and schools, hospitals and health organizations, civic organizations, United Way and Red Cross, and religious activities. **Priorities:** *Arts & Humanities:* 15%. Supports historical societies, arts groups, and museums. *Civic & Public Affairs:* 4%. Supports civic groups. *Education:* 51%. Funds colleges, universities, and precollege educational institutions. *Environment:* 12%. Gives to united funds and youth groups. *International:* 6%. Gives to hospitals, hospices, and medical research. *Note:* Total contributions made in 1999. **Typ. Recipients:** Alzheimers Disease, Cancer, Children's Health/Hospitals, Family Planning, Health Funds, Hospices, Hospitals, Medical Education, Medical Rehabilitation, Medical Research, People with Disabilities, Speech & Hearing, Substance Abuse, Trauma Treatment. **Geo. Dist:** nationally; Buffalo, NY.

★ 11962 ★ Sherman Fairchild Foundation, Inc.

5454 Wisconsin Ave. Suite 1205
Chevy Chase, MD 20815
Phone: (301)913-5990 **Fax:** (301)913-9444
Website: http://www.990pf.org
Bonnie Himmelman, President

Fnded: 1955. **Philosophy:** The foundation generally emphasizes the following areas: education, particularly colleges and universities; health and medical research; and, to a lesser extent, the arts and social services. **Priorities:** *Arts & Humanities:* 36%. Supports libraries, the performing arts, fine arts. *Civic & Public Affairs:* Approx. 1%. *Education:* 48%. Supports colleges, universities, school, and scholarship. *Environment:* 6%. Supports athletics and youth programs. *International:* 7%. Supports hospital and medical research. *Note:* Total contributions made in 2000. **Typ. Recipients:** Cancer, Children's Health/Hospitals, Clinics/Medical Centers, Health Funds, Hospitals, Medical Education, Medical Research. **Geo. Dist:** nationally; New York, NY, including metropolitan area.

★ 11963 ★ Shoreland Foundation

1 Comac Loop, Unit 9
Ronkonkoma, NY 11779-6816
Fax: (631)737-1974
Carol-Ann Mealy, Contact

Fnded: 1994. **Philosophy:** The foundation focuses on the arts, health care, and education. **Priorities:** *Arts & Humanities:* 24%. Large grant to the Metropolitan Museum of Art in New York, NY. *Civic & Public Affairs:* 2%. Funds women's issues and public safety. *Education:* 70%. Major grant to Wellesley College. *Environment:* 1%. Funds youth programs. *International:* Less than 1%. Funds single-disease health associations. *Religion:* Less than 1%. Supports natural history museum. *Note:* Total contributions made in 1999. **Typ. Recipients:** AIDS/HIV, Alzheimers Disease, Cancer, Children's Health/Hospitals, Eyes/Blindness, Geriatric Health, Health Organizations, Health-General, Hospitals, People with Disabilities, Substance Abuse. **Geo. Dist:** nationally.

★ 11964 ★ Shubert Foundation

234 W 44th St.
New York, NY 10036
Phone: (212)944-3777 **Fax:** (212)944-3767
Vicki Reiss, Executive Director

Fnded: 1945. **Philosophy:** The goal of the foundation's grants program "is to build and perpetuate the live performing arts, particularly the professional theatre, in the United States. Accomplishment of this goal involves support both of the theatrical institutions and of those other elements of the performing arts and related institutions that are necessary to maintain and support the theatre." Schubert Foundation fiscal 1999 IRS Form 990. Professional resident theater organizations in the United States are the major recipients of Shubert financial support. The foundation also supports "dance because it is a critical performing art form related to and supportive of the theater." The foundation also recognizes the importance of private graduate theater education. **Priorities:** *Arts & Humanities:* 92%. Primarily supports theater organizations. *Education:* 7%. Supports arts education. *Note:* Contributions made in fiscal 2001. **Typ. Recipients:** Clinics/Medical Centers, Hospitals (University Affiliated). **Geo. Dist:** nationally.

★ 11965 ★ Sid W. Richardson Foundation

309 Main St.
Fort Worth, TX 76102
Phone: (817)336-0494 **Fax:** (817)332-2176
Email: cjohns@sidrichardson.org
Website: http://www.sidrichardson.org
Mr. Valleau Wilkie, Jr., Executive Vice President

Fnded: 1947. **Philosophy:** The foundation believes it can best serve the state of Texas through its support of both tax-supported groups and nonprofit organizations. In education, it emphasizes support to public elementary and secondary schools, and faculty development programs. Health interests include preventive medicine and efforts to improve the delivery of efficient health care and research. In the areas of the arts, human services, and community projects, the foundation focuses on the needs of the Ft. Worth area. **Priorities:** *Arts & Humanities:* 16%. Art councils and symphony support. *Civic & Public Affairs:* 5%. Housing services, community initiatives and women's centers. *Education:* 36%. Primarily universities. *Environment:* 8%. Supports family services, elderly and youth programs. *International:* 29%. Medical research, universities, and healthcare programs. *Religion:* 1%. *Note:* Total contributions made in 2000. **Typ. Recipients:** Cancer, Children's Health/Hospitals, Clinics/Medical Centers, Diabetes, Emergency/Ambulance Services, Eyes/Blindness, Family Planning, Health Organizations, Health Policy/Cost Containment, Health-General, Heart, Hospitals, Hospitals (University Affiliated), Medical Education, Medical Research, Nursing Services, Outpatient Health Care, People with Disabilities, Prenatal Health Issues, Public Health, Research/Studies Institutes, Research/Studies Institutes, Substance Abuse. **Geo. Dist:** Ft. Worth, TX, some giving in other areas of Texas.

★ 11966 ★ Sidney J. Weinberg, Jr. Foundation

BCRS Associates LLC
100 Wall St., 11th Flr.
New York, NY 10005
Phone: (212)440-0800
Sydney Weinberg, Jr., Trustee

Fnded: 1979. **Philosophy:** The foundation makes most of its grants in the areas of health care, education, and civic affairs. Health care funding favors hospitals, cancer research, pediatrics, and single disease associations. Funding in education emphasizes colleges, universities, and business education. Support for civic affairs goes to the Carnegie Institute in Washington, DC, and economic development. The foundation also will fund the arts, religion, and social services. **Priorities:** *Arts & Humanities:* 6%. Museums, historic preservation. *Civic & Public Affairs:* 4%. *Education:* 48%. Precollege private education, colleges and universities, and business education. *Environment:* About 1%. *International:* 34%. Hospitals, Cystic Fibrosis research, aging research, and medical centers. *Religion:* 5%. Carnegie Institution and oceanography. *Note:* Total contributions made in fiscal 2001. **Typ. Recipients:** Cancer, Children's Health/Hospitals, Clinics/Medical Centers, Emergency/Ambulance Services, Family Planning, Geriatric Health, Health Funds, Health Organizations, Health-General, Heart, Hospices, Hospitals, Hospitals (University Affiliated), Medical Education, Medical Research, Mental Health, Nursing Services, People with Disabilities, Preventive Medicine/Wellness Organizations, Single-Disease Health Associations, Substance Abuse. **Geo. Dist:** nationally; New York, NY.

★ 11967 ★ Sidney Stern Memorial Trust

PO Box 893
Pacific Palisades, CA 90272
Phone: (310)459-2117
Peter Hoffenberg, Member, Board of Advisors

Fnded: 1974. **Philosophy:** The board of directors of the Sidney Stern Memorial Trust reviews all requests for grants. "The Board endeavors to support soundly managed charitable organizations which give service with broad scope, affect favorably their target populations, and contribute materially to the general welfare. The Board gives priority to the following areas: education, health and science, community service projects, youth, services to the physically and mentally disabled, the arts, and organizations and activities serving California." **Priorities:** *Arts & Humanities:* 1%. Primarily supports public broadcasting. *Civic & Public Affairs:* 12%. Funding for legal aid, public policy organizations, womens affairs, civil rights, zoos, Native American affairs. *Education:* 24%. Supports colleges and universities, special education, literacy, medical schools, religious education, and minority education. *Environment:* 20%. Emphasis on people with disabilities, family services, youth organizations, community services, food distribution programs, child welfare homes, family planning services, young men's christian association, and senior services. *International:* 18%. Supports hospitals, medical clinics, pediatric health, and medical research. *Note:* Total contributions made in fiscal 2000. **Typ. Recipients:** AIDS/HIV, Arthritis, Children's Health/Hospitals, Clinics/Medical Centers, Domestic Violence, Emergency/Ambulance Services, Eyes/Blindness, Family Planning, Health Organizations, Health-General, Hospitals, Kidney, Long-Term Care, Medical Education, Medical Education, Medical Research, Mental Health, Multiple Sclerosis, People with Disabilities, Prenatal Health Issues, Preventive Medicine/Wellness Organizations, Public Health, Research/Studies Institutes, Single-Disease Health Associations, Substance Abuse. **Geo. Dist:** nationally; CA.

★ 11968 ★ Siebert Lutheran Foundation

2600 North Mayfair Rd., Suite 390
Wauwatosa, WI 53226-1392
Phone: (414)257-2656 **Fax:** (414)257-1387
Email: siebertf@execpc.com
Website: http://www.SiebertFoundation.org
Ronald Jones, President

Fnded: 1952. **Philosophy:** The foundation concentrates its grant-making activities on the Lutheran community, primarily Lutheran churches and institutions in the state of Wisconsin. Currently, the foundation supports education, and training, community development and outreach, health care, child care, care for the aging, social services with a focus on inner-city service projects, and evangelism and youth. The foundation also sponsors a program which provides financial aid to congregations in Wisconsin on behalf of seminary students. **Priorities:** *Civic & Public Affairs:* 4%. Primarily for community services. *Education:* 57%. Primarily for religious education, private schools, and education associations. *Environment:* 6%. Emphasis on child welfare. *Note:* Total contributions made in 2000. **Typ. Recipients:** AIDS/HIV, Cancer, Clinics/Medical Centers, Geriatric Health, Hospitals, Long-Term Care, Nursing Services, People with Disabilities, Public Health. **Geo. Dist:** WI.

★ 11969 ★ Sierra Foundation

33 Witherspoon St., 3rd Floor
Princeton, NJ 08542-3209
Phone: (609)921-9071
Martin Deitchman, Treasurer

Fnded: 1994. **Priorities:** *Education:* 18%. Primarily supports universities. *International:* 61%. Supports medical research, vision services, and health foundations. *Note:* Total contributions made in fiscal 2000. **Typ. Recipients:** Alzheimers Disease, Eyes/Blindness, Geriatric Health, Health-General, Mental Health, Single-Disease Health Associations. **Geo. Dist:** NY.

★ 11970 ★ Sierra Health Foundation

1321 Garden Highway
Sacramento, CA 95833
Phone: (916)922-4755 **Fax:** (916)922-4024
Email: info@sierrahealth.org
Website: http://www.sierrahealth.org/
Len McCandliss, President & Chief Executive Officer

Fnded: 1984. **Philosophy:** "The foundation engages in an array of activities that support improved health for Northern Californians. Grantmaking, both in well-defined focus areas and for more general purposes, is a major function of the foundation. But equally important is the foundation's drive to stimulate collaboration, promote dialogue and share successful strategies throughout the region. By partnering with other foundations, grant recipients and community leaders, the foundation works to leverage resources and ensure effective outcomes." Currently, the foundation supports three key program areas: health grants, the Community Partnerships for Healthy Children (CPHC) Initiative, and the Conference Program. **Priorities:** *International:* 100%. Supports health and health-related activites in 26 northern California counties. The foundation focuses its giving on local and regional health-related programs and services, influencing public health policy and choices, and stimulating major improvements in California's health care system. *Note:* Total contributions made in 1999. **Typ. Recipients:** Adolescent Health Issues, AIDS/HIV, Cancer, Child Abuse, Children's Health/Hospitals, Clinics/Medical Centers, Domestic Violence, Emergency/Ambulance Services, Eyes/Blindness, Family Planning, Geriatric Health, Health Organizations, Health Policy/Cost Containment, Heart, Hospices, Hospitals, Long-Term Care, Medical Education, Medical Research, Mental Health, Nursing Services, Outpatient Health Care, People with Disabilities, Prenatal Health Issues, Public Health, Research/Studies Institutes, Respiratory, Single-Disease Health Associations, Trauma Treatment. **Geo. Dist:** CA, 26 counties in Northern California.

★ 11971 ★ Skillman Foundation

600 Renaissance Center, Suite 1700
Detroit, MI 48243
Phone: (313)393-1185 **Fax:** (313)393-1187
Email: mailbox@skillman.org
Website: http://www.skillman.org
Kari Schlachtenhaufen, President

Fnded: 1960. **Philosophy:** "The Skillman Foundation is a resource for improving the lives of children in Metropolitan Detroit. The Foundation funding priorities from 2001-2005 are: Quality pre-school experiences for very young children will be widely available, Families of newborns and very young children will be supported through home visits, Prenatal care will be normal for pregnant women, schools principals will be strong academic and community leaders, communities and schools will have high expectations for school performance and student achievement, Child friendly spaces (playgrounds, parks, community centers and housing) will be created in neighborhoods where there are lots of children and few positive activities or institutions, Neighborhood institutions such as churches, schools and nonprofits will be better able to support the full development of children, and Children's achievement is recognized and encouraged in the community and in the home." **Priorities:** *Arts & Humanities:* 17%. Supports libraries, public broadcasting, museums, and performing arts. *Civic & Public Affairs:* 14%. Funds juvenile justice concerns, youth development, minority affairs, and strengthening civic institutions. *Education:* 18%. Supports primary and secondary education with a focus on early childhood education and public school improvement. Also funds colleges, universities, and minority education. Provides college scholarships to individuals through the Skillman Scholars program. *Environment:* 33%. Supports children, youth, and family program areas. Also supports basic human needs causes and community services. The United Way also receives a contribution. *International:* 6%. Directs funding toward child and family health programs. *Religion:* 9%. Provides major funding for a science center. *Note:* Total contributions made in fiscal 2000. **Typ. Recipients:** Adolescent Health Issues, AIDS/HIV, Child Abuse, Children's Health/Hospitals, Domestic Violence, Family Planning, Health Organizations, Health Policy/Cost Containment, Hospitals, Medical Education, Medical Research, Mental Health, Nursing Services, People with Disabilities, Prenatal Health Issues, Preventive Medicine/Wellness Organizations, Public Health, Research/Studies Institutes, Respiratory, Substance Abuse, Trauma Treatment. **Geo. Dist:** MI, Wayne, Oakland, and Macomb Counties; Detroit, MI.

★ 11972 ★ Skirball Foundation

767 Fifth Ave., Suite 5001
New York, NY 10153
Phone: (212)832-8500 **Fax:** (212)593-6241
Martin Blackman, President

Fnded: 1950. **Philosophy:** The Skirball Foundation has had close ties with Hebrew Union College and the University of Southern California. The Skirballs helped fund the Hubbard Chair in British History, in honor of USC president emeritus John Hubbard. Mr. Skirball, a member and vice chairman of the board of governors at Hebrew Union College, was actively involved in the college's decision to accept then USC president Norman Topping's invitation to the college to locate its Los Angeles campus adjacent to the University The Skirball Cancer Pharmacology Laboratory is part of a major addition to the Kenneth Norris Jr. Cancer Hospital and Research Institute that opened in late 1991 on USC's Health Sciences Campus. The foundation is also a supporter of the arts and created the Skirball Museum at Hebrew Union College, one of the world's finest museums of Jewish culture. The Skirball Center serves biblical scholars, archaeologists, and students of biblical and ancient Near Eastern history, and preserves and exhibits the findings of excavations. The fund will also make possible a research and fellowships award program for study in the archaeology of the ancient Near East. **Priorities:** *Arts & Humanities:* 78%. Provides major support to the Skirball Cultural Center; also funds performing arts programs and centers. *Civic & Public Affairs:* 1%. Gives to legal aid organizations, urban development, and community organizations. *Education:* 9%. Funds colleges and universities. *Environment:* Less than 1%. *International:* 6%. Supports pediatric health funds and facilities, hospitals, medical centers, and single-disease health associations. *Note:* Total contributions made in 2000. **Typ. Recipients:** Arthritis, Cancer, Children's Health/Hospitals, Clinics/Medical Centers, Eyes/Blindness, Geriatric Health, Health Organizations, Health-General, Heart, Hospitals, Long-Term Care, Medical Education, Medical Research, People with Disabilities, Research/Studies Institutes, Single-Disease Health Associations, Speech & Hearing, Substance Abuse. **Geo. Dist:** Los Angeles, CA; New York, NY; Cincinnati, OH.

★ 11973 ★ Slemp Foundation

PO Box 5208 M.L. CN-WN-05EB
Cincinnati, OH 45201
Phone: (513)762-8878
Patricia Durbin, Trust Officer

Fnded: 1943. **Priorities:** *Arts & Humanities:* 8%. Supports art centers and libraries. *Civic & Public Affairs:* 1%. *Education:* 86%. Supports colleges, universities, and public schools. *Environment:* 4%. Primarily supports scouts. *International:* 1%. *Note:* Total contributions made in fiscal 2001. **Typ. Recipients:** Cancer, Child Abuse, Children's Health/Hospitals, Clinics/Medical Centers, Emergency/Ambulance Services, Hospices, People with Disabilities. **Geo. Dist:** VA, Lee County; VA, Wise County.

★ 11974 ★ Smart Family Foundation

74 Pin Oak Lane
Wilton, CT 06897-1329
Phone: (203)834-0400 **Fax:** (203)834-0412
Raymond Smart, President

Fnded: 1951. **Philosophy:** The foundation funds a wide variety of projects across all major categories. **Priorities:** *Arts & Humanities:* 28%. Supports museums, performing arts centers, libraries, music, and theater. *Civic & Public Affairs:* 13%. Supports civic and public affairs, municipalities. *Education:* 30%. Funds colleges, universities, primary and secondary schools, and educational programs. *Environment:* 5%. Funds YMHA, YWHA, youth councils. *International:* 1%. Supports health research, senior citizen's health. *Religion:* 2%. Supports the Aspen Center for Physics. *Note:* Total contributions made in 1999. **Typ. Recipients:** Clinics/Medical Centers, Eyes/Blindness, Family

Planning, Geriatric Health, Health Organizations, Hospitals, Hospitals (University Affiliated), Medical Education, Medical Research, Mental Health, People with Disabilities, Research/Studies Institutes, Substance Abuse. **Geo. Dist:** nationally.

★ 11975 ★ Smith Richardson Foundation
60 Jesup Rd.
Westport, CT 06880
Phone: (203)222-6222 **Fax:** (203)222-6282
Email: msteinmeyer@srf.org
Website: http://www.srf.org
Peter Richardson, President

Fnded: 1935. **Philosophy:** "The Smith Richardson Foundation supports programs that are consistent with the vision of its founder. H. Smith Richardson wrote that 'the need for the time and thought of able men is that they be applied to the increasingly weighty problems of government and the serious social questions which now confront us and will continue to press for solution in the future.' The Foundation's main objective, therefore, is the funding of pragmatic research and programs which seek to inform important public and foreign policy debates. In order to achieve this goal most effectively, the Foundation divides its grant making into two general program areas: international and domestic." "The Foundation's International Affairs program supports programs and research projects on security issues central to the interests of the United States. Such projects seek to define the important challenges facing the United States in the post-cold war security environment, to illuminate key issues affecting U.S. interests in Europe, the former Soviet Union, East Asia and the Middle East, and to underwrite historical research with clear implications or lessons for current policy." "The Foundation's Domestic program supports research on the public policy issues that affect children and families at risk. Accordingly, it supports projects that investigate 'what works' in social programs and that propose and evaluate models for more effective responses to the problems facing children and families in poverty. The Foundation also supports domestic public policy projects in such areas as education and government reform when such projects share similar qualities of pragmatism and applied scholarship." "Generally, the Foundation makes grants only to support research projects. However, a small portion of its funding is reserved for worthy direct service grants within the states of Connecticut and North Carolina, where the Foundation has its offices." **Priorities:** *Arts & Humanities:* 2%. *Civic & Public Affairs:* 44%. Primarily supports foreign public policy programs, domestic political and public policy institutes, and international security. *Education:* 44%. Supports educational research at universities. *Environment:* 5%. Supports family service organizations. *International:* 5%. Health research and hospitals. *Note:* Total contributions approved in 2000. **Typ. Recipients:** Cancer, Child Abuse, Children's Health/Hospitals, Domestic Violence, Family Planning, Health Policy/Cost Containment, Long-Term Care, Medical Education, Public Health, Single-Disease Health Associations. **Geo. Dist:** nationally; limited giving internationally.

★ 11976 ★ Sol Goldman Charitable Trust
640 5th Ave., 3rd Floor
New York, NY 10019
Phone: (212)265-2280 **Fax:** (212)265-2592
Amy Goldman, Trustee

Fnded: 1988. **Priorities:** *Education:* 54%. Supports educational initiatives. *Environment:* 5%. Community groups, children's services, and Special Olympics received funding. *International:* 29%. Supports hospitals, medical research, single-disease causes, and AIDS research. *Note:* Total contributions made in fiscal 1999. **Typ. Recipients:** AIDS/HIV, Cancer, Children's Health/Hospitals, Clinics/Medical Centers, Family Planning, Hospitals, Kidney, Medical Education, Medical Research, Mental Health, Multiple Sclerosis, People with Disabilities, Prenatal Health Issues, Research/Studies Institutes, Single-Disease Health Associations, Speech & Hearing. **Geo. Dist:** NY.

★ 11977 ★ Solon E. Summerfield Foundation, Inc.
1270 Ave. of the Americas
New York, NY 10020-1801
Phone: (212)218-7640
William Prager, Jr., President

Fnded: 1939. **Philosophy:** Education receives the majority of support from the Solon E. Summerfield Foundation. Jewish organizations and groups concerned with blindness and visual impairment also receive large grants from the foundation. Almost 80% of the foundation's funds are set aside for these and other pre-selected organizations. Generally, for new proposals, the foundation makes smaller contributions to many organizations with a wide variety of interests. **Priorities:** *Education:* 56%. Colleges and universities. *Environment:* 22%. Children's welfare organizations are primary recipients. *International:* 8%. Nurse services, hospitals, and foundation for the blind. *Note:* Total contributions made in 2000. **Typ. Recipients:** Child Abuse, Child Abuse, Clinics/Medical Centers, Domestic Violence, Emergency/Ambulance Services, Eyes/Blindness, Health Organizations, Hospitals, Long-Term Care, Medical Education, Medical Research, Mental Health, Nursing Services, People with Disabilities, Research/Studies Institutes. **Geo. Dist:** nationally; Northeast USA; New York, NY.

★ 11978 ★ Sosland Foundation
4800 Main St., Suite 100
Kansas City, MO 64112-2504
Phone: (816)756-1000 **Fax:** (816)756-0494
Debbie Sosland-Edelman, Executive Director

Fnded: 1955. **Philosophy:** The foundation supports a wide range of institutions, with at least half of the total awards going to Jewish philanthropies. The purpose of each grant "is to further the causes, whether they be civic, cultural, or religious, of each organization." Grants by the foundation are generally given for unrestricted general support. **Priorities:** *Arts & Humanities:* 15%. *Civic & Public Affairs:* 2%. *Education:* 11%. Focus on education funds, promary and secondary education, Jewish studies, and colleges and universities. *Environment:* 25%. United funds, child welfare, family services, and youth organizations. *International:* 16%. *Religion:* 8%. *Note:* Total contributions made in fiscal 1998. **Typ. Recipients:** AIDS/HIV, Children's Health/Hospitals, Clinics/Medical Centers, Emergency/Ambulance Services, Family Planning, Health Organizations, Hospitals, Medical Rehabilitation, Mental Health. **Geo. Dist:** Kansas City, KS, metropolitan area; Kansas City, MO, metropolitan area.

★ 11979 ★ South Texas Charitable Foundation
PO Box 2549
Victoria, TX 77902
Fax: (361)573-4383
Rayford Keller, Secretary-Treasurer

Fnded: 1981. **Philosophy:** The South Texas Charitable Foundation makes most of its grants to Christian religious organizations and social service organizations. Other interests include hospitals, religious education, community emergency services, and counseling. **Priorities:** *Arts & Humanities:* 1%. Performing arts center. *Civic & Public Affairs:* 4%. Supports fire departments. *Environment:* 35%. Supports food banks, elderly services, and social service groups. *International:* 16%. Contributes to hospitals and hospices. *Note:* Total contributions made in 2001. **Typ. Recipients:** Cancer, Children's Health/Hospitals, Domestic Violence, Emergency/Ambulance Services, Heart, Hospices, Hospitals, Long-Term Care, Medical Rehabilitation, People with Disabilities, Sexual Abuse, Single-Disease Health Associations, Substance Abuse. **Geo. Dist:** TX.

★ 11980 ★ Spencer Foundation
875 North Michigan Ave., Suite 3930
Chicago, IL 60611-1803
Phone: (312)337-7000 **Fax:** (312)337-0282
Email: information@spencer.org
Website: http://www.spencer.org
Paul Goren, Vice President

Fnded: 1962. **Philosophy:** "The Foundation has as its primary mission, by the intent of its founder, 'to investigate ways in which education can be improved, around the world.' To achieve this goal, the Foundation is committed to supporting high quality investigation of education through its research programs and to strengthening and renewing the educational research community through fellowship programs and related activities. The Foundation defines education broadly to include all the situations and institutions in which education proceeds, across the entire life span. An important expectation of the Foundation is that the activities it supports, taken together over the years, will contribute significantly to the enhancement of educational opportunity for all people." "The Foundation's programs are organized within three divisions: Research, Fellowships, and Training. In addition, a handful of programs are also operated out of the Office of the Vice President. Programs in the Research Division support work that shows promise of contributing new knowledge, understanding, and improvement of educational thought and practice. Programs in the Fellowship Division support educational researchers at different stages of their professional careers, providing resources to both beginning and senior researchers to pursue concentrated intellectual activity. Programs in the Training Division are aimed at improving the work and performance of agencies and institutions, mainly universities and graduate schools of education at universities, which hold a mission of training and apprenticing educational researchers. Funding programs within the Vice President's Office are experimental or developmental, spanning and augmenting the other divisions' programmatic objectives." 2000 Application and Review Information **Priorities:** *Education:* 99%. Supports colleges and universities, foreign schools, and research institutes. Within education, the foundation supports a broad range of disciplinary and interdisciplinary categories, primarily through the granting of fellowships and research grants. *Note:* Total contributions made in fiscal 2001. **Typ. Recipients:** Children's Health/Hospitals, Mental Health. **Geo. Dist:** internationally; nationally.

★ 11981 ★ Spencer T. and Ann W. Olin Foundation
7701 Forsyth Boulevard, Suite 1040
Saint Louis, MO 63105
Phone: (314)727-6202 **Fax:** (314)727-6157
Warren Shapleigh, President

Fnded: 1957. **Philosophy:** "The principal interests of the foundation are in the fields of higher education, medical education and research, health services and facilities, and environmental conservation...Support is also given to community needs in the metropolitan St. Louis area, including cultural, civic and welfare programs." **Priorities:** *Arts & Humanities:* 1% Supports performing and contemporary art primarily in St. Louis, MO, the symphony and theater. *Civic & Public Affairs:* 5% Supports community and public affairs, philanthropy, and botanical gardens. *Education:* 31% Supports educational programs and institutions, medical education, and arts/humanities education. *Environment:* 29% supports the United Way, youth and family services, the elderly, and disabled, animal protection, Young Men's Christian Association/Young Women's Christian Association and people with disabilities. *International:* 12% Supports hospice, research and treatment fund, Alzheimer's Association and other disease and disorder concerns. *Religion:* Less than 1%. *Note:* Contributions were made in 2001. **Typ. Recipients:** Alzheimers Disease, Arthritis, Cancer, Clinics/Medical Centers, Emergency/Ambulance Services, Family Planning, Geriatric Health, Hospices, Hospitals, Medical Education, Nursing Services, People with Disabilities, Preventive Medicine/Wellness Organizations. **Geo. Dist:** nationally.

★ 11982 ★ Spring/Close Foundation
1826 Second Baxter Crossing
Fort Mill, SC 29708
Phone: (803)548-2002 **Fax:** (803)548-1797
Angela McRae, President

Fnded: 1968. **Priorities:** *Arts & Humanities:* Less than 1%. Supports humanities. *Civic & Public Affairs:* 25%. Focus on community affairs. *Education:* 40%. Including a large grant to the University of South Carolina - Lancaster. *Environment:* 23%. Primarily supports athletics and recreation, animal protection, people with disabilities, and shelters. *International:* 10%. AIDS, clinics, hospitals. *Religion:* Less than 1%. Supports science councils. *Note:* Total contributions made in 2001. **Typ. Recipients:** AIDS/HIV, Alzheimers Disease, Clinics/Medical Centers, Diabetes, Emergency/Ambulance Services, Health-General, Hospices, Hospitals, Mental Health, People with Disabilities, Prenatal Health Issues, Substance Abuse. **Geo. Dist:** NC; Chester Township, SC; Fort Mill Township, SC; Lancaster County, SC.

★ 11983 ★ Springs Foundation, Inc.

1826 Second Baxter Crossing
Fort Mill, SC 29708
Phone: (803)548-2002 **Fax:** (803)548-1797
Angela McCrae, Jr., Executive Director

Fnded: 1942. **Philosophy:** The foundation was established to improve the lives of people in areas where Springs Industries plants were located. Colonel Springs was particularly interested in young people and helping them develop their greatest potential. The categories the founder determined to be the most basic to the well-being of individuals were recreation, health care, education, community service, and religion. The foundation continues to give in these five areas. In 1992, the foundation celebrated its 50th anniversary. **Priorities:** *Arts & Humanities:* 4%. Supports arts councils, libraries, and theater. *Civic & Public Affairs:* 1%. Supports clubs, towns, and housing. *Education:* 11%. Supports primary and secondary education and colleges and universities. *Environment:* 51%. Focus on recreation, community services, United Way, Young Men's Christian Association and camps. *International:* 32%. Supports Hospice and emergency services. *Note:* Total contributions made in 2000. **Typ. Recipients:** AIDS/HIV, Cancer, Clinics/Medical Centers, Emergency/Ambulance Services, Health Organizations, Hospices, Hospitals, Medical Education, Mental Health, Nutrition, Prenatal Health Issues, Substance Abuse. **Geo. Dist:** Chester Township, SC; Fort Mill Township, SC; Lancaster County, SC.

★ 11984 ★ Spunk Fund Inc.

780 3rd Ave., 24th Floor
New York, NY 10017
Phone: (212)980-8880 **Fax:** (212)980-8976
Email: sfi@spunkfund.com
Marianne Gerschel, President

Fnded: 1981. **Philosophy:** "The Spunk Foundation, Inc. is a private foundation created to support initiatives that contribute to the enrichment and well-being of children. Its goal is to fund programs, persons, institutions and ideas of outstanding quality and promise. "The Spunk Fund, Inc. focuses mainly on children's needs in the New York City metropolitan area. It also seeks well-conceived proposals of exceptional merit to benefit children in other nations and in other parts of the United States. Priority is given to programs which are well-integrated into the fabric of their communities and which draw upon existing public and private resources. The Spunk Fund, Inc. welcomes opportunities in which its own involvement will encourage or facilitate the participation of other grantmaking organizations. "While interested in initiatives which impact the overall world of the child, the Spunk Fund, Inc currently concentrates grants in four areas: programs directed toward medical and psychological problems of children; programs which contribute to the general education and cultural expression of children; programs aimed at the prevention and treatment of child abuse and neglect; and programs designed to enhance the quality of life and opportunities for less advantaged children overseas." Spunk Fund, Inc. Philosophy & Guidelines brochure **Priorities:** *Arts & Humanities:* 3% (Culture). Supports public broadcasting, photography, and performing arts. *Education:* 17%. Funds education initiatives focusing on teaching. *Environment:* 11% (Social Services & Policy). Supports services for children and under-served communities. *International:* 69% (Health/Medicine). Supports medical centers and schools of medicine. *Note:* Total contributions for fiscal 2001. Twenty-nine percent of total contributions went to internationally organizations. **Typ. Recipients:** Clinics/Medical Centers, Health Organizations, Heart, Hospitals (University Affiliated), Medical Education, Medical Research, Mental Health, Nutrition, People with Disabilities, Research/Studies Institutes, Substance Abuse. **Geo. Dist:** NY.

★ 11985 ★ Stackpole-Hall Foundation

44 South St. Marys St.
Saint Marys, PA 15857
Phone: (814)834-1845 **Fax:** (814)834-1869
William Conrad, Executive Secretary

Fnded: 1951. **Philosophy:** The foundation emphasizes local giving, with major priorities in the fields of education, social services, youth programs, and religious organizations. Educational support includes in-state universities, private education, and minority education funds. Some funding is given to civic causes, medical facilities, and the arts. **Priorities:** *Arts & Humanities:* 2%. Supports historic societies and arts councils. *Civic & Public Affairs:* 15%. Parks and community and municipal services, with major support to St. Mary's and Ridgway, Pennsylvania. *Education:* 40%. Supports schools, universities and religious education. *Environment:* 20%. Supports youth programs, Young Men's Christian Association, and scouting. *International:* 5%. Supports medical services in Pennsylvania. *Note:* Total contributions made in 2000. **Typ. Recipients:** Child Abuse, Children's Health/Hospitals, Clinics/Medical Centers, Emergency/Ambulance Services, Family Planning, Health-General, Hospices, Hospitals, Medical Education, Mental Health, Nursing Services, People with Disabilities, Public Health, Speech & Hearing, Substance Abuse. **Geo. Dist:** PA, Elk County.

★ 11986 ★ Stardust Foundation

6730 North Scottsdale Rd., Suite 230
Scottsdale, AZ 85253
Phone: (480)607-5800 **Fax:** (480)607-5801
Email: lkilgas@stardustco.com
Gerald Bisgrove, Chief Executive Officer/Chairman

Fnded: 1993. **Philosophy:** The foundation provides support for a local Habitat for Humanity, other civic concerns, community services, and education. The foundation promotes individuals responsibility and spiritual values in partnership with God and the community. **Priorities:** *Arts & Humanities:* 6%. Museums and theater. *Civic & Public Affairs:* 54%. Primarily for housing, municipalities, and safety organizations. *Education:* 7%. Leadership training and private, secondary education. *Environment:* 21%. Youth organizations, YMCAs, animal protection, and community services. *International:* 9%. Medical rehabilitation. *Religion:* 1%. Science center. *Note:* Total contributions made in 2000. **Typ. Recipients:** AIDS/HIV, Cancer, Domestic Violence, Family Planning, Health Organizations, Heart, Medical Rehabilitation, Medical Research, Public Health, Substance Abuse. **Geo. Dist:** AZ.

★ 11987 ★ Starr Foundation

70 Pine St., 14th Fl.
New York, NY 10270
Phone: (212)770-5202 **Fax:** (212)425-6261
Email: grants@starrfoundation.org
Website: http://fdncenter.org/grantmaker/starr/
Florence Davis, President

Fnded: 1955. **Philosophy:** The foundation's initial activities are "focused on education, particularly the provision of scholarships in the United States and Asia, and local assistance for international studies, community funds, and other civic organizations." This focus continued and grew through the 1970s. In 1980, the foundation added another area of funding: hospitals and health groups. The foundation's current interests are educational institutions and student aid. The foundation also funds health concerns, civic organizations, and cultural activities. **Priorities:** *Arts & Humanities:* 4%. Contributes to museums, libraries, arts councils, and the performing arts. *Civic & Public Affairs:* 2%. Gives to Habitat for Humanity, economic development organizations, ethnic associations, and public policy programs. *Education:* 37%. Funds colleges, universities, educational programs, and international studies; also provides scholarships. *Environment:* 2%. Gives to child welfare, youth programs, services for the disadvantaged, and senior services. *International:* 43%. Supports hospitals, medical centers, medical research, blood banks, AIDS research, and community health services. *Religion:* 1%. Scientific research centers receive support. *Note:* Total contributions made in 2000. **Typ. Recipients:** AIDS/HIV, Cancer, Children's Health/Hospitals, Emergency/Ambulance Services, Eyes/Blindness, Family Planning, Geriatric Health, Health Organizations, Health Policy/Cost Containment, Health-General, Heart, Hospices, Hospitals, Kidney, Long-Term Care, Medical Education, Medical Research, Medical Training, Nursing Services, People with Disabilities, Public Health, Single-Disease Health Associations, Substance Abuse, Transplant Networks/Donor Banks. **Geo. Dist:** internationally; nationally; nationally; internationally; New York, NY; New York, NY, metropolitan area.

★ 11988 ★ Statler Foundation

107 Delaware Ave., Suite 680
Buffalo, NY 14202
Phone: (716)852-1104 **Fax:** (716)852-3968
Edward Flynn, Chairman

Fnded: 1934. **Philosophy:** Following the interests of Mr. Statler, the foundation supports education, training, and research in the hotel and food industry. It contributes to educational institutions that teach hotel and food management, and food preparation. Its main emphasis is on scholarships. **Priorities:** *Education:* 100%. Includes universities, culinary institutes, and scholarships. *Note:* Total contributions made in 2000. **Typ. Recipients:** Children's Health/Hospitals, Hospitals, People with Disabilities. **Geo. Dist:** internationally; nationally; NY.

★ 11989 ★ Staunton Farm Foundation

650 Smithfield St., Suite 240
Pittsburgh, PA 15219
Phone: (412)281-8020 **Fax:** (412)232-3115
Website: http://www.stauntonfarm.org
Joni Schwager, Program Officer, Foundation Manager

Fnded: 1937. **Philosophy:** "The purpose of the foundation shall be to carry into effect the intent and purpose of the Last Will and Testament of Matilda S. McCready through grants to appropriate educational and charitable institutions, or by direct expenditures, for the study and treatment of persons suffering from curable neurotic functional disorders, mild mental and kindred ailments or recovery therefrom and for educational and charitable purposes in connection therewith. As interpreted by the Directors, the emphasis of the foundation is to award grants to non-profit organizations for mental health treatment, care and support through programming that purposes to restore individuals to their optimal functioning and productivity in society. The Staunton Farm Foundation's funding is limited to the ten-county region of southwestern Pennsylvania." Staunton Farm Foundation Mission Statement. **Priorities:** *Civic & Public Affairs:* 1%. *Education:* 12%. Mental health education programs. *Environment:* 58%. Counseling services, youth programs, and therapy. *International:* 23%. Mental health, AIDS, and therapeutic services. *Note:* Total contributions made in 2000. **Typ. Recipients:** AIDS/HIV, Children's Health/Hospitals, Clinics/Medical Centers, Domestic Violence, Eyes/Blindness, Family Planning, Health Funds, Health Organizations, Health-General, Hospices, Hospitals, Medical Education, Medical Rehabilitation, Mental Health, People with Disabilities, Public Health, Sexual Abuse, Single-Disease Health Associations, Substance Abuse. **Geo. Dist:** PA, Southwestern Pennsylvania.

★ 11990 ★ Steele Foundation, Inc.

PO Box 1112
Phoenix, AZ 85001-1112

Phone: (602)230-2038
Daniel Cracchiolo, President, Secretary, & Director

Fnded: 1980. **Philosophy:** Giving priorities are education and medical research. **Priorities:** *Arts & Humanities:* 21%. Phoenix Symphony, public libraries, and art museums. *Civic & Public Affairs:* 24%. *Education:* 27%. Mainly high schools and prep schools. *Environment:* 7%. Scouting and youth sports programs. *International:* 10%. Cancer treatment programs, heart research, and children's hospitals. *Religion:* 7%. Science centers and observatories. *Note:* Total contributions made in 2000. **Typ. Recipients:** AIDS/HIV, Arthritis, Cancer, Children's Health/Hospitals, Emergency/Ambulance Services, Eyes/Blindness, Health Organizations, Heart, Hospitals, Kidney, Medical Research, People with Disabilities, Prenatal Health Issues, Research/Studies Institutes, Sexual Abuse, Single-Disease Health Associations, Trauma Treatment. **Geo. Dist:** Phoenix, AZ.

★ 11991 ★ Steele-Reese Foundation

32 Washington Square West
New York, NY 10011
Phone: (212)557-7700 **Fax:** (212)286-8513
Website: http://www.davidsondawson.com
William Buice, III, Co-Trustee

Fnded: 1955. **Philosophy:** Eleanor Steele Reese established the foundation to honor her and her husband's families. "The attitude behind their giving was as firm and unsentimental as every aspect of their lives on the ranch: they wanted to help people and organizations to help themselves, and they knew that mere handouts often weakened the recipients more than helping them. In developing the foundation's grant policies, the trustees have tried to reflect the personal philosophies of the Reeses." The foundation has a strong preference for projects benefiting rural areas and those directly affecting the people served. "The foundation tends to favor modest, essential, local projects rather than large-scale, glamorous ones." Annual Report **Priorities:** *Arts & Humanities:* 14%. Funds opera, libraries, historical associations, and arts councils. *Civic & Public Affairs:* 20%. Gives to community foundations and rural affairs. *Education:* 21%. Focus on colleges, universities, and primary education. *Environment:* 22%. Supports child welfare, community service organizations, food banks, and an animal foundation. *International:* 17%. Hospitals, hospice, single-disease health associations, and health clinics. *Note:* Total contributions made in fiscal 2001. **Typ. Recipients:** AIDS/HIV, Alzheimers Disease, Child Abuse, Clinics/Medical Centers, Domestic Violence, Emergency/Ambulance Services, Family Planning, Health-General, Heart, Hospices, Hospitals, Long-Term Care, Medical Rehabilitation, Nursing Services, People with Disabilities, Public Health, Single-Disease Health Associations, Substance Abuse, Transplant Networks/Donor Banks. **Geo. Dist:** GA, Northern Georgia; ID; KY, Appalachian region of the state; MT; NC, Appalachian region of the state; TN, Appalachian region of the state; WA.

★ 11992 ★ Stella and Charles Guttman Foundation

445 Park Ave., 19th Floor
New York, NY 10022
Phone: (212)371-7082 **Fax:** (212)371-8936
Email: info@guttmanfdn.org
Website: http://www.fdncenter.org/grantsmaker/guttman/
Elizabeth Olofson, Executive Director

Fnded: 1959. **Philosophy:** "The Foundation grantmaking is focused on the following program areas: The Foundation funds efforts to improve the educational services available to New York City children and youth, from pre-school to high school. The Foundation also funds collaborative projects among public schools, non-profit education and community based agencies, and institutions of higher education that offer children, youth and their families additional academic and social support, in-school and after-school. The Foundation supports a wide range of traditional education, health and social service programs in Israel. In addition, the Foundation has in recent years supported social and educational programs for Arab Israelis and efforts to promote coexistence among Arabs and Jews in Israel. Through its special grants program, the Foundation is able to respond to project requests and address significant needs outside of its principal program areas. The Foundation also supports a number of cultural institutions that contribute to the quality of life in New York City." Funding Guidelines **Priorities:** *Arts & Humanities:* 6%. Supports public broadcasting, libraries, history, and journalism. *Civic & Public Affairs:* 4%. Supports safety, parks and botonical gardens. *Education:* 19%. Public education, education reform, minority education, faculty development, education, arts education and after school programs. *Environment:* 34%. Recreation and athletics, child welfare, youth organizations, Young Men's Christian Association, food distribution programs, emergency relief services, family planning services, and homes. *International:* 11%. Supports hospitals, AIDS, and emergency services. *Religion:* 2%. Supports science research. *Note:* Contributions made in 2000. **Typ. Recipients:** Adolescent Health Issues, AIDS/HIV, Alzheimers Disease, Cancer, Diabetes, Emergency/Ambulance Services, Family Planning, Geriatric Health, Health Policy/Cost Containment, Heart, Hospitals, Medical Education, Medical Research, Mental Health, Nutrition, People with Disabilities, Prenatal Health Issues, Public Health, Single-Disease Health Associations, Substance Abuse. **Geo. Dist:** New York, NY, including metropolitan area.

★ 11993 ★ Sterling-Turner Foundation

815 Walker St., Suite 1543
Houston, TX 77002-5724
Phone: (713)237-1117 **Fax:** (713)223-4638
Email: eyvonne@wt.net
Website: http://www.sterlingturnerfoundation.org
Eyvonne Moser, Executive Director

Fnded: 1956. **Philosophy:** The Sterling-Turner Foundation makes grants primarily in the areas of social services, the arts, and civic affairs. Social service funding favors recreation, youth organizations, the disabled, and child welfare. Funding for the arts includes opera, ballet, theater, and music; large grants are awarded to the Museum of Fine Arts in Houston, TX. Civic affairs interests include housing, zoos, and emergency services. The foundation funds other recipient areas on a limited basis. **Priorities:** *Arts & Humanities:* 14%. Supports arts and culture through museum of Fine Arts in Houston. *Education:* 24%. Supports schools, preschools, religious schools, education center and other education organizations. *Environment:* 27%. Provides funding for children and youth services, emergency services, family violence shelters and services. *International:* 12%. Funds local hospice, University of Texas Medical Center and health foundations. *Note:* Total contributions made in 2000. **Typ. Recipients:** AIDS/HIV, Cancer, Children's Health/Hospitals, Clinics/Medical Centers, Emergency/Ambulance Services, Eyes/Blindness, Family Planning, Health Organizations, Heart, Hospices, Hospitals, Medical Education, Medical Research, Mental Health, People with Disabilities, Research/Studies Institutes, Single-Disease Health Associations, Speech & Hearing, Substance Abuse. **Geo. Dist:** TX. **Frmly:** Turner Charitable Foundation.

★ 11994 ★ Stewardship Foundation

PO Box 1278
Tacoma, WA 98401-1278
Phone: (253)620-1340 **Fax:** (253)572-2721
Email: info@stewardshipfdn.org
Website: http://www.stewardshipfdn.org
Dr. Cary Paine, Executive Director

Fnded: 1962. **Philosophy:** The foundation's main objective is to support evangelical Christian institutions whose primary goal is "to bring people into a relationship with God through faith in Jesus Christ." **Priorities:** *Civic & Public Affairs:* 11%. Funds public policy organizations and the National Center for Law and Religious Freedom. *Education:* 13%. Supports colleges, religious education, and leadership development. *Environment:* 13%. Grants funds to Christian youth and family organizations and food distribution agencies. *International:* 1%. Provides funding for the Mercy Medical Airlift. *Note:* Total contributions made in 1999. **Typ. Recipients:** Domestic Violence, Emergency/Ambulance Services, Eyes/Blindness, Family Planning, Medical Research, Mental Health, People with Disabilities, Public Health, Substance Abuse. **Geo. Dist:** nationally.

★ 11995 ★ Stewart Huston Charitable Trust

Lukens Executive office Bldg.
50 S 1st Ave., 2nd Floor
Coatesville, PA 19320
Phone: (610)384-2666 **Fax:** (610)384-3396
Website: http://www.stewarthuston.org
Scott Huston, Executive Director

Fnded: 1989. **Philosophy:** "The purpose of the Trust is to supply funds, technical assistance and collaboration to corporations, of nonprofit associations, trusts, foundations and qualified organizations engaged exclusively in religious, charitable, or educational work; to extend opportunities to deserving, needy persons, and, in general, to promote the establishment of new and innovative religious, charitable, or educational projects." 2001 Annual Report Sixty percent of the annual distributions from the trust are made, as stipulated by Mr. Stewart Huston's will, for the benefit of Trinitarian/Evangelical activities. This includes activities carried on by Protestant churches and affiliated or related organizations that follow the Christian Gospel and exemplification of Christian principles through social welfare and other charitable endeavors. Forty percent of the annual distributions from the Trust are to be used for secular charitable activities within one 100 miles of Coatesville, PA. **Priorities:** *Arts & Humanities:* 9%. Supports historical societies and preservation, cultural heritage, and the performing and visual arts. *Civic & Public Affairs:* 15%. Supports community foundations, economic development, nonprofit interests, and public policy organizations. *Education:* 14%. Supports Christian day schools and colleges. *Environment:* 7%. Funds YMCAs. *International:* 8%. Funds healthcare access, outpatient and clinic care, public health, and rehabilitation services. *Note:* Total contributions made in 2001. **Typ. Recipients:** AIDS/HIV, Child Abuse, Children's Health/Hospitals, Clinics/Medical Centers, Family Planning, Geriatric Health, Health-General, Medical Rehabilitation, Mental Health, Nursing Services, People with Disabilities, Substance Abuse, Trauma Treatment. **Geo. Dist:** Savannah, GA; PA, Chester County.

★ 11996 ★ Stoddard Charitable Trust

370 Main St., 12th Floor
Worcester, MA 01608
Phone: (508)798-8621 **Fax:** (508)791-6454
Email: wfletcher@ftwlaw.com
Warner Fletcher, Chairman

Fnded: 1939. **Philosophy:** The trust does not have a fixed policy regarding the distribution of its funds. It makes grants to organizations in the areas of education, medicine, religion, science, social services, the arts, and civic affairs. Priorities among these areas are apt to vary significantly from year to year. **Priorities:** *Arts & Humanities:* 12%. Museums, theater, and public broadcasting. *Civic & Public Affairs:* 47%. Housing programs, community development, and horticulture. *Education:* 17%. Private schools, colleges and universities, and Junior Achievement. *Environment:* 11%. United funds, renovation projects, community centers, and youth programs. *International:* 7%. Biomedical research and health services and centers. *Note:* Total contributions made in 2000. **Typ. Recipients:** Cancer, Children's Health/Hospitals, Clinics/Medical Centers, Family Planning, Health Funds, Health Organizations, Health-General, Home-Care Services, Hospices, Medical Education, Medical Research, People with Disabilities, Public Health, Sexual Abuse, Substance Abuse. **Geo. Dist:** Worchester, MA.

★ 11997 ★ Strake Foundation

712 Main St., Suite 3300
Houston, TX 77002-3291
Phone: (713)216-2400 **Fax:** (713)216-2401

Email: foundation@strake.org
George Strake, Jr., President

Fnded: 1952. **Philosophy:** The foundation makes grants "primarily to Roman Catholic-affiliated associations, including hospitals and higher and secondary educational institutions; support also for the arts and social services, including programs for youth," primarily in Texas. Grants are made annually and are usually not long-term pledges. They are frequently made to projects whose funding is shared with other contributors. **Priorities:** *Arts & Humanities:* 13%. Cultural organizations. *Education:* 37%. Funds private secondary schools, colleges, and universities. *Environment:* 36%. Supports social services, youth programs, and the United Way. *International:* 10%. Supports hospitals, clinics, and single-disease associations. *Note:* Total contributions made in 2000. **Typ. Recipients:** Cancer, Children's Health/Hospitals, Clinics/Medical Centers, Health Organizations, Health Policy/Cost Containment, Heart, Hospices, Hospitals, Medical Education, Medical Rehabilitation, Medical Research, Mental Health, People with Disabilities, Prenatal Health Issues, Public Health, Single-Disease Health Associations, Speech & Hearing, Substance Abuse, Transplant Networks/Donor Banks. **Geo. Dist:** nationally; TX.

★ 11998 ★ Stranahan Foundation

4159 Holland-Sylvania Rd., Suite 206
Toledo, OH 43623
Phone: (419)882-5575 **Fax:** (419)882-2072
Email: proberts@stranahanfoundation.org
Website: http://www.stranahanfoundation.org
Pamela Roberts, Program Officer

Fnded: 1944. **Philosophy:** The foundation primarily supports education, health care, cultural organizations, and community initiatives in northwest Ohio. Preservation of the environment and public policy are secondary concerns. In addition, the foundation supports groups and institutions that give people the tools to become educated, healthy, self-reliant and contributing members of our society. **Priorities:** *Arts & Humanities:* 25%. Supports public broadcasting, music, museum, history, theater, and arts councils. *Civic & Public Affairs:* 32%. Supports clubs, safety, philanthropic organizations and community foundations. *Education:* 16%. Supports scholarship, technical education, after school/enrichment programs, medical education, tutoring, pre-school education, education funds, and minority education. *Environment:* 14%. Supports family planning services, united way, emergency relief, people with disabilities, child welfare, youth programs, and family services. *International:* 5%. Supports mental health, Alzheimers, hospital, hospice, preventative medicine, and medical research. *Note:* Total contributions made in 2000. **Typ. Recipients:** AIDS/HIV, Alzheimers Disease, Children's Health/Hospitals, Clinics/Medical Centers, Emergency/Ambulance Services, Eyes/Blindness, Family Planning, Geriatric Health, Health-General, Hospices, Hospitals, Medical Education, Medical Rehabilitation, Mental Health, People with Disabilities, Preventive Medicine/Wellness Organizations, Respiratory. **Geo. Dist:** OH, Northwest Ohio.

★ 11999 ★ Stratford Foundation

125 High St.
Boston, MA 02110
Phone: (617)248-7000 **Fax:** (617)248-7100
Peter Wilson, Executive Director

Fnded: 1983. **Philosophy:** The foundation makes grants "primarily to institutions closely associated with the donor and the donor's family. However, non-donor grants are also actively considered." **Priorities:** *Arts & Humanities:* 15%. Provides major support for a film festival and a public broadcasting station; also funds music, theater, museums, and historic preservation. *Civic & Public Affairs:* 18%. Gives to community foundations, housing, Native American reservations, and a zoo. *Education:* 23%. Funds colleges and universities, scholarship funds, and Christian secondary schools and colleges. *Environment:* 17%. Funds the United Way, child welfare organizations, shelters, food banks, and other social service agencies. *International:* 5%. Contributes to hospitals, pediatric health organizations, cancer research and treatment programs, and single-disease health associations. *Note:* Total contributions made in 2000. **Typ. Recipients:** Cancer, Cancer, Children's Health/Hospitals, Diabetes, Emergency/Ambulance Services, Health Funds, Health Organizations, Heart, Hospitals, Medical Research, People with Disabilities, Single-Disease Health Associations, Substance Abuse. **Geo. Dist:** Boston, MA.

★ 12000 ★ Strauss Foundation

123 Broad St., 16th Floor
Philadelphia, PA 19109-1199
Phone: (215)670-4226 **Fax:** (215)670-4236
Reginald Middleton, Vice President

Fnded: 1951. **Philosophy:** The Strauss Foundation makes grants across the major categories of support. In social services, interests include youth camps and youth organizations. Art support favors museums and art institutes. Health-care funding supports medical centers, pediatrics, and research. Religious giving supports Jewish organizations and temples. The foundation also supports civic affairs. **Priorities:** *Arts & Humanities:* 20%. Funds ballet, opera, other performing arts, and arts funds. *Civic & Public Affairs:* 6%. Gives to civil rights organizations, a zoological society, and philanthropic foundations. *Education:* 27%. Supports colleges, universities, private pre-college schools, and youth learning programs. *Environment:* 6%. Contributes to social services for young people. *International:* 9%. Funds medical centers, medical research, cancer centers, and single-disease organizations. *Note:* Total contributions made in 2000. **Typ. Recipients:** AIDS/HIV, Alzheimers Disease, Cancer, Clinics/Medical Centers, Diabetes, Health Organizations, Health Policy/Cost Containment, Health-General, Heart, Hospitals, Medical Education, Medical Research, People with Disabilities, Public Health, Single-Disease Health Associations, Substance Abuse, Transplant Networks/Donor Banks, Trauma Treatment. **Geo. Dist:** Los Angeles, CA; Palm Beach, FL; PA.

★ 12001 ★ Streisand Foundation

1460 Fourth St., Suite 212
Santa Monica, CA 90401
Phone: (310)535-3767 **Fax:** (310)395-9676
Email: stfnd@aol.com
Margery Tabankin, Treasurer & Secretary

Fnded: 1986. **Philosophy:** "Since its inception in 1986, the Streisand Foundation has made grants totaling over 12 million dollars. In the early years we provided assistance to national organizations working on the preservation of the environment, voter education, and the protection of civil liberties and civil rights, and nuclear disarmament." "In 1993, the Foundation added additional priorities and began focusing on women's, children's, and youth-related issues. Under these priorities, we provided assistance to an array of organizations, including those working on a national level to protect women's rights and those working locally in Los Angeles to provide aid and enrichment programs to economically at-risk children." "At this time, The Streisand Foundation only considers requests from United States based nonprofit organizations that are working on a national level to promote and support: environmental issues; women's issues, including choice and health-related concerns; civil rights and race relations; children's and youth-related issues, with a focus on the economically disadvantaged (Los Angeles only); and AIDS research, advocacy, service, and litigation." 2002-2003 Application Guidelines **Priorities:** *Arts & Humanities:* Funds museums, cinema, music, and literature. *Civic & Public Affairs:* Supports civil liberties, gay rights, women's advocacy, and democratic values. *Education:* Funds Teach for America and schools. *Environment:* Includes support for shelters, anti-violence projects, and human rights groups. *International:* Focus on women's health and single-disease organizations. **Typ. Recipients:** AIDS/HIV, Alzheimers Disease, Cancer, Children's Health/Hospitals, Domestic Violence, Emergency/Ambulance Services, Eyes/Blindness, Family Planning, Health Organizations, Health-General, Medical Research, Mental Health, Nutrition, Prenatal Health Issues, Research/Studies Institutes, Sexual Abuse, Transplant Networks/Donor Banks. **Geo. Dist:** nationally; nationally; Los Angeles, CA, for at-risk youth projects.

★ 12002 ★ Stuart Foundations

50 California St., Suite 3350
San Francisco, CA 94111
Phone: (415)393-1551 **Fax:** (415)393-1552
Email: info@stuartfoundation.org
Website: http://www.stuartfoundation.org
Theodore Lobman, President

Fnded: 1937. **Philosophy:** The Stuart Foundation supports efforts in California and Washington State to help children and youth become capable, responsible citizens. Grants are intended to improve policy and practice in the fields of public education, child welfare, and family services. Activities supported include evaluated demonstrations, technical assistance to implement reforms, policy analysis, and advocacy. The foundations generally do not provide capital or general operating support for individual agencies. Most grants are made within three programs. Under Strengthening the Public School System, grants emphasize enhancing student achievement. Grants for Strengthening Communities to Support Families focus on family support programs that allow children and youth to grow up in an environment that promotes their development. Grants for Strengthening the Child Welfare System are directed toward ensuring that children and youth facing abuse and neglect have a safe home. **Priorities:** *Civic & Public Affairs:* 8%. Funds economic development, law/justice organizations, community foundations, and nonprofit management programs. *Education:* 76%. Supports primary and secondary public schools; teacher training and professional development; educational improvement programs; literacy programs; and public colleges and universities. *Environment:* 5%. Focuses on family services, child welfare/child advocacy, and youth organizations. *International:* 11%. Funds health services for children. *Note:* Total contributions made in 2000. **Typ. Recipients:** Cancer, Child Abuse, Children's Health/Hospitals, Clinics/Medical Centers, Family Planning, Health Policy/Cost Containment, Medical Education, Medical Research, Public Health, Research/Studies Institutes, Sexual Abuse, Substance Abuse. **Geo. Dist:** CA; WA.

★ 12003 ★ Sulzberger Foundation

229 West 43rd St., 11th Floor
New York, NY 10036
Phone: (212)556-1755 **Fax:** (212)556-1434
Marian Heiskell, President

Fnded: 1956. **Philosophy:** The Sulzberger Foundation makes most of its grants to environmental organizations, zoos and botanical gardens, the arts, and education. Funding categorized as environmental supports think tanks, wilderness councils, and trusts. Contributions to the arts favor museums, the performing arts, libraries, public broadcasting, and arts funds. Educational support goes to medical training, private schools, and education funds. The foundation makes grants to other recipient areas on a limited basis. **Priorities:** *Arts & Humanities:* 23%. Supports museums, public broadcasting, libraries, and theater. *Civic & Public Affairs:* 12%. For foundations and community programs and botanical gardens parks *Education:* 22%. Universities, primary and secondary education, after school programs and study centers. *Environment:* 8%. Supports United Way, family planning services, food distribution programs, and day care. *International:* 5%. Supports cancer, medical centers, AIDS, and hospitals. *Religion:* 2%. Funds natural history museums. *Note:* Total contributions made in 2000. **Typ. Recipients:** AIDS/HIV, Cancer, Clinics/Medical Centers, Family Planning, Health Organizations, Hospitals, Kidney, Medical Education, Medical Research, Mental Health, People with Disabilities, Public Health, Sexual Abuse, Single-Disease Health Associations, Substance Abuse. **Geo. Dist:** nationally; internationally.

★ 12004 ★ Summit Charitable Foundation
2099 Pennsylvania Ave., NW
Suite 1000
Washington, DC 20006
Phone: (202)912-2900
Victoria Sant, President & Director

Fnded: 1991. **Priorities:** *Civic & Public Affairs:* 10%. Gives to public policy organizations, law & justice, consumer's rights, and women's affairs. *Education:* 12%. Primarily supports colleges and universities. *Environment:* 17%. Funds family planning, child welfare, and adoption organizations. *Note:* Total contributions made in 2000. **Typ. Recipients:** Family Planning, Health Organizations, Prenatal Health Issues, Public Health. **Geo. Dist:** Latin America and the Caribbean; nationally.

★ 12005 ★ Sunderland Foundation
PO Box 25900
Overland Park, KS 66225
Phone: (913)451-8900 **Fax:** (913)319-6191
Email: sunderlandfoundation@ashgrove.com
Website: http://www.sunderlandfoundation.org
James Sunderland, President

Fnded: 1945. **Philosophy:** The foundation primarily supports education, with emphasis on colleges and universities in the Midwest. Secondary interests include the arts, civic affairs, social services, religion, and hospitals. **Priorities:** *Arts & Humanities:* 19%. Museums, music, historical preservation, and art programs for youth. *Civic & Public Affairs:* 8%. Community and foundation grants, mostly in the Kansas City, Missouri area. *Education:* 29%. Colleges and universities, mainly in Missouri, Kansas, and Nebraska. *Environment:* 31%. Scouting, 4-H programs, children's homes, and YMCAs. *International:* 10%. Children's health and hospitals, the American Red Cross, and arthritis research. *Note:* Total contributions made in 2001. **Typ. Recipients:** Cancer, Children's Health/Hospitals, Clinics/Medical Centers, Domestic Violence, Eyes/Blindness, Family Planning, Health Organizations, Hospitals, Mental Health, Nursing Services, People with Disabilities, Research/Studies Institutes. **Geo. Dist:** AR; KS; MO; NE.

★ 12006 ★ Sunnen Foundation
7910 Manchester Ave.
Saint Louis, MO 63143
Phone: (314)781-2100 **Fax:** (314)781-1533
Website: http://www.sunnen.com
Kurt Kallaus, President

Fnded: 1953. **Philosophy:** Current primary interests are specific, goal-oriented projects that protect reproductive and First Amendment rights; and educational opportunities for the economically or physically disadvantaged. **Priorities:** *Arts & Humanities:* 11%. Supports historical societies and museums. *Civic & Public Affairs:* 6%. Funds public policy organizations. *Education:* 17%. Supports colleges, universities, Junior Achievement, and primary education. *Environment:* 62%. Contributions include Planned Parenthood, youth groups, and family services. *Note:* Total contributions made in 2000. **Typ. Recipients:** Cancer, Children's Health/Hospitals, Clinics/Medical Centers, Domestic Violence, Emergency/Ambulance Services, Family Planning, Health Organizations, Health Policy/Cost Containment, Medical Education, People with Disabilities, Single-Disease Health Associations, Speech & Hearing, Substance Abuse, Transplant Networks/Donor Banks. **Geo. Dist:** St. Louis, MO, metropolitan area & statewide.

★ 12007 ★ Surdna Foundation
330 Madison Ave., 30th Floor
New York, NY 10017-5001
Phone: (212)557-0010 **Fax:** (212)557-0003
Email: request@surdna.org
Website: http://www.surdna.org
Edward Skloot, Executive Director

Fnded: 1917. **Philosophy:** For many years, the principal beneficiary of the foundation was the Julia Dyckman Andrus Memorial, a children's home in Yonkers, NY, founded in 1928 in memory of Mrs. Andrus. Today, the foundation continues to provide support for the operations of the home, as well as for the John E. Andrus Memorial, a retirement home established in Hastings-on-Hudson, NY, in honor of Mr. Andrus. The foundation makes grants in four areas with the following objectives: *Environment*: to prevent irreversible damage to the environment; support government, private, and voluntary actions to sustain the environment; and foster a population of environmentally informed citizens. *Community Revitalization*: to increase the availability of affordable housing for low-income individuals; help the disadvantaged move from welfare dependence to economic independence; and strengthen families by enhancing and expanding early childhood initiatives for the zero-to-three population in both child care and parenting education. *Effective Citizenry*: to promote respect, empathy, fairness, and inclusivity in the way individuals and groups interact; motivate individuals to take active roles in their communities; help individuals work together effectively to create joint solutions to serious social and civic problems; and advance participatory decision making and governance in community institutions. *Arts*: to contribute to the ability of young people to explore both their identity and relationship to the world, through high-impact, long-term experiences with artists and the arts; and to deepen the ability of artists and arts organizations to contribute nationally to the needs of young people and educators. deepen the ability of artists and arts organizations to contribute nationally to the needs of young people and educators. **Priorities:** *Arts & Humanities:* 13%. Supports the performing arts, arts centers, and ats institutes. *Civic & Public Affairs:* 24%. Supports employment/job training, public policy, economic policy, business, community development, housing and ethnic organizations. *Education:* 24%. Supports arts/humainites education, education funds, leadership training, faculty development, public education. *Environment:* 7%. Supports youth programs, daycare, child welfare, at-risk youth. *Note:* Total contributions made in 1999. **Typ. Recipients:** Health Organizations, Long-Term Care, Research/Studies Institutes. **Geo. Dist:** nationally.

★ 12008 ★ Swalm Foundation
11511 Katy Freeway, Suite 430
Houston, TX 77079
Phone: (281)497-5280 **Fax:** (281)497-7340
Website: http://www.swalm.org
Dr. Billy Ward, President, CEO

Fnded: 1980. **Philosophy:** The Swalm Foundation makes most of its grants in the areas of social services and health care. Social service interests include youth organizations, retirement centers, family services, and drug counseling and rehabilitation. Funding for health care favors rehabilitation centers, mental health, and hospices. The foundation also provides scholarships for dyslexic students. **Priorities:** *Arts & Humanities:* 2%. Funds historical museum. *Civic & Public Affairs:* 19%. Supports job training programs, affordable housing, and Hispanic affairs. *Education:* 14%. Educational programs for at-risk youth, public precollege education, and literacy programs. *Environment:* 57%. Supports programs to prevent child abuse, camps, women's centers, and shelters for the homeless. *International:* 8%. Focus on cancer and AIDS research, children's health programs, and medical clinics for the underserved. *Note:* Contributions made in fiscal 2001. **Typ. Recipients:** AIDS/HIV, Alzheimers Disease, Cancer, Child Abuse, Children's Health/Hospitals, Clinics/Medical Centers, Domestic Violence, Emergency/Ambulance Services, Eyes/Blindness, Family Planning, Health-General, Hospices, Hospitals, Medical Rehabilitation, Mental Health, People with Disabilities, Public Health, Research/Studies Institutes, Speech & Hearing, Substance Abuse. **Geo. Dist:** TX.

★ 12009 ★ The Swig Foundation
220 Montgomery St.
San Francisco, CA 94104
Phone: (415)291-1100 **Fax:** (415)291-8373
Kent Swig, Trustee

Fnded: 1957. **Philosophy:** The foundation's main interest is promoting education, the arts, and schools for the arts. Other interests include zoological societies, recreational facilites and athletic foundations, and higher education. **Priorities:** *Arts & Humanities:* 16%. Major support to fine arts organization; also supports museums, opera, and art education. *Civic & Public Affairs:* 16%. Funds foundations, public policy. *Education:* 16%. Universities, theology, and precollege private education. *Environment:* 5%. Funds the United Way and other social service organizations. *International:* 19%. Medical centers and cancer research. *Note:* Contributions made in 1998. **Typ. Recipients:** Cancer, Child Abuse, Children's Health/Hospitals, Clinics/Medical Centers, Domestic Violence, Geriatric Health, Health Funds, Health Organizations, Hospitals, Hospitals (University Affiliated), Medical Research. **Geo. Dist:** CA; NY.

★ 12010 ★ T. J. Brown and C. A. Lupton Foundation
PO Box 1629
Fort Worth, TX 76101-1629
Sam Woodson, III, President

Fnded: 1942. **Philosophy:** The T. J. Brown and C. A. Lupton Foundation primarily supports education, particularly the Texas Christian University. Other educational support goes to legal training. Other interests include civic affairs, mainly zoos, and the arts. **Priorities:** *Arts & Humanities:* 29%. Supports the performing arts, the Fort Worth Symphony, and museums and opera. *Civic & Public Affairs:* 11%. The Fort Worth Zoological Society, philanthropic organizations and law & justice. *Education:* 50%. Major support is given to Texas Christian University, as well as schools and learning centers. *Environment:* 1%. Funds the Young Men's Christian Association, food banks, children's welfare, and shelters. *International:* 4%. Supports cancer, diabetes, and a health foundation. *Religion:* 5%. Supports a science museum. *Note:* Total contributions made in 2000. **Typ. Recipients:** Cancer, Diabetes, People with Disabilities, Public Health, Substance Abuse. **Geo. Dist:** Ft. Worth, TX.

★ 12011 ★ T. L. L. Temple Foundation
109 Temple Boulevard, Suite 300
Lufkin, TX 75901
Phone: (936)639-5197 **Fax:** (936)639-5199
Millard Zeagler, Assistant Executive Director

Fnded: 1962. **Philosophy:** The T. L. L. Temple Foundation looks favorably upon educational institutions located in the East Texas Pine Timber Belt area. The foundation also supports health care and human services, civic and public affairs, and provides limited funding for the arts. **Priorities:** *Arts & Humanities:* 2%. Supports museums and libraries. *Civic & Public Affairs:* 4%. Supports foundations and fire departments. *Education:* 35%. Supports adult education, colleges, and universities. *Environment:* 5%. Focus on substance abuse services, Special Olympics, women's services, and youth organizations. *International:* 42%. Supports hospitals, medical centers, and single-disease health associations. *Note:* Total contributions made in fiscal 2001. **Typ. Recipients:** Alzheimers Disease, Cancer, Children's Health/Hospitals, Clinics/Medical Centers, Domestic Violence, Emergency/Ambulance Services, Eyes/Blindness, Family Planning, Health Organizations, Heart, Hospices, Hospitals, Hospitals (University Affiliated), Kidney, Medical Education, Medical Rehabilitation, Medical Research, Mental Health, People with Disabilities, Prenatal Health Issues, Research/Studies Institutes, Single-Disease Health Associations, Substance Abuse, Transplant Networks/Donor Banks. **Geo. Dist:** TX, East Texas Pine Timber Belt area.

★ 12012 ★ Taconic Foundation
60 Wall St., 46th Fl.
New York, NY 10005
Phone: (212)789-5777 **Fax:** (212)648-5082
Hildy Simmons, Managing Director

Fnded: 1958. **Philosophy:** The foundation continues the Curriers' commitment to equal opportunity. Currently, it emphasizes programs related to housing opportunity, youth employment, economic development, and youth. The foundation's interests in housing and associated aspects of land use stem from Stephen Currier, who organized Urban America just three years before he died. He created this organization from the remnants of the old American Planning and Civic Association and the American Council to Improve Our Neighborhoods. Urban America merged with the Urban Coalition in the spring of 1970 to become the National Urban Coalition. Urban Coalition. **Priorities:** *Civic & Public Affairs:* 67%. Funds civic and community organizations focusing on housing opportunities, economic development and housing services. *Education:* 8%. Supports after-school education, education funds. *Environment:* 23%. Supports youth programs and services. *Note:* Total contributions made in 2000. **Typ. Recipients:** Children's Health/Hospitals, Family Planning. **Geo. Dist:** nationally; New York, NY.

★ 12013 ★ Teagle Foundation
10 Rockefeller Plaza, Room 920
New York, NY 10020-1903
Phone: (212)373-1970
John Chasltry, Chief Executive Officer & President

Fnded: 1944. **Philosophy:** The foundation's major interest is private higher education, including nursing education and theological education, which it supports with project and program grants aimed at strengthening institutions and enhancing the total educational experience of their students. Most grant recipients have relatively small enrollments and modest financial resources. The foundation sponsors a competitive program of college and graduate school scholarships for children of employees of Exxon Corporation and its affiliates. It also makes a few grants to New York City agencies serving youth and matches the gifts of directors and employees to various organizations. In December 1995, the foundation announced its $4 million, invitational Collaborative Ventures Program to encourage institutions of higher learning to work together to make more effective use of academic, administrative, finacial, and physical resources. The first grants, totaling almost $1.5 million, were made in November 1996. **Priorities:** *Education:* 92%. Supports colleges and universities. *Note:* Total contributions made in fiscal 2000. **Typ. Recipients:** Emergency/Ambulance Services, Hospitals, Hospitals (University Affiliated), Medical Education. **Geo. Dist:** nationally.

★ 12014 ★ Ted Mann Foundation
1801 Century Park East, Suite 1920
Los Angeles, CA 90067
Phone: (310)284-8528 **Fax:** (310)551-0604
Email: rkipper@mannfamilyoffice.com
Rich Kipper, Financial Advisor

Fnded: 1985. **Philosophy:** The foundation gives to broad purposes, with emphasis on educational organizations, health care, and youth welfare. **Priorities:** *Arts & Humanities:* 1%. Funds public broadcasting. *Civic & Public Affairs:* 65%. Supports community foundations, housing, and private foundations. *Education:* 21%. Support for higher education, the Mann Center for Education, and education funds. *Environment:* 4%. Supports animal protection, child welfare, family services, and food banks. *International:* 4%. Emphasis on hospitals and medical research at universities. *Note:* Total contributions made in fiscal 2000. **Typ. Recipients:** AIDS/HIV, Alzheimers Disease, Cancer, Clinics/Medical Centers, Diabetes, Eyes/Blindness, Heart, Hospitals, Long-Term Care, Medical Education, Medical Research, Multiple Sclerosis, Preventive Medicine/Wellness Organizations, Public Health,. Research/Studies Institutes, Single-Disease Health Associations, Speech & Hearing, Substance Abuse. **Geo. Dist:** nationally; Los Angeles, CA.

★ 12015 ★ Temple Hoyne Buell Foundation
1666 South University Boulevard, Suite B
Denver, CO 80210
Phone: (303)744-1688 **Fax:** (303)744-1601
Email: ssteele@buellfoundation.org
Website: http://www.buellfoundation.org
Susan Steele, Executive Director

Fnded: 1962. **Philosophy:** "The Temple Hoyne Buell Foundation is an active professional philanthropic organization supporting the healthy development of children, youth and families through grants and partnerships with other sectors of our community. In that regard, the foundation will focus primarily on the State of Colorado." "More emphasis will be placed on long-term programs or system changes that have demonstrated success in helping children thrive." Foundation Annual Report fiscal 1999. **Priorities:** *Arts & Humanities:* 3%. Includes a major grant to the Sangre de Cristo Arts and Conference Center and funding for children's arts & music education. *Civic & Public Affairs:* 8%. Primary support for the Cherokee Ranch and Castle Foundation. *Education:* 46%. Supports Head Start programs, 4-H, home schooling programs, Junior Achievement, and literacy. *Environment:* 32%. Funds programs promoting the social and emotional development of youth, and family stability. *International:* 6%. Emphasis on hospitals and medical centers that treat children and childhood diseases. *Note:* Total contributions made in fiscal 2000. **Typ. Recipients:** Cancer, Children's Health/Hospitals, Diabetes, Domestic Violence, Family Planning, Health Organizations, Heart, Hospitals, Kidney, Mental Health, People with Disabilities, Prenatal Health Issues, Preventive Medicine/Wellness Organizations, Public Health, Research/Studies Institutes, Single-Disease Health Associations, Speech & Hearing. **Geo. Dist:** CO.

★ 12016 ★ Thelma Doelger Charitable Trust
950 John Daly Boulevard, Suite 300
Daly City, CA 94015
Phone: (650)755-2333
Edward King, Trustee

Fnded: 1980. **Philosophy:** The trust traditionally supports California zoos and humane societies with large grants. **Priorities:** *Arts & Humanities:* 4%. Supports museum. *Civic & Public Affairs:* 35%. Supports San Francisco Zoological Society. *Education:* 5%. Supports Stanford University endowment. *Environment:* 35%. Supports animal protection organizations. *International:* 7%. Supports medical centers. *Note:* Total contributions made in 1999. **Typ. Recipients:** Clinics/Medical Centers, Hospitals, Speech & Hearing. **Geo. Dist:** CA, including Bay area.

★ 12017 ★ The Theodore H. Barth Foundation, Inc.
45 Rockefeller Plaza, Suite 2037
New York, NY 10111
Phone: (212)332-3466
Ellen Berelson, Vice President & Director

Fnded: 1953. **Philosophy:** The foundation's interests focus on higher education, including scholarships; health and hospitals; conservation; Lutheran churches; youth organizations; and the arts. **Priorities:** *Arts & Humanities:* 21%. Funds public library, music, museums, and performing arts in New York City. *Civic & Public Affairs:* 7%. Funds the botanical garden. *Education:* 13%. Supports higher education. *Environment:* 35%. Primarily youth groups. *International:* 20%. Supports hospitals and single-disease health associations. *Note:* Total contributions made in 2001. **Typ. Recipients:** Children's Health/Hospitals, Clinics/Medical Centers, Family Planning, Health Funds, Health Organizations, Hospices, Hospitals, Kidney, Medical Research, Mental Health, Nursing Services, People with Disabilities, Public Health, Research/Studies Institutes, Single-Disease Health Associations, Speech & Hearing, Transplant Networks/Donor Banks. **Geo. Dist:** MA; NY.

★ 12018 ★ Theodore and Vada Stanley Foundation
47 Richards Ave.
Norwalk, CT 06857
Theodore Stanley, Trustee

Fnded: 1985. **Priorities:** *Arts & Humanities:* 1%. Supports performing arts and a presidential museum & library. *Civic & Public Affairs:* Less than 1%. Gives to community foundations, economic public policy organizations, and a good citizenship organization. *Education:* 1%. Contributes to a statewide education program, a school for the mentally retarded, and a college. *Environment:* 5%. Funds child welfare, American refugee services, and poverty-fighting program. *International:* 89%. Supports medical research, organ donation programs, mental health organizations, hospitals, clinics, and family health. *Note:* Total contributions made in 2000. **Typ. Recipients:** Cancer, Eyes/Blindness, Family Planning, Health Organizations, Health Organizations, Health Policy/Cost Containment, Hospitals, Mental Health, People with Disabilities, Public Health, Single-Disease Health Associations, Substance Abuse. **Geo. Dist:** nationally; CT.

★ 12019 ★ Theresa A. Thomas Memorial Foundation
PO Box 1122
Richmond, VA 23218
Phone: (804)697-1373 **Fax:** (804)697-1399
James Roberts, President & Director

Fnded: 1975. **Philosophy:** The mission of the foundation is to support organizations providing medical care or assistance with emphasis on primary care provided to medically underserved and uninsured populations within 100 miles of the Richmond Metropolitan area. **Priorities:** *Education:* 51%. Supports medical training. *Environment:* 8%. Camps, senior services, and rescue squads. *International:* 41%. Primarily for clinics and hospitals. *Note:* Total contributions made in fiscal 2001. **Typ. Recipients:** Children's Health/Hospitals, Clinics/Medical Centers, Emergency/Ambulance Services, Family Planning, Health-General, Heart, Home-Care Services, Hospitals, Medical Education, Public Health, Single-Disease Health Associations. **Geo. Dist:** VA.

★ 12020 ★ Theresa and Edward O'Toole Foundation
One Wall St., 28th Fl.
New York, NY 10286
Phone: (212)408-4281
Estella Lau, Vice President

Fnded: 1971. **Philosophy:** The foundation is primarily interested in supporting Catholic churches and organizations. Some educational support goes to Catholic unions, universities, and schools. **Priorities:** *Education:* 63%. Primarily supports religious secondary schools and colleges. *International:* 34%. Supports hospitals, medical centers and programs. *Note:* Total contributions made in fiscal 2001. **Typ. Recipients:** Cancer, Clinics/Medical Centers, Health Organizations, Hospitals, Long-Term Care. **Geo. Dist:** nationally; NJ; NY.

★ 12021 ★ Thomas and Agnes Carvel Foundation
35 East Grassy Sprain Rd.
Yonkers, NY 10710
Phone: (914)793-7300 **Fax:** (914)793-7381
Ann McHugh, Contact

Fnded: 1976. **Philosophy:** The Thomas and Agnes Carvel Foundation makes most of its grants in the areas of health care and education. Health care funding favors cancer research, hospitals, and pediatric care. Funding for education emphasizes private secondary schools and religious education. **Priorities:** *Arts & Humanities:* 4%. Supports museums, theater, and music. *International:* 72%. Supports medical research, nursing, single-disease health associations, and hospitals. *Note:* Total contributions made in fiscal 2000. **Typ. Recipients:** Cancer, Children's Health/Hospitals, Clinics/Medical Centers, Domestic Violence, Emergency/Ambulance Services, Health-General, Hospices, Hospitals, Medical Rehabilitation, Medical Research, Nursing Services, Nutrition, Outpatient Health Care, Prenatal Health Issues, Prenatal Health Issues, Single-Disease Health Associations, Substance Abuse, Transplant Networks/Donor Banks. **Geo. Dist:** NY, Westchester County.

★ 12022 ★ Thomas Anthony Pappas Charitable Foundation
PO Box 463
Belmont, MA 02478-0004
Phone: (781)862-2802
John Pappas, Executive Director

Fnded: 1975. **Philosophy:** The foundation makes most of its grants in the areas of health, education, and the arts. Health interests include hospitals and single-disease associations. Educational funding favors dental schools, universities, technology, and law. Arts support goes primarily to performing arts centers. **Priorities:** *Arts & Humanities:* 1%. Focus on music, museums, and arts centers. *Education:* 53%. Supports colleges and specialized schools. *Environment:* 11%. Youth organizations and child welfare. *International:* 30%. Funds hospitals, single-disease health associations, and pediatric health. *Note:* Total contributions made in 2000. **Typ. Recipients:** Alzheimers Disease, Arthritis, Cancer, Children's Health/Hospitals, Clinics/ Medical Centers, Eyes/Blindness, Health Organizations, Health-General, Heart, Hospices, Hospitals, Kidney, Long-Term Care, Medical Education, Medical Rehabilitation, Medical Research, Nursing Services, People with Disabilities, Research/Studies Institutes, Respiratory, Single-Disease Health Associations, Substance Abuse. **Geo. Dist:** MA.

★ 12023 ★ Thomas and Dorothy Leavey Foundation
10100 Santa Monica Boulevard, Suite 610
Los Angeles, CA 90067
Phone: (310)551-9936 **Fax:** (310)551-9938
Kathleen McCarthy, President

Fnded: 1952. **Philosophy:** The foundation originally was established to provide college scholarships. They have broadened their grant-making program to include medical research, churches, and civic groups. **Priorities:** *Education:* 61%. Supports higher education and scholarships, with major support going to Loyola Marymount University, and religious pre-college education. *Environment:* 3%. Funds family services, including those for youth and the elderly. *International:* Less than 1%. Contributes to medical centers and hospitals. *Note:* Total contributions made in 2000. **Typ. Recipients:** AIDS/HIV, Cancer, Child Abuse, Children's Health/Hospitals, Clinics/Medical Centers, Domestic Violence, Emergency/Ambulance Services, Family Planning, Health Funds, Health Organizations, Hospitals, Long-Term Care, Medical Education, Medical Research, Nursing Services, People with Disabilities, Prenatal Health Issues, Public Health, Respiratory, Single-Disease Health Associations, Substance Abuse. **Geo. Dist:** Southern California, CA.

★ 12024 ★ Thomas F. and Kate Miller Jeffress Memorial Trust
PO Box 26688
Richmond, VA 23261-6688
Phone: (804)788-3698 **Fax:** (804)788-2700
Dr. Richard Brandt, Advisor

Fnded: 1981. **Priorities:** *Religion:* 100%. Funding went to Virginia colleges and universities. The foundation focused its funding toward younger scientists (assistant professors) and change in research directions. *Note:* Contribution made in fiscal 2001. **Typ. Recipients:** Medical Education, Medical Research, Research/Studies Institutes. **Geo. Dist:** VA.

★ 12025 ★ Thomas J. Emery Memorial
2120 US Bank
425 Walnut St.
Cincinnati, OH 45202
Phone: (513)621-3124 **Fax:** (513)651-8403
Lee Carter, President

Fnded: 1925. **Philosophy:** The memorial makes grants across the major categories of support. In social services, interests include united funds, homes, youth organizations, the disabled, child welfare, and community centers. Educational funding favors universities, high schools, day schools, and nursery schools in Cincinnati. Arts support goes to art institutes, museums, and public broadcasting. Health funding includes children's hospitals and hospices. The memorial also makes grants to other recipient areas. **Priorities:** *Arts & Humanities:* 22%. Supports art associations, theater, and performing arts. *Civic & Public Affairs:* 13%. Grants made to housing and economic development. *Education:* 23%. Funds public and private elementary schools, education funds, colleges, and day school. *Environment:* 29%. Gives to youth groups, shelters, united funds, and family services. *International:* 13%. Emphasis on hospitals, treatment centers, and children's health. *Note:* Total contributions made in 2000. **Typ. Recipients:** Cancer, Children's Health/Hospitals, Clinics/Medical Centers, Diabetes, Domestic Violence, Emergency/Ambulance Services, Eyes/Blindness, Family Planning, Health Organizations, Health-General, Hospices, Hospitals, Long-Term Care, Medical Rehabilitation, Mental Health, People with Disabilities, Prenatal Health Issues, Public Health, Research/Studies Institutes, Single-Disease Health Associations, Speech & Hearing, Substance Abuse, Transplant Networks/Donor Banks. **Geo. Dist:** Cincinnati, OH.

★ 12026 ★ Thomas J. Watson Foundation
293 South Main St.
Providence, RI 02903
Phone: (401)274-1952 **Fax:** (401)274-1954
Email: WatsonFoundation@Brown.edu
Website: http://www.WatsonFellowship.org
Tori Harding-Smith, Executive Director

Fnded: 1961. **Philosophy:** In 1968, in recognition of Mr. and Mrs. Watson's interests in education and world affairs, their children decided that a fellowship program should constitute the major activity of the foundation. The Watson Fellowship Program, administered in cooperation with 49 private colleges and universities throughout the United States, enables outstanding college graduates to engage in a year of independent study and travel abroad following graduation. **Priorities:** *Arts & Humanities:* 4%. Funds museums and literatary associations. *Education:* 62% Supports religious schools and the Watson Fellowship Program. *International:* 4%. Funds AIDS coalition. *Note:* Total contributions made in fiscal 2001. **Typ. Recipients:** AIDS/HIV, Children's Health/Hospitals. **Geo. Dist:** nationally.

★ 12027 ★ Thompson Charitable Foundation
4823 Old Kingston Pike
PO Box 10516
Knoxville, TN 37939-0516
Phone: (865)588-0491
Monica Luke, Foundation Manager

Fnded: 1987. **Philosophy:** The foundation's primary focus is health services and sciences, including hospitals and clinics, education, religion, culture, and human services. Major funding also supports capital campaigns and renovation projects for educational institutions. "Reflecting the concerns of the founder, the charitable trust supports programs that seek to improve the quality of life for individuals and communities." **Priorities:** *Arts & Humanities:* 19%. Supports theater groups and libraries. *Civic & Public Affairs:* 16%. Focus on Habitat for Humanity. *Education:* 16%. Community colleges, special education, and private precollege education. *Environment:* 21%. Family services, community services, and youth organizations. *International:* 28%. Clinics, hospice programs, hospitals, and public health. *Note:* Total contributions made in fiscal 2001. **Typ. Recipients:** AIDS/HIV, Cancer, Child Abuse, Children's Health/Hospitals, Clinics/Medical Centers, Family Planning, Geriatric Health, Health-General, Hospices, Hospitals, Medical Rehabilitation, Nursing Services, People with Disabilities, Prenatal Health Issues, Preventive Medicine/Wellness Organizations, Preventive Medicine/Wellness Organizations, Public Health. **Geo. Dist:** KY, Bell County; KY, Clay County; KY, Laurel County; KY, Leslie County; TN, Anderson County; TN, Blount County; TN, Knox County; TN, Scott County; VA, Buchanan County; VA, Tazewell County.

★ 12028 ★ Thoresen Foundation
2300 West Bay Drive
Largo, FL 33770-1945
Fax: (813)581-3625
Email: pvoconn@aol.com
Paul O'Connell, Trustee

Fnded: 1952. **Priorities:** *Arts & Humanities:* 3% Supports local art festival. *Civic & Public Affairs:* 5%. Supports community foundation. *Education:* 51%. Supports education foundations, colleges and universities, and schools. *Environment:* 15%. Supports services for the disabled, youth programs, and athletics. *International:* 8%. Supports emergency care and physician's groups. *Note:* Contributions were made in 2000. **Typ. Recipients:** Cancer, Clinics/Medical Centers, Emergency/Ambulance Services, Health Organizations, Health-General, Home-Care Services, People with Disabilities, Research/Studies Institutes, Respiratory. **Geo. Dist:** FL; IL; NC; VA.

★ 12029 ★ Timken Foundation of Canton
200 Market Ave, North, Suite 210
Canton, OH 44702-1437
Phone: (330)452-1144 **Fax:** (330)452-2306
Email: dickesd@timkenfoundation.org
Don Dickes, Secretary & Treasurer

Fnded: 1934. **Philosophy:** The foundation allocates major support for charitable organizations that will benefit the citizens in local areas, in the United States, Australia, Canada, France, Italy, Poland, Romania, South Africa, England, Germany, and Brazil where the Timken Company has manufacturing facilities. **Priorities:** *Arts & Humanities:* 7%. Makes donations to museums, art centers, and public libraries. *Education:* 45%. Funds colleges and universities and precollege education. *Environment:* 13%. Supports YMCAs, youth groups, and women's concerns. *International:* 11%. *Note:* Total contributions made in fiscal 1999. **Typ. Recipients:** Cancer, Clinics/Medical Centers, Domestic Violence, Emergency/Ambulance Services, Geriatric Health, Heart, Hospitals, Medical Education, Substance Abuse. **Geo. Dist:** internationally; nationally; operating locations; OH.

★ 12030 ★ Tinker Foundation
55 East 59th St., 21st Fl.
New York, NY 10022
Phone: (212)421-6858 **Fax:** (212)223-3326
Email: tinker@tinker.org
Website: http://fdncenter.org/grantmaker/tinker
Renate Rennie, President & Director

Fnded: 1959. **Philosophy:** "Tinker Foundation grants are awarded to organizations and institutions that promote the interchange and exchange of information within the community of those concerned with the affairs of Spain, Portugal, Ibero-America and Antarctica. (Ibero-America is defined here as the Spanish- and Portuguese-speaking countries of the Western Hemisphere.) Emphasis is placed on those activities that have strong public policy implications, offer innovative solutions to many of the problems facing these regions today, and incorporate new mechanisms for addressing environmental, economic and governance issues. Such activities may include, but are not limited to, research projects, conferences and short-term training workshops related to the Foundation's areas of interest. The Foundation encourages collaboration between organizations in the United States and Iberia or Latin America and among institutions in those regions." The Tinker Foundation Applicant Information. **Priorities:** *Civic & Public Affairs:* 16%. Funds foundations and public policy organizations. *Education:* 17%. Colleges and universities, projects and research. *Note:* Total contributions made in 2001. **Typ. Recipients:** Family Planning. **Geo. Dist:** internationally; nationally.

★ 12031 ★ Tisch Foundation
655 Madison Ave.
New York, NY 10021
Phone: (212)521-2943 **Fax:** (212)521-2983
Barry Bloom, Secretary & Treasurer

Fnded: 1957. **Philosophy:** The foundation was established in 1957 and emphasizes higher education and research programs. It supports Jewish organizations and welfare funds, museums, and secondary schools. It also supports institutions in Israel. **Priorities:** *Arts & Humanities:* 14%. Supports art museums, dance, orchestras, theater, public broadcasting, art funds, and historic preservation. *Civic & Public Affairs:* 5%. Gives to community foundations, zoos, parks, and urban development. *Education:* 52%. Supports colleges, universities, an arts school, and private academies. *Environment:* 6%. Funds YMHA/YWHA; United Way; child and family services organizations; and services for the homeless, hungry, and indigent. *International:* 7%. Funds HIV/AIDS, cancer, and colorectal health organizations; nurisng homes; medical research; women's health initiatives; and mental health associations. *Note:* Total contributions made in 2000. **Typ. Recipients:** AIDS/HIV, Cancer, Children's Health/ Hospitals, Clinics/Medical Centers, Diabetes, Emergency/Ambulance Services, Family Planning, Health Funds, Hospitals, Hospitals (University Affiliated), Long-Term Care, Medical Education, Medical Research, People with Disabilities, Research/Studies Institutes, Single-Disease Health Associations. **Geo. Dist:** nationally; New York, NY.

★ 12032 ★ Town Creek Foundation

PO Box 159
Oxford, MD 21654
Phone: (410)226-5315 **Fax:** (410)226-5468
Email: info@towncreekfdn.org
Website: http://www.towncreekfdn.org
Christine Shelton, Executive Director

Fnded: 1981. **Philosophy:** The Town Creek Foundation makes grants in the areas of conservation and the environment, public broadcasting, and the search for a peaceful and democratic society. Funding is also available for the improvement of economic and social conditions in Talbot County, Maryland, and its communities. The foundation no longer supports international efforts. Primary focus is on organizations dedicated to action and advocacy. **Priorities:** *Arts & Humanities:* 4%. Supports public broadcasting. *Civic & Public Affairs:* 28%. Supports public policy organizations, social research, and Talbot County organizations. *Education:* 5%. Supports education funds. *Environment:* 3%. *Religion:* About 1%. *Note:* Total contributions made in 2002. **Typ. Recipients:** Emergency/ Ambulance Services, Public Health, Respiratory. **Geo. Dist:** nationally; statewide or large regions; MD.

★ 12033 ★ Tozer Foundation

PO Box 64704
Saint Paul, MN 55164
Phone: (651)244-0958
Robert Davis, Director

Fnded: 1946. **Philosophy:** The foundation's primary focus is to provide scholarships for college students. Applications are made usually by seniors at their high school, and recipients are selected on the basis of ability and need by a scholarship committee appointed by the foundation. The scholarships may be renewed annually. Grants are made for educational and other charitable purposes, such as social service organizations and the arts. Most of the funding for social services is awarded to the United Way and youth organizations. Arts funding favors the performing arts in music and theater. The foundation also supports public school districts, civic affairs, health, and religion with smaller grants. **Priorities:** *Education:* About 80%. Supports scholarship programs at colleges and universities. *Note:* Total contributions made in fiscal 2001. **Typ. Recipients:** Clinics/Medical Centers, Hospitals, Medical Rehabilitation. **Geo. Dist:** MN, Kanabec County for scholarship program; MN, Pine County for scholarship program; MN, Washington County for scholarship program.

★ 12034 ★ The Trull Foundation

404 Fourth St.
Palacios, TX 77465
Phone: (361)972-5241 **Fax:** (361)972-1109
Email: info@trullfoundation.org
Website: http://www.trullfoundation.org
E. Purvis, Executive Director

Fnded: 1948. **Philosophy:** "For over forty years (the foundation has) been actively interested in various educational, religious, cultural and social programs, the majority of which have been in the State of Texas. (The foundation has) supported Presbyterian interests, without, however, being limited to those interests. The (foundation has) been concerned with people, with improving the quality of life, especially for those living in poor or oppressed conditions. Currently, the following priorities are set by the Trustees: °A concern for the needs of the Palacios area, where the Foundation has its roots. The senior citizens center, the city paving needs, the Marine Education Center, and other local projects were considered and supported.' °A concern for the pre-adolescent and their families, with special emphasis of family values. Grants were given to help direct and channel lives away from child abuse, from neglect, from hunger, and into an adolescence of good mental and physical growth.' °A concern for Hispanic issues, especially in South Texas. Grants have been made to help hurdle the language barrier, the poverty barrier, and a system which has consistently kept them poor, uneducated and unrepresented.' °A concern for those persons and families devastated by the results of substance abuse.'" 1995-1996 Annual Report **Priorities:** *Arts & Humanities:* 9%. Primary support for historical associations, public broadcasting, and libraries. *Education:* 22%. Focus on elementary and secondary education, colleges and universities, scholarships, and seminaries. *Environment:* (Welfare/Community Service) 43%. Supports family services, child welfare, youth organizations, municipalities, environmental organizations, and women's affairs. *International:* 7%. Supports hospitals. *Note:* Total contributions made in 2000. **Typ. Recipients:** AIDS/HIV, Cancer, Children's Health/Hospitals, Domestic Violence, Family Planning, Health Organizations, Health-General, Medical Education, Medical Rehabilitation, Medical Research, Mental Health, Nutrition, Preventive Medicine/Wellness Organizations, Public Health, Substance Abuse, Transplant Networks/Donor Banks. **Geo. Dist:** nationally, although Texas is given preference; TX.

★ 12035 ★ Trust for Mutual Understanding

30 Rockefeller Plaza
Room 5600
New York, NY 10112
Phone: (212)632-3405 **Fax:** (212)632-3409
Email: tmu@tmuny.org
Website: http://www.tmuny.org
Richard Lanier, Trustee

Fnded: 1984. **Philosophy:** The Trust for Mutual Understanding primarily is interested in supporting professional exchanges between the United States, the former Soviet Union, and East Central Europe in the areas of environmental conservation and the arts. "Approximately two-thirds of TMU's grants are awarded for exchanges in the visual and performing arts and one-third in environmental conservation and protection. Most are allocated specifically to help cover international travel, per diem, and related expenses of Russian, Eastern and Central European, and American participants in projects that involve the exchange of professionals and specialists in those fields." Trust for Mutual Understanding web site. **Priorities:** *Arts & Humanities:* 43%. Includes the visual and the performing arts, and exchanges eligible for consideration include exhibitions, performaces given in conjunction with lecture/demonstrations, creative collaborations, curatorial research projects, art conservation and historic preservation initiatives, arts management programs, and cultural documentation activities. *Civic & Public Affairs:* 8%. Funds business/nonprofit management and public policy. *Education:* 18%. Supports colleges and universities. *Religion:* 5%. Supports biological science/research. *Note:* Total contributions made in 1999. **Typ. Recipients:** AIDS/HIV, Health-General, Medical Education. **Geo. Dist:** nationally.

★ 12036 ★ Trustees of the Lowell Institute

Choate, Hall, & Stewart at Exchange Place
53 State St.
Boston, MA 02109
Phone: (617)248-5255 **Fax:** (617)248-4000
William Lowell, Administrator

Fnded: 1836. **Philosophy:** The Trustees of the Lowell Institute support education favoring technology, universities, and seminars and conferences. Public broadcasting and museums are also of interest. The institute places particular emphasis on programs dedicated to inner-city school children. **Priorities:** *Arts & Humanities:* 38%. Supports museums and art education programs. *Civic & Public Affairs:* 13%. Primarily supports aquariums. *Education:* 32%. Supports educational programs and universities. *International:* 1%. Supports a health clinic. *Religion:* 16%. Supports educational science programs and museums. *Note:* Contributions were made in fiscal 2001. **Typ. Recipients:** Clinics/Medical Centers. **Geo. Dist:** MA.

★ 12037 ★ Tudor Foundation, Inc.

1275 King St.
Greenwich, CT 06831
Phone: (203)863-6700
Andrew Paul, President & Director

Fnded: 1997. **Philosophy:** The Tudor Foundation makes grants to enhance children's health, welfare, and education. **Typ. Recipients:** Children's Health/ Hospitals, Health Organizations.

★ 12038 ★ Tull Charitable Foundation

Hurt Bldg.
50 Hurt Plaza, Suite 1245
Atlanta, GA 30303
Phone: (404)659-7079 **Fax:** (404)659-1223
Ms. Barbara Cleveland, Executive Director

Fnded: 1952. **Philosophy:** The foundation trustees prefer to make grants that will "have a significant and lasting impact on an organization as well as its community." The primary focus of the foundation is to respond to needs in Georgia, particularly in the Atlanta metropolitan area, that are strategically important to an organization's growth and capacity, enable the organization to more effectively address important community needs, and are cost-effective. The foundation's areas of primary interest are education, health and human services, civic and community affairs, youth development, and the arts. **Priorities:** *Arts & Humanities:* 3%. Funds arts and culture through history center and symphony orchestra. *Civic & Public Affairs:* 33%. Supports civic and community affairs through housing organizations, junior league and parks. *Education:* 34%. Supports education and youth development through schools, academies, colleges and universities. *Environment:* 19%. Supports boys and girls clubs, homes, youth services and United Way. *International:* 3%. Funds mental health and spinal health. *Religion:* 4%. Supports natural science centers. *Note:* Total contributions made in 2000. **Typ. Recipients:** Alzheimers Disease, Cancer, Children's Health/Hospitals, Clinics/Medical Centers, Domestic Violence, Emergency/Ambulance Services, Eyes/Blindness, Family Planning, Health Organizations, Hospitals, Long-Term Care, Medical Education, Medical Research, Mental Health, Nursing Services, People with Disabilities, Prenatal Health Issues, Public Health, Research/Studies Institutes, Single-Disease Health Associations, Substance Abuse. **Geo. Dist:** GA.

★ 12039 ★ Turner Foundation

One CNN Center
Suite 1090 South Tower
Atlanta, GA 30303
Phone: (404)681-9900 **Fax:** (404)681-0172
Email: turnerfi@turnerfoundation.org
Website: http://www.turnerfoundation.org
Mike Finley, President

Fnded: 1990. **Priorities:** *Arts & Humanities:* 1%. Gives to museums, public broadcasting, and historic preservation. *Civic & Public Affairs:* 11%. Funds women's rights, law/justice organizations, environmental and reproductive rights policy organizations, civic groups, and zoos. *Education:* 3%. Contributes to universities and university-conducted environmental and public interest research. *Environment:* 9%. Family planning and adolescent pregnancy prevention organizations receive support. *International:* Less than 1%. *Religion:* Less than 1%. *Note:* Total contributions made in 2001. **Typ. Recipients:** Adolescent Health Issues, Family Planning, Health Funds, Health Policy/Cost Containment, Hospitals, Medical Research, Mental Health, Preventive Medicine/Wellness Organizations, Research/Studies Institutes. **Geo. Dist:** nationally.

★ 12040 ★ Turrell Fund

21 Van Vleck St.
Montclair, NJ 07042-2358
Phone: (973)783-9358 **Fax:** (973)783-9283
Email: turrell@bellatlantic.net
Website: http://www.fdncenter.org/grantmaker/turrell
Dr. E. Williams, Executive Director & Secretary

Fnded: 1935. **Philosophy:** The Turrell Fund's principal interest is supporting organizations that help youth, with emphasis on needy youngsters. "Our purpose is to support activities that will contribute to the development of young persons from families which could not afford these services without help." These activities may be educational, vocational, recreational, and corrective; or they may be programs to provide care for the child. Programs to make such activities available to handicapped children are also eligible. Primary consideration is given to children age twelve or younger. The fund makes grants in the following program areas: Educational Programs, with emphasis on day care centers, day nurseries, elementary and intermediate schools, libraries, and museums; Social Support Services, with emphasis on children's aid and adoption services, community centers, family centers, neighborhood youth centers, and neighborhood organizations; Youth Activities, with emphasis on boys and girls clubs, boys and girls scouts, camps, and YM-YWCAs. **Priorities:** *Arts & Humanities:* 7%. Supports museums, libraries, music, and the performing arts. *Civic & Public Affairs:* 5%. Supports urban affairs and housing. *Education:* 37%. Primary support for elementary and secondary education. *Environment:* 45%. Supports youth organizations, child welfare, adoption services, community centers, family services, day care centers, and neighborhood organizations. *International:* Less than 1%. *Note:* Total contributions made in 2000. **Typ. Recipients:** Adolescent Health Issues, AIDS/HIV, Children's Health/Hospitals, Clinics/Medical Centers, Family Planning, Hospitals, Medical Education, Medical Rehabilitation, People with Disabilities, Preventive Medicine/Wellness Organizations, Research/Studies Institutes, Substance Abuse. **Geo. Dist:** NJ, Essex County; NJ, Hudson County; NJ, Passaic County; NJ, Union County; VT.

★ 12041 ★ Valley Foundation

16450 Los Gatos Boulevard, Suite 210
Los Gatos, CA 95032-5594
Phone: (408)358-4545 **Fax:** (408)358-4548
Website: http://www.valley.org
Ervie Smith, Executive Director

Fnded: 1984. **Philosophy:** "...the Highest priority...is to provide targeted funding for qualified charitable organizations serving the health care needs of lower income households in Santa Clara County...in the areas of medical research, higher education, social service, programs for youth, aid to senior citiziens, and the arts." The Valley Foundation 2000 Annual Report. **Priorities:** *Arts & Humanities:* 11%. Museums, theater, arts council, and music. *Education:* 28%. Supports health-related education. *Environment:* 39%. Youth programs, YMCA/YWCA, domestic violence, and family services. *International:* 22%. Hospice, wellness and medical research. *Note:* Contributions were made in fiscal 2001. **Typ. Recipients:** Adolescent Health Issues, AIDS/HIV, Alzheimers Disease, Cancer, Child Abuse, Children's Health/Hospitals, Clinics/Medical Centers, Diabetes, Domestic Violence, Emergency/Ambulance Services, Geriatric Health, Health Funds, Health Organizations, Health-General, Heart, Hospices, Medical Education, Medical Rehabilitation, Medical Research, Mental Health, Nutrition, People with Disabilities, Prenatal Health Issues, Preventive Medicine/Wellness Organizations, Public Health, Single-Disease Health Associations, Substance Abuse. **Geo. Dist:** CA, Santa Clara County.

★ 12042 ★ van Ameringen Foundation, Inc.

509 Madison Ave.
New York, NY 10022-5501
Phone: (212)758-6221 **Fax:** (212)688-2105
Website: http://www.vanamfound.org
Henry van Ameringen, President

Fnded: 1950. **Philosophy:** The foundation's primary interest is furthering "prevention, education, and direct care in the mental health field with an emphasis on those individuals and populations having a disadvantaged background and deprived opportunities." Priority interest areas include preventive and early-intervention strategies, particularly those which work in tandem with educational programs; programs to link existing resources for clients, particularly the mixing of public and private efforts; programs which increase the accessibility of the poor to mental health services; and programs which include a self-help model. Recently supported projects include programs dealing with parental stress, programs for abused children and their parents, crisis centers for runaways, services for the elderly, and education for minorities. Some funding is directed to arts projects related to mental health issues. **Priorities:** *Civic & Public Affairs:* 9%. Funds legal aid, government programs, housing, and career training and placement. *Environment:* 35%. Supports child welfare, child and family services, camps shelters, and incarceration alternatives programs. *International:* 38%. Supports mental health, hospitals and medical centers, clinics, and community health programs. *Note:* Total contributions made in 2000. **Typ. Recipients:** AIDS/HIV, Cancer, Children's Health/Hospitals, Clinics/Medical Centers, Domestic Violence, Emergency/Ambulance Services, Geriatric Health, Health Organizations, Health-General, Hospitals, Hospitals (University Affiliated), Long-Term Care, Medical Education, Medical Rehabilitation, Medical Research, Mental Health, People with Disabilities, Prenatal Health Issues, Preventive Medicine/Wellness Organizations, Single-Disease Health Associations, Substance Abuse. **Geo. Dist:** Northeastern USA.

★ 12043 ★ Victor E. Speas Foundation

Bank of America
PO Box 419119
Kansas City, MO 64141-6119
Phone: (816)979-7481 **Fax:** (816)979-7916
David Ross, Senior Vice President

Fnded: 1947. **Philosophy:** The foundation focuses on health and social service programs. It emphasizes the improvement of health-related services in the greater Kansas City metropolitan area. **Priorities:** *Civic & Public Affairs:* 18%. Neighborhood programs and programs that support business/free enterprise. *Education:* 7%. Support for colleges in Kansas City. *Environment:* 51%. Volunteer programs, Goodwill, and family projects, mainly in the Kansas City, MO, area. *International:* 13%. Health education, hospitals, and single-disease health organizations, with an emphasis on children. *Note:* Contributions made in 2000. **Typ. Recipients:** AIDS/HIV, Cancer, Children's Health/Hospitals, Children's Health/Hospitals, Clinics/Medical Centers, Emergency/Ambulance Services, Geriatric Health, Health Funds, Health Organizations, Health Policy/Cost Containment, Heart, Home-Care Services, Hospices, Hospitals, Kidney, Medical Education, Medical Rehabilitation, Mental Health, Nursing Services, Nutrition, People with Disabilities, Public Health, Research/Studies Institutes, Sexual Abuse, Single-Disease Health Associations, Speech & Hearing, Substance Abuse, Trauma Treatment. **Geo. Dist:** Kansas City, MO, metropolitan area.

★ 12044 ★ Victoria Foundation

946 Bloomfield Ave.
Glen Ridge, NJ 07028
Phone: (973)748-5300 **Fax:** (973)748-0016
Email: catherinemcfarland@victoriafoundation.org
Website: http://www.victoriafoundation.org
Catherine McFarland, Secretary & Executive Officer

Fnded: 1924. **Philosophy:** "At its 75th anniversary, the foundation's desire to help individuals in need reach their potential remains its core value. Whether providing emergency coal for needy families, treating rheumatic fever in children or helping Newark, NJ, become a shining City on the Hill, Victoria has worked to create greater access and opportunities for people and to improve the quality of life in the communities in which they live. Today, the foundation's efforts center on educational, urban development, and youth and family initiatives predominantly in Newark, NJ, as well as pressing environmental issues throughout the state. The foundation has grown from granting $2,000 in 1924 to approving more than $11 million in grants during 1999." 1999 Annual Report **Priorities:** *Arts & Humanities:* 26%. supports performing art center, public broadcasting, orchestra. *Civic & Public Affairs:* 14%. Supports libraries, public policy organizations, parks, job training, community foundations and housing initiatives. *Environment:* 9%. Supports food banks, family planning, scouting, community centers, YWCA. *International:* Approx. 1%. *Note:* Total contributions made in 2000. **Typ. Recipients:** Children's Health/Hospitals, Clinics/Medical Centers, Family Planning, Medical Education, People with Disabilities, Research/Studies Institutes, Substance Abuse. **Geo. Dist:** Newark, NJ.

★ 12045 ★ Vira I. Heinz Endowment

30 Dominion Tower
625 Liberty Ave.
Pittsburgh, PA 15222-3199
Phone: (412)281-5777 **Fax:** (412)281-5788
Email: info@heinz.org
Website: http://www.heinz.org
Maxwell King, President

Fnded: 1986. **Philosophy:** "Throughout their histories, the Howard and Vira I. Heinz Endowments have been privileged to enjoy a remarkable intimate relationship with the communities and organizations they serve. From this relationship continually emerge two of the Endowments' primary strengths: their sensitivity to the needs of their region, and their willingness to shoulder risks on its behalf. It has been characteristic of the Endowments to want to listen and respond personally to requests for help. We are neighbors, after all, not disinterested observers. For that reason, there has been a reluctance over the years to print formalized program guidelines, suggesting as they might an unfeeling institutionalization of process. We do not intend for that to happen. But we also appreciate how dramatically the philanthropic landscape has changed in recent years. With the demand for philanthropic resources increasing rapidly and with ever greater urgency, we must respond to the call from prospective grantseekers for guidance, specificity and direction... The Endowments' present grantmaking reflects over half a century of applied values and experiential learning. Three signature themes emerge from this rich history: leadership, cooperation and enterprise." *A Message from the Executive Director* **Priorities:** *Arts & Humanities:* 21%. Supports theater, history, museums of art, dance, the performing arts, libraries, opera, and arts councils. *Civic & Public Affairs:* 7%. Supports employment and job training, rural affairs, urban affairs, economic development, municipalities, and philanthropic organizations. *Education:* 36%. Supports schools, science education, colleges, universities, after-school programs, and economic education. *Environment:* 1%. *International:* 4%. Supports cancer research and hospitals. *Note:* Total contributions made in 2000. **Typ. Recipients:** Adolescent Health Issues, Cancer, Children's Health/Hospitals, Domestic Violence, Family Planning, Geriatric Health, Health Organizations, Health Policy/Cost Containment, Hospitals, Medical Education, Medical Research, Mental Health, Sexual Abuse, Single-Disease Health Associations, Substance Abuse. **Geo. Dist:** PA, Southwest Pennsylvania.

★ 12046 ★ Vollmer Foundation
PO Box 704
Butler, NJ 07405
Phone: (973)492-2309 **Fax:** (973)492-2309
Albert Ennist, Assistant Secretary & Assist. Treasurer

Fnded: 1965. **Philosophy:** The purpose of the Vollmer Foundation is "to make charitable distributions that will in some way benefit the people of Venezuela." The main areas of interest to the foundation are education, community foundations and scientific investigation. **Priorities:** *Civic & Public Affairs:* 11%. Funds Hispanic American Center for Economic Research. *Note:* Total contributions made in 2000. **Typ. Recipients:** Cancer.

★ 12047 ★ W. K. Kellogg Foundation
One Michigan Ave. East
Battle Creek, MI 49017-4058
Phone: (269)968-1611 **Fax:** (269)968-0413
Website: http://www.wkkf.org
Deborah Rey, Supervisor of Proposal Processing

Fnded: 1930. **Philosophy:** The W.K. Kellogg Foundation was established in 1930 "to help people help themselves through the practical application of knowledge and resources to improve their quality of life and that of future generations." Its programming activities center around the common visions of a world in which each person has a sense of worth; accepts responsibility for self, family, community, and societal well-being; and has the capacity to be productive, and to help create nurturing families, responsive institutions, and healthy communities. To achieve the greatest impact, the foundation targets its grants toward specific focal points or areas. These include health; food systems and rural development; youth development and education, and higher education; and philanthropy and volunteerism. When woven throughout these areas, funding also is provided for leadership; information systems/technology; efforts to capitalize on diversity; and family, neighborhood, and community development programming. Grants are concentrated in the United States, Latin America, the Caribbean, and southern Africa. **Priorities:** *Civic & Public Affairs:* 11%. Funds philanthropy, volunteerism, and social and economic development in the greater Battle Creek, MI area. *Education:* 24%. Funds colleges and universities; also supports public school systems, education foundations, leadership development, and private schools. *Environment:* 8%. Support youth services, food systems, and rural development. *International:* 15%. Supports healthcare systems organized around public health, prevention, and primary care. *Note:* Total contributions made in fiscal 2001. **Typ. Recipients:** Children's Health/Hospitals, Clinics/Medical Centers, Geriatric Health, Health Funds, Health Organizations, Health Policy/Cost Containment, Health-General, Hospices, Hospitals, Medical Education, Medical Research, Medical Training, Mental Health, Nursing Services, Nutrition, People with Disabilities, Prenatal Health Issues, Public Health, Research/Studies Institutes, Substance Abuse. **Geo. Dist:** nationally; Caribbean; Latin America; Southern Africa; nationally.

★ 12048 ★ W. M. Keck Foundation
550 South Hope St., Suite 2500
Los Angeles, CA 90071
Phone: (213)680-3833 **Fax:** (213)614-0934
Email: info@wmkeck.org
Website: http://www.wmkeck.org
Dr. Maria Pellegrini, Program Director

Fnded: 1954. **Philosophy:** "Consistent with Mr. Keck's vision, the Foundation primarily makes grants designed to provide far-reaching benefits for humanity in the fields of science, engineering, and medical research. Reflecting W.M. Keck's life as a pioneer, innovator and risk-taker, the Foundation seeks out research which opens new directions and could lead to breakthrough discoveries and the development of new technologies. Eligible institutions in these fields are accredited four-year colleges and universities, medical schools, and major, independent research institutions located within the United States. "The Foundation also wishes to help ensure that today's youth receive a high-quality, well-rounded education. To that end, it supports a program designed to promote innovative instruction and research at leading liberal arts colleges across the nation. "In addition to supporting the above purposes, the Foundation may from time to time consider special, major grants for potentially significant endeavors that the Foundation believes will ultimately benefit humankind." **Priorities:** *Arts & Humanities:* 3%. Funds public broadcasting. *Civic & Public Affairs:* Less than 1%. *Education:* 86%. Supports colleges and universities. *Environment:* 1%. *International:* 7%. Funds clinics and hospitals. *Religion:* 3%. Funds research laboratories. *Note:* Total contributions made in 2000. **Typ. Recipients:** Clinics/Medical Centers, Geriatric Health, Hospitals, Medical Education, Medical Rehabilitation, Medical Research, People with Disabilities, Speech & Hearing, Substance Abuse. **Geo. Dist:** nationally; CA, southern CA.

★ 12049 ★ W. O'Neil Foundation
5454 Wisconsin Ave., Suite 730
Chevy Chase, MD 20815
Phone: (301)656-5848
Helene O'Neil Cobb, President

Fnded: 1948. **Philosophy:** Grants are given primarily to Catholic organizations for international emergency relief and for programs that bring food, clothing, shelter, basic medical care, and basic education to the poor of the world, preferably though projects that help the poor to help themselves toward these goals. **Priorities:** *Civic & Public Affairs:* 6%. *Education:* 8%. Primarily for private schools. *International:* 5%. Medical clinics and mental health. *Note:* Total contributions made in 2000. **Typ. Recipients:** AIDS/HIV, Emergency/Ambulance Services, Geriatric Health, Health Funds, Health-General, Hospices, Hospitals, Hospitals (University Affiliated), Long-Term Care, Medical Education, Mental Health, People with Disabilities. **Geo. Dist:** nationally.

★ 12050 ★ W. W. Smith Charitable Trust
3515 West Chester Pike, Suite E
Newtown Square, PA 19073
Phone: (215)985-7917

Fnded: 1977. **Philosophy:** The trust supports four specific programs areas: medical research for heart disease, cancer, and AIDS; hospital indigent medical care; food, clothing, and shelter for children and the aged; and college financial aid. The trust funds research projects for heart disease, cancer, and AIDS that are new or are conducted by investigators before they have qualified for larger National Institutes of Health grants. In its program to provide medical care for the poor and needy, the trust supports hospitals in the cities of Chester and Philadelphia, with an explicit policy of accepting patients with no ability to pay. In its program to provide food, clothing, and shelter for children and the aged, the trust attempts to assist under-supported groups, including ethnic minorities, the elderly, orphans, and abused women and children. It is particularly interested in programs offering respite care to the elderly and in those benefiting older single women who live alone. The trust also supports financial aid programs for college students, prizes for college seniors, and scholarships through the Sea Education Association in Woods Hole, MA. **Priorities:** *Civic & Public Affairs:* 7%. Gives to women's and ethnic organizations, housing, and philanthropic organizations. *Education:* 65%. Provides scholarships and student aid for higher education. *Environment:* 7%. Supports programs and housing for seniors, food banks, shelters, and other social services. *International:* 15%. Supports cancer, heart, and AIDS research; other single-disease research; hospitals; medical centers; and maternity health care. *Note:* Total contributions made in fiscal 2000. **Typ. Recipients:** AIDS/HIV, Cancer, Diabetes, Domestic Violence, Emergency/Ambulance Services, Geriatric Health, Health Organizations, Heart, Home-Care Services, Hospitals, Long-Term Care, Medical Education, Medical Research, Nursing Services, People with Disabilities, Prenatal Health Issues, Single-Disease Health Associations. **Geo. Dist:** Philadelphia, PA, six-county Philadelphia regional area.

★ 12051 ★ W. W. W. Foundation
625 Fair Oaks Ave., Suite 360
South Pasadena, CA 91030
Phone: (626)441-5188 **Fax:** (626)441-3672
Linda Blinkenberg, Secretary & Director

Fnded: 1981. **Priorities:** *Civic & Public Affairs:* 1%. A Zoo. *Education:* 12%. Colleges and universities. *Environment:* 86%. Majority to Helen Woodward Animal Care Center, and the I Have a Dream Foundation. *International:* 1%. Medical research. *Note:* Total contributions made in fiscal 2001. **Typ. Recipients:** Child Abuse, Eyes/Blindness, Health-General, Hospitals, Medical Research, Single-Disease Health Associations, Substance Abuse. **Geo. Dist:** CA, Southern California.

★ 12052 ★ The Wagnalls Memorial Foundation
150 East Columbus St.
Lithopolis, OH 43136
Phone: (614)837-4765 **Fax:** (614)833-4767
Email: jneff@wagnalls.org
Website: http://www.wagnalls.org
Jerry Neff, Executive Director

Fnded: 1924. **Philosophy:** The Wagnalls Scholarship Fund, where most of the funding is given, was established "to encourage and assist student residents of Bloom Township and otherwise eligible to obtain a degree in higher education." The foundation makes grants for undergraduate and post-graduate study. **Priorities:** *Civic & Public Affairs:* 9%. Community projects. *Education:* 91%. Student aid for Lithopolis and Bloom Township, OH, residents. *Note:* Contributions made in fiscal 2000. **Typ. Recipients:** Medical Education. **Geo. Dist:** Bloom Township, OH; Lithopolis, OH.

★ 12053 ★ Waitt Family Foundation
PO Box 1948
La Jolla, CA 92038
Phone: (858)551-4839 **Fax:** (858)551-6871
Email: info@waittfoundation.org
Website: http://www.waittfoundation.org
Ted Waitt, Chairman & Director

Fnded: 1994. **Priorities:** *Civic & Public Affairs:* 7%. *Education:* 52%. Major support for a private school. *Environment:* 35%. Supports rehabilitation services, children's organizations, recreation, and social services. *Note:* Total contributions made in 1998. **Typ. Recipients:** Cancer, Children's Health/Hospitals, Emergency/Ambulance Services, Family Planning. **Geo. Dist:** IA.

★ 12054 ★ Wallace Alexander Gerbode Foundation
470 Columbus Ave., Suite 209
San Francisco, CA 94133-3930
Phone: (415)391-0911 **Fax:** (415)391-4587
Email: maildesk@gerbode.org
Website: http://fdncenter.org/grantmaker/gerbode
Thomas Layton, President

Fnded: 1953. **Philosophy:** The foundation is interested in programs and projects offering potential for significant impact. The primary focus is on the San Francisco Bay area and Hawaii. Interests generally fall under the following categories: arts and culture, environment, population, reproductive rights, citizen participation/building communities/inclusiveness, strength of the philanthropic process and the nonprofit sector, and special projects. **Priorities:** *Arts & Humanities:* 17%. Grants are made to dance, theater, and public broadcasting. *Civic & Public Affairs:* 36%. Issues related to reproductive rights, aid in dying, educational forums, ethnic organizations, and community foundations are funded. *Education:* 6%. Supports universities. *Environment:* 23%. Funding is provided to pro-choice organizations. *Note:* Total contributions made in 2000. **Typ. Recipients:** Children's Health/Hospitals, Domestic Violence, Family Planning, Health Organizations, Health Policy/Cost Containment, Health-General, Hospices, Long-Term Care, People with Disabilities, Public Health. **Geo. Dist:** San Francisco, CA, including Bay area; HI.

★ 12055 ★ Wallace Genetic Foundation
4900 Massachusetts Ave., Northwest, Suite 220
Washington, DC 20016
Phone: (202)966-2932 **Fax:** (202)966-3370
Email: wgfdn@aol.com
Website: http://www.wallacegenetic.org
Pat Lee, Co-Executive Director

Fnded: 1959. **Philosophy:** Grants are almost entirely limited to organizations associated with the personal interests of present or former trustees which include sustainable agriculture preservation of farmland nearcities, ecology, plant genetic research, biodiversity protection and environmental education. **Priorities:** *Civic & Public Affairs:* 18%. Supports botanical gardens, league of conservation voters, public policy organizations. *Environment:* 5%. Supports animal welfare organizations. *International:* 4%. Supports medical center, nutrition. *Note:* Total contributions made in 2000. **Typ. Recipients:** Cancer, Children's Health/Hospitals, Clinics/Medical Centers, Family Planning, Health Organizations, Health-General, Heart, Hospitals, Hospitals (University Affiliated), Medical Education, Medical Research, Nursing Services, Nutrition, Public Health, Respiratory, Single-Disease Health Associations. **Geo. Dist:** internationally; nationally.

★ 12056 ★ Wallis Foundation
1880 Century Park East, Suite 700
Los Angeles, CA 90067
Phone: (310)286-9777 **Fax:** (310)277-3411
Email: mark@mggcpa.com
Mark Augenstin, Chief Financial Officer & Director

Fnded: 1959. **Philosophy:** "The foundation's purpose of all grants and contributions is to aid and promote charitable, educational, scientific, literary and religious projects as well as the arts." 1996 **Priorities:** *Arts & Humanities:* 19%. Supports museums, music, orchestras, and ballet. *Civic & Public Affairs:* 5%. Supports zoos, police foundations, and gardens. *Education:* 13%. Supports private schools, universities, and education foundations. *Environment:* 3%. Funds Boys/Girls clubs, a food bank, and family planning. *International:* 3%. Supports hospitals. *Religion:* 11%. Supports a science museum. *Note:* Total contributions made in 1999. **Typ. Recipients:** AIDS/HIV, Cancer, Children's Health/Hospitals, Clinics/Medical Centers, Emergency/Ambulance Services, Health Organizations, Health-General, Hospices, Hospitals, Medical Education, Medical Rehabilitation, Medical Research, Mental Health, Single-Disease Health Associations, Substance Abuse. **Geo. Dist:** CA.

★ 12057 ★ Walter and Elise Haas Fund
1 Lombard St., Suite 305
San Francisco, CA 94111-1130
Phone: (415)398-4474 **Fax:** (415)986-4779
Email: brendan@haassr.org
Website: http://www.haassr.org
Pamela David, Executive Director

Fnded: 1953. **Philosophy:** "Responding to the growing challenges in public education, the Fund has developed a strong focus on K-12 schools, particularly in the areas of professional development for teachers and curricular interests in arts, civics, and environmental education. To address the profound problems facing the poor and disadvantaged members of our society, we have given increasing priority to grants in the area of human services that increase access to services and assist those in need to become financially and socially stable. In this area, there is a particular emphasis on the welfare of children and youth. Our funding in the field of Jewish Life illustrates the evolution of the Fund's interests. Building upon a long history of family support for Jewish institutions, the Fund has recently expanded its range of concern to include Jewish identity, tolerance and understanding, interfaith relations, volunteerism, and organizational excellence, as well as supporting more traditional services. The Fund's legacy of support for the arts has become focused in programs aimed at two primary goals: strengthening arts organizations through audience development grants and supporting the creation of new work. In the area of the environment, the Fund has built upon the founders' interests in parks and the outdoors to create a funding agenda emphasizing the preservation of parks and open space. Two of the Fund's priorities represent extensions of the founders' deeply held values of integrity, ethical behavior, and civic commitment. The professional ethics category addresses contemporary issues in the fields of corporate social responsibility and bioethics. In the area of community service and citizenship, the Fund supports projects that strengthen volunteerism and the other values of citizenship." Walter and Elise Haas Fund President's Statement **Priorities:** *Arts & Humanities:* 5%. Gives to art and children's museums, theater, orchestras, dance, opera, and art/cultural centers. *Civic & Public Affairs:* 25%. Supports urban affairs, women's affairs, nonprofit management, and community foundations. *Education:* 17%. Supports faculty development, public school, after-school programs, colleges, universities, and minority education. *Environment:* 4%. Funds community service organizations, sports and recreation programs, child welfare, family services, community centers, the United Way, food and clothing distribution, and shelters. *International:* 3%. Funds health funds, AIDS/HIV programs, health centers, and hospice programs. *Note:* Total contributions made in 2000. **Typ. Recipients:** AIDS/HIV, Children's Health/Hospitals, Clinics/Medical Centers, Diabetes, Domestic Violence, Family Planning, Health Organizations, Health-General, Hospitals, Long-Term Care, Mental Health, People with Disabilities, Prenatal Health Issues, Public Health, Substance Abuse. **Geo. Dist:** CA, Alameda County; CA, Marin County; CA, San Mateo County; San Francisco, CA, the Bay area.

★ 12058 ★ Walter and Josephine Ford Fund
100 Renaissance Center, 34th Floor
Detroit, MI 48243
Phone: (313)259-7777 **Fax:** (313)393-7579
David Hempstead, Secretary & Trustee

Fnded: 1951. **Philosophy:** The fund reports that "grants are generally limited to charitable organizations already favorably known to, and of interest to, the donors." The fund's designated categories of support are the arts, churches and religious organizations, community chests and other related organizations, hospitals and medical research, education, and miscellaneous organizations. **Priorities:** *Arts & Humanities:* 8%. Supports fine arts, performing arts, historical societies, public broadcasting, and libraries. *Civic & Public Affairs:* 19%. Supports neighborhood societies, community foundations, parks, and philanthropic organizations. *Education:* 37%. Funds support pre-college and higher education, both public and private, and minority education. *Environment:* 10%. Gives to boys and girls clubs, community services, animal causes, United Way, YMCA, and family services. *International:* 7%. Supports hospitals, single-disease associations, and medical centers. *Religion:* 2%. Funds scientific research. *Note:* Total contributions made in 2000. **Typ. Recipients:** Alzheimers Disease, Cancer, Clinics/Medical Centers, Family Planning, Health Organizations, Hospitals, Medical Research, Mental Health, Nursing Services, People with Disabilities, Public Health, Substance Abuse. **Geo. Dist:** ME; Detroit, MI, including metropolitan area; NY.

★ 12059 ★ Walter S. Johnson Foundation
525 Middlefield Rd., Suite 160
Menlo Park, CA 94025
Phone: (650)326-0485 **Fax:** (650)326-4320
Email: info@wsjf.org
Website: http://www.wsjf.org
Pancho Chang, Executive Director

Fnded: 1968. **Philosophy:** The foundation reflects the interests of Walter S. Johnson by focusing on strengthening public education, assisting young people in the transition from school to career, and enhancing the well-being of children, youth, and families. One of the foundation's highest priorities is enhancing the academic learning of children in the public elementary and secondary schools. The foundation feels that programs promoting the professional development of educators, especially in the context of whole school reform, will best help achieve this goal. The foundation is particularly interested in school reform efforts that feature school-to-career programs aiming to integrate challenging curricula with a real-world context. Working with social-service agencies toward solving problems facing children, adolescents, and families is another of the foundation's primary interests. The foundation gives high priority to projects seeking to promote positive youth development through programs promoting healthy social and emotional development, the prevention of teenage pregnancy, the strengthening of families, and the prevention of drug and alcohol abuse. **Priorities:** *Education:* 50%. Supports professional development of teachers and K-12 school reform. *Environment:* 25%. Supports youth development, family services, and social services. **Typ. Recipients:** Family Planning, Medical Research, Mental Health, Public Health, Research/Studies Institutes, Substance Abuse. **Geo. Dist:** CA, Northern California, including San Francisco Bay Area; Reno, NV, including Washoe County.

★ 12060 ★ Walton Family Foundation, Inc.
PO Box 2030
Bentonville, AR 72712
Phone: (479)464-1570 **Fax:** (501)464-1580
Website: http://www.wffhome.com
Buddy Philpot, Director

Fnded: 1987. **Philosophy:** The Foundation's main focus is systemic reform in education, with special emphasis on primary and secondary education. The Foundation also supports several university level programs that involve K-12 education and that address issues directly relating to children. The Foundation also currently funds three scholarship programs: Walton Scholarship–awarded to the children of Wal-Mart associates who are high school seniors and have exhibited superior standards academically and have been active in positions of leadership and responsibility. International Scholarship Program–recruits students from Belize, Costa Rica, El Salvador, Guatemala, Honduras, Mexico, Nicaragua, and Panama to attend college in the United States. Walton Delta Scholarship Program–awards grants to students from the Arkansas Delta region who are high school seniors interested in pursuing a career in teaching. The Foundation also has particular interest in the Mississippi River's delta region of Arkansas and Mississippi, concentrating on economic development in the area and on enhancing the educational opportunities for students and adults. **Priorities:** *Arts & Humanities:* 3%.Supports museums, performing arts, and art centers. *Civic & Public Affairs:* 10%. Focus on free enterprise, community affairs, and philanthropic organizations. *Education:* 83%. Supports private precollege education, colleges and universities, and education reform. *Environment:* 2%. Supports Big Brothers & Big Sisters. *Religion:* 2%. Supports Society of Natural History. *Note:* Total contributions made in 2000. **Typ. Recipients:** Cancer, Health Organizations, Long-Term Care, Mental Health, Research/Studies Institutes, Substance Abuse. **Geo. Dist:** AR.

★ 12061 ★ Washington Square Health Foundation
875 N Michigan Ave., Suite 3516
Chicago, IL 60611-1901
Phone: (312)664-6488 **Fax:** (312)664-7787
Email: wshf@aol.com
Website: http://www.wshf.org
Howard Nochumson, Executive Director

Fnded: 1985. **Philosophy:** "The Washington Square Health Foundation, Inc. grants funds in order to promote and maintain access to adequate healthcare for all people in the Chicagoland area regardless of race, sex, creed or financial need. The Foundation meets this goal through its grants for medical and nursing education, medical research and direct healthcare services." Washington Square Health Foundation General Guidelines. **Priorities:** *International:* 100%. Supports health services, purchases of medical equipment, medical and nursing education, and medical research. *Note:* Total contributions made in fiscal

1998. **Typ. Recipients:** AIDS/HIV, Children's Health/Hospitals, Clinics/Medical Centers, Domestic Violence, Geriatric Health, Health Organizations, Health Policy/Cost Containment, Health-General, Hospices, Hospitals, Hospitals (University Affiliated), Medical Education, Medical Rehabilitation, Medical Research, People with Disabilities, Prenatal Health Issues, Preventive Medicine/Wellness Organizations, Public Health, Respiratory, Sexual Abuse, Single-Disease Health Associations, Speech & Hearing. **Geo. Dist:** Chicago, IL.

★ 12062 ★ Wasie Foundation

4999 France Ave. South, Suite 250
601 Second Ave. South
Minneapolis, MN 55410
Phone: (612)332-3883 **Fax:** (612)455-6888
Rachel Pearson, Program Associate

Fnded: 1966. **Philosophy:** The Wasie Foundation strives to fulfill the interest of its donors by funding organizations whose goals and missions reflect the interests of the late Stanley and Marie Wasie: greater opportunity for young people of Polish descent through education; hope and recovery for people with schizophrenia; a higher quality of life for people with arthritis; a brighter future for children with medical problems and improved treatment and care for people with cancer. **Priorities:** *Civic & Public Affairs:* 29%. Supports associations of small foundations and general philanthropy. *Education:* 16%. Funds colleges, universities, scholarships, and medical education. *Environment:* 22%. Supports counseling, and services for seniors and children. *International:* 51%. Provides funding for organizations supporting cancer research, services for the mentally ill, cerebral palsy research, arthritis, and children's health. *Note:* Total contributions made in 2000. **Typ. Recipients:** Arthritis, Cancer, Children's Health/Hospitals, Clinics/Medical Centers, Health-General, Hospices, Long-Term Care, Medical Education, Medical Research, Mental Health, Research/Studies Institutes, Single-Disease Health Associations, Speech & Hearing. **Geo. Dist:** MN.

★ 12063 ★ Wasserman Foundation

10100 Santa Monica Blvd., Suite 1300
Los Angeles, CA 90067
Phone: (310)277-4657
Edward Landry, Contact

Fnded: 1956. **Philosophy:** The foundation generally supports arts groups, educational institutions, religious groups, and medical research. **Priorities:** *Arts & Humanities:* 9%. Supports performing arts centers, libraries, museums, and public broadcasting. *Civic & Public Affairs:* 12%. Supports foundations and legal aid groups. *Education:* 36%. Mostly supports colleges and universities. *Environment:* 9%. Focus on the disabled, child welfare, and food banks. *International:* 17%. Supports medical centers, AIDS research, diseases that affect women, and diabetes. *Note:* Total contributions made in 2000. **Typ. Recipients:** AIDS/HIV, Cancer, Children's Health/Hospitals, Clinics/Medical Centers, Domestic Violence, Emergency/Ambulance Services, Eyes/Blindness, Family Planning, Health Organizations, Hospitals, Medical Education, Medical Research, Multiple Sclerosis, People with Disabilities, Single-Disease Health Associations, Speech & Hearing, Substance Abuse. **Geo. Dist:** Los Angeles, CA; New York, NY.

★ 12064 ★ Wayne and Gladys Valley Foundation

1939 Harrison St., Suite 510
Oakland, CA 94612-3532
Phone: (510)466-6060 **Fax:** (510)466-6067
Stephen Chandler, President & Director

Fnded: 1977. **Philosophy:** The foundation has established four areas of interest. The areas include the following: Education, including public and private universities' research programs in oceanography; eye diseases; vascular defects, learning disabilities, and physical or mental afflictions affecting children and young adults; medical research concerning the above mentioned health-related programs; community and social services (generally limited to smaller grants to East Bay area projects serving youth or provided by Catholic hospitals, social services, or health care groups); and special projects, which provides the foundation with flexibility in its grant program for worthy projects. The foundation seeks to support organizations that have committed, enthusiastic, and diligent leadership; specifically defined goals and purposes; and reasonable expectations of demonstrating measurable progress and results. The foundation also favors grant requests contingent on receiving matching funding from other sources. Grants generally are payable only in one year. **Priorities:** *Arts & Humanities:* About 12%. Libraries, museums, and public television. *Education:* 22%. Supports science, legal, and mathematical education. *Environment:* 43%. Food banks, childrens services, care centers. *International:* 23%. Cancer research, blindness, and heart disease. *Note:* Total contributions made in fiscal 2001. **Typ. Recipients:** Alzheimers Disease, Cancer, Children's Health/Hospitals, Domestic Violence, Eyes/Blindness, Health Organizations, Heart, Hospitals, Medical Research, Mental Health, People with Disabilities, Prenatal Health Issues, Research/Studies Institutes, Single-Disease Health Associations, Speech & Hearing. **Geo. Dist:** CA, Alameda County; CA, Alameda and Contra Costa county; CA, Contra Costa County; CA, East Bay area; CA, Santa Clara County.

★ 12065 ★ Weeden Foundation

747 Third Ave., 34th Floor
New York, NY 10017
Phone: (212)888-1672 **Fax:** (212)888-1354
Email: weedenfdn@weedenfdn.org
Website: http://www.weedenfdn.org
Don Wheeden, Executive Director

Fnded: 1963. **Philosophy:** "Prior to his death in 1984, Frank Weeden, the Foundation's founder and chief benefactor, asked that the resources of the Weeden Foundation be used to address the adverse impact of growing human populations and overuse of natural resources on the biological fabric of the planet. From its inception in 1963, the Foundation embraced the protection of biodiversity as its main priority. Population growth, particularly in the United States, has also evolved into a major program interest. Organizations supported to date range from those that protect ecosystems and wildlife to those that raise the status of women and increase awareness about family planning. The Foundation financed the first debt-for-nature swap protecting the Beni Biosphere Reserve in Bolivia and is particularly interested in new and innovative efforts that help to develop sustainable models for conservation action. Projects that serve as catalysts inducing others to lend support receive priority consideration." **Priorities:** *Note:* Contributions made in fiscal 2001. **Typ. Recipients:** Family Planning, Health Funds. **Geo. Dist:** nationally.

★ 12066 ★ Weezie Foundation

345 Park Ave., 6th Fl.
New York, NY 10154
Phone: (212)464-1936
Shannon Hennessey, Contact

Fnded: 1961. **Philosophy:** The Weezie Foundation makes most of its grants in the areas of social services and education. Social service funding favors employment and job training and youth organizations. Funding for education goes to private schools and specialty colleges. The foundation also supports hospitals as a secondary interest. Other support areas are funded on a limited basis. **Priorities:** *Arts & Humanities:* 3%. Library. *Civic & Public Affairs:* 15%. Support community associations, Pittsburgh Zoo, libraries and MA Horticultural Society. *Education:* 30%. Provides supports to Massachusetts elementary schools and academies. *Environment:* 36%. Funds youth and family services. *International:* 11%. Supports local hospital and physical therapy program. *Note:* Total contributions made in 2000. **Typ. Recipients:** Clinics/Medical Centers, Eyes/Blindness, Hospitals, Hospitals (University Affiliated), Medical Education, Medical Rehabilitation, Mental Health, People with Disabilities, Substance Abuse. **Geo. Dist:** Northeastern USA.

★ 12067 ★ Wege Foundation

PO Box 6388
Grand Rapids, MI 49516
Phone: (616)957-0480
Peter Wege, President

Fnded: 1967. **Typ. Recipients:** Cancer, Diabetes, Emergency/Ambulance Services, Family Planning, Health Organizations, Health-General, Hospitals, Medical Rehabilitation, Multiple Sclerosis, Substance Abuse. **Geo. Dist:** MI, Greater Kent County; Grand Rapids, MI.

★ 12068 ★ Weill Family Foundation

399 Park Ave., 3rd Fl.
New York, NY 10022
Phone: (212)816-8868
Sanford Weill, Trustee

Fnded: 1967. **Priorities:** *Arts & Humanities:* 85%. Supports dance, the Carnegie Hall Society, museums and ballet. *Civic & Public Affairs:* 2%. Aids an indiana living project. *Education:* 6%. Public schools and universities receive funding. *Environment:* 1%. *International:* 5%. Funds cancer research and hospitals. *Note:* Total contributions made in 1999. **Typ. Recipients:** Cancer, Clinics/Medical Centers, Health Organizations, Health-General, Hospitals, Long-Term Care, Medical Education, Preventive Medicine/Wellness Organizations, Transplant Networks/Donor Banks.

★ 12069 ★ Weingart Foundation

1055 West 7th St., Suite 3050
Los Angeles, CA 90017
Phone: (213)688-7799 **Fax:** (213)688-1515
Email: info@weingartfnd.org
Website: http://www.weingartfnd.org
Fred Ali, President

Fnded: 1951. **Philosophy:** "The Weingart Foundation's primary area of interest in grant making, is to assist credible agencies and institutions serving children and youth in the Southern California area. "A secondary area of interest lies in supporting those agencies and institutions providing services that benefit the entire community regardless of age or other factors. " Preferential attention will be given to the support of well-conceived experimental or demonstration projects that promise significant positive results and are likely to produce long-term multiplier effects." 1999 Annual Report **Priorities:** *Arts & Humanities:* 6%. Funds music centers, museums, and the donor adivsed, dance companies. *Civic & Public Affairs:* 13%. Provided major grant to the San Diego Foundation to create Weingart-price fund; supports libraries and zoos. *Education:* 30%. Provides funding for private colleges and universities, and K-12 schools. *Environment:* 20%. Supports youth organizations, domestic violence, substance abuse prevention/ treatment programs, the homeless and community centers. *International:* 25%. Supports hospital, health and hospital foundations. *Religion:* 3%. Supports San Diego Space and Science foundation. *Note:* Total contributions made in fiscal 2000. **Typ. Recipients:** AIDS/HIV, Cancer, Child Abuse, Children's Health/Hospitals, Clinics/Medical Centers, Diabetes, Domestic Violence, Emergency/Ambulance Services, Eyes/Blindness, Health Organizations, Health-General, Hospices, Hospitals, Long-Term Care, Medical Education, Medical Research, Mental Health, Nursing Services, Outpatient Health Care, People with Disabilities, Prenatal Health Issues, Prenatal Health Issues, Preventive Medicine/Wellness Organizations, Public Health, Speech & Hearing, Substance Abuse. **Geo. Dist:** CA, seven counties in Southern California.

★ 12070 ★ Welfare Foundation

100 W 10th St., Suite 1109
Wilmington, DE 19801
Phone: (302)654-2477 **Fax:** (302)654-2323
Peter Morrow, Executive Secretary

Fnded: 1930. **Philosophy:** The foundation supports social welfare organizations, civic associations, the arts, and educational institutions. **Priorities:** *Arts & Humanities:* 18%. Suppots contemporary arts, museums, opera. *Civic & Public Affairs:* 14%. Supports zoo, libraries, riverfront development organization. *Education:* 26%. Supports colleges and universities, elementary and preschools, after-school programs. *Environment:* 33%. Supports scouting, youth services, food bank, housing, senior services, family planning. *International:* 5%. Supports single-disease health associationss. *Note:* Total contributions made in 2000. **Typ. Recipients:** AIDS/HIV, Cancer, Children's Health/Hospitals, Clinics/Medical Centers, Emergency/Ambulance Services, Family Planning, Health Funds, Health Organizations, Hospices, Hospitals, Long-Term Care, Medical Education, People with Disabilities, Prenatal Health Issues, Preventive Medicine/Wellness Organizations, Public Health, Single-Disease Health Associations, Substance Abuse. **Geo. Dist:** Wilmington, DE, including surrounding communities; PA, Southern Chester County.

★ 12071 ★ Wenner-Gren Foundation for Anthropological Research

220 Fifth Ave., 16th Fl.
New York, NY 10001-7708
Phone: (212)683-5000 **Fax:** (212)683-9151
Email: inquiries@wennergren.org
Website: http://www.wennergren.org
Dr. Richard Fox, President & Secretary

Fnded: 1951. **Philosophy:** The foundation's interest is the support of basic research in all branches of anthropology, including social/cultural anthropology, ethnology, biological/physical anthropology, archaeology, and anthropological linguistics, and in closely related disciplines concerned with human origins, development, and variation. The foundation particularly invites projects employing comparative perspectives or integrating two or more subfields of anthropology. The foundation supports small grants of up to $20,000 for general anthropological research; predoctoral grants to aid doctoral dissertation or thesis research; Richard Carley Hunt Memorial Postdoctoral Fellowships of up to $15,000 for scholars within five years of receipt of the doctorate; Developing Countries Training Fellowships of up to $12,500 per year, for periods from six months to three years, for scholars from developing countries seeking additional training in anthropology; and conference support in the form of grants to conference organizers and the foundation's own sponsored conferences. The foundation runs an International Collaborative Research Grants Program. This program awards up to $25,000 to assist anthropological research projects undertaken by two or more investigators from different countries. The foundation also has Historical Archives grants program to assist individuals holding significant records and personal papers with the expenses of preparing and transferring them for archival deposit and to assist individuals conducting oral history interviews. This program awards up to $15,000. **Priorities:** *Education:* 99%. Supports research and promotion of anthropological issues through fellowships and scholarships. *Note:* Total contributions made in 2000. **Typ. Recipients:** AIDS/HIV, Children's Health/Hospitals, Prenatal Health Issues. **Geo. Dist:** nationally.

★ 12072 ★ Whitaker Foundation

1700 North Moore St., Suite 2200
Arlington, VA 22209
Phone: (703)528-2430 **Fax:** (703)528-2431
Email: info@whitaker.org
Website: http://www.whitaker.org
Peter Katona, President

Fnded: 1975. **Philosophy:** The foundation will spend all its assets, primarily in support of education and research programs in biomedical engineering, and then go out of business at the end of 2006. The Biomedical Engineering Research Grants program supports research projects that enable investigators to establish academic careers in biomedical engineering or a closely related field. ...the foundation's Graduate Fellowship program...is designed to support top students in their pursuit of a biomedical engineering-based doctorate. In 1999 the foundation merged its two major programs for building education infrastructure - the Leaderships Awards and Development Awards programs. The goal of the Leadership Development Awards program is to support major initiatives to enhance the field of biomedical engineering at research universities in the United States. Since 1992, the foundation's Special Opportunity's Awards program has encouraged innovations in biomedical engineering research and education program development. The goal of the foundation's Industrial Internship program is to support internships and cooperate with education programs that smooth the way from student life to company employment. The Teaching Materials Program, is designed to enhance the education of biomedical engineers through the development of quality teaching materials. The Biomedical Engineering Summer Internships Program (BESIP), a joint enterprise between the foundation and the National Institute of Health, pairs undergraduate biomedical engineering students with mentors at various NIH laboratories. The foundation supports conferences that enhance the field of biomedical engineering in a new and innovative way. This usually excludes the general support of a conference in an ongoing series. The foundation operates regional programs in the Harrisburg, PA, and Naples, FL, areas. **Priorities:** *Arts & Humanities:* 7%. Supports science and art center. *Civic & Public Affairs:* Approx. 1%. *Education:* 88%. Supports graduate fellowships. *International:* 28%. Supports biomedical engineering research and other biomedical engineering programs. *Religion:* 1%. Supports Biomedical Engineering Society. *Note:* Total contributions made in 2000. **Typ. Recipients:** Cancer, Children's Health/Hospitals, Clinics/Medical Centers, Eyes/Blindness, Geriatric Health, Heart, Hospices, Hospitals, Hospitals (University Affiliated), Medical Education, Medical Rehabilitation, Medical Research, Mental Health, Prenatal Health Issues, Preventive Medicine/Wellness Organizations, Public Health, Research/Studies Institutes, Respiratory, Speech & Hearing. **Geo. Dist:** Harrisburg; for research, special opportunity, and other grant programs; Naples, FL, for regional programs.

★ 12073 ★ Whitehall Foundation

PO Box 3423
Palm Beach, FL 33480
Phone: (561)655-4474 **Fax:** (561)659-4978
Email: Email@Whitehall.org
Website: http://www.whitehall.org
George Moffett, II, President & Treasurer

Fnded: 1937. **Philosophy:** The foundation's policy is to assist areas of basic biological research that are not heavily supported by federal agencies or other specialized foundations. The foundation's current areas of interest are scholarly research in invertebrate and vertebrate neurobiology, specifically investigations of neural mechanisms involved in sensory, motor, and other complex functions of the whole organism as they relate to behavior. Research grants are available to established scientists working in accredited institutions in the United States. The foundation's grants-in-aid program is designed for researchers at the assistant professor level or higher who experience difficulty in competing for research funds, but grants are also available to senior scientists. Funds may be used for personnel, scientific equipment, scientific materials and supplies, publication costs, travel for research purposes, or overhead (limited indirect expenses). The foundation regularly reassesses its areas of interest. However, major changes in programs only occur after several years of consideration and evaluation. **Priorities:** *Education:* 3%. Provides scholarships. *International:* 97%. Medical research. *Religion:* Supports medical research, primarily at American universities and hospitals. *Note:* Contributions made in 2001. **Typ. Recipients:** Cancer, Children's Health/Hospitals, Clinics/Medical Centers, Hospitals, Medical Education, Medical Research, Substance Abuse. **Geo. Dist:** nationally.

★ 12074 ★ Whitehead Foundation

100 Wall St., 11th Fl.
New York, NY 10005
Phone: (212)440-0800 **Fax:** (212)751-5924

Fnded: 1982. **Philosophy:** The Whitehead Foundation makes grants across the major categories of support. In civic affairs, interests include environmental affairs, economic development, national security, international affairs, housing, and public policy. Educational support goes to colleges and universities, and economic and business education. Social service support favors child welfare, youth organizations, the disabled, and employment and job training. Arts funding goes to historic preservation, theaters, galleries, and museums. **Priorities:** *Arts & Humanities:* 9%. Supports libraries, museums, and theater. *Civic & Public Affairs:* 28%. Primary support for philanthropy. *Education:* 24%. Supports colleges, universities, and educational initiatives. *Environment:* 15%. Funds volunteer groups and services for the disabled. *International:* 6%. Focus on medical research. *Note:* Total contributions made in fiscal 2001. **Typ. Recipients:** Cancer, Hospitals, Medical Research, People with Disabilities, Single-Disease Health Associations, Substance Abuse. **Geo. Dist:** nationally; New York, NY.

★ 12075 ★ Wieboldt Foundation

53 West Jackson Boulevard, Suite 838
Chicago, IL 60604
Phone: (312)786-9377 **Fax:** (312)786-9232
Email: reginamc@corecomm.net
Carmen Prieto, Assistant Director

Fnded: 1921. **Philosophy:** Over 15 years ago, the directors adopted a creed that states the central purpose and direction of the foundation: "Our recognition of community organizing or community action as the foundation's prime concern is promoted by our conviction that a sense of powerlessness and the apathy and alienation bred of this sense are at the root of many of the ills of our time. We believe that funding those efforts that give people hope that they can exercise a degree of control over their lives and that involve them working together toward jointly defined ends is an important contribution to the resolution of social ills." The Wieboldt Foundation has three noteworthy characteristics: a grant-making program aimed at developing the capacity of local citizens in Chicago's poorest neighborhoods, a board of directors directly involved in the work of the foundation, and a propensity to fund new areas of interest. Community organizing has been a steadily increasing focus over the past 15 years. Grants have been awarded to organizations in low-income neighborhoods that foster leadership development and get neighborhood citizens involved in problem solving. The foundation recognizes that the difficulty of such efforts requires long-term commitment. A majority of grants, therefore, are renewals. The foundation also funds groups that develop policy, advocate, carry on research, and bring their technical expertise to the service of community groups. Such civic groups have been especially active in issues of equality and justice. Since 1988, the board has been deeply involved with school reform. It also focused on deepening its understanding of community organizations by greatly increasing the number of on-site visits and by holding board meetings in neighborhood settings with community leaders. The foundation also developed a Program Related Investments initiative. This initiative makes available loans, loan guarantees, and equity investments to housing, community development, and community service organizations. In 1992, the foundation in conjunction with the Woods Charitable Fund, established an annual "Community Organizing" award to recognize excellent and effective community organizing in the Chicago area. The award will be an unrestricted grant of $10,000 to $15,000. **Priorities:** *Arts & Humanities:* 4%. Supports video and literary projects. *Civic & Public Affairs:* 66%. Funds community foundations, economic development, civil liberties, neighborhood organizations, leadership development, and ethnic groups. *Education:* 6%. Supports school reform and primary and secondary school enrichment programs. *Environment:* 13%. Supports family services, senior and youth organizations, and homeless shelters. *International:* Less than 1%. *Note:* Total contributions made in 2000. **Typ. Recipients:** Health Policy/Cost Containment, Medical Rehabilitation, Medical Rehabilitation, Public Health. **Geo. Dist:** Chicago, IL, including metropolitan area.

★ 12076 ★ Wilbur May Foundation

2716 Ocean Park Blvd, Ste. 2011
Santa Monica, CA 90405

Phone: (310)314-2400 **Fax:** (310)314-2401
Dorothy Duffy May, Vice President & Section

Fnded: 1948. **Philosophy:** The foundation focuses its giving on programs for the young and hospitals. **Priorities:** *Arts & Humanities:* 2%. Supports libraries, music, and film & video. *Civic & Public Affairs:* 3%. Supports community foundations and clubs. *Education:* About 41%. Supports colleges and universities, scholarships, and education associations. *Environment:* 26%. Emphasis on parks and recreation, child welfare, youth organizations, scouts, Young Men's Christian Association, United Way, and camps. *International:* About 28%. Focus on an eye institute, single-disease health associations, and hospitals. *Note:* Total contributions made in fiscal 1997. **Typ. Recipients:** AIDS/HIV, Cancer, Child Abuse, Children's Health/Hospitals, Children's Health/Hospitals, Clinics/Medical Centers, Diabetes, Eyes/Blindness, Health Organizations, Heart, Hospitals, Medical Education, Medical Rehabilitation, Medical Research, People with Disabilities, Prenatal Health Issues, Public Health, Research/Studies Institutes, Respiratory, Single-Disease Health Associations, Substance Abuse. **Geo. Dist:** CA, Southern California; Los Angeles, CA; Reno, NV.

★ 12077 ★ Wilf Family Foundation
820 Morris Turnpike
Short Hills, NJ 07078
Phone: (973)467-5000 **Fax:** (973)467-0550
Joseph Wilf, Trustee

Fnded: 1964. **Philosophy:** The Wilf Family Foundation primarily supports Jewish organizations in education and religion. Most of the religious organizations are located in New York. Jewish education is supported both at the university and secondary levels. The foundation also supports a number of other recipient areas with Jewish interests. **Priorities:** *Arts & Humanities:* Less than 1%. *Civic & Public Affairs:* 2%. Funds community and justice organizations. *Education:* 1%. *Environment:* 1%. *International:* 2%. Supports hospitals and single-disease health associations. *Note:* Total contributions made in fiscal 2001. **Typ. Recipients:** Cancer, Children's Health/Hospitals, Clinics/Medical Centers, Eyes/Blindness, Heart, Hospitals, Long-Term Care, Medical Education, Medical Research, Respiratory, Trauma Treatment. **Geo. Dist:** nationally; New York, NY.

★ 12078 ★ Willard L. Eccles Charitable Foundation
PO Box 628
Salt Lake City, UT 84110
Phone: (801)463-9580
Clark Giles, Contact

Fnded: 1981. **Philosophy:** "The specific charitable purposes of the Foundation are to promote, encourage and make available to the public health care services, to aid charitable non-profit hospitals in acquiring appropriate medical equipment for research and for rendering health care services, and to further medical education and research. The Foundation is directed to provide this health care-medical assistance primarily in Utah and particularly in the Ogden area." "In addition to making grants for the above described health care-medical purposes, the Foundation provides funding to charitable organizations for other community charitable purposes and distributes limited grants to qualified charitable organizations as directed by members of the Advisory Committee. These grants are not based on requests submitted to the Foundation without the prior approval of a member of the Advisory Committee." **Priorities:** *Arts & Humanities:* 14%. Focus on theater, libraries, public broadcasting. *Civic & Public Affairs:* 3%. Funds community development. *Education:* 30%. Colleges and universities, and primary and secondary education. *Environment:* 7%. Emphasis on youth organizations and community services. *International:* 4%. Public health care, hospitals, pediatric health, and single-disease health associations. *Note:* Total contributions made in fiscal 2000. **Typ. Recipients:** AIDS/HIV, Alzheimers Disease, Cancer, Children's Health/Hospitals, Clinics/Medical Centers, Domestic Violence, Emergency/Ambulance Services, Eyes/Blindness, Eyes/Blindness, Family Planning, Health Organizations, Health-General, Hospices, Hospitals, Medical Education, Medical Research, Medical Training, Mental Health, Multiple Sclerosis, Nursing Services, People with Disabilities, Prenatal Health Issues, Preventive Medicine/Wellness Organizations, Public Health, Respiratory, Single-Disease Health Associations. **Geo. Dist:** UT, primarily Salt Lake City and Ogden.

★ 12079 ★ Willard and Pat Walker Charitable Foundation
PO Box 5000
Springdale, AR 72765
Tommy Karr, Contact

Fnded: 1990. **Philosophy:** The foundation places emphasis on the arts, health, and human services within Arkansas. **Priorities:** *Arts & Humanities:* 7%. Museum. *Education:* 82%. Colleges and universities. *Environment:* 4%. Primarily for family services. *Note:* Total contributions made in 2000. **Typ. Recipients:** Cancer, Clinics/Medical Centers, Single-Disease Health Associations. **Geo. Dist:** AR.

★ 12080 ★ Willard T. C. Johnson Foundation
630 5th Ave., Suite 1510
New York, NY 10111
Phone: (212)332-7500 **Fax:** (212)332-7510
Email: tjici1@tjinc.com
Neil Burmeister, President

Fnded: 1979. **Philosophy:** The foundation primarily supports the Arthritis Foundation, Juvenile Diabetes Foundation International, other health organizations, and educational institutions. Other recipients include Opera Festival New Jersey, religious organizations, and social services. **Priorities:** *Arts & Humanities:* 3%. Supports the June Opera Festival of New Jersey. *Civic & Public Affairs:* 18%. Supports the Robin Hood Foundation. *Education:* 18%. Funds a private school. *Environment:* 2%. Funds the Best Friends Foundation. *International:* 60%. Supports the Alliance for Lupus Research. *Note:* Total contributions made in 1999. **Typ. Recipients:** AIDS/HIV, Arthritis, Diabetes, Emergency/Ambulance Services, Family Planning, Health Organizations, Hospitals, Long-Term Care, Medical Research, Single-Disease Health Associations. **Geo. Dist:** Washington, DC; NJ; New York, NY.

★ 12081 ★ William Bingham Foundation
20325 Center Ridge Rd., Suite 629
Rocky River, OH 44116-3554
Phone: (440)331-6350
Email: www.info@wbinghamfoundation.org
Website: http://www.fdncenter.org/grantmaker/bingham/
Laura Gilbertson, Director

Fnded: 1955. **Philosophy:** "As a family foundation, The William Bingham Foundation furthers the charitable purposes of its founder, Elizabeth Bingham Blossom, in the fields of education, health and human services, science, and the arts; seeks to strengthen civil society and its institutions; works for a world that is environmentally self-sustaining; educates family members and others in the values and practices of philanthropy, community service, and stewardship; and seeks to build a sense of community among ourselves and with the world we share." William Bingham Foundation Mission Statement. contribute to a wide variety of organizations in the areas of education, the arts, health, and welfare, reflecting the diverse interests of the trustees and the needs of the communities in which they live. **Priorities:** *Arts & Humanities:* 20%. Funds theater, orchestras, museums, art associations, and historic preservation. *Civic & Public Affairs:* 9%. Contributes to grantmaker associations, parks, women's affairs, housing, and economic development. *Education:* 35%. Supports universities, arts and environmental education, and college prep and nursery schools. *Environment:* 32%. Supports Young Men's Christian Association, youth groups, and food and shelter programs. *International:* 2%. Funds health centers. *Note:* Total contributions made in 2001. **Typ. Recipients:** Cancer, Clinics/Medical Centers, Diabetes, Domestic Violence, Hospices, Hospitals, Medical Rehabilitation, Multiple Sclerosis, Nursing Services, People with Disabilities, Public Health, Sexual Abuse, Substance Abuse. **Geo. Dist:** United States only; CA; DC; NY; OH; RI.

★ 12082 ★ William Bingham Second Betterment Fund
330 Madison Ave. Rm. 3500
New York, NY 10017
Phone: (212)557-7700 **Fax:** (212)286-8513
Anna Mosquera, Administrator

Fnded: 1955. **Philosophy:** "Although the traditional recipients of Mr. Bingham's benefactions continue to be of special interest and scholarship support continues to be a major activity, the Betterment Fund views the areas of health and education broadly. The Fund will consider requests from qualified institutions and organizations whose activities promote health improvement and education which have the potential for a significant impact on the life of Maine residents in these areas. In recent years the Fund has expanded its areas of concern to include programs which support local communities in their own efforts to increase their capacity to improve the quality of life for residents and programs for the preservation and responsible use of Maine's natural resources." 1997 Statement of Grant Policies and Procedures **Priorities:** *Arts & Humanities:* 14%. Supports libraries, public broadcasting, and historic preservation. *Civic & Public Affairs:* 17%. Funds economic policy, community development, law & justice, and job training. *Education:* 35%. Funds primary and secondary schools, colleges and universities, education associations, literacy, technical colleges, scholarships. *Environment:* 6%. Supports homes, food banks, and community service programs. *International:* 13%. Supports hospitals, medical centers, oral health, public health, medical research, and visiting nurses. *Note:* Total contributions made in 2000. **Typ. Recipients:** Cancer, Children's Health/Hospitals, Clinics/Medical Centers, Diabetes, Family Planning, Health Funds, Health Organizations, Home-Care Services, Hospitals, Long-Term Care, Medical Education, Medical Research, Nursing Services, Preventive Medicine/Wellness Organizations, Public Health, Respiratory, Substance Abuse. **Geo. Dist:** Western Mountain region; ME.

★ 12083 ★ William E. Schrafft and Bertha E. Schrafft Charitable Trust
One Financial Center, 26th Floor
Boston, MA 02111-2662
Phone: (617)350-6100 **Fax:** (617)350-0038
Website: http://www.schrafftcharitabletrust.org
Karen Faulkner, Executive Director

Fnded: 1946. **Philosophy:** "The aim of the Schrafft Charitable Trust continues to be on making a difference in the educational and cultural opportunities for young people in Greater Boston's inner city." The FND's primary focus is on organizations that are involved with the education of indigent or disadvantaged youth in Boston. *Shcrafft Charitable Trust 2000 Annual Report* **Priorities:** *Arts & Humanities:* 15%. Supports dance, theater, music, museums, and fine art. *Civic & Public Affairs:* 17%. Gives to nonprofit management, job training, and an aquarium. *Education:* 25%. Funds scholarships, colleges and universities, charter and alternative schools, and art education. *Environment:* 43%. Supports United Way, youth clubs, camps and organizations, and homeless shelters. *Note:* Total contributions made in 2000. **Typ. Recipients:** Clinics/Medical Centers, Family Planning, Hospitals, Nursing Services, People with Disabilities, Single-Disease Health Associations, Substance Abuse. **Geo. Dist:** Boston, MA.

★ 12084 ★ William E. Simon Foundation
310 South St., PO Box 1913
Morristown, NJ 07962-1913
Phone: (973)898-0290 **Fax:** (973)898-4733
Website: http://www.wesimonfoundation.org
William Simon, Jr., Co-Chairman

Fnded: 1967. **Philosophy:** Named after its principal benefactor, the William E. Simon Foundation supports programs that are intended to strengthen the free enterprise system and the moral and spiritual values on which it rests: individual freedom, initiative, thrift, self-discipline, and faith in God. The mission of the Foundation reflects the unique accomplishments of the individual for whom it is named, and the principles of a free society that have made these accomplishments possible. The main charitable purpose of the Foundation is to assist those in need by providing the means through which they may help themselves. The charitable philosophy guiding the Foundation draws heavily on the thoughts expressed a century ago by Andrew Carnegie in *The Gospel of Wealth,* where he wrote: "In bestowing charity, the main consideration should be to help those who will help themselves; to provide part of the means by which those who desire to improve may do so; to give those who desire to rise the aids by which they may rise; to assist, but rarely or never to do all." In implementing this philosophy, and the Foundation seeks to fund programs which are effective in promoting independence and personal responsibility among those in need. **Priorities:** *Civic & Public Affairs:* 8%. Gives to community foundations and housing development. *Education:* 54%. Supports colleges, universities, and parochial secondary schools. *Environment:* 7%. Funds shelters, food banks, and other services for the needy. *International:* 16%. Funds health foundations and hospitals. *Religion:* 2%. A sea research organization receives support. *Note:* Total contributions made in 2000. **Typ. Recipients:** Cancer, Clinics/Medical Centers, Family Planning, Health Funds, Health Organizations, Hospices, Hospitals, Medical Rehabilitation, Medical Research, Multiple Sclerosis, Nursing Services, People with Disabilities, Public Health, Research/Studies Institutes, Single-Disease Health Associations, Substance Abuse, Transplant Networks/Donor Banks. **Geo. Dist:** nationally, with emphasis in New York Metro, Los Angeles, and the San Francio Bar metropolitan areas. **Frmly:** William E. and Carol G. Simon Foundation.

★ 12085 ★ William and Flora Hewlett Foundation

2121 Sand Hill Rd.
Menlo Park, CA 94025
Phone: (650)234-4500 **Fax:** (650)234-4501
Email: info@hewlett.org
Website: http://www.hewlett.org
Paul Brest, President

Fnded: 1966. **Philosophy:** "In defining programs and establishing objectives that show promise of realizing the aspirations of the founders, the foundation has restricted its attention to the fields of education, population, conflict resolution, environment, performing arts, family and community development, and U.S.-Latin American relations. A special projects category also was established to provide the foundation with flexibility to respond to proposals of special interest to the board. A large portion of funding has been for the general support of institutions, rather than for project support. Funding has been provided to increase the stability of performing arts organizations, and to strengthen international scholarship and training on university campuses. Institutional recipients have included research universities, liberal arts colleges, and organizations involved in conflict resolution, the environment, and population. In pursuing the development of public policy options, the foundation has supported institutions and organizations with a record of objective policy research. Some of these grants have gone to public policy organizations working in areas of program interest such as the environment, population, and the urban community. The foundation also has supported community development organizations, youth employment projects, historically black colleges, and a program to increase minority representation in science and engineering. The issues of homelessness and affordable housing are also of interest to the foundation. The foundation has a strong commitment to the voluntary, nonprofit sector. It will therefore assist efforts to improve the financial base and efficiency of organizations and institutions in this category. Proposals that show promise of stimulating private philanthropy are particularly welcome. The foundation's interest in international affairs is reflected primarily in its population program, which supports organizations providing family planning services in less-developed countries and in American population centers. The Hewlett Foundation also supports international and area studies at major research universities." **Priorities:** *Arts & Humanities:* 7%. Supports music, theater, opera, dance, film, and public broadcasting. *Civic & Public Affairs:* 11%. Contributes to community development, community foundations, employment initiatives, and public policy organizations. *Education:* 32%. Supports higher education, elementary education, and secondary education; education reform; teacher development; and education councils. *Environment:* 8%. Funds family services, family planning, and conflict resolution programs. *International:* 14%. Primarily funds women's and reproductive health. *Religion:* 4%. Gives to scientific research in the behavioral sciences and health. *Note:* Total contributions made in 2000. **Typ. Recipients:** Adolescent Health Issues, AIDS/HIV, Family Planning, Health Organizations, Health Policy/Cost Containment, Public Health, Research/Studies Institutes. **Geo. Dist:** internationally; nationally; San Francisco, CA, Bay area.

★ 12086 ★ William G. Baker, Jr. Memorial Fund

Latrobe Bldg., 9th Floor
2 East Read St.
Baltimore, MD 21202
Phone: (410)332-4171 **Fax:** (410)837-4701
Melissa Warlon, Contact

Fnded: 1964. **Philosophy:** The William G. Baker, Jr., Memorial Fund donates funds for "charitable purposes such as and limited to religious, charitable, scientific, literary, or educational purposes." **Priorities:** *Arts & Humanities:* 26%. Supports performing arts, museums, and historical societies. *Civic & Public Affairs:* 12%. Gives to neighborhood concerns, economic development, and community foundations. *Education:* 22%. Supports schools, accen programs, and universities. *Environment:* 23%. Supports children, family, and human needs. *International:* 7%. Supports health, and mental health projects. *Note:* Total contributions made in 2000. **Typ. Recipients:** Child Abuse, Children's Health/Hospitals, Clinics/Medical Centers, Emergency/Ambulance Services, Eyes/Blindness, Health Funds, Health Organizations, Health-General, Heart, Hospices, Hospitals, Medical Research, Mental Health, People with Disabilities, Public Health, Speech & Hearing, Substance Abuse. **Geo. Dist:** Baltimore, MD.

★ 12087 ★ William G. Irwin Charity Foundation

235 Montgomery St., Suite 711
San Francisco, CA 94104
Phone: (415)362-6954
Michael Gorman, Executive Director

Fnded: 1919. **Philosophy:** "The foundation is particularly interested in medical facilities, secondary schools, and cultural and community projects." **Priorities:** *Arts & Humanities:* 13%. Supports museums, history, opera, and music, ballet and theater. *Civic & Public Affairs:* less than 1%. *Education:* 57%. Supports school, religious education, and colleges and medicine education. *Environment:* 5%. Funds United Way, Young Men's Christian Association and youth centers. *International:* 14%. Supports medical research, medical centers, multiple sclerosis, and hospitals. *Note:* Contributions were made in 2000. **Typ. Recipients:** Alzheimers Disease, Arthritis, Cancer, Children's Health/Hospitals, Clinics/Medical Centers, Emergency/Ambulance Services, Eyes/Blindness, Geriatric Health, Health Organizations, Health Organizations, Heart, Hospitals, Long-Term Care, Medical Education, Medical Rehabilitation, Medical Research, Multiple Sclerosis, People with Disabilities, Research/Studies Institutes, Single-Disease Health Associations, Speech & Hearing, Transplant Networks/Donor Banks. **Geo. Dist:** CA; HI.

★ 12088 ★ William G. McGowan Charitable Fund

PO Box 40515
Washington, DC 20016-0515
Phone: (202)364-5030 **Fax:** (202)364-3382
Email: goodric@aol.com
Website: http://www.mcgowanfund.org
Bernard Goodrich, Executive Director

Fnded: 1992. **Philosophy:** The foundation primarily supports organizations engaging in healthcare research, promoting or providing educational opportunities, especially in the business field, or developing the critical skills of undereducated and underdeveloped youth. **Priorities:** *Civic & Public Affairs:* 3%. Supports employment/job training, housing and womens affairs. *Education:* 74%. Colleges and universities, international studies, public education, private secondary education, special education, religious education, student aid and scholarship. *Environment:* 2%. Youth organizations, people with disabilities, homes, united way, at risk youth. *International:* 17%. Supports heart and cancer research, artificial organ development, and transplant networks. *Note:* Total contributions made in fiscal 1997. **Typ. Recipients:** Cancer, Diabetes, Domestic Violence, Health-General, Heart, Medical Education, People with Disabilities, Public Health, Speech & Hearing, Transplant Networks/Donor Banks. **Geo. Dist:** CA, Central, North of San Luis; Washington, DC; Chicago, IL; Kansas City, KS; Baltimore, MD; NY, Western; PA, Northern; Dallas, TX; Houston, TX; San Antonio, TX.

★ 12089 ★ William G. Selby and Marie Selby Foundation

1800 Second St., Suite 750
Sarasota, FL 34236
Phone: (941)957-0442 **Fax:** (941)957-3135
Website: http://www.selbyfdn.org
Debra Jacobs, President

Fnded: 1955. **Philosophy:** The purpose of the foundation is to "make grants which will result in the improvement of life in the Sarasota community." Emphasis is placed on social services and education. Organizations and programs serving youth, and programs for the handicapped and the elderly are stressed. The foundation also maintains an extensive scholarship program. Funds are provided to Florida colleges and universities which, in turn, grant scholarships to individuals on the basis of academic excellence and financial need. **Priorities:** *Arts & Humanities:* 25%. Supports the performing arts, public broadcasting, and museums. *Civic & Public Affairs:* 15%. Supports legal aid, the botantical garden, Inc., *Education:* 18%. Supports student aid programs. *Environment:* 27%. Supports family YMCA, Boy Scouts of America, senior and youth centers, and United Way. *International:* 3%. Supports child development and Community AIDS Network, Inc. *Religion:* 4%. Supports Monte Marine Laboratory. **Typ. Recipients:** AIDS/HIV, Cancer, Children's Health/Hospitals, Domestic Violence, Emergency/Ambulance Services, Family Planning, Hospices, Medical Research, Mental Health, People with Disabilities, Prenatal Health Issues, Research/Studies Institutes, Single-Disease Health Associations, Substance Abuse. **Geo. Dist:** Sarasota, FL, Manatee, Charlotte, DeSoto Florida counties.

★ 12090 ★ William H. Donner Foundation, Inc.

500 Fifth Ave., Suite 1230
New York, NY 10110
Phone: (212)719-9290 **Fax:** (212)302-8734
Email: rhgregg@donner.org
Website: http://www.donner.org
Rachel Gregg, Program Officer

Fnded: 1961. **Philosophy:** In 1998, the foundation reported that its giving philosophy has changed. **Priorities:** *Arts & Humanities:* 6%. Supports film and arts. *Civic & Public Affairs:* 36%. Supports public policy and community affairs organizations. *Education:* 23%. Supports universities and education organizations. *Environment:* 21%. Supports youth services and animal welfare. *International:* 5%. Funds hospitals and mental health organizations. *Religion:* 7%. Funds science, natural history, marine research. *Note:* Total contributions made in 2001. **Typ. Recipients:** Adolescent Health Issues, Cancer, Child Abuse, Clinics/Medical Centers, Domestic Violence, Geriatric Health, Health Organizations, Health Policy/Cost Containment, Hospices, Hospitals, Medical Research, Mental Health, People with Disabilities, Prenatal Health Issues. **Geo. Dist:** nationally.

★ 12091 ★ William K. Bowes, Jr. Foundation

2180 Sand Hill Rd., Suite 300
Menlo Park, CA 94025
Phone: (650)926-7714
William Bowes, Jr., President

Fnded: 1992. **Priorities:** *Arts & Humanities:* 10%. Supports museums, a music conservatory and theater. *Civic & Public Affairs:* 4%. Aids foundations and a justice conference. *Education:* 41%. Funds universities, schools and an exploratorium. *Environment:* 35%. Funds children's services. *International:* 2%. Supports cancer research, multiple sclerosis society and hospitals. *Note:* Total contributions made in 1999. **Typ. Recipients:** Cancer, Children's Health/Hospitals, Clinics/Medical Centers, Health Organizations, Hospitals, Kidney, Medical Research, Multiple Sclerosis, Single-Disease Health Associations. **Geo. Dist:** CA.

★ 12092 ★ William K. Warren Foundation

PO Box 470372
Tulsa, OK 74147-0372
Phone: (918)492-8100 **Fax:** (918)481-7935
W. Lissau, President & Director

Fnded: 1945. **Philosophy:** The foundation reports that it gives preference to "local Catholic health care facilities." Its designated areas of interest are hospitals and medical research centers; churches and related organizations; educational institutions; and other (including youth-related causes, substance abuse prevention, human services, and single-disease health associations). **Priorities:** *Arts & Humanities:* Less than 1%. *Education:* 1%. Funds universities, parochial schools, and educational programs. *Environment:* 1%. Supports senior services, child welfare organizations, family and children's services, and youth programs/activities. *International:* 96%. Provides major support to a medical research center; also funds nursing homes, single-disease health associations, health systems, hospitals, and mental health organizations. *Note:* Total contributions made in 2000. **Typ. Recipients:** Alzheimers Disease, Arthritis, Cancer, Child Abuse, Children's Health/Hospitals, Clinics/Medical Centers, Clinics/Medical Centers, Diabetes, Emergency/Ambulance Services, Eyes/Blindness, Health Organizations, Heart, Hospitals, Medical Rehabilitation, Medical Research, Mental Health, Multiple Sclerosis, People with Disabilities, Prenatal Health Issues, Respiratory, Single-Disease Health Associations, Substance Abuse, Trauma Treatment. **Geo. Dist:** Tulsa, OK.

★ 12093 ★ William and Mary Greve Foundation

630 Fifth Ave., Suite 1750
New York, NY 10111
Phone: (212)307-7850 **Fax:** (212)262-8340
Anthony Kiser, Chairman

★ 12094 ★ William Penn Foundation

2 Logan Sq., 11th Fl.
100 N 18th St.
Philadelphia, PA 19103-2757
Phone: (215)988-1830 **Fax:** (215)988-1823
Email: moreinfo@williampennfoundation.org
Website: http://www.wpennfdn.org/
Kathryn Engebretson, President

Fnded: 1945. **Philosophy:** The Foundation's mission is "To improve quality of life in the Philadelphia region through efforts that strengthen children's futures, foster rich cultural expression, and deepen connections to nature and the community. In partnership with others, we work to advance a vital, just, and caring community." 2001 Annual Report. The foundation makes grants in three categories: Children, Youth and Families; Environment and Communities; and Arts and Culture. The foundation also has an initiative grantmaking program to address issues of broad community concerns. Through this program the foundation works in partnership with nonprofits exploring ideas and collaborating on long-term solutions to persistent problems of Philadelphia and the region. **Priorities:** *Arts & Humanities:* (Arts and Culture) 16%. Focus is fostering an environment in which arts and culture flourish, and in which artists are valued and enabled to undertake a wide range of creative pursuits and investigations. Supports historic preservation, museums, and the performing arts. *Civic & Public Affairs:* (Environment and Communities) 26%. Supports protecting and restoring watersheds and related ecosystems; revitalizing and stabilizing targeted communities around existing infrastructure; and promoting smart growth and livable communities within the region. *Environment:* (Children, Youth and Families) 46%. Focus is promoting the full development of children and youth to become capable adults and productive citizens, with a special emphasis on key transitions in their lives. Grants support the following priorities: Opportunity to Learn: promoting early care and family support to enhance school readiness and success in school; Opportunity to Succeed: promoting youth development opportunities during and after school to help young people make a successful transition to adult life. *Note:* Total contributions made in 2001. **Typ. Recipients:** Child Abuse, Children's Health/Hospitals, Clinics/Medical Centers, Domestic Violence, Emergency/Ambulance Services, Family Planning, Geriatric Health, Health Organizations, Medical Education, Nursing Services, Prenatal Health Issues, Public Health. **Geo. Dist:** Philadelphia, PA, including Bucks, Camden, Chester, Delaware, Montgomery, and Philadelphia counties.

★ 12095 ★ William Randolph Hearst Foundation

888 7th Ave., 45th Floor
New York, NY 10106-0057
Phone: (212)586-5404 **Fax:** (212)586-1917
Website: http://hearstfdn.org
Robert Frehse, Jr., Executive Director & Vice President

Fnded: 1948. **Philosophy:** "Within a general policy of assisting institutions to provide access and opportunity to underrepresented, low-income and minority populations, the Directors of the Hearst Foundations have established the following priorities: The Foundations' primary focus is support of undergraduate education through the establishment of endowed scholarships at private liberal arts colleges and universities. In addition, endowed scholarship support is provided for professional study in teaching, medicine, nursing, engineering, math, science and the health care professions, at the undergraduate and graduate levels. A limited number of proposals are also accepted from K-12 independent schools with outstanding academic programs, and demonstrated track records of outreach to economically disadvantaged students. In general grants are not made to public schools. However, private organizations or coalitions seeking improvement of public education and broadening access to education may be considered. The Foundations' interests in the health field seek to improve and increase health care, while facilitating wellness, prevention, and rehabilitation. Working largely through leading regional hospitals and medical centers, the Foundations support programs which increase access for underserved urban and rural populations. Areas of interest include perinatology, pediatrics, cancer, stroke, aging, women's health issues, and research. In social services, preference is given to well-established, larger agencies, providing comprehensive services. Requests for technical assistance, management training, and leadership development, designed to help non-profit agencies deliver services more efficiently and effectively are also considered. The Foundations' priority in the arts is to increase access and educational opportunities for diverse populations and underserved communities. The major portion of funds endows arts education and/or community outreach programs through major cultural institutions. Special attention is given to programs which enrich the lives of young people through exposure to the arts." *Guidelines for Grant Applications.* **Priorities:** *Arts & Humanities:* 29%. Supports music, arts centers, ballet, museum, opera, theater, arts festivals and public broadcasting. *Education:* 37%. Funds scholarship, colleges and universities, schools, religious education, minority education, journalism/media education, and medical education. *Environment:* 16%. Supports scouts, child welfare, Big Brothers/Big Sisters, Young Men's Christian Association/Young Women's Christian Association, domestic violence, and family services. *International:* 17%. Supports medical research, hospitals, AIDS, medical centers, heart, and eyes/blindness. *Note:* Contributions analysis provided by foundation. Analysis represents five years of contributions ending with 2000. **Typ. Recipients:** Cancer, Children's Health/Hospitals, Clinics/Medical Centers, Emergency/Ambulance Services, Eyes/Blindness, Geriatric Health, Health Funds, Health Organizations, Home-Care Services, Hospitals, Hospitals (University Affiliated), Medical Education, Medical Rehabilitation, Medical Research, Medical Training, People with Disabilities, Prenatal Health Issues, Public Health, Research/Studies Institutes, Single-Disease Health Associations, Substance Abuse, Transplant Networks/Donor Banks. **Geo. Dist:** nationally.

★ 12096 ★ William Rosenwald Family Fund

666 3rd Ave., 29th Fl.
New York, NY 10017
Phone: (212)476-8088 **Fax:** (212)476-8000
David Steinmann, President & Treasurer

Fnded: 1938. **Philosophy:** The William Rosenwald Family Fund primarily supports Jewish religious organizations. The fund also supports Jewish education and various other interests on a limited basis. **Priorities:** *Arts & Humanities:* 9%. Historical societies, film, and music. *Civic & Public Affairs:* 8%. Crime prevention, urban parks, and foundations. *Education:* 13%. Secondary schools and colleges. *Environment:* 9%. Youth and family programs. *International:* 9%. Medical schools and health centers. *Note:* Total contributions made in 2000. **Typ. Recipients:** AIDS/HIV, Alzheimers Disease, Cancer, Children's Health/Hospitals, Clinics/Medical Centers, Emergency/Ambulance Services, Eyes/Blindness, Family Planning, Geriatric Health, Health-General, Hospices, Hospitals, Hospitals (University Affiliated), Medical Education, Medical Research, Mental Health, People with Disabilities, Research/Studies Institutes, Single-Disease Health Associations, Substance Abuse, Transplant Networks/Donor Banks. **Geo. Dist:** NY.

★ 12097 ★ William S. Paley Foundation, Inc.

1 East 53rd St.
New York, NY 10022
Phone: (212)888-2520 **Fax:** (212)308-7845
Email: wspf@asan.com
Patrick Gallagher, Executive Director

Fnded: 1936. **Philosophy:** The founder, William S. Paley, enjoyed strong relationships with a number of charitable organizations during his lifetime. He founded the Museum of Broadcasting in New York, and the foundation continues its support to the organization. Also, the foundation supports the Museum of Modern Art in New York, where Mr. Paley had once served as president. Other art museums and art programs are also of interest to the foundation. **Priorities:** *Arts & Humanities:* 95%.Major support for the Museum of Television and Radio. *Civic & Public Affairs:* 3%. Funds parks and municipalities. *Education:* about 1%. Gives to colleges and universities and to primary and secondary education. *Environment:* Approx. 1%. *International:* Approx. 1%. *Note:* Total contributions made in 2000. **Typ. Recipients:** Alzheimers Disease, Cancer, Children's Health/Hospitals, Clinics/Medical Centers, Family Planning, Health Organizations, Hospices, Hospitals, Hospitals (University Affiliated), Medical

Education, Single-Disease Health Associations, Substance Abuse. **Geo. Dist:** New York, NY.

★ 12098 ★ William Stamps Farish Fund
10000 Memorial Drive, Suite 920
Houston, TX 77024
Phone: (713)686-7373
Martha Gary, President

Fnded: 1951. **Philosophy:** The fund primarily gives to local primary education, arts and humanities, social services, and medical research. **Priorities:** *Arts & Humanities:* 11%. Funds art, cultural, and children's museums; orchestras, ballet, photography, youth art programs, and art festivals. *Civic & Public Affairs:* 1%. Gives to community foundations, festivals, career counseling, and sustainable development programs. *Education:* 46%. Supports private secondary education, medical education, colleges, and universities. *Environment:* 20%. Supports Planned Parenthood, child welfare organizations, sexual abuse and violence prevention, substance abuse centers, and youth organizations. *International:* 16%. Funds medical centers, cancer research, hospitals, and eyes/blindness research and treatment. *Religion:* 5%. Supports scientific research laboratories, science centers, and natural history museums. *Note:* Total contributions made in fiscal 2000. **Typ. Recipients:** Cancer, Child Abuse, Clinics/Medical Centers, Emergency/Ambulance Services, Eyes/Blindness, Family Planning, Health Funds, Health Organizations, Health-General, Hospices, Hospitals, Hospitals (University Affiliated), Medical Education, Medical Research, Mental Health, People with Disabilities, Prenatal Health Issues, Public Health, Sexual Abuse, Single-Disease Health Associations, Speech & Hearing, Substance Abuse. **Geo. Dist:** Lexington, KY; NY; Houston, TX.

★ 12099 ★ William T. Grant Foundation
570 Lexington, 18th Floor
New York, NY 10022-6837
Phone: (212)752-0071 **Fax:** (212)752-1398
Email: nrivera@wtgrantfdn.org
Website: http://www.wtgrantfoundation.org

Fnded: 1936. **Priorities:** *Education:* (Faculty Scholars Program) 13%. Supports promising post-doctoral scholars from different disciplines, whose research deepens and broadens the knowledge base in areas that contribute to the foundation's mission. *Environment:* (Youth Service Grants) 6%. Supports programs that actively engage young people in the New York Tri-state area, and enable them to reach their full potential. *Note:* Total contributions made in 2002. **Typ. Recipients:** Adolescent Health Issues, AIDS/HIV, Cancer, Child Abuse, Children's Health/Hospitals, Clinics/Medical Centers, Family Planning, Hospitals, Medical Education, Medical Research, Mental Health, Prenatal Health Issues, Prenatal Health Issues, Public Health, Research/Studies Institutes, Respiratory, Substance Abuse. **Geo. Dist:** internationally, for major grants; nationally, for major grants; CT, youth services grants; NJ, youth services grants; NY, youth services grants.

★ 12100 ★ William T. Kemper Charitable Trust
PO Box 419692
Kansas City, MO 64141
Phone: (816)860-1933 **Fax:** (816)860-5690
Website: http://www.umb.com
Patty Glass, Trust Administrative

Fnded: 1989. **Philosophy:** The William T. Kemper Charitable Trust primarily supports the arts, with an emphasis on museums and the performing arts. Civic and community affairs and education are also of interest to the trust. **Priorities:** *Arts & Humanities:* 68%. Supports the Kemper Museum. *Civic & Public Affairs:* 7%. Supports parks and zoos. *Education:* 2%. Supports higher education. *Environment:* 8%. Supports children's centers. *International:* 1%. Supports hospitals. *Note:* Total contributions made in 2000. **Typ. Recipients:** Children's Health/Hospitals, Clinics/Medical Centers, Hospitals, Research/Studies Institutes. **Geo. Dist:** Kansas City, MO.

★ 12101 ★ William T. Kemper Foundation
PO Box 13095
Kansas City, MO 64199-3095
Phone: (816)234-2985 **Fax:** (816)234-8690
Michael Fields, Executive Director

Fnded: 1989. **Philosophy:** "The Foundation is dedicated to continuing Mr. Kemper's lifelong interest in improving the human condition and quality of life. Preference is given to projects located in the Midwest, with particular emphasis on his home state of Missouri and the surrounding area." "The philanthropic efforts of the William T. Kemper Foundation concentrate on four broad areas–education, health and human services, civic and economic development, and the arts." 2000 Brochure **Priorities:** *Arts & Humanities:* 43%. Principal support for museums. *Civic & Public Affairs:* 4%. Major support for a botanical garden, urban and community affairs organizations. *Education:* 35%. Primarily support for colleges and universities, primary and secondary education, and arts education. *Environment:* 7%. Youth organizations, child welfare, and community service organizations. *International:* 7%. Hospitals, single-disease health associations, medical research, and pediatric health. *Note:* Total contributions made in fiscal 2000. **Typ. Recipients:** Cancer, Children's Health/Hospitals, Clinics/Medical Centers, Domestic Violence, Eyes/Blindness, Family Planning, Health Organizations, Hospitals, Hospitals (University Affiliated), Medical Education, Medical Research, Mental Health, Nursing Services, Research/Studies Institutes, Sexual Abuse. **Geo. Dist:** MO.

★ 12102 ★ William T. Morris Foundation
230 Park Ave., Suite 622
New York, NY 10169-0622
Phone: (212)986-8036 **Fax:** (212)370-1962
Edward Antonelli, President and CEO

Fnded: 1937. **Philosophy:** The foundation supports general philanthropy, particularly in the areas of education, health, culture, and youth. **Priorities:** *Arts & Humanities:* 19%. Contributes to music and performing arts. *Civic & Public Affairs:* 5%. Supports other foundations and professional associations. *Education:* 40%. Supports higher education. *Environment:* 1%. Gives to youth groups. *International:* 26%. Funds hospitals, ear and eye research, and medical centers. *Religion:* 1%. Science museums. *Note:* Total contributions made in fiscal 1999. **Typ. Recipients:** Alzheimers Disease, Arthritis, Arthritis, Cancer, Clinics/Medical Centers, Emergency/Ambulance Services, Eyes/Blindness, Health Funds, Heart, Hospitals, Medical Education, Medical Rehabilitation, Medical Research, Multiple Sclerosis, People with Disabilities, Respiratory, Single-Disease Health Associations, Speech & Hearing. **Geo. Dist:** CT; NY; PA.

★ 12103 ★ Windham Foundation
PO Box 70
Grafton, VT 05146
Phone: (802)843-2211 **Fax:** (802)843-2205
Email: winfound@sover.net
Website: http://www.windham-foundation.org
Arthur Schubert, Vice President

Fnded: 1963. **Philosophy:** "The Foundation has a particular interest in innovative programs and furthering proven academic programs that could be replicated in other Vermont locations." "As of January 1, 1998, the Windham Foundation will institute a new grant policy. The Foundation will limit its grant interests to Vermont elementary and secondary education." **Priorities:** *Arts & Humanities:* 26%. Symphonies, historical preservation, and museums. *Civic & Public Affairs:* 27%. *Education:* 13%. Colleges and universities, high schools, and environmental education. *Environment:* 13%. Youth organizations, food programs, and family services. *International:* 3%. Hospice programs, hospitals, and cancer research and treatment. *Religion:* 3%. *Note:* Total contributions made in fiscal 2001. **Typ. Recipients:** Arthritis, Cancer, Diabetes, Domestic Violence, Emergency/Ambulance Services, Family Planning, Health Organizations, Health-General, Home-Care Services, Hospices, Hospitals, Kidney, Prenatal Health Issues, Public Health, Trauma Treatment. **Geo. Dist:** VT, emphasis on Windham County.

★ 12104 ★ Winthrop Rockefeller Foundation
308 East Eighth St.
Little Rock, AR 72202-3999
Phone: (501)376-6854 **Fax:** (501)374-4797
Website: http://www.wrockefellerfoundation.org
Dr. Sybil Hampton, President

Fnded: 1973. **Philosophy:** The underlying goal of the Winthrop Rockefeller Foundation is to improve the quality of life in Arkansas by creating an environment that makes development and improvement possible. Mr. Rockefeller believed economic conditions in Arkansas would improve only through the creation of opportunity within the state. To support economic development, the foundation has chosen to focus on strengthening local economies; providing access to capital, management, and technical assistance for small businesses; strengthening agriculture; developing leadership; supporting organizations that can improve the economic status of Arkansas; and improving the economic status of women and minorities. In the area of civic affairs, the foundation supports efforts to improve the effectiveness of government and private service providers; to focus attention on and promote discussion of public policy issues; to identify and develop leaders at the state, local, and institutional levels; and to improve civic opportunities for minority and disadvantaged citizens. Improving the quality of education is another major focus. The foundation has made a long-term commitment to eliminate educational barriers by supporting efforts to restructure schools, encourage parental involvement, increase minority participation, and identify issues and problems. The foundation also supports organizations promoting literacy. Community incentive grants of up to $10,000 are available for special assistance to community-based organizations for general operating support, construction funds, or equipment purchases. To be eligible for a community incentive grant, an organization must serve a minority or disadvantaged population, and must not be a previous grantee of the foundation. Minigrants of up to $2,000 are made at the discretion of the foundation president for technical assistance, organizational development, or program planning. Such grants also are made to educators. The foundation often develops initiatives to address an area of concern, particularly in education, and supports or initiates in-house public policy projects focusing on important issues in economic development, civic affairs, or education. Other goals are to strengthen the capacity of local communities to break the cycle of poverty by supporting local economic development, and nurture strong leadership through the development of community-based organizations. **Priorities:** *Arts & Humanities:* 23%. Funds historical groups, museums, music, and the performing arts. *Civic & Public Affairs:* 64%. Funds community development, community foundations, economic interests, community services, and employment. *Education:* 9%. Supports public schools, scholarships, arts education, and educational organizations. *Environment:* 5%. Supports United Way and services for youth and families. *Religion:* Less than 1%. *Note:* Total contributions made in 2000. **Typ. Recipients:** AIDS/HIV, Medical Education, People with Disabilities. **Geo. Dist:** AR.

★ 12105 ★ Wollenberg Foundation
6114 LaSalle Ave., PMB 275
Oakland, CA 94611-2802
Phone: (510)625-9049
Marc Monheimer, Trustee

Fnded: 1952. **Philosophy:** The foundation is primarily interested in education and educational funds. Science, medical, and business schools at the university level are supported in addition to public school systems. The foundation also supports a variety of social service programs and civic interests. **Priorities:** *Arts & Humanities:* 1%. Supports the symphony. *Civic & Public Affairs:* 4%. Supports urban affairs, civil rights. *Education:* 86%. Supports education fund, education organizations, colleges, and public elementary school programs. *Environment:* 3%. Supports emergency relief and youth services. *International:* 3%. *Religion:* 2%. Supports a science museum. *Note:* Total contributions made in 2000. **Typ. Recipients:** Domestic Violence, Emergency/Ambulance Services, Family Planning, Hospices, Medical Education, People with Disabilities, Single-Disease Health Associations. **Geo. Dist:** nationally.

★ 12106 ★ Woods Charitable Fund

PO Box 81309
Lincoln, NE 68501
Phone: (402)436-5971 **Fax:** (402)436-4128
Email: pbaker@woodscharitable.org
Website: http://www.woodscharitable.org
Pam Baker, Executive Director & Secretary

Fnded: 1941. **Philosophy:** The fund provides support to nonprofit organizations working to improve living conditions and opportunities for disadvantaged urban residents. A principal goal is to encourage citizen involvement in building a sense of community and in seeking long-term solutions for problems facing Lincoln, NE. The fund is interested in programs that explore policy options in the public interest, and it continues to support cultural and educational programs. Lincoln funding emphasizes education; community development and housing; children, youth, and families; and the arts and humanities. The fund's program for children, youth, and families includes direct-service and policy programs focused on child care, single parenthood, the elderly, family planning, shelter, troubled families, and others. The fund gives special consideration to programs addressing the areas of youth and family violence. The education program looks forward to reviewing proposals from existing educational institutions and from creative new programs to meet the challenge of preparing individuals of all ages for a rapidly changing society. The community development and housing program supports projects that empower less advantaged Lincoln residents to participate in the economic system and that foster community participation and responsibility, thus joining people to solve problems and improve opportunities for all. The program recognizes the growing need in Lincoln for affordable housing and supports projects that expand its availability. Advocacy groups and neighborhood, citizen, and community organizations are avenues to promote citizen involvement and strengthen neighborhoods. The need for individuals to achieve self-sufficiency, including helping people earn an adequate income, has also been identified as a primary community concern. The fund encourages submission of proposals that suggest creative approaches to address this concern. The fund also supports programs in the arts and humanities that enhance or develop the common aesthetic spirit through education, creation, or performance. **Priorities:** *Arts & Humanities:* 27%. Supports performing arts centers, arts councils and associations, orchestras, and public broadcasting. *Civic & Public Affairs:* 8%. Supports leadership organizations and housing. *Education:* 11%. Supports literacy, humanities education, and after-school programs. *Environment:* 52%. Supports youth and family services, food banks, and planned parenthood. *Note:* Total contributions made in 2000. **Typ. Recipients:** AIDS/HIV, Alzheimers Disease, Child Abuse, Clinics/Medical Centers, Domestic Violence, Family Planning, Medical Rehabilitation, Mental Health, People with Disabilities, Public Health, Single-Disease Health Associations, Substance Abuse. **Geo. Dist:** Lincoln, NE.

★ 12107 ★ Woods Fund of Chicago

360 N Michigan, Suite 1600
Chicago, IL 60601
Phone: (312)782-2698 **Fax:** (312)782-4155
Email: info@woodsfund.org
Todd Dietterle, Vice President

Fnded: 1993. **Philosophy:** "Woods Fund of Chicago is a grantmaking foundation whose goal is to increase opportunities for less advantaged people and communities in the metropolitan area, including the opportunity to contribute to decisions affecting them. The foundation works primarily as a funding partner with nonprofit organizations. Woods supports nonprofits in their important roles of engaging people in civic life, addressing the causes of poverty and other challenges facing the region, promoting more effective public policies, reducing barriers to equal opportunity, and building a sense of community and common ground." 1998 Annual Report. **Priorities:** *Arts & Humanities:* Less than 1%. *Civic & Public Affairs:* 59%. Supports organizations for community leadership, economic development, public housing, job training. *Education:* 14%. Funds after-school programs, pre-schools, and colleges and universities. *Environment:* 17%. Supports family and youth programs, the elderly, and programs for the hungry and the homeless. *International:* 6%. Supports adolescent health organizations and medical centers. *Note:* Total contributions made in 2000. **Typ. Recipients:** Adolescent Health Issues, Clinics/Medical Centers, Medical Rehabilitation, Medical Rehabilitation, Prenatal Health Issues. **Geo. Dist:** Chicago, IL.

★ 12108 ★ Wortham Foundation

2727 Allen Parkway, Suite 1570
Wortham Tower
Houston, TX 77019
Phone: (713)526-8849 **Fax:** (713)526-7222
Barbara Snyder, Grants Administrator

Fnded: 1958. **Philosophy:** Prior to the 1969 Tax Reform Act, the foundation was involved primarily with a research project in cattle fertility. The foundation now carries out its founders' interests in "cultural arts and civic beautification projects and to those projects which benefit the citizens of Houston, Harris County, Texas." Wortham Foundation fiscal 1998 Form 990. **Priorities:** *Arts & Humanities:* 55%. Focus on the performing arts and museums. Also supports public broadcasting and historic preservation. *Civic & Public Affairs:* 19%. Supports parks/recreation organizations, with a focus on civic beautification projects. *Environment:* 11%. Supports youth organizations, YMCA, and United Way. *Religion:* 9%. *Note:* Total contributions made in fiscal 2000. **Typ. Recipients:** Cancer, Children's Health/Hospitals, Clinics/Medical Centers, Emergency/Ambulance Services, Hospitals, Medical Education, Public Health. **Geo. Dist:** Houston, TX.

★ 12109 ★ Wyomissing Foundation

12 Commerce Drive
Wyomissing, PA 19610
Phone: (610)376-7494 **Fax:** (610)372-7626
Ned Diefenderfer, Secretary

Fnded: 1929. **Philosophy:** The Wyomissing Foundation makes most of its grants in the areas of education, the arts, civic affairs, and social services. Educational funding favors colleges and universities, special education, and literacy. Support for the arts goes to museums, festivals, ballet, libraries, and public broadcasting. Civic affairs support includes environmental affairs and zoos. The majority of the social service funding goes to united funds. Other recipient areas are also supported. **Priorities:** *Arts & Humanities:* 9%. Music, museums, public television, libraries, opera. and historic preservation. *Civic & Public Affairs:* 28%. Community foundations, housing, clubs and safety. *Education:* 9%. Reading/literacy programs, and colleges and universities. *Environment:* 32%. Food banks, scouting, United Way, and youth programs. *International:* 2%. Nursing services. *Note:* Total contributions made in 2000. **Typ. Recipients:** AIDS/HIV, Emergency/Ambulance Services, Family Planning, Health Funds, Home-Care Services, Hospitals, Medical Rehabilitation, Nursing Services, People with Disabilities, Prenatal Health Issues. **Geo. Dist:** PA, Berks County and contiguous counties.

★ 12110 ★ Y. and H. Soda Foundation

2 Theatre Square, Suite 211
Orinda, CA 94563-3346
Phone: (925)253-2630 **Fax:** (925)253-1814
Email: Judyed@PacBell.net
Mrs. Judith Murphy, President & Chief Executive Officer

Fnded: 1964. **Philosophy:** The foundation focuses on organizations providing the following services in Alameda and Contra Costa Counties, CA: religious welfare (primarily Catholic), health care, human services, youth development, and education. The foundation "seeks to enhance the quality of life for the disadvantaged, to promote their health and welfare, to provide opportunities for education and to support those organizations whose religious philosophy strengthens the spiritual and temporal well-being of those whom they serve." **Priorities:** *Arts & Humanities:* 1%. Supports a museum. *Civic & Public Affairs:* 6%. Funds housing associations, minority affairs, and community organizations. *Education:* 81%. Funds preschool and childcare programs, primary and secondary public and private schools, higher education, and job training programs. *Environment:* 5%. Supports youth development, including services for abused and disadvantaged youth, athletic and mentoring programs, vocational training, camps, and clubs. *International:* 5%. Funds medical centers and hospice. *Note:* Total contributions made in 2000. **Typ. Recipients:** AIDS/HIV, Cancer, Children's Health/Hospitals, Clinics/Medical Centers, Domestic Violence, Geriatric Health, Health Organizations, Hospices, Hospitals, Long-Term Care, People with Disabilities, Prenatal Health Issues, Public Health, Research/Studies Institutes, Sexual Abuse, Single-Disease Health Associations, Speech & Hearing, Substance Abuse. **Geo. Dist:** CA, Alameda and Contra Costa Counties.

★ 12111 ★ Yawkey Foundation II

990 Washington St.
Dedham, MA 02026
Phone: (781)329-7470 **Fax:** (781)329-8195
John Harrington, Executive Director & Trustee

Fnded: 1983. **Priorities:** *Arts & Humanities:* 7%. Supports museums, music, libraries, the performing arts, public broadcasting, and historic preservation. *Civic & Public Affairs:* 7%. Funds community services, housing, community organizations, and aquariums. *Education:* 34%. Supports colleges, secondary schools, scholarship funds, and universities. *Environment:* 38%. Supports youth and family services, athletics/recreation, homes, and people with disabilities. *International:* 7%. Funds medical research, single-disease associations, and hospitals. *Religion:* Less than 1%. *Note:* Total contributions made in fiscal 2000. **Typ. Recipients:** AIDS/HIV, Alzheimers Disease, Cancer, Children's Health/Hospitals, Clinics/Medical Centers, Emergency/Ambulance Services, Eyes/Blindness, Health Organizations, Hospitals, Medical Research, People with Disabilities, Single-Disease Health Associations. **Geo. Dist:** MA; Boston, MA, metropolitan area.

★ 12112 ★ Z. Smith Reynolds Foundation

147 S Cherry St., Suite 200
Winston-Salem, NC 27101
Phone: (336)725-7541 **Fax:** (336)725-6069
Email: info@zsr.org
Website: http://www.zsr.org
Thomas Ross, Executive Director

Fnded: 1936. **Philosophy:** The foundation's original donors intentionally left the terms of its charter broad so that trustees might make grants for a wide array of projects. The foundation is limited, however, to making grants exclusively within the state of North Carolina. The purpose of the foundation, in its own words, is "to enhance the quality of life in North Carolina." It fulfills this broad-based role by seeking out needy aspects of North Carolina life, and "places higher value on developing new, quality programs, rather than in sustaining well-established, well-funded ones." Areas of interest include economic and community development, pre-collegiate education, minority issues, women's issues, and protection of the environment. In the area of education, priorities are preschool education, teacher education, literacy, and the development of local public school foundations. The foundation also is committed to encouraging the emergence of community development corporations. The foundation's concern in minority affairs focuses on the need to bolster black family life; improve the academic performance of, and opportunities for, black youth; increase political participation; and foster new leadership in the black community. Particular emphasis is placed on programs for unemployed heads-of-households, efforts to improve parenting skills and parental participation in school life, job-training programs, and programs to provide training for political candidates. The foundation's concern for women's issues includes eliminating barriers to women's career progress, and raising women's income level. The foundation also is concerned with women in crisis and in the provision of shelters, counseling, and support groups for them. The overall goals of the foundation in the environmental area are to protect North Carolina's land, waters, and air, and to give special attention to the needs of the state's ecologically sensitive areas. The foundation has sponsored conferences in criminal justice, childhood education, housing, black issues, environmental concerns, and the future of rural North Carolina, in order to bring together people with needs and others with knowledge or solutions. **Priorities:** *Arts & Humanities:* 16%. Supports historic preservation and public broadcasting. *Civic & Public Affairs:* 35%. Funds community development initiatives, public policy, housing, self-help programs, and legal aid. *Education:* 32%. Supports literacy programs, alternative learning centers, elementary and middle schools, and colleges and universities. *Environment:* 5%. Funds youth programs, volunteerism, child advocacy programs, domestic violence prevention, and food banks. *Religion:* 2%. *Note:* Total contributions made in 2000. **Typ. Recipients:** Adolescent Health Issues, Alzheimers Disease, Child Abuse, Domestic Violence, Family Planning, Health Policy/Cost Containment, People with Disabilities, Prenatal Health Issues, Public Health, Substance Abuse. **Geo. Dist:** NC.

★ 12113 ★ Zarrow Family Foundation
401 S Boston, 900
Tulsa, OK 74103
Phone: (918)295-8004 **Fax:** (918)295-8049
Email: jgillert@zarrow.com
Website: http://www.zarrow.com
Jeanne Gillert, Manager

Fnded: 1988. **Priorities:** *Arts & Humanities:* 3%. Supports music, museums and the local community ballet theater. *Civic & Public Affairs:* 2%. Supports philanthropy, clubs, community organizations, and zoos. *Education:* 13%. Supports private schools (precollege), colleges, and universities, education reform and funds, business education, and medical education. *Environment:* 34%. Major support is awarded to Goodwill Industries. Other recipients include community service organizations, youth organizations, senior services, people with disabilities, and food distribution centers. *International:* 16%. Interests include single-disease health associations, mental health foundations, emergency services, clinics and medical centers, and hospitals. *Note:* Total contributions made in 2000. **Typ. Recipients:** Alzheimers Disease, Cancer, Children's Health/Hospitals, Clinics/Medical Centers, Diabetes, Emergency/Ambulance Services, Eyes/Blindness, Geriatric Health, Health Funds, Health Organizations, Heart, Hospices, Hospitals, Medical Education, Medical Research, Mental Health, Multiple Sclerosis, People with Disabilities, Prenatal Health Issues, Respiratory, Single-Disease Health Associations, Substance Abuse. **Geo. Dist:** nationally; Tulsa, OK, supports preselected organizations only.

★ 12114 ★ Zellerbach Family Fund
120 Montgomery St., Suite 1550
San Francisco, CA 94104
Phone: (415)421-2629 **Fax:** (415)421-6713
Linda Howe, Program Executive

Fnded: 1956. **Philosophy:** "In 1997, the Fund focused its efforts on programs that: enhance the ability of public systems and institutions to better serve families and children; increase and build upon the strengths and capacities within neighborhoods as residents work together to reduce shared problems; foster the ability of immigrants and refugees to successfully participate in American society; promote culture in its many varieties and traditions; and promote the healthy development of youth." 1997 Annual Report. Grants from the fund are directed largely to needs within the San Francisco Bay Area. The fund is affiliated with the Northern California Grantmakers, and it joins with other foundations, corporations, and nonprofit organizations to be more aware of and responsive to community needs. **Priorities:** *Arts & Humanities:* 24%. Supports ballet, opera, the symphony, and community art organizations. *Civic & Public Affairs:* 23%. Funds botanical gardens, small business development, and urban affairs. *Education:* 16%. Supports education reform and universities. *Environment:* 30%. Supports family services and youth development organizations. *International:* 6%. Supports education reform and universities. *Note:* Total contributions made in 2000. **Typ. Recipients:** AIDS/HIV, Cancer, Child Abuse, Children's Health/Hospitals, Clinics/Medical Centers, Domestic Violence, Health Organizations, Mental Health, People with Disabilities, Prenatal Health Issues, Public Health, Research/Studies Institutes, Trauma Treatment. **Geo. Dist:** San Francisco, CA, Bay Area.

★ 12115 ★ Zemurray Foundation
228 Saint Charles, Suite 1024
New Orleans, LA 70130
Phone: (504)522-1024 **Fax:** (504)571-1024

Fnded: 1951. **Philosophy:** The Zemurray Foundation makes most of its grants in the areas of education, civic affairs, and the arts in New Orleans. Educational giving favors colleges and universities. Civic affairs support is given primarily to environmental and regional foundations. The New Orleans Museum of Art is a major recipient along with other art organizations. Minor grants are given to other recipient areas. **Priorities:** *Arts & Humanities:* 22%. Supports art councils, art centers, literary organizations, and museums. *Civic & Public Affairs:* Less than 1%. *Education:* 44%. Supports academics, schools, colleges, and universities. *Environment:* Less than 1%. *Religion:* 2%. *Note:* Total contributions made in 2000. **Typ. Recipients:** Cancer, Clinics/Medical Centers, Family Planning, Health-General, Hospitals, Medical Research, People with Disabilities, Prenatal Health Issues. **Geo. Dist:** nationally, with some New Orleans, LA.

Corporate Foundations

★ 12116 ★ A.O. Smith Foundation, Inc.
PO Box 245001
Milwaukee, WI 53224-9501
Phone: (414)359-4100 **Fax:** (414)359-4064
Edward O'Connor, Secretary

Fnded: 1955. **Priorities:** *Arts & Humanities:* 16%. Supports museums, libraries, and theater. *Civic & Public Affairs:* 3%. Funds public safety, zoos, and memorials. *Education:* 27%. Emphasis on colleges and universities and independent college funds. *Environment:* 41%. Major emphasis on the United Way. Also supports human services and youth organizations. *International:* 10%. Supports hospitals and single-disease associations. *Note:* Total contributions made in 2000. **Typ. Recipients:** Emergency/Ambulance Services, Hospitals, Medical Education, Medical Rehabilitation, Mental Health, People with Disabilities, Public Health, Substance Abuse. **Geo. Dist:** communities where company has manufacturing facilities.

★ 12117 ★ ABB, Inc.
1455 Pennsylvania Ave. Suite 210
Washington, DC 20004
Phone: (202)639-4061 **Fax:** (202)737-1414
Fruzsina Harsanyi, Senior Vice President, Public Affairs

Typ. Recipients: Hospitals, Substance Abuse. **Geo. Dist:** headquarters and operating communities.

★ 12118 ★ Abbott Laboratories Fund
Department 379, Bldg. AP6D-2
100 Abbott Park Rd.
Abbott Park, IL 60064-6048
Phone: (847)937-7075 **Fax:** (847)935-5051
Website: http://abbott.com/community/lab_fund.html
Cindy Schwab, Vice President

Fnded: 1951. **Priorities:** *Arts & Humanities:* 11%. *Civic & Public Affairs:* 16%. *Education:* 28%. *Environment:* 33%. *International:* 9%. *Religion:* 4%. *Note:* Total contributions made in 2001. **Typ. Recipients:** AIDS/HIV, Cancer, Children's Health/Hospitals, Clinics/Medical Centers, Emergency/Ambulance Services, Geriatric Health, Health Organizations, Health-General, Heart, Hospices, Hospitals, Hospitals (University Affiliated), Kidney, Medical Education, Medical Rehabilitation, Medical Research, Medical Training, Nursing Services, Nutrition, People with Disabilities, Public Health, Research/Studies Institutes, Sexual Abuse, Single-Disease Health Associations, Substance Abuse. **Geo. Dist:** headquarters and operating communities.

★ 12119 ★ ABC Foundation
Bank of America Pl., NC1-002-11-18
Charlotte, NC 28255
Phone: 800-401-2635
Mr. Terry Weatherford, Secretary

Priorities: *Arts & Humanities:* 10%. Supports the United Arts Council of North Carolina. *Civic & Public Affairs:* 4%. Favors textile foundations, business foundations, and community organizations. *Education:* 30%. Provides scholarships to college students. Supports colleges, public education, vocational technical schools, and literacy. *Environment:* 50%. Primarily supports various United Ways located in North Carolina and South Carolina. Other support goes to YMCA and youth organizations. *International:* Less than 1%. Supports public health and hospice programs. *Note:* Total foundation contributions made in fiscal 2002. Giving percentages provided by foundation. **Typ. Recipients:** Emergency/Ambulance Services, Health Organizations, Health-General, Hospices, Multiple Sclerosis, People with Disabilities, Substance Abuse. **Geo. Dist:** operating locations; NC, Rutherford County; Greensboro, NC; Carlisle, SC, and surrounding area.

★ 12120 ★ Abel Foundation
PO Box 80268
Lincoln, NE 68501
Phone: (402)434-1212 **Fax:** (402)434-1799
Website: http://www.abelfoundation.org
J. McCown, Vice President

Fnded: 1951. **Priorities:** *Arts & Humanities:* 18%. Supports local arts organizations, the performing arts, libraries, and historical societies. *Civic & Public Affairs:* Less than 1%. Supports professional organizations and community foundations. *Education:* 11%. More than half of education grants support Lincoln, NE, area colleges and universities. Also supports public education. *Environment:* 49%. Supports the United Way, scouts, food banks, and community and family services organizations. *International:* 2%. Supports health facilities and the American Red Cross. *Note:* Total contributions made in 2001. **Typ. Recipients:** Children's Health/Hospitals, Domestic Violence, Emergency/Ambulance Services, Family Planning, Health Organizations, Health-General, Heart, Hospitals, Mental Health, People with Disabilities, Research/Studies Institutes, Transplant Networks/Donor Banks. **Geo. Dist:** NE.

★ 12121 ★ Ace Hardware Foundation
2200 Kensington Court
Oak Brook, IL 60523-2100
Phone: (630)990-6444 **Fax:** (630)990-1742
Email: pthom@memo.acehardware.com
Website: http://www.acehardware.com/corp/index.jsp?page=community
Rita Kahle, Manager, Corporate Communications

Priorities: *Civic & Public Affairs:* Less than 1%. *Environment:* 19%. *International:* 81%. *Note:* Total foundation contributions made in 2001. **Typ. Recipients:** Children's Health/Hospitals, Emergency/Ambulance Services, Medical Research. **Geo. Dist:** nationally.

★ 12122 ★ Adolph Coors Co.
PO Box 4030, NH 420
Golden, CO 80401-0030
Phone: (303)277-6204 **Fax:** (303)277-6132
Email: buck.boze@coors.com
Website: http://coors.com/community/philanthropy.asp
Buck Boze, Corporate Contributions Manager

Priorities: *Voluntarism:* Company supports Volunteers in Community Enrichment (VICE) program. Contact Crystal Adams at (303) 277-3736 for more information. **Typ. Recipients:** AIDS/HIV, Domestic Violence, Emergency/Ambulance Services, Health Funds, Health Organizations, Hospices, Hospitals, Medical Rehabilitation, Mental Health, People with Disabilities, Respiratory, Single-Disease Health Associations, Substance Abuse. **Geo. Dist:** Denver, CO; Memphis, TN; Elkton, VA.

★ 12123 ★ AEGON U.S.A. Charitable Foundation
1111 N Charles St.
Baltimore, MD 21201
Phone: (410)576-4576 **Fax:** (410)347-8685
Rosmary Kostmayer, Director, Public Relations

Fnded: 1988. **Priorities:** *Arts & Humanities:* 13%. *Civic & Public Affairs:* 5%. *Education:* 6%. *Environment:* 53%. *International:* 19%. *Note:* Total foundation contributions made in 2001. **Typ. Recipients:** Alzheimers Disease, Arthritis, Cancer, Children's Health/Hospitals, Clinics/Medical Centers, Diabetes, Domestic Violence, Health-General, Heart, Hospitals, Prenatal Health Issues, Public Health, Single-Disease Health Associations. **Geo. Dist:** headquarters and operating communities; IA, eastern; KY; MD, central.

★ 12124 ★ Aetna Foundation
151 Farmington Ave., RE2R
Hartford, CT 06156-3180
Phone: (860)273-6382
Website: http://www.aetna.com/foundation
Marilda Gandara, President & Executive Director

Priorities: *Arts & Humanities:* 53%. Supports museums, art funds, theater, and the performing arts. *Civic & Public Affairs:* 18%. Supports justice, chambers of commerce, business foundations, and ethnic organizations. *Education:* 7%. Supports colleges, universities, and educational programs. *Environment:* 12%. Supports the United Way, volunteer services, and crime prevention. *International:* 10%. Supports medical associations, health organizations, and single-disease health foundations. *Voluntarism:* The company sponsors the Aetna Volunteers! Program, which makes grants up to $500 to nonprofits where company employees volunteer; grants are initiated by the employee. Also supports the Aetna Volunteer Council, which matches employees with volunteer opportunities. *Note:* Total foundation contributions made in 2000. **Typ. Recipients:** AIDS/HIV, Cancer, Child Abuse, Children's Health/Hospitals, Clinics/Medical Centers, Diabetes, Domestic Violence, Emergency/Ambulance Services, Health Organizations, Health-General, Heart, Hospices, Hospitals, Medical Education, Nursing Services, Nutrition, People with Disabilities, Prenatal Health Issues, Public Health, Respiratory, Single-Disease Health Associations. **Geo. Dist:** principally near operating locations and to national organizations; Hartford, CT.

★ 12125 ★ AFLAC Foundation, Inc.
1932 Wynnton Rd.
Columbus, GA 31999
Phone: (706)323-3431 **Fax:** (706)320-2288
Website: http://www.aflac.com
Wendy Hogan, Administrator, Corp. Contributions

Priorities: *Arts & Humanities:* Less than 1%. *Civic & Public Affairs:* 6%. *Education:* 6%. *Environment:* 19%. *International:* 68%. *Note:* Total contributions made in 2001. **Typ. Recipients:** Arthritis, Cancer, Children's Health/Hospitals, Health Organizations, Health-General, Hospices, Medical Research, Single-Disease Health Associations, Substance Abuse. **Geo. Dist:** GA.

★ 12126 ★ AGL Resources Private Foundation
817 West Peachtree St. NW, 10th Floor
Atlanta, GA 30308
Phone: (404)584-3311 **Fax:** (404)584-3479
Website: http://www.aglresources.com/content/community_involvement/aglr_cominv.shtml
Harriet Watkins, Vice President Community Affairs

Priorities: *Arts & Humanities:* 33%. *Civic & Public Affairs:* 21%. *Education:* 5%. *Environment:* 13%. *International:* 12%. *Religion:* 1%. *Note:* Total foundation contributions made in 2001. **Typ. Recipients:** AIDS/HIV, Health Organizations, Health-General, Hospices, Medical Research, Mental Health, Nutrition, People with Disabilities, Public Health, Substance Abuse. **Geo. Dist:** GA.

★ 12127 ★ Agrilink Foods/Pro-Fac Foundation
PO Box 20670
Rochester, NY 14602-0670
Phone: (585)264-3155 **Fax:** (585)383-1606
Website: http://www.agrilinkfoods.com/corp/about/community/index.html
Susan Riker, Secretary

Priorities: *Arts & Humanities:* 14%. Supports museums, galleries, libraries, public broadcasting, and theater. *Civic & Public Affairs:* 7%. Supports parks, career development, and community foundations. *Education:* 19%. Supports arts/humanities education, scholarships, colleges, universities, and literacy. *Environment:* 52%. Supports people with disabilities, youth programs, United Way, scouting, Young Men's Christian Association, camps, shelters, and family services. *International:* 7%. Supports medical centers and single-disease health associations. *Religion:* 1%. Supports a museum and science center. *Note:* Total contributions made in fiscal 2001. **Typ. Recipients:** Cancer, Children's Health/Hospitals, Clinics/Medical Centers, Domestic Violence, Emergency/Ambulance Services, Family Planning, Geriatric Health, Health Organizations, Heart, Hospices, Hospitals, Medical Rehabilitation, Mental Health, Nursing Services, People with Disabilities, Public Health, Single-Disease Health Associations, Substance Abuse. **Geo. Dist:** headquarters and operating communities.

★ 12128 ★ AIG American General Corp.
2929 Allen Parkway
Houston, TX 77019
Phone: (713)522-1111 **Fax:** (713)831-3889
Email: virginia_tomlinson@agfg.com
Website: http://www.americangeneral.com
Virginia Tomlinson, Director, Community Relations

Priorities: *Arts & Humanities:* 15% to 20%. *Civic & Public Affairs:* 10% to 15%. *Education:* 25% to 30%. *Environment:* 45% to 50%. United Way and health care. *Voluntarism:* StepUp is American General's employee volunteer program centered on a companywide commitment to America's Promise. Employees are given time off to volunteer during the work week, allowing them to tutor, mentor, and carry out the goals of America's Promise. **Typ. Recipients:** Health-General.

★ 12129 ★ Air Products Foundation
7201 Hamilton Boulevard
Allentown, PA 18195-1501
Phone: (610)481-9627 **Fax:** (610)481-6642
Website: http://www.airproducts.com/social_responsibilities/
M.B. Gabriel, Contact

Priorities: *Arts & Humanities:* (Art and Culture) 2%. Supports museums, music, and the performing arts. Other areas of interest include theaters, festivals, and public broadcasting. *Civic & Public Affairs:* (Community and Economic Development) 11%. Economic development is a major concern, as are business and free enterprise organizations, and housing rehabilitation. Also supports safety organizations. *Education:* (Precollege and Higher Education) 21%. Supports engineering and business departments of colleges and universities. Also interested in independent college funds and minority, economic, and arts education. Majority of education funds are in the form of matching gifts. *Environment:* (United Way) 28%. The majority of United Way giving is through matching gifts. *International:* (Fitness, Health, and Welfare) Health interests include single-disease health associations and emergency services. *Voluntarism:* Seventy percent of employees volunteer in community activities. Volunteerism is encouraged and recognized by the company, but it does not have a formal volunteer program. *Note:* Above percentages represent fiscal 2001 foundation contributions only. Direct giving program priorities are similar. Matching gifts are included in the analysis. **Typ. Recipients:** Cancer, Children's Health/Hospitals, Domestic Violence, Emergency/Ambulance Services, Health Organizations, Heart, Multiple Sclerosis, Nutrition, People with Disabilities, Single-Disease Health Associations, Substance Abuse. **Geo. Dist:** headquarters and select operating communities.

★ 12130 ★ Airborne Express
PO Box 662
Seattle, WA 98111-0662
Phone: (206)285-4600 **Fax:** (206)830-4438
Website: http://www.airborne.com
Liz Paquette, Administrative Assistant

Priorities: *Arts & Humanities:* 10%. *Civic & Public Affairs:* 10%. *Education:* 20%. *Environment:* 55%. **Typ. Recipients:** Health-General. **Geo. Dist:** WA, western Washington.

★ 12131 ★ AK Steel Foundation
703 Curtis St.
Middletown, OH 45043
Phone: (513)425-2991 **Fax:** (513)425-5683
Brian Coughlin, Government Affairs Manager

Fnded: 1990. **Priorities:** *Arts & Humanities:* 1%. Funds community arts and art festivals. *Civic & Public Affairs:* 37. Support is directed to community foundations and housing. *Education:* 6%. Primary interests include colleges and universities, secondary education, Junior Achievement, and education associations. Also sponsors a scholarship program for children of employees. *Environment:* 42%. Primary support includes funding for the United Way in Ohio, Pennsylvania, Indiana, and Kentucky. *International:* 1%. Supports a healthcare foundation, emergency response, cancer research, and America Red Cross. *Voluntarism:* The foundation gives volunteer support donations to community organizations where employees volunteer their time and services. *Note:* Total contributions made in 2000. **Typ. Recipients:** Cancer, Child Abuse, Clinics/Medical Centers, Emergency/Ambulance Services, Health Organizations, Heart, Hospices, Hospitals, People with Disabilities, Public Health, Single-Disease Health Associations, Substance Abuse. **Geo. Dist:** operating locations.

★ 12132 ★ Alabama Power Foundation
600 N 18th St.
Birmingham, AL 35291-0011
Phone: (205)257-2508 **Fax:** (205)257-1860
William Johnson, President

Fnded: 1990. **Priorities:** *Arts & Humanities:* 9%. *Civic & Public Affairs:* 25%. *Education:* 24%. *Environment:* 31%. *International:* 6%. *Note:* Total foundation contributions made in 2001. **Typ. Recipients:** Cancer, Children's Health/Hospitals, Diabetes, Eyes/Blindness, Health Organizations, Heart, Mental Health, People with Disabilities, Single-Disease Health Associations, Substance Abuse. **Geo. Dist:** headquarters and operating communities.

★ 12133 ★ Albany International Corp.
PO Box 1907
Albany, NY 12201-1907
Phone: (518)445-2200 **Fax:** (518)447-6343
Email: ken_pulver@albint.com
Website: http://www.albint.com
Ken Pulver, Vice President, Corporate Communications

Priorities: *Arts & Humanities:* Funds cultural organizations that further the fine and performing arts. *Education:* Supports capital campaigns for colleges and universities, and paper schools from which company draws employees; also provides scholarships. *Environment:* Funds United Way and human service organizations. *International:* Supports hospital capital campaigns. **Typ. Recipients:** Hospices. **Geo. Dist:** headquarters and operating communities.

★ 12134 ★ Albertson's Inc.

PO Box 20
Boise, ID 83726
Phone: (208)395-6200 **Fax:** (208)395-4382
Website: http://www.albertsons.com/corporate/
Judy McLaughlin, Community Relations Coordinator

Priorities: *Education:* Seeks to assure the availability of a pool of trained and educated men and women from which to draw employees and to promote standards of educational excellence. Support includes assistance to public and private higher education institutions, employee matching grants, scholarship programs and related organizations, as well as youth development programs. *Environment:* Supports hunger relief programs in operating areas. Albertson's distribution centers and suppliers collect and donate products for food banks, churches, and other community-based hunger-relief services. *International:* Goals are to assure the availability of adequate health care and human service support for employees and other corporate constituents. Support includes assistance to health and nutrition-oriented programs that improve the availability of health care and human services; and supports organizations that provide education and services to help customers and employees maintain good health, fitness, and nutrition practices. Programs that bring health and nutrition resources to Albertson's stores are of primary interest. *Voluntarism:* The company sponsors the Warren E. McCain Community Volunteer Award. The program annually recognizes employees for volunteer efforts, donating $500 in the name of ten grand award winners to the charity of his/her choice. The company also selects an award winner from each of its operating divisions and donates $250 to each winner's charity of choice. **Typ. Recipients:** Emergency/Ambulance Services, Geriatric Health, Hospitals, Medical Rehabilitation, Mental Health, Public Health, Substance Abuse. **Geo. Dist:** headquarters and operating communities.

★ 12135 ★ Alcoa Foundation

201 Isabella St.
Pittsburgh, PA 15212-5858
Phone: (412)553-2348 **Fax:** (412)553-4532
Website: http://www.alcoa.com/site/community/homepage/community.asp
Kathleen Buechel, President

Fnded: 1952. **Priorities:** *Arts & Humanities:* 2%. *Civic & Public Affairs:* 23%. *Education:* 19%. *Environment:* 20%. *International:* 4%. *Note:* Total contributions made in 2000. About 15% of the foundation's annual giving is to international organizations that fall within the above categories of giving. **Typ. Recipients:** AIDS/HIV, Cancer, Children's Health/Hospitals, Clinics/Medical Centers, Domestic Violence, Emergency/Ambulance Services, Family Planning, Geriatric Health, Health Funds, Health Organizations, Health Policy/Cost Containment, Health-General, Heart, Hospices, Hospitals, Medical Education, Medical Rehabilitation, Medical Research, Medical Training, Mental Health, People with Disabilities, Prenatal Health Issues, Public Health, Single-Disease Health Associations, Speech & Hearing, Substance Abuse. **Geo. Dist:** principally near operating locations and to national organizations.

★ 12136 ★ Alcon Foundation

6201 South Freeway
Fort Worth, TX 76134-2099
Phone: (817)293-0450 **Fax:** (817)568-7000
Email: Mary.Dulle@alconlabs.com
Website: http://www.alconlabs.com
Mary Dulle, Director, Corporate Communications

Fnded: 1962. **Priorities:** *Arts & Humanities:* 12%. Major support goes to theaters, music, and symphonies in the Ft. Worth area. Also contributes to libraries and public broadcasting. *Civic & Public Affairs:* 7%. Supports a variety of community organizations. *Education:* 33%. Funding supports colleges, universities, and education associations for ophthalmic or optometric research. Also funds minority education, and secondary public and private education, Junior Achievement, and the Adopt-a-School program. *Environment:* 4%. Supports a variety of social service organizations in the Ft. Worth, TX, area with grants ranging from $250 to $1,000. Majority of contributions fund child welfare and youth organizations. Other priorities include community centers, food distribution, homes, shelters, and religious welfare. *International:* 43%. Majority of contributions support eye-related health funds and health associations. *Religion:* 2%. *Note:* Total contributions in 2000. **Typ. Recipients:** Cancer, Cancer, Children's Health/Hospitals, Clinics/Medical Centers, Emergency/Ambulance Services, Eyes/Blindness, Health Funds, Health Organizations, Hospitals, Medical Education, Medical Research, Mental Health, People with Disabilities, Prenatal Health Issues, Public Health, Single-Disease Health Associations. **Geo. Dist:** nationally; Ft. Worth, TX.

★ 12137 ★ Alexander & Baldwin Foundation

PO Box 3440
Honolulu, HI 96801-3440
Phone: (808)525-6642 **Fax:** (808)525-6677
Email: lhowe@abinc.com
Website: http://www.alexanderbaldwin.com/abf/index.htm
Ms. Meredith Ching, Vice President

Fnded: 1992. **Priorities:** *Arts & Humanities:* 15%. Recipients include the performing arts, theater, historical societies, and museums. *Civic & Public Affairs:* 9%. Supports local civic affairs, including economic development, housing, safety programs, minorities, and cultural festivals. *Education:* 24%. Contributes to colleges and universities and private and public education. *Environment:* 38%. Emphasis on United Way. Also supports youth organizations, child welfare, and the disabled. *International:* 8%. Support for hospitals, health services, and single-disease organizations. *Note:* Total foundation contributions made in 2001. **Typ. Recipients:** AIDS/HIV, Children's Health/Hospitals, Clinics/Medical Centers, Emergency/Ambulance Services, Health Organizations, Heart, Hospices, Hospitals, Medical Rehabilitation, Mental Health, Nutrition, Single-Disease Health Associations, Substance Abuse. **Geo. Dist:** west coast; San Francisco, CA, including bay area; HI.

★ 12138 ★ Alliant Energy Foundation, Inc.

4902 North Biltmore Ln.
PO Box 77007
Madison, WI 53701-1007
Phone: (608)458-3311 **Fax:** (608)283-6991
Website: http://alliantenergy.com/community/charity.htm
JoAnn Healy, Foundation Administrator

Priorities: *Arts & Humanities:* 21%. Cultural interests include history, museums, and libraries. Art interests include performing arts events, music, dance, community ensembles, small theaters, arts and crafts centers, and visual arts. *Civic & Public Affairs:* 1%. Supports neighborhood improvement, community business funds, parks and environmental projects, community affairs, and fire safety. *Education:* 39%. Supports colleges and universities in areas where the company operates, and funds agricultural and technical programs. Supports matching gifts and scholarship funds. *Environment:* 33%. Most support goes to social services, with about one-third awarded to united fund drives in local communities. Also supports youth organizations and family services. *International:* 2%. Contributes to health foundations, hospitals, and other health causes. *Religion:* 4%. Funds science centers. *Note:* Total foundation contributions made in 2000. **Typ. Recipients:** Cancer, Children's Health/Hospitals, Clinics/Medical Centers, Emergency/Ambulance Services, Health Organizations, Hospitals, Nursing Services, People with Disabilities, Public Health, Single-Disease Health Associations. **Geo. Dist:** IL; IA; MN; WI, near headquarters and service areas (central and south central Wisconsin). **Frmly:** Wisconsin Power & Light Foundation, Inc.

★ 12139 ★ Alliant Techsystems Community Investment Foundation

5050 Lincoln Dr.
Edina, MN 55436-1097
Phone: (952)351-3000
Website: http://www.atk.com
Nancy Darbut, Foundation Section

Fnded: 1992. **Priorities:** *Civic & Public Affairs:* (Community Relationships) 4%. Recipients include minority associations, public affairs, civic leagues, management improvement, economic development, and recreation. *Education:* (Increase Pool/Equip Teachers) 30%. Supports business, economic, math, and science education. Public education, colleges and universities, and scholarship funds are other recipients. Focus is on programs that overcome education barriers and equip math and science teachers to improve student performance. Also supports Junior Achievement. *Environment:* (Eliminate Barriers) 43%. Supports organizations and programs that resolve human services issues are barriers to learning. *Note:* Total contributions made in fiscal 2000. **Typ. Recipients:** Cancer, Children's Health/Hospitals, Emergency/Ambulance Services, Medical Education, Medical Research, People with Disabilities, Single-Disease Health Associations. **Geo. Dist:** headquarters and operating communities; Minneapolis, MN; Magna, UT; Seattle, WA.

★ 12140 ★ Allianz Life Insurance Co. of North America

5701 Golden Hills Drive
Minneapolis, MN 55416
Phone: (763)765-6500 **Fax:** (763)765-6299
Website: http://www.allianzlife.com
Julie Letner, Vice President, Human Resources

Typ. Recipients: Health Organizations, Heart, Hospitals, People with Disabilities. **Geo. Dist:** near headquarters only.

★ 12141 ★ Allied Waste Industries

5757 Oats Rd.
Houston, TX 77078
Phone: (713)671-1507 **Fax:** (713)671-1555
Maryann McGuire, Director Corporate Affairs

Typ. Recipients: Health Funds, Health Organizations, Hospices, Single-Disease Health Associations. **Geo. Dist:** headquarters and operating communities.

★ 12142 ★ Allmerica Financial Charitable Foundation, Inc.

440 Lincoln St.
Worcester, MA 01653
Phone: (508)855-1000 **Fax:** (508)855-6332
Michael Buckley, President

Fnded: 1991. **Priorities:** *Arts & Humanities:* 1%. *Civic & Public Affairs:* 13%. *Education:* 16%. *Environment:* 55%. *International:* 12%. *Voluntarism:* The company sponsors a Volunteer Incentive Program. *Note:* Total foundation contributions made in 2001. **Typ. Recipients:** AIDS/HIV, Cancer, Children's Health/Hospitals, Clinics/Medical Centers, Domestic Violence, Emergency/Ambulance Services, Eyes/Blindness, Health Organizations, Health-General, Heart, Hospitals, Hospitals (University Affiliated), Medical Education, Medical Research, Nursing Services, Public Health, Sexual Abuse, Single-Disease Health Associations, Substance Abuse. **Geo. Dist:** Boston, MA; Worcester, MA; Howell, MI.

★ 12143 ★ Allstate Foundation

2775 Sanders Rd., Suite F-4
Northbrook, IL 60062-6127

Phone: (847)402-2794 **Fax:** (847)326-7517
Email: allfound@allstate.com
Website: http://www.allstate.com/foundation
Jan Epstein, Executive Director

Priorities: *Arts & Humanities:* 2%. *Civic & Public Affairs:* 50%. *Education:* 17%. *Environment:* 25%. *Voluntarism:* Allstate's formal volunteer program, Helping Hands, provides opportunities for employees and agents to volunteer in the community. More than 200 committees nationally and 54 percent of employees and agents partake in volunteer activities. Nonprofit organizations at which Allstate employees volunteer may be eligible for Helping Hands grants from the Allstate Foundation. *Note:* Total contributions made in 2001. **Typ. Recipients:** Children's Health/Hospitals, Children's Health/Hospitals, Clinics/Medical Centers, Domestic Violence, Emergency/Ambulance Services, Health Funds, Health Organizations, Health Policy/Cost Containment, Hospitals, Hospitals (University Affiliated), Medical Education, Medical Research, Prenatal Health Issues, Public Health, Substance Abuse, Trauma Treatment. **Geo. Dist:** nationally.

★ 12144 ★ AMCORE Foundation
501 7th St., PO Box 1537
Rockford, IL 61110
Phone: (815)968-2241 **Fax:** (815)961-7530
Website: http://www.amcore.com
James Waddell, Chairman

Priorities: *Arts & Humanities:* 15%. Provides major support to the Coronado theater. Also funds museums, historic preservation, libraries, and art fests. *Civic & Public Affairs:* 25%. Provides a major donation to the Zion Development Corp. for neighborhood building and development of low-income housing. Also funds a community Fourth of July festival and community foundations. *Education:* 6%. Gives to Junior Achievement, literacy initiatives, public schools, and educational enrichment programs. *Environment:* 47%. Primarily funds a local United Way agency. Also supports youth organizations, a substance abuse treatment facility, food distribution, senior living, and other social service organizations. *International:* 7%. Funds hospice, single-disease health associations, and other health programs. *Note:* Total contributions made in 2001. **Typ. Recipients:** AIDS/HIV, Alzheimers Disease, Cancer, Clinics/Medical Centers, Domestic Violence, Emergency/Ambulance Services, Health Organizations, Health-General, Hospices, Hospitals, Long-Term Care, Medical Education, Medical Rehabilitation, Mental Health, Nursing Services, Nutrition, People with Disabilities, Public Health, Single-Disease Health Associations, Substance Abuse. **Geo. Dist:** Rockford, IL, including surrounding communities.

★ 12145 ★ AMD, Inc.
5204 E Ben White Boulevard
MailStop 529
Austin, TX 78741
Phone: (512)602-5501 **Fax:** (512)602-6985
Email: allyson.peerman@AMD.com
Website: http://www.amd.com
Allyson Peerman, Manager, Corporate Community Affairs

Priorities: *Civic & Public Affairs:* 3%. Funds community development. *Education:* 55%. Supports K-12 education, university education, and workforce development. *Environment:* 34%. Focus is on basic needs. Includes health and human services funding. *Voluntarism:* AMD organizes group volunteer activities that provide hundreds of AMD employees with the opportunity to participate in local community events. The company's Grant Incentives for Volunteer Efforts (GIVE) program provides grants to eligible organizations for which AMD employees volunteer. *Note:* Total contributions made in 2000. **Typ. Recipients:** Clinics/Medical Centers, Hospitals, People with Disabilities. **Geo. Dist:** Gives internationally in Dresden, Germany; Singapore; Bangkok, Thailand; Penang, Malaysia; and Suzhou, China; Sunnyvale, CA; Austin, TX. **Frmly:** Advanced Micro Devices Charitable Foundation.

★ 12146 ★ Ameren Corp. Charitable Trust
PO Box 66149, Mail Code 100
Saint Louis, MO 63166-6149
Phone: (314)554-4740 **Fax:** (314)554-2888
Email: ocowan@ameren.com
Website: http://www.ameren.com/community/adc_com_homepage.asp
Otis Cowan, Manager, Community Relations

Priorities: *Arts & Humanities:* 12%. Supports theater, opera, and the Arts and Education fund. *Civic & Public Affairs:* 4%. Supports botanical gardens, parks, and economic development. *Education:* 35%. The majority supports the "Ameren Scholarship" program. *Environment:* 40%. Principal support goes to the United Way of Greater St. Louis. Also supports youth organizations and social/cot services for children and families. *International:* 3%. Funds hospitals, a health foundation, and single-disease health organizations. *Religion:* 2%. Gives to a science center. *Voluntarism:* Ameren Helping Hands where employees and their families volunteer. VIP/TEAMS Program in which small grants ($50-$500) are given to nonprofits for which Ameren employees volunteer. The company also supports the "Ameren Helping Hands" program which involves group volunteer projects at local nonprofit organizations. *Note:* Total contributions made in 2000. **Typ. Recipients:** AIDS/HIV, Children's Health/Hospitals, Clinics/Medical Centers, Domestic Violence, Emergency/Ambulance Services, Health Funds, Health Organizations, Multiple Sclerosis, People with Disabilities. **Geo. Dist:** the company's local district offices; Peoria, IL; Springfield, IL; St. Louis, MO.

★ 12147 ★ American Century Companies Foundation
PO Box 418210
Kansas City, MO 64141
Phone: (816)531-5575
Email: communityinvestments@americancentury.com
Website: http://www.americancentury.com/welcome/community.jsp
Mary Browne, Contact

Fnded: 2000. **Priorities:** *Arts & Humanities:* 18%. *Civic & Public Affairs:* 14%. *Education:* 24%. *Environment:* 30%. *International:* 7%. *Note:* Total contributions made in 2001. **Typ. Recipients:** AIDS/HIV, Alzheimers Disease, Children's Health/Hospitals, Domestic Violence, Health Organizations, Medical Rehabilitation. **Geo. Dist:** Mountain View, CA; Denver, CO; Kansas City, MO; New York, NY.

★ 12148 ★ American Express Foundation
World Financial Center
200 Vesey St.
New York, NY 10285-4803
Phone: (212)640-5660 **Fax:** (212)693-1033
Website: http://home3.americanexpress.com/corp/philanthropy/
Anne Wickham, Director, Cultural Heritage Program

Priorities: *Arts & Humanities:* (Cultural Heritage) 29%. *Civic & Public Affairs:* (Economic Independence) 26%. Support is given to economic education, college funds, the Urban League, and global initiatives. *Education:* 15%. *Environment:* (Community Service) 45%. Supports foundations, hospitals and health causes, the Red Cross, YWCAs and YMCAs, United Way, children's concerns, homeless shelters, and domestic peace. *International:* 12%. *Note:* Total contributions made in 1999. **Typ. Recipients:** AIDS/HIV, Children's Health/Hospitals, Domestic Violence, Emergency/Ambulance Services, Health Organizations, Hospitals, Hospitals (University Affiliated), Medical Education, People with Disabilities, Single-Disease Health Associations, Substance Abuse. **Geo. Dist:** headquarters and operating communities; internationally committees South Pacific, South Asia, East Asia, Europe, Middle East, Africa and Latin America/Caribbean; AZ; CA; DC; FL; GA; IL; MA; MN; NY; NC; TX; UT.

★ 12149 ★ American Fidelity Corp. Founders Fund
2000 Classen Center
PO Box 25523
Oklahoma City, OK 73125
Phone: (405)523-5008 **Fax:** (405)523-5421
Joella Ramsey, Secretary

Priorities: *Arts & Humanities:* 21%. *Civic & Public Affairs:* 4%. *Education:* 20%. *Environment:* 40%. *International:* 1%. *Note:* Total contributions made in 2001. **Typ. Recipients:** AIDS/HIV, Arthritis, Cancer, Child Abuse, Children's Health/Hospitals, Clinics/Medical Centers, Emergency/Ambulance Services, Health Organizations, Heart, Hospitals, Hospitals (University Affiliated), Medical Rehabilitation, People with Disabilities, Prenatal Health Issues, Single-Disease Health Associations, Substance Abuse. **Geo. Dist:** OK.

★ 12150 ★ American General Finance Foundation
601 NW Second St.
Evansville, IN 47708
Phone: (812)468-5854 **Fax:** (812)468-5682
Website: http://www.agc.com/agfg2000/agfgweb.nsf
Michelle Dixon, Community Relations Coordinator

Fnded: 1958. **Priorities:** *Arts & Humanities:* 10%. Supports Evansville area performing arts organizations, including dance, theater, and the philharmonic. Also supports public broadcasting. *Civic & Public Affairs:* 2%. Supports community organizations that promote civic pride, as well as improved housing. *Education:* 18%. Primarily supports Indiana colleges and universities and Evansville public schools. Secondary support is allocated to scholarships for children of employees and a matching gifts program. *Environment:* 52%. More than half supports the United Way and related agencies. Also provides support to a company-sponsored employee volunteer program. The remainder goes to youth organizations. *International:* 4%. Supports local chapters of national single-disease health organizations and the America Red Cross. *Religion:* 6%. Supports museums. *Voluntarism:* The company's Community Spirit Awards program recognizes employees who demonstrate outstanding volunteer service. Award recipients designate $2,500 grants to the organizations they serve. *Note:* Total contributions made in 2000. **Typ. Recipients:** AIDS/HIV, Alzheimers Disease, Arthritis, Cancer, Children's Health/Hospitals, Children's Health/Hospitals, Diabetes, Domestic Violence, Emergency/Ambulance Services, Heart, Hospices, Hospitals, Medical Rehabilitation, Medical Research, Mental Health, People with Disabilities, Prenatal Health Issues, Single-Disease Health Associations, Substance Abuse. **Geo. Dist:** Evansville, IN, including tri-state area.

★ 12151 ★ American Savings Foundation
PO Box 10
New Britain, CT 06050-0010
Phone: (860)827-2556 **Fax:** (860)827-2547
Robert Kennedy, Chairman, Chief Executive Officer

Fnded: 1997. **Priorities:** *Civic & Public Affairs:* 16%. Funds women's affairs, community projects, and job training/placement. *Education:* 5%. Gives to universities, Junior Achievement, and public schools. *Environment:* 75%. Supports youth organizations, recreation programs, family and child services, teen pregnancy prevention, and drug abuse prevention. *Religion:* 4%. A science center receives foundation funds. *Note:* Total contributions made in 1999. **Typ. Recipients:** Family Planning. **Geo. Dist:** CT, principally near operating locations and to national organizations.

★ 12152 ★ American Standard Foundation
One Centennial Ave.
Piscataway, NJ 08855-6820
Phone: (732)980-6000 **Fax:** (732)980-6121
G. D'Aloia, President

Priorities: *Arts & Humanities:* Less than 1%. *Civic & Public Affairs:* 7%. *Education:* 40%. Supports scholarship funds, career programs, and education foundations. *Environment:* 56%. Provides major support to the United Way; also funds Young Men's Christian Association and Special Olympics. *International:* 1%. Gives to a local Cerebral Palsy Association office. *Note:* Total contributions made in 2000. **Typ. Recipients:** Emergency/Ambulance Services, Heart, Single-Disease Health Associations. **Geo. Dist:** headquarters and operating communities.

★ 12153 ★ American Stock Exchange, Inc.

86 Trinity Place
10th Fl.
New York, NY 10006-1881
Phone: (212)306-1000 **Fax:** (212)306-1152
Website: http://www.amex.com
Mike D'Emic, Controller

Priorities: *Arts & Humanities:* Museums and the performing arts. *International:* Health care, child welfare, and youth organizations. **Typ. Recipients:** Health-General. **Geo. Dist:** New York, NY, including the metropolitan area.

★ 12154 ★ Ameritas Charitable Foundation

PO Box 81889
Lincoln, NE 68501
Phone: (402)467-1122 **Fax:** (402)467-7939
Scott Stuckey, Assistant Vice Pres. of Corporate Comm.

Fnded: 1985. **Priorities:** *Arts & Humanities:* 12%. Supports music, museums, film, and performing art centers. *Civic & Public Affairs:* 9%. Supports economic development, neighborhood organizations, housing, and community foundations. *Education:* 45%. Supports colleges, universities, secondary education, Junior Achievement, and education associations in Nebraska. *Environment:* 19%. Supports YMCA, recreation, scouts, homes, child welfare, and family services. *International:* 6%. Supports health foundations and community health services. *Note:* Total contributions made in 2000. **Typ. Recipients:** AIDS/HIV, Children's Health/Hospitals, Clinics/Medical Centers, Emergency/Ambulance Services, Health Organizations, Hospitals, Medical Education, Medical Research, Multiple Sclerosis, People with Disabilities, Public Health, Research/Studies Institutes, Single-Disease Health Associations, Substance Abuse, Transplant Networks/Donor Banks. **Geo. Dist:** Lincoln, NE.

★ 12155 ★ AmerUs Group Charitable Foundation

699 Walnut St., 20th Fl.
Des Moines, IA 50309
Phone: (515)557-3910 **Fax:** (515)283-3269
Website: http://www.amerus.com/about/community.html
Jonna LaToure, Assistant Director

Priorities: *Arts & Humanities:* 14%. *Civic & Public Affairs:* 8%. *Education:* 25%. *Environment:* 50%. *International:* Less than 1%. *Religion:* 1%. *Note:* Total contributions made in 2001. **Typ. Recipients:** Health-General, Hospices, Substance Abuse. **Geo. Dist:** IA.

★ 12156 ★ AMETEK Foundation

37 North Valley Rd., Bldg. 4
PO Box 1764
Paoli, PA 19301-0801
Phone: (610)647-2121
Kathryn Londra, Secretary, Treasurer

Fnded: 1960. **Priorities:** *Arts & Humanities:* 18%. Supports libraries and visual and performing arts. *Civic & Public Affairs:* 7%. Supports parks and community foundations. *Education:* 32%. Primarily funds colleges and universities, and technical and engineering institutions and organizations. Other interests include student aid, private secondary education, education funds, and literacy. *Environment:* 20%. Funds the United Way, YMCA, and services for the disabled. *International:* 15%. Health services, cancer centers, single-disease health associations, and hospitals. *Religion:* 1%. Supports science museums. *Note:* Total contributions made in 2000. **Typ. Recipients:** Cancer, Clinics/Medical Centers, Diabetes, Emergency/Ambulance Services, Health Funds, Health Organizations, Hospitals, Medical Education, Medical Rehabilitation, Medical Research, Mental Health, People with Disabilities, Preventive Medicine/Wellness Organizations, Public Health, Single-Disease Health Associations. **Geo. Dist:** headquarters and operating communities; nationally.

★ 12157 ★ Amgen Foundation

One Amgen Center Drive
Thousand Oaks, CA 91320-1799
Phone: (805)447-1000
Website: http://www.amgen.com/community/
Elizabeth Malkerson, President and Chief Executive Officer

Priorities: *Arts & Humanities:* 14%. Gives to museums, visual and performing arts, history museums, and arts councils. *Civic & Public Affairs:* 2%. Funds zoos and festivals. *Education:* 48%. Supports precollege and higher education, with a focus on biological science. *Environment:* 12%. Funds senior concerns, the United Way, and youth programs. *International:* 18%. Supports free clinics, the Red Cross, hospice, single-disease health organizations. *Religion:* 3%. *Voluntarism:* The Amgen Staff Community Involvement Program (SCIP) makes the services of Amgen staff available to nonprofit organizations or needy individuals for community improvement. *Note:* Total contributions made in 2000. **Typ. Recipients:** AIDS/HIV, Alzheimers Disease, Cancer, Child Abuse, Children's Health/Hospitals, Clinics/Medical Centers, Emergency/Ambulance Services, Health Organizations, Heart, Hospices, Hospitals, Medical Education, Medical Research, People with Disabilities, Preventive Medicine/Wellness Organizations, Public Health, Single-Disease Health Associations. **Geo. Dist:** headquarters; nationally.

★ 12158 ★ Amon G. Carter Star Telegram Employees Fund

PO Box 17480
Fort Worth, TX 76102
Phone: (817)332-3535
Nenetta Carter Tatum, President

Fnded: 1945. **Priorities:** *Arts & Humanities:* 28%. Supports museums, arts councils, dance, music, and community theater. *Civic & Public Affairs:* 16%. Supports housing, philanthropic organizations, zoos, and community foundations. *Education:* 5%. Supports universities, educational programs, learning centers, and schools. *Environment:* 45%. Supports community centers, senior services, Big Brothers/Sisters, child welfare, people with disabilities, food distribution, shelters, and YMCA. *International:* 5%. Supports children's hospitals, health organizations, and single-disease health associations. *Note:* Total foundation contributions made in fiscal 2001. **Typ. Recipients:** AIDS/HIV, Cancer, Children's Health/Hospitals, Domestic Violence, Eyes/Blindness, Family Planning, Health Organizations, Heart, Hospitals, Hospitals (University Affiliated), Medical Research, Mental Health, Nursing Services, People with Disabilities, Public Health, Research/Studies Institutes, Single-Disease Health Associations, Substance Abuse, Transplant Networks/Donor Banks. **Geo. Dist:** TX, Tarrant County.

★ 12159 ★ AMR/American Airlines Foundation

PO Box 619616
Mail Drop 5656
Dallas, TX 75261-9616
Phone: (817)967-3540
Website: http://www.amrcorp.com/corpinfo.htm
Timothy Doke, Secretary

Priorities: *Arts & Humanities:* (Cultural) 3%. Funds activities that exemplify excellence in the visual and/or performing arts, including performances or programs that promote a higher level of understanding of the arts from countries where AMR/American Airlines has a presence. Also aids specific programs designed to highlight the world's diversity of cultures, ethnic background, and national origins. Also gives to art funds that make a significant contribution to the creation of high quality art programs in local communities. *Civic & Public Affairs:* (Civic) 36%. Funds educational programs aimed at increasing awareness and involvement in recycling and other environmental protection activities and projects designed to preserve environmentally sensitive property throughout the world. Partners with environmental organizations, such as the Nature Conservancy. Also sponsors initiatives that promote economic development in company's communities. *Education:* 11%. Supports programs aimed at providing higher education and business career training opportunities to minorities, in particular those that support American's existing national partnership with the United Negro College Fund. Supports efforts to create greater understanding and cooperation between various ethnic groups and activities aimed at educating young adults about world geography. *Environment:* (Health/Welfare) 46%. Funds social services, youth services, meals on wheels, volunteerism, and the United Way. Funding also supports the American Cancer Society, American Red Cross, and Give the Kids the World Foundation. *Voluntarism:* Company reports that no formal volunteer program exists, other than a volunteer recycling program aboard flights and in offices. *Note:* Total contributions made in 1999. **Typ. Recipients:** AIDS/HIV, Cancer, Children's Health/Hospitals, Clinics/Medical Centers, Diabetes, Emergency/Ambulance Services, Eyes/Blindness, Family Planning, Health Funds, Health Organizations, Heart, Hospitals, Hospitals (University Affiliated), Kidney, Medical Education, Medical Research, Multiple Sclerosis, People with Disabilities, Public Health, Single-Disease Health Associations, Single-Disease Health Associations, Substance Abuse, Transplant Networks/Donor Banks. **Geo. Dist:** nationally and internationally.

★ 12160 ★ AmSouth Foundation

PO Box 13906
Jackson, MS 39236-3906
Phone: (601)949-8958
James Moore, President & Executive Director

Priorities: *Arts & Humanities:* 7%. Funds a state history organization and a cultural exchange program. *Civic & Public Affairs:* 19%. Funding supports housing, community development, and minority business development. *Education:* 25%. Supports Mississippi colleges and universities, scholarship funds, public schools, and school volunteerism/community involvement. *Environment:* 21%. Supports family services, parenting centers, crime prevention programs, food banks, child welfare organizations, and youth programs. *International:* 9%. Gives to the American Red Cross. *Voluntarism:* AmSouth employees are encouraged to volunteer time to United Way agencies, the Salvation Army, Junior Achievement, and Young Men's Christian Association. *Note:* Total foundation contributions made in 2000. **Typ. Recipients:** Children's Health/Hospitals, Diabetes, Emergency/Ambulance Services, Health Organizations, Health-General, Hospitals, Mental Health, People with Disabilities, Single-Disease Health Associations, Substance Abuse, Transplant Networks/Donor Banks. **Geo. Dist:** headquarters and operating communities. **Frmly:** Deposit Guaranty Foundation.

★ 12161 ★ Amsted Industries Foundation

205 North Michigan Ave., 44th Floor
Chicago, IL 60601
Phone: (312)645-1700
Website: http://www.amsted.com
Shirley Whitsell, Contact

Fnded: 1953. **Priorities:** *Arts & Humanities:* 9%. Supports opera, orchestras, historic preservation, museums, and dance. *Civic & Public Affairs:* 9%. Supports legal services, public services, parks, gardens, and zoos. *Education:* 26%. Supports private precollege schools, education foundations, and colleges and universities. *Environment:* 38%. Supports United Way, food distribution, child welfare, and youth organizations. *International:* 16%. Supports rehabilitation, health organizations, and single-disease health associations. *Note:* Total foundation contributions made in fiscal 2001. **Typ. Recipients:** Alzheimers Disease,

Clinics/Medical Centers, Diabetes, Emergency/Ambulance Services, Family Planning, Health Organizations, Hospitals, Medical Rehabilitation, Medical Research. **Geo. Dist:** headquarters and operating communities; Chicago, IL.

★ 12162 ★ Analog Devices, Inc.

One Technology Way
PO Box 9106
Norwood, MA 02062-9106
Phone: (781)329-4700 **Fax:** (781)461-4483
Email: martha.giansanti@analog.com
Website: http://www.analog.com
Marriane Naumann, Administration Assistant, Contributions

Priorities: *Civic & Public Affairs:* 10% of contributions. Supports a wide variety of local organizations in the arts, social services, civic and public affairs,and health. *Education:* 90% of contributions. Supports higher education in the areas of electrical engineering and computer science with the purpose of increasing the number of engineering and computer science graduates. Emphasis on graduate level programs. Supports professorships, graduate student fellowships, facilities renovation, equipment purchases, sponsored research, and summer institutes. Also sponsors programs for employee education, cooperative students, summer interns, and matching gifts. **Typ. Recipients:** Hospitals. **Geo. Dist:** near company's major research and manufacturing sites.

★ 12163 ★ Anderson Foundation

608 Madison Ave., Suite 1540
Toledo, OH 43604
Phone: (419)243-1706
Ms. Fredi Heywood, Foundation Services Administrator

Priorities: *Arts & Humanities:* 14%. Primarily supports orchestras and theater. Also funds libraries, museums, historic associations, and arts associations. *Civic & Public Affairs:* 2%. Supports economic development, zoos, botanical gardens, and local and community organizations. *Education:* 18%. Supports colleges and universities. Also funds public and private precollege education and agricultural education. *Environment:* 54%. Almost half of the foundation's funding goes to the United Way under Community Chest funding. Also supports scouts, Young Men's Christian Association, food distribution, and family services. *International:* Less than 1%. Funds single-disease health organizations, hospitals, and medical centers. *Note:* Total contributions made in 2000. **Typ. Recipients:** Clinics/Medical Centers, Diabetes, Emergency/Ambulance Services, Eyes/Blindness, Health Organizations, Hospices, Hospitals, Medical Research, Mental Health, Nursing Services, People with Disabilities, Preventive Medicine/Wellness Organizations, Single-Disease Health Associations. **Geo. Dist:** headquarters and operating communities, including plant locations.

★ 12164 ★ Andrews McMeel Universal Foundation

4520 Main St., Suite 700
Kansas City, MO 64111
Phone: (816)932-6700 **Fax:** (816)531-5323
Email: kandrews@amuniversal.com
Kathleen Andrews, Vice President & Secretary

Fnded: 1991. **Priorities:** *Arts & Humanities:* 30%. Supports museums, music, dance, libraries, theater, and public broadcasting. *Civic & Public Affairs:* 7%. Gives to business/free enterprise programs, housing, professional journalism associations, women's affairs, and legal aid. *Education:* 47%. Funds colleges and universities, educational programs, journalism education, and scholarship funds. *Environment:* 6%. Supports youth organizations, camps, family services, and crime prevention. *International:* Less than 1%. *Note:* Total contributions made in 2001. **Typ. Recipients:** Clinics/Medical Centers, Domestic Violence, Health Organizations, Kidney, Medical Research, People with Disabilities, Prenatal Health Issues, Single-Disease Health Associations. **Geo. Dist:** nationally; KS; MO; Kansas City, MO, metropolitan area.

★ 12165 ★ Anheuser-Busch Foundation

USBank
PO Box 387, FL-TW-16IT
Saint Louis, MO 63166-0587
Phone: (314)418-2168 **Fax:** (314)577-3251
Jayne Nicholson, Specialist, Charitable Contributions

Fnded: 1975. **Priorities:** *Arts & Humanities:* 16%. Supports libraries, historic preservation, history organizations, and the performing arts. *Civic & Public Affairs:* 8%. Funds urban and community affairs. *Education:* 45%. Primarily supports colleges and universities near company's major facilities. *Environment:* 25%. Primarily supports the United Way, programs for the disabled, and organizations serving youth. *International:* 1%. Gives to hospitals and single-disease health organizations. *Religion:* 3%. *Voluntarism:* Through the Anheuser-Busch Employee Volunteer Grant Program, the company supports and recognizes its employees who actively volunteer their time and talents to nonprofit organizations by making grants to these organizations for unusual or special projects. An Employee Matching Gifts Program for educational institutions is also offered through the company's charitable foundation. *Note:* Total contributions made in 2000. **Typ. Recipients:** AIDS/HIV, Alzheimers Disease, Cancer, Children's Health/Hospitals, Emergency/Ambulance Services, Health Organizations, Health Policy/Cost Containment, Heart, Hospitals, Medical Education, Medical Research, People with Disabilities, Public Health, Single-Disease Health Associations, Substance Abuse. **Geo. Dist:** principally near operating locations and to national organizations.

★ 12166 ★ Anthem Blue Cross/Blue Shield

120 Monument Circle
Indianapolis, IN 46204
Phone: (317)488-6216 **Fax:** (317)488-6306
Email: anthem.corporate.communications@anthem.com
Connie Molland, Director Community Relations

Typ. Recipients: Health-General. **Geo. Dist:** CO, CT, IN, KY, ME, NH, NV, OH.

★ 12167 ★ Anthem Foundation, Inc.

120 Monument Circle
Indianapolis, IN 46204
Phone: 800-563-5465
Connie Molland, Contact

Fnded: 1990. **Priorities:** *Arts & Humanities:* 7%. Supports arts funds. *Civic & Public Affairs:* 9%. Funds leadership development and women's affairs organizations. *Education:* 13%. Supports higher education and matching gifts. *Environment:* 29%. Funds the United Way and youth and human services. *International:* 42%. Supports health education, community health initiatives, and single-disease associations. *Note:* Total contributions in 2000. **Typ. Recipients:** AIDS/HIV, Cancer, Child Abuse, Children's Health/Hospitals, Clinics/Medical Centers, Diabetes, Emergency/Ambulance Services, Health Organizations, Health-General, Heart, Hospitals, Medical Education, Medical Rehabilitation, Multiple Sclerosis, Nursing Services, Prenatal Health Issues, Preventive Medicine/Wellness Organizations, Public Health, Respiratory, Single-Disease Health Associations, Substance Abuse, Trauma Treatment. **Geo. Dist:** KY.

★ 12168 ★ AOL Time Warner Foundation

22000 AOL Way
Dulles, VA 20166-9323
Phone: (703)265-2282
Email: aoltwfoundation@aol.com
Website: http://aoltwfoundation.org

Priorities: *Arts & Humanities:* 4%. Gives to art and culture foundations, photography and video arts, and museums. *Civic & Public Affairs:* 28%. Funds labor, professional, and trade associations; public policy groups; community foundations; city planning; nonprofit management; and ethnic organizations. *Education:* 42%. Supports primary and secondary public schools, education associations, literacy programs, mentoring programs, and leadership education. *Environment:* 8%. Supports social welfare groups, the elderly, violence prevention, and youth organizations. *International:* 16%. Funds single-disease health associations and health care foundations. *Note:* Total contributions made in 2000, excluding gifts to individuals. **Typ. Recipients:** Cancer, Children's Health/Hospitals, Health Organizations, Health-General, Medical Education, People with Disabilities, Public Health, Transplant Networks/Donor Banks. **Geo. Dist:** nationally. **Frmly:** Time Warner Foundation.

★ 12169 ★ Aon Foundation

200 East Randolph St.
Chicago, IL 60601
Phone: (312)381-3549 **Fax:** (312)701-4533
Carolyn Labutka, Executive Director

Priorities: *Arts & Humanities:* 24%. Supports art museums, historical societies, and performing arts groups. Interests include symphonies, theater, and dance. *Civic & Public Affairs:* 11%. Funds economic and community development, urban affairs, business/professional organizations, and a zoo. *Education:* 26%. Colleges and universities, science, economic and insurance education, private precollege schools, and scholarship funds. *Environment:* 26%. Supports the United Way, child welfare organizations, volunteer groups, youth groups, services for the disabled, and various community service programs. *International:* 5%. Gives to hospitals, single-disease health organizations, pediatric health initiatives, medical research, and health funds. *Note:* Total contributions made in 2000. **Typ. Recipients:** AIDS/HIV, Alzheimers Disease, Cancer, Children's Health/Hospitals, Clinics/Medical Centers, Diabetes, Emergency/Ambulance Services, Health Funds, Hospitals, Hospitals (University Affiliated), Medical Rehabilitation, Medical Research, Multiple Sclerosis, People with Disabilities, Single-Disease Health Associations. **Geo. Dist:** internationally; operating locations.

★ 12170 ★ Appleton Papers, Inc.

825 East Wisconsin Ave.
PO Box 359
Appleton, WI 54912
Phone: (920)991-7448 **Fax:** (920)991-8407
Email: dkolb@appletonideas.com
Website: http://www.appletonideas.com
Donna Kolb, Contribution Committee

Typ. Recipients: Domestic Violence, People with Disabilities, Single-Disease Health Associations, Substance Abuse. **Geo. Dist:** headquarters and operating communities; Dayton, OH; Roaring Spring, PA; Appleton, WI.

★ 12171 ★ APS Foundation, Inc.

PO Box 53999
M/S 8010
Phoenix, AZ 85072-3999
Phone: (602)250-2888 **Fax:** (602)250-2113
Website: http://www.aps.com/my_community/default.html
Ms. Charlie Thompson, Manager, Community Relations

Priorities: *Arts & Humanities:* 18%. Recipients include local theaters, dance companies, museums, historical societies, and arts councils. *Civic & Public Affairs:* 24%. Supports community initiatives, leadership organizations, neighborhood organizations, and a botanical garden. *Education:* 15%. Gives to Junior Achievement, Arizona universities and colleges, and a learning center. *Environment:* 15%. Supports food banks, youth groups, scouts, and animal welfare organizations. *International:* 16%. Supports hospitals, health foundations, and medical centers. *Religion:* 4%. Funds an observatory and a science center. *Voluntarism:* The company matches employee volunteer hours given to nonprofit organizations that provide a service in one of their giving areas. Each hour an APS employee or retiree volunteers is matched at $5, if at least 25 hours in single calendar year have been spent volunteering. *Note:* Total contributions made in 2000. **Typ. Recipients:** Cancer, Children's Health/Hospitals, Clinics/Medical Centers, Domestic Violence, Emergency/Ambulance Services, Eyes/Blindness, Health Funds, Health Organizations, Health-General, Heart, Hospices, Hospitals, Medical Education, Medical Research, People with Disabilities, Prenatal Health Issues, Public Health, Research/Studies Institutes, Single-Disease Health Associations. **Geo. Dist:** near Four Corners Power Plant; AZ, primarily Arizona and New Mexico, near the Four Corners Power Plant; NM.

★ 12172 ★ Archer-Daniels-Midland Foundation

4666 Faries Parkway
PO Box 1470
Decatur, IL 62525
Phone: (217)424-5957 **Fax:** (217)424-5581
Website: http://www.admworld.com
Lori Magnussen, Contact

Fnded: 1953. **Priorities:** *Arts & Humanities:* 6%. Gives to arts councils, libraries, and orchestras. *Civic & Public Affairs:* 12%. Funds community foundations, professional and agricultural trade associations, public policy organizations, and civic groups. *Education:* 6%. Majority supports colleges and universities. Also supports religious, agricultural, business, and engineering education; public and parochial pre-college schools; and education funds and associations. *Environment:* 42%. Major support goes to united funds and youth organizations. Other interests include child and family welfare, emergency relief, senior services, food distribution, and community athletic and recreation programs. *International:* Less than 1%. Contributes to hospitals, single-disease organizations, hospice programs, and children's health services. *Religion:* 28%. Funds a science museum. *Note:* Total contributions in fiscal 2001, excluding matching gifts. **Typ. Recipients:** Cancer, Children's Health/Hospitals, Emergency/Ambulance Services, Family Planning, Health Organizations, Hospices, Hospitals, Medical Education, Mental Health, People with Disabilities, Prenatal Health Issues, Substance Abuse. **Geo. Dist:** nationally, principally near operating locations and to national organizations.

★ 12173 ★ ARCO Foundation

333 South Hope St.
Los Angeles, CA 90071
Phone: (213)486-3342 **Fax:** (213)486-0113
Website: http://ntlf.com/html/grants/5977.htm
Russell Sakaguchi, President

Priorities: *Arts & Humanities:* 53%. Supports museums, music, libraries, opera, and art foundations. *Civic & Public Affairs:* 19%. Supports economic development, business associations, ethnic organizations, aquariums, and community foundations. *Education:* 19%. Supports educational programs, colleges, universities, Junior Achievement, and scholarships. Pre-college organizations supported are aimed at promoting: readiness-for-school services, including parent training and early childhood curricula for at-risk children; academic achievement through improvements in school attendance, grades and school-completion levels; increased interest and achievement in mathematics and science resulting in higher enrollment and success rates in college preparatory course-work and in plans to pursue math/science careers; parent effectiveness through increased involvement in public school education, especially among low-income families; professional staff preparation and development through programs that incorporate school restructuring issues as part of the curriculum for teachers, counselors and administrators; programs that improve the qualifications and effectiveness of math and science teachers; and teacher-training curricula on language development and English-language acquisition. Supported higher education programs include special projects at selected research universities and programs that increase the number of minority students entering and completing degree programs in fields related to the energy industry. *Environment:* 6%. Supports United Way, food distribution, youth organizations and scouts. *Voluntarism:* Through company's Employee Volunteer Grants Program, employees may request grants of up to $500 for nonprofit organizations to which they give at least 12 hours per month of their own time. *Note:* Total foundation contributions made in 2000. **Typ. Recipients:** Children's Health/Hospitals, Domestic Violence, Research/Studies Institutes. **Geo. Dist:** Southwestern United States; Western United States; AK.

★ 12174 ★ Arison Foundation

3655 NW 87th Ave.
Miami, FL 33178-2428
Phone: (305)599-2600
Madelon Rosenberg, Assistant to the President

Fnded: 1981. **Priorities:** *Arts & Humanities:* 2%. Funds film. *Civic & Public Affairs:* 3%. Funds civic foundations. *Education:* 12%. Supports scholarships, secondary and higher education. *Environment:* 29%. Majority of funding supports United Way International. Also supports senior services and recreational facilities for the disabled. *International:* 33%. Funds Jewish hospitals, medical centers, and medical research organizations in America and Israel. *Religion:* 18%. Major grant to American Committee for Weizmann Institute of Science. *Note:* Total contributions made in 2000. **Typ. Recipients:** Cancer, Children's Health/Hospitals, Clinics/Medical Centers, Eyes/Blindness, Geriatric Health, Health Organizations, Health-General, Hospices, Hospitals, Medical Education, Medical Research, People with Disabilities, Public Health, Single-Disease Health Associations. **Geo. Dist:** Miami, FL, including surrounding area. **Frmly:** Arison Foundation.

★ 12175 ★ Armstrong Foundation

2500 Columbia Ave.
Lancaster, PA 17603
Phone: (717)396-2446
Website: http://www.armstrongfoundation.com
Cathy Witmer, Contributions Administrator

Priorities: *Arts & Humanities:* 1%. Support emphasizes libraries and historic preservation. *Civic & Public Affairs:* 36%. Funding supports chambers of commerce, civic associations, and public policy institutions. *Education:* 23%. Funding supports the National Merit Scholarship Corporation, universities, colleges and educational foundations. *Environment:* 26%. Funding supports various United Way chapters, local youth organizations, and local family support services. *International:* 3%. *Religion:* 1%. *Note:* Total contributions made in 2000. **Typ. Recipients:** Cancer, Clinics/Medical Centers, Emergency/Ambulance Services, Eyes/Blindness, Family Planning, Health Organizations, Hospices, Hospitals, Medical Education, Medical Research, Nursing Services, People with Disabilities, Public Health, Single-Disease Health Associations, Substance Abuse. **Geo. Dist:** Lancaster, PA.

★ 12176 ★ ASARCO Foundation

156 West 56th St., 19th Floor
New York, NY 10019
Kevin McCaffrey, Secretary

Fnded: 1956. **Priorities:** *Education:* 100%. Funding supports higher education. Also funds science and technology education and private secondary schools through grants and matching gifts. *Note:* Total contributions made in 2000. **Typ. Recipients:** Cancer, Hospices, People with Disabilities. **Geo. Dist:** headquarters and operating communities.

★ 12177 ★ Ashland Inc. Foundation

50 East RiverCenter Boulevard
PO Box 391
Covington, KY 41012-0391
Phone: (859)815-3333 **Fax:** (859)815-4496
Email: sgrice@ashland.com
Website: http://www.ashland.com

Priorities: *Arts & Humanities:* 6%. Funding supports art centers, funds, associations, museums, public broadcasting, and music. *Civic & Public Affairs:* 7%. Funding supports economic development; community affairs; and law and justice. *Education:* 62%. Funding supports colleges, universities, and secondary schools, primarily in operating areas, with a focus on schools preparing students for a career in the industry. Literacy, educational foundations, and community and junior colleges are also of interest. Foundation sponsors scholarships for children of employees, employee matching gifts program to educational institutions, and runs print and broadcast ads promoting education. *International:* 22%. Funds United Way; other recipients include youth organizations, groups concerned with the aged and child welfare, community centers and service agencies, and hospitals and health groups. *Voluntarism:* The company encourages employee volunteerism through activities such as the annual River Sweep, a clean-up of the Ohio River. *Note:* Total contributions made in 1999. **Typ. Recipients:** Cancer, Clinics/Medical Centers, Health Organizations, Hospitals, People with Disabilities, Single-Disease Health Associations, Speech & Hearing. **Geo. Dist:** headquarters and operating communities; Atlanta, GA; KY; Dublin, OH.

★ 12178 ★ Associated Banc-Corp Foundation

1305 Main St.
PO Box 13307
Stevens Point, WI 54481
Phone: (715)341-0400
Jonathon Drayna, Contact

Fnded: 1977. **Priorities:** *Civic & Public Affairs:* 100%. Primary support made to ABC Foundation Charitable. *Note:* Total foundation contributions made in 2001. **Typ. Recipients:** AIDS/HIV, Cancer, Children's Health/Hospitals, Clinics/Medical Centers, Domestic Violence, Family Planning, Geriatric Health, Health Funds, Hospitals, Medical Research, Nursing Services, People with Disabilities, Public Health, Single-Disease Health Associations. **Geo. Dist:** IL, areas of business; WI, areas of business. **Frmly:** First Financial Foundation.

★ 12179 ★ Associated Food Stores Charitable Foundation

122-20 Merrick Blvd.
Jamaica, NY 11434
Phone: (718)978-0764
Harry Laufer, President & Chief Executive Officer

Fnded: 1987. **Priorities:** *Arts & Humanities:* 1%. Primary support made to an art museum. *Civic & Public Affairs:* 26%. Supports community foundations and human rights organizations. *Education:* 16%. Supports secondary schools, and educational academies. *Environment:* Less than 1%. *International:* 1%. Supports hospitals and single-disease health associations. *Note:* Total foundation contributions made in 2001. **Typ. Recipients:** Cancer, Children's Health/Hospitals, Clinics/Medical Centers, Diabetes, Eyes/Blindness, Geriatric Health, Hospitals, Long-Term Care, Medical Research, Nursing Services, People with Disabilities, Single-Disease Health Associations. **Geo. Dist:** NY, including metropolitan area.

★ 12180 ★ AT&T Foundation

32 Ave. of the Americas
New York, NY 10013
Phone: (212)387-6557 **Fax:** (212)387-5098
Website: http://www.att.com/foundation
Vivian Nero, Operations & Local Grants

Priorities: *Arts & Humanities:* 8%. Supports museums, the performing arts, and libraries. Supports nationally and internationally recognized arts and cultural institutions that foster communication and promote cross-cultural understanding. Organizations must have been professionally managed for at least five years and compensate both artistic and managerial personnel. National arts service organizations are also funded, particularly those that offer technical assistance or professional services to foundation-eligible institutions. Particular interest in the creation, production, and presentation of new work and initiatives that provide access to the arts to all segments of society by bringing the work of women and artists of diverse cultures to wider audiences. The foundation supports two invitation-only initiatives: AT&T: OnStage, for theatrical works; and AT&T: NEAT (New Experiments in Art and Technology), supporting children's and science museums. *Civic & Public Affairs:*

20%. Supports women's affairs, political and economic organizations, ethnic organizations, employment services, and community foundations. Supports organizations and projects that enhance the effectiveness of the nonprofit sector and promote public policy formulation in matters of children and families, accessibility of health and social services to those in need, the advancement of diversity, and the protection of the environment. Projects should serve as models for other organizations and lend themselves to measurable evaluation, with results that can be disseminated to a wide audience. *Education:* 49%. Supports universities, schools, educational programs, institutes, and education foundations. Supports projects that assist and facilitate lifelong learning, teacher training, and parent participation in education. Emphasis is on initiatives that use technology to connect students, teachers, and institutions of learning; and which stimulate student interests and involvement in mathematics, science and engineering. Through the AT&T Learning Network, funding is provided to organizations that help teachers, students, parents and communities capitalize on technology to enhance education. As part of this effort, funding is provided for the innovative use of technology to foster family involvement in education and provide professional development opportunities for preparation of new teachers. Collaboration among institutions and across communities to promote lifelong learning is encouraged. Invitational grants go to projects that address issues of technology in public policy; education reform; academic standards, assessment and accountability; and access to educational opportunities by all segments of society. *Environment:* 21%. Supports the United Way, youth organizations, and recreation. *International:* 2%. Primarily supports health organizations. *Voluntarism:* Supports the AT&T CARES program, which makes grants to organizations where employees volunteer, and the Telephone Pioneers of America, a volunteer service organization. *Note:* Total foundation contributions made in 2000. **Typ. Recipients:** Children's Health/Hospitals, Emergency/Ambulance Services, Health Policy/Cost Containment, Hospitals, Medical Education, People with Disabilities, Speech & Hearing, Substance Abuse. **Geo. Dist:** headquarters and operating communities; nationally and internationally.

★ 12181 ★ Atofina Chemicals Foundation

2000 Market St.
Philadelphia, PA 19103-3222
Phone: (215)419-7000 **Fax:** (215)419-5494
George Hagar, Executive Secretary

Fnded: 1957. **Priorities:** *Arts & Humanities:* 27%. Supports public broadcasting, music, museums, and theaters. *Civic & Public Affairs:* 25%. Supports aquariums, zoos, police/public safety, and community foundations. *Education:* 33%. Supports universities and colleges. *Environment:* 10%. Supports United Way and YMCA. *Religion:* 5%. Supports the Chemical Heritage Foundation and science institutes. *Note:* Total foundation contributions made in 2000. **Typ. Recipients:** Clinics/Medical Centers, Emergency/Ambulance Services, Hospitals, Medical Rehabilitation, Medical Research, People with Disabilities. **Geo. Dist:** nationally; operating location communities.

★ 12182 ★ AUL Foundation Inc.

One American Square
PO Box 368
Indianapolis, IN 46206-0368
Phone: (317)285-1609 **Fax:** (317)285-1979
James Freeman, Chairman, Committee

Priorities: *Arts & Humanities:* 4%. Supports music, museums, and art foundations. *Civic & Public Affairs:* 1%. Primarily supports clubs. *Education:* 57%. Supports universities, educational funds, colleges, and Junior Achievement. *Environment:* 34%. Supports YWCA, youth homes, athletic organizations, veterans, day care, and scouts. *International:* 2%. Primary support made to rehabilitation centers. *Note:* Total foundation contributions made in 2000. **Typ. Recipients:** AIDS/HIV, Cancer, Domestic Violence, Health Organizations, Hospitals, Medical Education, Medical Rehabilitation, Medical Research, Medical Training, Mental Health, Nursing Services, People with Disabilities, Public Health, Single-Disease Health Associations, Substance Abuse. **Geo. Dist:** headquarters and operating communities; IN.

★ 12183 ★ Aventis Pharmaceuticals Foundation

Corporate Relations SC4-305A
400 Somerset Corporate Boulevard, Tax Department, Rm. SC4-42
Bridgewater, NJ 08807
Phone: (908)243-6000
Website: http://www.aventispharma-us.com/main/0.003.EN-US-28551-50426-00.html
Phillip St. James, Corp. Relations Mgr.

Priorities: *Arts & Humanities:* 3%. Gives to orchestras and museums. *Civic & Public Affairs:* 6%. Funds municipalities, community and urban affairs, economic development, and business associations. *Education:* 6%. Contributes to public schools, charter schools, teachers organizations, and science education programs. *Environment:* 10%. Funds the United Way, child welfare, shelters, and wish fulfillment for critically ill children. *International:* 70%. Provides major support to a children's hospital. Also supports hospitals, medical centers, bioethics research, hospice programs, pediatric health organizations, and the American Medical Association. *Religion:* 2%. Science centers and educational programs receive support. *Note:* Total foundation contributions made in fiscal 2001. **Typ. Recipients:** AIDS/HIV, Clinics/Medical Centers, Domestic Violence, Health Organizations, Health-General, Kidney, Medical Education, Research/Studies Institutes.

★ 12184 ★ Avery Dennison Foundation

150 North Orange Grove Boulevard
Pasadena, CA 91103
Phone: (626)304-2000 **Fax:** (626)577-9587
Email: joyce.reid@averydennison.com
Website: http://www.averydennison.com/corporate.nsf/PG/L3B1C9
Joyce Reid, Director, Corporate Programs

Priorities: *Arts & Humanities:* 21%. Supports a music center. *Education:* 45%. Supports educational funds and foundations. *Environment:* 29%. Funds United Way. *Note:* Total contributions made in 2001. **Typ. Recipients:** Children's Health/Hospitals, Health-General. **Geo. Dist:** headquarters and operating communities.

★ 12185 ★ Avon Products Foundation, Inc.

1345 Ave. of the Americas
New York, NY 10105-0196
Phone: (212)282-5517 **Fax:** (212)282-6049
Website: http://www.avoncompany.com/women/
Mary Quinn, Assistant Secretary & Director

Fnded: 1955. **Priorities:** *Arts & Humanities:* About 1%. Supports a variety of art interests, including arts associations and centers, dance, theater, music, museums, and youth performing art programs. *Civic & Public Affairs:* (Community and Social Services) 4%. Funds programs concerned with civil rights, minority affairs, and women's business development. Also supports united fund drives, and social services for women and children. *Education:* 3%. Primarily supports scholarships to students attending high schools in certain corporate operating locations and scholarship programs targeting women and minorities. Interests also include general support to colleges and universities; education funds; organizations concerned with youth leadership development; minority, business, and economic education; and literacy. *Environment:* 4%. *International:* 92%. Funds women's health organizations; programs that deal with research and early detection of breast cancer; single-disease health organizations; and hospitals. *Note:* Total foundation contributions made in 2000. **Typ. Recipients:** Cancer, Child Abuse, Children's Health/Hospitals, Clinics/Medical Centers, Domestic Violence, Emergency/Ambulance Services, Health Funds, Health Organizations, Health-General, Hospices, Hospitals, Medical Education, Medical Rehabilitation, Medical Research, Mental Health, Outpatient Health Care, People with Disabilities, Prenatal Health Issues, Single-Disease Health Associations, Substance Abuse. **Geo. Dist:** headquarters and operating communities.

★ 12186 ★ B.F. Goodrich Foundation, Inc.

Four Coliseum Center
2730 W Tyvola Rd.
Charlotte, NC 28217-4578
Phone: (704)423-7080 **Fax:** (704)423-7069
Website: http://www.goodrich.com/giving.asp
Jan Locke, Manager, Community Affairs

Priorities: *Arts & Humanities:* 15% to 25%. Supports a variety of interests in major plant communities, including the performing arts, public radio and television, museums, orchestras, ballet, art exhibitions, preservation organizations, and historical societies. Sponsors matching gifts programs for cultural organizations located in communities where employees live or work. *Civic & Public Affairs:* 15% to 25%. Supports the Civic and Community giving area, emphasizing the improvement of, or the economic environment of, communities in which company employees live and work. Funds projects and programs that strive to preserve or enhance the historic or economic development of communities and the economic vitality of a region. Grants have supported municipalities, trade associations, civic and nonacademic public policy research organizations in plant communities. *Education:* 30% to 40%. Supports higher education, with a focus on selected institutions where the company recruits for its workforce or where technical research is conducted; also funds science and engineering education for the technical workforce. Funds elementary and secondary education proposals designed to restructure the educational system to better educate all students; supports efforts that take a comprehensive approach to education reform rather than addressing issues on a piecemeal basis. Pre-college education support focuses on math and science initiatives. Supports adult education and welfare-to-work training and education. Also supports an employee matching gift program. *Environment:* (Health and Human Services/United Way) 20% to 30%. Emphasis on United Ways in communities where company has operating facilities. Also supports capital requests for hospitals and specialized health care providers. *International:* 10%. *Religion:* 1%. *Voluntarism:* Foundation sponsors a Bonus Volunteer Match program in addition to its Donors Match program. The foundation will make an extra 1 to 1 match of employee gifts to eligible organizations for which the employee volunteers, to a maximum of $1,000. The company also sponsors a school partnership in Charlotte, NC. *Note:* Total contributions made in 2001. **Typ. Recipients:** Cancer, Children's Health/Hospitals, Emergency/Ambulance Services, Geriatric Health, Health Organizations, Hospices, Hospitals, Nursing Services, People with Disabilities, People with Disabilities, Substance Abuse. **Geo. Dist:** nationally; operating locations.

★ 12187 ★ B. Thomas Golisano Foundation

One Fishers Rd.
Pittsford, NY 14534
Phone: (716)340-1200
Website: http://www.golisanofoundation.org

Priorities: *Civic & Public Affairs:* 5%. *Education:* 4%. *Environment:* 61%. *International:* 19%. *Note:* Total contributions made in 2001. **Typ. Recipients:** AIDS/HIV, Arthritis, Geriatric Health, Health Organizations, Health-General, Hospitals, Medical Rehabilitation, People with Disabilities. **Geo. Dist:** NY.

★ 12188 ★ Badger Meter Foundation

4545 West Brown Deer Rd.
Milwaukee, WI 53223
Phone: (414)371-5704 **Fax:** (414)371-5956
Beth McCallister, Secretary

Priorities: *Arts & Humanities:* 15%. Interests include festivals, opera, music, the performing arts, and theater. *Civic & Public Affairs:* 5%. Supports a diverse group of community services, including youth organizations, homes, children's centers, museums, and youth recreational activities. *Education:* 24%. Foundation supports colleges, universities, day schools, education funds, engineering education, continuing education, and scholarship funds. *Environment:* 44%. Recipients include rescue missions, aid for the mentally retarded, and food and clothing distribution. Majority of support funds Goodwill Industries. *International:* 4%. Support favors single-disease health associations and hospitals. Also supports pediatric health care, emergency services, community hospitals, and health organizations. *Religion:* Less than 1%. Supports a science museum. *Note:* Total contributions made in 2000. **Typ. Recipients:** Arthritis, Cancer, Domestic Violence, Health Organizations, Heart, Hospitals, Medical Education, Medical Research, Mental Health, People with Disabilities, Preventive Medicine/Wellness Organizations, Single-Disease Health Associations, Speech & Hearing, Substance Abuse, Transplant Networks/Donor Banks. **Geo. Dist:** Milwaukee, WI.

★ 12189 ★ Baker & Baker Foundation

PO Box 12397
Columbia, SC 29211-2397
Phone: (803)254-8987
John Baker, President

Priorities: *Arts & Humanities:* 3%. Funds art museums and arts councils. *Education:* 2%. Gives to an education foundation, a college, and Communities in Schools. *Environment:* 1%. Contributes to the United Way, youth organizations, a children's home, and services for the blind. *International:* Less than 1%. *Note:* Total contributions made in 2000. **Typ. Recipients:** Alzheimers Disease, Arthritis, Cancer, Children's Health/Hospitals, Clinics/Medical Centers, Diabetes, Diabetes, Domestic Violence, Emergency/Ambulance Services, Eyes/Blindness, Family Planning, Health Organizations, Hospitals, Multiple Sclerosis, People with Disabilities, Prenatal Health Issues, Respiratory, Single-Disease Health Associations. **Geo. Dist:** Columbia, SC.

★ 12190 ★ Baker Hughes Foundation

3900 Essex Lane, Suite 210
Houston, TX 77027-5133
Phone: (713)439-8600
Website: http://www.bakerhughes.com/bakerhughes/communityaffairs/impact_team.htm
Isaac Kerridge, Executive Director

Priorities: *Arts & Humanities:* 7%. Supports art museums, music, art associations, and dance. *Civic & Public Affairs:* 3%. Provides funding for urban, minority, and women's affairs. *Education:* 28%. Supports colleges and universities, private colleges and schools, technical education, international education, high schools, and Junior Achievement. *Environment:* 46%. Supports United Way, family services, Boys & Girls Clubs, child welfare organizations, substance abuse treatment and prevention, youth organizations, and animal welfare. *International:* 12%. Gives to single-disease health associations, hospitals, and pediatric health. *Religion:* 3%. Funds science museums. *Note:* Total contributions made in 2000. **Typ. Recipients:** Medical Research. **Geo. Dist:** Houston, TX, greater metro area.

★ 12191 ★ Ball Corp.

10 Longs Peak Dr.
Broomfield, CO 80021-2510
Phone: (303)469-5511 **Fax:** (303)460-2127
Harold Sohn, Vice President, Corporate Relations

Typ. Recipients: Health-General. **Geo. Dist:** CO.

★ 12192 ★ Bandag, Inc.

2905 N Hwy. 61
Muscatine, IA 52761-5886
Phone: (319)262-1400 **Fax:** (319)262-1069
Cindy Hank, Employee Services Generalist

Priorities: *Arts & Humanities:* Less than 5%. Supports arts associations, the performing arts, and community art programs. *Civic & Public Affairs:* About 30%. Contributes to environmental efforts, AfricanAmerican and Hispanic affairs, women's issues, and safety and urban concerns. *Education:* About 40%. Funding is awarded to colleges and universities, business and engineering educational programs, and public education and student aid programs. *International:* About 30%. Supports single-disease health organizations and issues, public health, health care cost containment, and hospitals. Additional support is for community activities and services, child welfare, counseling, and the United Way. **Typ. Recipients:** Adolescent Health Issues, Children's Health/Hospitals, Clinics/Medical Centers, Domestic Violence, Eyes/Blindness, Health Funds, Health Organizations, Health Policy/Cost Containment, Health-General, Hospices, Hospitals, Hospitals (University Affiliated), Prenatal Health Issues, Preventive Medicine/Wellness Organizations, Public Health, Speech & Hearing, Substance Abuse. **Geo. Dist:** headquarters and operating communities.

★ 12193 ★ Bandai Foundation

c/o The Carmen Group
1299 Pennsylvania Ave. NW, Eighth Fl.
Washington, DC 20004
Website: http://www.bandai.com/about/bandai_foundation.cfm
Alison Miller, Contributions Advisor

Fnded: 1994. **Priorities:** *Arts & Humanities:* 2%. Supports art funds and preservation of archived films. *Civic & Public Affairs:* 3%. *Education:* 17%. Supports schools, academies, and educational programs. *Environment:* 23% Supports children's social services and substance abuse programs. *International:* 58%. Supports health funds, children's health care and research, hospitals, and clinics. *Note:* Total foundation contributions made in 2000. **Typ. Recipients:** AIDS/HIV, Arthritis, Cancer, Children's Health/Hospitals, Clinics/Medical Centers, Hospitals (University Affiliated), Medical Education, Medical Research, Single-Disease Health Associations, Substance Abuse. **Geo. Dist:** nationally; CA.

★ 12194 ★ Banfi Vintners Foundation

1111 Cedar Swamp Rd.
Old Brookville, NY 11545
Phone: (516)626-9200
Frank Savino, Foundation Contact

Fnded: 1982. **Priorities:** *Arts & Humanities:* 8%. Supports ballet, art museums, music, public broadcasting, and a symphony orchestra. *Civic & Public Affairs:* 47% Funds professional associations and Italian American organizations. *Education:* 35%. Supports colleges, universities, primary and secondary schools, and specialty schools nationwide, with a focus on wine and food education. *Environment:* 3%. Supports people with disabilities, and family services. *International:* 4%. Gives to hospitals and disease research and prevention. *Note:* Total contributions made in 2000. **Typ. Recipients:** Alzheimers Disease, Cancer, Diabetes, Eyes/Blindness, Geriatric Health, Health Organizations, Heart, Hospitals, Medical Research, Multiple Sclerosis, People with Disabilities, Sexual Abuse, Single-Disease Health Associations, Substance Abuse, Trauma Treatment. **Geo. Dist:** nationally; New York, NY, Metropolitan Area.

★ 12195 ★ Bank of America Foundation

100 North Tryon St.
NC1-007-18-01
Charlotte, NC 28255-0001
Phone: (704)388-3183
Website: http://www.bankofamerica.com/foundation
Paula Fraher, Corporate Initiatives Executive

Priorities: *Arts & Humanities:* 10%. *Civic & Public Affairs:* 10%. *Education:* 20%. *Environment:* 60%. *Voluntarism:* The company sponsors the Volunteer Time for Schools program, which allows each full-time associate to volunteer at a public or private school for up to two hours of paid time per week. The company also sponsors a Volunteer Grants Program. If an associate volunteers 50 or more hours at a nonprofit organization in a calendar year, Bank of America donates $250 to that organization in the associates name; the donation is increased to $500 for those who volunteer 100 or more hours. In addition, the company maintains the Team Bank of America Volunteer Network, which provides volunteer opportunities for Bank of America associates wishing to get involved in any of the approximately 3,000 volunteer events the company sponsors each year. *Note:* Total contributions made in 2000. **Typ. Recipients:** Child Abuse, Children's Health/Hospitals, Clinics/Medical Centers, Emergency/Ambulance Services, Health Organizations, Hospitals, Medical Education, Medical Research, People with Disabilities, Prenatal Health Issues, Substance Abuse. **Geo. Dist:** headquarters and operating communities, except in Washington State.

★ 12196 ★ Bank of Hawaii Charitable Foundation

PO Box 3170
Honolulu, HI 96802-3170
Phone: (808)538-4540 **Fax:** (808)538-4647
Cheryl Ritchie, Contact

Fnded: 1981. **Priorities:** *Arts & Humanities:* 21%. Supports memorials, museums, public broadcasting, and performing arts. *Civic & Public Affairs:* 15%. Funds community loan funds, economic development, small business services, housing, and ethnic organizations. *Education:* 27%. Equally supports colleges, private academies, and public education. Additional support goes to scholarship funds and education foundations. *Environment:* 14%. Supports scouts and other youth organizations, family services, Young Men's Christian Association, and Special Olympics. *International:* 16%. Funds hospitals, medical centers, and health foundations. *Note:* Total contributions made in 2000. **Typ. Recipients:** Cancer, Children's Health/Hospitals, Clinics/Medical Centers, Domestic Violence, Emergency/Ambulance Services, Health Organizations, Hospices, Hospitals, Medical Rehabilitation, Mental Health, Multiple Sclerosis, People with Disabilities. **Geo. Dist:** Honolulu, HI.

★ 12197 ★ Bank of Louisville Charities

500 W Broadway
PO Box 1101
Louisville, KY 40201
Phone: (502)589-3351 **Fax:** (502)562-5403
Beth Paxton-Klein, Sr. Vice President, Community Relations

Fnded: 1973. **Priorities:** *Arts & Humanities:* 41%. Supports art funds, ballet, visual and performing arts, and public broadcasting. *Civic & Public Affairs:* 11%. Supports organizations working toward economic development and community improvement projects. *Education:* 11%. Primarily supports public education. *Environment:* 31%. Supports the United Way, family services, youth organizations, senior services, and organizations assisting the disabled. *International:* 1%. Funds hospitals and single-disease health associations. *Religion:* 1%. Funds science centers. *Voluntarism:* Company encourages employee volunteerism; Laura Hillerich is the Employee Activities Coordinator. *Note:* Total contributions made in 2000. **Typ. Recipients:** Cancer, Children's Health/Hospitals, Domestic Violence, Emergency/Ambulance Services, Eyes/Blindness, Health-General, Heart, Hospitals, Medical Rehabilitation, Multiple Sclerosis, Nursing Services, People with Disabilities, Prenatal Health Issues, Sexual Abuse. **Geo. Dist:** KY, Jefferson County; Oldham, KY.

★ 12198 ★ Bank of New York Co., Inc.

1 Wall St.
31st Floor
New York, NY 10286
Phone: (212)635-1787 **Fax:** (212)635-1799
Email: gschneider@bankofny.com
Website: http://bankofny.com/pages/acdb_bnyinthecomm.htm
Pat Bicket, Vice President and Assistant Secretary

Priorities: *Arts & Humanities:* About 20%. Support goes to museums, culturalgroups, historic preservation and restoration, public broadcasting, libraries, and the performing arts. *Civic & Public Affairs:* About 60%. Emphasis is on grants supporting housing, youth organizations, drug and alcohol abuse programs, and family and community services. Less than 5%. Emphasis on economic development, civil rights, business and free enterprise, international affairs, and national security. *Education:* About 20%. Private educational institutions receive considerable funding through the company's matching gift program. Support also goes to educational associations, elementary, minority, and liberal arts education. *International:* Less than 5%. Especially supports hospitals, health organizations and nursing services. **Typ. Recipients:** Health Organizations, Hospitals, Nursing Services, Single-Disease Health Associations, Substance Abuse. **Geo. Dist:** DE; NJ; NY.

★ 12199 ★ Bank of Oklahoma Foundation

PO Box 2300
Tulsa, OK 74192
Phone: (918)588-6831
Leslie Paris, Contact

Fnded: 1997. **Priorities:** *Arts & Humanities:* 5%. Supports music, theater, and museums. *Civic & Public Affairs:* 21%. Funds community foundations, festivals, housing, and philanthropy. *Education:* 15%. Funds higher education and public schools. *Environment:* 53%. Supports United Way and services for children and youth. *International:* 4%. *Note:* Total contributions made in 1999. **Typ. Recipients:** Alzheimers Disease, Arthritis, Cancer, Clinics/Medical Centers, Health-General, Prenatal Health Issues. **Geo. Dist:** operating communities.

★ 12200 ★ Bank One Foundation

1 Bank One Plaza, Suite 0308
Chicago, IL 60670
Phone: (312)407-8052 **Fax:** (312)732-2437
James Donovan, Treasurer

Priorities: *Arts & Humanities:* 17%. *Civic & Public Affairs:* 24%. *Education:* 8%. *Environment:* 49%. *International:* 2%. *Note:* Total foundation contributions made in 2000. **Typ. Recipients:** Children's Health/Hospitals, Clinics/Medical Centers, Hospitals, People with Disabilities. **Geo. Dist:** nationally.

★ 12201 ★ Bank One, Texas-Houston Office

910 Travis TX2-4240
Houston, TX 77002
Phone: (713)751-3526 **Fax:** (713)751-3870
Website: http://www.bankone.com
Barbara Harris, Charitable Contributions Coordinator

Priorities: *Arts & Humanities:* About 15%. Contributes to performing arts programs, museums, public radio and television, and cultural programs. *Civic & Public Affairs:* About 10%. Interests include business, voter registration and education, civil rights, justice and law, and non-academic research. About 10%. Supports programs and projects in the areas of community and neighborhood improvement, community development, housing and urban revitalization, community-based education, and economic development in low- to moderate-income neighborhoods. *Education:* About 20%. Interests include primary and secondary schools, public and private higher education institutions, adult education programs, scholarship programs, public library systems, and other related organizations. Also operates employee matching gift program to educational institutions. *International:* About 40% of total contributions. Includes assistance to federated drives such as United Way; hospitals; local health and welfare groups; health research organizations; and youth agencies. Also supports nonprofit drug abuse and rehabilitation programs in Houston, and a matching gift program for employee contributions to health and welfare organizations. **Typ. Recipients:** Health Organizations, Health-General, Hospitals, Medical Research, Substance Abuse. **Geo. Dist:** Houston, TX.

★ 12202 ★ BankAtlantic Foundation

PO Box 8608
Fort Lauderdale, FL 33310-8608
Phone: (954)760-5458
Website: http://www.bankatlantic.com/communityinvestment/bafoundation.asp
Shelley Levan-Margolis, Executive Director

Fnded: 1994. **Priorities:** *Arts & Humanities:* 29%. Supports fine arts, libraries, museums, and music. *Civic & Public Affairs:* 37%. Supports urban/community affairs, housing, civil rights, legal affairs, and community foundations. *Education:* 22%. Supports continuing studies, literacy programs, and higher education. *Environment:* 10%. Supports child and youth services, elder care, and human services. *International:* 1%. Supports prenatal health, children's health, and hearing & deaf services. *Religion:* 1%. Funds science museums. *Note:* Total contributions made in 2000. **Typ. Recipients:** AIDS/HIV, Domestic Violence, Emergency/Ambulance Services, People with Disabilities, Prenatal Health Issues. **Geo. Dist:** FL, Southern Florida.

★ 12203 ★ Banta Corp. Foundation

PO Box 8003
Menasha, WI 54952-8003
Phone: (920)751-7777 **Fax:** (920)751-7790
Donald Belcher, Vice President

Fnded: 1953. **Priorities:** *Arts & Humanities:* 33%. Supports libraries, public broadcasting, a children's museum, theater, and orchestras. *Civic & Public Affairs:* 17%. Supports municipalities, housing, and community development. *Education:* 30%. Funds scholarship programs, colleges, universities, and parochial schools. *Environment:* 16%. Supports youth organizations and services, family social services, scouting, counseling services, and food distribution. *International:* 1%. Contributes to mental health centers, hospice, and Make-a-Wish Foundation. *Note:* Total contributions made in 2001. **Typ. Recipients:** AIDS/HIV, Cancer, Children's Health/Hospitals, Clinics/Medical Centers, Domestic Violence, Emergency/Ambulance Services, Heart, Hospitals, Medical Education, Mental Health, Nursing Services, People with Disabilities, Substance Abuse. **Geo. Dist:** operating locations; WI.

★ 12204 ★ Barclays Capital

222 Broadway, 10th Floor
New York, NY 10038
Phone: (212)412-3825 **Fax:** (212)412-7300
Linda Wynns, Assoc. Dir., Corporate Communications

Priorities: *Arts & Humanities:* 33%. Donates to performing arts. *Civic & Public Affairs:* 7%. Focuses on improving the community through local community organizations, and neighborhood sports teams. *Education:* 42%. Primarily supports through matching gifts. Also donates to universities, specialized art schools and Junior Achievement. *Environment:* 5%. Majority of support goes to family services and youth organizations. *International:* 11%. Funds the Amyotropic Lateral Sclerosis Association, other disease-specific groups, and hospitals. *Note:* Total contributions in 1997. **Typ. Recipients:** AIDS/HIV, Cancer, Children's Health/Hospitals, Diabetes, Hospices, Hospitals, Medical Research, Single-Disease Health Associations. **Geo. Dist:** New York, NY. **Frmly:** Barclays Bank Foundation.

★ 12205 ★ Barden Foundation, Inc.

1146 Barnum Ave.
Bridgeport, CT 06610
Phone: (203)336-7531 **Fax:** (203)336-6440
Thomas Loughman, Treasurer & Trustee

Fnded: 1959. **Priorities:** *Arts & Humanities:* 1%. Primary support made to a theater. *Civic & Public Affairs:* 1%. Primary support made to Connecticut Zoological Society. *Education:* 6%. Supports colleges, universities, institutes, education funds, and Junior Achievement. *Environment:* 45%. Supports YMCA, child welfare, recreation, people with disabilities, scouts, Special Olympics, homes, and United Way. *International:* 46%. Supports health centers, nursing services, medical centers, hospitals, clinics, and health organizations. *Note:* Total foundation contributions in fiscal 2001. **Typ. Recipients:** Cancer, Children's Health/Hospitals, Clinics/Medical Centers, Emergency/Ambulance Services, Health Organizations, Hospices, Hospitals, Medical Rehabilitation, Nursing Services, Nursing Services, People with Disabilities, Single-Disease Health Associations. **Geo. Dist:** Bridgeport, CT; Danbury, CT; Winsted, CT.

★ 12206 ★ Barnes Group Foundation Inc.

123 Main St.
PO Box 489
Bristol, CT 06011-0489
Phone: (860)583-7070 **Fax:** (860)589-7466
Thomas Barnes, Secretary

Priorities: *Arts & Humanities:* 11%. Contributes to arts centers, museums, theaters, music, and public broadcasting. *Civic & Public Affairs:* 8%. Recipients include urban affairs, municipalities, leadership councils, and community foundations. *Education:* 40%. About three-fifths of funds supports Citizens Scholarship Foundation for college tuition for children of employees. Also supports colleges and universities, private education, business education, religious high schools, and college funds. *Environment:* 12%. Supports youth organizations, homes for children, guide dogs for the blind, Focus Hope, and family services. Also supports United Way. *International:* 26%. Funds hospitals, cancer centers, and health organizations. *Note:* Total contributions made in 2000. **Typ. Recipients:** Cancer, Children's Health/Hospitals, Clinics/Medical Centers, Emergency/Ambulance Services, Hospitals, Medical Research, People with Disabilities, Single-Disease Health Associations, Substance Abuse, Trauma Treatment. **Geo. Dist:** operating communities.

★ 12207 ★ Barry Foundation

PO Box 129
Columbus, OH 43216-0129
Marilyn Thomas, Corporate Finance Administrator

Fnded: 1963. **Priorities:** *Arts & Humanities:* Less than 1%. Supports museums and cultural programs. *Civic & Public Affairs:* 2%. Gives to community foundations. *Education:* 32%. Supports higher education and educational programs. *Environment:* 11%. Funds youth and social services. *International:* 3%. Funds health care organizations and concerns. *Note:* Total contributions made in 2000. **Typ. Recipients:** AIDS/HIV, Cancer, Children's Health/Hospitals, Diabetes, Emergency/Ambulance Services, Family Planning, Health Funds, Health Organizations, Health-General, Medical Research, People with Disabilities, Single-Disease Health Associations, Speech & Hearing, Substance Abuse. **Geo. Dist:** nationally.

★ 12208 ★ Bassett Furniture Industries Foundation

PO Box 626
Bassett, VA 24055-0626
Phone: (540)629-6200
Robert Spilman, Jr., President

Fnded: 1993. **Priorities:** *Arts & Humanities:* 9%. *Civic & Public Affairs:* 1%. *Education:* 43%. *Environment:* 35%. *Note:* Total contributions made in fiscal 2001. **Typ. Recipients:** Cancer, Emergency/Ambulance Services, Single-Disease Health Associations. **Geo. Dist:** GA; NC; VA.

★ 12209 ★ Bausch & Lomb Foundation, Inc.

One Bausch & Lomb Place
Rochester, NY 14604-2701
Phone: (585)338-6000 **Fax:** (585)338-6007
Barbara Kelley, Vice President

Priorities: *Arts & Humanities:* 9%. *Civic & Public Affairs:* 10%. *Education:* 42%. *Environment:* 35%. *International:* 3%. *Religion:* 1%. *Note:* Total contributions made in 2001. **Typ. Recipients:** Clinics/Medical Centers, Geriatric Health, Medical Rehabilitation,

Nursing Services, People with Disabilities. **Geo. Dist:** Rochester, NY.

★ 12210 ★ Baxter Allegiance Foundation
One Baxter Parkway
Deerfield, IL 60015-4633
Phone: (847)948-4604 **Fax:** (847)948-4026
Email: pat_a_morgan@baxter.com
Website: http://www.baxter.com
Ms. Patricia Morgan, Executive Director & Secretary

Priorities: *Civic & Public Affairs:* 4%. *Education:* 17%. *Environment:* 48%. *International:* 24%. *Voluntarism:* Supports Dollars for Doers program, which provides grants to organizations where employees volunteer. *Note:* Total contributions made in 2001. **Typ. Recipients:** AIDS/HIV, Child Abuse, Children's Health/Hospitals, Clinics/Medical Centers, Domestic Violence, Emergency/Ambulance Services, Eyes/Blindness, Health Organizations, Health Policy/Cost Containment, Health-General, Heart, Home-Care Services, Hospices, Hospitals, Hospitals (University Affiliated), Long-Term Care, Medical Education, Medical Rehabilitation, Medical Research, Mental Health, Nursing Services, People with Disabilities, Prenatal Health Issues, Preventive Medicine/Wellness Organizations, Public Health, Research/Studies Institutes, Respiratory, Sexual Abuse, Substance Abuse. **Geo. Dist:** nationally; Europe; Latin America; Puerto Rico; Chicago, IL.

★ 12211 ★ Bay State Federal Savings Charitable Foundation
1299 Beacon St.
Brookline, MA 02446-5242
Phone: (617)739-9577
Susan Kelliher, Contact

Fnded: 1999. **Priorities:** *Arts & Humanities:* 8%. *Civic & Public Affairs:* 15%. *Education:* 6%. *Environment:* 36%. *International:* 30%. **Typ. Recipients:** Cancer, Children's Health/Hospitals, Emergency/Ambulance Services, Geriatric Health, Health Organizations, Heart, Hospitals, Medical Research, Prenatal Health Issues, Single-Disease Health Associations. **Geo. Dist:** Bank's market area, or subject to approval.

★ 12212 ★ Bayer Foundation
100 Bayer Rd.
Pittsburgh, PA 15205-9741
Phone: (412)777-5791 **Fax:** (412)778-4432
Website: http://www.bayerus.com/about/community/index.html
Rebecca Lucore, Executive Director

Priorities: *Arts & Humanities:* 13%. *Civic & Public Affairs:* 20%. *Education:* 45%. *Environment:* 20%. *Religion:* 1%. *Note:* Total contributions made in 2001. **Typ. Recipients:** Clinics/Medical Centers, Diabetes, Health Funds, Health Organizations, Health-General, Hospitals, Medical Education, People with Disabilities, Single-Disease Health Associations. **Geo. Dist:** headquarters and operating communities.

★ 12213 ★ Bayport Foundation
White Pine Bldg.
342 Fifth Ave., North
Bayport, MN 55003-0204
Phone: (651)439-1557 **Fax:** (651)439-9480
Email: chloettehaley@scenicriver.org
Website: http://www.scenicriver.org
Chloette Haley, Grants Consultant

Priorities: *Arts & Humanities:* 13%. *Civic & Public Affairs:* 14%. *Education:* 10%. *Environment:* 23%. *International:* 15%. *Religion:* 1%. *Note:* Total foundation contributions made in fiscal 2001. **Typ. Recipients:** Cancer, Children's Health/Hospitals, Clinics/Medical Centers, Emergency/Ambulance Services, Eyes/Blindness, Family Planning, Health Funds, Health Organizations, Hospitals, Kidney, Medical Rehabilitation, Medical Research, People with Disabilities, Public Health, Single-Disease Health Associations, Speech & Hearing, Substance Abuse. **Geo. Dist:** MN, East Metro area; MN, Washington County; WI, Barron County; WI, Burnett County; WI, Dunn County; WI, Pierce County; WI, Polk County; WI, St. Croix County.

★ 12214 ★ BB&T Corp.
351 South Churton St.
PO Box 1269
Hillsboro, NC 27278
Phone: (919)644-2000
Website: http://www.bbandt.com
Crystal Cole, Financial Center Manager

Typ. Recipients: Health-General. **Geo. Dist:** NC; SC; VA.

★ 12215 ★ BD
1 Becton Dr.
Franklin Lakes, NJ 07417
Phone: (201)847-7065 **Fax:** (201)847-5305
Website: http://www.bd.com/responsibility/
Jennifer Farrington, Manager, Community Partnerships

Priorities: *Voluntarism:* BD employees and retirees who volunteer their time to charitable organizations are honored through the company's Community Service Awards Program. The program provides financial contributions to the non-profit organization to which BD associates have donated their time. **Typ. Recipients:** Hospitals, Medical Education, Medical Research, Medical Training, Nursing Services. **Geo. Dist:** principally near operating locations and to national organizations.

★ 12216 ★ Bechtel Foundation
50 Beale St.
San Francisco, CA 94105
Phone: (415)768-7158 **Fax:** (415)768-0263
Email: lmlang@bechtel.com
Website: http://www.bechtel.com/bechfoun.html
LeeAnne Lang, Assistant Secretary

Priorities: *Arts & Humanities:* 1%. Gives to performing arts and museums. *Civic & Public Affairs:* 7%. Funds professional engineering associations and philanthropic organizations. *Education:* 75%. Focus on math, science, and engineering education. Support is given for educational enrichment programs such as local science fairs, special educational activities, or regional museum programs in math or science for young people around the world; and engineering and business schools at selected colleges and universities around the world (divided between unrestricted support and support for scholarship programs). *Environment:* 10%. Primarily supports the United Way or similar campaigns in the communities with Bechtel offices or major projects. Other interests include youth programs and drug abuse prevention. *International:* 2%. Funds hospitals and single-disease health associations. *Religion:* 1%. *Note:* Total contributions made in 2000. **Typ. Recipients:** Adolescent Health Issues, AIDS/HIV, Cancer, Children's Health/Hospitals, Emergency/Ambulance Services, Hospitals, Medical Education, Prenatal Health Issues, Research/Studies Institutes, Substance Abuse. **Geo. Dist:** internationally, in major operating locations.

★ 12217 ★ Beckman Coulter, Inc.
4300 N Harbor Boulevard
PO Box 3100
C-30-B
Fullerton, CA 92835-3100
Phone: (714)871-4848 **Fax:** (714)773-7743
Email: communityaffairs@beckman.com
Website: http://www.beckman.com/hr/ourcompany/oc_communityRelations.asp
Tracy Hatt, Manager, Community Affairs

Priorities: *Education:* Scientific education, science, and research-related healthcare. **Typ. Recipients:** AIDS/HIV, Alzheimers Disease, Arthritis, Cancer, Diabetes, Heart, Kidney, Medical Research, Multiple Sclerosis, Respiratory. **Geo. Dist:** headquarters and operating communities.

★ 12218 ★ Belchatov Foundation
11755 Wilshire Blvd., Suite 1350
Los Angeles, CA 90025
Phone: (310)477-5252
Harry Faversham, President

Priorities: *Arts & Humanities:* 2%. Funds theater, music, and public broadcasting. *Civic & Public Affairs:* 93%. Major grant to the California Community Foundation. *Education:* 1%. Funds a school. *Note:* Total contributions made in fiscal 2001. **Typ. Recipients:** Cancer, Diabetes, Health-General, Hospices, Hospitals, Long-Term Care, Medical Education, Medical Research, Multiple Sclerosis, Research/Studies Institutes. **Geo. Dist:** headquarters and operating communities; Los Angeles, CA, Los Angeles. **Frmly:** National Metal & Steel Foundation.

★ 12219 ★ Belk Foundation
2801 West Tyvola Rd.
Charlotte, NC 28217-4500
Phone: (704)357-1000 **Fax:** (704)357-1883
Website: http://belk.com/main/about_philanthropic.jsp?bmUID=1029805668286
Paul Wyche, Jr., Trustee

Fnded: 1988. **Priorities:** *Arts & Humanities:* 11%. *Civic & Public Affairs:* 6%. *Education:* 59%. *Environment:* 13%. *Note:* Total contributions in fiscal 1999. **Typ. Recipients:** Arthritis, Cancer, Children's Health/Hospitals, Emergency/Ambulance Services, Family Planning, Health Funds, Health Organizations, Heart, Hospitals, Hospitals (University Affiliated), Medical Education, Medical Rehabilitation, Substance Abuse. **Geo. Dist:** GA; NC; SC.

★ 12220 ★ BellSouth Foundation
1155 Peachtree St., NE, Room 7H08
Atlanta, GA 30309-3610
Phone: (404)249-2396 **Fax:** (404)249-5696
Email: grants.manager@bellsouth.com
Website: http://www.bellsouthfoundation.org
Greg Norton, Grants Administrator

Fnded: 1986. **Priorities:** *Civic & Public Affairs:* 5%. *Education:* 100%. The foundation has the sole priority of improving the quality of education in its Southeastern service area and in Latin America. The foundation conducts a target requests for proposals process accepted for two special initiatives; limited funds are available for Opportunity Grants, or unsolicited requests that address the two initiatives. The first initiative is Closing the Divides: an equity agenda for student learning and achievement and for community well-being. Supported projects are for disadvantaged high school students, college-bound minorities, and technology-disadvantaged communities. The second initiative is Forging New Paths: a capacity-building agenda for innovation and opportunity. Supported projects benefit Latin America's children, teachers and leaders, and technology and learning. *Environment:* 3%. *Note:* Company also maintains a substantial direct giving program, which makes contributions within the company's service area in the categories of education, 51%; health and human services, 29%; arts and culture, 13%; civic and community, 6%; and miscellaneous interests, 1%. **Typ. Recipients:** Health-General, Medical Education. **Geo. Dist:** principally near operating locations and to national organizations.

★ 12221 ★ Belo Foundation
PO Box 655237
Dallas, TX 75265-5237
Phone: (214)977-6661 **Fax:** (214)977-6620
Website: http://www.belo.com/aboutbelo/philanthropy.html
Becky Odlozil, Executive Director

Fnded: 1952. **Priorities:** *Arts & Humanities:* 12%. *Civic & Public Affairs:* 8%. *Education:* 65%. *Environment:* 11%. *International:* 4%. *Note:* Total foundation contributions made in 2001. **Typ. Recipients:** AIDS/HIV, Diabetes, Family Planning, Health Organizations, Hospitals. **Geo. Dist:** Claremont, CA; Oakland, CA; Pasadena, CA; Washington, DC; Atlanta, GA; Boise, ID; Chicago, IL; Louisville, KY; New York, NY; Austin, TX; Dallas, TX; Ft. Worth, TX; Arlington, VA; Reston,

VA. **Frmly:** Dallas Morning News-WFAA Foundation A. H. Belo Corp. Foundation.

★ 12222 ★ Bemis Co. Foundation
222 South 9th St., Suite 2300
Minneapolis, MN 55402
Phone: (612)376-3093
Email: ajkirchner@bemis.com
Gene Seashore, Trustee

Priorities: *Arts & Humanities:* (Culture and Civic) 5%. Gives to art museums, orchestras, opera, theater, historical societies, and fire and police departments. *Education:* 45%. Supports employee educational matching gifts, scholarship programs for children of employees, and independent college associations in states where company facilities are located. *Environment:* (Social Welfare & Health) 50%. Major support goes to united fund drives in operating locations. Another priority is food shelves and food banks (the company also sponsors an employee matching gifts program to food banks). Other social welfare interests include child welfare and youth organizations, the aged, employment, and community service organizations. Health interests include hospitals and single-disease health organizations. *Note:* Total foundation contributions made in 2001, excluding matching gifts to miscellaneous organizations. **Typ. Recipients:** Clinics/Medical Centers, Diabetes, Domestic Violence, Emergency/Ambulance Services, Family Planning, Health Funds, Health Organizations, Health Policy/ Cost Containment, Health-General, Hospitals, Medical Education, Mental Health, Nursing Services, People with Disabilities, Prenatal Health Issues, Public Health, Single-Disease Health Associations, Speech & Hearing, Substance Abuse. **Geo. Dist:** principally near operating locations and to national organizations; Minneapolis, MN.

★ 12223 ★ Ben & Jerry's Foundation
30 Community Drive
South Burlington, VT 05403-6828
Phone: (802)651-9600 **Fax:** (802)846-1610
Website: http://www.benjerry.com/foundation
Lisa Pendolino, Executive Director

Fnded: 1977. **Priorities:** *Arts & Humanities:* 11%. *Civic & Public Affairs:* 63%. *Education:* 3%. *Environment:* 5%. *Note:* Total foundation contributions made in 2001. **Typ. Recipients:** AIDS/HIV, Cancer, Medical Rehabilitation, Mental Health, People with Disabilities. **Geo. Dist:** U.S.-based organizations; VT, focusing on Community Action Teams.

★ 12224 ★ Benjamin Jacobson & Sons Foundation
40 Wall St., 45th Floor
Suite 201
New York, NY 10005
Phone: (212)952-1012 **Fax:** (212)952-0920
Robert Jacobson, Sr., President

Priorities: *Arts & Humanities:* 13%. Supports public broadcasting, performing arts, museums, and theaters. *Civic & Public Affairs:* 8%. Supports philanthropic organizations, research funds, and community affairs. *Education:* 18%. Supports colleges, universities, and schools. *Environment:* 11%. Supports YMCA, child welfare, homes, people with disabilities, and athletic funds, family services, and community services organizations. *International:* 16%. Supports cancer research, hospitals, single-disease health associations, and health organizations. *Note:* Total foundation contributions made in fiscal 2001. **Typ. Recipients:** Arthritis, Cancer, Children's Health/Hospitals, Clinics/ Medical Centers, Diabetes, Emergency/Ambulance Services, Health Organizations, Hospitals, Long-Term Care, Medical Education, Medical Research, Multiple Sclerosis, People with Disabilities, Public Health, Single-Disease Health Associations, Substance Abuse. **Geo. Dist:** nationally; New York, NY.

★ 12225 ★ Berwind Group
3000 Centre Square West
1500 Market St.
Philadelphia, PA 19102
Phone: (215)563-2800 **Fax:** (215)563-1493
Email: mlarue@berwind.com
Website: http://www.berwind.com
Mary LaRue, Chairperson, Contributions Committee

Typ. Recipients: Family Planning, Health-General, Hospitals. **Geo. Dist:** headquarters area only.

★ 12226 ★ Best Buy Children's Foundation
c/o Community Relations Department
PO Box 9312
Minneapolis, MN 55440-9312
Phone: (952)947-2000
Website: http://www.bestbuy.com/About/CommunityRelations/ChildrensFoundation.asp
Richard Schulze, Chairman, Director

Fnded: 1995. **Priorities:** *Arts & Humanities:* Less than 1%. Gives to libraries and community arts. *Civic & Public Affairs:* 4%. Supports women's affairs and civic groups. *Education:* 28%. Funds alternative schools, community involvement in schools, Junior Achievement, colleges, and universities. *Environment:* 67%. Supports child and family services, youth organizations, scouts, senior services, domestic violence services, and shelters. *Note:* Total contributions made in fiscal 2001. **Typ. Recipients:** Sexual Abuse.

★ 12227 ★ Binney & Smith, Inc.
PO Box 431
1100 Church Ln.
Easton, PA 18044-0431
Phone: (610)559-6607 **Fax:** (610)559-6691
Email: mvoden@binney-smith.com
Website: http://www.binney-smith.com
Mary Ellyn Volden, Director, Global Philanthropy

Priorities: *Arts & Humanities:* Supports art organizations that help ensure a higher quality of life for all citizens. Considers requests to organizations that stress excellence and community participation, especially with children. Also considers support for performing arts and public broadcasting. *Civic & Public Affairs:* Funds organizations that encourage a better working relationship between business and the community. Also funds local environmental and ecological issues. *Education:* Focus on early childhood development and quality arts in education initiatives. Grants may be made for start-up programs. Limited support for special programs. Assistance is given to programs for the physically and mentally disabled. *International:* Majority of contributions go to the United Way. Limited support towards preventive health measures. Funding also given to human service programs, services for children, the elderly and the disabled, and programs that assist disadvantaged children. *Voluntarism:* The company provides volunteers for special events. **Typ. Recipients:** Children's Health/Hospitals, Domestic Violence, Emergency/Ambulance Services, Health-General, Sexual Abuse, Speech & Hearing. **Geo. Dist:** Easton, PA.

★ 12228 ★ Binswanger Foundation
2 Logan Square, 4th Floor
Philadelphia, PA 19103
Phone: (215)448-6000 **Fax:** (215)448-6238
Email: info@cbbi.com
John Binswanger, President

Priorities: *Arts & Humanities:* 9%. Supports public broadcasting, music, literature, libraries, theaters, historic preservation, and the performing arts. *Civic & Public Affairs:* 9%. Supports public parks, community funds, voting rights, economic development, and legal assistance organizations. *Education:* 11%. Supports universities, schools, and colleges. *Environment:* 12%. Supports United Way, athletic and recreational organizations, and child welfare. *International:* 30%. Supports hospitals, cancer research, children's health and medical centers. *Religion:* 2%. Supports science centers and institutes. *Note:* Total foundation contributions made in 2000. **Typ. Recipients:** Cancer, Children's Health/Hospitals, Emergency/Ambulance Services, Eyes/Blindness, Family Planning, Health Organizations, Hospitals, Hospitals (University Affiliated), Medical Research, Mental Health, People with Disabilities, Public Health, Single-Disease Health Associations, Substance Abuse. **Geo. Dist:** PA.

★ 12229 ★ Blade Foundation
541 N Superior St.
Toledo, OH 43604
Phone: (419)245-6210
William Block, Jr., President

Priorities: *Arts & Humanities:* 38%. Supports music, theater, libraries, art centers, dance, public broadcasting, literary arts, and historic preservation. *Civic & Public Affairs:* 13%. Supports urban affairs, parks, local initiatives, zoos, and community foundations. *Education:* 11%. Supports schools, literacy, colleges, and Junior Achievement. *Environment:* 28%. Supports United Way and family planning. *International:* 6%. Supports medical centers, health foundations, hospitals, and single-disease health associations. *Voluntarism:* Company actively promotes employee volunteerism through participation in the United Way, Read for Literacy, and in activities with the Sherman School, its adopted school. *Note:* Total foundation contributions made in 2000. **Typ. Recipients:** Alzheimers Disease, Arthritis, Children's Health/Hospitals, Clinics/Medical Centers, Emergency/Ambulance Services, Family Planning, Health Organizations, Medical Education, Multiple Sclerosis, Preventive Medicine/Wellness Organizations, Respiratory, Single-Disease Health Associations. **Geo. Dist:** Toledo, OH.

★ 12230 ★ Blue Bell Foundation
PO Box 21488
Greensboro, NC 27420
Phone: (910)373-3412
Charles Conkin, Vice President Human Resources

Priorities: *Arts & Humanities:* 16%. Supports museums and libraries. *Civic & Public Affairs:* 6%. Recipients include municipalities, environmental efforts, and community affairs organizations. *Education:* 41%. Emphasis is on the National Merit Scholarship Corporation, colleges and universities. Also supports preschools, high schools (public and private), education funds, and community education programs. The foundation operates a large matching gift program for company employees who wish to contribute to educational institutions. *Environment:* 34%. Supports United Way chapters and community service organizations. Housing, food distribution, and youth activities are also major priorities. *International:* 2%. Funds single-disease health associations, Ronald McDonald House, dental health, and health centers. *Note:* total contributions made in 2000. **Typ. Recipients:** Cancer, Child Abuse, Children's Health/Hospitals, Clinics/Medical Centers, Diabetes, Domestic Violence, Emergency/ Ambulance Services, Heart, Hospices, Hospitals, Medical Rehabilitation, Medical Research, People with Disabilities, Prenatal Health Issues, Public Health, Respiratory, Single-Disease Health Associations, Substance Abuse. **Geo. Dist:** principally near operating locations and to national organizations.

★ 12231 ★ Blue Cross & Blue Shield of Michigan Foundation
600 Lafayette E, X520
Detroit, MI 48226-2927
Phone: (313)225-8706 **Fax:** (313)225-7730
Email: nmaloy@bcbsm.com
Website: http://www.bcbsm.com/foundation
Nancy Szydlowski, Executive Assistant

Priorities: *Civic & Public Affairs:* 1%. *Education:* 3%. Supports student awards program in public health, medicine, and health policy. *Environment:* 26%. Funds went to projects that addressed domestic violence, through the Request for Proposals Program. *International:* 76%. Goals for giving are to enhance the quality and appropriate use of healthcare services, improve access to appropriate health services, and control healthcare costs. Supports the following programs: the Investigator Initiated Research Program, which supports healthcare researchers interested in finding ways to improve healthcare in Michigan by funding projects which address healthcare costs, quality, and access to services; the Matching Initiative Program, which supports a variety of innovative health service projects and attempts to foster collaboration among foundations and other funding organizations, and which matches grants for conferences and seminars; the Request for Proposals Program; the Physician Investigator Research Award, for projects that include physician-led pilot studies, feasibility studies, or small research studies in clinical or health services research; the Student Award Program, which offers one-year grants for health-care research to doctoral and medical students in Michigan universities; the Proposal Development Award, which helps community nonprofit organizations develop proposals for improving health-care delivery; and the Excellence in Research Awards, which honors researchers who make significant contributions toward improving health care delivery in Michigan. *Note:* Total foundation contributions made in 2000. **Typ. Recipients:** AIDS/HIV, Cancer, Children's Health/Hospitals, Diabetes, Domestic Violence, Geriatric Health, Health Organizations, Health Policy/Cost Containment, Health-General, Heart, Hospitals, Medical Education, Medical Research, Mental Health, People with Disabilities, Prenatal Health Issues, Preventive Medicine/Wellness Organizations, Single-Disease Health Associations. **Geo. Dist:** MI.

★ 12232 ★ Blue Cross & Blue Shield of Minnesota Foundation Inc.

PO Box 64560
Saint Paul, MN 55164-0560
Phone: (651)662-2566 **Fax:** (612)662-1570
Email: community@bluecrossmn.com
Website: http://www.bluecrossmn.com
Daniel Johnson, Director, Community Affairs

Fnded: 1986. **Priorities:** *Arts & Humanities:* 4%. *Civic & Public Affairs:* 6%. *Education:* Less than 1%. *Environment:* 55%. *International:* Supports programs and organizations that reduce tobacco use, particularly use by youths; help individuals with chronic illness to navigate the health care system; promote fitness, nutrition, and safety; increase childhood immunization; and other miscellaneous health objectives. *Voluntarism:* Volunteer Council manages employee volunteer efforts. *Note:* Giving analysis provided by foundation. **Typ. Recipients:** AIDS/HIV, Cancer, Children's Health/Hospitals, Clinics/Medical Centers, Diabetes, Domestic Violence, Emergency/Ambulance Services, Health Funds, Health Organizations, Health Organizations, Health Policy/Cost Containment, Health-General, Heart, Hospices, Hospitals, Kidney, Medical Education, Medical Rehabilitation, Medical Research, Medical Training, Mental Health, Multiple Sclerosis, Nursing Services, Nutrition, People with Disabilities, Prenatal Health Issues, Preventive Medicine/Wellness Organizations, Public Health, Respiratory, Single-Disease Health Associations, Trauma Treatment. **Geo. Dist:** MN.

★ 12233 ★ The Boeing Co. Charitable Trust

PO Box 3707 MS 17-MJ
Seattle, WA 98124-2207
Phone: (206)655-1131 **Fax:** (206)655-2000
Website: http://www.boeing.com/companyoffices/aboutus/community/guidelines.htm
Antoinette Bailey, Vice President, Community Relations

Fnded: 1964. **Priorities:** *Arts & Humanities:* 18%. Supports arts, music, drama, and dance. Especially interested in projects that explore the relationships between art, science, and technology. Contributions include grants for capital campaigns, performance scholarships and outreach programs, and one-time special grants. *Civic & Public Affairs:* 7%. Includes environmental grants. Funds initiatives concerned with long-term community growth, sustainable economic development, affordable housing, and free enterprise. Also interested in projects that aid communities and the environment at the same time. Contributions generally support capital campaigns, seed money for new programs that address community needs and priorities, and one-time grants for equipment purchases or special projects. *Education:* 41%. Supports K-12 and higher education. K-12 support focuses on schools with an emphasis on high academic standards, commitment to improving student achievement, effective school-to-work strategies, and the Tech Prep program. Higher education grants support engineering, business, technology, math, and selected science education; faculty preparation and development; collaborative academic programs; curriculum development; laboratory equipment that directly supports learning and academic performance; scholarships; and minority and women's programs. Two-year colleges are supported through the Tech Prep program. Favors innovative proposals in the following areas: aviation maintenance, manufacturing and engineering technologies, information technology, telecommunications/networks, business technologies or disciplines, electronics, machine tool maintenance, machine shop technology, quality assurance, and evaluation (learning assessment). The company recognizes excellence in higher education teaching with the annual Boeing Outstanding Educator Award. *International:* 34%. Includes human service organizations and United Way. Supports agencies that ease mental and physical suffering, addiction or substance abuse, and family problems. Funds basic needs for housing and nutrition, boys and girls clubs, and programs for the homeless. *Religion:* 36%. *Note:* Total contributions made in 2000. **Typ. Recipients:** Clinics/Medical Centers, Domestic Violence, Emergency/Ambulance Services, Hospices, Mental Health, People with Disabilities, Substance Abuse. **Geo. Dist:** headquarters and operating communities where Boeing employees work and reside; nationally.

★ 12234 ★ Boise Cascade Corp.

1111 West Jefferson St.
PO Box 50
Boise, ID 83728-0001
Phone: (208)384-7673 **Fax:** (208)384-7224
Connie Weaver, Manager,Community Relations

Typ. Recipients: Emergency/Ambulance Services, Hospitals, Substance Abuse. **Geo. Dist:** headquarters and operating communities.

★ 12235 ★ Bolick Foundation

PO Box 307
Conover, NC 28613
Phone: (828)464-0311 **Fax:** (828)464-0460
Jerome Bolick, Chairman, President & CEO

Fnded: 1967. **Priorities:** *Arts & Humanities:* 12%. *Civic & Public Affairs:* 7%. *Education:* 8%. *Environment:* 5%. *International:* 3%. *Note:* Total contributions made in 2001. **Typ. Recipients:** Cancer, Family Planning, Health Organizations, Heart, Hospices, Long-Term Care, Medical Research, Prenatal Health Issues. **Geo. Dist:** NC.

★ 12236 ★ Borden Foundation, Inc.

180 East Broad St.
24th Floor
Columbus, OH 43215-3799
Phone: (614)225-4580 **Fax:** (614)225-4066
Colleen Nissl, President

Fnded: 1944. **Priorities:** *Arts & Humanities:* 1%. *Civic & Public Affairs:* 76%. *Education:* 7%. *Environment:* 15%. *International:* 2%. *Note:* The foundation focuses on funding direct services and programs for disadvantaged youth across all program areas. Total contributions made in 2001. **Typ. Recipients:** AIDS/HIV, Arthritis, Cancer, Children's Health/Hospitals, Diabetes, Domestic Violence, Emergency/Ambulance Services, Eyes/Blindness, Hospitals, Medical Education, Medical Research, Mental Health, People with Disabilities, Prenatal Health Issues, Public Health, Single-Disease Health Associations, Speech & Hearing. **Geo. Dist:** principally near operating locations and to national organizations.

★ 12237 ★ Borman's Inc. Fund

20500 Civic Center Drive, Suite 2750
Southfield, MI 48076
Phone: (248)350-0300 **Fax:** (248)350-2920
Paul Borman, President

Priorities: *Education:* 6%. Gives to a Jewish day school. *Environment:* 16%. Contributes to children's charities and an animal welfare organization. *International:* 29%. Primarily funds single-disease health organizations, and cancer and eye care institutes. *Note:* Total foundation contributions made in 2000. **Typ. Recipients:** AIDS/HIV, Alzheimers Disease, Alzheimers Disease, Cancer, Children's Health/Hospitals, Diabetes, Domestic Violence, Emergency/Ambulance Services, Eyes/Blindness, Family Planning, Geriatric Health, Health Organizations, Hospices, Hospitals, Long-Term Care, Mental Health, Multiple Sclerosis, People with Disabilities, Single-Disease Health Associations, Substance Abuse. **Geo. Dist:** MI, Southeastern Michigan.

★ 12238 ★ Boston Globe Foundation

135 Morrissey Boulevard, 2nd Floor
Boston, MA 02107
Phone: (617)929-3467 **Fax:** (617)929-2041
Email: foundation@globe.com
Website: http://bostonglobe.com/community/index.stm
Mrs. Bailey, Contact

Priorities: *Education:* 6%. Supports scholarship funds, internships, student aid, colleges and universities. *Environment:* 41%. Supports the Globe Santa Fund, for the purchase and distribution of holiday gifts for needy children. Also supports the United Way and human service agencies. *Note:* Total foundation contributions made from July 31, 1999 through December 31, 2000. **Typ. Recipients:** AIDS/HIV, Children's Health/Hospitals, Clinics/Medical Centers, Domestic Violence, Health Organizations, Hospitals, Medical Education, Medical Research, Mental Health, Nutrition, People with Disabilities, Substance Abuse. **Geo. Dist:** Boston, MA; Cambridge, MA; Chelsea, MA; Somerville, MA.

★ 12239 ★ Boswell Foundation, Inc.

1078 South Jefferson
Lebanon, MO 65536
Phone: (417)588-4151 **Fax:** (417)588-3344
Paul Walker, Secretary

Fnded: 1985. **Priorities:** *Arts & Humanities:* 22%. *Civic & Public Affairs:* 22%. *Education:* 39%. *Environment:* 3%. *International:* 1%. *Note:* Total contributions made in fiscal 2001. **Typ. Recipients:** Arthritis, Cancer, Family Planning, Health-General, Medical Education, Prenatal Health Issues, Public Health, Single-Disease Health Associations. **Geo. Dist:** nationally; Palm Beach, FL; Lebanon, MO.

★ 12240 ★ Bourns Foundation

1200 Columbia Ave.
Riverside, CA 92507
Phone: (909)781-5084 **Fax:** (909)781-5203
Gordon Bourns, President

Priorities: *Civic & Public Affairs:* 6%. *Education:* 81%. *Environment:* 1%. *International:* 12%. *Note:* Total foundation contributions made in fiscal 2001. **Typ. Recipients:** Cancer, Children's Health/Hospitals, Diabetes, Health-General, Hospices, Hospitals, Mental Health. **Geo. Dist:** CA, focusing on Inland Empire area of Southern California; UT.

★ 12241 ★ Bowater, Inc.

55 East Camperdown Way
Greenville, SC 29601-3597
Phone: (864)271-7733 **Fax:** (864)282-9594
Gordon Manuel, Director, Government Affairs

Priorities: *Arts & Humanities:* 10% to 15%. Museums, libraries, community arts, theater, and the performing arts. *Civic & Public Affairs:* About 5%. Supports economic development, environmental affairs, urban and community affairs, and zoos and botanical gardens. *Education:* About 25%. Colleges, universities, community colleges, continuing education programs, economic education, business education, and education for minorities. *International:* 45% to 50%. Hospitals, hospices, health organizations, aid for the disabled, community centers, drug abuse programs, shelters, and community service organizations. A large portion of funds in this category support the United Way. **Typ. Recipients:** Health Organizations, Hospitals. **Geo. Dist:** headquarters and operating communities.

★ 12242 ★ BP Amoco Foundation
200 East Randolph Drive
Chicago, IL 60601
Phone: (312)856-3147 **Fax:** (312)616-0826
Website: http://synergos.org/globalphilanthropy/organizations/bpamoco.htm
Sonya Jackson, President

Priorities: *Arts & Humanities:* 1%. Supports museums and theaters. *Civic & Public Affairs:* 77%. Supports ethnic organizations, philanthropic organizations, community development, and community foundations. *Education:* 9%. Supports universities, colleges, learning centers, schools, and education funds. To foster an effective educational system and adequate workforce pool that reflects the diversity of the people in Amoco communities. Supports university programs that target disciplines required in Amoco's business; precollege programs that focus on math, science, and economic education; programs that promote minority participation in technical fields; and national and local school reform efforts. Also supports precollege and higher education through matching gifts and volunteer efforts. *Environment:* 9%. Supports United Way, child welfare, recreation, and community service organizations. *International:* 1%. Supports health organizations and single-disease health associations. *Note:* Total foundation contributions made in 2000. **Typ. Recipients:** Cancer, Children's Health/Hospitals, Clinics/Medical Centers, Domestic Violence, Emergency/Ambulance Services, Health-General, Hospitals, Mental Health, People with Disabilities, Public Health, Research/Studies Institutes, Single-Disease Health Associations. **Geo. Dist:** headquarters and operating communities, nationally and internationally. **Frmly:** Amoco Foundation.

★ 12243 ★ Brayton Wilbur Foundation
345 California St., 27th Floor
San Francisco, CA 94104-2644
Phone: (415)772-4006 **Fax:** (415)772-4005
Brayton Wilbur, Jr., President

Fnded: 1947. **Priorities:** *Arts & Humanities:* 88%. *Civic & Public Affairs:* 7%. *Education:* Less than 1%. *Environment:* Less than 1%. *International:* 4%. *Note:* Total foundation contributions made in 2001. **Typ. Recipients:** Clinics/Medical Centers, Emergency/Ambulance Services, Family Planning, Health Organizations, Health-General, Hospices, Hospitals, People with Disabilities, Single-Disease Health Associations, Substance Abuse, Substance Abuse. **Geo. Dist:** headquarters and operating communities.

★ 12244 ★ The Bridgestone/Firestone Trust Fund
50 Century Boulevard
Nashville, TN 37214
Phone: (615)872-1415 **Fax:** (615)872-1414
Email: bfstrustfund@bfsusa.com
Bernice Csaszar, Administrator

Fnded: 1952. **Priorities:** *Arts & Humanities:* 15%. *Civic & Public Affairs:* 19%. *Education:* 24%. *Environment:* 30%. *International:* 5%. *Religion:* 1%. *Note:* Total foundation contributions made in 2001. **Typ. Recipients:** Children's Health/Hospitals, Emergency/Ambulance Services, Family Planning, Health Organizations, Health Policy/Cost Containment, Hospices, Hospitals, Medical Education, Medical Research, Nursing Services, People with Disabilities, Single-Disease Health Associations, Substance Abuse. **Geo. Dist:** headquarters and operating communities. **Frmly:** Bridgestone/Firestone, Inc.

★ 12245 ★ Briggs & Stratton Corp. Foundation
12301 West Wirth St.
Wauwatosa, WI 53222
Phone: (414)259-5333 **Fax:** (414)259-5773
Robert Heath, Secretary & Treasurer

Priorities: *Arts & Humanities:* 20%. Supports the United Performing Arts Fund, museums, theater, and music. *Civic & Public Affairs:* 4%. Supports community and economic development projects in Milwaukee, public policy, business and free enterprise, and industry concerns. *Education:* 40%. Support includes funding for scholarships to employees' children. Other interests include colleges and universities, schools in communities where the company has plants, precollege programs, and agricultural education. *Environment:* (Health and Welfare) 36%. Majority of support goes to the United Way; also funds human services for families and youth. Also supports children's health organizations. *Note:* Total foundation contributions made in fiscal 2001. **Typ. Recipients:** Children's Health/Hospitals, Health Funds, Health Organizations, Health-General, Heart, Long-Term Care, Medical Education, Nursing Services, Speech & Hearing, Substance Abuse, Trauma Treatment. **Geo. Dist:** principally near operating locations and to national organizations; Milwaukee, WI.

★ 12246 ★ Bristol-Myers Squibb Foundation Inc.
345 Park Ave.
New York, NY 10154
Phone: (212)546-4000
Website: http://www.bms.com/aboutbms/founda/data/index.html
John Damonti, Foundation Coordinator

Fnded: 1990. **Priorities:** *Arts & Humanities:* 1%. *Civic & Public Affairs:* 20%. *Education:* 19%. *Environment:* 45%. *International:* 3%. *Note:* Total foundation giving in 2000. **Typ. Recipients:** AIDS/HIV, Cancer, Children's Health/Hospitals, Clinics/Medical Centers, Diabetes, Emergency/Ambulance Services, Geriatric Health, Health Organizations, Health-General, Heart, Hospitals, Medical Education, Medical Rehabilitation, Medical Research, Medical Training, Mental Health, Nutrition, People with Disabilities, Public Health, Research/Studies Institutes, Substance Abuse, Transplant Networks/Donor Banks. **Geo. Dist:** headquarters and operating communities; internationally; nationally.

★ 12247 ★ Brown Shoe Co. Charitable Trust
c/o Suntrust Bank, Atlanta
PO Box 4655
Atlanta, GA 30302
Phone: (314)854-4000
Email: tmalecek@brownshoe.com
Thomas Malecek, Secretary, Board of Control

Priorities: *Arts & Humanities:* 20%. Supports music, art foundations, theaters, historic preservation, public broadcasting, and museums. *Civic & Public Affairs:* 21%. Supports botanical gardens, festivals, zoos, community foundations, and economic development. *Education:* 16%. Supports universities, colleges, education funds, and Junior Achievement. Matches employee gifts to private colleges and universities. *Environment:* 38%. Supports United Way and people with disabilities. *International:* 1%. Primary support made to health organizations. *Religion:* 1%. Primary support made to science centers. *Note:* Total foundation contributions made in 2001. **Typ. Recipients:** Alzheimers Disease, Children's Health/Hospitals, Domestic Violence, Emergency/Ambulance Services, Eyes/Blindness, Hospitals, Medical Research, Multiple Sclerosis, People with Disabilities, Prenatal Health Issues, Preventive Medicine/Wellness Organizations. **Geo. Dist:** principally near operating locations and to national organizations; St. Louis, MO.

★ 12248 ★ Brown & Williamson Tobacco Corp.
Brown & Williamson Tower 200
401 S Fourth St.
PO Box 35090
Louisville, KY 40202
Phone: (502)568-7451 **Fax:** (502)568-8262
Website: http://www.bw.com
Gail Strange, Sr. Mgr., Corp. and Community Relations

Typ. Recipients: Substance Abuse. **Geo. Dist:** headquarters and operating communities.

★ 12249 ★ Brunswick Foundation
One North Field Court
Lake Forest, IL 60045
Phone: (847)735-4667
Carol Stame, President

Priorities: *Arts & Humanities:* 1%. Support given to cultural arts and music. *Civic & Public Affairs:* 3%. Supports economic development and community foundations. *Education:* 86%. Supports colleges, universities, economic education programs, and scholarships to children of company employees. *Environment:* 6%. Supports YMCA, homes, family services, and Big Brothers/Sisters. *International:* 4%. Primarily supports single-disease health associations. *Note:* Total foundation contributions made in 2000. **Typ. Recipients:** Cancer, Children's Health/Hospitals, Clinics/Medical Centers, Diabetes, Emergency/Ambulance Services, Family Planning, Health Organizations, Heart, Hospices, Hospitals, Mental Health, Nursing Services, People with Disabilities, Prenatal Health Issues, Single-Disease Health Associations, Substance Abuse. **Geo. Dist:** principally near operating locations and to national organizations.

★ 12250 ★ The BTM Foundation
1251 Ave. of the Americas, 15th Fl.
New York, NY 10020-1104
Phone: (212)782-4627 **Fax:** (212)782-6420
Email: bgilroy@btmna.com
Beth Gilroy, Vice President

Priorities: *Civic & Public Affairs:* 76%. *Education:* 8%. *Environment:* 15%. *Note:* Total contributions made in 2001. **Typ. Recipients:** Substance Abuse. **Geo. Dist:** New York, NY, headquarters area only.

★ 12251 ★ Bucyrus-Erie Foundation
1020 N Broadway
Milwaukee, WI 53202
Phone: (414)272-5805 **Fax:** (414)290-7344
Email: cwilson@greatermkefdn.org
Carol Wilson, Scholarship Administrator

Priorities: *Arts & Humanities:* 29%. Funds museums, performing arts, public broadcasting, and libraries. *Civic & Public Affairs:* 9%. Supports public policy, environmental affairs, business/free enterprise, and urban and community affairs. *Education:* 11%. Emphasis on higher education institutions. Interests include technical and engineering education at the university level. Also supports scholarships, education funds, arts education, student aid, literacy programs, and public and private precollege education. *Environment:* 48%. Majority of funding supports united funds, youth programs, and community service organizations in Milwaukee County. Other interests include the handicapped, the prevention of domestic violence, homes, employment programs, and family service organizations. *International:* 2%. Focus on hospitals, pediatric health, and single-disease associations. *Note:* Total foundation contributions made in 2000. **Typ. Recipients:** Children's Health/Hospitals, Clinics/Medical Centers, Domestic Violence, Health Organizations, Hospitals, Long-Term Care, Medical Education, Medical Rehabilitation, Medical Research, People with Disabilities, Single-Disease Health Associations, Substance Abuse. **Geo. Dist:** WI, Milwaukee County; Milwaukee, WI, South Milwaukee.

★ 12252 ★ Burlington Industries Foundation
PO Box 21207
Greensboro, NC 27420-1207
Phone: (336)379-2303 **Fax:** (336)379-4504
Dolores Sides, Executive Director

Priorities: *Arts & Humanities:* 4%. Supports art councils, music, and museums. *Civic & Public Affairs:* 5%. *Education:* 46%. Supports colleges, universities, schools, and educational institutes. Primarily supports colleges and universities located in areas where there is a high concentration of employees and from which the company recruits. Interests include textiles-related education, and technological, engineering, and business education. Education associations and funds, public secondary education, university libraries, economic, arts, fashion design, and math education all receive funding. Grants in this field, awarded in the Southeast and nationally, generally range between $1,000 and $10,000. *Environment:* 37%. Supports United Way, family services, and scouts. *International:* 8%. Supports hospitals, hospices, and single-disease health associations. *Voluntarism:* Company does not have a formal employee volunteer program, but it provides meeting space on the premises or time off to individual employees who volunteer for Junior Achievement. Company also sponsors two Red Cross Blood Drives annually. *Note:* Total foundation contributions made in fiscal 2000. **Typ. Recipients:** AIDS/HIV, Children's Health/Hospitals, Clinics/Medical Centers, Emergency/Ambulance Services, Health Organizations, Hospices, Hospitals, Multiple Sclerosis, Outpatient Health Care, People with Disabilities, Preventive Medicine/Wellness Organizations, Respiratory, Single-Disease Health Associations, Substance Abuse. **Geo. Dist:** principally near operating locations and to national organizations; NC; SC; VA.

★ 12253 ★ Burlington Resources Foundation

5051 Westheimer, Suite 1400
Houston, TX 77056-5604
Phone: (817)347-2000
Gavin Smith, President

Priorities: *Arts & Humanities:* 4%. Interests include libraries, theater, performing arts, visual arts, and other related activities. *Civic & Public Affairs:* 3%. Supports affordable housing, zoos, municipalities, and crime prevention. *Education:* 66%. Gives to colleges and universities, with an emphasis on medical centers and medical research; supports primary and secondary schools. Also matches employee gifts to institutions of higher learning. *Environment:* 2%. Primarily supports United Way, child welfare, youth camps and organizations, services for the disabled, community service organizations, and athletics/recreation programs. *International:* 21%. Supports hospitals, cancer and heart centers, hospices, pregnancy centers, and single-disease health associations. *Religion:* 2%. Gives to the Houston Museum of Natural Science. *Note:* Total foundation contributions made in 2001. **Typ. Recipients:** Alzheimers Disease, Child Abuse, Children's Health/Hospitals, Emergency/Ambulance Services, Heart, Hospices, Medical Education, Medical Research, Nursing Services, People with Disabilities, Prenatal Health Issues, Preventive Medicine/ Wellness Organizations, Public Health, Single-Disease Health Associations.

★ 12254 ★ Business Men's Assurance Co. of America

700 Karnes Boulevard
BMA Tower, PO Box 419458
Kansas City, MO 64141-6458
Phone: (816)751-5742 **Fax:** (816)751-5710
Simonetta Balzer, Chair for Community Giving

Typ. Recipients: Health-General. **Geo. Dist:** headquarters; Kansas City, MO, metropolitan area.

★ 12255 ★ Butler Manufacturing Co. Foundation

1540 Genessee St.
Kansas City, MO 64141-0917
Phone: (816)968-3208 **Fax:** (816)968-6501
Email: blfay@butlermfg.org
Barbara Fay, Foundation Administrator

Priorities: *Arts & Humanities:* 28%. *Civic & Public Affairs:* 2%. *Education:* 26%. *Environment:* 43%. *International:* 1%. *Note:* Contributions analysis represents typical annual charitable contributions. Total contributions made in 2001. **Typ. Recipients:** Cancer, Children's Health/Hospitals, Children's Health/Hospitals, Clinics/Medical Centers, Emergency/Ambulance Services, Health Organizations, Health Policy/Cost Containment, Heart, Hospitals, Medical Education, Medical Rehabilitation. **Geo. Dist:** Kansas City, MO.

★ 12256 ★ C.R. Bard Foundation

114 W 47th St.
New York, NY 10036
Phone: (212)852-3834
Email: linda.hrevnack@crbard.com
Website: http://www.crbard.com/about/foundation.html

Fnded: 1988. **Priorities:** *Arts & Humanities:* 3%. Funds symphonies and theater. *Civic & Public Affairs:* 14%. Supports civic foundations. *Education:* 35%. Supports colleges, universities, and independent college funds. Focus on medical education and research, and programs which benefit the health-care industry. *Environment:* 19%. Supports United Way, shelters, children's services, camps and other youth organizations. *International:* 29%. Funds health-care associations, hospitals, emergency services, and single-disease health associations *Religion:* Less than 1%. Funds a science center. *Note:* Total contributions made in 2000. **Typ. Recipients:** AIDS/HIV, Cancer, Children's Health/Hospitals, Clinics/Medical Centers, Diabetes, Domestic Violence, Emergency/Ambulance Services, Geriatric Health, Health Funds, Health Organizations, Health-General, Heart, Hospices, Hospitals, Hospitals (University Affiliated), Kidney, Medical Education, Medical Rehabilitation, Medical Research, People with Disabilities, Preventive Medicine/Wellness Organizations, Public Health, Single-Disease Health Associations, Speech & Hearing, Substance Abuse. **Geo. Dist:** headquarters and operating communities.

★ 12257 ★ Cabot Corp. Foundation

Two Seaport Ln., Ste. 1300
Boston, MA 02210
Phone: (617)342-6004 **Fax:** (617)342-6312
Email: dorothy_forbes@cabot-corp.com
Dorothy Forbes, Executive Director, Vice President

Priorities: *Arts & Humanities:* 4%. Supports museums that promote science education and community arts organizations, including visual and performing arts groups in company operating communities. *Civic & Public Affairs:* 10%. Includes civic, health and welfare concerns. Priority is given to community projects involving company employees and retirees. Typical recipients include youth organizations, urban and community affairs groups, safety organizations, the handicapped, and hospitals. *Education:* 28%. Supports higher educational science and technology programs, placing priority on mathematics, physics, chemistry, and special disciplines, including ceramics, materials and polymer sciences, and chemical and metallurgical engineering. Special interest is in schools that encourage research by students and junior faculty. Also supports secondary school science and mathematics education, particularly programs focused on gifted students. Other interests include colleges and universities in company operating communities; skills development and occupational retraining, especially for minorities, women, and the handicapped; and, to a lesser degree, applied economics programs at all levels of education. Also supports educational public broadcasting and Junior Achievement. *Environment:* 23%. Supports child and youth services, and the United Way. *International:* 2%. Supports hospitals, medical centers and single-disease concerns. *Religion:* 11%. Supports American Association for the Advancement of Science; Massachusetts State Science Fair. *Note:* Total contributions in 1999. **Typ. Recipients:** Cancer, Child Abuse, Children's Health/Hospitals, Clinics/Medical Centers, Diabetes, Domestic Violence, Health Organizations, Health-General, Heart, Hospitals, Medical Education, People with Disabilities, Prenatal Health Issues, Public Health, Substance Abuse. **Geo. Dist:** principally near operating locations and to national organizations.

★ 12258 ★ California Bank & Trust

Community Development Department
11622 El Camino Real, Suite 200
San Diego, CA 92130
Phone: (858)793-7470 **Fax:** (858)793-7438
Website: http://www.calbanktrust.com/
Lynda Buckner, Vice President and Manager

Priorities: *Voluntarism:* Employees are encouraged to become involved in their communities through participation in local civic and government groups and whose primary focus is to improve economic development in the community. **Typ. Recipients:** Health Organizations, People with Disabilities. **Geo. Dist:** headquarters area only; CA, Supports organizations within the state of California with priority given to those with whom we have a banking relationship.

★ 12259 ★ Callaway Golf Co. Foundation

2180 Rutherford Rd.
Carlsbad, CA 92008-7328
Phone: (760)930-8686 **Fax:** (760)929-9780
Website: http://www.callawaygolf.com
Janet Hebert, Contact

Fnded: 1994. **Priorities:** *Arts & Humanities:* 3%. Supports a museum. *Civic & Public Affairs:* 7%. Supports entrepreneurship and technical training. *Education:* 16%. Funds literacy, scholarships, technical schools, and mentoring programs. *Environment:* 44%. Major support for at-risk youth. Also funds family violence prevention and services, counseling, shelters, and programs for the disabled. *International:* 27%. Supports dental care, clinics, hospitals, and hospice, with a focus on children's health. *Religion:* 2%. *Voluntarism:* Committee supports the Callaway Golf Community Program, which organizes one community services project per month for employee volunteers. *Note:* Total foundation contributions made in 2000. **Typ. Recipients:** Alzheimers Disease, Cancer, Child Abuse, Children's Health/Hospitals, Domestic Violence, Emergency/Ambulance Services, Eyes/ Blindness, Health Organizations, Health-General, Hospices, Medical Rehabilitation, Medical Research, People with Disabilities, Prenatal Health Issues, Public Health, Single-Disease Health Associations. **Geo. Dist:** CA, San Diego County.

★ 12260 ★ Calvin Klein Foundation

205 West 39th St.
New York, NY 10018
Phone: (212)719-2600 **Fax:** (212)292-9787
Joel Semel, Foundation Manager

Priorities: *Arts & Humanities:* 17%. Funds art museums, performing arts, photography, dance, and historic preservation. *Civic & Public Affairs:* 21%. Supports women's and gay/lesbian affairs, fashion trade organizations and charities, and urban development. *Education:* 9%. Gives to colleges and universities, and institutions providing fashion design education. *Environment:* 30%. Funds youth organizations, food/clothing distribution, substance abuse treatment, services for the disabled, animal welfare, and recreational and athletic associations. *International:* 18%. Supports medical centers, children's health, and single-disease health associations with a focus on cancer and AIDS research and treatment. *Note:* Total contributions made in fiscal 2001. **Typ. Recipients:** AIDS/HIV, Alzheimers Disease, Cancer, Children's Health/Hospitals, Clinics/Medical Centers, Diabetes, Health Organizations, Health-General, Hospitals, Long-Term Care, Medical Research, Mental Health, Multiple Sclerosis, People with Disabilities, Prenatal Health Issues, Single-Disease Health Associations, Substance Abuse.

★ 12261 ★ Campbell Soup Foundation

Campbell Place
Camden, NJ 08103-1799
Phone: (856)342-4800
Website: http://www.campbellsoupcompany.com/community_center.asp
J. Buckley, Chairman

Priorities: *Arts & Humanities:* 7%. Gives to arts centers and performing arts in Camden and plant communities. *Civic & Public Affairs:* 24%. Supports trade associations, housing, economic development, and minority affairs. *Education:* 8%. Emphasis on Camden area public education. Also supports colleges and universities that specialize in medical, engineering, and business education. *Environment:* 53%. Supports Camden youth organizations, the United Way, family services, recreation, community centers, homelessness programs, and people with disabilities. *International:* 4%. Funds medical research, pediatric health care, and eye care center. *Voluntarism:* Foundation operates a Dollars for Doers fund to support and reward company employees who volunteer in their communities; also supports a program in which employees tutor disadvantaged youth. Giving to the United Way is determined by employee involvement. *Note:* Total foundation contributions made in fiscal 2001. **Typ. Recipients:** Cancer, Children's Health/Hospitals, Clinics/Medical Centers, Diabetes, Emergency/Ambulance Services, Eyes/Blindness, Health-General, Heart, Hospitals, Kidney, Medical Education, Medical Research, Nutrition, Single-Disease Health Associations. **Geo. Dist:** headquarters and operating communities.

★ 12262 ★ Capital Group Companies Charitable Foundation

11100 Santa Monica Boulevard, 9th Floor
Los Angeles, CA 90025-3384
Phone: (310)996-6188
Roberta Conroy, Secretary

Fnded: 1998. **Typ. Recipients:** Children's Health/Hospitals, Medical Research, Substance Abuse.

★ 12263 ★ Cargill Foundation

PO Box 5650
Minneapolis, MN 55440-5650
Phone: (952)742-6290
Email: toni_green@cargill.com
Website: http://www.cargill.com/commun/found.htm
Toni Green, Senior Program Officer

Priorities: *Arts & Humanities:* 10%. Gives to music, theater, museums, art centers, libraries, and historical societies. *Civic & Public Affairs:* 11%. Supports minority affairs, urban and economic development, neighborhood associations, housing, municipalities, and community foundations. *Education:* 48%. Funds higher education, public schools, early learning programs, and programs for the learning disabled. *Environment:* 29%. Supports United Way, Young Men's Christian Association, family and youth services, and community centers. *International:* Less than 1%. Primarily supports national single-disease health associations. *Religion:* Less than 1%. A science museum receives funding. *Note:* Total foundation contributions in 2001. **Typ. Recipients:** AIDS/HIV, Cancer, Children's Health/Hospitals, Clinics/Medical Centers, Domestic Violence, Emergency/Ambulance Services, Eyes/Blindness, Family Planning, Health Organizations, Hospitals, Medical Education, People with Disabilities, Substance Abuse. **Geo. Dist:** headquarters and operating locations; internationally; nationally; Minneapolis, MN, including western and northern suburbs.

★ 12264 ★ Caring Foundation

c/o Blue Cross and Blue Shield of Alabama
450 Riverchase Pkwy. East
Birmingham, AL 35244-2858
Phone: (205)220-2100
Website: http://www.bcbsal.org/community/index.html
Mr. Terry Kellogg, Contact

Priorities: *Arts & Humanities:* 9%. Emphasis on the symphony, ballet, and opera. *Civic & Public Affairs:* 11%. Supports community foundations, Rotary Clubs, and a poison control center. *Education:* 14%. Provides major support to the University of Alabama. Also funds other institutions of higher education, Junior Achievement, education foundations, and public pre-college schools. *Environment:* 45%. Supports youth agencies, child welfare, and the United Way. *International:* 21%. Primarily supports single-disease health organizations. *Note:* Total contributions in 2000. **Typ. Recipients:** AIDS/HIV, Alzheimers Disease, Arthritis, Cancer, Children's Health/Hospitals, Diabetes, Domestic Violence, Emergency/Ambulance Services, Eyes/Blindness, Health Organizations, Health-General, Heart, Hospitals, Kidney, Medical Research, Multiple Sclerosis, People with Disabilities, Prenatal Health Issues, Public Health, Respiratory, Single-Disease Health Associations, Speech & Hearing, Substance Abuse, Trauma Treatment. **Geo. Dist:** nationally; AL.

★ 12265 ★ Carrier Corp.

PO Box 4808
Syracuse, NY 13221
Phone: (315)432-6000 **Fax:** (315)432-7898
Dan Fessenden, Director, Community Relations

Priorities: *Arts & Humanities:* 13%. Interests include performing arts groups, museums, arts education, dance, opera, historical societies, arts centers, orchestras, libraries, theater, and public broadcasting. *Civic & Public Affairs:* 13%. Support goes to community and public policy groups. *Education:* 33%. Supports various colleges and universities, professional and technical schools, and non-public secondary schools that include at least grades 9-12. *Environment:* 24%. Supports united funds, health organizations, rehabilitation, and programs for the mentally retarded. Emphasis is also on geriatric care and programs for the disabled. Some support is provided for youth groups and community service organizations. *Note:* Total contributions made in 2000. **Typ. Recipients:** Health Organizations, Hospitals, Medical Rehabilitation, Mental Health, People with Disabilities. **Geo. Dist:** principally near operating locations and to national organizations.

★ 12266 ★ Carris Corp. Foundation

PO Box 696
Rutland, VT 05702-0696
Phone: (802)773-9111
Karen O'Brien, Foundation Bookkeeper

Fnded: 1990. **Priorities:** *Arts & Humanities:* 38%. Supports fine arts studios, museums, and art councils. *Civic & Public Affairs:* 12%. Supports housing initiatives, community festivals, civil rights organizations, and community foundations. *Education:* 10%. Supports academies, schools, colleges, and youth education programs. *Environment:* 28%. Supports YMCA, domestic violence programs, United Way, Special Olympics, family services, animal protection, food distribution, volunteer groups, camps, and Big Brothers/Sisters. *International:* 10%. Supports nursing, health organizations, and single-disease health associations. *Note:* Total foundation contributions made in 2001. **Typ. Recipients:** AIDS/HIV, Cancer, Child Abuse, Children's Health/Hospitals, Diabetes, Domestic Violence, Emergency/Ambulance Services, Health Organizations, Health Organizations, Health-General, Heart, Hospitals, Nursing Services, People with Disabilities, Prenatal Health Issues, Public Health, Single-Disease Health Associations, Substance Abuse. **Geo. Dist:** headquarters and operating communities.

★ 12267 ★ Carter-Wallace Foundation

1345 Ave. of the Americas
New York, NY 10105-0302
Phone: (212)339-5010 **Fax:** (212)339-5100
Mr. James Wagar, Vice President & Treasurer

Priorities: *Arts & Humanities:* 13%. Supports opera and other music-oriented organizations, performing arts centers, libraries, public broadcasting, and museums. *Civic & Public Affairs:* 2%. Primarily supports parks. *Education:* 28%. Supports colleges and universities, education funds, and Junior Achievement. *Environment:* 10%. Supports United Way, people with disabilities, athletics, family planning, substance abuse programs, and crime prevention. *International:* 46%. Supports hospitals, medical centers, and single-disease health associations. *Religion:* 1%. Primary support made to science museums. *Note:* Total foundation contributions made in fiscal 2001. **Typ. Recipients:** Arthritis, Cancer, Children's Health/Hospitals, Clinics/Medical Centers, Eyes/Blindness, Family Planning, Health Organizations, Hospitals, Hospitals (University Affiliated), Medical Education, Medical Research, Mental Health, People with Disabilities, Public Health, Single-Disease Health Associations, Speech & Hearing, Substance Abuse. **Geo. Dist:** CT; Decatur, IL; NJ; NY.

★ 12268 ★ Castle & Cooke Inc.

PO Box 898900
Mililani, HI 96789-8900
Phone: (808)548-4811 **Fax:** (808)548-6662
Email: bmhayashi@castlecooke.com
Beverly Hayashi, Secretary to Management Committee

Typ. Recipients: Health-General. **Geo. Dist:** HI.

★ 12269 ★ Caterpillar Foundation

100 NE Adams St.
Peoria, IL 61629-1480
Phone: (309)675-4464 **Fax:** (309)675-5815
Website: http://www.cat.com/foundation
Henry Holling, Vice President

Fnded: 1952. **Priorities:** *Arts & Humanities:* 11%. Provides capital and operating grants to orchestras, opera, public broadcasting, museums, theater, and art associations. Also sponsors matching gifts program, which accounts for the largest share of cultural giving. *Civic & Public Affairs:* 9%. The majority of funding in this area is awarded directly by the company and primarily goes to public policy issues, urban affairs, communities, and economic development programs. *Education:* 42%. Supports colleges and universities, business, economic, and engineering education; student aid; universities and colleges; and education funds. *Environment:* 23%. United Ways in plant communities receive the majority of funding. Also supports youth organizations, programs for drug and alcohol abuse prevention, violence prevention programs, Young Men's Christian Association, scouts, and services for the disabled. *International:* 6%. Provides grants to local health institutions, the American Red Cross, physical rehabilitation centers, and single-disease associations. *Note:* Total contributions made in 2001. **Typ. Recipients:** Cancer, Domestic Violence, Emergency/Ambulance Services, Health Organizations, Hospices, Hospitals, Medical Education, Medical Rehabilitation, Mental Health, People with Disabilities, Sexual Abuse, Single-Disease Health Associations, Substance Abuse. **Geo. Dist:** operating locations; educational matching gifts program is international.

★ 12270 ★ CBS Foundation

51 West 52nd St.
New York, NY 10019
Phone: (212)975-3773
Ken Silverman, Foundation Contact

Priorities: *Arts & Humanities:* 36%. Supports public broadcasting, theaters and performing arts centers, film, art museums, film/broadcasting museums, and libraries. *Civic & Public Affairs:* 29%. Funds broadcasting and entertainment industry professional organizations, community organizations, minority affairs, and public policy groups. *Education:* 28%. Funds minority education, colleges and universities, foundations promoting higher education, and broadcasting education. *Environment:* 7%. Gives to Young Men's Christian Association, youth organizations, child welfare programs, and a radio reading service. *Note:* Total contributions made in 2000. **Typ. Recipients:** People with Disabilities. **Geo. Dist:** markets where CBS has major ownership presence.

★ 12271 ★ CCB Foundation

PO Box 931
Durham, NC 27702-0931
Phone: (919)683-7251 **Fax:** (919)682-3870
John Ramsey, President

Fnded: 1985. **Priorities:** *Arts & Humanities:* 22%. Supports historic preservation, museums, arts councils, theater, dance, libraries, orchestras, and public broadcasting. *Civic & Public Affairs:* 6%. Gives to urban affairs, economic development, affordable housing programs, chambers of commerce, parks, counties and municipalities. *Education:* 22%. Funds universities, colleges, education foundations, scholarship funds, and a teacher recruitment program. *Envi-*

ronment: 45%. Provides major funding to the United Way in communities where the company has a presence. Also supports Young Men's Christian Association, community centers, recreation/athletic programs, foundation's assets and contributions figures fall below established criteria.me prevention, child welfare/abuse prevention, and shelters. *International:* 2%. Hospitals, single-disease health associations, and public health programs receive support. *Religion:* 3%. Contributes to a science museum. *Note:* Total contributions made in 2000. **Typ. Recipients:** Cancer, Emergency/Ambulance Services, Health Organizations, Health-General, Hospitals. **Geo. Dist:** headquarters area only.

★ 12272 ★ Centex Corp.

PO Box 199000
Dallas, TX 75219
Phone: (214)981-5000 **Fax:** (214)981-6859
Website: http://www.centex.com/Community_Service/
Amy Nation, Secretary to the Chairman & CEO

Priorities: *Arts & Humanities:* 15%. *Civic & Public Affairs:* 59%. The Company supports Habitat for Humanity and Hearts and Hammers. *Education:* 12%. *International:* 14%. **Typ. Recipients:** Health-General. **Geo. Dist:** Dallas, TX, including metropolitan area.

★ 12273 ★ Central Maine Power Co.

83 Edison Dr.
Augusta, ME 04336
Phone: (207)623-3521 **Fax:** (207)623-5908
John Carroll, Community Relations Specialist

Priorities: *Civic & Public Affairs:* (United Funds & United Way) About 30%. Company favors contributions to organizations such as United Ways which channel assistance to agencies active in service area. Employee involvement, number of customers served, population density, plus the number of organizations, communities, and services provided by each United Way will determine amount of support. 5% to 10%. General support to groups improving the quality of life in areas where employees work and live. *Education:* About 15%. Supports colleges, universities, and technical schools in Maine on a case-by-case basis. Also supports educational programs outside Maine offering programs of interest to company, such as: energy seminars; secondary schools, including public and private institutions for special programs; economic education; and a limited scholarship program. *Environment:* Less than 5%. Supports youth organizations and activities that guide, counsel, and enrich the lives of young people. Recipients include 4-H, community centers, scouting, Junior Achievement, summer camps, camps for disabled children, child welfare, and children's homes. *International:* About 20%. Supports capital campaigns conducted by hospitals and health care centers in service area for new facilities, expansion or renovation, or specialized equipment. Also supports annual operating gifts, single-disease health associations, and health organizations active in service area. *Note:* Company reports that 15% of its contributions budget is given at the discretion of its local divisions. **Typ. Recipients:** Domestic Violence, Emergency/Ambulance Services, Family Planning, Geriatric Health, Health Organizations, Health-General, Hospices, Hospitals, Medical Rehabilitation, Mental Health, Nutrition, People with Disabilities, Public Health, Single-Disease Health Associations, Substance Abuse. **Geo. Dist:** ME, primarily central and southern Maine.

★ 12274 ★ Central Newspapers Foundation

care of Gannett Co., Inc.
1100 Wilson Boulevard
Arlington, VA 22234
Phone: (317)633-1299 **Fax:** (317)656-1435
Sandy Harless, Executive Director

Fnded: 1935. **Priorities:** *Education:* 100%. The majority of the foundation's support goes to grants and scholarship programs in journalism education at major colleges and universities in Indiana and Arizona. Also provides higher education scholarships to children of employees and paper carriers. *Note:* Total foundation contributions made in fiscal 2001. **Typ. Recipients:** Cancer, Eyes/Blindness, People with Disabilities, Preventive Medicine/Wellness Organizations. **Geo. Dist:** AZ; IN.

★ 12275 ★ Central Vermont Public Service Corp.

77 Grove St.
Rutland, VT 05701
Phone: (802)747-5672 **Fax:** (802)747-2188
Email: above@cvps.com
Website: http://www.cvps.com
Andrea Bove, Exec. Asst.

Typ. Recipients: Mental Health. **Geo. Dist:** VT.

★ 12276 ★ Century 21 Associates Foundation

22 Cortlandt St.
New York, NY 10007
Abraham Gindi, Trustee

Fnded: 1982. **Priorities:** *Education:* 2%. *Environment:* 1%. *International:* 12%. Funds medical centers, cancer research, hospitals, and other medical research. *Note:* Total contributions made in 1999. **Typ. Recipients:** Cancer, Diabetes, Hospitals, Hospitals (University Affiliated), Long-Term Care, People with Disabilities. **Geo. Dist:** NJ; NY.

★ 12277 ★ Cessna Foundation, Inc.

PO Box 7706
Wichita, KS 67277-7706
Phone: (316)517-7810 **Fax:** (316)517-7812
Marilyn Richwine, Secretary & Treasurer

Fnded: 1952. **Priorities:** *Arts & Humanities:* 9%. Supports arts associations, museums, history, music, and theater. *Education:* 49%. Funding supports colleges and universities, primarily in Kansas. Other interests include vocational, economic, and medical education. Administers employee matching gifts program to education, and administers Del Roskam Scholarship program for children or grandchildren of Cessna employees. *Environment:* 39%. Funding supports united funds and youth organizations. Other interests include athletic programs, people with disabilities, emergency relief, and food and clothing distribution. *International:* 3%. Funding supports health, including mental health and single disease health associations. *Note:* Total foundation contributions made in 2000. **Typ. Recipients:** AIDS/HIV, Cancer, Children's Health/Hospitals, Clinics/Medical Centers, Emergency/Ambulance Services, Health Funds, Health Organizations, Heart, Hospices, Hospitals, Medical Education, Multiple Sclerosis, People with Disabilities, Preventive Medicine/Wellness Organizations, Single-Disease Health Associations, Substance Abuse. **Geo. Dist:** principally near operating locations and to national organizations; Wichita, KS, including surrounding area.

★ 12278 ★ The Charitable Foundation of Frost National Bank of San Antonio

100 W Houston St.
San Antonio, TX 78205
Phone: (210)220-4449 **Fax:** (210)220-5144
William Clyborne, Executive Committee

Fnded: 1981. **Priorities:** *Arts & Humanities:* 22%. *Civic & Public Affairs:* 8%. *Education:* 27%. *Environment:* 36%. *International:* 5%. *Note:* Total contributions made in 2001. **Typ. Recipients:** Cancer, Children's Health/Hospitals, Domestic Violence, Health Organizations, Hospices, Hospitals, Medical Education, Medical Rehabilitation, Medical Research, Mental Health, People with Disabilities, Public Health, Single-Disease Health Associations, Substance Abuse. **Geo. Dist:** TX.

★ 12279 ★ Charles Schwab Corp. Foundation

101 Montgomery St., 28th Floor
MS-SF120KNY-28-353
San Francisco, CA 94104
Phone: 877-408-5438 **Fax:** (415)636-3262
Email: CIS@schwab.com
Website: http://www.aboutschwab.com/sstory/communityservices.html
Ms. Elinore Robey, Sr. Mgr., Community Investor Services

Priorities: *Arts & Humanities:* 7%. Emphasis on educational and community-based arts programs. Funds opera, museums, dance, theater, libraries, film, historic preservation/history organizations, and arts funds. *Civic & Public Affairs:* 16%. Supports housing, community initiatives, gay and lesbian affairs, nonprofit management, legal aid, women's/minority affairs, zoos, and philanthropic organizations. *Education:* 8%. Contributions support K-12 education especially school-to-career programs and literacy. Also provides limited support to institutions of higher learning and scholarship funds. *Environment:* 16%. Supports children and youth programs, food banks, animal welfare, senior services, community services, and the United Way. *International:* 48%. Supports AIDS/HIV programs, pediatric health and children's hospitals, cancer organizations, and public health initiatives. *Voluntarism:* The company has a formal employee volunteer program and sponsors various volunteer programs during the year throughout the U.S., including Habitat for Humanity and Christmas in April. *Note:* Total foundation contributions made in fiscal 2000. **Typ. Recipients:** AIDS/HIV, Cancer, Children's Health/Hospitals, Clinics/Medical Centers, Diabetes, Domestic Violence, Emergency/Ambulance Services, Family Planning, Health Organizations, Heart, Home-Care Services, Hospices, Kidney, Medical Research, Mental Health, Multiple Sclerosis, Nursing Services, People with Disabilities, Prenatal Health Issues, Single-Disease Health Associations, Transplant Networks/Donor Banks. **Geo. Dist:** communities where there are Schwab branch offices; San Francisco, CA.

★ 12280 ★ Charter Manufacturing Co. Foundation

411 East Wisconsin Ave., Suite 2040
Milwaukee, WI 53202-4497
Phone: (414)277-5000
Linda Mellowes, President

Priorities: *Arts & Humanities:* 1%. *Civic & Public Affairs:* Less than 1%. *Education:* 64%. *Environment:* 26%. *International:* 4%. *Note:* Total contributions in 2001. **Typ. Recipients:** Cancer, Children's Health/Hospitals, Domestic Violence, Family Planning, Health Organizations, Health-General, Hospitals, Medical Education, Medical Research, People with Disabilities, Single-Disease Health Associations, Transplant Networks/Donor Banks. **Geo. Dist:** WI, WI.

★ 12281 ★ Chemed Foundation

255 East 5th St., 2600 Chemed Center
Cincinnati, OH 45202
Phone: (513)762-6912
Sandra Laney, President & Director

Fnded: 1993. **Priorities:** *Arts & Humanities:* 7%. Supports arts funds, museums, music, theater, and public broadcasting. *Civic & Public Affairs:* 2%. Funds civic councils, legal aid, and justice issues. *Education:* 47%. Supports colleges, universities, schools, and Junior Achievement. *Environment:* 22%. Funds scouting and youth organizations, services for the disabled, food banks, and the United Way. *International:* 5%. Supports hospitals, health groups, and single-disease health associations. *Voluntarism:* Company employees help rehabilitate homes for community housing projects. *Note:* Total foundation contributions made in 2001. **Typ. Recipients:** Cancer, Children's Health/Hospitals, Diabetes, Emergency/Ambulance Services, Eyes/Blindness, Health-General, Medical Education, Multiple Sclerosis, People with Disabilities, Single-Disease Health Associations, Speech & Hearing. **Geo. Dist:** Cincinnati, OH, headquarters and operating communities.

★ 12282 ★ Chesapeake Corp. Foundation
PO Box 2350
Richmond, VA 23218
Phone: (804)697-1000 **Fax:** (804)697-1199

Priorities: *Arts & Humanities:* 14%. Funding emphasizes libraries and museums; also supports arts councils and performing arts. *Civic & Public Affairs:* 7%. Supports municipal initiatives, housing coalitions, women's issues, and other community services. *Education:* 8%. Funds educational funds; and higher education through scholarships for children of employees, an employee matching gifts program for education; and direct grants to colleges and universities. *Environment:* 36%. Supports scouts, and United Way. *International:* 17%. Supports hospitals and medical centers, emergency response services, and single-disease health associations. *Religion:* 17%. Funds a science museum. *Note:* Total contributions made in 2001. **Typ. Recipients:** Cancer, Children's Health/Hospitals, Clinics/Medical Centers, Diabetes, Domestic Violence, Emergency/Ambulance Services, Health Organizations, Hospitals, Medical Rehabilitation, Mental Health, Multiple Sclerosis, People with Disabilities, Research/Studies Institutes. **Geo. Dist:** operating locations.

★ 12283 ★ ChevronTexaco Corp.
Worldwide Headquarters
575 Market St.
San Francisco, CA 94105
Phone: (925)842-1000 **Fax:** (415)894-3583
Email: comment@chevrontexaco.com
Website: http://www.chevronTEXACO.com/social_responsibility/community/annual_contributions.asp

Priorities: *Arts & Humanities:* 6%. Supports visual, literary, performing arts and cultural institutions in communities where company has significant operations, principally in California. Also supports local arts funds and councils, community concerts, historic preservation, libraries, national and regional art associations, cultural centers, and theaters. *Civic & Public Affairs:* (Civic and Employee Involvement) 9%. Contributes to policy research and planning organizations and business/free enterprise groups; organizations that deal with individual initiatives, volunteerism, and philanthropy; and groups that promote community involvement and civic pride, law and justice, better government, and public safety. Other interests include urban planning and development programs and agricultural expositions and fairs. *Education:* 26%. Colleges and universities in fields of science, engineering, computer science, business, economics, communications, human resource development, equal access and quality in schools, and other disciplines of interest to the company. Funds are for scholarships, fellowships, department support, and research. Also supports a variety of educational organizations and funds. While most contributions continue to go to higher education, support for targeted programs that improve the quality of public education at the primary and secondary levels is increasing. Provides support for disadvantaged and under-represented minority students requiring accelerated instruction in grades K-12. Also matches gifts to education. instruction in grades K-12. Also matches gifts to education. *International:* (Health and Human Services) 18%. Health funding emphasizes hospitals and various local health organizations. Human services includes youth organizations; united funds; social welfare organizations that meet the needs of the homeless and abused and neglected children; groups that promote equal opportunity, equity, and access to the mainstream of society; job-readiness and employment programs; and programs targeted to the elderly. *Note:* Total contributions made in 2000. **Typ. Recipients:** AIDS/HIV, Clinics/Medical Centers, Domestic Violence, Emergency/Ambulance Services, Health Funds, Health Organizations, Health Policy/Cost Containment, Hospices, Hospitals, Medical Rehabilitation, Mental Health, People with Disabilities, Public Health, Single-Disease Health Associations, Substance Abuse. **Geo. Dist:** corporate operating locations nationally and internationally.

★ 12284 ★ Chicago Sun-Times Charity Trust
401 N Wabash Ave.
Chicago, IL 60611
Phone: (312)321-2213 **Fax:** (312)321-0629
Email: pdudek@hollingerintl.com
Website: http://www.suntimes.com
Patricia Dudek, Manager, Community & Client Services

Fnded: 1936. **Priorities:** *Arts & Humanities:* 8%. *Civic & Public Affairs:* 70%. *Education:* 2%. *Environment:* 17%. *International:* 3%. *Note:* Total contributions in fiscal 2001. **Typ. Recipients:** AIDS/HIV, Cancer, Child Abuse, Children's Health/Hospitals, Domestic Violence, Health-General, People with Disabilities. **Geo. Dist:** Chicago, IL, including metropolitan area.

★ 12285 ★ Chicago Title and Trust Co. Foundation
171 N Clark St., 9TF
Chicago, IL 60601-3294
Phone: (312)335-9386
Eileen Hughes, Treasurer

Fnded: 1951. **Priorities:** *Arts & Humanities:* 27%. Supports major cultural institutions such as theaters, art institutes, festivals, and libraries. Also operates an Employee Matching Gift for PBS Programs with grants to Chicago stations and others throughout the United States. *Civic & Public Affairs:* 24%. Focus on strengthening the social and economic position of the community. Funds housing projects, services for the disadvantaged through job training, mentoring, and help programs. Supports parks, cultural diversity, and economic development. *Education:* 10%. Supports higher education, primarily through an employee matching gift program. Other education support includes Junior Achievement, grants for improvement of existing facilities, and for specific objectives with established needs evidenced by stable or growing enrollment. *Environment:* 37%. Emphasis on supporting youth by developing mentoring programs and youth groups. Recipients include United Way, youth programs, and Planned Parenthood. *International:* 2%. Limited funding supports American Red Cross, disease-specific organizations, and hospitals. *Religion:* Less than 1%. *Note:* Total foundation contributions made in 2000. **Typ. Recipients:** Cancer, Child Abuse, Children's Health/Hospitals, Clinics/Medical Centers, Diabetes, Emergency/Ambulance Services, Eyes/Blindness, Family Planning, Health Organizations, Hospitals, Long-Term Care, Medical Education, Multiple Sclerosis, Respiratory, Single-Disease Health Associations, Trauma Treatment. **Geo. Dist:** Chicago, IL.

★ 12286 ★ Chicago Tribune Foundation
435 N Michigan Ave., Suite 200
Chicago, IL 60611-4041
Phone: (312)222-4300 **Fax:** (312)222-3751
Email: ctcommunityrelations@tribune.com
Website: http://www.chicagotribune.com/extras/comrel/
Frank Gihan, President

Priorities: *Arts & Humanities:* 38%. *Civic & Public Affairs:* 34%. *Education:* 21%. *Environment:* 5%. *International:* 1%. *Voluntarism:* The company's TribUnity program directs volunteer efforts toward reading and hunger issues. *Note:* The company also helps raise money for Chicago area causes through the Chicago Tribune Charities Program by sponsoring local fundraising events. The program works in partnership with the Robert R. McCormick Tribune Foundation; focuses are employment and literacy. The Chicago Tribune Holiday Fund generates contributions from the public to address basic human needs for children, people with developmental disabilities, the homeless, and the hungry. Total contributions made in 2001. **Typ. Recipients:** AIDS/HIV, Child Abuse, Children's Health/Hospitals, Domestic Violence, Emergency/Ambulance Services, Health Organizations, People with Disabilities, Prenatal Health Issues, Substance Abuse, Transplant Networks/Donor Banks. **Geo. Dist:** Chicago, IL, including metropolitan area.

★ 12287 ★ CHS Cooperatives Foundation
5500 Cenex Drive
Inver Grove Heights, MN 55077
Phone: (651)451-5481 **Fax:** (651)451-5073
Email: wnels@chsco-ops.com
Website: http://www.cenexharveststates.com/nav/indexABOUTCHS.htm
William Nelson, President

Fnded: 1947. **Priorities:** *Civic & Public Affairs:* 32%. *Education:* 67%. *Environment:* 1%. *Note:* Total contributions made in 2001. **Typ. Recipients:** Emergency/Ambulance Services, Health-General, Medical Research, People with Disabilities. **Geo. Dist:** CO; ID; IA; KS; MN; MT; NE; ND; OR; SD; UT; WA; WA; WI.

★ 12288 ★ CIGNA Foundation
Tax Department
1601 Chestnut St., TL06B
Philadelphia, PA 19192
Phone: (215)761-1000 **Fax:** (215)761-5632
Email: deborah.veney-robinson@cigna.com
Website: http://www.cigna.com/general/about/community/index.html
Deborah Veney-Robinson, Director, Civic Affairs

Priorities: *Arts & Humanities:* 17%. *Civic & Public Affairs:* 25%. *Education:* 13%. *Environment:* 37%. *International:* 6%. *Religion:* 1%. *Voluntarism:* Foundation sponsors three "Employee Recognition Awards," which acknowledge employee volunteer efforts. Through the "Grants for Givers" program, employees and retirees who volunteer a significant amount of their time to qualifying nonprofits can request foundation grants of $100 for their organizations. If three or more employees volunteer for the same project, the organization could receive up to $5,000 through the CIGNA Team Award. The Volunteer of the Month award recognizes superior employee volunteer efforts with a $500 grant to the organization benefiting from the employee's volunteerism. *Note:* Total foundation contributions made in 2001. **Typ. Recipients:** Adolescent Health Issues, Cancer, Children's Health/Hospitals, Clinics/Medical Centers, Health Organizations, Health-General, Hospitals, Medical Education, People with Disabilities, Prenatal Health Issues, Public Health. **Geo. Dist:** Hartford, CT, including metropolitan area; Philadelphia, PA, including metropolitan area.

★ 12289 ★ Cincinnati Bell Foundation, Inc.
201 East Fourth St.
Rm 102-840
Cincinnati, OH 45202
Phone: (513)397-7862 **Fax:** (513)723-9815
Kim Sheehy, Contact

Priorities: *Arts & Humanities:* 33%. *Civic & Public Affairs:* 8%. *Education:* 20%. *Environment:* 30%. *International:* 5%. *Note:* Total foundation contributions made in 2001. **Typ. Recipients:** Cancer, Children's Health/Hospitals, Clinics/Medical Centers, Emergency/Ambulance Services, Hospices, Hospitals, Medical Education, People with Disabilities, Public Health, Single-Disease Health Associations, Speech & Hearing. **Geo. Dist:** areas where employees live and work.

★ 12290 ★ Cinergy Foundation
139 E 4th St.
Cincinnati, OH 45202
Phone: (513)287-1251 **Fax:** (513)651-9196
Email: kking@cinergy.com
Website: http://www.cinergy.com/Community/default.asp
Karol King, Foundation Manager

Fnded: 1992. **Priorities:** *Arts & Humanities:* Supports visual and performing arts, cultural programs, and arts education in company's service area. *Civic & Public Affairs:* Supports projects that help communities help themselves. Supports the environment through environmental education, park development and enhancement, resource preservation, reforestation, and recycling; and youth development. *Education:* Supports two primary areas: workforce development and staff development. Workforce development projects create a fundamental, seamless, results-based system that enhances the way youth are prepared to meet the demands of a highly skilled workforce, including school-to-work and career development initiatives; increase academic standards; and encourage lifelong learning. Staff development projects encourage continuous improvement in teaching and expanded leadership roles for all teachers, including providing peer assistance and review; training for teachers to take on new roles within the school as mentors, facilitators, community liaisons,curriculum development and assessment experts; enhance educators' ability to observe exemplary teaching practices, conduct and review research, plan for school improvement, and integrate technlogy; individualize instruction; and facilitate schools' efforts to reach out effectively to parents and the community. *International:* Supports health and social service programs which promotehealthy lifestyles and preventative medical care. Major support to the United Way. **Typ. Recipients:** Children's Health/Hospitals, Emergency/Ambulance Services, Health-General, Hospitals, Mental Health, People with Disabilities, Prenatal Health Issues, Single-Disease Health Associations, Substance Abuse. **Geo. Dist:** IN, company service area; KY, Northern Kentucky (company service area); OH, company service area. **Frmly:** PSI Energy Foundation.

★ 12291 ★ Circuit City Foundation

9950 Mayland Drive
Richmond, VA 23233
Phone: (804)527-4000 **Fax:** (804)527-4173
Jane Gurganus, Contact

Priorities: *Arts & Humanities:* 10%. Major emphasis is on public broadcasting; also supports museums, the performing arts, arts centers, and historical societies. *Civic & Public Affairs:* 8%. Funding is provided to community affairs organizations, police agencies and volunteer fire departments, economic development, job training, botanical gardens, African-American affairs, and women's groups. *Education:* 22%. Foundation focused its education giving to concentrate on public education reform; support also goes to higher education. *Environment:* 50%. Supports YMCA, United Way, youth organizations, family services, and aid to persons with disabilities. *International:* 1%. Grants generally benefit hospitals, single-disease health organizations, and the American Red Cross. *Religion:* 1%. Funds science museums. *Note:* Total contributions made in fiscal 2001. **Typ. Recipients:** Emergency/Ambulance Services, Heart, Multiple Sclerosis, People with Disabilities, Sexual Abuse, Single-Disease Health Associations, Transplant Networks/Donor Banks. **Geo. Dist:** communities where employees live and work.

★ 12292 ★ CIRI Foundation

2600 Cordova St., Suite 206
Anchorage, AK 99503
Phone: (907)265-5900 **Fax:** (907)263-5588
Email: tcf@ciri.com
Website: http://www.ciri.com/about_ciri/tcs
Lydia Hays, Contact

Fnded: 1982. **Priorities:** *Education:* 100%. Major support is given to scholarships and higher education. *Note:* Total foundation contributions made in 2000. **Typ. Recipients:** Medical Education. **Geo. Dist:** national.

★ 12293 ★ Cisco Systems Foundation

170 West Tasman Drive
San Jose, CA 95134
Phone: (408)526-4000
Website: http://www.cisco.com/warp/public/750/philanthropy/
Lynne Elliott, Contact

Typ. Recipients: AIDS/HIV, Cancer, Children's Health/Hospitals, Clinics/Medical Centers, Domestic Violence, Health Organizations, Hospices, People with Disabilities, Single-Disease Health Associations, Substance Abuse. **Geo. Dist:** San Jose area, CA; MA; NY; NC.

★ 12294 ★ CIT Group Foundation

1211 Ave. of the Americas
New York, NY 10036
Phone: (973)740-5200 **Fax:** (973)740-5264
Website: http://www.cit.com/about_us/corp_giving.html
Kelley Gibson, Contact

Priorities: *Arts & Humanities:* 15%. Supports music, performing arts, libraries, historical preservation, and museums. *Civic & Public Affairs:* 3%. Emphasis is on economic development, minority affairs, and industry concerns. *Education:* 33%. Supports scholarships, schools, business education, student aid, private education, and education reform. Other interests include minority education, enrichment programs, and education funds. Also supports matching gifts to colleges and universities. *Environment:* 28%. Majority of funding supports United Way and youth organizations. Also supports community centers, people with disabilities, and substance abuse organizations. *International:* 20%. Supports clinics, hospitals, hospice, single-disease associations, emergency care, and children's healthcare. *Note:* Total foundation contributions made in 2000. **Typ. Recipients:** AIDS/HIV, Arthritis, Cancer, Children's Health/Hospitals, Clinics/Medical Centers, Diabetes, Emergency/Ambulance Services, Health Organizations, Heart, Hospitals, Medical Research, Mental Health, Nursing Services, People with Disabilities, Single-Disease Health Associations, Substance Abuse, Transplant Networks/Donor Banks, Trauma Treatment. **Geo. Dist:** nationally, with an emphasis on headquarters area only.

★ 12295 ★ Citigroup Foundation

850 Third Ave., 13th Floor
New York, NY 10043
Phone: (212)559-9163 **Fax:** (212)793-5944
Email: citigroupfoundation@citigroup.com
Website: http://www.citigroup.com
Charles Raymond, President

Priorities: *Arts & Humanities:* 2%. *Civic & Public Affairs:* 58%. *Education:* 19%. *Environment:* 12%. *International:* 1%. *Religion:* 1%. *Voluntarism:* The corporation's volunteer incentive program provides up to $500 for organizations to which employees volunteer. *Note:* Total foundation contributions and corporate direct giving in 1999. **Typ. Recipients:** Children's Health/Hospitals, Emergency/Ambulance Services, Health Organizations, Health Policy/Cost Containment, Hospices, Hospitals, Hospitals (University Affiliated), Medical Research, People with Disabilities, Single-Disease Health Associations, Substance Abuse, Transplant Networks/Donor Banks. **Geo. Dist:** headquarters and operating communities; New York, NY.

★ 12296 ★ Citizens Bank-Flint

328 South Saginaw St.
Flint, MI 48502
Phone: (810)766-7500 **Fax:** (810)766-7634
Website: http://www.citizensonline.com
David Albert, Assistant Vice President

Typ. Recipients: Adolescent Health Issues, Children's Health/Hospitals, Clinics/Medical Centers, Family Planning, Health-General, Medical Education, People with Disabilities. **Geo. Dist:** headquarters and operating communities.

★ 12297 ★ Citizens Banking Corp. Charitable Foundation

328 S Saginaw St., 001051
Room 001051
Flint, MI 48502
Phone: (810)766-7789

Fnded: 1999. **Priorities:** *Arts & Humanities:* 2%. Gives to arts councils, libraries, music, historical societies, public broadcasting, and museums. *Civic & Public Affairs:* 46%. Supports community and economic development, community foundations, festivals, business associations, and affordable housing. *Education:* 8%. Contributes to colleges, universities, scholarship funds, public schools, 4-H, Junior Achievement, and economic education. *Environment:* 34%. Funds youth organizations, scouting, Young Men's Christian Association, camps, senior services, soup kitchens and food banks, family and children's services, community centers, and the United Way. *International:* 10%. Gives to single-disease health associations, hospitals, medical centers, nursing homes, hospice, and health foundations. *Note:* Total contributions made in 2002. **Typ. Recipients:** Cancer, Emergency/Ambulance Services, Health-General, Heart, Hospitals. **Geo. Dist:** IA; MI; WI.

★ 12298 ★ Citizens Charitable Foundation

1 Citizens Plaza
Providence, RI 02903-1339
Phone: (401)456-7285 **Fax:** (401)456-7644
D. Sanders, Senior Vice President

Priorities: *Arts & Humanities:* 8%. Supports museums, music, and the performing arts. *Civic & Public Affairs:* 28%. Supports economic development organizations, a tax clinic, low-income housing, minority affairs, and business groups. *Education:* 19%. Funds colleges and universities, medical schools, economic education, and programs for community education. Also provides scholarships. *Environment:* 38%. Supports United Way, child welfare, youth organizations, community centers, day care, and community service organizations. *International:* 1%. Supports medical information dissemination and general medical organizations. *Note:* Total contributions made in 2000. **Typ. Recipients:** AIDS/HIV, Children's Health/Hospitals, Clinics/Medical Centers, Emergency/Ambulance Services, Geriatric Health, Health Organizations, Hospices, Hospitals, Medical Education, Medical Rehabilitation, Medical Research, Mental Health, Nursing Services, People with Disabilities, Prenatal Health Issues, Public Health, Sexual Abuse, Single-Disease Health Associations, Substance Abuse. **Geo. Dist:** RI.

★ 12299 ★ CLARCOR Foundation

2323 6th St.
Rockford, IL 61125
Phone: (815)962-8867 **Fax:** (815)962-0417
David Lindsay, Chairman

Priorities: *Arts & Humanities:* 15%. Includes support for music, theater, historic preservation projects, and dance groups. *Civic & Public Affairs:* 7%. Gives to economic development and neighborhood/community enhancement projects. *Education:* 25%. Supports business education and colleges and universities. *Environment:* 39%. Supports the United Way, child welfare and youth organizations, veterans groups, and family services. *International:* 1%. Recipients include health organizations, hospitals, and mental health centers. *Religion:* 2%. *Note:* Total contributions made in 2000. **Typ. Recipients:** Cancer, Clinics/Medical Centers, Clinics/Medical Centers, Emergency/Ambulance Services, Health Funds, Health Organizations, Hospices, Hospitals, Long-Term Care, Mental Health, Nursing Services, People with Disabilities, Public Health, Respiratory, Single-Disease Health Associations, Substance Abuse. **Geo. Dist:** operating locations only.

★ 12300 ★ The Cleveland-Cliffs Foundation

1100 Superior Ave. East
Cleveland, OH 44114-2589
Phone: (216)694-5700 **Fax:** (216)694-6741
Website: http://www.cleveland-cliffs.com/GeneralInformation
Dana Byrne, Vice President, Assistant Treasurer

Priorities: *Arts & Humanities:* 17%. Supports museums, music, theater, public libraries, and art funds. *Civic & Public Affairs:* 21%. Interests include municipalities, urban leagues, legal foundations, better business, botanical gardens, zoological parks, and economic development. *Education:* 27%. Education foundations and college funds, including business, economic, minority, private, and public education. Supports matching gifts to education institutions. *Environment:* 27%. Supports United Way, emergency relief, family services, and child welfare. *International:* 3%.

Recipients include health foundations, clinics, and hospitals. *Religion:* 2%. Supports a science center and minerals groups. *Note:* Total contributions made in 2001. **Typ. Recipients:** Cancer, Children's Health/Hospitals, Clinics/Medical Centers, Emergency/Ambulance Services, Health Organizations, Heart, Hospitals, People with Disabilities, Preventive Medicine/Wellness Organizations, Public Health. **Geo. Dist:** nationally; Washington, DC; MI; OH; nationally.

★ 12301 ★ Cline Foundation
PO Box 3768
Greenville, SC 29608
Phone: (864)233-7104
Nesbit Cline, Sr., Chairman, President & CEO

Priorities: *Environment:* 97%. *Note:* Total contributions made in 1999. **Typ. Recipients:** Emergency/Ambulance Services. **Geo. Dist:** Greenville, SC.

★ 12302 ★ Clorox Co. Foundation
1221 Broadway, 13th Floor
Oakland, CA 94612-1888
Phone: (510)271-2199 **Fax:** (510)271-7757
Email: community.relations@clorox.com
Website: http://www.clorox.com/company/foundation
Carmella Johnson, Contributions Manager

Fnded: 1980. **Priorities:** *Arts & Humanities:* 10%. Funding is awarded to music, theater, community arts, and dance organizations in California. Other interests include museums, opera, painting/sculpture, ethnic arts, and arts festivals and centers. *Civic & Public Affairs:* 10%. Civic interests include civil rights, low-income housing, law and justice, economic development, parks and the environment, technical assistance, volunteer development, and conflict resolution programs. *Education:* 49%. Emphasis is on quality of education for all young people from kindergarten through college, particularly public school reform with attention to minority and low-income youth. Education grants will increasingly focus on K-12, as well as preschool and early childhood development programs that emphasize prevention and intervention through mentoring, tutoring, and parent involvement. Of special interest are drop-out prevention, programs designed to help students develop tools for learning, programs that actively involve parents and the community in the educational process, job readiness and career development, and programs that provide for and nurture students from infancy through high school and beyond. Matches employee contributions to higher education. Funds the Clorox Partners Scholarships for college education. *Environment:* 25%. Primarily funds United Way and youth organizations. Supports family counseling, and programs which promote positive relationships among youth from diverse cultural and ethnic groups. Includes support for employee matching gifts. *International:* 2%. Supports disaster relief. *Religion:* 1%. Contributes to science centers. *Voluntarism:* The company reports that more than one-third of employees in its General Offices and its Technical Center volunteer time at more than 375 agencies. The Clorox Employee Volunteer Program identifies volunteer opportunities, disseminates information about community agencies and programs to employees, and helps match volunteers with organizations. Company awards $200 grants to organizations where employees volunteer. *Note:* Foundation contributions made in fiscal 2001, excluding program-related investments and matching gifts. **Typ. Recipients:** Children's Health/Hospitals, Clinics/Medical Centers, Domestic Violence, Emergency/Ambulance Services, Family Planning, Geriatric Health, Health Funds, Health Organizations, Hospices, Hospitals, Mental Health, People with Disabilities, Prenatal Health Issues, Public Health, Research/Studies Institutes, Single-Disease Health Associations, Substance Abuse. **Geo. Dist:** operating locations; Oakland, CA; San Francisco, CA, including metropolitan area.

★ 12303 ★ CNA Foundation
CNA Plaza
Chicago, IL 60685
Andrea Sinisi, Executive Director

Fnded: 1995. **Priorities:** *Arts & Humanities:* 10%. Provides funding to a variety of causes, including music, theater, and art institutes. *Civic & Public Affairs:* 31%. Grants support professional organizations (especially those related to the insurance industry) and encourage community economic development and the advancement of sound civic policy. Funds programs that address affordable housing, leadership development, job creation and overall economic development in depressed neighborhoods. *Education:* 31%. The company encourages pre-collegiate education programs that strengthen public schools and school reform through the advancement of basic curriculum, enhanced learning opportunities and faculty development. Another area of interest is pre-collegiate mathematics and science. Emphasis is placed on programs that encourage innovations in the teaching and learning of mathematics and science. Provides matching gifts to higher education institutions. *Environment:* 22%. Primary support for the United Way. Also funds child welfare and youth organizations, food distribution, and other social services. *International:* 1%. Supports health organizations located in communities where the company has a presence. *Note:* Total contributions in 2000. **Typ. Recipients:** AIDS/HIV, Child Abuse, Children's Health/Hospitals, Diabetes, Emergency/Ambulance Services, Health Organizations, Health-General, Heart, Hospitals, Medical Research, Mental Health, People with Disabilities. **Geo. Dist:** in communities where co. has a presence.

★ 12304 ★ CNF Transportation, Inc.
3240 Hillview Ave.
Palo Alto, CA 94304
Phone: (650)494-2900 **Fax:** (650)813-0164
Susan Allen, Manager, Corporate Contributions

Priorities: *Civic & Public Affairs:* Supports organizations involved in the community and public well-being similar to United Way. *Education:* Supports scholarship programs. **Typ. Recipients:** People with Disabilities. **Geo. Dist:** nationally, with an emphasis on areas where company operates.

★ 12305 ★ Coachmen Industries, Inc.
PO Box 3300
Elkhart, IN 46515
Phone: (574)262-0123 **Fax:** (574)206-0063
Email: blenhart@coachmen.com
Bill Lenhart, Senior Vice President, Human Resources

Typ. Recipients: Health-General. **Geo. Dist:** headquarters area only.

★ 12306 ★ Coca-Cola Foundation
One Coca-Cola Plaza NW
Atlanta, GA 30313
Phone: (404)676-3525 **Fax:** (404)676-8804
Website: http://www2.coca-cola.com/citizenship/foundation.html
Ingrid Jones, Chairman

Fnded: 1984. **Priorities:** *Arts & Humanities:* 5%. *Civic & Public Affairs:* 5%. *Education:* 83%. *Environment:* 3%. *Religion:* 1%. *Voluntarism:* Company sponsors an employee volunteer reaching-out program. *Note:* Total foundation contributions made in 2001. **Typ. Recipients:** Medical Education. **Geo. Dist:** internationally; nationally.

★ 12307 ★ Colgate-Palmolive Co.
300 Park Ave.
New York, NY 10022
Phone: (212)310-2175 **Fax:** (212)310-2873
Website: http://colgate.com/cp/corp.class/colgate_cares/index.jsp
Sally Phipps, Contributions Manager

Typ. Recipients: Health-General.

★ 12308 ★ Collins & Aikman Foundation
701 McCullough Drive
Charlotte, NC 28232
Phone: (704)548-2389 **Fax:** (704)548-2391
Arlene Bookman, Administrator

Priorities: *Arts & Humanities:* 1%. Major interests are music, arts outreach programs, and performing arts. *Civic & Public Affairs:* 4%. Supports community foundations, urban affairs, zoos, fire departments, and civic groups. *Education:* 10%. Majority of grants benefit colleges and universities, with limited support to Junior Achievement. Also supports educational matching gifts and scholarship funds. *Environment:* 36%. Majority of funding supports United Ways in various communities. Remaining funds generally support youth organizations and family services. *International:* 5%. Funding supports hospitals, an ophthalmology institute, and cancer organizations. *Religion:* 43%. Provides a major grant to the Institute of Textile Technology. Also funds a science museum. *Note:* Total contributions made in 2001. **Typ. Recipients:** AIDS/HIV, Cancer, Clinics/Medical Centers, Eyes/Blindness, Health Organizations, Hospices, Hospitals, Medical Research, Nursing Services, People with Disabilities, Public Health, Single-Disease Health Associations, Substance Abuse, Trauma Treatment. **Geo. Dist:** operating locations.

★ 12309 ★ Colonial Foundation
PO Box 576
Savannah, GA 31402
Phone: (912)236-1331
Francis Brown, Vice President, Finance & CFO

Fnded: 1986. **Priorities:** *Arts & Humanities:* 14%. Supports historic preservation, museums, public broadcasting, and performing arts. *Civic & Public Affairs:* 3%. Funds citizen advocacy groups, low-income housing, legal aid, and chambers of commerce. *Education:* 38%. Funds higher education, scholarship programs, Junior Achievement, family literacy, and private pre-college education. *Environment:* 31%. Primarily funds United Way, Young Men's Christian Association, food banks, family services, and youth groups. *International:* 11%. Gives to hospice and single-disease health associations. *Religion:* Less than 1%. Funds a science museum. *Note:* Total contributions in 2001. **Typ. Recipients:** Arthritis, Cancer, Children's Health/Hospitals, Diabetes, Emergency/Ambulance Services, Health Organizations, Health-General, Hospices, Long-Term Care, People with Disabilities, Prenatal Health Issues, Respiratory, Sexual Abuse, Single-Disease Health Associations. **Geo. Dist:** GA.

★ 12310 ★ Colonial Life & Accident Insurance Co.
1200 Colonial Life Blvd.
PO Box 1365
Columbia, SC 29202
Phone: (803)213-5634 **Fax:** (803)213-7461
Email: dcnortham@unum.com
Website: http://www.coloniallife.com/about/ColonialCares.asp
Donna Northam, Assistant Vice President

Priorities: *Arts & Humanities:* About 20%. Favors local ballet, symphony, and museums. *Civic & Public Affairs:* 20%%. Supports better government, economic development, housing, community affairs, and national security. *Education:* 20%. Interests include teacher training and development programs, college scholarships, K-12 mentoring programs, and colleges, universities, and community colleges. *International:* 30%. Interests include homeless shelters, AIDS and drug abuse education projects, child abuse prevention, and elder-care. **Typ. Recipients:** Domestic Violence, Emergency/Ambulance Services, Family Planning, Geriatric Health, Health Policy/Cost Containment, Hospices, Hospitals, Medical Research, Medical Training, Mental Health, Nursing Services, People with Disabilities, Public Health, Single-Disease Health Associations, Substance Abuse. **Geo. Dist:** SC.

★ 12311 ★ Columbia/HCA Healthcare Foundation
PO Box 570
Nashville, TN 37202
Phone: (615)344-2509 **Fax:** (615)344-5722
Website: http://www.hcacaring.org
Lois Abrams, Foundation Administrative Coordinator

Priorities: *Civic & Public Affairs:* 15%. *Education:* 39%. *Environment:* 28%. *International:* 15%. *Note:* Total contributions made in 2001. **Typ. Recipients:** Cancer, Children's Health/Hospitals, Clinics/Medical Centers, Emergency/Ambulance Services, Health-General, Hospitals, Medical Education, Medical Rehabilitation, Prenatal Health Issues. **Geo. Dist:** headquarters and operating communities; Louisville, KY; TN.

★ 12312 ★ Comerica Charitable Foundation

500 Woodward Ave.
Detroit, MI 48226-3352
Phone: (313)222-3571 **Fax:** (313)222-8720
Email: caroline_chambers@comerica.com
Website: http://Comerica.com/cma/cda/main/0.1555.1_A_1472.00.html
Caroline Solomon-Chambers, Corporate Contributions Vice President

Fnded: 1997. **Priorities:** *Arts & Humanities:* 20%. Recipients include museums, opera, arts centers and institutes, and libraries. *Civic & Public Affairs:* (Housing & Neighborhood Revitalization) 33%. Contributes to revitalize the cities near operating locations, including projects to rehabilitate or construct housing in low- to moderate-income neighborhoods, and efforts to stimulate business growth. *Education:* 9%. Supports minority and independent college funds, colleges and universities, United Negro College Fund, public broadcasting, science centers, and business and free enterprise education programs for youth. Matches employee gifts to higher education. *Environment:* 28%. Supports United Way and federated campaigns, youth organizations, and food banks. *International:* 7%. Recipients include hospitals and single-disease health associations. *Religion:* 2%. *Voluntarism:* Company offers Comerica Cares program in which employees participate in volunteer activities of community organizations. *Note:* Total foundation contributions made in 2000. **Typ. Recipients:** Cancer, Children's Health/Hospitals, Emergency/Ambulance Services, Health Organizations, Health Organizations, Hospices, Hospitals, Medical Rehabilitation, Mental Health, People with Disabilities, Single-Disease Health Associations. **Geo. Dist:** CA; FL; MI, especially southeastern MI; TX. **Frmly:** Comerica Foundation.

★ 12313 ★ Commerce Bancshares Foundation

PO Box 13095
Kansas City, MO 64199-3095
Phone: (816)234-2985
Michael Fields, President

Fnded: 1952. **Priorities:** *Arts & Humanities:* 10% to 15%. Supports Kansas City arts organizations, including music, public television, and a museum. *Civic & Public Affairs:* 10% to 15%. Supports housing and economic development, civil rights, public protection, employment, and local civic organizations. *Education:* 10% to 15%. Supports institutions of higher education in Missouri, including colleges, universities, military schools, and education funds. Provides some support for public education. Also supports science and social science programs. *Environment:* 60% to 65%. Primarily supports the United Way, recreation, youth development, food distribution, and other human service organizations. *International:* 3%. *Religion:* 1%. *Voluntarism:* The company actively encourages employee volunteerism. Employees and executives also are active in United Way, Habitat for Humanity, and numerous community organizations. *Note:* Total contributions made in 2001. **Typ. Recipients:** Cancer, Children's Health/Hospitals, Clinics/Medical Centers, Domestic Violence, Emergency/Ambulance Services, Family Planning, Health Organizations, Health-General, Hospitals, Public Health, Single-Disease Health Associations, Substance Abuse. **Geo. Dist:** West Central, IL; KS; MO.

★ 12314 ★ Commercial Intertech Foundation

PO Box 239
Youngstown, OH 44501
Phone: (330)746-8011 **Fax:** (330)746-0422
Mary Tanner, Executive Assistant to CEO

Priorities: *Arts & Humanities:* 8%. Supports symphonies, art associations, public radio, and public television. *Civic & Public Affairs:* 6%. *Education:* 28%. Gives to colleges and universities, primarily in Ohio. *Environment:* 50%. Primarily gives to United Way; also supports drug abuse prevention. *International:* 7%. Supports hospices and medical centers. **Typ. Recipients:** Cancer, Children's Health/Hospitals, Children's Health/Hospitals, Clinics/Medical Centers, Diabetes, Domestic Violence, Emergency/Ambulance Services, Family Planning, Health Organizations, Health-General, Heart, Home-Care Services, Hospices, Hospitals, Long-Term Care, Multiple Sclerosis, People with Disabilities, Public Health, Single-Disease Health Associations, Speech & Hearing, Substance Abuse. **Geo. Dist:** OH.

★ 12315 ★ Commonwealth Edison Co.

PO Box 767
Chicago, IL 60690
Phone: (312)394-4361 **Fax:** (312)394-3552
Email: leslie.jackson@exeloncorp.com
Steve Salomon, Corporate Affairs Associate

Priorities: *Arts & Humanities:* 12%. Supports a wide variety of activities; largest contributions are awarded to major institutions within service area. Offers modest contributions to broad range of smaller organizations. *Civic & Public Affairs:* 35%. Primarily United Funds & United Way with emphasis on Metropolitan Crusade of Mercy. Other interest include urban development, particularly in low-income areas of northern Illinois. *Education:* 32%. Priority is higher education, particularly private institutions within company's service area. *Environment:* 18%. Supports various welfare and community organizations. *International:* 3%. Emphasis is on hospitals, which generally receive only capital support; also limited support for other health activities. *Note:* Total contributions made in 1997. **Typ. Recipients:** Health Organizations, Hospitals, Single-Disease Health Associations, Substance Abuse. **Geo. Dist:** Chicago, IL, including surrounding area.

★ 12316 ★ Compass Bank Foundation

PO Box 10566
15 S 20th St.
Birmingham, AL 35296
Phone: (205)933-3960 **Fax:** (205)933-3336
Jerry Powell, Jr., Contact

Fnded: 1981. **Priorities:** *Arts & Humanities:* 12%. Supports fine arts, children's theater, festivals, opera, orchestras, and arts councils. *Civic & Public Affairs:* 21%. Funds public affairs, urban revitalization programs, and community foundations. *Education:* 18%. Funds higher education, scholarships, and Junior Achievement. *Environment:* 43%. Primarily supports United Way, youth and social services. *International:* 5%. Funds community health, hospice, American Red Cross, and single-disease associations. *Note:* Total contributions made in 2001. **Typ. Recipients:** Cancer, Children's Health/Hospitals, Clinics/Medical Centers, Diabetes, Emergency/Ambulance Services, Health Funds, Health Organizations, Heart, Hospices, Hospitals, Kidney, Mental Health, Multiple Sclerosis, People with Disabilities, Speech & Hearing, Transplant Networks/Donor Banks. **Geo. Dist:** AL; AZ; FL; TX.

★ 12317 ★ Computer Associates International, Inc.

1 Computer Associates Plaza
Islandia, NY 11749
Phone: (631)342-6225 **Fax:** (631)342-5737
Email: communityrelations@ca.com
Website: http://www.ca.com/community/
Bonnie Burk, Administrative Assistant

Priorities: *Environment:* Provides community grants in support of programs for children in pre-K through grade 12. Also awards diversity grants to fund initiatives that benefit children of diverse cultural and ethnic backgrounds and children with developmental disabilities. **Typ. Recipients:** Health-General. **Geo. Dist:** nationally.

★ 12318 ★ ConAgra Foods Foundation

1 ConAgra Drive
Omaha, NE 68102-5001
Phone: (402)595-4000 **Fax:** (402)595-4595
Website: http://www.conagra.com/conagra_foundation.jsp
Lynn Phares, Vice President, Corporate Relations

Priorities: *Arts & Humanities:* 27%. Supports theater, museums, arts festivals, opera. *Civic & Public Affairs:* 13%. Supports housing, safety, municipalities/towns, botanical centers. *Education:* 29%. Supports scholarships, colleges, universities, literacy, schools, and minority education. *Environment:* 27%. Supports United Way, scouting, shelters, food banks, child welfare, Special Olympics, Young Men's Christian Association. *International:* 3%. *Note:* Total contributions made in 1999. **Typ. Recipients:** Clinics/Medical Centers, Emergency/Ambulance Services, Health Organizations, Hospices, Nursing Services, Nutrition, People with Disabilities, Substance Abuse. **Geo. Dist:** primarily in locations where there are major ConAgra facilities. **Frmly:** ConAgra Foundation.

★ 12319 ★ Connecticut Energy Foundation, Inc.

10 State House Square, 6th Floor
PO Box 1500
Hartford, CT 06144-1500
Phone: (860)727-3102 **Fax:** (860)727-3064
Website: http://www.cngcorp.com/community_center/index.html
William Reis, Trustee

Priorities: *Arts & Humanities:* 12%. Funds history organizations. *Education:* 88%. Supports a college. *Note:* Total contributions made in fiscal 2001. **Typ. Recipients:** People with Disabilities. **Geo. Dist:** Avon, CT; Berlin, CT; Bloomfield, CT; Canton, CT; East Granby, CT; East Hartford, CT; Farmington, CT; Glastonbury, CT; Granbury, CT; Greenwich, CT; Hartford, CT; Manchester, CT; Mansfield, CT; Marlborough, CT; New Britain, CT; Newington, CT; Portland, CT; Rocky Hill, CT; Simsbury, CT; West Hartford, CT; Wethersfield, CT; Windsor, CT.

★ 12320 ★ ConocoPhillips

600 N Dairy Ashford
3130 Marland Bldg.
Houston, TX 77079
Phone: (281)293-1000 **Fax:** (281)293-1440
Website: http://www.conocophillips.com/about/contributions.asp
Clara Bradley, Administrator, Corporate Contributions

Priorities: *Civic & Public Affairs:* (Civic & the Arts) 15%. Supports organizations involved with energy industry-related issues, tourism in operating communities, and international relations and trade. Funds arts associations, including almost one-third to educational television. Other interests include art centers, theater, and historical societies. Programs which introduce K-12 students to the arts and humanities are favored. *Education:* (Education & Youth) 48%. Primarily reflects the interests of the company, such as engineering and geoscience. Fellowship and research grants account for about one-tenth of this support and encompass agronomy and graduate education and research in chemistry, engineering, geophysics, geology, combustion, and polymer science. Significant support also goes to colleges and universities for miscellaneous purposes including scholarships; programs in chemistry, science, and technology; and unrestricted operating support. Educational contributions are limited to schools or organizations whose location, facilities, or curricula are beneficial to the communities from which the company recruits. Company also sponsors a matching gifts program and a scholarship program for employees' children. Also funds educational film series to promote interest in mathematics and science careers. Supports youth organizations, including child welfare programs, boys' and girls' clubs, Junior Achievement, and boy and girl scouts in locations where company operates. *International:* (Health & Safety) 23%. United funds, community services, substance abuse prevention, and health agencies. Emphasis on Oklahoma and Texas. *Note:* Total contributions made during the period 2000-2001. The company reports that Health & Safety giving was larger than normal during this period due to a substantial contributions made to assist the victims of the September 11 terrorist attacks. **Typ. Recipients:** Clinics/Medical Centers, Domestic Violence, Geriatric Health, Health Organizations, Hospitals, Medical Education, Medical Rehabilitation, Medical Research, Mental Health, Nutrition, People with Disabilities, Public Health, Substance Abuse. **Geo. Dist:** headquarters and operating communities.

★ 12321 ★ Consolidated Products Foundation

36 S Pennsylvania St., Suite 500
Indianapolis, IN 46204-3630
Phone: (317)633-4100

Fnded: 1995. **Priorities:** *Civic & Public Affairs:* 1%. Gives to public policy organizations and an urban league. *Education:* 55%. Supports public universities and a learning academy. *Environment:* 43%. Funds local United Ways. *International:* 1%. Contributes to single-disease health associations. *Note:* Total contributions made in fiscal 2001. **Typ. Recipients:** Cancer, Single-Disease Health Associations. **Geo. Dist:** headquarters and operating communities.

★ 12322 ★ Constellation Energy Group, Inc.

PO Box 1475
Baltimore, MD 21203-1475
Phone: (410)783-3273 **Fax:** (410)783-3279
Email: Malinda.B.Small@constellation.com
Website: http://www.constellation.com/about/givingfocus.asp
Malinda Small, Director, National-State Affairs

Fnded: 1986. **Priorities:** *Arts & Humanities:* 19%. Funds art galleries and museums, historical societies, and performing arts organizations. *Civic & Public Affairs:* 1%. Gives to economic development and community foundations. *Education:* 29%. Supports institutions of higher learning. *Environment:* 35%. Provides major support to the United Way; also funds child and family services. *International:* 7%. Contributes to health foundations, hospitals, and medical centers. *Religion:* 2%. Gives to an academy of sciences. *Voluntarism:* The company sponsors an employee volunteer program aimed at increasing pride, motivation, and participation by allowing volunteers to direct their own program. *Note:* Total contributions made by Baltimore Gas & Electric Foundation in 2000. Constellation Energy Group's priorities differ from those of the foundation. See Philosophy (below) for additional information. **Typ. Recipients:** Child Abuse, Clinics/Medical Centers, Health Organizations, Hospices, Hospitals, Medical Education, People with Disabilities, Public Health. **Geo. Dist:** headquarters and operating communities.

★ 12323 ★ Consumers Energy Foundation

One Energy Plaza
Jackson, MI 49201
Phone: (517)788-0432 **Fax:** (517)788-2281
Email: foundation@consumersenergy.com
Website: http://www.consumersenergy.com/welcome.htm
Carolyn Bloodworth, Secretary/Treasurer

Priorities: *Arts & Humanities:* Interests include museums, symphonies, and theater. *Civic & Public Affairs:* Supports economic development and job training, housing, and public affairs. *Education:* Supports Michigan colleges and universities, K-12 education, specialized educational foundations, and programs that improve the curricula for business, economics, engineering, math, and the natural and physical sciences. *Environment:* Majority of support goes to the United Way. *International:* Supports American Red Cross and cancer research. *Note:* Total contributions made in 2001. **Typ. Recipients:** Alzheimers Disease, Cancer, Children's Health/Hospitals, Emergency/Ambulance Services, Hospitals, People with Disabilities, Substance Abuse. **Geo. Dist:** nationally; MI.

★ 12324 ★ ContiGroup Companies Foundation

277 Park Ave.
New York, NY 10172-0003
Phone: (212)207-5879 **Fax:** (212)207-5163
Susan McIntyre, Assistant Secretary

Priorities: *Arts & Humanities:* 21%. Supports performing arts, museums, and The Library of Congress. *Civic & Public Affairs:* 7%. Funds leadership development and community development. *Education:* 35%. Supports colleges and universities, business education, scholarship funds, and education foundations. *Environment:* 20%. Supports youth organizations, including YMCAs and Girl Scouts councils. *International:* 2%. Gives to single-disease health organizations. *Note:* Total contributions made in fiscal 2001. **Typ. Recipients:** Alzheimers Disease, Cancer, Children's Health/Hospitals, Clinics/Medical Centers, Emergency/Ambulance Services, Hospitals, Multiple Sclerosis, Nursing Services, People with Disabilities, Single-Disease Health Associations, Substance Abuse. **Geo. Dist:** Midwest; NY.

★ 12325 ★ Conwood Charitable Trust

701 Main St.
Memphis, TN 38101
Phone: (901)523-6200
David Simpson, III, General Counsel

Fnded: 1952. **Priorities:** *Arts & Humanities:* 9%. Funds museums and arts councils, public broadcasting, and ballet. *Civic & Public Affairs:* 10%. Supports housing, leadership, and gardens. *Education:* 15%. Colleges, universities, public grade schools, and Junior Achievement are funded. *Environment:* 25%. Youth organizations, food banks, and the United Way receive support. *International:* 16%. Supports hospitals and single-disease associations with a pediatric health focus. *Note:* Total contributions in 2000. **Typ. Recipients:** Children's Health/Hospitals, Clinics/Medical Centers, Diabetes, Health-General, Kidney, Medical Research, People with Disabilities, Single-Disease Health Associations. **Geo. Dist:** headquarters area only. **Frmly:** American Snuff Co. Charitable Trust.

★ 12326 ★ Cooper Industries Foundation

PO Box 4446
Houston, TX 77210-4446
Phone: (713)209-8607 **Fax:** (713)209-8982
Website: http://www.cooperindustries.com/about/index.htm
Jennifer Evans, Director, Community Affairs

Priorities: *Arts & Humanities:* 13%. Supports opera, symphonies, museums, public broadcasting, art leagues, theaters, and dance. *Civic & Public Affairs:* 5%. Funds public safety, fire prevention, zoos, parks, housing, and special projects. *Education:* 17%. Supports scholarships, Junior Achievement, vocational education, alumni associations, and higher education. *Environment:* (Health and Human Services) 52%. Funds United Way, child care, charitable medical programs, disease prevention, disaster relief, homeless shelters, hospitals, scouting, YMCA, sports, and Special Olympics. *International:* 5%. *Voluntarism:* The company sponsors a volunteer Spirit Awards program at all of its international locations. In 1996, Cooper recognized 31 volunteers in nine countries, enabling them to direct cash contributions totaling $46,500 to the nonprofit organizations of their choice. *Note:* Total contributions made by the foundation in 2001. **Typ. Recipients:** Cancer, Children's Health/Hospitals, Emergency/Ambulance Services, Health Funds, Health Organizations, Heart, Hospices, Hospitals, Medical Education, Mental Health, People with Disabilities, Single-Disease Health Associations, Substance Abuse. **Geo. Dist:** operating locations.

★ 12327 ★ Cooper Tire & Rubber Foundation

701 Lima Ave.
Findlay, OH 45840
Phone: (419)423-1321 **Fax:** (419)424-4212
Website: http://www.cooperindustries.com/about/index.htm
Philip Weaver, Trustee

Priorities: *Arts & Humanities:* 5%. Supports arts associations, public broadcasting, and museums. *Civic & Public Affairs:* 10%. Supports job training and trade associations. *Education:* 44%. Funding supports universities, technical colleges, secondary education, and business education. *Environment:* 39%. Emphasis is on united funds, youth organizations, and senior services. *International:* 1%. Funds single-disease health organizations and hospitals. *Religion:* 1%. *Note:* Total contributions made in 2000. **Typ. Recipients:** Cancer, Clinics/Medical Centers, Emergency/Ambulance Services, Health-General, Hospitals, Medical Rehabilitation, People with Disabilities, Public Health. **Geo. Dist:** operating locations; OH.

★ 12328 ★ Copolymer Foundation

PO Box 2591
Baton Rouge, LA 70821
Phone: (225)267-3400 **Fax:** (225)267-3623
Larry Powell, Chairman, President & CEO

Priorities: *Arts & Humanities:* 15%. Supports public broadcasting and historic associations. *Civic & Public Affairs:* 22%. Supports community foundations and minority organizations. *Education:* 44%. Supports made to colleges, universities, and scholarship funds. *Environment:* 18%. Supports Special Olympics, food distribution, and crime prevention programs. *International:* 1%. Primarily supports single-disease health associations. *Note:* Total contributions made in fiscal 2001. **Typ. Recipients:** Arthritis, Cancer, Child Abuse, Domestic Violence, Hospices, Medical Research, Single-Disease Health Associations. **Geo. Dist:** LA.

★ 12329 ★ Corning Inc. Foundation

MP-LB-02
Corning, NY 14831
Phone: (607)974-8719 **Fax:** (607)974-4756
Email: martinkc@corning.com
Website: http://www.corning.com/inside_corning/foundation.asp
Kristin Swain, President

Priorities: *Arts & Humanities:* 29%. Emphasis is on cultural programs that support art preservation, art museums, performing arts, opera, and art workshops. Usually supports large cultural organizations. Support to cultural organizations includes art education, arts organizations, libraries, museums, and public broadcasting. *Civic & Public Affairs:* 32%. Community and civic issues funding includes youth organizations including scouts and Boys & Girls Clubs, community foundations, public policy research, natural disaster relief, emergency relief, and international organizations that directly benefit the US. Supports U.S.-based organizations with an international focus. Interests include community development in the Third World and foreign policy and international relations. *Education:* 28%. Recipients include colleges and universities, private elementary and secondary schools and public schools. Program supports the engineering grants-in-aid project, which provides assistance to women and other minority students enrolled at selected colleges of engineering. Also supports engineering education and career development projects, predoctoral science fellowships and special projects, with emphasis on the physical sciences. *Environment:* 11%. Supports the United Way. *Religion:* 5%. *Note:* Total contributions made in 2001. **Typ. Recipients:** Clinics/Medical Centers, Emergency/Ambulance Services, Family Planning, Hospices, Hospitals (University Affiliated), Medical Rehabilitation, Substance Abuse. **Geo. Dist:** headquarters and operating communities and nationally; internationally to U.S.-based organizations.

★ 12330 ★ Courts Foundation
1530 SunTrust Tower
25 Park Pl., NE
Atlanta, GA 30303-2917
Phone: (404)658-9066 **Fax:** (404)659-4802
John Stephenson, Executive Director

Fnded: 1950. **Priorities:** *Arts & Humanities:* 9%. Funds arts centers and festivals, museums, and dance. *Civic & Public Affairs:* 29%. Supports community foundations, a botanical garden, economic development, and legal affairs. *Education:* 43%. Funds pre-college and higher education. *Environment:* 6%. Supports United Way, scouting, and family services. *International:* 2%. Supports hospitals, hospice, and single-disease health associations. *Religion:* Less than 1%. *Note:* Total foundation contributions made in 2000. **Typ. Recipients:** Cancer, Children's Health/Hospitals, Clinics/Medical Centers, Diabetes, Emergency/Ambulance Services, Eyes/Blindness, Health Organizations, Heart, Hospices, Hospitals, Medical Education, Mental Health, People with Disabilities. **Geo. Dist:** headquarters and operating communities.

★ 12331 ★ Cowen Foundation
1221 Ave. of the Americas
New York, NY 10020
Robert Greenberger, Director, Taxes

Fnded: 1990. **Priorities:** *Arts & Humanities:* 2%. Supports museums and music. *Civic & Public Affairs:* 2%. *Education:* 42%. Supports colleges, universities, schools, and educational funds. *Environment:* 18%. Supports United Way, scouting, youth programs, and human services. *International:* 21%. Supports medical centers, hospitals, and medical research. *Note:* Total foundation contributions made in 2000. **Typ. Recipients:** AIDS/HIV, Cancer, Children's Health/Hospitals, Clinics/Medical Centers, Diabetes, Emergency/Ambulance Services, Eyes/Blindness, Health Organizations, Heart, Hospitals, Hospitals (University Affiliated), Long-Term Care, People with Disabilities, Single-Disease Health Associations, Transplant Networks/Donor Banks. **Geo. Dist:** NY; PA.

★ 12332 ★ CP&L Foundation
Posee Statement 2
Raleigh, NC 27602-1551
Phone: (919)546-4112 **Fax:** (919)546-4338
Website: http://www.progress-energy.com/community/
Tammy Brown, Manager, Corporate Community Relations

Priorities: *Arts & Humanities:* 11%. Supports local arts groups, museums, music, and dance. *Civic & Public Affairs:* 15%. Funds business and free enterprise, legal affairs, community foundations, and parks. *Education:* 53%. Supports engineering, minority, liberal arts, science, and math education at colleges, universities, and schools. *Environment:* 11%. Supports United Way, food banks, and athletics and recreation. *International:* 3%. Funds medical foundations. *Religion:* 2%. Funds science museums. *Note:* Total foundation contributions made in 2000. **Typ. Recipients:** Child Abuse, Emergency/Ambulance Services, Health Organizations, Hospitals, Single-Disease Health Associations. **Geo. Dist:** principally near operating locations and to national organizations. **Frmly:** CP&L Foundation.

★ 12333 ★ CPI Corp. Philanthropic Trust
1706 Washington Ave.
Saint Louis, MO 63103
Phone: (314)231-1575 **Fax:** (314)231-2398
Fran Scheper, Exec. Vice President, Human Resources

Priorities: *Arts & Humanities:* 22%. *Civic & Public Affairs:* 6%. *Education:* 20%. *Environment:* 45%. *International:* 5%. *Note:* Total contributions made in fiscal 2002. **Typ. Recipients:** Children's Health/Hospitals, Domestic Violence, Eyes/Blindness, Geriatric Health, Health Organizations, Health-General, Hospitals, Multiple Sclerosis, People with Disabilities, Respiratory. **Geo. Dist:** near headquarters.

★ 12334 ★ Crane & Co. Fund
30 South St.
Dalton, MA 01226
Phone: (413)684-2600 **Fax:** (413)684-1820
Liz Pomeroy, Executive Secretary

Fnded: 1953. **Priorities:** *Arts & Humanities:* 36%. Supports museums, theater, historic preservation, music, and the performing arts. *Civic & Public Affairs:* 3%. Supports business organizations, Native American affairs, community affairs, and local trade associations. *Education:* 20%. Funds the Zenas Crane Fund for Student Aid. Colleges and universities and educational programs also receive funding. *Environment:* 22%. Majority supports youth organizations. Additional recipients include organizations for people with disabilities, religious welfare, and community centers. *International:* 12%. A local medical center, health organizations, and emergency services receive funding. *Note:* Total contributions made in 2000. **Typ. Recipients:** Cancer, Child Abuse, Children's Health/Hospitals, Clinics/Medical Centers, Diabetes, Emergency/Ambulance Services, Eyes/Blindness, Health Funds, Health Organizations, Health-General, Heart, Hospices, Hospitals, Hospitals (University Affiliated), Kidney, People with Disabilities, Public Health, Respiratory, Single-Disease Health Associations, Substance Abuse. **Geo. Dist:** MA, Berkshire County and near headquarters.

★ 12335 ★ Crane Foundation
100 First Stamford Pl.
Stamford, CT 06902
Phone: (203)363-7268 **Fax:** (203)363-7295
Email: crfdn@craneco.com
Gil Dickoff, Treasurer

Fnded: 1951. **Priorities:** *Arts & Humanities:* 11%. Supports arts councils, libraries, museums, historical preservation, and the performing arts. *Civic & Public Affairs:* 16%. Legal affairs, municipalities, zoos and parks receive support. *Education:* 45%. Funds colleges, universities, and private pre-college education. *Environment:* 9%. Funds family services and athletic organizations. *International:* 12%. Supports hospitals, medical services, and healthcare. *Note:* Total foundation contributions made in 2000. **Typ. Recipients:** Cancer, Child Abuse, Diabetes, Domestic Violence, Emergency/Ambulance Services, Eyes/Blindness, Health Organizations, Hospitals, Medical Research, Mental Health, Multiple Sclerosis, People with Disabilities, Public Health, Single-Disease Health Associations, Substance Abuse, Transplant Networks/Donor Banks. **Geo. Dist:** headquarters and operating communities.

★ 12336 ★ Cranston Foundation
1381 Cranston St.
Cranston, RI 02920
Phone: (401)943-4800 **Fax:** (401)943-3971
Email: cpw@cpw.com
Carolyn Lake, Administrator

Priorities: *Arts & Humanities:* 1%. Interests include museums, libraries, music, historic preservation, and arts councils. *Civic & Public Affairs:* 1%. Favors housing projects, youth organizations, and ambulance and fire safety services. *Education:* 80%. Majority of funding supports scholarships to colleges and universities, primarily for children of company employees. Also, a few direct grants are given to education. Foundation also operates matching grants program. *Environment:* 11%. Supports United Way and Young Men's Christian Association. *International:* 6%. Focus on hospitals. *Note:* Total contributions made in fiscal 2001. **Typ. Recipients:** Emergency/Ambulance Services, Hospitals, Kidney, Medical Education, Prenatal Health Issues. **Geo. Dist:** FL; MA; NY; RI.

★ 12337 ★ Credit Suisse First Boston Foundation Trust
11 Madison Ave.
New York, NY 10010
Phone: (212)325-2389 **Fax:** (212)538-4633
Email: casey.karel@csfb.com
Website: http://www.csfb.com/about_csfb/company_information/foundation/index.shtml
Ms. Casey Karel, Vice President

Fnded: 1959. **Priorities:** *Arts & Humanities:* 7%. Support is for major nationally oriented groups and community-based organizations. Supports museums, music, theater, dance, and performing arts centers. *Civic & Public Affairs:* 57%. Supports ethnic organizations and community development projects. Major grant to Robin Hood Foundation ($1,000,000). *Education:* 33%. Grants support educational initiatives and inner-city youth programs. *Environment:* 54%. Supports organizations in the New York area or in cities where company has branch offices. Interests include shelters for the homeless, child welfare, volunteer services, sports and recreation, and youth development, including those organizations serving at-risk youth. *International:* 6%. Supports single-disease associations, nutrition, and children's health. *Voluntarism:* The company encourages employee volunteerism in programs such as Publicolor, Habitat for Humanity, Everybody Wins, and Big Brothers/Big Sisters. *Note:* Total contributions made in 2001. **Typ. Recipients:** Cancer, Children's Health/Hospitals, Clinics/Medical Centers, Emergency/Ambulance Services, Hospitals, Medical Research, Mental Health, People with Disabilities, Prenatal Health Issues, Single-Disease Health Associations, Transplant Networks/Donor Banks. **Geo. Dist:** headquarters and operating communities; nationally; New York, NY.

★ 12338 ★ Crestar Foundation
Care of Suntrust Bank
PO Box 27385
Richmond, VA 23261-7385
Phone: (804)782-7907 **Fax:** (804)782-5191
Website: http://iath.virginia.edu/readings/crestar.html
Brenda Skidmore, President

Priorities: *Arts & Humanities:* 19%. Supports museums, performing arts and literary groups, historic preservation, and arts funds and centers. Public broadcasting and libraries are also of interest. Includes matching gifts. *Civic & Public Affairs:* 27%. Economic development in operating communities is primary focus. Also supports national organizations that promote public understanding of economics and free enterprise. *Education:* 26%. Primarily supports private colleges and universities through independent college funds. Supports private secondary and elementary schools that are important to communities served by SunTrust. Support is also provided in the form of employee matching gifts. *Environment:* 31%. Major emphasis is on United Way organizations serving SunTrust communities. Also funds YMCA, relief funds, and youth organizations including scouting. *International:* (Health and Human Services) 28%. Major emphasis is on United Way organizations serving SunTrust communities. Awards capital and other grants to hospitals, religious welfare organizations such as the Salvation Army, youth homes, and scouting. *Religion:* 4%. Supports science museums. *Note:* Total contributions made in 2001. **Typ. Recipients:** AIDS/HIV, Cancer, Children's Health/Hospitals, Clinics/Medical Centers, Domestic Violence, Emergency/Ambulance Services, Eyes/Blindness, Health Funds, Health Organizations, Health Policy/Cost Containment, Heart, Hospices, Hospitals, Medical Education, Mental Health, Multiple Sclerosis, People with Disabilities, Speech & Hearing. **Geo. Dist:** headquarters and operating communities; DC; MD; VA. **Frmly:** Crestar Foundation.

★ 12339 ★ Croft-Leominster Foundation
Canton House, 300 Water St.
Baltimore, MD 21202
Phone: (410)576-0100 **Fax:** (410)576-8232
Website: http://www.croftleo.com/profile/
L. Croft, Vice President

Fnded: 1990. **Priorities:** *Arts & Humanities:* Less than 1%. *Civic & Public Affairs:* 4%. Supports foundations, volunteer programs, and housing. *Education:* 81%. Supports colleges, universities, and education organizations. *Environment:* 1%. Supports community programs for the hungry, for senior citizens, and for families. *International:* Less than 1%. *Note:* Total foundation contributions made in 2000. **Typ. Recipients:** Alzheimers Disease, Emergency/Ambulance Services, Health-General, Heart, Hospitals, Single-Disease Health Associations, Substance Abuse. **Geo. Dist:** Baltimore, MD.

★ 12340 ★ CSX Corp.

1 James Ctr.
901 E Cary St.
Richmond, VA 23219-5629
Phone: (904)359-3161
Adam Hollingsworth, Vice President, General Counsel

Typ. Recipients: Health-General. **Geo. Dist:** nationally.

★ 12341 ★ Cummings Properties Foundation

200 West Cummings Park
Woburn, MA 01801
Phone: (617)935-8000
Email: leasing@cummings.com
Website: http://www.cummings.com/mck_info.html
Rob Nigro, Managing Trustee

Fnded: 1986. **Priorities:** *Arts & Humanities:* 4%. Funds museums, societies, and collections. *Civic & Public Affairs:* 6%. Funds civic associations. *Education:* 19%. Funds colleges and universities. *Environment:* 30%. Supports youth organizations, human services, and United Way. *International:* 7%. Supports hospitals and single-disease health organizations. *Religion:* 2%. *Note:* Total contributions in 1999. **Typ. Recipients:** Cancer, Children's Health/Hospitals, Clinics/Medical Centers, Diabetes, Health Organizations, Heart, Hospices, Hospitals, Medical Education, Medical Research, Nursing Services, People with Disabilities, Respiratory, Single-Disease Health Associations, Substance Abuse. **Geo. Dist:** Woburn, MA.

★ 12342 ★ Cummins Foundation

Box 3005, Mail Code 60909
Columbus, IN 47202-3005
Phone: (812)377-3746 **Fax:** (812)377-3265
Website: http://www.cummins.com/na/pages/en/whoweare/foundation.cfm
Tracy Souza, President

Priorities: *Arts & Humanities:* 10%. Gives to museums, cultural and humanities centers, arts councils, and performing arts. *Civic & Public Affairs:* 19%. Funds minority affairs organizations, legal defense programs, public policy organizations, municipal services, housing projects, and dispute resolution centers. Also distributes funds to Cummins operating facilities for local community support. *Education:* 13%. Supports private, public, and religious elementary and secondary education, colleges, universities, and minority education. Provides scholarships and matches employee gifts. *Environment:* 42%. Supports United Way, child and family services, child care, senior services, and shelters. *International:* 3%. Funds public health programs and hospitals. *Note:* Total foundation giving in 2000. **Typ. Recipients:** Children's Health/Hospitals, Domestic Violence, Eyes/Blindness, Family Planning, Heart, Hospices, Hospitals, Mental Health, Preventive Medicine/Wellness Organizations, Public Health, Research/Studies Institutes, Substance Abuse. **Geo. Dist:** operating locations. **Frmly:** Cummins Engine Foundation.

★ 12343 ★ CUNA Mutual Group Foundation, Inc.

5910 Mineral Point Rd.
Madison, WI 53701
Phone: (608)231-7908 **Fax:** (608)236-7908
Website: http://www.cunamutual.com/cmg/freeFormDetail/0.1248.888.00.html
Terri Fiez, Executive Director

Priorities: *Arts & Humanities:* 9%. Supports theater, orchestras, pubic broadcasting, libraries, and history organizations. *Civic & Public Affairs:* 8%. Funds housing, legal and economic concerns, civic institutions and events, and a botanical society. *Education:* 8%. Emphasis on minority vocational training, fields related to CUNA Mutual business, employee recruitment, quality projects that do not receive tax support, and projects that link business need with educational development. Also supports colleges and universities. *Environment:* 63%. Majority of funding supports United Way. Emphasis is on basic resources (food/shelter/clothing), minority and underprivileged youth, transportation, and community assistance. *International:* 10%. Emphasis is on cost containment, wellness and prevention, family support and services access, and local-level services. Also supports single-disease health associations. *Voluntarism:* The company's Dollars for Doers program provides cash grants to qualifying nonprofit organizations for which employees and company board members volunteer. *Note:* Total contributions made in 2000. **Typ. Recipients:** AIDS/HIV, Cancer, Children's Health/Hospitals, Clinics/Medical Centers, Diabetes, Emergency/Ambulance Services, Geriatric Health, Health Organizations, Health Policy/Cost Containment, Health-General, Hospitals, Medical Rehabilitation, Medical Research, Mental Health, Nursing Services, People with Disabilities, Prenatal Health Issues, Public Health, Single-Disease Health Associations. **Geo. Dist:** generally in communities where CUNA Mutual is located; Rancho Cucamonga, CA, primary location; Duluth, GA, secondary location; Waverly, IA, primary location; Southfield, MI, secondary location; Bloomington, MN, secondary location; Albany, NY, secondary location; Dallas, TX, secondary location; Madison, WI, primary location. **Frmly:** CUNA Mutual Foundation, Inc.

★ 12344 ★ Curtis L. Carlson Family Foundation

301 Carlson Parkway, Suite 102
Minnetonka, MN 55305
Phone: (952)404-5600 **Fax:** (952)404-5601
Ms. Donna Snyder, Secretary

Fnded: 1959. **Priorities:** *Arts & Humanities:* 3%. *Civic & Public Affairs:* 12%. *Education:* 60%. *Environment:* 24%. *International:* 2%. *Note:* Total foundation contributions made in 2001. **Typ. Recipients:** AIDS/HIV, Cancer, Children's Health/Hospitals, Clinics/Medical Centers, Diabetes, Emergency/Ambulance Services, Eyes/Blindness, Health Organizations, Heart, Hospitals, Medical Research, Multiple Sclerosis, People with Disabilities, Public Health, Research/Studies Institutes, Single-Disease Health Associations, Substance Abuse. **Geo. Dist:** MN.

★ 12345 ★ Cutco Foundation, Inc.

1116 East State St.
Olean, NY 14760
Phone: (716)372-3111
Email: sgrey@cutco.com
Website: http://www.cutcofoundation.org/cutco.htm
James Stitt, Contact

Fnded: 1996. **Priorities:** *Education:* 68%. Supports colleges and universities. *Environment:* 22%. Supports youth programs and emergency relief. *International:* 10%. Supports a hospital and rehabilitation foundation. *Note:* Total contributions made in 2001. **Typ. Recipients:** Hospitals, Medical Rehabilitation. **Geo. Dist:** nationally; NY.

★ 12346 ★ D.B. Reinhart Family Foundation

PO Box 2228
La Crosse, WI 54602-2228
Phone: (608)782-4999 **Fax:** (608)782-5084
Nancy Hengel, Manager

Priorities: *Arts & Humanities:* 1%. Supports arts funds, music, and children's museums. *Civic & Public Affairs:* 5%. Funds community and economic development, community centers, and clubs. *Education:* 62%. Supports colleges, universities, and middle and high schools. *Environment:* 14%. Supports United Way, community services, traditional youth organizations, and children's services. *International:* 15%. Supports medical research, hospitals, emergency care, single-disease associations, and medical institutes. *Note:* Total foundation contributions made in fiscal 2001. **Typ. Recipients:** Cancer, Children's Health/Hospitals, Clinics/Medical Centers, Diabetes, Emergency/Ambulance Services, Eyes/Blindness, Heart, Hospitals, Medical Education, Medical Research, People with Disabilities, Prenatal Health Issues, Public Health, Single-Disease Health Associations, Substance Abuse. **Geo. Dist:** WI.

★ 12347 ★ DaimlerChrysler Corp. Fund

CIMS: 485-10-94
1000 Chrysler Dr.
Auburn Hills, MI 48326-2766
Phone: (248)512-2500 **Fax:** (248)512-2503
Website: http://www.daimlerchrysler.com/company/dccfund/dccfund_e.htm
Brian Glowiak, Vice President & Secretary

Fnded: 1953. **Priorities:** *Arts & Humanities:* 29%. Supports local and national cultural organizations, with emphasis on the performing arts. Recipients include performing arts centers, historical societies, music groups, libraries, museums, and public broadcasting. *Civic & Public Affairs:* 14%. Supports organizations that work for improvement of the economy and community vitality operating communities. Other interests include economic research and development, traffic safety, public policy, trade-related issues, minority and women's affairs, and groups that fight racism and bigotry. *Education:* 28%. About one-half of education support reaches precollege education programs and institutions, K-12 education, and community colleges. The other half supports colleges and universities, with special emphasis on business, automotive design, and engineering programs; state associations of colleges and universities; tax and economic education, minority education programs; and national educational organizations. Also provides scholarships for employees' children and matching gifts. The goal of the fund's educational spending is to prepare the future workforce. *Environment:* 25%. Provides major funding to the United Way in operating communities; also funds organizations serving youth and the disadvantaged, and community centers. *International:* Less than 1%. Supports the American Red Cross, single-disease health organizations and medical research. *Religion:* 4%. Supports science centers. *Note:* Total contributions made by DaimlerChrysler Corporation Fund in 2001. **Typ. Recipients:** Cancer, Diabetes, Emergency/Ambulance Services, Eyes/Blindness, Health Organizations, Hospices, Hospitals, People with Disabilities, Speech & Hearing, Substance Abuse. **Geo. Dist:** headquarters and operating communities and nationally.

★ 12348 ★ Dain Rauscher Foundation

60 South 6th St.
Minneapolis, MN 55402
Phone: (612)371-2711 **Fax:** (612)371-7933
Website: http://www.rbcdain.com
Sherry Koster, Program Manager

Fnded: 1961. **Priorities:** *Arts & Humanities:* 46%. Interests include art institutes, associations, and centers; public broadcasting; theater; music; and programs that generate an appreciation of diverse cultures. *Civic & Public Affairs:* 4%. Funds economic development, professional associations, housing, and civic organizations. *Education:* 17%. Emphasizes helping young people understand our country's economic system and helping disadvantaged youth. Supports K-12 programs that impact students of color or the economically disadvantaged. *Environment:* 25%. Supports the United Way, family and children's services, child welfare, youth organizations, domestic violence concerns, and food distribution. Focuses on fostering economic independence, self-sufficiency, breaking the cycle of poverty, and strengthening the family. *International:* 3%. Supports pediatric health organizations, hospitals, and single-disease health associations. *Voluntarism:* The company sponsors the Volunteer Involvement Program (VIP), which encourages employees to volunteer at various Twin Cities OrganizationS. *Note:* Total foundation contributions made in 2000. **Typ. Recipients:** AIDS/HIV, Cancer, Children's Health/Hospitals, Clinics/Medical Centers, Diabetes, Domestic Violence, Emergency/Ambulance

Services, Family Planning, Health Organizations, Health-General, Heart, Hospices, Hospitals, Kidney, Medical Rehabilitation, Medical Research, People with Disabilities, Prenatal Health Issues, Public Health, Research/Studies Institutes, Sexual Abuse, Single-Disease Health Associations, Substance Abuse. **Geo. Dist:** headquarters and operating communities; Minneapolis, MN; Saint Paul, MN.

★ 12349 ★ Dana Corp. Foundation
PO Box 1000
Toledo, OH 43697
Phone: (419)535-4601 **Fax:** (419)535-4896
Email: danainfo@dana.org
Website: http://dana.org/about/foundation/
Ed McNeal, Administrator

Priorities: *Arts & Humanities:* 9%. Emphasis on public broadcasting, arts associations, libraries, museums, theater, and music. *Civic & Public Affairs:* 8%. Interests include business and free enterprise, public policy, and zoos and botanical gardens. Other areas of concern include civil rights, environmental affairs, and urban and community affairs. *Education:* 13%. Funding primarily supports colleges and universities. Also supports private, public, and precollege education, and medical and technical education. *Environment:* 64%. Majority of funding supports united funds. Other interests include youth organizations, child welfare, community centers, community service organizations, drug and alcohol programs, and senior services, shelters, and food banks. *International:* 2%. Supports hospitals, hospices, health organizations, and pediatric health. *Religion:* 1%. The Edison Institute receives support. *Note:* Total contributions in fiscal 2001. **Typ. Recipients:** AIDS/HIV, Alzheimers Disease, Cancer, Emergency/Ambulance Services, Eyes/Blindness, Family Planning, Health Organizations, Hospices, Hospitals, Medical Education, Mental Health, People with Disabilities, Preventive Medicine/Wellness Organizations, Single-Disease Health Associations, Substance Abuse. **Geo. Dist:** principally near operating locations and to national organizations.

★ 12350 ★ Danis Foundation
Two River Place
PO Box 725
Dayton, OH 45401
Phone: (937)228-1225
Michael Matzko, Contact

Fnded: 1957. **Priorities:** *Arts & Humanities:* 42%. Supports museums, music, historic preservation, and the performing arts. *Civic & Public Affairs:* 2%. Funds urban affairs, economic and community development, and festivals. *Education:* 9%. Supports schools, colleges, and universities. *Environment:* 6%. Supports United Way and scouts. *International:* 29%. Supports hospitals, health foundations, medical centers, and single-disease health associations. *Religion:* 5%. Primarily supports science centers. *Note:* Total foundation contributions made in 2000. **Typ. Recipients:** Alzheimers Disease, Arthritis, Cancer, Children's Health/Hospitals, Clinics/Medical Centers, Health Funds, Health Organizations, Heart, Hospices, Hospitals, Medical Education, Medical Research, People with Disabilities, Public Health, Single-Disease Health Associations. **Geo. Dist:** OH.

★ 12351 ★ Darden Restaurants Foundation
PO Box 593330
Orlando, FL 32859-3330
Phone: (407)245-5213 **Fax:** (407)245-4462
Email: pdeyoung@darden.com
Website: http://www.darden.com/darden.asp?community=yes
Patty DeYoung, Asst. Dir. /Admin.

Typ. Recipients: Domestic Violence. **Geo. Dist:** Orange, Seminole, Osceola Coun; FL.

★ 12352 ★ Dayton Power and Light Co. Foundation
PO Box 20331
Dayton, OH 45420
Phone: (937)258-8841 **Fax:** (937)259-7245
Website: http://www.waytogo.com/support_community.html
Virginia Strausburg, Executive Director

Priorities: *Arts & Humanities:* 12%. Supports arts centers, opera, dance, theater, and orchestras. *Civic & Public Affairs:* 35%. Supports economic development efforts, community improvement, cities, clubs, parks, and crime prevention. *Education:* 16%. Support includes colleges and universities, public schools, scholarships, and public pre-college education. *Environment:* 22%. Supports united funds, domestic violence prevention, food banks, senior services, and youth organizations. *International:* 1%. *Religion:* 1%. *Note:* Total foundation contributions made in 2000. **Typ. Recipients:** Alzheimers Disease, Cancer, Children's Health/Hospitals, Domestic Violence, Heart, People with Disabilities, Substance Abuse, Transplant Networks/Donor Banks. **Geo. Dist:** headquarters and operating communities.

★ 12353 ★ Delta Air Lines Foundation
Hartsfield Atlanta International Airport
1020 Delta Boulevard
Department 979
Atlanta, GA 30354-1989
Phone: (404)715-7922 **Fax:** (404)715-5876
Website: http://www.delta-air.com/inside/community/index.jsp
Michael Young, Vice President, Community Affairs

Priorities: *Arts & Humanities:* 22%. Funds performing arts and museums of fine art. *Civic & Public Affairs:* 9%. *Education:* 31%. Supports colleges, universities, an education center, and aeronautics education. Also funds a matching gifts program. *Environment:* 14%. Supports youth fitness/recreation programs and social services. *International:* 33%. Contributes to hospitals, the American Red Cross, pediatric health programs, and organizations aiding those with juvenile diabetes. *Religion:* Less than 1%. *Note:* Total contributions in 2000. **Typ. Recipients:** AIDS/HIV, Child Abuse, Children's Health/Hospitals, Clinics/Medical Centers, Diabetes, Emergency/Ambulance Services, Health Organizations, Heart, Hospitals, Medical Education, People with Disabilities. **Geo. Dist:** headquarters and operating communities.

★ 12354 ★ Deluxe Corp. Foundation
PO Box 64235
Saint Paul, MN 55164-0235
Phone: (651)483-7111 **Fax:** (651)481-4371
Email: jenny.anderson@deluxe.com
Website: http://www.deluxe.com/dlxab/deluxe-foundation.jsp
Jennifer Anderson, Director of Foundations

Fnded: 1952. **Priorities:** *Arts & Humanities:* 15%. Supports public broadcasting, museums, theater, arts associations and centers, music, dance, and arts appreciation. *Civic & Public Affairs:* 9%. *Education:* 25%. Funding supports colleges and universities, education in the arts, student aid, education funds, and scholarships that are administered through the National Merit Scholarship Corporation, National Hispanic Scholarship Fund, and the United Negro College Fund. Also supports literacy initiatives, primary and secondary education, and Junior Achievement. *Environment:* 48%. Major support goes to the United Way. Also supports youth programs, with emphasis on at-risk youth; programs that serve the mentally challenged, with a special focus on employment programs; programs that serve people who are physically challenged; programs for senior citizens e.g., home delivered meals, companionship, chore services and other programs that enable seniors to remain in their homes; programs for victims of domestic abuse; transitional housing programs; programs that provide emergency needs, e.g., clothing, food, housing; programs that assist financially disadvantaged people; and programs that serve people of color. Also provides some funding for health organizations. *International:* 13%. *Religion:* 2%. *Voluntarism:* Deluxe's Time is Money program is geared toward encouraging company employees and retirees to volunteer at K-12 schools. The Deluxe Foundation matches 12 hours of volunteerism at a school with a $200 donation to that school's library. *Note:* Contributions analysis represents the foundation's typical annual funding allocation as reported by the Deluxe Foundation in 2002. **Typ. Recipients:** AIDS/HIV, Cancer, Children's Health/Hospitals, Clinics/Medical Centers, Domestic Violence, Emergency/Ambulance Services, Eyes/Blindness, Health Organizations, Medical Education, Medical Rehabilitation, People with Disabilities, Single-Disease Health Associations, Substance Abuse. **Geo. Dist:** headquarters and operating communities; Anniston, AL; Phoenix, AZ; Antelope Valley, CA; Chatsworth, CA; San Jose, CA; Colorado Springs, CO; Des Plaines, IL; Kansas City, KS; Shoreview, MN; Mountain Lakes, NJ; Syracuse, NY; Greensboro, NC; Streetsboro, OH; Pittsburgh, PA; Dallas, TX; Salt Lake City, UT.

★ 12355 ★ Demoulas Foundation
286 Chelmsford St.
Chelmsford, MA 01824
Phone: (978)224-1024 **Fax:** (978)640-8392
Telemachus Demoulas, Trustee

Fnded: 1964. **Priorities:** *Arts & Humanities:* 4%. Supports ballet, operas, music, arts centers, historical societies, libraries, cultural centers, and museums. *Civic & Public Affairs:* 38%. Provides major support for the Lowell (MA) Plan. Also supports urban affairs, revitalization projects, and philanthropic organizations. *Education:* 10%. Majority of funding supports colleges and universities in the New England area. Also supports scholarship funds, religious education, and private secondary education. *Environment:* 4%. Funds youth groups and recreation programs, services for the elderly and the disabled, and food/clothing distribution. *International:* 7%. Funds hospitals, medical centers, nursing homes, pediatric health, hospice programs, and single-disease health associations. *Note:* Total contributions in 2000. **Typ. Recipients:** Cancer, Children's Health/Hospitals, Diabetes, Geriatric Health, Health Organizations, Hospices, Hospitals, Long-Term Care, Medical Education, Medical Rehabilitation, Medical Research, People with Disabilities, Respiratory, Single-Disease Health Associations, Substance Abuse, Trauma Treatment. **Geo. Dist:** primarily New England.

★ 12356 ★ Deutsch Foundation
2444 Wilshire Blvd., Ste. 600
Santa Monica, CA 90403
Phone: (310)453-0055 **Fax:** (310)453-6467
Lester Deutsch, Executive Vice President

Priorities: *Arts & Humanities:* 7%. Interests include music centers, museums, dance societies, and public broadcasting. *Civic & Public Affairs:* 5%. Supports women's affairs, gardens, community foundations, and environmental concerns. *Education:* 13%. Supports colleges and universities, public and private precollege education, art schools, and education associations. *Environment:* 10%. Youth organizations are major recipients. Other interests include sexual abuse issues, substance abuse prevention programs, aid for the homeless, athletics, and animal welfare. *International:* 16%. Interests include single-disease health organizations, pediatric and geriatric medicine, and health centers. *Note:* Total contributions in fiscal 1999. **Typ. Recipients:** Arthritis, Cancer, Children's Health/Hospitals, Clinics/Medical Centers, Eyes/Blindness, Family Planning, Geriatric Health, Health Organizations, Health-General, Hospitals, Hospitals (University Affiliated), Long-Term Care, Medical Rehabilitation, Medical Research, Mental Health, People with Disabilities, Public Health, Research/Studies Institutes, Sexual Abuse, Single-Disease Health Associations, Speech & Hearing, Substance Abuse, Trauma Treatment. **Geo. Dist:** CA, including southern California.

★ 12357 ★ Dickson Foundation
301 South Tryon St., Suite 1800
Charlotte, NC 28202

Phone: (704)372-5404 **Fax:** (704)372-6409
Susan Patterson, Secretary & Treasurer

Priorities: *Arts & Humanities:* 8%. Funds visual arts centers, museums, and the Arts and Sciences Council. *Civic & Public Affairs:* 11%. Funds business and free enterprise, minority affairs, municipalities, and community affairs. *Education:* 42%. Primarily supports colleges and universities in North Carolina, specifically the University of North Carolina, Wake Forest University, and North Carolina University. Also supports education funds, faculty development, medical education, and secondary schools. *Environment:* 12%. Supports United Way and family and youth services. *International:* 10%. Supports medical centers, hospitals, and hospices; single-disease health associations also receive support. *Religion:* 1%. *Note:* Contributions made in 2000. **Typ. Recipients:** Cancer, Clinics/Medical Centers, Health Organizations, Health-General, Heart, Hospices, Hospitals, Medical Education, Medical Research, Preventive Medicine/Wellness Organizations, Single-Disease Health Associations, Substance Abuse. **Geo. Dist:** FL; GA; NC; SC; TN.

★ 12358 ★ Diebold, Inc.

PO Box 3077
5995 Mayfair Rd.
North Canton, OH 44720-8077
Phone: (330)490-4000 **Fax:** (330)490-4024
Email: scheurc@diebold.com
Charles Scheurer, Vice President, Human Resources

Typ. Recipients: Health-General. **Geo. Dist:** headquarters and operating communities.

★ 12359 ★ Dixie Yarns Foundation, Inc.

PO Box 751
Chattanooga, TN 37401
Phone: (423)698-2501 **Fax:** (423)493-7450
Ms. Starr Klein, Secretary, Treasurer & Trustee

Priorities: *Arts & Humanities:* 12%. Supports public broadcasting and art funds. *Civic & Public Affairs:* 14%. Supports housing for the disadvantaged, community foundations, urban development, and a conference center. *Education:* 38%. Supports educational organizations, colleges, universities, minority education, private precollege education, and Junior Achievement. *Environment:* 35%. Supports United Way, scouts, and youth organizations. *International:* 1%. Supports medical research and health foundations. *Note:* Total foundation contributions made in 2000. **Typ. Recipients:** Children's Health/Hospitals, Clinics/Medical Centers, Health Organizations, Hospitals, Medical Research, Mental Health, Substance Abuse. **Geo. Dist:** Chattanooga, TN.

★ 12360 ★ Dominion

PO Box 26532
Richmond, VA 23261
Phone: (804)819-2580 **Fax:** (804)819-2217
Email: reneejohnson@dom.com
Website: http://www.dom.com/about/community/index.jsp
Renee Johnson, Contributions Coordinator

Priorities: *Arts & Humanities:* 10% to 15%. Supports theater, ballet, symphonic and choral music, opera, art councils, museums, multicultural arts associations, and public broadcasting. *Education:* 15% to 20%. Supports early childhood and precollege basics programs, accredited private colleges and universities, independent college funds, job creation and training programs. *International:* 40% to 50%. Supports United Way, health care groups, volunteer fire and rescue squads, Red Cross, civic groups, neighborhood improvement, cultural diversity groups, shelters, programs for older Americans, literacy programs, and programs for the homeless. **Typ. Recipients:** Emergency/Ambulance Services, Health Organizations, Hospices, Hospitals, Mental Health, People with Disabilities, Substance Abuse. **Geo. Dist:** operating locations.

★ 12361 ★ Domino's Pizza, Inc.

PO Box 997
Ann Arbor, MI 48106
Phone: (734)930-3674 **Fax:** (734)668-1946
Email: ryanh@dominos.com
Holly Ryan, Public Affairs Director

Typ. Recipients: Cancer, Children's Health/Hospitals, People with Disabilities. **Geo. Dist:** nationally for religion-oriented grants; MI, including southeast Michigan.

★ 12362 ★ Donaldson Foundation

PO Box 1299 MS 100
Minneapolis, MN 55440
Phone: (612)703-4999 **Fax:** (952)887-3005
Email: donaldsonfoundation@mail.donaldson.com
Website: http://www.donaldson.com/en/about/community/foundation.html/html
Norman Linnell, President & Trustee

Priorities: *Civic & Public Affairs:* 26%. Funds urban affairs, civic groups, community action, parks, and women's affairs. *Education:* 29%. Support goes to the foundation's scholarship program. Other interests include minority education funds, colleges and universities, Junior Achievement, and public pre-college schools. *Environment:* 40%. Supports United Way, community services, and YMCAs. *International:* 1%. Clinics and medical centers receive support. *Note:* Total contributions made in fiscal 2001. **Typ. Recipients:** Children's Health/Hospitals, Clinics/Medical Centers, Domestic Violence, Emergency/Ambulance Services, Family Planning, Health Funds, Health Organizations, Hospices, Hospitals, Medical Rehabilitation, Mental Health, People with Disabilities, Preventive Medicine/Wellness Organizations, Public Health, Substance Abuse. **Geo. Dist:** headquarters and operating communities.

★ 12363 ★ Dow Chemical Co. Foundation

47 Bldg.
Midland, MI 48667
Phone: (989)636-6891 **Fax:** (989)638-7238
Website: http://www.dow.com/about/corp/social/social.htm
Mr. Jerold Ring, Executive Director

Priorities: *Arts & Humanities:* 7%. *Civic & Public Affairs:* 12%. *Education:* 51%. *Environment:* 24%. *International:* 1%. *Religion:* 1%. *Note:* Percentages reflect foundation grants made in 2001. Through direct giving programs, company and divisions disburse approximately 60% of support to Education, 30% to Health and Community Betterment, about 5% to Arts and Culture, and the remaining 5% to miscellaneous recipients. Company operating divisions administer independent contributions programs. Divisions support community projects (United Way and groups concerned with child welfare, health care, drug abuse prevention, etc.) and cultural activities in areas in which they are located. **Typ. Recipients:** Domestic Violence, Emergency/Ambulance Services, Geriatric Health, Hospitals. **Geo. Dist:** nationally.

★ 12364 ★ Dow Corning Foundation

CO2210
Midland, MI 48686-0994
Phone: (989)496-1863 **Fax:** (989)496-4393
Email: a.m.deboer@dowcorning.com
Website: http://www.dowcorning.com/content/about/aboutcomm/aboutcomm_guidelines1.asp
Anne DeBoer, Executive Director

Priorities: *Arts & Humanities:* 5%. Supports arts centers. *Civic & Public Affairs:* 13%. Supports job training, parks, zoos, community foundations, and fire departments. *Education:* 47%. Supports both privately endowed and tax-supported colleges and universities. The majority of aid to education is directed toward institutions that have been sources of new employees, have strong, effective minority programs, or provide science and math improvements in K-12 education. *Environment:* 32%. Funds family and community centers, youth organizations, recreation, and shelters. *Note:* Total contributions made in 2000. **Typ. Recipients:** Child Abuse, Medical Research. **Geo. Dist:** headquarters and operating communities.

★ 12365 ★ Dow Jones Foundation

PO Box 300
Princeton, NJ 08543
Phone: (609)520-5143 **Fax:** (609)520-5180
Leonard Doherty, Administrative Officer

Priorities: *Arts & Humanities:* 4%. Museums, libraries, art councils, and theaters. *Civic & Public Affairs:* 5%. Supports neighborhoods, botanical gardens, African and Asian American organizations, and women's affairs. Majority of giving supports the Dow Jones Newspaper Fund in a single grant. Professional and trade associations, primarily in journalism, also receive significant support. Other interests include organizations concerned with First Amendment issues and civil rights. *Education:* 67%. Supports universities and scholarships. Journalism education is also of significant interest. Other support goes to minority education and independent college funds. *Environment:* 21%. Primarily supports united funds. Also supports child welfare, youth groups and community service organizations. *International:* 3%. Supports hospitals and medical centers. *Note:* Total foundation contributions made in 2000. **Typ. Recipients:** Clinics/Medical Centers, Hospitals, Hospitals, People with Disabilities. **Geo. Dist:** principally near operating locations and to national organizations.

★ 12366 ★ Doyon Foundation

1 Doyon Pl., Suite 300
Fairbanks, AK 99701
Phone: (907)459-2040 **Fax:** (907)459-2065
Email: foundation@doyon.com
Miranda Wright, Director

Fnded: 1988. **Priorities:** *Education:* 100%. Supports scholarships and training. *Note:* Total contributions made in fiscal 2001. **Typ. Recipients:** Medical Education. **Geo. Dist:** AK.

★ 12367 ★ Drugstore.com Foundation

13920 SE Eastgate Way Ste. 300
Bellevue, WA 98005-4440
Phone: (425)372-3200 **Fax:** (425)372-3800
Email: foundation@drugstore.com
Website: http://www.shareholder.com/drugstore/support.cfm
Cynthia Hoppner, Contact

Fnded: 2001. **Priorities:** *Civic & Public Affairs:* 12%. *Education:* 10%. *Environment:* 28%. *International:* 50%. **Typ. Recipients:** AIDS/HIV, Cancer, Children's Health/Hospitals, Domestic Violence, People with Disabilities. **Geo. Dist:** WA, western area; NJ.

★ 12368 ★ DTE Energy Foundation

2000 Second Ave., Rm. 1046 WCB
Detroit, MI 48226-1279
Phone: (313)235-9416 **Fax:** (313)235-0285
Email: hallk@dteenergy.com
Website: http://www.dteenergy.com/community/foundation/index.html
Karla Hall, Secretary & Director

Priorities: *Arts & Humanities:* 16%. Primarily supports region's major cultural institutions. Interests include music, theater, arts centers and funds, libraries, museums, historical societies, and public broadcasting. Youth educational programs and event or project sponsorship are preferable to general operating support. *Civic & Public Affairs:* 29%. Interests include economic development, crime prevention, race relations, ethnic organizations, public policy research, zoos, and neighborhood revitalization. Urban and community development coalitions are a high priority. The foundation has a particular interest in local citizen and community self-help initiatives and projects where funds can complement support from the public sector. *Education:* 19%. Funds school readiness (pre-school), K-12 education improvement, vocational education, school-to-work and career awareness programs, citizenship education, environmental education, and higher education. In higher education, emphasis is placed on business and engineering and programs that increase student participation and retention, including pre-college math and science enrichment programs, and student tutoring and mentoring programs. *Environment:* 31%. Supports the United Way, emergency food and shelter, teen pregnancy prevention and parenting skills. *International:* 2%. Funds community health programs and single-disease health associations. *Religion:* 2%. Contributes to a science center. *Note:* Total foundation contributions made in 2000. **Typ. Recipients:** Children's Health/Hospitals, Emergency/Ambulance Services, Eyes/Blindness, Health Funds, Health Organizations, Hospices, Hospitals, Medical Education, Mental Health, Public Health, Single-Disease Health Associations, Substance Abuse. **Geo. Dist:** MI, headquarters and operating communities; Detroit, MI.

★ 12369 ★ Duke Energy Foundation
422 S Church St.
Charlotte, NC 28202-1904
Phone: (704)373-6885
Website: http://www.duke-energy.com/company/community/foundation/
Sabrina Austin, Executive Director, Secretary

Priorities: *Arts & Humanities:* 21%. *Civic & Public Affairs:* 10%. *Education:* 38%. *Environment:* 4%. *International:* 16%. *Voluntarism:* Community Volunteer Grants provide $1,000 for materials for employees and retirees who volunteer time to one-time, hands-on projects, and $1,000 grants to organizations where employees help achieve significant strategic objectives. *Note:* Total foundation contributions made in 2001. **Typ. Recipients:** Adolescent Health Issues, Child Abuse, Domestic Violence, Emergency/Ambulance Services, Family Planning, Health Organizations, Health Policy/Cost Containment, Health-General, Hospices, Hospitals, Medical Education, Mental Health, Nutrition, People with Disabilities, Single-Disease Health Associations, Substance Abuse. **Geo. Dist:** headquarters and operating communities; NC; SC. **Frmly:** Duke Power Co. Foundation.

★ 12370 ★ Dun & Bradstreet Corp. Foundation, Inc.
1 Diamond Hill Rd.
Murray Hill, NJ 07974
Phone: (908)665-8052 **Fax:** (908)665-5022
Rosanne Miller, Contact

Priorities: *Arts & Humanities:* Areas of interest include music, art centers, libraries, museums, and the performing arts. *Civic & Public Affairs:* Areas of interest include business, economics, civil rights, law and justice, and public policy. *Education:* Interests include independent and minority college funds, higher education associations, and business education. *Environment:* Majority of funding supports United Way campaigns. Other areas of interest include child welfare, youth groups, and community service organizations. *International:* Supports the American Red Cross, AIDS research, and single-disease health associations. **Typ. Recipients:** AIDS/HIV, Cancer, Emergency/Ambulance Services, Health Organizations, Hospitals, Mental Health, People with Disabilities, Single-Disease Health Associations, Speech & Hearing, Substance Abuse. **Geo. Dist:** nationally.

★ 12371 ★ Duquesne Light Co.
Cherrington Corporate Center
411 7th Ave. 16-4
Pittsburgh, PA 15219
Phone: (412)393-1517 **Fax:** (412)393-6110
Website: http://www.duquesnelight.com/community/fundpri.htm
Pamela Coats, Manager, Community Relations

Typ. Recipients: Health-General, Hospitals. **Geo. Dist:** PA, Allegheny County; PA, Beaver County.

★ 12372 ★ Duracell International
Research Drive
Berkshire Corporate Park
Bethel, CT 06801
Phone: (203)796-4000 **Fax:** (203)796-4483
Jane Steiner, Corporate Contributions Administration

Typ. Recipients: Health-General. **Geo. Dist:** principally near operating locations and to national organizations.

★ 12373 ★ Dynamet, Inc.
101 West Burn St.
Reading, PA 19601
Phone: (610)208-2000 **Fax:** (610)736-6232
Website: http://www.cartech.com
Katharine Marshall, Director of Communications

Priorities: *Arts & Humanities:* 3%. Supports museums, cultural resources, performing arts, music, and theater. *Education:* 52%. Funds educational programs, and colleges and universities. *Environment:* 3%. Supports handicapped services, volunteer services, senior care, people with mental disabilities, YM/YWCA, and youth services. *International:* 5%. Supports hospitals, rehabilitation centers, and single-disease concerns. *Religion:* 1%. Funds the Carnegie Institute, for scientific research. *Note:* Total contributions in 1998. **Typ. Recipients:** Cancer, Children's Health/Hospitals, Clinics/Medical Centers, Diabetes, Emergency/Ambulance Services, Eyes/Blindness, Health Organizations, Hospices, Hospitals, Kidney, Medical Rehabilitation, Medical Research, Mental Health, People with Disabilities, Single-Disease Health Associations, Substance Abuse. **Geo. Dist:** Pittsburgh, PA.

★ 12374 ★ E.I. du Pont de Nemours & Co.
Corporate Contributions Office
1007 Market St.
Wilmington, DE 19898
Phone: (302)774-2036 **Fax:** (302)773-2919
Website: http://www1.dupont.com/NASApp/dupontglobal/corp/index.jsp?page=/content/US/en_US/social/outreach/index.html
Pat Eggert, Contributions Coordinator

Priorities: *Arts & Humanities:* 5% to 10%. Supports local museums, libraries, and other cultural organizations. A limited number of high visibility national organizations also receive funding. *Civic & Public Affairs:* Focus on neighborhood revitalization, economic development, and minority businesses. *Education:* About 45%. Almost all grants are made at the initiative of the Committee on Educational Aid, not in response to proposals or requests. Most support falls within six main categories: University Science and Engineering Grants, supporting undergraduate business, science, and engineering departments and interdisciplinary programs in such areas as occupational and environmental health; Minority Education Grants, to colleges and universities for scholarships and programs to advance the science and engineering education of minorities and to K-12 programs to help prepare minority students for engineering and technical careers; Young Faculty Grants, for research assistants; College Science Grants, to liberal arts colleges producing significant numbers of graduates who go on to advanced studies in science; Business and Economic Grants, supporting training and research at business schools; and Secondary School Grants, emphasizing improvement of teaching in science and economics. The bulk of funding is awarded in the first two categories listed above. The educational program emphasizes physical and life sciences, with grants awarded on the basis of scope, quality of institution's teaching and research, and company's research and recruitment needs. The goals of the program include the following: stimulating applied and basic research; improving higher, secondary, and special educational support programs for minorities in science, engineering, and business management; increasing the number of top graduates, minority scholars, and prospective employees in the fields of company enterprise; and promoting programs to improve the national science policy. Additional areas funded in recent years include energy policy, materials science, and computer-based science applications. Other educational support activities include sponsorship of visiting and adjunct professorships and postdoctoral appointments in DuPont research labs. Does not award direct grants to individuals; endowment and capital grants do not fall within preferred areas of giving. giving. *International:* 15% to 20%. Primarily supports United Way programs. Strong support is also given to hospital capital campaigns and health projects in operating locations. Other contributions go toward occupational medicine, the elderly, and the disabled. **Typ. Recipients:** Domestic Violence, Emergency/Ambulance Services, Geriatric Health, Health Organizations, Health Policy/Cost Containment, Hospices, Hospitals, Medical Rehabilitation, Medical Research, Medical Training, Mental Health, People with Disabilities, Single-Disease Health Associations, Substance Abuse. **Geo. Dist:** headquarters and operating communities.

★ 12375 ★ E.L. Craig Foundation
PO Box 1404
Joplin, MO 64802-1404
Phone: (417)624-6644
Ethel Mae Humphreys, President

Fnded: 1960. **Priorities:** *Civic & Public Affairs:* 69%. Supports right to work organizations, policy groups and think-tanks. *Education:* 31%. Funds the Institute for Humane Studies and economic education. *Note:* Total contributions made in fiscal 2001. **Typ. Recipients:** Cancer, Hospitals, People with Disabilities, Public Health, Single-Disease Health Associations. **Geo. Dist:** nationally; Joplin, MO.

★ 12376 ★ Eastern Bank Charitable Foundation
217 Essex St.
Salem, MA 01970
Phone: (978)740-6319 **Fax:** (978)740-6329
Website: http://www.easternbank.com/a_charitable_foundation.html
Sumner Jones, Executive Vice President

Fnded: 1985. **Priorities:** *Arts & Humanities:* 12%. Supports libraries, museums, performing arts, and historic preservation. *Civic & Public Affairs:* 19%. Supports housing, free enterprise, ethnic organizations, and community and economic development. *Education:* 20%. Supports scholarship funds, colleges and universities, and public and private elementary and secondary schools. *Environment:* 37%. Supports YMCAs, counseling centers, United Way, children and family services, shelters, and youth organizations. *International:* 5%. Supports medical centers, single-disease associations, and health funds. *Note:* Total foundation contributions made in 2000. **Typ. Recipients:** AIDS/HIV, Cancer, Children's Health/Hospitals, Clinics/Medical Centers, Domestic Violence, Health Organizations, Health-General, Heart, Hospices, Hospitals, Medical Education, Mental Health, People with Disabilities, Preventive Medicine/Wellness Organizations, Single-Disease Health Associations. **Geo. Dist:** MA, market area.

★ 12377 ★ Eastman Chemical Co.
PO Box 431
Kingsport, TN 37662
Phone: (423)229-1413 **Fax:** (423)229-8280
Website: http://www.eastman.com
Paul Montgomery, Manager, Community Relations

Typ. Recipients: Health-General. **Geo. Dist:** headquarters and operating communities.

★ 12378 ★ Eastman Kodak Charitable Trust
343 State St.
Rochester, NY 14650-0517
Phone: (716)724-2434 **Fax:** (716)724-1376
Website: http://www.kodak.com/US/en/corp/community.shtml
Essie Calhoun, Director

Priorities: *Arts & Humanities:* 9%. Funds museums, film and photography institutes, and the performing arts. *Civic & Public Affairs:* 6%. Supports community revitalization programs that improve the standard of living of low-income residents; programs that improve employment skills; economic development activities (particularly minority owned and operated) to enhance the economy of a community; and programs that provide unbiased, third-party acquisition and distribution of information on issues of mutual concern to the company and the community. *Education:* 27%. Supports colleges, universities, preschool, umbrella education funds, diversity initiatives, special grants, and K-12 educational programs nationwide, with emphasis on science and engineering education. University funding is focused on recruitment, diversity, technology, and market development; it includes seed money or start-up grants for research in the areas of U.S. manufacturing competitiveness, optics, imaging science, biotechnology, electronics, and material processing. Also provides scholarships. Kodak Fellows program provides grants to graduate students and specific departments of science and engineering. Educational organizations supported include minority and independent college funds, economics, and minority engineering associations. On the precollege level, focuses on academic opportunities in scientific, mathematics, and technical disciplines. Sponsors partnerships between the company and precollege educational institutions in local Kodak communities to improve science and mathematics achievement for all students. Also funds school-based initiatives that aim at acquainting students with opportunities in manufacturing. *Environment:* (Health and Human Services) 58%. Principally supports the United Way. Youth groups, local and national health organizations, homes and shelters, child welfare, and services for the aged and the handicapped are also supported. Priority and international support is given to organizations delivering health and human services in Kodak communities. National organizations that address key issues of interest to Kodak are also funded. *International:* 6%. *Religion:* 1%. *Voluntarism:* Company offers "Dollars for Doers" program through which it makes small donations to nonprofit organizations where company employees serve as volunteers; supports Global Service Day; when all employees are encouraged to volunteer in their communities. *Note:* Total contributions made by the company and foundation in 2001. **Typ. Recipients:** Adolescent Health Issues, Cancer, Clinics/Medical Centers, Emergency/Ambulance Services, Health Organizations, Health-General, Hospitals, Medical Rehabilitation, Mental Health, Nursing Services, People with Disabilities, Single-Disease Health Associations. **Geo. Dist:** nationally, especially in operating locations.

★ 12379 ★ Eaton Charitable Fund

1111 Superior Ave.
Cleveland, OH 44114-2584
Phone: (216)523-4944 **Fax:** (216)479-7013
Email: jamesmason@eaton.com
Website: http://www.eaton.com/about/report.html
James Mason, Vice Pres., Public & Community Affairs

Fnded: 1953. **Priorities:** *Arts & Humanities:* 18%. *Civic & Public Affairs:* 32%. Within Eaton's Community Improvement giving area, the foundation contributes to organizations that help people become self-sufficient, strengthen families, encourage neighborhood and economic development, and enhance the qualify of life through civic, cultural and arts programs. Contributes to housing, shelters and social services, youth activities, health care facilities, and visual and performing arts institutions, public radio and television, civic improvements, and humanitarian efforts. *Education:* 20%. Gifts go to educational institutions for programs that help students prepare for careers in business and industry, particularly in engineering. Supports programs that attract students at all grade levels to the study of math, science, and technology. Contributes to programs that help students overcome barriers to academic achievement and complete their education. Awards scholarships for minority engineering students. *Environment:* 35%. Supports the United Way, primarily in Eaton operating communities. *International:* 12%. *Religion:* 2%. *Voluntarism:* Volunteer services of all types are encouraged. Volunteers support many causes including teaching reading to the illiterate, coaching little league softball, organizing school aid programs, serving food at hunger centers, building houses for the needy, and chairing United Way campaigns. Company sponsors the James R. Stover Awards to recognize employee volunteers, and makes cash grants to organizations where employees contribute their time and talents. *Note:* Total contributions made in 2001. **Typ. Recipients:** Cancer, Clinics/Medical Centers, Emergency/Ambulance Services, Health Funds, Health Organizations, Health Policy/Cost Containment, Hospices, Hospitals, Hospitals (University Affiliated), Medical Education, Nursing Services, People with Disabilities, Public Health, Single-Disease Health Associations. **Geo. Dist:** corporate operating locations.

★ 12380 ★ Ebsco Industries, Inc.

PO Box 1943
Birmingham, AL 35201
Phone: (205)991-1197 **Fax:** (205)995-1517
Email: wdimon@ebsco.com
Website: http://www.ebsco.com
Dell Brooke, Corp. Sec.

Typ. Recipients: Health-General. **Geo. Dist:** AL.

★ 12381 ★ Echoing Green Foundation

60 E 42nd St.
New York, NY 10165
Phone: (212)689-1165 **Fax:** (212)689-9010
Website: http://www.echoinggreen.org
Cheryl Dorsey, Contact

Fnded: 1987. **Priorities:** *Arts & Humanities:* 4%. Supports music and the literary arts. *Civic & Public Affairs:* 48%. Supports career services, civil and human rights organizations, women's affairs, economic development, and community foundations. *Education:* 13%. Supports schools, student funds, education centers, and college programs. *Environment:* 24%. Supports youth programs, counseling services, shelters, domestic violence programs, child welfare, and community service foundations. *International:* 3%. Primary support made to cancer funds. *Note:* Total foundation contributions made in fiscal 2000. **Typ. Recipients:** AIDS/HIV, Cancer, Child Abuse, Domestic Violence, Emergency/Ambulance Services, Health Organizations, Heart, Medical Education, Mental Health, People with Disabilities, Public Health, Substance Abuse. **Geo. Dist:** NY, emphasis on New York.

★ 12382 ★ Eckerd Corp. Foundation

PO Box 4689
Clearwater, FL 33758
Phone: (727)395-6289
Tami Alderman, Community and Public Relations Mgr.

Priorities: *Arts & Humanities:* 1%. Supports performing arts. *Civic & Public Affairs:* 4%. Supports regional community foundations. *Education:* 20%. Supports colleges and universities. *Environment:* 63%. Supports United Way, children's organizations, disability services, and recreation and athletics. Also supports the Children's Miracle Network. *International:* 12%. Funds national health organizations and hospitals. *Note:* Total contributions made in fiscal 2001. **Typ. Recipients:** Arthritis, Cancer, Clinics/Medical Centers, Diabetes, Emergency/Ambulance Services, Family Planning, Health Funds, Health Organizations, Heart, Hospices, Hospitals, Medical Education, Multiple Sclerosis, People with Disabilities, Prenatal Health Issues, Public Health. **Geo. Dist:** CT; DE; FL; GA; KS; LA; MD; MS; MO; NJ; NY; NC; OH; OK; PA; SC; TN; TX; VA; WV.

★ 12383 ★ Ecolab Foundation

370 North Wabasha St. N
Saint Paul, MN 55102
Phone: (651)293-2658 **Fax:** (651)225-3123
Website: http://www.ecolab.com/companyprofile/foundation/default.asp
Lois West Duffy, Director, Community & Public Relations

Priorities: *Arts & Humanities:* (Arts & Culture) 15%. Supports major performing arts groups, mid-size arts organizations, museums, and theaters. *Civic & Public Affairs:* (Civic & Community Development) 13%. Contributions are set aside to fund community relations task forces and contingencies. Funds community service organizations, community foundations, leadership development, and family services. Ecolab also donates products in cases of national disaster through disaster relief organizations. *Education:* (Youth & Education) 38%. Supports programs for at-risk youth, teacher grants, and colleges and universities. *Environment:* (Community-based Contributions) 30%. Provides contributions to the United Way and to health and human services organizations in Ecolab communities. *International:* 3%. *Religion:* 2%. *Voluntarism:* Employees volunteer as classroom speakers and with Business/Education Partnership. Company also provides technical assistance and coordinates volunteer projects for two weekends of the United Way's Week of Caring, Volunteer Fair, and provides contributions to nonprofit organizations to reward employee volunteers. *Note:* Contributions analysis provided by foundation in 2001. **Typ. Recipients:** AIDS/HIV, Cancer, Children's Health/Hospitals, Clinics/Medical Centers, Emergency/Ambulance Services, Family Planning, Hospitals, Long-Term Care, Medical Rehabilitation, Nutrition, People with Disabilities, Public Health, Speech & Hearing, Substance Abuse. **Geo. Dist:** areas where company has a major presence, and large numbers of employees live and work; St. Paul, MN.

★ 12384 ★ Edison International

Edison International
2244 Walnut Grove Ave. Room 100 G04
PO Box 800
Rosemead, CA 91770
Phone: (626)302-9853 **Fax:** (626)302-8114
Email: Lucia.Galindo@.sce.com
Website: http://www.edison.com
Lucia Galindo, Manager, Corporate Contributions

Typ. Recipients: Geriatric Health, Health Organizations, Hospices, Hospitals, Nursing Services, People with Disabilities, Substance Abuse. **Geo. Dist:** CA, primarily in company's Southern CA service area; strategic giving outside traditional service territory.

★ 12385 ★ EDS Foundation

5400 Legacy Dr., H3-6F-47
Plano, TX 75024-3105
Phone: (972)605-8429
Email: diane.spradlin-eds@eds.com
Website: http://www.eds.com/foundation/index.shtml
Diane Spradlin, Executive Director

Fnded: 2000. **Priorities:** *Arts & Humanities:* 19%. Funds a museum and an orchestra. *Civic & Public Affairs:* 34%. *Education:* 62%. Supports technology education in primary and secondary schools; public and urban schools; Junior Achievement and other programs aimed at encouraging youth to consider careers in business and technology. *Environment:* 9%. Contributes to a children's center. *International:* 15%. *Religion:* 7%. *Voluntarism:* The company sponsors a Global Volunteer Day annually to encourage and recognize employee volunteerism. *Note:* Total contributions made in 2002. **Typ. Recipients:** Health-General, Sexual Abuse, Single-Disease Health Associations. **Geo. Dist:** headquarters and operating communities.

★ 12386 ★ Edward D. Jones & Co. Foundation

12555 Manchester Rd.
Saint Louis, MO 63131
Phone: (314)515-2000 **Fax:** (314)515-3269
John Bachmann, Chairman

Fnded: 1992. **Priorities:** *Education:* 57%. Supports colleges and universities. *Environment:* 29%. Supports the United Way. *Note:* Total contributions made in 2000. **Typ. Recipients:** Emergency/Ambulance Services. **Geo. Dist:** Claremont, CA; St. Louis, MO.

★ 12387 ★ Edward F. Redies Foundation

118 E Michigan Ave.
Saline, MI 48176
Phone: (734)429-0154

Fnded: 1981. **Priorities:** *Arts & Humanities:* 2%. *Civic & Public Affairs:* 11%. *Education:* 49%. *Environment:* 29%. *International:* 10%. *Note:* Total contributions made in 2001. **Typ. Recipients:** Children's Health/Hospitals, Clinics/Medical Centers, Emergency/Ambulance Services, Health Organizations, Hospitals, Kidney, Long-Term Care, Medical Rehabilitation, Nursing Services, People with Disabilities, Public Health. **Geo. Dist:** MI.

★ 12388 ★ El Paso Energy Foundation

1001 Louisiana St.
Houston, TX 77002
Phone: (713)420-5192
Gloria Moritz, Community Relations Coordinator

Fnded: 1992. **Priorities:** *Arts & Humanities:* 8%. Supports opera, music foundations, and museums. *Civic & Public Affairs:* 5%. Supports economic and community development, housing, civil rights, and women's affairs. *Education:* 38%. Supports universities, scholarships, and institutes. Generally, contributions are directed toward the improvement of the quality of education. *Environment:* 45%. Supports United Way, youth organizations, programs assisting runaway youth, scouting, clubs, YMCA/YWCA, and child abuse prevention. *International:* 4%. *Note:* Total foundation contributions made in 2000. **Typ. Recipients:** Alzheimers Disease, Cancer, Child Abuse, Clinics/Medical Centers, Domestic Violence, Hospices, Hospitals (University Affiliated), Medical Rehabilitation, Medical Research, Nursing Services, People with Disabilities, Prenatal Health Issues, Public Health, Substance Abuse. **Geo. Dist:** nationally; AZ; CA; CO; NM; TX, western area.

★ 12389 ★ Eli Lilly Foundation

Tax Division
Lilly Corporate Center
Indianapolis, IN 46285
Phone: (317)276-3743 **Fax:** (317)277-6719
Email: tom@lilly.com
Website: http://www.lilly.com/about/community/foundation/cash/index.html
Thomas King, President

Priorities: *Arts & Humanities:* 7%. *Civic & Public Affairs:* 2%. *Education:* 35%. *Environment:* 35%. *International:* 17%. *Note:* Percentages reflect cash grants made in 2000 by the foundation and through corporate direct giving. Product donations and cash grants provided through Lilly International and other components are not included in the annual report. **Typ. Recipients:** AIDS/HIV, Cancer, Children's Health/Hospitals, Diabetes, Emergency/Ambulance Services, Health Organizations, Health Policy/Cost Containment, Heart, Medical Education, Medical Research, Mental Health, Mental Health, People with Disabilities, Prenatal Health Issues, Public Health, Single-Disease Health Associations, Trauma Treatment. **Geo. Dist:** headquarters and operating communities; international organizations; national organizations.

★ 12390 ★ Emerson Charitable Trust

8000 West Florissant Ave.
PO Box 63136
Saint Louis, MO 63136
Phone: (314)553-3722
Ms. Joann Harmon, Senior Vice President

Priorities: *Arts & Humanities:* 18%. *Civic & Public Affairs:* 16%. *Education:* 37%. *Environment:* 22%. *International:* 4%. *Note:* Foundation giving accounts for 80% of contributions; direct giving, 20%. Above priorities reflect foundation giving in fiscal 2000. **Typ. Recipients:** AIDS/HIV, Alzheimers Disease, Children's Health/Hospitals, Eyes/Blindness, Health Organizations, Hospitals, Long-Term Care, Medical Education, Medical Research, People with Disabilities, Single-Disease Health Associations, Substance Abuse. **Geo. Dist:** nationally, emphasizing operating locations.

★ 12391 ★ EMI Music Publishing

1290 Ave. of the Americas
New York, NY 10104
Phone: (212)492-1200 **Fax:** (212)492-1750
Website: http://www.emimusicpub.com
Ann Roche, Director

Typ. Recipients: Domestic Violence, Medical Research, People with Disabilities, Substance Abuse. **Geo. Dist:** nationally.

★ 12392 ★ Employers Insurance of Wausau, A Mutual Co.

2000 Westwood Dr.
PO Box 8017
Wausau, WI 54402-8017
Phone: (715)845-5211 **Fax:** (715)843-3690
Email: brad.zweck@wausau.com
Website: http://www.wausau.com
Brad Zweck, Manager, Communication

Typ. Recipients: Health-General. **Geo. Dist:** primarily at headquarters and operating communities.

★ 12393 ★ Employers Mutual Charitable Foundation

PO Box 712
Des Moines, IA 50303-0712
Phone: (515)280-2171
Website: http://www.emcins.com/about/communityinvolvement.htm
Joe Smith, Manager, Executive Director

Priorities: *Arts & Humanities:* 33%. *Civic & Public Affairs:* 9%. *Education:* 14%. *Environment:* 36%. *International:* 6%. *Religion:* 1%. *Note:* Total contributions made in 2001. **Typ. Recipients:** Cancer, Children's Health/Hospitals, Diabetes, Emergency/Ambulance Services, Eyes/Blindness, Health Policy/Cost Containment, Health-General, Hospices, Hospitals, Multiple Sclerosis, People with Disabilities. **Geo. Dist:** IA.

★ 12394 ★ Ensign-Bickford Foundation

10 Grist Mill Rd.
Simsbury, CT 06070
Phone: (860)658-4411 **Fax:** (860)843-2805
Website: http://www.e-bind.com/community.html
Linda Angelastro, Exec. Director, Corporate Communications

Fnded: 1952. **Priorities:** *Arts & Humanities:* 1%. Supports theater, music, and art councils. *Civic & Public Affairs:* 30%. Supports municipalities and towns, parks, safety, clubs, chambers of commerce, and community development. *Education:* 33%. Supports public and private schools, universities, and Junior Achievement. *Environment:* 6%. Supports athletics and recreation, food distribution, people with disabilities, and scouts. *International:* 12%. Supports hospitals and single-disease health associations. *Religion:* 13%. Primarily supports science centers. *Note:* Total foundation contributions made in 2000. **Typ. Recipients:** Cancer, Children's Health/Hospitals, Diabetes, Health Organizations, Heart, Hospitals, Medical Education, Medical Research, Multiple Sclerosis, Nursing Services, People with Disabilities, Single-Disease Health Associations. **Geo. Dist:** primarily in areas of company operations; Avon, CT; Simsbury, CT.

★ 12395 ★ Entergy Corp.

PO Box 61000
New Orleans, LA 70161
Phone: (504)576-5785 **Fax:** (504)576-2190
Email: karnold@entergy.com
Website: http://www.entergy.com/contributions
Kay Arnold, Vice President Public Affairs

Priorities: *Voluntarism:* Entergy sponsors Community Connectors, an employee volunteer program. Employees and retirees who volunteer as Connectors can earn grants through their volunteer hours (up to $250 on an individual basis and $500 per team) and designate those grants to a qualified organization of their choice. *Note:* Dollar for dollar matching funds must be secured for the requested grant amount. **Typ. Recipients:** Health-General. **Geo. Dist:** company's service area; AR; LA; MS; TX.

★ 12396 ★ Enterprise Rent-A-Car Foundation

600 Corporate Park Drive
Saint Louis, MO 63105
Phone: (314)512-2754 **Fax:** (314)512-4754
Email: cconrad@erac.com
JoAnn Kindle, President

Priorities: *Arts & Humanities:* 7%. Gives to symphonies, orchestras, and operas. Also supports art museums, art fairs, historical societies, and public broadcasting. Generally, giving for the arts has been limited to the St. Louis, MO, area. *Civic & Public Affairs:* 5%. Areas of interest include urban renewal, housing, community festivals, and zoos. *Education:* 24%. Primarily supports colleges and universities within Missouri. Also supports technology education and college preparation. *Environment:* 62%. Supports United Ways, projects designed to aid children, parent and family services, and Special Olympics. *International:* 1%. Supports single-disease health associations, medical centers, and children's hospitals and health organizations. *Religion:* 2%. *Voluntarism:* All employees are encouraged to participate in community and national programs. *Note:* Total contributions in fiscal 2000. **Typ. Recipients:** Alzheimers Disease, Cancer, Children's Health/Hospitals, Clinics/Medical Centers, Diabetes, Domestic Violence, Emergency/Ambulance Services, Family Planning, Health Organizations, Hospitals, Mental Health, Multiple Sclerosis, Preventive Medicine/Wellness Organizations, Single-Disease Health Associations.

★ 12397 ★ Equifax Foundation

1550 Peachtree St. NW, Drop H-46
Atlanta, GA 30309
Phone: (404)885-8000 **Fax:** (404)885-8215
Email: kirby.thompson@equifax.com
Website: http://www.equifax.com
Kirby Thompson, Contact

Priorities: *Arts & Humanities:* 16%. *Civic & Public Affairs:* 25%. *Voluntarism:* The Hearts and Hands program recognizes employees for volunteer efforts in their communitys. Employees who reach milestones in hours of service are rewarded with Hearts and Hands shirts, event tickets, etc. Volunteers may participate in company-organized activities or may initiate activities on their own. *Note:* Total contributions made in 2001. Giving percentages provided by foundation. **Typ. Recipients:** Cancer, Children's Health/Hospitals, Emergency/Ambulance Services, Health Organizations, Health-General, Heart, Hospices, Hospitals, Kidney, Medical Education, Medical Rehabilitation, Multiple Sclerosis, Nursing Services, People with Disabilities, Prenatal Health Issues, Public Health, Research/Studies Institutes, Single-Disease Health Associations, Substance Abuse. **Geo. Dist:** Atlanta, GA, primarily metro area.

★ 12398 ★ Equitable Resources, Inc.

One Oxford Center 3300
301 Grant St.
Pittsburgh, PA 15219
Phone: (412)553-7739 **Fax:** (412)553-5757
Website: http://www.eqt.com/about_EQT/Community.asp
Estelle Christian, Executive Assistant to CEO

Priorities: *Education:* Focuses support on education. *Environment:* Primary support to United Way. **Typ. Recipients:** Arthritis, Children's Health/Hospitals, Domestic Violence, Health-General, Hospitals, Hospitals (University Affiliated), Medical Education, People with Disabilities. **Geo. Dist:** headquarters area only.

★ 12399 ★ Erb Foundation

PO Box 458
Bloomfield Hills, MI 48303-0458
Phone: (248)644-6222
Fred Erb, President

Priorities: *Arts & Humanities:* 8%. Supports art museums, the performing arts, and public broadcasting. *Civic & Public Affairs:* 1%. Supports community foundations, zoos, and parks. *Education:* 1%. Supports colleges, universities and private educational institutions. *Environment:* 4%. Funds youth organizations, violence prevention, and United Way. *International:* 83%. Supports hospitals, single-disease health orgs, and hospice programs. *Religion:* 1%. Funds the Cranbrook Institute of Science. *Note:* Total contributions made in 2000. **Typ. Recipients:** Alzheimers Disease, Cancer, Children's Health/Hospitals, Eyes/Blindness, Family Planning, Hospices, Hospitals, Medical Research, Mental Health, People with Disabilities, Prenatal Health Issues, Substance Abuse. **Geo. Dist:** MI.

★ 12400 ★ Ethyl Corp.
330 S 4th St.
Richmond, VA 23219
Phone: (804)788-5522 **Fax:** (804)788-5636
Email: contributions@ethyl.com
Website: http://www.ethyl.com/contact/contributions.html
Diane Hazelwood, Contact

Priorities: *Arts & Humanities:* About 25%. Supports programs to improve the quality of life, particularly those designed to make a community more attractive to prospective employees. *Civic & Public Affairs:* 5% to 10%. Emphasis is on economic education and better government organizations. *Education:* 40% to 45%. Supports public and private institutions, with emphasis on those that serve as a potential source of employees or those which are of significance to employee family members. Administers matching gifts program and scholarship program for employee family members. Supports secondary, undergraduate, and graduate level study. *International:* About 25%. Emphasizes programs of direct benefit to employees in the areas of health, social services,recreation, and physical fitness. Includes support for United Way. **Typ. Recipients:** Emergency/Ambulance Services, Health Organizations, Hospitals. **Geo. Dist:** headquarters and operating communities.

★ 12401 ★ Excel Corp.
151 North Main St.
Wichita, KS 67202
Phone: (316)291-2500 **Fax:** (316)291-3499
Email: contactexcel@cargill.com
Scott Eilert, Excel Cargill Cares Chairperson

Typ. Recipients: Health-General, Medical Rehabilitation. **Geo. Dist:** headquarters and operating communities.

★ 12402 ★ Exelon
10 South Dearborn St., 37th Floor
PO Box 805379
Chicago, IL 60690-3005
Phone: (312)394-7398

Priorities: *Arts & Humanities:* Dance, music, opera, and general arts funding. *Civic & Public Affairs:* Supports civic and public affairs. *Education:* Supports education initiatives. *Environment:* Focus on crime prevention, youth organizations. *International:* Supports various health and welfare programs. *Note:* Supports traditional funding categories across the board. **Typ. Recipients:** Hospitals. **Geo. Dist:** PA, Bucks County; PA, Chester County; PA, Delaware County; PA, Montgomery County; PA, York County.

★ 12403 ★ Extendicare Foundation
111 W Michigan St.
Milwaukee, WI 53203
Phone: (414)908-8230
Website: http://www.extendicare.com/aboutus/Charitable.html
Dr. Ronald Retzke, Vice President, Community Relations

Fnded: 1985. **Priorities:** *Education:* 10%. Supports colleges and universities. *Environment:* 36%. Supports senior services, homes, and family foundations. *International:* 54%. Supports geriatric centers, nursing services, and Alzheimer's associations. *Note:* Total contributions made in 2000. **Typ. Recipients:** Alzheimers Disease, Geriatric Health, Health Organizations, Health Policy/Cost Containment, Long-Term Care, Mental Health, Nursing Services, Public Health. **Geo. Dist:** headquarters and operating communities.

★ 12404 ★ Exxon Mobil Foundation
5959 Las Colinas Boulevard
Irving, TX 75039-2298
Phone: (972)444-1104 **Fax:** (972)444-1405
Email: contributions@exxonmobil.com
Website: http://www2.exxonmobil.com/Corporate/Newsroom/Publications/c_cc_02/index.htm
Edward Ahnert, Manager, Contributions

Priorities: *Arts & Humanities:* 1%. *Civic & Public Affairs:* 12%. *Education:* 42%. *Environment:* 32%. *International:* 2%. *Religion:* 2%. *Note:* Total contributions made in 2001. **Typ. Recipients:** Cancer, Clinics/Medical Centers, Emergency/Ambulance Services, Health Organizations, Hospitals, Hospitals, Medical Education, Medical Rehabilitation, Medical Research, Medical Training, Nursing Services, Public Health, Substance Abuse. **Geo. Dist:** internationally; nationally. **Frmly:** Exxon Education Foundation.

★ 12405 ★ F.K. Bemis Family Foundation
PO Box 901
Sheboygan Falls, WI 53085-0901
Phone: (920)467-4621 **Fax:** (920)467-8573
Email: corp@BemisMfg.com
Richard Bemis, President

Fnded: 1953. **Priorities:** *Arts & Humanities:* 20%. Funds arts centers, theater, museums, historic preservation, and public broadcasting. *Civic & Public Affairs:* 25%. Gives to municipalities, job training initiatives, and civic groups such as Jaycees. *Education:* 37%. Supports colleges and universities and junior achievement. *Environment:* 14%. Supports United Way, Young Men's Christian Association, activities for youth, and athletics. *International:* 4%. Funds medical centers, single-disease associations, and American Red Cross. *Note:* Total contributions made in 2001. **Typ. Recipients:** Cancer, Children's Health/Hospitals, Clinics/Medical Centers, Emergency/Ambulance Services, Hospitals, Medical Research. **Geo. Dist:** MA; WI, Sheboygan County.

★ 12406 ★ Fabri-Kal Foundation
Plastics Place
Kalamazoo, MI 49001-4880
Phone: (616)385-5050 **Fax:** (616)385-0197
Robert Kittredge, Chairman & Chief Executive Officer

Priorities: *Arts & Humanities:* 2%. Supports arts councils. *Civic & Public Affairs:* 11%. Funds parks, community organizations and municipalities. *Education:* 19%. Funds educational grants for the children of company employees and educational initiatives. *Environment:* 50%. Funds the United Way, children's organizations, and human services. *International:* 16%. Supports hospice. *Note:* Total contributions made in 2000. **Typ. Recipients:** Emergency/Ambulance Services, Health-General, Hospices, Medical Education, Nursing Services, People with Disabilities, Substance Abuse. **Geo. Dist:** Kalamazoo, MI; Hazleton, PA; Greenville, SC.

★ 12407 ★ Fannie Mae Foundation
North Tower, Suite One
4000 Wisconsin Ave., NW
Washington, DC 20016-2804
Phone: (202)274-8062 **Fax:** (202)274-8111
Email: grants@fanniemaefoundation.org
Website: http://www.fanniemaefoundation.org

Fnded: 1979. **Priorities:** *Arts & Humanities:* 1%. *Civic & Public Affairs:* 70%. *Education:* 18%. *Environment:* 9%. *Note:* Total contributions made in 2000. **Typ. Recipients:** Child Abuse, Nursing Services, Single-Disease Health Associations. **Geo. Dist:** national organizations; operating locations; Washington, DC.

★ 12408 ★ Farber Foundation
1845 Walnut St., Suite 800
Philadelphia, PA 19103
Phone: (215)569-9900 **Fax:** (215)569-9979
Jack Farber, Chairman & President

Priorities: *Arts & Humanities:* 9%. Supports performing arts, public broadcasting, and music. *Civic & Public Affairs:* 4%. Funds community based organizations, economic development, and careers. *Education:* 44. Funds scholarship program for employees and through Thomas Jefferson University. *Environment:* 3%. Funds food distribution, athletics, and youth organizations. *International:* 1%. Primarily supports single-disease causes. *Religion:* Less than 1%. Supports a science institute. *Note:* Total contributions made in 2001. **Typ. Recipients:** Alzheimers Disease, Arthritis, Cancer, Children's Health/Hospitals, Diabetes, Emergency/Ambulance Services, Health Policy/Cost Containment, Hospitals, Kidney, Long-Term Care, Medical Rehabilitation, Medical Research, Multiple Sclerosis, People with Disabilities, Single-Disease Health Associations, Substance Abuse. **Geo. Dist:** PA.

★ 12409 ★ FBW Foundation
8403 Colesville Rd., No. 900
Silver Spring, MD 20910-4704
Phone: (301)273-6000

Fnded: 1994. **Priorities:** *Arts & Humanities:* 4%. Gives to opera, theater, arts centers, choral groups, and museums. *Civic & Public Affairs:* 8%. Funds affordable housing programs, city councils, and an aquarium. *Education:* 25%. Supports colleges, universities, business education, parochial schools, reading programs, scholarship funds, and public schools. *Environment:* 29%. Supports local United Way offices, youth activities, senior services, food distribution, animal welfare organizations, services for the disabled, family services, and child welfare organizations. *International:* 33%. Funds wellness programs, hospitals and medical centers, single-disease health associations, and hospice programs. *Note:* Total contributions made in fiscal 2001. **Typ. Recipients:** Alzheimers Disease, Cancer, Clinics/Medical Centers, Heart, Hospices, People with Disabilities, Preventive Medicine/Wellness Organizations. **Geo. Dist:** MD; VA; Washington, WA; WV.

★ 12410 ★ FC Foundation
44 First Alabama Plaza
Montgomery, AL 36104
Phone: (334)832-8619
A.J. Smith, Contact

Fnded: 1992. **Typ. Recipients:** AIDS/HIV, Arthritis, Cancer, Children's Health/Hospitals, Clinics/Medical Centers, Domestic Violence, Emergency/Ambulance Services, Family Planning, Health Organizations, Heart, Kidney, Medical Research, Mental Health, Respiratory. **Geo. Dist:** AL; AR; GA; LA; MS; NY; NY; OH; SC; TN; TX.

★ 12411 ★ Federated Department Stores Foundation
7 West Seventh St.
Cincinnati, OH 45202
Phone: (513)579-7569 **Fax:** (513)579-7185
Email: dbarker@fds.com
Website: http://www.fds.com/community
Dixie Barker, Executive Director of Foundation

Priorities: *Arts & Humanities:* 16%. *Civic & Public Affairs:* 17%. *Education:* 3%. *Environment:* 57%. *International:* 7%. *Voluntarism:* Partners in Time program established in 1989 as a vehicle to organize and stimulate volunteerism activities. Multi divisional projects involve employees from divisions in the same city working together on a unified project. *Note:* Total contributions made in fiscal 2001. **Typ. Recipients:** AIDS/HIV, Cancer, Children's Health/Hospitals, Domestic Violence, Eyes/Blindness, Family Planning, Health Funds, Hospices, Hospitals, Medical Education, People with Disabilities, Preventive Medicine/Wellness Organizations, Public Health, Single-Disease Health Associations, Substance Abuse. **Geo. Dist:** headquarters and operating communities. **Frmly:** Robert Campeau Family Foundation (U.S.) Ilse and Robert Campeau Family Foundation.

★ 12412 ★ Federated Mutual Insurance Foundation
121 E Park Sq.
Owatonna, MN 55060
Phone: (507)455-5200
Brian Brose, Contact

Priorities: *Arts & Humanities:* 5%. Funds community arts, performing arts, arts centers and institutes, and libraries. *Civic & Public Affairs:* 5%. Supports community foundations, housing, and professional trade organizations. *Education:* 11%. Supports colleges and universities and afterschool enrichment programs. *Environment:* 77%. Supports causes under the foundation's Human Services and Youth programs. Major support to disaster relief. *International:* 2%. Funds health and wellness organizations. *Note:* Total contributions made in 2001. **Typ. Recipients:** Cancer, Children's Health/Hospitals, Emergency/Ambulance Services, Geriatric Health, Health Organizations, Health Policy/Cost Containment, Health-General, Heart, Home-Care Services, Medical Rehabilitation, Medical Research, People with Disabilities, Public Health, Substance Abuse. **Geo. Dist:** operating locations, mainly MN.

★ 12413 ★ FedEx Corp.
PO Box 727- Dept 1850
Memphis, TN 38194
Phone: (901)395-5006 **Fax:** (901)346-1013
Patrick Melancon, Manager, Community Relations

Priorities: *Arts & Humanities:* 10% to 15%. Supports organizations that foster the arts on a broad, nonexclusive basis. Support includes public broadcasting, arts councils, and museums. *Civic & Public Affairs:* About 15%. Supports issue-oriented groups engaged in activities including civil rights, conservation, crime prevention, urban affairs, and community development. Also supports public policy organizations and business groups involved in matters such as transportation safety and business excellence, mostly in the company's headquarters area. *Education:* 20% to 25%. Emphasizes higher education institutions in headquarters area. The company has taken an increasingly active role in supporting secondary school education in recent years. The Adopt-a-School Program is among the company's recipients in this area. *International:* 50% to 55%. Makes capital grants in support of community service organizations, with emphasis on people-to-people assistance programs that have broad, nonexclusive community impact. Makes capital grants to operating support (including building funds) in communities in which a significant number of employees are concentrated. Considers both capital and operating support of agencies that provide medical and health research materials. Areas of interest include united funds, youth organizations (including Junior Achievement), food banks, the handicapped, the elderly, the homeless, and hospitals. *Voluntarism:* Volunteer teams work with many organizations in various areas: Children and Youth; Adopt-a-School programs; Junior Achievement; Deaf United for the Community; Civic Affairs; and promotion of the arts. **Typ. Recipients:** Health Organizations, People with Disabilities, Single-Disease Health Associations. **Geo. Dist:** headquarters; nationally.

★ 12414 ★ Ferro Foundation
1000 Lakeside Ave.
Cleveland, OH 44114-1147
Phone: (216)614-8580 **Fax:** (216)696-5803
James Hill, Secretary & Treasurer

Fnded: 1959. **Priorities:** *Arts & Humanities:* 17%. Supports performing arts, museums, music, public broadcasting, and historical preservation. Recipients include Musical Arts Association, Playhouse Square Foundation and Western Reserve Historical Association. *Civic & Public Affairs:* 15%. Supports employment and job training, towns and municipalities, and economic development. Recipients include Urban League of Northern Cleveland and Cleveland Technical Services Council. *Education:* 17%. Supports private precollege education and college and universities. *Environment:* 48%. Supports united funds, youth programs, and family services. *International:* 2%. *Religion:* 3%. *Note:* Total foundation contributions made in fiscal 2000. **Typ. Recipients:** Alzheimers Disease, Cancer, Children's Health/Hospitals, Clinics/Medical Centers, Diabetes, Emergency/Ambulance Services, Health-General, Hospitals, Hospitals (University Affiliated), Medical Rehabilitation, Mental Health, Multiple Sclerosis, Nursing Services, People with Disabilities, Prenatal Health Issues, Substance Abuse. **Geo. Dist:** Washington, DC; Cleveland, OH, and surrounding area.

★ 12415 ★ Fidelity Foundation
82 Devonshire St. S3
Boston, MA 02109
Phone: (617)563-6806 **Fax:** (617)476-4234
Website: http://www.fidelityfoundation.org
Margaret Morton, Vice President, Program

Priorities: *Arts & Humanities:* 41%. Supports museums, music, theaters, dance, art institutes, and historic preservation. *Civic & Public Affairs:* 13%. Community development interests include neighborhood housing services, economic development, non-profit management, civic foundations, women's issues, zoos, and aquariums. *Education:* 27%. Majority of support goes to matching gifts. Also supports universities, colleges, secondary education, and educational funds. *Environment:* 9%. Funds youth organizations, shelters, recreation, and volunteerism. *International:* 6%. Supports medical research in health organizations and hospitals. *Religion:* 1%. Funds museums. *Note:* Total foundation contributions made in 2000. **Typ. Recipients:** Cancer, Child Abuse, Children's Health/Hospitals, Clinics/Medical Centers, Health Organizations, Hospices, Hospitals, Medical Research, Mental Health, Nursing Services, People with Disabilities. **Geo. Dist:** Covington, KY; Boston, MA; Marlborough, MA; Merrimack, NH; New York, NY; Smithfield, RI; Dallas, TX; Ft. Worth, TX; Salt Lake City, UT; Toronto, ON. **Frmly:** Fidelity Investments Charitable Gift Fund Foundation, Inc.

★ 12416 ★ Fifth Third Foundation
38 Fountain Square Plaza
Maildrop 1090D7
Cincinnati, OH 45263
Phone: (513)579-6034 **Fax:** (513)579-5461
Lawra Baumann, Foundation Officer

Priorities: *Arts & Humanities:* 21%. Major support for music, arts funds, museums, and arts centers. Historic preservation, the performing arts, theater, and public broadcasting are also supported. *Civic & Public Affairs:* 25%. Funds housing, law and justice, chambers of commerce, economic development, city and regional planning, minority interests, and community foundations. *Education:* 15%. Majority of funding goes to colleges and universities. Other areas of interest include arts education, education funds, and youth, medical, precollege, economic, and religious education. *Environment:* 33%. Majority of funding supports United Way chapters. Major grants are also made to various youth organizations, especially those supporting scouting. Other interests include the aged, the disabled, and family services. *International:* 3%. Supports disease control, hospitals, clinics, single-disease health associations, and organizations that provide behavioral health and drug rehabilitation services. *Note:* Total contributions in fiscal 2001. **Typ. Recipients:** Children's Health/Hospitals, Emergency/Ambulance Services, Health Funds, Health Organizations, Hospices, Hospitals, Medical Education, Medical Rehabilitation, People with Disabilities, Single-Disease Health Associations, Speech & Hearing. **Geo. Dist:** Cincinnati, OH, including metropolitan area.

★ 12417 ★ Fireman's Fund Foundation
777 San Marin Drive
Novato, CA 94998-1406
Phone: (415)899-2757 **Fax:** (415)899-2012
Ms. Barbara Friede, Secretary & Director

Fnded: 1953. **Priorities:** *Arts & Humanities:* 28%. *Civic & Public Affairs:* 12%. *Education:* 4%. *Environment:* 40%. *International:* 5%. *Religion:* 1%. *Note:* Total foundation contributions made in 2001. **Typ. Recipients:** AIDS/HIV, Alzheimers Disease, Domestic Violence, Health Organizations, Home-Care Services, Hospitals, Medical Rehabilitation, Mental Health, People with Disabilities, Preventive Medicine/Wellness Organizations, Substance Abuse. **Geo. Dist:** CA, Marin and Sonoma Counties.

★ 12418 ★ First American Financial Foundation
1 First American Way
Santa Ana, CA 92707
Phone: (714)800-3312
Email: tklemens@firstam.com
Thomas Klemens, Vice President & Chief Financial Officer

Priorities: *Arts & Humanities:* 42%. Supports ballet, choir, opera, theater, and history organizations. *Civic & Public Affairs:* 11%. Gives to business/industry associations. *Education:* 23%. Primarily funds universities. *Environment:* 9%. Funds youth organizations. *International:* 15%. Contributes to hospitals, single-disease health associations, and an ear institute. *Note:* Total contributions made in fiscal 2000. **Typ. Recipients:** Diabetes, Health-General, Hospitals. **Geo. Dist:** CA.

★ 12419 ★ First American Foundation
First American Center
315 Deaderick St., 4th Floor
Nashville, TN 37237
Phone: (615)736-6679
Ashley Webster, Contact

Fnded: 1993. **Priorities:** *Arts & Humanities:* 28% Supports museums, opera, dance, and the performing arts. *Civic & Public Affairs:* 10%. Public policy, zoos, aquariums, parks, historical sites, and community foundations are supported. *Education:* 9%. Focus is on colleges and universities. *Environment:* 48%. Supports United Way, YMCA and YWCA, athletics, community centers, and youth organizations. *International:* 5%. Supports Ronald McDonald House, hospice and a children's hospital. *Religion:* 1%. *Note:* Total foundation contributions made in 2000. **Typ. Recipients:** Children's Health/Hospitals, Clinics/Medical Centers, Health Organizations, Hospices, Hospitals, Hospitals (University Affiliated), Medical Education, Public Health. **Geo. Dist:** headquarters and operating communities. **Frmly:** First American Foundation.

★ 12420 ★ First Hawaiian Foundation
999 Bishop St., 29th Floor
Honolulu, HI 96813
Phone: (808)525-7766 **Fax:** (808)525-7750
Lily Yao, President

Priorities: *Arts & Humanities:* 10%. Supports museums, arts centers, film, and music. *Civic & Public Affairs:* 4%. Supports housing and civic foundations. *Education:* 39%. Funds colleges and universities. Private and public precollege education receives most support through capital campaigns and grants used to renovate or refurbish facilities. *Environment:* 34%. Majority of giving supports united funds. Funds are also provided for services for youth, YMCA, community centers, shelters and food banks, and drug prevention. *International:* 8%. Supports health clinics, hospitals, single-disease health associations, and health foundations. *Voluntarism:* Company supports employee volunteerism through the YesTeam. *Note:* Total foundation contributions made in 2000. **Typ. Recipients:** Cancer, Children's Health/Hospitals, Clinics/Medical Centers, Domestic Violence, Emergency/Ambulance Services, Health Organizations, Hospices, Hospitals, Medical Rehabilitation, People with Disabilities, Research/Studies Institutes, Single-Disease Health Associations, Substance Abuse. **Geo. Dist:** HI.

★ 12421 ★ First National Bank in Wichita Charitable Trust
PO Box One
Wichita, KS 67201
Phone: (316)383-1004 **Fax:** (316)383-5879
Email: rdpitts@intrustbank.com

Website: http://www.intrustbank.com
Rodney Pitts, Senior Vice President

Priorities: *Arts & Humanities:* 7%. Supports museums, music, and art centers. *Civic & Public Affairs:* 2%. Supports community foundations and clubs. *Education:* 9%. Primarily supports universities. *Environment:* 60%. Supports YMCA, United Way, and youth organizations. *International:* 6%. Supports health centers and organizations. *Religion:* 16%. Primary support made to science centers. *Voluntarism:* INTRUST recruits employees to volunteer in school classrooms during regular work hours. *Note:* Total foundation contributions made in 2001. **Typ. Recipients:** Cancer, Children's Health/Hospitals, Health Organizations, Health-General, Hospices, Hospitals, Mental Health, People with Disabilities, Preventive Medicine/Wellness Organizations, Single-Disease Health Associations. **Geo. Dist:** operating locations.

★ 12422 ★ First Niagara Bank Foundation

6950 S Transit Rd.
PO Box 514
Lockport, NY 14095-0514
Phone: (716)625-7500

Fnded: 1998. **Priorities:** *Arts & Humanities:* 11%. *Civic & Public Affairs:* 22%. *Education:* 26%. *Environment:* 29%. *International:* 4%. *Note:* Total contributions made in 2002. **Typ. Recipients:** Hospitals, Multiple Sclerosis, Substance Abuse. **Geo. Dist:** NY.

★ 12423 ★ First Source Foundation

Care of First Source Bank
PO Box 1602
South Bend, IN 46601
Phone: (219)235-2790 **Fax:** (219)235-2771
Mary Sonneborn, Trust Officer

Fnded: 1952. **Priorities:** *Arts & Humanities:* 35%. Supports art museums, performing arts, and fine arts foundations and councils. *Civic & Public Affairs:* 8%. Funds community foundations, local community activities, and fire departments. *Education:* 12%. Gives to high schools, Junior Achievement, scholarship funds, colleges and universities. *Environment:* 41%. Supports local United Ways, Boys and Girls Clubs, animal welfare organizations, and rescue missions. *International:* 2%. Funds hospice programs, hospitals, and a health foundation. *Note:* Total contributions in 2000. **Typ. Recipients:** Alzheimers Disease, Child Abuse, Children's Health/Hospitals, Diabetes, Health Funds, Health Organizations, Hospices, Hospitals, Kidney, Medical Education, Mental Health, People with Disabilities, Preventive Medicine/Wellness Organizations, Public Health, Substance Abuse. **Geo. Dist:** IN.

★ 12424 ★ First Tennessee Foundation

165 Madison
Memphis, TN 38103
Phone: (901)523-4380
Email: jtlee@ftb.com
J. Lee, Sr. Vice Pres., Corporate Communications

Priorities: *Arts & Humanities:* 18%. *Civic & Public Affairs:* 18%. *Education:* 23%. *Environment:* 36%. *International:* 1%. *Voluntarism:* Company sponsors Volunteerbank. *Note:* Focus of priorities is shifting toward emphasis on education and parental involvement in education. Total contributions made in 2001. **Typ. Recipients:** Children's Health/Hospitals, Hospitals. **Geo. Dist:** TN, headquarters and operating communities.

★ 12425 ★ First Union National Bank, NA

Widener Bldg.
PA 4385
1339 Chestnut
Philadelphia, PA 19107
Phone: (267)321-7663 **Fax:** (267)321-7662
Website: http://www.wachovia.com
Kevin Dow, Vice President, Contributions

Priorities: *Arts & Humanities:* Interests include arts institutions which promote the Philadelphia area as a business location, and cultural institutions with a broad audience appeal. Recipients include arts centers, ethnic arts, libraries, museums, performing arts, and public broadcasting. *Civic & Public Affairs:* Prefers to support organizations that enhance the business and economic climate of the area it serves. Recipients include better government, economics, housing, and the environment. *Education:* Company reports that education is its top giving priority. Supports local four-year colleges and universities, an employee matching gift program, and economic education. *International:* Recipients include hospitals that are able to make a strong documented case of service to First Fidelity employees, their families, and customers, or that serve a special need in the community not adequately met by others. Youth agencies serving inner-city youth, children, or customers in more than one area of First Union's market are also funded. **Typ. Recipients:** Domestic Violence, Family Planning, Geriatric Health, Hospices, Substance Abuse. **Geo. Dist:** operating locations; PA.

★ 12426 ★ Firstar Foundation, Inc.

US Bank Place
225 South 6th St.
Minneapolis, MN 55402
Kathleen Toay, Foundation Director

Priorities: *Arts & Humanities:* 30%. Primarily supports a performing arts fund. Also gives to museums, ballet, historic preservation, opera, symphonies, and libraries. *Civic & Public Affairs:* 5%. About one-half supports economic and community development in Milwaukee. The remainder supports a variety of interests, including civil rights, professional organizations, public policy, nonprofit management, and zoos. *Education:* 14%. Supports colleges and universities, exclusively in the state of Wisconsin. *Environment:* 47%. Recipients include youth organizations, religious welfare groups, community centers, child welfare, and programs for the aged. *International:* 3%. Supports single-disease health associations, medical research, nursing services, and health funds. *Voluntarism:* The Company has an active employee volunteer program. *Note:* Total contributions made in 1998. **Typ. Recipients:** Children's Health/Hospitals, Clinics/Medical Centers, Emergency/Ambulance Services, Family Planning, Health Organizations, Health-General, Heart, Hospices, Hospitals, Medical Education, Nursing Services, People with Disabilities, Single-Disease Health Associations, Substance Abuse, Transplant Networks/Donor Banks. **Geo. Dist:** Milwaukee, WI. **Frmly:** Firstar Milwaukee Foundation.

★ 12427 ★ FirstEnergy Corp.

76 South Main St.
Akron, OH 44308-1890
Phone: (330)761-4246 **Fax:** (330)761-4203
Email: valentined@firstenergycorp.com
Website: http://www.firstenergycorp.com/community
Donna Valentine, Director of Contributions

Priorities: *Arts & Humanities:* 21%. Supports museums, orchestras, art centers, libraries, historical societies. *Civic & Public Affairs:* 14%. Funds community groups, zoos, botanical gardens, community festivals, business development and international affairs. *Education:* 14%. Gives to colleges and universities, secondary schools, Junior Achievement programs, and specialized education, including business and performing arts education programs. *Environment:* 51%. Supports scouts, hospitals and clinics, youth services, United Way, YMCA, and volunteer programs. *Note:* Total contributions made in 1999. **Typ. Recipients:** Health-General. **Geo. Dist:** headquarters and operating communities.

★ 12428 ★ Fisher Brothers Foundation, Inc.

299 Park Ave.
New York, NY 10017
Phone: (212)752-5000 **Fax:** (212)940-6207
Mr. Richard Fisher, Director

Fnded: 1981. **Priorities:** *Arts & Humanities:* 29%. Supports performing arts, museums, art associations, and public broadcasting. *Civic & Public Affairs:* 2%. Funds urban affairs, public safety/law enforcement, and other civic organizations. *Education:* 2%. Provides grants for colleges and universities, and private secondary education. *Environment:* 1%. Supports local United Way agencies, YMCA/YWCA, and Boy Scouts of America. *International:* 1%. Supports cancer care and medical research. *Religion:* Less than 1%. *Note:* Total contributions made in 2000. **Typ. Recipients:** AIDS/HIV, Cancer, Children's Health/Hospitals, Diabetes, Geriatric Health, Health-General, Heart, Hospitals, Medical Education, People with Disabilities, Single-Disease Health Associations, Transplant Networks/Donor Banks. **Geo. Dist:** MD; New York, NY, metropolitan area.

★ 12429 ★ Fleet Charitable Trust of New York

c/o Fleet Financial Group
75 State St.
Boston, MA 02109
Phone: (617)346-4534
Martha Buchanan-Forte, Contact

Priorities: *Arts & Humanities:* 7%. Supports performing arts. *Civic & Public Affairs:* 19%. Funds community development, urban affairs, and housing. *Education:* 26%. Funds schools, literacy, and colleges. *Environment:* 44%. Focus on United Way; also funds organizations serving children, youth, and families. *International:* 2%. *Note:* Total contributions made in fiscal 2000. **Typ. Recipients:** Arthritis, Children's Health/Hospitals, Clinics/Medical Centers, Health Organizations, Health-General, Hospices, Hospitals, Medical Rehabilitation, Nursing Services, People with Disabilities, Single-Disease Health Associations. **Geo. Dist:** NY.

★ 12430 ★ FleetBoston Financial Foundation

100 Hundred Federal St.
Boston, MA 02110
Phone: (617)434-2629 **Fax:** (617)434-6072
Website: http://www.fleet.com
Gail Snowdon, President

Priorities: *Arts & Humanities:* Funding in this area includes sponsorship of initiatives from major exhibits to community and grassroots performances; educational outreach to low- and moderate-income youth; and projects that promote increased access to the arts. *Civic & Public Affairs:* Funding in civic and public affairs focuses on economic opportunity, with a particular focus on community development programs; microenterprise, entrepreneurial, and small business development; job creation and employment training; affordable housing initiatives and homebuyer seminars; and selected programs that serve low- and moderate-income individuals. *Education:* Funds public education programs, emphasizing programs that support literacy programs, business and finance education, transition from school to career, and long-term education reform efforts. *Environment:* Supports youth development, including programs that promote healthy development, adult mentoring support, job readiness and skill building, and leadership skills through community service. *Note:* Contribution priorities were derived from the foundation's Grantmaking Guidelines. **Typ. Recipients:** AIDS/HIV, Children's Health/Hospitals, Clinics/Medical Centers, Domestic Violence, Emergency/Ambulance Services, Family Planning, Heart, Hospices, Hospitals, Hospitals (University Affiliated), Medical Research, Nutrition, People with Disabilities, Prenatal Health Issues, Substance Abuse. **Geo. Dist:** CT; FL, in limited areas; ME; MA; NH; NJ; NY; RI.

★ 12431 ★ Florida Rock Industries Foundation

PO Box 4667
Jacksonville, FL 32201
Phone: (904)355-1781 **Fax:** (904)366-1866
John Milton, Jr., Secretary

Priorities: *Civic & Public Affairs:* 9%. Supports urban leagues and public policy associations. *Education:*

42%. Funds scholarships and universities. *Environment:* 41%. Supports the United Way, youth organizations, and homeless centers. *International:* 2%. Supports single-disease health organizations. *Religion:* 3%. Supports a science and history museum. *Note:* Total contributions made in fiscal 2001. **Typ. Recipients:** Alzheimers Disease, Cancer, Children's Health/Hospitals, Clinics/Medical Centers, Family Planning, Geriatric Health, Health Organizations, Medical Research, Multiple Sclerosis, People with Disabilities, Single-Disease Health Associations. **Geo. Dist:** FL.

★ 12432 ★ Fluor Foundation
One Enterprise Dr., F2C
Aliso Viejo, CA 92656-2606
Phone: (949)349-6797
Email: community.relations@fluordaniel.com
Website: http://fluor.com/community/involvement.asp
Ms. Suzanne Esber, Manager Community Relations

Priorities: *Arts & Humanities:* 1%. *Civic & Public Affairs:* 2%. *Education:* 84%. Supports colleges, universities, and scholarship programs, with emphasis on science and technology education. Other interests include engineering education and minority education. Also sponsors employee matching gifts program. *Environment:* 16%. Supports YMCA. *International:* 9%. *Religion:* 1%. *Voluntarism:* "The Fluor Community Involvement Team," is a corporate volunteer program in which employees, retirees, and their family and friends carry out service projects in local communities. Employees also volunteer for many education programs: Junior Achievement, school partnerships, mentoring, and classroom presentations. *Note:* Total foundation contributions made in 2000. **Typ. Recipients:** AIDS/HIV, Cancer, Children's Health/Hospitals, Clinics/Medical Centers, Diabetes, Emergency/Ambulance Services, Hospitals, Medical Education, Substance Abuse. **Geo. Dist:** operating locations.

★ 12433 ★ FMC Foundation
1735 Market St.
Philadelphia, PA 19103
Phone: (215)299-6000
Judith Smeltzer, Contact

Priorities: *Arts & Humanities:* 12%. Museums, libraries, and performing arts supported. *Civic & Public Affairs:* 14%. Supports civic organizations that address recreational needs and environmental, urban, and governmental issues. *Education:* 12%. Generally, almost half of foundation's education contributions are made through employee matching gifts program. In addition, supports student associations at colleges and universities across the country that graduate a significant number of future employees. Grants are made to minority programs in fields relevant to company. Also supports free enterprise and economic education through colleges, universities, and other organizations for younger students. *Environment:* 50%. United Way, Salvation Army, and youth organizations are supported. *International:* 4%. Primarily funds single-disease associations. *Religion:* 4%. Supports research and science museums. *Voluntarism:* Through the Dollars for Doers program, the company matches up to $500 of employees' volunteer time at qualifying organizations. *Note:* Total contributions made in fiscal 2000. **Typ. Recipients:** Children's Health/Hospitals, Emergency/Ambulance Services, Health Funds, Health Organizations, Health Policy/Cost Containment, Heart, Hospitals, Medical Education, Medical Rehabilitation, Public Health, Single-Disease Health Associations. **Geo. Dist:** nationally; operating locations.

★ 12434 ★ Forbes Foundation
60 5th Ave.
New York, NY 10011
Phone: (212)620-2248 **Fax:** (212)633-1958
Mr. Leonard Yablon, Secretary & Treasurer

Fnded: 1979. **Priorities:** *Arts & Humanities:* 10%. Funds arts associations, museums, libraries, and historical preservation. *Civic & Public Affairs:* 14%. Business, law enforcement, public policy, and professional organizations receive support. *Education:* 70%. Colleges, universities, medical education, and private pre-college education are funded. *Environment:* 2%. Supports athletics, human services, and youth organizations. *International:* Less than 1%. Supports hospitals, medical research, and pediatric health. *Note:* Total contributions made in 2000. **Typ. Recipients:** AIDS/HIV, Arthritis, Cancer, Clinics/Medical Centers, Diabetes, Emergency/Ambulance Services, Family Planning, Health Funds, Health Organizations, Hospices, Hospitals, Medical Education, Medical Research, Mental Health, Nursing Services, Single-Disease Health Associations, Substance Abuse. **Geo. Dist:** New York, NY, including metropolitan area.

★ 12435 ★ Ford Meter Box Foundation
PO Box 443
775 Manchester Ave.
Wabash, IN 46992
Phone: (260)563-3171
Marta Gidley, Secretary

Fnded: 1988. **Priorities:** *Arts & Humanities:* 1%. Museums, opera, music, and arts associations receive funding. *Civic & Public Affairs:* 88%. Supports community-oriented philanthropic organizations and business and free enterprise. *Education:* 5%. Focus on higher education, education funds, and public education. *Environment:* 5%. Funds youth organizations, homes, child welfare, and counseling organizations. *International:* About 1%. Hospitals and single-disease health associations are funded. *Note:* Total contributions made in 2001. **Typ. Recipients:** Cancer, Child Abuse, Children's Health/Hospitals, Domestic Violence, Emergency/Ambulance Services, Eyes/Blindness, Geriatric Health, Health Organizations, Heart, Hospices, Hospitals, Medical Research, Mental Health, Outpatient Health Care, Prenatal Health Issues, Single-Disease Health Associations, Substance Abuse. **Geo. Dist:** IN, Wabash County and surrounding area.

★ 12436 ★ Ford Motor Co. Fund
One American Rd.
PO Box 1899
Dearborn, MI 48126
Phone: 888-313-0102
Website: http://www.ford.com/en/ourCompany/corporateCitizenship/fordMotorCompanyFund/defaul t.htm
Sandra Ulsh, Vice President, Executive Director

Priorities: *Arts & Humanities:* 19%. Large part of this support goes to performing arts groups in areas such as music, opera, dance, and theater, mostly in the Detroit area. The remainder primarily supports museums, libraries, public broadcasting, and arts councils and centers. Major support goes to the Edison Institute. *Civic & Public Affairs:* 15%. Emphasis on community improvement, which includes economic development, urban groups, and business associations. Other priorities are public policy research and youth groups. Employment training, traffic safety, housing, and education related to the free enterprise and economics also are of interest. Major grant to the Detroit Zoological Society ($2,000,000) and the Detroit Centennial Celebration ($2,000,000). *Education:* 27%. Major support goes to engineering, scientific, and technical education. Other priorities include business education, state and national education associations and funds, minority education, and general education (including, colleges and universities, public schools, and other organizations). Company also sponsors employee matching gifts program in this area, makes student loans to children of employees, and sponsors a program to promote scientific research. Support is also made to secondary education. *Environment:* 10%. Majority of support goes to United Way. The remainder supports social service groups such as food banks, shelters, recreation programs, and organizations serving children, the elderly, and the disabled. Also supports organizations serving youth. *International:* 5%. Interests include hospitals, health service organizations, cancer centers, and other health organizations. *Religion:* 1%. Supports a science center. *Voluntarism:* Ford Motor Company offers every Ford salaried employee 16 hours of paid time off per year to volunteer in teams of co-workers at various agencies. *Note:* Total contributions made in 2000. Above priorities are those of the Ford Motor Company Fund. Company also sponsors a direct giving program. Company reports that direct giving goes to a variety of organizations, but priorities are similar to those of the fund. **Typ. Recipients:** Cancer, Emergency/Ambulance Services, Health Organizations, Health Policy/Cost Containment, Hospices, Hospitals, Kidney, People with Disabilities, Prenatal Health Issues, Public Health, Substance Abuse. **Geo. Dist:** nationally; headquarters and operating communities; nationally.

★ 12437 ★ Forest City Enterprises Charitable Foundation, Inc.
50 Public Square, Suite 1100
Cleveland, OH 44113-2203
Phone: (216)621-6060 **Fax:** (216)263-6208
Allan Krulak, Vice President

Fnded: 1976. **Priorities:** *Arts & Humanities:* 17%. Supports orchestras, theater, art museums, and historical societies. *Civic & Public Affairs:* 2%. Funds organizations concerned with economic development, civil rights, youth, urban affairs, crime prevention, and employment. *Education:* 23%. Majority supports scholarships. High priorities include science and technology education and religious education. *Environment:* 11%. *International:* (Health and Welfare) 58%. Welfare funding supports the United Way and a variety of other social service groups, including religious welfare organizations. Majority of health support focuses on hospitals. Interests also include medical research and single-disease health associations. *Note:* Total contributions made in fiscal 2000. **Typ. Recipients:** AIDS/HIV, Alzheimers Disease, Arthritis, Cancer, Children's Health/Hospitals, Clinics/Medical Centers, Diabetes, Emergency/Ambulance Services, Eyes/Blindness, Health Organizations, Health-General, Hospices, Hospitals, Multiple Sclerosis, Prenatal Health Issues, Public Health, Sexual Abuse, Single-Disease Health Associations, Substance Abuse. **Geo. Dist:** operating locations; New York, NY, including metropolitan area; OH; Cleveland, OH, including metropolitan area.

★ 12438 ★ Fortis Foundation
1 Chase Manhattan Plaza, 41st Floor
New York, NY 10005
Phone: (212)859-7000 **Fax:** (212)859-7010
Website: http://www.fortisfoundation.com
Jackie Gentile, Directory

Fnded: 1982. **Priorities:** *Arts & Humanities:* 7%. Supports libraries, museums, and art funds. *Civic & Public Affairs:* 4%. *Education:* 61%. *Environment:* 33%. *International:* 2%. *Note:* Total foundation contributions made in 2001. **Typ. Recipients:** AIDS/HIV, Cancer, Children's Health/Hospitals, Emergency/Ambulance Services, Family Planning, Medical Education, Multiple Sclerosis, Single-Disease Health Associations, Transplant Networks/Donor Banks. **Geo. Dist:** nationally health-related organizations; NY.

★ 12439 ★ Fortis Insurance Foundation
501 West Michigan Ave.
Milwaukee, WI 53203-3050
Phone: (414)299-8557 **Fax:** (414)299-6900
Dawn Krautkramer, Secretary

Fnded: 1973. **Priorities:** *Arts & Humanities:* 28%. Funds museums, libraries, and art programs. *Civic & Public Affairs:* 5%. Gives to economic and community development organizations and a zoo. *Education:* 6%. Supports economic education and a middle school. *Environment:* 27%. Supports Young Men's Christian Association, food banks, community centers, and children's services. *International:* 19%. Supports single-disease associations. *Voluntarism:* The foundation supports employee volunteer activities, with special consideration given to organizations where employees volunteer that fall within the foundation's focus areas. The foundation does consider grants to organizations where employees volunteer but are not within the foundation focus. However, grants of this nature are limited to $100 per organization, with priority given to programs providing education, training, and direct services. *Note:* Total contributions in 2001. **Typ. Recipients:** AIDS/HIV, Alzheimers Disease, Alzheimers Disease, Children's Health/Hospitals, Clinics/Medical Centers, Domestic Violence, Family Planning,

Geriatric Health, Health Organizations, Health Policy/Cost Containment, Hospitals, Medical Rehabilitation, Medical Research, Mental Health, Nutrition, People with Disabilities, Public Health, Respiratory, Single-Disease Health Associations, Substance Abuse. **Geo. Dist:** WI, Southeastern Wisconsin. **Frmly:** Fortis Insurance Foundation.

★ 12440 ★ Fortune Brands International, Inc.

1700 East Putnam Ave.
Old Greenwich, CT 06870
Fax: (203)698-5577
Joan McGrath, Contributions Administrator

Typ. Recipients: Emergency/Ambulance Services, Health Organizations, Hospitals, Medical Research, People with Disabilities, Public Health, Single-Disease Health Associations, Substance Abuse. **Geo. Dist:** headquarters and operating communities.

★ 12441 ★ Foundation of the Litton Industries

1840 Century Park East
Los Angeles, CA 90067
Phone: (310)201-3323
Sandra Evers-Manly, President

Priorities: *Arts & Humanities:* 32%. Interests include community television, music, museums, and the performing arts. *Civic & Public Affairs:* 1%. Interests include law, ethics, and minorities. *Education:* 63%. Emphasis on math, engineering, and science. Supports universities and public and private schools at the elementary and secondary levels. Also supports minorities and students with military ties. *Environment:* 2%. Supports organizations for children and youth. *International:* 2%. Funds single-disease associations. *Note:* Above percentages reflect fiscal 2001 foundation priorities only. The company also operates a scholarship program for higher education. **Typ. Recipients:** People with Disabilities, Single-Disease Health Associations, Single-Disease Health Associations. **Geo. Dist:** nationally; Los Angeles, CA, national and regional appeals centered in metropolitan area.

★ 12442 ★ Fox Entertainment Group, Inc.

PO Box 900
Beverly Hills, CA 90213
Phone: (310)369-3029
Ms. Robin Corley, Director, Corporate Communications

Priorities: *Voluntarism:* The company sponsors an employee volunteer program that supports various activities, including an adopt-a-school relationship with Locke High School in South Central Los Angeles and events organized by the Permanent Charities Committee of the Entertainment Industries. **Typ. Recipients:** Health-General, Hospitals. **Geo. Dist:** headquarters area only.

★ 12443 ★ FPL Group Foundation, Inc.

9250 West Flagler St.
Miami, FL 33174
Phone: (305)552-4806 **Fax:** (305)552-4722
Email: John_Kitchens@fpl.com
Website: http://www.fpl.com
John Kitchens, Contributions Administrator

Fnded: 1989. **Priorities:** *Arts & Humanities:* 7%. Supports performing arts centers, museums, and music. *Civic & Public Affairs:* 9%. Funds economic development, community affairs, and municipalities. *Education:* 27%. Sponsors a matching gifts program to schools and universities; funding also goes to community colleges, and technology institutes. *Environment:* 52%. Supports United Way organizations and emergency relief, low-income family services and youth services. *International:* 7%. Funds diabetes and cancer research. *Religion:* 3%. *Note:* Total contributions in 2001. **Typ. Recipients:** AIDS/HIV, Cancer, Emergency/Ambulance Services, Geriatric Health, Health Organizations, Medical Rehabilitation, People with Disabilities. **Geo. Dist:** company service areas.

★ 12444 ★ Franklin Electric, Edward J. Schaefer, and T. W. KehoeCharitable and Educational Foundation

400 E Spring St.
Bluffton, IN 46714
Phone: (219)824-2900 **Fax:** (219)827-5530
William Lawson, President

Priorities: *Arts & Humanities:* 14$. Funds arts councils, performing arts, historic preservation, and museums. *Civic & Public Affairs:* 7%. Supports chambers of commerce, festivals, public safety, and economic development. *Education:* 44%. Provides scholarships. *Environment:* 31%. Supports community centers, youth organizations, food banks, and the United Way. *International:* 3%. Supports health centers and single-disease health organizations. *Religion:* 1%. Supports a science center. *Note:* Total contributions made in 2001. **Typ. Recipients:** Cancer, Children's Health/Hospitals, Hospitals, Multiple Sclerosis, Prenatal Health Issues, Preventive Medicine/Wellness Organizations. **Geo. Dist:** AR; Bluffton, IN, including surrounding area; MI.

★ 12445 ★ Fred C. and Mary R. Koch Foundation, Inc.

PO Box 2256
Wichita, KS 67201
Phone: (316)828-7483 **Fax:** (316)828-5739
Email: ramseyer@kochind.com
Website: http://www.kochind.com/community/default.asp
Roger Ramseyer, Director, Community Relations

Priorities: *Arts & Humanities:* 14%. Supports arts centers music, museums, opera, and theater. *Civic & Public Affairs:* 35%. Supports youth entrepreneurs. *Education:* 25%. Supports universities, colleges and scholarship funds in Kansas. Particularly funds programs involving economic and scientific problem solving. *Environment:* 16%. Funds Young Men's Christian Association and Goodwill. *International:* 4%. Funds a mental health association. *Note:* Total contributions made in 2000. **Typ. Recipients:** Cancer, Children's Health/Hospitals, Hospices, Mental Health, People with Disabilities, Preventive Medicine/Wellness Organizations, Single-Disease Health Associations. **Geo. Dist:** KS.

★ 12446 ★ Freddie Mac Foundation

8250 Jones Branch Drive
Mailstop A-40
McLean, VA 22102-3110
Phone: (703)918-8888 **Fax:** (703)918-8895
Email: freddiemac_foundation@freddiemac.com
Website: http://www.freddiemacfoundation.org
Renette Oklewicz, Foundation Contact

Fnded: 1990. **Priorities:** *Civic & Public Affairs:* 9%. Supports numerous child welfare and advocacy groups/programs, legal aid, and philanthropic associations. *Education:* 16%. Focus on early childhood education programs that address the developmental needs of children ages: 0-6 and prepare them for learning; elementary school years 6-12 to help them perform better in school; junior high and high school years 12-18 to help them prepare for college and explore career and work experiences. Includes early intervention services, strengthening day care and home day care systems; efforts to stimulate parental involvement in their child's educational development; school-based services for families, particularly pregnant or parenting teens; programs that enhance academic performance; initiatives to reform public education systems and advocate for stronger schools, including professional development opportunities and training for teachers; and programs that help children envision a successful future by providing teachers; and programs that help children envision a successful future by providing training and/or exposure to career opportunities. *Environment:* 61%. Focus on prevention of abuse (physical, sexual, emotional) and neglect. Targets factors leading to child abuse, including poor parenting skills, young inexperienced parents, stressful living situations and financial hardship, domestic violence, and substance abuse. Encourages grant requests in the following areas: parent training, education and support groups, home visitor programs, public awareness campaigns, comprehensive family support services, mental health services, teenage pregnancy prevention, services to parents and children who are victims of domestic violence, father involvement programs, support services to parents who are substance abusers, treatment programs that enable families to stay together during the treatment period, and advocacy and system reform initiatives related to preventing child abuse through the strengthening of families and communities, as well as professional development opportunities for social workers. *International:* 9%. Funding supports hospitals, health centers, and single-disease organizations. *Note:* Total contributions made in 2000. **Typ. Recipients:** AIDS/HIV, Child Abuse, Children's Health/Hospitals, Clinics/Medical Centers, Domestic Violence, Family Planning, Health Organizations, Health-General, Heart, Hospices, Mental Health, People with Disabilities, Prenatal Health Issues, Public Health, Substance Abuse. **Geo. Dist:** nationally; Washington, DC, including metropolitan area; MD, Charles County; MD, Frederick County; MD, Howard County; MD, Montgomery County; MD, Prince Georges County; VA, Fairfax County; VA, Loudoun and Prince William Counties; Alexandria, VA; Alexandria, VA; Arlington, VA; Falls Church, VA; Leesburg, VA; Manassas Park, VA.

★ 12447 ★ Freeport-McMoRan Foundation

1615 Poydras St.
New Orleans, LA 70112
Phone: (504)582-4000 **Fax:** (504)582-4028
Nancy Adkerson, Executive Director

Priorities: *Arts & Humanities:* 9%. Supports museums, opera, libraries, historic preservation, and art centers. *Civic & Public Affairs:* 16%. Supports community foundations, housing, civil rights, botanical gardens, and anti-crime activities. *Education:* 17%. Supports universities, schools, and educational foundations. *Environment:* 45%. Supports the homeless, United Way, crime prevention, child welfare, and animal protection. *International:* 5%. Supports medical foundations, nutrition programs, and single-disease health associations. *Note:* Total contributions made in 2000. **Typ. Recipients:** AIDS/HIV, Cancer, Cancer, Children's Health/Hospitals, Clinics/Medical Centers, Domestic Violence, Emergency/Ambulance Services, Eyes/Blindness, Health Organizations, Health-General, Heart, Hospitals, Medical Research, Mental Health, Nutrition, People with Disabilities, Prenatal Health Issues, Single-Disease Health Associations, Substance Abuse. **Geo. Dist:** principally near operating locations and to national organizations.

★ 12448 ★ Frito-Lay, Inc.

7701 Legacy Dr.
Plano, TX 75024
Phone: (972)334-2725 **Fax:** (972)334-2045
Email: kathy.cloud@fritolay.com
Website: http://www.fritolay.com/sitemap.html
Kathy Cloud, Public Affairs Coordinator

Typ. Recipients: Health-General. **Geo. Dist:** Dallas, TX; Fort Worth, TX.

★ 12449 ★ G.D. Searle and Co. Charitable Trust

PO Box 1045
Skokie, IL 60076
Phone: (847)581-6769 **Fax:** (847)581-4032
Dr. William Greener, Jr., Trust Administrator

Priorities: *Arts & Humanities:* 11%. Supports museums, historical societies, and the performing arts and fine arts. *Civic & Public Affairs:* 13%. Supports zoos, botanical gardens, parks, legal and urban issues, and community foundations. *Education:* 10%. Provides funding for medical education, primary and secondary education, and junior achievement. *Environment:* 21%. Supports family services, homeless shelters, and youth foundations. *International:* 41%. Funds single-disease health organizations, patient rights, and medical research. *Religion:* 3%. *Note:* Total foundation contributions made in 2001. **Typ. Recipients:** AIDS/HIV, Cancer, Child Abuse, Children's Health/Hospitals, Clinics/Medical Centers, Health Organizations, Health-General, Heart, Hospitals, Hospitals (University Affiliated), Long-Term Care, Medical Education, Medical Research, Nursing Services, People with Disabilities, Public Health, Single-Disease Health Associations. **Geo. Dist:** nationally, with emphasis on operating communities.

★ 12450 ★ Galter Foundation

55 E Superior
3rd Floor
Chicago, IL 60611
Phone: (312)664-5370
Dollie Galter, Director

Fnded: 1943. **Priorities:** *Arts & Humanities:* 1%. Supports public broadcasting and theaters. *Civic & Public Affairs:* 4%. *Education:* 32%. Primary support made to Northwestern University. *Environment:* 3%. Supports seniors, people with disabilities, Special Olympics, day care, camps, youth services, and animal protection. *International:* 56%. Supports hospitals, medical research, and single-disease health associations. *Note:* Total foundation contributions made in 2000. **Typ. Recipients:** AIDS/HIV, Arthritis, Cancer, Children's Health/Hospitals, Clinics/Medical Centers, Diabetes, Emergency/Ambulance Services, Health Organizations, Heart, Home-Care Services, Hospitals, Hospitals (University Affiliated), Kidney, Medical Education, Medical Rehabilitation, Medical Research, Multiple Sclerosis, People with Disabilities, Prenatal Health Issues, Public Health, Respiratory, Single-Disease Health Associations. **Geo. Dist:** Chicago, IL.

★ 12451 ★ Gannett Foundation

7950 Jones Branch Drive
McLean, VA 22107
Phone: (703)854-6000 **Fax:** (703)854-2002
Email: isimpson@gannett.com
Website: http://www.gannettfoundation.org
Irma Simpson, Manager

Priorities: *Arts & Humanities:* 16% Supports arts and culture organizations (11%) and media (5%). *Civic & Public Affairs:* 12%. *Education:* 15%. *Environment:* 16%. *International:* 9%. *Note:* Total contributions made in 2000. **Typ. Recipients:** Mental Health, People with Disabilities, Single-Disease Health Associations. **Geo. Dist:** operating locations.

★ 12452 ★ Gap Foundation

2 Folsom St., 14th Floor
San Francisco, CA 94105
Phone: (415)427-2000
Website: http://www.gapinc.com/social_resp/social_resp.htm

Fnded: 1969. **Priorities:** *Arts & Humanities:* 3%. The performing arts and museums receive funding. *Civic & Public Affairs:* 9%. Contributes to community development, housing, job training programs, minority affairs, and community foundations. *Education:* 38%. Supports educational programs for youth, public and private pre-college schools, school volunteerism, and business education. *Environment:* 34%. Supports Boys & Girls Clubs, youth programs, child and family services, and services for disadvantaged and abused women and children. *International:* 11%. Funds HIV/AIDS organizations, children's health programs, and single-disease health associations. *Religion:* 1%. Contributes to a space and science center. *Voluntarism:* The company sponsors an employee volunteer effort, wherein headquarters employees receive five hours per month of paid leave to volunteer, and field staff participate in on-going special volunteer projects. *Note:* Total contributions made in fiscal 2001. **Typ. Recipients:** AIDS/HIV, Cancer, Clinics/Medical Centers, Domestic Violence, Emergency/Ambulance Services, Eyes/Blindness, Health Funds, Health Organizations, Health-General, Hospices, Hospitals, Medical Education, Medical Research, Prenatal Health Issues, Preventive Medicine/Wellness Organizations, Public Health, Research/Studies Institutes, Single-Disease Health Associations, Transplant Networks/Donor Banks, Trauma Treatment. **Geo. Dist:** headquarters and operating locations; Los Angeles, CA; San Francisco, CA; Chicago, IL; New York, NY.

★ 12453 ★ Gates Corp.

PO Box 5887
31-1-1-A1
Denver, CO 80217-5887
Phone: (303)744-5228 **Fax:** (303)744-4443
Email: mhoppe@gates.com
Website: http://www.gates.com
Marje Hoppe, Asst. to Vice Pres. of Human Resources

Typ. Recipients: Health-General. **Geo. Dist:** Denver, CO, including immediate metropolitan area.

★ 12454 ★ GATX Corp.

500 West Monroe St.
Chicago, IL 60661-3676
Phone: (312)621-6222 **Fax:** (312)621-6665
Email: communityaffairs@gatx.com
Website: http://www.gatx.com
Jesse Kane, Supervisor, Community Affairs

Priorities: *Education:* Supports a variety of educational programs for economically disadvantaged children and youth. Programs focus on intellectual and emotional development, academic and social preparation for high school and college, academic support to youth in higher education, arts education, and adult literacy education. *Environment:* Supports programs that provide adults with skills training and placement services, prevent domestic and community violence, provide families with access to quality health care, enhance family communications and improve parenting capabilities, and work to provide affordable housing to families. *Voluntarism:* GATX employees nationwide are recognized for volunteer efforts from tutoring students to building playgrounds. GATX presents its Spirit of Volunteerism Award twice a year to honor those whose best exemplify principles of community service, teamwork, and good corporate citizenship. Unions service projects during work hours with work release time for eligible employees. **Typ. Recipients:** AIDS/HIV, Cancer, Child Abuse, Clinics/Medical Centers, Domestic Violence, Geriatric Health, Health Organizations, Hospices, Hospitals, Medical Rehabilitation, Mental Health, Nutrition, People with Disabilities, Public Health, Single-Disease Health Associations, Substance Abuse. **Geo. Dist:** operating locations; Chicago, IL.

★ 12455 ★ GE Capital Corp.

500 West Monroe St.
Chicago, IL 60661
Phone: (312)441-6748 **Fax:** (312)441-7710
Leslie Krohn, Vice President Communications

Priorities: *Voluntarism:* The company has a volunteer committee, an incentive program, and has adopted a public school. **Typ. Recipients:** Mental Health. **Geo. Dist:** headquarters and operating communities.

★ 12456 ★ GE Foundation

3135 Easton Turnpike
Fairfield, CT 06828
Phone: (203)373-3216 **Fax:** (203)373-3029
Email: gefoundation@ge.com
Website: http://www.gefoundation.com
Marc Saperstein, President

Priorities: *Arts & Humanities:* (Arts in Education) 10%. Program objective is to further arts education, particularly through partnerships of arts organizations with public schools. *Civic & Public Affairs:* (Public Policy) 8%. Funding in this category is focused on public policy organizations promoting workforce development, international trade, the environment, and the non-profit sector. *Education:* 65%. Higher education funding (about 45% of total giving) focuses on the disciplines of engineering, information technology, and quantitative business. Initiatives include Math Excellence and GE Fund Scholars. Pre-college education (about 20% of total giving) focuses on college bound programs, an early years initiative, and teacher quality and administrative leadership. Other initiatives include increased educational opportunities for women and minorities, with emphasis on engineering, management, and finance. Support includes sponsorship of a minority engineering scholarship program, funding for Hispanic scholarship programs, scholarships for first-year female engineering students, and aid for minority educational associations and institutions (including schools of engineering and faculty development). Grants on the precollege level emphasize improving math and science teaching and curricula and raising students' abilities in these subject areas. Also, the foundation supports school projects involving GE volunteers. Much support is in *Environment:* 3%. *Voluntarism:* GE supports the United Way and United Way-sponsored agencies where GE volunteers perform a variety of services, including agency clean-ups, refurbishing day care centers, and building houses through Habitat for Humanity. GE also supports Elfun, a global organization of GE employees and retirees who work to improve the company and communities through volunteerism, leadership, and camaraderie. GE volunteer hours approach $500,000 in billable hours. *Note:* Total contributions made in 2001. Contributions analysis excludes matching gifts, the STAR/ACE Scholarship Program (for children of GE employees), and donations to the United Way. **Typ. Recipients:** Clinics/Medical Centers, Emergency/Ambulance Services, Health Organizations, Health Policy/Cost Containment, Hospitals, Hospitals (University Affiliated), Medical Education, Medical Research, People with Disabilities, Substance Abuse. **Geo. Dist:** headquarters and operating communities; international organizations; national organizations. **Frmly:** GE Foundations GE Fund.

★ 12457 ★ GEICO Philanthropic Foundation

5260 Western Ave.
Chevy Chase, MD 20815
Phone: (301)986-3802 **Fax:** (301)718-5239
Website: http://www.geico.com/infocenter/goodworks.htm
David Schindler, Contact

Priorities: *Arts & Humanities:* 1%. Supports performing arts, public television, museums, and historical societies. *Civic & Public Affairs:* 54%. Majority of funding supports the National Safety Association and other safety programs. Other grants support environmental projects, professional organizations, and groups promoting better government. *Education:* 31%. Supports colleges and universities, with emphasis on business education. Also matches employee gifts to higher education. Other recipients include educational fundraising organizations and scholarship foundations. *Environment:* 6%. Primarily supports united funds. Other major recipients include child welfare and recreation groups, programs for the mentally retarded and disabled, and family services. *International:* 8%. Funds go primarily to hospitals and single-disease research organizations. Some support goes to hospices and other facilities. *Note:* Total foundation contributions made in 2000. **Typ. Recipients:** Cancer, Children's Health/Hospitals, Diabetes, Emergency/Ambulance Services, Heart, Hospices, Hospitals, Medical Rehabilitation, Medical Research, Mental Health, Multiple Sclerosis, People with Disabilities, Public Health, Single-Disease Health Associations, Substance Abuse. **Geo. Dist:** organizations serving operating locations.

★ 12458 ★ GenAmerican Foundation

700 Market St.
Saint Louis, MO 63101
Phone: (314)444-0434 **Fax:** (314)444-0681
Email: cendicott@genam.com
Website: http://www.genamerica.com
Cheryl Endicot, Contributions Specialist

Priorities: *Arts & Humanities:* 15%. Interests orchestras, theater, opera, ballet, museums, and historical societies. *Civic & Public Affairs:* 10%. A variety of causes are supported, including nonprofit management organizations, urban affairs, minority business development, and zoos. *Education:* 22%. Emphasis on colleges and universities. Interests include medical, business, and insurance education, public schools, minority education, and Junior Achievement. *Environ-*

ment: 47%. Primarily supports United Way. Also funds youth organizations and services for the disabled. *International:* 2%. Gives to biomedical research and AIDS, cancer, and poison control programs. *Religion:* 1%. Funds a science center. *Voluntarism:* Company executives and associates have assumed leadership roles in a variety of civic and charitable causes. *Note:* Total contributions made in fiscal 2000. **Typ. Recipients:** AIDS/HIV, Alzheimers Disease, Cancer, Children's Health/Hospitals, Clinics/Medical Centers, Diabetes, Domestic Violence, Emergency/Ambulance Services, Family Planning, Heart, Hospitals, Hospitals (University Affiliated), Medical Education, Medical Rehabilitation, Medical Research, People with Disabilities, Preventive Medicine/Wellness Organizations, Public Health, Single-Disease Health Associations, Substance Abuse. **Geo. Dist:** St. Louis, MO. **Frmly:** General American Foundation.

★ 12459 ★ Genentech Foundation for Biomedical Sciences
1 DNA Way
South San Francisco, CA 94080
Phone: (650)225-2487 **Fax:** (650)225-2414
Website: http://www.gene.com/gene/about/community/initiatives-scholarships/gfbs/
Bunnie Jack, Foundation Coordinator

Fnded: 1988. **Priorities:** *Arts & Humanities:* 2%. Funds a museum. *Education:* 76% of total contributions. Funds science and matches education programs in the San Francisco Bay area. Typical recipients include the University of California and Mills College. Also supports scholarship programs for math and science education. *Environment:* 18%. *International:* 4%. *Note:* Contributions made in fiscal 2000. **Typ. Recipients:** Kidney, Medical Education. **Geo. Dist:** CA, northern California.

★ 12460 ★ General Dynamics Corp.
3190 Fairview Park Drive
Falls Church, VA 22042
Phone: (703)876-3000 **Fax:** (703)876-3600
Website: http://www.generaldynamics.com
Diane Mossler, Director of Contributions and Government

Priorities: *Civic & Public Affairs:* About 55%. Public policy and international exchange organizations. *Education:* About 25%. Higher education, minority education, and education associations. *International:* About 10%. United Way, hospitals, drug abuse programs, family service organizations, and YWCA. **Typ. Recipients:** Medical Education, People with Disabilities. **Geo. Dist:** nationally and in company operating areas.

★ 12461 ★ General Mills Foundation
PO Box 1113
Minneapolis, MN 55440
Phone: (612)540-2579 **Fax:** (612)540-4114
Website: http://www.generalmills.com/corporate/about/community/
Chris Shea, President and Executive Director

Fnded: 1954. **Priorities:** *Arts & Humanities:* 17%. *Civic & Public Affairs:* 13%. *Education:* 26%. *Environment:* 43%. *Religion:* 1%. *Voluntarism:* General Mills' Volunteer Connection and Retirement PLUS programs promote employee volunteerism by matching volunteers with projects, and the Volunteer Advisory Board Steers Company involvement in volunteer endeavors. *Note:* Total contributions made in 2001. **Typ. Recipients:** Cancer, Children's Health/Hospitals, Clinics/Medical Centers, Domestic Violence, Emergency/Ambulance Services, Family Planning, Geriatric Health, Health Organizations, Health Policy/Cost Containment, Hospitals, Medical Education, Medical Rehabilitation, Medical Research, Mental Health, Nutrition, People with Disabilities, Substance Abuse. **Geo. Dist:** nationally; operating locations.

★ 12462 ★ General Motors Foundation
300 Renaissance Center
MC 482-C16-D25
Detroit, MI 48265-3000
Phone: (313)665-4085 **Fax:** (313)665-0746
Website: http://www.gm.com/company/gmability/philanthropy/
Deborah Dingell, Vice Chairman

Priorities: *Arts & Humanities:* 3%. *Civic & Public Affairs:* 38%. *Education:* 22%. *Environment:* 24%. *International:* 11%. *Voluntarism:* The GM Volunteer PLU$ program recognizes and rewards employees for the time they spend volunteering with charities and allows employees to direct a monetary gift from the GM Foundation to local charities for which they regularly volunteer. *Note:* A high percentage of grants are awarded through domestic and international subsidiaries and divisions, which have decision-making autonomy for gifts of less than $5,000. Total foundation contributions made 2000. **Typ. Recipients:** Alzheimers Disease, Cancer, Children's Health/Hospitals, Clinics/Medical Centers, Emergency/Ambulance Services, Health Organizations, Hospices, Hospitals, Medical Rehabilitation, Medical Training, Mental Health, People with Disabilities, Public Health, Single-Disease Health Associations, Substance Abuse, Transplant Networks/Donor Banks. **Geo. Dist:** nationally; operating locations.

★ 12463 ★ General Reinsurance Corp.
Financial Centre
PO Box 10351
Stamford, CT 06904
Phone: (203)328-5000 **Fax:** (203)328-5603
Email: rmanz@gcr.com
Website: http://www.gcre.com
Richard Manz, Assistant Vice President

Priorities: *Civic & Public Affairs:* 25% to 30%. Supports economic development through job training, environmental affairs, and women's affairs. *Education:* 25% to 30%. Funds colleges and universities, especially those with interest in medical education or liberal arts education. *International:* 25% to 40%. Supports hospitals and hospices, medical research and training, and mental health. **Typ. Recipients:** Emergency/Ambulance Services, Health Organizations, Health Policy/Cost Containment, Hospices, Hospitals, Medical Rehabilitation, Medical Research, Medical Training, Mental Health, People with Disabilities, Public Health, Substance Abuse. **Geo. Dist:** principally near operating locations and to national organizations.

★ 12464 ★ Genesis Foundation
2600 Kettering Tower
Dayton, OH 45423
Phone: (937)910-9300
Robert Reithman, Treasurer

Fnded: 1952. **Priorities:** *Arts & Humanities:* 31%. Supports music, dance, libraries, public television, and art institutes. *Civic & Public Affairs:* 7%. Supports minority business, parks, and community foundations. *Education:* 27%. Supports schools, community colleges, and scholarship funds. *Environment:* 16%. Supports YMCA, Boy Scouts of America, United Way, and Big Brothers/Big Sisters. *International:* 15%. Supports hospitals and health funds. *Religion:* 1%. Supports science Olympiad. *Note:* Total foundation contributions made in 2000. **Typ. Recipients:** Cancer, Children's Health/Hospitals, Clinics/Medical Centers, Clinics/Medical Centers, Emergency/Ambulance Services, Hospices, Hospitals, Long-Term Care, People with Disabilities, Transplant Networks/Donor Banks. **Geo. Dist:** NY; OH.

★ 12465 ★ George Kress Foundation
1700 N Webster Ave.
Green Bay, WI 54301
Phone: (920)433-5113
John Kress, Secretary & Treasurer

Fnded: 1953. **Priorities:** *Arts & Humanities:* 13%. Funds symphonic and performing arts, creativity programs, and art and historical museums. *Civic & Public Affairs:* 10%. Supports botanical gardens/parks, community foundations, economic development, and professional and trade associations. *Education:* 40%. Funds colleges and universities, minority education funds, literacy initiatives, and scholarship funds. *Environment:* 17%. Supports the United Way, animal protection, children's programs, volunteer services, and family services. *International:* 13%. Supports hospitals, single-disease health associations, and public health. *Note:* Total contributions made in 2000. **Typ. Recipients:** Children's Health/Hospitals, Emergency/Ambulance Services, Health Organizations, Hospitals, Hospitals (University Affiliated), Medical Education, People with Disabilities, Public Health, Single-Disease Health Associations. **Geo. Dist:** occasionally to state aside from Wisconsin; WI, primarily Green Bay.

★ 12466 ★ Georgia-Pacific Foundation
133 Peachtree St. Northeast
Atlanta, GA 30303
Phone: (404)652-4000 **Fax:** (404)584-1470
Website: http://www.gp.com/center/community/index.html
Curley Dossman, Jr., President

Priorities: *Arts & Humanities:* 18%. Special interest in art museums and music. Also supports arts associations, and historic preservation and history groups. *Civic & Public Affairs:* 18%. Provided a major grant to Habitat for Humanity. Also supports minority affairs, job training and placement, botanical gardens, community parks, and zoos. *Education:* 32%. Sponsors Georgia-Pacific Foundation Merit Scholarships. Other areas of interest include colleges and universities, literacy programs, school-to-work programs, higher education funds and associations, public schools, Junior Achievement, and technology education. *Environment:* 21%. Foundation generally emphasizes United Way chapters. Other recipients include programs for the disabled and recreational activities for youth. *International:* Less than 1%. *Voluntarism:* Employee volunteers serve such organizations as United Way, American Red Cross, Boy Scouts of America, Girl Scouts, Better Business Bureaus and councils, and Keep America Beautiful. *Note:* Total foundation contributions made in 2000. **Typ. Recipients:** Child Abuse, Children's Health/Hospitals, Emergency/Ambulance Services, Eyes/Blindness, Health Funds, Health Organizations, Health-General, Hospitals, Hospitals (University Affiliated), Medical Education, Medical Rehabilitation, Medical Research, People with Disabilities, Single-Disease Health Associations, Substance Abuse. **Geo. Dist:** operating locations.

★ 12467 ★ Georgia Power Foundation
Bin 10131
241 Ralph McGill Boulevard NE
Atlanta, GA 30308-3374
Phone: (404)506-6784 **Fax:** (404)506-1485
Judy Anderson, Foundation President

Fnded: 1930. **Priorities:** *Arts & Humanities:* 11%. *Civic & Public Affairs:* 8%. *Education:* 22%. *Environment:* 56%. *International:* 50%. *Voluntarism:* Company sponsors the Citizens of Georgia Power, a group of employees that volunteers with nonprofit groups throughout the state. The Ambassadors is the same type of program for retired employees. OrganizationS supported include Habitat for Humanity, the March of Dimes, and the American Red Cross. *Note:* Analysis provided by foundation. Total contributions made in 2001. **Typ. Recipients:** Alzheimers Disease, Cancer, Child Abuse, Children's Health/Hospitals, Clinics/Medical Centers, Emergency/Ambulance Services, Eyes/Blindness, Family Planning, Geriatric Health, Health Organizations, Hospices, Hospitals, Medical Education, Medical Rehabilitation, Medical Research, Mental Health, People with Disabilities, Public Health, Single-Disease Health Associations, Substance Abuse. **Geo. Dist:** GA, operating locations and service area.

★ 12468 ★ Gerber Foundation
4747 W 48th St., Suite 153
Fremont, MI 49412
Phone: (231)924-3175 **Fax:** (231)924-7906
Email: tgf@ncisd.net
Website: http://www.gerberfoundation.org
Cathy Obits, Contact

Priorities: *Arts & Humanities:* 4%. *Civic & Public Affairs:* Supports minority affairs, and local initiatives. *Education:* 22%. Supports programs which promote responsible parenting, beginning at young ages and extending to adulthood. Supports formal and informal instruction in such areas as parenting skills, infant and young child care, nutrition and development training, child abuse prevention, school readiness and early school success, and avoidance of too-early child bearing. Funds health research at accredited colleges and universities. *Environment:* 19%. Funds programs that ensure access to health and human services by infants and young children across all spectra of American society. *International:* 30%. Supports teaching hospitals, and independent research institutions for research projects in the areas of nutrition, health, and development of infants and young children. Priority is given to projects which have the potential of resulting in publication of findings with broad applicability for the public good. *Religion:* 23%. Supports accredited colleges and universities, teaching hospitals, and independent research institutions for research projects in the areas of nutrition, health, and development of infants and young children. Priority is given to projects which have the potential of resulting in publication of findings with broad applicability for the public good. *Note:* Analysis provided by foundation. **Typ. Recipients:** AIDS/HIV, Arthritis, Cancer, Child Abuse, Children's Health/Hospitals, Clinics/Medical Centers, Diabetes, Domestic Violence, Eyes/Blindness, Health Organizations, Health Policy/Cost Containment, Health-General, Heart, Hospices, Hospitals, Medical Education, Medical Rehabilitation, Medical Research, Medical Training, Mental Health, Nursing Services, Nutrition, People with Disabilities, Prenatal Health Issues, Preventive Medicine/Wellness Organizations, Public Health, Speech & Hearing. **Geo. Dist:** nationally.

★ 12469 ★ Giant Eagle Foundation

101 Kappa Drive
Pittsburgh, PA 15238
Phone: (412)963-6200 **Fax:** (412)963-2540
Jody Clark, Administrator

Priorities: *Arts & Humanities:* 8%. Funding supports performing arts organizations, museums, symphony, opera, ballet, theater, and dance. *Civic & Public Affairs:* 6%. Supports community development, municipalities, and zoos. *Education:* 17%. Favors educational foundations and the University of Pittsburgh. Other recipients include private precollege education, Junior Achievement, and minority education funds. Provides scholarships to children of employees. *Environment:* 7%. Contributes to youth organizations including Big Brothers and Big Sisters and scouting; supports family services, food banks, and the United Way. *International:* 5%. Supports AIDS concerns, pediatric health-care facilities, medical rehabilitation, cancer organizations, and medical research. *Note:* Total contributions in fiscal 2000. **Typ. Recipients:** AIDS/HIV, Cancer, Children's Health/Hospitals, Diabetes, Domestic Violence, Emergency/Ambulance Services, Geriatric Health, Health Organizations, Heart, Hospitals, Kidney, Medical Education, Medical Rehabilitation, Medical Research, Mental Health, People with Disabilities, Prenatal Health Issues, Public Health, Sexual Abuse, Single-Disease Health Associations, Substance Abuse. **Geo. Dist:** Pittsburgh, PA.

★ 12470 ★ Giant Food Foundation

6300 Sheriff Rd.
Landover, MD 20785
Phone: (301)341-4171 **Fax:** (301)618-4972
Website: http://www.giantfood.com/community.htm
Richard Baird, President

Fnded: 1950. **Priorities:** *Arts & Humanities:* 3%. Supports public broadcasting, art centers, museums, and performing arts. *Civic & Public Affairs:* 11%. Supports justice services, housing, and community foundations. *Education:* 13%. Supports colleges, universities, and private schools. *Environment:* 47%. Supports United Way, youth organizations, counseling services, child welfare, scouts, and food distribution programs. *International:* 4%. Supports health foundations, hospices, medical centers, hospitals, and single-diseases health associations. *Note:* Total foundation contributions made in fiscal 2001. **Typ. Recipients:** Alzheimers Disease, Cancer, Children's Health/Hospitals, Clinics/Medical Centers, Geriatric Health, Health Organizations, Heart, Hospices, Hospitals, Medical Education, Mental Health, People with Disabilities, Prenatal Health Issues, Single-Disease Health Associations, Substance Abuse. **Geo. Dist:** DE; DC; MD; NJ; VA.

★ 12471 ★ Giddings & Lewis Foundation

142 Doty St.
Fond du Lac, WI 54935
Phone: (920)921-9400
Heike Franke, Treasurer

Fnded: 1952. **Priorities:** *Arts & Humanities:* 1%. *Civic & Public Affairs:* 5%. Supports community development and foundations. *Education:* 50%. Supports scholarships, colleges, schools, universities. *Environment:* 35%. Supports community centers, scouts, youth organizations, homes, athletics and recreation, United Way, and YMCA. *International:* 4%. Supports hospitals, health clinics, and single-disease health associations. *Note:* Total foundation contributions made in 2000. **Typ. Recipients:** AIDS/HIV, Cancer, Clinics/Medical Centers, Emergency/Ambulance Services, Heart, Hospices, Hospitals, Multiple Sclerosis, Nursing Services, People with Disabilities, Prenatal Health Issues, Single-Disease Health Associations, Substance Abuse, Transplant Networks/Donor Banks. **Geo. Dist:** CA; MI; OH; WI.

★ 12472 ★ Gilbert and Ildiko Butler Foundation, Inc.

745 Fifth Ave.
New York, NY 10151
Phone: (212)980-0606
Gilbert Butler, President

Fnded: 1988. **Priorities:** *Arts & Humanities:* 37%. Funds museums, libraries, historic preservation, and performing arts. *Civic & Public Affairs:* 8%. Supports parks and botanical gardens. *Education:* 19%. Supports colleges, universities, and private pre-college schools. *Environment:* 4%. Primarily supports the United Way. *International:* 8%. Contributes to hospitals, medical research organizations, and nursing services. *Note:* Total foundation contributions made in 2000. **Typ. Recipients:** Cancer, Children's Health/Hospitals, Eyes/Blindness, Hospitals, Mental Health. **Geo. Dist:** headquarters area only.

★ 12473 ★ Gillette Co.

Prudential Tower Bldg., 49th Floor
Boston, MA 02199-8004
Phone: (617)463-8608 **Fax:** (617)421-8484
Email: royall_mack@gillette.com
Website: http://www.gillette.com/community/corpcontributions.asp
Royall Mack, Director, Civic Affairs

Priorities: *Voluntarism:* Company employees volunteer with Making Strides for Breast Cancer, Walk for Hunger, and the AIDS Walk. The Gillette Retiree Outreach Program (GROUP) is a retiree managed program that administers a variety of volunteer activities ranging from literacy programs to blood drives. **Typ. Recipients:** Clinics/Medical Centers, Emergency/Ambulance Services, Hospitals. **Geo. Dist:** operating locations; Boston, MA.

★ 12474 ★ Glickenhaus Foundation

100 Dorchester Rd.
Scarsdale, NY 10583
Phone: (212)953-7800 **Fax:** (212)983-8436
Nancy Pier, President

Fnded: 1960. **Priorities:** *Arts & Humanities:* 17%. Supports craft museums and councils, theater, orchestras, opera, and museums of fine art. *Civic & Public Affairs:* 6%. Funds legal awareness and services, and community affairs and projects. *Education:* 42%. Primarily funds colleges and universities, as well as educational foundations and funds. Also funds secondary schools. *Environment:* 6%. Supports youth services, family planning, United Way, and senior funds. *International:* 13%. Supports single-disease health associations, psychotherapy organizations, medical research, and medical centers and hospitals throughout New York. *Religion:* 1%. Funds a museum of natural history. *Note:* Total contributions made in fiscal 2000. **Typ. Recipients:** AIDS/HIV, Cancer, Children's Health/Hospitals, Clinics/Medical Centers, Emergency/Ambulance Services, Family Planning, Geriatric Health, Health Organizations, Health-General, Hospitals, Kidney, Medical Education, Medical Research, Mental Health, People with Disabilities, Single-Disease Health Associations. **Geo. Dist:** nationally; NY.

★ 12475 ★ Global Community Partnerships

One Franklin Plaza
PO Box 7929
Philadelphia, PA 19101-7929
Phone: (215)751-4668 **Fax:** (215)751-7655
Email: community.partnership@gsk.com
Website: http://corp.gsk.com/community/
Doug Bauer, Director, Global Community Partnerships

Fnded: 2001. **Priorities:** *Education:* A variety of education programs receive company support. A primary initiative is the Partners With Education program, through with GlaxoSmithKline creates partnerships with agencies that can help develop young people's knowledge, understanding, technical, and personal skills in a variety of fields, and enhance youth's interest in science. *Environment:* Product donations are made to support humanitarian relief efforts around the world. *International:* Health funding focuses on enhancing health care and improving, "...the quality of human life by enabling people to do more, feel better and live longer." Disease prevention, treatment, and education is a primary concern. The company has developed major initiatives aimed at the Elimination of Lymphatic Filariasis, Positive Action on HIV/AIDS, and The Fight Against Malaria. *Voluntarism:* The company maintains an employee volunteering support scheme. *Note:* GlaxoSmithKline Global Community Partnerships program priorities in 2002. **Typ. Recipients:** AIDS/HIV, Cancer, Children's Health/Hospitals, Clinics/Medical Centers, Diabetes, Emergency/Ambulance Services, Health Funds, Health Organizations, Hospitals, Long-Term Care, Medical Education, Medical Research, People with Disabilities, Single-Disease Health Associations, Substance Abuse. **Geo. Dist:** internationally; nationally.

★ 12476 ★ Globe Foundation

6730 North Scottsdale Rd., Suite 250
Scottsdale, AZ 85253-4424
Phone: (480)991-0500 **Fax:** (480)991-1912
James Johnson, Treasurer & Assistant Secretary

Fnded: 1958. **Priorities:** *Arts & Humanities:* 19%. Support goes to historical preservation, art museums, ballet, and other performing arts. *Civic & Public Affairs:* 10%. Gives to community and historical foundations, zoos, and botanical gardens. *Education:* 40%. Supports schools, Junior Achievement, colleges and universities, religious education, and medical education. *Environment:* 5%. Supports United Way, YMCA, youth organizations, and humane societies. *International:* 24%. Funding goes to a variety of causes including health foundations, hospitals, medical research, and education. *Note:* Total foundation contributions made in 2000. **Typ. Recipients:** AIDS/HIV, Arthritis, Cancer, Children's Health/Hospitals, Clinics/Medical Centers, Diabetes, Domestic Violence, Eyes/Blindness, Family Planning, Health Funds, Health Organizations, Health-General, Heart, Hospices, Hospitals, Medical Education, Medical Rehabilitation, Medical Research, Nursing Services, People with Disabilities, Public Health, Research/Studies Institutes, Single-Disease Health Associations. **Geo. Dist:** AZ; IL.

★ 12477 ★ Gold Kist Foundation

PO Box 2210
Atlanta, GA 30301
Phone: (770)393-5317
Paul Brower, Contact

Priorities: *Arts & Humanities:* 1%. *Civic & Public Affairs:* 25%. *Education:* 54%. *Environment:* 14%. *International:* 2%. *Note:* Total contributions made in

2001. **Typ. Recipients:** Cancer, Health-General, Single-Disease Health Associations. **Geo. Dist:** headquarters and operating communities.

★ 12478 ★ Goldman Sachs Foundation
375 Park Ave., Suite 1008
New York, NY 10152
Phone: (212)902-5402
Website: http://gs.com/our_firm/the_culture/social_responsibility/gs_foundation.html
Stephanie Bell-Rose, President

Priorities: *Education:* 87%. Supports universities, Junior Achievement, scholarships and educational funds. *Voluntarism:* The company encourages employee volunteerism through its Community TeamWorks program, which allows employees to spend a day working at a charitable organization of their choice while receiving full salary. *Note:* Total foundation contributions made in fiscal 2000. **Typ. Recipients:** Emergency/Ambulance Services, Hospitals, Hospitals (University Affiliated), Medical Education. **Geo. Dist:** nationally and internationally.

★ 12479 ★ Golub Foundation
PO Box 1074
Schenectady, NY 12301
Phone: (518)356-9450
Melissa Pabis, Foundation Administrator

Fnded: 1981. **Priorities:** *Arts & Humanities:* 9%. Supports theaters, performing arts centers, and music. *Civic & Public Affairs:* About 2%. Contributes to Haven. *Education:* 17%. Major interest in public education. Also supports colleges, literacy, and technology programs. Operates scholarship program for students attending colleges in New York, Massachusetts, Pennsylvania, Connecticut, Vermont, and New Hampshire. *Environment:* 9%. Favors community centers, united funds, community recreation and athletics, the disabled, and family services. *International:* 9%. Contributes to hospitals, medical centers, children's health, and single-disease health associations. *Note:* Contributions made in fiscal 2001. **Typ. Recipients:** Arthritis, Cancer, Children's Health/Hospitals, Clinics/Medical Centers, Eyes/Blindness, Health Organizations, Hospices, Hospitals, Medical Education, Medical Rehabilitation, People with Disabilities, Prenatal Health Issues, Single-Disease Health Associations. **Geo. Dist:** headquarters and operating communities.

★ 12480 ★ Gordon V. and Helen C. Smith Foundation
8716 Crider Brook Way
Potomac, MD 20854
Phone: (301)469-8597
Gordon Smith, Contact

Priorities: *Arts & Humanities:* 1%. *Education:* 52%. Funds higher education. *Environment:* 6%. YMCA receives funding. *Note:* Total contributions made in 1999. **Typ. Recipients:** Heart.

★ 12481 ★ Gosiger Foundation
108 McDonough St.
Dayton, OH 45402
Phone: (937)228-5174 **Fax:** (937)463-7718
Mrs. J. Haley, President

Fnded: 1992. **Priorities:** *Arts & Humanities:* 22%. Supports theater, museums, and art institute. *Civic & Public Affairs:* 5%. Funds economic development, parks, and civic festivals. *Education:* 43%. Focus is on universities and schools. *Environment:* 5%. Funds Young Women's Christian Association and youth organizations. *International:* 12%. Funds single-disease health associations. *Religion:* 8%. Funds a natural history society. *Note:* Contributions made in 2000. **Typ. Recipients:** Alzheimers Disease, Cancer, Children's Health/Hospitals, Heart. **Geo. Dist:** headquarters area only.

★ 12482 ★ Graco Foundation
PO Box 1441
Minneapolis, MN 55440-1441
Phone: (612)623-6684 **Fax:** (612)623-6944
Website: http://www.graco.com/Internet/Corp.nsf
Robert Mattison, Vice President & Secretary

Priorities: *Civic & Public Affairs:* 14%. Supports housing, neighborhood organizations, economic development, employment services, and refugee support. *Education:* 32%. Gives to scholarship funds, colleges and universities, economic education, private schools, and alternative schooling. *Environment:* 50%. Supports youth organizations, day care, and United Way. Achievement and the Business Economics Education Foundation. *International:* 2%. Supports single-disease health associations. *Voluntarism:* In the past, employees have volunteered time for education associations such as Junior Achievement and the Business Economics Education Foundation. Graco's program also included year-round volunteer assignments (on boards, etc.) with Junior Achievement, the United Way, Metro Paint-a-Thon, and other events of interest to employees. The company has a Volunteer Coordinator. *Note:* Total contributions in 2000. **Typ. Recipients:** AIDS/HIV, Alzheimers Disease, Cancer, Children's Health/Hospitals, Clinics/Medical Centers, Diabetes, Domestic Violence, Emergency/Ambulance Services, Health Organizations, Hospitals, Medical Education, Medical Rehabilitation, People with Disabilities, Research/Studies Institutes, Single-Disease Health Associations. **Geo. Dist:** operating locations; MN; Sioux Falls, SD.

★ 12483 ★ Graham Foundation
PO Box 1104
York, PA 17405
Phone: (717)849-4001
William Kerlin, Jr., Trustee

Fnded: 1986. **Priorities:** *Arts & Humanities:* 16%. Funds museums, historical preservation, and the performing arts. *Civic & Public Affairs:* 3%. *Education:* 46%. Funds colleges and universities, literacy and education councils, and private education. *Environment:* 27%. Supports United Way and children's and social services. *International:* 4%. *Note:* Total contributionss in fiscal 1998. **Typ. Recipients:** Cancer, Children's Health/Hospitals, Emergency/Ambulance Services, Family Planning, Health Organizations, Health-General, Heart, Home-Care Services, Hospices, Hospitals, Medical Research, Mental Health, Nursing Services, People with Disabilities, Public Health, Single-Disease Health Associations. **Geo. Dist:** headquarters area only.

★ 12484 ★ Grand Marnier Foundation
80 Route 4 East, 1st Floor
Paramus, NJ 07652
Phone: (201)368-9500
Jerry Ciraulo, Treasurer

Priorities: *Arts & Humanities:* 63%. Supports performing arts, public television, museums, libraries, and opera. *Civic & Public Affairs:* 11%. Supports women's organizations and community foundations. *Education:* 20%. Supports educational institutes, colleges, and universities. *Environment:* 3%. Supports youth and child services, food distribution, and social services. *International:* 1%. Supports health foundations and single-disease organizations. *Note:* Total foundation contributions made in 2000. **Typ. Recipients:** AIDS/HIV, Alzheimers Disease, Cancer, Child Abuse, Children's Health/Hospitals, Clinics/Medical Centers, Emergency/Ambulance Services, Health Organizations, Heart, Hospitals, Medical Education, Medical Research, Nutrition, Single-Disease Health Associations. **Geo. Dist:** nationally; CA; MD; NY.

★ 12485 ★ Grand Victoria Foundation
60 South Grove Ave.
Elgin, IL 60120
Phone: (847)289-8575 **Fax:** (847)289-8576
Email: info@grandvictoriafdn.org
Website: http://www.grandvictoriafdn.org
Nancy Fishman, Executive Director

Priorities: *Arts & Humanities:* 3%. *Civic & Public Affairs:* 52%. *Education:* 3%. *Environment:* 14%. *International:* 2%. *Religion:* 7%. *Note:* Giving percentages vary depending upon applications received. Total contributions made in 2002. **Typ. Recipients:** Children's Health/Hospitals, Hospitals. **Geo. Dist:** IL.

★ 12486 ★ Graybar Foundation
PO Box 7231
Saint Louis, MO 63177
Phone: (314)573-9200 **Fax:** (314)512-9216
T. Dowd, Vice President & Secretary

Priorities: *Arts & Humanities:* 20%. Gives to art centers, art museums, art councils, and performing arts. *Civic & Public Affairs:* 20%. Funds business associations, botanical gardens, legal aid, and public safety programs. *Education:* 31%. Supports education foundations, Junior Achievement, minority scholarship funds, colleges, and universities. *Environment:* 25%. Supports Boy and Girl Scouts, food distribution, children's services, programs for the disabled, and community services. *International:* 4%. Contributes to single-disease health associations, children's hospitals, and Paraquad. *Religion:* 2%. *Note:* Total contributions made in fiscal 2000. **Typ. Recipients:** Alzheimers Disease, Arthritis, Cancer, Children's Health/Hospitals, Emergency/Ambulance Services, Health Organizations, Health-General, Hospitals, Mental Health, Multiple Sclerosis, People with Disabilities, Preventive Medicine/Wellness Organizations, Single-Disease Health Associations, Substance Abuse. **Geo. Dist:** headquarters area only.

★ 12487 ★ Grede Foundation
9898 West Bluemound Rd.
Milwaukee, WI 53226-0499
Phone: (414)257-3600
Burleigh Jacobs, President

Priorities: *Arts & Humanities:* 4%. Supports art funds, museums, libraries. *Civic & Public Affairs:* 11%. Supports public policy, legal issues, taxpayer and worker rights, clubs, housing, and economic research. *Education:* 19%. Supports colleges and universities, educational foundations, medical, technology, and engineering education; and private pre-college education. *Environment:* 36%. Supports YMCA, United Way, volunteer services, and people with disabilities. *International:* 9%. Supports nursing, hospitals, and medical research. *Note:* Total foundation contributions made in 2001. **Typ. Recipients:** Cancer, Children's Health/Hospitals, Clinics/Medical Centers, Hospitals, Medical Education, Medical Research, Nursing Services, People with Disabilities, Single-Disease Health Associations, Speech & Hearing, Transplant Networks/Donor Banks. **Geo. Dist:** WI.

★ 12488 ★ Greenpoint Foundation
90 Park Ave., 4th Floor
New York, NY 10016-1303
Phone: (212)834-1215 **Fax:** (212)834-1406
Email: gperry@GreenPoint.com
Website: http://www.greenpoint.com/Index.cfm?spPathName=static/com-home.htm
Gwen Perry, Vice President & Foundation Manager

Fnded: 1997. **Priorities:** *Arts & Humanities:* Less than 1%. Museums, preservation, public broadcasting, and other cultural organizations receive support. *Civic & Public Affairs:* 28%. Funds philanthropic organizations, housing programs, neighborhood associations, housing, economic development, minority affairs, parks, and police and fire fighter organizations. *Education:* 32%. Supports education and scholarship foundations, primary and secondary schools, colleges, and universities. *Environment:* 36%. Supports the United Way, youth organizations/activities, child care, family services, food distribution, and child welfare. *International:* 2%. Gives to single-disease health associations, medical research organizations, hospitals and medical centers, and the American Red Cross. *Note:* Total contributions made in fiscal 2001. **Typ. Recipients:** Emergency/Ambulance Services. **Geo. Dist:** NY.

★ 12489 ★ Griffith Laboratories Foundation
1 Griffith Ctr.
Alsip, IL 60803-3495
Phone: (708)371-0900 **Fax:** (708)371-4783
Joseph Maslick, Chief Financial Officer

Priorities: *Civic & Public Affairs:* 3%. Gives to an executive outreach program. *Environment:* 35%. Supports a community center and Special Olympics. *International:* 6%. Single-disease health associations and children's health programs receive support. *Note:* Total contributions made in fiscal 2001. **Typ. Recipients:** Alzheimers Disease, Children's Health/Hospitals, Diabetes, Health Organizations, Multiple Sclerosis, Research/Studies Institutes, Single-Disease Health Associations.

★ 12490 ★ Group Health Foundation
36 Four Seasons Center, 274
Chesterfield, MO 63017
Phone: (314)205-0115
Dr. Robert Swanson, Secretary & Vice President

Fnded: 1986. **Priorities:** *Education:* 34%. Supports medical education programs and provides nursing scholarships. *Environment:* 13%. Funds family services and services for the mentally disabled. *International:* 53%. Supports health centers, infant health, childhood immunization, and promotion of healthy lifestyles. *Note:* Total contributions made in fiscal 2000. **Typ. Recipients:** Adolescent Health Issues, AIDS/HIV, Alzheimers Disease, Arthritis, Cancer, Children's Health/Hospitals, Clinics/Medical Centers, Diabetes, Emergency/Ambulance Services, Eyes/Blindness, Geriatric Health, Health Organizations, Health Policy/Cost Containment, Health-General, Heart, Hospices, Hospitals, Hospitals (University Affiliated), Kidney, Long-Term Care, Medical Education, Medical Rehabilitation, Medical Research, Medical Training, Mental Health, Multiple Sclerosis, Nursing Services, Nutrition, People with Disabilities, Prenatal Health Issues, Preventive Medicine/Wellness Organizations, Public Health, Respiratory, Single-Disease Health Associations, Speech & Hearing, Substance Abuse, Transplant Networks/Donor Banks, Trauma Treatment. **Geo. Dist:** headquarters and operating communities.

★ 12491 ★ Guardian Life Insurance Co. of America
7 Hanover Square
New York, NY 10004-2616
Phone: (212)598-7499 **Fax:** (212)919-2944
Email: karen_olvany@glic.com
Website: http://www.glic.com
Karen Olvany, Assistant Corporate Secretary

Priorities: *Arts & Humanities:* About 7%. Funding supports libraries, museums, and public broadcasting. *Civic & Public Affairs:* 6%. Supports economic development through free enterprise organizations, urban youth programs, homeless aid, and community development. *Education:* 22%. Includes 13% of total through matching gifts to colleges and universities. Also supports inner city youth education, insurance/actuarial education, scholarship programs, literacy, and work force development. *Environment:* 58%. Recipients include united funds and youth organizations. *International:* About 6%. Recipients include medical research, nutrition, drug-abuse programs, and safety. *Note:* Total contributions made in 2001. Analysis provided by foundation. **Typ. Recipients:** Health Policy/Cost Containment, Hospices, Medical Research, Single-Disease Health Associations, Substance Abuse. **Geo. Dist:** headquarters and operating communities; Bethlehem, PA; Spokane, WA; Appleton, WI.

★ 12492 ★ Gucci America, Inc.
50 Hartz Way
Secaucus, NJ 07094
Phone: (212)379-8596 **Fax:** (212)379-8679
Website: http://www.gucci.com
Charlotte Sprintis, Director, Public Relations

Priorities: *Note:* All of the donations are in the form of merchandise. **Typ. Recipients:** Hospitals, Medical Research, Single-Disease Health Associations, Substance Abuse. **Geo. Dist:** primarily headquarters and operating communities.

★ 12493 ★ Guess? Foundation
1444 South Alameda St.
Los Angeles, CA 90021
Phone: (213)765-3100 **Fax:** (213)765-5927
Website: http://guess.com/guesssinc.asp?section=foundation2&page=foundation
Maia Pilapil, Guess? Foundation

Fnded: 1995. **Priorities:** *Arts & Humanities:* 3%. Primarily supports a fashion museum. *Civic & Public Affairs:* 11%. Funds women's affairs, law and justice concerns, and philanthropic organizations. *Education:* 14% Gives to schools, vocational training, and scholarship programs, with a focus on clothing/fashion design education. *Environment:* 7%. Funds child welfare organizations, youth programs, child mentoring, and volunteer services. *International:* 48%. Supports single-disease organizations, clinics, hospitals, and AIDS/HIV. *Note:* Total contributions made in 2000. **Typ. Recipients:** Adolescent Health Issues, AIDS/HIV, Cancer, Clinics/Medical Centers, Diabetes, Geriatric Health, Health Organizations, Heart, Medical Education, Medical Research, Multiple Sclerosis, People with Disabilities, Prenatal Health Issues, Public Health, Single-Disease Health Associations, Substance Abuse. **Geo. Dist:** limited to headquarters area only.

★ 12494 ★ Guidant Foundation Inc.
111 Monument Circle, Suite 2900
Indianapolis, IN 46204-5129
Phone: (317)971-2000
Website: http://www.guidant.com/foundation/
Thomas Peterson, Contact

Fnded: 1996. **Typ. Recipients:** Diabetes, Health Organizations, Heart, Hospitals, Medical Education.

★ 12495 ★ GuideOne Foundation
Mailstation A27
1111 Ashworth Rd.
West Des Moines, IA 50265
Phone: 877-448-4331
Website: http://www.guideone.com/AboutUs/foundation.htm
Mark McDougal, Foundation Coordinator

Priorities: *Environment:* 100% of funds go toward eliminating drinking and driving, and underage drinking prevention programs. **Typ. Recipients:** Substance Abuse. **Geo. Dist:** nationally.

★ 12496 ★ Gulf Power Foundation
1 Energy Place
Pensacola, FL 32520-0786
Phone: (850)444-6806
John Hodges, Jr., Chairman

Fnded: 1987. **Priorities:** *Arts & Humanities:* 13%. Supports libraries, museums, music, historical societies, and arts councils. *Civic & Public Affairs:* 13%. Supports chambers of commerce, parks, and community organizations. *Education:* 29%. Supports scholarships, colleges and universities, and education associations. *Environment:* 40%. Supports United Way, homes, food distribution, scouts, substance abuse programs, and child welfare. *International:* 3%. Supports single-disease health associations, hospice programs, and health organizations. *Voluntarism:* Company reports that it supports, "Junior Achievement, (charity) runs and holiday shopping." *Note:* Total foundation contributions made in 2001. **Typ. Recipients:** Cancer, Children's Health/Hospitals, Emergency/Ambulance Services, Health Organizations, Health Organizations, Hospices, Hospitals, People with Disabilities, Prenatal Health Issues, Public Health, Single-Disease Health Associations, Substance Abuse. **Geo. Dist:** Northwest Florida.

★ 12497 ★ H.B. Fuller Co. Foundation
PO Box 64683
Saint Paul, MN 55164-0683
Phone: (651)236-5207
Website: http://www.hbfuller.com/About_Us/Community/index.shtml
Karen Muller, Director of Community Affairs

Priorities: *Arts & Humanities:* 14%. Supports performing arts, libraries, theaters, museums, opera, public broadcasting, and art centers. *Civic & Public Affairs:* 9%. *Education:* 15%. Supports schools, universities, and programs for economically disadvantaged youth which provide the basics in literacy and vocational training. *Environment:* 50%. Supports child welfare, family services, YMCA, counseling programs, United Way, the homeless, shelters, and Special Olympics. *International:* 2%. Primary support made to clinics and programs which provide activities and health care for disadvantaged youth, with the dual purpose of involving community adults and the development of local youth. *Note:* Total contributions made in 2001. **Typ. Recipients:** Child Abuse, Clinics/Medical Centers, Domestic Violence, Emergency/Ambulance Services, Health Organizations, Mental Health, People with Disabilities, Research/Studies Institutes, Substance Abuse. **Geo. Dist:** internationally; headquarters and operating communities; nationally.

★ 12498 ★ H.J. Heinz Co. Foundation
PO Box 57
Pittsburgh, PA 15230-0057
Phone: (412)456-5772 **Fax:** (412)456-7868
Email: heinz_foundation@hjheinz.com
Website: http://www.heinz.com/jsp/foundation.jsp
Loretta Oken, Program Director

Fnded: 1951. **Priorities:** *Arts & Humanities:* 19%. Funds ballet, opera, theater, symphonies, public broadcasting, arts centers, and history groups, primarily in the Pittsburgh area. *Civic & Public Affairs:* 2%. Funds community and economic development organizations and professional organizations, especially those associated with the food industry. *Education:* 22%. Includes support to pre-college and college education, educational foundations, with a focus on food science and restaurant education. *Environment:* 23%. Supports the United Way, youth and family services, substance abuse treatment and awareness, food banks, and animal welfare. *International:* 9%. Supports hospital foundations, children's health concerns, medical centers, hospice, and community health centers. *Religion:* 4%. *Note:* Total contributions made in 2000. **Typ. Recipients:** AIDS/HIV, Cancer, Children's Health/Hospitals, Clinics/Medical Centers, Family Planning, Health Organizations, Heart, Home-Care Services, Hospices, Hospitals, Medical Education, Medical Rehabilitation, Medical Research, Nutrition, People with Disabilities, Public Health, Single-Disease Health Associations, Substance Abuse. **Geo. Dist:** principally near operating locations and to national organizations.

★ 12499 ★ Habig Foundation
1600 Royal St.
Jasper, IN 47549
Phone: (812)482-1600 **Fax:** (812)482-8166
Website: http://www.free-4u.com/habig.htm
Douglas Habig, Chairman & Chief Executive Officer

Fnded: 1951. **Priorities:** *Arts & Humanities:* 6%. Supports public broadcasting and art funds. *Civic & Public Affairs:* 9%. Supports legal foundations, ethnic organizations, safety, parks, and community foundations. *Education:* 45%. Supports colleges, universities, elementary and secondary schools, and Junior Achievement. *Environment:* 7%. Supports athletics, child welfare, counseling, and youth organizations. *International:* 5%. Supports health organizations and Cancer funds. *Note:* Total foundation contributions made in fiscal 2001. **Typ. Recipients:** Cancer, Emergency/Ambulance Services, Home-Care Services, Hospices, Hospitals, Medical Education, Mental Health. **Geo. Dist:** headquarters and operating communities.

★ 12500 ★ Halliburton Foundation, Inc.
3600 Lincoln Plaza
500 N Akard St.
Dallas, TX 75201
Phone: (214)978-2600 **Fax:** (214)978-2611
Website: http://www.halliburton.com/corp/about.asp
Margaret Carriere, Vice President & Secretary

Priorities: *Arts & Humanities:* 1%. Gives to the Oklahoma City Memorial Foundation. *Education:* 89%. Primarily supports faculty, equipment acquisition, and content development initiatives within engineering, technical or business departments of major colleges and universities. Limited unrestricted support. *Environment:* 5%. A small number of grants support youth organizations and the United Way. *Religion:* 2%. Supports a natural science museum. *Note:* Contributions made in 1999. **Typ. Recipients:** Cancer, Hospitals, Medical Education, Substance Abuse. **Geo. Dist:** Southwest; TX.

★ 12501 ★ Hallmark Corporate Foundation
PO Box 419580
Department 323
Kansas City, MO 64141-6580
Phone: (816)274-8515 **Fax:** (816)274-8547
Karen Bartz, Vice President

Priorities: *Arts & Humanities:* 44%. *Civic & Public Affairs:* 4%. *Education:* 5%. *Environment:* 45%. *International:* Less than 1%. *Voluntarism:* Supports the Volunteer Involvement Pays Program, through which a $200 grant is contributed to a 501(c)3 organization that has benefited from employee volunteers. Grant applications are employee initiated, and employees must volunteer at least 25 hours of service within a six-month period. *Note:* Company prefers to respond to requests on a case-by-case basis and has not established target levels for contribution categories. Total contributions made in 2001. **Typ. Recipients:** AIDS/HIV, Cancer, Children's Health/Hospitals, Domestic Violence, Emergency/Ambulance Services, Health Organizations, Hospices, Hospitals, Long-Term Care, Mental Health, People with Disabilities, Public Health, Sexual Abuse, Substance Abuse. **Geo. Dist:** headquarters; principally near operating locations and to national organizations; Metamora, IL; Leavenworth, KS; Topeka, KS; Kansas City, MO; Liberty, MO.

★ 12502 ★ H&R Block Foundation
4400 Main St.
Kansas City, MO 64111
Phone: 800-869-9220 **Fax:** (816)753-1585
Email: foundation@hrblock.com
Website: http://www.hrblockfoundation.org
David Miles, President

Fnded: 1974. **Priorities:** *Arts & Humanities:* 10%. *Civic & Public Affairs:* 42%. *Education:* 25%. *Environment:* 17%. *International:* 2%. *Voluntarism:* Individual H&R Block associates actively participate in community programs such as Habitat for Humanity and United Way. The foundation provides strategic support, rewards, and recognition for volunteer efforts. *Note:* Total contributions made in 2001. **Typ. Recipients:** AIDS/HIV, Cancer, Children's Health/Hospitals, Clinics/Medical Centers, Domestic Violence, Family Planning, Geriatric Health, Health Funds, Health Organizations, Heart, Home-Care Services, Hospices, Hospitals, Medical Education, Medical Rehabilitation, Mental Health, Multiple Sclerosis, People with Disabilities, Prenatal Health Issues, Public Health, Research/Studies Institutes, Single-Disease Health Associations, Substance Abuse. **Geo. Dist:** Kansas City, MO.

★ 12503 ★ Hannaford Charitable Foundation
PO Box 1000
Portland, ME 04104
Phone: (207)883-2911
Website: http://www.hannaford.com/community/charitable.htm
Donna Boyce, Secretary

Fnded: 1994. **Priorities:** *Arts & Humanities:* 9%. *Civic & Public Affairs:* 1%. *Education:* 27%. *Environment:* 39%. *International:* 6%. *Religion:* 1%. *Note:* Total foundation contributions made in 2001. **Typ. Recipients:** AIDS/HIV, Alzheimers Disease, Cancer, Children's Health/Hospitals, Clinics/Medical Centers, Emergency/Ambulance Services, Health Organizations, Heart, Home-Care Services, Hospices, Hospitals, Hospitals (University Affiliated), Medical Research, Research/Studies Institutes. **Geo. Dist:** headquarters and operating communities.

★ 12504 ★ Harcourt General Charitable Foundation
1280 Boylston St., Suite 100
Chestnut Hill, MA 02467-2112
Phone: (617)278-5213 **Fax:** (617)731-2354
Kay Kilpatrick, Director of Corporate Giving

Fnded: 1990. **Priorities:** *Arts & Humanities:* 12%. Supports the performing arts, including theater, music and dance; also supports museums. *Civic & Public Affairs:* 1%. *Education:* 33%. Funds colleges and universities, medical and business education, and public pre-college education, including reform efforts. *Environment:* 18%. Funds Boys and Girls Clubs, scouting, shelters, and the YMCA. *International:* 10%. Supports hospitals and cancer research. *Religion:* 26%. Supports science centers and museums. *Note:* Total foundation contributions made in fiscal 2000. **Typ. Recipients:** Cancer, Children's Health/Hospitals, Clinics/Medical Centers, Diabetes, Domestic Violence, Eyes/Blindness, Health Funds, Health Organizations, Health-General, Hospices, Hospitals, Hospitals (University Affiliated), Medical Education, Medical Research, People with Disabilities, Prenatal Health Issues, Research/Studies Institutes, Substance Abuse. **Geo. Dist:** Boston, MA, including metropolitan area.

★ 12505 ★ Harley-Davidson Foundation
3700 West Juneau Ave.
Milwaukee, WI 53208
Phone: (414)343-4001
Mary Martiny, Manager

Fnded: 1993. **Priorities:** *Arts & Humanities:* 17%. Supports public broadcasting, performing arts programs, and museums. *Civic & Public Affairs:* 18%. Supports community foundations, development, and housing. *Education:* 10%. Funds universities, colleges, and educational programs. *Environment:* 43%. Primarily funds the United Way and youth organizations. *International:* 10%. Supports single-disease associations and hospitals. *Religion:* 1%. Funds a science center. *Note:* Total foundation contributions made in 2000. **Typ. Recipients:** Cancer, Children's Health/Hospitals, Clinics/Medical Centers, Diabetes, Emergency/Ambulance Services, Family Planning, Health Organizations, Mental Health, Nursing Services, People with Disabilities, Public Health, Single-Disease Health Associations, Substance Abuse. **Geo. Dist:** AL; AL, headquarters and operating communities; MO; PA, headquarters and operating communities; WI, headquarters and operating communities.

★ 12506 ★ Harnischfeger Industries Foundation
PO Box 554
Milwaukee, WI 53201-0554
Phone: (414)319-8506 **Fax:** (414)319-8520
Sandy McKenzie, Executive Assistant

Fnded: 1989. **Priorities:** *Arts & Humanities:* 19%. Supports museums, performing arts, libraries, the orchestra, and the theater. *Civic & Public Affairs:* 10%. Funds programs for ethnic and racial minorities, women's groups, foundations, and city offices. *Education:* 7%. Supports education programs, colleges, and secondary schools. *Environment:* 49%. Major grant to the United Way. Also gives to programs for the blind, youth clubs, Special Olympics, and community athletic and social clubs. *International:* 11%. Funds single-disease health organizations and organizations focusing on pediatric health/pediatric disease. *Religion:* 1%. Funds Discovery World - The James Lovell Museum of Science, Economic, and Technology. *Note:* Total contributions made in fiscal 2000. **Typ. Recipients:** AIDS/HIV, Cancer, Children's Health/Hospitals, Clinics/Medical Centers, Diabetes, Domestic Violence, Emergency/Ambulance Services, Health Organizations, Heart, Long-Term Care, Medical Education, Medical Research, Mental Health, People with Disabilities, Prenatal Health Issues, Single-Disease Health Associations. **Geo. Dist:** AZ; DC; IL; MD; MI; MN; NY; PA; TX; VA; WI.

★ 12507 ★ Harold Simmons Foundation, Inc.
5430 LBJ Freeway, Suite 1700
Dallas, TX 75240-2697
Phone: (972)991-2400 **Fax:** (972)448-1456
Lisa Simmons Epstein, President

Fnded: 1988. **Priorities:** *Arts & Humanities:* 3%. *Civic & Public Affairs:* 12%. *Education:* 38%. *Environment:* 29%. *International:* 5%. *Note:* Total contributions made in 2001. **Typ. Recipients:** AIDS/HIV, Cancer, Children's Health/Hospitals, Clinics/Medical Centers, Domestic Violence, Family Planning, Health Organizations, Hospitals, Hospitals (University Affiliated), Kidney, Medical Education, Medical Research, Mental Health, Multiple Sclerosis, Nursing Services, People with Disabilities, Prenatal Health Issues, Public Health, Single-Disease Health Associations, Substance Abuse, Transplant Networks/Donor Banks. **Geo. Dist:** Dallas, TX, including metropolitan area.

★ 12508 ★ Harris Bank Foundation
111 W Monroe St.
PO Box 755
Chicago, IL 60690-0755
Phone: (312)461-5193 **Fax:** (312)987-4702
Donna Streibich Curtis, Secretary & Treasurer

Fnded: 1953. **Priorities:** *Arts & Humanities:* 19%. Focus on promoting cultural diversity while providing access to the arts for under served communities. Supports both the major cultural institutions and smaller art groups in Chicago, including museums, dance, theater, music, and zoos and parks. *Civic & Public Affairs:* 42%. Civic focus is on race relations, business and economic issues, infrastructure concerns, and strategic planning efforts. Community revitalization grants support programs which increase or improve housing for low/moderate income people in Chicago, and which promote commercial and industrial activity in low income neighborhoods. *Education:* 14%. Supports higher education in the Chicago area. Also supports organizations advocating for training and/or public school reform; technical and science education; urban education; and opportunities for inner-city youth. *Environment:* 16%. Grants go to new projects or programs which provide direct services to under served, financially disadvantaged populations. Includes youth organizations, Young Men's Christian Associations, scouting, and community centers. *International:* 1%. Grants are designed to improve hospitals and health care delivery systems. *Religion:* 4%. Supports museums and a planetarium. *Note:* Above priorities are for foundation giving in 2000. The company and its subsidiaries also make cash and nonmonetary donations; priorities vary according to community needs. **Typ. Recipients:** Clinics/Medical Centers, Domestic Violence, Health Organizations, Hospices, Medical Rehabilitation, Mental Health, People with Disabilities. **Geo. Dist:** Chicago, IL, Chicagoland area.

★ 12509 ★ Harris Foundation
1025 West NASA Boulevard, MS-16
Melbourne, FL 32919
Phone: (321)727-9253 **Fax:** (321)727-9222
Richard Ballantyne, Secretary

Priorities: *Arts & Humanities:* 17%. Funds the performing arts, museums, and art funds. *Civic & Public Affairs:* 1%. Gives to housing programs, women's affairs, professional associations, civic organizations, and a zoo. *Education:* 62%. Funds public universities. Also supports a matching gift program for secondary and higher education institutions. *Environment:* 17%. Supports the United Way, child welfare, scouts, food and clothing distribution, and services for victims of domestic violence. *International:* Less than 1%. Contributes to single-disease health associations and nursing services. *Religion:* 1%. Funds a marine institute. *Note:* Above percentages reflect foundation giving in fiscal 2000. Company administers a direct giving program and a foundation. Both programs direct funds to eligible nonprofit organizations in Brevard County, FL, primarily through united funds, civic organizations, and various community service organizations. **Typ. Recipients:** Cancer, Children's Health/Hospitals, Clinics/Medical Centers, Diabetes, Domestic Violence, Emergency/Ambulance Services, Eyes/Blindness, Health Organizations, Hospitals, Nursing Services, Prenatal Health Issues, Substance Abuse. **Geo. Dist:** principally near operating locations and to national organizations; FL.

★ 12510 ★ Harsco Corp. Fund

PO Box 8888
Camp Hill, PA 17001-8888
Phone: (717)763-7064
Website: http://www.harsco.com/about1/community.html
Robert Yocum, Chairman & Trustee

Priorities: *Arts & Humanities:* 23%. *Civic & Public Affairs:* 4%. *Education:* 40%. *Environment:* 18%. *International:* 11%. *Religion:* 3%. *Note:* Total foundation contributions made in 2001. **Typ. Recipients:** Cancer, Children's Health/Hospitals, Clinics/Medical Centers, Diabetes, Emergency/Ambulance Services, Family Planning, Health Organizations, Hospices, Hospitals, Medical Education, Medical Research, Mental Health, People with Disabilities, Public Health, Sexual Abuse, Single-Disease Health Associations, Substance Abuse. **Geo. Dist:** headquarters and operating communities.

★ 12511 ★ Hartford Financial Services Group, Inc.

Hartford Place
690 Asylum Ave.
T-12-56
Hartford, CT 06115
Phone: (860)547-4995 **Fax:** (860)547-6393
Email: Jennifer.Kasparian@thehartford.com
Website: http://www.thehartford.com/about/affairs.html
Mrs. Jennifer Kasparian, Grants Program Specialist

Priorities: *Arts & Humanities:* 25%. Supports arts and cultural opportunities for people living in Greater Hartford's diverse communities. Examples of institutions supported include museums, public television, arts programs, and orchestras. *Civic & Public Affairs:* (Economic and Community Development) 8%. Funds programs that provide employment, training, and job creation. Focuses on programs aimed at improving the economic stability and vitality of Hartford's neighborhoods, with a special emphasis on the Asylum Hill neighborhood. *Education:* 40%. Hartford's top corporate contributions priority is to have a positive impact on public K-12 education. The company's primary focus is on programs that improve educational opportunities for students in the Hartford Public School system, with emphasis on those residing in Hartford's Asylum Hill neighborhood. Scholarships are an important part of The Hartford's education grants. The Alliance for Academic Achievement-The Hartford Straight A Program is aimed at top scholars in the three Hartford high schools and provides scholarships to Howard University, the University of Connecticut, and Trinity College, and summer employment and mentors at The Hartford. The company's oldest and most successful continuous initiative, The STAG (Skills Training Advancement Group) work-study program, provides students from Hartford area high schools the opportunity to earn money while they learn basic workplace skills. Qualified STAG graduates planning to attend college are eligible for a STAG scholarship. The Donald R. Frahm Hartford Scholar Program targets students pursuing a master's degree in business administration. The company also maintains a variety of other scholarship programs, the recipients of which are selected by the company rather than by an individual application process. Employee matching gifts to colleges and universities amount to nearly one third of all educational grants. *Environment:* 7%. The company's Aid to Individuals with Disabilities (5%) makes grants for programs that help people with disabilities become self-sufficient. The Aid to Mature Americans program (2%) emphasizes programs that help people utilize their experience and skills to remain independent and live productive lives. *Voluntarism:* The company sponsors a Reading Buddies Program with a local middle elementary school. Approximately 100 employees volunteer for this program. *Note:* Total contributions made in 2001. **Typ. Recipients:** AIDS/HIV, Children's Health/Hospitals, Clinics/Medical Centers, Domestic Violence, Eyes/Blindness, Geriatric Health, Health Organizations, Health Policy/Cost Containment, Hospices, Hospitals, Medical Education, Medical Rehabilitation, Medical Research, People with Disabilities, Prenatal Health Issues, Preventive Medicine/Wellness Organizations, Public Health, Substance Abuse. **Geo. Dist:** principally near operating locations and to national organizations, grants are allocated based on the size of the operation in the; Hartford, CT, Greater Hartford area.

★ 12512 ★ Hartmarx Charitable Foundation

101 North Wacker Drive, 23rd Floor
Chicago, IL 60606
Phone: (312)357-5331
Website: http://www.hartmarx.com
Kay Nalbach, President

Priorities: *Arts & Humanities:* 20%. Supports music, museums, arts festivals, dance, public broadcasting, libraries, history organizations, and theater. *Civic & Public Affairs:* 5%. Supports business organizations, community development, housing, professional associations, public policy, women's and minority affairs, zoos, and aquariums. *Education:* 17%. Supports colleges, universities, education associations, minority education, and education funds. Also sponsors an educational matching gifts program. *Environment:* 47%. Supports United Ways, youth organizations, and food distribution. *International:* 4%. Supports medical centers, single-disease health organizations, hospitals, and pediatric health. *Note:* Total foundation contributions made in fiscal 2000. About 60% of contributions are made from corporate headquarters; 40% is allocated and disbursed through operating companies. **Typ. Recipients:** AIDS/HIV, Arthritis, Cancer, Child Abuse, Children's Health/Hospitals, Clinics/Medical Centers, Diabetes, Domestic Violence, Emergency/Ambulance Services, Family Planning, Health Organizations, Heart, Hospitals, Multiple Sclerosis, Nursing Services, People with Disabilities, Prenatal Health Issues, Prenatal Health Issues, Public Health, Respiratory, Sexual Abuse, Single-Disease Health Associations. **Geo. Dist:** headquarters and operating communities.

★ 12513 ★ Hartzell-Norris Charitable Trust

c/o Fifth Third Bank, Trustee
PO Box 630858
Cincinnati, OH 45263
Phone: (513)579-5310
Website: http://www.hartzellindustries.com/community.htm

Fnded: 1943. **Priorities:** *Arts & Humanities:* 9%. Funds arts councils and art and children's museums. *Civic & Public Affairs:* 18%. Gives to community foundations, chambers of commerce, civic groups, fire departments, and affordable housing initiatives. *Education:* 45%. Supports colleges, universities, public high schools, and schools for children with behavioral and emotional problems. Also provides colleges scholarships. *Environment:* 18%. Supports YMCAs, child welfare, food distribution, services for the disabled, the United Way, recreation/athletic programs, and scouts. *International:* 4%. Funds medical rehabilitation, cancer research, public health programs, and emergency medical services. *Note:* Total contributions made in fiscal 2001. **Typ. Recipients:** Cancer, Child Abuse, Domestic Violence, Emergency/Ambulance Services, Geriatric Health, Health Organizations, Heart, Hospitals, Medical Rehabilitation, Respiratory, Single-Disease Health Associations, Substance Abuse. **Geo. Dist:** some giving nationally; AR; IL; IN; KY; MI; OH; WI.

★ 12514 ★ Harvest Charities

1426 Main St.
Columbia, SC 29226
Phone: (803)765-3677
C. Lane, Contact

Fnded: 1944. **Priorities:** *Arts & Humanities:* 3%. Supports music and art funds. *Education:* 60%. Supports schools, colleges, universities, and education funds. *Environment:* 6%. Supports YWCA, United Way, senior services, shelters, food distribution, and child welfare. *International:* 3%. Supports medical research and clinics, and single-disease health associations. *Note:* Total foundation contributions made in 2001. **Typ. Recipients:** Cancer, Clinics/Medical Centers, Diabetes, Emergency/Ambulance Services, Health Organizations, Hospitals, Medical Education, Medical Research, Sexual Abuse, Single-Disease Health Associations. **Geo. Dist:** headquarters and operating communities. **Frmly:** Belk Simpson Foundation.

★ 12515 ★ Harvey Hubbell Foundation

PO Box 549
584 Derby-Milford Rd.
Orange, CT 06477-4024
Phone: (203)799-4100 **Fax:** (203)799-4333
Harry Rowell, Trustee

Fnded: 1959. **Priorities:** *Arts & Humanities:* 1%. Funds museums. *Civic & Public Affairs:* 37%. Supports parks and recreational facilities, festivals, safety. *Education:* 26%. Contributes to several universities, and also supports medical education, scholarship programs, and schools. *Environment:* 22%. Majority supports various United Way agencies in Connecticut. Other recipients include boys clubs and homes, scouting programs, community centers, and food and clothing distribution. *International:* 14%. Interests include single disease health associations. *Note:* Total contributions made in 2001. **Typ. Recipients:** Cancer, Children's Health/Hospitals, Domestic Violence, Emergency/Ambulance Services, Health Organizations, Hospices, Hospitals, Hospitals (University Affiliated), Medical Education, Medical Rehabilitation, Mental Health, Nursing Services, People with Disabilities, Public Health, Respiratory, Single-Disease Health Associations. **Geo. Dist:** principally near operating locations and to national organizations.

★ 12516 ★ Hasbro Charitable Trust Inc.

1027 Newport Ave.
Pawtucket, RI 02862
Phone: (401)431-8151 **Fax:** (401)721-7275
Website: http://www.hasbro.org
Karen Davis, Director

Priorities: *Arts & Humanities:* 9%. Funds museums, public art, and history organizations/monuments. *Civic & Public Affairs:* 15%. Supports community and neighborhood associations, economic development, public parks/playgrounds, and urban, minority, and legal affairs. *Education:* 10%. Funds higher education, public education, and Junior Achievement in Rhode Island. *Environment:* 51%. Funds United Way, scouting, children's services, food banks, community centers, recreation programs, and services for the disabled. *International:* 10%. Funds children's health, the Red Cross, hospitals and rehabilitation centers, and single-disease health associations. *Note:* Total foundation giving in 2000. **Typ. Recipients:** AIDS/HIV, Alzheimers Disease, Cancer, Child Abuse, Children's Health/Hospitals, Clinics/Medical Centers, Diabetes, Emergency/Ambulance Services, Eyes/Blindness, Family Planning, Geriatric Health, Health Organizations, Heart, Hospices, Hospitals, Hospitals (University Affiliated), Kidney, Medical Education, Medical Rehabilitation, Medical Research, Multiple Sclerosis, Nursing Services, People with Disabilities, Prenatal Health Issues, Public Health, Research/Studies Institutes, Sexual Abuse, Single-Disease Health Associations, Single-Disease Health Associations, Substance Abuse, Transplant Networks/Donor Banks. **Geo. Dist:** headquarters and operating communities.

★ 12517 ★ Hasbro Children's Foundation
10 Rockefeller Plaza, 16th Fl.
New York, NY 10020
Phone: (212)713-7654
Website: http://www.hasbro.org/hcf/
Jane Englebardt, Executive Director

Typ. Recipients: Hospitals, Mental Health, Nutrition, People with Disabilities. **Geo. Dist:** nationally.

★ 12518 ★ Hawaiian Electric Industries Charitable Foundation
900 Richards St.
Honolulu, HI 96813
Phone: (808)543-7350
Website: http://www.heicf.org/heicf.html
Curtis Harada, Treasurer

Priorities: *Arts & Humanities:* 11%. Supports public broadcasting, museums, arts festivals, and historical societies. *Civic & Public Affairs:* 6%. Supports economic development, housing, and legal aid. *Education:* 16%. Education funds are directed to programs at Hawaiian colleges, universities, and secondary schools. Also supports the Citizens Scholarship Foundation of America. *Environment:* 57%. Supports youth organizations, food banks, Special Olympics, volunteer services, community centers, Young Men's Christian Association and Young Women's Christian Association, and United Way. *International:* 5%. Contributes to the American Heart Association, American Cancer Society, and hospitals and medical centers. *Voluntarism:* Company sponsors an employee volunteerism program, including the Great Aloha Run, and the Special Olympics; small grants are awarded to nonprofits where employees volunteer through the Volunteer Recognition Program. *Note:* Total contributions made in 2000. **Typ. Recipients:** AIDS/HIV, Cancer, Children's Health/Hospitals, Clinics/Medical Centers, Emergency/Ambulance Services, Health Organizations, Heart, Hospices, Hospitals, Medical Rehabilitation, Mental Health, People with Disabilities, Public Health, Single-Disease Health Associations, Speech & Hearing, Substance Abuse. **Geo. Dist:** CA; HI.

★ 12519 ★ HCR Manor Care Foundation
333 North Summit St.
PO Box 10086
Toledo, OH 43699-0086
Phone: (419)252-5989 **Fax:** (419)252-5521
Email: jsteiner@hcr-manorcare.com
Website: http://www.hcr-manorcare.org
Jennifer Steiner, Executive Director

Priorities: *Arts & Humanities:* 5%. Primary support made to public broadcasting. *Education:* 5%. Primarily supports medical colleges. *Environment:* 28%. Supports senior and family services. *International:* 57%. Supports the medical research, hospitals, health and medical centers, hospices, mental health programs, and single-disease health associations. *Note:* Total foundation contributions made in fiscal 2001. **Typ. Recipients:** Alzheimers Disease, Arthritis, Children's Health/Hospitals, Clinics/Medical Centers, Emergency/Ambulance Services, Geriatric Health, Heart, Home-Care Services, Hospices, Long-Term Care, Medical Education, Medical Rehabilitation, Mental Health, Nursing Services, Preventive Medicine/Wellness Organizations, Public Health, Research/Studies Institutes. **Geo. Dist:** the 32 states in which the company operates. **Frmly:** Manor Care Health SVS, Inc.

★ 12520 ★ Heinz Foundation
PO Box 185
Pittsburgh, PA 15230-9897
Phone: (412)234-5255
Email: heinz.foundation@hjheinz.com
Website: http://www.heinz.com/jsp/foundation.jsp
Tammy Aupperle, Program Directory

Priorities: *Arts & Humanities:* 5%. *Civic & Public Affairs:* 15%. *Education:* 31%. *Environment:* 26%. *International:* 14%. *Religion:* 4%. *Note:* Total contributions made in 2001. **Typ. Recipients:** Children's Health/Hospitals, Hospitals, Medical Education, Nutrition. **Geo. Dist:** headquarters and operating communities.

★ 12521 ★ Helene Curtis Industries, Inc.
325 North Wells St.
Chicago, IL 60610
Phone: (312)661-2920 **Fax:** (312)661-1437
Website: http://www.unilever.com
Maureen Collins, Director/Community Relations

Typ. Recipients: Health-General. **Geo. Dist:** IL.

★ 12522 ★ Henkel Loctite
1001 Troutbrook Crossing
Rocky Hill, CT 06067-3910
Phone: (860)571-5100 **Fax:** (860)571-5294
Email: don.atencio@loctite.com
Marshall Kearns, Director of Human Resources

Priorities: *Arts & Humanities:* About 10%. *Civic & Public Affairs:* Less than 5%. *Education:* About 65%. About one-third of educational funding supports pre-high school education, including infant and pre-kindergarten programs. *International:* About 20% **Typ. Recipients:** Health-General. **Geo. Dist:** areas where the company has offices.

★ 12523 ★ Hercules, Inc.
1313 N Market St.
Wilmington, DE 19894-0001
Phone: (302)594-5137 **Fax:** (302)594-6909
Shaun O'Hara, Community Relations Representative

Typ. Recipients: Health-General. **Geo. Dist:** principally near operating locations and to national organizations; DE.

★ 12524 ★ Herman O. West Foundation
101 Gordon Drive
Lionville, PA 19353
Phone: (610)594-2905 **Fax:** (610)594-3011
Email: maureen.goebel@westpharma.com
Maureen Goebel, Administrator

Priorities: *Arts & Humanities:* 30%. *Civic & Public Affairs:* 16%. *Education:* 44%. *International:* 8%. *Note:* Total contributions made in 2002. **Typ. Recipients:** Cancer, Children's Health/Hospitals, Emergency/Ambulance Services, Family Planning, Health Organizations, Hospitals, Medical Education, Medical Rehabilitation, Medical Research, Nursing Services, People with Disabilities, Prenatal Health Issues, Public Health, Substance Abuse, Trauma Treatment. **Geo. Dist:** headquarters and operating communities; FL; NE; NJ; NC; PA. **Frmly:** Herman O. West Foundation.

★ 12525 ★ Hershey Foods Corp.
100 Crystal A Dr.
PO Box 810
Hershey, PA 17033-0810
Phone: (717)534-7880 **Fax:** (717)534-7015
Website: http://www.hersheys.com/about/contributions.shtml
Jennifer Goss, Corporate Contributions Dept.

Typ. Recipients: Clinics/Medical Centers, Hospitals, Nutrition, People with Disabilities, Substance Abuse. **Geo. Dist:** limited to manufacturing site communities.

★ 12526 ★ Hewlett-Packard Co. Foundation
PO Box 10301
Palo Alto, CA 94304-0890
Phone: (650)857-2982
Email: bess_stephens@hp.com
Website: http://www.hp.com/go/grants
Mr. Bess Stephens, Executive Director

Priorities: *Civic & Public Affairs:* 5%. *Education:* 16%. *Environment:* 78%. *Note:* Total foundation contributions made in 2001. **Typ. Recipients:** Emergency/Ambulance Services, Eyes/Blindness, Health-General, Hospitals, Medical Education, Public Health, Single-Disease Health Associations, Substance Abuse. **Geo. Dist:** internationally principally near operating locations and to national organizations; nationally; U.S. principally near operating locations and to national organizations.

★ 12527 ★ Hickory Tech Corp. Foundation
221 E Hickory St.
PO Box 3248
Mankato, MN 56002-3248
Phone: (507)387-1866 **Fax:** (507)625-9191
Jane Rush, Administrator

Fnded: 1963. **Priorities:** *Arts & Humanities:* About 4%. Supports local music and theater groups. *Civic & Public Affairs:* 18%. Supports the chamber of commerce and community-school partnerships. *Education:* 41%. Supports public and private colleges and universities in company's headquarters area. The foundation also provides scholarships for children of employees, accounting for approximately one-third of education support, and has established scholarship programs at local universities. *Environment:* 29%. Primarily supports the United Way. Also supports youth organizations, shelters, clothes distribution and food distribution. *International:* 8%. *Note:* Contributions made in fiscal 2000. **Typ. Recipients:** Alzheimers Disease, Cancer, Children's Health/Hospitals, Clinics/Medical Centers, Emergency/Ambulance Services, Health-General, Heart, Hospitals, Medical Rehabilitation, Multiple Sclerosis, Prenatal Health Issues, Public Health, Trauma Treatment. **Geo. Dist:** Mankato, MN.

★ 12528 ★ High Meadow Foundation
PO Box 955
Stockbridge, MA 01262
Phone: (413)243-1474 **Fax:** (413)243-1067
John Fitzpatrick, President

Priorities: *Arts & Humanities:* 68%. Support theater and performing arts, chamber music, operas, symphonies, museums, art associations, dance, and public broadcasting. *Civic & Public Affairs:* 7%. Supports community service organizations, women's organizations, and community foundations. *Education:* 12%. The majority of giving supports private and public precollege education. Also donates to colleges and universities, including scholarships, agricultural education, arts education, educational associations and funds, international studies, legal education, and minority education. *Environment:* 6%. Funds United Way, child welfare, services for people with disabilities, family planning and services, shelters, and united funds. *International:* 5%. Funds home healthcare and hospitals. *Note:* Total contributions made in fiscal 2001. **Typ. Recipients:** AIDS/HIV, Children's Health/Hospitals, Clinics/Medical Centers, Emergency/Ambulance Services, Family Planning, Hospices, Hospitals, Nursing Services, People with Disabilities, Public Health. **Geo. Dist:** MA, Berkshire County, MA.

★ 12529 ★ Hitachi Foundation
1509 22nd St., NW
Washington, DC 20037-1073
Phone: (202)457-0588 **Fax:** (202)296-1098
Website: http://www.hitachi.org

Fnded: 1985. **Priorities:** *Arts & Humanities:* 6%. Supports film, children's museum, and art foundations. *Civic & Public Affairs:* 29%. Foundation is interested in helping to develop a wider definition of and vision for communities and community development. Supports projects that enable people and organizations to identify their collective needs and then develop strategies for addressing those needs. In this area, the foundation does not support single-issue community development approaches such as small business development, commercial revitalization, and neighborhood beautification; housing development or housing specific programming in isolation from other community development efforts; leadership development programs disconnected from specific problem identification and solving efforts; or social service provision in isolation from larger community building strategies. The company sponsors the yearly Yoshiyama Award to high school seniors for exemplary service to community. *Education:* 45%. Foundation encourages projects that support children, youth, adults, and educators as they learn to participate in an increasingly pluralistic and complex society. Projects that further these goals include those that foster an understanding of diversity and global issues across disciplines, connect learning objectives with community service, and work force development. The majority of the foundation's education dollars are targeted toward the pre-collegiate level, with support at the post-secondary level directed mainly toward assisting institutions to build collaborative and cooperative programs with communities or the K-12 schools. Education projects that receive support reflect the necessity to prepare individuals to participate more fully as citizens and productive members of society; recognize that schools can play a significant role in building and stabilizing communities; improve and develop the connections between schools, parents, and communities; recognize the diversity of learning styles and pedagogical approaches needed to educate all of America's students; incorporate the arts or museums as an educator and provider of increased opportunities for creativity and problem solving; link education to economic opportunity; and utilize community resources, such as arts organizations, corporations, churches and synagogues, and community service organizations. In the area of education, the foundation does not support math and science programs that are not interdisciplinary and do not build upon emerging and existing research on teaching and learning; projects that focus on schools, teachers, and students in a vacuum, seeing them as separate from the community; or efforts to "internationalize" curricula, programs, or institutions at the post-secondary level. *Environment:* 17%. Support goes to youth organizations, violence prevention, and volunteerism. *Religion:* 3%. Foundation makes grants to organizations for support programs that address technology-related issues in education and community development. Grants are not solely for acquisition or use of technology, nor for equipment purchase. **Typ. Recipients:** Domestic Violence, Domestic Violence, Medical Education, People with Disabilities, Substance Abuse. **Geo. Dist:** continental United States; parent company gives internationally.

★ 12530 ★ Hoffer Foundation

500 Collins St.
South Elgin, IL 60177
Phone: (847)741-5841
Robert Hoffer, Chairman, President & CEO

Fnded: 1966. **Priorities:** *Arts & Humanities:* 19%. Supports museums, music, and public broadcasting. *Education:* 32%. Supports higher education and primary and secondary schools. *Environment:* 44%. Supports United Way, community centers, Young Men's Christian Association, and day care. *International:* 2%. Supports single-disease health associations. *Note:* Total contributions made in fiscal 2001. **Typ. Recipients:** Children's Health/Hospitals, Hospitals. **Geo. Dist:** IL.

★ 12531 ★ Hoffmann-La Roche Foundation

PO Box 278
Nutley, NJ 07110-0278
Phone: (973)562-2055 **Fax:** (973)562-2999
Website: http://www.rocheusa.com
Vivian Beetle, Director Corporate Relations

Fnded: 1945. **Priorities:** *Arts & Humanities:* 2%. Primarily supports performing art centers. *Civic & Public Affairs:* 3%. Supports job training and community foundations. *Education:* 51%. Supports universities and college funds. Also funds educational programs that encourage math and science literacy. *Environment:* 38%. Supports United Way and senior organizations. *International:* 6%. Supports health care foundations, Cancer centers, hospitals, and medical research. *Note:* Total foundation contributions made in 2001. Company also sponsors a direct giving program, which is considerably larger than the foundation program. Financial data for the direct giving program is not available; interests include health promotion and education, and math and science literacy, with emphasis on site communities. **Typ. Recipients:** AIDS/HIV, Cancer, Children's Health/Hospitals, Emergency/Ambulance Services, Health Organizations, Health Policy/Cost Containment, Hospices, Hospitals, Hospitals, Medical Education, Medical Research, Medical Training, Mental Health, People with Disabilities, Public Health, Single-Disease Health Associations, Substance Abuse, Transplant Networks/Donor Banks. **Geo. Dist:** NJ.

★ 12532 ★ Hofmann Foundation

PO Box 907
Concord, CA 94520-4912
Phone: (925)682-4830
Lisa Hofmann Seeno, Secretary

Fnded: 1963. **Priorities:** *Arts & Humanities:* 1%. Most funding supports theater, public broadcasting, symphonies, and museums. *Civic & Public Affairs:* 13%. Supports philanthropic organizations and Rotary Clubs. *Education:* 16%. Funds a variety of institutions, ranging from high schools and elementary schools to colleges and universities, that demonstrate a profound desire to challenge and improve the hearts and minds of their students. Both public and private schools are supported, as well as scholarship funds. *Environment:* 21%. Supports organizations providing child welfare, youth programs, family services, animal welfare, and volunteer services. *International:* 5%. Supports the local medical and health community as well as single-disease health associations including cancer, Alzheimer's, and heart disease. *Note:* Total contributions made in fiscal 2001. **Typ. Recipients:** AIDS/HIV, Alzheimers Disease, Cancer, Children's Health/Hospitals, Clinics/Medical Centers, Diabetes, Domestic Violence, Emergency/Ambulance Services, Health Organizations, Heart, Hospices, Hospitals, Medical Education, Medical Research, People with Disabilities, Preventive Medicine/Wellness Organizations, Public Health, Respiratory, Single-Disease Health Associations. **Geo. Dist:** CA, Bay Area organizations only.

★ 12533 ★ Home Savings Charitable Foundation

PO Box 1111
Youngstown, OH 44501-1111
Phone: (330)742-0500
Website: http://www.homesavings.com
Darlene Pavlock, Executive Director

Fnded: 1992. **Priorities:** *Arts & Humanities:* 6%. Gives to public broadcasting, community theater, arts councils, historical societies, and museums. *Civic & Public Affairs:* 29%. Supports chambers of commerce, business associations, community foundations, public parks and gardens, civic groups, citizen's/voter's organizations, and police and fire departments. *Education:* 11%. Contributes to colleges, universities, literacy programs, and public schools. *Environment:* 41%. Supports youth organizations, community centers, athletic/recreation organizations, the United Way, human service agencies, substance abuse organizations, and animal welfare. *International:* 13%. Funds single-disease health associations, hospitals, the American Red Cross, hospice, health foundations, and a hearing & speech center. *Note:* Total contributions made in 2000. **Typ. Recipients:** Cancer, Children's Health/Hospitals, Diabetes, Domestic Violence, Emergency/Ambulance Services, Health-General, Hospices, People with Disabilities, Speech & Hearing. **Geo. Dist:** OH, various counties in the northern region of the state.

★ 12534 ★ HON Industries Charitable Foundation

414 East Third St.
Muscatine, IA 52761-0071
Phone: (563)264-7400 **Fax:** (563)264-7217
Website: http://www.honi.com/CorporateResponsibility.htm
Susan Cradick, Secretary-Treasurer

Fnded: 1985. **Priorities:** *Arts & Humanities:* 3%. *Civic & Public Affairs:* 19%. *Education:* 39%. *Environment:* 33%. *International:* 3%. *Note:* Total foundation contributions made in fiscal 2001. **Typ. Recipients:** Cancer, Children's Health/Hospitals, Domestic Violence, Emergency/Ambulance Services, Health Organizations, Hospitals, Preventive Medicine/Wellness Organizations, Public Health, Speech & Hearing. **Geo. Dist:** headquarters and operating communities; Muscatine, IA.

★ 12535 ★ Honda of America Foundation

24000 Honda Pkwy.
Marysville, OH 43040-9251
Phone: (937)645-6883
Lourene Hoy, Admin. Coord., Company Communications

Fnded: 1981. **Priorities:** *Arts & Humanities:* 10%. Contributes to historical associations and theater. *Civic & Public Affairs:* 16%. Funds economic development and job placement. *Education:* 54%. Supports colleges, universities, literacy programs, and Japanese language schools. *Environment:* 7%. *Religion:* 33%. *Voluntarism:* The company maintains the Honda Hero Volunteer program, through which the company will donate $200 to eligible organizations to which employees volunteer a minimum of 50 hours. *Note:* Total contributions made in 2000. **Typ. Recipients:** Health-General, People with Disabilities. **Geo. Dist:** OH, 15-county hiring area.

★ 12536 ★ Honeywell Foundation

101 Columbia Rd.
Morristown, NJ 07962
Phone: (973)455-5876
Website: http://www.honeywell.com/about/foundation.html
Andre Lewis, President

Priorities: *Arts & Humanities:* 9%. Provides capital grants, general support, and employee matching gifts to public radio and television. Other interests include theaters, arts centers and associations, and music and dance groups. Focuses on major arts organizations and a select group of new and emerging arts programs. *Civic & Public Affairs:* 37%. The foundation's contributions support affordable housing, crime prevention in the neighborhood, and training and employment preparedness. Disbursements outside of Minneapolis are determined by the individual community needs. *Education:* 33%. Emphasis on early childhood development and elementary and secondary education programs in major Honeywell locations. Other interests include business, engineering, and increased educational opportunities for women and minorities in technical disciplines. Grant types include scholarship funds (to institutions, not individuals), general support, endowment, and employee matching gifts. Also supports independent college and minority education funds, education associations, and precollegiate programs in technological sciences. *Environment:* 20%. Foundation supports United Ways in operating areas. Also funds food banks, family and youth services. *International:* Less than 1%. *Voluntarism:* The company encourages employees to volunteer through the Honeywell Employee Launched Projects grant-making initiative (HELP), which makes contributions of $100 to $500 to efforts in which Honeywell employees, retirees, or their families are involved. Honeywell also encourages involvement in a paint-a-thon, a Foodshare program, and Habitat for Humanity. *Note:* Total contributions made in 2000. **Typ. Recipients:** Adolescent Health Issues, Cancer, Children's Health/Hospitals, Domestic Violence, Family Planning, Health Organizations, Hospitals, Hospitals (University Affiliated), Mental Health, People with Disabilities, Prenatal Health Issues, Public Health, Research/Studies Institutes, Substance Abuse. **Geo. Dist:** major principally near operating locations and to national organizations; MN, organizations in Minnesota receive about 50% of total contributions.

★ 12537 ★ Household International Inc.

2700 Sanders Rd.
Prospect Heights, IL 60070
Phone: (847)564-6010 **Fax:** (847)564-7094
Email: dmfunk@household.com
Website: http://www.household.com/corp/hioc_community_commit.jsp
Donna Funk, Dir., Employee & Philanthropic Services

Priorities: *Arts & Humanities:* 5%. Focus is on headquarters community. Nonprofit groups in this category must demonstrate how their organization and its programming efforts enhance the quality of life, educational readiness, or economic vitality of the community. *Civic & Public Affairs:* 38%. Company takes particular interest in the economic vitality and physical rehabilitation of key communities around the nation where customers and employees live and work. Funded programs focus on helping those who need assistance in basic skills and job training; stabilizing or improving housing; and revitalizing neighborhoods. Also supports diversity initiatives for women, minorities, and young people, as well as work and family programs. *Education:* 31%. Supports economic education, strengthening consumer education, and preparing students and adults to be financially responsible. Funds efforts of local school systems to improve education in operating communities. It does not provide direct operating grants to secondary or elementary schools. Scholarship awards and financial aid is available for the children of company employees. The company also allocates a portion of its company-wide education budget for grants to select colleges and universities from which it recruits its employees, and for institutions that maintain outstanding research departments in topics of relevance to its industry. Unsolicited proposals from post-secondary institutions are not accepted. Company takes interest in the direct delivery of health care and human services and may make grants to community-based agencies which address the diverse needs of children and their families, the physically disabled, and senior citizens. Funds United Ways in operating communities. *Voluntarism:* Co. supports a Volunteer Incentive Plan that provides $100 grants to organizations where employees volunteer; also supports United for Hope Campaign and Junior Achievement Program. Household employees volunteer at a broad range of nonprofits annually. *Note:* Total domestic contributions made in 2000. **Typ. Recipients:** Health Organizations, Medical Rehabilitation, Mental Health, People with Disabilities, Substance Abuse. **Geo. Dist:** headquarters area only.

★ 12538 ★ Housen Foundation

120 E Main St.
Erving, MA 01344
Phone: (978)544-3335 **Fax:** (978)544-2865
Denis Emmett, Treasurer

Fnded: 1968. **Priorities:** *Arts & Humanities:* 1%. Gives to a community arts fund. *Civic & Public Affairs:* 17%. Supports community foundations, parks, and a fire department. *Education:* 65%. Primary interest in Brandeis University. Also funds a community college, elementary schools, and scholarships. *Environment:* 3%. Gives to the United Way and YMCAs. *International:* Less than 1%. Funds the Franklin Medical Center. *Note:* Total contributions made in 2000. **Typ. Recipients:** Cancer, Child Abuse, Children's Health/Hospitals, Clinics/Medical Centers, Domestic Violence, Emergency/Ambulance Services, Health-General, Heart, Home-Care Services, Hospices, Hospitals, Hospitals (University Affiliated), Medical Education, Preventive Medicine/Wellness Organizations. **Geo. Dist:** MA.

★ 12539 ★ HSB Group, Inc.

70 Pine St. 36F
New York, NY 10270
Phone: (212)770-7000 **Fax:** (212)770-6786
Email: ed.lee@aig.com
Ed Lee, Assistant Vice President

Priorities: *Education:* 100%. The company matches employee gifts to accredited colleges and independent secondary and elementary shools. Interests also include business education, literacy programs, and education funds. **Typ. Recipients:** AIDS/HIV, Emergency/Ambulance Services, Health Organizations, Hospitals, Medical Rehabilitation, People with Disabilities, Substance Abuse. **Geo. Dist:** headquarters area only.

★ 12540 ★ HSBC in the Community (USA) Inc. Foundation

One HSBC Center, 16th Fl.
452 Fifth Ave.
Buffalo, NY 14203-2885
Phone: 800-284-5866
Website: http://www.us.hsbc.com
Kristen Alvanson, Assistant VP Group Public Affairs

Priorities: *Arts & Humanities:* 14%. *Civic & Public Affairs:* Provides some support for Community and Economic Development, with a focus on the needs of low-to-moderate income people in HSBC communities. Funding interests include community-based organizations that develop affordable housing, create business opportunities, and address other important community needs, and local and national organizations that help such community-based organizations succeed; organizations that provide small business loans or technical assistance to small business/entrepreneurs; city and county-wide nonprofit organizations that provide technical assistance to community-based groups that serve low and moderate income people, and community-based groups that provide homeownership counseling to this target population. *Education:* Supports underprivileged young people and schools in economically deprived areas; K-12 public schools and post secondary institutions; and adult education. K-12 education funding may target students, teachers, or parents. Higher education grants give priority to scholarship programs, especially those that support disadvantaged students. Schools, colleges, universities, and other educational institutions also receive support. *Environment:* 1%. *Religion:* 1%. *Note:* Total contributions made in 2001. **Typ. Recipients:** Health-General. **Geo. Dist:** headquarters and operating communities.

★ 12541 ★ Hubbard Foundation

3415 University Ave.
Saint Paul, MN 55114
Phone: (651)642-4305 **Fax:** (612)642-4103
Kathryn Hubbard-Rominski, Executive Director

Priorities: *Arts & Humanities:* 14%. *Civic & Public Affairs:* 12%. *Education:* 33%. *Environment:* 18%. *International:* 16%. *Note:* Total foundation contributions made in fiscal 2001. **Typ. Recipients:** Arthritis, Cancer, Children's Health/Hospitals, Diabetes, Family Planning, Health Funds, Health Organizations, Heart, Hospitals, Kidney, Medical Education, Medical Rehabilitation, Medical Research, Mental Health, People with Disabilities, Preventive Medicine/Wellness Organizations, Research/Studies Institutes, Single-Disease Health Associations, Speech & Hearing, Substance Abuse. **Geo. Dist:** nationally; principally near operating locations and to national organizations.

★ 12542 ★ Hudson River Bancorp Inc. Foundation

One Hudson City Centre
PO Box 76
Hudson, NY 12534
Phone: (518)828-4600
Website: http://www.hudsonriverbank.com/html/foundation_hrbt.html
Holly Rappleyea, Secretary & Treasurer

Fnded: 1999. **Priorities:** *Arts & Humanities:* 14%. Gives to libraries, historic preservation, arts councils, museums, arts centers, performing arts, and public broadcasting. *Civic & Public Affairs:* 18%. Funds job placement services, community revitalization, parks, fire departments, an agricultural society, economic development, municipalities, and housing. *Education:* 13%. Contributes to scholarship funds, colleges, public schools, and private schools. *Environment:* 24%. Funds children's athletic leagues, scouting, youth programs, disaster relief, food banks, family services, and United Way. *International:* 25%. Supports medical centers and hospitals; mental health; health centers; and single-disease associations. *Note:* Total contributions made in fiscal 2002. **Typ. Recipients:** Clinics/Medical Centers, Emergency/Ambulance Services, Health-General, Hospitals, People with Disabilities, Single-Disease Health Associations. **Geo. Dist:** NY.

★ 12543 ★ Huffy Foundation, Inc.

225 Byers Rd.
Miamisburg, OH 45342
Phone: (937)865-5481 **Fax:** (937)865-5484
Pamela Booher, Secretary

Priorities: *Arts & Humanities:* 2%. Supports art institutes, dance, classical music, and theater. *Civic & Public Affairs:* (Civic & Community) 53%. Supports local community affairs, historical societies, parks, housing, and women's and minority affairs. Also supports public policy, the Red Cross, and public broadcasting. *Education:* 17%. Supports colleges and universities. Minor support for secondary education. Provides scholarships to children of employees. *Environment:* 27%. Supports the United Way, combined charities, and United Cerebral Palsy. Less than 5%. Supports sports, Boys and Girls Clubs, scouting, and Junior Achievement. *International:* 1%. Supports hospitals, research, hospices, community health, and single-disease health associations. *Note:* Total contributions made in 2000. **Typ. Recipients:** Alzheimers Disease, Cancer, Children's Health/Hospitals, Emergency/Ambulance Services, Family Planning, Health Funds, Health Organizations, Health-General, Hospices, Hospitals, Medical Research, People with Disabilities, Single-Disease Health Associations, Substance Abuse. **Geo. Dist:** headquarters; principally near operating locations and to national organizations; Dayton, OH.

★ 12544 ★ Humana Foundation

500 West Main St.
Louisville, KY 40202
Phone: (502)580-3613 **Fax:** (502)580-1256
Email: BWright@Humana.com
Website: http://www.humanafoundation.org
Virginia Kelly-Judd, Contact

Priorities: *Arts & Humanities:* 19%. Supports art associations, theaters, historic preservation, and public broadcasting. *Civic & Public Affairs:* 6%. Supports homes, zoos, women's affairs, clubs, economic development, business and free enterprise, philanthropic organizations, and urban and community affairs. *Education:* 63%. Supports schools, colleges, universities, Junior Achievement, and scholarship foundations. *Environment:* 8%. Supports YMCA, community centers, United Way, homes, child welfare, and scouts. *International:* 1%. Supports health organizations and single-disease health associations. *Religion:* 3%. Primary support made to science centers. *Note:* Total foundation contributions made in 2000. **Typ. Recipients:** AIDS/HIV, Cancer, Children's Health/Hospitals, Clinics/Medical Centers, Diabetes, Emergency/Ambulance Services, Eyes/Blindness, Family Planning, Health Organizations, Health-General, Heart, Hospitals, Medical Education, Medical Research, Mental Health, Nursing Services, People with Disabilities, Prenatal Health Issues, Public Health, Respiratory, Single-Disease Health Associations. **Geo. Dist:** principally near operating locations and to national organizations; Birmingham, AL; Claremont, CA; Pine, CO; New Haven, CT; Washington, DC; Lexington, KY; Louisville, KY; Murray, KY; St. Peter, MN; Princeton, NJ; New York, NY; Chapel Hill, NC; Columbia, SC; Memphis, TN; Middlebury, VT; Green Bay, WI.

★ 12545 ★ Humanitas Foundation

1114 Ave. of the Americas, 28th Floor
New York, NY 10036
Phone: (212)704-2304 **Fax:** (212)704-2301
Peter Robinson, Executive Director, Vice President

Fnded: 1979. **Priorities:** *Arts & Humanities:* 2%. *Civic & Public Affairs:* 2%. *Education:* 17%. *Environment:* 9%. *International:* 2%. *Note:* Total contributions made in 2001. **Typ. Recipients:** AIDS/HIV, Children's Health/Hospitals, Clinics/Medical Centers, Domestic Violence, Family Planning, Geriatric Health, Health Organizations, Health-General, Long-Term Care, Medical Education, Outpatient Health Care, Prenatal Health Issues, Public Health. **Geo. Dist:** nationally.

★ 12546 ★ Hunt Corp.
1 Commerce Sq.
2005 Market St.
Philadelphia, PA 19103-7085
Phone: (215)841-2398 **Fax:** (215)656-3714
Email: cheryl_walmsley@Hunt-Corp.com
Cheryl Walmsley, Grant Administrator

Priorities: *Arts & Humanities:* 25%. Supports programs which enable young people in low-income neighborhoods t participate in creative activities in their respective neighbothoods so far as such opportunities are either inadequate or non-existent. *Civic & Public Affairs:* 50%. Supports selected civic organizations which provide leadership on issues of importance to Philadelphians. Also contributes to programs where significant Hunt employee involvement has been demonstrated. Unusual approaches to problems outside of the above priority areas such as research projects or public policy forums are also considered. *Education:* 25%. Foundation places special emphasis on educational inititiatives which provide art-related educational programs to lower-income and/or educationally disadvantaged populations at the elementary and secondary levels, promote literacy, or contribute to curriculum development, specific skills training and/or educational innovation. *Note:* Total contributions made in 1998. **Typ. Recipients:** AIDS/HIV, Child Abuse, Children's Health/Hospitals, Domestic Violence. **Geo. Dist:** headquarters.

★ 12547 ★ Hunt Oil Co.
1445 Ross Ave.
Dallas, TX 75202-2785
Phone: (214)978-8000 **Fax:** (214)978-8888
Email: publicaffairs@.huntoil.com
Jim Oberwetter, Vice Pres., Government & Public Affairs

Typ. Recipients: Health-General. **Geo. Dist:** headquarters area only.

★ 12548 ★ Huntington Bancshares, Inc.
41 S High St.
Columbus, OH 43215
Phone: (614)480-8300 **Fax:** (614)480-4970
Email: elfi.dibella@huntington.com
Elfi DiBella, Executive Vice President

Typ. Recipients: Alzheimers Disease, Arthritis, Cancer, Children's Health/Hospitals, Eyes/Blindness, Geriatric Health, Health-General, Heart, Hospices, Hospitals, Hospitals (University Affiliated), Long-Term Care, Medical Research, Multiple Sclerosis, Respiratory, Speech & Hearing. **Geo. Dist:** headquarters area only; States where company has business locations.

★ 12549 ★ IBM International Foundation
New Orchard Rd.
Armonk, NY 10504
Phone: (914)765-1900 **Fax:** (914)499-7624
Website: http://www.ibm.com/ibm/ibmgives
Paula Baker, Director, Corporate Community Relations

Fnded: 1985. **Priorities:** *Civic & Public Affairs:* 88%. *Education:* 44%. Through the Reinventing Education Program, the company's K-12 focus, IBM promotes fundamental school restructuring and broad-based systemic change to improve student performance. The program motivates and enables districts to use technology to teach as well as restructure. Also promotes adult education, job training, literacy, and helping disadvantaged youth acquire education and skill technology. Contributions take place within the context of large-scale, district-wide reform efforts initiated locally. The program offers equipment, technical and consultant services and volunteer support. Also funds the KidSmart Early Learning Program and Project FIRST initiatives. and Project FIRST initiatives. In 2000, grants given through foundation fellowships for students pursuing PhDs in engineering and/or computer science and through the Reinventing Education Project to enhance student achievement through improved teacher performance. *Environment:* Corporate and employee contributions of cash and equipment aid local United Way and other community-based organizations. Areas of support include child care, substance abuse, hunger and homelessness, illiteracy and education, physical and developmental disabilities, children and youth at risk, the elderly, as well as disaster relief. *Voluntarism:* The IBM Fund for Community Service recognizes and encourages the involvement of IBM employees and their spouses as volunteers in their local communities. Through the Fund, IBM makes financial and IBM product grants to specific projects of eligible community organizations and schools, provided an employee, retiree or spouse is actively involved on a continuing basis. *Note:* Total contributions made in 2000. **Typ. Recipients:** Health Organizations, Health Policy/Cost Containment, Hospitals, Mental Health, People with Disabilities, Single-Disease Health Associations, Substance Abuse. **Geo. Dist:** principally near operating locations and to national organizations. **Frmly:** IBM South Africa Project Fund.

★ 12550 ★ IBP Foundation
PO Box 515
Dakota City, NE 68731
Phone: (605)235-2061
Gene Leman, Chairman, Board of DirectorS

Fnded: 1979. **Priorities:** *Arts & Humanities:* 28%. Supports theaters and libraries. *Civic & Public Affairs:* 22%. Supports housing, community groups, and public safety organizations. *Environment:* 49%. Supports YMCA, United Way, athletics and recreation, and family services. *International:* 1%. Primarily supports emergency health services. *Note:* Total foundation contributions made in 2000. **Typ. Recipients:** Children's Health/Hospitals, Clinics/Medical Centers, Emergency/Ambulance Services, Hospitals, Prenatal Health Issues. **Geo. Dist:** Boise, ID; Joslin, IL; Logansport, IN; Columbus Junction, IA; Denison, IA; Perry, IA; Sioux City, IA; Storm Lake, IA; Waterloo, IA; Emporia, KS; Garden City, KS; Dakota City, NE; Lexington, NE; Madison, NE; South Sioux City, NE; West Point, NE; Amarillo, TX; Pasco, WA.

★ 12551 ★ Idaho Power Co.
Idaho Power Corporate Contributions Committee
1221 Idaho St.
PO Box 70
Boise, ID 83707
Phone: (208)388-2530 **Fax:** (208)388-6903
Email: fmartin@idahopower.com
Website: http://www.idahopower.com
Fran Martin, Executive Assistant

Priorities: *Arts & Humanities:* Funds historic preservation and cultural centers. *Civic & Public Affairs:* Supports housing, animal welfare, and community recreation. *Environment:* Social services organizations receive funding. *Voluntarism:* Co. supports employee volunteerism and notifies employees of community events and projects. **Typ. Recipients:** Health-General. **Geo. Dist:** headquarters and operating communities; ID, Southern Idaho; OR, Eastern Oregon.

★ 12552 ★ IFF Foundation Inc.
521 West 57th St.
New York, NY 10019
Phone: (212)765-5500 **Fax:** (212)708-7144
Website: http://www.iff.com/Internet.nsf/WebCP/$First!OpenDocument
Douglas Wetmore, Treasurer

Priorities: *Arts & Humanities:* 28%. Supports fine art institutions, with major support benefiting the Whitney Museum of American Art. Also supports opera, ballet, art festivals, and historic preservation. *Civic & Public Affairs:* 29%. Supports women's affairs, ethnic organizations, safety, and community foundations. *Education:* 8%. Supports colleges and universities, and private precollege education. Th company also supports an employee matching gifts program for educational institutions. *Environment:* 3%. Supports YMCA, substance abuse programs, homes, scouts, and senior services. *International:* 24%. Supports cancer research, hospitals, medical centers, single-disease health associations, and fundraising events for health organizations. *Note:* Total foundation contributions made in 2000. **Typ. Recipients:** AIDS/HIV, Cancer, Child Abuse, Clinics/Medical Centers, Diabetes, Domestic Violence, Emergency/Ambulance Services, Eyes/Blindness, Family Planning, Health Policy/Cost Containment, Heart, Hospitals, Medical Research, Mental Health, People with Disabilities, Single-Disease Health Associations, Substance Abuse, Trauma Treatment. **Geo. Dist:** New York, NY.

★ 12553 ★ IKON Office Solutions Foundation, Inc.
70 Valley Stream Parkway
Malvern, PA 19355
Phone: (610)408-7285 **Fax:** (610)408-7022
Website: http://www.ikon.com
Kathy Fortebono, Manager, Strategic Services

Priorities: *Civic & Public Affairs:* 2%. Supports justice organizations and community foundations. *Education:* 52%. Supports universities, colleges, schools, and matching education gifts. *Environment:* 21%. Supports United Way, athletic organizations, and the homeless. *International:* 23%. Supports hospitals and single-disease health organizations. *Note:* Total contributions made in 2001. **Typ. Recipients:** AIDS/HIV, Alzheimers Disease, Cancer, Children's Health/Hospitals, Diabetes, Emergency/Ambulance Services, Health Funds, Health Organizations, Heart, Hospitals, Multiple Sclerosis, Nursing Services, Prenatal Health Issues, Sexual Abuse, Single-Disease Health Associations, Substance Abuse. **Geo. Dist:** nationally; Philadelphia, PA, including greater metropolitan area.

★ 12554 ★ Illinois Tool Works Foundation
3600 West Lake Ave.
Glenview, IL 60025
Phone: (847)657-4092 **Fax:** (847)657-4505
Email: mmallahan@itw.com
Website: http://itw.com/itw_foundation.html
Mary Mallahan, Manager, Community Relations

Priorities: *Arts & Humanities:* 11%. Primarily supports the Chicago Symphony Orchestra, Newberry Library, and the Chicago Historical Society. Museums, theater, music, dance, and public broadcasting also receive funding. *Civic & Public Affairs:* 11%. Supports the Commercial Club of Chicago Foundation and the Shedd Aquarium. Also makes matching grants to various civic organizations. Other interests include economic development, government improvement, professional and business organizations, and zoos. *Education:* 25%. Colleges and universities receive the majority of funds, many in the form of matching grants. Other interests include education associations and funds and student aid. *Environment:* 34%. Primarily supports united funds; youth organizations also receive substantial support. Other interests include child welfare, volunteer services, and community centers. *International:* 7%. Supports hospitals and medical centers. *Religion:* 11%. Supports museums and a planetarium. *Note:* Total contributions made in fiscal 2001. **Typ. Recipients:** Cancer, Children's Health/Hospitals, Clinics/Medical Centers, Family Planning, Heart, Hospitals, Medical Rehabilitation, Medical Research, Mental Health, Nursing Services, People with Disabilities, Substance Abuse. **Geo. Dist:** principally near operating locations and to national organizations; IL.

★ 12555 ★ IMMI Word and Deed Foundation
PO Box 408
18881 US Hwy 31 North
Westfield, IN 46074-0408
Phone: (317)896-9531 **Fax:** (317)867-0311
Email: dboyle@imminet.com
Website: http://www.imminet.com
Donald Boyle, Director

Fnded: 1991. **Priorities:** *Arts & Humanities:* 1%. *Civic & Public Affairs:* 4%. *Education:* 1%. *Environment:* 3%. *International:* 1%. *Note:* Total contributions in fiscal 2000. **Typ. Recipients:** Health Organizations, Long-Term Care.

★ 12556 ★ Indiana Energy Foundation Inc.

20-24 NW Fourth St.
Evansville, IN 47741
Phone: (812)491-4202
Website: http://www.vectren.com
Ron Christian, Vice President and Secretary

Fnded: 1995. **Priorities:** *Arts & Humanities:* 5%. Contributes to historic preservation, museums, arts councils, and a philharmonic orchestra. *Civic & Public Affairs:* 11%. Funds Urban Leagues, economic development, housing, minority affairs, and community leadership development. *Education:* 34%. Supports colleges, universities, public education, and Junior Achievement. *Environment:* 41%. Funds the United Way, scouts, food banks, and youth recreation and athletics programs. *International:* 9%. Gives to single-disease health associations and hospice. *Note:* Total contributions made in 2001. **Typ. Recipients:** Diabetes, Heart. **Geo. Dist:** IN; OH.

★ 12557 ★ Ing Foundation

5780 Powers Ferry Rd. NW
Atlanta, GA 30327
Phone: (770)980-6580
Website: http://ing-usa.com/about/connect/index.html
Audria Benn, Foundation Director

Priorities: *Arts & Humanities:* 7%. *Civic & Public Affairs:* 16%. *Education:* 23%. *Environment:* 47%. *Voluntarism:* ReliaStar offers employees a variety of opportunities to volunteer their time and talents to help others in the community. These programs include tutoring, food and clothing distribution, and community cleanup. *Note:* Total contributions made in 2001. **Typ. Recipients:** Health Funds, People with Disabilities. **Geo. Dist:** near headquarters and subsidiaries, and to a limited number of national organizations in health fields. **Frmly:** Reliastar Foundation.

★ 12558 ★ Ingram Industries, Inc.

4400 Harding Rd., 9th Fl.
Nashville, TN 37205
Phone: (615)298-7604 **Fax:** (615)298-7696
Email: dolanm@ingramindustries.com
Website: http://www.ingrambook.com/
Margaret Dolan, Manager Community Relations

Typ. Recipients: Health-General. **Geo. Dist:** TN, limited to Middle Tennessee.

★ 12559 ★ Inman-Riverdale Foundation

PO Box 207
Inman, SC 29349
Phone: (803)472-2121
Patricia Robbins, Secretary

Priorities: *Arts & Humanities:* 6%. Supports community arts organizations and music. *Civic & Public Affairs:* 5%. Gives to county foundations, affordable housing, community parks, and civic organizations. *Education:* 34%. Funds colleges and universities, private precollege schools, adult education, and scholarship funds. *Environment:* 23%. Favors United Way, food banks, youth organizations, scouting programs, and the disabled. *International:* 7%. Supports hospitals and medical centers, a free clinic, and single-disease associations. *Religion:* 1%. Supports a children's science museum. *Note:* Total contributions made in 2000. **Typ. Recipients:** AIDS/HIV, Clinics/Medical Centers, Emergency/Ambulance Services, Health Organizations, Heart, Hospices, Medical Research, People with Disabilities, Research/Studies Institutes, Single-Disease Health Associations. **Geo. Dist:** SC.

★ 12560 ★ Intel Foundation

5200 NE Elam Young Parkway, AG6-601
Hillsboro, OR 97124-6497
Phone: (503)696-8080
Email: intel.foundation@intel.com
Website: http://www.intel.com/education/
Lisa Siewert, Program Administrator

Fnded: 1988. **Priorities:** *Arts & Humanities:* 8%. *Civic & Public Affairs:* (Community) 9%. Community programs, the Intel Computer Clubhouse Network, disaster relief efforts, arts organizations, and environmental causes are supported under the Community Organizations program area. *Education:* 91%. Of all education grants, 56% went to higher education and 35% went to K-12 education. Supports colleges and universities through equipment donations, research grants, a visiting faculty program, Distinguished Lectures in Technology Series, and employee matching gifts. Goals are to enhance education in math and science, increase the use of technology in community schools, and develop a future work force that represents the diversity of operating communities. Grants support curriculum development that involves math, science, and technology. *Environment:* 2%. *Religion:* 22%. *Voluntarism:* Intel sponsors a Volunteer Matching Grant Program; for every 20 hours of volunteer time donated to local schools by Intel employees, Intel gives the school $200. *Note:* Total contributions made in 2001. **Typ. Recipients:** Emergency/Ambulance Services, Emergency/Ambulance Services, Medical Education. **Geo. Dist:** headquarters and operating communities; nationally; operating locations; AZ; CA; CO; MA; NM; OR; TX; UT; WA.

★ 12561 ★ International Multifoods Charitable Foundation

110 Cheshire Ln., Suite 300
Minnetonka, MN 55305-1060
Phone: (952)594-3568 **Fax:** (952)594-3377
Karen Anderson, Foundation Administrator

Priorities: *Arts & Humanities:* 3% to 5%. Supports art groups with strong touring companies and educational outreach in company communities. *Civic & Public Affairs:* 3% to 5%. Funds programs involving youth leadership, community involvement, and urban affairs. *Education:* 30% to 35%. Recipients include educational institutions and associations that prepare youth to become responsible adults. Also sponsors an employee matching gift program. *Environment:* 50% to 60%. Funding supports the United Way and independent programs throughout the country. Also funds organizations that target the problems of hunger and nutrition among youth. Special Funding grants focus on organizations that meet the needs of youth in selected operating locations. Employee committees solicit proposals from local nonprofits, and financial contributions are leveraged with employee volunteers. *Voluntarism:* Company donates to nonprofit organizations where employees volunteer through its Employee Volunteer Bonus program. Additionally, the company sponsors the Employee Board Member Bonus where employees serve on nonprofit boards. **Typ. Recipients:** Diabetes, Medical Education, People with Disabilities, Substance Abuse. **Geo. Dist:** Major principally near operating locations and to national organizations; Minneapolis, MN; St. Paul, MN.

★ 12562 ★ International Paper Co. Foundation

400 Atlantic St.
Stamford, CT 06921
Phone: (901)763-6000
Website: http://www.internationalpaper.com
Phyllis Epp, Executive Director

Priorities: *Arts & Humanities:* 12%. *Civic & Public Affairs:* 28%. *Education:* 23%. *Environment:* 11%. *International:* 2%. *Religion:* 17%. *Note:* Grants analysis provided by foundation. Total foundation contributions made in 2000. Company direct giving is about the same amount as foundation giving. Priorities are health and human services, United Way, professional and trade associations relating to company's business interests, local youth and community organizations, hospitals, civic organizations, and arts groups. **Typ. Recipients:** Children's Health/Hospitals, Clinics/Medical Centers, Emergency/Ambulance Services, Health Organizations, Hospitals, Substance Abuse. **Geo. Dist:** nationally; principally near operating locations and to national organizations.

★ 12563 ★ Interpublic Group of Companies Inc.

640 5th Ave.
New York, NY 10019
Phone: (212)445-8129 **Fax:** (212)445-8104
Email: nnichols@webershandwick.com
Nancy Nichols, Senior Vice President External Affairs

Priorities: *Arts & Humanities:* 50%. Supports the arts. *Civic & Public Affairs:* 10%. *Education:* 25%. *International:* Supports cancer research. **Typ. Recipients:** Health-General. **Geo. Dist:** headquarters area only.

★ 12564 ★ Invacare Foundation

One Invacare Way
Elyria, OH 44036
Phone: (440)329-6102 **Fax:** (440)365-4558
Debra Warden, Assistant Secretary

Fnded: 1994. **Priorities:** *Arts & Humanities:* 2%. Funds music and theater. *Civic & Public Affairs:* 2%. Job training, municipalities, and parks. *Education:* 8%. Gives to colleges, private secondary schools, public schools, and school-sponsored activities. *Environment:* 21%. Supports local United Way agencies, senior services, youth organizations, and people with disabilities. *International:* 66%. Primarily for single-disease health associations. *Religion:* 1%. *Voluntarism:* Company participates in the United Way Day of Sharing. *Note:* Total contributions made in 2000. **Typ. Recipients:** Alzheimers Disease, Arthritis, Cancer, Children's Health/Hospitals, Clinics/Medical Centers, Diabetes, Health Funds, Health-General, Heart, Hospices, Hospitals, Hospitals (University Affiliated), Medical Education, Medical Rehabilitation, Multiple Sclerosis, Nursing Services, People with Disabilities, Prenatal Health Issues, Respiratory, Single-Disease Health Associations. **Geo. Dist:** headquarters and operating communities.

★ 12565 ★ J.C. Penney Co. Fund

PO Box 10001
Dallas, TX 75301-8101
Phone: (972)431-1341 **Fax:** (972)431-1355
Email: jsiegel@jcpenney.com
Website: http://www.jcpenney.net/company/commrel/index.htm
Robin Caldwell, Executive Director, President

Priorities: *Arts & Humanities:* 4%. *Civic & Public Affairs:* 21%. *Education:* 28%. *Environment:* 21%. *International:* 25%. *Voluntarism:* In order to enhance employees' volunteer activities, the company sponsors the James Cash Penney Award for Community Service, which provides grants to organizations for which employees volunteer. *Note:* Total foundation contributions made in fiscal 2001. **Typ. Recipients:** Children's Health/Hospitals, Clinics/Medical Centers, Emergency/Ambulance Services, Health Organizations, Hospices, Hospitals, People with Disabilities, Substance Abuse, Transplant Networks/Donor Banks. **Geo. Dist:** headquarters and operating communities.

★ 12566 ★ J.D. Edwards Foundation

One Technology Way
Denver, CO 80237
Phone: (303)334-4807 **Fax:** (303)799-1705
Email: leslie_testa@jdedwards.com
Idella Kercher, Foundation Assistant

Fnded: 1991. **Priorities:** *Civic & Public Affairs:* 13%. Supports housing, employment initiatives, and urban affairs. *Education:* 26%. Supports private education, tutoring, and economic education. *Environment:* 19%. Supports youth programs, child welfare, and family planning. *International:* 11%. Supports health centers and foundations. *Voluntarism:* Company provides employee volunteers for the Habitat for Humanity Summer Build Program. *Note:* Total foundation contributions made in 2000. **Typ. Recipients:** Cancer, Children's Health/Hospitals, Clinics/Medical Centers, Emergency/Ambulance Services, Family Planning, Health-General, People with Disabilities, Prenatal Health Issues, Public Health, Substance Abuse. **Geo. Dist:** Denver, CO.

★ 12567 ★ J. F. Shea Co. Foundation

655 Brea Canyon Rd.
Walnut, CA 91789
Phone: (909)594-0941 **Fax:** (909)869-0849
Ronald Lakey, Chief Financial Officer

Fnded: 1967. **Priorities:** *Arts & Humanities:* 1%. Focus on museums, libraries, public broadcasting, and arts outreach. *Civic & Public Affairs:* 3%. Women's affairs, community affairs, and job training receive support. *Education:* 52%. Majority of funding supports school districts in California and Arizona. *Environment:* 32%. Emphasis on United Way, youth organizations, domestic violence, and family services. *International:* 8%. Supports single-disease health organizations, hospitals, and children's health. *Note:* Total contributions in 1998. **Typ. Recipients:** Arthritis, Cancer, Children's Health/Hospitals, Domestic Violence, Emergency/Ambulance Services, Eyes/Blindness, Health-General, Heart, Hospices, Hospitals, Hospitals (University Affiliated), Kidney, Mental Health, Multiple Sclerosis, Nutrition, People with Disabilities, Respiratory, Single-Disease Health Associations, Speech & Hearing, Transplant Networks/Donor Banks. **Geo. Dist:** AZ; CA.

★ 12568 ★ J.M. Smucker Co.

Strawberry Lane
Orrville, OH 44667
Phone: (330)682-0015 **Fax:** (330)684-3951
Email: info@smucker.com
Website: http://www.smucker.com
Maribeth Badertscher, Community Initiatives Manager

Priorities: *Arts & Humanities:* 5% to 10%. Supports business-sponsored arts funds, performing arts centers, libraries, public broadcasting, and the visual and performing arts. *Civic & Public Affairs:* About 35%. Supports national public policy research organizations and community improvement efforts. *Education:* About 50%. Supports accredited institutions of higher education, state and local education fund-raising associations, minority education funds, and economic education. *International:* Less than 5%. Support includes national health and human service organizations such as the American Cancer Society, the American Red Cross, and the National Committee to Prevent Child Abuse. **Typ. Recipients:** Health Organizations. **Geo. Dist:** emphasis on five-county area surrounding headquarters; operating locations.

★ 12569 ★ J.P. Morgan Charitable Trust

60 Wall St., 46th Floor
New York, NY 10260
Phone: (212)648-9673 **Fax:** (212)648-5082
Website: http://www.jpmorganchase.com/cm/cs?pagename=Chase/Href&urlname=jpmc/community/cdg/ grants
Hildy Simmons, Managing Director, Community Relations

Priorities: *Arts & Humanities:* 10%. Supports art foundations, music, museums, theaters, and performing arts. Supports both major cultural institutions and smaller, less established programs. Trust promotes groups which bring the arts to new audiences, particularly under-served populations and neighborhoods that lack cultural enrichment. Also supports those organizations that enrich the quality of life in New York City and encourage cultural diversity. *Civic & Public Affairs:* 39%. Supports community and economic development organizations, housing, employment services, civil rights, and ethnic organizations. Supports organizations that seek to improve the quality of life in New York City. *Education:* 20%. Supports colleges and universities. Supports colleges and universities from which company recruits its workforce, that provide educational opportunities for disadvantaged students, or that work collaboratively with the New York City public school system. Foundation matches gifts to education organizations. Foundation matches gifts to education organizations. *Environment:* 24%. Supports children and youth services, food distribution, family planning, YMCA, United Way, and basic social services *International:* 4%. Supports medical research, hospitals, and general health funds. *Voluntarism:* Employee volunteers work with social service agencies, educational institutions, arts organizations, and hospitals. Company administers two volunteer-support programs: "Volunteer Center," which assists employees in finding suitable volunteer work, and "Volunteer Involvement Fund," which enhances employee volunteer efforts with cash grants of $100 to $1,000. *Note:* Total foundation contributions made in 2000. **Typ. Recipients:** Cancer, Clinics/Medical Centers, Domestic Violence, Emergency/Ambulance Services, Family Planning, Geriatric Health, Health Organizations, Health Policy/Cost Containment, Hospitals, Medical Education, Medical Research, People with Disabilities, Public Health, Sexual Abuse, Transplant Networks/Donor Banks. **Geo. Dist:** some funding internationally; some funding nationally; New York, NY.

★ 12570 ★ J.P. Morgan Chase Foundation

Care of The Corporate Tax Department
245 Park Ave., 8th Floor
New York, NY 10167
Phone: (212)270-8055
Steven Gelston, Secretary

Priorities: *Arts & Humanities:* 7%. *Civic & Public Affairs:* 28%. *Education:* 28%. *Environment:* 32%. *International:* 4%. *Religion:* 1%. *Voluntarism:* Several thousand company employees volunteer in programs serving the communities in which they live and work, in a diverse set of activities that range from serving as mentors for at-risk teenagers to working as "huggers" for hospital boarder babies, from delivering meals to the homebound elderly to serving on numerous nonprofit boards. *Note:* Total contributions made in 2002. **Typ. Recipients:** AIDS/HIV, Cancer, Children's Health/Hospitals, Clinics/Medical Centers, Diabetes, Domestic Violence, Emergency/Ambulance Services, Eyes/Blindness, Family Planning, Geriatric Health, Health Organizations, Health Policy/Cost Containment, Hospitals, Medical Education, Medical Rehabilitation, Mental Health, People with Disabilities, Prenatal Health Issues, Public Health, Sexual Abuse, Substance Abuse, Transplant Networks/Donor Banks. **Geo. Dist:** internationally; nationally; primarily headquarters and operating communities; AZ; CA; CT; DE; FL; MA; NJ; NY; OH.

★ 12571 ★ J.R. Simplot Co. Foundation, Inc.

PO Box 27
Boise, ID 83707
Phone: (208)336-2110
Website: http://www.simplot.com/company/community.cfm
Connie Shields, Executive Secretary, Public Relations

Priorities: *Arts & Humanities:* 96%. Supports philharmonic associations and opera. *Environment:* 2%. Supports senior recreation and athletic funds. *Religion:* 2%. Primary support made to science centers. *Note:* Total foundation contributions made in fiscal 2001. **Typ. Recipients:** Cancer, Clinics/Medical Centers, Diabetes, Diabetes, Health Organizations, Prenatal Health Issues. **Geo. Dist:** headquarters and operating communities.

★ 12572 ★ J.T. Tai and Co. Foundation, Inc.

18 E 67th St.
New York, NY 10021
Phone: (212)288-5242 **Fax:** (212)737-4105
Y. Chen, Secretary

Priorities: *Arts & Humanities:* 1%. *Civic & Public Affairs:* 3%. Supports community programs. *Education:* 57%. Primarily supports colleges, universities, and medical schools throughout the country. *Environment:* 3%. Focuses on at-risk youth and community service organizations. *International:* 26%. Supports cancer research, other single-disease health organizations, and hospitals. *Note:* Total foundation contributions made in 2000. **Typ. Recipients:** Cancer, Children's Health/Hospitals, Clinics/Medical Centers, Emergency/Ambulance Services, Health Organizations, Heart, Hospitals, Hospitals (University Affiliated), Medical Education, Medical Research, People with Disabilities, Public Health. **Geo. Dist:** Northeastern United States; NY.

★ 12573 ★ J.W. Burress Foundation

380 Knollwood St., Suite 610
Winston-Salem, NC 27103
Phone: (336)725-7992
Email: jwburress@jwburress.com
John Burress, III, President & Treasurer

Fnded: 1986. **Priorities:** *Arts & Humanities:* 7%. Funds arts councils, music, historic preservation, and a children's museum. *Civic & Public Affairs:* 11%. *Education:* 73%. Supports colleges and universities, a military institute, and private pre-college education. *Environment:* 10%. Gives to the United Way, a children's home, senior services, and community centers. *International:* 37%. *Note:* Total contributions made in 2000. **Typ. Recipients:** Cancer, Child Abuse, Children's Health/Hospitals, Clinics/Medical Centers, Eyes/Blindness, Hospices, Mental Health, Single-Disease Health Associations, Transplant Networks/Donor Banks. **Geo. Dist:** NC; VA.

★ 12574 ★ J. Walter Thompson Co. Fund

466 Lexington Ave.
New York, NY 10017
Phone: (212)210-7000 **Fax:** (212)210-6852
Donald Gammon, Secretary

Priorities: *Civic & Public Affairs:* 45%. Supports The Advertising Council. *Education:* 44%. Funds scholarship funds. *Environment:* 11%. Supports child welfare organizations. *Note:* Requests in areas other than the arts and education are considered by the relevant offices of the co. Such contributions in most cases are made to organizations that in some way are connected with the co.'s business or because the request is client-related. Total contributions made in 2001. **Typ. Recipients:** Cancer, Clinics/Medical Centers, Diabetes, Health-General, Heart, Hospitals, Medical Education, Medical Rehabilitation, Medical Research, Single-Disease Health Associations, Speech & Hearing, Substance Abuse. **Geo. Dist:** nationally.

★ 12575 ★ Jack and Bessie Fiterman Foundation

5600 N Highway 169
Minneapolis, MN 55428
Phone: (612)536-6636 **Fax:** (612)536-6694
Email: davidlenzen@libertydiversified.com
Linda Fiterman, Executive Vice President

Fnded: 1966. **Priorities:** *Education:* 1%. Supports universities, education funds, and Junior Achievement. *Environment:* 24%. Supports youth organizations, family services, Big Brothers/Sisters, YMCA, United Way, and social service organizations. *International:* 4%. Supports medical research, hospices, and single-disease health associations. *Note:* Total foundation contributions made in fiscal 2001. **Typ. Recipients:** AIDS/HIV, Alzheimers Disease, Arthritis, Cancer, Children's Health/Hospitals, Diabetes, Health Organizations, Hospices, Long-Term Care, Medical Research, People with Disabilities, Substance Abuse. **Geo. Dist:** MN.

★ 12576 ★ Jacobs Engineering Foundation

1111 South Arroyo Parkway
Pasadena, CA 91105
Phone: (626)449-2171 **Fax:** (626)578-6837
John Prosser, Jr., Senior Vice President, Finance

Priorities: *Arts & Humanities:* 7%. Supports public broadcasting, art funds, and historic preservation. *Civic & Public Affairs:* 23%. Supports community foundations, minority funds, business organizations, and public policy. *Education:* 17%. Supports educational programs, universities, school associations, and education foundations. *Environment:* 43%. Supports United Way, scouts, youth programs, people with disabilities, senior services, and athletic organizations. *International:* 9%. Supports health funds, medical research, and hospitals. *Note:* Total foundation contributions made in 2001. **Typ. Recipients:** Alzheimers

Disease, Cancer, Children's Health/Hospitals, Clinics/Medical Centers, Emergency/Ambulance Services, Health Organizations, Health-General, Heart, Hospices, Hospitals, Medical Research, Multiple Sclerosis, People with Disabilities, Preventive Medicine/Wellness Organizations, Public Health, Research/Studies Institutes, Single-Disease Health Associations, Substance Abuse. **Geo. Dist:** headquarters area only.

★ 12577 ★ James M. Cox Foundation
PO Box 105357
Atlanta, GA 30348
Phone: (404)843-5000 **Fax:** (404)843-5599
Email: LeighAnn.Launius@cox.com
Leigh Launius, Assistant Secretary

Priorities: *Arts & Humanities:* 42%. *Civic & Public Affairs:* 20%. *Education:* 7%. *Environment:* 8%. *International:* 8%. *Religion:* 1%. *Note:* Total foundation contributions made in 2001. **Typ. Recipients:** Arthritis, Cancer, Child Abuse, Children's Health/Hospitals, Clinics/Medical Centers, Emergency/Ambulance Services, Health Policy/Cost Containment, Health-General, Hospices, Hospitals, Medical Education, Medical Rehabilitation, Multiple Sclerosis, Preventive Medicine/Wellness Organizations, Public Health, Single-Disease Health Associations, Transplant Networks/Donor Banks. **Geo. Dist:** headquarters and operating communities; Atlanta, GA.

★ 12578 ★ James S. Copley Foundation
PO Box 1530
La Jolla, CA 92038-1530
Phone: (858)454-0411

Priorities: *Arts & Humanities:* 60%. Support goes to San Diego area arts organizations such as the symphony, opera, and museum of art. The remainder, in grants generally less than $5,000, supports arts funds and festivals, historical societies, theaters, and dance. *Civic & Public Affairs:* 4%. Gives to zoos, police organizations, and community foundations. *Education:* 6%. Funds colleges and universities, private precollege education, scholarship programs, and education associations; supports journalism education and literacy. Also gives matching gifts. *Environment:* 24%. Primarily supports united funds and youth organizations. Also funds recreation, senior programs, assistance for the disadvantaged and various community service organizations. Supports religious organizations that help the disadvantaged. *International:* 4%. Funds hospitals and hospices. Occasionally gives to single-disease health associations and blood banks. *Religion:* 10%. *Note:* Total contributions made in 2000. **Typ. Recipients:** AIDS/HIV, Alzheimers Disease, Child Abuse, Children's Health/Hospitals, Clinics/Medical Centers, Health-General, Hospices, Hospitals, Medical Education, Medical Rehabilitation, Mental Health, People with Disabilities, Preventive Medicine/Wellness Organizations, Public Health, Research/Studies Institutes, Single-Disease Health Associations, Substance Abuse, Transplant Networks/Donor Banks. **Geo. Dist:** in immediate circulation areas only.

★ 12579 ★ James S. Kemper Foundation
One Kemper Drive
Long Grove, IL 60049-0001
Phone: (847)320-2000 **Fax:** (847)320-7996
Email: thellie@kemperinsurance.com
Website: http://jskemperfoundation.org
Thomas Hellie, Executive Director

Priorities: *Arts & Humanities:* 9%. Supports dance, theaters, art foundations, and music. *Civic & Public Affairs:* 1%. Primary support made to festivals. *Education:* 71%. Supports educational foundations, colleges, and universities. The Kemper Scholars grant program is offered in partnership with specific colleges and universities. The Foundation's Nursing Student grants are presently administered at Baylor University, Crouse-Irving Memorial Hospital School of Nursing, Massachusetts General Hospital Institute of Health Professions, and the University of Texas Austin. Fellowships are also supported at certain universities. *Environment:* 19%. Supports athletics, recreation, YMCA, and youth organizations. *Note:* Total foundation contributions made in fiscal 2000. **Typ. Recipients:** Emergency/Ambulance Services, Hospitals, Medical Education, Medical Rehabilitation, Medical Research, People with Disabilities, Single-Disease Health Associations, Substance Abuse. **Geo. Dist:** nationally; Chicago, IL, including metropolitan area.

★ 12580 ★ Jefferson Smurfit Corp. Charitable Trust
PO Box 66820
Saint Louis, MO 63166
Phone: (314)746-1151 **Fax:** (314)746-1259
Lyle Meyer, Administrative Committee

Fnded: 1951. **Priorities:** *Arts & Humanities:* 21%. Funds arts councils and foundations, museums, historical societies, orchestras, and children's art programs. *Civic & Public Affairs:* 5%. Contributes to economic/public policy, community services, employment programs, parks, clubs, and community festivals/parades. *Education:* 14%. Colleges, universities, literacy programs, and private pre-college schools receive support. *Environment:* 41%. Supports the United Way, Young Men's Christian Association, youth activities, crime prevention, and services for the disabled. *International:* 8%. Interests include single-disease health associations, pediatric health organizations, and hospitals. *Religion:* 1%. Science institutes are funded. *Note:* Total foundation contributions made in 2001. **Typ. Recipients:** Alzheimers Disease, Cancer, Children's Health/Hospitals, Diabetes, Emergency/Ambulance Services, Home-Care Services, Hospices, Mental Health, Multiple Sclerosis, Respiratory, Single-Disease Health Associations. **Geo. Dist:** St. Louis, MO.

★ 12581 ★ Jeld-wen Foundation
PO Box 1329
Klamath Falls, OR 97601
Phone: (541)882-3451 **Fax:** (541)885-7454
Carol Chesnut, Contact

Priorities: *Arts & Humanities:* 22%. Recipients include the performing arts, museums, libraries, and arts associations. *Civic & Public Affairs:* 12%. Grants support community organizations, clubs, business and economic associations, Native American organizations, and housing. *Education:* 13%. Most grants support higher education, including community colleges and universities; provides scholarships. Some funding supports secondary institutions, such as preparatory schools. *Environment:* 33%. United Way contributions account for the majority of grants in this category. Also funds children's organizations, community centers such as YMCAs, and recreational and athletic groups. *International:* 12%. Recipients include family and child health, medical centers, and the American Red Cross; also supports healthcare policy organizations. *Note:* Total foundation contributions made in 2000. **Typ. Recipients:** Children's Health/Hospitals, Clinics/Medical Centers, Domestic Violence, Emergency/Ambulance Services, Health Organizations, Health Policy/Cost Containment, Health-General, Hospices, Hospitals, Medical Rehabilitation, Medical Research, People with Disabilities, Prenatal Health Issues, Public Health, Substance Abuse. **Geo. Dist:** major principally near operating locations and to national organizations.

★ 12582 ★ The Jochum-Moll Foundation
PO Box 368022
Cleveland, OH 44136-9722
Phone: (216)642-3342 **Fax:** (330)225-0896
Chris Proto, Executive Administrator

Priorities: *Arts & Humanities:* 1%. Supports museums and music. *Civic & Public Affairs:* 4%. Supports civic institutes, housing, and economic development. *Education:* 33%. Supports colleges, universities, religious education, schools, and educational funds. *Environment:* 9%. Supports recreation, scouts, and United Way. *International:* 14%. Supports hospitals, clinics, medical centers, and single-disease health associations. *Note:* Total foundation contributions made in fiscal 2000. **Typ. Recipients:** Cancer, Clinics/Medical Centers, Diabetes, Health Organizations, Hospitals, People with Disabilities, Prenatal Health Issues, Research/Studies Institutes, Sexual Abuse. **Geo. Dist:** OH.

★ 12583 ★ John Deere Foundation
1515 River Drive
Moline, IL 61265
Phone: (309)765-4137 **Fax:** (309)765-9855
Email: DP51104@deere.com
Website: http://www.deere.com/en_US/compinfo/johndeere_foundations/contributions_index.html ?sidenavstate=00000000001
Judy Chistison, Mgr. Contrib. and Community Relations

Priorities: *Arts & Humanities:* 2%. Primary supports made to art funds. *Civic & Public Affairs:* 12%. Supports organizations concerned with public policy, business and free enterprise, civil rights, law and justice, and economic development. *Education:* 33%. Supports colleges, universities, higher education, K-12 programs, minority education associations, and economic, science, and technical education. Emphasis is on recruiting, research, and retraining programs. *Environment:* 38%. Supports United Way, athletics, and recreation. *International:* 6%. Primary support made to American Red Cross. *Religion:* 3%. Primary support made to science museums. *Note:* Total foundation contributions made in fiscal 2000. **Typ. Recipients:** Domestic Violence, Emergency/Ambulance Services, Health Organizations, Health Policy/Cost Containment, Health-General, Hospices, Outpatient Health Care, People with Disabilities, Public Health, Substance Abuse, Transplant Networks/Donor Banks. **Geo. Dist:** principally near operating locations and to national organizations.

★ 12584 ★ John Hancock Financial Services
Box 111, T-58
Boston, MA 02117
Phone: (617)572-0451 **Fax:** (617)572-6290
Email: cfulp@jhancock.com
Carol Fulp, Vice President of Community Relations

Priorities: *Arts & Humanities:* 12%. In general, supports arts programs that have special initiatives for inner-city residents. Music, dance, community arts, and performing arts are of interest. Boston, MA, area. *Education:* 34%. Supports public schools through partnerships in Boston, MA. Emphasizes career/vocational training, and programs for the advancement of women, minorities, and the handicapped. *Environment:* 40%. Funds youth organizations, hunger/housing/homelessness programs, human services, and violence prevention. *International:* 10%. Supports local hospitals, neighborhood health centers, and emergency services. *Voluntarism:* Supports HERO (Hancock Employees Reaching Out), a program which organizes group volunteer projects. Outreach programs include Community Sports Initiative; educational programs, such as Operation Math Corps, Adopt-a-Class, Summer of Opportunity, and Financial Wizard Program; and community service programs, including the Incredible Sandwich Making Event (for food banks), Habitat for Humanity building projects, and holiday relief efforts. *Note:* Contributions analysis provided by the company. Beginning in 2000, giving will focus on programs that serve Boston's youth, particularly educational, after-school and recreational programs. **Typ. Recipients:** Health Policy/Cost Containment, Hospitals, Medical Education, Medical Research, Nutrition, People with Disabilities, Public Health, Single-Disease Health Associations, Substance Abuse. **Geo. Dist:** Boston, MA.

★ 12585 ★ John Wiley & Sons, Inc.
111 River St.
Hoboken, NJ 07030
Phone: (201)748-6000 **Fax:** (201)748-6940
Deborah Wiley, Senior Vice President Corp. Comm.

Priorities: *Voluntarism:* Volunteerism is promoted through the Corporate ServiceMatch Program, through which the company provides small grants to organizations where employees volunteer (for 12 to 30 hours in six months, $250; for 30 or more hours, $500). Each employee is limited to two ServiceMatch grants per year. **Typ. Recipients:** AIDS/HIV, Diabetes, Medical Education. **Geo. Dist:** headquarters area only.

★ 12586 ★ Johnson Controls Foundation
5757 N Green Bay Ave.
PO Box 591
Milwaukee, WI 53201-0591
Phone: (414)524-2296 **Fax:** (414)524-3200
Website: http://www.johnsoncontrols.com/corpvalues/foundation.htmfoundation
Valerie Adisek, Foundation Coordinator

Priorities: *Arts & Humanities:* 34%. Primarily to Milwaukee-based arts organizations. Priorities include public broadcasting, museums, ballet, and visual, performing, and literary arts organizations and funds. Sponsors matching gifts program. *Civic & Public Affairs:* 4%. Mainly supports community and neighborhood development, parks, justice and law, civil rights and equal opportunity, citizenship, safety, and environmental affairs. *Education:* 8%. Primarily supports public and private colleges and universities. Other interests include adult education, education associations, and programs that seek to increase public knowledge of economics. Supports a matching gifts program. *Environment:* 48%. Major support to the United Way. Youth organizations are also a primary concern. Other interests include child welfare, the disabled, homes, the aged, and family and community centers. Also matches employee gifts to United Ways. *International:* 2%. Primarily supports hospitals and single-disease health associations. Will consider grants to capital fund programs supporting hospitals only if programs have been approved by appropriate health planning agencies. *Religion:* 1%. Science museums. *Note:* Total contributions made in 2000. **Typ. Recipients:** Cancer, Children's Health/Hospitals, Clinics/Medical Centers, Health Organizations, Heart, Hospices, Hospitals, Medical Education, Medical Research, People with Disabilities, Public Health, Single-Disease Health Associations, Substance Abuse, Transplant Networks/Donor Banks. **Geo. Dist:** in areas where company has a significant presence.

★ 12587 ★ Johnson & Johnson Family of Companies Contribution Fund
One Johnson & Johnson Plaza
New Brunswick, NJ 08933
Phone: (732)524-3255 **Fax:** (732)524-3300
Website: http://www.johnsonandjohnson.com/who_is_jnj/sr_index.html
Michael Bzdak, Director, Corporate Contributions

Priorities: *Arts & Humanities:* 6%. Supports the arts worldwide, with an emphasis on operating locations. *Civic & Public Affairs:* 11%. Supports urban, women's, and minority affairs and public policy. Also supports law and justice, public safety, and economic development. *Education:* 21%. Supports higher education, particularly medical and minority education. Also supports early learning programs and math and science education. *International:* About 45%. Supports health and medical research. *Note:* Total contributions made in 1999. **Typ. Recipients:** Cancer, Clinics/Medical Centers, Diabetes, Geriatric Health, Health Organizations, Hospitals, Hospitals (University Affiliated), Hospitals (University Affiliated), Medical Education, Medical Research, People with Disabilities, Public Health, Single-Disease Health Associations, Substance Abuse. **Geo. Dist:** internationally; nationally; principally near operating locations and to national organizations.

★ 12588 ★ The Jostens Foundation Inc.
5501 Norman Center Dr.
Minneapolis, MN 55437
Phone: (612)830-8461 **Fax:** (612)897-4116
Website: http://www.jostens.com
Lynda Michielutti, Executive Director

Priorities: *Arts & Humanities:* 5%. Interests include arts associations and centers, music, and theater. Emphasis is on programs for youth. *Civic & Public Affairs:* 10%. *Education:* 25%. Funds economic and business education. Supports education funds, public education, and minority grants. Also supports the Junior Achievement and Reading Is Fundamental programs. Sponsors the Jostens Scholars and Holt Memorial Programs for dependents of employees and sales agents. *Environment:* 28%. Supports the United Way. *International:* 2%. Supports youth organizations, disability centers, pediatric health clinics, single-disease health associations, and drug and substance abuse services. *Note:* Above priorities reflect foundation giving. The company also supports regional giving, directed by employees on Plant Contribution Committees. The company supports Jostens Renaissance Program, designed to recognize academic achievement through a business approach to education. Contributions made in 1998. **Typ. Recipients:** AIDS/HIV, Arthritis, Cancer, Child Abuse, Children's Health/Hospitals, Clinics/Medical Centers, Diabetes, Emergency/Ambulance Services, Eyes/Blindness, Health-General, Heart, Hospices, Hospitals, Medical Education, Mental Health, Multiple Sclerosis, People with Disabilities, Prenatal Health Issues, Public Health, Single-Disease Health Associations, Substance Abuse, Trauma Treatment. **Geo. Dist:** principally near operating locations and to national organizations.

★ 12589 ★ Journal-Gazette Foundation, Inc.
701 South Clinton St.
Fort Wayne, IN 46802-1883
Phone: (260)424-5257 **Fax:** (219)426-0949
Richard Inskeep, President

Fnded: 1985. **Priorities:** *Arts & Humanities:* 15%. *Civic & Public Affairs:* 17%. *Education:* 19%. *Environment:* 40%. *International:* 6%. *Note:* Total contributions made in 2001. **Typ. Recipients:** AIDS/HIV, Cancer, Child Abuse, Children's Health/Hospitals, Clinics/Medical Centers, Emergency/Ambulance Services, Family Planning, Geriatric Health, Health Organizations, Health-General, Hospices, Hospitals, Kidney, Medical Education, Mental Health, People with Disabilities, Research/Studies Institutes, Single-Disease Health Associations, Substance Abuse. **Geo. Dist:** IN, Northeast Indiana; OH, Northwest Ohio.

★ 12590 ★ JSJ Foundation
700 Robbins Rd.
Grand Haven, MI 49417-2603
Phone: (616)842-6350 **Fax:** (616)847-3112
Email: sherwoodl@jsjcorp.com
Lynne Sherwood, Secretary & Trustee

Priorities: *Arts & Humanities:* 5%. Supports arts, museums, and music. *Civic & Public Affairs:* 20%. Supports civic programs, libraries, and a diversity program. *Education:* 36%. Supports higher education. *Environment:* 33%. Supports humane society, united funds and United Way, and youth services. *International:* 6%. Supports hospice. *Note:* Total contributions made in 2000. **Typ. Recipients:** Cancer, Health Organizations, Health Policy/Cost Containment, Hospices, Substance Abuse, Transplant Networks/Donor Banks. **Geo. Dist:** CA, southern; FL; MI; TX; WI.

★ 12591 ★ Julius and Ray Charlestein Foundation
3600 Horizon Drive
King of Prussia, PA 19406
Phone: 888-773-6872 **Fax:** (610)239-6172
Ellyn Phillips, Contact

Fnded: 1963. **Priorities:** *Arts & Humanities:* 3%. Supports museums. *Civic & Public Affairs:* 2%. Supports ethnic organizations. *Education:* 17%. Supports religious day schools and colleges and universities. *Environment:* 6%. Supports United Way, athletics, and youth organizations. *International:* 38%. Funds health centers, rehabilitation, eyes/blindness, geriatrics, and single diseases health associations. *Note:* Total contributions made in fiscal 2001. **Typ. Recipients:** Alzheimers Disease, Children's Health/Hospitals, Clinics/Medical Centers, Diabetes, Eyes/Blindness, Family Planning, Geriatric Health, Health Organizations, Health-General, Hospitals (University Affiliated), Medical Education, Medical Rehabilitation, Medical Rehabilitation, Medical Research, Nursing Services, People with Disabilities, Public Health, Single-Disease Health Associations. **Geo. Dist:** nationally; Philadelphia, PA, and surrounding area.

★ 12592 ★ Kaman Corp.
PO Box 1
Bloomfield, CT 06002
Phone: (860)243-7100 **Fax:** (860)243-6365
Website: http://www.kaman.com
Russell Jones, Vice President & Treasurer

Priorities: *Arts & Humanities:* 10%. *Civic & Public Affairs:* 4%. *Education:* 10%. *Environment:* 75%. Supports organizations that serve the disabled and disadvantaged. *International:* 1%. **Typ. Recipients:** Health-General, People with Disabilities. **Geo. Dist:** headquarters and operating communities.

★ 12593 ★ Katten, Muchin & Zavis Foundation
525 West Monroe St., Suite 1600
Chicago, IL 60661-3693
Phone: (312)902-5200
Mark Broutman, Contributions

Fnded: 1982. **Priorities:** *Arts & Humanities:* 9%. Supports museums, opera, theater, and local arts organizations. *Civic & Public Affairs:* 19%. Primarily funds legal aid organizations for minorities, women, and the disadvantaged. Also supports community groups, civil rights organizations, and business/professional organizations. *Education:* 8%. Supports business education and colleges and universities. *Environment:* 6%. Supports youth organizations, the United Way, senior services, food banks, and various community services. *International:* 7%. Primarily supports hospitals, health care, pediatric health organizations, and local chapters of single-disease health associations. *Note:* Total contributions made in 2000. **Typ. Recipients:** AIDS/HIV, Alzheimers Disease, Cancer, Child Abuse, Children's Health/Hospitals, Clinics/Medical Centers, Diabetes, Emergency/Ambulance Services, Health Organizations, Hospitals, Kidney, Medical Research, Mental Health, Multiple Sclerosis, People with Disabilities, Public Health, Single-Disease Health Associations, Substance Abuse. **Geo. Dist:** nationally and internationally; Chicago, IL.

★ 12594 ★ Kellogg Co. Twenty-Five Year Employees' Fund Inc.
c/o Managing Decisions Inc.
400 Orchard Ave.
Battle Creek, MI 49017
Phone: (616)961-3125 **Fax:** (616)961-3494
Timothy Knowlton, President & Trustee

Priorities: *Civic & Public Affairs:* 100% Primary support made to community foundations. *Environment:* Less than 1%. *Note:* Total foundation contributions made in 2000. **Typ. Recipients:** Clinics/Medical Centers, Emergency/Ambulance Services, Health Organizations, Hospices, Hospitals, People with Disabilities, Substance Abuse. **Geo. Dist:** internationally; nationally; MI.

★ 12595 ★ Kellwood Foundation
600 Kellwood Parkway
Chesterfield, MO 63017
Phone: (314)576-3431 **Fax:** (314)576-3439
Terri Wise, Secretary, Treasurer & Director

Fnded: 1965. **Priorities:** *Arts & Humanities:* 2%. Supports museums and art councils. *Civic & Public Affairs:* 2%. Supports community foundations and botanical gardens. *Education:* 41%. Supports colleges, universities, and educational funds. *Environment:* 48%. Supports YMCA, United Way, day care, scouts, food distribution, youth centers, and people with disabilities. *International:* 2%. Supports single-disease health associations and general health organizations. *Note:* Total foundation contributions made in fiscal 2001. **Typ. Recipients:** AIDS/HIV, Cancer, Children's Health/Hospitals, Diabetes, Emergency/Ambulance Services, Eyes/Blindness, Health-General, People with Disabilities, Single-Disease Health Associations, Substance Abuse, Transplant Networks/ Donor Banks. **Geo. Dist:** St. Louis, MO, including greater metropolitan area.

★ 12596 ★ Kelly Services Foundation

999 W Big Beaver
Troy, MI 48084
Phone: (248)244-5419 **Fax:** (248)244-5516
Email: kennelb@kellyservices.com
Lori Beirne-Kennedy, Foundation Administrator

Fnded: 1994. **Priorities:** *Arts & Humanities:* 2%. *Civic & Public Affairs:* 18%. *Education:* 30%. *Environment:* 19%. *International:* 26%. *Note:* Total foundation contributions made in 2001. **Typ. Recipients:** Alzheimers Disease, Alzheimers Disease, Cancer, Children's Health/Hospitals, Clinics/Medical Centers, Emergency/Ambulance Services, Eyes/Blindness, Geriatric Health, Health Organizations, Health-General, Heart, Home-Care Services, Hospices, Hospitals, Long-Term Care, Medical Research, People with Disabilities. **Geo. Dist:** MI.

★ 12597 ★ Kendall International, Inc.

15 Hampshire St.
Mansfield, MA 02048
Phone: (508)261-8000 **Fax:** (508)261-8105
Email: allen.todres@tycohealthcare.com
Website: http://www.tycohealthcare.com
Allen Todres, Vice President, Human Resources

Typ. Recipients: Health-General. **Geo. Dist:** headquarters area only.

★ 12598 ★ Kennametal Foundation

PO Box 231
Route 981 South
Latrobe, PA 15650
Phone: (724)539-5203 **Fax:** (724)539-5024
Richard Gibson, Secretary & Treasurer

Priorities: *Arts & Humanities:* 15%. Supports public broadcasting, theaters, music, museums, opera, historic preservation, and libraries. *Civic & Public Affairs:* 8%. Supports community foundations, business organizations and free enterprise, and chambers of commerce. *Education:* 49%. Supports universities, colleges, institutes, and scholarships. *Environment:* 24%. Supports camps, veteran's organizations, and community service foundations. *Religion:* 3%. Primarily supports science institutes. *Note:* Total foundation contributions made in fiscal 2001. **Typ. Recipients:** Cancer, Diabetes, Health Organizations, Heart, Hospitals, Medical Research, Mental Health, People with Disabilities, Single-Disease Health Associations. **Geo. Dist:** East coast.

★ 12599 ★ Kerr-McGee Foundation

PO Box 25861
Kerr McGee Center
Oklahoma City, OK 73102
Phone: (405)270-1313 **Fax:** (405)270-3940
Martha Brady, Administrator, Contributions

Priorities: *Arts & Humanities:* 18%. *Civic & Public Affairs:* 56%. *Education:* 18%. *Environment:* 7%. *Note:* Total contributions made in 2001. **Typ. Recipients:** Health Funds, Health Organizations, Hospices, Hospitals, Medical Research, Medical Training, People with Disabilities, Prenatal Health Issues, Single-Disease Health Associations, Transplant Networks/Donor Banks. **Geo. Dist:** operating locations; Oklahoma City, OK. **Frmly:** Kerr-McGee Foundation Corp.

★ 12600 ★ Key Foundation

127 Public Square
Mailcode OH-01-27-1305
Cleveland, OH 44114-1306
Phone: (216)689-4517
Email: key_foundation@keybank.com
Website: http://keybank.com/templates/t-ak2.jhtml?nodeID=A-12
Margot Copeland, Contact

Priorities: *Arts & Humanities:* 13%. Funds art museums, libraries, art associations, historical societies, and the performing arts. *Civic & Public Affairs:* 6%. Gives to economic development organizations, community partnerships, community foundations, business associations, and housing programs. *Education:* 13%. Supports colleges and universities, scholarship programs, and public and private pre-college schools. *Environment:* 49%. Provides major support to the United Way. Also supports children's and youth organizations; child, family, and senior services; substance abuse programs; services for the homeless and the disabled; and animal welfare organizations. *International:* 13%. Contributes to hospitals, clinics, single-disease health associations, emergency medical services, and health care foundations. *Voluntarism:* Company employees volunteer at Neighbors Make The Difference Day, a program where key closes its office for one afternoon and send its employees to perform volunteer services. *Note:* Total contributions made in 2000. **Typ. Recipients:** Alzheimers Disease, Cancer, Children's Health/Hospitals, Hospitals, Mental Health, Multiple Sclerosis, People with Disabilities, Prenatal Health Issues. **Geo. Dist:** primarily service area.

★ 12601 ★ KeySpan Foundation

52 Second Ave.
Waltham, MA 02451
Phone: (781)466-5101 **Fax:** (781)290-4899
Email: foundation@keyspanenergy.com
Website: http://www.keyspanenergy.com/corpinfo/community/index_all_all.jsp

Fnded: 1998. **Priorities:** *Arts & Humanities:* 15%. Supports musical performance, libraries, art museums, public broadcasting, and other cultural organizations. *Civic & Public Affairs:* 10%. Funds community development, legal aid, and botanical gardens. *Education:* 13%. Supports colleges and universities, business and arts education, public schools, and literacy initiatives. *Environment:* 42%. Supports the United Way, food distribution, boy and girl scouts, and the Salvation Army. *International:* 8%. Gives to organizations that address cancer, heart, and birth defect issues. *Note:* Total contributions made in 2000. **Typ. Recipients:** Cancer, Health Organizations, Heart, Hospices, Hospitals, Kidney, Mental Health, People with Disabilities, Prenatal Health Issues, Single-Disease Health Associations.

★ 12602 ★ Kiewit Companies Foundation

1000 Kiewit Plaza
Omaha, NE 68131-3374
Phone: (402)271-2950 **Fax:** (402)943-1302
Email: mike.faust@kiewit.com
Website: http://www.kiewit.com
Michael Faust, Foundation Administrator

Fnded: 1963. **Priorities:** *Arts & Humanities:* 5%. Funds art museums, symphonies, and a children's museum. *Civic & Public Affairs:* 49%. Supports business and free enterprise, housing and community development, civil rights, and women's affairs. *Education:* 32%. Majority of education funds are provided to colleges and universities. Other interests include private precollege education, education funds, economic education, university athletic programs, and higher education in engineering. *Environment:* 8%. Primarily supports united funds in operating areas. Also supports youth organizations, religious welfare, and family planning. *International:* 2%. Supports single-disease health organizations and children's hospitals. *Note:* Total contributions made in 2000. Figures based on partial grants list. **Typ. Recipients:** Arthritis, Clinics/Medical Centers, Health Organizations, People with Disabilities. **Geo. Dist:** operating locations; Omaha, NE.

★ 12603 ★ Kimberly-Clark Foundation

PO Box 619100
Dallas, TX 75261-9100
Phone: (972)281-1200 **Fax:** (972)281-1490
Website: http://www.kimberly-clark.com/aboutus/comm_involvement.asp
Carolyn Mentesana, Vice President

Priorities: *Arts & Humanities:* 2%. *Civic & Public Affairs:* 25%. Supports legal services, civil and human rights, zoos, safety, botanical gardens, and community foundations. *Education:* 44%. Supports educational programs, universities, college funds, and scholarships. *Environment:* 10%. Supports YMCA, United Way, substance abuse programs, youth organizations, food distribution, and family services. *International:* 20%. Supports nursing associations, medical foundations, and health organizations. *Voluntarism:* Foundation makes grants to organizations where employees and their spouses volunteer through the Community Partners program. *Note:* Total foundation contributions made in 2000. **Typ. Recipients:** Adolescent Health Issues, Cancer, Children's Health/Hospitals, Clinics/Medical Centers, Diabetes, Domestic Violence, Emergency/Ambulance Services, Geriatric Health, Health Funds, Health Organizations, Health-General, Hospitals, Hospitals (University Affiliated), Medical Education, Medical Research, Multiple Sclerosis, Nursing Services, People with Disabilities, Public Health, Single-Disease Health Associations, Substance Abuse. **Geo. Dist:** nationally; operating locations.

★ 12604 ★ Kinder Morgan Foundation

370 Van Gordon St.
Lakewood, CO 80228-8304
Phone: (303)989-1740 **Fax:** (303)984-3306
Email: maureen_bulkley@kindermorgan.com
Website: http://www.kindermorgan.com/community/km_foundation.cfm
Maureen Bulkley, **** Administrator

Fnded: 1990. **Priorities:** *Arts & Humanities:* 5%. *Civic & Public Affairs:* 19%. *Education:* 26%. *Environment:* 32%. *International:* 5%. *Voluntarism:* The Foundation funds the KM for Kids program, through which youth programs throughout Kinder Morgan's retail communities receive funding and volunteer support. *Note:* Total foundation contributions made in 2001. **Typ. Recipients:** Children's Health/Hospitals, Clinics/Medical Centers, Emergency/Ambulance Services, Family Planning, Health Organizations, Health-General, Hospices, Hospitals, Multiple Sclerosis, People with Disabilities, Public Health. **Geo. Dist:** AR; CO; IL; IA; KS; LA; MO; MT; NE; NM; ND; OK; TX; UT; WY.

★ 12605 ★ Kingsbury Fund

Box 2020
80 Laurel St.
Keene, NH 03431-7020
Phone: (603)352-5212 **Fax:** (603)357-1955
Website: http://www.kingsburycorp.com
James O'Neil, Executive Trustee

Fnded: 1952. **Priorities:** *Arts & Humanities:* 17%. Historic preservation, public broadcasting, art centers, visual and performing arts, and museums. *Civic & Public Affairs:* 5%. *Education:* 27%. Colleges and universities, scholarship funds, and secondary education. *Environment:* 52%. United Ways, YMCAs, youth organizations, and athletic programs. *International:* 4%. Hospice and health care foundations. *Note:* Total contributions made in 2000. **Typ. Recipients:** AIDS/HIV, Cancer, Children's Health/Hospitals, Clinics/Medical Centers, Emergency/Ambulance Services, Health Organizations, Heart, Hospices, Medical Research, Substance Abuse. **Geo. Dist:** ME; MA; NH, especially Cheshire County; VT.

★ 12606 ★ Kirkland & Ellis Foundation

200 E Randolph Drive
Chicago, IL 60601
Phone: (312)861-2038 **Fax:** (312)861-2200
Willard Fraumann, President

Fnded: 1981. **Priorities:** *Arts & Humanities:* 7%. Opera, museums, and theater. *Civic & Public Affairs:* 23%. Legal aid, civil rights, public policy, and minority affairs. *Education:* 63%. Majority of funding supports legal education. Also supports minority education and colleges. *International:* 4%. Single-disease health organizations. **Typ. Recipients:** Cancer, Health-General, Substance Abuse. **Geo. Dist:** headquarters and operating communities.

★ 12607 ★ Knight Ridder Fund
50 West San Fernando St., Suite 1500
San Jose, CA 95113
Phone: (408)938-7838 **Fax:** (408)938-7766
Polk Laffoon, Vice President & Corporate Secretary

Priorities: *Arts & Humanities:* 26%. *Civic & Public Affairs:* 23%. *Education:* 16%. *Environment:* 28%. *International:* 5%. *Religion:* Less than 1%. *Voluntarism:* The company sponsors a variety of employee-led volunteer efforts. *Note:* Total foundation contributions made in 2001. **Typ. Recipients:** Cancer, Medical Rehabilitation, Substance Abuse. **Geo. Dist:** headquarters and operating communities.

★ 12608 ★ Koch Foundation
10 South 11th Ave.
Evansville, IN 47744
Phone: (812)465-9800 **Fax:** (812)465-9613
Website: http://www.kochenterprises.com/corporate/foundation.htm
Edward Koch, II, President

Fnded: 1945. **Priorities:** *Arts & Humanities:* 1%. *Civic & Public Affairs:* 3%. *Education:* 48%. *Environment:* 12%. *International:* 7%. *Religion:* 1%. *Note:* Total contributions made in 2001. **Typ. Recipients:** Cancer, Children's Health/Hospitals, Clinics/Medical Centers, Emergency/Ambulance Services, Hospitals, Medical Education, Medical Rehabilitation, Mental Health, People with Disabilities, Public Health, Single-Disease Health Associations, Substance Abuse. **Geo. Dist:** IN; KY, especially western KY. **Frmly:** George Koch Sons Foundation.

★ 12609 ★ Kraft Foods, Inc.
Three Lakes Drive
Northfield, IL 60093-2753
Phone: (847)646-2000
Website: http://www.kraft.com
Wanda Goin, Director, Corp. Contributions

Typ. Recipients: Health Organizations, Medical Research. **Geo. Dist:** nationally and in operating communities. **Frmly:** Kraft General Foods Foundation.

★ 12610 ★ The Kroger Co. Foundation
1014 Vine St.
Cincinnati, OH 45202-1100
Phone: (513)762-4000 **Fax:** (513)762-1295
Website: http://www.kroger.com/corpnewsinfo_charitablegiving.htm
Janet Ausdenmoore, Administrator

Priorities: *Arts & Humanities:* 1%. *Civic & Public Affairs:* 6%. *Education:* 10%. *Environment:* 76%. *International:* 5%. *Note:* Kroger targets its giving program to domestic problems related to food and pharmaceuticals by donating products to emergency community services, food banks, soup kitchens, and shelters for the homeless; drug abuse prevention and education programs; and nutrition consumer education. Contributions were made in 2001. **Typ. Recipients:** Arthritis, Cancer, Children's Health/Hospitals, Diabetes, Emergency/Ambulance Services, Eyes/Blindness, Health Organizations, Health-General, Hospices, Hospitals, Medical Education, Medical Rehabilitation, Medical Research, Nutrition, People with Disabilities, Prenatal Health Issues, Single-Disease Health Associations, Substance Abuse. **Geo. Dist:** headquarters and operating communities. **Frmly:** Kroger Co. Foundation.

★ 12611 ★ Kupferberg Foundation
131-38 Sanford Ave.
Flushing, NY 11352
Phone: (718)461-7000
Max Kupferberg, President

Fnded: 1961. **Priorities:** *Arts & Humanities:* 19%. *Civic & Public Affairs:* 1%. *Education:* 17%. *Environment:* 16%. *International:* 17%. *Religion:* 16%. *Note:* Total contributions made in fiscal 1998. **Typ. Recipients:** Cancer, Children's Health/Hospitals, Clinics/Medical Centers, Diabetes, Emergency/Ambulance Services, Eyes/Blindness, Geriatric Health, Health Funds, Health Organizations, Hospitals, Hospitals (University Affiliated), Mental Health, Nursing Services, People with Disabilities, Single-Disease Health Associations, Substance Abuse. **Geo. Dist:** Flushing, NY; New York, NY, metropolitan area; Queens, NY.

★ 12612 ★ L.L. Bean, Inc.
15 Casco St.
Freeport, ME 04033
Phone: (207)865-4761 **Fax:** (207)552-6821
Janet Wyper, Manager, Community Relations

Priorities: *Arts & Humanities:* Limited funding is available for local Maine cultural and arts organizations, such as the Portland Museum of Art and the Maine State Music Theater. *Education:* Educational reform in local public schools (K-12) in Maine is the second priority. Focus is on curriculum development and restructuring efforts to improve the quality of education and life choices of children of employees and their neighbors. Organizations that have been supported include Junior Achievement and the Maine Career Advantage Program. *Environment:* Support is also given to health and human services in the local area, primarily through gifts to the United Way. **Typ. Recipients:** Hospitals. **Geo. Dist:** nationally (for conservation/environment); Brunswick, ME; Freeport, ME; Lewiston, ME; Portland, ME.

★ 12613 ★ La-Z-Boy Foundation
1284 N Telegraph Rd.
Monroe, MI 48162
Phone: (734)242-1444 **Fax:** (734)457-2005
Donald Blohm, Administrator/Treasurer

Fnded: 1953. **Priorities:** *Arts & Humanities:* (Humanities-Art-Cultural) 5%. Supports arts centers and public television. *Civic & Public Affairs:* (Public Benefit) 35%. Supports economic development, community foundations, and clubs. *Education:* (Education-Libraries) 19%. Supports schools and colleges. *Environment:* (Human Services) 34%. United funds, YMCA's, and youth groups receive majority of funding. *International:* 6%. Major grants benefit hospitals and the American Red Cross. *Note:* Total contributions made in 2001. **Typ. Recipients:** Children's Health/Hospitals, Clinics/Medical Centers, Diabetes, Emergency/Ambulance Services, Health Organizations, Hospices, Hospitals, Single-Disease Health Associations. **Geo. Dist:** operating locations; Siloam Springs, AR; Redlands, CA; Monroe, MI; Leland, MS; Newton, MS; Neosho, MO; Lincolnton, NC; Florence, SC; Dayton, TN; Tremonton, UT.

★ 12614 ★ Laclede Gas Charitable Trust
720 Olive St., Suite 1528
Saint Louis, MO 63101
Phone: (314)342-0503 **Fax:** (314)421-1979
Email: mkullman@lacledegas.com
Website: http://www.lacledegas.com/about/cs_charitable.htm
Mary Kullman, Secretary, Charitable Contributions

Priorities: *Arts & Humanities:* 8%. Supports arts councils, music, and the performing arts. *Civic & Public Affairs:* 13%. Supports community development, housing, parks, and clubs. *Education:* 11%. Supports colleges and universities, schools, and education prgs. *Environment:* 64%. Major support for the United Way; also funds youth organizations and serves for the disabled and disadvantaged. *International:* 2%. Funds single-disease health associations. *Religion:* 1%. Funds a science center. *Note:* Total foundation contributions in fiscal 2000. **Typ. Recipients:** Children's Health/Hospitals, Hospitals, Mental Health, People with Disabilities, Prenatal Health Issues, Respiratory, Single-Disease Health Associations. **Geo. Dist:** MO, St. Louis area.

★ 12615 ★ Ladish Co. Foundation
5481 South Packard Ave.
PO Box 8902
Cudahy, WI 53110
Phone: (414)747-2863 **Fax:** (414)747-2915
Jim Miller, Trustee

Priorities: *Arts & Humanities:* 3%. Supports arts funds and museums. *Civic & Public Affairs:* 9%. Funds zoos, public policies, and fire departments. *Education:* 43%. Majority of funding supports the Wisconsin Foundation of Independent Colleges and scholarships. The remainder funds colleges, universities, and secondary schools in Wisconsin. *Environment:* 24%. Primarily supports the United Way of Milwaukee, WI. Also supports YMCA, youth organizations, food distribution, child welfare, the disabled, and community service organizations. *International:* 17%. Supports hospitals and healthcare foundations in Milwaukee, WI, and organizations for blindness and disease prevention. *Note:* Total contributions made in fiscal 2000. **Typ. Recipients:** Alzheimers Disease, Arthritis, Cancer, Children's Health/Hospitals, Clinics/Medical Centers, Diabetes, Diabetes, Emergency/Ambulance Services, Eyes/Blindness, Health Organizations, Heart, Hospitals, Medical Research, Multiple Sclerosis, Nursing Services, People with Disabilities, Prenatal Health Issues, Respiratory, Single-Disease Health Associations, Speech & Hearing, Substance Abuse, Transplant Networks/Donor Banks. **Geo. Dist:** Cudahy, WI; Milwaukee, WI.

★ 12616 ★ Lancaster Lens Foundation
37 West Broad St.
Suite 530
Columbus, OH 43215
Phone: (614)224-7141 **Fax:** (614)469-8219
Clarence Clapham, Secretary

Fnded: 1953. **Priorities:** *International:* 100%. Total support made to Children's Hospital Foundation. *Note:* Total foundation contributions made in fiscal 2001. **Typ. Recipients:** Cancer, Children's Health/Hospitals, Heart, Medical Research, Respiratory, Single-Disease Health Associations, Substance Abuse. **Geo. Dist:** OH.

★ 12617 ★ Lance Foundation
PO Box 32368
Charlotte, NC 28232-2368
Phone: (704)554-5529 **Fax:** (704)556-5636
Mr. Zean Jamison, Jr., Director

Priorities: *Arts & Humanities:* 14%. Arts councils, theater, and music. *Civic & Public Affairs:* 14%. Supports community affairs, parks and gardens, zoos, housing, women's affairs, trade associations, and safety issues. *Education:* 20%. Supports colleges and universities, education funds, and Junior Achievement. *Environment:* 49%. Supports United Way, youth homes and services, scouts, family centers. *International:* 2%. Primarily supports single-disease health organizations. *Religion:* 1%. Primary support made to science centers. *Note:* Total foundation contributions made in fiscal 2001. **Typ. Recipients:** Adolescent Health Issues, Cancer, Diabetes, Emergency/Ambulance Services, Family Planning, Health Organizations, Medical Research, Mental Health, Multiple Sclerosis, Nutrition, People with Disabilities, Single-Disease Health Associations, Substance Abuse, Transplant Networks/Donor Banks, Trauma Treatment. **Geo. Dist:** NC.

★ 12618 ★ Land O'Lakes Foundation
PO Box 64150
Saint Paul, MN 55164-0150
Phone: (651)481-2212 **Fax:** (651)481-2000
Email: bbbass@landolakes.com
Website: http://foundation.landolakes.com
Bonnie Bassett, Executive Director

Priorities: *Arts & Humanities:* 9%. Supports arts and culture to improve the quality of life for individuals and community, with a focus on programs in under-served rural areas or on touring and outreach programs. *Civic & Public Affairs:* 24%. Supports organizations active in addressing and solving community problems, and programs that work toward the preservation and wise use of water and soil resources between the environment, agriculture, and global food needs. Rural and general agricultural programs also receive special consideration. *Education:* 36%. Supports youth and education, primarily to leadership development opportunities for rural youth, agricultural and business education. *Environment:* 26%. Supports human services organizations, especially programs working to alleviate hunger. Federated giving organizations, such as the United Way, received funds to help provide the community infrastructure. *International:* 12%. *Religion:* 1%. *Voluntarism:* Supports a Dollars for Doers program, which provides cash donations to organizations where employees volunteer. At many company plants and offices, Community Involvement Councils organize and coordinate community activities for employees. The company also supports Expanding Community and Horizon Outreach for Seniors (ECHOS), a volunteer program for company retirees. *Note:* Total foundation contributions made in 2001. **Typ. Recipients:** Children's Health/Hospitals, Clinics/Medical Centers, Domestic Violence, Emergency/Ambulance Services, Geriatric Health, Health Organizations, People with Disabilities. **Geo. Dist:** CA; ID; IA; MN; MT; NE; ND; OR; PA; SD; WA; WI; CO; AR; IN; OH; VA; MD; MI.

★ 12619 ★ LandAmerica Foundation

c/o Lawyers Title Insurance Corp.
PO Box 27567
Richmond, VA 23261
Phone: (804)267-8330 **Fax:** (804)267-8827
Email: rpurcell@landam.com
W. Riker Purcell, Trustee

Priorities: *Arts & Humanities:* 7%. *Civic & Public Affairs:* 30%. Supports community foundations, business foundations, and housing. *Education:* 22%. Supports schools, colleges, universities, and Junior Achievement. *Environment:* 40%. Supports YWCA/YMCA, family planning, United Way, Special Olympics, athletic funds, and youth organizations. *International:* 7%. Supports hospitals, health funds, and single-disease health associations. *Religion:* 1%. *Voluntarism:* Co. encourages its employees to volunteer on a housing project with local colleges. *Note:* Total foundation contributions made in 2000. **Typ. Recipients:** Cancer, Children's Health/Hospitals, Clinics/Medical Centers, Clinics/Medical Centers, Diabetes, Emergency/Ambulance Services, Family Planning, Health Organizations, Heart, Hospitals, Medical Research, Single-Disease Health Associations. **Geo. Dist:** operating locations.

★ 12620 ★ Landmark Communications Foundation

150 W Brambleton Ave.
Norfolk, VA 23510
Phone: (757)446-2016 **Fax:** (757)446-2489
Email: Lhyatt@Lcimedia.com
Linda Hyatt, Executive Director

Priorities: *Arts & Humanities:* 17%. Supports public broadcasting, music, museums, and art funds. *Civic & Public Affairs:* 13%. Primarily supports community foundations. *Education:* 27%. Supports colleges, schools, universities, and educational foundations. *Environment:* 39%. Supports shelters, United Way, youth organizations, family services, food distribution, YMCA, and scouts. *International:* 3%. *Note:* Total foundation contributions made in 2000. **Typ. Recipients:** Emergency/Ambulance Services, Health-General, Hospitals, People with Disabilities, Research/Studies Institutes. **Geo. Dist:** MD; Las Vegas, NV; Greensboro, NC; TN; VA.

★ 12621 ★ Lee Foundation

215 North Main St.
Davenport, IA 52801
Phone: (319)383-2102 **Fax:** (319)326-2972
Carl Schmidt, Secretary & Director

Fnded: 1962. **Priorities:** *Arts & Humanities:* 10%. Supports museums and art centers. *Civic & Public Affairs:* 37%. Community foundations, clubs, botanical gardens, aquariums, zoos, parks, urban and community affairs, and economic development. *Education:* 23%. Supports colleges, universities, and scholarship funds. *Environment:* 25%. Supports YMCA, United Way, athletic funds, youth organizations, and Big Brothers/Sisters. *International:* 4%. Supports nursing services and health organizations. *Note:* Total foundation contributions made in fiscal 2001. **Typ. Recipients:** Children's Health/Hospitals, Clinics/Medical Centers, Emergency/Ambulance Services, Family Planning, Geriatric Health, Health-General, Hospitals, Medical Education, Nursing Services, Public Health, Single-Disease Health Associations. **Geo. Dist:** IL; IA; MT; ND; OR; WI.

★ 12622 ★ Lehigh Cement Co.

7660 Imperial Way
Allentown, PA 18195
Phone: (610)366-4764 **Fax:** (610)366-4684
Email: chirst@lehighcement.com
Website: http://www.lehighcement.com
Corliss Hirst, communications coordinator

Typ. Recipients: Cancer, Children's Health/Hospitals, Domestic Violence, Emergency/Ambulance Services, Health Organizations, Health-General, Heart, Hospices, Hospitals, People with Disabilities, Prenatal Health Issues, Sexual Abuse, Substance Abuse, Transplant Networks/Donor Banks. **Geo. Dist:** headquarters and operating communities. **Frmly:** Lehigh Portland Cement Co.

★ 12623 ★ Lennox Foundation

PO Box 799900
Dallas, TX 75379-9900
Phone: (805)963-6503 **Fax:** (972)497-5268
Dorothy Henson, Contact

Priorities: *Arts & Humanities:* 8%. Supports public broadcasting and symphonies. *Civic & Public Affairs:* 5%. Supports an arboretum. *Education:* 29%. Funds colleges and universities. Other support goes to the National Merit Scholarship Corporation and American Camping Association scholarship. *Environment:* 8%. Primarily to community service organizations and family planning. *International:* 3%. Supports women's health and emergency airlift services. *Religion:* 2%. Supports a natural history museum. *Note:* Contributions made in 2000. **Typ. Recipients:** Diabetes, Emergency/Ambulance Services, Family Planning, Health Funds, Health Organizations, Hospitals, Public Health, Single-Disease Health Associations. **Geo. Dist:** nationally.

★ 12624 ★ Leo Burnett Co. Charitable Foundation

35 West Wacker Drive
Chicago, IL 60601
Phone: (312)220-5959 **Fax:** (312)220-6523
Christian Kimball, Vice President

Priorities: *Arts & Humanities:* 3%. Supports art institutes, museums, art funds, and groups such as symphonies and theater players in the Chicago area. *Civic & Public Affairs:* 1%. Contributions go to groups in the field of advertising and organizations that benefit the Chicago area, including anti-defamation groups and projects devoted to urban safety and improvement. *Education:* 14%. Funds support colleges, universities, and business education. Also supports educational funds, high schools and other institutes in the Chicago region, and independent programs such as literacy promotion campaigns. Emphasis is placed on programs that support the field of advertising. *Environment:* 29%. Majority of funds support United Way. Also supports youth recreation and welfare organizations. *International:* 6%. Funds health organizations, hospitals, and single-disease associations. *Religion:* 2%. *Voluntarism:* Company sponsors "Give Back Day," a day when about 500 employees volunteer in local schools. *Note:* Total foundation contributions made in 2000. **Typ. Recipients:** AIDS/HIV, Arthritis, Cancer, Children's Health/Hospitals, Clinics/Medical Centers, Emergency/Ambulance Services, Family Planning, Health Organizations, Heart, Hospices, Hospitals, Medical Education, Medical Research, Mental Health, Multiple Sclerosis, People with Disabilities, Single-Disease Health Associations. **Geo. Dist:** Chicago, IL.

★ 12625 ★ Levi Strauss Foundation

1155 Battery St., 7th Fl.
Levi Plaza
San Francisco, CA 94111-1230
Phone: (415)501-6579 **Fax:** (415)501-6575
Email: lsf@levi.com
Website: http://www.levistrauss.com/responsibility/foundation/
Theresa Fay-Bustillos, Executive Director

Fnded: 1952. **Priorities:** *Arts & Humanities:* 1%. Primarily supports art centers. *Civic & Public Affairs:* 20%. *Education:* 23%. *Environment:* 11%. *International:* 21%. *Note:* Total foundation contributions made in 2002. **Typ. Recipients:** AIDS/HIV, Cancer, Clinics/Medical Centers, Domestic Violence, Emergency/Ambulance Services, Family Planning, Health Organizations, Health-General, Long-Term Care, People with Disabilities, Public Health, Research/Studies Institutes, Respiratory, Sexual Abuse. **Geo. Dist:** internationally; operating communities; Little Rock, AR; San Francisco, CA, Bay area; FL, Dade and Broward counties; Chicago, IL; Hebron/Florence, KY; Canton, MS; St. Louis, MO; St. Louis, MO; Henderson, NV; New York, NY; Eugene, OR; Dallas, TX; Milwaukee, WI.

★ 12626 ★ Leviton Foundation New York

59-25 Little Neck Parkway
Little Neck, NY 11362-2531
Phone: (718)229-4040
Email: hleviton@leviton.com
Harold Leviton, President

Fnded: 1952. **Priorities:** *Arts & Humanities:* Less than 1%. Funds a children's museum and the World War II Memorial Fund. *Civic & Public Affairs:* 9%. Gives to community foundations, parades, and other civic causes. *Education:* 21%. Supports colleges, universities, college/scholarship funds. *Environment:* 22%. Provides major support to the United Way of Southeastern New England. Also supports youth organizations and family services. *International:* 24%. Supports hospitals, medical centers, and single-disease associations. *Note:* Total contributions made in 2000. **Typ. Recipients:** Arthritis, Cancer, Children's Health/Hospitals, Emergency/Ambulance Services, Heart, Hospices, Hospitals, Hospitals, Kidney, Medical Education, Medical Research, Multiple Sclerosis, Respiratory, Single-Disease Health Associations. **Geo. Dist:** NY; RI.

★ 12627 ★ LG&E Energy Foundation

PO Box 32030
Louisville, KY 40232
Phone: (502)627-2000 **Fax:** (502)217-2672
Website: http://lgeenergy.com/communityrelations/lgesupport.htm
Elaine Ashcraft, Grants Administrator

Fnded: 1994. **Priorities:** *Arts & Humanities:* 16%. *Civic & Public Affairs:* 7%. *Education:* 25%. *Environment:* 42%. *International:* Less than 1%. *Religion:* Less than 1%. *Note:* Total foundation contributions in 2001. Percentage analysis provided by foundation. **Typ. Recipients:** Children's Health/Hospitals, Emergency/Ambulance Services, Geriatric Health, Heart. **Geo. Dist:** headquarters and operating communities; Louisville, KY.

★ 12628 ★ Liberty Corp. Foundation

PO Box 789
Greenville, SC 29602
Phone: (864)609-8398 **Fax:** (864)241-5401
Email: svergas@libertycorp.com
Sophia Vergas, Secretary

Priorities: *Arts & Humanities:* 4%. Primarily supports historic preservation. *Civic & Public Affairs:* 31%. Supports economic development, gardens, urban affairs, and business concerns. *Education:* 20%. Supports colleges, universities, schools, and educational funds. *Environment:* 41%. Supports United Way, YMCA, and community service foundations. *Note:* Total foundation contributions made in fiscal 2000. **Typ. Recipients:** Cancer, Children's Health/Hospitals, Clinics/Medical Centers, Emergency/Ambulance Services, Health Organizations, Hospitals, People with Disabilities, Research/Studies Institutes, Single-Disease Health Associations. **Geo. Dist:** nationally; SC.

★ 12629 ★ Liberty Mutual Insurance Co.
175 Berkeley St.-10B
Boston, MA 02117
Phone: (617)357-9500 **Fax:** (617)574-6688
Email: melissa.macdonnell@libertymutual.com
Melissa MacDonnell, Dir & Assistant Sec. Corp Public Affairs

Priorities: *Arts & Humanities:* 9%. Supports the orchestra, museums, and arts institutes. *Civic & Public Affairs:* 3%. Supports community and neighborhood service. *Education:* 14%. Supports universities and colleges. *Environment:* 46%. Supports child and youth services, and the United Way. *Note:* Contributions analysis provided by the company. **Typ. Recipients:** Health-General. **Geo. Dist:** headquarters and operating communities.

★ 12630 ★ Lieberman-Okinow Foundation
9549 Penn Ave. S
Minneapolis, MN 55431
Phone: (952)887-5208 **Fax:** (952)881-8286
David Lieberman, Vice President

Fnded: 1961. **Priorities:** *Arts & Humanities:* 4%. Supports music, art centers, theater, and public broadcasting. *Civic & Public Affairs:* 2%. Primarily supports civil rights, and civic affairs. *Education:* 2%. Supports schools, universities, and educational programs. *Environment:* 3%. Supports child welfare, athletics, and family planning. *Note:* Total contributions made in fiscal year ending September 30, 2002. **Typ. Recipients:** Diabetes, Emergency/Ambulance Services, Health Organizations, Medical Education, Medical Rehabilitation, Single-Disease Health Associations. **Geo. Dist:** MN.

★ 12631 ★ Lincoln Electric Foundation
22801 St. Clair Ave.
Cleveland, OH 44117
Phone: (216)481-8100 **Fax:** (216)486-6476
Website: http://www.lincolnelectric.com
Paul Beddia, Contact

Priorities: *Arts & Humanities:* 6%. *Civic & Public Affairs:* 7%. *Education:* 23%. *Environment:* 42%. *International:* 15%. *Religion:* 4%. *Note:* Total contributions in 2001. **Typ. Recipients:** Cancer, Children's Health/Hospitals, Clinics/Medical Centers, Diabetes, Emergency/Ambulance Services, Family Planning, Health Organizations, Hospitals, Long-Term Care, Medical Education, Medical Rehabilitation, Mental Health, Multiple Sclerosis, Nursing Services, People with Disabilities, Preventive Medicine/Wellness Organizations, Public Health, Respiratory, Single-Disease Health Associations, Substance Abuse. **Geo. Dist:** Cleveland, OH, Northeast Ohio.

★ 12632 ★ Lincoln Financial Group Foundation
1300 South Clinton St.
PO Box 7863
Fort Wayne, IN 46801-7863
Phone: (260)455-3879 **Fax:** (260)455-4004
Email: ao'neill@LNC.com
Website: http://www.lfg.com
Angeloa O'Neill, Program Manager

Priorities: *Arts & Humanities:* 25% to 30%. Support covers cultural spectrum: dance, museums, art exhibits, orchestras, theater, and historic preservation. *Education:* 15% to 20%. Focus on higher education. Supports colleges and universities, higher education associations. Also gives to the Local Education Fund, Junior Achievement, and preschool education. Provides matching gifts to higher education. *Environment:* 55% to 60%. Supports united funds, community services, the elderly, domestic violence, and youth programs. Also funds food banks, homeless shelters, drug treatment programs, and AIDS education programs. *International:* Less than 5%. Supports medical research, with focus on AIDS. *Voluntarism:* Volunteer Involvement Program retains a liaison linking employees with community non-profit organizations and activities. **Typ. Recipients:** AIDS/HIV, Domestic Violence, Medical Research, Mental Health, Single-Disease Health Associations, Substance Abuse. **Geo. Dist:** communities where their employees live and work.

★ 12633 ★ Lipton Foundation
800 Sylvan Ave.
Englewood Cliffs, NJ 07632
Phone: (201)894-7405 **Fax:** (201)871-8198
Suzanne Cuff, Contact

Fnded: 1952. **Priorities:** *Arts & Humanities:* 5% to 10%. Arts centers and institutes, historic preservation, museums, libraries, public broadcasting, and the performing arts. Also matches employee contributions to arts organizations. *Civic & Public Affairs:* About 30%. Community groups, environmental affairs, civil rights organizations, and others. *Education:* About 30%. National scholarship programs, higher education institutions, food sciences and nutrition, and technology and business education. Also sponsors matching gifts program. *International:* About 30%. Nutrition programs, united funds, youth organizations, legal aid agencies, family planning, recreation and athletics, community service organizations, hospitals, single-disease health organizations, and medical research groups. *Note:* Priorities remain flexible in an effort to respond to community needs. **Typ. Recipients:** Cancer, Children's Health/Hospitals, Clinics/Medical Centers, Diabetes, Family Planning, Health Funds, Health Organizations, Heart, Hospices, Hospitals, Medical Education, Medical Rehabilitation, Medical Research, Medical Training, Mental Health, Multiple Sclerosis, Nutrition, People with Disabilities, Prenatal Health Issues, Single-Disease Health Associations, Substance Abuse. **Geo. Dist:** primarily near corporate headquarters and plant locations.

★ 12634 ★ Liz Claiborne Foundation
1441 Broadway Ave.
New York, NY 10018
Phone: (212)626-5767 **Fax:** (212)626-8060
Website: http://www.lizclaiborne.com/lizinc/foundation
Melanie Lyons, Director

Fnded: 1981. **Priorities:** *Arts & Humanities:* 14%. Supports museums, libraries, public broadcasting, and the performing arts. *Civic & Public Affairs:* 31%. Supports housing, parks, clubs, women's affairs, economic development, and community foundations. Primarily helps women and families in need gain their self -sufficiency through long-term, broad-based solutions to poverty; improve opportunities for women through multi-dimensional job readiness, adult education, vocational training, career advancement, and enterprise development programs. *Education:* 13%. Supports schools, educational programs and organizations. *Environment:* 27%. Supports YWCA, homes, counseling services, child and family services, day care, and the homeless. Also supports organizations that provide comprehensive services to aid abused women and children in their recovery; address the causes of violence and abuse against women and children, and work toward prevention. To expand opportunities for economically disadvantaged children and teens to meet their full potential through innovative child care and educational approaches, and through exceptional programs providing solid preparation for higher education and the world of work. *International:* 4%. Supports medical centers, health organizations, and AIDS health associations. Primarily works to enhance services to meet the special needs of HIV-positive women and their children; increase access to effective education and prevention programs targeting women and girls. *Religion:* 1%. Primary support made to science centers. *Note:* Total foundation contributions made in 2000. **Typ. Recipients:** AIDS/HIV, Cancer, Child Abuse, Clinics/Medical Centers, Domestic Violence, Eyes/Blindness, Health Organizations, Hospitals, Long-Term Care, Medical Education, Prenatal Health Issues, Public Health, Single-Disease Health Associations. **Geo. Dist:** Montgomery, AL; NJ, Hudson County; New York, NY; Mount Pocono, PA.

★ 12635 ★ Lockheed Martin Corp. Foundation
6801 Rockledge Drive
Bethesda, MD 20817
Phone: (301)897-6292 **Fax:** (301)897-6252
Email: David_E_Phillips@ccmail.orl.mme.com
Website: http://lockheedmartin.com/about/community_relations.html
David Phillips, Manager, Corporate Philanthropy

Fnded: 1995. **Priorities:** *Arts & Humanities:* 4%. Funds museums, performing arts, and public broadcasting. *Civic & Public Affairs:* 4%. Gives to community foundations, law/justice organizations, business associations, job training and placement, nonprofit management, and minority affairs. *Education:* 86%. Supports colleges, universities, scholarship funds, technical schools/programs, and engineering programs. Provides scholarships to children of employees. *Environment:* (Health and Human Services) 3%. Funds the United Way, scouts, services for children and seniors, disaster relief organizations, hospice, and single-disease health associations. *International:* 1%. *Religion:* 3%. Contributes to science centers and a natural history museum. *Note:* Total foundation contributions made in 2000. **Typ. Recipients:** AIDS/HIV, Emergency/Ambulance Services. **Geo. Dist:** national organizations; principally near operating locations and to national organizations; Washington, DC; MD.

★ 12636 ★ Loews Foundation
667 Madison Ave.
New York, NY 10021
Phone: (212)521-2950 **Fax:** (212)521-2329
Peter Keegan, Senior Vice President & CFO

Fnded: 1957. **Priorities:** *Arts & Humanities:* 5%. Support goes to museums, libraries, public broadcasting, arts organizations, music, dance, and theater groups. *Civic & Public Affairs:* 21%. Interests include professional and trade associations, economic development groups, consumer affairs groups, housing, parks, and zoological societies. *Education:* 14%. Supports higher education and school reform; provides scholarships and matching gifts. *Environment:* 5%. Funds the United Way, family planning, neighborhood organizations, and youth concerns. *International:* 2%. Supports hospitals, single-disease associations, and medical research. *Religion:* 2%. Supports American Museum of Natural History. *Note:* Total contributions made in 2000. **Typ. Recipients:** AIDS/HIV, Cancer, Children's Health/Hospitals, Clinics/Medical Centers, Diabetes, Emergency/Ambulance Services, Family Planning, Geriatric Health, Health Organizations, Health-General, Hospitals, Hospitals (University Affiliated), Medical Education, Medical Rehabilitation, Medical Research, Medical Research, Mental Health, Multiple Sclerosis, Nutrition, People with Disabilities, Prenatal Health Issues, Public Health, Research/Studies Institutes, Single-Disease Health Associations, Speech & Hearing. **Geo. Dist:** operating locations; NY.

★ 12637 ★ Louisiana-Pacific Foundation
111 Southwest Fifth Ave.
Portland, OR 97204
Phone: (503)221-0800 **Fax:** (503)821-5322
Kim Miller, Contact

Priorities: *Education:* 100%. Virtually all funding supports a foundation-sponsored scholarship program for dependents of company employees. Limited support to public education and junior colleges, as well as to the Horatio Alger Association, a youth education and scholarship program. *Note:* Total contributions made in 2000. **Typ. Recipients:** Cancer, Children's Health/Hospitals, Emergency/Ambulance Services, Health Organizations, Heart, Hospices, Hospitals, Medical Research, People with Disabilities, Prenatal Health Issues, Public Health, Single-Disease Health Associations, Substance Abuse. **Geo. Dist:** primarily headquarters and operating communities.

★ 12638 ★ Lowe's Charitable and Educational Foundation
PO Box 1111
North Wilkesboro, NC 28656
Phone: (336)658-4221
Marlowe Foster, Contact

Priorities: *Arts & Humanities:* 2%. *Civic & Public Affairs:* 51%. *Education:* 18%. *Environment:* 29%. *Note:* Total contributions made in fiscal 2001. **Typ. Recipients:** Cancer, Children's Health/Hospitals, Domestic Violence, Emergency/Ambulance Services, Health-General, Hospices, Hospitals, Medical Education, People with Disabilities, Substance Abuse. **Geo. Dist:** headquarters and operating communities.

★ 12639 ★ The Lubrizol Foundation
29400 Lakeland Boulevard
Drop 053A
Wickliffe, OH 44092-2298
Phone: (440)943-4200 **Fax:** (440)347-1858
Email: kmi@lubrizol.com
Website: http://www.lubrizol.com/Foundation/default.asp
Kenneth Iwashita, President & Chief Operating Officer

Priorities: *Arts & Humanities:* 2%. Funds museums, music, dance, theater, historic preservation, and public broadcasting. *Civic & Public Affairs:* 3%. Supports community foundations, neighborhood and economic development, job training, clubs, and parks. *Education:* 40%. Major support for higher education. Through the scholarship program, the foundation selects the colleges and universities and designates the fields of study. Emphasis is on chemistry, chemical engineering, and mechanical engineering. Also makes grants for capital and operating purposes to colleges and universities and private and secondary schools. Grants are also made to educational programs and combined educational funds. *Environment:* 19%. Supports united funds and human services groups providing basic human needs. Supports organizations which grant youth the opportunity to enjoy healthy recreation and experience leadership and responsible citizenship. *International:* 8%. Provides direct capital and operating support for health organizations in its primary communities. Grants go to hospitals and specialized health care providers. *Religion:* 2%. Supports science museums. *Voluntarism:* The company has an employee volunteer program called The Explorers. *Note:* Contributions made in 2001. **Typ. Recipients:** AIDS/HIV, Alzheimers Disease, Children's Health/Hospitals, Clinics/Medical Centers, Emergency/Ambulance Services, Eyes/Blindness, Geriatric Health, Health Organizations, Hospices, Hospitals, Long-Term Care, Medical Rehabilitation, Mental Health, Nursing Services, People with Disabilities, Public Health, Sexual Abuse, Single-Disease Health Associations. **Geo. Dist:** Greater Cleveland, OH, metropolitan area; Deer Park, TX; Houston, TX, metropolitan area.

★ 12640 ★ Luck Stone Foundation
PO Box 29682
Richmond, VA 23229
Phone: (804)784-6300
Charles Luck, III, President

Fnded: 1966. **Priorities:** *Arts & Humanities:* 17%. Gives to museums and historical societies. *Civic & Public Affairs:* 13%. Funds fire departments, rescue squads, and community parks. *Education:* 54%. Provides major support for a military institute; also funds colleges, literacy initiatives, and parochial schools. *Environment:* 16%. Supports youth activities and the United Way. *Note:* Total contributions made in fiscal 2000. **Typ. Recipients:** Cancer, Child Abuse, Children's Health/Hospitals, Emergency/Ambulance Services, Health Organizations, Multiple Sclerosis, Public Health. **Geo. Dist:** VA.

★ 12641 ★ Lyman Lumber Co. Foundation
300 Morse Ave.
Excelsior, MN 55331-3016
Phone: (952)470-3600
Thomas Lowe, President

Fnded: 1997. **Priorities:** *Arts & Humanities:* Less than 1%. *Civic & Public Affairs:* 38%. Supports citizens groups, chambers of commerce, fire departments, housing, clubs, and employment services. *Education:* 17%. Funds colleges, universities, Junior Achievement, scholarship funds, business education, and academies. *Environment:* 41%. Supports distribution of food and essential items, shelters, community centers, athletic programs, emergency services, substance abuse treatment, and the United Way. *International:* 1%. Gives to single-disease associations and a mental health center. *Note:* Total contributions made in 2002. **Typ. Recipients:** Cancer, Clinics/Medical Centers, Diabetes, Emergency/Ambulance Services, Health Organizations, Heart, Multiple Sclerosis, Single-Disease Health Associations. **Geo. Dist:** MN, Primarily MN and WI; TX; WI.

★ 12642 ★ MacMillan Bloedel Foundation
c/o MacMillan Bloedel Packaging Inc.
PO Box 336
Pine Hill, AL 36769
Phone: (334)963-4391 **Fax:** (334)963-2762
Email: rcraig@mbpi.com
Lynn Jonakin, President

Fnded: 1989. **Priorities:** *Arts & Humanities:* 9%. Supports libraries, theaters, and the performing arts. *Civic & Public Affairs:* 5%. Supports festivals and community foundations. *Education:* 75%. Supports schools, learning centers, literacy programs, scholarship, and public education. *Environment:* 6%. Supports family resource centers, community centers, and youth centers. *Note:* Total foundation contributions made in fiscal 1999. **Typ. Recipients:** Emergency/Ambulance Services, Heart, Home-Care Services. **Geo. Dist:** headquarters area only.

★ 12643 ★ Macy's East, Inc.
151 West 34th St., Room 1825
New York, NY 10001
Phone: (212)494-4342
Website: http://www.macys.com
Tom Zapf, Director, Consumer Affairs

Priorities: *Arts & Humanities:* 20% to 25%. Supports museums, the performing arts, publicbroadcasting, and other arts organizations. Cultural organizations are eligible for matching gifts. *Civic & Public Affairs:* 20% to 25%. Urban and community affairs, civil rights, public policy, community development, and business and free enterprise organizations are among areas of interest. *Education:* 10% to 15%. Supports colleges and universities with interests in economic, minority, vocational, business, and journalism education. Also supports education funds, community and junior colleges, and adult education programs. *International:* 35% to 40%. Areas of interest include united funds, community service organizations, youth and child welfare, employment, the aged, and the disabled. Also supports hospitals, local and national health organizations, medical research, and mental health. Health care institutions are eligible for matching gifts. **Typ. Recipients:** Emergency/Ambulance Services, Health Funds, Health Organizations, Hospitals, Medical Education, Medical Rehabilitation, Medical Research, Medical Training, Mental Health, People with Disabilities, Public Health, Substance Abuse. **Geo. Dist:** company operating locations.

★ 12644 ★ Madison Gas & Electric Foundation
PO Box 1231
Madison, WI 53701-1231
Phone: (608)252-7279
Bonnie Juul, Grants Coordinator

Fnded: 1966. **Priorities:** *Arts & Humanities:* 5%. Supports theaters, libraries, music, and museums. *Civic & Public Affairs:* 19%. Supports botanical gardens, business organizations, community foundations, zoos, economic development, clubs, and minority organizations. *Education:* 52%. Supports universities, schools, educational funds, literacy, and scholarships. *Environment:* 18%. Supports United Way, homes, food distribution, scouts, family services, and community service organizations. *International:* 4%. Supports health organizations, rehabilitation programs, hospices, and single-disease health associations. *Note:* Total foundation contributions made in 2001. **Typ. Recipients:** AIDS/HIV, Cancer, Children's Health/Hospitals, Domestic Violence, Health Organizations, Heart, Hospices, Hospitals, Medical Rehabilitation, Medical Research, People with Disabilities, Prenatal Health Issues, Public Health, Single-Disease Health Associations. **Geo. Dist:** WI.

★ 12645 ★ Mallinckrodt, Inc.
675 McDonnel Blvd.
PO Box 5840
Saint Louis, MO 63134
Phone: (314)654-2000 **Fax:** (314)654-5381
Website: http://www.mallinckrodt.com
June Fowler, Senior Director Corporate Communication

Typ. Recipients: Hospitals, People with Disabilities, Substance Abuse. **Geo. Dist:** headquarters and operating communities.

★ 12646 ★ Mamiye Foundation
PO Box 320
Keasbey, NJ 08832
Phone: (732)417-9400 **Fax:** (732)346-3694
Charles Mamiye, Vice President

Fnded: 1982. **Priorities:** *Civic & Public Affairs:* 2%. *International:* 1%. *Note:* Total foundation contributions made in 2000. **Typ. Recipients:** AIDS/HIV, Cancer, Children's Health/Hospitals, Geriatric Health, Health Organizations, Hospitals, Medical Research, Single-Disease Health Associations. **Geo. Dist:** NJ.

★ 12647 ★ M&T Charitable Foundation
1 M&T Plaza, 6th Floor
Buffalo, NY 14240
Phone: (716)842-5110 **Fax:** (716)848-7318
Website: http://rin.buffalo.edu/s_fina/foun/m-t.html
Debbie Pringle, Charitable Contributions Coordinator

Fnded: 1994. **Priorities:** *Arts & Humanities:* 27%. Supports opera, historic preservation, museums, art centers, theaters, music, and performing arts. *Civic & Public Affairs:* 26%. Funds community development, job training, housing, zoos, and parks. *Education:* 29%. Supports schools, scholarships, colleges, and educational programs. *Environment:* 11%. Supports United Way, youth organizations, and people with disabilities. *International:* 3%. Supports health foundations and medical research. *Religion:* 3%. Primarily supports science museums. *Note:* Total foundation contributions made in 2000. **Typ. Recipients:** Cancer, Children's Health/Hospitals, Health Organizations, Hospitals, Medical Research, People with Disabilities, Public Health, Single-Disease Health Associations. **Geo. Dist:** headquarters and operating communities.

★ 12648 ★ Manpower Foundation
5301 N Ironwood Rd.
PO Box 2053
Milwaukee, WI 53201
Phone: (414)961-1000
Jeffrey Joerres, President

Priorities: *Arts & Humanities:* 24%. Supports the performing arts and museums. *Civic & Public Affairs:* 15%. Supports business, urban affairs, minority organizations, junior achievement, and welfare to work. *Education:* 4%. Supports scholarships and Junior Achievement. *Environment:* 51%. Supports the United Way, YMCA, and children's organizations. *International:* 3%. *Religion:* 2%. *Note:* Total contributions made in 2000. **Typ. Recipients:** Arthritis, Cancer, Children's Health/Hospitals, Clinics/Medical Centers, Diabetes, Domestic Violence, Heart, Medical Education, Mental Health, Multiple Sclerosis, Single-Disease Health Associations. **Geo. Dist:** WI.

★ 12649 ★ Manulife Financial
73 Tremont St., Suite 1300
Boston, MA 02108

Phone: (617)854-4345 **Fax:** (617)854-4438
Rebecca Schulman, Community Relations Manager

Typ. Recipients: Arthritis, Cancer, Health Organizations, Health-General, Heart, Hospitals, Medical Research, Public Health, Single-Disease Health Associations. **Geo. Dist:** headquarters and operating communities.

★ 12650 ★ Marcus Corp. Foundation
250 East Wisconsin Ave., Suite 1700
Milwaukee, WI 53202-4209
Phone: (414)905-1503
Stephen Marcus, President

Priorities: *Arts & Humanities:* 43%. *Civic & Public Affairs:* 13%. *Education:* 10%. *Environment:* 21%. *International:* 11%. *Note:* Contributions made in 2001. **Typ. Recipients:** AIDS/HIV, Alzheimers Disease, Arthritis, Cancer, Child Abuse, Children's Health/Hospitals, Clinics/Medical Centers, Diabetes, Domestic Violence, Health Organizations, Heart, Hospitals, Kidney, Medical Education, Medical Research, Multiple Sclerosis, People with Disabilities, Prenatal Health Issues, Public Health, Respiratory, Single-Disease Health Associations, Transplant Networks/Donor Banks, Trauma Treatment. **Geo. Dist:** Milwaukee, WI.

★ 12651 ★ Maritz, Inc.
1375 North Highway Drive
Fenton, MO 63099
Phone: (636)827-4000 **Fax:** (636)827-5505
Email: tom.tener@maritz.com
Website: http://www.maritz.com/maritz-community-involvement.html
Tom Tener, Sr. Vice Pres., Corporate Communications

Priorities: *Arts & Humanities:* About 20%. Supports a broad spectrum of community arts organizations, including libraries, museums, the performing arts, theater, and public broadcasting. *Civic & Public Affairs:* About 15%. Interests include economic development, business and free enterprise, civil rights, environmental affairs, public policy, and municipalities. *Education:* 30% to 35%. Interests include colleges and universities, economic education, literacy, minority education, and precollege education at all levels. *Environment:* About 5% of contributions. Focus on the United Way and Toys for Tots. *International:* 25% to 30%. Major support to youth organizations. Also supports child welfare, drug and alcohol prevention, united funds, food and clothing distribution, and employment and job training. **Typ. Recipients:** Domestic Violence, Health-General, Hospitals, Mental Health, People with Disabilities, Substance Abuse. **Geo. Dist:** headquarters and operating communities.

★ 12652 ★ Marriott International, Inc.
1 Marriott Drive
Washington, DC 20058
Phone: (301)380-7430 **Fax:** (301)380-2843
Website: http://www.marriott.com
Judi Hadfield, Vice President Community Relations

Priorities: *Arts & Humanities:* 5% to 10%. Supports the performing arts, arts organizations, public broadcasting, and historic preservation in headquarters area or programs which are national in scope. *Civic & Public Affairs:* 10% to 15%. Grants disbursed primarily in headquarters area. Interests are professional and tradeorganizations, urban and community affairs, cultural diversity, and minority affairs. *Education:* About 30%. Most contributions are made at the university level, supporting schools where company actively recruits, with interest in the hospitality industry. Contributions at the secondary level are national in scope and promote cultural diversity or serve minority or disadvantaged students. *International:* About 50%. Primarily supports the United Way in operating communities. The remaining funds support health and human service organizations in headquarters community and select national organizations, with focus on people with disabilities and hunger relief. **Typ. Recipients:** Health Funds, Health Organizations, People with Disabilities, Single-Disease Health Associations. **Geo. Dist:** organizations near headquarters and some giving nationally.

★ 12653 ★ Marshall & Ilsley Foundation, Inc.
770 North Water St.
Milwaukee, WI 53202
Phone: (414)765-7805 **Fax:** (414)765-7899
Rebecca Lonergan, Assistant Secretary

Fnded: 1958. **Priorities:** *Arts & Humanities:* 22%. *Civic & Public Affairs:* 4%. *Education:* 26%. *Environment:* 33%. *International:* 8%. *Note:* Total foundation contributions made in 2001. **Typ. Recipients:** Cancer, Children's Health/Hospitals, Clinics/Medical Centers, Family Planning, Health Organizations, Hospitals, Long-Term Care, Medical Education, Medical Research, Medical Training, Mental Health, Multiple Sclerosis, Nursing Services, People with Disabilities, Research/Studies Institutes, Single-Disease Health Associations, Transplant Networks/Donor Banks, Trauma Treatment. **Geo. Dist:** WI, emphasis on Milwaukee.

★ 12654 ★ Masco Corp. Foundation
21001 Van Born Rd.
Taylor, MI 48180
Phone: (313)274-7400 **Fax:** (313)792-6262
Website: http://www.masco.com
Karyn Lewish, Contact

Priorities: *Arts & Humanities:* (Culture/Arts) 28%. Supports museums, historical societies, opera, and arts organizations. *Civic & Public Affairs:* (Civic/Community) 30%. Supports accounting aid, economic development, and community groups. *Education:* 12%. Funds private schools, colleges and universities, minority education and education foundations. *Environment:* (Health & Human Services) 10%. Gives to health-care systems, cancer research, youth organizations, food distribution, and the United Way. *Voluntarism:* The company sponsors a Habitat for Humanity/Masco Home Build volunteer program. *Note:* Total of foundation and corporate giving contributions made in 2000. Does not include giving by subsidiaries. **Typ. Recipients:** Cancer, Health Organizations, Hospitals, Hospitals (University Affiliated), Medical Education, Medical Research, Public Health. **Geo. Dist:** some giving nationally; MI, Southeastern Michigan.

★ 12655 ★ The MassMutual Foundation for Hartford, Inc.
140 Garden St.
ATTN: H356
Hartford, CT 06154
Phone: (860)987-2085 **Fax:** (860)987-2493
Email: rcopes@massmutual.com
Website: http://massmutual.com/mmfg/about/community.html
Ronald Copes, Executive Director

Priorities: *Arts & Humanities:* 19%. Supports music, libraries, theater, and fine arts institutions which educate, inspire, and enrich the lives of Springfield and Hartford residents. *Civic & Public Affairs:* 27%. Emphasizes violence prevention, youth leadership development, clean streets, civic pride, ethnic and cultural diversity, youth activities, employment, and downtown events in Springfield and Hartford. Goal is to improve the economic and residential viability of neighborhoods. Promotes small business growth and first-time home ownership. Supports the Urban League, housing, and youth employment. *Education:* 8%. Supports business and school partnerships, teacher and student training, incentives for academic achievement in Springfield and Hartford schools, and colleges through scholarships. Grants emphasize school improvement, including academic excellence, safety, and scholarship opportunities. *Environment:* 35%. Supports the United Way, Salvation Army, family services, child welfare, and shelters. *International:* 10%. *Voluntarism:* Company sponsors volunteer activities, such as Junior Achievement, literacy, and tutor/mentor programs. Supports the volunteers in Action Program, which awards cash grants to organizations where employees actively volunteer. *Note:* Total foundation contributions in 2000. **Typ. Recipients:** AIDS/HIV, Children's Health/Hospitals, Clinics/Medical Centers, Hospitals, Medical Research, Multiple Sclerosis, People with Disabilities, Substance Abuse. **Geo. Dist:** Hartford, CT, and surrounding area.

★ 12656 ★ Mattel Foundation
333 Continental Blvd.
Mail Stop M1-1418
El Segundo, CA 90245-5012
Phone: (310)252-3530 **Fax:** (310)252-3802
Website: http://www.mattel.com
Paul Millman, Foundation Directory

Priorities: *Arts & Humanities:* 10%. Supports music, museums, historic preservation, and performing arts. *Civic & Public Affairs:* 2%. Supports philanthropic organizations and community foundations. *Education:* 22%. Supports schools, colleges, and universities. Supports the Mattel Family Learning Program, which promotes computer literacy, and the Hand in Hand program, which promotes volunteerism in school systems. *Environment:* 44%. Supports athletics, recreation, volunteer organizations, United Way, special olympics, and child welfare. *International:* 19%. Supports medical research, hospitals, and single-disease health associations. Major support for the Mattel Children's Hospital at UCLA. *Religion:* 1%. *Voluntarism:* Employees may apply for Employee Volunteer Grants. Grants amounts are linked to the length of service of requesting employee, and by number of other Mattel employees volunteering within the organization. The Foundation coordinates more than 30 volunteer activities annually to encourage employee volunteerism. *Note:* Total foundation contributions made in 2000. **Typ. Recipients:** AIDS/HIV, Cancer, Children's Health/Hospitals, Clinics/Medical Centers, Diabetes, Geriatric Health, Health Funds, Health Organizations, Heart, Hospitals, Medical Education, Medical Rehabilitation, Multiple Sclerosis, People with Disabilities, Prenatal Health Issues, Public Health, Single-Disease Health Associations, Substance Abuse. **Geo. Dist:** Southern California and Western New York; Los Angeles, CA.

★ 12657 ★ Maytag Corp. Foundation
403 W 4th St. N
PO Box 39
Newton, IA 50208
Phone: (641)787-8524 **Fax:** (641)787-8170
Website: http://www.maytagcorp.com
Janis Cooper, Director, Foundation Programs

Priorities: *Civic & Public Affairs:* (Community Betterment) 38%. Supports innovative community problem solving and community development. Supports organizations concerned with business and free enterprise, and community-wide arts and culture, including historical organizations, music, museums, and public broadcasting. *Education:* 24%. Major support is given to colleges through college funds and the foundation's gift-matching plan. Direct student aid is given through scholarships and career education awards to the children of U.S. employees. Supports school-to-work training and technical skills. *Environment:* (Families and Early Childhood) 17%. Supports United Way, YMCA, recreation, and community centers. *Note:* Total foundation contributions made in 2001. **Typ. Recipients:** People with Disabilities. **Geo. Dist:** Galesburg, IL; Herrin, IL; Newton, IA; Concord, NH; North Canton, OH; Quakertown, PA; Williston, SC; Cleveland, TN; Jackson, TN; El Paso, TX; Burlington, VT; Williston, VT.

★ 12658 ★ Mazda Foundation (USA), Inc.
1025 Connecticut Ave., Suite 910
Washington, DC 20036
Phone: (202)467-5088 **Fax:** (202)233-6490
Website: http://www.mazdafoundation.org
Barbara Nocera, Program Director

Priorities: *Education:* 67%. Supports schools, universities, literacy programs, scholarship funds, and organizations that promote study abroad. *Environment:* 12%. Supports community and volunteer service foundations. *International:* 3%. Supports the Juvenile Diabetes Foundation and an organization that addresses mental/emotional health issues for minority children. *Note:* Total foundation contributions made in fiscal 2001. **Typ. Recipients:** Children's Health/Hospitals, Diabetes, Medical Research, People with Disabilities, Substance Abuse. **Geo. Dist:** headquarters and operating communities.

★ 12659 ★ MBIA, Inc.
113 King St.
Armonk, NY 10504
Phone: (914)273-4545 **Fax:** (914)765-3375
Email: sue.voltz@mbia.com
Susan Voltz, Director

Priorities: *Arts & Humanities:* About 10%. Funds arts associations, historic preservation, libraries, museums, and the performing arts. *Civic & Public Affairs:* About 20%. Recipients include ethnic and minority affairs, housing programs, municipalities, and women's affairs. *Education:* About 30%. Supports business, elementary, and legal education. Also funds colleges and universities. Employee matching gift program supports institutions of higher education. *International:* About 40%. Interests include geriatric health, health organizations, medical research, single-disease associations, family services, community service organizations, volunteer services, youth organizations, and other social services. *Note:* Primary focus is on programs for children, which receive half of all contributions. **Typ. Recipients:** Family Planning, Geriatric Health, Health Organizations, Health-General, Medical Research, People with Disabilities, Single-Disease Health Associations, Substance Abuse. **Geo. Dist:** generally in tri-state area where employees live.

★ 12660 ★ The MBNA Foundation
1100 N King St.
Wilmington, DE 19884
Phone: 800-441-7048
Website: http://www.mbnafoundation.org
W. Schroeder, Executive Director

Fnded: 2000. **Priorities:** *Arts & Humanities:* 6%. *Civic & Public Affairs:* 3%. *Education:* 47%. *Environment:* 15%. *International:* 19%. *Voluntarism:* The Community Partnership Program matches MBNA businesses with charitable organizations and schools for volunteer opportunities. The company provides financial contributions to nonprofit organizations for which MBNA employees have volunteered more than 40 hours of their personal time during a calendar year. MBNA also sponsors the Francis X. Norton Community Service award to recognize outstanding volunteerism among MBNA employees. *Note:* Total contributions made in 2001. **Typ. Recipients:** Children's Health/Hospitals, Health Organizations, Hospitals, Long-Term Care. **Geo. Dist:** DE; ME; Cleveland, OH.

★ 12661 ★ McCormick & Co., Inc.
18 Loveton Circle
Sparks, MD 21152-6000
Phone: (410)771-7310 **Fax:** (410)527-8289
Allen Barrett, Jr., Vice President, Corporate Communications

Priorities: *Arts & Humanities:* Limited support goes to museums, historic preservation, and public broadcasting. *Civic & Public Affairs:* Supports professional and trade associations and programs promoting economic development and the free enterprise system. *Education:* Primary support is given to colleges and universities, with an emphasis on business education programs. Supports scholarship programs. *Environment:* The highest priority, with an emphasis on united fund drives and volunteer service programs. Also supports family and community service organizations and youth activities. **Typ. Recipients:** Family Planning, Health Organizations, Medical Research, Nutrition. **Geo. Dist:** headquarters and operating communities.

★ 12662 ★ McDermott International, Inc.
1450 Poydras St.
New Orleans, LA 70112-6058
Phone: (504)587-4411 **Fax:** (504)587-6150
Email: dmcelestin@mcdermott.com
Dona Celestin, Corporate Training Coordinator

Typ. Recipients: Hospitals. **Geo. Dist:** nationally; operating locations.

★ 12663 ★ McDonald Investments Foundation
800 Superior Ave.
Cleveland, OH 44114-2603
Phone: (216)443-2981 **Fax:** (216)689-3865
Email: karen_a_white@keybank.com
Website: http://www.key.com
Karen White, Administrator

Priorities: *Arts & Humanities:* 13%. Supports museums, theater, music, and art. *Civic & Public Affairs:* 27%. Supports community and neighborhood development, clubs, and community foundations. *Education:* 13%. Funds higher education, education foundations, and education programs. *Environment:* 22%. Supports youth services, the disabled, social services, and United Way. *International:* 15%. Supports hospitals, medical centers, single-disease associations, and AIDS prevention. *Religion:* 1%. *Note:* Total contributions made in fiscal 1999. **Typ. Recipients:** AIDS/HIV, Alzheimers Disease, Cancer, Children's Health/Hospitals, Diabetes, Domestic Violence, Emergency/Ambulance Services, Eyes/Blindness, Family Planning, Health Organizations, Health-General, Hospices, Hospitals, Medical Research, Mental Health, Multiple Sclerosis, Nursing Services, People with Disabilities, Prenatal Health Issues, Sexual Abuse, Single-Disease Health Associations, Speech & Hearing, Substance Abuse. **Geo. Dist:** headquarters and operating communities.

★ 12664 ★ McDonald's Corp. Charitable Foundation
One Kroc Drive
Oak Brook, IL 60523
Phone: (630)623-7048 **Fax:** (630)623-7488
Ken Barun, Executive Vice President

Typ. Recipients: Hospitals, Nutrition, People with Disabilities, Single-Disease Health Associations, Substance Abuse. **Geo. Dist:** nationally and in local operating areas.

★ 12665 ★ McGraw-Hill Companies, Inc.
1221 Ave. of the Americas, 47th Floor
New York, NY 10020-1095
Phone: (212)512-6480 **Fax:** (212)512-3611
Email: swallman@mcgraw-hill.com
Website: http://www.mcgraw-hill.com/community/community/html
Susan Wallman, Manager, Corporate Contributions

Typ. Recipients: AIDS/HIV, Clinics/Medical Centers, Eyes/Blindness, Health Organizations, Hospitals, Hospitals (University Affiliated), People with Disabilities, Substance Abuse, Transplant Networks/Donor Banks. **Geo. Dist:** nationally; primarily headquarters and operating communities; New York, NY.

★ 12666 ★ McKesson Foundation
1 Post St.
San Francisco, CA 94104
Phone: (415)983-9325 **Fax:** (415)983-7590
Website: http://www.mckesson.com/community.html
Ms. Marcia Argyris, President

Priorities: *Arts & Humanities:* 5%. Supports museums, symphonies, and the performing arts in the San Francisco Bay Area. *Civic & Public Affairs:* 11%. Employee committees in operating communities evaluate and recommend grants. 5% to 10%. Supports volunteer centers and public broadcasting. Less than 5%. Primarily encourages and supports employee volunteers. The company has created special grant programs: the Community Action Team Fund Grant program, which supports nonprofit organizations in which five or more McKesson employees and retirees are involved on a volunteer basis (grants range from $500 to $5,000); the Community Action Fund Grant program, which funds nonprofits with grants for specific items or special programs (grants range up to $1,000 and are limited to organizations where employees, retirees, or their spouses volunteer); and the Neil Harlan Award for Community Service program, which awards grants to organizations appointed by chosen employees who are being honored for community service (grants to nonprofits range from $300 to $5,000 and employees must work for company for one year). *Education:* 27%. Contributions support colleges, universities, and other educational institutions, both in the form of grants and through the employee matching gifts program. Supports scholarships with a focus on the children of employees. The foundation also funds youth educational enrichment programs, especially those that deal with the prevention of substance abuse, development of decision-making skills, exploration of career directions, after-school community service projects, and K-12 public school education. *Environment:* 32%. Supports Youth with Special Needs, comprised of Learning Exchange (a tutoring program), Work Experience Program, and Summer Youth Employment Program. Emphasis is on pre-teen and adolescent age groups. Also funds Human Services, including emergency services for families in crisis, including emergency food programs, services for runaway youth, and shelter for mothers and children in temporary crisis situations. The Youth and Families Initiative, a regional program, focuses on youth services and medical care. mothers and children in temporary crisis situations. mothers and children in temporary crisis situations. *International:* 17%. Supports health programs for at-risk children. *Note:* Total contributions made in fiscal 2001. **Typ. Recipients:** AIDS/HIV, Children's Health/Hospitals, Clinics/Medical Centers, Emergency/Ambulance Services, Health Organizations, Health-General, Hospitals, Medical Education, People with Disabilities, Prenatal Health Issues, Preventive Medicine/Wellness Organizations, Public Health, Single-Disease Health Associations, Substance Abuse. **Geo. Dist:** communities where company has a sizable employee representation; CA, San Francisco Bay area.

★ 12667 ★ McWane Foundation
2900 Highway 280, Suite 300
Birmingham, AL 35223
Phone: (205)414-3100 **Fax:** (205)414-3180
Jeanette Sommers, Corporate Secretary

Fnded: 1961. **Priorities:** *Arts & Humanities:* 6%. Supports dance, historical preservation, libraries, the performing arts, and music. *Civic & Public Affairs:* 3%. Supports community development, free enterprise, housing, and civil rights organizations. *Education:* 79%. Supports colleges, universities, scholarships, Junior Achievement, and educational foundations. *Environment:* 3%. Supports YWCA, athletics and recreation, counseling services, substance abuse programs youth organizations, and family services. *International:* 8%. Primarily supports single-disease health associations. *Note:* Total foundation contributions made in 2000. **Typ. Recipients:** Arthritis, Cancer, Children's Health/Hospitals, Diabetes, Emergency/Ambulance Services, Health Organizations, Heart, Hospitals, Mental Health, Multiple Sclerosis, Single-Disease Health Associations, Substance Abuse. **Geo. Dist:** AL.

★ 12668 ★ MDU Resources Foundation
PO Box 5650
Bismarck, ND 58506-5650
Phone: (701)222-7828 **Fax:** (701)222-7607
Email: robert.wood@mduresources.com
Website: http://www.mdu.com/corp-fdtn.html
Robert Wood, President

Priorities: *Arts & Humanities:* 10%. Supports public broadcasting, dance, opera, museums, historic preservation. *Civic & Public Affairs:* 18%. Supports civic parks, zoos, free enterprise, and community foundations. *Education:* 20%. Supports schools, scholarships, universities, colleges, and educational foundations. *Environment:* 34%. Supports United Way, scouts, food distribution, recreational organizations, YMCA, Special Olympics, and homes. *International:* 16%. Supports hospitals, medical foundations, emergency services, and health centers. *Note:* Total foundation contributions made in 2001. **Typ. Recipients:** Alzheimers Disease, Children's Health/Hospitals, Clinics/Medical Centers, Domestic Violence, Emergency/

Ambulance Services, Eyes/Blindness, Health Organizations, Health Policy/Cost Containment, Health-General, Hospitals, Long-Term Care, Medical Education, Medical Rehabilitation, Mental Health, People with Disabilities, Public Health, Research/Studies Institutes. **Geo. Dist:** near operating locations.

★ 12669 ★ Mead Witter Foundation, Inc.

PO Box 39
Wisconsin Rapids, WI 54495-0039
Phone: (715)424-3004 **Fax:** (715)424-1314
Susan Feith, President

Fnded: 1951. **Priorities:** *Arts & Humanities:* 10%. Supports public broadcasting, public libraries, arts councils, historic preservation, history organizations, and the performing arts. *Civic & Public Affairs:* 3%. Gives to municipalities; community development initiatives; botanical gardens; and professional/trade organizations for the timber, paper, and pulp industries. *Education:* 72%. Primarily supports independent, accredited four-year colleges and universities in Wisconsin. Support includes unrestricted and capital grants. Special interests include science, technology, and engineering education relating to the pulp and paper industry. Also supports minority and independent college funds and merit scholarship programs. *Environment:* 5%. Contributes to youth services, youth athletics and recreation programs, food and clothing distribution, women's shelters, and the United Way. *International:* Less than 1%. *Note:* Total contributions made in 2000. **Typ. Recipients:** AIDS/HIV, Emergency/Ambulance Services, Eyes/Blindness, Family Planning, Health Organizations, Hospices, Hospitals, Medical Education, Medical Rehabilitation, People with Disabilities, Preventive Medicine/Wellness Organizations, Trauma Treatment. **Geo. Dist:** WI, headquarters and operating communities.

★ 12670 ★ Meadwestvaco Corp. Foundation

Courthouse Plaza, Northeast
Dayton, OH 45463
Phone: (937)495-3428 **Fax:** (937)495-4103
Website: http://www.meadwestvaco.com/corporate.nsf/company/foundation
Ronald Budzik, Executive Director

Fnded: 1957. **Priorities:** *Arts & Humanities:* 4%. *Civic & Public Affairs:* 47%. *Education:* 21%. *Environment:* 23%. *International:* 1%. *Note:* Total contributions made in 2001. **Typ. Recipients:** Diabetes, Domestic Violence, Emergency/Ambulance Services, Health-General, Hospices, Medical Rehabilitation, People with Disabilities, Public Health, Respiratory. **Geo. Dist:** operating locations; Cottonton, AL; Lanett, AL; Phenix City, AL; Alisa Viejo, CA; Buena Park, CA; Garden Grove, CA; Huntington Beach, CA; Irvine, CA; Los Angeles, CA; Pasadena, CA; San Francisco, CA; Boulder, CO; Denver, CO; Enfield, CT; Norwich, CT; Stamford, CT; Newark, DE; Wilmington, DE; Washington, DC; Coral Gables, FL; Tampa, FL; Atlanta, GA; Greenville, GA; Smyrna, GA; Chicago, IL; Franklin Park, IL; Jacksonville, IL; Melrose Park, IL; Schaumburg, IL; Overland Park, KS; Louisville, KY; Wickliffe, KY; DeRidder, LA; Rumford, ME; Laurel, MD; Luke, MD; Pittsfield, MA; South Lee, MA; Springfield, MA; Brooklyn Park, MI; Detroit, MI; Escanaba, MI; St. Joseph, MO; St. Louis, MO; East Rutherford, NJ; Pine Brook, NJ; Potsdam, NY; Sidney, NY; Garner, NC; Grover, NC; Mebane, NC; Chillicothe, OH; Cincinnati, OH; Cleveland, OH; Dayton, OH; Fremont, OH; Portland, OR; Alexandria, PA; Warrington, PA; Williamsburg, PA; North Charleston, SC; Summerville, SC; Dallas, TX; Evadale, TX; Garland, TX; Houston, TX; Silsbee, TX; Covington, VA; Louisa, VA; Low Moor, VA; Richmond, VA; Seattle, WA; Rupert, WV; Kenosha, WI.

★ 12671 ★ Medic Computer Systems Foundation

PO Box 3099
Winston-Salem, NC 27150-6732
Phone: (336)732-5252

Fnded: 1997. **Priorities:** *Civic & Public Affairs:* 39%. Supports a private foundation. *Education:* 55%. Supports higher education through grants and scholarships. *International:* 3%. Supports a children's hospital. *Note:* Total contributions made in 2001. **Typ. Recipients:** Children's Health/Hospitals. **Geo. Dist:** nationally.

★ 12672 ★ Medtronic Foundation

710 Medtronic Parkway
MS LC110
Minneapolis, MN 55432-5604
Phone: (763)505-2640 **Fax:** (763)505-2648
Website: http://www.medtronic.com/foundation
Penny Hunt, Foundation Executive Director

Priorities: *Arts & Humanities:* 10%. *Civic & Public Affairs:* 27%. Community grants are made to strengthen communities and specifically to improve the lives of people who are socioeconomically disadvantaged through grants to selected human service, arts and culture, and civic programs. Supports human service programs outside of the Twin Cities that benefit disadvantaged children and youth and their families; civic organizations that address the needs of the disadvantaged; and cultural organizations that make significant contributions to the life of the community. *Education:* 30%. Supports K-12 education, with focus on kindergarten through grade 12 science education programs under STAR (Science and Technology Are Rewarding), a grant initiative designed to stimulate and sustain the interest of young people in science. Post-secondary education is supported with grants in programs that benefit those traditionally underrepresented in science, technology, engineering or health, socioeconomically disadvantaged students and women. *Environment:* 18%. *International:* 43%. Grants are provided to programs and projects that directly impact the lives of community members who are most in need. Supports projects that: serve economically disadvantaged people, cultural communities, and those most vulnerable in operating communities; adress the need to strengthen the capacity of communities, violence, access to health care, and developing and maintaining healthy lifestyles; involve the people most affected by the problem in defining and then delivering the solutions; emphasize prevention of health problems, including outreach efforts, support groups, health education, and supportive services; and include partnerships and collaborations in the sponsorship of programs. Special consideration is given to projects that focus on diseases or conditions that are addressed by Medtronic as a business, including: heart disease, neurological disorders, incontinence, sleep apnea, and chronic pain. The Full Life Patient Partnership engages patients, providers, and policymakers to improve the quality of health care for people with chronic disease through three national programs: Patient Link, Health Leadership Grants, and HeartRescue. Medtronic also supports the Healthy Countries initiative, providing funding for disease prevention and treatment in parts of China, India, Mexico, and Eastern Europe. *Religion:* 3%. *Voluntarism:* The foundation's Medtronic Time-n-Talent Fund donates $500 to qualifying nonprofit organizations at which an employee or retiree volunteers at least 40 hours per year. If a volunteer who has donated 40 hours and also makes a financial contribution of $25 to $500 to the same organization, the foundation will match the contribution. *Note:* Total contributions made in fiscal 2001. **Typ. Recipients:** Adolescent Health Issues, AIDS/HIV, Cancer, Children's Health/Hospitals, Clinics/Medical Centers, Emergency/Ambulance Services, Geriatric Health, Health Organizations, Health Policy/Cost Containment, Health-General, Heart, Hospices, Hospitals, Long-Term Care, Medical Education, Medical Research, Multiple Sclerosis, Nursing Services, Preventive Medicine/Wellness Organizations, Public Health, Research/Studies Institutes, Single-Disease Health Associations, Trauma Treatment. **Geo. Dist:** internationally in Medtronic plant communities; nationally in Medtronic plant communities; Minneapolis, MN, metropolitan area; St. Paul, MN, metropolitan area.

★ 12673 ★ Mellon Financial Corp. Foundation

PO Box 185
Pittsburgh, PA 15230-9897
Phone: (412)234-1443 **Fax:** (412)234-0831
Website: http://www.mellon.com/communityaffairs/charitablegiving.html
James McDonald, Vice President

Priorities: *Arts & Humanities:* 17%. Supports museums, arts centers and festivals, music groups, and programs concerned with historic preservation. Matches employee gifts to arts and cultural organizations. *Civic & Public Affairs:* 24%. Favors community initiatives that attract and develop business and jobs. Also supports efforts to promote affordable housing, homeownership, and economic development in low and moderate income areas. *Education:* 25%. Interests include business education, literacy and minority education funds. Matches employee gifts to colleges and universities. *Environment:* 34%. Primarily funds United Way and, in 2001, disaster relief related to the September 11 terrorist attacks. Also typically provides some funding for organizations concerned with the disabled, drug and alcohol abuse, and food distribution. *International:* 11%. *Religion:* 1%. *Voluntarism:* Mellon Volunteer Professionals - a volunteer program that supports nonprofit initiatives at certain Mellon communities. Mellon also has an active Retiree Volunteer program in its Pittsburgh location. *Note:* Total contributions made in 2001. **Typ. Recipients:** AIDS/HIV, Cancer, Emergency/Ambulance Services, Health Organizations, Health-General, Hospitals, People with Disabilities, Single-Disease Health Associations. **Geo. Dist:** retail location areas; DE; Boston, MA; Philadelphia, PA; Pittsburgh, PA.

★ 12674 ★ Memphis Light Gas & Water Division

PO Box 430
Memphis, TN 38101-0430
Phone: (901)528-4151 **Fax:** (901)528-4321
Email: corpcomm@mlgw.com
Website: http://www.mlgw.com
Doris Douglas, Administration Assistant

Priorities: *Voluntarism:* Company sponsors volunteer involvement program and community involvement council, and employees volunteer their time with United Way. *Note:* Most giving is through employee campaigns and fundraising efforts. **Typ. Recipients:** Cancer, Children's Health/Hospitals, Health-General, Mental Health, Prenatal Health Issues, Transplant Networks/Donor Banks. **Geo. Dist:** Memphis, TN.

★ 12675 ★ Menasha Corp. Foundation

PO Box 367
Neenah, WI 54957-0367
Phone: (920)751-1217 **Fax:** (920)751-1236
Steven Kromholz, President

Priorities: *Arts & Humanities:* 11%. Supports museums, theater, historical societies and history organizations, public broadcasting, and opera. *Civic & Public Affairs:* 18%. Interests include urban and community affairs and local clubs, chambers of commerce, parks, and municipalities, with a focus on community redevelopment. *Education:* 10%. Funds universities and colleges in Wisconsin, economic education, education funds, minority education, literacy programs, public and private precollege schools, and youth educational programs. *Environment:* 49%. Supports local United Way agencies, senior services, and youth organizations including YMCAs, Boys and Girls Clubs, and scouting. *International:* 7%. Gives to medical centers, residency programs, medical foundations, hospice, and single-disease health associations. *Voluntarism:* Foundation gives Employee Volunteer Awards, donating cash grants to select organizations where employees volunteer. *Note:* Total foundation contributions made in 2000. **Typ. Recipients:** Cancer, Child Abuse, Children's Health/Hospitals, Clinics/Medical Centers, Diabetes, Domestic Violence, Emergency/Ambulance Services, Health Organizations, Health-General, Hospices, Hospitals, Nursing Services, People with Disabilities, Public Health, Sexual Abuse, Substance

Abuse. **Geo. Dist:** headquarters and operating communities.

★ 12676 ★ Mentor Graphics Corp. Foundation

8005 SW Boeckman Rd.
Wilsonville, OR 97070-9733
Phone: (503)685-7000 **Fax:** (503)682-6972
Marti Brown, Vice President

Fnded: 1985. **Priorities:** *Arts & Humanities:* 45%. Funds a variety of organizations in Oregon. Interests include ballet, public broadcasting, and symphonies. Also funds dance, a historical society, and the literary arts. *Civic & Public Affairs:* Less than 1%. Funds zoological associations and urban affairs. *Education:* 33%. Supports colleges and universities, college funds, and business education. *Environment:* 9%. Supports child welfare, youth organizations, and community service. *International:* 5%. Supports pediatric health, nursing associations, and single-disease health associations. *Religion:* 8%. Primarily supports science museums and scientific centers and institutes. *Note:* Total contributions made in 2000. **Typ. Recipients:** AIDS/HIV, Alzheimers Disease, Cancer, Children's Health/Hospitals, Clinics/Medical Centers, Diabetes, Domestic Violence, Family Planning, Medical Research, Multiple Sclerosis, Single-Disease Health Associations, Substance Abuse. **Geo. Dist:** CA, Silicon Valley area; Portland, OR.

★ 12677 ★ Merck Co. Foundation

PO Box 100, WS2F-96
Whitehouse Station, NJ 08889-0100
Phone: (908)423-2043 **Fax:** (908)423-1987
Website: http://www.merck.com/about/cr/policies_performance/social/philanthropy.html
John Taylor, Executive Vice President

Priorities: *Arts & Humanities:* 5%. *Civic & Public Affairs:* (Civics, Culture & Environment/Health Care & Social Services) About 40%. Funds social services through the United Way, and health interests such as hospitals, medical centers, and children's health; the arts and the environment receive minor support. Some civic groups also receive funding. (Public Policy) About 10%. Mainly supports groups concerned with health policy issues. Also supports organizations dealing with the pharmaceutical business, economics, and health care cost containment. *Education:* About 40%. Supports programs designed to increase knowledge of medicine and science. Also emphasizes the creation of education opportunities for minorities. Support to secondary and primary science education in selected locations. *Environment:* 38%. *International:* 11%. *Note:* Total contributions made in 2001. **Typ. Recipients:** AIDS/HIV, Cancer, Children's Health/Hospitals, Clinics/Medical Centers, Emergency/Ambulance Services, Geriatric Health, Health Organizations, Health Policy/Cost Containment, Health-General, Heart, Hospitals, Hospitals (University Affiliated), Medical Education, Medical Research, Medical Training, Public Health, Research/Studies Institutes, Respiratory, Single-Disease Health Associations, Substance Abuse. **Geo. Dist:** internationally; nationally; primarily headquarters and operating communities.

★ 12678 ★ Meredith Corp. Foundation

1716 Locust St.
Des Moines, IA 50309-3023
Phone: (515)284-2656 **Fax:** (515)284-3153
Gail Stilwill, Foundation Manager

Priorities: *Arts & Humanities:* 12%. *Civic & Public Affairs:* 24%. *Education:* 21%. *Environment:* 38%. *International:* 2%. *Religion:* 1%. *Voluntarism:* Employees who volunteer a minimum of 20 hours at one agency within a 12-month period between July 1 and June 30 are eligible to apply for a grant to that agency. Matches range from a minimum of $200 for 20 to 29 volunteer hours, to a maximum of $500 for 50 or more hours. A maximum of $1,500 is awarded to any one nonprofit within each fiscal year, regardless of the number of employees or hours volunteered. An employee may request one grant per year, and must apply within three months of the last day he or she volunteered. *Note:* Total foundation contributions made in fiscal 2001. **Typ. Recipients:** Arthritis, Children's Health/Hospitals, Hospices, People with Disabilities. **Geo. Dist:** Des Moines, IA, metropolitan area.

★ 12679 ★ Merrill Lynch & Co. Foundation Inc.

200 Union Ave.
Cresskill, NJ 07626
Phone: (201)871-0350
Website: http://www.ml.com
Eddy Bayardelle, Director, Philanthropic Programs

Fnded: 1950. **Priorities:** *Arts & Humanities:* 22%. Major areas of support include music, ethnic and folk museums, arts centers and institutes, dance theaters, libraries, history organizations and memorials, and botanical gardens. *Civic & Public Affairs:* 14%. Interests include business organizations, civil rights, job training, urban and community affairs, housing initiatives, and women's and minority affairs. *Education:* 33%. Supports education reform, minority education, student aid, colleges and universities, and business and technical education. Additionally, awards scholarships to children of employees based both on merit and need. *Environment:* 22%. Gives to a variety of local and national social service organizations, with emphasis on youth and community service organizations. Other interests include substance abuse programs, YMCAs, and people with disabilities. About 3% of total contributions is provided to the United Way. *International:* 9%. Donations fund single-disease health associations, hospitals and health organizations, clinics and medical centers, geriatric health groups, children's health concerns, and emergency services. *Voluntarism:* The company sponsors an Employee Community Involvement Program, which provides grants of $100 to $1,000 to organizations where employees volunteer. *Note:* Total contributions made in 2001. **Typ. Recipients:** AIDS/HIV, Cancer, Children's Health/Hospitals, Clinics/Medical Centers, Emergency/Ambulance Services, Geriatric Health, Health Organizations, Heart, Hospitals, Medical Education, Medical Research, People with Disabilities, Research/Studies Institutes, Single-Disease Health Associations, Substance Abuse, Transplant Networks/Donor Banks. **Geo. Dist:** national organizations; primarily in areas where Merrill Lynch & Co. maintains offices; New York, NY, metropolitan area.

★ 12680 ★ MetLife Foundation

1 Madison Ave.
New York, NY 10010-3690
Phone: (212)578-7049 **Fax:** (212)685-1435
Website: http://www.metlife.org
Sibyl Jacobson, President & Chief Executive Officer

Priorities: *Arts & Humanities:* 16%. *Civic & Public Affairs:* 13%. *Education:* 16%. *Environment:* 29%. *International:* 22%. *Religion:* 1%. *Voluntarism:* Recognizes company volunteers with the MetLife Volunteer ServiceAwards; also sponsors an employee volunteer program that helps employees find volunteer opportunities with nonprofits, schools, and other public agencies. There is a full-time volunteer coordinator at the headquarters location, and several branch offices have structured volunteer programs. Company makes small grants to organizations where employees actively volunteer, through the Volunteer Ventures program. *Note:* Total contributions made in 2001. **Typ. Recipients:** AIDS/HIV, Alzheimers Disease, Cancer, Children's Health/Hospitals, Clinics/Medical Centers, Geriatric Health, Health Funds, Health Organizations, Health Policy/Cost Containment, Heart, Hospitals, Medical Education, Medical Research, Medical Training, Mental Health, Nursing Services, Nutrition, Prenatal Health Issues, Public Health, Research/Studies Institutes, Respiratory, Substance Abuse, Transplant Networks/Donor Banks. **Geo. Dist:** nationally; special consideration to communities in which Metropolitan has a major presence.

★ 12681 ★ Metris Companies Foundation

10900 Wayzata Blvd.
Minnetonka, MN 55305-1534
Phone: (652)525-5020
Website: http://www.metriscompanies.com/Community/index.html
Anne Morrow, Director of Community Relations

Fnded: 2000. **Priorities:** *Arts & Humanities:* 1%. *Civic & Public Affairs:* 17%. *Education:* 20%. *Environment:* 45%. *International:* 17%. *Voluntarism:* The company participates in volunteer programs with charities in its operating communities. *Note:* Total contributions made in 2001. **Typ. Recipients:** Health Organizations, People with Disabilities, Public Health, Single-Disease Health Associations, Substance Abuse. **Geo. Dist:** Scottsdale, AZ; Jacksonville, FL; Orlando, FL; White Marsh, MD; Duluth, MN; Tulsa, OK.

★ 12682 ★ MGIC Investment Corp.

PO Box 488
Milwaukee, WI 53202
Phone: (414)347-6577 **Fax:** (414)347-4866
Email: john_ludwick@mgic.com
John Ludwick, Vice President Human Resources

Priorities: *Arts & Humanities:* 25%. *Civic & Public Affairs:* 20%. *Education:* 15%. *International:* 40%. Funds health and welfare organizations. **Typ. Recipients:** Domestic Violence, Hospitals, Single-Disease Health Associations, Substance Abuse. **Geo. Dist:** Milwaukee, WI.

★ 12683 ★ Micron Technology Foundation, Inc.

Mailstop 407, PO Box 6
Boise, ID 83707-0006
Phone: (208)368-4000 **Fax:** (208)368-4435
Email: mtf@micron.com
Chris Earphman, Corp. Affairs

Typ. Recipients: Emergency/Ambulance Services, Public Health. **Geo. Dist:** ID, Giving limited to communities where Micron has manufacturing facilities.

★ 12684 ★ Microsoft Corp.

One Microsoft Way
Redmond, WA 98052-6399
Phone: (425)882-8080 **Fax:** (425)936-7329
Email: giving@microsoft.com
Website: http://www.microsoft.com/Giving
Bruce Brooks, Director, Community Affairs

Priorities: *Arts & Humanities:* 6%. Funds theater, orchestras, and other arts organizations. *Civic & Public Affairs:* 4%. Supports community efforts including civic affairs, technology and the arts. *Education:* 28%. Donates cash and software to colleges and universities, educational funds, and awards programs. Also supports local elementary education, and provides scholarships to employees' children. Makes Access to Technology grants, and Instructional Grant software licenses to colleges and universities to support innovative uses of technology in academic areas such as computer science, business information technologies, engineering, and math. *Environment:* 47%. Includes employee programs and matching gifts. *Note:* Total contributions made in fiscal 2000. **Typ. Recipients:** AIDS/HIV, Cancer, Children's Health/Hospitals, Domestic Violence, Emergency/Ambulance Services, Kidney, Medical Rehabilitation, People with Disabilities, Single-Disease Health Associations, Transplant Networks/Donor Banks. **Geo. Dist:** some national initiatives; WA.

★ 12685 ★ Mid-American Foundation

4700 Westown Parkway, Suite 303
West Des Moines, IA 50266
Phone: (515)244-3600
Joe Pierce, President

Priorities: *Arts & Humanities:* 14%. Supports art museums, art festivals, performing arts, libraries, history organizations, and public broadcasting. *Civic & Public Affairs:* 7%. Funds minority affairs, civic centers, zoos, law & justice, and economic and urban development. *Education:* 51%. Supports a Jewish academy, scholarship funds, minority education, and universities. *Environment:* 14%. Supports the United Way, family services, family planning, youth organizations, and sports and recreation. *International:* 8%.

Supports alternative medicine, pediatric disease and mental health organizations, and national single-disease associations. *Note:* Total contributions made in 2001. **Typ. Recipients:** Alzheimers Disease, Cancer, Children's Health/Hospitals, Clinics/Medical Centers, Diabetes, Emergency/Ambulance Services, Eyes/Blindness, Family Planning, Health Organizations, Health-General, Heart, Multiple Sclerosis, People with Disabilities, Prenatal Health Issues. **Geo. Dist:** headquarters and operating communities.

★ 12686 ★ Midland Co. Foundation

7000 Midland Blvd.
Amelia, OH 45102
Phone: (513)943-7100
John Von Lehman, Vice President & Secretary

Priorities: *Arts & Humanities:* 5%. Gives to ballet, theater, arts funds, libraries, museums, and public broadcasting. *Civic & Public Affairs:* 2%. Parks, fire and police departments, clubs, employment services, and economic development are supported. *Education:* 66%. Supports public schools, education funds, economic education, Junior Achievement, colleges, and universities. *Environment:* 19%. Funds senior services, youth organizations, scouting, family services, food banks, sports and recreation, substance abuse treatment, and United Way. *International:* 8%. Contributes to single-disease associations, hospitals, children's hospitals, hospice, cancer research, wellness programs, and mental health organizations. *Note:* Total contributions made in 2002. **Typ. Recipients:** Cancer, Children's Health/Hospitals, Diabetes, Eyes/Blindness, Heart, Hospices, Hospitals, Multiple Sclerosis, Prenatal Health Issues. **Geo. Dist:** Cincinnati, OH.

★ 12687 ★ Milacron Foundation

2090 Florence Ave.
Cincinnati, OH 45206
Phone: (513)487-5662 **Fax:** (513)487-5586
John Francy, Assistant Treasurer

Priorities: *Arts & Humanities:* 7%. Gives to museums, opera, and arts funds. *Civic & Public Affairs:* 8%. Supports urban development, organizations that promote racial equality, employment services, public safety, and zoos. *Education:* 26%. Supports higher education with an emphasis on technology, engineering, and science education. Also funds a school for the deaf. *Environment:* 55%. Majority of funding supports United Way campaigns near operating locations. Other interests include youth organizations and services for senior citizens. *International:* 3%. Funds a children's hospital and wellness initiatives. *Religion:* 1%. Gives to a science fair. *Note:* Total contributions made in 2000. **Typ. Recipients:** Cancer, Children's Health/Hospitals, Emergency/Ambulance Services, Health Organizations, Hospices, People with Disabilities, Preventive Medicine/Wellness Organizations. **Geo. Dist:** principally near operating locations and to national organizations. **Frmly:** Cincinnati Milacron Inc.

★ 12688 ★ Milliken Foundation

153 E 53rd St.
New York, NY 10043
Jim Hamrick, Executive Director

Fnded: 1945. **Priorities:** *Arts & Humanities:* 11%. Supports arts associations, libraries, museums, and historic preservation. *Civic & Public Affairs:* 10%. Supports towns, economic development, employment services, legal services, and community organizations. *Education:* 29%. Supports Junior Achievement, colleges, institutes, literacy associations, educational academies, universities, and education funds. *Environment:* 31%. Supports YMCA, United Way, youth services, people with disabilities, substance abuse programs, food distribution, scouts, Special Olympics, and athletics. *International:* 16%. Supports medical clinics, hospices, health organizations, and single-disease health associations. *Note:* Total foundation contributions made in 2000. **Typ. Recipients:** Alzheimers Disease, Cancer, Children's Health/Hospitals, Clinics/Medical Centers, Emergency/Ambulance Services, Family Planning, Hospices, Hospitals, Medical Education, Medical Rehabilitation, Mental Health, People with Disabilities, Prenatal Health Issues, Public Health, Single-Disease Health Associations, Substance Abuse. **Geo. Dist:** headquarters and operating communities; nationally.

★ 12689 ★ The Millipore Foundation

80 Ashby Rd.
Bedford, MA 01730-2271
Phone: (781)533-2210 **Fax:** (781)533-3301
Email: Charleen_Johnson@millipore.com
Website: http://www.millipore.com/foundation
Charleen Johnson, Executive Director

Priorities: *Arts & Humanities:* 11%. Supports public libraries, performing arts, museums, and fine arts. *Civic & Public Affairs:* 9%. Supports employment services, public policy, aquariums, and community foundations. *Education:* 39%. Supports selected organizations, schools, universities, institutes, colleges, and teaching hospitals engaged in research and training, primarily in the fields of chemistry, biochemistry and engineering. Supports programs in minority education (national organizations that extend opportunities for minorities at all educational levels), and awards scholarships each year to employees' children. *Environment:* 22%. Supports food distribution, youth homes, child services, and youth development, especially regional programs that provide employment and self-development, particularly for inner-city youth. Additionally, employees and others are matched with nonprofit agencies and organizations that can benefit from their specific skills, talent and knowledge. *International:* 12%. Supports hospitals, medical centers, single-disease health associations, and biomedical research. *Religion:* 5%. Primary support made to science museums. *Voluntarism:* Under the Voluntary Service Grant Program, employees who are currently doing volunteer work in their communities can petition the foundation for funds to support a special need or program of the organization where they volunteer. The program now provides a grant of up to $5,000 to support specific projects of eligible community organizations in which the Millipore employee is actively involved. The SkillsBank program is open to current employees, retirees, and family members who want to get involved in volunteer work. SkillsBank is a computerized program linked to the United Way's Voluntary Action Center, The Massachusetts Volunteer Network, and local charitable organizations. It acts as a clearinghouse between 500 agencies and the volunteers. Employees and others are matched with nonprofit agencies and organizations that can benefit from their specific skills, talent and knowledge. *Note:* Total foundation contributions made in fiscal 2001. **Typ. Recipients:** AIDS/HIV, Cancer, Children's Health/Hospitals, Clinics/Medical Centers, Diabetes, Emergency/Ambulance Services, Health Organizations, Home-Care Services, Hospitals, Medical Education, Medical Research, Medical Training, Mental Health, People with Disabilities, Public Health, Respiratory, Single-Disease Health Associations, Substance Abuse. **Geo. Dist:** matching gifts awarded nationally; MA, cash grants made primarily in Massachusetts.

★ 12690 ★ Mine Safety Appliances Co. Charitable Foundation

PO Box 426
Pittsburgh, PA 15230
Phone: (412)967-3000 **Fax:** (412)967-3367
Website: http://www.msanet.com
Dennis Zeitler, Vice President

Priorities: *Arts & Humanities:* 8%. Funds music, ballet, opera, theater, museums, and libraries. *Civic & Public Affairs:* 20%. Emphasis on economic development and public policy. Supports business, professional, and industrial and public safety organizations in addition to those with an emphasis on urban and community affairs. *Education:* 8%. Pittsburgh area colleges and universities receive funding, with a focus on economic, engineering, and minority education and independent college funds. *Environment:* 58%. Primarily supports united funds. Also funds shelters, youth organizations, emergency relief, child welfare, and the disabled. *International:* 3%. Supports hospitals, single-disease health associations, and the American Red Cross. *Note:* Total foundation contributions made in 2001. **Typ. Recipients:** AIDS/HIV, Alzheimers Disease, Children's Health/Hospitals, Diabetes, Emergency/Ambulance Services, Health Funds, Health Organizations, Hospitals, Kidney, Long-Term Care, Medical Rehabilitation, Mental Health, Multiple Sclerosis, People with Disabilities, Respiratory, Single-Disease Health Associations. **Geo. Dist:** operating location communities; Pittsburgh, PA.

★ 12691 ★ Minnesota Mutual Foundation

400 Robert St. North
Saint Paul, MN 55101-2098
Phone: (651)665-3501 **Fax:** (651)665-3551
Email: lori.koutsky@minnesotamutual.com
Website: http://www.minnesotamutual.com/about/community.asp
Lori Koutsky, Manager

Priorities: *Arts & Humanities:* 24%. Supports chamber orchestras, theaters, music, public broadcasting, historic preservation, libraries, and united arts funds. *Civic & Public Affairs:* 9%. Supports women's affairs, housing, zoos, civic groups in operating locations, particularly business-related causes. *Education:* 20%. Supports colleges, universities, business and economic education, literacy, and science education. *Environment:* 38%. Supports United Way, YMCA, homes, scouts, and youth organizations. *International:* 2%. Supports health programs and nursing services. *Religion:* 4%. Primary support made to science museums. *Voluntarism:* Company conducts a special program that recognizes employee volunteerism with $100 donations to organizations where employees volunteer their time. *Note:* Total foundation contributions made in 2000. **Typ. Recipients:** AIDS/HIV, Child Abuse, Children's Health/Hospitals, Domestic Violence, Emergency/Ambulance Services, Health Funds, Health-General, Hospices, Hospitals, Long-Term Care, Medical Rehabilitation, Medical Research, Nursing Services, People with Disabilities, Prenatal Health Issues, Public Health, Research/Studies Institutes, Substance Abuse. **Geo. Dist:** Minneapolis, MN, metropolitan area; St. Paul, MN, metropolitan area.

★ 12692 ★ Mississippi Power Foundation, Inc.

PO Box 4079
Gulfport, MS 39502-4079
Phone: (228)865-5904 **Fax:** (228)865-5876
Ms. Domenica Plitt, Contact

Fnded: 1997. **Priorities:** *Education:* 54%. Supports colleges and universities. *Environment:* 38%. Supports United Way. *International:* 3%. Supports the American Red Cross. *Note:* Total contributions made in 2001. **Typ. Recipients:** Cancer, Emergency/Ambulance Services. **Geo. Dist:** MS.

★ 12693 ★ Mitsubishi Electric America Foundation

1560 Wilson Boulevard, Suite 1150
Arlington, VA 22209
Phone: (703)276-8240 **Fax:** (703)276-8260
Email: rayna.aylward@meus.mea.com
Website: http://www.meaf.org
Rayna Aylward, Executive Director

Fnded: 1991. **Priorities:** *Arts & Humanities:* 4%. *Civic & Public Affairs:* 8%. *Education:* 32%. *Environment:* 100%. Funding supports a range of projects addressing the needs of people with disabilities. Grants have supported internships of visually impaired students, exploration of career opportunities, online meeting places for children with disabilities, and training for teachers to improve their ability to assist disabled students. *International:* 11%. *Voluntarism:* To recognize growing interest in volunteerism among Mitsubishi Electric America employees, the foundation administers the MEA Foundation Starfish Enterprise Award program. The foundation also donates $10 per volunteer hour contributed to eligible projects by employees, their friends, and family members. *Note:* Total contributions made in 2002. **Typ. Recipients:** AIDS/HIV, Cancer, Children's Health/Hospitals, Children's Health/Hospitals, Diabetes, Eyes/Blindness, Health Organizations, Heart, Medical Rehabilitation, People with Disabilities, Prenatal Health Issues, Single-Disease Health Associations, Speech & Hearing. **Geo. Dist:** nationally; operating locations.

★ 12694 ★ Mizuho U.S.A. Foundation, Inc.

1251 Ave. of the Americas
New York, NY 10020-1104
Phone: (212)282-4192 **Fax:** (212)282-4250
Email: mizuho.usa.foundation@mizuhocbus.com
Ms. Lesley Harris Palmer, Executive Directory

Priorities: *Arts & Humanities:* Less than 1%. *Civic & Public Affairs:* 59%. *Education:* 18%. *Environment:* 21%. *International:* 1%. *Note:* Total contributions made in 2001. **Typ. Recipients:** Cancer, Children's Health/Hospitals, Domestic Violence, Heart, Home-Care Services, Mental Health, People with Disabilities, Transplant Networks/Donor Banks. **Geo. Dist:** Los Angeles, CA; Chicago, IL; New York, NY, primarily gives in NY. **Frmly:** IBJ Foundation.

★ 12695 ★ Modine Manufacturing Co. Foundation Inc

1500 DeKoven Ave.
Racine, WI 53403
Ernest Thomas, Vice President & Treasurer

Fnded: 1995. **Typ. Recipients:** Hospices, Medical Research. **Geo. Dist:** IL; KY; MO; VA; WI.

★ 12696 ★ Monroe Auto Equipment Co. Foundation

c/o Comerica Bank
PO Box 75000
MC 3462
Detroit, MI 48275-3462
Phone: (313)222-5067
Jane Ostrander, Director, Corporate Communications

Priorities: *Arts & Humanities:* 11%. Funds museums. *Civic & Public Affairs:* 9%. Funds housing and civic foundations. *Education:* 31%. Funds schools, colleges, and universities. *Environment:* 48%. Funds United Way and recreation. *International:* 35%. *Note:* Total contributions made in 2000. **Typ. Recipients:** Cancer, Children's Health/Hospitals, Clinics/Medical Centers, Emergency/Ambulance Services, Health Organizations, Home-Care Services, Hospices, Hospitals, Substance Abuse. **Geo. Dist:** headquarters and operating communities; Chicago, IL; Detroit, MI.

★ 12697 ★ Monsanto Fund

800 N Lindbergh Boulevard
Saint Louis, MO 63167
Phone: (314)694-1000 **Fax:** (314)694-7658
Email: monsanto.fund@monsanto.com
Website: http://www.monsantofund.org
Deborah Patterson, President

Priorities: *Arts & Humanities:* 4%. *Civic & Public Affairs:* 8%. *Education:* 5%. *Environment:* 12%. *International:* 3%. *Religion:* 58%. *Note:* Total fund contributions made in 2001. **Typ. Recipients:** AIDS/HIV, Alzheimers Disease, Cancer, Children's Health/Hospitals, Clinics/Medical Centers, Diabetes, Domestic Violence, Emergency/Ambulance Services, Health Organizations, Health Policy/Cost Containment, Hospitals, Medical Research, Research/Studies Institutes, Substance Abuse. **Geo. Dist:** operating facilities.

★ 12698 ★ Montana Power Foundation

130 North Main St.
Butte, MT 59701
Phone: (406)497-5468
Website: http://www.northwesternenergy.com/aboutus/community_relations.htm
Kathy Vogelsang, Contact

Fnded: 1985. **Priorities:** *Arts & Humanities:* 14%. Supports local museums, libraries, music, and historic preservation. *Civic & Public Affairs:* 5%. Supports business organizations, housing, employment initiatives, community activities, special events, and civic improvement. *Education:* 42%. Supports universities, colleges, and schools. Funds are applied to higher education at public and private colleges, universities, and vocational and technical programs within the state. Additional grants were made for capital programs, matching gifts, and scholarships to these same schools and additional primary and secondary schools in the state in the fields of math, science, and youth leadership. *Environment:* 29%. Supports food distribution, Big Brothers/Sisters, scouts, community services, Special Olympics, child welfare, services for seniors, United Way, and YMCA. *International:* 10%. Supports hospitals, health centers, and single-disease health associations. *Note:* Total foundation contributions made in 2000. **Typ. Recipients:** Cancer, Children's Health/Hospitals, Clinics/Medical Centers, Diabetes, Domestic Violence, Emergency/Ambulance Services, Family Planning, Health Organizations, Health-General, Hospitals. **Geo. Dist:** headquarters and operating communities.

★ 12699 ★ MONY Foundation

1740 Broadway
New York, NY 10019
Phone: (212)708-2377 **Fax:** (212)708-2001
Website: http://www.mony.com/AboutMONY/Inside-MONY/Foundation
Lynn Stekas, President

Priorities: *Arts & Humanities:* 3%. *Civic & Public Affairs:* 11%. *Education:* 19%. *Environment:* 49%. *International:* 12%. *Religion:* 1%. *Voluntarism:* The company sponsors the Volunteer Incentive at MONY (VIM) program, which encourages employee volunteerism at nonprofit organizations by providing semi-annual grants to those served by MONY Group volunteers. Another program, the Volunteer Incentive Award Program (VIP), makes an annual monetary award to a nonprofit social service agency in the community of each of its two major sites to encourage volunteer programs that effectively maximize their recourses by creatively utilizing employed volunteers. *Note:* Total contributions in 2001. **Typ. Recipients:** AIDS/HIV, Cancer, Clinics/Medical Centers, Emergency/Ambulance Services, Family Planning, Health Organizations, Health-General, Hospices, Medical Research, Mental Health, People with Disabilities, Prenatal Health Issues, Public Health, Research/Studies Institutes, Single-Disease Health Associations, Substance Abuse. **Geo. Dist:** headquarters and operating communities; New York, NY; Syracuse, NY. **Frmly:** MONY Life Insurance of New York.

★ 12700 ★ Morgan Stanley Foundation

1221 Ave. of the Americas, 27th Floor
New York, NY 10020
Phone: (212)762-6484 **Fax:** (212)762-7790
Email: whatadifference@morganstanley.com
Website: http://www.morganstanley.com/about/inside/community.html

Fnded: 1961. **Priorities:** *Arts & Humanities:* 1%. *Civic & Public Affairs:* 20%. *Education:* 27%. *Environment:* 49%. *International:* 1%. *Voluntarism:* Morgan Stanley employees are associated with several organizations addressing critical human service needs. Programs include employment training for the homeless, shelters for homeless women, scholarships for students from Chicago's housing projects, shelters in San Francisco, summer vacations for NYC youngsters, mental illness services, camps for youngsters, employment programs for runaways, and educational services to Chicago public schools. The company sponsors a Volunteer Incentive Program (VIP) which provides grants to health and human service charities where employees are active and ongoing volunteers. Grants through VIP typically range from $500 to $5,000. *Note:* Total contributions made in 2001. **Typ. Recipients:** AIDS/HIV, Cancer, Children's Health/Hospitals, Family Planning, Home-Care Services, Hospitals, Hospitals (University Affiliated), Medical Rehabilitation, Mental Health, Multiple Sclerosis, Prenatal Health Issues, Substance Abuse. **Geo. Dist:** Los Angeles, CA, branch locations; San Francisco, CA, branch locations; Chicago, IL, branch locations; New York, NY, branch locations. **Frmly:** Morgan Stanley Dean Witter Foundation.

★ 12701 ★ Motorola Foundation

1303 E Algonquin Rd.
Schaumburg, IL 60196
Phone: (847)576-6200 **Fax:** (847)576-3997
Website: http://fdncenter.org
Judy Adkins, Program Administrator

Priorities: *Arts & Humanities:* 5%. *Civic & Public Affairs:* 39%. *Education:* 30%. *Environment:* 19%. *International:* 1%. *Religion:* 1%. *Voluntarism:* The company sponsors volunteer programs that enable employees to support local organizations and schools in their communities. The foundation sponsors a volunteer grants program. *Note:* Total contributions made in 2001. **Typ. Recipients:** Emergency/Ambulance Services, Hospices, Hospitals, People with Disabilities, Single-Disease Health Associations, Substance Abuse. **Geo. Dist:** headquarters community, plant locations, and to select national organizations.

★ 12702 ★ Muriel F. Siebert Foundation

885 3rd Ave.
New York, NY 10022
Phone: (212)644-2400
Muriel Siebert, Chairman & President

Priorities: *Arts & Humanities:* 6%. Focus on museums. *Civic & Public Affairs:* 21%. Funds foundations and a women's center. *Education:* 17%. Supports literacy, public schools, and academics. *Environment:* 3%. Supports athletic activities and scouting. *International:* 44%. The Cancer Institute, cancer research and medicine. *Note:* Total contributions made in 1999. **Typ. Recipients:** Cancer, Clinics/Medical Centers, Health-General, Hospitals, Medical Education, Medical Rehabilitation, Medical Research, Single-Disease Health Associations. **Geo. Dist:** CA; CO; Washington, DC; FL; MI; NY; San Antonio, TX.

★ 12703 ★ Murphy Oil Corp.

200 Peach St.
El Dorado, AR 71730
Phone: (870)864-6222 **Fax:** (870)864-6231
Email: Betty_LeBrescu@murphyoilcorp.com
Betty LeBrescu, Manager, Community & Public Relations

Typ. Recipients: Hospitals. **Geo. Dist:** headquarters and operating communities.

★ 12704 ★ Mutual of Omaha Insurance Co.

Mutual of Omaha Plaza
Omaha, NE 68175
Phone: (402)342-5263 **Fax:** (402)351-2407
Website: http://www.mutualofomaha.com/about/community/contributions2002.html
Pam Shafer, Community Affairs & Corp. Contributions

Priorities: *Arts & Humanities:* 20%. *Civic & Public Affairs:* 20%. Distributed equally among the arts, health and human services, and civic organizations. *Education:* 40%. *International:* 20%. **Typ. Recipients:** AIDS/HIV, Domestic Violence, Health-General, Heart, Hospices, People with Disabilities. **Geo. Dist:** major business locations; mainly eastern Nebraska and western Iowa.

★ 12705 ★ National City Bank Foundation

PO Box 1919,
Minneapolis, MN 55480-1919
Phone: (612)904-8000 **Fax:** (612)904-8016
Donna DeMatteo, Secretary

Fnded: 1970. **Priorities:** *Arts & Humanities:* 12%. *Civic & Public Affairs:* 24%. *Education:* 3%. *Environment:* 56%. *International:* 3%. *Note:* Total contributions in 2001. **Typ. Recipients:** AIDS/HIV, Children's Health/Hospitals, Emergency/Ambulance Services, Family Planning, Health Organizations, Kidney, Medical Rehabilitation, Research/Studies Institutes, Substance Abuse, Transplant Networks/Donor Banks. **Geo. Dist:** Minneapolis, MN.

★ 12706 ★ National City Bank of Indiana
One National City Center Suite 400 East
Indianapolis, IN 46255
Phone: (317)267-3910 **Fax:** (317)267-7040
Email: darwinmay@nationalcity.com
Website: http://www.nationalcity.com/communityrelations
Darwin May, Senior Vice President
Typ. Recipients: Health-General. **Geo. Dist:** IN.

★ 12707 ★ National City Bank of Ohio
1900 E 9th St.
Locator 2157
Cleveland, OH 44114
Phone: (216)222-2995 **Fax:** (216)222-2670
Joanne Clark, Vice President, Corporate Public Affairs
Priorities: *Arts & Humanities:* 12%. Supports museums, theaters, galleries, and orchestras. *Civic & Public Affairs:* 25%. Funds community members in need, neighborhood revitalization, historical landmarks, and developing better community resources. *Education:* 20%. Supports high schools, colleges, scholarships, and career development programs. *Environment:* 20%. Funds United Way. *International:* (Health and Human Services) 23%. Supports health, safety, and supportive services. *Voluntarism:* The Heartbeat program provides small ($100 - $500) grants to nonprofit organizations where employees volunteer. *Note:* Total contributions made in 2001. **Typ. Recipients:** Health Organizations, Health-General, Hospitals. **Geo. Dist:** operating community.

★ 12708 ★ National City Bank of Pennsylvania
20 Stanwix, 25-146
Pittsburgh, PA 15222-4802
Phone: (412)644-8086 **Fax:** (412)644-8099
Website: http://www.nationalcity.com
Angie Longa, Vice President, Public Affairs
Priorities: *Arts & Humanities:* Supports local museums, theater, and arts festivals. *Civic & Public Affairs:* Emphasis on revitalization of low-to-modrate-income housing and neighborhoods. *Education:* Provides scholarships to children of employees. Matches employee contributions to secondary schools and colleges and universities. *Environment:* Supports the United Way and a variety of community service programs. *International:* Priorities include children's health and health services for the indigent. **Typ. Recipients:** Health-General. **Geo. Dist:** PA, headquarters and operating communities in western PA.

★ 12709 ★ National City Corp.
c/o Corporate Public Affairs Department
PO Box 5756
Cleveland, OH 44101
Phone: (216)575-2994 **Fax:** (216)222-2670
Website: http://nationalcity.com/communityrelations/default.asp
Bruce McCrodden, Senior Vice President
Priorities: *Arts & Humanities:* 12%. *Civic & Public Affairs:* 30%. *Education:* 21% *Environment:* 37%. *Note:* Total contributions made in 2002. **Typ. Recipients:** Cancer, Children's Health/Hospitals, Clinics/Medical Centers, Emergency/Ambulance Services, Geriatric Health, Hospices, Hospitals, Hospitals (University Affiliated), Medical Rehabilitation, Mental Health, Prenatal Health Issues, Public Health, Substance Abuse. **Geo. Dist:** considers national organizations on an individual basis; IL; IN; KY; MI; OH; PA.

★ 12710 ★ National City Corp. Charitable Foundation II
Care of National City Bank Cleveland
PO Box 5756
Cleveland, OH 44101
Phone: (216)575-2994
Bruce McCrodden, Contact
Fnded: 1996. **Priorities:** *Arts & Humanities:* 10%. *Civic & Public Affairs:* 21%. *Education:* 19%. *Environment:* 43%. *International:* 8%. *Note:* Total contributions made in 2001. **Typ. Recipients:** Cancer, Emergency/Ambulance Services, Health Organizations, Hospitals, Medical Education.

★ 12711 ★ National Fuel Gas Co.
10 Lafayette Square
Buffalo, NY 14203
Phone: (716)857-7861 **Fax:** (716)857-7413
Julie Cox, Senior Manager
Priorities: *Arts & Humanities:* Arts associations and centers, historic preservation, museums, music, public broadcasting, and theater. *Civic & Public Affairs:* Interests include better government, civil rights, consumer affairs, the environment, housing, safety, and zoos. *Education:* Supports colleges and universities; education associations; engineering, elementary, minority, and health education; and literacy. *Environment:* Supports programs for the aged, animal protection, community centers, drug and alcohol programs, employment and job training, the disabled, youth organizations, and united funds. *International:* Funds geriatric health, cost containment, hospitals and hospices, mental health, and single-disease associations. *Voluntarism:* The company reports that it participates in volunteer programs in conjunction with the United Way, and sponsors a mentoring program at specific schools. **Typ. Recipients:** Hospices, Hospitals, Mental Health, People with Disabilities, Substance Abuse. **Geo. Dist:** headquarters and operating communities.

★ 12712 ★ National Life Group
One National Life Dr.
Montpelier, VT 05604
Phone: (802)229-3333 **Fax:** (802)229-7006
Brian Vachon, Vice President, Communications
Priorities: *Voluntarism:* Company promotes employee volunteerism by providing support to organizations at which employees volunteer, as well as by allowing time off during the work day. **Typ. Recipients:** Domestic Violence, Health-General, Medical Research, Mental Health, Single-Disease Health Associations, Substance Abuse. **Geo. Dist:** VT, Central Vermont.

★ 12713 ★ National Machinery Foundation, Inc.
161 Greenfield St.
Tiffin, OH 44883
Phone: (419)447-5211 **Fax:** (419)443-2380
Don Bero, Assistant Secretary
Priorities: *Arts & Humanities:* 53%. *Civic & Public Affairs:* 1%. *Education:* 19%. *Environment:* 11%. *International:* 12%. *Note:* Total foundation contributions made in 2001. **Typ. Recipients:** AIDS/HIV, Cancer, Children's Health/Hospitals, Clinics/Medical Centers, Domestic Violence, Emergency/Ambulance Services, Geriatric Health, Health Organizations, Health-General, Heart, Hospices, Hospitals, Medical Rehabilitation, Nursing Services, Single-Disease Health Associations, Substance Abuse. **Geo. Dist:** OH, Seneca County.

★ 12714 ★ National Service Foundation
1420 Peachtree St., NE
Atlanta, GA 30309-3002
Phone: (404)853-1000 **Fax:** (404)858-1015
Carol Morgan, Contact
Fnded: 1969. **Priorities:** *Arts & Humanities:* 15%. Supports arts centers, the performing arts, art councils, and libraries. *Civic & Public Affairs:* 13%. Funds economic development, community foundations, and civic organizations. *Education:* 9%. Supports colleges and universities, minority education, and Junior Achievement. *Environment:* 37%. Funds United Way and youth concerns. *International:* 8%. Funds hospitals and single-disease health associations. *Note:* Total contributions made in fiscal 2001. **Typ. Recipients:** Arthritis, Cancer, Child Abuse, Clinics/Medical Centers, Diabetes, Domestic Violence, Heart, Hospitals, Medical Education, Medical Rehabilitation, Medical Research, Multiple Sclerosis, People with Disabilities, Prenatal Health Issues. **Geo. Dist:** Eastern US; GA.

★ 12715 ★ National Starch & Chemical Foundation
10 Finderne Ave.
Bridgewater, NJ 08807
Phone: (908)685-5001 **Fax:** (908)685-5096
Carmen Ortiz, Contact
Fnded: 1968. **Priorities:** *Arts & Humanities:* 4%. Supports theater and performing arts, musical groups such as symphonies, museums and historical societies, and arts associations and festivals. *Civic & Public Affairs:* 9%. Funds professional associations, public policy, urban leagues, business groups, and environmental organizations. *Education:* 25%. Elementary and secondary schools, colleges and universities, and Junior Achievement receive funding. Also supports math and science education programs for minorities. Matching gifts constitute a large number of grants to colleges. Foundation provides scholarships to the children of employees. *Environment:* 48%. Funds United Way organizations in various company-operating communities, child welfare and recreational groups, volunteer organizations, food banks, and services for the elderly and disabled. *International:* 12%. Supports hospitals, research, foundations, and single-disease health organizations. *Voluntarism:* In the counties surrounding company headquarters in Bridgewater, NJ, National actively supports the Science Alliance Program. Senior staffers devote their time and expertise to help teach middle school and high school students about science in an interesting and hands-on fashion. In Woodruff, SC, employees help nurture the growth and aspirations of children by serving as positive role models, confidants and supporters. Volunteerism extends to international National Starch and Chemical employees in England, Italy, and South Africa. *Note:* Total contributions made in 2000. **Typ. Recipients:** Cancer, Clinics/Medical Centers, Emergency/Ambulance Services, Health Funds, Health Organizations, Hospitals, Medical Rehabilitation, Medical Training, Nursing Services, People with Disabilities, Public Health, Substance Abuse. **Geo. Dist:** primarily in headquarters and operating communities.

★ 12716 ★ Nationwide Foundation
1 Nationwide Plaza
Mail Drop 1-26-05
Columbus, OH 43215-2220
Phone: (614)249-5095 **Fax:** (614)677-0320
Website: http://www.nationwide.com/about_us/involve/fndatn.htm
Stephen Rish, President
Fnded: 1959. **Priorities:** *Arts & Humanities:* 11%. Supports libraries, musical performance, ballet, theater, art councils, museums, and history. *Civic & Public Affairs:* 14%. Funds urban affairs, public safety, economic development, housing initiatives, and community organizations. *Education:* 20%. Supports colleges, universities, economic education, education funds, scholarships, and literacy. *Environment:* 51%. Supports child abuse programs, youth programs, shelters, food banks, YMCAs, family planning services and major support to United Way. *International:* 2%. Supports hospitals and health organizations. *Religion:* 1%. Primarily supports science centers. *Note:* Total foundation contributions made in 2000. **Typ. Recipients:** AIDS/HIV, Alzheimers Disease, Cancer, Child Abuse, Children's Health/Hospitals, Emergency/Ambulance Services, Eyes/Blindness, Family Planning, Health Organizations, Heart, Hospitals, Long-Term Care, Medical Research, Mental Health, Nursing Services, People with Disabilities, Single-Disease Health Associations, Speech & Hearing, Substance Abuse. **Geo. Dist:** OH, Central Ohio and near state operating locations. **Frmly:** Nationwide Insurance Enterprise Foundation.

★ 12717 ★ Nationwide Provident
1000 Chesterbrook Boulevard
Berwyn, PA 19312
Phone: (610)407-1674
Email: crbrown@nationwideprovident.com
Craig Brown, Communication Manager

Typ. Recipients: Health-General. **Geo. Dist:** Philadelphia, PA, metropolitan area.

★ 12718 ★ Navcom Charities Foundation
9815 Godwin Drive
Manassas, VA 20110-4156
Phone: (703)361-0884
Liz Johnson, Administrative Assistant to the Pres.

Fnded: 1992. **Typ. Recipients:** AIDS/HIV. **Geo. Dist:** headquarters area only.

★ 12719 ★ NCR Foundation
1700 S Patterson Boulevard
Dayton, OH 45479
Phone: (937)445-6779 **Fax:** (937)445-0636
Mary Karr, Vice President & Director

Fnded: 1953. **Priorities:** *Arts & Humanities:* 4%. *Civic & Public Affairs:* 43%. *Education:* 18%. *Environment:* 32%. *International:* Less than 1%. *Note:* Total contributions made in 2001. **Typ. Recipients:** Cancer, Emergency/Ambulance Services, Health Organizations, Hospices. **Geo. Dist:** headquarters and operating communities; Dayton, OH.

★ 12720 ★ NCS Pearson, Inc.
5601 Green Valley Dr.
Bloomington, MN 55437
Phone: (952)681-3000 **Fax:** (952)681-3066
Carol Johnson, Assistant Secretary

Priorities: *Arts & Humanities:* 20%. Supports arts and humanities, including art appreciation, art centers, and art institutes. Focus is on larger, established, highly-visible institutions. *Civic & Public Affairs:* 20%. Contributions fund economic development, professional associations, nonprofit management, public policy, environmental affairs, and urban affairs. *Education:* 25%. Recipients include arts education, business education, career/vocational education, and colleges and universities. *International:* 35%. Supports public health, hospitals, health care cost containment, and health maintenance services. Additional funding goes to child welfare agencies, chemical abuse treatment centers, employment programs for the handicapped, community services, youth and family organizations, shelters, united funds, and volunteer action. *Voluntarism:* Company sponsors the Jumpstart volunteer program. *Note:* Giving analysis provided by foundation. **Typ. Recipients:** Domestic Violence, Family Planning, Health Policy/Cost Containment, Health-General, Hospices, Hospitals, Nutrition, People with Disabilities, Public Health, Single-Disease Health Associations, Substance Abuse. **Geo. Dist:** headquarters and operating communities.

★ 12721 ★ Nestle U.S.A., Inc.
800 North Brand Boulevard
Glendale, CA 91203
Phone: (818)549-6000 **Fax:** (818)549-6952
Website: http://www.nestleusa.com

Fnded: 1952. **Priorities:** *Civic & Public Affairs:* The company's Community Care campaigns support community activities through corporate direct and employee matching gifts. Typical recipients include women's groups, children's charities, health education, food banks, and animal welfare programs. *Education:* Nestle U.S.A. makes a significant contribution to national education organizations and educational programs in company operating communities. Major support is provided to Reading is Fundamental, the United Negro College Fund, the National Hispanic Scholarship fund, and Teach for America. Nestle's Community Affairs bureau publishes and distributes a series of books that introduce young people to inspirational role models. The company's Adopt-a-School program enables employee volunteers to contribute time to local schools. *Environment:* Food donations play a large role in the company's charitable contributions program. Through America's Second Harvest program, Nestle products are distributed to food banks, soup kitchens, shelters, children's hunger programs, and other food distribution organizations. The company's pet food operation donates to and fosters partnerships with animal welfare organizations to promote responsible pet ownership. The United Way is supported via an employee matching gift program. **Typ. Recipients:** Clinics/Medical Centers, Emergency/Ambulance Services, Hospitals, Nutrition, People with Disabilities, Preventive Medicine/Wellness Organizations. **Geo. Dist:** manufacturing facility areas.

★ 12722 ★ New Balance Foundation
20 Guest St.
Boston, MA 02135-2088
Phone: (617)783-4000
Anne Davis, Trustee

Priorities: *Arts & Humanities:* 25%. *Civic & Public Affairs:* 8%. *Education:* 31%. *Environment:* 29%. *International:* 7%. *Note:* Total contributions made in fiscal 2001. **Typ. Recipients:** Alzheimers Disease, Arthritis, Cancer, Children's Health/Hospitals, Clinics/Medical Centers, Diabetes, Health Organizations, Hospitals, Mental Health, People with Disabilities, Single-Disease Health Associations, Substance Abuse. **Geo. Dist:** ME; MA.

★ 12723 ★ New England Bio Labs Foundation
32 Tozer Rd.
Beverly, MA 01915
Phone: (978)927-2404 **Fax:** (978)921-1350
Email: cataldo@nebf.org
Website: http://www.nebf.org
Martine Kellett, Executive Director

Fnded: 1982. **Priorities:** *Arts & Humanities:* 12%. Supports music, dance, and community arts organizations, primarily in Massachusetts. *Education:* 7%. Funds the reuse of textbooks in international locations, and a college of art. *Environment:* 5%. Supports self-sufficiency, youth, and health initiatives internationally, and funds youth and family services domestically. *Note:* Contributions analysis provided by foundation. Total contributions made in fiscal 2001. The foundation reports that 73% of its grants were made to international organizations and 27% were made to domestic community organizations. **Typ. Recipients:** Clinics/Medical Centers, Eyes/Blindness, Health Organizations, Health-General, Nutrition, Prenatal Health Issues, Preventive Medicine/Wellness Organizations, Public Health. **Geo. Dist:** internationally; nationally.

★ 12724 ★ New Haven Savings Bank Foundation, Inc.
195 Church St.
New Haven, CT 06510-2009
Phone: (203)784-5057
Website: http://www.nhsb.com/foundation/default.asp
Kim Healey, Vice President

Fnded: 1998. **Priorities:** *Arts & Humanities:* 16%. *Civic & Public Affairs:* 27%. *Education:* 11%. *Environment:* 40%. *International:* 7%. *Note:* Total contributions made in 2001. **Typ. Recipients:** Hospitals, Nursing Services, Single-Disease Health Associations.

★ 12725 ★ New Jersey Natural Gas Foundation
PO Box 1464
Wall, NJ 07719
Phone: (732)938-1134 **Fax:** (732)938-7183
Website: http://www2.njng.com/community/
Tom Kononowitz, Vice President

Priorities: *Civic & Public Affairs:* 3%. Supports community safety initiatives, Urban Leagues, minority affairs, law enforcement organizations, parks, environmental organizations, and community foundations. *Education:* 25%. Supports colleges, universities, community colleges, and programs that assist minority students. *Environment:* 45%. Supports the United Way, youth organizations, scouts, family services, and drug abuse prevention. Company also sponsors a "Gift of Warmth" program. *International:* 27%. Gives to medical centers, hospitals, single-disease health associations, American Red Cross, health care foundations, and pediatric health. *Note:* Total contributions made in fiscal 2000. **Typ. Recipients:** Cancer, Children's Health/Hospitals, Clinics/Medical Centers, Diabetes, Emergency/Ambulance Services, Health Organizations, Health-General, Hospitals, People with Disabilities, Prenatal Health Issues, Public Health, Single-Disease Health Associations, Single-Disease Health Associations, Substance Abuse. **Geo. Dist:** company's service area; NJ, Monmouth County; NJ, Ocean County; NJ, portions of Morris County. **Frmly:** New Jersey Resources Foundation, Inc.

★ 12726 ★ New York Life Foundation
51 Madison Ave., Room 604
New York, NY 10010-1655
Phone: (212)576-6902
Email: NYLFoundation@newyorklife.com
Website: http://www.newyorklife.com/foundation
Peter Bushyeager, President

Priorities: *Arts & Humanities:* 4%. Supports libraries, the performing arts, public broadcasting, and theaters. *Civic & Public Affairs:* 12%. Supports community development programs, civil rights, housing, and philanthropic organizations. *Education:* 24%. Supports universities, scholarships, literacy, Junior Achievement, and matching gifts to educational institutes. *Environment:* 59%. Supports the United Way, scouts, Big Brothers/Sisters, child welfare, recreation, YWCA, single-disease health associations, and volunteer groups. *International:* 1%. Supports AIDS and health organizations. *Voluntarism:* Provides grants to local grassroots organizations where employees volunteer. *Note:* Total foundation contributions made in 2000. **Typ. Recipients:** AIDS/HIV, Clinics/Medical Centers, Domestic Violence, Emergency/Ambulance Services, Eyes/Blindness, Geriatric Health, Health Organizations, Hospitals, Medical Education, Medical Rehabilitation, Medical Research, Medical Training, Mental Health, Nursing Services, People with Disabilities, Single-Disease Health Associations, Substance Abuse. **Geo. Dist:** nationally; San Francisco/San Ramon, CA; Tampa, FL; Atlanta, GA; Minneapolis, MN; New York, NY; Cleveland, OH; Dallas, TX.

★ 12727 ★ New York Mercantile Exchange Charitable Foundation
Executive Committee
1 North End Ave.
World Financial Center, Room 1440
New York, NY 10282-1101
Phone: (212)299-2517
Email: charitablefoundation@nymex.com
Website: http://www.nymex.com/jsp/about/cs_relief_fund.jsp
Madeline Boyd, Chairman Executive Committee

Fnded: 1989. **Priorities:** *Arts & Humanities:* 3%. Supports public broadcasting and a music outreach program. *Civic & Public Affairs:* 6%. Funds public parks and community resource foundations. *Education:* 7%. Gives to education foundations, universities, precollege education, and a school for autistic children. *Environment:* 43%. Supports disaster relief efforts, summer camps, and services for families, youth, seniors. *International:* 26%. Supports single-disease health organizations, hospitals and medical centers, and pediatric health initiatives. *Note:* Total contributions made in 2000. **Typ. Recipients:** AIDS/HIV, Cancer, Children's Health/Hospitals, Clinics/Medical Centers, Diabetes, Domestic Violence, Emergency/Ambulance Services, Health-General, Hospitals, Medical Education, Medical Rehabilitation, Multiple Sclerosis, People with Disabilities, Public Health, Research/Studies Institutes, Single-Disease Health Associations, Substance Abuse, Trauma Treatment. **Geo. Dist:** principally near operating locations and to national organizations.

★ 12728 ★ New York Stock Exchange Foundation, Inc.
11 Wall St., 6th Floor
New York, NY 10005
Phone: (212)656-5057 **Fax:** (212)656-5629
Robert Zito, Contact

Priorities: *Arts & Humanities:* 21%. Supports public broadcasting, the performing arts, libraries, museums, theaters, opera, and historic preservation. *Civic & Public Affairs:* 17%. Supports public policy, community affairs, civil rights, safety, parks, and economic development. *Education:* 14%. Supports universities, colleges, Junior Achievement and other national educational programs and organizations. *Environment:* 22%. Supports United Way, camps, food distribution, YMCA, crime prevention, people with disabilities, youth organizations, and recreation programs. *International:* 26%. Supports hospitals, medical centers, and single-disease health associations. *Note:* Total foundation contributions made in 2000. **Typ. Recipients:** Adolescent Health Issues, Cancer, Hospitals, Medical Education, People with Disabilities. **Geo. Dist:** Washington, DC; New York, NY.

★ 12729 ★ New York Times Co. Foundation
229 W 43rd St.
New York, NY 10036-3959
Phone: (212)556-1091 **Fax:** (212)556-4450
Website: http://nytco.com/company/foundation/index.html
Jack Rosenthal, President

Priorities: *Arts & Humanities:* 32%. Majority supports the performing arts, particularly the Metropolitan Museum of Art and Lincoln Center and its constituent institutions. Other interests include museums, libraries, public broadcasting, and literary arts. *Civic & Public Affairs:* 13%. Supports urban and economic development, community clubs, food distribution, youth services, foreign and domestic policy, a police foundation, civil rights, minority and women's affairs, and services for the elderly. *Education:* 40%. Particular interest in minority education, arts and journalism programs, scholarships, and precollege education. Supports colleges and universities near operating locations, particularly New York. *Environment:* 5%. *International:* 1%. *Religion:* 11%. *Note:* Total contributions made in 2000. **Typ. Recipients:** Children's Health/Hospitals, Substance Abuse. **Geo. Dist:** communities served by company affiliates; some internationally; some nationally; New York, NY, metropolitan area.

★ 12730 ★ Newman's Own Foundation
246 Post Rd. East
Westport, CT 06880-3615
Phone: (203)222-0136 **Fax:** (203)227-5630
Website: http://www.newmansown.com/5_good.html
Joan Williams, Contact

Fnded: 1989. **Priorities:** *Note:* Total contributions made in fiscal 2001. **Typ. Recipients:** Arthritis, Child Abuse, Children's Health/Hospitals, Domestic Violence, Health Funds, Hospices, Hospitals, Medical Rehabilitation, People with Disabilities, Single-Disease Health Associations. **Geo. Dist:** internationally, where Newman's Own is sold.

★ 12731 ★ Niagara Mohawk Foundation
300 Erie Boulevard
Syracuse, NY 13202
Phone: (315)428-5691
Carolyn May, Contact

Priorities: *Arts & Humanities:* 9%. Support goes to public broadcasting, libraries, art museums, and the performing arts. *Civic & Public Affairs:* 8%. Supports local initiatives and community services. *Education:* 15%. Supports universities and colleges. *Environment:* 40%. Major support for the United Way; also funds youth organizations and human services. *International:* 21%. Funds American Red Cross, hospice, and hospitals. *Religion:* 1%. Supports museums of science and technology. *Voluntarism:* Sponsors a volunteer grant program and a community action team. *Note:* Total foundation contributions made in 2000. **Typ. Recipients:** Cancer, Children's Health/Hospitals, Clinics/Medical Centers, Emergency/Ambulance Services, Health-General, Heart, Hospices, Hospitals, People with Disabilities, Prenatal Health Issues, Trauma Treatment. **Geo. Dist:** service areas; NY, Upstate New York.

★ 12732 ★ Nike Foundation
1 Bowerman Dr., NRB-1
Beaverton, OR 97005
Phone: (503)532-0265 **Fax:** (503)532-0418
Website: http://www.nikebiz.com/community
Robert Speltz, Global Giving Manager

Priorities: *Arts & Humanities:* (Arts/Culture) 3%. Supports arts institutions, mainly near headquarters area. *Civic & Public Affairs:* (Community) 31%. Supports various civic and community organizations. *Education:* 9%. Supports mentoring programs, scholarship funds, colleges and universities, and public education. *Environment:* 23%. Supports disaster relief efforts. *International:* 4%. Supports research and single-disease organizations. A major focus is AIDS. *Voluntarism:* Company encourages employee volunteerism, particularly through mentoring and coaching under-served children. Nike matches employee volunteer time at $10 per hour, up to $5,000 annually per employee. *Note:* Contributions analysis is based on giving program figures provided by Nike in 2001. **Typ. Recipients:** Cancer, Emergency/Ambulance Services. **Geo. Dist:** nationally & internationally; emphasis on headquarters and operating communities.

★ 12733 ★ Nissan Foundation
PO Box 191
Gardena, CA 90248-0191
Phone: (310)771-3161
Website: http://www.nissandriven.com/insidenissan/corporateoutreach/

Fnded: 1992. **Priorities:** *Arts & Humanities:* 50%. Supports a symphony association. *Education:* 50%. Supports The Accelerated School. *Note:* Total foundation contributions made in fiscal 2001. **Typ. Recipients:** Adolescent Health Issues, Children's Health/Hospitals, Clinics/Medical Centers, Health Funds, Health Organizations. **Geo. Dist:** Los Angeles, CA, South Central LA.

★ 12734 ★ NMC Foundation
1 1st Ave.
Sterling, IL 61081
Phone: (815)625-1320 **Fax:** (815)625-1333
Email: jlbittorf@natman.com
Joseph Bittorf, Chairperson

Typ. Recipients: Cancer, Emergency/Ambulance Services, Heart, Hospices, Public Health, Substance Abuse. **Geo. Dist:** headquarters area only.

★ 12735 ★ Nomura America Foundation
2 World Financial Center, Bldg. B
New York, NY 10281-1198
Phone: (212)667-9433
Chris Becker, Assistant Secretary

Fnded: 1994. **Priorities:** *Civic & Public Affairs:* 25%. Supports women's affairs and Empower Organization. *Education:* 18%. Funds colleges and universities and private precollege education. *Environment:* 54%. Typically supports youth organizations. Majority of 2001 social services support was granted to September 11 causes, with funds provided by Nomura employees. *International:* 2%. Gives to visiting nurse services. *Note:* Total contributions made in 2001. **Typ. Recipients:** Arthritis, Cancer, Children's Health/Hospitals, Emergency/Ambulance Services, Health Funds, Hospitals, Medical Education, Multiple Sclerosis, People with Disabilities, Single-Disease Health Associations, Transplant Networks/Donor Banks. **Geo. Dist:** headquarters and operating communities.

★ 12736 ★ Nordson Corp. Foundation
28601 Clemens Rd.
Westlake, OH 44145-1148
Phone: (440)892-1580 **Fax:** (440)892-9507
Email: kladiner@nordson.com
Website: http://www.nordson.com/corporate/grants.html
Constance Haqq, Executive Director

Priorities: *Arts & Humanities:* 24%. Funding is given to established arts organizations that actively seek to broaden their audience bases in Nordson communities. Supports museums, musical groups, art programs, public broadcasting, performing arts, and enhanced multicultural awareness. *Civic & Public Affairs:* 21%. Supports minority affairs, housing, economic development, and job training and placement. Efforts to involve citizens in community improvement are also a priority. *Education:* 35%. Supports education reform, colleges, minority education, student aid, and secondary public and private education. *Environment:* 12%. Funding supports organizations that promote prevention, crisis intervention, life transition opportunities, and systemic policy change. Also, supports family services and united funds. Other interests include services for the aged, and youth organizations. Each year, two or three organizations are chosen to receive intense assistance for one year in the form of grant money, emergency funding, equipment donations, and volunteer time. *International:* 5%. Funds clinics, hearing and speech and blindness organizations, and nursing associations. *Religion:* 1%. Supports a hands-on science museum. *Voluntarism:* Company operates the Time'n Talent (T'nT) program, which links employees with volunteer opportunities in the community and generates new community service projects. *Note:* Total contributions made in fiscal 2000. **Typ. Recipients:** Clinics/Medical Centers, Domestic Violence, Emergency/Ambulance Services, Hospices, Medical Education, Medical Research, Mental Health, Nursing Services, People with Disabilities, Single-Disease Health Associations, Speech & Hearing, Substance Abuse. **Geo. Dist:** headquarters and operating communities; CA, San Diego County; Atlanta, GA; MA, Southeastern Massachusetts; OH; RI.

★ 12737 ★ Norfolk Southern Foundation
Three Commercial Place
Norfolk, VA 23510-2191
Phone: (757)629-2640 **Fax:** (757)629-2361
Email: dhwyld@nscorp.com
Website: http://www.nscorp.com
Kathryn McQuade, Vice President & Executive Officer

Priorities: *Arts & Humanities:* 25%. Supports music, theater and performing arts. *Civic & Public Affairs:* 21%. Urban affairs and community foundations. *Education:* 29%. Supports scholarship programs and education funds. *Environment:* 25%. Supports United Way. *Note:* Total contributions made in 1999. **Typ. Recipients:** Cancer, Children's Health/Hospitals, Emergency/Ambulance Services, Health Organizations, Heart, Hospitals, Medical Education, Medical Research, Research/Studies Institutes, Single-Disease Health Associations. **Geo. Dist:** headquarters and operating communities within the company's 22-state territory.

★ 12738 ★ North American Royalties Foundation
1418 Winding Way
Chattanooga, TN 37405
Phone: (423)265-0295

Priorities: *Arts & Humanities:* 27%. *Civic & Public Affairs:* 7%. *Education:* 51%. *Environment:* 8%. *International:* Less than 1%. *Note:* Total contributions made in 2001. **Typ. Recipients:** Cancer, Clinics/Medical Centers, Health-General, People with Disabilities, Respiratory. **Geo. Dist:** Chattanooga, TN.

★ 12739 ★ North Carolina Foam Foundation
PO Box 1528
Mount Airy, NC 27030
Phone: (910)789-9161
J. Barnhardt, Jr., President

Priorities: *Arts & Humanities:* 7%. Supports museums and libraries. *Civic & Public Affairs:* 6%. Supports community center and development. *Education:* 9%. Supports schools and universities. *Environment:* 41%. Supports youth organizations and United Way. *International:* 10%. Supports research organizations and blood banks. *Religion:* 1%. *Note:* Total contributions made in 1999. **Typ. Recipients:** Cancer, Children's Health/Hospitals, Clinics/Medical Centers, Emergency/Ambulance Services, Health Funds, Health Organizations, Health-General, Hospices, Hospitals, People with Disabilities, Public Health. **Geo. Dist:** NC.

★ 12740 ★ Northeast Utilities Foundation
107 Seldon St.
Berlin, CT 06037
Phone: (860)721-4063 **Fax:** (860)721-4331
Website: http://www.nu.com
Teresa Hopkins-Staten, Executive Director

Priorities: *Arts & Humanities:* 26%. *Civic & Public Affairs:* 7%. *Education:* 54%. *Environment:* 1%. *International:* 6%. *Religion:* 1%. *Note:* Total contributions made in 2001. **Typ. Recipients:** Cancer, Domestic Violence, Emergency/Ambulance Services, Hospitals, Mental Health, Nutrition, People with Disabilities, Substance Abuse. **Geo. Dist:** company service areas.

★ 12741 ★ Northern Indiana Public Service Co.
801 E 86th Ave.
Merrillville, IN 46410
Phone: (219)647-6388 **Fax:** (219)647-6380
Email: rbiddings@nisource.com
Website: http://www.nipsco.com
Regina Biddings, Dir., Communications and Community Rel.

Priorities: *Arts & Humanities:* 5%. Symphonies, united arts organizations, art centers, science exhibits and fairs, museums, performing arts, and historic preservation. *Civic & Public Affairs:* 10%. Civic organization membership. Funds also support nature preservation through assistance to wildlife organizations, and humane societies. *Education:* 10%. Schools, colleges, and universities, including agricultural education, engineering, literacy, vocational education, liberal arts, science and technology, and student aid. *International:* 55%. Organizations promoting health and safety, as well as individuals and families confronted with various health issues, including cancer, arthritis, heart disease, and lung disease. Includes social service funding that supports services for the good of the community, including youth organizations, food and clothing distribution, community service organizations, civil rights advocacy, and community centers. **Typ. Recipients:** Hospices, Hospitals, Nursing Services, People with Disabilities, Single-Disease Health Associations. **Geo. Dist:** headquarters and operating communities; IN, northern third of Indiana.

★ 12742 ★ Northern Trust Co. Charitable Trust
Community Affairs Division
50 S LaSalle St., M-5
Chicago, IL 60675
Phone: (312)444-4059
Email: eta1@ntrs.com
Website: http://www.ntrs.com/aboutus/community/index.html
Eleanor Alcantara, Contact

Priorities: *Arts & Humanities:* 10%. Priority is given to programs which reach out to the community, making cultural opportunities more accessible for hard-to-reach and disadvantaged populations. Art museums; music, dance, and theater organizations; and libraries receive support. *Civic & Public Affairs:* 15%. Supports projects designed to serve communities which have both limited local resources and the potential for significant development. Priority is given to programs which improve and increase affordable housing for low-income Cook County residents, and promote commercial and industrial development that creates and sustains jobs in low and moderate income neighborhoods. Recipients include community development organizations; zoos, aquariums, and horticultural societies; and minority organizations. *Education:* 12%. Contributes to higher education in the Chicago area, and nationally through the employee matching gifts program. Other priorities are groups which focus on prevention of school failure through early intervention, initiatives to improve the Chicago public school system, and programs that help the economically disadvantaged stay in school and further their education. *Environment:* 49%. Priority is given to programs that help the unemployed and underemployed break out of the cycle of poverty and public dependency, and that provide services to victims of domestic abuse. Youth groups, United Way, services for families and the disabled, substance abuse treatment facilities, community centers, and shelters receive support. *International:* 12%. Priority is given to programs which make primary healthcare services more accessible and affordable to low-income Cook County residents. Primarily funds hospitals, medical centers, and health foundations. *Religion:* 2%. Supports science centers and museums, and a planetarium. *Voluntarism:* Company supports a volunteer grants program which makes grants to organizations where employees volunteer. *Note:* Total contributions made in 2000. **Typ. Recipients:** Adolescent Health Issues, AIDS/HIV, Children's Health/Hospitals, Clinics/Medical Centers, Domestic Violence, Emergency/Ambulance Services, Family Planning, Health Funds, Health Organizations, Hospices, Hospitals, Medical Rehabilitation, Medical Training, Mental Health, Multiple Sclerosis, Nutrition, People with Disabilities, Public Health, Research/Studies Institutes, Sexual Abuse, Substance Abuse. **Geo. Dist:** Chicago, IL, metropolitan area, with priority given to Cook County.

★ 12743 ★ Northrop Grumman Corp.
1840 Century Park E, 131/cc
Los Angeles, CA 90067-2199
Phone: (310)553-6262 **Fax:** (310)556-4510
Website: http://www.northgrum.com
Cheryl Horn, Community Relations Manager

Typ. Recipients: Health-General. **Geo. Dist:** emphasis on company plants and employee living areas.

★ 12744 ★ Northwest Natural Gas Co.
220 Northwest 2nd Ave.
Portland, OR 97209
Phone: (503)226-4211 **Fax:** (503)220-2584
Email: george.richardson@nwnatural.com
Marie Krasnow, Administrative Assistant

Priorities: *Arts & Humanities:* 5%. Supports arts centers and funds, museums, music, performing arts, and visual arts. *Civic & Public Affairs:* 15%. Funding goes to economic development, housing, urban and community affairs, environmental concerns, and women's affairs. *Education:* 10%. Primary support goes to business education, colleges and universities, elementary education, and minority education. *Environment:* 45%. United Way. *International:* 15%. Supports hospices and hospitals, medical rehabilitation, mental health, the aged, child welfare, community centers, the disabled, food and clothing distribution, and traditional youth groups. **Typ. Recipients:** Health Organizations, Health-General, Hospices, Hospitals, Medical Rehabilitation, Mental Health, People with Disabilities, Single-Disease Health Associations, Substance Abuse. **Geo. Dist:** headquarters and operating communities.

★ 12745 ★ Novartis US Foundation
608 Fifth Ave.
New York, NY 10020
Phone: (212)307-1122 **Fax:** (212)246-0185
Website: http://www.novartis.com/corporate_citizenship/en/index.shtml
Sheldon Jones, Contact

Priorities: *Civic & Public Affairs:* 9%. *Education:* 50%. *Environment:* 6%. *International:* 34%. *Note:* Total contributions made in 2001. **Typ. Recipients:** Health Organizations, Nutrition. **Geo. Dist:** principally near operating locations and to national organizations.

★ 12746 ★ NYSEG Foundation, Inc.
PO Box 3287
Ithaca, NY 14852
Phone: (607)347-2530 **Fax:** (607)347-2417
Email: ptkarakantas@energyeast.com
Website: http://www.nyseg.com/nysegweb/ComCalendar.nsf/events?OpenView
Paul Karakantas, Treasurer/Secretary

Priorities: *Arts & Humanities:* 6%. Supports arts councils, living history centers, community arts organizations, opera, and libraries. *Civic & Public Affairs:* 5%. Gives to community foundations, The American Ireland Fund, and community initiatives. *Education:* 8%. Funding goes to schools for higher learning. *Environment:* 65%. Primarily supports the American Red Cross and United Ways. Also funds YMCAs and youth organizations. *International:* 8%. Funds medical centers and hospitals, hospice programs, and health foundations. *Religion:* 6%. Supports the Paleontological Research Institute and science centers. *Note:* Total contributions made in fiscal 2000. **Typ. Recipients:** Emergency/Ambulance Services, Health-General. **Geo. Dist:** headquarters and operating communities; Binghamton, NY; Ithaca, NY.

★ 12747 ★ Ohio National Foundation
PO Box 237
Cincinnati, OH 45201
Phone: (513)794-6594
Anthony Esposito, Vice President, Human Resources

Fnded: 1987. **Priorities:** *Arts & Humanities:* 15%. Funds public broadcasting, performing arts, arts funds, and museums. *Civic & Public Affairs:* 21%. Supports urban affairs, law/justice organizations, housing, police, community foundations, parks, and zoos. *Education:* 11%. Education foundations, colleges and universities, business and economic education programs, and parochial schools are supported. *Environment:* 41%. Majority of support goes to the United Way. Also funds Young Men's Christian Association, youth programs, Special Olympics, substance abuse prevention programs, and family services. *International:* 8%. Funds a children's hospital, single-disease health associations, home health care, and a hospice program. *Note:* Total contributions made in 2001. **Typ. Recipients:** AIDS/HIV, Alzheimers Disease, Cancer, Children's Health/Hospitals, Clinics/Medical Centers, Diabetes, Eyes/Blindness, Health Policy/Cost Containment, Health-General, Heart, Home-Care Services, Hospices, Hospitals, Medical Rehabilitation, Medical Research, Multiple Sclerosis, People with Disabilities, Public Health, Substance Abuse. **Geo. Dist:** Cincinnati, OH.

★ 12748 ★ Oklahoma Gas & Electric Co. Foundation
Box 321
Oklahoma City, OK 73101
Phone: (405)553-3196 **Fax:** (405)553-3567
Erma Elliot, Secretary & Treasurer

Fnded: 1957. **Priorities:** *Arts & Humanities:* 16%. Supports historic preservation, museums, music, and arts funds. *Civic & Public Affairs:* 6%. Economic and community development are typical areas of funding, with support also going to environmental, urban, and community affairs. *Education:* 56%. Supports colleges and universities, public and private secondary schools. Large grants consistently are given to Oklahoma City University, the University of Oklahoma, and Oklahoma State University. *Environment:* 18%. Supports YWCA, community services, family planning, food distribution, and scouts. *International:* 4%. Supports hospitals, health centers, medical research, and pediatric health. *Note:* Total foundation contributions made in 2000. **Typ. Recipients:** Children's Health/Hospitals, Clinics/Medical Centers, Emergency/Ambulance Services, Family Planning, Health Organizations, Health-General, Heart, Hospitals, Medical Education, Medical Research, People with Disabilities, Public Health. **Geo. Dist:** headquarters and operating communities; OK.

★ 12749 ★ The Oklahoman Foundation
PO Box 25125
Oklahoma City, OK 73125
Phone: (405)475-3200 **Fax:** (405)475-3128
Email: lbrown@oklahoman.com
Linda Brown, Executive Assistant

Fnded: 1990. **Priorities:** *Arts & Humanities:* 36%. Supports the National Cowboy Hall of Fame and Western Heritage Museum, and various art funds.

Civic & Public Affairs: 5%. *Education:* 31%. Primarily supports Oklahoma universities. *Environment:* 18%. Supports the United Way and US Olympic Committee. *International:* 11%. Primary support made to health organizations. *Religion:* 4%. Supports the Omniplex Science Museum. *Note:* Total foundation contributions made in 2000. **Typ. Recipients:** Child Abuse, Children's Health/Hospitals, Clinics/Medical Centers, Emergency/Ambulance Services, People with Disabilities, Public Health. **Geo. Dist:** Oklahoma City, OK.

★ 12750 ★ Old National Bank Charitable Trust

PO Box 718
Evansville, IN 47705
Phone: (812)461-9706 **Fax:** (812)465-0623
Email: cyndi_ozaki@oldnational.com
Cyndi Ozaki, Public Relations Representative

Fnded: 1957. **Priorities:** *Arts & Humanities:* 7%. Gives to Evansville area arts organizations, including museums, theaters, music, and historic preservation organizations. *Civic & Public Affairs:* 8%. Funds community beautification, housing, civic groups, minority affairs, and economic development. *Education:* 42%. Major support goes to colleges and universities. Other interests include private and public education at the elementary and secondary school levels. *Environment:* 24%. Primarily supports the United Way, youth organizations, and senior services. *International:* 13%. Supports medical rehabilitation, health centers, pregnancy care, and various single-disease health organizations. *Voluntarism:* The company encourages employee volunteerism through an informal volunteer program. *Note:* Total contributions made in 2001. **Typ. Recipients:** Adolescent Health Issues, Cancer, Children's Health/Hospitals, Clinics/Medical Centers, Emergency/Ambulance Services, Family Planning, Health Organizations, Health-General, Home-Care Services, Hospitals, Medical Education, Medical Rehabilitation, Medical Research, Multiple Sclerosis, People with Disabilities, Respiratory, Single-Disease Health Associations, Substance Abuse. **Geo. Dist:** IN, Gibson County; IN, Perry County; IN, Posey County; IN, Spencer County; IN, Vanderburg County; IN, Wabash County; IN, Warrick County; IN, White County; KY, Henderson County.

★ 12751 ★ Olin Corp. Charitable Trust

501 Merritt 7
PO Box 4500
Norwalk, CT 06856-4500
Phone: (203)750-3301 **Fax:** (203)750-3065
Email: cpiacentini@corp.olin.com
Website: http://www.olin.com/about/charitable.asp
Carmella Piacenini, Administrator

Priorities: *Arts & Humanities:* 7%. Major support for the Buffalo Bill Memorial Association. Also supports theaters, the performing arts, museums, libraries, ballet, and art centers. Predominant means of arts support is matching gifts program. *Civic & Public Affairs:* 13%. Recipients include local community affairs associations; minority and urban affairs groups; economics, business, free enterprise, and public policy organizations; municipal beautification projects; and an aquarium. *Education:* 39%. Primary support to higher education institutions, with emphasis on engineering, science, and technology. Private secondary schools are supported through matching gifts. Minority and pre-college programs also supported. The remainder supports educational associations, including scholarship programs. Sponsors matching gifts program for higher and secondary educational institutions. *Environment:* 23%. Primarily supports the United Way. Also funds youth groups and children's charities. *International:* 12%. Primary interests are hospitals and medical centers. Also supports single-disease health associations and ambulatory services. *Religion:* 1%. Funds a science museum. *Voluntarism:* Supports programs which include employee volunteers. Also awards Volunteer Recognition grants; organizations where employees volunteer receive grants of $500 to $3,000. *Note:* Total foundation contributions made in 2000. **Typ. Recipients:** Cancer, Children's Health/Hospitals, Clinics/Medical Centers, Emergency/Ambulance Services, Geriatric Health, Health Organizations, Hospices, Hospitals, Medical Education, Medical Rehabilitation, Mental Health, Nursing Services, Public Health, Single-Disease Health Associations, Substance Abuse. **Geo. Dist:** communities where employees work and live; some support for national organizations.

★ 12752 ★ OMNOVA Solutions Foundation

175 Ghent Rd.
Fairlawn, OH 44333-3300
Phone: (330)869-4000 **Fax:** (330)869-4345
Email: theresa.carter@omnova.com
Website: http://omnova.com/commfr.htm
S. Theresa Carter, Director

Fnded: 1999. **Priorities:** *Arts & Humanities:* 9%. Provides limited support to arts and cultural institutes and activities that promote cultural diversity and that broaden awareness and appreciation for the arts. *Civic & Public Affairs:* 30%. Supports urban renewal projects, crime prevention and safety, and community awareness of key issues and community educational opportunities. *Education:* 44%. Supports schools K-12, reading and economic literacy programs, math and science, school-to-work readiness, initiatives that encourage professional development for teachers, parental involvement, programs that advance status of the art technologies, state and local organizations that support and encourage educational excellence, and adult literacy programs where employees take an active role as tutors and volunteers. Provides technology partnership grants, student achievement awards, and scholarships. *Environment:* 14%. Primary support to the United Way; also funds disaster relief programs, youth organizations, and human services organizations focused on education or health, and supportive of clearly-defined community needs. *International:* 2%. Funds hospitals. *Voluntarism:* Company provides Community Leadership Awards to recognize employee involvement; supports Akron Reads literacy program. *Note:* Total contributions made in fiscal 2001. **Typ. Recipients:** Children's Health/Hospitals, Emergency/Ambulance Services.

★ 12753 ★ Omron Foundation

1 East Commerce Dr.
Schaumburg, IL 60173
Phone: (847)843-7900 **Fax:** (847)843-7931
Nicholas Hahn, Director

Fnded: 1988. **Priorities:** *Arts & Humanities:* 4%. Funds public broadcasting and an arts festival. *Civic & Public Affairs:* 11%. Funds civic foundations. *Education:* 39%. Funds universities and colleges. *Environment:* Funds Young Men's Christian Associations, hunger relief, and children's welfare. *International:* 17%. Funds single-disease health associations. *Note:* Total contributions made in fiscal 2001. **Typ. Recipients:** Alzheimers Disease, Cancer, Children's Health/Hospitals, Clinics/Medical Centers, Emergency/Ambulance Services, Family Planning, Health Organizations, Heart, Hospitals, Medical Research, Multiple Sclerosis, People with Disabilities, Prenatal Health Issues, Public Health, Respiratory, Single-Disease Health Associations. **Geo. Dist:** IL.

★ 12754 ★ ONDEO Nalco Foundation

1 ONDEO Nalco Center
Naperville, IL 60563-1198
Phone: (630)305-1566 **Fax:** (630)305-2896
Email: foundation@ondeo-nalco.com
Website: http://www.ondeo-nalco.com
Ellen DeLordo, President

Priorities: *Arts & Humanities:* 10%. Funds go to art institutes, community theater, performing arts, the symphony, and public broadcasting. *Civic & Public Affairs:* 30%. Supports boys and girls clubs, housing assistance, career training, and youth issues. *Education:* 35%. Supports junior achievement, pre-college and college education, arts education, training for disabled, and scholarship awards. *Environment:* 30%. *International:* 25%. Support goes to AIDs programs, single-disease research, equipment needs, substance abuse programs, care for the disabled, hospitals, and medical centers. *Religion:* 2%. *Note:* Total contributions made in 2001. **Typ. Recipients:** AIDS/HIV, Alzheimers Disease, Cancer, Children's Health/Hospitals, Clinics/Medical Centers, Domestic Violence, Emergency/Ambulance Services, Geriatric Health, Health Organizations, Health Policy/Cost Containment, Heart, Home-Care Services, Hospices, Hospitals, Hospitals (University Affiliated), Medical Education, Medical Rehabilitation, Medical Research, Mental Health, People with Disabilities, Prenatal Health Issues, Preventive Medicine/Wellness Organizations, Public Health, Single-Disease Health Associations, Substance Abuse, Trauma Treatment. **Geo. Dist:** Carson, CA; IL, DuPage County; Chicago, IL, metropolitan area; Garyville, LA; Freeport, TX; Sugarland, TX.

★ 12755 ★ One Valley Bank Foundation

BB & T
PO Box 1793
Charleston, WV 25326
Phone: (304)348-7000
Michael Stajduhar, Senior Vice President

Priorities: *Arts & Humanities:* 1%. Funds a library. *Civic & Public Affairs:* 1%. Funds a municipal leadership center. *Education:* 42%. Funds universities, colleges, and other educational groups. *Environment:* 43%. Funds United Way, shelters, food distribution, and scouting. *International:* 4%. Funds healthcare and hospice. *Note:* Total contributions made in 2000. **Typ. Recipients:** Children's Health/Hospitals, Clinics/Medical Centers, Health Organizations, Health Policy/Cost Containment, Health-General, Hospices, Hospitals, People with Disabilities, Single-Disease Health Associations. **Geo. Dist:** WV.

★ 12756 ★ OneBeacon Charitable Trust

One Beacon St.
Tax U.S. Department of B05-02
Boston, MA 02108-3107
Phone: (617)725-7529
Tom Ford, Vice President of Association Relations

Fnded: 1987. **Priorities:** *Civic & Public Affairs:* Less 7%. *Education:* 2%. Gives to private schools and seminaries. Also supports colleges, universities, education funds, and high schools. *Environment:* 91%. Funds scouting, youth organizations, and United Way. *Note:* Total foundation contributions made in 2000. **Typ. Recipients:** Cancer, Children's Health/Hospitals, Clinics/Medical Centers, Diabetes, Emergency/Ambulance Services, Health-General, Hospitals, Long-Term Care, Medical Research, Multiple Sclerosis, People with Disabilities, Prenatal Health Issues, Single-Disease Health Associations, Substance Abuse. **Geo. Dist:** nationally. **Frmly:** General Accident Charitable Trust CGU Charitable Trust.

★ 12757 ★ ONEOK, Inc.

PO Box 871
Tulsa, OK 74102-0871
Phone: (918)588-7000 **Fax:** (918)588-7490
Ginny Creveling, Administrator, Corporate Responsibility

Typ. Recipients: Health-General.

★ 12758 ★ Orange & Rockland Utilities, Inc.

1 Blue Hill Plaza
Pearl River, NY 10965
Phone: (845)577-2545 **Fax:** (845)577-6913
Email: fegerl@oru.com
Website: http://www.oru.com/community/
Linda Vessa-Feger, Manager, Corporate Programs

Typ. Recipients: Cancer, Health-General, Heart, Hospitals, Medical Research, People with Disabilities, Respiratory. **Geo. Dist:** headquarters and operating communities.

★ 12759 ★ Orscheln Industries Foundation, Inc.
PO Box 698
Moberly, MO 65270
Phone: (816)263-4377 **Fax:** (816)269-3520
Gerald Orscheln, Director

Fnded: 1968. **Priorities:** *Arts & Humanities:* 9%. Supports theaters and the performing arts. *Civic & Public Affairs:* 4%. Primarily supports community foundations. *Education:* 35%. Supports local schools and colleges, as well as religious colleges. Also sponsors scholarship awards program for Randolph County High School seniors, and provides scholarships to children of employees. *Environment:* 15%. Supports United Way, day care, community service centers, and youth organizations. *International:* 2%. Supports single-disease health associations and health centers. *Note:* Total foundation contributions in fiscal 2001. **Typ. Recipients:** Alzheimers Disease, Arthritis, Cancer, Clinics/Medical Centers, Health Funds, Health Organizations, Hospitals, Medical Education, Prenatal Health Issues, Public Health, Single-Disease Health Associations. **Geo. Dist:** MO, especially Randolph County.

★ 12760 ★ OSG Foundation
511 5th Ave.
New York, NY 10017-4093
Phone: (212)953-4100 **Fax:** (212)578-1832
Luis Alicea, Secretary

Priorities: *Arts & Humanities:* 1%. Supports museums, symphonies, dance, and public broadcasting. *Civic & Public Affairs:* 4%. Supports human rights, business interests, and ethnic organizations. *Education:* 4%. Majority of grants benefit colleges and universities. Also funds Junior Achievement. *Environment:* 3%. Supports children's organizations and recreation. *International:* 67%. Highest grants were given to Mount Sinai Medical Center. Remaining funds benefit medical centers, medical research, and single-disease health organizations. *Note:* Total contributions made in 2000. **Typ. Recipients:** AIDS/HIV, Cancer, Children's Health/Hospitals, Clinics/Medical Centers, Diabetes, Geriatric Health, Health Policy/Cost Containment, Heart, Hospitals, Medical Education, Medical Research, Mental Health, People with Disabilities, Respiratory, Single-Disease Health Associations, Substance Abuse, Transplant Networks/Donor Banks. **Geo. Dist:** New York, NY, metropolitan area.

★ 12761 ★ Oshkosh B'Gosh Foundation Inc.
112 Otter Ave.
Oshkosh, WI 54901
Phone: (920)231-8800 **Fax:** (920)231-8621
Website: http://www.oshkoshbgosh.com
Michael Wachtel, Executive Vice President

Priorities: *Arts & Humanities:* 15%. The Paine Art Center and Arboretum in Oshkosh, WI, receives major support. Music festivals, opera, orchestras, and arts funds are also supported. *Education:* 27%. Funds colleges, universities and educational foundations and programs. About 20% of total giving is devoted to scholarships, awarded to high school graduates from cities with company operating locations. *Environment:* 30%. United Way funding comprises about 20% of total giving. Additional funds support community service organizations and youth activities. *International:* 27%. Supports hospitals, health societies, and single-disease health associations. *Note:* Total contributions made in 2001. **Typ. Recipients:** Cancer, Child Abuse, Children's Health/Hospitals, Clinics/Medical Centers, Diabetes, Domestic Violence, Emergency/Ambulance Services, Eyes/Blindness, Health Organizations, Heart, Medical Education, Medical Rehabilitation, Mental Health, People with Disabilities, Respiratory, Sexual Abuse, Single-Disease Health Associations, Speech & Hearing. **Geo. Dist:** operating locations.

★ 12762 ★ Oshkosh Truck Foundation
2307 Oregon St.
PO Box 2566
Oshkosh, WI 54903-2566
Phone: (920)235-9151
Robert Bohn, Jr., President

Fnded: 1960. **Priorities:** *Arts & Humanities:* 5%. Supports art centers, music, and historic preservation. *Civic & Public Affairs:* 8%. *Education:* 18%. Supports schools, and educational foundations. *Environment:* 76%. Supports YMCA, United Way, substance abuse programs, and youth organizations. *International:* 1%. Primarily supports health organizations. *Religion:* Less than 1%. *Note:* Total contributions made in fiscal 2000. **Typ. Recipients:** Cancer, Clinics/Medical Centers, Domestic Violence, Emergency/Ambulance Services, Heart, People with Disabilities, Public Health, Sexual Abuse, Substance Abuse. **Geo. Dist:** Oshkosh, WI, and surrounding area.

★ 12763 ★ Owens Corning Foundation, Inc.
One Owens Corning Parkway
Toledo, OH 43659
Phone: (419)248-8000 **Fax:** (419)248-5689
Email: em.ross@owenscorning.com
Website: http://www.owenscorning.com/acquainted/support/
Mr. Emerson Ross, President & Treasurer

Priorities: *Arts & Humanities:* (Arts & Culture) 10%. Supports museums and galleries, music, and the performing arts. Also gives to arts associations and community arts groups. *Civic & Public Affairs:* (Civic & Community) 14%. Primary interests are business and free enterprise organizations and civil rights groups. Also supports organizations concerned with safety, public policy, and environmental, urban, and women's affairs. *Education:* 27%. Emphases include colleges and universities; business, economic, and engineering education; public and private precollege education programs; at-risk children's achievement programs; junior achievement; and minority education. Other interests include faculty development, literacy, community and junior colleges, and science and technology education. *Environment:* (Health & Human Services) 49%. Priority is affordable housing. Supports human service organizations in communities with major employee populations. Also supports united funds, community centers, organizations concerned with domestic violence and substance abuse, youth organizations, family services, the aged, delinquency and crime, health organizations, hospitals, and health-care cost containment. *International:* 7%. *Voluntarism:* The company sponsors the Owens Corning Volunteer of the Year award to recognize employee and retiree volunteer efforts. The Owens Corning Foundation provides grants in honor of the Volunteer of the Year finalists to charities of their choice. *Note:* Total contributions made in 2000. **Typ. Recipients:** Cancer, Medical Research, Mental Health, People with Disabilities, Preventive Medicine/Wellness Organizations, Respiratory, Substance Abuse. **Geo. Dist:** headquarters and operating communities; principally near operating locations and to national organizations.

★ 12764 ★ Owens-Illinois Inc.
1 Seagate
Toledo, OH 43666
Phone: (419)247-1386 **Fax:** (419)247-1436
Email: cheryl.johnson@usa.o-i.com
Cheryl Johnson, Contributions Administrator

Priorities: *Note:* Support for minority education is given only in areas of company operation. **Typ. Recipients:** Health-General. **Geo. Dist:** headquarters and operating communities.

★ 12765 ★ PACCAR Foundation
PO Box 1518
Bellevue, WA 98009-1518
Phone: (425)468-7400
Website: http://www.paccar.com/corp/foundation.asp
Norm Proctor, Vice President & General Manager

Fnded: 1951. **Priorities:** *Arts & Humanities:* 10%. Supports arts councils, orchestras, and art museums. *Civic & Public Affairs:* 5%. Supports community foundations, business and free enterprises, and public policy groups. *Education:* 20%. Primarily supports colleges and universities, including major support to independent college foundations. Also awards matching gifts and supports economic education. *Environment:* 57%. Major support for the United Way and Boy Scout troops; also funds youth organizations, child welfare, adult daycare services, and family services. *International:* 3%. Funds cancer organizations and cancer research, medical centers, and single-disease health associations addressing diseases that affect children. *Religion:* 3%. Supports science centers. *Note:* Total contributions made in 2000. **Typ. Recipients:** AIDS/HIV, Cancer, Children's Health/Hospitals, Clinics/Medical Centers, Emergency/Ambulance Services, Health Organizations, Hospitals, Medical Research, Mental Health, People with Disabilities, Research/Studies Institutes, Substance Abuse. **Geo. Dist:** headquarters and operating communities.

★ 12766 ★ Pacific Life Foundation
700 Newport Center Drive
Newport Beach, CA 92660-6397
Phone: (949)219-3787
Website: http://www.pacificlife.com/AboutPacificLife/FoundationorCommunity/index.htm
Robert Haskell, President

Priorities: *Arts & Humanities:* (Arts and Culture) 12%. Supports museums, symphonies, ballets, gardens and musical endeavors. *Civic & Public Affairs:* (Civic, Community, and Environment) 11%. Includes support for cultural diversity programs, urban affairs, community development organizations, and ecological and environmental concerns. *Education:* 32%. Supports universities, graduate schools, and drop-out programs. Also includes matching gifts to institutions of higher learning. *International:* (Health and Human Services) 45%. Supports the United Way, shelters, hospitals and single disease organizations such as the American Cancer Society and the American Heart Association. Funding also goes to children's advocacy groups and AIDS education/home care. *Voluntarism:* Company supports employee volunteerism through the Good Guys program, steering volunteers to local community projects. *Note:* Total contributions made in 2001. **Typ. Recipients:** AIDS/HIV, Alzheimers Disease, Cancer, Child Abuse, Children's Health/Hospitals, Domestic Violence, Emergency/Ambulance Services, Eyes/Blindness, Family Planning, Geriatric Health, Health Organizations, Health Policy/Cost Containment, Heart, Hospices, Hospitals, Medical Education, Medical Research, Medical Training, Mental Health, Multiple Sclerosis, Nutrition, People with Disabilities, Public Health, Single-Disease Health Associations, Speech & Hearing, Substance Abuse, Trauma Treatment. **Geo. Dist:** primarily to organizations in areas with large concentrations of company employees; some funding nationally; Phoenix, AZ; CA, Orange County, and some statewide organizations.

★ 12767 ★ PacifiCare Health System Foundation
3120 Lake Center Dr.
Mail Stop LC01-320
PO Box 25186
Santa Ana, CA 92799
Phone: (714)825-5233 **Fax:** (714)825-5028
Riva Gebel, Director

Fnded: 1996. **Priorities:** *Arts & Humanities:* 3%. *Civic & Public Affairs:* 5%. Supports clubs and community foundations. *Education:* 3%. Supports schools and educational programs. *Environment:* 14%. Supports the United Way, youth and family services, prevention of rape and child abuse, community counseling organizations, food distribution, shelters, and senior services. *International:* 76%. Supports health services and centers, single-disease health associations, hospices, hospitals, and medical centers. *Note:* Total foundation contributions made in 2000. **Typ. Recipients:** Adolescent Health Issues, AIDS/HIV, Alzheimers Disease, Arthritis, Cancer, Child Abuse, Children's Health/Hospitals, Clinics/Medical Centers, Diabetes, Domestic Violence, Emergency/Ambulance Services, Geriatric Health, Health Funds, Health Organizations, Health-General, Heart, Hospices, Hospitals, Long-Term Care, Medical Rehabilitation, People with Disabilities, Prenatal Health Issues, Preventive Medicine/

Wellness Organizations, Public Health, Sexual Abuse, Single-Disease Health Associations. **Geo. Dist:** AZ, within company service areas; CA, within company service area; CO, within company service areas; NV, within company service areas; OK, within company service area; OR, within company service area; TX, within company service areas; WA, within company service areas; within company service areas.

★ 12768 ★ PacifiCorp Foundation
825 NE Multnomah, Suite 2000
Portland, OR 97232-4116
Phone: (503)813-7257 **Fax:** (503)813-7249
Website: http://www.pacificorpfoundation.org/
Ernest Bloch, II, Executive Director

Fnded: 1988. **Priorities:** *Arts & Humanities:* 18%. Supports the performing arts, the visual arts, historic preservation, and public broadcasting. *Civic & Public Affairs:* 10%. Funds community chests, parks, recreation facilities, crime prevention, gardens, ethnic funds, and an aquarium. *Education:* 39%. Provides funds to educational and research institutions, both public and private, from elementary through university level. Also funds learning-related programs by special arrangement in alliance with others. *Environment:* 30%. Funds youth organizations, United Way, runaway youth services, domestic violence treatment and prevention, scouting, and Young Men's Christian Association. *Religion:* 3%. Supports a natural history museum. *Note:* Total contributions made in fiscal 2001. **Typ. Recipients:** Children's Health/Hospitals, Emergency/Ambulance Services, Family Planning, Health Organizations, Hospitals, People with Disabilities, Public Health. **Geo. Dist:** CA, Northern California; ID; NV; OR; UT; WA; WY.

★ 12769 ★ Paine Webber Foundation
1000 Harvard Boulevard
Weehawken, NJ 07086
Phone: (201)352-4324
Paul Greene, Foundation Contact

Fnded: 1879. **Priorities:** *Arts & Humanities:* 44%. Major support for the New York Public Library; also supports art museums. *Education:* 7%. Funds mentoring and educational programs. *Environment:* 31% Emphasis on the homeless and youth organizations. *International:* 18%. Major support for the New York Foundling Hospital. *Voluntarism:* The company sponsors a national volunteer initiative through which employees can access volunteer opportunities at local and national nonprofit organizations via the PaineWebber's Intranet system. *Note:* Total contributions in 1999. **Typ. Recipients:** AIDS/HIV, Arthritis, Cancer, Children's Health/Hospitals, Diabetes, Emergency/Ambulance Services, Health Organizations, Hospices, Hospitals, Medical Research, People with Disabilities, Public Health, Single-Disease Health Associations, Substance Abuse, Transplant Networks/Donor Banks. **Geo. Dist:** New York, NY.

★ 12770 ★ Pan-American Life Insurance Co.
Pan-American Life Center
601 Poydras St.
New Orleans, LA 70130
Phone: (504)566-3621 **Fax:** (504)566-3381
Todd Schexnayder, Senior Vice President Human Resources

Typ. Recipients: Medical Rehabilitation, Medical Research. **Geo. Dist:** headquarters area only.

★ 12771 ★ Park National Corp. Foundation
PO Box 3500
Newark, OH 43058-3500
Phone: (614)349-8451
Stuart Parsons, Trust Officer

Priorities: *Arts & Humanities:* 10%. Funds history organizations, arts centers, arts councils, and an orchestra. *Civic & Public Affairs:* 19%. Supports community festivals, parks, housing, and business and community development, and community foundations. *Education:* 14%. Contributes to colleges and universities, learning centers, public schools, private pre-college schools, and PTAs. *Environment:* 53%. Majority of social services funding is for local United Ways. Also funds scouting, YMCAs, and youth sports and recreation programs. *International:* 4%. Gives to health foundations, the American Red Cross, and United Cerebral Palsy. *Note:* Total contributions made in 2001. **Typ. Recipients:** Cancer, Domestic Violence, Emergency/Ambulance Services, Hospitals, Mental Health, Prenatal Health Issues, Public Health, Single-Disease Health Associations, Substance Abuse. **Geo. Dist:** OH.

★ 12772 ★ Park Place Entertainment Corp.
3930 Howard Hughes Parkway
Las Vegas, NV 89109
Phone: (702)699-5233 **Fax:** (702)691-2702
Website: http://www.parkplace.com
Brenda O'Boyle-Haynes, Director of Community Affairs

Typ. Recipients: Health-General. **Geo. Dist:** headquarters and operating communities.

★ 12773 ★ Parker Hannifin Foundation
6035 Parkland Boulevard
Cleveland, OH 44124-1290
Phone: (216)896-3000 **Fax:** (216)896-4057
Chris Semik, Administrative Assistant

Priorities: *Arts & Humanities:* 10%. Major support goes to theater groups. Other recipients include arts centers, museums, and music and dance groups. *Civic & Public Affairs:* 27%. Emphasis is on economic development organizations. Other recipients include environmental affairs organizations and police and fire departments in plant communities. *Education:* 34%. Funds matching gifts to educational institutions. Major support is provided to colleges, universities, and funds for higher education. Focus on economic education. *Environment:* 24%. Majority of funds go to United Way drives in plant communities. Also provides substantial support to youth organizations, particularly to local Boy Scouts/Girl Scouts, YMCA/YWCA, and Junior Achievement chapters. Other recipients include organizations concerned with child welfare, the handicapped, and recreation and athletics, as well as local chapters of the Salvation Army and the Red Cross. *International:* 1%. Focus is on hospitals and medical centers. Other interests include single-disease health organizations, and clinics. Remaining funds support ambulance services, pediatric health, mental health, and medical research programs. *Religion:* 4%. Supports science centers and museums. *Note:* Total contributions made in fiscal 2001. **Typ. Recipients:** Children's Health/Hospitals, Emergency/Ambulance Services, Health Funds, Health Organizations, Hospitals, Medical Research, Mental Health, Nursing Services, Outpatient Health Care, Single-Disease Health Associations, Substance Abuse. **Geo. Dist:** nationally.

★ 12774 ★ Patagonia, Inc.
PO Box 150
Ventura, CA 93002-0150
Phone: (805)643-8616 **Fax:** (805)667-4740
Email: jil_zilligen@patagonia.com
Jil Zilligen, Vice President Environmental Initiatives

Priorities: *Note:* Contributions made in fiscal 2000. **Typ. Recipients:** Family Planning. **Geo. Dist:** nationally; Europe.

★ 12775 ★ Paul R. Gingher State Auto Insurance Cos. Foundation
518 E Broad St.
Columbus, OH 43215-3976
Phone: (614)464-5000
Noreen Johnson, Director, Technology Communications

Fnded: 1989. **Priorities:** *Arts & Humanities:* 2%. Supports music, museums, and dance. *Civic & Public Affairs:* 27%. Supports housing, community development, zoos, festivals, and community foundations. *Education:* 12%. Supports universities, colleges, academies, and educational funds. *Environment:* 58%. Supports United Way, youth organizations, child welfare, food distribution, and scouts. *International:* 1%. Primary support made to hospices. *Note:* Total foundation contributions made in 2001. **Typ. Recipients:** Child Abuse, Family Planning, Hospices, People with Disabilities.

★ 12776 ★ Pella Rolscreen Foundation
102 Main St.
Pella, IA 50219
Phone: (641)621-6224
Email: mavzante@pella.com
Mary Van Zante, Secretary

Priorities: *Arts & Humanities:* 3%. Primarily supports historical organizations, public broadcasting, museums, libraries, and performing arts. *Civic & Public Affairs:* 70%. Interests include economic development, municipalities, and housing. *Education:* 16%. Majority of education funds support colleges and universities in Iowa in the form of scholarship and capital grants. Also sponsors a scholarship program for children of company employees. *Environment:* 2%. Most contributions are made to recreational and athletic programs and centers, child welfare, community service organizations, and united funds. *International:* 3%. *Religion:* 1%. *Note:* Total foundation contributions made in 2000. **Typ. Recipients:** AIDS/HIV, Cancer, Child Abuse, Clinics/Medical Centers, Emergency/Ambulance Services, Health Policy/Cost Containment, Hospices, Hospitals, Outpatient Health Care, People with Disabilities, Substance Abuse, Transplant Networks/Donor Banks. **Geo. Dist:** IA, central and western Iowa.

★ 12777 ★ PEMCO Foundation
325 Eastlake Ave. E
Seattle, WA 98109
Phone: (206)628-5760
Stan McNaughton, Foundation Administrator

Priorities: *Arts & Humanities:* 7%. *Civic & Public Affairs:* 2%. *Education:* 31%. *Environment:* 33%. *International:* 19%. *Religion:* 2%. *Note:* Total contributions made in fiscal 2002. **Typ. Recipients:** Cancer, Children's Health/Hospitals, Clinics/Medical Centers, Domestic Violence, Emergency/Ambulance Services, Emergency/Ambulance Services, Geriatric Health, Health Funds, Health Organizations, Health-General, Heart, Home-Care Services, Hospices, Hospitals, Kidney, Medical Rehabilitation, Multiple Sclerosis, People with Disabilities, Research/Studies Institutes, Respiratory, Single-Disease Health Associations, Trauma Treatment. **Geo. Dist:** WA.

★ 12778 ★ Penn Mutual Life Insurance Co.
C3A
600 Dresher Rd.
Horsham, PA 19044
Phone: (215)956-8060 **Fax:** (215)956-8347
Donna Beath, Contributions Coordinator

Priorities: *Voluntarism:* Employee volunteers support United Way related events. **Typ. Recipients:** Health-General. **Geo. Dist:** DE; NJ; NY; PA.

★ 12779 ★ Pentair Foundation
1500 County Rd. B2 West
Saint Paul, MN 55113-3105
Phone: (651)636-7920 **Fax:** (651)639-5203
Website: http://www.pentair.com/foundation.html
Michelle Murphy, Foundation Manager

Priorities: *Arts & Humanities:* 11%. Funds programs that provide a solid cultural base and offer opportunities to experience art in many different forms. Encourages development and preservation of artistic and cultural traditions; broadening and expanding the audience base for the arts so they are accessible for all; and development and expansion of programs that offer educational and developmental opportunities in literature, music, and theater. *Civic & Public Affairs:* 29%. Supports mentoring and tutoring opportunities for youth, together with general guidance and recreation; programs which encourage economic self-reliance among individuals; job training for youth, the disadvantaged, and the disabled; and low-income housing. *Education:* 19%. Supports elementary, secondary, and higher education programs that provide innovative education opportunities for youth; target socially and economically disadvantaged youth; bring business concepts, practices, and principles into the classroom; and provide a trade curriculum to add skilled workers to the work force. *Environment:* 33%. Funds United Ways, disaster relief organizations, youth organizations, services for the disabled, Girl and Boy Scouts, and senior centers. *International:* 5%. Supports programs which ensure access to adequate health care and health care education, including rehabilitation services for the disabled, particularly youth; effective, low-cost health care services for those who are unable to afford adequate health care; and educational information and promotion of sound physical and mental health and development. *Religion:* 1%. Supports a science museum. *Note:* Total contributions made in 2000. **Typ. Recipients:** Emergency/Ambulance Services, Family Planning, Health Organizations, Health-General, Medical Rehabilitation. **Geo. Dist:** headquarters and operating communities; Minneapolis, MN, metropolitan area; St. Paul, MN, metropolitan area; OH.

★ 12780 ★ Peoples Energy Corp.
130 E Randolph Dr.
Chicago, IL 60601
Phone: (312)240-7516 **Fax:** (312)240-4389
Richard Turner, Manager, Corporate Contributions

Priorities: *Arts & Humanities:* Supports performance and visual arts, historical societies, libraries, museums, and cultural institutions. *Civic & Public Affairs:* Supports neighborhood development interests that address community and economic development efforts; housing programs; job development and job training; community organizing; and leadership development. *Education:* Education priorities include organizations and programs that address system and system-wide issues; basic literacy and school readiness; professional development for teachers and school personnel; relationships between community residents and local schools; partnerships and collaborative efforts with business and volunteers; assistance to help economically disadvantaged students further their education; and early intervention designed to prevent failing grades. *International:* Supports organizations that make quality health care affordable and accessible, including neighborhood medical care, prevention efforts, and educational programming. Priority is placed on projects that focus on the health of high risk populations; access to quality healthcare for low-income families; and outreach to promote, develop, and maintain a healthy lifestyle. *Voluntarism:* Company sponsors an employee volunteer program at a local childcare agency and in annual community service projects. *Note:* Contributions analysis provided by foundation. **Typ. Recipients:** Health Organizations, Hospitals. **Geo. Dist:** company service area.

★ 12781 ★ Pepco Holdings, Inc.
701 9th NW, Suite 1003
Washington, DC 20068
Phone: (202)872-3488 **Fax:** (202)872-2472
Website: http://www.pepco.com
Pamela Holman, Contributions Coordinator

Priorities: *Arts & Humanities:* 30% to 35%. Nationally known performing arts centers in Washington, D.C. commonly receive large grants. Interests also include music and opera, theater, public broadcasting, libraries, and historic preservation. *Education:* 15% to 20%. Extensive support is given to colleges anduniversities; also supports education funds, minority and scientific education, student aid, and literacy. *Environment:* 35% to 40%. Main priority is united funds. The remainder supports organizations dealing with youth, the elderly, drug and alcohol abuse, the disabled, and employment. *International:* 5% to 10%. Interests include hospitals, hospices, health organizations, and pediatric health. **Typ. Recipients:** Health Organizations, Hospices, Hospitals, Medical Research, People with Disabilities, Single-Disease Health Associations, Substance Abuse. **Geo. Dist:** Washington, DC, company service area of greater Washington DC.

★ 12782 ★ PepsiCo Foundation, Inc.
700 Anderson Hill Rd.
Purchase, NY 10577
Phone: (914)253-3153 **Fax:** (914)253-3553
Jacqueline Millan, Vice President, Contributions

Fnded: 1962. **Priorities:** *Arts & Humanities:* 5%. Supports opera, dance, theater, museums, and historical societies. *Civic & Public Affairs:* 11%. Funds the National Urban League, community and neighborhood affairs. *Education:* 57%. Support is given to major colleges and universities; education programs for minorities, including scholarships and leadership development; and scholarships for children of employees. *Environment:* 24%. Provides major support to the United Way. Also supports youth organizations, senior services and other social service organizations. *International:* 1%. *Voluntarism:* Contributions are matched dollar for dollar to institutions and organizations that are determined tax-exempt by the I.R.S. When an employee volunteers in addition to a financial contribution, the foundation will double the match. Employee Community Involvement Grants are made to non-profit organizations where employees volunteer. *Note:* Total contributions made in 1999, excluding matching gifts. **Typ. Recipients:** Cancer, Children's Health/Hospitals, Clinics/Medical Centers, Emergency/Ambulance Services, Family Planning, Health Organizations, Hospitals, Medical Education, Multiple Sclerosis, People with Disabilities, Substance Abuse. **Geo. Dist:** headquarters and operating communities.

★ 12783 ★ Pfizer Foundation
235 East 42nd St.
New York, NY 10017-5755
Phone: 800-733-4717
Email: Grant.Info@Pfizer.com
Website: http://www.pfizer.com/pfizerinc/philanthropy
Rick Luftglass, Grants Coordinator

Priorities: *Arts & Humanities:* 8%. Priority is given to arts and cultural organizations identified as making a positive contribution to the cultural life of a Pfizer operating community. Primary focus is on New York City. Cultural organizations eligible for funding include, but are not limited to, art education programs, museums, performing arts organizations, and cultural and performing arts centers. Programs that strive to develop working relationships between business and the arts community also are funded. *Civic & Public Affairs:* 12%. Focus is on New York City. Grants support programs such as community organizations and development, botanical gardens, aquariums, and non-profit management assistance providers. Through this fund, the company invests in nonprofit organizations dedicated to breaking the cycle of poverty through innovative, entrepreneurial programs that create wealth in local communities. Funds organizations that address urgent community needs, seek long-term solutions to community issues, and strengthen to cultural vitality of diverse communities. *Education:* 38%. Preference given to schools at which Pfizer recruits; to schools located in Pfizer facility communities; and to educational programs that relate to the company's business operations in math and science-based disciplines. Focus is on science and math K-12 education, especially improving understanding of scientific principles and the importance of scientific innovation. Supports organizations that develop and apply systematic, sustainable strategies to improve teaching and learning, such as implementation of hands-on, inquiry-based science curricula, teacher training, and the upgrading of labs. Supports exhibits and educational outreach programs at various science-rich institutions as well as collaborations between Pfizer sites and local schools. *Environment:* 5%. *International:* 44%. Supports patient education programs; programs that help people live healthier, more productive lives; therapeutic programs including those targeting hypertension, diabetes and depression; community health centers; social service providers; technical assistance providers; health communications technology to provide access to up-to-date health information; projects for changing the health care system; maternal and child health; and women's health issues. Focus is on community-based efforts to improve the health of those at greatest risk for poor health outcomes. *Religion:* 1%. *Voluntarism:* The company sponsors the Pfizer Volunteer Program (PVP) which provides grants of $1,000 to nonprofit organizations with which the company's employees and retirees are regularly involved. *Note:* Total contributions made in 2001. **Typ. Recipients:** Adolescent Health Issues, AIDS/HIV, Alzheimers Disease, Arthritis, Arthritis, Cancer, Child Abuse, Children's Health/Hospitals, Clinics/Medical Centers, Diabetes, Emergency/Ambulance Services, Eyes/Blindness, Geriatric Health, Health Funds, Health Organizations, Health Policy/Cost Containment, Health-General, Home-Care Services, Hospices, Hospitals, Medical Education, Medical Rehabilitation, Medical Research, Mental Health, People with Disabilities, Preventive Medicine/Wellness Organizations, Public Health, Single-Disease Health Associations, Substance Abuse, Transplant Networks/Donor Banks. **Geo. Dist:** principally near operating locations and to national organizations; New York, NY.

★ 12784 ★ Phelps Dodge Foundation
2600 N Central Ave.
Phoenix, AZ 85004-3014
Phone: (602)366-8100 **Fax:** (602)234-8082
Email: phx-communityaffairs@phelpsdodge.com
Website: http://www.phelpsdodge.com/index-community.html
Ann Gibson, Community Affairs

Priorities: *Arts & Humanities:* 17%. Supports symphonies, opera, museums, performing arts, and historic preservation. Limited support to art funds and centers. *Civic & Public Affairs:* 3%. Primarily supports zoos. *Education:* 56%. Primarily supports scholarships to colleges and universities. Funding also emphasizes scientific, technological, mining, and business education. Interests include minority and independent college funds, community colleges, and medical education. *Environment:* 3%. Supports family planning and domestic violence shelters. *International:* 21%. Supports children's health centers, electrical safety, hospitals, crisis nurseries, prevention of domestic violence, and public health and safety. *Religion:* 1%. *Note:* Total foundation contributions made in 2000. **Typ. Recipients:** Cancer, Child Abuse, Children's Health/Hospitals, Clinics/Medical Centers, Domestic Violence, Emergency/Ambulance Services, Family Planning, Geriatric Health, Health Funds, Health Organizations, Hospitals, Kidney, Medical Education, Medical Research, Medical Training. **Geo. Dist:** communities where company maintains major operating facilities.

★ 12785 ★ Philips Electronics North America Corp.
1251 Ave. of the Americas
New York, NY 10020
Phone: (212)536-0500

Priorities: *Education:* 100%. The company's charitable activities go directly to support a scholarship program. *Note:* Total contributions made in 1998. **Typ. Recipients:** Hospitals, Medical Education. **Geo. Dist:** operating areas.

★ 12786 ★ Phoenix Foundation
1 American Row
Hartford, CT 06102-5056
Phone: (860)403-5863 **Fax:** (860)403-5755
Email: Tina.Muzzy@phoenixwm.com
Website: http://www.phoenixwm.com
Jane Driscoll, Vice President

Priorities: *Arts & Humanities:* 23%. *Civic & Public Affairs:* 13%. *Education:* 33%. *Environment:* 21%. *International:* 9%. *Note:* Total contributions made in 2001. **Typ. Recipients:** AIDS/HIV, Cancer, Children's Health/Hospitals, Emergency/Ambulance Services, Health-General, Hospices, Hospitals, Prenatal Health Issues, Single-Disease Health Associations. **Geo. Dist:** nationally.

★ 12787 ★ Phoenix Foundation
1945 The Exchange, Suite 300
Atlanta, GA 30339-2029
Phone: (770)953-0304

Fnded: 1957. **Priorities:** *Arts & Humanities:* 9%. Primarily supports museums and art centers. *Civic & Public Affairs:* 4%. Supports justice, community foundations, and professional organizations. *Education:* 40%. Supports education councils and higher education. *Environment:* 17%. Supports Boy Scouts, United Way, and family services. *International:* 2%. Supports recovery centers. *Note:* Total contributions made in 2000. **Typ. Recipients:** Preventive Medicine/Wellness Organizations, Public Health. **Geo. Dist:** GA. **Frmly:** Phoenix Foundation.

★ 12788 ★ Physicians Mutual Insurance Co. Foundation
2600 Dodge St.
Omaha, NE 68131
Phone: (402)633-1000 **Fax:** (402)633-1096
Jerome Coon, Secretary/Treasurer

Priorities: *Arts & Humanities:* 4. Supports public broadcasting, theater, museums, and music. *Civic & Public Affairs:* 7%. Supports community foundations, professional organizations, justice, and civic policy. *Education:* 37%. Supports colleges, universities, and secondary and primary education. *Environment:* 49%. Supports food banks, family services, veterans organizations, scouting, disabilities organizations, and United Way. *International:* 2%. Funds single-disease health associations and hospitals. *Note:* Total contributions made in fiscal 2001. **Typ. Recipients:** Alzheimers Disease, Arthritis, Cancer, Children's Health/Hospitals, Diabetes, Emergency/Ambulance Services, Health Organizations, Health Policy/Cost Containment, Health-General, Heart, Hospices, Hospitals, Long-Term Care, Medical Research, Multiple Sclerosis, Nursing Services, People with Disabilities, Public Health, Respiratory, Single-Disease Health Associations, Substance Abuse. **Geo. Dist:** NE; Alexandria, VA.

★ 12789 ★ Piedmont Charitable Foundation
7 Piedmont Center, Suite 100
Atlanta, GA 30305
Phone: (404)816-5205 **Fax:** (404)816-3537
J. Robinson, President

Fnded: 1957. **Priorities:** *Arts & Humanities:* 8%. Historic preservation and art centers are funded. *Civic & Public Affairs:* 4%. Funds chambers of commerce and business forums. *Education:* 67%. Supports higher education, literacy, and educational enrichment. *Environment:* 11%. Supports services for youth. *International:* 1%. *Note:* Total contributions in 1999. **Typ. Recipients:** Cancer, Children's Health/Hospitals, Clinics/Medical Centers, Geriatric Health, Hospitals, Public Health, Single-Disease Health Associations. **Geo. Dist:** GA.

★ 12790 ★ Pieper Power Foundation, Inc.
5070 North 35th St.
Milwaukee, WI 53209-5302
Phone: (414)462-7700 **Fax:** (414)462-7711
Website: http://www.pieperpower.com
Donna Ebert, Executive Secretary

Priorities: *Arts & Humanities:* 12%. *Civic & Public Affairs:* 7%. *Education:* 22%. *Environment:* 55%. *International:* 2%. *Note:* Total contributions made in 2001. **Typ. Recipients:** Children's Health/Hospitals, Clinics/Medical Centers, Domestic Violence, Emergency/Ambulance Services, Eyes/Blindness, Family Planning, Heart, Multiple Sclerosis, People with Disabilities, Research/Studies Institutes, Single-Disease Health Associations, Speech & Hearing. **Geo. Dist:** Milwaukee, WI. **Frmly:** Pieper Power Foundation, Inc.

★ 12791 ★ Pillsbury Co. Foundation
200 South, 6th St.
Minneapolis, MN 55402-1464
Phone: (612)330-5046
William Birtcil, Executive Director

Fnded: 1957. **Priorities:** *Civic & Public Affairs:* 8%. Supports community foundations, and organizations and programs that offer educational and employment skills young people need to achieve self-sufficiency. Typically funds career awareness/work readiness, life skills, and employment programs. *Education:* 6%. Supports universities, schools, and educational programs. Funds public and private precollege and higher education. Also provides scholarships to children of employees. *Environment:* 82%. Supports United Way, youth groups, family services, food distribution, YWCA, and organizations that build and sustain ongoing relationships with caring adults and at-risk young people. *International:* Less than 1%. *Voluntarism:* Company offers employee volunteer opportunities, and gives priority to organizations where employees volunteer. *Note:* Total foundation contributions in fiscal 2001. **Typ. Recipients:** Children's Health/Hospitals, Clinics/Medical Centers, Family Planning, Hospitals, Medical Rehabilitation, Nutrition, Prenatal Health Issues. **Geo. Dist:** headquarters and operating communities.

★ 12792 ★ Pioneer Investments Management USA, Inc.
60 State St., 5th Fl.
Boston, MA 02109
Phone: (617)742-7825 **Fax:** (617)422-4293
Susan Bullock, Sr. Corporate Paralegal

Typ. Recipients: Clinics/Medical Centers, Health-General. **Geo. Dist:** headquarters and operating communities.

★ 12793 ★ Pitney Bowes Inc.
1 Elmcroft Rd.
Stamford, CT 06926-0700
Phone: (203)351-6669 **Fax:** (203)351-6303
Email: polly.obrien@pb.com
Website: http://www.pb.com
Polly O'Brien, Director, Community Investment

Priorities: *Voluntarism:* Employee volunteerism is encourage through the company's National Week of Caring and PB People: Building Stronger Communities programs. **Typ. Recipients:** Hospitals. **Geo. Dist:** headquarters and operating communities.

★ 12794 ★ Pittway Corp. Charitable Foundation
200 S Wacker Dr., Suite 3900
Chicago, IL 60606-5802
Phone: (312)831-4130 **Fax:** (312)382-0722
Paul Gauvreau, Treasurer

Priorities: *Arts & Humanities:* 10%. Emphasis on public broadcasting, museums, history, and arts institutes. *Civic & Public Affairs:* 4%. Funds economic development, business and free enterprise, promotion of democracy, and urban and community programs. *Education:* 34%. Supports colleges and universities, early education, literacy programs, and education funds. *Environment:* 35%. Focuses on programs working to break the intergenerational transmission of poverty. Family planning and family services receive much of this funding, as well as united funds. Child welfare, food and clothing distribution, and youth organizations are also supported. *International:* 10%. Funds support hospitals, various single-disease health organizations, pediatric health, and other facilities. *Religion:* 1%. Funds laboratories and institutes specializing in biological, cancer, neurobiology and plant genetics research. *Note:* Total foundation contributions made in fiscal 2000. **Typ. Recipients:** Alzheimers Disease, Cancer, Children's Health/Hospitals, Clinics/Medical Centers, Family Planning, Health Funds, Hospices, Hospitals, Medical Education, Medical Rehabilitation, Medical Research, Mental Health, Nursing Services, People with Disabilities, Prenatal Health Issues, Single-Disease Health Associations, Substance Abuse. **Geo. Dist:** emphasis on communities near company's manufacturing sites.

★ 12795 ★ Playboy Foundation
680 N Lake Shore Dr.
Chicago, IL 60611
Phone: (312)751-8000 **Fax:** (312)266-8506
Email: cleow@playboy.com
Website: http://www.playboyenterprises.com/foundation
Cleo Wilson, Executive Director

Typ. Recipients: Domestic Violence, Family Planning, Medical Research, People with Disabilities, Single-Disease Health Associations. **Geo. Dist:** nationally.

★ 12796 ★ PNC Foundation
One PNC Plaza, 29th Floor
249 Fifth Ave.
Pittsburgh, PA 15222
Phone: (412)762-7076 **Fax:** (412)705-1062
Email: foundations@pncbank.com
Website: http://www.pnc.com/aboutus/pncfoundation.html
Mia Hallett, Vice President and Manager

Fnded: 1970. **Priorities:** *Arts & Humanities:* 18%. Supports local symphony organizations and music groups, public broadcasting, libraries, museums, opera, and arts associations, festivals, and arts centers. *Civic & Public Affairs:* 25%. Primary support to economic development and urban affairs. Other interests include international affairs, public policy, economics, civil rights, women's interests, and business and free enterprise. *Education:* 11%. Major support goes to local colleges and universities. Also gives to public and private precollege education, minority education, and education funds. *Environment:* (Health and Human Services) 24%. Supports the United Way in southwestern Pennsylvania. Also contributes to organizations concerned with youth, the elderly, the disabled, food distribution, community and family services, and emergency relief. Health concerns include local hospitals, single-disease health associations, health funds, medical rehabilitation, and pediatric health. *International:* 1%. *Note:* Total contributions made in 2001. **Typ. Recipients:** Cancer, Children's Health/Hospitals, Clinics/Medical Centers, Domestic Violence, Health Organizations, Heart, Home-Care Services, Hospices, Hospitals, Long-Term Care, Medical Rehabilitation, People with Disabilities, Single-Disease Health Associations. **Geo. Dist:** areas served by PNC Bank Corp. and affiliates. **Frmly:** PNC Bank Foundation.

★ 12797 ★ PNM Foundation
Alvarado Sq., MS 2708
Albuquerque, NM 87158-2708
Phone: (505)241-2237
Chandra Manning, Sr. Community Relations Representative

Fnded: 1983. **Priorities:** *Arts & Humanities:* 12%. Supports music and art programs. *Civic & Public Affairs:* 21%. Primarily supports community foundations. *Education:* 56%. Supports literacy, schools, and educational funds. *Environment:* 11%. Supports homes and recreation. *International:* 7%. *Note:* Total contributions made in 1999. **Typ. Recipients:** Cancer, Diabetes, Health Organizations, Hospices, Hospitals, Prenatal Health Issues, Preventive Medicine/Wellness Organizations, Respiratory, Speech & Hearing, Transplant Networks/Donor Banks. **Geo. Dist:** NM.

★ 12798 ★ Polaroid Foundation
784 Memorial Drive
Cambridge, MA 02139
Phone: (781)386-9400 **Fax:** (781)386-9818
Email: polaroid.foundation@polaroid.com
Website: http://www.polaroid.com/polinfo/foundation
Donna Eidson, Executive Director

Priorities: *Arts & Humanities:* 12%. *Civic & Public Affairs:* 73%. *International:* 15%. *Voluntarism:* Polaroid employees who volunteer 50+ hours of personal time per calendar year at a nonprofit organization can apply to the Polaroid Foundation for a $1,000 grant for that organization. Information on Polaroid's Volunteer Action Program is available from (800)480-4438. Polaroid employees also have the opportunity to volunteer on grantmaking committees; on company time, employee volunteers review grant proposals, visit agencies, and make funding recommendations under the direction of foundation staff members. *Note:* Total contributions made in 2001. **Typ. Recipients:** AIDS/HIV, Clinics/Medical Centers, Diabetes, Domestic Violence, Eyes/Blindness, Heart, Hospices, Hospitals, Medical Education, Medical Research, Mental Health, Nursing Services, People with Disabilities, Public Health, Speech & Hearing. **Geo. Dist:** internationally for product donations; nationally for product donations; nationally: considers funding outside of Massachusetts to historically black educational institutions; Boston, MA, metropolitan area; Cambridge, MA; New Bedford, MA, including surrounding area; Waltham, MA.

★ 12799 ★ Post and Courier Foundation

134 Columbus St.
Charleston, SC 29403-4800
Phone: (843)937-5789
J. Donehue, Administrator

Priorities: *Arts & Humanities:* 14%. Museums, historic foundations, music, ballet, and art associations receive support. *Civic & Public Affairs:* 6%. Primary support goes to ethnic affairs, trade associations, and community affairs. *Education:* 10%. Recipients include South Carolina colleges, secondary schools, and educational organizations. *Environment:* 19%. Majority of funding supports Carolina Youth Development Center and the United Way. *International:* 16%. Supports health care centers, single-disease associations, and hospice. *Note:* Total contributions made in 1999. **Typ. Recipients:** Cancer, Health-General, Hospices, Medical Education, Medical Rehabilitation, People with Disabilities, Preventive Medicine/Wellness Organizations, Speech & Hearing. **Geo. Dist:** headquarters area only.

★ 12800 ★ PPG Industries Foundation

One PPG Pl.
Pittsburgh, PA 15272
Phone: (412)434-2788
Website: http://corporate.ppg.com/PPG/corporate/AboutUs/PPGIndustriesFoundation/default.htm
Jeffrey Gilbert, Executive Director

Priorities: *Arts & Humanities:* (Culture) 8%. Pittsburgh arts organizations, including symphonies, libraries, and museums. Also supports local performing arts organizations and public broadcasting. *Civic & Public Affairs:* (Civic & Community Affairs) 3%. Research, education, and the dissemination of information related to the areas of economic education and development, and public policy issues. Large grants are awarded to support economic development and public policy groups. Other recipients include business and free enterprise, and civil rights groups. *Education:* 29%. Most grants support higher education, with emphasis on private colleges and universities, especially those in plant communities and those with engineering and science programs. Of special interest are science-based efforts that attract students to chemistry, business, and engineering; education for minorities; and support of students achieving high academic standards. Other areas receiving major gifts include college funds, minority engineering and other education associations, and precollege education. Awards include capital and operating support. *Environment:* (Human Services) 27%. Primarily United Way campaigns, which receive about two-thirds of human service funds. Other grants are allocated for capital projects and special programs to provide support for new facilities and changing services. *International:* (Health & Safety) 2%. Improved patient care, effective delivery of services, and educational programs. *Voluntarism:* Sponsors the GIVE Program to recognize employee involvement in volunteerism. Employees may apply for one grant of $250 annually to benefit an eligible non-profit organization for whom they volunteer. *Note:* Total contributions made in 2001. **Typ. Recipients:** Clinics/Medical Centers, Emergency/Ambulance Services, Eyes/Blindness, Health Organizations, Health Policy/Cost Containment, Hospitals, Long-Term Care, Medical Rehabilitation, Mental Health, Nursing Services, People with Disabilities, Public Health, Single-Disease Health Associations. **Geo. Dist:** headquarters and operating communities; nationally; Pittsburgh, PA.

★ 12801 ★ Praxair Foundation

39 Old Ridgebury Rd.
Danbury, CT 06810-5113
Phone: (203)837-2000 **Fax:** (203)837-2550
Nigel Muir, President & Director

Fnded: 1995. **Priorities:** *Arts & Humanities:* 3%. Funds public libraries. *Civic & Public Affairs:* 24%. Supports minority/women's organizations and professional associations (particularly associations of engineers and scientists), gardens, municipalities, economic development, and public policy. *Education:* 23%. Primarily supports universities and colleges, especially those that focus on science, technology, and engineering education. *Environment:* 4%. Supports scouts, youth sports and recreation programs, YMCAs, United Way, and youth welfare organizations. *International:* 41%. Funds hospice programs, single-disease health organizations, and medical centers, with cancer, AIDS, and multiple sclerosis organizations receiving significant funding. *Religion:* 2%. Supports science institutes and museums. *Note:* Total contributions made in fiscal 2000. **Typ. Recipients:** AIDS/HIV, Cancer, Children's Health/Hospitals, Clinics/Medical Centers, Emergency/Ambulance Services, Health-General, Heart, Hospices, Hospitals, Medical Education, Medical Rehabilitation, Multiple Sclerosis, Single-Disease Health Associations, Transplant Networks/Donor Banks.

★ 12802 ★ Premcor

8182 Maryland Ave.
Saint Louis, MO 63105
Phone: (314)854-9804 **Fax:** (314)854-1580
Website: http://www.premcor.com
Paula Novack, Charitable Contributions Coordinator

Typ. Recipients: AIDS/HIV, Alzheimers Disease, Arthritis, Cancer, Children's Health/Hospitals, Clinics/Medical Centers, Diabetes, Eyes/Blindness, Health-General, Multiple Sclerosis. **Geo. Dist:** headquarters and operating communities.

★ 12803 ★ Presto Foundation

3925 North Hastings Way
Eau Claire, WI 54703
Phone: (715)839-2119 **Fax:** (715)839-2122
Norma Jaenke, Executive Director

Priorities: *Arts & Humanities:* 29%. Primarily supports public television stations. Also supports libraries, historical museums, theater, dance, and symphonies. *Civic & Public Affairs:* 16%. Funds community development, job training, and advocacy issues. *Education:* 38%. Supports colleges and universities, scholarships to employee's children, career/vocational education, and public pre-college education. *Environment:* 7%. Primarily supports the United Way. Also funds organizations concerned with personal growth, such as Special Olympics, youth recreation and athletic activities, and Big Brothers/Big Sisters. *International:* 8%. Supports hospitals, pediatric health, and single-disease health associations. *Note:* Total contributions made in fiscal 2001. **Typ. Recipients:** Cancer, Children's Health/Hospitals, Emergency/Ambulance Services, Health Funds, Heart, Hospitals, Medical Research, Multiple Sclerosis, People with Disabilities, Single-Disease Health Associations. **Geo. Dist:** headquarters and operating communities; WI, Northwestern Wisconsin, especially Eau Claire and Chippewa Falls.

★ 12804 ★ Principal Financial Group Foundation, Inc.

711 High St.
Des Moines, IA 50392-0001
Phone: (515)247-5091 **Fax:** (515)246-5475
Website: http://www.principal.com/about/giving/index.htm
Michele Walstrom, Contributions Consultant

Fnded: 1987. **Priorities:** *Arts & Humanities:* 15%. Support of the greater Des Moines area and selected visual and performing arts organizations, museums, cultural centers, public television, arts-related organizations, and other cultural groups. *Civic & Public Affairs:* 18%. Supports civic and public policy. *Education:* 20%. Support of local universities and colleges, the Iowa College Foundation, various actuarial scholarships and programs at select universities, economic education programs, and education-related organizations. Supports education matching gifts program for employees and qualified agents/brokers of The Principal Financial Group. *Environment:* 44%. Support of human services organizations, youth organizations, family services, Young Men's Christian Associations, the United Way, and special projects. *International:* Less than 1%. Primarily supports single-disease health associations. *Religion:* Supports a science museum. *Note:* Total contributions made in 2000. **Typ. Recipients:** AIDS/HIV, Alzheimers Disease, Cancer, Children's Health/Hospitals, Emergency/Ambulance Services, Family Planning, Health Organizations, Health Policy/Cost Containment, Health-General, Hospices, Medical Research, Mental Health, People with Disabilities, Respiratory, Single-Disease Health Associations, Substance Abuse. **Geo. Dist:** occasional nationally and internationally; operating locations; Des Moines, IA.

★ 12805 ★ Procter & Gamble Cosmetics Foundation

11050 York Rd.
Hunt Valley, MD 21030
Phone: (410)785-7300 **Fax:** (410)316-8025
Marian Lubbert, Administrator

Fnded: 1951. **Priorities:** *Arts & Humanities:* 28%. Supports art museums, music, theater, and community arts organizations. *Civic & Public Affairs:* 6%. Supports community youth organizations and civic organizations. *Education:* 38%. Funds colleges and universities, Catholic colleges and precollege schools, arts education, and scholarship funds. *Environment:* 22%. Supports youth organizations, zoos, community organizations, nonprofit management, and long-term commitments to theaters, libraries, a medical center, and educational organizations. *International:* 4%. Supports hospitals and single-disease health associations, with a focus on pediatric health. *Religion:* 2%. *Note:* Total contributions made in 2001. **Typ. Recipients:** AIDS/HIV, Cancer, Children's Health/Hospitals, Clinics/Medical Centers, Diabetes, Domestic Violence, Emergency/Ambulance Services, Health Organizations, Hospitals, Medical Education, Medical Rehabilitation, Mental Health, Nursing Services, People with Disabilities, Public Health, Respiratory, Single-Disease Health Associations, Substance Abuse. **Geo. Dist:** some support to nationally organizations with local chapters; NY: New York City; Baltimore, MD, metropolitan area.

★ 12806 ★ Procter & Gamble Fund

PO Box 599
Cincinnati, OH 45201-0599
Phone: (513)945-8454
Website: http://www.pg.com/about_pg/corporate/community/community_submain.jhtml
Carol Talbot, Secretary

Priorities: *Arts & Humanities:* 11%. Promotes cultural enrichment, educational programs, and entertainment. Supports museums, theater, dance, music, and the visual arts. *Civic & Public Affairs:* 22%. Goals are to promote economic stimulation and enrichment for all parts of the community. Supports youth programs, chambers of commerce, the Urban League, zoos, community foundations, parks, and economic policy and development. *Education:* 28%. Major support to scholarship programs and grants to public and private colleges and universities. Also supports employee matching gifts; economic education organizations; scholarships for employees' children, and K-12 initiatives. *Environment:* 35%. Supports United Way, scouting, food banks, and youth services. *International:* 2%. Funds hospitals. *Note:* Total contributions made in 2000. **Typ. Recipients:** Cancer, Emergency/Ambulance Services, Health Organizations, Health-General,

Hospitals, Nutrition, People with Disabilities, Substance Abuse. **Geo. Dist:** headquarters and operating communities, nationally and internationally.

★ 12807 ★ Providence Journal Charitable Foundation
75 Fountain St.
Providence, RI 02902-9985
Phone: (401)277-7597 **Fax:** (401)277-7529
Email: mary_ellen_ahern@projo.com
Mary Ahern, Community Services Director

Priorities: *Arts & Humanities:* 26%. Supports performing arts groups, libraries, public broadcasting, museums, orchestras, and historic preservation. *Civic & Public Affairs:* 14%. Funds community festivals, economic development, urban planning, responsible growth programs, minority affairs. *Education:* 25%. Local colleges and universities, preparatory schools, education funds, civics education, and Junior Achievement receive support. *Environment:* 20%. Supports youth organizations, the United Way, food banks and shelters, traveler's aid, and women's and family services. *International:* 8%. Funds hospitals, mental health centers, and the American Red Cross. *Note:* Total contributions made in 2000. **Typ. Recipients:** Adolescent Health Issues, AIDS/HIV, Cancer, Emergency/Ambulance Services, Family Planning, Geriatric Health, Health Organizations, Hospices, Hospitals, Long-Term Care, Medical Rehabilitation, Mental Health, Nursing Services, People with Disabilities, Research/Studies Institutes, Sexual Abuse, Single-Disease Health Associations, Substance Abuse. **Geo. Dist:** RI.

★ 12808 ★ Prudential Foundation
213 Washington St.
Newark, NJ 07102
Phone: (973)802-3780 **Fax:** (973)802-3345
Email: community.resources@prudential.com
Website: http://www.prudential.com/community
Lata Reddy, Secretary

Priorities: *Arts & Humanities:* 6%. *Civic & Public Affairs:* (Ready to Work) 15% to 20%. Promotes job entry skills that are acquired through initiatives that focus on school-to-work transition, workforce development and welfare-to-work; job creation strategies that include access to capital, nonprofit/for-profit ventures, adult and youth entrepreneurship, financial training, business attraction/development/retention; decent, affordable housing that is created through programs that focus on either housing strategies or neighborhood-based activities. Housing strategies include investment/grant partnerships with Prudential's Social Investment Program, community development financial institutions, or technical assistance to Community Housing Development Organizations. Neighborhood-based activities include community organizing, neighborhood strategic planning, leadership development, and community security. *Education:* (Ready to Learn) 15% to 20%. Supports education efforts that strengthen early childhood education initiatives; support professional development for preK-3 teachers; build strong school leadership, with a particular emphasis on parental involvement; provide school-based health and human services that reduce the barriers to learning; or create safe school environments through conflict resolution programs. Within this framework, the foundation emphasizes the creation of model schools, arts education, and literacy. *Environment:* (Ready to Live) 25% to 30%. Supports community health and safety efforts that include community-based culture/arts programs in New Jersey; initiatives that build healthy families; community-based health care and human services for economically disadvantaged populations; high-impact national projects that address major health or human services issues affecting children and families; and youth development programs that foster leadership skills. Also supports the Greater Newark AIDS Initiative. *International:* 19%. *Voluntarism:* Company supports Prudential CARES (Community, Action Renewal Efforts) which provides individual and team building volunteer programs for Prudential employees and retirees at local nonprofits. Also supports Global Volunteer Day. *Note:* Total contributions made in 1999. **Typ. Recipients:** AIDS/HIV, Child Abuse, Children's Health/Hospitals, Clinics/Medical Centers, Emergency/Ambulance Services, Family Planning, Geriatric Health, Health Organizations, Health Policy/Cost Containment, Hospitals, Medical Education, Medical Rehabilitation, Medical Training, Mental Health, People with Disabilities, Public Health, Research/Studies Institutes, Substance Abuse. **Geo. Dist:** headquarters and operating communities; nationally; Phoenix, AZ; Los Angeles, CA; Jacksonville, FL; Atlanta, GA; Minneapolis, MN; NJ, particularly Newark; Philadelphia, PA; Houston, TX.

★ 12809 ★ Prudential Securities Foundation
One New York Plaza
New York, NY 10292
Phone: (212)214-4884 **Fax:** (212)214-5541
Email: liz_longley@prusec.com
Elizabeth Longley, Vice President

Priorities: *Arts & Humanities:* 39%. Supports museums, libraries, dance, orchestras, opera, and arts associations. *Civic & Public Affairs:* 16%. Supports community development, housing, employment, and parks. *Education:* 35%. Funds colleges and universities, literacy programs, schools, and education associations. *Environment:* 8%. Primarily supports youth organizations and children's services. *International:* 2%. Contributes to a hospital. *Note:* Total contributions made in fiscal 2001. **Typ. Recipients:** Arthritis, Children's Health/Hospitals, Emergency/Ambulance Services, Health Organizations, Heart, Hospitals, Medical Research, Mental Health, Outpatient Health Care, People with Disabilities, Single-Disease Health Associations, Substance Abuse, Transplant Networks/Donor Banks. **Geo. Dist:** NY.

★ 12810 ★ Public Service Co. of Oklahoma
PO Box 201
Tulsa, OK 74102
Phone: (614)223-1697 **Fax:** (614)223-1682
Website: http://www.aep.com
Ms. Rody Woischke, Contributions Administrator

Typ. Recipients: Health-General. **Geo. Dist:** OK, Southeastern and Southwestern Oklahoma.

★ 12811 ★ Public Service Electric & Gas Foundation
80 Park Plaza, Mail Code T-10
Newark, NJ 07101
Phone: (973)430-5763 **Fax:** (973)297-1480
Email: william.walsh3@pseg.com
Website: http://www.pseg.com/community
William Walsh, President

Priorities: *Civic & Public Affairs:* 4%. *Education:* 16%. *Environment:* 41%. *International:* 2%. *Religion:* 37%. *Voluntarism:* Company supports Dollars for Doers and Recognizing Excellence programs. *Note:* Total foundation contributions made in 2001. **Typ. Recipients:** Cancer, Emergency/Ambulance Services, Hospitals, People with Disabilities, Substance Abuse. **Geo. Dist:** nationally for education grants; primarily in service area. **Frmly:** Public Service Electric & Gas Foundation.

★ 12812 ★ Publix Supermarkets Charities
PO Box 407
Lakeland, FL 33802
Phone: (863)686-8754
Website: http://www.publix.com/servlet/MainController?action=prepareCommunityInvolvement
Carol Barnett, Chairperson

Fnded: 1967. **Priorities:** *Civic & Public Affairs:* 1%. Supports Florida Olympic campaign, public affairs, the Florida aquarium, and civic organizations. *Education:* 13%. Supports colleges, universities, public schools and educational programs in Florida. *Environment:* 80%. Majority of social service funding is donated to the United Way; also supports youth services, YMCA, the homeless, family services, and the handicapped. *International:* 1%. Funds clinics, hospitals, and single-disease health associations. *Note:* Contributions were made in 2000. **Typ. Recipients:** Cancer, Clinics/Medical Centers, Emergency/Ambulance Services, Family Planning, Geriatric Health, Hospices, Hospitals, People with Disabilities, Single-Disease Health Associations, Substance Abuse, Transplant Networks/Donor Banks. **Geo. Dist:** AL; FL; GA; SC.

★ 12813 ★ Pulitzer Foundation
900 North Tucker Boulevard
Saint Louis, MO 63101
Phone: (314)340-8440 **Fax:** (314)340-3133
Alan Silverglat, Secretary & Treasurer

Priorities: *Arts & Humanities:* 20%. Primarily supports St. Louis area cultural institutions. Funds the St. Louis Symphony, history organizations, music, and theater. *Civic & Public Affairs:* 7%. Funds press associations, First Amendment issues, parks, and a zoo. *Education:* 23%. Supports colleges and universities, principally in St. Louis and elsewhere in Missouri. Remaining funds support journalism studies, education funds and student aid. Scholarships are limited to St. Louis area minority students who are either high school graduates or in junior college. Scholarships are for students attending the University of Missouri Journalism School. *Environment:* 48%. Majority of funding goes to the United Way, including a substantial gift to the September 11 Fund. Also supports traditional youth organizations and sports programs. *Note:* Total foundation contributions made in 2001. **Typ. Recipients:** AIDS/HIV, Cancer, Children's Health/Hospitals, Emergency/Ambulance Services, Family Planning, Home-Care Services, Hospices, Hospitals, Long-Term Care, Medical Education, Mental Health, Multiple Sclerosis, Respiratory, Single-Disease Health Associations. **Geo. Dist:** St. Louis, MO, metropolitan area.

★ 12814 ★ Putnam Investors Fund
c/o Public Relations
1 Post Office Square, Mail Stop A-4-E
Boston, MA 02109
Phone: (617)292-1000 **Fax:** (617)760-8048
Margaret Leipsitz, Manager, Community Relations

Priorities: *Arts & Humanities:* 10%. Boston area arts and cultural organizations receive funding. Interests include the fine arts, museums, public broadcasting, music, and dance. *Civic & Public Affairs:* 5%. Supports housing, city improvement projects, charitable gift funds, a taxpayer's foundation, and organizations that provide job skills training. *Education:* 24%. Primarily supports colleges and universities, particularly highly recognized business schools; technology education; scholarship funds; and literacy initiatives. *Environment:* 55%. Supports youth organizations, the United Way, family services, homeless shelters, and organizations assisting the disabled and at-risk. *International:* 1%. Funds hospitals, pediatric health, and cancer research and treatment. *Note:* Total foundation contributions made in 2000. **Typ. Recipients:** AIDS/HIV, Arthritis, Cancer, Child Abuse, Children's Health/Hospitals, Clinics/Medical Centers, Diabetes, Heart, Hospices, Hospitals, Medical Research, Multiple Sclerosis, People with Disabilities, Prenatal Health Issues, Single-Disease Health Associations. **Geo. Dist:** Boston, MA; Quincy, MA.

★ 12815 ★ Quaker Chemical Foundation
Elm and Lee St.s
Conshohocken, PA 19428
Phone: (610)832-4127 **Fax:** (610)832-4282
Kathleen Lasota, Secretary

Priorities: *Arts & Humanities:* 20%. Supports arts outreach, opera, arts funds, library funds, art centers, and performing arts. *Civic & Public Affairs:* 16%. Emphasis on job training, community affairs, and parks and zoos. *Education:* 41%. One third of education contributions are in the form of scholarships to employees and individuals in the community. Focus is on chemistry and the physical sciences. Other funding supports colleges, universities, and primary and secondary education. One third of contributions are matching gifts. *Environment:* 16%. Supports disabilities, youth organizations, food distribution, and family services. *International:* 4%. Funding supports hospice foundations, nursing services, and health organizations. *Religion:* 3%. Supports science institutes. *Note:* Total foundation contributions made in fiscal 2001. **Typ. Recipients:** Eyes/Blindness, Health Organizations, Heart, Home-Care Services, Hospices, Hospitals, Medical Research, Nursing Services, Nutrition, People with Disabilities, Sexual Abuse, Single-Disease Health Associations. **Geo. Dist:** headquarters and operating communities.

★ 12816 ★ Quanex Foundation

1900 West Loop S, Suite 1500
Houston, TX 77027
Phone: (713)961-4600
Sandy Hatcher, Director Corporate Communications

Fnded: 1951. **Priorities:** *Arts & Humanities:* 15%. Supports museums, art centers, and libraries. *Civic & Public Affairs:* 15%. Supports festivals, housing, and community development. *Education:* 21%. Supports scholarships funds, colleges and universities, schools, and Junior Achievement. *Environment:* 40%. Funds United Way, shelters, scouting, athletics, and emergency relief. *International:* 7%. Supports hospice and single-disease health associations. *Note:* Total foundation contributions made in 2001. **Typ. Recipients:** AIDS/HIV, Cancer, Children's Health/Hospitals, Clinics/Medical Centers, Diabetes, Emergency/Ambulance Services, Eyes/Blindness, Health Organizations, Heart, Hospices, Hospitals, Kidney, Medical Research, Nutrition, People with Disabilities, Public Health, Research/Studies Institutes, Single-Disease Health Associations. **Geo. Dist:** TX.

★ 12817 ★ Questar Corp.

180 East 1st South St.
PO Box 45433
Salt Lake City, UT 84145-0433
Phone: (801)324-5435 **Fax:** (801)324-5483
Email: janb@questar.com
Janice Bates, Director, Community Affairs

Priorities: *Arts & Humanities:* 25%. Funding goes to dance and music, historic preservation, museums and galleries, and performing arts. *Civic & Public Affairs:* 15%. Funds programs for better government and economic development. *Education:* 30%. Business education, colleges and universities, and economic education are all supported. *International:* 30%. Support goes to hospitals, single-disease health associations, child welfare, community service organizations, traditional youth groups, the United Way, and food and clothing distribution. **Typ. Recipients:** Health Organizations, Hospitals, People with Disabilities. **Geo. Dist:** CO, limited funding; OK, limited funding; TX, limited funding; UT; WY.

★ 12818 ★ R. J. Reynolds Tobacco Co. Foundation

PO Box Box 2959
Winston-Salem, NC 27102-2959
Phone: (336)741-0049
Vivian Turner, Contact

Fnded: 1996. **Typ. Recipients:** Hospices, People with Disabilities, Substance Abuse. **Geo. Dist:** NC.

★ 12819 ★ R.K. Laros Foundation

76 South Main St.
Nazareth, PA 18064
Phone: (610)746-7312
Robert Spillman, Trustee

Fnded: 1952. **Priorities:** *Arts & Humanities:* 17%. Funds art museums and theater. *Civic & Public Affairs:* 33%. Supports community action, municipalities, and minority affairs. *Education:* 14%. Gives to colleges and medical education. *Environment:* 25%. Supports child care and youth groups. *International:* 1%. Gives to a visiting nurse organization. *Note:* Total contributions made in 2000. **Typ. Recipients:** Emergency/Ambulance Services, Health Organizations, Hospitals, Medical Education, Nursing Services, People with Disabilities, Substance Abuse. **Geo. Dist:** headquarters and operating communities.

★ 12820 ★ R.R. Donnelley & Sons Co.

77 West Wacker Drive
Chicago, IL 60601-1696
Phone: (312)326-8102 **Fax:** (312)326-8262
Email: susan.levy@rrd.com
Website: http://www.rrdonnelley.com/cportal/public/home/publicaffairs/index.jsp
Susan Levy, Vice President

Priorities: *Arts & Humanities:* 10% to 15%. Interests include museums, libraries, and literary and performing arts. Matches employee gifts to cultural institutions. *Civic & Public Affairs:* About 10%. Supports better government groups, and conservation and environmental projects. Other interests include civil rights and economic development. Main focus of national giving is public policy organizations. *Education:* 20% to 25%. Emphasis is on higher education, especially independent college funds and educational institutions located in operating communities. Precollegiate education is also of interest. Matches employee gifts to higher and secondary education and provides scholarships to employees' children. *Environment:* 55% to 60%. Company contributes to organizations serving operating locations, including united funds and groups concerned with youth, the disabled, and minorities. *Voluntarism:* The company sponsors the Donnelley Dollars for Doers program, which provides grants to organizations for which Donnelley employees or retirees volunteer. Grant amounts are based on the number of hours donated by the employee or retiree, to a maximum of $500 per employee and $5,000 to any one organization. *Note:* Total contributions made in 1999. Donations are given either as special purpose grants, to support initiatives that require defined funds to launch or develop a major program, or as general operating grants, for ongoing assistance to local organizations. An overall company priority is organizations which promote the written word, including libraries and literary organizations. **Typ. Recipients:** Domestic Violence, Hospitals, Mental Health, People with Disabilities. **Geo. Dist:** principally near operating locations and to national organizations.

★ 12821 ★ Ralph's-Food 4 Less Foundation

PO Box 54143
Los Angeles, CA 90054
Phone: (310)884-6250 **Fax:** (310)884-2590
Website: http://ralphs.com/corpnewsinfo_charitable-giving_art5.htm
Jan Golleher, Executive Director

Fnded: 1992. **Priorities:** *Arts & Humanities:* Less than 1%. Supports music, the performing arts, libraries, and arts funds/foundations. *Civic & Public Affairs:* 10%. Funds urban leagues, public safety, minority affairs, and legal aid. *Education:* 14%. Supports colleges and universities, and educational programs for pre-college education. *Environment:* 49%. Supports day care, food distribution, family services, scouting, community sports, and violence and substance abuse prevention. *International:* 18%. Supports children's health organizations, medical centers, and single-disease health organizations. *Religion:* 1%. *Note:* Total foundation contributions made in 2000. **Typ. Recipients:** AIDS/HIV, Cancer, Child Abuse, Children's Health/Hospitals, Clinics/Medical Centers, Diabetes, Domestic Violence, Emergency/Ambulance Services, Eyes/Blindness, Family Planning, Health Organizations, Heart, Hospitals, Medical Education, Mental Health, Multiple Sclerosis, People with Disabilities, Prenatal Health Issues, Single-Disease Health Associations, Substance Abuse. **Geo. Dist:** CA, southern California.

★ 12822 ★ Ralston Purina Trust Fund

Checkerboard Square
Saint Louis, MO 63164-0001
Phone: (314)982-3234 **Fax:** (314)982-2752
Website: http://Purina.com/company/profile/profile_articles.asp?article=367
Fred Perabo, Secretary

Priorities: *Arts & Humanities:* 6%. Supports museums, music, and public broadcasting. *Civic & Public Affairs:* 7%. Supports urban affairs, community development, parks, and chambers of commerce. *Education:* 20%. Supports colleges and universities, scholarship programs, and Junior Achievement. *Environment:* 54%. Supports the United Way, humane societies, youth concerns, and service groups. *International:* 1%. Funds the Alzheimer's Association and the March of Dimes. *Note:* Total foundation contributions made in fiscal 2000. **Typ. Recipients:** Alzheimers Disease, Children's Health/Hospitals, Domestic Violence, Family Planning, Health Organizations, Health Policy/Cost Containment, Hospices, Hospitals, Medical Education, Medical Research, Nursing Services, People with Disabilities, Single-Disease Health Associations, Substance Abuse. **Geo. Dist:** headquarters and operating communities; St. Louis, MO.

★ 12823 ★ Raymond Foundation

PO Box 1273E
Greene, NY 13778
Phone: (607)656-8897
Theresa Brant, Assistant Executive Secretary

Fnded: 1964. **Typ. Recipients:** Cancer, Cancer, Children's Health/Hospitals, Clinics/Medical Centers, Emergency/Ambulance Services, Eyes/Blindness, Health Organizations, Heart, Hospices, Hospitals, Kidney, Respiratory, Single-Disease Health Associations. **Geo. Dist:** CA, limited to areas of company operations; NY, limited to areas of company operations.

★ 12824 ★ Rayonier Foundation

50 North Laura St., Suite 1900
Jacksonville, FL 32202
Phone: (904)357-9100
Jay Fredericksen, Vice President

Fnded: 1952. **Priorities:** *Arts & Humanities:* 3%. Supports museums and music. *Civic & Public Affairs:* 3%. Supports community organizations, chambers of commerce, fire departments, and free enterprise. *Education:* 55%. Supports individual scholarship programs including the Black Scholar Awards, the Four Year Scholarship Program, the Timber County Scholarship Program, and the Rayonier College Scholarship. Other areas of interests include colleges and universities, elementary and secondary schools, and Head Start programs. *Environment:* 34%. Supports United Way, YMCA, youth organizations, volunteer programs, and shelters. *International:* 1%. Contributes to hospitals and health-care organizations. *Religion:* 2%. Supports a museum. *Note:* Total contributions made in 2000. **Typ. Recipients:** Child Abuse, Children's Health/Hospitals, Domestic Violence, Hospices, Hospitals, Mental Health, People with Disabilities, Substance Abuse. **Geo. Dist:** headquarters area only.

★ 12825 ★ Reader's Digest Foundation

1 Reader's Digest Rd.
Pleasantville, NY 10570
Phone: (914)244-5370 **Fax:** (914)244-7642
Email: carolyn.malile@readersdigest.com
Website: http://www.rd.com/corporate/
Claudia Edwards, Executive Director

Priorities: *Arts & Humanities:* 31%. Primarily supports libraries. *Civic & Public Affairs:* 21%. Supports community services. *Education:* 23%. The company supports such initiatives as the Putnam Valley School's early intervention reading program, the Links to Literacy program, the Westchester Education Coalition, and the Horizons Student Summer Enrichment program. The company also maintains a national scholarship program and the Tall Tree Initiative for Libraries. *Environment:* 2%. *International:* 24%. Supports children's health organizations and a clinic. *Voluntarism:* Reader's Digest employees, employee spouses, and retirees can receive grants for nonprofit groups where they actively volunteer. The company operates a Double-Match Gift Program where employees and retirees may give up to $10,000 per year to charities of their choice. *Note:* Contributions made in 1998. Percentages exclude matching gifts, scholarship, and volunteer program investments. **Typ. Recipients:** Cancer, Children's Health/Hospitals, Clinics/Medical Centers, Single-Disease Health Associations. **Geo. Dist:** nationally.

★ 12826 ★ Red Wing Shoe Co. Foundation
314 Main St.
Red Wing, MN 55066-2300
Phone: (651)388-8211 **Fax:** (651)385-1760
Stacy Crownhart, Secretary

Priorities: *Arts & Humanities:* 2%. Supports arts associations, historic preservation, orchestral music, theater, and public broadcasting. *Civic & Public Affairs:* 21%. Supports community development, municipalities, an auditorium, and parks. *Education:* 21%. Major support for Red Wing School District No. 256; colleges, economic education, and education reform receive minor funding. *Environment:* 53%. Primarily supports the YMCA and United Way. Youth organizations, family services, and Special Olympics also receive support. *International:* 1%. Health organizations, single disease associations, and medical centers. *Religion:* 1%. Science Museum of Minnesota. *Note:* Total foundation contributions made in 2000. **Typ. Recipients:** Cancer, Children's Health/Hospitals, Clinics/Medical Centers, Emergency/Ambulance Services, Health Organizations, Hospices, Medical Rehabilitation, People with Disabilities, Preventive Medicine/Wellness Organizations, Single-Disease Health Associations, Substance Abuse. **Geo. Dist:** Danville, KY; Minneapolis, MN; Red Wing, MN; St. Paul, MN; Potosi, MO.

★ 12827 ★ The Reebok Human Rights Foundation
1895 J.W Foster Blvd.
Canton, MA 02021
Phone: (781)401-5000 **Fax:** (781)401-4806
Website: http://www.reebok.com/x/us/humanRights/text-only/foundation/
David Pace, Manager

Priorities: *Arts & Humanities:* 3%. *Civic & Public Affairs:* Company supports human rights organizations. The majority of company's international giving is through its Human Rights Award. Foundation supports a short list of major national organizations devoted to furthering the achievement of social and economic equality of communities of color. Grants are made by invitation only. *Education:* 6%. *Environment:* Contributions go to organizations in Boston serving the needs of underserved youth population, especially programs that educate, improve self-esteem, and protect the rights of African-American, Hispanic and Asian people. New proposals are not currently being accepted for this program. *International:* 3%. *Note:* Total contributions made in 2001. **Typ. Recipients:** Children's Health/Hospitals, Clinics/Medical Centers, Diabetes, Domestic Violence, Health Organizations, Medical Education, Public Health. **Geo. Dist:** internationally through Human Rights Awards; principally near operating locations and to national organizations; Boston, MA. **Frmly:** The Reebok Foundation.

★ 12828 ★ Regions Financial Corp.
PO Box 10247
Birmingham, AL 35202
Phone: (205)326-7206 **Fax:** (205)326-7099
Ms. Artist McMicken, Assistant Corporate Chairperson

Typ. Recipients: Health-General. **Geo. Dist:** headquarters and operating communities; AL, especially small communities.

★ 12829 ★ Regis Foundation
7201 Metro Boulevard
Minneapolis, MN 55439-2103
Phone: (952)947-7777 **Fax:** (952)947-7900
Website: http://www.regiscorp.com/corporate/communityInvolve.html
Mr. Myron Kunin, President

Fnded: 1981. **Priorities:** *Arts & Humanities:* 14%. Supports art museums and a theater. *Civic & Public Affairs:* 1%. Supports housing initiatives and other civic causes. *Education:* 32%. Funds universities and scholarship funds. *Environment:* 1%. Supports United Way. *Note:* Total contributions in 1998. **Typ. Recipients:** Cancer, People with Disabilities. **Geo. Dist:** Minneapolis, MN, and surrounding area.

★ 12830 ★ Reilly Foundation
300 North Meridian St., Suite 1500
Indianapolis, IN 46204-1763
Phone: (317)248-6464 **Fax:** (317)248-6472
Rand Brooks, Trustee

Fnded: 1962. **Priorities:** *Arts & Humanities:* 13%. Supports museums, art councils, and the performing arts. *Civic & Public Affairs:* 5%. Supports neighborhood organizations, leadership development, and a zoological park. *Education:* 49%. Supports colleges and universities, education funds and associations. Foundation offers scholarships and an employee matching gifts program. *Environment:* 30%. Funding primarily supports the United Way. Other interests include youth activities, child welfare, homelessness, food distribution, and athletics. *International:* 1%. Supports community clinics and Ronald McDonald House. *Religion:* Less than 1%. Supports a chemical foundation. *Note:* Total foundation contributions made in 2001. **Typ. Recipients:** Cancer, Children's Health/Hospitals, Clinics/Medical Centers, Family Planning, Health Organizations, Hospitals, Long-Term Care, Medical Rehabilitation, Medical Research, People with Disabilities, Public Health, Transplant Networks/Donor Banks. **Geo. Dist:** company operating locations, mainly Indianapolis, IN.

★ 12831 ★ Reily Foundation
640 Magazine St.
New Orleans, LA 70130
Phone: (504)524-6131 **Fax:** (504)539-5417
H. Reily, Director

Priorities: *Arts & Humanities:* 12%. Emphasis on arts funds, museums, orchestras, historic preservation, and public broadcasting. *Civic & Public Affairs:* 15%. Majority of funding supports community foundations, public policy, botanical gardens, and professional trade associations in New Orleans. *Education:* 42%. Supports universities; public and private, secondary and elementary education; education reform; minority education; and Junior Achievement. *Environment:* 16%. Provides funding for United Way, youth groups, family services, crime prevention, and food distribution. Also supports criminal rehabilitation and at-risk youth. *International:* 1%. Single-disease health organizations, hospitals, and clinics receive support. *Note:* Total foundation contributions made in 2000. **Typ. Recipients:** AIDS/HIV, Clinics/Medical Centers, Family Planning, Health Organizations, Hospitals, Medical Education, Medical Education, People with Disabilities, Single-Disease Health Associations. **Geo. Dist:** New Orleans, LA, and surrounding area.

★ 12832 ★ Reliant Resources Foundation
PO Box 4567
Houston, TX 77210
Phone: (713)207-5155 **Fax:** (713)207-0207
Website: http://www.reliantenergy.com/company/community/
Robert Gibbs, Director, Corporate Community Relations

Fnded: 1997. **Priorities:** *Arts & Humanities:* 3%. Funds theater, music, and radio. *Civic & Public Affairs:* 36%. Supports community festivals; organizational programs, foundations, housing, local rodeo, parks, city beautification, Junior Achievement, and neighborhood centers. Major grant to Houston Livestock Show and Rodeo ($1,216,300). *Education:* 27%. Funds scholarships, college funds, and universities. Major grant to the Texas A&M Foundation ($1,000,000). *Environment:* 26%. Provides support to child advocates, scouting, family centers, Young Men's Christian Associations, United Way, and food banks. *International:* 5%. Supports hospitals and single-disease health associations. *Note:* Total contributions made in 2000. **Typ. Recipients:** Cancer, Children's Health/Hospitals, Diabetes, Emergency/Ambulance Services, Health Organizations, Heart, Hospitals, Medical Education, Medical Research, Mental Health, People with Disabilities, Single-Disease Health Associations, Substance Abuse. **Geo. Dist:** headquarters and operating communities, mainly TX. **Frmly:** Houston Industries, Inc. Reliant Energy Foundation.

★ 12833 ★ Revlon Foundation Inc.
625 Madison Ave.
New York, NY 10022
Phone: (212)527-5000 **Fax:** (212)527-6977
Website: http://www.revlon.com/corporate/corp_philanthopic.asp
Joan Horton, Corporate Events

Fnded: 1955. **Priorities:** *Arts & Humanities:* 2%. Supports a performing arts center. *Civic & Public Affairs:* 3%. Gives to African-American affairs groups and to urban affairs. *Education:* 83%. Supports colleges and universities. Matching grants also are made in the area of education. *International:* 12%. Support goes to medical centers. *Note:* Total contributions made in 1997. **Typ. Recipients:** AIDS/HIV, Cancer, Clinics/Medical Centers, Hospitals, Medical Education, People with Disabilities, Single-Disease Health Associations. **Geo. Dist:** headquarters and operating communities; nationally.

★ 12834 ★ Rexford Fund
1 Whitehall St., 17th Floor
New York, NY 10004
Phone: (212)483-1500 **Fax:** (212)363-7265
Douglas Schloss, Chairman & Chief Executive Officer

Fnded: 1967. **Priorities:** *Arts & Humanities:* 11%. Funds art and history museums, theater and other performing arts, and libraries. *Civic & Public Affairs:* 7%. Supports parks and conservatories, community clubs, and community loan funds. *Education:* 57%. Funds colleges and universities, nursery and primary education, and scholarship funds. *Environment:* 14%. Supports family and youth centers. *International:* 1%. Supports a hospital. *Note:* Total contributions made in 2001. **Typ. Recipients:** Adolescent Health Issues, Cancer, Clinics/Medical Centers, Emergency/Ambulance Services, Family Planning, Health Organizations, Hospices, Hospitals, Mental Health, Multiple Sclerosis, People with Disabilities, Public Health, Single-Disease Health Associations, Substance Abuse. **Geo. Dist:** CT; ME; MA; NY; VA.

★ 12835 ★ Reynolds & Reynolds Co. Foundation
PO Box 2608
Dayton, OH 45401-2608
Phone: (937)485-2309 **Fax:** (937)485-3831
Email: alice_davisson@reyrey.com
Website: http://www.reyrey.com/about/community.asp
Alice Davisson, Administrator

Priorities: *Arts & Humanities:* 16%. Foundation supports a variety of arts and cultural organizations that enrich the quality of life for area residents. Funds museums, theater, and music. *Civic & Public Affairs:* 17%. Grants encourage strategic community economic development in company's operating areas, including community foundations and urban affairs. *Education:* 17%. Funding emphasizes support for programs geared toward at-risk children in grades K-12. Foundation allocates funds to educational institutions and nonprofit organizations that help keep children in school and prepare them for employment, college, technical training, or the military. *Environment:* 50%. Majority of support reaches the United Way; also funds YMCA and youth organizations. *Voluntarism:* Employee "Spirit Award" offered to employees dedicating 50+ hours per calendar year to a non-profit agency. Agency receives $200 grant in employee's name. *Note:* Total foundation contributions made in fiscal 2000. **Typ. Recipients:** Arthritis, Cancer, Children's Health/Hospitals, Emergency/Ambulance Services, Health Organizations, Hospices, Trauma Treatment. **Geo. Dist:** OH.

★ 12836 ★ Rich Family Foundation
PO Box 245
Buffalo, NY 14240-0245

Phone: (716)878-8363 **Fax:** (716)878-8775
David Rich, Executive Director

Fnded: 1961. **Priorities:** *Arts & Humanities:* 8%. Contributes to music and the performing arts. *Civic & Public Affairs:* 4%. Supports business concerns. *Education:* 67%. Supports the University of Buffalo Foundation in New York, NY, and other regional colleges and universities, scholarship funds, and schools. *Environment:* 9%. The United Way receives the majority of grants. Also supports child welfare organizations. *International:* 3%. Funds hospitals and single-disease associations. *Note:* Total foundation contributions made in 2000. **Typ. Recipients:** Alzheimers Disease, Cancer, Children's Health/Hospitals, Clinics/Medical Centers, Diabetes, Emergency/Ambulance Services, Health Organizations, Health-General, Heart, Hospitals, Medical Rehabilitation, Medical Research, Multiple Sclerosis, Prenatal Health Issues, Public Health, Single-Disease Health Associations, Substance Abuse, Substance Abuse. **Geo. Dist:** Buffalo, NY.

★ 12837 ★ Riggs Bank NA

800 17th St., NW, 2nd Floor
Washington, DC 20006
Phone: (202)835-4495 **Fax:** (202)835-5184
Marybeth Jones, Corporate Events Manager

Priorities: *Arts & Humanities:* Supports organizations that provide artistic enrichment to the community or reach underserved audiences, including museums and visual and performing arts groups. *Civic & Public Affairs:* Supports organizations committed to the safety, welfare, and well-being of the community. Physical revitalization of the community; economic development; groups with monitor legal, consumer, and governmental issues; boys and girls clubs; and community associations are supported. Supports organizations dedicated to affordable housing initiatives, neighborhood development, small-business development and enhancement, and job training and development programs. *Education:* Supports formal education and community-based organizations for educational purposes. *International:* Supports mental and physical medical care and basic human services. Supports hospitals, clinics, food banks, shelters for the homeless, and federated campaigns. **Typ. Recipients:** Clinics/Medical Centers, Kidney, Single-Disease Health Associations. **Geo. Dist:** Washington, DC, metropolitan area.

★ 12838 ★ Rinker Companies Foundation, Inc.

1501 Belvedere Rd.
West Palm Beach, FL 33406
Phone: (561)833-5555 **Fax:** (561)820-8359
Frank LaPlaca, Administrator

Fnded: 1957. **Priorities:** *Arts & Humanities:* 2%. Supports the Raymond F. Kravis Center. *Civic & Public Affairs:* 5%. Supports community foundations and other civic organizations. *Education:* 59%. Funds universities and colleges. *Environment:* 27%. Supports United Way, scouts, and substance abuse initiatives. *International:* 1%. Gives to single-disease health associations. *Note:* Total foundation giving made in fiscal 2001. **Typ. Recipients:** Cancer, Children's Health/Hospitals, Substance Abuse. **Geo. Dist:** FL, Dade County; FL, Palm Beach County. **Frmly:** CSR America Company Foundation, Inc.

★ 12839 ★ Robbins and Myers Foundation

1400 Kettering Tower
Dayton, OH 45423
Phone: (937)222-2610
Gerald Connelly, President & Chief Executive Officer

Priorities: *Arts & Humanities:* 21%. Supports dance, music, historic preservation, and art institutes. *Civic & Public Affairs:* 10%. Supports civic organizations, and community foundations. *Education:* 43%. Supports schools, colleges, and scholarships. *Environment:* 26%. Primarily supports United Way. *Religion:* 4%. *Note:* Total contributions made in 1999. **Typ. Recipients:** Alzheimers Disease, Cancer, Emergency/Ambulance Services, Health Organizations, Hospices, People with Disabilities, Sexual Abuse. **Geo. Dist:** headquarters and operating communities; OH.

★ 12840 ★ Robert I. Wishnick Foundation

1 American Lane
Greenwich, CT 06831
Phone: (212)371-1844
William Wishnick, President & Director

Priorities: *Arts & Humanities:* 17%. Supports art associations, dance, opera, theaters, music, and museums. *Civic & Public Affairs:* 13%. Supports Native American issues, peace initiatives, parades, safety organizations, heritage foundations, and civil rights funds. *Education:* 18%. Supports colleges, universities, private secondary education, and art, science and math education programs. *Environment:* 12%. Supports athletic foundations, counseling programs, family planning, people with disabilities, the homeless, and animal welfare. *International:* 3%. Supports hospitals, health centers, and single-disease health foundations. *Note:* Total foundation contributions made in 2001. **Typ. Recipients:** AIDS/HIV, Cancer, Children's Health/Hospitals, Clinics/Medical Centers, Emergency/Ambulance Services, Family Planning, Geriatric Health, Home-Care Services, Hospitals, Medical Education, Medical Research, Multiple Sclerosis, People with Disabilities, Sexual Abuse, Single-Disease Health Associations. **Geo. Dist:** operating communities.

★ 12841 ★ Robert W. Baird & Co. Foundation

777 East Wisconsin Ave., 28th Floor
Milwaukee, WI 53202
Phone: (414)765-3500 **Fax:** (414)765-3600
Website: http://www.rwbaird.com/about/fr3_ab_ic_home.asp
G. Kasten, Jr., Chairman & Chief Executive Officer

Fnded: 1967. **Priorities:** *Arts & Humanities:* 20%. Funding goes to art institutions and museums, the performing arts, theaters, and libraries. Also funds events under the category of "entertainment," including cultural festivals and parades. *Civic & Public Affairs:* 12%. Supports community and economic development, gardens, clubs, and urban affairs. *Education:* 24%. Supports business education, colleges and universities, education reform, minority education and private education. *Environment:* 37%. Supports the United Way, YMCA, child welfare issues, scouting, youth organizations, and delinquency and criminal rehabilitation. *International:* 4%. Funding goes to cancer research, children's health issues, health organizations, hospitals, and medical research. *Note:* Total contributions made in 2000. **Typ. Recipients:** Cancer, Children's Health/Hospitals, Diabetes, Domestic Violence, Emergency/Ambulance Services, Eyes/Blindness, Health Organizations, Health-General, Heart, Hospitals, Medical Education, Medical Rehabilitation, Medical Research, Mental Health, People with Disabilities, Public Health. **Geo. Dist:** headquarters and operating communities.

★ 12842 ★ Rochester Gas & Electric Corp.

89 East Ave.
Rochester, NY 14649-0001
Phone: (585)546-1100 **Fax:** (716)724-8799
Lydia Boddie-Neal, Manager Corporate Contributions

Priorities: *Civic & Public Affairs:* 5%. *Education:* 25%. *International:* (Health & Welfare) 70%. *Voluntarism:* The company Dollars for Deeds program encourages employee volunteerism. **Typ. Recipients:** Hospitals. **Geo. Dist:** NY, Finger Lakes region.

★ 12843 ★ Rockwell International Corp. Trust

777 E Wisconsin Ave., Suite 1400
Milwaukee, WI 53202
Phone: (414)212-5258
Website: http://rockwellautomation.com/about_us/citizenship.html
Christine Rodriguez, Contact

Priorities: *Arts & Humanities:* 8%. Supports museums; public broadcasting; arts alliances; the performing arts, including theater, music, and opera; and historic preservation. *Civic & Public Affairs:* 15%. Supports chambers of commerce, law and justice, civil rights, public policy, Native American Affairs, ethnic organizations, and housing. *Education:* 37%. Supports colleges, universities, education reform, educational associations, minority education, scholarships, and education funds. *Environment:* 32%. Supports United Way, Young Men's Christian Association, youth programs, scouting, and volunteer services. *International:* 1%. Funds hospitals and single-disease health associations. *Religion:* 6%. Supports museums. *Note:* Total foundation contributions made in fiscal 2000. **Typ. Recipients:** Cancer, Children's Health/Hospitals, Domestic Violence, Emergency/Ambulance Services, Health Organizations, Health Policy/Cost Containment, Hospices, Hospitals, Medical Rehabilitation, Mental Health, People with Disabilities, Public Health, Single-Disease Health Associations, Substance Abuse. **Geo. Dist:** headquarters and operating communities; nationally to education.

★ 12844 ★ Rodman Ford Sales Charitable Trust

Route One
Foxboro, MA 02035-9800
Phone: (508)543-1590
Donald Rodman, Contact

Fnded: 1987. **Typ. Recipients:** Cancer, Diabetes, Single-Disease Health Associations.

★ 12845 ★ Rohm & Hass Corp.

100 Independence Mall West
Philadelphia, PA 19106-2399
Phone: (215)592-3644 **Fax:** (215)592-6808
Email: asamuels@rohmhaas.com
Website: http://www.rohmhaas.com/community/giving/guideline.htm
Alexandra Samuels, Manager, Civic & Philanthropic Affairs

Priorities: *Arts & Humanities:* 17%. Funding primarily supports Philadelphia arts organizations, including public broadcasting stations, music groups, and museums. *Civic & Public Affairs:* 11%. Typically funds organizations concerned with civil rights, urban affairs, business and free enterprise, *Education:* 39%. Support for higher education includes programs that encourage minority youths to enter the fields of chemistry and engineering. Also supports career and vocational training programs, economic education, and matching gifts to precollege and higher education. *International:* 32% of total annual contributions. Primarily supports united funds in company operating locations, the handicapped and youth. *Voluntarism:* Dollars for Doers; Team Doers; J.A. **Typ. Recipients:** Health-General. **Geo. Dist:** principally near operating locations and to national organizations; where employees live.

★ 12846 ★ Rouse Co. Foundation

10275 Little Patuxent Pkwy.
Columbia, MD 21044
Phone: (410)992-6000 **Fax:** (410)992-6363
Website: http://therousecompany.com/whoweare/community/index.html
Margaret Mauro, Executive Director

Fnded: 1967. **Priorities:** *Arts & Humanities:* 36%. Supports the performing arts, film, arts councils, museums, and literary arts. *Civic & Public Affairs:* 18%. Funds housing, civic groups, job training & placement, economic enterprise, regional foundations, and public policy organizations. *Education:* 7%. Gives to education foundations, colleges and universities, scholarship funds, with an emphasis on arts education. *Environment:* 33%. Supports the United Way, sports/recreation programs, food banks, children & family services, and services for the developmentally disabled. *International:* 1%. Supports single-disease health organizations, hospitals and medical centers, hospice programs, and health care for the disadvantaged. *Religion:* 1%. Funds science centers. *Voluntarism:* The company encourages its employees to volunteer time to nonprofit groups and organizations through its Volunteer Contributions Program. Through this program, the company provides grants of up to $1,000 to nonprofit organizations at which the Rouse employees volunteer. Volunteer grants are awarded in the fields of health, education, human services, arts and humanities, community affairs, museums, conservation and preservation. *Note:* Total foundation contributions made in 2000. **Typ. Recipients:** Cancer, Clinics/Medical Centers, Domestic Violence, Hospices, Hospitals, Hospitals (University Affiliated), People with Disabilities, Prenatal Health Issues, Preventive Medicine/Wellness Organizations, Sexual Abuse, Single-Disease Health Associations, Substance Abuse. **Geo. Dist:** MD, Central Maryland.

★ 12847 ★ Royal & SunAlliance Insurance Foundation, Inc.

9300 Arrowpoint Blvd.
Charlotte, NC 28201-1000
Phone: (704)522-2056 **Fax:** (704)522-2055
Fred Dabney, Executive Director

Fnded: 1989. **Priorities:** *Arts & Humanities:* 21%. *Civic & Public Affairs:* 2%. *Education:* 20%. *Environment:* 30%. *International:* 28%. *Religion:* Less than 1%. *Voluntarism:* Company actively encourages employee volunteerism, including an Education Week. Special consideration is given to requests for funding if an employee is involved in the organization in a meaningful voluntary capacity. *Note:* Total contributions in 2001. **Typ. Recipients:** Adolescent Health Issues, AIDS/HIV, Cancer, Child Abuse, Children's Health/Hospitals, Emergency/Ambulance Services, Geriatric Health, Health Funds, Health Organizations, Health-General, Heart, Home-Care Services, Hospices, Hospitals, Mental Health, People with Disabilities, Public Health, Single-Disease Health Associations, Substance Abuse. **Geo. Dist:** areas where producers, employees, and customers reside.

★ 12848 ★ Russer Foods/Zemsky Family Trust

6420 SE Harbor Circle
Stuart, FL 34996-1958
Phone: (407)225-1602
Sam Zemsky, Manager

Fnded: 1987. **Priorities:** *Arts & Humanities:* 32%. Supports museums, performing arts, libraries, public broadcasting, music, dance, and theaters. *Civic & Public Affairs:* 2%. Supports justice organizations, zoos, and community foundations. *Education:* 10%. Supports schools, institutes, and Junior Achievement. *Environment:* 12%. Supports family planning, homes, scouts, senior services, and community funds. *International:* 9%. Support single-disease health associations and general health organizations. *Note:* Total foundation contributions made in 2001. **Typ. Recipients:** Alzheimers Disease, Arthritis, Cancer, Children's Health/Hospitals, Diabetes, Domestic Violence, Family Planning, Geriatric Health, Health Organizations, Heart, Hospices, Hospitals, Medical Research, Mental Health, Multiple Sclerosis, People with Disabilities, Prenatal Health Issues, Public Health, Research/Studies Institutes, Respiratory, Single-Disease Health Associations, Substance Abuse. **Geo. Dist:** Buffalo, NY.

★ 12849 ★ Ryder System Charitable Foundation

3600 NW 82nd Ave.
Miami, FL 33166
Phone: (305)500-3031 **Fax:** (305)593-4579
Email: ray_goode@ryder.com
R. Goode, Executive Director

Priorities: *Arts & Humanities:* 7%. *Civic & Public Affairs:* 9%. *Education:* 20%. *Environment:* 62%. *Voluntarism:* Company actively supports employee volunteerism, and encourages management to volunteer in organizations it supports. *Note:* Total foundation contributions made in 2001. **Typ. Recipients:** Cancer, Children's Health/Hospitals, Hospitals, People with Disabilities, Research/Studies Institutes, Single-Disease Health Associations, Substance Abuse. **Geo. Dist:** Los Angeles, CA, through community initiative program; FL, Dade County; Miami, FL, metropolitan area Miami; Atlanta, GA, through community initiative program; St. Louis, MO, through community initiative program; Cincinnati, OH, through community initiative program; Dallas, TX, through community initiative program.

★ 12850 ★ S.C. Johnson Fund

1525 Howe St.
Racine, WI 53403
Phone: (262)260-2119 **Fax:** (262)260-2652
Website: http://www.scjohnson.com/community/
Colleen Cribari, Program Administrator

Priorities: *Arts & Humanities:* 10%. Supports music, museums, dance, and theater. *Civic & Public Affairs:* 23%. Funds community development, urban centers, municipalities, housing, gardens, and justice concerns. *Education:* 23%. Majority of funding supports scholarships and fellowships for employee children, and minority students in a variety of fields. Also supports capital campaigns and specific programs at local colleges and universities. Education funds, associations, high schools, and INROADS/Wisconsin's Racine Youth Leadership Academy receive funding as well. *Environment:* 6%. Supports Young Men's Christian Association, food banks, human service agencies, and women's centers. *International:* Less than 1%. *Note:* Total contributions made in fiscal 2000. Priorities based on contributions made by S.C. Johnson Fund only. Corporation also sponsors the Johnson Foundation, a private operating foundation. The Johnson Foundation hosts conferences (known as Wingspread conferences) devoted to the improvement of society in several key areas: international understanding, educational excellence, improvement of the human environment, and intellectual and cultural growth. The foundation carries out program extension activities and publications through which it shares with a wider audience the information generated in these conferences. The corporation also offers limited direct contributions. Direct contributions are made to worthy causes for education, social welfare, culture and the arts, youth activities, health and medical concerns, preservation of the environment, emergency and disaster relief, and the disadvantaged. **Typ. Recipients:** AIDS/HIV, Cancer, Children's Health/Hospitals, Clinics/Medical Centers, Health Organizations, Hospitals, Medical Education, Medical Research, Medical Training, Nutrition, People with Disabilities, Single-Disease Health Associations, Substance Abuse. **Geo. Dist:** headquarters and operating communities; Racine, WI. **Frmly:** S.C. Johnson Wax Fund, Inc.

★ 12851 ★ SAFECO Corp.

SAFECO Plaza
Seattle, WA 98185
Phone: (206)545-6279 **Fax:** (206)545-5730
Email: roslin@safeco.com
Website: http://www.safeco.com/safeco/about/giving/giving.asp
Rose Lincoln, Assistant Vice President

Priorities: *Arts & Humanities:* 10% to 15%. Interests include theater, music, dance, museums, arts federations, visual arts, and community festivals. *Civic & Public Affairs:* About 30%. Supports economic development, public safety, civic improvement and neighborhood development. *Education:* About 20%. Interests include job readiness and consumer education in financial areas. *Environment:* 12%. Major support goes to United Way in operating communities. *Voluntarism:* Company has a Volunteer Awards Program through which over 11,000 employees nationwide can participate. *Note:* Total contributions made in 2001. **Typ. Recipients:** Health Organizations, Health Policy/Cost Containment, Mental Health, Nutrition, People with Disabilities, Public Health, Single-Disease Health Associations, Substance Abuse. **Geo. Dist:** headquarters and operating communities in the United States.

★ 12852 ★ Safeguard Scientifics Foundation

800 Safeguard Bldg.
435 Devon Park Drive
Wayne, PA 19087
Phone: (610)293-0600
Gerald Hogan, Director, Corporate Administration

Priorities: *Arts & Humanities:* 16%. *Civic & Public Affairs:* 6%. *Education:* 38%. *Environment:* 21%. *International:* 4%. *Religion:* 11%. *Note:* Total foundation contributions made in 2001. **Typ. Recipients:** AIDS/HIV, Cancer, Children's Health/Hospitals, Diabetes, Emergency/Ambulance Services, Health Funds, Health Organizations, Heart, Hospices, Hospitals, Medical Education, Medical Rehabilitation, Multiple Sclerosis, People with Disabilities, Single-Disease Health Associations.

★ 12853 ★ Saint-Gobain Corp. Foundation

PO Box 860
Valley Forge, PA 19482-0101
Phone: (610)341-7000 **Fax:** (610)341-7777
Dorothy Wackerman, Vice President

Fnded: 1955. **Priorities:** *Arts & Humanities:* 26%. *Civic & Public Affairs:* 8%. *Education:* 24%. *Environment:* 14%. *International:* 8%. *Note:* Approximately 42% of total contributions are for matching gifts. Total foundation contributions made in 2001. **Typ. Recipients:** Alzheimers Disease, Cancer, Child Abuse, Children's Health/Hospitals, Clinics/Medical Centers, Domestic Violence, Emergency/Ambulance Services, Health Organizations, Heart, Hospices, Hospitals, Medical Education, Medical Research, Multiple Sclerosis, People with Disabilities, Prenatal Health Issues, Public Health, Single-Disease Health Associations, Substance Abuse. **Geo. Dist:** principally near operating locations and to national organizations. **Frmly:** CertainTeed Corp. Foundation.

★ 12854 ★ St. Paul Companies Inc. Foundation

385 Washington St.
Saint Paul, MN 55102-1396
Phone: (651)310-7911 **Fax:** (651)310-2327
Website: http://www.stpaul.com
Mary Pickard, President & Executive Director

Priorities: *Arts & Humanities:* 25%. Supports a variety of art groups to ensure expression of diverse cultures and to enhance efforts in education and neighborhood development. Funding includes annual operating support on a three-year basis, capital support (excluding endowment) and special project funds for activities that advance the company's other community affairs goals. Interests include museums, music and art funds, which combine resources to support small- and medium-sized organizations. *Civic & Public Affairs:* (Community Development) 18%. Focus on low-income housing opportunities, leadership skills, and economic viability of city neighborhoods. Interests include philanthropic organizations, neighborhood development, neighborhood-based health clinics, housing, ethnic/minority organizations, and youth organizations. *Education:* 23%. General operating support to private colleges and secondary schools in Minnesota through federated fund drives; support of private college capital and endowment fund drives in Minnesota; support of community-based education, including early childhood development, K-12 initiatives, and employment programs, and support of opportunities for minorities and under-served populations. *Environment:* 22%. *Religion:* 1%. *Voluntarism:* Company-sponsored volunteer projects have included: Junior Achievement, Metro Paint-A-Thon, Voluntary Action Center, Wilson Hi-Rise, Retiree Volunteer Program, Special Olympics, Habitat for Humanity, and school pairing projects. *Note:* Total contributions made in 2001. **Typ. Recipients:** Adolescent Health Issues, AIDS/HIV, Cancer, Clinics/Medical Centers. **Geo. Dist:** select areas where company has large business presence; MD, Baltimore area; Minneapolis, MN; St. Paul, MN.

★ 12855 ★ Salomon Smith Barney Holdings, Inc.
New York, NY 10048
Phone: (718)248-1656 **Fax:** (212)783-4262
Jane Heffner, Vice President, Corporate Contributions

Priorities: *Arts & Humanities:* 27%. Supports the Old Station House Association. *Civic & Public Affairs:* 1%. Grants were given to The Fulbright Foundation and the Japan Society. *Education:* 6%. Awards given to the Capital Partners for Education and The Inner City Scholarship Foundation. *Environment:* 12%. Funds given to the YMCA of Greater New York, and the National Committee to Prevent Child Abuse. *International:* 6% Grant given to The Hartford Hospital. *Note:* Total contributions made in 1997. Contributions were made by the Traveler's Foundation. The company now gives directly through the Salomon Smith Barney Community Investment Program. **Typ. Recipients:** Family Planning, Hospitals, Medical Research, Single-Disease Health Associations, Substance Abuse. **Geo. Dist:** headquarters and operating communities; nationally. **Frmly:** Salomon Foundation Traveler's Group Foundation Traveler's Foundation.

★ 12856 ★ Samuel and Julia Bernstein Foundation
25 Melville Park Rd.
Melville, NY 11747
Phone: (631)752-6178
Joan Marcello, Contact

Fnded: 1946. **Priorities:** *Arts & Humanities:* 30%. Supports opera, galleries, and art associations. *Civic & Public Affairs:* 3%. Primarily supports community foundations. *Education:* 9%. Primary support made to universities. *Environment:* 1%. Supports YWCA and United Way. *International:* 9%. Supports health organizations and single-disease health associations. *Note:* Total contributions made in 2000. **Typ. Recipients:** Arthritis, Cancer, Diabetes, Heart, Hospitals, Medical Rehabilitation, Multiple Sclerosis, People with Disabilities, Prenatal Health Issues, Public Health, Single-Disease Health Associations. **Geo. Dist:** New York, NY.

★ 12857 ★ S&T Bancorp Charitable Foundation
Main Office
PO Box 190
Indiana, PA 15701-0190
Phone: (724)465-1443
James Miller, President

Fnded: 1993. **Priorities:** *Arts & Humanities:* 7%. Supports museums, libraries, and art centers. *Civic & Public Affairs:* 7%. Supports community and economic development, fire departments, public safety, and community fairs and festivals. *Education:* 8%. Supports universities, school funds, and scholarships. *Environment:* 28%. Supports senior services, Big Brothers/Sisters, scouts, United Way, homes, athletic and recreation funds, YMCA, child welfare. *International:* 50%. Supports hospitals, health and medical centers, and single-disease health associations. *Note:* Total foundation contributions made in 2001. **Typ. Recipients:** Cancer, Children's Health/Hospitals, Clinics/Medical Centers, Diabetes, Emergency/Ambulance Services, Heart, Hospitals, Nursing Services, People with Disabilities, Public Health, Single-Disease Health Associations. **Geo. Dist:** headquarters and operating communities.

★ 12858 ★ Sanford C. Bernstein & Co. Foundation, Inc.
767 5th Ave., 22nd Fl.
New York, NY 10153
Phone: (212)486-5800 **Fax:** (212)486-8430
Lewis Sanders, Trustee

Priorities: *Arts & Humanities:* 13%. Supports historical societies, arts associations, museums, and performing arts. *Civic & Public Affairs:* 10%. Funds immigrant services, community projects, and community foundations. *Education:* 20%. Primarily supports pre-college education, including public, private, and Jewish schools; tutoring programs, and special education. *Environment:* 22%. Supports youth programs with emphasis on disadvantaged youth; child welfare programs; shelters; senior services; and volunteer services. *International:* 16%. Support favors hospitals, medical research, single-disease associations, nursing homes, camps for the disabled, and AIDS/HIV health services. *Note:* Total foundation contributions in 2001. **Typ. Recipients:** AIDS/HIV, Arthritis, Cancer, Child Abuse, Children's Health/Hospitals, Clinics/Medical Centers, Diabetes, Eyes/Blindness, Family Planning, Geriatric Health, Health Organizations, Heart, Hospices, Hospitals, Long-Term Care, Medical Research, Nursing Services, People with Disabilities, Prenatal Health Issues, Preventive Medicine/Wellness Organizations, Single-Disease Health Associations, Speech & Hearing. **Geo. Dist:** Los Angeles, CA; San Francisco, CA; CT; FL; NJ; NY; Dallas, TX.

★ 12859 ★ Sara Lee Foundation
3 First National Plaza
49th Floor
Chicago, IL 60602-4260
Phone: (312)558-8426 **Fax:** (312)419-3192
Website: http://www.saraleefoundation.org
Robin Tryloff, President, Executive Director

Priorities: *Arts & Humanities:* 64%. Provides cash support for new, emerging arts groups as well as for major, established institutions in Chicago. Funds performing arts, libraries, art institutes and the visual arts, and culture and the humanities. *Civic & Public Affairs:* 8%. Supports housing, women's causes, community services, and employment. *Education:* 8%. Supports educational programs, minority education and scholarship programs, colleges, and universities. *Environment:* 17%. Gives to organizations that aid the homeless, hungry, youth, and victims of family violence. Also provides major support to the United Way. *International:* 4%. *Religion:* 2%. Funds the Field Museum of Natural History, the Museum of Science and Industry, and food industry related research. *Voluntarism:* Company maintains a 15 to 20 person "Employee Volunteerism Committee," which is responsible for organizing approximately eight programs per year. Also sponsors a "Board Placement Program," through which company executives in the Chicago area are recruited to serve on nonprofit boards. These organizations also may be eligible for a $1,000 grant. *Note:* Total foundation contributions made in fiscal 2000. In addition to foundation's programs, operating companies and divisions administer giving programs based on assessment of needs in the communities where they operate. They contribute cash and product donations to local and national organizations. Divisions and employees also participate in community-based projects. **Typ. Recipients:** AIDS/HIV, Cancer, Domestic Violence, Family Planning, Health Organizations, Hospitals, Nutrition, People with Disabilities, Prenatal Health Issues, Public Health, Research/Studies Institutes, Substance Abuse. **Geo. Dist:** principally near operating locations and to national organizations; Chicago, IL, metropolitan area.

★ 12860 ★ SBC Foundation
130 Travis St., Suite 350
San Antonio, TX 78205
Phone: 800-591-9663 **Fax:** (210)351-2259
Website: http://www.sbc.com/Community/SBC_Foundation
Laura Sanford, President

Priorities: *Arts & Humanities:* 27%. *Civic & Public Affairs:* 6%. *Education:* 23%. *Environment:* 33%. *International:* 7%. *Religion:* 3%. *Note:* Total contributions made in 2001. **Typ. Recipients:** AIDS/HIV, Alzheimers Disease, Cancer, Children's Health/Hospitals, Emergency/Ambulance Services, Health Organizations, Health-General, Hospitals, Medical Education, Medical Research, Mental Health, People with Disabilities, Public Health. **Geo. Dist:** nationally; AR; CA; CT; Washington, DC; IL; IN; KS; MI; MO; NV; NY; OH; OK; TX; VA; WI. **Frmly:** Southwestern Bell Foundation.

★ 12861 ★ SCANA Corp.
1426 Main St.
Columbia, SC 29201
Phone: (803)217-9394 **Fax:** (803)217-9469
Website: http://www.scana.com/SCANA/ForLiving/default.htm
Joann Butler, Manager, Corp. Affairs

Priorities: *Civic & Public Affairs:* Emphasis on community development. *Education:* Focus on primary education. Sponsors programs such as Homework Centers, First Steps, Downtown as Classroom, and Communities in Schools. **Typ. Recipients:** Health-General. **Geo. Dist:** SC, only in company operating locations in central SC.

★ 12862 ★ Schering-Plough Foundation
2000 Galloping Hill Rd.
Kenilworth, NJ 07033-1310
Phone: (908)298-7232 **Fax:** (908)298-7349
Website: http://www.sch-plough.com/cr/philanthropy.html
Christine Fahey, Assistant Secretary

Priorities: *Arts & Humanities:* 11%. *Civic & Public Affairs:* 10%. *Education:* 38%. *Environment:* 6%. *International:* 35%. *Voluntarism:* Provides small grants through its Dollar for Volunteer program most used by employees and their families, American Red Cross, health-care services to low-income working people, and university schools of pharmacy. *Note:* Total foundation contributions made in 2001. **Typ. Recipients:** Alzheimers Disease, Cancer, Children's Health/Hospitals, Clinics/Medical Centers, Domestic Violence, Emergency/Ambulance Services, Geriatric Health, Health Organizations, Health Policy/Cost Containment, Health-General, Hospices, Hospitals, Hospitals (University Affiliated), Long-Term Care, Medical Education, Medical Rehabilitation, Medical Research, Medical Training, Mental Health, People with Disabilities, Public Health, Research/Studies Institutes, Single-Disease Health Associations, Single-Disease Health Associations, Substance Abuse, Transplant Networks/Donor Banks. **Geo. Dist:** principally near operating locations and to national organizations.

★ 12863 ★ Schlumberger Foundation
153 E 53 St., 57th Floor
New York, NY 10022
Phone: (212)350-9400 **Fax:** (212)350-9440
Website: http://www.slb.com/seed/
Arthur Alexander, Executive Director

Priorities: *Civic & Public Affairs:* 2%. *Education:* 84%. *Environment:* 10%. *International:* 2%. *Note:* Total contributions made in 2001. **Typ. Recipients:** Alzheimers Disease, Cancer, Children's Health/Hospitals, Eyes/Blindness, Family Planning, Hospices, Hospitals, Medical Education, Medical Research, People with Disabilities, Single-Disease Health Associations, Substance Abuse. **Geo. Dist:** nationally to education; New York, NY.

★ 12864 ★ Schoeneckers Foundation
PO Box 1610
Minneapolis, MN 55440
Phone: (612)835-4800 **Fax:** (612)844-4033
L. Schoenecker, President

Fnded: 1979. **Priorities:** *Civic & Public Affairs:* 2%. Supports philanthropic organizations and community foundations. *Education:* 94%. Primary support made to universities. *Environment:* 2%. Supports YMCA, United Way, athletic organizations, and youth services. *International:* 2%. Primary support made to health associations. *Note:* Total foundation contributions made in fiscal 2001. **Typ. Recipients:** Alzheimers Disease, Cancer, Children's Health/Hospitals, Diabetes, Emergency/Ambulance Services, Health Organizations, Heart, Hospices, Hospitals, Multiple Sclerosis, Respiratory, Single-Disease Health Associations. **Geo. Dist:** MN.

★ 12865 ★ Schurz Communications Foundation
225 West Colfax Ave.
South Bend, IN 46624
Phone: (219)287-1001 **Fax:** (219)236-1765
Todd Schurz, President

Fnded: 1940. **Priorities:** *Arts & Humanities:* 20%. *Civic & Public Affairs:* 11%. *Education:* 3%. *Environment:* 53%. *International:* 5%. *Note:* Total contributions made in 2001. **Typ. Recipients:** Hospices. **Geo. Dist:** South Bend, IN, and surrounding area.

★ 12866 ★ Schwebel Family Foundation
PO Box 6018
Youngstown, OH 44501-6018
Phone: (330)783-2860
Paul Schwebel, Trustee

Fnded: 1989. **Priorities:** *Arts & Humanities:* 5%. Funds arts councils and a theater. *Civic & Public Affairs:* 4%. Supports Junior League and other civic organizations. *Education:* 25%. Supports colleges and universities, public schools, and arts education. *Environment:* 22%. Supports the United Way, youth organizations, YMCAs, substance abuse organizations, planned parenthood, and food distribution services. *International:* 22%. Supports single-disease health organizations, hospitals, hospice, and health funds. *Note:* Total contributions made in 1998. **Typ. Recipients:** Cancer, Children's Health/Hospitals, Diabetes, Family Planning, Health Organizations, Health-General, Heart, Hospices, Hospitals, Multiple Sclerosis, People with Disabilities, Single-Disease Health Associations, Speech & Hearing. **Geo. Dist:** OH.

★ 12867 ★ Scientific-Atlanta, Inc.
5030 Sugarloaf Pkwy.
Lawrenceville, GA 30042
Phone: (770)236-4607 **Fax:** (770)236-4725
Email: bill.mccargo@sciatl.com
Bill McCargo, Directory, Community Relations

Priorities: *Arts & Humanities:* 15%. *Civic & Public Affairs:* 15%. *Education:* 40%. *International:* 30%. **Typ. Recipients:** Health-General. **Geo. Dist:** headquarters and operating communities.

★ 12868 ★ Scripps Howard Foundation
312 Walnut St.
PO Box 5380
Cincinnati, OH 45201-5380
Phone: (513)977-3035 **Fax:** (513)977-3800
Email: cottingham@scripps.com
Website: http://www.scripps.com/foundation
Judith Clabes, President & CEO

Priorities: *Arts & Humanities:* 7%. *Civic & Public Affairs:* 38%. The Fund supports various charitable organizations that improve the quality of life in operating areas through the Community Fund and the Greater Cincinnati Fund. Supports educational institutions that produce potential employees, readers or viewers; or that promote strong community conscience and encourage alternatives in education. Social welfare organizations which make significant contributions to the disadvantaged are supported, including the United Way, the Salvation Army, food banks, and scouting and Big Brothers. Supports civic organizations that promote leadership, community involvement, good government, sound public policy, free speech or journalism. Company also awards grants up to $1,000 to qualifying organizations where employees volunteer, and encourages employees to become involved in the communities where they live and work. *Education:* 21%. Awards scholarships, fellowships, and internships to full-time students preparing for careers in journalism. Preference is given to students with continuing interest and work in the field of journalism, prior recipients, and students residing in or attending schools located in communities served by company operations. The Robert P. Scripps Graphic Arts Grant is awarded to graphic arts majors who, in the opinion of college authorities, have the potential for becoming newspaper production administrators. Also provides grants to organizations that promote literacy, and matches employee gifts to educational institutions. *Environment:* 6%. *International:* 3%. *Note:* Total contributions made in 2001. **Typ. Recipients:** Children's Health/Hospitals, Emergency/Ambulance Services, Geriatric Health, People with Disabilities, Prenatal Health Issues, Preventive Medicine/Wellness Organizations, Substance Abuse. **Geo. Dist:** nationally, with emphasis on operating locations; particularly Greater Cincinnati, OH; OH, operating locations; Cincinnati, OH, metropolitan area.

★ 12869 ★ Sealaska Heritage Foundation
1 Sealaska Plz., Suite 201
Juneau, AK 99801
Phone: (907)586-9261
Rosita Worl, Executive Director

Typ. Recipients: Health Organizations. **Geo. Dist:** AK.

★ 12870 ★ Security Benefit Life Insurance Co. Charitable Trust
700 Southwest Harrison St.
Topeka, KS 66636-0001
Phone: (785)431-3215
Howard Fricke, Contact

Fnded: 1976. **Priorities:** *Arts & Humanities:* 20%. Supports performing arts, theaters, museums, and libraries. *Civic & Public Affairs:* 6%. Supports zoos, women's affairs, and community foundations. *Education:* 31%. Supports schools, education associations, colleges, and universities. *Environment:* 28%. Supports YWCA, volunteer services, United Way, senior organizations, food distribution, scouts, shelters, homes, and Big Brothers/Sisters. *International:* 8%. Supports hospitals and health foundations. *Note:* Total foundation contributions made in 2001. **Typ. Recipients:** Cancer, Children's Health/Hospitals, Diabetes, Emergency/Ambulance Services, Family Planning, Health Organizations, Hospices, Medical Education, Mental Health, People with Disabilities, Prenatal Health Issues, Single-Disease Health Associations. **Geo. Dist:** Topeka, KS, some giving in other areas of Kansas.

★ 12871 ★ Sega Youth Education & Health Foundation
650 Townsend St., Suite 650
San Francisco, CA 94103-5633
Phone: (415)701-3725
Steve Choy, Director

Fnded: 1992. **Priorities:** *Arts & Humanities:* 1%. *Education:* 32%. The foundation contributes to educational programs that seek to integrate technology into the curriculum and school culture, programs that supplement school curriculum and improve learning, and teacher development programs. Applicants should be prepared to demonstrate project's impact on systemic change efforts. While classroom use of technology is a high priority, the foundation prefers to fund comprehensive technology programs, not necessarily the purchase of hardware. The foundation also supports youth HIV/AIDS programs, primarily focusing on education and prevention. *Environment:* 34%. Funds programs to prevent child abuse, Boys and Girls Clubs, and other youth-related social services. *International:* 32%. Supports health programs that provide medical services to children, preferably in the context of enduring and meaningful access to care, and programs that improve pediatric care through resources and training for pediatricians, nurses, and others who care for children. Another area of focus is the pediatric AIDS crisis. *Note:* Total contributions in 1998. **Typ. Recipients:** AIDS/HIV, Cancer, Child Abuse, Children's Health/Hospitals, Clinics/Medical Centers, Diabetes, Family Planning, Health Organizations, Heart, Hospitals, Prenatal Health Issues, Respiratory, Single-Disease Health Associations, Substance Abuse. **Geo. Dist:** nationally–some foundation-initiated programs may be national in scope; San Francisco Bay area of Contra Costa County; CA, San Francisco Bay Area of Alamedo County; CA, San Francisco Bay Area of Santa Clara County; CA, San Francisco Bay area of San Francisco; CA, San Francisco Bay area of San Mateo County.

★ 12872 ★ Sempra Energy
101 Ash St.
San Diego, CA 92101-3017
Phone: (619)696-4297 **Fax:** (619)696-1868
Email: community@sempra.com
Website: http://sempra.com/community/
Molly Cartmill, Director Corporate Community Relations

Priorities: *Arts & Humanities:* About 15%. Supports arts appreciation, art associations, art centers, visual arts, opera and music, and historic preservation. Special preference is given to efforts that create cultural dialog and promote a greater understanding of diversity. The company is a partner in Disney Hall in Los Angeles. *Civic & Public Affairs:* About 20%. Funds community leadership and events. Supports consumer affairs, economic development, environmental affairs, urban and community affairs, and ethnic and minority affairs. Emphasis is on crime prevention. *Education:* 25% to 30%. Supports programs that motivate students to be prepared for higher education; that promote technology-based learning; and that encourage success in the fields of engineering, technology, business, or international relations. Also funds the Sempra Scholars program, developed to attract outstanding undergraduates to the fields of engineering and information technology. *International:* (Health and Human Services) 35% to 40%. Funds programs that lead to lifelong fitness, healthy lifestyles, and human wellness. Also supports efforts to help those in need, such as the homeless or hungry. Supports the aged and geriatric health, hospices and hospitals, medical research, single-disease health associations, child welfare, community centers and community service organizations, family services, and traditional youth organizations. Major emphasis is on drug abuse prevention. *Voluntarism:* The company promotes employee volunteerism through Team San Diego Gas & Electric, a group of nearly 1,200 employees and family members who volunteer in hands-on community service projects. **Typ. Recipients:** Geriatric Health, Health Organizations, Hospices, Hospitals, Medical Education, Medical Research, Mental Health, People with Disabilities, Single-Disease Health Associations, Substance Abuse. **Geo. Dist:** CA, Southern California.

★ 12873 ★ Sentry Insurance Foundation Inc.
1800 N Point Drive
Stevens Point, WI 54481
Phone: (715)346-6000 **Fax:** (715)346-6405
Margie Coker-Nelson, Executive Director, Vice President

Priorities: *Arts & Humanities:* 2%. Funds cultural groups and public broadcasting. *Civic & Public Affairs:* 5%. Supports community industries and commerce. *Education:* 43%. Supports scholarships and higher education, and matching gifts. *Environment:* 48%. Supports the United Way and human service organizations. *International:* 1%. Supports medical research. *Note:* Total foundation contributions made in 2001. **Typ. Recipients:** Cancer, Domestic Violence, Health Organizations, Heart, Hospitals, Medical Research, People with Disabilities, Public Health, Substance Abuse. **Geo. Dist:** nationally; areas with large employee populations.

★ 12874 ★ Servco Foundation
PO Box 2788
Honolulu, HI 96803
Phone: (808)521-6511 **Fax:** (808)523-3937
Website: http://www.servco.com/community/
Sandra Wong, Corporate Secretary

Fnded: 1986. **Typ. Recipients:** Cancer, Child Abuse, Clinics/Medical Centers, Diabetes, Emergency/Ambulance Services, Health Organizations, Health-General, Heart, Hospitals, Medical Rehabilitation, Single-Disease Health Associations, Substance Abuse. **Geo. Dist:** nationally; HI.

★ 12875 ★ ServiceMaster Foundation
2300 Warrenville Rd.
Downers Grove, IL 60515

Phone: (630)271-1300
C. Pollard, President & Director

Fnded: 1987. **Priorities:** *Arts & Humanities:* 4%. *Civic & Public Affairs:* 30%. *Education:* 31%. *Environment:* 15%. *Note:* Total contributions in 2001. **Typ. Recipients:** Family Planning, Health-General, Hospitals. **Geo. Dist:** headquarters area only.

★ 12876 ★ Shaw Industries, Inc.
PO Box 2128
Dalton, GA 30722
Phone: (706)278-3812 **Fax:** (706)275-1139
Gerald Embry, Vice President, Administration

Typ. Recipients: Health-General. **Geo. Dist:** headquarters and operating communities.

★ 12877 ★ Shaw's Supermarkets Charitable Foundation
140 Laurel St.
PO Box 600
East Bridgewater, MA 02333
Phone: (508)350-3316 **Fax:** (508)350-3112
Website: http://www.shaws.com/Public/about_us/community_commitment.cfm
Bernard Rogan, Corporate Communications Director

Fnded: 1959. **Priorities:** *Arts & Humanities:* 7%. *Civic & Public Affairs:* 1%. *Environment:* 87%. *International:* 5%. *Note:* Total contributions in fiscal 2001. **Typ. Recipients:** Children's Health/Hospitals, Clinics/Medical Centers, Emergency/Ambulance Services, Eyes/Blindness, Geriatric Health, Health Funds, Health Organizations, Hospitals, Nursing Services, Public Health, Single-Disease Health Associations. **Geo. Dist:** headquarters and operating communities; CT; ME; MA; NH; RI; VT.

★ 12878 ★ Shell Oil Co. Foundation
One Shell Plaza
PO Box 2099
Houston, TX 77252
Phone: (713)241-4480 **Fax:** (713)241-3329
Email: SOCFoundation@shellus.com
Website: http://www.countonshell.com/community/involvement/shell_foundation.html
Betty McHam, vice president

Fnded: 1953. **Priorities:** *Arts & Humanities:* About 10%. Primarily gives in communities where company employees live. Supports a variety of disciplines, with emphasis on cultural centers, music, museums, opera, public TV/radio, dance, art councils, performing arts, theaters, and libraries. *Civic & Public Affairs:* 3%. Interest in national and local development, community improvement, research organizations, environmental efforts, public policy, justice and law, and minority needs. *Education:* 45% to 50%. Emphasis on support of higher education through established programs (by invitation only). Shell Doctoral Fellowships encourage outstanding students to seek teaching careers in engineering and the sciences. Shell Faculty Career Initiation Funds support untenured faculty in science and engineering research. Shell Departmental Grants are designed to strengthen activities in specified areas related to teaching and/or research. Shell Career Counseling Grants are used to enhance career counseling and placement activities in colleges and universities with well-established programs. Precollege programs focus on math and science programs. Shell Incentive Funds are targeted to undergraduate minority students, with emphasis on technology and business education. National education funds, education organizations, and economic education receive substantial support. Also sponsors matching gifts program, and scholarships for children of employees. *Environment:* 50%. *International:* About 33%. Primary support goes to united funds. Support also goes to national health agencies, national welfare agencies, youth organizations and local health and welfare agencies. A priority is hospitals which serve employees, particularly through capital support. *Religion:* Less than 1%. *Voluntarism:* Company sponsors "Shell Employees and Retirees Volunteerism Effort" (SERVE), through which company employees and retirees have participated in housing rehabilitation projects, educational television solicitations, school clothing drives, and picnics for mentally handicapped children. Employees also serve on the boards of various organizations and loaned executives work with United Way campaigns. *Note:* Total contributions made in fiscal 2000 as reported by the foundation. **Typ. Recipients:** Children's Health/Hospitals, Clinics/Medical Centers, Eyes/Blindness, Health Funds, Health Organizations, Heart, Hospices, Hospitals, Hospitals, Hospitals (University Affiliated), Medical Education, Medical Rehabilitation, Medical Research, Mental Health, People with Disabilities, Single-Disease Health Associations, Substance Abuse. **Geo. Dist:** nationally, with emphasis on communities where Shell employees are located.

★ 12879 ★ Shelter Insurance Foundation
1817 West Broadway
Columbia, MO 65218
Phone: (573)214-4290 **Fax:** (573)446-5727
Raymond Jones, Secretary & Director

Fnded: 1981. **Priorities:** *Arts & Humanities:* 1%. *Civic & Public Affairs:* 3%. *Education:* 91%. Almost all funding went towards scholarships. *Environment:* 2%. Supports scouting, crime prevention, and programs for the elderly. *International:* 2%. *Note:* Total contributions in fiscal 2001. **Typ. Recipients:** AIDS/HIV, Alzheimers Disease, Cancer, Children's Health/Hospitals, Heart, Medical Education, Medical Research, People with Disabilities, Single-Disease Health Associations. **Geo. Dist:** AK; CO; IL; IN; IA; KS; KY; LA; MS; MO; Columbia, MO; NE; OK; TN.

★ 12880 ★ Sherman-Standard Register Foundation
600 Albany St., PO Box 1167
Dayton, OH 45408
Phone: (937)443-1540 **Fax:** (937)221-3431
Kathryn Lamme, Corporate Vice President

Fnded: 1955. **Priorities:** *Arts & Humanities:* 3%. Supports an art center. *Civic & Public Affairs:* 3%. Supports women's causes. *Education:* 11%. Provides funds for a high school and children's learning center. *Environment:* 49%. Supports the United Way, scouting, YMCA, and youth organizations. *International:* 4%. Funds neuroscience and the American Red Cross. *Religion:* 4%. Funds a natural history museum. *Note:* Total contributions made in fiscal 2001. **Typ. Recipients:** Cancer, Children's Health/Hospitals, Clinics/Medical Centers, Emergency/Ambulance Services, Health Funds, Health-General, Hospices, Hospitals, Public Health, Research/Studies Institutes, Transplant Networks/Donor Banks. **Geo. Dist:** OH.

★ 12881 ★ Sherwin-Williams Foundation
101 Prospect Ave. NW
Cleveland, OH 44115
Phone: (216)566-2000 **Fax:** (216)566-3266
Barbara Gadosik, Director, Corporate Contributions

Priorities: *Arts & Humanities:* 10%. Supports museums, art associations, and performing arts associations in Cleveland, OH, area. *Civic & Public Affairs:* 28%. Funds community/neighborhood development programs, manufacturing associations, and matching gifts for volunteer leaders. *Education:* 29%. About half of education support is given in the form of matching gifts. Also supports 4-H, universities, independent college funds, and scholarship programs. *Environment:* 27%. Funds the United Way in operating locations. Youth, the disabled, and other human services organizations also receive support. *International:* 3%. Supports hospitals, single-disease health associations, and the American Red Cross. *Note:* Total foundation contributions made in 2000. **Typ. Recipients:** Cancer, Diabetes, Emergency/Ambulance Services, Hospices, Hospitals, Hospitals (University Affiliated), Long-Term Care, Medical Education, Medical Education, Medical Rehabilitation, People with Disabilities, Preventive Medicine/Wellness Organizations, Public Health, Single-Disease Health Associations. **Geo. Dist:** headquarters and operating communities, primarily Cleveland.

★ 12882 ★ Sierra Pacific Foundation
PO Box 496028
Redding, CA 96049-6028
Phone: (530)378-8000 **Fax:** (530)378-8109
Email: foundation@spi-ind.com
Website: http://www.sierrapacificind.com/Company/SPFoundation.htm
Stephanie Donham, Contact

Fnded: 1978. **Priorities:** *Arts & Humanities:* 11%. *Civic & Public Affairs:* 25%. *Education:* 29%. *Environment:* 18%. *Note:* Total foundation contributions made in fiscal 2002. **Typ. Recipients:** Cancer, Emergency/Ambulance Services, Health Organizations, Heart, Hospices, Hospitals, Medical Research, Nutrition, Single-Disease Health Associations, Transplant Networks/Donor Banks. **Geo. Dist:** headquarters and operating communities.

★ 12883 ★ Sierra Pacific Resources Charitable Foundation
PO Box 30150
Reno, NV 89520
Phone: (702)579-1589
Email: kfoster@sppc.com
Website: http://www.sierrapacific.com/comenv/comrel/foundation/
Karen Foster, Secretary, Treasurer

Fnded: 1988. **Priorities:** *Arts & Humanities:* 16%. Supports art museums and foundations, classical music, humanities councils, libraries, public broadcasting, and an opera house. *Civic & Public Affairs:* 11%. Gives to municipalities, minority and women's affairs, economic development, and state sponsored events, including a rodeo. *Education:* 34%. Primarily supports colleges and universities, with an emphasis on technology, mining and geology, and environmental science. Also supports science fairs and pre K-12 education schools and programs. *Environment:* 32%. Mainly supports youth organizations including scouting, Boys & Girls Clubs, YMCAs and athletic/recreational activities. Also funds senior services, food distribution, and the United Way. *International:* 1%. Primarily funds national health organizations and single-disease associations. *Voluntarism:* Company employees are active in the community, participating in the Day of Caring, blood drives, and events such as the Special Olympics and the March of Dimes WalkAmerica. *Note:* Total contributions made in 2000. **Typ. Recipients:** Alzheimers Disease, Cancer, Children's Health/Hospitals, Diabetes, Emergency/Ambulance Services, Family Planning, Heart, Hospitals, Mental Health, People with Disabilities, Public Health, Respiratory, Single-Disease Health Associations. **Geo. Dist:** headquarters and operating communities; CA, Northeastern California; NV, Northern Nevada.

★ 12884 ★ Simpson Fund
1301 5th Ave., No. 2800
Seattle, WA 98101
Phone: (206)224-5198 **Fax:** (206)436-1852
Email: cmusgra@simpson.com
Website: http://www.simpson.com
Colleen Musgrave, Administrator

Priorities: *Arts & Humanities:* 8%. Gives to museums, performing arts, and art councils. *Civic & Public Affairs:* 20%. Funds civic and community organizations, including volunteer fire departments, economic development organizations, business associations, community foundations, and civic clubs. *Education:* 37%. Supports colleges and universities, primary and secondary schools, and public school districts. *Environment:* 27%. Most support goes to united funds, shelters, and food banks. Supports some health organizations. *Voluntarism:* The company sponsors a United Way "Day of Caring" program where employees volunteer their time to help a designated United Way organization. *Note:* Total contributions made in 2000. **Typ. Recipients:** Arthritis, Child Abuse, Children's Health/Hospitals, Clinics/Medical Centers, Emergency/Ambulance Services, Geriatric Health, Health Organizations, Hospices, Hospitals, Nursing Services, Sexual Abuse, Substance Abuse, Transplant Networks/Donor Banks, Trauma Treatment. **Geo. Dist:** CA, Del Norte County; CA, Humboldt

County; OR, Lincoln County; OR, Tillamook County; WA, Grays Harbor County; WA, King County; WA, Mason County; WA, Pierce County; WA, Thurston County.

★ 12885 ★ Simpson Investment Co.
1301 5th Ave., Suite 2800
Seattle, WA 98101
Phone: (206)224-5198 **Fax:** (206)436-1852
Email: cmusgra@simpson.com
Colleen Musgrave, Coordinator

Typ. Recipients: Hospitals, Medical Research, Single-Disease Health Associations. **Geo. Dist:** CA, Del Norte County and Humboldt County; OR, Lincoln County and Tillamook County; WA, Mason County, Grays Harbor County, and Thurston County; Seattle, WA; Tacoma, WA.

★ 12886 ★ SIT Investment Associates Foundation
90 S 7th St., Ste. 4600
Minneapolis, MN 55402-4130
Phone: (612)332-3223 **Fax:** (612)342-2018
Paul Rasmussen, Chief Financial Officer

Priorities: *Arts & Humanities:* 53%. Funds music, theater, historic societies, museums, and public broadcasting. *Civic & Public Affairs:* 3%. Funds housing, civic organizations, leadership foundations, and professional organizations. *Education:* 24%. Mainly supports colleges and universities. *Environment:* 12%. Supports shelters, food banks, United Way, and youth organizations. *International:* 3%. Funds medical foundations, emergency services, and single-disease health associations. *Note:* Total contributions made in 2000. **Typ. Recipients:** Children's Health/Hospitals, Emergency/Ambulance Services, Health Organizations, Heart, Hospices, Medical Rehabilitation, People with Disabilities, Single-Disease Health Associations, Substance Abuse. **Geo. Dist:** IN; MN; NY.

★ 12887 ★ Slant/Fin Foundation
100 Forest Dr.
Greenvale, NY 11548
Phone: (516)484-2600 **Fax:** (516)484-8906
M. Dubin, Controller

Fnded: 1985. **Priorities:** *Arts & Humanities:* 2%. Interests include art associations, museums, music, and performing arts. *Civic & Public Affairs:* 2%. Emphasis on community development and civic affairs. *Education:* 6%. Supports colleges, universities, and foundations. *Environment:* 1%. *International:* 3%. Supports hospitals, medical centers, and single-disease health associations. *Note:* Total contributions made in 1998. **Typ. Recipients:** Alzheimers Disease, Cancer, Children's Health/Hospitals, Clinics/Medical Centers, Geriatric Health, Health-General, Hospices, Hospitals, Medical Education, Medical Rehabilitation, Medical Research, People with Disabilities, Public Health, Single-Disease Health Associations. **Geo. Dist:** nationally; NY.

★ 12888 ★ SMBC Global Foundation, Inc.
277 Park Ave.
New York, NY 10172
Phone: (212)224-4031
Naoyuki Kawamoto, President

Fnded: 1995. **Priorities:** *Arts & Humanities:* 30%. *Civic & Public Affairs:* 5%. *Education:* 42%. *Environment:* 12%. *Note:* Total contributions made in 2001. **Typ. Recipients:** Children's Health/Hospitals, Domestic Violence, Substance Abuse. **Geo. Dist:** internationally, with emphasis on Asian countries.

★ 12889 ★ Solo Cup Foundation
1700 Old Deerfield Rd.
Highland Park, IL 60035
Phone: (847)831-4800 **Fax:** (847)831-5849
Ronald Whaley, Foundation Administrator

Fnded: 1959. **Priorities:** *Civic & Public Affairs:* 2%. Supports volunteer organizations and civic initiatives. *Education:* 13%. Funds private precollege education. *Environment:* 7%. Supports United Way, homes for the disabled, substance abuse recovery programs, religious welfare, and youth groups. *International:* 7%. Supports hospitals and medical research. *Note:* Total foundation contributions made in fiscal 2001. **Typ. Recipients:** Cancer, Children's Health/Hospitals, Clinics/Medical Centers, Hospices, Hospitals, People with Disabilities, Prenatal Health Issues, Public Health, Single-Disease Health Associations, Substance Abuse. **Geo. Dist:** IL.

★ 12890 ★ Sonoco Foundation
One North 2nd St., Mail Stop A09
Hartsville, SC 29550
Phone: (843)383-7000 **Fax:** (843)383-7008
Email: joyce.beasley@sonoco.com
Website: http://www.sonoco.com/sonoco_foundation.htm
Joyce Beasley, Manager, Community Affairs

Priorities: *Arts & Humanities:* 3%. Supports historic preservation, museums, arts councils, and arts festivals. *Civic & Public Affairs:* 7%. Majority of giving supports urban and community development projects designed to improve and revitalize communities, and promote the general well-being of all citizens. *Education:* 64%. Primarily supports colleges and universities, college funds, private and public secondary education, business education, and humanities education. Focus is on institutions from which the company recruits. *Environment:* 22%. Emphasis on YMCAs, youth organizations, and the United Way. *International:* 1%. Single-disease health associations. *Religion:* 3%. Supports a museum. *Note:* Total contributions made in 2000. **Typ. Recipients:** Cancer, Children's Health/Hospitals, Domestic Violence, Emergency/Ambulance Services, Eyes/Blindness, Health Organizations, Health-General, Heart, Hospitals, Medical Rehabilitation, Medical Research, Mental Health, Multiple Sclerosis, People with Disabilities, Research/Studies Institutes, Single-Disease Health Associations, Substance Abuse. **Geo. Dist:** counties in which employees reside; SC.

★ 12891 ★ Sony U.S.A. Foundation Inc.
550 Madison Ave., 33rd Floor
New York, NY 10022
Phone: (212)833-6873 **Fax:** (212)833-6854
Website: http://www.sony.com/SCA/philanthropy.shtml
Ann Morfogen, President

Priorities: *Arts & Humanities:* 1%. Supports music, opera, museums, and public broadcasting in New York City. *Civic & Public Affairs:* 19%. Supports urban and community affairs including civic organizations, foundations, and employment training. Includes efforts to promote the advancement and recognition of minorities. *Education:* 29%. Funding supports institutions and programs that bring commitment and innovation to the task of strengthening education at the primary and secondary school levels, with consideration also given to selected higher education initiatives. Also supports efforts that promote literacy and basic educational competency, and encouragement of the technical and scientific skills required of tomorrow's work force. Also funds arts education. Scholarships are awarded to the children of employees. *Environment:* 41%. Majority of funds support the United Way. Additional funding supports youth organizations and other human services. *International:* 10%. Supports hospitals and healthcare organizations. *Religion:* 1%. *Note:* Above priorities are for Sony USA Foundation in 2000. Sony Corp. of America subsidiaries run independent giving programs. **Typ. Recipients:** Cancer, Child Abuse, Children's Health/Hospitals, Diabetes, Emergency/Ambulance Services, Eyes/Blindness, Health Organizations, Heart, Hospitals, Medical Rehabilitation, Mental Health, Multiple Sclerosis, People with Disabilities, Prenatal Health Issues, Preventive Medicine/Wellness Organizations, Public Health. **Geo. Dist:** headquarters and operating communities; nationally.

★ 12892 ★ Southwest Gas Corp. Foundation
5241 Spring Mountain Rd.
PO Box 98510
Las Vegas, NV 89193-8510
Phone: (702)876-7247 **Fax:** (702)876-7037
Suzanne Farinas, Assistant to the Chief Executive Officer

Priorities: *Arts & Humanities:* 8%. Support includes local orchestras, symphonies, museums, public broadcasting, and performing arts. *Civic & Public Affairs:* 14%. Funding supports a variety of legal and business associations, community service, housing, and public safety. *Education:* 22%. Education program emphasizes universities, colleges, scholarship funds, and literacy. *Environment:* 43%. Major support for the United Way. Also supports community service organizations, a volunteer center, seniors, low-income services, shelters and food banks, and emergency relief. Supports youth agencies and scouting. *International:* 7%. Funds single-disease health associations and university medical centers. *Religion:* 2%. Supports museums and science centers. *Voluntarism:* The company sponsors an employee volunteer team that works on various projects. *Note:* Total contributions made in 2001. **Typ. Recipients:** Arthritis, Cancer, Children's Health/Hospitals, Clinics/Medical Centers, Diabetes, Domestic Violence, Emergency/Ambulance Services, Eyes/Blindness, Heart, Hospices, Hospitals, Medical Research, People with Disabilities, Prenatal Health Issues, Respiratory, Single-Disease Health Associations. **Geo. Dist:** AZ, Southern and Central Arizona; CA; KS; NV, Northern and Southern Nevada (except Reno); WA.

★ 12893 ★ Sovereign Bank Foundation
Two Aldwyn Center
Lancaster Ave. & Route 30
Villanova, PA 19085
Phone: (610)526-6226
Joseph Schupp, Foundation Manager

Priorities: *Civic & Public Affairs:* 70%. Supports community, economic, and neighborhood development, housing, ethnic organizations and business services. *Education:* 4%. Supports universities, institutes, and academies. *Environment:* 23%. Supports YMCA, senior services, homeless shelters, and youth organizations. *Note:* Total foundation contributions made in 2001. **Typ. Recipients:** AIDS/HIV, Clinics/Medical Centers, Domestic Violence, Family Planning, Health-General, Hospitals, People with Disabilities, Public Health, Sexual Abuse, Single-Disease Health Associations. **Geo. Dist:** bank or service areas; NJ, Mercer County.

★ 12894 ★ Spang & Co. Charitable Trust
PO Box 751
Butler, PA 16003-0751
Phone: (724)287-8781
K. McKnight, Contact

Priorities: *Arts & Humanities:* 16%. Supports libraries, theaters, music, symphony, public broadcasting, and opera. *Civic & Public Affairs:* 22%. Supports safety, zoos, community foundations and development, and fire departments. *Education:* 15%. Supports private schools and educational funds. *Environment:* 21%. Supports United Way, scouts, animal protection, senior services, and camps. *International:* 26%. Funds hospitals, medical institutes, and single-disease associations. *Note:* Total foundation contributions made in 2000. **Typ. Recipients:** Cancer, Children's Health/Hospitals, Clinics/Medical Centers, Domestic Violence, Eyes/Blindness, Heart, Hospitals, Hospitals (University Affiliated), Kidney, Medical Education, Medical Research, Nursing Services, People with Disabilities, Single-Disease Health Associations. **Geo. Dist:** PA.

★ 12895 ★ Spartan Stores, Inc.
1020 Ford St.
Maumee, OH 43537
Phone: (616)878-8513 **Fax:** (419)891-4907
Email: pat_nowak@spartansstores.com

Priorities: *Arts & Humanities:* About 20%. Contributes to art associations, museums, community and folk arts, libraries, performing arts, and public broadcasting. *Civic & Public Affairs:* About 15%. Primary support for philanthropic organizations. *Education:* About 10%. Colleges and universities, elementary education, and literacy programs are the primary recipients. *Environment:* About 25%. Supports child services and youth organizations, community centers, drug rehabilitation programs, homeless shelters and recreation programs. *International:* About 10%. Support for hospitals and health organizations with emphasis on geriatric health. **Typ. Recipients:** Domestic Violence, Geriatric Health, Health Organizations, Hospitals, Nutrition, Substance Abuse. **Geo. Dist:** headquarters area only; MI, Southeastern Michigan; OH, Northwest Ohio.

★ 12896 ★ Springs Industries, Inc.

PO Box 70
Fort Mill, SC 29716
Phone: (803)547-1500 **Fax:** (803)547-3740
Ted Matthews, Vice President, Corporate Contributions

Priorities: *Arts & Humanities:* About 10%. Priorities include arts associations and historic preservation. Other interests include a museum, galleries, and community arts. *Civic & Public Affairs:* 25%. Primary interest is organizations concerned with business or free enterprise. Interests also include economic development, professional and trade associations, and public policy organizations. *Education:* 55%. Major priorities include improvement in higher education and adult education. Other interests include business education, elementary and secondary education, economic education, and public and private education organizations. *International:* 10%. Major welfare interests include community service, family service, and youth organizations. Major health interests include hospitals and single disease health associations. Smaller contributions go to organizations promoting health care cost containment, child welfare, drug and alcohol abuse prevention, and united funds. **Typ. Recipients:** Hospices, Hospitals, Single-Disease Health Associations, Substance Abuse. **Geo. Dist:** principally near operating locations and to national organizations.

★ 12897 ★ Sprint Foundation

6330 Sprint Parkway
Overland Park, KS 66251
Phone: (913)762-4555 **Fax:** (913)624-3490
Website: http://www.sprint.com/sprint/overview/commun.html
David Thomas, Executive Director

Priorities: *Arts & Humanities:* 17%. Supports major visual and performing arts organizations, museums and other cultural organizations, and activities which have effective outreach programs that broaden the cultural experience of the general public and bring cultural opportunity to the economically disadvantaged. *Civic & Public Affairs:* 23%. Supports economic development, legal and women's issues, and civic organizations. Special project grants targeted to encourage resource-sharing efforts among not-for-profit agencies are also considered. *Education:* 30%. Supports activities that will prepare people for the challenges of the workplace and enable them to be productive participants in the economy by addressing educational needs and initiatives covering the childhood through early adult years. Targets public school renewal and reform, programs that enhance educational opportunities for minorities and/or the disadvantaged, excellence in teaching and retention of quality educators, encourages employee and public support of education, and the use of new communications technology in education. Also sponsors matching gifts program. *Environment:* 29%. Supports youth organizations with drug and alcohol education, minority youth endeavors, community youth activities, and United Way. *International:* 2%. Supports medical centers. *Note:* Total contributions in 1998. **Typ. Recipients:** Cancer, Children's Health/Hospitals, Emergency/Ambulance Services, Heart, Public Health. **Geo. Dist:** principally near operating locations and to national organizations; also to areas where the company's subsidiaries have major concentrations of employees.

★ 12898 ★ SPX Foundation

700 Terrace Point Drive
Muskegon, MI 49443-3301
Phone: (231)724-5121 **Fax:** (231)724-5720
Tina Betlejewski, President

Fnded: 1984. **Priorities:** *Arts & Humanities:* Less than 1%. *Civic & Public Affairs:* 58%. *Education:* 18%. *Environment:* 11%. *International:* 6%. *Note:* Total contributions made in 2001. **Typ. Recipients:** Cancer, Child Abuse, Children's Health/Hospitals, Diabetes, Emergency/Ambulance Services, Family Planning, Health Organizations, Health-General, Hospitals, Multiple Sclerosis, People with Disabilities, Single-Disease Health Associations, Substance Abuse. **Geo. Dist:** primarily in plant communities.

★ 12899 ★ Square D Foundation

1415 South Roselle Rd.
Palatine, IL 60067
Phone: (847)397-2600 **Fax:** (847)397-2804
Harry Wilson, Secretary

Priorities: *Arts & Humanities:* 2%. *Civic & Public Affairs:* 13%. *Education:* 45%. *Environment:* 30%. *International:* 8%. *Religion:* 2%. *Note:* Total contributions made in 2001. **Typ. Recipients:** Cancer, Children's Health/Hospitals, Clinics/Medical Centers, Emergency/Ambulance Services, Health Funds, Hospitals, Long-Term Care, Medical Research, Mental Health, People with Disabilities, Single-Disease Health Associations. **Geo. Dist:** manufacturing facility communities.

★ 12900 ★ Stanley Works

1000 Stanley Drive
New Britain, CT 06053
Phone: (860)827-3566 **Fax:** (860)827-3581

Typ. Recipients: Cancer, Children's Health/Hospitals, Emergency/Ambulance Services, Hospitals, Medical Research, People with Disabilities, Substance Abuse. **Geo. Dist:** operating location communities.

★ 12901 ★ Star Tribune Foundation

425 Portland Ave.
Minneapolis, MN 55488-0002
Phone: (612)673-7314 **Fax:** (612)673-7020
Email: sfleitman@startribune.com
Website: http://startribune.com/company/ic/home/community/foundation.htm
Sandra Fleitman, Assistant Secretary

Priorities: *Arts & Humanities:* 26%. Support goes to major organizations that form the core of the cultural community, primarily in the Twin Cities. Also funds smaller organizations that have demonstrated promise or community interest. Recipients include theaters, orchestral and music groups, the visual arts, and organizations concerned with literature and writing. *Civic & Public Affairs:* 20%. Funds organizations concerned with neighborhood development, both socially and economically. Also supports programs that help people understand world issues and that encourage people to participate in important civic issues. Sponsors an employee matching gifts program for civic and cultural organizations that have a company employee on the governing board. Also supports journalism and media professional associations. *Education:* 12%. Emphasis is on preeminent institutions of higher learning and on writing-related programs that also enlighten social consciousness. Support is directed to educational organizations concerned with the First Amendment and to policy issues in journalism and communications, and to professional education programs. Recipients include: journalism education programs, particularly for minorities; the Minnesota Newspaper Foundation, conferences concerned with newspapers, reports, and editors; and groups interested in libel and freedom of the press. *Environment:* 36%. Funds organizations which assist people to move from dependence to self-reliance; in particular, those organizations which help create opportunities, aid self-reliance, assist people to meet basic needs, and respond to current and future needs. Supports local United Way chapter in the headquarters area; a portion of this funding is in matching gifts. Also supports organizations concerned with adolescents, youth groups, teen pregnancy and parenting. Aids emergency services such as food distribution and matches employee gifts to the Emergency Food Shelf. *International:* 5%. Contributes to the American Red Cross, as well as women's and children's health programs. *Religion:* 1%. Funds a science museum. *Note:* Total foundation contributions in fiscal 2000. **Typ. Recipients:** AIDS/HIV, Domestic Violence, Emergency/Ambulance Services, Family Planning, Medical Rehabilitation, People with Disabilities, Substance Abuse. **Geo. Dist:** Minneapolis-St. Paul, MN. **Frmly:** Cowles Media Foundation.

★ 12902 ★ Starwood Hotels & Resorts Worldwide, Inc.

1111 Westchester Ave.
White Plains, NY 10604
Phone: (914)640-8198 **Fax:** (914)640-8134
Email: Katherine.Condits@starwoodhotels.com
Website: http://www.starwoodhotels.com/corporate/company_values_comm.html
Katherine Condits, Senior Vice President Corporate Affairs

Priorities: *Arts & Humanities:* Supports a variety of local arts groups, centers, and funds. Also supports museums and public broadcasting. *Civic & Public Affairs:* Sponsors awards and assistance program to recognize and support ideas for local civic improvement. Also supports civil rights and minority affairs groups and urban affairs organizations. *Education:* Highest priority. Areas of interest include independent and minority college funds, business education, and education associations. Also supports programs in creative management and computer technology. Administers matching gifts program. *Environment:* Emphasis on youth programs. Also supports organizations concerned with the disabled, emergency relief, alcohol and drug abuse, the aged, community service, and delinquency and crime. *International:* Supports a variety of medical research programs, as well as hospitals and other health organizations. **Typ. Recipients:** Domestic Violence, Emergency/Ambulance Services, Geriatric Health, Hospices, Hospitals, Medical Research, Nutrition, People with Disabilities, Single-Disease Health Associations, Substance Abuse. **Geo. Dist:** headquarters and operating communities.

★ 12903 ★ State Farm Companies Foundation

One State Farm Plaza, SC3
Bloomington, IL 61710-0001
Phone: (309)766-9739 **Fax:** (309)766-2314
Website: http://www.statefarm.com/foundati/foundati.htm
Lori Manning, Contact

Fnded: 1963. **Priorities:** *Arts & Humanities:* 3%. Supports arts and culture organizations with an emphasis on history museums and societies. *Civic & Public Affairs:* 1%. Funds leadership foundations, law organizations and women's organizations. *Education:* 66%. Supports colleges and universities, insurance education, fellowships, and doctoral awards. *Environment:* 27%. Supports the United Way, youth activities, and a wide variety of health and human service organizations. *International:* 3%. Funds medical programs. *Voluntarism:* Company-sponsored volunteer programs include loaned executives for United Way campaigns, Junior Achievement advisors, and Red Cross Blood drives. Interested employees complete a questionnaire, then receive a newsletter of volunteer activities. Employees participate in activities on their own initiative. *Note:* Total contributions made in 1998. **Typ. Recipients:** Cancer, Children's Health/Hospitals, Clinics/Medical Centers, Hospitals, Medical Education, Medical Rehabilitation, Public Health, Substance Abuse. **Geo. Dist:** near major offices.

★ 12904 ★ State Street Foundation
225 Franklin St.
Boston, MA 02110-2804
Phone: (617)664-3381 **Fax:** (617)451-6315
Email: gabowman@statestreet.com
George Bowman, Jr., Vice President, Community Affairs

Priorities: *Civic & Public Affairs:* (Neighborhood Revitalization) 12%. Funds programs to increase housing availability for low and moderate income persons and make their neighborhoods safer, more prosperous places to live and work. *Education:* (Education and Job Skills Training) 30%. Supports initiatives to improve educational quality and opportunities for students in areas where State Street has operations. Funds programs that help students succeed and prepare for advancement to higher education, and that increase jobs and job opportunities. Funds adult/family literacy and job skills training and development initiatives that help prepare under-employed and displaced workers to participate successfully in the changing workforce. *Environment:* (Youth Programs) 14%. Funds initiatives addressing high school dropout prevention and teen pregnancy and parenting issues. *International:* (Health and Human Needs) 31%. Supports hospitals, medical centers, single-disease health associations, and other health-related organizations. Provides funding for human services, including child and family services, youth organizations, and major support for the United Way. *Voluntarism:* State Street Global Outreach is a company-wide volunteer program that encourages employee participation in company-sponsored programs, pairs employees who are interested in volunteer opportunities with non-profit organizations with missions that are of interest to the employees, and offers each employee one work day a year for volunteer efforts. *Note:* Total foundation contributions in 2001. **Typ. Recipients:** Adolescent Health Issues, AIDS/HIV, Cancer, Child Abuse, Children's Health/Hospitals, Clinics/Medical Centers, Diabetes, Domestic Violence, Eyes/Blindness, Geriatric Health, Health Funds, Health Organizations, Health Policy/Cost Containment, Hospitals, Medical Education, Medical Rehabilitation, Mental Health, People with Disabilities, Public Health. **Geo. Dist:** Boston, MA, including the metro area.

★ 12905 ★ Stauffer Communications Foundation
PO Box 936
Augusta, GA 30903-0936
Phone: (706)823-3462
William Morris, IV, Trustee

Priorities: *Arts & Humanities:* 19%. Primarily for the literary arts. *Civic & Public Affairs:* 38%. Support for a community foundation, philanthropic organizations, public policy groups, and civil rights causes. *Education:* 17%. Colleges and universities, medical education, public and private secondary education, and vocational education. *Environment:* 15%. Community centers, YM/YWCAs, scouting, child welfare, and youth organizations. *International:* 2%. *Religion:* 8%. *Note:* Total contributions made in 1998. **Typ. Recipients:** Alzheimers Disease, Cancer, Child Abuse, Children's Health/Hospitals, Clinics/Medical Centers, Emergency/Ambulance Services, Health Organizations, Hospitals, Medical Education, People with Disabilities, Public Health. **Geo. Dist:** KS; OK.

★ 12906 ★ Steelcase Foundation
PO Box 3636
Grand Rapids, MI 49501-3636
Phone: (616)653-0364 **Fax:** (616)475-2200
Email: sbroman@steelcase.com
Susan Broman, Executive Director

Priorities: *Arts & Humanities:* 9%. *Civic & Public Affairs:* 6%. *Education:* 23%. *Environment:* 34%. *International:* 10%. *Note:* Total foundation contributions made in fiscal 2001. **Typ. Recipients:** AIDS/HIV, Arthritis, Child Abuse, Children's Health/Hospitals, Clinics/Medical Centers, Domestic Violence, Emergency/Ambulance Services, Family Planning, Geriatric Health, Health Organizations, Health Policy/Cost Containment, Health-General, Hospices, Medical Rehabilitation, Mental Health, Nutrition, People with Disabilities, Prenatal Health Issues, Public Health, Single-Disease Health Associations, Substance Abuse. **Geo. Dist:** principally near operating locations and to national organizations.

★ 12907 ★ Steiner Foundation
505 East South Temple
Salt Lake City, UT 84102
Phone: (801)328-8831
Kevin Steiner, President

Fnded: 1959. **Priorities:** *Arts & Humanities:* 26%. Funds music, dance, and theater. *Civic & Public Affairs:* 5%. Funds a zoo and civil society. *Education:* 54%. Supports schools, colleges and universities, educational programs, and literacy. *Environment:* 7%. Funds athletics and homes. *International:* 3%. *Religion:* 3%. *Note:* Total contributions made in fiscal 2000. **Typ. Recipients:** Adolescent Health Issues, Arthritis, Cancer, Children's Health/Hospitals, Domestic Violence, Hospitals, Nursing Services, Single-Disease Health Associations. **Geo. Dist:** UT.

★ 12908 ★ Stone & Webster, Inc.
100 Technology Ctr. Dr.
Stoughton, MA 02072
Phone: (617)589-2023 **Fax:** (617)589-2156

Priorities: *Note:* Minimally supports civic and public affairs, health and human services, and arts organizations. **Typ. Recipients:** Health Organizations. **Geo. Dist:** MA; New York, NY.

★ 12909 ★ Stonecutter Foundation
Dallas St.
PO Box 157
Spindale, NC 28160
Phone: (828)286-2341
Van Lonon, Staff Assistant

Priorities: *Civic & Public Affairs:* 5%. Supports employee legal affairs, economic development, and housing. *Education:* 84%. Supports colleges, universities, and private secondary education. *Environment:* 3%. Supports United Way, recreation, youth and family centers, and scouts. *International:* 2%. Supports hospices, medical research, and health centers. *Religion:* 1%. Primarily supports science centers. *Note:* Total foundation contributions made in fiscal 2001. **Typ. Recipients:** Domestic Violence, Hospices, Hospitals, Medical Research, Preventive Medicine/Wellness Organizations. **Geo. Dist:** NC.

★ 12910 ★ StorageTek Foundation
One StorageTek Drive
Louisville, CO 80028-4305
Phone: (303)673-6833 **Fax:** (303)673-8876
Website: http://www.storagetek.com/home/about/foundation/
Arlyce Lewis, Manager, Community Relations

Priorities: *Arts & Humanities:* 8%. Supports orchestras, outreach programs, arts education, and children's programs. Supports projects that extend cultural opportunities that benefit a broad population base and enhance the quality of life. *Education:* 29%. Supports Junior Achievement, scholarships, leadership and outreach programs, women and minority engineering programs, computer labs and networking, educational media, matching gifts, and Boulder Valley public schools. Focus is on innovative programs that strengthen the educational process in the areas of science, math, engineering, management, and technology. Supports literacy, including computer literacy and reading skills. *Environment:* 61%. Support includes health and human services. Major support to the YMCA in Boulder, CO. *Voluntarism:* Employees actively volunteer for a variety of corporate-sponsored activities, including Meals on Wheels, Boy Scouts, community hospitals, food banks, high schools and elementary schools, 4-H clubs, and wildlife and rescue groups. The company initiated the Volunteers in Partnership with the Community (VIP.COM) program in 1998. The program not only encourages employees to volunteer commitments, but also generates additional funds from the company for nonprofit organizations to which employees dedicate time. *Note:* Total contributions made in 1998. **Typ. Recipients:** Arthritis, Cancer, Children's Health/Hospitals, Clinics/Medical Centers, Domestic Violence, Emergency/Ambulance Services, Health Funds, Health Organizations, Health-General, Heart, Hospices, Hospitals, Medical Rehabilitation, Mental Health, Multiple Sclerosis, Nutrition, People with Disabilities, Public Health, Single-Disease Health Associations, Substance Abuse, Transplant Networks/Donor Banks. **Geo. Dist:** headquarters area only.

★ 12911 ★ Strear Family Foundation
6825 E Tennessee Ave., Suite 235
Denver, CO 80224
Phone: (303)399-4631 **Fax:** (303)388-9125
Leonard Strear, Chairman, President & CEO

Fnded: 1987. **Priorities:** *Arts & Humanities:* 2%. *Civic & Public Affairs:* 19%. *Education:* 3%. *Environment:* 3%. *International:* 10%. *Religion:* 2%. *Note:* Total foundation contributions made in fiscal 2002. **Typ. Recipients:** Alzheimers Disease, Cancer, Children's Health/Hospitals, Diabetes, Emergency/Ambulance Services, Health Organizations, Health-General, Hospices, Hospitals, Medical Research, Multiple Sclerosis, People with Disabilities, Speech & Hearing, Substance Abuse. **Geo. Dist:** CO.

★ 12912 ★ Stride Rite Foundation
400 Atlantic Ave.
Boston, MA 02110
Phone: (617)574-4169 **Fax:** (617)574-6595
Website: http://www.strideritecorp.com/pages/philanthropic/index.asp
Ellen Sahl, Treasurer & Director

Fnded: 1953. **Priorities:** *Arts & Humanities:* 1%. Grants often support museums, art centers, theater, dance, operas, and symphonies. *Civic & Public Affairs:* 22%. Recipients include civic and public affairs groups and community organizations. Supports other grantmaking foundations. *Education:* 27%. Majority of funding supports precollege education. *Environment:* 48%. Supports United Way, Big Brothers/Big Sisters, and children and family social service organizations. Recipients also include child recreational groups, including volunteer groups and community centers. *International:* 1%. *Note:* Total foundation contributions made in fiscal 2000. **Typ. Recipients:** Cancer, Child Abuse, Children's Health/Hospitals, Clinics/Medical Centers, Diabetes, Hospitals, Nursing Services, People with Disabilities, Prenatal Health Issues, Public Health, Substance Abuse. **Geo. Dist:** operating locations; Boston, MA; Cambridge, MA.

★ 12913 ★ Stupp Brothers Bridge & Iron Co. Foundation
120 S Central Ave., Suite 1650
Saint Louis, MO 63105
Phone: (314)638-5000 **Fax:** (314)721-6334
Robert Stupp, Trustee

Priorities: *Arts & Humanities:* 4%. Supports historical societies, arts councils, museums, archaeology, and public broadcasting. *Civic & Public Affairs:* 12%. Funds community beautification, zoos, parks, botanical gardens, community festivals, and philanthropic organizations. *Education:* 48%. Colleges, universities, and secondary schools receive support, as well as education funds and foundations. *Environment:* 24%. Major support is given to the United Way. Other interests include traditional youth organizations, sports and recreation programs, community services, and child welfare. *International:* 4%. Funds children's hospitals, pediatric health care, hospice, single-disease health associations. *Religion:* 2%. Contributes to science centers. *Note:* Total foundation contributions made in fiscal 2001. **Typ. Recipients:** Cancer, Children's Health/Hospitals, Family Planning, Health Organizations, Hospices, Hospitals, Medical Research, People with Disabilities, Public Health, Single-Disease Health Associations, Substance Abuse. **Geo. Dist:** MO.

★ 12914 ★ Subway Sandwich Shops, Inc.
325 Bic Drive
Milford, CT 06460
Phone: (203)877-4281 **Fax:** (203)783-7302
Email: klotzer_m@subway.com
Website: http://www.subway.com/subwayroot/about-subway
Michele Klotzer, Corp. Communications
Typ. Recipients: Multiple Sclerosis, People with Disabilities. **Geo. Dist:** headquarters; nationally.

★ 12915 ★ Sun Microsystems Foundation, Inc.
Mail Stop PAL 1-462
901 San Antonio Rd.
Palo Alto, CA 94303
Phone: (650)336-0545 **Fax:** (650)856-2114
Email: corpaffrs@sun.com
Website: http://www.sun.com/aboutsun/comm_invest/giving/foundation.html
Andrea Gooden, Executive Director
Fnded: 1990. **Priorities:** *Arts & Humanities:* Less than 1%. *Civic & Public Affairs:* 11%. *Education:* 29%. *Environment:* 39%. *International:* Less than 11%. *Voluntarism:* Sun Microsystem's Community Action Volunteer Program provides employees with a wide range of volunteer opportunities. Through the Open Gateways program, employees volunteer to provide technical support and training for schools and teachers to make meaningful use of technology in the classroom. The Community Partnership Program provides financial support for organizations where employees volunteer; the company and organization form a yearlong partnership. Employee volunteers also participate in the Sun Foundation's grant review process. Worldwide Volunteer Week allows for more concentrated efforts by company volunteers. *Note:* Total foundation contributions made in fiscal 2001. **Typ. Recipients:** AIDS/HIV, Cancer, Children's Health/Hospitals, Diabetes, Emergency/Ambulance Services, Health Organizations, Heart, Hospitals, Multiple Sclerosis, People with Disabilities, Single-Disease Health Associations. **Geo. Dist:** South San Francisco, CA, Bay Area; Denver, CO, the Front Page Communities (up to and including Longmont); MA, Merrimack Valley; West Lothian District.

★ 12916 ★ Sunoco Inc.
Ten Penn Center
1801 Market St.
Philadelphia, PA 19103
Phone: (215)977-3924
Website: http://www.sunocoinc.com/aboutsunoco/contributions.htm
Ed Hazzouri, Director Public Affairs
Typ. Recipients: Hospitals, People with Disabilities, Public Health, Substance Abuse. **Geo. Dist:** operating locations; Philadelphia, PA.

★ 12917 ★ SunTrust Bank Atlanta Foundation
Mail Code 041
PO Box 4418, Mail Code 041
Atlanta, GA 30302
Phone: (404)588-8246 **Fax:** (404)230-5550
William Bowdoin, Jr., First Vice President/Secretary
Priorities: *Arts & Humanities:* 20%. Supports major Atlanta arts organizations and centers through direct grants and arts funds. Interests include dance, history, and public broadcasting. *Civic & Public Affairs:* 9%. Interests include urban and community affairs, economic development, municipalities, philanthropic organizations, botanical gardens, and zoos. *Education:* 17%. Primarily supports colleges and universities. Private schools are also major recipients, including religious institutions. The remainder supports business and economic education, minority education, international studies, and secondary education. Also sponsors matching gifts program. *Environment:* 52%. Supports human service organizations primarily through the United Way of Metropolitan Atlanta. Other interests include youth organizations, child welfare, community service organizations, family services, and recreation and athletics. *International:* Less than 1%. *Note:* Total foundation contributions made in 2000. **Typ. Recipients:** Alzheimers Disease, Children's Health/Hospitals, Clinics/Medical Centers, Domestic Violence, Emergency/Ambulance Services, Geriatric Health, Health Organizations, Hospitals, Medical Education, Medical Rehabilitation, Medical Training, Mental Health, Nursing Services, People with Disabilities, Public Health, Single-Disease Health Associations, Substance Abuse. **Geo. Dist:** Atlanta, GA, metropolitan area.

★ 12918 ★ SunTrust Banks Foundation
PO Box 3838
Orlando, FL 32802
David Hanson, Contact
Priorities: *Arts & Humanities:* 9%. *Civic & Public Affairs:* 20%. Funds a statewide leadership organization and a zoo. *Education:* 14%. Supports an educational foundation and Florida community colleges. *Environment:* 9%. Funds services for families, youth, and the disabled. *International:* 57%. Supports Florida medical centers and hospitals. *Note:* Total contributions made in 2000. **Typ. Recipients:** Cancer, Clinics/Medical Centers, Hospices, Hospitals, People with Disabilities, Research/Studies Institutes, Substance Abuse. **Geo. Dist:** FL.

★ 12919 ★ SuperValu Foundation
PO Box 990
Minneapolis, MN 55440
Phone: (612)828-4000 **Fax:** (952)828-4838
Website: http://www.supervalu.com/community/comm_main.html
Frank O'Keefe, Vice President, Assistant Treasurer
Fnded: 1993. **Priorities:** *Arts & Humanities:* 4%. Funds arts councils, children's art programs, theaters, art museums and centers, and orchestras. *Civic & Public Affairs:* 10%. Gives to citizen's leagues, ethnic organizations, cities, zoos and parks, chambers of commerce, and job training/self sufficiency. *Education:* 47%. Supports business, political, and cooperative education programs; programs designed to build knowledge and leadership skills of youth; and urban projects relating to the employability of youth. Also supports colleges and universities. *Environment:* 35%. Supports the United Way in the headquarters area; organizations providing assistance to minority, physically challenged, disabled, and disadvantaged persons; and hunger relief efforts. Also supports organizations and programs aimed at promotion of nutrition and organizations established to educate and train people to enter the workforce. *International:* 4%. Primarily supports single-disease health associations. *Note:* Total foundation contributions made in fiscal 2001. Percentages provided by foundation. **Typ. Recipients:** Arthritis, Cancer, Emergency/Ambulance Services, Health-General, People with Disabilities, Single-Disease Health Associations, Substance Abuse. **Geo. Dist:** nationally; organizations in the company's general service area; Minneapolis-St. Paul, MN.

★ 12920 ★ Susquehanna-Pfaltzgraff Foundation
140 East Market St.
York, PA 17401
Phone: (717)848-5500 **Fax:** (717)771-1440
John Finlayson, Vice President, Finance & Administration
Fnded: 1966. **Priorities:** *Arts & Humanities:* 50%. *Civic & Public Affairs:* 7%. *Education:* 8%. *Environment:* 28%. *International:* 4%. *Voluntarism:* The company provides employee volunteer opportunities with the United Way, Junior Achievement, Boy Scouts, Adopt-A-House, blood drives, walk-a-thons, and a variety of other charities and fundraising events. *Note:* Total contributions made in 2001. **Typ. Recipients:** Cancer, Children's Health/Hospitals, Eyes/Blindness, Health-General, Hospitals, People with Disabilities, Public Health, Single-Disease Health Associations. **Geo. Dist:** headquarters and operating communities.

★ 12921 ★ Sverdrup Corp. Charitable Trust
13723 Riverport Drive
Maryland Heights, MO 63043
Phone: (314)466-3439
Thomas Wehrle, Treasurer
Fnded: 1951. **Priorities:** *Arts & Humanities:* 23%. Supports performing arts and arts councils. *Civic & Public Affairs:* 14%. Funds professional trade organizations, county fairs, and the Better Business Bureau. *Education:* 33%. Supports scholarship funds, colleges and universities, technical and engineering education, and Junior Achievement. *Environment:* 24%. Supports the United Way and Goodwill Industries. *International:* Less than 1%. Supports Race for the Cure. *Note:* Total contributions made in 2000. **Typ. Recipients:** Cancer, Children's Health/Hospitals, People with Disabilities, Single-Disease Health Associations. **Geo. Dist:** nationally; Saint Louis, MO.

★ 12922 ★ Synetic Foundation
PO Box 359
Elmwood Park, NJ 07407-0359
Phone: (858)759-3508
Cynthia Young, Executive Director
Fnded: 1991. **Priorities:** *Civic & Public Affairs:* 10%. Funds community services. *Education:* 7%. Supports schools. *Environment:* 13%. Supports programs for youth and family services. *International:* 70%. Supports public health issues and children's health. *Note:* Total contributions made in fiscal 2000. **Typ. Recipients:** Adolescent Health Issues, AIDS/HIV, Alzheimers Disease, Cancer, Children's Health/Hospitals, Clinics/Medical Centers, Family Planning, Health Organizations, Health Policy/Cost Containment, Health-General, Hospitals, Medical Research, Public Health. **Geo. Dist:** CA; NJ. **Frmly:** Medco Containment Services Foundation.

★ 12923 ★ Synovus Charitable Trust
PO Box 120
Columbus, GA 31902
Phone: (706)649-2679 **Fax:** (706)649-5986
William Slaughter, Jr., Manager
Priorities: *Arts & Humanities:* Less than 1%. *Civic & Public Affairs:* 18%. *Education:* 12%. *Environment:* 55%. *International:* 7%. *Religion:* 2%. *Note:* Total foundation contributions made in 2001. **Typ. Recipients:** Alzheimers Disease, Arthritis, Cancer, Child Abuse, Children's Health/Hospitals, Clinics/Medical Centers, Domestic Violence, Emergency/Ambulance Services, Eyes/Blindness, Family Planning, Geriatric Health, Health Organizations, Health-General, Heart, Hospices, Hospitals, Long-Term Care, Medical Education, Medical Rehabilitation, Mental Health, Multiple Sclerosis, Outpatient Health Care, Single-Disease Health Associations, Substance Abuse. **Geo. Dist:** Columbus, GA.

★ 12924 ★ T/A Frontier Corp. Educational Fund
On HSBC Center, 16th Fl.
Buffalo, NY 14203-2885
Phone: 800-284-5866
Pat Grover, Contact
Priorities: *Education:* 100%. Supports scholarships. *Voluntarism:* Company supports the Genesee Chapter of the Telephone Pioneers. **Typ. Recipients:** People with Disabilities. **Geo. Dist:** company's service areas.

★ 12925 ★ T. Rowe Price Associates Foundation
100 E Pratt St., 8th Fl.
Baltimore, MD 21202
Phone: (410)345-3603 **Fax:** (410)345-2848
A. Hubbard, Jr., President
Priorities: *Arts & Humanities:* 24%. Supports theaters, museums, galleries, music, art associations, and historic preservation. *Civic & Public Affairs:* 24%. Funds environmental affairs, and urban and community affairs. *Education:* 33%. Supports colleges and universities, public and private schools for precollege

education, art education, business education, literacy, after-school and summer education programs, education scholarship funds and minority education. *Environment:* (Human Services) 19%. Supports United Way chapters, community and family service organizations, child welfare, shelters for abused women and children, food distribution, mentoring programs for at-risk children, homeless shelters, welfare-to-work programs, and low-income housing. *International:* 1%. *Religion:* 1%. *Voluntarism:* The foundation sponsors several volunteer events per year, including: New Song Investment Academy Program, in partnership with a local inner-city school; Habitat for Humanity, employees volunteer on a weekly basis throughout the year to build or renovate a sponsored house; United Way Day of Caring, in conjunction with the corporate United Way campaign; Dollars for Doers, matches employee's volunteer hours with a financial donation; Susan G. Komen Race for the Cure, with over 350 employee participants; Dragon Boat Race, employees practice more than 800 hours to race for a local charity; Holiday Giving Program, with employee donations for the needy; and Red Cross Blood Drive, to encourage participation in blood donation. *Note:* Total contributions in 2000. Contributions analysis provided by foundation. **Typ. Recipients:** Child Abuse, Emergency/Ambulance Services, Health Organizations, Heart, Hospitals, Medical Education, Mental Health, People with Disabilities, Single-Disease Health Associations. **Geo. Dist:** headquarters and operating communities.

★ 12926 ★ Taco Bell Foundation

17901 Von Karman Ave., MD 1207
Irvine, CA 92614
Phone: (949)863-3970 **Fax:** (949)863-2246
Email: lgannon@tacobell.com
Website: http://www.teensupreme.org/main.html
Laurie Gannon, Manager, Public Affairs

Fnded: 1993. **Priorities:** *Environment:* 100%. **Typ. Recipients:** Emergency/Ambulance Services, Health Organizations. **Geo. Dist:** CA, Southern California.

★ 12927 ★ Tanner Foundation

PO Box 1139
Rutherfordton, NC 28139
Phone: (828)287-4205 **Fax:** (828)286-2072
George Clayton, III, Treasurer

Typ. Recipients: Emergency/Ambulance Services, Eyes/Blindness, Health Organizations, Health-General, Heart, Hospices, Hospitals, People with Disabilities, Prenatal Health Issues, Single-Disease Health Associations. **Geo. Dist:** NC, Rutherford County.

★ 12928 ★ Target Foundation

1000 Nicollet Mall, TPS30
Minneapolis, MN 55403
Phone: (612)696-6098 **Fax:** (612)696-5088
Email: bridget.mcginnis@target.com
Website: http://www.target.com/target_group/community/community_main.jhtml

Fnded: 1918. **Priorities:** *Arts & Humanities:* 37%. Supports professional nonprofit arts organizations in all disciplines. Typically supported are arts centers and museums, public broadcasting, orchestras and opera, theater, and children's arts organizations. *Civic & Public Affairs:* 11%. Funds community volunteer resources, chambers of commerce, economic and neighborhood development, housing, minority affairs, job training, nonprofit management, public parks, and other civic interests. *Education:* 10%. Contributes to scholarship funds, colleges and universities, primary school programs, and literacy initiatives. *Environment:* 35%. Supports the United Way, youth and family services, prevention of child abuse, disaster relief, community services, and recreation programs. *International:* 6%. Funds hospitals, medical centers, and camps for children with cancer and terminal illnesses and single-disease health organizations. *Voluntarism:* Each division of the company has its own volunteer program. Company-wide, Target Corp. jointly sponsors "Day of Giving" in the spring/summer. *Note:* Total foundation contributions made in fiscal 2001. Target stores (Mervyn's California, Target, Dayton's, Hudson's, and Marshall Field's) also support giving programs. See Additional Information for information on these giving programs. **Typ. Recipients:** AIDS/HIV, Children's Health/Hospitals, Domestic Violence, Family Planning, Health Organizations, People with Disabilities, Research/Studies Institutes. **Geo. Dist:** headquarters and operating communities. **Frmly:** Dayton Hudson Corporate.

★ 12929 ★ TCF Foundation

200 Lake St. East (EXO-02-C)
Wayzata, MN 55391-1693
Phone: (952)745-2757 **Fax:** (952)745-2775
Email: ksack@tcfbank.com
Ms. Kelly Sack, **** Officer

Priorities: *Civic & Public Affairs:* 11%. Supports employment initiatives. *Environment:* 89%. Supports YMCA. *Voluntarism:* The company encourages employee volunteerism through local divisions, including programs such as March of Dimes, paint-a-thons, and home-repair days. *Note:* Total foundation contributions made in 2000. **Typ. Recipients:** Children's Health/Hospitals, Clinics/Medical Centers, Health Funds, Health Organizations, Health-General, Heart, Hospitals, Medical Rehabilitation, Public Health, Substance Abuse. **Geo. Dist:** MN, headquarters and operating communities.

★ 12930 ★ Teichert Foundation

3500 American River Dr.
Sacramento, CA 95864-5802
Phone: (916)484-3011
Email: info@teichertfoundation.org
Website: http://www.teichertfoundation.org
Frederick Teichert, Executive Director

Fnded: 1990. **Priorities:** *Arts & Humanities:* 20%. Supports benefit productions, libraries, historical societies, opera, and the arts. *Civic & Public Affairs:* 9%. Funds women's services and neighborhood development and housing, community foundations. *Education:* 21%. Supports universities, public schools, and educational programs. *Environment:* 34%. Funds youth services, the needy, food banks, and animal welfare. *International:* 2%. Funds single-disease health associations. *Religion:* 1%. Supports the Explorit Science Center. *Note:* Total contributions made in 1998. **Typ. Recipients:** Children's Health/Hospitals, Clinics/Medical Centers, Emergency/Ambulance Services, Family Planning, Heart, Mental Health, Multiple Sclerosis, People with Disabilities, Prenatal Health Issues, Public Health. **Geo. Dist:** headquarters and operating communities.

★ 12931 ★ Tektronix Foundation

PO Box 500, MS 55-715
Beaverton, OR 97077-0001
Phone: (503)627-7111
Website: http://www.tektronix.com
Karen Montague, Administrator

Priorities: *Arts & Humanities:* 17%. Majority supports arts outreach programs, which combine arts and education. Also supports Oregon arts groups, with an emphasis on Portland. Matches gifts to art and culture. *Civic & Public Affairs:* 15%. Supports the Portland Metro Zoo and minority and employment programs. *Education:* 41%. Major support is awarded to colleges and universities emphasizing technical, business, and computer science education. Also supports K-12 education, focusing on math, physical sciences, and supplementary programs. Matches gifts to education, and provides scholarships for employees' children. *Environment:* 27%. Majority supports the United Way; also funds youth organizations. *Note:* Total contributions made in 2000. **Typ. Recipients:** Emergency/Ambulance Services, Hospitals. **Geo. Dist:** OR, Northwestern Oregon; WA, Southwestern Washington.

★ 12932 ★ Telcordia Technologies

445 South St., Room 1A301B
Morristown, NJ 07960
Phone: (973)829-2177 **Fax:** (973)829-2159
Ron Reichmann, Manager, Corporate Contributions

Fnded: 1984. **Priorities:** *Arts & Humanities:* About 10%. Supports arts associations. *Civic & Public Affairs:* 10% to 15%. Includes grants to professional and trade associations. *Education:* Approximately 50%. Focus is on colleges and universities. *International:* About 25%. Primarily supports the United Way, hospitals, and emergency services. **Typ. Recipients:** Emergency/Ambulance Services, Hospitals. **Geo. Dist:** headquarters area only.

★ 12933 ★ Teleflex Foundation

630 West Germantown Pike, Suite 461
Plymouth Meeting, PA 19462
Phone: (610)831-6301
Email: foundation@teleflex.com
Website: http://www.teleflex.com/foundation/
Thelma Fretz, Executive Director

Priorities: *Arts & Humanities:* 4%. Funds a children's museum and a musical concert series. *Civic & Public Affairs:* 32%. Supports zoos, women's affairs, public safety, community foundations, career training, and free enterprise. *Education:* 27%. Funds major universities, private precollege schools, and Junior Achievement. *Environment:* 19%. Supports youth organizations, substance abuse education, child welfare, food banks, senior services, volunteer corps, Special Olympics, and animal welfare. *International:* 11%. Supports hospice, children's health, burn treatment, poison control, hospitals, and single-disease associations. *Note:* Total contributions made in 2000. **Typ. Recipients:** Children's Health/Hospitals, Health-General, Hospices, Nursing Services, People with Disabilities, Public Health, Single-Disease Health Associations, Substance Abuse. **Geo. Dist:** headquarters and operating communities.

★ 12934 ★ Temple-Inland Foundation

303 South Temple Drive
Diboll, TX 75941
Phone: (936)829-7950
Website: http://www.templeinland.com
M. Warner, Vice President

Priorities: *Arts & Humanities:* 5%. Under the Arts program area, the foundation supports libraries, historical societies, public broadcasting, performing arts, and art museums/centers. *Civic & Public Affairs:* 20%. Funds civic groups, community programs, and municipalities under the foundation's Cultural program area. *Education:* 27%. Supports institutions of higher learning and private schools, and provides scholarships for children of company employees. *Environment:* 33%. Supports services for the disabled, child welfare initiatives, recreational youth programs that contribute to healthy growth, substance abuse councils, adoption, and United Way. *International:* 13%. Funds single-disease health associations. *Note:* Total contributions made in fiscal 2001. Grant awards comprise 55% to 60% of total foundation giving; employee scholarships and other scholastic awards, 20% to 25%; and matching gifts, 15% to 20%. **Typ. Recipients:** Cancer, Children's Health/Hospitals, Clinics/Medical Centers, Health Organizations, Hospices, Hospitals, Medical Research, People with Disabilities, Prenatal Health Issues, Substance Abuse. **Geo. Dist:** headquarters.

★ 12935 ★ Tenet Healthcare Foundation

3820 State St.
Santa Barbara, CA 93105
Phone: (805)563-6845 **Fax:** (805)898-9104
Email: foundation@tenethealth.com
Website: http://etenet.com/GeneralInfo/thf.asp
Barbara Luton, Secretary, Executive Director

Priorities: *Arts & Humanities:* 2%. Provides some support for arts organizations. *Civic & Public Affairs:* 6%. Funds civic and community organizations. *Education:* 26%. Funding goes to general education programs and to programs leading to careers in medicine, nursing, or health care administration; institutions that train future health care professionals, and provide continuing education of health care professionals; and programs to support advancement and improvement of health care education. *Environment:* 14%. Funds human service programs and United Way. *International-*

al: 51%. Majority of support goes to health care projects and programs, including organizations that improve the efficiency of the healthcare delivery system; organizations that promote individual and community education in health; organizations and institutions the develop medical research programs, publications, conferences and seminars; organizations that seek to develop cures for debilitating diseases and conditions; and human service programs that benefit the aging, the handicapped, and persons unable to obtain adequate medical care. *Note:* Total contributions made in fiscal 2001. **Typ. Recipients:** Health Organizations, Medical Education, Medical Research, Medical Training, Mental Health, Nursing Services, People with Disabilities, Single-Disease Health Associations. **Geo. Dist:** principally near operating locations and to national organizations.

★ 12936 ★ TENNANT Co. Foundation

PO Box 1452
Minneapolis, MN 55440
Phone: (763)540-1209 **Fax:** (763)540-1616
Email: carol.vanlith@tennantco.com
Carol A. Van Lith, Secretary/Administrator

Fnded: 1973. **Priorities:** *Arts & Humanities:* 13%. Supports Minneapolis/St. Paul area arts organizations. Interests include the performing arts, opera, music, museums, and public broadcasting. *Civic & Public Affairs:* 4%. Supports housing, shelters, neighborhood improvement projects, citizens groups, and women's issues. *Education:* 4%. Supports public and private higher education and education organizations. Company also sponsors a scholarship program for eligible children of employees. *Environment:* 51%. Main support goes to United Way. Also supports children services, shelters, YMCA, and food for the hungry. *International:* 1%. Funds crisis health centers. *Religion:* 1%. Supports a museum. *Voluntarism:* The Volunteer Gift-Matching Program was established to recognize the volunteer work of company employees. The program matches 40 hours or more per year of volunteer hours to a single agency with a $200 gift, if that agency would otherwise be eligible for foundation grants. In 2001, the program supported over 760 hours of volunteer work by Tennant employees. *Note:* Total foundation contributions made in 2001. **Typ. Recipients:** Clinics/Medical Centers, Domestic Violence, Family Planning, Health Organizations, Health Policy/Cost Containment, Medical Rehabilitation, Mental Health, People with Disabilities, Prenatal Health Issues, Single-Disease Health Associations, Substance Abuse. **Geo. Dist:** headquarters and operating communities.

★ 12937 ★ Tension Envelope Foundation

819 East 19th St., 3rd Floor
Kansas City, MO 64108
Phone: (816)471-3800 **Fax:** (816)283-1498
Eliot Berkley, Secretary

Fnded: 1954. **Priorities:** *Arts & Humanities:* 5%. Supports theaters, public broadcasting, dance, art centers, and museums. *Civic & Public Affairs:* 1%. Supports civic foundations, businesses, and entrepreneurial organizations. *Education:* 20%. Supports colleges, universities, education funds, and Junior Achievement. *Environment:* 32%. Supports United Way, domestic violence programs, shelters, and family and youth services. *International:* 1%. Primary support made to health centers. *Note:* Total foundation contributions made in fiscal 2001. **Typ. Recipients:** Clinics/ Medical Centers, Domestic Violence, Family Planning, Health Organizations, Hospices, Hospitals, Mental Health, People with Disabilities, Public Health, Substance Abuse, Transplant Networks/Donor Banks. **Geo. Dist:** MO.

★ 12938 ★ Tesoro Petroleum Corp.

300 Concord Plaza Drive
San Antonio, TX 78216-6999
Phone: (210)283-2801 **Fax:** (210)283-2345
Website: http://www.tesoropetroleum.com
Tara Ford, Investor's Services

Priorities: *Arts & Humanities:* 10%. Emphasis is on music, public broadcasting, and museums and art galleries. Interests also include arts associations and centers, historic preservation and restoration, and the performing arts. *Civic & Public Affairs:* 4%. *Education:* 14%. Primarily funds colleges and universities through matching, capital, and general support grants. Other interests include international studies and business, economic, and engineering education. Company also administers a scholarship program for children of employees. *Environment:* 54%. Interests include United Way, community service organizations, shelters, and family services. Health support is directed primarily toward hospitals and single-disease associations. Other interests include public health, nutrition, and health maintenance. Supports youth organizations and groups concerned with child welfare. *International:* 1%. *Voluntarism:* Tesoro Petroleum encourages employees to volunteer in community organizations and company-sponsored events through its Team Tesoro volunteer program. The company reports that it donates more than 5,000 volunteer hours annually. *Note:* Total contributions made in 1998. **Typ. Recipients:** Cancer, Children's Health/Hospitals, Clinics/Medical Centers, Emergency/Ambulance Services, Eyes/ Blindness, Health Policy/Cost Containment, Hospices, Hospitals, Mental Health, Nutrition, People with Disabilities, Substance Abuse. **Geo. Dist:** headquarters and operating communities; Northern Great Plains; AK; CA, California Bay Area; HI; ND; Houston/Gulf Coast, TX; Salt Lake City/Intermountain, UT; WA. **Frmly:** BHP Hawaii Foundation.

★ 12939 ★ Texas Instruments Foundation

PO Box 660199, M/S 8656
Dallas, TX 75266-0199
Phone: (214)480-3221 **Fax:** (214)480-6820
Website: http://www.ti.com/corp/docs/company/citizen/index.shtml
Ann Minnis, Grants Administrator

Priorities: *Arts & Humanities:* 2%. Funds performing arts, music and cultural centers. *Civic & Public Affairs:* 1%. Funds minority affairs, job training programs, zoos, and arboretums. *Education:* 76%. Supports educational programs, colleges and universities. *Environment:* 21%. Major support given to United Way; also supports child welfare, youth organizations, and drug abuse treatment. *International:* Less than 1%. *Religion:* Less than 1%. Supports science museums. *Note:* Total foundation contributions made in 2000. **Typ. Recipients:** Clinics/Medical Centers, Hospitals, Hospitals (University Affiliated), Medical Education, Medical Research, Nursing Services, People with Disabilities, Research/Studies Institutes, Substance Abuse. **Geo. Dist:** nationally; TX, emphasis on Texas-based organizations; Dallas, TX.

★ 12940 ★ Textron Charitable Trust

40 Westmintster St.
Providence, RI 02903
Phone: (401)457-2430
Website: http://www.textron.com/profile/community.html
Cate Roberts, Director, Community Affairs

Priorities: *Arts & Humanities:* 19%. Arts centers and music receive primary support. Other interests include art associations, dance, historic preservation, libraries, and museums. Also includes matching gifts to arts institutions and organizations. *Civic & Public Affairs:* 30%. Supports community foundations, chambers of commerce, and organizations involved in civil rights, women's issues and urban development. *Education:* 36%. Majority of funding consists of matching grants. Substantial amounts also support student aid organizations, such as the National Merit Scholarship program and College Scholarship Service. Limited support goes to colleges, universities, and minority education. *Environment:* 4%. Support typically includes scouting organizations, children and family services, youth employment services, and YMCA/YWCAs and united funds. *International:* 11%. Hospitals receive the largest amount of health care funds, through both general support and matching grants. Health organizations, single-disease health associations, hospices, and pediatric health also are supported. *Note:* Total contributions made in 2000. **Typ. Recipients:** Cancer, Children's Health/Hospitals, Emergency/Ambulance Services, Family Planning, Health Organizations, Health Policy/Cost Containment, Hospices, Hospitals, Medical Education, Medical Rehabilitation, People with Disabilities, Prenatal Health Issues, Single-Disease Health Associations, Substance Abuse. **Geo. Dist:** headquarters and operating communities.

★ 12941 ★ Thomasville Furniture Industries Foundation

PO Box 339
Thomasville, NC 27360
Phone: (336)472-4000 **Fax:** (336)472-4085
Email: vholder@thomasville.com
Vickie Holder, General Manager

Fnded: 1960. **Priorities:** *Education:* 11%. Provides scholarships for higher education and funds elementary school programs. *Environment:* 89%. Major support is awarded to the United Way and Young Men's Christian Association. *Voluntarism:* Thomasville employees volunteer in Communities in Schools and Chamber programs and in local school systems and YMCA's. *Note:* Total contributions made in 2001. **Typ. Recipients:** Emergency/Ambulance Services, Hospitals, Medical Research. **Geo. Dist:** NC.

★ 12942 ★ 3M Foundation

Contributions Program
3M Center, Bldg. 225-01-S-23
Saint Paul, MN 55144-1000
Phone: (651)733-0144 **Fax:** (651)737-3061
Email: cfkleven@mmm.com
Website: http://www.3M.com/about3m/community
Cynthia Kleven, Manager Contributions

Fnded: 1953. **Priorities:** *Arts & Humanities:* 11%. *Civic & Public Affairs:* 6%. *Education:* 31%. *Environment:* 24%. *International:* 9%. *Religion:* 1%. *Voluntarism:* The 3M GIVES (Grants Initiated by Volunteer Service) program matches 25 hours of employee/ retiree volunteer service with $200 to the volunteer's designated nonprofit organization. The company also supports a Community Volunteer Award program through which it selects 25 exceptional employee/ retiree volunteers annually and awards $1,000 to a nonprofit organization selected by each winner. Volunteer programs contact is Anne E. Mazurowski. *Note:* Total contributions made in 2001. **Typ. Recipients:** Clinics/Medical Centers, Domestic Violence, Emergency/Ambulance Services, Geriatric Health, Health Organizations, Health Policy/Cost Containment, Hospices, Hospitals, Medical Education, Medical Rehabilitation, Mental Health, People with Disabilities, Public Health, Substance Abuse, Transplant Networks/Donor Banks. **Geo. Dist:** headquarters and operating communities.

★ 12943 ★ Times Mirror Foundation

202 W First St.
Los Angeles, CA 90053
Phone: (213)237-3005 **Fax:** (213)237-2116
Kim McCleary La France, President

Priorities: *Arts & Humanities:* 20%. Primary beneficiaries include community television and public radio stations, museums, music centers, and major performing arts centers. Other interests include symphonies and orchestras, theater, arts festivals, American folk arts, community arts groups, and libraries. *Civic & Public Affairs:* 30% to 35%. Special interests include journalism, the press, First Amendment, and other media-related concerns. Other recipients in this category include conservation groups, civil rights and women's affairs organizations, public policy research organizations, zoos, and business and free enterprise groups. *Education:* 25% to 30%. Communications, the arts, teaching, computers, independent and minority college funds, educational youth organizations, precollege schools, arts institutes, and minority scholarship assistance. *International:* 10% to 15%. Primarily supports united funds. Other community service concerns include youth agencies, shelters for homeless women and youth, child welfare, community centers, religious welfare, services for the disabled, and family planning. Health interests include hospitals, mental health, medical schools, and health organizations. *Note:* Above priorities reflect combined foundation and direct giving priorities. Subsidiaries give both directly and through the foundation in their operating areas; other direct and foundation grants concentrate on Southern California organizations. Foundation grants typically range from $2,500 to $25,000, while company grants are usually $2,500 or less. Also provides matching gifts in the areas of education,cultural, conservation, and hospitals. **Typ. Recipients:** Cancer, Diabetes, Domestic Violence, Emergency/Ambulance Services, Eyes/Blindness, Health-General, People with Disabilities, Respiratory. **Geo. Dist:** headquarters and operating communities; CA, nonprofits located in Southern CA.

★ 12944 ★ The Timken Co. Charitable Trust
1835 Dueber Ave. Southwest
Canton, OH 44706
Phone: (330)471-4062 **Fax:** (330)471-4041
Mr. Ward Timken, Trust Advisor

Priorities: *Arts & Humanities:* 8%. *Civic & Public Affairs:* 6%. *Education:* 66%. *Environment:* 20%. *Note:* Total contributions made in 2001. **Typ. Recipients:** Alzheimers Disease, Arthritis, Emergency/Ambulance Services, Health Organizations, Substance Abuse. **Geo. Dist:** communities where company operates plants, with an emphasis on Ohio.

★ 12945 ★ Tippins Foundation
1090 Freeport Rd.
Pittsburgh, PA 15238
Phone: (412)784-8804 **Fax:** (412)782-7210
George Tippins, Trustee

Priorities: *Arts & Humanities:* 13%. Supports museums, opera, theater, film, dance, historical preservation, and public broadcasting. *Civic & Public Affairs:* 7%. Supports women's affairs, economic development, philanthropy, and parks and zoos. *Education:* 25%. Supports schools, colleges, and universities. *Environment:* 10%. Supports shelters, scouting, human service organizations, and animal welfare. *International:* 40%. Supports single-disease health associations, and hospitals. *Note:* Total foundation contributions made in 2001. **Typ. Recipients:** Alzheimers Disease, Alzheimers Disease, Arthritis, Cancer, Children's Health/Hospitals, Clinics/Medical Centers, Diabetes, Emergency/Ambulance Services, Health Organizations, Health-General, Heart, Hospitals, Kidney, Medical Rehabilitation, People with Disabilities, Public Health, Respiratory, Single-Disease Health Associations. **Geo. Dist:** PA.

★ 12946 ★ Titan Industrial Foundation
555 Madison Ave., 10th Fl.
New York, NY 10022
Phone: (212)421-6700
Jerome Siegel, President & Treasurer

Fnded: 1951. **Priorities:** *Arts & Humanities:* 6%. Supports museums, art centers, music, libraries, and performance centers. *Civic & Public Affairs:* 8%. Gives to civil rights organizations and minority affairs. *Education:* 57%. Funds institutions of higher learning, leadership development for educators, and major support to Sarah Lawrence College. *Environment:* 12%. Supports Big Brothers/Big Sisters, volunteer programs, shelters, food banks, family planning, and YMCA. *International:* 6%. Supports hospitals, medical centers, and single-disease health associations. *Religion:* 1%. Supports the American Museum of Natural History. *Note:* Total contributions made in fiscal 2001. **Typ. Recipients:** AIDS/HIV, Cancer, Clinics/Medical Centers, Eyes/Blindness, Family Planning, Health Organizations, Hospitals, Mental Health, People with Disabilities, Research/Studies Institutes, Single-Disease Health Associations. **Geo. Dist:** Washington, DC; NY. **Frmly:** Titan Industrial Foundation.

★ 12947 ★ TJX Foundation, Inc.
770 Cochituate Rd., Route J5S
Framingham, MA 01701
Phone: (508)390-3199 **Fax:** (508)390-2091
Email: christy_strickland@tjx.com
Website: http://www.tjmaxx.com
Christine Strickland, Foundation Manager

Priorities: *Arts & Humanities:* 7%. Proposals that bring art or artists to new audiences; also supports initiatives that encourage people, especially the handicapped, elderly, young, or disadvantaged, to express themselves through art. *Civic & Public Affairs:* 15%. Supports programs which promote improved race relations, community development and housing. *Education:* 10%. Funds programs that benefit children of preschool age through college, which provide scholarship or vocational education for the disadvantaged; strengthen leadership in public schools; teach people to speak, read, and write English; and encourage collaboration between community agencies and schools. *Environment:* 43%. Families and children are main beneficiaries. Priority is given to programs that strengthen the family unit, help single-parent families, encourage families to adopt or accept foster children, and help the physically impaired; also funds programs that provide shelter for victims of domestics violence. *International:* 21%. Supports health care initiatives for underserved populations; seeks programs that provide early and comprehensive prenatal services, immunizations and health screening for children who lack them, and preventative care and alternatives to hospitalization. *Note:* Total contributions made in fiscal 2001. **Typ. Recipients:** AIDS/HIV, Cancer, Child Abuse, Children's Health/Hospitals, Clinics/Medical Centers, Diabetes, Domestic Violence, Emergency/Ambulance Services, Health Organizations, Health-General, Heart, Hospices, Hospitals, Medical Education, Medical Rehabilitation, Medical Research, Mental Health, Nursing Services, People with Disabilities, Prenatal Health Issues, Public Health, Single-Disease Health Associations, Substance Abuse. **Geo. Dist:** principally near operating locations and to national organizations; Boston, MA.

★ 12948 ★ Tomkins Corp. Foundation
4801 Springfield St.
Dayton, OH 45431
Phone: (937)476-0359 **Fax:** (937)476-0439
Greg Kirchhoff, Vice President

Fnded: 1989. **Priorities:** *Civic & Public Affairs:* 1%. Supports legal foundations, botanical organizations, and community foundations. *Education:* 48%. Supports scholarships, public and private education, colleges, universities, and Junior Achievement. *Environment:* 33%. Supports United Way, Special Olympics, animal protection, scouts, and family services. *International:* 13%. Supports health foundations, medical research, hospitals, hospices, and single-disease health associations. *Note:* Total foundation contributions made in fiscal 2001. **Typ. Recipients:** Alzheimers Disease, Cancer, Child Abuse, Children's Health/Hospitals, Clinics/Medical Centers, Diabetes, Emergency/Ambulance Services, Eyes/Blindness, Family Planning, Health Organizations, Hospices, Hospitals, Medical Research, People with Disabilities, Prenatal Health Issues, Public Health, Single-Disease Health Associations, Substance Abuse. **Geo. Dist:** Dayton, OH. **Frmly:** Philips Industries Foundation.

★ 12949 ★ Torchmark Corp.
2001 3rd Ave. South
Birmingham, AL 35233
Phone: (205)325-4243 **Fax:** (205)325-4198
Email: cmccoy@torchmarkcorp.com
Carol McCoy, Associate Counsel & Secretary

Priorities: *Education:* About 30%. Colleges and universities. *Environment:* About 35%. United appeals in communities where home office and district offices are located. *International:* About 20%. Health organizations in the Birmingham area. **Typ. Recipients:** Health Organizations, Hospitals, Medical Rehabilitation, People with Disabilities, Single-Disease Health Associations. **Geo. Dist:** Birmingham, AL.

★ 12950 ★ Toro Foundation
8111 Lyndale Ave. South
Bloomington, MN 55420-1196
Phone: (952)887-8911 **Fax:** (952)887-7291
Email: stacy.bogart@toro.com
Stacy Bogart, President

Fnded: 1989. **Priorities:** *Arts & Humanities:* 5%. Supports music, museums, and theaters. *Civic & Public Affairs:* 7%. Supports economic development, municipalities, and foundation councils. *Education:* 18%. Supports higher education and schools. *Environment:* 49%. Primary support for the United Way; also supports food banks. *International:* 2%. Primarily supports hospitals and cancer institutions. *Voluntarism:* The company launched an employee volunteer program in 2003. *Note:* Total fnd contributions made in 2000. **Typ. Recipients:** AIDS/HIV, AIDS/HIV, Cancer, Diabetes, Emergency/Ambulance Services, Health-General, Heart, Hospitals, People with Disabilities, Public Health, Substance Abuse. **Geo. Dist:** headquarters and operating communities.

★ 12951 ★ Toyota U.S.A. Foundation
19001 South Western Ave., A-404
Torrance, CA 90509
Phone: (310)468-6766
Website: http://www.toyota.com/about/community/index.html

Fnded: 1987. **Priorities:** *Arts & Humanities:* 23%. Funds public broadcasting and cultural and children's museums. *Education:* 62%. Supports science and math education at universities; math, science, and environmental precollege educational programs; and teacher development and training in math, science, and environmental curricula. *Environment:* 5%. Gives to youth organizations. *Note:* Total foundation contributions made in fiscal 2001. **Typ. Recipients:** Health Organizations, Nutrition, People with Disabilities, Substance Abuse. **Geo. Dist:** nationally for foundation contributions; major operating facility areas for corporate contributions.

★ 12952 ★ Tribune New York Foundation
450 West 33rd St., 3rd Floor
New York, NY 10001
Phone: (212)210-2100
John Campi, Vice President, Promotions

Fnded: 1958. **Priorities:** *Arts & Humanities:* 62%. Supports the theater, music, dance, museums, film, and arts centers, including broadcasting. *Civic & Public Affairs:* 15%. Funds minority and journalism interests. *Education:* 8%. Supports schools and higher education through employee matching. *Environment:* 5%. Supports meals-on-wheels, and drug use prevention and rehabilitation. *International:* 3%. Supports single-disease health associations through employee matching. *Religion:* 5%. Funds museums. *Note:* Total contributions made in 2000. **Typ. Recipients:** Cancer, Family Planning, Hospitals, Long-Term Care, Medical Research, People with Disabilities, Single-Disease Health Associations, Substance Abuse. **Geo. Dist:** CT; NJ; New York, NY. **Frmly:** Daily News Foundation.

★ 12953 ★ True Foundation
PO Box 2360
Casper, WY 82602
Phone: (307)237-9301
Jean True, Trustee

Priorities: *Arts & Humanities:* 21%. Supports history organizations, museums, arts councils, and an orchestra. *Civic & Public Affairs:* 17%. Funds legal aid, business services organizations, and public policy. *Education:* 10%. Contributes to colleges, universities, and public pre-college schools. Also funds economic, agricultural, and civics education programs. *Environment:* 32%. Provides support to united funds, hunger relief, activities for children and youth, community centers, and child welfare organizations. *International:* 12%. Medical rehabilitation centers, single-disease health associations, cancer treatment centers, hospitals, and medical centers. *Note:* Total contributions made in fiscal 2001. **Typ. Recipients:** Alzheimers Disease, Cancer, Cancer, Children's Health/Hospitals, Clinics/Medical Centers, Diabetes, Emergency/Ambulance Services, Health Funds, Hospitals, Medical Rehabilitation, Medical Research, Public Health, Respiratory, Single-Disease Health Associations. **Geo. Dist:** WY.

★ 12954 ★ Truland Foundation
3330 Washington Blvd., 7th Fl.
Arlington, VA 22201
Phone: (703)524-4900
Robert Truland, President & Chief Executive Officer

Fnded: 1954. **Priorities:** *Arts & Humanities:* 54%. Funds museums. *Civic & Public Affairs:* 4%. Funds civic programs. *Education:* 7%. Funds primary schools, universities. *International:* 35%. Funds health foundations and groups. *Note:* Total contributions made in fiscal 2000. **Typ. Recipients:** Cancer, Children's Health/Hospitals, Health-General, Hospices, Hospitals, Hospitals (University Affiliated), Mental Health, People with Disabilities, Public Health.

★ 12955 ★ Trustmark Foundation
400 Field Drive
Lake Forest, IL 60045
Phone: (847)615-1500 **Fax:** (847)615-5860
Warren Schreier, Trustee

Priorities: *Arts & Humanities:* 4%. Gives to museums, art festivals, historical societies, and libraries. *Civic & Public Affairs:* 9%. Funds community initiatives and a zoo. *Education:* 19%. Supports various colleges and universities, mostly within Illinois, Wisconsin, and Indiana; and programs associated with technology, finance or actuarial studies, and minority scholarships and endowments. *Environment:* 46%. Supports family and youth services, United Way and sexual assault prevention programs *International:* 19%. Funds hospitals; clinics; and heart, diabetes, cancer, and AIDS organizations. *Voluntarism:* The company encourages employee volunteerism by loaning executives to the United Way and through Community IMPACT, a program in which volunteers teach seventh graders about healthy lifestyles. *Note:* Total contributions made in 2001. **Typ. Recipients:** Adolescent Health Issues, AIDS/HIV, Cancer, Clinics/Medical Centers, Diabetes, Domestic Violence, Health-General, Heart, Hospices, Hospitals, Medical Research, People with Disabilities, Prenatal Health Issues, Preventive Medicine/Wellness Organizations, Sexual Abuse, Single-Disease Health Associations, Substance Abuse. **Geo. Dist:** headquarters and operating communities.

★ 12956 ★ Trustmark National Bank
248 East Capitol St.
Jackson, MS 39201
Phone: (601)208-5942 **Fax:** (601)208-2313
Vicki Mason, Vice President

Priorities: *Arts & Humanities:* 10%. *Civic & Public Affairs:* About 50%. *Education:* 10%. *International:* 30%. **Typ. Recipients:** Health-General. **Geo. Dist:** headquarters and operating communities.

★ 12957 ★ TRW Foundation
1900 Richmond Rd.
Cleveland, OH 44124
Phone: (216)291-7164 **Fax:** (216)291-7632
Terri Preskar, Foundation Administrator

Priorities: *Arts & Humanities:* 21%. Supports the performing arts, museums, theaters, arts centers, and dance and music groups. *Civic & Public Affairs:* 21%. Supports professional trade associations, economic development, and urban and community affairs. *Education:* 28%. Supports colleges and universities. Special interests include mathematics, engineering, computer science, and business administration. Also funds minority education and scholarship programs. *Environment:* 19%. Supports United Ways in company operating locations and in areas with a significant number of TRW employees. Also funds YMCA and youth organizations. *International:* 5%. Supports research institutes, emergency services, hospitals, youth organizations, and volunteer services. *Religion:* 6%. Funds science centers. *Note:* Total foundation contributions made in 2000. In addition to foundation giving, the company also makes direct grants. Foundation generally represents about 90% of the total TRW contributions program. Direct giving priorities are the same as those of the foundation. **Typ. Recipients:** Alzheimers Disease, Children's Health/Hospitals, Clinics/Medical Centers, Emergency/Ambulance Services, Health Organizations, Health Policy/Cost Containment, Hospices, Hospitals, Hospitals (University Affiliated), Medical Rehabilitation, Mental Health, People with Disabilities, Research/Studies Institutes. **Geo. Dist:** principally near operating locations and to national organizations and internationally.

★ 12958 ★ Tyco Electronics Foundation
MS 140-10
PO Box 3608, M/S 176-42
Harrisburg, PA 17105-3608
Phone: (717)592-4869 **Fax:** (717)592-3043
Email: mjrakocz@tycoelectronics.com
Website: http://www.tycoelectronics.com/about/foundation
Mary Rakoczy, Jr., Administrator

Priorities: *Arts & Humanities:* 20%. *Civic & Public Affairs:* 19%. *Education:* 31%. *Environment:* 20%. *International:* 9%. *Religion:* 1%. *Voluntarism:* After employees complete 100 hours of volunteer services in a calendar year with a nonprofit organization, the Dollars for Doers program will authorize a $250 contribution from the Foundation to that organization. This is a yearly maximum of $2,000 to one eligible organization. *Note:* Total contributions made in 2001. **Typ. Recipients:** Cancer, Child Abuse, Children's Health/Hospitals, Clinics/Medical Centers, Emergency/Ambulance Services, Health Organizations, Health-General, Hospices, Hospitals, Mental Health, People with Disabilities, Single-Disease Health Associations, Substance Abuse. **Geo. Dist:** headquarters and operating communities; Triad, NC; PA, central Pennsylvania; VA. **Frmly:** AMP Foundation.

★ 12959 ★ Tyson Foundation, Inc.
PO Box 2020
Springdale, AR 72765
Phone: (479)290-4999 **Fax:** (479)290-7984
Email: comments@tysonfoundation.org
Website: http://www.tysonfoundation.org
Shelby Rogers, President

Priorities: *Arts & Humanities:* 3%. Funds arts centers and music. *Civic & Public Affairs:* 3%. Supports towns and fire departments. *Education:* 72%. Support goes to a large scholarship program, colleges and universities. *Environment:* 22%. Supports family services. *Note:* Total foundation contributions made in 2000. **Typ. Recipients:** Children's Health/Hospitals, Emergency/Ambulance Services, Health Organizations, Heart, Medical Education, Sexual Abuse, Single-Disease Health Associations, Substance Abuse. **Geo. Dist:** AR.

★ 12960 ★ Ukrop Foundation
9030 Stony Point Pkwy., Ste. 350
Richmond, VA 23235
Phone: (804)327-7521 **Fax:** (804)379-7368
Gail Long, Assistant to the President

Fnded: 1983. **Priorities:** *Arts & Humanities:* 15%. Primarily supports historic preservation. *Civic & Public Affairs:* 26%. Major support to business and economic development organizations. Also supports community affairs organizations, professional organizations, cities and counties, and housing. *Education:* 28%. Funds colleges and universities, with emphasis on business education; community-school partnerships; and literacy. *Environment:* 22%. Major support goes to the United Way. Also supports recreation, athletics programs, community service organizations, and the disabled. *International:* 1%. Supports a free clinic and single-disease health associations. *Religion:* 1%. *Note:* Total contributions made in fiscal 1999. **Typ. Recipients:** Cancer, Clinics/Medical Centers, Emergency/Ambulance Services, Hospitals, Medical Education, Medical Research, Public Health, Single-Disease Health Associations. **Geo. Dist:** Richmond, VA.

★ 12961 ★ Unilever United States Foundation
Care of UNUS Tax Department
700 Sylvan Ave.
Englewood Cliffs, NJ 07632
Phone: (201)567-8000
Website: http://www.unilever.com/so/co.html
John Gould, Jr., Director, Corporate Affairs

Fnded: 1952. **Priorities:** *Arts & Humanities:* 2%. *Civic & Public Affairs:* 55%. *Education:* 30%. *Environment:* 10%. *International:* 3%. *Note:* Total foundation contributions made in 2001. **Typ. Recipients:** Cancer, Children's Health/Hospitals, Clinics/Medical Centers, Diabetes, Emergency/Ambulance Services, Health Organizations, Heart, Hospitals, Medical Education, Medical Research, People with Disabilities, Prenatal Health Issues, Respiratory, Single-Disease Health Associations, Substance Abuse, Trauma Treatment. **Geo. Dist:** headquarters and operating communities.

★ 12962 ★ Union Pacific Foundation
1416 Dodge St., Room 738
Omaha, NE 68179
Phone: (402)271-5000 **Fax:** (402)271-5477
Website: http://www.up.com/found/
Darlynn Herweg, Director

Priorities: *Arts & Humanities:* 15%. Supports opera, music, museums, historic preservation, libraries, and the performing arts. *Civic & Public Affairs:* 6%. Supports zoos, economic development, and community foundations. *Education:* 34%. Supports private colleges and universities and independent college funds. Also supports a variety of programs through capital projects, annual giving funds, scholarships, and special research projects related to company business. *Environment:* 43%. Supports United Way, community centers, and youth organizations. *International:* 1%. Primary support made to hospitals. *Religion:* 1%. Primarily supports science centers. *Note:* Total foundation contributions made in 2000. **Typ. Recipients:** Alzheimers Disease, Cancer, Children's Health/Hospitals, Clinics/Medical Centers, Domestic Violence, Emergency/Ambulance Services, Health Organizations, Hospices, Hospitals, Long-Term Care, Medical Rehabilitation, Medical Research, Mental Health, People with Disabilities, Prenatal Health Issues, Public Health, Substance Abuse. **Geo. Dist:** AR; CA; CO; DE; Washington, DC; FL; GA; ID; IL; IN; IA; KS; LA; MD; MI; MN; MS; MT; NE; NV; NJ; NM; NY; NC; OH; OK; OR; PA; TN; TX; UT; VA; WA; WI.

★ 12963 ★ United Airlines Foundation
PO Box 66100
Chicago, IL 60666
Phone: (847)700-5714 **Fax:** (847)700-7345
Email: uafoundation@UAL.com
Caryn Cross, Secretary

Priorities: *Arts & Humanities:* 24%. Supports museums, music, libraries, historic preservation, art institutes, and literary arts. *Civic & Public Affairs:* 4%. Supports aquariums and civil and human rights. *Education:* 6%. Supports schools and literacy programs. *Environment:* 48%. Supports youth organizations and United Way. *International:* 11%. Supports Muscular Dystrophy associations, hospital foundations, and medicine research. Also funds programs that help individuals with disabilities and disease through grants, airline tickets for medical transport, and employee volunteerism. *Religion:* 7%. Primarily supports science centers and museums. *Voluntarism:* Co. sponsors employee volunteer programs such as: Believers Program-an educational mentoring and tutoring program; Habitat for Humanity; Take Your Community to Work Day; and AIDS walks. Through its United We Care Program, co. also awards grants to organizations where employees volunteer. *Note:* Total foundation contributions made in 2000. **Typ. Recipients:** Alzheimers Disease, Cancer, Children's Health/Hospitals, Heart, Hospitals, Medical Research, Single-Disease Health Associations. **Geo. Dist:** internationally; focusing on major cities served by the company.

★ 12964 ★ United Illuminating Foundation

157 Church St.
PO Box 1564
New Haven, CT 06506-0901
Phone: (203)499-2000
Mary Cody, Trustee

Fnded: 1990. **Priorities:** *Arts & Humanities:* 7%. Supports the symphony. *Civic & Public Affairs:* 2%. Funds leadership activities. *Education:* 4%. *Environment:* 87%. Supports the United Way, boys and girls clubs, and the YMCA. *International:* 2%. *Note:* Total contributions made in 1998. **Typ. Recipients:** Children's Health/Hospitals, Clinics/Medical Centers, Hospitals.

★ 12965 ★ U.S. Bancorp Foundation

222 S Ninth St.
Minneapolis, MN 55402
Phone: (612)342-5501 **Fax:** (612)342-6085
Website: http://www.piperjaffray.com/about/community_involve.html
Marina Lyon, Director, Public Affairs

Fnded: 1993. **Priorities:** *Arts & Humanities:* 2%. Funds art museums, opera, public radio, film institute, and performing art. *Civic & Public Affairs:* 25%. Funds urban leagues, economic development, employment initiatives, and neighborhood services. *Education:* 30%. Funds educational programs, literacy initiatives, parent involvement in education, preparatory schools, and colleges. *Environment:* 32%. Funds youth services, YMCA/YWCAs, and food banks. *Note:* Total foundation contributions made in fiscal 2000. **Typ. Recipients:** Cancer, Children's Health/Hospitals, Domestic Violence, Emergency/Ambulance Services, Family Planning, Hospitals, Long-Term Care, Medical Rehabilitation, Multiple Sclerosis, People with Disabilities, Public Health. **Geo. Dist:** headquarters; MN, Twin Cities area. **Frmly:** Piper Jaffray Companies Inc. U.S. Bancorp Piper Jaffray Foundation.

★ 12966 ★ U.S. Bancorp Foundation Inc.

601 Second Ave. South
Minneapolis, MN 55402-4302
Phone: (612)973-1789 **Fax:** (612)973-4392
Website: http://www.usbank.com/comm_relations
Reza Aghamirzadeh, Contact

Priorities: *Arts & Humanities:* 15%. Major arts and cultural institutions, with operating budgets over 2 million. *Civic & Public Affairs:* Less than 2%. *Education:* 74%. Public education, adult education, especially in distressed areas. *Environment:* About 5%. Funds youth services, animal services, and social services. *International:* 2%. Majority of funds support the American Red Cross. Other funds support children's health, and AIDS awareness. *Note:* Total contributions made in 1999. **Typ. Recipients:** AIDS/HIV, Children's Health/Hospitals, Clinics/Medical Centers, Diabetes, Emergency/Ambulance Services, Medical Rehabilitation, Multiple Sclerosis, People with Disabilities, Prenatal Health Issues, Research/Studies Institutes. **Geo. Dist:** operating locations; Minneapolis, MN.

★ 12967 ★ U.S. Steel Foundation

600 Grant St., Rm. 685
Pittsburgh, PA 15219-2800
Phone: (412)433-5237 **Fax:** (412)433-6847
Website: http://www.ussteel.com/corp/ussfoundation/ussfound.htm
Craig Mallick, General Manager

Priorities: *Arts & Humanities:* (Public, Cultural, and Scientific Affairs) 16%. Public Affairs support is allocated to public policy, legal, business, and community organizations. Cultural Affairs funding focuses on capital and operating support for major performing arts organizations and cultural institutions. Scientific Affairs grants are geared toward science and environmental organizations that relate to the business interest of U.S. Steel. *Civic & Public Affairs:* 2%. *Education:* 53%. Supports higher educational programs focusing on engineering, science, and business. Also supports scholarship programs for children of employees, and an employee matching gifts program for colleges and universities. *Environment:* (Health and Human Services) 31%. A large portion of Human Services is provided to the United Way. Also funds single-disease health associations, pediatric health, substance abuse treatment, community centers, and youth groups. *Note:* Total contributions made in 2001. **Typ. Recipients:** Health Organizations, Medical Rehabilitation, Mental Health, People with Disabilities, Single-Disease Health Associations, Substance Abuse, Trauma Treatment. **Geo. Dist:** nationally, with emphasis on communities where U.S. Steel Corp. operates. **Frmly:** USX Foundation.

★ 12968 ★ United States Sugar Corp. Charitable Trust

PO Box 1207
Clewiston, FL 33440
Phone: (863)983-8121 **Fax:** (863)983-9827
Website: http://www.ussugar.com/aboutus/aboutus_frame.html
James Terrill, CO-Trustee

Fnded: 1952. **Priorities:** *Arts & Humanities:* 4%. Supports history organizations, museums and libraries. *Civic & Public Affairs:* 14%. Supports municipalities, community development projects, and business programs. *Education:* 54%. Supports schools, educational foundations, and Junior Achievement. *Environment:* 27%. Supports homes, athletics and recreation, child welfare, and scouts. *Note:* Total foundation contributions made in fiscal 2001. **Typ. Recipients:** Alzheimers Disease, Cancer, Children's Health/Hospitals, Clinics/Medical Centers, Diabetes, Emergency/Ambulance Services, Eyes/Blindness, Health Organizations, Heart, Hospices, Hospitals, Medical Rehabilitation, Mental Health, People with Disabilities, Public Health, Single-Disease Health Associations, Substance Abuse. **Geo. Dist:** headquarters and operating communities.

★ 12969 ★ U.S. Trust Corp. Foundation

114 West 47th St.
New York, NY 10036-1532
Phone: (212)852-1400 **Fax:** (212)852-1341
Email: foundation@ustrust.com
Carol Strickland, Chair, Corp. Contributions Committee

Priorities: *Arts & Humanities:* 36%. Contributions are equally distributed between cultural jewels of New York City and institutions supporting the work of emerging artists. U.S. Trust is interested in institutions which make their art accessible to all New Yorkers. *Civic & Public Affairs:* 8%. Supports economic development and community and neighborhood organizations. *Education:* 40%. Supports private pre-college education, colleges, and universities. Most funding to education is provided through employee participation in the matching gift program. *Environment:* 11%. A substantial portion of the trust's support for human services is allocated through the United Way system. Also funds organizations serving children and the disadvantaged. *International:* 5%. Supports children's health and services for seniors. *Note:* Total foundation contributions made in 2000. **Typ. Recipients:** AIDS/HIV, Cancer, Children's Health/Hospitals, Geriatric Health, Health Funds, Health Organizations, Health Policy/Cost Containment, Hospitals, Long-Term Care, Medical Rehabilitation, Nursing Services, Nutrition, People with Disabilities, People with Disabilities, Substance Abuse. **Geo. Dist:** Costa Mesa, CA; Larkspur, CA; Los Angeles, CA; Palo Alto, CA; San Francisco, CA; Essex, CT; Greenwich, CT; Stamford, CT; West Hartford, CT; Wilmington, DE; Washington, DC; Boca Raton, FL; Naples, FL; Palm Beach, FL; Vero Beach, FL; Minneapolis, MN; St. Paul, MN; Jersey City, NJ; Morristown, NJ; Princeton, NJ; Garden City, NY; New York, NY; Charlotte, NC; Greensboro, NC; Raleigh, NC; Portland, OR; Wayne, PA; Dallas, TX; Houston, TX; McLean, VA; Tacoma, WA.

★ 12970 ★ United Stationers Foundation

2200 E Golf Rd.
Des Plaines, IL 60016-1267
Phone: (847)699-5000 **Fax:** (847)699-8046
Brian Cooper, Treasurer

Priorities: *Arts & Humanities:* 4%. Supports a field museum. *Civic & Public Affairs:* 7%. Funds urban and defense leagues. *Education:* 28%. Supports a community college. *Environment:* 44%. Supports United Way, YWCA/YMCA, and social welfare. *International:* 13%. Supports cancer, multiple sclerosis, AIDS, and public health. *Note:* Total contributions made in fiscal 2000. **Typ. Recipients:** AIDS/HIV, Alzheimers Disease, Cancer, Clinics/Medical Centers, Diabetes, Eyes/Blindness, Health-General, Medical Research, Multiple Sclerosis, People with Disabilities, Research/Studies Institutes, Single-Disease Health Associations. **Geo. Dist:** principally near operating locations and to national organizations.

★ 12971 ★ United Technologies Corp.

One Financial Plaza
MS 503
Hartford, CT 06101
Phone: (860)728-7943 **Fax:** (860)728-7041
Email: krista.pilot@utc.com
Website: http://www.utc.com/social/community/grants.htm
Krista Pilot, Manager Corporate Contributions

Priorities: *Arts & Humanities:* 10%. Contributes to national touring museum exhibitions, art education, dance companies, opera, historical societies, art centers, libraries, museums, public radio and television, and historic architectural restoration projects. *Civic & Public Affairs:* 15%. Primarily funds organizations involved in community development activities in operating locations. Supports civic projects, minority and women's programs, and public policy organizations. Particular interest in agencies willing to form alliances with other groups to improve the community. *Education:* 37%. Colleges and universities, including company's 22 "focus" schools, receive company support. Emphasis is on institutions from which company recruits employees and quality engineering programs, including those directed at women and minorities. Other interests include basic research related to company's fields of business and continuing education for company employees. Additional support provided through precollegiate math and science programs and teacher enrichment programs. Education is the company's major priority. *International:* (Health & Human Services) 28%. Major support to United Ways and hospitals. Also supports preventive medical treatment groups and activities for the mentally and physically handicapped, senior citizens, youth groups, and health care cost containment. Some funding seeks to establish links between traditional funding areas; for example, funding for a human service organization might be contingent on help they provide an educational or civic group. Grants favored in states where company has operations. *Note:* Total contributions made in 2002. **Typ. Recipients:** Health Organizations, Health Policy/Cost Containment, Hospitals, People with Disabilities, Substance Abuse. **Geo. Dist:** communities with major facilities and substantial employee residence population; East Hartford, CT; Hartford, CT; Middletown, CT; Stratford, CT; Windsor Lock, CT; Washington, DC; Palm Beach, FL; Bloomington, IN; Dearborn, MI; Syracuse, NY.

★ 12972 ★ United Wisconsin Services Foundation

401 West Michigan St.
Milwaukee, WI 53203
Phone: (414)226-5756
Thomas Hefty, Chairman & President

Fnded: 1984. **Priorities:** *Arts & Humanities:* 20%. Supports performing arts, art museums, and art associations. *Civic & Public Affairs:* 16%. Funds community foundations, business/professional associations, urban affairs, community development, and programs encouraging public education and involvement in government. *Education:* 12%. Contributes to universities, colleges, and economic education. *Environment:* 29%. Major support given to the United Way. Also funds Young Men's Christian Association, youth programs, and child welfare issues. *International:* 21%. Supports single-disease health associations, children's health programs, clinics, hospitals, nursing programs, and senior health. **Typ. Recipients:** Alzheimers Disease, Arthritis, Cancer, Children's Health/Hospitals, Clinics/Medical Centers, Diabetes, Eyes/Blindness, Geriatric Health, Health Organizations, Health Policy/Cost Containment, Heart, Medical Education, Medical Research, Mental Health, People with Disabilities, Prenatal Health Issues, Public Health, Respiratory, Single-Disease Health Associations, Substance Abuse. **Geo. Dist:** WI.

★ 12973 ★ Universal Foods Foundation
777 East Wisconsin Ave.
Milwaukee, WI 53202-5304
Phone: (414)271-6755
Stephen Rolfs, Secretary & Treasurer

Priorities: *Arts & Humanities:* (Culture & Art) 21%. Supports historic preservation, art museums, public broadcasting, libraries, and performing arts. *Civic & Public Affairs:* (Civic Activity) 21%. Recipients include chambers of commerce, job training, law enforcement and fire departments, economic development programs, community festivals and activities, women's affairs, zoos, and community foundations. *Education:* 24%. Major support goes to colleges and universities, with some emphasis on medical and education. Other recipients include literacy groups and education funds. *Environment:* (Health and Welfare) 34%. Supports the United Way and youth organizations. Primarily supports hospitals, but funding also goes to medical research and United Way agencies. *Note:* Total contributions made in fiscal 2000. **Typ. Recipients:** Cancer, Children's Health/Hospitals, Clinics/Medical Centers, Emergency/Ambulance Services, Health-General, Heart, Hospitals, Medical Education, Medical Research, Multiple Sclerosis, People with Disabilities, Single-Disease Health Associations, Transplant Networks/Donor Banks. **Geo. Dist:** headquarters and operating communities.

★ 12974 ★ Universal Leaf Foundation
PO Box 25099
Richmond, VA 23260
Phone: (804)359-9311 **Fax:** (804)254-3594
Nancy Powell, Manager, Corporate Relations

Priorities: *Arts & Humanities:* 9%. Supports theater, art and history museums, symphonies, dance, and events promoting the arts. *Civic & Public Affairs:* 19%. Funds community foundations, professional women's organizations, fire departments, minority affairs, and economic and community development. *Education:* 33%. Supports scholarship funds, universities, middle schools, high schools, literacy programs, and business education. *International:* (Health & Welfare) 38%. Contributes to single-disease health associations, pediatric health and pediatric disease research, hospice programs, youth groups and activities, and United Way agencies. *Note:* Total foundation contributions made in fiscal 2001. **Typ. Recipients:** Children's Health/Hospitals, Clinics/Medical Centers, Emergency/Ambulance Services, Eyes/Blindness, Family Planning, Health Funds, Health Organizations, Hospices, Kidney, Multiple Sclerosis, People with Disabilities, Single-Disease Health Associations, Transplant Networks/Donor Banks. **Geo. Dist:** headquarters and operating communities; NC; VA.

★ 12975 ★ Universal Studios Foundation
100 Universal City Plaza
Universal City, CA 91608
Phone: (818)777-1208
Website: http://www.universalstudios.com/homepage/html/about_us/
Helene Giambone, Foundation Contact

Fnded: 1956. **Priorities:** *Arts & Humanities:* 32%. Supports theater/performing arts, film and filmmaker organizations, and history organizations. *Civic & Public Affairs:* 9%. Provides funding for economic development organizations and the Greater Los Angeles Zoo. *Education:* 31%. Funds colleges, universities, and a scholarship fund. *Environment:* 6%. Funds child welfare, youth programs, and a women's shelter/counseling program. *International:* 19%. Supports hospitals, medical centers, medical research, the Cystic Fibrosis Foundation, and the American Red Cross. *Voluntarism:* The company holds a company-wide annual Volunteer Day during which employees volunteer to work in food banks, build houses with Habitat for Humanity, beautify schools and parks, and provide books to school libraries. In addition, the company sponsors Education is Universal, through which employee volunteers tutor children in schools, provide students with job shadowing opportunities, and hold career days to introduce students to careers within the entertainment industry. *Note:* Total contributions made in fiscal 2001. **Typ. Recipients:** Cancer, Children's Health/Hospitals, Clinics/Medical Centers, Diabetes, Emergency/Ambulance Services, Eyes/Blindness, Family Planning, Health Organizations, Health-General, Hospitals, Medical Education, Medical Research, Mental Health, Multiple Sclerosis, People with Disabilities, Public Health, Research/Studies Institutes, Single-Disease Health Associations, Substance Abuse. **Geo. Dist:** Los Angeles, CA.

★ 12976 ★ Unocal Foundation
14141 Southwest Freeway
Sugar Land, TX 77478
Phone: (281)287-7917
Stephen Hayes, Vice President

Priorities: *Arts & Humanities:* 2%. *Civic & Public Affairs:* 40%. Supports economic and social progress initiatives in communities throughout the world where Unocal operates. *Education:* 39%. Education grants are also disbursed through the company's matching gifts program for employees, retirees, and company directors. Also gives graduate and undergraduate scholarships and fellowships that aim to strengthen student interest in disciplines vital to the petroleum industry. Supports regional associations of independent colleges. Awards scholarships to children of employees. *Environment:* 3%. Funds disaster relief efforts. *International:* 9%. Gives to health clinics, the American Red Cross, and a variety of other health organizations. *Religion:* 1%. *Note:* Total contributions made in fiscal 2001. **Typ. Recipients:** AIDS/HIV, Arthritis, Children's Health/Hospitals, Clinics/Medical Centers, Diabetes, Emergency/Ambulance Services, Health Organizations, Hospitals, Medical Education, Medical Rehabilitation, Medical Research, Medical Training, Mental Health, People with Disabilities, Single-Disease Health Associations, Substance Abuse. **Geo. Dist:** nationally, with preference given to locations with Unocal corporate facilities.

★ 12977 ★ UNUM Foundation
2211 Congress St.
Portland, ME 04122
Phone: (207)575-4478
Sheila Coyne, Grant Administrator

Priorities: *Arts & Humanities:* 11%. Supports public broadcasting and historic preservation. *Civic & Public Affairs:* 4%. Supports legal services, economic development, and clubs. *Education:* 81%. Supports schools, universities, scholarships, colleges, and education foundations. Focus is on long-term, systemic restructuring K-12 public schools that are committed to outcome-based education, accountability, and community involvement. *Environment:* 3%. Supports YWCA, United Way, and animal welfare. *Voluntarism:* Company provides cash grants to nonprofits where employees volunteer. Also supports Heart-to-Heart, an employee-managed volunteer program that researches, develops, and coordinates activities for employees. *Note:* Total foundation contributions made in 2001. **Typ. Recipients:** AIDS/HIV, Alzheimers Disease, Cancer, Clinics/Medical Centers, Domestic Violence, Emergency/Ambulance Services, Health Policy/Cost Containment, Medical Rehabilitation, Medical Research, People with Disabilities. **Geo. Dist:** Portland, ME.

★ 12978 ★ UPS Foundation
55 Glenlake Pkwy. NE
Atlanta, GA 30328
Phone: (404)828-6374 **Fax:** (404)828-7435
Website: http://www.community.ups.com
Ms. Evern Cooper, Executive Director

Priorities: *Arts & Humanities:* 5%. Supports historical societies, art and history museums, and libraries. *Civic & Public Affairs:* 22%. Funds women's groups, ethnic and minority organizations, urban leagues, municipalities, economic development, job training and placement, and affordable housing initiatives. *Education:* 23%. Supports academic research, programs that raise the level of educational effectiveness, enhance the quality of instruction, family learning opportunities, literacy, and school involvement projects. Scholarship programs include The Citizen's Scholarship Foundation of America, Inc. and The National Merit Scholarship Corporate. *Environment:* 48%. Primarily funds United Way. Also supports programs for families and children in crisis, food shelters, the economically or culturally disadvantaged, the physically or mentally challenged, community development programs, YMCAs, and organizations dealing with domestic violence. *International:* 1%. *Voluntarism:* The UPS Neighbor to Neighbor program matches employees and their family members interested in volunteer opportunities with community service projects based upon their interests, skills, and schedules. UPS volunteers also nominate organizations for grants through the region/district grant program. *Note:* Total foundation contributions made in 2000. **Typ. Recipients:** AIDS/HIV, Child Abuse, Domestic Violence, Family Planning, Long-Term Care, Medical Education, Medical Rehabilitation, Nursing Services, People with Disabilities, Single-Disease Health Associations, Trauma Treatment. **Geo. Dist:** nationally.

★ 12979 ★ US Bank
1420 5th Ave., Suite 800
PO Box 720 PD-WA-T8CR
Seattle, WA 98111-0720
Phone: (206)344-2360 **Fax:** (206)340-8554
Email: mary.moore@usbank.com
Website: http://www.usbank.com/comm_relations
Mary Moore, Vice Pres. & Manager, Comm. Relations

Priorities: *Arts & Humanities:* 25%. Funds organizations and programs that build audiences of arts organizations; bring the arts to underserved populations; bring select and limited civic amenities to underserved, rural communities; and promote the arts in education. *Civic & Public Affairs:* 25%. Funds economic opportunity by supporting affordable housing, welfare-to-work transitioning, and employment and skills training. Also supports small business development and expansion, commercial revitalization, and job creation. *Education:* 25%. Funds organizations that work in collaboration with K-12 schools (public or private) that develp and/or deliver innovative programs addressing dropout prevention, economic education, mentoring, and curriculum innovation. *Environment:* 25%. United Way. **Typ. Recipients:** Adolescent Health Issues, AIDS/HIV, Cancer, Children's Health/Hospitals, Domestic Violence, Health-General, Hospices, Mental Health, People with Disabilities, Prenatal Health Issues, Sexual Abuse, Substance Abuse. **Geo. Dist:** WA.

★ 12980 ★ USAA Foundation, A Charitable Trust
9800 Fredericksburg Rd.
San Antonio, TX 78288-0026
Phone: 800-531-8159 **Fax:** (210)498-9490
Website: http://www.usaaedfoundation.org
Barbara Gentry, Community Affairs, D-3-E

Fnded: 1994. **Priorities:** *Arts & Humanities:* 7%. Gives to music, museums, libraries, history organizations, and public broadcasting. *Civic & Public Affairs:* 22%. Supports housing programs, community foundations, community development, and law and justice. *Education:* 23%. Funds scholarships, religious education, colleges and universities, insurance education, and educational programs. *Environment:* 30%. Supports the United Way, family services, crime prevention, animal protection, child welfare, youth programs, community service organizations, and relief agencies. *International:* 12%. Supports preventative medicine, single-disease health associations, health foundations, hospitals, pediatric health care, medical research, and the American Red Cross. *Note:* Total contributions made in 2001. **Typ. Recipients:** Cancer, Children's Health/Hospitals, Emergency/Ambulance Services, Emergency/Ambulance Services, Health

Funds, Hospitals, Medical Research. **Geo. Dist:** headquarters and operating communities.

★ 12981 ★ USG Foundation

PO Box 6721
Chicago, IL 60680-6721
Phone: (312)606-4297 **Fax:** (312)606-5316
Website: http://www.usg.com/USG_Profile/6_5_2_social_respon.asp
Peter Maitland, President

Priorities: *Arts & Humanities:* 18%. Supports performing arts, museums, and historical preservation. Matches employee contributions to the arts. *Civic & Public Affairs:* 16%. Funds crime prevention, legal and justice issues, urban affairs, housing, parks, and economic development. *Education:* 21%. Funds organizations committed to educational improvement, colleges and universities, and scholarship programs. Matches employee contributions to education. *Environment:* 35%. Funds family services, youth organizations, and services for the disabled. *International:* 8%. Supports hospice, hospitals, health education, and single-disease associations. *Note:* Total foundation contributions made in 2000. **Typ. Recipients:** AIDS/HIV, Cancer, Children's Health/Hospitals, Clinics/Medical Centers, Diabetes, Eyes/Blindness, Health Organizations, Heart, Hospices, Hospitals, Long-Term Care, Medical Research, Medical Training, Mental Health, People with Disabilities, Public Health, Single-Disease Health Associations, Substance Abuse. **Geo. Dist:** IL, nationally, with emphasis on corporate operating locations.

★ 12982 ★ UST, Inc.

100 W Putnam Ave.
Greenwich, CT 06830
Phone: (203)661-1100 **Fax:** (203)863-7259
Email: mminton@usthq.com
Website: http://www.ustinc.com/content.cfm?id=34
Mary Minton, Manager, Corporate Contributions

Typ. Recipients: Domestic Violence, Health Organizations, Medical Research, Substance Abuse. **Geo. Dist:** headquarters and operating communities; on rare occasions will consider awards to national organizations.

★ 12983 ★ Valero Energy Corp.

1 Valero Pl.
San Antonio, TX 78212
Phone: (210)370-2000 **Fax:** (210)370-2327
Website: http://www.valero.com/con1.php@p=communityinvolvement
Mary Brown, Sr. Vice President Corporate Comm.

Typ. Recipients: Emergency/Ambulance Services. **Geo. Dist:** headquarters and operating communities.

★ 12984 ★ Valmont Foundation

One Valmont Plaza
Omaha, NE 68154-5215
Phone: (402)963-1000 **Fax:** (402)963-1095
Robert Daugherty, Director

Fnded: 1976. **Priorities:** *Arts & Humanities:* 3%. Funds museums, history organizations, and the performing arts. *Civic & Public Affairs:* 15%. Supports community foundations, economic development, zoos, and fairs/festivals. *Education:* 41%. Funds colleges and universities, and public and private secondary educational institutions. *Environment:* 35%. Supports the United Way and youth groups, and family services. *International:* 3%. Gives to single-disease health organizations and hospitals. *Note:* Total contributions made in fiscal 2000. **Typ. Recipients:** AIDS/HIV, Arthritis, Children's Health/Hospitals, Diabetes, Domestic Violence, Emergency/Ambulance Services, Heart, Hospitals, Kidney, Medical Rehabilitation, Nutrition, People with Disabilities, Single-Disease Health Associations, Substance Abuse. **Geo. Dist:** limited giving nationally; NE.

★ 12985 ★ Valspar Foundation

1700 Foshay Tower
821 Marquette Ave.
Minneapolis, MN 55402
Phone: (612)337-5903 **Fax:** (612)337-5904
Email: gleifeld@valspar.com
Website: http://www.valspar.com/av/av_cr.htm
Gwen Leifeld, Administrator

Priorities: *Arts & Humanities:* 19%. Funds public broadcasting, theater, opera, orchestras, art museums, and art centers. *Civic & Public Affairs:* 28%. Supports housing, community development, zoos, and an arboretum. *Education:* 8%. Provides scholarships to children of Valspar employees. Also funds institutions of higher learning and some pre-college educational programs. *Environment:* 35%. Supports United Way, Young Men's Christian Association, Big Brothers/Big Sisters, and criminal rehabilitation programs. *International:* 4%. Funds women's and children's cancer organizations. *Religion:* 5%. Contributes to the Science Museum of Minnesota. *Note:* Total contributions made in fiscal 2001. **Typ. Recipients:** Cancer, Hospitals, Medical Research, People with Disabilities, Single-Disease Health Associations. **Geo. Dist:** communities with manufacturing facilities only.

★ 12986 ★ Vanguard Group Foundation

PO Box 2600 (V38)
Valley Forge, PA 19482-2600
Phone: (610)669-6331
Tami Wise, Manager

Fnded: 1994. **Priorities:** *Arts & Humanities:* 12%. *Civic & Public Affairs:* 3%. *Education:* 11%. *Environment:* 68%. *International:* 2%. *Religion:* 2%. *Note:* Total contributions made in 2001. **Typ. Recipients:** Cancer, Emergency/Ambulance Services, Health Funds, Health Funds, Heart, Hospitals, Medical Rehabilitation, Nursing Services, People with Disabilities, Public Health. **Geo. Dist:** PA, Delaware Valley.

★ 12987 ★ Varian Medical Systems, Inc.

3100 Hansen Way
Palo Alto, CA 94304
Phone: (650)424-6444 **Fax:** (650)424-6822
Email: giving@varian.com
Website: http://www.varian.com/com/ctz000.html

Typ. Recipients: Health Organizations, Mental Health, People with Disabilities, Public Health. **Geo. Dist:** headquarters and operating communities.

★ 12988 ★ Verizon Delaware, Inc.

901 Tatnall St., 2nd Floor
Wilmington, DE 19801
Phone: (302)576-5322 **Fax:** (302)777-0491
Email: lauren.a.petrusky@verizon.com
Website: http://www.verizon.com/foundation
Lauren Petrusky, Co-Manager, Corporate Contributions

Typ. Recipients: Health-General. **Geo. Dist:** DE; DC; ME; MD; MA; NH; NJ; NY; PA; RI; VT; VI; WV.

★ 12989 ★ Verizon Foundation

1095 Ave. of the Americas
New York, NY 10036
Phone: (212)395-2295 **Fax:** (212)398-0951
Website: http://foundation.verizon.com
Suzanne DuBose, President

Fnded: 2000. **Priorities:** *Arts & Humanities:* 31%. *Civic & Public Affairs:* 9%. *Education:* 22%. *Environment:* 37%. *Religion:* 1%. *Voluntarism:* The Verizon Incentive Program recognizes employees' contribution of time and talent to nonprofit organizations where they live and work. Under the program, employees apply for a grant for the qualified organization where they volunteered at least 50 hours in a 12 month period. The foundation rewards them with a $500 check for presentation to the designated organization. Employees may request VIP grants on behalf of two separate organizations in a 12 month period for a total of $1,000. The Verizon Team Incentive Program rewards teams of ten or more eligible employees to collectively raise funds for nonprofit organizations across the country through organized pledge-a-thons, such as walk-a-thons or bike-a-thons. Under the program, the foundation matches funds collected by each team up to $25,000 per team to qualified nonprofit organizations. *Note:* Total contributions made in 2000. **Typ. Recipients:** Domestic Violence, Emergency/Ambulance Services, Geriatric Health, Health Policy/Cost Containment, Hospitals, People with Disabilities, Substance Abuse. **Geo. Dist:** operating locations.

★ 12990 ★ Verizon - West Virginia

1500 MacCorkle Ave., Room 500
Charleston, WV 25314
Phone: (304)344-7445 **Fax:** (304)344-6123
Email: hugh.s.cavendish@verizon.com
Website: http://foundation.verizon.com/
Stan Cavindish, Director, External Affairs

Typ. Recipients: Health-General. **Geo. Dist:** WV.

★ 12991 ★ Vesper Foundation

8223 Brecksville Rd., Suite 100
Brecksville, OH 44141
Phone: (440)838-4700 **Fax:** (440)838-4702
John Curci, Trustee

Priorities: *Arts & Humanities:* 7%. Contributes to libraries, museums, historic preservation, and the literary and performing arts. *Civic & Public Affairs:* 39%. Supports zoos, parks, botanical gardens, fire and police departments, and community foundations. *Education:* 11%. Funds private colleges and universities, education foundations, and private and parochial primary and secondary schools. *Environment:* 34%. Primarily supports United Way, youth organizations, sports and recreation programs. *International:* Less than 1%. *Note:* Total contributions made in 2001. **Typ. Recipients:** Cancer, Cancer, Emergency/Ambulance Services, Hospitals, Hospitals (University Affiliated), Respiratory, Single-Disease Health Associations. **Geo. Dist:** nationally, focusing on the Northeast USA.

★ 12992 ★ Viad Corp. Fund

15501 North Dial Boulevard
Scottsdale, AZ 85260-1619
Phone: (480)754-4090
Website: http://www.dialcorp.com/index.cfm?page_id=17
Cindy Demers, Vice President, Corp./Gov. Affairs

Fnded: 1987. **Priorities:** *Arts & Humanities:* 5%. Supports museums and music. *Civic & Public Affairs:* 14%. Supports economic development, urban and community affairs, and public policy. *Education:* 4%. Supports colleges, universities, and schools. *Environment:* 45%. Supports youth organizations, family services, and community service organizations. *International:* 23%. Supports hospitals and single-disease health associations. *Note:* Total contributions in 2001. **Typ. Recipients:** Alzheimers Disease, Arthritis, Cancer, Child Abuse, Children's Health/Hospitals, Diabetes, Domestic Violence, Emergency/Ambulance Services, Eyes/Blindness, Family Planning, Health Funds, Health Organizations, Health-General, Heart, Hospices, Hospitals, Kidney, Medical Rehabilitation, People with Disabilities, Prenatal Health Issues, Preventive Medicine/Wellness Organizations, Respiratory, Sexual Abuse, Single-Disease Health Associations, Substance Abuse. **Geo. Dist:** AZ, statewide; Phoenix, AZ.

★ 12993 ★ Victorinox-Swiss Army Knife Foundation

645 Madison Ave., Suite 500
New York, NY 10022-1010
Phone: (212)888-4004
Louis Marx, Jr., President & Director

Fnded: 1993. **Priorities:** *Arts & Humanities:* 12%. Supports a presidential library. *Education:* 10%. Funds the University of Alabama. *Environment:* 73%. Supports child welfare organizations, foundations for children, and Special Olympics. *International:* 5%. Gives to the Cystic Fibrosis Foundation. *Note:* Total contributions made in 2000. **Typ. Recipients:** Cancer, Medical

Research, Single-Disease Health Associations. **Geo. Dist:** nationally.

★ 12994 ★ The Visteon Fund
5500 Auto Club Dr.
PO Box 6200
Dearborn, MI 48126
Phone: (313)755-9500
Peter Look, Trustee

Fnded: 2001. **Priorities:** *Arts & Humanities:* 2%. *Civic & Public Affairs:* 4%. *Education:* 15%. *Environment:* 72%. *International:* 5%. *Note:* Total contributions made in 2001. **Typ. Recipients:** Children's Health/Hospitals, Diabetes, Eyes/Blindness, Medical Rehabilitation, People with Disabilities.

★ 12995 ★ Vivendi Universal Foundation
375 Park Ave., 5th Floor
New York, NY 10152-0192
Phone: (212)572-7240
Website: http://publicaffairs.vivendiuniversal.com/publicaffairsweb/pa/start.html
Nancy Morgan, Contact

Fnded: 1951. **Priorities:** *Arts & Humanities:* 8%. Funds museums, history, music, opera, and theater. *Civic & Public Affairs:* 6%. Supports housing and urban affairs and nature centers. *Education:* 25%. Supports Jewish studies, colleges and universities, public schools, and educational projects. *Environment:* 4%. Youth organizations and camps receive the majority of funding. Also supports United Way. *International:* 1%. Funds hospitals and AIDS research. *Note:* Total foundation contributions made in fiscal 2001. **Typ. Recipients:** AIDS/HIV, Cancer, Clinics/Medical Centers, Medical Education, Medical Research, Mental Health, Substance Abuse. **Geo. Dist:** New York, NY.

★ 12996 ★ Vodaphone-US Foundation
2999 Oak Rd., 9th Floor
Walnut Creek, CA 94597
Phone: (925)210-3870
Sam Ginn, Chairman & President

Fnded: 1993. **Priorities:** *Arts & Humanities:* 33%. Supports art funds, music, theater, museums, dance, opera, and the performing arts. *Civic & Public Affairs:* 9%. Supports women's affairs, zoos, legal aid, economic policy, and community foundations. *Education:* 7%. Supports educational foundations, mentoring programs, and schools. *Environment:* 32%. Supports YMCA, United Way, and scouts. *International:* 5%. Supports hospitals, health organizations, and single-disease health associations. *Religion:* 2%. Primarily supports science centers. *Voluntarism:* Company actively promotes and encourages volunteerism, both through its grantmaking and internal policies. *Note:* Total foundation contributions made in 2000. **Typ. Recipients:** AIDS/HIV, Cancer, Child Abuse, Children's Health/Hospitals, Emergency/Ambulance Services, Eyes/Blindness, Family Planning, Public Health, Research/Studies Institutes. **Geo. Dist:** areas where company provides cellular and paging operations; AZ; CA; San Francisco, CA; Walnut Creek, CA; CO; Washington, DC; Atlanta, GA; ID; IA; MI; MN; NE; NM; ND; OH; OR; Dallas, TX; UT; WA; WY. **Frmly:** Airtouch Communications Foundation.

★ 12997 ★ Vulcan Materials Co. Foundation
PO Box 385014
Birmingham, AL 35253-5014
Phone: (205)298-3229 **Fax:** (205)298-2960
Website: http://www.vulcanmaterials.com
Mary Russom, Manager Community Programs

Priorities: *Arts & Humanities:* 18%. *Civic & Public Affairs:* 9%. *Education:* 27%. *Environment:* 36%. *International:* 5%. *Note:* Total contributions made in fiscal 2002. **Typ. Recipients:** Cancer, Children's Health/Hospitals, Clinics/Medical Centers, Emergency/Ambulance Services, Health Organizations, Health-General, Mental Health, People with Disabilities, Substance Abuse. **Geo. Dist:** states in which company has operations.

★ 12998 ★ The Wachovia Foundation, Inc.
100 North Main St.
Winston-Salem, NC 27102-7203
Phone: (336)732-5252
Email: contact.community@wachovia.com
Website: http://www.wachovia.com/inside/page/0,,139,00.html

Priorities: *Arts & Humanities:* 14%. Recipients include festivals, art museums, living history sites, performing arts, and community arts organizations. *Civic & Public Affairs:* 12%. Supports chambers of commerce, business organizations, economic and community development, and community organizations. *Education:* 27%. Funds colleges and universities, precollege programs and schools, school readiness programs, and community involvement in schools. *Environment:* 36%. Supports traditional youth organizations, senior services, food distribution, and other human welfare agencies. Major support goes to united funds in North Carolina. *International:* 3%. Supports single-disease health organizations, public health, and medical research. **Typ. Recipients:** Emergency/Ambulance Services, Family Planning, Health Funds, Health Organizations, Hospices, Hospitals, Medical Education, People with Disabilities, Respiratory, Substance Abuse. **Geo. Dist:** GA; NC; SC.

★ 12999 ★ Wachtell, Lipton, Rosen & Katz Foundation
51 West 52nd St.
New York, NY 10019
Phone: (212)403-1000 **Fax:** (212)403-2000
Hillary Rappaport, Coordinator, Charitable Contributions

Fnded: 1981. **Priorities:** *Civic & Public Affairs:* 2%. Gives to law & justice organizations. *Education:* 61%. Provides major support to New York University; also funds college preparatory programs. *Environment:* 1%. *International:* 4%. *Note:* Total contributions made in fiscal 2000. **Typ. Recipients:** Cancer, Geriatric Health, Hospitals (University Affiliated), Long-Term Care, Medical Education, Speech & Hearing. **Geo. Dist:** New York, NY, metropolitan area.

★ 13000 ★ Waffle House Foundation, Inc.
5986 Financial Drive
PO Box 6450
Norcross, GA 30071
Phone: (770)729-5700 **Fax:** (770)729-5900
Alice Johnson, President

Priorities: *Arts & Humanities:* 2%. Gives to theater, historic preservation, and a fine arts center. *Civic & Public Affairs:* 9%. Funds housing, community foundations, community development, civic clubs, and philanthropic organizations. *Education:* 10%. Contributes to K-12 education and literacy efforts. *Environment:* 53%. Supports family services, child welfare organizations, services for victims of domestic violence and rape, and fundraising events. *International:* 19%. Single-disease associations, clinics, and a mental health foundation receive support. *Religion:* Less than 1%. *Note:* Total contributions made in fiscal 2001. **Typ. Recipients:** AIDS/HIV, Alzheimers Disease, Arthritis, Cancer, Child Abuse, Children's Health/Hospitals, Clinics/Medical Centers, Domestic Violence, Emergency/Ambulance Services, Eyes/Blindness, Health Organizations, Heart, Hospices, Hospitals, Medical Rehabilitation, Mental Health, Multiple Sclerosis, Nursing Services, People with Disabilities, Prenatal Health Issues, Preventive Medicine/Wellness Organizations, Sexual Abuse, Single-Disease Health Associations, Speech & Hearing, Trauma Treatment. **Geo. Dist:** Atlanta, GA, including metropolitan area.

★ 13001 ★ Wal-Mart Foundation
702 Southwest Eighth St.
Bentonville, AR 72716-0150
Phone: (479)273-8510
Email: fndatn@wal-mart.com
Website: http://www.walmartfoundation.org
Brad Fisher, Senior Manager, Wal-Mart Foundation

Priorities: *Education:* 29%. *Environment:* 45%. *International:* 22%. *Note:* Total contributions made in fiscal 2001. **Typ. Recipients:** Cancer, Children's Health/Hospitals, Domestic Violence, Emergency/Ambulance Services, Eyes/Blindness, Geriatric Health, Health Funds, Health Organizations, Hospices, Hospitals, Medical Education, Medical Rehabilitation, Medical Research, Mental Health, Nutrition, People with Disabilities, Public Health, Single-Disease Health Associations, Substance Abuse. **Geo. Dist:** headquarters and operating communities; Giving is done through operating locations in all states including Puerto Rico. The foundation reports that it does not accept unsolicited proposals for funds.

★ 13002 ★ Waldbaum's Supermarkets, Inc.
1 Hemlock St.
Central Islip, NY 11722
Phone: (631)582-9300
Website: http://www.waldbaums.com
Bill Clark, V. P. /Personnel

Typ. Recipients: Domestic Violence, People with Disabilities. **Geo. Dist:** principally near operating locations and to national organizations.

★ 13003 ★ Walgreen Benefit Fund
200 Wilmot Rd.
Mail Stop 2255
Deerfield, IL 60015-4681
Phone: (847)914-3550 **Fax:** (847)914-3417
Email: ed.king@walgreens.com
Website: http://www.walgreens.com
Edward King, Vice President

Priorities: *Arts & Humanities:* 4%. Funds museums and music. *Civic & Public Affairs:* 1%. *Education:* 1%. *Environment:* 6%. Focus is on youth organizations. *International:* 12%. Supports single-disease associations. *Note:* Total foundation contributions made in fiscal 2000. **Typ. Recipients:** AIDS/HIV, Cancer, Children's Health/Hospitals, Health-General, Hospitals, Medical Research, Mental Health, People with Disabilities, Single-Disease Health Associations, Substance Abuse. **Geo. Dist:** company operating locations; Chicago, IL, including metropolitan area.

★ 13004 ★ Walt Disney Co. Foundation
500 South Buena Vista St.
Burbank, CA 91521-0987
Phone: (818)560-1006
Ms. Tillie Baptie, Executive Director

Priorities: *Arts & Humanities:* 42%. *Civic & Public Affairs:* 11%. *Education:* 8%. *Environment:* 7%. *International:* 12%. *Religion:* 3%. *Note:* Total foundation contributions made in fiscal 2001. **Typ. Recipients:** Cancer, Children's Health/Hospitals, Clinics/Medical Centers, Diabetes, Domestic Violence, Emergency/Ambulance Services, Eyes/Blindness, Health Organizations, Health-General, Hospitals, Medical Education, Medical Rehabilitation, Mental Health, People with Disabilities, Public Health, Single-Disease Health Associations, Substance Abuse. **Geo. Dist:** headquarters and operating communities; CA, Los Angeles County; CA, Orange County; FL, Orange County; FL, Osceola County.

★ 13005 ★ Walter Foundation
1500 North Dale Mabry
PO Box 31601
Tampa, FL 33631-3601
Phone: (813)871-4168 **Fax:** (813)871-4094
W. Baker, Trustee

Fnded: 1966. **Priorities:** *Arts & Humanities:* 2%. Supports literary art and the performing arts. *Civic & Public Affairs:* 7%. Supports zoos, ethnic clubs, botanical organizations, community foundations and neighborhood improvement. *Education:* 65%. Supports schools, universities, and educational foundations. *Environment:* 14%. Supports United Way, youth groups, and scouts. *International:* 3%. Supports hospices, hospitals, clinics, health centers, and single-disease health associations. *Note:* Total foundation contributions made in fiscal 2001. **Typ. Recipients:** Cancer, Children's Health/Hospitals, Children's Health/Hospitals, Clinics/Medical Centers, Emergency/Ambulance Services, Health Organizations, Heart, Hospices, Hospitals, Medical Research, People with Disabilities, Prenatal Health Issues, Respiratory, Single-Disease Health Associations, Substance Abuse. **Geo. Dist:** headquarters and operating communities; Tampa, FL.

★ 13006 ★ Warren Alpert Foundation

27 Warren Way, PO Box 72743
Providence, RI 02907
Phone: (401)781-9900
John Dziedzic, Treasurer

Fnded: 1988. **Priorities:** *Civic & Public Affairs:* 1%. Supports a charitable foundation. *Education:* 56%. Foundation makes awards to individuals, selected after consultation with a panel of medical experts in concert with the faculty of Harvard Medical School. Also funds medical research. *International:* 34%. Supports medical centers, hospitals, and long-term care. *Note:* Total contributions made in 2001. **Typ. Recipients:** Cancer, Eyes/Blindness, Heart, Hospitals, Long-Term Care, Medical Education.

★ 13007 ★ Washington Group Foundation, Inc.

One Morrison Knudsen Plaza
Boise, ID 83729
Phone: (208)386-5201
Marlene Puckett, Administrator, Director, Secretary

Priorities: *Arts & Humanities:* 9%. *Civic & Public Affairs:* 2%. *Education:* 53%. *Environment:* 12%. Supports child welfare, Boy Scouts, food distribution, shelters, and senior centers. *International:* 1%. *Religion:* 2%. *Note:* Total foundation contributions made in 2000. **Typ. Recipients:** Alzheimers Disease, Cancer, Children's Health/Hospitals, Clinics/Medical Centers, Diabetes, Domestic Violence, Emergency/Ambulance Services, Health Organizations, Health-General, Hospices, Hospitals, Long-Term Care, Medical Rehabilitation, Medical Research, Multiple Sclerosis, People with Disabilities, Public Health, Respiratory, Single-Disease Health Associations. **Geo. Dist:** nationally; operating locations; ID.

★ 13008 ★ Washington Mutual Foundation

999 Third Ave., FIS2913
Seattle, WA 98104
Phone: (206)490-3249
Website: http://wamu.com

Priorities: *Arts & Humanities:* 7%. *Civic & Public Affairs:* 32%. *Education:* 41%. *Environment:* 19%. *Voluntarism:* Employees who work 20 hours or more per week are eligible to receive up to four hours of paid time off each month to do volunteer work through the company's Volunteer Release Time program. *Note:* Total foundation contributions made in 2001. **Typ. Recipients:** AIDS/HIV, Cancer, Children's Health/Hospitals, Clinics/Medical Centers, Domestic Violence, Emergency/Ambulance Services, Long-Term Care, Mental Health, Public Health. **Geo. Dist:** company operating areas; AZ; CA; CO; FL; ID; IL; MA; NV; NY; OR; TX; UT; WA. **Frmly:** Washington Mutual Bank Foundation.

★ 13009 ★ Waste Management Inc.

1001 Fannin, Suite 4000
Houston, TX 77002
Phone: (713)512-6200 **Fax:** (713)287-2616
Marilyn Brown, Director, Community Relations

Typ. Recipients: Health Funds, Hospitals, Medical Research, Mental Health, Single-Disease Health Associations. **Geo. Dist:** principally near operating locations and to national organizations.

★ 13010 ★ Wausau Insurance Companies

2000 Westwood Drive
Wausau, WI 54401
Phone: (715)845-5211 **Fax:** (715)843-3690
Website: http://www.wausau.com
Brad Zweck, Manager, Public Relations

Priorities: *Arts & Humanities:* 10% to 15%. Local art centers and activities involving youths. *Civic & Public Affairs:* 60% to 65%. Includes United Way. *Education:* 15% to 20%. Local education. *Note:* Health care, although not represented in a separate category, has gained importance in recent years. **Typ. Recipients:** Health-General. **Geo. Dist:** some giving nationally; WI; WI, Marathon County; WI, Wausau County.

★ 13011 ★ Wausau Paper Mills Foundation

1244 Kronenwetter Drive
Mosinee, WI 54455-9099
Phone: (715)962-2024
Thomas Howatt, Foundation Officer

Priorities: *Arts & Humanities:* 18%. *Civic & Public Affairs:* 12%. *Education:* 10%. *Environment:* 55%. *International:* 5%. *Note:* Total foundation contributions made in 2001. **Typ. Recipients:** Cancer, Children's Health/Hospitals, Health Organizations, Heart, Hospitals, Public Health, Respiratory. **Geo. Dist:** WI. **Frmly:** Wausau Paper Mills Foundation, Inc.

★ 13012 ★ Weil, Gotshal & Manges Foundation

767 5th Ave.
New York, NY 10153
Phone: (212)310-8000
Jesse Wolff, Treasurer & Director

Fnded: 1983. **Priorities:** *Arts & Humanities:* 2%. Supports performing arts, museums, symphonies, and libraries. *Civic & Public Affairs:* 33%. Primarily supports legal aid, clubs, parks, economic development, and urban affairs. *Education:* 13%. Focus is on law schools and private primary and secondary education. *Environment:* 17%. Funds the United Way, family services, and youth organizations. *International:* 3%. Funds single-disease associations, blood centers, and Make-a-Wish Foundation. *Religion:* 2%. Funds science and technology centers. *Note:* Total foundation contributions made in 2000. **Typ. Recipients:** AIDS/HIV, Cancer, Children's Health/Hospitals, Emergency/Ambulance Services, Family Planning, Heart, Medical Education, Medical Research, Prenatal Health Issues, Public Health, Single-Disease Health Associations, Transplant Networks/Donor Banks. **Geo. Dist:** NY.

★ 13013 ★ Weldon F. Osborne Foundation

Krystal Bldg.
1 Union Square, Suite 210
Chattanooga, TN 37402-2501
Phone: (423)267-0931 **Fax:** (423)267-0931
Glenn Stophel, Executive Director

Priorities: *Arts & Humanities:* 2%. *Civic & Public Affairs:* 32%. Priorities include: community revitalization, the police force, foundations, community centers, and self monitoring neighborhood programs. *Education:* 14%. Supports colleges and private primary and secondary schools. *Environment:* 10%. Funds the United Way, YMCA, food banks, and youth programs. *International:* 4%. Funding supports children's hospitals, homes, and medical foundations. *Note:* Total foundation contributions made in 2001. **Typ. Recipients:** Children's Health/Hospitals, Health-General, Hospitals. **Geo. Dist:** TN; Chattanooga, TN.

★ 13014 ★ Wellmark Foundation

636 Grand Ave., Station 150
Des Moines, IA 50309-2502
Phone: (515)245-4706 **Fax:** (515)235-4445
Email: wmfoundation@wellmark.com
Website: http://www.wellmark.com/community/wellmark_foundation/wellmark_foundation.htm
Dr. Sheila Riggs, Executive Director

Fnded: 1991. **Priorities:** *Civic & Public Affairs:* 10%. *Education:* 7%. *Environment:* 32%. *International:* 52%. *Note:* Total contributions made in 2001. **Typ. Recipients:** Alzheimers Disease, Arthritis, Cancer, Child Abuse, Children's Health/Hospitals, Clinics/Medical Centers, Domestic Violence, Emergency/Ambulance Services, Eyes/Blindness, Family Planning, Health Organizations, Health-General, Home-Care Services, Hospices, Hospitals, Hospitals (University Affiliated), Medical Education, Mental Health, Multiple Sclerosis, Nursing Services, People with Disabilities, Prenatal Health Issues, Preventive Medicine/Wellness Organizations, Public Health, Respiratory, Substance Abuse. **Geo. Dist:** IA; SD.

★ 13015 ★ Wells Fargo Bank Nebraska, N.A.

1919 Douglas St., MAC N8000-020
Omaha, NE 68103
Phone: (402)536-2650 **Fax:** (402)536-2509
Email: Jane.Braden@wellsfargo.com
Website: http://www.wellsfargo.com/about/charitable/index.jhtml
Jane Braden, Contributions Administrator

Priorities: *Arts & Humanities:* 10% to 15%. Contributes to theaters, arts festivals, ballet, symphonies, and arts centers. *Civic & Public Affairs:* About 15%. Supports parades and community arts events. 5% to 10%. Primarily supports philanthropic associations and economic development. *Education:* 20% to 25%. Supports colleges and universities, public high schools, education foundations, religious colleges, and Junior Achievement programs. *Environment:* 40% to 45%. Majority of funds support United Way agencies throughout Nebraska. Also supports religious organizations, community service organizations, scouting and other youth organizations, Planned Parenthood, and community centers. **Typ. Recipients:** Family Planning, Health Organizations, Mental Health, People with Disabilities, Public Health, Single-Disease Health Associations. **Geo. Dist:** operating communities.

★ 13016 ★ Wells Fargo Foundation

550 California St., 7th Floor
San Francisco, CA 94163
Phone: (415)222-5235 **Fax:** (415)975-6260
Website: http://www.wellsfargo.com/about/charitable.jhtml
Tim Hanlon, Contact

Priorities: *Arts & Humanities:* 23%. Funds music, art museums, libraries, public broadcasting, theater, cultural centers, historic preservation, historical societies, and arts associations. *Civic & Public Affairs:* 26%. Programs that help provide affordable housing for low and moderate income individuals; promote economic development by financing small businesses or small farms that meet size eligibility standards for the SBA's Development Company Program or have gross annual revenues of $1,000,000 or less; provide job training programs that assist low and moderate income individuals to find and retain employment; or help revitalize or stabilize low and moderate income communities. *Education:* 16%. Pre-kindergarten through twelfth grade institutions, as well as for nonprofits whose primary focus is to assist them, when the primary purpose of the grant is to promote academic achievement to low and moderate income students in the areas of math and science, literacy, and history of the American West. Also considers support of programs that work to encourage school partnerships with parents/guardians, the community in which the school is located, and the business community, as well as to programs that provide staff training for teachers and administrators working with low and moderate income students. *Environment:* 29%. Organizations whose work primarily benefits low and moderate income individuals. Issues of interest include child care, and basic needs assistance. *International:* 3%. Gives to single-disease health associations, health foundations, clinics, medical centers, and other community health services. *Religion:* 1%. An observatory and science center receives support. *Note:* Total foundation contributions made in 2000. **Typ. Recipients:** AIDS/HIV, People with Disabilities, Single-Disease

Health Associations. **Geo. Dist:** AZ; CA, headquarters and operating communities; CO; ID; NV; NM; OR; TX; UT; WA.

★ 13017 ★ West Bend Mutual Charitable Trust

1900 S 18th Ave.
West Bend, WI 53095-8796
Phone: (414)334-5571
John Dedrick, Trustee

Fnded: 1994. **Priorities:** *Civic & Public Affairs:* 18%. Supports municipalities, community foundations, and county facilities. *Education:* 16%. Funds medical education, Junior Achievement, and scholarship funds. *Environment:* 33%. Supports the United Way, YMCAs, and youth athletics. *International:* 20%. Hospitals, health care services, and the American Red Cross receive support. *Note:* Total contributions made in 2000. **Typ. Recipients:** Health-General, Heart, Hospitals, Public Health. **Geo. Dist:** Washington, DC; MD; WI.

★ 13018 ★ Westar Energy Foundation

818 South Kansas Ave.
Topeka, KS 66612
Phone: (785)575-1544 **Fax:** (785)575-6399
Email: cynthia_a_mccarvel@wr.com
Website: http://www.wstnres.com/westar_foundation.html
Cynthia McCarvel, President

Fnded: 1991. **Priorities:** *Arts & Humanities:* 17%. Funds museums, theater, music, and festivals. *Civic & Public Affairs:* 3%. Supports local public affairs and employment programs. *Education:* 56%. Funds colleges and universities; major support for scholarships through matching funds. *Environment:* 18%. United Way and youth programs, especially those dealing with employment opportunity enhancement. Also contributes to groups dealing with the problems of aging. *International:* 3%. Supports hospitals, hospice, and emergency relief. *Voluntarism:* Community Partners is a voluntary program for active and retired Western Resources employees. *Note:* Total contributions made in 2000. **Typ. Recipients:** Public Health. **Geo. Dist:** headquarters and operating communities; KS. **Frmly:** Western Resources Foundation.

★ 13019 ★ Western-Southern Foundation, Inc.

400 Broadway
Cincinnati, OH 45202-3341
Phone: (513)629-2121
Richard Taulbee, Assistant Treasurer

Fnded: 1990. **Priorities:** *Arts & Humanities:* 11%. *Civic & Public Affairs:* 16%. *Education:* 39%. *Environment:* 24%. *International:* 4%. *Note:* Total foundation contributions made in 2001. **Typ. Recipients:** Cancer, Children's Health/Hospitals, Diabetes, Emergency/Ambulance Services, Health Organizations, Home-Care Services, Hospices, Hospitals, Long-Term Care, Mental Health, Multiple Sclerosis, People with Disabilities, Prenatal Health Issues, Single-Disease Health Associations. **Geo. Dist:** OH. **Frmly:** Western-Southern Enterprise Fund, Inc.

★ 13020 ★ Weyerhaeuser Co. Foundation

CH1 L32
PO Box 9777
Federal Way, WA 98063-9777
Phone: (253)924-3159 **Fax:** (253)924-3658
Website: http://www.weyerhaeuser.com/citizenship/philanthropy/
Elizabeth Crossman, Vice President

Priorities: *Arts & Humanities:* 10%. *Civic & Public Affairs:* 16%. *Education:* 31%. *Environment:* 37%. *International:* 2%. *Note:* Total contributions made in 2001. **Typ. Recipients:** Children's Health/Hospitals, Clinics/Medical Centers, Emergency/Ambulance Services, Hospices, Hospitals, People with Disabilities, Public Health, Substance Abuse. **Geo. Dist:** nationally, with emphasis on communities, particularly remote communities, in which company has significant numbers of employees; AL; AR; MS; NC; OK; OR; WA.

★ 13021 ★ Whirlpool Foundation

2000 North M-63
Benton Harbor, MI 49022
Phone: (616)923-5583 **Fax:** (616)923-3214
Website: http://www.whirlpoolcorp.com/whr/foundation/index.html
Barbara Hall, Foundation Contact

Priorities: *Arts & Humanities:* (Arts & Culture) 1%. Primarily gives to museums, operas, orchestras, theater, arts councils, and public broadcasting. *Civic & Public Affairs:* (Civic & Community/Contemporary Family Life) 23%. Supports cultural diversity organizations, affordable housing, women's affairs, economic development, chambers of commerce, community leadership programs, municipalities, and civic and community groups. *Education:* (Colleges & Universities/Lifelong Learning) 25%. Supports colleges and universities, with interests in science, technological, business, and arts and humanities education, as well as minority education organizations and higher education associations. Funds education foundations, school systems, and institutions of higher learning that offer lifelong learning opportunities. Also provides scholarships for children of employees who exhibit exceptional academic achievement. *Environment:* 25%. Provides major support for the United Way. *International:* (Health & Human Services) 4%. Funds children's and family services, single-disease health organizations, hospitals, health centers/foundations, and programs for the handicapped, the needy, the elderly, and children. *Note:* Total contributions made in fiscal 2001. **Typ. Recipients:** Cancer, Clinics/Medical Centers, Domestic Violence, Emergency/Ambulance Services, Family Planning, Health Organizations, Hospitals, Medical Education, People with Disabilities, Public Health, Sexual Abuse, Substance Abuse. **Geo. Dist:** operating locations.

★ 13022 ★ Whitman Corp. Foundation

3501 Algonquin Rd.
Rolling Meadows, IL 60008
Phone: (847)818-5000 **Fax:** (847)818-5046
Karen Golden, President

Priorities: *Arts & Humanities:* 1%. Supports the symphony. *Civic & Public Affairs:* 14%. Urban and community affairs. *Education:* 80%. Includes matching gifts to educational institutions. Majority of funding supports colleges and universities nationwide. *Environment:* 4%. United funds, YMCA's youth organizations, and child welfare. *International:* 1%. Emergency relief, health policy, hospitals, and single-disease health associations. *Note:* Total contributions in 1998. **Typ. Recipients:** Cancer, Child Abuse, Children's Health/Hospitals, Diabetes, Emergency/Ambulance Services, Eyes/Blindness, Health Organizations, Health Policy/Cost Containment, Hospitals, Hospitals (University Affiliated), Kidney, Medical Rehabilitation, People with Disabilities, Prenatal Health Issues, Single-Disease Health Associations. **Geo. Dist:** nationally; Chicago, IL.

★ 13023 ★ William Blair & Co. Foundation

222 West Adams St.
Chicago, IL 60606
Phone: (312)236-1600
E. Coolidge, III, Chief Executive Officer

Fnded: 1980. **Priorities:** *Arts & Humanities:* 17%. Supports arts institutes, dance, museums, historical societies, opera, and theater. *Civic & Public Affairs:* 24%. Primarily funds community affairs programs, business development, zoos, and a horticultural society. *Education:* 17%. Emphasis is on colleges and universities, secondary schools, and education associations. *Environment:* 19%. Focus is on youth organizations, child welfare, and recreation projects. *International:* 13%. Hospitals, medical centers, single-disease associations, and medical rehabilitation receive support. *Religion:* 3%. Funds planetariums. *Note:* Total contributions for fiscal 2001. **Typ. Recipients:** Cancer, Children's Health/Hospitals, Clinics/Medical Centers, Diabetes, Health Organizations, Health-General, Hospitals, Hospitals (University Affiliated), Medical Rehabilitation, Medical Research, People with Disabilities, Single-Disease Health Associations, Substance Abuse. **Geo. Dist:** Chicago, IL.

★ 13024 ★ The Williams Companies Foundation

One Williams Center
MD 49-3
Tulsa, OK 74172
Phone: (918)573-2106
Email: communityrelationstulsa@williams.com
Website: http://www.williams.com/community/
Ms. Sylvia Schmidt, Director, Community Relations

Priorities: *Environment:* 100%. *Note:* Above giving reflects corporate donations. In 2000, the foundation donated 95% of funds to a community foundation, and 5% to higher education. Total contributions made in 2001. **Typ. Recipients:** AIDS/HIV, Children's Health/Hospitals, Clinics/Medical Centers, Domestic Violence, Family Planning, Health Funds, Health Organizations, Hospitals, People with Disabilities, Prenatal Health Issues, Single-Disease Health Associations, Substance Abuse. **Geo. Dist:** areas near company headquarters and operating communities.

★ 13025 ★ Williams Companies Inc.

2800 Post Oak Boulevard
Houston, TX 77056
Phone: (713)215-3132 **Fax:** (713)215-4269
Email: helen.m.dworsky@williams.com
Website: http://www.williams.com/community
Helen Dworsky, Administrative Assistant to President

Priorities: *Arts & Humanities:* About 15%. Programs that benefit the greatest number of people in the community. *Civic & Public Affairs:* 10% to 15%. Organizations that address diverse contemporary issues and challenges facing society, including conservation and preservation, crime prevention, community revitalizations, and thedevelopment of public policy. *Education:* About 35%. Direct grants to colleges and universities where the company actively recruits and to those institutions that provide education to their employees; K-12 education with focus on adopt-a-school programs, character education, math, science, and technology education, and literacy; and economic education programs that promote the understanding of economics and the free enterprise systems. Additionally, the company matches employee gifts to eligible educational institutions and sponsors a scholarship program for employee children. *Environment:* About 35%. Majority to United Way. Also supports disaster relief efforts, programs for the disabled, prevention of child abuse, and youth organizations. *International:* Less than 5%. Organizations where employees are directly involved and hospitals near operating locations. **Typ. Recipients:** Domestic Violence, Hospices, Medical Research, Mental Health, People with Disabilities, Substance Abuse. **Geo. Dist:** headquarters and operating communities.

★ 13026 ★ Winn-Dixie Stores Foundation

PO Box B
Jacksonville, FL 32203-0297
Phone: (904)783-5000 **Fax:** (904)783-5235
Website: http://www.winn-dixie.com/company/about_wd/community_commitment.asp
August Toscano, President & Director, Matching Gifts

Priorities: *Arts & Humanities:* 1%. *Civic & Public Affairs:* 14%. *Education:* 29%. *Environment:* 31%. *International:* 21%. *Note:* About half of foundation giving is in the form of employee matching gifts. Total contributions made in 2001. **Typ. Recipients:** Alzheimers Disease, Cancer, Children's Health/Hospitals, Clinics/Medical Centers, Clinics/Medical Centers, Diabetes, Emergency/Ambulance Services, Heart, Hospices, Hospitals, Medical Education, Mental Health, Multiple Sclerosis, People with Disabilities, Prenatal Health Issues, Public Health, Single-Disease Health Associations, Substance Abuse. **Geo. Dist:** primarily in the company's 14-state trade area; generally within the Southern United States; AL; FL; GA; IN; KY; LA; MS; NC; OH; OK; SC; TN; TX; VA.

★ 13027 ★ Wiremold Foundation
60 Woodlawn St.
West Hartford, CT 06110
Phone: (860)233-6251 **Fax:** (860)523-3699
John Murphy, President

Fnded: 1967. **Priorities:** *Arts & Humanities:* 16%. Supports public broadcasting, music, dance, arts councils, music, and historic preservation. *Civic & Public Affairs:* 9%. Supports housing, job training services, and community development. *Education:* 10%. Supports colleges, school foundations, Junior Achievement, scholarships, and schools for the deaf and blind. *Environment:* 20%. Supports United Way, youth organizations, scouts, camps, family services, senior services, YMCA, food distribution, homes, and people with disabilities. *International:* 39%. Supports rehabilitation and health organizations. *Religion:* 1%. Primarily supports science centers. *Note:* Total foundation contributions made in 2000. **Typ. Recipients:** AIDS/HIV, Cancer, Children's Health/Hospitals, Clinics/Medical Centers, Emergency/Ambulance Services, Health Organizations, Health-General, Hospitals, People with Disabilities, Prenatal Health Issues, Public Health. **Geo. Dist:** headquarters area only.

★ 13028 ★ Wisconsin Energy Corp. Foundation, Inc.
231 West Michigan St.
Milwaukee, WI 53203
Phone: (414)221-2106 **Fax:** (414)221-2412
Website: http://foundation.wisconsinenergy.com
Carolyn Simpson, Foundation Coordinator

Priorities: *Arts & Humanities:* 21%. Supports the performing arts, community arts, and arts centers. Museums also receive significant support. *Civic & Public Affairs:* 4%. Funds community/economic development initiatives, civil rights, and business and free enterprise groups. *Education:* 34%. Majority of education support is given to general programs at colleges and universities in Wisconsin. Other recipients include education reform programs, education funds, engineering programs, minority education, and business education projects. Also sponsors an employee matching gifts program for contributions to higher education institutions. *Environment:* 38%. Provides major support to the United Way in Wisconsin communities. Also supports youth groups and community centers. Other interests include the aged and community service organizations. *Religion:* 2%. Funds a science museum. *Voluntarism:* Company actively promotes volunteerism through the Employee Volunteer Program, including mentoring programs, a speakers bureau, and other volunteer activities. *Note:* Total contributions made in 2000. **Typ. Recipients:** Children's Health/Hospitals, Clinics/Medical Centers, Health Organizations, Hospitals, Medical Education, Medical Rehabilitation, Medical Research, Mental Health, People with Disabilities, Public Health, Respiratory, Single-Disease Health Associations, Trauma Treatment. **Geo. Dist:** headquarters and operating communities.

★ 13029 ★ Wm. Jr. Wrigley Co. Foundation
410 North Michigan Ave.
Chicago, IL 60611
Phone: (312)645-3950 **Fax:** (312)661-1267
William Piet, President

Priorities: *Arts & Humanities:* 2%. Primary support made to public broadcasting. *Civic & Public Affairs:* 34%. Supports NAACP, parks, clubs, and neighborhood and community development. *Education:* 10%. Supports universities, colleges, Junior Achievement, groups concerned with minority education, education and scholarship funds. *Environment:* 27%. Supports United Way, food distribution, shelters, youth and family services, child welfare, and social services. *International:* 19%. Supports medical centers, health care, and single-disease health associations. *Religion:* 1%. Primary support made to Chicago Academy of Science. *Note:* Total foundation contributions made in 2000. **Typ. Recipients:** AIDS/HIV, Alzheimers Disease, Cancer, Child Abuse, Clinics/Medical Centers, Clinics/Medical Centers, Diabetes, Domestic Violence, Eyes/Blindness, Health Funds, Health Organizations, Heart, Hospitals, Medical Education, Nursing Services, People with Disabilities, Prenatal Health Issues, Public Health, Single-Disease Health Associations, Substance Abuse. **Geo. Dist:** nationally; Chicago, IL.

★ 13030 ★ Wolfe Associates, Inc.
770 Twin Rivers Drive
Columbus, OH 43215
Phone: (614)460-3782
Email: comrel@dispatch.com
Website: http://www.dispatch.com
Rita Wolfe Hoag, Vice President & Trustee

Fnded: 1973. **Priorities:** *Arts & Humanities:* 6%. Funds organizations which perform and promote public appreciation of music, drama and dance, and those institutions which provide public access to the visual arts; institutions, such as museums, libraries, and historical societies dedicated to the preservation of and providing public access to the political, social and cultural heritage of the United States; and programs dedicated to arts and humanities, history, language, and literature. *Civic & Public Affairs:* 12%. Supports programs dedicated to improving quality of life in operating communities and programs promoting minority opportunities, including community foundations and organizations addressing economic development, legal aid, affordable housing, community parks/public spaces, and minority affairs. *Education:* 16%. Contributions are designed to provide opportunities for advanced study to those unable to procure funds. Scholarship grants are not made directly to individuals, but to the endowment of chaired professorships at colleges and universities. Public and private institutions of higher learning which offer students of high scholastic achievement the opportunity to pursue their studies, and programs dedicated to adult continuing education, adult literacy, and special education are given high priority. *Environment:* 33%. Provides major support to the United Way. Also funds organizations and groups providing social services to children, families, and the elderly, who through misfortune, disability, or other adversity, are deprived of basic living needs. *International:* 15%. Funds groups organized on a statewide/national basis, as well as local chapters, committed to research in and treatment of a variety of catastrophic diseases; hospitals and health care institutions dedicated to delivering quality health care services to the communities they serve; programs dedicated to mental health, health education, substance abuse, public health and medical care. *Religion:* 8%. Funds science centers. *Note:* Total foundation contributions made in fiscal 2001. **Typ. Recipients:** Cancer, Children's Health/Hospitals, Clinics/Medical Centers, Emergency/Ambulance Services, Family Planning, Health Funds, Health-General, Heart, Hospices, Hospitals, Long-Term Care, Medical Rehabilitation, Medical Research, People with Disabilities, Single-Disease Health Associations. **Geo. Dist:** OH, Central Ohio and other areas in which the corporate donors have a substantial presence.

★ 13031 ★ Wolff Shoe Foundation
1705 Larkin Williams Rd.
Fenton, MO 63026
Phone: (636)343-7770 **Fax:** (636)343-7371
William Wolff, Manager

Priorities: *Education:* 9%. Gives to private day schools and a university. *International:* 22%. Funds wellness initiatives, medical centers, single-disease health associations, and medical research. *Note:* Total contributions made in 2000. **Typ. Recipients:** Cancer, Children's Health/Hospitals, Clinics/Medical Centers, Diabetes, Health Organizations, Hospitals, Kidney, Medical Research, Preventive Medicine/Wellness Organizations, Public Health, Single-Disease Health Associations. **Geo. Dist:** Palm Beach, FL; St. Louis, MO; New York, NY.

★ 13032 ★ Woodward Governor Co. Charitable Trust
5001 N Second St.
Rockford, IL 61125
Phone: (815)877-7441 **Fax:** (815)639-6033
Pam Johnson, Contributions Committee Chairman

Priorities: *Arts & Humanities:* 9%. Supports the arts, including symphonies, theater, arts councils, and various museums. *Civic & Public Affairs:* 3%. Gives to regional partnering programs, community foundations, and parks. *Education:* 34%. Supports colleges, universities, education foundations, and Junior Achievement. *Environment:* 48%. Supports food banks, community services, youth organizations, United Way, day care, and various programs for child welfare. *International:* 5%. Funds clinics, medical centers, hospice programs, mental health, and single-disease health associations. *Religion:* 1%. Funds science museums. *Note:* Total contributions made in 2001. **Typ. Recipients:** Alzheimers Disease, Cancer, Children's Health/Hospitals, Clinics/Medical Centers, Emergency/Ambulance Services, Geriatric Health, Health Organizations, Health-General, Hospices, Hospitals, Medical Rehabilitation, Medical Research, Mental Health, People with Disabilities, Public Health, Research/Studies Institutes, Single-Disease Health Associations, Speech & Hearing, Substance Abuse, Transplant Networks/Donor Banks. **Geo. Dist:** headquarters and operating communities.

★ 13033 ★ Woronoco Savings Charitable Foundation
31 Court St.
Westfield, MA 01086-0978
Phone: (413)564-6241
Website: http://www.woronoco.com/home/sponsors.php
Debra Murphy, Senior Vice President & CFO

Fnded: 2000. **Priorities:** *Arts & Humanities:* 19%. Funds museums, historic preservation, historical societies, libraries, theater, and a music festival. *Civic & Public Affairs:* 6%. Gives to housing, gardens, police departments, and philanthropic organizations. *Education:* 27%. Supports state, private and community colleges; public schools; Junior Achievement; a school for the deaf; and scholarships. *Environment:* 22%. Supports scouting, emergency relief, veterans affairs, Young Men's Christian Association, and Boys & Girls Clubs. *International:* 26%. Contributes to hospitals, nursing services, services for cancer patients, and children's hospitals. *Voluntarism:* The company encourages employee volunteerism. Woronoco Savings Bank employees contribute approximately 6,500 volunteer hours annually. *Note:* Total contributions made in 2001. **Typ. Recipients:** Hospices, Hospitals. **Geo. Dist:** MA, western area.

★ 13034 ★ WPS Resources Foundation, Inc.
PO Box 19001
Green Bay, WI 54307-9001
Phone: (920)433-1103 **Fax:** (414)433-1693
Website: http://www.wpsr.com/foundat/index.html
Larry Weyers, President

Priorities: *Arts & Humanities:* 5%. Supports museums, historical societies, libraries, arts councils, music, theater, and public broadcasting. *Civic & Public Affairs:* 20%. Funds cities, community foundations, community development, parks, and public affairs organizations. *Education:* 27%. Major support is for colleges and universities. Also funds technical and engineering education, and provides scholarships. *Environment:* 34%. Supports united funds, family services, and youth organizations including clubs, camps, sports, YMCA. *International:* 9%. Supports hospitals, medical centers, mental health, single-disease health associations. *Voluntarism:* The company sponsors employee volunteer programs in association with the United Way at Work Committee, Adopt-a-Classroom, and the Lyle Kingston Environmental Group. *Note:* Total contributions made in 2000. **Typ. Recipients:** Children's Health/Hospitals, Clinics/Medical Centers, Domestic Violence, Emergency/Ambulance Services, Health Organizations, Health-General, Hospitals, Medical Education, Medical Rehabilitation, Mental Health, People with Disabilities, Prenatal Health Issues, Single-Disease Health Associations, Substance Abuse. **Geo. Dist:** MI, Northern Michigan; WI, Northeast Wisconsin. **Frmly:** Wisconsin Public Service Foundation, Inc.

★ 13035 ★ WPWR-TV Channel 50 Foundation

2151 N Elston Ave.
Chicago, IL 60614-3999
Phone: (773)292-5016 **Fax:** (773)276-6477
Email: mail@wpwr50fund.org
Laura Sampson, Program Officer

Fnded: 1992. **Priorities:** *Arts & Humanities:* 57%. Supports museums, ballet, theater, arts councils, and public broadcasting. *Civic & Public Affairs:* 16%. Funds law and justice issues, advocacy, and parks. *Education:* 14%. Funds colleges and universities and arts education. *Environment:* 6%. Funds United Way, youth organizations, and services for immigrants and the disadvantaged. *International:* 6%. Supports AIDS research. *Note:* Total foundation contributions made in fiscal 2000. **Typ. Recipients:** AIDS/HIV, Cancer, Health Policy/Cost Containment. **Geo. Dist:** Chicago, IL, including metropolitan area; IN, Northwest part of the state.

★ 13036 ★ Wyman-Gordon Foundation

370 Main St., Suite 1100
Worcester, MA 01608
Phone: (508)798-8621 **Fax:** (508)791-6454
Warner Fletcher, Jr., Director

Priorities: *Arts & Humanities:* 27%. *Civic & Public Affairs:* 4%. *Education:* 4%. *Environment:* 63%. *International:* 2%. *Religion:* Less than 1%. *Note:* Total contributions made in 2001. **Typ. Recipients:** AIDS/HIV, Cancer, Children's Health/Hospitals, Diabetes, Emergency/Ambulance Services, Health Organizations, Health-General, Hospices, Hospitals, Medical Research, Multiple Sclerosis, Nursing Services, People with Disabilities, Public Health. **Geo. Dist:** principally near operating locations and to national organizations.

★ 13037 ★ Xcel Energy Foundation

800 Nicollet Mall Suite 2900
Minneapolis, MN 55402
Phone: (612)330-5500 **Fax:** (612)330-6947
Email: foundation@xcelenergy.com
Website: http://www.xcelenergy.com/XLWEB/CDA/0,2914,1-1-1_4359_847-0-0_0-0,00.html
James Rhodes, Contribution Specialist

Priorities: *Arts & Humanities:* 8%. Contributions provide opportunities for all individuals and families to learn and grow from the arts. Supports a broad spectrum of cultural activities, including theater, dance, music and arts organizations. Historic preservation and museums also supported. Emphasis on programs designed to increase accessibility to community performances for special populations. *Civic & Public Affairs:* 35%. Contributions build stronger neighborhoods by providing opportunities for members of the community to rebuild their neighborhoods. Interests include urban and community affairs. 10% to 15%. Generally smaller grants made at the local level. Priorities will vary according to community needs. *Education:* 14%. Contributes to education-focused programs to provide access to life-long learning, and opportunities for youth and adults to become contributing members of the workforce. Primarily supports post-secondary scholarship and financial assistance programs for low-income groups, minorities, and women. Emphasis on learning-disabled children and adults. Capital grants awarded to higher education institutions. Also sponsors matching gifts program in education. *Environment:* 31%. Contributions focus on building the capacity of families and individuals of all ages to become stronger, more independent and self sufficient members in the community. Major support for programs that remove barriers for the economically or socially disadvantaged, including social services to special population groups; employment assistance; and short-term and crisis assistance programs such as food shelves, battered women's shelters, and crisis nurseries. Youth organizations, community centers, and organizations concerned with the elderly are also supported, as well as health care for under-served population groups. **Typ. Recipients:** AIDS/HIV, Cancer, Clinics/Medical Centers, Domestic Violence, Health Organizations, Hospitals, Mental Health, Nursing Services, People with Disabilities, Single-Disease Health Associations, Substance Abuse. **Geo. Dist:** near headquarters and service areas only.

★ 13038 ★ Xerox Foundation

PO Box 1600
800 Long Ridge Rd.
Stamford, CT 06904
Phone: (203)968-3445 **Fax:** (203)968-3330
Mr. Joseph Cahalan, Vice President

Priorities: *Education:* 18%. Supports higher education, colleges and universities located in communities where company has facilities, and sponsors employee matching gifts. *Voluntarism:* The company encourages employee volunteerism through the Social Service Leave and Community Involvement programs. *Note:* Total foundation contributions made in 2001. **Typ. Recipients:** Domestic Violence, Health Policy/Cost Containment, People with Disabilities, Substance Abuse. **Geo. Dist:** nationally, with emphasis on operating locations.

★ 13039 ★ Yellow Corp. Foundation

10990 Roe Ave.
Overland Park, KS 66211-1213
Phone: (913)696-6123 **Fax:** (913)696-6116
William Martin, Vice President

Priorities: *Arts & Humanities:* 2%. Primarily supports museums. *Education:* 23%. Supports colleges and universities. Major interests include education concerned with traffic and logistics, business education, and arts education. *Environment:* 72%. Supports child welfare, homeless services, and United Way. *International:* 3%. Supports health funds. *Note:* Total foundation contributions made in 2001. **Typ. Recipients:** Cancer, Children's Health/Hospitals, Domestic Violence, Health Organizations, Heart, Multiple Sclerosis, Public Health. **Geo. Dist:** headquarters and operating communities; Kansas City, MO.

★ 13040 ★ York Federal Savings & Loan Foundation

c/o York Federal Savings & Loan Foundation
101 South George St.
York, PA 17401
Phone: (717)815-4501 **Fax:** (717)846-5590
Robert Pullo, Chairman & Chief Executive Officer

Priorities: *Arts & Humanities:* 27%. Supports theater, performing arts, libraries, community art projects, and art funds. *Civic & Public Affairs:* 7%. Interests include immigrant services and community foundations. *Education:* 24%. Funds Penn State York, public and private preK-12 schools, scholarship funds, and Junior Achievement. *Environment:* 25%. Major funding for the United Way; also supports youth organizations and social service agencies. *International:* 13%. Supports hospitals, a mental health association, and single-disease health associations. *Note:* Total contributions made in fiscal 2000. **Typ. Recipients:** Cancer, Children's Health/Hospitals, Clinics/Medical Centers, Emergency/Ambulance Services, Health Organizations, Health-General, Heart, Hospices, Hospitals, Mental Health, Multiple Sclerosis, People with Disabilities, Prenatal Health Issues, Public Health, Sexual Abuse, Single-Disease Health Associations, Substance Abuse. **Geo. Dist:** York, PA.

★ 13041 ★ Young & Rubicam Foundation

1114 Ave. of the Americas, 12th Floor
125 Park Ave.
New York, NY 10036
Phone: (212)798-1039

Fnded: 1955. **Priorities:** *Arts & Humanities:* 32%. Supports museums, theaters, opera, orchestras, and libraries. *Civic & Public Affairs:* 13%. Funds The Advertising Council, with other funding directed to professional associations and community and economic development. *Education:* 21%. Majority of education funding is in the form of employee matching gifts. Remaining support goes to education funds and schools in New York, NY. *Environment:* 25%. Supports the United Way of New York City, youth and family services, YMCA/YWCA, scouts, victim services, and disaster relief. *International:* 5%. Funds hospitals, community service programs, and disease-specific foundations. *Note:* Total contributions made in 2000. **Typ. Recipients:** AIDS/HIV, Arthritis, Cancer, Children's Health/Hospitals, Clinics/Medical Centers, Diabetes, Emergency/Ambulance Services, Family Planning, Geriatric Health, Heart, Hospitals, Medical Education, Medical Research, Multiple Sclerosis, Nursing Services, People with Disabilities, Prenatal Health Issues, Public Health, Respiratory, Single-Disease Health Associations, Substance Abuse, Transplant Networks/Donor Banks. **Geo. Dist:** NY.

★ 13042 ★ The Zachry Foundation

310 South St. Mary's St., Suite 2500
San Antonio, TX 78205
Phone: (210)554-4663 **Fax:** (210)554-4605
Pamela O'Connor, Executive Director

Fnded: 1960. **Priorities:** *Arts & Humanities:* 8%. Funds performing arts, libraries, and museums and galleries. *Civic & Public Affairs:* 2%. Gives to nonprofit management, a zoo, and other civic organizations. *Education:* 41%. Supports public education, colleges and universities, and private/parochial schools. *Environment:* 8%. Supports child welfare, scouts, youth programs, and family services. *International:* 30%. Supports hospitals, health systems, cancer research, and the American Red Cross. *Religion:* 2%. Funds a natural science museum. *Note:* Total contributions made in 2000. **Typ. Recipients:** Cancer, Children's Health/Hospitals, Clinics/Medical Centers, Diabetes, Domestic Violence, Emergency/Ambulance Services, Health Organizations, Health-General, Hospices, Hospitals, Hospitals (University Affiliated), Medical Education, Medical Rehabilitation, Medical Research, People with Disabilities, Public Health, Speech & Hearing, Substance Abuse. **Geo. Dist:** TX, higher education grants are given throughout the state; San Antonio, TX.

★ 13043 ★ Zenith Electronics Corp.

2000 Milbrook Dr.
Lincolnshire, IL 60069
Phone: (847)941-8184 **Fax:** (847)941-8177
John Taylor, Vice President, Public Affairs

Priorities: *Arts & Humanities:* Less than 5%. Preference to public radio and television stations. *Civic & Public Affairs:* (United Funds & United Way) Around 40% of budget. Supports United Ways and other federated campaigns in Chicago and other plant communities. Between 10% and 15%. Preference given to organizations that serve and involve minorities, the handicapped, and youth. *Education:* Between 20% and 25%. Contributes to institutions where company recruits employees or with which there are significant corporate relationships, such as joint research projects, board leadership by Zenith executives, and employee involvement or benefits. Generally does not support precollegiate educational institutions. *International:* Between 15% and 20%. Priority given to hospitals serving Zenith plant communities or significant numbers of employees and their families. **Typ. Recipients:** Hospitals, People with Disabilities. **Geo. Dist:** nationally; preference is given to organizations located near corporate operating locations.

★ 13044 ★ Zilkha Foundation, Inc.

767 5th Ave., Suite 4605
New York, NY 10153-0002
Phone: (212)758-7750 **Fax:** (212)758-7803
Ezra Zilkha, President & Treasurer

Fnded: 1948. **Priorities:** *Arts & Humanities:* 82%. Supports operas, libraries, museums, ballet, and historic preservation. *Civic & Public Affairs:* 6%. Funds public policy organizations, foundations, and the American Society of the French Legion of Honor.

Education: 4%. Gives to universities, music schools, and foreign language/cultural exchange institutions. *Environment:* 1%. Support goes to the disabled, youth organizations, and animal welfare. *International:* 1%. Supports hospitals, medical centers, and single-disease health associations. *Religion:* Less than 1%. Gives to biology research and a natural history museum. *Note:* Total contributions made in fiscal 2000. **Typ. Recipients:** AIDS/HIV, Alzheimers Disease, Cancer, Clinics/Medical Centers, Emergency/Ambulance Services, Eyes/Blindness, Geriatric Health, Hospitals, Hospitals (University Affiliated), Medical Education, Medical Research, People with Disabilities, Public Health, Research/Studies Institutes, Substance Abuse, Transplant Networks/Donor Banks. **Geo. Dist:** New York, NY.

Other Funding Organizations

★ 13045 ★ A-T Medical Research Foundation

c/o Pam Smith
5241 Round Meadow Rd.
Hidden Hills, CA 91302
Phone: (818)703-0151 **Fax:** (818)703-0176
Email: Becca4435@aol.com
Website: http://www.gspartners.com/at
George Smith, Chm.

Desc: Works to fund medical research to find a cure for Ataxia-Telangiectasia (A-T), a degenerative genetic disease of the nervous system. Sponsors pioneering research as well as advanced work. **Awards:** Grant to support research.

★ 13046 ★ Academy of Osseointegration (AO)

85 W Algonquin Rd., Ste. 550
Arlington Heights, IL 60005-4460
Phone: (847)439-1919 **Free:** 800-656-7736
Fax: (847)439-1569
Email: academy@osseo.org
Website: http://www.osseo.org
Kevin P. Smith, Exec. Dir.

Desc: Works for the advancement of osseointegration among dentists, physicians and related professionals. Conducts research and educational programs; disseminates information to the public and medical agencies; provides a forum for interdisciplinary discussions. **Awards:** Osseointegration Foundation Implant Research Grant (annual); Osseointegration Foundation Patient Care Grants.

★ 13047 ★ Academy of Pharmaceutical Research and Science (APRS)

American Pharmaceutical Association
2215 Constitution Ave. NW
Washington, DC 20037-2985
Phone: (202)628-4410 **Free:** 800-237-2742
Fax: (202)783-2351
Email: apha-aprs@mail.aphanet.org
Website: http://www.aphanet.org/about/aprs.html
Arthur H. Kibbe, Pres.

Desc: A part of American Pharmaceutical Association. Pharmaceutical scientists from industry and academia. Objective is to serve the profession of pharmacy by developing knowledge and integrating the process of science into the profession. Sponsors national meetings to provide a forum for presentation and discussion of original research, controversial topics, and continuing communication. Provides consultation and advice to: pharmacists on scientific matters as they relate to policy; congressional committees on bills of interest to pharmaceutical scientists; governmental agencies. **Awards:** Best Published Paper in the Economic, Social, and Administrative Sciences (annual); Ebert Prize (annual); Kilmer Prize (annual); Postgraduate Best Paper Awards (annual); Research Achievement Award (annual); Takeru Higuchi Research Prize (triennial).

★ 13048 ★ Academy of Surgical Research (ASR)

13355 10th Ave. N, Ste. 108
Minneapolis, MN 55441-5510
Phone: (763)765-2300 **Fax:** (763)765-2329
Email: director@surgicalresearch.org
Website: http://www.surgicalresearch.org
Patricia Nolt, Exec. Dir.

Desc: Individuals, organizations, and corporations with an interest in surgical research. Seeks to advance surgical techniques and equipment through improved research. Facilitates cooperation and exchange of information among members; fosters interdisciplinary transfer of ideas to advance surgical research. **Awards:** Barry Sauer Award (annual); C. William Hall Award (annual); Markowitz Award (annual) various; Von Recum Award (annual).

★ 13049 ★ Alexander Graham Bell Association for the Deaf and Hard of Hearing (AGBELL)

3417 Volta Pl. NW
Washington, DC 20007
Phone: (202)337-5220 **Fax:** (202)337-8314
Email: info@agbell.org
Website: http://www.agbell.org
K. Todd Houston, PhD, Exec. Dir.

Desc: An international membership organization and resource center on hearing loss and spoken language approaches and related issues. Founded in 1890 by Alexander Graham Bell, the association offers members a wide range of programs and services and provides to all inquirers information on a vast array of issues pertaining to hearing loss. Members include parents of children with hearing loss, educators, adults with hearing loss, and hearing health professionals. Publishes books and provides financial aid to qualifying applicants for mainstreamed, auditory-based education at pre-school, school-age and university levels. Provides governmental and education advocacy services through its national office and state chapters, children's rights coordinators and international affiliates. **Awards:** Recognition; scholarship (annual) for oral deaf students.

★ 13050 ★ Alpha Omega International Dental Fraternity

500 Commonwealth Dr.
Warrendale, PA 15086
Phone: (724)778-3419 **Free:** 800-677-8468
Fax: (724)772-8349
Email: headquarters@ao.org
Website: http://www.ao.org/
Susan Branscum, Ch. Staff Off.

Desc: Professional fraternity - dentistry. Encourages fraternalism and monitors discrimination in dental schools. Maintains the Alpha Omega Foundation, which sends funds to dental schools in Israel and the U.S. Holds continuing education seminars. **Awards:** Grant for post-graduate dental students; recognition (annual) for students with superior scholastic standing.

★ 13051 ★ Alpha Tau Delta (ATD)

150 Cruickshank Dr.
Folsom, CA 95630
Phone: (916)984-9150
Email: kerrik@atdnursing.org
Website: http://www.atdnursing.org
Kerri L. Kaye, Pres.

Desc: Professional fraternity - nursing. Seeks to further educational standards for the nursing profession. Maintains scholarship program for members only. **Awards:** Miriam Furlong Grant (annual) for member students; National Advisor of the Year (annual); National Member of Year (annual); PRN Grant (annual) for alummi members.

★ 13052 ★ Alzheimer's Association (ADRDA)

919 N Michigan Ave., Ste. 1100
Chicago, IL 60611-1676
Phone: (312)335-8700 **Free:** 800-272-3900
Fax: (312)335-1110
Email: info@alz.org
Website: http://www.alz.org
Patricia Pinkowski, Dir. Library

Desc: Alzheimer's disease is a progressive, degenerative brain disease in which changes occur in the central nervous system and regions of the brain causing memory loss and other changes in thought, personality, and behavior. Promotes research to find the cause, treatment, and cure for the disease; provides educational programs for the public, media, and health care and medical professionals; represents the continuing care needs of the affected population before government and social service agencies. Seeks to destroy the myth that what were once called "senile behaviors" are a natural part of aging. Works to develop family support systems for relatives of persons with the disease. Sponsors educational forums; operates speakers' bureau. Compiles statistics. Library available. **Awards:** Grant (annual) for research.

★ 13053 ★ Ambucs Resource Center

3315 North Main St.
High Point, NC 27265
Phone: (336)869-2166 **Fax:** (336)887-8451
Email: ambucs@ambucs.com
Website: http://www.ambucs.com

Desc: Dedicated to creating independence and opportunities for people with disabilities. Conducts service projects designed to give children with disabilities their first set of wheels. **Awards:** AMBUCS Scholars (annual) for PT, OT, Speech or Audiology students in junior year or higher.

★ 13054 ★ America Society of Plastic Surgeons (ASPS)

444 E Algonquin Rd.
Arlington Heights, IL 60005
Phone: (847)228-9900 **Free:** 888-4-PLASTIC
Fax: (847)228-9131
Website: http://www.plasticsurgery.org
James Wells, MD, Pres.

Desc: Plastic surgeons. Dedicated to quality patient care and to maintain professional and ethical standards through education, research, and advocacy of socioeconomic and other professional activities. **Awards:** Circle of Excellence Media Awards (annual) offered to newspapers, magazines, radio, television, news services, and news web sites.

★ 13055 ★ American Academy of Addiction Psychiatry (AAAP)

7301 Mission Rd., Ste. 252
Prairie Village, KS 66208
Phone: (913)262-6161 **Fax:** (913)262-4311
Email: info@aaap.org
Website: http://www.aaap.org
Becky Stein, Exec. Dir.

Desc: Psychiatrists and other health care and mental health professionals treating people with addictive behaviors. Promotes accessibility to highest quality treatment for all who need it; promotes excellence in clinical practice in addiction psychiatry; educates the public to influence public policy regarding addictive illness; provides continuing education for addiction professionals; disseminates new information in the field of addiction psychiatry; and encourages research on the etiology, prevention, identification, and treatment of the addictions. **Awards:** Founders Award (annual); Medical Student Scholarships (annual); monetary (annual); Resident Scholarships (annual).

★ 13056 ★ American Academy of Allergy, Asthma and Immunology (AAAAI)

611 E Wells St.
Milwaukee, WI 53202
Phone: (414)272-6071 **Fax:** (414)272-6070
Email: membership@aaaai.org

Website: http://www.aaaai.org
Audrey Mudek, Membership Service Mgr.

Desc: Professional society of physicians specializing in allergy and allergic diseases. Sponsors annual two-day postgraduate course and three-day scientific session. Conducts research and educational programs. Maintains speakers' bureau; operates placement service; compiles statistics. **Awards:** Grant (annual); recognition for research.

★ 13057 ★ American Academy of Esthetic Dentistry (AAED)

401 N Michigan Ave.
Chicago, IL 60611
Phone: (312)321-5121 **Fax:** (312)673-6952
Email: aaed@sba.com
Website: http://www.estheticacademy.org/
Ronald I. Maitland, DMD, Pres.

Desc: Dentists seeking to advance the art and science of esthetic dentistry (dentistry concerned with restorative procedures of natural teeth). **Awards:** AAED Research Grant (annual).

★ 13058 ★ American Academy of Facial Plastic and Reconstructive Surgery (AAFPRS)

310 S Henry St.
Alexandria, VA 22314
Phone: (703)299-9291 **Free:** 800-332-FACE
Fax: (703)299-8898
Email: info@aafprs.org
Website: http://www.facemd.org
Stephen C. Duffy, Exec. VP

Desc: Physicians specializing in facial plastic surgery. Promotes research and study in the field. Maintains speakers' bureau. Conducts educational and charitable programs; compiles statistics. **Awards:** Ben Shuster Memorial (annual) for the most outstanding research paper by a resident or fellow in trainig on any clinical work or research in facial plastc and reconstructive surgery delivered at a national meeting (or its equivalent) between March 1 and February 28; Bernstein Award (annual) for an AAFPRS Fellow member who is conducting original research which will advance facial plastic and reconstructive surgery; Community Service (annual) for any member who has distinguished himself/herself by providing and/or making possible free medical service to the poor in his/her community; F. Mark Rafaty Memorial (annual) for any member who has made outstanding contributions to facial plastic and reconstructive surgery; Investigator Development Award (annual) for AAFPRS member who is conducting significant clinical or labo ratory research and for the training of resident surgeons in research; Ira Tresley Research Award (annual) for the best original research in facial plastic surgery by an AAFPRS member who has been board certified for at least three years; John Dickinson Teacher (annual) for a Fellow member for sharing knowledge about facial plastic surgery with the effective use of audiovisuals over a number of years; John Orlando Roe (annual) for the graduate fellow who submits the best scholarly paper written during fellowship; Resident Research Award (annual) for residents who are AAFPRS members; Sir Harold Delf Gillies (annual) for the graduate fellow who submits the best research paper written during fellowship; William Wright (annual) for a member who has made outstanding contributions to facial plastic and reconstructive surgery.

★ 13059 ★ American Academy of Fixed Prosthodontics (AAFP)

PO Box 1409
Bodega Bay, CA 94923-1409
Phone: (707)875-3040 **Free:** 800-785-9188
Fax: (707)875-2927
Email: secaafp@monitor.net
Website: http://www.prosthodontics.org/aafp
Dr. Robert S. Staffanou, Sec.

Desc: Dentists. Provides 2-day professional continuing education course in the specialty of fixed prosthodontics. **Awards:** Stanley D. Tylman (annual) bestowed upon six graduate students for outstanding research in fixed prosthodontics.

★ 13060 ★ American Academy of the History of Dentistry (AAHD)

c/o Aletha A. Kowitz
100 S Vail Ave.
Arlington Heights, IL 60005-1866
Phone: (847)670-7561
Aletha A. Kowitz, Sec. -Treas.

Desc: Seeks to stimulate interest, study, and research in the history of dentistry and promote the teaching of dental history. **Awards:** Bremner Award (annual) for dental students only.

★ 13061 ★ American Academy of Neurology (AAN)

1080 Montreal Ave.
Saint Paul, MN 55116-2325
Phone: (651)695-2717 **Free:** 800-879-1960
Fax: (651)695-2791
Email: memberservices@aan.com
Website: http://www.aan.com
Catherine M. Rydell, Exec. Dir.

Desc: Professional society of medical doctors specializing in brain and nervous system diseases. Maintains placement service. Sponsors research and educational programs. Compiles statistics. Publishes scientific journal. **Awards:** Bruce S. Schoenberg International Award and Lecture in Neuroepidemiology (annual) for a young investigator from a developing country; Founder's Award (annual) for a junior member who is the senior author of a research-based manuscript; John Jay Dystel Prize (annual) for multiple sclerosis research; Lawrence C. McHenry Award (annual) for excellence in research in the history of neurology; Medical Student Essay Awards (annual); Potamkin Prize (annual) for research in Pick's, Alzheimer's, and related diseases; S. Weir Mitchell Award (annual) for research by a junior member.

★ 13062 ★ American Academy of Oral and Maxillofacial Radiology (AAOMR)

PO Box 55722
Jackson, MS 39296
Phone: (601)984-6060 **Fax:** (601)984-6086
Email: mocarroll@sod.umsmed.edu
Website: http//www.aaomr.org
Dr. M. Kevin O Carroll, Exec. Dir.

Desc: Dentists and other professionals who specialize in oral and maxillofacial rediology in clinical practice, teaching or research. Serves as authoritative body on radiation hygiene and hazards for the American Dental Association. **Awards:** Albert G. Richards Graduate Student Research Grant (annual) applied research in radiology; Charles R. Morris Student Research Award (annual); Howard R. Raper Oral and Maxillofacial Radiology Award (annual) academic achievement in graduate studies and potential for a career in academia.; Radiology Centennial Scholarship (annual) performance during first year of graduate study; Student Award for senior dental students for achievement in oral and maxillofacial radiology; William H. Rollins Award (annual) basic research in radiology.

★ 13063 ★ American Academy of Orthopaedic Surgeons (AAOS)

6300 N River Rd.
Rosemont, IL 60018-4262
Phone: (847)823-7186 **Free:** 800-346-AAOS
Fax: (847)823-8125
Email: custserv@aaos.org
Website: http://www.aaos.org
Dr. William Tipton, Exec. VP

Desc: Professional society of orthopedic surgeons certified by the American Board of Orthopedic Surgery to practice orthopedic (bone and joint) surgery. Promotes physician education and skills enhancement by offering textbooks, clinical videotapes, courses and self-assessment exams. **Awards:** Humanitarian Award (annual); International Award (annual); Kappa Delta (annual); National Award (annual).

★ 13064 ★ American Academy of Otolaryngology - Head and Neck Surgery (AAO-HNS)

1 Prince St.
Alexandria, VA 22314-3357
Phone: (703)836-4444 **Fax:** (703)683-5100
Email: webmaster@entnet.org
Website: http://www.entnet.org
David R. Nielsen, MD, Exec. VP

Desc: Professional society of medical doctors specializing in otolaryngology (diseases of the ear, nose, and throat) and head and neck surgery. Represents otolaryngology in governmental and socioeconomic areas and provides high-quality medical education for otolaryngologists. Coordinates Combined Otolaryngological Spring Meetings for ten national otolaryngological societies. Operates job information exchange service and museum. **Awards:** Grant for research; Honor Award (annual); Humanitarian Efforts Award (annual); Presidential Award (annual).

★ 13065 ★ American Academy of Physician Assistants (AAPA)

950 N Washington St.
Alexandria, VA 22314-1552
Phone: (703)836-2272 **Fax:** (703)684-1924
Email: aapa@aapa.org
Website: http://www.aapa.org
Timi Agar-Barwick, Exec. Dir.

Desc: Physician assistants and other interested parties. Seeks to promote quality, cost-effective, and accessible healthcare, and the professional and personal development of PAs. Provide services for members. Organizes annual National PA Day. Develops research and education programs; compiles statistics. **Awards:** Scholarship.

★ 13066 ★ American Academy on Physician and Patient

6728 Old McLean Village Dr.
Mc Lean, VA 22101
Phone: (703)556-9222 **Fax:** (703)556-8729
Email: aappatient@degnon.org
Website: http://www.physicianpatient.org

Desc: Research and education professionals. Dedicated to research, education and improving professional standards in doctor-patient communication. Sponsors scholarships and grants. **Awards:** Grant; scholarship.

★ 13067 ★ American Academy of Professional Coders (AAPC)

309 West 700 South
Salt Lake City, UT 84101-2608
Free: 800-626-2633 **Fax:** (801)236-2258
Email: info@aapc.com
Website: http://www.aapc.org
Lan C. England, Exec. Dir.

Desc: Certified professional coders. Promotes high standards of physician and outpatient facility coding through education and cerification. **Awards:** Coder of the Year (annual) for excellence in medical coding; Networker of the Year (annual) for connecting coders together for discussion leading to correct solutions of reimbursement problems.

★ 13068 ★ American Action Fund for Blind Children and Adults (AAFBCA)

1800 Johnson St., Ste. 100
Baltimore, MD 21230
Phone: (410)659-9315 **Fax:** (410)685-5653
Email: acc@roudley.com
Website: http://www.actionfund.org

Desc: Works to assist blind persons in securing reading material, to educate the public about blindness, to give aid to the deaf-blind and to improve the quality of life for blind persons. Provides information and referral services on Social Security Disability Insurance, employment, civil rights, products and aids, education of blind children and public rehabilitation agencies; disseminates information on Braille and sign language; distributes publications free of charge to libraries and schools. **Awards:** Kenneth Jernigan Scholarship (annual).

★ 13069 ★ American Art Therapy Association (AATA)
1202 Allanson Rd.
Mundelein, IL 60060-3808
Phone: (847)949-6064 **Free:** 888-290-0878
Fax: (847)566-4580
Email: info@arttherapy.org
Website: http://www.arttherapy.org
Shaun McNiff, Pres.

Desc: Art therapists, students, and individuals in related fields. Supports the progressive development of therapeutic uses of art, the advancement of research, and improvements in the standards of practice. Has established specific professional criteria for training art therapists. Facilitates the exchange of information and experience. Compiles statistics. **Awards:** Cay Drachnik Minorities Fund (annual) bestowed to members of a minority group who are enrolled in an AATA approved program and who can demonstrate financial need; Distinguished Service Awards (annual); Gladys Agell Award for Excellence in Research (annual) bestowed to the most outstanding project, completed within the past year, by an art therapist using a statistical measure in the area of applied art therapy; Myra Levick Scholarship Fund (annual) bestowed to students who demonstrate financial need, acceptance into an AATA approved graduate art therapy program, and an undergraduate GPA of at least 3.0; Rawley Silver Scholarship Fund (annual) bestowed to persons whose academic record or prior experience is deemed excellent and who are enrolled in an AATA approved art therapy program.

★ 13070 ★ American Association for Cancer Research (AACR)
615 Chestnut St., 17th Fl.
Philadelphia, PA 19106
Phone: (215)440-9300 **Fax:** (215)440-9313
Email: membership@aacr.org
Website: http://www.aacr.org
Margaret Foti, PhD, CEO

Desc: Works to facilitate communication and dissemination of information among scientists and others dedicated to cancer research; seeks to advance understanding of cancer etiology, prevention, diagnosis and treatment throughout the world. Fosters research on cancer, public and science education and training. **Awards:** American Cancer Society Award (annual); Bruce F. Cain Memorial Award (annual); G.H.A. Clowes Memorial Award (annual); Gertrude Elion Cancer Research Award (annual); Joseph H. Burchenal Clinical Research Award (annual); Landon-AACR Prize in Basic Cancer Research (annual) for medical or graduate students; Landon-AACR Prize in Translational Cancer Research (annual); Pezcoller Foundation-AACR International Award for Cancer Research (annual); Travel Award-Scientific Meetings (annual) for medical or graduate students.

★ 13071 ★ American Association for Chronic Fatigue Syndrome (AACFS)
34693 Bookhammer Landing Rd.
Lewes, DE 19958
Phone: (302)947-9634
Email: info@aacfs.org
Website: http://www.aacfs.org
Dharam V. Ablashi, DVM, Pres.

Desc: Research scientists, physicians and other health care professionals, and institutions with and interest in chronic fatigue syndrome (CFS). Seeks to advance the diagnosis and treatment of CFS. Facilitates exchange of information among members; sponsors research; serves as a clearinghouse on CFS diagnosis and patient care. Maintains speakers' bureau. **Awards:** Junior Investigator Award (biennial); Rudy Perpich Award (biennial).

★ 13072 ★ American Association of Colleges of Osteopathic Medicine (AACOM)
5550 Friendship Blvd., Ste. 310
Chevy Chase, MD 20815-7231
Phone: (301)968-4100 **Fax:** (301)968-1554
Email: ckearns@aacom.org
Website: http://www.aacom.org
Douglas L. Wood, PhD,DO, Pres.

Desc: Osteopathic medical colleges. Operates centralized application service; monitors and works with Congress and other government agencies in the planning of health care programs. Gathers statistics on osteopathic medical students, on innovations in medical education, faculty, administers federal contract, develops national communication programs on behalf of member colleges. **Awards:** Sherry R. Arnstein Minority Student Scholarship (annual) qualifying current or incoming minority student at a U.S. collegeof osteopathic medicine.

★ 13073 ★ American Association for Dental Research (AADR)
1619 Duke St.
Alexandria, VA 22314-3406
Phone: (703)548-0066 **Fax:** (703)548-1883
Email: research@iadr.org
Website: http://www.iadr.com/IADR_AADR/About/AADR/default.htm
Robert Collins, DDS, Interim Exec. Dir.

Desc: A division of the International Association for Dental Research. Dentists, researchers, dental schools, and dental products manufacturing companies. Seeks to promote better dental health and research activities. Presents current research information at annual meeting. Sponsors competitions; sponsors seminars. **Awards:** Distinguished Scientist Award (triennial) Outstanding scientific achievement; Research Fellowship (annual).

★ 13074 ★ American Association of Equine Practitioners (AAEP)
4075 Iron Works Parkway
Lexington, KY 40511
Phone: (859)233-0147 **Free:** 800-443-0177
Fax: (859)233-1968
Email: aaepoffice@aaep.org
Website: http://www.aaep.org
David L. Foley, Exec. Dir.

Desc: Veterinarians who specialize in equine medicine and surgery. Disseminates the latest scientific information relative to the practice of equine medicine; promotes research on horses. Maintains 10 professional committees. **Awards:** AAEP/American Live Stock Insurance Co. (annual); AAEP Research Program (annual); AAEP/United States Pony Club (annual).

★ 13075 ★ American Association of Feline Practitioners (AAFP)
200 4th Ave. N, No. 900
Nashville, TN 37219
Phone: (615)257-7788 **Free:** 800-204-3514
Fax: (615)254-7047
Email: aafp@walkermgmt.com
Website: http://www.aafponline.org
Dr. Joanna Guglielmino, Pres.

Desc: Doctors of veterinary medicine who specialize or have a general interest in the field of feline medicine and surgery. Works to promote the interests and improve the public stature of feline practice and to increase the knowledge of veterinarians in the field. Cooperates with other veterinary and cat fancier organizations. **Awards:** Grant for feline research; recognition for student achievement.

★ 13076 ★ American Association of Gynecological Laparoscopists (AAGL)
13021 E Florence Ave.
Santa Fe Springs, CA 90670-4505
Phone: (562)946-8774 **Free:** 800-554-2245
Fax: (562)946-0073
Email: generalmail@aagl.com
Website: http://www.aagl.com
Linda Michels, Exec. Dir.

Desc: Physicians who specialize in obstetrics and gynecology and who are interested in gynecological endoscopic procedures. Purposes are to: teach; demonstrate; exchange ideas; distribute literature; stimulate interest in gynecological laparoscopy; maintain and improve medical standards in medical schools and hospitals regarding gynecological laparoscopy; maintain and improve the ethics, practice, and efficiency of the medical practice pertaining to obstetrics and laparoscopy. Conducts seminars and workshops. **Awards:** Circon ACMI Golden Hysteroscope Award (annual) presented to best submitted paper on hysteroscopy by a physician; Olympus Golden Laparoscope Award (annual) presented to best submitted surgical video/film on gynecologic endoscopy by a physician.; Postgraduate Prize Paper (annual) presented to best submitted paper on gynecologic endoscopy by a resident or fellow physician. Must have proof of training status.

★ 13077 ★ American Association for Hand Surgery (AAHS)
20 N Michigan Ave., Ste. 700
Chicago, IL 60602
Phone: (312)236-3307 **Fax:** (312)782-0553
Email: contact@handsurgery.org
Website: http://www.handsurgery.org
Laura Downes Leeper, CAE, Asst. VP

Desc: Plastic, orthopedic, general surgeons, and physical and occupational therapists having a specific interest in hand surgery; individuals in the medical profession, basic sciences, or allied services interested in the improvement of hand surgery. Purpose is to advance hand surgery. Conducts symposia; offers specialized education. **Awards:** Research Grants (annual) based on proposal submission.

★ 13078 ★ American Association of Hip and Knee Surgeons (AAHKS)
704 Florence Dr.
Park Ridge, IL 60068-2104
Phone: (847)698-1200 **Fax:** (847)825-9294
Email: helpdesk@aahks.org
Website: http://www.aahks.org
Priscilla Majewski, Exec. Dir.

Desc: Provides current educational, research and communication opportunities to promote quality management of arthritic disorders of the hip and knee. **Awards:** Research Grant (annual).

★ 13079 ★ American Association for Marriage and Family Therapy (AAMFT)
112 S Alfred St.
Alexandria, VA 22314
Phone: (703)838-9808 **Fax:** (703)838-9805
Email: exec@aamft.org
Website: http://www.aamft.org
Mary Hotvedt, PhD, Pres.

Desc: Professional society of marriage and family therapists. Assumes a major role in developing & maintaining the highest standards of excellence in this field. Has 76 accredited training programs throughout the U.S. Sponsors educational and research programs. **Awards:** Cumulative Contribution to Family Therapy Research Award (annual); Distinguished Leadership Award (annual); Distinguished Professional Contribution to Family Therapy Award (annual); Divisional Contribution Award (annual); Ethnic Minority Fellowships Awards; Ethnic Minority Honorable Mention Awards; Graduate Student Research Grant Award (annual); Organizational Contribution Award (annual); Outstanding Scholarly Publication in Family Therapy Research Award (annual); Significant Contribution to the Field of Marriage and Family Therapy Award (annual).

★ 13080 ★ American Association of Medical Assistants (AAMA)

20 N Wacker Dr., Ste. 1575
Chicago, IL 60606-2963
Phone: (312)899-1500 **Free:** 800-228-2262
Fax: (312)899-1259
Website: http://www.aama-ntl.org
Donald A. Balasa, Exec. Dir.

Desc: Medical assistants are allied health professionals who work primarily in anbilatory (out patient) settings and perform clinical and administrative procedures. Activities include a certification program consisting of study and an examination, passage of which entitles the individual to become credentialed as a Certified Medical Assistant. Conducts accreditation of one- and two-year programs in medical assisting in conjunction with the commission on Accreditation of Allied Health Education Programs. Provides assistance and information to institutions of higher learning desirous of initiating courses for medical assistants. Awards continuing education units for selected educational programs. **Awards:** Maxine Williams Scholarship.

★ 13081 ★ American Association of Oral and Maxillofacial Surgeons (AAOMS)

9700 W Bryn Mawr Ave.
Rosemont, IL 60018-5701
Phone: (847)678-6200 **Free:** 800-822-6637
Fax: (847)678-6286
Email: inquiries@aaoms.org
Website: http://www.aaoms.org
Dr. Robert Rinaldi, Asst. Exec. Dir.

Desc: Dentists specializing in disease diagnosis and surgical, adjunctive, and esthetic treatment of diseases, injuries, and defects of the oral and maxillofacial region (jaw deformities, dental implants, infections, and oral cancer). **Awards:** Committeeman of the Year (annual); Distinguished Service Award; fellowship (annual) bestows $25,000 for research; fellowship bestows $30,000 for clinical surgery; Foundation Fellowship bestows $23,000 for one year; grant (annual) bestows two research grants of $35,000; monetary (annual) bestows up to five research awards of $1,000 each; recognition (annual) for research.

★ 13082 ★ American Association of People with Disabilities (AAPD)

1819 H St. NW, Ste. 330
Washington, DC 20006
Phone: (202)457-0046 **Free:** 800-840-8844
Fax: (202)457-0473
Email: aapd@aol.com
Website: http://www.aapd-dc.org
Helena Berger, COO

Desc: Promotes economic and political empowerment of persons with disabilities; educating businesses and general public about disability issues. **Awards:** Paul G Heane/AAPD Leadership Awards (annual) for leadership achievements that show a positive impact on the community of people with disabilities or within their area of disability interest.

★ 13083 ★ American Association of Small Ruminant Practitioners (AASRP)

1910 Lyda Ave., No. 200
Bowling Green, KY 42104
Phone: (270)793-0781 **Fax:** (270)782-0188
Email: aasrp@assrp.org
Website: http://www.aasrp.org
Richard W. Stobaeus, Jr., Pres.

Desc: Practicing veterinarians and veterinary students; associate members are producers, feeders, hobbyists, and others interested in sheep, goats, llamas, deer, and exotic small ruminants. Aims are to: elevate standards of practice in the field; further research programs that will assist in solving small ruminant health problems; foster communication between veterinarians, owners, and researchers in order to improve small ruminant health management programs. Sponsors specialized education programs. Conducts educational programs. Maintains speakers' bureau. **Awards:** George McConnell Award (biennial) professional service; Sam Guss Memorial Awards for student research and extern purposes.

★ 13084 ★ American Association for Women Podiatrists (AAWP)

c/o Dr. Marlene Reid, DPM, Pres.
6601 S Cass Ave.
Westmont, IL 60559
Phone: (630)852-8640 **Fax:** (630)852-8612
Email: rwoodfoot@aol.com
Website: http://www.aawpinc.com
Dr. Marlene Reid, DPM, Pres.

Desc: Promotes the advancement of the educational, political, financial and social well-being of members. Provides networking opportunities, consulting and financial assistance to student members. Maintains speakers' bureau **Awards:** Founders Scholarship (annual) Female student member of AAWP.

★ 13085 ★ American Auditory Society (AAS)

352 Sundial Ridge Cir.
Dammeron Valley, UT 84783-5196
Phone: (435)574-0062 **Fax:** (435)574-0063
Email: amaudsoc@aol.com
Website: http://www.amauditorysoc.org
Wayne J. Staab, PhD, Sec. -Treas.

Desc: Audiologists, otolaryngologists, scientists, hearing aid industry professionals, and educators of hearing impaired people; individuals involved in industries serving hearing impaired people, including the amplification systems industry. Works to increase knowledge and understanding of: the ear, hearing, and balance; disorders of the ear, hearing, and balance; prevention of these disorders; habilitation and rehabilitation of individuals with hearing and balance dysfunction. **Awards:** Carhart Memorial Lecturer (annual) for contribution to goals of the society; Lifetime Achievement Award (periodic) for contributions to the discipline of hearing.

★ 13086 ★ American Autoimmune Related Diseases Association (AARDA)

22100 Gratiot Ave.
East Detroit, MI 48021-2227
Phone: (586)776-3900 **Free:** 800-598-4668
Fax: (586)776-3903
Email: aarda@aarda.org
Website: http://www.aarda.org
Virginia Ladd, Exec. Dir.

Desc: Promotes national focus and collaborative efforts among state and national volunteer health groups on autoimmunity, the major cause of serious chronic diseases. Offers research and educational programs; maintains speakers' bureau. **Awards:** Grant for nonprofit organizations and foundations doing work on autoimmunity and basic autoimmunity research.

★ 13087 ★ American Board for Occupational Health Nurses (ABOHN)

201 E Ogden Ave., Ste. 114
Hinsdale, IL 60521-3652
Phone: (630)789-5799 **Free:** 888-842-2646
Fax: (630)789-8901
Email: info@abohn.org
Website: http://www.abohn.org
Mary Amann, RN,MSN, Exec. Dir.

Desc: Occupational health nurses. Establishes standards and confers initial and ongoing certification in occupational health nursing. Conducts semiannual certification examination. **Awards:** ABOHN Employer Award (annual) for firms that promote certification of occupational health nurses; ABOHN Research Award (annual) for research related to occupational health; Marguerite Ahern Graff Excellence Award (annual) for the Candidate Receiving the highest score on the COHN certification exam; Mayrose Snyder Excellence Award (annual) for the candidate receiving the highest score on the COHN-S certification exam.

★ 13088 ★ American Board of Veterinary Toxicology (ABVT)

School of Veterinary Medicine
382 W St. Rd.
Kennett Square, PA 19348
Phone: (610)444-5800 **Fax:** (610)925-8117
Email: roder@cox-internet.com
Website: http://www.abvt.org
Robert H. Poppenga, Pres.

Desc: Seeks to: further education and scientific progress in veterinary toxicology; encourage research and training; establish and maintain the highest possible standards of training and experience for qualification in toxicology; recognize qualified specialists through certification. Conducts annual examination. **Awards:** Lloyd Laboratories Pfizer Student Paper Award (annual) for best paper relating to veterinary toxicology.

★ 13089 ★ American Brain Tumor Association (ABTA)

2720 River Rd., Ste. 146
Des Plaines, IL 60018
Phone: (847)827-9910 **Free:** 800-886-2282
Fax: (847)827-9918
Email: info@abta.org
Website: http://www.abta.org
Naomi Berkowitz, Exec. Dir.

Desc: Seeks to eliminate brain tumors through research and meet the needs of brain tumor patients and their families. **Awards:** Research Awards for Post-Doctorates (annual) for post-doctoral candidates whose intent is to pursue a career in brain tumor research; Research Awards for Post-Doctorates (annual) for post-doctorates conducting brain tumor research.

★ 13090 ★ American Broncho-Esophagological Association (ABEA)

c/o Kim Davis, MD, Sec.
Division of Otolaryngology
University of Utah
50 N Medical Cr., 3C120SOM
Salt Lake City, UT 84132-0002
Phone: (801)587-7678 **Fax:** (801)585-5744
Email: peak.woo@mountsinai.org
Website: http://www.abea.net/
Peak Woo, Pres.

Desc: Professional society of otolaryngologists, chest specialists, thoracic surgeons, and gastroenterologists engaged in the practice of broncho-esophagology (diseases and injuries of the respiratory system and upper digestive tract). Conducts program on study of foreign bodies. **Awards:** Broyles-Maloney Award (annual) for outstanding manuscripts, a thesis, or accomplishments in endoscopy, bronchology, esophagology, laryngology, and related science; Resident Essay Award (annual) for the best original paper on research in clinical bronchoesophagology, physiology, or pathology of the larynx, tracheobronchial tree, or esophagus written by a resident or fellow in training; Seymour R. Cohen Award (annual) for the resident, fellow, or practicing physician who submits the best original paper in either basic research or clinical investigation in pediatric laryngology and bronchoesophagology.

★ 13091 ★ American Burn Association (ABA)

c/o National Headquarters Office
625 N Michigan Ave., Ste. 1530
Chicago, IL 60611
Phone: (312)642-9260 **Free:** 800-548-2876
Fax: (312)642-9130
Email: info@ameriburn.org
Website: http://www.ameriburn.org
Marion H. Jordan, MD, Pres.

Desc: Physicians, nurses, physical therapists, occupational therapists, dietitians, biomedical engineers, social service workers, and researchers interested in the care of burn injuries. Objective is the improvement of the care and treatment of burns, which includes a program of prevention of burn injuries. Sponsors visiting professorship, education, and awards. **Awards:** Burn Prevention Award for contributions having worldwide, nationwide, or statewide impact; contributions at a local level serving as a model prevention effort; collection and reporting of epidemiological data; or for individuals who have shaped the careers of others; Carl A. Moyer Resident Award for the best paper submitted by a medical doctor who has not yet completed his/her formal training; Curtis P. Artz Distinguished Service Award (annual) for a nonphysician member of the ABA for his/her outstanding contributions in the burn field; Education Exchange Program for OT's, PT's, RN's, and other non-physician individuals to visit another (or other) burn center; Everett Idris Evans Memorial Lecture Award for an outstanding scientist in the burn field outside the U.S.; Harvey Stuart Allen Distinguished Service Award for an outstanding U.S. scientist for his/her contributions in the burn field; International Association of Fire Fighters Burn Foundation Research Grant for burn-injury related research; Presidents Continuing Education Grant for an ABA member other than a physician who has made significant contributions to the care of burned patients; Robert A. Lindberg Award for the best scientific paper submitted by a non-physician; Traveling Fellowship Award (annual) for a physician or postdoctoral fellow who has given evidence of a continuing interest and productivity in the field of burn care, teaching, and/or research; Visiting Professor Program for a physician, educator, or specialist to visit a specified school, hospital, or community and present his/her expertise in the burn field.

★ 13092 ★ American Chiropractic Association (ACA)

1701 Clarendon Blvd.
Arlington, VA 22209
Phone: (703)276-8800 **Free:** 800-986-4636
Fax: (703)243-2593
Email: memberinfo@amerchiro.org
Website: http://www.amerchiro.org
Garrett F. Cuneo, HCD, Exec. VP

Desc: Enhances the philosophy, science, and art of chiropractic, and the professional welfare of individuals in the field. Promotes legislation defining chiropractic health care and improves the public's awareness and utilization of chiropractic. Conducts chiropractic survey and statistical study; maintains library. Sponsors Correct Posture Week in May and Spinal Health Month in October. Chiropractic colleges have student ACA groups. **Awards:** Scholarship (periodic) to students at chiropractic colleges.

★ 13093 ★ American College of Angiology (ACA)

295 Northern Blvd., Ste. 104
Great Neck, NY 11021-4701
Phone: (516)466-4055 **Fax:** (516)466-4099
Email: aca@collegeofangiology.org
Website: http://www.collegeofangiology.org
H. E. Shaftel, MD, Meeting Chm.

Desc: Scientists from 27 countries interested in the field of vascular medicine and surgery and dedicated to scientific advancement and continued education in angiology (the study of the circulatory, or vascular system). Seeks to: define, represent, and foster the growth and development of the specialty practice of angiology; improve patient care by advising physicians on recent developments in the field; provide a common forum for the exchange of ideas, technical research, and clinical experiences. Conducts continuing medical education programs. Disseminates original research findings related to cerebrovascular, cardiovascular, and peripheral vascular diseases, diagnostic methods, therapeutic procedures, clinical and laboratory research, and case reports. Holds clinical, diagnostic, and therapeutic symposia and seminars. **Awards:** Young Investigators Award (annual).

★ 13094 ★ American College of Cardiology (ACC)

9111 Old Georgetown Rd.
Bethesda, MD 20814-1699
Phone: (301)897-5400 **Free:** 800-253-4636
Fax: (301)897-9745
Email: exec@acc.org
Website: http://www.acc.org
Christine W. McEntee, CEO

Desc: Professional society of physicians, surgeons, and scientists specializing in cardiology (heart) and cardiovascular (circulatory) diseases. Operates Heart House Learning Center. Maintains numerous committees. **Awards:** ACC/Bristol-Myers Squibb Affiliate Travel Awards (annual) bestowed to 20 Affiliate-In-Training members of the American College of Cardiology to attend the American College of Cardiology annual scientific session; ACC/Merck Adult Cardiology Research Fellowship Awards bestowed to 6 cardiology trainees enrolled in adult cardiology fellowship training to support advanced research fellowship training in adult cardiology.

★ 13095 ★ American College of Chest Physicians (ACCP)

3300 Dundee Rd.
Northbrook, IL 60062
Phone: (847)498-1400 **Free:** 800-343-ACCP
Fax: (847)498-5460
Email: accp@chestnet.org
Website: http://www.chestnet.org
Alvin Lever, Exec. VP/CEO

Desc: Professional society of physicians and surgeons specializing in diseases of the chest (heart and lungs). Promotes undergraduate and postgraduate medical education and research in the field. Sponsors forums. Maintains placement service; conducts educational programs. **Awards:** Grant; recognition; scholarship.

★ 13096 ★ American College of Chiropractic Orthopedists (ACCO)

c/o Dr. Jesse Rothenberger
1030 Broadway, Ste. 101
El Centro, CA 92243
Phone: (760)370-9106
Website: http://www.accoweb.org
Dr. Jesse Rothenberger, Pres.

Desc: Certified (426) and noncertified (304) chiropractic orthopedists; students enrolled in a postgraduate chiropractic orthopedic program (100). Seeks to establish and maintain optimal educational and clinical standards within the field of chiropractic orthopedics. Sponsors educational programs. **Awards:** F. Maynard Lipe Scholarship (annual); recognition.

★ 13097 ★ American College of Foot and Ankle Surgeons (ACFAS)

515 Busse Hwy.
Park Ridge, IL 60068
Phone: (847)292-2237 **Free:** 800-421-2237
Fax: (847)292-2022
Email: mail@acfas.org
Website: http://www.acfas.org/
Thomas R. Schedler, CAE, Exec. Dir.

Desc: Objectives are to: promote and disseminate information on podiatric surgery among the public, podiatric surgeons, and other health professionals; encourage and publish research findings and related literature; provide intensive programs for clinical and experimental research to improve podiatric surgery and to promote our members' professional and socio-economic activities. **Awards:** Abstract Award (annual); Journal Article Award (annual); Research Award (annual).

★ 13098 ★ American College of Legal Medicine (ACLM)

1111 N Plaza Dr., Ste. 550
Schaumburg, IL 60173
Phone: (847)969-0283 **Free:** 800-433-9137
Fax: (847)517-7229
Email: info@aclm.org
Website: http://www.aclm.org
Miles Zaremski, Pres.

Desc: Persons who hold degrees in medicine, dentistry, law and nursing. Promotes and advances the field of legal medicine or medical jurisprudence; arranges for meetings with medical, legal, and professional groups and legislative, judicial, and enforcement bodies interested in any province where law and medicine are contiguous; fosters and encourages centers for study and research in the field of legal medicine and publishes materials pertaining to legal medicine. **Awards:** Hirsh Award (annual) bestowed to a dentistry, podiatry, nursing, pharmacy, health science or health care administration student for outstanding original paper on legal medicine; Letourneau Award (annual) bestowed to a law student for outstanding original paper on legal medicine; Schwartz Award (annual) bestowed to a medical student for outstanding original paper on legal medicine.

★ 13099 ★ American College of Medical Physics (ACMP)

11250 Roger Bacon Dr., Ste. 8
Reston, VA 20190-5202
Phone: (703)481-5001 **Fax:** (703)435-4390
Email: lrowland@drohanmgmt.com
Website: http://www.acmp.org
Laureen Rowland, Exec. Dir.

Desc: Covers socioeconomic aspects of practice, management issues, reimbursement, licensure, and practice standards. **Awards:** ACMP Graduate Scholarship Award (annual).

★ 13100 ★ American College of Medical Toxicology (ACMT)

PO Box 356
Hershey, PA 17033
Phone: (602)239-2353 **Free:** 888-633-5784
Fax: (425)645-6139
Email: hmiller@pamedsoc.org
Website: http://www.acmt.net
Michael J. Kosnett, Pres.

Desc: Seeks to advance the science, study and practice of medical toxicology by fostering the development of medical toxicology in its provision of emergency, consultation, forensic, legal, community and industrial services; and by otherwise striving to advance and elevate the science, study and practice of medical toxicology. **Awards:** ACMT Research Award (annual).

★ 13101 ★ American College of Osteopathic Emergency Physicians (ACOEP)

142 E Ontario St., Ste. 1250
Chicago, IL 60611
Phone: (312)587-3709 **Free:** 800-521-3709
Fax: (312)587-9951
Email: jwachtler@acoep.org
Website: http://www.acoep.org
Janice Wachtler, Exec. Dir.

Desc: Provides and evaluates postdoctoral and continuing education for osteopathic emergency physicians; encourages and implements the training of emergency physicians; promotes the coordination of community emergency care facilities and personnel. Sponsors Emergency Medicine CME Program for Accreditation. Conducts research and educational programs. Maintains speakers' bureau. **Awards:** Fellowship; Resident Research Award (annual).

★ 13102 ★ American College of Osteopathic Obstetricians and Gynecologists (ACOOG)

900 Auburn Rd.
Pontiac, MI 48342-3365
Phone: (248)332-6360 **Free:** 800-875-6360
Fax: (248)332-4607
Email: acoog@acoog.com
Website: http://www.acoog.com
Jaki K. Holzer, Admin.

Desc: Osteopathic physicians and surgeons specializing in obstetrics and gynecology. Conducts educational programs, and reviews osteopathic obstetric and gynecologic residency training programs. Holds annual postgraduate course and annual convention.

Awards: Annual ORTHO-ACOOG Resident Thesis Competition (annual) for research papers.

★ 13103 ★ American College of Osteopathic Pain Management and Sclerotherapy (ACOPMS)

303 S Ingram Ct.
Middletown, DE 19709
Phone: (302)376-8080 **Free:** 800-471-6114
Fax: (302)376-8081
Email: admin@acopms.com
Website: http://acopms.com
Linda J. Pavina, Exec. Sec.

Desc: Osteopathic medical therapists. Seeks to improve the practice of and disseminate knowledge about Sclerotherapy. Supports research and education. **Awards:** Scholarship (annual) for the osteopathic medical student submitting the best paper on Sclerotherapy.

★ 13104 ★ American College of Phlebology (ACP)

100 Webster St., Ste. 101
Oakland, CA 94607-3724
Phone: (510)834-6500 **Fax:** (510)832-7300
Email: acp@amsinc.org
Website: http://www.phlebology.org
Bruce A. Sanders, Exec. Dir.

Desc: Physicians and medical students with an interest in the evaluation and management of patients with varicose veins, thrombophlebitis, thrombosis, and venous leg ulcers. Seeks to advance the study, teaching, and practice of phlebology; promotes continuing professional development of members. Serves as a network facilitating cooperation and exchange of information among medical professionals with an interest in phlebology; conducts educational programs; functions as a clearinghouse on medical techniques and technologies applicable to the practice of phelbology. **Awards:** BSN-JOBST Research Grant (annual); Walter DeGroot Fellowship Award (annual).

★ 13105 ★ American College of Surgeons (ACS)

633 N Saint Clair St.
Chicago, IL 60611-3211
Phone: (312)202-5000 **Fax:** (312)202-5001
Email: postmaster@facs.org
Website: http://www.facs.org
Thomas R. Russell, MD, Exec. Dir.

Desc: Professional association of surgeons worldwide organized primarily to improve the quality of care for surgical patients by elevating the standards of surgical education and practice. Conducts nationwide programs to improve emergency medical services and hospital cancer programs. Sponsors continuing education and self-assessment courses for surgeons in practice. **Awards:** Australia/New Zealand Traveling Fellowship (periodic); Distinguished Service Award (annual); International Guest Scholarship (periodic) surgeons from overseas; Research Scholarship (periodic).

★ 13106 ★ American College of Veterinary Dermatology (ACVD)

c/o Alexis Borich, Exec. Sec.
5610 Kearny Mesa Rd., Ste. B
San Diego, CA 92111
Phone: (858)560-9393 **Fax:** (858)560-0206
Website: http://www.acvd.org
Dr. Donna W Angarano, Pres.

Desc: Specialists in veterinary dermatology who have satisfied examination requirements; individuals with national reputation and standing are charter diplomates. promotes veterinary dermatology enhances the competencey of professionals in the field. Seeks to develop guidelines for postdoctoral education and to establish experience prerequisites for certification in veterinary dermatology. Administers examinations and certifies veterinarians as veterinary dermatology specialists. Encourages research and other contributions in areas of pathogenesis, diagnosis, therapy, prevention, and control of diseases affecting the skin of animals. Authorizes training programs in the field. **Awards:** ACVD Award of Excellence (annual) for excellence in research, teaching, and service in the field of veterinary dermatology.

★ 13107 ★ American College of Veterinary Radiology (ACVR)

c/o Dr. M. Bernstein
PO Box 87
Glencoe, IL 60022
Phone: (847)251-5517 **Fax:** (847)446-8618
Email: tgnyland@usdavis.edu
Website: http://www.acvr.ucdavis.edu/
Dr. M. Bernstein, Exec. Dir.

Desc: Diplomate members (215) are veterinarians certified by the college in veterinary radiology; associate members (6) are individuals distinguished in radiological science but who are not certified veterinary radiologists. Educational association working to advance the art and science of radiology. Certifies candidates who have demonstrated proficiency in veterinary radiology. Encourages the development of teaching personnel and training facilities in veterinary radiology. Aids in the evaluation of residencies and fellowships in veterinary radiology under consideration by the Council on Education of the American Veterinary Medical Association. Advises veterinarians who desire certification in veterinary radiology. Conducts continuing education seminars in conjunction with other veterinary organizations. **Awards:** Research Grant (annual) publishes in Journal Veterinary Radiology and Ultrasound; Resident Authored Paper (annual) for best resident-authored paper.

★ 13108 ★ American Contact Dermatitis Society (ACDS)

233 E Erie, No. 700
Chicago, IL 60611
Phone: (312)988-7700 **Fax:** (312)988-7759
Email: info@contactderm.org
Website: http://www.contactderm.org/about.html

Desc: Promotes information about contact dermatitis and occupational skin disease. **Awards:** ACDS Mentoring Award to medical residents and fellows; Alexander A. Fisher Resident Award to resident or medical student; Clinical Research Fellows; Howard Maibach Travel Award to investigators outside U.S.

★ 13109 ★ American Council of the Blind (ACB)

1155 15th St. NW, Ste. 1004
Washington, DC 20005
Phone: (202)467-5081 **Free:** 800-424-8666
Fax: (202)467-5085
Email: info@acb.org
Website: http://www.acb.org
Charles Crawford, Exec. Dir.

Desc: Blind and visually impaired persons. Serves as a national information clear Security and supplemental security income programs, radio reading services, special library services, eye research, and low vision technology. Offers group insurance plans, professional assistance in public interest, class action litigation, and public education about blindness and the abilities of visually impaired people. **Awards:** Floyd Qualls Memorial Scholarships (annual) for blind postsecondary students; scholarship.

★ 13110 ★ American Diabetes Association (ADA)

1701 N Beauregard St.
Alexandria, VA 22311
Phone: (703)549-1500 **Free:** 800-DIABETES
Fax: (703)549-6995
Email: askada@diabetes.org
Website: http://www.diabetes.org
John H. Graham, IV, CEO

Desc: Physicians, laypersons, and health professionals interested in diabetes mellitus. Promotes research, information and advocacy to find a prevention and cure for diabetes and to improve the lives of all people with diabetes. Promotes public awareness of diabetes as a serious disease. Conducts educational programs and provides information to people with diabetes and the health professionals who care for them. Administers research grants. **Awards:** Career Development Award (semiannual) for promising new investigators who hold an assistant professor or justified equivalent academic position within his/her institution. The award supports salary and the research project; Clinical Research Grant (semiannual) for investigators whose studies directly involve humans and focus on human subjects in which the effect of a change in the individual's external or internal environment is evaluated; Lions SightFirst Retinopathy Research Award (annual) for clinical or applied research in diabetic retinopathy; Medical Student Diabetes Research Fellowships (annual) for medical students to conduct a 3-6 month diabetes research project. The applicant must have a qualified sponsor; Mentor-Based Postdoctoral Fellowships (annual) for established diabetes investigators to provide stipend support of postdoctoral fellows who will train with them in diabetes research; Research Award (semiannual) for investigators who are conducting studies in diabetes research.

★ 13111 ★ American Dietetic Association (ADA)

120 S Riverside Plz.
Chicago, IL 60606
Phone: (312)899-0040 **Free:** 800-877-1600
Fax: (312)899-1979
Email: membrshp@eatright.org
Website: http://www.eatright.org
Ronald Moen, CEO

Desc: Food and nutrition professionals. Promotes nutrition, health and well-being. **Awards:** Recognition; scholarship.

★ 13112 ★ American Federation for Aging Research (AFAR)

70 W 40th St.
New York, NY 10018
Phone: (212)703-9977 **Free:** 800-330-4660
Fax: (212)997-0330
Email: amfedaging@aol.com
Website: http://www.afar.org
Hadley C. Ford, Chair

Desc: Physicians, scientists, and other individuals involved or interested in research in aging and associated diseases. Purpose is to stimulate and fund research on aging. Facilitates communication among scientists in the field. Fosters public education regarding the need for support of related research. **Awards:** AFAR Research Grant (annual) to individuals conducting research; Irving Wright Distinghished Achievement Award (annual); Merck/AFAR Fellows in Gevatric Clinical Pharmacology (annual) to individual; Paul Beeson Physician Faculty Scholar in Aging Research.

★ 13113 ★ American Foundation for Aging Research (AFAR)

North Carolina State University
Biochemistry Department
128 Polk Hall
Raleigh, NC 27695-7622
Phone: (919)515-5679 **Fax:** (919)515-2047
Email: afar_office@ncsu.edu
Website: http://www4.ncsu.edu/unity/users/a/agris/afar/afar.htm
Dr. Paul F. Agris, Pres.

Desc: Supports basic research and educational opportunities for the study of age-related diseases and the biology of aging. Supports projects emphasizing modern biological, genetic, biochemical, and biophysical techniques and approaches to the problems of age-associated diseases and the understanding of aging. **Awards:** AFAR Fellowship (annual) for graduate students; Cecille Gould Memorial Fund for Cancer Research (annual); Glaxo Wellcome Fellowship (annual); MaWren Wilson Fulton Memorial Scholarship (annual) for undergraduates.

★ 13114 ★ American Foundation for the Blind (AFB)

11 Penn Plz., Ste. 300
New York, NY 10001
Phone: (212)502-7600 **Free:** 800-232-5463
Fax: (212)502-7777
Email: afbinfo@afb.net
Website: http://www.afb.org
Carl R. Augusto, Pres.

Desc: Mission is to eliminate the inequities faced by the ten million Americans who are blind or visually impaired; Helen Keller dedicated 40 years of her life to the organization. Develops, collects, and disseminates information that benefits people who are blind or visually impaired, their families and friends, professionals in the blindness field, and the general public. Takes a leadership role in identifying issues critical to people who are blind or visually impaired; conducts research, and acts as a catalyst for change. Educates the public and policymakers as to the needs and capabilities of people who are blind or visually impaired; records and duplicates Talking Books for the Library of Congress and other audio materials for various corporations and organizations; and develops public education programs. Maintains offices in Atlanta, Chicago, Dallas and San Francisco, and a governmental relations office in Washington, DC. **Awards:** Delta Gamma Foundation Memorial Scholarship (annual) to undergraduate juniors, seniors, or graduate students who are legally blind, of good character, have exhibited academic excellence, and are studying in the field of rehabilitation and/or education of persons who are visually impaired or blind; Ferdinand Torres AFB Scholarship (annual) to a full-time post-secondary student who is legally blind and who presents evidence of economic need; Frederick A. Downes Scholarship to persons who are 22 years of age or younger, legally blind, and enrolled in a course of study leading to credentials in a profession or vocation; Gladys C. Anderson Memorial Scholarship to a woman who is legally blind, studying religious or classical music at the college level; Rudolph Dillman Memorial Scholarship (annual) to graduate and undergraduate students who are legally blind and studying in the field of rehabilitation and/or education of persons who are visually impaired or blind; Telesensory Scholarship to a full-time undergraduate student who is legally blind and does not meet criteria for other AFB scholarships.

★ 13115 ★ American Foundation for Suicide Prevention (AFSP)

120 Wall St., Fl. 22
New York, NY 10005
Phone: (212)363-3500 **Free:** 888-333-AFSP
Fax: (212)363-6237
Email: inquiry@afsp.org
Website: http://www.afsp.org
Robert Gebbia, Exec. Dir.

Desc: Medical professionals, community leaders, and suicide survivors. Provides funding for research on the causes and prevention of suicide. Trains professionals in the treatment of suicidal individuals; offers support programs for suicide survivors. **Awards:** AFSP Institutional Grants (annual) for research centers exploring innovative ideas in the prevention of suicide; Established Researcher Award (annual) for senior researchers in suicidology investigating new aspects of the field; Post-Doctoral Research Fellowship (annual) for full-time research by an investigator who has received a Ph.D. degree within the previous 5 years but has not had 3 years of fellowship support.

★ 13116 ★ American Foundation for Surgery of the Hand (AFSH)

6300 N River Rd., Ste. 600
Rosemont, IL 60018-4256
Phone: (847)384-8300 **Fax:** (847)384-1435
Email: info@hand-surg.org
Website: http://www.assh.org
Mark Anderson, Exec. Dir.

Desc: Awards grants to medical, educational, research, and public education programs related to the field of hand and upper extremity surgery. **Awards:** Grant bestowed to medical, educational, research, and public education programs related to the field of hand and upper extremity surgery.

★ 13117 ★ American Foundation for Vision Awareness (AFVA)

243 N Lindbergh Blvd.
Saint Louis, MO 63141
Free: 800-927-2382 **Fax:** (314)991-4101
Email: afva@aol.com

Desc: Seeks to educate people of all ages about their vision; to create awareness of quality eye and vision care; and to support vision-related scientific research. **Awards:** Grant for postgraduate study and research; recognition.

★ 13118 ★ American Gastroenterological Association (AGA)

7910 Woodmont Ave., 7th Fl.
Bethesda, MD 20814
Phone: (301)654-2055 **Fax:** (301)652-3890
Email: webinfo@gastro.org
Website: http://www.gastro.org
Robert Greenberg, Exec. VP

Desc: Physicians of internal medicine certified in gastroenterology; radiologists, pathologists, surgeons, and physiologists with special interest and competency in gastroenterology. Studies normal and abnormal conditions of the digestive organs and problems connected with their metabolism; conducts scientific research; offers placement services. **Awards:** Advanced Research Training Award (annual) for advanced fellow, usually in second full research year; Elsevier Research Initiative Award for junior faculty, senior faculty, or established investigator; Fiterman Clinical Research Award (annual) for senior faculty or established investigator; Funderberg Scholar Award for junior faculty, senior faculty, or established investigator; Industry Research Scholar Award (annual) for junior faculty; International Travel Award for junior faculty, senior faculty, or established investigator; Sponsored Symposia (biennial) for senior faculty or established investigator; Student Abstract Prize for high school, undergraduate, medical, and graduate students; Student Research Fellowship Award (annual) for high school undergraduate, medical, and graduate students.

★ 13119 ★ American Geriatrics Society (AGS)

350 5th Ave., Ste. 801
New York, NY 10118
Phone: (212)308-1414 **Free:** 800-247-4779
Fax: (212)832-8646
Email: info.amger@americangeriatrics.org
Website: http://www.americangeriatrics.org
Linda Hiddemen Barondess, Exec. VP

Desc: Professional society of physicians and other health care professionals interested in problems of the aged. Encourages and promotes the study of geriatrics; stresses the importance of medical research in the field of aging. Conducts seminars. **Awards:** Edward Henderson Student Award (annual); Milo D. Leavitt Student Award (annual); Nascher/Manning Award (biennial) for excellence in clinical geriatrics; New Investigator Award (annual); Student Travel Stipend (annual).

★ 13120 ★ American Guild for Infant Survival (AGIS)

301 Eastwood Cir., Ste. 200
Virginia Beach, VA 23454-4014
Phone: (757)463-3845
Email: afgisinc@ivilliage.com
Scott Hessek, Pres.

Desc: Works to reduce infant mortality, especially Sudden Infant Death Syndrome. Develops low-tech innovations to reduce infant mortality, such as the AFGIS test, which scores risk categories of infants and fetuses. Promotes the home monitoring program. Conducts educational and research programs. Compiles statistics. Maintains speakers' bureau. Offers children's services. **Awards:** Grant (annual) for research.

★ 13121 ★ American Head and Neck Society (AHNS)

601 N Caroline, Rm. 6221
Baltimore, MD 21287
Phone: (412)647-2227 **Fax:** (412)647-8944
Email: rwagner@pitt.edu
Website: http://www.headandneckcancer.org
Paul A. Levine, MD, Pres.

Desc: Otolaryngologists and other physicians with board certification whose primary interest is head and neck oncology. Associate membership is for other other practioners who treat head and neck cancer. Seeks to advance knowledge relevant to treatment of diseases of the head and neck, including reconstruction and rehabilitation. Promotes development of programs of training in head and neck oncology. **Awards:** Research Award (annual) competition for best head and neck cancer research; Resident Awards.

★ 13122 ★ American Health Care Association (AHCA)

1201 L St. NW
Washington, DC 20005
Phone: (202)842-4444 **Fax:** (202)842-3860
Website: http://www.ahca.org
Dr. Charles H. Roadman, II, CEO

Desc: Federation of state associations of long-term health care facilities. Promotes standards for professionals in long-term health care delivery and quality care for patients and residents in a safe environment. Focuses on issues of availability, quality, affordability, and fair payment. Operates as liaison with governmental agencies, Congress, and professional associations. Compiles statistics. **Awards:** James Durante Nurse Scholarship (annual) for nursing student working in a long term care facility.

★ 13123 ★ American Holistic Nurses Association (AHNA)

PO Box 2130
Flagstaff, AZ 86003-2130
Phone: (520)526-2196 **Free:** 800-278-2462
Fax: (520)526-2752
Email: communications@ahna.org
Website: http://www.ahna.org
Michael French, Communications Admin.

Desc: The AHNA is a 501(c) (3) non-profit educational organization whose membership is open to nurses and other individuals interested in holistically-oriented health care practices throughout the United States and the world. ASHNA supports the education of nurses, allied health practitioners, and the general public on health-related issues. The American Holistic Nurses' Association embraces nursing as a lifestyle and a profession and provides a means to create bonds within the nursing community. Because true healing comes from within, the AHNA recognizes that nurses must first heal themselves before they can facilitate the healing of others. **Awards:** Scholarship (annual).

★ 13124 ★ American Institute for Cancer Research (AICR)

1759 R St., NW
Washington, DC 20009
Phone: (202)328-7744 **Free:** 800-843-8114
Fax: (202)328-7226
Email: aicrweb@aicr.org
Website: http://www.aicr.org

Desc: Fosters research on diet, nutrition and cancer prevention and educates the public about the results. **Awards:** AICR Research Grants (semiannual).

★ 13125 ★ American Institute of the History of Pharmacy (AIHP)

777 Highland Ave.
Madison, WI 53705
Phone: (608)262-5378
Email: aihp@aihp.org

Website: http://www.aihp.org
Gregory J. Higby, Dir.

Desc: Pharmacists, firms, and organizations interested in historical and social aspects of the pharmaceutical field. Maintains pharmaceutical Americana collection; conducts research programs. **Awards:** Fischelis Grants; Graduate Study in the History of Pharmacy Grants.

★ 13126 ★ American Institute of Ultrasound in Medicine (AIUM)

14750 Sweitzer Ln., Ste. 100
Laurel, MD 20707-5906
Phone: (301)498-4100 **Free:** 800-638-5352
Fax: (301)498-4450
Email: admin@aium.org
Website: http://www.aium.org
Carmine M. Valente, PhDCAE, CEO

Desc: A multidisciplinary organization dedicated to advancing the art and science of ultrasound in medicine through its educational, scientific, literary and professional activities. Membership comprises professionals from many medical specialties, as well as basic scientists, engineers, manufacturers, nurses, physicists, radiologic technologists, sonographers and veterinarians involved with diagnostic medical ultrasound. **Awards:** Joseph Holmes Pioneer (annual); Memorial Hall of Fame (annual); Research Grants (annual); Sonographer (annual); William Fry (annual).

★ 13127 ★ American Lithotripsy Society (ALS)

305 Second Ave., Ste. 200
Waltham, MA 02451
Phone: (781)895-9098 **Fax:** (781)895-9088
Email: als@lithotripsy.org
Website: http://www.lithotripsy.org
Kenneth G. Scholl, Jr., Pres.

Desc: Promotes trade and public awareness of Lithotripsy. (Lithotripsy is a non-invasive procedure to treat kidney stones and gall stones.) Disseminates information; conducts educational programs, quality improvement and certification programs. **Awards:** Distinguished Guest Lecturer (annual).

★ 13128 ★ American Lyme Disease Foundation (ALDF)

Mill Pond Offices
293 Rte. 100
Somers, NY 10589
Phone: (914)277-6970 **Free:** 800-876-LYME
Fax: (914)277-6974
Email: inquire@aldf.com
Website: http://www.aldf.com
David L. Weld, Contact

Desc: Health care professionals and other individuals with an interest in Lyme Disease, a disorder transmitted to humans by the deer tick. Works to control the spread of Lyme Disease, and to improve treatments for the disorder. Maintains physician referral service; produces educational materials and conducts public and professional education programs; supports Lyme Disease research. **Awards:** Research Fund (annual) for prevention and control of tick-borne diseases.

★ 13129 ★ American Medical Student Association (AMSA)

1902 Association Dr.
Reston, VA 20191
Phone: (703)620-6600 **Free:** 800-767-2266
Fax: (703)620-5873
Email: amsa@www.amsa.org
Website: http://www.amsa.org
Eric Hodgson, Pres.

Desc: Medical students; local, state, and national organizations; premedical students, interns, and residents. Seeks to improve medical education by making it relevant to today's needs and by making the process by which physicians are trained more humanistic. Contributes to the improvement of health care of all people; involves its members in the social, moral, and ethical obligations of the profession of medicine. Serves as a mechanism through which students may actively participate in the fields of community health through various student health programs. Addresses political issues relating to the nation's health care delivery system and other medical and health issues. Maintains action committees and interest groups which publish newsletters, organize educational workshops, and initiate special projects. **Awards:** Paul R. Wright Excellence in Medical Education Award (annual).

★ 13130 ★ American Neurotology Society (ANS)

c/o Paul Lambert, MD, Chairman
Medical University of South Carolina
Box 250582
Charleston, SC 29425
Phone: (843)792-7161 **Fax:** (843)792-0546
Email: lambert@musc.edu
Website: http://itsa.ucsf.edu/~ajo/ANS/ANS.html
Newton J. Coker, MD, Pres.

Desc: Physicians and audiologists interested in the diagnosis and treatment of hearing and balance disorders. Promotes education and research in the field of neurotology. **Awards:** Monetary (annual).

★ 13131 ★ American Nouthetic Psychology Association (ANPA)

PO Box 801
Hardwick, GA 31034
Email: biblespy@alltel.net
Website: http://www.alltel.net/~biblepsy
Dr. David M. Carnrike, Pres.

Desc: Psychologists and other individuals with an interest in nouthetic psychology. Promotes high standards of training, ethics, and practice in the field. Conducts research and educational programs. **Awards:** Alice M. Camp Award (annual) for first year college psychology students.

★ 13132 ★ American Nurses Foundation (ANF)

600 Maryland Ave. SW, Ste. 100W
Washington, DC 20024-2571
Phone: (202)651-7227 **Fax:** (202)651-7354
Email: anf@ana.org
Website: http://www.nursingworld.org/anf
Leo Schargorodski, Dir.

Desc: Research, education, and charitable arm of the American Nurses' Association. Promotes nursing and consumers wherever nurses practice. Mission accomplished through four major functions: fundraising, Nursing Research Grants, grant development and management, and American Nurses Publishing. **Awards:** Distinguished Contribution to Nursing Science Award (semiannual); grant for nurse researchers.

★ 13133 ★ American Occupational Therapy Association (AOTA)

4720 Montgomery Ln.
PO Box 31220
Bethesda, MD 20824-1220
Phone: (301)652-2682 **Free:** 800-377-8555
Fax: (301)652-7711
Email: praota@aota.org
Website: http://www.aota.org
Joseph C. Isaacs, Exec. Dir.

Desc: Occupational therapists and occupational therapy assistants who provide services to people whose lives have been disrupted by physical injury or illness, developmental problems, the aging process, or social or psychological difficulties. Occupational therapy focuses on the active involvement of the patient in specially designed therapeutic tasks and activities to improve function, performance capacity, and the ability to cope with demands of daily living. **Awards:** Scholarship (annual) awardee must be accepted in an occupational therapy education program.

★ 13134 ★ American Occupational Therapy Foundation (AOTF)

4720 Montgomery Lane
PO Box 31220
Bethesda, MD 20824-1220
Phone: (301)652-6611 **Fax:** (301)656-3620
Email: aotf@aotf.org
Website: http://www.aotf.org
Martha Kirkland, Exec. Dir.

Desc: Encourages practice, research and scholarship in occupation and occupational therapy. Educates the public and professionals about occupation and occupational therapy. **Awards:** Scholarship (annual).

★ 13135 ★ American Optometric Foundation (AOF)

6110 Executive Blvd., Ste. 506
Rockville, MD 20852
Phone: (301)984-4734 **Free:** 800-368-6AOF
Fax: (301)984-4737
Email: christine@aapotom.org
Website: http://www.aaopt.org/aof/about/index.asp
Christine Armstrong, Dir.

Desc: Optometrists, optometric organizations, corporations, and the public. Promotes research, education, literature, and professional advancement in the visual sciences. Supports fellowships in graduate research. **Awards:** Vincent Salierno Memorial Scholarship (annual) to colleges and institutions; Vistaken Research Grants (annual) for optometric research in soft disposable contact lenses; William Ezell Fellowship (annual) for post-graduate research.

★ 13136 ★ American Organization of Nurse Executives (AONE)

325 Seventh St. NW
Washington, DC 20004
Phone: (202)626-2240 **Fax:** (202)638-5499
Email: aone@aha.org
Website: http://www.aone.org
Pamela Thompson, RN, Exec. Dir.

Desc: Provides leadership, professional development, advocacy, and research to advance nursing practice and patient care, promote nursing leadership and excellence, and shape healthcare public policy. Supports and enhances the management, leadership, educational, and professional development of nursing leaders. Offers placement service through Career Development and Referral Center. **Awards:** Research Award (annual); scholarship.

★ 13137 ★ American Orthopaedic Foot and Ankle Society (AOFAS)

2517 Eastlake Ave. E, Ste. 200
Seattle, WA 98102
Phone: (206)223-1120 **Free:** 800-235-4855
Fax: (206)223-1178
Email: aofas@aofas.org
Website: http://www.aofas.org
Richard Cantrall, Exec. Dir.

Desc: Members of American Academy of Orthopaedic Surgeons interested in research on, education in, and care of the foot and ankle. Sponsors continuing medical education courses. **Awards:** Goldner Award (annual); Kenneth Johnson MD Memorial Lectureship (annual); Roger Mann MD Award (annual).

★ 13138 ★ American Orthopaedic Society for Sports Medicine (AOSSM)

6300 N River Rd., Ste. 200
Rosemont, IL 60018
Phone: (847)292-4900 **Free:** 877-321-3500
Fax: (847)292-4905
Email: irv@aossm.org
Website: http://www.sportsmed.org
Irvin E. Bomberger, Exec. Dir.

Desc: Promotes sports medicine education, research, communication and fellowship; disseminates information to orthopaedic surgeons working in sports medicine. **Awards:** Excellence in Research (annual).

★ 13139 ★ American Osteopathic Association (AOA)
142 E Ontario St.
Chicago, IL 60611
Phone: (312)202-8000 **Free:** 800-621-1773
Fax: (312)202-8200
Email: info@aoa-net.org
Website: http://www.aoa-net.org
John B. Crosby, JD, Exec. Dir.

Desc: Osteopathic physicians, surgeons, and graduates of approved colleges of osteopathic medicine. Associate members include teaching, research, administrative, and executive employees of approved colleges, hospitals, divisional societies, and affiliated organizations. Forms (with its affiliates) an officially recognized structure of the osteopathic profession. Promotes the public health, to encourage scientific research, and to maintain and improve high standards of medical education in osteopathic colleges. Inspects and accredits colleges and hospitals; conducts a specialty certification program; sponsors a national examining board satisfactory to state licensing agencies; maintains mandatory program of continuing medical education for members. Compiles statistics on location and type of practice of osteopathic physicians. Sponsors research activities through Bureau of Research in osteopathic colleges and hospitals. Maintains Physician Placement Service. Produces public service radio and television programs; maintains 2000 item library and biographical archives on osteopathic medicine and history. Offers speakers' bureau. **Awards:** Grant; scholarship.

★ 13140 ★ American Osteopathic Foundation (AOF)
c/o Leda Hanin
142 East Ontario
Chicago, IL 60611
Phone: (312)202-8230 **Free:** 800-621-1773
Fax: (312)202-8216
Email: Sdowney@aoa-net.org
Website: http://www.osteopathic.org
Steve Downey, Deputy Dir.

Desc: Osteopathic physicians and laypersons interested in raising and administering funds for osteopathic medical education, research, colleges, and hospitals. Functions as philanthropic affiliate of the American Osteopathic Association; seeks to foster understanding of osteopathic principles and practice. **Awards:** Bristol-Myers Squibb Outstanding Resident Award (annual) for a 2nd or 3rd yr. osteopathic medical resident in Family Practice, Internal Medicine, or Pediatrics; Donna Jones Moritsugu Award (annual) for a spouse of a fourth-year osteopathic medical student; Russell C. McCaughan Education Fund Scholarship (annual) for a rising second-year student at each of the osteopathic colleges; Zeneca Pharmaceuticals Underserved Healthcare Grant (annual) for one or two student in the colleges of osteopathic medicine, demonstrating commitment to practice in underserved or minority populations.

★ 13141 ★ American Pediatric Surgical Nurses Association (APSNA)
PO Box 200585
Boston, MA 02120
Phone: (203)457-1275
Email: info@apsna.com
Website: http://www.apsna.com/
Laura Flanigan, RN, Pres.

Desc: Supports the practice of pediatric surgical nurses through continuing education, networking and mentoring. **Awards:** Founders Award (annual); Research and Scholarship Gift Fund.

★ 13142 ★ American Podiatric Medical Writers Association (APMWA)
PO Box 750129
Forest Hills, NY 11375
Phone: (718)897-9700 **Fax:** (718)896-5747
Email: bblock@prodigy.net
Dr. Barry H. Block, Exec. Dir.

Desc: Podiatric medical writers. Promotes the improvement of writing on podiatric topics. **Awards:** Elizabeth H. Roberts Award (annual); Golden Quill Award (annual); Student Writers Award (annual).

★ 13143 ★ American Polarity Therapy Association (APTA)
PO Box 19858
Boulder, CO 80308
Phone: (303)545-2080 **Fax:** (303)545-2161
Email: hq@polaritytherapy.org
Website: http://www.polaritytherapy.org
Ellie Simmons, RPP, Exec. Dir.

Desc: Dedicated to the advancement of polarity therapy. (Polarity therapy is a non-diagnostic holistic health system supplementing and supporting medical treatment. Polarity techniques include bodywork, diet, exercise and self awareness for health maintenance.) Develops and disseminates educational and support materials; registers practitioners; holds competitions. **Awards:** Dr. Stone Award (annual).

★ 13144 ★ American Porphyria Foundation (APF)
PO Box 22712
Houston, TX 77227
Phone: (713)266-9617 **Fax:** (713)871-1788
Email: porphyrus@aol.com
Website: http://www.porphyriafoundation.com/
Yvette Strange, Office Admin.

Desc: Persons interested in advancing awareness and treatment of the porphyrias; affected patients. Porphyria is a class of seven rare (and usually inherited) metabolic disorders of varying severity affecting the nervous system or the skin. It is characterized by a deficiency of an enzyme used in making heme (a ring-shaped molecule called a porphyrin), which in turn is used in making hemoglobin. One of porphyria's recurrent though not requisite symptoms is purple-red urine. The foundation's purposes are to: provide financial support for researchers in porphyria; improve the diagnosis and treatment of porphyria through educational programs; locate porphyria patients. Maintains a lending library of videotapes, papers, and pamphlets. **Awards:** Research Grant (annual).

★ 13145 ★ American Psychoanalytic Foundation (APF)
1636 Connecticut Ave. NW, 2nd Fl.
Washington, DC 20009
Phone: (202)667-6363 **Fax:** (202)667-4477
Email: apf@cyberpsych.org
Website: http://www.cyberpsych.org/apf/contactus.htm

Desc: Dedicated to the advancement of psychoanalysis through community outreach, education, research, clinical programs. **Awards:** Grant.

★ 13146 ★ American Psychological Society (APS)
1010 Vermont Ave. NW, Ste. 1100
Washington, DC 20005-4907
Phone: (202)783-2077 **Fax:** (202)783-2083
Email: akraut@aps.washington.dc.us
Website: http://www.psychologicalscience.org
Alan G. Kraut, Exec. Dir.

Desc: Scientists and academics. Works for the advancement of the discipline of psychology and the promotion of human welfare through research and application. Conducts research programs; educates policy makers on the role human behavior plays in societal problems; offers liability insurance plans. **Awards:** William James Fellow (annual).

★ 13147 ★ American Psychopathological Association (APPA)
Department of Psychiatry
Washington University School of Medicine
4940 Children's Pl.
Saint Louis, MO 63110
Email: zorumskc@psychiatry.wustl.edu
Website: http://www.appassn.org
Chuck Zorumski, MD, Pres.

Desc: Physicians and scientists interested in the field of psychopathology. To investigate scientific problems of abnormal psychology including: study of phenomena arising from abnormal mental processes; study of organic pathological conditions directly connected with abnormal mental processes; study of means which may remove or modify social or individual factors operating in the production of mental disease; study of relationship between psychopathological and social or cultural problems. **Awards:** Paul Moch Award (annual) for academy distinction; Samuel Hamilton Award (annual); Zubin Award (annual).

★ 13148 ★ American Radiological Nurses Association (ARNA)
7794 Grow Dr.
Pensacola, FL 32514
Phone: (850)474-7292 **Free:** (866)486-2762
Fax: (850)484-8762
Email: arna@puetzamc.com
Website: http://www.arna.net
Belinda Puetz, Exec. Dir.

Desc: Radiological nurses. Seeks to provide, promote, and maintain continuity of quality patient care through education, standards of care, professional growth, and collaboration with other health care providers. **Awards:** Dorothy Budnek Scholarship (annual).

★ 13149 ★ American Roentgen Ray Society (ARRS)
44211 Slatestone Ct.
Leesburg, VA 20176-5109
Phone: (703)729-3353 **Free:** 800-438-2777
Fax: (703)729-4839
Email: rdunnick@umich.edu
Website: http://www.arrs.org
N. Reed Dunnick, Pres.

Desc: Trade association for radiologists worldwide. Offers many educational programs. **Awards:** ARRS Scholar (annual) for a practicing radiologist.

★ 13150 ★ American School Health Association (ASHA)
PO Box 708
7263 State Route 43
Kent, OH 44240
Phone: (330)678-1601 **Free:** 800-445-2742
Fax: (330)678-4526
Email: asha@ashaweb.org
Website: http://www.ashaweb.org
Susan Wooley, Exec. Dir.

Desc: School physicians, school nurses, dentist, nurses, nutritionists, health educators, dental hygienist, school-based professionals and public health workers. Promotes coordinated school health programs that include health education, health services, a healthful school environment, physical education, nutrition services, and psycho-social health services offered in schools collaboratively with families and other members of the community. Offers professional reference materials. Conducts pilot programs that inform materials development, provides technical assistance to school professionals, advocates for school health, and complies statistics. **Awards:** ASHA Scholarship (annual) for college juniors, seniors, and graduate students majoring in health education, nursing, adolescent/pediatric medicine, or dentistry; Distinguished Service Award (annual) for outstanding contributions to the child health field through ASHA; William A. Howe Award (annual) for distinguished service in school health.

★ 13151 ★ American Skin Association (ASA)
346 Park Ave. S
New York, NY 10010
Phone: (212)889-4858 **Free:** 800-499-SKIN
Email: info@skinassn.org

Website: http://www.americanskin.org

Desc: Supports research on all skin diseases. Promotes public education on prevention and treatment of skin disorders. Created School Skin Health Education Program, K-12, with the New York Academy of Medicine. **Awards:** Research Achievement Awards (annual) for original research in psoriasis, vitiligo, pigment cell biology, autoimmune/inflammatory skin disorders and skin cancer/melanoma; Research Grants (annual) for dermatologi research on psoriasis, melanoma/skin cancer, vitiligo, childhood diseases/disfigurement, autoimmune, and inflammatory diseases; Research Scholar Awards (annual) to young research investigators.

★ 13152 ★ American Society for Bariatric Surgery (ASBS)

7328 W University Ave., Ste. F
Gainesville, FL 32607
Phone: (352)331-4900 **Fax:** (352)331-4975
Email: info@asbs.org
Website: http://www.asbs.org
Georgeann Mallory, Exec. Dir.

Desc: Works to advance the art and science of bariatric surgery. Supports clinical and laboratory investigations; promotes guidelines for ethical patient care; conducts educational programs for physicians, paramedicals and lay people; provides a forum for the exchange of ideas. **Awards:** Resident/Trainee Award (annual) for a resident or trainee in the field of bariatric surgery.

★ 13153 ★ American Society of Clinical Hypnosis - Education and Research Foundation (ASCH-ERF)

140 N Bloomingdale Rd.
Bloomingdale, IL 60108-1017
Phone: (630)980-4740 **Fax:** (630)351-8490
Email: info@asch.net
Website: http://www.asch.net
Philip R. Appell, PhD, Pres.

Desc: Teaching and research arm of the American Society of Clinical Hypnosis. Physicians, dentists, and psychologists. Underwrites workshops in the U.S. and Canada to train professionals in hypnosis and broaden their knowledge of psychotherapy. Basic section is designed to familiarize physicians, psychologists, and dentists with hypnosis and its applications to problems of the psychologically normal patient including preparation for childbirth, comfort in the dental chair, and other problems and complaints complicated by emotional conflicts, such as smoking and obesity. Advanced section deals with techniques that can be used in addition to hypnotherapy in treating patients. **Awards:** Mutter Fund for ASCH Regional Workshops for financial hardship students.

★ 13154 ★ American Society for Clinical Investigation (ASCI)

35 Research Dr., Ste. 300
Ann Arbor, MI 48103
Phone: (734)222-6050 **Fax:** (734)222-6058
Email: asci@the-jci.org
Website: http://www.asci-jci.org
Dr. Chi Van Dang, Pres.

Desc: Physician scientists with meritorious original clinical investigations. Active members are doctors under age 50; senior members are those over age 50. Promotes cultivation of clinical research by methods of natural sciences, correlation of science with the art of medical practice, encouragement of scientific investigation by medical practitioners, and publication of papers on the methods and results of clinical research. **Awards:** ASCI Award (annual) to society member, under 56 years of age.

★ 13155 ★ American Society for Clinical Laboratory Science (ASCLS)

6701 Democracy Blvd., Ste. 300
Bethesda, MD 20817
Phone: (301)657-2768 **Fax:** (301)657-2909
Email: ascls@ascls.org
Website: http://www.ascls.org
Elissa Passiment, EdM, Exec. VP

Desc: Primarily clinical laboratory personnel who have an associate or baccalaureate degree and clinical training and specialists who hold at least a master's degree in one of the major fields of clinical laboratory science such as bacteriology, mycology, or biochemistry; also includes technicians, specialists, and educators with limited certificates and students enrolled in approved programs of clinical laboratory studies and military medical technology schools. Promotes and maintains high standards in clinical laboratory methods and research and advances standards of education and training of personnel. Conducts educational program of seminars and workshops. Sponsors award competition to encourage the writing of scientific papers. Approves programs of continuing education and maintains records on participation in continuing education programs for members. **Awards:** Scholarship for training in clinical laboratory science.

★ 13156 ★ American Society of Clinical Psychopharmacology (ASCP)

PO Box 2257
New York, NY 10116
Phone: (212)696-1088 **Free:** 800-248-4344
Fax: (212)696-0563
Website: http://www.ascpp.org
J. Craig Nelson, MD, Pres.

Desc: Works to encourage clinical research in psychopharmacology and provide continuing education for members. Sponsors research; facilitates exchange of information; conducts professional educational programs and; provides educational programs on the treatment of psychiatric disorders for patients and families; develops relationships with mental health advocacy groups; advocates public policies which promote research and the delivery of high quality care. **Awards:** Residency Travel Award (annual) goes to 4 outstanding psychiatry residents.

★ 13157 ★ American Society of Cytopathology (ASC)

400 W 9th St., Ste. 201
Wilmington, DE 19801
Phone: (302)429-8802 **Fax:** (302)429-8807
Email: asc@cytopathology.org
Website: http://www.cytopathology.org
Elizabeth A. Jenkins, Exec. Admin.

Desc: Physicians, Cytotechnologists and scientists dedicated to the cytologic method of diagnostic pathology. **Awards:** Papanicoluau Award (annual) for a cytopathologist selected by committee.

★ 13158 ★ American Society of Echocardiography (ASE)

1500 Sunday Dr., Ste. 102
Raleigh, NC 27607
Phone: (919)861-5574 **Fax:** (919)787-4916
Email: rbarry@asecho.org
Website: http://www.asecho.org
Robin L. Barry, Exec. Dir.

Desc: Physicians and sonographers specializing in ultrasound heart imaging and diagnosis. Promotes excellence in the ultrasonic examination of the heart and assists in establishing standards for education of physicians and cardiac- sonographers in echocardiography. Sponsors educational activities including distribution of self-testing materials, continuing education calendar, and annual scientific sessions. Maintains liaison with governmental agencies and other professional groups. **Awards:** Outcomes Research Grants (annual); Research Awards (annual).

★ 13159 ★ American Society of Electroneurodiagnostic Technologists (ASET)

426 West 42nd St.
Kansas City, MO 64111
Phone: (816)931-1120 **Fax:** (816)931-1145
Email: sheila@aset.org
Website: http://www.aset.org
Sheila R. Navis, CAE, Exec. Dir.

Desc: Persons engaged in clinical electroencephalographic (EEG) technology, evoked potential responses, nerve conduction studies, and polysomnography (sleep studies). Objective is the advancement of electroneurodiagnostic technology education and practice standards. **Awards:** Maureen Berkeley Memorial Award (annual) for the best article by an EEG technologist published in the *American Journal of Electroneurodiagnostic Technology*; scholarship (quarterly) for members for expenses in attending the annual meeting and short courses.

★ 13160 ★ American Society of Extra-Corporeal Technology (AmSECT)

503 Carlisle Dr. No. 125
Herndon, VA 20170-4838
Phone: (703)435-8556 **Fax:** (703)435-0056
Email: gcate@amsect.org
Website: http://www.amsect.org
George M. Cate, Exec. Dir.

Desc: Perfusionists, technologists, doctors, nurses, and others actively employed and using the applied skills relating to the practice of extracorporeal technology (involving heart-lung machines); student members. Disseminates information necessary to the proper practice of the technology. Conducts programs in continuing education and professional-public liaison and hands-on workshops. Maintains placement service. **Awards:** Recognition (annual); Research Grant Award (annual); scholarship.

★ 13161 ★ American Society for Healthcare Food Service Administrators (ASHFSA)

One N Franklin
Chicago, IL 60606
Phone: (312)422-3870 **Fax:** (312)422-4581
Email: ashfsa@aha.org
Website: http://www.ashfsa.org
Patricia Burton, Exec. Dir.

Desc: Serves individuals with healthcare food service management responsibilities, educators, suppliers and consultants to the profession, is the driving force in the healthcare food service industry and provides healthcare professionals with the resources to compete and succeed. **Awards:** Dorothy Killian Scholarship hotel, restaurant, food management or dietetics programs.

★ 13162 ★ American Society for Healthcare Risk Management (ASHRM)

One N Franklin
Chicago, IL 60606
Phone: (312)422-3989 **Fax:** (312)422-4580
Email: esummy@aha.org
Website: http://www.ashrm.org
Elizabeth Summy, Exec. Dir.

Desc: Employees actively involved in the risk management functions of hospitals or other health care providers, and others involved in insurance, brokerage, and consulting. Purposes are to: promote professional development of hospital risk managers; provide educational resources and programs on healthcare risk management; address risk management issues affecting the health care industry, particularly patient safety and risk financing. **Awards:** Innovation and Research Awards (annual).

★ 13163 ★ American Society for Investigative Pathology (ASIP)

9650 Rockville Pke.
Bethesda, MD 20814-3993
Phone: (301)634-7130 **Fax:** (301)634-7990
Email: asip@asip.org
Website: http://www.asip.org
Mark E. Sobel, MD,PhD, Exec. Off.

Desc: Experimental research pathologists who have made significant contributions to the knowledge of disease. **Awards:** Chugai Award for Excellence in Mentoring and Scholarship for a member of the ASIP with a distinguished career that especially links excellence in mentoring and education with outstanding research achievements in experimental and investigative pathology; Experimental Pathologist-in-Training Award for individuals who have excelled in their investigative efforts as trainees in studying mechanisms of disease; Gold Headed Cane Award for recognition of long-term contributions to pathology, including meritorious research, outstanding teacher and general excellence; Minority Trainee Travel Awards to promote the entry of under-represented minority scientists and minority-serving institutions into the mainstream of the basic science community; Pfizer Outstanding Investigator Award (annual) for an ASIP member under age 43 at time of meeting for meritorious research in experimental pathology; Rous-Whipple Award for a pathologist age 50 years or older with a distinguished career in research and continued productivity at the time of the award; Trainee Travel Awards to promote the entry of young scientists into the mainstream of the basic science community; Young Pathologist Fellowship offers 12 graduate students in pathology an opportunity to attend symposia, lectures and poster sessions, network with career pathologists and explore career pathways at the Experimental Biology Meeting.

★ 13164 ★ American Society for Laser Medicine and Surgery (ASLMS)
2404 Stewart Ave.
Wausau, WI 54401
Phone: (715)845-9283 **Fax:** (715)848-2493
Email: information@aslms.org
Website: http://www.aslms.org
Richard O. Gregory, MD, Sec.

Desc: Physicians, physicists, and other scientists; nurses, dentists, podiatrists, veterinarians, and other paramedical personnel; technicians and commercial representatives concerned with the medical applications of lasers. Facilitates exchange of information concerning lasers. **Awards:** Grant.

★ 13165 ★ American Society of Master Dental Technologists (ASMDT)
PO Box 640248
Oakland Gardens, NY 11364
Phone: (718)347-1239 **Fax:** (718)347-3113
Email: info@asmdt.com
Website: http://www.asmdt.com
Sue Heppenheimer, Exec. Sec.

Desc: Dental lab technicians. Dedicated to the upgrading of dental technology. Seeks to provide educational resources such as texts, instructors, and guidance for technicians interested in becoming master dental technologists. Conducts associate and master level courses in conjunction with New York University School of Dentistry, Dept. of Continuing Education. **Awards:** Irving Sutla Award (annual) for best tooth carving; NGS (Northeastern Grathological Society) Award (annual) for best student in courses.

★ 13166 ★ American Society of Maxillofacial Surgeons (ASMS)
4900B S 31st. St.
Arlington, VA 22206-1656
Phone: (703)820-7400 **Fax:** (703)931-4520
Email: admin@maxface.org
Website: http://www.maxface.org
Thomas F. Fise, Exec. Dir.

Desc: Professional society of doctors of medicine and doctors of dental surgery who have at least five years of recognized graduate training and experience in maxillofacial surgery. Seeks to stimulate and advance knowledge of the science and art of maxillofacial surgery and improve and elevate the standard of practice. **Awards:** Research Grant Awards (annual).

★ 13167 ★ American Society of Nuclear Cardiology (ASNC)
9111 Old Georgetown Rd.
Bethesda, MD 20814-1699
Phone: (301)493-2360 **Fax:** (301)493-2376
Email: admin@asnc.org
Website: http://www.asnc.org
Ernest V. Garcia, Pres.

Desc: Physicians, scientists, technologist, biomedical engineers and health care workers. Seeks to foster optimal delivery of nuclear cardiology services and promote research. Provides continuing medical education opportunities; establishes guidelines and standards for training and practice; provides information on licensure requirements. **Awards:** ASNC/Amersham Clinical Research in Nuclear Cardiology (annual).

★ 13168 ★ American Society of Ophthalmic Administrators (ASOA)
4000 Legato Rd., No. 850
Fairfax, VA 22033
Phone: (703)591-2220 **Free:** 800-451-1339
Fax: (703)591-0614
Email: asoa@asoa.org
Website: http://www.asoa.org
Lucy Santiago, Exec. Dir.

Desc: A division of the American Society of Cataract and Refractive Surgery . Persons involved with the administration of an ophthalmic office or clinic. Facilitates the exchange of ideas and information in order to improve management practices and working conditions. Offers placement services. **Awards:** William A. Rose Pinnacle Award (annual) to ophthalmology practices demonstrating exemplary effort to eliminate potential abusive billing practices and maintain compliance with government regulations.

★ 13169 ★ American Society for Parenteral and Enteral Nutrition (ASPEN)
8630 Fenton Ste., No. 412
Silver Spring, MD 20910-3805
Phone: (301)587-6315 **Fax:** (301)587-2365
Email: aspen@nutr.org
Website: http://www.nutritioncare.org
Robin Kriegel, Exec. Dir.

Desc: Physicians, dietitians, nurses, pharmacists, and members of the industry. Works to promote quality patient care, education, and research in the field of nutrition and metabolic support in all health care settings. Educates health care professionals. Conducts postgraduate courses and research programs; compiles statistics. **Awards:** Discipline Research Awards (annual) for research by nurse, dietitian, and pharmacist members of ASPEN; Dudrick Research Scholar Award (annual) for past research accomplishments of a young investigator in the field of nutrition support; RHOADS Foundation Research Award (annual) for nutrition researchers in the early stages of their careers, to encourage research in the fields of nutrition and metabolic support and related areas of clinical nutrition; Vars Award (annual) for best research by a young investigator at each Clincial Congress.

★ 13170 ★ American Society of Plastic Surgeons and Plastic Surgery Education Foundation (ASPRS)
444 E Algonquin Rd.
Arlington Heights, IL 60005
Phone: (847)228-9900 **Free:** 888-4-PLASTIC
Fax: (847)228-9131
Website: http://www.plasticsurgery.org
James Wells, MD, Pres.

Desc: Professional society of plastic surgeons. Works in cooperation with the Plastic Surgery Educational Foundation to promote optimal care for plastic surgery patients through research, service, and education activities. Sponsors public/patient education program, clinical symposia, and professional development workshops. Acts as a liaison between members and government and medical organizations. Conducts charitable activities; maintains speakers' bureau; compiles statistics. **Awards:** Circle of Excellence Journalism Award (annual) to newspapers, wire services, magazines, radio, or TV.

★ 13171 ★ American Society of Plastic Surgical Nurses (ASPSN)
E Holly Ave.
Box 56
Pitman, NJ 08071
Phone: (856)256-2340 **Fax:** (856)589-7463
Email: asprsn@ajj.com
Rick Grimes, Exec. Dir.

Desc: Registered nurses, licensed practical nurses, and licensed vocational nurses working with plastic surgeons or interested in plastic and reconstructive nursing. Objectives are: to enhance leadership qualities of nurses in the field of plastic surgery; to increase the skills, knowledge, and understanding of personnel in plastic surgery nursing through continuing education; to study existing practices and new developments in the field; to encourage participation and interest in professional organizations; to cooperate with others in the profession. **Awards:** Grant (annual).

★ 13172 ★ American Society of Podiatric Dermatology (ASPD)
c/o Dr. Steven Berlin
1901 Sulfer Spring Rd.
Baltimore, MD 21227-0378
Fax: (410)247-7329
Dr. Richard Chase, Contact

Desc: Doctors of podiatric medicine with demonstrated expertise in foot dermatology (100); candidates for D.P.M. degrees in colleges of podiatric medicine (400). Fosters research in podiatric dermatology; supports college-affiliated study groups; conducts semiannual continuing education programs; sponsors student affiliates. Maintains speakers' bureau; conducts research programs; sponsors competitions. **Awards:** Ortho Pharmaceutical Award (annual) for best paper on podiatric dermatology by a podiatric resident or medical student.

★ 13173 ★ American Society of Podiatric Medical Assistants (ASPMA)
2124 S Austin Blvd.
Cicero, IL 60804
Phone: (708)863-6303 **Free:** 888-88ASPMA
Fax: (708)863-5375
Email: mmalone@aspma.org
Website: http://www.aspma.org
Sandra Lohrentz, PMAC, Exec. Dir.

Desc: Podiatric assistants. Purposes are to hold educational seminars and to administer certification examinations. **Awards:** Scholarship; Zelda W. Vicha Memorial Scholarship Fund financial need and academic standing.

★ 13174 ★ American Society of Regional Anesthesia and Pain Medicine (ASRA)
2209 Dickens Rd.
PO Box 11086
Richmond, VA 23230-1086
Phone: (804)282-0010 **Fax:** (804)282-0090
Email: asra@societyhq.com
Website: http://www.asra.com
James C. Eisenach, MD, Pres.

Desc: Physicians and research Ph.D.s. Conducts educational workshops. Sponsors annual refresher course. **Awards:** Gaston Labat Award (annual); Koller Research Grant.

★ 13175 ★ American Society of Transplantation (ASTA)
17000 Commerce Pkwy., Ste. C
Mount Laurel, NJ 08054
Phone: (856)439-9986 **Fax:** (856)439-9982
Email: ast@ahint.com
Website: http://www.a-s-t.org/
Susan J. Nelson, MD, Exec. Dir.

Desc: Promotes and encourages education and research with respect to transplantation medicine and immunology; provides a forum for exchange of scientific information related to transplantation across solid organ specialties. **Awards:** AST Fujisawa Fellowship in Transplantation (annual); AST President's Award (annual); AST Sandoz Fellowship in Transplantation (biennial); Faculty Development (annual); Novartis Fellowship in Transplantation (annual); Roche New Investigator Award (annual); Upjohn Young Investigators Award.

★ 13176 ★ American Spinal Injury Association (ASIA)

345 E Superior, Rm. 1436
Chicago, IL 60611
Phone: (312)238-1242 **Fax:** (312)238-0869
Email: mars@northwestern.edu
Website: http://www.asia-spinalinjury.org
Marianne G. Kaplan, Exec. Sec.

Desc: Medical doctors and Allied Health Care professionals who have been trained in the care of spinal injury patients and who are either actively engaged in the field and acknowledged to be competent by their peers or who have made a significant contribution to the advancement of the basic sciences or one of the clinical fields of practice as they are applicable to the treatment of spinal cord injury. Purposes are to: develop knowledge and investigation of the causes, cure, and prevention of spinal injury and related trauma; pursue excellence in spinal injury patient care; promote and exchange ideas between professionals in the field; standardize medical terminology in spinal cord injury; foster and encourage basic research in the field; develop teaching and educational material; foster education of the medical profession and laity in the prevention and proper management of spinal injury, including the necessity for specialized regional spinal injury centers, provision for educational and vocational training, removal of architectural barriers, and promotion of a society more sensitive to the physically inconvenienced individual, including adequate housing and transportation; establish criteria for centers and/or systems of total spinal injury management so as to provide optimal care of the spinal injured person. Conducts annual scientific sessions. Sponsors G. Heiner Sell Distinguished Lectureship. **Awards:** G. Heiner Sell Educational Award (annual).

★ 13177 ★ American Surgical Association (ASA)

c/o Robert P. Jones, Jr., Ed.D.
13 Elm St.
Manchester, MA 01944-1314
Phone: (978)526-8330 **Fax:** (978)526-7521
Email: asa@prri.com
Carlos A. Pellegrini, MD, Sec.

Desc: Surgeons organized to promote the science and art of surgery. Bestows medallion for scientific achievement. **Awards:** American Surgical Association Foundation Fellowship (annual) US citizen or permanent resident with a M.D. or equivalent medical degree who has completed an ACGME approved residency and hold a faculty appointment in an accredited medical school or similar medical institution.

★ 13178 ★ American Tinnitus Association (ATA)

PO Box 5
Portland, OR 97207-0005
Phone: (503)248-9985 **Free:** 800-634-8978
Fax: (503)248-0024
Email: Tinnitus@ata.org
Website: http://www.ata.org
Cheryl McGinnis, Exec. Dir.

Desc: Dedicated to tinnitus research and educating patients, and professionals through conferences, books, brochures, videos and the quarterly journal Tinnitus Today. ATA is the national champion of tinnitus awareness, prevention and treatment. Under its guiding principles Education, Advocacy, Research and Support - the ATA offers prevention programs in schools, urges governmental and private organizations to support hearing conservation, funds the nation's brightest researchers and facilitates self-help groups around the country. **Awards:** ATA Research Grants (semiannual) for research.

★ 13179 ★ American Urogynecologic Society (AUGS)

2025 M St. NW, Ste. 800
Washington, DC 20036
Phone: (202)367-1167 **Fax:** (202)367-2167
Email: augs@dc.sba.com
Website: http://www.augs.org
Steven C. Kemp, Exec. Dir.

Desc: Physicians and health professionals actively engaged in providing quality urogynecologic care to women. Dedicated to research and education in urogynecology and to improved care for women with lower urinary tract disorders. **Awards:** Health Science Award (annual).

★ 13180 ★ American Venous Forum (AVF)

c/o Robin Hoyle, J.D.
13 Elm St.
Manchester, MA 01944
Phone: (978)526-8330 **Fax:** (978)526-8330
Email: avf@prri.com
Website: http://www.venous-info.com
Robin Hoyle, Exec. Dir.

Desc: Board-certified vascular surgeons. Provides a forum intent on improving the quality care to patients suffering venous and lymphatic disorders. Assists in research and offers guidelines for clinical trials. **Awards:** BSN-Jobst, Inc. Fellowship (annual); Siquaris Traveling Fellowship (annual).

★ 13181 ★ American Veterinary Society of Animal Behavior (AVSAB)

c/o Steven Feldman
1535 Rugby Cir.
Thousand Oaks, CA 91360
Email: avsabe@yahoo.com
Website: http://www.avma.org/avsab/
Steve Feldman, Sec. /Treas.

Desc: Veterinarians and veterinary students. Promotes inquiry and research into animal behavior. Seeks to advance ethological knowledge regarding the care and utilization of captive, domesticated, and free-living animals. Promotes and facilitates the exchange of information among those concerned with animal behavior and well-being; encourages discussion on veterinary aspects of animal behavior and the publication of materials in the field. **Awards:** Student Excellence in Applied Animal Research (annual).

★ 13182 ★ Amyotrophic Lateral Sclerosis Association (ALSA)

27001 Agoura Rd. Suite 150
Calabasas Hills, CA 91301-5104
Phone: (818)880-9007 **Free:** 800-782-4747
Fax: (818)880-9006
Email: alsinfo@alsa-national.org
Website: http://www.alsa.org
Michael W. Havlicek, Pres. /CEO

Desc: Patients; relatives and friends of patients; doctors, neurologists, physical therapists, nurses, and professional organizations dedicated to finding the cause, prevention, and cure for amyotrophic lateral sclerosis (ALS). Offers help and information to ALS patients and their families. Funds ALS-specific research at major medical institutions. Works with other agencies, including the government, to increase their involvement on a priority basis in ALS research. Conducts patient meetings. **Awards:** Grant (annual) for ALS research.

★ 13183 ★ Anesthesia Patient Safety Foundation (APSF)

4246 Colonial Park Dr.
Pittsburgh, PA 15227-2621
Phone: (412)882-8040
Email: info@apsf.org
Website: http://gasnet.med.yale.edu/apsf/

Desc: Promotes safer anesthesia, fosters investigations to provide understanding of preventable anesthetic injuries. **Awards:** Grant.

★ 13184 ★ Animal Health Foundation (AHF)

3615 Bassett Rd.
Pacific, MO 63069
Website: http://www.animalhealthfoundation.com

Desc: Individuals interested in finding the causes, treatments, and cure for the crippling equine disease laminitis/founder syndrome. (Laminitis is an inflammation of the laminae, the semi-rigid internal supporting structures of the horse's foot; founder is the crippling result of laminitis in which the coffin bone in the horse's foot puts pressure on the sole of the foot, and sometimes actually penetrates the sole.) These ailments affect horses of any age or breed, and are counted by the AHF as the second ranking disease leading to the need to euthanize horses. Supports extensive research and collects a range of related data. **Awards:** Grant.

★ 13185 ★ Aplastic Anemia and MDS International Foundation (AAFA)

PO Box 613
Annapolis, MD 21404-0613
Free: 800-747-2820 **Fax:** (410)867-0240
Email: help@aamds.org
Website: http://www.aplastic.org
Marilyn Baker, Exec. Dir.

Desc: Serves as an information source for persons with aplastic anemia and myelodysplastic syndromes. (Aplastic anemia is an often fatal disease in which the bone marrow fails to produce new blood cells.) Provides free educational materials and medical information. Financially supports research. Hosts annual International Patient Conferences presenting the latest in medical research findings and networking opportunities for patients and their families. **Awards:** New Research Award (annual).

★ 13186 ★ ASHP Foundation

7272 Wisconsin Ave.
Bethesda, MD 20814
Phone: (301)657-3000 **Fax:** (301)657-8817
Email: foundation@ashp.org
Website: http://www.ashpfoundation.org
Stephen J. Allen, Sec.

Desc: Established for pharmaceutical care and research purposes. Offers research grants, awards; and anticoagulation, asthma, stem cell transplantation, diabetes, pain management, oncology, and traineeships. **Awards:** Fellowship for the study of practice areas such as oncology drug therapy, psychiatric drug therapy, clinical pharmacokinetics, cardiovascular drug therapy, critical care, drug information, and pharmacy nutritional support; grant for research and special projects; recognition (annual) for the most significant contributions to literature in the areas of research and practice.

★ 13187 ★ Associated Professional Sleep Societies (APSS)

1 West Brook Corp. Ctr., Ste. 920
Westchester, IL 60154
Phone: (708)492-0930 **Fax:** (708)492-0943
Email: info@aasmet.org
Website: http://www.apss.org
Jerry Barrett, Exec. Dir.

Desc: Members are the Sleep Research Society and American Academy of Sleep Medicine . Works to facilitate sleep research and development of sleep disorder medicine by encouraging cooperation and exchange of information among members. **Awards:** Dement/Kleitman/Hatfield (annual) academic achievement/distinguished service/public policy.

★ 13188 ★ Association for Advancement of Behavior Therapy (AABT)

305 7th Ave., Ste. 16A
New York, NY 10001-6008
Phone: (212)647-1890 **Free:** 800-685-AABT
Fax: (212)647-1865
Email: mjeimer@aabt.org

Website: http://www.aabt.org/
Mary Jane Eimer, CAE, Exec. Dir.

Desc: Psychologists primarily, but also psychiatrists, social workers, counselors, physicians, dentists, nurses, students, and other professionals interested in the issues, problems, and development of the field of behavior therapy and cognitive behavior therapy, with specific emphasis on research and clinical applications. Sponsors training programs and lectures for professionals; maintains speakers' bureau; handles referrals for the public to locate behavior therapists in their area; facilitates communication between behavior therapists interested in specific problems or information. AABT local affiliates hold training meetings, workshops, seminars, case demonstrations, and discussion groups. discussion groups. **Awards:** Career/ Lifetime Achievement (annual); Distinguished Friend to Behavior Therapy (annual); Distinguished/Outstanding Contribution by an Individual for Education/ Training (triennial); Elsie Ramos Awards (annual) for the best student poster submitted at annual convention; Outstanding Training Program (annual); President's New Researcher Award (annual); Virginia A. Roswell Student Dissertation Award (annual).

★ 13189 ★ Association for Applied Psychophysiology and Biofeedback (AAPB)

10200 W 44th Ave., Ste. 304
Wheat Ridge, CO 80033
Phone: (303)422-8436 **Free:** 800-477-8892
Fax: (303)422-8894
Email: fbutler@resourcecenter.com
Website: http://www.aapb.org
Francine Butler, PhD, Pres.

Desc: Persons interested in the "interrelationship of external feedback systems, states of consciousness, and the physiological mechanisms involved." Promotes rapid interchange of ideas and information among members. Offers Continuing Education Training Programs. Maintains numerous committees. **Awards:** AAPB Foundation Award; Distinguished Scientist Award; Mary Brazier Scholarship; Student Travel Scholarship.

★ 13190 ★ Association of Bone and Joint Surgeons (ABJS)

6300 N River Rd., Ste. 727
Rosemont, IL 60018-4226
Phone: (847)698-1636 **Fax:** (847)823-4921
Email: abjs@aaos.org
Website: http://www.abjs.org
Colette I. Hohimer, Exec. Dir.

Desc: Orthopedic surgeons interested in clinical aspects of orthopedics and in training of leaders in the specialty. **Awards:** Marshall R. Urist Award; Nicolas Andry Award (annual).

★ 13191 ★ Association for Child Psychoanalysis (ACP)

PO Box 253
Ramsey, NJ 07446
Phone: (201)825-3138 **Fax:** (201)825-3138
Email: childanalysis@compuserve.com
Nancy Hall, Admin.

Desc: Child psychoanalysts united to provide a forum for discussion and dissemination of information in their field. Conducts national and international scientific meetings. **Awards:** Monetary (annual).

★ 13192 ★ Association of Chiropractic Colleges (ACC)

c/o David S. O'Bryon
4424 Montgomery Ave., Ste. 102
Bethesda, MD 20814
Phone: (301)652-5066 **Fax:** (301)913-9146
Email: Info@ChiroColleges.org
Website: http://www.chirocolleges.org
David S. O'Bryon, CAE, Exec. Dir.

Desc: Presidents of chiropractic colleges that are members of the Council on Chiropractic Education. Objective is to provide a cooperative base that assists members in the search for and promotion of the practices and concepts most effective in the academic and continuing education of doctors of chiropractic. Serves as a clearinghouse for information related to opportunities and advancement in research as they affect chiropractic education and health care. Seeks to enhance services to the consumer of chiropractic education and to the public. **Awards:** Student Scholarships in Chiropractic (annual).

★ 13193 ★ Association for Glycogen Storage Disease (AGSD)

PO Box 896
Durant, IA 52747
Phone: (563)785-6038 **Fax:** (563)785-6038
Email: maryc@agsdus.org
Website: http://www.agsdus.org
Hollie Swain, Pres.

Desc: Individuals afflicted with glycogen storage disease; families of GSD sufferers; health care professionals. (GSD is a hereditary condition characterized by a lack of or deficiency in any of the enzymes used by the body to break down glycogen, resulting in hypoglycemia and related disorders, and requiring diet modifications and frequent or continual feeding, and in extreme cases resulting in death.) Acts as a forum for the discussion of GSD, its treatment, and the problems faced by parents raising children with GSD. Disseminates medical information; fosters communication between the families of GSD patients and health care professionals. Conducts fundraising drive. Aids members in obtaining equipment necessary for home care of GSD patients; provides referral services for individuals seeking GSD treatment facilities. **Awards:** AGSD Grant (annual) for work with GSD.

★ 13194 ★ Association for the Help of Retarded Children

200 Park Ave. S
New York, NY 10003
Phone: (212)780-2500
Email: sbstein@ahrcnyc.org
Website: http://www.ahrcnyc.org

Desc: Developmentally disabled children and adults; their families; interested individuals. Provides support services, training programs, clinics, schools, and residential facilities to the developmentally disabled. **Awards:** Scholarship (annual).

★ 13195 ★ Association of Medical Illustrators (AMI)

5475 Mark Dabling Rd., Ste. 108
Colorado Springs, CO 80918-3847
Phone: (719)598-8622 **Fax:** (719)599-3075
Email: ami@capsys.com
Website: http://www.ami.org
Janet McAndless, Exec. Dir.

Desc: Medical illustrators and individuals engaged in related pursuits. Promotes the study and encourages the advancement of medical illustration and allied fields of visual education. Works to advance medical education and to promote understanding and cooperation with medical and related professions; accredits six postgraduate medical illustration programs. Offers continuing education program; provides professional certification; compiles statistics. **Awards:** Recognition; scholarship.

★ 13196 ★ Association of Nurses in AIDS Care (ANAC)

80 S Summit St.
500 Courtyard Sq.
Akron, OH 44308
Phone: (330)762-5739 **Free:** 800-260-6780
Fax: (330)762-5813
Email: anac@anacnet.org
Website: http://www.anacnet.org/
Adele Webb, Exec. Dir.

Desc: Nurses and other health care professionals involved in caring for people who are HIV-infected or have AIDS. Functions as a network and provides leadership and educational services for members. Promotes public awareness of AIDS issues; advocates for HIV-infected individuals. Plans to develop a national standard for care of people with AIDS. **Awards:** Monetary (annual).

★ 13197 ★ Association of Occupational and Environmental Clinics (AOEC)

1010 Vermont Ave. NW, Ste. 513
Washington, DC 20005
Phone: (202)347-4976 **Fax:** (202)347-4950
Email: aoec@aoec.org
Website: http://www.aoec.org
Katherine H. Kirkland, Exec. Dir.

Desc: Seeks to enhance the practice of occupational and environmental medicine. Shares information. Provides educational and research programs. **Awards:** Grant.

★ 13198 ★ Association of Pediatric Oncology Nurses (APON)

4700 W Lake Ave.
Glenview, IL 60025-1485
Phone: (847)375-4724 **Fax:** 877-734-8755
Email: info@apon.org
Website: http://www.apon.org/
CJ Hutto, RNCPON, Pres.

Desc: Scientific and educational association seeking to establish lines of communication among nurses caring for children and adolescents with cancer. Encourages updating of literature and development of standards of care for children with cancer. Plans annual conference. **Awards:** APON Excellence in Pediatric Oncology Nursing Practice Award to registered professional nurse; Casey Hooke Distinguished Service Award; Dr. Patricia Greene Leadership Award; Jean Fergusson Excellence in Pediatric Oncology Nursing Education Award to registered professional nurse; Patient/Family Educational Materials Award to registered professional nurse.

★ 13199 ★ Association of Physician Assistant Programs (APAP)

950 N Washington St.
Alexandria, VA 22314-1552
Phone: (703)548-5538 **Fax:** (703)684-1924
Website: http://www.apap.org
David P. Asprey, Pres.

Desc: Represents physician assistant (PA) educational programs in the United States. Assists PA educational programs-institutions with training programs for physician assistants to primary care and surgical physicians. Assists in the development and organization of educational curricula for PA programs to assure the public of competent PAs. Contributes to defining the roles of PAs in the field of medicine to maximize their benefit to the public; serves as a public information center on the profession; coordinates program logistics such as admissions and career placements; and is currently initiating a centralized application service for PA applicants. Sponsors the Annual Survey of Physician Assistant Educational Programs in the United States. Conducts and sponsors research projects; compiles statistics; offers ongoing training for PA leadership and faculty. **Awards:** APAP Partnership Award (annual) for contribution to excellence in PA education by an individual or institution outside of PA program circles; J. Peter Nyquist Student Writing Award Competition (annual) for student submissions dealing with clinical medicine or us issues impacting the PA profession; Master Teacher Award (annual) for excellence in clinical or classroom teaching, scholarship and/or professional service; Outstanding Service Award (annual) for exceptional service or leadership to APAP, or contributions to the profession through scholarly, teaching or advocate activit.

★ 13200 ★ Association of Polysomnographic Technologists (APT)

PO Box 14861
Lenexa, KS 66285-1991
Phone: (913)541-1991 **Fax:** (913)599-5340
Email: soneal@goamp.com

Website: http://www.aptweb.org
Sheila O'Neal, Exec. Dir.

Desc: Individuals who practice polysomnography in research or clinical settings. (Polysomnographic technology deals with the measurement and recording of multiple physiological activity, such as eye movement and heart rate, during sleep.) Seeks to establish standards for polysomnographic technology and provide education and training for people entering in the field. Acts as a forum for communication among members. **Awards:** Carskadon Research (annual).

★ 13201 ★ Association of Rehabilitation Nurses (ARN)

4700 W Lake Ave.
Glenview, IL 60025-1485
Phone: (847)375-4710 **Free:** 800-229-7530
Fax: 877-734-9384
Email: info@rehabnurse.org
Website: http://www.rehabnurse.org
Paul Nathenson, Pres.

Desc: Registered nurses concerned with or actively engaged in the practice of rehabilitation nursing; others interested in rehabilitation. Works to advance the quality of rehabilitation nursing practice through educational opportunities and to facilitate the exchange of ideas. Committees involve members in issues of organizational, local, and national importance and provide an avenue to effect change. Has formed the Rehabilitation Nursing Foundation to promote, develop, and engage in scientific research in the rehabilitation field. **Awards:** MaryAnn Mikulic Scholarship (annual); RNF Research Grant (annual).

★ 13202 ★ Association for Research in Otolaryngology (ARO)

c/o Susan Whitehouse
19 Mantua Rd.
Mount Royal, NJ 08061
Phone: (856)423-0041 **Fax:** (856)423-3420
Email: headquarters@aro.org
Website: http://www.aro.org
Darla Dobson, Headquarter Admin. Mgr.

Desc: Medical professionals, scientists, and researchers with an interest in otolaryngology. Promotes increased understanding of basic science and clinical practice associated with hearing, speech, balance, the senses of taste and smell, and diseases of the head and neck. Conducts educational programs; facilitates exchange of information among members. **Awards:** Midwinter Meeting Travel Award (annual).

★ 13203 ★ Association for Surgical Education (ASE)

SIU School of Medicine
Department of Surgery
PO Box 19655
Springfield, IL 62794-9655
Phone: (217)545-3835 **Fax:** (217)545-2431
Email: membershipo@surgicaleducation.com
Website: http://www.surgicaleducation.com
Susan Kepner, Exec. Dir.

Desc: Surgeons and individuals involved or interested in undergraduate surgical education. Purpose is to develop and disseminate information on motivation, techniques, research, and applications for presenting curricula in undergraduate surgical education. Acts as forum for research in surgical education; serves as information clearinghouse. Compiles statistics; maintains speakers' bureau. Conducts educational programs. **Awards:** Best Paper Award (annual); Presidential Teaching Award (annual) for research in surgical education.

★ 13204 ★ Association of Surgical Technologists (AST)

7108-C S Alton Way
Englewood, CO 80112-2106
Phone: (303)694-9130 **Fax:** (303)694-9169
Email: bteutsch@ast.org
Website: http://www.ast.org
William J. Teutsch, Exec. Dir.

Desc: Individuals who have received specific education and training to deliver surgical patient care in the operating room. Membership categories are available for both certified and student surgical technologists. Emphasis is placed on encouraging members to participate actively in a continuing education program. Aims are: to study, discuss, and exchange knowledge, experience, and ideas in the field of surgical technology; to promote a high standard of surgical technology performance in the community for quality patient care; to stimulate interest in continuing education. Local groups sponsor workshops and institutes. Conducts research. **Awards:** AST Scholarship (annual) for students enrolled in CAAHEE accredited programs.

★ 13205 ★ Association for Women in Psychology (AWP)

c/o Cassandra Nichols, AWP Treas.
PO Box 641065
Pullman, WA 99164-1065
Email: support@awpsych.org
Website: http://www.awpsych.org
Dr. Susan Rose, Contact

Desc: Seeks to: end the role that the association feels psychology has had in perpetuating unscientific and unquestioned assumptions about the "natures" of women and men; encourage unbiased psychological research on sex and gender in order to establish facts and expose myths; encourage research and theory directed toward alternative sex-role socialization, child rearing practices, life-styles, and language use; educate and sensitize the science and psychology professions as well as the public to the psychological, social, political, and economic rights of women; combat the oppression of women of color; encourage research on issues of concern to women of color; achieve equality of opportunity for women and men within the profession and science of psychology. Conducts business and professional sessions at meetings of regional psychology associations. Maintains Hall of Fame and speakers' bureau. Monitors sexism in the American Psychological Association. **Awards:** Distinguished Publication Award (annual) selection by committee; Jewish Women's Caucus Award for Scholarship (annual) for projects and papers published, also unpublished documents; Lesbian Psychologies Unpublished Manuscript Award (annual); Student Research Prize (annual) for research on women and gender; Women of Color Psychologies Award (annual).

★ 13206 ★ Association for Women Veterinarians (AWV)

c/o Magnolia Association Management Affiliates
310 North Indian Hill Blvd., Box 337
Claremont, CA 91711-4611
Email: lapancho@ra.msstate.edu
Website: http://www.awv-women-veterinarians.org
Dr. Marilyn Waldhalm, Exec. Sec.

Desc: Works to support veterinary medicine by providing leadership in women's issues. **Awards:** AWV Service Award (annual) to individual contributing to the advancement of women in veterinary medicine; Outstanding Woman Veterinarian (annual) for contributions to veterinary medicine; Student Scholarship (annual) for second or third year veterinary students.

★ 13207 ★ Association of Women's Health, Obstetric and Neonatal Nurses (AWHONN)

2000 L St. Nw, Ste. 740
Washington, DC 20036
Phone: (202)261-2400 **Free:** 800-673-8499
Fax: (202)728-0575
Email: gailk@awhonn.org
Website: http://www.awhonn.org
Gail Kincaide, Exec. Dir.

Desc: Members are registered nurses; associate members are allied health workers with an interest in obstetric, women's health, and neonatal (OGN) nursing. Promotes and establishes the highest standards of OGN nursing practice, education, and research; cooperates with all members of the health team; stimulates interest in OGN nursing. Sponsors educational meetings, audiovisual programs, and continuing education courses. **Awards:** Research Award (periodic).

★ 13208 ★ Association of Zoo Veterinary Technicians

White Oak Conservation Center
3823 Owens Rd.
Yulee, FL 32097
Phone: (336)879-7636 **Fax:** (336)879-7637
Email: cheryl_purnell@ncmail.net
Website: http://www.AZVT.org
Cheryl Purnell, Exec. Dir.

Desc: Zoo veterinary technicians. **Awards:** Laurie Page-Peck Scholarship (annual) for veterinary technician students with interest in zoo medicine; must write a paper for presentation at annual conference.

★ 13209 ★ Asthma and Allergy Foundation of America (AAFA)

1233 Twentieth St. NW, Ste. 402
Washington, DC 20036
Phone: (202)466-7643 **Free:** 800-7-ASTHMA
Fax: (202)466-8940
Email: info@aafa.org
Website: http://www.aafa.org
William McLin, Exec. Dir.

Desc: Dedicated to finding a cure for and controlling asthma and allergic diseases. AAFA serves the estimated 50 million Americans with asthma and allergic diseases through the support of research, patient and public education programs, public and governmental advocacy, and a nationwide network of chapters and education/support groups. **Awards:** Investigator Grants (annual) researchers referred by NIH.

★ 13210 ★ Attention Deficit Information Network (AD-IN)

58 Prince St.
Needham, MA 02492
Phone: (781)455-9895
Email: adin@gis.net
Website: http://www.addinfonetwork.com
Libby Ostrofsky, Contact

Desc: People with Attention Deficit Disorders (ADD), their families, and other individuals with an interest in ADD. Promotes improved quality of life for people with ADD. Works to expand home, school, and work-based strategies for aiding people with ADD; advocates for improved responsiveness to the needs of people with ADD by schools, businesses, and organizations. Provides support and information to families of people with ADD; conducts educational programs; maintains speakers' bureau. **Awards:** AD-IN Scholarship (annual).

★ 13211 ★ Auxiliary to the American Osteopathic Association (AAOA)

142 E Ontario St.
Chicago, IL 60611
Phone: (312)202-8192 **Free:** 800-621-1773
Fax: (312)202-8218
Email: bprice@aoa-net.org
Website: http://www.aux-aoa.org
Bridget L. Price, Exec. Dir.

Desc: Immediate family members of osteopathic physicians; spouses of students of osteopathic medicine. Promotes public health education; provides funds for scholarships for the training of osteopathic physicians and surgeons, and for research and other activities at osteopathic colleges; encourages establishment and continuation of volunteer service organizations in nonprofit osteopathic hospitals; participates in national and community health programs. Sponsors summer seminars. **Awards:** Scholarship (annual) for sophomores attending an accredited osteopathic college.

★ 13212 ★ Auxiliary to the National Medical Association (ANMA)
1012 10th St. NW
Washington, DC 20001
Phone: (202)371-9008 **Fax:** (202)289-2662
Email: info@anma-online.org
Website: http://www.anma-online.org
Mrs. Maurce W. Ayton, Pres.

Desc: Spouses of active members of the National Medical Association (see separate entry); widows and widowers of former members. Purposes are to: create a greater interest in the NMA; assist and encourage the medical profession in its efforts to educate and serve the public in matters of sanitation and health; develop and promote a national program on health and education with subcategories in community needs, legislation, and human relations. Conducts workshops on teenage pregnancy, breast self-examinations, high blood pressure screening, and sickle cell anemia screening. Plans and implements an annual youth forum under the auspices of the March of Dimes Birth Defects Foundation . Provides youth with professional guidance and the opportunity for peer exchange in the areas of mental and physical health; deals with the health of newborns, health services, nutrition, and teenage pregnancy. Also conducts programs for youth on parenting, socially transmitted diseases, nutrition, birth defects, and continued education after pregnancy. **Awards:** Alma Wells Givens Scholarship (annual) to medical students; Omega Mason Memorial Scholarship to outstanding student nurses.

★ 13213 ★ Batten Disease Support and Research Association (BDSRA)
120 Humphries Dr., Ste. 2
Reynoldsburg, OH 43068
Phone: (740)927-4298 **Free:** 800-448-4570
Email: bdsra1@bdsra.org
Website: http://www.bdsra.org
Lance W. Johnson, Exec. Dir.

Desc: Families of children afflicted with Batten Disease; health care professionals; interested others. (Batten Disease, is a degenerative neurological disease affecting children, causing seizures, dementia, loss of motor skills, and blindness.) Represents the interest of individuals with Batten; seeks to educate the public and professional community concerning the needs of Battens Disease patients. Provides information and referral services. Conducts support group activities. Maintains registry. **Awards:** Batten Disease Research (annual) for pertinent research.

★ 13214 ★ Benign Essential Blepharospasm Research Foundation (BEBRF)
PO Box 12468
Beaumont, TX 77726-2468
Phone: (409)832-0788 **Fax:** (409)832-0890
Email: bebrf@ih2000.net
Website: http://www.blepharospasm.org/
Bob Campbell, Contact

Desc: Victims of benign essential blepharospasm (BEB), a rare disorder of unknown cause characterized by an involuntary forcible closure of the eyelids. Purpose is to undertake, promote, and develop research into the cause and cure of BEB and related disorders and infirmities of the facial musculature, such as Meige's Syndrome (involving muscle spasms of the eyes, lower face, mouth, tongue, throat, and respiratory system). Seeks to foster public awareness of the disorder in order to guarantee detection at the onset of symptoms. Encourages continuity and cooperation among neurologists, neuro-ophthalmologists, ophthalmologists, plastic surgeons, psychologists, psychiatrists, and other medical professionals in rendering correct diagnoses, implementing effective treatment, improving surgical procedure, and discovering a cure. Organizes seminars, clinical studies, and other programs in continuing education; sponsors fundraising activities. Endeavors to locate sufferers of the disorder and to compile data in order to determine the incidence of BEB and to advise on available treatment. Carries out research activities in areas such as brain tissue collection and experimental treatments. **Awards:** Grant (annual) for research.

★ 13215 ★ Bill and Melinda Gates Foundation
PO Box 23350
Seattle, WA 98102
Phone: (206)709-3140
Email: libraryinfo@gatesfoundation.org
Website: http://www.gatesfoundation.org
Richard Akeroyd, Exec. Dir.

Desc: Strives to help improve people's lives through health and learning and looks for strategic opportunities to extend the benefits of modern science and technology to people around the world. **Awards:** Grant.

★ 13216 ★ Biomagnetic Therapy Association (BTA)
PO Box 394
Lyons, CO 80540
Phone: (303)823-0307
Email: info@biomagnetic.org
Website: http://www.biomagnetic.org
Suzy Balliett, Contact

Desc: Health care professionals and other individuals with an interest in biomagnetic therapy. Biomagnetic therapy is the art and science of applying and removing magnetic fields for health benefits. Seeks to advance the study and practice of biomagnetic therapy; promotes increased use of biomagnetic therapy in the treatment of a wide variety of disorders. Serves as a clearinghouse on biomagnetic and related therapies; conducts continuing professional education programs; sponsors research. **Awards:** William Philpott (annual) to member.

★ 13217 ★ Blind Service Association (BSA)
22 W Monroe, 11th Fl.
Chicago, IL 60603
Phone: (312)236-0808 **Fax:** (312)236-8679
Email: blindsrvc@aol.com
Debbie Grossman, Exec. Dir.

Desc: Organization that has supported the independence of blind and partially blind Chicago residents since 1924. The association maintains reading rooms for daily oral readings of textbooks and work-related material primarily to blind students, senior citizens, and business and professional people; records textbooks on cassette tapes for blind people's home, study, work and leisure needs; supplies visual aids, field trips, and other assistance to blind and visually handicapped children in Chicago, IL schools; operates senior program and a consortium of blind computer users. **Awards:** Grant for blind college students; Harry G. Hershenson Memorial Award for outstanding contribution to blind people; scholarship (annual).

★ 13218 ★ Blinded Veterans Association (BVA)
477 H St. NW
Washington, DC 20001
Phone: (202)371-8880 **Free:** 800-669-7079
Fax: (202)371-8258
Email: bva@bva.org
Website: http://www.bva.org
Thomas H. Miller, Exec. Dir.

Desc: Veterans who lost their sight as a result of military service in the armed forces of the U.S.; associate members are veterans whose loss of sight was not connected with military service. Assists blinded veterans in attaining benefits and employment and with reestablishing themselves as adjusted, active, and productive citizens in their communities. Offers placement service; supports research programs; compiles statistics. Constructs initiatives designed to improve blind rehabilitation programs for veterans. **Awards:** Kathern F. Gruber Scholarship (annual) for spouses and dependent children of blinded veterans; Major General Melvin T. Maas Achievement Award (annual) for service-connected blinded veteran.

★ 13219 ★ Boston International Foundation for Medical Exchange
c/o Joseph J. Vitale, MD
784 Massachusetts Ave.
Boston, MA 02118-2317
Phone: (617)414-4829
Email: jjvitale@bu.edu
Website: http://www.bifme.org
Joseph J. Vitale, Chm.

Desc: Supports senior medical students, medical and surgical residents and junior faculty from Harvard, Tufts and Boston University, who successfully complete a minimum two to six month elective at a foreign medical center acceptable to the respective medical school administration and the foundation. Support is intended to defray travel and living expenses. Believes this experience provides useful and practical insight into cultural, moral and ethnic perceptions of health care in our multi-ethnic and multi-cultural society. **Awards:** Scholarship (3/year) 4th year medical student completing a 2-3 month overseas elective.

★ 13220 ★ Brain Injury Association of America
105 N Alfred St.
Alexandria, VA 22314
Phone: (703)236-6000 **Free:** 800-444-6443
Fax: (703)236-6001
Email: publicrelations@biausa.org
Website: http://www.biausa.org/Pages/splash.html
Allan I. Bergman, Pres. & CEO

Desc: National organization working for and with people with brain injury and their families. Seeks to create a better future through brain injury prevention, research, education and advocacy. **Awards:** Founders Award (annual) for outstanding contributions in building and strengthening the BIA, enabling it to fulfill its mission; Jim and Sarah Brady Public Service Award (annual) for an individual who has enhanced the understanding of brain injury through public service and education at the national level; Sheldon Berrol Clinical Service Award (annual) for individual who, through clinical service, has made outstanding contributions to improving quality of care, professional training, and/or education; Silvio O. Conte Award (annual) for outstanding contributions in affecting national policy as it relates to brain injury; William Fields Caveness Award (annual) for individual who, through research, has made outstanding contributions toward bettering the lives of persons who have sustained traumatic brain injuries; a cash award of $2,000 is given to further the work of the recipient; Young Investigator Award (annual) for an individual within five years of completing professional training.

★ 13221 ★ The Brain Tumor Society (TBTS)
124 Watertown St., Ste. 3-H
Watertown, MA 02472
Phone: (617)924-9997 **Free:** 800-770-8287
Fax: (617)924-9998
Email: info@tbts.org
Website: http://www.tbts.org
Neal P. Levitan, Exec. Dir.

Desc: Strives to improve the quality of life of brain tumor patients by providing support for them and their families. Raises funds for research in order to find a cure for brain tumors. **Awards:** Grant (annual) for scientific research.

★ 13222 ★ Cancer Federation (CFI)
PO Box 1298
Banning, CA 92220-0009
Phone: (909)849-4325 **Free:** 800-207-2873
Fax: (909)849-0156
Email: cancerfederation@yahoo.com
Website: http://www.cancerfed.com
Karen Alene, Admin.

Desc: Physicians, scientists, nurses, and laymen (both cancer patients and nonpatients). Promotes research and education in the field of cancer immunology. Seeks to discover appropriate cancer therapies using natural biological modifiers. Funds research at major centers throughout the U.S., including the University of California (Riverside and Santa Barbara), University of Hawaii, and University of Pittsburgh, on biological modifiers, such as lymphokines; killer cells; Interleukin I and II; diet; and psychological aspects of cancer. Compiles statistics; conducts research and education in cancer therapy, including vaccines, and in psychological programming for patients. Offers counseling program for cancer patients and their families. Sponsors public medical conferences and in-service courses for nurses on the psychology of cancer, and research projects at many universities and hospitals in the field of immunology. Sponsors charitable program. **Awards:** Scholarship (annual) for high school and college seniors in the field of microbiology; Science, Communication, and Service Awards (annual).

★ 13223 ★ Cancer Research Foundation of America

1600 Duke St., Ste. 110
Alexandria, VA 22314
Phone: (703)836-4412 **Free:** 800-227-2732
Fax: (703)836-4413
Website: http://www.preventcancer.org

Desc: Foundations, individuals and companies. Aims to prevent cancer through research and education. Sponsors grants and fellowships, publishes educational materials. **Awards:** Fellowship; grant.

★ 13224 ★ Catholic Association of Persons With Visual Impairment (CAPVI)

c/o Msgr. Paul M. Lackner
111 Perrymont Ave.
Pittsburgh, PA 15237
Phone: (412)687-1409 **Fax:** (212)826-8377
Msgr. Paul Lackner, Pres.

Desc: To assist, support, and further the vocational, spiritual, and social integration of blind and visually impaired persons in local parishes and in the community. CAPVI focuses on: raising awareness of the ability and spiritual needs, promotes active participation in the spiritual and social life of the church and within the community; exchanges ideas, resources and other pertinent information, assists in obtaining religious material in accessible format; and works toward establishing programs within dioceses to serve this group. activities; instructs volunteers to act as guides. Assists in obtaining audiotapes and religious materials printed in Braille and large type. large type. A national CAPVI office is open in New York City. **Awards:** Koch Foundation (annual).

★ 13225 ★ CFIDS Association of America

PO Box 220398
Charlotte, NC 28222-0398
Free: 800-442-3437 **Fax:** (704)365-9755
Email: cfids@cfids.org
Website: http://www.cfids.org
Jon Sterling, Chm.

Desc: Individuals with chronic fatigue and immune dysfunction syndrome (chronic viral illness associated with dysfunction of the immune system; formerly called chronic Epstein-Barr virus); doctors, nurses, and government officials. Advocates continued research into the cause and cure of the syndrome. Funds pilot medical research projects. **Awards:** Grant for research.

★ 13226 ★ Chi Eta Phi Sorority

3029 13th St. NW
Washington, DC 20009
Phone: (202)232-3858 **Fax:** (202)232-3460
Email: chietaphi@erols.com
Website: http://www.chietaphi.com
Carolyn Mosley, Pres.

Desc: Professional sorority - registered and student nurses. Objectives are to: encourage continuing education; stimulate friendship among members; develop working relationships with other professional groups for the improvement and delivery of health care services. Sponsors leadership training seminars every two years and holds additional seminars at the local, regional, and national levels. Offers educational programs for entrance into nursing and allied health fields. Maintains health screening and consumer health education programs; volunteers assistance to senior citizens; sponsors recruitment and retention programs for minority students in nursing. Operates speakers' bureau on health education. **Awards:** Scholarship students.

★ 13227 ★ Childhood Brain Tumor Foundation

20312 Watkins Meadow Dr.
Germantown, MD 20876
Phone: (301)515-2900 **Free:** 877-217-4166
Email: cbtf@childhoodbraintumor.org
Website: http://www.childhoodbraintumor.org/
Jeanne Young, Pres.

Desc: Committed to raising funds for scientific research and public awareness of brain tumors in children; works to improve prognosis and quality of life. **Awards:** Grant (annual).

★ 13228 ★ Children of Deaf Adults (CODA)

Box 30715
Santa Barbara, CA 93130
Phone: (805)682-0997 **Fax:** (617)789-3801
Email: coda@coda-international.org
Website: http://www.coda-international.org
Millie Brother, Founder

Desc: Hearing children of deaf parents who are interested in sharing experiences with others of similar backgrounds. Provides information to professional organizations, libraries, community agencies, researchers, and other interested persons. Acts upon issues regarding deafness; provides support to deaf parent/hearing child families. Serves as clearinghouse for deaf parent/hearing children families. **Awards:** Millie Brother Scholarship (annual).

★ 13229 ★ Children's Brain Tumor Foundation (CBTF)

274 Madison Ave., No. 1301
New York, NY 10016
Phone: (212)448-9494 **Free:** (866)228-HOPE
Fax: (212)448-1022
Email: info@cbtf.org
Website: http://www.cbtf.org
Judy Hurley, Exec. Dir.

Desc: Works to improve the outlook for children with brain and spinal cord tumors. Raises funds for research; provides counseling, education and support services for families and survivors. **Awards:** Fellowship for young physicians studying pediatric neuro-oncology; grant for research scientists.

★ 13230 ★ Children's Leukemia Research Association (NLA)

585 Stewart Ave., Ste. LL18
Garden City, NY 11530
Phone: (516)222-1944 **Fax:** (516)222-0457
Email: clra@erols.com
Website: http://www.childrensleukemia.org/
Allan D. Weinberg, Exec. Dir.

Desc: Promotes leukemia research and public awareness of the disease. Provides financial aid to leukemia patients and their families, based on need. **Awards:** Grant (annual) for research; recognition.

★ 13231 ★ Children's PKU Network (CPN)

3790 Via De La Valle, Ste. 120
Del Mar, CA 92014
Phone: (858)509-0767 **Free:** 800-377-6677
Fax: (858)509-0768
Email: pkunetwork@aol.com
Website: http://www.pkunetwork.org

Desc: Works to address the special needs of all people involved in the treatment of Phenylketonuria (PKU), a genetic metabolic disease whereby the body is unable to process the amino acid phenyalanine. Networks families and individuals with each other; provides discount dietary aids; offers financial assistance and support groups; provides crisis intervention; advocates mandatory guidelines for insurance carriers to cover expenses of medical food treatment of PKU individuals; conducts fundraisers; endows research benefiting PKU and other metabolic disorders. **Awards:** Children's PKU Network Annual Scholarship (annual) students with PKU.

★ 13232 ★ Chinese American Medical Society (CAMS)

c/o Dr. H.H. Wang
281 Edgewood Ave.
Teaneck, NJ 07666
Phone: (201)833-1506 **Fax:** (201)833-8252
Email: hw5@columbia.edu
Website: http://www.camsociety.org
Dr. Daisy Saw, MD, Pres.

Desc: Physicians of Chinese origin residing in the U.S. and Canada. Seeks to advance medical knowledge, scientific research, and interchange of information among members and to promote the health status of Chinese Americans. Conducts educational meetings; supports research. Maintains placement service. Sponsors limited charitable program. **Awards:** Scholarship (annual); Scientific Award (annual) for member with highest scholastic achievements.

★ 13233 ★ Christian Pharmacists Fellowship International (CPFI)

PO Box 1717
501 5th St.
Bristol, TN 37621-1717
Phone: (423)764-6000 **Free:** 888-253-6885
Fax: (423)764-4490
Email: info@cpfi.org
Website: http://www.cpfi.org
Allan Sharp, P.D., Admin. Dir.

Desc: To promote and maintain fellowship among Christian pharmacists. Establishes clubs and chapters at universities, colleges, schools, hospitals, and in communities; sponsors activities and retreats for Christian pharmacists and their families. Encourages active Christian witness and evangelism; teaches pharmacists how to share and present the Gospel of Jesus Christ in their practice; disseminates information among Christian pharmacists; identifies areas of service for pharmacists in missions worldwide and sponsors missionaries in the field. Provides and promotes Christian pharmacist-speakers. speakers at state and national pharmacy meetings. **Awards:** Scholarship Award (annual).

★ 13234 ★ Christian Record Services (CRS)

4444 S 52nd St.
Lincoln, NE 68516-1302
Phone: (402)488-0981 **Fax:** (402)488-7582
Email: info@christianrecord.org
Website: http://www.christianrecord.org
Ron Bowes, Contact

Desc: Assists blind, visually impaired individuals. Sponsors Bible correspondence courses. Representatives visit about 40,000 blind people annually. Conducts glaucoma screening clinics in cooperation with local physicians and organizations; provides home visitation program. Sponsors National Camps for Blind Children; maintains speakers' bureau. **Awards:** Scholarship bestowed to qualified individuals who cannot obtain finacial assistance from other sources.

★ 13235 ★ Christopher Reeve Paralysis Foundation

500 Morris Ave.
Springfield, NJ 07081
Phone: (973)379-2690 **Free:** 800-225-0292
Fax: (973)912-9433
Website: http://www.christopherreeve.org
David R. Landrey, Chair/Exec. Committee

Desc: Seeks to encourage and support research to find a cure for paralysis caused by spinal cord injury and other central nervous system disorders. **Awards:** Grant to research laboratories and individuals for postgraduate study; grant to physicians and scientists conducting research on the spinal cord and central nervous system.

★ 13236 ★ Cleft Palate Foundation

104 S Estes Dr., Ste. 204
Chapel Hill, NC 27514-2866
Phone: (919)933-9044 **Free:** 800-242-5338
Fax: (919)933-9604
Email: info@cleftline.org
Website: http://www.cleftline.org
Nancy C. Smythe, Exec. Dir.

Desc: Enhances the quality of life for individuals with facial birth defects through education, research support, and facilitation of family-centered care. Provides research programs and information services. **Awards:** Parent-Patient Leadership Award (annual) outstanding contribution by individual or parent affected by facial birth defects.

★ 13237 ★ Clinical Immunology Society (CIS)

611 E Wells St.
Milwaukee, WI 53202
Phone: (414)224-8095 **Fax:** (414)272-6070
Email: cis@execinc.com
Website: http://www.clinimmsoc.org
Lynda J. Patterson, CAE, Exec. Dir.

Desc: Investigators and clinicians concerned with immunologic diseases. Promotes research on: the causes and mechanisms of immunologic diseases; improved treatment, evaluation, and prevention of diseases related to immunity. Facilitates exchange of ideas and findings; fosters excellence in research and medical practice. Works to increase public awareness and knowledge of immunologically-mediated diseases. Conducts scientific, educational programs. **Awards:** CIS Science Recognition Award for New Investigators (annual) based on abstract submissions.

★ 13238 ★ Clinical Laboratory Management Association (CLMA)

989 Old Eagle School Rd., Ste. 815
Wayne, PA 19087
Phone: (610)995-9580 **Fax:** (610)995-9568
Email: rneri@lcma.org
Website: http://www.clma.org
Robert A. Neri, Exec. VP

Desc: Individuals holding managerial or supervisory positions with clinical laboratories; persons engaged in education of such individuals; manufacturers or distributors of equipment or services to clinical laboratories. Objectives are: to enhance management skills and promote more efficient and productive department operations; to further exchange of professional knowledge, new technology, and colleague experience; to encourage cooperation among those engaged in management or supervisory functions. Activities include: workshops, seminars, and expositions; dissemination of information about legislation and other topics. **Awards:** Chapter of the Year (annual); Educational Scholarship (annual); Industry Awards (annual); Sterling Service (annual).

★ 13239 ★ Clinical Ligand Assay Society (CLAS)

3139 S Wayne Rd.
Wayne, MI 48184
Phone: (734)722-6290 **Fax:** (734)722-7006
Email: clas@clas.org
Website: http://www.clas.org
Daisy S. McCann, PhD, Exec. Dir.

Desc: Seeks to establish and promote high standards in the science and application of ligand assay technology by encouraging research, education practitioners, and fostering communication and cooperation among individuals in laboratories in medicine, academia, and industry. Sponsors job placement service. **Awards:** CLAS Distinguished Scientist Award (semiannual) distinguished record in ligand assay technology.

★ 13240 ★ Clinical Magnetic Resonance Society (CMRS)

4550 Post Oak Pl., Ste. 342
Houston, TX 77027
Phone: (713)623-8336 **Free:** 877-841-2522
Fax: (713)960-0488
Email: cmrs@one.net
Website: http://www.cmrs.com
Darcee Brown, Acct. Exec.

Desc: Offers experience-based credentialing for physicians who practice MRI. Provides a forum for networking among members. Defines procedure protocols and safety information. **Awards:** Recognition (annual); scholarship (annual) for physicians in training.

★ 13241 ★ Cochlear Implant Association

5335 Wisconsin Ave. NW, Ste. 440
Washington, DC 20015-2052
Phone: (202)895-2781 **Fax:** (202)895-2782
Email: info@cici.org
Website: http://www.cici.org
John McCelland, Pres.

Desc: Cochlear implant users, candidates for cochlear implant, and their families and friends; health care professionals. Provides support services including advocacy for the hearing impaired. Promotes improved cochlear implant technology and research on hearing impairment. Serves as an information clearinghouse. Conducts educational programs and childrens' services; operates speakers' bureau. **Awards:** Dr. Bill House (biennial) child who overcomes his/her hearing loss and shows good response to cochlear implant.

★ 13242 ★ Complementary Medicine Association (CMA)

c/o Mary Wolken
4649 E Malvern
Tucson, AZ 85711-4249
Fax: (520)323-0264
Email: compmeded@aol.com
Website: http://www.compmed.com
Mary Wolken, Exec. Dir.

Desc: Provides education and supports cooperation between all medical disciplines. Fosters and teaches cost effective and more natural systems of medicine to professionals and the public. Focuses on homeopathic, acupuncture, herbal medicines, kinesiology and learning/memory improvement research and education. **Awards:** AIDS Education (annual).

★ 13243 ★ Concern Foundation

8383 Wilshire Blvd., Ste. 337
Beverly Hills, CA 90211
Phone: (310)724-5333 **Fax:** (310)858-1474
Email: info@concernfoundation.org
Website: http://www.concernfoundation.org/

Desc: Dedicated to funding basic cancer research. **Awards:** Grant to independent investigators.

★ 13244 ★ Consultant Dietitians in Health Care Facilities (CDHCF)

2219 Cardinal Dr.
Waterloo, IA 50701
Phone: (319)235-0991 **Fax:** (319)235-7224
Email: cdhcf@cdhcf.org
Website: http://www.cdhcf.org
Marolyn Steffani, RD, LD, Chm.

Desc: A special interest group of the American Dietetic Association. Dietitians employed in extended care facilities, nursing homes, homecare, and a variety of food service operations. Disseminates information; assists in solving their problems in the field. Conducts workshops; offers networking opportunities for professionals. **Awards:** CDHCF Horizon Award (annual); CDHCF Scholarship Award (annual); Gaynold Jenson Education Stipend (annual).

★ 13245 ★ Contact Lens Association of Ophthalmologists (CLAO)

c/o John S. Massare, PhD
721 Papworth Ave., Ste. 206
Metairie, LA 70005
Phone: (504)835-3937 **Fax:** (504)833-5884
Email: eyes@clao.org
Website: http://www.clao.org
John S. Massare, PhD, Exec. Dir.

Desc: To advance quality medical eyecare for the public by providing comprehensive ophthalmologists and other eye care professionals with education and training in contact lenses, refractive surgery, and related eyecare science. **Awards:** Grant bestowed to residents for traveling.

★ 13246 ★ Cooley's Anemia Foundation (CAF)

129-09 26th Ave., No. 203
Flushing, NY 11354
Phone: (718)321-2873 **Free:** 800-522-7222
Fax: (718)321-3340
Email: info@cooleysanemia.org
Website: http://www.cooleysanemia.org
Jayne Restivo, National Exec. Dir.

Desc: Dedicated to advancing the treatment and cure of Coley's Anemia (also known as Thalassemia). Conducts national programs that provide medical research patient services, awareness and education. Sponsors the Thalassemia Action Group, a support group for patients and families. Provides information about the condition referrals to local medical sources, brochures, newsletters and other information. Provides medical supplies to patients in need. anemia or other thalassemias. Sponsors Thalassemia Action Group, a networking task force of young adult victims of thalassemia. Operates speakers' bureau. Conducts blood drives. **Awards:** Fellowship Grant (annual) for fellowships and innovative and promising research projects; Humanitarian Achievement; Patient Scholarship (annual) for patients pursuing undergraduate and graduate degrees; recognition for scientific and humanitarian achievement.

★ 13247 ★ Council of Citizens With Low Vision (CCLV)

c/o American Council of the Blind
1155 15th St. NW, Ste. 1004
Washington, DC 20005
Phone: (202)467-5081 **Free:** 800-733-2258
Email: badkron@aol.com
Website: http://www.cclvi.org
Ken Stewart, Pres.

Desc: Partially sighted and low-vision individuals, their families, and professional workers. Provides a vehicle through which partially sighted people may voice their needs, preferences, and interests. Promotes the concept that partially sighted and low-vision individuals are not blind and that they have the right to maximize the use of residual vision through the use of any visual aid, service, or technology. Keeps abreast of all developments benefiting partially sighted persons. Promotes educational, engineering, medical, rehabilitative, scientific, and social research that facilitates the lives of individuals with residual vision. Supports the development of pre-service professional training programs for the establishment and expansion of multidisciplinary low-vision services. Strives to educate the public about the existence, capabilities, and needs of such individuals. Establishes outreach programs to insure access to available services for partially sighted persons. Maintains speakers' bureau. **Awards:** Carl Foley Scholarship (annual); Telesensory Scholarship (annual).

★ 13248 ★ Crohn's and Colitis Foundation of America (CCFA)

386 Park Ave. S, 17th Fl.
New York, NY 10016-8804
Phone: (212)685-3440 **Free:** 800-932-2423
Fax: (212)779-4098
Email: info@ccfa.org

Website: http://www.ccfa.org
Rodger L. DeRose, CEO

Desc: Supports research to find the cause and cure of Crohn's Disease (ileitis) and ulcerative colitis. Provides educational programs for patients, physicians, and the public, support groups, chapter newsletters, a national magazine, informational brochures and books, professional medical forums, and research publications, and a website. **Awards:** Research Fellowship (semiannual) for training; Research Grant (semiannual) for research.

★ 13249 ★ Cyclic Vomiting Syndrome Association USA/Canada (CVS)

3585 Cedar Hill Rd. NW
Canal Winchester, OH 43110
Phone: (614)837-2586 **Fax:** (614)837-2586
Email: waitesd@cvsaonline.org
Website: http://www.cvsaonline.org/
Debra Waites, Exec. Dir.

Desc: Provides patients, families and professionals opportunities to offer and receive support and share knowledge about CVS; promotes research. **Awards:** Joan Butta Burkhardt Fund.

★ 13250 ★ Cystic Fibrosis Foundation (CFF)

6931 Arlington Rd.
Bethesda, MD 20814
Phone: (301)951-4422 **Free:** 800-344-4823
Fax: (301)951-6378
Email: info@cff.org
Website: http://www.cff.org
Robert J. Beall, PhD, Pres. & CEO

Desc: Supports medical research, professional education, and care centers to benefit patients with cystic fibrosis (CF), an inherited fatal disease among children and adults. With this disease a thick mucus clogs the lungs, creating breathing difficulties and high susceptibility to infection; the digestive system and other organs are also affected. More than 113 care centers affiliated with the foundation provide patient services. Medical programs provide support for a national network of multidisciplinary basic and clinical research grants. **Awards:** Fellowship for clinical or research training, professional education, accreditation, and development of treatment centers; grant for the study and treatment of CF.

★ 13251 ★ Cystinosis Foundation (CF)

604 Vernon St.
Oakland, CA 94610
Free: 800-392-8458 **Fax:** (209)222-7997
Email: jd2hotz@qnis.net
Website: http://www.cystinosisfoundation.org
Jean Hotz, Pres.

Desc: Parents, relatives, and friends of cystinotic children; interested members of the medical community and the public. (Cystinosis is a genetic metabolic disease in which abnormal amounts of the amino acid cystine collect in the cells, leading to kidney failure.) Purposes are to increase public awareness about cystinosis; to act as a support group to parents of children with the disease; to raise funds for research. Maintains speakers' bureau. **Awards:** Grant for research; Volunteer of the Year Award.

★ 13252 ★ Deafness Research Foundation (DRF)

1050 17th St. NW, Ste701
Washington, DC 20036
Phone: (202)289-5850 **Free:** 800-829-5934
Fax: (202)293-1805
Email: drf@drf.org
Website: http://www.drf.org
Kromeklia Bryant, Off. Mgr.

Desc: Participates in the National Temporal Bone and Balance Pathology Resource Registry Program of the National Institute on Deafness and Other Communication Disorders. Approximately 1000 physicians and other professionals in ear medicine and research and 52 medical societies underwrite the foundation's fundraising costs through membership in the Centurions of the Deafness Research Foundation; approximately 300 other interested individuals raise funds through membership in the Deafness Research Foundation Alliance. **Awards:** Otologic Fellowship (annual) for third-year medical students to allow research for one year; Otologic Research Grant (annual) for 1-3 years of support to promising new research projects related to hearing disorders and ear diseases.

★ 13253 ★ Delta Society (DS)

580 Naches Ave. SW, No. 101
Renton, WA 98055
Phone: (425)226-7357 **Fax:** (425)235-1076
Email: info@deltasociety.org
Website: http://www.deltasociety.org
Michelle Cobey, Contact

Desc: Doctors, nurses, veterinarians, therapists, nursing home personnel, animal trainers and breeders, pet owners, academicians, and students of gerontology, psychology, therapeutic recreation, and other health fields. Assesses the role of animal companions in society and the effect of human-animal interaction on the mental and physical well-being of people. Seeks to establish an interdisciplinary approach to studying human-animal interactions, and to increase awareness of these interactions among health and social care professionals. Provides training to for persons seeking to establish and maintain programs that involve animals in animal-assisted activities/therapy. Operates National Service Dog Center serving people with disabilities in conjunction with the American Humane Association; and Pet Partners, a national registration for volunteers and animals involved in programs. Creating Service Dog Education System to train trainers of service dogs. Distributes information on research, programs, and legislation concerning human-animal relationships. Maintains collection of article reprints. **Awards:** Delta Society Beyond Limits Service and Therapy Animals Awards (annual); Harris Sweatt Travel Grant (annual).

★ 13254 ★ Depression and Related Affective Disorders Association (DRADA)

Johns Hopkins Hospital Meyer 3-181
600 N Wolfe St.
Baltimore, MD 21287-7381
Phone: (410)955-4647 **Fax:** (410)614-3241
Email: drada@jhmi.edu
Website: http://www.drada.org
Cathy Pollock, Dir.

Desc: Individuals with affective disorders, their families and friends, and mental health professionals. (Affective disorders include depressive illnesses and manic-depression.) Provides support services including referrals, educational programs, networking, and consultation. Encourages and facilitates the formation of local support groups for those with affective disorders; provides training for support group leaders. Cosponsors with Johns Hopkins annual mood disorders symposium. Maintains speakers' bureau. **Awards:** Scholarship (annual) bestowed to a research student.

★ 13255 ★ Diabetes Action Research and Education Foundation

426 C St. NE
Washington, DC 20002
Website: http://www.daref.org/
Pat DeVoe, Pres.

Desc: Works to improve quality of life for those affected by diabetes and its complications. **Awards:** Grant to medical experts and researchers.

★ 13256 ★ Diabetes Exercise and Sports Association (DESA)

PO Box 1935
Litchfield Park, AZ 85340
Phone: (623)535-4593 **Free:** 800-898-4322
Fax: (623)535-4741
Email: desa@diabetes-exercise.org
Website: http://www.diabetes-exercise.org
Paula Harper, RN, CDE, Pres.

Desc: Individuals with diabetes and healthcare professionals. Promotes the participation of individuals with diabetes in sports activities. Provides a network and support group for athletes with diabetes. Conducts educational programs to increase self care skills for individuals with diabetes and counseling skills for healthcare professionals. Offers blood sugar screenings; sponsors volunteer services and speakers' bureau. Conducts children's services. **Awards:** Lifescan Prize for Athletic Achievement (annual) athletic achievements, potential for further success in endeavors potential for grant to assist in goal, how prize will be used to promote value of exercise for people w/ diabetes.

★ 13257 ★ Donald W. Reynolds Foundation

1701 Village Center Cir.
Las Vegas, NV 89134
Phone: (702)804-6000 **Fax:** (702)804-6099
Email: generalquestions@dwrf.org
Website: http://www.dwreynolds.org

Desc: Works to provide support for cardiovascular clinical research and aging and quality of life programs. **Awards:** Grant.

★ 13258 ★ Drug Information Association (DIA)

800 Enterprise Rd., Ste. 200
Horsham, PA 19044
Phone: (215)442-6100 **Fax:** (215)442-6199
Email: dia@diahome.org
Website: http://www.diahome.org
Joseph R. Assenzo, PhD, Exec. Dir.

Desc: Provides neutral, global forum promoting exchange of information critical to professional performance and achievement in the discovery, development, regulation, surveillance, or marketing of pharmaceuticals or related products. **Awards:** Research Award Grant (annual).

★ 13259 ★ Dysautonomia Foundation

633 3rd Ave., 12th Fl.
New York, NY 10017
Phone: (212)949-6644 **Fax:** (212)682-7625
Email: dys212@aol.com
Website: http://www.familialdysautonomia.org/
Lenore F. Roseman, Exec. Dir.

Desc: Parents, relatives, friends, and benefactors of children afflicted with Familial dysautonomia, a Jewish genetic disease of the autonomic nervous system. Now that the FD Gene has been located and there is a carrier available, we must now fund research into discovering the function the gene plays within the body. **Awards:** Research Grants (annual) for post doctoral research into FD.

★ 13260 ★ Dystonia Medical Research Foundation

1 E Wacker Dr., Ste. 2430
Chicago, IL 60601-1905
Phone: (312)755-0198 **Free:** 800-377-DYST
Fax: (312)803-0138
Email: dystonia@dystonia-foundation.org
Website: http://www.dystonia-foundation.org
Robert McAlister, PhD., Exec. Dir.

Desc: Dystonia patients and their families; medical personnel; health agencies; interested individuals. Promotes and funds research and encourages increased public awareness of dystonia, a neurologic muscular disorder causing muscles to jerk and contract into abnormal positions. Disseminates information concerning dystonia. Sponsors patient and family support groups. **Awards:** Research Grant (annual) Dystonia research.

★ 13261 ★ Dystrophic Epidermolysis Bullosa Research Association of America (DEBRA)
5 W 36th St., No. 404
New York, NY 10018
Phone: (212)868-1573 **Free:** (866)332-7276
Fax: (212)868-9296
Email: debra.nurse@mindspring.com
Website: http://www.debra.org
Martin Hassner, Exec. Dir.

Desc: People with Epidermolysis Bullosa and their families; other interested individuals. (Epidermolysis Bullosa represents a group of inherited disorders of the skin characterized by formation of blisters resulting from the most minimal trauma.) To raise funds to promote and support research into the cause, nature, and treatment of EB in all its forms; to relieve the physical and mental distress of victims by providing practical advice, guidance, support, and other assistance. Distributes educational material to the public and medical professionals. Works for federal funding for biomedical research of EB and related disorders. Offers children's services; conducts educational programs. conducts educational programs. **Awards:** Debra Research Grants (annual) scientific research in EB.

★ 13262 ★ Ear Foundation (EF)
1817 Patterson St.
Nashville, TN 37203
Phone: (615)627-2724 **Fax:** (615)627-2728
Email: earfound@earfoundation.org
Website: http://www.theearfound.com
Suzane Wyatt, Exec. Dir.

Desc: Benefactors dedicated to advance medical knowledge concerning ear diseases and to encourage public understanding of such disorders. Offers professional and public education programs; research directed towards Eustachian tube disorders, ear diseases, and related disorders such as hearing loss, tinnitus, and vertigo. **Awards:** Minnie Pearl Scholarship.

★ 13263 ★ Elizabeth Glaser Pediatric AIDS Foundation
2950 31st St., No. 125
Santa Monica, CA 90405
Phone: (310)314-1459 **Free:** 888-499-HOPE
Fax: (310)314-1469
Email: info@pedaids.org
Website: http://www.pedaids.org

Desc: Devoted to pediatric AIDS research leading to new/better treatments and prevention of HIV infection in infants and children, to reduce and prevent HIV transmission from mother to child. **Awards:** Elizabeth Glaser Scientist Award (annual) to outstanding scientists; Research Grants (1 & 2 year) to investigators; Scholar Awards to young investigators; Short-Term Awards for travel and short-term study at U.S. institution; Student Intern Award to students.

★ 13264 ★ Elton John AIDS Foundation (EJAIDSF)
PO Box 17139
Beverly Hills, CA 90209-3139
Phone: (310)535-1775
Email: AmgejAIDSF@ejaf.org
Website: http://ejaf.org
Alexandra Crane, Contact

Desc: Individuals and organizations. Promotes increased access to, and improved quality of, patient care services for people with AIDS. Provides financial assistance to AIDS care programs and prevention projects; conducts fundraising activities. **Awards:** Service and Prevention Grants (quarterly).

★ 13265 ★ Emergency Nurses Association (ENA)
915 Lee St.
Des Plaines, IL 60016
Phone: 800-900-9659 **Free:** 800-243-8362
Fax: (847)460-4001
Email: enainfo@ena.org
Website: http://www.ena.org
Donna Nowakowski, Exec. Dir.

Desc: Registered nurses, licensed practical nurses, and licensed vocational nurses; emergency medical technicians or nurses and members of allied health fields engaged or interested in emergency patient care. Objectives are: to promote emergency nursing and to establish standards in the field; to work with other health-related organizations toward the improvement of emergency care; to serve as a resource for emergency nursing education and research. Seeks to identify and address emergency nursing issues. Disseminates educational and research information in the field. Sponsors: Emergency Nursing Core Curriculum; Standards of Emergency Nursing Practice; Emergency Nursing Pediatric Course; Trauma Nursing Core Course; Concepts in Advanced Trauma Nursing Course. **Awards:** Grant (annual); recognition (annual) for contributions of members; scholarship (annual).

★ 13266 ★ Entertainment Industries Council (EIC)
c/o Government Liaison and Administrative Office
1760 Reston Pky., Ste. 415
Reston, VA 20190-3303
Phone: (703)481-1414 **Fax:** (703)481-1418
Email: eic@eiconline.org
Website: http://eiconline.org
Brian Dyak, Pres.

Desc: Corporations and representatives of the entertainment industry including actors, agents, publicists, producers, directors, and writers. Goal is to utilize the power and influence of the entertainment industry in a national campaign to combat and deglamorize substance abuse, especially among young people. Seeks to identify and provide celebrity role models for young people. Hopes to increase youth awareness of drug abuse through television, radio, music, and motion pictures. Develops projects to aid in eliminating substance abuse problems within the entertainment industry. Conducts seminars and training sessions on drug abuse prevention; also conducts radio interview series, television specials, outreach programs, and employee assistance and fundraising programs. Collects and disseminates information on progress made by the entertainment industry in drug abuse prevention. In conjunction with IMMEDIA Foundation, coordinates network of 400 radio stations involved in public affairs projects designed to discourage substance abuse. Provides celebrity speakers' bureau on drug prevention, seat belt awareness, and intravenous drug use/AIDS. Bestows EIC Drug Prevention Award annually to a leader from entertainment industry contributing to drug awareness. **Awards:** Prism Awards (annual); Prism Generation Next (annual).

★ 13267 ★ Epilepsy Foundation (EFA)
4351 Garden City Dr.
Landover, MD 20785
Phone: (301)459-3700 **Free:** 800-332-1000
Fax: (301)577-4941
Email: postmaster@efa.org
Website: http://www.epilepsyfoundation.org/
Eric R. Hargis, Pres. /CEO

Desc: National voluntary health agency which serves as the "focal point for the fight against epilepsy in the United States." Augmented by 64 affiliates in the U.S. committed to preventing and controlling epilepsy and improving the lives of those who have it. Provides federal government liaison. The foundation supports medical, social, rehabilitational, legal, employment, and information, education, and advocacy programs. Sponsors research in causes of epilepsy, prevention, psychosocial needs, and improved methods of treatment. Provides research and training grants and fellowships to students and professionals. Assistance and counseling for epilepsy patients and their families is provided through local organizations and the National Information Center on Epilepsy. Annual projects include National Epilepsy Month (November), School Alert (a national educational program for schools), selection of the Epilepsy Poster Child, and a continuing professional and public education and information program. Maintains a resource center. Provides members with access to mail order pharmacy program. Compiles statistics; maintains placement program. **Awards:** Grant (annual) for epilepsy research.

★ 13268 ★ Eye Bank Association of America (EBAA)
1015 18th St., NW, Ste. 1010
Washington, DC 20036
Phone: (202)775-4999 **Fax:** (202)429-6036
Email: patricia@restoresight.org
Website: http://www.restoresight.org
Patricia Aiken-O'Neill, Pres.

Desc: Eye banks working to restore sight through the promotion and advancement of eye banking. Makes possible over 46,000 corneal transplants annually. Establishes standards for the procurement and distribution of eyes and corneal tissue. Offers training and certification programs for eye banking personnel. Compiles statistics; maintains speakers' bureau. Conducts research and educational programs. **Awards:** Gift of Sight Award (annual); Heise Award (annual); Paton Award (annual); Scientific Award (annual).

★ 13269 ★ Facioscapulohumeral (FSH) Society
3 Westwood Rd.
Lexington, MA 02420
Phone: (781)860-0501 **Fax:** (781)860-0599
Email: info@fshsociety.org
Website: http://www.fshsociety.org
Daniel Paul Perez, Pres.

Desc: Individuals, families, and medical and business professionals interested in Facioscapulohumeral Muscular Dystrophy. (FSHD is an inheritable disease that causes a progressive loss of skeletal muscle with weakness of facial, scapular, and upper arm muscles.) Promotes research, solicits contributions and grants, and disperses information on FSHD. Offers support groups, acts as clearinghouse for researchers, clinicians and patients to facilitate participation in FSHD studies. Funds Research on FSHD. **Awards:** Marjorie Bronfman Grant (semiannual) FSHD research; 1 Delta Railroad Construction Fellowship (annual) FSHD Research.

★ 13270 ★ Family Therapy Section of the National Council on Family Relations (FTSNCFR)
3989 Central Ave. NE, No. 550
Minneapolis, MN 55421
Phone: (763)781-9331 **Free:** 888-781-9331
Fax: (763)781-9348
Email: kbriggs@okstate.edu
Website: http://www.oakland.edu/~blume/ncfr/
Kathleen Briggs, Ch.

Desc: A section of the National Council on Family Relations. Practicing family therapists and family therapy supervisors, educators, and researchers. Seeks to improve the practice of family therapy through the development of theory, research, and training. Promotes communication between family therapy researchers and clinicians; functions as a network for family therapy research projects; conducts educational programs. **Awards:** Family Therapy Section Awards (annual) to student members.

★ 13271 ★ Fanconi Anemia Research Fund (FARF)
1801 Willamette St., Ste. 200
Eugene, OR 97401
Phone: (541)687-4658 **Free:** 800-828-4891
Fax: (541)687-0548
Email: info@fanconi.org
Website: http://www.fanconi.org
Mary Ellen Eiler, Exec. Dir.

Desc: Families with children afflicted with Fanconi anemia, a genetic disorder. Seeks to offer support to families, help them network, and keep them apprised of research relating to Fanconi anemia; assists research on this disorder. Operates support group. Conducts fundraising for research through public awareness programs and special projects. Funds research projects. **Awards:** Grant.

★ 13272 ★ Fellowship of Associates of Medical Evangelism (FAME)

PO Box 34800
Indianapolis, IN 46234
Phone: (317)272-5937 **Free:** 800-379-4351
Fax: (317)272-5940
Email: medicalmissions@fameworld.org
Website: http://www.fameworld.org
Rick Wolford, Exec. Dir.

Desc: Builds hospitals and clinics and provides mobile medical units for Christian missionaries outside the U.S.; secures and ships medicine and medical supplies. Conducts charitable programs; maintains speakers' bureau. **Awards:** Scholarship for individuals who have been accepted into medical school and are committed to missionary work.

★ 13273 ★ Flower Essence Society (FES)

PO Box 459
Nevada City, CA 95959
Phone: (530)265-9163 **Free:** 800-736-9222
Fax: (530)265-0584
Email: mail@flowersociety.org
Website: http://www.flowersociety.org
Patricia A. Kaminski, Pres.

Desc: Project of Earth-Spirit Inc. Health centers, holistic health practitioners, and interested individuals. Seeks to increase public awareness of Nature and the evolving spiritual relationship between human beings and the earth. Promotes the use of flower essences as catalysts to health and important tools "for personal and planetary evolution." Seeks to establish a worldwide network among health practitioners and others using flower essences. Encourages intuitive and scientific investigation of the essences and the creation of a center for educational and research programs. Organizes introductory weekends and annual weeklong intensives for professional and lay health practitioners. Sponsors lectures and research, educational, and experimental activities on topics concerning scientific and spiritual approaches to nature, preparation and use of flower essences, practical skills for flower essence practitioners, and recent developments in the field. Maintains library and referral service. Conducts seven-day professional training seminar and wildflower preservation and naturalist program. **Awards:** Scholarship (annual) for our certification program.

★ 13274 ★ Forward Face

317 E 34th St., Ste. 901A
New York, NY 10016
Phone: (212)684-5860 **Fax:** (212)684-5864
Email: linda@forwardface.org
Website: http://www.forwardface.org/
Barbara Robertson, Pres.

Desc: Individuals with craniofacial disorders, their families and friends, and health care professionals. Provides medical, psychological, and financial support services. Facilitates communication and cooperation between patients and health care professionals; operates referral service. Offers workshops; conducts networking activities and children's services; Also includes a support group, Inner Faces, specifically for teenagers and young adults; activities include communications workshops theatre productions and social functions. Operates family assistance fund to assist families with expenses not covered by insurance, such as lodging and transportation. **Awards:** Forward Face (annual) for members; The John McNeil Burns Scholarship (annual) for educational purposes.

★ 13275 ★ Foundation of American College of Health Care Administrators (FACHCA)

300 N Lee St., No. 301
Alexandria, VA 22314-2807
Phone: (703)739-7900 **Free:** 888-88A-CHCA
Fax: (703)739-7901
Email: mtn@achca.org
Website: http://www.achca.org
Mary Tellis-Nayak, Pres. /CEO

Desc: Individuals dedicated to the improvement of the administration of long-term care facilities. Conducts professional training programs and research in administration. **Awards:** Administrator in Training Scholarship (annual) for an administrator-in-training in a long-term care facility; Director of Nursing Award (annual); Research Award (annual) for research pertaining to long-term care.

★ 13276 ★ Foundation for Chiropractic Education and Research (FCER)

380 Wright Rd.
Norwalk, IA 50211
Phone: (515)981-9888 **Free:** 800-622-6309
Fax: (515)981-9427
Email: fcer@fcer.org
Website: http://www.fcer.org
DeAnna L. Beck, Dir.

Desc: Chiropractors and laymen. Provides funding for scientific research and research training that will "enhance the knowledge and practice of chiropractic as a conservative approach to health care restoration, maintenance, and disease prevention." **Awards:** Fellowship for postdoctorate students; grant for research in clinical science; grant for dissertations in biomechanics and public health.

★ 13277 ★ Foundation for Hand Research and Education

8501 Harcourt Rd.
PO Box 80434
Indianapolis, IN 46280-0434
Phone: (317)471-4340 **Free:** 800-888-HAND
Fax: (317)876-0462
Email: information@indianahandcenter.com
Website: http://www.indianahandcenter.com
Tony O'Connell, MALS, Fnd. Mgr.

Desc: Promotes the advancement of hand surgery and research. Aims to improve the quality of life of persons with injuries or disorders of the hands and upper extremities. Conducts educational programs. **Awards:** Research Grant (annual) board certified hand surgeons engaged in research.

★ 13278 ★ Foundation for Ichthyosis and Related Skin Types (FIRST)

650 N Cannon Ave., Ste. 17
Lansdale, PA 19446
Phone: (215)631-1411 **Free:** 800-545-3286
Fax: (215)631-1413
Email: info@scalyskin.org
Website: http://www.scalyskin.org
Jean R. Pickford, Exec. Dir.

Desc: Dedicated to helping persons affected with ichthyosis, a rare genetic skin disease characterized by dry, cracked, scaling and thickened skin, and related diseases. **Awards:** Dermatology Foundation (annual).

★ 13279 ★ Foundation for Physical Therapy (FPT)

c/o American Physical Therapy Association
1111 Fairfax St.
Alexandria, VA 22314-1488
Phone: (703)683-6743 **Free:** 800-875-1378
Fax: (703)684-7343
Email: foundation@apta.org
Website: http://www.apta.org/Foundation
Christine A. Williams, COO

Desc: Supports the physical therapy profession's research needs by funding scientific and clinically-relevant physical therapy research. **Awards:** Doctoral Opportunities for Clinicians and Scholars (annual) for physical therapists who have completed one full year of doctoral coursework.; Research Grants for individuals and groups of researchers to pursue scientifically based and clinically related physical therapy research.

★ 13280 ★ Foundation for Science and Disability (FSD)

236 Grand St.
Morgantown, WV 26501-7509
Phone: (304)293-5201 **Fax:** (304)293-6363
Email: ekeller@wvu.edu
Website: http://www.as.wvu.edu/~scidis/organize/fsd.html
E. C. Keller, Jr., Treas.

Desc: Disabled scientists and interested individuals. Offers consultation and advice concerning problems faced by persons with disabilities in scientific fields. **Awards:** Disabled Graduate Students in Science (annual) for U.S. graduate students with disabilities.

★ 13281 ★ Frontier Nursing Service (FNS)

132 FNS Dr.
Wendover, KY 41775
Phone: (606)672-2317 **Fax:** (606)672-3022
Website: http://www.frontiernursing.org
Barb Gibson, Exec. Asst.

Desc: Provides health care to persons in approximately 1000 square miles of eastern Kentucky using a 40-bed hospital, two primary care centers, three rural health clinics, and a home health agency. Operates Frontier School of Midwifery and Family Nursing. Provides social and ancillary services; conducts research on health services; compiles statistics; offers educational programs. Maintains a hall of fame and museum. **Awards:** Scholarship for nurses in higher education.

★ 13282 ★ Fund for Podiatric Medical Education (FPME)

9312 Old Georgetown Rd.
Bethesda, MD 20814
Phone: (301)581-9200 **Fax:** (301)530-2752
Email: mpgaujean@apma.org
Website: http://www.apma.org/fpme/fundmain.htm
Steven J. Berlin, Pres.

Desc: Open to all People who wish to join. Offers financial support to third and fourth year podiatric medical students. Awards scholarships. **Awards:** Scholarship (annual) offers financial support to third and fourth year podiatric medical students with highest financial and academic qualifications.

★ 13283 ★ Gazette International Networking Institute (GINI)

4207 Lindell Blvd., No. 110
Saint Louis, MO 63108-2915
Phone: (314)534-0475 **Fax:** (314)534-5070
Email: gini_intl@msn.com
Website: http://www.post-polio.org
Joan L. Headley, Dir.

Desc: Polio survivors, ventilator users, other individuals with neuromuscular diseases, health care personnel, insurance agencies, government agencies, independent living centers, and interested others. Works to inform, encourage, dignify, and sustain people with disabilities. Seeks to create a communications network to provide information on issues related to disabilities. Serves as clearinghouse for information on polio, ventilators, neuromuscular diseases, and independent living. Sponsors seminars. Coordinates International Polio Network and International Ventilator Users Network. **Awards:** Research Awards (periodic).

★ 13284 ★ Glaucoma Foundation

116 John St., Ste. 1605
New York, NY 10038
Phone: (212)285-0080 **Fax:** (212)651-1888
Email: info@glaucomafoundation.org
Website: http://www.glaucomafoundation.org/
Scott R. Christensen, Pres. /CEO

Desc: Individuals who have been affected by glaucoma and interested others. Works to increase public awareness and to provide research funding. Provides information about glaucoma to the medical and lay communities. Targets and funds the following areas for research: optic nerve regeneration; molecular genetics. Sponsors scientific research. **Awards:** Award of Merit; grant.

★ 13285 ★ Glaucoma Research Foundation

490 Post St., Ste. 1427
San Francisco, CA 94102
Phone: (415)986-3162 **Free:** 800-826-6693
Fax: (415)986-3763
Email: info@glaucoma.org
Website: http://www.glaucoma.org
Rita Loskill, Dir. of Education

Desc: Dedicated to protecting the sight and independence of individuals with glaucoma through research and education, with the ultimate goal of finding a cure. Funds pilot project grants. **Awards:** Catalyst (annual); Pilot Project (annual) for research.

★ 13286 ★ Gluten Intolerance Group of North America (GIGNA)

15110 10th Ave., SW
Ste. A
Seattle, WA 98116-1820
Phone: (206)246-6652 **Fax:** (206)246-6531
Email: info@gluten.net
Website: http://www.gluten.net
Cynthia Kupper, CRD, CDE, Exec. Dir.

Desc: Persons with gluten-sensitive enteropathy (celiac sprue) or dermatitis herpetiformis, family members, physicians, dietitians, and celiac sprue societies. (Gluten is a protein found in wheat, rye, oats, and barley. Gluten-sensitive enteropathy is an inherited disorder characterized by gluten-related destruction of the small intestine. Symptoms include diarrhea, weight loss, fatigue, and anemia.) Works to educate patients, health care personnel, and the public; to offer psychological support to celiac sprue patients and their families in dealing with the adjustment and nutritional limitations of the disease; to conduct research into the causes. Promotes practical application in specific food research, such as recipe development and information on gluten content of products. Offers children's services and group and individual counseling. **Awards:** Campership (annual); Membership (annual).

★ 13287 ★ Gray Panthers (GP)

733 15th St. NW, Ste. 437
Washington, DC 20005
Phone: (202)737-6637 **Free:** 800-280-5362
Fax: (202)737-1160
Email: info@graypanthers.org
Website: http://www.graypanthers.org
Tim Fuller, Exec. Dir.

Desc: Consciousness-raising activist group of older adults and young people. Aims to combat ageism - the discrimination against persons on the basis of chronological age. Believes that both the old and the young have much to contribute to make our society more just and humane. Advises, acts as acatalyst for, and organizes local groups of young, middle-aged, and older persons to work on issues of their choosing. Conducts work on eight national interests: national health care, affordable housing, environmental preservtion, peace, ending discrimination, education, economic and tax justice, and social justice. **Awards:** Mahler Grant (semiannual).

★ 13288 ★ Healthcare Information and Management Systems Society (HIMSS)

230 E Ohio St., Ste. 500
Chicago, IL 60611-3269
Phone: (312)664-4467 **Fax:** (312)664-6143
Email: himss@himss.org
Website: http://www.himss.org/
H. Stephen Lieber, CAE, Pres.

Desc: Persons who, by education and/or appropriate experience, are professionally qualified to engage in the analysis, design, and operation of health care information systems, management engineering, telecommunications, and clinical systems professions. Also, corporate members include companies with information technology solutions for health care organizations. Provides leadership in health care for the management of systems, information, and change, while striving for high quality, efficient and effective patient care through analysis and technology implementation. Maintains speakers' bureau. Offers placement service. **Awards:** CIO of the Year Award (annual); John E. Gall Award (annual); Richard P. Covert Scholarship (annual) for student member in field of study consistent with HIMSS service areas.

★ 13289 ★ Healthcare Forum

180 Montgomery St., Ste. 1520
San Francisco, CA 94104-4230
Kathryn E. Johnson, CEO & Pres.

Desc: Healthcare leaders and executives. Promotes visionary leadership and motivation in healthcare. Conducts leadership development education programs; produces computer based educational materials. Sponsors research activities. **Awards:** Healthier Communities (annual).

★ 13290 ★ Helene Fuld Health Trust

452 Fifth Ave., 17th Fl.
New York, NY 10018
Phone: (212)525-2418 **Fax:** (212)681-1335
Email: www.mail@fuldtrust.org
Website: http://www.fuldtrust.org
Jina Piak, Grants Mgr.

Desc: Strives to support the improvement of the health, welfare, and education of student nurses. **Awards:** Grant.

★ 13291 ★ Hellenic American Dental Society (HADS)

PO Box 4803
Oak Brook, IL 60523-4803
Phone: (773)763-3600
Email: info@hads.com
Website: http://www.hads.com/
Dr. Athina Danigeles, Pres.

Desc: Dentists, dental hygienists and dental technicians of Greek descent, promoting Hellenic heritage. **Awards:** Scholarship (annual).

★ 13292 ★ Hepatitis Foundation International

c/o Martha Young
504 Blick Dr.
Silver Spring, MD 20904
Phone: (301)622-4200 **Free:** 800-891-0707
Fax: (301)622-4702
Email: hfi@comcast.net
Website: http://www.hepfi.org
Thelma King Thiel, Chm. and C. E. O.

Desc: Individuals concerned about those with hepatitis. Provides education and information for distribution to the general public, patients, educators, and medical professionals about the diagnosis, treatment, and prevention of viral hepatitis. Maintains database of hepatitis support groups and website information. Conducts train-the-trainer programs for those interested in the topic. **Awards:** Career Development Award (annual) for epidemiology and outcomes research of viral hepatitis.

★ 13293 ★ Hereditary Disease Foundation (HDF)

1303 Pico Blvd.
Santa Monica, CA 90405-1553
Phone: (310)450-9913 **Fax:** (310)450-9532
Email: cures@hdfoundation.org
Website: http://www.hdfoundation.org
Leslie P. Weiner, Chair

Desc: To fund basic biomedical research on the causes, prevention, diagnosis, treatment, and cure of genetic disorders and in particular Huntington's Disease, an inherited neurological disorder. Maintains grant programs to support scientific projects in major medical and basic science laboratories throughout the U.S. Offers grants and postdoctoral fellowships. Sponsors a series of interdisciplinary workshops to stimulate new ideas and approaches to understanding hereditary problems. Helps maintain two tissue banks for research purposes. Disseminates information to organizations and individuals. **Awards:** John J. Wasmuth Award postdoctoral fellowships; Lieberman Award (annual) innovative research for treatment or cure of huntington's disease; Milton Wexler Award postdoctoral fellowships.

★ 13294 ★ Herpes Resource Center - American Social Health Association (HRC)

PO Box 13827
Research Triangle Park, NC 27709
Phone: (919)361-8488 **Fax:** (919)361-8425
Email: phidra@ashastd.org
Website: http://www.ashastd.org/hrc

Desc: Individuals with recurrent genital herpes infections; individuals interested in the dissemination of information about genital herpes. (Herpes is a sexually transmitted disease which is as yet incurable.) Works to give emotional support to individuals, and to provide current information about herpes. Maintains the National HPV Hotline. Offers referrals to local support groups (HELP) throughout the U.S. and Canada for people living with herpes; HELP groups provide a safe, confidential environment in which to obtain accurate information about HPV and share experiences with other people concerned about herpes. Compiles statistics. **Awards:** Fellowship; grant.

★ 13295 ★ HIKE Fund

c/o Shirley R. Terrill
10115 Cherry Hill Pl.
Spring Hill, FL 34608-7116
Phone: (352)688-2579 **Fax:** (352)688-2579
Email: ceterrilli@aol.com
Website: http://www.missouriiojd.org/MO-HIKE/HIKE.htm
Carol Mentges, Pres.

Desc: Supported by the International Order of Job's Daughters. Works for complete equality and integration of the hearing impaired in society. Provides support and information services. Provides hearing devices for children (up to the age of 20) with financial need. **Awards:** The HIKE Fund (monthly).

★ 13296 ★ The Hip Society

c/o Karen V. Andersen
951 Old County Rd., No. 182
Belmont, CA 94002
Phone: (650)596-6190 **Fax:** (650)508-2039
Website: http://www.hipsoc.org/
Karen V. Andersen, Exec. Dir.

Desc: Dedicated to the advancement of knowledge relating to the hip joint. **Awards:** Frank Stinchfield Award (annual) to resident or fellow in training; John Charnley Award (annual); Otto Aufranc Award (annual).

★ 13297 ★ Hispanic Dental Association

188 W Randolph St., Ste. 415
Chicago, IL 60601
Phone: (312)577-4013 **Free:** 800-852-7921
Fax: (312)577-4013
Email: hdassoc@aol.com
Website: http://www.hdassoc.org
Sandy Reed, Exec. Dir.

Desc: Provides leadership and represents professionals who share a common commitment to improve the oral health of the Hispanic community. **Awards:** HDA Foundation for entry-level dental school students, and other programs.

★ 13298 ★ Histiocytosis Association of America

72 E Holly Ave., Ste. 101
Pitman, NJ 08071
Phone: (856)589-6606 **Fax:** (856)589-6614
Email: histiocyte@aol.com

Website: http://www.histio.org/association/index.shtml
Jeffrey M. Toughill, Pres.

Desc: Patients, families, and friends of those suffering from histiocytic disorders; physicians, oncologists, and hematologists working in the field of histiocytosis research. (Histiocytosis is a rare disease that causes histiocytes, a type of white blood cell, to multiply and attack organs, body systems, or bones.) Works to provide support for patients and their families and friends. Funds research on the cause and treatment of histiocytosis. Acts as a referral service. Maintains speakers' bureau. **Awards:** Medical Research (annual).

★ 13299 ★ Hospice Foundation of America (HFA)

2001 S St. NW, Ste. 300
Washington, DC 20009
Free: 800-854-3402 **Fax:** (202)638-5312
Email: david@hospicefoundation.org
Website: http://www.hospicefoundation.org
David Abrams, Pres.

Desc: Works to promote the philosophy and application of hospice care for terminally ill people and improve the American health system. Advocates the hospice concept of care; offers professional development and educational programs; sponsors research on ethical issues; participates in public policy initiatives; provides technical assistance to hospices **Awards:** Grant.

★ 13300 ★ Hospitalized Veterans Writing Project (HVWP)

5920 Nall, Rm. 105
Mission, KS 66202
Phone: (913)432-1214
Barbara Sauvan, Pres.

Desc: Individuals and organizations united to encourage hospitalized U.S. veterans to write for pleasure and rehabilitation during their hospital stay. Maintains speakers' bureau and slide program with commentary. Conducts writing sessions in hospitals. **Awards:** Monetary (3/year) for prose, poetry, cartoon and drawing, and photographs.

★ 13301 ★ Howard Hughes Medical Institute (HHMI)

4000 Jones Bridge Rd.
Chevy Chase, MD 20815-6789
Phone: (301)215-8500
Email: webmaster@hhmi.org
Website: http://www.hhmi.org

Desc: Works to help enhance biomedical science education at all levels. Conducts research. **Awards:** Grant.

★ 13302 ★ Huntington's Disease Society of America (HDSA)

158 W 29th St., 7th Fl.
New York, NY 10001-5300
Phone: (212)242-1968 **Free:** 800-345-4372
Fax: (212)239-3430
Email: hdsainfo@hdsa.org
Website: http://www.hdsa.org
Barbara T. Boyle, Exec. Dir., CEO

Desc: Individuals and groups of volunteers concerned with Huntington's disease, an inherited and terminal neurological condition causing progressive brain and nerve deterioration. Goals are to: identify HD families; educate the public and professionals, with emphasis on increasing consumer awareness of HD; promote and support basic and clinical research into the causes and cure of HD; maintain patient services program, coordinated with various community services, to assist families in meeting the social, economic, and emotional problems resulting from HD. Is working to change the attitude of the working community toward the HD patient, enhance the HD patient's lifestyle, and promote better health care and treatment, both in the community and in facilities. Has launched nationwide campaign in support of federal and state legislation establishing clinics, genetic counseling and screening centers, and diagnostic and treatment centers for HD patients and those suffering from other chronic, debilitating diseases. Actively cooperates with researchers in ongoing studies; cosponsors and supports workshops and symposia; provides grants to individual researchers; sponsors brain donor program. Crisis intervention and other support services are available. **Awards:** Grant (periodic) Researchers investigating a treatment or cure for Huntington's Disease.

★ 13303 ★ Hydrocephalus Association (HA)

870 Market St., Ste. 705
San Francisco, CA 94102
Phone: (415)732-7040 **Free:** 888-598-3789
Fax: (415)732-7044
Email: info@hydroassoc.org
Website: http://www.hydroassoc.org
Emily Fudge, Exec. Dir.

Desc: People with hydrocephalus and their families, health care professionals with an interest in hydrocephalus, and interested businesses and foundations. Works to improve the quality of life of people with hydrocephalus through education. Conducts training for families of people with hydrocephalus; sponsors social gatherings; facilitates networking among families of people with hydrocephalus and between organizations representing people with hydrocephalus. **Awards:** Anthony Abbene Scholarship; Gerard Fudge Memorial Scholarship (3/year) for a person ages 18 to 30 with hydrocephalus; Morris L. Ziskind Memorial Scholarship.

★ 13304 ★ Immune Deficiency Foundation (IDF)

40 W Chesapeake Ave., Ste. 308
Towson, MD 21204
Phone: (410)321-6647 **Free:** 800-296-4433
Fax: (410)321-9165
Email: idf@primaryimmune.org
Website: http://www.primaryimmune.org
Thomas L. Moran, Pres.

Desc: Immune deficiency patients, their families, and medical professionals. Promotes education and research in primary immune deficiency diseases. Holds medical symposia; bestows patient scholarship and research awards. **Awards:** Immune Deficiency Foundation Scholarship (annual) primary immune deficiency diagnosis; Novartis Fellowship (annual).

★ 13305 ★ International Anesthesia Research Society (IARS)

2 Summit Park Dr., Ste. 140
Cleveland, OH 44131-2571
Phone: (216)642-1124 **Fax:** (216)642-1127
Email: iarshq@iars.org
Website: http://www.iars.org

Desc: Anesthesiologists and other doctors of medicine and dentistry interested in the specialty of anesthesiology; associate members are registered nurses, physician assistants, and respiratory therapists. Fosters progress and research in all phases of anesthesiology. **Awards:** Ben Covino Research Award (biennial) research relating to the use of local anesthetics; Clinical Scholar Research Award (annual); Frontiers in Anesthesia Research Award (biennial).

★ 13306 ★ International Association for Dental Research (IADR)

1619 Duke St.
Alexandria, VA 22314
Phone: (703)548-0066 **Fax:** (703)548-1883
Email: research@iadr.org
Website: http://www.iadr.com
Robert Collins, DDS, Interim Exec. Dir.

Desc: Individuals engaged or interested in advancing research in the various aspects of dental and related sciences. **Awards:** Edward H. Hatton Award for winners of Junior Investigators competition; H. Trendley Dean Memorial Award for research in epidemiology and public health; Young Investigator Award for basic research in all dental research disciplines.

★ 13307 ★ International Association for Hospice and Palliative Care (IAHPC)

c/o Josefina B. Magno
5535 Memorial Dr., Ste. F-PMB 509
Houston, TX 77007
Phone: (713)880-2940 **Fax:** (713)880-2948
Email: info@iahpc.com
Website: http://www.hospicecare.com/
Liliana DeLima, MHA, Exec. Dir.

Desc: Promotes availability and access to high quality hospice and palliative care for patients and families in order to alleviate physical and psychosocial suffering associated with progressive, incurable illness throughout the world. Provides communication and education for patients, professionals, health care providers and policy makers. **Awards:** Individual Recognition Awards (annual); Institutional Recognition Awards (annual); Scholarships (quarterly); Traveling Fellowships (quarterly).

★ 13308 ★ International Atherosclerosis Society (IAS)

6550 Fannin, Ste. 1211
Houston, TX 77030-2704
Phone: (713)797-9620 **Fax:** (713)797-9507
Email: ias@bcm.tmc.edu
Website: http://www.athero.org
Ann S. Jackson, MBA, Exec. Dir.

Desc: Scientists and other professionals involved in research in the field of atherosclerosis; corporations and firms supporting aims of the IAS. Promotes the advancement of science, research, and teaching in the field of atherosclerosis throughout the world. (Atherosclerosis is a form of arteriosclerosis characterized by the deposition of fatty substances in and fibrosis of the inner layer of the arteries.) Advocates an interdisciplinary approach to the study of atherosclerosis and related diseases. Facilitates international communication and exchange of knowledge among scientists in the field. Assists in the organization of exchange visits among scientists at various research centers. Fosters and encourages young researchers by arranging contacts, and offering travel support to world gatherings in the field. Coordinates activities in atherosclerosis research. **Awards:** Scholarship; Visiting Fellowship Award (semiannual).

★ 13309 ★ International College of Applied Kinesiology - U.S.A. (ICAK-U.S.A.)

6405 Metcalf Ave., Ste. 503
Shawnee Mission, KS 66202-3929
Phone: (913)384-5336 **Fax:** (913)384-5112
Email: icak@dci-kansascity.com
Website: http://www.icakusa.com
Andria Dibbern, Membership Services

Desc: Promotes the science of applied kinesiology. Applied Kinesiology is the system of evaluating the structural, chemical, and mental aspect of human heath, involving muscle health, nutrition, manipulation, diet, acupressure, and exercise. Conducts educational programs, research programs, and training seminars. **Awards:** Scholarship (annual).

★ 13310 ★ International College of Prosthodontists

PO Box 99119
San Diego, CA 92169-1119
Phone: (858)270-1814
Email: res-inc@msn.com
Website: http://www.icp-org.com
Eben Yancy, Exec. Dir.

Desc: Prosthodontists. **Awards:** Young Prosthodontists Award (biennial).

★ 13311 ★ International Federation of Societies for Histochemistry and Cytochemistry (IFSHC)
c/o Dr. Denis G. Baskin
Department of Biological Structure
Univ. of Washington
PO Box 357420
Seattle, WA 98195-9420
Phone: (206)616-5894 **Fax:** (206)616-5842
Email: baskindg@u.washington.edu
Website: http://www.ifshc.org
Prof.Dr. Denis G. Baskin, Sec. Gen.

Desc: National societies for histochemistry and cytochemistry. Seeks to promote communication and cooperation among scientists throughout the world and establish histochemistry and cytochemistry institutes. Promotes histochemistry and cytochemistry as basic, independent sciences and advocates their teaching in universities. Appoints committees for the study of scientific matters requiring international collaboration. **Awards:** David Glick Lectureship (quadrennial) for significant contribution to histochemistry; Young Histochemist Awards (quadrennial) for new investigators from societies with paid-up dues to travel to International Congress of Histochemistry & Cytochemistry.

★ 13312 ★ International Life Sciences Institute - North America (ILSINA)
One Thomas Cir. NW, 9th Fl.
Washington, DC 20005
Phone: (202)659-0074 **Fax:** (202)659-3859
Email: ilsi@ilsi.org
Website: http://www.ilsi.org
PhD Richard Black, PhD, Exec. Dir.

Desc: Advances the understanding of scientific issues related to the nutritional quality and safety of the food supply, as well as health issues related to consumer self-care products. Sponsors relevant research programs, professional education programs and workshops, seminars, and publications, as well as providing a neutral forum for government, academic, and industry scientists to discuss and resolve scientific issues of common concern for the well-being of the general public. Fosters career development of outstanding new scientists. Programs are supported primarily by its industry membership. **Awards:** Future Leader Awards (annual) to a resident of North America with a doctoral degree within the past 7 years.

★ 13313 ★ International Myeloma Foundation (IMF)
12650 Riverside Dr., Ste. 206
North Hollywood, CA 91607
Phone: (818)487-7455 **Free:** 800-452-CURE
Fax: (818)487-7454
Email: theimf@myeloma.org
Website: http://www.myeloma.org
Susie Novis, Pres.

Desc: The International Myeloma Foundation is a non-profit organization dedicated to the education, treatment and research of multiple myeloma, a little-known cancer of the bone marrow. We provide a variety of patient and physician education and support programs and services. **Awards:** Brian D. Novis Research Grant (annual) for a doctor or researcher actively working on multiple myeloma; Junior and Senior Grants.

★ 13314 ★ International Nurses Society on Addictions (NNSA)
PO Box 10752
Raleigh, NC 27605
Phone: (919)821-1292 **Fax:** (919)833-5743
Email: snow@uta.edu
Website: http://www.intnsa.org
Diane Snow, Pres.

Desc: Promotes quality nursing care for persons addicted to alcohol and other drugs, and their families. Fosters continuing education and development of skills among nurses involved in the field; works to enhance the professional image of addictions nurses. Participates in public policy and social issues related to alcohol or chemical abuse. Serves as liaison between members and professional groups with common goals. Represents members' interests before national organizations. Regional groups sponsor workshops. Provides certification program. **Awards:** Grant (periodic).

★ 13315 ★ International Rett Syndrome Association (IRSA)
9121 Piscataway Rd.
Clinton, MD 20735
Phone: (301)856-3334 **Free:** 800-818-RETT
Fax: (301)856-3336
Email: irsa@rettsyndrome.org
Website: http://www.rettsyndrome.org
Kathy Hunter, Pres.

Desc: Parents of children with Rett Syndrome; interested professionals and supporters. (A child afflicted with Rett Syndrome, which strikes predominately in females, seems normal until 7 to 18 months of age, when a regression leads to loss of psychomotor and communication skills. Autistic-like withdrawal often sets in; though this symptom eases in time, higher brain functions are compromised. The child also loses purposeful use of her hands, wringing them in a constant "hand-washing" movement in front of the face or chest. The syndrome is named for Dr. Andreas Rett, of Vienna, Austria, who described it in 1966. The cause of Rett Syndrome has been traced to a defective gene, called the MeCP2 on the X chromosome.) Provides support to parents; encourages research; collects and disseminates information. Assists in identifying patients; conducts activities aimed at the prevention, treatment, and eventual eradication of Rett Syndrome. **Awards:** Research Grant (annual) for individuals approved by a Professional Advisory board.

★ 13316 ★ International Society of Arthroscopy, Knee Surgery and Orthopaedic Sports Medicine (ISAKOS)
145 Town and Country Dr., Ste. 106
Danville, CA 94526-3963
Phone: (925)314-7920 **Fax:** (925)314-7922
Email: isakos@isakos.com
Website: http://www.isakos.com
Barry R. Tietjens, Pres.

Desc: Orthopaedic surgeons specializing in problems of the knee, arthoscopy, orthopaedic sports medicine. **Awards:** Albert Trillot Award (biennial); John T. Joyce Award (biennial).

★ 13317 ★ International Society for Experimental Hematology (ISEH)
2025 M St. NW, Ste. 800
Washington, DC 20036
Phone: (202)367-1183 **Fax:** (202)367-2183
Email: iseh@dc.sba.com
Website: http://www.iseh.org
Thomas Reiser, Exec. Dir.

Desc: Scientists and health care professionals in the field of experimental hematology. Seeks to advance the science and practice of hematology; promotes professional development of members. Serves as a forum for the exchange of information on experimental hematology and related topics; sponsors research and educational programs. **Awards:** Young Investigators Awards (annual) for depth of research in abstracts.

★ 13318 ★ International Society for Heart and Lung Transplantation (ISHLT)
14673 Midway Rd., Ste. 200
Addison, TX 75001
Phone: (972)490-9495 **Fax:** (972)490-9499
Email: ishlt@ishlt.org
Website: http://www.ishlt.org
Amanda W. Rowe, Exec. Dir.

Desc: Medical doctors, Ph.D.s, nurses, researchers, and others interested in artificial hearts and in heart and heart-lung failure and transplantation. Provides a center for discussion, exchange of information, and activities that promote the interests of heart and lung transplantation. Seeks to heighten awareness of public and governmental agencies regarding developments in the field. Maintains the International Heart and Lung Transplantation Registry. **Awards:** Caves Award (annual) best abstract by student/resident; Ortho Biotech/ISHLT Research Fellowship Award (annual) for young researchers; Roche/ISHLT Research Fellowship Award (annual) for young researchers.

★ 13319 ★ International Society for Magnetic Resonance in Medicine
2118 Milvia St., Ste. 201
Berkeley, CA 94704
Phone: (510)841-1899 **Fax:** (510)841-2340
Email: info@ismrm.org
Website: http://www.ismrm.org
Jane Tiemann, Exec. Dir.

Desc: Devoted to furthering the development and application of MRI and its techniques in medicine and biology. Sponsors educational and research programs. **Awards:** Young Investigator's Award/Student Stipends (annual).

★ 13320 ★ International Society for Mountain Medicine (ISMM)
c/o Peter Hackett, MD
610 Sabeta Dr.
Ridgway, CO 81432-9335
Phone: (970)626-2477 **Fax:** (970)626-2467
Email: hackett@ismmed.org
Website: http://www.ismmed.org
Peter Hackett, MD, Contact

Desc: Brings together scientists and physicians, and allied trade professionals interested in mountain medicine. Encourages research on all aspects of mountains, mountain peoples and mountaineers. **Awards:** ISMM Research Prize (biennial) for scientific merit.

★ 13321 ★ International Society for Neuroimmunomodulation
c/o Craig C. Smith
National Institute of Health
36 Convent Dr., Rm. 1A23/MSC 4020
Bethesda, MD 20892-4020
Phone: (301)496-4561 **Fax:** (301)496-6095
Email: ccs@codon.nih.gov
Website: http://www.isnim.org
Craig C. Smith, Exec. Dir.

Desc: Professional society for scientists involved in interdisciplinary research in the molecular and cellular aspects of neurobiology, neuroendocrinology, immunology, and the behavioral sciences. Interests focus on discerning the integrative elements underlying communication and modulation between the central nervous, endocrine, and immune systems, and upon related disease states. **Awards:** Novera Herbert Spector Lectureship (annual) for significant contributions in both leadership and research to the field of Neuroimmunomodulation.

★ 13322 ★ International Society of Neurovirology
c/o Brian Wigdahl, Dept. of Microbiology and Immunology Penn State College of Medicine
500 University Dr.
PO Box 850
Hershey, PA 17033
Phone: (717)531-8258 **Fax:** (717)531-5580
Email: bwigdahl@psu.edu
Website: http://www.isnv.org
Brian Wigdahl, PhD, Pres.

Desc: Neurovirologists. **Awards:** Pioneer Award (annual) for outstanding contribution to the field of neurovirology.

★ 13323 ★ International Society of Nurses in Genetics (ISONG)
c/o Jean Anderson, RN, MA, CPNP
2593 W 15th St. S
Newton, IA 50208
Phone: (641)831-9230
Email: janderson@isong.us

Website: http://www.isong.org
Jean Anderson, RN,MA, Exec. Dir.

Desc: Case managers, administrators, coordinators of public and private programs, educators in the field of nursing and/or genetics, genetic counselors, researchers. Committed to incorporating the knowledge of human genetics into nursing practice, education and research activities. **Awards:** Research Award (annual).

★ 13324 ★ International Society of Psychiatric Mental Health Nurses (ISPN)

1211 Locust St.
Philadelphia, PA 19107
Phone: (215)545-2843 **Free:** 800-826-2950
Fax: (215)545-8107
Email: ispn@nursecominc.com
Website: http://www.ispn-psych.org
Joseph Broden, Exec. Dir.

Desc: Psychiatric and mental health nurses. Seeks to advance the study, teaching, and practice of psychiatric and mental health nursing. Represents members' professional and economic interests. **Awards:** Robert O. Gilbert Foundation Research Award (annual).

★ 13325 ★ International Transactional Analysis Association (ITAA)

436 14th St. Ste. 1301
Oakland, CA 94612-2710
Phone: (510)625-7720 **Fax:** (510)625-7725
Email: itaa@itaa-net.org
Website: http://www.itaa-net.org
Gordon B. Hewitt, PhD, Pres.

Desc: Educational corporation of persons in medical and behavioral sciences, including psychiatrists, psychologists, social workers, nurses, educators, marriage and family counselors, clergy, and organizational consultants. Maintains standards of practice and teaching of transactional analysis, which involves group therapy, social dynamics, and personality theory based on analysis of the "transactions" or interactions between persons. (The book, *Games People Play*, covers basic transactional analysis theory; its author, Dr. Eric Berne, was ITAA founder.) **Awards:** Eric Berne Memorial Award (annual) scientific research in transactional analysis; Eric Berne Research Grant.

★ 13326 ★ International Transplant Nurses Society (ITNS)

1739 E Carson St., No. 351
PO Box 351
Pittsburgh, PA 15203-1700
Free: (412)343-ITNS **Fax:** (412)343-3959
Email: itns@msn.com
Website: http://www.itns.org
Beth Kassalen, MBA, Exec. Dir.

Desc: Nurses, LVNs, LPNs, and others involved in patient care for organ transplantation. Works to encourage cooperation among all medical disciplines involved in transplantation, disseminate information, and establish certification for this nursing specialty. **Awards:** Nursing Research (annual) grant proposal.

★ 13327 ★ International Trauma Anesthesia and Critical Care Society (ITACCS)

PO Box 4826
Baltimore, MD 21211
Fax: (410)235-8084
Email: info@nwas.com
Website: http://www.trauma.itaccs.com
Christopher M. Grande, MD,MPH, Exec. Dir.

Desc: Healthcare professionals involved in trauma and critical care anesthesiology. Works to gain recognition for trauma anesthesiology as a discipline within anesthesiology and critical care medicine. Promotes cooperation and information sharing among healthcare professionals. Sponsors seminars and workshops; conducts research and educational programs; provides children's services; holds competitions; maintains speakers' bureau and placement service. **Awards:** ITACCS Research Award (annual) Application packet available.

★ 13328 ★ International Union of Nutritional Sciences (IUNS)

c/o Prof. Osman M. Galal
UCLA School of Public Health
International Health Program
PO Box 951772
Los Angeles, CA 90095-1772
Phone: (310)206-9639 **Fax:** (310)794-1805
Email: ogalal@ucla.edu
Website: http://www.iuns.org
Prof. O.M. Galal, Sec. Gen.

Desc: National nutritional societies. Promotes international cooperation in the scientific study of nutrition and its applications. Encourages research and the exchange of scientific information. Cooperates with the Food and Agriculture Organization of the United Nations, the United Nations Educational, Scientific and Cultural Organization, and the World Health Organization. Maintains 9 task forces. **Awards:** IUNS Award (quadrennial); IUNS Fellow (quadrennial).

★ 13329 ★ International Veterinary Acupuncture Society (IVAS)

PO Box 271395
Fort Collins, CO 80527-1395
Phone: (970)266-0660 **Fax:** (970)266-0777
Email: office@ivas.org
Website: http://www.ivas.org/
Edward C. Boldt, Jr., Exec. Dir.

Desc: Veterinarians and veterinary students. Encourages knowledge and research of the philosophy, technique, and practice of veterinary acupuncture. Fosters high standards in the field; promotes scientific investigation. Accumulates resources for scientific research and education; collects data concerning clinical and research cases where animals have been treated with acupuncture; disseminates information to veterinary students, practitioners, other scientific groups, and the public. Offers 100 contact hour basic veterinary acupuncture course; administers certification examination. **Awards:** Research Grant (annual).

★ 13330 ★ Interplast

300-B Pioneer Way
Mountain View, CA 94041-1506
Phone: (650)962-0123 **Free:** 888-467-5278
Fax: (650)962-1619
Email: ipnews@interplast.org
Website: http://www.interplast.org
Susan W. Hayes, Pres. /CEO

Desc: Provides free reconstructive plastic surgery for needy children around the world, with more than 47,000 free surgeries performed since 1969. Seeks to ensure access to reconstructive plastic surgery in developing countries worldwide by sending teams of medical volunteers overseas and providing advanced medical training and support to host-country medical partners. **Awards:** Medical Scholar Program (annual) medical scholarship for foreign medical personnel.

★ 13331 ★ Interstitial Cystitis Association (ICA)

110 N Washington St., No. 340
Rockville, MD 20850-2239
Phone: (301)610-5300 **Free:** 800-HEL-PICA
Fax: (301)610-5308
Email: icamail@ichelp.org
Website: http://www.ichelp.org
Nicole Mehall, Admin. Mgr.

Desc: Support network for patients suffering or suspected of suffering from interstitial cystitis, an inflammation of the bladder wall that primarily affects women; its cause and cure are unknown. Works to inform the public and especially the medical profession about the seriousness of IC. Raises funds for research into treatments and cures; maintains a medical advisory board. Is establishing a national registry to record facts about IC. **Awards:** Pilot Award for worthy research connected.

★ 13332 ★ Iron Overload Diseases Association (IOD)

433 Westwind Dr.
North Palm Beach, FL 33408-5123
Phone: (561)840-8512 **Fax:** (561)842-9881
Email: iod@ironoverload.org
Website: http://www.ironoverload.org
Roberta Crawford, Pres.

Desc: Physicians and patients. Purposes are to: serve hemochromatosis patients and families; encourage research and public information; press for earlier diagnosis and more effective treatment. (Hemochromatosis is a genetic condition of iron overload in which excess iron damages organs and tissues, producing varying late-stage symptoms including liver cirrhosis, diabetes, heart failure, arthritis, and skin pigmentation, leading to death unless diagnosed early and treated adequately.) Specific plans are: to develop a public relations plan, television interviews, and press releases; to sponsor screening programs and patient referral service; prepare diagnosis sheets for doctors and medical schools. Current emphasis is on alerting the public to the dangers of excess iron, since the disease is more prevalent than previously believed, and most susceptible individuals are unaware of the hazard. Authorities believe that five in 1000 carry both genes and that one in eight carries a single gene. Acts as a clearinghouse for doctors to call on for research materials. Sponsors fundraising program. Is also in the process of setting up an index of laboratory research in progress. Conducts programs; compiles statistics; maintains speakers' bureau; conducts research programs. **Awards:** Grant for research.

★ 13333 ★ Islamic Medical Association of North America (IMANA)

950 75th St.
Downers Grove, IL 60516
Phone: (630)852-2122 **Fax:** (630)435-1429
Email: imana@aol.com
Website: http://www.imana.org
Abdul Rauf Mir, MD, Pres.

Desc: Muslim physicians and allied health professionals. Unites Muslim physicians and allied health professionals in the U.S. and Canada for the improvement of professional and social contact; provides assistance to Muslim communities worldwide. Charitable programs include: donation of books, journals, and educational and research materials to medical institutions; donation of medical supplies and equipment to charity medical institutions in Muslim countries. Maintains speakers' bureau to present Islamic viewpoints on medical topics; sponsors placement service; offers assistance in orientation. **Awards:** Scholarship.

★ 13334 ★ Jewish Alcoholics, Chemically Dependent Persons and Significant Others (JACS)

850 Seventh Ave.
New York, NY 10019
Phone: (212)397-4197 **Fax:** (212)399-3525
Email: jacs@jacsweb.org
Website: http://www.jacsweb.org
Arnie Goldfein, Pres.

Desc: Jewish alcoholics and addicts, family members, and concerned friends. Acts as an additional resource to promote and enhance recovery from chemical dependency. Provides research and information on chemical addiction in the Jewish community. Maintains speakers' bureau. **Awards:** Retreat Scholarships (semiannual) for recovering alcoholics, addicts, family members in financial need.

★ 13335 ★ John A. Hartford Foundation

55 E 59th St., 16th Fl.
New York, NY 10022-1178
Phone: (212)832-7788 **Fax:** (212)593-4913
Email: mail@jhartford.org

Website: http://www.jhartfound.org
Corinne H. Rieder, Exec. Dir.

Desc: Works to promote health care, training, research, and service related to older adults. **Awards:** Grant.

★ 13336 ★ Juvenile Diabetes Research Foundation International (JDFI)

120 Wall St.
New York, NY 10005-4001
Phone: (212)785-9500 **Free:** 800-533-CURE
Fax: (212)785-9595
Email: info@jdf.org
Website: http://www.jdrf.org
Peter Van Etten, Pres. /CEO

Desc: World's leading nonprofit, nongovernmental funder of diabetes research. Mission is to find a cure for diabetes and its complications through the support of research. Sponsors international workshops and conferences for biomedical researchers. Individual chapters offer support groups and other activities for families affected by diabetes. **Awards:** Fellowship for research; grant; recognition (annual) for scientific and humanitarian achievements, and for public service.

★ 13337 ★ Klingenstein Third Generation Foundation

787 Seventh Ave., 6th Fl.
New York, NY 10019-6016
Phone: (212)492-6179 **Fax:** (212)492-7007
Email: sally@ktgf.org
Website: http://www.ktgf.org/
Sally Klingenstein, Exec. Dir.

Desc: Strives to improve the lives of families afflicted by clinical depressions; addresses childhood and adolescent depression as well as Attention Deficit/Hyperactivity Disorder. **Awards:** Grant.

★ 13338 ★ Laboratory Animal Management Association (LAMA)

7300 Metro Blvd., Ste. 585
Edina, MN 55439
Phone: (952)250-6201 **Fax:** (952)835-4774
Email: imartinez@rcm.upr.edu
Website: http://www.lama-online.org
Ivette Martinez-Palma, Pres.

Desc: Laboratory animal facility managers. Seeks to evaluate and update basic and advanced management techniques and to educate laboratory animal facility managers. Makes available resource material; coordinates exchange programs for management personnel. Offers consulting on management techniques. **Awards:** Charles River Medallion for distinguished contributions to the field by an administrator/manager who is a current member of LAMA and engaged in laboratoryanimal management; LAMA Foundation Award to qualified members within laboratory animal management for the futherance of his or her education in the field; U. Kristina Stephens Award awarded to a LAMA Member for outstanding and exceptional service to LAMA.

★ 13339 ★ Lamaze International

2025 M St., NW, Ste. 800
Washington, DC 20036
Phone: (202)367-1128 **Free:** 800-368-4404
Fax: (202)367-2128
Email: lamaze@dc.sba.com
Website: http://www.lamaze-childbirth.com
Linda L. Harmon, Exec. Dir.

Desc: Physicians, nurses, nurse-midwives, certified teachers of psychoprophylatic (Lamaze) method of childbirth, other professionals, parents, and others interested in Lamaze childbirth preparation and family-centered maternity care. Disseminates information about the theory and practical application of psychoprophylaxis in obstetrics; administers teacher training courses and certifies qualified Lamaze teachers; provides educational lectures, public forums, films, and written materials; maintains national and local teacher and physician referral service. Also presents materials to prospective parents concerning the demands of childrearing. National office serves as information clearinghouse. **Awards:** Elisabeth Bing Award (annual) for members enrolled in Lamaze Childbirth Educator Program who demonstrate financial need; Lamaze Childbirth Educator Program Schoolarship (annual) for members enrolled in Lamaze Childbirth Educator Program who demonstrate financial need; Marjorie Karmel Award (annual); President's Award (annual).

★ 13340 ★ Lesbian Health Fund (LHF)

459 Fulton St., Ste. 107
San Francisco, CA 94102
Phone: (415)255-4547 **Fax:** (415)255-4784
Email: info@glma.org
Website: http://www.glma.org/

Desc: Works to recognize the unique healthcare needs of lesbians; seeks to strengthen the health of lesbians and their families through health and medical research grants and education. **Awards:** Lesbian Health Research Grant (semiannual).

★ 13341 ★ Leukemia and Lymphoma Society

1311 Mamaroneck Ave.
White Plains, NY 10605
Phone: (914)949-5213 **Free:** 800-955-4572
Fax: (914)949-6691
Email: infocenter@leukemia-lymphoma.org
Website: http://www.leukemia-lymphoma.org
Dwayne Howell, PhD, Pres. /CEO

Desc: Dedication to curing leukemia, lymphoma, Hodgkinson's disease and myeloma; seeks to improve the quality of life of patients and their families. Sponsors medical symposia and research; provides financial aid for patients; provides free information, support groups, teleconferences, and Web conferences for patients and families. **Awards:** Specialized Center of Research Grant; Translational Research PRG.

★ 13342 ★ Lifegain Institute (LI)

115 Dunder Rd.
Burlington, VT 05401
Phone: (802)862-8855 **Fax:** (802)862-6389
Email: info@healthyculture.com
Website: http://www.healthyculture.com
Judd Allen, PhD, Pres.

Desc: People who work with health promotion programs in hospitals, corporations, colleges, and communities. Promotes healthy practices such as exercise, nutrition, safety, and the reduction or curtailment of smoking and alcohol consumption through health promotion programs that provide a supportive environment. Maintains speakers' bureau. Compiles data on improvements cultural support nationwide. **Awards:** Robert F. Symbol of HOPE Award (annual) for health promotion contribution to underserved populations.

★ 13343 ★ Lowe Syndrome Association (LSA)

222 Lincoln St.
West Lafayette, IN 47906
Phone: (765)743-3634
Email: info@lowesyndrome.org
Website: http://www.lowesyndrome.org
Kaye McSpadden, Dir. of Public & Scientific Affairs

Desc: Parents, friends, and relatives of individuals with Lowe syndrome; medical, educational, and social service professionals and agencies. Fosters communication among families; provides medical and educational information; promotes a better understanding of Lowe syndrome; supports and encourages medical research. **Awards:** Medical Research Grant (annual) potential to further the understanding of Lowe syndrome or lead to better treatments.

★ 13344 ★ Lymphatic Research Foundation (LRF)

39 Pool Dr.
Roslyn, NY 11576-2038
Phone: (516)625-9675 **Fax:** (516)625-9410
Email: lrf@lymphaticresearch.org
Website: http://www.lymphaticresearch.org
Wendy Chaite, Esq., Pres.

Desc: Health care professionals, scientists, and researchers with an interest in lymphatic diseases and related disorders. Seeks to advance the prevention, diagnosis, and treatment of lymphatic diseases. Serves as a clearinghouse on lymphatic research; facilitates exchange of information among members; advocates the creation of a nationally supported lymphatic research program; functions as a liaison linking public and private-sector lymphatic research institutions and programs. **Awards:** Andrew Moisoff Young Investigator Award (periodic) for lymphatic research.

★ 13345 ★ March of Dimes Birth Defects Foundation (MDBDF)

1275 Mamaroneck Ave.
White Plains, NY 10605
Phone: (914)428-7100 **Free:** 888-663-4637
Fax: (914)428-8203
Website: http://www.marchofdimes.com
Dr. Jennifer L. Howse, Pres.

Desc: Founded by President Franklin D. Roosevelt as the National Foundation for Infantile Paralysis. Promotes prevention of birth defects by focusing on maternal and child health issues including low birthweight, infant mortality, prenatal care, and maternal substance abuse. Offers public and professional health education and community service programs to improve maternal and newborn health. Works with other national and local organizations to initiate and implement community programs of prenatal care education and service. Operates the Pregnancy and Newborn Health Education Center which provides information on pregnancy, birth defects, genetic disorders and related topics. Develops and distributes educational materials for health professionals and the public. **Awards:** Grant to hospitals and universities for clinical research; grant for professionals concerned with prevention of birth defects; grant for improved perinatal and genetic services; monetary for promising young scientists and medical students.

★ 13346 ★ Maternity Center Association (MCA)

281 Park Ave. S, 5th Fl.
New York, NY 10010
Phone: (212)777-5000 **Fax:** (212)777-9320
Email: info@maternitywise.org
Website: http://www.maternitywise.org
Maureen Corry, Exec. Dir.

Desc: Laypersons, physicians, nurses, nurse-midwives, childbirth educators, and public health workers interested in improvement of maternity care, maternal and infant health, and family life. A national nonprofit health organization for over 800 years, MCA's goals are to expand access to family-centered maternity care through collaborative practice, education, publications, consultation services, public policy initiatives and demonstration programs. Sponsors research; administers nurse-midwifery student assistance fund. Co-sponsors community-based Nurse-Midwifery Education Program. Sponsors research; administers nurse-midwifery student assistance fund. Co-sponsors community-based Nurse-Midwifery Education Program. **Awards:** Hazel Corbin Grant (annual) open to individuals who are enrolled in ACNM accredited certification programs.

★ 13347 ★ Medical Group Management Association (MGMA)

104 Inverness Terr. E
Englewood, CO 80112-5306
Phone: (303)799-1111 **Free:** 877-275-6462
Fax: (303)643-4439
Email: infocenter@mgma.com
Website: http://www.mgma.com
William F. Jessee, MD, CEO

Desc: For professionals involved in the business management of groups in medical practice. Products and services include education, benchmarking, surveys, national advocacy and networking opportunities for members. **Awards:** Recognition (annual); scholarship (annual).

★ 13348 ★ Mid-Atlantic States Association of Avian Veterinarians (MASAAV)
Memorial Bldg., Ste. 291
610 N Main St.
Blacksburg, VA 24060-3311
Phone: (540)951-2559 **Fax:** (540)953-0230
Email: office@masaav.org
Website: http://www.masaav.org
Keath L. Marx, DVM, Exec. Dir.

Desc: Works to address the needs of the avian veterinarian and technicians. innovative veterinary medicine and surgery to improve the health of avian patients. Conducts educational programs; makes donations for avian research; keeps members informed regarding legislation of interest to the profession. **Awards:** E. L. Stubbs Research Grant (periodic) researchers in avian medicine and surgery; Pamela Slack Award for Excellence (annual) veterinary college junior.

★ 13349 ★ Milton H. Erickson Foundation (MHEF)
3606 N 24th St.
Phoenix, AZ 85016
Phone: (602)956-6196 **Fax:** (602)956-0519
Email: office@erickson-foundation.org
Website: http://www.erickson-foundation.org
Jeffrey K. Zeig, Dir.

Desc: Seeks to promote and advance the contributions made to health sciences by Milton H. Erickson, M.D. (1901-1980), regarded as an authority on hypnotherapy and brief strategic therapy. Dedicated to the training of health and restricted to mental health professionals. **Awards:** Lifetime Achievement Award (periodic); scholarship (periodic).

★ 13350 ★ Movement Disorder Society (MDS)
611 E Wells St.
Milwaukee, WI 53202
Phone: (414)276-2145 **Fax:** (414)276-3349
Email: info@movementdisorders.org
Website: http://www.movementdisorders.org
Gail Bast, Exec. Dir.

Desc: Provides international forums and research to disseminate information on recent advances in clinical and basic science pertinent to movement disorders, enhance education of physicians and public, and enrich the quality of care to patients. **Awards:** Abstract Awards (annual); Honorary Member Award (annual).

★ 13351 ★ Multidisciplinary Association for Psychedelic Studies (MAPS)
2105 Robinson Ave.
Sarasota, FL 34232
Phone: (941)924-6277 **Free:** 888-868-6277
Fax: (941)924-6265
Email: info@maps.org
Website: http://www.maps.org
Dr. Rick Doblin, Pres.

Desc: Promotes the development of beneficial, socially sanctioned uses of psychedelic drugs and marijuana. Helps researchers design, obtain government approval for, fund, conduct and report on psychedelic research in human volunteers; funds MDMA psychotherapy studies; facilitates research and FDA approval for marijuana to be prescribed for medical uses. **Awards:** Grant.

★ 13352 ★ Muscular Dystrophy Association (MDA)
3300 E Sunrise Dr.
Tucson, AZ 85718
Phone: (520)529-2000 **Free:** 800-572-1717
Fax: (520)529-5300
Email: mda@mdausa.org
Website: http://www.mdausa.org
Bob Mackle, Dir. Public Information

Desc: National voluntary health agency fostering research into the cause and cure of neuromuscular diseases in the following 8 categories. Muscular dystrophies: Becker; congenital; distal; Duchenne (pseudohypertrophic); Emery-Dreifuss; facioscapulohumeral (Landouzy-Dejerine); limb-girdle; myotonic (Steinert's disease); oculopharyngeal. Motor Neuron Diseases: adult spinal muscular atrophy (Aran-Duchenne type); amyotrophic lateral sclerosis (ALS); infantile progressive spinal muscular atrophy (type 1, Werdnig-Hoffmann disease); intermediate spinal muscular atrophy (type 2); juvenile spinal muscular atrophy (type 3, Kugelberg-Welander disease), Spinal Bulbar Muscular Atrophy (SBMA). Inflammatory Myopathies: dermatomyositis; polymyositis; inclusion body myositis. Diseases of Neuromuscular Junction: Eaton-Lambert (myasthenic) syndrome;congenital myasthenic syndrome; myasthenia gravis. Diseases of the Peripheral Nerve: Dejerine-Sottas disease; Friedreich's ataxia; Charcot-Marie-Tooth disease (peroneal muscular atrophy). Metabolic Diseases of Muscle: acid maltase deficiency (Pompe's disease); carnitine deficiency; carnitine palmityl transferase deficiency; Debrancher enzyme deficiency (Cori'sor Forbes' disease); lactate dehydrogenase deficiency; mitochondrial myopathy; myoadenylate deaminase deficiency; phosphofructokinase deficiency (Tarui's disease); phosphoglycerate kinase deficiency; phosphoglycerate mutase deficiency; phosphorylase deficiency (McArdle's disease). Myopathies due to Endocrine Abnormalities: hyperthyroid myopathy; hypothyroid myopathy. Other myopathies: central core disease; myotonia congenita; myotubular myopathy; nemaline myopathy; paramyotonia congenita; periodic paralysis. Supports international programs of some 350 research awards, major university-based neuromuscular disease research/clinical centers, and 230 outpatient clinics in hospitals in the U.S. and Puerto Rico. Awards grants for neuromuscular disease research to individual scientific investigators. Renders services to patients locally through its chapters, including: diagnostic examinations; follow-up medical evaluations; wheelchairs; leg braces; physical therapy; flu shots; summer camps. Maintains 28 centers across the nation offering research and care for persons affected by Lou Gehrig's disease. **Awards:** Neuromuscular disease research grants (semiannual) must meet eligibility requirements set by MDA.

★ 13353 ★ Myasthenia Gravis Foundation of America
5841 Cedar Lake Rd., Ste. 204
Minneapolis, MN 55416
Phone: (952)545-9438 **Free:** 800-541-5454
Fax: (952)545-6073
Email: myastheniagravis@msn.com
Website: http://www.myasthenia.org
Debora K. Boelz, CEO

Desc: Persons suffering from myasthenia gravis; their families, doctors, and nurses; others dedicated to the detection, treatment, and cure of MG. Raises funds for research and for professional and public education programs. Provides literature. Lay and professional materials available upon request. **Awards:** Henry R. Viets Students Medical Students Fellowships (annual); Nurse's Fellowship (annual) for research related to myasthenia gravis; Postdoctural Research Grants (annual).

★ 13354 ★ NADD - An Association for Persons with Developmental Disabilities and Mental Health Needs
c/o Robert Fletcher
132 Fair St.
Kingston, NY 12401-4802
Phone: (845)331-4336 **Free:** 800-331-5362
Fax: (845)331-4569
Email: thenadd@aol.com
Website: http://www.thenadd.org
Dr. Robert Fletcher, Dir.

Desc: People with developmental disabilities and mental health care needs; mental health professionals; other interested individuals. Promotes public and professional interest in developmental disability; seeks to improve access to mental health care. Supports research programs; facilitates exchange of information among mental health professionals and consumers; conducts advocacy to insure implementation of effective public mental health policies and legislation. Holds educational programs; maintains speakers' bureau. **Awards:** Menolacino Award (annual); Merck Award (annual).

★ 13355 ★ Narcolepsy Network
10921 Reed Hartman Hwy.
Cincinnati, OH 45242
Phone: (513)891-3522 **Fax:** (513)891-3836
Email: narnet@aol.com
Website: http://www.websciences.org/narnet
Robert L. Cloud, Exec. Dir.

Desc: Individuals with narcolepsy, their friends and families, sleep professionals, and interested others. Seeks to improve the quality of life of individuals who have narcolepsy. Works to educate members and the general public about narcolepsy. Fosters communication among members. Offers referral service. Supports research; disseminates information. **Awards:** Grant (periodic) for research.

★ 13356 ★ National Academy of Clinical Biochemistry (NACB)
c/o Charles D. Hawker
Laboratories
500 Chipeta Way
Salt Lake City, UT 84108
Phone: (801)584-5261 **Fax:** (801)584-5207
Email: hawkercd@aruplab.com
Website: http://www.nacb.org/

Desc: Dedicated to advancing the science and practice of clinical laboratory medicine through research, education, professional development. **Awards:** Fellowships; George Grannis Award for Excellence in Research and Scientific Publication (annual); NACB Distinguished Scientist Award (annual); Professor Alvin Dubin Award (annual).

★ 13357 ★ National AIDS Fund
1030 15th St. NW, Ste. 860
Washington, DC 20005-2208
Phone: (202)408-4848 **Free:** 800-234-AIDS
Fax: (202)408-1818
Email: info@aidsfund.org
Website: http://www.aidsfund.org
Candy Ferree, CEO

Desc: Promotes leadership and generates resources for effective community responses to HIV/AIDS. **Awards:** Scholarship activists to participate in conference/training.

★ 13358 ★ National Alliance for Autism Research (NAAR)
99 Wall St., Research Park
Princeton, NJ 08540
Phone: (609)430-9160 **Free:** 888-777-NAAR
Fax: (609)430-9163
Email: naar@naar.org
Website: http://www.naar.org
Glenn R. Tringali, COO

Desc: Dedicated to finding the causes, prevention, effective treatment and, ultimately, cure of the autism spectrum disorders. **Awards:** NAAR Autism Research (annual).

★ 13359 ★ National Alliance of Breast Cancer Organizations (NABCO)
9 E 37th St., 10th Fl.
New York, NY 10016
Phone: (212)889-0606 **Free:** 888-80-NABCO
Fax: (212)689-1213
Email: NABCOinfo@aol.com
Website: http://www.nabco.org
Amy Langer, Exec. Dir.

Desc: The National Alliance of Breast Cancer Organization (NABCO) is the leading non-profit information and education resource on breast cancer in the U.S. NABCO provides information to medical professionals and their organizations and to patients and their families, and advocates for beneficial regulatory change and legislation. With public and corporate partners, NABCO has collaborated on programs that have reached a national audience, heightening public awareness and connecting women with needed services. Services are free of charge. **Awards:** Within Our Reach (a NABCO program) (annual) for community programs serving poor and medically underserved women.

★ 13360 ★ National Alliance of Methadone Advocates (NAMA)

435 2nd Ave.
New York, NY 10010
Phone: (212)595-6262 **Fax:** (212)595-6262
Email: nama4u@mail-x-change.com
Website: http://www.methadone.org/
Joycelyn Woods, Pres.

Desc: Methadone maintenance patients and supporters of methadone maintenance treatment. Promotes quality methadone maintenance treatment as the most effective modality for the treatment of opiate addiction. **Awards:** National Methadone Conference (periodic) to patient or family member interested in methadone advocacy.

★ 13361 ★ National Alliance for Research on Schizophrenia and Depression (NARSAD)

60 Cutter Mill Rd., Ste. 404
Great Neck, NY 11021
Phone: (516)829-0091 **Free:** 800-829-8289
Fax: (516)487-6930
Email: info@narsad.org
Website: http://www.narsad.org/
Constance Lieber, Pres.

Desc: Raises funds for research on schizophrenia, depression, and other mental illnesses. **Awards:** Lieber Prize (annual) for established scientific investigator; Young Investigators (annual) for scientific research.

★ 13362 ★ National Alopecia Areata Foundation (NAAF)

PO Box 150760
San Rafael, CA 94915-0760
Phone: (415)472-3780 **Fax:** (415)472-5343
Email: info@naaf.org
Website: http://www.naaf.org
Vicki Kalabokes, CEO

Desc: Individuals concerned about alopecia areata, a disease causing partial scalp hair loss, total scalp hair loss (alopecia totalis), or total loss of body hair (alopecia universalis); cause and cure are unknown and the course of the disease is unpredictable. Objectives are to: develop public awareness of the disease; provide a support network; raise funds for research; keep patients medically informed with explanations about AA and the latest treatments. Maintains medical advisory board; operates information booth at meetings of the American Academy of Dermatology. **Awards:** National Alopecia Areata Foundation Research Grants (annual) for research on Alopecia Areata.

★ 13363 ★ National AMBUCS

3315 N Main St.
High Point, NC 27265
Phone: (336)869-2166 **Fax:** (336)887-8451
Email: ambucs@ambucs.com
Website: http://www.ambucs.com
Tom Fender, Pres.

Desc: Dedicated to creating opportunities for independence for people with disabilities. Performs community service; provides physically challenged children with tricycles that can be operated by hand, foot or both: operates the Living Endowment Fund. **Awards:** Scholarships for Therapists (annual) for students majoring in occupational, physical, therapy, speech pathology, hearing audiology.

★ 13364 ★ National Amputee Golf Association (NAGA)

11 Walnut Hill Rd.
Amherst, NH 03031-1713
Phone: (603)672-6444 **Free:** 800-633-6242
Fax: (603)672-2987
Email: info@nagagolf.org
Website: http://www.nagagolf.org
Bob Wilson, Dir.

Desc: Individuals who have lost a hand, foot, or a combination thereof at a major joint. Purpose is to promote the mental and physical rehabilitation of amputees through the sport of golf. Conducts first swing program for therapists. Organizes local, regional, national, and international tournaments. Compiles statistics. **Awards:** Recognition; scholarship bestowed to college students demonstrating financial need.

★ 13365 ★ National Association of Child Care Professionals

PO Box 90723
Austin, TX 78709
Free: 800-537-1118 **Fax:** (512)301-5080
Email: admin@naccp.org
Website: http://www.naccp.org
Sherry Workman, Exec. Dir.

Desc: Child care supervisors and individuals involved in decision making at a child care facility. Offers networking opportunities and support services to child care professionals. Dedicated to the professional development of child care directors. Conducts educational programs. **Awards:** National Child Care Director of the Year Award (annual) recipient for exceptional contributions to the child care industry.

★ 13366 ★ National Association of Clinical Nurse Specialists (NACNS)

3969 Green St.
Harrisburg, PA 17110
Phone: (717)234-6799 **Fax:** (717)234-6798
Email: info@nacns.org
Website: http://www.nacns.org
Christine Carson Filipovich, Exec. Dir.

Desc: Clinical Nurse Specialists. **Awards:** CNS of the Year (annual) per jury of peers; Graduate Student Scholarship (annual) based on manuscript submission.

★ 13367 ★ National Association for Continence

PO Box 8310
Spartanburg, SC 29305-8310
Phone: (864)579-7900 **Free:** 800-BLA-DDER
Fax: (864)579-7902
Email: memberservices@nafc.org
Website: http://www.nafc.org
Nancy Muller, Exec. Dir.

Desc: Works to help individuals who have bladder control problems. Acts as a clearinghouse of information involving incontinence and assistive devices for consumers and their families as well as medical, nursing, and social service organizations. **Awards:** Continence Care Champion (periodic).

★ 13368 ★ National Association of the Deaf (NAD)

814 Thayer Ave., Ste. 250
Silver Spring, MD 20910-4500
Phone: (301)587-1788 **Fax:** (301)587-1791
Email: nadinfo@nad.org
Website: http://www.nad.org
Nancy J. Bloch, Exec. Dir.

Desc: Safeguards accessibility and civil rights of America's deaf population in areas of education, employment, healthcare, and telecommunications. **Awards:** Stokoe Scholarship (annual) for deaf graduate student pursuing studies in field related to sign language or the deaf community.

★ 13369 ★ National Association of Dental Assistants (NADA)

900 S Washington St., No. G-13
Falls Church, VA 22046
Phone: (703)237-8616 **Fax:** (703)533-1153
R. Ludeman, Dir.

Desc: Professional dental auxiliaries. Seeks to: bring added stature and purpose to the profession through continuing education; make available to dental assistants the special benefits normally limited to members of specialized professional and fraternal groups. **Awards:** Scholarship (annual).

★ 13370 ★ National Association of Directors of Nursing Administration in Long Term Care (NADONA/LTC)

10101 Alliance Rd., No. 140
Cincinnati, OH 45242
Phone: (513)791-3679 **Free:** 800-222-0539
Fax: (513)791-3699
Email: info@nadona.org
Website: http://www.nadona.org
Joan C. Warden-Saunders, R.N., Exec. Dir. & Founder

Desc: Directors, assistant directors, and former directors of nursing in long term care. Goals are: to create and establish an acceptable ethical standard for practices in long term care nursing administration and to promote and encourage research in the profession; to develop and provide a consistent program of education and certification for the positions of director, associate director, and assistant director; to promote a positive image of the long term health care industry. Encourages members to share concerns and experiences; sponsors research programs. Advocates legislation pertaining to the practice of professional nursing. Maintains speakers' bureau. nursing. Maintains speakers' bureau. **Awards:** Above and Beyond (annual) upon request; Caring (annual) members conference; Upward Bound (annual).

★ 13371 ★ National Association for the Dually Diagnosed (NADD)

132 Fair St.
Kingston, NY 12401
Phone: (845)331-4336 **Free:** 800-331-5362
Fax: (845)331-4569
Email: rfletcher@thenadd.org
Website: http://www.thenadd.org
Dr. Robert J. Fletcher, Founder/Exec. Dir.

Desc: Promotes understanding of and services for individuals with developmental disabilities and mental health needs. **Awards:** Research Award (annual); scholarship (annual) Menolascino Award for Excellence.

★ 13372 ★ National Association of Federal Veterinarians (NAFV)

1101 Vermont Ave. NW, Ste. 710
Washington, DC 20005-6308
Phone: (202)289-6334 **Fax:** (202)842-4360
Email: dboyle@nafv.org
Website: http://users.erols.com/nafv/
Dr. Joe Yearous, Pres.

Desc: Professional society of veterinarians employed by the U.S. Government. Maintains speakers' bureau. **Awards:** Dr. Daniel E. Salmon Award (annual) for federally employed veterinarians with no more than 10 years service.

★ 13373 ★ National Association for Healthcare Quality (NAHQ)

4700 W Lake Ave.
Glenview, IL 60025-1485
Phone: (847)375-4720 **Free:** 800-966-9392
Fax: 877-218-7939
Email: dsimmons@nahq.com
Website: http://www.nahq.org
Diane K. Simmons, Exec. Dir.

Desc: Healthcare professionals in quality assessment and improvement, utilization and risk management, case management, infection control, managed care, nursing, and medical records. Objectives are: to encourage, develop, and provide continuing education for all persons involved in health care quality; to give the patient primary consideration in all actions affecting his or her health and welfare; to promote the sharing of knowledge and encourage a high degree of professional ethics in health care quality. Offers accredited certification in the field of healthcare quality, utilization, and risk management. Facilitates communication and cooperation among members, medical staff, and health care government agencies. Conducts educational seminars and conferences. **Awards:** Award for Association Excellence (annual); Clare Glover Distinguished Member Award (annual); Stumph Award for Excellence in Publication (annual).

★ 13374 ★ National Association of Health Services Executives (NAHSE)

8630 Fenton St., No. 126
Silver Spring, MD 20910
Phone: (202)628-3953
Email: nationalHQ@nahse.org
Dr. Sandra Gould, PhD, Pres.

Desc: Black health care executive managers, planners, educators, advocates, providers, organizers, researchers, and consumers participating in academic ventures, educational forums, seminars, workshops, systems design, legislation, and other activities. Conducts National Work-Study Program and sponsors educational programs. **Awards:** Haynes Rice Scholarship (annual) for students majoring in healthcare; Humanitarian Award (annual) for outstanding service in the field of human services; NAHSE Scholarship (annual).

★ 13375 ★ National Association of Hispanic Nurses (NAHN)

1501 Sixteenth St. NW
Washington, DC 20036
Phone: (202)387-2477 **Fax:** (202)483-7183
Email: thehispanicnurses@earthlink.net
Website: http://www.thehispanicnurses.org/
Nilda Peragallo, Pres.

Desc: Nurses on all educational levels, from all Hispanic subgroups; non-Hispanic nurses concerned about the health delivery needs of the Hispanic community; nursing students. Serves the nursing and health care delivery needs of the Hispanic community and the professional needs of Hispanic nurses. Provides a forum in which Hispanic nurses can analyze, research, and evaluate the health care needs of the Hispanic community. Disseminates findings of that research to local, state, and federal agencies so as to affect policy-making and resource allocation. Aims to ensure that Hispanic nurses have equal access to educational, professional, and economic opportunities. Identifies Hispanic nurses throughout the nation to determine the size of the work force available to provide culturally sensitive nursing care to Hispanics. **Awards:** Henrietta Villaescusa Award; Ildaura Murillo-Rhode Awards; scholarship.

★ 13376 ★ National Association for Holistic Aromatherapy

4509 Interlake Ave., N, No. 233
Seattle, WA 98103
Phone: (314)963-2071 **Free:** 888-ASK-NAHA
Fax: (206)547-2680
Email: info@naha.org
Website: http://www.naha.org/
Jade Shutes, Pres.

Desc: Seeks to establish and promote the art and science of aromatherapy as a health care alternative. Works to elevate and maintain high standards of aromatherapy eduction. Works to raise public awareness of the benefits of aromatherapy. Fosters communication and exchange among members. Offers educational programs. Maintains speakers' bureau. **Awards:** Student Education Scholarship (annual).

★ 13377 ★ National Association of Medical Minority Educators (NAMME)

c/o Iral D. Porter
Health Careers Pathways Program
University of Kansas Medical Center
3007 Student Center Bldg, 39th & Rainbow
Kansas City, KS 66103
Phone: (212)843-3701 **Fax:** (212)650-3925
Email: premed@premed.edu
Website: http://www.namme-hpe.org
Ms. Iral D. Porter, M.B.A., Membership Chairperson

Desc: Educators, administrators, and practitioners of medicine, osteopathic medicine, dentistry, veterinary medicine, optometry, podiatry, public health, and allied health. Promotes the increase of medical minority personnel; admissions of minority students to health professionals schools; retention and graduation of minority students in health profession schools; recruitment and development of minority faculty administrators and managerial personnel in the health professions; delivery of quality health care for minority populations; and recruitment, retention, and development of minority students in pre-health profession programs. Sponsors workshops for high school counselors and junior high and high school science teachers; provides training for minority affairs workers and officers. Offers annual student development sessions and recruitment fairs. Conducts research programs and systematic studies. **Awards:** Scholarship.

★ 13378 ★ National Association of Pediatric Nurse Practitioners (NAPNAP)

20 Brace Rd., Ste. 200
Cherry Hill, NJ 08034
Phone: (856)857-9700 **Fax:** (856)857-1600
Email: info@napnap.org
Website: http://www.napnap.org
Cathy Van Horn, Off. Mgr.

Desc: Pediatric, school, and family nurse practitioners and interested persons. Seeks to improve the quality of infant, child, and adolescent health care by making health care services accessible and providing a forum for continuing education of members. Facilitates and supports legislation designed to promote the role of pediatric nurse practitioners; promotes salary ranges commensurate with practitioners' responsibilities; facilitates exchange of information between prospective employers and job seekers in the field. Supports research programs; compiles statistics. **Awards:** NAPNAP/McNeil Scholarship (semiannual) for students entering pediatric nurse practitioner programs; recognition.

★ 13379 ★ National Association of Physician Nurses (NAPN)

900 S Washington St., No. G-13
Falls Church, VA 22046
Phone: (703)237-8616 **Fax:** (703)533-1153
Susan Young, Dir.

Desc: Physicians' nurses united to bring added stature and purpose to their profession and to create for themselves the benefits normally limited to members of specialized professional and fraternal groups. **Awards:** Scholarship.

★ 13380 ★ National Association for Pseudoxanthoma Elasticum (NAPE)

8764 Manchester Rd., Ste. 200
Saint Louis, MO 63144
Phone: (314)962-0100 **Fax:** (314)962-0100
Website: http://www.pxenape.org
Frances Benham, PhD, Board Chair

Desc: People who have Pseudoxanthoma Elasticum (PXE), as well as interested others(Pseudoxanthoma elasticum is a rare connective tissue disorder that can affect eyes, skin, and organs). Provides educational information about PXE. Compiles statistics. Serves to unite PXE patients with professionals who treat the disease and others who have the disease. Maintains database of patients with PXE. **Awards:** Grant to scientists studying PXE; monetary to finance low-vision devices for affected members.

★ 13381 ★ National Association of Vascular Access Networks (NAVAN)

11441 S State St., Ste. A, No. 113
Draper, UT 84020-9131
Phone: (801)576-1824 **Free:** 888-576-2826
Fax: (801)553-9137
Email: info@navannet.org
Website: http://www.navannet.org
Mary Lea Nations, Exec. Dir.

Desc: Physicians, pharmacists, nurses, and manufacturers involved in the care and management of patients with vascular access devices. Seeks to advance the effectiveness of vascular access devices; promotes professional development of members. Serves as a network linking members; conducts educational programs. **Awards:** NAVAN/Suzanne LaVere Herbst Award (annual).

★ 13382 ★ National Ataxia Foundation (NAF)

2600 Fernbrook Ln. N, No. 119
Minneapolis, MN 55447
Phone: (763)553-0020 **Fax:** (763)553-0167
Email: naf@mail.ataxia.org
Website: http://www.ataxia.org
Donna Gruetzmacher, Exec. Dir.

Desc: Membership is open to any individual who wishes to contribute to the eradication of ataxia (a genetic disease characterized by the degeneration of the nerves of the spinal cord and the cerebellum, causing a loss of coordination and disturbance in gait and related conditions such as peroneal muscular atrophy, hereditary spastic paraplegia, and hereditary tremor. Ataxia may be inherited as a recessive or dominant trait and may strike persons from a very early age up to and even beyond 50 years of age. Ataxia is very similar to multiple sclerosis; however, multiple sclerosis is not inherited and has a different origin.) Objectives are: to make an early diagnosis of ataxia by locating all potential victims and encouraging them to have an examination; to educate the public and the helping professions about ataxia; to initiate basic research and coordinate efforts of worldwide research centers. Emphasis is on locating and understanding the genes responsible. Provides services and information to ataxia victims and their families. **Awards:** Ataxia Research Grant (annual).

★ 13383 ★ National Black Leadership Initiative on Cancer (NBLIC)

PO Box 34828
Las Vegas, NV 89133
Phone: (702)655-3752 **Fax:** (702)655-3762
Email: dot.blic@yahoo.com
Dorothy M. Johnson, Chair

Desc: African-Americans and health care professionals concerned with the prevention, diagnosis, and treatment of people with cancer, particularly those of African-American descent. Seeks to facilitate "closing the gap in cancer incidence and mortality and increasing survival from cancer" by increasing awareness among African-AMRs of cancer and its prevention and treatment. Conducts educational programs to develop volunteer leaders in African-American communities, with emphasis on increasing understanding of breast, colorectal, and prostate cancer and the role played by diet in their prevention. **Awards:** Scholarship (periodic).

★ 13384 ★ National Blood Foundation (NBF)

8101 Glenbrook Rd.
Bethesda, MD 20814-2749
Phone: (301)215-6552 **Fax:** (301)907-6895
Email: nbf@aabb.org
Website: http://www.aabb.org

Desc: Promotes the safety and adequacy of America's blood supply by supporting research and education for blood banking and transfusion medicine. **Awards:** Scientific Research Grants Program (annual) one or two year grants to prepare or support new investigators in the fields of blood banking, transfusion medicine, and tissue transplantation.

★ 13385 ★ National Board of Medical Examiners (NBME)
3750 Market St.
Philadelphia, PA 19104-3190
Phone: (215)590-9500 **Fax:** (215)590-9555
Email: webmail@nbme.org
Website: http://www.nbme.org
Donald E. Melnick, MD, Pres.

Desc: Purposes are: to prepare and administer qualifying examinations either independently or in conjunction with other organizations, of such high quality that legal agencies governing the practice of medicine within each state may, in their discretion, grant a license without further examination for those who have successfully completed such examinations; to cooperate with and, where appropriate, to make its specialized services available to the examining boards of the states, specialty boards, and other organizations concerned with the education and qualification of personnel in the fields of health; to assist medical schools, hospitals and related organizations and institutions in evaluation of the effectiveness of their educational programs; to initiate, develop, and participate in research designed to evaluate the effectiveness of educational programs and techniques, and to assess ever more precisely the knowledge, competence, and qualification of professionals in public health care; to provide educational opportunities for professional personnel in the methods, techniques, and values of testing methods related to knowledge and competence in the broad field of medicine. **Awards:** Medical Education Research Fund (annual).

★ 13386 ★ National Brain Tumor Foundation (NBTF)
414 13th St., Ste. 700
Oakland, CA 94612-2603
Phone: (510)839-9777 **Free:** 800-934-CURE
Email: nbtf@braintumor.org
Website: http://www.braintumor.org
Janis Brewer, Exec. Dir.

Desc: Medical researchers, doctors, brain tumor patients, and relatives working together to improve the quality of life for brain tumor patients and their families and find a cure through research. Raises funds for brain tumor research; offers patient services such as educational materials, a toll-free brain tumor information line, a quarterly newsletter, information about support groups and patient networks, and national and regional conferences. **Awards:** Grant (annual) for research.

★ 13387 ★ National Catholic AIDS Network (NCAN)
PO Box 960
Occidental, CA 95465
Phone: (707)874-3031 **Fax:** (707)874-1433
Email: info@ncan.org
Website: http://www.ncan.org
Fr. Rodney DeMartini, Exec. Dir.

Desc: Provides support and exchange of information among Roman Catholic HIV/AIDS service workers and pastoral ministers. Disseminates educational materials on HIV/AIDS. **Awards:** Lumina Award (annual) for creative and effective pastoral leadership in HIV/AIDS ministry; monetary (annual) for an individual with HIV from an economically impoverished area or service providers who qualify to attend annual ministry conference.

★ 13388 ★ National Caucus and Center on Black Aged (NCBA)
1220 L St. NW, Ste. 800
Washington, DC 20005
Phone: (202)637-8400 **Fax:** (202)347-0895
Email: info@ncba-aged.org
Website: http://www.ncba-aged.org
Karyne J. Conley, Pres. /CEO

Desc: Seeks to improve living conditions for low-income elderly Americans, particularly blacks. Advocates changes in federal and state laws in improving the economic, health, and social status of low-income senior citizens. Promotes community awareness of problems and issues effecting low-income aging population. Operates an employment program involving 2000 older persons in 14 states. Sponsors, owns, and manages rental housing for the elderly. Conducts training and intern programs in nursing home administration, long-term care, housing management, and commercial property maintenance. **Awards:** Recognition; scholarship.

★ 13389 ★ National Center for Complementary and Alternative Medicine (NCCAM)
PO Box 7923
Gaithersburg, MD 20898-7923
Phone: (301)519-3153 **Free:** 888-644-6226
Fax: (866)464-3616
Email: info@nccam.nih.gov
Website: http://nccam.nih.gov/
Stephen E. Straus, MD, Dir.

Desc: Committed to exploring complementary and alternative healing practices, including but not limited to acupuncture, herbs, homeopathy, therapeutic massage, and traditional oriental medicine; trains CAM researchers; conducts biomedical research; disseminates information. Programs focus on evaluating the safety and efficacy of natural products, supporting pharmacological studies to determine potential interactive effects with standard treatment medications, evaluates CAM practices such as acupuncture and chiropractic. Acts as the NCCAM Clearinghouse. **Awards:** National Research Service Award Institutional Training Grants to eligible institutions to develop or enhance research training in specified areas of biomedical and behavioral research.

★ 13390 ★ National Center for FarmWorker Health
1770 FM 967
Buda, TX 78610
Phone: (512)312-2700 **Free:** 800-531-5120
Fax: (512)312-2600
Email: info@ncfh.org
Website: http://www.ncfh.org
E. Roberta Ryder, Chief Exec. Officer

Desc: Seeks to make quality primary health care accessible to migrant and seasonal farm workers. Supports the establishment of a national network of migrant health centers through the production, processing, and distribution of information, including information on health problems specific to or more prevalent in the migrant community. Works to provide technical assistance for health development and research. Develops collaborative working relationship between agencies serving migrant farmworkers. Maintains job/resume bank, biographical archives, and library. Bestows awards; operates placement service; compiles statistics. biographical archives, library, and speakers' bureau. Bestows awards; operates placement service; compiles statistics. **Awards:** Migrant Health Scholarship (annual) work in migrant health center.

★ 13391 ★ National CFIDS Foundation
103 Althea Rd.
Needham, MA 02492
Phone: (781)449-3535 **Fax:** (781)449-8606
Email: info@ncf-net.com
Website: http://www.ncf-net.org
Gail R. Kansky, Pres.

Desc: Provides education, advocacy and fundraising for research. **Awards:** B&D for research into causal matters.

★ 13392 ★ National Child Care Association (NCCA)
1016 Rosser St.
Conyers, GA 30012
Free: 800-543-7161 **Fax:** (770)388-7772
Website: http://www.nccanet.org
Lynn L. White, Exec. Dir.

Desc: Works to promote and safeguard the interest of quality child care in the United States. Focuses on licensed, private providers of child care and preschool services. Conducts lobbying activities; offers casualty insurance programs; conducts educational and research programs; provides networking opportunities. **Awards:** National Early Childhood Program Accreditation; scholarship.

★ 13393 ★ National Children's Eye Care Foundation (NCECF)
c/o American Association for Pediatric Ophthalmology and Strabismus
PO Box 193832
San Francisco, CA 94119-3832
Phone: (415)561-8505 **Fax:** (415)561-8531
Email: aapos@aao.org
Website: http://med-aapos.bu.edu
Denise De Losada Wilson, Admin.

Desc: Seeks to optimize the quality of life of infants, children, and families by fostering normal development and protection of vision through promoting programs of prevention, detection, treatment, research and education. **Awards:** Fellowship Loans (annual) to fund fellowships in pediatric opthalmology; grant (annual) for research in children's eye disorders and diseases.

★ 13394 ★ National Chronic Fatigue Syndrome and Fibromyalgia Association (NCFSFA)
PO Box 18426
Kansas City, MO 64133
Phone: (816)313-2000 **Fax:** (816)524-6782
Email: information@ncfsfa.org
Website: http://www.ncfsfa.org
Orvalene Prewitt, Contact

Desc: Individuals suffering from chronic fatigue syndrome and Fibromyalgia health care professionals. Chronic fatigue syndrome, also known as Chronic Epstein-Barr Virus syndrome, is characterized by persistent, recurring feelings of general weakness; other symptoms include sore throat, unexplained muscle pain, new headaches, devastating fatigue, impaired memory or concentration, tender lymph nodes, unrefreshing sleep and post-exertion malaise. Fibromyalgia is characterized as pain, generally felt all over, and can be compounded by fatigue, sleep disturbances, changes in mood, headaches and gastro-intestinal problems. Sponsors educational programs. Maintains speakers' bureau. **Awards:** Research Grant (annual).

★ 13395 ★ National Dental Association (NDA)
3517 16th St., NW
Washington, DC 20010
Phone: (202)588-1697 **Fax:** (202)588-1244
Email: admin@ndaonline.org
Website: http://www.ndaonline.org
Dr. Romell J. Madison, Pres.

Desc: Professional society for dentists. Aims to provide quality dental care to the unserved and underserved public and promote knowledge of the art and science of dentistry. Advocates the inclusion of dental care services in health care programs on local, state, and national levels. Fosters the integration of minority dental health care providers in the profession, and promotes dentistry as a viable career for minorities through support programs. Conducts research programs. Group is distinct from the former name of the American Dental Association. **Awards:** Recognition; scholarship bestowed to minorities for dentistry careers.

★ 13396 ★ National Dental Hygienists' Association (NDHA)
c/o Barbara Seldon, Trustee
28315 Kalong Cir. W
Southfield, MI 48034
Email: ndha@aol.com
Website: http://www.ndaonline.org/auxillary.htm
Diane Lane-Tyson, Pres.

Desc: Minority dental hygienists. To cultivate and promote the art and science of dental hygiene and to enhance the professional image of dental hygienists. Attempts to meet the needs of society through educational, political, and social activities while giving the minority dental hygienist a voice in shaping the profession. Encourages cooperation and mutual support among minority professionals. Seeks to increase opportunities for continuing education and employment in the field of dental hygiene. Works to improve individual and community dental health. Sponsors annual seminar, fundraising events, and scholarship programs; participates in career orientation programs; counsels and assists students applying for or enrolled in dental hygiene programs. Maintains liaison with American Dental Hygienists' Association. **Awards:** NDHA Scholarship (annual) for an African American individual.

★ 13397 ★ National EMS Pilots Association (NEMSPA)

526 King St., Ste. 415
Alexandria, VA 22314-3143
Phone: (703)836-8930 **Fax:** (703)836-8920
Email: dmancuso@aams.org
Website: http://www.nemspa.org

Desc: Pilots in the air medical industry and interested individuals. Works to help the air medical industry prosper safely and enhance the delivery of health care. Facilitates the exchange of information; evaluates new equipment; conducts educational programs; monitors governmental organizations; supports research; offers legal assistance. **Awards:** EMS Pilot of the Year (annual).

★ 13398 ★ National Federation of the Blind (NFB)

1800 Johnson St.
Baltimore, MD 21230
Phone: (410)659-9314 **Fax:** (410)685-5653
Email: nfb@nfb.org
Website: http://www.nfb.org
Marc Maurer, Pres.

Desc: Federation of state (50 plus Washington, DC and Puerto Rico) and local (700) organizations representing over 50,000 blind people. Seeks the complete equality and integration of the blind into society. Monitors all legislation affecting the blind; evaluates present programs for the blind; stimulates and assists in promoting needed services. Supports and conducts scholarly research and publication of results. Works to improve policies toward the blind in such places as the U.S. Office of Personnel Management. Sponsors National White Cane Week annually for fundraising and educational purposes. Distributes information. Maintains National Blindness Information Center. **Awards:** Hermione Grant Calhoun Scholarship (annual) for blind women students; Howard Brown Rickard Scholarship for blind students of the professions; recognition for greatest contribution to the welfare of the blind; scholarship for blind postsecondary students; scholarship given to blind students.

★ 13399 ★ National Foundation for Ectodermal Dysplasias (NFED)

410 E Main
Box 114
Mascoutah, IL 62258
Phone: (618)566-2020 **Fax:** (618)566-4718
Email: info@nfed.org
Website: http://www.nfed.org
Mary Kaye Richter, Exec. Dir.

Desc: Families of ectodermal dysplasia patients and the medical community. (Ectodermal dysplasia is a genetic birth defect usually resulting in an abnormal development of the outer layer of cells in the embryo. The disorder may be characterized by absent or poorly functioning sweat glands, sparse hair follicles, abnormal hair texture, absence of hair and skin oils, disfigured finger and toe nails, hearing or sight deficiencies, abnormalities of the limbs and cleft palate. With proper medical care, ED patients can live fairly normal lives.) Locates patients and provides them with support and information. Assists the medical community in acquiring the necessary information for treating an ED patient, locates treatment facilities and provides referral services. Makes funds available to qualified applicants for dental and other necessary care. Conducts educational meetings and assists with research projects. Provides children's services; compiles statistics. Supports researchers financially and through access to patients when approved. **Awards:** Kenneth S. Brown, MD Research Award (periodic) for outstanding research with history of research and results applicable to ED; Outstanding Service Award; Research Awards (annual) for outstanding research with history of research and results applicable to ED.

★ 13400 ★ National Foundation for Infectious Diseases (NFID)

4733 Bethesda Ave., Ste. 750
Bethesda, MD 20814
Phone: (301)656-0003 **Fax:** (301)907-0878
Email: info@nfid.org
Website: http://www.nfid.org
Susan J. Rehm, MD, Pres.

Desc: Supports research into the causes and cures of infectious diseases; assists in the education of both professionals and the public in infectious diseases. Conducts programs in prevention of infectious diseases. **Awards:** Jimmy & Rosalynn Carter Award for Humanitarian Contributions (annual) for humanitarian contributions to the health of humankind; Maxwell Finland Award for Scientific Achievement (annual) for scientific achievements which contribute to improving medical research; New Investigator Matching Grants (annual); NFID Postdoctoral Fellowships (annual) for physicians specializing in infectious diseases.

★ 13401 ★ National Foundation for Jewish Genetic Diseases (NFJGD)

250 Park Ave., Ste. 1000
New York, NY 10177
Phone: (212)371-1030 **Fax:** (212)319-5808
Website: http://www.nfjgd.org
George Crohn, Pres.

Desc: Individuals concerned with the eradication of the seven known genetic diseases that affect children of predominantly Ashkenazi Jewish heritage. (These diseases include Gaucher's disease, Dystonia, Dysautonomia, Tay-Sachs, Bloom's Syndrome, Niemann-Pick, and Mucolipidosis IV.) Seeks to accomplish its goal by establishing carrier identification tests, providing genetic counseling which includes prenatal testing procedures, and conducting a nationwide education campaign to inform the public that these diseases exist and attack without warning. Supports basic medical research in the prevention and cure of these diseases. Acts as referral agency. Has sponsored symposia on chromosome breakage and neoplasia, Gaucher's disease, and cellular molecular biology of neuronal development. **Awards:** Scholarship.

★ 13402 ★ National Foundation for Transplants (NFT)

1102 Brookfield, Ste. 200
Memphis, TN 38119
Phone: (901)684-1697 **Free:** 800-489-3863
Fax: (901)684-1128
Email: jhill@transplants.org
Website: http://www.transplants.org
Gary McMahan, Dir.

Desc: Works to guide and assist fundraising for transplant patients and their families. Offers grants for smaller emergency transplants and medication needs. Provides financial support and advocacy. **Awards:** Medications Grants and Emergency Grants (monthly) transplant candidates or transplant recipients with one-time (not ongoing) need for medications or other transplant-related emergencies. Must be verified by a medical professional.

★ 13403 ★ National Gaucher Foundation (NGF)

5410 Edson Ln., Ste. 260
Rockville, MD 20852
Phone: (301)816-1515 **Free:** 800-GAU-CHER
Fax: (301)816-1516
Email: ngf@gaucherdisease.org
Website: http://www.gaucherdisease.org
Rhonda P. Buyers, Exec. Dir.

Desc: Persons with Gaucher Disease; interested medical professionals and individuals. Gaucher Disease, one of the most common inherited metabolic disorders, is caused by an enzyme deficiency which renders the body unable to break down and dispose of complex lipids (fat-like substances). These lipids accumulate in the spleen, liver, and bone marrow, causing enlargement of the organs and intermittent pain of varying severity. Gaucher is treatable through enzyme replacement therapy. (The disease is named for Phillippe C.E. Gaucher, a French physician who described it in 1882.) One in 14 Jews of E. European descent is a carrier and one in 450 has Gaucher Disease. Sponsors direct funding of and support for research and clinical programs at medical centers in the U.S. and abroad to develop a cure and/or treatment for Gaucher Disease. Seeks to help persons with the disorder by providing them the opportunity to share experiences and feelings on a confidential, personal basis. Disseminates technical and nontechnical information concerning the disease. Advocates increased screening for carriers and availability of prenatal diagnosis for families at risk. **Awards:** Grant.

★ 13404 ★ National Gerontological Nursing Association

7794 Grow Dr.
Pensacola, FL 32514
Phone: (850)473-1174 **Free:** 800-723-0560
Fax: (850)484-8762
Email: ngna@puetzamc.com
Website: http://www.ngna.org
Belinda E. Puetz, RN,PHD, Contact

Desc: Gerontological nurses. Seeks to effectively improve the care and well-being of older adults. Provides a forum in which gerontological nursing issues are identified and explored. Develops and supports educational programs for nurses, health providers, and the general public. Disseminates information. **Awards:** Innovations in Practice Award (annual); Judith V. Braun Research Award (annual); Mary Opal Wolanin Scholarship (annual).

★ 13405 ★ National Institute of Neurological Disorders and Stroke (NINDS)

Financial Management Branch
Bldg. 31, Rm. 8A34
31 Center Dr.
Bethesda, MD 20892-2350
Phone: (301)496-4927
Email: giftfunds@ninds.nih.gov
Website: http://www.ninds.nih.gov/about_ninds/mission.htm

Desc: Works to identify the causes and to prevent, diagnose and treat neurological disorders and stroke. **Awards:** Fellowship; Grants-in-aid to public and private institutions.

★ 13406 ★ National Marfan Foundation (NMF)

22 Manhasset Ave.
Port Washington, NY 11050-2023
Phone: (516)883-8712 **Free:** 800-862-7326
Fax: (516)883-8040
Email: support@marfan.org
Website: http://www.marfan.org
Karen Wolk, CSW, Dir. Support Svcs.

Desc: Persons affected with the Marfan syndrome and related connective tissue disorders; families of affected persons; genetic counselors; cardiologists, ophthalmologists, orthopedists, and other medical professionals. (Marfan syndrome is a heritable disorder of the connective tissue affecting the skeleton, lungs, eyes, heart, and blood vessels.) Objectives are to: disseminate accurate and timely information on Marfan syndrome; act as support network and provide a means for patients and relatives to share experiences; improve medical care. Supports and fosters research. **Awards:** NMF Research Grant (annual) for basic and clinical research on Marfan Syndrome and related connective tissue disorders.

★ 13407 ★ National Medical Fellowships (NMF)

5 Handover Sq., 15th Fl.
New York, NY 10004
Phone: (212)483-8880 **Fax:** (212)483-8897
Email: info@nmfonline.org
Website: http://www.nmfonline.org
Vivian Fox, Pres. /CEO

Desc: Promotes education of minority students in medicine. Provides need-based scholarships, special merit awards, and leadership opportunities to medical students of African American, Native American, Mexican American and mainland Puerto Rican heritage. **Awards:** Recognition (annual) for third- and fourth-year minority medical students; scholarship (annual).

★ 13408 ★ National MedPeds Residents' Association (NMPRA)

c/o Renee Gaines
Department of Internal Medicine
1542 Tulane Ave., Rm. 447
New Orleans, LA 70112
Fax: (270)596-5951
Email: nmpra@medpeds.org
Website: http://www.medpeds.org/\
David Kendrick, MD, Pres.

Desc: Promotes the practice of MedPeds, combined internal medicine and pediatrics; educates and serves MedPeds residency and serves as a resource for medical students interested in MedPeds. **Awards:** Scholarship.

★ 13409 ★ National Minority AIDS Council (NMAC)

1931 13th St. NW
Washington, DC 20009
Phone: (202)483-6622 **Fax:** (202)483-1135
Email: info@nmac.org
Website: http://www.nmac.org
Paul A. Kawata, Exec. Dir.

Desc: Public health departments and AIDS service organizations. Serves as a clearinghouse of information on AIDS as it affects minority communities in the U.S. Facilitates discussion among national minority organizations about AIDS. Maintains Project Health, Education, and AIDS Leadership, which provides computer usage, strategic planning, financial management, and volunteer program development assistance to AIDS service organizations, and Project Volunteer Information, Technical Assistance, and Leadership, which provides technical assistance in volunteer program development and maintenance. Conducts training conferences. Offers educational and research programs; compiles statistics. Maintains speakers' bureau. **Awards:** Recognition; scholarship.

★ 13410 ★ National MPS Society

45 Packard Dr.
Bangor, ME 04401
Phone: (207)947-1445 **Fax:** (207)990-3074
Email: info@mpssociety.org
Website: http://www.mpssociety.org
Barbara Wedehase, Exec. Dir.

Desc: Professionals and families devoted to educating the public and discovering and aiding families of MPS and ML children. Mucopolysaccharidoses (MPS) and mucolipidoses (ML) are extremely rare hereditary diseases caused by particular enzyme deficiencies and range in severity from strictly bone and joint involvement to massive complications in all organ systems. Helps to facilitate diagnosis and treatment through referrals to doctors and hospitals. Maintains parent referral service to direct families with newly diagnosed MPS and ML children to other members. **Awards:** MPS & ML Research (annual).

★ 13411 ★ National Network for the Disabled

c/o Linda Walls
PO Box 3574
Gardena, CA 90247-7274
Phone: (310)638-5717 **Fax:** (310)638-5986
Linda Walls, Founder-Pres.

Desc: Provides support, companionship, and networking opportunities for elderly individuals and parents of disabled children. Conducts research. Sponsors education on such topics as assertiveness, resources, and medical options. Provides transportation and emergency services, including a food program through which meals are delivered to homes. Conducts special events for parents and children, including picnics and field trips; special programs on nutrition and accessible travel with groups. **Awards:** Scholarship.

★ 13412 ★ National Neurofibromatosis Foundation (NNFF)

95 Pine St., 16th Fl.
New York, NY 10005
Phone: (212)344-6633 **Free:** 800-323-7938
Fax: (212)747-0004
Email: nnff@nf.org
Website: http://www.nf.org/
W. John Radziejewski, Dir. of Pub. Ed.

Desc: The leading resource on neurofibromatosis, a genetic disorder that causes tumors to grow along nerves throughout the body. Provides direct services to children and adults with NF, as well as information and resources to the public and medical professionals via a toll-free number and a website. **Awards:** Basic Grant (annual) for research in neurofibromatosis; Young Investigator Grant (annual) for research in neurofibromatosis.

★ 13413 ★ National Neurotrauma Society

c/o Linda Garcia
PO Box 143060
Gainesville, FL 32608
Phone: (352)271-1169 **Fax:** (352)271-3060
Email: lindahou@aol.com
Website: http://www.neurotrauma.org
Linda Garcia, Contact

Desc: Conducts scientific research in neurotrauma field. **Awards:** Student Travel Award (annual).

★ 13414 ★ National Niemann Pick Disease Foundation (NPD)

c/o Barb Vorpahl
415 Madison Ave.
PO Box 49
Fort Atkinson, WI 53538
Phone: (920)563-0930 **Free:** 877-287-3672
Fax: (920)563-0931
Email: webmaster@nnpdf.org
Website: http://www.nnpdf.org
Barb Vorpahl, Chm.

Desc: Parents, medical and educational professionals, and friends. Works to promote medical research on Niemann-Pick Disease (NPD), a disorder which prevents metabolizing of the sphingomyelin lipid or cholesterol. Provides medical and educational information; offers support to families of children with NPD; facilitates genetic counseling for parents; supports legislation that affects patients and families with NPD; sponsors medical research. **Awards:** Grant for research of Niemann Pick Disease.

★ 13415 ★ National Nursing Staff Development Organization

7794 Grow Dr.
Pensacola, FL 32514
Phone: (850)474-0995 **Free:** 800-489-1995
Fax: (850)484-8762
Email: nnsdo@puetzamc.com
Website: http://www.nnsdo.org
Belinda E. Puetz, PhD, Exec. Dir.

Desc: Advances the specialty practice of staff development for the enhancement of quality healthcare outcomes. Staff development, as a specialty of nursing practice, is defined by standards, based on research critical to quality patient and organizational outcomes. Provides a forum for networking among staff development educators. **Awards:** Affiliate Excellence in Quality Programs Awards (annual); Belinda E. Puetz Award (annual); Excellence Awards (quarterly); grant (annual).

★ 13416 ★ National Organization for Associate Degree Nursing (N-OADN)

c/o Sharon L. Bernier
Montgomery College
7600 Takoma Ave.
Takoma Park, MD 20912
Phone: (301)650-1355 **Fax:** (301)650-1346
Email: sbernier@aol.com
Website: http://www.noadn.org
Sharon L. Bernier, Pres.

Desc: Individuals interested in retaining current competency level examinations and endorsement of RN licensure from state to state for associate degree nursing graduates. Represents and advances the status of associate degree nursing education and practice. Provides networking among members to facilitate the exchange of legislative information and support. Offers clearinghouse for interpretation of legal issues and liability insurance. **Awards:** Naomi Brack (annual) student.

★ 13417 ★ National Organization of Nurse Practitioners Faculties

1522 K St. NW, Ste. 702
Washington, DC 20005
Phone: (202)289-8044 **Fax:** (202)289-8046
Email: nonpf@nonpf.org
Website: http://www.nonpf.com
Kathryn Werner, MPA, Exec. Dir.

Desc: Works to promote public health by developing and implementing nurse practitioner education. Disseminates research related to nurse practitioner education; provides a forum for the exchange of information; works to influence policy affecting nurse practitioners; and develops national guidelins and criteria for nurse practitioner educational programs. **Awards:** Achievement in Research Award (annual); Outstanding Group Faculty Practice Award (annual); Outstanding Nurse Practitioner Educator Award (annual); Small Grant Research Award (annual).

★ 13418 ★ National Organization for Rare Disorders (NORD)

PO Box 1968
Danbury, CT 06813-1968
Phone: (203)744-0100 **Free:** 800-999-6673
Fax: (203)798-2291
Email: orphan@rarediseases.org
Website: http://www.rarediseases.org
Susan Olivo, Admin. Assistant

Desc: Doctors, professionals, academics, voluntary health organizations, and individuals interested in rare disorders. Serves as a clearinghouse for information concerning rare disorders. Objectives are: to monitor the Orphan Drug Act; to link individuals with rare disorders together for mutual support; to stimulate research on rare diseases; to foster communication among voluntary agencies, health-related industries, and government bodies. (Orphan drugs are used in the treatment of rare disorders. Since their use is not widespread, most drug companies cannot expect to profit from the development and manufacture of these drugs. The Orphan Drug Act gives financial assistance and tax incentives to drug companies that develop these drugs.) Provides information on rare disorders and referrals to organizations. **Awards:** NORD Research Grant (biennial) bestowed to scientists for clinical research on new treatments for rare diseases; recognition (annual) bestowed to individuals and corporations for outstanding service in health or orphan drug development.

★ 13419 ★ National Ovarian Cancer Coalition (NOCC)
500 NE Spanish River Blvd., Ste. 14
Boca Raton, FL 33431
Phone: (561)393-0005 **Free:** 888-OVA-RIAN
Fax: (561)393-7275
Email: noccnat@ovarian.org
Website: http://www.ovarian.org

Desc: Individuals with ovarian cancer and their families; health care professionals treating people with ovarian cancer. Seeks to advance the prevention, diagnosis, and treatment of ovarian cancer. Serves as a clearinghouse on ovarian cancer; provides support and services to members; conducts educational programs. **Awards:** Research Fund (annual).

★ 13420 ★ National Parkinson Foundation (NPF)
1501 NW 9th Ave.
Bob Hope Parkinson's Research Center
Miami, FL 33136-1494
Phone: (305)547-6666 **Free:** 800-327-4545
Fax: (305)548-4403
Email: mailbox@parkinson.org
Website: http://www.parkinson.org
Herbert C. Zemel, Pres.

Desc: Doctors, nurses, scientists, pharmacologists, and therapists who research, diagnose, and treat Parkinsonism. Supports basic and clinical research for Parkinsonism and related neurological disorders and provides physical, speech, and occupational therapy. NPF is associated with the University of Miami School of Medicine, and supports the National Parkinson Institute, which provides diagnosis, treatment, care, and rehabilitation. Conducts educational programs. Distributes literature to medical libraries, nurses training schools, health clinics, physicians, and patients. Sponsors regional patient self-support groups where problems are discussed and experiences are exchanged under guidance of physicians, social workers, and psychologists. Maintains offices at 122 E. 42nd St., New York, NY 10017 and 4929 Wilshire Blvd., Los Angeles, CA 90010. **Awards:** Research Grants (annual).

★ 13421 ★ National Perinatal Association (NPA)
3500 E Fletcher Ave., Ste. 205
Tampa, FL 33613
Phone: (813)971-1008 **Free:** 888-971-3295
Fax: (813)971-9306
Email: npa@nationalperinatal.org
Website: http://www.nationalperinatal.org
Shelia S. Sorkin, Exec. Dir.

Desc: Organizations and individuals interested in perinatal health care. Purpose is to promote improved patient care, education, research, advocacy and delivery systems for perinatal health. **Awards:** National Perinatal Association Award (annual) for contribution to maternal/child health; Stanley N. Graven Leadership Award (annual); State Initiative (annual).

★ 13422 ★ National Rehabilitation Administration Association (NRAA)
c/o National Rehabilitation Association
633 S Washington St.
Alexandria, VA 22314
Phone: (703)836-0850 **Fax:** (703)836-0848
Email: info@nationalrehab.org
Website: http://www.nationalrehab.org

Desc: Nonprofit rehabilitation instructors, state agency vocational rehabilitation instructors, and private instructors. Promotes continuing professional development of members. Conducts professional training sessions. **Awards:** Grant (periodic) Professional programs in the fields of rehabilitation administration and supervision.

★ 13423 ★ National Rosacea Society
800 S Northwest Hwy., Ste. 200
Barrington, IL 60010
Free: 800-NO-BLUSH **Fax:** (847)382-5567
Email: rosaceas@aol.com
Website: http://www.rosacea.org
Day Olney, Contact

Desc: Mission is to improve the lives of people with rosacea by raising awareness, providing public health information and supporting research on this widespread but little-known disorder. **Awards:** Medical and Scientific Grants for Research (annual).

★ 13424 ★ National Service Dog Center (NSDC)
c/o Delta Society
580 Naches Ave. SW, No. 101
Renton, WA 98055
Phone: (425)226-7357 **Fax:** (425)235-1076
Email: info@deltasociety.org
Website: http://www.deltasociety.org
Nancy Kedward, Contact

Desc: A joint program of the American Humane Association and the Delta Society. Provides a national service dog education, advocacy and referral service. Promotes the health benefits of service animals for people with disabilities. **Awards:** Service Animals of the Year (annual) for outstanding work by animals trained to help people with disabilities.

★ 13425 ★ National Sjogren's Syndrome Association (NSSA)
PO Box 22066
Beachwood, OH 44122-0066
Phone: (216)292-3866 **Free:** 800-395-6772
Fax: (216)292-4955
Email: nickofohio@aol.com
Website: http://www.sjogrenssyndrome.org/
Barbara Henry, Exec. Dir.

Desc: Promotes public awareness of Sjogren's Syndrome; encourages research into the cause and cure of the disorder. (Sjogren's Syndrome is an autoimmune disorder characterized by dryness of all mucous membranes resulting from deficient secretion of the glands. Approximately 50% of Sjogren's Syndrome patients also have rheumatoid arthritis.) Sponsors chapters and offers information to the medical community. Conducts educational and research programs; maintains speakers' bureau. **Awards:** Fellow in Rheumatology (annual); Student of Ophotolomology (annual).

★ 13426 ★ National Sleep Foundation
1522 K St., NW, Ste. 510
Washington, DC 20005
Phone: (202)347-3471 **Fax:** (202)347-3472
Email: nsf@sleepfoundation.org
Website: http://www.sleepfoundation.org
James K. Walsh, PhD, Pres.

Desc: Works to improve the quality of life of people suffering from sleep disorders and to prevent accidents related to sleep disorders. (Sleep disorders include: insomnia, narcolepsy, sleep apnea syndrome, sudden infant death syndrome, stroke, epilepsy, and other disorders of sleep and daytime alertness.) Educates health care professionals and the public about the existance and treatment of sleep disorders. Promotes the development of patient services, community resources, and support groups for individuals affected by sleep disorders. Sponsors educational and research programs. **Awards:** Pickwick Club and Narcolepsy Fellowships (annual); scholarship.

★ 13427 ★ National Society of Genetic Counselors (NSGC)
c/o Bea Leopold
233 Canterbury Dr.
Wallingford, PA 19086-6617
Phone: (610)872-7608 **Fax:** (610)872-1192
Email: fyi@nsgc.org
Website: http://www.nsgc.org
Bea Leopold, Exec. Dir.

Desc: The leaing voice, authority and advocate for the genetic counseling profession. **Awards:** Jane Engelberg Memorial Fellowship (annual); Natalie Weissberger Paul National Achievement Award (annual); Special Project Fund (annual).

★ 13428 ★ National Society for Histotechnology (NSH)
4201 Northview Dr., Ste. 502
Bowie, MD 20716-2604
Phone: (301)262-6221 **Fax:** (301)262-9188
Email: histo@nsh.org
Website: http://www.nsh.org
Lena Spencer, Pres.

Desc: Histology laboratory technicians, pathologists, laboratory equipment manufacturers' representatives, and interested individuals. Encourages the professional growth and advancement of histoprofessionals and promotes the exchange of ideas and knowledge significant to histotechnology. Assists in the establishment and mutual understanding of related societies. Provides continuing education training courses. Investigates health hazards in the laboratory; ensures the safety of the laboratory; and participates in formulating federal laboratory regulations. **Awards:** Histotechnologist of the Year Award (annual); J.B. McCormick Award (annual); Newsletter of the Year Award (annual); scholarship.

★ 13429 ★ National Stroke Association (NSA)
9707 E Easter Ln.
Englewood, CO 80112
Phone: (303)649-9299 **Free:** 800-STR-OKES
Fax: (303)649-1328
Email: info@stroke.org
Website: http://www.stroke.org
Andrew J. Beck, Sec.

Desc: Stroke survivors and their families; health care professionals and institutions; the lay community. Seeks to reduce the incidence and impact of stroke by promoting research, educating the public, and providing a network for stroke survivors and concerned persons. Serves as an information referral clearinghouse on stroke; makes available educational materials on stroke prevention, treatment, rehabilitation, resocialization, and research. Offers guidance in the development of stroke support groups and clubs. Maintains speakers' bureau and Stroke Information and Referral Center; compiles statistics. Conducts educational symposiums/meetings. **Awards:** Community Education Award (annual) for medical facilities and community Organization; Research Fellowship Award in Cerebrovascular Disease (annual) for doctors dedicated to the field of stroke as a career.

★ 13430 ★ National Student Nurses' Association (NSNA)
45 Main St., Ste. 606
Brooklyn, NY 11201
Phone: (718)210-0705 **Fax:** (718)210-0710
Email: nsna@nsna.org
Website: http://www.nsna.org
Diane J. Mancino, Ed.D., RN CAE, Exec. Dir.

Desc: Students enrolled in state-approved schools for the preparation of registered nurses. Seeks to aid in the development of the individual nursing student and to urge students of nursing, as future leaders and health professionals, to be aware of and to contribute to improving the health care of all people. Encourages programs and activities in state groups concerning nursing, health, and the community. Provides assistance for state board review, as well as materials for preparation for state RN licensing examination. Cooperates with nursing organizations in recruitment of nurses and in professional, community, and civic programs. Sponsors Foundation of the National Student Nurses' Association in memory of Frances Tompkins to award scholarships to student nurses. **Awards:** Scholarship (annual).

★ 13431 ★ National Tay-Sachs and Allied Diseases Association (NTSAD)
2001 Beacon St., Ste. 204
Brighton, MA 02135

Phone: (617)277-4463 **Free:** 800-906-8723
Fax: (617)277-0134
Email: ntsad-boston@att.net
Website: http://www.ntsad.org
Jayne C. Gershkowitz, Exec. Dir.

Desc: Supports educational, prevention, family service, and research programs concerning Tay-Sachs and allied degenerative lysosomal and leukodystrophy and neurological diseases occurring in infants, children, and adults. Provides educational literature on Tay-Sachs and allied diseases; serves as a referral agency for the layperson and professional on all aspects of Tay-Sachs and related diseases; promotes mass screening programs and appropriate legislation locally and nationally. Sponsors International Laboratory Quality Control and Reference Sample Center for TSD laboratories. Offers support groups and services for parents of children with Tay-Sachs and related diseases, grandparents and extended family members. Compiles statistics; operates speakers' bureau. **Awards:** Research Initiative (annual).

★ 13432 ★ National Wellness Institute
PO Box 827
Stevens Point, WI 54481-0827
Phone: (715)342-2969 **Free:** 800-243-8674
Fax: (715)342-2979
Email: nwi@nationalwellness.org
Website: http://www.nationalwellness.org
Anne Helmke, Dir. Member Services

Desc: Purposes are to provide national leadership in the wellness movement; to assist professionals working in health and wellness promotion in all types of settings; and organizations with planning, development, implementation, and evaluation of wellness programs; and to assist in the development of high quality wellness products and services. Acts as clearinghouse on wellness information. Provides consultations; offers professional development conferences. Sponsors National Wellness Association. **Awards:** National Wellness Institute Research Merit Award (annual) for original research in health and wellness not yet published.

★ 13433 ★ Neuro-Developmental Treatment Association (NDTA)
1540 S Coast Hwy., Ste. 203
Laguna Beach, CA 92651
Free: 800-869-9295 **Fax:** (949)376-3456
Email: membership@ndta.org
Website: http://www.ndta.org
Brad Lund, Principal Dir.

Desc: Physical and occupational therapists, speech pathologists, special educators, physicians, parents, and others interested in neurodevelopmental treatment. (NDT is a form of therapy for individuals who suffer from central nervous system disorders resulting in abnormal movement. Treatment attempts to initiate or refine normal stages and processes in the development of movement.) Informs members of new developments in the field and with ideas that will eventually improve fundamental independence. Locates articles related to NDT. Regional groups maintain libraries. **Awards:** Award of Excellence (annual); Certificate of Appreciation; Research Grant Award (annual).

★ 13434 ★ Neurofibromatosis (NF)
9320 Annapolis Rd., Ste. 300
Lanham, MD 20706-3123
Phone: (301)918-4600 **Free:** 800-942-6825
Fax: (301)918-0009
Email: info@nfinc.org
Website: http://www.nfinc.org
Brenda Duffy, Pres.

Desc: Organizations providing support for individuals with neurofibromatosis (NF) and their families, physicians, and other health care providers. (NF is a genetic neurological disorder that can cause tumors to form on nerves and is linked to learning disabilities, hearing loss, vision impairment, epilepsy, and cancer.) Increases public awareness of NF through information dissemination; informs federal, state, and local legislators of the needs of NF families. Promotes, supports, and funds medical, clinical, educational, and sociological research that addresses the need to diagnose, treat, cure, and prevent NF. Identifies local NF support and peer counseling groups; offers referrals to medical resources and scientifically-evaluated research. Participates in networking of voluntary health organizations. **Awards:** NF Inc. Scholar (annual) for contribution to the NF cause.

★ 13435 ★ Neuropathy Association
Lincoln Bldg.
60 E 42nd St., Ste. 942
New York, NY 10165
Phone: (212)692-0662 **Free:** 800-247-6968
Fax: (212)692-0668
Email: info@neuropahty.org
Website: http://www.neuropathy.org
Catherine Law, CFO

Desc: Offers support to persons suffering from disorders affecting the peripheral nerves; provides patient support and education, advocates for patients' interests, promotes research into the causes and cure for peripheral neuropathies. **Awards:** Grant (periodic).

★ 13436 ★ North American Menopause Society (NAMS)
PO Box 94527
Cleveland, OH 44101
Phone: (440)442-7550 **Fax:** (440)442-2660
Email: info@menopause.org
Website: http://www.menopause.org
Wulf H. Utian, MD,PhD, Exec. Dir.

Desc: Physicians, scientists, research and clinical personnel, and other health care professionals are active members; student or physicians serving residencies or fellowships are associate members. Promotes understanding of menopause in women. Advances the exchange of research plans and experience between members. Offers educational programs. **Awards:** Grant (annual).

★ 13437 ★ North American Society for Cardiac Imaging (NASCI)
930 Edgecliff Way
Redwood City, CA 94061
Phone: (650)216-6621 **Fax:** (650)556-1678
Email: info@nasci.org
Website: http://www.nasci.org
Joan Oefner, CAE, Exec. Dir.

Desc: Approved individuals engaged in the practice and advancement of cardiac and vascular imaging are active members; medical students, other individuals, and corporations with an interest in cardiac imaging are sponsors. Seeks to advance the practice of cardiac imaging and to develop improved medical imaging technologies. Serves as a forum for the exchange of information among individuals and corporations with an interest in cardiac imaging; sponsors educational programs; maintains NASCI Research and Education Fund. **Awards:** AHA Council of Cardiovascular Radiology (annual); Berlex Poster Awards (annual); Young Investigator's Awards (annual).

★ 13438 ★ North American Spine Society (NASS)
22 Calendar Ct., 2nd Fl.
La Grange, IL 60525
Phone: (708)588-8080 **Free:** 877-SPI-NEDR
Fax: (708)588-1080
Email: info@spine.org
Website: http://www.spine.org
Eric J. Muehlbauer, CAE, Exec. Dir.

Desc: Organization of physicians, osteopaths, orthopedists, neurosurgeons, physiatrists, radiologists, and other professionals that advances quality spine care through education, research and advocacy. Works to improve the quality of scientific practice in spinal disorders; exchange ideas and disseminate scientific information about clinical techniques; investigate and propagate methods by which malfunction of the spine can be corrected. Makes inquiries into practice characteristics, language usage and terminology, and treatment methods. **Awards:** Research Grant (annual) quality research on spinal care.

★ 13439 ★ Nurse Healers Professional Associates International (NH-PAI)
3760 Highland Dr., No. 429
Salt Lake City, UT 84106
Phone: (801)273-3399 **Fax:** (509)693-3537
Email: nh-pai@therapeutic-touch.org
Website: http://www.therapeutic-touch.org
Rebecca M. Good, MA, RN, LPC, Coor.

Desc: Official organization for Therapeutic Touch (TT). Healthcare professionals and lay persons united to promote a holistic approach to healing and health maintenance and nontraditional healing methods. Disseminates information on therapeutic touch. Maintains speakers' bureau; conducts research and educational programs for Therapeutic Touch. Sets standards and scope of practice for TT and recognition program for Qualified Therapeutic Touch teachers and practitioners. **Awards:** Healer's Award (annual); scholarship (annual) outstanding accomplishments in working for the advancement of complementary therapies and therapeutic touch through research, practice, education and/or publications.

★ 13440 ★ Nurses Educational Funds (NEF)
304 Park Ave. S, No. 11F
New York, NY 10010-4301
Phone: (212)399-1428 **Fax:** (212)581-2368
Email: bbnef@aol.com
Barbara Butler, Exec. Dir.

Desc: Seeks to establish, maintain, and administer funds to provide financial assistance to registered nurses studying for advanced degrees; masters/doctoral level only formulate policies for the administration of such funds; collect and manage all funds contributed to it. Masters study must be full-time only GRE/or MAT scores are required. **Awards:** Scholarship for RN, member of professional nursing, full-time student at Master's Level, full or part-time at doctoral level, U.S. Citizen, enrolled in or applying to NLNAC or CCNE accredited nursing masters program or at doctoral level; for academic and service leader.

★ 13441 ★ Opticians Association of America (OAA)
PO Box 6600
Springfield, VA 22150-6600
Phone: (703)916-8856 **Free:** 800-443-8997
Fax: (703)916-7966
Email: oaa@opticians.org
Website: http://www.opticians.org
Earl M. Cleveland, Pres.

Desc: Retail dispensing opticians who fill prescriptions for glasses or contact lenses written by a vision care specialist. Works to advance the science of ophthalmic optics. Conducts research and educational programs. Maintains museum and speakers' bureau. Compiles statistics. **Awards:** Russell Fritz Memorial Scholarship (annual) for a first-year student in an opticianry program accredited by the Commission on Opticianry Accreditation.

★ 13442 ★ Oral Health America
410 N Michigan Ave., Ste. 352
Chicago, IL 60611-4211
Phone: (312)836-9900 **Free:** 800-523-3438
Fax: (312)836-9986
Email: liz@oralhealthamerica.org
Website: http://www.oralhealthamerica.org
Robert J. Klaus, Pres. & CEO

Desc: Funds dental education, research, and service programs. Operates speakers' bureau. **Awards:** Dental Education Fellowship (annual) for dental teacher training; Dental Laboratory Technology Scholarship (annual) for dental laboratory technology; grant for research and dental health projects; Hillenbrand Fellowship in Oral Health Policy (biennial) for dental administrator; Minority Dental Student Scholarship (annual) for minority dental students.

★ 13443 ★ Orthopedic Foundation for Animals (OFA)
2300 Nifong Blvd.
Columbia, MO 65201-3856
Phone: (573)442-0418 **Fax:** (573)875-5073
Email: ofa@offa.org
Website: http://www.offa.org
Dr. G.G. Keller, Project Dir.

Desc: National and local dog clubs and individual breeders. Acts as a clearinghouse for information on orthopedic diseases of animals, particularly hip dysplasia in dogs (a hereditary condition resulting in abnormal development of the hip joints). Is attempting to develop a national control program through monitoring animals and conducting selective breeding and research. Conducts educational seminars; compiles statistics; sponsors a national referral service for animal breeders. Maintains library of all breed canine pelvic radiographs. **Awards:** Grant for research.

★ 13444 ★ OsteoArthritis Research Society International (OARSI)
2025 M St., Ste.800
Washington, DC 20036
Phone: (202)367-1177 **Fax:** (202)367-2177
Email: oarsi@orsi.org
Website: http://www.oarsi.org

Desc: Researchers and health care professionals with an interest in osteoarthritis. Seeks to promote and encourage fundamental and applied research on osteoarthritis and its treatment. Gathers and disseminates information on osteoarthritis and related research; sponsors educational programs. **Awards:** OARSI Award in Osteoarthritis Research (annual); Student Scholarship (periodic).

★ 13445 ★ Osteogenesis Imperfecta Foundation (OIF)
804 W Diamond Ave., Ste. 210
Gaithersburg, MD 20878
Phone: (301)947-0083 **Free:** 800-981-2663
Fax: (301)947-0456
Email: bonelink@oif.org
Website: http://www.oif.org
Ms. Mary Beth Huber, Information & Resource Dir.

Desc: Osteogenesis Imperfecta Foundation, Inc. is a voluntary national health organization dedicated to helping people cope with osteogenesis imperfecta. The mission of the OI Foundation is to improve the quality of life for individuals affected by OI through education, awareness, mutual support and research into the treatment and potential cure of the disorder. Information is provided to individuals who have OI and their families, medical professionals and other members of the community. Resources and programs include a quarterly newsletter, a physician information service, written literature, informative videos, national conferences and local support groups. Compiles statistics. support groups. Compiles statistics. **Awards:** Michael Geisman Memorial Fellowship and Seed Awards (annual) for research contribution; monetary for OI research projects.

★ 13446 ★ Oxalosis and Hyperoxaluria Foundation (OHF)
5727 Westcliffe Dr.
Saint Louis, MO 63129
Phone: (618)281-9450 **Free:** 888-721-2432
Fax: (618)281-9452
Email: bdjrk@aol.com
Website: http://www.ohf.org
Brett Rosen, Pres.

Desc: Individuals affected by oxalosis and hyperoxaluria; health care professionals. Hyperoxaluria is a metabolic disease affecting the kidneys. Oxalosis occurs when calcium crystals have deposited elsewhere in the body, often the eyes, bones, and joints. Provides support services and information regarding the conditions and their affects. Encourages research. Operates referral service. **Awards:** Grant (annual) for hyperoxaluria and oxalosis researchers.

★ 13447 ★ Pain Management and Sclerotherapy
303 S Ingram Ct.
Middletown, DE 19709-7935
Phone: (302)996-0300 **Free:** 800-471-6114
Fax: (302)996-5300
Linda Pavina, Exec. Sec.

Desc: Dedicated to improving the practice of and disseminating knowledge about sclerotherapy. (The academy defines sclerotherapy as the stimulation of the formation of fibrous-connective tissues by the body, in a specific location, by the specific application of a sclerosing modality.) The most frequently used modality is the injection of certain medications, known as sclerosants. Primary studies involve the treatment of: unstable joints, venous abnormalities, and tendeno-osseous points of hyper-irritability. Supports research program; maintains speakers' bureau. **Awards:** Scholarship (annual) bestowed to an osteopathic medical student submitting best paper on sclerotherapy; student is invited to present paper at academy convention.

★ 13448 ★ Pan-American Association of Ophthalmology (PAAO)
1301 S Bowen Rd., Ste. 365
Arlington, TX 76013
Phone: (817)265-2831 **Fax:** (817)275-3961
Email: info@paao.org
Website: http://www.paao.org
Dr. Rubens Belfort, Jr., Pres.

Desc: Ophthalmologists throughout the Western Hemisphere. Seeks to improve the treatment of eye diseases and prevention of blindness in the Americas through the exchange of ideas and treatments. **Awards:** Benjamin F. Boyd Humanitarian Award (biennial) for ophthalmological service and blindness prevention activities; fellowship; Gillingham - Pan American Fellowship (annual) for education.

★ 13449 ★ Pan American Medical Association (PAMA)
c/o William E. Sorrel, M.D. Pres.
263 W End Ave., Ste. 1A
New York, NY 10023
William E. Sorrel, M.D., PhD, Pres.

Desc: Fosters the exchange of medical information and research results among physicians in Western Hemisphere countries. **Awards:** P.A.M.A. Medal for distinguished medical service; Postgraduate Medical Fellowship (annual) for postgraduate students with M.D. degree.

★ 13450 ★ Pediatric/Adolescent Gastroesophageal Reflux Association (PAGER)
PO Box 1153
Germantown, MD 20875-1153
Phone: (301)601-9541
Email: gergroup@aol.com
Website: http://www.reflux.org
Beth Anderson, Exec. Dir.

Desc: Provides information and support to parents, patients and doctors about Gastroesophageal Reflux. **Awards:** Hereditary GERD Research Award (annual).

★ 13451 ★ Pediatric AIDS Foundation
2950 31st St., No. 125
Santa Monica, CA 90405
Phone: (310)314-1459 **Free:** 888-499-HOPE
Fax: (310)314-1469
Email: info@pedAIDS.org
Website: http://www.pedaids.org
Kate Carr, CEO & Pres.

Desc: Confronts medical problems unique to children infected with HIV/AIDS, and focuses on finding medical answers that will bring hope. Identifies and funds critically needed pediatric AIDS research worldwide. Provides funds to hospitals around the country which serve children with HIV/AIDS through an Emergency Assistance Program. Encourages students to enter the field of pediatric AIDS through a Student Intern Award Program. Develops and distributes national Parent Education Program for parents of elementary and pre-school age children. **Awards:** Research Grant; Student Internship.

★ 13452 ★ Pediatric Brain Tumor Foundation of the United States (PBTFUS)
302 Ridgefield Ct.
Asheville, NC 28806
Phone: (828)665-6891 **Free:** 800-253-6530
Fax: (828)665-6894
Email: pbtfus@pbtfus.org
Website: http://www.pbtfus.org
Mike Traynor, Pres.

Desc: Seeks to find the cause and cure of brain tumors in children. Supports medical research; promotes public awareness of the disease; aids in early detection and treatment of childhood brain tumors. **Awards:** Grant for research.

★ 13453 ★ Pediatric Endocrinology Nursing Society (PENS)
PO Box 2933
Gaithersburg, MD 20886-2933
Website: http://www.pens.org

Desc: Pediatric endocrine nurses. Promotes professional responsibility, accountability, ethics and respect; dedicated to the advancement of the art and science of pediatric endocrine nursing; establishes and maintains standards of practice; enhances nursing research, clinical expertise and recognition of excellence in nursing. **Awards:** Academic Education Scholarships for nursing academic programs (BSN, MSN, PhD); Continuing Education Scholarships to assist members attending PENS annual conference; Manual Chapter Author Grant provides financial support to active members authoring an original or revised chapter for the manual; Poster Presentation Grant for materials necessary to create a poster presentation for the PENS annual conference; Research grants to support pediatric endocrinology nursing research projects.

★ 13454 ★ Pediatric Orthopaedic Society of North America (POSNA)
6300 N River Rd., Ste. 727
Rosemont, IL 60018-4226
Phone: (847)698-1692 **Fax:** (847)823-0536
Email: goldberg@aaos.org
Website: http://www.posna.org
Sharon Goldberg, Exec. Dir.

Desc: Pediatric orthopedic surgeons. Purpose is to provide continuing education to members. Conducts tutorial programs. **Awards:** Huene Award (annual) for past and future research in pediatric orthodpaedics - publishable material.

★ 13455 ★ Phi Chi Medical Fraternity (PCMF)
2039 Ridgeview Dr.
Floyds Knobs, IN 47119
Phone: (812)948-0581 **Free:** 800-800-7442
Fax: (812)941-8850
Email: phichi@phi-chi.org
Website: http://www.phi-chi.org
Daniel H. Cannon, MD, Chm., Exec. Trustees

Desc: Professional fraternity - medicine. Maintains Phi Chi Welfare Association, which accepts voluntary contributions to a student loan fund and other services. **Awards:** Recognition (annual); scholarship (annual).

★ 13456 ★ Phlebology Society of America (PSA)
c/o Denise M. Rossignol, Exec. Dir.
5 Daremy Ct.
Nesconset, NY 11767-1547
Phone: (631)366-1429 **Fax:** (631)366-3609

Email: denisemrossignol@cs.com
Dr. John B. Chang, Bd. Chm.

Desc: Physicians and scientists with an interest in phlebitis and other diseases of the vascular system. Seeks to advance the diagnosis and treatment of peripheral vascular disease. Serves as a certifying board for professional phlebologists; functions as a clearinghouse on phlebology; facilitates exchange of information among members. Conducts educational programs. **Awards:** Young Investigator Award (annual) presentation and originality of research.

★ 13457 ★ Plastic Surgery Educational Foundation (PSEF)

444 E Algonquin Rd.
Arlington Heights, IL 60005
Phone: (847)228-9900 **Free:** 888-4-PLASTIC
Fax: (847)228-9131
Email: memserv@plasticsurgery.org
Website: http://www.plasticsurgery.org
Paul Pomerantz, CAE, Exec. Dir.

Desc: Plastic and reconstructive surgeons. Purpose is to identify and respond to the educational needs of members and their patients. Sponsors regional and national demonstrations, lectures, educational seminars, symposia, and workshops focusing on plastic surgery techniques and procedures. Conducts annual in-service and self-assessment examinations dealing with topics such as aesthetic and breast surgery, hand and extremities, integument, maxillofacial surgery, and pediatric plastic surgery. Administers Visiting Professors Program; compiles statistics; sponsors charitable programs. **Awards:** Scholarship bestowed in basic science, clinical research, and senior categories.

★ 13458 ★ Polycystic Ovarian Syndrome Association

PO Box 80517
Portland, OR 97280
Phone: (856)218-4815 **Free:** 877-775-PCOS
Fax: (413)751-4866
Email: info@pcosupport.org
Website: http://www.pcosupport.org
Kristin Rencher, Exec. Dir.

Desc: Chapters worldwide provide support, education and advocacy for women suffering from polycystic ovary syndrome (PCOS). Host educational events combining lectures with support sessions. Advocate for women with PCOS in the media and medical community by attending and speaking at professional meetings as well as hosting exhibit booths. **Awards:** Chair's Award (annual) for outstanding service of an individual volunteer; Director's Award (annual) for outstanding service of an individual volunteer; Founder's Award (annual) for outstanding service of an individual volunteer; scholarship (periodic) given to those who indicate need.

★ 13459 ★ Postpartum Support International (PSI)

c/o Laurence Kruckman
Indiana-University of Pennsylvania
Department of Anthropology
Indiana, PA 15705
Phone: (724)357-3935 **Fax:** (724)357-7637
Email: kruckman@iup.edu
Website: http://www.postpartum.net/
Laurence Kruckman, PhD, Pres. Elect

Desc: Promotes international awareness, prevention and treatment of mental health issues related to childbearing. **Awards:** Susan Hickman Memorial Research Award (annual) to member who is also a masters, doctoral, or post-doctoral student, or junior research faculty member.

★ 13460 ★ Prader-Willi Foundation

267 Oxford St.
Rochester, NY 14607
Phone: (716)442-1655 **Free:** 800-442-1655
Fax: (716)271-2782
Email: alliance@proder-willi.org
Sheldon L. Tarakan, Pres.

Desc: Devoted to serving individuals with Prader-Willi Syndrome. Provides information on subjects related to Prader-Willi Syndrome. Finances related projects such as residential development, family support, behavioral research, and awareness. Works with other Prader-Willi organizations. **Awards:** Grant for other Prader-Willi organizations for development and publication.

★ 13461 ★ Prescription Foot Orthotic Laboratory Association (PFOLA)

c/o Jay Skoog, Exec.Dir.
36 S Last Chance Gulch, Ste. A
Helena, MT 59601
Free: 800-347-6585 **Fax:** (406)443-4614
Email: jskoog@rmsmanagement.com
Website: http://www.nvo.com/pfola
Jay Skoog, Exec. Dir.

Desc: Works to promote and improve the efficacy of custom, prescription foot orthoses. **Awards:** Grant.

★ 13462 ★ Prevent Blindness America

500 E Remington Rd.
Schaumburg, IL 60173-5611
Phone: (847)843-2020 **Free:** 800-331-2020
Fax: (847)843-8458
Email: info@preventblindness.org
Website: http://www.preventblindness.org
Hugh R. Parry, Pres. /CEO

Desc: Charitable organization committed to preventing blindness and preserving sight through nationwide comprehensive programs of public and professional education, research, industrial, and community services. Services include promotion and support of local glaucoma screening programs, preschool vision testing, industrial eye safety, and collection of statistical and other data on nature and extent of causes of blindness and defective vision. Operates a toll-free information center dealing with eye health and safety topics. Through the Fight for Sight Research Division, the organization awards student fellowships, postdoctoral awards and grants in aid for medical research. Sponsors Wise Owl Program to promote widespread use of safety eyewear for various activities and occupations. Compiles statistics. **Awards:** Grant-In-Aid (annual) for funding of research in vision and ophthalmology; Postdoctoral Fellowship (annual) for basic or clinical research in vision and ophthalmology; Student Fellowship (annual) for undergraduate, graduate, and medical students interested in eye-related basic or clinical research.

★ 13463 ★ Preventive Cardiovascular Nurses Association (PCNA)

613 Williamson St., Ste. 205
Madison, WI 53703
Phone: (608)250-2440 **Fax:** (608)250-2410
Email: info@pcna.net
Website: http://www.pcna.net
Sue Koob, Exec. Dir.

Desc: Works to develop and promote the role of nurses in managing of patients with cardiovascular disease. Defines a certification process; disseminates information to increase consumer awareness; funds a training grant; seeks to have preventive cardiology designated a nursing specialty. **Awards:** Grant.

★ 13464 ★ Psi Beta

1027 Westbridge Ln.
Chattanooga, TN 37405
Phone: (423)265-6555 **Free:** 888-PSI-BETA
Fax: (423)265-0033
Email: carol@psibeta.org
Website: http://www.psibeta.org
Carol Tracy, Exec. Dir.

Desc: Honor society - community, and junior college psychology students. Participates in psychology conventions. Provides means for contact with professors in students' areas of interest. Conducts educational programs and sponsors national awards. Promotes excellence in scholarship, leadership, research and community service. **Awards:** Allyn & Bacon Research Paper Award (annual) for 3 original emperical research papers written in APA style; Ann G. Robinson College Life (annual) for a unique promotion of the quality of 2-year college life that advances psychology and Psi Beta's mission; Carol Tracy Community Service Award (annual) for outstanding community service project; Harcourt College Publishers National Chapter Award (annual) active chapter that demonstrates outstanding programming; Virginia Sexton Faculty Advisor Award (annual) for outstanding service as faculty advisor.

★ 13465 ★ Psychohistory Forum (PF)

627 Dakota Trail
Franklin Lakes, NJ 07417
Phone: (201)891-7486
Email: pelovitz@aol.com
Website: http://cliospsyche.org
Paul H. Elovitz, PhD, Dir.

Desc: Psychologists, psychiatrists, Psychotherapists, social workers, historians, psychohistorians, and laypeople having a scholarly interest in the integration of depth psychology and history. (Psychohistory is the study of psychobiography, group process, the mechanisms of defense, the history of childhood, creativity, dreams, and the difference between stated intention and actual behavior). Seeks to further psychohistory through the exchange of information. Conducts bimonthly workshops on topics related to psychohistory and training seminars on dream analysis, innovation, teaching, and methodology. Aids individuals in psychohistorical research. Holds lecture series. lecture series. lecture series. **Awards:** Halpern Award for the Best Psychohistorical Idea (annual); Halpern Graduate Student Award (annual) for the best psychohistorical idea; Student Award year's membership.

★ 13466 ★ Psychometric Society (PS)

c/o Dr. Terry Ackerman
UNCG
207 Curry Bldg.
Greensboro, NC 27402-6171
Phone: (336)334-3474 **Fax:** (336)334-4120
Email: taackerm@uncg.edu
Website: http://www.psychometricsociety.org/
Dr. Terry Ackerman, Sec.

Desc: Persons interested in development of quantitative models for psychological phenomena and quantitative methodology in the social and behavioral sciences. **Awards:** Psychometric Society Dissertation Award (annual) review of dissertation by a committee of three past presidents.

★ 13467 ★ Pulmonary Hypertension Association (PHA)

850 Sligo Ave., No. 800
Silver Spring, MD 20910
Phone: 800-748-7274 **Fax:** (301)565-3994
Email: pha@phassociation.org
Website: http://www.phassociation.org
Rino Aldrighetti, Exec. Dir.

Desc: Patients with pulmonary hypertension (PH) and primary pulmonary hypertension (PPH); families and physicians of patients; researchers. Provides fellowship and educational support for members and the public on PH and PPH, including current research and findings, early detection, resource organizations, organ transplantation, and support networks. Conducts support group meetings. Funds medical research **Awards:** Outstanding Physician Award (biennial); Outstanding Volunteer Award (biennial); Research Fellowships (annual) proposal.

★ 13468 ★ Purine Research Society

c/o Tahma Metz
5424 Beech Ave.
Bethesda, MD 20814-1730
Phone: (301)530-0354 **Fax:** (301)564-9597
Email: purine@erols.com
Website: http://www2.dgsys.com/~purine/
Tahma Metz, Exec. Dir.

Desc: Dedicated to funding research and treatment of diseases resulting from errors in purine metabolism, specifically purine autism, the largest single subgroup of autism. As with other metabolic diseases, purine disorders are caused by a defective gene that results in the production of an enzyme with too little or too much catalytic activity. Purine metabolic diseases include gout, Lesch-Nyhan syndrome, purine autism, ADA deficiency and others. We are supporting research to find the defective enzyme(s) responsible for purine overproduction in purine autism, particularly, and to find effective screening and treatment methods, including newborn screening, so that symptoms will never occur. **Awards:** Grant.

★ 13469 ★ PXE International

c/o Sharon F. Terry
23 Mountain St.
Sharon, MA 02067-2234
Phone: (781)784-3817 **Fax:** (781)784-6672
Email: pxe@pxe.org
Website: http://www.pxe.org
Sharon F. Terry, Exec. Dir.

Desc: Dedicated to supporting those affected by Pseudoxanthomas elasticum (PXE) and to research into its causes, treatments, and cure. (Pseudoxanthomas elasticum is a heritable connective tissue disorder causing calcification of connective tissue, potentially affecting the skin, arteries, gastro-intestinal tissue, and the retina.) Provides information and support to patients, their families, and clinicians on diagnosis, effects, and treatment. Through a consortium of researchers worldwide, supports research by providing to researchers monetary grants and samples from its confidential Blood and Tissue Bank. Initiates and conducts epidemiological studies and other research. **Awards:** Excellence in PXE Research (annual) for special contributions to PXE research; grant (periodic).

★ 13470 ★ The Radiance Technique International Association

PO Box 40570
Saint Petersburg, FL 33743
Phone: (727)347-2106 **Fax:** (727)347-2106
Email: trtia@aol.com
Website: http://www.trtia.org
Shoshanna Shay, Dir. Office Services

Desc: Protects and preserves the science known as The Radiance Technique, an Authentic Reiki "science of universal energy which harmonizes and aligns the mind-body-spirit dynamic." Provides a network for those interested in The Radiance Technique. Maintains speakers' bureau. Compiles statistics and conducts research on the effectiveness of The Radiance Technique. Creates and promotes Radiant Peace Projects and sponsors the International Day of Radiant Peace on June 22 every year. **Awards:** Peace Education Awards (annual) for elementary-school children writing on the selected theme about peace; Peace Profiles for people and organizations who have made a definite contribution towards peace locally or globally.

★ 13471 ★ Radiological Society of North America (RSNA)

820 Jorie Blvd.
Oak Brook, IL 60523-2251
Phone: (630)571-2670 **Fax:** (630)571-7837
Email: informat@rsna.org
Website: http://www.rsna.org
Lise Steg Swanson, Account Exec.

Desc: Radiologists and scientists in fields closely related to radiology. Promotes study and practical application of radiology, radium, electricity, and other branches of physics related to medical science. **Awards:** Grant (annual); Research and Education Fund (annual); RSNA Gold Medal (annual) for outstanding contribution in radiology field.

★ 13472 ★ Reflex Sympathetic Dystrophy Association of America (RSDSA)

PO Box 502
Milford, CT 06460
Phone: (203)877-3790 **Free:** 877-662-7737
Fax: (203)882-8362
Email: jwbroatch@aol.com
Website: http://www.rsds.org
James Broatch, MSW, Exec. Dir.

Desc: People with Reflex Sympathetic Dystrophy Syndrome, also known as Complex Regional Pain Syndrome Type I and Type II; health care professionals treating RSDS patients. (RSDS is a disorder of the autonomic nervous system whose onset is usually preceded by a minor trauma such as a muscle sprain; symptoms of RSDS include severe pain, loss of muscle motion and use, swelling, skin and nail changes, and softening of the bones in affected areas.) Promotes increased awareness of RSDS among health care professionals and the public; conducts media campaigns; maintains national network of physicians involved in RSDS treatment and research. Encourages and supports RSDS research; has a national data bank for the coordination of RSDS research and treatment information. Aids in the formation of support groups for people with RSDS; develops in-service programs and seminars for use at hospitals and educational institutions. Makes available referral services. Conducts educational programs; maintains speakers' bureau; compiles statistics, funds research, has published clinical practice guidelines for diagnosis, treatment, and management of RSDS/CRPS. **Awards:** RSDSA Fellowship Grant (annual) for research.

★ 13473 ★ Registry of Interpreters for the Deaf (RID)

333 Commerce St.
Alexandria, VA 22314
Phone: (703)838-0030 **Fax:** (703)838-0454
Email: admin@rid.org
Website: http://www.rid.org
Clay Nettles, Exec. Dir.

Desc: Advocates sign language and oral interpreters. programs. Maintains 34 committees. Compiles statistics. **Awards:** Elizabeth Benson Scholarship (annual) Desc: For a student member who has completed at least one semester of a related program.

★ 13474 ★ Renal Pathology Society (RPS)

c/o Guillermo Herrera
Department of Pathology
LSUMC Shreveport
1501 Kings Hwy
Shreveport, LA 71130-3932
Phone: (318)675-5878 **Fax:** (318)675-7662
Email: gherre@lsuhsc.edu
Website: http://www.renalpathsoc.org
Dr. Guillermo A. Herrerame, Sec. -Treas.

Desc: Works to spread and increase knowledge of pathology of the kidney and seeks to develop renal pathology as a subspecialty. Conducts research and educational programs. **Awards:** Jacob Churg Award (annual); Young Investigator Award (biennial).

★ 13475 ★ Research to Prevent Blindness (RPB)

645 Madison Ave.
New York, NY 10022-1010
Phone: (212)752-4333 **Free:** 800-621-0026
Fax: (212)688-6231
Email: info@rpbusa.org
Website: http://www.rpbusa.org/hc2/index.asp
James V. Romano, PhD, COO

Desc: National voluntary health foundation supported by foundations, corporations, and voluntary gifts and bequests from individuals. Established to stimulate basic and applied research into the causes, prevention, and treatment of blinding eye diseases. Grants funds for equipment, eye research professorships with up to 7 year salary support, assistance in financing construction campaigns for eye research laboratory facilities, and travel expenses for international scholars for short-term collaborative research in the U.S. Through seminars and other means, encourages communication among scientists, practicing ophthalmologists, and the public. Maintains scientific advisory panel. **Awards:** Career Development Award to young physicians and scientists who wish to conduct eye research; grant (annual) for eye research to departments of ophthalmology at university medical schools; Jules and Doris Stein Professorship for outstanding basic scientists from other disciplines who conduct relevant clinical research in ophthalmology; Lew R. Wasserman Merit Award for mid-career scientists who hold primary positions within departments of ophthalmology and who are actively engaged in eye research; Physician-Scientist Award for nationally recognized and established M.D.'s engaged in clinical eye research; Senior Scientific Investigator Award for investigators who have deeply influenced the course of eye research; Special Research Scholars Award for outstanding young scientists conducting research of exceptional merit and promise.

★ 13476 ★ Retirement Research Foundation (RRF)

8765 W Higgins Rd., Ste. 430
Chicago, IL 60681-4170
Phone: (773)714-8080 **Fax:** (773)714-8089
Email: info@rrf.org
Website: http://www.rrf.org
Edward J. Kelly, Chm.

Desc: Works to promote aging and retirement issues. Supports efforts that improve care for the aging, and enable older adults to live at home or in residential settings that facilitate independent living. **Awards:** Grant.

★ 13477 ★ RGK Foundation

1301 W 25th St., Ste. 300
Austin, TX 78705-4236
Phone: (512)474-9298 **Fax:** (512)474-7281
Website: http://www.rgkfoundation.org
Gregory A. Kozmetsky, Pres.

Desc: Works to promote medical research. **Awards:** Grant.

★ 13478 ★ Royal Society of Medicine Foundation (RSMF)

207 E Westminster Rd. Ste. 201
Lake Forest, IL 60045
Phone: (847)234-6382 **Fax:** (847)234-6511
Email: RSMFIL@aol.com
Website: http://www.rsm.ac.uk
Dr. Richard S. Wilbur, Pres.

Desc: Serves as a forum for the discussion of topics relevant to the medical community in the U.S. and the United Kingdom. Sponsors conference series and exchange programs in conjunction with the Royal Society of Medicine. **Awards:** Hewitt (semiannual) lifetime achievement.

★ 13479 ★ Ruth Jackson Orthopaedic Society (RJOS)

c/o Mary Gebhardt
6300 N River Rd., Ste. 727
Rosemont, IL 60018
Phone: (847)698-1637 **Fax:** (847)823-0536
Email: gebhardt@aaos.org
Website: http://www.rjos.org
Mary Gebhardt, Contact

Desc: Women orthopaedic surgeons, residents, fellows, and medical students. Seeks to advance the science of orthopaedic surgery and to provide support for women orthopaedic surgeons. Named for practicing orthopaedic surgeon Dr. Ruth Jackson (1902-94), the first woman certified by the American Board of Orthopaedic Surgery and the first female member of the American Academy of Orthopaedic Surgeons. Conducts educational programs; operates placement service and speakers' bureau, holds biennial meeting, sponsors mentoring program, offers traveling fellowship and resident research award. **Awards:** Resident Research Award (annual); RJOS Traveling Fellowship (annual) for interest in promoting the general cause of women in orthopaedics.

★ 13480 ★ Scleroderma Foundation (SF)
12 Kent Way, Ste. 101
Byfield, MA 01922
Phone: (978)463-5843 **Free:** 800-722-4673
Fax: (978)463-5809
Email: sfinfo@sclerdoma.org
Website: http://www.scleroderma.org
Elaine Furst, Chm.

Desc: Scleroderma organizations. Promotes medical research to find a cure for scleroderma, a chronic systemic disease affecting all organs resulting from uncontrolled growth of connective tissue. Seeks to foster an understanding of the disease through media and outreach programs; raises funds. Provides patients with educational materials and referrals to local organizations and medical specialists. Offers encouragement and consultation services towards the formation and development of local support groups. Acts as a clearinghouse for information about scleroderma research, drugs, and therapies. Conducts accredited programs for professionals. Maintains speakers' bureau; compiles statistics. Funds one million dollars a year in new research. **Awards:** Grant (annual) for medical research.

★ 13481 ★ Scleroderma Research Foundation (SRF)
2320 Bath St., Ste. 315
Santa Barbara, CA 93105
Phone: (805)563-9133 **Free:** 800-441-CURE
Fax: (805)563-2402
Email: srfcure@srfcure.org
Website: http://www.srfcure.org/
Luke Evnin, Chm.

Desc: Seeks to find a cure for scleroderma, a life-threatening and degenerative illness. Funds and facilitates research and public awareness. **Awards:** Thomas Jefferson University Grant for research projects.

★ 13482 ★ Scoliosis Research Society (SRS)
611 E Wells St.
Milwaukee, WI 53202
Phone: (414)289-9107 **Fax:** (414)276-3349
Email: jschaper@execinc.com
Website: http://www.srs.org
Tressa Goulding, Exec. Dir.

Desc: Orthopedic surgeons and physicians. Furthers research and education in spinal deformities, particularly scoliosis, a twisting of the spine to one side. Most cases are of unknown cause, though scoliosis can result from a birth defect, polio, or spinal injury and usually develops in children during the growth spurt between ages ten and 15. Early detection followed with use of a brace and exercise can halt the curvature and prevent deformity. **Awards:** Grant (periodic).

★ 13483 ★ Seventh-Day Adventist Dietetic Association (SDADA)
6100 Leoni Rd.
Box 400
Grizzly Flats, CA 95636-0400
Phone: (916)782-5200 **Fax:** (916)782-5458
Email: rubyh@rsvl.ah.com

Desc: Seventh-Day Adventist registered dietitians; dietitians working in Seventh-Day Adventist institutions. Strives to motivate members to attain high professional standards and to actively promote Seventh-Day Adventist health principles. Provides resources and guidance concerning vegetarian lifestyles to dietitians. Disseminates nutrition information. **Awards:** Dietetic Studetn Scholarship Awards; scholarship for Seventh-Day adventist dietetic students.

★ 13484 ★ Sigma Phi Alpha
University of Texas, Health Science Center
Houston, Dental B
PO Box 20068
Houston, TX 77225
Phone: (713)500-4085
Patricia Campbell, Treas.

Desc: Honorary society, dental hygiene. **Awards:** Scholarship bestowed to individuals in dental hygiene; Sigma Phi Alpha Award (annual) for dental hygiene students in their final semester.

★ 13485 ★ Sjogren's Syndrome Foundation (SSF)
8120 Woodmont Ave., No. 530
Bethesda, MD 20814
Phone: (301)718-0300 **Free:** 800-475-6473
Fax: (301)718-0322
Email: ssf@sjogrens.org
Website: http://www.sjogrens.com
Suzanne Stone, Exec. Dir.

Desc: Individuals who have Sjogren's Syndrome, xerostomia (dry mouth), or keratoconjunctivitis sicca (dry eyes); specialists, internists, immunologists, rheumatologists, otolaryngologists, opthalmologists, gynecologists, gastroenterologists, pulmonologists, dermatologists, neurologists, urologists, pharmaceutical companies, and dentists. (Sjogren's Syndrome is a disorder marked by dryness of all mucous membranes, resulting from deficient secretion of the glands, particularly the lacrimal and salivary glands, those of the upper respiratory tract, the sweat glands, and the vaginal area. Approximately 50% of Sjogren's Syndrome patients also have rheumatoid arthritis, lupus, or scleroderma.) Objectives are to increase public awareness and medical knowledge about Sjogren's Syndrome, educate patients and their families, and allow patients to share information on coping with the syndrome. Supports research. Sponsors support groups with meetings in which doctors speak on aspects of the syndrome. Compiles statistics. **Awards:** Research Fellowship (annual) for research in the field; Research Grant (periodic).

★ 13486 ★ Skin Cancer Foundation (SCF)
245 5th Ave., Ste. 1403
New York, NY 10016
Phone: (212)725-5176 **Free:** 800-SKIN-490
Fax: (212)725-5751
Email: info@skincancer.org
Website: http://www.skincancer.org
Perry Robins, MD, Pres.

Desc: Sponsors medical symposia and public education programs on the prevention and early recognition of skin cancer. Grants its Seal of Recommendation to sunscreen products that meet the criteria and standards established by the SCF as effective aids in the prevention of sun-induced damage to the skin. **Awards:** The Frederic E. Mohs Award (annual) bestowed to qualified researchers and institutions; The Henry W. Menn Memorial Award (annual); The Henry W. Shotmeyer Award (annual).

★ 13487 ★ Society of Air Force Clinical Surgeons
839 W Lincoln Ave., No. 716
Woodland, CA 95695
Phone: (530)661-0352 **Fax:** (530)661-0352
Email: rosepreuit@aol.com
Website: http://www.atech.org/SAFCS/about/history.htm
Rose A. Thomas, Exec. Dir.

Desc: Air Force Clinical Surgeons. Promotes excellence in surgery within the Air Force, serves as a forum for the presentation of scientific papers, fosters esprit de corps, and promulgates military surgical objectives. **Awards:** Clinical Surgeons Award (annual) for the best original paper written and presented by a resident or fellow at the annual meeting; Excaliber Award for outstanding Active Duty member who has made significant contributions to academic or clinical Air Force surgery and exemplifies the highest dedication, process, competence, character and vis ion of a career Air Force Officer; Paul W. Myers Award for Excellence in Resident Research; Trauma/Critical Care Award (annual) for the best scientific and best clinical paper presented.

★ 13488 ★ Society of Cardiovascular Anesthesiologists (SCA)
2209 Dickens Rd.
PO Box 11086
Richmond, VA 23230-1086
Phone: (804)282-0084 **Fax:** (804)282-0090
Email: sca@societyhq.com
Website: http://www.scahq.org
Heather A. Spiess, Chief Staff Exec.

Desc: Anesthesiologists who specialize in cardiovascular surgical conditions. Purpose is to further medical education of cardiovascular anesthesiologists. Establishes goals and objectives for education of trainees in cardiovascular anesthesia; promotes personnel exchange between the U.S. and other countries; reviews related literature; maintains workshops; conducts research competitions. Sponsors Anesthesia Grand Rounds: Case Presentations as a section of the annual meeting. **Awards:** Research Starter Grant (annual) for a SCA member.

★ 13489 ★ Society for Clinical Vascular Surgery
13 Elm St.
Manchester, MA 01944-1314
Website: http://www.vascsurg.org/doc/Jvonliebig.html

Desc: Academic and community vascular surgeons. Promotes vascular surgery in the U.S. **Awards:** William J. von Liebig Foundation Award for Excellence in Vascular Surgical Research (annual) to individuals early in their training to pursue a career in research.

★ 13490 ★ Society of Critical Care Medicine (SCCM)
701 Lee St., Ste. 200
Des Plaines, IL 60016
Phone: (847)827-6869 **Fax:** (847)827-6886
Email: info@sccm.org
Website: http://www.sccm.org
David Julian Martin, CEO/Exec. VP

Desc: Physicians, nurses, scientists, technicians, respiratory therapists, engineers, pharmacists, and physicians assistants involved in the field of critical care medicine. Purposes are: to improve care for acute life-threatening illnesses and injuries; to promote development of optimal care facilities; to guarantee high educational standards in critical care medicine. SCCM has initiated self-assessment testing program in an effort to establish core curriculum and assist physicians in self-evaluation. SCCM established American College of Critical Care Medicine in 1988. **Awards:** American College of Critical Care Medicine Distinguished Investigator Award (annual) honors the meritorious and pioneering research of an SCCM established clinical investigator with a $10,000 award; Christer Grenvik Memorial Award (annual) honors an SCCM member who has promoted the ethical and humane delivery of critical care medicine with a $1000 cash award; ICU Design Citation (annual) honors a critical care unit that combines functional ICU design with the humanitarian delivery of critical care with a $1500 award; In-Training Fellow Award (annual) honors an author participating in a critical care fellowship training program or who has completed a program not more than a year before the annual Symposium with a $3000 cash award; Norma J. Shoemaker Award (annual) award of $1000 presented to the nurse member who demonstrates excellence in clinical practice, education, and/or administration; Norma J. Shoemaker Grant (annual) $15,000 nursing research award; Young Investigator's Award.

★ 13491 ★ Society for Disability Studies
c/o Carol J. Gill, PhD
University of Illinois at Chicago, MC626
Department of Disability and Human Development
1640 W Roosevelt Rd., No. 236
Chicago, IL 60608-6904
Phone: (312)996-4664 **Fax:** (312)996-7743
Email: cg16@uic.edu
Website: http://www.uic.edu/orgs/sds/
Carol J. Gill, PhD, Exec. Officer

Desc: Social scientists and scholars studying the problems of disabled people in society. Strives to develop theoretical and practical knowledge about disability and promotes equal participation in society for individuals with disabilities. **Awards:** Irving Kenneth Zola Emerging Scholar Award (annual); recognition.

★ 13492 ★ Society of Environmental Toxicology and Chemistry (SETAC)
1010 N 12th Ave.
Pensacola, FL 32501-3367
Phone: (850)469-1500 **Fax:** (850)469-9778
Email: setac@setac.org
Website: http://www.setac.org
Jeffery A. Foran, Pres.

Desc: Professionals in the fields of chemistry, toxicology, biology, and ecology; atmospheric, health, and earth sciences; and environmental engineering. Promotes the use of multidisciplinary approaches to examine the impacts of chemicals and technology on the environment. Strives to balance the interests of academia, business, and government. Conducts workshops and symposia on research topics of interest to members. **Awards:** Exceptional Service Award (annual) to an individual who has performed long-term, exceptionally high quality service for SETAC; Founders Award (annual) for outstanding career with clearly identifiable contributions in the environmental sciences consistent with the goals of SETAC; Rachel Carson Award (periodic) for substantially increasing public awareness and understanding of critical environmental issues; SETAC-ABC Laboratories Environmental Education Award (annual) for individuals, organizations, or corporations making significant contributions to environmental education; SETAC - Procter & Gamble Pre-Doctoral Fellowship (annual) for pursuit of a Ph.D. degree in environmental toxicology, chemistry, or related disciplines; SETAC/Roy F. Weston Award (annual) for individuals under the age of 35, selection based on the significance of contribution of published papers to the field of environmental chemistry; SETAC/ Taylor Francis Award (annual) for pre- or postdoctoral scholars conducting research in an area related to environmental toxicology, chemistry or ecological risk assessment.

★ 13493 ★ Society of Geriatric Cardiology (SGC)
Heart House
9111 Old Georgetown Rd.
Bethesda, MD 20814
Phone: (301)581-3449 **Fax:** (301)581-3408
Email: rpallott@sgcard.org
Website: http://www.sgcard.org
Rose Pallotta, Mgr.

Desc: Geriatric cardiologists and physicians in related fields are fellows; medical practitioners certified in specialties other than geriatrics or cardiologists are members; other individuals with an interest in geriatric cardiology are nonphysician members. Works to improve the clinical and therapeutic management of older individuals with cardiovascular disease; encourages use of preventive measures to avert the onset of cardiovascular aging and disease. Promotes more effective public policy and education regarding cardiac health. Conducts educational programs for physicians, other health care professionals, and the public. Supports research into cardiovascular aging and diseases relevant to older people. Serves as a clearinghouse on geriatric cardiology. Sponsors competitions. **Awards:** Merck Geriatric Cardiology Award (annual) for applicant reviewed by Research Committee.

★ 13494 ★ Society for Gynecologic Investigation (SGI)
409 12th St. SW
Washington, DC 20024-2188
Phone: (202)863-2544 **Fax:** (202)863-0739
Email: sgiava@aol.com
Website: http://sgionline.org/
Ava A. Tayman, Exec. Dir.

Desc: Present and former faculty members of institutions interested or engaged in fundamental gynecologic research. Purpose is to stimulate, encourage, assist, and conduct gynecologic research. **Awards:** Solvay/ Joseph Mortoln Research Grant (annual).

★ 13495 ★ Society of Infectious Diseases Pharmacists (SIDP)
502 E 11th St., Ste. 400
Austin, TX 78701-2656
Phone: (512)708-0611 **Fax:** (512)708-0627
Email: sidp@aams-texas.com
Website: http://www.sidp.org/
Charles H. Ballow, FCCP, Pres.

Desc: Pharmacists with a primary interest and practice in infectious diseases pharmacotherapy, and who have spent at least two years performing pharmacotherpeutic research are active members; pharmacists and other individuals not meeting the requirements for active membership, but who share an interest in infectious diseases pharmacotherapy, are associate members. Seesk to advance the study and practice of infectious diseases pharmacotherapy, and to enhance the professional status of members. Serves as a forum for discussion and exchange of information among members. Encourages pharmacotherapeutic research. **Awards:** SIDP/Abbott Award for Outcomes Research (annual) for established researcher making a significant contribution to the field of infectious diseases pharmacotherapy; SIDP/Ortho McNeil Scientist Preceptorship Award (annual) for research groups wishing to visit their collaborators; SIDP Young Investigator's Award (annual) for outstanding young pharmacotherapeutic researcher.

★ 13496 ★ Society of Interventional Radiology (SIR)
10201 Lee Hwy., Ste. 500
Fairfax, VA 22030
Phone: (703)691-1805 **Free:** 800-488-7284
Fax: (703)691-1855
Email: info@sirweb.org
Website: http://www.sirweb.org
Pete Lauer, Exec. Dir.

Desc: Physicians who are leaders in the field of interventional radiology. Facilitates exchange of new ideas and techniques and provides educational courses for all physicians working in the field. Conducts annual postgraduate course. Conducts Interventional Radiology Political Action. **Awards:** Young Investigator Award (annual).

★ 13497 ★ Society for Maternal Fetal Medicine (SMFM)
409 12th St. SW
Washington, DC 20024-2188
Phone: (202)863-2476 **Fax:** (202)554-1132
Email: info@smfm.org
Website: http://www.smfm.org
Patricia Stahr, Exec. Dir.

Desc: Obstetricians specializing in maternal-fetal medicine. Works to improve perinatal care through promotion and expansion of education in obstetrical perinatology. Provides a forum for exchange between members. **Awards:** SMFM Scholarship Award (annual) for research.

★ 13498 ★ Society for Medical Decision Making (SMDM)
1211 Locus St.
Philadelphia, PA 19107
Phone: (215)545-7697 **Fax:** (215)545-8107
Email: smdm-office@lists.smdm.org
Website: http://www.smdm.org
Daniel E. Reichard, Admin. Dir.

Desc: Individuals with an interest in "developing rational and systematic approaches" to medical decision making, including educators, clinicians, managers, and policy makers. Promotes improvement in all aspects of medical decision making. Evaluates decision making applications and disseminates conclusions. Facilitates multidisciplinary scholarship and research; conducts continuing professional education programs. **Awards:** Career Achievement Award (annual); Distinguished Service Award (annual); Lee B. Lusted Student Prizes (annual) outstanding research presented at SMDM annual meeting; Outstanding Short Course; Young Investigator Award (annual).

★ 13499 ★ Society for Menstrual Cycle Research (SMCR)
10559 N 104th Pl.
Scottsdale, AZ 85258
Phone: (480)451-9731 **Fax:** (480)451-9731
Email: maryannafriederich@msn.com
Website: http://www.pop.psu.edu/smcr
Mary Anna Friederich, MD, Sec. -Treas.

Desc: Physicians, nurses, endocrinologists, geneticists, physiologists, psychologists, sociologists, researchers, educators, students, and others interested in the health needs of women as related to the menstrual cycle. Goals are: to identify research priorities, recommend research strategies, and promote interdisciplinary research on the menstrual cycle; to establish a communication network for facilitating interdisciplinary dialogue on menstrual cycle events; to disseminate information and promote discussion of issues among public groups. **Awards:** Linda McKeever Student Prize (biennial) for student who presents paper at meeting.

★ 13500 ★ Society for Obstetric Anesthesia and Perinatology (SOAP)
1910 Byrd Ave., Ste. 100
PO Box 11086
Richmond, VA 23230-1086
Phone: (804)282-5051 **Fax:** (804)282-0090
Email: soap@societyhq.com
Website: http://www.soap.org
Joy L. Hawkins, MD, Pres.

Desc: Physicians and scientists interested in perinatal health care. Purpose is to improve the health care of pregnant women and their unborn children. Conducts specialized education programs; compiles statistics. **Awards:** OAPEF/SOAP Research Starter Grant for young members who wish to launch an academic career in obstretic anesthesia.

★ 13501 ★ Society for Occlusal Studies (SOS)
c/o Dr. Bernard Williams
4601 W 109th St. Ste. 225
Overland Park, KS 66211-1314
Fax: (816)941-4832
Dr. Bernard Williams, Pres.

Desc: Dentists and laboratory technicians who have completed the society's continuing education course in occlusion (bringing opposing surfaces of the teeth of the two jaws into contact). Promotes effective occlusal treatment. Conducts Principles of Occlusion Seminar, Advanced Restorative Seminar, laboratory technician program, and practice management program. **Awards:** Scholarship for paper presented on occlusion.

★ 13502 ★ Society of Otorhinolaryngology and Head/Neck Nurses (SOHN)
116 Canal St., Ste. A
New Smyrna Beach, FL 32168
Phone: (904)428-1695 **Fax:** (904)423-7566
Email: info@sohnnurse.com
Website: http://www.sohnnurse.com/
Sandra L. Schwartz, R.N., Exec. Dir.

Desc: Registered nurses specializing in otorhinolaryngology (the study of the ear, nose, and throat) and the head and neck. Seeks to: promote awareness of professional techniques and new developments in the field; enhance professional standards; create a channel for the exchange of ideas, concerns, and information; develop interaction with similar groups. Offers programs and seminars that have been approved for continuing education credits by the American Nurses' Association. **Awards:** Recognition; scholarship.

★ 13503 ★ Society of Pediatric Nurses (SPN)

7794 Grow Dr.
Pensacola, FL 32514
Phone: (850)494-9467 **Free:** 800-723-2902
Fax: (850)484-8762
Email: spn@puetzamc.com
Website: http://www.pedsnurses.org
Belinda E. Puetz, PhD RN, Contact

Desc: Registered pediatric nurses are regular members; nursing students and other professionals with an interest in pediatric nursing are associate members. Promotes quality health and nursing care of children. Conducts advocacy campaigns to improve access to affordable care for children; works to advance techniques of pediatric nursing and health care. Sponsors research and educational programs for members; formulates standards of practice and ethics; fosters collaboration between members and other health care professionals, child health care advocates, and related organizations. **Awards:** Corinne J. Barnes Research Grant (annual); Educational Scholarship Award (annual); Excellence in Advanced Practice Award (annual); Excellence in Clinical Practice Award (annual); Excellence in Education Award (annual); Excellence in Research Award (annual).

★ 13504 ★ Society for Physician Assistants in Pediatrics (SPAP)

950 N Washington St.
Alexandria, VA 22314-1552
Free: 800-596-4398 **Fax:** (703)684-1924
Email: jrv1007@aol.com
Website: http://www.geocities.com/spap_peds1
Tom Moreno, Membership Coor.

Desc: Designed to gather and disseminate information affecting the practice of pediatric physician assistants, collect demographic data to share within the profession or with other organizations, assist in developing guidelines for physician assistant utilization in clinical settings, and to enhance the relationship with the American Academy of Pediatrics. **Awards:** Scholarship (annual) PA student with documented interest in pediatric practice.

★ 13505 ★ Society for Prevention Research (SPR)

1300 I St. NW, Ste. 250 West
Washington, DC 20005
Phone: (202)216-9670 **Fax:** (202)216-9671
Email: info@preventionresearch.org
Website: http://www.preventionresearch.org
Jennifer Lewis, Admin. Dir.

Desc: Scientists, practitioners, advocates, administrators, and policy makers concerned with the prevention of social, physical and mental health problems and the promotion of health, safety and well-being. Promotes the advancement of science-based prevention programs and policies through empirical research. Facilitates communication and cooperation among prevention interventionists working in fields that include etiology, epidemiology, and the social sciences. **Awards:** Community, Culture, and Prevention Science Award (annual) to individual or team; Early Career Award (annual) to individual early in career in prevention; Federal Achievement Award; Friend of ECPN Award (annual) to mid-career or senior preventionist; International Collaborative Prevention Research Award (annual) to individual or team; Lifetime Achievement Award; Nan Tobler Award for Review of the Prevention Science Literature (annual) to individual or team; Presidential Award (annual) to individual or team; Prevention Science Award (annual) to individual or team for research; Public Service Award (annual) to individual or team; Science to Practice Award (annual) to individual or team; Service to SPR Award; Society for Prevention Research Award; State Achievement Award; Travel scholarships (annual).

★ 13506 ★ Society for the Psychological Study of Lesbian, Gay and Bisexual Issues (SPSLGBI)

c/o American Psychological Association
750 First St. NE
Washington, DC 20002
Phone: (202)336-6041 **Free:** 800-374-2721
Fax: (202)336-6040
Email: mdelong@apa.org
Website: http://www.apa.org/divisions/div44
James Fitzgerald, PhD, Pres.

Desc: Psychologists, graduate students in psychology, and others interested in the psychological study of lesbian, gay, and bisexual issues and the delivery of affirmative mental health services to gay, lesbian, and bisexual individuals. Promotes scholarship in the study of psychology as it relates to bisexual, gay, and lesbian issues; provides training for psychologists in the field. Cooperates with other groups sharing similar goals, including other divisions of the American Psychological Association. Conducts scholarly programs. **Awards:** Distinguished Contributions Awards (annual); Malyon-Smith Scholarship Award (annual) for graduate student research.

★ 13507 ★ Society for the Psychological Study of Social Issues (SPSSI)

208 I St. NE
Washington, DC 20002
Phone: (202)223-5100 **Fax:** (202)223-5555
Email: spssi@spssi.org
Website: http://www.spssi.org
Shari Miles, PhD, Exec. Dir.

Desc: Psychologists, sociologists, anthropologists, psychiatrists, political scientists, and social workers. Works to: obtain and disseminate to the public scientific knowledge about social change and other social processes; promote psychological research on significant theoretical and practical questions of social issues; encourage application of findings to problems of society. **Awards:** Award for Best Paper (annual); Internship research grant (annual); Research Grants (annual).

★ 13508 ★ Society of Radiologists in Ultrasound (SRU)

44211 Slatestone Ct.
Leesburg, VA 20176-5109
Phone: (703)858-9210 **Fax:** (703)729-4839
Email: info@sru.org
Website: http://www.sru.org
Carol B. Benson, MD, Pres.

Desc: Board certified and Board eligible radiologists interested in ultrasound imaging. Promotes the interests of radiologists in ultrasound. Funds research; educates non-physician health care professionals. **Awards:** Grant (annual) for clinical ultrasound research.

★ 13509 ★ Society of Reproductive Surgeons (SRS)

1209 Montgomery Hwy.
Birmingham, AL 35216-2809
Phone: (205)978-5000 **Fax:** (205)978-5005
Email: cfinch@asrm.org
Website: http://www.reprodsurgery.org

Desc: Reproductive surgeons. Gathers and disseminates information on reproductive surgery; conducts continuing education programs for members. Makes available referrals list. **Awards:** SRS Prize Paper (annual) based on peer review.

★ 13510 ★ Society for a Science of Clinical Psychology

c/o Raymond P. Lorion
University of Pennsylvania
Graduate School of Education
Psychology in Education Division
3700 Walnut St.
Philadelphia, PA 19104-6216
Phone: (215)898-7367 **Fax:** (215)573-2115
Email: lorion@gse.upenn.edu
Website: http://pantheon.yale.edu/~tat22/
Thomas D. Borkovec, PhD, Pres.

Desc: Promotes the integration of the scientist and the practitioner in training, research and applied undertakings in the field of clinical psychology. **Awards:** Dissertation Grant Awards; Distinguished Scientist Award; Outstanding Dissertation Award.

★ 13511 ★ Society for the Scientific Study of Sexuality (SSSS)

c/o David L. Fleming
PO Box 416
Allentown, PA 18105
Phone: (610)530-2483 **Fax:** (610)530-2485
Email: thesociety@inetmail.att.net
Website: http://www.sexscience.org
David L. Fleming, Exec. Dir.

Desc: Dedicated to advancing knowledge of sexuality. Support for research, and an interdisciplinary network of collaborating scholars. **Awards:** Student Research Grant (3/year).

★ 13512 ★ Society for Surgery of the Alimentary Tract (SSAT)

13 Elm St.
Manchester, MA 01944
Phone: (978)526-8330 **Fax:** (978)526-4018
Email: ssat@prri.com
Website: http://www.ssat.com
Robert P. Jones, Jr., Exec. Dir.

Desc: Licensed physicians with an interest in surgical aspects of digestive diseases. Seeks to advance the study, teaching, and practice of surgery of the alimentary tract; promotes continuing professional development of members. Serves as a forum for the discussion of new alimentary surgical techniques; encourages training opportunities and funding for alimentary surgical research. **Awards:** Career Development Award (annual) to young researchers.

★ 13513 ★ Society of Surgical Oncology (SSO)

c/o Rick Slawny
85 W Algonquin Rd., Ste. 550
Arlington Heights, IL 60005
Phone: (847)427-1400 **Fax:** (847)427-1294
Website: http://www.surgonc.org/
Rick Slawny, Exec. Dir.

Desc: Physicians and scientists working in the field of cancer. **Awards:** Monetary for outstanding cancer basic scientist; monetary for outstanding clinical scientist; monetary for outstanding clinical layman; recognition (annual) for medical resident who is performing an original research project.

★ 13514 ★ Society of Toxicologic Pathology (STP)

1767 Business Center Dr., Ste. 302
Reston, VA 20190
Phone: (703)438-7508 **Fax:** (703)438-7508
Email: stp@toxpath.org
Website: http://www.toxpath.org
Clarissa Wilson, Exec. Dir.

Desc: Promotes the advancement of the Individuals interested in toxicology and toxicologic pathology from industry, academic institutions, and government. **Awards:** Student Investigator Awards (annual).

★ 13515 ★ Society for Ultrastructural Pathology

c/o Joseph M. Harb, PhD
14655 East View Ct.
Brookfield, WI 53005
Phone: (414)781-6703
Email: khewanl@zappa.ultrakohl.com
Website: http://sup.ultrakohl.com/
Joseph Harb, PhD, Treas.

Desc: Promotes the art and science of diagnostic electron microscopy. Fosters the application of electron microscopy in the diagnosis and research of human diseases. Also provides an opportunity for the exchange of information, particularly ultrastructural and immunohistochemical, relevant to diagnostic pathology. Relevance of molecular pathology techniques to tumor pathology is also a focus. **Awards:** Pathologist in Training Award (annual) for best poster with ultrastructural study at U.S.-Canadian Academy of Pathology.

★ 13516 ★ Society for Vascular Nursing (SVN)
7794 Grow Dr.
Pensacola, FL 32514
Phone: (850)474-6963 **Free:** 888-536-4SVN
Fax: (850)484-8762
Email: svn@puetzamc.com
Website: http://www.svnnet.org
Belinda Puetz, PhD, RN , Exec. Dir.

Desc: Nurses and other health care professionals interested in providing comprehensive care for persons with vascular disease. Seeks to educate public about prevention of PVD. Provides educational programs; conducts research. **Awards:** Distinguished Service Award (annual); scholarship (annual).

★ 13517 ★ Society for Vascular Ultrasound (SVU)
4601 Presidents Dr., Ste. 260
Lanham, MD 20706-4831
Phone: (301)459-7550 **Free:** 800-788-8346
Fax: (301)459-5651
Email: info@svunet.org
Website: http://www.svunet.org
Steve Haracznak, Exec. Dir.

Desc: Vascular technologists and others in the field of noninvasive vascular technology. (Noninvasive vascular technology is a highly technical and specialized method of monitoring the blood flow in arms and legs and veins and arteries away from the heart in order to better diagnose disease and blood clots.) Seeks to establish an information clearinghouse providing reference and assistance in matters relating to noninvasive vascular technology; facilitate cooperation among noninvasive vascular facilities and other health professions; provide continuing education for individuals in the field; represents members on various regulatory issues. **Awards:** Pioneer Award (annual).

★ 13518 ★ Society of Women in Urology
c/o Wendy J. Weiser
1111 N Plaza Dr., Ste. 550
Schaumburg, IL 60173-4946
Phone: (847)517-7225 **Fax:** (847)517-7229
Email: swiu@wjweiser.com
Wendy Weiser, Contact

Desc: Women working in the field of urology. **Awards:** Elisabeth Pickett Research Award (annual) for urology based.

★ 13519 ★ Society for Women's Health Research
1828 L St. NW, Ste. 625
Washington, DC 20036
Phone: (202)223-8224 **Fax:** (202)833-3472
Email: info@womenshealth.org
Website: http://www.womens-health.org
Phyllis Greenberger, MSW, Exec. Dir.

Desc: Seeks to improve the health of women by promoting equity in research. Advocates policies which promotes the inclusion of women in clinical trials; informs government agencies and private industry of issues affecting women's health and sex-based biology; educates women consumers on conditions that affect women; promotes funding for women's health research. **Awards:** Excellence in Media (annual) for excellence in reporting research on women's health.

★ 13520 ★ Speak Easy International Foundation (SEIF)
233 Concord Dr.
Paramus, NJ 07652
Phone: (201)262-0895 **Fax:** (201)262-0895
Email: bob-antoinette@worldnet.att.net
Antoinette Gathman, Exec. Dir.

Desc: Support group and information source for individuals with a speech dysfluency (stuttering). Seeks to instill confidence in stutterers and reinforce fluency in their speech. Educates public, families, and friends on the problems of speech dysfluent individuals. **Awards:** Scholarship (periodic).

★ 13521 ★ Stickler Involved People (SIP)
15 Angelina Dr.
Augusta, KS 67010
Phone: (316)775-2993
Email: sip@stickler.org
Website: http://sticklers.org/sip/
Pat Houchin, Coord.

Desc: Dedicated to early diagnosis and treatment of Stickler Syndrome; provides support, medical information and offers ways in which to cope. **Awards:** Dr. Gunnar B. Stickler Scholarship (annual) to high school senior with Stickler Syndrome diagnosis.

★ 13522 ★ Sturge-Weber Foundation (SWF)
PO Box 418
Mount Freedom, NJ 07970
Phone: (973)895-4445 **Free:** 800-627-5482
Fax: (973)895-4846
Email: swf@sturge-weber.com
Website: http://www.sturge-weber.com
Joseph G. Morelli, MD, Chm.

Desc: Persons with Sturge-Weber syndrome and their families; concerned professionals and supporters. Serves as an information clearinghouse on Sturge-Weber syndrome, port-wine stains, and Klippel-Trenaunay Weber syndrome. (Sturge-Weber syndrome is a congenital neurological disorder characterized by facial port-wine stains, seizures, glaucoma, and loss of motor control, accompanied in rare cases by internal organ irregularities.) Disseminates information; offers support to afflicted persons. Maintains speakers' bureau; compiles statistics. Funds research. **Awards:** Grant (annual) for research into port wine stains, glaucoma, and Sturge-Weber.

★ 13523 ★ Stuttering Foundation of America (SFA)
3100 Walnut Grove Rd., Ste. 603
PO Box 11749
Memphis, TN 38111-0749
Phone: (901)452-7343 **Free:** 800-992-9392
Fax: (901)452-3931
Email: stutter@stutteringhelp.org
Website: http://www.stutteringhelp.org
Jane Fraser, Pres.

Desc: Provides comprehensive materials, including videotapes, books and brochures, on stuttering to both the public and professionals. Seeks to bring together speech pathologists concerned with the prevention and treatment of stuttering. Provides referrals to speech-language pathologists specializing in stuttering. Provides support for research into the causes of stuttering. **Awards:** SFA Award for Excellence in Reporting (annual).

★ 13524 ★ Surfer's Medical Association
PO Box 1210
Aptos, CA 95001
Phone: (831)684-0916 **Fax:** (831)684-0916
Email: smacentral@aol.com
Website: http://www.damoon.net/sma/
Paula Smith, Exec. Dir.

Desc: Surfer-health professionals and surfers interested in the health and medical aspects of surfing. Works to educate surfers and medical practitioners on the unique health problems of surfers. Represents the sport of surfing in the fields of medicine and science and also works to preserve the environment of beaches and oceans. Established the first international network of surfing health professionals. Sponsors members' research in this field. **Awards:** Scholarship (periodic) to a fijian village student.

★ 13525 ★ Susan G. Komen Breast Cancer Foundation (SGKF)
5005 LBJ, Ste. 250
Dallas, TX 75244
Phone: (972)855-1600 **Free:** 800-IM-AWARE
Fax: (972)855-1605
Email: helpline@komen.org
Website: http://www.komen.org
Susan Braun, CEO/Pres.

Desc: Breast cancer patients, health care professionals, and other interested individuals. Works to: increase the recovery and survival rates of breast cancer patients; heighten public awareness of the risks of breast cancer and the need for early detection. Establishes breast screening and training in self-examination procedures; provides funding through grants for research and screening programs. Sponsors educational programs. Bestows awards; sponsors competitions; maintains speakers' bureau. **Awards:** Fellowship (annual); grant (annual).

★ 13526 ★ Tissue Banks International (TBI)
815 Park Ave.
Baltimore, MD 21201-4887
Phone: (410)783-0183 **Free:** 800-756-4824
Fax: (410)454-4457
Email: tbi@tbionline.org
Website: http://www.tbionline.org
Gerald Cole, Pres. /CEO

Desc: A non-profit network of medical eye and tissue banks. Provides eye tissue for sight-restoring corneal transplant surgery. Also distributes bone, skin, and other soft tissues. Assists members with operational areas. Provides grants for research into the causes and cures of blindness. Distributes information on eye, tissue, and organ donation. Conducts educational and charitable programs. **Awards:** Grant.

★ 13527 ★ Tourette Syndrome Association (TSA)
42-40 Bell Blvd.
Bayside, NY 11361-2820
Phone: (718)224-2999 **Fax:** (718)279-9596
Email: ts@tsa-usa.com
Website: http://www.tsa-usa.org/
Fred Cook, VP

Desc: People with Tourette Syndrome (TS) and their families and friends; physicians, nurses, teachers, psychologists, social workers, and other professionals; organizations such as mental health agencies. (TS is characterized by involuntary muscular movements and utterances of sounds or words, and is often undiagnosed or misdiagnosed.) Develops and disseminates educational materials to families, professionals, and agencies involved in health care, education, and governments. Schedules meetings and seminars for professionals and families to explore the latest information on TS. Stimulates support for research into the nature and causes of the disorder. Apprises members of rights, services, and benefits provided by the government and other organizations. Provides lists of doctors experienced in treating the disorder. Operates support groups and other services to help persons with TS and their families. Maintains sources for advocacy referral services in the areas of education, employment, and housing. **Awards:** Permanent Research Fund Award (annual) for research.

★ 13528 ★ Transplant Recipients International Organization (TRIO)
2117 L St. NW, Ste. 353
Washington, DC 20037-1524
Phone: (202)293-0980 **Free:** 800-TRIO-386
Fax: (703)820-3948
Email: trionintt@saol.com

Website: http://www.trioweb.org
Elizabeth Rubin, Pres.

Desc: Transplant candidates, recipients, family members, donor families, and medical personnel. Provides support and medical information to patients and their families. Conducts educational programs. **Awards:** Scholarship (annual); Thomas Starzl Humanitarian Award (annual) for a person who has greatly influenced the field of transplantation.

★ 13529 ★ Tuberous Sclerosis Alliance (TSAlliance)

801 Roeder Rd., Ste. 750
Silver Spring, MD 20910
Phone: (301)562-9890 **Free:** 800-225-6872
Fax: (301)562-9870
Email: mleongini@tsalliance.org
Website: http://www.tsalliance.org
Michael Coburn, Pres. /CEO

Desc: Encourages and provides grants for research into the diagnosis, cause, management, and cure of tuberous sclerosis. (Tuberous sclerosis is a genetic disease characterized by one or more of the following: epileptic seizures, mental retardation, behavioral problems, non-malignant tumors, or skin lesions.) Provides support to families affected by the disease through a nationwide network of volunteer area representatives and the distribution of informational packets. Conducts educational programs for medical and allied professionals. **Awards:** Gomez Award for research; Rothberg Courage Award for research; TS Champion Award.

★ 13530 ★ United Mitochondrial Disease Foundation (UMDF)

8085 Saltsburg Rd., Ste. 201
Pittsburgh, PA 15239
Phone: (412)793-8077 **Fax:** (412)793-6477
Email: info@umdf.org
Website: http://www.umdf.org
Antoinette Renda Beasley, Fin. Svcs. Coord.

Desc: Patients, parents or guardians, friends, relatives, medical professionals, hospitals, and other organizations. Promotes research for cures and treatments of mitochondrial disease; provides support to patients and families. Patient registry database includes information from symptoms and treatment to diagnostic methods and specific disorders. **Awards:** Research Award (annual).

★ 13531 ★ United Ostomy Association (UOA)

19772 MacArthur Blvd., Ste. 200
Irvine, CA 92612-2405
Free: 800-826-0826 **Fax:** (949)660-9262
Email: director@uoa.org
Website: http://www.uoa.org
Nancy Italia, Exec. Dir.

Desc: Individuals who have lost the normal function of their bowel or bladder necessitating colostomy, ileostomy, ileal conduit, or ureterostomy surgery, known as ostomy. Aids in rehabilitation of these persons through mutual aid, moral support, and exchange of practical information in managing the stoma and its necessary prosthetic appliances; sponsors visiting program allowing patients to ask non-medical questions of individuals who have experienced a similar condition. Works to educate the public as to the nature of ostomy, with a view to ending job and insurance discrimination. Encourages research on management of ostomy and prosthetic equipment and appliances; also encourages study of the costs for rehabilitating ostomy patients. Prepares exhibits for medical conventions. Maintains speakers' bureau; compiles statistics. **Awards:** AVET Scholarship (semiannual).

★ 13532 ★ U.S. Association for Blind Athletes (USABA)

33 N Institute St.
Colorado Springs, CO 80903
Phone: (719)630-0422 **Fax:** (719)630-0616
Email: usaba@usa.net
Website: http://www.usaba.org/
Dr. Charly Huebner, Exec. Dir.

Desc: Visually impaired athletes; fully sighted physical educators, coaches, and special education teachers; interested volunteers. Aims to develop individual independence through sports opportunities and athletic competition. Promotes sports for the legally blind and visually impaired, organizes regional, national, and international competitions; works with other international organizations to promote goodwill and independence through friendly competition. Sports contested include alpine skiing, goalball, gymnastics, judo, Nordic skiing, powerlifting, speed skating, 5-side football, swimming, tandem cycling, track and field and wrestling. Sponsors coaches' training seminars, panel discussions, and training groups. Offers children's services; compiles statistics. **Awards:** Copland Scholarship.

★ 13533 ★ United States and Canadian Academy of Pathology

3643 Walton Way Extension
Augusta, GA 30909
Phone: (706)733-7550 **Fax:** (706)733-8033
Email: iap@uscap.org
Website: http://www.uscap.org
Fred Silva, MD, Sec. -Treas.

Desc: Works for the advancement of pathology teaching, practice, and research. Disseminates information to members. Sponsors educational programs to serve the needs of pathologists of various levels of experience. Presents Maude Abbott Lectureship to a recognized and respected person in contemporary pathology. **Awards:** Benjamin Castleman Award (annual) for a pathologist or pathologist-in-training under 40 years old who has written an outstanding paper on human pathology in English; Council's Distinguished Pathologist Award for an individual who has made a major contribution to pathology over the years; F. K. Mostofi Distinguished Service Award (annual) for a member who has rendered outstanding service to the Academy and the International Academy of Pathology; Stowell-Orbison Awards for Pathologists-in-Training for authors of outstanding papers.

★ 13534 ★ Velo-Cardio-Facial Syndrome (VCFS)

c/o Dr. Robert J. Shprintzen
Upstate Medical University
University Hospital
708 Jacobsen Hall (CDU)
750 E Adams St.
Syracuse, NY 13210
Phone: (315)464-6590 **Fax:** (315)464-6593
Email: info@vcfsef.org
Website: http://www.vcfsef.org
Dr. Robert J. Shprintzen, Exec. Dir.

Desc: Committed to educating the lay and professional public, offers family programs, provides parent-to-parent networking; promotes the diagnosis and treatment of individuals with VCF; distributes educational materials about Velo-Cardio-Facial (also known as Shprintzen Syndrome, DiGeorge Sequence, and Catch 22); and distributes questionnaire regarding the medical diagnosis and management of individuals with this disorder. **Awards:** Caitlin Lynch Memorial Fund Award (annual); Tony Lipson Memorial Fund Award (annual) helps members from Australia attend annual meetings.

★ 13535 ★ Veterinary Orthopedic Society (VOS)

PO Box 313
Newmarket, NH 03857-0313
Phone: (603)659-7989 **Fax:** (603)659-7989
Email: vosclarkmt@aol.com
Website: http://www.landscapesearch.com
Mary Tuson Clark, Exec. Sec.

Desc: Veterinarians interested in orthopedic surgery. Promotes education and research in veterinary orthopedic surgery. Provides a forum for the exchange of ideas among veterinarians in academia, research, and practice. **Awards:** Hohn-Johnson Research Awards (annual) for research; Mark S. Blomberg Memorial Resident Research Award (annual) outstanding resident abstract submitted to the VOS scientific program.

★ 13536 ★ VHL Family Alliance (VHLFA)

171 Clinton Rd.
Brookline, MA 02445
Phone: (617)277-5667 **Free:** 800-767-4VHL
Fax: (617)734-8233
Email: info@vhl.org
Website: http://www.vhl.org
Joyce Graff, Chair

Desc: Patients affected by Von Hippel-Lindau Disease; their families; medical professionals; interested others. Von Hippel-Lindau Disease is a genetic disorder involving abnormal growth forming "knots" of blood vessels in the retina, brain, or spinal cord areas. These knots are hemangiomas, a kind of tumor. Promotes education of the medical community, patients, and the general public about the disease. Provides an international support network to families affected by VHL. Conducts research and educational programs; funds research on VHL; maintains speakers' bureau. **Awards:** Minster Volunteer Award (annual); Research Award (annual) for a proposal approved by research board.

★ 13537 ★ Vietnamese Medical Association of the U.S.A.

c/o B.S. NguyenleHieu, M.D.
Shelton Medical Clinic
302 C St.
PO Box 476
Shelton, NE 68876
Phone: (308)647-6828 **Fax:** (308)647-5219
B.S. Nguyenlehieu, MD, Contact

Desc: Vietnamese-American medical professionals. Promotes mutual support and fellowship among its members, while fostering and maintaining medical ethics. Assures the provision of equal educational and professional opportunities for its members and the welfare of the general Vietnamese community. Supports and assists the Vietnamese victims of the Vietnamese communist regime. **Awards:** Pham bieu Tam MD Award (biennial) for contribution to advancing medical knowledge for Vietnamese.

★ 13538 ★ Visually Impaired Data Processors International (VIDPI)

c/o American Council of the Blind
1155 15th St. NW, Ste. 1004
Washington, DC 20005
Phone: (202)467-5081 **Free:** 800-424-8666
Email: rrrogers@one.net
Website: http://www.acb.org/vidpi/
Robert R. Rogers, Pres.

Desc: Visually impaired electronic data processing employees; those seeking employment; employers, instructors, manufacturers, and students in the electronic data processing field. Advocates high standards in training visually impaired students. Seeks to increase employment opportunities; encourages the exchange of work technique ideas and the development of new equipment. Works with agencies to increase the availability of braille and recorded materials. Supports a speakers' bureau. **Awards:** Kelly Cannon Scholarship (annual).

★ 13539 ★ Vocational Evaluation and Work Adjustment Association (VEWAA)

PO Box 26273
Colorado Springs, CO 80936
Phone: (719)638-4787 **Fax:** (719)638-6153
Email: info@vewaa.org
Website: http://www.vewaa.org
Robin Cook, Pres.

Desc: Specialists in vocational evaluation and work adjustment whose goals are to improve and advance the field and to promote high ethical practices through training and research. Conducts educational programs at state, regional, and national levels. Works with other organizations to develop a certification program for vocational evaluators and work adjustment personnel. Keeps legislators informed of the needs of persons with disabilities; promotes adequate funding of state and federal programs benefiting persons with disabilities. Disseminates employment information to members. **Awards:** Grant to members for small research projects; Paul R. Hoffman Service Award.

★ 13540 ★ Voice Foundation (VF)

1721 Pine St.
Philadelphia, PA 19103
Phone: (215)735-7999 **Fax:** (215)735-9293
Email: voicefound@onrampcom.com
Website: http://www.voicefoundation.org
Robert T. Sataloff, Chm.

Desc: Sponsors research and education on the causes, prevention, and treatment of voice disorders. Sponsors educational programs. Holds fundraising events. **Awards:** Grant; recognition; scholarship.

★ 13541 ★ W.M. Keck Foundation

550 S Hope St., Ste. 2500
Los Angeles, CA 90071
Phone: (213)680-3833
Website: http://www.wmkeck.org
Robert A. Day, Pres.

Desc: Works to support medical research, science, and engineering. **Awards:** Grant.

★ 13542 ★ Western Surgical Association (WSA)

c/o Richard C. Thirlby, MD
Virginia Mason Medical Clinic
1100 Ninth Ave., C6-GSUR
Seattle, WA 98111
Phone: (206)223-6636 **Free:** 800-354-9527
Fax: (206)625-7245
Email: Richard.Thirlby@vmmc.org
Website: http://www.westernsurg.org
Dr. Richard Thirlby, MD, Sec.

Desc: Surgeons who have contributed to surgical education and advancement. Objectives are: to cultivate, promote, and diffuse knowledge of the art and science of surgery; to sponsor and maintain the highest standards of practice; to deliver the best possible care to all people. **Awards:** J. Bradley Aust Award (annual) for best paper presented by a new member.

★ 13543 ★ William H. Donner Foundation

500 Fifth Ave., Ste. 1230
New York, NY 10110-0180
Phone: (212)719-9290 **Fax:** (212)302-8734
Website: http://www.donner.org

Desc: Strives to fund thoughtful and creative medical-related projects. **Awards:** Grant.

★ 13544 ★ Williams Syndrome Association (WSA)

PO Box 297
Clawson, MI 48017-0297
Phone: (248)244-2229 **Fax:** (248)244-2230
Email: tmonkaba@aol.com
Website: http://www.williams-syndrome.org
Terry Monkaba, Exec. Dir.

Desc: Individuals with Williams Syndrome and their families; medical and health care professionals; educators. (Williams Syndrome is characterized by similar facial features, low birth weight, heart disorders, hearing sensitivity, talkative personality, mild to severe learning disabilities, and developmental delays.) Provides support and assistance to families with a WS child. Conducts networking in the medical, scientific, educational, and professional communities for referral and study of newly-diagnosed WS individuals. Encourages medical behavior and supports research into all aspects of the syndrome. Compiles statistics. **Awards:** Chloe Reisig Music Scholarship (annual) for interest and ability in music and financial need; monetary; Research Grant (periodic).

★ 13545 ★ World Allergy Organization (WAO)

611 E Wells St.
Milwaukee, WI 53202
Phone: (414)276-1791 **Fax:** (414)276-3349
Email: info@worldallergy.org
Website: http://www.worldallergy.org/
Denise Lemke, Exec. Dir.

Desc: Umbrella organization for 56 international allergy associations representing 38,000 health professionals. **Awards:** Lectureship Grant (annual) to hold a national scientific meeting.

★ 13546 ★ World Federation of Neurosurgical Societies (WFNS)

c/o Dr. Edward Laws
University of Virginia Health Systems
Department of Neuro-Societies
PO Box 800212
Charlottesville, VA 22908
Phone: (434)924-2650 **Free:** 800-650-2650
Fax: (434)924-5894
Website: http://www.wfns.org
Dr. Edward Laws, Pres.

Desc: National neurosurgical societies representing approximately 17,400 neurosurgeons. Works for the advancement of neurological surgery. **Awards:** Gold Medal of Honor (quadrennial) for excellence in neurosurgery; Scoville Award (quadrennial) for excellence in nuerosurgery; Young Neurosurgeons Award (quadrennial) for excellence in neurosurgery.

★ 13547 ★ World Organization and Public Education Corp. of the National Association for the Advancement of Psychoanalysis

80 8th Ave., Ste. 1501
New York, NY 10011-5126
Phone: (212)741-0515 **Fax:** (212)366-4347
Email: naap72@aol.com
Website: http://www.naap.org
Margery Quackenbush, Admin.

Desc: Works for public education for the National Association for the Advancement of Psychoanalysis. **Awards:** Gradiva Awards (annual) for work that advances psychoanalysis; Vision Awards (annual) for work that advances psychoanalysis.

★ 13548 ★ Wound, Ostomy and Continence Nurses Society: An Association of E.T. Nurses (WOCN)

4700 W Lake Ave.
Glenview, IL 60025
Phone: (847)375-6730 **Free:** 888-224-9626
Fax: (866)615-8560
Email: membership@wocn.org
Website: http://www.wocn.org
Dionne Wilson, Sr. Mgr.

Desc: Enterostomal therapy (ET) nurses, wound, ostomy and continence care nurses in 10 countries trained in WOCN accredited schools; individuals interested in objectives of the association who hold a valid license in medicine or nursing; health-related firms. Seeks to support ET, wound, ostomy, and continence, nurses by promoting educational, clinical, and research opportunities and to guide the delivery of expert health care to individuals with wounds, ostomies, and incontinence. **Awards:** ET/WOC Nursing Education Programs and Advanced Degree Scholarships (quarterly).

★ 13549 ★ Xi Psi Phi

c/o Dr. Keith W. Dickey
1623 Washington Ave., No. 300
Alton, IL 62002
Phone: (618)463-1889 **Fax:** (618)463-1882
Email: gobux@attbi.com
Website: http://www.xipsiphi.org
Dr. Keith W. Dickey, Sec. -Treas.

Desc: Professional dental fraternity - dentistry. Maintains Hall of Fame. Conducts educational programs. **Awards:** Reagan Scholarship (annual).

★ 13550 ★ Yes I Can Foundation for Exceptional Children

1110 N Glebe Rd., Ste. 300
Arlington, VA 22201-5704
Phone: (703)264-3660 **Free:** 800-224-6830
Fax: (703)264-9494
Email: yesican@cec.sped.org
Website: http://yesican.sped.org
Christine Mason, Acting Dir.

Desc: The Council for Exceptional Children. Advocates for quality education for all individuals with physical disabilities, multiple disabilities, and special health care needs served in schools, hospitals, or home settings. The council also advocates for gifted and talented children and youth. Operates the ERIC Clearinghouse on Disabilities and Gifted Education, and the National Clearinghouse for Professions in Special Education. Develops programs to help teachers, administrators, and related services professionals improve their practice. **Awards:** Business Award (annual); Clarissa Hug Teacher of the Year (annual); Elizabeth Wetzel Scholarship (annual); J.E. Wallace Wallin Special Education Lifetime Achievement (annual); Joan Wald Baaken Award (annual); Outstanding Leadership (annual); Outstanding Public Service Award (annual); Special Education Research (annual).

Chapter 4
Consultants & Consulting Organizations

Entries in this chapter are arranged alphabetically by states, then by cities, then by consultant names. For additional information, see the "User's Guide" located at the front of the directory.

X123Q8

★ 13551 ★ HealthShare Lactation Services Inc.
Free: 800-887-5428
Email: info@hsls.com
Website: http://hsls.com

Activities: Experts in workplace lactation. Offers onsite corporate lactation program consulting, or a do-it-yourself Business Lactation Program. Offers promotional materials, lactation room selection and setup, interior design, breast pump selection, breastfeeding education, and a breastfeeding resource center.

Alabama

Birmingham

★ 13552 ★ Chris Frings & Associates
633 Winwood Dr.
Birmingham, AL 35226-2837
Phone: (205)823-5044 **Fax:** (205)823-4283
Email: cfrings@compuserve.com

Fnded: 1978. **Activities:** Provides expert testimony and consultation for court and arbitration regarding abused drug testing. Consultant to industry and labor relations attorneys with abused drug testing needs and problems. Also offers seminars and workshops and keynote speeches on management issues. Geographic Area Served: United States.

★ 13553 ★ King & Associates Inc.
2477 Valleydale Rd., Ste. B-1
Birmingham, AL 35244
Phone: (205)988-4222 **Fax:** (205)988-4101
Email: marieking@writeme.com

Fnded: 1980. **Activities:** Offers services in the area of healthcare, including reimbursement, documentation, and administration. Geographic Area Served: Southeastern United States.

Fultondale

★ 13554 ★ Management Institute
1712 Decatur Hwy.
PO Box 564
Fultondale, AL 35068
Phone: (205)841-7675 **Fax:** (205)841-7644
Email: mgtinst@bellsouth.net

Fnded: 1975. **Activities:** Three-phase program for small businesses. A leadership training institute offers specialized business training, career consulting and small business consulting. Primary areas of management and supervisory fundamentals, professional program planning and introductions, communication and public speaking, sales, women in leadership, stress, and harassment management. Geographic Area Served: Alabama.

Mobile

★ 13555 ★ B.G. Brogdon, MD
University of South Alabama
2451 Fillingim St.
Mobile, AL 36617
Phone: (251)471-7868 **Fax:** (251)471-7882
Email: gbrogdon@usouthal.edu

Fnded: 1996. **Activities:** Forensic radiology consultant specializing in individual and mass identification matters, child abuse, trauma and gunshot evaluation excessive torez, missed diagnoses and malpractice, and personal injury cases. Prepares courtroom exhibits. **Remarks:** Author or co-author of 270 publications. Geographic Area Served: United States.

Montgomery

★ 13556 ★ Drug Research and Analysis Corp.
PO Box 240308
Montgomery, AL 36124-0308
Phone: (334)265-2700 **Free:** 800-372-2669
Fax: (334)265-2704
Email: hfrazer@drugresearch.com
Website: http://www.drugresearch.com

Fnded: 1978. **Activities:** Offers pharmaceutical/device product development service which provides support to pharmaceutical and healthcare industries in areas of clinical research, new product development, and regulatory affairs. Clinical safety/efficacy studies and clinical pharmacology studies can be conducted using in-house facilities or management/monitoring on a multi-center basis. Consultation services available on product research and development issues and on regulatory affairs. **Remarks:** Experience: 23 years, 400 protocols, 40 drug companies, 50 approved NDAs. Geographic Area Served: United States.

★ 13557 ★ T.R. McDougal & Associates Inc.
4150 Carmichael Ct.
Montgomery, AL 36106
Phone: (334)260-8600 **Free:** 800-826-9410
Fax: (334)260-0023

Fnded: 1990. **Activities:** Firm offers expertise in healthcare consulting and management. Serves hospitals, physicians, assisted living facilities and commercial concerns. Geographic Area Served: Southeastern United States.

Tuscaloosa

★ 13558 ★ Ronald D. Hood & Associates - Toxicology Consultants
Box 870344 University of Alabama
Tuscaloosa, AL 35487-0344
Phone: (205)348-1817 **Fax:** (205)348-1786
Email: rhood@bsc.as.ua.edu

Fnded: 1978. **Activities:** Specializes in toxicology, especially developmental toxicology (teratology), reproductive toxicology, epidemiology and environmental toxicology. Provides data interpretation, hazard assessment, literature review, and litigation support. Also preclinical study design and monitoring study report review and preparation of manuscrpits for publication. Special expertise offered in the toxicology and pharmacology of arsenicals. Clients served include: state and federal agencies, especially the Environmental Protection Agency, law firms, and a wide variety of industrial clients. Geographic Area Served: United States.

Arizona

Chandler

★ 13559 ★ Quality Systems Group Inc.
25 S Arizona Pl. Ste. 570
Chandler, AZ 85225
Phone: (480)821-9116 **Fax:** (480)899-6026
Website: http://www.qsginc.com

Activities: A healthcare consulting company. Consulting services include management consulting, regulatory assistance, and interim staffing.

Green Valley

★ 13560 ★ Tingstad Associates Inc.
1243 W Camino de la Oca
Green Valley, AZ 85614
Phone: (520)648-1568 **Fax:** (520)648-6779

Fnded: 1984. **Activities:** Human resource development consulting firm offering organization, management and staff development programs on topics such as career development, conflict/resolution, negotiation styles, time management. Specializes in consulting for technical management. Particular emphasis is focused on teaching consumer skills to employees about healthcare thereby benefiting employer and worker. Provides customized group programs.

Mesa

★ 13561 ★ Alternatives: Consultation, Training and Development
PO Box 21177
Mesa, AZ 85277
Phone: (602)832-8876 **Fax:** (602)832-8985
Email: Jjalter@aol.com
Website: http://www.alternativesconsult.com

Activities: Specialists in behavioral health accreditation and the improvement of organizational systems and documentation.

Peoria

★ 13562 ★ R&G Medical Consultants Inc.
19243 N 88th Ave.
Peoria, AZ 85382
Phone: (602)566-3333 **Free:** 888-486-2245
Fax: (602)566-3438
Email: RnGMedCons@aol.com
Website: http://www.rngmedcons.com

Fnded: 1992. **Activities:** A team of professionals specialized in all areas of medicine. Provides medical records summaries and analysis. Researches case specific medical issues. Locates expert witnesses. Develops trial exhibits. Offers review of interrogatories, assistance with depositions, and scheduling of independent medical evaluations. Also offers technical trial consulting services. **Remarks:** 2003 appointed co-chair to the Business Advisory Council to the White House. Geographic Area Served: Worldwide.

Phoenix

★ 13563 ★ Arthur Sitelman, MD
Phoenix Memorial Hospital
Pathology Department
1201 S 7th Ave.
Phoenix, AZ 85007
Phone: (602)824-3235 **Fax:** (602)824-3139
Email: sitelman.path@worldnet.att.net

Activities: Specializes in surgical pathology, cancer and tumor diagnosis, anatomic and clinical pathology, autopsy pathology, cytopathology, clinical pathology consultations, and hematopathology. Services include expert witness, depositions, independent review, case preparation consultant, literature review, court testimony, and private autopsies. Geographic Area Served: United States.

★ 13564 ★ Behavioral Health Systems Inc.
3618 N 24th St.
Phoenix, AZ 85016-6509
Phone: (602)268-8404 **Fax:** (602)268-5396

Fnded: 1974. **Activities:** Offers direct and consulting services to consumers and providers of behavioral health programming. Direct services include outpatient individual and group psychotherapy. Also offers social development and psychotherapeutic services to the physically handicapped. Other services include statewide behavioral health planning, training, program design and evaluation as well as executive assessment and career counseling assessment to management personnel in transitional positions.

★ 13565 ★ Lifemark
7600 N 16th St., Ste. 150
Phoenix, AZ 85020
Phone: (602)331-5100 **Free:** 800-377-2055
Fax: (602)331-5199
Email: info@lifemarkcorp.com
Website: http://www.lifemarkcorp.com

Fnded: 1989. **Activities:** Offer managed care, HMO and Medicaid consulting services. Industries served: HMO's, Medicaid health plans, hospitals, and physicians. Geographic Area Served: United States.

★ 13566 ★ R.S. McQuate & Associates Inc.
3636 E Columbine Dr.
Phoenix, AZ 85032
Phone: (602)788-5651 **Fax:** (602)788-5655
Email: mcquate@aol.com

Fnded: 1987. **Activities:** Provides technical regulatory assistance with emphasis on FDA approvals and compliance issues associated with foods and medical devices. Offers particular expertise with food and color additives, food labeling, and in vitro diagnostic products. Develop and implement technology commercialization strategies, featuring alliance, partnerships and licensing. Industries served: foods and food ingredients; medical device manufacturers and distributors. Geographic Area Served: Pacific Rim countries and western states.

★ 13567 ★ Whitehall Management
PO Box 23482
Phoenix, AZ 85063
Phone: (623)934-2108 **Fax:** (623)934-6902
Email: Info@whitehallmgt.com
Website: http://www.whitehallmgt.com

Activities: Consulting team provides strategic practice planning services for dentists and other health care professionals.

Scottsdale

★ 13568 ★ The Conference Connection
c/o Community Resource Associates
8338 E Buena Terra Way
Scottsdale, AZ 85250
Phone: (602)949-8472 **Fax:** (602)949-2894
Website: http://www.conferenceconnection.org

Fnded: 1982. **Activities:** Offers meeting planning and conference coordination; board and volunteer development through training and education; development of corporate wellness programs; and management and leadership development programs. Industries served: private industries, government agencies, and religious organizations. Geographic Area Served: Worldwide, but primarily southwest, western, and northeast United States.

★ 13569 ★ Kelly/LaCoy & Associates
5019 N 86th Pl.
Scottsdale, AZ 85250
Phone: (480)941-5988 **Fax:** (480)945-0313
Email: dlacoy@concentric.net

Fnded: 1981. **Activities:** Management consultants provide staff performance appraisals. Industries served: foodservice, lodging, and retail, grocery stores and banking industry. Geographic Area Served: United States.

★ 13570 ★ Practice Systems Halstead Management
14439 N 73rd St.
Scottsdale, AZ 85260
Phone: (602)991-3319 **Fax:** (602)368-8754

Fnded: 1985. **Activities:** Offers medical/chiropractic practice management counsel.

Sierra Vista

★ 13571 ★ NAFC/BodyBasics
PO Box 67
Sierra Vista, AZ 85636
Phone: (520)452-8712 **Free:** 800-324-8315
Fax: (520)452-1320
Email: bodybasics@body-basics.com
Website: http://www.body-basics.com

Fnded: 1987. **Activities:** Speaks professionally on the training of fitness instructors; Certification Programs for Fitness Instructors and Personal Trainers.

Sun City

★ 13572 ★ Robert S. Pogrund
11022 Windsor Dr.
Sun City, AZ 85351-3339
Phone: (623)977-2940
Email: bobfind@juno.com

Fnded: 1974. **Activities:** Specialist in occupational and environmental health and safety with consulting expertise in environmental physiology and toxicology, occupational or industrial hygiene, human factors (ergonomics, man-machine integration), nutrition, public health and preventive medicine, human health effects of air and water pollution, and pesticides. Legal expert testimony provided for toxic occupational exposures; specialty in carbon monoxide toxicity, low level ionizing radiation, and ELF (extremely low frequency) radiation. Serves private industries as well as government agencies. Geographic Area Served: Southwestern United States.

Tempe

★ 13573 ★ BioQuest Medical Product Development Ltd.
2211 W 1st St., Ste. 106
Tempe, AZ 85281
Phone: (480)350-9944 **Fax:** (480)350-9966
Email: bioquestmed@qwest.net

Fnded: 1993. **Activities:** BioQuest is a medical product development corporation. The principal business is product design and introduction. Primary functions include design, prototyping, regulatory affairs, patents, intellectual property, project management, package design, technology assessment, research and development, mechanical testing, new business development, acquisition due diligence, distribution, marketing research, and strategic global marketing. Geographic Area Served: United States.

Tucson

★ 13574 ★ Cessna Consulting
13401 N Rancho Vistoso Blvd., Ste. 79
Tucson, AZ 85737
Phone: (520)544-7636 **Free:** 800-548-3141
Fax: (520)797-9671
Email: cessnaconsulting@aol.com
Website: http://cessnaconsulting.com

Fnded: 1987. **Activities:** Firm offers expertise in medical management and training. Geographic Area Served: Worldwide.

★ 13575 ★ Emergency Medicine Litigation Analysts Inc.
5189 N Marlin Canyon Pl.
Tucson, AZ 85750
Phone: (520)615-5412 **Free:** 888-335-3652
Fax: (520)615-5413
Email: questions@ERexperts.com
Website: http://www.erexperts.com/

Activities: Cost-effective impartial analysis of emergency medicine cases; review of duty, breach, causation, damages; strategic planning; database searches; expert witness services by board-certified, full-time emergency physicians; and complete litigation support.

★ 13576 ★ Falter & Associates Inc.
10560 N Stargazer Dr.
Tucson, AZ 85737
Phone: (520)531-8252 **Fax:** (520)531-8982
Email: bfalteraz@comcast.net

Fnded: 1990. **Activities:** Adjunct Professor at University of Arizona and Georgetown University.

★ 13577 ★ Humor Horizons
4745 S Paseo Melodioso
Tucson, AZ 85730
Phone: (520)370-2203 **Free:** 888-206-2203
Email: dj@humorhorizons.com
Website: http://www.humorhorizons.com/

Fnded: 1993. **Activities:** Consults on the use of humor techniques to improve stress management skills and to reduce stress and illness in the work environment. Consultant will conduct "playshops" and is available for speaking assignments.

★ 13578 ★ Jacquelyn St. Germaine
1641 E Prince Rd
Tucson, AZ 85719
Phone: (520)325-6097 **Fax:** (520)795-3670
Website: http://www.drstgermaine.com/

Fnded: 1987. **Activities:** An expert witness and consultant to attorneys involved in litigation related to psychiatric hospitals, addiction treatment centers, mental health centers, psychologists, and other mental health and addiction professionals. Geographic Area Served: United States.

★ 13579 ★ LaCasse Inc.
6727 Quartzite Canyon Pl.
Tucson, AZ 85718
Phone: (520)299-6171 **Fax:** (520)299-4362

Fnded: 1983. **Activities:** Involved in regulatory matters concerning the food and drug industry, both domestic and foreign, including food additive petitions,

NADAs, NDAs, ANDAs, INDs, and pesticide and fungicide regulation. Consults in the development of drugs and their approval by the FDA. Develops protocols on all aspects of pre-clinical and clinical studies, both animal and human. Advises on establishing a pharmaceutical presence in the U.S. for foreign pharmaceutical companies. Expert in generic drug industry. Geographic Area Served: North and South America, Europe, and Japan.

Arkansas

Little Rock

★ 13580 ★ Drug Free Inc.
100 S University Ave., Ste. 401
Little Rock, AR 72205-5213
Phone: (501)664-4434 **Fax:** (501)664-8886
Fnded: 1989. **Activities:** Consulting firm managing and administering drug treatment programs for business in the U.S.

★ 13581 ★ Jimmie L. Valentine, PhD
University of Arkansas for Medical Sciences
Department of Pediatrics & Pharmacology
800 Marshall St.
Little Rock, AR 72202
Phone: (501)320-2802 **Fax:** (501)320-3551
Email: valentinejimmiel@exchange.uams.edu
Activities: Specializes in drug abuse cases, accidents and medical malpractice, and forensic toxicology.

★ 13582 ★ P.A. Hames & Associates Inc.
PO Box 17083
Little Rock, AR 72222
Phone: (501)221-0984 **Fax:** (501)228-0591
Email: pathames@aristotle.net
Activities: Medical and legal consultants specializing in life care planning and American's with Disabilities Act (ADA).

Rogers

★ 13583 ★ Anita Thibeault & Associates
100 N Dixieland Rd., Ste. D2-287
Rogers, AR 72756
Phone: (501)750-3827 **Fax:** (501)443-6634
Fnded: 1986. **Activities:** Provides quality assurance and regulatory affairs support for medical device manufacturers.

California

Agoura

★ 13584 ★ Office Workouts
31400 Lobo Canyon Rd.
Agoura, CA 91301
Phone: (818)991-6256 **Free:** 800-442-9255
Fax: (818)991-9315
Email: denise@officeworkouts.com
Website: http://www.officeworkouts.com
Activities: Corporate wellness programs consulting firm offers the design and development of comprehensive, educational, and fun programs to client's employees. A corporate fitness and wellness program provider. Specializes in on-site exercise classes. Provides full fitness center management and long or short term staffing services.

Alameda

★ 13585 ★ Industrial Sensors & Actuators
Alameda, CA 94501
Phone: (510)814-1943 **Free:** 800-644-3628
Activities: Designs and constructs prototypes of special purpose sensors and related instrumentation systems for process monitoring and control, nondestructive evaluation, and medical diagnostics. Also specializes in design and fabrication of ultrasonic and sonic based instruments; ultrasonic transducers and EMATs; custom packaging of ultrasonic electronics; piezoelectric actuators and arrays; magnetic sensor arrays, magnetic field mapping instruments; and magnetic flux leakage systems.

Alta Loma

★ 13586 ★ Nancy Green, R.N., M.S.N., Stress Management Consultant
5861 Sacramento Ave.
Alta Loma, CA 91701
Phone: (909)987-5157 **Fax:** (909)987-9347
Fnded: 1982. **Activities:** Offers stress management consultation and seminars to all businesses and industries, as well as government agencies. Geographic Area Served: Worldwide.

Anaheim

★ 13587 ★ Anaheim Orthopedic Surgery
1741-F W Romneya Dr.
Anaheim, CA 92801
Phone: (714)776-7920 **Fax:** (714)776-3786
Activities: Provides expert witness testimony in the areas of orthopedic surgery, arthroscopy spine surgery, and hand surgery.

★ 13588 ★ The Thomas Group Ltd.
130 Chaparral Ct., Ste. 200
Anaheim, CA 92808
Phone: (714)279-1000 **Fax:** (714)279-1011
Email: info@tgltd.com
Website: http://www.tgltd.com
Activities: A consulting firm specializing in providing professional business management assistance to manufacturers, distributors, and service organizations in the healthcare, managed care, and general business communities. Business services offered include global business development, strategic, operational, and tactical planning, acquisition and merger activities, candidate identification and due diligence activities, market research and analysis, training and development, conflict management, team building, cost containment strategies, offering insight into acquisition practices, PACS acquisition and integration, identifying opportunities, risk, and feasibility, and strategic partnering.

★ 13589 ★ Werlinger & Associates Inc.
1371 N Red Gum St.
Anaheim, CA 92806-5932
Phone: (714)688-1280 **Free:** 800-227-5610
Fax: (714)688-1270
Email: info@werlinger.com
Website: http://www.werlinger.com
Fnded: 1974. **Activities:** Engineering firm offering expertise in electronics equipment and loss prevention to insurance companies and law firms worldwide.

Apple Valley

★ 13590 ★ Back in the Saddle: Long-term Residential Services for Head Injured Adults
9775 Mockingbird Ave.
Apple Valley, CA 92308
Phone: (760)240-3217 **Fax:** (760)240-3274
Email: staff@thesaddle.com
Website: http://www.thesaddle.com
Fnded: 1994. **Activities:** A residential and transitional program design for adult head injured. Specializes in head injury, CVA, spinal injury and other catastrophic rehabilitation pictures. Geographic Area Served: North America.

Applegate

★ 13591 ★ Criterion Systems Inc.
100 Crother Rd.
Applegate, CA 95703
Phone: (916)878-6689 **Fax:** (916)878-6585
Fnded: 1978. **Activities:** Health services consulting firm focusing on medical equipment. Industries served: hospitals and medical office buildings. Geographic Area Served: Worldwide.

Arcata

★ 13592 ★ Karen Zimbelman
PO Box 399
Arcata, CA 95518
Phone: (707)445-4849 **Fax:** (707)445-1808
Email: kz@tidepool.com
Fnded: 1987. **Activities:** Management consulting firm with dual focus: (1) employee benefits consulting for small/medium-sized businesses implementing retirement plans, self-insuring medical insurance benefits, wellness plans, etc.; and (2) cooperative business training programs and management consulting. Specialty in board of directors training program design and delivery, public relations, publications design, editing and distribution for company (internal and external) communications. Industries served: various -primarily served consumer-owned, worker-owned and nonprofit businesses thus far, including government agencies. Geographic Area Served: United States.

Atascadero

★ 13593 ★ Rogers & Associates
2026 Alturas Rd.
Atascadero, CA 93422
Phone: (805)466-2972 **Fax:** (805)462-2110
Email: rrogers@cali.net
Fnded: 1994. **Activities:** Certified Management Consultant offers services in reengineering, strategic planning, organizational assessment, employee counseling, and teambuilding, (surveys, studies, and seminars), executive coaching. Industries served: industry in general and government agencies. Geographic Area Served: California.

Atherton

★ 13594 ★ Neil Sheehan
1 Southgate St.
Atherton, CA 94027
Phone: (650)363-0913 **Fax:** (650)363-0923
Email: neiljs@aol.com
Fnded: 1992. **Activities:** A consulting engineer specializing in medical device design and development. Emphasis on disposables, intravenous systems and components, hemodialysis, catheters, electrodes, pipettors, including manufacturing processes (injection molding, compression molding, vacuum forming, die cutting). An expert witness in patent infringement, and product liability cases. Provides demonstrative evidence and litigation graphics. Geographic Area Served: United States.

Avery

★ 13595 ★ Bill Senger & Associates
PO Box 369
Avery, CA 95224
Phone: (209)795-5192 **Fax:** (209)795-5346
Email: billsenger@compuserve.com
Fnded: 1986. **Activities:** Specializes in concept, design, research, organization, development and production of communication tools for the healthcare industry. Projects serve primarily as customer education, public education, and sales training tools for pharmaceutical, animal health, and telecommunications companies; software developers; engineering firms; and medical instrument, reagent, and diagnostic equipment manufacturers. Services include development of printed materials, videos, slides, overheads, poster sessions, and computer-based training pro-

grams. Also designs and produces newsletters, brochures, logos, and information booklets. Geographic Area Served: Continental United States.

Bakersfield

★ 13596 ★ BC Laboratories Inc.

4100 Atlas Ct.
Bakersfield, CA 93308
Phone: (661)327-4911 **Fax:** (661)327-1918
Website: http://www.bclabs.com

Fnded: 1949. **Activities:** Analytical consulting laboratory working in the areas of petroleum testing (oil, water, gas and geochemical analysis), environmental pollutants (purgeable halocarbons, and volatile organics), GC/MS, and ICAP/MS. Geographic Area Served: California and neighboring states.

★ 13597 ★ Ben W. Laverty III, PhD, REA, CEI

4909 Stockdale Hwy., Ste. 132
Bakersfield, CA 93309
Phone: (661)283-8300 **Free:** 800-833-0373
Fax: (661)283-8313
Email: cstc@cstcsafety.com
Website: http://www.cstcsafety.com/cstc

Fnded: 1986. **Activities:** Offers safety standards training programs, including Business Safety Check, Pesticide Awareness, Safety and Environmental Audit, Pesticide Hazard Communication, Ag Hazard Materials Training, Injury and Illness Prevention Program, Confined Space, Hazardous Materials Business Plan, Respirator Training, Emergency Action Plan, Equipment Operator Training, Process Safety Management, Worker Protection Standard, Monthly Safety Classes, Hazardous Material Communication, Drug Free Workplace, Blood Borne Pathogens Training, CPR and First Aid Classes, and SCBA Training (Self Contained Breathing Apparatus). **Remarks:** Cross Compliance Training Credits (sm). Geographic Area Served: United States.

Belmont

★ 13598 ★ IFM Data Services

951-2 Old County Rd., Ste. 311
Belmont, CA 94002
Phone: (415)570-5742 **Fax:** (415)578-1325

Fnded: 1988. **Activities:** Information research and reporting consultancy specializing in the biotechnical industry. Also specializes in environmental business and technical information. For the healthcare and biotechnical industry, the firm collects and manages financial, federal, demographic, sales and marketing data. Industries served: biomedical, biotechnical, pharmaceutical, and environmental, worldwide.

Berkeley

★ 13599 ★ American Medical Forensic Specialists

2640 Telegraph Ave.
Berkeley, CA 94704-3322
Phone: (510)549-1693 **Free:** 800-275-8903
Fax: (510)486-1255
Email: medicalexperts@amfs.com
Website: http://www.amfs.com/

Activities: In-house case analysis by Board-certified physicians who designate medical experts from a panel of 4,000 pre-screened medical specialists nationwide.

★ 13600 ★ Berkeley Therapy Institute

1749 Martin Luther King Way
Berkeley, CA 94709
Phone: (510)841-8484 **Fax:** (510)540-1707
Email: office@bti.org
Website: http://www.bti.org

Activities: General psychiatry assessment of injuries and disability, fitness for duty, mental competence, and testamentary capacity. Evaluates professionals whose hospital privileges or licenses are being challenged. Offer both plaintiff and defense testimonials.

★ 13601 ★ Freedom Workshop

PO Box 5881
540 Alcatraz Ave., Ste.205
Berkeley, CA 94705
Phone: (510)428-1184

Fnded: 1981. **Activities:** Interpersonal communication consultant specializing in neurolinguistic programming, Yoga, food and sugar addictions, self-hypnosis, personal development, human relations, family relations, library services, indexing, planning for aging, and women's concerns. Industries served: companies wanting stress relief for their employees, adult schools, recreation departments, libraries, authors and publishing companies desiring indexes, counselors starting practice. Geographic Area Served: Northern California, primarily Bay area.

★ 13602 ★ Robert A. Epstein MD

2702 Dana St.
Berkeley, CA 94705
Phone: (510)848-0900 **Fax:** (510)848-7495

Activities: Provides forensic psychiatric consultation, independent medical evaluations, and psychiatric evaluation and testimony. Specializes in child, adolescent and adult psychiatric disorders, psychological trauma, child custody, and physical and sexual abuse.

★ 13603 ★ Thomas Stern, MD

2636 Telegraph Ave.
Berkeley, CA 94704-3322
Phone: (510)841-1647 **Fax:** (510)848-4924

Fnded: 1974. **Activities:** Provides medical-legal evaluations and expert testimony for personal injury, workers' compensation, and medical malpractice. **Remarks:** Assistant Clinical Professor, UC San Francisco Medical School; Preceptor, USC School of Medicine; Member of Expert Witness Panel. Geographic Area Served: United States for expert witness work, Northern California for injury treatment.

★ 13604 ★ Womanhood Media

1909 Cedar St., Ste. 107
PO Box 9373
Berkeley, CA 94709-2035
Phone: (510)549-2970

Fnded: 1975. **Activities:** Consultant in academic affirmative management, with specializations in areas of women's studies/women's services, aging and ageism, media, libraries, and community college, through counseling in research structure and projects, course and program innovation, and staff and professional development. Professional development services include tailor-made training and workshops mainly for women in academe and in management. Also offer book reviews and video reviews. Geographic Area Served: Worldwide.

Beverly Hills

★ 13605 ★ Avner I. Feldman, MD

1130 Maytor Pl.
Beverly Hills, CA 90210-2605
Phone: (310)674-0873 **Fax:** (310)412-7948

Activities: Specializes in neurosurgery, head and spine trauma, tumors, aneurysms, disc surgery, and peripheral nerve injury. Provides industrial, personal injury and malpractice evaluations, and reports and medical record reviews. Offers consultation and expert witness testimony.

★ 13606 ★ Carole Lieberman, MD

247 S Beverly Dr., Ste. 202
Beverly Hills, CA 90212
Phone: (310)278-5433
Website: http://www.drcarole.com

Activities: An expert witness and legal consultant in forensic psychiatry, specializing in high-profile cases, sexual harassment, entertainment law, divorce, custody, psychiatric malpractice, sports injuries, criminal behavior, violence, and work/personal injury law. Media consultant. **Remarks:** Also fluent in French. Geographic Area Served: United States.

★ 13607 ★ Intercontinental Enterprises Ltd.

256 S Robertson, No. 3194
Beverly Hills, CA 90211-2898
Phone: (310)276-6525 **Fax:** (310)276-6595
Email: gsr@mindspring.com
Website: http://www.internationalexpert.indexl.html

Fnded: 1976. **Activities:** Consultants in international business and technology transfer. Specializes in finding and supervising foreign distributors, licensees, and joint-venture partners; identifying markets; preparing market studies; and implementing sales programs. Assists firms in setting up international operations. Acts as the client company's "International Department" at home, and its "Local Office" abroad. Assists in negotiating technology transfers, mergers, and acquisitions. Industries served: healthcare, personal care products, pharmaceuticals, computer software, medical devices and laboratory equipment. Conducts seminars and management training courses on corporate organization, management development, franchising, cross-cultural joint ventures and strategic planning. Geographic Area Served: United States, Canada, Europe (including Eastern Europe), Asia, Australia and Brazil.

★ 13608 ★ Jon A. Perlman, MD

414 N Camden Dr., Ste. 800
Beverly Hills, CA 90210
Phone: (310)854-0031 **Fax:** (310)275-5079
Email: jonap@ucla.edu
Website: http://www.plasticsurgerybeverlyhills.com

Fnded: 1980. **Activities:** Specializes in plastic surgery, cosmetic surgery, liposuction, nasal and facial injuries and scars. Geographic Area Served: West Los Angeles and Beverly Hills.

★ 13609 ★ Steven M. Simons, MD

435 N Roxbury, Ste. 311
Beverly Hills, CA 90210
Phone: (310)274-7303 **Fax:** (310)274-8572
Email: simons@cshs.org
Website: http://www.simonsmd.com

Activities: Offers expert witness testimony in the medical matters, including pulmonary, internal medicine, critical care, asthma, pulmonary embolism, ventilator management, pneumonia, pleural effusion, and bronchoscopy.

Boulder Creek

★ 13610 ★ Braun Science & Engineering Inc.

955 Kings Hwy.
Boulder Creek, CA 95006-9213
Phone: (408)338-7857 **Fax:** (408)338-7844
Email: cbraun@bseng.com
Website: http://www.bseng.com

Activities: Offers systems research, design, and development, including embedded systems: medical and sientific, ATE, and DSP. Develops display processors for avionics, navigation, and military applications; and computer peripherals. Experienced in digital hardware, firmware, software, and custom CPU design; Intel microcontrollers and microprocessors; programmable logic, and FPGA. Has complete development lab facilities.

Boulevard

★ 13611 ★ Medi-Legal Services

38160 Highway 94
Boulevard, CA 91905-9543
Phone: (619)579-2135 **Free:** 800-343-2135
Fax: (619)766-4900
Website: http://www.autopsy-organretrieval.com

Fnded: 1973. **Activities:** Offers evaluation of potential medical, dental and legal malpractice cases. Immediate autopsy services by Certified Pathologists also available in any type case, civil or criminal. Provides highly qualified medical and legal experts to testify in meritorious cases. Types of cases involve medical malpractice, personal injury, worker's compensation, medical product liability, drug related liability issues, legal malpractice and other professional liability litigation. Experts available include physicians, osteopaths, surgeons, dentists, attorneys, nurses, chiropractors, podiatrists, and accountants. Serves plaintiff and defense. Industries served: attorneys, hospitals, governmental agencies, medical societies, news media and insurance companies. Geographic Area Served: United States and Canada.

Burlingame

★ 13612 ★ Basil R. Meyerowitz, MD Inc.
1828 El Camino Real, Ste. 601
Burlingame, CA 94010
Phone: (650)342-1289
Email: pischer1@earthlink.net

Activities: Specializes in bariatric surgery (for morbid obesity) and malpractice and quality assurance. Geographic Area Served: California; Western States.

★ 13613 ★ Worldwide Promedica Inc.
577 Airport Blvd., Ste. 130
Burlingame, CA 94010
Phone: (650)344-6242 **Fax:** (650)344-3217

Fnded: 1984. **Activities:** Consulting firm offers marketing research expertise for medical products and services. Industries served: healthcare (pharmaceuticals, diagnostics, biotech). Woman owned firm.

Campbell

★ 13614 ★ Lewis Bass International Inc.
621 E Campbell Ave., Ste. 11A
Campbell, CA 95008
Phone: (408)374-4453 **Fax:** (408)374-0295
Email: lewbass@lewisbass.com
Website: http://www.lewisbass.com

Fnded: 1978. **Activities:** Offers product, occupational and environmental safety consulting to industrial and consumer goods manufacturers. Services include safe product design, safe work practices, expert witness testimony, and seminars and training in system safety and product liability prevention.

★ 13615 ★ Reginald Hamer
1313 Virginia Ave.
Campbell, CA 95008
Phone: (408)370-9545

Fnded: 1984. **Activities:** Involved in medical electronic product design, development and testing. Specializes in microprocessor, digital and analog circuits, and transducers and instrumentation. Services include safety analysis, failure modes and effects analysis, and regulatory agency investigations. Serves electronics and medical electronics industries.

Carlsbad

★ 13616 ★ PRO Inc./Professional Recruiting Offices Inc.
2558 Roosevelt St., Ste. 200
Carlsbad, CA 92008
Phone: (760)400-0123 **Free:** 800-748-6474
Fax: (760)400-0100
Email: info@proinc.com
Website: http://www.proinc.com

Fnded: 1981. **Activities:** Human resource development consulting firm offers particular expertise in executive search. Industries served: employee benefits, managed care, insurance, and healthcare and banking legal in the U.S.

Carmel by the Sea

★ 13617 ★ Doctors Professional Consulting
PO Box S-PMB 3061
Carmel by the Sea, CA 93921-0589
Phone: (805)490-2799 **Fax:** (760)416-8911

Fnded: 1987. **Activities:** Serves as advisor to optometrists and ophthalmologists, covering both the technical and administrative aspects. Primary interest is the evaluation of the value of practices. Serves as troubleshooter for doctors who have management problems and concerns. Certified by the courts as an expert witness. Geographic Area Served: United States.

Carmichael

★ 13618 ★ Arterial & Venous Diagnosis & Treatment Center
6357 Coyle Ave.
Carmichael, CA 95608
Phone: (916)965-5050 **Fax:** (916)965-4040

Activities: An examiner and expert consultant for the Medical Board of California. Specializes in both venous and arterial pathology, including phlebitis, varicose veins, thrombotic disorders, chronic venous insufficiency, arterial occlusion, carotid stenosis, aortic aneurysm, doppler ultrasound and other vascular disorders.

Castro Valley

★ 13619 ★ DWSmothers and Associates
3111 Castro Valley Blvd., Ste. 210
Castro Valley, CA 94546
Phone: (510)728-9861 **Fax:** (510)788-9874

Fnded: 1978. **Activities:** Provides investigative consulting regarding loss prevention in areas of personnel safety and physical security. Active in systems and procedures design as well as development of same. Serves private industries as well as government agencies. Geographic Area Served: Western United States.

Chico

★ 13620 ★ Narad and Associates
3110 Hidden Creek Dr.
Chico, CA 95973-5846
Phone: (530)893-5907

Fnded: 1985. **Activities:** Offers emergency medical services and disaster medical services planning, implementation, and evaluation. Industries served: healthcare and local government. Geographic Area Served: California.

Costa Mesa

★ 13621 ★ Steven Hirsch & Associates
950 S Coast Dr., Ste. 106
Costa Mesa, CA 92626
Phone: (714)962-2800 **Free:** 800-624-3750
Fax: (714)962-3800
Email: stevenhirsch@shassociates.com
Website: http://www.shassociates.com

Fnded: 1987. **Activities:** Offers healthcare administration expertise in these areas: hospital regulatory compliance, Medicare certification, licensing, and joint commission, quality improvement, infection control, safety management, and staff support. Industries served: hospitals, ambulatory healthcare providers, and long-term care facilities in the United States.

Coto De Caza

★ 13622 ★ National Contracts Inc.
31111 Via Consuelo
Coto De Caza, CA 92679-4017
Phone: (714)589-6500 **Fax:** (714)589-9600

Fnded: 1986. **Activities:** Professional practice management firm consults on medical national account services. Works closely with major healthcare purchasing organizations, networks/alliances and HMOs. Firm can also serve as a manufacturer's corporate account department, advising on negotiation strategies, selection of sales mechanisms, and distribution channels for a manufacturer's products and services. Also provides executive search services. Industries served: medical. Geographic Area Served: United States.

Crestline

★ 13623 ★ The Sensenbrenner Corp.
PO Box 5098
Crestline, CA 92325-5098
Phone: (909)338-0858 **Fax:** (909)338-9079
Email: wysiwyg51@earthlink.net

Activities: Specializes in medical device applications, safety and training, medical equipment, surgical instrumentation, physiologic monitoring, endoscopic technologies and instrumentation, anesthesia equipment, clinical equipment management and maintenance, repair and service, device testing and evaluation, clinical engineering, and intra-operative incident evaluation. Geographic Area Served: Worldwide.

Cupertino

★ 13624 ★ Antioch Systems
10285 Colby Ave.
Cupertino, CA 95014
Phone: (408)446-9451 **Fax:** (240)359-5575
Email: dick@antiochsys.com
Website: http://www.antiochsys.com/

Activities: Provides biomedical optical systems design, troubleshooting, and packaging. Uses 3-D AutoCAD in packaging design. Emphasizes cost effective designs and on-going cost reduction programs. Also experienced in biotechnical writing regarding restriction analysis, PCR, miniprep, and ELISA. Offers patent services and other protection of intellectual property. UL, VDE, FCC, and FDA assist with approvals.

★ 13625 ★ B. Meredith Burke
22996 Standing Oak Ct.
Cupertino, CA 95014
Phone: (408)973-0963

Fnded: 1970. **Activities:** Offers demographic, economic, and health policy/research services. As a private sector market researcher and strategic planner has surveyed Fortune 500 marketing directors, directors of off-shore assembly operations, and medical professionals on product/biotech development and manpower issues. Has prepared business and demographic forecasts for banks, industry groups, and international organization. Field experience in the Caribbean, Southern Africa, and Australia; expertise on Japanese economy. Has assessed community and maternal and child health needs for local, national, and international agencies. Evaluated family planning programs and social marketing schemes and developed policy statements. Industries served: health policy and planning/service delivery firms, international development agencies, environmental and manpower analysis firms. Geographic Area Served: Worldwide.

Danville

★ 13626 ★ Advanced Biosearch Associates Inc.
3880 Blackhawk Rd.
Danville, CA 94506-4617
Phone: (510)736-2500 **Fax:** (510)736-2800

Activities: Provides management services for the health and medical fields.

Diamond Bar

★ 13627 ★ JMPM Health and Residential Care Facility Consultants
22875 Hilton Head, No. 237
Diamond Bar, CA 91765

Phone: (909)860-0981 Free: 800-860-0920
Fax: (909)860-3387
Email: jmpm@earthlink.net
Website: http://www.jmpm.com/

Fnded: 1990. **Activities:** Designed to help residential care facilities realize and attain optimum quality care and services. Offers assistance with the application for licensure; on-site evaluation and in-service training prior to annual evaluator inspection; preparation of customized facility policies and procedures manual; assistance with appeal procedures; representation in informal hearings; license violation plan of corrections; advice and pre-inspection in the sale or transfer of property of a home or an existing facility; response to complaints reported to the department of social services; on-site review of the overall facility operation and management in accordance with the Health and Safety Code Regulations: Title 22 and Title 17; training and review of documentation requirements; assistance with facility upgrade and specialization of services; and assistance with program proposals to obtain a vendor license from the regional center (Levels 1 through 4). Geographic Area Served: State of California.

★ 13628 ★ Miraflor & Associates
858 N Diamond Bar Blvd.
Diamond Bar, CA 91765
Phone: (909)861-6761 **Free:** 800-994-4404
Fax: (909)860-1514
Email: info@miraflor.com
Website: http://www.miraflor.com

Fnded: 1987. **Activities:** A provider of consultation services to acute care hospitals and health clinics in the areas of utilization management, risk management, healthcare accreditation, licensure and HCFA revalidation. Services include temporary staffing, case management, utilization management, quality management, discharge planning / social services, clinical staffing, infection control, medical coding, quality / chart auditing, claims analysis, bill auditing, and medical records. Geographic Area Served: California, Nevada and Arizona.

Dobbins

★ 13629 ★ Inkwell
PO Box 178
Dobbins, CA 95935-0178
Phone: (530)692-1581 **Free:** 800-242-8545
Fax: (530)692-1581
Email: inkwell@oro.net
Website: http://inkwellbooks.com

Fnded: 1989. **Activities:** Offers publishing expertise specializing in areas of book illustration; disabilities and architectural barriers; artists and authors profile writing; art reviews; metaphysics. Geographic Area Served: Worldwide.

Dublin

★ 13630 ★ Chemical Data Management Systems
6515 Trinity Ct., Ste. 201
Dublin, CA 94568
Phone: (925)551-7300 **Free:** 800-735-1761
Fax: (925)829-3886
Email: info@cdms.com
Website: http://www.cdms.com

Fnded: 1988. **Activities:** Specializes in environmental and health and safety compliance support services. Provides advice on hazardous material and OSHA regulations.

El Cerrito

★ 13631 ★ Ellis Eye & Laser Medical Center
6500 Fairmount Ave., Ste. 2
El Cerrito, CA 94530
Phone: (510)525-2600
Email: drellis@elliseye.com
Website: http://www.elliseye.com

Activities: Specializes in eye disability evaluation and rehabilitation, vision loss and related emotional effects; toxicology, pharmacological and chemical injury, radial keratotomy, cataract surgery, retroactive surgery, and diseases and surgery of the eyes and eyelids. Offers expert testimony and records analysis in workers' compensation, ophthalmic product liability, and medical malpractice.

★ 13632 ★ Probe Scientific-Toxicology
2109 Pinehurst Ct.
El Cerrito, CA 94530-1879
Phone: (510)233-2300 **Fax:** (510)233-2300
Email: kenparker@kenparker.com
Website: http://www.kenparker.com

Fnded: 1973. **Activities:** Serves attorneys, insurance companies, and individuals with forensic toxicology consulting and laboratory services. Emphasizes DUI-DUID cases; alcohol and drug use and abuse; human factors vs. driving skills; disorders and errors with breath, urine, and blood tests; correct diagnosis of intoxication, dose related to blood alcohol or drug concentration and action and effects on persons. Industries served: non-governmental companies' programs for employee drug use prevention, detection, forensic urine drug testing (FUDT), and consultation for certification of laboratory FUDT by College of American Pathologists. Also serves government agencies. **Remarks:** Toxicology - personal and professioanl services. Geographic Area Served: Primarily the West Coast of United States, specifically, the Greater San Francisco Bay Area.

El Segundo

★ 13633 ★ SEAL Laboratories
250 N Nash St.
El Segundo, CA 90245
Phone: (310)322-2011 **Free:** 888-SEALLAB
Fax: (310)322-2243
Email: akumar@seallabs.com
Website: http://www.seallabs.com

Fnded: 1971. **Activities:** A failure analysis laboratory with Metallurgists and Chemists available to perform failure analysis and to determine cause of failures of aircraft and automobile components, machinery, tools, medical devices, implants, etc., Expert witnesses for product liability and patent infringement litigation support. Geographic Area Served: United States, Canada, Europe, Japan.

Emeryville

★ 13634 ★ The Genser Group
2200 Powell St., Ste. 890
Emeryville, CA 94608
Phone: (510)237-6916 **Fax:** (510)236-9851
Email: genser@lawecon.com
Website: http://www.lawecon.com

Activities: Provides services for lawyers to increase effectiveness of economic testimony in litigation, including identifying economic issues which might enhance or threaten a case; locating appropriate economists to act as consultants or expert witnesses; translating the legal standards so economist understands the constraints; interpreting economist's analysis and opinions; defending expert's deposition and deposing opponent's economist; assisting in the presentation of economic issues to the trier of fact.

Encinitas

★ 13635 ★ Clin/Regs Associates
162 S Rancho Santa Fe Rd.
Encinitas, CA 92024
Phone: (760)634-3100 **Fax:** (760)634-3168

Activities: Specializes in all aspects of biotech/biopharmaceuticals new product development, including research, pre-clinical, clinical, regulatory, quality control, manufacturing practices, FDA interactions, immunology, pathology, cancer, viral diseases, monoclonal antibodies, cytokines, recombinant proteins, and gene therapy.

Fair Oaks

★ 13636 ★ Nutrition For You
4125 Temescal, Ste. J
Fair Oaks, CA 95628
Phone: (916)965-4012 **Fax:** (916)965-4012
Email: judy@judyfields.com
Website: http://judyfields.com

Fnded: 1985. **Activities:** Nutrition counseling services designed for the individual including: personalized meal planning, recipes and informational brochures, behavior modification, exercise guidelines, body composition analysis, breath acetone levels, and image mirror with picture to illustrate weight goals. Serves private industries as well as government agencies. Geographic Area Served: Solano, Yolo, Sacramento, Placer, El Dorado counties.

Foster City

★ 13637 ★ iManage Collaboration Software
950 Tower Ln., Ste. 500
Foster City, CA 94404
Phone: (650)356-1166 **Fax:** (650)627-8751
Website: http://collaboration.imanage.com

Activities: Provides collaboration software for business, commerce, and supply chain collaboration solutions.

Fremont

★ 13638 ★ Richard Feinberg, PhD
38950 Blacow Rd., Ste. D
Fremont, CA 94536
Phone: (510)794-2800 **Fax:** (510)791-8572
Email: drfeinberg@fremontpsych.com
Website: http://www.fremontpsych.com

Activities: Specializes in clinical and forensic psychology. Offers expert witness testimony in both, civil and criminal cases, including workers' compensation. Provides psychological assessments and psychotherapy for adults and children.

Fresno

★ 13639 ★ MooreInfo Inc.
1212 W Paul Ave.
Fresno, CA 93711
Phone: (914)572-6879 **Fax:** (914)591-6748
Email: dsmoore@mooreinfo.com
Website: http://www.mooreinfo.com

Fnded: 1986. **Activities:** Provides medical information service for professionals and consumers including scientific and medical-legal research. Services include manuscript consultation, grant writing and fundraising, medical-legal research, training programs, and childbirth preparation, including Lamaze instruction. Industries served: medical, pharmaceutical, educational, and government agencies. Geographic Area Served: Worldwide.

Glendale

★ 13640 ★ Circuit Technology
1426 Sunshine Dr.
Glendale, CA 91208
Phone: (818)242-6925
Email: george.dodson@prodigy.net

Fnded: 1982. **Activities:** Consultants in analog circuits, switching power supplies, instrumentation, data acquisition, power magnetics, spice modeling, worst case circuit analysis, nuclear event and radiation hardending. Industries served: military aerospace, commercial and medical electronics, and telcom. Geographic Area Served: Southwestern United States.

★ 13641 ★ Sterling Management Systems
316 W Wilson Ave.
Glendale, CA 91203
Phone: (818)241-1144 **Free:** 800-933-7538

Email: info@sterling-management.com
Website: http://www.sterling-management.com

Activities: Firm offers business consulting and management training for accountants and health care professionals. Offers on-site training and consulting.

Granada Hills

★ 13642 ★ Humanomics Ins Services Inc.

15650 Devonshire St., Ste. 212
Granada Hills, CA 91344
Phone: (818)830-5600 **Fax:** (818)895-2352
Email: info@humanomics.com
Website: http://www.humanomics.com

Fnded: 1981. **Activities:** Provides innovative and cost effective human resources and organizational development products and services for international and domestic organizations. Areas of expertise include organizational development, open book management, training and development, strategic staffing, compensation and benefit solutions, customized communications, proactive employee relations, HR compliance, workers' compensation, and Intranet development.

Irvine

★ 13643 ★ Irvine Orthopaedic Associates

16300 Sand Canyon Ave., Ste. 511
Irvine, CA 92618
Phone: (949)727-3636 **Fax:** (949)727-9515

Activities: Offers consulting and expert witness testimony in civil and criminal litigation in the area of orthopedics. Provides case evaluations and independent medical evaluation.

★ 13644 ★ SK&A Information Services Inc.

2601 Main St., Ste. 650
Irvine, CA 92614
Phone: (714)476-2051 **Free:** 800-752-5478
Fax: (714)476-2168
Email: skasales@skainfo.com

Activities: Firm develops and rents medical mailing lists and provides consulting on the marketing of pharmaceutical products.

La Jolla

★ 13645 ★ Devon Hill Associates

1535 El Paso Real
La Jolla, CA 92037
Phone: (858)459-4446 **Fax:** (858)459-4447
Email: mlgerber@san.rr.com

Activities: Cardiac surgeon/attorney with over 2700 open heart procedures, as well as extensive operative experience in thoracic (chest and lung) surgery and peripheral vascular surgery. Provides expert case evaluation for attorneys at the various stages of the litigation process.

★ 13646 ★ The Reference Desk - Research Services

PO Box 12122
La Jolla, CA 92039
Email: ezyroff@yahoo.com

Fnded: 1983. **Activities:** Information retrieval projects in all fields also provides instruction in research techniques and issues in information science. Provides information and referral services, photocopies, and document retrieval. Serves the following industries: advertising, aerospace, architecture, agriculture, banking and finance, biomedical, data processing, and education, electronics, engineering, environmental protection, food, geology, healthcare, insurance, journalism, libraries, manufacturing, marketing, medicine, mental health, nonprofits, patents, pharmaceutical, psychology, publishing, government, legal profession, and trademarks. served: national and international. Geographic Area Served: Worldwide.

Lafayette

★ 13647 ★ John H. Devor, MD

970 Dewing Ave., Ste. 200
Lafayette, CA 94549
Phone: (925)284-5100 **Fax:** (925)284-5551
Email: jdevor@aol.com

Activities: Specializes in general orthopedics; occupational and forensic orthopedics; neck and lower back problems; provides medical-legal evaluations for personal injury and workers' compensation. Offers medical record review/analysis; reviews myelograms, MRIS and CT scans; gives expert witness testimony.

★ 13648 ★ Mirfak Associates Inc.

201 Lafayette Cir., Ste. 100
Lafayette, CA 94549-4370
Phone: (925)283-4100 **Free:** 800-634-6445
Fax: (925)283-9549
Email: info@mirfak.com
Website: http://www.mirfak.com

Activities: Pain resolution consultant handling physical and psychiatric injuries, head injuries, severe and complex medical cases, work injuries, personal injuries.

★ 13649 ★ Soyfoods Consulting Services

PO Box 234
Lafayette, CA 94549
Phone: (925)283-2991 **Fax:** (925)283-9091
Website: http://www.thesoydaily.com

Fnded: 1976. **Activities:** Specializes in consulting related to all aspects of traditional, low-technology soyfoods, especially market research, production, starting a new soyfoods company, developing and launching new products, integrating soyfoods into an existing product line, entering a new market, modernizing a national soyfoods industry, and starting a new soyfoods industry. Geographic Area Served: Worldwide.

Laguna Beach

★ 13650 ★ Victor White International

30100 Town Center Dr., Ste. 220
PO Box 3318
Laguna Beach, CA 92654-3318
Phone: (949)380-4800 **Fax:** (949)380-7477
Email: vic@victorwhite.com
Website: http://www.victorwhite.com

Fnded: 1984. **Activities:** A resource management group in the medical device, bioscientific, and pharmaceutical marketplace. Key emphasis is on capital resourcing, technology acquisition or transfer, and strategic recruitment.

Laguna Hills

★ 13651 ★ Arnold D. Purisch, PhD

24422 Ave. de la Carlota
Laguna Hills, CA 92653-3648
Phone: (949)829-8141 **Fax:** (949)829-8215
Email: APurisch@aol.com

Activities: Provides neuropsychological evaluation, psychometric testing, areas include forensic psychology and forensic neuropsychology for criminal behavior and workers' compensation cases. Provides neuropsych/psychological evaluation.

Laguna Niguel

★ 13652 ★ Allen-Jeffers Associates

23716 Marlin Cove
Laguna Niguel, CA 92677
Phone: (949)495-1096 **Fax:** (949)495-5009
Email: bobjeffers@aol.com

Fnded: 1978. **Activities:** Executive and technical recruiting in the medical industry. Placement specialists with Fortune 500 through entrepreneurial venture firms.

★ 13653 ★ In-Sync Solutions Inc.

24232 Mimosa Dr.
Laguna Niguel, CA 92677
Phone: (949)363-9448 **Fax:** (949)362-9450
Website: http://www.in-syncsolutions.com

Fnded: 1984. **Activities:** Specializes in computer-enhanced facilitated meeting projects designed to help companies make smarter decisions in a significantly shorter time frame. The process provides a means of achieving consensus on issues ranging from strategic planning to move forward smoothly after major reorganizations, to improving an organization's creativity. The computer process generates a large amount of information in minutes. All input and ranking of ideas is anonymous, which encourages honest participation and ensures the same quality of feedback from outgoing and quiet members alike. The unbiased trained facilitator guides the group to reach the predetermined goals.

★ 13654 ★ The Remington Report Inc.

30100 Town Center Dr., Ste. 421
Laguna Niguel, CA 92677-2064
Free: 800-247-4781 **Fax:** (949)715-1797
Website: http://www.remingtonreport.com

Fnded: 1982. **Activities:** Advises healthcare industry in the United States.

Larkspur

★ 13655 ★ Benefits Planning & Insurance Agency Inc.

101 Larkspur Landing Cir., Ste. 120
Larkspur, CA 94939-1749
Phone: (415)461-8383 **Fax:** (415)925-2077
Email: bpi@bpihq.com
Website: http://www.bpihq.com

Fnded: 1978. **Activities:** Insurance brokerage and consulting firm offering professional services related to employee benefit programs. Specializes in employee healthcare plan management. Management service includes plan analysis, design, funding, installation, communication and administration. Arranges insured, partially self-funded, fully self-funded, and split-funded/minimum premium programs. Services also extend to executive benefits, group and long-term disability, group life, business travel, and other corporate benefit needs relative to clients' objectives.

★ 13656 ★ O'Rourke & Associates

PO Box 512
Larkspur, CA 94977
Phone: (415)924-3350 **Fax:** (415)924-3341
Email: morourke@jong.com

Fnded: 1975. **Activities:** Firm provides management and education services for rethinking health care delivery systems that improve operational effectiveness and role productivity of managers and staff. Expertise includes organizational and role redesign; team building; program development; managerial and staff role clarification; organizational transition and cultural change management; establishing interdisciplinary, collaborative work environments; creating learning environments that motivate members of an organization; and assisting executive leadership in aligning strategic effort with business/operational goals and succession strategy. Geographic Area Served: United States.

Long Beach

★ 13657 ★ American Podiatric Medical Association-La County

2333 Pacific Ave.
Long Beach, CA 90806
Phone: (562)427-7443 **Fax:** (562)424-3395

Activities: Offers foot and ankle medical evaluations and consultations. Provides personal injury evaluation; footprint identification, and medical record review. Offers expert testimony in workers comp and personal injury cases. Reviews insurance claims.

★ 13658 ★ Eliezer Nussbaum, MD, FAAP, FCCP, FCCM
2801 Atlantic Ave., 3dr Fl.
Long Beach, CA 90801-1428
Phone: (562)933-8740 **Fax:** (562)933-8744
Email: enussbaum@memorialcare.org
Activities: Specializes in pediatrics, pediatric pulmonary, pediatric critical care, and emergency medicine. Offers expert testimony.

★ 13659 ★ First Consulting Group
111 W Ocean Blvd., Ste. 1000
Long Beach, CA 90802
Phone: (562)624-5200 **Free:** 800-345-0957
Fax: (562)432-5774
Email: info@fcg.com
Website: http://www.fcg.com
Fnded: 1980. **Activities:** A leading provider of consulting, integration and management services to healthcare, pharmaceutical, and other life sciences organizations. Geographic Area Served: North America and Europe.

★ 13660 ★ Litigation Management & Training Services Inc.
301 E Ocean Blvd., Ste. 220
Long Beach, CA 90802
Phone: (562)495-0098 **Free:** 800-LIT-MGMT
Fax: (562)495-1786
Email: patricia@preventlitigation.com
Website: http://preventlitigation.com
Fnded: 1987. **Activities:** Consults with private industry employers and government agencies on proactive legal management of the workplace, including sexual harassment prevention, legal aspects of human resources management, how to hire, fire and manage employees legally. Special programs for adopting and enforcing e-mail and internet abuse policies. Also trains on avoiding liabilities for design and delivery of training programs, health and safety regulatory compliance issues and legal aspects of violence prevention and workplace security. Personnel policey development, internal discrimination and misconduct investigations. Geographic Area Served: Worldwide.

★ 13661 ★ Malloy & Associates Inc.
354 Whites Landing
Long Beach, CA 90803-6823
Phone: (562)494-1632 **Fax:** (562)494-2842
Email: jjmalloy3@cs.com
Fnded: 1986. **Activities:** Provides guidance to medical device manufacturers in the area of U.S. Food and Drug Administration and International Standards Organization requirements. Areas of expertise include good manufacturing practices (GMP), International Standards (ISO 9001), and operation audits: 510(k), IDE, PMA, and other submissions to the U.S. Food and Drug Administration. The firm also presents GMP, ISO, and software development seminars. Clients include start-ups, large corporations, international firms, and government agencies worldwide. Geographic Area Served: Worldwide.

★ 13662 ★ RX 4 Law
3591 Thornlake Ave.
Long Beach, CA 90808-3353
Phone: (562)430-7839 **Fax:** (562)493-6999
Email: jearsley@earthlink.net
Activities: Offers consulting services in medical and hospital malpractice. Provides expert witness consultation and testimony regarding critical care, medical/surgical nursing, or telemetry.

Los Altos

★ 13663 ★ George E. Bolduc, Jr., MD
27160 Moody Rd.
Los Altos, CA 94022
Phone: (650)559-9764 **Fax:** (415)388-3732
Activities: Provides expert witness testimony in forensic pathology for both: criminal and civil law cases. Geographic Area Served: California, Arizona, Washington, New York, and Tennessee.

Los Angeles

★ 13664 ★ Animal Behavior Counseling Services Inc.
2288 Manning Ave.
Los Angeles, CA 90064
Phone: (310)474-3776 **Free:** 800-605-2227
Fax: (310)475-9659
Email: dr.polsky@verizon.net
Website: http://www.dogexpert.com
Activities: Dog behavior specialist. Provides assessment and reconstruction of dog-related injuries, including dog bites. Answers questions such as: Was the dog provoked? Was the owner faulty in the management of the dog? Did the dog possess dangerous behavioral propensities? Did the injury occur as the plaintiff claims it did? Was the incident a foreseeable event? Assists in the utilization of behavioral arguments. Prepares declarations and reports. Inspects the dog and premises. Renders deposition trial and testimony. Geographic Area Served: California, Nevada, Arizona, Oregon, and Texas.

★ 13665 ★ Cadvan O. Griffiths Jr., MD
11645 Wilshire Blvd., Fl. 6
Los Angeles, CA 90025
Activities: Offers medical-legal consultation and malpractice review related to cosmetic and reconstructive surgery involving the head, neck, hands, and extremities. Geographic Area Served: Worldwide.

★ 13666 ★ Conomikes Associates Inc.
12233 W Olympic Blvd., Ste. 116
Los Angeles, CA 90064
Free: 800-421-6512 **Fax:** (310)571-4178
Email: information@conomikes.com
Website: http://www.conomikes.com
Fnded: 1970. **Activities:** Offers medical management consulting services. Focus is on the following areas: improving medical practice management, mergers and acquisitions, valuations for practice sales or mergers, strategic planning, income and expense sharing arrangements, and coding and reimbursement review. Industries served: medical practices. Geographic Area Served: United States.

★ 13667 ★ Digestive Diseases Foundation
8737 Beverly Blvd.
Los Angeles, CA 90048
Phone: (310)659-5088 **Free:** 800-900-5650
Fnded: 1975. **Activities:** Specializes in stomach, intestine, colon, and liver diseases. Consultant to Department of Corporations State of California (HMO oversight). Consultant to Medical Board of California (Doctor oversight). Medico Legal Consulation. Consultant Gersman-Lehmann Group. Geographic Area Served: Worldwide.

★ 13668 ★ Edward R. Ritvo, MD
10570 Rocca Way
Los Angeles, CA 90077
Phone: (310)825-0220
Activities: Specializes in child and adult psychiatry, results of head trauma, mental retardation, psychiatric disability, developmental disabilities, learning disabilities, and autism.

★ 13669 ★ Evaluation & Training Institute
12300 Wilshire Blvd., Ste. 420
Los Angeles, CA 90025
Phone: (310)820-8521 **Fax:** (310)207-2964
Fnded: 1974. **Activities:** Specializes in policy development with expertise in program evaluation, management, and applied research. Provides consulting for public and private sector. Previous studies and projects have covered organizational, educational and social policy issues in such areas as employment training, management audits, affirmative action, health management, and criminal justice. Geographic Area Served: United States.

★ 13670 ★ Gardenswartz & Rowe
12658 W Washington Blvd., Ste. 105
Los Angeles, CA 90066
Phone: (310)823-2466 **Fax:** (310)823-3923
Email: mail@gardenswartzrowe.com
Website: http://www.gardenswartzrowe.com
Fnded: 1980. **Activities:** Provides consultation to organizations and training and development on diversity, stress management, managing change, team-building, and train the trainer. Industries served: healthcare, government, insurance, entertainment, newspaper, aerospace, and utilities. Geographic Area Served: United States.

★ 13671 ★ Gerontological Planning Associates
3041 Queensbury Dr.
Los Angeles, CA 90064
Phone: (310)838-9400 **Fax:** (310)838-6069
Fnded: 1974. **Activities:** Offers consulting services including planning, programming, and design of homes for the elderly. Services include assessment of existing facilities and services, new program implementation, and marketing to the consumer. Expertise is based upon the knowledge and experience of the needs and desires of older persons, derived from surveys and interviews of 400,000 senior citizens. Geographic Area Served: United States, Europe, and Asia.

★ 13672 ★ Jules Stein Eye Institute
100 Stein Plz., UCLA
Los Angeles, CA 90095-7000
Phone: (310)825-5000
Website: http://www.jsei.org
Activities: Specializes in the diagnosis and medical and surgical treatment of eye diseases, including glaucoma. Performs clinical research in ophthalmology.

★ 13673 ★ Michael Peck, PhD & Associates
10642 Santa Monica Blvd., Ste. 300
Los Angeles, CA 90025
Phone: (310)475-3018 **Fax:** (310)475-3018
Email: m_peck@msn.com
Website: http://www.michaelpeckphd.com
Activities: Specializes in clinical psychology assessment and consultation. Forensic psychology services in wrongful death, suicide and accident, alcohol and drug abuse, personal injury, and medical malpractice (psychology).

★ 13674 ★ Murray Grossan, MD
Cedars Sinai Medical Towers
8631 W 3rd St., Ste. 440E
Los Angeles, CA 90048
Phone: (310)659-1006 **Fax:** (310)652-9906
Email: entconsult@aol.com
Website: http://www.ent-consult.com.members.aol.com/ent16law
Activities: Specializes in problems that involve hearing loss, tinnitus, and dizziness (both ENT and VAT). Provides audiograms, tinnitus diagnosis and treatment, electronystagmography, brain stem auditory evoked response, otoacoustic emissions for objective hearing loss/damage recording, sinus and nasal evaluation for toxic exposure, objective measurements of mucocilliary impairment, and scar evaluation. **Remarks:** Bibliography includes 35 peer review articles. Medical editor of www.allergybuyersclub.com. Geographic Area Served: Greater Los Angeles and United States.

★ 13675 ★ Nachman Brautbar, MD
6200 Wilshire Blvd., Ste. 1000
Los Angeles, CA 90048
Phone: (323)634-6500 **Fax:** (323)634-6501
Email: brautbar@aol.com
Activities: Medical doctor specializing in internal medicine, nephrology, pharmacology, occupational medicine, toxicology, internal medicine, and nephrology. Offers consultations, assessments, review records, and expert opinion testimony. Geographic Area Served: Worldwide.

★ 13676 ★ Reid Product Development
12701 Woodgreen Ave.
Los Angeles, CA 90066
Phone: (310)390-1573 **Fax:** (310)390-4853
Website: http://reidpd.com
Fnded: 1987. **Activities:** Professional firm develops a broad range of small equipment products and disposables for the medical, laboratory, food and beverage, and consumer markets. Technical specialties are pneumatics, fluid metering, position control, electronics interface, opto-mechanical packaging, injection-molded components, material selection, and precision-engineered assemblies. Services include program management, innovative design, mechanical engineering, prototypes, production engineering drawings, and confidential vendor sourcing (OEM components, secondary processes, and fabrication equipment). Client products include robotic clinical sample processor, clinical reagent dispensers, surgical equipment and disposables, non- invasive medical diagnostic equipment and disposables, and hospital sterilizers. Other expertise includes engineering development of durable equipment products for anesthesia, respiratory therapy, intravenous fluid delivery, and beverage-carbonation. **Remarks:** Our clients are entrepreneurs (at the angel and VC funding stages), owners (of private businesses), and key management (of small public companies and major coporate divisions). Geographic Area Served: Primarily western United States.

★ 13677 ★ Ronald E. Saul, MD
3575 Cahuenga Blvd. W
Los Angeles, CA 90068-1366
Phone: (323)512-8701 **Fax:** (323)851-2658
Activities: Provides neurological and neuropsychiatric evaluation limited to adult-adolescent cases of suspected brain injury, head trauma, epilepsy, dementia, anoxia, toxic exposure, and stroke. Provides expert witness testimony for personal injury cases.

★ 13678 ★ Tower Urology Medical Group
8631 W 3rd St., Ste. 915E
Los Angeles, CA 90048
Phone: (310)854-9898 **Fax:** (310)854-0267
Website: http://www.towerurology.com
Activities: Specializes in pediatric and adult urology. Geographic Area Served: United States.

★ 13679 ★ UCLA Statistical/ Biomathematical Consulting Clinic
AV-516 CHS
10833 LeConte Ave.
Box 951766
Los Angeles, CA 90095-1766
Phone: (310)825-3296 **Fax:** (310)825-8685
Email: gornbein@ucla.edu
Website: http://www.biomath.medsch.ucla.edu
Activities: Biomathematical services include clinical trial preparation, study design, statistical analysis, data management, data form design, help with reports and publications, mathematical modeling, help with research grant preparation (methods section), survey sampling, statistical graphics and custom mini-courses. Expertise in descriptive statistical methods, regression, correlation and analysis of variance, discrimination and classification/classification trees, logistic regression and categorical analysis, survival analysis, power and sample size calculations, nonlinear regression, and structural equation modeling.

Los Gatos

★ 13680 ★ Charles Jacobson Associates
433 Alberto Way
Los Gatos, CA 95032
Phone: (408)996-9989
Fnded: 1980. **Activities:** Offers consulting services in optical systems design engineering and development. Areas of experience include: laser systems and laser optics, fiber optics, medical laser instrumentation, photographic and holographic instrumentation, product development, custom instrumentation for manufacturing and quality assurance, and office copy machine optical systems.

Manhattan Beach

★ 13681 ★ Drucker Health & Safety Management Inc.
505 N Sepulveda Blvd., Ste. 16
PO Box 3515
Manhattan Beach, CA 90266
Phone: (310)372-8686 **Fax:** (310)318-1450
Email: mdrucker@druckerhealthsafety.com
Website: http://www.druckerhealthsafety.com
Fnded: 1984. **Activities:** Specialists on compliance and cost-effective solutions related to occupational and environmental health and safety and hazardous materials control. Develops programs which help to avoid costly accidents, escalating workers' compensation premiums, lost productivity, class-action suits, and adverse publicity. Also provides expert witness testimony. Serves private industries as well as government agencies. Geographic Area Served: United States.

Marina del Rey

★ 13682 ★ Paul K. Bronston, MD
1 Jib St., Ste. 202
Marina del Rey, CA 90292
Phone: (310)301-9426 **Fax:** (310)823-2433
Email: drprotec@attbi.com
Activities: Acts as plaintiff or defense expert consultant or witness in medical insurance bad faith evaluations; medical quality assurance evaluations; utilization review; liability evaluations; medical malpractice evaluations; emergency medicine and quality assurance and utilization review; hospital liability; and HMO/ managed care liability evaluation. **Remarks:** National chairman of the Ethics & Professional Policy Committee of the American College of Medical Quality. Geographic Area Served: United States.

Meadow Vista

★ 13683 ★ Jean Zimmermann
PO Box 934
Meadow Vista, CA 95722
Phone: (530)878-8553
Fnded: 1982. **Activities:** Offers consulting services in psychiatric and mental health nursing, nursing leadership, and the nursing process. Serves hospitals, businesses, individuals, government agencies, institutions, and firms in stress management, interpersonal relationships, leadership, nursing process and evaluation, psychiatric and mental health crises, and drug and alcohol counseling. Also provides advertising evaluations from the consumer's view point. Geographic Area Served: United States and Canada.

Mill Valley

★ 13684 ★ Green Dog Campaign Strategies Group
173 E Blithedale, Ste. 3
Mill Valley, CA 94941
Phone: (415)383-3715 **Fax:** (415)383-3718
Activities: Specializes in consulting with neighborhood and citizens' groups on environmental issues. Gives workshops for activists focusing on the specific needs of the group. Has trained activists in lobbying legislators, building coalitions, dealing with the media, recruiting and keeping volunteers and direct action techniques.

★ 13685 ★ Hugh H. West
10 Morning Sun
Mill Valley, CA 94941
Phone: (415)383-2301 **Fax:** (415)383-2388
Activities: Specialties include: Emergency Medicine; Emergency Department performance of Physicians, Consultants, and Ancillary staff (Nursing, Respiratory, Social Services, etc.); Pre-hospital Care performance of Paramedics and first responders (Police, Fire Department, etc.); Transfers and stabilization (COBRA/EMTALA issues); Trauma (Verified Level II Trauma Center experience); Ultrasound (Emergency Medicine performed/interpreted); Additional formal background training in Neurology and Neurosurgery; Administration (former Medical Director, Associate Medical Director, credentials, etc.). **Remarks:** Degrees/ Licenses: M.D., FAAEM (Fellow American Academy of Emergency Medicine); FACEP (Fellow American College of Emergency Physicians); ABEM Diplomate; Former ABEM Examiner (American Board of Emergency Medicine); Current University Faculty (UC San Francisco Medial Center), SAEM (Society for Academic Emergency Medicine). Geographic Area Served: United States.

★ 13686 ★ Mark I. Levy, MD
655 Redwood Hwy., Ste. 271
Mill Valley, CA 94941
Phone: (415)388-8040 **Fax:** (415)388-1225
Email: mark@levymd.com
Website: http://www.levymd.com
Activities: Specializes in post traumatic stress disorder, including witnessing or sustaining injury from disaster, violence, bereavement, torture, terrorization, auto/aircraft/industrial accidents, severe pain, rape, divorce, anxiety, work/school performance, sleep disturbance, depression, fearfulness, sexual dysfunction, psychotic states, molestation, sexual harassment, drug/alcohol abuse, job stress/violence/harassment, and psychiatric malpractice.

Montclair

★ 13687 ★ John L. Carrigan - Library and Information Services
PO Box 28
Montclair, CA 91763
Phone: (909)621-5225 **Fax:** (909)498-7302
Email: carrigan@attglobal.net
Fnded: 1976. **Activities:** Offers database searching and library research, as well as document delivery in the areas of science, medicine, law, and business. Search capabilities on the following database systems: Dialog, Lexis, Nexis, National Library of Medicine, STN, and Biosis. Industries served: all. Geographic Area Served: Worldwide.

Mountain View

★ 13688 ★ Ina K. Bendis, MD
2204 Grant Rd., Ste. 102
Mountain View, CA 94040
Phone: (650)941-4100
Activities: Specializes in internal medicine, pulmonary diseases, geriatrics, psychosomatics, HMO benefits denials, and claims fraud. Performs Record reviews, examinations, reports, detailed case analyses, and testimony.

★ 13689 ★ Retina Vitreous Associates Inc.
Orchard Pavilion, 2485 Hospital Dr., Ste. 200
Mountain View, CA 94040
Phone: (415)988-7480 **Fax:** (415)988-7482
Website: http://www.mdidocs.com/retina-vitreous.htm
Activities: Offers consulting on vision and automobile driving and medical malpractice.

Napa

★ 13690 ★ Dr. Mathis & Associates
3435 Valle Verde Dr., Ste. C
Napa, CA 94558
Phone: (707)252-2151 **Fax:** (707)252-1349
Email: rmathis1@aol.com
Website: http://www.mathisassociates.com

Activities: Specializes in clinical and industrial psychology. Offers expert witness testimony for personnel and wrongful termination, discrimination (sexual, age, etc.), and personal injury cases. Offers social security, disability, workers' compensation, stress management and post-traumatic stress, and medical malpractice evaluation and assessment, and abuse valuations.

Newport Beach

★ 13691 ★ Institute for Applied Management and Law Inc.
610 Newport Center Dr., Ste. 1060
Newport Beach, CA 92660
Phone: (949)760-1700 **Free:** 800-521-4265
Fax: (949)760-8192
Email: iaml@iaml.com
Website: http://iaml.com

Fnded: 1979. **Activities:** The Institute produces practically-oriented seminars, materials and videotapes for professionals requiring timely and accurate information in employment and employee benefits law, environmental law, health and safety law, and human resources management. The Institute also specializes in customized, in-house training programs, ranging from one-day seminars to full five-day certificate programs. Geographic Area Served: United States.

★ 13692 ★ Spiehler & Associates
422 Tustin Ave.
Newport Beach, CA 92663
Phone: (949)642-0574 **Fax:** (949)642-2852
Email: spiehleraa@aol.com

Activities: Specializes in pharmacology, pharmacokinetics and toxicology of cocaine, morphine and heroin, amphetamines, phencyclidine, alcohol, pharmaceuticals, poisons and drugs of abuse, immunoassay development and FDA submissions. Reviews employee drug testing, QA/QC, postmortem toxicology and drug testing in hair, saliva or sweat. Also specializes in drugs and DUI, memory, drug concentrations, combinations, time and cause of death.

★ 13693 ★ The Trizetto Group Inc.
567 San Nicolas Dr., Ste. 360
Newport Beach, CA 92660
Phone: (949)719-2200 **Free:** 800-569-1222
Fax: (949)219-2197
Website: http://www.trizetto.com

Activities: The Trizetto Group offers information technology staffing, claims processing, billing and receivable management, and consulting services.

North Hollywood

★ 13694 ★ Dana Productions
6249 Babcock Ave.
North Hollywood, CA 91606
Phone: (818)508-5331

Fnded: 1972. **Activities:** Produces educational materials specializing in audiovisual programs. Focuses on drug and substance abuse programs. These programs are used in human resources development to promote better productivity in corporations, government agencies, correctional institutions, and hospitals.

★ 13695 ★ QualityCare
5723 Ensign Ave.
North Hollywood, CA 91601
Free: 800-341-0404 **Fax:** (818)760-4577
Email: qualitycare@compuserve.com
Website: http://quality-care.org

Fnded: 1989. **Activities:** Firm offers extensive knowledge in nursing homes consulting. Geographic Area Served: California.

Novato

★ 13696 ★ Bundy, Gale & Shields L.L.C.
44 School Ter.
Novato, CA 94945
Phone: (415)897-8133 **Free:** 800-229-7773
Fax: (415)897-1263
Email: galesafe@a.crl.com-galesafe@atdial.net
Website: http://www.Fireexperts.com

Activities: Provides fire and explosion investigations industrial safety, hazardous materials, and loss prevention services. **Remarks:** Litigation support and expert witness services. Geographic Area Served: Worldwide.

Oakland

★ 13697 ★ John D. Warbritton III, MD
350 - 30th St., Ste. 530
Oakland, CA 94609
Phone: (510)839-5564 **Fax:** (510)839-1692

Activities: Specializes in orthopedic surgery. Provides medi-legal evaluations and consultations. A Spanish language translator.

★ 13698 ★ Joseph B. Marzouk MD
350 30th St., Ste. 511
Oakland, CA 94609
Phone: (510)835-6225 **Fax:** (510)834-8206
Email: jobm@aol.com
Website: http://infectiousdiseasemd.com

Activities: Specializes in infectious diseases, infection control; AIDS; food poisoning. Provides independent medical evaluations. Offers medical malpractice testimony. Geographic Area Served: United States.

★ 13699 ★ Mothertongue Institute for Creative Development
PO Box 16217
Oakland, CA 94610
Phone: (510)273-2463

Activities: Specializes in stress reduction. Other areas of expertise include youth work, writing and creativey, and alcohol/drug issues with a focus on harm reduction.

★ 13700 ★ Paul Perchonock, MD
461 34th St.
Oakland, CA 94609
Phone: (510)452-1390 **Fax:** (510)452-0834
Email: prpmd@aol.com
Website: http://perchonockmd.com

Activities: Performs record review to establish preexisting conditions/apportionment of treatment, to establish prognosis and future medical costs, and to establish medical necessity and reasonableness of care. Review of records to determine standard of care issues on Emergency Medicines. Verbal and written reports. IMEs on request. Geographic Area Served: San Francisco Bay Area, Northern California.

Orange

★ 13701 ★ David A. Lombardi, MD
1467 N Wanda Rd., Ste. 165
Orange, CA 92867
Email: David_Lombardi@msn.com

Activities: A board certified neurologist and medical evaluator specializing workers' compensation.

★ 13702 ★ Max A. Schneider, MD Inc.
3311 E Kirkwood Ave.
Orange, CA 92869-5211
Phone: (714)639-0062 **Fax:** (714)639-0987
Email: masmdinc@aol.com
Website: http://www.addictionsexpert.com

Fnded: 1981. **Activities:** A consultant on substance abuse issues. An expert witness in court cases involving alcohol and other mood altering drugs in criminal, civil, and malpractice issues. Lectures, seminars provided on all phases of substance use/abuse; author of educational videos. Also: physician health, impaired physicians. Geographic Area Served: Worldwide.

Orinda

★ 13703 ★ Cameron Bruce Associates
301 Village Sq.
Orinda, CA 94563
Phone: (925)253-9220 **Fax:** (925)253-9223
Email: cba@prodigy.net
Website: http://www.c-b-a.net

Activities: A healthcare consulting firm specializing in Environment of Care Practices. Experienced in the development of house-wide and department specific policy and procedure manuals. The firm has created, rewritten, or consulted in over 60 manuals, offering full production capabilities ranging from process review to a volume delivery of manuals.

★ 13704 ★ Robert H. Dailey, MD
29 Charles Hill Cir.
Orinda, CA 94563
Phone: (925)980-2459 **Fax:** (925)253-8373
Email: yeliad57@hotmail.com

Activities: Expert in emergency medicine and medicolegal experience, including court appearances. Geographic Area Served: Worldwide.

Pacific Palisades

★ 13705 ★ Center for Management Effectiveness Inc.
PO Box 1202
Pacific Palisades, CA 90272
Phone: (310)459-6052 **Free:** 888-819-0200
Fax: (310)459-9307
Email: info@cmeinc.org
Website: http://www.cmeinc.org

Fnded: 1978. **Activities:** The Center specializes in publishing training materials in he areas of, managing stress, managing disagreement & conflict, risk taking and decision-making. Principal training is provided via on-site workshops, and using thoroughly tested assessment instruments. Programs are designed to serve the specific needs of each client. Extensive training for Fortune 500 companies, government agencies and nonprofit organizations worldwide. E-learning versions available. Geographic Area Served: Worldwide.

Palo Alto

★ 13706 ★ Charles W. Casella, M.D.
701 Welch Rd., Ste. 211
Palo Alto, CA 94304
Phone: (650)326-6638 **Fax:** (650)326-1994
Email: casella1@pacbell.net
Website: http://www.member.expertpages.com/cwcasella

Fnded: 1971. **Activities:** Medical-legal consultant specializing in legal psychiatry, occupational psychiatry, and psychiatric disability evaluation. Industries served: insurance, legal, peace officers, government agencies, and all employees. Geographic Area Served: United States.

★ 13707 ★ Daniel W. Meub
1101 Welch Rd., Ste. C-9
Palo Alto, CA 94304
Phone: (415)327-9373 **Fax:** (415)327-1942
Email: dmeub@earthlink.net

Activities: Active practicing neurosurgeon providing arbitration appearances in personal injury and medical malpractice cases. Geographic Area Served: California, Vermont.

★ 13708 ★ IPT Corp.
1076 E Meadow Cir.
Palo Alto, CA 94303
Phone: (415)494-7500 **Free:** 800-656-8876
Fax: (415)494-2758
Email: steve@iptcorp.com
Website: http://www.IPTWeb.com
Fnded: 1974. **Activities:** Fully integrated contract product development and manufacturing company specializing in medical, diagnostic and biotechnology products. Firm is active in electronic product design, design and manufacture of medical instruments, UNIX and CI programming, and microprocessor systems design. Serves private industries as well as government agencies.

★ 13709 ★ Mary O'Leary
1788 Oak Creek Dr., Ste. 201
Palo Alto, CA 94304
Phone: (650)853-7487
Email: mmoleary@att.net
Fnded: 1980. **Activities:** Serves medical and health-care institutions and government agencies in the following areas: nursing administration, continuing education and patient/family education; psychiatric administration with focus on managed care contracting, product/service line development, research/development, marketing and patient/family mental health education. Geographic Area Served: Worldwide.

Petaluma

★ 13710 ★ Dow Pharmaceutical Sciences
1330A Redwood Way
Petaluma, CA 94954
Phone: (707)793-2600 **Free:** 877-369-7476
Fax: (707)793-0145
Email: info@dowpharmsci.com
Website: http://www.DowPharm.com
Fnded: 1973. **Activities:** Provides contract product development and clinical trial materials (CTMs) services. Corporate capabilities can be utilized as part of a complete development program, or individually to meet your specific project needs. Topical Pharmaceutics specializes in topical formulation development for dermatological, ophthalmic, nasal, otic, vaginal, intra-oral and intra-rectal products. Analytical Services offers method development and validation for all dosage forms with ICH stability and photostability studies. Strategic Planning and Consulting for your topical product development project is another core competency. Topicals Manufacturing provides cGMP laboratory and pilot-scale batches of non-sterile semi-solids, liquids and suppositories. Clinical Labeling and Packaging offers comprehensive labeling services for CTMs with distribution (including refrigeration), returned drug accountability and destruction with full GMP documentation. Industries served: dermatological, pharmaceutical, and biotechnology. Geographic Area Served: Primarily the continental United States, with some international clients.

Playa del Rey

★ 13711 ★ Nutritional Consultants Group Inc.
6806 Vista del Mar Ln.
Playa del Rey, CA 90293
Phone: (310)821-6456 **Fax:** (310)821-0780
Email: ncgroup@ix.netcom.com
Fnded: 1982. **Activities:** Specialists in nutritional supplements, and food product and pharmaceutical formulation and development with emphasis on nutritional needs in different life periods, different occupations and different health status. Industries served: food processing, pharmaceutical, health food, and Orange County government agencies. Geographic Area Served: United States, Europe and Asia.

Pleasant Hill

★ 13712 ★ Buckman Co. Inc.
200 Gregory Ln., Ste. C-100
Pleasant Hill, CA 94523
Phone: (925)356-2640 **Free:** 800-358-8785
Fax: (925)356-2654
Email: bcj@fda-help.com
Website: http://www.fda-help.com
Fnded: 1983. **Activities:** Services include medical device regulatory planning/evaluation, study design, study monitoring, 510(K) submissions, I.D.E. design/development, PMAA preparation and filing, and FDA panel presentations. Industries served: medical device manufacturers, and in-vitro diagnostic manufacturers. Geographic Area Served: Worldwide.

★ 13713 ★ Deedee Jenson Consulting
19 Dudley Ct.
Pleasant Hill, CA 94523
Phone: (925)943-7546 **Fax:** (925)943-1671
Activities: A trainer and facilitator working primarily with human service agencies.

★ 13714 ★ Sara Scientific Co.
295 Stevenson Dr.
Pleasant Hill, CA 94523
Phone: (925)934-1331 **Fax:** (530)548-7315
Fnded: 1960. **Activities:** Firm specializes in ultrasonicology and performs research and problem-solving in ultrasound; emphasis is on the use of ultrasound in biology and medical research. Provides consulting to entrepreneurial non-corporate stand-alone inventors in areas of patent protection and marketing. Industries served: medical, marine, fisheries, food processing, industrial cleaning for quality control, plating, as well as government agencies. Geographic Area Served: United States and Canada.

Pleasanton

★ 13715 ★ King Design Associates Beta Medical
1724 Beachwood Way
Pleasanton, CA 94566
Phone: (925)484-0843 **Fax:** (925)485-1797
Email: dakdakdak@aol.com
Activities: Designs electronic products from concept to production, concentrating on medical instrumentation. Skilled in project management; embedded systems design; and analog and digital circuit design. Programs firmware in C and Assembly. Develops battery operated, low power electronics, stepper motors, sensors, and transducers.

★ 13716 ★ Optical Design & Engineering
1742 Beechwood Way
Pleasanton, CA 94566
Phone: (925)425-9425 **Fax:** (925)398-8609
Email: epwoptic@attbi.com
Fnded: 1974. **Activities:** Designs optical components and systems, including UV, visible, IR, refracting, reflecting, catadioptric; and optical systems tolerancing. Has broad knowledge of current resources for optics and coating, both prototypes and production.

★ 13717 ★ Spinal Health Center
2340 Santa Rita Rd., Ste. 3
Pleasanton, CA 94566
Phone: (925)484-2558 **Fax:** (925)484-3951
Website: http://www.drstevenhickey.com
Activities: Specializes in work, auto, sports, and recreational injuries. X-ray and physiotherapy services available.

Point Reyes Station

★ 13718 ★ Shirley M. Kison, RN
12088 State Rte. One
PO Box 1018
Point Reyes Station, CA 94956-1018
Phone: (415)663-8343 **Fax:** (415)663-1260
Activities: Specializes in nursing home and medical records review, organization, and summary. Assists in and general discovery. Serves as an expert witness in industry standards for nursing homes, residential care facilities, and adult day care. Reviews medical literature.

Port Hueneme

★ 13719 ★ The Wilson Group
475 W Channel Islands Blvd.
Port Hueneme, CA 93041
Phone: (805)444-8777 **Fax:** (805)984-0507
Email: mailbox@the-wilsongroup.com
Website: http://www.the-wilsongroup.com
Fnded: 1973. **Activities:** Human resource management consulting service conducting evaluations and management training. Additional emphasis on internet assessment & travel & tourism services. Provides expertise in contracts administration and procurement training programs. Serves private industries as well as government agencies. Geographic Area Served: United States.

Portola Valley

★ 13720 ★ Samuel R. Phillips, Consulting Engineer
5 Joaquin Rd.
Portola Valley, CA 94028-8114
Phone: (650)851-4628 **Fax:** (650)851-5546
Fnded: 1971. **Activities:** Helps manufacturing companies' production and engineering departments work together to design and manufacture vital new products and improved mature ones.

Redwood City

★ 13721 ★ Auditory Rehabilitation Engineering
1302 Hopkins Ave., Ste. 8
Redwood City, CA 94062
Phone: (650)364-2127
Email: ghaasaudio@aol.com
Fnded: 1979. **Activities:** Consultancy specializing in audiology research and development, field testing and selection, and fitting procedures of hearing aids with new signal processing schemes; improvement of noisy communication channels; and hearing conservation and design of active hearing protection devices. Also offers expert witness services. Serves private industries as well as government agencies. Geographic Area Served: Worldwide.

★ 13722 ★ Lingane and Associates
735 Loma Ct.
Redwood City, CA 94062
Phone: (650)299-9390 **Fax:** (650)299-9391
Email: engineering@lingane.com
Website: http://www.lingane.com/eng
Fnded: 1992. **Activities:** Medical product design involving electronics, optics, disposables, and software. Expertise in point-of-care and battery-powered systems. Specializes in bringing complete engineering solutions to start-up organizations. Projects range from meeting short-term needs to full instrument development.

Reedley

★ 13723 ★ Forensic Addiction Medical Associates
1311 11th St.
Reedley, CA 93654
Free: 800-974-3578 **Fax:** (559)638-6703

Email: deutsch1998@msn.com
Website: http://www.forensicaddiction.medem.com

Activities: Serves as an expert witness specializing in the correlation of behavior with laboratory and clinical evidence of toxicity; characterological and personality disorders involving drugs and the law; and fetal alcohol syndrome.

Richmond

★ 13724 ★ The Center for Applied Local Research

5200 Huntington Ave., Ste. 200
Richmond, CA 94804
Phone: (510)558-7930 **Fax:** (510)558-7940
Email: admin@cal-research.org
Website: http://www.cal-research.org

Fnded: 1985. **Activities:** Designs, manages, and participates in short- and long-term evaluations and needs assessments throughout California. Also writes and oversees consultants' writing of federal, state, and local grant proposals and applications. Geographic Area Served: State of California.

★ 13725 ★ Richard A. Rubenstein, MD

3220 Blume Dr., Ste. 151
Richmond, CA 94806
Phone: (415)924-1340 **Free:** 800-426-9558
Fax: (415)924-5259
Email: rr@rrubenstein.com
Website: http://www.rrubenstein.com

Activities: Neurologist providing worker's compensation disability evaluations and personal and bodily injury evaluations.

Rodeo

★ 13726 ★ Spivey Chiropractic Clinic

667 Parker Ave.
Rodeo, CA 94572
Phone: (510)799-3112 **Fax:** (510)799-9013

Activities: Provides chiropractic, IDE, QME, services, chiropractic treatment, and permanent and stationary evaluation. Geographic Area Served: Northern California.

Sacramento

★ 13727 ★ Benchmark Administrative Services Co.

601 University Ave., Ste. 225
Sacramento, CA 95825
Phone: (916)920-2272 **Free:** 800-458-1261
Fax: (916)920-2515
Email: pcasey@benchmarkadmin.com
Website: http://www.benchmarkadmin.com

Activities: Independent healthcare professionals and related consultants. Provides professional, cost effective administrative support and case management services in all areas of medicolegal forensic, and legal consulting. Geographic Area Served: California, Nevada, Oregon, Washington and Hawaii.

★ 13728 ★ Fair Oaks Psychiatric Associates

2100 Northrup Ave., No. 700
Sacramento, CA 95825
Phone: (916)567-6622 **Fax:** (916)567-6620
Email: mmohit@aol.com

Activities: Acts as an expert medical witness specializing in neuropsychiatry and psychopharmacology for civil and criminal cases, including medical malpractice, personal injury, workers' compensation, and employee assistance.

★ 13729 ★ Health Management Systems Inc.

10831 Old Placerville Rd.
Sacramento, CA 95827
Phone: (916)414-5500 **Free:** 800-882-7777
Fax: (916)852-2669
Website: http://www.hmsy.com

Fnded: 1990. **Activities:** Offers expertise regarding medical billing.

Salinas

★ 13730 ★ Bloom, Reid and Associates

344 Salinas St.
Salinas, CA 93901
Phone: (408)759-9081 **Fax:** (408)759-8631
Email: bloomreid@msn.com

Fnded: 1987. **Activities:** Provides management consultation to acute, skilled/long term, home health, facilities and other healthcare and industrial organizations. Also offers expertise in system analysis, policy/procedures, quality assurance, risk management, disaster planning, hazardous materials, and educational services. Additional specialization extended to areas of in-house education for management, nursing personnel, and ancillary personnel. Industries served: healthcare and related industries including government agencies.

San Anselmo

★ 13731 ★ Ann Goforth & Associates

20 Brookmont Cir.
San Anselmo, CA 94960
Phone: (415)459-3303 **Fax:** (415)459-4441

Fnded: 1989. **Activities:** Independent/medical analysis of records for attorneys and insurance companies. Provides chronology, summary and evaluation of medical records. Geographic Area Served: United States.

★ 13732 ★ Martin Blinder, MD

130 Melville Ave.
San Anselmo, CA 94960
Phone: (415)453-8920

Fnded: 1967. **Activities:** Offers expert testimony in claims of emotional distress and psychic trauma, sexual harassment and molestation, wrongful death, post traumatic stress disorder, closed head injury, and psychogenic pain syndromes. Offers detection of malingering and eyewitness fallibility. Distinguishes authentic from false psychological claims. Provides disability assessments. Geographic Area Served: United States.

★ 13733 ★ New Hypnosis Institute

PO Box 633
San Anselmo, CA 94979
Phone: (415)454-2500 **Free:** 800-449-4422
Website: http://www.newpsycho.com/coaching

Activities: Provides specialized training and consulting services to hospitals and other medial institutions through anodyne awareness and process coaching se rvices. Geographic Area Served: USA & Canada.

San Carlos

★ 13734 ★ L & M Electronics Inc.

541 Taylor Way, No. 10
San Carlos, CA 94070-6254
Phone: (650)631-3758

Fnded: 1955. **Activities:** Electronics consulting firm serving the medical field in public and private sector as well as internationally.

San Clemente

★ 13735 ★ Biomedical Consulting Services

3551 Camino Mira Costa
San Clemente, CA 92672-3508
Phone: (949)640-1701

Activities: Performs medical device and equipment evaluation, as well as medical equipment testing and incident analysis. Offers technology risk management and expert witness services.

San Diego

★ 13736 ★ Bill Miller & Associates Inc.

12696 N Pacato Cir.
San Diego, CA 92128-2370
Phone: (858)487-2455 **Fax:** (858)487-2611
Email: la_jolla@usa.net
Website: http://www.bma-inc-online.com

Fnded: 1975. **Activities:** Recruits senior executives and management teams for healthcare industry, telecommunications, engineering and M.I.S., attorneys and finance, hotel and casino management. **Remarks:** Can provide world champion martial artists for any occasion. Men & women for spectacular demonstrations or instruction. One on one, or group training. Geographic Area Served: Nationwide.

★ 13737 ★ CAL/OSHA Consultation Services

7575 Metropolitan Dr., Ste. 204
San Diego, CA 92108
Phone: (619)767-2060
Website: http://www.dir.ca.gov/dosh

Fnded: 1973. **Activities:** The CAL/OSHA Consultation Service is a government funded, technical assistance program designed to help employers protect their workers from accidents and illness on the job through hazard identification and control, education and training, and development of effective on-the-job safety and health programs. Geographic Area Served: San Diego and Imperial County.

★ 13738 ★ Clark Smith, MD, Forensic Psychiatry

9750 Miramar Rd., Ste. 214
San Diego, CA 92126
Phone: (619)298-0518 **Fax:** (619)298-1613
Email: DoctrClark@aol.com

Fnded: 1982. **Activities:** Specializes in Forensic and Addiction Psychiatry in personal injury, malpractice, wrongful death, workers' compensation, employment, alcohol and drug abuse, PTSD, impulse control, disability, diminished actuality, insanity, drug and alcohol abuse, intoxication, and death penalty. Geographic Area Served: United States.

★ 13739 ★ Martin Associates

11835 Carmel Mountain Rd., No. 1304-362
San Diego, CA 92128
Phone: (858)385-0034

Fnded: 1993. **Activities:** Provides consulting services to healthcare providers, managed care organizations, regulatory agencies and consumer groups. Areas of specialization include quality management, marketing, operational audits, strategic business planning, process improvement and training in the following healthcare areas: behavioral health, complementary health/integrative medicine and laboratory medicine. Geographic Area Served: United States.

★ 13740 ★ Raymond Fox & Associates

5090 Shoreham Pl., Ste. 100
San Diego, CA 92122
Phone: (619)296-4595 **Fax:** (619)296-1838

Fnded: 1984. **Activities:** Architecture firm specializes in medical facilities. Geographic Area Served: United States, Europe, Mexico, Canada.

★ 13741 ★ Terry L. Schmidt Inc. - Hospital Terrorism Preparedness

7770 Regents Rd., Ste. 113-611
San Diego, CA 92122
Phone: (858)597-8888 **Fax:** (858)597-8890
Email: terry@terryschmidt.com
Website: http://www.terryschmidt.com

Fnded: 1974. **Activities:** Physician practice management; assists clients in maximizing their reimbursement for health and medical services under various third-party reimbursement systems and marketing programs. The firm is heavily involved in healthcare reimbursement issues pending before the Health Care Financing Administration including Medicare and Medicaid, emergency physician practice management, hospital contract negotiations, medical group organization and reorganization. Clients include individual physician practices; physician group practices; hospitals; medical centers; individual providers and groups.

★ 13742 ★ Wintriss Engineering Corp.
6344 Ferris Sq.
San Diego, CA 92121
Phone: (858)550-7300 **Free:** 800-550-7300
Fax: (858)550-0373
Email: weco@weco.com
Website: http://www.weco.com

Fnded: 1989. **Activities:** Develops and manufactures imaging and measurement systems, including SMART, High resolution, charge-coupled device cameras for manufacturing surface inspection. Also provides custom engineering services, specializing in microprocessor/DSP applications, imaging systems (including machine version), factory automation, and continuous web inspection. Geographic Area Served: Worldwide.

San Francisco

★ 13743 ★ Accreditation Compliance Group
1700 Montgomery St., Ste. 111
San Francisco, CA 94111
Phone: (415)835-9481 **Free:** 800-575-2185
Fax: (415)954-7199
Email: info@surveyready.com

Activities: Provides accreditation and management support to hospitals, ambulatory, health system networks, private offices, and other healthcare organizations and facilities with associates.

★ 13744 ★ Bruce S. Victor, MD
1819 Union St.
San Francisco, CA 94123
Phone: (415)346-7025 **Fax:** (415)346-0931

Activities: Specializes in mood and anxiety disorders and ethics violations. Offers expert testimony and consultation in malpractice litigation.

★ 13745 ★ Charles B. Warren
2033 Powell St.
San Francisco, CA 94133
Phone: (415)433-0959 **Fax:** (415)982-1441
Email: cwarren@batnet.com
Website: http://www.batnet.com/cwarren

Activities: Firm specializes in forensic appraisal, land economic/feasibility studies, economic geography, and assessment/assessment appeals. Unusual properties a specialty-damaged, contaminated, wetlands; also small craft harbors, hazardous seismic analyses, and other maritime related property. Geographic Area Served: Most consultation and valuation work in the Western United States Education and training in economic geography, appraisal and assessment available worldwide.

★ 13746 ★ The Children's Psychological Health Center
2024 Divisadero St.
San Francisco, CA 94115
Phone: (415)474-0955 **Fax:** (415)474-7514
Email: gil.kliman@cphc-sf.org
Website: http://www.cphc-sf.org

Fnded: 1992. **Activities:** Treats those with psychological trauma claimed from stressors including institutional negligence, vehicular and aviation accidents, wrongful death in the family, rape, molestation, fire, explosion, flood, earthquake, loss of parents, terrorism, kidnapping, disfiguring events, emotional damage from social work, medical malpractice or defective products. Provides evaluation and reports to referring professionals. Experienced in forensic consultation and testimony. Geographic Area Served: United States.

★ 13747 ★ Donald P. Cliggett, PhD
2340 Sutter St., Ste. 210
San Francisco, CA 94109-6710
Phone: (415)346-3761 **Fax:** (415)479-6539

Activities: Consultation services include use and limitations of psychological and neuropsychological testing and psychological testing/assessment. Provides expert testimony in cases such as mental competence, criminal responsibility, child custody, post-traumatic stress disorder, chronic pain, personal injury, psychological disability, job stress, sexual abuse or harassment, and fitness-for-duty/practice for firefighters, police, airline personnel and attorneys.

★ 13748 ★ E. David Manace, MD
California Pacific Medical Ctr.
2100 Webster St., Ste. 200
San Francisco, CA 94115
Phone: (415)923-3133 **Fax:** (415)931-5849
Email: edmanace@hotmail.com

Activities: Specializes in otolaryngology (ear, nose and throat, laryngeal and voice disorders). **Remarks:** Workers Compensation and expert witness specialist authority. Geographic Area Served: San Francisco Bay area.

★ 13749 ★ Fred Rosenthal
825 Van Ness Ave., Ste. 411
San Francisco, CA 94109
Phone: (415)346-4608 **Fax:** (415)885-5815

Activities: Provides expert witness testimony in legal cases and medical-legal evaluations. Areas include criminal behavior, sexual harassment, workers' compensation, divorce, custody, violence. Performs record review, psychiatric evaluations and psychological testing.

★ 13750 ★ The Health Services Group & Disability Management Group
333 Kearny St., Ste. 506
San Francisco, CA 94108
Phone: (415)391-5338 **Fax:** (415)391-1543

Activities: HSG is a company of health professionals including physical therapists, nurses, physicians, rehabilitation consultants, and allied health professionals who have joined together to offer multiple services including injury prevention, disability management and cost containment programs.

★ 13751 ★ Health Watch International
25 Hinckley Walk
San Francisco, CA 94115-2381
Phone: (415)956-5670 **Fax:** (415)956-8950
Email: rschmidt@sfsu.edu

Activities: Provides health assessments in the areas of morbidity, mortality, prediction, longevity, quality of life, and function. Consultation on estimated survival, effective function, and job-related productivity. Assists in claims preparation, discovery, depositions. Reviews medical records. Gives patient interviews, physical examinations, and comparative productivity estimates.

★ 13752 ★ Kenneth Associates Inc.
2014 Judah St.
San Francisco, CA 94122
Phone: (415)665-6500 **Fax:** (415)664-6400
Email: bobjimm@aol.com

Fnded: 1971. **Activities:** Consultants for hospitals.

★ 13753 ★ Michael S. Stulbarg MD
University of California Medical Ctr., Box 0111
Rm. M-1093
505 Parnassus Ave.
San Francisco, CA 94143-0111
Phone: (415)476-0631 **Fax:** (415)476-5172
Email: michae@itsa.ucsf.edu

Activities: Serves as an expert witness. Specializes in pneumonia, asthma, asbestosis, pleural effusion, shortness of breath, pulmonary embolism, inhalation injury, respiratory failure, malignancy, malpractice, unusual pulmonary problems, and critical care. Geographic Area Served: United States.

★ 13754 ★ Pan Pacific Urology
2100 Webster St., Ste. 309
San Francisco, CA 94115
Phone: (415)202-0250 **Fax:** (415)202-0255

Activities: Specializes in prostate diseases, prostate cancer, male infertility, impotence, sexual dysfunction, penile prostheses, vasectomy, vasectomy reversal, incontinence, urinary stones, and general urology.

★ 13755 ★ Practice & Liability Consultants
461 2nd St., Ste. 229
San Francisco, CA 94107
Phone: (415)764-4800 **Fax:** (415)764-4802
Email: plcsanfran@aol.com
Website: http://practiceconsultants.net

Fnded: 1985. **Activities:** Provides malpractice prevention and practice management services for the healthcare field including: hospitals, outpatient surgery centers, physicians, medical groups and dentists. Seminar programs for physicians, nurses, office staff, and dentists and dental staff. Many programs have CE credit approval. Serves private industries as well as government agencies. Geographic Area Served: United States.

★ 13756 ★ Richard J. Cohen, MD
3838 California St., Ste. 707
San Francisco, CA 94118
Phone: (415)668-0160 **Fax:** (415)752-4635
Email: rcohen3@aol.com

Fnded: 1968. **Activities:** A consultant in medical oncology and hematology. Special expertise in cancers of breast, colon, lung, lymphomas, and melanoma. Geographic Area Served: Bay area and Northern California.

★ 13757 ★ Richard Lieberman, MD
2112 Divisadero St.
San Francisco, CA 94115
Phone: (415)346-9333 **Fax:** (415)346-8170

Activities: Provides expert witness testimony and psychiatric-legal evaluations, in matters that include criminal behavior, sexual harassment, workers' compensation, divorce, custody, psychiatric malpractice, post-traumatic stress disorders, false memory syndromes, and violence.

★ 13758 ★ Richard M. Krieg, MD
University of California, San Francisco
505 Parnassus Ave., Rm. L-08
PO Box 0226
San Francisco, CA 94143-0226
Phone: (415)353-8900 **Fax:** (415)353-9883
Email: krieg@radonc17.ucsf.edu

Activities: Specializes in radiation oncology brachytherapy, lymphoma, breast cancer, rectal and anal cancer.

★ 13759 ★ Roger Freed, MD
3020 Fillmore St.
San Francisco, CA 94123
Phone: (415)567-8908 **Fax:** (415)435-0220
Email: freed@forensicpsychexpert.com
Website: http://ForensicPsychExpert.com

Activities: Superior and federal courts: civil and criminal; IME consultations; Bar Association and Attorney Office Seminars. Specializes in forensic psychiatry and pain management. Provides medical-legal evaluations in workers' compensation and personal injury cases, child abuse, criminal behavior, and post-traumatic stress. Offers social security and disability evaluations. Offers expert witness testimony in industrial psychiatry and medical malpractice cases. **Remarks:** ABPN Board Certified in Adult and Child Psychiatry; Added Qualifications in Forensic Psychiatry. Geographic Area Served: California.

★ 13760 ★ Ronald H. Roberts, PhD., ABPP
Northpoint Centre
2351 Powell St., Ste. 530
San Francisco, CA 94133-1443
Phone: (415)362-8202 **Fax:** (415)362-8242
Activities: Clinical psychologist/neuropsychologist specializing in personal injury, automobile accidents, head injuries, chronic pain, toxic exposure, discrimination, post-traumatic stress, disability, back injuries, and criminal law. **Remarks:** Board Certified in Forensic Psychology, American Board of Professional Psychology, and the American College of Forensic Psychology.

★ 13761 ★ San Francisco Sports Medicine
Davies Medical Ctr.
45 Castro, Ste. 117
San Francisco, CA 94102
Phone: (415)861-9966 **Fax:** (415)861-0174
Activities: Orthopedic surgeons and board certified medical-legal evaluators. Provide medical record reviews, expert witness testimony, and Spanish and German translation.

★ 13762 ★ Science, Toxicology & Technology and AIL Laboratories
1 Embarcadero Ctr., Ste. 500
PO Box 470116
San Francisco, CA 94147
Phone: (415)441-2163 **Free:** 800-869-4636
Fax: (415)441-3204
Email: toxinfo@aol.com
Website: http://www.toxinfo.com
Fnded: 1983. **Activities:** Provides consultant and expert services in medical toxicology (adverse reactions to chemicals or drugs), leaders in dietary supplement toxicology and clinical research for safety and efficiency and lab review/design, veterinary toxicology (food chain contamination), and pharmacology (efficacy and safety). Areas covered include industrial, occupational and environmental toxicology (including "sick building" syndrome); drug/chemical risk assessment and management; veterinary, dietary and environmental chemical exposures; drug regulation and promotion; hospital and pharmacy risk management; terato and carcinogenesis research; and medicolegal evaluation. Industries served: insurance, corporate (industrial and manufacturing), pharmaceutical, pharmacies, legal, public utilities, and state governments. Geographic Area Served: United States, Canada, Mexico, Europe, and Taiwan.

★ 13763 ★ Stuart J. Eisendrath, MD
University of California, San Francisco
School of Medicine
401 Parnassus
San Francisco, CA 94143-0984
Phone: (415)476-7868 **Fax:** (415)476-7657
Email: eisen@itsa.ucsf.edu
Activities: Provides psychiatric consultation. Specializes in psychosomatic medicine, psychiatric aspects of medical illness, factitious disorders, hysterical conversion, post-traumatic stress disorder, and Munchausen syndrome. Provides claim analysis, depositions, and trial testimony.

★ 13764 ★ Thomas L. Engel, MD
California Pacific Medical Ctr., California Campus
3838 California St., Ste. 505
San Francisco, CA 94118
Phone: (415)751-4914 **Fax:** (415)751-1414
Activities: Specializes in otolaryngology, head and neck surgery, and pediatric otolaryngology.

★ 13765 ★ UCSF Psoriasis & Skin Treatment Center
515 Spruce St.
San Francisco, CA 94118
Phone: (415)476-4701 **Fax:** (415)502-4126
Activities: Specializes in dermatology, psychodermatology, phototherapy, psoriasis treatment, transcultural psychiatry, and stress-induced skin conditions.

★ 13766 ★ William S. Breall, MD
St. Francis Memorial Hospital
1150 Bush St., Ste. 4A
San Francisco, CA 94109
Phone: (415)775-2277
Activities: Specializes in cardiology, cardiovascular disease, peripheral vascular disease, cerebrovascular disease, and hypertension.

★ 13767 ★ Work Return
333 Kearny St.
San Francisco, CA 94108
Phone: (415)391-8435 **Fax:** (415)391-1543
Activities: A certified vocational rehabilitation counselor with experience in vocational rehabilitation and economic wage loss. Testifies in all types of civil litigation. Provides vocational evaluation, testing labor market regarding job availability, salaries, trends, employment, wage loss and economic ramifications, job site analysis, medical management, job placement, career counseling, and out-placement services. Geographic Area Served: Will travel anywhere in the United States, related countries.

San Jose

★ 13768 ★ Anna Kuramoto
1617 Koch Ln.
San Jose, CA 95125
Phone: (408)723-9361 **Fax:** (408)723-0623
Email: Kuramoto@ix.netcom.com
Fnded: 1985. **Activities:** Health enhancement consultant offers services for corporate wellness, associations and groups, and individuals. Provides consultation in health risk assessment, stress management, back care and injury prevention, weight control and management, personalized exercise programs, workshops and presentations. Geographic Area Served: Northern California.

★ 13769 ★ Beverly Morgan, IBCLC, CLE
4653 Park Sutton Pl.
San Jose, CA 95136
Phone: (408)629-6455 **Fax:** (408)225-5816
Email: feedback@milkywaypress.com
Website: http://www.milkywaypress.com
Fnded: 1997. **Activities:** Provides breastfeeding help to mothers and infants, as well as education for health care providers. Geographic Area Served: San Francisco Bay Area.

★ 13770 ★ Circuit Solutions
6125 Prospect Rd.
San Jose, CA 95129-4739
Phone: (408)996-2166 **Fax:** (408)446-9471
Email: RHamstra@CirSol.com
Website: http://www.cirsol.com
Activities: Offers low noise, high speed circuit and instrument design, including analog IBM PC data acquisition and control: electronic temperature, motor, motion, light, etc. Also designs digital glue logic ECL, TTL, CMOS; x-ray CAT, CCD, and Reticon cameras, and photodetector instruments. Provides precision noise measurement service from 1 mHz to 30 kHz. Designs with in-house SPICE, OrCAD, C, and FORTRAN.

★ 13771 ★ Clinimetrics Inc.
5285 Hellyer Ave.
San Jose, CA 95138-1002
Phone: (408)452-8215 **Fax:** (408)452-0912
Email: info@clinimetrics.com
Website: http://www.clinimetrics.com
Fnded: 1988. **Activities:** Clinical research consultants specialize in the development and management of clinical research trials (phase II through IV) on drugs, biologics and medical devices. Consulting services are offered in the following specific areas: clinical research management, clinical trial monitoring, clinical trial design/development, data management, and regulatory compliance monitoring. Industries served: pharmaceutical, biotechnology, and medical device. Geographic Area Served: North and South America and Europe and Australia.

★ 13772 ★ Enviro Safetech Inc.
2455 Autumnvale Dr.
San Jose, CA 95148-4002
Phone: (408)941-9393 **Fax:** (408)941-9345
Email: jayjam@envirosafetech.com
Website: http://www.envirosafetech.com
Fnded: 1989. **Activities:** Environmental health and safety consultants. Safety equipment sales and rental. Industries served: bio tech, semiconductor, high tech, government. Geographic Area Served: Worldwide.

★ 13773 ★ Exactum
2787 Moorpark Ave.
San Jose, CA 95128
Phone: (408)358-0362 **Fax:** (408)351-9009
Email: info@exactum.com
Website: http://www.exactum.com
Activities: Experienced in machine design involving precision mechanisms, tooling, and fixtures. Designs production automation, including selection and integration of specialized equipment, automatic machinery, and material handling systems. Develops automated test equipment prototypes and pre-production development from concept through production, assembly, and test.

★ 13774 ★ International Nutrition Consultants Inc.
101 Quail Hollow Dr.
San Jose, CA 95128
Free: 800-249-4554
Website: http://www.inc-inc.com
Fnded: 1995. **Activities:** A nutritional education and analysis services company providing California state licensed home study nutrition courses. Offers in-depth health status reports and laboratory analyses for our graduates and individuals and on-line vitamin deficiency analysis software to health enthusiasts. Offers an Nutritional Counseling Course, which provides nutritional foundation, carries a diploma, and is licensed by the State of California. Analysis services complement educational programs. Available to graduates who become consultants are analysis services that include in-depth symptomology questionnaires as well as laboratory services, such as, tissue mineral analysis, blood testing and a DHEA saliva analysis. Geographic Area Served: California, Nevada.

★ 13775 ★ Paradigm Group Inc.
97 E Brokaw Ave., Ste. 220
San Jose, CA 95112
Phone: (408)451-4646 **Free:** 800-367-6745
Fax: 800-441-9006
Email: info@pgimedical.com
Website: http://www.pgimedical.com
Activities: Develops systems and services that expedite communications between patients, doctors, imaging centers, attorneys and insurance carriers. Established an integrated medical imaging network. Diagnostic imaging services include MRI, CT, Nuclear Medicine, Bone Analysis, Ultrasound, Mammogram, General Rad., R/F, Neurological exams (EMG, EEG), and numerous special procedures. Geographic Area Served: California, Nevada, Texas.

★ 13776 ★ Phyllis M. Connolly
Health Bldg. 416
San Jose, CA 95120
Phone: (408)924-3144 **Fax:** (408)924-3135
Email: connolly@sjsuvm1.sjsu.edu

Fnded: 1981. **Activities:** Offers counseling on individual, group, family, and organizational interpersonal relationships, conflict resolution, crisis intervention, assertiveness training, and collaboration partnership models. Also active in nursing research, TQI activities, and organizational development. Industries served: education, healthcare, and government. **Remarks:** Has won awards and recognitions, including a nomination for Outstanding Professor, College of Applied Arts and Sciences.

★ 13777 ★ Robert L. Weinmann, MD
2040 Forest Ave., Ste. 4
San Jose, CA 95128
Phone: (408)292-0802 **Fax:** (408)292-9574

Activities: Specializes in neurology, soft tissue, back and neck, head injury, alterations in consciousness (epilepsy, seizure disorders), cervical and lumbar radiculitis, post-concussion headache, wrongful death from brain injury, post-traumatic head syndrome, brain death, carpal tunnel syndrome, and chronic pain management. Serves as an expert witness. Provides QME- AME Evaluations.

San Luis Obispo

★ 13778 ★ Sequest Consulting Inc.
2267 Augusta St.
San Luis Obispo, CA 93401
Phone: (805)788-0200 **Fax:** (805)788-0300
Website: http://www.sequestconsulting.net

Fnded: 1983. **Activities:** Offers management and accreditation consultation services to U.S. hospitals and other healthcare facilities, including redesign of work flow and business processes. **Remarks:** Extensive experience on JCAHO accreditation including trading, consultation, and mock surveys. Geographic Area Served: Worldwide.

San Mateo

★ 13779 ★ Charles S. Syers, DDS MA
PO Box 1879
San Mateo, CA 94401-9991
Phone: (650)347-2614 **Fax:** (650)347-2680

Fnded: 1965. **Activities:** Specializes in temporomandibular joint injury, dento-facial nerve injury, dentofacial trauma, dental implants, dental pain, and orthognathic surgery. Also works with work compensation cases. Standard of care determination as it is applied to professional negligence. Geographic Area Served: San Francisco, United States, and Canada.

★ 13780 ★ Karlene Sugarman, M.A.
490 Mariners Island Blvd., No. 319
San Mateo, CA 94404
Phone: (650)341-1492 **Fax:** (650)375-0653
Email: karsug@pathlink.com

Fnded: 1993. **Activities:** Consultant specializes in sport psychology, team building, performance enhancement, and stress management.

★ 13781 ★ Marvin Firestone
730 Polhemus, Ste. 200
San Mateo, CA 94402
Phone: (650)212-4900 **Fax:** (650)212-4905
Email: mdjd@paratas.net

Activities: A brain injury assessment specialist. Serves as a consultant in cases involving head injuries, brain dysfunction, and mental distress. Also specializes in clinical psychiatry, psychopharmacology, forensic psychiatry, legal medicine, and neuropsychiatry.

San Rafael

★ 13782 ★ Joan Heidenreich and Associates
454 Las Gallinas, Ste. 249
San Rafael, CA 94903
Phone: (415)491-4234 **Fax:** (415)472-4722

Activities: A medical legal consultant nurse/attorney providing record review and analysis, standard of care and causation evaluation, preparation of treatment chronologies, research of medical issues, and defining of medical terminology and pathology. Geographic Area Served: Worldwide.

★ 13783 ★ Johnson Hershey Corp.
4340 Redwood Hwy., Ste. 16
San Rafael, CA 94903
Phone: (415)479-1099 **Fax:** (415)479-0601

Activities: Consultant provides business loss claim analysis. Analyzes lost income, business profits, business value, opportunity. Specialist in retailing, distribution, health care, food service. Discovery, deposition, trial preparation and courtroom graphic support services.

★ 13784 ★ Snyder Research Co.
509 Miller Creek Rd.
San Rafael, CA 94903-1319
Phone: (415)499-3463

Fnded: 1988. **Activities:** Snyder Research Company (SRC) assists clients needing technical and regulatory information concerning environmental, health, and safety issues. Typical subjects include: health effects of chemicals; remedial technologies; hazardous waste site locations; and regulations. SRC uses extensive government and commercial online database resources to perform fast and comprehensive research. Consulting services include formulation of research strategies, research using electronic and hard copy resources or personal contacts, preparation of reports and bibliographies, and retrieval of copies of documents. Also trains people to perform their own research using online databases and bulletin board systems (BBSs) and assists with setting up computer modem hardware and software. Industries served: commercial and industrial companies involved with hazardous materials or hazardous waste, or having other environmental health, and safety concerns; environmental consultants; attorneys; and government agencies. Geographic Area Served: United States.

★ 13785 ★ Stens Corp.
3020 Kerner Blvd., Ste. D
San Rafael, CA 94901
Email: sales@stens-biofeedback.com
Website: http://www.stens-biofeedback.com

Fnded: 1979. **Activities:** Biofeedback Sales and training plus a large inventory of books, tapes, videos, and medical supplies. Offers consulting and training on the use of biofeedback equipment. Industries served: healthcare. Geographic Area Served: Worldwide.

★ 13786 ★ Systems Applications International
101 Lucas Valley Rd., Ste. 230
San Rafael, CA 94903
Phone: (415)507-7164 **Fax:** (415)507-7272
Website: http://uamv.saintl.com

Fnded: 1968. **Activities:** Provides advanced, analytic compliance services to government agencies, electric utilities, and the petroleum and chemical industries in the areas of environmental and health sciences. Specializes in human exposure assessments, statistical analysis of air pollution, photochemical modeling of air pollution, analysis of control strategies, and meteorological modeling. Geographic Area Served: Worldwide.

San Ramon

★ 13787 ★ Visual Forensics
130 Ryan Industrial Ct., Ste. 105
San Ramon, CA 94583
Phone: (925)837-2083 **Free:** 800-426-6872
Fax: (925)837-0139
Email: inquiry@visualforensics.com
Website: http://www.visualforensics.com

Activities: Provides consultation in visibility analysis and human factors, particularly analysis for vision-related accidents (aviation, highway, vehicular, personal injury, pedestrian, industrial and sports). Provides research, statistical, experimental, and pictorial analysis of personal functional vision loss, including simulation studies, 2 and 3-d animation, day and night driving simulation, and vision functional analysis for accidents. Specializes in investigating visual disorders or eye disease including drugs, AIDS, and toxic elements.

Santa Ana

★ 13788 ★ Curt Deckert Associates Inc. - Technical & Management Consulting
18061 Darmel Pl.
Santa Ana, CA 92705-1923
Phone: (714)639-0746 **Free:** 800-394-0748
Fax: (714)639-0746
Email: curt@cdeckert.com
Website: http://www.cdeckert.com

Fnded: 1976. **Activities:** Provides technical management services for conceptual and prototype design in optical and related areas; research and development; and technological review. Industries served: medical, computer, aerospace, instrumentation, optical, manufacturing, and research. **Remarks:** Certified Management Consultant, Pro Savvy listing, IEEE listing and OSA listing. Geographic Area Served: United States and Canada.

★ 13789 ★ Lawrence Ball Consulting
1008 N Olive St.
Santa Ana, CA 92703
Phone: (714)542-9525 **Fax:** (714)836-0475

Activities: Provides expert witness consultation in the areas of: age, race, sex, & disability harassment; discrimination; discipline; termination; wrongful discharge; recruitment; selection; placement; layoff; policies & procedures, and management practices.

Santa Barbara

★ 13790 ★ Apollo Managed Care Consultants
860 Ladera Ln.
Santa Barbara, CA 93108
Phone: (805)969-2606 **Fax:** (805)969-3749
Email: mbischel@apollomanagedcare.com
Website: http://www.apollomanagedcare.com

Fnded: 1987. **Activities:** Specializes in healthcare strategic planning, utilization, and quality management for managed healthcare, hospitals, and physicians' practices. Serves public and private sector in the U.S. Publishes extensive lists of managed care, proactive management and disease state management manuals. Geographic Area Served: United States.

Santa Clara

★ 13791 ★ Healthstyles Consulting Group
1707 Civic Center Dr.
Santa Clara, CA 95050
Phone: (408)984-1892

Fnded: 1983. **Activities:** Human resources development consultants offering programs in stress management, health promotion, risk factor identification, peak performance training, and communications training to any business, organization, corporation, or government agencies.

Santa Cruz

★ 13792 ★ Alan Buchwald, MD Inc.
PO Box 2009
Santa Cruz, CA 95063
Phone: (831)761-0260 **Fax:** (831)761-0260
Email: albuchwald955@pol.net
Website: http://www.mydoctor.com/buchwald

Fnded: 1981. **Activities:** Medical consultant specializing in medical toxicology, poisoning, overdose, envenomation, industrial/occupational injuries, environmental, hazardous materials, agricultural, food toxicology, and indoor air problems. **Remarks:** CV available and fees, on request. Geographic Area Served: California primarily.

★ 13793 ★ Jest for the Health of It Services
PO Box 8484
Santa Cruz, CA 95061-8484
Phone: (831)475-9570 **Fax:** (831)475-9569
Email: pwooten@jesthealth.com
Website: http://www.jesthealth.com

Fnded: 1982. **Activities:** Develops and presents seminars, keynotes, and skill shops about the power of humor. Provides consulting services for development of humor rooms and comedy carts in hospitals. Conducts training for clowns to make visits in hospitals and nursing homes. Industries served: health professionals and businesses wishing to educate staff about healthy lifestyle choices. Geographic Area Served: United States, Canada, England, and Australia.

★ 13794 ★ Phillips & Fenwick
343 Soquel Ave., Ste. 273
Santa Cruz, CA 95062-2305
Phone: (831)457-5640 **Fax:** (831)457-5644
Website: http://www.pandf.com

Fnded: 1988. **Activities:** Offers medical services, specializing in women's healthcare. Industries served: hospitals in United States and Canada.

Santa Maria

★ 13795 ★ Edward A. Smith, MD Inc.
426 E Barcellus, Ste. 202
Santa Maria, CA 93454
Phone: (805)922-8346 **Free:** 800-638-7674
Fax: (805)925-5151

Fnded: 1975. **Activities:** A neurologic surgeon specializing in acute and chronic head injury evaluation and treatment; brain injury; post-traumatic pain syndromes; and spinal injuries. Gives medical record reviews, written reports, and expert testimony. Provides impartial analysis for both plaintiff and defense. Geographic Area Served: United States.

Santa Monica

★ 13796 ★ Irwin Intl.
853 - 18th St., Ste. 6
Santa Monica, CA 90403
Phone: (310)828-7328 **Fax:** (310)828-9781

Activities: Experienced in outplacement, wrongful termination, age/gender discrimination, sexual harassment, interviewing and performance assessment, layoff, selection, placement, recruitment, discipline, and plaintiff or defense testimony.

★ 13797 ★ M.L. McManus & Associates
1148 4th St., Ste. 202
Santa Monica, CA 90401
Phone: (310)451-3118 **Fax:** (310)393-7988

Fnded: 1958. **Activities:** Conducts psychological appraisals and developmental planning for key managers and executives. Work includes critical incident stress debriefing, workman's compensation evaluations (psychological), and return to work evaluations.

★ 13798 ★ Thomas Mintz, M.D.
1500 Montana Ave., Ste. 201
Santa Monica, CA 90403
Phone: (310)394-3010 **Fax:** (310)393-4939

Activities: Psychiatrist and psychoanalyst specializing in testimony and evaluation on all medical-psychiatric issues, including diagnosis, treatment, supervision, standards of care, medical malpractice, stress disorders, custody issues, boundary and ethical violations, competency, pre-trial case evaluation and analysis, sexual exploitation and harassment, wrongful death, wrongful termination, employment discrimination, witness and expert preparation, and jury-selection. **Remarks:** Also a lawyer. Geographic Area Served: California.

Simi Valley

★ 13799 ★ Jeff Bray Associates Inc.
PO Box 1570
Simi Valley, CA 93062
Free: 800-367-1521

Fnded: 1981. **Activities:** Provides sales and marketing services for the medical device industry.

Sonoma

★ 13800 ★ William A. Markey
866 Princeton Dr.
Sonoma, CA 95476
Phone: (707)996-2212 **Fax:** (707)939-8960

Fnded: 1984. **Activities:** Health care consultant offering advice on hospital management improvement programs, middle management involvement in strategic planning, goal setting, professional practice enhancement, implementation, and IPA, PPO, and HMO networking. Geographic Area Served: Primarily northern California.

South San Francisco

★ 13801 ★ Jo Anne Powell
228 Pinehurst Way
South San Francisco, CA 94080
Phone: (650)875-1721

Fnded: 1977. **Activities:** Independent nursing administration consultant in staff development and executive coaching primarily within the healthcare delivery system.

Stockton

★ 13802 ★ International Consulting Associates Inc.
1020 N Commerce
Stockton, CA 95202
Phone: (209)460-0622 **Fax:** (209)938-0416
Email: goss09@aol.com
Website: http://www.carlosabonilla.com

Fnded: 1988. **Activities:** Offers human resources development and management consulting in three principal areas: (1) education: dropout prevention, illiteracy, and Hispanic workers; (2) health-related issues: stress reduction in the workforce, cardiovascular medicine and others; and (3) workforce-related issues: training and education of underskilled workers, etc. Industries served: all except the military or defense agencies in the U.S. and Puerto Rico; and Korea, Japan, Europe, and South and Central America; child development; early childhood education; behavioral psychology. Geographic Area Served: Worldwide.

Sunset Beach

★ 13803 ★ A & A Medical Case Review
PO Box 1555
Sunset Beach, CA 90742
Phone: (310)592-5650

Activities: Provides medical-legal reviews in medical/nursing malpractice, personal injury, products liability, and good/bad faith insurance cases. To save time and money, initial reviews are done by an experienced registered nurse, followed by MD consultation. Offers screening, analysis, summaries, chronologies and indexing of medical reviews.

Tarzana

★ 13804 ★ Sound Feelings Publishing
18375 Ventura Blvd., Ste. 8000
Tarzana, CA 91356-4218
Phone: (818)757-0600
Email: info@soundfeelings.com
Website: http://www.soundfeelings.com

Fnded: 1984. **Activities:** Firm's approach is to incorporate music and music awareness as a tool to help gain control over worksite stress. This may be used alone or as a complement to other stress management programs. Firm's "entrainment" music tapes provide a unique non-hypnotic/non-subliminal tool as a self-study technique. Provides consulting, lectures, seminars, and tape programs for corporations, hospitals, insurance companies, as well as government agencies. Geographic Area Served: United States.

Temecula

★ 13805 ★ World Botanical Associates
PO Box 880
Temecula, CA 92593-0880
Phone: (750)742-0345 **Free:** 800-772-7216
Fax: (661)589-5369
Email: richspjut@aol.com
Website: http://www.worldbotanical.com

Fnded: 1983. **Activities:** Consulting biological scientists who: provide botanical/chemical guidance for discovery of potential compounds for medicinal therapies; provide plant samples of indigenous plants for medicinal research; provide resources to conduct floristic inventories; and conduct research on taxonomy of various terrestrial plants. Industries served: government agencies, universities, and pharmaceutical companies. Geographic Area Served: North America, Latin America, Asia, and Africa.

Torrance

★ 13806 ★ Children's Eye Care Medical Group
3565 Torrance Blvd., Ste. A
Torrance, CA 90501
Phone: (310)543-1310 **Fax:** (310)316-8148
Email: rls@bigfoot.com

Activities: Specializes in pediatric ophthalmology and strabismus; children's eye surgery and diseases; adult disorders of eye muscles, double vision and cosmetic misalignments of the eye; retinopathy of prematurity; visual difficulties in children; surgical and medical problems of children's and infant's eyes; surgical and medical complications in children and adult strabismus surgery; and ocular birth defects.

★ 13807 ★ Keenan & Associates
2355 Crenshaw Blvd., Ste. 200
Torrance, CA 90501-3325
Phone: (310)212-3344 **Free:** 800-654-8102
Fax: (310)328-6793
Email: info@keenanassoc.com
Website: http://www.keenanassoc.com

Fnded: 1972. **Activities:** Firm is active in welfare plan consulting. Services include plan design, insurer/broker selection consulting, evaluation of other service providers, healthcare and other types of claims administration, and risk management consulting.

★ 13808 ★ Robert J. Marshall & Associates Inc.
1010 Crenshaw Blvd., Ste. 170
Torrance, CA 90501-2055
Phone: (310)787-8751 **Fax:** (310)320-8930

Fnded: 1975. **Activities:** Provides nutrition information and consulting.

★ 13809 ★ **Yeast Consulting Services**
PO Box 11157
Torrance, CA 90510-1157
Phone: (310)375-1073 **Fax:** (310)791-1363
Email: drcrandall@aol.com
Website: http://www.yeastconsulting.com
Fnded: 1988. **Activities:** Provides confidential telephone counseling of Candida patients, an information packet about yeast infections, public seminars, scientific lectures with slide presentations, review of medical records, referrals for testing and healthcare, offers expert witness testimony, and research and development of antifungals and diagnostics. Clients served: patients, physicians, attorneys, health insurance companies, pharmaceutical firms, diagnostic companies, nonprofit health organizations, health book publishers, and manufacturers. Geographic Area Served: United States and English-speaking clients worldwide.

Tustin

★ 13810 ★ **Performance Management Services Inc.**
13522 Newport Ave., Ste. 200
Tustin, CA 92780-3707
Phone: (714)731-3414 **Fax:** (714)731-4620
Email: office@pmsi-pbds.com
Website: http://www.pmsi-pbds.com

Ventura

★ 13811 ★ **Peter G. Gaal, MD**
145 N Brent St., Ste. 102
Ventura, CA 93003
Phone: (805)643-2375 **Fax:** (805)643-3511
Activities: Specializes in thoracic and cardiovascular surgery. Reviews medical-legal matters for lawsuits.

Walnut Creek

★ 13812 ★ **Thomas H. Milby, M.D.**
1399 Yganacio Valley Rd., Ste. 25
Walnut Creek, CA 94598
Phone: (510)284-4944 **Fax:** (510)256-4617
Email: tmilby@aol.com
Website: http://www.lawinfo.com/biz/milby/index.html
Activities: A physician-toxicologist and medical-legal consultant specializing in the effects of toxic chemical exposures, spills, air and water pollution, hazardous dumps, molds and workplace exposures. Geographic Area Served: Worldwide.

Westlake Village

★ 13813 ★ **Roundtable of Toxicology Consultants**
31308 Via Colinas, Ste. 107
Westlake Village, CA 91362
Phone: (818)706-2410 **Fax:** (818)706-2413
Website: http://lawinfo.com/biz/toxicology/index.html
Fnded: 1980. **Activities:** Provides general toxicology consulting by experienced doctoral-level scientists. Specialty areas include: legal support in product liability cases, new drug applications, FDA approvals, OSHA and EPA standards, pesticides, food additives, workplace safety, animal testing for regulatory approval, expert testimony, EPA compliance, and many related areas. Offers expert reviews in toxicology, medical, chemical, and other scientific databases. Industries served: attorneys, pharmaceutical, chemical, government, general manufacturing, as well as government agencies. **Remarks:** Free list of each consultant's expertise available. Contact them directly: no fee. Geographic Area Served: Worldwide.

★ 13814 ★ **Toxicology Consultants Roundtable**
31308 Via Colinas, Ste. 107
Westlake Village, CA 91362
Phone: (818)706-2410 **Fax:** (818)706-2413
Email: jabudny@earthlink.net
Website: http://lawinfo.com/biz/toxicology/index.html
Activities: Toxicology consultants.

Woodland Hills

★ 13815 ★ **Alpha Consulting Associates**
4741 Larkwood Ave.
Woodland Hills, CA 91364-3737
Phone: (818)224-4224 **Free:** 800-898-1354
Fax: (818)224-4343
Email: fm@alphaconsulting.net
Website: http://www.alphaconsulting.net
Fnded: 1985. **Activities:** Counsels on healthcare, specializing in strategic and market planning, product development business planning and development, feasibility studies, and new venture start-ups. Expertise with providers, payers, manufacturers, distributors and vendors. Industries served: healthcare and government in the U.S. and Canada. Geographic Area Served: Worldwide.

★ 13816 ★ **Lees-Haley Corp.**
21331 Costanso St.
Woodland Hills, CA 91364
Phone: (818)887-2874 **Fax:** (818)887-9034
Fnded: 1988. **Activities:** Specialists in the evaluation of mass injury claims and fear of future illness claims, environmental and toxic claims, psychological and neuropsychological injury claims, sexual harassment claims, and numerous other types of personal injury claims. Provides training and consulting to risk managers, claims managers, and attorneys. Offers in-house lectures for self-insured companies, insurers and reinsurers, and literature reviews in complex litigation. Industries served: chemical, oil, insurance, medical device manufacturers - almost any industry involved in litigation. Geographic Area Served: United States.

★ 13817 ★ **Ray Stammire, D.C.**
6325 Topanga Canyon Blvd., Ste. 111
Woodland Hills, CA 91367
Phone: (818)716-6112 **Fax:** (818)716-1810
Activities: Provides workers' compensation and private investigation. Evaluation and treatment. Offers case reviews and expert testimony. **Remarks:** State appointed Q.M.E.; Certified W.C.D.E./I.D.E.; Fellow A.F.I.C.C.

Yorba Linda

★ 13818 ★ **SpecialTeam Medical Services Inc.**
22445 E La Palma Ave., Ste. F
Yorba Linda, CA 92887
Phone: (714)694-0348 **Fax:** (714)694-0171
Email: spetm@aol.com
Website: http://www.specialteam.com
Fnded: 1996. **Activities:** Provides contract assembly, packaging, sterilization, and sterile package design for medical manufacturers. The company offers design, assembly, and packaging services for syringes and anesthesiology and respiratory single-use sterile disposable products. Technical knowledge of medical devices and expertise focusing on cleanroom processing and manufacturing-systems development related to sterile medical disposable products. Geographic Area Served: United States and Europe.

Yucaipa

★ 13819 ★ **Medically Speaking**
13507 Big Sky Ct.
Yucaipa, CA 92399
Free: 800-762-9778 **Fax:** (909)446-8870
Email: medspkg@aol.com
Website: http://www.medicallyspeaking.com
Fnded: 1988. **Activities:** Organizes, reviews and analyzes medical records. Provides chronological summaries, expert referral, and medical literature research. Identifies areas for impeachment. Identifies issues, discrepancies, beneficial and detrimental aspects, compliance, and pre-existing conditions. Identifies liability and damages, answers questions for deposition and trial. Provides medical bill audits. Demonstrative exhibits. Defines medical terms and procedures. Geographic Area Served: United States and Canada.

Colorado

Arvada

★ 13820 ★ **Diamond Decisions Inc.**
8972 W 81st Ln.
Arvada, CO 80005
Phone: (303)423-5570 **Fax:** (303)423-8367
Fnded: 1995. **Activities:** Consultants for the health care industry specializing in improving business operations with technology, including streamlining business operations for greater profit and improved efficiencies, purchasing a new information system, introducing a new product, or needing project management.

Aurora

★ 13821 ★ **Colorado Orthopedic Consultants P.C.**
1411 S Potomac St., Ste. 400
Aurora, CO 80012-4540
Phone: (303)695-6060 **Fax:** (303)369-7776
Activities: A group of accredited orthopedic surgeons in private practice. Scope of practice ranges throughout the spectrum of surgical and non-surgical care for disorders affecting the musculoskeletal system. Interests range from sports injuries, and reconstructive surgery of the shoulder, hip, knee, ankle, and foot to micro- vascular and reconstrucive nerve surgery of the hand. Geographic Area Served: Colorado.

Boulder

★ 13822 ★ **Environmental Acoustical Research Inc.**
PO Box 18888
Boulder, CO 80308
Phone: (303)447-2619 **Free:** 800-525-2690
Fax: (303)447-2637
Email: garry@earinc.com
Website: http://www.earinc.com
Fnded: 1971. **Activities:** Offers counsel on instrumentation for sound and hearing evaluation. Sales and service for specialized hearing systems. Conducts marketing for hearing protection systems. Industries served: industrial, medical, recreational, educational, governmental, recreational firearms industry, audiology, otology, industrial, and hearing conservation. Geographic Area Served: Worldwide.

★ 13823 ★ **Franklin D. Aldrich**
1094 Quince Ave.
Boulder, CO 80304
Phone: (303)443-2316 **Fax:** (303)938-9420
Fnded: 1977. **Activities:** Comprehensive consulting practice of environmental/clinical toxicology includes field investigations, hazard reviews, product liability and medicolegal litigation support. Expertise includes indoor air quality, office technologies, agricultural chemicals, industrial chemical processes, and microelectronics. Industries served: industries, healthcare institutions, and attorneys. Geographic Area Served: Worldwide.

★ 13824 ★ **Michele L. Gerard, PhD**
1750-1 30th St., Ste. 224
Boulder, CO 80301
Phone: (303)939-9650 **Fax:** (303)939-9677
Email: braindr2@aol.com
Fnded: 1990. **Activities:** Specializes in brain injury medical cases. Offers expert witness testimony in the areas of neuropsychology; neurology, and neurosurgery for personal injury cases; ADA cases; and return to work evaluation. Geographic Area Served: Boulder/ Denver.

★ 13825 ★ Preventive Measures Inc.
PO Box 315
Boulder, CO 80306
Phone: (303)440-9095 **Fax:** (303)440-9095
Email: prevmeas@aol.com

Fnded: 1984. **Activities:** Stress assessment and stress-management consultants offer complete materials and assistance for implementing a stress-management program. Computerized stress assessment generates individual narrative reports. Stress-management book referenced in report teaches coping skills. Participant workbooks and audiotapes available. Free statistical summaries and group/corporate reports generated from data users provided. Workshop outlines and training assistance available. Industries served include: education, government as an industry, mental healthcare, insurance, and nonprofits.

★ 13826 ★ Reed Group Ltd.
4041 Hanover Ave., 2nd Fl.
Boulder, CO 80305-5942
Phone: (303)247-1860 **Free:** 800-347-7443
Fax: (303)247-1863
Website: http://www.rgl.net

Fnded: 1981. **Activities:** Offers medical disability case management and occupational health and medical services.

Buena Vista

★ 13827 ★ SCAN - Sports, Cardiovascular and Wellness Nutritionists
PO Box 4995
Buena Vista, CO 81211
Phone: (719)395-9271 **Fax:** (719)395-5615
Email: scan@nutrifit.org
Website: http://www.nutrifit.org

Fnded: 1982. **Activities:** Nutrition consultants offering the following services: nutrition education for public via clinics, hospitals, health clubs, physicians' offices; clinical nutrition counseling via clinics, hospitals, cardiac rehab and eating disorders programs; and preventive and wellness program design and implementation. **Remarks:** Leaders in promoting the role of nutrition in physical performance, cardiovascular health, wellness, and disordered eating. Geographic Area Served: United States.

Colorado Springs

★ 13828 ★ Northview Health Associates
5526 N Academy Blvd., Ste. 106
Colorado Springs, CO 80918
Phone: (719)594-9997 **Fax:** (719)594-4152

Fnded: 1982. **Activities:** Rehabilitation and disability management specialists offering the following services: income impairment, vocational rehabilitation evaluation/services, labor market analysis, transferrable skill analysis, and displaced homemaker evaluation. Conducts aptitude, interest, and abilities testing. Additional services are; adoption studies, family counseling, marriage counseling, and custody evaluations. Serves private industries as well as government agencies. Geographic Area Served: Southern Colorado.

Conifer

★ 13829 ★ J & JG Associates
10742 Timothys Rd.
Conifer, CO 80433
Phone: (303)838-7533
Email: jgreyson@mstg.net

Fnded: 1982. **Activities:** Provides chemical and biotechnology consultation specializing in research and development program development and product transfer to manufacturing and sales. Specific expertise in analytical instrumentation and production equipment. Also provides consultation on analytical instruments and procedures for environmental monitoring and consultation on analytical methods for home-use clinical diagnostics. Serves private industries as well as government agencies. Geographic Area Served: United States.

Denver

★ 13830 ★ Alexander Mead
900 Lincoln St., No. 781
Denver, CO 80203-2712
Phone: (303)313-2866
Email: ammd@well.com
Website: http://www.well.com/user/vamead/

Activities: A medical review consultant specializing in medical-legal case review and malpractice screening. Provides attorneys, insurers, and institutions with prompt, cost-effective case review – potential medical malpractice, quality and utilization concerns, medical-legal issues – across a broad spectrum of adult medicine, surgery, and injury.

★ 13831 ★ Association of Operating Room Nurses Inc.
2170 S Parker Rd., Ste. 300
Denver, CO 80231-5711
Phone: (303)755-6300 **Fax:** (303)755-5494
Website: http://www.aorn.org

Fnded: 1954. **Activities:** AORN consultation services cover organizational efficiency of the surgical suite (operating room) in the areas of space and facility utilization, management, technical practices, staffing, scheduling, and interpersonal relationships of the surgical team members. Industries served: healthcare and government agencies.

★ 13832 ★ Bardwell Consulting Ltd.
2245 S Stuart St.
Denver, CO 80219
Phone: (303)934-3851 **Fax:** (303)934-3881

Activities: Provides statistical consulting for business, law and government. Specializing in sampling, probability models, & customized statistical programming. Experienced in litigation support, including class action and discrimination cases, and criminal probability modeling.

★ 13833 ★ HealthStream Education Design
2170 S Parker Rd., Ste. 140
Denver, CO 80231
Phone: (303)745-5996 **Free:** 800-832-5115
Fax: (303)745-5856
Website: http://www.healthstream.com

Fnded: 1980. **Activities:** Offers education and consultation to hospitals and surgery centers and professional associations. Firm works with the Association of Perioperative Registered Nurses. Works with medical industry in the area of education and marketing of products. Accredited as a sponsor of CME, pharmacy, podiatry and nursing education. Geographic Area Served: Worldwide.

★ 13834 ★ Rocky Mountain Health Care Corp.
700 Broadway
Denver, CO 80273
Phone: (303)831-2131 **Fax:** (303)830-0887
Website: http://www.bcbsco.com

Fnded: 1987. **Activities:** Offers healthcare and benefits services, business administration, and education to businesses statewide.

★ 13835 ★ Tim Gard
4150 Ireland St.
Denver, CO 80249-8098
Phone: (303)932-9835 **Free:** 800-865-9939
Fax: (303)932-0990
Website: http://www.timgard.com

Fnded: 1985. **Activities:** Develops humor plans for work for good business and to protect supervisors and managers.

Englewood

★ 13836 ★ Rocky Mountain Professional Consultants Inc.
770 W Hampden Ave., Ste. 325
Englewood, CO 80110
Email: thompsongw@aol.com

Fnded: 1969. **Activities:** Consulting services for the medical, dental, healthcare practitioner include: management, consultations for office facilities and layout, new practice development, marketing plan, physician recruitment, practice valuations, purchase and sale of medical practices and practice network. Geographic Area Served: Continental United States.

Evergreen

★ 13837 ★ Reyer & Associates
27336 Mountain Park Rd.
Evergreen, CO 80439
Phone: (303)674-7490 **Fax:** (303)674-7490

Fnded: 1986. **Activities:** Offers consultation to hospitals and medical care groups in developing new program strategies and alternative delivery systems for government agencies. Geographic Area Served: Continental United States.

Fort Collins

★ 13838 ★ Baretich Engineering Inc.
PO Box 469
Fort Collins, CO 80522-0469
Phone: (970)493-8239 **Free:** 877-795-2738
Fax: (970)493-8269
Website: http://www.baretich.com

Activities: Provides a wide range of consulting services related to the environment of care. Also offers incident/investigation services where a medical device or building system may have contributed to an adverse event and equipment planning primarily for medical equipment.

★ 13839 ★ Metcalf & Associates
7965 Bayside Dr.
Fort Collins, CO 80528
Phone: (970)226-0610 **Free:** 800-LIT-ENUP
Email: metco@verinet.com
Website: http://www.litenup.org

Fnded: 1980. **Activities:** Offers programs to corporate, healthcare, government and education industry clients focusing on humor, risk, and change adaptation; creativity; communication; and health and humor. Geographic Area Served: Worldwide.

★ 13840 ★ Rocky Mountain Instrumental Laboratories Inc.
108 Corondo Ct.
Fort Collins, CO 80525
Phone: (970)266-8108 **Fax:** (303)530-1169
Email: rklantz@rockylab.com
Website: http://www.rockylab.com

Fnded: 1978. **Activities:** Provides the following consulting services: pharmacologic and pharmacokinetic drug and toxin studies, forensic analysis in toxicology and serology, and product and method development in analytical chemistry and toxicology. Also provides expert witness testimony in state and federal courts. Serves pharmaceutical, forensic, chemical, as well as government agencies. Geographic Area Served: United States, Canada, and Europe.

Golden

★ 13841 ★ Dialysis Management Inc.
23731 Willowherb Ln.
Golden, CO 80401-9180
Phone: (303)526-0168 **Free:** 800-526-0168
Fax: (303)526-2585
Email: lmday@att.net

Fnded: 1979. **Activities:** Provides medical practice management services to physicians and hospitals in the United States.

Littleton

★ 13842 ★ Lerch, Bates and Associates Inc.
8089 S Lincoln Ave., Ste. 205
Littleton, CO 80122
Phone: (303)795-7956 **Fax:** (303)797-7109
Email: busdev@lerchbates.com
Website: http://lerchbates.com

Fnded: 1947. **Activities:** Independent elevator, escalator, materials handling and materials management consulting organization providing client-focused services relative to new installations, modernizations and ongoing maintenance programs. New and modernization related services consit fo conceptual/schematic design, CAD drawings, bid documents, bidding assistance, installation administration and project close-out. Maintenance related services consist of auditing the existing equipment maintenance and establishing a proactive program with the maintenance provider to correct observed deficiencies. Preventive maintenance monitoring is also available. We provide integrity, quality, value and client satisfaction. Geographic Area Served: Worldwide.

★ 13843 ★ SLBA
PO Box 260797
Littleton, CO 80163-0797
Phone: (303)790-1884 **Fax:** (303)790-1885
Email: beckley@slba.com
Website: http://www.aescon.com/slba

Activities: Specializes in student health care delivery and finance. Provides program reviews, strategic planning, and student health insurance and financing consultation. Works exclusively with institutions of higher education.

Steamboat Springs

★ 13844 ★ Gregory F. O'Brien
33875 County Rd. 38
Steamboat Springs, CO 80487
Phone: (970)879-6439
Email: gfobrien@pol.net

Activities: Over fifteen years experience as a surveyor for the JCAHO and is a surveyor for the American College of Surgeons Commission on Cancer. Has extensive experience providing educational and consultative services to rural and urban Hospitals, Networks, single-specialty and multi-specialty groups with special focus on medical staff leadership development.

Telluride

★ 13845 ★ Creative Team Consulting
226 W Colorado Ave.
PO Box 3258
Telluride, CO 81435
Phone: (970)728-5234 **Fax:** (970)728-5234

Fnded: 1975. **Activities:** Organizational effectiveness consulting firm offers the following services: needs assessments; systems change process: centralization, decentralization; systems reorganizations (board of trustees, administrative); action plans; performance appraisal systems installation; workshops, communication skills training; leadership and management styles; stress management; life planning; evaluation, vocational, educational; personnel screening and selection; team building; handling negative feedback; and burnout. Industries served: major hospitals, small businesses, medical corporations, communities, schools, government, and industry. States and international. Geographic Area Served: Worldwide.

Connecticut

Bethel

★ 13846 ★ Holistic Chiropractic, Dr. Keith Erwin
24 Grassy Plain St.
Bethel, CT 06801
Phone: (203)798-7930

Fnded: 1985. **Activities:** Teaches professionals in chiropractic, medicine, dentistry and osteopathy how to identify the basic cause of spinal pain - the intervertebral cartilage (disc) lesion. Also involved in advertising, marketing, and sports medicine. Industries served: health insurance firms. Geographic Area Served: Worldwide.

Bridgewater

★ 13847 ★ Parker Medical Inc.
137 New Milford Rd. E
Bridgewater, CT 06752
Phone: (203)350-4304 **Fax:** (203)350-3432

Fnded: 1984. **Activities:** Consultants on radiologic procedures and equipment; x-ray equipment components such as high voltage cables, x-ray tube cooling units, x-ray tube shields, and x-ray tubes. Expertise in equipment design and manufacture.

Cheshire

★ 13848 ★ Pivirotto Consulting
949 Waterbury Rd.
PO Box 787
Cheshire, CT 06410-1936
Phone: (203)272-9204 **Fax:** (203)271-2070
Email: h.pivirotto@alon.com

Fnded: 1986. **Activities:** Offers healthcare and financial management services to businesses in Connecticut.

Clinton

★ 13849 ★ Richard Clare
27 Janes Ln.
Clinton, CT 06413
Phone: (860)664-3877 **Fax:** (860)349-9506
Email: rclare@snet.net

Fnded: 1981. **Activities:** Marketing researcher specializing in medical devices. Offers the following services: gathering information on market size and competition; evaluating product selling features for United States and foreign markets; investigating United States market for overseas clients; developing criteria for new products and for new domestic and international markets; finding new products and new product ideas; identifying relevant standards and government regulations; and arranging international sales and licensing. Industries served: medical devices and related high technology fields. Geographic Area Served: Worldwide.

Danbury

★ 13850 ★ Steffen, Steffen and Associates Inc.
107 Newtown Rd.
Danbury, CT 06810
Phone: (203)792-1000 **Fax:** (203)748-2290
Email: rjsteffen@aol.com
Website: http://www.ssainternational.com

Fnded: 1975. **Activities:** Dedicated to the purpose of helping companies increase their customer loyalty, revenue and profit while assisting the individual contributors in that company to increase their own job satisfaction. This is accomplished by developing and implementing programs in the area of creating the very satisfied customer, "Optimization Mission-Critical Relationships, Successful Partnering and Time Mastery". Geographic Area Served: Worldwide.

Essex

★ 13851 ★ Dole Associates
20 Hemlock Dr.
PO Box 409
Essex, CT 06426
Phone: (860)767-0773 **Fax:** (860)767-7832

Fnded: 1967. **Activities:** Offers consulting services in marketing, industrial design, product design, and production and manufacturing engineering. Projects have included consumer medical/scientific and consumer products. Industries served: industrial, consumer, and high-tech. Geographic Area Served: Worldwide.

Fairfield

★ 13852 ★ Occupational Health Registry & Consulting Service Inc.
1734 Stratfield Rd.
Fairfield, CT 06432
Phone: (203)372-3768 **Fax:** (203)371-7240

Fnded: 1980. **Activities:** Offers consultation regarding medical services and agencies.

Glastonbury

★ 13853 ★ Healthcare Forecasting Inc.
110 National Dr.
Glastonbury, CT 06033
Phone: (860)659-4077

Fnded: 1984. **Activities:** Pharmaceutical industry consultants. Industries served: pharmaceuticals, medical supply, and biotechnology. Geographic Area Served: Worldwide.

★ 13854 ★ The Pharmacy Group L.L.C.
12 E Lake Shore Trl.
PO Box 129
Glastonbury, CT 06033
Phone: (860)633-0062 **Fax:** (860)659-1598
Email: perrycohen@compuserve.com

Fnded: 1997. **Activities:** A healthcare consulting company representing a consortium of managed care professionals with diverse expertise in all facets of managed pharmacy programs. This firm provides creative solutions to managed care companies and healthcare providers managing the cost of the pharmacy benefit. Geographic Area Served: Worldwide.

★ 13855 ★ Vianna Zimbel Consulting
114 Goodrich Rd.
Glastonbury, CT 06033
Phone: (860)657-9530 **Fax:** (860)659-5863
Email: viannaz@vzimbel.com
Website: http://www.vzimbel.com

Activities: Provides assessment compliance levels with JCAHO standards and requirements. Also provides expert review of quality/risk issues. Methods for improvement are offered. Performs warehouse and facility inspection, equipment maintenance records review, delivery vehicle inspections, and education and preparation of staff for the survey questions.

Greenwich

★ 13856 ★ Marjorie Roberts
101 River W
Greenwich, CT 06831
Phone: (203)531-7795 **Fax:** (914)594-4541

Fnded: 1982. **Activities:** Editorial services specialist focuses expertise on medical writing and editing, preferably for the consumer. Geographic Area Served: Westchester, Fairfield counties (NY & Conn.)

Hartford

★ 13857 ★ Murtha Cullina L.L.P.
CityPlace I, 29th Fl.
Hartford, CT 06103-3469
Phone: (860)240-6000 **Fax:** (860)240-6150

Website: http://www.murthalaw.com

Fnded: 1937. **Activities:** Litigation support firm offers legal services in the areas of corporate and banking, labor, environmental, commercial finance, bankruptcy, real estate, public utility, healthcare, government affairs, and estate planning and settlement. Industries served: agriculture, banking, closely held businesses, computer software, construction, defense, healthcare, environmental, manufacturing, public utility, resource recovery, telecommunications, and government agencies. Geographic Area Served: Connecticut, Massachusetts.

Huntington

★ 13858 ★ Baker Hewett & Associates Inc.

42 Timberlane Dr.
Huntington, CT 06484
Phone: (203)929-9186 **Fax:** (203)929-6562
Email: webteam@bakerhewett.com
Website: http://www.bakerhewett.com

Fnded: 1987. **Activities:** Small business management consulting firm providing strategic and long range planning, venture capital planning, market research, conflict resolution, restructuring, process improvement, business finance planning, and marketing services. Geographic Area Served: Connecticut, Massachusetts, Rhode Island, New York.

Killingworth

★ 13859 ★ Matrix Public Health Consultants Inc.

79 Laurel Ridge Trl.
Killingworth, CT 06419
Phone: (860)663-0451 **Fax:** (860)663-1185
Email: stevens@matrixphc.com
Website: http://www.matrixphc.com

Activities: Experienced in diverse areas of health, including strategic planning, promotion & training on evidence-based practices, evaluation, assessment, project management, health policy, design & implementation of public health programs, training & technical assistance, and public health emergency preparedness. Provides the planning, development, facilitation and implementation of complex projects and programs as well as sophisticated statistical analyses. Specialty areas include: evidence-based research to practice; behavioral health of adults and children including substance abuse; women's health; HIV/AIDS; crime; poverty; access to care and social services; and psychiatric/medical comorbidity.

Madison

★ 13860 ★ Nolan & Bober Associates

44 Sunny Hill Dr.
Madison, CT 06443
Phone: (203)318-0894 **Fax:** (203)318-0837

Fnded: 1989. **Activities:** Health administration consulting specialists provide services to the healthcare industry, specialty hospitals and physicians. Areas include financial, investment planning, and operations. Industries served: hospital, physician practice. Geographic Area Served: United States.

Middletown

★ 13861 ★ Qualidigm

100 Roscommon Dr.
Middletown, CT 06457-1591
Phone: (860)632-2008 **Fax:** (860)632-5865
Email: communications@qualidigm.org
Website: http://www.qualidigm.org

Fnded: 1983. **Activities:** Offers quality improvement consulting, health services utilization and needs assessment statistical analysis services, and support of health services research. Geographic Area Served: United States.

Milford

★ 13862 ★ Dietary Management Services L.L.C.

284 Quarry Rd.
Milford, CT 06460
Phone: (203)874-6019 **Fax:** (203)877-5918
Email: cag@eaglesol.com

Fnded: 1984. **Activities:** Offers wholistic health options and nutritional consulting services to individuals, families, and industry. Emphasis is placed on assessment of health and wellness status and developing a lifestyle program suited to each client. Programs enforce dietary variation and modification reflecting the client's needs including weight management, diabetes, cholesterol, infectious disease, and hypertension counseling. Also offers preconceptual and maternal nutritional counseling. Consultant to: manufacturing, hospitals, and healthcare programs. **Remarks:** Yoga and Tai Qi classes available on-site. Geographic Area Served: Fairfield and New Haven counties, Connecticut.

Mystic

★ 13863 ★ Mariner Health At Pendleton

44 Maritime Dr.
Mystic, CT 06355
Phone: (860)572-1700 **Fax:** (860)572-7830

Fnded: 1986. **Activities:** Health care consultants.

New Haven

★ 13864 ★ Corporate Health Strategies Inc.

157 Church St.
New Haven, CT 06510
Phone: (203)781-5100 **Free:** 800-367-2427
Fax: (203)624-7935

Fnded: 1981. **Activities:** Company consults with employers regarding the performance of their health benefit plans and opportunities to implement demand management, and lifestyle or disease management programs. Serves private industries as well as government agencies. **Remarks:** Subsidiary of United Health Care Corporation. Geographic Area Served: United States.

New Milford

★ 13865 ★ Paul D. Ellner Associates Inc.

2 Rustic Hill Ln.
New Milford, CT 06776
Phone: (860)354-8155 **Fax:** (860)354-8447
Email: pde1@columbia.edu
Website: http://ellner.com

Activities: Specializes in clinical microbiology and infectious disease. Acts as a testifying witness or litigation consultant in medical malpractice, product liability, or disputes. Geographic Area Served: Worldwide.

Norwalk

★ 13866 ★ Weatherby Health Care

25 Van Zant St.
Norwalk, CT 06855
Phone: (203)866-1144 **Free:** 800-365-8900
Fax: (203)853-3154
Email: lstewart@whcmail.com
Website: http://www.weatherbyhealthcare.com

Fnded: 1972. **Activities:** Executive search for the health care industry. Special emphasis placed on recruitment of physicians and professionals in the areas of healthcare administration. Geographic Area Served: United States.

Redding

★ 13867 ★ Aejes L.L.C.

88 Peaceable St.
Redding, CT 06896
Phone: (203)544-9901 **Free:** 877-463-8093
Fax: (203)544-7193
Email: skorwin@aejes.com
Website: http://www.aejes.com/

Fnded: 1991. **Activities:** Provides quality management services to health care and related organizations. Offers organizational self-assessment, strategic planning, and performance improvement. Helps senior managers create supporting structures for process improvement efforts to achieve desired outcomes. Geographic Area Served: North America.

Ridgefield

★ 13868 ★ Bruce J. Sobol

275 Ridgebury Rd.
Ridgefield, CT 06877
Phone: (203)438-3650

Fnded: 1983. **Activities:** Offers medical writing expertise including clinical summaries for submission to the FDA, clinical trial reports for scientific journals, critiquing and writing research protocols, and medical articles for lay publications. Industries served: pharmaceutical and marketing.

Rocky Hill

★ 13869 ★ Health Care Resources Inc.

2360 Main St.
Rocky Hill, CT 06067-2599
Phone: (860)563-4566 **Fax:** (860)257-4004

Fnded: 1973. **Activities:** Advises state agencies, healthcare providers and corporations on healthcare management; medicare/medicaid regulations, billing, cost reporting, and appeal representation; recovering state and federal reimbursements feasibility studies and special studies. Geographic Area Served: Countrywide.

Stamford

★ 13870 ★ Compliance Consultants

1151 Hope St.
Stamford, CT 06907
Phone: (203)329-2700 **Fax:** (203)329-2345
Email: c2fda@aol.com

Fnded: 1988. **Activities:** A consultancy with expertise in regulatory engineering, product development, and medical devices. Firm advises manufacturers of regulatory requirements and submits detailed engineering facts and marketing reports to obtain market approval from FDA (Federal Drug Administration). Serves domestic and foreign clients who wish to market products in the U.S. Geographic Area Served: Worldwide technologies companies.

★ 13871 ★ First Management Services Inc.

1780 Newfield Ave.
Stamford, CT 06903
Phone: (203)329-0853 **Free:** 800-455-1213
Fax: (203)968-2223
Website: http://www.firstmanagement.com

Fnded: 1981. **Activities:** Designer and developer of training program custom-solutions for executives, managers and line staff across a wide range of management and individual development topics. Programs are interactive, providing practical approaches to real work situations. Services include: organizational analysis, needs assessment, assessment of managerial skill, executive coaching and customized development of strategic planning meetings, offsites and retreats. Developing of AAPS compensation plans, benefit packages, recruitment and retention strategies. Geographic Area Served: Worldwide.

★ 13872 ★ Gastroenterology Consultants

166 W Broad St., Ste. 303
Stamford, CT 06902
Phone: (203)967-2100 **Fax:** (203)967-4872
Website: http://www.gastro.com/

Fnded: 1989. **Activities:** Medical practice in gastroenterology and liver disease, providing information on and treating symptoms and conditions in chest pain, heartburn, liver diseases, jaundice, gallstones, colitis, diarrhea, abdominal pain, ulcers, ulcerative colitis, Crohn's disease, nervous stomach, hemochromatosis, lactose intolerance, hepatitis, hemorrhoids, constipation, and bleeding.

★ 13873 ★ MGA Systems Inc.
24 Richmond Hill Ave.
Stamford, CT 06901
Phone: (203)325-1010 **Fax:** (203)967-9272
Website: http://www.sfa-us.com/mga

Fnded: 1986. **Activities:** Contract programming, contract human resource, contract accounting, contract nursing consultants. Industries served: banking, hospitals, nursing homes, and software companies. **Remarks:** Xerox and IBM Business Partners. Geographic Area Served: Tri-state area of New York, Connecticut, and New Jersey.

★ 13874 ★ Pape & Associates
1177 High Ridge Rd.
Stamford, CT 06905
Free: 800-736-0503 **Fax:** 800-736-9096
Website: http://members.aol.com/brianpape/index.html

Fnded: 1986. **Activities:** Offers toxicology consulting services. **Remarks:** Expert testimony: toxicology. Geographic Area Served: United States, North East, Mid-Atlantic.

Trumbull

★ 13875 ★ Joe Bean & Associates Inc.
171 Edison Rd.
Trumbull, CT 06611
Phone: (203)459-0121
Email: beansafe@aol.com

Fnded: 1989. **Activities:** Safety management consulting firm specializes in OSHA-type inspections, OSHA compliance training - all subjects, long or short-term safety management, OSHA defense, accident investigation and reconstruction, process safety management, expert witnessing, and total loss control. Fully written compliance programs and safety manuals. Industries served: all special expertise in the automotive, pulp and paper industry and lockout/tagout. Geographic Area Served: Worldwide.

West Hartford

★ 13876 ★ Health Consultants Group L.L.C.
20 Hurlbut St.
West Hartford, CT 06110
Phone: (860)953-0509 **Free:** 800-367-2482
Fax: (860)953-0543
Website: http://www.healthconsultantsgroup.com

Fnded: 1992. **Activities:** Offers comprehensive review of current benefits, market analysis of competitive programs, and employee benefit services. Geographic Area Served: New England.

Westport

★ 13877 ★ Joseph J. Okon Associates
46 Post Rd. E
Westport, CT 06880
Phone: (203)341-3394 **Free:** 800-367-6566
Fax: (203)341-3393
Email: info@jjoa.com
Website: http://www.jjoa.com

Fnded: 1982. **Activities:** Provides a variety of services to medical schools, hospitals and graduate medical education programs, ranging from assistance with grant and accreditation applications to help with resident and faculty recruitment. Can also provide planning and management strategies for ambulatory care, long-term care, prepaid plans, faculty practice, marketing and facilities improvement. Industries served: hospitals, medical schools, foundations, ambulatory care facilities, professional organizations and law firms, and other healthcare institutions. Geographic Area Served: United States.

Wilton

★ 13878 ★ Juran Institute Inc.
115 Old Ridgefield Rd.
PO Box 811
Wilton, CT 06897
Phone: (203)834-1700 **Free:** 800-338-7726
Fax: (203)834-9891
Email: jdefeo@juran.com
Website: http://www.juran.com

Fnded: 1979. **Activities:** Juran Institute's Training Consulting Practice has had success with organizations from a variety of industries, from manufacturing to distribution centers, to internal and external services provided by blue chip companies. The team has enabled clients to achieve bottom-line results. Juran Consulting, supported by our global resources, can provide your organization with expert guidance, analysis, training, and ongoing support to achieve six sigma results by offering the following services: Juran's Six Sigma Breakthrough, Strategic Cost Improvement, Creating a Lean Enerprise, Benchmarking Best Practices, Supply Chain Optimization, Strategic Deployment and a Balanced Scorecard, Business Process Improvement, Strategic Systems Integration, Achieving International Quality Systems Certification. Geographic Area Served: Worldwide.

★ 13879 ★ XL Communications Inc.
44 Old Ridgefield Rd., Ste. 217
Wilton, CT 06897
Phone: (203)761-8841 **Fax:** (203)761-9276
Website: http://www.xlcommunications.com

Activities: Firm provides human resources, employment, and communication-related services to hospitals and healthcare development organizations. Geographic Area Served: Pacific Northwest.

District of Columbia

Washington

★ 13880 ★ The Advisory Board Co.
600 New Hampshire Ave. NW
Washington, DC 20037
Phone: (202)672-5600 **Fax:** (202)672-5700
Email: website@advisory.com
Website: http://www.advisory.com

Fnded: 1982. **Activities:** Researches the best and worst demonstrated practices in the health system. Publishes major studies and handles executive inquiry research briefs on progressive management practices.

★ 13881 ★ Alpha Center For Healthcare Planning Inc.
2055 L St. NW
Washington, DC 20036
Phone: (202)296-1818 **Fax:** (202)296-1825

Fnded: 1976. **Activities:** Medical consultants.

★ 13882 ★ Brian Crowley, MD
5225 Connecticut Ave., NW, Ste. 215
Washington, DC 20015
Phone: (202)537-3300 **Fax:** (301)365-8644
Email: bcrowleymd@aol.com
Website: http://www.drcrowley.yourmd.com

Fnded: 1962. **Activities:** Provides forensic psychiatry consultation and expert testimony for civil and criminal cases: malpractice cases, including personal injury, pain and suffering, sexual harassment and abuse, and sexual misconduct by professionals. Also specializes in post-traumatic stress disorder; professional ethics and peer review; hospital and outpatient treatment standards; recovered memories; workplace violence; sanity; trial competency; and diminished capacity. Geographic Area Served: United States.

★ 13883 ★ Consultants in Toxicology, Risk Assessment, and Product Safety
560 N St. SW, Ste. N707
Washington, DC 20024
Phone: (202)484-7707 **Fax:** (202)484-8019
Email: ctraps@radix.net
Website: http://www.ctraps.org

Fnded: 1981. **Activities:** Firm consists of six professionals who provide biomedical research services to the private sector in the area of human health, including toxicology and epidemiology. Approximately one half of firm's practice involves the construction of simulation models, both physiologically-based kinetic and dynamic (biological mechanism) models. The other half focuses on the safety of specific products. Geographic Area Served: Worldwide.

★ 13884 ★ The Foundation For International Human Relations
2020 Pennsylvania Ave. NW, Ste. 806
Washington, DC 20006
Phone: (202)429-2851 **Fax:** (202)429-2852
Email: rhhamden@hotmail.com
Website: http://www.cmcdubai.com

Fnded: 1976. **Activities:** Human resources consultancy offering services in international healthcare, political psychology, organization development, training and development, personnel selection, leadership and management, cross-cultural dynamics, terrorism, employee relations, motivation, and communications. Industries served: health, aviation security, smokestack industry, and government agencies. Geographic Area Served: Worldwide.

★ 13885 ★ Health Management Inc.
1707 L St. NW, Ste. 900
Washington, DC 20036
Phone: (202)887-8110 **Fax:** (202)659-8983
Email: info@hmi-usa.com
Website: http://www.hmi-usa.com

Fnded: 1983. **Activities:** Healthcare consultants experienced with programs in management consultation; management of healthcare institutions; staff development and training; management development and training; operations of hospitals, nursing homes, and clinics; institutional research and feasibility studies; corporate fitness program development; patient and public relations; and healthcare service organizational analysis and change management. Industries served: hospital referrals from Washington, DC, including government. Geographic Area Served: Washington, DC, and Maryland.

★ 13886 ★ Health Policy Alternatives Inc.
400 N Capitol St. NW, Ste. 799
Washington, DC 20001
Phone: (202)737-3390 **Fax:** (202)628-3607

Fnded: 1978. **Activities:** Advises healthcare associations in the United States on federal healthcare policy.

★ 13887 ★ Health Systems Research Inc.
1200 18th St. NW, Ste. 700
Washington, DC 20036-4992
Phone: (202)828-5100 **Fax:** (202)728-9469
Website: http://www.hsrnet.com

Fnded: 1981. **Activities:** Advises government agencies worldwide on healthcare and financial management.

★ 13888 ★ Kaludis Consulting
1919 M St. NW, Ste. 440
Washington, DC 20036
Phone: (202)331-3650 **Fax:** (202)331-1428
Email: info@kaludisconsulting.com
Website: http://www.kaludisconsulting.com

Fnded: 1977. **Activities:** Management and educational consultants for the medical and healthcare industries, as well as colleges and universities in the U.S.

★ 13889 ★ Karch & Associates Inc.
1701 K St. NW, Ste. 1000
Washington, DC 20006-1503
Phone: (202)463-0400 **Fax:** (202)463-0502
Fnded: 1982. **Activities:** Consultants on toxicology, epidemiology and risk assessment. Other services include regulatory/litigation support in relevant cases as well as hazards communications policies and procedures. Industries served: chemical, paper, plastics, and pharmaceutical industries; law firms; trade associations; and federal government.

★ 13890 ★ LaScola Qualitative Research
3900 Connecticut Ave., Ste. 101F
Washington, DC 20008
Phone: (202)363-9367 **Fax:** (202)244-1623
Email: lindalascola@compuserve.com
Fnded: 1984. **Activities:** Provides qualitative research, including focus groups, in-depth interviewing and analysis. Specializes in health and mental health, public affairs, human resources, and social issues. Has expertise with exploratory studies, sensitive topics and difficult respondents. Serves private industries as well as government agencies. Geographic Area Served: Washington DC, and national.

★ 13891 ★ Mary C. Roberts
3333 Wisconsin Ave. NW
Washington, DC 20016
Phone: (202)244-7077 **Fax:** (202)362-1213
Fnded: 1983. **Activities:** Health care communications consulting firm offering full service marketing, public relations and advertising services to the healthcare industry. Clients include hospitals, nursing homes, health associations, agencies, HMOs and health businesses. Geographic Area Served: Primarily mid-Atlantic states, but also out-of-state clients.

★ 13892 ★ Mindy B. Feirman
2440 M St. NW
Washington, DC 20037
Phone: (202)296-0777 **Fax:** (202)251-7050
Fnded: 1984. **Activities:** Presents nutrition counseling and education programs presented to business, industry, and government, including Culinary Hearts Kitchen program developed by American Heart Association. Nutrition and health-promotion services also provided to individuals and groups. Nutrition topics include cardiovascular disease, weight management, gastrointestinal disorders, sports nutrition, eating disorders, prenatal and postnatal nutrition, and infant and pediatric nutrition. Serves private industries as well as government agencies. Geographic Area Served: Washington, DC, and Baltimore, Maryland, metropolitan areas.

★ 13893 ★ Pacific Bridge Inc.
1155 Connecticut Ave. NW, Ste. 850
Washington, DC 20036
Phone: (202)467-8585 **Fax:** (202)833-2279
Email: pacificbridge@erols.com
Website: http://www.pacificbridge.com
Fnded: 1988. **Activities:** Consulting company that helps American medical manufacturers with business development in the Asian market, Assists medical manufacturers sell their products and services, set up joint ventures, conduct market research, and deal with regulatory issues. Services China, Hong Kong, Indonesia, Japan, Korea, Malaysia, the Philippines, Singapore, Taiwan, Thailand, and Vietnam.

★ 13894 ★ Pettsons Inc.
545 8th St. SE
Washington, DC 20003
Phone: (202)543-5500 **Fax:** (202)562-2011
Fnded: 1984. **Activities:** Advises government and private sector worldwide on home healthcare.

★ 13895 ★ Population Connection
1400 16th St. NW, Ste. 320
Washington, DC 20036
Phone: (202)332-2200 **Free:** 800-666-1956
Fax: (202)332-2302
Email: info@populationconnection.org
Website: http://www.populationconnection.org
Fnded: 1968. **Activities:** National nonprofit population and environmental education and advocacy organization.

★ 13896 ★ Sarah Greene Burger
3403 Woodley Rd. NW
Washington, DC 20016
Phone: (202)966-3025
Fnded: 1976. **Activities:** Nursing consultant in management and supervision of long-term patient care facilities. Works with individuals and families making decisions about the combination of services needed for long-term care in the community or in institutions.

★ 13897 ★ Washington Occupational Health Associates Inc.
1120 19th St. NW, Ste. 410
Washington, DC 20036
Phone: (202)463-6698 **Free:** 800-777-WOHA
Fax: 800-865-6525
Email: kchase@woha.com
Website: http://www.woha.com
Fnded: 1980. **Activities:** Occupational health consultants offering clinical, epidemiologic, industrial hygiene and toxicologic services in the areas of occupational and environmental health. Typical activities include toxic substance monitoring, audiometric testing and evaluation, respirator certification programs, epidemiologic surveys, expert opinion formulation and preplacement and in-service physical examination programs throughout the U.S. Geographic Area Served: North America.

★ 13898 ★ The Weinberg Group Inc.
1220 19th St. NW, Ste. 300
Washington, DC 20036
Phone: (202)833-8077 **Fax:** (202)833-7057
Website: http://www.weinberggroup.com
Fnded: 1983. **Activities:** Environmental consultants, drug development, medical devices, regulatory issues, foods, technology management, and audits.

Florida

Boca Raton

★ 13899 ★ Best Insurance Consultants
Boca Raton, FL 33487
Phone: (561)994-2581 **Fax:** (561)997-8517
Email: best1@gate.net
Website: http://webcast1.com/best/
Activities: Offers affordable health care solutions for every age group. Assists clients select plans to fit their needs. Specializes in major medical insurance, HMOs, PPOs, and dental insurance, as well as L.T.N. care, Medicare supplements, nursing home and home health care policies for senior citizens. Offers free consultations. Geographic Area Served: Florida (Palm Beach and Broward counties).

★ 13900 ★ Gail Becker Associates of Florida
4920 Conference Way S, Ste. 8
Boca Raton, FL 33431
Free: 800-422-2160 **Fax:** (561)241-8222
Email: info@gbafl.com
Website: http://www.gbafl.com
Fnded: 1975. **Activities:** Experts in product publicity, media campaigns, special events, and professional and consumer communications, including 800-number consumer information systems. Maintains a staff of dietitians and home economists skilled in creating marketing, promotional, and educational materials that effectively communicate health, food, and nutritional issues in a variety of media to companies of all sizes.

Cape Coral

★ 13901 ★ TYPE 1 Solutions
166 SE 18th. Ter.
Cape Coral, FL 33990
Phone: (941)574-8318 **Free:** 877-368-4645
Fax: (941)574-8814
Email: AEJBBK@aol.com
Activities: A JCAHO consulting practice which provides mock survey services and regulatory agency compliance to acute care hospitals, home health care, ambulatory care, long term care, psychiatric facilities and other specialty areas.

Coral Springs

★ 13902 ★ Gropper & Associates Inc.
4155 NW 90th Ave., Ste. 201
Coral Springs, FL 33065
Phone: (954)255-5772 **Fax:** (954)255-0299
Email: EGropper@aol.com
Activities: Organization providing accreditation assessment and preparation regulatory compliance review; documentation streamlining (integrated documentation systems) change management; turnaround and new program start up; and staff development. These services are provided to acute and long-term hospitals, nursing homes, behavioral health organizations, home health agencies and ambulatory care centers. Geographic Area Served: United States.

★ 13903 ★ National Search Inc.
2902 University Dr.
Coral Springs, FL 33065
Free: 800-935-4355 **Fax:** (954)755-7913
Email: recruiter@nationalsearch.com
Website: http://www.nationalsearch.com
Fnded: 1983. **Activities:** A contingency search firm for the insurance and healthcare industries. Geographic Area Served: United States.

DeLand

★ 13904 ★ Primary Resources Inc.
PO Box 2091
DeLand, FL 32721-2091
Phone: (904)738-0405
Website: http://www.primaryresourcesinc.com
Activities: Providing comprehensive consulting services to the ambulatory healthcare industry. Services include accreditation, licensure, Medicare, quality management/performance improvement programs, organizational development, management strategies, and equipment budget and selection. Emphasis on systemic application and use of policies and procedures through installation of a computer program that provides immediate and constant access to any policy/procedure.

Delray Beach

★ 13905 ★ Leon Services L.L.C.
6591 Skyline Dr.
Delray Beach, FL 33446-2201
Phone: (561)498-3954 **Fax:** (561)865-8670
Fnded: 1971. **Activities:** An association of individual scientists, engineers, technicians, managers, and several specialty consulting companies. Offer clients access to the following areas of expertise and services: biomedical chemistry, pharmaceutical veterinary, analytical and diagnostic instrumentation, reagent development and production, management, quality control, regulatory affairs, toxicological studies, clinical trials and marketing. Extensive expertise in instrument design (analytical), including replectumetry and chromatography, particularly linked to diagnostic clinical chemistry. Geographic Area Served: Worldwide.

Flagler Beach

★ 13906 ★ Judith Moylan
2119 Joyce Ave.
PO Box 5057
Flagler Beach, FL 32136-3439
Phone: (386)439-3103 **Fax:** (386)439-3103
Fnded: 1967. **Activities:** Consultant dietitian and nutritionist in healthcare to hospitals, nursing homes, adult congregate living facilities, and government agencies. Also performs book reviews and provides expert legal witness services. Additional expertise in governmental compliance. Serves as a licensed consultant dietitian, adjunt professor, and specializes in kitchen design. Geographic Area Served: United States.

Fort Myers

★ 13907 ★ National Hospital Network Systems Group
4458 Cleveland Ave.
Fort Myers, FL 33901-9010
Phone: (239)275-2666 **Fax:** (239)936-3380
Fnded: 1975. **Activities:** Advises healthcare industry worldwide on employment staffing needs and qualifications. **Remarks:** FO-40EM/Corp. coverage (24-7). Geographic Area Served: Worldwide.

Gainesville

★ 13908 ★ George G. Feussner, MD
7106 NW 11th Pl.
Gainesville, FL 32605
Phone: (352)331-6430 **Fax:** (352)371-2338
Activities: Specializes in neurology, chronic pain management, and disability analysis. Acts as a medical expert witness.

★ 13909 ★ MedEdit Associates
5429 SW 80th St.
Gainesville, FL 32608
Phone: (352)376-3071 **Fax:** (352)336-8377
Email: BarbCox@aol.com
Fnded: 1985. **Activities:** Consultant and editor/writer in biomedical communications. Activities include editing/writing of biomedical research publications for physicians and other health professionals who publish in medical journals; and preparation of patient education materials for pharmaceutical companies. Consultant also teaches seminars and workshops in biomedical writing and publishing to physicians and other health professionals. Industries served: pharmaceutical companies, academic departments of medical schools, physicians in private practice, hospitals, medical publishers, and government agencies. Geographic Area Served: United States, Canada, Western Europe.

Hernando

★ 13910 ★ RFK Associates Inc.
658 W Chase St.
Hernando, FL 34442
Phone: (352)344-8076
Email: rfka@yahoo.com
Website: http://24.129.184.120
Fnded: 1983. **Activities:** Provides application of emerging IT Technologies. Industries served: All. Geographic Area Served: United States.

Hialeah

★ 13911 ★ Pal-Med Health Services
7150 W 20th Ave., Ste. 412
Hialeah, FL 33010
Phone: (305)362-1986 **Fax:** (305)556-6028
Fnded: 1985. **Activities:** Advises local businesses on healthcare management.

Jacksonville

★ 13912 ★ Ray Howard and Associates
3350 Kori Rd.
Jacksonville, FL 32257
Phone: (904)268-0787 **Fax:** (904)268-0846
Email: rha@rayhowardassociates.com
Fnded: 1974. **Activities:** Provides in-depth management assistance to the healthcare field. Also performs time management studies and salary surveys for general industry. Geographic Area Served: United States.

Kissimmee

★ 13913 ★ Medical Planning & Consultants Inc.
405 Lake Butler Dr.
Kissimmee, FL 34759
Fnded: 1979. **Activities:** Specialists in the development of healthcare facilities including ambulatory surgical centers, cardiology, diagnostic imaging, home IV therapy, and radiation therapy centers. Consulting focuses on business development, financing/leasing, program planning, and facility design and construction. Geographic Area Served: Eastern United States.

Lake Wales

★ 13914 ★ The Bottom Line Medical Administrative Consultants Inc.
Administrative Consultants Inc.
PO Box 1618
Lake Wales, FL 33859
Phone: (863)696-3792 **Fax:** (863)696-3654
Email: bottomline@ithink.net
Website: http://www.bottomlinemedicalconsultants.com
Fnded: 1996. **Activities:** Firm provides services in operations and clinical resource management and physician organization and management. Offers comprehensive evaluations or focus on key areas of concern such as accounts receivable and front desk management, reimbursement optimization and managed care. Geographic Area Served: United States.

Largo

★ 13915 ★ Women's Wellness Center
1301 Seminole Blvd.
Largo, FL 33770
Phone: (813)581-6479 **Fax:** (813)585-4089
Fnded: 1977. **Activities:** Involved in promotion of wellness and health promotion programs at the worksite and at the Women's Wellness Center to improve employee morale and productivity and reduce costs due to employee illness, absenteeism and turnover. Conducts stress management and support groups for executive women. Provides low cost wellness and health promotion resources including: company newsletters, self-help tapes, wellness selfassessments and healthy living booklets. Provides consultation for corporations to develop their own newsletters. Geographic Area Served: Northeast and southeast United States.

Loxahatchee

★ 13916 ★ Professional Safety Inc.
2319 Palm Deer Dr.
Loxahatchee, FL 33470
Phone: (561)790-2050 **Free:** 800-562-7233
Fax: (561)795-9833
Email: profsafety@profsafety.com
Website: http://www.profsafety.com
Fnded: 1988. **Activities:** Maintains a national network of more than 1500 certified and degreed consultants and experts, specializing in safety, security services, and health and vocational rehabilitation. Through the network, firm covers the entire safety spectrum: product/occupational safety, industrial hygiene, human factors engineering, recreational safety, risk management/loss control, environmental safety, and vocational rehabilitation. Geographic Area Served: United States and Canada.

Marco Island

★ 13917 ★ Bob Olson
900 Montego Ct.
Marco Island, FL 34145
Phone: (239)394-2000
Email: bob@bigplanet.com
Fnded: 1980. **Activities:** Provides knowledge to general health industries. Geographic Area Served: Worldwide.

Miami

★ 13918 ★ COMPUTERx Consulting
9719 S Dixie Hwy., Ste. 1
Miami, FL 33156
Phone: (305)666-7100 **Fax:** (305)662-9756
Email: jnadeau@computerx-consulting.com
Website: http://computerx-consulting.com
Fnded: 1974. **Activities:** Services include assessment/feasibility studies, preparation of a comprehensive computer produced "request for proposal", quantitative systems evaluation, systems selection and recommendations, contract negotiations, implementation monitoring assistance, staff screening and selection, on-going management audits, and long-range planning. Application areas are all hospital financial management and clinical areas. Geographic Area Served: United States.

★ 13919 ★ Thomas J. Zaydon, Jr., MD
3661 S Miami Ave., Ste. 509
Miami, FL 33133
Phone: (305)856-3030 **Fax:** (305)285-9423
Email: tzaydon@pol.net
Website: http://cosmeticsurgeryinstituteofmiami.com
Activities: Evaluates and manages scars and other deformities resulting from accidents. Geographic Area Served: Florida Region.

Miami Beach

★ 13920 ★ Brennan Counsulting Inc.
7955 Biscayne Point Cir.
Miami Beach, FL 33141
Phone: (305)864-7070 **Fax:** (305)864-4140
Email: Michael.Brennan@poboxes.com
Fnded: 1984. **Activities:** Provides expert witness services for legal and insurance firms regarding compliance with the Americans with Disabilities Act. Facility/property assessments degree of compliance with access determined. Geographic Area Served: Florida.

New Port Richey

★ 13921 ★ Applicant Insight Ltd.
5396 School Rd.
New Port Richey, FL 34652
Free: 800-771-7703 **Fax:** 800-890-6454
Website: http://www.emc-corp.com/
Activities: Offers employee screening services, including a variety of applicant screening programs, background investigations, drug testing services, and physical examination programs.

★ 13922 ★ Lifespan Services Inc.
5207 Trouble Creek Rd.
New Port Richey, FL 34652
Phone: (727)847-0069 **Fax:** (727)530-5433
Email: lifespan@lifespanservices.com
Website: http://www.lifespanservices.com
Fnded: 1982. **Activities:** Nursing care consultant whose activities include consultation, managed care services, education, workshops, support groups for staff, individual counseling, group counseling, and marital counseling. Serves healthcare industries, nursing services, insurance companies, and colleges. Geographic Area Served: United States.

Nokomis

★ 13923 ★ Risk & Quality Solutions
1204 Laurel Pines Cir.
Nokomis, FL 34275
Phone: (941)485-9872
Website: http://www.rqsolutions.com
Activities: Offers personalized consulting services for ambulatory surgery centers, endoscopy centers, ambulatory centers and physician practices. Provides risk, quality and customer service program development, and AAAHC and JCAHO accreditation preparation.

North Miami Beach

★ 13924 ★ Julien Nutrition Institute
2627 NE 203rd St., Ste. 116
North Miami Beach, FL 33180
Phone: (305)932-9155 **Fax:** (305)932-3989
Fnded: 1978. **Activities:** Offers consulting in nutrition for athletes, weight control, diabetes, failure to thrive, cholesterol reduction, eating disorders, renal heart disease, and pediatrics. Specializes in the development of wellness programs. Industries served: law enforcement, education, banking, private and public sector industry in southern Florida.

Plantation

★ 13925 ★ Basic Learning Systems Inc.
600 SW 75th Ter.
Plantation, FL 33317
Phone: (954)792-4698 **Free:** 888-204-3600
Fax: (954)791-5004
Email: admin@basic-learning.com
Website: http://www.basic-learning.com
Fnded: 1980. **Activities:** Provides courses to improve verbal and written communication skills; to cope with change, stress, and time management; and to enhance management, organizational, and professional development. Offers professional, management, and organizational development services. Experienced in pinpointing performance needs. **Remarks:** Free business writing tips- via e-mail offered.

Port Charlotte

★ 13926 ★ Sweetland Associates
PMB 61
2200 Kings Hwy., Ste. 3L
Port Charlotte, FL 33980
Phone: (941)629-2630 **Fax:** (941)629-3832
Fnded: 1985. **Activities:** Firm offers healthcare management and facilities consultation.

Saint Petersburg

★ 13927 ★ Albright and Associates L.L.C.
Vinoy Pl., Unit 1021
555 5th Ave. NE
Saint Petersburg, FL 33701
Phone: (727)821-9233 **Fax:** (727)821-9033
Website: http://www.albrightandassociates.com/
Activities: Experts on consultation and case strategy development. Specific deposition and testimony skills concerning all aspects of institutional management and standard of care issues. Also experts in reviewing medical cases for assessment of merit, liability, damages and standard of care deviations.

★ 13928 ★ The DRB Group Inc.
PO Box 23176
Saint Petersburg, FL 33742
Phone: (813)568-0088 **Fax:** (813)568-9776
Fnded: 1990. **Activities:** Medical equipment consultants provide service and maintenance.

★ 13929 ★ Grobmyer Associates Inc.
111 2nd Ave. NE, Ste. 804
Saint Petersburg, FL 33701-3441
Phone: (727)822-8900 **Free:** 800-525-3480
Fax: (727)821-7238
Email: info@grobmyerassociates.com
Website: http://www.grobmyerassociates.com
Fnded: 1985. **Activities:** Firm specializes in assisting health systems, hospitals, and physician clients with strategic direction assessments (including the options of stand along, affiliation, form change, sale and merger); operations assessments governance assessments; interim management and turnaround; physician/hospital and physician/physician integration; physician practice management assessments and valuations; and business development. Geographic Area Served: United States.

★ 13930 ★ The Sports Performance Institute
PO Box 66189
Saint Petersburg, FL 33736-6189
Phone: (813)360-7200 **Fax:** (813)367-7227
Fnded: 1987. **Activities:** Provides sports performance services for professional and university teams. **Remarks:** Affiliated with The Sports Marketing Institute.

★ 13931 ★ Swain and Associates
5075 54th Way N
Saint Petersburg, FL 33709
Phone: (727)526-6605
Email: info@snaconsulting.com
Website: http://www.snaconsulting.com
Fnded: 1985. **Activities:** Provides education and consultation in areas of JCAHO accreditation and other regulations such as HCFA's Conditions of Participation. Provides support in safety management, administrative and staffing issues, medical record and HIPAA preparation, LTC, home care and medical equipment.

Sanibel

★ 13932 ★ Jass Associates
3347 Twin Lakes Ln.
Sanibel, FL 33957
Phone: (239)395-0791 **Fax:** (239)472-8073
Fnded: 1976. **Activities:** Active in the development, monitoring, and conduct of preclinical and clinical studies. Offers expertise with investigational new drug and new drug application development, label review, and regulatory services (FDA and FTC). Also provides expert witness testimony in area of skin treatment products, liability, new product development programs, and acquisition aid. Particularly accommodating to foreign firms attempting to market drugs and cosmetics in the U.S. Industries served: pharmaceutical and cosmetic. Geographic Area Served: Worldwide.

Sarasota

★ 13933 ★ CEBRAL Inc.
PO Box 5850
Sarasota, FL 34277-5850
Phone: (941)923-3268 **Fax:** (941)923-5579
Email: CEBRAL@home.com
Fnded: 1986. **Activities:** Senior pharmaceutical executives providing creative consulting services to the Pharmaceutical, Biotech and Chemical Industries. Services include drug discover, development and licensing, evaluation of new pharmaceutical products/technologies/services, and access to the pharmaceutical industry. **Remarks:** Extensive network of contacts. Geographic Area Served: Worldwide.

★ 13934 ★ Interactive Solutions Inc.
6448 Parkland Dr.
Sarasota, FL 34243
Phone: (941)753-5000
Email: support@myicommunicator.com
Website: http://www.isi-icommunicator.com
Fnded: 1984. **Activities:** Provides marketing and technical support for all of the major medical software publishers, as well as IBM multimedia system hardware. Consults with healthcare training institutions to determine how computer-based training can be utilized as part of their educational programs. Industries served: healthcare in southeastern U.S.

Seminole

★ 13935 ★ Chiro Alliance Corp.
PO Box 3340
Seminole, FL 33775
Phone: (727)319-2434 **Fax:** (727)319-0372
Email: chiroipa@tampabay.rr.com
Website: http://chiroalliance.com
Fnded: 1993. **Activities:** Assists independent chiropractic practitioner in obtaining provider status in various managed care companies, in negotiating contracts for them, in case management, and claims submission and collection of their professional fees. Geographic Area Served: Florida.

Sun City Center

★ 13936 ★ Human Resources Management Services Inc.
1713 W Del Webb Blvd.
Sun City Center, FL 33573
Phone: (813)633-0875 **Fax:** (813)634-6123
Email: hiteatsuncity@juno.com
Fnded: 1990. **Activities:** Offers professional human resources and safety mangement to business and industry. Services include: personnel administration, personnel policies/procedures, wage/salary administration, employee relations, labor relations, labor negotiations, job analysis/classification, staffing and recruitment, safety and health, and equal employment opportunity.

Tallahassee

★ 13937 ★ Larry J. Overton & Associates Inc.
101 E College Ave., Ste. 302
Tallahassee, FL 32301-7703
Phone: (850)224-2859 **Fax:** (850)561-6311
Fnded: 1988. **Activities:** Provides healthcare services to U.S. businesses.

Tampa

★ 13938 ★ Occupational Health Conservation Inc.
5118 N 56th St., Ste. 215
Tampa, FL 33610-5427
Phone: (813)626-8156 **Free:** 800-229-8156
Fax: (813)623-6702
Email: gschlossnagle@ohcnet.com
Website: http://ohcnet.com/
Fnded: 1983. **Activities:** Offers industrial hygiene, safety standards, lead abatement, and air testing services to businesses, public utilities, and state government agencies. Geographic Area Served: Florida and Georgia.

★ 13939 ★ Physician Executive Management Center
3403 W Fletcher Ave.
Tampa, FL 33618
Phone: (813)963-1800 **Fax:** (813)264-2207
Email: info@physicianexecutive.com
Website: http://www.physicianexecutive.com
Fnded: 1983. **Activities:** Specialists in physician executive search for health care delivery organizations such as health systems, hospitals, group practice and managed care. **Remarks:** Because of our specialty, we present only physician executives to our client organizations. Geographic Area Served: United States.

★ 13940 ★ Sortor Occupational Safety Consulting
6327 S Queensway Dr.
Tampa, FL 33617
Phone: (813)988-7493 **Fax:** (813)988-7493
Email: sortor@safestyle.com
Website: http://www.safestyle.com
Activities: Safety & health consulting, training and expert witness services. See web site for useful safety & health resources, including the Safestyle.com bookstore, compliance software, professional articles, job postings, a bulletin board, and valuable links. Geographic Area Served: United States.

★ 13941 ★ Thornton Laboratories Inc.
1145 E Cass St.
Tampa, FL 33601
Phone: (813)223-9702 **Fax:** (813)223-9332
Fnded: 1922. **Activities:** An independent testing laboratory with capability to test and consult in areas such as: sampling and surveying of bulk, liquid, or containerized cargo; Lead-in-paint assessments; compliance testing for governmental regulations in water, sludge, wastes; confined space; laboratory quality assurance; and industrial chemical product quality. Industries served: engineering, consultants, government, fertilizer, food processors, and construction worldwide.

Venice

★ 13942 ★ Agrippa Enterprises Inc.
PO Box 175
Venice, FL 34284-0175
Phone: (941)355-7876
Activities: A health care consultant. Offers physician network design, development, and management. Provides Internet web page consulting, grant proposals preparation, and technology assessments. Researches issues involving the Department of Insurance.

West Palm Beach

★ 13943 ★ Edge Group, Consultants, Planners & Architects
444 Bunker Rd.
West Palm Beach, FL 33405
Phone: (561)585-9307 **Fax:** (561)585-9628
Fnded: 1960. **Activities:** Offers consulting and planning services for the design, construction, and correction of buildings. Specializes in healthcare facilities; planning, programming and design of healthcare facilities of any type, and safety correction and remodeling of healthcare facilities. Industries served: government agencies, hospitals, psychiatric hospitals, medical offices, clinics, nursing homes, and long-term care facilities. Geographic Area Served: southeastern and middle southwestern United States, and Caribbean.

★ 13944 ★ Matlock Academy
2491 Homewood Rd.
West Palm Beach, FL 33406
Phone: (561)687-0327 **Fax:** (561)684-3935
Fnded: 1994. **Activities:** Firm specializes in youth and human services, and adolescent stress management. Offers advice on how to respond to clients' lack of resources, including the rendering of unbiased evaluations or judgments, and to deal with sensitive matters within organizations. Undertakes staff development for innovative programs. D. Grad is bilingual in English and Hebrew. Industries served: education, youth services, and health and human services for small businesses.

Weston

★ 13945 ★ The Electronic Librarian Inc.
16870 Crestview Ln.
Weston, FL 33326
Phone: (954)446-6466 **Fax:** (954)446-6480
Fnded: 1987. **Activities:** Researches and retrieves information (online/manual) for the insurance, medical malpractice attorneys, healthcare, and pharmaceutical industries in Florida. Also provides desktop publishing and PC consulting services.

Winter Park

★ 13946 ★ The Farris Group
3300 University Blvd., Ste. 140
Winter Park, FL 32792
Fnded: 1994. **Activities:** Offers healthcare management services to healthcare providers and managed care organizations in the United States.

★ 13947 ★ The PM Group Orlando
1752 Howell Branch Rd.
Winter Park, FL 32789-1120
Phone: (407)645-1150 **Free:** 800-329-1150
Fax: (407)645-2178
Email: mbrosius@cfl.rr.com
Website: http://www.accountantwebs.com/websites/12691/3.htm
Fnded: 1979. **Activities:** Advises general public on healthcare management in central Florida.

Georgia

Alpharetta

★ 13948 ★ The Dogwood Institute Inc.
1640 Mid-Broadwell Rd., Ste. 200
Alpharetta, GA 30004
Phone: (770)751-9571 **Free:** 800-533-2440
Fax: (770)751-9572
Email: information@dogwoodinstitute.com
Website: http://dogwoodinstitute.com
Fnded: 1970. **Activities:** Provides training for healthcare professionals, particularly for physical therapists and orthopaedic specialists. Training covers both management and clinical physical therapy related topics. Industries served: physical therapists, rehabilitation managers and administrators, hospital physical therapy directors, private practice owners, and office managers.

Atlanta

★ 13949 ★ A.M. Wolven Inc.
175 W Wieuca Rd., Ste. 118
Atlanta, GA 30342
Phone: (404)252-6377 **Fax:** (404)303-0052
Fnded: 1978. **Activities:** Involved in regulatory compliance: EPA, FDA, FHSA (CPSC), OSHA, product development, GLP's, GMP's, quality assurance audits, claim substantiation, planning and contract proposals, PRG-clinical and clinical studies, in vitro technology, and risk assessment. Industries served: chemical, cosmetic, toiletries, food, household products, medical device, and pharmaceuticals. Geographic Area Served: United States and Europe.

★ 13950 ★ Abbey Information Systems
1002 Citadel Dr.
Atlanta, GA 30324
Phone: (404)633-7446 **Fax:** (404)634-1174
Email: LAbbey@LAbbey.com
Website: http://www.labbey.com
Fnded: 1988. **Activities:** Offers computer access to over a dozen health science databases. Traditional library-based research is provided as well. Areas of expertise include bibliographies, current awareness, document delivery, on-line searching, patent searching, information retrieval, patent documentation, background reports, expert witness location, litigation support, medical-legal research, medical library management, microforms, and library security. Industries served: no limitations; most frequently medical, legal, engineering, library, pharmacology, psychology, healthcare administration, health devices, and government agencies. Geographic Area Served: Worldwide.

★ 13951 ★ American Health Consultants
3525 Piedmont Rd., Bldg. 6, Ste. 400
Atlanta, GA 30305
Phone: (404)262-7436 **Free:** 800-688-2421
Fax: 800-284-3291
Website: http://www.ahcpub.com
Activities: An information resource designed to present information and opinion to professionals in health care-related fields. The largest publisher of health care newsletters in the world. Also publishes dozens of sourcebooks in a variety of health care topics. Holds conferences in key areas from emergency medicine to hospital case management.

★ 13952 ★ Dave M. Davis, M.D., F.A.P.A
1938 Peachtree Rd. NW, Ste. 505
Atlanta, GA 30309-1253
Phone: (404)355-2914 **Fax:** (404)355-2917
Fnded: 1976. **Activities:** Offers nationwide consultations for psychiatric/mental health facilities in program development, planning, troubleshooting, and conflict resolution. Also provides forensic psychiatric services for criminal, civil, and probate cases. **Remarks:** Physician board certified in subspecialty area of psychiatry. Geographic Area Served: United States.

★ 13953 ★ Fowler Healthcare Affiliates Inc.
2000 RiverEdge Pky., Ste. 920
Atlanta, GA 30328
Phone: (770)261-6363 **Free:** 800-784-9829
Fax: (770)261-6361
Email: fha@mindspring.com
Website: http://www.fowler-consulting.com
Fnded: 1984. **Activities:** Goal is to improve the profitability and quality of care for health care systems and hospitals through effective and appropriate and quality care of care for health care systems and hospitals through effective and appropriate use of acute care, post acute levels of care and senior services. Through their expertise, clients have learned how to develop, strategically grow, and operationally enhance all facets of post acute including home health and senior care, long term acute care programs (LTAC), subacute/skilled care, acute rehabilitation, ambulatory centers and services, medical day programs and assisted living. The bottom line has stayed healthy using FHA's unique approach at development, repositioning and integration of the post acute and senior care services. **Remarks:** Intoducing a compliance program for post acute services in the fall 1999. Geographic Area Served: Worldwide.

★ 13954 ★ Frank Strickland & Associates
3525 Piedmont Rd. NE
Atlanta, GA 30303
Phone: (404)261-6362 **Fax:** (404)261-6770
Email: sci6362@aol.com
Fnded: 1981. **Activities:** Helps healthcare professionals manage change. Physicians, hospitals and ancillary healthcare providers utilize consulting and management services in the areas of strategic planning for managed care, merger/acquisition and alliances, practice valuation, physician buy-in/buy-out, network strategy/development, practice management services systems and staff efficiencies evaluation and physician career strategies. Geographic Area Served: United States.

★ 13955 ★ Garrett Associates Inc.
PO Box 53359
Atlanta, GA 30355
Phone: (404)364-0001 **Fax:** (404)364-0726
Email: gaisearch@comcast.net
Website: http://www.garrettassociatesinc.com
Fnded: 1982. **Activities:** Garrett Associates Inc. is a retained executive search firm specializing in coast-to-coast healthcare recruiting since 1982. We recruit for all management levels from CEOs to director level for hospitals and healthcare related organizations. Geographic Area Served: United States.

★ 13956 ★ Gates, Moore & Co.
Tower Pl. 100, Ste. 600
3340 Peachtree Rd., NE
Atlanta, GA 30326-1065
Phone: (404)266-9876 **Fax:** (404)266-2669
Email: postmaster@gatesmoore.com
Website: http://www.gatesmoore.com
Fnded: 1982. **Activities:** Firm provides management consulting and accounting services to medical practices, hospital owned practices, staff model managed care organizations, IPA;s, MSO's, PO, and PHO's. Services include comprehensive operational assessments, managed care negotiations, practice start-ups and expansion, development of MSO's, strategic planning, mergers, cost accounting analysis, practice valuations, income division plans, medical record documentation and coding reviews, expert witness testimony, patient satisfaction surveys and corporate compliance planning. Geographic Area Served: United States.

★ 13957 ★ Independent Rehabilitation Consultants Inc.
3475 Lenox Rd. NE, Ste. 400
Atlanta, GA 30326-1232
Phone: (404)238-0520 **Fax:** (404)240-7201
Fnded: 1982. **Activities:** Provides case management, life care planning, medical and vocational rehabilitation and medical-legal consulting services. Industries served: insurance, self-insured companies, and attorneys. Geographic Area Served: Georgia and Alabama.

★ 13958 ★ Jennings Ryan & Kolb
17 Executive Park Dr., Ste. 500
Atlanta, GA 30329
Phone: (404)634-7162 **Fax:** (404)634-7661
Email: atlanta@jrk.com
Website: http://www.jrk.com
Activities: Provides professional management consulting services to the health care industry. Management services include: strategy development, strategic planning, business and service planning, planning retreats and facilitation, integrated delivery system planning, hospital integration/affiliation, continuum of care planning, physician practice/organizational planning, managed care planning, strategy development, risk sharing readiness assessment, contract review and advisory services, financial analyses, financial planning, acquisition and divestiture analysis, financial feasibility assessment, regulatory planning, certificate of need preparation, and expert testimony.

★ 13959 ★ Kurt Salmon Associates Health Care Consulting Group
1355 Peachtree St. NE, Ste. 900
Atlanta, GA 30309-0900
Phone: (404)892-3436 **Fax:** (404)898-9590
Website: http://www.kurtsalmon.com
Fnded: 1935. **Activities:** The health care consulting group of Kurt Salmon Associates specializes in providing management advisory services in strategy, facilities, and information technology to hospitals and physician practices. Geographic Area Served: United States.

★ 13960 ★ Medical Communications Center Inc.
5825 Glenridge Dr., Bldg. 2, Ste. 211
Atlanta, GA 30328
Phone: (404)257-1251 **Fax:** (404)252-8328
Email: medcomctr@pol.net
Website: http://www.medcomctr.com
Fnded: 1975. **Activities:** Sales Rep. training and value added marketing programs for the pharmaceutical, medical product and service companies. Geographic Area Served: United States.

★ 13961 ★ Medirisk Inc.
2 Piedmont Ctr., Ste. 400
3565 Piedmont Rd.
Atlanta, GA 30305-1502
Phone: (404)364-6700 **Free:** 800-955-5056
Fax: (404)364-6710
Website: http://www.medirisk.com
Fnded: 1983. **Activities:** Provides healthcare information services to consumers and to medical and insurance industries in the U.S. and Puerto Rico.

★ 13962 ★ Outreach Inc.
825 Cascade Ave. SW
Atlanta, GA 30311-5410
Phone: (404)755-6700 **Fax:** (404)752-9969
Website: http://www.outreachatlanta.org
Fnded: 1986. **Activities:** Educates HIV positive patients and alcohol and substance abusers in healthcare techniques regionally.

★ 13963 ★ R.G.M. Decker
5035 Riverview Rd. NW
Atlanta, GA 30327-4237
Phone: (770)818-9935
Fnded: 1978. **Activities:** International healthcare consultant who assists management teams at treatment facilities worldwide. Experienced, multi-lingual resource person with competency in technical/clinical areas and management, specializing in Eastern Europe. Expertise in all phases of hospital commissioning, needs analysis and problem solving, cost control, program development (including preventive health/fitness), budgeting, nursing research, technical training, quality assurance, infection control, talent search, and marketing new products. Industries served: governments, industry, hospitals, and individuals. Offers nursing escort services worldwide.

★ 13964 ★ Successful Solutions Inc.
3565 Piedmont Rd. NE, Ste. 400
Atlanta, GA 30305
Fnded: 1985. **Activities:** Firm specializes in offering expertise in management and medical and health institutions to commercial concerns in the Southeast area.

★ 13965 ★ Susan Y. Stevens
3573 Chelsea Cres. NE
Atlanta, GA 30319
Phone: (404)256-4350
Email: susanystevens@yahoo.com
Fnded: 1976. **Activities:** Nursing administration consultant and educator serving schools of nursing, hospital education services, and healthcare institutions. Services include improving nursing's image, curriculum development and planning for nursing schools, nursing education for nursing homes, and general consulting on creating better healthcare environments. Serves private industries as well as government agencies. Geographic Area Served: Worldwide.

★ 13966 ★ Sylvia M. Sultenfuss - Human Relations Consultation
Piedmont Ct.
3098 Piedmont Rd. NE, Ste. 430
Atlanta, GA 30305
Phone: (404)237-7130 **Fax:** (404)237-6654
Email: sylvia@sylviasays.com
Website: http://www.sylviasays.com
Fnded: 1980. **Activities:** Offers organizational consultation and programs such as specialized management training, excellence in productivity, stress management program team building working together with different styles of communication, stress reduction program, leadership effectiveness, team building, conflict resolution, corporate wellness programs, and employee assistance programs. The focus is on small businesses or divisions where personnel issues/development are the target need. Serves private industries as well as government agencies. Geographic Area Served: United States, primarily southeast, and international including developing countries.

★ 13967 ★ Tyler & Co.
375 Northridge Rd., Ste. 400
Atlanta, GA 30350-3299
Phone: (770)396-3939 **Free:** 800-989-6789
Fax: (770)396-6693
Email: info@tylerandco.com
Website: http://www.tylerandco.com
Fnded: 1978. **Activities:** Retained executive search for the healthcare, food, market research, manufacturing and insurance industries. Geographic Area Served: Searches conducted nationwide.

Augusta

★ 13968 ★ MAG Mutual Healthcare Consultants
1054 Claussen Rd., Ste. 307
Augusta, GA 30907
Phone: (706)738-2078 **Free:** 800-738-7495
Fax: (706)738-9839
Email: ask@magmutual.com
Website: http://www.magmutual.com
Fnded: 1988. **Activities:** Offers hospital and physician services regarding managed care and fees and coding issues.

Decatur

★ 13969 ★ Oncology Solutions L.L.C.
150 E Ponce de Leon Ave., Ste. 120
Decatur, GA 30030
Phone: (404)836-2000 **Fax:** (404)836-2002
Email: consulting@oncsolutions.com
Website: http://www.oncsolutions.com
Fnded: 1973. **Activities:** Health care firm offers medical schools, hospital and physician consulting for cancer programs and facilities. **Remarks:** CDP Services and Cancer Care Point merged 1/1/01 to from Oncology Solutions. Geographic Area Served: Worldwide.

★ 13970 ★ Southern Pain Control Center
2786 N Decatur Rd., Ste. 200
Decatur, GA 30033-5928
Phone: (770)997-7655 **Fax:** (770)991-1843
Activities: Specializes in multi-disciplinary pain management, physical therapy, nerve blocks, epidural injections, and bio feedback therapy.

Duluth

★ 13971 ★ Gale A. Sloan
510 Bell Grove Point
Duluth, GA 30097
Phone: (770)495-8778 **Fax:** (770)495-8778
Fnded: 1986. **Activities:** Registered nurse and freelance writer and editor. Performs medical research, and health and fitness writing and editing services for a variety of clients. Also performs medical research for law firms specializing in medical malpractice and personal injury. Serves private industries as well as government agencies. Geographic Area Served: Continental United States.

Evans

★ 13972 ★ Augusta Nutrition Consultants
PO Box 799
Evans, GA 30809-0799
Phone: (706)860-8935 **Fax:** (706)860-8932
Fnded: 1985. **Activities:** Provides nutrition consultation for individuals, groups, businesses, health departments, hospitals, private physicians, health maintenance organizations, and prepaid group plans.

Hoschton

★ 13973 ★ Quality Management Resources Ltd.
5802 Chalet Way
Hoschton, GA 30548-4023
Phone: (770)967-0700 **Free:** 800-762-1967
Fax: (770)967-3070
Email: qmr@eqmr.com
Website: http://www.eqmr.com
Fnded: 1988. **Activities:** Firm offers expertise in medicine, healthcare, and quality assurance. Serves hospitals, insurance companies, doctors, and HMO's in the U.S.

Marietta

★ 13974 ★ International Healthcare Consultants Inc.
3657 Canton Rd.
PO Box 7029
Marietta, GA 30065-1029
Phone: (770)926-0062 **Fax:** (770)926-0437
Email: Ira@ihcatl.com
Website: http://www.ihcatl.com
Fnded: 1985. **Activities:** Offers healthcare consulting for insurance companies; provides engineering and biomechanical analysis of accidents; accident reconstruction; scheduling of independent medical evaluations. Geographic Area Served: National.

Norcross

★ 13975 ★ Angelica Textile Services Inc.
655 Engineering Dr., Ste. 370.
Norcross, GA 30092
Phone: (678)421-1700 **Fax:** (678)969-0684
Website: http://www.angelica.com/ATS/
Fnded: 1876. **Activities:** Specialists in hospital and healthcare laundry/linen management offering linen distribution and inventory control systems; laundry/linen program cost reductions through linen usage, linen loss control and labor-saving programs; laundry and linen base costing and cost projections; production requirements and hospital laundry contract management. Consulting services include: review and audit surveys; in-depth cost studies; on-going program implementation and support services.

★ 13976 ★ Pathogen Control Associates Inc.
270 Scientific Dr., Ste. 3
Norcross, GA 30092
Phone: (770)446-0540 **Fax:** (770)446-0610
Website: http://www.pathcon.com
Fnded: 1986. **Activities:** Applied microbiology problems: microbiological/air quality issues, sick building syndrome, Legionella and air quality testing, prevention and control of food-related pathogens and diarrheal diseases, hazard analysis, prevention strategies, medical, epidemiological, public health evaluations, seminars, courses, laboratory evaluations, and expert witness testimony. Industries served: buildings indoor air quality, heating/air conditioning, poultry industry, and government agencies. Geographic Area Served: Worldwide.

Smyrna

★ 13977 ★ A Friend of the Family
3964 Atlanta Rd. SE
Smyrna, GA 30080
Phone: (770)725-2748
Email: judim@afriend.com
Website: http://www.afriend.com
Fnded: 1983. **Activities:** Human resource development consultants for personal care services as part of employee benefit programs. Programs include: childcare, elder care, home secretaries, shopping and errand services. Serves private industries as well as government agencies. Geographic Area Served: Metro-Atlanta.

Stone Mountain

★ 13978 ★ Isenberg & Associates Inc.
1316 Rockbridge Rd., Ste. J
Stone Mountain, GA 30087
Phone: (770)381-0359 **Fax:** (770)381-5226
Email: isenb@bellsouth.net
Fnded: 1981. **Activities:** Professionals to assist in providing cost containment services, including claims administration audits, hospital audits, medical case management/home healthcare reviews, consulting services, disability programs and psychiatric peer reviews; and to assist in evaluation, development and administration of benefit programs. Industries served: corporations, insurance companies/brokers, third party administrators, and government agencies, and managed health care organization, credentialing administration, physician office site review, medical record review, hedis and research data collection. Geographic Area Served: United States.

Tucker

★ 13979 ★ Aubrey Daniels International
3531 Habersham at Northlake
Tucker, GA 30084
Phone: (770)493-5080 **Free:** 800-223-6191
Fax: (770)493-5095
Email: lglass@aubreydaniels.com
Website: http://www.aubreydaniels.com
Fnded: 1978. **Activities:** Behavior-based change management, public seminars, consulting, online reinforcement systems. Geographic Area Served: Worldwide.

Valdosta

★ 13980 ★ Kaare Lovoll
204 Fairway Dr.
Valdosta, GA 31605
Phone: (229)242-5051 **Fax:** (229)253-9147
Email: lov1021@aol.com
Website: http://member.expertpages.com/klovoll/
Activities: Comprehensive record/case review with medico/legal opinion.

Woodstock

★ 13981 ★ Wiederhold & Associates
12195 Hwy. 92, Ste. 114
Box 347
Woodstock, GA 30188
Free: 800-618-2650 **Fax:** (770)592-7598
Email: wiedman43@mindspring.com
Activities: A healthcare recruiting and career consulting firm specializing in operational and executive management. Geographic Area Served: United States.

Hawaii

Honolulu

★ 13982 ★ INALAB Inc.
3615 Harding Ave., Ste. 308
Honolulu, HI 96816
Phone: (808)735-0422 **Fax:** (808)735-0047
Email: inalab@msn.com
Website: http://www.inalab.com
Fnded: 1978. **Activities:** Provides professional consultation in analytical chemistry and the application of scientific methodology to clients' needs (arson, forensics, drugs/narcotics). Evaluates workers' occupational environment and provides board-certified industrial hygiene services. Provides expert witness testimony. Industries served: insurance, contractors (general), asbestos and lead abatement contractors, attorneys, other laboratories, environmental agencies, building managers and owners, military, architects and engineers, and government agencies. **Remarks:** A.I.H.A. accredited laboratory (industrial hygiene). Geographic Area Served: Pacific Basin.

★ 13983 ★ Kuakini Pathologists L.L.C.
347 N Kuakini St.
Honolulu, HI 96817
Phone: (808)547-9139 **Fax:** (808)547-9497
Fnded: 2000. **Activities:** Professional medical consultants in the fields of medical pathology or diseases including occupational and environmental disease; anatomic pathology, clinical pathology, and forensic pathology; legal medicine; accidental and industrial fatalities for insurance, industry, and legal profession; and epidemiology of cancer in the Pacific. Serves private industries as well as government agencies. Geographic Area Served: City and county of Honolulu, Hawaii.

Kaneohe

★ 13984 ★ Medical Litigation Consultants
PO Box 1306
Kaneohe, HI 96744-1306
Phone: (808)599-2444 **Free:** 800-763-3548
Fax: (808)538-1833
Email: info@medmal-inc.com
Website: http://www.medmal-inc.com/
Fnded: 1978. **Activities:** Firm offers comprehensive litigation support services for attorneys in cases involving complex medical issues, primarily medical malpractice and catastrophic personal injury cases. Geographic Area Served: Worldwide.

Illinois

Arlington Heights

★ 13985 ★ Access Medical Group Ltd.
3395 N Arlington Heights Rd., Ste. A
Arlington Heights, IL 60004
Phone: (847)392-2227 **Fax:** (847)392-2257
Email: access@access-medical.com
Website: http://www.access-medical.com
Fnded: 1991. **Activities:** A professional medical communications organization. Offers scientific and medical marketing consulting. Assists product managers in the commercialization of new chemical entities.

Aurora

★ 13986 ★ C-A-B Consultants Inc.
2287 Tanglewood Dr.
Aurora, IL 60506-4423
Phone: (630)859-2221 **Fax:** (630)859-2255
Email: c-a-b@c-a-b.net
Website: http://www.cab.net
Fnded: 1985. **Activities:** Safety, OSHA related, Workers Compensation and Occupational Health. Geographic Area Served: Chicago matropolitan area but will travel.

Bannockburn

★ 13987 ★ Irvine Consulting Inc.
2207 Lakeside Dr.
Bannockburn, IL 60015-1265
Phone: (847)615-0040 **Free:** 800-229-0040
Fax: (847)615-0192
Email: irves224@msn.com
Website: http://www.irvineconsultinginc.com
Fnded: 1987. **Activities:** Firm provides expertise in marketing research to the healthcare industry nationwide.

Barrington

★ 13988 ★ Toxdata Systems Inc.
380 Sutton Rd.
Barrington, IL 60010-9378
Phone: (847)382-5291 **Fax:** (847)382-9406
Email: cbenk@attglobal.net
Fnded: 1981. **Activities:** Offers consultation or expert testimony in lawsuits in the area of industrial and regulatory toxicology. Also specializes in MSDS; product labels; product safety; industrial chemicals and

pharmaceuticals; and cancer causation. Provides: case analysis; alternative causation; online computer searches (medical and business databases); document retrieval; database management; and data summaries.

Buffalo Grove

★ 13989 ★ Tyson Consulting Group
612 White Pine Rd.
Buffalo Grove, IL 60089-3330
Phone: (847)459-9189 **Fax:** (847)215-6141
Fnded: 1978. **Activities:** Product and market development consultants offer: technology assessment - investigation of current and new technologies, their commercial potential, and business compatibility; market analysis - market potential and competitor intelligence studies with emphasis on trends and niches; product development - concept testing and feasibility studies, determination of optimum specifications, features and benefits; and sales planning development and implementation of sales and distribution programs. Industries served: healthcare, including biotechnology, medical devices, and pharmaceuticals, as well as government agencies. **Remarks:** Developed and manage website for healthcare organization in the medical device field. Geographic Area Served: United States and Europe.

Capron

★ 13990 ★ Willowcreek MedCom Consultants
8132 Hunter Rd.
Capron, IL 61012
Phone: (815)569-2642
Email: arctblis@gte.net
Website: http://home1.gte.net/arctblis
Fnded: 1978. **Activities:** Prepares biomedical documentation (brochures, books, summaries), literature searches and interpretation, abstracting, presentations, lectures, seminars, and educational materials. Also offers expertise in advertising, translation from German and French, clinical study protocol design, and the coordinating and monitoring of clinical studies. Will interpret medical literature for legal profession and insurance industry. Industries served: pharmaceutical industry, medical education industry, insurance/legal, medico-legal, and medical research groups. Geographic Area Served: Worldwide.

Champaign

★ 13991 ★ Health Services Consultants Inc.
4102 Belmont Pt.
Champaign, IL 61822
Phone: (217)398-0754 **Fax:** (217)398-0944
Website: http://www.ryle.com
Fnded: 1988. **Activities:** Offers healthcare management services to the general public in Illinois.

Chicago

★ 13992 ★ Altman Information Systems
118 N Clinton St., Ste. L-1200
Chicago, IL 60661-2385
Phone: (312)441-1234 **Fax:** (312)382-0614
Fnded: 1980. **Activities:** Offers expertise in investment management and medical office management systems. Services involve investment technology including securities and portfolio accounting and measurement systems; analyst evaluations management information reports (investment applications); portfolio performance financial modeling; indices - option evaluation, selection, and spreads; stock data bases (creation, maintenance, updates); online portfolio pricing systems securities screening and selection; and equipment selection communication. Industries served: banks, insurance companies, and publishers.

★ 13993 ★ Ambulatory Systems Development
625 N Michigan St., Ste. 500
Chicago, IL 60611
Phone: (312)540-0662 **Fax:** (312)540-0663
Email: joezasa@woodrumasd.com
Website: http://www.asdconsulting.com
Activities: Specializes in ambulatory and outpatient care services. Offers strategic services, operational analysis, financial feasibility analysis, development services, and management services. Provides strategic healthcare provider realignment.

★ 13994 ★ American College of Chiropractic Consultants
28 E Jackson Bldg., Fl. 10, Ste. 1020
Chicago, IL 60604
Phone: (708)895-3141 **Fax:** (708)895-2268
Email: dcox152565@aol.com
Website: http://www.ACCC-chiro.com
Fnded: 1975. **Activities:** Independent contractors who provide advisory consulting services with expertise in independent medical examinations, educational training, medicolegal, risk management, and healthcare administration activities. Geographic Area Served: United States.

★ 13995 ★ Bensinger Du Pont & Associates Inc.
20 N Wacker Dr., Ste. 920
Chicago, IL 60606
Phone: (312)726-8620 **Free:** 800-227-8620
Fax: (312)726-1061
Email: marie.apke@bensingerdupont.com
Website: http://www.bensingerdupont.com
Fnded: 1982. **Activities:** Offers expertise regarding drug, alcohol, substance abuse, and violence in the workplace; employee assistance programs; drug testing; security and fitness for duty audits; and gambling addiction.

★ 13996 ★ Care Communications Inc.
205 W Wacker Dr., Ste. 1900
Chicago, IL 60606-1214
Phone: (312)551-3100 **Free:** 800-458-3544
Fax: (312)422-0106
Email: info@care-communications.com
Website: http://www.carecommunications.com
Fnded: 1976. **Activities:** Care Communications, a temporary health information staffing services company, provides comprehensive solutions for HIM functions including coding (on or remote), abstracting, clerical functions, interim management, operations review/planning, reengineering, coding/DRG validation improvement, compliance reviews, coding training, Master Patient Index clean-up, and other consulting services related to health information management. Cancer/trauma registry services include outsourcing or temporary staffing for abstracting, staging, survey preparation, studies, and annual reports. Technology that enables hospitals to implement their own remote coding program. Geographic Area Served: United States.

★ 13997 ★ Diversified Health Resources Inc.
875 N Michigan Ave., Ste. 3250
Chicago, IL 60611
Phone: (312)266-0466 **Fax:** (312)266-0715
Fnded: 1979. **Activities:** Offers healthcare consulting for hospitals, nursing homes (including homes for the aged), and other health-related facilities and companies. Specializes in planning and marketing. Also conducts executive searches for top level healthcare administrative positions. Serves private industries as well as government agencies. Geographic Area Served: United States.

★ 13998 ★ Donald Radcliffe/ Communications Consultant
1528 W Morse Ave.
Chicago, IL 60626
Phone: (773)465-1536
Fnded: 1966. **Activities:** Provides consulting services and educational programs in writing, editing, and company communications for business and health-oriented institutions.

★ 13999 ★ GTCR Golder, Rauner L.L.C.
6100 Sears Tower
Chicago, IL 60606-6402
Phone: (312)382-2200 **Fax:** (312)382-2201
Website: http://www.gtcr.com
Fnded: 1980. **Activities:** A private equity investment firm and long-term strategic partner for management teams. Currently manages more than $2 billion in equity capital invested in a wide range of companies and industries. Primary industry focus includes marketing services, distribution, healthcare services, information technology services, outsourced business services and transaction processing.

★ 14000 ★ Mark M. Rasenick
Department of Physiology & Biophysics
Univ. of Illinois, College of Medicine
901 S Wolcott
Chicago, IL 60612-7342
Phone: (312)996-6641 **Fax:** (312)996-1414
Email: raz@uic.edu
Website: http://www.uic.edu/depts/mcpb/pages/rasenick/rasenick.htm
Activities: Offers consultation on various aspects of neuropharmacology and psychopharmacology, especially those relating to GTP-binding proteins and neuronal signal transduction. Serves as expert witness for all drug effects upon the central nervous system, especially antidepressant drugs and treatments. Provides consultation for the preparation of research grant applications. Industries served: biomedical, scientific, legal applications, and government agencies. Also provides consultation on the interface between Biomedical R & D and also provides Government policy. Geographic Area Served: Worldwide.

★ 14001 ★ Mary J. Dyra, Registered Dietitian
c/o Association of Internal Medicine
211 E Chicago Ave., Ste. 930
Chicago, IL 60611
Phone: (312)944-6677 **Fax:** (312)944-3346
Email: mjd@aol.com
Fnded: 1977. **Activities:** Applied clinical nutritionist provides individual consultation on nutrition and conducts weight loss classes as well as cholesterol screening program for corporations.

★ 14002 ★ MEBS Industrial Services Inc.
1525 E 53rd St., Ste. 401
Chicago, IL 60615-4530
Phone: (773)752-1400 **Fax:** (773)752-7235
Fnded: 1973. **Activities:** Provides a range of consultant services in the areas of psychosocial services, educational services, personnel services, recruitment services, and clinical services covering a broad range of human needs. Clients include social service agencies, educational agencies, and private industry clinics. Services are provided to both staff and clients of facilities.

★ 14003 ★ Mikki Williams Unltd.
1749 N Wells St.
Chicago, IL 60614
Phone: (312)664-8447 **Fax:** (312)664-8460
Email: mikki@mikkiwilliams.com
Website: http://www.mikkiwilliams.com
Fnded: 1988. **Activities:** International management consulting firm specializing in speaking, training, and consulting. Offers keynote addresses, seminars, workshops in personal and professional development, and

business dynamics. Industries served: entrepreneurs, insurance, healthcare, hospitality, women, corporations, associations, human resources, pharmaceutical, government and educational institutions. Geographic Area Served: Worldwide.

★ 14004 ★ Sheldon I. Dorenfest & Associates Ltd.
515 N State St., Ste. 1801
Chicago, IL 60610
Phone: (312)464-3000 **Fax:** (312)464-3030
Email: info@dorenfest.com
Website: http://www.dorenfest.com

Fnded: 1976. **Activities:** Helps integrated healthcare delivery systems, as well as individual acute care hospitals, ambulatory clinics, long-term care facilities, and physician offices develop and implement successful information systems strategies that maximize the benefits of automation. Consulting services include: competitive analysis studies, strategic planning, vendor evaluation and selection, contract negotiations, managing implementation of new systems, process reengineering, benefits realizations, networking strategies, and education. Also assists suppliers shape better products for the health care information systems industry. Geographic Area Served: Worldwide.

★ 14005 ★ SMG Marketing Group Inc.
875 N Michigan Ave., Ste. 3100
Chicago, IL 60611
Phone: (312)642-3026 **Free:** 800-678-3026
Fax: (312)642-3597
Website: http://www.verispan.com

Fnded: 1976. **Activities:** An international management consulting and marketing services company working exclusively with manufacturers, suppliers and hospitals in the healthcare field. Offers specialized market potential indexes, sales territory analyses, market research and computer-driven analytical models for sales management allocations and sales call activity programs. Also offers complete marketing programs and market research and analysis for hospitals to increase physician and patient utilization of the hospital. Geographic Area Served: United States.

★ 14006 ★ Solucient
2731 N Marshfield
Chicago, IL 60614
Phone: (773)871-3929
Email: info@solucient.com
Website: http://www.solucient.com

Fnded: 1984. **Activities:** Develops computer software for the healthcare industry in the U.S.

★ 14007 ★ U.S. Occupational Health Inc.
205 W Randolph St., Ste. 720
Chicago, IL 60606
Phone: (312)641-1449 **Fax:** (312)641-1714
Email: info@usohclinic.com
Website: http://usohclinic.com

Fnded: 1986. **Activities:** Occupational health consultants and health testing. Particular expertise available in OSHA medical compliance exams including: asbestos or respirator wearer - certification at time of exam, benzene, coke oven, hearing conservation (audio), and HAZMAT and emergency response. Serves private industries as well as government agencies. Geographic Area Served: Chicago metropolitan area.

★ 14008 ★ Woodrum Inc.
175 N Harbor Dr.
Chicago, IL 60601
Phone: (312)540-0662 **Fax:** (312)540-0663
Email: dwoodrum@msn.com

Fnded: 1990. **Activities:** Firm provides consulting and implementation services exclusively to the health care industry. Services include merger and acquisition services, network integration, joint ventures between health care organizations and personal providers, community care networks and short-term management turnaround and workout services. Geographic Area Served: United States.

Clarendon Hills

★ 14009 ★ Physician Management Resources Inc.
PO Box 188
Clarendon Hills, IL 60514
Phone: (630)655-0731 **Fax:** (630)655-0729
Website: http://www.sandragill.com

Fnded: 1980. **Activities:** Provides a variety of consulting services and workshops to accelerate the development of leadership skills among physician managers, trustees, and executive leaders. Services include: medical staff organizational assessments, meeting design and facilitation, strategic planning and transition management, and retreat planning and implementation. Active exclusively with the healthcare industry. Geographic Area Served: United States.

Deerfield

★ 14010 ★ TechnoClin Consulting Inc.
830 Warwick Rd.
Deerfield, IL 60015
Phone: (847)945-0030 **Fax:** (847)945-0124
Email: dgriffin@technoclin.com
Website: http://www.technoclin.com

Fnded: 1990. **Activities:** Consultants on laboratory management and radiology, combining management skills with knowledge of laboratory technologies, procedures, and operations.

★ 14011 ★ W-F Professional Associates Inc.
400 Lake Cook Rd., Ste. 207
Deerfield, IL 60015
Phone: (847)945-8050 **Free:** 800-323-4305
Fax: (847)945-5037
Email: info@wfprofessional.com
Website: http://www.wfprofessional.com

Fnded: 1977. **Activities:** Consulting firm conducts pharmacy continuing education programs.

Des Plaines

★ 14012 ★ The Joseph Group
1933 Locust St.
Des Plaines, IL 60018
Phone: (847)299-7145 **Fax:** (847)299-7145

Fnded: 1993. **Activities:** Highly-specialized public relations and public affairs marketing firm with unique healthcare communications expertise, provides consulting services to pharmaceutical, biotechnology, medical devices and health association clients. Firm's special forte is medical media relations and marketing for new products as well as crisis communications and identity programs. Geographic Area Served: United States and Europe.

Downers Grove

★ 14013 ★ ServiceMaster Home Health Care Services Inc.
1 ServiceMaster Way
Downers Grove, IL 60515-1700
Free: 800-333-6678 **Fax:** (630)271-5724

Activities: Offers consultative services in the area of home health care operational, regulatory, financial and clinical areas. Services include regulatory support and research, training and education, business reviews, regulatory survey-support/ education, clinical support and research, customization and development of programs/ pathways, development of a home health care compliance plan, quality improvement consultation, policy and procedure customization advice, participation in educational seminars and conferences, accreditation consultation, and reimbursement strategies.

Evanston

★ 14014 ★ Ada P. Kahn
2562 Wellington Ct.
Evanston, IL 60201-4975
Phone: (847)328-4512 **Fax:** (847)328-1695
Email: adapkahn@aol.com
Website: http://www.keepingthebeat.com

Fnded: 1980. **Activities:** Offers writing services for health related fields and public relations for pharmaceutical and medical products. Geographic Area Served: Worldwide.

★ 14015 ★ KAM Healthcare Consulting Inc.
1847 Lincoln St.
Evanston, IL 60201
Phone: (847)869-6934 **Fax:** (847)869-0838

Fnded: 1990. **Activities:** Health care research and consulting. Industries served: pharmaceuticals, diagnostics, OTC manufacturers, healthcare advertising agencies, and consumer advertising agencies. Geographic Area Served: United States; international subcontractors.

★ 14016 ★ Medicus Systems Corp.
1 American Plz.
Evanston, IL 60201
Phone: (847)570-7518 **Free:** 800-257-2805
Fax: (847)570-7597

Fnded: 1969. **Activities:** Offers consulting services to healthcare providers in the U.S. and Canada. Areas of expertise include case management, clinical pathway automation/management, computer information systems management, cost containment, fiscal managemnet, flexible budgeting, patient care workload measurement, patient care productivity management, and nurse staffing/scheduling.

★ 14017 ★ Morley Brickman & Associates Ltd.
9221 Drake Ave., Unit 410
Evanston, IL 60203-1626
Phone: (847)674-2664 **Fax:** (847)674-0096
Email: mbrickman@engineer.com

Fnded: 1986. **Activities:** Occupational safety and health consultants provide forensic services primarily to construction and manufacturing industry. Serves private industry and the private sector. Geographic Area Served: Worldwide, primarily the Midwest.

★ 14018 ★ Women's Healthcare Consultants Inc.
1603 Orrington Ave.
Evanston, IL 60201-4623
Phone: (847)869-1200 **Fax:** (847)328-9056

Fnded: 1984. **Activities:** Provides women's healthcare services to hospitals and institutions in the United States.

★ 14019 ★ Wordscope Associates Inc.
2562 Wellington Ct.
Evanston, IL 60201-4975
Phone: (847)328-4512 **Fax:** (847)328-1695
Email: adapkahn@aol.com
Website: http://www.keepingthebeat.com

Fnded: 1980. **Activities:** Editorial specialist providing written materials for pharmaceutical company's product launches, assisting physicians in publishing articles and books; preparing book-length manuscripts; writing proposals for public relations agencies and corporate clients; expediting projects; and HMO marketing and public relations. Serves private sector and government agencies worldwide. Minority and woman-owned firm. Geographic Area Served: United States.

Glen Ellyn

★ 14020 ★ M - D Management Associates
PO Box 2997
Glen Ellyn, IL 60138-2997
Phone: (630)918-6741 **Fax:** (630)790-0054
Fnded: 1977. **Activities:** Professional practice management consultants for the healthcare professional. Services provided on an as needed basis include basic accounting, administration, systems management (to include electronic communications systems), financial and marketing systems. Industries served: medical and healthcare professions primarily and other small businesses (variety). Geographic Area Served: Metropolitan Chicago, Illinois area.

★ 14021 ★ PRISM Healthcare Consulting
Bldg. 4, Ste. 317
799 Roosevelt Rd.
Glen Ellyn, IL 60137-5908
Phone: (630)790-1265 **Fax:** (630)790-2696
Email: prism@consultprism.com
Website: http://www.consultprism.com
Fnded: 1992. **Activities:** Firm offers a personalized consulting process focusing on strategic planning, business development, financial analysis, medical staff integration and development, board development, and facilities planning. Geographic Area Served: United States.

Glenview

★ 14022 ★ InfoScript Inc.
2100 Pfingsten Rd.
Glenview, IL 60025
Email: Susan@InfoScript.com
Website: http://www.InfoScript.com
Activities: A company focused on management resource information and the prescription for meaningful application of that information. Specializing in emergency department consultation.

★ 14023 ★ Walsh Consulting Group Inc.
Carillon Sq.
1500 Waukegan Rd., Ste. 230
Glenview, IL 60025-2123
Phone: (847)998-8282 **Fax:** (847)998-4634
Email: wcg@wcg-inc.com
Website: http://wcg-inc.com
Fnded: 1995. **Activities:** Firm provides medical equipment consulting to the healthcare industry. Services include equipment planning for construction projects, CON budgeting, technology assessments, capital asset planning, merger/acquisition analysis (relating to equipment), equipment valuation and activation/occupancy planning. Servicing community hospitals, academic medical centers, health systems and other providers. Geographic Area Served: United States.

Highland Park

★ 14024 ★ B. Howard Zirn and Associates Inc.
366 Seven Pines Cir.
Highland Park, IL 60035-4548
Phone: (847)433-2249 **Fax:** (847)433-6205
Email: bhzassocs@msn.com
Fnded: 1977. **Activities:** A management consulting firm specializing in developing/implementing strategic plans and marketing programs for the human healthcare industry. The firm provides complete programs leading to growth through product development, acquisitions or cost/performance improvement. Geographic Area Served: North America.

★ 14025 ★ The Detwiler Group
396 Vine Ave.
Highland Park, IL 60035
Phone: (847)432-9575 **Fax:** (847)432-9577
Email: sdetwiler@detwiler.com
Website: http://www.detwiler.com
Fnded: 1985. **Activities:** Analyzes health and business internet content for traditional and dot-com companies. Presents findings in concise, footnoted reports in these categories: Quick-Answer Service; Market Overviews; Competitor Intelligence Reports; Summarized Literature Reviews; and Interactive Databases tailored to client needs. Also provides marketing, sales, and strategic planning services. Industries served: healthcare, medical device, pharmaceutical, and biotech worldwide.

Hinsdale

★ 14026 ★ Occupational & Environmental Health Consulting Services
635 Harding Rd.
Hinsdale, IL 60521-4814
Phone: (630)325-2083 **Fax:** (630)325-2098
Website: http://www.safety-epa.com
Fnded: 1984. **Activities:** Provides consulting to industry on safety program development and implementation, industrial hygiene monitoring programs, occupational health nursing, wellness programs, medical monitoring, accident trending and statistics, emergency response planning, multilingual training, right-to-know compliance and training, hazardous waste management, radon monitoring and mitigation, asbestos school inspection, and project management. Also offers indoor air quality, expert witnessing service. Geographic Area Served: United States, Europe, Mexico, Canada, Puerto Rico.

Joliet

★ 14027 ★ Healy & Associates
3033 W Jefferson St., Ste. 205
Joliet, IL 60435-6449
Phone: (815)741-0102 **Fax:** (815)744-5412
Fnded: 1982. **Activities:** Personal development consultant with experience in alcoholism and family treatment; employee assistance program consultation and implementation; health promotion programming on stress, smoking cessation, weight control; alcohol and drug related prevention and educational programming; and individual, group and family counseling. Serves private industries as well as government agencies. Geographic Area Served: Chicago metropolitan area.

★ 14028 ★ Murer Group
58 N Chicago St., Ste. 7
Joliet, IL 60432-4375
Phone: (815)727-3355 **Fax:** (815)727-3360
Website: http://www.murer.com
Fnded: 1984. **Activities:** Offers healthcare management services to healthcare networks, hospitals, and physicians' groups in all areas of post acute care, including rehabilitation, subacute care, outpatient, and home health. Geographic Area Served: Worldwide.

La Grange

★ 14029 ★ Herman Smith Associates Internation
5311 Edgewood Ave.
La Grange, IL 60525
Phone: (708)352-6584 **Fax:** (708)352-6547
Email: customersupport@herman-smith.com
Website: http://www.hostjordan.com
Fnded: 1947. **Activities:** Hospital and healthcare consulting division of Coopers & Lybrand L.L.P. offering services in strategic planning and marketing, facilities and equipment planning, management, clinical operations, physician/hospital integration, system planning studies,and organizational development. Industries served: hospitals, healthcare providers, long-term care providers, and government agencies. Geographic Area Served: Worldwide.

Lake Forest

★ 14030 ★ Management Planning Associates Inc.
222 Wisconsin Ave., Ste. 207B
Lake Forest, IL 60045
Phone: (847)535-9740 **Fax:** (847)535-9441
Email: pgdickey@medplannet.com
Website: http://www.medplannet.com
Fnded: 1975. **Activities:** Provides strategic/marketing planning, evaluation of acquisitions/mergers/divestitures, new product analysis, market forecasting, technology assessment, market research, and corporate planning for the healthcare industry. Industries served: pharmaceuticals, biotechnology, diagnostics, healthcare instrumentation and devices. Geographic Area Served: United States and Europe.

★ 14031 ★ Medical Directions Inc.
PO Box 923
Lake Forest, IL 60045
Phone: (847)735-8900 **Fax:** (847)735-8914
Fnded: 1977. **Activities:** Full-service marketing communications agency and marketing consultant. Services include: writing monographs, brochures, mail, ads, sales brochures and sales training programs; marketing consultation for new and established healthcare providers; and developing and producing sponsored publications and newsletters. Industries served: pharmaceuticals, hospital products, diagnostic instruments and tests, and home care services. Geographic Area Served: Worldwide.

★ 14032 ★ Scott Group
250 E Illinoise Rd.
Lake Forest, IL 60045-1969
Phone: (847)295-8979 **Fax:** (847)934-1290
Fnded: 1989. **Activities:** Focuses on acute care hospitals and systems seeking to serve senior (elderly) needs; these systems include nursing home administration, in-home life care, housing with services for the elderly, and senior care networks.

Lake Zurich

★ 14033 ★ James J. Gadwood
590 Pheasant Ridge Dr.
Lake Zurich, IL 60047
Phone: (847)438-0528
Email: jimgadwood@aol.com
Website: http://hometown.rd.com/jimgadwood/nayhomepage/resume.html
Fnded: 1996. **Activities:** Offers consulting services in areas that include chemical and coatings plant management, chemicals, coatings, resins, pigments, aerosols, environmental safety, quality maintenance, and union negotiating expert witnesses - Chemical Plant and Safety Management. Geographic Area Served: United States.

Lombard

★ 14034 ★ MedEval Corp.
1920 S Highland Ave.
Lombard, IL 60148
Phone: (630)629-5900 **Fax:** (630)629-5960
Fnded: 1982. **Activities:** Provides medical recommendations to companies that self administer their income continuation plans. The firm is a cost continuation corporation specializing in disability plans. As a part of its medical services, the firm will medically review and submit appropriate recommendations for disability covering employees for Accident/Sickness and Short-term Disability plans; locate and set-up second opinions with Board Certified M.D. Physicians; locate Board Certified M.D. Internists for executive physical exam programs; and act as a general medical consultant.

Mundelein

★ 14035 ★ Pharmaceutical Systems Inc.
909 Orchard St.
Mundelein, IL 60060-3826
Phone: (847)566-9229 **Fax:** (847)566-4960
Website: http://www.pharmsystems.com
Fnded: 1988. **Activities:** Offers legal, contract auditing, regulatory compliance, lab research, business planning, technology, sterility assurance and quality assurance services to U.S. healthcare medical device and pharmaceutical industries. Geographic Area Served: Worldwide.

★ 14036 ★ Research Oriented Biostatistics Inc.
375 Banbury Rd.
Mundelein, IL 60060-1108
Phone: (847)949-5901 **Fax:** (847)949-9851
Email: kkborden@juno.com
Fnded: 1994. **Activities:** Our company designs studies to support clinical utility claims of new tumor markers and other diagnostic medical devices; performs statistical analyses for all types of research, marketing, and clinical studies; prepares and reviews FDA PMA, and 510 (k) submissions; prepares and reviews articles for journal publication; and provides onsite statistical training. Geographic Area Served: United States, Canada, Europe, Asia/Pacific.

Naperville

★ 14037 ★ Association Management Resources
1151 E Warrenville Rd.
Naperville, IL 60566
Phone: (630)505-7777 **Fax:** (630)505-4693
Website: http://www.ihatoday.org
Fnded: 1979. **Activities:** Specialists in solving problems in the healthcare environment. Clients include hospitals, extented care facilities, and physicians' offices. Geographic Area Served: Statewide.

New Lenox

★ 14038 ★ Stan A. Huber Consultants Inc.
200 N Cedar Rd.
New Lenox, IL 60451-1751
Phone: (815)485-6161 **Free:** 800-383-0468
Fax: (815)485-4433
Email: sahci@aol.com
Website: http://www.sahci.com
Activities: Provides radiation safety/health physics support services for a wide variety of facilities that use radioactive materials, including hospitals, universities, research laboratories, manufacturing and industrial facilities. Services include radiation safety consulting services and audits, licensing and regulatory compliance, nuclear equipment calibrations and leak testing services, and decontamination-decommissioning services. Consultants are experienced in all facets of health physics consulting services. Geographic Area Served: United States.

Northbrook

★ 14039 ★ AccuStar Labs
3334 Commercial Ave.
Northbrook, IL 60062-1909
Phone: (847)205-0110 **Free:** 800-206-0110
Fax: (847)205-0114
Email: info2@remradon.com
Website: http://www.REMRadon.com
Fnded: 1985. **Activities:** Offers consultation for radon testing surveys and mitigation system planning and design, radon evaluation project design for wide geographic surveys, schools, soil studies and public outreach. Mitigation system design for schools and large commercial and public buildings. Radon resistant construction archives. Industries served: medical, industrial and government agencies. Geographic Area Served: Worldwide.

★ 14040 ★ Morell and Associates Inc.
One Northbrook Pl.
5 Revere Dr., Ste. 200
Northbrook, IL 60062-8000
Phone: (847)498-7363 **Fax:** (847)205-5330
Email: Morellasso@aol.com
Fnded: 1990. **Activities:** Works with healthcare organizations to provide strategic direction, consulting on medical staff development and physician relationships. Also assist clients with issues of organization and governance.

★ 14041 ★ Northview Laboratories Inc.
1880 Holste Rd.
Northbrook, IL 60062
Phone: (847)564-8181 **Fax:** (847)564-8269
Email: info@northviewlabs.com
Website: http://www.northviewlabs.com
Fnded: 1972. **Activities:** An independent laboratory offering comprehensive testing capabilities in microbiology, sterility testing services, analytical chemistry and toxicology for the medical device, pharmaceutical, food and feed, cosmetic, specialty chemical, and consumer product industries. **Remarks:** FDA registered; ISO 9002 Certified (BSI registered); AAALAC accredited. Geographic Area Served: United States, Canada, Japan, Europe.

Northfield

★ 14042 ★ Kaufman, Hall & Associates Inc.
1 Northfield Plz., Ste. 240
Northfield, IL 60093
Phone: (847)441-8780 **Fax:** (847)441-3288
Email: info@kaufmanhall.com
Website: http://www.kaufmanhall.com
Fnded: 1985. **Activities:** Provides capital advisory services to healthcare organizations, which includes financial and capital planning, debt acquisitions, merger and acquisition analysis, valuation, and capital allocation. Geographic Area Served: United States.

★ 14043 ★ KaufmanHall
1 Northfield Plz., Ste. 240
Northfield, IL 60093-1214
Phone: (847)441-8780 **Fax:** (847)441-3288
Email: KKaufman@Kaufmanhall.com
Website: http://www.kaufmanhall.com
Fnded: 1985. **Activities:** Firm provides financial planning and capital advisory services to healthcare organizations. Services include strategic financial and capital planning, financial advisory services to debt transactions, financial consultation to mergers, acquisitions, and divestitures and the design and implementation of capital allocation strategies. Geographic Area Served: United States.

Oak Brook

★ 14044 ★ Witt/Kieffer, Ford, Hadelman & Lloyd
2015 Spring Rd., Ste. 510
Oak Brook, IL 60523
Phone: (630)990-1370 **Fax:** (630)990-1382
Website: http://www.wittkieffer.com
Fnded: 1969. **Activities:** Witt/Kieffer is leading national executive search firm and the single largest that specializes in hospitals and health systems, including those with faith-based sponsors, as well as managed care and insurance companies; specialty, venture-capital-backed and e-Health corporations; physician group practices; colleges and universities and not-for-profit community service and cultural organizations. The firm has 13 offices across the country, an extensive database of executive talen nationwide and a variety of on line networking resources. Geographic Area Served: Worldwide.

Orland Park

★ 14045 ★ Aantia Kersey Phd & Associates
8318 W 138th Pl.
Orland Park, IL 60462
Phone: (708)460-6060 **Fax:** (708)460-6060
Email: antia@juno.com
Fnded: 1972. **Activities:** Human resources development consultants offering employee assistance programs in alcohol and substance abuse for employees with problems, psychological services to industry and public and private organizations, and on-the-spot or by-mail psychological testing programs for selection, promotion, and transfer of employees. Serves private industries as well as government agencies. Geographic Area Served: United States.

Palatine

★ 14046 ★ Diversified Biomedical Technologies Inc.
1110 Thackeray Dr., Ste. 170
Palatine, IL 60067
Phone: (847)496-5172 **Fax:** (847)934-8125
Email: info@dbtco.com
Website: http://www.dbtco.com
Fnded: 1987. **Activities:** Regulatory compliance consulting for the medical device and diagnostic industry. Includes strategic development of quality systems, CE mark, compliance and product approvals, validations, and analytical and clinical laboratory services. Geographic Area Served: Worldwide.

★ 14047 ★ Ventrone Ltd.
20278 N Rand Rd.
Palatine, IL 60074-2051
Phone: (847)550-9814 **Fax:** (847)438-9931
Fnded: 1985. **Activities:** Serves the healthcare industry in the areas of revenue enhancements, operational improvements, accounts receivable management, and productivity.

Rolling Meadows

★ 14048 ★ TriBrook Healthcare Consultants/American Express Tax & Business Services
1600 Golf Rd., Ste. 400
Rolling Meadows, IL 60008
Phone: (847)378-4400 **Free:** 800-323-7310
Fax: (847)378-4500
Email: douglas.r.rich@aexp.com
Website: http://www.tribrook.com
Fnded: 1972. **Activities:** National healthcare consulting practice active in strategic planning, managed care strategy, facilities and equipment planning, ambulatory care planning, mergers, acquisitions and affliations, and operations improvement. Geographic Area Served: United States.

Rosemont

★ 14049 ★ Metis Advisory Group Ltd.
10255 E Higgins Rd., Ste. 840
Rosemont, IL 60018
Phone: (847)993-0180 **Fax:** (847)993-0188
Email: metisltd@ metisltd.com
Website: http://www.metisltd.com
Fnded: 1984. **Activities:** Specializes in healthcare facilities planning, including long-range master facility planning, functional and space programming, departmental space planning and design, equipment planning and code and compliance reviews. Serves healthcare facilities in the U.S. and worldwide.

Schaumburg

★ 14050 ★ Impact Leadership Consultants Inc.
1701 E Woodfield Rd., Ste. 1095
Schaumburg, IL 60173
Phone: (847)240-2211 **Fax:** (847)240-2418
Email: pmc@impactleaders.com
Website: http://www.impactleaders.com
Fnded: 1992. **Activities:** An executive performance and leadership development firm that assists top management to enhance their leadership skills, ensure appropriate candidate selection and create a cultural reality consistent with organizational goals. Believes that achieving organizational health is integral to accomplishing organizational development goals and achieving sustained performance. Services include: leadership development, pre-hire selection, organizational effectiveness/culture evaluations, executive coaching, team retreats and leadership trainings. Industries served: Business, Managed Care, and Healthcare. **Remarks:** Unique backgrounds in psychology and psychiatry. Members of the Academy of Organizational and Occupational Psychiatry and Society of Industrial and Organizational Psychology. Geographic Area Served: United States, primarily Chicago area.

Skokie

★ 14051 ★ Dynamic Healthcare Consultant Inc.
3359 W Main St.
Skokie, IL 60076
Phone: (847)679-8219 **Fax:** (847)679-7377
Fnded: 1984. **Activities:** Healthcare consulting firm specialing in bookkeeping and accounting services to the medical and healthcare industries in Illinois.

South Elgin

★ 14052 ★ Safety & Loss Control Associates
PO Box 611
South Elgin, IL 60177-0611
Phone: (847)622-1690 **Fax:** (847)622-1695
Email: donneslund@aol.com
Website: http://www.safetyandlosscontrolassoc.com
Fnded: 1984. **Activities:** Assists contractors and industrial operators in reducing worker injuries and illnesses. Safety and training consulting includes employee training, supervisor and management seminars, OSHA compliance audits, pre-job inspections, expert witness work, accident investigation and reconstruction. Also provides expertise in ladders/scaffolds, fall protection, drugs/alcohol in work place, confined space entry, blasting and man produced vibration, driving, trench safety, Hazcom, and lockout/tagout. Serves the construction, insurance, legal profession, and manufacturing industries. Geographic Area Served: United States.

Tinley Park

★ 14053 ★ Infinitec, United Cerebral Palsy Association of Greater Chicago
7400 183rd St.
Tinley Park, IL 60477
Phone: (708)444-4202
Website: http://www.infinitec.org
Fnded: 1951. **Activities:** Information and referral services on assistive technology products and services for people with disabilities and their families, healthcare and rehabilitation professionals, funders and insurers, employers, and human relations professionals. Geographic Area Served: United States, primarily Illinois.

Westmont

★ 14054 ★ Police Consultants Inc.
825 N Cass Ave., Ste. 210
Westmont, IL 60559-1132
Phone: (630)325-2336 **Fax:** (630)325-3318
Fnded: 1968. **Activities:** Consultants specialize in police and fire testing for entrace and promotion. Offers in-depth psychological exams. Geographic Area Served: United States.

★ 14055 ★ Surgical Resource Management Inc.
582 Revere Ave.
Westmont, IL 60559-1237
Phone: (630)323-0540 **Fax:** (630)323-0576
Fnded: 1983. **Activities:** Specializes in surgical services in the following areas: operating rooms, post anesthesia care units, ambulatory surgery, and endoscopy.

Winnetka

★ 14056 ★ Hermann Associates
117 Church Rd.
Winnetka, IL 60093
Phone: (847)446-7640
Email: hygieology@aol.com
Fnded: 1963. **Activities:** Offers counsel in the recognition, evaluation, and control of occupational health hazards. Activities include environmental and occupational toxicology, industrial and municipal waste treatment problems, industrial hygiene of oil refining, chemical processing, and hearing conservation. Provides expert witness testimony. Serves private industries as well as government agencies. **Remarks:** Toxicity, photosynthetic/chemosynthetic waste treatment, hearing conservation, thresholds. Geographic Area Served: United States.

Indiana

Brownsburg

★ 14057 ★ Med-Rec Systems Inc.
23 Blvd. Motif St.
Brownsburg, IN 46112
Phone: (317)852-9733 **Fax:** (317)852-9733
Email: medrec@msn.com
Fnded: 1984. **Activities:** Specializes in providing quality medical record consulting to long-term care facilities, ambulatory care centers, and physicians' offices. Experienced Registered Record Administrators (R.R.A.'s) and Accredited Record Technicians (A.R.T.'s) assist in the design and development of effective medical record systems for healthcare settings. Also routinely assists facilities in monitoring the quality of required healthcare documentation.

Carmel

★ 14058 ★ Medical Communicators
11078 Huntington Ct.
Carmel, IN 46033
Phone: (317)843-2065 **Fax:** (317)843-1914
Email: Kurtullman@sprintmail.com
Website: http://home.sprintmail.com/~kurtullman
Fnded: 1987. **Activities:** Public relations consultancy for hospitals, physicians and other healthcare-related businesses. Assists in preparation of medical newsletters and magazines. Also assists in production of conferences and seminars. Utilizes audiovisual services for patient teaching, referral source recruitment, public relations presentation, and support for lectures, talks, and meetings. Geographic Area Served: Indiana, Ohio, Michigan, Illinois, and Kentucky.

Delphi

★ 14059 ★ Noteworthy Creations Inc.
209 N Connelly St.
Delphi, IN 46923
Phone: (765)564-4167 **Free:** 800-305-4167
Fax: (765)564-4280
Email: mayfield@funwithfood.com
Website: http://www.funwithfood.com
Fnded: 1992. **Activities:** Offers nutritional assessment and dietary education consultation to individuals and groups. Makes presentations to all age groups on nutrition-related topics. Also sells nutrition education curricula, books, and tapes. Geographic Area Served: Primarily United States but some international business as well.

Evansville

★ 14060 ★ Environmental Management Consultants Inc.
427 Main St.
Evansville, IN 47708
Phone: (812)424-7768 **Fax:** (812)424-7797
Email: emc@emcevv.com
Website: http://www.emcevv.com
Fnded: 1988. **Activities:** Offers environmental consulting in the following areas: air and water quality monitoring; environmental site assessments; training; underground and aboveground storage tanks; industrial regulatory compliance; and hazardous materials cleanups. Serves all industries in Indiana, Kentucky, and Illinois areas. Geographic Area Served: IN, KY, TN, IL, and OH.

Indianapolis

★ 14061 ★ Artekna
321 E New York St.
Indianapolis, IN 46204
Phone: (317)579-5300 **Free:** 888-479-5300
Fax: (317)579-5301
Email: tfrank@artekna.com
Website: http://www.artekna.com
Fnded: 1988. **Activities:** Architectural firm specializing in healthcare facilities.

★ 14062 ★ Continuum Solutions Consulting
9365 Counselors Row, Ste. 300
Indianapolis, IN 46240
Phone: (317)819-7666 **Fax:** (317)819-7288
Email: dmiesle@continuumsolutions.com
Website: http://www.continuumsolutions.com
Activities: A healthcare management and planning consulting firm. Specializes in facility planning; asset and facility management; strategic planning; and operations management. Geographic Area Served: United States.

★ 14063 ★ Health Care Services Inc.
Prospective Medicine Ctr.
6220 Lawrence Dr.
Indianapolis, IN 46226
Phone: (317)549-3600 **Fax:** (317)549-3670
Fnded: 1976. **Activities:** Health care consulting group provides expertise in health wellness programs and health hazard appraisal and analysis. **Remarks:** Firm is affiliated with Beacon Services and Medical Research Consortium Inc. Beacon Services. Geographic Area Served: United States.

★ 14064 ★ HMO Executive Search
3500 Depauw Blvd.
Indianapolis, IN 46268
Phone: (317)872-1056 **Free:** 800-729-1056
Fax: (317)879-1233
Email: mail@searchprogroup.com
Website: http://www.hmoexecutivesearch.com
Fnded: 1976. **Activities:** HMO Executive Search personnel consultants service the general recruitment needs of all HMOs, PPOs, TPAs and all managed care firms in the U.S. Also provide retained and contingency search. Geographic Area Served: Worldwide.

★ 14065 ★ Jack J. Bulloff Consulting and Expert Witness Services
8140 Township Line Rd.
Indianapolis, IN 46260-5866
Phone: (317)824-0014 **Fax:** (317)824-0589

Fnded: 1968. Activities: Chemical and environmental consultant and expert witness offers expertise in the following areas: occupational and environmental safety and health, hazardous chemicals and waste management/disposal, research and development and innovation information development, environmental impact/technology assessment, technological forecasting, and planning. Particular specialization offered in metallic soaps, polymer thickeners, drag reducers, photoultra microminiaturization/MOVCD, heteropoly oxyionic electrolytes and solid-state conductors, photomaterials, radcure materials, etchants and corrosives, flammable and/or explosive vapors and mixtures, biohazards, radio hazards, carboxymethyl dextrans and celluloses, odor control agents, and toxic materials. Additional assistance provided in compliance/litigation regarding federal, state and local laws and regulations compliances, product and process defects, liabilities, and patents. Industries served: chemical and allied products and processes and related industries (SIC 20-36 inclusive), graphic arts and related industries (printing, duplicating, and copying); hazardous wastes management and remediation industries; and phototechnologies. Polymath bibliography, bibliotechnology, and electronic information for any of the foregoing if requested. Patent disclosure agreement included. Geographic Area Served: Worldwide, but limited to English-speaking countries or enterprises.

★ 14066 ★ Karl Manders, MD
c/o Neurosurgical Associates of Indiana
7369 Shadeland Sta., Ste. 100
Indianapolis, IN 46256
Phone: (317)577-3900 **Fax:** (317)579-7459
Activities: Medico-legal consultancy offers expertise in neurological surgery, review, depositions, and trial testimony. **Remarks:** Board certified in pain medicine and neurological surgery. Geographic Area Served: Worldwide.

★ 14067 ★ Lawson & Associates
2625 N Meridian, No. 1011
Indianapolis, IN 46208
Phone: (317)283-1031 **Fax:** (317)283-6732
Email: mhslawson@aol.com
Fnded: 1972. **Activities:** Human resources consultants with expertise in personnel management, organization and management development, corporate culture, corporate wellness programming, and career guidance. Industries served: manufacturing, service, hospitals, banking, nonprofits, and government agencies. Geographic Area Served: United States.

★ 14068 ★ Medical Research Consortium Inc.
6220 Lawrence Dr.
Indianapolis, IN 46226
Phone: (317)549-3131 **Fax:** (317)549-3670
Fnded: 1993. **Activities:** Conduct and consult on research studies and clinical trials. **Remarks:** Firm is affiliated with Medical Research Consortium, Inc. and Health Care Services, Inc. Beacon Services, LLC. Geographic Area Served: United States.

★ 14069 ★ National Federation of Medical/Legal Networks Inc.
840 Spring Mill Ln.
Indianapolis, IN 46260
Phone: (317)253-9080 **Free:** 800-727-7966
Fax: (317)257-2375
Fnded: 1987. **Activities:** Provides consultative advice and renders expert medical opinions to attorneys, hospitals and insurance companies involving medical-legal problems, i.e., medical malpractice litigation and risk management problems. Primary expertise involves pediatric patients (age 0-21 years) with special interest in areas of infectious diseases, newborn, pulmonary and kidney problems. Also provides "networking" service for attorneys who desire non-pediatric medical experts and non-medical experts as the case merits it. Offers additional consultative advice on risk management for ambulatory medical settings. Geographic Area Served: Primarily the Midwest.

★ 14070 ★ Schick & Affiliates Inc.
320 E 45th, Ste. 100
Indianapolis, IN 46205-1752
Phone: (317)283-2262
Fnded: 1984. **Activities:** Firm provides general management consulting services to the healthcare industry. Areas of specialized knowledge include systems for quantification of nursing care requirements in a variety of settings. Microcomputer based software supports results of projects. Geographic Area Served: United States.

Lebanon

★ 14071 ★ Occupational Health & Hygiene Corp. of America
419 Ransdell Rd.
Lebanon, IN 46052-2348
Phone: (765)482-7652 **Free:** (866)203-3197
Fax: (765)482-7658
Website: http://www.ohhca.com
Fnded: 1989. **Activities:** Counsels in industrial health, offering mobile/industrial and environmental health testing. Industries served: manufacturing and utilites in the United States. Geographic Area Served: United States.

Mount Vernon

★ 14072 ★ Toxicology Pathology Services Inc.
10424 Middle Mt. Vernon Rd.
Mount Vernon, IN 47620
Phone: (812)985-5900 **Free:** 800-837-8771
Fax: (812)985-3403
Email: tps@toxpath.com
Fnded: 1975. **Activities:** Evaluates animal safety data including toxicology, body weight, clinical pathology, gross and microscopic pathology, organ weights, clinical signs and statistics for the pharmaceutical, chemical, petrochemical, and agricultural industries. Emphasis is on product safety through animal research. Geographic Area Served: United States.

Muncie

★ 14073 ★ Nicki C. Turner, M.D.
4009 W Cornbread Rd.
Muncie, IN 47302
Phone: (765)286-2111 **Fax:** (765)286-2134
Activities: More than 15 years experience in: critical care, adults 17 years; clinical nutrition, including that of hospitalized, critically ill patients; EHA; and complex internal medicine.

Noblesville

★ 14074 ★ Professional Counseling Centers of Indiana
543 Coventry Way
Noblesville, IN 46060-9024
Phone: (317)846-7999 **Fax:** (317)574-5063
Activities: Business counselors offer expertise in the following areas: employee assistance, managed care, alcohol and drug treatment, labor and union consultation, and industrial mental health.

Notre Dame

★ 14075 ★ Security Audit Inc.
PO Box 1005
Notre Dame, IN 46556
Phone: (574)277-2560 **Fax:** (574)277-2560
Email: secaudit@mindspring.com
Website: http://www.iapsc.org/rmurphy
Fnded: 1977. **Activities:** A management consulting firm specializing in security. Areas of expertise include security management and loss prevention security. Serves healthcare, financial and educational institutions, businesses and industrial firms. Geographic Area Served: United States.

Terre Haute

★ 14076 ★ Ann Marriner-Tomey
c/o Indiana State University, School of Nursing
8th & Chestnut
Terre Haute, IN 47809
Phone: (812)234-8072 **Fax:** (812)237-4300
Email: A-Tomey@indstate.edu
Website: http://mama.indstate.edu/users/tomey
Fnded: 1976. **Activities:** Human resource consultant providing leadership, management, conflict management, decision making, performance appraisal, time management, and motivation theory for educational and healthcare agencies, including hospitals, public health organizations, and government agencies. Geographic Area Served: Worldwide.

Iowa

Cedar Falls

★ 14077 ★ Key Automation
201 Washington St.
Cedar Falls, IA 50613
Website: http://www.keyauto.com
Fnded: 1988. **Activities:** Provides engineering knowledge to consumer goods manufacturers, food producers, and pharmaceutical companies in the U.S.

Cedar Rapids

★ 14078 ★ Michael L. Bradnan & Associates Ltd.
5750 Country Ln. NE
Cedar Rapids, IA 52411
Phone: (319)395-0395 **Fax:** (319)395-0395
Fnded: 1977. **Activities:** Food service design consultants specializing in creative solutions for planning, design and management problems in food service. Services include the following skills: design equipment selection, specifications, facilities layout, and decor; management - employee training, menu planning, including recipe formulation, testing, food specification, nutrition, portioning and packaging, and simplified cooking methods, and troubleshooting; planning - market research, feasibility studies, concept planning, and marketing studies. Clients include health centers, hotels, country clubs, school feeding programs, restaurants, government facilities, and correctional institutions. Geographic Area Served: United States and Europe -Mid East and Far East.

Decorah

★ 14079 ★ Human Development Center
220 E Water St.
Decorah, IA 52101
Phone: (319)382-3713
Email: sayer@rconnect.com
Fnded: 1977. **Activities:** Distress and tension management consultants advising on how to enhance personal effectiveness, productivity, creativity, and health; and to affect these qualities in others. Programs are designed for upper management, the nursing profession, designated participants, and the general public. Geographic Area Served: Worldwide.

Des Moines

★ 14080 ★ Sue Roberts Health Concepts
1515 Linden St.
Des Moines, IA 50309
Phone: (515)247-0014 **Fax:** (515)247-0016
Email: sue@healthconceptsinc.com
Website: http://www.healthconceptsinc.com
Fnded: 1981. **Activities:** Nutrition consultants providing individual patient consulting: group seminars and workshops; development and implementation of em-

ployee wellness programs for business and industry; and consultation to food producers, processors and marketers. Serves private industries as well as government agencies. Geographic Area Served: United States.

Indianola

★ 14081 ★ Herbert R. Heinicke
1302 W Boston Ave.
Indianola, IA 50125
Phone: (515)961-8933 **Fax:** (515)961-8903
Email: rayheinicke@compuserve.com
Fnded: 1971. **Activities:** Technical consultant to pet food, food, and feed industries in such areas as product and ingredient development, quality assurance, nutritional evaluation, government and regulatory compliance, and production trouble shooting services. Serves private industries as well as government agencies. Geographic Area Served: Worldwide.

Kansas

Leawood

★ 14082 ★ Klein Consultant Services
12726 Overbrook Rd.
Leawood, KS 66209
Phone: (913)338-3001 **Fax:** (913)338-3039
Email: kleinmarkettest@aol.com
Fnded: 1977. **Activities:** Full service market research company specializes in package goods, medical services, pharmaceuticals and small city research. Serves private industries as well as government agencies. Geographic Area Served: United States with focus on small towns.

★ 14083 ★ Telemedicine Today
5101 College Blv. No. 206
Leawood, KS 66211-1619
Phone: (913)338-1496 **Fax:** (913)338-3631
Email: info@telemedtoday.com
Website: http://www.telemedtoday.com
Fnded: 1993. **Activities:** Dr. Allen provides strategic planning, workshops, and other expert services in telemedicine. He has been a principal with the U. of Kansas-affiliated Telemedicine Project since 1992. Has widely lectured in North America, Europe, and Latin America; organized and participated in dozens of telemedicine workshops and seminars. Serves university and private hospitals, governmental agencies, and private corporations worldwide.

Mission

★ 14084 ★ Helios Inc.
6820 W 52nd Pl., Ste. 1A
Mission, KS 66202
Phone: (913)262-6520 **Fax:** (913)262-6520
Email: cdstout2@email.msn.com
Fnded: 1988. **Activities:** Offers education programs, fundraising, program development and enhancement, case management, legal compliance, complaint handling skills and techniques, ombudsman program support, public benefit program development, mediation and resolution; document review: inconsistencies, authenticity and corroboration of facts; techniques: interviewing people to secure maximum information, deposition questions formulated; and resources identified. Serves private industry as well as government agencies. Geographic Area Served: Worldwide.

Neosho Rapids

★ 14085 ★ Helen Tredway
1638 Rd. W
Neosho Rapids, KS 66864-8700
Phone: (620)343-3637 **Fax:** (620)342-8175
Fnded: 1982. **Activities:** Nursing consultant to nursing homes. Services include inservice education.

Olathe

★ 14086 ★ NCES Inc.
1904 E 123rd
Olathe, KS 66061
Free: 888-545-5653 **Fax:** 800-251-9349
Email: info@ncescatalog.com
Website: http://www.ncescatalog.com
Fnded: 1980. **Activities:** Nutrition consultants who offer mail order book services. Geographic Area Served: United States.

Overland Park

★ 14087 ★ C.L. Gerwick & Associates Inc.
10560 Barkley, Ste. 340
Overland Park, KS 66212
Phone: (913)383-3464 **Free:** 888-383-3464
Fax: (913)383-3729
Email: info@clgerwick.com
Website: http://www.clgerwick.com
Fnded: 1965. **Activities:** Consulting dietitians provide service to small hospitals, extended care facilities, group homes, government agencies. Develops educational materials. Geographic Area Served: Kansas Missouri.

Salina

★ 14088 ★ Wellplan Inc.
617 E Elm
Salina, KS 67401
Phone: (785)825-8224 **Fax:** (785)825-0644
Email: wellplan@comcarepa.com
Website: http://www.comcarepa.com
Fnded: 1981. **Activities:** Offers consultation on health maintenance and improvement through positive lifestyles. Individual counseling on disease prevention and maintenance through medical nutrition and exercise therapy. Group programs are also offered. Geographic Area Served: Salina Region.

Shawnee Mission

★ 14089 ★ KAYTRON
12015 Pawnee Ln.
Shawnee Mission, KS 66209
Phone: (913)663-5298 **Fax:** (913)663-5298
Email: rplous@worldnet.att.net
Website: http://www.kaytron.to
Activities: A healthcare consulting firm that focuses on the integration of medical and engineering principles to the healthcare industry. Functions as a virtual engineering consulting firm. The range of services spans all medical and operational disciplines within the healthcare delivery system.

★ 14090 ★ Pharmaceutical Consultants Inc.
PO Box 7003
Shawnee Mission, KS 66207-0003
Phone: (913)491-9825 **Fax:** (913)491-9829
Email: beth@pharmconsult.com
Website: http://www.pharmconsult.com
Fnded: 1985. **Activities:** Regulatory and Clinical Consultants in the areas of Research and Development of Drugs and Devices. Geographic Area Served: United States.

Topeka

★ 14091 ★ Hatcher Consultants Inc.
2955 SW Wanamaker Dr.
Topeka, KS 66614
Phone: (785)271-5557 **Fax:** (785)271-8333
Activities: A consulting group composed of experienced individuals in the substance abuse program field. Provides substance abuse consulting. Evaluates existing substance abuse programs and make them more effective and cost-efficient. Develops new programs. Trains employees to detect the earliest stage of drug abuse and, if appropriate, identify a program of treatment. Conducts training workshops.

Westwood

★ 14092 ★ Virden Associates
1900 W 47th Pl., Ste. 218
Westwood, KS 66205
Phone: (913)362-2813 **Fax:** (913)362-2813
Email: mvirden@virdenassociates.com
Website: http://www.virdenassociates.com
Fnded: 1987. **Activities:** Marketing consultancy provides expertise in strategic planning, market research, site analysis, demographic studies, and housing market studies geared to health and safety related industries. Industries served: healthcare, retirement housing, school districts, and real estate development. Geographic Area Served: Primary: midwest; secondary: United States.

Wichita

★ 14093 ★ Ed Greif and Co. Inc.
4110 N Tara Cir.
Wichita, KS 67226-3301
Phone: (316)636-5515 **Fax:** (316)236-6701
Fnded: 1983. **Activities:** Sales and marketing consultant with expertise in the development and marketing of sophisticated products and techniques, including microsurgery scopes and instruments, laser surgery, silicone implants, radiation diagnostics and oncology, video technology, and computers. Also offers sales and management workshops and seminars ranging from one hour to three days, tailored to the specific needs and frame of reference of the audience. The goal: to get everyone to share the same vision simultaneously. Industries served: medical, pharmaceutical, high-tech and healthcare providers (including hospitals, HMO's, associations, etc.). Geographic Area Served: Worldwide.

Kentucky

Owenton

★ 14094 ★ Irene Bilyeu
110 E Adair St., Ste. 101
Owenton, KY 40359-3062
Phone: (502)484-2149
Fnded: 1982. **Activities:** Nursing service consultant who assists providers of healthcare in the effective use of their assets, helps them to visualize potential growth, and minimize or eliminate deficiencies. Serves hospitals, nursing homes, and home health agencies throughout the state of Kentucky. Serves private industries as well as government agencies. Limiting activities to family based problems in residence and today's problems in the family, schools, and community at no charge. Geographic Area Served: Kentucky.

Prestonsburg

★ 14095 ★ Medisin Inc., Medical Waste/ Environmental Consulting
5032 Kentucky Rte. 321
Prestonsburg, KY 41653
Phone: (606)886-6955 **Fax:** (606)886-0450
Fnded: 1989. **Activities:** Environmental consulting firm focuses primarily on medical waste.

Louisiana

Alexandria

★ 14096 ★ Amedisys Inc.
5503 John Eskew Blvd.
Alexandria, LA 71303-3725
Phone: (318)442-3100
Activities: A provider and manager of alternate site health care services. Offers home health care consulting services.

Baton Rouge

★ 14097 ★ Encore Associates Inc.
3851 S Sherwood Forest Blvd., Ste. 500
Baton Rouge, LA 70816
Phone: (225)291-7080 **Free:** 800-321-0059
Fax: (225)291-7392
Email: encore21@encore21.com
Website: http://www.encore21.com
Fnded: 1984. **Activities:** Firm provides software development services for medical practices.

Covington

★ 14098 ★ V-Labs Inc.
423 N Theard St.
Covington, LA 70433
Phone: (985)893-0533 **Fax:** (985)893-0517
Email: v-labs@v-labs.com
Website: http://www.v-labs.com
Fnded: 1979. **Activities:** Offers analytical service for carbohydrates and polysaccharides. Performs contract research and consulting for biotechnology, pharmaceutical, chemical, and food companies. Services include analysis of sugar processing products, dietary fiber determination, custom synthesis and polysaccharide modification, and computerized data acquisition and reporting. Geographic Area Served: Worldwide.

Gretna

★ 14099 ★ Kroll Laboratory Specialists Inc.
1111 Newton St.
Gretna, LA 70053
Phone: (504)361-8989 **Fax:** (504)361-1530
Email: info@krollworldwide.com
Website: http://www.kroll-labs.com
Fnded: 1978. **Activities:** Provides consulting services for industry and business requiring drug screens and confirmations of drug usage in employees. Offers four basic types of programs: for cause, preemployment, accident related, and random screens. Services include expert legal testimony.

Metairie

★ 14100 ★ Drug Education Associates Inc.
4729 Trenton St.
Metairie, LA 70006
Phone: (504)454-6933 **Fax:** (504)454-6934
Email: Customer_Service@globalsafety.net
Website: http://www.globalsafety.net
Fnded: 1981. **Activities:** Develops, designs, and implements corporate, government and educational institutions' response to drug abuse prevention, detection and suppression. Provides assistance in policy and procedure design, training, education and establishment of setting of employer-based drug prevention and detection programs, especially involving drug testing, searches, use of drug detector dogs, undercover approaches, honesty testing and traditional investigative means. Principals have expertise in areas of drug enforcement, law, pharmacology, toxicology, research and behavior; and have testified as expert witnesses in many courts. Geographic Area Served: Worldwide.

★ 14101 ★ Global Safety & Security Inc.
4729 Trenton St.
Metairie, LA 70006
Phone: (504)454-6933 **Free:** 800-938-3782
Fax: (504)454-6934
Email: Customer_Service@globalsafety.net
Website: http://www.globalsafety.net
Fnded: 1983. **Activities:** Designs, develops and delivers drug abuse detection programs, including: drug investigators, drug detector dogs, drug screen urinalysis, and urine sample collection. Serves private industries as well as government agencies.

★ 14102 ★ Nursing Knowledge Inc.
2540 Severn Ave., Ste. 206
Metairie, LA 70002
Phone: (504)887-0401 **Free:** 800-359-5114
Email: nursknow@aol.com
Fnded: 1979. **Activities:** Consultants in continuing education programs for nurses principally in hospitals, other healthcare agencies, and colleges. Also serves government agencies. Additionally provides courses on instructional media production and use. Geographic Area Served: United States.

Monroe

★ 14103 ★ H.M. Mehendale
The University of Louisiana at Monroe
College of Pharmacy
Department of Toxicology
Monroe, LA 71209-0495
Phone: (318)342-1691 **Fax:** (318)342-1686
Email: pymehendale@ulm.edu
Website: http://www.ulm.edu.pharmacy/mehendale.default.htm
Fnded: 1990. **Activities:** Toxicology specialist. Areas of expertise include chemical toxicology, pesticides, solvents, and other industrial chemicals; cancer; regulatory affairs; occupational or accidental exposures and short- or long-term hazards; hazardous wastes; forensic toxicological analysis of extraneous evidence; body fluids and tissues, drugs, and intoxicants; and exposure to single or combinations of chemicals; chemical interactions; and toxicological data interpretations. Error in medications and related issues. Geographic Area Served: Worldwide.

New Orleans

★ 14104 ★ JLN, MD Associates L.L.C.
4939 Chestnut St.
New Orleans, LA 70115-2941
Phone: (504)899-7893 **Fax:** (504)899-7557
Email: jln@jln-md.com
Website: http://jln-md.com
Activities: Consultant in infectious diseases, disease/demand management, healthcare quality assurance, NCQA/regulatory compliance, and an expert witness.

★ 14105 ★ Marcantelli Group
PO Box 29744
New Orleans, LA 70130
Phone: (504)522-5111
Fnded: 1981. **Activities:** Specializes in investigations attorney services, asset searches, skip tracing, certified fraud investigations, security consulting, and travel security consulting for Mexico, Central and South America. Geographic Area Served: North America, Central & South America, Southeast Asia.

★ 14106 ★ Methodist Health System Foundation Inc.
5620 Read Blvd.
New Orleans, LA 70127-3154
Phone: (504)244-5962 **Fax:** (504)244-4585
Fnded: 1981. **Activities:** Advises regional hospitals on healthcare management.

Port Allen

★ 14107 ★ Kathleen Babbitt
1590 Court St., No. 50
Port Allen, LA 70767-2500
Phone: (225)343-5539
Activities: Provides consultations on alternate healing processes to health problems and health issues using a natural healing approach instead of drugs and surgery. Serves all industries in all geographic locations.

Thibodaux

★ 14108 ★ Gordon Whyte & Associates
216 Lafourche Dr.
Thibodaux, LA 70301-2518
Phone: (985)447-8592 **Free:** 800-232-9550
Fax: (985)447-1614
Fnded: 1990. **Activities:** Wide variety of hands-on experience in the marketing and management of healthcare facilities. Can provide professional consultation and services or can facilitate workshops, seminars and conferences in each of the following areas: strategic planning, marketing research, survey and focus group research, organizational marketing audits, board retreats, and staff/management development. Industries served: healthcare and long term care. Geographic Area Served: Southeastern and southwestern United States.

Maine

Bangor

★ 14109 ★ Affiliated Healthcare Management
925 Union St., Ste. 2
PO Box 811
Bangor, ME 04402-0811
Phone: (207)973-6700 **Fax:** (207)973-6725
Fnded: 1977. **Activities:** Management consulting firm specializes in serving the healthcare industry.

Bridgton

★ 14110 ★ Western Maine Nutrition Counseling
48 Main St.
Bridgton, ME 04009
Phone: (207)647-3517 **Fax:** (207)647-3517
Fnded: 1987. **Activities:** Provides individualized therapeutic and weight loss diet counseling. Conducts group weight loss programs. Acts as a resource and referral person for physicians. Geographic Area Served: Oxford and Cumberland Counties, Maine.

Portland

★ 14111 ★ Stroudwater NHG
443 Congress St.
Portland, ME 04101
Phone: (207)756-6090 **Free:** 800-947-5712
Fax: (207)828-0821
Email: jreuthe@stroudwaternhg.com
Website: http://www.stroudwaternhg.com
Fnded: 1985. **Activities:** Offers a multi-faceted approach to medical management consulting. Specializes in network development performance improvement, relationship building, strategic and program planning.

Skowhegan

★ 14112 ★ Occupational Health Research
28 Research Dr.
PO Box 900
Skowhegan, ME 04976
Phone: (207)474-8432 **Free:** 800-444-8432
Fax: (207)474-6398
Email: consult-ed@systoc.com
Website: http://www.systoc.com
Fnded: 1985. **Activities:** OHR offers a cost effective approach to occupational health program development, product enhancement and operational improvement. Our consulting associates provide a broad range of services to help health care organizations establish high quality, competitive occupational health programs tailored to their market areas. Each project is unique and our consultants always create client-specific solutions. No assessment or report is ever produced using standardized forms, templates, or methods. **Remarks:** We offer quarterly journal, The Occupational Health Tracker, which provides 24

pages of professional articles. Call to subscribe. Geographic Area Served: United States.

South Portland

★ 14113 ★ Diets Limited
527 Sawyer St.
South Portland, ME 04106
Phone: (207)799-6394 **Fax:** (207)799-7695
Email: rxnutriton@aol.com

Fnded: 1978. **Activities:** Provides professional healthcare counseling, specializing in nutrition and diet modification for individuals of all ages, groups, healthcare professionals, business/industry, and the media. Also offers food service management to institutions. Geographic Area Served: Southern Maine Cumberland and York counties.

Topsham

★ 14114 ★ Smith Diabetes Research
PO Box 543
Topsham, ME 04086
Phone: (207)725-4899 **Fax:** (207)729-3219

Fnded: 1993. **Activities:** Offers information to doctors, patients, and lawyers on a correlation between THORAZINE (chlorpromazine, LARGACTIL), a psychiatric drug, and insulin-dependent diabetes. Seeks to substantiate the working hypothesis that CPZ causes diabetes and death generally. **Remarks:** Affiliated with United States Department of Justice and the Courts (under the False Claims Act). Geographic Area Served: Worldwide.

Vinalhaven

★ 14115 ★ The Haystack Group Inc.
15 High St.
PO Box 823
Vinalhaven, ME 04863-0823
Phone: (207)863-2793 **Fax:** (207)863-9916
Email: islandman@haystack-group.com
Website: http://www.haystack-group.com

Fnded: 1994. **Activities:** A retained executive search consultancy providing exhaustive executive search and search research services to firms withing the medical device, biotechnology, pharmaceutical, and health-care information technology industries.

Westbrook

★ 14116 ★ Northeast Test Consultants
587 Spring St.
Westbrook, ME 04092
Phone: (207)854-3939 **Free:** 800-888-3911
Fax: (207)854-3659
Email: info@netest.com
Website: http://www.netest.com

Fnded: 1983. **Activities:** Industrial test consultants offer expertise in asbestos testing, lead testing, and industrial hygiene.

Maryland

Baltimore

★ 14117 ★ Air Analysis Associates of America Inc.
1005 W 36th St.
Baltimore, MD 21211-2416
Phone: (410)366-0250 **Fax:** (410)235-6240

Fnded: 1987. **Activities:** Full service industrial hygiene and environmental consultation firm. Conducts indoor air quality surveys, building surveys and inspections, comprehensive air monitoring and sampling, asbestos and hazardous substance abatement monitoring and planning, and lead paint surveys. Also offer Phase I and Phase II environmental site assessments, specification design, safety and health programs, worker right-to-know programs, total project oversight, accident investigation, expert testimony, training services, and in-house laboratory capabilities. Industries served: banking, government agencies, health, legal, real estate, and private sector. Geographic Area Served: United States.

★ 14118 ★ Block, McGibony, Bellmore and Associates
3609 Woodvalley Dr.
Baltimore, MD 21208
Phone: (410)486-1092 **Free:** 800-554-7200
Fax: (410)484-9884

Fnded: 1958. **Activities:** Hospital administration consultants focusing on four areas: (1) strategic planning, to strengthen the hospital's competitive and financial position; (2) market development, to identify market segments in which the client has distinct competencies, establishing specific market share objectives for each segment, and applying marketing techniques to achieve these objectives; (3) regulatory agency activities, to prepare and defend certificates of need or changes; and (4) litigation support, to prepare technical analyses and expert testimony at the request of the hospital's counsel.

★ 14119 ★ Bolton Offutt Donovan Inc.
575 S Charles St., Ste. 500
Baltimore, MD 21201-2428
Phone: (410)547-0500 **Fax:** (410)685-1924
Email: info@boltonpartners.com
Website: http://www.bodgroup.net

Activities: Employee benefit planning firm offers particular expertise with retirement and health insurance benefits. Geographic Area Served: United States.

★ 14120 ★ C.M. Citrenbaum & Assoc.
2 Hamill Rd., Ste. 322
Baltimore, MD 21210
Phone: (410)433-6555 **Fax:** (410)433-6565
Email: ccitren@aol.com
Website: http://www.headmenders.com

Fnded: 1978. **Activities:** Psychological services and training in leadership, management and communication skills; wellness/habit control and stress management programs. Geographic Area Served: United States, primarily mid-Atlantic.

★ 14121 ★ Dodge-Marck Associates
8 S Broadway
Baltimore, MD 21231
Phone: (410)276-8775
Email: granitewyo@aol.com

Fnded: 1987. **Activities:** Develops and conducts informative and entertaining seminars for a broad spectrum of audiences ranging from active business managers to retired persons from all walks of life. Subjects range from re-building husband and wife teams to regenerating corporate management. The core of each seminar focuses on personal growth and the use of humor, among several instruments, to stimulate a new outlook on life.

★ 14122 ★ EpiHealth
7904 Starburst Dr.
Baltimore, MD 21208-3033
Phone: (410)484-9133 **Free:** 800-969-1441
Fax: (410)484-9515
Email: ehacorporate@msn.com
Website: http://www.epihealth.com/

Fnded: 1980. **Activities:** A consulting firm specializing in providing environmental health, public health and infectious disease epidemiological investigation and litigation support services to an international clientele in the legal, insurance and business fields. Conducts a detailed investigation of the premises and facilities involved, including sampling and laboratory testing. Analyzes technical information to determine its impact on case or claim, including providing effective expert witness testimony.

★ 14123 ★ The Haner Group Inc.
1507 Druid Hill Ave.
Baltimore, MD 21217
Phone: (410)383-3337 **Fax:** (410)383-3338

Fnded: 1991. **Activities:** Registered dietitians who counsel patients referred by physicians regarding nutrition. Also plan menus for healthcare institutions and sometimes train staff. Conduct continuing education activities for dietitians also. Industries served: pregnant Medicaid recipients, diabetic Medicaid recipients, pediatric Medicaid recipients from birth through age 20, and subscribers to Travelers Managed Care Services are covered; other clients are expected to pay at the time of service. Geographic Area Served: Baltimore, Maryland, and surrounding counties.

★ 14124 ★ Heritage Theatre Artists Censortion
116 W University Pky., Penthouse 3
Baltimore, MD 21210
Phone: (410)235-4457 **Fax:** (410)235-4457
Email: hlynn@h-t-a-c.com
Website: http://www.h-t-a-c.com

Fnded: 1985. **Activities:** Human resource development group promotes excellence in the workplace through programs, print and video services. Offers communications training and on-camera skills. An employee wellness program (Alive and Well) consists of over 15 training topics to boost productivity, reduce stress, and reduce healthcare costs. Also designs employee/patient education materials (four-color/print); healthcare related videos, and coordinate and produce special events. Industries served: health, service, and government agencies in Maryland, Washington DC, and Northern Virginia. **Remarks:** Subsidary of Communications Health/Network, Inc. Geographic Area Served: Worldwide.

★ 14125 ★ Insect Control & Research Inc.
1330 Dillon Heights Ave.
Baltimore, MD 21228
Phone: (410)747-4500 **Fax:** (410)747-4928
Email: icr@erols.com
Website: http://www.icrlab.com

Fnded: 1946. **Activities:** Pesticide registration, testing (GLP & Non-GLP), and screening specialists offer consulting on vector borne diseases and household and public health pests. Industries served: chemical, pest control, pharmaceutical, and government agencies. Geographic Area Served: Worldwide.

★ 14126 ★ MEC Health Care Inc.
100 Park Ave.
Baltimore, MD 21201
Phone: (410)752-1981 **Free:** 800-766-4393
Fax: (410)752-1990

Fnded: 1986. **Activities:** Managed healthcare firm devotes itself to eliminating unnecessary medical costs in eye care while promoting superior quality care. Firm has formulated a successful model incorporating customized software, utilization review, credentialing, quality assurance, claims and billings, authorizations and triage.

★ 14127 ★ SHR Associates Inc.
3700 Koppers St., Ste. 204
Baltimore, MD 21227
Phone: (410)644-0772

Fnded: 1981. **Activities:** Advises on shared health resources, assisting physicians, hospitals, and nursing homes in Illinois, Michigan, New York, New Jersey, Maryland, and Washington D.C.

★ 14128 ★ Solucient L.L.C.
300 E Lombard St., Ste. 1600
Baltimore, MD 21202
Phone: (410)576-9600 **Free:** 800-568-3282
Fax: (410)576-9429
Website: http://www.solucient.com

Fnded: 1985. **Activities:** Provides comparative/normative information concerning the cost and quality of healthcare. Specific areas of expertise include review of patterns of patient care, drug and clinical service utilization, and approaches for quality improvement and utilization management, primarily for acute care facilities. Industries served: education, government agencies, healthcare, nonprofit organizations, and pharmaceutical. Geographic Area Served: Worldwide.

★ 14129 ★ SPA Inc.
203 W 11th Ave.
Baltimore, MD 21225
Phone: (410)789-5888 **Fax:** (410)636-7310
Email: stan@spainco.com
Website: http://spainco.com
Fnded: 1981. **Activities:** Provides research analysis and consultative services in the areas of safety, health, human factors engineering, and risk management to private industry, insurance and legal communities, government, and trade organizations. These services include, but are not limited to analysis of facilities, products, operations, and equipment; programs to detect programmatic, physical or environmental hazards/failures, coupled with recommendations of needed solutions/methods to mitigate or eliminate hazardous and/or high risk conditions and/or lower insurance and worker compensation costs; and seminar development production.

★ 14130 ★ STAR Associates Inc.
The BeuMar Bldg.
12 W Montgomery St.
Baltimore, MD 21230
Phone: (410)727-1558 **Free:** 877-708-7827
Fax: (410)752-2579
Email: barbara@starassociatesinc.com
Website: http://www.starassociatesinc.com
Fnded: 1985. **Activities:** Provide In-home aide health care to the senior population. Also provide transportation services for the Department of Aging. Provide training and certification as Certified Nursing Assistants. Provide training for all related healthcare industry needs. Provide residential group homes for youth between the ages of 13 and 18 years. Diversity and leadership training and development programs for women. **Remarks:** Barbara A. Robinson is the president and founder of STAR and its sister company, SelfPride, Incorporated. Barbara is an author and her fourth book "Somebody Is Now," an inspiration and motivational book will be available later this year. Barbara is a radio talk show host, inducted into the Maryland Women Hall of Fame, a 1995 Avon Women of Enterprise winner, a 1996 Entrepreneur of the year, and honored at the White House by President Bill Clinton for the work her company has done in welfare reform. Geographic Area Served: Worldwide.

★ 14131 ★ Toby Drews
PO Box 19910
Baltimore, MD 21211
Phone: (410)243-8352 **Fax:** (410)243-8558
Email: Tdrews3879@aol.com
Website: http://www.gettingthemsober.com
Activities: Acts as expert witness and offers consultation in the field of substance abuse and addiction. Industries served: legal, healthcare, and government. **Remarks:** Specializing in telephone consultations, based philosophically on her "Getting Them Sober" million-selling books. Please see award-winning website www.gettingthemsober.com. Geographic Area Served: Nationwide & Canada.

★ 14132 ★ Uttenreither Health Care Consulting
8348 Streamwood Dr.
Baltimore, MD 21208
Free: 800-533-2834 **Fax:** (410)521-7590
Activities: Offers healthcare consulting services.

★ 14133 ★ Yale H. Caplan, PhD
3411 Philips Dr.
Baltimore, MD 21208
Phone: (410)486-7486 **Fax:** (410)653-4824
Email: fortox@aol.com
Fnded: 1974. **Activities:** Consultant in toxicology, drug and chemical analysis, workplace drug testing, and interpretation of toxicologic information. Serves as expert witness in drunk driving and drug testing cases. Geographic Area Served: United States.

Bethesda

★ 14134 ★ BEMW Inc. Counseling and Training for the Workplace
7984-D Old Georgetown Rd.
Bethesda, MD 20814
Phone: (301)657-8922 **Fax:** (301)657-8924
Fnded: 1976. **Activities:** Human resource development specialists provide counseling programs in the following areas: employee assistance, career management, and outplacement. Provides vocational assessment and expert testimony. Industries served: government, telecommunications, real estate, high-tech, and universities. Geographic Area Served: Washington DC metropolitan area.

★ 14135 ★ Dynamic Physicians Management L.L.C.
7232 Swansong Way
Bethesda, MD 20817
Phone: (301)610-6666 **Fax:** (301)294-0508
Email: jeffp@dynamicpm.com
Website: http://www.dynamicpm.com
Activities: Consulting firm specializes in physician practice management.

★ 14136 ★ Edison Technical Services
5101 River Rd.
Bethesda, MD 20816
Phone: (301)654-1515 **Fax:** (301)654-1414
Email: algriff@griffex.com
Website: http://www.griffex.com
Fnded: 1960. **Activities:** Consultants serving the plastics industry (especially extrusion, agriculture, thermoforming, blow molding), the packaging industry (especially food and beverage packaging), construction (manufacturing and use of plastic products), and government agencies. Extensive experience in international industry-information services, Third World development (especially Latin America), food and nutrition problems, and food processing. Also offers patent and other legal assistance (as technical expert). Maintains extensive files on plastics extrusion and food/beverage packaging, including patents.

★ 14137 ★ MacKeen Consultants Ltd.
4903 Sangamore Rd.
Bethesda, MD 20816
Phone: (301)229-7445 **Fax:** (301)229-3541
Email: dmackeen@mackeen.com
Website: http://www.mackeen.com
Fnded: 1980. **Activities:** Health services consulting firm focuses on medical product development. Specializing in ophthalmic drugs and devices. Also skilled with medical and non-medical laser interactions with regulatory agencies.

★ 14138 ★ Medical Care Management Corp.
5272 River Rd., Ste. 650
Bethesda, MD 20816-1405
Phone: (301)652-1818 **Fax:** (301)652-1250
Email: mcman@mcman.com
Website: http://www.mcman.com
Fnded: 1992. **Activities:** Provides information for health care decision-making. Services include case reviews (both external reviews of health plan coverage denials and advisory opinions to inform coverage decisions and to forestall costly litigation or mandatory appeals), and expert analyses (e.g., of coverage, practice, and technology guidelines), expert assessments (e.g., of medical technology). Geographic Area Served: Worldwide.

★ 14139 ★ Research Associates
4949 Battery Ln., Ste. 112
Bethesda, MD 20814
Phone: (301)652-1924 **Fax:** (301)652-1637
Email: info@researchassociates.com
Website: http://www.researchassociates.com
Fnded: 1985. **Activities:** Information broker for major pharmaceutical companies. Provides various information services for companies, law firms or individuals. Industries served: pharmaceutical companies and law firms. Geographic Area Served: Worldwide.

★ 14140 ★ Richard B. Edelman, PhD
8515 Whittier Blvd.
Bethesda, MD 20817
Phone: (301)469-9575 **Free:** 800-257-8626
Activities: Provides economic analysis for the determination of lost income in personal injury, wrongful death, and wrongful discharge cases. Also performs the valuation of businesses, pensions, and securities for divorce, contract disputes, and churning cases.

Cheverly

★ 14141 ★ Paulette Thompson
3117 Belleview Ave.
Cheverly, MD 20785
Phone: (301)772-5831 **Fax:** (301)618-4968
Fnded: 1782. **Activities:** Consulting nutritionist in the Chesapeake Bay area and registered dietitian in private practice. Geographic Area Served: Washington area.

Chevy Chase

★ 14142 ★ CDM Group Inc.
5530 Wisconsin Ave., Ste. 1600
Chevy Chase, MD 20815-4301
Phone: (301)654-6740 **Fax:** (301)656-4012
Activities: Consulting firm provides management services and consults on healthcare issues.

★ 14143 ★ Connie Badillo
5530 Wisconsin Ave., Ste. 1400
Chevy Chase, MD 20815
Phone: (301)656-9170 **Fax:** (301)654-5893
Email: badillo@erols.com
Activities: Consulting nutritionist in the Chesapeake Bay area and registered dietitian in private practice.

Columbia

★ 14144 ★ Cook International Inc.
5659 Thicket Ln
PO Box 2128
Columbia, MD 21044-2557
Phone: (301)596-0462 **Fax:** (410)992-7318
Fnded: 1983. **Activities:** Offers both consultation and operational field services for both basic and complex security problems required by government and private industry. Services include security surveys and vulnerability studies, personnel background investigations, security guard training, preboard screening for airlines, internal/external investigations, building security planning and design, and drug abuse programs. Industries served: automobile dealers, retail stores, U.S. and local governments, and military installations. Geographic Area Served: United States.

★ 14145 ★ FMAS Corp.
9170 Rumsey Rd.
Columbia, MD 21045
Phone: (410)964-9117 **Fax:** (410)964-9133
Fnded: 1980. **Activities:** Provides clients with healthcare management information concerning quality and cost effectiveness of services they pay for, deliver, or

receive. Offers services focusing on company's ability to manage data derived from clinical care process reliably and efficiently. Includes developing clinical practice profiles through measurement of medical care processes, outcomes, and costs; health information management services; professional liability consulting; and professional education. Evaluations can range from one to thousands of medical records.

Ellicott City

★ 14146 ★ Koffel Associates Inc.
3300 N Ridge Rd., Ste. 275
Ellicott City, MD 21043
Phone: (410)750-2246　**Fax:** (410)750-2588
Email: wkoffel@koffel.com
Website: http://www.koffel.com
Fnded: 1986. **Activities:** Independent firm providing fire protection engineering and code consulting services. Offers a broad range of services including fire protection engineering surveys, fire protection system design and analysis, fire loss investigations, product testing and development, community fire defense planning, seminars, and building and fire code consulting. Although services are offered for a variety of occupancies, the firm has specialized experience in healthcare facilities. Industries served: architectural, building owners, developers, engineering, fire service, legal, manufacturers, municipalities, and producers. **Remarks:** W.E. Koffel - President-Elect, Society of Fire Protection Engineers. Geographic Area Served: Worldwide.

★ 14147 ★ Occu-Health Inc.
24 Frederick Rd.
Ellicott City, MD 21043-4710
Phone: (410)418-8205　**Fax:** (410)381-9249
Email: occu@pop.erols.com
Fnded: 1991. **Activities:** Advises government and private sector organizations on occupational healthcare; industrial hygiene; quality assurance; wellness programs; and drug testing. Geographic Area Served: Maryland, Virginia, and Washington D.C.

Frederick

★ 14148 ★ Automation Counselors Inc.
5728 Industry Ln. Rear
PO Box 3917
Frederick, MD 21704
Phone: (301)663-3700　**Free:** 800-966-6725
Fax: (301)663-6692
Fnded: 1970. **Activities:** Furnishes data processing consulting, encompassing the following specialty areas: biomedical systems design and design of government financial systems. Industries served: primarily government. Geographic Area Served: United States.

Gaithersburg

★ 14149 ★ Beverly Celotta, Ph.D
13517 Haddonfield Ln.
Gaithersburg, MD 20878
Phone: (301)330-8803
Fnded: 1983. **Activities:** Provides a variety of psychological/educational services to organizations serving children or parents. Services include: needs assessments, program design, program implementation (e.g. run groups, provide conflict mediation), research, report writing, curricula and materials design, and training. Will train employees, administrators, professionals, staff/parent in areas such as communication skills, decision making, problem solving, stress prevention, self esteem enhancement, leadership, counseling skills, parenting, crisis intervention, suicide prevention, and program development. Available for speaking engagements. Industries served: educational, health, large and small businesses, professional groups, and local governments. Geographic Area Served: Maryland, Virginia, and Washington DC.

★ 14150 ★ Carol Tilford
9910 Brink Rd.
Gaithersburg, MD 20879
Phone: (301)926-6751　**Fax:** (301)924-1844
Activities: Consulting nutritionist in the Chesapeake Bay area and registered dietitian in private practice.

★ 14151 ★ Norbert P. Page
17601 Stoneridge Ct.
Gaithersburg, MD 20878
Phone: (301)948-9408　**Fax:** (301)948-9408
Fnded: 1984. **Activities:** Provides consultation on toxicology; risk assessment of chemicals and radiation; expert testimony; literature compilation and evaluation; design of toxicology studies; compliance with TSCA, FIFRA, international law; new drug applications; toxicology data and experiment evaluation; and report preparation. **Remarks:** Faculty, University of Maryland.

★ 14152 ★ Ruth Devoe
17708 Parkridge Dr.
Gaithersburg, MD 20878
Phone: (301)330-3944
Activities: Consulting nutritionist in the Chesapeake Bay area and registered Dietitian in private practice.

★ 14153 ★ T.M. Osborn Associates Inc., Facility Planning and Architecture
481 N Frederick Ave., No. 400
Gaithersburg, MD 20877
Phone: (301)840-0606　**Fax:** (301)840-0320
Email: tosborn@tmosborn.com
Website: http://www.tmosborn.com
Fnded: 1984. **Activities:** Healthcare strategic facility planning and architecture. Assessment, focused facility plan, master facility plan, functional program, concept design, space planning; project consultation, equipment plan, architectural services, CADFM Database, Construction Management Audit, Design/Built Process Management. **Remarks:** International work combines health and medical education into the facility development process. Geographic Area Served: Worldwide.

Glen Arm

★ 14154 ★ Charlotte Eliopoulos Considine, PhD
11104 Glen Arm Rd.
Glen Arm, MD 21057
Phone: (410)668-7055　**Fax:** (410)668-7718
Email: charlotte@healthed.net
Website: http://www.chronicpractice.com
Fnded: 1978. **Activities:** Offers holistic-focused consultation and educational programs to long-term care facilities and geriatric care agencies. Services include workshop presentation, assistance in integrating alternative complementary therapies, and planning and development of new programs. Industries served: long-term care facilities, assisted living, and hospitals. Geographic Area Served: Worldwide.

Glen Burnie

★ 14155 ★ Arundle Psycotherapy Associates
1406-B Crain Hwy. S, Ste. 301
Glen Burnie, MD 21061-4094
Phone: (410)760-5588　**Fax:** (410)760-9727
Fnded: 1983. **Activities:** Offers individualized consulting services ranging from stress management to enhancing self-image. Covers the psychology of individual and group in families, the workplace or the community. Some experience with sales training. Works with corporations and government social service agencies.

Grasonville

★ 14156 ★ The Fitness Movement Inc.
4 Bateau Landing
Grasonville, MD 21638
Phone: (410)827-8324　**Fax:** (410)827-8324
Website: http://www.acepro.org/optimumwellness
Fnded: 1982. **Activities:** Designs and assists in implementation of major lifestyle changes for optimum health and wellness, including nutrition, exercise, stress management, and communication skills. Creates comprehensive programs for integrated mind-body wellness. Prevention of and lifestyle management of eating disorders, weight management, hypertension, adult on-set diabetes, premenstrual syndrome, coronary artery disease, osteoporosis, and post-traumatic stress disorder, and other lifestyle-related issues. Industries served: individuals, groups, corporations, schools, colleges, and community organizations. Geographic Area Served: Howard County/Baltimore; Washington, DC, area; and Anne Arundel County.

Greenbelt

★ 14157 ★ Changing Weighs
7219D Hanover Pky.
Greenbelt, MD 20770
Phone: (301)474-2499　**Fax:** (301)474-5943
Email: info@dietitianoffice.com
Website: http://www.dietitianoffice.com
Activities: Consulting nutritionist in the Chesapeake Bay area and registered dietitian in private practice.

Hanover

★ 14158 ★ United Auto Credit Corp.
7250 Parkway Dr., Ste. 510
Hanover, MD 21076
Phone: (410)712-4110　**Free:** 800-325-4177
Fax: (410)712-4424
Fnded: 1979. **Activities:** Diversified communications company providing a wide range of educational services for healthcare professionals. These services include: seminars and workshops, in-house/in-service programs, national conferences, publications, management services, corporate health, and consultation services.

Hunt Valley

★ 14159 ★ Special Response Corp. Inc.
10612 Beaver Dam Rd.
Hunt Valley, MD 21030
Phone: (410)785-1212　**Free:** 800-717-8243
Fax: (410)785-9025
Email: martinherman@specialresponse.com
Website: http://www.specialresponse.com
Activities: Firm provides special knowledge in health and safety issues. Geographic Area Served: United States.

Ijamsville

★ 14160 ★ Merlin & Associates Inc.
3501 Big Woods Rd.
Ijamsville, MD 21754
Phone: (301)831-9151　**Fax:** (301)865-6464
Email: merlin@fred.net
Fnded: 1989. **Activities:** Merlin can use its expertise in the education, curriculum development, and training fields to help increase marketability, expand programs, improve employee productivity, morale and commitment. Firm can provide market reviews, curriculum and workshop materials, and unique participatory learning experiences. Industries served: banking, retail, service organizations, government agencies, schools, manufacturing, and insurance. Geographic Area Served: United States, willing to do foreign business.

Landover

★ 14161 ★ Health Management Resources Inc.
8401 Corporate Dr., Ste. 400
Landover, MD 20785
Phone: (301)429-2300 **Fax:** (301)429-2314
Email: hmrinfo@healthman.com
Website: http://www.healthman.com

Fnded: 1983. **Activities:** Health care consultants. Industries served: healthcare. Geographic Area Served: Worldwide.

Laurel

★ 14162 ★ Gerontological Nursing Ventures
8369 Cherry Ln.
Laurel, MD 20707
Phone: (301)470-4345 **Free:** 888-701-4345
Fax: (301)776-5800
Email: info@jwgnv.com
Website: http://www.jwger-nurseventures.com

Fnded: 1988. **Activities:** Works on behalf of geriatric health care providers. Specializes in crisis intervention, staff enhancement and quality management. An allied professional gerontological nursing specialist.

★ 14163 ★ Integrated Healthcare Auditing and Services
14435 Cherry Lane Ct., Ste. 418
Laurel, MD 20707
Phone: (301)206-2006 **Fax:** (301)369-3454
Email: ihasinc@ihas.com
Website: http://www.ihas.com

Fnded: 1987. **Activities:** Health care consultants.

Marriottsville

★ 14164 ★ Yurow Health Care Consultants
1905 Stone Haven Ct.
Marriottsville, MD 21104
Phone: (410)795-5507 **Fax:** (410)653-1296

Fnded: 1990. **Activities:** Offers a variety of healthcare management consulting services that include but are not limited to: physician networking, hospital/physician ventures, capitation/HMO agreements, mergers/practice acquisitions, practice reviews, accounts receivable management, facility planning, and cost containment strategies for purchasers of healthcare. Industries served: physicians, hospitals, and other sectors of the healthcare industry. Geographic Area Served: Mid-Atlantic.

Owings Mills

★ 14165 ★ Genesis Technology
11403 Cronhill Dr., Ste. B
Owings Mills, MD 21117
Phone: (410)654-0090 **Fax:** (410)654-0138
Email: info@genesismedical.com
Website: http://www.genesismedical.com

Fnded: 1994. **Activities:** Designs and develops medical products; and instrumentation.

★ 14166 ★ Maximum Potential Inc.
4500 Chaucer Way, Ste. 401
Owings Mills, MD 21117-6605
Phone: (410)581-0817 **Fax:** (410)581-3293
Email: ho@harryolson.com
Website: http://www.harryolson.com

Fnded: 1981. **Activities:** Offers consultation and training in human resource development, personal counseling, career counseling, public speaking coaching, and speaker's bureau. Primary areas include managing competition, human productivity, stress management, leadership development, communications, and appraisal-assessment. Serves private industries as well as government agencies. Geographic Area Served: Worldwide.

Potomac

★ 14167 ★ Estrin Consulting Group Inc.
9109 Copenhaver Dr.
Potomac, MD 20854
Phone: (301)279-2899 **Fax:** (301)294-0126
Email: estrin@yourfdaconsultant.com
Website: http://yourfdaconsultant.com

Fnded: 1990. **Activities:** Emphasis on medical device regulatory submissions (510(k), PDP, PMA, IDE). Regulatory strategy development, labeling compliance, litigation support and special projects. Industries served: medical device, drug, and cosmetic. ECG also advises clients in business entrepreneurial areas. Acts as agent and official correspondent for foreign companies. **Remarks:** Awarded the RAPS Special Recognition Award. Received the cosmetic industry's two highest honors for contributions to cosmetic science. Served for nine years on the Board of Trustees of the National Health Museum under Former Surgeon General, C. Everett Koop. Also served on the Boards of Director's of Discovery Pharmaceuticals Inc., Chantal Pharmaceuticals Inc and NCCLS. Was former Vice President of the Cosmetic, Toiletry and Fragrance Association. Dr. Estrin was awarded a doctorate in physical-organic chemistry from Florida State University. Geographic Area Served: United States, Europe, Asia.

★ 14168 ★ Perry Hookman, MD
9605 Halter Ct.
Potomac, MD 20854
Email: hookman@hookman.com
Website: http://www.hookman.com

Activities: Specialist in evaluation and/or testimony and/or mediation in medical malpractice, alleged health care fraud and abuse, utilization review, medical malpractice and quality assurance. Geographic Area Served: United States.

Reisterstown

★ 14169 ★ John A. Donaho and Associates Inc.
6600 Deer Park Rd.
Reisterstown, MD 21136
Phone: (410)833-1780 **Fax:** (410)833-3077
Email: Donassoc@bellatlantic.net

Fnded: 1953. **Activities:** Offers counsel to corporate and government officials on organization, methods, personnel, budgeting and finance, purchasing, planning, and data processing. Additional expertise in public works, public welfare, resource management, inventory control, insurance and healthcare management. Principally active in the United States, Asia and the Far East.

Rockville

★ 14170 ★ BAE SYSTEMS - Technologies Services Sector
1601 Research Blvd.
Rockville, MD 20850-3173
Phone: (301)838-6000 **Fax:** (301)738-4643
Website: http://www.tst.tracor.com

Fnded: 1955. **Activities:** Offers environmental, health, and safety services including environmental assessments of properties, abatement of hazardous materials, and evaluation of workplace environment. Specializes in bio-medical and health communications and publications. Conducts workplace drug abuse screening programs. Also assists with battery evaluation and testing. Industries served: property managers and owners, architectural and engineering firms, painting contractors, heavy manufacturing industry, ship yards, schools, public housing authorities, and federal, state, and local governments. Geographic Area Served: United States.

★ 14171 ★ BioSciCon Inc.
14905 Forest Landing Cir.
Rockville, MD 20850-3924
Phone: (301)610-9130 **Fax:** (301)610-7662
Email: bioscicon@netscape.net

Fnded: 1996. **Activities:** Sponsoring development of the MARK-PAP™ Technology of the Pap test accuracy via introduction of a new biomarker that enhances visibility of abnormal cells on Pap smears or monolayers of cervical cells obtained in solution. Conducts clinical trials for assessment of the test efficacy and safety, manufactures research tools (kit, accessories) for conduct of trials, and markets IP to license manufacturing, marketing, sales and distribution rights of the new technology line of products. **Remarks:** Looking for well established manufacturers of in vitro diagnostic medical devices with access to cytopathology laboratories, women's health centers, and cancer prevention centers. Geographic Area Served: Worldwide.

★ 14172 ★ Creative Stress Management
822 Fordham St.
Rockville, MD 20850
Phone: (301)251-0538

Fnded: 1981. **Activities:** Offers occupational health and stress management consulting. Emphasis is on training employees of client corporations to avoid professional burnout with the development of the skills and techniques to counter stressful situations with a positive approach. Serves private industries as well as government agencies. Geographic Area Served: United States.

★ 14173 ★ Decision Systems Technologies Inc.
7361 Calhoun Pl., Ste. 600
Rockville, MD 20855
Phone: (301)315-9200 **Fax:** (301)762-7727
Email: busdev@dsti.com
Website: http://www.dsti.com

Fnded: 1986. **Activities:** Professional services consulting firm supportive of the Federal Government and private sector in the areas of Information Technology, Engineering Services, and Science Support. Competencies include enterprise systems management, IV&V, seat management, web-based technologies, system engineering and integration, complete logistics support, remote sensing instrumentation, research, modeling and simulation, and algorithm development. Firm possesses both SEI Level II processes and ISO 9001 certification. Geographic Area Served: Maryland, Virginia, District of Columbia, New Jersey, Ohio, Missouri, Texas.

★ 14174 ★ ELM Services Inc.
11600 Nebel St., Ste. 201
Rockville, MD 20852
Phone: (301)984-1242 **Fax:** (301)770-1949
Website: http://www.elmservices.com

Fnded: 1976. **Activities:** For the past 20 years, ELM Services, Inc., has been the leader in guiding, advising, and supporting the practice and delivery of oncology nationwide. ELM has influence the art, business, and science of this industry as it continues to undergo radical change and transformation. ELM, oncology's premier consulting firm, is assisting hospitals, physicians, health care systems, and academic/university programs in the development of whole new approaches to cancer program management. Geographic Area Served: United States.

★ 14175 ★ First Seminar Service
129 S Van Buren St.
Rockville, MD 20850
Phone: (301)762-3003

Fnded: 1988. **Activities:** The firm provides training and consulting concerned with the establishment and maintenance of a drug-free workplace. Programs are offered on the following major topics: policy development/compliance, education/prevention, testing, employee assistance programs, legal issues, corporate/government programs, treatment, science/research, role of the medical review officer, and workplace wellness. Industries served: human resource managers, business owners, health and wellness coordinators, corporate and government mangers. Also provide training & consulting concerned with workplace wellness issues, i.e. safe and healthy workplace. Geographic Area Served: East Coast (Primary market).

★ 14176 ★ H. Daniel Roth Associates Inc.
6115 Executive Blvd.
Rockville, MD 20852-3901
Phone: (301)770-4405 **Fax:** (301)770-9248
Fnded: 1975. **Activities:** Statistical consulting. Designs, conducts, and analyzes data from epidemiological, economic, highway safety, environmental, and statistical studies. Industries served include: automotive, food and beverage, utilities (electric and gas), trade associations, non-profit research, oil and coal, petrochemical, mining, metals, appliances, computer, health service and care, construction, pharmaceuticals, chemical, and governments (federal, state, local and foreign). Specializes in providing legal support and expert witness testimony. Geographic Area Served: Worldwide.

★ 14177 ★ KAI
6001 Montrose Rd., Ste. 920
Rockville, MD 20852-4801
Phone: (301)770-2730 **Free:** 800-710-8053
Fax: (301)770-4183
Email: kai@kai-research.com
Website: http://www.kai-research.com
Fnded: 1986. **Activities:** Offers extensive expertise regarding clinical research, health research data management, clinical information systems and data management, and life quality assessment tools and studies. Services include clinical studies, coordinating center services, surveys, focus groups, and evaluation studies. Industries served: pharmaceutical, healthcare, rehabilitation, and government agencies worldwide. Geographic Area Served: North America, Europe, Asia.

★ 14178 ★ National Medical Advisory Service Inc.
6001 Montrose Rd., Ste. 400
Rockville, MD 20852
Phone: (301)230-2999 **Free:** 800-258-0014
Fax: (301)230-2996
Fnded: 1975. **Activities:** National insurance claims and litigation support practice uniquely integrates medical, occupational health and technical environmental services. Primary expertise involves complex personal injury claims, multi-party toxic waste and environmental matters, workers' compensation and medical malpractice cases. Special interests consist of chemical exposure/poisoning, clinical ecology, sick building syndrome and multiple chemical sensitivity claims. Most popular services include medical causation reviews, exposure assessment, risk communication, product stewardship programs (product risk analysis), industrial hygiene and environmental testing for insurers, law firms, government, associations and industry. Scientific specialties: medicine, toxicology, industrial hygiene, chemical engineering, environmental science and other related disciplines. Geographic Area Served: United States.

★ 14179 ★ R.O.W. Sciences Inc.
1700 Research Blvd., Ste. 400
Rockville, MD 20850
Phone: (301)294-5400 **Fax:** (301)294-5401
Website: http://www.rowsciences.com
Fnded: 1983. **Activities:** Performs biomedical and health services research and consulting. Also provides computer and telecommunications services.

★ 14180 ★ R.P. Chiacchierini & Associates L.L.C.
15825 Shady Grove Rd., Ste. 30
Rockville, MD 20850
Phone: (240)683-3738 **Fax:** (240)683-9236
Website: http://www.rpcaconsulting.com
Activities: Provides comprehensive medical and regulatory affairs services to executives and regulatory affairs professionals at medical device, in vitro diagnostic, and biologic corporations. Services include regulatory strategic planning and implementation; clinical trial and study management; statistical design, analysis, and interpretation; regulatory submissions; and compliance assistance and training.

★ 14181 ★ Stephen D. Bruck Associates Inc.
255 N Washington St., Ste. 501
Rockville, MD 20850
Fnded: 1997. **Activities:** Provides services including technological assessments, product planning, and consulting in regulatory requirements for biomaterials, implants, medical devices, and therapeutic drug-carrier systems. Especially knowledgeable in toxicity, biocompatibility, blood compatibility, and physical properties of materials in biomedical applications. Geographic Area Served: Worldwide.

★ 14182 ★ Technical Resources International Inc.
3203 Tower Oaks Blvd.
Rockville, MD 20852
Phone: (301)564-6400 **Fax:** (301)897-7400
Website: http://www.tech-res-intl.com
Fnded: 1980. **Activities:** Biomedical and environmental consultant. Geographic Area Served: Worldwide.

★ 14183 ★ ToxNetwork.com
14317 Bauer Dr.
Rockville, MD 20853
Phone: (301)871-6714 **Fax:** (301)871-5586
Website: http://www.toxnetwork.com
Activities: An internationally recognized consulting and expert witness practice serving law firms and the chemical and pharmaceutical industries in the areas of toxicology and chemical carcinogenesis as well as safety, hazard and risk assessments.

Salisbury

★ 14184 ★ The National Academy of Television Journalists
207 W Main St.
Salisbury, MD 21803
Phone: (410)548-5343 **Fax:** (410)543-0698
Website: http://www.angelfire.com/md/NATJ/index.html
Fnded: 1988. **Activities:** Provides counseling services in a broad range of areas including: marriage and family relationships, pre-marital counseling, child custody and divorce mediation, marriage reconciliation, loss and bereavement, stress and anxiety management, chemical abuse and co-dependency, and building self-esteem. For businesses and other organizations, firm offers organizational and management development consulting to include teambuilding, managing cross-cultures, and career transition counseling. Serves private industries as well as government agencies. Geographic Area Served: Maryland, Virginia, and Washington DC.

Silver Spring

★ 14185 ★ American Institutes for Research - Prospect Center
10720 Columbia Pke., Ste. 500
Silver Spring, MD 20901-4449
Phone: (301)592-8600 **Fax:** (301)593-9433
Website: http://www.air.org
Fnded: 1979. **Activities:** A health sciences research and communications firm which provides support to scientific, health and technical clients to help them combat and solve the nation's foremost health problems. Prospect offers particular expertise and experience on such issues as AIDS; cancer; heart, lung, and blood diseases; diabetes; digestive diseases; kidney and urologic diseases; arthritis; mental disorders; dental problems; and concerns of the aging population. Communications services include support in health education, mass media, minority health, and public affairs. Scientific support includes services in research and evaluation, information services, and biomedical and behavioral sciences. Information services are also offered which include integrated support in information services and management, computer applications, and library services. Prospect specializes in the dissemination of health and scientific information to consumers and professionals. Support services such as conference logistics, graphics support, word processing, data processing, publications management, editorial services, messenger service, warehousing and distribution, and clerical and administrative support are also available. Industries served: government agencies, universities and other nonprofit organizations, foundations and associations, and private industry. Small women-owned firm.

★ 14186 ★ Birch & Davis Associates Inc.
8905 Fairview Rd., Ste. 200
Silver Spring, MD 20910
Phone: (301)589-6760 **Fax:** (301)650-0398
Fnded: 1976. **Activities:** Services include consultation in healthcare program development, operations, and financing; management information systems; financial management and accounting; and conference management. Other activities include commercial activity reviews (Federal OMB Circular a-76), internal control reviews and vulnerability assessments; managed care program development and operations; large-scale survey and data collection efforts; and epidemiologic surveillance systems. Clients include private industry; federal, state, and local governments; and government and private sector organizations in Africa, the Middle East and the Caribbean. Minority owned, women-owned firm.

★ 14187 ★ ERNACO Inc.
3740 Capulet Ter.
PO Box 6522
Silver Spring, MD 20906
Phone: (301)598-5025
Fnded: 1979. **Activities:** Provides expert services in the biomedical, health and environmental sciences. Also offers specialized programs in biological and biomedical topics for professionals. Industries served: pharmaceutical, health, environmental; nonprofit organizations; and federal, state, and local government. Geographic Area Served: United States, primarily mid-Atlantic states.

★ 14188 ★ Feola & Kornbluh Associates
1939 Hiskory Hill Ln.
Silver Spring, MD 20906
Phone: (301)871-5753
Activities: Management consultant experienced in organization and management development. While specializing in the healthcare environment, consultant has provided strategic planning, teambuilding, and management training to medical and dental practices, hospitals, engineering and pharmaceutical firms, as well as government agencies.

★ 14189 ★ Humor Communication Co.
8902 Maine Ave.
Silver Spring, MD 20910
Phone: (301)588-3561 **Fax:** (301)588-3561
Email: gliner@erols.com
Fnded: 1974. **Activities:** Activities include consulting with individuals and organizations on the uses of humor to improve communication, enhance creativity and help cope with stress and burnout. Serves private industries as well as government agencies. **Remarks:** Please call before transmitting fax. Geographic Area Served: United States.

★ 14190 ★ Johnson, Bassin & Shaw Inc.
8630 Fenton St., Ste. 1200
Silver Spring, MD 20910
Phone: (301)495-1080 **Fax:** (301)587-4352
Email: gbassin@jbs1.com
Website: http://www.jbs1.com

Fnded: 1985. **Activities:** Health and social services issues-oriented consulting firm. Geographic Area Served: United States.

★ 14191 ★ Mankind Research Foundation
8720 Georgia Ave., Ste. 303
Silver Spring, MD 20910-3614
Phone: (301)587-8686 **Fax:** (301)587-8688

Fnded: 1973. **Activities:** Established to provide an organization for scientific development and application of technology that could have positive impact on the health, education, and welfare of mankind. MRF is organized so as to seek and apply futuristic solutions to current problems. Provides services in the areas of advanced sciences, biotechnical, bionic, biocybernetic, biomedical, holistic health, bioimmunology, solar energy, accelerated learning, and sensory aids for handicapped. Current specific activities involve research in AIDS, drug abuse, affordable housing, food for the hungry, and literacy and remedial education. Industries served: agriculture and forestry, education, electronics, energy and government as industries, healthcare, nonprofit organizations, pharmaceutical, transportation, and service industries. Geographic Area Served: Worldwide.

★ 14192 ★ Multi Consultants Associates
8484 Georgia Ave., Ste. 320
Silver Spring, MD 20910-5604
Phone: (301)565-4020 **Fax:** (301)565-5112

Fnded: 1984. **Activities:** Health care consultants offer consulting expertise in the following areas: technical assistance, information technology services, publications, conference management, logistics support, and clearinghouse operations. Industries served: information service. Geographic Area Served: United States.

★ 14193 ★ SoftMed Systems Inc.
12215 Plum Orchard Dr.
Silver Spring, MD 20904
Phone: (301)572-3800 **Free:** 800-234-0422
Fax: (301)572-3809
Website: http://www.softmed.com

Fnded: 1983. **Activities:** Software company offers various areas of computer expertise particularly with regard to document management and medical record field. Serves healthcare industry.

Timonium

★ 14194 ★ Behavioral Science Training Associates
114 Oakway Rd.
Timonium, MD 21093
Phone: (410)339-5370 **Fax:** (410)339-5374

Fnded: 1994. **Activities:** Services include organizational development, strategic planning, educational training for businesses and governmental agencies in the areas of education, mental health, health, business management, and social services, human resources. Geographic Area Served: United States.

Towson

★ 14195 ★ Oleen Healthcare Information Management Inc.
8600 LaSalle Rd., Ste. 624
Towson, MD 21286
Phone: (410)296-9602 **Free:** 800-466-4760
Fax: (410)296-9699
Website: http://www.oleen.com

Fnded: 1988. **Activities:** A managed healthcare consulting firm that develops software and supports management information systems for local or national HMO's.

Upper Marlboro

★ 14196 ★ Takacs Techniques
1310 Wembley Dr.
Upper Marlboro, MD 20774
Phone: (301)350-7474
Website: http://polaris.umuc.edu/~gtakacs/

Fnded: 1984. **Activities:** Consulting firm offering the following services: training programs, problem solving, organizational development, management techniques and needs assessment. Services also include vocational counseling and remedial education in such basic skills as math, reading and grammar; team building and performance appraisal; customer service training; stress management and supervisor training, and analysis of organizational behavior problems. Serves private industries as well as government agencies.

Massachusetts

Acton

★ 14197 ★ Margaret L. Mikkola
5 Nashoba Rd.
Acton, MA 01720
Phone: (978)264-9040 **Fax:** (978)264-9040

Fnded: 1982. **Activities:** Nutrition consultant provides expertise for individuals and groups regarding food/health related issues.

Andover

★ 14198 ★ Philips Medical Systems
3000 Minuteman Rd.
Andover, MA 01810-1099
Phone: (978)687-1501
Website: http://www.medical.philips.com

Activities: Medical doctor offering services in medical interface design; electronic medical records; UML workflow modeling.

Bedford

★ 14199 ★ Millipore Corp.
80 Ashly Rd.
Bedford, MA 01730
Phone: (781)533-6000 **Free:** 800-645-5476
Fax: (781)533-3110
Website: http://www.millipore.com

Activities: Product and market development firm as well as worldwide leader in the separation of liquids, combining chromatographic and electrophoretic instrumentation, column and membrane chemistries, and information processing. Firm solves applications ranging from the synthesis and sequencing of peptides, and the assurance of product formulations in the chemical industry, to the search for new pharmaceuticals.

Belmont

★ 14200 ★ Larry H. Strasburger
527 Concord Ave.
Belmont, MA 02478
Phone: (617)484-8271

Fnded: 1961. **Activities:** Consults with attorneys, governmental agencies, insurance companies, hospitals, physicians and individuals regarding legal-psychiatric issues.

Beverly

★ 14201 ★ Behavioral Health Care Consultants Inc.
12 Windham Ln.
Beverly, MA 01915-1568
Phone: (978)921-5968 **Fax:** (978)921-9085
Email: mlkat@prodigy.net

Fnded: 1994. **Activities:** Support and clinical service specialists (behavioral health care) offers clients a full range of consulting services specific to the behavioral health and substance abuse areas. Strategic planning, new business development, operational restructuring, organization change facilitation, physician/hospital integration, physician practice valuation and financial analysis and feasibility studies are among services offered. Firm has developed specific expertise in the development of local and regional integrated delivery systems for behavioral healthcare providers, including managed care contract development physician practice management structures. Also provides interim management support for clients in need of turnaround or new program start-up assistance. Geographic Area Served: United States.

Billerica

★ 14202 ★ Design Technology Corp.
101 Billerica Ave., Bldg. 3
Billerica, MA 01821
Phone: (978)663-7000 **Fax:** (978)663-6841

Fnded: 1968. **Activities:** Design and build automated equipment for processing, assembly, inspection and packaging of medical devices and disposables. Product design and package design, process development for medical and drug-delivery devices. Also develop robotic systems for processing, assembly, packaging, inspection, and testing of biologicals, medical devices, pharmaceuticals, drug-delivery devices and disposables. Geographic Area Served: United States.

Bolton

★ 14203 ★ HC Associates
PO Box 856
Bolton, MA 01740
Phone: (978)365-2701 **Fax:** (978)365-7513
Email: info@hcassoc.com
Website: http://www.hcassoc.com

Fnded: 1995. **Activities:** Sales of Telecom/Datacom test equipment and timing devices. Geographic Area Served: New England, United States.

Boston

★ 14204 ★ BD Healthcare Consulting and Services
101 Arch St., Ste. 1765
Boston, MA 02110
Phone: (617)737-7575 **Free:** 800-394-7171
Fax: (617)737-0202
Email: maryann_ciampa@bd.com
Website: http://www.bd.com/consulting

Fnded: 1998. **Activities:** Firm offers cost management and operational improvement services for materials management, pharmacy, surgical services, and clinical laboratory. Assessment, planning, and implementation services provide for a full solution continuum. Staff of highly experienced healthcare professionals ensure services deliver financially sound and clinical sensitive solutions that deliver bottom line results. Geographic Area Served: United States.

★ 14205 ★ Boston Medical Center, Occupational and Environmental Medicine
Preston F-5, 732 Harrison Ave.
Boston, MA 02118
Phone: (617)638-8400 **Fax:** (617)638-8406
Email: barbanel@bu.edu

Fnded: 1989. **Activities:** Provides occupational and environmental medicine services. **Remarks:** Provides 24-hour on-call drug and alcohol testing. Geographic Area Served: Greater Boston Area.

★ 14206 ★ Cheryl Barbanel, M.D.
Boston Medical Center
88 E Newton St.
Boston, MA 02118-2393
Phone: (617)638-8400 **Fax:** (617)638-8406
Email: barbanel@bu.edu

Activities: Occupational medicine, toxicology, environmental medicine, biological monitoring, and medical surveillance, and drug testing. Geographic Area Served: Greater Boston area.

★ 14207 ★ Hazard Management Consulting Inc.
88 Broad St.
Boston, MA 02110
Phone: (617)695-1695 **Fax:** (617)695-1795
Fnded: 1986. **Activities:** Environmental management consulting firm.

★ 14208 ★ John Snow Inc.
44 Farnsworth St.
Boston, MA 02210-1211
Phone: (617)482-9485 **Fax:** (617)482-0617
Email: jsinfo@jsi.com
Website: http://www.jsi.com
Fnded: 1978. **Activities:** Advises hospitals and government agencies on public healthcare practices worldwide.

★ 14209 ★ Management Sciences For Health Inc.
165 Allandale Rd.
Boston, MA 02130-3400
Phone: (617)524-7799 **Fax:** (617)524-2825
Email: development@msh.org
Website: http://www.msh.org
Fnded: 1971. **Activities:** Nonprofit public health management organization. Manages the Family Planning Management Development project, and the National Pharmaceutical Management and Rational Pharmaceutical Management Projects, both of which are funded by the U.S. Agency for International Development.

★ 14210 ★ Susan B. DeCristofaro
44 Binney St.
Boston, MA 02115
Phone: (617)632-4880 **Fax:** (617)632-6053
Email: susan_decristofaro@dfcl.harvard.edu
Activities: Consultant in healthcare administration and oncology nursing serving hospitals and other healthcare organizations. Also consults on complementary therapies (i.e. homeopathy, creative art, and reiki). Geographic Area Served: United States, Canada, Europe.

★ 14211 ★ Victoria International Corp.
187 W Brookline St.
Boston, MA 02118
Phone: (617)247-4100 **Fax:** (617)247-0038
Fnded: 1968. **Activities:** Management consultants providing supervisory, customer relations, and Total Quality Management training. Serves diversified industries but specializes in the hospitality and healthcare fields. Geographic Area Served: Americas, Asia.

Brookline

★ 14212 ★ Micro Management Technologies Inc.
165 Winchester St.
Brookline, MA 02446
Phone: (617)731-3737 **Fax:** (617)738-8601
Email: custserv@micromanagesoft.com
Website: http://www.micromanagesoft.com
Fnded: 1979. **Activities:** Business software solutions, databases, office suites, productivity, security software, cotract programmers/analysts, consulting and network solutions, installation and on-site support. Geographic Area Served: New England.

Burlington

★ 14213 ★ Applied Management Systems Inc.
3 New England Executive Pk.
Burlington, MA 01803
Phone: (781)272-8001 **Fax:** (781)272-5666
Website: http://www.aboutams.com
Fnded: 1967. **Activities:** Health care consultants providing management engineering, reengineering, nursing management, operations improvement, product cost identification, information systems, health information management, materials management, accounts receivables management, and facilities design to the healthcare industry. Geographic Area Served: Nationwide.

Cambridge

★ 14214 ★ Cambridge Research Institute
929 Massachusetts Ave., Ste. 02B
Cambridge, MA 02139
Phone: (617)492-3800 **Fax:** (617)492-3840
Email: crimail@criconsult.com
Website: http://www.criconsult.com
Fnded: 1976. **Activities:** Management consultants specializing in strategy and organization design for the healthcare industry.

★ 14215 ★ Harold J. Bursztajn, MD
96 Larchwood Dr.
Cambridge, MA 02138-4639
Phone: (617)492-8366 **Fax:** (617)441-3195
Email: Harold_bursztajn@hmsharvard.edu
Website: http://www.forensic-psych.com
Activities: An expert consultant, risk management and witness resource specializing in forensic psychiatry and medicine; managed medical care, medical and psychiatric malpractice; and informed consent; sexual misconduct in professional relationships; supervisory responsibility psychiatric and medical disability evaluation; ADA workers' compensation; and premises liability. **Remarks:** Nationally distinguished Harvard Medical School graduate, and senior faculty active clinician in patient practice. Geographic Area Served: United States.

★ 14216 ★ Hypnosis Authority Inc.
955 Massachusetts Ave., Ste. 268
Cambridge, MA 02139
Phone: (212)330-6886 **Fax:** (212)591-6886
Email: mail@hypnosisauthority.com
Website: http://www.hypnosisauthority.com
Fnded: 2002. **Activities:** Performance consulting firm offers services to virtually any type of business. Services include stress management programs, sales coaching, leadership development, and peak performance training. Provides speakers, seminar leaders, and motivational entertainers for college events, association meetings, conventions, and corporate training sessions, dealing with subjects in areas of self-hypnosis, stress management, mental conditioning, and personal development. Geographic Area Served: United States, Asia, Australia, Europe.

Chestnut Hill

★ 14217 ★ David M. Benjamin, PhD
77 Florence St., Ste. 107
Chestnut Hill, MA 02467
Phone: (617)969-1393 **Fax:** (617)969-4285
Email: medlaw@channel1.com
Website: http://www.channel1.com/users/medlaw
Fnded: 1986. **Activities:** Develops educational and risk management programs for physicians, hospitals, healthcare professionals and the pharmaceutical industry. Areas of expertise include drug information, root cause analysis, preparation of IND and New Drug Applications (NDAs), development of clinical research studies, medical-legal case review, and alternative dispute resolution. Industries served: healthcare professionals, pharmaceutical industry, insurance companies, and legal professionals. **Remarks:** Alternative Dispute Resolution of law suits including early neutral evaluation, medication and arbitration. Specialized training programs to prepare for your disposition or day in court.

Dedham

★ 14218 ★ V. T. Regina & Associates
24 Rosen Rd.
Dedham, MA 02026-6244
Phone: (781)326-4480 **Fax:** (781)634-0415
Email: vince@vtregina.com
Website: http://www.vtregina.com
Fnded: 1981. **Activities:** Firm provides services in healthcare information technology systems management. Geographic Area Served: United States and Canada.

East Bridgewater

★ 14219 ★ Healthcare Compliance Specialists L.L.C.
20 Country Farm Rd.
East Bridgewater, MA 02333
Phone: (508)378-2114 **Free:** 800-777-6932
Fax: (508)378-2130
Email: m.baldassarre@prodigy.net
Website: http://member.expertpages.com/hccs
Activities: Licensed and certified professionals. Expertise in nursing home litigation, investigations, case review, depositions and court testimony. Professional experts and consultants ready to assist you with any nursing home litigation that requires clinical, financial, operational or regulatory analysis.

Haverhill

★ 14220 ★ Veterinary Healthcare Consultants L.L.C.
200 Merrimack St., Ste. 301
Haverhill, MA 01830
Phone: (978)372-7600 **Free:** 800-467-0627
Fax: (978)372-7644
Email: info@vhc.biz
Website: http://www.vhc.biz
Fnded: 1997. **Activities:** Firm is dedicated to providing innovative and resourceful business solutions for veteranary professionals, animal-related companies, and humane organizations. Geographic Area Served: Worldwide.

Lexington

★ 14221 ★ The Bristol Group Inc.
1050 Waltham St., Ste. 500
Lexington, MA 02421-8094
Phone: (781)863-5658 **Fax:** (781)863-5657
Email: amacnulty@bristolgroup.com
Website: http://www.bristolgroup.com
Fnded: 1985. **Activities:** Provides counsel to healthcare organizations, including hospitals and physician groups. Geographic Area Served: United States.

★ 14222 ★ J. H. Clausen
PO Box 400
Lexington, MA 02420
Phone: (781)862-9391
Fnded: 1969. **Activities:** Provides technical solutions in the fields of occupational and environmental health, industrial hygiene, chemical hazard evaluation and control, hazardous substances/wastes management, product and process evaluation, product safety and labeling, chemical aspects of litigation, and liaison between client and regulatory agencies. Technical management consulting in the areas of marketing, technology commercialization, strategic planning, and corporate policy formation assessment of the impact of regulations on processes and products. Also offers hazard communication/community relations training programs. Additional services include: emergency planning and spill prevention, toxicity and waste reduction, exposure and risk assessment, MSDS (Material Safety Data Sheet) and labels preparation and review, state-of-the-art reviews, and program development/implementation/review. Industries served: chemical, pharmaceutical, rubber, plastics, electronics, computers, biomedical/biotechnology,

general manufacturing/business, insurance, facilities management, real estate, and instrumentation. Geographic Area Served: National, but most services provided east of Mississippi River.

Lincoln

★ 14223 ★ UNICA Technologies Inc.
55 Old Bedford Rd.
Lincoln, MA 01773-1125
Phone: (781)259-5900 **Free:** 877-864-2261
Fax: (781)259-5901
Email: unica@unica-usa.com
Website: http://www.unica-usa.com

Fnded: 1992. **Activities:** Offers data mining and database marketing consulting. Services include: problem analysis, data preparation, modeling, model deployment, market campaign planning and design, development of campaign testing and measurement metrics, campaign optimization, campaign management process development. Geographic Area Served: North America.

Lynnfield

★ 14224 ★ Health Care Management Associates Inc.
200 Broadway, Ste. 301
Lynnfield, MA 01940-2349
Phone: (781)596-0122 **Fax:** (781)595-3540
Email: hcmai@att.net

Fnded: 1979. **Activities:** Advises nursing homes and hospitals on healthcare management practices. Geographic Area Served: New York, New Jersey, and New England.

Medfield

★ 14225 ★ John F. Tomera, PhD
354 South St.
Medfield, MA 02052-3127
Phone: (508)359-4072 **Fax:** (508)359-4072
Email: johntomera@prodigy.net
Website: http://pages.prodigy.net/johntomera/home.htm

Fnded: 1986. **Activities:** Consulting pharmacologist with experience in the following client markets: pharmaceutical, nutraceutical, chemical, agricultural, cosmetic, medical device, medical diagnostic, environmental toxicology, contract research and health maintenance organizations, and medical scientific publishers. Significant expertise in medical applications in vivo and in vitro, with therapeutic experience in cardiovascular, breast cancer, biochemical, immusuppression, pharmacoeconomics, trauma research, clinical trial study designa nd analysis. **Remarks:** Biography in Who's Who in the East; American Men and Women of Science, and Strathmore's Who's Who. Active Member of the American Physiology Society. Ph.D. in Pharmacology. Former Faculty Member at Harvard Medical School. Geographic Area Served: Worldwide.

★ 14226 ★ Robert Luttman & Associates
53 Colonial Rd.
Medfield, MA 02052
Phone: (508)359-9630
Email: rluttman@robertluttman.com
Website: http://www.robertluttman.com

Fnded: 1995. **Activities:** A healthcare improvement consultant, lecturer, and trainer. Provides training in: Clinical pathways, Variance management systems , Next Generation Quality: using pathways, variance systems, and continuous improvement to go beyond accreditation compliance, Tools and Techniques of Quality Management for Healthcare, Statistical Process Control Tools for Healthcare, Statistical Quality Assessment Using the Baldrige Criteria, Statistical Quality Assessment Implementation.

Medway

★ 14227 ★ Raphaela Rozanski, Registered Dietitian, Licensed Dietitian/Nutritionist
5 Virginia Rd.
Medway, MA 02053
Phone: (508)533-8560
Email: rrozanski@juno.com

Fnded: 1966. **Activities:** Consulting nutritionist offers dietetic expertise in areas of management, education, and for clinical settings to individuals, groups, long-term care institutions, and corporations. Particular counsel provided in products or healthcare benefits. Medical Nutriotion Therapy Medicare Participant.

Natick

★ 14228 ★ International Technology Group
36 Bradford Rd.
Natick, MA 01760
Phone: (508)651-0140 **Fax:** (508)653-0759
Email: itgplus@earthlink.net
Website: http://inventing-solutions.com

Fnded: 1987. **Activities:** Provides practical Inventions-By-Request™ and at no cost or obligations. Client can obtain license for inventions and intellectual property. Uses special intellectual filter to identify inventions with strong commercial potential. Uses both high and low technology solutions. Experience shows that the lowest technology solutions give the highest profit. Also reviews patents for clients to determine how to use better technology to bypass the patent claims. Also helps make client patents "bulletproof" and stronger. Consults in confidence for companies, law firms, investors, and financial organizations. Helps in implementation of technology based inventions and businesses. Shares royalties with individuals who identify clients who want specific Inventions-By-Request™. Senior advisor on intellectual property. **Remarks:** Consultant has held part-time appointments as a staff member at M.I.T., and as a lecturer at Harvard Medical School. In addition to his consulting activities, he was a (part-time) visiting research professor in the Bioengineering Department of Boston University.

Needham

★ 14229 ★ National Pediculosis Association
50 Kearney Rd.
Needham, MA 02494
Phone: (781)449-6487 **Free:** 800-446-4672
Fax: (781)449-8129
Email: npa@headlice.org
Website: http://www.headlice.org

Fnded: 1982. **Activities:** Consultants in head lice and scabies management, treatment, prevention, and education. Specializes in monitoring health policy administration in schools and trends in the treatment of head lice. Emphasis is on educational activities. Industries served: schools, health professionals, medical professionals, child care centers, health departments, hospitals, HMO's, clinics, libraries, parents, PTA's, camps, military bases, and churches. **Remarks:** Reporting Registry toll free number: (800)446-4NPA (for reporting lice and scabies outbreaks, treatment failures, and adverse reactions to products). Geographic Area Served: Worldwide.

Newton

★ 14230 ★ Education Development Center
Healthy Human Development Programs
55 Chapel St.
Newton, MA 02458
Phone: (617)969-7100 **Free:** 800-225-4276
Fax: (617)527-4096
Website: http://www.edc.org/hhd

Fnded: 1958. **Activities:** Non-profit organization; Health and Human Development Programs division specializes in promoting health and justice across the life cycle in many settings. HHD conducts research, evaluation, program development and professional development activities. Geographic Area Served: Worldwide; primarily U.S.

★ 14231 ★ Medical Records Institute
567 Walnut St.
PO Box 600770
Newton, MA 02460
Phone: (617)964-3923 **Fax:** (617)964-3926
Website: http://www.medrecinst.com

Fnded: 1979. **Activities:** Provides consulting to healthcare institutions on medical record audits, automation, space management, microfilm and optical disk systems. Specializes in the following areas: feasibility studies for Optical Disk Systems (electronic imaging), developing a strategy for information and records management, integrating MIS and records management, development of a corporate indexing and database system, and management systems for information assets. Offers additional consulting on clinical computing systems and conversions.

★ 14232 ★ Scheur Management Group Inc.
255 Washington St., Ste. 100
Newton, MA 02458-1611
Phone: (617)969-7500 **Fax:** (617)969-7508
Email: smgnow@scheur.com
Website: http://www.scheur.com

Fnded: 1988. **Activities:** A specialized healthcare operations management and business revitalization consulting firm. Offers the following services: managed care environmental assessment and strategic planning; managed care readiness analysis for hospital and medical staffs; managed care product development, design, packaging and marketing; integrated delivery systems for PHOs - organization, business plan pre-operational development, marketing analysis and management; HMOs: feasibility, licensure, development and operation; MSOs - feasibility, development and operation; structuring of managed care contracts and HMO joint ventures among payers, physicians and hospitals; training and education seminars; physician group practice development and mergers.

★ 14233 ★ TRO/The Ritchie Organization
80 Bridge St.
Newton, MA 02458
Phone: (617)969-9400 **Fax:** (617)527-6753
Email: info@troarch.com
Website: http://www.troarch.com

Fnded: 1909. **Activities:** Architectural, planning, interior design, and engineering consulting firm that has specialized in healthcare facilities for over 40 years. The firm possesses exceptional design expertise in the areas of acute care, ambulatory services, laboratories, rehabilitation medicine, cancer treatment research facilities, and facilities for the elderly. Serves private industries as well as government agencies. Geographic Area Served: Worldwide.

★ 14234 ★ Whole Systems International
255 Washington St., No. 190
Newton, MA 02458
Phone: (617)928-1555 **Fax:** (617)928-1585

Fnded: 1980. **Activities:** Specializes in serving the training and education needs of the healthcare industry, so that these companies may maximize their marketing and sales strategies. Has served most major pharmaceutical firms worldwide with effective multimedia training systems for a wide spectrum of human resource development applications. Multimedia development capability includes self-instructional text, audiotape, videotape, computer-based tutorials and assessments, computer-based interactive video, and applied workshop programs. Offers standard (off-the-shelf) and customized learning systems for new hire training, continuing education, product launches, management training, and sales training. Each program integrates the development of desired knowledge, skills, and performance in a competency-based structure.

Newton Center

★ 14235 ★ Creative Success
10 Langley Rd., Ste. 401
Newton Center, MA 02459
Phone: (617)323-1442 **Fax:** (617)323-1963
Email: gail@creativesuccess.com
Website: http://www.creativesuccess.com
Fnded: 1982. **Activities:** Career and creativity consultin and coaching services, human resources projeccts, stress management workshop-on-audiotape, writing projects. Geographic Area Served: United States.

Norwell

★ 14236 ★ Beacon Partners Inc.
200 Cordwainer Dr., Ste. 300
Norwell, MA 02061
Phone: (781)982-8400 **Free:** 800-4BE-ACON
Fax: (781)982-8469
Email: cra@beaconpartners.com
Website: http://www.beaconpartners.com
Fnded: 1989. **Activities:** A health care management consulting firm with. Provides health care organizations with a wide range of client-focused consulting services, including strategic planning, business operations management, enterprise security and HIPAA compliance, e-solutions, clinical solutions, information systems and technical solutions. Geographic Area Served: United States.

★ 14237 ★ Jay M. Portnow
36 Farrar Farm Rd.
Norwell, MA 02061
Phone: (781)659-2521 **Fax:** (781)659-5858
Email: jportnow@hotmail.com
Fnded: 1987. **Activities:** Offers consultation on establishing rehabilitation services in hospital, ambulatory or home care setting, case management of high cost cases, and level of care decisions and alternative care options. Available for subacute programs. Additional expertise available on establishing home care programs, coordination and clinical concerns. Industries served: insurance companies, government agencies, and private organizations in the U.S. Development of case management programs and services. Geographic Area Served: Worldwide.

Peabody

★ 14238 ★ Spectrum Consulting
4 Harvard St.
Peabody, MA 01960-1304
Phone: (978)531-0939 **Fax:** (978)531-0939
Email: iarons@erols.com
Website: http://www.expertsinternational.com/arons
Fnded: 1989. **Activities:** Provides technology assessments and market projections on technology and applications for medical lasers and ophthalmic devices and refractive surgery. Serves vision care and medical industries worldwide. Publishes monthly newsletter, Executive Laser Briefing, for medical laser executives. Geographic Area Served: Worldwide.

Springfield

★ 14239 ★ Naomi Volain, MS, RD
34 Virginia St.
Springfield, MA 01108-2623
Phone: (413)785-1792
Email: naomi.vo@verizon.net
Fnded: 1986. **Activities:** Registered dietitian and Certified Biology teacher (grades 9-12) offering advertising copywriting, specializing in pharmaceuticals, patient education, medical instrumentation, and nutrition. Also writes advertising copy, promotional materials, feature articles, direct mail patient educational and public relations material. Serves the consumer and healthcare industries in addition to those mentioned above. Geographic Area Served: Northeastern United States.

Sudbury

★ 14240 ★ Joan Salge Blake
300 Old Lancaster Rd.
Sudbury, MA 01776
Phone: (508)443-0172 **Fax:** (508)443-0172
Email: salgeblake@aol.com
Fnded: 1987. **Activities:** Offers nutrition and weight loss counseling, blood pressure reduction, cholesterol lowering, pre and post pregnancy care, nutrition planning for athletes, and meal planning for busy families.

Taunton

★ 14241 ★ Consulting & Technical Services Inc.
40 Myles Standish Blvd.
Taunton, MA 02780-1026
Phone: (508)880-6915 **Fax:** (508)880-6916
Fnded: 1984. **Activities:** Medical manufacturing consulting firm specializes in medical equipment sterilization worldwide.

Vineyard Haven

★ 14242 ★ Oberfest Associates Inc.
Tisbury Wharf
Vineyard Haven, MA 02568
Phone: (508)693-6650 **Free:** 800-693-6650
Fax: (508)693-6780
Fnded: 1978. **Activities:** Specializes in strategic and market planning for the healthcare industry. Provides the following services: market studies, business planning, medical staff planning, facility planning, project development and coordination, assistance with regulatory reviews and data systems development.

Waban

★ 14243 ★ Bargar and Associates
137 Pine Ridge Rd.
Waban, MA 02468
Phone: (617)527-5225 **Fax:** (617)527-4913
Email: nelsonbargar@msn.com
Website: http://member.expertpages.com/robertbargar/
Activities: Involved in healthcare quality assurance and utilization review. Helps attorneys evaluate the care provided to clients by all of their physicians and the institutions in which they practice - to identify where failures in systems and procedures resulted in injury. A consultant to the health insurance and managed care industries.

Waltham

★ 14244 ★ Boston Biomedical Consultants Inc.
1000 Winter St., Ste. 1600
Waltham, MA 02451
Phone: (781)890-5060 **Fax:** (781)890-6746
Email: mdaley@bostonbiomed.com
Fnded: 1976. **Activities:** Offers strategic management services to the biomedical industry, including business strategy formulation, strategic market planning, technology assessment, business development planning, design of new product portfolios, and due diligence searches. Conducts appraisals of potential acquisition, and licensing and divestiture candidates for investment organizations. Primarily serves manufacturers and distributors of human diagnostic and therapeutic products and life science instruments and reagents. Geographic Area Served: Worldwide.

★ 14245 ★ KMI/PAREXEL Inc.
195 West St.
Waltham, MA 02451
Phone: (781)434-4800 **Fax:** (781)487-0525
Website: http://www.kminc.com
Fnded: 1989. **Activities:** Firm of engineering professionals and former FDA investigators provide validation and compliance services to pharmaceuticals, biotech, and medical device clients worldwide. Has expertise in process, process control, and IS/IT. Services include training, consulting, and full validation implementation for projects ranging from unit operations and expansion projects to complete new facilities. Also offers Information Systems Consulting Services. Geographic Area Served: Worldwide.

★ 14246 ★ Massachusetts Health Data Consortium Inc.
460 Totten Pond Rd., Ste. 385
Waltham, MA 02451
Phone: (781)890-6040 **Fax:** (781)768-2510
Email: info@mahealthdata.org
Website: http://www.mahealthdata.org
Fnded: 1978. **Activities:** Offers healthcare management services to medical institutions in the eastern United States.

★ 14247 ★ PAREXEL International Corp.
195 West St.
Waltham, MA 02451-1163
Phone: (781)487-9900 **Free:** 800-PAR-EXEL
Fax: (781)487-0525
Website: http://www.parexel.com
Fnded: 1983. **Activities:** A pharmaceutical outsourcing organization providing a broad range of knowledge-based contract research, medical marketing and consulting services to the worldwide pharmaceutical, biotechnology and medical device industries. With a commitment to providing solutions that expedite time-to-market and peak market penetration, PAREXEL has developed significant expertise in clinical trials management, data management, biostatistical analysis, medical marketing, clinical pharmacology, regulatory and medical consulting, industry training and publishing and other drug development consulting services. Geographic Area Served: Worldwide.

★ 14248 ★ Telecommunications Management Corp.
1 Pleasant St.
Waltham, MA 02452-6107
Phone: (781)647-1112 **Fax:** (781)899-2143
Email: fhimss@msn.com
Website: http://www.go-tmc.com
Fnded: 1992. **Activities:** An independent consulting firm specializing in telecommunications analysis and design particularly for the healthcare industry. Also works with college and universities, state and local governments, utilities, and private industry. Geographic Area Served: United States.

Wayland

★ 14249 ★ Lehmann Consulting
15 Training Field Rd.
Wayland, MA 01778-1415
Phone: (508)358-9555 **Fax:** (508)358-4517
Fnded: 1995. **Activities:** Industry-experienced physician services for development strategy, market creation, technology assessment and due diligence, optimal clinicals and submissions, and scientific product support.

★ 14250 ★ Medical Opinions Associates Inc.
31 Rich Valley Rd.
Wayland, MA 01778
Free: 800-874-7677 **Fax:** (508)358-9921
Website: http://members.aol.com/medopins/title.html
Activities: Board-certified physicians evaluate medical records, write opinion letters, and are available for

consultation, deposition, and trial testimony. Geographic Area Served: North America.

Westborough

★ 14251 ★ BioPolymer Technologies International Inc.
PO Box 84
Westborough, MA 01581
Phone: (508)366-4089 **Free:** 800-246-7668
Fax: (508)836-3862
Email: biopolti@aol.com
Fnded: 1995. **Activities:** Offers a range of expertise in the area of analysis, chemistry, biochemistry, biotechnology, pharmakinetics, and preclinical studies for commercial uses. Also provides market studies and multiclient surveys. Industries served: foods, biotechnology, pharmaceuticals, and specialty chemicals worldwide. Geographic Area Served: North America/Europe.

Weston

★ 14252 ★ Health Advances L.L.C.
9 Riverside Rd.
Weston, MA 02493
Phone: (781)647-3435 **Fax:** (781)392-1484
Email: rec@healthadvances.com
Website: http://www.healthadvances.com
Fnded: 1992. **Activities:** A strategy consulting firm specializing in the commercialization of new health care technologies. Examples of the types of services provided include market assessments, competitive analysis, technology evaluations, and health economic studies. In addition to consulting services, Health Advances actively engages in evaluating and starting up new businesses in the health care field on our own account. Geographic Area Served: Worldwide.

Woburn

★ 14253 ★ Biotek Inc.
21 Olympia Ave., Ste. C
Woburn, MA 01801
Phone: (781)938-0938 **Fax:** (781)938-8939
Email: moreinformation@BIOTEK-INC.com
Website: http://www.biotek-inc.com
Fnded: 1980. **Activities:** Privately-owned medical research corporation.

Worcester

★ 14254 ★ HMA Behavioral Health Inc.
PO Box 706
Worcester, MA 01613
Phone: (508)757-2290 **Free:** 800-248-9908
Fax: (508)754-3616
Website: http://www.hmabh.com
Fnded: 1982. **Activities:** Offers services in psychiatric and substance abuse managed care network development.

★ 14255 ★ Jernberg Corp.
10 Chestnut St.
Worcester, MA 01608
Phone: (508)754-1770 **Fax:** (508)753-0902
Fnded: 1978. **Activities:** Human resources consultants specializing in employee assistance programs, healthcare cost-containment systems, and managed disability.

Michigan

Ann Arbor

★ 14256 ★ Biopharmaceutical Research Consultants
PO Box 2506
Ann Arbor, MI 48106
Phone: (734)426-2820 **Fax:** (734)426-2849
Email: BRCI@compuserve.com
Website: http://ourworld.compuserve.com/homepages/brci/homepage.htm
Activities: Firm provides pharmaceutical research services including clinical trial monitoring, data management, statistical analysis and report writing. Geographic Area Served: North America and Europe.

★ 14257 ★ CCHB: Communications Consultants in Health Care and Business
821 Hewett Dr.
Ann Arbor, MI 48103
Phone: (734)665-0296 **Fax:** (734)665-0296
Fnded: 1984. **Activities:** Editorial specialists in the preparation of all kinds of publishable materials with emphasis on the medical field. Technical advisor to providers on coding, nomenclature, and Medicare Resource-Based Relative Value Scale (RBRVS). Industries served: physician's groups, publishing houses, periodicals, government agencies, hospitals, medical centers, and universities. Geographic Area Served: Worldwide.

★ 14258 ★ Elan Systems Inc.
415 Detroit St., Ste. 200
Ann Arbor, MI 48104-1117
Phone: (734)668-6738 **Fax:** (734)668-0182
Fnded: 1976. **Activities:** Advises U.S. hospitals in medical management and planning. Geographic Area Served: United States and Canada.

★ 14259 ★ Emergency Physicians Medical Group P.C.
2000 Green Rd., Ste. 300
Ann Arbor, MI 48105-1571
Phone: (734)995-3764 **Free:** 800-466-EPMG
Fnded: 1976. **Activities:** A full service, regional medical group with a traditional commitment to providing excellence in emergency and unscheduled ambulatory care. Focus is on physician staffing and management services for emergency departments, urgent care centers, occupational health facilities, and inpatient services. Services include risk management, quality improvement, occupational medicine, information management, medical transcription, clinical decision units, managed care services, physician extender and mid-level provider programs.

★ 14260 ★ Human Networks Inc.
210 Crest Ave.
Ann Arbor, MI 48103
Phone: (734)665-1220 **Fax:** (734)665-1220
Email: aa@exclte.com
Website: http://www.humannet.com
Fnded: 1983. **Activities:** Provides the following consulting services: training in the areas of stress management, team building, supervisory skills, and leadership skills (management); and consultation regarding organizational climate assessment and improvement. Industries served include automotive, banking, small business, school, universities, and human service agencies.

★ 14261 ★ Medical Physics Consultants Inc.
2309 Shelby Ave.
Ann Arbor, MI 48103
Phone: (313)662-3197 **Free:** 800-321-2207
Fax: (313)662-9224
Email: mpc@medphyscon.com
Website: http://www.medphyscon.com
Fnded: 1978. **Activities:** Medical consulting group provides hospitals with nuclear medicine and radiological physics support. Industries served: medical and industrial using radiation. Geographic Area Served: Michigan, Ohio, Indiana, and Kentucky, Wisconsin, Utah.

★ 14262 ★ The MEDSTAT Group Inc.
777 E Eisenhower Pky.
Ann Arbor, MI 48108
Phone: (734)913-3000 **Fax:** (734)913-3500
Email: medstat@medstat.com
Website: http://www.medstat.com
Fnded: 1981. **Activities:** The MEDSTAT Group (www.medstat.com) is a health information company that provides decision support systems, market intelligence, benchmark databases, and research for managing the purchase, administration, and delivery of health services and benefits. It serves more than 1,000 organizations including many of the nation's leading employers, providers, pharmaceutical companies, government organizations, and health plans and insurance companies. Headquartered in Ann Arbor, Mich., MEDSTAT has a 20-year track record of delivering results for customers through innovative products, superior customer service, and outstanding people. MEDSTAT is part of The Thomson Corporation (www.thomson.com), a global e-information and solutions company in the business and professional marketplace with 2000 revenues of approximately US$6.0 billion. The company's common shares are listed on the Toronto and London stock exchanges (TSE:TOC).

★ 14263 ★ The Nova Group
4654 Bayberry Cir.
PO Box 130327
Ann Arbor, MI 48105
Phone: (734)662-7149 **Fax:** (734)662-8820
Email: NVAGrp@aol.com
Fnded: 1982. **Activities:** Provides personnel and training consulting services. Training programs and materials are available to meet the specific needs of corporations, hospitals, long-term care facilities, insurance, government agencies, and manufacturing. Nova develops personnel policies for organizations throughout the United States and Canada. Also offers performance appraisal systems designed to suit the organization's needs.

★ 14264 ★ Rudy Richardson Sc.D., DABT
1420 Washington Hts.
Ann Arbor, MI 48109-2029
Phone: (734)936-0769 **Fax:** (734)647-9770
Email: rjrich@umich.edu
Website: http://www.umich.edu/~neurosci/faculty/richardson.htm
Activities: Consulting toxicologist offers expertise on health effects of environmental chemicals, especially organophosphorus compounds and of pharmaceuticals, e.g. neuroprotective drugs. Provides advice on evaluation of data and design of studies for registration of pesticides. Experience includes specialized laboratory work such as in vitro inhibition of ACHE, BCHE, and NTE; delayed neurotoxicity studies. Industries served: chemical, agricultural, pharmaceutical, legal, health, and government agencies. **Remarks:** University-industry research collaborations. Geographic Area Served: Worldwide.

★ 14265 ★ Span Corp.
1505 White St.
Ann Arbor, MI 48104-4306
Phone: (734)623-7726 **Fax:** (734)769-6268
Website: http://www.spancorp.com
Fnded: 1988. **Activities:** Assists healthcare providers and employers in all areas of occupational medicine, employee health, and workers' compensation cost containment. Develops and manages primary care occupational medicine facilities; counsels on ergonomics, toxicology, preventive services, rehabilitation case management, and other provider based disability management services. Conducts independent medical evaluations, early return-to-work programs, and advises on OSHA regulatory compliance. Industries served: healthcare, manufacturing, and transportation in the continental United States, primarily the Midwest. **Remarks:** Span is actively seeking hospital and large group practice partners for the joint development and

management of Occupational Health and Safety Service delivery.

★ 14266 ★ Terrance E. Baulch
103 E Liberty, Ste. 207
Ann Arbor, MI 48104
Phone: (734)930-0800 **Fax:** (734)930-0801
Fnded: 1987. **Activities:** Healthcare management consultant specializing in financial and economic analysis including changes in third party payment systems and other operating issues for the healthcare industry.

★ 14267 ★ Vector Research Inc.
PO Box 1506
Ann Arbor, MI 48106
Phone: (734)973-9210 **Fax:** (734)973-7845
Fnded: 1969. **Activities:** Broad-based operations research and data-processing effort with sharp focus on solving complex healthcare planning and delivery problems for private industry and government, including Department of Defense, Veterans Administration and Public Health Service. Consulting experience spans large-scale computer modeling of healthcare demand and demographics of physician supply, automated quality-of-care monitoring, medical database management and information quality engineering, site-specific economic analyses, software development for integrated hospital information systems, and graduate medical education.

Belleville

★ 14268 ★ Richard Hamer Associates Inc.
48910 Denton Rd.
Belleville, MI 48111
Email: rhamer@hamerassoc.com
Website: http://www.hamerassoc.com
Fnded: 1983. **Activities:** Active in the development of premarket approval strategies for new drug and medical device products; preparation, and submission and approval monitoring of investigational and/or premarketing approval applications (IND, IDE, NDA, ANDA, PMA, 510(k), etc.); monitoring of preclinical and clincial studies for GLP and GCP compliance; and review of labeling, advertising and promotional materials. Conducts comprehensive facility audits to evaluate GMP compliance, develops practical standard operation procedures and documentation systems to facilitate GMP compliance, and provides effective representation of clients' interests during FDA site inspections or meetings with regulatory agencies. Offers continuous monitoring of regulatory developments and provides recommendations for dealing with issues of specific interest. Industries served: pharmaceuticals, medical devices, cosmetics, and food. Geographic Area Served: United States, Canada, Western Europe, and Far East.

Bloomfield Hills

★ 14269 ★ Healthcare Management Consultants Inc.
5856 Sutters Ln.
Bloomfield Hills, MI 48301
Phone: (810)851-4980 **Fax:** (810)851-0943
Activities: Services include utilization review and quality assurance, pre-admission review, and audit preparation. Consultants assist hospitals with improving coding and documentation procedures in order to achieve accurate billing. Industries served: hospitals and third party payers.

★ 14270 ★ Marilyn LeVasseur
2595 Hickory Grove
Bloomfield Hills, MI 48302
Phone: (248)338-1016 **Fax:** (248)338-1016
Email: marlevbri@aol.com
Fnded: 1984. **Activities:** Provides seminars, programs or individual consultation for home healthcare, either Medicare/Medicaid, private pay or other insurances. The emphasis ranges from agency start-up and encompasses any area of the home care agency: i.e., financial, management, nursing, marketing, and public relations. Serves government agencies also. Geographic Area Served: United States and Canada.

Cement City

★ 14271 ★ Placement Associates Ltd.
14222 Blarney Cir.
Cement City, MI 49233
Phone: (517)688-4637 **Fax:** (517)688-4235
Email: expertpa@direcway.com
Website: http://expertpages.com/cv/mooney.htm
Fnded: 1992. **Activities:** Physician's assistant experienced in family medicine, emergency medicine and urgent care medicine. Provides medical record review, written opinion, deposition and trial testimony concerning medical malpractice cases involving physician assistant practice. Experienced in recruitment of physician assistants. Knowledge of laws concerning the scope of practice and rules and regulations concerning physician assistant practice. For additional physician assistants and nurse practitioners on a nationwide basis see http://www.panp.com. Geographic Area Served: United States.

Clarkston

★ 14272 ★ Medical Technology Management Inc.
PO Box 808
Clarkston, MI 48346
Phone: (248)620-3646 **Fax:** (248)625-9473
Email: mtminc@prodigy.net
Website: http://mtminc.org
Fnded: 1992. **Activities:** Firm provides clinical, biomedical and radiology engineering and clinical equipment asset (service) management program evaluation and development, with emphasis on quantifying options available to the hospital (and/or hospital systems) for equipment service cost reduction and program quality improvements. Consulting programs include equipment maintenance cost of service benchmarks; in-house and outsourced equipment service program evaluations; clinical, biomedical and radiology engineering program development; equipment acquisitions; equipment service and insurance based program consolidations; PAC's and telemedicine system design; JCAHO equipment management program survey preparation. Geographic Area Served: United States.

Detroit

★ 14273 ★ AIDS Partnership Michigan
2751 E Jefferson, Ste. 301
Detroit, MI 48207
Phone: (313)446-9800 **Free:** 800-872-AIDS
Fax: (313)446-9039
Email: info@aidspartnership.org
Website: http://www.aidspartnership.org
Fnded: 1983. **Activities:** Offers customized advice to corporations on the effects of HIV & AIDS in the workplace. Covers strategies for dealing with HIV/AIDS in work situations. Focus is on infected employee rights, co-worker rights, and employer responsibilities. Serves all industries. Geographic Area Served: Southeastern Michigan.

★ 14274 ★ Osei Akoto
2926 Stanley St.
Detroit, MI 48208
Phone: (313)895-4325 **Fax:** (313)832-4290
Fnded: 1993. **Activities:** Specialist in holistic health and community services development and administration. Geographic Area Served: Regional.

Farmington Hills

★ 14275 ★ Alder Associates Inc.
35560 Grand River Ave., Ste. 350
Farmington Hills, MI 48335
Phone: (248)473-0906 **Fax:** (248)473-0949
Email: gdalder@msn.com
Fnded: 1988. **Activities:** Record management, information systems and reimbursement issues consulting services consist of the following: department operation analysis, database management, record processing and data retrieval, physician office management, and management consulting services and special projects. Industries served: healthcare, (hospitals, HMO's, clinics), physician's offices, legal, attorneys, insurance companies, industry, and government agencies. Geographic Area Served: United States.

★ 14276 ★ American Institute for Preventive Medicine
30445 Northwestern Hwy., Ste. 350
Farmington Hills, MI 48334
Phone: (248)539-1800 **Fax:** (248)539-1808
Website: http://www.healthylife.com
Fnded: 1983. **Activities:** Firm offers expertise in health promotion, wellness, and medical self care. Publishes 21 self care guides that address the needs of families, women, men, seniors, children, Hispanics, and Medicaid recipients. Geographic Area Served: Worldwide.

★ 14277 ★ Fitness Rx
28575 Wintergreen
Farmington Hills, MI 48331
Phone: (248)488-9830 **Fax:** (248)488-9828
Email: fitnessrx@netquest.com
Website: http://www.fitnessrxonline.com
Activities: Fitness and weight management consultants offering personal training and dietary, nutrition, exercise, and wellness counseling. Yoga Pilates Spinning Weight Training and Kickboxing classes offered. Geographic Area Served: Metro Detroit.

★ 14278 ★ Gerald S. Kirzner
29992 Northwestern Hwy.
Farmington Hills, MI 48334
Phone: (248)851-8505 **Free:** 800-THERAPIST
Fax: (248)851-8698
Email: drkirz@aol.com
Fnded: 1985. **Activities:** Productivity motivators offering the following range of professional consulting services to assist the individual and the corporation: treatment of personal and attitude problems on an individual basis or within a group setting; stress management and wellness training; career, relocation, outplacement and cessation counseling; assessment and screening of individuals selected for leadership positions, and executive assistance programs focusing on chemical dependency or morale problems. Also works with corporate groups focusing on corporate executive's identification and understanding of life-disrupting stress factors among employees. Geographic Area Served: North Oakland County, Michigan.

★ 14279 ★ Mercy Health Services
34605 W 12 Mile Rd.
Farmington Hills, MI 48331
Phone: (248)489-6000 **Fax:** (248)489-6690
Fnded: 1986. **Activities:** Offers organizational development and management services to NASA and U.S. Air Force healthcare providers.

Flint

★ 14280 ★ Harvey A. Swanebeck
3929 W Court St.
Flint, MI 48532
Phone: (810)233-6322 **Fax:** (810)233-7604
Fnded: 1980. **Activities:** Medical management specialist in professional practice management for physicians and dentists. Geographic Area Served: Mid-Michigan.

Grand Rapids

★ 14281 ★ Catastrophic & Rehabilitation Management Inc.
4163 Clyde Park SW, Ste. 201
Grand Rapids, MI 49509
Phone: (616)531-4040 **Free:** 800-531-9634
Fax: (616)531-4070
Email: cbs@catastrophicrehabmgt.com
Website: http://www.catastrophicrehabmgt.com
Fnded: 1991. **Activities:** Specializes in catastrophic case management, medical case management, home modification assessment, home care coordination, job modification, health care education, life care planning and geriatric long term care assessments. Geographic Area Served: Western Michigan.

★ 14282 ★ Employee Assistance Associates L.L.C.
900 Victors Way, Ste. 350
Grand Rapids, MI 49503
Phone: (616)459-9180 **Fax:** (616)788-8630
Website: http://www.employeeassistanceassoc.com
Fnded: 1981. **Activities:** Provides comprehensive employee assistance programs to workplaces on a contract basis. Assists employees and family members with personal problems. Primary aim is early intervention so personal problems will not affect job performance. Major emphasis is placed on cost containment of mental health, substance abuse, and other insurance costs by providing case management services. Industries served: manufacturing, paint and chemicals, publishing and printing, high-tech, government, retail, service, banking and insurance, and healthcare and human service. Geographic Area Served: Southeast Michigan, northern Ohio with a network throughout the United States.

★ 14283 ★ Human Resource Associates
161 Ottawa NW, Ste. 300C
Grand Rapids, MI 49503
Phone: (616)458-0692 **Free:** 800-237-2673
Fax: (616)458-8129
Email: hrainfo@iserv.net
Website: http://www.hresource.com
Fnded: 1972. **Activities:** Offers the following consulting services for business, industry and hospitals: management consultation, executing coaching, evaluation of new employees for hire and current employees for promotion, and employee outplacement. For individuals, consulting services include evaluation and counseling to children, adolescents and adults, and treatment for addictions. Also offers consultation on forensic psychology to attorneys. Geographic Area Served: Michigan.

★ 14284 ★ The La Penna Group
2110 Enterprise St. SE, Ste. 300
Grand Rapids, MI 49508-5325
Phone: (616)281-2882 **Free:** 800-LAP-ENNA
Fax: (616)281-0573
Email: lapenna@lapenna.com
Website: http://www.lapenna.com
Activities: A consultative group that assists its clients through the development and implementation of strategies to foster growth. Specializes in the health care field – hospitals, health systems, physicians, group practices and networks. Assignments include research, analysis and planning but firm specializes in "hands on" implementation. Geographic Area Served: United States.

Hillsdale

★ 14285 ★ Dow Leadership Center
Hillsdale College
22 E Galloway Dr.
Hillsdale, MI 49242
Phone: (517)437-3311 **Fax:** (517)437-0558
Email: dow.center@hillsdale.edu
Website: http://www.hillsdale.edu/dowcenter
Fnded: 1952. **Activities:** The Center's professional staff is equipped to consult in many areas, including needs analysis, organizational analysis and development, evaluation, research and training. Expertise areas include organizational change, team-building and team-problem-solving, participative management, peer counseling, motivation, management effectiveness, communication, stress processing, conflict resolution, and family business issues. Serves private industries as well as government agencies. Geographic Area Served: Worldwide.

Howell

★ 14286 ★ Lance Associates
Howell, MI 48843
Phone: (517)548-1228 **Fax:** (517)548-3574
Email: lanceasc@ismi.net
Website: http://www.ismi.net/lryassoclegal
Fnded: 1978. **Activities:** Provides services to long-term care and senior housing businesses. Helps facilities in financial and/or regulatory peril. Projects include roles in receivership, temporary management, and monitoring for the State of Michigan.

Lansing

★ 14287 ★ Health Management Associates Inc.
120 Washington Sq. N, Ste. 705
Lansing, MI 48933-1608
Phone: (517)482-9236 **Free:** 800-678-2299
Fax: (517)482-0920
Email: info@healthmanagement.com
Website: http://www.healthmanagement.com
Fnded: 1985. **Activities:** Provides expertise in the areas of health and human services policy, finance and economics, evaluation, and health data analysis. Serves public and private sector health and human services clients in the U.S., primarily Michigan. Geographic Area Served: United States.

★ 14288 ★ Medical Management Systems of Michigan Inc.
1701 Lake Lansing Rd., Ste. 100
Lansing, MI 48912-3708
Phone: (517)485-0001 **Fax:** (517)485-2622
Email: maxine@mmsm.com
Website: http://www.mmsm.com
Fnded: 1983. **Activities:** Advises physicians and hospitals in Michigan on healthcare management, billing, and documentation billing and coding audits. Geographic Area Served: Michigan.

Livonia

★ 14289 ★ John E. Levis Associates Inc.
32945 Indiana St., Ste. B
Livonia, MI 48150-3766
Phone: (734)422-8029 **Free:** 800-400-5171
Fax: (734)525-8302
Fnded: 1992. **Activities:** Firm has experience in healthcare and medical information research services. Also provides competitor intelligence service.

Midland

★ 14290 ★ Sandra Simmons
90 Seeley Dr.
Midland, MI 48640
Phone: (517)839-1764 **Fax:** (517)839-1796
Fnded: 1966. **Activities:** Emphasis on organizational structure, staff utilization, financial management, change. Primary agency focus-skilled home care. Secondary agency focus-hospice. Geographic Area Served: United States, primarily Great Lakes and Midwest.

Monroe

★ 14291 ★ Maplewood Manor
3250 N Monroe St.
Monroe, MI 48162-9297
Phone: (734)457-0746 **Free:** 800-932-5202
Fax: (313)432-6788
Fnded: 1985. **Activities:** Health services consultants offer expertise in elderly care services, wound care, home health care, private duty services, hospice care, skilled nursing, physical, speech & occupational therapy in, home x-ray, medical social workers, diabetes management, spiritual care, grief counseling, pain management.

Okemos

★ 14292 ★ Rehabilitation Case Management Consultants Inc.
PO Box 1006
Okemos, MI 48805-1006
Phone: (517)349-8221 **Free:** 800-968-4087
Fax: (517)349-1290
Email: rcmc-ssc@ix.netcom.com
Website: http://www.seniorcitizencns.com
Fnded: 1989. **Activities:** Specializes in case management services for catastrophic accident and auto accident victims, group health, and short- and long-term disability and worker compensation claimants. Also provides care management services for senior citizens both privately and through long term care insurance companies. Geographic Area Served: Michigan.

Plymouth

★ 14293 ★ Knopf Co. Inc.
1126 S Main St.
Plymouth, MI 48170-2214
Phone: (734)455-4343 **Free:** 800-420-4343
Fax: (734)455-0015
Email: knopf1@ameritech.net
Website: http://www.knopfcompany.com
Fnded: 1984. **Activities:** Advises businesses and school districts, and general public locally on health issues in the areas of substance abuse, prevention programs, conflict resolution programs. Meeting and conference planning services. Geographic Area Served: United States and Canada for training and consulting services.

Redford

★ 14294 ★ Anne Sullivan Smith
24831 Ross Dr.
Redford, MI 48239
Phone: (313)532-0464
Fnded: 1982. **Activities:** Offers healthcare expertise in the areas of development, refinement, and evaluation of services and programs of community health and social service agencies, hospitals, ambulatory care programs, and senior citizen facilities and services. Serves public and private sector in the U.S.

Southfield

★ 14295 ★ Acton Sell Associates
21415 Civic Center Dr., Ste. 211
Southfield, MI 48076
Phone: (248)357-1426 **Free:** 800-473-5460
Fax: (248)357-3745
Email: steveatasa@aol.com
Fnded: 1982. **Activities:** Advises on health services management, specializing in physician recruiting and general healthcare employment and interviewing. Geographic Area Served: Continental United States.

★ 14296 ★ Bernie Hoffmann Associates Inc.
15565 Northland Dr., Ste. 800 E
Southfield, MI 48075

Phone: (248)557-9340 **Free:** 800-685-2600
Fax: (248)557-8282
Fnded: 1978. **Activities:** Human resources development consultants serving the healthcare industry, including hospitals, nursing homes, clinics, and physicians practices. Experienced in executive and physician searches, executive and hourly pay systems, organization and management development, and employee relations in a union free environment. Also offers expertise in outplacement and downsizing.

★ 14297 ★ Claudenia Buford, MSW
28220 Franklin Rd.
Southfield, MI 48034
Phone: (248)355-1452
Fnded: 1986. **Activities:** Provides on-site workshops, training, and seminars to assist in continuing education of staff. Offers presentations and can tailor a program to fit the specific needs of an organization. **Remarks:** Psychotherapy services as well as employee assistance offered.

★ 14298 ★ Consultants in Opthalmic Plastic Surgery
Comerica Southfield Twr.
29201 Telegraph Rd., Ste. 305
Southfield, MI 48034
Phone: (248)357-5100 **Fax:** (248)746-0683
Website: http://www.facialworks.com
Activities: Offers plastic surgery on the eyes and the latest advances in laser resurfacing. Specific problems seen by consultants in ophthalmic plastic surgery include ptosis-drooping of upper eyelid, entropion-eyelid rolling inward, ectropion-sagging of lower eyelid, tearing-due to injury or disease, skin cancers (basal cell, melanoma, squamous cell, etc.), tumors and cysts-growth of eyelids and surrounding tissues, orbital fractures, trauma, congenital problems (lids or tearing), cosmetic surgery, and laser resurfacing. Surgical counselors are available to answer questions regarding proposed procedures including pre-op and post-opcare, surgical facilities, and transportation.

★ 14299 ★ Wellness Group Inc.
29201 Telegraph Rd., Ste. 420
Southfield, MI 48034
Phone: (248)351-7890 **Fax:** (248)351-7896
Email: wgi@wellnessgroup.net
Website: http://www.wellnessgroup.net
Fnded: 1982. **Activities:** Human Resources consulting firm provides expertise in: employee assistance programs, counseling, seminars, stress management, medical expert witness, accident reconstruction, independent medical exams and organizational development. Geographic Area Served: United States.

Traverse City

★ 14300 ★ Lillian E. Smith
19367 Whispering Trl.
Traverse City, MI 49686-9771
Phone: (231)223-4817 **Fax:** (231)223-4827
Fnded: 1987. **Activities:** Provides nutrition consulting for individuals, corporations, educational institutions, and private sector. Geographic Area Served: United States.

West Bloomfield

★ 14301 ★ Equity Funding & Associates Inc.
7071 Orchard Lake Rd., Ste. 300
West Bloomfield, MI 48322
Phone: (248)932-3040 **Free:** 800-444-7763
Fax: (248)932-0827
Email: equityfund@earthlink.net
Fnded: 1987. **Activities:** Credit rehabilitational consultants. **Remarks:** First licensed in Michigan as a credit service organization. Geographic Area Served: Michigan.

Whitmore Lake

★ 14302 ★ Bio-Sentry Engineering Inc.
9205 Main St.
Whitmore Lake, MI 48189-9411
Phone: (313)449-4407 **Fax:** (313)449-8408
Fnded: 1971. **Activities:** Offers medical equipment engineering design and repair services to healthcare and medical equipment manufacturing industries in the United States.

Minnesota

Bloomington

★ 14303 ★ Health Fitness Corp.
3500 W 80th St., Ste. 130
Bloomington, MN 55431
Phone: (952)831-6830 **Fax:** (952)831-7264
Fnded: 1981. **Activities:** Health Fitness Corporation, a former division of Abbott Northwestern Hospital in Minneapolis, Minnesota, is a consulting and management company that specializes in the start-up, development and operation of hospital and corporate fitness centers. Consulting services include conducting comprehensive feasibility studies, facility and program planning and design, developing business/marketing plans and developing operational strategies. Offers a turn-key approach to developing onsite fitness and PT centers and comprehensive wellness programs. Industries served: corporations, communitites and hospitals in the U.S. Geographic Area Served: United States.

Burnsville

★ 14304 ★ J Miller Associates
12319 Oak Leaf Ct., Ste. 4
Burnsville, MN 55337-2969
Phone: (952)890-2071 **Free:** 800-766-1664
Fax: (952)890-2072
Email: jm@jmillerassociates.com
Website: http://www.jmillerassociates.com
Fnded: 1981. **Activities:** Training and development focusing on management and staff development issues. Serves nonprofit, for-profit and public sector businesses. Provides conference speaking and seminars, needs assessment, and custom-designed training programs, as well as off-the-shelf materials and programs. **Remarks:** Provides a "cafeteria" of HRD resources through the collaborative talents of their many associates. Tailored for customer satisfaction. Geographic Area Served: Worldwide.

★ 14305 ★ MacNeil Environmental Inc.
12257 C Nicollet Ave. S
Burnsville, MN 55337
Phone: (952)890-3452 **Fax:** (952)890-2991
Email: jmacneil@mac-env.com
Website: http://www.mac-env.com
Fnded: 1987. **Activities:** Provides environmental engineering, health, and safety support to businesses in the Midwest. Geographic Area Served: Midwest (MN, WI, IO, IL, IN, MI, KT).

Duluth

★ 14306 ★ J.P. Consulting Inc.
355 Kenilworth Ave.
PO Box 3053
Duluth, MN 55803
Activities: Specializes in valuation of lost earnings from death or injury, valuation of lost business profits and property, market and financial assessment, and business start up.

Eden Prairie

★ 14307 ★ James Bissonett & Associates Inc.
7901 Flying Cloud Dr., Ste. 154
Eden Prairie, MN 55344-5411
Phone: (952)944-7117 **Fax:** (952)944-7056
Fnded: 1982. **Activities:** Assists businesses in the purchasing and managing of group insurance and corporate retirement plans. Geographic Area Served: Minnesota, Arizona, and Nevada.

Edina

★ 14308 ★ International Medical Products Inc.
4503 Moorland Ave.
Edina, MN 55424
Phone: (612)835-4018 **Fax:** (612)832-5806
Email: impc@msn.com
Fnded: 1981. **Activities:** Health services consulting firm specializes in medical products, clinical trials and FDA approvals for medical devices. Industries served: medical device. Geographic Area Served: United States, Europe, Canada, and Asia.

★ 14309 ★ REM Inc.
6921 York Ave. S
Edina, MN 55435
Phone: (952)925-5067 **Fax:** (952)925-0739
Website: http://www.reminc.com
Fnded: 1967. **Activities:** Firm provides consultation and training in the areas of home health care, health-related training, rehabilitation therapy, services for senior citizens, including independent living and assisted living, community living, including medical and vocational/recreation services for people with developmental and other types of disabilites, psychological assessment and behavioral therapy for children, adults and families, and management and financial consultation. Geographic Area Served: Has services in 17 states including: Minnesota, North Dakota, Iowa, Montana, Wisconsin, Utah, Nevada, Colorado, Arizona, Indiana, Ohio, West Virginia, Oklahoma, New Jersy, Maryland, Pennsylvania, and Connecticut.

Inver Grove Heights

★ 14310 ★ Scott Loss, MD
5270 Greystone Dr., Ste. 109
Inver Grove Heights, MN 55077
Phone: (651)554-1423 **Fax:** (651)554-1429
Activities: Board-certified internist with 9 years experience in HIV/AIDS. Experience with medical case review, and deposition.

Minneapolis

★ 14311 ★ Braley Consulting Services Inc.
2500 39th Ave. NE, Ste. 210
Minneapolis, MN 55421
Phone: (612)781-4434 **Fax:** (612)782-8668
Email: gbraley@braley.com
Website: http://www.braley.com
Fnded: 1978. **Activities:** Assists hospitals and clinics with analysis and evaluation of real-time computerized medical systems in a variety of applications such as clinical laboratory, pharmacy, admissions and communications/order entry. Services include preliminary investigations and needs assessment, system selection, and installation. Geographic Area Served: United States.

★ 14312 ★ Clark/Bardes Consulting - Healthcare Group
225 S 6th St., Ste. 1200
Minneapolis, MN 55402
Phone: (612)339-0919 **Free:** 800-327-9335
Fax: (612)339-2569
Email: hg-info@clarkbardes.com

Website: http://www.clarkbardes.com/healthcare

Fnded: 1958. **Activities:** The largest compensation consulting firm in the U.S. Consulting assignments consist of designing and installing all aspects of executive compensation plans, executive level benefits plans, and physician compensation design and implementation. Provides all forms of compensation planning in both the executive and physician areas including employment agreements, severance agreements, board compensation, leadership transition planning, retention incentive plans, deferred compensation planning, and substantial retirement planning. Geographic Area Served: United States.

★ 14313 ★ Community Intervention Inc.
529 S 7th St., Ste. 570
Minneapolis, MN 55415
Phone: (612)332-6537 **Free:** 800-328-0417
Fax: (612)342-2388
Email: service@communityintervention.com
Website: http://www.communityintervention.com

Fnded: 1979. **Activities:** A national organization dedicated to helping communities deal with the problems of youth. Community Intervention helps concerned adults mobilize into cohesive teams with clearly defined roles, goals and objectives; empowers those teams with the organization, skills and knowledge necessary to turn concerns into positive action; and supports teams with a variety of valuable services and resources. Geographic Area Served: United States and Canada.

★ 14314 ★ Comprehensive Reimbursement Consultants
8990 Springbrook Dr. NW, Ste. 200
Minneapolis, MN 55433-5880
Phone: (763)785-4400 **Fax:** (763)656-2512

Fnded: 1984. **Activities:** CRC provides a full array of quality and innovative reimbursement consulting services designed to expedite payer recognition, ensure long term favorable coverage policies, and improve access to healthcare. CRC offers the following services: Strategic Reimbursement Planning and Implementation; New Products Introductions and Advocacy; Market Research and Due Diligence; Sales Training and Education Programs; Customer Support Programs; and Reimbursement Program Summaries. Geographic Area Served: United States.

★ 14315 ★ Creative Health Care Management Inc.
1701 E 79th St., Ste. 1
Minneapolis, MN 55425-1151
Phone: (952)854-9015 **Free:** 800-728-7766
Fax: (952)854-1866
Website: http://www.chcm.com

Fnded: 1978. **Activities:** Offers organization and management of professional services in all healthcare settings including patient care delivery systems, work redesign, executive and management team building, leadership development, competency, professional practice and case management. Geographic Area Served: Canada, United States, Japan, United Kingdom, Australia, Brazil.

★ 14316 ★ Grace Management Inc.
6225 42nd Ave. N
Minneapolis, MN 55422
Phone: (763)544-9934 **Fax:** (763)544-9858
Website: http://www.gracemanagement.com

Fnded: 1984. **Activities:** Offers management and marketing consulting services to developers, owners, and operators of seniors housing communities. Expertise includes planning, market research and analysis, building design, financing, auditing, accounting, budgets, management, information systems, specialized marketing, kitchen design and equipment specifications, food service, personnel hiring, training, insurance, cost control, safety, and activities programs. Industries served: congregate for independent and assisted living seniors communities, as well as government agencies.

★ 14317 ★ Hans Tronnes Associates
4311 Cedarwood Rd., Ste. 106
Minneapolis, MN 55416-3828
Phone: (952)926-3488 **Fax:** (952)924-9211
Email: tronnes@consultant.com
Website: http://www.hanstronnes.com

Fnded: 1986. **Activities:** Works with healthcare leaders in strategic planning, physician/hospital integration, consolidation of hospitals, master planning, and programming. Geographic Area Served: United States and Canada.

★ 14318 ★ Hilleren & Associates Inc.
3800 W 80th St., Ste. 880
Minneapolis, MN 55431
Phone: (612)956-9090 **Fax:** (612)956-9009
Website: http://www.hilleren.com

Fnded: 1983. **Activities:** Provides executive search services in sales, marketing and management in the medical and pharmaceutical manufacturing industry. Geographic Area Served: Worldwide.

★ 14319 ★ Medallion Laboratories
9000 Plymouth Ave.
Minneapolis, MN 55427
Phone: (612)540-4453 **Free:** 800-245-5615
Fax: (612)540-4010
Website: http://www.medlabs.com

Fnded: 1974. **Activities:** Firm specializes in the fields of analytical testing, microbiological testing, pesticides, and physical testing. Innovative technology, superior customer service, and a staff of over 40 analysts and consultants provide the flexibility and expertise to meet a client's analytical needs.

★ 14320 ★ Medtronic Inc.
710 Medtronic Pky.
Minneapolis, MN 55432-5604
Phone: (763)574-4000 **Free:** 800-328-2518
Fax: (763)574-4879
Website: http://www.medtronic.com

Fnded: 1949. **Activities:** Works with industrial and government agencies to develop procedures to test chemicals and drugs or medical device products to meet federal regulations for Food and Drug Administration, Environmental Protection Agency, Department of Transportation, and other regulatory agencies. **Remarks:** Medtronic is the world's leading medical technology company, providing lifelong solutions for people with chronic disease. With deep roots in the treatment of heart disease, Medtronic now provides a wide range of products and therapies that help physicians treat the most challenging, life-limiting medical problems & restore health, extend life and alleviate pain.

★ 14321 ★ Nutrition & Food Associates
PO Box 47007
Minneapolis, MN 55447
Phone: (763)550-9475 **Fax:** (763)559-3675
Email: patgodfrey@worldnet.att.net
Website: http://www.nutriform.com

Fnded: 1984. **Activities:** Nutritional consultants specializing in product regulations, nutrition labeling, nutritional recipe analysis and nutrition copy for product labels, national magazines and publishing companies. The purpose is to provide the nutrition information for recipes and products. Also offers food-styling and photography services, as well as nutritional and medical communication services. The purpose is to provide accurate nutrition and medical information copy for magazines and publishers. Industries served: food manufacturers, restaurants, bakeries, and grocers worldwide.

★ 14322 ★ Pathways to Performance Inc.
14475 23rd Ave. N
Minneapolis, MN 55447
Phone: (763)745-7907 **Free:** 800-661-8767
Fax: (763)473-0083
Email: info@pathways-to-performance.com
Website: http://www.ztraining.com

Fnded: 1979. **Activities:** A consortium of trainers and consultants specializing in creating custom designed professional developoment seminars. Provides training resources and educational products for the purpose of increasing people's motivation, morale, productivity and satisfaction. Also consults with firms in areas of employee selection to effectively place people in appropriate jobs to obtain and maintain maximum performance. Administers and interprets a battery of assessments to determine behavioral styles, value systems, role perceptions, and influencing modes. Industries served: business, manufacturing, government, hospitals, churches, educational institutions, and professional associations. Geographic Area Served: United States.

Minnetonka

★ 14323 ★ Corporate Benefit Services of America Inc.
10159 Wayzata Blvd.
Minnetonka, MN 55305
Phone: (952)541-0444 **Fax:** (952)545-6235
Email: cbsa@cbsainc.com
Website: http://www.cbsainc.com

Fnded: 1976. **Activities:** Provides third party health administration. Geographic Area Served: United States.

★ 14324 ★ The Edumed Corp.
5610 Rowland Rd., Ste. 165
Minnetonka, MN 55343
Phone: (612)932-9922 **Free:** 800-338-6339
Fax: (612)932-9939
Website: http://www.edumed.com

Fnded: 1988. **Activities:** Offers consulting to medical startup companies, physicians, and healthcare organizations in medical diagnostics for the PC and software systems with a particular focus on nursing and radiology. Industries served: healthcare and biotechnology in the U.S.

Robbinsdale

★ 14325 ★ Heinemann Associates Inc.
4538 Quail Ave. N
Robbinsdale, MN 55422
Phone: (763)504-2559 **Fax:** (763)537-1469
Email: caheinemann@attbi.com

Fnded: 1988. **Activities:** Specialists in planning medical facilities and equipment. Serves healthcare clients in the U.S. and overseas.

Saint Louis Park

★ 14326 ★ M.H. Katz Consulting Inc.
3630 Phillips Sky., Ste. 609
Saint Louis Park, MN 55426
Phone: (952)929-9004

Fnded: 1980. **Activities:** Consultant in food science and technology and flavor chemistry. Offers development and problem solving services in areas related to: protocept development to reduce new concepts to practice, flavor problems, odor control problems, product formulation, process development, ingredient system functionality, product stability, ingredient cost reduction, quality improvement, ingredient quality and safety specifications, product quality and safety specifications, and ingredient and nutritional labeling information. Industries served: flavor manufacturers and food manufacturers.

Saint Paul

★ 14327 ★ Damberg Ltd.
433 Otis Ave., Ste. MG
Saint Paul, MN 55104
Phone: (612)646-1044 **Fax:** (612)646-1995

Activities: Experienced facility planner consultant for healthcare institutions.

★ 14328 ★ **Emeritus Corp.**
1919 University Ave., Ste. 160
Saint Paul, MN 55104
Phone: (651)645-5300 **Fax:** (651)645-0976
Activities: Health care consulting firm offers mental health management services.

★ 14329 ★ **Ivan Engineering Ltd.**
1117 Benton Way
Saint Paul, MN 55112-3755
Phone: (651)483-2071 **Fax:** (651)483-2071
Email: jsyd@pclink.com
Fnded: 1982. **Activities:** Registered professional engineering consultant offering mechanical and bio-medical engineering service. Research and development, product improvement, and failure analyses in the area of material evaluation, electro-mechanical, and bio-medical engineering. Geographic Area Served: Minnesota and nationwide.

Stillwater

★ 14330 ★ **Paladin Medical Inc.**
PO Box 560
Stillwater, MN 55082-0560
Phone: (715)549-6035 **Fax:** (715)549-5380
Email: duncan@paladinmedical.com
Website: http://www.paladinmedical.com
Fnded: 1987. **Activities:** Offers a full range of medical product regulatory, clinical, and technical contract services including total quality system implementation, design control procedures and review, pre-clinical and biocompatibility qualification, and clinical study design/management. The company specializes in 510 (k)s, IDEs, and PMAs, as well as ISO/CE marking and international regulatory requirements.

Winona

★ 14331 ★ **Nursing Consultation Inc.**
PO Box 255
498 Kerry Ct.
Winona, MN 55987
Phone: (507)454-1680
Fnded: 1975. **Activities:** Offers mental health consultations and workshop development. All services arranged by client request. Services related to human relations and interpersonal communication are provided to individuals, families, nonprofit associations and organizations, the healthcare field, and government as an industry. Geographic Area Served: United States.

Mississippi

Jackson

★ 14332 ★ **Malloy Associates**
177 St. Andrews Dr.
Jackson, MS 39211-2532
Phone: (601)957-9991 **Fax:** (601)957-3626
Email: jmalloy@son.umsmed.edu
Fnded: 1991. **Activities:** Firm involved in strategic planning for integrated delivery systems disease management as a cost savings tool; managed care alternative strategies and positioning; IPA development and implementation; physician recruiting; long term care facility business planning; and physician-directed HMO development and operations. Geographic Area Served: United States.

Water Valley

★ 14333 ★ **Billie Winters RHIT Medical Record Consultant**
PO Box 549
Water Valley, MS 38965
Phone: (601)473-1480 **Fax:** (601)473-1458
Email: winters@watervalley.net
Fnded: 1975. **Activities:** Medical records consultant to nursing homes, hospitals, and other healthcare institutions. Provides training programs, as well as training tapes and manuals for health information managers in all types of facilities. Industries served: nursing homes, home health organizations, health departments, and mental health facilities (hospitals LTC) In service on PPS Documentation. Geographic Area Served: Tennessee, Mississippi, Alabama, Louisiana, Texas.

Missouri

Independence

★ 14334 ★ **Practice Support Resources Inc.**
4230 Phelps Rd., Ste. E
Independence, MO 64055
Phone: (816)478-8766 **Free:** 800-967-7790
Fax: (816)478-8914
Email: info@practicesupport.com
Website: http://www.practicesupport.com
Fnded: 1986. **Activities:** Emphasis in working with hospitals to develop and expand their physician support services. Offers Practice Management Bookstore, Practice Management Training Programs, and Compliance Audits. Geographic Area Served: United States.

Kansas City

★ 14335 ★ **Brady & Associates - Consultants to Health Care Management**
7667 NW Prarie View Rd., Ste. 204
Kansas City, MO 64151
Phone: (816)587-2120 **Fax:** (816)587-1698
Email: brady@bradyinc.com
Website: http://www.bradyinc.com
Fnded: 1983. **Activities:** Business purpose is to help hospitals achieve optimum results in all critical outcome areas. Provides comparative staffing data, identifies solutions, conducts on-site management training workshops, and supplies assistance to departments with special needs. Geographic Area Served: United States.

★ 14336 ★ **Exemplar Internationab Inc.**
1600 Genessee, Ste. 700
Kansas City, MO 64102
Phone: (816)471-3900 **Free:** 800-946-7228
Fax: (816)471-1929
Website: http://www.healtheval.com
Fnded: 1969. **Activities:** Offers occupational safety and health counseling services to a wide range of industries relative to workers compensation and OSHA activities. Also offers a full range of environmental monitoring services and a full line of health screening equipment. Geographic Area Served: United States.

★ 14337 ★ **Healthcare Administrative Services Inc.**
10301 Hickman Mills Dr.
Kansas City, MO 64137
Phone: (816)763-5446 **Fax:** (816)523-2355
Fnded: 1988. **Activities:** Advises physicians in private practice on administrative, accounting, and billing processes. Geographic Area Served: Kansas City and St. Louis, Missouri.

Platte City

★ 14338 ★ **Fitch & Associates L.L.C.**
303 Marshall Rd., Ste. 5
Platte City, MO 64079
Phone: (816)431-2600 **Fax:** (816)431-2653
Website: http://www.fitchassoc.com
Fnded: 1984. **Activities:** Offers emergency medical services counsel to private and public ambulence services, medical institutions, and government agencies in the United States, Canada, Latin America, Europe and Middle East. Geographic Area Served: Worldwide.

Saint Louis

★ 14339 ★ **ASI Food Safety Consultants Inc.**
7625 Page Ave.
Saint Louis, MO 63133
Free: 800-477-0778
Website: http://www.asifood.com
Fnded: 1934. **Activities:** Advises food stores, restaurants, processors, warehouses and distributors on government regulations (GMP and HACCP). Inspects, instructs and advises food processing, handling and storage facilities to minimize contamination risks. Trains employees and management in practices and techniques that will make the facility safer and more profitable. Geographic Area Served: North America with consultants positioned throughout the United States and Canada.

★ 14340 ★ **Birenbaum & Associates**
917 Locust, Ste. 1100
Saint Louis, MO 63101-1419
Phone: (314)241-1445 **Fax:** (314)241-1449
Email: birenbaum@birenbaum.org
Website: http://www.aab.org
Fnded: 1968. **Activities:** Multi-association management firm and industrial relations specialists offering consultation to management in public and private sectors. Experienced also in meeting management. Clients in manufacturing, service industry, fire protection districts, and government throughout the U.S.

★ 14341 ★ **First Class Solutions Inc.**
2060 Concourse Dr.
Saint Louis, MO 63146
Phone: (314)997-8998 **Free:** 800-274-1214
Fax: (314)997-0400
Email: info@firstclasssolutions.com
Website: http://www.firstclasssolutions.com
Fnded: 1988. **Activities:** First Class Solutions, Inc. is a diversified computer and healthcare consulting firm, serving clients throughout the United States. Computer consulting services include: complete Internet services, website design and host, network design, installation services and sales, software installation, hardware sales, and system design. Healthcare consulting services include: temporary management and operational assessments of medical records, transcription, business office, quality assurance and utilization review services, JCAHO preparation, temporary staffing for coding activities, coding proficiency and compliance audits, DRG validation studies, and HMO/PPO provider network development. Industries served: all industries, with emphasis on hospitals, physicians, insurance companies, and clinics. Geographic Area Served: United States.

★ 14342 ★ **Harshman & Associates**
2510 S Brentwood Blvd., Ste. 204
Saint Louis, MO 63144
Phone: (314)961-9676 **Fax:** (314)961-9678
Email: info@harshman.com
Website: http://www.harshman.com
Fnded: 1980. **Activities:** Assists organizations through customized strategies to develop organizational change process, personnel assessment, labor-management partnerships, and organizational communication strategies. Offers training and development programs in leadership, facilitation skills, stress management, business team meetings, and listening and communication skills.

★ 14343 ★ **Health Capital Consultants**
9666 Olive Blvd., Ste. 375
Saint Louis, MO 63132-3013
Phone: (314)994-7641 **Free:** 800-FYI-VALU
Fax: (314)991-3435
Email: info@healthcapital.com
Website: http://www.healthcapital.com/
Activities: A Healthcare Consulting firm specializing in valuation, litigation support, provider integration, mergers and acquisitions, financial analysis/forecast-

ing, and research for healthcare providers and their advisors.

★ 14344 ★ Health Technologies Inc.
8446 Page Ave.
Saint Louis, MO 63130
Phone: (314)423-0579 **Free:** 800-544-3059
Fax: (314)423-9825
Email: info@ht-ss.com
Website: http://ht-ss.com
Fnded: 1984. **Activities:** Advises hospitals and long-term care facilities on nutrition and food service. Geographic Area Served: United States.

★ 14345 ★ L.A. Direct
8342 Olive Blvd.
Saint Louis, MO 63132
Phone: (314)997-3452 **Fax:** (314)727-0552
Fnded: 1986. **Activities:** Specializing in medical, dental, nursing and allied health markets. Serves companies seeking to direct market services (advertising, co-ops, mailings, and telemarketing), to physicians, allied health professionals, and those employed in legal, accounting, insurance, and banking industries. Specializes in medical device promotion and launches, start-up and integration of direct mail sales into existing sales organizations, solo mailing (planning through execution), sales lead programs, and mailing list research and acquisition. Geographic Area Served: Worldwide.

★ 14346 ★ Mattson Jack Group Inc.
11960 Westline Industrial Dr., Ste. 180
Saint Louis, MO 63146
Phone: (314)469-7600 **Fax:** (314)469-6794
Email: info@mattsonjack.com
Website: http://www.mattsonjack.com
Fnded: 1986. **Activities:** Consults on growth strategy to the pharmaceutical and healthcare industry. MJG specializes in Product Forecasting & Portfolio Analysis, Corporate Development Services (Valuations, Licensing, M&A, and Alliances), Strategic Analysis and Planning, Assessment (Science & Technology and Market Research), Pharmaceutical, Return on Investment (ROI) services and Brand Optimization/ Life Cycle Management. Geographic Area Served: North America, Europe, Japan Pacific Rim.

★ 14347 ★ The Riner Group Inc.
1034 S Brentwood Blvd., Ste. 1640
Saint Louis, MO 63117
Phone: (314)727-7098 **Fax:** (314)727-2735
Website: http://www.rinergroup.com
Fnded: 1981. **Activities:** Provides health care advisory and management services, specializing in strategic planning, organizational development, professional medical practice/hospital mergers and acquisitions, and new business development. Educational efforts are focused on hospital-medical staff organizational structure and board structures and new business development. Industries served: healthcare private medical practices, universities, health systems, pharmaceutical and medical device manufacturers, law firms, accounting firms, other consultancies, government in the U.S. and worldwide. **Remarks:** Special focus on Cardiovascular Service Line development/ heart institute and heart center development and evolution. Geographic Area Served: United States.

Springfield

★ 14348 ★ Consulting Nutritionists
1501 S Essex
Springfield, MO 65809
Phone: (417)882-7575 **Fax:** (417)882-7875
Email: dansued@msn.com
Fnded: 1984. **Activities:** Nutrition consultant for nursing homes and small hospitals and residented facilities. Geographic Area Served: Southwestern Missouri.

★ 14349 ★ Medical Consulting Group L.L.C.
3058 S Delaware
Springfield, MO 65804
Phone: (417)889-2040 **Fax:** (417)889-2041
Email: info@MedCGroup.com
Website: http://www.medcgroup.com
Fnded: 1995. **Activities:** Specialization in the eyecare industry, with a wide range of services including developing and implementing strategies for efficiency and growth for individual practices and corporations. Develop clinics and ambulatory surgical centers from the ground up. In-house creative agency produces specialized and targeted advertising campaigns along with formulating brand imaging strategies and solutions. Geographic Area Served: U.S. & Canada.

Union

★ 14350 ★ Pharma-Tech Industries Inc.
1310 Stylemaster Dr.
PO Box 638
Union, MO 63084
Phone: (314)583-8664 **Fax:** (314)583-5373
Activities: Offers counsel on packaging of over-the-counter drugs, cosmetics, food and veterinary products.

Warrensburg

★ 14351 ★ World Safety Organization Inc.
106 E Young Ave., Ste. G
PO Box 518
Warrensburg, MO 64093
Phone: (660)747-3132 **Fax:** (660)747-2647
Email: wsowmc@socket.net
Website: http://www.worldsafety.org
Fnded: 1975. **Activities:** The purpose of our professional Organizations is to internationalize and promote all safety fields including occupational, environmental and public safety & health, etc.; and to disseminate throughout the world the practices, skills, arts and technologies of safety and accident prevention fields. The primary objective is to protect people, property, environment and its resources. We are an international organization with Consultative status Category II (non-governmental) to the economic and Social Council of the United Nations. We have consultants that work in fire, industrial hygiene, hazardous materials, nuclear incidents, expert witnesses, etc. These consist of certified safety executives, certified safety managers, certified safety specialists, certified safety and security directors, certified safety technicians, certified hazardous materials technicians level I & II, certified hazardous materials supervisors, certified hazardous materials executives, certified safety instructors, certified governmental environmental officers, and certified governmental safety officers. Industries served: any type of industrial operations where safety, security, health, etc. is involved including both light and heavy industries, plus public operations such as schools, government, hospitals, etc. Geographic Area Served: 180 member countries.

Montana

Billings

★ 14352 ★ Ned Tranel - Neuropsychology Services
1645 Ave. D, Ste. E
Billings, MT 59102-3043
Phone: (406)252-6620 **Fax:** (406)252-0151
Fnded: 1974. **Activities:** Consulting service designed to assist with personnel selection and development of general management strategies. Areas of service include: applicant evaluation, personnel motivation, long-range planning, communications skills, assertiveness training, leadership potential, stress management, time management, and marriage, family and individual counseling. Serves private industries as well as government agencies. Geographic Area Served: Montana, Wyoming, and North Dakota.

Missoula

★ 14353 ★ American Diversified Products
207 Pattee Creek Dr.
Missoula, MT 59801
Phone: (406)543-8548 **Fax:** (406)728-2846
Email: adp@bigsky.net
Fnded: 1981. **Activities:** Establishes distribution networks for American medical companies who want to sell to hospitals in the Far East and Pacific Region. Company also assists medical companies in the U.S. who want to establish their own international divisions. Geographic Area Served: Pacific, Far East countries.

★ 14354 ★ PharmaMedical Consultants International L.L.C.
5725 Eastwood Ln.
Missoula, MT 59803-3015
Phone: (406)251-5098 **Free:** 800-248-5101
Fax: (406)251-5099
Website: http://missoula.bigsky.net/pmci
Activities: Company provides medical consulting services to pharmaceutical/biotech companies, CROs and managed care groups. Also provides full CRO services through Clinical Consulting Alliance LLC, a joint venture with International Quantitative Consultants Inc. Geographic Area Served: North America, Europe, Australia, Mid-East.

Nebraska

Lincoln

★ 14355 ★ Chiropractic Associates
5540 South St., Ste. 200
Lincoln, NE 68506
Phone: (402)488-1500 **Free:** 800-552-6347
Fax: (402)488-6651
Activities: Evaluates office ergonomics, and counsels on health and wellness, performance, and safety issues. Geographic Area Served: United States and Canada.

Omaha

★ 14356 ★ Aureus Group
11825 Q St.
Omaha, NE 68137-3503
Phone: (402)397-2980 **Free:** 800-574-9829
Fax: (402)397-1122
Email: info@aureusgroup.com
Website: http://www.aureusgroup.com
Fnded: 1969. **Activities:** Executive search and recruiting consultants specializing in six areas: accounting/finance, data processing, aerospace, engineering, manufacturing, and medical professionals. Industries served: hospitals, all mainframe computer shops, and all areas of accounting. Geographic Area Served: Middle section of the United States, healthcare nationally.

★ 14357 ★ Joni Stinson Enterprises
PO Box 21
14541 Webster Cir.
Omaha, NE 68154
Phone: (402)496-0167
Fnded: 1982. **Activities:** Primarily a consulting firm specializing in the field of long term care food service management and dietetics. Firm's kitchen design department provides expert consultation on the design, layout, and equipment for new construction and renovation projects. Offers systems design services including: food cost accounting systems, purchasing programs, cost effective menus and recipe services, policy and procedure development, nutritional assessment and quality assurance programs. The A La Carte Division is the Nutrition Education Division providing group and individual nutrition education and counsel-

ing programs. Geographic Area Served: Midwestern United States.

★ 14358 ★ Radiology Consultants
13918 Gold Cir.
Omaha, NE 68144
Phone: (402)330-6550
Website: http://www.RadiologyConsultants.com
Activities: Specializes in documentation of brain injury with positron emission tomography (PET scan). Experience in personal injury, including workers' compensation.

★ 14359 ★ Sister Mary Christelle Macaluso, The Fun Nun
College of St. Mary
1901 72nd St.
Omaha, NE 68124-2377
Phone: (402)399-2474 **Fax:** (402)399-2686
Email: funnun@csm.edu
Website: http://www.funnun.com
Fnded: 1980. **Activities:** Professional speaker, author, and Certified Laughter Leader (CLL). Member of the National Speakers Association (NSA) and Association for Applied and Therapeutic Humor. Convention, seminar, in-service, banquet presenter on humor, stress and self-image. Presents to business, health, education, government, social and religious groups. Geographic Area Served: Worldwide.

Nevada

Las Vegas

★ 14360 ★ David Buanno
4560 S Eastern Ave., Ste. 15
Las Vegas, NV 89119
Phone: (702)735-2311 **Fax:** (702)731-1767
Activities: Offers chiropractic consulting. Geographic Area Served: Nevada.

★ 14361 ★ Managing Partners Inc.
Las Vegas, NV 89101
Phone: (702)939-5398 **Fax:** (702)221-0904
Fnded: 1999. **Activities:** Emphasis is to bring about significant change and substantial bottom line profit improvements through continuing education and cost savings. Offers customized education, sales, compliance and management programs. **Remarks:** MPI runs a completely virtual office with professional staff that services every major city in the United States. All Corporate Affairs are handled via our Corporate Headquarters (Las Vegas, NV) and all Sales and Operations are coordinated from our Arizona Regional Office. Geographic Area Served: Worldwide.

★ 14362 ★ Medical Association of Billers
2441 Tech Center Ct., Ste. 110
Las Vegas, NV 89128
Phone: (702)240-8519 **Fax:** (702)243-0359
Email: medassocb@aol.com
Website: http://www.physicianswebsites.com
Fnded: 1994. **Activities:** Specializes in improving healthcare office efficiency and financial results. Capabilities include medical billing and coding training, custom billing and coding training, Certification preparation, Office Assessments, HIPAA Compliance assessments, medical billing services, accounts receivable collections, revenue enhancement. Geographic Area Served: United States.

New Hampshire

Bedford

★ 14363 ★ Rehabinc East Corp.
9 Cedarwood Dr.
Bedford, NH 03110
Phone: (603)669-7833 **Fax:** (603)669-1224
Fnded: 1986. **Activities:** Advises insurance companies on rehabilitation services, focusing on workers' compensation injuries. Geographic Area Served: New England.

Candia

★ 14364 ★ Les A. Cartier & Associates Inc.
PO Box 559
Candia, NH 03034
Phone: (603)483-2180 **Free:** 800-639-7703
Fax: (603)483-8986
Fnded: 1985. **Activities:** An environmental service company comprised of scientists and engineers offers an eight-hour Health and Safety Refresher Course and a forty-hour Health and Safety Course as part of their Hazardous Materials Management Series. Industries served: manufacturing. Geographic Area Served: United States, specifically New England.

Nashua

★ 14365 ★ SAS Management Consultants
92 Walden Pond Dr.
Nashua, NH 03064-2877
Phone: (603)880-7621 **Fax:** (603)886-3302
Fnded: 1991. **Activities:** Offers management consulting services in organizational development. Services include organizational and cultural change; leadership coaching and development; team building; conflict resolution; and design and facilitation of retreats. **Remarks:** Practice dedicated to healthcare. Geographic Area Served: United States.

New Ipswich

★ 14366 ★ J. Crow Co.
PO Box 172
New Ipswich, NH 03071
Free: 800-878-1965 **Fax:** 800-878-1965
Email: jcrow@jcrow.mv.com
Website: http://www.jcrows.com
Activities: Consultant specializing in practices and techniques for health and wellness, including aromatherapy.

New London

★ 14367 ★ The Nutrition Counselling Center
The Gallery, Ste. 202
46 Newport Rd.
New London, NH 03257
Phone: (603)526-2078 **Fax:** (603)526-0214
Email: hdamon@tds.net
Fnded: 1987. **Activities:** Offers individual nutrition counselling for weight control and therapeutic diets (low cholesterol, diabetic, prenatal, etc.); also provides group nutrition programs for business, industry and community groups (weight control, heart healthy eating). Diabetes education services. Geographic Area Served: predominantly the Dartmouth-Lake Sunapee area of New Hampshire.

North Stratford

★ 14368 ★ Northern Consultants Inc.
17 Western Ave., RR No. 1
PO Box 558
North Stratford, NH 03590
Phone: (603)636-9914 **Fax:** (603)636-9924
Email: alcjdb@ncia.net
Fnded: 1975. **Activities:** Specializes in executive search, career counseling, and operational audits in the plastics, packaging, machinery, and healthcare industries. Geographic Area Served: Midwest, northeastern and southeastern United States.

Somersworth

★ 14369 ★ Northeast Pain Consultation and Management Inc.
255 Rte. 108
Somersworth, NH 03878
Phone: (603)692-3166 **Free:** 800-660-4004
Fax: (603)692-3168
Email: info@painmd.com
Website: http://www.painmd.com
Fnded: 1992. **Activities:** Patient care services include spinal catheters and pump implants; medication management; home care pain supervision; diagnostic work-up to determine the exact cause of the pain; nerve blocks and trigger point injections; assistance in restoring functional status; pain coping strategies such as hypnosis, biofeedback, music; and emotional support. Professional consulting services covers the full spectrum of professional pain practice management, including all aspects of financial and medical practice, development. Geographic Area Served: New England and United States.

New Jersey

Bedminster

★ 14370 ★ Yelenik & Associates Inc.
298 Enclave Ln.
Bedminster, NJ 07921
Phone: (908)781-7400
Email: yelenik@webex.net
Website: http://expertpages.com/cv/yelenik.htm
Activities: Expertise in managed care, Medicaid managed care, integrated delivery systems, health and hospital administration.

Boonton

★ 14371 ★ Food-Tek Inc.
50 Intervale Rd.
Boonton, NJ 07005
Phone: (973)257-4000 **Free:** 800-648-8114
Fax: (973)257-5555
Email: info@foodtek.com
Website: http://www.foodtek.com
Fnded: 1972. **Activities:** Specialists in solving technical problems relating to food preparation. Experienced in product development and/or reformulation, cost control, regulatory guidance, nutrition labeling, pilot and prototype production, and other specialized areas. Whether for a totally new product, new product line, or a reformulation, services emphasize minimizing ingredient costs, streamline processing and maintaining quality.

Bridgewater

★ 14372 ★ Cantox Health Sciences International
1011 Hwy. 22 W, Ste. 200
Bridgewater, NJ 08807
Phone: (908)429-9202 **Fax:** (908)429-9260
Email: dridley@cantox.com
Website: http://www.cantox.com
Fnded: 1985. **Activities:** Provides scientific and global regulatory consulting services for human health and safety-related issues involving chemical and biological agents. Our experience and expertise includes food ingredients, food additives, novel foods, nutraceuticals, dietary supplements, OTC and Rx pharmaceuticals, cosmetics, medical devices, pesticides and industrial chemicals. Our strength is in providing innovative solutions to complex toxicology, developmental and regulatory issues. Geographic Area Served: United States, Europe, and Asia.

Clifton

★ 14373 ★ Oxford Research International Corp.
1425 Broad St.
Clifton, NJ 07013-4221
Phone: (201)777-2800 **Fax:** (201)777-9847
Fnded: 1979. **Activities:** Provides medical, legal, and statistical services to pharmaceutical and healthcare industry worldwide.

Edison

★ 14374 ★ Health Communications Inc.
292 Fernwood Ave.
Edison, NJ 08837
Phone: (732)346-0027 **Fax:** (732)346-0442
Website: http://www.hcomm.com
Fnded: 1984. **Activities:** The company's activities focuses on medical writing for pharmaceuticals, producing principally clinical manuscripts, scientific exhibits, regulatory support documents, product monographs, and related projects. The firm offers a complete range of pre-marketing and post-marketing services, including symposium development as well as audiovisual and other specialized programs. Industries served: healthcare, pharmaceutical, and medical device manufacturers. Geographic Area Served: United States and Europe.

★ 14375 ★ J.L. Shapiro Associates Inc.
292 Fernwood Ave.
Edison, NJ 08837-3839
Phone: (732)346-0444 **Fax:** (732)346-0442
Email: info@jlshapiro.com
Website: http://www.jlshapiro.com
Fnded: 1974. **Activities:** A healthcare communications and marketing firm servicing the pharmaceutical and allied health industry. Offers a wide range of services in medical communications, educational programs, electronic media, and medical publishing. Includes preparing preclinical and clinical manuscripts for publication, product monographs, formulary kits integrating print and video, retrospective studies, product backgrounders, IND/NDA submissions, scientific exhibits, and developing, coordinating, and conducting symposia and medical meetings. Also offers medical education videos and computer programs, audioconfering, Internet programs, laptop computer and CD-ROM training programs, patient education videos, and interactive multimedia display.

★ 14376 ★ Morrisy & Co. Inc.
3840 Park Ave., Ste. 208
Edison, NJ 08820
Phone: (732)906-8863 **Free:** 888-492-7638
Fax: (732)906-9138
Email: solutions@hwcsoft.com
Website: http://www.hwcsoft.com
Fnded: 1987. **Activities:** Offers financial and data processing services to hospital and healthcare industries.

Englewood

★ 14377 ★ HLA Systems
163 Engle St.
Englewood, NJ 07631
Phone: (201)569-1953 **Free:** 800-447-7899
Fax: (201)569-1793
Email: hlasystems@aol.com
Fnded: 1977. **Activities:** Consultants in surgical and special care facilities and systems for hospitals. Industries served: healthcare - surgical and special care facilities and systems. Geographic Area Served: Worldwide.

★ 14378 ★ Zelner and Badner Inc.
163 Engle St.
Englewood, NJ 07631
Phone: (201)569-5522 **Free:** 800-447-7899
Fax: (201)569-1793
Email: hlasystems@aol.com
Website: http://www.hlasystems.com
Fnded: 1969. **Activities:** Provides materials handling, physical distribution, and cost reduction consulting services for healthcare and industrial organizations. Health care services include facilities programming and systems improvement studies for surgical, nursing, other special care and other support areas. Industrial services include: functional facility design and cost reduction studies for warehousing and manufacturing materials handling operations; automation and work simplification studies; significant activity in food processing layout and equipment studies. Industries served: healthcare, distribution, and food processing. **Remarks:** Zelner and Badner, Inc. is affiliated with HLA Systems and provides healthcare consulting services for the partnership. Geographic Area Served:

Fanwood

★ 14379 ★ Lehecka Pratt Associates Inc.
380 North Ave.
Fanwood, NJ 07023
Phone: (908)889-8162 **Fax:** (908)889-8162
Email: lpassociates@comcast.net
Website: http://www.lpa-training.com
Fnded: 1986. **Activities:** Firm specializes in innovative technical training and documentation consulting for the pharmaceutical industry. Services include design, production and presentation of training programs, design of training aids and manuals, SOP writing, in-house seminars, packaged training programs and aids, and custom training projects. Industries served: pharmaceutical, medical device, and chemical industries, including government agencies. Geographic Area Served: United States, Canada, and international affiliates.

Flanders

★ 14380 ★ Toxcor Associates Inc.
PO Box 454
Flanders, NJ 07836
Phone: (973)252-0204 **Fax:** (973)252-4424
Email: kaminsky@toxcor-associates.com
Website: http://toxcor-associates.com
Fnded: 1995. **Activities:** Provides consulting in regulatory toxicology and product safety assessment. Also products liability and toxic tort litigation support/expert witness. Industries served: Pharmaceutical, consumer product, chemical, and cosmetic. Geographic Area Served: Worldwide.

Flemington

★ 14381 ★ Med League Support Services
260 Rte. 202-31
Liberty Ct., Ste. 200
Flemington, NJ 08822
Phone: (908)788-8227 **Fax:** (908)806-4511
Email: mail@medleague.com
Website: http://www.medleague.com
Fnded: 1989. **Activities:** Provides services to personal injury, malpractice and product liability attorneys. Explains anatomy, physiology, medical terminology, and standards of care. Summarizes the plaintiff's pain and suffering. Suggestions for interrogatory, requests for production, and demonstrative evidence. Develops a chronology of pertinent events. Prepares questions for deposing medical experts. Locates medical and nursing expert witnesses. Reviews medical literature for key facts and use as learned treatises. Obtains and summarizes literature written by expert witnesses. Geographic Area Served: United States.

Franklin Lakes

★ 14382 ★ Telesis
795 Franklin Ave.
Franklin Lakes, NJ 07417-1368
Phone: (201)848-9544 **Fax:** (201)848-8335
Email: telesis@bellatlantic.net
Fnded: 1982. **Activities:** Offers pre-merger consultation, business valuations, and independent analysis relating to mergers and acquisition primarily in the home healthcare industry. Mr. Roa is qualified as an expert witness in several court jurisdictions relative to going concern issues, evaluations and business appraisals. Industries served: home healthcare including physician supply, home medical equipment distributors, home IV therapy providers, and surgical supply companies. **Remarks:** Specializing in the home health care industry. Geographic Area Served: United States.

Glen Rock

★ 14383 ★ TechnoBusiness Solutions
48 Pinelynn Rd.
Glen Rock, NJ 07452-3037
Phone: (201)652-6668 **Fax:** (201)652-5569
Website: http://www.technobusiness-solutions.com/index.html
Fnded: 1990. **Activities:** Helps clients achieve desired results in the medical device and pharmaceutical industries. Offers services in research and development, packaging, technology transfer, manufacturing, quality, reliability, and productivity improvement programs. These include: product invention and feasibility; product and process design/development; material failure analysis; experimental design; process scale-up; process troubleshooting; control and validation; product quality improvement; manufacturing productivity improvement; and quality, productivity, and assessment audits. It serves all industries worldwide.

Hamburg

★ 14384 ★ Millenium
38 Bourne Cir.
Hamburg, NJ 07419
Phone: (978)372-6003 **Fax:** (978)521-5083
Fnded: 1980. **Activities:** Offers organizational development and training on the following topics: management development, quality and customer satisfaction, performance management, train-the-trainer, stress management, employee selection and management, and training documentation. Specializes in business, government, and industry. Geographic Area Served: United States.

Hawthorne

★ 14385 ★ Xenopore Corp.
299 Wagaraw Rd.
Hawthorne, NJ 07506
Phone: (973)423-2400 **Fax:** (973)423-2401
Website: http://www.xenopore.com
Fnded: 1988. **Activities:** Firm provides consulting services to the pharmaceutical and biotechnological industries.

Hillsborough

★ 14386 ★ Chris Flahive Associates
566 Southwoods Rd.
PO Box 63
Hillsborough, NJ 08844
Phone: (908)281-7000 **Fax:** (908)281-7245
Email: flahive@ix.netcom.com
Fnded: 1989. **Activities:** Offers support to the medical device industry in the assessment, design, development, and implementation of FDA and EC quality systems. Specializes in compliance solutions; quality system documentation; auditing; ISO 9000/EN 46000/MDD registration preparation and pre-assessments; supplier and service quality; design control; on-site training in FDA/ISO/EN quality systems, EC directives and auditing; validation; and sterilization technology.

Jersey City

★ 14387 ★ Altura & Altura Consultants
31-1003 River Ct.
Jersey City, NJ 07310
Phone: (718)270-2618 **Fax:** (718)270-3103

Fnded: 1984. **Activities:** Cardiovascular and nutritionist consultants specializing in the etiology and treatment of cardiovascular disease processes. Investigates the role of magnesium in health and nutrition. Conducts research on the effects of alcohol, cocaine, and PCP on brain and cardiovascular system. Offers expertise in the mechanisms and treatment of shock-trauma, and the toxicological effects of substances of abuse. Also serve as editorial consultants in biomedical publishing. Industries served: pharmaceutical, biomedical research establishments, universities, colleges, medical centers, biomedical publishers, and government agencies. Geographic Area Served: United States, Canada, Europe, and Asia.

Lawrenceville

★ 14388 ★ MIIX Healthcare Group

2 Princess Rd.
Lawrenceville, NJ 08648-2382
Phone: (609)219-1111 **Free:** 800-234-MIIX
Fax: (609)219-6727
Website: http://www.miix.com

Fnded: 1996. **Activities:** Firm provides comprehensive healthcare consulting services and unique products designed to assist physicians, and healthcare organizations meet the challenges of a managed care environment. Consulting services range from practice management to network formation and marketing, practice valuations, practice mergers and acquisitions, and compliance. Geographic Area Served: United States.

Lindenwold

★ 14389 ★ Enviromed Corp.

555 Blackwood-Clementon Rd.
Lindenwold, NJ 08021
Phone: (856)435-7200 **Free:** 800-521-5051
Fax: (856)435-4599
Email: rstepkin@protectyourhearing.com
Website: http://www.protectyourhearing.com

Fnded: 1977. **Activities:** Industrial audiologist consults on the development and implementation of effective hearing conservation programs for industry. Services include mobile audiometry, audiogram interpretation, educational training, noise surveys, hearing protection programs, computerization, custom audiometric software sales, and expert testimony. Geographic Area Served: New Jersey, New York, Connecticut, Rhode Island, New Hampshire, Maine, Vermont, Massachusetts, Virginia, Maryland, Delaware, Pennsylvania, West Virginia, North Carolina, and South Carolina.

Livingston

★ 14390 ★ Hyman W. Fisher Inc.

121 E Northfield Rd.
Livingston, NJ 07039-4506
Phone: (973)994-9480 **Fax:** (973)535-8741
Email: hwfisher@pol.net

Fnded: 1980. **Activities:** Performs market research, organizes and moderates panels and symposia, recruits expert panels, prepares sales training programs, and advises on pharmaceuticals and medical products development. Other areas of expertise include advertising and promotion, continuing education, and professional service programs. Serves pharmaceutical, medical products, healthcare advertising, public relations, and other industries.

Long Branch

★ 14391 ★ Professional Healthcare Associates Inc.

422 Morris Ave., Ste. 1
Long Branch, NJ 07740
Phone: (732)229-4545 **Free:** 800-634-2498
Fax: (732)229-9647
Email: czagury@vistapubl.com
Website: http://www.vistapubl.com

Fnded: 1989. **Activities:** Offers healthcare consulting services in the areas of geriatric service development; grant funding research, development and application preparation; and system development and strategic planning for nursing. Additional work in education and training for healthcare professionals in management training, clinical areas, and writing skills. Other services include manuscript development, editing, publishing and marketing of books, journals and articles related to healthcare, human services and women's issues. Industries served: healthcare, long term care, human services, and municipal government agencies. **Remarks:** Sister company, Vista Publishing, Inc., publishes books and manuals related to nursing and general healthcare issues. Geographic Area Served: United States.

Maywood

★ 14392 ★ Rowin Group Inc.

25 E Spring Valley Ave.
Maywood, NJ 07607
Phone: (201)843-9400 **Fax:** (201)909-8707
Email: d.phadnis@rowingroup.com
Website: http://www.rowingroup.com

Fnded: 1976. **Activities:** Independent consulting company exclusively serving the health industry. Conducts multi- and single-client studies in the following areas: new product introduction; new market development, including confidential representation, company analysis, technology transfer, and diversification. Also actively involved in harnessing web technology for dissemination of healthcare information. Targeted segments are international, industry executives, sales training, consumer education and medical professional education. Geographic Area Served: Worldwide.

Morganville

★ 14393 ★ Leonard Flynn Consulting

254 Tennent Rd.
Morganville, NJ 07751
Phone: (732)591-1328

Fnded: 1985. **Activities:** Provides scientific and regulatory consultation for the pharmaceutical, personal products, and other manufacturing industries. Services include document preparation of scientific reports and submissions to regulatory agencies and review of compliance with federal and state regulatory requirements. Industries served: manufacturers and importers of pharmaceutical, medical device and related health and personal/consumer products plus their raw material suppliers. Geographic Area Served: Worldwide.

Morristown

★ 14394 ★ Pharmaceutical Patent Attorneys L.L.C.

55 Madison Ave., 4th Fl.
Morristown, NJ 07960-6397
Phone: (973)984-0076 **Fax:** (973)984-6159
Email: mark.pohl@licensinglaw.net
Website: http://www.licensinglaw.net

Fnded: 1991. **Activities:** Legal counsel for patents, pharmaceutical business development transactions, co-marketing contracts, research joint ventures, drug licensing transactions. Industries served: pharmaceutical and biotechnology. Geographic Area Served: Has clients worldwide, and counsels on United States law only.

Newark

★ 14395 ★ John D. Bogden, PhD

UMDNJ - New Jersey Medical School
Department of Preventive Medicine
185 S Orange Ave.
Newark, NJ 07103-2714
Phone: (973)972-5432 **Fax:** (973)972-7625
Email: bogden@umdnj.edu

Activities: An environmental toxicology and nutrition consultant, specializing in mineral and trace element nutrition and toxicology, including lead poisoning, chromium toxicity, overdoses of minerals and trace elements, air, soil and water pollutants, and environmental toxins. Analyzes body tissues and fluids. Provides expert reports, deposition and court testimony experience. Geographic Area Served: United States.

★ 14396 ★ Michael Schulder, MD

Section of Neurological Surgery
New Jersey Medical School
90 Bergen St., Ste. 8100
Newark, NJ 07103-2499
Phone: (973)972-2907 **Fax:** (973)972-2333
Email: schulder@umdnj.edu

Activities: Specializes in neurosurgery, treatment of head and spinal injury, and treatment of brain tumors.

Ocean

★ 14397 ★ Phil-Lu Inc.

1206 Herbert Ave.
Ocean, NJ 07712
Phone: (732)531-6338 **Fax:** (732)531-3045
Email: philluinc@aol.com
Website: http://www.philluinc.com

Fnded: 1970. **Activities:** A research corporation specializing in the engineering and making of medical mechanical electronic prototypes. Also has extensive expertise in the development of special instruments, devices, and implants. Industries served: medical, healthcare, safety, new products for all industries, and government agencies. Geographic Area Served: Worldwide.

Parsippany

★ 14398 ★ Bogart Delafield Ferrier Inc.

9 Campus Dr.
Parsippany, NJ 07054
Phone: (973)898-9800 **Free:** 800-732-4221
Fax: (973)267-3681
Email: info@bdf.com
Website: http://www.bdf.com

Fnded: 1981. **Activities:** Management consulting firm focuses on serving the healthcare industry, specializes in pharmaceuticals, devices and diagnostics.

★ 14399 ★ CommonHealth

30 Lanidex Plz. W
Parsippany, NJ 07054
Phone: (973)884-2200 **Fax:** (973)884-2487
Email: mgiegerich@commonhealth.com
Website: http://www.commonhealth.com

Fnded: 1992. **Activities:** Provides a full spectrum of products and services, from traditional healthcare advertising to strategic planning to disease management research. CommonHealth handles healthcare and nutritional products in almost every therapeutic category. Geographic Area Served: Parsippany, NJ; Wayne, NJ; New York, NY; Washington, DC; London, England; Sidney, Australia; Paris, France; Tokyo, Japan; Newport Beach, CA.

Perth Amboy

★ 14400 ★ Management-Plus

791 May Ave.
Perth Amboy, NJ 08861-1618
Phone: (732)826-8061

Fnded: 1976. **Activities:** Offers in-house training in all management areas; related services in needs assessments programs, Quality Circles, attitudinal problems, and job related stress reduction. Serves private industries as well as government agencies. Geographic Area Served: Northeastern United States.

Piscataway

★ 14401 ★ Johnson & Johnson Health Care Systems Inc.

425 Hoes Ln.
Piscataway, NJ 08855
Free: 800-456-5427
Website: http://www.jjhcs.com

Fnded: 1976. **Activities:** Provides medical management, legal counsel, and contract services to physicians, hospitals, and healthcare operations in the United States.

Princeton

★ 14402 ★ Health Science Inc.
418 Wall St.
Princeton, NJ 08540
Phone: (609)924-7616 **Free:** 800-841-8923
Fax: (609)921-0483
Email: healthscience@erols.com
Website: http://www.healthscience.bigstep.com

Fnded: 1984. **Activities:** Specialists in rehabilitation technology for speech disorder and physically disabled persons. Offers demonstrations, evaluations and sales of the following types of equipment: augmentative speech communication systems, adaptive switches and specialty controls, and computer access devices. Industries served: hospitals and rehabilitation centers, schools, and special service organizations such as United Cerebral Palsy Association, Department of Human Services, etc. Geographic Area Served: New Jersey, New York, Pennsylvania, Delaware, Connecticut, Maryland, and Massachusetts.

★ 14403 ★ Princeton Health Systems Inc.
9 Mercer St.
Princeton, NJ 08540
Phone: (609)924-7799 **Free:** 800-437-6668
Fax: (609)497-0739

Fnded: 1981. **Activities:** Offers consulting services in the evaluation, planning, implementation and assessment of medical care services to employees, including cost containment strategies and health and fitness programs. Geographic Area Served: Continental United States.

Princeton Junction

★ 14404 ★ Purdue Associates
4 Canoe Brook Dr.
Princeton Junction, NJ 08550
Phone: (609)799-0330 **Fax:** (609)275-3810
Email: robertoi@aol.com

Fnded: 1971. **Activities:** Offers pharmaceutical research and product development expertise in oral and topical dosage forms, applied nutrition and emulsion technology. Also provides expertise in biotechnology, patents, licensing, technology assessment and transfer. Additional assistance in human resources management and training. Industries served: pharmaceutical, biotechnology, technology-transfer and venture capital, as well as government agencies. Geographic Area Served: New Jersey, New York, and Pennsylvania.

★ 14405 ★ Theradex Systems Inc.
14 Washington Rd.
Princeton Junction, NJ 08550-1028
Phone: (609)799-7580 **Fax:** (609)799-4148
Website: http://www.theradex.com

Fnded: 1982. **Activities:** Pharmaceutical consultants. Geographic Area Served: Worldwide.

Randolph

★ 14406 ★ Network Inc.
1572 Sussex Tpke.
Randolph, NJ 07869
Phone: (973)442-2990 **Free:** 800-523-1394
Fax: (973)442-2883

Fnded: 1977. **Activities:** Firm offers management expertise to medical institutions and hospitals. Serves boards of education in New York and New Jersey. Geographic Area Served: United States and Canada.

Red Bank

★ 14407 ★ Center for Children of Alcoholics Inc.
205 Broad St.
PO Box 8640
Red Bank, NJ 07701
Phone: (732)530-8513 **Fax:** (732)758-8228
Email: KEHerrick@aol.com
Website: http://www.adult-child.com

Activities: Provides information and consultations on issues such as abusive and addictive behaviors.

★ 14408 ★ Microscopy Laboratories
61 W St.
PO Box 338
Red Bank, NJ 07701
Phone: (908)747-6228 **Fax:** (908)758-9142
Email: micro@mail.superlink.net
Website: http://www.microscopylab.com

Fnded: 1977. **Activities:** Specializes in application of electron microscopy to problems in research and development, manufacturing, and quality control. Equipped for scanning electron microscopy (SEM/EDS/BS) and transmission electron microscopy (TEM/STEM/EDS), and maintains the necessary support instrumentation for sample preparation and photography. Offers high-resolution imprint replicas of "live" samples or selected areas of large specimens; cryofracturing; backscattered electron imaging; and energy dyspersive spectroscopy. Provides general sample preparation, ultra-thin sections, shadowing, replication, negative staining, autoradiography, enzyme- and immunocytochemistry, freeze fracture, and histology services. Designs and sets up electron microscopy facilities to assist and train in electron microscopy. Also provides EM and related equipment. Industries served: public and private sector.

Ridgewood

★ 14409 ★ Biomedical Information Center Inc.
219 Phelps Rd.
PO Box 1298
Ridgewood, NJ 07451
Phone: (201)670-7446 **Fax:** (201)670-8836
Email: kminer1@idt.net

Fnded: 1987. **Activities:** Medical writing, including scientific papers for publication, clinical reports for regulatory submissions (NDA, INDs), abstracting and indexing. Therapeutic areas of expertise include: cardiovascular disease, cancer, infectious disease, CNS disorders, inflammation and immunology.

★ 14410 ★ Reed C. Perron, MD
1200 E Ridgewood Ave., 2nd Fl.
Ridgewood, NJ 07450
Phone: (201)444-0868 **Fax:** (201)444-7363

Activities: Specializes in medical malpractice involving diagnosis and management of stroke, hemorrhage, injury, infection of brain, spine or peripheral nerves.

River Vale

★ 14411 ★ Forensic Toxicology Associates
638 Debchar Ct.
River Vale, NJ 07675
Phone: (201)391-0015 **Fax:** (201)908-9229
Email: k.verebey@att.net
Website: http://www.home.att.net/~k.verebey/

Fnded: 1998. **Activities:** Specializes in alcohol and drugs of abuse testing, including disputes of laboratory results. Interprets psychopharmacology and clinical pharmacology laboratory and behavioral data. Interprets drugs and/or alcohol induced behavior based on drug concentration and time/action parameters, and toxicology of alcohol, drugs, and metals. **Remarks:** Qualifications: PhD, Pharmacology, Biochemistry minor, Cornell University Medical College; Diplomat American Board of Forensic Toxicology; Fellow America Academy of Forensic Sciences; Society of Forensic Toxicologists; International Association of Forensic Toxicology; Former Chief Toxicologist for the City of New York, Licensed Clinical Laboratory Director (NY, NJ, PA, etc). Board certification by American Board of Bioanalysis as High Complexity Clinical Laboratory Director. Geographic Area Served: NJ, NY, CT, FL, and other as available.

Roseland

★ 14412 ★ Urban Health Institute Inc.
101 Eisenhower Pky.
Roseland, NJ 07068-1028
Phone: (973)228-9000 **Fax:** (973)228-3128

Fnded: 1973. **Activities:** Assists hospitals, healthcare operations, and government agencies in healthcare management planning. Geographic Area Served: New York, New Jersey, and Connecticut.

Roselle Park

★ 14413 ★ Celsis Laboratory Group Laboratory Division
123 Hawthorne St.
Roselle Park, NJ 07204-0206
Phone: (908)245-1933 **Free:** 800-523-LABS
Fax: (908)245-6253

Fnded: 1939. **Activities:** Offers consulting in animal toxicology, in-vitro toxicology, microbiology and chemical analysis to the pharmaceutical, cosmetic, toiletry, medical device, bacteriocide, pesticide, coatings, graphic arts, and specialty chemical industries. Also serves government agencies. Geographic Area Served: New Jersey, New York, Pennsylvania, and Connecticut.

Secaucus

★ 14414 ★ Concentra Medical Centers
405 County Ave.
Secaucus, NJ 07094-2606
Phone: (201)319-0952 **Free:** 800-851-0034
Fax: (201)319-1611

Fnded: 1991. **Activities:** Advises businesses on environmental and occupational healthcare issues. Geographic Area Served: New Jersey.

Short Hills

★ 14415 ★ K. David Steidley, PhD
50 Baltusrol Way
Short Hills, NJ 07078
Phone: (973)322-5625 **Fax:** (973)533-5648
Email: steidley@nac.net

Fnded: 1965. **Activities:** Radiation health and safety consultant offering expert witness services and relevant safety surveys. Geographic Area Served: Worldwide.

Springfield

★ 14416 ★ The Gloria Rose Gourmet Long Life Cooking School
48 Norwood Rd.
Springfield, NJ 07081
Phone: (201)376-0942 **Fax:** (201)352-2855

Fnded: 1984. **Activities:** Registered dieticians assist with the operation of nutritional schools teaching those with hypertension, high cholesterol, diabetes, and obesity (as well as a preventative healthy lifestyle) how to prepare delicious meals without the use of oils, fats, sugar, or salt. Provide individual attention upon request; with fine restaurants, hotels, and gourmet chefs. Serving physicians, hospitals, as well as large corporations in the New Jersey and New York. **Remarks:** Grant by AARP to Salvation Army for G. Rose to create a specialized low fat, low sodium food program for senior citizens. G. Rose is a national spokesperson for Chicken of the Sea seafood products.

Summit

★ 14417 ★ ARIA Chem-Services
24 Bedford Rd.
Summit, NJ 07901
Phone: (908)273-6729 **Fax:** (908)273-6729

Fnded: 1983. **Activities:** Provides assistance to makers and users of industrial and consumer chemicals in matters of safety, toxicity, and environmental effects. Offers assistance in interpreting government regulations of chemicals, and counsels attorneys in litigation concerning chemicals and chemistry. Industries served: chemical, law, export-import firms, and government agencies.

★ 14418 ★ Equipment Planners Inc.
557 Morris Ave.
Summit, NJ 07901-1308
Phone: (908)273-1616 **Fax:** (908)273-7411
Email: info@equipmentplanners.com
Website: http://www.equipmentplanners.com

Fnded: 1981. **Activities:** Specialists in the management and purchase of fixed and moveable medical equipment. Works with healthcare institutions to provide accurate and pertiennt information during the various phases of new construction and renovations.

Tenafly

★ 14419 ★ Healthcare Affiliates Inc.
121 County Rd.
Tenafly, NJ 07670-1838
Phone: (201)568-4011 **Fax:** (201)568-9031
Email: DRNO230@aol.com

Fnded: 1985. **Activities:** Medical and Dental consultants/expert witnesses to the legal profession. Medical and Dental malpractice case analysis and consultations, including examinations before trial for litigants. Serves both plaintiffs and defendants. Questioned documents analysis, motor vehicle evaluation and fraud investigation, mass fatality victim identification, affiliations with numerous local, county, and state law enforcement agencies; federal anti-terrorism task force. Industries served: legal profession and government agencies. Verification and evaluation of injuries, including temporo-mandibular joint (TMJ) dysfunction syndrome, and secondary to personal injury insurance claims. All medical and dental specialties represented or accessible. Geographic Area Served: United States.

Trenton

★ 14420 ★ GA Environmental Services Inc.
15 W State St.
Trenton, NJ 08608
Phone: (609)393-4089 **Fax:** (609)393-7304

Fnded: 1987. **Activities:** Specializes in environmental audits; remediation planning and coordination; asbestos and lead based paint inspection, abatement, and monitoring; and occupational health investigation and monitoring. The firm serves governments, school boards, commercial building owners, realtors, lending institutions, and attorneys. Geographic Area Served: North Eastern United States.

Union

★ 14421 ★ Pharm Rx Consultants Inc.
1238 Stuyvesant Ave.
Union, NJ 07083
Phone: (908)686-2063 **Fax:** (908)686-8473
Email: bartonf@msn.com

Fnded: 1983. **Activities:** Pharmacy consultants for nursing homes and pharmacy and nursing educational programs. Geographic Area Served: NJ, PA, and MD.

Warren

★ 14422 ★ Human Potential Institute Inc.
45 Washington Valley Rd.
Warren, NJ 07059

Activities: A consulting organization experienced in experiential learning, facilitation, and field support. Offers services in customized curriculum development, team development, and population research and assessments. Seminars offered in addition issues, choice making, and diversity issues among others.

Wayne

★ 14423 ★ Boron, LePore & Associates Inc.
1800 Valley Rd.
Wayne, NJ 07470-2047
Phone: (201)791-7272 **Fax:** (201)791-1121

Whitehouse Station

★ 14424 ★ People Management Associates Inc.
9 Van Pelt Dr.
Whitehouse Station, NJ 08889
Phone: (908)534-6335 **Fax:** (908)534-6335

Fnded: 1981. **Activities:** Human Resource Consultants specializing in creation and integration of Human Resource strategies, programs and policies that fosters employee commitment. We help our clients achieve corporate goals by thorough reviews and analysies of current human resource strategies and programs including preventative healthcare; benefits; employment; employee relations; performance management; compensation and job evaluation; creation of policies and procedures; leadership training; and EEO/AAP/legal requirements. We also provides development and delivery of Team and Individual Effectiveness sessions that reduce conflict, improve communications and lead to the establishment of creative and successful solutions to business issues; interactive employee communications programs, and management of "crisis" situations. Geographic Area Served: Worldwide.

Woodbine

★ 14425 ★ Jerold S. Cohen
287 Hands Mill Rd.
Woodbine, NJ 08270
Phone: (609)364-3712 **Fax:** (856)785-2570
Email: jcohen287@aol.com

Fnded: 1975. **Activities:** Consultant in home health care, hospice, adult day care, disease management; case management, and nursing management. HIPAA, Regulatory compliance and accreditation are specialties. Also provide interim management services. Geographic Area Served: United States.

New Mexico

Albuquerque

★ 14426 ★ Ducks in a Row by Lenfest & Associates
3600 Eubank Blvd. NE
PO Box 16021
Albuquerque, NM 87111
Phone: (505)292-5780 **Fax:** (505)844-6161
Email: lenfest@swcp.com

Fnded: 1982. **Activities:** Independent contractor works in intelligent systems and robotics, writing and editing all manner of professional and technical documents. Offers proficiency in financial systems designing, editing, and writing help screens for a 300 plus screen system. Also performs work for Environmental Safety and Health, writing numerous documents. Has launched award-winning Ducks-In-A-Row, service to design and implement web pages. Geographic Area Served: Primarily Southwest, but will travel when necessary.

★ 14427 ★ Medical Data Systems
12001 Lomas Blvd. NE
PO Box 11879
Albuquerque, NM 87192-0879
Phone: (505)292-3699

Fnded: 1977. **Activities:** Provides technical and professional services relating primarily to healthcare data systems to state and federal governmental agencies, commercial insurance carriers, institutions, institutional consortiums, group and solo practices, clinics, and professional medical societies in: claims processing, systems design and development, Medicaid Management Information Systems, systems testing and evaluation, statistical analysis, systems reports development, production of applications and systems software, systems troubleshooting and consultation, and contract monitoring and project management services. Geographic Area Served: United States.

New York

Albany

★ 14428 ★ Jean M. Bigaouette
460 Krumkill Rd.
Albany, NY 12203
Phone: (518)482-8704

Fnded: 1976. **Activities:** Nutritionist and registered dietitian offering private counseling in nutrition. Services include nutritional assessment of dietary intake and body composition analysis. Provides dietary counseling for obesity, underweight, eating disorders, hypertension, high cholesterol, elevated triglycerides, vitamin and mineral deficiencies and excesses, pregnancy, lactation vegetariarism, adolescence, body builders, and professional athletes. Serves private industries as well as government agencies. Geographic Area Served: Tri-city area of New York (Albany, Schenetady, and Troy).

Bay Shore

★ 14429 ★ William H. Bloom, MD
75 Shore Ln.
Bay Shore, NY 11706
Phone: (631)665-6685 **Fax:** (631)665-6686
Website: http://www.claims.com

Activities: Provides expert testimony on neurological and medical matters.

Bronx

★ 14430 ★ Beth Abraham Management Solutions Inc.
612 Allerton Ave.
Bronx, NY 10467
Phone: (718)881-3000 **Free:** 888-BETH-ABE
Fax: (718)519-4010
Email: info@bethabe.org
Website: http://www.bethabe.org

Fnded: 2000. **Activities:** Expert management, outsourcing and consulting services to continuing care retirement communities, nursing facilities, housing programs, assisted living facilites, adult day health service programs and home care programs. Geographic Area Served: New York, New Jersey, Connecticut.

Bronxville

★ 14431 ★ Life-Line
PO Box 482
Bronxville, NY 10708
Phone: (914)423-3531 **Fax:** (914)423-3531
Email: healthie1@aol.com
Website: http://www.joanfriedrich.com

Fnded: 1985. **Activities:** Alternative healthcare, nutraceutical consulting. Services include research, writing, educational programs, and media presentations on various health and nutrition related areas. Seminars and workshops conducted on topics such as family health, wellness, stress management, osteoporosis, aging, immunity and others. Presentations given to hospitals, corporations, colleges, schools and special groups. Industries served: health, nutrition, public relations, education, and government agencies. Geographic Area Served: Worldwide.

Brooklyn

★ 14432 ★ Center for Thanatology Research and Education Inc.

391 Atlantic Ave.
Brooklyn, NY 11217
Phone: (718)858-3026 **Fax:** (718)852-1846
Email: rhalporn@pipeline.com
Website: http://www.thanatology.org

Fnded: 1981. **Activities:** Serves the publishing industry in editorial and sale of books, and media on death and dying; serves the public and academics in selecting materials on these topics for their own use; helps libraries develop collections on these topics. Also acts as a small press, specializing in Death & Dying publications. Produces two journals in this field. Consults with educators about the methods of using cemetaries to teach history and art. Geographic Area Served: Worldwide.

★ 14433 ★ Comprehensive Resources Inc.

1675 E 16th St.
Brooklyn, NY 11229-1259
Phone: (718)998-0200 **Fax:** (718)339-4172
Email: nursing@comprehensivenet.com
Website: http://www.comprehensivenet.com

Buffalo

★ 14434 ★ John M. Wadsworth MD

313 Summer St.
Buffalo, NY 14222
Phone: (716)883-5367 **Fax:** (716)884-7260

Fnded: 1973. **Activities:** Psychiatric forensic work in areas that include competency, sanity, disability, stress and workers' compensation. Offers expert witness testimony. Geographic Area Served: Western New York.

Chatham

★ 14435 ★ Health Systems Management Network Inc.

170 Daley Rd.
PO Box 366
Chatham, NY 12037
Phone: (518)392-6610 **Free:** 888-280-4766
Fax: (518)392-6606
Website: http://www.hsmn.com

Fnded: 1977. **Activities:** Healthcare management consultants with extensive experience in hospital/clinical operations, utilization, finance, medical records and quality assurance.

Commack

★ 14436 ★ Newman Technical Services Inc.

2193 Jericho Tpke.
Commack, NY 11725
Phone: (631)462-8550 **Fax:** (631)462-8551

Fnded: 1982. **Activities:** Offers electronics design and development for commercial and medical industries. Specializes in computer interfacing and programming, technical project management, and technical manual preparation and documentation development. Geographic Area Served: Northeast United States.

Crugers

★ 14437 ★ Food Science Associates Inc.

PO Box 525
Crugers, NY 10521-0525
Phone: (914)739-7541 **Fax:** (914)739-7541
Email: info@foodconsult.com

Fnded: 1956. **Activities:** Technical, management and implementation consultants to the food industry. Specializing in product development, nutritional labeling, quality contorl and HACCP, package development and graphc design, co-pacher sourcing and start-up guidance and implementation and food regulations. Experts in development of nutrifoods, dietary supplements and medical foods. Processing authority in frozen and extended shelf life chilled foods. Geographic Area Served: North America and Western Europe.

Douglaston

★ 14438 ★ NRH Nutrition Consultants Inc.

334 Hollywood Ave.
Douglaston, NY 11363
Phone: (718)229-0606 **Fax:** (718)631-4336
Email: anandjh@aol.com
Website: http://thenutritionexperts.com

Fnded: 1975. **Activities:** Registered dietitians and nutritionists providing services as translators of nutrition concepts and information. To this end, they prepare educational and audiovisual materials; prepare, implement and evaluate research; conduct seminars, conferences, and in-service education programs; represent and/or advise clients at conferences and meetings; interpret theoretical nutrition information into practical material to enhance promotion and sales of a product, concept or service; and serve as a resource to other medical specialties. Serves private industries as well as government agencies. Geographic Area Served: United States, located in New York metropolitan area.

East Hills

★ 14439 ★ Pall Corp.

2200 Northern Blvd.
East Hills, NY 11548
Phone: (516)484-5400 **Free:** 800-645-6532
Fax: (516)484-5228
Website: http://www.pall.com

Fnded: 1946. **Activities:** Offers the widest range of hydrophilic and hydrophobic materials for use in diagnostic, health-care, and industrial applications.

Elmhurst

★ 14440 ★ RBH Associates Inc.

91-31 Queens Blvd., Ste. 404
Elmhurst, NY 11373
Phone: (718)426-5131 **Free:** 800-461-9227
Fax: (718)426-5980
Email: rbh@mindspring.com
Website: http://www.rbhonline.com

Fnded: 1993. **Activities:** Provides customized resources drawing together talents of independent specialists to address specific client needs. Services include strategic thinking and creative development; successful new products and product repositioning; client presentations; scientific review and analysis of medical communications ideas and materials; effective publication development for products; advisory and editorial board development from medical opinion leaders; writing expanded into new clinical areas; electronic, video, and slides applied to educational, promotional, and sales training programs; and cost effectiveness studies.

Fishkill

★ 14441 ★ Hudson Valley Eye Surgeons P.C.

200 Westage Business Center Dr.
Fishkill, NY 12524
Phone: (845)896-9280 **Fax:** (845)896-0246
Email: eyes@hves.com
Website: http://hves.com

Activities: Specializes in ophthalmology and ophthalmic surgery. Geographic Area Served: Northwest United States.

Garden City

★ 14442 ★ Medical Marketing Development Inc.

601 Franklin Ave.
Garden City, NY 11530
Phone: (516)616-5000 **Fax:** (516)616-5007

Fnded: 1986. **Activities:** Provides medical marketing, management, and practice development services to radiology facilities and other medical practices in the New York Metro area and New Jersey.

Great Neck

★ 14443 ★ MDI Consultants Inc.

55 Northern Blvd., Ste. 200
Great Neck, NY 11021
Phone: (516)482-9001 **Fax:** (516)482-0186
Email: info@mdiconsultants.com
Website: http://www.mdiconsultant.com

Fnded: 1978. **Activities:** Management consulting company assisting companies to comply with FDA regulations, quality assurance programs, ISO certification (9000, 13485, 14000), strategic partnering, strategic planning. Specializing in medical devices, pharmaceutical and food regulations. Act as United States Agent for foreign manufactureres exporting to the United States. Assist with HAACP programs for food companies. Geographic Area Served: Worldwide.

Greenfield Center

★ 14444 ★ Templin Management Associates

265 Locust Grove Rd.
Greenfield Center, NY 12833
Phone: (518)893-7760 **Free:** 888-836-7546
Fax: (518)893-2215
Email: info@templin.com
Website: http://www.templin.com

Fnded: 1986. **Activities:** Templin primarily serves two healthcare sectors, hospitals and healthcare systems, and medical device and instrument suppliers. Services include operations analysis, systems improvement, patient care and workflow redesign, ED & OR turnaround and throughput studies, productivity measurement and monitoring, resource utilization analyses, patient classification system installation and evaluation. Geographic Area Served: United States.

Hamburg

★ 14445 ★ Educational Services

6748 Boston State Rd.
Hamburg, NY 14075
Phone: (716)649-1350 **Free:** 800-724-9866
Fax: (716)649-1959
Email: edsers@buffnet.net
Website: http://www.educationalservices.org

Fnded: 1981. **Activities:** Consultants in critical care nursing, complementary therapies, herbs, pharmcology, and general management programs providing educational services for nurses seeking continuing education units and certification in nursing. Geographic Area Served: United States.

Larchmont

★ 14446 ★ AINSLIE

27 Pine Ridge Rd.
Larchmont, NY 10538-2616
Phone: (914)833-2649 **Fax:** (914)833-5037
Email: broadwin@ainslie.com
Website: http://www.lawinfo.com/biz/ainslie

Fnded: 1993. **Activities:** A design and litigation consultant specializing in patent and technology evaluation and regulatory compliance assessment of ISO and GMP quality systems. Evaluates the adequacy of medical devices and disposables. Assists in discovery and depositions as a fact or expert witness. Offers engineering and due diligence investigations and surgeon/hospital interface. Reviews clinical and technical reports. Geographic Area Served: Worldwide.

★ 14447 ★ William M. Bisordi
151 Rockland Ave.
Larchmont, NY 10538
Phone: (914)834-8426 **Fax:** (914)834-8426
Activities: Board-certified gastroenterologist with 20 years experience. Experience in medical record review and testimony.

Mamaroneck

★ 14448 ★ Carol B. Greenbaum, R.D., C.D.E.
490 Bleeker Ave.
Mamaroneck, NY 10543
Phone: (914)698-4743 **Fax:** (914)698-4743
Fnded: 1986. **Activities:** Provides nutrition counseling for all therapeutic needs; weight reduction and maintenance; and guidance for normal nutrition for all ages, sports, etc., MD-referred or verified. Consultant is a Certified Diabetes Educator. Serves individuals or groups (lecture or round-table). Geographic Area Served: Westchester County, New York.

Massapequa Park

★ 14449 ★ Sports and Recreation Consultants Inc.
18 Scott St.
Massapequa Park, NY 11762
Phone: (516)938-0600 **Fax:** (516)931-6344
Email: sberheim@ntr.net
Website: http://www.ntr.net/~sbernheim
Fnded: 1990. **Activities:** Accident analysis/sports liability consultant. Expert in a variety of sports injury negligence suits against schools, and recreational facilities, including sports and recreational accidents caused by faulty equipment, improper supervision, poor facilities, non-adherence to standards, human error. Provides sports risk management. Geographic Area Served: United States and Canada.

Melville

★ 14450 ★ Sandler Occupational Medicine Associates Inc.
125 Baylis Rd., Ste. 120
Melville, NY 11747-4801
Phone: (631)756-2204 **Fax:** (631)756-2213
Email: info@somaonline.com
Website: http://www.somaonline.com
Fnded: 1983. **Activities:** Advises U.S. businesses in the fields of occupational and environmental health.

★ 14451 ★ The Whitman Group
145 Pinelawn Rd.
Melville, NY 11747
Phone: (631)777-2710 **Fax:** (631)777-2714
Email: info@whitmangroup.com
Website: http://www.whitmangroup.com
Fnded: 1985. **Activities:** Nationally recognized consultation and management firm assisting hospitals, nursing facilities, and other healthcare organizations in identification, analysis, design, development, implementation, and management of programs and services for senior adults and chronic care populations. The organization's multidisciplinary expertise spans the areas of clinical gerontology, subacute facility contract management, financial analysis (including Medicare reimbursement of subacute units), expert witness testimony, long-term care continuum planning, and assisted living. Serves hospitals, nursing facilities, subacute care providers, rehabilitation hospitals, physicians, attorneys, government agencies, and professional healthcare organizations (as speakers) in the U.S. and worldwide.

Mount Kisco

★ 14452 ★ The Hermann Group
23 Peck Rd.
Mount Kisco, NY 10549
Phone: (914)241-8714 **Fax:** (914)666-0919
Email: hermanngroup@compuserve.com
Fnded: 1988. **Activities:** Offers public relations, communications and marketing consultation in nutrition and healthcare. Industries served: public relations, pharmaceutical, food, publishing, and healthcare. Geographic Area Served: Metropolitan New York based; active nationwide.

★ 14453 ★ Valley Cardiovascular
12 Rolling Ridge Ct.
Mount Kisco, NY 10549-4750
Phone: (914)565-7399 **Free:** 877-565-7399
Fax: (914)565-7402
Website: http://valleycardiovascular.com/medheart/
Activities: An actively practicing Interventional Cardiologist with extensive courtroom experience, impeccable credentials, and unshakable testimony.

New City

★ 14454 ★ Professional Resource Systems
31 Beaumont Dr.
New City, NY 10956
Phone: (845)638-9227 **Fax:** (845)638-4323
Website: http://www.proresourcesystems.com
Activities: Provides pre-employment screening assessments that measure honesty & substance abuse. Job specific assessments for managers, sales, customer service, call center, team analysis, and career coaching.

New York

★ 14455 ★ AIG Consultants Inc.
70 Pine St., Fl. 10
New York, NY 10270
Phone: (212)770-7000 **Free:** 888-285-7780
Fax: (212)742-1564
Fnded: 1979. **Activities:** Consulting company with extensive experience in containing and solving a wide range of industrial and commercial problems related to risk management, loss control, and quality improvement. Provides clients with analyses of current or potential risks, recommendations for corrective actions and follow-up assessment to contain risk and ensure profitability. Areas of expertise include environmental services (property transfer assessments, hospital medical waste plans, compliance audits, environmental risk assessments, hazardous materials/waste management); healthcare services (quality improvement, accreditation, peer review, risk management consulting); industrial hygiene (asbestos abatement); and property conservation (casualty, fleet, ergonomics, products liability, construction). Industries served: all manufacturing and service industries, as well as government agencies. Geographic Area Served: Worldwide through affiliates.

★ 14456 ★ AM Medica Communications Ltd.
305 E 46th St., 7th Fl.
New York, NY 10017
Phone: (212)751-1818 **Fax:** (212)751-2005
Email: action@ammadelphi.com
Fnded: 1986. **Activities:** Medical consulting.

★ 14457 ★ American Business Training Inc.
2109 Broadway
New York, NY 10023-2106
Phone: (917)441-8914 **Fax:** (917)233-6607
Fnded: 1992. **Activities:** Various subjects.

★ 14458 ★ Beverly L. Daniel - Consulting Nutritionist
865 W End Ave., Ste. 14B
New York, NY 10025
Phone: (212)663-4830
Fnded: 1988. **Activities:** Provides individualized nutrition consultation. Receives referrals from health professionals, physicians, and psychologists, as well as self-referrals. Expertise in special medical problems. Serves government agencies also. Geographic Area Served: New York City and vicinity primarily; available elsewhere upon request.

★ 14459 ★ Corporate Psychological Services P.C.
2166 Broadway, No. 6D
New York, NY 10024
Phone: (212)832-0477 **Fax:** (212)371-6102
Email: DrGlazer@att.net
Activities: Specializes in discrimination, harassment, wrongful termination, and disability. Geographic Area Served: United States.

★ 14460 ★ Cybertec Consulting Group Inc.
444 E 86th St., Ste. 36B
New York, NY 10028-6464
Phone: (212)772-7592 **Fax:** (212)772-7692
Email: muben@aol.com
Fnded: 1982. **Activities:** Management consultants specializing in strategic planning, organizational development, environmental management, and sustainable development. Geographic Area Served: Worldwide.

★ 14461 ★ DaSilva Black Calcagni Chesser, Architects P.C.
37 W 28th St., 5th Fl.
New York, NY 10001
Phone: (212)889-1840 **Fax:** (212)696-1986
Fnded: 1977. **Activities:** An architectural and planning firm, specializing in health facility consultation. Services range from program needs, costs and scheduling analysis; through long-range plans, programming, design and construction administration; to interior design, medical equipment selection and specification. Activities include consultation on reuse, retrofit and reconfiguration of existing plants. Serves private industries as well as government agencies. Geographic Area Served: NY, NJ, CT, ME, and PA.

★ 14462 ★ Fisher-Todd Associates
535 5th Ave., Ste. 701
New York, NY 10017
Phone: (212)986-9052 **Fax:** (212)682-1742
Email: rfranz@winstonstaffing.com
Website: http://www.winstonresources.com
Fnded: 1967. **Activities:** Specializes in nationwide recruiting of mid to senior level executives in human resources, marketing management, sales, sales promotion, market research and direct response/data base marketing for virtually all product and service industries. Geographic Area Served: United States.

★ 14463 ★ Greenbaum Eye Associates
40 Park Ave.
New York, NY 10016
Phone: (212)686-6075 **Fax:** (212)532-1192
Activities: Ophthalmology surgeon specializing in cataracts, the cornea, glaucoma, laser vision correction, and ophthalmic anesthesia. **Remarks:** Dr. Greenbaum specializes in eye surgery and anesthesia techniques related to eye surgery. Dr. Greenbaum past president of the ophthalmic anesthesia society. Geographic Area Served: Northeastern United States.

★ 14464 ★ In-Flight Radiation Protection Services Inc.
211 E 70th St., Ste. 12G
New York, NY 10021
Phone: (212)288-7201
Email: robbarish@aol.com
Website: http://robbarish.tripod.com
Fnded: 1988. **Activities:** Provides education and training regarding cosmic ray radiation exposure of airline crew members. Produces seminars and briefing

sessions for airline executives. Provides monitoring instrument for radiation dose measurements on airplanes. Industries served: aviation and government agencies. Geographic Area Served: Worldwide.

★ 14465 ★ Industrial Testing Laboratories
50 Madison Ave.
New York, NY 10010
Phone: (212)685-8788 **Fax:** (212)689-8742
Fnded: 1887. **Activities:** Analytical and consulting chemists to the pharmaceutical, petroleum, food, cosmetic, and chemical industries. Also provides forensic consulting including analysis of biological fluids and fire investigations, as well as courtroom testimony.

★ 14466 ★ J. Friedman Communications Inc.
18 E 48th St., 20th Fl.
New York, NY 10017
Phone: (212)980-1217 **Fax:** (212)980-1239
Fnded: 1987. **Activities:** Marketing and communications consultants providing expertise to the food and healthcare companies to reach health professionals and the health concerned consumer. Special areas of expertise: wellness, health promotion, home healthcare, aging, nutrition, packaged goods and special nutritionals, managed care, healthcare and financial services, and health services marketing. Industries served: manufacturers of healthcare and home care products and services, food, pharmaceutical, and proprietary drug. Geographic Area Served: North America, Europe and Far East.

★ 14467 ★ Jay P. Goldsmith, DMD
121 E 60th St.
New York, NY 10022
Phone: (212)838-5895 **Fax:** (212)838-6007
Activities: Specializes in oral and maxillofacial surgery.

★ 14468 ★ Joseph M. Jabbour, MD
2 5th Ave.
New York, NY 10011-8856
Phone: (212)674-5200 **Fax:** (212)674-5801
Website: http://www.plasticsurgery.org/md/jabbour.htm
Activities: A board certified plastic and reconstructive surgeon providing expert witness testimony.

★ 14469 ★ Klein Biomedical Consultants Inc.
215 W 90th St.
New York, NY 10024
Phone: (212)362-0579 **Fax:** (212)362-1028
Email: kleinbiomed@aol.com
Fnded: 1980. **Activities:** General business consultant to the medical equipment field. Provides a wide range of consulting services in the following areas: market studies, corporate strategy and long-range planning, new product evaluation, mergers and acquisitions, and venture capital. Geographic Area Served: United States, Europe, and Japan.

★ 14470 ★ Laszlo Bodak Engineer
45 W 36th St., Fl. 3
New York, NY 10018-7638
Phone: (212)643-1444 **Fax:** (212)764-1591
Email: engineers@laszlobodale.com
Fnded: 1985. **Activities:** Provides HVAC, electrical, plumbing, and fire protection engineering for commercial, industrial, institutional, and residential building projects. Recent experience with environmental investigations for building air quality as well as intelligent building consulting. Clients served: architects, owners, developers, builders, and government. Geographic Area Served: United States and Europe.

★ 14471 ★ Marion Gindes & Associates
19 W 34th St. Penthouse
New York, NY 10001
Phone: (212)947-7111 **Fax:** (914)833-1602
Activities: Psychologist offering evaluations, plaintiff/defendant testimony; HR & case consultation, training, and coaching. Also specializes in employment discrimination, sexual harassment, diversity, wrongful termination, workplace conflict and family law-custody disputes.

★ 14472 ★ Medilex Inc.
175 E 96th St., Ste. 8H
New York, NY 10128-6204
Phone: (212)860-8700 **Fax:** (212)860-8263
Website: http://www.medilex.net
Fnded: 1992. **Activities:** Medical-legal case review, consultation and expert testimony. Provides high quality, cost-effective medical and scientific expertise. Specializes in malpractice, toxic tort, forensic pathology, products liability and behavioral science matters. Geographic Area Served: Primarily East Coast to Midwest, but will begin accepting cases from further west.

★ 14473 ★ medQuest Ltd.
116 E 30th St.
New York, NY 10016
Phone: (212)725-8000 **Free:** 800-633-6251
Fax: (212)725-5090
Email: info@medQuestLtd.com
Website: http://www.medQuestLtd.com
Fnded: 1974. **Activities:** Expert referral service for medical malpractice and other tort litigation, offering prompt access to an unparalleled group of experts nationwide. Has provided evaluation and testimony in more than 40,000 cases.

★ 14474 ★ National Health Plan Corp.
11 Penn Plz., Ste. 330
New York, NY 10001
Phone: (212)279-3232 **Free:** 800-647-2677
Fax: (212)629-0749
Fnded: 1975. **Activities:** Provides national health plan administration, PPO, and cost containment services.

★ 14475 ★ The Nierenberg Group
420 E 51st St., Ste. 12D
New York, NY 10022
Phone: (212)980-0930 **Fax:** (212)980-4185
Email: andrean@selfmarketing.com
Website: http://www.selfmarketing.com
Fnded: 1993. **Activities:** A communications, training, and performance consulting company that specializes in sales training for all levels as well as presentation skills, stress management, and customer service. Emphasis is on personal motivation, implementing change, and improving performance in the workplace. Industries served: publishing, education, securities, financial, manufacturing, pharmaceutical, and associations. Geographic Area Served: Worldwide.

★ 14476 ★ Norman Weiss, MD
55 E 87 St., Ste. 1J
New York, NY 10028
Phone: (917)492-2400 **Fax:** (914)723-4343
Activities: Clinical and medico-legal psychiatry consultation and expert witness testimony.

★ 14477 ★ O'Toole-Ewald Art Associates Inc.
1133 Broadway
New York, NY 10010
Phone: (212)989-5151 **Fax:** (212)242-1629
Email: ele@otoole-ewald.com
Website: http://www.otoole-ewald.com
Fnded: 1932. **Activities:** Appraisal experts and consultants specializing in damage/loss/fraud cases relating to fine/decorative art. Expertise in painting, sculpture, antiques, Asian art, ethnographic art, works on paper, ceramics and glassware, rugs and textiles, silver, etc., Provides forensic appraisals, fully documented and with photographs, adhering to USPAP standards. Geographic Area Served: United States.

★ 14478 ★ Pharmaceutical Recruiters Inc.
271 Madison Ave., Ste. 1200
New York, NY 10016
Phone: (212)557-5627 **Fax:** (212)557-5866
Email: pharmrec@aol.com
Website: http://www.pharmrecruit.com
Activities: Firm recruits medical professionals for clinical research positions.

★ 14479 ★ PJB Medical Publications Inc.
1775 Broadway, Ste. 511
New York, NY 10019
Phone: (212)262-8320 **Fax:** (212)262-8234
Website: http://www.thetareports.com
Fnded: 1968. **Activities:** Provides in-depth technology off-the-shelf and custom research studies in the medical, pharmaceutical, electronics, instrumentation, and biotechnology industries. Specializes in healthcare and biotechnology market analysis, competitor profiles, and market share analysis. Geographic Area Served: Worldwide.

★ 14480 ★ Rational Effectiveness Training Systems
45 E 65th St.
New York, NY 10021
Phone: (212)535-0822 **Free:** 800-323-IRET
Fax: (212)249-3582
Website: http://www.rebt.org
Fnded: 1985. **Activities:** RETS is the corporate services division of the Albert Ellis Institute, a nonprofit educational organization. RETS provides: on-site workshops and seminars to enhance work performance, facilitate decision making, improve communications; full-service employee counseling; advanced training for employee assistance professionals; and training materials especially designed for the workplace. Provides professional training; research; counseling and therapy services; psycho-educational workshops, speakers for community organizations; self-help pamphlets; and books and tapes. Serves private industries as well as government agencies. Geographic Area Served: Worldwide.

★ 14481 ★ Richard B. Krueger, MD
210 E 68th St., Ste. 1-H
New York, NY 10021-6024
Phone: (212)517-6624 **Fax:** (212)517-4073
Email: rbk1721305@aol.com
Activities: Assesses and treats sex offenders and forensic populations, as well as neuropsychiatry and head injury. Oversees a program for treating sex offenders and for treating professionals accused of professional sexual misconduct. Specializes in psychopharmacology, malpractice, forensic psychiatry, competency, criminal responsibility, PTSD, and psychiatric disability.

★ 14482 ★ Robert J. Barish
211 E 70th St., Ste. 12G
New York, NY 10021
Phone: (212)288-7201
Email: robbarish@aol.com
Fnded: 1981. **Activities:** Consultant in radiological physics and radiation safety. Specializes in radiation therapy calibrations, planning, architectural design, equipment selection, and medical-legal aspects of radiology including expert opinion in malpractice suits. Serves private industries as well as government agencies. Geographic Area Served: Worldwide.

★ 14483 ★ Robinson Institute for Addictions
1841 Broadway, Ste. 201
New York, NY 10023-7603
Phone: (212)459-8900 **Fax:** (212)459-8959

Fnded: 1990. **Activities:** Offers intensive outpatient treatment program for drugs, alcohol and eating disorders. Provides dual-diagnosis psychiatric and addiction counseling. Conducts relapse prevention training. Many programs nationally are based on the philosophy and methodology of treatment utilized at the Institute for food addictions. Industries served: unlimited but have served automotive, transportation, educational, and government agencies. Geographic Area Served: New York City metropolitan area.

★ 14484 ★ Sandra Fisher Consulting
535 E 86th St.
New York, NY 10028
Phone: (212)744-5900 **Fax:** (212)879-0032
Email: sfisherfit@aol.com

Fnded: 1985. **Activities:** Offers expertise as consultant, speaker, seminar leader, writer and coach on marketing and promotion; people and organizations; communication and presentation skills; stress management, women's issues and travel. Geographic Area Served: United States and Nordic countries.

★ 14485 ★ Standpoint Inc.
77 W 15th St., Ste. 1-T
New York, NY 10011
Phone: (212)929-7521 **Fax:** (212)627-5432
Email: contact@standpointinc.com
Website: http://www.standpointinc.com

Fnded: 1985. **Activities:** Firm maintains a Speakers Bureau that addresses the business issues of healthcare for the manufacturers, providers, and payers of healthcare products and services. The Speakers Bureau recruits pro bono and paid speakers who speak on business issues facing the U.S. healthcare industry. It arranges engagements for its speakers on conference programs conducted by industry associations, private conference organizers, healthcare alliances, investors, and educational institutions. Industries served: pharmaceutical, biotechnology, diagnostics, medical devices, managed care, hospitals, health systems, insurers, and other provider organizations. Geographic Area Served: United States.

★ 14486 ★ Sutton Associates
300 E 51st St., Ste. 4C
New York, NY 10022
Phone: (212)753-7068

Fnded: 1983. **Activities:** Communications consultant on pharmaceutical, medical device, and healthcare management for problem solving, promotion, marketing strategy, industrial psychology, and FDA matters. Offers additional focus as literary agent consultant.

★ 14487 ★ The Swain Consulting Group
420 E 72nd St.
New York, NY 10021
Phone: (212)717-2556 **Fax:** (212)717-2566
Email: mbswain@aol.com

Fnded: 1978. **Activities:** Specializing in organizational development, communications, teambuilding, executive coaching, conflict resolution, leadership development and assessments. Industries served: all. Geographic Area Served: United States, England, Europe, and Asia.

★ 14488 ★ Taylor Clark Architects Inc.
149 5th Ave., Fl. 10
New York, NY 10010-6801
Phone: (212)460-8840 **Fax:** (212)505-8184

Fnded: 1945. **Activities:** Architectural consultants specializing in the design of healthcare facilities (hospitals, nursing homes, medical office buildings, clinics, etc.) and research laboratories. Services include master planning and programming, certificate of need applications, interior design, 2D/3D CADD, and medical equipment planning and selection.

★ 14489 ★ Theresa Incagnoli, PhD, A.B.P.P.
240 Central Park S, Ste. 24-C
New York, NY 10019
Phone: (212)757-0375 **Fax:** (212)757-0376

Activities: Specialist in neuropsychology. Offers particular expertise in the evaluation of brain damage. Services include medical-legal work for plaintiff and defense. Experience in testifying. Geographic Area Served: New York, New Jersey, Connecticut.

★ 14490 ★ The Wilkerson Group Inc.
590 Madison Ave., 10th Fl.
New York, NY 10022
Phone: (212)745-4500 **Fax:** (212)745-4555

Fnded: 1968. **Activities:** Strategy consulting and technology/market opportunity identification and assessment for worldwide pharmaceutical, medical supply/equipment/device, biotechnology, and similar healthcare companies. Activities include product/market opportunity assessment, strategy development, acquisition/diversification planning, due diligence analyses, and sales/research and development organization and related implementation studies. Industries served: medical products, healthcare services, and medical investment. Geographic Area Served: Worldwide.

★ 14491 ★ WPP Group PLC
125 Park Ave., Fl. 4
New York, NY 10017-5529
Phone: (212)632-2200 **Fax:** (212)632-2249
Email: mljuljdjuraj@wpp.com
Website: http://www.wpp.com

Fnded: 1976. **Activities:** Offers services in healthcare marketing/development of new health systems; healthcare mergers and acquisitions, and healthcare properties. Industries served: healthcare, general corporate, and real estate development in the U.S.

★ 14492 ★ ZOL Consultants Inc.
340 W 57th St.
New York, NY 10019
Phone: (212)957-8029
Email: saul@ssr.com

Fnded: 1982. **Activities:** Specialist in the investigation of health frauds, offering scientific evaluation of unproved or questionable medical treatments particularly for cancer and AIDS. Also offers scientific evaluation of proposals to venture capitalists or individuals interested in setting up bioengineering companies and cancer research projects. Serves attorneys, insurance companies, and government agencies. Geographic Area Served: United States.

Oceanside

★ 14493 ★ South Shore Nutritional Consultants
2723 Aldred Ave.
Oceanside, NY 11572
Phone: (516)536-7885 **Fax:** (516)536-4108

Fnded: 1982. **Activities:** Offers nutritional counseling.

Palisades

★ 14494 ★ Lillian Langseth, Dr. PH
PO Box 700
Palisades, NY 10964
Phone: (914)359-8282 **Fax:** (914)359-1229
Email: l.langseth@att.net

Fnded: 1980. **Activities:** Consultants who produce technical documents in biomedical science, specializing in clinical nutrition, nutrition, food safety, and toxicology. Serves private industries as well as government agencies. Geographic Area Served: Worldwide.

★ 14495 ★ Lyda Associates Inc.
PO Box 700
Palisades, NY 10964
Phone: (914)359-8282 **Fax:** (914)359-1229
Email: l.langseth@worldnet.att.net

Fnded: 1980. **Activities:** Offers consulting services in clinical nutrition, food safety, toxicology, and health sciences. Provides technical writing, editing, technical documents, and ghost writing services. Specializes in newsletters. Industries served: food, food supplements, vitamins and minerals, food-related trade organizations, as well as government agencies. Geographic Area Served: Worldwide.

Peekskill

★ 14496 ★ VMC Consulting Service
8 S Division St.
Peekskill, NY 10566
Phone: (914)737-1977 **Fax:** (914)838-2331

Fnded: 1986. **Activities:** Social issues counseling offered on family problems, dysfunctional disorders, and drug and alcohol abuse. Also provides expertise to companies including EAP consulting and assessment-referral services. Training extended to human resource management and staff on substance abuse problems.

Penfield

★ 14497 ★ Rx: Medical Expertise
PO Box 0166
Penfield, NY 14526
Phone: (585)388-8760 **Fax:** (585)388-8983
Email: info@rxmedicalexpertise.com
Website: http://www.rxmedicalexpertise.com

Activities: Expertise witness testimony and medical resource providing case consultation.

Poughkeepsie

★ 14498 ★ Natalie R. Dickstein, Dietician, Cert., Diabetes Educator
56 Clover Hill Dr.
Poughkeepsie, NY 12603-3202
Phone: (845)462-3113

Fnded: 1968. **Activities:** Provides nutrition counseling for individuals and groups. Specializes in weight control, diabetes, sports, cardiovascular system, and wellness. Geographic Area Served: Dutchess and Ulster County, New York.

Rochester

★ 14499 ★ The DeWolff Partnership
151 St. Paul St.
Rochester, NY 14604
Phone: (716)454-5860 **Fax:** (716)454-5268
Email: tdp_main@dewolff.com
Website: http://www.dewolff.com

Fnded: 1963. **Activities:** Firm provides architectural services including master planning, programming and design of corporate, commercial, recreational, educational, medical, surgical and eldercare facilities.

★ 14500 ★ Russell Phillips & Associates Inc.
1099 Jay St., Ste. J-200
Rochester, NY 14611-1153
Phone: (716)621-3700 **Fax:** (716)621-7300
Email: rphillips@medsafe.com

Fnded: 1976. **Activities:** Team of professional fire protection and emergency preparedness procedure experts offers facility inspections, evacuation system design and staff training, code review, and statements of condition and fire safety evaluation systems. Industries served: healthcare and government agencies. Geographic Area Served: Worldwide.

★ 14501 ★ The Writing Doctor
NYH HealthCare Communications Group
16 San Rafael Dr.
Rochester, NY 14618
Phone: (585)385-1515 **Fax:** (585)385-3858
Email: nywriter@rochester.rr.com
Website: http://www.nyhwriter.com
Fnded: 1985. **Activities:** Writes, collaborates, edits, and consults on writing of medical and scientific books, articles for peer-reviewed medical journals, patient education materials. Does speechwriting, editing, and lecturing on all phases of health care. Seminar leader conducts health care symposia for physicians and scientists on better medical writing, better physician-to-physician communication, and better doctor-to-patient communication. Focuses on primary and secondary prevention of heart disease, breast, prostate, and colon cancer; encouraging patient adherence to recommendations, diagnosis and treatment of disease, treatment of pain devising strategies for patients on coping with disease; geratrics, palliative care, and end-of-life care; sex over 50; sex after surgery for cancer; changing a Type A personality to Type A–(we're realists); helping patients cope with prostate, colon and breast cancer and hypertensive cardiovascular disease. Available for short-term and long-term projects all over the world. Geographic Area Served: Worldwide.

Rye

★ 14502 ★ Poul Sherman and Associates
411 Theodore Fremd Ave.
Rye, NY 10580
Phone: (914)967-5395 **Free:** 800-548-1259
Fax: (914)967-5132
Fnded: 1979. **Activities:** Human resource development firm consults on employee assistance programs, case management, and chemical dependency programs.

Scarsdale

★ 14503 ★ Advanced Dermaceuticals International
PO Box 209
Scarsdale, NY 10583
Phone: (914)723-5536 **Fax:** (914)725-3774
Email: mh.adi@worldnet.att.net
Fnded: 1988. **Activities:** A consumer-oriented technical/marketing consulting firm with experience in research and development management and problem solving. Areas of special expertise include: developing creative new ideas and concepts including product development; technical marketing; efficacy and safety testing for cosmetics, toiletries and drugs, OTC and prescription. Has worked in the international technical/marketing areas for cosmetic and toiletries; and does competitive technical/marketing analysis and technology forecasting/transfer. Industries served: cosmetics, toiletries, and over-the-counter drug manufacturers. Geographic Area Served: United States, Canada, Europe, Asia.

★ 14504 ★ Harry Schwartz and Associates
50 Argyle Rd.
PO Box 1169
Scarsdale, NY 10583
Phone: (914)725-1642 **Fax:** (914)725-1134
Fnded: 1979. **Activities:** Provides public relations and marketing assistance to many entities in the healthcare field, including physician groups, hospitals, manufacturers and sellers of pharmaceuticals and hospital supplies. Geographic Area Served: United States.

★ 14505 ★ Kassalow Training & Development Inc.
17 Continental Rd.
Scarsdale, NY 10583
Phone: (914)472-5918 **Fax:** (914)723-4276
Email: ktdinc@aol.com
Fnded: 1976. **Activities:** Consultants in human resource development who provide custom-designed seminars and provide corporate business coaching. Emphasis is on helping to motivate employees to pursue a standard of professional excellence; to empower personnel to take initiative; to build effective working relationships with managers, supervisors, coworkers and subordinates; to develop leadership skills and styles; to manage their time effectively; to decrease stress; and to communicate more effectively. Industries served: banking, law, service, travel, advertising, research firms, financial, retail, and government and manufacturing. **Remarks:** Available for sale-Survival For the Fittest(sm) Kit-A comprehensive package of techniques for handling the 12 most critical topics addressed in business seminars today. Kit includes desktop flip chart, 60-minute audiotape, fun stress releaser star-burst. Geographic Area Served: Worldwide.

Smithtown

★ 14506 ★ Glass & Inserra
309 Middle Country Rd.
Smithtown, NY 11787
Phone: (516)360-2200 **Fax:** (516)360-1328
Fnded: 1990. **Activities:** Offers medical consulting for insurance companies, including second opinions for orthopaedic surgery. Industries served: health, medicine, and safety (particularly insurance and orthopaedics), including government agencies. Geographic Area Served: Long Island, New York (primarily Suffolk County).

Somers

★ 14507 ★ MICOR
61 Driftwood Dr.
Somers, NY 10589
Phone: (914)276-0755 **Fax:** (914)276-0755
Email: micor@earth.execnet.com
Fnded: 1987. **Activities:** Consults on design and performance enhancements of automated medical diagnostic instrumentation. Specializes in micro hydraulics. Industries Served: medical, clinical, scientific instrumentation. Geographic Area Served: Worldwide.

South Salem

★ 14508 ★ Psychotherapy Associates
40 Old Pond Rd.
South Salem, NY 10590-1018
Phone: (914)763-5916 **Fax:** (914)763-6567
Fnded: 1986. **Activities:** Nutritional consultants with expertise in weight reduction or maintenance and stress-related modification. Offers a weight modifying program based on an eclectic approach consisting of medical, psychological and nutritional services. Also provide a stress reduction program utilizing this eclectic approach. Additional areas of expertise include: post traumatic stress disorders and electric burn trauma. Geographic Area Served: North Westchester County, New York; and Ridgefield, New Cannan, and Greenwich, Connecticut.

Spring Valley

★ 14509 ★ J.R.D. McCormick
19 Pomona Ln.
Spring Valley, NY 10977-1112
Phone: (845)354-9149 **Fax:** (845)354-9640
Email: mccormick_jrd@att.net
Fnded: 1983. **Activities:** Provides research planning and problem solving by the application of chemical and biochemical principles to the fields of industrial microbiology, fermentation, and the fermentation-like industries, including constructive reviews of existing research programs. Specialist in tetracycline antibiotics and in methodology of screening soil microorganisms. Industries served: Pharmaceuticals and fine chemicals, the fermentation industry, and government agencies. **Remarks:** Particular personal interest on alternative energy and waste paper utilization. Also available through Teltech™network of experts.

Staten Island

★ 14510 ★ Gianpaolo Maestrone
4 Sophia Ln.
Staten Island, NY 10304
Phone: (718)987-5010
Fnded: 1987. **Activities:** Professional veterinarian with Board Certification in Veterinary Microbiology, plus twenty-five years experience in human and veterinary pharmaceutical industry. Conducts feasibility studies, development and clearance of animal health products for systemic, topical, anti-mastitic and growth promotion uses. Specializes in selection, evaluation and registration of fish health products. Serves the aquaculture, agriculture, and pharmaceutical industries.

Stony Brook

★ 14511 ★ Steven Jonas, M.D., M.P.H., M.S.
Department of Preventive Medicine
School of Medicine
State University of New York
Stony Brook, NY 11794-8036
Phone: (631)444-2147 **Fax:** (631)444-7525
Email: sjonas@notes.cc.sunysb.edu
Fnded: 1968. **Activities:** Specialized expertise in wellness, health promotion, disease prevention, educational program planning and development, drug abuse policy, and health policy. Industries served: health services industry, higher education, and not-for-profit health care-related agencies. Geographic Area Served: Northeast, Mid-Atlantic, and Rocky Mountain regions.

Valhalla

★ 14512 ★ Associations Plus
8 Madison Ave.
Valhalla, NY 10595
Phone: (914)946-3802 **Fax:** (914)946-2674
Email: mtrossi@aol.com
Fnded: 1977. **Activities:** Human resource development experts specializing in sales training, support staff training, trade show selling, time management skills, and stress management training. Geographic Area Served: United States, Canada, and Europe.

West Chazy

★ 14513 ★ Thought Technology Ltd.
8396 Rte. 9
West Chazy, NY 12992
Phone: (518)489-8251 **Free:** 800-361-3651
Fax: (518)489-8255
Email: mail@thoughttechnology.com
Website: http://www.thoughttechnology.com
Fnded: 1974. **Activities:** Personal development specialists train individuals in stress control, taking tests with confidence, weight control, sleeping well, smoking cessation, athletic peak performance, flying free of fear, evaluation of alcohol and drug abuse, public speaking with confidence, breathing for health, and pain control for medical, educational, athletic, corporate and military markets. Geographic Area Served: Worldwide.

Westbury

★ 14514 ★ Cambridge Network
900 Merchants Concourse, Ste. 112
Westbury, NY 11590-5114
Phone: (516)832-7000 **Free:** 800-245-8931
Fax: (516)832-7993
Fnded: 1995. **Activities:** PPO Network. Geographic Area Served: New York.

★ 14515 ★ Jordan Services Inc.
900 Merchants Concourse, Ste. 112
Westbury, NY 11590-5114

Phone: (516)683-0100 Free: 800-767-1616
Fax: (516)683-0259
Email: information@jordanservices.com
Website: http://www.jordanservices.com

Fnded: 1975. **Activities:** Provides private and vocational case management services. Also provides medical auditing services including hospital, provider bills and peer review. Geographic Area Served: New York, New Jersey, Eastern Pennsylvania, Connecticut.

★ 14516 ★ Northeast M.E.D.S. P.C.
900 Merchants Concourse, Ste. 114
Westbury, NY 11590-5114
Phone: (516)683-0255 **Free:** 800-366-0255
Fax: (516)683-0538
Website: http://www.northeastmeds.com

Fnded: 1975. **Activities:** Independent medical exams, second opinion and peer reviews. Serves private industries, insurance carriers, employees as well as government agencies. Geographic Area Served: United States.

White Plains

★ 14517 ★ Arthur S. Goldenberg, DDS
151 E Post Rd.
White Plains, NY 10601
Phone: (914)682-8883

Activities: Provides consultation concerning pain of dental and non-dental origin; also provides case reviews and assessments and expert opinion testimony.

Yonkers

★ 14518 ★ Charles M. Mathis Associates Inc.
45 S Broadway, Ste. 206
Yonkers, NY 10701
Phone: (914)476-0454 **Fax:** (914)476-1932

Fnded: 1986. **Activities:** Medical management consultants serving community healthcare centers.

North Carolina

Asheville

★ 14519 ★ HAZCOM Inc.
31 College Pl., Ste. 306D
Asheville, NC 28801
Phone: (828)258-9919 **Fax:** (828)258-9913

Fnded: 1987. **Activities:** Hazcom, Inc. was formed to address the accelerating pace of environmental and worker safety responsibilities for business, and offers a complete array of services to provide the information, preventative planning, and technical support needed to ensure cost effective compliance. Specific services include hazardous waste materials consulting and management, remediation plans and management, PCB testing and consulting, emergency response plans, spill response plans, storm water permitting programs, safety audits, accident investigation, hazard communications compliance, safety plans, infectious disease control programs, asbestos inspection noise assessment and consulting, indoor air quality assessments, employee exposure monitoring, and naturally occuring radioactive materials programs. Serves private industries as well as government agencies. Geographic Area Served: United States.

★ 14520 ★ Thomas J. Berger
25 Crowningway Dr.
Asheville, NC 28804
Phone: (828)252-5152 **Fax:** (828)252-5148
Email: bladesmn@aol.com
Website: http://member.expertpages.com/heartofyourcase/

Activities: An expert in medicine involving cardiology. Board-certified Forensic Examiner; Fellow, American College of Surgeons; Fellow, American College of Chest Physicians.

Cary

★ 14521 ★ The Copernicus Group
118 MacKenan Dr., Ste. 400
Cary, NC 27511
Free: 888-303-2224
Email: irb@copernicusgroup.com
Website: http://www.copernicusgroup.com

Fnded: 1996. **Activities:** Assists researchers meet the increasing regulatory demands of clinical trials. Focus is on responsibly addressing regulatory and ethical concerns to protect the rights of human subjects taking part in research.

★ 14522 ★ Innovative Health Group Inc.
100 Chalon Dr.
Cary, NC 27511-6469
Phone: (919)467-6100 **Fax:** (919)481-3818
Email: bvaughn794@aol.com

Fnded: 1984. **Activities:** Provides market research, feasibility studies, and strategic planning expertise and development services to healthcare industry with a focus on assisted living, retirement and long-term care, primarily in North and South Carolina and Virginia.

★ 14523 ★ Inveresk Research Inc.
11000 Weston Pky., Ste. 100
Cary, NC 27513
Email: inveresk@aol.com

Fnded: 1974. **Activities:** Project management, strategic development, clinical trial monitoring, regulatory affairs are tailored to the sponsors needs for manufacturers of medical devices, diagnostics, pharmaceuticals, and cosmetics. Geographic Area Served: Worldwide.

Charlotte

★ 14524 ★ Bright Associates Inc.
5701 Camelot Dr.
Charlotte, NC 28270-0498
Phone: (704)844-6226 **Fax:** (704)844-6226
Email: dbright@worldnet.att.net

Fnded: 1990. **Activities:** A professional consulting firm dedicated to serving the pharmaceutical, medical device and related industries in specialized areas of regulatory affairs and quality assurance. Geographic Area Served: Worldwide.

★ 14525 ★ Corporate Benefits Service Inc.
145 Scaleybark Rd., Ste. B
Charlotte, NC 28209
Phone: (704)373-0447 **Fax:** (704)342-2777
Website: http://www.corbenser.com

Fnded: 1990. **Activities:** Administers third party medical reimbursement and employment benefits programs for businesses in the eastern United States.

★ 14526 ★ Maxwell Group Inc.
8393 Providence Rd.
Charlotte, NC 28277-9753
Phone: (704)544-9055 **Free:** 800-366-7024
Fax: (704)544-9057
Email: info@Maxwell-Investments.com
Website: http://www.maxwell-investments.com

Fnded: 1989. **Activities:** Services include marketing-oriented home builder management; financial packaging for real estate projects; retirement community marketing, development, and financing; and merger and acquisition assistance for long-term care providers and for owners of retirement communities. Industries served: real estate, long-term care, and government agencies. Geographic Area Served: United States and Canada.

★ 14527 ★ Preferred Medical Marketing Corp.
7400 Carmel Executive Pk., Ste. 240
Charlotte, NC 28226
Phone: (704)543-8103 **Fax:** (704)543-8106
Website: http://www.pmmconline.com

Fnded: 1987. **Activities:** Health care consultants.

★ 14528 ★ SunHealth Inc.
PO Box 668800
Charlotte, NC 28266-8800
Phone: (704)529-3324 **Fax:** (704)527-3654

Fnded: 1969. **Activities:** Provides management consulting services to healthcare providers. The purpose of these services is to assist healthcare providers to become high quality, cost effective providers of healthcare. Geographic Area Served: 15 states, primarily southeastern region.

Clayton

★ 14529 ★ Expert Medico-Legal Opinions
PO Box 1306
Clayton, NC 27520
Phone: (919)550-3229 **Fax:** (919)550-3229
Email: DrGuha@ExpertMedLegOpinions.com
Website: http://www.expertmedlegopinions.com/

Activities: Physician-operated medical case review firm, providing board-certified physicians to analyze cases in their areas of expertise.

Garner

★ 14530 ★ Barry Page Consulting
1304 Buckingham Rd.
Garner, NC 27529-4706
Phone: (919)779-3037 **Fax:** (919)779-9682
Email: bfjpage@aol.com

Fnded: 1993. **Activities:** Provides consulting for laboratory operations, product and process troubleshooting, technical file preparation, and product submissions. Expert knowledge of domestic and international standards and requirements for risk assessment, material characterization, biological evaluation, product sterilization, sterilization residuals, and the changing regulatory requirements for medical devices. On-site supervision and training for laboratory operations.

Greenville

★ 14531 ★ Helen Merrill Brinson
313 Pinewood Rd.
Greenville, NC 27858
Phone: (252)756-4104
Email: brinsonh@mail.ecu.edu

Fnded: 1982. **Activities:** Provides management consulting services to the healthcare education field. Geographic Area Served: United States.

Raleigh

★ 14532 ★ Francis M. Esposito, PhD
8613 Abbotsbury Ct.
Raleigh, NC 27615
Phone: (919)676-8779
Email: pegmo@hotmail.com

Activities: Specializes in forensic toxicology, including blood alcohol interpretation, and blood and urine drug interpretation; board certified forensic toxicologist. Estimates blood alcohol levels and/or amount of alcohol consumed based on laboratory result or drinking history. Predicts impairment based on blood alcohol or blood drug level. Gives expert witness testimony.

★ 14533 ★ North Carolina Fair Share
530 N Person St.
Raleigh, NC 27604-1264
Phone: (919)832-7130 **Fax:** (919)832-4635

Fnded: 1982. **Activities:** Social services firm consults on community organizing and (local) lobbying for health issues.

Wake Forest

★ 14534 ★ National Toxicology Consultants

501 Vista Del Lago Ln.
Wake Forest, NC 27587
Phone: (919)570-9630 **Free:** 800-250-7780
Email: rryan@nationaltoxicology.com
Website: http://www.nationaltoxicology.com

Fnded: 1992. **Activities:** A full-service professional consulting firm, providing service related to all aspects of assessment of hazards associated with various metals and chemicals. Functions as a "partner" to plaintiff, defense, and insurance clients to help clients solve their problems through scientific work. Staff possess professional board certifications in areas including toxicology, occupational and environmental medicine, emergency medicine, pathology, industrial hygiene, and medical toxicology. Areas of expertise include biological monitoring, expert witness testimony/ litigation support, occupational/ environmental exposure assessment, geology/environmental toxicology, chemical/ metal exposure, risk assessment, groundwater contamination, hazardous waste, alcohol and drug abuse, groundwater microbiology, and geochemical toxicology. Geographic Area Served: North Carolina and Georgia.

Waxhaw

★ 14535 ★ Weichinger Computer Consultants Inc.

1515 Waxhaw-Indian Trl. Dr.
Waxhaw, NC 28173
Phone: (704)843-2414 **Free:** 800-859-2241
Fax: (704)843-1093

Fnded: 1976. **Activities:** Offers custom programming design and software development with expertise in computer network planning and bar code applications. Industries served: healthcare. Geographic Area Served: United States.

Ohio

Centerville

★ 14536 ★ Monica A. Cengia

7707 Paragon Rd., Ste. 105
Centerville, OH 45459
Phone: (937)436-1985

Fnded: 1985. **Activities:** Registered dietitian offers nutritional assessments and consultations. Also provides individualized nutrition counseling, wellness programs, nutrition education programs, long-term healthcare counseling, and media presentations. Industries served: long-term healthcare, hospitals, universities, private businesses, health clubs/spas, physicians' offices, food industry, radio, television, and newspaper. Geographic Area Served: Geater Dayton Cincinnati Area.

Cincinnati

★ 14537 ★ Beta Associates

915 Greenville Ave.
Cincinnati, OH 45246
Phone: (513)772-9296 **Fax:** (513)772-9296
Website: http://www.betaassociates.com

Fnded: 1981. **Activities:** Offers occupational health and safety consulting on solving complex industrial hygiene and environmental exposure problems. Performs feasibility studies and design services for noise control and ventilation systems. Also has extensive experience in hazardous waste assessments, air pollution permits, worker's compensation investigations, management and employee training, and compliance plans for OSHA regulations. Provides expert testimony in these areas. Emphasis on development and use of microcomputers to implement industrial hygiene, safety, medical and chemical information database management systems. Geographic Area Served: Worldwide.

★ 14538 ★ Denise A. Sadowski

7312 Plainfield Rd.
Cincinnati, OH 45236
Phone: (513)791-9439

Fnded: 1988. **Activities:** Clinical nurse specialist provides educational classes, lectures and seminars to hospitals, schools of nursing and medical companies. Also offers consulting to medical companies for new product development as well as conducting research on their new products in the clinical area. Primary areas include burns, wounds. Industries served: hospitals and medical companies. Geographic Area Served: continental United States.

★ 14539 ★ Hill Top Research Inc.

PO Box 429501
Cincinnati, OH 45242
Phone: (513)831-3114 **Fax:** (513)831-1217
Email: info@hill-top.com
Website: http://www.hill-top.com

Fnded: 1947. **Activities:** Specialists in protocol design, study execution, and statistical analysis and interpretation, and conduct of testing programs for safety, efficacy, and registration of cosmetics, OTC drugs, personal care and household products, specialty chemicals, paper products, nonwovens, medical devices, and oral care products. Provides complete clinical trial services and is a valued partner to hundreds of pharmaceutical companies and contract research organizations. Founded in 1947, Hill Top Research is the world's leading clinical research services company with 12 research centers throughout North America and Europe. Hill Top Research provides safety and efficacy, microbiology, and CRO services for personal care, oral care, and health care companies. More information about the company can be found on the company's website at www.hill-top.com. Geographic Area Served: Worldwide.

★ 14540 ★ The Nutter Group

PO Box 46352
Cincinnati, OH 45246-0352
Phone: (513)771-1848 **Free:** 800-529-9847
Fax: (513)772-6270
Email: roger@nuttergroup.com
Website: http://www.thenuttergroup.com

Fnded: 1988. **Activities:** Specializes in executive search, administrative and management recruitment; employee attitude surveys, training/development, and customer satisfaction measurement. Created Videoview-videotaped candidate interviews. Geographic Area Served: United States.

Cleveland

★ 14541 ★ D/E3 Inc.

18234 S Miles Pky.
Cleveland, OH 44128-4232
Phone: (216)663-1500 **Fax:** (216)663-1501

Fnded: 1984. **Activities:** Environmental engineers serving as liaison for clients. Aid in preparation of environmental impact statements and related reports. Advise on corrective process changes, pollution abatement treatment and/or equipment. Consult on safety and hazardous waste hazards, management and control. Survey and test radon and asbestos hazards, plus other indoor gases and materials. Industries served: primary and secondary steel, nonferrous, chemical, government agencies, industrial and commercial buildings, plus colleges, universities and schools. Geographic Area Served: Northeast Ohio.

★ 14542 ★ Strategic Change Consulting Inc.

23230 Chagrin Blvd., Ste. 305
Cleveland, OH 44122
Phone: (216)831-5055 **Free:** 877-566-3020
Fax: (216)831-5871
Email: info@wireless-managers.com
Website: http://www.wireless-managers.com

Fnded: 1986. **Activities:** Offers expertise in strategic analysis and planning, financial planning, marketing management development, labor relations, employee benefits, job classifications, salary grade systems, organizational development, engineering and operations, and process control systems. Financial services include payroll deduction flexible premium life insurance, healthcare claims administration, managed care dental plans, managed care pharmaceutical plans, medical case management, auditing of claims administration, and healthcare benefit planning and cost management. Also offers outplacement services, service recognition programs, job and compensation structuring, telecommunication planning and audits, information systems development, Request for Proposal (RFP) services, Wireless Assets Management, supply chain improvement, mergers & acquisitions, software inventory & licensing. Geographic Area Served: Worldwide.

Columbus

★ 14543 ★ Advanced Laser Services Corp.

819 Phillipi Rd.
Columbus, OH 43228
Phone: (614)351-8321 **Free:** 800-795-2737
Fax: (614)351-8328

Fnded: 1985. **Activities:** Offers expertise on the medical and surgical applications of lasers.

★ 14544 ★ Barbara H. McSheffery

2720 Tremont Rd.
Columbus, OH 43085
Phone: (614)481-8465 **Fax:** (614)487-8635
Email: bmcsheff@aol.com
Website: http://eatright.com

Fnded: 1981. **Activities:** Offers individualized nutrition and diet consultation services for all age groups and health levels, well or with medical diagnosis. Serves private industries as well as government agencies. **Remarks:** Call before faxing. Geographic Area Served: Franklin County-Central Ohio.

★ 14545 ★ Battelle Environmental Systems and Technology

505 King Ave.
Columbus, OH 43201
Phone: (614)424-6424 **Free:** 800-201-2011
Fax: (614)424-3404

Activities: Firm specializes in strategic environmental health and safety management, environmental restoration, waste management, decommissioning and decontamination, atmospheric science and applied technology, statistics and data analysis, and pollution prevention.

★ 14546 ★ Battelle Memorial Institute

505 King Ave.
Columbus, OH 43201-2693
Phone: (614)424-6424 **Free:** 800-201-2011
Fax: (614)424-5263
Email: solutions@battelle.org
Website: http://www.battelle.org

Fnded: 1929. **Activities:** Battelle conducts science and technology research, helping customers develop and commercialize products and services in the areas of medical products, pharmaceuticals, consumer products, agrochemicals, chemicals, energy, automotive, and digital transactions. Battelle also provides hundreds of federal, state, and local government agencies with technology solutions in the areas of national security, environment, transportation, health and human services, and NASA technology. In addition, Battelle provides on-site technical assistance to clients and manages large technical programs. **Remarks:** Established in 1929, Battelle has helped companies develop thousands of products, including: the plastic

6-pack beverage holder, abrasion-resistant golf ball coatings, the photographic process that became Xerox, tamper-resistant packages for a wide variety of products, a smart card system that electronically logs store discounts onto a computer chip, a device for Mr. Coffee that separates one coffee filter at a time from a stack of filters. Geographic Area Served: Worldwide.

★ 14547 ★ Education Consultants
255 Oakland Park Ave.
Columbus, OH 43214
Phone: (614)267-6020
Fnded: 1984. **Activities:** Nursing consultants primarily serving the healthcare industry through product flow studies, organizational evaluations, staff education, management enhancement, and employee health programs. Also serves government and industry primarily through employee health enhancement programs such as cardiovascular health, positive communication skills, stress reduction, and exercise. Geographic Area Served: East of Mississippi.

★ 14548 ★ Karlsberger Companies
99 E Main St.
Columbus, OH 43215-5189
Phone: (614)461-9500 **Fax:** (614)461-6324
Email: columbus@karlsberger.com
Website: http://www.karlsberger.com
Fnded: 1928. **Activities:** A multidisciplinary organization of architects, hospital consultants, interior and graphic designers, landscape architects and others. The firm specializes in hospital and related health facilities planning and design as well as other institutional type projects including laboratories, research and development, colleges and justice facilities. **Remarks:** Karlsberger Companies is the parent company of Karlsberger Architecture Inc., Karlsberger Planning Inc., and KA International Inc. Geographic Area Served: North America.

Cuyahoga Falls

★ 14549 ★ Medical Integrated Services Inc.
2000 Chestnut Blvd.
Cuyahoga Falls, OH 44223
Phone: (216)928-0706 **Free:** 800-828-0706
Fax: (216)928-0077
Website: http://www.misinc.org
Fnded: 1973. **Activities:** Provides clinical/professional engineering consulting, preventive maintenance, and repair services to client hospitals. Also provides environmental testing, thermography, medical gas systems verification, anesthesia, laboratory, EtO waste gas, vapor testing, computer/data processing, codes and standards, and JCAHO consulting services to hospital clients. Industries served: healthcare and construction. Geographic Area Served: Ohio, Michigan, Kentucky, West Virginia, and Pennsylvania.

Dayton

★ 14550 ★ Bright Future
6540 Cedarview Ct.
Dayton, OH 45459-1214
Phone: (937)438-9458 **Fax:** (937)438-3229
Email: lindaj@bflrc.com
Website: http://www.bflrc.com/bflrc.htm
Activities: Consults with governments, hospitals and clinics who want to build policies and programs for helping mothers breastfeed. Acts as a distribution center for information, education, and services related to breastfeeding and lactation management. Offers professional consultations, lectures, courses, professional coaching, teaching materials, printed materials, promotional items, and networking information.

★ 14551 ★ John D. Bullock, MD
Department of Ophthalmology
Wright State University
500 Lincoln Park Blvd., Ste. 104
Dayton, OH 45429-3492
Phone: (937)297-7676
Activities: Ophthalmologist and forensic examiner experienced in medical-legal investigations, depositions, and court appearances. Specializes in medical malpractice, accident reconstruction and analysis, product liability (including contact lenses and pharmaceuticals), malingering, biophysics of ocular and orbital trauma, post-operative blindness, optometric liability, forensic ocular and orbital microbiology, and insurance/Medicare billing, coding, and fraud. Geographic Area Served: Worldwide.

Dublin

★ 14552 ★ McKenzie Management Inc.
PO Box 3276
Dublin, OH 43016
Phone: (614)889-0246 **Free:** 800-288-1877
Fax: (614)889-5934
Fnded: 1980. **Activities:** Provides business, clinical, hygiene, marketing, and management services. Industries served: dental profession. Geographic Area Served: United States and Canada.

★ 14553 ★ Medical Strategies Inc.
7000 Cardinal Pl.
Dublin, OH 43017
Phone: (614)274-0200 **Free:** 800-825-3742
Fax: (614)529-1259
Fnded: 1986. **Activities:** Advises U.S. drug manufacturers on healthcare issues, marketing, and advertising; and develops computer software.

Kettering

★ 14554 ★ Wyonna Stiffler - Doreen White
1496 Bowman Ave.
Kettering, OH 45409
Phone: (937)294-8855 **Fax:** (937)294-8855
Fnded: 1984. **Activities:** Offers community-based specialized nursing care for persons with an ostomy, draining wounds, fistulas, drains, and ulcers. Also provides patient care consults, product evaluation, continuing education courses, and program development. Industries served: healthcare. **Remarks:** Female-owned firm.

Martins Ferry

★ 14555 ★ Gabriel E. Sella
92 N 4th St., Ste. 12
Martins Ferry, OH 43935
Phone: (740)633-4485 **Fax:** (740)633-4141
Email: paris10@aol.com
Website: http://www.gesellamd.com
Fnded: 1987. **Activities:** Consulting physician provides independent medical evaluations, examinee evaluation, file review, trial preparation for insurance or attorneys, and data research. Available for expert witness testimony. Industries served: insurance, industrial enterprises, attorneys, and judges. Geographic Area Served: United States and Canada.

Maumee

★ 14556 ★ Professional Alternatives Inc.
320 Conant St.
Maumee, OH 43537
Phone: (419)891-9068 **Fax:** (419)891-0696
Email: info@compscreen.com
Website: http://www.compscreen.com
Fnded: 1990. **Activities:** Human resources consulting firm specializes in substance and alcohol abuse programs.

Mentor

★ 14557 ★ ABC Consultants
7677 Lucretia Ct.
not found
Mentor, OH 44060
Phone: (440)266-0441 **Fax:** (440)266-0442
Email: celamyakelam@aol.com
Fnded: 1978. **Activities:** Health consultants who identify, develop, educate, and initiate programs for staff development, patient education, performance evaluation (hospital), and patient and family education (outpatient areas). Also designs educational programs for nursing homes. Additional expertise on meeting requirements of state and federal guidelines on nursing homes and home health agencies. Industries served: health services (administration, management, healthcare programs), home healthcare, (LTC) nursing homes, and hospitals. Geographic Area Served: United States, primarily Ohio.

Middleburg Heights

★ 14558 ★ MedSearch Staffing Services Inc.
7271 Engle Rd., Ste. 115
Middleburg Heights, OH 44130
Phone: (440)243-6363 **Fax:** (440)243-9117
Email: mhts@medsearchonline.com
Website: http://www.medstaffing.com
Fnded: 1981. **Activities:** Provides specialized recruitment of sales, marketing and management personnel. Also involved in top-level hospital management consulting and physician recruitment, interim/temporary staffing. Industries served: healthcare manufacturers and institutions in the United States.

New Albany

★ 14559 ★ Veronica K. Casey
4598 Neiswander Sq.
New Albany, OH 43054
Phone: (614)933-0829 **Fax:** (614)933-0829
Email: caseydong@aol.com
Fnded: 1971. **Activities:** Maternal-child healthcare nurse specialist. Geographic Area Served: New England.

North Canton

★ 14560 ★ John Smithkey, III, RN
1271 Overland Ave. NE
North Canton, OH 44720-1731
Phone: (330)494-3729
Activities: Specializes in public and occupational health, HIV/AIDS education and prevention programs, grant and proposal writing, and programs for businesses and employees.

Northwood

★ 14561 ★ NAMSA
2261 Tracy Rd.
Northwood, OH 43619
Phone: (419)666-9455 **Free:** 888-666-9455
Fax: (419)666-2954
Email: info@NAMSA.com
Website: http://www.namsa.com
Fnded: 1967. **Activities:** Specialists in biological safety testing of medical devices, raw materials, biomaterials. component parts, and plastics.

Painesville

★ 14562 ★ Saponaro Inc.
2168 Mentor Ave.
Painesville, OH 44077
Phone: (440)639-1413 **Free:** 800-327-3026
Fax: (440)639-1013
Fnded: 1974. **Activities:** A consulting firm that provides objective evaluations of medical care, medical literature research, and experts for plaintiff and defense, attorneys, and hospitals. Geographic Area Served: United States and Canada.

Parma

★ 14563 ★ Carol K. Revilock
1004 Tuxedo Ave.
Parma, OH 44134
Phone: (216)749-2293

Fnded: 1984. **Activities:** Offers healthcare consulting services, specializing in the following areas: home healthcare, geriatrics, non-profit organizations, and staff development.

Solon

★ 14564 ★ Health Action Council
33610 Solon Rd., Ste. 4
Solon, OH 44139
Phone: (440)248-2559 **Fax:** (440)248-5830
Email: contact@healthactioncouncil.com
Website: http://www.healthactioncouncil.org

Fnded: 1983. **Activities:** Conducts management training sessions.

Springfield

★ 14565 ★ Adcare Health Systems Inc.
5057 Troy Rd.
Springfield, OH 45502-9032
Phone: (937)964-8974 **Fax:** (937)964-8961
Email: info@adcarehealth.com
Website: http://www.adcarehealth.com

Fnded: 1986. **Activities:** Consulting firm offers expertise in the areas of healthcare systems management. Focus is on senior housing (retirement communities, asorted living and nursing homes), movement feasibility and Medicare/Medicaid reimbursement.

Watertown

★ 14566 ★ Betty M. Neuman
PO Box 77
Watertown, OH 45787
Phone: (740)749-3322 **Fax:** (740)749-3322

Fnded: 1974. **Activities:** Nursing curriculum consultant for implementation of the Neuman Systems Model into both educational and nursing practice settings. Also offers organizational development assistance with emphasis on conflict resolution and leadership skill development. Geographic Area Served: Worldwide.

Oklahoma

Bethany

★ 14567 ★ Intelemed
5810 Philip J. Rhoads Ave.
Bethany, OK 73008
Phone: (405)789-3889 **Free:** 800-428-9288
Fax: (918)621-2154

Fnded: 1995. **Activities:** Medical systems integration, telemedicine consulting services, telemedicing networks, connectivity, and intranets. Geographic Area Served: United States.

Stillwater

★ 14568 ★ Nutrition Counseling Service
311 S Duck St.
Stillwater, OK 74074
Phone: (405)624-1343 **Fax:** (405)377-5561

Fnded: 1978. **Activities:** Provides nutrition counseling for both individuals and group in central Oklahoma.

Tulsa

★ 14569 ★ Donna Lee Wong
7535 S Urbana Ave.
Tulsa, OK 74136-6113
Phone: (918)496-0544 **Fax:** (918)496-8344
Website: http://www.mosby.com/WOW

Fnded: 1975. **Activities:** Pediatric nurse consultant specializing in management of complex nursing care problems, family counseling related to childhood adjustment disorders and grief therapy, and in pain assessment and management. Consultant authors publications and conducts workshops and seminars on these topics; schedule available upon request. Geographic Area Served: Worldwide.

★ 14570 ★ Fry, Hughes, and Associates - Professional Management Consultants
1516 S Boston, Ste. 212
Tulsa, OK 74119
Phone: (918)582-4000 **Free:** 877-582-4400
Fax: (918)582-4000
Email: mfrydumas@yahoo.com

Fnded: 1970. **Activities:** A financial consulting and small business advisory organization providing financial planning, estate planning, tax planning, tax preparation, accounting and personnel systems and procedures. Also offers services in the area of financial and practice management for the medical and dental professions. Industries served: primarily the healthcare industry. Geographic Area Served: United States and selected foreign countries.

Oregon

Beaverton

★ 14571 ★ Animal School Inc.
7850 SW Nimbus Ave.
Beaverton, OR 97008
Phone: (503)646-3060 **Fax:** (503)643-8963

Activities: Consultant behaviorist for pets, specializing in animal behavior therapy, applied animal behavior, human animal interaction, psychology/pet behavior, pet training, and animal/human bonding.

Forest Grove

★ 14572 ★ Brown-Spath & Associates
PO Box 721
Forest Grove, OR 97116
Phone: (503)357-9185 **Fax:** (503)357-9267
Email: patrice@brownspath.com
Website: http://www.brownspath.com

Activities: Offers educational resources for healthcare quality and resource management professionals.

Klamath Falls

★ 14573 ★ Cell Tech/Priscilla Reynolds
1300 Main St.
Klamath Falls, OR 97601-5900
Phone: (541)882-5406

Fnded: 1982. **Activities:** To make our Super Blue Green products available to everyone and to create a generation of leaders, guided by a global vision of health, environmental integrity, economic abundance, and incredible quality of life for everyone. Geographic Area Served: Worldwide.

Lake Oswego

★ 14574 ★ The Walker Co.
4848 Hastings Dr.
Lake Oswego, OR 97035
Phone: (503)534-9461 **Fax:** (503)534-9462
Email: lw@walkercompany.com
Website: http://www.walkercompany.com

Activities: Provides a range of healthcare strategic planning services, including board and staff retreats, development of mission, values and vision statements, board performance self-assessments, market research, focus groups, communications assessments, and goal, objective and strategy development.

Medford

★ 14575 ★ BWR Associates Inc.
920 Mason Way
Medford, OR 97501-1343
Phone: (541)779-2646 **Fax:** (541)779-1174

Fnded: 1971. **Activities:** Environmental consultants active in the following areas: source evaluation, stack testing, ambient air testing and monitoring, water and wastewater analysis, process evaluation, control device efficiency testing, compliance tests, laboratory analysis, and microscopy. Additional areas of expertise include: asbestos consulting and project design, building surveys, bulk analysis, environmental audits, site assessments, hazardous materials, and wetlands consulting. Geographic Area Served: Western United States.

Portland

★ 14576 ★ Carol Lange, R.D.
1012 SW King
Portland, OR 97205
Phone: (503)221-1793 **Fax:** (503)221-1793

Fnded: 1976. **Activities:** Provides full-spectrum nutrition counseling to bring about comfortable, permanent lifestyle changes. This includes private clients and physican referrals for general nutrition, compulsive eating, all weight problems, diabetes, hypoglycemia, high cholesterol and triglycerides, vegetarian diets, maternal nutrition, and food allergies. Combines expertise in nutrition, psychology, counseling, and education.

★ 14577 ★ Digital Vision Inc.
6805 SE Milwaukie Ave.
Portland, OR 97202-5619
Phone: (503)231-6606

Fnded: 1983. **Activities:** Offers optical laboratory research and services, and related computer support to government and private sector industries on the West Coast.

Pennsylvania

Bensalem

★ 14578 ★ Stelex-TVG
3331 St. Rd., Ste. 300
Bensalem, PA 19020
Phone: (215)638-9700 **Fax:** (215)638-9333
Email: sales@stelex-tvg.com
Website: http://www.stelex-tvg.com

Fnded: 1994. **Activities:** Provides full regulatory compliance and validation services to the Pharmaceutical, Bulk Pharmaceutical, Biotech, Medical Device, and Veterinary industries. Geographic Area Served: Worldwide.

Berwick

★ 14579 ★ Medical Management Services Inc.
1651 W Front St.
Berwick, PA 18603-2305
Phone: (570)759-7619 **Free:** 800-982-0886
Fax: (570)759-7613

Fnded: 1981. **Activities:** Business related health services firm provides expertise on billing services for doctors offices.

Bethel Park

★ 14580 ★ Allegheny Podiatry Foot
6040 Library Rd.
Bethel Park, PA 15102
Phone: (412)833-0511

Activities: Firm provides comprehensive assessments, home care, care plans, nursing home and personal care home placement. Coordinates and monitors services. Also offers crisis intervention, management services for out of town care givers, and counseling. Geographic Area Served: Southwestern PA.

★ 14581 ★ Applied Health Physics Inc.
2986 Industrial Blvd.
Bethel Park, PA 15102-2536
Phone: (412)835-9555 **Free:** 800-332-6648
Fax: (412)835-9559
Email: ahp@icubed.com
Website: http://www.appliedhlth.qpg.com
Fnded: 1962. **Activities:** Provides radiation services for industry academic, research, medical and nuclear users in the United States. licensing, renewals, amendments, compliance, audits. **Remarks:** 24 hour emergency response, calibration and sales. Sealed source leak testing and analysis. Geographic Area Served: Worldwide.

Blue Bell

★ 14582 ★ Adult Day Care Group
3 Ramsgate Ct.
Blue Bell, PA 19422
Phone: (610)941-0340 **Fax:** (610)834-0459
Website: http://www.adultdaycaregroup.com
Fnded: 1993. **Activities:** Professional adult day care consultants, specializing in adult day care services for adult day care centers, nursing homes, assisted living facilities, retirement communities, and hospitals. Geographic Area Served: United States, Canada, Europe, and Asia.

★ 14583 ★ ComputerTalk Associates Inc.
492 Norristown Rd., Ste. 160
Blue Bell, PA 19422-2355
Phone: (610)825-7686 **Fax:** (610)825-7641
Email: maggie@computertalk.com
Website: http://www.computertalk.com
Fnded: 1980. **Activities:** Data processing consultants serving the healthcare market: end users such as pharmacists and physicians as well as companies considering these vertical markets.

★ 14584 ★ Medical Marketing Group Inc.
512 Township Line Rd., 2-800
Blue Bell, PA 19422-2701
Phone: (215)641-2900
Activities: Pharmaceutical marketing and consulting company.

★ 14585 ★ The Medical Phone Co.
1777 Sentry Pky. W, Dublin Hall, Ste. 300
Blue Bell, PA 19422
Phone: (215)643-2500 **Free:** 800-866-8672
Fax: (215)643-7000
Fnded: 1988. **Activities:** Health care marketing communications firm. Geographic Area Served: United States.

Butler

★ 14586 ★ Strategic Controls Inc.
332 South Main St.
Butler, PA 16001
Phone: (724)282-1066 **Free:** 888-206-8325
Email: gorourke7@earthlink.net
Website: http://www.securityexpert.ws
Activities: Offers security and litigation support in matters that concern co-ops, condominiums, malls, parking lots, commercial and residential high rise, transportation, air-ground, hotels, casinos, public events, concerts, educational institutions, security training, court security.

Chester

★ 14587 ★ Emergency & Safety Programs
Main St., Ste. 911
Chester, PA 19015-2902
Phone: (610)872-7447 **Fax:** (610)872-5727
Fnded: 1979. **Activities:** Healhcare consulting firm offering expertise in emergency medical training and emergency response planning & evaluation to business and government agencies worldwide.

Conshohocken

★ 14588 ★ Longshore & Simmons Inc.
625 Ridge Pke., Ste. 410
Conshohocken, PA 19428
Phone: (610)941-3400 **Free:** 800-346-8397
Fax: (610)941-2424
Fnded: 1979. **Activities:** Firm offers expertise on healthcare-related issues: strategic planning, departmental reviews, compensation issues, medical staff planning, and valuations. Geographic Area Served: United States.

Danville

★ 14589 ★ Geisinger Medical Management Corp
100 N Academy Ave.
Danville, PA 17822-2412
Phone: (570)271-8120 **Free:** 800-275-6401
Fax: (570)271-5964
Website: http://www.geisinger.org
Fnded: 1978. **Activities:** Business management firm specializing in healthcare consulting to medical institutions and nursing homes by providing human resource, financial, clinical, and administrative services. Geographic Area Served: A 45-county service area covering Northern, Central, and Southern regions of Pennsylvania.

Duboistown

★ 14590 ★ Lycoming Analytical Laboratories
2687 Euclid Ave.
Duboistown, PA 17702
Phone: (570)323-5001 **Fax:** (570)323-0009
Email: cnilsen@lycominganalytical.com
Website: http://www.lycominganalytical.com
Fnded: 1989. **Activities:** Provides technical consultation to chemical and pharmaceutical industries. Services include problem-solving, management plan development and compliance advice for the analytical chemical laboratory, and analytical testing servi es, including pharmaceutical raw material and finished dosage form testing: assays, monograph testing, stability, methods development and validation, analytical R&D and process and cleaning validation support. Also offered is laboratory-management computer software, custom written for clients. Geographic Area Served: Ireland, Puerto Rico. Canada.

Eldred

★ 14591 ★ Ensanian Physicochemical Institute
Barden Brook Rd.
PO Box 98
Eldred, PA 16731
Phone: (814)225-3296
Fnded: 1963. **Activities:** Industrial engineering consultants active in nondestructive testing of metals, failure analysis of metals, robotics quantium physics, and artificial intelligence. Also works in areas of electronic diagnostic medicine, manufacturing in space (zero gravity), electrochemistry, solid state physics and chemistry, and surface phenomena. Industries served: aerospace, metalworking, marine, automotive, electronics, biomedical, bioengineering, government, sports medicine, healthcare, and cosmetics. Geographic Area Served: Worldwide.

Fairless Hills

★ 14592 ★ Pharmaceutical Information Associates Ltd.
333 N Oxford Valley Rd., Ste. 404
Fairless Hills, PA 19030
Phone: (215)949-0490 **Fax:** (215)949-2594
Activities: Company communicates scientific information to regulatory and healthcare professionals.

Gordonville

★ 14593 ★ Personal Care Resource Center Inc.
41 Londonvale Rd.
Gordonville, PA 17529
Phone: (717)768-7271 **Free:** 800-725-7395
Fax: (717)768-8553
Email: royeby@aol.com
Activities: Residential healthcare consultants provide training programs.

Harleysville

★ 14594 ★ Outsource Technology Associates Inc.
159 Ruth Rd.
Harleysville, PA 19438
Phone: (215)256-6848 **Fax:** (215)256-4906
Email: RobtHaluska@aol.com
Fnded: 1996. **Activities:** Consultant to the pharmaceutical and chemical industries with a focus on controlled-release formulation technology from a product and business development perspective, as well as customer technical service. Extensive experience in technical communications/training, opportunity analysis, external resource identification and liaison, patent and regulatory compliance matters, organization development and project planning/management. Geographic Area Served: Americas and Europe.

Huntingdon Valley

★ 14595 ★ Andrew Newman, MD
2030 County Line Rd.
Huntingdon Valley, PA 19006
Phone: (610)660-0805 **Fax:** (610)660-9270
Activities: Orthopedist, consultant, and expert witness specializing in workers' compensation and medical malpractice.

Ingomar

★ 14596 ★ Radiological Science Associates Inc.
PO Box 677
Ingomar, PA 15127
Phone: (412)232-7805 **Fax:** (412)232-5753
Email: ushab@aol.com
Fnded: 1984. **Activities:** Radiological physicists offer consulting expertise. Geographic Area Served: Penn-Ohio.

Jenkintown

★ 14597 ★ Consultants in Medical Imaging
820 Fox Chase Rd.
Jenkintown, PA 19046-4437
Phone: (215)663-2450
Website: http://www.cmixray.com
Activities: A radiology consultation service providing independent film reviews and second opinion radiology interpretations to the legal community and insurance companies.

★ 14598 ★ Einstein Consulting Group Inc.
501 Washington Ln., Ste. 302
Jenkintown, PA 19046
Phone: (215)886-4622 **Free:** 800-765-9975
Fax: (215)886-4640

Fnded: 1985. **Activities:** Firm offers expertise in healthcare consulting.

★ 14599 ★ Habitat Consultants
1139 Sewell Ln.
PO Box 212
Jenkintown, PA 19046
Phone: (215)576-1359 **Fax:** (215)576-1404
Email: thebutterflylady@juno.com

Fnded: 1990. **Activities:** Provide services to schools, mental health facilities, hospitals, senior centers, museums, and nature centers concerning establishment of habitats to attract and sustain butterflies. Provide information and programs about interactions of people, animals, and environment including pet visitation programs to health facilities. Geographic Area Served: United States, Canada, and Mexico.

Kennett Square

★ 14600 ★ Center for Animal Health and Productivity
School of Veterinary Medicine, University of Pennsylvania
New Bolton Ctr.
382 W St. Rd.
Kennett Square, PA 19348-1692
Phone: (610)444-5800 **Fax:** (610)925-8123
Website: http://cahpwww.nbc.upenn.edu/

Fnded: 1986. **Activities:** Mission is to develop, communicate and apply knowledge needed for improvement of the health productivity of food animal populations. Implements teaching, research and service programs directed toward the improvement of health and productivity in food animal herds and flocks. Programs involve an integrated approach employing expertise in disciplines such as clinical nutrition, reproduction, health economics, and computer science in addition to conventional specialties in veterinary medicine. Educational activities include instruction of veterinary students in production systems medicine, postgraduate training and continuing education for food animal practitioners. Provides an infrastructure for applied research and directly supports specific research and development projects pertaining to the health management of food animal populations. Provides health management services for animal populations and conducts field investigation of herd and flock problems which pose a threat to the economic productivity of animal agriculture. Constitutes an important line of early defense against the spread of economically important disease among food animal populations. Geographic Area Served: Pennsylvania.

King of Prussia

★ 14601 ★ BioChem Technology Inc.
100 Ross Rd., Ste. 201
King of Prussia, PA 19406-2100
Phone: (610)768-9360 **Fax:** (610)768-9363
Email: sales@biochemtech.com
Website: http://www.biochemtech.com

Fnded: 1977. **Activities:** Consultants in wastewater treatment processes specializing in evaluation and optimization of biological nutrient removal facilities. On-line process monitoring and control of wastewater treatment processes as well as yeast, bacterial or fungal fermentation. Experience in biochemical process development, wastewater treatment process design, fermentation system design, process and plant design, biochemical engineering research and a variety of engineering specialities. Undertakes a wide variety of projects which range from preliminary feasibility studies to the development and optimization of a biological process. Geographic Area Served: Southern United States, Pacific Northwest, Mid-Atlantic states.

Lancaster

★ 14602 ★ David G. Polin, MD
2110 Harrisburg
Lancaster, PA 17601-2644
Phone: (717)399-4364 **Fax:** (717)392-8160

Activities: Specializes in brain injury, spinal cord injury, amputations, reflex sympathetic dystrophy, myopascial pain, and EMG testing.

Lansdale

★ 14603 ★ Winifred S. Hayes Inc.
157 S Broad St., Ste. 200
Lansdale, PA 19446
Phone: (215)855-0615 **Fax:** (215)855-5218
Website: http://www.hayesinc.com

Fnded: 1989. **Activities:** Offers healthcare services, focusing on environment health. Industries served: healthcare, insurance, and businesses regionally.

Latrobe

★ 14604 ★ P R S Inc. - Pharmacy Services
PO Box 852
Latrobe, PA 15650
Phone: (412)539-7820 **Free:** 800-338-3688
Fax: (412)539-1388
Email: harryl@prsrx.com
Website: http://www.prsrx.com

Fnded: 1983. **Activities:** Pharmacy consultants. Industries served: grocery, retail pharmacy, and hospital pharmacy. Geographic Area Served: United States.

Lemoyne

★ 14605 ★ Irene C. Berman-Levine - Nutrition Program Planning
650 N 12th St.
Lemoyne, PA 17043
Phone: (717)763-1798 **Fax:** (717)238-5147

Fnded: 1986. **Activities:** Develops educational programs on the topics of nutrition and health. Frequently speaks on subjects such as diet and cancer and diet and oils in coronary heart disease. Expertise in consumer food purchasing patterns, nutrition labeling, and development/evaluation of nutrition education materials. Geographic Area Served: Harrisburg, Central Pennsylvania, Philadelphia/Baltimore.

Malvern

★ 14606 ★ AREUFIT Health Services Inc.
270 W Lancaster Ave., Ste. J-2
Malvern, PA 19355
Phone: (610)993-9123 **Fax:** (610)993-9125

Activities: Health promotion, wellness, and physiological testing company. Services include employee testing, wellness programs, health related seminars, osteoporosis testing and education, influenza vaccination programs, bloodborne pathogen compliance training, CPR/First Aid training, stress management seminars, smoking cessation programs, and fitness evaluations. Geographic Area Served: Philadelphia, Lancaster County, Southern New Jersey, Delaware, and Maryland.

Mechanicsburg

★ 14607 ★ Cocciardi & Associates Inc.
4 Kacey Ct.
Mechanicsburg, PA 17055
Phone: (717)766-4500 **Free:** 800-377-3024
Fax: (717)766-3999
Email: jcocciardi@cocciardi.com
Website: http://www.cocciardi.com

Fnded: 1988. **Activities:** Firm provides safety, health and environmental consulting and training. It handles such issues as Hazardous Waste Operations and Emergency Response Regulation (HAZWOPER), asbestos and lead training (for licensing requirements), environmental auditing, and health and safety investigations. It serves all industries worldwide. Geographic Area Served: Worldwide.

Merion Station

★ 14608 ★ Ralph M. Myerson
310 Maplewood Ave.
Merion Station, PA 19066
Phone: (610)664-0406
Email: mdralph@aol.com

Fnded: 1985. **Activities:** Provides freelance writing and consultation services to pharmaceutical industries and health career establishments by supplying data such as patient information and manuscripts for use in health journals for promotional and educational purposes. Industries served: publishing and pharmaceutical. Geographic Area Served: Worldwide.

Moon Twp

★ 14609 ★ Augmentative Communication Consultants Inc.
280-B Moon Clinton Rd.
Moon Twp, PA 15108
Phone: (412)264-6121 **Free:** 800-982-2248
Fax: (412)269-0923
Email: acci@usacr.net
Website: http://www.ACClinc.com

Fnded: 1987. **Activities:** Represents more than a dozen manufacturers of augmentative communication and other assistive technologies, offering demonstrations, workshops and consultation. Geographic Area Served: United States.

Narberth

★ 14610 ★ The Right Connection Inc.
PO Box 513
Narberth, PA 19072
Phone: (610)664-7374

Fnded: 1984. **Activities:** Advertising and marketing consulting group has expertise in microbiology and antimicrobial chemotherapy. Industries served: pharmaceutical and communication media. Geographic Area Served: Greater Philadelphia, Pennsylvania; New Jersey; New York; and south Florida.

Newtown

★ 14611 ★ Scott-Levin
60 Blacksmith Rd.
Newtown, PA 18940
Phone: (215)860-0440 **Fax:** (215)860-5477
Website: http://www.scottlevin.com

Fnded: 1982. **Activities:** Firm offers expertise in healthcare and pharmaceutical consulting.

★ 14612 ★ VirSci Corp.
PO Box 760
Newtown, PA 18940
Phone: (215)504-4164 **Fax:** (215)504-4164
Email: infovirsci@virsci.com
Website: http://www.virsci.com

Activities: Specializes in the design and development of medical and pharmaceutical web sites. Helps clients bring and market their medical communications online. Clients include medical societies, pharmaceutical companies, medical publishers, and other medical information providers.

Philadelphia

★ 14613 ★ The Center for Forensic Economic Studies
1608 Walnut St., Ste. 1200
Philadelphia, PA 19103
Phone: (215)546-5600 **Fax:** (215)732-8158
Email: cfes@cfes.com
Website: http://www.cfes.com

Fnded: 1980. **Activities:** Provides economic and statistical analysis in litigation, including personal injury, commercial, employment and civil rights matters: as well as business valuations. Geographic Area Served: United States and other countries.

★ 14614 ★ Edith Schwager
4404 Sherwood Rd.
Philadelphia, PA 19131-1526
Phone: (215)877-1137 **Fax:** (215)877-1137
Email: edieschwager@cs.com

Fnded: 1981. **Activities:** Editorial consultant specializing in English usage, medicine, and pharmaceuticals. Conducts workshops and seminars on medical editing and on English usage and abusage for physicians and nurses, publishing houses, pharmaceutical corporations, universities and colleges, government agencies and other organizations. **Remarks:** Call before faxing. Geographic Area Served: Worldwide.

★ 14615 ★ Herbert L. Goldberg, DDS
528 Delancey St.
Philadelphia, PA 19106-4106
Phone: (215)925-9551 **Fax:** (215)627-7417

Activities: A certified dental consultant. Diplomat of the Academy of Forensic Dentistry. Provides orofacial pain, dental, and temporomandibular evaluations with expert witness testimony. Geographic Area Served: PA, NJ, DE, and MD.

★ 14616 ★ Joshua H. Werblowsky
Presidential Ste. D-111
Philadelphia, PA 19131
Phone: (215)878-3954 **Fax:** (610)667-1691

Fnded: 1971. **Activities:** Forensic psychiatric consultant for civil, family, and criminal cases with particular expertise in workmen's compensation and personal injury. Geographic Area Served: Philadelphia, PA.

★ 14617 ★ Marc S. Micozzi, MD, PhD
19 S 22nd St.
Philadelphia, PA 19103
Phone: (215)563-3737 **Fax:** (215)575-3499
Email: micozzi@collphyphil.org
Website: http://www.c3r.org/Advisory/Micozzi-Marc.htm

Fnded: 1984. **Activities:** General health services consultant offers expertise in the following areas: public health, medicine, medical technology, public health organization and policy, diet and nutrition, forensic science, and anthropology. Also provides preparation and presentation of seminars, lectures, articles, workshops, case review and preparation. Industries served: health industry manufacturers, pharmaceuticals, food, legal, print and broadcast media, museums, education and entertainment. Geographic Area Served: United States.

★ 14618 ★ Perfecseal
9800 Bustleton Ave.
Philadelphia, PA 19115
Phone: (215)673-4500 **Free:** 888-673-4100
Fax: (215)676-1311
Email: perfecseal@bemis.com
Website: http://www.perfecseal.com

Activities: Dedicated to flexible packaging for the medical and healthcare markets. A global supplier of high-performance materials including PerfecSeal heat-seal-coated Tyvek, PerfeCraft heat-seal-coated paper, and PerfecFlex multiple-layer coextruded and oriented films, vacuum-metallized laminates, peel pouches, tubing, header polybag packaging, PerfedForm custom thermoformed trays and die-cut lids, pharmaceutical labels, eight-color flexo and rotogravure printing. Perfecseal is ISO 9000 certified worldwide.

★ 14619 ★ R.D. Network Inc.
303 Shawmont Ave., Ste. D
Philadelphia, PA 19128-4238
Phone: (215)482-4461 **Free:** 877-482-4991
Fax: (215)482-9947
Email: rd-network@msn.com
Website: http://www.rdnetwork.com

Fnded: 1983. **Activities:** Dietitians, diet technicians, and certified dietary managers available nationwide and worldwide through an international registry (over 2000 members) for consulting positions to wellness/employee education programs, drug/alcohol rehabilitation, hospital, LTC, nutrition/labeling communications, nutrition consultation, weight control classes, healthcare staff supplementation, media and program development, and all nutrition and food-related needs. Expert witness and speakers bureau also available. Industries served: healthcare, food industry, food service, restaurateurs, corrections, supermarkets, pharmaceutical companies, home health agencies, insurance companies, HMOs, and government agencies.

★ 14620 ★ RMC Medical
3019 Darnell Rd.
Philadelphia, PA 19154-3201
Phone: (215)824-4100 **Free:** 800-322-0672
Fax: (215)824-1371
Email: rmcmedical@cs.com
Website: http://www.rmcmedical.com

Fnded: 1969. **Activities:** Offers training in Chemical/Biological and Hazardous management and treatment to U.S. industries. Geographic Area Served: United States.

★ 14621 ★ RX-OTC Consultants Inc.
1500 Locust St., Ste. 3805
Philadelphia, PA 19105
Phone: (215)732-8994 **Fax:** (215)732-8422
Email: RXOTC1@aol.com

Fnded: 1989. **Activities:** Provides Out-licensing, In-licensing, Partner Selection and marketing assistance in pharmaceutical industry. Geographic Area Served: United States.

★ 14622 ★ TRG Healthcare L.L.C.
1601 Market St., Ste. 550
Philadelphia, PA 19103
Phone: (267)256-0726 **Fax:** (267)256-0728
Website: http://www.trghealthcare.com

Fnded: 1999. **Activities:** Firm provides critical financial performance improvement services to various types of healthcare organizations. Services include time critical financial performance improvement implementation; interim management for executive positions; facilitation of mergers or corporate separations; bankruptcy "workouts". Related services include strategic positioning, managed care alignment, physician organization improvement, information systems planning and improvement, organizational behavioral change, and alignment and integration of organizations. Geographic Area Served: United States.

Pittsburgh

★ 14623 ★ Consad Research Corp.
121 N Highland Ave.
Pittsburgh, PA 15206
Phone: (412)363-5500 **Fax:** (412)363-5509
Email: info@consad.com
Website: http://www.consad.com

Fnded: 1962. **Activities:** Performs basic and applied social science research such as technology assessment and transfer, environmental risk assessment, health and safety planning, drug abuse policy and programs, urban planning, environmental and physical planning, law and criminal justice, economics, science policy issues, transportation, management and public administration, computer sciences, energy policy and program analysis, regulation and deregulation, military manpower issues, and mineral economics.

★ 14624 ★ Daniel Stern and Associates Ltd.
Duff Commercial Ctr.
10 Duff Rd., Ste. 215
Pittsburgh, PA 15235
Phone: (412)244-6434 **Free:** 800-892-2781
Fax: 800-438-2476
Email: sternd@danielstern.com
Website: http://www.danielstern.com

Fnded: 1970. **Activities:** Expertise in Physician Contracts, Compensation, Benefits, Staff Employment and staffing issues. Specail Experts in Emergency Medicine and its allied concerns. National and Regional Salary Surveys Available. Geographic Area Served: United States.

★ 14625 ★ Health Evaluation Systems
130 7th St., Ste. 1140
Pittsburgh, PA 15222-3409
Phone: (412)281-8727 **Fax:** (412)281-8728

Fnded: 1987. **Activities:** Offers expertise in health evaluation. Industries served: insurance, transportation, certified medical/review offices (all safety sensitive areas for drug and alcohol testing, workers compensation issues). Geographic Area Served: United States.

★ 14626 ★ Lawson Bernstein
PO Box 81977
Pittsburgh, PA 15217
Phone: (412)422-9240 **Fax:** (412)422-5203

Activities: A certified forensic neuropsychiatrist with expertise in brain injury, stroke, toxic environmental exposure, drug and alcohol abuse, PTSD and other related areas in neurology and psychiatry.

★ 14627 ★ Madalon O. Amenta
5512 Northumberland St.
Pittsburgh, PA 15217
Phone: (412)687-3852 **Fax:** (412)687-9095

Fnded: 1982. **Activities:** Offers healthcare consultation including hospice programs (all aspects), nursing policy, medical and nursing writing projects (editorial and writing), nursing research, and quality assurance in hospice care and nursing. Geographic Area Served: United States.

★ 14628 ★ Omega Communications Inc.
Acacia Bldg., Ste. 275
875 Greentree Rd.
Pittsburgh, PA 15220-3503
Phone: (732)733-0550

Fnded: 1976. **Activities:** Provides health management, marketing, and sales training to pharmaceutical industry in the United States and Canada.

★ 14629 ★ Spindle Publishing Co.
4136 Library Rd., Ste. 200
Pittsburgh, PA 15234
Phone: (412)531-9742 **Fax:** (412)531-2004
Email: info@spindlepub.com
Website: http://www.spindlepub.com

Fnded: 1976. **Activities:** Publishes an online guide for international patients on locating U.S. hospitals, health clinics, and medical practices.

★ 14630 ★ Susquehanna American Inc.
733 Washington Rd., Ste. 100
Pittsburgh, PA 15228
Phone: (412)344-7250 **Fax:** (412)344-7272

Fnded: 1976. **Activities:** Offers medical management specializing in nursing home services and administration; and third party reimbursement.

Plymouth Meeting

★ 14631 ★ Dr. Gerald S. Brenner
3007 Oakwood Dr.
Plymouth Meeting, PA 19462

Phone: (610)279-3944 **Fax:** (610)279-3944
Email: gsbrenner@erols.com
Fnded: 1994. **Activities:** Consultant to pharmaceutical, chemical, biotechnologyg, medical device and allied industries. Development and validation of processes for bulk pharmaceuticals. Physical/Chemical characterization of drug substances and raw materials. Drug development troubleshooting: stability, solubility, bioavailability. Analytical methods development and validation. Stability protocols and data review. Specification development. Formulation development: composition and process, CMC preparation and review. SOP preparation and review. Regulatory compliance, DAI preparation, 483 responses. Patent preparation and review. Expert witness. Geographic Area Served: Worldwide.

★ 14632 ★ ECRI
5200 Butler Pke.
Plymouth Meeting, PA 19462-1298
Phone: (610)825-6000 **Fax:** (610)834-1275
Email: info@ecri.org
Website: http://www.ecri.org
Fnded: 1955. **Activities:** Offers assistance in healthcare technology including, strategic planning, management consulting, assessment, evaluation, specification and acquisition of medical devices and systems, healthcare facilities and equipment planning, risk management, accident investigation, and forensic engineering. Additional services include healthcare and environmental management. Also offers expertise in medical technology assessment, medical equipment acquisition, and medical equipment purchasing. Industries served: healthcare institutions, healthcare insurers and government. Geographic Area Served: Worldwide.

★ 14633 ★ The Health Care Group Inc.
140 W Germantown Pke., Ste. 200
Plymouth Meeting, PA 19462
Phone: (610)828-3888 **Free:** 800-473-0032
Fax: (610)828-3658
Website: http://www.healthcaregroup.com
Fnded: 1970. **Activities:** Provides consulting services in practice management, marketing, business and health law and financial planning for physicians, and other health care professionals. Geographic Area Served: United States.

★ 14634 ★ Mary Anne Clairmont
3127 Colony Ln.
Plymouth Meeting, PA 19462
Phone: (610)941-9429 **Fax:** (610)941-9995
Email: Fse452@erols.com
Fnded: 1985. **Activities:** Consultant in nutrition and health to hospitals and long-term care facilities, schools, colleges and private industry. Areas covered include: all topics of general nutrition, wellness, sports topics, weight loss programs, vegetarianism, nutrition over fifty, drug and alcohol rehabilitation, and long-term care regulations for dietary departments. Consultant to weight loss groups. Also offers presentations to groups, on limited or ongoing basis. Industries served: individuals, groups, hospitals, health centers, nursing homes, colleges, schools, and government agencies.

Pottstown

★ 14635 ★ Jeffrey S. Yablon
1600 E High St.
Chestmont Bldg., 3rd Fl.
Pottstown, PA 19464
Phone: (610)327-7514
Email: jydoc11@aol.com
Website: http://www.yablon.com/
Activities: An actively practicing, board-certified neurosurgeon with extensive experience in neurosurgical case review, personal injury claims, and medical malpractice issues. Specializes in diseases of the central nervous system, cervical and lumbar disc disease, carotid endarterectomy, peripheral nerve surgery including carpal tunnel syndrome, non-surgical and surgical treatment of complex pain problems, and medical-legal expert testimony.

Richboro

★ 14636 ★ Dr. Mark Shapiro
26 Legacy Oaks Dr.
Richboro, PA 18954
Phone: (215)364-2822 **Fax:** (215)443-8587
Fnded: 1976. **Activities:** Provides real-time software services for mini and micro computers including scientific applications and operating system internals. Active primarily with medical and pharmaceutical industries.

Southampton

★ 14637 ★ AddVal Inc.
1300 Industrial Blvd., Ste. 202
Southampton, PA 18966
Phone: (215)396-8972 **Fax:** (215)364-2187
Email: mmcfarla@addvalinc.com
Website: http://www.addvalinc.com
Fnded: 1995. **Activities:** Experienced in the credentialing processes. Provides outsourcing of the verification process and oversight audits. Experienced in quality improvement. Geographic Area Served: United States.

Springfield

★ 14638 ★ Crozer-Keystone Health System
196 W Sproul Rd., Ste. 105
Springfield, PA 19064-2045
Phone: (610)328-8800 **Fax:** (610)892-8030
Email: crozer@crozer.org
Website: http://www.crozer.org
Fnded: 1990. **Activities:** Health services specialists in hospital administration and integrated healthcare systems.

Swarthmore

★ 14639 ★ John E. Hoover - Consultant
363 Riverview Rd.
Swarthmore, PA 19081
Phone: (610)328-9786
Email: hoovjohn@netscape.net
Fnded: 1978. **Activities:** Consultant in bio-medical communications; offers editorial and writing services for wide variety of clients in pharmaceutical, medical, and other healthcare fields. Geographic Area Served: United States.

Upper Darby

★ 14640 ★ Grief Counseling & Support Services
8600 W Chester Pke., Ste. 304
Upper Darby, PA 19082
Phone: (610)789-7707 **Fax:** (610)469-9499
Email: jkharry@voicenet.com
Fnded: 1984. **Activities:** Specializing in consulting and training services for organizations dealing with loss and grief issues. These services may include management consultations, crisis intervention, educational programming, policy development, program design, group process work, individual counseling or other support services. Training and support services also provided for loss issues for mental retardation service providers. Serves private industries as well as government agencies.

Wayne

★ 14641 ★ Armstrong, Doyle & Carroll Inc.
4 Glenhardie Corporate Ctr.
1255 Drummers Ln., Ste. 300
Wayne, PA 19087
Phone: (610)971-2100 **Fax:** (610)971-0660
Email: adc@adcbenefits.com
Website: http://www.adcbenefits.com
Fnded: 1955. **Activities:** Offers expertise on health and welfare plans, employee benefits, including profit sharing, and pensions for businesses (profit and non-profit). Geographic Area Served: United States.

★ 14642 ★ Kalogredis, Sansweet, Dearden and Burke Ltd.
987 Old Eagle School Rd., Ste. 704
Wayne, PA 19087-1708
Phone: (610)687-4013 **Free:** 800-688-8314
Fax: (610)687-8402
Email: admin@KSDBHEALTHLAW.com
Website: http://www.ksdbhealthlaw.com
Fnded: 1981. **Activities:** Provides consulting for healthcare providers in the areas of employment agreements, health law matters (3rd party disputes, antitrust, HMO/PPO), joint ventures, pension profit sharing administration, practice management/mergers/acquisitions/sales or liquidations, practice valuation, and reimbursement and coding analysis. Geographic Area Served: Eastern United States.

West Chester

★ 14643 ★ National Technomics Inc.
814 Sunset Hollow Rd.
West Chester, PA 19380
Phone: (610)436-4551 **Fax:** (610)436-0255
Email: jimccrea@chesco.com
Fnded: 1983. **Activities:** Specializes in organizational development, education and training in health services industries. Industries served: hospitals, services, government agencies, and civilian employees of the U.S. Army, Navy, Marine Corps, and Veterans Administration in the United States. Geographic Area Served: United States and Canada.

★ 14644 ★ Nursing Technomics
814 Sunset Hollow Rd.
West Chester, PA 19380
Phone: (610)436-4551 **Fax:** (610)436-0255
Fnded: 1983. **Activities:** Administrative nursing consultants offer expertise in the design and implementation of customized software applications for departments of nursing, organizational design and implementation, and executive nurse search. Also specializes in department staffing, scheduling and nurse recruitment. Serves private industries as well as government agencies. Geographic Area Served: United States and Canada.

★ 14645 ★ Westwood Research Laboratory Inc.
24 S Church St.
PO Box 3126
West Chester, PA 19381-3126
Phone: (610)692-6933
Fnded: 1957. **Activities:** Offers consulting in the dental field in vitro testing and product development. Industries served: dental and medical organizations, and government agencies. Geographic Area Served: Worldwide.

Williamsport

★ 14646 ★ Providence Ventures Inc.
1100 Crampian Blvd.
Williamsport, PA 17701-1909
Phone: (570)320-7696 **Fax:** (570)321-7780
Fnded: 1986. **Activities:** Provides medical management services including shared mobile services.

Willow Grove

★ 14647 ★ MEDCO Inc.
PO Box 617
Willow Grove, PA 19090-0617
Phone: (215)659-9311 **Fax:** (215)659-9406
Email: medco@voicenet.com

Website: http://www.consultmedco.com

Fnded: 1977. **Activities:** Management consulting firm provides operations, customer service excellence, organizational change management, and physician practice management assistance services to health-care organizations. Operations services include: productivity assessment and analysis, benchmarking assessment, operational analysis, and productivity and cost accounting systems and implementation. Customer Service Excellence services include programs to assess service culture competencies and to educate, and train management and staff in delivering and maintaining a culture of service excellence. Organization transformation and change management, and management training and development programs and workshops are provided to support culture and organization development. Services also include, financial projections and practice valuations. Also provides software products to support productivity, cost accounting and facility utilization. Serves the healthcare field. Geographic Area Served: United States.

★ 14648 ★ National Medical Services Inc.
3701 Welsh Rd.
Willow Grove, PA 19090
Phone: (215)657-4900 **Free:** 800-522-6671
Fax: (215)657-2631
Website: http://www.nmslab.com

Fnded: 1970. **Activities:** Forensic-, clinical-, analytical toxicology and criminalistics. Specializes in toxic tort and occupational chemical product liability; worker's compensation and disability claims; referee drug testing; dram shop and social host liability; life insurance claims; pharmacological malpractice and therapeutic misadventure; driving under the influence of alcohol and/or drugs; forensic abuse substance testing; criminalistics; product tampering and product integrity; employee drug and alcohol testing; forensic toxicology; occupational toxicology; community and ecological toxicology; forensic hair testing for drugs and other toxicants. Geographic Area Served: United States.

Worcester

★ 14649 ★ West Point Pharmaceutical Consulting
2250 Berks Rd.
PO Box 221
Worcester, PA 19490
Phone: (215)699-1703 **Fax:** (215)699-5698

Activities: Practice is dedicated to serving customer drug development needs by providing: insight, corrective strategies and targeted training. Core services include: outsourcing support including due diligence, project transfer and management, and in-depth evaluation of contractor capabilities; analytical data evaluation; regulatory submission strategy and communication; and customized training services.

York

★ 14650 ★ Healthcare Management Associates Ltd.
209 N Beaver St.
PO Box 5047
York, PA 17403-5321
Phone: (717)854-7857 **Fax:** (717)846-2594

Fnded: 1984. **Activities:** Health services consulting firm specializes in nursing homes and retirement facilities.

★ 14651 ★ Ralph E. Duncan, MD, FACS
25 Monument Rd., Ste. 100
York, PA 17403-5060
Phone: (717)741-4785 **Fax:** (717)741-4696

Activities: Specializes in urologic surgery, uroradiology, and adult and pediatric urology. Provides expert witness testimony in urology for plaintiff and defense in medical-legal cases. Gives medical-legal reviews, peer reviews, second opinion consultations, and quality assurance consultations. Board certified fellow, American College of Surgeons. Geographic Area Served: United States.

Rhode Island

Warwick

★ 14652 ★ Medhat A. Kader, MD Inc.
300 Toll Gate Rd.
Warwick, RI 02886
Phone: (401)734-9980 **Fax:** (401)734-9987

Fnded: 1976. **Activities:** Provides consultation, medical records review, and expert testimony in orthopedics. Geographic Area Served: United States.

South Carolina

Columbia

★ 14653 ★ Sue P. Heiney
108 Greengate Dr.
Columbia, SC 29223
Phone: (803)736-6117 **Fax:** (803)865-9227
Email: heart.stories@attglobal.net

Fnded: 1983. **Activities:** Offers expertise in assessment, skill building, and evaluation of educational services related to increasing productivity through personal development. Experienced with personnel in healthcare. Geographic Area Served: United States.

★ 14654 ★ Terrance L. Baker
226 Lame Horse Rd.
Columbia, SC 29223
Phone: (803)736-7422
Email: terrancelbakermd@prodigy.net

Fnded: 1992. **Activities:** Case review, narrative reports, consultations, testimony for both plaintiff and defense. Board Certified in emergency medicine, family practice geriatrics and forensic medicine.

Greenville

★ 14655 ★ ClaimsWare Inc.
PO Box 6125
Greenville, SC 29606-6125
Phone: (803)234-8200 **Free:** 800-992-8088
Fax: (803)234-8202
Email: wbuser@claimsware.com
Website: http://www.claimsware.com

Fnded: 1986. **Activities:** Offers health services administration, specializing in benefit administration systems, including medical, dental, disability, and flexible spending accounts. Geographic Area Served: United States.

★ 14656 ★ HealthCare Concepts Inc.
531 S Main St.
Greenville, SC 29601
Phone: (864)370-4770 **Fax:** (864)458-9422
Email: hccinc@ix.netcom.com
Website: http://www.hccinc.com

Fnded: 1977. **Activities:** A healthcare consulting firm dedicated to rendering professional services in the areas of strategic planning, marketing plan development and implementation, facility planning, systems development and implementation, and management assistance in areas of strategic and operational plans for hospitals and related healthcare centers. **Remarks:** Special expertise in women's and children's planning. Geographic Area Served: United States.

Hilton Head Island

★ 14657 ★ Tempo Personnel Services
PO Box 22448
Hilton Head Island, SC 29926
Phone: (843)681-9066 **Fax:** (843)689-6477

Fnded: 1985. **Activities:** Full service employment agency that includes local temporary and permanent placements, medical home health provider and regional and national hospitality placement. Industries served: locally: administrative and clerical, home health; regionally: food and beverage and hospitality. Geographic Area Served: Hilton Head Island and Beaufort County on the local level; Georgia, Florida, South Carolina and North Carolina on a regional level.

Johns Island

★ 14658 ★ David W. Seignious
4208 Chisolm Rd.
Johns Island, SC 29455
Phone: (843)559-3500
Email: DTSeig@worldnet.att.net
Website: http://member.expertpages.com/dseignious/

Activities: A practicing internal medicine/geriatrician available for consulting assignments in areas of geriatric medicine, nursing home and hospital standards of care, and personal and occupational injury.

Lexington

★ 14659 ★ Source Atlantic Inc.
4766 Sunset Blvd., Ste. 1
Lexington, SC 29072-9252
Phone: (803)957-4646 **Fax:** (803)957-3607
Email: w.mcgowan@sourceatlantic.com
Website: http://www.sourceatlantic.com

Fnded: 1978. **Activities:** Specializes in medical equipment planning and management for healthcare facilities. The scope of services includes space design guidance, budget development, long-range equipment replacement plans, inventory evaluation, and procurement assistance. The firm assists administrators, physicians, technologists and equipment users to establish need, analyze alternatives, and recommend practical, cost effective solutions. Industries served: medical facilities and government agencies in the U.S.

Manning

★ 14660 ★ National Board of Forensic Chiropractors
601 S Mill St.
PO Box 356
Manning, SC 29102
Phone: (803)435-5078 **Free:** 800-692-2256
Fax: (803)435-8096
Email: omyback@gte.net

Fnded: 1996. **Activities:** Administers exams and designates qualifying chiropractic physicians as having the credential of Certified Independent Forensic Chiropractic Medical Examiner™, or CIFCME™. After receiveing this credentail, a doctor is qualified to assist insurance companies, workers' compensation commissions, social security boards, employres, police departments, and attorneys by providing independnet assessments of challenging bodily injury cases. The purpose of the NBOFC is to advance the profession of forensic examination and consultation throughout the chiropractic profession by elevating standards through education, and advanced training, and certification. The Board serves as a national center for this purpose and disseminates information and knowledge by coordinating lectures, seminars, conferences, workshops, Internet, continuing education courses and publications. Geographic Area Served: United States, Canada, Australia, and Europe.

Saint Helena

★ 14661 ★ Concerns, Counseling & Consultation Firm
A106 Cedar Reef VLG
Saint Helena, SC 29920
Email: conc@penn.com

Fnded: 1980. **Activities:** Consultants on a variety of social issues and concerns for both individuals and businesses. Topics covered include: Employee Assistance Programs (E.A.P.), interpersonal communication, stress management, assertiveness training, addictions training for clinical settings, family violence counselor training, life change management, and emergency personnel training in handling victims of rape and violence, i.e., police, EMTs, emergency room personnel. Also advises on the establishment of DUI (Driving Under the Influence) education and intervention programs. Active with manufacturing firms, police departments, and hospitals. Serves private industries as well as government agencies. Geographic Area Served: Northeastern United States.

Spartanburg

★ 14662 ★ Pharmacy Consultants Inc.
348 E Blackstock Rd., Ste. A
Spartanburg, SC 29301-3741
Phone: (864)574-5220 **Fax:** 800-842-2238

Fnded: 1976. **Activities:** Medication consultation services to long-term care facilities, nursing homes, residential-care facilities, group homes for the mentally retarded, prison systems, and trauma recovery centers.

Tennessee

Brentwood

★ 14663 ★ Brim HealthCare Inc.
105 Westwood Pl., Ste. 300
Brentwood, TN 37027
Phone: (615)309-6053 **Fax:** (615)370-2859
Website: http://www.brimhealthcare.com

Fnded: 1971. **Activities:** A diversified healthcare services company offering management and consulting services to the healthcare industry including direct management services, healthcare planning and full development. Services include full-service management, interim administrative management, fiscal services management, accounts receivable recovery, operational assessment, strategic planning, and quality assurance. Geographic Area Served: United States.

Chattanooga

★ 14664 ★ C.J. Enterprises Inc.
7010 Lee Hwy., Ste. 214
Chattanooga, TN 37421
Phone: (423)899-1770 **Fax:** (423)894-4484
Email: info@cjeonline.com
Website: http://www.cjeonline.com

Fnded: 1980. **Activities:** Consulting firm which specializes in developing record and information management systems. Industries served: commercial business, healthcare industry and government agencies. Geographic Area Served: United States.

Clarksville

★ 14665 ★ Occupational and Environmental Health Consultants Inc.
1498 Madison St., Ste. 1
Clarksville, TN 37040
Phone: (931)552-4655 **Free:** 888-287-4655
Fax: (931)552-7596
Email: sales@healthconsultantsusa.com
Website: http://www.healthconsultantsUSA.com

Fnded: 1986. **Activities:** Specialists in occupational safety, health and environmental. Industries served: manufacturing. Geographic Area Served: United States.

Cookeville

★ 14666 ★ Birman & Associates Inc.
502 Gould Dr.
Cookeville, TN 38506
Phone: (931)432-6314 **Fax:** (931)432-6536

Activities: Consulting firm offers expertise in the healthcare field.

Knoxville

★ 14667 ★ Doctors Management
10401 Kingston Pke.
Knoxville, TN 37922
Phone: (865)531-0176 **Free:** 800-635-4040
Fax: (865)531-0722
Email: info@doctors-management.com
Website: http://www.doctors-management.com

Fnded: 1956. **Activities:** Have served clients in 46 states since 1956. Full management services with specialty departments including human resources, coding, reimbursement, OSHA, CLIA, customer care, accounting, and marketing. Geographic Area Served: United States.

★ 14668 ★ Health Advancement Inc.
PO Box 53444
Knoxville, TN 37902
Phone: (865)691-4689 **Fax:** (865)602-2594

Fnded: 1990. **Activities:** Health care consultants offer computerized health risk appraisals, health education workshops, corporate health fairs, health education consultation, and flu vaccinations. Serves private industries as well as government agencies. Geographic Area Served: East Tennessee Region.

★ 14669 ★ Southeastern Accreditation Consultants
Knoxville, TN
Email: consultvol@aol.com

Activities: Assists healthcare organizations in preparing for J.C.A.H.O accreditation, Experienced in current survey process and have a wide variety of clinical and administrative experiences.

Madison

★ 14670 ★ Advanced Receivables Services Inc.
101 Cumberland Ave., Ste. 1000
Madison, TN 37115
Phone: (615)860-9999 **Fax:** (615)860-8911

Fnded: 1981. **Activities:** Specializes in accounts receivable management and collection assistance. Experienced in working with hospitals, physicians and retail credit. Services include short assessments of key receivable areas through complete management of business offices.

Memphis

★ 14671 ★ Eurofins Scientific Inc.
1331 Union Ave., Ste. 1500
Memphis, TN 38104
Phone: (901)272-7511 **Free:** 800-880-1038
Fax: (901)272-2926
Email: eurofinsus@eurofins.com
Website: http://www.eurofins.com

Fnded: 1933. **Activities:** Designs and develops tests for evaluating efficacy and safety of products and provides guidance for claims substantiation. Also advises on subjects related to analytical chemistry, microbiology, quality control, toxicology, nutrition, and product labeling. Geographic Area Served: United States, Canada, Mexico, Europe, and Japan.

★ 14672 ★ Harber & Associates, Performance Consulting Inc.
4646 Poplar Ave., Ste. 425
Memphis, TN 38117-4434
Phone: (901)761-9953 **Fax:** (901)761-9951
Email: harberinc@aol.com

Fnded: 1979. **Activities:** Organization development, executive coaching, leadership training, stress management, communication, conflict management, and time management. Industries served:service industries, such as architects, lawyers, property managers, medical practices and small manufacturing companies. Geographic Area Served: Tennessee, Arkansas, and Mississippi, Mid-America and the Southeastern United States.

★ 14673 ★ Healthcare Concepts Inc.
266 S Front St.
Memphis, TN 38103-3213
Phone: (901)527-7701 **Free:** 800-442-4346
Fax: (901)529-9101
Email: hcc@wspice.com
Website: http://www.healthcareconcepts.com

Fnded: 1980. **Activities:** Provides compliance assessments, compliance programming and monitoring, accreditation preparation and mock surveys, program development, temporary and permanent executive placement, operational assessments and training for home health and related organizations. Geographic Area Served: Worldwide.

★ 14674 ★ Insurance Consulting Group Inc.
5865 Ridgeway Center Pky., Ste. 105
Memphis, TN 38120-4006
Phone: (901)795-8444 **Fax:** (901)795-8555
Email: info@employeebenefits.com
Website: http://www.employeebenefits.com

Fnded: 1979. **Activities:** An employee benefits firm that offers assistance in the design, implementation, and administration of employee benefit programs. Services include health insurance strategic plan and design, provider network evaluation and selection, and utilization and cost comparisons. Geographic Area Served: TN, AR, MS employers.

Nashville

★ 14675 ★ Campus Health Services
2021 21st Ave. S, Ste. B-105
Nashville, TN 37212
Phone: (615)383-4830 **Fax:** (615)383-0475
Website: http://www.campushs.org

Fnded: 1997. **Activities:** Third-party billing and insurance reimbursement; physician contracting and credentialing; accreditation, facility design, and financing; and issues related to student health services, such as immunization projects. **Remarks:** Billing system.

★ 14676 ★ Diversified Health Management Inc.
4015 Travis Dr.
Nashville, TN 37211
Phone: (615)781-0666 **Fax:** (615)781-0138

Activities: Health Care - Home Health Medicare & Private Duty & Staffing. Geographic Area Served: Middle & West TN.

★ 14677 ★ K & S Associates Inc.
1926 Elm Tree Dr.
Nashville, TN 37210-3718
Phone: (615)883-9760 **Free:** 800-522-2325
Fax: (615)871-0856
Email: ksinfo@kslab.com
Website: http://www.kslab.com

Fnded: 1974. **Activities:** A privately owned precision calibration laboratory offering a full range of specialized radiation measurement calibrations for medical, nuclear, and industrial applications. K & S also provides medical and health physics consulting services including radiation shielding design, on-site physics services, and specialized analysis services. Geographic Area Served: United States.

★ 14678 ★ MDL Information Services Inc., OHS Authorizing, Reference and Hazard Communication
1281 Murfreesboro Rd., Ste. 300
Nashville, TN 37217
Phone: (615)366-2000 **Free:** 800-738-4765
Fax: (615)360-9538
Email: ohs@mdl.com
Website: http://www.mdli.com/ohs

Fnded: 1978. **Activities:** Product MSDS Authoring, Hazards Communication, and Custom Data services for environmental health and safety. Industries served: chemical, pharmaceutical, utilities, petroleum, metals, food, paper, government and public service agencies, and academic institutions. Geographic Area Served: Worldwide.

★ 14679 ★ National Safety Alliance Corp.
1421 Elm Hill Pk.
PO Box 159060
Nashville, TN 37210
Phone: (615)777-3681 **Fax:** (615)832-0054

Fnded: 1988. **Activities:** Offers health services counsel, specializing in substance abuse programs, administration, testing, research, legal support, and education. Industries served: U.S. businesses.

★ 14680 ★ THA Consulting Solutions
500 Interstate Blvd. S
Nashville, TN 37210-4634
Phone: (615)256-8240 **Free:** 800-258-9541
Fax: (615)248-4836
Email: webmaster@tha.com
Website: http://www.tha.com

Activities: Specializes in strategic planning, operations analysis, re-engineering, management engineering, and managed care. **Remarks:** Subsidiary of the Tennessee Hospital Association specializing in Health Care Consulting. Geographic Area Served: Tennessee.

Springfield

★ 14681 ★ Health Resources Unlimited
449 Ott Wilson Rd.
Springfield, TN 37172
Phone: (615)384-7760 **Free:** 888-654-3363
Fax: (615)384-2868
Email: educate@hru.net

Activities: Provides education, consulting, seminars and coaching services for health care providers and organizations.

Texas

Austin

★ 14682 ★ Audit Express Inc.
3724 Executive Center Dr., Ste. 101
Austin, TX 78731
Phone: (512)338-9196 **Fax:** (512)338-4972

Fnded: 1991. **Activities:** Offers business related health services, providing auditing expertise for workmen's compensation claims for Texas workers. Also offers cost containment services. Industries served: businesses and municipal governments in Texas.

★ 14683 ★ Delphi Groupe Inc.
2211 S IH-35, Ste. 400
Austin, TX 78741-3802
Phone: (512)462-1181 **Fax:** (512)462-1187
Email: info@delphigroupe.com
Website: http://www.delphigroupe.com

Fnded: 1988. **Activities:** Management consulting, project management, software application design and support, engineering design, environmental engineering, health and safety, health physics, regulatory compliance, licensing, and operational readiness, facility management and emergency preparedness. Geographic Area Served: United States and limited International support.

★ 14684 ★ Dydek Environmental Consulting
11506 Knipp Cove
Austin, TX 78739
Phone: (512)280-5477 **Fax:** (512)280-8900
Email: dydek@tox-expert.com
Website: http://www.tox-expert.com

Fnded: 1994. **Activities:** Environmental toxicologist and engineer specializing in toxicological/human health risk analyses for community/occupational exposures to metals, solvents, pesticides, and other chemicals; Superfund risk assessments; and air quality. Provides expert witness litigation support and trainings in toxicology and risk assessment. **Remarks:** Board Certified Environmental Toxicologist, Licensed Professional Engineer. Geographic Area Served: United States.

★ 14685 ★ PageSoutherlandPage
606 West Ave.
Austin, TX 78701-2725
Phone: (512)472-6721 **Fax:** (512)477-3211
Email: aus@psp.com
Website: http://www.psp.com

Fnded: 1898. **Activities:** Provides architectural, engineering, and interior design services for advanced technology, corporate R&D, health care, interior architecture, education, and public facilities worldwide. Specializes in masterplanning and designing hospitals, clinics, medical office buildings, convention centers, high-tech/industrial manufacturing facilities, and airport passenger terminals. Also offers facilities management, space planning, and interior design. Geographic Area Served: Worldwide.

★ 14686 ★ Trans-Century
8140 N Mopac Expy.
Westpark III, Ste. 200
Austin, TX 78759
Phone: (512)345-0280 **Fax:** (512)345-6231
Email: Mary@Trans-Century.com
Website: http://www.Trans-Century.com

Fnded: 1982. **Activities:** Firm specializes in managed care market analysis, development, management and operational assessment of PHOs and IPAs, provider contracting, NCQA and URAC credentialing and Utilization Management programs. Services include provider reimbursement analysis, contract negotiations, management, Medicare and Medicaid program development, Clinical Practice guideline development, CPT Cost Analysis for physicians, managed care educational program seminars, and human resource assistance to hospitals and physicians. Geographic Area Served: United States.

Bedford

★ 14687 ★ expertwitness.com Inc.
1902 Central Dr.
Bedford, TX 76021
Phone: (817)509-1919 **Fax:** (817)509-1999
Email: management@expertwitness.com
Website: http://www.expertwitness.com

Activities: Provides forensic, biomechanical, and medical analysis of causation and prevention of accidental injury, including vehicular, industrial, sport, construction and other accident environments. Evaluates protective devices and safety systems, including seat belts and helmets. Evaluates work place hazards. Offers computer reconstruction and animation.

Corpus Christi

★ 14688 ★ Pathways To Wellness
13845 Flintlock Dr.
Corpus Christi, TX 78418
Phone: (361)949-4790 **Fax:** (361)949-4627
Email: path2wellness@earthlink.net
Website: http://www.path2wellness.com

Fnded: 1988. **Activities:** Offer natural holistic health counseling, yoga classes and teachers training programs for individuals and companies. R.Y.T.500 and R.Y.Training Center through the Yoga Alliance. Hatha Yoga style is traditional and includes all aspects of yoga from jnana, bhakti, karma, and hatha for all levels of student. Health counseling includes nutritional guidance, kinesiology, iridology, reflexology, energy healing, massage therapy and reflexology, herbal and supplemental direction, creative visualization and meditation. Teachers training program will qualify students for registry with the Yoga Alliance. Geographic Area Served: Worldwide.

Dallas

★ 14689 ★ ACS Healthcare Solutions
2828 N Haskell Ave.
Bldg 5, Fl. 6
Dallas, TX 75204
Free: 800-845-5530 **Fax:** (214)584-5084
Email: healthcaresolutions@acs-inc.com
Website: http://www.acs-inc.com/healthcare/

Activities: A provider of management information systems to major healthcare providers. Offers services in the areas of business process solutions, technology solutions, systems integration and professional services, and elecronic commerce.

★ 14690 ★ Arthur L. Rice and Associates
5612 Ursula Ln.
Dallas, TX 75229-6428
Phone: (214)369-3739 **Fax:** (214)691-3212

Fnded: 1965. **Activities:** Business management consultants specializing in the healthcare field. Emphasis is on development of new companies. Involved in limited partnership design and organization, debt and equity financing for emerging firms, and tax shelters.

★ 14691 ★ Aspartame Consumer Safety Network
PO Box 780634
Dallas, TX 75378
Phone: (214)352-4268 **Free:** 800-969-6050
Fax: (214)352-2480
Website: http://web2.airmail.net/marystod

Fnded: 1987. **Activities:** Maintains a network of consultants with expertise regarding the safety of aspartame. Provides in-house consulting services and speeches and will conduct seminars and workshops. Also offers referrals of expert witnesses for trial lawyers. Industries served: Fortune 500 companies and others. **Remarks:** Collecting adverse reaction reports from health care professionals and consumers. Invaluable resource for Media. (Broadcase and Print) Routinely provides support and background information for assignments editors, producers and writers. Will write articles for publication, if asked. Founder, Mary Nash Stoddard has been interviewed thousands of times by media all over the world. Geographic Area Served: Worldwide.

★ 14692 ★ Earnhart & Associates Inc.
5905 TreeShadow Pl., Ste. 1200
Dallas, TX 75252-5101
Phone: (972)713-6626 **Free:** 800-720-5742
Fax: (972)713-6611
Email: corporate@earnhart.com
Website: http://www.earnhart.com

Fnded: 1985. **Activities:** A healthcare consulting firm specializing in the development and management of ambulatory surgery centers. Core business is putting hospitals and physicians into a joint venture partnership in a for-profit, freestanding ambulatory surgery center. Services include evaluating the feasibility of developing an ambulatory surgery center for hospitals or physicians via a comprehensive feasibility study; providing turnkey ASC development services of the operating entity for hospitals or private physician groups or in a joint venture; managing new or existing ASCs owned either by a hospital, a private physician group, corporate entity, or combination.

★ 14693 ★ Jirousek and Jirousek Inc., Healthcare Facilities Consultants
4207 Shady Bend Dr.
Dallas, TX 75244-7346
Phone: (972)484-8448 **Fax:** (972)484-1445

Activities: Specialists in the design of healthcare facilities with experience in space evaluation and planning, equipment listing and inventory, and project management.

★ 14694 ★ Landauer Realty Group Inc.
14785 Preston Rd.
1000 Signature Place II
Dallas, TX 75240
Phone: (972)450-3267
Email: lauri.conway@grubb-ellis.com
Website: http://www.landauer.com

Fnded: 1946. **Activities:** Appraises commercial real estate with a specialty in complex or portfolio transactions. Provides analytical and technical assistance to the legal profession. Financial services group provides debt and equity financing. Geographic Area Served: United States, Canada, Mexico, Europe, and Australia.

★ 14695 ★ Lige B. Rushing, Jr.
8210 Walnut Hill Ln., Ste. 120
Dallas, TX 75231
Phone: (214)368-3611 **Fax:** (214)696-3695

Activities: Board-certified in rheumatology, geriatrics, internal medicine, and as an independent medical examiner. Experienced in nursing homes, disability, & personal injury. Over 20 years full-time private practice, reviews, reports, and testimony.

★ 14696 ★ Medical Cities Inc.
7777 Forest Ln., Ste. C840
Dallas, TX 75230-2505
Phone: (972)566-8800 **Free:** 800-633-7305
Fax: (972)566-8882
Email: scottsmith@medicalcity.com

Fnded: 1972. **Activities:** Offers medical facilities planning and real estate development. Industries served: healthcare regionally. Geographic Area Served: Worldwide with heavy emphasis on the United States.

Denison

★ 14697 ★ Lone Star Orthopaedics
2805 Pyramid Cir.
Denison, TX 75020
Phone: (903)465-5714 **Free:** 800-632-5159
Fax: (903)465-4185
Email: info@zakin.com
Website: http://www.zakin.com/legal.html

Activities: Willing to consult, do research and testify as an expert witness on a full range of medical and surgical issues, emphasizing extremity disease and injury.

Flower Mound

★ 14698 ★ Shotwell & Carr Inc.
3535 Fire Wheel Dr., Ste. A
Flower Mound, TX 75028
Phone: (972)355-9700 **Free:** 888-326-3311
Fax: (972)355-9984
Email: pwcarr@shotcarr.com
Website: http://www.shotcarr.com

Fnded: 1974. **Activities:** Specializes in maximizing cost effectiveness in development, approval, production, and distribution of animal and human drugs, medical devices, and in vitro diagnostics worldwide.

Fort Worth

★ 14699 ★ EA Plus Inc.
PO Box 101805
Fort Worth, TX 76185
Phone: (817)989-7400 **Free:** 800-297-1872
Fax: (817)853-5800
Email: ea2000@usa.net
Website: http://www.eaplus.com

Fnded: 1984. **Activities:** Career consultants providing contingent contract and retained searel. Additional services includes providing employee assistance and employment services, and confidential assistance to troubled employees. Supports managers in the resolution of job performance problems. Conducts reemployment workshops, for displaced workers. Offers inplacement and outplacement services for executive officers. Implements change management and survivor training programs for managers. Assists senior management find the "best" candidates for the organization. Addresses employee problems that pose a threat to employee health and corporate profits, including: alcohol and drug abuse, stress, anxiety, and depression, financial and legal concerns, emotional issues, family difficulties, and job loss and employment related crises. Primary activities: executive search and career transition services. **Remarks:** Caters to the hitech financial services, healthcare, aerospace and electronics industries. Geographic Area Served: United States.

★ 14700 ★ First Fitness Equipment International
4750 Bryant Irvin Rd., Ste. 808-229
Fort Worth, TX 76132
Phone: (817)569-9700 **Free:** 800-922-3488
Fax: (817)569-9705
Email: sales@firstfitnessequipment.com
Website: http://www.firstfitnessequipment.com

Fnded: 1983. **Activities:** Serving the fitness industry. Firm aids health/exercise club owners (nonprofit organizations, corporations, hospitals, government agencies, and schools) in saving time and money through involvement with facility design, exercise equipment purchase and layout, membership marketing, and club management. **Remarks:** Fitness facilities owner 1976-1982, Consultant since 1982. Geographic Area Served: Worldwide.

Houston

★ 14701 ★ Applied Logic Associates Inc.
5615 Kirby Dr., Ste. 710
Houston, TX 77005-2495
Phone: (713)529-4747 **Fax:** (713)529-4924
Website: http://www.alogic.com/

Fnded: 1987. **Activities:** Consulting firm for pharmaceutical, medical device, and biotechnology companies in the areas of clinical/regulatory affairs, clinical study management, information management, and biostatistical analysis and health care economics. Provides services from the conceptual stage to product approval. Provides assistance in clinical data management, statistical analysis, and regulatory affairs.

★ 14702 ★ Appraisal & Mentor Group L.L.C.
PO Box 820889
Houston, TX 77282-0889
Phone: (281)496-7777 **Fax:** (281)496-9574
Website: http://internetappraisal.net

Fnded: 2000. **Activities:** Advises physicians on professional practice management in the United States. Also mentors, advises start-ups on funding. Geographic Area Served: United States.

★ 14703 ★ Biomedical Engineering Consultants
1111 Hermann Dr., Ste. 12B
Houston, TX 77004
Phone: (713)522-6666 **Fax:** (713)522-6686
Email: ydavid@texaschildrenshospital.org
Website: http://www.biomedeng.com

Fnded: 1982. **Activities:** Tests, evaluates, services, and repairs of medical devices and accessories. Devices range from infusion pumps to anesthesia machines and from lasers to telemedicine. Directs large biomedical engineering program within hospital and home-care environments. Failure analysis and regulatory compliance, and EMI testing. **Remarks:** Member of FDA advisory panel and standards writing committees. Geographic Area Served: Worldwide.

★ 14704 ★ Debra F. Latimer Nutrition Associates
2626 S Loop W, Ste. 306
Houston, TX 77054
Phone: (713)795-0876 **Fax:** (713)432-7989
Email: dfldiet@earthlink.net

Fnded: 1981. **Activities:** Provides medical nutrition therapy on individual and group bases. Plans and conducts corporate wellness programs. Consultant to service and food manufacturing industries, as well as government agencies. Specializes in diabetes and renal education and management, weight management, and compulsive eating disorders. Geographic Area Served: Greater Houston.

★ 14705 ★ Frank D. Stevens, PhD
12714 La Belle Ln.
Houston, TX 77015
Phone: (713)455-2288 **Fax:** (713)455-2288

Activities: Specializes in toxic chemical exposure, testimony, consultation, and investigations, as well as industrial hygiene, occupational health, and epidemiology air quality.

★ 14706 ★ Gastroenterology Associates of Memorial City
Memorial City Professional Bldg.
10565 Katy Fwy., Ste. 305
Houston, TX 77024
Phone: (713)932-8651 **Fax:** (713)465-1940
Email: klein@insync.net
Website: http://www.driraklein.com

Fnded: 1978. **Activities:** Offers consulting services regarding medical malpractice in gastroenterology and internal medicine.

★ 14707 ★ Goddard Management Resources
333 N Sam Houston Pky. E, Ste. 400
Houston, TX 77060
Phone: (281)359-4996 **Fax:** (281)359-3341

Fnded: 1983. **Activities:** Specializes in financial planning, staffing/budgeting, organization and leadership development. Provides systems for healthcare organizations and professionals. Geographic Area Served: North America and Europe.

★ 14708 ★ Healthcare Management Consulting Services
5723 Benning St.
Houston, TX 77096
Phone: (713)723-0297 **Fax:** (713)723-0297
Email: hmcmarn@flash.net
Website: http://www.prosavvy.com/affiliates/healthcaremgtconsulting

Fnded: 1991. **Activities:** Offers healthcare consulting services in such areas as: pharmaceutical market research and market analysis, utilization and case management integration, quality management, wellness program/3-health, Disease Management program assessment/development, clinical risk management and patient safety consulting. Geographic Area Served: United States.

★ 14709 ★ Huiras & Associates International Training
13815 Ella Lee Ln., Ste. 100
Houston, TX 77077
Phone: (281)496-9044 **Fax:** (281)496-3671
Email: dhuiras@huirasassoc.com
Website: http://www.huirasassoc.com

Fnded: 1981. **Activities:** Executive, business, and team coaching. Accredited in Insights Learning & Development an International Psychometric Assessment tool for personal, business, sales, management, team effectiveness and learning styles. **Remarks:** International speaker for conferences and conventions. Topics: Interpersonal Communication Styles; How Men and Women Communicate; Putting Humor in the Workplace. Geographic Area Served: Worldwide.

★ 14710 ★ K & T Safety Service Inc.
800 Wilcrest Dr., No. 205
Houston, TX 77042-6301
Phone: (713)974-4394 **Fax:** (713)974-4396
Email: ktsafetyhkana@email.msn.com

Fnded: 1981. **Activities:** Safety and environmental consultants active in the following areas: asbestos inspection and management services, environmental Phase I and II site assessments, expert testimony, and indoor air quality surveys. Involved in development of safety manuals and programs, construction safety services, safety audits, and reviews. Clients are schools, hospitals, universities, and private industry. Geographic Area Served: Texas, New Mexico, and Colorado.

★ 14711 ★ Langley, Johnson & Associates P.C.
100 Glenborough Dr., Ste. 930
Houston, TX 77067
Phone: (281)873-5320 **Fax:** (281)873-5216

Fnded: 1980. **Activities:** Medical management consulting firm.

★ 14712 ★ Lehrer Financial and Economic Advisory Services
5555 Del Monte Dr., Ste. 802
Houston, TX 77056
Phone: (713)972-7912 **Free:** (866)275-4958
Fax: (713)964-0444
Email: drken@lehecoserv.com
Website: http://www.lehecoserv.com

Fnded: 1982. **Activities:** All aspects of economic consulting with emphasis on economics in the real estate, banking and medical industries. Assignments include real estate finance, economic damages, non-public business valuations, institutional loan presentations, market and feasibility analysis, fairness opinions, investment and portfolio analysis, business plans in corporate finance, and expert witness for court testimony. Primary emphasis is to act as a "full service" economic consulting group, capable of fulfilling the complete economic/financial needs of corporations, banks, attorneys, insurance companies, pension funds, medical groups and other investment organizations. **Remarks:** Since the company accepts engagements nationwide, we have adopted a policy of NOT charging for travel time. Geographic Area Served: United States and the Marshall Islands.

★ 14713 ★ Linda McDonald Associates Inc.
11102 Lakeside Forest Ln.
Houston, TX 77042-1032
Phone: (713)978-6960 **Free:** 888-577-2889
Fax: (713)978-7044
Email: linda@supermarketsavvy.com
Website: http://www.supermarketsavvy.com

Fnded: 1984. **Activities:** Specializes in providing nutrition support for the food industry -processors, producers and food service. Solutions start with the dedevelopment or reformulation of products, continue through the labeling process, and provide expertise to position products in the health conscious marketplace. Expertise in the health and medical fields can help position products for the best results. Also experienced in media and material development for the consumer and health professional. Mrs. McDonald is also available as a speaker on related nutrition topics. Geographic Area Served: Worldwide.

★ 14714 ★ Locke Bryan Productions Inc.
800 Bering Dr., Ste. 101
Houston, TX 77057-2130
Phone: (713)977-5989 **Free:** 800-624-6778
Fax: (713)977-0419
Email: camille@lbp1.com
Website: http://www.lbp1.com

Fnded: 1986. **Activities:** Communications firm provides video training films and tapes targeted at supervisors and covering a wide range of human resource topics. Topics include drug abuse prevention, conflict management, labor relations, safety and security training, and wellness. Production staff provides "off-the-shelf" video tapes as well as custom products designed and filmed for individual organizations. Also provide free catalogs upon request. Serves private industries as well as government agencies. Geographic Area Served: United States.

★ 14715 ★ Med-Expertise L.L.C.
7000 Regency Sq., Ste. 225
Houston, TX 77036
Phone: (713)914-0112 **Fax:** (713)914-0162
Email: wjcouch@med-expertise.com
Website: http://www.med-expertise.com/

Activities: Medical Expert Witness referral service, screens physicians and nurses for attorneys, government agencies, insurance-case merit review, medical-legal strategy. Daubert Standard Testimony. Firm saves time and reduces costs for clients by screening medical malpractice, personal injury and workers' compensation cases for merit to save time wasted on frivolous and marginal lawsuits; analyzing issues pertinent to damages and liability; organizing and analyzing medical records-vital steps in verifying case allegations; defining applicable standards of care and pinpointing any deviations from these standards; locating and interviewing prospective expert witnesses whose authoritative testimony will meet Daubert standards.

★ 14716 ★ MSCH
2600 N Loop W, Ste. 250
Houston, TX 77092
Phone: (713)683-2900 **Fax:** (713)683-2929

Fnded: 1984. **Activities:** Health care-related consulting firm.

★ 14717 ★ N.J. Vaughan & Associates Inc.
11501 Chimney Rock Rd.
Houston, TX 77035
Phone: (713)729-5310

Fnded: 1977. **Activities:** Offers consulting services in health administration.

★ 14718 ★ Peggy Morrow & Associates
15810 Brook Forest Dr.
Houston, TX 77059
Phone: (281)280-8190 **Free:** 800-375-1982
Fax: (281)286-9477
Email: info@peggymorrow.com
Website: http://www.peggymorrow.com/

Fnded: 1982. **Activities:** Presentation consultant offers expertise and customized in-house programs on customer service, time management, interpersonal and communication skills, stress management, conflict management, and professionalism. Geographic Area Served: Worldwide.

★ 14719 ★ Safety Short Production Inc.
650 Gemini St.
Houston, TX 77058
Phone: (281)956-1028

Activities: Firm offers video and computer-based training programs designed to reduce accident rates, meet with OSHA training regulations, and reduce liability exposures through employee and management training. **Remarks:** Call for free video and catalog.

★ 14720 ★ Social Health Inc.
5610 Warm Springs Rd.
Houston, TX 77035
Phone: (713)729-8869 **Fax:** (713)729-7618

Fnded: 1969. **Activities:** Nonprofit agency which offers consulting services and materials to organizations and individuals concerning the establishing of public health and social welfare programs. These programs enable groups and individuals to achieve and sustain wellness in the personal, family, work, spiritual, recreational and/or other areas of their life. Focus is prevention of social behaviors that affect health and interventions to prevent disease. Works with large population groups.

Irving

★ 14721 ★ Merritt Hawkins & Associates
5001 Statesman Dr.
Irving, TX 75063
Phone: (469)524-1400 **Free:** 800-876-0500
Fax: (469)524-1421
Email: info@mhagroup.com
Website: http://www.merritthawkins.com

Fnded: 1988. **Activities:** Physician recruitment firm. Industries served: healthcare. Geographic Area Served: United States.

★ 14722 ★ Trigon Health Ventures Inc.
5215 N O'Connor Blvd., Ste. 970
Irving, TX 75039-3707
Phone: (214)869-6565 **Fax:** (214)869-6530

Fnded: 1987. **Activities:** Offers healthcare services emphasizing provider-based managed care programs, including turnkey development and ongoing management. Industries served: physicians and hospitals worldwide.

Lago Vista

★ 14723 ★ Caring Options Residential Experts
2306 American Dr.
Lago Vista, TX 78645
Phone: (512)267-3439 **Fax:** (512)267-2193
Email: chucklesn@aol.com

Activities: Counsels in long-term care, Medicare, and Medicaid. Serves Geriatric in Texas.

League City

★ 14724 ★ Medical Liability Consultants
2015 Enterprise Ave.
League City, TX 77573
Phone: (281)334-5166 **Fax:** (281)334-7712
Email: advice@malpractice.us.com
Website: http://mlc.getwebnet.com

Activities: Provides evaluations, fee assessments, and expert testimony in medical negligence and personal injury claims. **Remarks:** Now entering our 3rd decade of specialized service. Geographic Area Served: United States.

Lubbock

★ 14725 ★ The MED Group
3223 S 289 Loop, Ste. 600
Lubbock, TX 79423
Phone: (806)793-8421 **Free:** 800-825-5633
Fax: (806)793-6480
Website: http://www.medgroup.com

Fnded: 1968. **Activities:** The MED Group offers a wide range of consulting services. MED consultants assist HME providers with accreditation, reimbursement, activity based costing, resource management, and inventory control to name a few. **Remarks:** The MED Group is more than a group purchasing organization. MED is a "difference maker." With a diverse selection of consulting services and education/trining services, The MED Group is truly posed to partner with providers to enhance their success. Geographic Area Served: The MED Group is a 600 location home care provider network serving all fifty states and Puerto Rico.

New Braunfels

★ 14726 ★ Institute for Management Success Inc.
800 W San Antonio St., Ste. B
New Braunfels, TX 78130
Phone: (830)608-0033 **Fax:** (830)608-0036
Activities: Provides management consulting and training, pre-employment testing, interviewing, and screening, and career counseling. Offers team building seminars in problem solving, goal setting, and stress, conflict, and time management. Offers resume writing and supervisory training.

Plano

★ 14727 ★ Center for Lifestyle Enhancement - Columbia Medical Center of Plano
3900 American Dr., Ste. 202
Plano, TX 75075-6135
Phone: (972)519-1207 **Fax:** (972)519-1299
Email: mcp.cle@hcahealthcare.com
Website: http://www.medicalcenterofplano.com
Fnded: 1982. **Activities:** Provides professional health counseling in the areas of general nutrition for weight management, eating disorders, diabetic education, cholesterol reduction, and adolescent weight management. Offers work site health promotion and preventive services. Also coordinates speaker's bureau, cooking classes, and physician referrals. Industries served: education, insurance, healthcare, retail/wholesale, data processing, and manufacturing in Dallas, Ft. Worth, and Collin County, Texas.

★ 14728 ★ Health Equipment Logistics & Planning Inc.
850 Central Pky. E, Ste. 260
Plano, TX 75074
Phone: (972)985-1313 **Fax:** (972)423-2398
Email: slowe@helpintl.com
Website: http://www.helpintl.com
Fnded: 1983. **Activities:** Medical equipment consultants and planners. Industries served: healthcare. Geographic Area Served: North America, Central America and Mexico.

San Antonio

★ 14729 ★ Ear Medical Group
4410 Medical Dr., Ste. 550
San Antonio, TX 78229
Phone: (210)614-6070 **Fax:** (210)615-6814
Email: eardoc@swbell.net
Website: http://www.earmedicalgroup.com
Activities: Provides evaluation and treatment of hearing and balance disorders.

★ 14730 ★ Eytek Consulting Co.
210 Bluff Knoll, Ste. 1
San Antonio, TX 78216-1915
Phone: (210)496-9663 **Fax:** (210)496-3481
Email: eytek@sbcglobal.net
Fnded: 1981. **Activities:** Offers technical management and biomedical engineering expertise to attorneys, medical device manufacturers and importers, insurance companies, hospitals, and other healthcare facilities. Provides inspection, evaluation, and testing services related to the design, manufacture, labeling, maintenance, regulatory compliance, and pre-use readiness of medical devices. These services include incident and failure analysis, forensic engineering studies, and hazard and risk analyses. Geographic Area Served: North America and Europe.

★ 14731 ★ Medical Audit Consultants
12915 Jones Maltsberger Rd.
PO Box 160368
San Antonio, TX 78247-4282
Phone: (210)494-1167 **Fax:** (210)494-8332
Email: info@med-audit.com
Website: http://www.med-audit.com
Fnded: 1982. **Activities:** Provides accounting services, specializing in the auditing of healthcare facilities. Industries served: commercial concerns in the United States.

★ 14732 ★ Medical Business Consultants Inc.
6800 Park Ten Blvd., Ste. 110 N
San Antonio, TX 78213-4211
Phone: (210)734-4358 **Fax:** (210)734-4329
Fnded: 1977. **Activities:** Professional practice management firm assists physician offices in maximizing revenues. Industries served: medical. Geographic Area Served: Texas.

★ 14733 ★ Moore Management Consulting
7600 Blanco Rd., Apt. 4708
PO Box 171363
San Antonio, TX 78217
Phone: (210)525-8310 **Fax:** (210)349-8118
Fnded: 1986. **Activities:** Business management and personnel consulting firm specializing in finding solutions to management and employee problems, strategic planning, and corporate engineering services including an increase of profit and productivity by identifying problem areas, discovering solutions, obtaining innovative ideas, and gaining other valuable information through employees and Activity Based Costing. Commercial real estate consulting including site selection, acquisition and disposition.

Victoria

★ 14734 ★ Ruth Constant Inc.
4800 N Navarro St., Ste. 103-A
Victoria, TX 77904
Phone: (361)578-0762 **Free:** 800-338-1608
Fax: (361)578-1567
Email: drc@rchh.com
Website: http://www.rchh.com
Fnded: 1983. **Activities:** Offers organizational management and organizational image improvement consulting primarily related to home health service. Industries served: state and national healthcare associations, banking, corporations, and associations.

Wharton

★ 14735 ★ Healthcare Technology Group Inc.
625 N Fulton St.
Wharton, TX 77488-3941
Phone: (979)282-8808 **Fax:** (979)282-8809
Email: schulze@neosoft.com
Fnded: 1992. **Activities:** Specializing in the collection, analysis, and presentation of information on technology adoption trends in the health-care industry.

Wichita Falls

★ 14736 ★ Radiology Associates of Wichita Falls P.A.
808 Brook Ave.
Wichita Falls, TX 76301
Phone: (940)766-0217 **Fax:** (940)691-4305
Email: sutton@wf.net
Website: http://www.wf.net/~sutton
Activities: Specializes in diagnostic radiology, angiography, mammography, myelography, computed tomography. Provides film and case reviews and expert witness services.

The Woodlands

★ 14737 ★ Alliance Search Management Inc.
1717 Woodstead Ct., Ste. 106
The Woodlands, TX 77380
Phone: (281)367-8630 **Free:** 800-444-0573
Fax: (281)419-0335
Email: kathy@alliancesearch.com
Website: http://www.alliancesearch.com
Fnded: 1988. **Activities:** Offers healthcare executive recruitment in the U.S. Special emphasis on financial leadership, medically based fitness & wellness, integrated delivery systems, physician leadership and marketing professionals. Geographic Area Served: United States.

Utah

Murray

★ 14738 ★ 3M Health Information Systems
575 W Murray Blvd.
Murray, UT 84123
Phone: (801)265-4400
Website: http://www.3mhis.com
Fnded: 1987. **Activities:** Provides healthcare and computer counsel to government and private sector in the United States.

Pleasant Grove

★ 14739 ★ Time Masters - The Institute for Personal Excellence
776 South 980 East
Pleasant Grove, UT 84062-9531
Phone: (801)785-1105 **Fax:** (801)785-5035
Fnded: 1988. **Activities:** Employs a telephone coaching approach to teaching personal productivity, one-on-one, to any location in the world. Focus is on implementation and application of success principles over four months. Gives guarantee on in the course. Training course focuses on motivation, personal leadership, time management, sales, and entrepreneurship.

Salt Lake City

★ 14740 ★ DFW Enterprises/IDT
223 W 700 S
Salt Lake City, UT 84101-2715
Phone: (801)328-4027 **Free:** 800-561-4231
Fax: (801)530-1550
Fnded: 1995. **Activities:** Firm provides consulting services to private businesses and public sector entities on the establishment of drug- and alcohol-free workplace policies and programs. Will write policy and procedures manuals, provide training and technical assistance, design and manage drug-testing programs and provide expert witness testimony throughout the U.S. National drug and alcohol collection. Geographic Area Served: United States.

★ 14741 ★ Richard C. Webber
3760 S Highland Dr., Ste. 431
Salt Lake City, UT 84106
Phone: (801)273-3322 **Fax:** (801)273-3321
Email: rickcwebber@cs.com
Website: http://icscareers.com
Fnded: 1981. **Activities:** Human resources development consultant specializing in the development and presentation of drug and substance abuse programs, as well as executive and employee development programs. Areas of expertise include: instructor development (train-the- trainer), curriculum design/development, presentation skills/stage fright coping skills, and media relations. Leadership and motivation seminars are offered for both middle management and executives. Industries served: city, county, state, and federal law enforcement agencies; energy/oil; aerospace/aircraft; motion picture; and government agencies. **Remarks:** Expert witness in Law Enforcement/Public Safety/Security. Geographic Area Served: United States; overseas assignments considered.

★ 14742 ★ Wallace B. Brown, DDS
1955 S 1300 E, Ste. 6
Salt Lake City, UT 84105
Phone: (801)487-0758 **Fax:** (801)487-0750
Email: percha@earthlink.net

Fnded: 1973. **Activities:** Endodontist providing diagnosis and treatment of pain of dental origin; as well as malpractice evaluation. **Remarks:** Diplomate - American Board of Endodonties; Diplomate - American Board of Forensic Dentistry; Fellow - International College of Dentists.

Tooele

★ 14743 ★ J.E. Lincoln & Associates
Federal Bldg.
65 N Main, Ste. 101
PO Box 154
Tooele, UT 84074-0154
Phone: (435)882-4655 **Free:** 888-882-4655
Fax: (435)882-4669
Email: jel@trilobyte.net
Website: http://www.jelincoln.com

Fnded: 1995. **Activities:** Serving the medical device industry (Fortune 100 to start-up) for more than 18 years. Engineering, plastics selection, molding, design, assembly, project management, systems design, implementation, new product development to market, GMP/OS regulation/regulatory, import/export, agency submissions/responses, SOPs, training, failure analysis/FMEA, defect reduction, SPC/control chart, quality systems, and validations. Geographic Area Served: Worldwide.

Vermont

Bomoseen

★ 14744 ★ Continuing Education Consulting
PO Box 600
Bomoseen, VT 05732
Phone: (802)468-3200 **Fax:** (802)468-8989
Email: sunshinebirdie@aol.com

Fnded: 1979. **Activities:** Consultant for healthcare systems. Services include analysis, planning and management services for health clinics, ambulance services, hospitals, and nursing homes. Geographic Area Served: New England.

Randolph

★ 14745 ★ Theken Associates Inc.
Ridge Rd.
PO Box 307
Randolph, VT 05060
Phone: (802)728-3145 **Fax:** (802)728-5996

Fnded: 1980. **Activities:** Executive search firm for nursing administrators. Consulting services include emphasis on organizational development in the healthcare field and interim leadership in patient care services across the continuum. Geographic Area Served: Worldwide.

Woodstock

★ 14746 ★ Health Information Referral System
RR1 Box 850
Woodstock, VT 05091
Phone: (802)457-3455

Activities: Specializes in aspects of healthcare.

Virginia

Alexandria

★ 14747 ★ Accredited Podiatry P.C.
Seminary Professional Village
5256 Dawes Ave.
Alexandria, VA 22311
Phone: (703)578-3899

Fnded: 1982. **Activities:** Professional practice management specialist provides consultation for opening medical offices. Offers particular expertise for opening, running, and upgrading podiatric medical offices. Also assists with courtroom testimony regarding podiatric care. Additional counseling extended to insurance companies regarding validity of claims. Assistance provided to authors and editors of health-related publications.

★ 14748 ★ Institute for Alternative Futures
100 N Pitt St., Ste. 235
Alexandria, VA 22314-3134
Phone: (703)684-5880 **Fax:** (703)684-0640
Email: futurist@altfutures.com
Website: http://www.altfutures.com

Fnded: 1977. **Activities:** Counsels in the areas of healthcare, information/communications technology, the environment, work, and the future in general. Geographic Area Served: Worldwide.

★ 14749 ★ Phyllis M. Barrier, MS, RD, CDE
1701 N Beauregard St.
Alexandria, VA 22311
Phone: (703)299-2067 **Fax:** (703)683-1839
Email: pbarrier@diabetes.org

Activities: Registered dietitian in private practice, specializing in diabetes, weight management, dislipidemia, and eating disorders. Geographic Area Served: Maryland, Virginia and District of Columbia metropolitan areas.

★ 14750 ★ Steinman Associates
1033 N Fairfax St., 4th Fl.
Alexandria, VA 22314
Phone: (703)836-2686 **Fax:** (703)836-4084
Email: stevsa1@aol.com

Fnded: 1982. **Activities:** Provides consulting services to drug development companies, biotechnology companies, and fully integrated pharmaceutical firms regulated under the Federal Food, Drug, and Cosmetic Act. The firm possess expertise in quality assurance, government affairs, drug manufacturing, data management, biostatistics, clinical trials management. Steinman Associates will draft and produce IND applications, New Drug Applications, and Biological Product Licenses. Geographic Area Served: United States, Europe, and Japan.

★ 14751 ★ WWRice Healthcare
PO Box 7007
Alexandria, VA 22307-7007
Phone: (703)960-0009 **Fax:** (703)960-0900
Email: wwricehealthcare@aol.com
Website: http://www.ricehealth.com

Fnded: 1992. **Activities:** Firm provides solutions in strategic planning assignments. Assists clients in protecting and developing market share through assessment, research and activation planning. Business and financial planning are provided to insure client success. Firm has capital facilities planning credentials and stresses flexible solutions for tomorrow's needs. Specializes in oncology planning, development, and operations. Consulting practice also revolves around new information technologies and new clinical technologies including infertility/reproduction, cardiology, and diagnostic imaging. Geographic Area Served: United States.

Annandale

★ 14752 ★ JWK International Corp.
7617 Little River Tpke., Ste. 800
Annandale, VA 22003-2689
Phone: (703)750-0500 **Fax:** (703)256-1986
Website: http://www.jwk.com

Fnded: 1973. **Activities:** Provides instructional systems development, scientific research support and analysis, nutritional guidance, survey design and execution, and training program development and support. Also offers computer-based instructional development in health, environment, and personnel development. Industries served: federal, state, and local governments as prime or subcontractor; foreign governments. Geographic Area Served: Worldwide.

Arlington

★ 14753 ★ Wilma J. Winter - Medical Communications
2111 Jefferson Davis Hwy., Apt. 513 N
Arlington, VA 22202
Phone: (703)415-0610

Fnded: 1984. **Activities:** Provides research and writing expertise on medical affairs. Attends and summarizes science seminars. Writes and researches clinical papers, drug brochures, audiovisuals on drugs, and salesperson's mail pieces. Summarizes pharmacologic and clinical data for government application and review. Industries served: pharmaceutical firms, federal government, medical journals, and local TV (cable). Geographic Area Served: United States.

Chantilly

★ 14754 ★ Health Cost Consultants Inc.
14120 Newbrook Dr., Ste. 140
Chantilly, VA 20151-2273
Phone: (703)995-6300 **Fax:** (703)488-9663
Website: http://www.66.84.18.45/index.htm

Fnded: 1993. **Activities:** Advises businesses and public healthcare organizations on health costs and economics. Geographic Area Served: Washington, D.C. Metro area.

Charlottesville

★ 14755 ★ Anne D. Brown
Albemarle Center for Family Medicine
535 Westfield Rd., Ste. 200
Charlottesville, VA 22901
Phone: (434)973-4040 **Fax:** (434)974-1780

Fnded: 1982. **Activities:** Provides nutritional consultation for individuals referred by physician. All areas of nutrition addressed with primary emphasis on low cholesterol diets, weight reduction, gestational diabetes, as well as prudent diet restrictions.

★ 14756 ★ C. Knight Aldrich M.D.
905 Cottage Ln.
Charlottesville, VA 22903
Phone: (434)296-4816

Fnded: 1982. **Activities:** Offers administrative consultations, on a single or continuing basis, with mental health centers and similar organizations for planning, staff development, and trouble-shooting. Also provides editorial services for assistance in the preparation of psychiatric and medical articles, books, and other materials. Serves private industries as well as government agencies. Geographic Area Served: United States.

★ 14757 ★ Occupational Health Strategies Inc.
901 Preston Ave., Ste. 400
Charlottesville, VA 22903-4491
Phone: (434)977-3784 **Fax:** (434)977-8570
Email: OHS@HealthySelf.org
Website: http://www.healthyself.org

Fnded: 1984. **Activities:** Offers expertise in the areas of occupational medicine; regulatory compliance; planning and development; and safety programs to manufacturers worldwide, but primarily in the United States.

Fairfax

★ 14758 ★ Consolidated Safety Services Inc.
10335 Democracy Ln., Ste. 202
Fairfax, VA 22030
Phone: (703)691-4612 **Free:** 800-888-4612
Fax: (703)691-4615
Website: http://www.consolidatedsafety.com
Fnded: 1988. **Activities:** Provides services in occupational health and safety; industrial hygiene; transportation safety; information services; and testing and certification of bio-hazard safety cabinets, clean rooms, and fume hoods. Industries served: government agencies, transportation, manufacturing, construction, and institutions in the United States.

★ 14759 ★ Drug Testing Consultants Inc.
10875 Main St., Ste. 107
PO Box 706
Fairfax, VA 22030-0706
Phone: (703)273-1757 **Fax:** (703)352-7124
Fnded: 1987. **Activities:** Conducts workplace drug testing programs for government and private sector in the United States.

★ 14760 ★ Food, Drug, Chemical Services
3771 Center Way
Fairfax, VA 22033
Phone: (703)352-5913 **Fax:** (703)255-6434
Fnded: 1976. **Activities:** Provides scientific, regulatory, and management consulting services for a wide variety of product lines and industries including pharmaceutical, industrial and agricultural chemicals, biotechnology, toiletries and cosmetics, food additives, diagnostics, and devices. Areas of expertise include product integrity, scientific affairs, management, medical communications, environmental science, pharmacology and toxicology, clinical studies, FDA liaison, and product licensing. Geographic Area Served: Worldwide.

Fairfax Station

★ 14761 ★ Health Systems Technology Corp.
11701 Yates Ford Rd.
Fairfax Station, VA 22039-1507
Phone: (703)978-2084 **Fax:** (703)978-2197
Fnded: 1990. **Activities:** Provides healthcare and case management services to businesses in the United States.

Falls Church

★ 14762 ★ Aldo M. Rosemblat, MD
6316 Castle Pl., Ste. 200
Falls Church, VA 22044
Phone: (703)241-8989 **Fax:** (703)532-6247
Activities: Specializes in surgery of the brain, spine, spinal cord and peripheral nerves. Provides disability evaluations for workers' compensation, personal injury and social security pertaining to the neurological system and to the joint and muscular skeletal systems. Geographic Area Served: Falls Church, VA; Woodbridge, VA.

★ 14763 ★ Pragma Corp.
116 E Broad St.
Falls Church, VA 22046-4501
Phone: (703)237-9303 **Fax:** (703)237-9326
Email: pragma@pragmacorp.com
Website: http://www.pragmacorp.com
Fnded: 1977. **Activities:** Offers expertise in the fields of finance, corporate governance, agriculture and agribusiness,training and education, health environment and urban development, municipal development, systems and technology,Clients include: U.S. and international private firms; development institutions; non-governmentaland private voluntary organizations; and academic institutions.

★ 14764 ★ Quintiles BRI
3130 Fairview Park Dr., Ste. 800
Falls Church, VA 22042
Fnded: 1971. **Activities:** Consults on pharmaceuticals and medical devices.

★ 14765 ★ Team Placement Service Inc.
5113 Leesburg Pke., Ste. 510
Falls Church, VA 22041
Phone: (703)820-8618 **Free:** 800-495-6767
Fax: (703)820-3368
Website: http://www.teamplace.com
Fnded: 1983. **Activities:** Full-service personnel consultants provide placement for healthcare staff, physician and dentist, private practice, and hospitals. Conduct interviews, tests, and reference checks to select the top 20% of applicants. Survey applicants' skill levels, provide back-up information on each candidate, select compatible candidates for consideration, and insure the hiring process minimizes potential legal liability. Industries served: healthcare and government agencies providing medical, dental, biotech, laboratory, hospitals, and physician search. Geographic Area Served: Washington metro area.

Front Royal

★ 14766 ★ Medical Device Assistance Inc.
PO Box 296
272 Trent Trail Ct.
Front Royal, VA 22630
Phone: (540)636-2509 **Free:** 888-571-1148
Fax: (540)636-2787
Email: info@mdassist.com
Website: http://www.mdassist.com
Fnded: 1995. **Activities:** Former chief medical officer, CDRH, FDA. Provides medical products and FDA evaluation, including grandfathered devices, safety and effectiveness, labeling, FDA's instructor pre-clinical and clinical trials, good manufacturing practices (GMP), health risk assessment, and medical device reporting (MDR). Certified pathologist with background in medical practice and forensics. Knowledgeable in all aspects of FDA regulation. Geographic Area Served: Worldwide.

Hampton

★ 14767 ★ Holmes-Tucker International Inc.
2101 Executive Dr.
Hampton, VA 23666
Phone: (757)838-1930 **Fax:** (757)642-1568
Fnded: 1989. **Activities:** Engineering and management consulting firm that offers training, software documentation, requirements management (including requirements linking and tracking), business process reengineering, and process analysis, redesign, and improvement. Serves private industries as well as government agencies. Geographic Area Served: United States, Canada, and Europe.

McLean

★ 14768 ★ Apache Medical System/ National Health Advisors Ltd.
1650 Tysons Blvd., Ste. 300
McLean, VA 22102
Phone: (703)883-0400 **Fax:** (703)847-1401
Website: http://www.apache-msi.com/psdx.shtml
Fnded: 1981. **Activities:** A management consulting firm specializing in strategic management in today's healthcare industry. Emphasis on diversification and development, merger and acquisition planning, trustee education, and corporate reorganization. The firm has provided services to independent hospitals, multi-institutional arrangements and networks, and health-related companies in over 30 states throughout the United States.

★ 14769 ★ Barbara J. Barbu, RD, LD
6506 Deidre Ter.
McLean, VA 22101
Phone: (703)848-8110 **Fax:** (703)848-8110
Email: bbarbu@hotmail.com
Activities: Registered dietitian in private practice. Consultant to companies, health care and medical facilities. Board Member of the Northern District, Virginia Dietetic Association Member of Consulting Nutritionist in the Chesapeake Bay Area Association. **Remarks:** Offer cooking demostrations and nutrition consultations at corporate health fairs. Geographic Area Served: Washington D.C. Metro Area

★ 14770 ★ Cambridge Consulting Corp.
7901 Jones Branch Dr., No. 110
McLean, VA 22102-3301
Phone: (703)917-8560 **Fax:** (703)917-8603
Email: admin@ccc-mclean.com
Website: http://www.ccc-mclean.com
Fnded: 1985. **Activities:** An international health, management, and research organization. Serves private industries as well as government agencies. Geographic Area Served: Worldwide.

★ 14771 ★ The Center for Corporate Health Inc.
8201 Greenboro Dr., Ste. 500
McLean, VA 22102
Phone: (703)394-7600 **Free:** 800-745-1333
Fax: (703)394-7585
Fnded: 1984. **Activities:** Consultants on integrated health promotion programs. Offers a variety of products and services to educate people on taking better care of themselves and using medical services wisely. Products include health-oriented newsletters, health counseling, medical self-care books, and health risk appraisals. Works with individual organizations to assess healthcare cost management and tailor a program for client company. Industries served: human resources/employee benefits executives, managed care organizations, and government agencies. Geographic Area Served: United States.

★ 14772 ★ Consumer Health Information Corp.
8300 Greensboro Dr., Ste. 1220
McLean, VA 22102-3604
Phone: (703)734-0650 **Fax:** (703)734-1459
Email: chic@consumer-health.com
Website: http://www.consumer-health.com
Fnded: 1983. **Activities:** Internationally recognized for development of patient programs that improve patient compliance with prescription drugs and increase ROI; customized patient compliance strategies integrated into product marketing strategy; FDA-approved Patient Package Inserts (PPIs); DTC educational materials for consumers that are understandable and motivational; Phase III Informed Consent and patient materials that meet FDA requirements for patient comprehension; drug information specialists; affiliated with more than 30 universities and a teaching site. Experts in Transtheoretical Model of Change and behavior modification. Award-winning design. **Remarks:** Specialists in Drug Information, 32 University Affiliations in U.S., Member of Board of Directors National Council on Patient Information and Education. Geographic Area Served: Worldwide.

Norfolk

★ 14773 ★ Damsey & Associates Ltd.
420 N Center Dr.
Norfolk, VA 23502
Phone: (757)455-5554 **Fax:** (757)455-5558
Fnded: 1982. **Activities:** Offers medical management services, including operations audits, marketing plans, managed care contracting, administration, mergers,

management recruitment, professional practice setup, cost controls, productivity enhancement, and coding issues. Serves more than 1,500 physicians and hospitals in fourteen states. Serves three medical schools.

★ 14774 ★ Frank Westmeyer, MD
957 W 21st St.
Norfolk, VA 23517
Phone: (757)622-4613 **Fax:** (757)627-0258
Activities: Provides expert witness testimony in cases involving primary care, internal medicine, and emergency medicine.

★ 14775 ★ Joseph L. Kelly
309 W Freemason St., No. 2
Norfolk, VA 23510
Phone: (757)624-2083
Email: jlkmd@exis.net
Website: http://member.expertpages.com/jlkmd/
Activities: Expert medical opinions in all areas of internal medicine, hospital practice, long term care, emergency medicine and outpatient practice.

★ 14776 ★ Tidewater Emergency Medical Services Council Inc.
855 W Brambleton Ave.
Norfolk, VA 23510
Phone: (757)446-5179 **Fax:** (757)446-5906
Email: tidewater@vaems.org
Website: http://tidewater.vaems.org
Fnded: 1974. **Activities:** Emergency medical training organization consults on appropriate training and EMS system development. Geographic Area Served: Primarily southeastern Virginia.

Portsmouth

★ 14777 ★ Atlantic Rehabilitation Services Inc.
307 County St., Ste. 210
Portsmouth, VA 23704
Phone: (757)399-0900 **Free:** 800-476-4394
Fax: (757)399-8043
Email: admin@atlanticrehabservices.com
Website: http://www.atlanticrehabservices.com
Fnded: 1989. **Activities:** A private vocational rehabilitation company that provides services to attorneys, insurance companies, and government agencies on the vocational impact of injuries and the need for vocational rehabilitation services. Firm routinely testifies as vocational experts. Geographic Area Served: Eastern United States, Virginia, and northern North Carolina.

Potomac Falls

★ 14778 ★ Frida Theros
20328 Burnley Sq.
Potomac Falls, VA 20165-6455
Phone: (703)404-2547
Activities: Consulting nutritionist in the Chesapeake Bay area and registered dietitian in private practice.

Reston

★ 14779 ★ Lammers & Gershon Associates
1801 Alexander Graham Bell
Reston, VA 20190
Phone: (703)476-8400 **Fax:** (703)476-8541
Fnded: 1979. **Activities:** A healthcare consulting firm that specializes in planning and development services. The firm has a national practice and offers a comprehensive range of consultative assistance to healthcare providers, including: strategic and program planning, marketing, market research, facility evaluations, master planning, functional/space programming, and materials management. Geographic Area Served: United States.

Roanoke

★ 14780 ★ TJL Associates Inc.
6781 Mount Chestnut Rd.
Roanoke, VA 24018
Phone: (540)314-8004 **Fax:** (540)989-6819
Email: tom@tjlassociatesinc.com
Website: http://www.tjlassociatesinc.com
Fnded: 1974. **Activities:** Specialist in emulsion technology and surface chemistry. Serves manufacturers of cosmetics, personal care products, and pharmaceutical products.

Vienna

★ 14781 ★ Medical Review Foundation Inc.
120 Beulah Rd. NE, Ste. 200
Vienna, VA 22180
Free: 800-336-0332 **Fax:** (703)255-6134
Email: medexperts@aol.com
Website: http://www.malpracticeexperts.com
Fnded: 1976. **Activities:** A large medical-legal consulting firm made up of more than 5000 independent, board certified medical experts, in all specialities. Consultants review medical records, prepare written reports and testify. Offers free case evaluations.

Virginia Beach

★ 14782 ★ Miles & Associates
PO Box 6249
Virginia Beach, VA 23456
Phone: (757)721-3332 **Free:** 800-922-0866
Fax: (757)721-2892
Email: info@dentalmanagementu.com
Website: http://www.DentalManagementU.com
Fnded: 1978. **Activities:** Offers practice management services to dentists. Geographic Area Served: United States, Australia, and Canada.

Woodbridge

★ 14783 ★ Douglas E. Heritage, MD
2026A Opitz Blvd., Ste. A
Woodbridge, VA 22191-3306
Phone: (703)491-7155 **Fax:** (703)690-3958
Fnded: 1978. **Activities:** Private practice of obstetrics and gynecology. Special qualifications in GYN laser surgery, laparoscopic surgery, pelvic microsurgery. Experience in treatment of endometriosis, abnormal PAP smears, and pelvic pain. Offers expert witness testimony.

Washington

Anacortes

★ 14784 ★ Beverly Ann Benedict
2414 16th St.
Anacortes, WA 98221
Phone: (360)293-9086 **Fax:** (360)299-9151
Fnded: 1993. **Activities:** How To Start a Newspaper On a Shoestring and How to Write and Publish a Cookbook. Geographic Area Served: Worldwide.

★ 14785 ★ George M. Johnson & Associates
11746 McCorkle Pl.
Anacortes, WA 98221
Email: johns.me@ix.netcom.com
Fnded: 1982. **Activities:** Provides medical device technical consulting, R&D program assessment, project management, product development, technology transfer, individual and group R&D management training, project troubleshooting, business development, and R&D strategic planning.

Edmonds

★ 14786 ★ Center for Counseling & Health Resources Inc.
547 Dayton Ave.
Edmonds, WA 98020
Phone: (425)771-5166 **Free:** 888-771-5166
Fax: (425)670-2807
Email: thecenterinc@aplaceofhope.com
Website: http://www.aplaceofhope.com
Fnded: 1983. **Activities:** Consulting services of the Center include education and training, as well as counseling and treatment programs concerning family relationships, eating disorders, weight loss, and addictions and compulsions. Emphasis is on health programs and nutrition.

★ 14787 ★ Pat Ford HealthCare Consulting
17207 76th Ave. W
Edmonds, WA 98026
Phone: (425)743-0576 **Fax:** (425)787-2774
Email: pat@pfhc.com
Website: http://www.pfhc.com
Activities: Primary areas of expertise are project management, process redesign, program development and implementation. Specializes in NCQA and URAC survey preparation, quality management and improvement, utilization and case management, disease management, credentialing, development of processes to increase HEDIS compliance, and medical record review. Also provides interim staffing for medical management positions while searches are being conducted for a permanent person.

Gig Harbor

★ 14788 ★ Center for Leadership Development
PO Box 2447
Gig Harbor, WA 98335
Phone: (206)295-6694 **Free:** 800-832-6360
Fax: (253)851-1158
Website: http://teamcld.com
Activities: The Center designs and conducts a wide variety of personal and professional improvement seminars. These seminars may be conducted either publicly or in-house. The Center also provides a full range of organizational development consulting services, such as training needs assessments, employee relations, action planning, strategic and operational planning, position profiling, leadership development, team building, and experiencial outdoor programs. Geographic Area Served: United States and Canada.

★ 14789 ★ Peter F. Hampl, DDS
7898 Greyhawk Ave.
Gig Harbor, WA 98335-4926
Phone: (253)853-1984
Email: peter@phampl.com
Website: http://www.phampl.com
Activities: Dentistry services include Human Identification; Bite Mark Analysis; Dental Liability in malpractice; mass disaster prepardness; human abuse.

Issaquah

★ 14790 ★ Flemming & Wickett Inc.
26428 SE 160th St.
Issaquah, WA 98027
Phone: (425)392-9791 **Fax:** (425)392-4670
Fnded: 1980. **Activities:** Firm provides food processing consulting, from hourly contract work to turnkey plants. Offers expertise on frozen, fresh, and canned processing of fish, fruits, vegetables, cereals, surimi plants, and wine. Geographic Area Served: United States.

Kirkland

★ 14791 ★ Charles Pearson Associates
12014 86th Ave. NE
Kirkland, WA 98034
Phone: (206)517-4300

Fnded: 1979. **Activities:** Management consultant offers hospital and health system management services with major focus on restructuring hospital-physician contractual relationships. Geographic Area Served: United States.

★ 14792 ★ Miller.Miller L.L.C.
PO Box 3088
Kirkland, WA 98083
Phone: (425)822-3145 **Free:** 800-820-1055
Fax: (425)827-9194
Email: info@millermiller.com
Website: http://millermiller.com

Fnded: 1989. **Activities:** An executive search service that supports biotechnology and medically related industries.

Olympia

★ 14793 ★ Nutrition Entrepreneurs
9212 Delphi Rd. SW
Olympia, WA 98502
Phone: (360)956-1367 **Fax:** (360)956-1367
Email: nedpg@aol.com
Website: http://www.nutritionentrepreneurs.org

Fnded: 1977. **Activities:** Serves as the clearinghouse for nutrition entrepreneurs throughout the U.S. and Canada. Members provide consultation to a variety of clients which include consumers, medical clinics, physician's offices, outpatient departments of hospitals, restaurants, corporations, long-term care facilities, television, radio-television-print media, supermarkets, and food companies. In addition, many members produce and market nutrition related products. Industries served: acute and long term healthcare settings, all forms of media, consumer and professional education, corporate wellness, entrepreneurial production and marketing of products for consumers and/or professionals.

Pasco

★ 14794 ★ Bob Greenwell
515 W Clark St.
Pasco, WA 99301-5521
Phone: (509)547-5551 **Fax:** (509)547-8085

Fnded: 1970. **Activities:** A licensed insurance brokerage. Individual offerings include life insurance (a variety of both term and permanent, cash value life insurance products); health insurance (traditional major medical and managed care plans); disability insurance (to provide monthly income in the event of illness, injury, or inability to work); Medicare supplements (standardized plans A, B, C, E, F, and I available); nursing home insurance (aka long term care insurance); Individual Retirement Accounts (IRA). Employee benefits offerings include health insurance (traditional major medical, Preferred Provider Organizations (PPO), and Managed Care Plans); life insurance (group term life and key person); retirement plans (401(k), SEP-IRA, and non-qualified retirement plans); and dental and vision plans. Geographic Area Served: Eastern Washington.

Renton

★ 14795 ★ PRO-FIT
12012 156th Ave. SE
Renton, WA 98059-6317
Phone: (425)255-3817 **Fax:** (425)255-0478
Email: alice@exercisexpress.com
Website: http://www.exercisexpress.com

Fnded: 1983. **Activities:** Health fitness consultant offers expertise on simple steps to start doing what's good for you. Consultant stresses correct techniques of exercise and their importance. Topics include: aerobics for real people, back fitness, nutrition, stretching, food fats, office exercises, correct exercise form, physiology facts, principles of adult exercise and exercise abuse. Will also discuss client/requested topic at public presentations. Programs designed and operated in occupationally pertinent fitness programs for physically demanding careers. Geographic Area Served: Focus on Pacific Northwest - travels nationwide.

Richland

★ 14796 ★ Health Metrics Inc.
2031 Greenbrook Blvd.
Richland, WA 99352
Phone: (509)628-0215 **Free:** 800-878-3466
Fax: (509)628-9215
Email: healthmetrics@aol.com
Website: http://www.healthmetrics.com

Fnded: 1976. **Activities:** A consulting, research and occupational health service firm specializing in human factors applications with expertise and capabilities in human factors research, work physiology, biomechanics, occupational health, medical information management, and program development. The principal areas of service and research include: applied physiology, occupational health, preventive medicine, job/task analysis, human nutrition, health and fitness program development, biomechanics, physical fitness assessment, medical/physical standards, and sports medicine. Projects have included: design of job-related physical ability tests ,studies on the effects of physical fitness programs on overall occupational health, development of physical performance standards for public safety workers, military physical performance task analysis, expert testimony in litigation and occupational health hearings, development of fitness testing and training centers, and design and instruction of exercise leadership classes. Geographic Area Served: United States and Canada.

★ 14797 ★ Thomas C. Hall, M.D.
1323 Thayer Dr.
Richland, WA 99352-3253
Phone: (509)943-3310 **Fax:** (360)738-6711
Email: all4halls@earthlink.net

Fnded: 1970. **Activities:** Offers medical consultation services related to medical malpractice, medical disability, and general medico-legal problems, with special emphasis on cancer cases. Serves private industries as well as government agencies. **Remarks:** Good backup resources in pathology, radiology, pelliative care, treatment of cancer. Geographic Area Served: United States and Canada.

Seattle

★ 14798 ★ ECG Management Consultants Inc.
1111 3rd Ave., Ste. 2700
Seattle, WA 98101-3201
Phone: (206)689-2200 **Fax:** (206)689-2209
Email: ecg@ecgmc.com
Website: http://www.ecgmc.com

Fnded: 1973. **Activities:** Company provides a wide range of professional services in the following areas: academic healthcare management consulting, general healthcare management consulting and healthcare information technology consulting. Provide healthcare organizations with strategic and implementation assistance in the following areas: organization and planning; physician group practice plan organization and enhancement; development of integrated delivery systems; formulation of strategies that address market objectives, academic objectives; medical education planning; development of clinical and academic affiliations, mergers, and acquisitions; redesign of organizational/operational structures; preparation of strategic and business plans; and IT planning, selection and implementation. Geographic Area Served: United States.

★ 14799 ★ EMISAR
1023 32nd Ave. E
Seattle, WA 98112
Phone: (206)323-2820 **Fax:** (206)325-5180
Email: mcooper@emisar.com
Website: http://www.emisar.com

Fnded: 1985. **Activities:** Works with CEO's and senior executives in organizational and executive performance throughout the United States, Europe and the Far East. **Remarks:** All information and conditions for a consulting relationship noted on the website.

★ 14800 ★ Health Sciences Center for Educational Resources
University of Washington
Box 357161, Room T252
Seattle, WA 98195-7161
Phone: (206)685-1156 **Fax:** (206)543-8051

Activities: Specialists in biomedical education offer generic consultation, planning, and production.

★ 14801 ★ Jacobson Engineers
5220 Roosevelt Way NE
Seattle, WA 98105
Phone: (206)522-5511 **Fax:** (206)522-5512

Fnded: 1967. **Activities:** Offers engineering design and analysis and prototype fabrication and testing. Specializes in mechanical, hydraulic, and electrical systems; biomedical applications; forensic engineering; and accident reconstruction.

★ 14802 ★ The Joyce Institute
1107 NE 45th St.
Seattle, WA 98105
Phone: (206)632-9720

Fnded: 1981. **Activities:** Ergonomics Consulting services include assessments, evaluations and design projects for industrial, office and laboratory workplaces, product design consulting, and ergonomic program plan development. Ergonomists offer training programs for engineers, managers, supervisors, health/safety professionals which include video workshops and problem solving activities for industrial environments. Office courses are designed for facilities managers and supervisors, and incorporate office design guidelines and criteria for furniture, accessories, equipment and job design. VDT user training teaches "do-it-yourself" ergonomics. Industries served: all types of office, industrial and laboratory environments, including government agencies.

★ 14803 ★ Medical Consultants Network
901 Boren Ave., Ste. 1400
Seattle, WA 98104
Phone: (206)621-9097 **Free:** 888-626-4637
Fax: (206)623-4956
Email: network@mcn.com
Website: http://www.mcn.com

Fnded: 1985. **Activities:** Provides Medical Judgment services nationwide. Services include Independent Medical Evaluations (IME), Peer Reviews, and Medical Case Management. MCN has a network of over 60,000 consulting physicians across the nation. Geographic Area Served: Worldwide.

★ 14804 ★ Milliman USA
1301 5th Ave., Ste. 3800
Seattle, WA 98101-2605
Phone: (206)624-7940 **Fax:** (206)340-1380
Email: seattle.office@milliman.com
Website: http://www.milliman.com

Fnded: 1947. **Activities:** Evaluator of risks and opportunities for clients in four major areas healthcare, employee benefits, life insurance/financial services, and property and casualty insurance for over 50 years. Internationally, M&R is a founding member of Woodrow Milliman, a network of consulting firms with more than 100 offices in over 30 countries. Geographic Area Served: Worldwide.

★ 14805 ★ Peter Fisher, MD
2100 3rd Ave., Ste. 2302
Seattle, WA 98121
Phone: (206)728-9997 **Fax:** (206)728-1460
Activities: Evaluates the biodynamics and medical aspects of aviation, industrial, criminal, civil and slip and fall injuries, and highway injuries, including the relationship of vehicle damage and claimed passenger injuries, multiple impacts, motorcycle, bicycle and pedestrian injuries, child seats and the role of safety belts, helmets, airbags and vehicular design. Analyzes the role of alcohol and other drugs in driver performance and accident occurrence, roadside hazards, and product liability. Geographic Area Served: United States and Canada.

★ 14806 ★ Schorr Communications
201 Queen Anne Ave. N, Ste. 400
Seattle, WA 98109-4824
Phone: (206)284-5730 **Fax:** (206)233-0236
Fnded: 1986. **Activities:** Provides consulting services to the healthcare/medical industries regarding the application of visual media to meet sales, marketing, public relations, and training needs. With expertise especially in video production and broadcast media relations, the firm assists with strategic planning in these areas and implements these plans through the production of top-quality visual communications products. Industries served: primarily healthcare and medical industries, including pharmaceuticals, medical manufacturers, healthcare providers, and consumer products related to healthcare; government agencies. Geographic Area Served: Worldwide.

Tacoma

★ 14807 ★ American Institute for Biosocial and Medical Research Inc. - AIBMR Life Sciences Div.
PO Box 1174
Tacoma, WA 98401-1174
Phone: (253)286-2888 **Fax:** (253)286-2886
Email: info@aibmr.com
Website: http://www.aibmr.com
Fnded: 1980. **Activities:** Prepares comprehensive databases on any area concerning public health issues. Examines products in the healthcare-giving marketplace. Conducts in-service training programs on public health topics for insurance companies, government agencies (federal, state, and local), and universities and colleges. Prepares scientific papers for publication to assist researchers desiring to submit manuscripts for publication. Industries served: insurance companies, hospitals, federal, state and local government agencies, colleges and universities, food processors, food distributors, food manufacturers, and informational database developers. Geographic Area Served: Worldwide.

★ 14808 ★ Final Analysis Forensics
PO Box 6888
Tacoma, WA 98407-0385
Phone: (253)627-2739 **Fax:** (253)627-0350
Email: finalanalysis@msn.com
Website: http://www.finalanalysisforensics.com
Fnded: 1985. **Activities:** Forensic science investigative consultant specializing in death & medical investigation, including cause, manner of death, investigation of scenes, histories; criminalistics, including trace evidence, organic/inorganic identifications, comparisons, ballistics; scene investigation, including bloodstain pattern analysis, evidence collection, event/accident reconstruction; forensic analysis; and analysis of scientific evidence, including chain of custody, recognition/collection issues, assess limitations/scope of sciences applied, assessment of omissions, opinions, and investigation and evaluation of expert testimony. Geographic Area Served: Worldwide.

Winlock

★ 14809 ★ Sturza Enterprises Inc.
376 Avery Rd. W
Winlock, WA 98596
Phone: (360)262-3202 **Fax:** (360)740-0387
Activities: Specializes in product liability, compliance inspections, safety code development, accident investigation, forest road design and inspection, logging system analyses, code interpretation, forest products, and logging and sawmills.

West Virginia

Huntington

★ 14810 ★ ErgoTek Inc.
729 Ninth Ave., Ste. 196
Huntington, WV 25701
Free: 877-374-6835 **Fax:** 877-374-6329
Activities: Specializes in ergonomics, occupational hazards and medicine, human factors and safety engineering, accident reconstruction, personal injury, and slips and falls.

Martinsburg

★ 14811 ★ Hollingsworth Med X-Press Rehabilitation & Consulting Services Inc.
442 Winchester Ave.
Martinsburg, WV 25401
Phone: (304)263-3400 **Free:** 800-734-2238
Fax: (304)263-3860
Email: hrcs@intrepid.net
Fnded: 1990. **Activities:** Provides medical and vocational coordination services regarding the legal medical, and vocational issues inherent in the rehabilitation process of the industrially injured. Also Med X-Press provides transportation. Geographic Area Served: Virginia, Maryland, and West Virginia.

Morgantown

★ 14812 ★ Norma E. Simbra - Diet Counseling Service
1189 Pineview Dr.
PO Box 4423
Morgantown, WV 26504-4423
Phone: (304)599-1555 **Fax:** (304)599-1555
Email: normasimbra@aol.com
Fnded: 1983. **Activities:** Nutrition consulting work in hospitals, clinics, long-term care, drug rehab centers, and home health agencies. Provides diet counseling on various areas such as weight control, pre-admission surgical diets, hypertension, diabetes education, allergies, sports nutrition, kidney disease, digestive disorders, general nutrition, and pre-natal care. Provides workshops and seminars on weight loss, eating disorders, and general nutrition, as well as cooking demonstrations. Geographic Area Served: West Virginia and Pennsylvania, MD.

★ 14813 ★ U.S. Industrial Medicine Corp.
3041 University Ave.
Morgantown, WV 26505-2815
Phone: (304)599-6367 **Fax:** (304)599-0400
Fnded: 1980. **Activities:** Specializes in occupational medicine, training, and development. Industries served: manufacturing in the United States.

Wisconsin

Brookfield

★ 14814 ★ Far Cliffs Consulting Inc.
2290 Brittany Ct.
Brookfield, WI 53045
Phone: (262)827-0355 **Free:** 800-592-6448
Fax: (262)827-0356
Email: farcliffs@aol.com
Website: http://www.farcliffs.com
Fnded: 1986. **Activities:** Firm provides human resources expertise through training, management development, and assessment for the peak performance of individuals and organizations. Primary activities are educational: programs to analyze information for individual and organizational decision-making, and management training programs for professional development. **Remarks:** Human Resources Research, a division of the firm, offers expertise in substance abuse and compulsive gambling. Geographic Area Served: Worldwide.

★ 14815 ★ Heartland Home Healthcare
13255 W Bluemound Rd., Ste. 100
Brookfield, WI 53005
Free: 800-236-2331
Fnded: 1961. **Activities:** Advises Wisconsin healthcare industry on management issues.

★ 14816 ★ Professional Resources Management Inc.
15850 W Bluemound Rd., Ste. 300
Brookfield, WI 53005
Phone: (262)784-6777 **Free:** 800-272-2777
Fax: (262)784-0727
Activities: Consulting specialists in medical and healthcare/physician recruiting. Geographic Area Served: United States.

★ 14817 ★ U.S. Counseling Services Inc.
120 Bishops Way, Ste. 100
Brookfield, WI 53008
Free: 800-558-6377 **Fax:** (262)784-5779
Email: info@uscounselingservices.com
Website: http://www.uscounselingservices.com
Fnded: 1969. **Activities:** Equipment technology management company helping U.S. healthcare organizations manage their capital investment through a series of services designed to reduce expenses associated with the purchase, maintenance, and operation of medical equipment. Geographic Area Served: United States.

Cedarburg

★ 14818 ★ Smith—Pigg Consulting Inc.
1928 Fairhaven Dr.
Cedarburg, WI 53012
Phone: (414)377-8938
Fnded: 1978. **Activities:** Musculoskeletal (arthritis and orthopedics) product line development.

Columbus

★ 14819 ★ Hospital Maintenance Consultants Inc.
479 Fuller St.
Columbus, WI 53925-1652
Phone: (920)623-5718 **Free:** 800-513-3832
Fax: (920)623-5721
Email: mob@gdinet.com
Fnded: 1972. **Activities:** Experts in the field of hospital maintenance. Industries served: hospitals, multi-hospital groups, medical and scientific manufacturers, leasing companies, shared clinical engineering services, and independent service companies. Geographic Area Served: United States and Canada.

Glendale

★ 14820 ★ Healics Worksite Wellness
PO Box 170925
Glendale, WI 53217
Phone: (414)963-8889 **Free:** 800-432-5427
Email: healics@execpc.com
Website: http://www.healics.net
Activities: HEALICS stands for HEALth Information Computer System. Offers Health Risk Appraisals (HRA's) as an annual employer paid health benefit.

Madison

★ 14821 ★ Bioenergetics Inc.
PO Box 259141
Madison, WI 53725
Phone: (608)255-4028 **Free:** 800-203-4028
Fax: (608)251-0658

Fnded: 1973. **Activities:** Offers technical counsel on chemical toxicology for forensic problems. Consultant has done numerous studies for insurance companies, legal firms, and others on a wide spectrum of problems, including paint identification, fuel and lubricant contaminants, identification of flammable solvents, Breathalyzer, Intoxilyzer and blood testing, and other chemical and biochemical problems. Also experienced with gender issues including sexual harassment defense. **Remarks:** Subsidaries: Forensic Associates, Enterprise Real Estate of Madison (WI). Geographic Area Served: Primarily Midwestern United States.

★ 14822 ★ HealthChoice, a Carequest Inc. Co.
583 D'Onofrio Dr., Ste. 103
Madison, WI 53719
Phone: (608)833-7988 **Free:** 800-327-7138
Fax: (608)833-7540
Email: info@carequestplus.com
Website: http://www.healthchoice.com/who.cfm

Fnded: 1989. **Activities:** Work and Family Life and Long-term care employee assistance program (EAP) offering Eldercare Plus and Information Line. It serves all industries, including unions and some associations, in the U.S. Maintains a branch office in Minneapolis, Minnesota, Neenah Wisconsin and 7 regional branch sales offices. Geographic Area Served: United States.

★ 14823 ★ Lowell Hokin
University of Wisconsin Medical School
1300 University Ave.
Madison, WI 53706
Phone: (608)224-2190 **Fax:** (608)262-1257
Email: lehokin@facstaff.wisc.edu

Activities: Performs pharmacology research on psychoactive drugs. Skilled in forensic pharmacology and psychopharmacology. Geographic Area Served: U.S.A.

★ 14824 ★ Mitchell Health Cost Consultants
5138 Stage House Trl.
Madison, WI 53714-2767
Phone: (608)249-0300

Fnded: 1987. **Activities:** Consultant will advise corporations on health cost management, including cost control, value enhancement, and design and development of health promotion programs. Also develops and writes marketing/promotional materials, professional reports, position papers, and policies/procedures. Additional duties include long-range health planning and conducting research/analytical studies of fiscal, budget, administrative and policy matters. Industries served: public, private, nonprofit agencies, and businesses. Geographic Area Served: Primarily midwest, although will travel nationwide.

Marshfield

★ 14825 ★ Marshfield Clinic Inc.
1000 N Oak Ave.
Marshfield, WI 54449-5703
Phone: (715)387-5511 **Free:** 800-782-8581
Fax: (715)387-5240
Website: http://www.marshfieldclinic.org

Fnded: 1978. **Activities:** Medical education specialists serving physicians, nurses, laboratories, and allied healthcare organizations, as well as various government agencies. Produces audiovisual and other educational programs as well as numerous supplemental medical evaluation videotapes ranging in subject content from allergies to cost containment topics of urology and rheumatology; available in single or series format. Geographic Area Served: United States and Canada.

★ 14826 ★ National Farm Medicine Center
1000 N Oak Ave.
Marshfield, WI 54449-5790
Phone: (715)387-9298 **Free:** 800-662-6900
Fax: (715)389-4950
Email: webmaster@marshfieldclinic.org
Website: http://www.marshfieldclinic.org/nfmc

Activities: Offers a variety of research, education, and service projects focusing on clinical health issues affecting farm workers and families. Special focus areas include: respiratory disease, noise-induced hearing loss, and degenerative joint disease. Industries served: rural Americans and healthcare workers and educators who provide services to the rural community.

Milwaukee

★ 14827 ★ Kowalski-Dickow Associates Inc.
PO Box 170678
Milwaukee, WI 53217-8056
Phone: (262)241-7060 **Fax:** (262)241-7067
Email: kda@kdaconsult.com
Website: http://www.kdaconsult.com

Fnded: 1979. **Activities:** Materials management specialists serving primarily healthcare providers/hospitals by assisting in the development of strategies and programs to increase services and productivity of limited resources, as well as reducing operating expenses. Materials management methods are applied to non-clinical support services to achieve optimum efficiency, productivity, quality, and control.

★ 14828 ★ Shared Care Research & Education Consulting Inc.
2821 N 4th St., Ste. 410
Milwaukee, WI 53212
Phone: (414)374-2733 **Free:** 800-962-7787
Fax: (414)374-9927
Email: sharedcare@aol.com
Website: http://sharedcare.net

Fnded: 1985. **Activities:** Develops and sells video tutored courses and services for healthcare professionals. Also supplies healthcare/medical equipment. Current specialties: training volunteers and professionals in proper blood pressure measurement technique. Maintains certification database for anti-hypertensive research. Clinical trial consultant. **Remarks:** Shared care has set the standard for Human BP Measurement Standardization in Pharmaceutical trial for a decade. Geographic Area Served: Worldwide.

Pewaukee

★ 14829 ★ Dr. Rebecca Cogwell Anderson, PhD
1104 Riverway Ct.
Pewaukee, WI 53072
Phone: (262)454-5464 **Fax:** (262)454-5464
Email: Rander5727@aol.com

Activities: A psychologist specializing in the areas of women's health issues, breast cancer adjustment, depression, wellness, stress management, post traumatic stress disorder, silicone breast implants/issues and adjustments, chronic disease, adjustment to loss of function and disfigurement, and parenting issues.

Richfield

★ 14830 ★ Advanced Health Care Concepts
3799 Turnwood Dr.
Richfield, WI 53076-9633
Phone: (262)628-9007 **Fax:** (262)628-3590

Fnded: 1980. **Activities:** Consulting and continuing education for nurses/aides/emergency medical technicians. Consulting services to nursing service departments in hospitals, nursing homes, HMOS, and public health facilities.

Wyoming

Cheyenne

★ 14831 ★ Options & Choices
2232 Dell Range Blvd., Ste. 300
Cheyenne, WY 82009-4005
Phone: (307)635-3777 **Fax:** (307)634-0828
Email: info@oci.com
Website: http://www.optis.com

Fnded: 1985. **Activities:** Offers health education expertise to businesses on dealing with disabilities. Geographic Area Served: Wyoming, Maryland, Tennessee, and Washington, D.C.

Chapter 5
Peer Review Organizations

The following is a state listing of peer review organizations. Consult the "User's Guide" located at the front of this directory for additional information.

Alabama

★ 14832 ★ Alabama Quality Assurance Foundation, Inc.
1 Perimeter Park S, Ste. 200 N
Birmingham, AL 35243-2354
Phone: (205)970-1600 **Fax:** (205)970-1616
Website: http://www.agaf.com
Henry W. Koehler, CEO

Alaska

★ 14833 ★ PRO-WEST
721 Sesame St., Ste. 1A
Anchorage, AK 99503
Phone: (907)562-2252 **Fax:** (907)562-2149
Website: http://www.pro-west.org
Jonathan Sugarman, MD, CEO & Pres

Arizona

★ 14834 ★ Health Services Advisory Group, Inc.
301 E Bethany Home Rd., Ste. B-157
Phoenix, AZ 85012
Phone: (602)264-6382 **Fax:** (602)241-0757
Website: http://www.hsag.com/
Lawrence J. Shapiro, MD, CEO & Pres

Arkansas

★ 14835 ★ Arkansas Foundation for Medical Care, Inc.
2201 Brooken Hill Dr.
PO Box 180001
Fort Smith, AR 72918-0001
Phone: (501)649-8501 **Fax:** (501)649-8180
Website: http://www.afmc.org
Russell G. Brasher, PhD, CEO

California

★ 14836 ★ California Medical Review, Inc.
1 Sansome St., Ste. 600
San Francisco, CA 94104
Phone: (415)677-2000 **Fax:** (415)677-2195
Website: http://www.cmri-ca.org
Jo Ellen H. Ross, CEO & Pres

Colorado

★ 14837 ★ Colorado Foundation for Medical Care
2851 S Parker Rd., Ste. 1000
Aurora, CO 80014-2713
Phone: (303)695-3300 **Fax:** (303)695-3350
Website: http://www.cfmc.org
Arja P. Adair, Jr, CEO & Pres

Connecticut

★ 14838 ★ Qualidigm Connecticut Peer Review Organization, Inc.
100 Roscommon Dr., Ste. 200
Middletown, CT 06457
Phone: (860)632-2008 **Fax:** (860)632-5865
Marcia K. Petrillo, CEO

Delaware

★ 14839 ★ Quality Insights of Delaware
Plaza III, 1847 Marsh Rd.
Wilmington, DE 19810
Phone: (302)475-8100 **Fax:** (302)475-7317
John C. Wiesendanger, CEO

District of Columbia

★ 14840 ★ Delmarva Foundation for Medical Care, Inc.
1620 L St., NW, Ste. 1275
Washington, DC 20036
Phone: (202)293-9650 **Fax:** (202)293-7317
Website: http://www.dfmc.org
Thomas J. Schaefer, CEO

Florida

★ 14841 ★ Florida Medical Quality Assurance, Inc.
4350 W Cypress St., Ste. 900
Tampa, FL 33607
Phone: (813)354-9111 **Fax:** (813)354-0737
Website: http://www.fmqai.com
Logan Malone, EdD, CEO

Georgia

★ 14842 ★ Georgia Medical Care Foundation
57 Executive Park S, Ste. 200
Atlanta, GA 30329
Phone: (404)982-0411 **Fax:** (404)982-7584
Website: http://www.gmcf.org
Tom W. Williams, CEO

Hawaii

★ 14843 ★ Mountain-Pacific Quality Health Foundation
1360 S Beretania St., Ste. 501
Honolulu, HI 96814
Phone: (808)545-2550 **Fax:** (808)440-6030
Dee Dee Nelson, Director

Idaho

★ 14844 ★ PRO-West/Idaho
720 Park Blvd., Ste. 120
Boise, ID 83712-7756
Phone: (208)343-4617 **Fax:** (208)343-4705
Website: http://www.pro-west.org
Jonathan R. Sugarman, MD, CEO

Illinois

★ 14845 ★ Illinois Foundation for Medical Care
2625 Butterfield Rd., Ste. 104S
Oak Brook, IL 60521
Phone: (630)571-5540 **Fax:** (630)571-5611
Fred Ferree, Exec VP

Indiana

★ 14846 ★ Health Care Excel, Inc.
2901 Ohio Blvd.
PO Box 3713
Terre Haute, IN 47803
Phone: (812)234-1499 **Fax:** (812)232-6167
Sharon Pygman, CEO

Iowa

★ 14847 ★ Iowa Foundation for Medical Care/The Sunderbruch Corp.
6000 Westtown Parkway, Ste. 350E
West Des Moines, IA 50266-7771
Phone: (515)223-2900 **Fax:** (515)222-2407
Website: http://www.ifmc.org/
Fred A. Ferree, Exec VP

★ 14848 ★ The Sunderbruch Corp., Nebraska
6000 Westtown Parkway, Ste. 350E
West Des Moines, IA 50266-7771
Phone: (515)223-2900 **Fax:** (515)222-2407
Fred A. Ferree, Exec VP

Kansas

★ 14849 ★ Kansas Foundation for Medical Care, Inc.
2947 SW Wanamaker Dr.
Topeka, KS 66614
Phone: (785)273-2552 **Fax:** (785)273-5130
Website: http://www.kfmc.org
Larry Pitman, CEO & Pres

Kentucky

★ 14850 ★ Health Care Excel, Inc.
9300 Shelbyville Rd.
Hurstburg Place, Ste. 600
Louisville, KY 40222
Phone: (502)339-7442 **Fax:** (502)339-8641
Sharon Pygman, CEO

Louisiana

★ 14851 ★ Louisiana Health Care Review, Inc.
8591 United Plaza Blvd., Ste. 270
Baton Rouge, LA 70809
Phone: (504)926-6353 **Fax:** (504)923-0957
Website: http://www.lhcr.org
Leo Stanley, CEO

Maryland

★ 14852 ★ Delmarva Foundation for Medical Care, Inc.
9240 Centreville Rd.
Easton, MD 21601
Phone: (410)822-0697 **Fax:** (410)822-9572
Website: http://www.dfmc.org
Thomas J. Schaefer, CEO

Massachusetts

★ 14853 ★ Massachusetts Peer Review Organization, Inc.
235 Wyman St.
Waltham, MA 02451
Phone: (781)890-0011 **Fax:** (781)487-0083
Website: http://www.masspro.org
Kathleen E. McCarthy, CEO & Pres

Michigan

★ 14854 ★ Michigan Peer Review Organization
40600 Ann Arbor Rd., Ste. 200
Plymouth, MI 48170-4495
Phone: (734)459-0900 **Fax:** (734)454-7301
Website: http://www.mpro.org
Carli Meister, CEO

Minnesota

★ 14855 ★ Stratis Health
2901 Metro Dr., Ste. 400
Bloomington, MN 55425
Phone: (612)854-3306 **Fax:** (612)853-8503
Website: http://www.stratishealth.org
Patricia Riley, CEO

Mississippi

★ 14856 ★ Information and Quality Healthcare
385 Highland Colony Parkway, Ste. 120
Ridgeland, MS 39157
Phone: (601)957-1575 **Fax:** (601)956-1713
Website: http://www.iqh.org/
James McIlwain, MD, President

Missouri

★ 14857 ★ Missouri Patient Care Review Foundation
3425 Constitution Court, Ste. E
Jefferson City, MO 65109
Phone: (573)893-7900 **Fax:** (573)893-5827
Website: http://www.mpcrf.org
Richard A. Royer, CEO

Montana

★ 14858 ★ Mountain-Pacific Quality Health Foundation
3404 Cooney Dr.
Helena, MT 59602
Phone: (406)443-4020 **Fax:** (406)443-4585
Website: http://www.mt.net/~mtwy/
Janice Connors, Exec Director

Nevada

★ 14859 ★ HealthInsight
500 S Rancho Dr., Ste. C-17
Las Vegas, NV 89106
Phone: (702)385-9923 **Fax:** (702)385-4586
Website: http://www.healthinsight.org/
Marc Bennett, CEO & Pres

New Hampshire

★ 14860 ★ Northeast Health Care Quality Foundation
15 Old Rollinsford Rd., Ste. 302
Dover, NH 03820-2830
Phone: (603)749-1641 **Fax:** (603)749-1195
Website: http://www.medicarequality.org
Robert A. Aurilio, CEO

New Jersey

★ 14861 ★ The Peer Review Organization of New Jersey, Inc.
557 Cranbury Rd., Ste. 21
East Brunswick, NJ 08816
Phone: (732)238-5570 **Fax:** (732)238-7766
Martin P. Margolies, CEO

New Mexico

★ 14862 ★ New Mexico Medical Review Association
2340 Menaul Blvd. NE, Ste. 300
PO Box 3200
Albuquerque, NM 87190-3200
Phone: (505)998-9898 **Fax:** (505)998-9899
Dan Jaco, CEO

New York

★ 14863 ★ Island Peer Review Organization, Inc.
1979 Marcus Ave., 1st Fl.
Lake Success, NY 11042-1002
Phone: (516)326-7767 **Fax:** (516)328-2310
Website: http://www.ipro.org
Theodore O. Will, Exec VP

North Carolina

★ 14864 ★ Medical Review of North Carolina, Inc.
5625 Dillard Dr., Ste. 203
Cary, NC 27511-9227
Phone: (919)851-2955 **Fax:** (919)851-8457
Website: http://www.carolinaqio.org
Charles J. Riddick, Exec Director

North Dakota

★ 14865 ★ North Dakota Health Care Review, Inc.
800 31st Ave. SW
Minot, ND 58701
Phone: (701)852-4231 **Fax:** (701)838-6009
Website: http://www.ndhcri.org/
David Remillard, CEO

Ohio

★ 14866 ★ Ohio KePRO, Inc.
Rock Run Center
5700 Lombardo Center Dr., Ste. 100
Seven Hills, OH 44131
Phone: (216)447-9604 **Fax:** (216)447-7925
Website: http://www.kepro.org/
Marcia Rynearson, Exec Director

Oklahoma

★ 14867 ★ Oklahoma Foundation for Medical Quality, Inc.
5801 Broadway Extension
The Paragon Bldg., Ste. 400
Oklahoma City, OK 73118-7489
Phone: (405)840-2891 **Fax:** (405)840-1343
Website: http://www.ofmq.com
Jim L. Williams, CEO & Pres

Oregon

★ 14868 ★ Oregon Medical Professional Review Organization
2020 SW 4th Ave., Ste. 520
Portland, OR 97201-4960
Phone: (503)279-0100 **Fax:** (503)279-0190
Website: http://www.ompro.org/
Robert S. Kinoshita, CEO & Pres

Pennsylvania

★ 14869 ★ Keystone Peer Review Organization, Inc.
777 E Park Dr.
PO Box 8310
Harrisburg, PA 17105-8310
Phone: (717)564-8288 **Fax:** (717)564-3862
Website: http://www.kepro.org
John DiNardi, III, Exec Director

Puerto Rico

★ 14870 ★ Quality Improvement Professional Research Organization
Mercantile Plaza Bldg., Ste. 605
San Juan, PR 00918
Phone: (787)641-1240 **Fax:** (787)641-1248
Website: http://www.netdial.caribe.net/~qipro/~qi-pro.html
Jose Robles, CEO

Rhode Island

★ 14871 ★ Rhode Island Quality Partners, Inc.
9 Hayes St.
Providence, RI 02908
Phone: (401)528-3200 **Fax:** (401)528-3210
Marsha K. Petrillo, Exec Director

South Carolina

★ 14872 ★ Carolina Medical Review
250 Berryhill Rd., Ste. 101
Columbia, SC 29210
Phone: (803)731-8225 **Fax:** (803)731-8229
Website: http://www.carolinaqio.org
Diana M. Zona, Contact

South Dakota

★ 14873 ★ South Dakota Foundation for Medical Care
1323 S Minnesota Ave.
Sioux Falls, SD 57105
Phone: (605)336-3505 **Fax:** (605)336-0270

Website: http://www.sdfmc.org/
Mark Hoven, CEO

Tennessee

★ 14874 ★ Mid-South Foundation for Medical Care, Inc.
3175 Lenox Park Blvd., Ste. 309
Memphis, TN 38119
Phone: (901)682-0381 **Fax:** (901)761-3786
Website: http://www.tnproqio.com/
Albert J. Grobmyer III, MD, CEO

Texas

★ 14875 ★ Texas Medical Foundation
901 Mopac Expwy. S
Barton Oaks Plaza 2, Ste. 200
Austin, TX 78746-5799
Phone: (512)329-6610 **Fax:** (512)327-7159
Website: http://www.tmf.org
Philip K. Dunne, CEO

Utah

★ 14876 ★ HealthInsight
348 E 4500 South, Ste. 300
Salt Lake City, UT 84107
Phone: (801)892-0155 **Fax:** (801)892-0160
Website: http://www.healthinsight.org/
Marc Bennett, CEO & Pres

Virgin Islands

★ 14877 ★ Virgin Islands Medical Institute, Inc.
1AD Estate Diamond Ruby
PO Box 5989
St Croix, VI 00823-5989
Phone: (340)712-2400 **Fax:** (340)712-2449
Website: http://www.networkvi.com/vimi
Patrick Peterson, CEO

Virginia

★ 14878 ★ Virginia Health Quality Center
1604 Santa Rosa Rd., Ste. 200
Richmond, VA 23288-0070
Phone: (804)289-5320 **Fax:** (804)289-5324
Website: http://www.vhqc.org
Joy Hogan Rozman, CEO

Washington

★ 14879 ★ PRO-West
10700 Meridian Ave. N, Ste. 100
Seattle, WA 98133-9075
Phone: (206)364-9700 **Fax:** (206)368-2427
Website: http://www.pro-west.org
Jonathan Sugarman, CEO

West Virginia

★ 14880 ★ West Virginia Medical Institute, Inc.
3001 Chesterfield Pl.
Charleston, WV 25304
Phone: (304)346-9864 **Fax:** (304)346-9863
Website: http://www.wvmi.org
John Wiesendanger, CEO

Wisconsin

★ 14881 ★ MetaStar, Inc.
2909 Landmark Pl.
Madison, WI 53713
Phone: (608)274-1940 **Fax:** (608)274-5008
Website: http://www.metastar.com
Greg E. Simmons, CEO & Pres

Wyoming

★ 14882 ★ Mountain-Pacific Quality Health Foundation
1950 Bluegrass Cir., Ste. 280
Cheyenne, WY 82009
Phone: (307)778-8404 **Fax:** (307)778-9161
Janice Connors, Exec Director

Chapter 6
Medical Ethics and History Organizations

Listed below are organizations, centers, and educational programs specializing in biomedical ethics and medical history. Entries are arranged alphabetically by organization or program name. For additional information, see the "User's Guide" located at the front of this directory.

★ 14883 ★ Advocate Luthern General Hospital
Center for Clinical Ethics
1775 Dempster St.
Park Ridge, IL 60068
Phone: (847)696-7847 **Fax:** (847)723-6667
Email: clint.moore@advocatehealth.com
John La Puma, MD, Director

★ 14884 ★ American Academy of Medical Ethics
4205 Mcauley Blvd., Ste. 420
Oklahoma City, OK 73120
Phone: (405)751-6111 **Fax:** (405)751-0479
Curtis E. Harris, MD, Director

★ 14885 ★ American Institute of Medical Ethics
409 Encina Ave.
Davis, CA 95616
Phone: (530)758-0739
John F. Monagle, PhD, Director

★ 14886 ★ American Medical Association Council on Ethical and Judicial Affairs
515 N State St.
Chicago, IL 60610
Phone: (312)464-4823 **Fax:** (312)464-4799
Website: http://www.ama-assn.org/go/ceja
Linda L. Emanuel, MD, Contact

★ 14887 ★ American Society of Law, Medicine and Ethics
765 Commonwealth Ave., 16th Fl.
Boston, MA 02215
Phone: (617)262-4990 **Fax:** (617)437-7596
Email: info@aslme.org
Website: http://www.aslme.org
Lawrence Gostin, Director

★ 14888 ★ Ankara Medical Faculty
Department Of Deontology
Sihhiye
TR-06100 Ankara, Turkey
Phone: 90 4 3103010 **Fax:** 90 4 3106370
Email: arda@dialup.ankara.edu.tr
Website: http://www.ankara.edu.tr
Yaman Ors, MD, Contact

★ 14889 ★ Applied Research Ethics National Association (ARENA)
126 Brookline Ave., Ste. 202
Boston, MA 02115
Phone: (617)423-4112 **Fax:** (617)423-1185
Email: info@arena.org
Website: http://www.primr.org
Jeffrey Cohen, Director

★ 14890 ★ ASEAN Institute for Health Development (AIHD)
25/5 Phutthamonthon 4
Salaya
Nakhon Chaisri
Nakhon Pathom 73170, Thailand
Phone: 662 441 9040 **Fax:** 662 441 9044
Email: direct@mahidol.ac.th
Website: http://www.mahidol.ac.th
Dr. Som-arch Wongkhomthong, Director
Remarks: The institute provides long and short-term trainings in the field of health and health care ethics.

★ 14891 ★ Australian Catholic Hospital/ Saint Vincent's Hospital
Plunkett Centre for Ethics in Health Care
Victoria St.
Darlinghurst, NSW 2010, Australia
Phone: 61 02 3612869 **Fax:** 61 02 3610975
Email: plunkett@plunkett.edu.au
Website: http://www.acu.edu.au/plunkett/
Dr. Bernadette Tobin, Director

★ 14892 ★ Ball State University
Department of Biology
Human Genetics and Bioethics Education Lab
2000 University Ave.
Muncie, IN 47306
Phone: (765)285-8840 **Fax:** (765)285-8804
Email: 01JRHendrix@bsuvc.BSU.Edu
Jon R. Hendrix, Director

★ 14893 ★ Baylor College of Medicine
Center for Medical Ethics and Health Policy
One Baylor Plaza
IREL, Rm. 401
Houston, TX 77030
Phone: (713)798-6290 **Fax:** (713)798-5678
Website: http://www.bcm.tmc.edu/ethics/
Baruch Brody, PhD, Director

★ 14894 ★ Ben-Gurion University of the Negev
Lord Immanuel Jakobovits Center for Jewish Medical Ethics
PO Box 653
IL-84105 Beer-Sheva, Israel
Phone: 972 76477415 **Fax:** 972 76477633
Email: gshimon@bgumail.bgu.ac.il
Prof. Shimon Glick, Director
Dr. Yeruham Leavitt, Director

★ 14895 ★ Beth Israel Hospital
Ethics Program
330 Brookline Ave.
Boston, MA 02215
Phone: (617)667-8000 **Fax:** (617)735-4393
Rabbi Terry R. Bard, Director

★ 14896 ★ Bioethics Centre
University of Otago
PO Box 913
Dunedin, New Zealand
Phone: 64 3 4747977 **Fax:** 64 3 4747601
Email: bioethics@otago.ac.nz
Website: http://www.otago.ac.nz/bioethics
Donald Evans, Director

★ 14897 ★ Bioethics Resource Group
1112 Harding Place, No. 200
Charlotte, NC 28204
Phone: (704)332-4421 **Fax:** (704)376-3173
Email: regionalnet@brg.org
Website: http://www.meckmed.org/bioethics
Bill Porter, MD, Director

★ 14898 ★ Bioethics Studies Centre
A. Humberto Delgad 444
P-3030-327 Coimbra, Portugal
Phone: 239712806
Email: jbiscaia@mail.telepac.pt
Dr. Jorge Biscaia, Director
Fnded: 1988. **Remarks:** Members of the center include philosophers, lawyers, doctors, theologians, psychologists, and biologists. It organizes 4-5 meetings a year and publishes a journal and various books.

★ 14899 ★ Borja Institute of Bioethics (Institut Borja de Bioetica)
Llaseres 30
08190 Sant Cugat del Valles
Barcelona, Spain
Phone: 34 93 674 47 66 **Fax:** 34 93 674 79 80
Email: ibbioetica@bioinsbor.org
Website: http://www.bioinsbor.org
Francesc Abel, MD/PhD, Director

★ 14900 ★ Boston University Schools of Medicine and Public Health
Law, Medicine, and Ethics Program
715 Albany St. T3w
Boston, MA 02118
Phone: (617)638-4626 **Fax:** (617)638-5299
George J. Annas, Director

★ 14901 ★ Bowling Green State University
Department of Philosophy
Social Philosophy and Policy Center
305 Shatzel Hall
Bowling Green, OH 43403-0222
Phone: (419)372-2117 **Fax:** (419)372-8191
Website: http://www.bgsu.edu/offices/sppc/journal.htm
Thomas Attig, PhD, Director

★ 14902 ★ Brown University Program in Biomedical Ethics
54 College St.
Providence, RI 02912
Phone: (401)863-2718 **Fax:** (401)863-2719
Prof. Sumner B. Twiss, Director

★ 14903 ★ Cambridge Medical Ethics Forum
Churchill College
Storey's Way
Cambridge CB3 0DS, United Kingdom
Dr. Richard Grove, Director

★ 14904 ★ Canadian Bioethics Society (CBS)
A.NR. 222, 8220 - 114 St.
Edmunton, AB, Canada T6G 2J3
Phone: (780)492-6676 **Fax:** (780)492-0673
Bartha M. Knoppers, PhD, Director

★ 14905 ★ Canadian Medical Association Department of Ethics and Legal Affairs
1867 Alta Vista Dr.
Ottawa, ON, Canada K1G 3Y6
Phone: (613)731-9331 **Free:** 800-267-9703
Fax: (613)731-9013
John R. Williams, PhD, Director

★ 14906 ★ Cardiff University Centre for Applied Ethics
PO Box 94
Cardiff CF10 3XB, United Kingdom
Phone: 44 29 20874025 **Fax:** 44 29 20874618
Email: philosophy@cardiff.ac.uk
Ruth Chadwick, Director
Frmly: University of Wales College of Cardiff.

★ 14907 ★ Caroline Chisholm Centre for Health Ethics
166 Gipps St.
East Melbourne, VIC 3002, Australia
Phone: 61 03 9270 2681 **Fax:** 61 03 9270 2682
Email: ccche@mercy.com.au
Rev. Norman Ford, Director
Remarks: The Centre publishes a quarterly journal, proceedings of conferences, and ethics-related kits.

★ 14908 ★ Catholic Health Association Division of Theology, Mission and Ethics
4455 Woodson Rd.
Saint Louis, MO 63134
Phone: (314)427-2500 **Fax:** (314)427-0029
Rev. Joseph Kukura, Director

★ 14909 ★ Catholic Health Association of Canada
1247 Kilborn
Ottawa, ON, Canada K1H 6K9
Phone: (613)731-7148 **Fax:** (613)731-7797
Email: sdeliencourt@cyberus.ca
Website: http://www.chac.ca
Rev. Everett MacNeil, Director

★ 14910 ★ Catholic Institute of Lille / Polytechnical University of Lille Centre D'Ethique Medicale (CEM)
56 Rue Du Port
59046 Lille Cedex, France
Phone: 33 20 134046 **Fax:** 33 20 782645
Email: secretariat.cem@fupl.asso.fr
Website: http://www.fupl.asso.fr
Prof. Marie-Louise Lamau, Director

★ 14911 ★ Catholic Medical Association
N 27th W 23957 Paul Rd.
PO Box 757
Pewaukee, WI 53072-0757
Phone: (262)523-6201 **Fax:** (262)523-6211
Email: info@cathmed.org
Website: http://www.cathmed.org
Charles Hermes, MD, Director
Frmly: National Federation of Catholic Physician's Guilds.

★ 14912 ★ Catholic University of Chile School of Medicine Bioethics Unit
PO Box 114-D
Santiago 1, Chile
Phone: 56 2 332051 **Fax:** 56 2 2225515
Fernando Jose R. da Rocha, Director

★ 14913 ★ Catholic University of Louvain Bioethics Studies Center
1, place de l'Universite
B-1348 Louvain la Neuve, Belgium
Phone: 32 10472111
Website: http://www.ucl.ac.be/
Jean-Francois Malherbe, Director

★ 14914 ★ Catholic University of Nijmegen Department of Ethics, Philosophy and History of Medicine European Society for Philosophy of Medicine and Health Care (ESPMH)
PO Box 9101
NL-6500 HB Nijmegen, Netherlands
Phone: 31 243 615320 **Fax:** 31 243 540254
Email: h.tenhave@efg.kun.nl
H. Ten Have, MD, Director
Remarks: The Department offers research programs in the ethics of genetics and the ethics of palliative care; summer course in bioethics; advanced courses in ethics and genetics and ethics and pallative care; and European Masters in Bioethics. The Society holds an annual conference. **Pub:** *Medicine, Health Care and Philosophy.*

★ 14915 ★ Catholic University of Nijmegen Department of Ethics, Philosophy and History of Medicine International Program in Bioethics Education and Research (IPBER)
PO Box 9101
NL-6500 HB Nijmegen, Netherlands
Phone: 31 80 615320 **Fax:** 31 80 540254
Henk A.M.J. ten Have, Director

★ 14916 ★ Catholic University of Sacro Cuore A. Gemelli Faculty of Medicine and Surgery Bioethics Center / Institute of Bioethics
Largo Francesco Vito, 1
I-00168 Rome, Italy
Phone: 39 6 30154960 **Fax:** 39 6 3051149
Email: istbio@uni.net
Website: http://www.centrobioetica.org
Antonio G. Spagnolo, MD, Contact
Remarks: The Center has postgraduate courses in bioethics and publishes a journal.

★ 14917 ★ Catholic University of Uruguay Institute of Bioethics
Av. 8 de Octubre No. 2738
11600 Montevideo, Uruguay
Phone: 598 2 4872717 **Fax:** 598 2 4870323
Email: etica@ucu.edu.uy
Website: http://www.ucu.edu.uy
Omar Franca, MD, Director
Remarks: The Bioethics Service engages in bioethics documentation, research, and teaching.

★ 14918 ★ Center of Documentation in Health Sciences Ethics National Consulting Committee of Health and Life Sciences Ethics
101 rue de Tolbiac
F-75013 Paris, France
Phone: 33 1 44236015
Marie-Helene Lhuguenot, Director

★ 14919 ★ Center for Ethics Washington Hospital Center
110 Irving St. NW, Rm. EB 3108
Washington, DC 20010-2975
Phone: (202)877-0246 **Fax:** (202)877-3898
Email: nneka.o.mokwunuye@medstar.net
Janicemarie K. Vinicky, MD, Director

★ 14920 ★ Center for Ethics and Advocacy in Health Care
PO Box 525
2001 Waukegan Rd.
Techny, IL 60082
Phone: (847)509-9130
Email: PMcdonn702@aol.com
M. Margaret McDonnell, Director

★ 14921 ★ Central Ethical Committee of the Ministry of Health of the Czech Republic
Palaokeo 4
128 01 Prague 2, Czech Republic
Phone: 42 2 295343 **Fax:** 42 2 290092
Milan Kment, MD, Director

★ 14922 ★ Centre for Biomedical Ethics Development
J1. Kramat VI/7
Jakarta, Indonesia
Phone: 62 021 3140455 **Fax:** 62 021 326044
Email: perdhaki@cbn.net.id
Program(s): Guidance & Counseling

★ 14923 ★ Centre Sevres Department of Biomedical Ethics
12, rue d'Assas
F-75006 Paris, France
Phone: 33 1 45441899 **Fax:** 33 1 45449020
Patrick Verspieren, Director

★ 14924 ★ Children's National Medical Center Office of Ethics
111 Michigan Ave.
Washington, DC 20010
Phone: (202)884-3201 **Fax:** (202)884-3630
Email: tsilber@cnmc.org
Website: http://www.cnmc.org/
Sanford L. Leikin, MD, Director

★ 14925 ★ Chinese Academy of Social Sciences Institute of Philosophy Programs in Bioethics
5 Jianguomennei Ave.
Beijing, People's Republic of China
Phone: 86 1 5122025 **Fax:** 86 1 5137828
Prof. Qiu Renzong, Director

★ 14926 ★ Christian Medical and Dental Society
Medical Ethics Commission
PO Box 7500
Bristol, TN 37621
Phone: (423)844-1000 **Fax:** (423)844-1005
Email: main@christian-doctors.com
Robert D. Orr, MD, Director

★ 14927 ★ Cleveland Clinic Foundation
Department of Bioethics
Department of Bioethics, NA10
9500 Euclid Ave.
Cleveland, OH 44195
Phone: (216)444-8720 **Fax:** (216)444-9275
Website: http://www.clevelandclinic.org/bioethics
George J. Agich, PhD, Director

★ 14928 ★ Cleveland State University
Department of Philosophy
Bioethics Program
Euclid Ave. at E 24th St.
Cleveland, OH 44115
Phone: (216)687-3900
Email: b.orgovan@csuohio.edu
Mary Ellen Waithe, PhD, Director

★ 14929 ★ Clinical Research Institute of Montreal
Centre for Bioethics
110 Pine Ave. West
Montreal, QC, Canada H2W 1R7
Phone: (514)987-5617 **Fax:** (514)987-5695
Email: royd@ircm.qc.ca
Website: http://www.ircm.qc.ca/bioethique/english/index.html
Dr. David J. Roy, Director

★ 14930 ★ Columbia University
College of Physicians and Surgeons
Center for Study of Society and Medicine
P&S Box 11
630 W 168th St.
New York, NY 10032
Phone: (212)305-4184 **Fax:** (212)305-6416
Email: tfr7@columbia.edu
Website: http://www.societyandmedicine.org
David Rothman, PhD, Director

★ 14931 ★ Columbian Association of Faculties of Medicine
Medical Ethics Center
Calle 39A, No. 28-63
Santa Fe de Bogota, D.E., Colombia
Phone: 57 1 2973601 **Fax:** 57 1 2699584
Email: jlopez@ascofame.org.co
Website: http://www.ascofame.org.co
Dr. Julio Enrique Ospina, Director

★ 14932 ★ Consumers for Ethics in Research (CERES)
PO Box 1365
London N16 0BW, United Kingdom
Phone: 44 81 8028231

★ 14933 ★ Costa Rica University
Institute of Philosophy Studies, Faculty of Letters
City University Rodrogo Facio'
Bioethics Investigations Program
San Pedro de Montes de Oca
San Jose, Costa Rica
Phone: 506 535323 **Fax:** 506 342347
Email: cgolcher@ucrvm2
Dr. Cristian Golcher-Carranza, Director

★ 14934 ★ Council of Europe
Steering Committee for Bioethics
Piece 2004
F-67006 Strasbourg Cedex, France
Phone: 33 88 412013
Octavi Quintana, Director

★ 14935 ★ Council for International Organizations of Medical Sciences (CIOMS)
c/o World Health Organization
CH-1211 Geneva 27, Switzerland
Phone: 41 22 791 34 06 **Fax:** 41 22 791 31 11
Email: idanpaanj@who.ch
Dr. Zbigniew Bankowski, Secretary-General
Remarks: The council publishes guidelines and publications in the fields of drug safety, bioethics/healthcare ethics, disease nomenclature and other fields of biomedicine and health.

★ 14936 ★ Council for Responsible Genetics (CRG)
5 Upland Rd., Ste. 3
Cambridge, MA 02140
Phone: (617)868-0870 **Fax:** (617)491-5344
Email: crg@gene-watch.org
Website: http://www.gene-watch.org
Nachama Wikler, Director

★ 14937 ★ Creighton University
Center for Health Policy and Ethics
2500 California Plaza
Omaha, NE 68178
Phone: (402)280-2017 **Fax:** (402)280-5735
Charles J. Dougherty, PhD, Director

★ 14938 ★ Danish Council on Ethics
Ravnsborggade, 2-4
DK-2200 Copenhagen N, Denmark
Phone: 45 35375833 **Fax:** 45 35375755
Email: etiskraad@etiskraad.dk
Website: http://www.etiskraad.dk
O. Munster, Director

★ 14939 ★ Department of Bioethics
Case Western Reserve University
10900 Euclid Ave.
Cleveland, OH 44106-4976
Phone: (216)368-6196 **Free:** 800-773-2633
Fax: (216)368-8713
Email: bioethics@cwru.edu
Website: http://www.cwru.edu/med/bioethics/bioethics.html
Thomas Murray, PhD, Director

★ 14940 ★ Dietrich Bonhoeffer International Institute for Bioethical Studies
GPO Box 588
Adelaide, SA 5001, Australia
Phone: 61 8 8297 0022 **Fax:** 61 8 8371 1391
Email: rjpollnitz@esc.net.au
Website: http://www.bio-ethics.com
Dr. Robert Pollnitz, Contact

★ 14941 ★ Division of Medical Ethics
641 Huntington Ave.
Boston, MA 02115
Phone: (617)432-2570 **Fax:** (617)432-3721
Email: dme@hms.harvard.edu
Lynn M. Peterson, MD, Director

★ 14942 ★ Division of Medical Ethics
LDS Hospital/University of Utah SOM
8th Ave. and C. St.
Salt Lake City, UT 84143
Phone: (801)408-1135 **Fax:** (801)408-5171
Email: ldjacob@ihc.com
Website: http://uuhsc.utah.edu/ethics
Jay A. Jacobson, MD, Director

★ 14943 ★ Dr. G.A. Lindeboom Institute
Center for Medical Ethics
Oude Kerkweg 100
PO Box 224
NL-6710 BE Ede, Netherlands
Phone: 318 696333 **Fax:** 318 696334
Email: lindinst@che.nl
Website: http://www.che.lindeboominstituut.nl
Prof. Dr. G.A. Lindeboom, PhD, Director
Remarks: The center is involved in the study, publication, education, and advise in the area of health care ethics.

★ 14944 ★ Dr. Jose Maria Mainetti Foundation
Bioethics and Medical Humanities Institute
Bioethics Center
calle 508 no. 2200 e/16 y 18
M.B. Gonnet
1897 Buenos Aires, Argentina
Phone: 54 221 471 1160 **Fax:** 54 221 471 2222
Email: elabe@satlink.com
Website: http://www.fundacionmainetti.org.ar
Dr. Jose Alberto Mainetti, Director
Liliana Barletta, Contact
Remarks: The center maintains a bioethics database and conducts continuing education courses in bioethics.

★ 14945 ★ East Carolina University
School of Medicine
Department of Medical Humanities
2 S-17 Brody Medical Sciences Bldg.
Greenville, NC 27858-4354
Phone: (252)816-2797 **Fax:** (252)816-2319
Email: kopelmanlo@med.ecu.edu
Website: http://www.med.ecu.edu/medhum/
Loretta M. Kopelman, PhD, Director

★ 14946 ★ Edinboro University of Pennsylvania
Bio-Medical Ethics Project
c/o Dr. James F. Drane
Edinboro, PA 16444
Phone: (814)732-2604 **Fax:** (814)732-2883
Email: whitney@edinboro.edu
James F. Drane, PhD, Contact

★ 14947 ★ Endocrinology Institute
Bioethics Committee of the Academy of Medicine
Bd. Aviatorilor, 34
Bucharest, Romania
Phone: 40 0 335751
Dr. C. Maximilian, Director

★ 14948 ★ Ersta Institute for Health Care Ethics
Box 4619
S-116 91 Stockholm, Sweden
Phone: 46 8 7146100 **Fax:** 46 8 6416671
Email: goran.lantz@teol.uu.se
Website: http://www.ersta.se
Goran Lantz, Director
Jana Vanova, Contact

★ 14949 ★ Espace Ethique (Observatoire et Institut) De L'Assistance Publique - Hopitaux De Paris
1, ave. Claude Vellefaux
75475 Paris, France
Phone: 33 1 44841757 **Fax:** 33 1 44841758
Email: espace.ethique@sls.ap-hop-paris.fr
Website: http://www.espace-ethique.org
Prof. Emmanuel Hirsch, Director

★ 14950 ★ Ethics Forum Inc.
1360 Beverly Rd., Ste. 201
McLean, VA 22101
Phone: (703)790-3480 **Fax:** (703)790-3460
Kurt Darr, Director

★ 14951 ★ The Ethox Centre
University of Oxford
Old Rd.
Oxford OX3 7LF, United Kingdom
Phone: 44 1865 226936 **Fax:** 44 1865 226938
Email: admin@ethox.ox.ac.uk
Tony Hope, PhD, Director

★ 14952 ★ Eubios Ethics Institute
PO Box 125
Tsukuba Science City 305-0005, Japan
Phone: 81 298 53 4662 **Fax:** 81 298 53 6614
Email: macer@biol.tsukuba.ac.jp
Website: http://www.biol.tsukuba.ac.jp/~macer/index.html
Darryl Macer, PhD, Director

★ 14953 ★ European Association of Centres of Medical Ethics (EACME)
Center for Biomedical Ethics and Law
Kapucijnenvoer 35
B-3000 Leuven, Belgium
Phone: 32 16 336951 **Fax:** 32 16 336952
Email: Paul.Schotsmans@med.kuleuven.ac.be
Website: http://www.kuleuven.ac.be/cbmer
Paul Schotsmans, Contact

★ 14954 ★ European Medical Students Association
Committee on Medical Ethics
54 Lochaline St.
London W6 9SH, United Kingdom
Miguel J. de Arbide, Contact

★ 14955 ★ Federal University of Rio Grande do Sul
Department of Philosophy
Ave. Bento Goncalves, 9500
91509-900 Porto Alegre, Brazil
Phone: 55 51 316 6897 **Fax:** 55 51 316 6616
Email: fjrr@ifch.ufrgs.br
Fernando Jose R. da Rocha, Contact

★ 14956 ★ Flinders Medical Centre
Medical Ethics Unit
404 Flinders Dr.
Bedford Park, SA 5042, Australia
Phone: 61 8 8204 5386 **Fax:** 61 8 8204 4639
Email: Brian.Stoffell@flinders.edu.au
Website: http://som.flinders.edu.au/hsmdu.html
Brian Stoffell, Director
Program(s): The Centre has a masters program in Health Services Management.

★ 14957 ★ Florida Bioethics Network
University of Miami
c/o Bioethics Program
PO Box 016960 (M-825)
Miami, FL 33101
Phone: (305)243-5723 **Fax:** (305)243-6416
Email: kggoodman@miami.edu
Esther Sanger, Director

★ 14958 ★ Free University of Brussels
Bioethics Center
Pleinlaan 2
B-1050 Brussels, Belgium
Phone: 32 2 6413408 **Fax:** 32 2 6413389
Email: scharles@vnet3.vub.ac.be
Prof. Charles Susanne, Director

★ 14959 ★ Free University of Brussels
Interdisciplinary Research Center in Bioethics
145, Ave. Adolphe Buyl
CP 188
B-1050 Brussels, Belgium
Phone: 32 2 6502628 **Fax:** 32 2 6503647
Prof. Gilbert Hottois, Director

★ 14960 ★ French Society of Bioethics Studies
30 rue d'Auteuil
F-75016 Paris, France
Dr. Marie-Helene Congourdeau, Director

★ 14961 ★ Gateway Catholic Ethics Network
6626 Mardel Ave.
Saint Louis, MO 63109
Phone: (314)994-7721 **Fax:** (314)994-7862
Email: michael_panicola@ssmhc.com
William Longust, Director

★ 14962 ★ Georg August University at Gottingen
Department of Ethics and History of Medicine
((Georg-August-Universitat Gottingen) Abteilung fur Ethik und Geschichte der Medizin)
Humboldtallee 36
D-37073 Gottingen, Germany
Phone: 49 551 399006 **Fax:** 49 551 399554
Website: http://www.gwdg.de/paracelsus
Dr. Stella Reiter-Theil, Director

★ 14963 ★ George Mason University
Center for Health Policy Research and Ethics
4400 University Dr.
Fairfax, VA 22030-4444
Phone: (703)993-1931 **Fax:** (703)993-1953
Email: chpre@gmu.edu
Website: http://www.chpre.gmu.edu
Mary Wakefield, PhD, Director

★ 14964 ★ Georgia Health Decisions
1720 Peachtree St., Ste. 1029
Atlanta, GA 30309
Phone: (404)874-9327 **Free:** 800-544-5751
Fax: (404)874-9327
Website: http://www.critical-conditions.org
Beverly A. Tyler, Director

★ 14965 ★ Goteborg University
Center for Research Ethics
Box 700
SE 405 30 Goteborg, Sweden
Phone: 46 31 7734934 **Fax:** 46 31 7734863
Email: swelin@cre.gu.se
Website: http://www.cre.gu.se/homepage
Stellan Welin, Director
Eiua Hagberg, Secretary
Remarks: Publishes booklets on research ethics and participates in PhD courses.

★ 14966 ★ Graduate Theological Union
Center for Ethics and Social Policy (CESP)
2400 Ridge Rd.
Berkeley, CA 94709
Phone: (510)649-2560 **Fax:** (510)649-2565
Email: cesp@gtu.edu
Website: http://www.gtu.edu/centers/CESP/cesp.html
Robert N. Bellah, Director

★ 14967 ★ Hellenic Society for Medical Ethics
42 Amalias St.
GR-105 58 Athens, Greece
Phone: 30 1 3236783 **Fax:** 30 1 3238807
Dr. Meropi Violaki, Director

★ 14968 ★ Hiram College
Department of Biology
Biomedical Humanities Program
PO Box 67
Hiram, OH 44234
Phone: (330)569-3211
Email: madarsi@hiram.edu
Website: http://www.hiram.edu/acad/general.asp?dept=BIOM
Colleen Fried, Coordinator
Sandy Madar, Coordinator

★ 14969 ★ Holy Apostles College and Seminary
Pope John Paul II Bioethics Center
33 Prospect Hill Rd.
Cromwell, CT 06416-2005
Phone: (860)632-3033 **Free:** 800-330-7272
Fax: (860)632-3075
Website: http://www.holyapostles.edu
Very Rev. Douglas L. Mosey, PhD, Director

★ 14970 ★ Hospital for Sick Children
Department of Bioethics
555 University Ave.
Toronto, ON, Canada M5G 1X8
Phone: (416)813-5000 **Fax:** (416)813-4967
Abbyann Lynch, Director

★ 14971 ★ Hungarian Academy of Sciences
Institute of Experimental Medicine
Commission Nationale de Bioethique de Hongria
1083 Szigony u 43
PO Box 167
H-1450 Budapest, Hungary
Phone: 36 1 1137616 **Fax:** 36 1 1141866
Dr. Vizi, Director

★ 14972 ★ International Federation of Catholic Medical Associations
Biomedical Ethics Center
St. Pius X College
Aarey Rd., Goregaon E
Bombay, India
Phone: 69 12 17
Dr. E.J. De Souza, Director

★ 14973 ★ International Institute of Ethics Studies-Juridiques sur la Nouvelle Biologie
Villa Eolian
Via Cappuccini
I-90057 Milazzo, Italy
Phone: 39 90 9282912 **Fax:** 39 90 9286565
Prof. Marado Milani-Comparetti, Director

★ 14974 ★ Iowa State University
Department of Philosophy
Bioethics Program
402 Catt Hall
Iowa State University
Ames, IA 50011
Phone: (515)294-5400 **Fax:** (515)294-0780
Email: bperri@iastate.edu
Website: http://grad.admin.iastate.edu/bioethics
Brad Pierri, Contact

★ 14975 ★ Johns Hopkins University School of Public Health Department of Health Policy and Management Program in Law, Ethics and Health
Baltimore, MD 21205
Phone: (410)955-3018
Website: http://www.med.jhu.edu/bioethics_institute
Ruth R. Faden, PhD, Director

★ 14976 ★ Kasteel Heyendael Catholic University Department of Medical Ethics
Geert Grooteplein Noord 9
NL-6525 EZ Nijmegen, Netherlands
Phone: 31 80 513104
C.J. Beemer, Director

★ 14977 ★ Keele University Centre for Professional Ethics
Keele Hall
Staffordshire ST5 5BG, United Kingdom
Phone: 44 1782 584084 **Fax:** 44 1782 584239
Email: ethics@keele.ac.uk
Website: http://www.keele.ac.uk/ethics
Adam Goldberg, Contact
Program(s): The Centre offers flexible part-time diploma and MA courses in: medical ethics and law healthcare ethics, research, and biotechnology ethics of cancer and palliative care ethics of social welfare.

★ 14978 ★ King's College London Centre of Medical Law and Ethics
Strand
London WC2R 2LS, United Kingdom
Phone: 44 020 7848 2382 **Fax:** 44 020 7848 2575
Email: cmle.eng@kcl.ac.uk
Website: http://www.kcl.ac.uk/
Richard Else, Director
Remarks: The centre provides postgraduate and professional courses and publishes a newsletter and occasional papers.

★ 14979 ★ Kingswood Centre for Applied Ethics
Hampden Rd.
Crawley, WA 6009, Australia
Phone: 61 09 3890389 **Fax:** 61 09 3890389
Colin Honey, Director

★ 14980 ★ Kitasato University School of Medicine Institute of Medical Humanities
1-15-1 Kitasato
Sagamihara, Japan
Koichi Bai, Director

★ 14981 ★ Kyoto Women's University Institute of Religion and Culture International Bioethics Research Center
35 Kita-Hioshi-machi Imakumano
Higashiyamaku, Japan
Phone: 81 75 5317221 **Fax:** 81 75 5317215
Kazumasa Hoshino, MD, Director

★ 14982 ★ L.J. Goody Bioethics Centre
39 Jugan St.
Glendalough, WA 6016, Australia
Phone: 61 08 9242 4066 **Fax:** 61 08 9242 4067
Email: ljgbc@iinet.net.au
Website: http://members.iinet.net.au/ljgbc
Dr. Joe C. Parkinson, Director
Dr. Walter K. Black, Sr. Consultant

★ 14983 ★ Lahey Clinic Medical Center Section of Medical Ethics
41 Mall Rd.
Burlington, MA 01805
Phone: (781)273-8400 **Fax:** (781)273-5245
Website: http://www.lahey.org
David Steinberg, MD, Director

★ 14984 ★ Laval University Philosophy Department Medical Ethics Research Group
Quebec City, QC, Canada G1K 7P4
Phone: (418)656-2244 **Fax:** (418)656-7267
Email: cz53@musica.McGill.ca
Marie-Helene Parizeau, Director

★ 14985 ★ Law of Ethics of the Medical Services
95, Boulevard Pinel
F-69677 Bron Cedex, France
Phone: 33 7 272358710 **Fax:** 33 7 272358740
Dr. Nicole Lery, Director

★ 14986 ★ Lawrence University Program in Biomedical Ethics
PO Box 599
Appleton, WI 54912-0599
Phone: (920)832-6670 **Fax:** (920)832-6944
Website: http://www.lawrence.edu/academics/biomed
John M. Stanley, Director

★ 14987 ★ Leuven Catholic University Faculty of Medicine Center for Biomedical Ethics and Law
Kapucijnenvoer 35
B-3000 Leuven, Belgium
Phone: 32 16 336951 **Fax:** 32 16 336952
Email: paul.schotsmaus@med.kuleuven.ac.be
Website: http://www.kuleuven.ac.be/cbmer
DR. Paul Schotsmans, Director

★ 14988 ★ Linacre Centre for Healthcare Ethics
60 Grove End Rd.
St. John's Wood
London NW8 9NH, United Kingdom
Phone: 44 20 7086 4088 **Fax:** 44 20 7266 5424
Email: admin@linacre.org
Website: http://www.linacre.org
Dr. Helen Watt, Director
Remarks: This Roman Catholic Centre publishes papers and books and sponsors conferences relating to health care ethics.

★ 14989 ★ Lincoln Medical Center Association Nebraska Health Decisions
4600 Valley Rd.
Lincoln, NE 68510
Phone: (402)483-7537
Jay Upright, Director

★ 14990 ★ Loma Linda University Center for Christian Bioethics
Coleman Pavilion Rm. 11121-S
Loma Linda, CA 92350
Phone: (909)558-4956 **Fax:** (909)558-0336
Email: hmorrison@ethicscenter.llu.edu
Website: http://www.llu.edu/llu/bioethics
David Larson, PhD, Director

★ 14991 ★ Louis-Jeantet de Medecine Foundation
Case Postale 227
CH-1211 Geneva 17, Switzerland
Phone: 41 22 7043636 **Fax:** 41 22 7043637
Email: info@jeantet.ch
Website: http://www.jeantet.ch
Alex Mauron, PhD, Contact

★ 14992 ★ Loyola University of Chicago Neiswanger Institute of Bioethics and Health Policy
2160 S 1st Ave.
Maywood, IL 60153
Phone: (708)327-9219 **Fax:** (708)327-9209
Email: ssom_bioethics@egroups.com
Website: http://bioethics.lumc.edu
David C. Thomasma, Director
Frmly: Medical Humanities Program.

★ 14993 ★ Loyola University of Chicago Philosophy Department Master's Degree Program in Health Care Ethics
6525 N Sheridan Rd.
Chicago, IL 60626
Phone: (773)508-2291 **Fax:** (773)508-2292
Email: mwaymac@luc.edu
Website: http://www.luc.edu/depts/philosophy/hcema.htm
David Ozar, Contact

★ 14994 ★ Lund University Department of Medical Ethics
Solvegatan 9
S-223 62 Lund, Sweden
Phone: 46 46 104040 **Fax:** 46 46 104045
Goran Hermeren, PhD, Director

★ 14995 ★ Massachusetts Health Decisions
PO Box 417
Sharon, MA 02067-0417
Phone: (781)784-1966
David B. Clarke, Director

★ 14996 ★ Max Planck Institute for Foreign and International Criminal Law Research in Ethics and Rights in Medicine
Gunderstrasse 73
D-79100 Freiburg, Germany
Phone: 49 761 7081223
Hans-Georg Koch, Contact

★ 14997 ★ McGill University McGill Centre for Medicine, Ethics and Law
3690 Peel St.
Montreal, QC, Canada H3A 1W9
Phone: (514)398-7400 **Fax:** (514)398-4668
Margaret A. Somerville, Director

★ 14998 ★ Medical College of Wisconsin Center for the Study of Bioethics
8701 Watertown Plank Rd.
PO Box 26509
Milwaukee, WI 53226-0509
Phone: (414)456-8498 **Fax:** (414)456-6511
Email: bioethics@mcw.edu
Website: http://www.mcw.edu/bioethics/
Robyn S. Shapiro, JD, Director

★ 14999 ★ Medical Ethics Resource Network of Michigan Michigan State University Center for Ethics and Humanities
C-208 E Fee Hall
East Lansing, MI 48824-1316
Phone: (517)355-7550 **Fax:** (517)353-3289
Email: mern@msu.edu
Website: http://www.mern.org
James Turrant, Director

★ 15000 ★ Michigan State University Center for Ethics and Humanities in the Life Sciences
C-208 E Fee Hall
East Lansing, MI 48824-1316
Phone: (517)355-7550 **Fax:** (517)353-3289
Email: center@msu.edu
Website: http://www.bioethics.msu.edu
Howard Brody, MD, Director

★ 15001 ★ Midwest Bioethics Center
1021-1025 Jefferson St.
Kansas City, MO 64105
Phone: (816)221-1100 **Free:** 800-344-3829
Fax: (816)221-2002
Email: bioethic@midbio.org
Website: http://www.midbio.org
Myra Christopher, Director

★ 15002 ★ Ministry of Health Bioethics Consultative Committee
Merchants St.
Valletta, Malta
Phone: 356 675683 **Fax:** 356 225028
Email: mcau@synapse.net.mt
Website: http://www.synapse.net.mt/bioethics
M.N. Cauchi, Director
Dr. P. Mallia, Secretary
Remarks: The Committee advises the Ministry of Health, organizes bioethics seminars, and provides representation at the Council of Europe Bioethics Committees.

★ 15003 ★ Minnesota Center for Health Care Ethics College of Saint Catherine
601 25th Ave. S
Minneapolis, MN 55454
Phone: (651)690-7895 **Fax:** (651)690-7774
Email: MNETHX@stkate.edu
Website: http://www.stkate.edu/mnethx
Karen G. Gervais, PhD, Director

★ 15004 ★ Monash University Centre for Human Bioethics
Clayton
Melbourne, VIC 3168, Australia
Phone: 61 3 5654000 **Fax:** 61 3 5653279
Email: SECHB@arts.cc.monash.edu.au
Dr. Helga Kuhse, Director

★ 15005 ★ Monash University Centre for Human Bioethics International Association of Bioethics
Clayton, VIC 3168, Australia
Phone: 61 3 5654279 **Fax:** 61 3 5653279
Email: HUB116E@vaxc.cc.monash.edu.au
Prof. Peter Singer, Contact

★ 15006 ★ Nanjing Railway Medical College Center for Bioethics
87 Dingjiaqiao Rd.
Nanjing, People's Republic of China
Phone: 306257 2481
Website: http://www.njrmc.edu.cn/
Dr. He Lun, Director

★ 15007 ★ National Academy of Medicine Columbian Institute of Bioethics Studies
Calle 65, No. 9-39, Of. 202
Bogota 2, D.E., Colombia
Phone: 57 1 2353896 **Fax:** 57 1 2881310
Dr. Fernando Sanchez Torres, Director

★ 15008 ★ National Catholic Bioethics Center
159 Washington St.
Brighton, MA 02135
Phone: (617)787-1900 **Fax:** (617)787-4900
Email: postmaster@NCBCenter.org
Website: http://www.NCBCenter.org
Rev. Russell E. Smith, Director
Frmly: Pope John XXIII Medical-Moral Research and Education Center.

★ 15009 ★ National Center for Bioethics
2960 Vecino Dr.
Sacramento, CA 95833
Phone: (916)921-2205
Bruce Hilton, Director

★ 15010 ★ National Center of Scientific Research Center for Research on Meaning, Ethics and Society
IRESCO 59-61 rue Pouchet
F-75849 Paris Cedex 17, France
Phone: 33 1 40251075 **Fax:** 33 1 60251271
Email: cerses@iresco.fr
Simone Bateman, Contact

★ 15011 ★ National Committee of Bioethics
Via Dei Villini 16
Rome, Italy
Phone: 39 6 4404282

★ 15012 ★ National Council on Ethics in Human Research (NCEHR)
774 Echo Dr.
Ottawa, ON, Canada K1S 5N8
Phone: (613)730-6225 **Free:** 800-668-3740
Fax: (613)730-8251
Email: office@ncehr-cnerh.org
Website: http://ncehr-cnerh.org
Richard Carpentier, Exec Director

★ 15013 ★ National Council on Medical Ethics
Box 60-204
S-104 01 Stockholm, Sweden
Phone: 46 8 7297111 **Fax:** 46 8 7297108
Gunnar Bengtsson, Director

★ 15014 ★ National Counsel of Life Sciences Ethics
Rua Professor Gomes
Teixeira, No. 3
P-1300 Lisboa, Portugal
Phone: 351 1 6670006 **Fax:** 351 1 602600
M. Riaposo, Director

★ 15015 ★ National Health and Medical Research Council (NHMRC) Australian Health Ethics Committee
MDP 100, GPO Box 9848
Canberra, ACT 2601, Australia
Phone: 61 02 6289 9807 **Fax:** 61 02 6289 9898
Email: ahec.nhmrc@nhmrc.gov.au
Website: http://www.nhmrc.gov.au/

★ 15016 ★ National Institutes of Health Department of Clinical Bioethics
10 Center Dr.
Bldg. 10, Rm. 1C118
Bethesda, MD 20892-1156
Phone: (301)496-2429 **Fax:** (301)496-0760
Email: bioethics@nih.gov
Website: http://www.bioethics.nih.gov
Frederick Bonkovsky, PhD, Director

★ 15017 ★ National Reference Center for Bioethics Literature Kennedy Institute of Ethics Georgetown University
Washington, DC 20057-1212
Phone: (202)687-3885 **Free:** 800-BIO-ETHX
Fax: (202)687-6770
Email: medethx@georgetown.edu
Website: http://bioethics.georgetown.edu
Robert M Veatch, PhD, Director

★ 15018 ★ New Hampshire Ethics Network
Concord Family Medicine
141 E Side Dr.
Concord, NH 03301
Phone: (603)228-0071
Randy Hayes, MD, Contact

★ 15019 ★ New York Medical College Bioethics Institute
Administration Bldg.
Valhalla, NY 10595
Phone: (914)594-4060 **Fax:** (914)594-4145
Website: http://www.nymc.edu/bioethics
Michael Herman, MD, Director
Frmly: Alfred E. Smith Institute of Human Values in Medical Ethics.

★ 15020 ★ Northeastern Ohio Universities College of Medicine Human Values in Medicine Program
PO Box 95
Rootstown, OH 44272
Phone: (330)325-2511
Martin Kohn, PhD, Director
Remarks: The program also sponsors the Center for Literature, Medicine, and the Health Care Professions in collaboration with Hiram College.

★ 15021 ★ Northridge Hospital Medical Center Bioethics Institute
18300 Roscoe Blvd.
Northridge, CA 91328
Phone: (818)885-5479
Alyce Vrolyh, Director

★ 15022 ★ Northwest Ethics Institute
2729 Ne 87th St.
Seattle, WA 98115-3455
Phone: (206)623-1572 **Fax:** (206)517-4734
Ray T. Cole, PhD, Director

★ 15023 ★ Northwestern University Feinberg School of Medicine Medical Humanities and Bioethics Program
750 N Lake Shore Dr., Ste. 625
Chicago, IL 60611
Phone: (312)503-7962 **Fax:** (312)503-0574
Email: kmontgomery@northwestern.edu
James F. Bresnahan, Director

★ 15024 ★ Norwegian Research Council for Science and the Humanities National Committee for Medical Research Ethics
Gaustadalleen 21
N-0371 Oslo 3, Norway
Phone: 47 22958780 **Fax:** 47 22698471
Prof. Jarle Ofstad, MD, Director

★ 15025 ★ Nuffield Council on Bioethics
28 Bedford Square
London WC1B 3JS, United Kingdom

Phone: 44 20 76819619 **Fax:** 44 20 76371712
Email: bioethics@nuffieldfoundation.org
Website: http://www.nuffieldbioethics.org
Dr. Sandy Thomas, Director
Prof. Bob Hepple, QC, Chairman

★ 15026 ★ Oklahoma Bioethics Center
Schusterman Health Sciences Center
University of Oklahoma
4502 E 41st St., Ste. 2H11
Tulsa, OK 74135-2512
Phone: (918)660-3212 **Fax:** (918)660-3205
Email: bioethics-center@ouhsc.edu
Website: http://www.tulsa.ouhsc.edu/medicine/ouh-sci.htm
G. Kevin Donovan, MD, Director

★ 15027 ★ Oregon Health & Science University
Center for Ethics in Health Care
3181 Sw Sam Jackson Park Rd., UHN-86
Portland, OR 97239-3098
Phone: (503)494-4466 **Fax:** (503)494-1260
Email: ethics@ohsu.edu
Website: http://www.ohsu.edu/ethics
Susan W. Tolle, MD, Director

★ 15028 ★ Pacific Center for Health Policy and Ethics
Keck School of Medicine and School of Law
University of Southern California
Los Angeles, CA 90089-0071
Phone: (213)740-2541 **Fax:** (213)740-5502
Email: pacific.center@law.usc.edu
Website: http://www.usc.edu/dept/law/pacific_center
David Goldstein, MD, Director

★ 15029 ★ Pacific School of Religion
Program in Bioethics
1798 Scenic Ave.
Berkeley, CA 94709
Phone: (510)848-0528 **Fax:** (510)845-8948
Karen Lebacqz, PhD, Director

★ 15030 ★ Park Ridge Center for Health, Faith, and Ethics
205 W Touhy Ave., Ste. 203
Park Ridge, IL 60068-4202
Phone: (847)384-3504 **Fax:** (847)384-3557
Website: http://www.parkridgecenter.org
Laurence J. O'Connell, PhD, Director

★ 15031 ★ Pennsylvania State University College of Medicine
Milton S. Hershey Medical Center
Department of Humanities, H134
500 University Dr.
Hershey, PA 17033
Phone: (717)531-8779 **Fax:** (717)531-3894
Website: http://www.collmed.psu.edu
David Barnard, PhD, Director

★ 15032 ★ Princeton University
University Center for Human Values
Louis Marx Hall
Princeton, NJ 08544
Phone: (609)258-4798 **Fax:** (609)258-2729
Email: values@princeton.edu
Website: http://www.princeton.edu/values/
Amy Gutmann, Director

★ 15033 ★ Public Responsibility in Medicine and Research (PRIM&R)
132 Boylston St., 4th Fl.
Boston, MA 02116
Phone: (617)423-4112 **Fax:** (617)423-1185
Email: info@primr.org
Website: http://www.primr.org
Joan Rachlin, Director

★ 15034 ★ Queensland Bioethics Centre
PO Box 3343
South Brisbane, QLD 4101, Australia
Phone: 61 7 448708 **Fax:** 61 7 8408142
Email: ehepburn@maver.org.au
Linda Reardon, Director

★ 15035 ★ Royal College of Physicians and Surgeons of Canada
Biomedical Ethics Committee
774 Echo Dr.
Ottawa, ON, Canada K1S 5N8
Phone: (613)730-6212 **Fax:** (613)730-8260
Gilles D. Hurteau, MD, Director

★ 15036 ★ Royal Free Hospital School of Medicine
Department of Public Health and Primary Care
Royal Free Ethics Group
Rowland Hill St.
London NW3 2PF, United Kingdom
Phone: 44 071 7940500 **Fax:** 44 071 7941224
Website: http://www.ucl.ac.uc/primcare-popsci
Dr. Margaret Lloyd, Director

★ 15037 ★ Royal Netherlands Medical Sciences Group
Commission of Medical Ethics
Postbus 20051
NL-3502 LB Utrecht, Netherlands

★ 15038 ★ Ruhr University-Bochum
Center for Medical Ethics
Universitatstrasse 150
D-44801 Bochum, Germany
Phone: 49 234 32 22749 **Fax:** 49 234 32 14598
Email: med.ethics@ruhr-uni-bochum.de
Website: http://www.ruhr-uni-bochum.de/zme/
Herbert Viefhues, MD, Director

★ 15039 ★ Russian Academy of Sciences
Russian National Committee on Bioethics (RNCB)
Volkhonka 14
Moscow, Russia
Phone: 7 95 2039169 **Fax:** 7 95 2039169
Dr. Ivan Frolov, Director

★ 15040 ★ Saint Louis University Health Sciences Center
Center for Health Care Ethics
3545 Lafayette Ave.
Saint Louis, MO 63104
Phone: (314)977-6660 **Fax:** (314)977-5150
Email: magill@slu.edu
Website: http://www.chce.slu.edu
Kevin O'Rourke, Director

★ 15041 ★ Saint Mary's Hospital Medical Ethics Forum
Medical School
Norfolk Place
London W2, United Kingdom
Jonathan Hoare, Director

★ 15042 ★ San Francisco Medical Society
Bay Area Network of Ethics Committees (BANEC)
1409 Sutter St.
San Francisco, CA 94109
Phone: (415)561-0870 **Fax:** (415)561-0834
Steve Heilig, Director

★ 15043 ★ Scientific Institute San Raffaele Hospital
Institute of Human Sciences and Medicine
Bioethics Center
I-20132 Milan, Italy
Phone: 39 02 21702767
Dr. Paolo Cattorini, Director

★ 15044 ★ Scientific Institute San Raffaele Hospital
Institute of Human Sciences and Medicine
Committee on Medical Ethics
Via Olgettina, 60
I-20132 Milan, Italy
Phone: 39 02 21702476
Dr. Rocco Mangia, Director

★ 15045 ★ Seattle Veterans Affairs Medical Center
Northwest Ethics Center for Veterans Health Care
1660 S Columbian Way
Grecc F-182 Va Puget Sound Healthcare Systems
Seattle, WA 98108
Phone: (206)764-2308 **Fax:** (206)764-2569
Robert A. Pearlman, MD, Director

★ 15046 ★ Sioux Valley Hospital and Health System
Center for Ethics and Caring
1305 W 18th St.
Sioux Falls, SD 57117-5039
Phone: (605)333-6381
Email: info@siouxvalley.org
Website: http://www.siouxvalley.org
Ellen Schellinger, CNT, Director

★ 15047 ★ South East Asian Center for Bioethics
St. Martin Porres Bldg., Rm. 226, UST
Espana Manila, Philippines
Phone: 63 2 7313101
Angeles Tan Alora, MD, Director

★ 15048 ★ Southern Cross Bioethics Institute
PO Box 206
Plympton, SA 5038, Australia
Phone: 61 8 2970022 **Fax:** 61 8 82970022
Email: scbi@bioethics.org.au
Website: http://www.bio-ethics.com
Dr. John Fleming, Director
Rosanne Parker, Administrative Assistant
Pub: *Bioethics Research Notes.*

★ 15049 ★ Southern Illinois University School of Medicine
Department of Medical Humanities
PO Box 19603
Springfield, IL 62794-9603
Phone: (217)782-4261 **Fax:** (217)557-8749
Website: http://www.siumed.edu/lib
Glen W. Davidson, PhD, Director

★ 15050 ★ Stanford University
Center for Biomedical Ethics
701 Welch Rd., Ste. 1105
Palo Alto, CA 94304
Phone: (650)723-5760 **Fax:** (650)725-6131
Email: scbe-info@med.stanford.edu
Website: http://www.scbe.stanford.edu
Thomas A. Raffin, MD, Director

★ 15051 ★ SunnyBrook and Women's College
Health Sciences Centre
Clinical Ethics Centre
2075 Bayview Ave., Rm. E228b
Toronto, ON, Canada M4N 3M5
Phone: (416)480-4818 **Fax:** (416)480-6899
Email: clinical.ethics@sw.ca
Scott Berry, MD, Director

★ 15052 ★ Swedish Delegation for Medical Ethics
PO Box 738
S-101 35 Stockholm, Sweden
Phone: 46 8 243350 **Fax:** 46 8 244248
Prof. Jan-Otto Ottosson, Director

★ 15053 ★ Swiss Academy of Medical Sciences
Ethics Commission
Petersplatz 13
CH-4051 Basel, Switzerland
Phone: 41 61 2699030 **Fax:** 41 61 2699039
Email: mail@samw.ch
Website: http://www.samw.ch
Walter H. Hitzig, MD, Director

★ 15054 ★ Swiss Society of Biomedical Ethics
Ospedale Civico
Via Tesserete 46
CH-6900 Lugano, Switzerland
Phone: 41 79 301 44 69 **Fax:** 41 91 805 61 42
Email: sseb@bluewin.ch
Roberta Wullschleger, Contact

★ 15055 ★ Texas Medical Center
Institute of Religion
1129 Wilkens
Houston, TX 77030-2805
Phone: (713)797-0600 **Fax:** (713)797-9199
Website: http://www.tmc.edu/institutions/irel.html
Rev. Allen Verhey, PhD, Director
Dr. William L. Turner, Pres & Chm Bd

★ 15056 ★ Theology Faculty of Sicily
Sicilian Institute of Bioethics
((Facolta Teologica de Sicilia)
Istituto Siciliano do Bioetica)
Piazza S Domenico
I-95024 Acireale, Italy
Phone: 39 95 7631324 **Fax:** 39 95 7634931
Email: salpriisb@mail.get.it
Website: http://www.gte.it/isb

★ 15057 ★ Uniformed Services University of Health Sciences
Program in Medical Ethics
4301 Jones Bridge Rd.
Bethesda, MD 20814
Phone: (301)295-3097 **Fax:** (301)295-1536
Edmund G. Howe, MD, Director

★ 15058 ★ United Nations Educational, Scientific and Cultural Organizations
International Committee Bioethics (IBC)
7, Pl. de Fontenoy
F-75700 Paris, France
Phone: 33 1 45683814 **Fax:** 33 1 45685515
Email: o.iebe@unesco.org
Website: http://www.unesco.org/ibc
Noelle Lenoir, Director

★ 15059 ★ U.S. Conference of Catholic Bishops
Secretariat for Prolife Activities
3211 4th St., Ne
Washington, DC 20017
Phone: (202)541-3070 **Fax:** (202)541-3054
Website: http://www.usccb.org/prolife
Gail Quinn, Director

★ 15060 ★ University of Alberta
John Dossetor Health Ethics Centre
8220 114th St.
222 Aberhart Centre Two
Edmonton, AB, Canada T6G 2J3
Phone: (780)492-6676 **Fax:** (780)492-0673
Email: dossetorcentre@ualberta.ca
Website: http://www.ualberta.ca/BIOETHICS
John B. Dossetor, Director

★ 15061 ★ University of Alberta
St. Joseph's College Ethics Centre
402,8215-112 St.
Edmonton, AB, Canada T6G 2C8
Phone: (780)439-2422 **Fax:** (780)432-0245
Email: ethics@connect.ab.ca
Website: http://www.connect.ab.ca/~ethics/
Dr. Mary Lou Cranston, Director

★ 15062 ★ University of Arkansas for Medical Sciences
Division of Medical Humanities
4301 W Markham
Slot 646
Little Rock, AR 72205
Phone: (501)661-7970 **Fax:** (501)661-7967
Email: Hacklerchris@uams.edu
Website: http:/www.uams.edu/humanities
Chris Hackler, PhD, Director

★ 15063 ★ University of Calgary
Faculty of Medicine
Medical Ethics Research Program
3330 Hospital Dr., NW
Calgary, AB, Canada T2N 4N1
Phone: (403)220-7990 **Fax:** (403)283-8524
Email: omb@ucalgary.ca
Douglas Kinsella, Director

★ 15064 ★ University of California at San Francisco
School of Medicine
Program in Medical Ethics
521 Parnassus Ave., Rm. C 126
San Francisco, CA 94143-0903
Phone: (415)476-6240 **Fax:** (415)476-5020
Bernard Lo, MD, Director

★ 15065 ★ University of Capetown
Department of Medicine
Bioethics Centre
Cape Town Observatory
Cape Town 7925, Republic of South Africa
Phone: 27 021 4066115 **Fax:** 27 021 4486815
S.R. Benatar, Director

★ 15066 ★ University of Chicago
Department of Medicine
Center for Clinical Medical Ethics
5841 S Maryland Ave.
Mc-6098
Chicago, IL 60637-1470
Phone: (773)702-1453 **Fax:** (773)702-0900
Mark Siegler, MD, Director

★ 15067 ★ University of Connecticut Health Center
School of Medicine
Department of Community Medicine and Health Care
Division of Medical Humanities, Health Law, and Ethics
263 Farmington Ave.
Farmington, CT 06032-6325
Phone: (860)679-5495 **Fax:** (860)679-5464
Email: lazzarini@nso.uchc.edu
Website: http://www.commed.uchc.edu/medicalhumanities/
Joseph M. Healey, Director

★ 15068 ★ University of Florida
College of Medicine
Program In Bioethics, Law, and Medical Professionalism
Box 103588
Gainesville, FL 32610
Phone: (352)265-7204 **Fax:** (352)265-8045
Email: allen@chfm.ufl.edu
Website: http://www.med.ufl.edu/chfm/ethics/
Ray Moseley, PhD, Director

★ 15069 ★ University of Genova
Center Study on Contemporary Philosophy
National Research Advisory Board
Via Lomellini, 8/8
Genoa, Italy
Phone: 39 10 293511 **Fax:** 39 10 2471184
Prof. Evandro Agazzi, PhD, Director

★ 15070 ★ University of Glasgow
Institute of Law and Ethics in Medicine
Stair Bldg.
Glasgow G12 8QQ, United Kingdom
Phone: 44 41 3303688 **Fax:** 44 41 3304698
Email: a.mooney@law.gla.ac.uk
Website: http://www.law.gla.ac.uk/medlaw
Annabelle Mooney, Contact
Remarks: The Institute offers research degrees up to the PhD level. It also offers two taught degrees with a research component, a masters degree in Law and Ethics in Medicine, and a masters degree in medical law.

★ 15071 ★ University of Illinois at Chicago
Department of Medical Education
Medical Humanities
Department of Medical Education (MC 591)
808 S Wood St., 986 CME
Chicago, IL 60612-7309
Phone: (312)996-6738 **Fax:** (312)413-2048
Website: http://www.uic.edu/com/mcme/humanities.htm
Timothy F. Murphy, PhD, Director

★ 15072 ★ University of Iowa
College of Medicine
Program in Biomedical Ethics and Medical Humanities
1-106 Medical Education Bldg.
Iowa City, IA 52242
Phone: (319)335-6706 **Fax:** (319)335-8515
Website: http://www.medicine.uiowa.edu/bemh/
Robert Weir, PhD, Director

★ 15073 ★ University of Manchester
School of Law
United Kingdom Forum for Health Care Ethics and Law
Oxford Rd.
Manchester M13 9PL, United Kingdom
Phone: 44 161 2757703 **Fax:** 44 161 2757704
Email: CSEP@Man.ac.uk
Website: http://les.man.ac.uk/law/ethicspol.htm
Margaret Brazier, Contact

★ 15074 ★ University of Maryland
School of Law
Maryland Healthcare Ethics Committee Network
Law and Health Care Program
515 W Lombard St.
Baltimore, MD 21201
Phone: (410)706-4457 **Fax:** (410)706-4045
Email: aoneil@law.umaryland.edu
Website: http://www.law.umaryland.edu
Dianne E. Hoffmann, Director

★ 15075 ★ University of Miami
Bioethics Program
PO Box 016960 (M-825)
Miami, FL 33101
Phone: (305)243-5723
Email: ethics@miami.edu
Website: http://www.miami.edu/ethics
Kenneth Goodman, PhD, Director

★ 15076 ★ University of Minnesota
BioEthics Program
410 Church St. SE, Ste. N504
Minneapolis, MN 55455-0392
Phone: (612)624-9440 **Fax:** (612)624-9108
Email: bioethx@tc.umn.edu
Website: http://www.bioethics.umn.edu/
Arthur L. Caplan, PhD, Director

★ 15077 ★ University of Montreal
Centre De Recherche En Droit Public
Public Law Research Centre
C.P. 6128, Succursale Centre-Ville
Montreal, QC, Canada H3C 3J7
Phone: (514)343-7210 **Fax:** (514)343-7508
Website: http://www.crdp.umontreal.ca
Pierre Trudel, Director

★ 15078 ★ University of New Mexico
Institute of Public Law
Center for Health, Law and Ethics
1117 Stanford Ne
Albuquerque, NM 87131
Phone: (505)277-5006 **Fax:** (505)277-7064
Joan McIver Gibson, PhD, Director

★ 15079 ★ University of New South Wales
School of Community Medicine
Australian Bioethics Association
Sydney, NSW 2052, Australia
Phone: 61 2 9385 2516 **Fax:** 61 2 9313 6185
Email: paul.mcneill@unsw.edu.au
Paul McNeill, Contact

★ 15080 ★ University of North Dakota
Department of Community Medicine and Rural Health
School of Medicine
501 N Columbia Rd.
Grand Forks, ND 58203
Phone: (701)777-2344 **Fax:** (701)777-2389

★ 15081 ★ University of Oslo
Center for Medical Ethics
Box 1130 Blindern
N-0318 Oslo, Norway
Phone: 47 22844660 **Fax:** 47 22844661
Email: j.h.solbakk@medetikk.uio.no
J.H. Solbakk, Director

★ 15082 ★ University of South Florida
College of Medicine
Department of Internal Medicine
Division of Medical Ethics and Humanities
12901 Bruce B. Downs Blvd., M.D.C. Box 19
Tampa, FL 33612
Phone: (813)974-5300
Robert M. Walker, MD, Director

★ 15083 ★ University of Technology, Sydney
Centre for Bioethics and Health Care
Kuring-gai Campus
PO Box 123
New South Wales 2007, Australia
Phone: 61 2 3305137 **Fax:** 61 2 3305513
Michael Walsh, Director

★ 15084 ★ University of Tennessee
Department of Philosophy
Center for Applied and Professional Ethics
801 McClung Tower
Knoxville, TN 37996-0480
Phone: (865)974-3255 **Fax:** (865)974-3509
Email: jhardwig@utk.edu
Website: http://www.web.utk.edu/~philosop/
Glen Graber, PhD, Director

★ 15085 ★ University of Tennessee at Memphis
College of Medicine
Department of Human Values and Ethics
956 Court St.
Rm. B324 Coleman Bldg.
Memphis, TN 38163
Phone: (901)448-5686 **Fax:** (901)448-1291
Terrance Ackerman, PhD, Director

★ 15086 ★ University of Texas Medical Branch
Institute for the Medical Humanities
301 University Blvd.
Galveston, TX 77555-1311
Phone: (409)772-2376 **Fax:** (409)772-5640
Email: sgoodwin@utmb.edu
Website: http://www.utmb.edu/imh
Ronald A. Carson, PhD, Director

★ 15087 ★ University of Toronto
Centre for Bioethics
88 College St.
Toronto, ON, Canada M5G 1L4
Phone: (416)978-2709 **Fax:** (416)978-1911
Website: http://www.utoronto.ca/jcb/
Arnold Aberman, Chairman of the Board

★ 15088 ★ University of Trondheim
Department of Medicine
Resource Center for Teaching of Bioethics
Regionsykehuset
N-7000 Trondheim, Norway
Phone: 47 7598801 **Fax:** 47 7598802
John Mauritzen, Director

★ 15089 ★ University of Virginia
Health Sciences Center
Center for Biomedical Ethics
Box 800758
Charlottesville, VA 22908
Phone: (434)924-5974 **Fax:** (434)982-3971
Email: cg2b@virginia.edu
Website: http://www.med.virginia.edu/bioethics
John D. Moreno, PhD, Director

★ 15090 ★ University of Wales—Swansea
School of Health Science
Centre for Philosophy and Health Care
Singleton Park
Swansea SA2 8PP, United Kingdom
Phone: 44 792 295611 **Fax:** 44 792 295612
Email: cphc@swansea.ac.uk
Emrys Jenkins, Contact

★ 15091 ★ University of Washington
School of Medicine
Department of Medical History and Ethics
A-204 Health Sciences Center, Box 357120
Seattle, WA 98195-7120
Phone: (206)543-5145 **Fax:** (206)685-7515
Email: mheinfo@u.washington.edu
Website: http://www.depts.washington.edu/mhe/dept/
James C. Wharton, PhD, Director

★ 15092 ★ University of Wisconsin
Department of Medical History and Bioethics
1300 University Ave.
1420 Medical Sciences Center
Madison, WI 53706-1532
Phone: (608)263-3414 **Fax:** (608)262-2327
Email: medhisteth@med.wisc.edu
Website: http://www.medsch.wisc.edu/medhist/eth-main.html
Norman Fost, MD, Director

★ 15093 ★ University of Zagreb
School of Medicine
Medical Center for Human Rights
Center for Global Development and Cooperation
Salata 3
CT-41000 Zagreb, Croatia
Phone: 384 1 271304 **Fax:** 384 1 271251
Danijal Derezic, Dir of Merchandising

★ 15094 ★ Utrecht University
Center for Bioethics and Health Law
Heidelberglaan 2
Postbus 80.105
Utrecht, Netherlands
Phone: 31 30 2534399 **Fax:** 31 30 2539410
Email: cbg@theo.uu.nl
Mrs. E. Eckelboom, LLM, Director
Remarks: The Centre is an independent academic institute offering short-term advice and research; it organizes courses and provides training sessions. Within the Centre, physicians, veterinarians, ethicists, philosophers, lawyers, and theologians work together in areas of applied ethics and education and judicial research. Topics of particular interest to the Centre are ethical and legal aspects of biotechnology and genetic modification of humans, animals, and plants.

★ 15095 ★ Vanderbilt University
School of Medicine
Center for Clinical and Research Ethics
Vanderbilt University Medical Center
319 Oxford House
Nashville, TN 37232-4350
Phone: (615)936-2686 **Fax:** (615)436-3800
Email: medethics@vanderbilt.edu
Website: http://www.mc.vanderbilt.edu/ethics
Richard M. Zaner, PhD, Director

★ 15096 ★ Vermont Ethics Network
89 Main St.
Drawer 20
Montpelier, VT 05620-3601
Phone: (802)828-2909 **Fax:** (802)828-6558
Email: ven@bishca.state.vt.us
Website: http://www.vtethicsnetwork.org
Jean B. Mallary, Director

★ 15097 ★ Waseda University
Advanced Research Center for Human Sciences
Bioethics Research Project
1-6-1, Nishiwaseda, Shinjuky-ku
Tokyo 169-50, Japan
Phone: 81 3 32034141 **Fax:** 81 429 484314
Rihito Kimura, Director

★ 15098 ★ West Virginia University
Health Sciences Center
Center for Health Ethics and the Law
1195 Health Sciences North
PO Box 9022
Morgantown, WV 26506-9022
Phone: (304)293-7618 **Free:** 877-209-8086
Fax: (304)293-7442
Email: lmcmillen@hsc.wvu.edu
Website: http://www.wvethics.org
Alvin H. Moss, MD, Director

★ 15099 ★ Western Michigan University
Philosophy Department
Medical Ethics Program
1201 Oliver St.
Kalamazoo, MI 49008-3899
Phone: (616)387-3113 **Fax:** (616)387-4390
Email: hyuni@wmich.edu
Arthur Falk, PhD, Director

★ 15100 ★ Youngstown State University
Department of Philosophy and Religious Studies
Bioethics Network of Ohio (BENO)
One University Plaza
Youngstown, OH 44555-3448
Phone: (330)742-1624
Email: FR134701@YSU.EDU
Brendan Minogue, PhD, Director

Chapter 7
Hospital Management Companies

Entries listed below are arranged alphabetically by company names. For additional information, see the "User's Guide" located at the front of this directory.

★ 15101 ★ Accord Health Care Corp.
3696 Ulmerton Rd.
Clearwater, FL 33762
Phone: (727)573-1755 **Fax:** (727)572-0185
Stephen H. Noble, President
Ransom Stigleman, III, Vice President
Hospitals: 2. **Beds:** 72.

★ 15102 ★ American MedTrust Corp. (AMT)
3700 Crestwood Parkway
Duluth, GA 30096
Phone: (770)923-6500 **Fax:** (770)923-7800
Website: http://www.medtrust.com
Tom McNaull, CEO & Pres
Hospitals: 2.**Beds:** 439.

★ 15103 ★ Ardent Health Services (ARHS)
102 Woodmont Boulevard, Ste. 800
Nashville, TN 37205
Phone: (615)269-3492 **Fax:** (615)269-5397
David T. Vandewater, CEO & Pres
Hospitals: 24. **Beds:** 2225.

★ 15104 ★ Associated Healthcare Systems, Inc. (AHS)
12230 Magnolia Circle
Alpharetta, GA 30005
Phone: (770)569-7173 **Fax:** (770)752-0962
Email: jim70@bellsouth.net
A. Ronald Turner, CEO & Pres
Hospitals: 2. **Beds:** 92.

★ 15105 ★ Associates Capital Group, LLC
PO Box 380995
Birmingham, AL 35242
Phone: (205)408-9095
Len Bryant, CEO
Hospitals: 1. **Beds:** 76.

★ 15106 ★ Bayou Healthcare Corp. (BHCC)
110 John Eskew Dr.
Alexandria, LA 71303
Phone: (318)445-5111 **Fax:** (318)442-2261
Joseph Rodriguez, CEO
Hospitals: 1. **Beds:** 70.

★ 15107 ★ Brown Schools, Inc.
900 Cummings Center, Ste. 310-U
PO Box 4088
Beverly, MA 01915
Phone: (978)922-3388 **Fax:** (978)922-0678
Thomas Riley, CEO
Sherry Thornton, President
Hospitals: 13. **Beds:** 1497.

★ 15108 ★ Cambridge International, Inc.
7505 Fannin, Ste. 510
PO Box 20624
Houston, TX 77225
Phone: (713)790-1153 **Fax:** (713)790-1302
Timothy Sharma, MD, President
Deo Shanker, Contact
Hospitals: 2. **Beds:** 232.

★ 15109 ★ Camelot Healthcare, LLC
416 Travis, Ste. 804
Shreveport, LA 71101
Phone: (318)226-8611 **Fax:** (318)226-8680
Website: http://www.camelothealthcare.com
Clifton L. Watson, Chairman of the Board
Robert R. Hicks, CEO & Pres
Hospitals: 4. **Beds:** 235.

★ 15110 ★ Cancer Treatment Centers of America
3150 Salt Creek Ln., Ste. 122
Arlington Heights, IL 60005-1087
Phone: (847)342-7400 **Fax:** (847)342-7477
Website: http://www.cancercenter.com
Richard J. Stephenson, Chairman of the Board
Robert W. Mayo, Chairman of the Board
Hospitals: 2. **Beds:** 389.

★ 15111 ★ Charles River Hospital, Inc. (CRH)
203 Grove St.
Wellesley, MA 02482-7413
Phone: (781)416-5300 **Fax:** (781)416-5334
Frederick J. Thacher, Chairman of the Board
Hospitals: 1. **Beds:** 62.

★ 15112 ★ Children's Comprehensive Services
Behavioral Services Division
3401 W End Ave., Ste. 400
Nashville, TN 37203-1042
Phone: (615)250-0000 **Free:** 800-844-0080
Fax: (615)250-1000
William J. Ballard, CEO & Chm Bd
Amy S. Harrison, Chairman of the Board
Hospitals: 11. **Beds:** 746.

★ 15113 ★ Clarent Hospital Corp. (CLHC)
515 West Greens Rd., Ste. 500
Houston, TX 77067
Phone: (281)774-5100 **Fax:** (281)774-5250
Robert L. Smith, CEO
Hospitals: 9. **Beds:** 1108.

★ 15114 ★ College Health Enterprises
8141 E 2cd. St., Ste. 500
Downey, CA 90241
Phone: (562)923-9449 **Fax:** (562)923-4030
Website: http://www.collegehospitals.com
Barry J. Weiss, CEO & Pres
Hospitals: 2. **Beds:** 247.

★ 15115 ★ Community Health Systems, Inc.
155 Franklin Rd., Ste. 400
PO Box 217
Brentwood, TN 37027-4646
Phone: (615)373-9600 **Fax:** (615)376-3438
Website: http://www.chs.net
Wayne T. Smith, Chairman of the Board
W. Larry Cash, Vice President
Hospitals: 58. **Beds:** 5575.

★ 15116 ★ Comprehensive Addiction Programs, Inc.
1175 Herndon Parkway, Ste. 250
Herndon, VA 20170-5532
Phone: (703)904-9300 **Fax:** 800-835-3903
Website: http://www.helpfinders.com
Jerome E. Rhodes, CEO
Steven Levine, Vice President
Hospitals: 5. **Beds:** 233.

★ 15117 ★ Diamond Healthcare Corp.
700 E Main St., Ste. 900
Richmond, VA 23219
Phone: (804)649-9340 **Fax:** (804)782-2286
Website: http://www.diamondhealth.com
John William Crews, Chairman of the Board
Thomas F. Hancock, Contact
Hospitals: 1. **Beds:** 30.

★ 15118 ★ Doctors Community Healthcare Corp.
6730 N Scottsdale Rd., Ste. 200
Scottsdale, AZ 85253
Phone: (602)348-9800 **Fax:** (602)348-9801
Website: http://www.doctorscommunity.com
Paul Tuft, CEO & Chm Bd
Mel Redman, President
Hospitals: 6. **Beds:** 1572.

★ 15119 ★ Essent Healthcare, Inc. (EHC)
3100 W End Ave., Ste. 900
Nashville, TN 37203
Phone: (615)312-5100 **Fax:** (615)312-5101
Website: http://www.essenthealthcare.com
Hud Connery, CEO
Hospitals: 2. **Beds:** 223.

★ 15120 ★ First Hospital Corp. (FHC)
240 Corporate Blvd.
Norfolk, VA 23502
Phone: (757)459-5100 **Fax:** (757)459-5219
Website: http://www.fhchealthsystems.com
Ronald I. Dozoretz, MD, Chairman of the Board
Elliot Gerson, President

Hospitals: 7. **Beds:** 730.

★ 15121 ★ Greenleaf Health Systems, Inc. (GHS)
1 Northgate Pk., Ste. 307
Chattanooga, TN 37415-6912
Phone: (423)870-9765 **Fax:** (423)870-5648
Website: http://www.greenleafhealth.org
Dan B. Page, Contact
Diana S. Gilbert, Contact
Hospitals: 1. **Beds:** 70.

★ 15122 ★ Hallmark Systems, Inc. (HSI)
300 Galleria Parkway, Ste. 650
Atlanta, GA 30339-0049
Phone: (770)933-5500 **Fax:** (770)933-1886
James T. McAfee, Jr., Chairman of the Board
Hospitals: 3. **Beds:** 210.

★ 15123 ★ HCA, Inc. (HCA)
PO Box 550
1 Park Plaza
Nashville, TN 37202-0550
Phone: (615)344-9551 **Fax:** (615)344-2291
Website: http://www.hcahealthcare.com
Jack O. Bovender, CEO & Chm Bd
Hospitals: 198. **Beds:** 43125.

★ 15124 ★ HCR Manor Care (HCRM)
333 N Summit St., Ste. 100
Toledo, OH 43604-2617
Phone: (419)252-5500 **Fax:** (419)252-5537
Website: http://www.hcr-manorcare.com
Paul A. Ormond, CEO & Pres
M. Keith Weikel, Contact
Hospitals: 1. **Beds:** 172.

★ 15125 ★ Health Management Associates, Inc. (HMA)
5811 Pelican Bay Blvd., Ste. 500
Naples, FL 34108
Phone: (941)598-3131 **Fax:** (941)597-5794
Website: http://www.hma-corp.com
William J. Schoen, Chairman of the Board
Joseph V. Vumbacco, CEO & Pres
Hospitals: 38. **Beds:** 5304.

★ 15126 ★ Health Systems America (HSA)
555 SW 148th Ave.
Sunrise, FL 33325
Phone: (954)915-0474 **Fax:** (954)915-0750
Michael Piercey, MD, CEO
Manuel R. Llano, Vice President
Hospitals: 2. **Beds:** 164.

★ 15127 ★ HealthMont, Inc. (HLM)
113 Seaboard Lane, Ste. C-200
Franklin, TN 37067
Phone: (615)250-7800 **Fax:** (615)250-7802
Website: http://www.healthmont.com
Timothy Hill, CEO
Hospitals: 5. **Beds:** 499.

★ 15128 ★ HEALTHSOUTH Corp. (HRC)
1 HealthSouth Pkwy.
Birmingham, AL 35243-2329
Phone: (205)967-7116 **Fax:** (205)969-3543
Website: http://www.healthsouth.com
Richard M. Scrushy, CEO & Chm Bd
William T. Owens, President
Hospitals: 101. **Beds:** 7775.

★ 15129 ★ Healthstar Corp. (HSR)
5560 Franklin Pike Circle
Brentwood, TN 37027
Phone: (615)373-7827 **Fax:** (615)373-7749
Website: http://www.healthstarcorp.net
Robert M. Martin, Chairman of the Board

★ 15130 ★ IASIS Healthcare Corp. (IHC)
113 Seaboard Lane, Ste. A200
Franklin, TN 37067
Phone: (615)846-2747 **Fax:** (615)846-3006
Website: http://www.iasishealthcare.com
David R. White, CEO & Chm Bd
Sandra K. McRee, Contact
Hospitals: 15. **Beds:** 2588.

★ 15131 ★ Integrated Health Services, Inc. (IHS)
910 Ridgebrrok Rd.
Sparks, MD 21152
Phone: (410)773-1000 **Fax:** (410)773-1044
John Heller, President
John Walton, Contact
Hospitals: 17. **Beds:** 781.

★ 15132 ★ Kindred Healthcare, Inc. (KIND)
680 South Fourth Ave.
Louisville, KY 40202
Phone: (502)596-7300 **Fax:** (502)596-4026
Website: http://www.kindredhealthcare.com
Edward L. Kuntz, Chairman of the Board
Hospitals: 55. **Beds:** 4812.

★ 15133 ★ Liberty Management Group, Inc. (LMG)
19 Spear Rd., Ste. 305
Ramsey, NJ 07446
Phone: (201)236-8880 **Fax:** (201)236-9117
Website: http://www.libertymgt.com
William J. Hartigan, CEO & Pres
Gerald A. Johnson, Contact
Hospitals: 5. **Beds:** 564.

★ 15134 ★ LifeCare Management Services, LLC (LCMS)
5700 Tennyson Parkway
Plano, TX 75024
Phone: (469)241-2100 **Fax:** (469)241-2197
Website: http://www.lifecare-hospitals.com
David LeBlanc, CEO & Pres
Jim Shelton, Contact
Hospitals: 19. **Beds:** 931.

★ 15135 ★ LifePoint Hospitals,Inc. (LPNT)
103 Powell Court, Ste. 200
Brentwood, TN 37027
Phone: (615)372-8500 **Fax:** (615)372-8586
Website: http://www.lifepointhospitals.com
Kenneth C. Donahey, CEO & Chm Bd
William F. Carpenter, III, Contact
Hospitals: 21. **Beds:** 2028.

★ 15136 ★ Mariner Post-Acute Network, Inc. (MPAN)
1 Ravinia Dr., Ste. 1500
Atlanta, GA 30346
Phone: (678)443-7000 **Fax:** (770)379-0753
Francis "Butch" Cash, Chairman of the Board
George Morgan, Contact
Hospitals: 11. **Beds:** 683.

★ 15137 ★ MedCath Inc. (MDTH)
10720 Sikes Place Ste. 300
Charlotte, NC 28277-8143
Phone: (704)541-3228 **Fax:** (704)541-2615
Website: http://www.medcath.com
Stephen R. Puckett, Chairman of the Board
David Crane, CEO & Pres
Hospitals: 8. **Beds:** 467.

★ 15138 ★ Mountain State Behavioral Health Services, LLC (MSBHS) dba River Park Hospital
PO Box 1875
Huntington, WV 25719-1875
Phone: (304)526-9100 **Fax:** (304)526-9140
Website: http://www.riverparkhospital.net
Scott Stamm, CEO
Hospitals: 1. **Beds:** 165.

★ 15139 ★ National Surgical Hospitals (NSH)
30 South Wacker Dr., Ste. 2302
Chicago, IL 60606
Phone: (312)627-8400 **Fax:** (312)474-1950
Website: http://www.nshinc.com
John G. Rex-Waller, CEO & Pres
Hospitals: 3. **Beds:** 62.

★ 15140 ★ Northeast Health Management, Inc. (NEHM)
1220 Butterworth Court
Stevensville, MD 21666
Phone: (410)643-3393 **Fax:** (410)643-9511
Harold A. McBee, Sr., President
Hospitals: 4. **Beds:** 230.

★ 15141 ★ Pacific Health Corp. (PAC)
14642 Newport Ave., Ste. 340
Tustin, CA 92780
Phone: (714)669-2085 **Fax:** (714)669-2059
James W. Young, CEO & Pres
Linda Bentley, Contact
Hospitals: 49. **Beds:** 9922.

★ 15142 ★ Park Health Management, Inc. (PHM)
149 Belle Forest Circle
Nashville, TN 37221
Phone: (615)662-2577 **Fax:** (615)662-7459
Website: http://www.newlifelodge.com
Jerry E. Gilliland, CEO & Pres
J. Kevin Duvall, Contact
Hospitals: 1. **Beds:** 65.

★ 15143 ★ Pioneer Behavioral Health (PIHC)
200 Lake St., Ste. 102
Peabody, MA 01960
Phone: (978)536-2777 **Fax:** (978)536-2677
Website: http://www.phc-inc.com
Bruce A. Shear, CEO & Pres
Robert H. Boswell, Contact
Hospitals: 3. **Beds:** 123.

★ 15144 ★ Preferred Management Corp. (PFMC)
2713 N Market
Shawnee, OK 74804
Phone: (405)878-0202 **Fax:** (405)273-6007
Jerry G. Hulin, President
Donald A. Freeman, Vice President
Hospitals: 4. **Beds:** 191.

★ 15145 ★ Progressions Group, Inc. (PGI)
450 Bethlehem Pike
Fort Washington, PA 19034
Phone: (215)641-5300 **Fax:** (215)641-6853
Nicholas Tenaglia, MD, CEO
Hospitals: 3. **Beds:** 316.

★ 15146 ★ Province Healthcare (PRHC)
105 Westwood Pl., Ste. 400
Brentwood, TN 37027

Phone: (615)370-1377 **Fax:** (615)377-9539
Martin S. Rash, CEO & Chm Bd
John M. Rutledge, President
Hospitals: 56. **Beds:** 4689.

★ 15147 ★ Quorum Health Resources, LLC (QHR)
105 Continental Place
Brentwood, TN 37027
Phone: (615)371-7979
James G. Stokes, President
David Dempsey, Contact
Hospitals: 180. **Beds:** 18201.

★ 15148 ★ Ramsay Health Care Australia (RHCA)
154 Pacific Hwy. - Level 9
Saint Leonards, NSW 2065, Australia
Paul Ramsay, Chairman of the Board
Michael S. Siddle, Contact
Hospitals: 11. **Beds:** 1312.

★ 15149 ★ Ramsay Youth Services, Inc. (RAM)
Columbus Center
1 Allhambra Plaza, Ste. 750
Coral Gables, FL 33134
Phone: (305)569-6993 **Fax:** (305)569-4647
Paul J. Ramsay, Chairman of the Board
Luis E. Lamela, CEO & Pres
Hospitals: 9. **Beds:** 834.

★ 15150 ★ Resurgence Health Group, LLC. (RHG)
PO Box 5
6652 Sweetwater Point
Flowery Branch, GA 30542
Phone: (770)967-1653 **Fax:** (770)967-1641
Website: http://www.resurgencehealthgroup.com
Phillip H. Eastman, III, President
Hospitals: 1. **Beds:** 40.

★ 15151 ★ Select Medical Corp. (SMC)
4718 Old Gettysburg Rd.
PO Box 2034
Mechanicsburg, PA 17055
Phone: (717)972-1100 **Fax:** (717)972-1042
Website: http://www.selctmediclcorp.com
Rocco A. Ortenzio, CEO & Chm Bd
Robert A. Ortenzio, President
Hospitals: 58. **Beds:** 2119.

★ 15152 ★ Southeastern Hospital Corp. (SEHC)
104 E Park Dr., Ste. 309
Brentwood, TN 37027
Phone: (615)371-6673 **Fax:** (615)371-6675
Larry F. McFall, CEO & Pres
Philip H. Sanderson, Contact
Hospitals: 1. **Beds:** 67.

★ 15153 ★ Springhill Health Services (SHS)
3632 Dauphin St.
Mobile, AL 36608
Phone: (334)460-5280 **Fax:** (334)460-5339
Website: http://www.springhillmemorial.com
Celia A. Wallace, CEO & Chm Bd
Randy A. Sucher, Contact
Hospitals: 1. **Beds:** 252.

★ 15154 ★ Sun Healthcare Group (SHG)
101 Sun Ave. NE
Albuquerque, NM 87109
Phone: (505)821-3355 **Fax:** (505)823-4136
Website: http://www.sunh.com
James R. Tolbert, III, Chairman of the Board
Mark G. Wimer, CEO & Pres
Hospitals: 9. **Beds:** 642.

★ 15155 ★ Sunlink Health Systems, Inc. (SLHC)
900 Circle 75 Parkway, Ste. 1300
Atlanta, GA 30339
Phone: (770)933-7000 **Fax:** (770)933-7010
Website: http://www.sunlinkhealth.com
Robert M. Thornton, Jr., CEO
Hospitals: 6. **Beds:** 333.

★ 15156 ★ Telecare Corp. (TCC)
1100 Manina Village Pkwy., Ste. 100
Alameda, CA 94501-1043
Phone: (510)337-7950 **Fax:** (510)337-7969
Website: http://www.telecarecorp.com
Anne Baker, CEO & Pres
Stacey Calhoun, Vice President
Hospitals: 13. **Beds:** 1090.

★ 15157 ★ Tenet Healthcare Corp. (THC)
3820 State St.
Santa Barbara, CA 93103
Phone: (805)563-7000 **Fax:** (805)593-6808
Website: http://www.tenethealth.com
Jeffrey C. Barbakow, CEO & Chm Bd
Thomas B. Mackey, President
Hospitals: 127. **Beds:** 29411.

★ 15158 ★ Timber Ridge Group (TRG)
4500 W Commercial Dr.
North Little Rock, AR 72116
Phone: (501)758-8799 **Fax:** (501)758-8778
Jack Robertson, PHD, President
Roger Carrillo, Vice President
Hospitals: 3. **Beds:** 114.

★ 15159 ★ Triad Hospitals, Inc. (TRIH)
13455 Noel Rd., Ste. 2000
Dallas, TX 75240
Phone: (972)789-2700 **Free:** 800-238-6006
Fax: (972)663-3945
Website: http://www.triadhospitals.com
James D. Shelton, CEO & Chm Bd
Michael J. Parsons, Contact
Hospitals: 47. **Beds:** 7795.

★ 15160 ★ United Medical Corp. (UMC)
603 Main St.
PO Box 1100
Windermere, FL 34786-1100
Phone: (407)876-2200 **Fax:** (407)876-5959
Donald R. Dizney, CEO & Chm Bd
James E. English, President
Hospitals: 9. **Beds:** 1127.

★ 15161 ★ Universal Health Services Inc. (UHS)
Universal Corporate Center
367 S Gulph Rd.
PO Box 61558
King of Prussia, PA 19406-0958
Phone: (610)768-3300 **Fax:** (610)768-3336
Website: http://www.uhsinc.com
Alan B. Miller, President
Kirk E. Gorman, Contact
Hospitals: 60. **Beds:** 8978.

★ 15162 ★ Vanguard Health Systems (VHS)
20 Burton Hills Blvd., Ste. 100
Nashville, TN 37215
Phone: (615)665-6000 **Fax:** (615)665-6099
Website: http://www.vanguardhealth.com
Charles N. Martin, Jr., CEO & Chm Bd
William Larry Hough, President
Hospitals: 9. **Beds:** 1878.

★ 15163 ★ Youth and Family Centered Services (YFCS)
1705 Capital of Texas Highway South, 5th Fl.
Austin, TX 78746
Phone: (512)327-1119 **Fax:** (512)327-4576
Website: http://www.yfcs.com
Kevin P. Sheehan, CEO & Pres
J. Mack Nunn, Vice President
Hospitals: 8. **Beds:** 794.

Chapter 8
Pharmaceutical and Related Healthcare Companies

Entries listed below are alphabetical by company names. For additional information, consult the "User's Guide" located at the front of this directory.

★ 15164 ★ A-T Surgical Manufacturing Co., Inc.
115 Clemente St.
Holyoke, MA 01040
Phone: (413)532-4551 **Free:** 800-225-2023
Fax: (413)532-0826
Email: sales@a-tsurgical.com
Website: http://www.a-tsurgical.com
Eugene P. Kirejczyk, President
Desc: Manufacturer of home healthcare; hospital equipment and supplies; orthopedic and prosthetic equipment and supplies; physical therapy and rehabilitation equipment and supplies; surgical supplies.

★ 15165 ★ Abbott Diagnostic Division
Division of Abbott Laboratories
5440 Patrick Henry Dr.
Santa Clara, CA 95054
Phone: (408)982-4800 **Free:** 800-933-5535
Fax: (408)982-4881
Website: http://www.abbott.com
John Morradian, Vice President
Desc: Manufacturer and distributor of diagnostic equipment and instruments; diagnostic reagents and test kits; and laboratory equipment.

★ 15166 ★ Abbott Hospital Products Division
Electronic Drug Delivery Systems
Division of Abbott Laboratories
200 Abbott Park Rd.
Bldg. AP30, Department 04EF
Abbott Park, IL 60064
Phone: (847)937-6100 **Free:** 800-ABBOTT-3
Fax: (847)938-6230
Website: http://www.abbotthosp.com
Patrick Keely, Contact

★ 15167 ★ Abbott Laboratories
Division of Pharmaceutical Products
200 Abbott Park Rd.
Abbott Park, IL 60064-3500
Phone: (847)937-6100 **Fax:** (847)938-3560
Website: http://www.abbott.com
Miles White, CEO & Chm Bd
Desc: Manufacturer/distributor of Rx/ethical pharmaceuticals, anesthesia equipment and products; diagnostic equipment and instruments; EMS equipment and supplies; hospital equipment and supplies; orthopedic and prosthetic equipment and supplies.

★ 15168 ★ Abbott Laboratories, MediSense Products
4A Crosby Dr.
Bedford, MA 01730
Phone: (781)276-6000 **Fax:** (781)276-6364
Website: http://www.medisense.com
Christopher Ludwig, Contact
Desc: Manufacturer of diagnostic reagents and test kits, home healthcare.

★ 15169 ★ Abgenix
6701 Kaiser Dr.
Fremont, CA 94555
Phone: (510)608-6500 **Fax:** (510)608-6589
Website: http://www.abgenix.com
R. Scott Greer, CEO & Chm Bd
Desc: Biotechnology company: biotechnology/biopharmaceutical products.

★ 15170 ★ Abkit, Inc.
207 E 94th St., Ste. 201
New York, NY 10128
Phone: (212)860-8358 **Free:** 800-226-6227
Fax: (212)860-8323
Email: info@abkit.com
Website: http://www.abkit.com
Claus Gehringer, PhD, President
Desc: Manufacturer of dietary, nutritional and vitamin supplements; skin/wound care products.

★ 15171 ★ Abodia Lighted Slide Storage Systems
Division of Elden Enterprises, Inc.
PO Box 3201
Charleston, WV 25332-3201
Phone: (304)344-2335 **Free:** 800-950-7775
Fax: (304)344-4764
Email: slides@abodia.com
Website: http://www.abodia.com
T. Elden, President
Desc: Manufacturer/distributor of audiovisual supplies and equipment; hospital equipment and supplies; hospital furniture; laboratory supplies; ophthalmic equipment; record keeping/archival; slide viewing systems.

★ 15172 ★ Accu-line Products, Inc.
379 Iyanough Rd.
PO Box 875
Hyannis, MA 02601
Phone: (508)771-8022 **Free:** 800-363-7740
Fax: (508)771-8022
Email: acculine@acculine.com
Website: http://www.acculine.com
Douglas J. Laviana, President
Desc: Manufacturer of cardiovascular supplies; disposable medical devices and supplies; hospital equipment and supplies; ophthalmic supplies; ostomy equipment and supplies; physicians' supplies; skin/wound care products; sterilization supplies; surgical disposables; surgical instruments; surgical supplies; X-ray supplies.

★ 15173 ★ Accurate Surgical & Scientific Instruments Corp.
300 Shames Dr.
Westbury, NY 11590
Phone: (516)333-2570 **Free:** 800-645-3569
Fax: (516)997-4948
Email: assi@accuratesurgical.com
Website: http://www.accuratesurgical.com
Marie Bonazinga, President
Desc: Manufacturer/distributor of disposable medical devices and supplies; hospital equipment and supplies; leeches, microsurgical instruments; ophthalmic equipment and supplies; orthopedic and prosthetic equipment and supplies; sterilization supplies; surgical disposables; surgical instruments; surgical supplies; veterinary products.

★ 15174 ★ Acme Medical Scale Co.
1801 Adams Ave.
San Leandro, CA 94577
Phone: (510)638-5040 **Free:** 800-233-5113
Fax: (510)638-5619
Email: information@acmescales.com
Website: http://www.acmescales.com
Lou Buran, President
Desc: Manufacturer of hospital equipment and supplies; hospital patient weighing scales.

★ 15175 ★ Acme-Monaco Corp.
75 Winchell Dr.
New Britain, CT 06052
Phone: (860)224-1349 **Fax:** (860)827-9982
Email: acmecorp@acmemonaco.com
Website: http://www.acmemonaco.com
Michael Karabin, President
Desc: Contract manufacturer of disposable medical devices and supplies.

★ 15176 ★ Acme of Precision Surgical Co., Inc.
485 S 21st St.
Irvington, NJ 07111
Phone: (973)373-6797 **Fax:** (973)373-1267
Rosa Auricchio, President
Desc: Manufacturer of surgical instruments.

★ 15177 ★ ACMI Corp.
Corporate Headquarters
Southborough Place
136 Turnpike Rd.
Southborough, MA 01772
Phone: (508)804-2600 **Free:** 888-524-7266
Fax: (508)804-2624
Website: http://www.circoncorp.com
Greg Barrett, CEO & Pres
Desc: Manufacturer/distributor of anesthesia equipment and products; diagnostic equipment and instruments; disposable medical devices and supplies; endoscopy products; hospital equipment and supplies; physicians' equipment; surgical disposables, instruments and supplies; urinary equipment.

★ 15178 ★ Action Labs, Inc.
2915 E Ricker Way
Anaheim, CA 92806
Phone: (714)630-5941 **Free:** 800-400-5696
Fax: (714)630-8221
Email: actionvit@aol.com
Website: http://www.actionlab.com
James R. Bailey, President

/DES Manufacturer/distributor of OTC/proprietary pharmaceuticals; dental supplies; dietary, nutritional and vitamin supplements.

★ 15179 ★ Action Technology Division of Tekni-Plex
18 Greenpond Rd.
Rockaway, NJ 07866
Phone: (973)625-9400 **Fax:** (973)625-9409
Joseph V. Raborn, Contact
Desc: Manufacturer of disposable medical devices and supplies.

★ 15180 ★ ACUSON Corp. a Siemens Co.
1220 Charleston Rd.
Mountain View, CA 94043
Phone: (650)969-9112 **Free:** 800-422-8766
Website: http://www.acuson.com
John Pavlidis, CEO
Desc: Manufacturer/distributor of cardiovascular equipment; diagnostic equipment and instruments; hospital equipment and supplies; ultrasonic equipment; ultrasound and electromedical equipment and supplies.

★ 15181 ★ ADC Hospital Equipment Division of Automatic Devices Co.
2121 S 12th St.
Allentown, PA 18103
Phone: (610)797-6000 **Fax:** (610)797-4088
Website: http://www.automaticdevices.com/hospital
John A. Samuels, President
Desc: Manufacturer of hospital equipment and supplies.

★ 15182 ★ ADH Health Products, Inc.
215 N Rte. 303
Congers, NY 10920
Phone: (845)268-0027 **Fax:** (845)268-2988
Email: info@adhhealth.com
Website: http://www.adhhealth.com
Balram Advani, Chairman of the Board
Desc: Manufacturer/distributor of dietary, nutritional and vitamin supplements.

★ 15183 ★ Adtech Filling Systems
Lincoln Center No. 2
Reetz and Lincoln Ave.s
Hulmeville, PA 19047
Phone: (215)891-9272 **Fax:** (215)891-9273
Email: maildrop@liquidfilling.com
Website: http://www.liquidfilling.com
Alan Miller, President
Desc: Manufacturer of liquids; sterile filling equipment; parenteral equipment.

★ 15184 ★ Advanced American Biotechnology (AAB)
1166 E Valencia Dr.
Unit 6C
Fullerton, CA 92831
Phone: (714)870-0290 **Free:** 800-927-2290
Fax: (714)870-6385
Email: aab@ix.netcom.com
Website: http://www.aabi.com
R.A. Zeineh, PhD, President
Desc: Manufacturer of laboratory equipment.

★ 15185 ★ Advanced Instrument Development, Inc.
1011 N 25th Ave.
Melrose Park, IL 60160
Phone: (708)343-7777 **Free:** 800-243-9729
Fax: (708)343-7795
Email: sales@aidxray.com
Website: http://www.aidxray.com
Lyle E. Packard, CEO & Chm Bd
Desc: Manufacturer of x-ray equipment.

★ 15186 ★ Advanced Instruments, Inc.
2 Technology Way
Norwood, MA 02062-2680
Phone: (781)320-9000 **Free:** 800-225-4034
Fax: (781)320-8181
Email: mail@aicompanies.com
Website: http://www.aicompanies.com
John Coughlin, President
Desc: Manufacturer of diagnostic reagents and test kits; laboratory equipment.

★ 15187 ★ Advanced Magnetics, Inc.
61 Mooney St.
Cambridge, MA 02138
Phone: (617)497-2070 **Fax:** (617)547-2445
Email: ami@aol.com
Website: http://www.advancedmagnetics.com
Jerome Goldstein, CEO & Chm Bd
Desc: Manufacturer/biotechnology company: Rx/ethical pharmaceuticals; biotechnology/biopharmaceutical products; magnetic resonance imaging.

★ 15188 ★ Advanced Medical Systems, Inc.
121 N Eagle St.
Geneva, OH 44041
Phone: (440)466-8005 **Fax:** (440)466-8629
Seymour S. Stein, PhD, President
Desc: Manufacturer of nuclear and radiological equipment; nuclear and radiological supplies.

★ 15189 ★ Advanced Neuromodulation Systems, Inc.
6501 Windcrest Dr.
Ste. 100
Plano, TX 75024
Phone: (972)309-8000 **Free:** 800-727-7846
Fax: (972)309-8150
Email: lifegetsbetter@ans-medical.com
Website: http://www.ans-medical.com
Christopher G. Chavez, CEO & Pres
Desc: Manufacturer of implantable device systems for pain management.

★ 15190 ★ Aesculap, Inc. Subsidiary of Aesculap AG of Germany
3773 Corporate Parkway
Center Valley, PA 18034
Free: 800-258-1946 **Fax:** (610)791-6880
Website: http://www.aesculap-usa.com
Desc: Distributor of diagnostic equipment and instruments; hospital equipment and supplies; orthopedic and prosthetic equipment and supplies; physicians' equipment; sterilization equipment; sterilization supplies; surgical disposables; surgical instruments.

★ 15191 ★ AFP Imaging Corp. Marketing Division
250 Clearbrook Rd.
Elmsford, NY 10523
Phone: (914)592-6100 **Free:** 800-592-6666
Fax: (914)592-6148
Website: http://www.afpimaging.com
David Vozick, Chairman of the Board
Manufacturer/distributor of dental equipment and supplies; diagnostic equipment and instruments; hospital equipment and supplies; nuclear and radiological equipment; physicians' equipment; surgical supplies; urinary supplies; veterinary products; X-ray equipment and supplies.

★ 15192 ★ AgFa Healthcare Healthcare Imaging
10 S Academy St.
Greenville, SC 29602
Phone: (864)421-1700 **Free:** 888-557-6100
Fax: (864)421-1622
Website: http://www.agfa.com/healthcare
Robert Pryor, President
Desc: Manufacturer/distributor of PACS supplier; X-ray equipment and supplies.

★ 15193 ★ Air Products and Chemicals, Inc.
7201 Hamilton Blvd.
Allentown, PA 18195-1501
Phone: (610)481-4911 **Free:** 800-654-4567
Fax: 800-272-4449
Email: gasinfo@apci.com
Website: http://www.airproducts.com
John P. Jones, Chairman of the Board
Desc: Manufacturer of laboratory equipment; laboratory gases, magnetic resonance imaging; respiratory therapy and/or cardiopulmonary supplies.

★ 15194 ★ Aircast, Inc.
PO Box 709
Summit, NJ 07902
Phone: (908)273-6349 **Free:** 800-526-8785
Fax: 800-457-4221
Website: http://www.aircast.com
Jim Johnson, President
Desc: Manufacturer/distributor of orthopedic and prosthetic equipment and supplies; skin/wound care products; physical therapy and rehabilitation equipment and supplies.

★ 15195 ★ AirSep Corp. Medical Products Division
401 Creekside Dr.
Buffalo, NY 14228-2085
Phone: (716)691-0202 **Free:** 800-874-0202
Fax: (716)691-4141
Email: marketing@airsep.com
Website: http://www.airsep.com
Ravinder Bansal, CEO & Chm Bd
Desc: Manufacturer of home healthcare; hospital equipment and supplies; oxlmetry system; respiratory therapy and/or cardiopulmonary equipment and supplies; sleep diagnostics/therapeutics; ultrasonic nebulizers.

★ 15196 ★ AIRWAY Division of Surgical Appliance Industries
3960 Roslyn Dr.
Cincinnati, OH 45209
Phone: (513)271-4594 **Free:** 800-888-0458
Fax: 800-309-9055
Email: airway@surgicalappliance.com
Website: http://www.surgicalappliance.com
Tom Applegate, CEO & Pres
Desc: Manufacturer/distributor of orthopedic and prosthetic equipment and supplies; patient aid products.

★ 15197 ★ AIV Systems, Inc
443 Commerce Lane
PO Box 458
Berlin, NJ 08009
Phone: (856)768-8370 **Free:** 800-922-0117
Fax: (856)768-1321
Email: whd@aivsystems.com
Website: http://www.aivsystems.com
Wallace Desjardins, President
Desc: Manufacturer of hospital equipment and supplies.

★ 15198 ★ Akorn, Inc.
2500 Millbrook Dr.
Buffalo Grove, IL 60089
Phone: (847)279-6100 **Free:** 800-932-5676
Fax: (847)279-6123
Email: you@akorn.com
Website: http://www.akorn.com
Antonio Pera, Sr., CEO & Pres
Desc: Manufacturer/distributor of Rx/ethical pharmaceuticals; OTC/proprietary pharmaceuticals; generic

pharmaceuticals; ophthalmic supplies; sterilization supplies; surgical disposables.

★ 15199 ★ Al Pharma Purpac USPD, Inc.
200 Elmora Ave.
Elizabeth, NJ 07207
Phone: (908)527-9100 **Free:** 800-432-8534
Fax: (908)659-2480
Website: http://www.alphapharmauspd.com
Michael Nestor, President
Desc: Manufacturer of generic pharmaceuticals.

★ 15200 ★ ALARIS Medical Systems, Inc.
10221 Wateridge Circle
San Diego, CA 92121-2733
Phone: (858)458-7000 **Free:** 800-854-7128
Fax: (858)458-7760
Website: http://www.alarismed.com
David Schlotterbeck, CEO & Pres
Desc: Manufacturer/distributor of disposable medical devices and supplies; home healthcare; hospital equipment and supplies; patient aid products; patient monitoring equipment.

★ 15201 ★ Alba Health Products Division of Alba-Waldensian, Inc.
425 N Gateway Ave.
Rockwood, TN 37854
Phone: (865)354-0410 **Free:** 800-262-2404
Fax: (865)354-1541
Email: info@alba1.com
Website: http://www.albahealth.com
Jeffrey Hale, Contact
Desc: Manufacturer of cardiovascular equipment; hospital equipment and supplies; patient aid products; physicians' supplies; surgical disposables; urinary equipment.

★ 15202 ★ Alcan Packaging Wheaton USA Inc.
1101 Wheaton Ave.
Millville, NJ 08332
Phone: (856)825-1400 **Free:** 800-257-8547
Fax: (856)765-2003
Website: http://www.alcan.com
Michael Rubenstein, Contact
Desc: Manufacturer of disposable medical devices and supplies; hospital equipment and supplies; laboratory equipment and supplies; parenteral supplies; personal care and cosmetics packaging; pharmaceutical packaging.

★ 15203 ★ Alcon Laboratories, Inc. Division of Nestle
6201 S Freeway
Fort Worth, TX 76134-2099
Phone: (817)293-0450 **Fax:** (817)568-7000
Website: http://www.alconlabs.com
Tim Sear, CEO & Pres
Desc: Manufacturer/distributor of Rx/ethical pharmaceuticals; OTC/proprietary pharmaceuticals; ophthalmic equipment; surgical disposables, instruments and supplies.

★ 15204 ★ Alcon Laboratories, Inc. Pharmaceutical Division
6201 S Freeway
Fort Worth, TX 76134-2099
Phone: (817)293-0450 **Free:** 800-451-3937
Fax: (817)551-9821
Website: http://www.alconlabs.com
Tim Sear, CEO
Desc: Manufacturer/distributor of Rx/ethical pharmaceuticals; OTC/proprietary pharmaceuticals; generic pharmaceuticals; ophthalmic supplies; surgical instruments and supplies.

★ 15205 ★ Alconox Inc.
30 Glenn St., Ste. 309
White Plains, NY 10603
Phone: (914)948-4040 **Fax:** (914)948-4088
Email: cleaning@alconox.com
Website: http://www.alconox.com
A. Zisman, MD, President
Desc: Manufacturer of biotechnology/biopharmaceutical products; dental supplies; laboratory supplies; nuclear and radiological supplies; parenteral supplies; pharmaceutical manufacturing supplies and equipment; physicians' supplies; renal dialysis supplies; respiratory therapy and/or cardiopulmonary supplies; surgical supplies; veterinary products.

★ 15206 ★ Alexander Technologies
PO Box 1508
Mason City, IA 50402
Phone: (641)423-8955 **Free:** 800-247-1821
Fax: (641)423-1644
Email: alexcust@jumpgate.net
Website: http://www.alexanderbatteries.com
John Casey, Chairman of the Board
Desc: Manufacturer of batteries; battery chargers; EMS equipment and supplies; hospital equipment and supplies.

★ 15207 ★ Alexion Pharmaceuticals Inc.
352 Knotter Dr.
Cheshire, CT 06410
Phone: (203)272-2596 **Fax:** (203)271-8197
Website: http://www.alxn.com
John H. Fried, PhD, Chairman of the Board
Desc: Biotechnology company: Rx/ethical pharmaceuticals; biotechnology/biopharmaceutical products.

★ 15208 ★ AliMed, Inc.
297 High St.
Dedham, MA 02026
Phone: (781)329-2900 **Free:** 800-225-2610
Fax: (781)329-8392
Email: alimed@alimed.com
Website: http://www.alimed.com
Jonathan Bretz, Vice President
Desc: Manufacturer/distributor: Alzheimer products; dysphagia products; home healthcare; hospital equipment and supplies; nuclear and radiological equipment and supplies; orthopedic and prosthetic equipment and supplies; patient aid products; patient monitoring equipment; physical therapy and rehabilitation equipment and supplies; skin/wound care products; speech therapy products; ultrasound and electromedical equipment and supplies; X-ray supplies.

★ 15209 ★ Allegiance Healthcare Corp. A Cardinal Health Co.
1500 Waukegan Rd.
McGaw Park, IL 60085
Phone: (847)578-2311
Website: http://www.cardinal.com
Ronald Labrum, President
Desc: Manufacturer/distributor of cardiovascular equipment and supplies; ophthalmic equipment and supplies; slide viewing systems; sterilization equipment and supplies; surgical disposables; urinary equipment.

★ 15210 ★ Allergan, Inc.
2525 Dupont Dr.
PO Box 19534
Irvine, CA 92623-9534
Phone: (714)246-4500 **Free:** 800-347-4500
Fax: (714)246-4800
Email: corpinfo@allergan.com
Website: http://www.allergan.com
David E. I. Pyott, CEO & Pres
Desc: Manufacturer/distributor of Rx/ethical pharmaceuticals; OTC/proprietary pharmaceuticals; ophthalmic equipment and supplies; Pharmaceutical manufacturing supplies and equipment.

★ 15211 ★ Allergan Skin Care
2525 DuPont Dr.
Irvine, CA 92623-9534
Phone: (714)246-4500 **Free:** 800-347-4500
Fax: (714)246-4764
Website: http://www.allergan.com
Bill Humpfries, Vice President
Desc: Manufacturer/distributor: Rx/ethical pharmaceuticals; OTC/proprietary pharmaceuticals; skin/wound care products.

★ 15212 ★ Allergan Surgical Division of Allergan, Inc.
2525 DuPont Dr.
Irvine, CA 92623
Phone: (714)246-4500 **Free:** 800-347-4500
Fax: (714)246-2440
Email: corpinfo@allergan.com
Website: http://www.allergan.com
Michael Ball, President
Desc: Manufacturer of Rx/ethical pharmaceuticals; ophthalmic equipment and supplies; surgical instruments.

★ 15213 ★ Alliant Medical Technologies
1400 Providence Hwy.
Bldg. 2
Norwood, MA 02062
Phone: (781)762-2080 **Free:** 800-433-5474
Fax: (781)762-2416
Email: sales@alliantmed.com
Website: http://www.alliantmed.com
Dan Muscatello, CEO & Pres
Desc: Manufacturer/Distributor/Biotechnology Company: disposable medical devices and supplies; radiation treatment planning software; radiopharmaceuticals; surgical disposables and instruments; ultrasound and electromedical equipment and supplies.

★ 15214 ★ Allied Diagnostic Imaging Resources, Inc. A CPAC Co.
5440 Oakbrook Parkway
Norcross, GA 30093
Phone: (770)448-0250 **Free:** 800-262-9333
Fax: (770)448-0257
Website: http://www.alliedautex.com
Brad Hendrickson, President
Desc: Manufacturer of dental accessories and supplies; X-ray accessories, equipment and supplies.

★ 15215 ★ Allied Healthcare Products, Inc.
1720 Sublette Ave.
Saint Louis, MO 63110
Phone: (314)771-2400 **Free:** 800-444-3954
Fax: (314)771-1242
Website: http://www.alliedhpi.com
Earl R. Refsland, President
Desc: Manufacturer of dental supplies; disposable medical devices and supplies; EMS equipment and supplies; home healthcare; hospital equipment and supplies; respiratory therapy and/or cardiopulmonary equipment and supplies; skin/wound care products.

★ 15216 ★ Allscripts, Inc.
2401 Commerce Dr.
Libertyville, IL 60048
Phone: (847)680-3515 **Free:** 800-654-0889
Fax: (847)680-3573
Email: info@allscripts.com
Website: http://www.allscripts.com
Glen Tullman, CEO
Desc: Distributor of Rx/ethical pharmaceuticals; OTC/proprietary pharmaceuticals; generic pharmaceuticals; medication management solutions; repackaged pharmaceuticals.

★ 15217 ★ Alpha Industries, Inc.
701 N Greenwood Ave.
PO Box 808
Clearwater, FL 33757
Phone: (727)443-2673 **Fax:** (727)443-2674
Email: alphainc@tampabay.rr.com
Loleta M. Magers, President
Desc: Manufacturer of cardiovascular supplies; renal dialysis supplies; surgical disposables; surgical instruments.

★ 15218 ★ Alpha Therapeutic Corp.
Division of Mitsubishi Pharma
5555 Valley Blvd.
Los Angeles, CA 90032
Phone: (323)225-2221 **Free:** 800-421-0008
Email: info@alphather.com
Website: http://www.alphather.com
Edward A. Colton, CEO & Pres
Desc: Manufacturer/distributor/biotechnology company: Rx/ethical pharmaceuticals; biotechnology/biopharmaceutical products.

★ 15219 ★ Alpharma
Alpharma Corporate Headquarters
1 Executive Dr.
Fort Lee, NJ 07024
Phone: (201)947-7774
Website: http://www.alpharma.com
Ingrid Wiik, CEO & Pres
Desc: Manufacturer/distributor: Rx/ethical pharmaceuticals; OTC/proprietary pharmaceuticals; generic pharmaceuticals; veterinary products.

★ 15220 ★ Alra Laboratories, Inc.
3850 Clearview Ct.
Gurnee, IL 60031
Phone: (847)244-9440 **Free:** 800-248-2572
Fax: (847)244-9464
Dr. Raj Bhutani, President
Desc: Manufacturer/distributor: Rx/ethical pharmaceuticals; OTC/proprietary pharmaceuticals; generic pharmaceuticals.

★ 15221 ★ Altana Inc.
Division of Altana A.G.
60 Baylis Rd.
Melville, NY 11747
Phone: (631)454-7677 **Free:** 800-432-6673
Fax: (631)454-6389
Website: http://www.savagelabs.com
George Cole, President
Desc: Manufacturer/distributor: Rx/ethical pharmaceuticals; OTC/proprietary pharmaceuticals; generic pharmaceuticals.

★ 15222 ★ AltaRex Corp.
610 Lincoln St.
Waltham, MA 02451
Phone: (781)672-0138 **Free:** 888-801-6665
Fax: (781)672-0142
Email: info@altarex.com
Website: http://www.altarex.com
Antoine A. Noujaim, PhD, Chairman of the Board
Desc: Biotechnology company: Rx/ethical pharmaceuticals; biotechnology/biopharmaceutical products.

★ 15223 ★ Alto Pharmaceuticals, Inc.
15810 Gulf Blvd.
Redington Beach, FL 33708
Phone: (727)319-2891 **Free:** 800-330-2891
Fax: (727)392-0692
Email: altopharm@aol.com
John J. Cullaro, Chairman of the Board
Desc: Distributor of Rx/ethical pharmaceuticals; OTC/proprietary pharmaceuticals; generic pharmaceuticals; dietary, nutritional and vitamin supplements.

★ 15224 ★ Altus Biologics, Inc.
625 Putnam Ave.
Cambridge, MA 02139-4807
Phone: (617)299-2900 **Free:** 888-ALT-CLEC
Fax: (617)299-2999
Email: info@altus.com
Website: http://www.altus.com
Peter Lanciano, President
Desc: Biotechnology company: biotechnology/biopharmaceutical products; pharmacy delivery.

★ 15225 ★ ALVA/AMCO Pharmacal Cos., Inc.
7711 N Merrimac Ave.
Niles, IL 60714
Phone: (847)663-0700 **Fax:** (847)663-1400
Email: alva-amco@aol.com
Website: http://www.alva-amco.com
Emile H. Gerchenson, Chairman of the Board
Desc: Distributor of OTC/proprietary pharmaceuticals.

★ 15226 ★ ALZA Corp.
1900 Charleston Rd.
Mountain View, CA 94043
Phone: (650)564-5000 **Fax:** (650)564-5151
Email: corpinfo@alza.com
Website: http://www.alza.com
Samuel Saks, Chairman of the Board
Desc: Manufacturer/distributor/biotechnology company: Rx/ethical pharmaceuticals; OTC/proprietary pharmaceuticals; biotechnology/biopharmaceutical products; diagnostic equipment and instruments; implants and infusions; patient aid products.

★ 15227 ★ Amano Enzyme U.S.A. Co., Ltd.
Division of Amano Pharmaceutical (Nagoya, Japan)
1157 N Main St.
Lombard, IL 60148
Phone: (630)953-1891 **Free:** 800-446-7652
Fax: (630)953-1895
Website: http://www.amano-enzyme.co.jp
Setsuko Jolly, CEO & Pres
Desc: Manufacturer/distributor/biotechnology company: biotechnology/biopharmaceutical products; diagnostic reagents and test kits; diagnostic enzymes.

★ 15228 ★ Ambulatory Monitoring, Inc.
731 Saw Mill River Rd.
PO Box 0609
Ardsley, NY 10502-0609
Phone: (914)693-9240 **Free:** 800-341-0066
Fax: (914)693-6604
Email: info@ambulatory-monitoring.com
Website: http://www.ambulatory-monitoring.com
William Gruen, Contact
Desc: Manufacturer/distributor: diagnostic equipment and instruments; hospital equipment and supplies; patient monitoring equipment; sleep diagnostics/therapeutics.

★ 15229 ★ AMD-Ritmed Inc.
175 Rano St.
Buffalo, NY 14207
Phone: (716)871-9164 **Free:** 800-445-0340
Fax: (716)871-3415
Email: amdsales@amdritmed.com
Website: http://www.amdritmed.com
Ian Levine, President
Desc: Manufacturer/distributor: apparel; dental supplies; disposable medical devices and supplies; home healthcare; hospital equipment and supplies; ophthalmic supplies; skin/wound care products; sterilization supplies; surgical disposables; surgical supplies.

★ 15230 ★ American Gas & Chemical Corp.
220 Pegasus Ave.
Northvale, NJ 07647
Phone: (201)767-7300 **Free:** 800-288-3647
Fax: (201)767-1741
Email: info@amgas.com
Website: http://www.amgas.com
Gerald L. Anderson, President
Desc: Manufacturer of hospital equipment and supplies; sterilization equipment.

★ 15231 ★ American Generics, Inc.
34 W Fulton St.
Gloversville, NY 12078
Phone: (518)725-1800 **Free:** 800-721-3784
Fax: (518)725-1869
V. Ravi Chandran, PhD, CEO & Pres
Desc: Manufacturer/distributor: Rx/ethical pharmaceuticals; OTC/proprietary pharmaceuticals; generic pharmaceuticals.

★ 15232 ★ American Medical Systems, Inc.
10700 Bren Rd. W
Minnetonka, MN 55343
Phone: (952)933-4666 **Free:** 800-328-3881
Fax: (952)930-6157
Website: http://www.visitams.com
Mary Strom, Contact
Desc: Manufacturer/biotechnology company: biotechnology/biopharmaceutical products; implants and infusion.

★ 15233 ★ American Regent Laboratories
Division of Luitpold Pharmaceuticals, Inc.
1 Luitpold Dr.
Shirley, NY 11967-4799
Phone: (631)924-4000 **Free:** 800-645-1706
Fax: (631)924-1731
Website: http://www.luitpold.com
Ralf Lange, CEO & Pres
Desc: Manufacturer of Rx/ethical pharmaceuticals; generic pharmaceuticals; home healthcare.

★ 15234 ★ American Ultraviolet Co.
212 S Mt. Zion Rd.
Lebanon, IN 46052
Phone: (765)483-9514 **Free:** 800-288-9288
Fax: (765)483-9525
Website: http://www.americanultraviolet.com
Meredith C. Stines, CEO
Desc: Manufacturer of sterilization equipment and supplies; UV.

★ 15235 ★ AmeriSourceBergen Corp.
1300 Morris Dr.
Ste. 100
Wayne, PA 19087
Phone: (610)727-7000 **Fax:** (610)727-3600
Email: sales@amerisourcebergen.net
Website: http://www.amerisource.com
R. David Yost, CEO & Pres
Desc: Distributor/biotechnology company: Rx/ethical pharmaceuticals; OTC/proprietary pharmaceuticals; generic pharmaceuticals; biotechnology/biopharmaceutical products; dietary, nutritional and vitamin supplements; disposable; EMS equipment and supplies; home healthcare; laboratory equipment and supplies; parenteral catheters and supplies; patient aid products; patient monitoring equipment; physical therapy and rehabilitation equipment and supplies; physicians' equipment and supplies; renal dialysis supplies; respiratory therapy and/or cardiopulmonary supplies; skin/wound care products. equipment and supplies; parenteral catheters, equipment and supplies; patient aid products; physical therapy and rehabilitation equipment and supplies; physicians' equipment and supplies; radiopharmaceuticals; renal dialysis equipment and supplies; respiratory therapy and/or cardiopulmonary equipment and supplies; skin/wound care prod-

ucts; sleep diagnostics/therapeutics; sterilization supplies; surgical disposables and supplies; urinary supplies; veterinary products; X-ray supplies.

★ 15236 ★ AmerisourceBergen Corp.
9900 J.EB. Sturat Pkwy
Glen Allen, VA 23060
Phone: (804)264-0444 **Free:** 800-262-8470
Fax: (804)533-1044
Website: http://www.amerisourcebergen.net
Rick Oyler, Contact

Desc: Distributor of Rx/ethical pharmaceuticals; OTC/proprietary pharmaceuticals; generic pharmaceuticals; dietary, nutritional and vitamin supplements.

★ 15237 ★ Amersham Biosciences, Inc.
800 Centennial Ave.
Piscataway, NJ 08855
Phone: (732)457-8000 **Free:** 800-526-3593
Fax: (732)457-8225
Email: info@amersham.com
Website: http://www.apbiotech.com
Andrew Carr, CEO

Desc: Manufacturer/distributor/biotechnology company: biotechnology/biopharmaceutical products; diagnostic reagents and test kits; laboratory equipment; nuclear and radiological supplies; sequencing instruments and reagents.

★ 15238 ★ Amersham Health
101 Carnegie Center
Princeton, NJ 08540
Phone: (609)514-6000 **Free:** 800-394-6926
Fax: (609)514-6580
Website: http://www.amersham.com
Daniel L. Peters, President

Desc: Manufacturer/distributor of contrast media; nuclear and radiological equipment and supplies; nuclear imaging; renal dialysis equipment.

★ 15239 ★ Amgen, Inc.
1 Amgen Center Dr.
Thousand Oaks, CA 91320
Phone: (805)447-1000 **Fax:** (805)447-1010
Website: http://www.amgen.com
Kevin Sharer, CEO & Chm Bd

Desc: Manufacturer/distributor/biotechnology company: Rx/ethical pharmaceuticals; biotechnology/biopharmaceutical products.

★ 15240 ★ Amigo Mobility International, Inc.
6693 Dixie Hwy.
Bridgeport, MI 48722
Phone: (517)777-0910 **Free:** 800-821-2710
Fax: (517)777-8184
Email: info@myamigo.com
Website: http://www.myamigo.com
Allan R. Thieme, President

Desc: Manufacturer of patient aid products.

★ 15241 ★ Amrex Electro-Therapy Equipment
641 E Walnut St.
Carson, CA 90746
Phone: (310)527-6868 **Free:** 800-221-9069
Fax: (310)366-7343
Email: amrex@amrex-zetron.com
Website: http://www.amrex-zetron.com
George L. Bell, CEO & Pres

Desc: Manufacturer of EMS equipment and supplies; pain management; physical therapy and rehabilitation equipment and supplies; ultrasonic equipment; ultrasound and electromedical equipment and supplies.

★ 15242 ★ Amzco/Surgical Devices Division of Amzura Enterprises, Inc.
198-200 N Main St.
Freeport, NY 11520
Phone: (516)378-3140 **Free:** 800-645-2848
Fax: (516)623-7679
Email: amzura@aol.com
Javaid Ratcher, President

Desc: Manufacturer/distributor: anesthesia equipment and products; diagnostic equipment and instruments; disposable medical devices and supplies; EMS equipment and supplies; home healthcare; hospital equipment and supplies; patient aid products; physicians' equipment and supplies; slide viewing systems; sterilization supplies; surgical disposables and instruments.

★ 15243 ★ Anabolic Laboratories, Inc.
17802 Gillette Ave.
PO Box C-19508
Irvine, CA 92710
Phone: (949)863-0340 **Fax:** (949)261-2928
Email: sales@anabolicinc.com
Website: http://www.anabolicinc.com
Steven R. Brown, President

Desc: Manufacturer of Rx/ethical pharmaceuticals; generic pharmaceuticals; dietary, nutritional and vitamin supplements.

★ 15244 ★ Analogic
Centennial Industrial Park
8 Centennial Dr.
Peabody, MA 01960
Phone: (978)977-3000 **Fax:** (978)977-6809
Email: corporate@analogic.com
Website: http://www.analogic.com
Bernard M. Gordon, CEO & Chm Bd

Desc: Manufacturer of cardiovascular equipment; hospital equipment and supplies; magnetic resonance imaging; nuclear and radiological equipment; patient monitoring equipment; ultrasound and electromedical equipment and supplies; X-ray equipment.

★ 15245 ★ Analox Instruments U.S.A.
PO Box 208
Lunenburg, MA 01462-0208
Phone: (978)582-9368 **Fax:** (978)582-9588
Email: info@analoxusa.com
Website: http://www.analoxusa.com
David Redstone, Chairman of the Board

Desc: Manufacturer/biotechnology company: biotechnology/biopharmaceutical products; diagnostic equipment and instruments; diagnostic reagents and test kits; laboratory equipment and supplies.

★ 15246 ★ Anchor Products Co.
52 Official Rd.
Addison, IL 60101
Phone: (630)543-9124 **Free:** 800-323-5134
Fax: (630)543-9131
Email: info@anchorsurgical.com
Website: http://www.anchorsurgical.com
Robert H. Thrun, President

Desc: Manufacturer/distributor: dental equipment and supplies; ophthalmic equipment and supplies; surgical instruments; veterinary products.

★ 15247 ★ Andrews Glass Comp.
3740 N West Blvd.
Vineland, NJ 08360
Phone: (856)692-4435 **Free:** 800-845-0026
Fax: (856)692-5357
Email: mail@andrews-glass.com
Website: http://www.andrews-glass.com
Dennis Courtney, President

Desc: Manufacturer of custom glass/quartz fabrication; laboratory supplies; OEM glass/quartz components.

★ 15248 ★ Andrx Corp.
4955 Orange Dr.
Davie, FL 33314
Phone: (954)217-4500 **Free:** 800-331-2632
Fax: (954)792-1034
Website: http://www.andrx.com
Alan P. Cohen, Contact

Desc: Manufacturer/distributor of Rx/ethical pharmaceuticals; generic pharmaceuticals; OTC/proprietary pharmaceuticals.

★ 15249 ★ Angelica Image Apparel Division of Angelica Corp.
700 Rosedale
Saint Louis, MO 63112
Phone: (314)889-1111 **Free:** 800-325-8032
Fax: (314)889-1146
Email: custadm@angelica.com
Website: http://www.angelica.com
Charles Molloy, President

Desc: Manufacturer/distributor of apparel.

★ 15250 ★ Antares Pharma, Inc.
161 Cheshire Lane North, Ste. 100
Minneapolis, MN 55441
Phone: (763)475-7700 **Free:** 800-328-3074
Fax: (763)476-1009
Email: needlefree@antarespharma.com
Website: http://www.antarespharma.com
Roger G. Harrison, PhD, CEO & Pres

Desc: Manufacturer of disposable medical devices and supplies; drug delivery equipment; pharmaceutical manufacturing supplies and equipment.

★ 15251 ★ Antek Instruments
300 Bammel Westfield Rd.
Houston, TX 77090
Phone: (281)580-0339 **Free:** 800-365-2143
Fax: (281)580-0719
Email: sales@antekhou.com
Website: http://www.antekhou.com
Tom E. McMullen, CEO & Pres

Desc: Manufacturer of biotechnology/biopharmaceutical products; HPLC and sulfur detectors; laboratory equipment; pharmaceutical manufacturing supplies and equipment; total nitrogen analyzers.

★ 15252 ★ Antibodies Inc.
PO Box 1560
Davis, CA 95617-1560
Phone: (530)758-4400 **Free:** 800-824-8540
Fax: (530)758-6307
Email: antiinc@aol.com
Website: http://www.antibodiesinc.com
Richard Krogsrud, PhD, CEO & Pres

Desc: Manufacturer/distributor/biotechnology company: biotechnology/biopharmaceutical products; contract manufacturing; diagnostic reagents and test kits.

★ 15253 ★ Antigenics Inc.
630 Fifth Ave.
Ste. 2100
New York, NY 10111
Phone: (212)332-4774 **Fax:** (212)332-4778
Email: ir@antigenics.com
Website: http://www.antigenics.com
Garo H. Armen, CEO & Chm Bd

Desc: Biotechnology company offering biotechnology/biopharmaceutical products.

★ 15254 ★ AO SOLA
2277 Pine View Way
PO Box 6006
Petaluma, CA 94954
Phone: (707)763-9911 **Free:** 800-358-8258
Fax: (707)765-1378
Website: http://www.sola.com
Mark Ashcroft, President

Desc: Manufacturer of ophthalmic supplies.

★ 15255 ★ Apex Medical Corp.
921 E Amidon St.
PO Box 1235
Sioux Falls, SD 57104

Phone: (909)941-2844 **Free:** 877-844-2739
Fax: (909)941-1292
Email: apexmed@apexmedical.com
Website: http://www.apexmedical.com
Brian Wicklow, Contact
Desc: Manufacturer/distributor: Disposable medical devices and supplies; home healthcare; patient aid products; veterinary products.

★ 15256 ★ Apotex Corp. Division of Apotex Inc.
2400 N Commerce Parkway
Ste. 400
Weston, FL 33326
Phone: (954)384-8007 **Free:** 800-706-5575
Fax: 800-706-5576
Email: usmarketing@apotexcorp.com
Website: http://www.apotexcorp.com
Tammy L. McIntire, MS,RPh, President
Desc: Manufacturer of generic pharmaceuticals.

★ 15257 ★ Apothecary Products
11750 12th Ave. S
Burnsville, MN 55337
Phone: (952)890-1940 **Free:** 800-328-2742
Fax: 800-328-1584
Email: pillminder@aol.com
Website: http://www.apothecaryproducts.com
Terry O. Noble, RPh, Chairman of the Board
Desc: Manufacturer/distributor: OTC/proprietary pharmaceuticals; generic pharmaceuticals; dental supplies; dietary, nutritional and vitamin supplements; disposable medical devices and supplies; home healthcare; hospital equipment and supplies; laboratory equipment and supplies; patient aid products; physical therapy and rehabilitation equipment and supplies; urinary equipment and supplies; veterinary products.

★ 15258 ★ Applied Biosystems Division of Applera Corp.
500 Old Connecticut Pth
Framingham, MA 01701
Phone: (508)383-7700 **Free:** 800-345-5224
Fax: (508)383-7880
Email: customer.service@appliedbiosystems.com
Website: http://www.appliedbiosystems.com
Tony L. White, CEO & Pres
Desc: Biotechnology company offering biotechnology/biopharmaceutical products; diagnostic reagents and test kits; pharmaceutical manufacturing supplies and equipment.

★ 15259 ★ APREX Division of AARDEX
2849-B Whipple Rd.
Union City, CA 94587
Phone: (510)476-1940 **Free:** 800-524-6833
Fax: (510)476-1946
Website: http://www.aprex.com
Jean-Michel Metry, CEO & Chm Bd
Desc: Manufacturer/distributor of patient monitoring equipment.

★ 15260 ★ AR-EX Ltd.
1282 Old Skokie Rd.
Highland Park, IL 60035
Phone: (847)579-1408 **Fax:** (847)579-1437
Perry Blatt, President
Remarks: Manufacturer of OTC/proprietary pharmaceuticals; skin/wound care products.

★ 15261 ★ Arista Surgical Supply Co.
67 Lexington Ave.
New York, NY 10010
Phone: (212)679-3694 **Free:** 800-223-1984
Fax: (212)696-9046
Email: aristasurgical@juno.com
Website: http://www.aristasurgical.com
Irving Horowitz, President
Desc: Distributor of diagnostic equipment and instruments; hospital equipment and supplies; physicians' equipment and supplies; skin/wound care products; sterilization equipment and supplies; surgical instruments and supplies; veterinary products.

★ 15262 ★ Arjo, Inc.
50 N Gary Ave.
Roselle, IL 60172
Phone: 800-323-1245 **Free:** 888-594-ARJO
Website: http://www.arjo.com
Lorena Chevrie, Contact
Desc: Manufacturer/distributor: bathing and hydrotherapy equipment; hospital equipment and supplies; patient aid products; patient lift transport; patient weighing equipment; skin/sound care products.

★ 15263 ★ Armstrong Medical Industries Inc.
575 Knightsbridge Parkway
PO Box 700
Lincolnshire, IL 60069
Phone: (847)913-0101 **Free:** 800-323-4220
Fax: (847)913-0138
Email: csr@armstrongmedical.com
Website: http://www.armstrongmedical.com
Warren G. Armstrong, CEO & Pres
Desc: Manufacturer/distributor: anesthesia equipment and products; cardiovascular equipment and supplies; diagnostic equipment and instruments; EMS equipment and supplies; hospital equipment and supplies; hospital furniture; respiratory therapy and/or cardiopulmonary equipment and supplies.

★ 15264 ★ Arrow International, Inc.
2400 Bernville Rd.
PO Box 12888
Reading, PA 19612-2888
Phone: (610)378-0131 **Free:** 800-233-3187
Fax: (610)374-5360
Website: http://www.arrowintl.com
Marlin Miller, Jr., Chairman of the Board
Desc: Manufacturer/distributor: anesthesia equipment and products; cardiovascular equipment and supplies; implants and infusion; parenteral catheters; radiopharmaceuticals; renal dialysis supplies; sterilizations supplies; surgical instruments.

★ 15265 ★ Arrow International, Inc.
9 Plymouth St.
Everett, MA 02149
Phone: (617)389-6400 **Free:** 800-343-3297
Fax: (617)387-2157
Website: http://www.arrowintl.com
Donald Kirkpatrick, Contact
Desc: Manufacturer/distributor of anesthesia equipment and products; cardiovascular equipment and supplies; disposable medical devices and supplies; hospital equipment and supplies; implants and infusion; surgical disposables.

★ 15266 ★ Artisan Technologies Dosimeter Products
5 Eastmans Rd.
Parsippany, NJ 07054
Phone: (973)887-7100 **Free:** 800-322-8258
Fax: (973)887-4732
Website: http://www.dosimeter.com
Carolyn Murat, Contact
Desc: Manufacturer/distributor of nuclear and radiological equipment and supplies; x-ray equipment.

★ 15267 ★ Ascendant Solutions, International
101 Merritt 7
Norwalk, CT 06856
Phone: (203)846-0203 **Free:** (866)846-0203
Fax: (203)846-0848
Email: sales@askasi.net
Website: http://www.askasi.net
Mike Oris, Contact
Desc: Manufacturer/distributor of biological and environmental safety products; document imaging supplies and equipment; invasive surgery; film processor.

★ 15268 ★ AstraZeneca
1800 Concord Pike
PO Box 15437
Wilmington, DE 19850-5437
Phone: (302)886-3000 **Fax:** (302)886-2972
Website: http://www.astrazeneca-us.com
David R. Brennan, CEO & Pres
Desc: Manufacturer of Rx/ethical pharmaceuticals.

★ 15269 ★ At Last Naturals
401 Columbus Ave.
Valhalla, NY 10595-1325
Phone: (914)479-0900 **Free:** 800-527-8123
Fax: (914)479-0901
Email: last@alast.com
Website: http://www.alast.com
Bruce M. Last, President
Desc: Manufacturer of OTC/proprietary pharmaceuticals.

★ 15270 ★ Athena Diagnostics Inc.
377 Plantation St.
4 Biotech Park
Worcester, MA 01605
Phone: (508)756-2886 **Free:** 800-394-4493
Fax: (508)753-5601
Email: info@athenadiagnostics.com
Website: http://www.athenadiagnostics.com
Robert E. Flaherty, CEO & Pres
Desc: Biotechnology company: neurological diagnostic laboratory testing.

★ 15271 ★ Atlantic Medco Division of St. Charles Manufacturing Co.
520 Kane St.
Scranton, PA 18505
Phone: (570)969-4066 **Free:** 800-203-8444
Fax: (570)969-2753
Email: stcharlesm@cs.com
Website: http://www.atlanticmedco.com
Leonard A. Mancuso, President
Desc: Manufacturer/distributor: contract manufacturing; hospital equipment and supplies; hospital furniture; laboratory equipment.

★ 15272 ★ Atlantic Ultraviolet Corp.
375 Marcus Blvd.
Hauppauge, NY 11788
Phone: (631)273-0500 **Fax:** (631)273-0771
Email: auv@atlanticuv.com
Website: http://www.atlanticuv.com
Hilary Boehme, President
Desc: Manufacture of hospital equipment and supplies; laboratory equipment; sterilization equipment.

★ 15273 ★ Aurora Biosciences Corp.
11010 Torreyana Rd.
San Diego, CA 92121
Phone: (858)404-6600 **Fax:** (858)404-6714
Email: info@aurorabio.com
Website: http://www.aurorabio.com
Thomas G. Klopack, PhD, Contact
Desc: Biotechnology company offering biotechnology/biopharmaceutical products and drug discovery.

★ 15274 ★ AutoImmune Inc.
1199 Madia St.
Pasadena, CA 91103
Phone: (626)792-1235 **Fax:** (626)792-1236
Website: http://www.autoimmuneinc.com
Robert C. Bishop, PhD, CEO & Chm Bd

Desc: Biotechnology company: Rx/ethical pharmaceuticals; biotechnology/biopharmaceutical products; dietary, nutritional and vitamin supplements.

★ 15275 ★ AVANIR Pharmaceuticals
11388 Sorrento Valley Rd.
Ste. 200
San Diego, CA 92121
Phone: (858)622-5200 **Fax:** (858)658-7447
Email: info@avanir.com
Website: http://www.avanir.com
Gerald J. Yakatan, CEO & Pres
Desc: Biotechnology company: Rx/ethical pharmaceuticals; OTC/proprietary pharmaceuticals; biotechnology/biopharmaceutical products.

★ 15276 ★ AVANT Immunotherapeutics, Inc.
119 Fourth Ave.
Needham, MA 02494
Phone: (781)433-0771 **Fax:** (781)433-0262
Email: info@avantimmune.com
Website: http://www.avantimmune.com
Una S. Ryan, PhD, CEO & Pres
Desc: Biotechnology company: biotechnology/biopharmaceutical products.

★ 15277 ★ Aventis Behring LLC
1020 First Ave.
King of Prussia, PA 19406-1310
Phone: (610)878-4000 **Free:** 800-683-1288
Fax: (610)878-4040
Website: http://www.aventisbehring.com/na
Ruedi Wager, PhD, CEO & Pres
Desc: Manufacturer/biotechnology company: biotechnology/biopharmaceutical products; skin/wound care products.

★ 15278 ★ Aventis Pasteur Inc.
Discovery Dr.
Swiftwater, PA 18370
Phone: (570)839-7187 **Free:** 800—VACCINE
Fax: (570)839-5415
Website: http://www.aventispasteur.com
David J. Williams, CEO & Pres
Desc: Manufacturer/distributor/biotechnology company: biotechnology/biopharmaceutical products.

★ 15279 ★ Aventis Pharmaceuticals
300 Somerset Corporate Blvd.
Bridgewater, NJ 08807
Phone: (908)243-6000
Gerald P. Belle, President
Desc: Manufacturer/biotechnology company: Rx/ethical pharmaceuticals; biotechnology/biopharmaceutical products.

★ 15280 ★ Axcan Pharma
597 Laurier Blvd.
Mont-Saint-Hilaire, QC, Canada J3H 6C4
Phone: (450)467-5138 **Free:** 800-565-3255
Fax: (450)464-9979
Email: axcan@axcan.com
Website: http://www.axcan.com
Leon F. Gosselin, Contact
Desc: Manufacturer/distributor of biotechnology/biopharmaceutical products; diagnostic reagents and test kits.

★ 15281 ★ Axcan Scandipharm Inc.
22 Inverness Center Parkway
Birmingham, AL 35242
Phone: (205)991-8085 **Free:** 800-950-8085
Fax: (205)991-9547
Website: http://www.axcanscandipharm.com
Leon Gosselin, Chairman of the Board
Desc: Manufacturer/distributor of Rx/ethical pharmaceuticals; dietary, nutritional and vitamin supplements; respiratory therapy and/or cardiopulmonary equipment.

★ 15282 ★ Axiom Medical Inc.
555 W Victoria St.
Rancho Dominguez, CA 90220
Phone: (310)898-1779 **Free:** 800-221-8569
Fax: (310)632-1326
Email: sales@axiommed.com
Website: http://www.axiommed.com
J. Rae Walker, MD, CEO & Chm Bd
Desc: Manufacturer of anesthesia equipment and products; cardiovascular supplies; contract manufacturing; disposable medical devices and supplies; laboratory equipment; parenteral catheters; renal dialysis supplies; surgical disposables and instruments; urinary supplies; veterinary products.

★ 15283 ★ B. Braun Biotech, Inc. Division of Sartorius AG
999 Postal Rd.
Allentown, PA 18109
Phone: (610)266-6262 **Free:** 800-258-9000
Fax: (610)266-9319
Email: bbusinfo@bioscripro.com
Website: http://www.bbraunbiotech.com
Leonard Goren, Contact
Desc: Manufacturer/distributor/biotechnology company: bioreactors; biotechnology/biopharmaceutical products; fermentors; laboratory equipment; pharmaceutical manufacturing supplies and equipment.

★ 15284 ★ B. Braun Medical Inc. Division of B. Braun of America
824 12th Ave.
Bethlehem, PA 18018
Phone: (610)691-5400 **Free:** 800-BBR-AUN2
Fax: (610)691-6249
Website: http://www.bbraunusa.com
Caroll H. Neubauer, CEO & Chm Bd
Desc: Manufacturer of Rx/ethical pharmaceuticals; anesthesia equipment and products; cardiovascular supplies; disposable medical devices and supplies; implants and infusion; parenteral catheters, equipment and supplies; skin/wound care products; sterilization supplies; surgical disposables.

★ 15285 ★ Bacti-Lab Inc.
PO Box 1179
Mountain View, CA 94042
Phone: (650)968-3815 **Fax:** (650)961-1020
Website: http://www.bactilab.com
Z. Fink, President
Desc: Manufacturer/distributor/biotechnology company: biotechnology/biopharmaceutical products; diagnostic reagents and test kits; laboratory equipment and supplies; physicians' supplies; ultrasound and electromedical equipment and supplies.

★ 15286 ★ Bailey Manufacturing
118 Lee St.
Lodi, OH 44254
Free: 800-321-8372 **Fax:** 800-224-5390
Email: baileymfg@baileymfg.com
Website: http://www.baileymfg.com
Larry Strimple, President
Desc: Manufacturer of home healthcare; hospital equipment and supplies; hospital furniture; physical therapy and rehabilitation equipment and supplies.

★ 15287 ★ Bajamar Chemical Co., Inc.
9609 Dielman Rock Island
Saint Louis, MO 63132
Phone: (314)997-3414 **Free:** 888-242-3414
Fax: (314)997-2948
Website: http://walden.mvp.net/~bmizes/bcc/bajamar.htm
Harvey Mizes, President
Desc: Distributor of Rx/ethical pharmaceuticals; OTC/proprietary pharmaceuticals; generic pharmaceuticals; dietary, nutritional and vitamin supplements; orthopedic and prosthetic equipment and supplies.

★ 15288 ★ The Baker Co., Inc.
161 Gatehouse Rd.
PO Drawer E
Sanford, ME 04073
Phone: (207)324-8773 **Free:** 800-992-2537
Fax: (207)324-3869
Email: bakerco@bakerco.com
Website: http://www.bakerco.com
Dennis Eagleson, President
Desc: Manufacturer/biotechnology company: biological and environmental safety products; biotechnology/biopharmaceutical products; hospital equipment and supplies; laboratory equipment; pharmaceutical manufacturing supplies and equipment.

★ 15289 ★ Banner Pharmacaps Inc.
4125 Premier Dr.
High Point, NC 27265
Phone: (336)812-4729 **Free:** 800-447-1140
Fax: (336)812-3719
Email: info@banpharm.com
Website: http://www.banpharm.com
Timothy B. Doran, Contact
Desc: Manufacturer of Rx/ethical pharmaceuticals; OTC/proprietary pharmaceuticals; generic pharmaceuticals; contract manufacturing; dietary, nutritional and vitamin supplements.

★ 15290 ★ Banta Healthcare Group Division of Banta Corp.
570 Enterprise Dr.
Neenah, WI 54957
Phone: 888-295-2502 **Free:** 800-521-1314
Fax: 800-837-7770
Email: service@bantahealthcare.com
Website: http://www.bantahealthcare.com
Kevin McNamara, Contact
Desc: Manufacturer of apparel; dental supplies; disposable medical devices and supplies; EMS equipment and supplies; home healthcare; hospital equipment and supplies; laboratory supplies; physicians' supplies; skin/wound care products; sterilization supplies; surgical supplies; veterinary products; X-ray supplies.

★ 15291 ★ Banyan International Corp.
2118 E Interstate 20
PO Box 1779
Abilene, TX 79604
Phone: (915)677-1874 **Free:** 800-351-4530
Fax: (915)677-1372
Email: customerservice@statkit.com
Website: http://www.statkit.com
John W. Michener, Jr., Chairman of the Board
Desc: Manufacturer/distributor: Rx/ethical pharmaceuticals; cardiovascular equipment; disposable medical devices and supplies; EMS equipment and supplies; physicians' equipment and supplies.

★ 15292 ★ Bar-Ray Products, Inc.
95 Monarch St.
Littlestown, PA 17340
Phone: (717)359-9100 **Free:** 800-359-6115
Fax: (717)359-9109
Email: info@bar-ray.com
Website: http://www.bar-ray.com
Jeff Stein, Vice President
Desc: Manufacturer of dental supplies; hospital equipment and supplies; nuclear and radiological supplies; veterinary products; X-ray supplies.

★ 15293 ★ Barnstead International
2555 Kerper Blvd.
Dubuque, IA 52001
Phone: (563)556-2241 **Free:** 800-553-0039
Fax: (563)589-0516
Email: mkt@barnstead.com

Website: http://www.barnsteadint.com
Duncan Ross, President
Desc: Manufacturer of laboratory equipment.

★ 15294 ★ Barnstead/Thermolyne Corp. Division of Apogent Technologies
2555 Kerper Blvd.
PO Box 797
Dubuque, IA 52004-0797
Phone: (319)556-2241 **Free:** 800-446-6060
Fax: (319)589-0516
Email: adv@barnsteadthermolyne.com
Website: http://www.barnsteadthermolyne.com
Duncan Ross, President
Desc: Manufacturer/biotechnology company: biological and environmental safety products; biotechnology/biopharmaceutical products; dental equipment and supplies; laboratory equipment; pharmaceutical manufacturing supplies and equipment; slide viewing systems; sterilization equipment; ultrasonic equipment.

★ 15295 ★ Barr Laboratories, Inc.
2 Quaker Rd.
Box 2900
Pomona, NY 10970
Phone: (845)362-1100 **Free:** 800-222-4043
Fax: (845)353-3843
Email: sales@barrlabs.com
Website: http://www.barrlabs.com
Bruce Downey, CEO & Chm Bd
Desc: Manufacturer/distributor of generic pharmaceuticals.

★ 15296 ★ Bausch & Lomb Pharmaceuticals, Inc. Division of Bausch & Lomb, Inc.
8500 Hidden River Pkwy.
Tampa, FL 33637
Phone: (813)975-7700 **Free:** 800-227-1427
Fax: (813)975-7774
Website: http://www.blpharm.com
Ron Zarella, CEO & Chm Bd
Desc: Manufacturer/distributor of Rx/ethical pharmaceuticals; OTC/proprietary pharmaceuticals; generic pharmaceuticals.

★ 15297 ★ Bausch & Lomb Surgical
180 Via Verde Dr.
San Dimas, CA 91773
Free: 800-338-2020 **Fax:** (909)971-5115
Email: info@blsurgical.com
Website: http://www.bausch.com
Mark Sieczkarek, Vice President
Desc: Manufacturer/distributor of Rx/ethical pharmaceuticals; OTC/proprietary pharmaceuticals; generic pharmaceuticals; diagnostic equipment and instruments; dietary, nutritional and vitamin supplements; disposable medical devices and supplies; implants and infusion; ophthalmic equipment and supplies; physicians' equipment; surgical disposables and instruments.

★ 15298 ★ Baxa Corp.
13760 E Arapahoe Rd.
Englewood, CO 80112-3903
Phone: (303)690-4204 **Free:** 800-567-BAXA
Fax: (303)690-4804
Email: baxamail@baxa.com
Website: http://www.baxa.com
Gregory Baldwin, CEO & Pres
Desc: Manufacturer/distributor of disposable medical devices and supplies; hospital equipment and supplies; parenteral equipment and supplies.

★ 15299 ★ Baxter Healthcare Corp. Anesthesia and Critical Care
95 Spring St.
New Providence, NJ 07974
Phone: (908)286-7000 **Fax:** (908)286-7260
Website: http://www.baxter.com
Ron Quadrel, Vice President
Desc: Manufacturer/distributor of Rx/ethical pharmaceuticals; generic pharmaceuticals; anesthesia equipment and products.

★ 15300 ★ Baxter Healthcare Corp. Baxter BioScience
1627 Lake Cook Rd.
Deerfield, IL 60015
Phone: (847)948-2000 **Free:** 800-241-9360
Fax: (847)940-6802
Website: http://www.baxter.com
Pete O'Malley, Vice President
Desc: Manufacturer/distributor/biotechnology company: Rx/ethical pharmaceuticals; biotechnology/biopharmaceuticals products; skin/wound care products.

★ 15301 ★ Baxter Healthcare Corp. Baxter BioScience
550 N Brand Blvd.
Glendale, CA 91203
Phone: (818)956-3200 **Fax:** (818)507-5596
Website: http://www.baxter.com
Thomas Glanzmann, President
Desc: Biotechnology company: Rx/ethical pharmaceuticals; biotechnology/biopharmaceutical products.

★ 15302 ★ Baxter Healthcare Corp. Medication Delivery
Rte. 120 and Wilson Rd.
Round Lake, IL 60073
Phone: (847)546-6311 **Fax:** (847)270-5562
Website: http://www.baxter.com
Dave Drohan, President
Desc: Manufacturer/distributor of anesthesia equipment and products; home healthcare; hospital equipment and supplies; parenteral equipment and supplies.

★ 15303 ★ Bayer Corp. Biotechnology Center
800 Dwight Way
PO Box 1986
Berkeley, CA 94701-1986
Phone: (510)705-5000 **Free:** 800-227-2720
Fax: (510)705-7889
Website: http://www.bayerus.com
Wolfe-Dieter Busse, Contact
Desc: Manufacturer/biotechnology company: Rx/ethical pharmaceuticals; biotechnology/biopharmaceutical products; generic pharmaceuticals.

★ 15304 ★ Bayer Corp. Consumer Care Division
36 Columbia Rd.
PO Box 1910
Morristown, NJ 07962-1910
Phone: (973)254-5000 **Free:** 800-331-4536
Fax: (973)254-4857
Website: http://www.consumercare.bayer.com
Gary Balkema, President
Desc: manufacturer of OTC/proprietary pharmaceuticals.

★ 15305 ★ Bayer Corp. Diagnostics Group
511 Benedict Ave.
Tarrytown, NY 10591-5097
Phone: (914)631-8000 **Free:** 800-431-1970
Fax: (914)524-2132
Website: http://www.bayerdiag.com
Rolf Classon, Contact
Desc: Manufacturer/distributor of diagnostic equipment and instruments; diagnostic reagents and test kits; hospital equipment and supplies; laboratory equipment.

★ 15306 ★ Bayer Corp. Pharmaceutical Division
400 Morgan Ln.
West Haven, CT 06516-4175
Phone: (203)812-2000 **Free:** 800-468-0894
Fax: (203)812-6547
Website: http://www.bayerus.com
Karen Dawes, Contact
Desc: Manufacturer/biotechnology company: Rx/ethical pharmaceuticals; generic pharmaceuticals; biotechnology/biopharmaceutical products.

★ 15307 ★ BD Biosciences-Discovery Labware
2 Oak Park
Bedford, MA 01730
Phone: (781)275-0004 **Free:** 800-343-2035
Fax: 800-743-6200
Email: labware@bd.com
Website: http://www.bdbiosciences.com/
Guy Page, Contact
Desc: Manufacturer of biotechnology/biopharmaceutical products; cell culture products; laboratory supplies; pharmaceutical manufacturing supplies and equipment.

★ 15308 ★ BD Consumer Healthcare Consumer Health Care
1 Becton Dr.
Franklin Lakes, NJ 07417-1884
Phone: (201)847-7100 **Free:** 800-526-0458
Fax: (201)847-5487
Website: http://www.bd.com/consumer
Kevin Siefert, Vice President
Desc: Manufacturer/distributor of diagnostic equipment and instruments; diagnostic reagents and test kits; disposable medical devices and supplies; home healthcare; laboratory supplies; physicians' supplies; skin/wound care products.

★ 15309 ★ BD Diagnostic Systems
7 Loveton Cir.
Sparks, MD 21152
Phone: (410)316-4000 **Free:** 800-638-8663
Fax: (410)316-4906
Website: http://www.bd.com/diagnostics
Michael Meehan, Vice President
Desc: Manufacturer of biotechnology/biopharmaceutical products; diagnostic equipment and instruments; diagnostic reagents and test kits; instruments; laboratory equipment and supplies; physicians' equipment and supplies.

★ 15310 ★ BD Medical Systems
1 Becton Dr.
Franklin Lakes, NJ 07417
Phone: (201)847-6800 **Free:** 888-237-2762
Fax: (201)847-4845
Website: http://www.bd.com
Gary M. Cohen, President
Desc: Manufacturer of hospital equipment and supplies; parenteral supplies; physicians' supplies; sterilization supplies; X-ray equipment.

★ 15311 ★ BD Medical Systems, Infusion Therapy
9450 S State St.
Sandy, UT 84070
Phone: (801)565-2592 **Free:** 800-453-4538
Fax: (801)565-2378
Website: http://www.bd.com/infusion
Beva Shelby, Contact
Desc: Manufacturer of anesthesia equipment and products; biological and environmental safety products; cardiovascular devices; disposable medical devices and supplies; home healthcare; parenteral catheters.

★ 15312 ★ BD-Preanalytical Solutions
1 Becton Dr.
Franklin Lakes, NJ 07417-1885
Phone: (201)847-6800 **Fax:** (201)847-4862
Website: http://www.bd.com/preanalytical
Richard O. Brajer, President
Desc: Manufacturer of biological and environmental safety products; disposable medical devices and supplies; home healthcare; hospital equipment and supplies; laboratory supplies; physicians' supplies; urinary equipment.

★ 15313 ★ Beach Pharmaceuticals
Division of Beach Products, Inc.
5220 S Manhattan Ave.
Tampa, FL 33611
Phone: (813)839-6565 **Free:** 800-322-8210
Fax: (813)837-2511
Richard Beach Jenkins, President
Manufacturer/distributor of Rx/ethical pharmaceuticals; OTC/proprietary pharmaceuticals; generic pharmaceuticals.

★ 15314 ★ Beckman Coulter
Primary Care Diagnostics
1050 Page Mill Rd., Bldg. 2B
PO Box 10200
Palo Alto, CA 94303-0803
Phone: (650)857-1227 **Free:** 800-877-6242
Fax: (650)845-3535
Website: http://www.beckmancoulter.com/pcd
Jack Wareham, President
Desc: Manufacturer of diagnostic equipment and instruments; diagnostic reagents and test kits.

★ 15315 ★ Beckman Coulter, Inc.
PO Box 8000
Brea, CA 92822-8000
Phone: (714)993-8369 **Free:** 800-526-3821
Fax: (714)961-4504
Website: http://www.beckmancoulter.com
Patrick Patterson, Contact
Desc: manufacturer of diagnostic reagents and test kits; hospital equipment and supplies; laboratory equipment.

★ 15316 ★ Beckman Coulter, Inc.
4300 Harbor Blvd.
Fullerton, CA 92835
Phone: (714)871-4848 **Free:** 800-526-3821
Fax: (714)773-8898
Website: http://www.beckmancoulter.com
John P. Wareham, CEO & Pres
Desc: Manufacturer/distributor/biotechnology company: diagnostic equipment and instruments; diagnostic reagents and test kits; hospital equipment and supplies; laboratory equipment and supplies.

★ 15317 ★ Bedford Laboratories
Division of Ben Venue Laboratories, Inc.
300 Northfield Rd.
Bedford, OH 44146
Phone: (440)232-3320 **Free:** 800-562-4797
Fax: (440)232-6264
Email: bedfordlabs@cle.boehringer-ingelheim.com
Website: http://www.bedfordlabs.com
Thomas Russillo, President
Desc: Manufacturer/biotechnology company: Rx/ethical pharmaceuticals; generic pharmaceuticals; biotechnology/biopharmaceutical products; contract manufacturing; diagnostic reagents and test kits; parenteral supplies; radiopharmaceuticals.

★ 15318 ★ BEI Medical Systems, Inc.
100 Hollister Rd.
Teterboro, NJ 07608-1139
Phone: (201)727-4900 **Fax:** (201)727-4998
Email: info@beimedical.com
Website: http://www.beimedical.com
Richard W. Turner, PhD, CEO & Pres
Desc: Manufacturer of diagnostic equipment and instruments; disposable medical devices and supplies; hospital equipment and supplies; physicians' equipment and supplies.

★ 15319 ★ Beiersdorf, Inc.
A subsidiary of Beiersdorf AG
187 Danbury Rd.
Wilton, CT 06897
Phone: (203)563-5800 **Fax:** (203)563-5890
Website: http://www.beiersdorf.com
James Kenton, President
Desc: Manufacturer/distributor of OTC/proprietary pharmaceuticals; home healthcare; hospital equipment and supplies; patient aid products; physical therapy and rehabilitation equipment and supplies; skin/wound care products.

★ 15320 ★ Bel-Art Products
6 Industrial Rd.
Pequannock, NJ 07440
Phone: (973)694-0500 **Free:** 800-4-BELART
Fax: (973)694-7199
Email: info@belart.com
Website: http://www.belart.com
Kurt Landsberger, Chairman of the Board
Desc: Manufacturer/biotechnology company: biotechnology/biopharmaceutical products; bottles; X-ray accessories; custom molding; laboratory equipment and supplies.

★ 15321 ★ Bell-Horn
7952 Zionsville Rd.
Indianapolis, IN 46268
Phone: (317)228-1144 **Free:** 800-226-4799
Fax: (317)228-1155
Email: info@bell-horn.com
Website: http://www.bell-horn.com
Todd Katz, President
Desc: Distributor of home healthcare; orthopedic and prosthetic equipment and supplies; ostomy equipment and supplies.

★ 15322 ★ Bellco Glass, Inc.
340 Edrudo Rd.
Vineland, NJ 08360
Phone: (856)691-1075 **Free:** 800-257-7043
Fax: (856)691-3247
Email: sales@bellcoglass.com
Website: http://www.bellcoglass.com
Steven Harker, CEO & Pres
Desc: Manufacturer/biotechnology company: biotechnology/biopharmaceutical products; laboratory equipment; laboratory supplies.

★ 15323 ★ Berlex Laboratories
Division of Berlex Laboratories, Inc.
340 Changebridge Rd.
PO Box 1000
Montville, NJ 07045
Phone: (973)487-2000 **Free:** 800-237-5392
Website: http://www.berlex.com
Dale Stringfellow, PhD, CEO & Pres
Desc: Manufacturer/distributor/biotechnology company: Rx/ethical pharmaceuticals; biotechnology/biopharmaceutical products; cardiovascular supplies; magnetic resonance imaging; nuclear and radiological supplies; radiopharmaceuticals.

★ 15324 ★ Berlex Oncology
Division of Berlex Laboratories, Inc.
15049 San Pablo Ave.
Richmond, CA 94804-0099
Phone: (510)262-5000 **Fax:** (510)262-7055
Website: http://www.berlex.com
Michael Quattro, Contact
Desc: Manufacturer of Rx/ethical pharmaceuticals.

★ 15325 ★ Berna Products Corp.
4216 Ponce de Leon Blvd.
Coral Gables, FL 33146
Phone: (305)443-2900 **Free:** 800-533-5899
Fax: 800-392-9490
Website: http://www.bernaproducts.com
Andres Murai, Jr., President
Desc: Manufacturer of Rx/ethical pharmaceuticals.

★ 15326 ★ Bernell
4016 N Home St.
Mishawaka, IN 46545-4308
Phone: (219)259-2070 **Free:** 800-348-2225
Fax: (219)259-2102
Website: http://www.bernell.com
Craig Andrews, OD, President
Desc: Distributor of ophthalmic equipment and supplies.

★ 15327 ★ Bertek Pharmaceuticals, Inc.
The Branded Product Division of Mylan Laboratories, Inc.
Research Triangle Park
530 Davis Dr.
Durham, NC 27713
Phone: (919)991-9800 **Free:** 888-5-BERTEX
Fax: (919)993-5901
Email: info@bertek.com
Website: http://www.bertek.com
Jim Mauzey, CEO & Pres
Desc: Manufacturer of Rx/ethical pharmaceuticals; OTC/proprietary pharmaceuticals; home healthcare; skin/sound care products.

★ 15328 ★ Best Industries, Inc.
7643 Fullerton Rd.
Springfield, VA 22153
Phone: (703)451-2378 **Free:** 800-336-4970
Fax: (703)451-5228
Website: http://www.best-medical.com
Krishnan Suthanthiran, President
Desc: Manufacturer/distributor of laboratory equipment and supplies; nuclear and radiological equipment and supplies; radiopharmaceuticals; surgical disposables.

★ 15329 ★ Beta Technology Inc.
2841 Mission St.
Santa Cruz, CA 95060
Phone: (831)426-5890 **Free:** 800-858-2382
Fax: (831)423-4644
Email: sales@beta-technology.com
Website: http://www.langecaliper.com
David Collette, Contact
Desc: Manufacturer of diagnostic equipment and instruments; metered chemical dosage equipment; patient monitoring equipment; pharmaceutical manufacturing equipment; physical therapy and rehabilitation equipment and supplies; physicians' equipment.

★ 15330 ★ Beutlich L.P.
1541 Shields Dr.
Waukegan, IL 60085
Phone: (847)473-1100 **Free:** 800-238-8542
Fax: (847)473-1122
Email: beutlich@beutlich.com
Website: http://www.beutlich.com
F.J. Beutlich, Contact
Desc: Distributor of OTC/proprietary pharmaceuticals; anesthesia equipment and products; dental supplies; dietary, nutritional and vitamin supplements; home healthcare; hospital equipment and supplies; physicians' supplies.

★ 15331 ★ Bio-Feedback Systems, Inc.
2736 47th St.
Boulder, CO 80301
Phone: (303)444-1411 **Fax:** (303)444-1412
Website: http://www.users.qwest.net/~pitchj
John B. Picchiottino, Chairman of the Board

Desc: Manufacturer/distributor/biotechnology company: biomedical/medical devices; contract manufacturing; diagnostic equipment and instruments; disposable medical devices and supplies; home healthcare; hospital equipment and supplies; patient aid products; patient monitoring equipment; physical therapy and rehabilitation equipment and supplies; physicians' equipment and supplies; sleep diagnostics/therapeutics; electro-uterograph equipment.

★ 15332 ★ Bio-Lok International Inc.
312 S Military Trail
Deerfield Beach, FL 33442
Phone: (954)698-9998 **Free:** 800-789-0830
Fax: (954)698-9925
Email: biolok@biolok.com
Website: http://www.biolok.com
Bruce L. Hollander, CEO & Pres

Desc: Manufacturer/distributor of implants; related prosthetics; tools and devices.

★ 15333 ★ Bio-Medical Products Corp.
10 Halstead Rd.
Mendham, NJ 07945
Phone: (973)543-7434 **Free:** 800-543-7427
Fax: (973)543-7497
Email: biomedicalproductscorp@msn.com
John Geppert, Contact

Desc: Manufacturer/distributor/biotechnology company: OTC/proprietary pharmaceuticals; biotechnology/biopharmaceutical products; diagnostic reagents and test kits; dietary, nutritional and vitamin supplements; disposable medical devices and supplies; home healthcare; laboratory supplies; urinary equipment and supplies; skin/wound care products.

★ 15334 ★ Bio-Pharm, Inc.
10 H Runway Rd.
Levittown, PA 19057
Phone: (215)949-3711 **Fax:** (215)949-3736
Email: info@bio-pharminc.com
Website: http://www.bio-pharminc.com
Umakant Shah, President

Desc: Manufacturer/distributor of Rx/ethical pharmaceuticals; OTC/proprietary pharmaceuticals; generic pharmaceuticals.

★ 15335 ★ Bio-Plexus, Inc.
129 Reservoir Rd.
Vernon, CT 06066
Phone: (860)870-6112 **Free:** 800-223-0010
Fax: (860)870-6118
Email: products@bio-plexus.com
Website: http://www.bio-plexus.com
John Metz, CEO & Pres

Desc: Manufacturer of disposable medical devices and supplies; hospital equipment and supplies; laboratory supplies;

★ 15336 ★ Bio-Rad Laboratories
6565 185th Ave., NE
Redmond, WA 98052
Phone: (425)881-8300 **Free:** 800-424-9117
Fax: (425)498-1650
Website: http://www.bio-rad.com
Donald Diamond, Jr., Contact

Desc: Manufacturer of diagnostic equipment and instruments; diagnostic reagents and test kits.

★ 15337 ★ Bio-Rad Laboratories, Inc. Clinical Diagnostics Group
4000 Alfred Nobel Dr.
Hercules, CA 94547
Phone: (510)724-7000 **Free:** 800-2-BIORAD
Fax: (510)742-5024
Website: http://www.bio-rad.com
James Bennett, Contact

Desc: Manufacturer/distributor of diagnostic equipment and instruments; diagnostic reagents and test kits; laboratory equipment and supplies; newborn screening reagents and instrumentation; patient monitoring equipment; physicians' equipment; quality control data management software.

★ 15338 ★ Bio-Technology General Corp.
70 Wood Ave. S
Iselin, NJ 08830
Phone: (732)632-8800 **Fax:** (732)632-8844
Email: information@btgc.com
Website: http://www.btgc.com
Sim Fass, PhD, CEO & Chm Bd

Desc: Manufacturer/biotechnology company: Rx/ethical pharmaceuticals; biotechnology/biopharmaceutical products; human healthcare; skin/wound care products.

★ 15339 ★ Bio-Tek Instruments
Highland Industrial Park
PO Box 998
Winooski, VT 05404
Phone: (802)655-4040 **Free:** 800-451-5171
Fax: (802)655-7941
Email: labcsr@biotek.com
Website: http://www.biotek.com
Briar Alpert, President

Desc: Manufacturer/biotechnology company: biotechnology/biopharmaceutical products; diagnostic equipment and instruments; diagnostic reagents and test kits; laboratory equipment.

★ 15340 ★ Biocell Laboratories, Inc.
2001 E University Dr.
Rancho Dominguez, CA 90220
Phone: (310)537-3300 **Free:** 800-222-8382
Fax: (310)637-3927
Email: info@biocell.com
Website: http://www.biocell.com
Marc M. McKonic, CEO & Pres

Desc: Manufacturer/biotechnology company: biotechnology/biopharmaceutical products; diagnostic reagents and test kits; skin/wound care products; sterilization supplies.

★ 15341 ★ Biogen, Inc.
14 Cambridge Center
Cambridge, MA 02142
Phone: (617)679-2000 **Fax:** (617)679-2617
Website: http://www.biogen.com
James L. Vincent, Chairman of the Board

Desc: Manufacturer/biotechnology company: biotechnology/biopharmaceutical products.

★ 15342 ★ Bioglan Pharma, Inc. Division of Bioglan Pharma PLC
7 Great Valley Parkway
Ste. 301
Malvern, PA 19355
Phone: (610)232-2000 **Fax:** (610)232-2020
Website: http://www.bioglanusa.com
Robert Moccia, President

Desc: Manufacturer/distributor of Rx/ethical pharmaceuticals; OTC/proprietary pharmaceuticals; skin/wound care products.

★ 15343 ★ Biomed Instruments, Inc.
1166 E Valencia Dr., No. 6C
Fullerton, CA 92831
Phone: (714)870-0290 **Free:** 800-927-2290
Fax: (714)870-6385
Email: aab@ix.netcom.com
Website: http://www.aabi.com
R.A. Zeineh, PhD, President

Desc: Biotechnology company: biotechnology/biopharmaceutical products; diagnostic equipment and instruments; medical research programming.

★ 15344 ★ Biomerica, Inc.
1533 Monrovia Ave.
Newport Beach, CA 92663
Phone: (949)645-2111 **Free:** 800-854-3002
Fax: (949)722-6674
Email: bmra@biomerica.com
Website: http://www.biomerica.com
Fran Capitanio, President

Desc: Manufacturer of OTC/proprietary pharmaceuticals; diagnostic reagents and test kits; home healthcare.

★ 15345 ★ bioMerieux
100 Rodolphe St.
Durham, NC 27712
Phone: (919)620-2000 **Free:** 800-682-2666
Fax: (919)620-2615
Email: customerservice@orgtek.com
Website: http://www.biomerieux-usa.com
Philippe Sans, CEO & Pres

Desc: Manufacturer of diagnostic equipment and instruments; diagnostic reagents and test kits; laboratory equiment.

★ 15346 ★ bioMerieux Inc. Division of bioMerieux SA
595 Anglum Rd.
Hazelwood, MO 63042-2320
Phone: (314)731-8500 **Free:** 800-634-7656
Fax: (314)731-8678
Email: usa@na.biomerieuz.com
Website: http://www.biomerieux-usa.com
Philippe Sans, President

Desc: Manufacturer of diagnostic equipment and instruments; diagnostic reagents and test kits; hospital equipment and supplies; laboratory equipment and supplies.

★ 15347 ★ Biomet, Inc.
56 E Bell Dr.
PO Box 587
Warsaw, IN 46581-0587
Phone: (219)267-6639 **Fax:** (219)267-8137
Email: biomet@biomet.com
Website: http://www.biomet.com
Dane A. Miller, PhD, CEO & Pres

Desc: Manufacturer/distributor of hospital equipment and supplies; implants and infusion; orthopedic and prosthetic equipment and supplies; patient aid products; physical therapy and rehabilitation equipment and supplies; physicians' supplies; sterilization supplies; surgical disposables; surgical instruments; ultrasonic equipment.

★ 15348 ★ Bion Enterprises Ltd.
455 State St.
Ste. 100
Des Plaines, IL 60016
Phone: (847)544-5044 **Fax:** (847)544-5051
Email: bion@bionenterprises.com
Website: http://www.bionenterprises.com
Edward Nowakowski, President

Desc: Manufacturer/distributor of diagnostic reagents and test kits.

★ 15349 ★ BioTransplant, Inc.
Bldg. 75, Third Ave.
Charlestown Navy Yard
Charlestown, MA 02129
Phone: (617)241-5200 **Fax:** (617)241-8780
Website: http://www.biotransplant.com
Elliot Lebowitz, PhD, CEO & Pres

Desc: Biotechnology company: Rx/ethical pharmaceuticals; biotechnology/biopharmaceutical products; diagnostic reagents and test kits; disposable medical devices and supplies.

★ 15350 ★ Biovest International
25 South St.
Hopkinton, MA 01748
Phone: (508)435-2000 **Fax:** (508)435-7779
Website: http://www.biovest.com
David Eansor, Contact

Desc: Manufacturer/biotechnology company offering biotechnology/biopharmaceutical products; diagnostic reagents and test kits; contract manufacturing; laboratory equipment.

★ 15351 ★ BioWhittaker, Inc.
A Cambrex Co.
8830 Biggs Ford Rd.
Walkersville, MD 21793-0127
Phone: (301)898-7025 **Free:** 800-654-4452
Fax: (301)845-4024
Email: sales@biowhittaker.com
Website: http://www.biowhittaker.com
David Eansor, Contact
Desc: Manufacturer/biotechnology company: biotechnology/biopharmaceutical products; diagnostic reagents and test kits; endotoxin detection reagents; laboratory supplies; pharmaceutical manufacturing supplies and equipment.

★ 15352 ★ Blaine Pharmaceuticals
1515 Production Dr.
Burlington, KY 41005
Phone: (859)283-9437 **Free:** 800-633-9353
Fax: (859)283-9460
Website: http://www.blainepharmaceuticals.com
Frank Manella, President
Desc: Manufacturer/distributor of Rx/ethical pharmaceuticals; OTC/proprietary pharmaceuticals.

★ 15353 ★ Blickman, Inc.
39 Robinson Rd.
Lodi, NJ 07644
Phone: (201)909-0807 **Free:** 800-247-5070
Fax: (201)909-0832
Email: info@blickman.com
Website: http://www.blickman.com
Ben Freedman, Chairman of the Board
Desc: Manufacturer of hospital equipment and supplies; hospital furniture; physicians' equipment.

★ 15354 ★ Blistex, Inc.
1800 Swift Dr.
Oak Brook, IL 60521
Phone: (630)571-2870 **Free:** 800-837-1800
Fax: (630)571-3437
Website: http://www.blistex.com
David C. Arch, CEO & Chm Bd
Desc: Manufacturer of OTC/proprietary pharmaceuticals.

★ 15355 ★ Blue M
4 Quality St.
Williamsport, PA 17701
Phone: (920)262-3916 **Free:** 800-216-7725
Fax: (920)262-3993
Email: webmaster@lindberg-bluem.com
Website: http://www.blue-m.com
Lisa Deinlein, Contact
Desc: Manufacturer of laboratory equipment; pharmaceutical manufacturing supplies and equipment.

★ 15356 ★ BMC Vision-Ease Lens
A subsidiary of BMC Industries
7100 Northland Circle
Ste. 312
Brooklyn Park, MN 55428-1500
Phone: (763)536-7885 **Free:** 800-633-5829
Fax: (763)536-8789
Website: http://vision-ease.com
Paul B. Burke, CEO & Pres
Desc: Manufacturer/distributor of ophthalmic equipment and supplies.

★ 15357 ★ Boehringer Ingelheim Pharmaceuticals, Inc.
A subsidiary of Boehringer Ingelheim Corp.
900 Ridgebury Rd.
PO Box 368
Ridgefield, CT 06877-0368
Phone: (203)798-9988 **Free:** 800-344-4095
Fax: (203)791-6234
Website: http://ww.boehringer-ingelheim.com
Werner Gerstenberg, President
Desc: Manufacturer of Rx/ethical pharmaceuticals.

★ 15358 ★ Boehringer Laboratories, Inc.
PO Box 870
Norristown, PA 19404
Phone: (610)278-0900 **Free:** 800-642-4945
Fax: (610)278-0907
Email: info@boehringerlabs.com
Website: http://www.boehringerlabs.com
John R. Boehringer, President
Desc: Manufacturer of anesthesia equipment and products; auto transfusion; blood diagnostics; blood processing equipment; cardiovascular equipment and supplies; diagnostic equipment and instruments; diagnostic reagents and test kits; disposable medical devices and supplies; implants and infusion; laboratory equipment; orthopedic equipment and supplies; respiratory and/or cardiopulmonary equipment and supplies.

★ 15359 ★ Boiron
A Division of Boiron SA
6 Campus Blvd.
Newtown Square, PA 19073
Phone: (610)325-7464 **Free:** 800-258-8823
Fax: (610)325-7480
Website: http://www.boiron.com
Thierry Boiron, President
Desc: Manufacturer/distributor of Rx/ethical pharmaceuticals; OTC/proprietary pharmaceuticals.

★ 15360 ★ Borda Products, Inc.
80 Bruckner Blvd.
Bronx, NY 10454
Phone: (718)665-0440 **Fax:** (718)292-6038
Zoltan Wieder, President
Desc: Distributor of home healthcare; hospital equipment and supplies; physicians' equipment; surgical disposables; surgical supplies.

★ 15361 ★ Boston Biomedica, Inc.
375 West St.
West Bridgewater, MA 02379
Phone: (508)580-1900 **Free:** 800-676-1881
Fax: (508)580-2202
Email: info@bbii.com
Website: http://www.bbii.com
Richard T. Schumacher, CEO & Chm Bd
Desc: Biotechnology company: biotechnology/biopharmaceutical products; diagnostic equipment and instruments; diagnostic reagents and test kits; laboratory equipment and supplies.

★ 15362 ★ Bosworth Co.
7227 N Hamlin Ave.
Skokie, IL 60076
Phone: (847)679-3400 **Free:** 800-323-4352
Fax: (847)679-2080
Email: hjbinfo@bosworth.com
Website: http://www.bosworth.com
Mildred Goldstein, President
Desc: Manufacturer of OTC/proprietary pharmaceuticals; dental equipment and supplies; laboratory supplies; sterilization equipment.

★ 15363 ★ Bracco Diagnostics Inc.
PO Box 5225
Princeton, NJ 08543-5225
Phone: (609)514-2200 **Free:** 800-631-5245
Fax: (609)514-2514
Website: http://www.bdi.bracco.com
Robert Aromando, Contact
Desc: Manufacturer/distributor of cardiovascular equipment; diagnostic equipment and instruments; magnetic resonance imaging; nuclear and radiological supplies; renal dialysis equipment; surgical supplies; X-ray equipment and supplies.

★ 15364 ★ Brain Power, Inc.
4470 SW 74th Ave.
Miami, FL 33155
Phone: (305)264-4465 **Free:** 800-327-2250
Fax: (305)264-1467
Email: bpi@callbpi.com
Website: http://www.callbpi.com
Herbert Wertheim, PhD, President
Desc: Manufacturer of ophthalmic equipment and supplies.

★ 15365 ★ Braintree Laboratories, Inc.
60 Columbian St. W
PO Box 850929
Braintree, MA 02185-0929
Phone: (781)843-2202 **Free:** 800-874-6756
Fax: (781)843-7932
Website: http://www.braintreelabs.com
Harry P. Keegan, President
Desc: Manufacturer of Rx/ethical pharmaceuticals.

★ 15366 ★ Brandt Industries, Inc.
4461 Bronx Blvd.
Bronx, NY 10470
Phone: (718)994-0800 **Free:** 800-221-8031
Fax: (718)325-7995
Neil Brandt, President
Desc: Manufacturer of dental equipment; home healthcare; hospital equipment and supplies; hospital furniture; ophthalmic equipment; physical therapy and rehabilitation equipment and supplies; physicians' equipment; veterinary products; x-ray equipment; x-ray equipment illuminated.

★ 15367 ★ Brasel Products, Inc.
715 Hunter Dr.
Batavia, IL 60510
Phone: (630)879-3759 **Fax:** (630)879-6912
Email: info@brasel.com
Website: http://brasel.com
Melody Brasel Davoust, President
Desc: Manufacturer of disposable medical devices and supplies; patient aid products; skin/wound care products; urinary supplies.

★ 15368 ★ Brasseler USA
1 Brasseler Blvd.
Savannah, GA 31419
Phone: (912)925-8525 **Free:** 800-841-4522
Fax: (912)927-8671
Email: brasseler@aol.com
Website: http://www.brasselerusa.com
Don Waters, CEO & Pres
Desc: Manufacturer/distributor of dental equipment and supplies; laboratory equipment and supplies.

★ 15369 ★ Breckenridge Pharmaceutical, Inc.
1141 S Rogers Circle
Ste. 3
Boca Raton, FL 33487
Phone: (561)443-3314 **Free:** 800-367-3395
Fax: (561)989-0819
Carol Bauer, Contact
Desc: Manufacturer of Rx/ethical pharmaceuticals; OTC/proprietary pharmaceuticals; generic pharmaceuticals.

★ 15370 ★ Brecon Knitting Mills, Inc.
994 Ironaton Rd.
PO Box 478
Talladega, AL 35160
Phone: (256)362-6141 **Free:** 800-841-2821
Fax: (256)362-6143
Website: http://www.breconknittingmill.com
Allen G. McMillan, III, President

Desc: Manufacturer of orthopedic and prosthetic equipment and supplies; patient aid products; sterilization supplies.

★ 15371 ★ Brennen Medical, Inc.
1290 Hammond Rd.
Saint Paul, MN 55110
Phone: (651)429-7413 **Free:** 800-328-9105
Fax: (651)429-8020
Email: brennenmedical@worldnet.att.net
Website: http://www.brennenmedical.com
Phil Lawin, CEO & Pres

Desc: Manufacturer of hospital equipment and supplies; skin/wound care products.

★ 15372 ★ The Brewer Co.
13901 Main St.
Menomonee Falls, WI 53051
Phone: (262)251-9530 **Free:** 800-558-8777
Fax: (262)251-1786
Email: sales@brewercompany.com
Website: http://www.brewercompany.com
Jeff Beischel, President

Desc: Manufacturer of dental equipment; diagnostic equipment and instruments; hospital equipment and supplies; hospital furniture; ophthalmic equipment, physicians' equipment; veterinary products.

★ 15373 ★ Brioschi, Inc.
19-01 Pollitt Dr.
Fair Lawn, NJ 07410
Phone: (201)796-4226 **Free:** 800-BRIOSCHI
Fax: (201)796-0391
Email: customerservice@brioschi-usa.com
Website: http://www.brioschi-usa.com
Marco A. Brizzolara, President

Desc: Manufacturer/distributor of OTC/proprietary pharmaceuticals.

★ 15374 ★ Bristol-Myers Squibb World Wide Medicines Group
PO Box 4500
Princeton, NJ 08543-4500
Phone: (609)897-2000
Website: http://www.bms.com
Peter R. Dolan, J, Chairman of the Board

Desc: Manufacturer/distributor of Rx/ethical pharmaceuticals; OTC/proprietary pharmaceuticals.

★ 15375 ★ Bristol Myers Squibb Medical Imaging
331 Treble Cove Rd.
North Billerica, MA 01862
Phone: 800-362-2668 **Free:** 800-225-1572
Fax: (978)436-7506
Website: http://www.radiopharm.com
Bob Gaffey, Contact

Desc: Manufacturer of radiopharmaceuticals.

★ 15376 ★ Britannia Limited
21 E 65th St.
New York, NY 10021
Phone: (212)734-5678 **Free:** 800-241-1447
Fax: (212)744-2288
Email: camchem@aol.com
Joseph Policar, President

Desc: Distributor of dietary, nutritional and vitamin supplements.

★ 15377 ★ Britt Medical Products Division of Britt Corp.
PO Box 547
Freehold, NJ 07728
Phone: (732)817-1122 **Fax:** (732)817-1123
Email: brittcorp@aol.com
Joal H. Britton, Chairman of the Board

Desc: Manufacturer of compression therapy for wound care; disposable medical devices and supplies; home healthcare; home medical equipment and supplies; hospital equipment and supplies.

★ 15378 ★ Brown Medical Industries
Lakes Business Park
1300 Lundberg Dr. W
Spirit Lake, IA 51360
Phone: (712)336-4395 **Free:** 800-843-4395
Fax: (712)336-2874
Email: info@brownmed.com
Website: http://www.brownmed.com
Ivan E. Brown, PhD, CEO & Pres

Desc: Manufacturer/distributor of cast protectors; contract manufacturing; home healthcare; hospital equipment and supplies; orthopedic and prosthetic equipment and supplies; physical therapy and rehabilitation equipment and supplies; physicians' supplies; skin/wound care products.

★ 15379 ★ BSD Medical Corp.
2188 W 2200 South
Salt Lake City, UT 84119
Phone: (801)972-5555 **Fax:** (801)972-5930
Email: info@bsdmc.com
Website: http://www.bsdmc.com
Paul Turner, Chairman of the Board

Desc: Manufacturer of hospital equipment and supplies; thermotherapy equipment for prostate diseases.

★ 15380 ★ BSN-Jobst, Inc. Subsidiary of Beiersdorf AG
5825 Carnegie Blvd.
Charlotte, NC 28209
Phone: (704)554-9933 **Free:** 800-876-3664
Fax: (704)551-8581
Website: http://www.jobst-usa.com
Claus-H. Wiegel, President

Desc: Manufacturer of disposable medical devices and supplies; home healthcare; hospital equipment and supplies; orthopedic and prosthetic equipment and supplies; patient aid products; skin/wound care products.

★ 15381 ★ Budget Buddy Co., Inc.
PO Box 590
Belton, MO 64012
Phone: (816)322-2290 **Free:** 800-208-3375
Fax: (816)322-6332
Email: office@budgetbuddy.com
Website: http://www.budgetbuddy.com
Ken Tompkins, President

Desc: Manufacturer/distributor of hospital furniture; physicians' equipment.

★ 15382 ★ Buffalo Dental Manufacturing Co., Inc.
99 Lafayette Dr.
Syosset, NY 11791
Phone: (516)496-7200 **Free:** 800-828-0203
Fax: (516)496-7751
Email: tech.support@bdm1.com
Website: http://www.buffalodental.com
Donald M. Nevin, President

Desc: Manufacturer of dental equipment and supplies.

★ 15383 ★ Burkhart Roentgen International Inc.
5201 Eighth Ave. S
Saint Petersburg, FL 33707
Phone: (727)327-6950 **Free:** 800-USA-XRAY
Fax: (727)327-3255
Email: cathlabx@gte.net
Website: http://www.usa-xray.com
George D. Burkhart, CEO & Pres

Desc: Manufacturer/distributor of apparel; biological and environmental safety products; cardiovascular equipment and supplies; contract manufacturing; dental supplies; diagnostic equipment and instruments; disposable medical devices and supplies; hospital equipment and supplies; laboratory equipment and supplies; lead protective wear; physicians' equipment and supplies; surgical supplies; ultrasound and electromedical equipment and supplies; veterinary products; X-ray equipment; X-ray supplies.

★ 15384 ★ Burrell Scientific
2223 Fifth Ave.
Pittsburgh, PA 15219
Phone: (412)471-2527 **Free:** 800-637-6074
Fax: (412)391-4231
Email: burrellsci@sprintmail.com
Website: http://www.procurenet.com/burrell
Loren R. Holmes, President

Desc: Manufacturer/distributor of laboratory equipment and supplies.

★ 15385 ★ Busse Hospital Disposables, Inc.
PO Box 11067
Hauppauge, NY 11788-0920
Phone: (631)435-4711 **Free:** 800-645-6526
Fax: (631)435-4721
Email: mail@busseinc.com
Website: http://www.busseinc.com
Emanuel Cardinale, President

Desc: Manufacturer of apparel; dental supplies; disposable medical devices and supplies; EMS equipment and supplies; hospital equipment and supplies; laboratory supplies; parenteral supplies; physicians' equipment; skin/wound care products; sterilization supplies.

★ 15386 ★ Buxco Electronics, Inc.
95 W Woods Rd., No. 2
Sharon, CT 06069
Phone: (860)364-5558 **Fax:** (860)364-5116
Email: support@buxco.com
Website: http://www.buxco.com
Joseph M. Lomask, President

Desc: Manufacturer/distributor/biotechnology company: biotechnology/biopharmaceutical products; cardiovascular equipment; data acquisition systems.

★ 15387 ★ C.B. Fleet Co., Inc.
4615 Murray Pl.
Lynchburg, VA 24506
Phone: (804)528-4000 **Free:** 800-999-9711
Fax: (804)847-4219
William R. Chambers, Chairman of the Board

Desc: Manufacturer/distributor of Rx/ethical pharmaceuticals; OTC/proprietary pharmaceuticals; physicians' supplies.

★ 15388 ★ C.R. Bard, Inc.
730 Central Ave.
Murray Hill, NJ 07974
Phone: (908)277-8000 **Free:** 800-367-2273
Fax: (908)277-8240
Website: http://www.crbard.com
William H. Longfield, CEO & Chm Bd

Desc: Manufacturer/distributor of diagnostic equipment and instruments; disposable medical devices and supplies; home healthcare; hospital equipment and supplies; implants and infusion; oncology; gastroenterology; hemostasis and abdominal repair products; parenteral catheters; patient monitoring equipment; physicians' equipment and supplies; renal dialysis supplies; skin/wound care products; surgical disposables and supplies; urinary equipment and supplies; vascular grafts.

★ **15389** ★ **C.R. Bard, Inc.**
Access Systems Division
5425 W Amelia Earhart Dr.
Salt Lake City, UT 84116
Phone: (801)595-0700 **Free:** 800-443-5505
Fax: (801)595-4969
Website: http://www.bardaccess.com
Amy Paul, President
Desc: Manufacturer of cardiovascular supplies; home healthcare; hospital equipment and supplies; implants and infusion; parenteral catheters; renal dialysis supplies; ultrasound and electromedical equipment and supplies.

★ **15390** ★ **C.R. Bard, Inc.**
Electrophysiology Division
55 Technology Dr.
Lowell, MA 01851
Phone: (978)441-6202 **Free:** 800-282-1332
Fax: (978)323-2340
Email: bardep@crbard.com
Stephen W. Sagon, President
Desc: Manufacturer/distributor of diagnostic equipment and instruments; disposable medical devices and supplies; laboratory equipment; patient monitoring equipment.

★ **15391** ★ **C.R. Bard, Inc.**
Endoscopic Technologies Division
129 Concord Rd.
Billerica, MA 01821
Phone: (978)663-8989 **Free:** 800-225-1332
Fax: (978)262-4992
Website: http://bardendoscopy.com
Bradford R. Gay, President
Desc: Manufacturer/distributor of sterilization supplies.

★ **15392** ★ **C.R. Bard, Inc.**
IMPRA Division
1625 W Third St.
Tempe, AZ 85281
Phone: (480)894-9515 **Free:** 800-321-4254
Fax: (480)966-7062
Website: http://www.crbard.com
John McDermott, President
Desc: Manufacturer/distributor of cardiovascular supplies; hospital equipment and supplies; implants and infusion; peripheral vascular devices; surgical instruments and supplies.

★ **15393** ★ **C.R. Bard, Inc.**
Medical Division
8195 Industrial Blvd.
Covington, GA 30014
Phone: (770)784-6100 **Free:** 800-526-4455
Fax: (770)784-6340
Website: http://www.bardmedical.com
Bill Midgette, President
Desc: Manufacturer/distributor of disposable medical devices and supplies; home healthcare; ostomy equipment and supplies; parenteral catheters; patient aid products; patient monitoring equipment; skin/sound care products; surgical disposables, instruments and supplies; urinary equipment and supplies.

★ **15394** ★ **C.R. Bard, Inc.**
Urological Division
8195 Industrial Blvd.
Covington, GA 30014
Phone: (770)784-6100 **Free:** 800-526-4455
Fax: (770)784-6966
Email: bud.customerservice@crbard.com
Burt S. Mirsky, President
Desc: Manufacturer of diagnostic equipment and instruments; diagnostic reagents and test kits; disposable medical devices and supplies; patient monitoring equipment; physicians' equipment and supplies; radiopharmaceuticals; surgical disposables, instruments and supplies; urinary equipment and supplies.

★ **15395** ★ **C.S. Dent & Co.**
Division of Grandpa Brands Co.
1820 Airport Exchange Blvd.
Erlanger, KY 41018
Phone: (859)647-0777 **Free:** 800-684-1468
Fax: (859)647-0778
Email: gbc@grandpabrands.com
Website: http://www.grandpabrands.com
Richard D. Oliver, CEO
Desc: Manufacturer of OTC/proprietary pharmaceuticals.

★ **15396** ★ **CAIRE, Inc.**
3505 County Rd. 42 W
Burnsville, MN 55306-3803
Phone: (952)882-5000 **Free:** 800-482-2473
Fax: (952)882-5172
Website: http://www.chart-ind.com
Jeff Dresow, Contact
Desc: Manufacturer of home healthcare; laboratory equipment; pharmaceutical manufacturing supplies and equipment; respiratory therapy and/or cardiopulmonary equipment.

★ **15397** ★ **Caligor**
Division of Micro Bio-Medics, Inc./Henry Schein
846 Pelham Parkway
Pelham Manor, NY 10803
Phone: (914)738-8400 **Free:** 800-225-9906
Fax: (914)738-9538
Website: http://www.caligor.com
Mike Raccioppi, President
Desc: Distributor/biotechnology company: Rx/ethical pharmaceuticals; OTC/proprietary pharmaceuticals; generic pharmaceuticals; biological and environmental safety products; biotechnology/biopharmaceutical products; cardiovascular equipment; diagnostic equipment and instruments; diagnostic reagent and test kits; disposable medical devices and supplies; EMS equipment and supplies; home healthcare; hospital equipment and supplies; laboratory equipment and supplies; office furniture and supplies; ophthalmic equipment and supplies; orthopedic and prosthetic equipment and supplies; ostomy equipment and supplies; parenteral catheters, equipment and supplies; patient aid products; patient monitoring equipment; physicians' equipment and supplies; renal dialysis supplies; skin/wound care products; slide viewing systems; sterilization equipment and supplies; surgical disposables; surgical instruments and supplies; ultrasonic equipment; ultrasound and electromedical equipment and supplies; urinary equipment and supplies; X-ray equipment and supplies.

★ **15398** ★ **Camp Healthcare**
PO Box 89
Jackson, MI 49203
Phone: (517)333-9700 **Free:** 800-492-1088
Fax: 800-245-3765
Email: info@camphealthcare.com
Website: http://www.camphealthcare.com
Pearce Daley, Contact
Desc: Manufacturer of home healthcare; orthopedic and prosthetic equipment and supplies; physical therapy and rehabilitation equipment and supplies; compression hosiery.

★ **15399** ★ **Candela Corp.**
530 Boston Post Rd.
Wayland, MA 01778
Phone: (508)358-7637 **Free:** 800-733-8550
Fax: (508)358-5602
Website: http://www.clzr.com
Gerard Puorro, CEO & Chm Bd
Desc: Manufacturer/distributor of hospital equipment and supplies; laser equipment; skin/wound care products; sterilization supplies; surgical disposables; ultrasound and electromedical equipment and supplies; medical devices.

★ **15400** ★ **Capintec, Inc.**
Medical Products Division
6 Arrow Rd.
Ramsey, NJ 07446
Phone: (201)825-9500 **Free:** 800-631-3826
Fax: (201)825-1336
Email: getinfo@capintec.com
Website: http://www.capintec.com
Arthur M. Weis, President
Desc: Manufacturer/distributor of cardiovascular equipment; diagnostic equipment and instruments; laboratory equipment and supplies; nuclear and radiological equipment and supplies; X-ray supplies.

★ **15401** ★ **Capricorn Products, Inc.**
301 US Rte. 1
Scarborough, ME 04074
Phone: (207)885-0480 **Fax:** (207)885-0494
Email: info@capricornproducts.com
Website: http://www.capricornproducts.com
Jane K. Havey, CEO & Pres
Desc: Manufacturer/distributor/biotechnology company: biotechnology/biopharmaceutical products; diagnostic reagents and test kits; purified antibodies; purified antigens.

★ **15402** ★ **Capsugel**
Division of Pfizer Pharmaceutical, Inc.
535 N Emerald Rd.
Greenwood, SC 29646
Phone: (864)223-2270 **Free:** 800-845-6973
Fax: (864)942-6516
Website: http://www.capsugel.com
Guido Driesen, President
Desc: Manufacturer of dietary, nutritional and vitamin supplements; filling equipment; gelatin and vegetarian capsules; pharmaceutical manufacturing supplies and equipment.

★ **15403** ★ **Caraco Pharmaceutical Laboratories, Ltd.**
1150 Elijah McCoy Dr.
Detroit, MI 48202-3344
Phone: (313)871-8400 **Free:** 800-818-4555
Fax: (313)871-8314
Email: nborkar@caraco.com
Website: http://www.caraco.com
Narendra Borkar, CEO
Desc: Manufacturer of generic pharmaceuticals.

★ **15404** ★ **Carapace**
DeRoyal-Master Distributor of Carapace Products
200 DeBusk Lane
Powell, TN 37849
Free: 888-938-7828 **Fax:** (865)362-6043
Email: jpmccormick@deroyal.com
Website: http://www.deroyal.com
Jim McCormick, Contact
Desc: Manufacturer/distributor of fracture walkers and softgoods; hospital equipment and supplies; orthopedic and prosthetic equipment and supplies; physicians' supplies; plaster of Paris and synthetic casting and splinting materials.

★ **15405** ★ **Cardinal Health**
7000 Cardinal Place
Dublin, OH 43017
Phone: (614)757-5000
Website: http://www.cardinal.com
Robert D. Walter, CEO & Chm Bd
Desc: Manufacturer/distributor/biotechnology company: Rx/ethical pharmaceuticals; OTC/proprietary pharmaceuticals; generic pharmaceuticals; anesthesia equipment and products; biotechnology/biopharmaceutical products; contract manufacturing; diagnostic equipment and instruments; dietary, nutritional and vitamin supplements; disposable medical devices and supplies; home healthcare; hospital equipment and supplies; patient aid products; pharmaceutical manu-

facturing supplies and equipment; physical therapy and rehabilitation equipment and supplies; physicians' supplies; radiopharmaceuticals; respiratory therapy and/or cardiopulmonary supplies; skin/wound care products; surgical disposables, instruments and supplies; urinary supplies; laboratory supplies.

★ 15406 ★ Cardinal Health Pharmaceutical Technologies & Services Group
645 Martinsville Rd.
Ste. 200
Basking Ridge, NJ 07920
Phone: (908)580-1500 **Free:** 888-636-1919
Fax: (908)580-9208
Email: pat.mccullough@rpscherer.com
Website: http://www.cardinal.com
Patricia McCullough, Contact
Desc: Manufacturer of Rx/ethical pharmaceuticals; OTC/proprietary pharmaceuticals; generic pharmaceuticals; biotechnology/biopharmaceutical products; contract manufacturing; dietary, nutritional and vitamin supplements; drug delivery systems; skin/wound care products; sterile processing and packaging.

★ 15407 ★ CardioCommand, Inc.
5660-H W Cypress St.
Tampa, FL 33607
Phone: (813)289-5555 **Free:** 800-231-6370
Fax: (813)289-5454
Website: http://www.cardiocommand.com
Dr. Maynard Ramsey, III, CEO & Pres
Desc: Manufacturer/distributor of anesthesia equipment and products; cardiovascular equipment and supplies; disposable medical devices and supplies; patient monitoring equipment.

★ 15408 ★ Cardiocontrol Inc.
207 Piaget Ave.
Clifton, NJ 07011
Phone: (973)340-8000 **Free:** 800-526-6046
Fax: (973)340-5522
Email: sales@ekgcharts.com
Website: http://www.ekgcharts.com
Chanoch Shiloh, CEO & Pres
Desc: Manufacturer/distributor of cardiovascular supplies; EMS equipment and supplies; medical paper supplies; patient monitoring equipment.

★ 15409 ★ Cardiodynamics International Corp.
6175 Nancy Ridge Dr.
Ste. 300
San Diego, CA 92121
Phone: (858)535-0202 **Free:** 800-778-4825
Fax: (858)535-0055
Email: mperry@cdic.com
Website: http://www.cardiodynamics.com
Michael K. Perry, CEO
Desc: Manufacturer of cardiovascular equipment; disposable medical devices and supplies; patient monitoring equipment.

★ 15410 ★ Care-Tech Laboratories, Inc. Division of Consolidated Chemicals, Inc.
3224 S Kingshighway Blvd.
Saint Louis, MO 63139
Phone: (314)772-4610 **Free:** 800-325-9681
Fax: (314)772-4613
Email: caretech@swbell.net
Website: http://www.caretechlabs.com
John C. Brereton, CEO
Desc: Biotechnology company: OTC/proprietary pharmaceuticals; biological and environmental safety products; biotechnology/biopharmaceutical products; home healthcare; hospital equipment and supplies; ostomy equipment and supplies; patient aid products; physicians' supplies; skin/wound care products; surgical disposables and supplies; veterinary products.

★ 15411 ★ Care Technologies, Inc.
10 Corbin Dr.
PO Box 82
Darien, CT 06820-0582
Phone: (203)655-9680 **Free:** 800-783-1919
Fax: (203)655-9682
Email: info@clearcare.com
Website: http://www.clearcare.com
Harry F. Upton, President
Desc: Manufacturer/distributor of OTC/proprietary pharmaceuticals.

★ 15412 ★ Carl Zeiss Opthalmic Systems, Inc. Humphrey Division
5160 Hacienda Dr.
Dublin, CA 94568
Phone: (925)557-4651 **Fax:** (925)557-4217
Email: info@humphrey.com
Website: http://www.humphrey.com
James Taylor, President
Desc: Manufacturer/distributor of diagnostic equipment and instruments; ophthalmic equipment.

★ 15413 ★ Carl Zeiss Surgical, Inc. Subsidiary of Carl Zeiss, Inc.
1 Zeiss Dr.
Thornwood, NY 10594
Phone: (914)747-1800 **Free:** 800-233-2343
Fax: (914)681-7409
Email: surgical@zeiss.com
Website: http://www.zeiss.com
James J. Kelly, CEO & Pres
Desc: Manufacturer/distributor of dental equipment; laboratory equipment; ophthalmic equipment and supplies; sterilization supplies; surgical disposables.

★ 15414 ★ Carma Laboratories
5801 W Airways Ave.
Franklin, WI 53132
Phone: (414)421-7707 **Fax:** (414)421-0737
Website: http://www.carma-labs.com or http://www.carmexlipbalm.com
Donald Woelbing, President
Desc: Manufacturer/distributor of OTC/proprietary pharmaceuticals.

★ 15415 ★ Carolina Medical, Inc.
PO Box 307
King, NC 27021
Phone: (336)983-5132 **Free:** 800-334-4531
Fax: (336)983-8992
Email: info@caromed.com
Website: http://www.caromed.com
Carroll Turner, President
Desc: Manufacturer/distributor of cardiovascular equipment; diagnostic equipment and instruments; laboratory equipment and supplies; surgical supplies; ultrasonic equipment; ultrasound and electromedical equipment and supplies; urinary equipment and supplies.

★ 15416 ★ Carrington Laboratories, Inc.
2001 Walnut Hill Lane
Irving, TX 75038
Phone: (972)518-1300 **Free:** 800-527-5216
Fax: (972)518-1020
Email: aloe@carringtonlabs.com
Website: http://www.carringtonlabs.com
George DeMott, Chairman of the Board
Desc: Manufacturer/distributor of OTC/proprietary pharmaceuticals; dental supplies; patient aid products; skin/sound care products; veterinary products; contract manufacturing; dietary, nutritional and vitamin supplements.

★ 15417 ★ Cavro Scientific Instruments, Inc. A Tecan Group Co.
2450 Zanker Rd.
San Jose, CA 95131
Phone: (408)953-3100 **Free:** 800-231-0711
Fax: (408)953-3107
Email: cavro@cavro.com
Website: http://www.cavro.com
Steve Levers, President
Desc: Manufacturer: contract manufacturing; diagnostic equipment and instruments; laboratory equipment; sample preparation equipment.

★ 15418 ★ Cellegy Pharmaceuticals Inc.
349 Oyster Point Blvd., Ste. 200
South San Francisco, CA 94080
Phone: (650)616-2200 **Fax:** (650)616-2222
Email: webmaster@cellegy.com
Website: http://www.cellegy.com
K. Michael Forrest, MD, CEO & Pres
Desc: Biotechnology company: Rx/ethical pharmaceuticals; OTC/proprietary pharmaceuticals; biotechnology/biopharmaceutical products; skin/wound care products.

★ 15419 ★ Celltech Pharmaceuticals, Inc.
755 Jefferson Rd.
PO Box 1766
Rochester, NY 14603
Phone: (585)475-9000 **Free:** 800-234-5535
Fax: (585)475-1016
Website: http://www.medeva.com
Ian Garland, Contact
Desc: Manufacturer/distributor of Rx/ethical pharmaceuticals; OTC/ proprietary pharmaceuticals; generic pharmaceuticals.

★ 15420 ★ Centocor, Inc.
200 Great Valley Parkway
Malvern, PA 19355-1307
Phone: (610)651-6000 **Fax:** (610)651-6100
Website: http://www.centocor.com
David P. Holveck, Chairman of the Board
Desc: Manufacturer/distributor/biotechnology company: Rx/ethical pharmaceuticals; biotechnology/biopharmaceutical products.

★ 15421 ★ Century Pharmaceuticals, Inc.
10377 Hague Rd.
Indianapolis, IN 46256
Phone: (317)849-4210 **Fax:** (317)849-4263
Email: info@centurypharmaceuticals.com
Ross A. Deardorff, RPh, President
Desc: Manufacturer/distributor of Rx/ethical pharmaceuticals; OTC/proprietary pharmaceuticals; generic pharmaceuticals; dental supplies; dietary, nutritional and vitamin supplements; home healthcare; patient aid products; skin/wound care products; veterinary products.

★ 15422 ★ Cephalon
4745 Wiley Post Way, Ste. 650
Salt Lake City, UT 84116
Phone: (801)344-0200 **Fax:** (801)344-7563
Website: http://www.cephalon.com
Dr. Frank Baldino, Jr., CEO & Chm Bd
Desc: Manufacturer of Rx/ethical pharmaceuticals; anesthesia equipment and products; biotechnology/biopharmaceutical products.

★ 15423 ★ Cervical Cap (CXC) Ltd.
430 Monterey Ave., 1B
Los Gatos, CA 95030-5323
Phone: (408)395-2100 **Fax:** (408)395-2103
Email: info@cervcap.com
Website: http://www.cervcap.com
Liz Summerhayes, President
Desc: Distributor of Rx/ethical pharmaceuticals.

★ 15424 ★ Cetylite Industries, Inc.
9051 River Rd.
PO Box 90006
Pennsauken, NJ 08110
Phone: (856)665-6111 **Free:** 800-257-7740
Fax: (856)665-5408
Email: cetylite@cetylit.com
Website: http://www.cetylite.com
Stanley L. Wachman, President
Desc: Manufacturer of Rx/ethical pharmaceuticals; dental supplies.

★ 15425 ★ Chase Scientific Glass, Inc.
234 Cardiff Valley Rd.
Rockwood, TN 37854
Phone: (865)354-1212 **Free:** 800-451-4351
Fax: (865)354-3853
Website: http://www.chasescientific.com
Steven E. Munzer, President
Desc: Manufacturer/distributor/biotechnology company: biotechnology/biopharmaceutical products; laboratory supplies; pharmaceutical manufacturing supplies and equipment; physicians' supplies; urinary supplies.

★ 15426 ★ Chattanooga Group, Inc.
PO Box 489
4717 Adams Rd.
Hixson, TN 37343
Phone: (423)870-2281 **Free:** 800-592-7329
Fax: (423)875-5497
Website: http://www.chattgroup.com
Paul Chapman, President
Desc: Manufacturer of OTC/proprietary pharmaceuticals; diagnostic equipment and instruments; home healthcare; hospital equipment and supplies; orthopedic and prosthetic equipment and supplies; patient aid products; physical therapy and rehabilitation equipment and supplies; physicians' equipment and supplies; ultrasonic equipment; ultrasound and electromedical equipment and supplies.

★ 15427 ★ Chattem, Inc.
1715 W 38th St.
Chattanooga, TN 37409
Phone: (423)821-4571 **Free:** 800-366-6077
Fax: (423)821-0395
Website: http://www.chattem.com
Zan Guerry, CEO & Chm Bd
Desc: Manufacturer/distributor of OTC/proprietary pharmaceuticals; dietary, nutritional and vitamin supplements.

★ 15428 ★ Chester Labs Inc.
1900 Section Rd., Ste. A
Cincinnati, OH 45237
Phone: (513)458-3840 **Free:** 800-354-9709
Fax: (513)458-3858
Website: http://www.chester-labs.com
John B. Armstrong, President
Desc: Manufacturer: contract manufacturing; disposable medical devices and supplies; hospital equipment and supplies; patient aid products; physicians' supplies; skin/wound care products; ultrasonic equipment; ultrasound and electromedical equipment and supplies.

★ 15429 ★ Chiron BioPharmaceuticals
A division of Chiron Corp.
4560 Horton St.
Emeryville, CA 94608
Phone: (510)655-8730 **Free:** 800-745-2388
Fax: (510)655-9910
Website: http://www.chiron.com
Craig A. Wheeler, President
Desc: Biotechnology company: Rx/ethical pharmaceuticals; OTC/proprietary pharmaceuticals; biotechnology/biopharmaceutical products.

★ 15430 ★ Chiron Corp.
4560 Horton St.
Emeryville, CA 94608
Phone: (510)655-8730 **Fax:** (510)655-9910
Email: corpcomm@chiron.com
Website: http://www.chiron.com
Seal P. Lance, , CEO & Chm Bd
Desc: Manufacturer/distributor/biotechnology company: Rx/ethical pharmaceuticals; biotechnology/biopharmaceutical products; skin/wound care products; surgical disposables.

★ 15431 ★ Chiron Vaccines USA
Division of Chiron Corp.
4560 Horton St.
Emeryville, CA 94608
Phone: (510)655-8730 **Free:** 800-745-2388
Fax: (510)658-3434
Website: http://www.chiron.com
John A. Lambert, President
Desc: Manufacturer/distributor/biotechnology company: Rx/ethical pharmaceuticals; biotechnology/biopharmaceutical products.

★ 15432 ★ Cho-Pat, Inc.
PO Box 293
Hainesport, NJ 08036
Phone: (609)261-1336 **Free:** 800-221-1601
Fax: (609)261-7593
Email: sales@cho-pat.com
Website: http://www.cho-pat.com
George R. Gauvry, President
Desc: Manufacturer/distributor of physicians' supplies.

★ 15433 ★ Cholestech Corp.
3347 Investment Blvd.
Hayward, CA 94545-3808
Phone: (510)732-7200 **Free:** 800-733-0404
Fax: (510)732-7227
Email: ctech_sales@cholestech.com
Website: http://www.cholestech.com
Warren E. Pinckert, II, CEO & Pres
Desc: Manufacturer/distributor of cardiovascular equipment and supplies; diagnostic equipment and instruments; diagnostic reagents and test kits; disposable medical devices and supplies; laboratory equipment; physicians' equipment and supplies.

★ 15434 ★ Chrono-Log Corp.
2 W Park Rd.
Havertown, PA 19083
Phone: (610)853-1130 **Free:** 800-247-6665
Fax: (610)853-3972
Email: webmail@chronolog.com
Website: http://www.chronolog.com
Arthur Freilich, President
Desc: Manufacturer of diagnostic equipment and instruments; diagnostic reagents and test kits; laboratory equipment and supplies.

★ 15435 ★ Chugai Biopharmaceuticals, Inc.
A subsidiary of Chugai Pharmaceutical Co., Ltd. of Tokyo
6275 Nancy Ridge Dr.
San Diego, CA 92121
Phone: (858)535-5900 **Fax:** (858)546-5977
Email: info@chugaibio.com
Website: http://www.chugaibio.com
Henry L. Nordhoff, CEO & Pres
Desc: Manufacturer of Rx/ethical pharmaceuticals; research and development.

★ 15436 ★ Church & Dwight Co., Inc.
Specialty Products Division
469 N Harrison St.
Princeton, NJ 08543-5297
Phone: (609)683-5900 **Free:** 800-221-0453
Fax: (609)497-7176
Email: arthur.esposito@churchdwight.com
Website: http://www.ahperformance.com
Art Esposito, Contact
Desc: Manufacturer of food products; food products/antislip; renal dialysis supplies.

★ 15437 ★ CIMA LABS INC.
10000 Valley View Rd.
Eden Prairie, MN 55344
Phone: (952)947-8700 **Fax:** (952)947-8770
Website: http://www.cimalabs.com
Terrence W. Glarner, Chairman of the Board
Desc: Manufacturer of Rx/ethical pharmaceuticals; drug delivery systems.

★ 15438 ★ Cincinnati Sub-Zero Products, Inc.
12011 Mosteller Rd.
Cincinnati, OH 45241
Phone: (513)772-8810 **Free:** 800-989-7373
Fax: (513)772-9119
Email: medsales@cszinc.com
Website: http://www.cszinc.com
Steve Berke, President
Desc: Manufacturer/distributor of hospital equipment and supplies; ultrasound and electromedical equipment and supplies.

★ 15439 ★ Cincinnati Surgical Co., Inc.
11256 Cornell Park Dr.
Cincinnati, OH 45242
Phone: (513)489-6640 **Free:** 800-544-3100
Fax: (513)489-6683
Email: csblades@cincinnatisurgical.com
Website: http://www.cincinnatisurgical.com
Richard F. Gregory, Jr., Contact
Desc: Distributor of dental supplies; laboratory supplies; physicians' supplies; surgical disposables and supplies; veterinary products.

★ 15440 ★ CIRCON SURGITEK
3037 Mt. Pleasant St.
Racine, WI 53404
Phone: (262)639-7205 **Free:** 800-942-2268
Fax: (262)681-4038
Website: http://www.circoncorp.com
Greg Barrett, President
Desc: Manufacturer/distributor of diagnostic equipment and instruments; disposable medical devices and supplies; sterilization equipment; surgical disposables, instruments and supplies; urinary equipment; biotechnology/ biopharmaceutical products.

★ 15441 ★ Clark Research and Development, Inc.
No. 13 Park Lane
Folsom, LA 70437
Phone: (504)796-5837 **Fax:** (504)796-8768
Website: http://www.clarkrd.com
William T. Clark, III, President
Desc: Manufacturer/distributor of hospital equipment and supplies; renal dialysis equipment; X-ray equipment.

★ 15442 ★ Clay Park Labs
1700 Bathgate Ave.
Bronx, NY 10457
Phone: (718)901-2800 **Free:** 800-933-5550
Fax: (718)960-0121
Giora Carni, CEO & Pres
Desc: Manufacturer of Rx/ethical pharmaceuticals; generic pharmaceuticals; private labeler of OTC topicals, creams and lotions.

★ 15443 ★ Clean Room Engineering
85 Orville Dr.
Bohemia, NY 11716
Phone: (631)218-2188 **Free:** 800-804-1273
Fax: (631)218-2209

Email: customerservice@cleanroomeng.com
Website: http://www.cleanroomeng.com
Christopher Young, President

Desc: Manufacturer/distributor of biological safety cabinets; clean rooms; clean room furniture and supplies; laminar flow clean benches.

★ 15444 ★ ClearMedical, Inc.

1776 136th Place, NE
Bellevue, WA 98005
Phone: (425)401-1414 **Free:** 800-426-1042
Fax: (425)401-1515
Email: info@clearmedical.com
Website: http://www.clearmedical.com
Sandra Rorem, CEO & Pres

Desc: Manufacturer/distributor of biological and environmental safety products; home healthcare; hospital equipment and supplies; implants and infusion; ostomy equipment and supplies; parenteral supplies; pasteurizing and drying equipment; patient aid products; reprocessing services; respiratory therapy and/or cardiopulmonary equipment; skin/wound care products.

★ 15445 ★ Coast Labs, Inc. d/b/a Green's Pharmaceuticals

521 W 17th St.
Long Beach, CA 90813
Phone: (562)432-7387 **Fax:** (562)436-0216
John T. Green, President

Desc: Distributor of Rx/ethical pharmaceuticals; OTC/proprietary pharmaceuticals; generic pharmaceuticals; physicians' supplies.

★ 15446 ★ Codman Division of Johnson & Johnson

325 Paramount Dr.
Raynham, MA 02767
Phone: (508)880-8100 **Fax:** (508)828-3027
David Hable, President

Desc: Manufacturer/distributor of hospital equipment and supplies; implants and infusion; patient monitoring equipment; sterilization supplies; surgical disposables and instruments; cardiovascular supplies; disposable medical devices and supplies; neurosurgery implants and instruments.

★ 15447 ★ Cole-Parmer Instrument Co.

625 E Bunker Ct.
Vernon Hills, IL 60061
Phone: (847)549-7600 **Free:** 800-323-4340
Fax: (847)247-2929
Email: info@coleparmer.com
Website: http://www.coleparmer.com
Nancy Spaulding, Contact

Desc: Distributor/biotechnology company: biotechnology/biopharmaceutical products; laboratory equipment and supplies.

★ 15448 ★ CollaGenex Pharmaceuticals, Inc.

41 University Dr.
Ste. 200
Newtown, PA 18940
Phone: (215)579-7388 **Free:** 800-613-7847
Fax: (215)579-8577
Email: bmg@collagenex.com
Website: http://www.collagenex.com
Brian M. Gallagher, PhD, CEO & Pres

Desc: Biotechnology company offering Rx/ethical pharmaceuticals.

★ 15449 ★ Collins Medical Inc.

220 Wood Rd.
Braintree, MA 02184
Phone: (781)843-0610 **Free:** 800-225-5157
Fax: (781)843-4024
Email: mail@collinsmedical.com
Website: http://www.collinsmedical.com
Terry Kirch, President

Desc: Manufacturer of diagnostic equipment and instruments; disposable medical devices and supplies; respiratory therapy and/or cardiopulmonary equipment and supplies.

★ 15450 ★ Coloplast Corp.

1955 W Oak Circle
Marietta, GA 30062
Phone: (770)281-8400 **Free:** 800-533-0464
Fax: (770)281-8504
Email: gamedweb@coloplast.com
Website: http://www.us.coloplast.com
Dave Hotchkiss, Contact

Desc: Manufacturer/distributor of OTC/proprietary pharmaceuticals; home healthcare; ostomy equipment and supplies; skin/wound care products; urinary supplies.

★ 15451 ★ Coltene/Whaledent Inc.

750 Corporate Dr.
Mahwah, NJ 07430
Phone: (201)512-8000 **Free:** 800-221-3046
Fax: (201)529-2118
Website: http://www.coltenewhaledent.com
Jerry Sullivan, CEO & Pres

Desc: Manufacturer of dental equipment and supplies; ultrasonic equipment; veterinary products.

★ 15452 ★ Combe Inc.

1101 Westchester Ave.
White Plains, NY 10604
Phone: (914)694-5454 **Fax:** (914)694-6320
Website: http://www.combe.com
Christopher B. Combe, Chairman of the Board

Desc: Manufacturer/distributor of OTC/proprietary pharmaceuticals.

★ 15453 ★ Cone Instruments, Inc.

5201 Naiman Parkway
Solon, OH 44139
Phone: (440)248-1035 **Free:** 800-321-6964
Fax: (440)248-9477
Email: info@coneinstruments.com
Website: http://www.coneinstruments.com
Patrick Beck, President

Desc: Distributor of cardiovascular equipment and supplies; diagnostic equipment and instruments; diagnostic reagents and test kits; magnetic resonance imaging; nuclear and radiological equipment and supplies; surgical supplies; ultrasonic equipment; ultrasound and electromedical equipment and supplies; veterinary products; X-ray equipment and supplies.

★ 15454 ★ CONMED Corp.

525 French Rd.
Utica, NY 13502
Phone: (315)797-8375 **Free:** 800-448-6506
Fax: (315)797-0321
Email: info@conmed.com
Website: http://www.conmed.com
Eugene R. Corasanti, CEO & Chm Bd

Desc: Manufacturer/distributor of cardiovascular supplies; disposable medical devices and supplies; EMS equipment and supplies; home healthcare; hospital equipment and supplies; I.V. controllers; I.V. stabilization dressings; orthopedic and prosthetic equipment and supplies; patient monitoring supplies; physicians' equipment and supplies; skin/wound care products; smoke plume management; surgical disposables, instruments and supplies.

★ 15455 ★ Connecticut Bioinstruments Inc.

PO Box 2567
Danbury, CT 06813
Phone: (203)744-7488 **Free:** 800-336-1935
Fax: (203)744-7488
Email: cbi@cbi-pace.com
Website: http://www.cbi-pace.com
Sidney Weinstein, Chairman of the Board

Desc: Manufacturer/distributor of diagnostic equipment and instruments; patient monitoring equipment; sensory monofilaments.

★ 15456 ★ Consolidated Stills and Sterilizers

76 Ashford St.
PO Box 297
Boston, MA 02134-0003
Phone: (617)782-6072 **Fax:** (617)787-5865
Email: info@consteril.com
Website: http://www.consteril.com
William A. Barnstead, CEO & Pres

Desc: Manufacturer of laboratory equipment and sterilization equipment.

★ 15457 ★ ConvaTec Division of Bristol-Myers Squibb Co.

PO Box 5254
Princeton, NJ 08543-5254
Phone: (908)904-2200 **Fax:** (908)904-2589
Website: http://www.convatec.com
David Johnson, Vice President

Desc: Manufacturer/distributor: contamination and infection control products; ostomy and continence products; ostomy equipment and supplies; skin/wound care products.

★ 15458 ★ CooperSurgical Division of The Cooper Cos., Inc.

95 Corporate Dr.
Trumbull, CT 06611
Phone: (203)601-5200 **Free:** 800-645-3760
Fax: 800-262-0105
Email: email@coopersurgical.com
Website: http://www.coopersurgical.com
Nicholas J. Pichotta, CEO & Pres

Desc: Manufacturer/distributor of diagnostic equipment and instruments; diagnostic reagents and test kits; disposable medical devices and supplies; hospital equipment and supplies; ophthalmic equipment and supplies; patient monitoring equipment; physicians' equipment and supplies; sterilization equipment and supplies; surgical disposables, instruments and supplies; ultrasonic equipment.

★ 15459 ★ CoorsTek, Inc.

16000 Table Mesa Pkwy.
Golden, CO 80403
Phone: (303)271-7000 **Fax:** (303)271-7009
Email: info@coorstek.com
Website: http://www.coorstek.com
John K. Coors, CEO & Pres

Desc: Manufacturer of biological and environemntal safety products; laboratory equipment and supplies; surgical disposables, instruments and supplies; contract manufacturing.

★ 15460 ★ Coral Biotechnology Division of Medquest Technologies

150 Vallecitos de Oro
San Diego, CA 92169
Phone: (760)736-4080 **Free:** 800-433-6105
Fax: (760)736-4084
Website: http://www.coralbiotech.com
Jeffrey D. Williams, PhD, President

Desc: Manufacturer/distributor/biotechnology company offering biotechnology/biopharmaceutical products; diagnostic equipment and instruments; diagnostic reagents and test kits.

★ 15461 ★ Cordis Corp.

14201 NW 60th Ave.
Miami Lakes, FL 33014
Phone: (786)313-2000 **Free:** 800-327-2490
Fax: (786)313-2020
Website: http://www.cordis.com
Robert W. Croce, Chairman of the Board

Desc: Manufacturer/biotechnology company: biotechnology/biopharmaceutical products; cardiovascular equipment and supplies.

★ 15462 ★ Corixa Corp.
Corporate Headquarters
1124 Columbia St.
Ste. 200
Seattle, WA 98104
Phone: (206)754-5711 **Free:** 800-548-7424
Fax: (206)754-5715
Email: info@corixa.com
Website: http://www.corixa.com
Steven Gillis, PhD, CEO & Chm Bd
Desc: Manufacturer/biotechnology company offering Rx/ethical pharmaceuticals; biotechnology/biopharmaceutical products.

★ 15463 ★ Corning Inc.
Life Sciences
45 Nagog Park
Acton, MA 01720
Phone: (978)635-2200 **Free:** 800-492-1110
Fax: (978)635-2476
Email: cccwebmail@corning.com
Website: http://www.corning.com/lifesciences
John W. Loose, Chairman of the Board
Desc: Manufacturer/biotechnology company: biotechnology/biopharmaceutical products; diagnostic reagents and test kits; laboratory equipment and supplies; pharmaceutical manufacturing supplies and equipment.

★ 15464 ★ Corvas International, Inc.
3030 Science Park Rd.
San Diego, CA 92121
Phone: (858)455-9800 **Fax:** (858)455-7895
Email: info@corvas.com
Website: http://www.corvas.com
Randall E. Woods, CEO & Pres
Desc: Biotechnology company: Rx/ethical pharmaceuticals; biotechnology/biopharmaceutical products.

★ 15465 ★ Crest Ultrasonics Corp.
Division of Crestek
Scotch Rd.
PO Box 7266
Trenton, NJ 08628
Phone: (609)883-4000 **Free:** 800-273-7822
Fax: (609)530-0923
Email: biomedical@crest-ultrasonics.com
Website: http://www.crest-ultrasonics.com
J. Michael Goodson, CEO & Pres
Desc: Manufacturer of ultrasonic equipment; ultrasonic cleaning equipment.

★ 15466 ★ Criticare Systems, Inc.
PO Box 26556
Milwaukee, WI 53226
Phone: (262)798-8282 **Fax:** (262)798-8290
Email: customerserv@csiusa.com
Website: http://www.csiusa.com
Emil Soika, CEO & Pres
Desc: Manufacturer of anesthesia equipment and products; diagnostic equipment and instruments; EMS equipment and supplies; hospital equipment and supplies; patient monitoring equipment; telemetery systems.

★ 15467 ★ Crosstex International
10 Ranick Rd.
Hauppauge, NY 11788-4209
Phone: (631)582-6777 **Free:** 888-CROSSTEX
Fax: (631)582-1726
Email: crosstex@crosstex.com
Website: http://www.crosstex.com
Richard Allen Orofino, President
Desc: Manufacturer of dental supplies; disposable medical devices and supplies; physicians' supplies; skin/wound care products; sterilization supplies; surgical disposables and supplies; veterinary products.

★ 15468 ★ Cryobiogenics Corp.
10 Halstead Rd.
Mendham, NJ 07945
Phone: (973)543-7434 **Fax:** (973)543-7497
Email: info@cryobiogenics.com
Website: http://www.cryobiogenics.com
Ari Marshall, President
Desc: Manufacturer/biotechnology company offering diagnostic reagents and test kits; implants and infusion; skin/wound care products; Xeno transplantation.

★ 15469 ★ CSC Scientific Co., Inc.
2810 Old Lee Hwy.
Fairfax, VA 22031
Phone: (703)876-4030 **Free:** 800-458-2558
Fax: (703)280-5142
Email: csc@cscscientific.com
Website: http://www.cscscientific.com
Arthur W. Gatenby, CEO & Pres
Desc: Manufacturer/distributor of laboratory equipment and supplies.

★ 15470 ★ Cumberland Pharmaceuticals
209 Tenth Ave. S
Ste. 332
Nashville, TN 37203
Phone: (615)255-0068 **Fax:** (615)255-0094
Email: info@cumberlandpharma.com
Website: http://www.cumberlandpharma.com
A.J. Kazimi, CEO
Desc: Manufacturer of Rx/ethical pharmaceuticals.

★ 15471 ★ Cyclin Pharmaceuticals, Inc.
1289 Deming Way
PO Box 259651
Madison, WI 53717
Phone: (608)833-7046 **Free:** 800-558-7046
Fax: 888-898-7412
Email: wha@womenshealth.com
Website: http://www.womenshealth.com
Marla Ahlgrimm, Chairman of the Board
Desc: Distributor of OTC/proprietary pharmaceuticals; dietary, nutritional and vitamin supplements; laboratory supplies; diagnostic reagents and test kits.

★ 15472 ★ Cygnus, Inc.
400 Penobscot Dr.
Redwood City, CA 94063
Phone: (650)369-4300 **Fax:** (650)599-2503
Website: http://www.cygn.com
John C. Hodgman, CEO & Pres
Desc: Manufacturer/biotechnology company: biotechnology/biopharmaceutical products; diagnostic equipment and instruments.

★ 15473 ★ Cymed Ostomy Co.
1336A Channing Way
Berkeley, CA 94702
Phone: (510)540-1926 **Free:** 800-582-0707
Fax: (510)540-6505
Email: cymed@cymed-ostomy.com
Website: http://www.cymed-ostomy.com
Dianne Eastman, President
Desc: Manufacturer of disposable medical devices and supplies; hospital equipment and supplies; medical disposable products; ostomy equipment and supplies.

★ 15474 ★ CYNACON/OCuSOFT, Inc.
PO Box 429
Richmond, TX 77406-0429
Phone: (281)342-3350 **Free:** 800-233-5469
Fax: (281)232-6015
Email: ocusoft@ocusoft.com
Website: http://www.ocusoft.com
Nat G. Adkins, Chairman of the Board
Desc: Manufacturer/distributor of Rx/ethical pharmaceuticals; OTC/proprietary pharmaceuticals; generic pharmaceuticals; ophthalmic equipment and supplies; sterilization equipment and supplies; surgical supplies.

★ 15475 ★ Cytogen Corp.
600 College Rd. E
Princeton, NJ 08540
Phone: (609)750-8200 **Free:** 800-833-3533
Email: cytoinfo@corpcomm.cytogen.com
Website: http://www.cytogen.com
H. Joseph Reiser, PhD, CEO & Pres
Desc: Manufacturer/biotechnology company: Rx/ethical pharmaceuticals; biotechnology/biopharmaceutical products; diagnostic imaging agent; radiopharmaceuticals.

★ 15476 ★ Cytovax Biotechnologies, Inc.
8223 Roper Rd.
Edmonton, AB, Canada T6E 6S4
Phone: (780)448-0621 **Fax:** (780)448-0624
Email: biotech@cytovax.com
Website: http://www.cytovax.com
Bin Huang, PhD, CEO & Pres
Desc: Biotechnology company: biotechnology/biopharmaceutical products.

★ 15477 ★ Dade Behring Inc.
SYVA Division
20400 Mariani Ave., M/S 9-21
Cupertino, CA 95014
Phone: (408)366-3811 **Fax:** (408)366-3749
Email: jamesteipen@dadbehring.com
Website: http://www.dadbehring.com
James Teipen, Vice President
Desc: Manufacturer/distributor of diagnostic equipment and instruments; diagnostic reagents and test kits.

★ 15478 ★ Dade MicroScan
Division of Dade Behring
1584 Enterprise Blvd.
West Sacramento, CA 95691
Phone: (916)372-1900 **Free:** 800-677-SCAN
Fax: (916)372-6418
Website: http://www.dadebehring.com
Bob Badal, Contact
Desc: Manufacturer of diagnostic equipment and instruments; diagnostic reagents and test kits; hospital equipment and supplies; laboratory equipment.

★ 15479 ★ Daiichi Pharmaceutical Corp.
11 Phillips Pkwy.
Montvale, NJ 07645
Phone: (201)573-7000 **Free:** 877-324-4244
Fax: (201)573-7619
Website: http://www.daiichius.org
Nicholas Marcellos, Contact
Desc: Manufacturer/distributor of Rx/ethical pharmaceuticals.

★ 15480 ★ Dako Corp.
Division of Dakopotts
6392 Via Real
Carpinteria, CA 93013
Free: 800-235-5743 **Fax:** (805)566-6688
Email: general@dakousa.com
Website: http://www.dakousa.com
Viggo G. Harboe, President
Desc: Manufacturer/distributor/biotechnology company: biotechnology/biopharmaceutical products; diagnostic reagents and test kits.

★ 15481 ★ Danker Laboratories
Ophthalmic Solutions Division
PO Box 1899
Sarasota, FL 34230
Phone: (941)758-7711 **Free:** 800-237-9641
Fax: (941)758-5965

Email: sales@dankerlabs.com
Website: http://www.dankerlabs.com
Frederick J. Danker, Chairman of the Board

Desc: Manufacturer/distributor of OTC/proprietary pharmaceuticals; ophthalmic equipment and supplies; contract manufacturing.

★ 15482 ★ Dartmouth Pharmaceuticals, Inc.
38 Church Ave., Ste 220
Wareham, MA 02571-2008
Phone: (508)295-2200 **Fax:** (508)291-6155
Email: info@ilovemynails.com
Website: http://www.ilovemynails.com
Michael J. Greco, Contact

Desc: Manufacturer/distributor of Rx/ethical pharmaceuticals; OTC/proprietary pharmaceuticals.

★ 15483 ★ Data Medical Associates, Inc.
845 Ave. G East
Arlington, TX 76011
Phone: (817)640-0965 **Free:** 800-433-7224
Fax: (817)649-2461
Website: http://www.dma-inc.com
Bret Hendzel, President

Desc: Manufacturer of diagnostic reagents and test kits; laboratory supplies.

★ 15484 ★ Datascope Corp.
14 Philips Parkway
Montvale, NJ 07645
Phone: (201)391-8100 **Free:** 800-288-2121
Fax: (201)995-8967
Website: http://www.datascope.com
Lawrence Saper, CEO & Chm Bd

Desc: Manufacturer of intra-aortic balloon pumps and catheters; patient monitoring equipment; vascular hemostasis sealing device.

★ 15485 ★ Datex - Ohmeda
Ohmeda Dr.
PO Box 7550
Madison, WI 53707-7550
Phone: (608)221-1551 **Free:** 800-345-2700
Fax: (608)223-2476
Website: http://www.datex-ohmeda.com
Lori Cross, President

Desc: Manufacturer of anesthesia equipment and products; disposable medical devices and supplies; home healthcare; patient monitoring equipment.

★ 15486 ★ David Clark Co., Inc.
PO Box 15054
360 Franklin St.
Worcester, MA 01615-0054
Phone: (508)751-5800 **Free:** 800-900-3434
Fax: (508)753-5827
Email: sales@davidclark.com
Website: http://www.davidclark.com
Robert Vincent, President

Desc: Manufacturer of cardiovascular equipment; EMS equipment and supplies; hospital equipment and supplies.

★ 15487 ★ DCI International
PO Box 228
Newberg, OR 97132
Phone: (503)538-8343 **Free:** 800-624-2793
Fax: (503)537-2489
Email: peggyf2@dcionline.com
Website: http://dcionline.com
John Spencer, CEO & Pres

Desc: Manufacturer of dental equipment; dental service parts and cabinetry; dental supplies; sterilization equipment and supplies; sterilizers.

★ 15488 ★ DEB SBS Inc.
1100 Hwy. 27 S
Stanley, NC 28164
Phone: (704)263-4240 **Free:** 800-248-7190
Fax: 800-367-7408
Email: cser@debsbs.com
Allen Soden, President

Desc: Manufacturer of hospital equipment and supplies; skin/wound care products.

★ 15489 ★ Del Mar Medical Systems
1621 Alton Pkwy.
Irvine, CA 92606
Phone: (949)250-3200 **Free:** 800-854-0481
Fax: (949)252-7692
Email: sales@delmarmedical.com
Website: http://www.delmarmedical.com
Raphael Henkin, PhD, President

Desc: Manufacturer of cardiovascular equipment and supplies; diagnostic equipment and instruments; disposable medical devices and supplies; hospital equipment and supplies; patient monitoring equipment; physical therapy and rehabilitation equipment and supplies; physicians' equipment and supplies; respiratory therapy and/or cardiopulmonary equipment and supplies.

★ 15490 ★ Del Pharmaceuticals, Inc.
A subsidiary of Del Laboratories, Inc.
178 EAB Plaza
Uniondale, NY 11556-0178
Phone: (516)844-2020 **Free:** 800-645-4664
Fax: 800-257-0205
Website: http://www.dellabs.com
Charles J. Hinkaty, President

Desc: Manufacturer of OTC/proprietary pharmaceuticals.

★ 15491 ★ Delasco
608 13th Ave.
Council Bluffs, IA 51501-6401
Phone: (712)323-3269 **Free:** 800-831-6273
Fax: (712)323-1156
Email: questions@delasco.com
Website: http://www.delasco.com
Deborah L. Grafelman, President

Desc: Distributor of Rx/ethical pharmaceuticals; OTC/proprietary pharmaceuticals; diagnostic equipment and instruments; diagnostic reagents and test kits; disposable medical devices and supplies; hospital equipment and supplies; laboratory supplies; patient aid products; physicians' equipment and supplies; skin/wound care products; slide viewing systems; sterilization equipment and supplies; surgical disposables, instruments and supplies; ultrasound and electromedical equipment and supplies.

★ 15492 ★ Delco Wire Winding Co.
57 St. Rd.
Newtown Square, PA 19073
Phone: (610)296-0350 **Fax:** (610)296-7809
Joseph Rubino, Chairman of the Board

Desc: Manufacturer/distributor of surgical supplies; surgical sutures; suture and implant wire.

★ 15493 ★ Den-Mat Corp.
2727 Skyway Dr.
PO Box 1729
Santa Maria, CA 93456
Phone: (805)922-8491 **Free:** 800-433-6628
Fax: (805)922-6933
Email: info@denmat.com
Website: http://www.rembrandt.com
Robert Ibsen, DDS, CEO & Pres

Desc: Manufacturer of dental restorative materials; Rembrandt oral care products; dental supplies.

★ 15494 ★ Dendreon Corp.
3005 First Ave.
Seattle, WA 98121
Phone: (206)256-4545 **Fax:** (206)256-0571
Website: http://www.dendreon.com
Christopher S. Henney, PhD, CEO & Chm Bd

Desc: Biotechnology Company: biotechnology/biopharmaceutical products; therapeutic cancer vaccines.

★ 15495 ★ DentalEZ Group
Valleybrooke Corporate Center
101 Lindenwood Dr., Ste. 225
Malvern, PA 19355
Phone: (610)725-8004 **Free:** (866)383-4636
Fax: (610)725-9898
Email: efficiency@dentalez.com
Website: http://www.dentalez.com
Carl E. Bretko, President

Desc: Manufacturer of dental equipment and supplies; diagnostic equipment and instruments; X-ray equipment.

★ 15496 ★ DentalEZ Group Equipment Division
2500 Hwy. 31 S
Bay Minette, AL 36507
Phone: (334)937-6781 **Free:** 888-DTE-INFO
Fax: (334)937-0461
Website: http://www.dentalez.com
Edward Holland, Vice President

Desc: Manufacturer/distributor of dental equipment; dental units/lights; doctor's stools; nurse stools; patient chairs.

★ 15497 ★ Dentsply Caulk
Division of Dentsply International, Inc.
38 W Clarke Ave.
Milford, DE 19963
Phone: (302)422-4511 **Free:** 800-532-2855
Fax: (302)422-5719
Website: http://www.caulk.com
John C. Miles, II, CEO & Chm Bd

Desc: Manufacturer of dental equipment and supplies; hospital equipment and supplies; laboratory supplies.

★ 15498 ★ Dentsply/Ceramco
Division of Dentsply International, Inc.
6 Terri Lane, Ste. 100
Burlington, NJ 08016
Phone: (609)386-8900 **Free:** 800-487-0100
Fax: (609)386-8282
Email: mkting@ceramco.com
Website: http://www.ceramco.com
Timothy Mack, Vice President

Desc: Manufacturer of dental equipment and supplies; laboratory equipment and supplies.

★ 15499 ★ Dentsply Professional
1301 Smile Way
PO Box 7807
York, PA 17404-0807
Phone: (717)767-8500 **Free:** 800-989-8825
Fax: (717)767-8252
Email: promarketing@dentsply.com
Website: http://www.professional.dentsly.com
James Mosch, Vice President

Desc: Manufacturer of dental equipment and supplies; surgical supplies.

★ 15500 ★ Dentsply Rinn/MPL Technologies
Division of Dentsply International, Inc.
1212 Abbott Dr.
Elgin, IL 60123-1819
Phone: (847)742-1115 **Free:** 800-323-0970
Fax: (847)742-1122
Website: http://www.rinncorp.com
Kimberly Clementz Brown, Contact

Desc: Manufacturer of dental equipment and supplies; x-ray equipment and supplies.

★ 15501 ★ Dentsply/Trubyte Division
570 W College Ave.
York, PA 17404

Phone: (717)845-7511 **Free:** 800-877-0020
Fax: (717)849-4628
Website: http://www.trubyte.com
Steven E. Jenson, Vice President

Desc: Manufacturer of dental equipment and supplies; laboratory supplies.

★ 15502 ★ DePuy ACE
Division of Johnson & Johnson
700 Orthopaedic Dr.
Warsaw, IN 46580
Phone: (219)267-8143 **Free:** 800-473-3789
Fax: (219)267-7098
Email: abalaity@dpyus.jnj.com
Website: http://www.depuyace.com
Andy Balaity, Vice President

Desc: Manufacturer of hospital equipment and supplies; implants and infusion; orthopedic and prosthetic equipment and supplies; orthopedic trauma products; surgical disposables and instruments.

★ 15503 ★ Derma Sciences, Inc.
214 Carnegie Center, Ste. 100
Princeton, NJ 08540
Phone: (609)514-4744 **Free:** 800-825-4325
Fax: (609)514-0502
Email: info@dermasciences.com
Website: http://www.dermasciences.com
Edward Quilty, CEO & Pres

Manufacturer of OTC/proprietary pharmaceuticals; skin/wound care products; surgical supplies.

★ 15504 ★ Dermik Laboratories, Inc.
Subsidiary of Aventis USA
1050 Westlakes Dr.
Berwyn, PA 19312
Phone: (484)595-2700
Website: http://www.dermik.com
Robert Bitterman, President

Desc: Manufacturer/distributor of Rx/ethical pharmaceuticals; OTC/proprietary pharmaceuticals.

★ 15505 ★ Dermozone Solutions, LLC
2040 Calumet St.
Clearwater, FL 33765
Phone: (727)446-6882 **Free:** 800-253-5115
Fax: (727)446-7322
Steve Oman, Contact

Desc: Manufacturer/distributor of OTC/proprietary pharmaceuticals; drug delivery technology; licensing; skin/wound care products.

★ 15506 ★ Despatch Industries
63 St. Anthony Parkway
Minneapolis, MN 55418
Phone: (612)781-5363 **Free:** 800-828-9903
Fax: (612)781-5353
Email: info@despatch.com
Website: http://www.despatch.com
Steve Oman, Contact

Desc: Manufacturer/biotechnology company: biotechnology/biopharmaceutical products; laboratory equipment; parenteral equipment; sterilization equipment.

★ 15507 ★ Detecto Scale Co.
366 N Broadway, Ste. 314
Jericho, NY 11753
Phone: (516)937-0500 **Fax:** (516)937-0524
Email: detecto@aol.com
Website: http://www.detectoscale.com
Harvey Schoener, Contact

Desc: Manufacturer of hospital equipment and supplies; physicians' equipment; scales.

★ 15508 ★ Dey, L.P.
Division of Merck KGaA, Darmstadt, Germany
2751 Napa Valley Corporate Dr.
Napa, CA 94558
Phone: (707)224-3200 **Free:** 800-755-5560
Fax: (707)224-0495
Website: http://www.deyinc.com
Charles A. Rice, CEO & Pres

Desc: Manufacturer/distributor of Rx/ethical pharmaceuticals; OTC/proprietary pharmaceuticals; generic pharmaceuticals; lung surfactants; respiratory therapy devices (non-disposable).

★ 15509 ★ DHD Healthcare
1 Madison St.
Wampsville, NY 13163
Phone: (315)363-2330 **Free:** 800-847-8000
Fax: (315)363-9625
Email: info@dhd.com
Website: http://www.dhd.com
Rex Niles, President

Desc: Manufacturer of disposable medical devices and supplies; respiratory therapy and/or cardiopulmonary supplies.

★ 15510 ★ Diack
Division of Auric Enterprises, Inc.
7755 Narrow Gauge Rd.
Beulah, MI 49617
Phone: (231)882-7251 **Fax:** (231)882-4804
Email: info@thornsmithlabs.com
Website: http://www.thornsmithlabs.com
Robert M. Brown, President

Desc: Manufacturer/distributor of dental supplies; hospital equipment and supplies; laboratory supplies; sterilization equipment.

★ 15511 ★ Diacrin, Inc.
Bldg. 96, 13th St.
Charlestown Navy Yard
Charlestown, MA 02129
Phone: (617)242-9100 **Fax:** (617)242-0070
Email: info@diacrin.com
Website: http://www.diacrin.com
Thomas Fraser, PhD, CEO & Pres

Desc: Biotechnology company: biotechnology/biopharmaceutical products.

★ 15512 ★ Diagnostic Products Corp.
5700 W 96th St.
Los Angeles, CA 90045-5997
Phone: (310)645-8200 **Free:** 800-444-5757
Fax: (310)645-9999
Email: info@dpconline.com
Website: http://www.dpcweb.com
Michael Ziering, CEO & Pres

Desc: Manufacturer/biotechnology company: biotechnology/biopharmaceutical products; diagnostic equipment and instruments; diagnostic reagents and test kits.

★ 15513 ★ Diagnostic Specialties
4 Leonard St.
PO Box 4338
Metuchen, NJ 08840
Phone: (732)549-4011 **Fax:** (732)549-4711
Email: dsmetuchen@aol.com
Praful K. Raja, President

Desc: Manufacturer/distributor/biotechnology company: biotechnology/biopharmaceutical products; diagnostic equipment and instruments; diagnostic reagents and test kits; laboratory equipment and supplies.

★ 15514 ★ Diagnostica Stago, Inc.
5 Century Dr.
Parsippany, NJ 07054
Phone: (973)631-1200 **Free:** 800-222-2624
Fax: (973)631-1618
Website: http://www.stago-us.com
Philippe Gadel, Contact

Desc: Distributor of diagnostic equipment and instruments; diagnostic reagents and test kits.

★ 15515 ★ Diamedix Corp.
Division of Ivax Corp.
2140 N Miami Ave.
Miami, FL 33127
Phone: (305)324-2300 **Free:** 800-327-4565
Fax: (305)324-2395
Email: diamedix@ivax.com
Website: http://www.diamedix.com
Giorgio D'Urso, CEO & Pres

Desc: Manufacturer of diagnostic equipment and instruments; diagnostic reagents and test kits.

★ 15516 ★ DiaSorin Inc.
1990 Industrial Blvd.
PO Box 285
Stillwater, MN 55082-0285
Phone: (651)439-9710 **Free:** 800-328-1482
Fax: (651)779-7847
Email: info@diasorin.com
Website: http://www.diasorin.com
John Walter, Contact

Desc: Manufacturer/distributor of diagnostic equipment and instruments; diagnostic reagents and test kits; laboratory equipment.

★ 15517 ★ Diffusan Sales, Inc.
99 W Hawthorne Ave.
Ste. 408
Valley Stream, NY 11580
Phone: (516)825-7736 **Free:** 800-645-2622
Fax: (516)825-7714
Robert Morris, President

Desc: Manufacturer/distributor of ostomy equipment and supplies; skin/wound care products.

★ 15518 ★ Digene Corp.
1201 Clopper Rd.
Gaithersburg, MD 20878
Phone: (301)944-7000 **Free:** 800-DIGENE-1
Fax: (301)944-7121
Email: inforeq@digene.com
Website: http://www.digene.com
Evan Jones, CEO

Desc: Manufacturer/distributor/biotechnology company: biotechnology/biopharmaceutical products; diagnostic equipment and instruments; diagnostic reagents and test kits.

★ 15519 ★ Digisonics, Inc.
3701 Kirby Dr., Ste. 930
Houston, TX 77098
Phone: (713)529-7979 **Free:** 800-940-3240
Fax: (713)529-7999
Email: service@digisonicsinc.com
Website: http://www.digisonicsinc.com
Diana McSherry, CEO

Desc: Manufacturer/distributor of medical software.

★ 15520 ★ Diosynth, Inc.
Division of Akzo Nobel Pharma
2136 S Wolf Rd.
Des Plaines, IL 60018
Phone: (847)635-0985 **Free:** 800-621-1509
Fax: (847)635-1320
Email: diosynth.inc@akzonobel.com
Website: http://www.diosynth.com
Geri Roman, Contact

Desc: Manufacturer/biotechnology company: Rx/ethical pharmaceuticals; OTC/proprietary pharmaceuticals; generic pharmaceuticals; biotechnology/biopharmaceutical products.

★ 15521 ★ Diversified Ophthalmics, Inc.
250 McCullough St.
Cincinnati, OH 45224
Phone: (513)321-7988 **Free:** 800-626-2281
Fax: (513)321-6355
Email: hefh@aol.com
Website: http://www.divopt.com
Harry Fagedes, OD, Contact

Desc: Distributor of ophthalmic equipment and supplies.

★ 15522 ★ dj Orthopedics, LLC
2985 Scott St.
Vista, CA 92083-8339
Phone: (760)734-4766 **Free:** 800-321-6569
Fax: (760)734-3595
Email: les.cross@djortho.com
Website: http://www.djortho.com
Les Cross, CEO & Pres
Desc: Manufacturer/distributor of cold therapy products; electromedical devices; orthopedic bracing products; othopedic and prosthetic equipment and supplies; physical therapy and rehabilitation equipment and supplies; soft goods and support products; surgical instruments.

★ 15523 ★ DNI Nevada, Inc.
Lionheart Technologies, Inc.
2000 Arrowhead Dr.
Carson City, NV 89706
Phone: (775)883-3400 **Free:** 800-648-7952
Fax: (775)883-9541
Email: sales@dninevada.com
Website: http://www.dninevada.com
Michael Erwrine, Contact
Desc: Manufacturer of biological and environmental safety products.

★ 15524 ★ Doak Dermatologics
Subsidiary of Bradley Pharmaceuticals, Inc.
383 Rte. 46 West
Fairfield, NJ 07004-2402
Phone: (973)882-1505 **Free:** 800-929-9300
Fax: (973)575-5366
Email: bradpharm@bradpharm.com
Website: http://www.bradpharm.com
Daniel Glassman, CEO & Chm Bd
Desc: Manufacturer/distributor of Rx/ethical pharmaceuticals; OTC/proprietary pharmaceuticals.

★ 15525 ★ Dolisos America, Inc.
3014 Rigel Ave.
Las Vegas, NV 89102
Phone: (702)871-7153 **Free:** 800-365-4767
Fax: (702)871-9670
Email: dolisos@skylink.net
Luc Clouatre, President
Desc: Manufacturer of Rx/ethical pharmaceuticals; OTC/proprietary pharmaceuticals; dietary, nutritional and vitamin supplements; pharmaceutical manufacturing supplies and equipment; veterinary products.

★ 15526 ★ Dornier Medtech America
1155 Roberts Blvd.
Kennesaw, GA 30144
Phone: (770)426-1315 **Free:** 800-DOR-NIER
Fax: (770)426-6115
Website: http://www.dornier.com
Brian Walsh, Contact
Desc: Manufacturer/distributor of diagnostic equipment and instruments; disposable medical devices and supplies; hospital equipment and supplies; lasers; lithotripters; X-ray equipment.

★ 15527 ★ Drager Medical, Inc.
3135 Quarry Rd.
Telford, PA 18969
Phone: (215)721-5400 **Free:** 800-462-7566
Fax: (215)721-9561
Website: http://www.draegermedical.com
Ruben Derderian, CEO & Pres
Desc: Manufacturer/distributor of anesthesia equipment and products; architectural systems; information systems; neonatal care systems; respiratory therapy and/or cardiopulmonary equipment.

★ 15528 ★ Dravon Medical, Inc.
11465 SE Hwy. 212
PO Box 69
Clackamas, OR 97015
Phone: (503)656-6600 **Free:** 800-654-1976
Fax: (503)655-5229
Email: dravon@mindspring.com
Website: http://www.dravon.com
Michael P. Napoli, CEO & Pres
Desc: Manufacturer: contract manufacturing; contract sterilization; custom medical bags; disposable medical devices and supplies; tube occluding clamps; towel clamps.

★ 15529 ★ DRG International, Inc.
1167 U.S. Hwy. 22
Mountainside, NJ 07092
Phone: (908)233-2075 **Free:** 800-321-1167
Fax: (908)233-0758
Email: corp@drg-international.com
Website: http://www.drg-diagnostics.de
C. Geacintov, PhD, CEO & Pres
Desc: Manufacturer/distributor of augiography digital software; biotechnology/biopharmaceutical products; cardiovascular equipment and supplies; dental equipment and supplies; diagnostic equipment and instruments; diagnostic reagents and test kits; hospital equipment and supplies; laboratory equipment and supplies; patient monitoring equipment; skin/wound care products; sleep diagnostics/therapeutics; surgical disposables; X-ray; ultra-sound software.

★ 15530 ★ Durex Consumer Products, Inc.
Division of SSL Americas, Inc.
3585 Engineering Dr., Ste. 200
Norcross, GA 30092
Phone: (770)582-2222 **Fax:** (770)582-2233
Website: http://www.durex.com
Ron Plumridge, Contact
Desc: Manufacturer of diagnostic reagents and test kits; disposable medical devices and supplies; home healthcare; skin/wound care products; surgical disposables.

★ 15531 ★ DuroMed Industries, Inc.
1788 W Cherry St.
Jesup, GA 31598
Phone: (912)427-7358 **Fax:** (912)427-2372
Email: duromed@jesup.net
Website: http://www.duro-med.com
Jeff Lazenby, Contact
Desc: Manufacturer/distributor of EMS equipment and supplies; home healthcare; hospital equipment and supplies; orthopedic equipment.

★ 15532 ★ Dynalab Corp.
350 Commerce Dr.
Rochester, NY 14623
Phone: (716)334-2060 **Free:** 800-828-6595
Fax: (585)334-0241
Email: info@dynalabcorp.com
Website: http://www.dynalabcorp.com
Martin Davies, Contact
Desc: Manufacturer/distributor of biological and environmental safety products; biotechnology/biopharmaceutical products; hospital equipment and supplies; laboratory equipment and supplies; contract manufacturing.

★ 15533 ★ Dynarex Corp.
40 Saw Mill River Rd.
Hawthorne, NY 10532
Phone: (845)345-1010 **Free:** 888-335-7500
Fax: (914)345-1011
Email: sales@dynarex.com
Website: http://www.dynarex.com
George Deutsch, President
Desc: Manufacturer/distributor of dental supplies; disposable medical devices and supplies; EMS equipment and supplies; home healthcare; hospital equipment and supplies; laboratory supplies; ostomy equipment and supplies; physicians' supplies; skin/wound care products; sterilization supplies.

★ 15534 ★ E-Z-EM, Inc.
717 Main St.
Westbury, NY 11590
Phone: (516)333-8230 **Free:** 800-544-4624
Fax: (516)333-8278
Email: webmaster@ezem.com
Website: http://www.ezem.com
Howard S. Stern, Chairman of the Board
Desc: Manufacturer/biotechnology company: biotechnology/biopharmaceutical products; cardiovascular equipment and supplies; contract manufacturing; diagnostic equipment and instruments; diagnostic reagents and test kits; disposable medical devices and supplies; hospital equipment and supplies; magnetic resonance imaging; physicians' supplies; surgical disposables and instruments; ultrasound and electromedical equipment and supplies; X-ray supplies.

★ 15535 ★ Eastman Kodak Co.
Health Imaging Division
343 State St.
Rochester, NY 14650-1132
Phone: (716)724-4000 **Free:** 800-336-4722
Fax: (716)724-9728
Email: webmaster@kodak.com
Website: http://www.kodak.com/go/health
Candy M. Obourn, Contact
Desc: Manufacturer of anesthesia equipment and products; cardiovascular equipment and supplies; dental supplies; hospital equipment and supplies; nuclear and radiological supplies; veterinary products; X-ray equipment and supplies.

★ 15536 ★ Eckstein Brothers, Inc.
4807 W 118th Pl.
Hawthorne, CA 90250
Phone: (323)772-6113 **Free:** 800-432-4913
Fax: (310)644-3869
Email: ebinc@jps.net
Isabelle Gordon, Contact
Desc: Manufacturer/distributor of bedside hearing amplifiers; hospital equipment and supplies; patient aid products; physical therapy and rehabilitation equipment and supplies.

★ 15537 ★ Ecolab Professional Products
Division of Ecolab Inc.
370 N Wabasha St.
Saint Paul, MN 55102
Phone: (651)293-2626 **Free:** 800-332-6522
Fax: (651)293-2959
Email: Ecolab@ecolab.com
Website: http://www.ecolab.com
Mel Yasis, Contact
Desc: Manufacturer of home healthcare; hospital equipment and supplies; infection control supplies; laboratory supplies; skin/wound care products; sterilization equipment and supplies.

★ 15538 ★ ECR Pharmaceuticals
Division of Claiborne Robins Co., Inc.
3969 Deep Rock Rd.
PO Box 71600
Richmond, VA 23255
Phone: (804)527-1950 **Free:** 800-527-1955
Fax: (804)527-1959
Email: ecrpharma@aol.com
Website: http://www.ecrpharmaceuticals.com
E. C. Robins, Jr., Chairman of the Board
Desc: Distributor of Rx/ethical pharmaceuticals; OTC/proprietary pharmaceuticals.

★ 15539 ★ Edwards Lifesciences Corp.
1 Edwards Way
Irvine, CA 92614
Phone: (949)250-2500 **Free:** 800-4AH-EART

Website: http://www.edwards.com
Michael A. Mussallem, Chairman of the Board
Desc: Manufacturer/distributor of cardiovascular equipment and supplies.

★ 15540 ★ Eigen, L.L.C.
848 Gold Flat Rd.
Nevada City, CA 95959
Phone: (530)265-2020
Email: marketing@eigen.com
Website: http://www.eigen.com
Michael Castorino, President
Desc: Manufacturer of cardiovascular equipment; diagnostic imaging.

★ 15541 ★ Eisai Inc.
500 Frank W Burr Blvd.
Teaneck, NJ 07666
Phone: (201)692-1100 **Fax:** (201)692-1804
Website: http://www.eisai.com
Soichi Matsuno, Chairman of the Board
Desc: Manufacturer of Rx/ethical pharmaceuticals.

★ 15542 ★ ELA Medical
2950 Xenium Lane North
Ste. 120
Plymouth, MN 55441
Phone: (763)519-9400 **Free:** 800-352-6466
Fax: (763)519-9440
Email: info@ela-usa.com
Website: http://www.elamedical.com
Russell D. Van Zandt, CEO & Pres
Desc: Distributor of cardiovascular equipment; pacemakers and related supplies; holter analysis recorders; ICD.

★ 15543 ★ Elan Diagnostics
2 Thurber Blvd.
Smithfield, RI 02917
Phone: (401)233-3526 **Fax:** (401)233-6483
Email: slsmktg@elandiagnostics.com
Website: http://www.elandiagnostics.com
Peter von Stein, Contact
Desc: Manufacturer of diagnostic equipment and instruments; diagnostic reagents and test kits; laboratory equipment; veterinary products.

★ 15544 ★ Elan Pharmaceuticals Member of the Elan Group
7475 Lusk Blvd.
San Diego, CA 92121-5796
Phone: (858)457-2553 **Free:** 800-859-8585
Fax: (858)457-2555
Website: http://www.elan.com
Dan Welch, President
Desc: Manufacturer/distributor/biotechnology company: Rx/ethical pharmaceuticals; OTC/proprietary pharmaceuticals; generic pharmaceuticals; biotechnology/biopharmaceutical products; diagnostic reagents and test kits.

★ 15545 ★ Electro-Med Health Industries
11601 Biscayne Blvd., Ste. 200A
North Miami, FL 33181
Phone: (305)892-2866 **Free:** 800-232-3644
Fax: (305)892-2980
Email: info@egs-emhi.com
Website: http://www.egs-emhi.com
Phyllis Lehman, President
Desc: Manufacturer/distributor of EMS equipment and supplies; physical therapy and rehabilitation equipment and supplies; disposable medical devices and supplies.

★ 15546 ★ Electrolyte Laboratories, Inc.
6803 E Bucknell Pl.
Denver, CO 80224
Phone: (303)757-8767 **Free:** 800-547-8767
Fax: (303)758-8140
Email: magmatrs@ecentral.com
James Landauer, President
Desc: Distributor of dietary, nutritional and vitamin supplements.

★ 15547 ★ Eli Lilly and Co.
Lilly Corporate Center
Indianapolis, IN 46285
Phone: (317)276-2000 **Fax:** (317)277-3354
Website: http://www.lilly.com
Sidney Taurel, Contact
Desc: Manufacturer of Rx/ethical pharmaceuticals; respiratory therapy and/or cardiopulmonary supplies.

★ 15548 ★ Elmed Inc.
60 W Fay Ave.
Addison, IL 60101
Phone: (630)543-2792 **Fax:** (630)543-2102
Email: medical@elmed.com
Website: http://www.elmed.com
Karl Hausner, President
Desc: Manufacturer/distributor of cardiovascular equipment and supplies; endoscopy instruments and equipment; hospital equipment and supplies; ophthalmic equipment; physical therapy and rehabilitation equipment and supplies; physicians' equipment; slide viewing systems; surgical disposables, instruments and supplies; ultrasound and electromedical equipment and supplies.

★ 15549 ★ EluSys Therapeutics, Inc.
10 Bloomfield Ave.
PO Box 102
Pine Brook, NJ 07058
Phone: (973)808-0222 **Fax:** (973)808-0322
Email: info@elusys.com
Website: http://www.elusys.com
William R. Miller, Chairman of the Board
Desc: Biotechnology/biopharmaceutical products.

★ 15550 ★ EM Industries, Inc. Affiliate of Merck KG-aA of Darmstadt, Germany
7 Skyline Dr.
Hawthorne, NY 10532
Phone: (914)592-4660 **Free:** 800-364-4535
Fax: (914)785-5815
Email: feedback@emindustries.com
Website: http://www.emindustries.com
Karin Maul, PhD, Contact
Desc: Manufacturer/distributor of biotechnology/biopharmaceutical products; dietary, nutritional and vitamin supplements; fine chemicals.

★ 15551 ★ Emergen, Inc.
390 Wakara Way
Salt Lake City, UT 84108
Phone: (801)883-0103 **Fax:** (801)883-0110
Email: info@emergenlabs.com
Website: http://www.emergenlabs.com
Kenneth Ward, Contact
Desc: Biotechnolgy company: Rx/ethical pharmaceuticals; biological and environmental safety products; diagnostic equipment and instruments; diagnostic reagents and test kits.

★ 15552 ★ Emisphere Technologies
765 Old Saw Mill River Rd.
Tarrytown, NY 10591
Phone: (914)347-2220 **Fax:** (914)347-2498
Email: info@emisphere.com
Website: http://www.emisphere.com
Michael Goldberg, MD, CEO & Chm Bd
Desc: Biotechnology company: Rx/ethical pharmaceuticals; OTC/proprietary pharmaceuticals; generic pharmaceuticals; biotechnology/biopharmaceutical products.

★ 15553 ★ Empi
599 Cardigan Rd.
Saint Paul, MN 55126-4099
Phone: (651)415-9000 **Free:** 800-328-2536
Fax: (651)415-8535
Website: http://www.empi.com
H. Philip Vierling, CEO & Pres
Desc: Manufacturer/distributor of orthopedic and prosthetic equipment and supplies; physical therapy and rehabilitation equipment and supplies; ultrasound and electromedical equipment and supplies; urinary equipment.

★ 15554 ★ ENOCHS Examining Room Furniture
PO Box 50559
Indianapolis, IN 46250
Phone: (317)580-2940 **Free:** 800-428-2305
Fax: (317)580-2944
Email: enochs@enochsmed.com
Website: http://www.enochsmed.com
Marla Foster, Contact
Desc: Manufacturer of examining room tables; physicians' equipment.

★ 15555 ★ Envirco Corp.
5601 Balloon Fiesta Parkway, NE
Albuquerque, NM 87113
Phone: (505)345-3561 **Fax:** (505)345-8875
Website: http://www.envirco.com
Rosemarie Stansbury, Contact
Desc: Manufacturer of biological and environmental safety products; hospital equipment and supplies; laboratory equipment; pharmaceutical manufacturing supplies and equipment; hospital surgical suite air systems.

★ 15556 ★ Environmental Growth Chambers Division of Integrated Development & Manufacturing Co.
PO Box 390
Chagrin Falls, OH 44022
Phone: (440)247-5100 **Free:** 800-321-6854
Fax: (440)247-8710
Email: sales@egc.com
Website: http://www.egc.com
A.O. Rule, III, President
Desc: Manufacturer of controlled environmental rooms; hospital equipment and supplies; laboratory equipment; pharmaceutical manufacturing supplies and equipment.

★ 15557 ★ Environmental Tectonics Corp.
125 James Way
Southampton, PA 18966-3877
Phone: (215)355-9100 **Fax:** (215)357-4000
Email: info@etcusa.com
Website: http://www.etcusa.com
William F. Mitchell, President
Desc: Manufacturer/distributor of pharmaceutical manufacturing supplies and equipment; sterilization equipment.

★ 15558 ★ Enzo Life Sciences Division of Enzo Biochem, Inc.
60 Executive Blvd.
Farmingdale, NY 11735
Phone: (631)694-7070 **Free:** 800-221-7705
Fax: (631)694-7501
Email: custserv@enzobio.com
Website: http://www.enzobio.com
Elazar Rabbani, CEO
Desc: Manufacturer/distributor of diagnostic reagents and test kits; research products/gene sequencing.

★ 15559 ★ Enzon, Inc.
20 Kingsbridge Rd.
Piscataway, NJ 08854-3998
Phone: (732)980-4500 **Fax:** (732)980-5911
Website: http://www.enzon.com
Susan Mesco, Contact
Desc: Manufacturer/distributor/biotechnology company: Rx/ethical pharmaceuticals; biotechnology/biopharmaceutical products.

★ 15560 ★ Eon Labs Manufacturing, Inc.
227 15 N Conduit Ave.
Laurelton, NY 11413
Phone: (718)276-8600 **Free:** 800-526-0225
Fax: (718)949-3120
Website: http://www.eonlabs.com
Bernhard Hampl, CEO & Pres
Desc: Manufacturer of generic pharmaceuticals.

★ 15561 ★ Epix Medical, Inc.
71 Rogers St.
Cambridge, MA 02142-1118
Phone: (617)250-6000 **Fax:** (617)250-6031
Email: info@epixmed.com
Website: http://www.epixmed.com
Michael D. Webb, CEO
Desc: Biotechnology company offering cardiovascular supplies; magnetic resonance imaging.

★ 15562 ★ Erie Medical
Division of Ocenco Inc.
Lakeview Corporate Park
10225 82nd Ave.
Pleasant Prairie, WI 53158
Phone: (262)947-9000 **Free:** 800-932-2293
Fax: (262)947-9020
Email: sales@eriemedical.com
Website: http://eriemedical.com
R.C. Rakers, Contact
Desc: Manufacturer of EMS equipment and supplies; home healthcare; hospital equipment and supplies; respiratory therapy and/or cardiopulmonary equipment and supplies; disposable medical devices and supplies.

★ 15563 ★ Erie Scientific Co.
Division of Apogent Technologies
175 Heritage Ave.
Portsmouth, NH 03801
Phone: (603)431-0146 **Free:** 800-662-0973
Fax: (603)427-0881
Email: productinfo@erisci.com
Website: http://www.eriesci.com
Mark F. Stuppy, Jr., Contact
Desc: Manufacturer of laboratory supplies.

★ 15564 ★ ESA Inc.
22 Alpha Rd.
Chelmsford, MA 01824-4171
Phone: (978)250-7000 **Fax:** (978)250-7090
Email: info@esainc.com
Website: http://www.esainc.com
Alvin V. Block, Chairman of the Board
Desc: Manufacturer/distributor of diagnostic equipment and instruments; diagnostic reagents and test kits; laboratory equipment; laboratory services; biotechnology/biopharmaceutical products.

★ 15565 ★ Escalon Medical Corp.
2440 S 179th St.
New Berlin, WI 53146
Phone: (262)821-9182 **Free:** 800-433-8197
Fax: (262)821-9927
Website: http://www.escalonmed.com
Rich DePiano, CEO
Desc: Manufacturer/distributor of disposable medical devices and supplies; ophthalmic equipment an supplies; surgical disposables and supplies; ultrasonic equipment; vascular devices.

★ 15566 ★ Eschenbach Optik
904 Ethan Allen Hwy.
Ridgefield, CT 06877
Phone: (203)438-7471 **Fax:** (203)438-1670
Email: info@eschenbach.com
Website: http://www.eschenbach.com
Geoffrey Moss, President
Desc: Manufacturer/distributor of diagnostic equipment and instruments; ophthalmic equipment.

★ 15567 ★ ESI Lederle
Division of Wyeth
PO Box 8299
Philadelphia, PA 19101-8299
Phone: (610)971-5400 **Fax:** (610)964-5683
Website: http://www.wyeth.com
Ron Warner, Contact
Desc: Manufacturer/distributor of generic pharmaceuticals.

★ 15568 ★ ETHEX Corp.
Division of KV Pharmaceutical Co.
10888 Metro Ct.
Hazelwood, MO 63043-2413
Phone: (314)567-3307 **Free:** 800-321-1705
Fax: (314)567-0701
Email: info@ethex.com
Website: http://www.ethex.com
Philip Vogt, President
Desc: Manufacturer/distributor of Rx/ethical pharmaceuticals; generic pharmaceuticals.

★ 15569 ★ ETHICON, Inc.
A Johnson & Johnson Co.
PO Box 151
Somerville, NJ 08876
Phone: (908)218-0707 **Free:** 800-255-2500
Website: http://www.ethiconinc.com
Clifford E. Holland, President
Desc: Manufacturer of surgical instruments.

★ 15570 ★ Ethox Corp.
251 Seneca St.
Buffalo, NY 14204
Phone: (716)842-4000 **Fax:** (716)842-4040
Email: info@ethoxcorp.com
Website: http://www.ethoxcorp.com
Salvatore J. Alagna, CEO & Pres
Desc: Manufacturer of cardiovascular supplies; disposable medical devices and supplies; EMS equipment and supplies; hospital equipment and supplies; parenteral catheters; surgical disposables.

★ 15571 ★ Eurand
845 Center Dr.
Vandalia, OH 45377
Phone: (937)898-9669
Email: bizdev@eurand.com
Website: http://www.eurand.com
Gearoid Faherty, CEO
Desc: Manufacturer of Rx/ethical pharmaceuticals; OTC/proprietary pharmaceuticals; generic pharmaceuticals; biotechnology/biopharmaceutical products; drug delivery; drug development.

★ 15572 ★ Ever Ready Thermometer Co., Inc.
228 Lackawanna Ave.
West Paterson, NJ 07424
Phone: (973)812-7474 **Free:** 800-453-7826
Fax: (973)812-7475
Website: http://www.ertco.com
Paul Stinson, Contact
Desc: Manufacturer of laboratory equipment and supplies; thermometers and hydrometers; data loggers; temperature recorders.

★ 15573 ★ Everett Laboratories, Inc.
29 Spring St.
West Orange, NJ 07052
Phone: (973)324-0200 **Free:** 800-964-9650
Fax: (973)324-0795
Email: evlabs@aol.com
Website: http://www.everettlabs.com
Everett G. Felper, President
Desc: Manufacturer of Rx/ethical pharmaceuticals; OTC/proprietary pharmaceuticals.

★ 15574 ★ Exocell, Inc.
3508 Market St., Ste. 420
Philadelphia, PA 19104
Phone: (215)222-5515 **Free:** 800-234-3962
Fax: (215)222-5325
Email: exocellinc@aol.com
Website: http://www.exocell.com
Margo P. Cohen, MD, President
Desc: Manufacturer/biotechnology company: biotechnology/biopharmaceutical products; diagnostic reagents and test kits.

★ 15575 ★ Fashion Seal Uniforms
Division of Superior Uniform Group, Inc.
10099 Seminole Blvd.
Seminole, FL 33772
Phone: (727)397-9611 **Fax:** (727)391-5401
Email: ssmc2@fashionseal.com
Website: http://www.superioruniformgroup.com
Gerald M. Benstock, CEO & Chm Bd
Desc: Apparel manufacturer.

★ 15576 ★ The Female Health Co.
875 N Michigan Ave., Ste. 3660
Chicago, IL 60611
Phone: (312)280-1119 **Free:** 800-635-0844
Fax: (312)280-9360
Email: info@femalehealth.com
Website: http://www.femalehealth.com
Mary Ann Leeper, PhD, President
Desc: Manufacturer/distributor of OTC/proprietary pharmaceuticals.

★ 15577 ★ Ferndale Laboratories, Inc.
780 W Eight Mile Rd.
Ferndale, MI 48220
Phone: (248)548-0900 **Free:** 888-548-0900
Fax: (248)548-8427
Email: conatctus@ferndalelabs.com
Website: http://www.ferndalelabs.com
Michael Burns, PhD, President
Desc: Manufacturer/distributor of Rx/ethical pharmaceuticals; OTC/proprietary pharmaceuticals; pharmaceutical manufacturing supplies and equipment; skin/wound care products.

★ 15578 ★ Ferno-Washington, Inc.
70 Weil Way
Wilmington, OH 45177
Phone: (937)382-1451 **Free:** 800-73-FERNO
Fax: (937)383-1157
Email: info@ferno.com
Website: http://www.ferno.com
Joe Bourgraf, President
Desc: Manufacturer of EMS equipment and supplies; hospital equipment and supplies; physical therapy and rehabilitation equipment and supplies; skin/wound care products.

★ 15579 ★ Ferraris Medical, Inc.
4 Centre Dr.
Orchard Park, NY 14127
Phone: (716)667-0100 **Free:** 800-205-7187
Fax: (716)667-0200
Email: ferrarisny@aol.com
Website: http://www.ferrarismedicalusa.com
Desc: Manufacturer of asthma management; home healthcare; respiratory therapy and/or cardiopulmonary equipment and supplies.

★ 15580 ★ Ferring Pharmaceuticals, Inc.
120 White Plains Rd., Ste. 400
Tarrytown, NY 10591
Phone: (914)333-8900 **Free:** 888-793-6367
Fax: (914)631-2237
Website: http://www.ferringusa.com
Wayne Anderson, CEO & Pres

Desc: Manufacturer/distributor/biotechnology company: Rx/ethical pharmaceuticals; generic pharmaceuticals; biotechnology/biopharmaceutical products.

★ 15581 ★ Ferris Manufacturing Corp.
16W300 83rd St.
Burr Ridge, IL 60527
Phone: (630)887-9797 **Free:** 800-POL-YMEM
Fax: (630)887-1008
Email: info@ferrispolymem.com
Website: http://www.ferrispolymem.com
Roy Carr, Vice President

Desc: Manufacturer of disposable medical devices and supplies; EMS equipment and supplies; home healthcare; hospital equipment and supplies; physical therapy and rehabilitation equipment and supplies; physicians' supplies; skin/wound care products.

★ 15582 ★ First Healthcare Products
6125 Lendell Dr.
Sanborn, NY 14132
Free: 800-854-8304 **Fax:** 800-542-7225
Email: info@firstproducts.com
Website: http://www.firstproducts.com
Paul Smith, President

Desc: Manufacturer/distributor of hospital equipment and supplies; medical charting equipment and supplies.

★ 15583 ★ Fischer Imaging Corp.
12300 N Grant St.
Denver, CO 80241
Phone: (303)452-6800 **Free:** 800-825-8434
Fax: (303)450-4335
Email: mnields@fischerimaging.com
Website: http://www.fischerimaging.com
Morgan W. Nields, Chairman of the Board

Desc: Manufacturer of cardiovascular equipment; digital mammography equipment; X-ray equipment.

★ 15584 ★ Fisher Hamilton LLC Subsidiary of Fisher Scientific International
1316 18th St.
PO Box 137
Two Rivers, WI 54241
Phone: (920)793-1121 **Fax:** (920)793-3084
Website: http://www.fisherhamilton.com
J. Michael Brown, President

Desc: Manufacturer of biological and environmental safety products; hospital furniture; laboratory equipment.

★ 15585 ★ Flanders Precisionaire
531 Flanders Filters Rd.
Washington, NC 27889
Phone: (252)946-8081 **Fax:** (252)946-3425
Website: http://www.precisionaire.com
Robert R. Amerson, President

Desc: Manufacturer of barrier isolators and glove boxes; hospital equipment and supplies; industrial ashrae and hepa filters and equipment; pharmaceutical manufacturing supplies and equipment.

★ 15586 ★ Fleming & Co.
1733 Gilsinn Lane
Fenton, MO 63026
Phone: (636)343-5306 **Fax:** (636)343-5322
Email: tjohnson@flemingcompany.com
Website: http://www.flemingcompany.com
Tom Johnson, Exec VP

Desc: Manufacturer/distributor of Rx/ethical pharmaceuticals; OTC/proprietary pharmaceuticals; dietary, nutritional and vitamin supplements.

★ 15587 ★ The Flinchbaugh Co., Inc.
390 Eberts Lane
York, PA 17403
Phone: (717)848-2418 **Free:** 800-326-2418
Fax: (717)843-7385
Email: flinchbaugh@earthlink.net
Website: http://www.flinchbaugh.com
Harry F. Miller, President

Desc: Manufacturer of durable medical equipment; wheel chair lifts.

★ 15588 ★ Florida Manufacturing Corp./ Flamanco International
501 Beville Rd.
Daytona Beach, FL 32119
Phone: (904)767-2372 **Free:** 800-447-2372
Fax: 800-447-6167
Email: info@flamanco.com
Website: http://www.flamanco.com
Tom Moore, Contact

Desc: Manufacturer of orthopedic and prosthetic equipment and supplies; orthopedic soft goods.

★ 15589 ★ FMI-Fluid Metering, Inc.
5 Aerial Way, Ste. 500
Syosset, NY 11791
Phone: (516)922-6050 **Free:** 800-223-3388
Fax: (516)624-8261
Email: pumps@fmipump.com
Website: http://www.fmipump.com
Harry E. Pinkerton, III, President

Desc: Manufacturer of dispensers; laboratory equipment; pharmaceutical manufacturing supplies and equipment; pumps.

★ 15590 ★ FONAR Corp.
110 Marcus Dr.
Melville, NY 11747
Phone: (631)694-2929 **Fax:** (631)249-3734
Email: sales@fonar.com
Website: http://www.fonar.com
Raymond Damadian, CEO & Pres

Desc: Manufacturer/distributor of magnetic resonance imaging.

★ 15591 ★ The Foredom Electric Co. Division of Blackstone Industries, Inc.
16 Stony Hill Rd.
Bethel, CT 06801
Phone: (203)792-8622 **Fax:** (203)796-7861
Email: info@foredom.com
Website: http://www.foredom.com
Willard P. Nelson, President

Desc: Manufacturer of dental equipment and supplies; laboratory equipment and supplies; ultrasonic equipment.

★ 15592 ★ Forest Laboratories, Inc.
909 Third Ave.
New York, NY 10022
Phone: (212)421-7850 **Fax:** (212)750-9152
Website: http://www.frx.com
Howard Solomon, CEO & Chm Bd

Desc: Manufacturer of Rx/ethical pharmaceuticals.

★ 15593 ★ Fort Dodge Animal Health Division of Wyeth
9401 Indian Creek Parkway, No. 1500
Overland Park, KS 66210
Phone: (913)664-7000 **Free:** 800-477-1365
Fax: (913)664-7227
Website: http://www.wyeth.com/divisions/fort_dodge.asp
E. Tom Corcoran, President

Desc: Manufacturer/biotechnology company: Rx/ethical pharmaceuticals; OTC/proprietary pharmaceuticals; anesthesia equipment and products; biotechnology/biopharmaceutical products; hospital equipment and supplies; implants and infusion; veterinary products; skin/wound care products; dietary, nutritional and vitamin supplements.

★ 15594 ★ Fortrad Eye Instruments Division of Fortrad Corp.
8 Franklin Rd.
Mendham, NJ 07945
Phone: (973)543-2371 **Fax:** (973)543-5446
Karl H. Grohn, President

Desc: Manufacturer of hand-held eye surgical instruments; ophthalmic equipment and supplies; steel, plastic and aluminum sterilization cases.

★ 15595 ★ FOTODYNE, Inc.
950 Walnut Ridge Dr.
Hartland, WI 53029-9388
Phone: (262)369-7000 **Free:** 800-362-3686
Fax: (262)369-7017
Email: fotodyne@execpc.com
Website: http://www.fotodyne.com
Brian P. Walsh, President

Desc: Manufacturer/distributor/biotechnology company: biotechnology/biopharmaceutical products; diagnostic equipment and instruments; laboratory equipment and supplies.

★ 15596 ★ Fougera Division of Altana Inc.
60 Baylis Rd.
Melville, NY 11747-3816
Phone: (631)454-6996 **Free:** 800-645-9833
Fax: (631)756-7017
Email: info@fougera.com
Website: http://www.fougera.com
George Cole, President

Desc: Manufacturer of generic pharmaceuticals.

★ 15597 ★ The Foxboro Co. Foxboro Analytical
38 Neponset Ave.
NO5-BA
Foxboro, MA 02035
Phone: (508)543-8750 **Free:** 888-FOXBORO
Fax: (508)549-4734
Email: kbrown@foxboro.com
Website: http://www.foxboro.com
Ken (K.B.) Brown, Contact

Desc: Manufacturer of ambient air analyzer; sensors and analyzers for PH, ORP, conductivity and resistivity; dissolved oxygen; hospital equipment and supplies; nuclear magnetic resonance.

★ 15598 ★ Freeman Manufacturing Co.
900 W Chicago Rd.
PO Box J
Sturgis, MI 49091
Phone: (616)651-2371 **Free:** 800-253-2091
Fax: (616)651-8248
Email: freeman@freemanmfg.com
Website: http://www.freemanmfg.com
Richard L. Freeman, CEO & Chm Bd

Desc: Manufacturer of orthopedic and prosthetic equipment and supplies; patient aid products; physical therapy and rehabilitation equipment and supplies.

★ 15599 ★ Friedrich & Dimmock, Inc.
2127 Wheaton Ave.
Millville, NJ 08332
Phone: (856)825-0305 **Free:** 800-524-1131
Fax: (856)327-4299
Website: http://www.fdglass.com
Robert E. Goffredi, President

Desc: Manufacturer/distributor of disposable medical devices and supplies; laboratory supplies.

★ 15600 ★ Fuji Film Medical Systems, USA, Inc.
Subsidiary of Fuji Photo Film Co., Ltd.
419 West Ave.
Stamford, CT 06902
Phone: (203)324-2000 **Free:** 800-431-1850
Fax: (203)327-6485
Email: info@fujimed.com
Website: http://www.fujimed.com
Takushi Nasu, President
Desc: Manufacturer/biotechnology company: biotechnology/biopharmaceutical products; diagnostic equipment and instruments; X-ray equipment and supplies.

★ 15601 ★ Fujinon Inc.
Division of Fuji Photo Optical Co., Ltd.
10 High Point Dr.
Wayne, NJ 07470
Phone: (973)633-5600 **Free:** 800-872-0196
Fax: (973)633-8818
Website: http://www.fujinon.co.jp
Toshihiro Nakamura, President
Desc: Manufacturer of endoscopy equipment; hospital equipment and supplies; physicians' equipment; veterinary products.

★ 15602 ★ Fujisawa Healthcare, Inc.
3 Parkway N
Deerfield, IL 60015
Phone: (847)317-8800 **Free:** 800-888-7704
Fax: (847)317-7296
Website: http://www.fujisawa.com
Hideo Fukumoto, CEO & Pres
Desc: Manufacturer of Rx/ethical pharmaceuticals; OTC/proprietary pharmaceuticals; skin/wound care products.

★ 15603 ★ Fulcrum, Inc.
23 Carol St.
Clifton, NJ 07014
Phone: (973)473-6900 **Free:** (866)473-6900
Fax: (973)472-0814
Email: fulcrum.inc@verizon.net
Website: http://www.fulcruminc.net
James Q. Maloy, CEO & Pres
Desc: Manufacturer of pharmaceutical balances; precision weight sets.

★ 15604 ★ Futura Medical Corp.
380 Stevens Ave.
Solana Beach, CA 92075
Phone: (858)350-0130 **Free:** 800-631-0076
Fax: (858)350-0136
Email: inquiries@futuramedical.com
Website: http://www.futuramedical.com
Harold Callicoat, CEO & Pres
Desc: Manufacturer of OTC/proprietary pharmaceuticals; disposable medical devices and supplies; home healthcare; hospital equipment and supplies; laboratory supplies; physicians' supplies; surgical disposables.

★ 15605 ★ Futuremed America, Inc.
15700 Devonshire St.
Granada Hills, CA 91344-7225
Phone: (818)830-2500 **Free:** 800-222-6780
Fax: (818)891-4755
Email: info@futuremedamerica.com
Website: http://www.futuremedamerica.com
Susan Lukenbill, President
Desc: Manufacturer/distributor of cardiovascular equipment and supplies; diagnostic equipment and instruments; EMS equipment and supplies; hospital equipment and supplies; physcians' equipment; respiratory therapy and/or cardiopulmonary equipment and supplies; sterilization equipment.

★ 15606 ★ G. E. Miller, Inc.
45 Sawmill River Rd.
Yonkers, NY 10701
Phone: (914)969-4036 **Free:** 800-431-2924
Fax: (914)969-3511
Email: gemill45@bellatlantic.net
Website: http://www.gemiller.com
George Miller, President
Desc: Distributor of biomagnetics; cardiovascular equipment; hospital equipment, supplies and furniture; patient aid products; physical therapy and rehabilitation equipment and supplies; skin/wound care products; surgical supplies; ultrasonic equipment; ultrasound and electromedical equipment and supplies; veterinary products.

★ 15607 ★ G.E. Ultrasound
175 Curtner Ave.
San Jose, CA 95125
Phone: (408)925-2121 **Free:** 800-952-2259
Fax: (408)925-2045
Website: http://www.geultrasound.com
Desc: Manufacturer of cardiovascular equipment; diagnostic equipment and instruments; ultrasonic equipment.

★ 15608 ★ G. Hartzell & Son
2372 Stanwell Circle
PO Box 5988
Concord, CA 94520
Phone: (925)798-2206 **Free:** 800-950-2206
Fax: (925)798-2053
Email: ghartzellandson@worldnet.att.net
Website: http://www.ghartzellandson.com
Andrew C. McIver, President
Desc: Manufacturer of dental equipment and supplies; hospital equipment and supplies; surgical disposables; veterinary products.

★ 15609 ★ G & W Laboratories, Inc.
111 Coolidge St.
South Plainfield, NJ 07080
Phone: (908)753-2000 **Free:** 800-922-1038
Fax: (908)753-1587
Email: gwlabs@gwlabs.com
Website: http://www.gwlabs.com
Burton G. Greenblatt, CEO & Chm Bd
Desc: Manufacturer of Rx/ethical pharmaceuticals; OTC/proprietary pharmaceuticals; generic pharmaceuticals.

★ 15610 ★ Galderma
14501 N Freeway
Fort Worth, TX 76177
Phone: (817)961-5000 **Fax:** (817)961-0035
Website: http://www.galderma.com
Stephen W. Clark, President
Desc: Manufacturer of Rx/ethical pharmaceuticals; OTC/proprietary pharmaceuticals.

★ 15611 ★ GAMBRO Renal Products
10810 W Collins Ave.
Lakewood, CO 80215
Phone: (303)232-6800 **Free:** 800-525-2623
Fax: (303)231-4915
Website: http://www.usa-gambro.com
Len Braganza, President
Desc: Manufacturer of renal dialysis equipment and supplies.

★ 15612 ★ Gammex RMI
2500 W Beltline Hwy. at University Ave.
PO Box 620327
Middleton, WI 53562-0327
Phone: (608)828-7000 **Free:** 800-GAMMEX-1
Fax: (608)828-7500
Email: info@gammex.com
Website: http://www.gammex.com
Charles Lescrenier, PhD, CEO & Chm Bd
Desc: Manufacturer/distributor of diagnostic equipment and instruments; hospital equipment and supplies; nuclear and radiological equipment and supplies; ultrasonic equipment; ultrasound and electromedical equipment and supplies; X-ray equipment.

★ 15613 ★ Garren Scientific, Inc.
15916 Blythe St.
Unit A
Van Nuys, CA 91406
Phone: (818)989-6340 **Free:** 800-342-3725
Fax: (818)908-9189
Email: info@garren-scientific.com
Website: http://www.garren-scientific.com
Steven Garren, President
Desc: Manufacturer/distributor of biological and environmental safety products; contract manufacturing; disposable medical devices and supplies; hospital equipment and supplies; laboratory equipment and supplies; physicians' equipment and supplies; sterilization supplies; urinary equipment.

★ 15614 ★ GATE Pharmaceuticals
Division of TEVA Pharmaceuticals, USA
1090 Horsham Rd.
North Wales, PA 19454
Free: 800-292-4283 **Fax:** (215)591-8801
Email: gangelil@tevausa.com
Website: http://www.gatepharma.com
Joseph Grotzinger, Contact
Desc: Manufacturer/distributor of Rx/ethical pharmaceuticals.

★ 15615 ★ GC America Inc.
3737 W 127th St.
Alsip, IL 60803
Phone: (708)597-0900 **Free:** 800-323-7063
Fax: (708)597-6222
Email: gca_sales@gcamerica.com
Website: http://www.gcamerica.com
Dominic Barraza, Contact
Desc: Manufacturer of dental supplies; laboratory equipment and supplies; sterilization supplies.

★ 15616 ★ GE Medical Systems Information Technologies
4502 Woodland Corporate Boulevard
Tampa, FL 33614
Phone: (813)887-2000 **Fax:** (813)887-2413
Email: ads@critikon.com
Website: http://www.gemedicalsystems.com
Scott R. Eibel, Contact
Desc: Manufacturer/distributor of anesthesia equipment and products; disposable medical devices and supplies; hospital equipment and supplies; patient monitoring equipment.

★ 15617 ★ GE Medical Systems Information Technologies
8200 W Tower Ave.
Milwaukee, WI 53223
Phone: (414)355-5000 **Free:** 800-558-5120
Fax: (414)355-3790
Website: http://www.gemedicalsystems.com
Desc: Manufacturer of diagnostic equipment and instruments; fetal monitoring systems; hospital equipment and supplies; patient monitoring equipment.

★ 15618 ★ Gebauer Co.
9410 St. Catherine Ave.
Cleveland, OH 44104
Phone: (216)271-5252 **Free:** 800-321-9348
Fax: (216)271-5335
Email: sales@gebauerco.com
Website: http://www.gebauerco.com
Ralph Stilphen, Contact
Desc: Manufacturer of Rx/ethical pharmaceuticals; OTC/proprietary pharmaceuticals; dental supplies; physical therapy and rehabilitation equipment and supplies.

★ 15619 ★ Geist Pharmaceuticals
20 N Meridian St.
Ste. 9500
Indianapolis, IN 46204
Phone: (317)833-0700 **Free:** 888-644-3478
Fax: (317)833-0707
Email: mcmains@mcmainsfoster.com
Website: http://www.geistrx.com
Michael McMains, CEO
Desc: Manufacturer of Rx/ethical pharmaceuticals; OTC/proprietary pharmaceuticals.

★ 15620 ★ GelTex Pharmaceuticals, Inc.
A Genzyme General Business Unit
153 Second Ave.
Waltham, MA 02451
Phone: (781)290-5888 **Fax:** (781)290-5890
Website: http://www.geltex.com
Timothy Noyes, Contact
Desc: Biotechnology company: biotechnology/biopharmaceutical products.

★ 15621 ★ Gem Refrigerator Co.
650 E Erie Ave.
Philadelphia, PA 19134
Phone: (215)426-8700 **Free:** 800-922-1422
Fax: (215)426-8731
Bruce Gruhler, CEO & Pres
Desc: Manufacturer of home healthcare; hospital equipment and supplies; laboratory equipment.

★ 15622 ★ Gen-Probe Inc.
Subsidiary of Chugai Pharmaceutical Co., Ltd. of Tokyo
10210 Genetic Center Dr.
San Diego, CA 92121
Phone: (858)410-8000 **Free:** 800-523-5001
Fax: (858)410-8625
Email: nordhoff@gen-probe.com
Website: http://www.gen-probe.com
Henry L. Nordhoff, CEO & Pres
Desc: Manufacturer/distributor/biotechnology company: biotechnology/biopharmaceutical products; diagnostic equipment and instruments; diagnostic reagents and test kits.

★ 15623 ★ Gen Trak, Inc.
PO Box 1290
Liberty, NC 27298
Phone: (336)622-5266 **Free:** 800-221-7407
Fax: (336)622-1750
Email: sfpresearc@aol.com
Steve Repp, CEO & Pres
Desc: Manufacturer of diagnostic reagents and test kits.

★ 15624 ★ Genaera Corp.
5110 Campus Dr.
Plymouth Meeting, PA 19462
Phone: (610)941-4020 **Fax:** (610)941-5399
Email: info@geneara.com
Website: http://www.geneara.com
Roy C. Levitt, MD, CEO & Pres
Desc: Biotechnology company: biotechnology/biopharmaceutical products.

★ 15625 ★ GenBio
15222 Ave. of Science, Ste. A
San Diego, CA 92128
Phone: (858)592-9300 **Free:** 800-288-4368
Fax: (858)592-9400
Email: genbio@genbio.com
Website: http://www.genbio.com
Fred Adler, President
Desc: Manufacturer/distributor/biotechnology company: biotechnology/biopharmaceutical products; diagnostic reagents and test kits; hospital equipment and supplies; laboratory supplies; physicians' supplies.

★ 15626 ★ Gendron, Inc.
400 Lugbill Rd.
Archbold, OH 43502
Phone: (419)445-6060 **Free:** 800-537-2521
Fax: (419)446-2631
Email: sales@gendronic.com
Website: http://www.gendroninc.com
Steven W. Cotter, Contact
Desc: Manufacturer of home healthcare; hospital equipment and supplies; patient aid products.

★ 15627 ★ Genelabs Technologies, Inc.
505 Penobscot Dr.
Redwood City, CA 94063
Phone: (650)369-9500 **Fax:** (650)368-0709
Email: investorinfo@genelabs.com
Website: http://www.genelabs.com
Irene Chow, PhD, Chairman of the Board
Desc: Manufacturer/distributor/biotechnology company: Rx/ethical pharmaceuticals; biotechnology/biopharmaceutical products.

★ 15628 ★ Genentech, Inc.
1 DNA Way
South San Francisco, CA 94080
Phone: (650)225-1000 **Fax:** (650)225-2021
Email: medinfo@gene.com
Website: http://www.gene.com
Arthur D. Levinson, PhD, CEO & Chm Bd
Desc: Manufacturer/biotechnology company: biotechnology/biopharmaceutical products.

★ 15629 ★ General Physiotherapy Inc.
Division of General Medventures International, Inc.
13222 Lakefront Dr.
Earth City, MO 63045
Phone: (314)291-1442 **Free:** 800-237-1832
Fax: (314)291-1485
Email: info@g5.com
Website: http://www.g5.com
Thomas Muchisky, CEO & Pres
Desc: Manufacturer of OTC/proprietary pharmaceuticals; disposable medical devices and supplies; home healthcare; hospital equipment and supplies; physical therapy and rehabilitation equipment and supplies; plastic surgery/dermatology equipment and supplies; respiratory therapy and/or cardiopulmonary equipment and supplies; skin/wound care products.

★ 15630 ★ Genesis Bio-Pharmaceuticals, Inc.
185 Linden St.
Hackensack, NJ 07601-4628
Phone: (201)488-0998 **Free:** 800-828-6941
Fax: (201)488-3968
Email: genesis01@genesisbio.com
Website: http://www.genesisbio.com
Jerrold Grossman, PhD, President
Desc: Distributor/biotechnology company: Rx/ethical pharmaceuticals; generic pharmaceuticals; biotechnology/biopharmaceutical products; home healthcare.

★ 15631 ★ Geneva Pharmaceuticals
Subsidiary of Novartis
2655 W Midway Blvd.
PO Box 446
Broomfield, CO 80038-0446
Phone: (303)466-2400 **Free:** 800-523-1808
Fax: (303)466-6378
Website: http://www.genevarx.com
John Sedor, CEO & Pres
Desc: Manufacturer/distributor of generic pharmaceuticals.

★ 15632 ★ Geneva Pharmaceuticals, Inc.
Subsidiary of Novartis
101 Morgan Lane
Second Floor
Plainsboro, NJ 08536
Phone: (609)750-4700 **Fax:** (609)750-4798
Email: joseph.renner@gx.novartis.com
Website: http://www.genevarx.com
Jon Sedor, CEO
Desc: Manufacturer/distributor of generic pharmaceuticals; Rx/ethical pharmaceuticals; OTC/proprietary pharmaceuticals.

★ 15633 ★ Genome Therapeutics Corp.
100 Beaver St.
Waltham, MA 02453
Phone: (781)398-2300 **Fax:** (781)893-9535
Website: http://www.genomecorp.com
Steven M. Rauscher, CEO & Pres
Desc: Biotechnology company: biotechnology/biopharmaceutical products; genomics; S-DNA sequencing.

★ 15634 ★ GenVec, Inc.
65 W Watkins Mill Rd.
Gaithersburg, MD 20878
Phone: (240)632-0740 **Fax:** (240)632-0735
Website: http://www.genvec.com
Herb Conrad, Chairman of the Board
Desc: Biotechnology company: biotechnology/biopharmaceutical products.

★ 15635 ★ Genzyme Corp.
1 Kendall Sq.
Cambridge, MA 02139
Phone: (617)252-7500 **Fax:** (617)252-7600
Website: http://www.genzyme.com
Henri A. Termeer, CEO & Pres
Desc: Biotechnology company: OTC/proprietary pharmaceuticals; biotechnology/biopharmaceutical products; cardiovascular equipment; diagnostic reagents and test kits; skin/wound care products; surgical disposables and instruments.

★ 15636 ★ George C. Bishop Co.
PO Box 684
Horsham, PA 19044
Phone: (215)672-1202 **Free:** 800-476-7374
George C. Bishop, Contact
Desc: Manufacturer/distributor of hospital equipment and supplies; orthopedic and prosthetic equipment and supplies; patient aid products; physical therapy and rehabilitation equipment and supplies.

★ 15637 ★ George Glove Co., Inc.
301 Greenwood Ave.
Midland Park, NJ 07432
Phone: (201)251-1200 **Free:** 800-631-4292
Fax: (201)251-8431
Email: georgeglove@quicksitemaker.com
Website: http://www.georgeglove.com
Clark Bullock, CEO
Desc: Manufacturer/distributor of Rx/ethical pharmaceuticals; OTC/proprietary pharmaceuticals; apparel; biological and environmental safety products; dental supplies; hospital equipment and supplies; laboratory supplies; physicians' supplies; skin/wound care products; sterilization equipment and supplies.

★ 15638 ★ George Tiemann & Co.
25 Plant Ave.
Hauppauge, NY 11788
Phone: (631)273-0005 **Free:** 800-843-6266
Fax: (631)273-6199
Email: richard@georgetiemann.com
Website: http://www.georgetiemann.com
Richard Moriarty, President
Desc: Manufacturer/distributor of surgical instruments.

★ 15639 ★ Gerhard Surgical, Inc.
1432 Hanley Industrial Ct.
Saint Louis, MO 63144
Phone: (314)918-8877 **Free:** 800-325-9685
Fax: (314)918-8853
Email: Gerhard@il.net
William M. Terry, President
Desc: Surgical instruments distributor.

★ 15640 ★ Geri-Care Pharmaceuticals Corp.
1650 63rd St.
Brooklyn, NY 11204
Phone: (718)382-5000 **Free:** 800-540-3765
Fax: (718)382-5001
Email: gericare@hotmail.com
Sheindy J. Shindler, President
Desc: Manufacturer of OTC/proprietary pharmaceuticals; generic pharmaceuticals; dietary, nutritional and vitamin supplements.

★ 15641 ★ Geritrex Corp.
144 E Kingsbridge Rd.
Mount Vernon, NY 10550-7954
Phone: (914)668-4003 **Free:** 800-736-3437
Fax: (914)668-4047
Email: geritrex@aol.com
Website: http://www.geritrex.com
Anthony A. Madaio, President
Desc: Manufacturer of OTC/proprietary pharmaceuticals; generic pharmaceuticals; biological and environmental safety products; contract manufacturing; dental supplies; home healthcare; hospital equipment and supplies; ostomy equipment and supplies; pharmaceutical manufacturing supplies and equipment; physicians' supplies; skin/wound care products; veterinary products.

★ 15642 ★ Germfree Laboratories, Inc. Purified Microenvironments Division
7435 NW 41st St.
Miami, FL 33166
Phone: (305)592-1780 **Free:** 800-888-5357
Fax: (305)591-7280
Email: info@germfree.com
Website: http://www.germfree.com
Jerome J. Landy, MD,PhD, President
Desc: Manufacturer of biological and environmental safety products; home healthcare; hospital and home healthcare IV pharmacy equipment; hospital equipment and supplies; laboratory equipment; parenteral equipment; pharmaceutical clean room equipment.

★ 15643 ★ Getinge/Castle, Inc.
1777 E Henrietta Rd.
Rochester, NY 14623
Phone: (716)475-1400 **Free:** 800-475-9040
Fax: (716)272-5033
Email: info@getingecastle.com
Website: http://www.getingecastle.com
Creighton White, CEO & Pres
Desc: Manufacturer/distributor of animal-care washers; biological and environmental safety products; contract manufacturing; hospital equipment and supplies; laboratory equipment; orthopedic and prosthetic equipment and supplies; pharmaceutical manufacturing supplies and equipment; sterilization equipment and supplies; surgical supplies; ultrasonic equipment; veterinary products.

★ 15644 ★ Gilbert Surgical Instruments, Inc.
115 Harding Ave.
PO Box 458
Bellmawr, NJ 08099
Phone: (856)933-2770 **Fax:** (856)931-1916
Website: http://www.gilbertsurgical.com
Gilbert Goldberg, President
Desc: Manufacturer of Frazier suction tubes; hospital equipment and supplies; Jackson trachea tubes; Sims uterine curettes; surgical instruments; Yankauer tubes.

★ 15645 ★ Gillead Sciences, Inc.
333 Lakeside Dr.
Foster City, CA 94404
Phone: (650)574-3000 **Free:** 800-GIL-EAD5
Fax: (650)522-5853
Email: corporate_communications@gilead.com
Website: http://www.gillead.com
John C. Martin, CEO & Pres
Desc: Manufacturer/biotechnology company: Rx/ethical pharmaceuticals; biotechnology/biopharmaceutical products.

★ 15646 ★ Gilson, Inc.
3000 W Beltline Hwy.
PO Box 620027
Middleton, WI 53562-0027
Phone: (608)836-1551 **Free:** 800-445-7661
Fax: (608)831-4451
Email: sales@gilson.com
Website: http://www.gilson.com
Warren E. Gilson, MD, Chairman of the Board
Desc: Manufacturer/biotechnology company: biotechnology/biopharmaceutical products; laboratory equipment; pharmaceutical manufacturing supplies and equipment.

★ 15647 ★ Gish Biomedical, Inc.
22942 Arroyo Vista
Rancho Santa Margarita, CA 92688
Phone: (949)635-6200 **Free:** 800-938-0531
Fax: (949)635-6299
Email: gish@gishbiomedical.com
Website: http://www.ishbiomedical.com
Kelly Scott, President
Desc: Manufacturer/distributor of cardiovascular equipment and supplies; disposable medical devices and supplies; hospital equipment and supplies; implants and infusion; parenteral catheters; surgical disposables.

★ 15648 ★ Glades Pharmaceuticals Division of Stiefel Laboratories
255 Alhambra Circle
Coral Gables, FL 33134
Phone: (305)567-1319 **Free:** 800-GLADES-1
Fax: (305)443-3467
Email: bmurphy@glades.com
Website: http://www.glades.com
Brendan Murphy, President
Desc: Manufacturer of Rx/ethical pharmaceuticals; OTC/proprietary pharmaceuticals; generic pharmaceuticals.

★ 15649 ★ Glas-Col Apparatus Co. Division of Templeton Coal Co., Inc.
PO Box 2128
Terre Haute, IN 47802
Phone: (812)235-6167 **Free:** 800-452-7265
Fax: (812)234-6975
Email: pinnacle@glascol.com
Website: http://www.glascol.com
Steve Sterrett, President
Desc: Manufacturer of combinatorial chemistry; laboratory equipment.

★ 15650 ★ GlaxoSmithKline
1 Franklin Plaza
PO Box 7929
Philadelphia, PA 19101
Phone: (215)751-4000 **Free:** 888-825-5249
Fax: (215)751-3400
Website: http://www.gsk.com
Jean-Pierre Garnier, CEO
Desc: Manufacturer/distributor/biotechnology company: Rx/ethical pharmaceuticals; OTC/proprietary pharmaceuticals; biotechnology/biopharmaceutical products.

★ 15651 ★ GlaxoSmithKline Consumer Healthcare
100 Beecham Dr.
PO Box 1467
Pittsburgh, PA 15230
Phone: (412)928-1000 **Fax:** (412)928-5864
Website: http://www.gsk.com
Manfred Scheske, President
Desc: Manufacturer/distributor/: OTC/proprietary pharmaceuticals.

★ 15652 ★ Glenwood, LLC
19 Empire Blvd.
South Hackensack, NJ 07606
Phone: (201)221-0050 **Free:** 800-542-0772
Fax: (201)221-0060
Email: info@glenwood-llc.com
Website: http://www.glenwood-llc.com
Christopher Fuhrmann, CEO
Desc: Manufacturer/distributor of Rx/ethical pharmaceuticals; OTC/proprietary pharmaceuticals; generic pharmaceuticals; dental equipment; veterinary products.

★ 15653 ★ Global Pharmaceuticals Division of IMPAX Laboratories
3735 Castor Ave.
Philadelphia, PA 19124
Phone: (215)289-2220 **Free:** 800-296-5227
Fax: (215)289-2223
Website: http://www.globalphar.com
Barry R. Edwards, Contact
Desc: Manufacturer of Rx/ethical pharmaceuticals; generic pharmaceuticals.

★ 15654 ★ Good-Lite Co., Inc.
865 Muirfield Dr.
Hanover Park, IL 60133
Phone: (630)529-9720 **Free:** 800-362-3860
Fax: (630)529-9293
Email: rob@good-lite.com
Website: http://www.good-lite.com
Robert D. Rogers, President
Desc: Manufacturer of ophthalmic equipment and supplies; physicians' equipment.

★ 15655 ★ Gottfried Medical, Inc.
4105 W Alexis Rd.
PO Box 8966
Toledo, OH 43623
Phone: (419)474-2973 **Free:** 800-537-1968
Fax: (419)474-8822
Email: sales@gottfriedmedical.com
Website: http://www.gottfriedmedical.com
Brent M. Gottfried, President
Desc: Manufacturer/distributor of custom surgical support garments; home healthcare; hospital equipment and supplies.

★ 15656 ★ Gould Instrument Systems, Inc. A ThermoSpectra Co.
8333 Rockside Rd.
Valley View, OH 44125
Phone: (216)328-7000 **Free:** 800-468-5365
Fax: (216)328-7403
Website: http://www.gouldis.com
John Milbandt, President
Desc: Manufacturer/biotechnology company: biotechnology/biopharmaceutical products; cardiovascular data acquisition; cardiovascular equipment and supplies; medical data acquisition; respiratory therapy and/or cardiopulmonary equipment.

★ 15657 ★ GPC Biotech AG
610 Lincoln St.
Waltham, MA 02451
Phone: (781)890-9007 **Fax:** (781)890-9005
Email: info@gpc-biotech.com

Website: http://www.biotech.com
Dr. Bernd R. Seizinger, PhD, CEO & Pres
Desc: Biotechnology company: Rx/ethical pharmaceuticals; biotechnology/biopharmaceutical products.

★ 15658 ★ Graham-Field Health Products
2935 Northeast Parkway
Atlanta, GA 30360
Phone: (770)447-1609 **Free:** 800-347-5678
Fax: (678)291-3232
Website: http://www.grahamfield.com
Michael Crouch, Contact
Desc: Manufacturer of home healthcare; hospital equipment and supplies; laboratory equipment and supplies; patient aid products; physical therapy and rehabilitation equipment and supplies.

★ 15659 ★ Graham-Field, Inc.
2935 Northeast Parkway
Atlanta, GA 30360
Phone: (770)447-1609 **Free:** 800-235-4661
Fax: (770)840-4797
Email: mail@grahamfield.com
Website: http://www.grahamfield.com
Michael Joffred, CEO & Pres
Desc: Manufacturer/distributor of dental supplies; diagnostic equipment and instruments; disposable medical devices and supplies; EMS equipment and supplies; home healthcare; hospital equipment and supplies; laboratory equipment and supplies; ophthalmic equipment and supplies; orthopedic and prosthetic equipment and supplies; patient aid products; patient monitoring equipment; physical therapy and rehabilitation equipment and supplies; physicians' equipment and supplies; respiratory therapy and/or cardiopulmonary equipment and supplies; slide viewing systems; sterilization equipment and supplies; surgical disposables, instruments and supplies; ultrasonic equipment; ultrasound and electromedical equipment and supplies; urinary equipment and supplies; veterinary products; X-ray equipment and supplies.

★ 15660 ★ Graham Medical Division of Little Rapids Corp.
2273 Larsen Rd.
PO Box 19100
Green Bay, WI 54307
Phone: (920)494-8701 **Free:** 800-558-6765
Fax: 800-494-7877
Email: grahammedical@littlerapids.com
Website: http://www.grahammedical.com
Jeff Anderson, Contact
Desc: Manufacturer of apparel; contract manufacturing; dental supplies; disposable medical devices and supplies; disposable paper products; hospital equipment and supplies; laboratory supplies; nuclear and radiological supplies; physicians' supplies; X-ray supplies.

★ 15661 ★ Grant Airmass Corp.
126 Chestnut Hill Rd.
Stamford, CT 06903
Phone: (203)321-3460 **Free:** 800-243-5237
Fax: (203)321-3465
Email: grant@grantairmass.com
Website: http://www.grantairmass.com
B.H. Grant, President
Desc: Manufacturer of alternating air pressure mattress overlay; home healthcare; hospital equipment and supplies; skin/wound care products.

★ 15662 ★ Grason-Stadler Inc.
5225-2 Verona Rd.
Madison, WI 53711
Free: 800-700-2282 **Fax:** (608)441-2234
Email: sales@grasonstadler.com
Website: http://www.grason-stadler.com
Chris Ingham, Contact
Desc: Manufacturer/distributor of diagnostic equipment and instruments; hospital equipment and supplies.

★ 15663 ★ Greer Laboratories, Inc.
639 NuWay Circle
PO Box 800
Lenoir, NC 28645
Phone: (828)754-5327 **Free:** 800-438-0088
Fax: (828)754-5320
Website: http://www.greerlabs.com
William White, Jr., Chairman of the Board
Desc: Manufacturer/distributor/biotechnology company: Rx/ethical pharmaceuticals; biotechnology/biopharmaceutical products; contract manufacturing; diagnostic equipment and instruments; diagnostic reagents and test kits; disposable medical devices and supplies; patient monitoring equipment; veterinary products.

★ 15664 ★ Gricks Ostomy Appliances & Q-T Products Division of Torbot Group, Inc.
1367 Elmwood Ave.
PO Box 3564
Cranston, RI 02910
Phone: (401)780-8737 **Free:** 800-545-4254
Fax: (401)780-8740
Email: torbot@worldnet.att.net
Website: http://www.torbot.com
Stephen Yarlas, President
Desc: Manufacturer/distributor of home healthcare; ostomy equipment and supplies; urinary equipment.

★ 15665 ★ Grieshaber Manufacturing Co., Inc.
7020 W Cullom Ave.
Norridge, IL 60706
Phone: (708)457-1551 **Fax:** (708)457-0810
Sharon Booth, President
Desc: Manufacturer/distributor of surgical instruments.

★ 15666 ★ Guardian Laboratories Division of United-Guardian Inc.
PO Box 18050
Hauppauge, NY 11788
Phone: (631)273-0900 **Free:** 800-645-5566
Fax: (631)273-0858
Email: evp@u-g.com
Website: http://www.u-g.com
Alfred R. Globus, CEO & Chm Bd
Desc: Manufacturer of Rx/ethical pharmaceuticals; OTC/proprietary pharmaceuticals.

★ 15667 ★ Gudebrod, Inc.
PO Box 357
Pottstown, PA 19464
Phone: (610)327-4050 **Fax:** (610)327-4588
Email: sales@gudebrod.com
Website: http://www.gudebrod.com
Edward F. John, CEO & Pres
Desc: Manufacturer/distributor of dental supplies; hospital equipment and supplies; physicians' supplies; surgical cords and supplies.

★ 15668 ★ Guidant Corp. Endovascular Solutions
1525 O'Brien Dr.
Menlo Park, CA 94025
Phone: (650)617-5000 **Free:** 800-457-8145
Fax: (650)470-6320
Website: http://www.guidant.com
Bev Huss, President
Desc: Manufacturer/distributor of surgical instruments.

★ 15669 ★ Guidant Corp. Vascular Intervention Group
3200 Lakeside Dr.
Santa Clara, CA 95054
Phone: (408)845-3000 **Free:** 800-633-3375
Fax: (408)845-3333
Website: http://www.guidant.com
John Capek, President
Desc: Manufacturer/distributor of cardiovascular equipment and supplies; disposable medical devices and supplies.

★ 15670 ★ Guilford Pharmaceuticals Inc.
6611 Tributary St.
Baltimore, MD 21224
Phone: (410)631-6300 **Fax:** (410)631-6485
Website: http://www.guilfordpharm.com
Craig R. Smith, Contact
Desc: Biotechnology company: biotechnology/biopharmaceutical products.

★ 15671 ★ Gulden Ophthalmics
225 Cadwalader Ave.
Elkins Park, PA 19027-2020
Phone: (215)884-8105 **Free:** 800-659-2250
Fax: (215)884-0418
Email: info@guldenindustries.com
Website: http://www.guldenindustries.com
Thomas Cockley, President
Desc: Manufacturer of ophthalmic equipment and supplies.

★ 15672 ★ Gynetics Inc.
3371 Route 1
Ste. 200
Lawrenceville, NJ 08648
Phone: (609)919-1931 **Free:** 800-311-7378
Fax: (609)919-9409
Email: info@gynetics.com
Website: http://www.gynetics.com or http://www.preven.com
Roderick L. Mackenzie, Chairman of the Board
Desc: Distributor of Rx/ethical pharmaceuticals; disposable medical devices and supplies; physicians' supplies.

★ 15673 ★ Gyrus ENT
2925 Appling Rd.
Bartlett, TN 38133
Phone: (901)373-0200 **Free:** 800-262-3540
Fax: (901)373-0220
Website: http://www.gyrus-ent.com
Jerry Dowdy, CEO & Pres
Desc: Manufacturer of disposable medical devices and supplies; implants and infusion; rhinology (nose) and laryngology (throat/ head, neck) surgical disposables; surgical instruments; surgical instruments and implants for otology (ear), surgical supplies.

★ 15674 ★ H.W. Naylor Co., Inc.
121 Main St.
PO Box 190
Morris, NY 13808
Phone: (607)263-5145 **Fax:** (607)263-2416
Howard N. Elliott, President
Desc: Manufacturer of veterinary products.

★ 15675 ★ Hacker Instruments Inc.
17 Sherwood Lane
PO Box 10033
Fairfield, NJ 07004
Phone: (973)226-8450 **Free:** 800-4-HACKER
Fax: (973)808-8281
Email: hackerlab@aol.com
Website: http://www.hackerinstruments.com
Elfi Hacker, President
Desc: Manufacturer/distributor of laboratory equipment and supplies.

★ 15676 ★ Haemo-Sol, Inc.
7301 York Rd.
Towson, MD 21204
Phone: (410)821-5676 **Free:** 800-821-5676
Fax: (410)828-8461
Email: haemosol@haemo-sol.com
Website: http://www.haemo-sol.com
William L. Hermann, Contact

Desc: Manufacturer of laboratory supplies; no-scrub detergents for removal of blood and other proteinaceous waste from dental, hospital, surgical and laboratory instruments and apparatus.

★ 15677 ★ Haemonetics Corp.
400 Wood Rd.
Braintree, MA 02184
Phone: (781)848-7100 **Free:** 800-225-5242
Fax: (781)356-3558
Email: info@haemonetics.com
Website: http://www.haemonetics.com
James L. Peterson, CEO & Pres
Desc: Manufacturer of automated blood processing systems; cardiovascular equipment and supplies.

★ 15678 ★ Hallcrest Inc.
1820 Pickwick Lane
Glenview, IL 60025
Phone: (847)998-8580 **Free:** 800-527-1419
Fax: (847)998-8051
Email: hcsales@hallcrest.com
Website: http://www.hallcrest.com
Patrick Van Minnen, CEO & Pres
Desc: Manufacturer of anesthesia equipment and products; disposable medical devices and supplies; hospital equipment and supplies.

★ 15679 ★ Halsey Drug Co., Inc.
695 N Perryville Rd.
Rockford, IL 61107
Phone: (815)399-2060 **Free:** 800-336-2750
Fax: (815)399-9710
Email: general@halseydrug.com
Website: http://www.halseydrug.com
Michael K. Reicher, CEO & Pres
Desc: Manufacturer of Rx/ethical pharmaceuticals; OTC/proprietary pharmaceuticals; generic pharmaceuticals.

★ 15680 ★ Hamilton Bell Co., Inc.
30 Craig Rd.
Montvale, NJ 07645
Phone: (201)391-4100 **Free:** 800-526-0864
Fax: (201)391-5994
Email: hamiltonbell@mindspring.com
Website: http://www.hamiltonbell.com
James N. San Vito, President
Desc: Manufacturer/distributor of hospital equipment and supplies; laboratory equipment and supplies; physicians' equipment; surgical instruments; protective eye wear; biology supplies and centrifuges.

★ 15681 ★ Hanford Pharmaceuticals
304 Oneida St.
PO Box 1017
Syracuse, NY 13201
Phone: (315)476-7418 **Free:** 800-234-4263
Fax: (315)476-7434
Email: info@hanford.com
Website: http://www.hanford.com
George R. Hanford, Chairman of the Board
Desc: Manufacturer/distributor of Rx/ethical pharmaceuticals; generic pharmaceuticals; veterinary products.

★ 15682 ★ Hanovia
825 Lehigh Ave.
Union, NJ 07083
Phone: (908)688-0050 **Free:** 800-229-3666
Fax: (908)686-8404
Email: hanovia@juno.com
Website: http://www.hanovia-uv.com
Bob Majka, Contact
Desc: Sterilization equipment manufacturer.

★ 15683 ★ Hard Manufacturing Co., Inc.
230 Grider St.
Buffalo, NY 14215
Phone: (716)893-1800 **Free:** 800-USE-HARD
Fax: (716)896-2579
Email: hardmfg@hardmfg.com
Website: http://www.hardmfg.com
William Godin, President
Desc: Manufacturer of hospital cribs; youth beds and furniture; hospital equipment and supplies; hospital furniture.

★ 15684 ★ Hardwood Products Co. LP
PO Box 149
Guilford, ME 04443
Phone: (207)876-3311 **Free:** 800-321-2313
Fax: 800-323-4153
Email: info@hwppuritan.com
Website: http://www.hwppuritan.com
Terry N. Young, Contact
Desc: Manufacturer of dental supplies; diagnostic equipment and instruments; disposable medical devices and supplies; hospital equipment and supplies; laboratory supplies; physicians' supplies; surgical disposables.

★ 15685 ★ Hardy Diagnostics
1430 W McCoy Lane
Santa Maria, CA 93455
Phone: (805)346-2766 **Free:** 800-266-2222
Fax: (805)614-9274
Email: sales@hardydiagnostics.com
Website: http://www.hardydiagnostics.com
Jay R. Hardy, President
Desc: Manufacturer/distributor of apparel; biological and environmental safety products; biotechnology/biopharmaceutical products; contract manufacturing; diagnostic equipment and instruments; diagnostic reagents and test kits; disposable medical devices and supplies; laboratory equipment and supplies; microbiology supplies; pharmaceutical manufacturing supplies and equipment; prepared culture media; slide viewing systems; sterilization equipment.

★ 15686 ★ Harmac Medical Products, Inc.
2201 Bailey Ave.
Buffalo, NY 14211-1797
Phone: (716)897-4500 **Fax:** (716)897-0016
Email: info@harmac.com
Website: http://www.harmac.com
John Somers, President
Desc: Manufacturer: contract manufacturing; disposable medical devices and supplies; hospital equipment and supplies; implants and infusion; laboratory supplies; ophthalmic supplies; surgical disposables.

★ 15687 ★ Harmony Laboratories, Inc.
1109 S Main St.
Landis, NC 28088
Phone: (704)857-0707 **Free:** 800-245-6284
Fax: (704)855-1090
Email: harlab@harmonylabs.com
J. Michael Gorman, CEO & Pres
Desc: Manufacturer of OTC/proprietary pharmaceuticals; generic pharmaceuticals; contract manufacturing.

★ 15688 ★ Hartmann-Conco Inc.
481 Lakeshore Pkwy.
Rock Hill, SC 29730
Phone: (803)325-7600 **Free:** 800-243-2294
Fax: (803)243-7606
Website: http://www.hartmann-conco.com
Jacques Lemmetti, President
Desc: Manufacturer of disposable medical devices and supplies; EMS equipment and supplies; home healthcare; hospital equipment and supplies; orthopedic and prosthetic equipment and supplies; patient aid products; physicians' supplies; skin/wound care products; veterinary products.

★ 15689 ★ Harvy Surgical Supply Corp.
34-35 Collins Pl.
Flushing, NY 11354-2790
Phone: (718)939-1122 **Free:** 800-221-0142
Fax: (718)939-1222
Email: harvyusa@aol.com
Gene Levy, Vice President
Desc: Manufacturer/distributor of home healthcare; hospital equipment and supplies; orthopedic and prosthetic equipment and supplies; patient aid products and supplies.

★ 15690 ★ Hausmann Industries, Inc.
130 Union St.
Northvale, NJ 07647
Phone: (201)767-0255 **Free:** 800-526-0289
Fax: (201)767-1369
Email: sales@hausmann.com
Website: http://www.hausmann.com
David Hausmann, CEO
Desc: Manufacturer of dental equipment; hospital equipment and supplies; hospital furniture; patient aid products; physical therapy and rehabilitation equipment and supplies; physicians' equipment.

★ 15691 ★ Health Factors International
429 S Siesta Lane
Tempe, AZ 85281
Phone: (480)921-1991 **Fax:** (480)921-2084
Kirk Neal, Contact
Desc: Manufacturer of dietary, nutritional and vitamin supplements.

★ 15692 ★ Health o Meter
Pelstar LLC
7400 W 100th Pl.
Bridgeview, IL 60455
Phone: (708)598-9100 **Free:** 800-815-6615
Fax: (708)233-5472
Website: http://www.healthometer.com
Paul Nizzere, President
Desc: Manufacturer: body fat analysis; home healthcare; hospital equipment and supplies; physicians' equipment; veterinary products.

★ 15693 ★ HealthFirst Corp.
22316 70th Ave. W, Unit A.
Mountlake Terrace, WA 98043
Phone: (425)771-5733 **Free:** 800-331-1984
Fax: (425)775-2374
Email: hfirst1@aol.com
Website: http://www.healthfirstcorp.com
Thomas J. Schulstad, President
Desc: Manufacturer/distributor of Rx/ethical pharmaceuticals; CPR emergency crash carts; diagnostic equipment and instruments; EMS equipment and supplies; pharmaceutical emergency kits; physicians' equipment.

★ 15694 ★ Healthmark Industries Co.
22522 E Nine Mile Rd.
Saint Clair Shores, MI 48080
Phone: (810)774-7600 **Free:** 800-521-6224
Fax: (810)774-6473
Email: healthmark@hmark.com
Website: http://www.hmark.com
Mark D. Basile, President
Desc: Distributor of anesthesia equipment and products; biological and environmental safety products; dental supplies; disposable medical devices and supplies; EMS equipment and supplies; hospital equipment and supplies; laboratory equipment and supplies; ophthalmic supplies; orthopedic and prosthetic equipment and supplies; pharmaceutical manufacturing supplies and equipment; physicians' equipment and supplies; respiratory therapy and/or cardiopulmonary equipment; sterilization equipment and supplies.

★ 15695 ★ HealthWatch Technologies, Inc.
1040 Joshua Way
Vista, CA 92083
Phone: (760)598-4333 **Free:** 800-223-5009
Fax: (760)598-4330
Website: http://healthwatchonline.com
Paul Harrison, CEO & Chm Bd
Desc: Manufacturer of cardiovascular equipment and supplies; diagnostic equipment and instruments; healthcare management software.

★ 15696 ★ Helena Laboratories
PO Box 752
Beaumont, TX 77704
Phone: (409)842-3714 **Free:** 800-231-5663
Fax: (409)842-6241
Website: http://www.helena.com
Tipton Golias, President
Desc: Manufacturer/distributor of laboratory equipment and supplies.

★ 15697 ★ Helix Scientific, Inc.
PO Box 2386
Warminster, PA 18974
Phone: (215)953-1990 **Fax:** (215)953-1991
Email: info@helixscientific.com
Steve Finlayson, President
Desc: Manufacturer of laboratory equipment; pharmaceutical manufacturing supplies and equipment.

★ 15698 ★ Heller Laboratories
100 W Ave. of the Colors
Sparks, NV 89434-9536
Phone: (775)342-2000 **Fax:** (775)342-0222
Robert E. Heller, Contact
Desc: Manufacturer of diagnostic equipment and instruments; laboratory equipment and supplies.

★ 15699 ★ Helmac Products Corp.
3440 Preston Ridge Rd.
Ste. 650
Alpharetta, GA 30005
Phone: (770)570-5000 **Free:** 800-521-5856
Fax: (770)570-5001
Email: customerserv@helmac.com
Website: http://www.helmac.com
Nick McKay, Jr., CEO
Desc: Manufacturer of hospital equipment and supplies; laboratory supplies; physicians' supplies; surgical disposables.

★ 15700 ★ Hemagen Diagnostics, Inc.
Virgo Products Division
9033 Red Branch Rd.
Columbia, MD 21045
Phone: (443)367-5500 **Free:** 800-436-2436
Fax: (410)992-7812
Email: info@hemagen.com
Website: http://www.hemagen.com
Jerry Ruyan, CEO & Chm Bd
Desc: Manufacturer: contract manufacturing; diagnostic equipment and instruments; diagnostic reagents and test kits; laboratory equipment; veterinary products.

★ 15701 ★ HEMCO International
111 Powell Rd.
Independence, MO 64056
Phone: (816)796-2900 **Free:** 800-779-4362
Fax: (816)796-3333
Email: info@hemcocorp.com
Website: http://www.hemcocorp.com
Ronald E. Hill, President
Desc: Manufacturer/distributor of biological and environmental safety products; hospital equipment and supplies; laboratory equipment; parenteral equipment.

★ 15702 ★ Her-Mar Inc.
1410 20th St., Ste. 202
Miami Beach, FL 33139
Phone: (305)532-5413 **Free:** 800-327-8209
Fax: (305)532-6803
Martin Mayer, President
Desc: Distributor of diagnostic equipment and instruments; home healthcare; hospital equipment and supplies; physicians' equipment and supplies; respiratory therapy and/or cardiopulmonary equipment; surgical instruments; ophthalmic equipment.

★ 15703 ★ Herculite Products, Inc.
PO Box 435
Emigsville, PA 17318
Phone: (717)764-1192 **Free:** 800-772-0036
Fax: (717)764-5211
Email: customercare@herculite.com
Website: http://www.herculite.com
William Wanner, Contact
Desc: Manufacturer of hospital equipment and supplies; hospital furniture; patient aid products.

★ 15704 ★ Hermell Products, Inc.
9 Britton Dr.
Bloomfield, CT 06002
Phone: (860)242-6550 **Free:** 800-233-2342
Fax: (860)243-0361
Email: hermell@hermell.com
Website: http://www.hermell.com
Ronald Pollack, President
Desc: Manufacturer: contract manufacturing; home healthcare; hospital equipment and supplies; orthopedic and prosthetic equipment and supplies; patient aid products; skin/wound care products; sleep diagnostics/therapeutics.

★ 15705 ★ Hermitage Hospital Products, Inc.
Division of Keilei International
38 Hope St.
Niantic, CT 06357
Phone: (860)739-5421 **Free:** 800-243-0741
Fax: (860)739-2804
Website: http://www.hermitageonline.com
Stephanie Shen, President
Desc: Manufacturer of apparel; dental supplies; home healthcare; hospital equipment and supplies; patient aid products; physicians' supplies; renal dialysis supplies; skin/wound care products; sterilization supplies; surgical instruments; urinary supplies; veterinary products; X-ray equipment; disposable medical devices and supplies; EMS equipment and supplies.

★ 15706 ★ High Chemical Co.
Division of National Generic Dist. Inc.
3901-A Nebraska St.
Levittown, PA 19056
Phone: (215)788-3113 **Free:** 800-447-8792
Fax: (215)788-3148
Website: http://www.sarapin.com
Nalin Parikh, President
Desc: Manufacturer of Rx/ethical pharmaceuticals.

★ 15707 ★ Hill Laboratories Co.
PO Box 2028
3 Bacton Hill Rd.
Frazer, PA 19355
Phone: (610)644-2867 **Fax:** (610)647-6297
Email: hah.hill@erols.com
Website: http://www.hilllabs.com
Howard A. Hill, President
Desc: Manufacturer of physical therapy and rehabilitation equipment and supplies; physicians' equipment.

★ 15708 ★ Hill-Rom
Architectural Products
1069 State Rte. 46 E
Batesville, IN 47006-9167
Phone: (812)934-7777 **Free:** 800-445-3730
Fax: (812)934-8465
Website: http://www.hill-rom.com
Tony Orsini, Contact
Desc: Manufacturer/distributor of hospital equipment and supplies; medical gas equipment and headwalls.

★ 15709 ★ Hill-Rom Air-Shields
A Hillenbrand Industry
330 Jacksonville Rd.
Hatboro, PA 19040-2211
Phone: (215)675-5200 **Free:** 800-523-5756
Fax: (215)675-8346
Website: http://www.hill-rom.com
Nancy St. Clair, Contact
Desc: Manufacturer of hospital equipment and supplies.

★ 15710 ★ Hill-Rom Co., Inc.
A Hillenbrand Industry
1069 State Rte. 46 E
Batesville, IN 47006
Phone: (812)934-7777 **Free:** 800-445-3720
Fax: (812)934-8329
Email: webops@hill-rom.com
Website: http://www.hill-rom.com
Ernest Waaser, CEO & Pres
Desc: Manufacturer of disposable medical devices and supplies; home healthcare; hospital equipment and supplies; hospital furniture; patient aid products; patient monitoring equipment; respiratory therapy and/or cardiopulmonary supplies; skin/wound care products; surgical instruments; ultrasound and electromedical equipment and supplies.

★ 15711 ★ Hitachi Chemical Diagnostics, Inc.
630 Clyde Ct.
Mountain View, CA 94043
Phone: (650)961-5501 **Free:** 800-233-6278
Fax: (650)969-2745
Email: info@hcdiagnostics.com
Website: http://www.hcdiagnostics.com
Tetsuo Odashiro, CEO & Pres
Desc: Manufacturer/distributor/biotechnology company offering biotechnology/biopharmaceutical products; diagnostic equipment and instruments; diagnostic reagents and test kits; hospital equipment and supplies; laboratory equipment.

★ 15712 ★ Hoffmann-La Roche, Inc.
Member of the Roche Group
340 Kingsland St.
Nutley, NJ 07110
Phone: (973)235-5000 **Free:** 800-526-0625
Fax: (973)235-7605
Website: http://www.rocheusa.com
George B. Abercrombie, CEO & Pres
Desc: Manufacturer of Rx/ethical pharmaceuticals.

★ 15713 ★ Hogil Pharmaceutical Corp.
2 Manhattanville Rd.
Purchase, NY 10577
Phone: (914)696-7600 **Fax:** (914)696-4600
Email: hogil@aol.com
Howard Wendy, CEO & Pres
Desc: Manufacturer of OTC/proprietary pharmaceuticals.

★ 15714 ★ Holles Laboratories, Inc.
30 Forest Notch
Cohasset, MA 02025
Phone: (781)383-0741 **Free:** 800-356-4015
Theodora Lelecas, President
Desc: Manufacturer of Rx/ethical pharmaceuticals; ophthalmic supplies.

★ 15715 ★ Hollister Inc.
2000 Hollister Dr.
Libertyville, IL 60048
Phone: (847)680-1000 **Free:** 800-323-4060
Fax: (847)680-2123
Website: http://www.hollister.com
Mary Ellen Buckley, Contact
Desc: Manufacturer of heel and elbow protectors; home healthcare; hospital equipment and supplies; patient monitoring equipment; physical therapy and rehabilitation equipment and supplies; restraint jackets and wrist holders; skin/wound care products.

★ 15716 ★ Home Access Health Corp.
2401 W Hassell Rd., Ste. 1510
Hoffman Estates, IL 60195-5200
Phone: (847)781-2500 **Free:** 800-HIV-TEST
Fax: (847)781-2560
Email: info@homeaccess.com
Website: http://www.homeaccess.com
Tracey T. Powell, CEO & Chm Bd
Desc: Manufacturer/distributor: call center; diagnostic reagents and test kits; home testing: HIV/hepatitis/cholesterol.

★ 15717 ★ Hooker Sales Co., Inc.
PO Box 491333
Leesburg, FL 34749
Phone: (352)728-1123 **Free:** 800-359-5180
Fax: (352)728-2600
Robert Hummell, President
Desc: Manufacturer/distributor of dental supplies; laboratory supplies; ophthalmic supplies; patient aid products.

★ 15718 ★ Horizon Medical Products, Inc.
1 Horizon Way
Manchester, GA 31816
Phone: (706)846-3126 **Free:** 800-472-5221
Fax: (706)846-3146
Email: email@hmpvascular.com
Website: http://www.hmpvascular.com
Bill Peterson, Contact
Desc: Manufacturer/distributor of anesthesia equipment and products; cardiovascular supplies and equipment; hemodialysis casters; implantable ports; implants and infusion; renal dialysis equipment and supplies.

★ 15719 ★ Hospital Marketing Services Co., Inc.
Naugatuck Industrial Park
162 Great Hill Rd.
PO Box 1217
Naugatuck, CT 06770
Phone: (203)723-1466 **Free:** 800-786-5094
Fax: (203)723-7248
Email: info@hmsmedical.com
Website: http://www.hmsmedical.com
Brian C. Hurley, Contact
Desc: Manufacturer of disposable medical devices and supplies; EMS equipment and supplies; hospital equipment and supplies; patient aid products; physicians' supplies; surgical disposables, instruments and supplies.

★ 15720 ★ Hotpack An SP Industries Co.
10940 Dutton Rd.
Philadelphia, PA 19154
Phone: (215)824-1700 **Free:** 800-523-3608
Fax: (215)637-0519
Email: sales@hotpack.com
Website: http://www.hotpack.com
Jay Silverman, President
Desc: Manufacturer/distributor of biological and environmental safety products; laboratory equipment; incubators; environmental rooms; freezers and refrigerators; sterilization equipment; washers and sterilizers.

★ 15721 ★ Houba, Inc. Division of Halsey Drug Co., Inc.
16235 State Rd. 17
Culver, IN 46511
Phone: (574)842-3305 **Free:** 877-942-5739
Fax: (574)842-2519
Website: http://wwww.halseydrug.com
Michael Reicher, CEO & Pres
Desc: Manufacturer of generic pharmaceuticals.

★ 15722 ★ Howmedica Osteonics Corp.
59 Route 17 S
Allendale, NJ 07401
Phone: (201)825-4900 **Fax:** (201)934-4369
Website: http://www.howost.com
Ned Lipes, President
Desc: Manufacturer/distributor of orthopedic and prosthetic equipment and supplies; surgical disposables.

★ 15723 ★ Hudson Industries, Inc.
5250 Klockner Dr.
Richmond, VA 23231
Phone: (804)226-1155 **Free:** 800-343-8112
Fax: (804)222-4308
Website: http://hudsonindustries.com
Gary C. Hudson, Contact
Desc: Manufacturer: contract manufacturing; disposable medical devices and supplies; home healthcare; hospital equipment and supplies; patient aid products.

★ 15724 ★ Hudson RCI
27711 Diaz Rd.
PO Box 9020
Temecula, CA 92589-9020
Phone: (909)676-5611 **Free:** 800-848-3766
Fax: (909)676-1578
Email: postmaster@hudsonrci.com
Website: http://www.hudsonrci.com
Charles French, CEO & Pres
Desc: Manufacturer of anesthesia equipment and products; EMS equipment and supplies; home healthcare; respiratory therapy and/or cardiopulmonary equipment and supplies; disposable medical devices and supplies; sleep diagnostics/therapeutics; veterinary products.

★ 15725 ★ Huntleigh Healthcare
40 Christopher Way
Eatontown, NJ 07724
Phone: 800-223-1218 **Free:** 888-223-1218
Fax: (732)578-9889
Website: http://www.huntleigh-healthcare.com
Robert Angel, CEO & Pres
Desc: Manufacturer/distributor of hospital equipment and supplies; physical therapy and rehabilitation equipment and supplies; physicians' equipment; ultrasonic equipment.

★ 15726 ★ Hycor Biomedical Inc.
7272 Chapman Ave.
Garden Grove, CA 92841
Phone: (714)933-3000 **Free:** 800-382-2527
Fax: (714)933-3222
Email: mjdeal@hycorbiomedical.com
Website: http://www.hycorbiomedical.com
Mary Joanne Deal, PhD, Contact
Desc: Manufacturer of diagnostic equipment and instruments; diagnostic reagents and test kits; laboratory equipment and supplies.

★ 15727 ★ Hydromer Inc./Biosearch Medical Products, Inc.
35 Industrial Parkway
Somerville, NJ 08876
Phone: (908)526-2828 **Free:** 800-326-5976
Fax: (908)526-3633
Email: rlee@hydromer.com
Website: http://www.hydromer.com
Manfred F. Dyck, CEO & Pres
Desc: Manufacturer offering contract manufacturing; cardiovascular supplies; disposable medical devices and supplies; GI/endoscopic medical devices; hospital equipment and supplies; ostomy equipment and supplies; skin/wound care products; urinary catheters, equipment and supplies.

★ 15728 ★ The Hygenic Corp.
1245 Home Ave.
Akron, OH 44310
Phone: (330)633-8460 **Free:** 800-321-2135
Fax: (330)633-9359
Email: feedback@hygenic.com
Website: http://www.hygenic.com
Nancy Hunter, Contact
Desc: Manufacturer: contract manufacturer; disposable medical devices and supplies; home healthcare; hospital equipment and supplies; laboratory supplies; physical therapy and rehabilitation equipment and supplies; surgical disposables.

★ 15729 ★ HYPAC, Inc.
Rte. 2, Box A-1
Flemingsburg, KY 41041
Phone: (606)849-2447 **Fax:** (606)849-2401
Email: hypac_inc@hotmail.com
Website: http://www.hypachydraulics.com
Benjamin J. Hill, Contact
Desc: Manufacturer of hospital equipment and supplies; laboratory equipment.

★ 15730 ★ Hypoguard Medisys Group Co.
7301 Ohms Lane, Ste. 200
Edina, MN 55439
Phone: (952)646-3200 **Free:** 800-818-8877
Fax: (952)646-3210
Email: info@hypoguard.com
Website: http://www.hypoguard.com
Loren Smith, Contact
Desc: Manufacturer/distributor of contract manufacturing; diagnostic equipment and instruments; diagnostic reagents and test kits; disposable medical devices and supplies; hospital equipment and supplies; patient monitoring equipment; veterinary products.

★ 15731 ★ Hyrex Pharmaceuticals
3494 Democrat Rd.
PO Box 18385
Memphis, TN 38118
Phone: (901)794-9050 **Free:** 800-238-5282
Fax: (901)794-9051
Email: hytuss@aol.com
James E. Baker, President
Desc: Manufacturer/distributor of Rx/ethical pharmaceuticals; OTC/proprietary pharmaceuticals; generic pharmaceuticals; dietary, nutritional and vitamin supplements; parenteral supplies; physicians' supplies.

★ 15732 ★ Hyseq Pharmaceuticals, Inc.
675 Almanor Ave.
Sunnyvale, CA 94085
Phone: (408)524-8100
Email: ir@sbh.com
Website: http://www.hyseq.com
George B. Rathmann, PhD, Chairman of the Board
Desc: Biotechnology company: Rx/ethical pharmaceuticals; OTC/ proprietary pharmaceuticals; biotechnology/biopharmaceutical products.

★ 15733 ★ IBA Worldwide
2015 Spring Rd.
Ste. 650
Oak Brook, IL 60523
Phone: (630)928-1700 **Free:** 800-811-4674
Fax: (630)928-1702
Email: info@iba-group.com
Website: http://www.iba-group.com
Mark McLoughlin, President

Desc: Manufacturer of analytical lab services; sterilization equipment; sterilization services.

★ 15734 ★ ICN Pharmaceuticals Diagnostics Division
13 Mountain View Ave.
Orangeburg, NY 10962
Phone: (845)359-2700 **Free:** 800-854-0530
Fax: (845)359-2188
Website: http://www.icnpharm.com
Bill Richardson, Contact
Desc: Manufacturer of diagnostic reagents and test kits.

★ 15735 ★ ICN Pharmaceuticals, Inc.
3300 Hyland Ave.
Costa Mesa, CA 92626
Phone: (714)545-0100 **Free:** 800-548-5100
Fax: (714)668-3139
Website: http://www.icnpharm.com
Mark Taylor, MD, Contact
Desc: Manufacturer of Rx/ethical pharmaceuticals; OTC/proprietary pharmaceuticals; diagnostic reagents and test kits; laboratory equipment and supplies; skin/wound care products; dermatology devices (lasers); physicians' equipment.

★ 15736 ★ IDEXX Laboratories, Inc.
1 IDEXX Dr.
Westbrook, ME 04092
Phone: (207)856-0300 **Free:** 800-551-0998
Fax: (207)856-0319
Email: investorrelations@idexx.com
Website: http://www.idexx.com
Jonathan W. Ayers, CEO
Desc: Manufacturer/distributor/biotechnology company: OTC/proprietary pharmaceuticals; biotechnology/biopharmaceutical products; diagnostic equipment and instruments; diagnostic reagents and test kits; laboratory equipment; pharmaceutical manufacturing supplies and equipment; veterinary products.

★ 15737 ★ Immunetics, Inc.
63 Rogers St.
Cambridge, MA 02142
Phone: (617)492-5416 **Free:** 800-227-4765
Fax: (617)868-7879
Email: info@immunetics.com
Website: http://www.immunetics.com
Andrew Levin, President
Desc: Manufacturer of diagnostic equipment and instruments; diagnostic reagents and test kits.

★ 15738 ★ Immunex Corp.
51 University St.
Seattle, WA 98101
Phone: (206)587-0430 **Free:** 800—IMMUNEX
Fax: (206)587-0606
Website: http://www.immunex.xom
Edward V. Fritzky, CEO & Chm Bd
Desc: Manufacturer/biotechnology company: Rx/ethical pharmaceuticals; biotechnology/biopharmaceutical products;

★ 15739 ★ Immuno Concepts N.A., Ltd.
9779-D Business Park Dr.
Sacramento, CA 95827
Phone: (916)363-2649 **Free:** 800-251-5115
Fax: (916)363-2843
Email: techservice@immunoconcepts.com
Website: http://www.immunoconcepts.com
Bert Williams, III, President
Desc: Manufacturer of diagnostic reagents and test kits.

★ 15740 ★ Immuno-Mycologics, Inc.
PO Box 1151
Norman, OK 73070
Phone: (405)288-2383 **Free:** 800-654-3639
Fax: (405)288-2228
Email: immy@immy.com
Website: http://www.immy.com
David S. Bauman, PhD, Chairman of the Board
Desc: Manufacturer/distributor of diagnostic reagents and test kits.

★ 15741 ★ ImmunoGen, Inc.
128 Sidney St.
Cambridge, MA 02139
Phone: (617)995-2500 **Fax:** (617)995-2510
Email: info@immunogen.com
Website: http://www.immunogen.com
Mitchel Sayare, CEO & Chm Bd
Desc: Biotechnology company offering Rx/ethical pharmaceuticals; biotechnology/biopharmaceutical products.

★ 15742 ★ Inhale Therapeutic Systems, Inc.
150 Industrial Rd.
San Carlos, CA 94070-6256
Phone: (650)631-3100 **Fax:** (650)631-3150
Email: inhale@inhale.com
Website: http://www.inhale.com
Robert B. Chess, Chairman of the Board
Desc: Manufacturer of Rx/ethical pharmaceuticals; generic pharmaceuticals; biotechnology/biopharmaceutical products.

★ 15743 ★ InKine Pharmaceutical Co., Inc.
1787 Sentry Parkway W, Bldg. 18
Ste. 440L
Blue Bell, PA 19422
Phone: (215)583-6850 **Fax:** (215)283-4600
Website: http://www.inkine.com
Leonard S. Jacob, CEO & Chm Bd
Desc: Biotechnology company offering Rx/ethical pharmaceuticals.

★ 15744 ★ Innapharma, Inc.
1 Maynard Dr.
Ste. 205
Park Ridge, NJ 07656
Phone: (201)505-1300 **Fax:** 877-711-8711
Email: innapharma@aol.com
Website: http://www.innapharma.com
John P. Feighner, MD, President
Desc: Manufacturer/distributor of Rx/ethical pharmaceuticals.

★ 15745 ★ Instromedix
6779 Mesa Ridge Rd.
Ste. 200
San Diego, CA 92121
Phone: (858)777-2200 **Free:** 800-633-3361
Fax: (858)777-2371
Website: http://www.instromedix.com
Robert White, CEO & Pres
Desc: Manufacturer/distributor of cardiovascular equipment and supplies; diagnostic equipment and instruments; home healthcare; hospital equipment and supplies; patient monitoring equipment; physicians' equipment; EMS equipment and supplies; respiratory therapy and/or cardiopulmonary equipment.

★ 15746 ★ Instrumentation Laboratory Division of C. H. Werfen
101 Hartwell Ave.
Lexington, MA 02421
Phone: (781)861-0710 **Free:** 800-955-9525
Fax: (781)861-1908
Website: http://www.ilww.com
Jose Manent, CEO
Desc: Manufacturer/distributor of diagnostic equipment and instruments; diagnostic reagents and test kits; laboratory equipment and supplies; respiratory therapy and/or cardiopulmonary equipment.

★ 15747 ★ Integrity Pharmaceutical Corp.
9084 Technology Dr.
Ste. 600
Fishers, IN 46038
Phone: (317)558-2820 **Free:** 800-823-6878
Fax: (317)558-2821
Email: info@integritypharma.com
Website: http://www.integritypharma.com
Keith D. Gates, CEO
Desc: Manufacturer/distributor of Rx/ethical pharmaceuticals; OTC/proprietary pharmaceuticals; generic pharmaceuticals.

★ 15748 ★ Interface Biomedical Laboratory Corp.
7600 Ridge Blvd.
Brooklyn, NY 11209
Phone: (718)238-5554 **Fax:** (718)238-0010
Philip N. Sawyer, MD, President
Desc: Manufacturer/distributor of cardiovascular supplies; sterilization supplies.

★ 15749 ★ Interferon Sciences, Inc.
783 Jersey Ave.
New Brunswick, NJ 08901
Phone: (732)249-3250 **Fax:** (732)249-6895
Email: info@interferonsciences.com
Website: http://www.interferonsciences.com
Samuel H. Ronel, PhD, Chairman of the Board
Desc: Manufacturer/biotechnology company: Rx/ethical pharmaceuticals; biotechnology/biopharmaceutical products.

★ 15750 ★ Intergen(r) Co.
The Centre at Purchase
2 Manhattanville Rd.
Purchase, NY 10577
Phone: (914)694-1700 **Free:** 800-431-4505
Fax: (914)694-1429
Website: http://www.intergenco.com
Robert J. Beckman, CEO & Pres
Desc: Manufacturer/biotechnology company: biotechnology/biopharmaceutical products; contract manufacturing; diagnostic reagents and test kits.

★ 15751 ★ Intermagnetics General Corp.
450 Old Niskayuna Rd.
PO Box 461
Latham, NY 12110-0461
Phone: (518)782-1122 **Fax:** (518)782-0900
Email: ir@igc.com
Website: http://www.igc.com
Carl H. Rosner, Chairman of the Board
Desc: Manufacturer of magnetic resonance imaging; superconducting magnet system for magnetic resonance imaging.

★ 15752 ★ InterMetro Industries Corp. Healthcare Division
651 N Washington St.
Wilkes Barre, PA 18705
Phone: (570)825-2741 **Free:** 800-433-2232
Fax: (570)824-2704
Email: moreinfo-hc@metro.com
Website: http://www.metro.com
John G. Nackley, CEO & Pres
Desc: Manufacturer of hospital equipment and supplies; hospital furniture; modular casework; storage and transport products.

★ 15753 ★ Intermune, Inc.
3280 Bayshore Blvd.
Brisbane, CA 94005
Fax: (415)466-2300
Email: ir@intermune.com
Website: http://www.intermune.com
Scott Harkonen, CEO & Pres
Desc: Biotechnology company offering Rx/ethical pharmaceuticals.

★ 15754 ★ International Biomedical, Inc.
8508 Cross Park Dr.
Austin, TX 78754-4557
Phone: (512)873-0033 **Free:** 800-433-5615
Fax: (512)873-9090
Website: http://www.int-bio.com
A. J. Segars, Contact
Desc: Manufacturer of home healthcare; hospital equipment and supplies; sleep diagnostics/therapeutics; surgical instruments; transport incubators; veterinary products.

★ 15755 ★ International Medication Systems, Ltd.
Division of Amphastar
1886 Santa Anita Ave.
South El Monte, CA 91733
Phone: (626)442-6757 **Free:** 800-423-4136
Fax: (626)579-2025
Email: info@ims-limited.com
Website: http://www.ims-limited.com
Jack Zhang, PhD, CEO & Pres
Desc: Manufacturer of Rx/ethical pharmaceuticals; generic pharmaceuticals; anesthesia equipment and products; contract manufacturing; EMS equipment and supplies; home healthcare; hospital equipment and supplies; surgical instruments; urinary equipment.

★ 15756 ★ Interneuron Pharmaceuticals, Inc.
99 Hayden Ave.
Ste. 200
Lexington, MA 02421
Phone: (781)861-8444 **Fax:** (781)861-3830
Email: bizdev@interneuron.com
Website: http://www.interneuron.com
Glenn L. Cooper, MD, Contact
Desc: Biotechnology company: Rx/ethical pharmaceuticals.

★ 15757 ★ Interpharm, Inc.
75 Adams Ave.
Hauppauge, NY 11788-3605
Phone: (631)952-0214 **Fax:** (631)952-9587
Email: mail@interpharmic.com
Website: http://www.interpharmic.com
Manu Sutaria, Chairman of the Board
Desc: Manufacturer of Rx/ethical pharmaceuticals; OTC/proprietary pharmaceuticals; generic pharmaceuticals.

★ 15758 ★ Invacare Corp.
1 Invacare Way
Elyria, OH 44035
Phone: (440)329-6000 **Free:** 800-333-6900
Fax: (440)329-6568
Email: info@invacare.com
Website: http://www.invacare.com
A. Malachi Mixon, III, CEO & Chm Bd
Desc: Manufacturer/distributor of home healthcare; hospital equipment and supplies; hospital furniture; patient aid products; patient monitoring equipment; physical therapy and rehabilitation equipment and supplies; respiratory therapy and/or cardiopulmonary equipment; sleep diagnostics/ therapeutics.

★ 15759 ★ Invacare Corp.
Invacare Retail Group
39400 Taylor Pkwy.
North Ridgeville, OH 44039
Phone: 800-343-6059 **Free:** 888-628-7672
Fax: (440)329-6270
Email: info@invacare.com
Website: http://invacare.com
Brig Carr, Contact
Desc: Manufacturer/distributor/biotechnology company: biotechnology/biopharmaceutical products; laboratory equipment and supplies.

★ 15760 ★ Invitrogen Corp.
1600 Farady Ave.
Carlsbad, CA 92008
Phone: (760)603-7200 **Free:** 800-955-6288
Fax: (760)603-7201
Website: http://www.invitorgen.com
Lyle Turner, CEO
Desc: Manufacturer/distributor/biotechnology company: biotechnology/biopharmaceutical products; laboratory equipment and supplies.

★ 15761 ★ Ipsen, Inc.
27 Maple St.
Milford, MA 01757
Phone: (508)478-8900 **Free:** 800-456-7322
Fax: (508)478-1883
Email: stephen.murdock@ipseninc.com
Stephen C. Murdock, Contact
Desc: Manufacturer/distributor of Rx/ethical pharmaceuticals.

★ 15762 ★ Isomedix Services
A STERIS Corp. Co.
5960 Heisley Rd.
Mentor, OH 44060-1834
Phone: (440)354-2600 **Free:** 800-548-4873
Fax: (440)639-4450
Website: http://www.steris.com
Desc: Manufacturer: contract sterilization services; sterilization services.

★ 15763 ★ ITC
Wholly owned subsidiary of Thoratec Corp.
8 Olsen Ave.
Edison, NJ 08820
Phone: (732)548-5700 **Free:** 800-631-5945
Fax: (732)548-8632
Website: http://www.itcmed.com
Larry Cohen, President
Desc: Manufacturer of Rx/ethical pharmaceuticals; cardiovascular equipment and supplies; diagnostic reagents and test kits; disposable medical devices and supplies; home healthcare; laboratory supplies; patient monitoring equipment; physicians' equipment; radiopharmaceuticals; renal dialysis supplies.

★ 15764 ★ IVAX Laboratories, Inc.
Formerly Wakefield Pharmaceuticals, Inc.
Division of IVAX Corp.
4400 Biscayne Blvd.
9th floor N
Miami, FL 33137
Phone: (305)575-6000 **Fax:** (305)575-6221
Email: david_bailey@ivax.com
Website: http://www.ivax.com
Frank E. Byington, President
Desc: Manufacturer/distributor of Rx/ethical pharmaceuticals.

★ 15765 ★ Ivax Pharmaceuticals, Inc.
Division of IVAX Corp.
4400 Biscayne Blvd.
Miami, FL 33137
Phone: (305)575-4100 **Free:** 800-327-4114
Fax: (305)575-4211
Website: http://www.ivaxpharmaceuticals.com
Phillip Frost, MD, CEO & Chm Bd
Desc: Manufacturer/distributor of Rx/ethical pharmaceuticals; OTC/proprietary pharmaceuticals; generic pharmaceuticals.

★ 15766 ★ Ivek Corp.
10 Fairbanks Rd.
North Springfield, VT 05150
Phone: (802)886-2238 **Free:** 800-356-4746
Fax: (802)886-8274
Email: ivek@ivek.com
Website: http://www.ivek.com
Mark N. Tanny, President
Desc: Manufacturer of diagnostic equipment and instruments; dispensing and metering equipment; laboratory equipment; pharmaceutical manufacturing supplies and equipment.

★ 15767 ★ J.H. Emerson Co.
22 Cottage Park Ave.
Cambridge, MA 02140
Phone: (617)864-1414 **Free:** 800-252-1414
Fax: (617)868-0841
Email: info@jhemerson.com
Website: http://www.jhemerson.com
George Emerson, President
Desc: Manufacturer of home healthcare; hospital equipment and supplies; physical therapy and rehabilitation equipment and supplies; respiratory therapy and/or cardiopulmonary equipment and supplies; sterilization supplies; disposable medical devices and supplies.

★ 15768 ★ J.R. Carlson Laboratories, Inc.
15 W College Ave.
Arlington Heights, IL 60004
Phone: (847)255-1600 **Free:** 800-323-4141
Fax: (847)255-1605
Email: carlson@carlsonlabs.com
Website: http://www.carlsonlabs.com
John R. Carlson, President
Desc: Manufacturer of dietary, nutritional and vitamin supplements.

★ 15769 ★ J.T. Posey Co.
5635 Peck Rd.
Arcadia, CA 91006
Phone: (626)443-3143 **Free:** 800-44-POSEY
Fax: (626)443-5014
Website: http://www.posey.com
Leanne Heriot, Contact
Desc: Manufacturer of orthopedic and prosthetic equipment and supplies; patient aid products; patient monitoring equipment; physical therapy and rehabilitation equipment and supplies; respiratory therapy and/ or cardiopulmonary equipment and supplies; skin/ wound care products.

★ 15770 ★ Janssen Pharmaceutica, Inc.
Division of Johnson & Johnson
1125 Trenton-Harbourton Rd.
PO Box 200
Titusville, NJ 08560-0200
Phone: (609)730-2000 **Fax:** (609)730-2616
Website: http://www.janssen.com
Alex Gorsky, President
Desc: Manufacturer of Rx/ethical pharmaceuticals.

★ 15771 ★ Jarit Surgical Instruments
9 Skyline Dr.
Hawthorne, NY 10532
Phone: (914)592-9050 **Free:** 800-431-1123
Fax: (914)592-8056
Email: info@jarit.com
Website: http://www.jarit.com
Howard Jamner, President
Desc: Surgical instruments distributor.

★ 15772 ★ Jason Pharmaceuticals Inc.
11445 Cronhill Dr.
Owings Mills, MD 21117
Phone: (410)581-8042 **Free:** 800-638-7867
Fax: (410)581-8070
Email: info@medifastdiet.com
Website: http://www.medifastdiet.com
Bradley T. MacDonald, CEO & Chm Bd
Desc: Manufacturer/distributor of Rx/ethical pharmaceuticals; dietary, nutritional and vitamin supplements.

★ 15773 ★ JCL Clinical Research
5433 Straw Plains Pike
Knoxville, TN 37914
Phone: (865)546-0654 **Fax:** (865)971-1969
Tommye A. Jordan, Contact
Desc: Manufacturer/distributor of diagnostic reagents and test kits.

★ 15774 ★ Jobri.LLC dba MorLoc, Accu-Back, BetterBody
615 W 33rd
Ada, OK 74820
Phone: (580)310-0079 **Free:** 800-432-2225
Fax: (580)310-0787
Email: support@jobri.com
Website: http://www.jobri.com
Jonathan Hulme, CEO
Desc: Manufacturer of home healthcare; hospital equipment and supplies; orthopedic and prosthetic equipment and supplies; physical therapy and rehabilitation equipment and supplies.

★ 15775 ★ Jodee Inc.
3100 N 29th Ave.
Hollywood, FL 33020
Phone: (954)926-1900 **Free:** 800-865-6333
Fax: (954)926-1926
Email: jod1006@aol.com
Steven Altman, CEO & Pres
Desc: Manufacturer/distributor of breast form prosthetics; mastectomy brassieres.

★ 15776 ★ John O. Butler Co.
4635 W Foster Ave.
Chicago, IL 60630
Phone: (773)777-4000 **Fax:** (773)777-5101
Website: http://www.jbutler.com
Michael G. Bava, President
Desc: Manufacturer of dental supplies; home healthcare.

★ 15777 ★ Johnson & Johnson Merck Consumer Pharmaceuticals Co.
Camp Hill Rd.
Fort Washington, PA 19034
Phone: (215)273-7700 **Fax:** (215)233-3307
Website: http://www.jnj-merck.com
Peter K. Miller, President
Desc: Manufacturer of OTC/proprietary pharmaceuticals.

★ 15778 ★ Jones Medical Instrument Co.
200 Windsor Dr.
Oak Brook, IL 60523
Phone: (630)571-1980 **Free:** 800-323-7336
Fax: (630)571-2023
Email: jonesmed1@aol.com
Website: http://www.jonesmedical.com
William Jones, Jr., Contact
Desc: Manufacturer of hospital equipment and supplies; physicians' equipment; respiratory therapy and/or cardiopulmonary equipment.

★ 15779 ★ Karl Storz Endoscopy-America, Inc.
600 Corporate Pointe
Culver City, CA 90230-7600
Phone: (310)338-8100 **Free:** 800-421-0837
Fax: (310)410-5527
Email: cwilhelm@ksea.com
Website: http://www.karlstorz.com
Charles Wilhelm, Contact
Desc: Manufacturer/distributor of anesthesia equipment and products; hospital equipment and supplies; orthopedic and prosthetic equipment and supplies; physicians' equipment and supplies; surgical disposables and instruments.

★ 15780 ★ Katena Products Inc.
4 Stewart Ct.
Denville, NJ 07834
Phone: (973)989-1600 **Free:** 800-225-1195
Fax: (973)989-8175
Email: globe@katena.com
Website: http://www.katena.com
Kate Tiedemann, President
Desc: Manufacturer/distributor of ophthalmic equipment and supplies; surgical disposables and instruments.

★ 15781 ★ Kay Elemetrics Corp.
2 Bridgewater Lane
Lincoln Park, NJ 07035-1488
Phone: (973)628-6200 **Free:** 800-289-5297
Fax: (973)628-6363
Email: sales@kayelemetrics.com
Website: http://www.kayelemetrics.com
John M. Crump, Contact
Desc: Manufacturer/biotechnology company: biotechnology/biopharmaceutical products; diagnostic equipment and instruments.

★ 15782 ★ KCI
8023 Vantage Dr.
San Antonio, TX 78230
Phone: (210)524-9000 **Free:** 800-531-5396
Fax: (210)255-6987
Website: http://www.kci1.com
Robert Jainich, Chairman of the Board
Desc: Manufacturer/distributor of disposable medical devices and supplies; home healthcare; hospital furniture; hospital specialty beds; nuclear and radiological supplies; patient aid products; respiratory therapy and/or cardiopulmonary equipment; skin/wound care products.

★ 15783 ★ Keeler Instruments Inc.
456 Parkway
Broomall, PA 19008
Phone: (610)353-4350 **Free:** 800-523-5620
Fax: (610)353-7814
Email: keeler@keelerusa.com
Website: http://www.keelerusa.com
David J. Keeler, President
Desc: Manufacturer/distributor of cardiovascular instruments; dental instruments; diagnostic equipment and instruments; hospital equipment and supplies; hospital furniture; ophthalmic instruments; orthopedic and prosthetic equipment and supplies; patient aid products; physicians' equipment and supplies; surgical disposables and instruments.

★ 15784 ★ KEM Kyoto Electronics Mfg.
2810 Old Lee Highway
Fairfax, VA 22031
Phone: (703)876-4030 **Free:** 800-458-2558
Fax: (703)280-5142
Email: kem@cscscientific.com
Website: http://www.kyoto-kem.com
Nob Yamanaka, Contact
Desc: Manufacturer of laboratory equipment.

★ 15785 ★ Kendall-LTP
2 Ludlow Park Dr.
Chicopee, MA 01022
Phone: (413)593-6400 **Free:** 800-669-1009
Fax: (413)593-6114
Website: http://www.kendall-ltp.com
Lee A. Carrier, President
Desc: Manufacturer of cardiovascular supplies; chart paper; disposable medical devices and supplies; EMS equipment and supplies; home healthcare; hospital equipment and supplies; laboratory supplies; obstetric and neonatal products; protection and safety products; radiology products; skin/wound care products; surgical disposables and supplies; ultrasound and electromedical equipment and supplies.

★ 15786 ★ The Kendrick Co., Inc.
6139 Germantown Ave.
Philadelphia, PA 19144
Phone: (215)438-1122 **Free:** 800-523-0178
Fax: (215)438-8065
Lesley DeVine, President
Desc: Manufacturer/distributor of belts; trusses and stockings; surgical supplies.

★ 15787 ★ Kent Elastomer Products, Inc.
1500 St. Clair Ave.
Kent, OH 44240
Phone: (330)673-1011 **Free:** 800-331-4762
Fax: (330)673-1351
Email: info@kentelastomer.com
Website: http://www.kentelastomer.com
Cindy Harry, Contact
Desc: Manufacturer of anesthesia equipment and products; dip molded components; disposable medical devices and supplies; surgical disposables; laboratory supplies; physical therapy and rehabilitation equipment and supplies; physicians' supplies; tubing.

★ 15788 ★ Kent Laboratories Inc.
777 Jorgensen Place
Bellingham, WA 98226
Phone: (360)398-8641 **Fax:** (360)954-6333
Email: kent@kentlabs.com
Website: http://www.kentlabs.com
Allan H. Jorgensen, Chairman of the Board
Desc: Manufacturer/biotechnology company: biotechnology/biopharmaceutical products; diagnostic equipment and instruments; diagnostic reagents and test kits; veterinary products.

★ 15789 ★ Kenwood Therapeutics Division of Bradley Pharmaceuticals, Inc.
383 Rte. 46 West
Fairfield, NJ 07004-2402
Phone: (973)882-1505 **Free:** 800-929-9300
Fax: (973)575-5366
Email: bradpharm@bradpharm.com
Website: http://www.bradpharm.com
Daniel Glassman, CEO & Chm Bd
Desc: Manufacturer/distributor of Rx/ethical pharmaceuticals; OTC/proprietary pharmaceuticals.

★ 15790 ★ Kewaunee Scientific Corp.
2700 W Front St.
Statesville, NC 28677
Phone: (704)873-7202 **Fax:** 800-932-3296
Email: marketing@kewaunee.com
Website: http://www.kewaunee.com
William A. Shumaker, CEO
Desc: Manufacturer of hospital furniture; laboratory equipment.

★ 15791 ★ Key Pharmaceuticals, Inc. Division of Schering-Plough Corp.
2000 Galloping Hill Rd.
Kenilworth, NJ 07033
Phone: (908)298-4000 **Fax:** (908)298-5661
Website: http://www.schering-plough.com
Richard J. Kogan, CEO & Chm Bd
Desc: Manufacturer/distributor of Rx/ethical pharmaceuticals.

★ 15792 ★ Kimble Glass, Inc.
1101 Laurel Oak Rd.
Ste. 100
Voorhees, NJ 08043
Phone: (856)782-6420 **Fax:** (856)309-9480
Website: http://www.kimble-kontes.com
Uwe Roehrhoff, CEO & Pres
Desc: Manufacturer of laboratory supplies; parenteral supplies; primary pharmaceutical packaging.

★ 15793 ★ King Pharmaceuticals, Inc.
501 Fifth St.
Bristol, TN 37620
Phone: (423)989-8000 **Free:** 800-336-7783
Website: http://www.kingpharm.com
John M. Gregory, Chairman of the Board
Desc: Manufacturer/distributor of Rx/ethical pharmaceuticals; OTC/proprietary pharmaceuticals; animal health products; skin/wound care products.

★ 15794 ★ Kingswood Laboratories, Inc.
10375 Hague Rd.
Indianapolis, IN 46256
Phone: (317)849-9513 **Free:** 800-968-7772
Fax: (317)849-4263
Email: sales@kingswood-labs.com
Website: http://www.kingswood-labs.com
Ross Deardorff, President
Desc: Distributor of OTC/proprietary pharmaceuticals; dental supplies; disposable medical devices and supplies; home healthcare; hospital equipment and supplies.

★ 15795 ★ Kipp & Zonen
125 Wilbur Pl.
Bohemia, NY 11716
Phone: (631)589-2065 **Free:** 800-645-1025
Fax: (631)589-2068
Email: kippzonen@usa.com
Website: http://www.kippzonen.com
Desc: Manufacturer/distributor of laboratory equipment.

★ 15796 ★ Kleen Test Products Division of Meridian Industries, Inc.
8225 W Parkland Ct.
Milwaukee, WI 53223
Phone: (414)357-7444 **Free:** 800-558-6842
Fax: (414)357-6355
Website: http://www.kleentest.com
Patrick J. Trottier, Contact
Desc: Manufacturer of OTC/proprietary pharmaceuticals; contract manufacturing; disposable medical devices and supplies; home healthcare; patient aid products; physicians' supplies; skin/wound care products; surgical disposables and supplies.

★ 15797 ★ KLI Corp.
1119 Third Ave., SW
Carmel, IN 46032
Phone: (317)846-7452 **Free:** 800-308-7452
Fax: (317)846-1676
Email: estr@inetdirect.net
Website: http://www.entertainers-secret.com
Gordon L. Schmitz, President
Desc: Distributor of OTC/proprietary pharmaceuticals; throat spray.

★ 15798 ★ KMC Systems, Inc. Subsidiary of Kollsman, Inc.
220 Daniel Webster Hwy.
Merrimack, NH 03054
Phone: (603)889-2500 **Fax:** (603)594-7022
Email: wgilde@kollsman.com
Website: http://www.kmcsystems.com
Walter Gilde, Contact
Desc: Manufacturer: contract manufacturing; diagnostic equipment and instruments; laboratory equipment; patient monitoring equipment; respiratory therapy and/or cardiopulmonary equipment.

★ 15799 ★ Komet Medical Division of Brasseler USA
1 Brasseler Blvd.
Savannah, GA 31419
Phone: (912)925-8525 **Free:** 800-535-6638
Fax: (912)921-7578
Website: http://www.kometmedical.com
Don Waters, CEO & Chm Bd
Desc: Manufacturer/distributor of dental supplies; hospital equipment and supplies.

★ 15800 ★ Konica Medical Imaging Division of Konica Corp.
411 Newark Pompton Turnpike
Wayne, NJ 07470
Phone: (973)633-1500 **Fax:** (973)633-5405
Email: corporate@konicamedical.com
Website: http://www.konicamedical.com
Wayne Thompson, Contact
Desc: Manufacturer/distributor of hospital equipment and supplies; medical imaging film and equipment.

★ 15801 ★ Konsyl Pharmaceuticals, Inc.
4200 S Hulen St., No. 513
Fort Worth, TX 76109
Phone: (817)763-8011 **Free:** 800-356-6795
Fax: (817)731-9389
Email: konsyl@flash.net
Website: http://www.konsyl.com
Frank X. Buhler, President
Desc: Manufacturer of OTC/proprietary pharmaceuticals; diagnostic equipment and instruments.

★ 15802 ★ KRKA, d.d. Novo mesto Representative Office, New York
12 E 52nd St.' 6th floor
New York, NY 10022
Phone: (212)838-1090 **Fax:** (212)838-0932
Website: http://www.krka.si/en
Barbara Bulc, Contact
Desc: Manufacturer/biotechnology company: Rx/ethical pharmaceuticals; OTC/proprietary pharmaceuticals; generic pharmaceuticals; biotechnology/biopharmaceutical products.

★ 15803 ★ Kuntz Mfg. Co., Inc. Automation Engineering Division
2614 S Rousselle St.
Santa Ana, CA 92707
Phone: (714)540-7370 **Fax:** (714)540-6287
Email: mail@kuntzautomation.com
Website: http://www.kuntzautomation.com
Axel M. Kuntz, Contact
Desc: Manufacturer of cardiovascular equipment and supplies; dental equipment and supplies; diagnostic equipment and instruments; diagnostic reagents and test kits; disposable medical devices and supplies; ophthalmic equipment and supplies; pharmaceutical manufacturing supplies and equipment; special automated equipment; surgical disposables; X-ray equipment and supplies; laboratory equipment; custom mfg. Systems.

★ 15804 ★ KV Pharmaceutical Co.
2503 S Hanley Rd.
Saint Louis, MO 63144-2555
Phone: (314)645-6600 **Fax:** (314)991-4215
Website: http://kvpharma.com
Marc S. Hermelin, Contact
Desc: Manufacturer of Rx/ethical pharmaceuticals; OTC/proprietary pharmaceuticals; generic pharmaceuticals; dietary, nutritional and vitamin supplements.

★ 15805 ★ Labconco Corp.
8811 Prospect Ave.
Kansas City, MO 64132-2696
Phone: (816)333-8811 **Free:** 800-821-5525
Fax: (816)363-0130
Email: labconco@labconco.com
Website: http://www.labconco.com
John N. McConnell, Chairman of the Board
Desc: Manufacturer of biological and environmental safety products; laboratory equipment.

★ 15806 ★ Ladd Research Industries Division of RAJ Communications, Ltd.
83 Holly Ct.
Williston, VT 05495
Phone: (802)658-4961 **Free:** 800-451-3406
Fax: (802)660-8859
Email: sales@laddresearch.com
Website: http://www.laddresearch.com
J.D. Arnott, President
Desc: Manufacturer/distributor of laboratory equipment and supplies.

★ 15807 ★ Laerdal Medical Corp.
167 Myers Corners Rd.
PO Box 1840
Wappingers Falls, NY 12590
Phone: (845)297-7770 **Free:** 800-431-1055
Fax: 800-227-1143
Email: customerservice@laerdal.com
Website: http://www.laerdal.com
Terje Aasen, CEO & Pres
Desc: Manufacturer/distributor of EMS equipment and supplies; hospital equipment and supplies; respiratory therapy and/or cardiopulmonary equipment and supplies.

★ 15808 ★ Lafayette Instrument Co.
PO Box 5729
Lafayette, IN 47903-5729
Phone: (765)423-1505 **Free:** 800-428-7545
Fax: (765)423-4111
Email: rehab@lafayetteinstrument.com
Website: http://www.lafayetteinstrument.com
Roger McClellan, President
Desc: Manufacturer of cardiovascular equipment; laboratory equipment; physical therapy and rehabilitation equipment and supplies; physicians' equipment.

★ 15809 ★ Lake City Medical Products
7745 Chillicothe Rd.
Mentor, OH 44060-7711
Phone: (440)974-0043 **Free:** 800-497-9874
Fax: (440)255-7955
Email: rcrakes@yahoo.com
Ken Rakes, Contact
Desc: Manufacturer/distributor of radiopharmaceuticals; renal dialysis supplies.

★ 15810 ★ Lake Consumer Products, Inc.
730 Corporate Woods Pkwy.
Vernon Hills, IL 60061
Phone: (847)793-0230 **Free:** 800-635-3696
Fax: (847)793-0247
Email: info@lakeconsumer.com
Website: http://www.lakeconsumer.com
Gary Burns, CEO & Pres
Desc: Manufacturer/distributor of OTC/proprietary pharmaceuticals; dietary, nutritional and vitamin supplements; feminine hygiene; skin/wound care products.

★ 15811 ★ Laminaire Corp.
960 E Hazelwood Ave.
Rahway, NJ 07065
Phone: (732)381-8200 **Free:** (866)381-8200
Fax: (732)381-4091
Email: laminaire@att.net
Website: http://www.laminaire.com
Antonio Garay, President
Desc: Manufacturer of biotechnology/biopharmaceutical products; clean room equipment; disposable clean packaging; laboratory equipment; ultrasonic equipment.

★ 15812 ★ Lannett Co., Inc.
9000 State Rd.
Philadelphia, PA 19136
Phone: (215)333-9000 **Free:** 800-325-9994
Fax: (215)333-9004
Email: info@lannett.com

Website: http://www.lannett.com
William Farber, Chairman of the Board
Desc: Manufacturer of Rx/ethical pharmaceuticals; OTC/proprietary pharmaceuticals; generic pharmaceuticals.

★ 15813 ★ Lansinoh Laboratories, Inc.
333 N Fairfax St.
Ste. 400
Alexandria, VA 22314
Phone: (703)299-1100 **Free:** 800-292-4794
Fax: (703)299-6201
Email: customerservice@lansinoh.com
Website: http://www.lansinoh.com
Resheda Hagen, CEO
Desc: Manufacturer of OTC/proprietary pharmaceuticals.

★ 15814 ★ The Larkotex Co.
1002 Olive St.
Texarkana, TX 75501
Phone: (903)793-4647 **Fax:** (903)793-4650
Email: info@larkotex.com
Website: http://www.larkotex.com
Fred R. Norton, Sr., Contact
Desc: Manufacturer: contract manufacturing; disposable medical devices and supplies; home healthcare; hospital equipment and supplies; orthopedic and prosthetic equipment and supplies; patient aid products; physical therapy and rehabilitation equipment and supplies.

★ 15815 ★ Laser, Inc.
2200 W 97th Pl.
PO Box 905
Crown Point, IN 46307
Phone: (219)663-1165 **Fax:** (219)663-1330
Email: laser-inc@mindspring.com
J.N. Allegretti, RPh, President
Desc: Distributor of Rx/ethical pharmaceuticals.

★ 15816 ★ Leedal Inc.
4025 S Western Blvd.
Chicago, IL 60609
Phone: (773)376-5900 **Fax:** (773)376-7844
Email: sink@leedal.com
Website: http://www.leedal.com
S. Levin, President
Desc: Manufacturer of dental equipment; laboratory equipment; X-ray equipment.

★ 15817 ★ Legend Health Systems, Inc. d/b/a Legend Pharmacies
1111 Rte. 110
Ste. 355
East Farmingdale, NY 11735
Phone: (631)630-4713 **Fax:** (631)630-4719
Email: headquaters@legendpharmacies.com
Website: http://www.legendpharmacies.com
John R. Marmero, CEO & Pres
Desc: Distributor of OTC/proprietary pharmaceuticals; patient aid products.

★ 15818 ★ Legere Pharmaceuticals Division of Preventics Inc.
7326 E Evans Rd.
Scottsdale, AZ 85260
Phone: (480)991-4033 **Free:** 800-528-3144
Fax: (480)483-0792
Email: legerephar@aol.com
Website: http://www.preventics.com
R. J. Legere, President
Desc: Manufacturer/distributor of Rx/ethical pharmaceuticals; OTC/proprietary pharmaceuticals; dietary, nutritional and vitamin supplements; parenteral supplies.

★ 15819 ★ Leica Microsystems Inc.
2345 Waukegan Rd.
Bannockburn, IL 60015
Phone: (847)405-0123 **Free:** 800-248-0123
Fax: (847)405-0164
Email: info@leica-microsystems.com
Website: http://www.leica-microsystems.com
Dr. Robert Wick, Contact
Desc: Manufacturer/distributor/biotechnology company: biotechnology/biopharmaceutical products; diagnostic equipment and instruments; hospital equipment and supplies; laboratory equipment; ophthalmic equipment and supplies; slide viewing systems; surgical instruments.

★ 15820 ★ LeMare Medical, Inc.
2829 Bird Ave.
Ste. 5, PMB No. 305
Miami, FL 33133
Phone: (305)775-9170 **Fax:** (305)594-5993
Email: lemaremed@aol.com
Julio E. Estay, Chairman of the Board
Desc: Distributor of cardiovascular supplies; diagnostic equipment and instruments; hospital equipment and supplies; surgical instruments; U.S.P. reference standards; urinary equipment and supplies; sterilization supplies.

★ 15821 ★ Level 1, Inc. Subsidiary of Smiths Group, plc
160 Weymouth St.
Rockland, MA 02370
Phone: (781)878-8011 **Free:** 800-553-8351
Fax: (781)878-8201
Email: info@smith-level1.com
Website: http://www.smiths-medical.com/mediweb
Bob James, Contact
Desc: Manufacturer/distributor of anesthesia equipment and products; disposable medical devices and supplies; hospital equipment and supplies; surgical supplies.

★ 15822 ★ LIFE Corp. OxygenPac Division
1776 N Water St.
Milwaukee, WI 53202
Phone: (414)272-4000 **Free:** 800-700-0202
Fax: (414)272-0000
Email: email@lifecorporation.com
Website: http://www.lifecorporation.com
John Kirchgeorg, President
Desc: Manufacturer of OTC/proprietary pharmaceuticals; biological and environmental safety products; cardiovascular equipment; EMS equipment and supplies; respiratory therapy and/or cardiopulmonary equipment.

★ 15823 ★ Lifemed of California
1216 S Allec St.
Anaheim, CA 92805-6301
Phone: (714)517-6900 **Free:** 800-LIF-EMED
Fax: (714)517-6911
Email: info@lifemedofcalifornia.com
Website: http://www.lifemedinc.com
Tom Hamon, CEO & Pres
Desc: Manufacturer/distributor: contract manufacturing; disposable medical devices and supplies; implants and infusion; renal dialysis suppliesand equipment.

★ 15824 ★ LifeScan, Inc. Division of Johnson & Johnson, Inc.
1000 Gibraltar Dr.
Milpitas, CA 95035
Phone: (408)263-9789 **Free:** 800-227-8862
Fax: (408)946-6070
Email: lifescan@lfsus.jnj.com
Website: http://www.lifescan.com
Eric Milledge, Contact
Desc: Manufacturer of diagnostic reagents and test kits; patient monitoring equipment.

★ 15825 ★ LifeSign LLC
PO Box 218
Somerset, NJ 08873
Phone: (732)246-3366 **Free:** 800-526-2125
Fax: (732)246-0570
Email: larry@lifesignmed.com
Website: http://www.lifesignmed.com
Larry Porter, President
Desc: Distributor of diagnostic reagents and test kits.

★ 15826 ★ Ligand Pharmaceuticals Inc.
10275 Science Center Dr.
San Diego, CA 92121
Phone: (858)550-7500 **Fax:** (858)550-7707
Email: investors@ligand.com
Website: http://www.ligand.com
David E. Robinson, Contact
Desc: Manufacturer/biotechnology company: Rx/ethical pharmaceuticals; biotechnology/biopharmaceutical products.

★ 15827 ★ Linvatec Corp. Division of ConMed Corp.
11311 Concept Blvd.
Largo, FL 33773
Phone: (727)392-6464 **Free:** 800-325-5900
Fax: (727)399-5290
Email: marketing@linvatec.com
Website: http://www.linvatec.com
Gerald Woodard, President
Desc: Manufacturer/distributor of disposable medical devices and supplies; hospital equipment and supplies; implants and infusion; orthopedic and prosthetic equipment and supplies; physicians' equipment; surgical disposables, instruments and supplies.

★ 15828 ★ Lionville Systems Inc.
311 Commerce Dr.
Exton, PA 19341
Phone: (610)363-9100 **Free:** 800-523-7114
Fax: (610)524-7934
Email: lionville@lionville.com
Website: http://www.lionville.com
E. Ford Williams, President
Desc: Manufacturer of hospital equipment and supplies.

★ 15829 ★ Lixi, Inc.
1438 Brook Dr.
Downers Grove, IL 60515
Phone: (630)620-4646 **Fax:** (630)620-7776
Email: lixi@lixi.com
Website: http://www.lixi.com
Brent Burns, President
Desc: Manufacturer of nuclear and radiological equipment; veterinary test equipment; X-ray equipment.

★ 15830 ★ LM Air Technology, Inc.
1467 Pinewood St.
Rahway, NJ 07065
Phone: (732)381-8200 **Fax:** (732)381-4091
Email: lmair@att.net
Website: http://www.lmairtech.com
Peter Daniele, President
Desc: Manufacturer of clean room equipment; laboratory equipment; pharmaceutical manufacturing supplies and equipment.

★ 15831 ★ Lofstrand Cane & Crutch Co. Division of Harvey Surgical Supply Co.
34-35 Collins Pl.
Flushing, NY 11354-2790
Phone: (718)939-1122 **Free:** 800-221-0142
Fax: (718)939-1222
Desc: Manufacturer/distributor of home healthcare; hospital equipment and supplies; patient aid products; surgical supplies.

★ 15832 ★ Lorad
A Hologic Co.
36 Apple Ridge Rd.
Danbury, CT 06810
Phone: (203)790-1188 **Fax:** (203)207-4501
Email: information@loradmedical.com
Website: http://www.loradmedical.com
John Cumming, CEO & Pres
Desc: Manufacturer/distributor of diagnostic equipment and instruments; nuclear and radiological equipment; patient monitoring equipment.

★ 15833 ★ Lossing Orthopedic
3230 Snelling Ave. S
PO Box 6224
Minneapolis, MN 55406
Phone: (612)724-2669 **Free:** 800-328-5216
Fax: (612)724-5089
Email: lossingortho@qwest.net
Website: http://www.lossingorthopedic.com
Gary Lossing, President
Desc: Manufacturer of physical therapy and rehabilitation equipment and supplies.

★ 15834 ★ Lumenis, Inc.
2400 Condensa St.
Santa Clara, CA 95051
Phone: (408)764-3000 **Free:** 800-635-1313
Fax: (408)764-3999
Email: information@lumenis.com
Website: http://www.lumenis.com
Jacob A. Frenkel, PhD, Chairman of the Board
Desc: Manufacturer/distributor of aesthetic equipment; dental equipment; ophthalmic equipment; surgical disposables and instruments; veterinary products.

★ 15835 ★ The Lumiscope Co., Inc.
122 Tices Lane
East Brunswick, NJ 08816
Phone: (732)254-3800 **Free:** 800-221-5474
Fax: (732)254-3401
Email: info@lumiscope.net
Website: http://www.lumiscope.net
Allen J. Beeber, CEO
Desc: Manufacturer/distributor of apparel; dental equipment; diagnostic equipment and instruments; home healthcare; hospital equipment and supplies; orthopedic and prosthetic equipment and supplies; patient aid products; respiratory therapy and/or cardiopulmonary equipment and supplies.

★ 15836 ★ Lunaire Environmental, Tenney Environmental, Gruenberg Oven Divisions of Lunaire Ltd.
2121 Reach Rd.
Williamsport, PA 17701
Phone: (570)326-1770 **Free:** 800-LUN-AIRE
Fax: (570)236-7304
Email: marketing@lunaire.com
Website: http://www.lunaire.com
Mike Grausam, President
Desc: Manufacturer/biotechnology company: biotechnology/biopharmaceutical products; laboratory equipment; pharmaceutical manufacturing supplies and equipment; sterilization equipment.

★ 15837 ★ M.J. Markell Shoe Co., Inc.
504 Saw Mill River Rd.
PO Box 246, Main Station
Yonkers, NY 10702-0246
Phone: (914)963-2258 **Fax:** (914)963-9293
Website: http://www.markellshoe.com
Richard A. Markell, President
Desc: Manufacturer/distributor of adult accommodative footwear; apparel; children's corrective footwear; contract manufacturing; home healthcare; hospital equipment and supplies; orthopedic and prosthetic equipment and supplies; patient aid products; physical therapy and rehabilitation equipment and supplies; physicians' equipment and supplies; skin/wound care products.

★ 15838 ★ Mada Medical Products Inc.
625 Washington Ave.
Carlstadt, NJ 07072
Phone: (201)460-0454 **Free:** 800-526-6370
Fax: (201)460-3509
Website: http://www.madainternational.com
Ralph A. Adam, PhD, President
Desc: Manufacturer/distributor of dental equipment; disposable medical devices and supplies; EMS equipment and supplies; home healthcare; hospital equipment and supplies; patient aid products; respiratory therapy and/or cardiopulmonary equipment and supplies; surgical supplies.

★ 15839 ★ Maddak, Inc.
Division of Bel-Art Products
6 Industrial Rd.
Pequannock, NJ 07440-1993
Phone: (973)628-7600 **Free:** 800-443-4926
Fax: (973)305-0841
Email: custservice@maddak.com
Website: http://www.maddak.com
Kurt Landsberger, Chairman of the Board
Desc: Manufacturer of home healthcare; hospital equipment and supplies; laboratory equipment; ostomy equipment and supplies; patient aid products; physical therapy and rehabilitation equipment and supplies.

★ 15840 ★ Maersk Medical
6001 S 35th St.
McAllen, TX 78503
Phone: (956)683-8472 **Free:** 800-634-6003
Fax: (956)683-8482
Email: usa@maersk-medical.com
Website: http://www.maersk-medical.com
Eric Nissen, President
Desc: Manufacturer of anesthesia equipment and products; disposable medical devices and supplies; EMS equipment and supplies.

★ 15841 ★ Mallinckrodt Inc.
Business Unit of Tyco Healthcare Imaging Division
675 McDonnell Blvd.
Saint Louis, MO 63140
Phone: (314)654-2000 **Free:** 888-744-1414
Fax: (314)654-3135
Email: customer.service-imaging@tycohealthcare.com
Website: http://www.imaging-mallinckrodt.com
Mark Thom, President
Desc: Manufacturer/distributor of cardiovascular equipment and supplies; diagnostic reagents and test kits; disposable medical devices and supplies; hospital equipment and supplies; implants and infusion; magnetic resonance imaging; nuclear and radiological supplies; parenteral equipment and supplies; pharmaceutical manufacturing supplies and equipment; physicians' equipment and supplies; radiopharmaceuticals; ultrasound and electromedical equipment and supplies; x-ray supplies. supplies; X-ray supplies.

★ 15842 ★ Mallinckrodt Inc.
Pharmaceutical Group
Dosage Products Division
675 McDonnell Blvd.
PO Box 5840
Saint Louis, MO 63134
Phone: (314)654-2000 **Free:** 800-325-8888
Fax: (314)654-8238
Email: dpharma@mkg.com
Website: http://www.mallinckrodt.com
Michael J. Collins, President
Desc: Manufacturer of Rx/ethical pharmaceuticals; generic pharmaceuticals; oral peptide delivery; specialty narcotics.

★ 15843 ★ Market Forge Industries Inc.
35 Garvey St.
Everett, MA 02149
Phone: (617)387-4100 **Fax:** 800-227-2659
Email: custserv@mfii.com
Website: http://www.mfii.com
Bob Stefka, President
Desc: Manufacturer of shelving; sterilization equipment.

★ 15844 ★ Marketing International, Inc.
PO Box 4835
Topeka, KS 66604-0835
Phone: (785)272-4773 **Free:** 800-447-0173
Fax: (785)272-4273
Email: mktgintl@inlandnet.net
Website: http://www.marketing-international.net
James H. Becker, President
Desc: Distributor of disposable medical devices and supplies; laboratory supplies.

★ 15845 ★ Markson Lab Sales
661 Rte. 23 S
Wayne, NJ 07470
Phone: (973)628-1535 **Free:** 800-528-5114
Fax: 800-858-2243
Email: custservice@markson.com
Website: http://www.markson.com
George Barnes, Contact
Desc: Distributor/biotechnology company: apparel; biological and environmental safety products; biotechnology/biopharmaceutical products; hospital equipment and supplies; laboratory equipment and supplies; slide viewing systems; sterilization equipment.

★ 15846 ★ Martec Pharmaceutical, Inc.
1800 N Topping
PO Box 33510
Kansas City, MO 64120-3510
Phone: (816)241-4144 **Free:** 800-822-6782
Fax: (816)483-5432
Email: officemrtc@aol.com
Website: http://www.martec-kc.com
Paul Sudhakar, CEO & Pres
Desc: Manufacturer/distributor of Rx/ethical pharmaceuticals; generic pharmaceuticals; contract manufacturing.

★ 15847 ★ Maxim Pharmaceuticals, Inc.
8899 University Center Ln.
Ste. 400
San Diego, CA 92122
Phone: (858)453-4040 **Fax:** (858)453-5005
Email: investorrelations@maxim.com
Website: http://www.maxim.com
Larry Stambaugh, Contact
Desc: Manufacturer/distributor of Rx/ethical pharmaceuticals.

★ 15848 ★ Maxxim Medical
PO Box 2425
Columbus, OH 39704
Phone: (614)327-8011 **Free:** 888-462-9822
Fax: (614)327-1881
Website: http://www.maximmedical.com
Gene Kirser, Contact
Desc: Manufacturer/distributor of ophthalmic supplies; surgical disposables.

★ 15849 ★ Mayer Laboratories, Inc.
646 Kennedy St., Bldg. C
Oakland, CA 94606
Phone: (510)437-8989 **Free:** 800-426-6366
Fax: (510)536-9912
Email: mayerlabs@aol.com
Website: http://www.mayerlabs.com
David Mayer, President
Desc: Manufacturer of condoms; latex and non-latex gloves; personal lubricants.

★ 15850 ★ McCarty's Sacro Ease, LLC
3329 Industrial Ave.
Coeur d'Alene, ID 83815
Phone: (208)765-8408 **Free:** 800-635-3557
Fax: (208)664-6891
Email: sacroease@aol.com
Website: http://www.mccartys.com
Kerry Standish, Contact
Desc: Manufacturer/distributor of home healthcare; hospital equipment and supplies.

★ 15851 ★ McNeil Consumer Healthcare Division of Johnson & Johnson
7050 Camp Hill Rd.
Fort Washington, PA 19034
Phone: (215)273-7000 **Fax:** (215)273-4193
Website: http://www.jnj.com
Brian D. Perkins, Contact
Desc: Manufacturer of OTC/proprietary pharmaceuticals.

★ 15852 ★ Mead Johnson Nutritionals A Bristol-Myers Squibb Co.
,
2400 W Lloyd Expressway
Evansville, IN 47721
Phone: (812)429-5000
Website: http://www.meadjohnson.com
Randall K. Alsman, President
Desc: Manufacturer/distributor of Rx/ethical pharmaceuticals; OTC/proprietary pharmaceuticals; dietary, nutritional and vitamin supplements.

★ 15853 ★ The Med-Design Corp.
2810 Bunsen Ave.
Ventura, CA 93003
Phone: (805)339-0375 **Fax:** (805)339-9751
Email: msimpson@med-design.com
Website: http://www.med-design.com
James M. Donegan, Contact
Desc: Manufacturer of cardiovascular supplies; dental supplies; disposable medical devices and supplies; home healthcare; hospital equipment and supplies; parenteral supplies; pharmaceutical manufacturing supplies and equipment; physicians' supplies; renal dialysis supplies; surgical supplies; anesthesia equipment and products.

★ 15854 ★ Med-E-Jet D
8092 Olmway Ave.
Olmsted Falls, OH 44138
Phone: (440)235-2279 **Free:** 800-231-4203
Fax: (440)235-2247
Donald J. Kuch, CEO
Desc: Manufacturer/distributor of hospital equipment and supplies; hypodermic jet injectors.

★ 15855 ★ Medcom Information Systems, Inc.
2117 Stonington Ave.
Hoffman Estates, IL 60195
Phone: (847)885-1553 **Free:** 800-213-2161
Fax: (847)885-1591
Email: medcom@emirj.com
Website: http://www.emirj
John M. Holub, President
Desc: Manufacturer/distributor of computerized patient records; laboratory equipment; laboratory information systems; physicians' equipment.

★ 15856 ★ Medex Medical
6250 Shier-Rings Rd.
Dublin, OH 43016-1295
Phone: (614)889-2220 **Free:** 800-848-1757
Fax: (614)889-2651
Website: http://www.medexmedical.com
Dominick Arena, President
Desc: Manufacturer of anesthesia equipment and products; cardiovascular supplies; disposable medical devices and supplies; home healthcare; hospital equipment and supplies; implants and infusion; parenteral catheters and supplies; patient monitoring equipment; surgical disposables.

★ 15857 ★ Medi Inc.
75 York Ave.
PO Box 302
Randolph, MA 02368
Phone: (781)961-1232 **Free:** 800-225-8634
Fax: (781)961-5750
W. J. McGilivray, CEO & Pres
Desc: Manufacturer/distributor of cardiovascular supplies; hospital equipment and supplies; laboratory supplies; parenteral catheters, equipment and supplies; patient aid products; physical therapy and rehabilitation equipment and supplies; physicians' supplies; respiratory therapy and/or cardiopulmonary supplies; urinary equipment.

★ 15858 ★ Medical Chemical Corp.
19430 Van Ness Ave.
Torrance, CA 90501
Phone: (310)787-6800 **Free:** 800-424-9394
Fax: (310)787-4464
Website: http://www.med-chem.com
Emmanuel R. Didier, CEO & Pres
Desc: Manufacturer/distributor of diagnostic reagents and test kits; hospital disinfectants and cold sterilants; parasitology kits and soaps; skin/wound care products.

★ 15859 ★ Medical Coaches Inc.
399 County Hwy. 58
PO Box 129
Oneonta, NY 13820
Phone: (607)432-1333 **Fax:** (607)432-8190
Website: http://www.medcoach.com
Geoffrey A. Smith, Contact
Desc: Manufacturer of dental equipment; home healthcare; hospital equipment and supplies; laboratory equipment; magnetic resonance imaging; mobile units; nuclear and radiological equipment; ophthalmic equipment; renal dialysis equipment; urinary supplies; veterinary products; X-ray equipment.

★ 15860 ★ Medical Illumination International
547 Library St.
San Fernando, CA 91340
Phone: (818)838-3025 **Free:** 800-831-1222
Fax: (818)838-3725
Email: medilum@ix.netcom.com
Website: http://medilum.com
William K. Schellenberg, President
Desc: Manufacturer of dental equipment, diagnostic equipment and instruments; hospital equipment and supplies; veterinary products.

★ 15861 ★ Medical Plastics Division of Allergan
2525 Pullman St.
Santa Ana, CA 92705
Phone: (714)246-4700 **Fax:** (714)246-6969
Email: timothy_lindsay@allergan.com
Website: http://www.allergan.com
Tim Lindsay, Contact
Desc: Manufacturer of molded plastic parts.

★ 15862 ★ Medicis Pharmaceutical Corp.
8125 N Hayden Rd.
Scottsdale, AZ 85258-2463
Phone: (602)808-8800 **Free:** 800-845-1313
Fax: (602)808-0822
Email: medicis@medicis.com
Website: http://www.medicis.com
Jonah Shacknai, CEO
Desc: Manufacturer/distributor of Rx/ethical pharmaceuticals; OTC/proprietary pharmaceuticals.

★ 15863 ★ MedImmune, Inc.
35 W Watkins Mill Rd.
Gaithersburg, MD 20878
Phone: (301)417-0770 **Fax:** (301)527-4207
Website: http://www.medimmune.com
Wayne T. Hockmeyer, PhD, Chairman of the Board
Desc: Biotechnology company: Rx/ethical pharmaceuticals; biotechnology/biopharmaceutical products; respiratory therapy and/or cardiopulmonary supplies.

★ 15864 ★ Medin Corp.
90 Dayton Ave.
Passaic, NJ 07055
Phone: (973)779-2400 **Free:** 800-922-0476
Fax: (973)779-2463
Email: traysrus@medin.com
Jay D. Schainholz, President
Desc: Manufacturer/distributor of hospital equipment and supplies; sterilization equipment.

★ 15865 ★ Medipoint, Inc.
72 E Second St.
Mineola, NY 11501
Phone: (516)294-8822 **Free:** 800-445-0525
Fax: (516)746-6693
Email: medipoint1@aol.com
Website: http://www.medipoint.com
Peter Gollobin, President
Desc: Manufacturer/distributor of disposable medical devices and supplies; first aid products; home healthcare; hospital equipment and supplies; laboratory supplies; physicians' supplies; skin/wound care products.

★ 15866 ★ Medovations, Inc.
102 E Keefe Ave.
Milwaukee, WI 53212
Phone: (414)265-7620 **Free:** 800-558-6408
Fax: (414)265-7628
Email: medo@medovations.com
Brant Stanford, President
Desc: Manufacturer: contract manufacturing; disposable medical devices and supplies; surgical disposables.

★ 15867 ★ Medrad, Inc. Subsidiary of Schering Berlin, Inc.
1 Medrad Dr.
Indianola, PA 15051-0780
Phone: (412)767-2400 **Free:** 800-633-7231
Fax: (412)767-4128
Email: info@medrad.com
Website: http://www.medrad.com
John P. Friel, CEO & Pres
Desc: Manufacturer of cardiovascular equipment; disposable medical devices and supplies; hospital equipment and supplies; injection systems: angiography/CT/MR; magnetic resonance imaging; ultrasonic equipment.

★ 15868 ★ Medtronic, Inc. Corporate Center
710 Medtronic Pkwy.
Minneapolis, MN 55432
Phone: (763)514-4000 **Free:** 800-328-2518
Fax: (763)514-4879
Website: http://www.medtronic.com
Bill George, Chairman of the Board
Desc: Manufacturer of cardiovascular equipment and supplies; implants and infusion; parenteral catheters; surgical disposables, instruments and supplies.

★ 15869 ★ Medtronic MiniMed
18000 Devonshire St.
Northridge, CA 91325-1219
Phone: (818)362-5958 **Free:** 800-933-3322
Fax: (818)362-3788
Website: http://www.minimed.com
Terrance Gregg, President

Desc: Manufacturer of Rx/ethical pharmaceuticals; disposable medical devices and supplies; home healthcare; implants and infusion.

★ 15870 ★ Medtronic Perfusion Systems
7611 Northland Dr.
Minneapolis, MN 55428
Phone: (763)391-9000 **Fax:** (763)391-9100
Website: http://medtronic.com
Bob Guezuraga, Contact
Desc: Manufacturer/distributor of orthopedic and prosthetic equipment and supplies.

★ 15871 ★ Medtronic Sofamor Danek Division of Medtronic, Inc.
1800 Pyramid Pl.
Memphis, TN 38132
Phone: (901)396-3133 **Fax:** (901)344-1555
Website: http://www.sofamordanek.com
Keith Williams, President
Desc: Manufacturer/distributor of orthopedic and prosthetic equipment and supplies.

★ 15872 ★ Medtronic Xomed Division of Medtronic, Inc.
6743 Southpoint Dr. N
Jacksonville, FL 32216
Phone: (904)296-9600 **Free:** 800-874-5797
Fax: (904)279-0970
Email: bblankemeyer@xomed.com
Website: http://www.xomed.com
Bob Blankemeyer, President
Desc: Manufacturer/distributor of ENT medical devices; hospital equipment and supplies; ophthalmic equipment and supplies; sterilization supplies; surgical disposables and instruments.

★ 15873 ★ Medworks
PO Box 581
Chatham, IL 62629
Phone: (217)698-3935 **Free:** 800-323-9790
Fax: (217)698-3928
Email: medworks@onebox.com
Website: http://www.medexamtools.com
Cynthia Heise-Swartz, President
Desc: Distributor of diagnostic equipment and instruments; neurological diagnostic tools; reflex hammers; stethoscopes; physical therapy and rehabilitation equipment and supplies; physicians' equipment; surgical instruments; surgical instruments for veterinarians; veterinary products.

★ 15874 ★ MEDX, Inc.
3456 N Ridge Ave., Ste. 100
Arlington Heights, IL 60004
Phone: (847)463-2020 **Free:** 800-323-MEDX
Fax: (847)463-2019
Email: info@medx-inc.com
Website: http://www.medx-inc.com
Floyd R. Rowan, Contact
Desc: Manufacturer of nuclear and radiological equipment.

★ 15875 ★ Menda Division of Desco Industries, Inc.
3651 Walnut Ave.
Chino, CA 91710
Phone: (909)627-2453 **Fax:** (909)755-8848
Email: menda@mendapump.com
Website: http://www.mendapump.com
Cheryl Uresti, Contact
Desc: Manufacturer of liquid pump dispensers.

★ 15876 ★ Mennen Medical Corp. Division of Mennen Medical Ltd.
10123 Main St.
Clarence, NY 14031
Phone: (716)759-6921 **Free:** 800-223-2201
Fax: (716)759-6237
Email: sales@mennenmedical.com
Website: http://www.mennenmedical.com
Michael Guzzetta, Contact
Desc: Manufacturer/distributor of cardiovascular equipment and supplies; diagnostic equipment and instruments; disposable medical devices and supplies; hemodynamic monitoring equipment; patient monitoring equipment.

★ 15877 ★ Mentor Corp.
201 Mentor Dr.
Santa Barbara, CA 93111
Phone: (805)879-6000 **Fax:** (805)964-2712
Website: http://www.mentorcorp.com
Christopher J. Conway, Contact
Desc: Manufacturer/distributor of diagnostic equipment and instruments; disposable medical devices and supplies; home healthcare; hospital equipment and supplies; implants and infusion; ostomy equipment and supplies; skin/wound care products; surgical disposables, instruments and supplies; ultrasonic equipment; urinary equipment and supplies.

★ 15878 ★ Merck & Co., Inc. U.S. Human Health
PO Box 1000
North Wales, PA 19454
Phone: (267)305-5000
Website: http://www.merck.com
David W. Anstice, Contact
Desc: Manufacturer of Rx/ethical pharmaceuticals.

★ 15879 ★ Merck & Co., Inc. Worldwide Human Health Marketing
PO Box 100
Whitehouse Station, NJ 08889-0100
Phone: (908)423-1000
Website: http://www.merck.com
Dr. Steven Nichtnerger, Contact
Desc: Manufacturer of Rx/ethical pharmaceuticals.

★ 15880 ★ Merck KGaA
Frankfurter Strasse 250
D-64293
Darmstadt, Germany
Email: service@merck.de
Website: http://www.merck.de
Dr. Bernhard Scheuble, CEO & Chm Bd
Desc: Manufacturer of Rx/ethical pharmaceuticals; OTC/proprietary pharmaceuticals; generic pharmaceuticals; biological and environmental safety products; biotechnology/biopharmaceutical products; cardiovascular equipment and supplies; diagnostic equipment and instruments; diagnostic reagents and test kits; dietary, nutritional and vitamin supplements; laboratory equipment and supplies; orthopedic and prosthetic equipment and supplies.

★ 15881 ★ Merck Vaccine Division Worldwide Marketing
PO Box 4
West Point, PA 19486
Phone: (215)652-5000
Website: http://www.merck.com
Adel Mahoud, MD, Contact
Desc: Manufacturer of Rx/ethical pharmaceuticals.

★ 15882 ★ Meridian Medical Technologies, Inc.
10240 Old Columbia Rd.
Columbia, MD 21046
Phone: (410)309-6830 **Free:** 800-638-8093
Fax: (410)309-1475
Email: info@meridianmt.com
Website: http://www.meridianmeds.com
James H. Miller, CEO & Chm Bd
Desc: Manufacturer/biotechnology company: Rx/ethical pharmaceuticals; generic pharmaceuticals; biotechnology/biopharmaceutical products; cardiovascular equipment and supplies; contract manufacturing; diagnostic equipment and instruments; EMS equipment and supplies; home healthcare; hospital equipment and supplies; parenteral equipment and supplies; patient monitoring equipment; pharmaceutical manufacturing supplies and equipment; respiratory therapy and/or cardiopulmonary equipment.

★ 15883 ★ Merit Medical Systems Inc.
1600 W Merit Parkway
South Jordan, UT 84095
Free: 800-356-3748 **Fax:** (801)253-1652
Website: http://www.merit.com
Fred Lampropoulos, President
Desc: Manufacturer/distributor of cardiovascular equipment and supplies.

★ 15884 ★ Merrick Medicine Co.
501 S Eighth St.
Waco, TX 76706
Phone: (254)753-3461 **Fax:** (254)753-3461
Email: percymedicine@aol.com
J. Reese Killion, President
Desc: Manufacturer/distributor of OTC/proprietary pharmaceuticals.

★ 15885 ★ Merz Pharmaceuticals, LLC
PO Box 18806
Greensboro, NC 27419
Phone: (336)856-2003 **Free:** 800-334-0514
Fax: (336)856-0107
Email: info@merzusa.com
Website: http://www.merzusa.com
Terry Conrad, CEO & Pres
Desc: Distributor of Rx/ethical pharmaceuticals; OTC/proprietary pharmaceuticals; dietary, nutritional and vitamin supplements; skin/wound care products.

★ 15886 ★ Metagenics Gig Harbor
5800 Soundview Dr.
Bldg. B
Gig Harbor, WA 98335
Phone: (253)851-3943 **Free:** 800-843-9660
Fax: (253)851-9749
Email: info@metagenics.com
Website: http://www.metagenics.com
Jeffrey S. Bland, PhD, President
Desc: Manufacturer/distributor of OTC/proprietary pharmaceuticals; dietary, nutritional and vitamin supplements; patient aid products.

★ 15887 ★ Mettler Electronics Corp.
1333 S Claudina St.
Anaheim, CA 92805
Phone: (714)533-2221 **Free:** 800-854-9305
Fax: (714)635-7539
Email: mail@mettlerelec.com
Website: http://www.mettlerelec.com
Stephen C. Mettler, President
Desc: Manufacturer of physical therapy and rehabilitation equipment and supplies; ultrasound and electromedical equipment and supplies.

★ 15888 ★ MGI PHARMA, Inc.
5775 Old Shakopee Rd.
Ste. 100
Bloomington, MN 55437
Phone: (952)346-4700 **Fax:** (952)346-4800
Website: http://www.mgipharma.com
Charles N. Blitzer, CEO & Pres
Desc: Distributor of Rx/ethical pharmaceuticals.

★ 15889 ★ Micro Essential Laboratory, Inc.
4224 Ave. H
PO Box 10824
Brooklyn, NY 11210
Phone: (718)338-3618 **Fax:** (718)692-4491
Email: custserv@microessentiallab.com

Website: http://www.microessentiallab.com
Joel Florin, President
Desc: Manufacturer/distributor of diagnostic reagents and test kits; hospital equipment and supplies; physicians' supplies; test paper (pH and Litmus); urinary supplies.

★ 15890 ★ MicroAire Surgical Instruments
1641 Edlich Dr.
Charlottesville, VA 22911
Phone: (804)975-8000 **Free:** 800-722-0822
Fax: (804)975-4144
Email: microair@microaire.com
Website: http://www.microaire.com
Francis Lavin, President
Desc: Manufacturer of burs and blades; powered surgical instruments; surgical disposables; surgical instruments.

★ 15891 ★ Microgenics Corp.
46360 Fremont Boulevard
Fremont, CA 94538
Phone: (510)979-5000 **Free:** 800-232-3342
Fax: (510)979-5498
Email: ytsay@microgenics.com
Website: http://www.microgenics.com
Yuh-Geng Tsay, President
Desc: Manufacturer/distributor/biotechnology company: biotechnology/biopharmaceutical products; diagnostic equipment and instruments; diagnostic reagents and test kits.

★ 15892 ★ Microtek Medical Inc. Division of ISOLYSER
602 Lehmberg Rd.
Columbus, MS 39702
Phone: (662)327-1863 **Free:** 800-844-0988
Fax: (662)327-5921
Email: info@microtekmed.com
Website: http://www.microtechmed.com
Dan R. Lee, CEO & Pres
Desc: Manufacturer/distributor of apparel; biological and environmental safety products; cardiovascular supplies; dental supplies; disposable medical devices and supplies; hospital equipment and supplies; ophthalmic supplies; surgical disposables and supplies; ultrasound and electromedical equipment and supplies.

★ 15893 ★ Midmark Corp.
60 Vista Dr.
PO Box 286
Versailles, OH 45380
Phone: (937)526-3662 **Free:** 800-MID-MARK
Fax: 800-365-8631
Email: webmaster@midmark.com
Website: http://www.midmark.com
Anne Eiting Klamar, MD, President
Desc: Manufacturer of cardiovascular equipment; dental equipment; laboratory equipment; ophthalmic equipment; physicians' equipment; sterilization equipment; veterinary products; diagnostic equipment and instruments.

★ 15894 ★ Midwest Glove Co., Inc. Security Medical Products Division
8088 McCormick Blvd.
Skokie, IL 60076
Phone: (847)674-8080 **Free:** 800-621-3861
Fax: (847)674-8181
Email: allied-glove@cyberlynk.net
Website: http://www.alliedglove.com
Sol Appelbaum, President
Desc: Manufacturer of apparel; biological and environmental safety products; dental supplies; disposable medical devices and supplies; nuclear and radiological supplies; surgical disposables; veterinary products; X-ray supplies.

★ 15895 ★ MII/Teltron Technologies, Inc.
2 Riga Lane
Birdsboro, PA 19508
Phone: (610)582-9450 **Free:** 800-835-8766
Fax: (610)582-0851
Email: miipgt@miipgt.com
Website: http://www.miipgt.com
Clyde A. Mock, Contact
Desc: Manufacturer/distributor of diagnostic equipment and instruments; X-ray equipment.

★ 15896 ★ Milex Products, Inc.
4311 N Normandy
Chicago, IL 60634
Phone: (773)736-5500 **Fax:** (773)736-5256
Website: http://www.milexproducts.com
H. T. Milgrom, President
Desc: Manufacturer of Rx/ethical pharmaceuticals; OTC/proprietary pharmaceuticals; gynecological devices; pharmaceutical manufacturing supplies and equipment; physicians' supplies; surgical disposables.

★ 15897 ★ Millar Instruments, Inc.
6001-A Gulf Freeway
Houston, TX 77023-5417
Phone: (713)923-9171 **Free:** 800-669-2343
Fax: (713)923-7757
Email: info@millarmail.com
Website: http://www.millarinstruments.com
Huntly D. Millar, President
Desc: Manufacturer of cardiovascular equipment; diagnostic equipment and instruments; laboratory equipment; patient monitoring equipment urinary equipment.

★ 15898 ★ Millennium Pharmaceuticals
75 Sidney St.
Cambridge, MA 02140
Phone: (617)679-7000 **Fax:** (617)374-7788
Email: info@mlnm.com
Website: http://www.mlnm.com
Mark J. Levin, CEO
Desc: Biotechnology/biopharmaceutical products.

★ 15899 ★ Millipore Corp.
80 Ashby Rd.
Bedford, MA 01730
Phone: (781)533-6000 **Free:** 800-645-5476
Fax: (781)533-3110
Website: http://www.millipore.com
Francis J. Lunger, Contact
Desc: Manufacturer/biotechnology company: biotechnology/biopharmaceutical products; laboratory equipment and supplies.

★ 15900 ★ Miltex, Inc.
700 Hicksville Rd.
Bethpage, NY 11714-3490
Phone: (516)349-0001 **Free:** 800-854-8300
Fax: (866)854-8400
Email: surgical@miltex.com
Website: http://www.miltex.com
T. Robert Perrett, CEO & Pres
Desc: Manufacturer/distributor of cardiovascular supplies; dental equipment and supplies; disposable medical devices and supplies; hospital equipment and supplies; laboratory supplies; ophthalmic supplies; physicians' supplies; sterilization supplies; surgical disposables, instruments and supplies; urinary supplies; veterinary products.

★ 15901 ★ Mine Safety Appliances Co. Medical Products Division
PO Box 427
Pittsburgh, PA 15230
Phone: (724)776-8600 **Free:** 800-851-4500
Fax: (724)776-8885
Email: info@msanet.com
Website: http://www.msanet.com
Steve Bayer, Contact
Desc: Manufacturer of EMS equipment and supplies; hospital equipment and supplies; respiratory therapy and/or cardiopulmonary equipment.

★ 15902 ★ Minntech Corp. dba Renal Systems, Fibercor, Unitrol
14605 28th Ave. N
Minneapolis, MN 55447
Phone: (763)553-3300 **Free:** 800-328-3345
Fax: (763)553-3387
Email: info@minntech.com
Website: http://www.minntech.com
Roy K. Malkin, CEO & Pres
Desc: Manufacturer/distributor of cardiovascular equipment and supplies; high purity water filters; laboratory equipment and supplies; renal dialysis equipment and supplies; sterilization equipment and supplies.

★ 15903 ★ MinXray, Inc.
3611 Commercial Ave.
Northbrook, IL 60062
Phone: (847)564-0323 **Free:** 800-221-2245
Fax: (847)564-9040
Email: info@minxray.com
Website: http://www.minxray.com
Keith R. Kretchmer, President
Desc: Manufacturer/distributor of dental equipment; diagnostic equipment and instruments; hospital equipment and supplies; X-ray equipment.

★ 15904 ★ Misonix, Inc.
1938 New Hwy.
Farmingdale, NY 11735
Phone: (631)694-9555 **Free:** 800-645-9846
Fax: (631)694-9412
Website: http://www.misonix.com
Mike McManus, CEO & Pres
Desc: Manufacturer of laboratory equipment and ultrasonic equipment.

★ 15905 ★ Mission Pharmacal Co.
PO Box 786099
San Antonio, TX 78278-6099
Phone: (210)696-8400 **Free:** 800-531-3333
Fax: (210)696-6010
Website: http://www.missionpharmacal.com
Bob Ganguzza, Contact
Desc: Manufacturer of Rx/ethical pharmaceuticals; OTC/proprietary pharmaceuticals; contract manufacturing; diagnostic reagents and test kits; dietary, nutritional and vitamin supplements.

★ 15906 ★ Miza Pharmaceuticals Inc.
4950 Yonge St., Ste. 2001
PO Box 118
Toronto, ON, Canada M2N 6K1
Phone: (416)927-0600 **Fax:** (416)927-0699
Email: info@miza.com
Website: http://www.miza.com
Jack Kachkar, MD, CEO & Pres
Desc: Manufacturer/distributor of Rx/ethical pharmaceuticals; OTC/proprietary pharmaceuticals; generic pharmaceuticals; contract manufacturing; dietary, nutritional and vitamin supplements; ophthalmic supplies; skin/wound care products.

★ 15907 ★ MMAR Medical Group, Inc.
9619 Yupondale Dr.
Houston, TX 77080
Phone: (713)465-2003 **Free:** 800-662-7633
Fax: (713)465-2818
Email: mmarmedical@earthlink.net
Website: http://www.mmarmedical.com
Charles D. Dillon, President
Desc: Manufacturer/distributor of orthopedic and prosthetic equipment and supplies; physical therapy and rehabilitation equipment and supplies.

★ 15908 ★ Moll Industries, Inc.
2100 SW 71st Terr.
Davie, FL 33317
Phone: (954)577-2660 **Free:** 800-275-6655
Fax: (954)474-5992
Email: chuck.schiele@mollindustries.com
Website: http://www.mollindustries.com
Charles B. Schiele, President
Desc: Manufacturer of cardiovascular equipment and supplies; dental equipment and supplies; diagnostic equipment and instruments; diagnostic reagents and test kits; disposable medical devices and supplies; hospital equipment and supplies; respiratory therapy and/or cardiopulmonary equipment; ultrasound and electromedical equipment and supplies; urinary equipment.

★ 15909 ★ Monarch Pharmaceuticals, Inc.
Subsidiary of King Pharmaceuticals
501 Fifth St.
Bristol, TN 37620
Phone: (423)989-8000 **Free:** 800-776-3637
Website: http://www.kingpharm.com
Joseph R. Gregory, CEO & Pres
Desc: Distributor of Rx/ethical pharmaceuticals; OTC/proprietary pharmaceuticals; skin/wound care products.

★ 15910 ★ Monticello Drug Co.
Subsidiary of The Monticellos Cos., Inc.
1604 Stockton St.
Jacksonville, FL 32204
Phone: (904)384-3666 **Free:** 800-735-0666
Fax: (904)388-6307
Website: http://www.monticellocompanies.com
Henry E. Dean, III, President
Desc: Distributor of OTC/proprietary pharmaceuticals; ostomy equipment and supplies.

★ 15911 ★ Morton Grove Pharmaceuticals, Inc.
6451 W Main St.
Morton Grove, IL 60053
Phone: (847)967-5600 **Free:** 800-346-6854
Fax: (847)967-5607
Website: http://www.mgp-online.com
Brian Tambi, Contact
Desc: Manufacturer of OTC/proprietary pharmaceuticals; generic pharmaceuticals.

★ 15912 ★ Muro Pharmaceutical, Inc.
890 East St.
Tewksbury, MA 01876-1496
Phone: (978)851-5981 **Free:** 800-225-0974
Fax: (978)851-7346
Website: http://www.muropharm.com
Colin W. Stewart, CEO & Pres
Desc: Manufacturer/distributor of Rx/ethical pharmaceuticals; OTC/proprietary pharmaceuticals; contract manufacturing.

★ 15913 ★ Mylan Laboratories
130 7th St.
1030 Century Bldg.
Pittsburgh, PA 15222
Phone: (412)232-0100 **Fax:** (412)232-0123
Email: investor_relations@mylan.com
Website: http://www.mylanlabs.com
Milan Puskar, CEO & Chm Bd
Desc: Manufacturer/distributor of Rx/ethical pharmaceuticals; OTC/proprietary pharmaceuticals; generic pharmaceuticals; biotechnology/biopharmaceutical products.

★ 15914 ★ Mylan Pharmaceuticals, Inc.
Generic Product Division of Mylan Laboratories, Inc.
781 Chestnut Ridge rd.
PO Box 4310
Morgantown, WV 26505
Phone: (304)599-2595 **Fax:** (304)598-3232
Website: http://www.mylanpharms.com
Milan Puskar, Chairman of the Board
Desc: Manufacturer of generic pharmaceuticals.

★ 15915 ★ Myron L Co.
6115 Corte del Cedro
Carlsbad, CA 92009
Phone: (760)438-2021 **Fax:** (760)931-9189
Email: sales@myronl.com
Website: http://www.myronl.com
Kathryn Robinson, Contact
Desc: Manufacturer of water quality test instruments; laboratory equipment.

★ 15916 ★ Nabi
5800 Park of Commerce Blvd.
Boca Raton, FL 33487
Phone: (561)989-5800 **Free:** 800-635-1766
Fax: (561)989-5899
Email: dgury@nabi.com
Website: http://www.nabi.com
David J. Gury, Contact
Desc: Manufacturer/distributor/biotechnology company: biotechnology/biopharmaceutical products; diagnostic reagents and test kits; pharmaceutical manufacturing supplies and equipment.

★ 15917 ★ Nalge Nunc International Corp.
An Apogent Technologies Co.
75 Panorama Creek Dr.
Rochester, NY 14625-2385
Phone: (716)586-8800 **Free:** 800-625-4327
Fax: (716)586-3294
Email: webmaster@nalgenunc.com
Website: http://www.nalgenunc.com
Robert Ahlgren, Contact
Desc: Manufacturer/biotechnology company: Biological and environmental safety products; biotechnology/biopharmaceutical products; disposable medical devices and supplies; laboratory equipment and supplies; pharmaceutical manufacturing supplies and equipment.

★ 15918 ★ NaPro BioTherapeutics, Inc.
6304 Spine Rd., Unit A
Boulder, CO 80301
Phone: (303)516-8500 **Fax:** (303)530-1296
Website: http://www.naprobio.com
Leonard P. Shaykin, Chairman of the Board
Desc: Manufacturer of Rx/ethical pharmaceuticals.

★ 15919 ★ Nasco
Division of Nasco International
901 Janesville Ave.
Fort Atkinson, WI 53538
Phone: (920)563-2446 **Free:** 800-558-9595
Fax: (920)563-8296
Email: info@enasco.com
Website: http://www.enasco.com
Phil Niemeyer, Contact
Desc: Manufacturer/distributor of hospital equipment and supplies; laboratory equipment and supplies.

★ 15920 ★ National Instrument Co., Inc.
4119 Fordleigh Rd.
Baltimore, MD 21215
Phone: (410)764-0900 **Free:** 800-526-1301
Fax: (410)764-7719
Email: sales@filamatic.com
Website: http://www.filamatic.com
Sidney Rosen, President
Desc: Manufacturer of Rx/ethical pharmaceuticals; OTC/proprietary pharmaceuticals; generic pharmaceuticals; anesthesia equipment and products; biotechnology/biopharmaceutical products; dental supplies; dietary, nutritional and vitamin supplements; laboratory equipment; parenteral equipment.

★ 15921 ★ Natren, Inc.
Professional Division
3105 Willow Ln.
Westlake Village, CA 91361
Phone: (805)371-4737 **Free:** 877-962-8736
Fax: (805)496-4039
Website: http://www.natren.com
Yordan Trenev, CEO
Desc: Manufacturer of dietary, nutritional and vitamin supplements; face cream or moisturizer; skin care products; veterinary products.

★ 15922 ★ Nature's Bounty, Inc.
90 Orville Dr.
Bohemia, NY 11716
Phone: (631)567-9500 **Free:** 800-244-2055
Fax: (631)244-2136
Email: info@naturesbounty.com
Website: http://www.naturesbounty.com
Scott Rudolph, Contact
Desc: Manufacturer/distributor of dietary, nutritional and vitamin supplements; hospital equipment and supplies.

★ 15923 ★ Neopharm, Inc.
150 Field Dr., Ste. 195
Lake Forest, IL 60045
Phone: (847)295-8678 **Fax:** (847)295-8854
Email: investorrelations@neophrm.com
Website: http://www.neophrm.com
John N. Kapoor, Chairman of the Board
Desc: Biotechnology/biopharmaceutical products; research and development.

★ 15924 ★ Neose Technologies, Inc.
102 Witmer Rd.
Horsham, PA 19044
Phone: (215)441-5890 **Fax:** (215)441-5896
Email: info@neose.com
Website: http://www.neose.com
C. Boyd Clarke, PhD, CEO & Pres
Desc: Manufacturer/biotechnology company: Rx/ethical pharmaceuticals; biotechnology/biopharmaceutical products; dietary, nutritional and vitamin supplements.

★ 15925 ★ Neurocrine Biosciences, Inc.
10555 Science Center Dr.
San Diego, CA 92121
Phone: (858)658-7600 **Free:** 800-876-3522
Fax: (858)658-7602
Email: info@neurocrine.com
Website: http://www.neurocrine.com
Joseph A. Mollica, Chairman of the Board
Desc: Biotechnology/biopharmaceutical products.

★ 15926 ★ Neutrogena Corp.
Dermatologics Division
5760 W 96th St.
Los Angeles, CA 90045
Phone: (310)642-1150 **Free:** 800-421-6857
Fax: (310)337-2156
Website: http://www.neutrogena.com
Michael McNamara, CEO & Pres
Desc: Manufacturer of Rx/ethical pharmaceuticals; OTC/proprietary pharmaceuticals; skin/wound care products.

★ 15927 ★ Neutron Products, Inc.
22301 Mt. Ephraim Rd.
PO Box 68
Dickerson, MD 20842

Phone: (301)349-5001 **Free:** 800-424-8169
Fax: (301)349-5007
Email: neutronprod@erols.com
J.A. Ransohoff, President
Desc: Manufacturer/distributor of nuclear and radiological equipment and supplies.

★ 15928 ★ Nexell Therapeutics Inc.
9 Parker
Irvine, CA 92618
Phone: (949)470-9011 **Fax:** (949)586-2420
Email: investor_relations@nexell.com
Website: http://www.nexell.com
Richard L. Dunning, Chairman of the Board
Desc: Biotechnology company offering biotechnology/biopharmaceutical products diagnostic equipment and instruments; diagnostic reagents and test kits; disposable medical devices and supplies.

★ 15929 ★ Neytech
Division of Degussa-Ney
65 W Dudleytown Rd.
Bloomfield, CT 06002
Phone: (860)242-6188 **Free:** 800-426-8834
Fax: (860)769-5050
Email: neyinfo@neydental.com
Website: http://www.neydental.com
Holger Meinicke, President
Desc: Manufacturer/distributor of dental equipment and supplies; laboratory equipment; surgical supplies; ultrasonic equipment.

★ 15930 ★ Niche Pharmaceuticals, Inc.
200 N Oak St.
Roanoke, TX 76262
Phone: (817)491-2770 **Free:** 800-677-0355
Fax: (817)491-3533
Email: niche@waymark.net
Website: http://www.niche-inc.com
Steve F. Brandon, CEO & Pres
Desc: Manufacturer of Rx/ethical pharmaceuticals; OTC/proprietary pharmaceuticals.

★ 15931 ★ Nicolet Biomedical Inc.
Division of VIASYS Healthcare
5225 Verona Rd., Bldg. 2
Madison, WI 53711-4495
Phone: (608)273-5000 **Free:** 800-356-0007
Fax: (608)273-5067
Email: mailbox@nicoletbiomedical.com
Website: http://www.nicoletbiomedical.com
Gerry Brew, President
Desc: Manufacturer/distributor of diagnostic equipment and instruments; hospital equipment and supplies; neurodiagnostic and monitoring instrumentation; patient monitoring equipment; physicians' equipment and supplies; sleep diagnostics/therapeutics; surgical supplies.

★ 15932 ★ Nihon Kohden America, Inc.
Division of Nihon Kohden Corp.
90 Icon St.
Foothill Ranch, CA 92610
Phone: (949)580-1555 **Free:** 800-325-0283
Fax: (949)580-1550
Email: info@nkusa.com
Website: http://www.nkusa.com
H. Adachi, President
Desc: Manufacturer/distributor of diagnostic equipment and instruments; hospital equipment and supplies; patient monitoring equipment; sleep diagnostics/therapeutics.

★ 15933 ★ Nikon Instruments Inc.
1300 Walt Whitman Rd.
Melville, NY 11747
Phone: (631)547-8500 **Free:** 800-52-NIKON
Fax: (631)547-0306
Email: biosales@nikonincmail.com
Website: http://www.nikonusa.com
Takeshi Hirai, CEO & Pres
Desc: Manufacturer/distributor of diagnostic equipment and instruments; laboratory equipment; ophthalmic equipment; physicians' equipment; veterinary products.

★ 15934 ★ Nobel Biocare USA, Inc.
Subsidiary of Nobel Biocare AB, Sweden
22715 Savi Ranch Parkway
Yorba Linda, CA 92887
Phone: (714)282-4800 **Fax:** (714)998-9236
Website: http://www.nobelbiocare.com
Martin J. Dymek, President
Desc: Dental equipment manufacturer.

★ 15935 ★ Nova Medical Systems, Inc.
6414 NW 82nd Ave.
Miami, FL 33166
Phone: (305)597-0322 **Fax:** (305)597-3914
Email: custserv@medicalsystems.com
Website: http://www.medicalsystems.com
Mardin Varela, President
Desc: Manufacturer/distributor of cardiovascular equipment and supplies; diagnostic equipment and instruments; hospital equipment and supplies; patient aid products; patient monitoring equipment; physicians' equipment; respiratory therapy and/or cardiopulmonary equipment.

★ 15936 ★ Novametrix Medical Systems, Inc.
5 Technology Dr.
PO Box 690
Wallingford, CT 06492
Phone: (203)265-7701 **Free:** 800-243-3444
Fax: (203)284-0753
Email: sales@novametrix.com
Website: http://www.novametrix.com
William J. Lacourciere, CEO & Chm Bd
Desc: Manufacturer/distributor of patient monitoring equipment; pulse oximetry; respiratory mechanics; noninvasive cardiac output.

★ 15937 ★ Novartis Consumer Health, Inc.
10401 Hwy. 6
PO Box 83288
Lincoln, NE 68501
Phone: (402)464-6311 **Fax:** (402)467-8833
Website: http://www.consumer-health.novartis.com
Mark Kurtenbach, Contact
Desc: Manufacturer/distributor of OTC/proprietary pharmaceuticals.

★ 15938 ★ Novartis Nutrition Corp.
Medical Nutrition Division
5320 W 23rd St.
PO Box 370
Minneapolis, MN 55440
Phone: (952)925-2100 **Free:** 800-999-9978
Fax: (952)593-7990
Website: http://www.novartisnutrition.com
Joe Heron, Contact
Desc: Manufacturer of dietary, nutritional and vitamin supplements; hospital equipment and supplies.

★ 15939 ★ Novartis Ophthalmics
11695 Johns Creek Parkway
Duluth, GA 30097-1556
Phone: (866)393-6336 **Fax:** (678)415-4000
Email: dan.myers@pharma.novartis.com
Website: http://www.novartisophthalmics.com
C. Daniel Myers, Contact
Desc: Manufacturer of Rx/ethical pharmaceuticals; OTC/proprietary pharmaceuticals.

★ 15940 ★ Novartis Pharmaceuticals Corp.
Division of Novartis AG
1 Health Plaza
East Hanover, NJ 07936-1080
Phone: (973)781-8300 **Free:** 800-644-8585
Fax: (973)781-7185
Email: paulo.costa@pharma.novartis.com
Website: http://www.novartis.com
Paulo Costa, CEO & Pres
Desc: Manufacturer/distributor of Rx/ethical pharmaceuticals.

★ 15941 ★ Novo Nordisk Pharmaceuticals, Inc.
Division of Novo Nordisk A/S
100 College Rd. W
Princeton, NJ 08540
Phone: (609)987-5800 **Fax:** (609)987-5394
Website: http://www.novonordisk-us.com
Martin Soeters, President
Desc: Manufacturer/distributor/biotechnology company: Rx/ethical pharmaceuticals; OTC/proprietary pharmaceuticals; biotechnology/biopharmaceutical products.

★ 15942 ★ NSG Precision Cells, Inc.
195 G Central Ave.
Farmingdale, NY 11735
Phone: (631)249-7474 **Fax:** (631)249-8575
Email: nsgpciny@aol.com
Website: http://www.nsgpci.com
Seymour Schoenfeld, President
Desc: Manufacturer/distributor of hospital equipment and supplies; laboratory equipment and supplies; refractometers; spectrophotometer cells; urinary supplies.

★ 15943 ★ Nu-Hope Laboratories, Inc.
PO Box 331150
Pacoima, CA 91333-1150
Phone: (818)899-7711 **Free:** 800-899-5017
Fax: (818)899-2079
Email: info@nu-hope.com
Website: http://www.nu-hope.com
Eugene Galindo, President
Desc: Manufacturer of ostomy equipment and supplies.

★ 15944 ★ Nuclear Associates
120 Andrews Rd.
Hicksville, NY 11801
Phone: (516)870-0100 **Free:** 888-466-8257
Fax: (516)870-0140
Email: sales@nuclr.com
Website: http://www.nucl.com
Art Swayhoover, Contact
Desc: Manufacturer/distributor of biological and environmental safety products; cardiovascular equipment and supplies; dental supplies; diagnostic equipment and instruments; disposable medical devices and supplies; hospital equipment and supplies; hospital furniture; laboratory equipment and supplies; magnetic resonance imaging; nuclear and radiological equipment and supplies; patient aid products; patient monitoring equipment; radiopharmaceuticals; skin/wound care products; ultrasound and electromedical equipment and supplies; urinary equipment; veterinary products; X-ray equipment and supplies.

★ 15945 ★ O.R. Marketing, Inc.
PO Box 815
Columbia, MD 21044
Phone: (410)799-7474 **Free:** 800-825-6073
Fax: (410)799-7749
Email: ormkt@rcn.com
Website: http://www.ormarketing.com
Paul Meola, President
Desc: Manufacturer/distributor of disposable medical devices and supplies; hospital equipment and sup-

plies; ophthalmic supplies; sterilization equipment and supplies; surgical disposables and instruments.

★ 15946 ★ Oakhurst Co.
Division of Woolfoam Corp.
3000 Hempstead Tpke.
Levittown, NY 11756
Phone: (516)731-5380 **Free:** 800-831-1135
Fax: (516)731-5607
Email: oakhurstco@aol.com
Website: http://www.oldmedicine.com
Stanley H. Roberts, President
Desc: Manufacturer/distributor of OTC/proprietary pharmaceuticals.

★ 15947 ★ OCG Technology, Inc.
56 Harrison St.
New Rochelle, NY 10801
Phone: (914)576-8457 **Fax:** (914)576-7821
Email: elevine@ocgt.com
Website: http://www.pcare.com
Edward C. Levine, Contact
Desc: Manufacturer of cardiovascular equipment; diagnostic equipment and instruments; PrimeCare (tm) Patient Management System; code complier (tm).

★ 15948 ★ Ohaus Corp.
19 Chapin Rd.
Pine Brook, NJ 07058
Phone: (973)377-9000 **Free:** 800-672-7722
Fax: (973)593-0359
Email: sales@ohaus.com
Website: http://www.ohaus.com
James Ohaus, President
Desc: Laboratory equipment manufacturer.

★ 15949 ★ Omnimed, Inc.
Beam Products
800 Glen Ave.
Moorestown, NJ 08057
Free: 800-257-2326 **Fax:** (856)359-2249
Email: info@omnimedbeam.com
Website: http://www.omnimedbeam.com
George Samanko, President
Desc: Manufacturer of hospital equipment and supplies.

★ 15950 ★ Omron Healthcare, Inc.
Medical Division
300 Lakeview Parkway
Vernon Hills, IL 60061
Phone: (847)680-6200 **Free:** 800-231-4030
Fax: (847)680-6269
Website: http://www.omronhealthcare.com
Kazuo Saito, CEO
Desc: Manufacturer/distributor of cardiovascular equipment; diagnostic equipment and instruments; disposable medical devices and supplies; EMS equipment and supplies; home healthcare; hospital equipment and supplies; physicians' equipment; respiratory therapy and/or cardiopulmonary equipment; sterilization supplies; surgical disposables.

★ 15951 ★ Oncogene Science
80 Rogers St.
Cambridge, MA 02142-1168
Phone: (617)492-7289 **Free:** 888-674-3424
Fax: (617)492-8438
Email: walter.carney.b@oncogene.com
Website: http://www.oncogene.com
Walter P. Carney, PhD, Contact
Desc: Manufacturer/biotechnology company: diagnostic reagents and test kits.

★ 15952 ★ Onyx Pharmaceuticals
3031 Research Dr.
Richmond, CA 94806
Phone: (510)222-9700 **Fax:** (510)222-9758
Website: http://www.onyx-pharm.com
Hollings Renton, CEO & Chm Bd
Desc: Biotechnology/biopharmaceutical products.

★ 15953 ★ Organogenesis, Inc.
150 Dan Rd.
Canton, MA 02021
Phone: (781)575-0775 **Fax:** (781)401-1299
Email: communications@organo.com
Website: http://www.organogenesis.com
Michael Sabolinski, MD, CEO & Pres
Desc: Manufacturer/biotechnology company providing cardiovascular supplies; skin/wound care products; tissue engineering.

★ 15954 ★ Organomation Associates, Inc.
266 River Rd. W
Berlin, MA 01503
Phone: (978)838-7300 **Free:** 888-838-7300
Fax: (978)838-2786
Email: sales@organomation.com
Website: http://www.organomation.com
Andrew McNiven, Chairman of the Board
Desc: Manufacturer of laboratory equipment; sample preparation instruments.

★ 15955 ★ Organon, Inc.
Division of Akzo Pharma
375 Mt. Pleasant Ave.
West Orange, NJ 07052
Phone: (973)325-4500 **Free:** 800-631-1253
Fax: (973)325-4589
Website: http://www.organoninc.com
Hans Rader, President
Desc: Manufacturer of Rx/ethical pharmaceuticals; anesthesia equipment and products.

★ 15956 ★ Ortec International, Inc.
3960 Broadway
New York, NY 10032
Phone: (212)740-6999 **Fax:** (212)740-6963
Email: ortechinfo@aol.com
Website: http://www.ortecinternational.com
Steven Katz, PhD, CEO & Chm Bd
Desc: Biotechnology company: biotechnology/biopharmaceutical products; skin/wound care products.

★ 15957 ★ Ortho Biotech, L.P.
A Johnson & Johnson Co.
700 U.S. Hwy. 202
PO Box 670
Raritan, NJ 08869
Phone: (908)704-5000 **Fax:** (908)526-7076
Website: http://www.orthobiotech.com
Gary Reedy, President
Desc: Manufacturer/biotechnology company providing Rx/ethical pharmaceuticals; biotechnology/biopharmaceutical products.

★ 15958 ★ Ortho-Clinical Diagnostics
A Johnson & Johnson Co.
1001 U.S. Hwy. 202
Raritan, NJ 08869
Phone: (908)218-1300 **Free:** 800-828-6316
Fax: (908)218-3893
Website: http://www.orthoclinical.com
Desc: Manufacturer/distributor of diagnostic equipment and instruments; diagnostic reagents and test kits.

★ 15959 ★ Ortho-McNeil Pharmaceutical
A Johnson & Johnson Co.
U.S. Rte. 202
PO Box 300
Raritan, NJ 08869
Phone: (908)218-6000 **Fax:** (908)218-1416
Website: http://www.orthomcneil.com
Seth H.Z. Fischer, President
Desc: Manufacturer/distributor of Rx/ethical pharmaceuticals.

★ 15960 ★ Ortho-Neutrogena
A Johnson & Johnson Co.
5760 W 96th St.
Los Angeles, CA 90045
Phone: (310)642-1150 **Free:** 800-421-6857
Fax: (310)337-2156
Website: http://www.orthoderm.com
Michael McNamara, CEO & Pres
Desc: Manufacturer/distributor of Rx/ethical pharmaceuticals; skin/wound care products.

★ 15961 ★ OSI Pharmaceuticals Inc.
58 S Service Rd.
Melville, NY 11747
Phone: (631)962-2000 **Fax:** (631)752-3880
Email: information@osip.com
Website: http://www.osip.com
Colin Goddard, PhD, CEO & Chm Bd
Desc: Biotechnology/biopharmaceutical products.

★ 15962 ★ OSMONICS, Inc.
5951 Clearwater Dr.
Minnetonka, MN 55343-8995
Phone: (952)933-2277 **Free:** 800-848-1750
Fax: (952)988-6056
Website: http://www.osmonics.com
D. Dean Spatz, CEO
Desc: Manufacturer of hospital equipment and supplies; laboratory equipment; renal dialysis equipment; sterilization equipment.

★ 15963 ★ Owens & Minor, Inc.
Headquarters
4800 Cox Rd.
Glen Allen, VA 23060
Phone: (804)747-9794 **Free:** 800-488-8850
Fax: (804)270-7281
Website: http://www.owens-minor.com
G. Gilmer Minor, III, CEO & Chm Bd
Desc: Distributor of anesthesia equipment and products; apparel; cardiovascular supplies; diagnostic equipment and instruments; hospital equipment and supplies; laboratory supplies; orthopedic and prosthetic equipment and supplies; ostomy equipment and supplies; patient aid products; patient monitoring equipment; physical therapy and rehabilitation equipment and supplies; physicians' equipment and supplies; respiratory therapy and/or cardiopulmonary equipment and supplies; skin/wound care products; sterilization equipment and supplies; surgical disposables and instruments; urinary equipment.

★ 15964 ★ Owl Separation Systems
55 Heritage Ave.
Portsmouth, NH 03801
Phone: (603)559-9297 **Free:** 800-242-5560
Fax: (603)559-9258
Email: sales@owlsci.com
Website: http://www.owlsci.com
Stephen Norton, President
Desc: Manufacturer/distributor/biotechnology company providing biotechnology/biopharmaceutical products; electrophoresis equipment and supplies; laboratory equipment and supplies.

★ 15965 ★ Oxford Instruments Medical, Inc.
12 Skyline Dr.
Hawthorne, NY 10532
Phone: (914)593-7100 **Free:** 800-438-8322
Fax: (914)593-7290
Email: sales@ms.oxinst.com
Website: http://www.oxford-instruments.com
M.P.R. Pattinson, CEO & Pres

Desc: Manufacturer/distributor of cardiovascular equipment; diagnostic equipment and instruments; disposable medical devices and supplies; fetal monitoring equipment; hospital equipment and supplies; neurophysiology monitoring equipment; sleep diagnostics/therapeutics.

★ 15966 ★ Oxis International, Inc.
6040 N Cutter Circle, Ste. 317
Portland, OR 97217
Phone: (503)283-3911 **Free:** 800-547-3686
Fax: (503)283-4058
Email: info@oxis.com
Website: http://www.oxis.com
Ray Rogers, Contact
Desc: Manufacturer/distributor/biotechnology company providing Rx/ethical pharmaceuticals; biotechnology/biopharmaceutical products; diagnostic reagents and test kits; laboratory supplies.

★ 15967 ★ Oxoid Inc.
800 Proctor Ave.
Ogdensburg, NY 13669
Free: 800-567-8378
Email: sales@oxoid.ca
Website: http://www.oxoid.ca
Greg Nyman, Contact
Desc: Manufacturer/distributor/biotechnology company providing biotechnology/biopharmaceutical products; diagnostic equipment and instruments; diagnostic reagents and test kits; laboratory equipment and supplies; fermendation media/peptones.

★ 15968 ★ Oxygen Delivery Systems, LLC
Division of Pharmaceutical Marketing Partners, LLC
317 ½ N Main St.
Galena, IL 61036
Phone: (815)777-9811 **Free:** 800-358-3852
Fax: (815)777-9822
Website: http://www.systemO2.com
Robert J. Gunter, CEO & Pres
Desc: Manufacturer of disposable medical devices and supplies; respiratory therapy and/or cardiopulmonary equipment and supplies.

★ 15969 ★ P.J. Noyes Co., Inc.
89 Bridge St.
Lancaster, NH 03584-3103
Phone: (603)788-4952 **Free:** 800-522-2469
Fax: (603)788-3873
Email: info@pjnoyes.com
Website: http://www.pjnoyes.com
David C. Hill, President
Desc: Manufacturer of OTC/proprietary pharmaceuticals; contract manufacturing; dietary, nutritional and vitamin supplements; skin/wound care products; veterinary products.

★ 15970 ★ Paddock Labs, Inc.
3940 Quebec Ave. N
Minneapolis, MN 55427
Phone: (763)546-4676 **Free:** 800-328-5113
Fax: (763)546-4842
Email: info@paddocklabs.com
Website: http://www.paddocklabs.com
Bruce G. Paddock, President
Desc: Manufacturer of Rx/ethical pharmaceuticals; OTC/proprietary pharmaceuticals; generic pharmaceuticals.

★ 15971 ★ Panasonic Industrial Co.
Division of Matsushita Electric Corp. of America
2 Panasonic Way
M.S 7E-6
Secaucus, NJ 07094
Phone: (201)348-5339 **Fax:** (201)392-4888
Website: http://www.panasonic.com
Joseph Taylor, President
Desc: Manufacturer of radiation measurement equipment.

★ 15972 ★ Paragon Vision Sciences
947 E Impala
Mesa, AZ 85204
Phone: (480)892-7602 **Free:** 800-528-8279
Fax: (480)926-7369
Email: info@paragonvision.com
Website: http://www.paragonvision.com
Joe Sicari, CEO & Pres
Desc: Manufacturer of ophthalmic equipment and supplies.

★ 15973 ★ Park Surgical Co., Inc.
5001 New Utrecht Ave.
Brooklyn, NY 11219
Phone: (718)436-9200 **Free:** 800-633-7878
Fax: (718)854-2431
Email: parksurgical@aol.com
Website: http://www.parksurgical.com
Daniel L. Dube, President
Desc: Distributor of Rx/ethical pharmaceuticals; OTC/proprietary pharmaceuticals; diagnostic equipment and instruments; diagnostic reagents and test kits; EMS equipment and supplies; home healthcare; hospital equipment and supplies; hospital furniture; ophthalmic supplies; ostomy equipment and supplies; parenteral catheters; physical therapy and rehabilitation equipment and supplies; physicians' equipment and supplies; skin/wound care products; slide viewing systems; sterilization equipment and supplies; surgical disposables, instruments and supplies; ultrasonic equipment; ultrasound and electromedical equipment and supplies; urinary equipment; X-ray equipment an supplies.

★ 15974 ★ Parkedale Pharmaceuticals, Inc.
Subsidiary of King Pharmaceuticals, Inc.
870 Parkedale Rd.
Rochester, MI 48307
Phone: (248)656-5400 **Fax:** (248)656-5508
Website: http://www.kingpharm.com
John M. Gregory, Chairman of the Board
Desc: Manufacturer of Rx/ethical pharmaceuticals.

★ 15975 ★ Parkell Products, Inc.
155 Schmitt Blvd.
Farmingdale, NY 11735
Phone: (631)249-1134 **Free:** 800-243-7446
Fax: (631)249-1242
Email: sales@parkell.com
Website: http://www.parkell.com
Bob Burke, Contact
Desc: Manufacturer/distributor of dental equipment and supplies.

★ 15976 ★ Parker Hannifin Corp.
100 Ames Pond Dr.
PO Box 1262
Tewksbury, MA 01876
Phone: (978)858-0505 **Free:** 800-343-4048
Fax: (978)858-0625
Website: http://www.parker.com/ags
Mindy Rutfield, Contact
Desc: Manufacturer of hospital equipment and supplies; laboratory equipment and supplies; sterilization equipment and supplies; pharmaceutical manufacturing supplies and equipment.

★ 15977 ★ Parker Hannifin Corp.
Veriflo Division
250 Canal Blvd.
PO Box 4034
Richmond, CA 94804-0034
Phone: (510)235-9590 **Free:** 800-962-4074
Fax: (510)232-7396
Email: info@veriflo.com
Website: http://www.veriflo.com
Brian Fussner, Contact
Desc: Manufacturer of anesthesia equipment and products; cardiovascular equipment; hospital equipment and supplies; laboratory equipment; pharmaceutical manufacturing supplies and equipment; pressure regulators; pharmaceutical and biotechnology; valves diaphragm.

★ 15978 ★ Parker Laboratories, Inc.
286 Eldridge Rd.
Fairfield, NJ 07004
Phone: (973)276-9500 **Free:** 800-631-8888
Fax: (973)276-9510
Email: parker@parkerlabs.com
Website: http://www.parkerlabs.com
Martin Buchalter, President
Desc: Manufacturer of cardiovascular supplies; disposable medical devices and supplies; hospital equipment and supplies; physicians' supplies; ultrasound and electromedical equipment and supplies; X-ray supplies.

★ 15979 ★ Parks Medical Electronics, Inc.
PO Box 5669
Aloha, OR 97006
Phone: (503)649-7007 **Free:** 800-547-6427
Fax: (503)591-9753
Email: leparks2@yahoo.com
Website: http://www.parksmed.com
Loren E. Parks, Contact
Desc: Manufacturer/distributor of cardiovascular equipment; diagnostic equipment and instruments.

★ 15980 ★ Parnell Pharmaceuticals, Inc.
PO Box 5130
Larkspur, CA 94977-5130
Phone: (415)256-1800 **Fax:** (415)256-8099
Email: mail@parnellpharm.com
Website: http://www.parnellpharm.com
Francis W. Parnell, MD, Contact
Desc: Manufacturer/distributor of Rx/ethical pharmaceuticals; OTC/proprietary pharmaceuticals; skin/wound care products.

★ 15981 ★ Pascal Co., Inc.
PO Box 1478
Bellevue, WA 98009-1478
Phone: (425)827-4694 **Free:** 800-426-8051
Fax: (425)827-6893
Email: pascaldental@pascaldental.com
Website: http://www.pascaldental.com
Benjamin Paschall, CEO & Chm Bd
Desc: Manufacturer/distributor of Rx/ethical pharmaceuticals; OTC/proprietary pharmaceuticals; dental equipment and supplies; sterilization supplies.

★ 15982 ★ Patheon, Inc.
2100 Syntex Ct.
Mississauga, ON, Canada L5N 7K9
Phone: (905)821-4001 **Free:** 888-PATHEON
Fax: (905)812-6791
Email: patheon@patheon.com
Website: http://www.patheon.com
Robert Tedford, CEO
Desc: Manufacturer/biotechnology company providing Rx/ethical pharmaceuticals; OTC/proprietary pharmaceuticals; biotechnology/biopharmaceutical products; contract manufacturing; dietary, nutritional and vitamin supplements.

★ 15983 ★ PCP Champion
Division of Surgical Appliance Industries, Inc.
300 Congress St.
Ripley, OH 45167
Phone: (937)392-4301 **Free:** 800-888-0867
Fax: 800-667-5984

Email: pcp-champion@surgicalappliance.com
Website: http://www.pcp-champion.com
Dave Scott, Contact

Desc: Manufacturer/distributor of orthopedic and prosthetic equipment and supplies; patient aid products.

★ 15984 ★ PediaMed Pharmaceuticals, Inc.
782 Springdale Dr.
Ste. 120
Exton, PA 19341
Phone: (484)875-9375 **Free:** (866)543-6337
Fax: (484)875-9380
Email: service@pediamedpharma.com
Website: http://www.pediamedpharma.com
Michael W. Speidel, CEO & Pres

Desc: Manufacturer of Rx/ethical pharmaceuticals; OTC/proprietary pharmaceuticals.

★ 15985 ★ Pedinol Pharmacal, Inc.
30 Banfi Plaza N
Farmingdale, NY 11735
Phone: (631)293-9500 **Free:** 800-PED-INOL
Fax: (631)293-7359
Email: sales@pedinol.com
Website: http://www.pedinol.com
Richard Strauss, RPh, CEO & Pres

Desc: Distributor of Rx/ethical pharmaceuticals; OTC/proprietary pharmaceuticals; generic pharmaceuticals; physicians' supplies; prescription/OTC pharmaceuticals; office use products; skin/wound care products; sterilization supplies.

★ 15986 ★ Penox Technologies, Inc.
1 Penox Plaza
Commerce Rd.
Pittston, PA 18640
Phone: (570)655-1421 **Free:** 800-233-3029
Fax: (570)655-2036
Website: http://www.penox.com
Jim Soroka, Contact

Desc: Manufacturer of home health care; oxygen equipment.

★ 15987 ★ Peregrine Pharmaceuticals
14272 Franklin Ave.
Tustin, CA 92780
Phone: (714)508-6000 **Fax:** (714)838-5817
Email: info@peregrineinc.com
Website: http://www.peregrine.com
Edward Legere, CEO & Pres

Desc: Biotechnology/biopharmaceutical products.

★ 15988 ★ PerkinElmer Instruments
710 Bridgeport Ave.
Shelton, CT 06484
Phone: (203)925-4600 **Free:** 800-762-4000
Fax: (203)944-4902
Email: info@perkinelmer.com
Website: http://www.perkinelmer.com
Stephen P. DeFalco, President

Desc: Manufacturer/biotechnology company providing laboratory equipment and supplies; pharmaceutical manufacturing supplies and equipment.

★ 15989 ★ PerkinElmer Life Sciences
549 Albany St.
Boston, MA 02118
Phone: (617)482-9595 **Free:** 800-551-2121
Fax: (617)482-1380
Email: techsupport@perkinelmer.com
Website: http://www.perkinelmer.com/lifesciences
John Engel, President

Desc: Manufacturer/distributor/biotechnology company offering biotechnology/biopharmaceutical products; diagnostic reagents and test kits; imaging systems; laboratory equipment and supplies.

★ 15990 ★ Perrigo Co.
515 Eastern Ave.
Allegan, MI 49010
Phone: (616)673-8451 **Fax:** (616)673-9128
Email: investor@perrigo.com
Website: http://www.perrigo.com
David T. Gibbons, CEO

Desc: Manufacturer of OTC/proprietary pharmaceuticals; contract manufacturing; diagnostic reagents and test kits; dietary, nutritional and vitamin supplements.

★ 15991 ★ Person & Covey, Inc.
616 Allen Ave.
PO Box 25018
Glendale, CA 91221-5018
Phone: (818)240-1030 **Free:** 800-423-2341
Fax: (818)547-9821
Email: helpdesk@personandcovey.com
Website: http://www.personandcovey.com
Frank Brisben, CEO & Pres

Desc: Manufacturer of Rx/ethical pharmaceuticals; OTC/proprietary pharmaceuticals; skin/wound care products.

★ 15992 ★ Personal Products Co.
Division of Johnson & Johnson
199 Grandview Rd.
Skillman, NJ 08558-9418
Phone: (908)874-1000 **Fax:** (908)874-2481
Website: http://www.jnj.com
Beth Burough, Contact

Desc: Manufacturer/distributor of OTC/proprietary pharmaceuticals.

★ 15993 ★ Pfeiffer Glass
Division of Fisher Scientific Co.
140 Bennington Dr.
Rochester, NY 14616
Phone: (716)865-1290 **Fax:** (716)865-1303
Email: pglass@frontiernet.net
Website: http://www.pfeiffer.com
Morris Lew, Contact

Desc: Manufacturer of hospital equipment and supplies; laboratory equipment and supplies.

★ 15994 ★ Pfeiffer Pharmaceuticals, Inc.
Division of S.S.S. Co.
71 University Ave. SW
Atlanta, GA 30315
Phone: (404)614-0255 **Free:** 800-342-6450
Fax: (404)614-0322
Website: http://www.pfeiffer.com
Charles M. Bentley, CEO & Pres

Desc: Manufacturer of OTC/proprietary pharmaceuticals.

★ 15995 ★ Pfizer Animal Health Group
150 E 42nd St.
New York, NY 10017
Phone: (212)573-2323
Website: http://www.pfizer.com/ahg
Pedro Lichtinger, President

Desc: Manufacturer of veterinary products.

★ 15996 ★ Pfizer Consumer Group
Division of Pfizer Inc.
201 Tabor Rd.
Morris Plains, NJ 07950
Phone: (973)385-2000 **Fax:** (973)385-2581
Website: http://www.pfizer.com
Maurice A. Renshaw, Contact

Desc: Manufacturer of OTC/proprietary pharmaceuticals.

★ 15997 ★ Pfizer Inc.
Pfizer Pharmaceutical Group
235 E 42nd St.
New York, NY 10017-5755
Phone: (212)573-2323 **Fax:** (212)573-7851
Website: http://www.pfizer.com
Karen Katen, President

Desc: Manufacturer of Rx/ethical pharmaceuticals.

★ 15998 ★ Pharmaceutical Associates Inc.
Subsidiary of Beach Products, Inc.
201 Delaware St.
Greenville, SC 29605
Phone: (864)277-7282 **Free:** 800-845-8210
Fax: (864)277-8045
Richard B. Jenkins, CEO

Desc: Manufacturer of Rx/ethical pharmaceuticals; OTC/proprietary pharmaceuticals; generic pharmaceuticals.

★ 15999 ★ Pharmaceutical Formulations, Inc.
460 Plainfield Ave.
PO Box 1904
Edison, NJ 08818-1904
Phone: (732)985-7100 **Fax:** (732)819-3330
Email: sales@chase-walton.com
Website: http://www.pfiotc.com
Jim Ingram, Contact

Desc: Manufacturer/distributor of OTC/proprietary pharmaceuticals; generic pharmaceuticals.

★ 16000 ★ Pharmaceutical Innovations, Inc.
897 Frelinghuysen Ave.
Newark, NJ 07114
Phone: (973)242-2900 **Fax:** (973)242-0578
Email: info@pharminnovations.com
Website: http://www.pharminnovations.com
Gilbert Buchalter, President

Desc: Manufacturer of cardiovascular supplies; diagnostic equipment and instruments; home healthcare; physical therapy and rehabilitation equipment and supplies; physicians' supplies; ultrasound and electromedical equipment and supplies; X-ray supplies.

★ 16001 ★ Pharmacia Corp.
100 Rte. 206 N
Peapack, NJ 07977
Phone: (908)901-8000 **Free:** 800-595-9051
Fax: (908)901-1840
Website: http://www.pharmacia.com
Fred Hassan, CEO & Chm Bd

Desc: Manufacturer of Rx/ethical pharmaceuticals; OTC/proprietary pharmaceuticals; animal health; bioscience; contract manufacturing; diagnostic equipment and instruments; hospital equipment and supplies; ophthalmic supplies; skin/wound care products; sleep diagnostics/ therapeutics; veterinary products.

★ 16002 ★ Pharmacyclics
995 E Arques Ave.
Sunnyvale, CA 94086
Phone: (408)774-0330 **Fax:** (408)774-0340
Email: info@pcyc.com
Website: http://www.pcyc.com
Richard Miller, MD, President

Desc: Biotechnology company: Rx/ethical pharmaceuticals; biotechnology/biopharmaceutical products.

★ 16003 ★ Pharmed Group Corp.
3075 NW 107th Ave.
Miami, FL 33172
Phone: (305)592-2324 **Free:** 800-683-7342
Fax: (305)591-0221
Website: http://www.pharmed.com
Carlos deCespedes, CEO & Chm Bd

Desc: Distributor/biotechnology company providing Rx/ethical pharmaceuticals; OTC/proprietary pharmaceuticals; generic pharmaceuticals; anesthesia equipment and products; apparel; biological and environmental safety products; biotechnology/biopharmaceutical products; cardiovascular equipment and supplies; contract manufacturing; diagnostic equipment and instruments; diagnostic reagents and test kits; dietary, nutritional and vitamin supplements; disposable medical devices and supplies; EMS equipment and supplies; home healthcare; hospital equipment and supplies; hospital furniture; laboratory equipment and supplies; magnetic resonance imaging; nuclear and radiological equipment and supplies; ophthalmic equipment and supplies; orthopedic and prosthetic equipment and supplies; ostomy equipment and supplies; parenteral catheters and equipment and supplies; patient aid products; patient monitoring equipment; physical therapy and rehabilitation equipment and supplies; physicians' equipment and supplies; radiopharmaceuticals; renal dialysis equipment and supplies; respiratory therapy and/or cardiopulmonary equipment and supplies; skin/wound care products; slide viewing systems; sterilization equipment and supplies; surgical disposables, instruments and supplies; ultrasonic equipment; ultrasound and electromedical equipment and supplies; urinary equipment and supplies; veterinary products; X-ray equipment and supplies.

★ 16004 ★ Philips Medical Systems North American Co.
595 Miner Rd.
Cleveland, OH 44143
Phone: (440)483-3000 **Fax:** (440)483-7571
Website: http://www.pmsna.com
Fred B. Parks, CEO & Pres
Desc: Manufacturer of cardiovascular equipment and supplies; diagnostic equipment and instruments; disposable medical devices and supplies; hospital equipment and supplies; laboratory supplies; magnetic resonance imaging; nuclear and radiological equipment and supplies; physicians' supplies; x-ray supplies.

★ 16005 ★ Phillips Medical Systems Cardiac and Monitoring Systems
3000 Minuteman Rd.
Andover, MA 01810
Phone: (978)687-1501 **Free:** 800-934-7372
Fax: (978)686-7262
Website: http://www.pmsna.com
Hans Barella, CEO & Pres
Desc: Manufacturer/distributor of cardiac and monitoring systems.

★ 16006 ★ Phillips Medical Systems, North America
22100 Bothell Everett Hwy.
Bothell, WA 98041-3027
Phone: (425)487-7000 **Free:** 800-982-2011
Fax: (425)485-6080
Website: http://www.pmsna.com
Tim Mickelson, Contact
Desc: Manufacturer of cardiovascular equipment; diagnostic equipment and instruments; diagnostic imaging and related services; disposable medical devices and supplies; hospital equipment and supplies; magnetic resonance imaging; nuclear and radiological equipment; surgical supplies; ultrasound and electromedical equipment and supplies; x-ray equipment.

★ 16007 ★ Physician Sales & Services, Inc.
4345 Southpoint Blvd.
Jacksonville, FL 32216
Phone: (904)281-0011
Website: http://www.pssd.com
Doug Harper, President
Desc: Distributor of Rx/ethical pharmaceuticals; diagnostic equipment and instruments; diagnostic reagents and test kits; disposable medical devices and supplies; hospital equipment and supplies; laboratory equipment and supplies; orthopedic and prosthetic equipment and supplies; parenteral supplies; patient aid products; physicians' equipment and supplies; respiratory therapy and/or cardiopulmonary supplies; skin/wound care products; sterilization equipment and supplies; surgical disposables, instruments and supplies; ultrasound and electromedical equipment and supplies; urinary equipment and supplies.

★ 16008 ★ Physitemp Instruments Inc.
154 Huron Ave.
Clifton, NJ 07013
Phone: (973)779-5577 **Free:** 800-452-8510
Fax: (973)779-5954
Email: physitemp@aol.com
Website: http://www.physitemp.com
Ronald R. Feller, Contact
Desc: Manufacture of laboratory equipment and patient monitoring equipment.

★ 16009 ★ Plantex U.S.A. Inc. Division of Teva Pharmaceutical Industries Ltd.
482 Hudson Terrace
Englewood Cliffs, NJ 07632
Phone: (201)567-1010 **Fax:** (201)567-7994
Email: plantex@carroll.com
Website: http://www.plantexusa.com
George Svokos, President
Desc: Manufacturer of generic pharmaceuticals.

★ 16010 ★ Plas-Labs, Inc.
917 E Chilson St.
Lansing, MI 48906
Phone: (517)372-7177 **Free:** 800-866-7527
Fax: (517)372-2857
Email: plaslabs@aol.com
Website: http://www.plas-labs.com
Dave L. Regan, President
Desc: Manufacturer/distributor/biotechnology company providing biological and environmental safety products; biotechnology/biopharmaceutical products; laboratory equipment; pharmaceutical manufacturing supplies and equipment; veterinary products.

★ 16011 ★ PML Microbiologicals Division of PML Inc.
PO Box 570
Wilsonville, OR 97070
Phone: (503)570-2500 **Free:** 800-547-0659
Fax: (503)570-2501
Email: inquiry@pmlmicro.com
Website: http://www.pmlmicro.com
Ken Minton, CEO & Pres
Desc: Manufacturer/distributor of diagnostic reagents and test kits; disposable medical devices and supplies; laboratory equipment and supplies; pharmaceutical manufacturing supplies and equipment.

★ 16012 ★ Polar Electro, Inc. Division of Polar Electro, OY (Finland)
370 Crossways Park Dr.
Woodbury, NY 11797
Phone: (516)364-0400 **Free:** 800-290-6330
Fax: (516)364-5454
Website: http://www.polarusa.com
Allison Herrforth, Contact
Desc: Manufacturer of cardiovascular equipment; home healthcare; hospital equipment and supplies; patient monitoring equipment; physical therapy and rehabilitation equipment and supplies; physicians' equipment and supplies; respiratory therapy and/or cardiopulmonary equipment.

★ 16013 ★ Polar Plastics NC, Inc. Division of The Polar Group
2500 Old Lexington Rd.
Winston-Salem, NC 27107
Phone: (336)784-8880 **Free:** 800-334-6229
Fax: (336)785-1815
Email: polar@polarplastic.com
Website: http://www.polarplastic.com
Eric Cohen, President
Desc: Manufacturer of disposable medicine cups; disposable specimen containers; hospital equipment and supplies.

★ 16014 ★ Polar Ware
2806 N 15th St.
Sheboygan, WI 53083
Phone: (920)458-3561 **Free:** 800-237-3655
Fax: (920)458-2205
Email: info@polarawre.com
Website: http://www.polarware.com
Jerry Baltus, Contact
Desc: Manufacturer of dental equipment and supplies; EMS equipment and supplies; hospital equipment and supplies; laboratory equipment and supplies; patient aid products; physicians' equipment and supplies; sterilization equipment and supplies; surgical instruments and supplies.

★ 16015 ★ Poly-Seal Corp.
1810 Portal St.
Baltimore, MD 21224
Phone: (410)633-1990 **Fax:** (410)633-6311
Email: pscapinfo@poly-seal.com
Website: http://www.poly-seal.com
William J. Herdrich, Contact
Desc: Manufacturer of dispensing plugs; dropper bulb assemblies; plastic closures and applicators.

★ 16016 ★ PolyMedica Pharmaceuticals (USA), Inc.
11 State St.
Woburn, MA 01801
Phone: (781)933-2020 **Fax:** (781)933-7992
Email: etzel@polymedica.com
Website: http://www.polymedica.com
Arthur A. Siciliano, PhD, President
Desc: Manufacturer of Rx/ethical pharmaceuticals; OTC/proprietary pharmaceuticals.

★ 16017 ★ Polysciences, Inc.
400 Valley Rd.
Warrington, PA 18976
Phone: (215)343-6484 **Free:** 800-523-2575
Fax: 800-343-3291
Email: polysci@tigger.jvnc.net
Website: http://www.polysciences.com
Michael Ott, President
Desc: Manufacturer/distributor/biotechnology company providing biotechnology/biopharmaceutical products; diagnostic reagents and test kits; laboratory equipment and supplies.

★ 16018 ★ Popper & Sons, Inc.
300 Denton Ave.
New Hyde Park, NY 11040
Phone: (516)248-0300 **Free:** 888-717-7677
Fax: 800-557-6773
Email: sales@popperandsons.com
Website: http://www.popperandsons.com
Joseph A. Popper, President
Desc: Manufacturer/biotechnology company providing anesthesia equipment and products; biotechnology/biopharmaceutical products; cardiovascular supplies; disposable medical devices and supplies; hospital equipment and supplies; hypodermic and specialty needles; custom needles; laboratory supplies; surgical instruments.

★ 16019 ★ Porex Bio Products Group
1120 Holm Rd.
Petaluma, CA 94954-1106
Phone: (707)762-6689 **Free:** 800-426-9595
Fax: (707)762-7198
Email: bio.info@porex.com
Website: http://www.porex.com/bio
Clive Wingar, President
Desc: Manufacturer of disposable medical devices and supplies; hospital equipment and supplies; laboratory supplies.

★ 16020 ★ Porex Surgical, Inc.
15 Dart Rd.
Newnan, GA 30265-1017
Phone: (678)479-1610 **Free:** 800-521-7321
Fax: (678)423-1435
Email: surgical.info@porex.com
Website: http://www.porex.com/surgical
L. Franklin Bost, President
Desc: Manufacturer/distributor of disposable medical devices and supplies; implants and infusion; surgical disposables, instruments and supplies.

★ 16021 ★ Portex Inc.
10 Bowman Dr.
Keene, NH 03431
Phone: (603)352-3812 **Free:** 800-258-5361
Fax: (603)352-3703
Email: webmaster@mail.portexusa.com
Website: http://www.portexusa.com
Jeff Spielman, President
Desc: Manufacture of anesthesia equipment and products; disposable medical devices and supplies; EMS equipment and supplies; hospital equipment and supplies; laboratory supplies; patient monitoring equipment; physicians' supplies; respiratory therapy and/or cardiopulmonary supplies; skin/wound care products.

★ 16022 ★ Porto-Lift Corp.
PO Box 5
Higgins Lake, MI 48627-0005
Phone: (989)821-6688 **Free:** 800-321-1454
Fax: (989)821-8084
Wayne H. Teeter, President
Desc: Manufacturer of home healthcare; hospital equipment and supplies; patient aid products.

★ 16023 ★ Postcraft Co.
625 W Rillito St.
Tucson, AZ 85705
Phone: (520)624-2531 **Free:** 800-528-4844
Fax: (520)884-0013
Email: sales@postcraft.com
Website: http://www.postcraft.com
Bruce S. Beyer, President
Desc: Manufacturer of hospital equipment and supplies.

★ 16024 ★ Powervar, Inc.
1450 Lakeside Dr.
Waukegan, IL 60085
Phone: (847)596-7000 **Free:** 800-369-7179
Fax: (847)596-7100
Email: georgel@powervar.com
Website: http://www.powervar.com
George Lannert, CEO & Pres
Desc: Manufacturer/distributor of hospital equipment and supplies.

★ 16025 ★ Praxair, Inc.
39 Old Ridgebury Rd.
Danbury, CT 06810-5113
Phone: (203)879-4077 **Free:** 800-PRA-XAIR
Fax: (203)879-2040
Email: info@praxair.com
Website: http://www.praxair.com/healthcare
Sally A. Savoia, Contact
Desc: Manufacturer/distributor of anesthesia equipment and products; diagnostic equipment and instruments; home healthcare; hospital equipment and supplies; MRI cryogens; nuclear and radiological supplies; respiratory gases and equipment; respiratory therapy and/or cardiopulmonary equipment and supplies; sleep diagnostics/therapeutics; sterilization supplies.

★ 16026 ★ Precise Optics/PME, Inc.
239 S Fehr Way
Bayshore, NY 11706
Phone: (631)242-6600 **Free:** 800-242-6604
Fax: (631)242-4421
Email: info@preciseoptics.com
Website: http://www.preciseoptics.com
Robert Corso, Contact
Desc: Manufacturer of cardiovascular equipment; diagnostic equipment and instruments; X-ray equipment.

★ 16027 ★ Precision Charts Inc.
130 Wilbur Pl.
Bohemia, NY 11716
Phone: (631)567-6100 **Free:** 800-645-5410
Fax: (631)567-6224
Email: pcicharts@worldnett.att.net
Website: http://www.pcicharts.com
Sol Lesh, CEO & Chm Bd
Desc: Manufacturer of cardiovascular supplies; surgical supplies; ultrasound and electromedical equipment and sales.

★ 16028 ★ Precision Dynamics Corp.
13880 Del Sur St.
San Fernando, CA 91340
Phone: (818)897-1111 **Free:** 800-772-1122
Fax: (818)899-4045
Email: info@pdcorp.com
Website: http://www.pdcorp.com
Walter W. Mosher, Jr., President
Desc: Manufacturer/biotechnology company providing biotechnology/biopharmaceutical products; disposable medical devices and supplies; EMS equipment and supplies; home healthcare; hospital equipment and supplies; laboratory supplies; parenteral catheters and supplies; patient aid products; patient monitoring equipment; skin/wound care products; surgical disposables; urinary supplies.

★ 16029 ★ Precision Scientific, Inc. Division of Jouan, Inc.
170 Marcel Dr.
Winchester, VA 22602
Phone: (540)869-9892 **Free:** 800-621-8820
Fax: (540)869-0130
Email: info@precisionsci.com
Website: http://www.precisionsci.com
Lyle E. Cady, Jr., President
Desc: Manufacturer of laboratory equipment and sterilization equipment; centrifuges.

★ 16030 ★ Precision Technology Inc.
50 Maple St.
Norwood, NJ 07648
Phone: (201)767-1600 **Fax:** (201)767-6739
Website: http://www.ptiplastics.com
Ira Housman, President
Desc: Manufacturer of implants and infusion; orthopedic and prosthetic equipment and supplies.

★ 16031 ★ Premier Dental Products Co.
1710 Romano Dr.
Plymouth Meeting, PA 19462
Phone: (610)239-6000 **Free:** 888-773-6872
Fax: 888-614-6646
Email: dentalinfo@premusa.com
Website: http://www.premusa.com
Gary Charlestein, CEO
Desc: Manufacturer of dental equipment and supplies.

★ 16032 ★ Prestige (tm) Medical Corp. Division of Rashman Corp.
8600 Wilbur Ave.
Northridge, CA 91324
Phone: (818)993-3030 **Free:** 800-762-3333
Fax: (818)993-4151
Email: prestigemed@gte.net
Website: http://www.prestigemed.com
Dennis Shick, Contact
Desc: Distributor of cardiovascular equipment; EMS equipment and supplies; home healthcare; hospital equipment and supplies; nursing supplies; physicians' supplies; surgical instruments.

★ 16033 ★ Pride Mobility Products Corp.
182 Susquehanna Ave.
Exeter, PA 18643
Phone: (570)655-5574 **Free:** 800-800-8586
Fax: 800-800-1636
Website: http://www.pridemobility.com
Scott Meuser, CEO & Chm Bd
Frmly: Pride Health Care, Inc. DES/ Manufacturer of home healthcare; hospital equipment and supplies; hospital furniture; patient aid products.

★ 16034 ★ Princeton Medical Products, Inc.
1189 Royal Links Dr.
Mount Pleasant, SC 29466
Phone: (843)849-0869 **Free:** 800-875-0869
Fax: (843)971-1600
Email: prnceton@aol.com
Joseph G. Frick, Contact
Desc: Distributor of cardiovascular equipment; hospital equipment and supplies; ophthalmic equipment; orthopedic and prosthetic equipment and supplies; sterilization equipment and supplies; surgical disposables, instruments and supplies.

★ 16035 ★ Principle Business Enterprise, Inc.
Pine Lake Industrial Park
PO Box 129
Dunbridge, OH 43414
Phone: (419)352-1551 **Free:** 800-467-3224
Fax: (419)352-8340
Email: info@gopeach.com
Website: http://www.gopeach.com
Charles A. Stocking, CEO & Pres
Desc: Manufacturer of apparel; disposable medical devices and supplies; hospital equipment and supplies; incontinence products (disposable adult briefs).

★ 16036 ★ Procter & Gamble Co.
PO Box 599
Cincinnati, OH 45201
Phone: (513)983-1100
Website: http://www.pg.com
Mark A. Collar, Contact
Desc: Manufacturer of Rx/ethical pharmaceuticals; OTC/proprietary pharmaceuticals.

★ 16037 ★ Products International Co.
2320 W Holly St.
Phoenix, AZ 85009
Phone: (602)257-0141 **Free:** 800-521-5123
Fax: (602)253-7148
Email: information@tabband.com
Website: http://www.tabband.com
Carl Twentier, President
Desc: Manufacturer/distributor of hospital equipment and supplies.

★ 16038 ★ Professional Compounding Centers of America
9901 S Wilcrest
Houston, TX 77099
Phone: (281)933-6948 **Free:** 800-331-2498
Fax: (281)933-6627
Website: http://www.pccarx.com
David Sparks, CEO & Pres
Desc: Distributor of Rx/ethical pharmaceuticals.

★ 16039 ★ Professional Disposables International Healthcare Division of Nice-Pak Products, Inc.
2 Nice Pak Park
Orangeburg, NY 10962

Phone: (845)365-1700 **Free:** 800-999-6423
Fax: (845)365-1729
Website: http://www.pdipdi.com
Robert P. Julius, CEO

Desc: Manufacturer of disposable medical devices and supplies; skin/wound care products.

★ 16040 ★ Profex Medical Products/ Professional Specialties Co.

PO Box 140669
Memphis, TN 38114
Free: 800-325-0196 **Fax:** (901)454-9850
Email: profexmed@aol.com
Website: http://www.profexmed.com
Stephen E. Zwick, President

Desc: Manufacturer of dental equipment and supplies; hospital equipment and supplies; hospital furniture; laboratory equipment and supplies; ophthalmic equipment; patient aid products; physical therapy and rehabilitation equipment and supplies; physicians' equipment.

★ 16041 ★ Purdue Pharma L.P.

1 Stamford Forum
Stamford, CT 06901-3431
Phone: (203)588-8000 **Free:** 800-745-7445
Fax: (203)588-8850
Website: http://www.purduepharma.com
Michael Friedman, Contact

Desc: Manufacturer/distributor of Rx/ethical pharmaceuticals; OTC/proprietary pharmaceuticals.

★ 16042 ★ Purified microEnvironments Division of Germfree Labs, Inc.

7435 NW 41st St.
Miami, FL 33166
Phone: (305)592-1780 **Free:** 800-888-5357
Fax: (305)591-7280
Email: info@purified.com
Website: http://www.purified.com
Jerome J. Landy, MD,PhD, President

Desc: Manufacturer of biological and environmental safety products; laboratory equipment; parenteral equipment; phamaceutical clean room equipment.

★ 16043 ★ Purity Life Health Products Ltd.

6 Commerce Crescent
Acton, ON, Canada L7J 2X3
Phone: (519)853-3511 **Free:** 800-265-2615
Fax: (519)853-4660
Email: sales@puritylife.com
Website: http://www.puritylife.com
David Chapman, President

Desc: Distributor of OTC/proprietary pharmaceuticals; dietary, nutritional and vitamin supplements; skin/wound care products.

★ 16044 ★ Qosina

150-Q Executive Dr.
Edgewood, NY 11717
Phone: (631)242-3000 **Fax:** (631)242-3230
Email: info@qosina.com
Website: http://www.qosina.com
Stuart Herskovitz, President

Desc: Distributor of cardiovascular supplies; dental supplies; diagnostic reagents and test kits; disposable medical devices and supplies; parenteral catheters and supplies; physicians' supplies; renal dialysis supplies; respiratory therapy and/or cardiopulmonary supplies; skin/wound care products; sterilization supplies; surgical disposables and supplies; urinary equipment and supplies; veterinary products.

★ 16045 ★ Quantimetrix Corp.

2005 Manhattan Beach Blvd.
Redondo Beach, CA 90278-1205
Phone: (310)536-0006 **Free:** 800-624-8380
Fax: (310)536-9977
Email: info@4qc.com
Website: http://www.4qc.com
Robert W. Ban, PhD, CEO & Chm Bd

Desc: Manufacturer of clinical controls; diagnostic reagents and test kits.

★ 16046 ★ Questar Corp.

6204 Ingham Rd.
New Hope, PA 18938
Phone: (215)862-5277 **Free:** 800-247-9607
Fax: (215)862-0512
Email: questar@questarcorporation.com
Website: http://www.questarcorporation.com
Donald J. Bandurick, CEO

Desc: Manufacturer/distributor of laboratory equipment and ophthalmic equipment.

★ 16047 ★ Questcor Pharmaceuticals, Inc.

3260 Whipple Rd.
Union City, CA 94587
Phone: (510)400-0700 **Fax:** (510)400-0799
Email: info@questcor.com
Website: http://www.questcor.com
Charles J. Casamento, Contact

Desc: Manufacturer of Rx/ethical pharmaceuticals; radiopharmaceuticals.

★ 16048 ★ Quidel Corp.

10165 McKellar Ct.
San Diego, CA 92121
Phone: (858)552-1100 **Free:** 800-874-1517
Fax: (858)453-4338
Website: http://www.quidel.com
Andre de Bruin, Chairman of the Board

Desc: Manufacturer/distributor of diagnostic reagents and test kits; veterinary products; biotechnology/biopharmaceutical products; diagnostic equipment and instruments; disposable medical devices and supplies; urinary equipment and supplies.

★ 16049 ★ Quinton Inc.

3303 Monte Villa Parkway
Bothell, WA 98021-8906
Phone: (425)402-2000 **Free:** 800-426-0337
Fax: (425)402-2001
Website: http://www.quinton.com
Ruediger Naumann-Etienne, PhD, CEO & Chm Bd

Desc: Manufacturer of cardiovascular equipment; diagnostic equipment and instruments; disposable medical devices and supplies; patient monitoring equipment; physical therapy and rehabilitation equipment and supplies.

★ 16050 ★ R.A. Fischer Co., Inc.

517 Commercial St.
Glendale, CA 91203
Phone: (818)241-1178 **Fax:** (323)245-2748
Email: info@rafischer.com
Website: http://www.rafischer.com
Mark Van Orden, President

Desc: Manufacturer/distributor of dermatologic equipment.

★ 16051 ★ The R. Schattner Co.

121 Congressional Lane
Rockville, MD 20852
Phone: (301)231-7700 **Fax:** (301)231-8165
Website: http://www.sporicidin.com
Robert I. Schattner, DDS, President

Desc: Manufacturer of OTC/proprietary pharmaceuticals; dental supplies; hospital equipment and supplies; laboratory supplies; ophthalmic supplies; physicians' supplies; renal dialysis supplies; sterilization equipment; surgical instruments; urinary equipment.

★ 16052 ★ R. Weinstein Pharmaceuticals & Medical Products Division of R. Weinstein, Inc.

846 Pohukaina St.
Honolulu, HI 96813
Phone: (808)591-8331 **Free:** 800-442-0639
Fax: (808)591-8339
Richard A. Weinstein, President

Desc: Distributor of Rx/ethical pharmaceuticals; OTC/proprietary pharmaceuticals; generic pharmaceuticals; diagnostic equipment and instruments; diagnostic reagents and test kits; disposable medical devices and supplies; hospital equipment and supplies; hospital furniture; laboratory equipment and supplies; ophthalmic supplies; physicians' equipment and supplies; skin/wound care products; slide viewing systems; sterilization equipment and supplies; surgical disposables and instruments.

★ 16053 ★ Radiation Dynamics, Inc.

151 Heartland Blvd.
Edgewood, NY 11717-8374
Phone: (631)254-6800 **Fax:** (631)254-6810
Email: sales@iba-rdi.com
Website: http://www.iba.rdi.com
Richard Galloway, Vice President

Desc: Sterilization equipment manufacturer.

★ 16054 ★ Radiometer America Inc. Subsidiary of Radiometer A/S (Copenhagen, Denmark)

810 Sharon Dr.
Westlake, OH 44145
Phone: (440)871-8900 **Free:** 800-736-0600
Fax: (440)871-2633
Email: info@radiometeramerica.com
Website: http://www.radiometeramerica.com
Johan Schroder, Chairman of the Board

Desc: Manufacturer of diagnostic equipment and instruments; patient monitoring equipment; respiratory therapy and/or cardiopulmonary equipment; respiratory therapy and/or cardiopulmonary supplies; skin/wound care products; sleep diagnostics/therapeutics.

★ 16055 ★ RAICHEM Division of Hemagen Diagnostics

8225 Mercury Ct.
San Diego, CA 92111-1203
Phone: (858)569-8009 **Free:** 800-438-6100
Fax: (858)569-6208
Email: sales@raichem.com
Website: http://www.hemagen.com
Ira Marks, President

Desc: Manufacturer/distributor of diagnostic equipment and instruments; diagnostic reagents and test kits; hospital equipment and supplies; laboratory equipment and supplies; veterinary products.

★ 16056 ★ Ramco Laboratories, Inc.

4100 Greenbriar Dr., Ste. 200
Stafford, TX 77477
Phone: (281)313-1200 **Free:** 800-231-6238
Fax: (281)313-1251
Email: ramcolab@aol.com
Clarence P. Alfrey, MD, Chairman of the Board

Desc: Manufacturer/distributor offering contract manufacturing; diagnostic reagents and test kits.

★ 16057 ★ Ranbaxy Pharmaceuticals, Inc. Division of Ranbaxy Laboratories, Ltd.

600 College Rd. E
Princeton, NJ 08540
Phone: (609)720-9200 **Free:** 888-726-2299
Fax: (609)720-1155
Email: dipakc@ranbaxy.com
Website: http://www.ranbaxy.com
Dipak Chattaraj, CEO

Desc: Manufacturer of Rx/ethical pharmaceuticals; generic pharmaceuticals.

★ 16058 ★ Ranfac Corp.
30 Doherty Ave.
Avon Industrial Park
Avon, MA 02322
Phone: (508)588-4400 **Free:** 800-272-6322
Fax: (508)584-8588
Email: info@ranfac.com
Website: http://www.ranfac.com
Barry Zimble, Vice President
Desc: Manufacturer/distributor of dental supplies; disposable medical devices and supplies; nuclear and radiological supplies; surgical disposables and instruments.

★ 16059 ★ Razel Scientific Instruments Inc.
100 Research Dr.
Stamford, CT 06906
Phone: (203)324-9914 **Fax:** (203)324-5568
Email: razelsci@aol.com
Website: http://www.razelscientific.com
Mo Nesin, Contact
Desc: Manufacturer/distributor of hospital equipment and supplies; laboratory equipment; parenteral equipment; renal dialysis equipment.

★ 16060 ★ Reckitt Benckiser Pharmaceuticals Inc.
Division of Reckitt Benckiser plc
1909 Huguenot Rd.
Richmond, VA 23235
Phone: (804)379-1090 **Free:** 800-444-7599
Fax: (804)379-1215
Email: charles.okeeffe@reckitt.com
Website: http://www.cortex.org
Charles B. O'Keeffe, CEO & Pres
Desc: Manufacturer of Rx/ethical pharmaceuticals; OTC/proprietary pharmaceuticals. **Frmly:** Reckitt & Colman Pharmaceuticals, Inc.

★ 16061 ★ Reckitt Benckiser Professional
1655 Valley Rd.
Wayne, NJ 07470
Phone: (973)633-3600 **Free:** 800-677-9218
Fax: (973)633-3593
Website: http:///www.reckittprofesional.com
Elio Leoni Sceti, President
Desc: Manufacturer of dental supplies; home healthcare; hospital equipment and supplies; laboratory supplies; physicians' supplies.

★ 16062 ★ Recordati Corp.
35 Walnut Ave.
Ste. 14
Clark, NJ 07066
Phone: (732)882-0880 **Fax:** (732)882-0316
Website: http://www.recordati.com
Giovani Recordati, CEO & Pres
Desc: Manufacturer/distributor of Rx/ethical pharmaceuticals; OTC/proprietary pharmaceuticals.

★ 16063 ★ Regeneron Pharmaceuticals, Inc.
777 Old Saw Mill River Rd.
Tarrytown, NY 10591-6707
Phone: (914)345-7400 **Fax:** (914)345-7797
Email: info@regn.com
Website: http://www.regeneron.com
P. Roy Vagelos, MD, Chairman of the Board
Desc: Biotechnology company offering biotechnology/biopharmaceutical products.

★ 16064 ★ Rehabilicare
1811 Old Hwy. 8
New Brighton, MN 55112
Phone: (651)631-0590 **Free:** 800-676-6489
Fax: (651)638-0476
Email: info@rehabilicare.com
Website: http://www.rehabilicare.com
David B. Kaysen, CEO & Pres
Desc: Manufacturer of OTC/proprietary pharmaceuticals; disposable medical devices and supplies; home healthcare; physical therapy and rehabilitation equipment and supplies; physicians' equipment and supplies; ultrasound and electromedical equipment and supplies.

★ 16065 ★ Reliance Medical Products
Division of Haag-Streit
3535 Kings Mills Rd.
Mason, OH 45040
Phone: (513)398-3937 **Free:** 800-735-0357
Fax: (513)398-0256
Website: http://www.reliance-medical.com
David Edenfield, Contact
Desc: Ophthalmic equipment manufacturer.

★ 16066 ★ Repligen Corp.
117 Fourth Ave.
Needham, MA 02494
Phone: (781)449-9560 **Free:** 800-622-2259
Fax: (781)453-0048
Email: sales@repligen.com
Website: http://www.repligen.com
Desc: Manufacturer/biotechnology company offering biotechnology/biopharmaceutical products; diagnostic reagents and test kits; laboratory supplies; pharmaceutical manufacturing supplies.

★ 16067 ★ Requa, Inc.
540 Barnum Ave.
PO Box 2384
Bridgeport, CT 06608
Phone: (203)345-0110 **Free:** 800-321-1085
Fax: (203)345-0108
Email: jgeils@requa.com
Website: http://www.requa.com
J.L. Geils, President
Desc: Manufacturer of OTC/proprietary pharmaceuticals; contract manufacturing; dietary, nutritional and vitamin supplements.

★ 16068 ★ Respironics, Inc.
Corporate Headquarters
1501 Ardmore Blvd.
Pittsburgh, PA 15221
Phone: (724)387-4000 **Free:** 800-345-6443
Fax: (412)473-5017
Website: http://www.respironics.com
James Liken, CEO & Pres
Desc: Manufacturer of home healthcare; patient monitoring equipment; respiratory therapy and/or cardiopulmonary equipment and supplies; sleep diagnostics/therapeutics; diagnostic equipment and instruments.

★ 16069 ★ Respironics Inc.
HealthScan Asthma and Allergy Products
41 Canfield Rd.
Cedar Grove, NJ 07009
Phone: (973)857-3414 **Free:** 800-962-1266
Fax: (973)857-9521
Email: susanlloyd@respironics.com
Website: http://www.respironics.com
Susan A. Lloyd, Vice President
Desc: Manufacturer of home healthcare; hospital equipment and supplies; patient monitoring equipment; respiratory therapy and/or cardiopulmonary equipment and supplies; disposable medical devices and supplies.

★ 16070 ★ Ribozyme Pharmaceuticals, Inc.
2950 Wilderness Pl.
Boulder, CO 80301
Phone: (303)449-6500 **Fax:** (303)449-6995
Website: http://www.rpi.com
Howard W. Robin, CEO & Pres
Desc: Biotechnology company offering biotechnology/biopharmaceutical products.

★ 16071 ★ Richard Wolf Medical Instruments Corp.
Division of Richard Wolf GMBH Germany
353 Corporate Woods Parkway
Vernon Hills, IL 60061-3110
Phone: (847)913-1113 **Free:** 800-323-9653
Fax: (847)913-1168
Email: sales&marketing@richardwolfusa.com
Website: http://www.richardwolf.com
Frau Burkhard, CEO
Desc: Manufacturer of diagnostic equipment and instruments; disposable medical devices and supplies; endoscopes; hospital equipment and supplies; physicians' equipment; slide viewing systems; sterilization supplies; surgical disposables and instruments; trocar systems; ultrasound and electromedical equipment and supplies; urinary supplies; veterinary products.

★ 16072 ★ Riley Medical, Inc.
L.A. Airport Park
27 Wrights Landing
Auburn, ME 04210
Phone: (207)786-2775 **Free:** 800-245-3300
Fax: (207)786-5553
Website: http://www.rileymed.com
Edward Riley, President
Desc: Sterilization equipment manufacturer.

★ 16073 ★ Robbins Instruments, Inc.
2 N Passaic Ave.
Chatham, NJ 07928
Phone: (973)635-8972 **Free:** 800-206-8649
Fax: (973)635-8732
Email: info@robbinsinstruments.com
Website: http://www.robbinsinstruments.com
George Mulvaney, President
Desc: Manufacturer/distributor of disposable medical devices and supplies; sterilization equipment and supplies; surgical disposables, instruments and supplies; ultrasonic equipment.

★ 16074 ★ Roche Diagnostics Corp.
9115 Hague Rd.
PO Box 50446
Indianapolis, IN 46250-0446
Phone: (317)845-2000 **Free:** 800-428-5074
Website: http://www.roche-diagnostics.com
Martin Madaus, CEO & Pres
Desc: Manufacturer/distributor of diagnostic equipment and instruments; diagnostic reagents and test kits.

★ 16075 ★ Roche Diagnostics Corp.
Roche Applied Science
9115 Hague Rd.
PO Box 50414
Indianapolis, IN 46250-0414
Phone: (317)849-9350 **Free:** 800-262-1640
Fax: 800-428-2883
Email: biochemts.us@roche.com
Website: http://www.roche-diagnostics.com
Suzanne Raehs, President
Desc: Manufacturer/biotechnology company providing biotechnology/biopharmaceutical products; laboratory supplies.

★ 16076 ★ The ROHO Group
100 N Florida Ave.
Belleville, IL 62221-5429
Phone: (618)277-9150 **Free:** 800-851-3449
Fax: (618)277-9561
Email: mail@therohogroup.com
Website: http://www.therohogroup.com
Tom Olesky, CEO & Pres
Desc: Manufacturer of home healthcare; physical therapy and rehabilitation equipment and supplies; skin/wound care products; wound care.

★ 16077 ★ Roloke Co.
127 W Hazel St.
Inglewood, CA 90302
Phone: (310)673-8300 **Free:** 800-533-8212
Fax: (310)673-7773
Email: lawalpin@pacbell.net
Lionel A. Walpin, MD, CEO
Desc: Manufacturer/distributor of bed wedges (adjustable); moist heat automatic cervical pillows; home healthcare; magnetic therapy products; patient aid products; sleep diagnostics/therapeutics.

★ 16078 ★ Ross Products Division
Division of Abbott Laboratories
625 Cleveland Ave.
Columbus, OH 43215-1724
Phone: (614)624-7677 **Fax:** (614)624-7030
Website: http://www.ross.com
Gary Flynn, President
Desc: Manufacturer of Rx/ethical pharmaceuticals.

★ 16079 ★ Rowley Biochemical Institute
Danvers Industrial Park
10 Electronics Ave.
Danvers, MA 01923
Phone: (978)739-4883 **Fax:** (978)739-5640
Email: rbi@transene.com
Martin E. Hecht, President
Desc: Manufacturer of diagnostic reagents and test kits.

★ 16080 ★ Roxane Laboratories, Inc.
Subsidiary of Boehringer Ingelheim Corp.
PO Box 16532
Columbus, OH 43216
Phone: (614)276-4000 **Free:** 800-848-0120
Fax: (614)274-0974
Website: http://www.roxane.com
Werner Gerstenberg, Contact
Desc: Manufacturer of Rx/ethical pharmaceuticals; generic pharmaceuticals.

★ 16081 ★ Royce Medical
742 Pancho Rd.
Camarillo, CA 93012
Phone: 800-487-5007 **Free:** 800-521-0601
Fax: 800-889-5722
Website: http://www.roycemedical.com
Jeff R. Haines, President
Desc: Manufacturer of orthopedic and prosthetic equipment and supplies.

★ 16082 ★ Rusch, Inc.
2450 Meadowbrook Parkway
Duluth, GA 30096
Phone: (770)623-0816 **Free:** 800-553-5214
Fax: (770)623-1829
Email: ruschinc@mindspring.com
Website: http://www.ruschinc.com
David Emm, President
Desc: Manufacturer/distributor of anesthesia equipment and products; disposable medical devices and supplies; EMS equipment and supplies; home healthcare; hospital equipment and supplies; laboratory supplies; ostomy equipment and supplies; parenteral catheters; physicians' supplies; respiratory therapy and/or cardiopulmonary equipment and supplies; surgical disposables; ultrasound and electromedical equipment and supplies; urinary equipment and supplies; surgical instruments.

★ 16083 ★ Rush Berivon, Inc.
PO Box 1851
Meridian, MS 39301
Phone: (601)693-6344 **Free:** 800-251-RUSH
Fax: (601)693-6348
Email: berivon@netdoor.com
Website: http://www.netdoor.com/com/berivon
L. Vaughan Rush, Jr., MD, Contact
Desc: Manufacturer of hospital equipment and supplies; orthopedic and prosthetic equipment and supplies.

★ 16084 ★ Rxtra Inc.
40 Richards Ave.
Norwalk, CT 06854
Phone: (203)831-9098 **Free:** 888-227-9872
Fax: (203)852-7268
Email: rxtra@aol.com
Allan R. Avery, President
Desc: Manufacturer of home healthcare and patient aid products.

★ 16085 ★ S & B Biomedics, Inc.
844 Dalworth Dr., Ste. 6
Mesquite, TX 75149
Phone: (972)288-3278 **Fax:** (972)288-3279
A.J. Segars, Contact
Desc: Manufacturer/distributor/biotechnology company offering biotechnology/biopharmaceutical products; cardiovascular equipment and supplies; diagnostic equipment and instruments; orthopedic and prosthetic equipment and supplies; patient monitoring equipment.

★ 16086 ★ S.S.S. Co.
71 University Ave. SW
PO Box 4447
Atlanta, GA 30302
Phone: (404)521-0857 **Free:** 800-237-3843
Fax: (404)880-0383
Email: sssco@bellsouth.net
Charles M. Bentley, CEO & Pres
Desc: Manufacturer of Rx/ethical pharmaceuticals; OTC/proprietary pharmaceuticals; generic pharmaceuticals; OTC/nonprescription pharmaceuticals.

★ 16087 ★ S & S X-Ray Products, Inc.
10625 Telge Rd.
Houston, TX 77095
Phone: (281)815-1300 **Free:** 800-347-XRAY
Fax: (281)815-1494
Email: info@ssxray.com
Website: http://www.ssxray.com
Norm Shoenfeld, MD, President
Desc: Manufacturer of nuclear and radiological supplies; X-ray equipment and supplies.

★ 16088 ★ SaatiTech Inc.
Division of SaatiGroup
247 Rte. 100
Somers, NY 10589
Phone: (914)767-0100 **Fax:** (914)767-0109
Email: info.us@saatitech.com
Website: http://www.saatitech.com
Gene Franks, President
Desc: Manufacturer of biotechnology/biopharmaceutical products; cardiovascular supplies; diagnostic reagents and test kits; disposable medical devices and supplies; laboratory supplies; pharmaceutical manufacturing supplies and equipment; respiratory therapy and/or cardiopulmonary supplies.

★ 16089 ★ Sage BioPharma, Inc.
135 Rtes. 202/206
Bedminster, NJ 07921
Phone: (908)306-5700 **Free:** 800-480-1985
Fax: (908)306-5722
Website: http://www.sagebiopharma.com
James Posillico, CEO & Pres
Desc: Manufacturer/distributor of Rx/ethical pharmaceuticals; OTC/proprietary pharmaceuticals.

★ 16090 ★ Saint Gobain Performance Plastics
460 Milltown Rd.
Bridgewater, NJ 08807
Free: 800-435-3992 **Fax:** (908)541-0025
Website: http://www.plastics.saint-gobain.com
Gerard Walsh, President
Desc: Manufacturer of laboratory supplies; pharmaceutical manufacturing supplies and equipment; respiratory therapy and/or cardiopulmonary supplies.

★ 16091 ★ St. Jude Medical
Cardiac Rhythm Management Division
15900 Valley View Ct.
Sylmar, CA 91342
Phone: (818)493-2826 **Free:** 800-777-2237
Fax: (818)362-8093
Website: http://www.sjm.com
Mike Coyle, CEO & Pres
Desc: Manufacturer/distributor of cardiovascular equipment and supplies.

★ 16092 ★ Salix Pharmaceuticals, Inc.
8540 Colonnade Center Dr.
Ste. 501
Raleigh, NC 27615
Phone: (919)862-1000 **Free:** 888-802-9956
Fax: (919)862-1096
Email: robert.ruscher@salixpharm.com
Website: http://www.salixpharm.com
Robert Ruscher, CEO & Pres
Desc: Manufacturer of Rx/ethical pharmaceuticals; gastroenterology products.

★ 16093 ★ Salk , Inc.
320 Washington St.
Brookline, MA 02445
Phone: (617)232-4030 **Free:** 800-343-4497
Fax: 800-343-0243
Email: salkco@aol.com
Website: http://www.salkcompany.com
Lawrence Salk, President
Desc: Manufacturer of apparel; home healthcare; hospital equipment and supplies; incontinence products; patient apparel; urinary equipment.

★ 16094 ★ Sammons Preston
An AbilityOne Co.
4 Sammons Ct.
Bolingbrook, IL 60440
Phone: (630)226-1300 **Free:** 800-323-5547
Fax: (630)226-1389
Email: sp@sammonspreston.com
Website: http://www.sammonspreston.com
Desc: Manufacturer/distributor of cardiovascular equipment; diagnostic equipment and instruments; home healthcare; hospital equipment and supplies; orthopedic and prosthetic equipment and supplies; patient aid products; physical therapy and rehabilitation equipment and supplies; skin/wound care products; ultrasound and electromedical equipment and supplies.

★ 16095 ★ SangStat, Inc.
6300 Dumbarton Circle
Fremont, CA 94555
Phone: (510)789-4300 **Fax:** (510)789-4400
Email: jbienaime@sangstat.com
Website: http://www.sangstat.com
Jean-Jacques Bienaime, Contact
Desc: Manufacturer/distributor of generic pharmaceuticals; biotechnology/biopharmaceutical products.

★ 16096 ★ Sankyo Parke Davis
Division of Sankyo Pharma Inc.
780 Third Ave.
4th Floor
New York, NY 10017
Phone: (212)884-8301 **Fax:** (212)308-2491
Email: jalexander@sankyopharma.com
Website: http://www.sankyopharma.com
John C. Alexander, President
Desc: Manufacturer/biotechnology company offering Rx/ethical pharmaceuticals and biotechnology/biopharmaceutical products.

★ 16097 ★ Sankyo Pharma Inc.
2 Hilton Ct.
Parsippany, NJ 07054
Phone: (973)359-2600 **Fax:** (973)359-2645
Website: http://www.sankyopharma.com
Joe Pieroni, President

Desc: Manufacturer/biotechnology company: Rx/ethical pharmaceuticals; biotechnology/biopharmaceutical products.

★ 16098 ★ Sanofi-Synthelabo, Inc.
Division of Sanofi-Synthelabo
90 Park Ave.
New York, NY 10016
Phone: (212)551-4000
Website: http://www.sanofi-synthelabous.com
Gordon Proctor, CEO & Pres

Desc: Manufacturer/distributor of Rx/ethical pharmaceuticals.

★ 16099 ★ Savage Laboratories
Division of Altanta Inc.
60 Baylis Rd.
Melville, NY 11747
Phone: (631)454-7677 **Free:** 800-231-0206
Fax: (631)454-0732
Email: savagelabs@altanainc.com
Website: http://www.savagelabs.com
George Cole, President

Desc: Manufacturer/distributor of Rx/ethical pharmaceuticals; skin/wound care products.

★ 16100 ★ Scale-Tronix, Inc.
200 E Post Rd.
White Plains, NY 10601
Phone: (914)948-8117 **Fax:** (914)948-0581
Website: http://www.scale-tronix.com
Carolyn Lepler, Contact

Desc: Manufacturer of hospital equipment and supplies; intensive care and neonatal care; physical therapy and rehabilitation equipment and supplies; renal dialysis supplies; scales for dialysis.

★ 16101 ★ Scanlan International, Inc.
1 Scanlan Plaza
Saint Paul, MN 55107
Phone: (651)298-0997 **Free:** 800-328-9458
Fax: (651)298-0018
Email: info@scanlangroup.com
Website: http://www.scanlangroup.com
Timothy M. Scanlan, CEO & Pres

Desc: Manufacturer of cardiovascular equipment and supplies; disposable medical devices and supplies; sterilization supplies; surgical disposables, instruments and supplies; hospital equipment and supplies.

★ 16102 ★ Scherer Laboratories, Inc.
120 Interstate N Parkway, Ste. 305
Atlanta, GA 30339
Phone: (770)933-1800 **Free:** 800-310-5357
Fax: (770)933-1880
Website: http://www.schererlabs.com
Robert P. Scherer, Jr., CEO & Chm Bd

Desc: Distributor of OTC/proprietary pharmaceuticals.

★ 16103 ★ Schering Laboratories
Division of Schering-Plough Corp.
2000 Galloping Hill Rd.
Kenilworth, NJ 07033
Phone: (908)298-4000
Website: http://www.schering-plough.com
Richard W. Zahn, President

Desc: Manufacturer of Rx/ethical pharmaceuticals.

★ 16104 ★ Schering-Plough Healthcare Products
Division of Schering-Plough Corp.
3 Connell Dr.
PO Box 603
Berkeley Heights, NJ 07922
Phone: (908)679-1640 **Fax:** (908)679-1840
Website: http://www.schering-plough.com
Mark Kirn-Slaboszewicz, President

Desc: Manufacturer of OTC/proprietary pharmaceuticals.

★ 16105 ★ Schleicher & Schuell, Inc.
10 Optical Ave.
PO Box 2012
Keene, NH 03431
Phone: (603)352-3810 **Free:** 800-245-4024
Fax: (603)357-3627
Email: techserv@s-and-s.com
Website: http://www.s-and-s.com
Gary Henricksen, President

Desc: Biotechnology company offering biological and environmental safety products; biotechnology/biopharmaceutical products; laboratory equipment and supplies.

★ 16106 ★ Schott Fiber Optics, Inc.
122 Charlton St.
Southbridge, MA 01550-1960
Phone: (508)765-9744 **Free:** 800-343-6120
Fax: (508)764-6273
Email: sfoinfo@us.schott.com
Website: http://www.us.schott.com/sfo
Donald A. Miller, President

Desc: Manufacturer offering contract manufacturing and fiber optic imaging components.

★ 16107 ★ Schwarz Pharma, Inc.
6140 W Executive Dr.
Mequon, WI 53092
Phone: (262)238-9994 **Free:** 800-558-5114
Fax: (262)238-0961
Website: http://www.schwarzpharma.com
Ron Stratton, PhD, Contact

Desc: Manufacturer/distributor of Rx/ethical pharmaceuticals and generic pharmaceuticals.

★ 16108 ★ Schwarz Pharma Manufacturing, Inc.
1101 W "C" Ave.
Freeman Field Industrial Park
Seymour, IN 47274
Phone: (812)523-3457 **Fax:** (812)523-1887
Website: http://www.schwarzusa.com
Patrick Schwarz-Schutte, Chairman of the Board

Desc: Manufacturer offering Rx/ethical pharmaceuticals; OTC/proprietary pharmaceuticals; contract manufacturing.

★ 16109 ★ Schwarzkof & Dep
2101 E Via Arado
Rancho Dominguez, CA 90220-6189
Phone: (310)604-0777 **Free:** 800-326-2855
Fax: (310)537-8438
Website: http://www.dep.com
Herman ter Haar, President

Desc: Manufacturer/distributor of OTC/proprietary pharmaceuticals; health and beauty aids; hospital equipment and supplies; Topol toothpaste.

★ 16110 ★ Scientific Industries, Inc.
70 Orville Dr.
Bohemia, NY 11716
Phone: (631)567-4700 **Free:** 888-850-6208
Fax: (631)567-5896
Email: info@scientificindustries.com
Website: http://www.scientificindustries.com
Lowell A. Kleiman, Contact

Desc: Manufacturer of hospital equipment and supplies; laboratory equipment.

★ 16111 ★ Scientific Instruments & Technology Corp.
470 Rte. 9
Englishtown, NJ 07726
Phone: (732)536-1550 **Fax:** (732)536-9179
Email: sitcorp@aol.com
Website: http://www.sitco-home.com
Yogi Shah, President

Desc: Manufacturer/distributor of Rx/ethical pharmaceuticals; OTC/proprietary pharmaceuticals; generic pharmaceuticals; dietary, nutritional and vitamin supplements; laboratory equipment and supplies; ophthalmic supplies; parenteral equipment and supplies; pharmaceutical manufacturing supplies and equipment.

★ 16112 ★ Scios Inc.
820 W Maude Ave.
Sunnyvale, CA 94085
Phone: (408)616-8200 **Free:** 800-522-9586
Fax: (408)616-8206
Email: investor_relations@sciosinc.com
Website: http://www.sciosinc.com
Richard B. Brewer, CEO & Pres

Desc: Biotechnology/biopharmaceutical products.

★ 16113 ★ Scott Health & Safety
Division of Scott Technologies Inc.
2206 W Roosevelt Blvd.
Monroe, NC 28110
Phone: (704)282-8400 **Fax:** (704)282-8424
Website: http://www.scottaviation.com
Jim Kaletta, Contact

Desc: Manufacturer of breathing equipment.

★ 16114 ★ Scott Specialties, Inc.
PO Box 508
Belleville, KS 66935-0508
Phone: (785)527-5627 **Free:** 800-255-7136
Fax: (785)527-5713
Email: customer.service@scottspecialties.com
Website: http://www.scottspecialties.com
Jim McDonald, President

Desc: Manufacturer of home healthcare; orthopedic and prosthetic equipment and supplies; patient aid products; physical therapy and rehabilitation equipment and supplies; physicians' supplies.

★ 16115 ★ SEBRA
100 N Tucson Blvd.
Tucson, AZ 85716
Phone: (520)881-6555 **Free:** 800-625-5550
Fax: (520)323-9055
Email: sales@sebra.com
Website: http://www.sebra.com
Alan Smith, President

Desc: Manufacturer of cardiovascular equipment; hospital equipment and supplies; laboratory equipment.

★ 16116 ★ Sechrist Industries, Inc.
4225 E La Palma Ave.
Anaheim, CA 92807
Phone: (714)579-8400 **Free:** 800-SECHRIST
Fax: (714)579-0814
Email: info@sechristind.com
Website: http://www.sechristind.com
J. Ronald Sechrist, CEO & Pres

Desc: Manufacturer of hyperbaric equipment; respiratory therapy and/or cardiopulmonary equipment; skin/wound care products.

★ 16117 ★ Seecor, Inc.
844 Dalworth Dr., Ste. 6
Mesquite, TX 75149

Phone: (972)288-3278 **Fax:** (972)288-3279
Jack E. Burroughs, Contact
Desc: Manufacturer/distributor/biotechnology company offering biotechnology/biopharmaceutical products; cardiovascular equipment and supplies; hospital equipment and supplies; patient monitoring equipment; physicians' equipment.

★ 16118 ★ SENETEK Drug Delivery Technologies, Inc.
Division of Senetek, PLC
620 Airpark Rd.
Napa, CA 94558
Phone: (707)226-3900 **Fax:** (707)226-3999
Website: http://www.senetekplc.com
Frank Massino, CEO
Desc: Manufacturer/distributor/biotechnology company offering Rx/ethical pharmaceuticals; generic pharmaceuticals; biotechnology/biopharmaceutical products; disposable medical devices and supplies; home healthcare.

★ 16119 ★ SensorMedics Corp.
Subsidiary of VIASYS Healthcare
22705 Savi Ranch Parkway
Yorba Linda, CA 92887
Phone: (714)283-2228 **Free:** 800-231-2466
Fax: (714)283-8439
Email: ed.pulwer@sensormedics.com
Website: http://www.sensormedics.com
Edward Pulwer, Contact
Desc: Manufacturer of cardiovascular equipment; diagnostic equipment and instruments; home healthcare; respiratory therapy and/or cardiopulmonary equipment and supplies; sleep diagnostics/therapeutics.

★ 16120 ★ Serono, Inc.
Affiliate of Serono, S.A.
1 Technology Pl.
Rockland, MA 02370
Phone: (781)982-9000 **Free:** 800-283-8088
Website: http://www.seronousa.com
Ernesto Bertaelli, Contact
Desc: Manufacturer/distributor of Rx/ethical pharmaceuticals; biotechnology/biopharmaceutical products.

★ 16121 ★ SF Medical
Division of Chase-Walton Elastomers, Inc.
19 Brent Dr.
Hudson, MA 01749
Phone: (978)568-0202 **Free:** 800-634-2000
Fax: (978)562-5178
Email: sales@chase-walton.com
Website: http://www.chase-walton.com
James C. Walton, Contact
Desc: Manufacturer/biotechnology company offering biotechnology/biopharmaceuticals products; disposable medical devices and supplies; laboratory supplies; ophthalmic supplies; parenteral catheters and supplies; pharmaceutical manufacturing supplies and equipment; renal dialysis equipment; skin/wound care products; sterilization equipment; surgical disposables and supplies; urinary equipment.

★ 16122 ★ SGD Pharma, Inc.
Division of Saint-Gobain Desjonqueres
750 Lexington Ave.
New York, NY 10022
Phone: (212)223-7100 **Fax:** (212)223-8371
Email: sgd.pharma@saint-gobain.com
Website: http://www.sgd-pharma.com
Jean-Pierre Floris, Contact
Desc: Manufacturer of molded glass for pharmaceutical packaging; parenteral supplies; pharmaceuticals manufacturing supplies and equipment.

★ 16123 ★ Shear/Kershman Laboratories, Inc.
701 Crown Industrial Ct.
Chesterfield, MO 63005
Phone: (636)519-8900 **Fax:** (636)215-2679
Email: jshear@shearkershman.com
Website: http://www.shearkershman.com
Jeff L. Shear, President
Desc: Manufacturer of Rx/ethical pharmaceuticals; OTC/proprietary pharmaceuticals; dietary, nutritional and vitamin supplements.

★ 16124 ★ Shercon, Inc.
10425 Slusher Dr.
Santa Fe Springs, CA 90670
Phone: (562)946-8555 **Fax:** (562)946-1015
Email: sherconla@aol.com
Website: http://www.shercon.com
Keith Ennis, CEO
Desc: Manufacturer of masking supplies.

★ 16125 ★ Shire US Inc.
PO Box 6497
Florence, KY 41022
Phone: (859)282-2100 **Free:** 800-536-7878
Fax: (859)282-2118
Website: http://www.shire.com
William Nuerge, CEO & Pres
Desc: Manufacturer/distributor of Rx/ethical pharmaceuticals; OTC/proprietary pharmaceuticals.

★ 16126 ★ SICOR Inc.
19 Hughes
Irvine, CA 92618
Phone: (949)455-4700 **Free:** 800-729-9991
Fax: (949)855-8210
Email: customer.service@gensiasicor.com
Website: http://www.sicorinc.com
Donald E. Panoz, Chairman of the Board
Desc: Manufacturer of Rx/ethical pharmaceuticals; generic pharmaceuticals; contract manufacturing.

★ 16127 ★ Siemens Medical Systems, Inc.
Electromedical Systems Division
16 Electronics Ave.
Danvers, MA 01923
Phone: (978)907-6300 **Free:** 800-333-8646
Fax: (978)907-6368
Website: http://www.siemensmedical.com
Michael Bunnell, Contact
Desc: Manufacturer of anesthesia equipment and products; cardiovascular equipment; diagnostic equipment and instruments; hospital equipment and supplies; patient monitoring equipment; respiratory therapy and/or cardiopulmonary equipment and supplies.

★ 16128 ★ Siemens Medical Systems, Inc.
Nuclear Medicine Group
2501 N Barrington Rd.
Hoffman Estates, IL 60195
Phone: (847)304-7700 **Fax:** (847)304-7712
Website: http://www.sms.siemens.com/nmg
Fahad Gaffoor, Contact
Desc: Manufacturer of diagnostic equipment and instruments; nuclear and radiological equipment and supplies.

★ 16129 ★ Siemens Medical Systems, Inc.
Oncology Care Systems Group
4040 Nelson Ave.
Concord, CA 94520-1271
Phone: (925)246-8200 **Free:** 800-318-5602
Fax: (925)246-8284
Website: http://www.sms.siemens.com/ocsg
Desc: Manufacturer/distributor of linear accelerators.

★ 16130 ★ Siemens Medical Systems, Inc.
Sales and Services Group
186 Wood Ave. S
Iselin, NJ 08830-2770
Phone: (732)321-4500 **Fax:** (732)494-2250
Website: http://www.siemensmedical.com
Thomas N. McCausland, CEO & Pres
Desc: Manufacturer of anesthesia equipment and products; cardiovascular equipment; diagnostic equipment and instruments; hearing aids; magnetic resonance imaging; nuclear and radiological equipment and supplies; patient monitoring equipment; radiation therapy devices; respiratory therapy and/or cardiopulmonary equipment and supplies; ultrasound and electromedical equipment and supplies; X-ray equipment and supplies.

★ 16131 ★ SIENCO, Inc.
11485 W 48th Ave.
Unit A
Wheat Ridge, CO 80033
Phone: (303)420-1148 **Free:** 800-432-1624
Fax: (303)420-2204
Email: sienco@sienco.com
Website: http://www.sienco.com/
Jon Henderson, President
Desc: Manufacturer of cardiovascular equipment; diagnostic equipment and instruments; diagnostic reagents and test kits; laboratory equipment and supplies.

★ 16132 ★ Sigma Diagnostics
Subsidiary of Sigma-Aldrich Corp.
545 S Ewing Ave.
Saint Louis, MO 63103
Phone: (314)771-5765 **Free:** 800-325-3424
Fax: (314)286-7813
Email: dbargiel@sial.com
Website: http://www.sigma-aldrich.com
Dana Bargiel, Contact
Desc: Manufacturer of diagnostic equipment and instruments; diagnostic reagents and test kits.

★ 16133 ★ SIGMA, Inc.
711 Park Ave.
Medina, NY 14103
Phone: (716)798-3901 **Free:** 800-356-3454
Fax: (716)798-3909
Email: customersupport@sigmapumps.com
Website: http://www.sigmapumps.com
Roger L. Hungerford, President
Desc: Manufacturer of home healthcare; hospital equipment and supplies; implants and infusion; parenteral equipment.

★ 16134 ★ Sigma-Tau Pharmaceuticals, Inc.
Division of Sigma-Tau S.p.A. of Rome, Italy
800 S Frederick Ave., Ste. 300
Gaithersburg, MD 20877
Phone: (301)948-1041 **Free:** 800-447-0169
Fax: (301)948-3194
Website: http://www.sigmatau.com
Claudio Cavazza, PhD, Contact
Desc: Distributor of Rx/ethical pharmaceuticals.

★ 16135 ★ Simmons Healthcare, Inc.
Division of Basic American Medical
2935 Northeast Parkway
Atlanta, GA 30360
Phone: (770)368-4700 **Free:** 800-334-8203
Fax: (770)368-4701
Jim Harkins, Contact
Desc: Manufacturer/distributor of hospital equipment and supplies; hospital furniture.

★ 16136 ★ SIMS Deltec, Inc.
1265 Grey Fox Rd.
Saint Paul, MN 55112
Phone: (651)633-2556 **Free:** 800-426-2448
Fax: (651)628-7459
Email: webmaster@deltec.com
Website: http://www.deltec.com
James Stitt, President
Desc: Manufacturer of disposable medical devices and supplies; home healthcare; hospital equipment and supplies; implants and infusion; parenteral catheters and equipment.

★ 16137 ★ Simulaids, Inc.
16 Dixon Ave.
PO Box 807
Woodstock, NY 12498
Phone: (845)679-2475 **Free:** 800-431-4310
Fax: (845)679-8996
Email: info@simulaids.com
Website: http://www.simulaids.com
Jack McNeff, Contact
Desc: Manufacturer/distributor of EMS equipment and supplies.

★ 16138 ★ Sklar Instrument Co.
889 S Matlack St.
West Chester, PA 19382
Phone: (610)430-3200 **Free:** 800-221-2166
Fax: (610)429-0500
Email: surgi@sklarcorp.com
Website: http://www.sklarcorp.com
Don Taylor, President
Desc: Manufacturer/distributor of dental equipment and supplies; diagnostic equipment and instruments; disposable medical devices and supplies; hospital equipment and supplies; ophthalmic equipment and supplies; physicians' equipment and supplies; sterilization equipment and supplies; surgical disposables, instruments and supplies; veterinary products.

★ 16139 ★ SkyePharma Inc.
10450 Science Center Dr.
San Diego, CA 92121
Phone: (858)625-2424 **Fax:** (858)625-2439
Email: john_longenecker@skyepharma.com
Website: http://www.skyepharma.com
John P. Longenecker, PhD, President
Desc: Manufacturer/biotechnology company offering Rx/ethical pharmaceuticals; biotechnology/biopharmaceutical products; drug delivery technology.

★ 16140 ★ Skytron
Division of KMW Group
5000 36th St., SE
Grand Rapids, MI 49512
Phone: (616)957-0500 **Free:** 800-SKY-TRON
Fax: (616)957-5053
Email: sales@skytronsurgical.com
Website: http://www.skytronsurgical.com
Dave Mehney, President
Desc: Manufacturer/distributor of anesthesia equipment and products; biological and environmental safety products; cardiovascular equipment; hospital equipment and supplies; imaging tables; vascular tables; ophthalmic equipment; orthopedic and prosthetic equipment and supplies; surgical and exam lights; power booms; ultrasonic equipment; urinary equipment.

★ 16141 ★ SmartPractice
3400 E McDowell Rd.
Phoenix, AZ 85008
Phone: (602)225-9090 **Fax:** (602)225-0599
Email: info@smartpractice.com
Website: http://www.smartpractice.com
Curtis P. Hamann, MD, CEO & Pres
Desc: Manufacturer/distributor of apparel; biological and environmental safety products; dental equipment and supplies; disposable medical devices and supplies; hospital equipment and supplies; patient aid products; physicians' supplies; skin/wound care products; slide viewing systems; sterilization equipment and supplies; urinary supplies; veterinary products; x-ray supplies.

★ 16142 ★ Smith & Nephew, Inc.
5825 Carnegie Blvd.
Charlotte, NC 28209
Phone: (704)331-0600 **Free:** 800-552-1157
Fax: (704)358-4558
Website: http://www.bsnmedical.com
Stuart Ashman, Contact
Desc: Manufacturer of orthopedic and prosthetic equipment and supplies; splinting and casting products.

★ 16143 ★ Smith & Nephew, Inc.
Endoscopy Division
160 Dascomb Rd.
Andover, MA 01810
Phone: (978)749-1000 **Free:** 800-343-8386
Fax: (978)749-1217
Website: http://www.endoscopy1.com
Ron Sparks, President
Desc: Manufacturer of arthroscopy/endoscopy surgical equipment and instrumentation; disposable medical devices and supplies; orthopedic and prosthetic equipment and supplies; powered surgical instruments; video cameras; surgical disposables and instruments.

★ 16144 ★ Smith & Nephew, Inc.
Rehabilitation Division
N104 W13400 Donges Bay Rd.
PO Box 1005
Germantown, WI 53022
Phone: (262)251-7840 **Free:** 800-228-3693
Fax: (262)251-7758
Website: http://www.smith-nephew.com
Jim McHargue, President
Desc: Manufacturer of disposable medical devices and supplies; home healthcare; hospital equipment and supplies; orthopedic and prosthetic equipment and supplies; patient aid products; physical therapy and rehabilitation equipment and supplies; skin/wound care products.

★ 16145 ★ Smith & Nephew, Inc.
Wound Management Division
11775 Starkey Rd.
Largo, FL 33773
Phone: (727)392-1261 **Free:** 800-289-1261
Fax: (727)399-3498
Website: http://www.smith-nephew.com
Rod Skaggs, President
Desc: Manufacturer of chronic wound care; IV site care; ostomy equipment and supplies; skin/wound care products.

★ 16146 ★ Solvay Pharmaceuticals, Inc.
901 Sawyer Rd.
Marietta, GA 30062
Phone: (770)578-9000 **Fax:** (770)578-5586
Website: http://www.solvay.com
Harold H. Shlevin, PhD, CEO & Pres
Desc: Manufacturer of Rx/ethical pharmaceuticals.

★ 16147 ★ Somerset Pharmaceuticals, Inc.
2202 NW Shore Blvd.
Ste. 450
Tampa, FL 33607
Phone: (813)288-0040 **Free:** 800-892-8889
Fax: (813)282-0287
Website: http://www.somersetpharm.com
Mel Sharoky, MD, CEO & Pres
Desc: Manufacturer of Rx/ethical pharmaceuticals; EMS equipment and supplies; sleep diagnostics/therapeutics.

★ 16148 ★ Southwest Technologies, Inc.
1746 Levee Rd.
North Kansas City, MO 64116
Phone: (816)221-2442 **Free:** 800-247-9951
Fax: (816)221-3995
Email: swtech@birch.net
Website: http://www.elastogel.com
Edward I. Stout, PhD, Contact
Desc: Manufacturer of dental supplies; disposable medical devices and supplies; EMS equipment and supplies; home healthcare; hospital equipment and supplies; orthopedic and prosthetic equipment and supplies; physical therapy and rehabilitation equipment and supplies; physicians' supplies; skin/wound care products; sterilization supplies; surgical supplies; veterinary products.

★ 16149 ★ Spacelabs Burdick
500 Burdick Parkway
Deerfield, WI 53531
Phone: (608)764-1919 **Free:** 800-777-1777
Fax: (608)764-7183
Email: slbinfo@slmd.com
Website: http://www.spacelabsburdick.com
Darryl Lustig, Contact
Desc: Manufacturer of cardiovascular equipment and supplies; diagnostic equipment and instruments; hospital equipment and supplies; patient monitoring equipment; physicians' equipment and supplies; respiratory therapy and/or cardiopulmonary equipment and supplies; ultrasound and electromedical equipment and supplies; sleep diagnostics/therapeutics; OXY 100 and OXY 200.

★ 16150 ★ Span-America Medical Systems, Inc.
PO Box 5231
Greenville, SC 29606
Phone: (864)288-8877 **Free:** 800-888-6752
Fax: (864)288-8692
Email: info@spanamerica.com
Website: http://www.spanamerica.com
Thomas Henrion, Chairman of the Board
Desc: Manufacturer of patient aid products; specialty mattresses and seat cushions; surgical positioners.

★ 16151 ★ Spectronics Corp.
956 Brush Hollow Rd.
PO Box 483
Westbury, NY 11590
Phone: (516)333-4840 **Free:** 800-274-8888
Fax: (516)333-4859
Email: uvuv@aol.com
Website: http://www.spectroline.com
Jonathan D. Cooper, President
Desc: Manufacturer/distributor/biotechnology company offering biotechnology/biopharmaceutical products; dental equipment; hospital equipment and supplies; laboratory equipment and supplies; nuclear and radiological supplies; ophthalmic equipment; veterinary products; X-ray supplies.

★ 16152 ★ Spectrum Laboratories Inc.
18617 Broadwick St.
Rancho Dominguez, CA 90220-6345
Phone: (310)885-4600 **Free:** 800-634-3300
Fax: (310)885-4666
Email: customerservice@spectrumlabs.com
Website: http://www.spectrumlabs.com
F. Jesus Martinez, President
Desc: Manufacturer/distributor/biotechnology company offering biotechnology/biopharmaceutical products; hospital equipment and supplies; laboratory equipment and supplies; physicians' supplies; surgical disposables.

★ 16153 ★ Spiral Biotech
An Advanced Instruments Co.
2 Technology Way
Norwood, MA 02062-2680

Phone: (781)320-9000 **Free:** 800-225-4034
Fax: (781)320-8181
Email: infosbi@spiralbiotech.com
Website: http://www.spiralbiotech.com
John Coughlin, President
Desc: Manufacturer of diagnostic equipment and instruments; diagnostic reagents and test kits.

★ 16154 ★ Spirometrics Medical Equipment Co.
22 Shaker Rd.
Gray, ME 04039
Phone: (207)657-6700 **Free:** 800-767-0004
Fax: (207)657-4123
Email: spiro@spirometrics.com
Website: http://www.spirometrics.com
Michael Kane, Contact
Desc: Manufacturer of diagnostic equipment and instruments; disposable medical devices and supplies; home healthcare; hospital equipment and supplies; physicians' equipment and supplies; respiratory therapy and/or cardiopulmonary equipment and supplies.

★ 16155 ★ Sporicidin International
121 Congressional Lane
Rockville, MD 20852
Phone: (301)231-7700 **Fax:** (301)231-8165
Email: info@sporicidin.com
Website: http://www.sporicidin.com
Robert I. Schattner, DDS, President
Desc: Manufacturer of dental supplies; ophthalmic supplies; physicians' supplies; sterilization supplies; veterinary products.

★ 16156 ★ Squire-Cogswell Co.
1111 Lakeside Dr.
Gurnee, IL 60031
Phone: (847)855-0500 **Free:** 800-662-5822
Fax: (847)855-6300
Email: info@healthcair.com
Website: http://www.healthcair.com
Carol Lewis, President
Desc: Manufacturer/distributor of hospital equipment and supplies.

★ 16157 ★ Stackhouse
Subsidiary of VIASYS Healthcare
1110 Bird Center Dr.
Palm Springs, CA 92262
Phone: (760)778-7300 **Free:** 800-325-0082
Fax: (760)778-6355
Email: stkhouse@viasyshealthcare.com
Website: http://www.stackhouseinc.com
Tom Kuhn, President
Desc: Manufacturer/distributor of apparel; biological and environmental safety products; biotechnology/biopharmaceutical products; cardiovascular equipment; dental equipment and supplies; disposable medical devices and supplies; hospital equipment and supplies; ophthalmic equipment; orthopedic and prosthetic equipment and supplies; patient monitoring equipment; pharmaceutical manufacturing supplies and equipment; surgical disposables; surgical helmet systems; surgical smoke evacuators; surgical supplies; ultrasound and electromedical equipment and supplies; veterinary products.

★ 16158 ★ STADA Pharmaceuticals, Inc.
5 Cedar Brook Dr.
Cranbury, NJ 08512
Phone: (609)409-5999 **Free:** 800-542-6482
Fax: (609)409-5995
Website: http://www.stada.com
Christian Scheiner, President
Desc: Manufacturer of OTC/proprietary pharmaceuticals; generic pharmaceuticals.

★ 16159 ★ Stanbio Laboratory
1261 N Main St.
Boerne, TX 78006
Phone: (830)249-0772 **Free:** 800-531-5535
Fax: (830)249-0851
Email: stanbio@stanbio.com
Website: http://www.stanbio.com
William R. Pippin, President
Desc: Manufacturer of diagnostic equipment and instruments; diagnostic reagents and test kits; laboratory supplies; physicians' equipment and supplies; urinary equipment and supplies.

★ 16160 ★ Standard Textile Co., Inc.
1 Knollcrest Dr.
Cincinnati, OH 45237
Phone: (513)761-9255 **Free:** 800-999-0400
Fax: (513)761-0467
Email: info@standardtextile.com
Website: http://www.standardtextile.com
Norman A. Frankel, Contact
Desc: Manufacturer/distributor of apparel; home healthcare; hospital equipment and supplies; skin/wound care products.

★ 16161 ★ Stanford Professional Products Corp.
1416 Union Ave.
Pennsauken, NJ 08110
Phone: (856)665-4054 **Free:** 800-345-3929
Fax: (856)665-3511
Email: info@stanfordproducts.com
Website: http://www.stanfordproducts.com
Lee F. Mueller, Contact
Desc: Manufacturer of dental supplies; hospital equipment and supplies; incontinence supplies; laboratory supplies; patient aid products; physicians' supplies.

★ 16162 ★ Star Pharmaceuticals
1990 NW 44th St.
Pompano Beach, FL 33064
Phone: (954)971-9704 **Free:** 800-845-7827
Fax: (954)971-7718
Email: info@starpharm.com
Website: http://www.starpharm.com
Scott L. Davidson, Contact
Desc: Manufacturer/distributor of Rx/ethical pharmaceuticals; OTC/proprietary pharmaceuticals; urologic pharmaceuticals.

★ 16163 ★ Star (tm) Dental Products
DentalEZ Group
1816 Colonial Village Lane
Lancaster, PA 17601
Phone: (717)291-1161 **Fax:** (717)291-3249
Email: jbrunozzi@dentalez.com
Website: http://www.dentalez.com
John Brunozzi, Contact
Desc: Manufacturer of dental equipment and supplies; X-ray equipment.

★ 16164 ★ Star X-Ray Co., Inc.
63 Ranick Dr.
Amityville, NY 11701
Phone: (631)842-3010 **Free:** 800-374-2163
Fax: (631)842-5901
Website: http://www.starxray.com
Erik Rosen, President
Desc: Manufacturer of dental equipment and supplies; veterinary products; X-ray equipment.

★ 16165 ★ Staveley Sensors, Inc.
Subsidiary of Staveley NDT Technologies Inc.
91 Prestige Park Circle
East Hartford, CT 06108
Phone: (860)289-5428 **Fax:** (860)289-3189
Email: staveley.sndt.xtals@snet.net
Website: http://www.staveleyndt.com
Joseph Zarrelli, Contact
Desc: Manufacturer/distributor of ultrasonic equipment; ultrasound and electromedical equipment and supplies.

★ 16166 ★ Steelcraft, Inc.
115 W Main St.
Millbury, MA 01527
Phone: (508)865-4445 **Fax:** (508)865-4600
Email: db@steelcraft-inc.com
Website: http://www.steelcraft-inc.com
Douglas J. Backman, President
Desc: Manufacturer of hospital equipment and supplies; laboratory equipment; patient aid products; physicians' equipment.

★ 16167 ★ Stellar Pharmacal Corp.
Subsidiary of Star Pharmaceuticals
1990 NW 44th St.
Pompano Beach, FL 33064
Phone: (954)972-6060 **Free:** 800-845-7827
Fax: (954)971-7718
Email: info@starpharm.com
Website: http://www.starpharm.com
Scott L. Davidson, Contact
Desc: Manufacturer/distributor of Rx/ethical pharmaceuticals; OTC/proprietary pharmaceuticals; brand name pharmaceuticals; OTC products.

★ 16168 ★ Steridyne Corp.
3725 Investment Lane
Riviera Beach, FL 33404
Phone: (561)844-3486 **Free:** 800-327-6185
Fax: (561)844-8415
Email: steridyn@bellsouth.net
Joseph L. Del Vecchio, President
Desc: Manufacturer of OTC/proprietary pharmaceuticals; home healthcare; hospital equipment and supplies; patient aid products; patient monitoring equipment; physicians' supplies.

★ 16169 ★ STERIS Corp.
5960 Heisley Rd.
Mentor, OH 44060-1834
Phone: (440)354-2600 **Free:** 800-548-4873
Fax: (440)350-7086
Website: http://www.steris.com
Les C. Vinney, Contact
Desc: Manufacturer/biotechnology company offering anesthesia equipment and products; hospital equipment and supplies; hospital furniture; laboratory equipment and supplies; ophthalmic equipment; orthopedic and prosthetic equipment and supplies; patient handling equipment; procedure chairs; stretcher; pharmaceutical manufacturing supplies and equipment; physical therapy and rehabilitation equipment and supplies; physicians' equipment; skin/wound care products; sterilization equipment and supplies; surgical beds, tables and lights; surgical disposables and supplies; ultrasonic equipment; X-ray equipment.

★ 16170 ★ Stiefel Laboratories, Inc.
255 Alhambra Circle
Ste. 1000
Coral Gables, FL 33134
Phone: (305)443-3800 **Fax:** (305)443-3467
Website: http://www.stiefel.com
Werner K. Stiefel, Chairman of the Board
Desc: Manufacturer of Rx/ethical pharmaceuticals; OTC/proprietary pharmaceuticals; generic pharmaceuticals.

★ 16171 ★ Stockwell Scientific
7325 E Evans Rd.
Scottsdale, AZ 85260
Phone: (480)951-1111 **Free:** 800-722-8920
Fax: (480)951-6117
Website: http://www.stockwellscientific.com
Joe Stockwell, President
Desc: Manufacturer/biotechnology company offering biotechnology/biopharmaceutical products; disposable

medical devices and supplies; hospital equipment and supplies; laboratory equipment and supplies; pharmaceutical manufacturing supplies and equipment; physicians' supplies.

★ 16172 ★ Stryker Corp.
PO Box 4085
Kalamazoo, MI 49003
Phone: (616)385-2600 **Fax:** (616)385-1062
Website: http://www.strykercorp.com
John W. Brown, Contact
Desc: Manufacturer of hospital equipment and supplies; hospital furniture; implants and infusion; sterilization supplies; surgical disposables and instruments.

★ 16173 ★ Stryker Instruments Division of Stryker Corp.
4100 E Milham Ave.
Kalamazoo, MI 49001
Phone: (616)323-7700 **Free:** 800-253-3210
Fax: 800-999-3811
Website: http://www.strykercorp.com
Si Johnson, Contact
Desc: Manufacturer/distributor of skin/wound care products; surgical disposables and instruments.

★ 16174 ★ Sultan Dental Products
242 S Dean St.
Englewood, NJ 07631
Phone: (201)894-5500 **Free:** 800-238-6739
Fax: (201)894-1539
Website: http://www.sultandental.com
Herb Wolfe, President
Desc: Manufacturer of dental equipment and supplies.

★ 16175 ★ Sulzer Carbomedics Inc. A company of Sulzer Medica USA Inc.
1300 E Anderson Lane
Austin, TX 78752
Phone: (512)435-3200 **Free:** 800-648-1579
Fax: (512)435-3395
Website: http://www.carbomedics.com
Terry L. Marlatt, President
Desc: Manufacturer/distributor of cardiovascular supplies.

★ 16176 ★ Sulzer Dental Inc.
1900 Aston Ave.
Carlsbad, CA 92008
Phone: (760)929-4300 **Free:** 800-854-7019
Fax: (760)431-7811
Email: marketing@sulzerdental.com
Website: http://www.sulzerdental.com
Steven Hanson, President
Desc: Manufacturer/distributor of dental implants and supplies; oral wound care products.

★ 16177 ★ Summit Hill Laboratories
1 Sheila Dr.
Tinton Falls, NJ 07724
Phone: (732)933-0800 **Free:** 800-922-0722
Fax: (732)933-0055
Email: vmstntnfls@aol.com
Charles W. Rahner, Jr., Contact
Desc: Manufacturer/distributor of Rx/ethical pharmaceuticals; OTC/proprietary pharmaceuticals; anesthesia equipment and products; dental equipment and supplies; hospital equipment and supplies; lasers; surgical instruments; ultrasonic equipment; veterinary products.

★ 16178 ★ Summit Industries, Inc. Creomulsion/Lantiseptic Division
839 Pickens Industrial Dr.
PO Box 7329
Marietta, GA 30065
Phone: (770)590-0600 **Free:** 800-241-6996
Fax: (770)590-0714
Website: http://www.summitinds.com
Arthur Howell, Chairman of the Board
Desc: Manufacturer of OTC/proprietary pharmaceuticals; skin/wound care products.

★ 16179 ★ Sunrise Medical
5001 Joerns Dr.
Stevens Point, WI 54481
Phone: (715)341-3600 **Free:** 800-826-0270
Fax: (715)341-3962
Email: info_ccg@sunmed.com
Website: http://www.sunrisemedical.com
Allen Traylor, Contact
Desc: Manufacturer/distributor of hospital equipment and supplies; hospital furniture; patient aid products; physical therapy and rehabilitation equipment and supplies; skin/wound care products.

★ 16180 ★ Sunrise Medical Inc.
7477 E Dry Creek Parkway
Longmont, CO 80503
Phone: (303)218-4600 **Free:** 800-333-4000
Fax: 800-300-7502
Website: http://www.sunrisemedical.com
John Kitts, President
Desc: Manufacturer of home healthcare; hospital equipment and supplies; hospital furniture; patient aid products; physical therapy and rehabilitation equipment and supplies; respiratory therapy and/or cardiopulmonary equipment and supplies; skin/wound care products; sleep diagnostics/therapeutics; surgical supplies; urinary supplies.

★ 16181 ★ Sunwest Vitamin Corp.
PO Box D 3700
Pomona, NY 10970
Phone: (845)354-8787 **Fax:** (845)354-8703
A.P. Bedrosian, JD, CEO & Pres
Desc: Manufacturer of Rx/ethical pharmaceuticals; OTC/proprietary pharmaceuticals; generic pharmaceuticals; dietary, nutritional and vitamin supplements; disposable medical devices and supplies; physicians' supplies; renal dialysis supplies; skin/wound care products; surgical disposables and instruments.

★ 16182 ★ Supelco
Supelco Park
Bellefonte, PA 16823
Phone: (814)359-3441 **Free:** 800-247-6628
Fax: (814)359-5459
Email: supelco@sial.com
Website: http://www.sigma-aldrich.com/supelco
Russel Gant, President
Desc: Manufacturer/distributor/biotechnology company offering biotechnology/biopharmaceutical products; diagnostic reagents and test kits; laboratory equipment and supplies; pharmaceutical manufacturing supplies and equipment.

★ 16183 ★ Superior Uniform Group, Inc.
10099 Seminole Blvd.
PO Box 4002
Seminole, FL 33772
Phone: (727)397-9611 **Fax:** (727)391-5401
Email: info@superioruniformgroup.com
Gerald M. Benstock, CEO
Desc: Manufacturer of apparel; patient aid products; sterilization supplies.

★ 16184 ★ SupratekPharma Inc.
455 Fenelon Blvd.
Ste. 104
Montreal, QC, Canada H9S 5T8
Phone: (514)849-6094 **Fax:** (514)282-1338
Email: info@supratek.com
Website: http://www.supratek.com
Oleg Romar, Contact
Desc: Biotechnology company offering Rx/ethical pharmaceuticals; biotechnology/biopharmaceutical products.

★ 16185 ★ Surgical Instrument Co. of America
1185 Edgewater Ave.
Ridgefield, NJ 07657
Phone: (201)941-6500 **Fax:** (201)941-6656
Email: sicoa@aol.com
Alfred G. Biberfeld, President
Desc: Manufacturer/distributor of dental equipment and supplies; diagnostic equipment and instruments; disposable medical devices and supplies; EMS equipment and supplies; hospital equipment and supplies; ophthalmic supplies; sterilization equipment; surgical disposables and instruments.

★ 16186 ★ Surgical Specialties Corp.
100 Dennis Dr.
Reading, PA 19606
Phone: (610)404-1000 **Free:** 800-523-3332
Fax: (610)404-4010
Email: info@surgicalspecialties.com
Website: http://www.surgspecialties.com
Steve Bryant, Contact
Desc: Manufacturer of cardiovascular supplies; dental supplies; surgical disposables and supplies.

★ 16187 ★ Swift Instruments, Inc. Scientific Instrument Division
1190 N Fourth St.
San Jose, CA 95112
Phone: (408)293-2380 **Free:** 800-523-4544
Fax: (408)292-7967
Email: sales@swiftoptics.com
Website: http://www.swiftmicroscope.com
Alison Swift, President
Desc: Manufacturer of hospital equipment and supplies; laboratory equipment; physicians' equipment; USB digital video microscopy.

★ 16188 ★ Syncor Pharmaceutical Services Division of Syncor International Corp.
6464 Canoga Ave.
Woodland Hills, CA 91367-2407
Phone: (818)737-4000 **Free:** 800-999-9098
Fax: (818)737-4676
Email: funarib@syncor.com
Website: http://www.syncor.com
Bob Funari, CEO & Pres
Desc: Distributor of magnetic resonance imaging; nuclear and radiological equipment and supplies; radiopharmaceuticals; renal dialysis equipment.

★ 16189 ★ Syncor Radiation Management
6045 Cochran Rd.
Cleveland, OH 44139
Phone: (440)248-9300 **Free:** 800-850-4608
Fax: (440)349-2307
Website: http://www.inovision.com
Tim Hansen, Contact
Desc: Manufacturer of diagnostic equipment and instruments; hospital equipment and supplies; quality assurance devices; radiation measurements.

★ 16190 ★ Synthes (U.S.A.)
1690 Russell Rd.
PO Box 1766
Paoli, PA 19301
Phone: (610)647-9700 **Fax:** (610)695-2475
Desc: Manufacturer/distributor of orthopedic implants; surgical instruments; veterinary products.

★ 16191 ★ Sysmex Corp. of America Subsidiary of Sysmex Corp. of Japan
6699 Wildlife Way
Long Grove, IL 60047
Phone: (847)726-3500 **Free:** 800-3-SYSMEX
Fax: (847)726-3559
Email: mktcom@sysmex.com

Website: http://www.sysmex.com
John Kershaw, Contact

Desc: Manufacturer of diagnostic equipment and instruments; diagnostic reagents and test kits; laboratory equipment and supplies; Sysmex UF-100 automated urinalysis analyzer; urinary equipment and reagents; urinary supplies.

★ 16192 ★ TAP Pharmaceutical Products Inc.
675 N Field Dr.
Lake Forest, IL 60045
Free: 800-348-2779 **Fax:** (847)582-4540
Website: http://www.tap.com
Tom Watkins, President

Desc: Manufacturer of Rx/ethical pharmaceuticals.

★ 16193 ★ Techne, Inc.
743 Alexander Rd.
Princeton, NJ 08540-6328
Phone: (609)452-9275 **Free:** 800-225-9243
Fax: (609)987-8177
Email: labproducts@techneusa.com
Website: http://www.techneusa.com
Neil R. Pope, President

Desc: Manufacturer/biotechnology company offering biotechnology/biopharmaceutical products; diagnostic equipment and instruments; hospital equipment and supplies; laboratory equipment and supplies.

★ 16194 ★ TeleDiagnostic Systems
1757 E Bayshore Rd., Ste. 24
Redwood City, CA 94063
Phone: (650)474-0424 **Free:** 800-227-3224
Fax: (650)474-0427
Email: info@telediagnostic.com
Website: http://www.telediagnostic.com
Larry Woodard, MD, President

Desc: Manufacturer of diagnostic equipment and instruments; home healthcare; hospital equipment and supplies; patient monitoring equipment; sleep diagnostics/therapeutics.

★ 16195 ★ Terumo Cardiovascular Systems
Capiox (r), Sarns (tm), and CDI (tm) Products
6200 Jackson Rd.
Ann Arbor, MI 48103-9300
Phone: (734)663-4145 **Free:** 800-521-2818
Fax: (734)663-7981
Website: http://www.terumo-cvs.com
Mark Sutter, CEO & Pres

Desc: Manufacturer/distributor of cardiovascular equipment and supplies; hospital equipment and supplies; patient monitoring equipment; surgical disposables.

★ 16196 ★ Terumo Medical Corp.
American Bloc Headquarters
2101 Cottontail Lane
Somerset, NJ 08873
Phone: (732)302-4900 **Free:** 800-283-7866
Fax: (732)302-4905
Website: http://www/terumomedical.com
Shogo Ninomiya, CEO & Pres

Desc: Manufacturer of cardiovascular supplies; dental supplies; disposable medical devices and supplies; home healthcare; hospital equipment and supplies; laboratory equipment and supplies; nuclear and radiological equipment and supplies; patient monitoring equipment; physicians' supplies; renal dialysis supplies; respiratory therapy and/or cardiopulmonary supplies; safety hypodermic supplies; interventional radiology supplies.

★ 16197 ★ Tetra Medical Supply Corp.
6364 W Gross Point Rd.
Niles, IL 60714-3916
Phone: (847)647-0590 **Free:** 800-621-4041
Fax: (847)647-9034
Email: sales@tetramed.com
Website: http://www.tetramed.com
Constance A. Shier, President

Desc: Manufacturer/distributor of disposable medical devices and supplies; EMS equipment and supplies; hospital equipment and supplies; orthopedic and prosthetic equipment and supplies; patient aid products; physical therapy and rehabilitation equipment and supplies; physicians' supplies; skin/wound care products; surgical disposables and instruments; ultrasound and electromedical equipment and supplies.

★ 16198 ★ TEVA Pharmaceutical Industries Ltd.
PO Box 1142
91010 Jerusalem, Israel
Phone: 011 97 22 589 2811 **Fax:** 011 97 22 589 2839
Email: pr@teva.co.il
Website: http://www.tevapharm.com
Meir Heth, Chairman of the Board

Desc: Manufacturer/distributor of Rx/ethical pharmaceuticals; OTC/proprietary pharmaceuticals; generic pharmaceuticals; biotechnology/biopharmaceutical products; dental supplies; diagnostic reagents and test kits; disposable medical devices and supplies; home healthcare; hospital equipment and supplies; pharmaceutical manufacturing supplies and equipment; renal dialysis equipment and supplies; veterinary products.

★ 16199 ★ TEVA Pharmaceuticals USA
1090 Horsham Rd.
North Wales, PA 19454
Phone: (215)591-3000 **Free:** 888-TEVA-USA
Fax: (215)591-8600
Email: info@tevausa.com
Website: http://www.tevapharmusa.com
George Barrett, CEO & Pres

Desc: Manufacturer of generic pharmaceuticals.

★ 16200 ★ Texas Biotechnology Corp.
7000 Fannin, 20th floor
Houston, TX 77030
Phone: (713)796-8822 **Fax:** (713)796-8232
Email: dmcwilliams@tbc.com
Website: http://www.tbc.com
John M. Pietruski, Chairman of the Board

Desc: Biotechnology company offering Rx/ethical pharmaceuticals.

★ 16201 ★ TFX Medical, Inc.
Division of Teleflex Inc.
50 Plantation Dr.
Jaffrey, NH 03452
Phone: (603)532-7706 **Free:** 800-548-6600
Fax: (603)532-6108
Email: info@tfx.com
Website: http://www.tfxmedical.com
Peter Rothe, President

Desc: Manufacturer of anesthesia equipment and products; cardiovascular supplies; contract manufacturing; disposable medical devices and supplies; parenteral catheters; surgical disposables.

★ 16202 ★ Thames Pharmacal Co.
2100 Fifth Ave.
Ronkonkoma, NY 11779
Phone: (631)737-1155 **Free:** 800-225-1003
Fax: (631)737-3185
Email: info@thamespharmacal.com
Mary B. Harmon, Chairman of the Board

Desc: Manufacturer/distributor of Rx/ethical pharmaceuticals; OTC/proprietary pharmaceuticals; generic pharmaceuticals.

★ 16203 ★ Therabite Corp.
1530 McDaniel Dr.
West Chester, PA 19380
Phone: (610)429-4545 **Free:** 800-322-2650
Fax: (610)429-4484
Email: rhorst@therabite.com
Website: http://www.therabite.com
Robert W. Horst, President

Desc: Manufacturer/distributor of disposable medical devices and supplies; home healthcare; MRI device; patient aid products; physical therapy and rehabilitation equipment and supplies.

★ 16204 ★ Theradyne Healthcare Products Division
Division of Kurt Manufacturing Co.
395 Ervin Industrial Dr.
Jordan, MN 55352
Phone: (612)502-6190 **Free:** 800-328-4014
Fax: 800-458-7864
Website: http://www.theradyne.com
Paul Lawson, Contact

Desc: Manufacturer offering contract manufacturing; home healthcare; hospital equipment and supplies; orthopedic and prosthetic equipment and supplies; physical therapy and rehabilitation equipment and supplies; cardiovascular equipment.

★ 16205 ★ THERAKOS
A Johnson & Johnson Co.
437 Creamery Way
Exton, PA 19341
Phone: (610)280-1000 **Fax:** (610)280-1087
Website: http://www.therakos.com
Roy Davis, President

Desc: Manufacturer of hospital equipment and supplies; disposable medical devices and supplies.

★ 16206 ★ Thermo Andersen Instruments, Inc.
500 Technology Ct.
Smyrna, GA 30082-5211
Phone: (770)319-9999 **Free:** 800-241-6898
Fax: (770)319-0336
Website: http://www.thermoandersen.com
Sam Lanasa, Contact

Desc: Manufacturer/biotechnology company: air monitoring equipment; biological and environmental safety products.

★ 16207 ★ Thermo Finnigan Corp.
355 River Oaks Parkway
San Jose, CA 95134
Phone: (408)965-6000 **Free:** 800-532-4752
Fax: (408)965-6010
Email: moreinfo@thermofinnigan.com
Website: http://www.thermofinnigan.com
Dr. Ian Jardine, President

Desc: Manufacturer of laboratory equipment and supplies.

★ 16208 ★ Thermo Forma
PO Box 649
Marietta, OH 45750
Phone: (740)373-4763 **Free:** 800-848-3080
Fax: (740)374-1817
Email: marketing@thermoforma.com
Website: http://www.thermoforma.com
Randy Andersen, Contact

Desc: Manufacturer of laboratory equipment.

★ 16209 ★ Thermo IEC
300 Second Ave.
Needham Heights, MA 02494
Phone: (781)449-8060 **Free:** 800-843-1113
Fax: (781)444-6743
Email: info@thermoeic.com
Website: http://www.labcentrifuge.com
Mark Shon, Contact

Desc: Manufacturer of laboratory equipment and supplies.

★ 16210 ★ Thermo NESLAB
PO Box 1178
Portsmouth, NH 03802-1178
Phone: (603)436-9444 **Free:** 800-258-0830
Fax: (603)436-8411
Email: thermoneslab@thermoneslab.com
Website: http://www.thermoneslab.com
Roland Schultner, CEO
Desc: Manufacturer of laboratory equipment.

★ 16211 ★ Thermo Orion
A Thermo Electron Business
500 Cummings Center
Beverly, MA 01915
Phone: (978)232-6000 **Free:** 800-225-1480
Fax: (978)232-6015
Email: webmaster@thermoorion.com
Website: http://www.thermoorion.com
James Barbookles, CEO & Pres
Desc: Manufacturer/biotechnology company offering biological and environmental safety products; biotechnology/biopharmaceutical products; diagnostic equipment and instruments; hospital equipment and supplies; laboratory equipment and supplies; pharmaceutical manufacturing supplies and equipment.

★ 16212 ★ Thermo Savant
100 Colin Dr.
Holbrook, NY 11741
Phone: (631)244-2929 **Free:** 800-634-8886
Fax: (631)244-0606
Email: savantec@savec.com
Website: http://www.thermosavant.com
Mark Shon, President
Desc: Manufacturer/biotechnology company offering biotechnology/biopharmaceutical products; laboratory equipment.

★ 16213 ★ Thermo Shandon
A Thermo Electron Business
171 Industry Dr.
Pittsburgh, PA 15275
Phone: 800-245-6212 **Free:** 800-547-7429
Fax: (412)788-1138
Email: thermoshandon@thermoshandon.com
Website: http://www.thermoshandon.com
Mark Zinsky, President
Desc: Manufacturer/distributor of autopsy/mortuary refrigerators and freezers; casework; hospital equipment and supplies; laboratory equipment and supplies; veterinary products.

★ 16214 ★ Thermo Westronics Inc.
Formerly Westronics
22001 N Park Dr.
Ste. 100
Kingwood, TX 77339-3804
Phone: (281)348-1800 **Fax:** (281)348-1288
Email: sales@thermowestronics.com
Website: http://www.thermowestronics.com
Desc: Manufacturer offering data acquisitions; laboratory equipment; recorders; chart recorders; video graphic recorders.

★ 16215 ★ Thomas Scientific
99 High Hill Rd. at I-295
PO Box 99
Swedesboro, NJ 08085
Phone: (856)467-2000 **Free:** 800-345-2100
Fax: (856)467-3087
Email: value@thomassci.com
Website: http://www.thomassci.com
G. Wesner, President
Desc: Distributor/biotechnology company offering biotechnology/biopharmaceutical products; diagnostic equipment and instruments; laboratory equipment and supplies; ultrasonic equipment.

★ 16216 ★ Thompson Surgical Instruments, Inc.
10170 E Cherry Bend Rd.
Traverse City, MI 49684
Phone: (231)922-0177 **Free:** 800-227-7543
Fax: (231)922-0174
Website: http://www.thompsonsurgical.com
Dan Farley, President
Desc: Surgical instruments manufacturer.

★ 16217 ★ Thought Technology, Ltd.
2180 Belgrave Ave.
Montreal, QC, Canada H4A 2L8
Phone: (514)489-8251 **Free:** 800-361-3651
Fax: (514)489-8255
Email: mail@thoughttechnology.com
Website: http://www.thoughttechnology.com
Hal K. Myers, PhD, President
Desc: Manufacturer of diagnostic equipment and instruments; patient aid products; patient monitoring equipment; physical therapy and rehabilitation equipment and supplies; physicians' equipment; respiratory therapy and/or cardiopulmonary equipment and supplies; sleep diagnostics/therapeutics; ultrasound and electromedical equipment and supplies; urinary equipment.

★ 16218 ★ 3M
3M Drug Delivery Systems Division
3M Center
Bldg. 275-3E-10
Saint Paul, MN 55144-1000
Phone: (651)736-3549 **Fax:** (651)737-5265
Website: http://www.3M.com/dds
Sue Thoreson, Contact
Desc: Manufacturer of Rx/ethical pharmaceuticals.

★ 16219 ★ 3M Health Care
3M Center, Bldg. 275-4E-01
Saint Paul, MN 55144-1000
Phone: (651)604-5599 **Free:** 800-228-3957
Fax: (651)633-2072
Email: healthcare@3m.com
Website: http://www.3M.com/healthcare
Desc: Manufacturer of Rx/ethical pharmaceuticals; OTC/proprietary pharmaceuticals; generic pharmaceuticals; dental equipment and supplies; diagnostic equipment and instruments; disposable medical devices and supplies; home healthcare; hospital equipment and supplies; ophthalmic supplies; ostomy equipment and supplies; patient aid products; patient monitoring equipment; pharmaceutical manufacturing supplies and equipment; physical therapy and rehabilitation equipment and supplies; physicians' equipment and supplies; skin/wound care products; sterilization equipment and supplies; surgical disposables and instruments; surgical tapes; veterinary products.

★ 16220 ★ 3M Pharmaceuticals
Division of 3M
3M Center, Bldg. 275-3W-01
Saint Paul, MN 55133-3275
Phone: (651)736-4930 **Free:** 800-328-0255
Fax: (651)736-8930
Website: http://www.3M.com/pharma
Thomas B. Harrison, Vice President
Desc: Manufacturer of Rx/ethical pharmaceuticals.

★ 16221 ★ 3M Unitek Corp.
Dental Products Division
2724 S Peck Rd.
Monrovia, CA 91016-5097
Phone: (626)574-4000 **Free:** 800-634-5300
Fax: (626)574-4892
Email: mrlane@mmm.com
Website: http://www.3Munitek.com
Michael Lane, Contact
Desc: Manufacturer of orthodontic supplies.

★ 16222 ★ TimeMed Labeling Systems, Inc.
144 Tower Dr.
Burr Ridge, IL 60527
Phone: (630)986-1800 **Free:** 800-323-4840
Fax: (630)986-0016
Website: http://www.timemed.com
John Nerad, CEO
Desc: Manufacturer of hospital equipment and supplies; pressure sensitive tapes and labels.

★ 16223 ★ Tobias Associates, Inc.
50 Industrial Dr.
PO Box 2699
Ivyland, PA 18974
Phone: (215)322-1500 **Free:** 800-877-3367
Fax: (215)322-1504
Email: tobias@densitometer.com
Website: http://www.densitometer.com
Philip E. Tobias, President
Desc: Manufacturer of hospital equipment and supplies; laboratory equipment; X-ray equipment.

★ 16224 ★ Tomey Corp. USA
300 Second Ave.
Waltham, MA 02451
Phone: (781)890-1515 **Free:** 800-358-6639
Fax: (781)290-5885
Email: sales@tomey.com
Website: http://www.tomey.com
Leslie Amodei, Contact
Desc: Ophthalmic equipment manufacturer.

★ 16225 ★ Tomtec Inc.
1000 Sherman Ave.
Hamden, CT 06514
Phone: (203)281-6790 **Fax:** (203)248-5724
Email: info@tomtec.com
Website: http://www.tomtec.com
Thomas W. Astle, President
Desc: Manufacturer/distributor of biotechnology/biopharmaceutical products; laboratory equipment and supplies; pharmaceutical manufacturing supplies and equipment.

★ 16226 ★ Toolmex Corp.
Medical Instruments and Equipment Division
1075 Worcester Rd.
Natick, MA 01760
Phone: (508)653-8897 **Free:** 800-992-4766
Fax: (508)653-5110
Email: arkadiusz.kielb@toolmex.com
Website: http://www.toolmex.com
Arkadiusz Kielb, President
Desc: Distributor of dental equipment and supplies; orthopedic and prosthetic equipment and supplies; surgical instruments; veterinary products.

★ 16227 ★ Topix Pharmaceuticals, Inc.
Dermatopics & Pharmatopics Divisions
5200 New Horizons Blvd.
North Amityville, NY 11701-1144
Phone: (631)225-5757 **Free:** 800-445-2595
Fax: (631)226-8588
Stanley Shaffer, Chairman of the Board
Desc: Manufacturer of OTC/proprietary pharmaceuticals; generic pharmaceuticals; skin/wound care products.

★ 16228 ★ TORBOT Group, Inc.
1367 Elmwood Ave.
PO Box 3564
Cranston, RI 02910
Phone: (401)780-8737 **Free:** 800-545-4254
Fax: (401)780-8740
Email: torbot@worldnet.att.net
Website: http://www.torbot.com
Stephen Yarlas, President

Desc: Manufacturer/distributor of disposable medical devices and supplies; home healthcare; ostomy equipment and supplies; patient aid products; skin/wound care products; surgical supplies; urinary equipment.

★ 16229 ★ Toshiba America Medical Systems, Inc.
2441 Michelle Dr.
Tustin, CA 92780
Phone: (714)730-5000 **Free:** 800-421-1968
Fax: (714)505-3076
Email: jburch@tams.com
Website: http://www.medical.toshiba.com
Jim Burch, Contact

Desc: Manufacturer of cardiovascular equipment; diagnostic equipment and instruments; magnetic resonance imaging; nuclear and radiological equipment; ultrasonic equipment; X-ray equipment.

★ 16230 ★ Triangle Pharmaceuticals
PO Box 50530
4611 University Dr.
No. 4 University Place
Durham, NC 27717
Phone: (919)493-5980 **Free:** 800-264-2142
Fax: (919)493-5925
Website: http://www.tripharm.com
David Barry, MD, CEO & Chm Bd

Desc: Biotechnology company: Rx/ethical pharmaceuticals; biotechnology/biopharmaceutical products.

★ 16231 ★ Tridak Division of Indicon, Inc.
144-B Old Brookfield Rd.
Danbury, CT 06811
Phone: (203)798-7471 **Free:** 800-289-8735
Fax: (203)798-8154
Email: tridak@tridak.com
Website: http://www.tridak.com
Paul S. Citrin, Contact

Desc: Manufacturer/biotechnology company offering biotechnology/biopharmaceutical products; dental equipment; diagnostic equipment and instruments; laboratory equipment; pharmaceutical manufacturing supplies and equipment.

★ 16232 ★ Trigen Laboratories, Inc. Division of Trinity Laboratories, Inc.
201 Kiley Dr.
PO Box 1818
Salisbury, MD 21801-1818
Phone: (410)860-8500 **Fax:** (410)860-2913
Email: sales@trigenlabs.com
Website: http://www.trigenlabs.com
A.P. Bedrosian, JD, CEO & Pres

Desc: Manufacturer of Rx/ethical pharmaceuticals; generic pharmaceuticals; contract manufacturing; cardiovascular supplies; physicians' supplies; renal dialysis supplies; skin/wound care products; surgical disposables, instruments, and supplies.

★ 16233 ★ Trimeris Inc.
3518 Westgate Dr.
3rd floor
Durham, NC 27707
Phone: (919)419-6050 **Fax:** (919)419-1816
Email: info@trimeris.com
Website: http://www.trimeris.com
Dr. Dani Bolognesi, Contact

Desc: Biotechnology company offering Rx/ethical pharmaceuticals; biotechnology/biopharmaceutical products.

★ 16234 ★ Trimline Medical Products Corp.
PO Box 40
Raritan, NJ 08869-0040
Phone: (908)429-0590 **Free:** 800-526-3538
Fax: (908)429-0536
Email: trimmed@infi.net
Website: http://www.trimlinemed.com
Rich Jacobson, President

Desc: Manufacturer of disposable medical devices and supplies; hospital equipment and supplies; physicians' supplies.

★ 16235 ★ Trinity Biotech USA
PO Box 1059
2823 Girts Rd.
Jamestown, NY 14702-1059
Phone: (716)483-3851 **Fax:** (716)488-1990
Website: http://www.trinitybiotech.com
Brendan Farrell, President

Desc: Manufacturer of diagnostic equipment and instruments; diagnostic reagents and test kits.

★ 16236 ★ Triton Consumer Products, Inc.
561 W Golf Rd.
Arlington Heights, IL 60005
Phone: (847)228-7650 **Fax:** (847)228-7691
Email: triton@intersccess.com
Website: http://www.mg217.com
Karen L. Shrader, Contact

Desc: Manufacturer of OTC/proprietary pharmaceuticals; skin/wound care products.

★ 16237 ★ Trueform-OTC Orthotics and Prosthetics Division of Surgical Appliance Industries
3960 Rosslyn Dr.
Cincinnati, OH 45209
Phone: (513)271-4594 **Free:** 800-888-0458
Fax: 800-309-9055
Email: trueform-otc@surgicalappliance.com
Website: http://www.surgicalappliance.com
Tom Applegate, CEO & Pres

Desc: Manufacturer/distributor of orthopedic and prosthetic equipment and supplies; patient aid products.

★ 16238 ★ Turner Designs
845 W Maude Ave
Sunnyvale, CA 94085
Phone: (408)749-0994 **Fax:** (408)749-0998
Email: sales@turnerdesigns.com
Website: http://www.turnerdesigns.com
Mike Mokelke, President

Desc: Manufacturer/biotechnology company offering biotechnology/biopharmaceutical products; diagnostic equipment and instruments; laboratory equipment.

★ 16239 ★ Tyco Healthcare Mallinckrodt Imaging
675 McDonnell Blvd.
PO Box 5840
Saint Louis, MO 63134
Phone: (314)654-8262 **Fax:** (314)654-3860
Website: http://www.mallinckrodt.com
John T. Friedl, Contact

Desc: Manufacturer of cardiovascular equipment; diagnostic equipment and instruments; disposable medical devices and supplies; hospital equipment and supplies; magnetic resonance imaging; radiological equipment and supplies; x-ray equipment and supplies.

★ 16240 ★ Tyco Healthcare Mallinckrodt
675 McDonnell Blvd.
PO Box 5840
Saint Louis, MO 63141
Phone: (314)654-2000 **Fax:** (314)654-5381
Website: http://www.tycohealthcare.com
Michael J. Collins, Contact

Desc: Manufacturer/distributor of disposable medical devices and supplies; EMS equipment and supplies; home healthcare; hospital equipment and supplies; implants and infusion; patient aid products; patient monitoring equipment; physical therapy and rehabilitation equipment and supplies; physicians' equipment and supplies; respiratory therapy and/or cardiopulmonary equipment and supplies; sleep diagnostics/therapeutics; ultrasound and electromedical equipment and supplies.

★ 16241 ★ U.M.A., Inc.
260 Main St.
PO Box 100
Dayton, VA 22821
Phone: (540)879-2040 **Free:** 800-842-5578
Fax: (540)879-2738
Email: umainc@rica.net
Website: http://www.umainstruments.com
Awad Da'Mes, President

Desc: Manufacturer of hospital equipment and supplies; medical test equipment.

★ 16242 ★ UCB Pharma, Inc.
1950 Lake Park Dr.
Smyrna, GA 30080
Phone: (770)437-5500 **Free:** 800-477-7877
Fax: (770)437-5514
Website: http://www.ucbepilepsy.com
Anthony G. Tebbutt, President

Desc: Manufacturer/distributor of Rx/ethical pharmaceuticals; OTC/proprietary pharmaceuticals.

★ 16243 ★ UDL Laboratories Inc. Subsidiary of Mylan Laboratories Inc.
1718 Northrock Ct.
Rockford, IL 61103
Phone: (815)282-1201 **Free:** 800-435-5272
Fax: (815)282-9391
Website: http://www.udllabs.com
Sherri MacDonald, Contact

Desc: Manufacturer/distributor of Rx/ethical pharmaceuticals; generic pharmaceuticals.

★ 16244 ★ Ulmer Pharmacal
1614 Industry Ave.
PO Box 408
Park Rapids, MN 56470
Phone: (218)732-2656 **Free:** 800-848-5637
Fax: (218)732-5300
Email: ulmer@unitelc.com
Al Trudeau, President

Desc: Manufacture of OTC/proprietary pharmaceuticals; skin/wound care products.

★ 16245 ★ Ulster Scientific, Inc.
83 S Putt Corners Rd.
New Paltz, NY 12561
Phone: (845)255-2200 **Fax:** (845)255-3299
Email: ulstersci@aol.com
Website: http://www.usi.ebz.com
Peter F. Lordi, Jr., President

Desc: Manufacturer/distributor of diagnostic equipment and instruments; laboratory equipment and supplies.

★ 16246 ★ Uni-Patch
1313 W Grant Blvd.
PO Box 271
Wabasha, MN 55981
Phone: (651)565-2601 **Free:** 800-328-9454
Fax: (651)565-3971
Email: sales@uni-patch.com
Website: http://www.uni-patch.com
Brian H. Wolfe, P, President

Desc: Manufacturer offering contract manufacturing; physical therapy and rehabilitation equipment and supplies; ultrasound and electromedical equipment and supplies; skin/wound care products; disposable medical devices and supplies.

★ 16247 ★ United Hospital Supply Corp.
PO Box 1238
Burlington, NJ 08016

Phone: (609)387-7580 Free: 800-486-8484
Fax: (609)387-0803
Email: jlyons3298@aol.com
Website: http://www.lab-design.com
Jonathan Lyons, Vice President

Desc: Manufacturer of hospital furniture; medication carts; pharmacy/ laboratory casework.

★ 16248 ★ United Research Labs/Mutual Pharmaceutical
1100 Orthodox St.
Philadelphia, PA 19124
Phone: (215)288-6500 Free: 800-523-3684
Fax: (215)807-1090
Website: http://www.urlmutual.com
Richard Roberts, PhD, CEO

Desc: Manufacturer/distributor of generic pharmaceuticals.

★ 16249 ★ U.S. Orthotics, Inc.
8605 Palm River Rd.
Tampa, FL 33619
Phone: (813)621-7797 Fax: (813)623-1055
Website: http://www.usorthotics.com
Anthony E. Velazquez, President

Desc: Manufacturer/distributor of orthopedic and prosthetic equipment and supplies.

★ 16250 ★ Unitron, Inc.
120- C Wilbur St.
PO Box 469
Bohemia, NY 11716
Phone: (631)589-6666 Fax: (631)589-6975
Email: info@unitronusa.com
Website: http://www.unitronusa.com
Thomas A. Zappetti, Contact

Desc: Manufacturer/distributor of laboratory equipment.

★ 16251 ★ Universal Surgical Appliance Co.
400 NE 191st St.
Miami, FL 33179
Phone: (305)652-0810 Free: 800-635-8319
Fax: (305)654-8485
David Lehman, Vice President

Desc: Manufacturer of orthopedic appliances.

★ 16252 ★ Universal Voltronics Corp.
57 Commerce Dr.
Brookfield, CT 06804
Phone: (203)740-8555 Fax: (203)740-8103
Website: http://www.voltronics.com
Leonard Braverman, PhD, President

Desc: Manufacturer of biological and environmental safety products; cardiovascular equipment; X-ray equipment and supplies.

★ 16253 ★ Upsher-Smith Laboratories, Inc.
14905 23rd Ave. N
Minneapolis, MN 55447
Phone: (763)475-3023 Free: 800-654-2299
Fax: (763)449-6612
Website: http://www.upsher-smith.com
Kenneth L. Evenstad, CEO & Chm Bd

Desc: Manufacturer of Rx/ethical pharmaceuticals; OTC/proprietary pharmaceuticals; generic pharmaceuticals; dietary, nutritional and vitamin supplements.

★ 16254 ★ Upsher-Smith Laboratories, Inc.
Denver Division
301 S Cherokee St.
Denver, CO 80223
Free: 800-445-8091 Fax: (303)733-8703
Website: http://www.upsher-smith.com

Desc: Manufacturer of Rx/ethical pharmaceuticals; OTC/proprietary pharmaceuticals; generic pharmaceuticals; dietary, nutritional and vitamin supplements.

★ 16255 ★ Urocare Products Inc.
2735 Melbourne Ave.
Pomona, CA 91767-1931
Phone: (909)621-6013 Free: 800-423-4441
Fax: (909)621-4436
Email: sales@urocare.com
Website: http://www.urocare.com
Friedhelm Franke, Contact

Desc: Manufacturer/distributor of disposable medical devices and supplies; home healthcare; physical therapy and rehabilitation equipment and supplies; skin/ wound care products; urinary equipment and supplies.

★ 16256 ★ Uroplasty, Inc.
2718 Summer St., NE
Minneapolis, MN 55413-2820
Phone: (612)378-1180 Fax: (612)378-2027
Email: info.usa@uroplasty.com
Website: http://www.uroplasty.com
Daniel Holman, CEO & Pres

Desc: Manufacturer of hospital equipment and supplies; implants and infusion.

★ 16257 ★ Utak Laboratories, Inc.
25020 Ave. Tibbitts
Valencia, CA 91355
Phone: (661)294-3935 Free: 800-235-3442
Fax: (661)294-9272
Email: utakcontrols@worldnet.att.net
Website: http://www.utaklabs.com
Judy H. Plutchak, President

Desc: Manufacturer of diagnostic reagents and test kits; OEM.

★ 16258 ★ v STAT-CHEK Co.
PO Box 25308
Seattle, WA 98125
Phone: (206)364-2174 Free: 800-248-6618
Fax: (206)364-5384
Email: stat-chek@worldnet.att.net
E. G. McFarling, President

Desc: Manufacturer/distributor of patient aid products.

★ 16259 ★ Vacudyne, Inc.
375 E Joe Orr Rd.
Chicago Heights, IL 60411
Phone: (708)757-5200 Fax: (708)757-7180
Email: info@vacudyne.com
Website: http://www.vacudyne.com
Bob Williams, Contact

Desc: Manufacturer of sterilization equipment.

★ 16260 ★ Valley Forge Scientific Corp.
136 Green Tree Rd.
PO Box 1179
Oaks, PA 19456
Phone: (610)666-7500 Fax: (610)666-7565
Jerry L. Malis, President

Desc: Manufacturer of disposable medical devices and supplies; hospital equipment and supplies; surgical disposables.

★ 16261 ★ Valleylab
Division of Tyco Healthcare Group LP
5920 Longbow Dr.
Boulder, CO 80301
Phone: (303)530-2300 Free: 800-255-8522
Fax: (303)530-6285
Website: http://www.valleylab.com
Richard Granger, President

Desc: Manufacturer of hospital equipment and supplies; surgical disposables, instruments and supplies; ultrasonic equipment.

★ 16262 ★ Varian Medical Systems/ Interay
3235 Fortune Dr.
North Charleston, SC 29418
Phone: (843)767-3005 Free: 800-468-3729
Fax: (843)760-0079
Email: interay.sales@varian.com
Website: http://www.varian.com
Robert Hibdon, Contact

Desc: Manufacturer of hospital equipment and supplies; rotating medical X-ray tubes; X-ray equipment.

★ 16263 ★ Varian X-Ray Products/Interay
3235 Fortune Dr.
North Charleston, SC 29418
Phone: (843)767-3005 Free: 800-468-3729
Fax: (843)760-0079
Email: steve.kimmel@varian.com
Website: http://www.varian.com
Steve Kimmel, Contact

Desc: Manufacturer of rotating medical X-ray tubes; X-ray equipment.

★ 16264 ★ Velcro USA Inc.
406 Brown Ave.
Manchester, NH 03108
Phone: (603)669-4880 Free: 800-225-0180
Fax: (603)669-9271
Email: marketing@velcro.com
Website: http://www.velcro.com
Lorrie Piper, Contact

Desc: Manufacturer of home healthcare; hospital equipment and supplies; patient aid products; surgical disposables.

★ 16265 ★ Ventura Enterprises
35 Lawton Ave.
Danville, IN 46122
Phone: (317)745-2989 Fax: (317)745-3179
Website: http://www.venturaenterprises.com
Linda L. Plunkett, Contact

Desc: Manufacturer of patient aid products.

★ 16266 ★ Venusa, Ltd.
31 Butterfield Trail, Ste. C
El Paso, TX 79906
Phone: (915)771-9112 Fax: (915)771-9107
Email: info@venusa.com
Website: http://www.venusa.com
Ross Magladry, Contact

Desc: Manufacturer offering contract manufacturing; disposable medical devices and supplies.

★ 16267 ★ Vertex Pharmaceuticals Inc.
130 Waverly St.
Cambridge, MA 02139-4242
Phone: (617)444-6100 Fax: (617)444-6680
Email: webmaster@vpharm.com
Website: http://www.vrtx.com
Joshua Boger, PhD, CEO & Chm Bd

Desc: Biotechnology company offering Rx/ethical pharmaceuticals.

★ 16268 ★ VH Technologies
185 E 85th St.
New York, NY 10028
Phone: (212)427-4859
Email: afreed1@nyc.rr.com
Anna B. Freed, Contact

Desc: Manufacturer of disposable medical devices and supplies; patient aid products.

★ 16269 ★ VIASYS Healhcare
1100 Bird Center Dr.
Palm Springs, CA 92262
Phone: (760)778-7200 Free: 800-937-3750
Fax: (760)778-7274
Website: http://www.viasyscriticalcare.com
Tony van den Berg, President

Desc: Manufacturer of hospital equipment and supplies; respiratory therapy and/or cardiopulmonary equipment and supplies.

★ 16270 ★ Virbac Corp.
3200 Meacham Blvd.
Fort Worth, TX 76137
Phone: (817)831-5030 **Free:** 800-338-3659
Fax: (817)831-8327
Website: http://www.virbac.com
Thomas Bell, CEO & Pres
Desc: Manufacturer/distributor of Rx/ethical pharmaceuticals; OTC/proprietary pharmaceuticals; veterinary products; dental supplies; dietary, nutritional and vitamin supplements.

★ 16271 ★ ViroPharma Inc.
405 Eagleview Blvd.
Exton, PA 19341
Phone: (610)458-7300 **Fax:** (610)458-7380
Email: medicalinfo@viropharma.com
Website: http://www.viropharma.com
Michael de Rosen, CEO & Pres
Desc: Manufacturer/biotechnology company: Rx/ethical pharmaceuticals; OTC/proprietary pharmaceuticals; biotechnology/biopharmaceutical products.

★ 16272 ★ VirTis
An SP Industries Co.
815 Rte. 208
Gardiner, NY 12525
Phone: (845)255-5000 **Free:** 800-431-8232
Fax: (845)255-5338
Email: sales@virtis.com
Website: http://www.virtis.com
S. G. Bart, Jr., President
Desc: Manufacturer/distributor of laboratory equipment; pharmaceutical manufacturing supplies and equipment.

★ 16273 ★ Viscot Industries, Inc.
32 West St.
PO Box 351
East Hanover, NJ 07936
Phone: (973)887-9273 **Free:** 800-221-0658
Fax: (973)887-3961
Email: info@viscot.com
Website: http://www.viscot.com
Vincent Muccione, President
Desc: Manufacturer of dental supplies; disposable medical devices and supplies; drapes and dental bibs; hospital equipment and supplies; male and female urinals; professional towels; sterilization supplies, sterilization wrap; surgical disposables; surgical skin markers; surgical supplies; urinary equipment and supplies.

★ 16274 ★ Vision-Sciences, Inc.
9 Strathmore Rd.
Natick, MA 01760
Phone: (508)650-9971 **Free:** 800-874-9975
Fax: (508)653-0533
Email: info@visionsciences.com
Website: http://www.vision-sciences.com
Katsumi Oneda, Contact
Desc: Manufacture of disposable medical devices and supplies; endoscopes; hospital equipment and supplies.

★ 16275 ★ Vita Needle Co.
919 Great Plain Ave.
Needham, MA 02492
Phone: (781)444-1780 **Fax:** (781)444-3956
Email: sales@vitaneedle.com
Website: http://www.vitaneedle.com
Frederick M. Hartman, President
Desc: Manufacturer of cardiovascular supplies; dental supplies; laboratory equipment and supplies; nuclear and radiological supplies; ophthalmic supplies; physicians' supplies; surgical disposables and instruments; urinary supplies; X-ray equipment.

★ 16276 ★ VIVUS, Inc.
1172 Castro St.
Mountain View, CA 94040
Phone: (650)934-5200 **Free:** 888-367-6873
Fax: (650)934-5389
Email: ir@vivus.com
Website: http://www.vivus.com
Leland Wilson, CEO & Pres
Desc: Manufacturer of Rx/ethical pharmaceuticals; OTC/proprietary pharmaceuticals.

★ 16277 ★ Vollrath Group
209 Vollrath Dr.
PO Box 228
Gallaway, TN 38036
Phone: (901)867-2951 **Free:** 800-233-1987
Fax: (901)867-8954
Email: email@vollrathgroup.com
Website: http://www.vollrathgroup.com
Jim Trautschold, Contact
Desc: Manufacturer of cardiovascular supplies; dental supplies; disposable medical devices and supplies; home healthcare; hospital equipment and supplies; laboratory equipment and supplies; patient aid products; physicians' supplies; skin/wound care products; sterilization equipment and supplies; surgical instruments; urinary equipment and supplies.

★ 16278 ★ Volu-Sol, Inc.
5095 W 2100 South
Salt Lake City, UT 84120
Phone: (801)974-9474 **Free:** 800-821-2495
Fax: (801)974-9553
Email: volu-sol@slkc.ufwest.net
Website: http://www.volusol.com
Bill Kirton, CEO
Desc: Manufacturer of diagnostic reagents and test kits.

★ 16279 ★ VuMax File Systems, Inc.
510 W Exchange St.
PO Box 181
Spring Lake, MI 49456
Phone: (616)847-0380 **Free:** 800-628-1945
Fax: (616)847-0980
Website: http://www.viewmax.com
Rich Robinson, CEO
Desc: Manufacturer of hospital furniture; shelves for files.

★ 16280 ★ VWR International
1310 Goshen Parkway
West Chester, PA 19380
Phone: (610)431-1700 **Free:** 800-932-5000
Email: solutions@vwr.com
Website: http://www.vwr.com
Walter Zywottek, CEO & Chm Bd
Desc: Distributor/biotechnology company offering apparel; biological and environmental safety products; biotechnology/biopharmaceutical products; laboratory equipment and supplies; sterilization equipment; surgical disposables and instruments; ultrasonic equipment; veterinary products; safety products for laboratory/industrial settings; skin/wound care products.

★ 16281 ★ W.A. Baum Co., Inc.
620 Oak St.
Copiague, NY 11726
Phone: (631)226-3940 **Free:** 888-281-6061
Fax: (631)226-3969
Email: info@wabaum.com
Website: http://www.wabaum.com
John C. Baum, President
Desc: Manufacturer of hospital equipment and supplies; physicians' equipment.

★ 16282 ★ W.F. Young, Inc.
302 Benton Dr.
East Longmeadow, MA 01028
Phone: (413)526-9999 **Free:** 800-628-9653
Fax: (413)526-8990
Email: marketing@absorbine.com
Website: http://www.absorbine.com
Tyler F. Young, CEO & Pres
Desc: Manufacturer of OTC/proprietary pharmaceuticals.

★ 16283 ★ Wako Chemicals USA, Inc.
BioProducts Division
1600 Bellwood Rd.
Richmond, VA 23237
Phone: (804)271-7677 **Free:** 800-922-WAKO
Fax: (804)271-7791
Email: bioproducts@wakousa.com
Website: http://www.wakousa.com
Hiroshi Shima, President
Desc: Manufacturer/distributor/biotechnology company offering biotechnology/biopharmaceutical products; diagnostic reagents and test kits; laboratory supplies.

★ 16284 ★ Wallace Laboratories
MedPointe Co.
265 Davidson Ave.
Ste. 300
Somerset, NJ 08875-6833
Phone: (732)564-2200
Website: http://www.medpointeinc.com
Anthony H. Wild, PhD, CEO & Chm Bd
Desc: Manufacturer/distributor of Rx/ethical pharmaceuticals.

★ 16285 ★ Walter Lorenz Surgical, Inc.
Wholly owned subsidiary of Biomet, Inc.
1520 Tradeport Dr.
Jacksonville, FL 32218
Phone: (904)741-4400 **Free:** 800-874-7711
Fax: (904)741-4500
Website: http://www.lorenzsurgical.com
Joel Pratt, President
Desc: Manufacturer of craniofacial products; surgical instruments.

★ 16286 ★ Wampole Laboratories
MedPointe Co.
2 Research Way
Half Acre Rd.
Princeton, NJ 08540
Free: 800-257-9525 **Fax:** 800-532-0295
Email: wampole@medpointeinc.com
Website: http://www.wampolelabs.com
Jean Zych, Contact
Desc: Manufacturer/distributor of diagnostic equipment and instruments; diagnostic reagents and test kits; laboratory equipment and supplies; physicians' equipment and supplies.

★ 16287 ★ Ware-Medics Glass Works, Inc.
Garnerville Holding Co.
55 W Railroad Ave., Bldg. 14
PO Box 368
Garnerville, NY 10923
Phone: (845)429-6950 **Fax:** (845)429-6951
Email: sales@waremedics.com
Ann Benitto, President
Desc: Manufacturer/distributor of dental equipment; hospital equipment and supplies; laboratory equipment and supplies; urinary equipment; veterinary products.

★ 16288 ★ Warner Chilcott Inc.
Division of Galen Pharmaceuticals
100 Enterprise Dr., No. 280
Rockaway, NJ 07866

Phone: (973)442-3200 **Free:** 800-521-8813
Fax: (973)442-3346
Website: http://www.wclabs.com
Roger M. Boissonneault, CEO
Desc: Manufacturer/distributor of Rx/ethical pharmaceuticals.

★ 16289 ★ WaterLoo Healthcare Division of Easton Enterprises, LLC
1821 Lincoln St.
Cedar Falls, IA 50613-0527
Phone: (319)277-6090 **Free:** 800-833-4419
Fax: (319)277-6091
Email: dwright@waterloohealthcare.com
Website: http://www.waterloohealthcare.com
Douglas Wright, Contact
Desc: Manufacturer of hospital equipment and supplies.

★ 16290 ★ Waterpik Technologies, Inc.
1730 E Prospect Rd.
Fort Collins, CO 80553-0001
Phone: (970)484-1352 **Free:** 800-525-2020
Fax: (970)221-8715
Email: service@waterpik.com
Website: http://www.waterpik.com
Robert A. Shortt, Contact
Desc: Manufacturer of dental equipment and supplies; diagnostic equipment and instruments.

★ 16291 ★ Waters Medical Systems Division of Waters Instruments, Inc.
2411 Seventh St., NW
Rochester, MN 55901
Phone: (507)252-3784 **Free:** 800-426-9877
Fax: (507)252-3700
Website: http://www.watersmed.com
Jerry Grabowski, President
Desc: Manufacturer/distributor of cardiovascular equipment and supplies; transplant devices and supplies.

★ 16292 ★ Watson Laboratories, Inc. Subsidiary of Watson Pharmaceuticals, Inc.
311 Bonnie Circle
Corona, CA 92880-2882
Phone: (909)270-1400 **Fax:** (909)270-1096
Website: http://www.watsonpharm.com
Susan Skara, Contact
Desc: Manufacturer of Rx/ethical pharmaceuticals; OTC/proprietary pharmaceuticals; generic pharmaceuticals.

★ 16293 ★ Watson Pharm, Inc. Wholly owned subsidiary of Watson Pharmaceuticals, Inc.
360 Mt. Kemble Ave.
Morristown, NJ 07962
Phone: (973)355-8300 **Fax:** (973)355-8301
Website: http://www.watsonpharm.com
Allen Chao, CEO & Chm Bd
Desc: Manufacturer/distributor of Rx/ethical pharmaceuticals; generic pharmaceuticals.

★ 16294 ★ Weck Closure Systems Division of Teleflex Inc.
1 Weck Dr.
PO Box 12600
Research Triangle Park, NC 27709
Phone: (919)544-8000 **Free:** 800-334-9751
Fax: (919)361-3914
Email: sholmes@weckclosure.com
Website: http://www.weckclosuresystems.com
J. Stephen Holmes, President
Desc: Manufacturer/distributor of disposable medical devices and supplies; implants and infusion; skin/wound care products; surgical disposables and instruments.

★ 16295 ★ Welch Allyn, Inc.
4341 State St. Rd.
Skaneateles Falls, NY 13153
Phone: (315)685-4100 **Free:** 800-535-6663
Fax: (315)685-3361
Email: info@welchallyn.com
Website: http://www.welchallyn.com
Lew F. Allyn, Chairman of the Board
Desc: Manufacturer of cardiovascular equipment; diagnostic equipment and instruments; disposable medical devices and supplies; EMS equipment and supplies; hospital equipment and supplies; ophthalmic equipment; patient monitoring equipment; physicians' equipment; respiratory therapy and/or cardiopulmonary equipment; surgical equipment; veterinary products.

★ 16296 ★ Wells Johnson Co.
8000 S Kolb Rd.
PO Box 18230
Tucson, AZ 85731-8230
Phone: (520)298-6069 **Free:** 800-528-1597
Fax: (520)885-1189
Email: sales@wellsgrp.com
Website: http://www.wellsgrp.com
John F. Wells, President
Desc: Manufacturer/distributor of apparel; diagnostic equipment and instruments; hospital equipment and supplies; patient monitoring equipment; sterilization equipment; surgical disposables; ultrasonic equipment.

★ 16297 ★ WellSpring Pharmaceutical Corp.
1430 Rte. 34
Neptune, NJ 07753
Phone: (732)983-5885 **Fax:** (732)751-9056
Website: http://www.wellspringpharma.com
Robert Vukovich, PhD, Contact
Desc: Manufacturer of Rx/ethical pharmaceuticals; OTC/proprietary pharmaceuticals.

★ 16298 ★ Wescor, Inc.
459 S Main
Logan, UT 84321
Phone: (435)752-6011 **Free:** 800-453-2725
Fax: (435)752-4127
Email: biomed@wescor.com
Website: http://www.wescor.com
Wayne K. Barlow, President
Desc: Manufacturer of diagnostic equipment and instruments; hospital equipment and supplies; laboratory equipment and supplies.

★ 16299 ★ West Pharmaceutical Services
101 Gordon Dr.
Lionville, PA 19353
Phone: (610)594-2900 **Free:** 800-345-9800
Fax: (610)594-3000
Email: webmaster@westpharma.com
Website: http://www.westpharma.com
William G. Little, CEO & Chm Bd
Desc: Manufacturer offering clinical services; contract laboratory; dental supplies; disposable medical devices and supplies; drug delivery; implants and infusion; laboratory supplies; ophthalmic supplies; parenteral supplies; pharmaceutical manufacturing supplies and equipment.

★ 16300 ★ Whatman Inc.
9 Bridewell Pl.
Clifton, NJ 07014
Phone: (973)773-5800 **Free:** 888—WHATMAN
Fax: (973)472-6949
Email: info@whatman.com
Website: http://www.whatman.com
Bodo Franz, President
Desc: Manufacturer of laboratory equipment and supplies; sterilization equipment.

★ 16301 ★ Wheaton, Inc. Division of Alcan
1101 Wheaton Ave.
Millville, NJ 08332
Phone: (856)825-0400 **Free:** 800-959-4328
Fax: (856)765-2004
Website: http://www.algroupwheaton.com
Rich Tobin, Contact
Desc: Manufacturer of parenteral supplies.

★ 16302 ★ Wheaton Science Products
1501 N 10th St.
Millville, NJ 08332
Phone: (856)825-1100 **Free:** 800-225-1437
Fax: (856)825-1368
Email: products@wheatonsci.com
Website: http://www.wheatonsci.com
Steve Drozdow, President
Desc: Manufacturer of electronic equipment; glass and plastic containers, equipment and apparatuses; laboratory equipment and supplies.

★ 16303 ★ Whitestone Acquisition Corp.
4265 W Vernal Pike
Bloomington, IN 47404
Phone: (812)332-3703 **Free:** 800-800-2042
Fax: (812)333-3270
Jamie Better, President
Desc: Manufacturer of home healthcare; patient aid products; urinary supplies.

★ 16304 ★ Wilder Manufacturing Co., Inc.
41 Mechanic St.
PO Box 1112
Port Jervis, NY 12771
Phone: (845)856-5188 **Free:** 800-832-1319
Fax: (845)856-1950
Website: http://www.winholt.com
Bruce Schwartz, Contact
Desc: Manufacturer of hospital equipment and supplies; laboratory equipment.

★ 16305 ★ Winco, Inc.
5516 SW First Lane
Ocala, FL 34474
Phone: (352)854-2929 **Free:** 800-237-3377
Fax: (352)854-9544
Email: sales@wincomfg.com.
Website: http://www.wincomfg.com
Don R. Frank, President
Desc: Manufacturer of home healthcare; hospital equipment and supplies; hospital furniture; patient aid products; physical therapy and rehabilitation equipment and supplies; physicians' equipment; renal dialysis supplies.

★ 16306 ★ Wisconsin Aluminum Foundry Co., Inc.
PO Box 246
Manitowoc, WI 54221-0246
Phone: (920)682-8627 **Fax:** (920)682-4090
Email: customerrelations@wafco.com
Website: http://www.wafco.com
Phillip Jacobs, Contact
Desc: Manufacturer of dental equipment; hospital equipment and supplies; laboratory equipment and supplies; sterilization equipment; veterinary products.

★ 16307 ★ World Heart, Inc.
7799 Pardee Lane
Oakland, CA 94621
Phone: (510)568-8338 **Fax:** (510)563-5005
Email: communications@worldheart.com
Website: http://www.worldheart.com
Dolg Hillier, Contact
Desc: Manufacturer/distributor of cardiovascular equipment and supplies; patient monitoring equipment.

★ 16308 ★ WR Medical Electronics Co.
123 N Second St.
Stillwater, MN 55082
Phone: (651)430-1200 **Free:** 800-321-6387
Fax: (651)439-9733
Email: info@wrmed.com
Website: http://www.wrmed.com
Patrick J. Anderson, President
Desc: Manufacturer of hospital equipment and supplies; patient monitoring equipment; physical therapy and rehabilitation equipment and supplies; physicians' equipment; surgical disposables.

★ 16309 ★ Wright Medical Technology, Inc.
5677 Airline Rd.
PO Box 100
Arlington, TN 38002
Phone: (901)867-9971 **Free:** 800-238-7188
Fax: (901)867-8249
Email: webmaster@wmt.com
Website: http://www.wmt.com
F. Barry Bays, CEO & Pres
Desc: Manufacturer/distributor of orthopedic and prosthetic equipment and supplies; orthopedic implants/products and instrumentation.

★ 16310 ★ Wyeth Consumer Healthcare
Division of Wyeth
5 Giralda Farms
Madison, NJ 07940-0871
Phone: (973)660-5500
Website: http://www.wyeth.com
Ulf Wiinberg, President
Desc: Manufacturer of OTC/proprietary pharmaceuticals; dietary, nutritional and vitamin supplements.

★ 16311 ★ Wyeth Genetics Institute
Division of Wyeth
87 Cambridge Park Dr.
Cambridge, MA 02140-2387
Phone: (617)876-1170 **Fax:** (617)665-8838
Jay Brack, Contact
Desc: Manufacturer/biotechnology company: Rx/ethical pharmaceuticals; biotechnology/biopharmaceutical products.

★ 16312 ★ Wyeth Pharmaceuticals
Division of American Home Products Corp.
PO Box 8299
Philadelphia, PA 19101
Phone: (610)902-1200
Website: http://www.wyeth.com
Bernard Poussot, President
Desc: Manufacturer of Rx/ethical pharmaceuticals; OTC/proprietary pharmaceuticals; generic pharmaceuticals.

★ 16313 ★ Wyeth Vaccines
A business unit of Wyeth Pharmaceuticals
280 King of Prussia Rd.
Radnor, PA 19087
Phone: (610)688-4400 **Fax:** (610)989-5700
Kevin L. Reilly, Contact
Desc: Manufacturer/biotechnology company offering Rx/ethical pharmaceuticals; biotechnology/biopharmaceutical products.

★ 16314 ★ X-Rite, Inc.
Medical Division
3100 44th St., SW
Grandville, MI 49418
Phone: (616)534-7663 **Free:** 888-826-3044
Fax: (616)534-8960
Website: http://www.x-rite.com
Bill Owens, Contact
Desc: Manufacturer of dental supplies; general radiography; nuclear and radiological equipment; veterinary products; X-ray equipment.

★ 16315 ★ Xillix Technologies Corp.
100-13775 Commerce Parkway
Richmond, BC, Canada V6V 2V4
Phone: (604)278-5000 **Free:** 800-665-2236
Fax: (604)278-3356
Email: info@xillix.com
Website: http://www.xillix.com
Pierre Leduc, Chairman of the Board
Desc: Biotechnology company offering biotechnology/biopharmaceutical products; diagnostic equipment and instruments; medical imaging.

★ 16316 ★ XOMA (US) LLC
2910 Seventh St.
Berkeley, CA 94710
Phone: (510)644-1170 **Fax:** (510)649-0315
Email: investorrelations@xoma.com
Website: http://www.xoma.com
John L. Castello, Contact
Desc: Manufacturer/biotechnology company offering biotechnology/biopharmaceutical products.

★ 16317 ★ Yamanouchi Pharma Technologies, Inc.
Division of Yamanouchi Pharmaceutical Co., Ltd.
1050 Arastradero Rd.
Stanford Research Park
Palo Alto, CA 94304
Phone: (650)849-8505 **Free:** 877-663-3643
Fax: (650)849-8565
Email: jfix@ypharma.com
Website: http://www.ypharma.com
Steve Kirnon, Contact
Desc: Manufacturer/distributor of Rx/ethical pharmaceuticals; OTC/proprietary pharmaceuticals; contract manufacturing; contract R & D; drug delivery systems.

★ 16318 ★ Yamanouchi USA, Inc.
S 61 Paramus Rd.
4th Floor
Paramus, NJ 07652
Phone: (201)291-2556 **Fax:** (201)291-7929
Website: http://www.yamanouchi.com
Gensei Kon, President
Desc: Manufacturer of Rx/ethical pharmaceuticals.

★ 16319 ★ YSI Inc.
1700/1725 Brannum Lane
Yellow Springs, OH 45387
Phone: (937)767-7241 **Free:** 800-765-4974
Fax: (937)767-9320
Email: info@ysi.com
Website: http://www.ysi.com
Malte von Matthiessen, CEO & Chm Bd
Desc: Manufacturer/biotechnology company offering biotechnology/biopharmaceutical products; cardiovascular equipment; diagnostic equipment and instruments; diagnostic reagents and test kits; laboratory equipment; patient monitoring equipment; pharmaceutical manufacturing supplies and equipment.

★ 16320 ★ Zambon Corp.
Subsidiary of Zambon Group, S.p.A.
Meadows Office Complex
301 Rte. 17
Ste. 205
Rutherford, NJ 07070
Phone: (201)939-4800 **Fax:** (201)939-4825
Website: http://www.zambongroup.com
Robert Rettani, , Chairman of the Board
Desc: Manufacturer of Rx/ethical pharmaceuticals; OTC/proprietary pharmaceuticals; home healthcare; generic pharmaceuticals.

★ 16321 ★ Zenex Corp.
850 Elmhurst Rd.
Elk Grove Village, IL 60007
Phone: (847)390-0700 **Fax:** (847)390-0706
Elias R. Zenkich, Contact
Desc: Manufacturer of hospital equipment and supplies.

★ 16322 ★ Zeus Scientific, Inc.
PO Box 38
Raritan, NJ 08869
Phone: (908)526-3744 **Free:** 800-526-3874
Fax: (908)526-2058
Email: info@zeusscientific.com
Website: http://www.zeusscientific.com
Donald R. Tourville, PhD, CEO & Chm Bd
Desc: Manufacturer/distributor of diagnostic reagents and test kits.

★ 16323 ★ Zimmer, Inc.
A Bristol-Myers Squibb Co.
PO Box 708
Warsaw, IN 46581-0708
Phone: (219)267-6131 **Fax:** (219)372-4206
Email: raymond.elliott@bms.com
Website: http://www.zimmer.com
J. Raymond Elliott, CEO
Desc: Manufacturer/distributor of hospital equipment and supplies; orthopedic and prosthetic equipment and supplies; physical therapy and rehabilitation equipment and supplies; skin/wound care products; surgical disposables.

★ 16324 ★ Zonagen Inc.
2408 Timberloch Place, B-4
The Woodlands, TX 77380
Phone: (281)367-5892 **Fax:** (281)363-8796
Website: http://www.zonagen.com
Joseph S. Podolski, CEO & Pres
Desc: Manufacturer/biotechnology company offering Rx/ethical pharmaceuticals; biotechnology/biopharmaceutical products.

★ 16325 ★ ZymeTx, Inc.
Affiliated with Oklahoma Medical Research Foundation
800 Research Parkway, Ste. 100
Oklahoma City, OK 73104
Phone: (405)271-1314 **Free:** 888-817-1314
Fax: (405)271-1944
Email: proulxn@zymetx.com
Website: http://www.zymetx.com
Norman R. Proulx, CEO & Pres
Desc: Manufacturer/distributor/biotechnology company offering Rx/ethical pharmaceuticals; biotechnology/biopharmaceutical products; diagnostic reagents and test kits; disposable medical devices and supplies; home healthcare; laboratory supplies; physicians' supplies; respiratory therapy and/or cardiopulmonary supplies.

Chapter 9
Dental Care Plans

The Delta Dental Plans listed below are arranged alphabetically by states, then by plan names. For additional information, consult the "User's Guide" located at the front of this directory.

Alabama

★ 16326 ★ Delta Dental Insurance Co.—Alabama
1 Perimeter Park S, Ste. 420N
Birmingham, AL 35243
Phone: (205)969-5755 **Free:** 800-521-2651
Fax: (205)969-5777
Website: http://www.deltadental.com
Robert Elliott, President

Arizona

★ 16327 ★ Delta Dental Plan of Arizona
PO Box 43000
Phoenix, AZ 85080-3000
Phone: (602)938-3131 **Free:** 800-352-6132
Fax: (602)588-3636
Website: http://www.deltadentalaz.com
Bernard Glossy, CEO

Arkansas

★ 16328 ★ Delta Dental Plan of Arkansas
100 Shadow Oaks Dr.
Sherwood, AR 72120-9310
Phone: (501)835-3400 **Free:** 800-462-5410
Fax: (501)834-6244
Website: http://www.deltadentalar.com

California

★ 16329 ★ Delta Dental Plan of California
PO Box 7736
San Francisco, CA 94120
Phone: (415)972-8300 **Free:** 888-335-8227
Fax: (415)543-4463
Website: http://www.deltadentalca.org
Gary Radine, CEO

Colorado

★ 16330 ★ Delta Dental Plan of Colorado
4582 S Ulster St., Ste. 800
Denver, CO 80237
Phone: (303)741-9300 **Fax:** (303)741-9350
Website: http://www.deltadentalco.com
Kate Paul, CEO

Florida

★ 16331 ★ Delta Dental Insurance Co.—Florida
258 S Hall Lane, Ste. 350
Maitland, FL 32751
Phone: (407)660-9034 **Free:** 800-662-9034
Fax: (407)660-2899
Website: http://www.deltadental.com
Robert Elliott, President

Georgia

★ 16332 ★ Delta Dental Insurance Co.—Georgia
1000 Mansell Exchange W, B100, No. 100
Alpharetta, GA 30022
Phone: (770)645-8700 **Free:** 800-521-2651
Fax: (770)518-4757
Website: http://www.deltadentalga.com
Mindy Broda, DDS, Contact

Idaho

★ 16333 ★ Delta Dental Plan of Idaho
555 E Parkcenter Blvd.
Boise, ID 83706
Phone: (208)344-4546 **Fax:** (208)344-4649
Website: http://www.deltadental.com
Hammer Bramstenner, CEO

Illinois

★ 16334 ★ Delta Dental Plan of Illinois
801 Ogden Ave.
Lisle, IL 60532
Phone: (630)964-2400 **Free:** 800-331-0538
Fax: (630)964-2596
Email: bschor@deltadentalil.com
Website: http://www.deltadentalil.com/
Robert D. Tranter, Chairman of the Board

Indiana

★ 16335 ★ Delta Dental Plan of Indiana
5875 Castle Creek Pkwy. N, No. 191
Indianapolis, IN 46250-4327
Phone: (317)842-4022 **Free:** 800-382-5404
Fax: (317)577-2361
Website: http://www.deltadentalmi.com
Thomas J. Fleszar, DDS, CEO & Pres

Iowa

★ 16336 ★ Delta Dental Plan of Iowa
2401 SE Tones Dr., Ste. 13
Ankeny, IA 50021
Free: 800-544-0718 **Fax:** (515)963-0373
Email: mail@deltadentalia.com
Website: http://www.deltadentalia.com/
Don Hutchinson, CEO

Kansas

★ 16337 ★ Delta Dental Plan of Kansas
PO Box 49198
Wichita, KS 67201-9198
Phone: (316)264-1099 **Fax:** (316)264-5912
Email: info@deltadentalks.com
Website: http://www.deltadentalks.com
Derek Bridges, CEO

Kentucky

★ 16338 ★ Delta Dental Plan of Kentucky, Inc.
PO Box 242810
Louisville, KY 40224-2810
Free: 800-955-2030 **Fax:** (502)327-5715
Website: http://www.deltadentalky.com/
Clifford T. Maesaka, Jr., CEO

Massachusetts

★ 16339 ★ Delta Dental Plan of Massachusetts
PO Box 9695
Boston, MA 02114-9695
Phone: (617)886-1000 **Free:** 800-451-1249
Fax: (617)886-1129
Website: http://www.deltadentalma.com/
Robert E. Hunter, CEO

Michigan

★ 16340 ★ Delta Dental Plan of Michigan
PO Box 30416
Lansing, MI 48909-7916
Phone: (517)349-6000 **Free:** 800-524-0149
Fax: (517)347-5327
Website: http://www.deltadentalmi.com/
Thomas J. Fleszar, DDS, CEO & Pres

Minnesota

★ 16341 ★ Delta Dental Plan of Minnesota
PO Box 9304
Minneapolis, MN 55440
Phone: (651)406-5900 **Free:** 800-328-1188
Fax: (651)406-5936
Website: http://www.deltadental.org/
Michael F. Walsh, CEO & Pres

Missouri

★ 16342 ★ Delta Dental Plan of Missouri
12399 Gravois Rd.
Saint Louis, MO 63127-1702
Phone: (314)656-3000 **Free:** 800-392-1167
Fax: (314)656-2900
Website: http://www.deltadentalmo.com
Steve Gall, Contact

Nebraska

★ 16343 ★ Delta Dental Plan of Nebraska
8601 W Dodge Rd., Ste. 116
Omaha, NE 68114
Free: 800-736-0710 **Fax:** (402)397-6401
Website: http://www.deltadental.com
Michael Walsh, CEO

Nevada

★ 16344 ★ Delta Dental Insurance Co. of Nevada
3012 W Charleston Blvd., Ste. 120
Las Vegas, NV 89102
Phone: (702)870-6860 **Fax:** (702)870-0644
Website: http:www.deltadental.com
Gary Radine, CEO

New Hampshire

★ 16345 ★ Northeast Delta Dental
Delta Dental Plan of New Hampshire
PO Box 2002
Concord, NH 03302-2002
Phone: (603)223-1000 **Free:** 800-832-5700
Fax: (603)223-1199
Email: nedelta@nedelta.com
Website: http://www.nedelta.com/
Tom Raffeo, CEO

New Jersey

★ 16346 ★ Delta Dental Plan of New Jersey
PO Box 222
Parsippany, NJ 07054
Phone: (973)285-4000 **Free:** 800-624-2633
Fax: (973)285-4139
Website: http://www.deltadentalnj.com/
Gerald A. Snydell, DDS, Chairman of the Board

New Mexico

★ 16347 ★ Delta Dental Plan of New Mexico
2500 Louisiana Blvd. NE, Ste. 300
Albuquerque, NM 87110
Free: 800-999-0963 **Fax:** (505)883-7444
Email: contact@deltadentalnm.com
Website: http://www.deltadentalnm.com
Walt Bolic, CEO

North Carolina

★ 16348 ★ Delta Dental Plan of North Carolina
333 E Six Forks Rd., Ste 180
Raleigh, NC 27609
Free: 800-662-8856 **Fax:** (919)832-6061
Website: http://www.deltadentalnc.org
Linda Smith, President

Ohio

★ 16349 ★ Delta Dental Plan of Ohio
PO Box 29979
Columbus, OH 43229
Phone: (614)890-1117 **Free:** 800-537-5527
Fax: (614)890-1274
Website: http://www.deltadentaloh.com/
Robert A. Anthony, DDS, Chairman of the Board

Oklahoma

★ 16350 ★ Delta Dental Plan of Oklahoma
PO Box 54709
Oklahoma City, OK 73154-1809
Free: 800-522-0188 **Fax:** (405)607-2190
Website: http://www.deltadental.com
John Gladden, CEO

Pennsylvania

★ 16351 ★ Delta Dental of Pennsylvania
1 Delta Dr.
Mechanicsburg, PA 17055
Free: 800-932-0783 **Fax:** (717)766-8719
Website: http://www.deltadentalpa.org
Gary Radine, CEO

Rhode Island

★ 16352 ★ Delta Dental of Rhode Island
PO Box 1517
Providence, RI 02901-1517
Free: 800-598-6684 **Fax:** (401)752-6060
Website: http://www.deltadentalri.com
Joseph Nagle, CEO

South Carolina

★ 16353 ★ Delta Dental Plan of South Carolina
111 Executive Center Dr., Ste. 242
Columbia, SC 29210
Free: 800-392-1167 **Fax:** (803)731-0273
Website: http://www.deltadental.com
Steve Gaal, CEO

South Dakota

★ 16354 ★ Delta Dental Plan of South Dakota
720 N Euclid Ave.
Pierre, SD 57501
Free: 800-627-3961 **Fax:** (605)224-0909
Website: http://www.deltadental.com

Tennessee

★ 16355 ★ Delta Dental Plan of Tennessee
240 Venture Circle
Nashville, TN 37228
Phone: (615)255-3175 **Free:** 800-223-3104
Fax: (615)244-8108
Website: http://www.deltadentaltn.com
Phil Wenk, DDS, CEO

Texas

★ 16356 ★ Delta Dental Insurance Co.—Texas
1431 Greenway Dr., Ste. 520
Irving, TX 75038
Phone: (972)580-1616 **Free:** 800-775-0523
Fax: (972)580-1333
Website: http://www.deltadental.com
Kim Volk, CEO & Pres

Utah

★ 16357 ★ Delta Dental Insurance Co.—Utah
257 East 200 South, Ste. 375
Salt Lake City, UT 84111
Phone: (801)575-5168 **Fax:** (801)575-5171
Website: http://www.dltadental.com
Gary Radine, CEO

Virginia

★ 16358 ★ Delta Dental Plan of Virginia
4818 Starkey Rd.
Roanoke, VA 24014
Phone: (540)989-8000 **Free:** 800-237-6060
Fax: (540)774-7574
Website: http://www.deltadentalva.com/
George A. Levicki, DDS, CEO

Washington

★ 16359 ★ Washington Dental Service
9706 Fourth Ave. NE
Seattle, WA 98115
Phone: (206)526-7685 **Free:** 800-342-8355
Fax: (206)525-2330
Email: info@ddpwa.com
Website: http://www.deltadentalwa.com/
James D. Dwyer, CEO

Wisconsin

★ 16360 ★ Delta Dental Plan of Wisconsin
PO Box 828
Stevens Point, WI 54481
Phone: (715)344-6087 **Free:** 800-236-3713
Fax: (715)344-2446
Website: http://www.deltadentalwi.com
Dennis Brown, CEO & Pres

Wyoming

★ 16361 ★ Delta Dental Plan of Wyoming
PO Box 29
Cheyenne, WY 82003-0029
Free: 800-735-3379 **Fax:** (307)632-7309
Website: http://www.deltadentalwy.org
Kerry Hall, CEO

Chapter 10
Blue Cross & Blue Shield Plans

Entries in this chapter are arranged alphabetically by states, then by plan names. For additional information, consult the "User's Guide" located at the front of this directory.

Alabama

★ 16362 ★ Blue Cross and Blue Shield of Alabama
450 Riverchase Pkwy. E
Birmingham, AL 35244
Phone: (205)220-2121 **Fax:** (205)444-6555
Website: http://www.bcbsal.org/index.html
H. L. Jones, CEO

Alberta

★ 16363 ★ Alberta Blue Cross Plan
10009 108th St. NW
Edmonton, AB, Canada T5J 3C5
Phone: (780)498-8297 **Fax:** (780)498-8383
V. George Ward, CEO & Pres

Arizona

★ 16364 ★ Blue Cross and Blue Shield Arizona
2444 W Las Palmaritas Dr.
Phoenix, AZ 85021
Phone: (602)864-4444 **Fax:** (602)864-4242
Website: http://www.bcbsaz.com
Robert B. Bulla, CEO

Arkansas

★ 16365 ★ Arkansas Blue Cross and Blue Shield
601 Gaines St.
Little Rock, AR 72201
Phone: (501)378-2242 **Fax:** (501)378-2037
Website: http://www.arkbluecross.com
Robert L. Shoptaw, CEO & Pres

California

★ 16366 ★ Blue Shield of California
California Physicians' Service Corp.
50 Beale St.
San Francisco, CA 94105
Phone: (415)229-5806 **Fax:** (415)229-5056
Website: http://www.blueshieldca.com
Bruce Bodaken, CEO & Chm Bd

★ 16367 ★ WellPoint Health Networks, Inc./BC California
21555 Oxnard St.
Woodland Hills, CA 91367
Phone: (805)557-6000
Leonard D. Schaeffer, CEO & Chm Bd

Colorado

★ 16368 ★ Blue Cross and Blue Shield Colorado
Rocky Mountain Hospital and Medical Service
700 Broadway
Denver, CO 80273
Phone: (303)831-2954 **Fax:** (303)830-0887
Email: webmaster@bcbsco.com
Website: http://www.bsbsco.com
Caroline S. Matthews, CEO

Connecticut

★ 16369 ★ Anthem Insurance Companies of Connecticut
Anthem Insurance Companies, Inc.
370 Bassett Rd.
North Haven, CT 06473
Phone: (317)488-6493
Website: http://www.anthem-inc.com
Marjorie Dorr, President

Delaware

★ 16370 ★ Blue Cross and Blue Shield Delaware
Care First, Inc.
1 Brandywine Gateway
Wilmington, DE 19899
Phone: (302)421-3210 **Fax:** (302)421-2089
Website: http://www.bcbsde.com
Paul C. King, Jr., President

District of Columbia

★ 16371 ★ CareFirst Blue Cross and Blue Shield
550 12th St. SW
Washington, DC 20065
Phone: (410)998-5252
Website: http://www.bcbsnca.com
William L. Jews, CEO

Florida

★ 16372 ★ Blue Cross and Blue Shield Florida, Inc.
4800 Deerwood Campus Parkway
Jacksonville, FL 32246
Phone: (904)905-6115 **Fax:** (904)905-6638
Website: http://www.bcbsfl.com
Michael Cascone, Jr., CEO

Georgia

★ 16373 ★ Blue Cross and Blue Shield Georgia
Wellpoint Health Networks, Inc.
3350 Peachtree Rd. NE
Atlanta, GA 30326
Phone: (404)842-8413 **Fax:** (404)842-8801
Rebecca Kapustay, CEO

Hawaii

★ 16374 ★ Blue Cross and Blue Shield Hawaii
Hawaii Medical Service Association
818 Keeaumoku St.
Honolulu, HI 96804
Phone: (808)948-5580 **Fax:** (808)948-5999
Website: http://www.hmsa.com
Robert P. Hiam, CEO

Idaho

★ 16375 ★ Blue Cross of Idaho Health Service, Inc.
3000 E Pine Ave.
Meridian, ID 83642
Phone: (208)331-8820 **Fax:** (208)331-7311
Ray Flachbart, CEO
Alt. Contact: PO Box 7408, Boise, ID, 83707.

★ 16376 ★ Regence BlueShield of Idaho
1602 21st Ave.
Lewiston, ID 83501
Phone: (208)798-2102
Website: http://www.medbbs.com
John Ruch, CEO

Illinois

★ 16377 ★ Blue Cross and Blue Shield Illinois
Health Care Service Corp.
300 E Randolph St.
Chicago, IL 60601
Phone: (312)653-6847 **Fax:** (312)819-1220
Website: http://www.bcbsil.com
Raymond F. McCaskey, CEO

Indiana

★ 16378 ★ Anthem Blue Cross and Blue Shield
Anthem Insurance Companies, Inc.
120 Monument Circle
Indianapolis, IN 46204
Phone: (317)488-6493 **Fax:** (317)488-6477
Larry Glasscock, CEO

Iowa

★ 16379 ★ Wellmark Blue Cross and Blue Shield of Iowa
Wellmark, Inc.
636 Grand Ave.
Des Moines, IA 50309
Phone: (515)245-4545 **Fax:** (515)245-5090
Website: http://www.wellmarkbcbs.com
John D. Forsyth, CEO

Kansas

★ 16380 ★ Blue Cross and Blue Shield Kansas
1133 SW Topeka Blvd.
PO Box 239
Topeka, KS 66629-0001
Phone: (785)291-8700
John W. Knack, CEO & Pres

Louisiana

★ 16381 ★ Blue Cross and Blue Shield Louisiana
Louisiana Health Service and Indemnity Co.
5525 Reitz Ave.
Baton Rouge, LA 70809-3802
Phone: (225)295-2266 **Fax:** (225)295-2054
Website: http://www.lablue.com
Kathryn Sullivan, CEO

Maine

★ 16382 ★ Blue Cross and Blue Shield Maine
Associated Hospital Service of Maine
2 Gannett Dr.
South Portland, ME 04106-6911
Phone: (207)822-7000 **Fax:** (207)822-7350
Keith W. Vangelson, CEO

Manitoba

★ 16383 ★ Manitoba Blue Cross
United Health Services Corp.
100A Polo Park Centre
1485 Portage Ave.
Winnipeg, MB, Canada R3C 2X7
Phone: (204)775-0161 **Fax:** (204)774-1761
Kerry V. Bittner, President

Maryland

★ 16384 ★ CareFirst Blue Cross and Blue Shield
10455 Mill Run Cir.
Owings Mills, MD 21117
Phone: (410)998-5252 **Fax:** (410)998-5576
Website: http://www.bcbsmd.com
William L. Jews, CEO

Massachusetts

★ 16385 ★ Blue Cross and Blue Shield Massachusetts
401 Park Dr.
Boston, MA 02215
Phone: (617)246-3300 **Fax:** (617)832-3353
Website: http://www.bcbsma.com
William C. Van Faasen, CEO & Pres

Michigan

★ 16386 ★ Blue Cross and Blue Shield Michigan
600 Lafayette E
Detroit, MI 48226-2998
Phone: (313)225-0443 **Fax:** (313)225-6239
Website: http://www.bcbsm.com
Richard E. Whitmer, CEO

Minnesota

★ 16387 ★ Blue Cross and Blue Shield Minnesota
Aware Integrated, Inc.
3535 Blue Cross Rd.
Saint Paul, MN 55122
Phone: (651)662-8438 **Fax:** (651)662-7767
Mark W. Banks, MD, CEO

Mississippi

★ 16388 ★ Blue Cross and Blue Shield Mississippi
3545 Lakeland Dr.
Jackson, MS 39208
Phone: (601)664-4200 **Fax:** (601)939-7035
Richard J. Hale, CEO

Missouri

★ 16389 ★ Blue Cross and Blue Shield Kansas City
2301 Main St.
Kansas City, MO 64108
Phone: (816)395-2016 **Fax:** (816)395-2035
John A. O'Rourke, CEO

★ 16390 ★ Blue Cross and Blue Shield Missouri
1831 Chestnut St.
Saint Louis, MO 63103-2275
Phone: (314)923-8991 **Fax:** (314)923-4809
Website: http://www.abcbs.com
John A. O'Rourke, CEO

Montana

★ 16391 ★ Blue Cross and Blue Shield Montana
560 N Park Ave.
Helena, MT 59601
Phone: (406)444-8216 **Fax:** (406)442-6946
Website: http://www.bcbsmt.com
Peter J. Babin, CEO

Nebraska

★ 16392 ★ Blue Cross and Blue Shield Nebraska
7261 Mercy Rd.
Omaha, NE 68180-0001
Phone: (402)390-1800 **Fax:** (402)392-2141
Website: http://www.bcbsne.com
Richard L. Guffey, CEO
Alt. Contact: 1233 Lincoln Mall, Lincoln, NE, 68508-2847, (402)458-4800; (800)562-6394. 1811 W. Second St., No. 105, Grand Island, NE, 68803, (308)381-6130; (800)373-9109.

Nevada

★ 16393 ★ Blue Cross and Blue Shield Nevada
Anthem Insurance Companies, Inc.
5250 S Virginia St.
Reno, NV 89502
Phone: (303)831-3234
C. David Kikumoto, CEO & Pres

New Brunswick

★ 16394 ★ Blue Cross of Atlantic Canada
644 Main St.
PO Box 220
Moncton, NB, Canada E1C 8L3
Phone: (506)853-1811 **Fax:** (506)867-4651
PierreYves Julian, CEO & Pres

★ 16395 ★ Blue Cross in Ontario, Moncton Office
644 Main St.
PO Box 220
Moncton, NB, Canada E1C 8L3
Phone: (506)853-1811 **Fax:** (506)867-4646
PierreYves Julian, CEO & Pres

New Hampshire

★ 16396 ★ Blue Cross and Blue Shield New Hampshire
Anthem Insurance Companies, Inc.
3000 Goffs Falls Rd.
Manchester, NH 03111-0001
Phone: (603)695-7064 **Fax:** (603)695-7304
David Jensen, CEO & Pres

New Jersey

★ 16397 ★ Horizon Blue Cross and Blue Shield of New Jersey, Inc.
Horizon Healthcare Services, Inc.
3 Penn Plaza East
Newark, NJ 07105
Phone: (973)466-8300 **Fax:** (973)466-8762
Website: http://www.bcbsnj.com
William J. Marino, CEO & Pres

New Mexico

★ 16398 ★ Blue Cross and Blue Shield New Mexico
12800 Indian School Rd. NE
Albuquerque, NM 87112
Phone: (505)816-4400
Norman P. Becker, CEO

New York

★ 16399 ★ Blue Cross and Blue Shield Central New York
Excellus, Inc.
344 S Warren St.
Syracuse, NY 13202
Phone: (315)448-3739 **Fax:** (315)448-4922
Howard F. Beacham, III, President

★ 16400 ★ Blue Cross and Blue Shield of the Rochester Area
Excellus, Inc.
165 Court St.
Rochester, NY 14647
Phone: (716)238-4351 **Fax:** (716)238-4400
David Klein, President

★ 16401 ★ Blue Cross and Blue Shield Utica-Watertown
Excellus, Inc.
12 Rhoads Dr.
Utica, NY 13502-6398
Phone: (315)731-9655 **Fax:** (315)797-4288
Howard F. Beacham, III, President

★ 16402 ★ Blue Cross and Blue Shield Western New York
1901 Main St.
Buffalo, NY 14240-0080
Phone: (716)887-6949 **Fax:** (716)887-8981
Thomas P. Hartnett, PhD, CEO

North Carolina

★ 16403 ★ Blue Cross and Blue Shield North Carolina
5901 Chapel Hill Rd.
PO Box 2291
Durham, NC 27707
Phone: (919)765-7831 **Fax:** (919)765-7105
Robert Grecyzn, CEO

North Dakota

★ 16404 ★ Blue Cross and Blue Shield North Dakota
Noridian Mutual Insurance Co.
4510 13th Ave. SW
Fargo, ND 58121-0001
Phone: (701)282-1327 **Fax:** (701)282-1866
Website: http://www.bcbsnd.com
Michael B. Unhjem, CEO

Ohio

★ 16405 ★ Anthem Blue Cross and Blue Shield
4361 Irwin Simpson Rd.
Mason, OH 45040
Phone: (317)488-6493
Larry C. Glasscock, CEO

Oklahoma

★ 16406 ★ Blue Cross and Blue Shield Oklahoma
1215 S Boulder Ave.
Tulsa, OK 74119-2800
Phone: (918)560-2195 **Fax:** (918)560-2095
Website: http://www.bcbsok.com
Ronald F. King, CEO

Ontario

★ 16407 ★ Blue Cross in Ontario, Ontario Office
185 The West Mall, Ste. 600
Etobicoke, ON, Canada M9C 5P1
Phone: (416)626-1688 **Fax:** (416)626-0997
Claude Bovin, President

Oregon

★ 16408 ★ Regence Blue Cross and Blue Shield Oregon
100 SW Market St.
Portland, OR 97201
Phone: (503)225-5206 **Fax:** (503)225-5232
Website: http://www.bcbso.com
Richard L. Woolworth, CEO & Pres

Pennsylvania

★ 16409 ★ Blue Cross Northeastern Pennsylvania
Hospital Service Association of Northeastern Pennsylvania
70 N Main St.
Wilkes Barre, PA 18711
Phone: (570)829-8801 **Fax:** (570)200-6860
Denise Cesare, CEO & Pres

★ 16410 ★ Capital Blue Cross
2500 Elmerton Ave.
Harrisburg, PA 17110
Phone: (717)541-7474 **Fax:** (717)541-7405
Website: http://www.capbluecross.com
James M. Mead, CEO
Alt. Contact: Mail Drop 4611, Harrisburg, PA, 17177-4611, (717)541-6915.

★ 16411 ★ Independence Blue Cross
1901 Market St.
Philadelphia, PA 19103
Phone: (215)241-2422 **Fax:** (215)241-3824
Website: http://www.ibx.com
G. Fred DiBona, Jr., CEO

★ 16412 ★ Pennsylvania Blue Shield Highmark, Inc.
120 5th Ave.
Pittsburgh, PA 15222-3099
Phone: (412)544-8202
Website: http://www.highmark.com
John S. Brouse, CEO

★ 16413 ★ Pennsylvania Blue Shield Highmark, Inc.
1800 Center St.
Camp Hill, PA 17089
Phone: (412)544-8208
John S. Brouse, CEO

Puerto Rico

★ 16414 ★ La Cruz Azul de Puerto Rico Independence Blue Cross
Carr. 1 Im 17.3
Rio Piedras, PR 00927
Phone: (787)272-7800
Rafael Santos Del Valle, Esq., CEO

★ 16415 ★ Triple-S Inc.
Triple-S Management Corp.
1441 F. D. Roosevelt Ave.
San Juan, PR 00920
Phone: (787)749-4114
Miguel A. Vasquez Deynes, CEO

Quebec

★ 16416 ★ Quebec Blue Cross Canassurance Hospital Service Association
550 Sherbrooke St. W, Ste. B-9
Montreal, QC, Canada H3A 1B9
Phone: (514)286-8482 **Fax:** (514)286-8475
Claude Bolvin, CEO & Pres

Rhode Island

★ 16417 ★ Blue Cross and Blue Shield Rhode Island
444 Westminster St.
Providence, RI 02903-3279
Phone: (401)459-1200 **Fax:** (401)459-1290
Website: http://www.bcbsri.com
Ronald A. Battista, CEO & Pres

Saskatchewan

★ 16418 ★ Saskatchewan Blue Cross
516 2nd Ave. N
PO Box 4030
Saskatoon, SK, Canada S7K 3T2
Phone: (306)244-1192 **Fax:** (306)664-1945
Terry R. Brash, CEO & Pres

South Carolina

★ 16419 ★ Blue Cross and Blue Shield South Carolina
I-20 East at Alpine Rd.
Columbia, SC 29219
Phone: (803)788-1039 **Fax:** (803)736-3420
M. Edward Sellers, CEO & Pres

South Dakota

★ 16420 ★ Wellmark Blue Cross and Blue Shield South Dakota
1601 W Madison St.
Sioux Falls, SD 57104
Phone: (515)245-4545
John D. Forsyth, CEO & Pres

Tennessee

★ 16421 ★ Blue Cross and Blue Shield of Tennessee
801 Pine St.
Chattanooga, TN 37402
Phone: (423)755-5620 **Fax:** (423)755-2178
Thomas Kinser, CEO

Texas

★ 16422 ★ Blue Cross and Blue Shield Texas
901 S Central Expwy.
Richardson, TX 75080
Phone: (972)766-6900 **Fax:** (972)766-8586
Website: http://www.bcbstx.com
Raymond F. McCaskey, President

Utah

★ 16423 ★ Regence Blue Cross and Blue Shield Utah
2890 E Cottonwood Pkwy.
Salt Lake City, UT 84130
Phone: (801)333-5630
Website: http://www.bcbsutah.com
John Ruch, CEO

Vermont

★ 16424 ★ Blue Cross and Blue Shield Vermont
445 Industrial Ln.
Berlin, VT 05602
Phone: (802)371-3770 **Fax:** (802)229-0511
William R. Milnes, Jr., CEO

Virginia

★ 16425 ★ Trigon Blue Cross and Blue Shield
Trigon Healthcare, Inc.
2015 Staples Mill Rd.
Richmond, VA 23230
Phone: (804)354-3510 **Fax:** (804)354-7044
Website: http://www.trigon.com
Thomas Snead, CEO

Washington

★ 16426 ★ Blue Cross and Blue Shield Alaska
Premera Blue Cross
PO Box 327
Seattle, WA 98111-0327
Phone: (425)670-5780 **Fax:** (425)670-4900
H. R. Brereton Barlow, CEO

★ 16427 ★ Northwest Washington Medical Bureau
1100 S 2nd St.
Mount Vernon, WA 98273
Phone: (360)336-9660
Karen J. Larson, CEO

★ 16428 ★ Regence Blue Shield
The Regence Group
1800 9th Ave.
Seattle, WA 98101-1322
Phone: (206)464-3624 **Fax:** (206)389-6778
Rich D. Nelson, CEO

West Virginia

★ 16429 ★ Mountain State Blue Cross and Blue Shield
Highmark Inc.
700 Market Sq.
PO Box 1948
Parkersburg, WV 26101
Phone: (304)424-7734 **Fax:** (304)424-7789
Gregory K. Smith, CEO

Wisconsin

★ 16430 ★ Blue Cross and Blue Shield United of Wisconsin
401 W Michigan St.
Milwaukee, WI 53203
Phone: (414)226-6295 **Fax:** (414)226-5488
Website: http://www.healthnet.connect.net
Thomas R. Hefty, CEO

Wyoming

★ 16431 ★ Blue Cross and Blue Shield Wyoming
4000 House Ave.
Cheyenne, WY 82001-2266
Phone: (307)432-2701
Tim J. Crilly, CEO

Chapter 11
Commercial Insurance Companies

The following entries are arranged alphabetically by company names. For additional information, see the "User's Guide" located at the front of this directory.

★ 16432 ★ A.G. Edwards Life Insurance Co.
1 N Jefferson
Saint Louis, MO 63103
Phone: (314)955-3000 **Fax:** (314)955-5043
Michael Scafati, President

★ 16433 ★ AAA Life Insurance Co.
AAA Life Group
17250 Newburgh Rd., Ste. 100
Livonia, MI 48152
Phone: (734)779-2085 **Fax:** (734)632-0678
Website: http://wwww.aaalife.com
Michael D. Daubenmier, CEO & Pres

★ 16434 ★ Abraham Lincoln Insurance Co.
United Trust, Inc. Group
PO Box 5147
Springfield, IL 62705-5147
Phone: (217)241-6300
Randall L. Attkisson, CEO & Pres
Larry E. Ryherd, Chairman of the Board

★ 16435 ★ Abundant Life Insurance Co.
PO Box 2187
Tulsa, OK 74171
Phone: (918)495-7536
George E. Fisher, President

★ 16436 ★ Acacia Life Insurance Co.
Ameritas Acacia Group
7315 Wisconsin Ave.
Bethesda, MD 20814
Phone: (301)280-1000 **Fax:** (301)280-1027
Website: http://www.acaciagroup.com
Haluk Ariturk, CEO & Pres

★ 16437 ★ Acacia National Life Insurance Co.
Ameritas Acacia Group
7315 Wisconsin Ave.
Bethesda, MD 20814
Phone: (301)280-1000 **Fax:** (301)280-1027
Website: http://www.acaciagroup.com
Haluk Ariturk, CEO & Pres

★ 16438 ★ Academy Life Insurance Co.
AEGON USA, Inc.
20 Moores Rd.
Frazer, PA 19355
Phone: (610)648-5000 **Fax:** (610)648-5326
Paul Reaburn, President

★ 16439 ★ Acadian Life Insurance Co.
PO Box 4669
Baton Rouge, LA 70801
Phone: (985)868-2630
Craig Anderson Netterville, President

★ 16440 ★ Acceleration Life Insurance Co.
Protective Life Corp.
2801 Hwy. 280 S
Birmingham, AL 35223
Phone: (314)275-5200 **Fax:** (314)275-5220
Website: http://www.protective.com
Roland G. Anderson, President
Robert J. Miller, Exec VP

★ 16441 ★ Access Dental Plan
555 University Ave., Ste. 182
Sacramento, CA 95825
Phone: (916)922-5000 **Fax:** (916)646-9000
Website: http://www.accessdental.com
Reza Abbaszadeh, DDS, CEO & Pres

★ 16442 ★ Adams Life Insurance Co.
PO Box 4562
Montgomery, AL 36103
Phone: (334)265-4359
Samuel Adams, President

★ 16443 ★ Admiral Life Insurance Co. of America
PO Box 30416
Lansing, MI 48909
Phone: (517)349-6000
C. Richard Seitz, President

★ 16444 ★ Advance Insurance Co.
Blue Cross & Blue Shield of Kansas Group
1133 SW Topeka Blvd.
Topeka, KS 66614-5326
Phone: (785)273-9804 **Fax:** (785)273-6121
Website: http://www.advanceinsurance.com
John D. Murrell, President

★ 16445 ★ Advanta Life Insurance Co.
PO Box 429
Spring House, PA 19477
Phone: (215)323-4135 **Free:** 877-250-6245
Fax: (215)232-4640
Website: http://www.Advanta.com
Mark Wlaz, President

★ 16446 ★ Advantage Dental Plan, Inc.
1813 W Harvard, Ste. 431
PO Box 1328
Roseburg, OR 97470
Phone: (541)677-7600
Carson Kendall, Chairman of the Board

★ 16447 ★ Aetna Health of California Inc.
980 Jolly Rd.
PO Box 1109
Blue Bell, PA 19422
Phone: (925)543-9000
Website: http://www.aetnaushc.com
Thomas R. Williams, President

★ 16448 ★ Aetna Health of the Carolinas Inc.
980 Jolly Rd.
PO Box 1109
Blue Bell, PA 19422
Free: 800-872-3862
Website: http://www.aetna.com
John J. Webb, President

★ 16449 ★ Aetna Health of Illinois Inc.
980 Jolly Rd.
PO Box 1109
Blue Bell, PA 19422
Phone: (312)928-3000
Website: http://www.aetna.com
Alicia H. Bolton, Vice President

★ 16450 ★ Aetna Health Inc. a Colorado Corp.
980 Jolly Rd.
PO Box 1109
Blue Bell, PA 19422
Free: 800-872-3862
Website: http://www.aetna.com
Charles T. Brown, President

★ 16451 ★ Aetna Health Inc. a Connecticut Corp.
980 Jolly Rd.
PO Box 1109
Blue Bell, PA 19422
Free: 800-872-3862
Website: http://www.aetna.com
Mary C. Bonner, President

★ 16452 ★ Aetna Health Inc. a Delaware Corp.
980 Jolly Rd.
PO Box 1109
Blue Bell, PA 19422
Free: 800-872-3862
Website: http://www.aetna.com
Felicia F. Norwood, President

★ 16453 ★ Aetna Health Inc. a Florida Corp.
980 Jolly Rd.
Blue Bell, PA 19422
Free: 800-872-3862
Website: http://www.aetna.com
John J. Webb, President

★ 16454 ★ Aetna Health Inc. a Georgia Corp.
980 Jolly Rd.
PO Box 1109
Blue Bell, PA 19422

Free: 800-872-3862
Website: http://www.aetna.com
John J. Webb, President

★ 16455 ★ Aetna Health Inc. a Maine Corp.
980 Jolly Rd.
PO Box 1109
Blue Bell, PA 19422
Free: 800-872-3862
Website: http://www.aetna.com
Mary C. Bonner, President

★ 16456 ★ Aetna Health Inc. a Maryland Corp.
980 Jolly Rd.
PO Box 1109
Blue Bell, PA 19422
Free: 800-872-3862
Website: http://www.aetna.com
Felicia F. Norwood, President

★ 16457 ★ Aetna Health Inc. a Massachusetts Corp.
980 Jolly Rd.
PO Box 1109
Blue Bell, PA 19422
Free: 800-872-3862
Website: http://www.aetna.com
Mary C. Bonner, President

★ 16458 ★ Aetna Health Inc. a Michigan Corp.
26933 Northwestern Hwy., Ste. 100
Southfield, MI 48034-4728
Phone: (248)208-8600
Website: http://www.aetna.com
Alicia H. Bolton, Vice President

★ 16459 ★ Aetna Health Inc. a Missouri Corp.
980 Jolly Rd.
PO Box 1109
Blue Bell, PA 19422
Phone: (314)567-6660
Website: http://www.aetna.com

★ 16460 ★ Aetna Health Inc. a New Hampshire Corp.
980 Jolly Rd.
PO Box 1109
Blue Bell, PA 19422
Free: 800-872-3862
Website: http://www.aetna.com
Mary C. Bonner, President

★ 16461 ★ Aetna Health Inc. a New Jersey Corp.
980 Jolly Rd.
PO Box 1109
Blue Bell, PA 19422
Free: 800-872-3862
Website: http://www.aetna.com
Felicia F. Norwood, President

★ 16462 ★ Aetna Health Inc. a New York Corp.
980 Jolly Rd.
PO Box 1109
Blue Bell, PA 19422
Phone: (516)794-6565 **Free:** 800-872-3862
Website: http://www.aetna.com
Mary C. Bonner, President

★ 16463 ★ Aetna Health Inc. a Pennsylvania Corp.
980 Jolly Rd.
PO Box 1109
Blue Bell, PA 19422
Free: 800-872-3862
Website: http://www.aetnaushc.com
Felicia F. Norwood, President

★ 16464 ★ Aetna Health Inc. a Tennessee Corp.
980 Jolly Rd.
PO Box 1109
Blue Bell, PA 19422
Phone: (615)322-1600
Website: http://www.aetna.com
John J. Webb, President

★ 16465 ★ Aetna Health Inc. a Texas Corp.
980 Jolly Rd.
PO Box 1109
Blue Bell, PA 19422
Phone: (713)350-2350
Website: http://www.aetna.com
Clarence C. King, II, President

★ 16466 ★ Aetna Health Inc. a Washington Corp.
980 Jolly Rd.
PO Box 1109
Blue Bell, PA 19422
Free: 800-872-3862
Website: http://www.aetna.com
Thomas R. Williams, President

★ 16467 ★ Aetna Health Inc. an Arizona Corp.
980 Jolly Rd.
Blue Bell, PA 19422
Phone: (602)427-2200
Website: http://www.aetna.com
Martin L. Block, President

★ 16468 ★ Aetna Health Inc. an Ohio Corp.
980 Jolly Rd.
PO Box 1109
Blue Bell, PA 19422
Phone: (330)659-8000
Website: http://www.aetna.com
Alicia H. Bolton, Vice President

★ 16469 ★ Aetna Health Inc. an Oklahoma Corp.
980 Jolly Rd.
PO Box 1109
Blue Bell, PA 19422
Free: 800-872-3862
Website: http://www.aetna.com
Clarence C. King, II, President

★ 16470 ★ Aetna Health and Life Insurance Co.
Aetna Inc. Group
151 Farmington Ave., MC 64
Hartford, CT 06156-0417
Phone: (708)245-4001 **Fax:** (708)245-4006
Frolly M. Boyd, President

★ 16471 ★ Aetna Health of North Texas Inc.
980 Jolly Rd.
PO Box 1109
Blue Bell, PA 19422
Phone: (214)200-8000
Website: http://www.aetna.com
Clarence C. King, II, President

★ 16472 ★ Aetna Healthcare Insurance Co. of Connecticut
151 Farmington Ave.
Hartford, CT 06156
Phone: (860)636-0602 **Fax:** (860)636-3871
Mary C. Bonner, President

★ 16473 ★ Aetna Healthcare Insurance Co. of New York
151 Farmington Ave.
Hartford, CT 06156
Phone: (516)794-6565 **Fax:** (215)283-6790
Mary C. Bonner, President

★ 16474 ★ Aetna Insurance Co. of Connecticut
Aetna Inc. Group
151 Farmington Ave.
Hartford, CT 06156-0147
Phone: (860)273-0123 **Fax:** (860)273-6348
Alan M. Bennett, President

★ 16475 ★ Aetna Life Insurance Co.
Aetna Inc. Group
151 Farmington Ave., MC 64
Hartford, CT 06156-0417
Phone: (860)273-0123 **Fax:** (860)273-1303
John W. Rowe, MD, President

★ 16476 ★ Aetna Life Insurance Co. of America
ING Group
151 Farmington Ave.
Hartford, CT 06156
Phone: (860)273-0123 **Fax:** (860)273-6348
Patrick S. C. Poon, President

★ 16477 ★ AF & L Insurance Co.
AF & L Group
PO Box 368
Warrington, PA 18976
Phone: (215)918-0515
Website: http://www.aflltc.com
Aloysius J. Abel, III, President

★ 16478 ★ AGC Life Insurance Co.
American International Group
American General Center
Nashville, TN 37250
Phone: (615)749-1000 **Fax:** (615)749-1251
Website: http://www.agla.com
Donald W. Britton, President

★ 16479 ★ AGL Life Assurance Co.
Phoenix Life Group
1 American Row
Hartford, CT 06115
Phone: (484)530-4800 **Fax:** (484)530-9272
Website: http://www.guar.com
John K. Hillman, CEO & Pres

★ 16480 ★ AIG Annuity Insurance Co.
American International Group
205 E 10th Ave.
Amarillo, TX 79101
Phone: (806)345-7400
Website: http://www.agannuity.com
Bruce R. Abrams, President
Frmly: American General Annuity Insurance Co.

★ 16481 ★ AIG Life Insurance Co.
American International Group
PO Box 667
Wilmington, DE 19899
Phone: (302)594-2000 **Fax:** (302)654-5436
Gerald W. Wyndorf, CEO & Pres

★ 16482 ★ AIG Life Insurance Co. of Puerto Rico
American International Group
PO Box 9172
San Juan, PR 00908-9172
Phone: (787)764-6200 **Fax:** (787)763-8630
Manual Rodriguez, President

★ 16483 ★ AIG SunAmerica Life Assurance Co.
American International Group
1 SunAmerica Ctr.
Los Angeles, CA 90067-6022
Phone: (310)772-6000 **Fax:** (310)772-6635
Website: http://www.sunamerica.com
Jay S. Wintrob, President
Frmly: Anchor National Life Insurance Co.

★ 16484 ★ Alabama Reassurance Co.
PO Box 020152
Tuscaloosa, AL 35402
Phone: (205)345-5600 **Fax:** (205)345-3937
Scott M. Phelps, President

★ 16485 ★ Alameda Alliance for Health
1240 S Luke Rd.
Alameda, CA 94502
Phone: (510)747-4500

★ 16486 ★ Alaska Vision Services, Inc.
Vision Services Group
3333 Quality Dr.
Rancho Cordova, CA 95670
Phone: (916)851-5000 **Fax:** (916)858-5388
Roger J. Valine, President

★ 16487 ★ Alfa Life Insurance Corp.
Alfa Insurance Group
2108 E South Blvd.
PO Box 11000
Montgomery, AL 36191-0001
Phone: (334)288-3900 **Fax:** (334)288-0905
Website: http://www.alfains.com
Jerry A. Newby, Chairman of the Board

★ 16488 ★ Alfa Life Insurance Corp.
Alfa Insurance Group
PO Box 11000
Montgomery, AL 36191-0001
Phone: (334)288-3900 **Fax:** (334)288-0905
Website: http://www.alfains.com
Roger J. Valine, President

★ 16489 ★ All American Life Insurance Co.
American International Group
PO Box 2074
Milwaukee, WI 53201-2074
Phone: (414)286-1500 **Fax:** (414)286-1550
Donald W. Britton, President

★ 16490 ★ All Savers Insurance Co.
Golden Rule Group
7440 Woodland Dr.
Indianapolis, IN 46278-1719
Phone: (317)297-4123
Website: http://www.goldenrule.com
John M. Whelan, President

★ 16491 ★ Allegiance Life Insurance Co.
Horace Mann Group
1 Horace Mann Plaza
Springfield, IL 62715
Phone: (217)789-2500 **Fax:** (217)535-7117
Website: http://www.horacemann.com
Louis G. Lower, II, President

★ 16492 ★ Alliance for Community Health
Tenet HealthSystem Hospitals Inc.
5615 Pershing Ave., No. 29
Saint Louis, MO 63112
Phone: (314)454-0055

★ 16493 ★ Alliance Health and Life Insurance Co.
2850 W Grand Blvd., 5th Fl.
Detroit, MI 48202-2692
Phone: (313)872-8100 **Fax:** (313)664-8566
Website: http://www.hapcorp.org
Cleve L. Killingsworth, Jr., President

★ 16494 ★ Allianz Life Insurance Co. of North America
Allianz Insurance Group
5701 Golden Hills Dr.
PO Box 1344
Minneapolis, MN 55440-1344
Phone: (763)765-6500 **Fax:** (763)765-6657
Website: http://www.allianzlife.com
Robert W. MacDonald, Chairman of the Board
Mark A. Zesbaugh, President

★ 16495 ★ Allied Financial Insurance Co.
6110 Pinemont, Ste. 215
Houston, TX 77092
Phone: (512)261-5132
Jim Hodge, President

★ 16496 ★ Allmerica Financial Life Insurance & Annuity Co.
Allmerica Financial Group
440 Lincoln St.
Worcester, MA 01653
Phone: (508)855-1000 **Fax:** (508)853-6332
Website: http://www.allmerica.com
Mark A. Hug, CEO & Pres

★ 16497 ★ Allstate Assurance Co.
Allstate Financial Group
3100 Sanders Rd.
Northbrook, IL 60062-7154
Phone: (847)402-5000
Website: http://www.allstate.com
Thomas J. Wilson, II, Chairman of the Board
Frmly: Provident National Assurance Co.

★ 16498 ★ Allstate Life Insurance Co.
Allstate Financial Group
3100 Sanders Rd.
Northbrook, IL 60062
Phone: (847)402-5000 **Fax:** (847)326-5052
Website: http://www.allstate.com
Thomas J. Wilson, II, President

★ 16499 ★ Allstate Life Insurance Co. of New York
Allstate Financial Group
3100 Sanders Rd.
Northbrook, IL 60062
Phone: (516)451-5300 **Fax:** (516)451-5329
Website: http://www.allstate.com
Thomas J. Wilson, II, President

★ 16500 ★ Aloha Care
1357 Kapiolani Blvd., Ste. 1250
Honolulu, HI 96814
Phone: (602)331-5100

★ 16501 ★ Alta Health & Life Insurance Co.
Great-West Life Group
8515 E Orchard Rd.
Greenwood Village, CO 80111
Phone: (303)737-3000 **Fax:** (303)737-4321
James D. Motz, President

★ 16502 ★ Altius Health Plans
Elan Health Partners
10421 S Jordan Gateway, Ste. 400
South Jordan, UT 84095
Phone: (801)933-3500

★ 16503 ★ Altus Dental Insurance Co.
10 Charles St.
Providence, RI 02904
Phone: (401)752-6000
Joseph A. Nagle, President

★ 16504 ★ Amalgamated Life and Health Insurance Co.
333 S Ashland Ave.
Chicago, IL 60607
Phone: (212)539-5939
Ronald Willis, President

★ 16505 ★ Amalgamated Life Insurance Co.
730 Broadway
New York, NY 10003
Phone: (212)539-5000 **Fax:** (212)473-1354
Website: http://www.amalgamatedlife.com
Ronald L. Minikes, CEO & Pres

★ 16506 ★ Ambassador Life Insurance Co.
1250 S Capital of Texas Hwy.
Austin, TX 78746
Phone: (512)328-6390
Jerry E. Finger, President

★ 16507 ★ AmCare Health Plans of Louisiana Inc.
AmCareCo Inc.
2707 N Loop W, Ste. 300
Houston, TX 77008
Phone: (713)293-3700

★ 16508 ★ AmCare Health Plans of Oklahoma Inc.
AmCareCo Inc.
2707 N Loop W, Ste. 300
Houston, TX 77008
Phone: (713)293-3700

★ 16509 ★ AmCare Health Plans of Texas Inc.
2707 N Loop W, Ste. 300
Houston, TX 77008
Phone: (713)293-3700
Thomas S. Lucksinger, President

★ 16510 ★ Amedex Insurance Co.
7001 SW 97th Ave.
Miami, FL 33173
Phone: (305)275-1400 **Fax:** (305)275-8484
Website: http://www.Amedex.com
Michael L. Carricarte, President

★ 16511 ★ Ameribest Life Insurance Co.
ING Group
5780 Powers Ferry Rd. NW
Atlanta, GA 30327
Phone: (515)698-7000 **Free:** 800-555-1910
Fax: (515)698-6973
Chris D. Schreier, President

★ 16512 ★ American-Amicable Life Insurance Co. of Texas
American Amicable Group
PO Box 2549
Waco, TX 76702-2549
Phone: (254)297-2777 **Fax:** (254)297-2784
S. Lanny Peavy, CEO & Pres

★ 16513 ★ American Bankers Life Assurance Co. of Florida
Fortis, Inc. Group
11222 Quail Roost Dr.
Miami, FL 33157
Phone: (305)253-2244 **Fax:** (305)252-6987
Website: http://www.assurant.com
Philip B. Camacho, CEO & Pres
Edward O'Hare, Chairman of the Board

★ 16514 ★ American Capital Life Insurance Co.
Health Care Service Corp.
1220 Huron Rd.
Cleveland, OH 44115-1700
Phone: (216)687-6800 **Fax:** (216)522-8702
Larry J. Newsom, CEO & Pres

★ 16515 ★ American Capitol Insurance Co.
American Capitol Group
PO Box 42814
Houston, TX 77242
Phone: (713)974-2242 **Fax:** (713)953-7920
John D. Cornett, President

★ 16516 ★ American Centurion Life Assurance Co.
American Express Financial Corp.
227 AXP Financial Ctr.
Minneapolis, MN 55474
Phone: (518)452-4150 **Free:** 800-504-0469
Fax: (518)452-3486
Website: http://www.americanexpress.com
Timothy V. Bechtold, President

★ 16517 ★ American Century Life Insurance Co.
4815 S Harvard, Ste. 280
Tulsa, OK 74135
Phone: (405)292-2120
Marlan K. Stumpff, President

★ 16518 ★ American Century Life Insurance Co. of Texas
7001 Grapevine Hwy., No. 434
North Richland Hills, TX 76180
Phone: (918)712-7770

★ 16519 ★ American Community Mutual Insurance Co.
American Community Group
39201 W Seven Mile Rd.
Livonia, MI 48152-1094
Phone: (734)591-4671 **Fax:** (734)591-4628
Website: http://www.american-community.com
Gerald E. Meach, President

★ 16520 ★ American Creditors Life Insurance Co.
PO Box 17748
Irvine, CA 92623-7748
Phone: (949)474-7600 **Fax:** (714)979-2658
Nelson Bobb, President

★ 16521 ★ American Enterprise Life Insurance Co.
American Express Financial Corp.
1114 AXP Financial Ctr.
Minneapolis, MN 55474
Phone: (612)671-1257 **Free:** 800-333-3437
Fax: (612)671-2154
Carol Ann Holton, President

★ 16522 ★ American Equity Investment Life Insurance Co.
PO Box 71216
Des Moines, IA 50325
Phone: (515)457-1714 **Fax:** (515)221-9989
Website: http://www.american-equity.com
David J. Noble, CEO & Chm Bd

★ 16523 ★ American Equity Investment Life Insurance Co. of New York
American Equity Investment Group
PO Box 71157
Des Moines, IA 50325
Phone: (515)457-1714 **Fax:** (515)221-9989
David J. Noble, Chairman of the Board

★ 16524 ★ American Exchange Life Insurance Co.
Universal American Financial Corp.
600 Courtland St.
Orlando, FL 32804
Phone: (407)628-1776 **Free:** 800-442-2223
Fax: (407)628-4227
Website: http://www.universalamericanfinancialcorp.com
Gary W. Bryant, CEO & Pres
Richard A. Barasch, Chairman of the Board

★ 16525 ★ American Family Life Assurance Co. of Columbus
AFLAC, Inc. Group
1932 Wynnton Rd.
Columbus, GA 31999
Phone: (706)323-3431 **Fax:** (706)596-3454
Daniel P. Amos, CEO & Pres

★ 16526 ★ American Family Life Assurance Co. of New York
AFLAC, Inc. Group
PO Box 15087
Albany, NY 12212
Phone: (518)438-0764 **Fax:** (518)438-0896
Daniel P. Amos, President

★ 16527 ★ American Family Life Insurance Co.
American Family Insurance Group
6000 American Pkwy.
Madison, WI 53783-0001
Phone: (608)249-2111 **Fax:** (608)243-4920
Website: http://www.amfam.com
David R. Anderson, President

★ 16528 ★ American Farm Life Insurance Co.
National Farm Group
PO Box 1486
Fort Worth, TX 76101-1486
Phone: (817)451-9550
Ronald G. Downing, President

★ 16529 ★ American Federated Life Insurance Co.
American Federated Group
PO Box 6000
Jackson, MS 39288-6000
Phone: (601)664-1000 **Fax:** (601)664-3805
James L. Martin, Jr., President

★ 16530 ★ American Fidelity Assurance Co.
American Fidelity Group
PO Box 25523
Oklahoma City, OK 73125-0523
Phone: (405)523-2000 **Fax:** (405)416-7879
Website: http://www.af-group.com
John W. Rex, President

★ 16531 ★ American Fidelity Life Insurance Co.
4060 Barrancas Ave.
Pensacola, FL 32507
Phone: (850)456-7401 **Fax:** (850)453-5440
Ruben E. Mauch, President

★ 16532 ★ American Financial Life Insurance Co.
Citigroup
307 W 7th St., Ste. 400
Fort Worth, TX 76102
Phone: (817)348-7565 **Free:** 800-316-5607
Fax: (817)348-7570
Darrell J. Gambero, President

★ 16533 ★ American Financial Security Life Insurance Co.
323 W 8th St., Ste. 202
Kansas City, MO 64105
Phone: (816)842-6605 **Fax:** (816)471-6421

★ 16534 ★ American Founders Life Insurance Co.
Vesta Insurance Group
PO Box 52121
Phoenix, AZ 85072-2121
Phone: (602)957-0778 **Fax:** (602)224-6884
Wayne A. Schreck, CEO & Pres
Kenneth Phillips, Chairman of the Board

★ 16535 ★ The American Franklin Life Insurance Co.
American International Group
1 Franklin Sq.
Springfield, IL 62713-0001
Phone: (217)528-2011 **Fax:** (217)528-3960
Website: http://www.thefranklin.com
Donald W. Britton, President

★ 16536 ★ American General Assurance Co.
American International Group
1000 Woodfield Rd.
Schaumburg, IL 60173-4793
Phone: (847)517-6000 **Fax:** (847)517-6005
William M. Keeler, CEO & Pres

★ 16537 ★ American General Life and Accident Insurance Co.
American International Group
American General Center
Nashville, TN 37250
Phone: (615)749-1000 **Fax:** (615)749-1251
Website: http://www.agla.com
Richard L. Bender, President

★ 16538 ★ American General Life Insurance Co.
American International Group
PO Box 1591
Houston, TX 77251-1591
Phone: (713)522-1111 **Fax:** (713)831-8269
Donald W. Britton, President

★ 16539 ★ American General Life Insurance Co. of New York
American International Group
PO Box 1456
Syracuse, NY 13202
Phone: (315)471-1121 **Fax:** (315)476-6520
Donald W. Britton, President

★ 16540 ★ American General Life Insurance Co. of Pennsylvania
American International Group
3600 Rte. 66
Neptune, NJ 07754-1580
Phone: (732)922-7000 **Fax:** (732)922-7194
Rodney O. Martin, Jr., Chairman of the Board

★ 16541 ★ American Guaranty Life Insurance Co.
3700 S Stonebridge Dr.
PO Box 8080
McKinney, TX 75070
Phone: (972)540-6516
Robert E. Richey, President

★ 16542 ★ American Health and Life Insurance Co.
Citigroup
307 W 7th St., Ste. 400
Fort Worth, TX 76102
Phone: (817)348-7500 **Free:** 800-316-5607
Fax: (817)348-7570
Darrell J. Gambero, President

★ 16543 ★ American Heritage Life Insurance Co.
Allstate Financial Group
3100 Sanders Rd.
Northbrook, IL 60062
Phone: (904)992-1776 **Fax:** (904)992-2658
Website: http://www.AHL1776.com
David A. Bird, CEO & Pres

★ 16544 ★ American Home Life Insurance Co.
PO Box 1497
Topeka, KS 66601-1497
Phone: (785)235-6276 **Fax:** (785)235-1037
Website: http://www.amhomelife.com
Steven S. Lobell, CEO & Pres

★ 16545 ★ American Home Life Insurance Co.
PO Box 715
North Little Rock, AR 72115-0715
Phone: (501)758-1778
Anne S. Powell Black, President

★ 16546 ★ American Income Life Insurance Co.
Torchmark Corp.
PO Box 2608
Waco, TX 76710
Phone: (254)761-6400 **Fax:** (254)751-8639
Website: http://www.ailins.com
Mark S. McAndrew, CEO & Pres

★ 16547 ★ American Independent Network Insurance Co. of New York
Penn Treaty American Corp.
3440 Lehigh St.
Allentown, PA 18103-7001
Phone: (607)732-3008
Website: http://www.penntreaty.com
Irving Levit, CEO & Pres

★ 16548 ★ American Insurance Co. of Texas
Ascent Assurance Inc.
110 W 7th St., Ste. 300
Fort Worth, TX 76102
Phone: (817)878-3300 **Fax:** (817)878-3672
Website: http://www.ascentassurance.com
Patrick J. Mitchell, CEO & Pres

★ 16549 ★ American International Life Assurance Co. of New York
American International Group
PO Box 727
Wall St. Station
New York, NY 10268
Phone: (212)770-7000 **Fax:** (212)514-6505
Gerald W. Wyndorf, CEO & Pres

★ 16550 ★ American Investors Life Insurance Co., Inc.
AmerUs Group
PO Box 2039
Topeka, KS 66601-2039
Phone: (785)232-6945 **Fax:** (785)232-3534
Mark V. Heitz, CEO & Pres

★ 16551 ★ American Life and Accident Insurance Co.
Torchmark Corp.
PO Box 2390
McKinney, TX 75070
Phone: (972)540-6516
Mark S. McAndrew, CEO & Pres

★ 16552 ★ American Life & Accident Insurance Co. of Kentucky
3 Riverfront Plaza
Louisville, KY 40202
Phone: (502)585-5347
Dinwiddie Lampton, Jr., President

★ 16553 ★ American Life and Annuity Co.
PO Box 11146
Knoxville, TN 37939
Phone: (865)588-5228
Stanley P. Brown, President

★ 16554 ★ American Life & Annuity Co.
PO Box 6011
Hot Springs, AR 71902
Phone: (501)623-7718
Phil Hale, President

★ 16555 ★ American Life and Health Insurance Co.
First Health Group Corp.
27725 Santa Margarita Pkwy., Ste. 220
Mission Viejo, CA 92691
Phone: (949)380-0233 **Fax:** (949)859-2815
Jane Hannabach, President
Lottie A. Kurcz, Vice President

★ 16556 ★ American Life Insurance Co.
208 S LaSalle St., Ste. 2070
Chicago, IL 60604
Phone: (312)372-5722 **Fax:** (312)372-5727
Robert T. Napier, President

★ 16557 ★ American Life Insurance Co.
American International Group
PO Box 2226
Wilmington, DE 19899
Phone: (302)594-2000 **Fax:** (302)428-6019
R. K. Nottingham, CEO & Chm Bd

★ 16558 ★ American Life Insurance Co. of New York
435 Hudson St.
New York, NY 10014
Phone: (212)741-9311 **Fax:** (212)741-9322
Shane Gleeson, President
David A. Smilow, CEO & Chm Bd

★ 16559 ★ American Maturity Life Insurance Co.
Hartford Life, Inc.
200 Hopmeadow St.
Simsbury, CT 06070
Phone: (860)525-8555 **Fax:** (860)843-5568
Website: http://www.thehartford.com
Thomas M. Marra, President

★ 16560 ★ American Mayflower Life Insurance Co. of New York
GE Financial Assurance Group
6604 W Broad St.
Richmond, VA 23230
Phone: (212)672-4200 **Fax:** (212)672-4299
Website: http://www.ge.com
Cheryl C. Whaley, CEO & Pres

★ 16561 ★ American Medical and Life Insurance Co.
35 Broadway
Hicksville, NY 11801
Phone: (516)822-8700 **Fax:** (516)931-1010
Dr. Jules V. Lane, President

★ 16562 ★ American Medical Security Insurance Co. of Georgia
American Medical Security Group, Inc.
PO Box 19032
Green Bay, WI 54307-9032
Free: 800-232-5432 **Fax:** (920)661-2132
Samuel V. Miller, CEO & Pres

★ 16563 ★ American Memorial Life Insurance Co.
Fortis, Inc. Group
PO Box 2730
Rapid City, SD 57709-2730
Phone: (605)719-0999 **Free:** 800-810-9046
Fax: (605)719-0853
John E. Wade, President

★ 16564 ★ American Modern Life Insurance Co.
American Modern Insurance Group
PO Box 5323
Cincinnati, OH 45201-5323
Phone: (513)943-7200 **Fax:** (513)943-7201
Website: http://www.midlandcompany.com
John W. Hayden, CEO & Pres

★ 16565 ★ American National Insurance Co.
American National Group
1 Moody Plaza, 17th Fl.
Galveston, TX 77550-7999
Phone: (409)763-4661 **Fax:** (409)766-6663
Website: http://www.anico.com
G. R. Ferdinandtsen, President

★ 16566 ★ American National Life Insurance Co. of Texas
American National Group
1 Moody Plaza, 17th Fl.
Galveston, TX 77550-7999
Phone: (409)763-4661 **Fax:** (409)766-6663
Website: http://www.anico.com
G. R. Ferdinandtsen, President

★ 16567 ★ American Network Insurance Co.
Penn Treaty American Corp.
3440 Lehigh St.
Allentown, PA 18103-7001
Phone: (610)965-2222
Website: http://www.penntreaty.com
Irving Levit, President

★ 16568 ★ American Partners Life Insurance Co.
American Express Financial Corp.
227 AXP Financial Ctr.
Minneapolis, MN 55474
Phone: (612)671-2154 **Fax:** (612)671-7543
Website: http://www.americanexpress.com
Gumer C. Alvero, President

★ 16569 ★ American Phoenix Life and Reassurance Co.
Phoenix Life Group
1 American Row
Hartford, CT 06115
Phone: (860)403-1000
David R. Pellerin, President

★ 16570 ★ American Pioneer Life Insurance Co.
Universal American Financial Corp.
600 Courtland St.
Orlando, FL 32804
Phone: (407)628-1776 **Fax:** (407)628-3679
Website: http://www.amerpion.com
Gary W. Bryant, CEO & Pres

★ 16571 ★ American Progressive Life & Health Insurance Co. of New York
Universal American Financial Corp.
600 Courtland St.
Orlando, FL 32804
Phone: (914)934-8300 **Free:** 800-332-3377
Fax: (914)934-1988
Website: http://www.amerprog.com
Richard A. Barasch, CEO & Pres

★ 16572 ★ American Public Life Insurance Co.
American Fidelity Group
PO Box 925
Jackson, MS 39205-0925
Phone: (601)936-6600 **Fax:** (601)939-2157
Website: http://www.ampublic.com
William M. Cameron, CEO & Pres

★ 16573 ★ American Republic Insurance Co.
PO Box 1
Des Moines, IA 50301
Phone: (515)245-2000 **Fax:** (515)245-2041
Website: http://www.aric.com
Michael E. Abbott, President

★ 16574 ★ American Reserve Life Insurance Co.
8200 Brookriver Dr., Ste. 600N
Dallas, TX 75247-4069
Free: 800-876-8776
Bradford A. Phillips, President

★ 16575 ★ American Resources Life Insurance Co.
NCMIC Life Insurance Group
PO Box 9118
Des Moines, IA 50306-9118
Phone: (515)222-1736 **Fax:** (515)222-2951
Patrick E. McNerneyi, President

★ 16576 ★ American Retirement Life Insurance Co.
American Financial Group
PO Box 5420
Cincinnati, OH 45201-5420
Phone: (605)719-0999 **Fax:** (605)719-0603
Charles R. Scheper, President

★ 16577 ★ American Savings Life Insurance Co.
935 E Main St., Ste. 100
Mesa, AZ 85203-8849
Phone: (480)835-5000
David K. Allen, President

★ 16578 ★ American Service Life Insurance Co.
Fidelity Security Group
3130 Broadway
Kansas City, MO 64111-2452
Phone: (816)756-1060 **Fax:** (816)968-0563
Richard F. Jones, President

★ 16579 ★ American Skandia Life Assurance Corp.
PO Box 883
Shelton, CT 06484-0883
Free: 800-628-6039
Website: http://www.americanskandia.com
Wade A. Dokken, President

★ 16580 ★ American Slovenian Catholic Union
2439 Glenwood Ave.
Joliet, IL 60435
Phone: (815)741-2001 **Fax:** (815)741-2002
Eugene Kogovsek, President

★ 16581 ★ American States Life Insurance Co.
SAFECO Life Group
PO Box 34690
Seattle, WA 98124-1690
Phone: (425)376-8000 **Fax:** (425)376-5818
Randall H. Talbot, President

★ 16582 ★ American Travelers Assurance Co.
20 Glover Ave.
Norwalk, CT 06850
Phone: (203)229-1000
Website: http://www.healthmarket.com
Gregory R. Morris, President

★ 16583 ★ American Underwriters Life Insurance Co.
American Underwriters Life Group
PO Box 9510
Wichita, KS 67277-0510
Phone: (316)794-2200 **Fax:** (316)794-8470
Website: http://www.IAI-Online.com
R. Kell Hawkins, President

★ 16584 ★ American United Life Insurance Co.
American United Life Group
PO Box 368
Indianapolis, IN 46206-0368
Phone: (317)285-1877 **Fax:** (317)285-1979
Website: http://www.aul.com
Jerry D. Semler, CEO & Pres
R. Stephen Radcliffe, Exec VP

★ 16585 ★ American Vanguard Life Insurance Co.
AmerUs Group
611 5th Ave.
Des Moines, IA 50309
Phone: (515)283-2371 **Fax:** (515)242-2385
Gary R. McPhail, CEO & Pres

★ 16586 ★ AmeriChoice of New Jersey Inc.
AmeriChoice Corp.
2 Gateway Ctr.
Newark, NJ 07102
Phone: (973)297-5500
Website: http://www.americhoice.com

★ 16587 ★ AmeriChoice of Pennsylvania Inc.
AmeriChoice Corp.
100 Penn Sq. E, Ste. 900
Philadelphia, PA 19107
Phone: (215)832-4500
Website: http://www.americhoice.com

★ 16588 ★ Americo Financial Life and Annuity Insurance Co.
Americo Life Group
PO Box 13487
Kansas City, MO 64199-3487
Phone: (816)391-2000 **Fax:** (816)391-2083
Gary L. Muller, CEO & Pres

★ 16589 ★ Americom Life and Annuity Insurance Co.
1001 Fleet St.
Baltimore, MD
Phone: (913)402-2300 **Fax:** (913)402-2344
Website: http://www.americomlife.com
Guy V. Barker, CEO & Chm Bd

★ 16590 ★ AMERIGROUP Illinois Inc.
AMERIGROUP Corp.
4425 Corporation Ln.
Virginia Beach, VA 23462
Phone: (757)473-2737

★ 16591 ★ AMERIGROUP Texas Inc.
AMERIGROUP Corp.
4425 Corporation Ln.
Virginia Beach, VA 23462
Phone: (757)490-6900

★ 16592 ★ AmeriHealth HMO Inc.
Independence Blue Cross
919 N Market St., Ste. 1200
Wilmington, DE 19801
Phone: (215)241-2400

★ 16593 ★ Amerihealth Insurance Co. of New Jersey
8000 Midlantic Dr., Ste. 333
Mount Laurel, NJ 08054-1560
Phone: (856)778-6598
G. Fred DiBona, Jr., President

★ 16594 ★ Ameritas Life Insurance Corp.
Ameritas Acacia Group
PO Box 81889
Lincoln, NE 68501
Phone: (402)467-1122 **Fax:** (402)465-6100
Website: http://www.ameritas.com
Kenneth C. Louis, CEO & Chm Bd

★ 16595 ★ Ameritas Managed Dental Plan Inc.
Ameritas Life Insurance Corp.
151 Kalmus Dr., Ste. J3
Costa Mesa, CA 92626-5988
Phone: (714)437-5966
David C. Moore, C, Contact

★ 16596 ★ Ameritas Variable Life Insurance Co.
Ameritas Acacia Group
PO Box 82550
Lincoln, NE 68501
Phone: (402)467-1122 **Fax:** (402)465-6100
Website: http://www.overturelife.com
William J. Atherton, President

★ 16597 ★ AmerUs Life Insurance Co.
AmerUs Group
611 5th Ave.
Des Moines, IA 50309
Phone: (515)283-2371 **Fax:** (515)241-4869
Website: http://www.amerus.com
Gary R. McPhail, CEO & Pres

★ 16598 ★ Amica Life Insurance Co.
Amica Insurance Companies
PO Box 6008
Providence, RI 02940-6008
Phone: (401)334-6000 **Free:** 800-242-6422
Fax: (401)333-9630
Website: http://www.amica.com
Thomas A. Taylor, CEO & Pres

★ 16599 ★ Amil International Insurance Co.
9229 Waterford Centre Blvd., Ste. 500
Austin, TX 78758
Phone: (512)349-4137

★ 16600 ★ Amil International (Texas) Inc.
9229 Waterford Centre Blvd., Ste. 500
Austin, TX 78758
Phone: (512)349-4137

★ 16601 ★ Annuity Investors Life Insurance Co.
American Financial Group
PO Box 5423
Cincinnati, OH 45201-5423
Phone: (513)357-3300 **Fax:** (513)357-3397
Website: http://www.gafri.com
Charles R. Scheper, CEO & Pres

★ 16602 ★ Annuity and Life Reassurance of America
280 Trumbull St., 21st Fl.
Hartford, CT 06103
Phone: (860)256-2122 **Fax:** (860)525-1200
Website: http://www.annuityandlifere.com
Bryan Featherstone, President

★ 16603 ★ Anthem Alliance Health Insurance Co.
Anthem Inc.
120 Monument Cir.
Indianapolis, IN 46204
Phone: (317)488-6000
William R. Vandervennet, Jr., President

★ 16604 ★ Anthem Health and Life Insurance Co. of New York
Anthem Inc.
1200 South Ave., Ste. 301
Staten Island, NY 10314
Phone: (718)370-5380
Carmine A. Morano, President

★ 16605 ★ Anthem Health Plans, Inc.
Anthem Inc.
370 Bassett Rd.
North Haven, CT 06473-4201
Phone: (203)239-4911
Website: http://www.anthem.com
Marjorie W. Dorr, President

★ 16606 ★ Anthem Health Plans of Maine
Anthem Inc.
2 Gannett Dr.
South Portland, ME 04106-6911
Phone: (207)822-7000 **Fax:** (207)822-7350
Website: http://www.mainebluecross.com
Keith W. Vangeison, President

★ 16607 ★ Anthem Health Plans of New Hampshire, Inc.
Anthem Inc.
300 Goffs Falls Rd.
Manchester, NH 03111-0001
Phone: (603)695-7000 **Fax:** (603)695-7304
Website: http://www.anthembcbsnh.com
Marjorie W. Dorr, President

★ 16608 ★ Anthem Insurance Companies, Inc.
Anthem Inc.
120 Monument Cir.
Indianapolis, IN 46204-4903
Phone: (317)488-6000 **Fax:** (317)488-6200
Website: http://www.anthem-inc.com
Larry C. Glasscock, CEO & Pres

★ 16609 ★ Anthem Life Insurance Co.
Anthem Inc.
1801 Watermark Dr., Ste. 200
Columbus, OH 43215
Phone: (614)436-0688 **Fax:** (614)438-3959
Website: http://www.anthem.com
John J. Gainor, President

★ 16610 ★ Appalachian Life Insurance Co.
United Trust, Inc. Group
PO Box 5147
Springfield, IL 62705-5147
Phone: (217)241-6300
Randall L. Attkisson, President
Larry E. Ryherd, CEO & Chm Bd

★ 16611 ★ Arbella Life and Health Insurance Co.
Arbella Insurance Group
1100 Crown Colony Dr.
Quincy, MA 02269
Phone: (617)328-2936
Website: http://www.arbella.com
John F. Donohue, Chairman of the Board

★ 16612 ★ Arista Insurance Co.
116 John St.
New York, NY 10038-3302
Phone: (212)964-2150 **Fax:** (212)608-6473
Website: http://www.aristacorp-tpa.com
Stanley S. Mandel, President

★ 16613 ★ Arkansas Bankers Life Insurance Co.
PO Box 1947
Texarkana, AR 75504-1947
Phone: (870)773-7221
James Barron, President

★ 16614 ★ Arkansas Life Insurance Co.
PO Box 30
Trumann, AR 72472
Phone: (870)483-6355 **Fax:** (870)483-6328
Ben R. Hyneman, President

★ 16615 ★ Arkansas National Life Insurance Co.
Forethought Group
Forethought Ctr.
Batesville, IN 47006-9170
Phone: (812)934-7139 **Fax:** (812)934-8564
Website: http://www.forethought.com
Stephen R. Lang, President

★ 16616 ★ Arnett HMO Inc.
415 N 26th St., Ste. 101
PO Box 6108
Lafayette, IN 47903-6108
Phone: (765)448-7400

★ 16617 ★ Ashley Life Insurance Co., Inc.
PO Box 571
Hamburg, AR 71646
Phone: (318)322-8181
Tex R. Kilpatrick, President

★ 16618 ★ Associated American Mutual Life Insurance Co.
36 S State St., Ste. 1000
Salt Lake City, UT 84111-1486
Phone: (801)442-5000
Steven R. Michel, President

★ 16619 ★ Associated Mutual Hospital Service of Michigan
25 Jefferson SE
Grand Rapids, MI 49503
Phone: (616)458-6327 **Fax:** (616)458-1486
John Jacobitz, President

★ 16620 ★ Associates Financial Life Insurance Co.
Citigroup
307 W 7th St., Ste. 400
Fort Worth, TX 76102
Phone: (817)348-7500
Darrell J. Gambero, President

★ 16621 ★ Associates Financial Life Insurance Co. of Texas
Citigroup
307 W 7th St., Ste. 400
Fort Worth, TX 76102
Free: 800-316-5607
Darrell J. Gambero, President

★ 16622 ★ Assured Investors Life Co.
Tenet Healthcare Corp.
1005 W Orangeburg, Ste. B
Modesto, CA 95350-4163
Free: 800-468-8600 **Fax:** (207)597-8751
Robert W. Mills, President

★ 16623 ★ Assurity Life Insurance Co.
Lincoln Insurance Group
PO Box 82533
Lincoln, NE 68501-2533
Phone: (402)476-6500 **Fax:** (402)437-4395
Website: http://www.assurity.com
Thomas D. Potter, CEO & Pres

★ 16624 ★ Athens Area Health Plan Select Inc.
Athens Regional Health Services Inc.
295 W Clayton St.
Athens, GA 30601
Phone: (706)549-0549

★ 16625 ★ Atlanta Life Insurance Co.
100 Auburn Ave. NE
Atlanta, GA 30303
Phone: (404)659-2100 **Fax:** (404)654-8808
Website: http://www.atlantalife.com
Charles H. Cornelius, CEO & Pres

★ 16626 ★ Atlantic Coast Life Insurance Co.
PO Box 20010
Charleston, SC 29413-0010
Phone: (843)763-8680 **Fax:** (843)763-8688
Y. W. Scarborough, III, CEO & Pres

★ 16627 ★ Atlantic Southern Insurance Co.
PO Box 362889
San Juan, PR 00936-2889
Phone: (787)767-9750 **Fax:** (787)751-2250
Robin Bolton, President

★ 16628 ★ Atrium Health Plan Inc.
Aware Integrated Inc.
3535 Blue Cross Rd.
PO Box 64179
Saint Paul, MN 55164-0179
Phone: (715)386-6886 **Fax:** (715)386-8326
Website: http://www.atriumhealthplan.com
George Emslie, Chairman of the Board

★ 16629 ★ AultCare HMO
Aultman Health Foundation
2600 6th St. SW
Canton, OH 44710
Phone: (330)438-6360

★ 16630 ★ Aurora National Life Assurance Co.
American International Group
1290 Silas Deane Hwy.
Wethersfield, CT 06109
Phone: (310)264-3200 **Free:** 800-513-6090
Fax: (310)264-3206
Website: http://www.auroralife.com
Steven W. Turner, President

★ 16631 ★ AUSA Life Insurance Co., Inc.
AEGON USA, Inc.
4 Manhattanville Rd.
Purchase, NY 10577
Phone: (914)697-8000
Tom Schlossberg, President

★ 16632 ★ Auto Club Life Insurance Co.
AAA Life Group
17250 Newburgh Rd., Ste. 100
Livonia, MI 48152
Phone: (734)591-9422 **Fax:** (734)632-0678
Website: http://www.aaalife.com
Steven D. Monahan, President

★ 16633 ★ Auto-Owners Life Insurance Co.
Auto-Owners Insurance Group
PO Box 30660
Lansing, MI 48909-8160
Phone: (517)323-1200 **Fax:** (517)391-1901
Website: http://www.auto-owners.com
John W. Fisher, President

★ 16634 ★ Automobile Club of Southern California Life Insurance Co.
AAA Life Group
17250 Newburgh Rd., Ste. 100
Livonia, MI 48152
Phone: (714)850-5111
Thomas V. McKernan, Jr., President

★ 16635 ★ AvMed Inc.
AvMed Group
PO Box 749
Gainesville, FL 32602-0749
Phone: (352)372-8400
Edward Peddie, President

★ 16636 ★ AXA Corporate Solutions Life Reinsurance Co.
AXA Group
17 State St.
New York, NY 10004-1501
Phone: (212)859-0555 **Fax:** (212)859-0511
Website: http://www.axa-corporatesolutions.com
Michael W. Pado, President
Robert Lippincott, III, Chairman of the Board

★ 16637 ★ Balboa Life Insurance Co.
Balboa Life Insurance Group
18581 Teller Ave.
Irvine, CA 92612
Phone: (949)553-0700 **Fax:** (949)553-5962
Website: http://www.balboainsurance.com
Dwight D. Cissell, President

★ 16638 ★ Balboa Life Insurance Co. of New York
Balboa Life Insurance Group
18581 Teller Ave.
Irvine, CA 92623-9702
Phone: (949)553-0700
Dwight D Cissell, President

★ 16639 ★ The Baltimore Life Insurance Co.
Baltimore Life Group
10075 Red Run Blvd.
Owings Mills, MD 21117-6050
Phone: (410)581-6600 **Fax:** (410)581-6612
Website: http://www.baltlife.com
L. John Pearson, CEO & Pres

★ 16640 ★ Banc One Kentucky Insurance Co.
Banc One Insurance Group
416 W Jefferson St.
Louisville, KY 40202
Phone: (502)566-2289 **Fax:** (502)566-2269
Glen Milesko, President

★ 16641 ★ Bankers Commercial Life Insurance Co.
5720 LBJ Fwy., Ste. 200
Dallas, TX 75240-6334
Phone: (972)980-1151 **Fax:** (972)980-4310
Sidney F. Rowland, Jr., President

★ 16642 ★ Bankers Fidelity Life Insurance Co.
Atlantic American/Delta Group
PO Box 105185
Atlanta, GA 30348
Phone: (404)266-5500 **Fax:** (404)266-5699
Website: http://www.atlam.com
Eugene Choate, President
J. Mack Robinson, Chairman of the Board

★ 16643 ★ Bankers Life and Casualty Co.
Conseco Insurance Group
11815 N Pennsylvania St.
Carmel, IN 46032
Phone: (312)396-6000 **Fax:** (317)817-2161
Website: http://www.conseco.com
Edward M. Berube, President
Stephen C. Hilbert, Chairman of the Board

★ 16644 ★ Bankers Life Insurance Co.
Bankers Insurance Group
360 Central Ave.
Saint Petersburg, FL 33701
Phone: (727)823-4000 **Fax:** (727)803-4095
Website: http://www.bankerslifeinsurance.com
Douglas B. Pierce, CEO & Pres

★ 16645 ★ Bankers Life Insurance Co. of America
4925 McKinney Ave.
Dallas, TX 75205
Phone: (254)744-3160
Mildred N. Bickel, President

★ 16646 ★ Bankers Life Insurance Co. of Illinois
Conseco Insurance Group
11815 N Pennsylvania St.
Carmel, IN 46032
Phone: (312)396-6000 **Fax:** (312)817-2161
Website: http://www.conseco.com
Edward M. Berube, President

★ 16647 ★ Bankers Life Insurance Co. of New York
AmerUs Group
65 Froehlich Farm Blvd.
Woodbury, NY 11797-9847
Phone: (516)364-5900 **Fax:** (516)364-5920
Website: http://www.blny.com
Stephen J. Shorrock, CEO & Pres

★ 16648 ★ Bankers Life of Louisiana
Life of the South Group
601 N Trenton St.
PO Box 2010
Ruston, LA 71273
Phone: (904)350-9660 **Fax:** (904)354-4525
Website: http://www.life-south.com
William C. Wardlaw, President

★ 16649 ★ Bankers National Life Insurance Co.
Conseco Insurance Group
11825 N Pennsylvania St.
Carmel, IN 46032
Phone: (317)817-6300 **Fax:** (317)817-2161
Website: http://www.conseco.com
Thomas J. Kilian, President
Elizabeth C. Georgakopoulos, Chairman of the Board

★ 16650 ★ Bankers Reserve Life Insurance Co. of Wisconsin
Life & Health Group
220 W Germantown Pike
Plymouth Meeting, PA 19462
Phone: (610)940-1477 **Fax:** (610)940-1478
Melvyn K. Miller, President

★ 16651 ★ Banner Life Insurance Co.
Legal & General America, Inc.
1701 Research Blvd.
Rockville, MD 20850
Phone: (301)279-4800 **Fax:** (301)279-4178
Website: http://www.lgamerica.com
David S. Lenaburg, CEO & Chm Bd

★ 16652 ★ BCBSD, Inc.
CareFirst of Maryland Inc.
1 Brandywine Gateway
Wilmington, DE 19801
Phone: (302)421-3000
Paul C. King, Jr., President

★ 16653 ★ Beacon Health Plans Inc.
Beacon Health Systems Inc.
2511 Ponce De Leon Blvd., 5th Fl.
PO Box 14-9080
Coral Gables, FL 33114-9080
Phone: (305)460-2000

★ 16654 ★ Benchmark Health Insurance Co.
2550 Charles St.
Rockford, IL 61108
Phone: (815)391-7350
Thomas E. Hecht, President

★ 16655 ★ Beneficial Life Insurance Co.
36 S State St.
Salt Lake City, UT 84136
Phone: (801)933-1100 **Fax:** (801)531-3306
Website: http://www.beneficiallife.com
Kent H. Cannon, CEO & Pres

★ 16656 ★ Benefit Capital Life Insurance Co.
203 Carondelet, Ste. 717
New Orleans, LA 70130
Phone: (504)522-3407
Randal M. Beach, President

★ 16657 ★ Benicorp Insurance Co.
PO Box 68917
Indianapolis, IN 46268-0917
Phone: (317)290-1205 **Fax:** (317)216-7857
Website: http://www.benicorp.com
Dennis W. Houchens, President

★ 16658 ★ Berkshire Hathaway Life Insurance Co. of Nebraska
Berkshire Hathaway Group
3024 Harney St.
Omaha, NE 68131-3580
Phone: (402)536-3000 **Fax:** (402)536-3030
Website: http://www.bhln.com
Donald F. Wurster, President

★ 16659 ★ Berkshire Life Insurance Co. of America
Guardian Life Group
7 Hanover Sq.
New York, NY 10004
Phone: (413)499-4321 **Fax:** (413)499-4831
Website: http://www.berkshirelife.com
James W. Zilinski, CEO & Pres

★ 16660 ★ Best Life & Health Insurance Co.
PO Box 19721
Irvine, CA 92623-9721
Phone: (949)253-4080 **Fax:** (949)222-1004
Website: http://www.bestins.com
Donald R. Lawrenz, CEO & Pres

★ 16661 ★ Best Meridian Insurance Co.
1320 S Dixie Hwy., 6th Fl.
Coral Gables, FL 33146
Phone: (305)443-2898 **Fax:** (305)668-3608
Website: http://www.bmicos.com
Brent Bush, CEO & Pres

★ 16662 ★ BHG Life Insurance Co.
Berkshire Hathaway Group
3024 Harney St.
Omaha, NE 68131-3580
Phone: (402)536-3000 **Fax:** (402)536-3050
Donald F. Wurster, President

★ 16663 ★ Big Sky Life Inc.
501 N Sanders St.
Helena, MT 59601
Phone: (406)442-1233
Thomas G. Walker, President

★ 16664 ★ Bluebonnet Life Insurance Co.
Blue Cross & Blue Shield of Mississippi Group
PO Box 22924
Jackson, MS 39225-2924
Phone: (601)932-8269 **Fax:** (601)664-5190
Richard J. Hale, CEO & Pres

★ 16665 ★ Bluegrass Family Health Inc.
Baptist Healthcare System Inc.
651 Perimeter Dr., Ste. 300
Lexington, KY 40517
Phone: (859)269-4475 **Fax:** (859)335-3375

★ 16666 ★ Booker T. Washington Insurance Co.
PO Box 697
Birmingham, AL 35201-0697
Phone: (205)328-5454 **Fax:** (205)251-6873
Walter Howlett, Jr., CEO & Pres

★ 16667 ★ Boston Mutual Life Insurance Co.
Boston Mutual Group
120 Royall St.
Canton, MA 02021-1098
Phone: (781)828-7000 **Fax:** (781)828-6584
Website: http://www.bostonmutual.com
Paul E. Petry, President

★ 16668 ★ Brandywine Life Insurance Co., Inc.
1100 N Market St.
Wilmington, DE 19890
Phone: (302)651-1504
Hugh D. Leahy, Jr., President

★ 16669 ★ Brokers National Life Assurance Co.
2100 W William Cannon, Ste. L
Austin, TX 78745
Phone: (512)383-0220 **Fax:** (512)383-8596
Website: http://www.bnlac.com
Kenneth Tobey, President

★ 16670 ★ Brooke Life Insurance Co.
Jackson National Group
1 Corporate Way
Lansing, MI 48951
Phone: (517)381-5500 **Fax:** (517)706-5524
Website: http://www.jacksonnational.com
Clark P. Manning, CEO & Pres

★ 16671 ★ BSH Life Insurance Co. Inc.
PO Box 379
Honolulu, HI 96809
Phone: (808)948-5145
John Jacobs, President

★ 16672 ★ Business Men's Assurance Co. of America
PO Box 419458
Kansas City, MO 64141
Phone: (816)753-8000 **Fax:** (816)751-5563
Website: http://www.bma.com
Robert T. Rakich, President
Giorgio Balzer, CEO & Chm Bd

★ 16673 ★ C.M. Life Insurance Co.
MassMutual Financial Group
1295 State St.
Springfield, MA 01111
Phone: (413)788-8411
Website: http://www.massmutual.com
Robert J. O'Connell, CEO & Pres

★ 16674 ★ Cambridge Life Insurance Co.
First Health Group Corp.
27725 Santa Margarita Pkwy., Ste. 220
Mission Viejo, CA 92691
Phone: (949)380-0233 **Fax:** (949)859-2815
Jane Hannabach, President
Lottie A. Kurcz, Vice President

★ 16675 ★ Cameron Life Insurance Co.
Cameron Mutual Group
214 McElwain Dr.
Cameron, MO 64429-1321
Phone: (816)632-3737
Darwin G. Copeman, President

★ 16676 ★ The Canada Life Assurance Co.
Canada Life Group
330 University Ave.
Toronto, ON, Canada M5G 1R8
Phone: (416)597-1456 **Fax:** (416)597-9876
Website: http://www.canadalife.com
D. A. Nield, CEO & Pres

★ 16677 ★ Canada Life Insurance Co. of America
Canada Life Group
6201 Powers Ferry Rd. NW
Atlanta, GA 30339
Phone: (770)953-1959 **Fax:** 888-670-4836
Website: http://www.canadalifeus.com
Ronald E. Beettam, President

★ 16678 ★ Canada Life Insurance Co. of New York
Canada Life Group
410 Saw Mill River Rd.
Ardsley, NY 10502
Phone: (914)693-2300 **Fax:** (914)674-2535
Website: http://www.canadalifeny.com
Paul R. McCadam, President

★ 16679 ★ Canada Life Insurance Co. of Puerto Rico, Inc.
Canada Life Group
Canada Life Plaza, Ste. A
St. 1, Corner Rd. 165
Rexco Industrial Park
Guaynabo, PR 00968

★ 16680 ★ Cape Health Plan Inc.
17421 Telegraph Rd.
Detroit, MI 48219
Phone: (313)537-0220

★ 16681 ★ Capital District Physicians' Health Plan, Inc.
Patroon Creek Corporate Ctr.
1223 Washington Ave.
Albany, NY 12206-1057
Phone: (518)641-3000
Joseph W. Monahan, MD, Chairman of the Board

★ 16682 ★ Capital Group Health Services of Florida, Inc.
Blue Cross & Blue Shield of Florida
4800 Deerwood Campus Pkwy., DCC1-6
Jacksonville, FL 32224
Phone: (850)383-3333
W. K. Boutwell, Jr., President

★ 16683 ★ Capital Health Plans, Inc.
820 Parish St.
Pittsburgh, PA 15220
Phone: (412)922-2803 **Fax:** (412)922-9071
Charles E. Davidson, President

★ 16684 ★ Capital Reserve Life Insurance Co.
PO Box 896
Jefferson City, MO 65102-0896
Phone: (573)636-3913
Joseph E. Warden, President

★ 16685 ★ Capitol Life & Accident Insurance Co.
PO Box 4216
Little Rock, AR 72214
Phone: (501)562-3894
Paul D. Eaton, President

★ 16686 ★ Capitol Mutual Insurance Co.
6522 Dogwood View Pkwy.
Jackson, MS 39213
Phone: (601)856-4367
Susan O. Snyder, President

★ 16687 ★ Capitol Security Life Insurance Co.
PO Box 982005
Fort Worth, TX 76182-8005
Phone: (817)284-4888

★ 16688 ★ Care Choices HMO
Care Choices Group
34605 12 Mile Rd.
Farmington Hills, MI 48331
Phone: (248)489-6321
Website: http://www.carechoices.com

★ 16689 ★ Care 1st Health Plan, Inc.
1000 S Fremont Ave., A-11, Unit 22
Alhambra, CA 91803
Phone: (626)299-4299

★ 16690 ★ CareAmerica Life Insurance Co.
Blue Shield of California Group
PO Box 7725
San Francisco, CA 94120-7725
Phone: (209)367-3408 **Fax:** (209)367-3450
Debra E. Bowles, CEO & Pres

★ 16691 ★ CareFirst BlueChoice Inc.
CareFirst of Maryland Inc.
550 12th St. SW
Washington, DC 20065
Phone: (202)479-8000

★ 16692 ★ CareFirst of Maryland, Inc.
10455 Mill Run Cir.
Owings Mills, MD 21117
Phone: (410)581-3000
William L. Jews, President

★ 16693 ★ Carelink Health Plans Inc.
Coventry Health Care Inc.
500 Virginia St. E, Ste. 400
Charleston, WV 25301
Phone: (304)348-2900
Website: http://www.cvty.com

★ 16694 ★ Caribbean American Life Assurance Co.
Fortis, Inc. Group
273 Ponce De Leon Ave.
Hato Rey, PR 00917-1838
Phone: (787)250-6470 **Fax:** (787)250-7680
Website: http://www.calac.com
Ivan C. Lopez, President

★ 16695 ★ Cariten Health Plan Inc.
PHP Companies Inc.
1420 Centerpoint Blvd.
Knoxville, TN 37932
Phone: (865)470-7470

★ 16696 ★ Cariten Insurance Co.
1420 Centerpoint Blvd.
Knoxville, TN 37932
Phone: (865)670-7282
Anthony L. Spezia, President

★ 16697 ★ Carolina Care Plan Inc.
Physicians Health Plan of South Carolina
201 Executive Ctr. Dr., Ste. 300
Columbia, SC 29210-8438
Phone: (803)750-7400

★ 16698 ★ Cass County Life Insurance Co.
102 W Main St.
Atlanta, TX 75551
Phone: (903)796-2833
H. Randy Hanner, President

★ 16699 ★ Catalina Life & Health Reinsurance Co.
6100 Niel Rd., Ste. 500
Sierra Plaza
Reno, NV 89511-1149
Phone: (651)714-4450
Robert W. Morey, President

★ 16700 ★ Catholic Family Life Insurance
PO Box 11563
Shorewood, WI 53211-0563
Phone: (414)961-0500 **Fax:** (414)961-0477
Website: http://www.cfli.org
Daniel T. Lloyd, CEO & Pres
Patrick J. Murphy, Chairman of the Board

★ 16701 ★ Catholic Knights
1100 W Wells St.
Milwaukee, WI 53233-2316
Phone: (414)273-6266 **Fax:** (414)273-2120
Website: http://www.catholicknights.com
Daniel J. Steininger, President

★ 16702 ★ Catholic Life Insurance Co.
1635 NE Loop 410
San Antonio, TX 78209-1694
Phone: (210)828-9921 **Fax:** (210)828-4629
Website: http://www.catholiclifeinsurance.com
J. Michael Belz, CEO & Pres

★ 16703 ★ Catholic Order of Foresters
PO Box 3012
Naperville, IL 60566-7012
Phone: (630)983-4900 **Fax:** (630)983-4057
Website: http://www.catholicforester.com
Robert Ciesla, President

★ 16704 ★ CDPHP Universal Benefits Inc.
1223 Washington Ave.
Albany, NY 12206-1057
Phone: (518)641-3000

★ 16705 ★ Celtic Insurance Co.
233 S Wacker Dr., Ste. 700
Chicago, IL 60606-6393
Phone: (312)332-5401 **Fax:** (312)441-0341
Website: http://www.celtic-net.com
Frederick J. Manning, CEO & Pres
James P. Daly, Exec VP

★ 16706 ★ Censtat Life Assurance Co.
Central States H & L Group
PO Box 34350
Omaha, NE 68134-0350
Phone: (402)397-1111 **Fax:** (402)399-3340
Website: http://www.cso.com
Thomas E. Kizer, President

★ 16707 ★ Central American Life Insurance Co.
PO Box 217
West Monroe, LA 71294-0217
Phone: (318)322-8181
Tex R. Kilpatrick, President

★ 16708 ★ Central Benefits Mutual Insurance Co.
716 Mt. Airyshire Blvd.
Columbus, OH 43235
Phone: (614)797-5200 **Fax:** (614)464-5768
Website: http://www.centralbenefits.com
John B. Reinhardt, Jr., CEO & Chm Bd

★ 16709 ★ Central Benefits National Life Insurance Co.
Central Benefits Mutual Insurance Co.
PO Box 16526
Columbus, OH 43216
Phone: (614)797-5200 **Fax:** (614)464-5768
Website: http://www.centralbenefits.com
John B. Reinhardt, Jr., CEO & Chm Bd

★ 16710 ★ Central Investors Life Insurance Co. of Illinois
Citizens, Inc. Group
400 E Anderson Ln.
Austin, TX 78752
Phone: (512)837-7100 **Fax:** (512)836-9785
Website: http://www.citizensinc.com
Rick D. Riley, President

★ 16711 ★ Central National Life Insurance Co. of Omaha
Presidential Life Corp.
69 Lydecker St.
Nyack, NY 10960
Free: 800-926-7599 **Fax:** (908)203-4229
Donald Barnes, President

★ 16712 ★ Central Oregon Independent Health Services Inc.
2650 NE Courtney Dr.
Bend, OR 97701
Phone: (541)382-5920
Website: http://www.clearchoicehp.com

★ 16713 ★ Central Reserve Life Insurance Co.
Ceres Group Inc.
17800 Royalton Rd.
Strongsville, OH 44136-5197
Phone: (440)572-2400 **Fax:** (440)572-4500

Website: http://www.centralreserve.com
Anthony J. Pino, CEO & Pres

★ 16714 ★ Central Security Life Insurance Co.
Insmark Group
PO Box 833879
Richardson, TX 75083-3879
Phone: (972)699-2770 **Fax:** (972)699-2788
Website: http://www.cslic.com
William H. Lewis, Jr., President

★ 16715 ★ Central States Health and Life Co. of Omaha
Central States H & L Group
PO Box 34350
Omaha, NE 68134-0350
Phone: (402)397-1111 **Fax:** (402)399-3530
Website: http://www.cso.com
Richard T. Kizer, CEO & Chm Bd

★ 16716 ★ Central United Life Insurance Co.
Central United Group
2727 Allen Pkwy., Ste. 500
Houston, TX 77019-2115
Phone: (713)529-0045 **Fax:** (713)529-8945
Website: http://www.centralunited.com
Dan George, President

★ 16717 ★ Centre Life Insurance Co.
Zurich Insurance Group
1 Chase Manhattan Plaza
New York, NY 10005
Phone: (212)898-5300
Website: http://www.masscasualty.com
Eileen M. Sweeney, President

★ 16718 ★ Centris Insurance Co.
HCC Insurance Group
13403 Northwest Freeway
Houston, TX 77040
Phone: (713)996-1200
Website: http://www.hcch.com
Michael J. Schell, President

★ 16719 ★ Centurion Life Insurance Co.
Centurion Insurance Group
206 8th St.
Des Moines, IA 50309
Phone: (515)243-2131 **Fax:** (515)557-7267
Steve R. Wagner, President

★ 16720 ★ Century Credit Life Insurance Co.
PO Box 789
Tupelo, MS 38802
Phone: (662)680-2407
Norman Bowen, President

★ 16721 ★ Century Life Assurance Co.
Century Holdings
101 N Broadway, Ste. 950
Oklahoma City, OK 73102-8409
Phone: (405)601-0099 **Fax:** (405)601-8237
Emmett D. Carter, CEO & Pres

★ 16722 ★ CGU Life Insurance Co. of America
CGU Group
108 Myrtle St.
North Quincy, MA 02171
Phone: (617)786-2324 **Free:** 800-343-5660
Fax: (617)786-2016
Website: http://www.cgulifeusa.com
Hans L. Carstensen, III, President
Robert C. Gowdy, Chairman of the Board

★ 16723 ★ CGU Life Insurance Co. of New York
CGU Group
108 Myrtle St.
North Quincy, MA 02171
Phone: (716)862-5600 **Fax:** (716)833-4134
Website: http://www.cgulifeusa.com
Hans Carstensen, III, President

★ 16724 ★ CHA HMO Inc.
CHA Service Co.
300 W Vine St., 16th Fl.
Lexington, KY 40507
Phone: (859)232-8686
Website: http://www.cha-health.com
Mark Birdwhistell, CEO

★ 16725 ★ Champions Life Insurance Co.
Insmark Group
PO Box 833879
Richardson, TX 75083-3879
Phone: (972)699-2770 **Fax:** (972)699-2788
William H. Lewis, Jr., President

★ 16726 ★ Charter National Life Insurance Co.
Allstate Financial Group
3100 Sanders Rd.
Northbrook, IL 60062
Phone: (847)402-5000 **Fax:** (847)402-0508
Website: http://www.allstate.com
Thomas J. Wilson, II, President

★ 16727 ★ Chase Life & Annuity Co.
CBD Holdings, Ltd.
500 Stanton-Christiana Rd.
2-OPS-1
Newark, DE 19713
Phone: (302)634-1453 **Fax:** (302)634-1475
Paul G. Petrylak, President

★ 16728 ★ Chase Life & Annuity Co. of New York
CBD Holdings, Ltd.
380 Madison Ave., 13th Fl.
New York, NY 10017
Phone: (212)622-3939 **Fax:** (302)576-6676
Paul G. Petrylak, President

★ 16729 ★ Cherokee National Life Insurance Co.
American United Life Group
PO Box 368
Indianapolis, IN 46206-0368
Phone: (478)477-0400 **Fax:** (478)477-1177
Website: http://www.cherokeenational.com
John R. Barton, President
E. Doyle Kelly, Vice President

★ 16730 ★ The Chesapeake Life Insurance Co.
United Insurance Companies Inc.
4001 McEwen Dr., Ste. 200
Dallas, TX 75244
Phone: (405)848-0179
Website: http://www.uici.net
Phillip J. Myhra, CEO & Pres

★ 16731 ★ Children's Mercy/Truman Medical
Children's Mercy Hospital/Truman Medical
215 W Pershing Rd., Ste. 600
Kansas City, MO 64108
Phone: (816)855-1870
Website: http://www.fhp.org

★ 16732 ★ Chiropractic Service Bureau
1202 E Main St.
Auburn, WA 98002
Phone: (206)329-4900

★ 16733 ★ Christian Fidelity Life Insurance Co.
AMERCO Group
5840 W Interstate Hwy. 20, Ste. 140
Arlington, TX 76017
Phone: (817)563-0048 **Fax:** (817)563-0299
Mark A. Haydukovich, CEO & Pres
James O. Strahan, Chairman of the Board

★ 16734 ★ Christiana Care Health Plans, Inc.
Christiana Care Corp.
11 Reads Way
New Castle, DE 19720
Phone: (302)327-7650
Website: http://www.christianacare.org

★ 16735 ★ Church Life Insurance Corp.
Church Pension Fund
445 5th Ave.
New York, NY 10016
Phone: (212)592-1800 **Fax:** (212)592-9424
Website: http://www.cpg.org
Alan F. Blanchard, President

★ 16736 ★ CIGNA HealthCare of Arizona Inc.
CIGNA Corp.
900 Cottage Grove Rd.
Hartford, CT 06152
Phone: (602)371-2437
Website: http://www.cigna.com
Clyde A. Wright, President

★ 16737 ★ CIGNA HealthCare of California Inc.
CIGNA Corp.
900 Cottage Grove Rd.
Hartford, CT 06152
Phone: (818)500-6284
Website: http://www.cigna.com
Leroy A. Volberding, President

★ 16738 ★ CIGNA HealthCare of Colorado Inc.
CIGNA Corp.
900 Cottage Grove Rd.
Hartford, CT 06152
Phone: (303)782-1500
Website: http://www.cigna.com
Daryl W. Edmonds, President

★ 16739 ★ CIGNA HealthCare of Connecticut Inc.
CIGNA Corp.
900 Cottage Grove Rd.
Hartford, CT 06152
Phone: (860)226-2300
Website: http://www.cigna.com
Kurt A. Weimer, President

★ 16740 ★ CIGNA HealthCare of Delaware Inc.
CIGNA Corp.
900 Cottage Grove Rd.
Hartford, CT 06152
Phone: (302)797-3700
Website: http://www.cigna.com
Vincent J. Sobocinski, President

★ 16741 ★ CIGNA HealthCare of Florida Inc.
CIGNA Corp.
5404 Cypress Ctr. Dr., Ste. 365
PO Box 24203
Tampa, FL 33609
Phone: (813)281-1000
Website: http://www.cigna.com
Andrew D. Crooks, President

★ 16742 ★ CIGNA HealthCare of Georgia Inc.
CIGNA Corp.
900 Cottage Grove Rd.
Hartford, CT 06152
Phone: (404)681-7000
Website: http://www.cigna.com
Robert A. Yungk, President

★ 16743 ★ CIGNA HealthCare of Illinois Inc.
CIGNA Corp.
900 Cottage Grove Rd.
Hartford, CT 06152
Phone: (312)648-2460
Website: http://www.cigna.com

★ 16744 ★ CIGNA Healthcare of Indiana Inc.
CIGNA Corp.
900 Cottage Grove Rd.
Hartford, CT 06152
Phone: (317)685-1133
Website: http://www.cigna.com
Mary L. Brandt, President

★ 16745 ★ CIGNA HealthCare of Maine Inc.
CIGNA Corp.
900 Cottage Grove Rd.
Hartford, CT 06152
Phone: (207)865-5000 **Fax:** (207)865-5632
Website: http://www.cigna.com
Mary L. Brandt, President

★ 16746 ★ CIGNA HealthCare of Massachusetts Inc.
CIGNA Corp.
900 Cottage Grove Rd.
Hartford, CT 06152
Phone: (508)849-4311
Website: http://www.cigna.com
Linda J. Johnson, President

★ 16747 ★ CIGNA HealthCare Mid-Atlantic Inc.
CIGNA Corp.
900 Cottage Grove Rd.
Hartford, CT 06152
Phone: (410)720-5850
Website: http://www.cigna.com
Matthew G. Manders, President

★ 16748 ★ CIGNA HealthCare of New Hampshire Inc.
CIGNA Corp.
900 Cottage Grove Rd.
Hartford, CT 06152
Phone: (603)268-7000
Website: http://www.cigna.com
Brian D. Wells, President

★ 16749 ★ CIGNA HealthCare of New Jersey Inc.
CIGNA Corp.
900 Cottage Grove Rd.
Hartford, CT 06152
Phone: (201)533-5001
Website: http://www.cigna.com
Kurt A. Weimer, President

★ 16750 ★ CIGNA HealthCare of New York Inc.
CIGNA Corp.
900 Cottage Grove Rd.
Hartford, CT 06152
Phone: (201)533-7000
Website: http://www.cigna.com
Kurt A. Weimer, President

★ 16751 ★ CIGNA HealthCare of North Carolina Inc.
CIGNA Corp.
900 Cottage Grove Rd.
Hartford, CT 06152
Phone: (704)556-5800
Website: http://www.cigna.com
Steven A. White, President

★ 16752 ★ CIGNA HealthCare of Ohio Inc.
CIGNA Corp.
900 Cottage Grove Rd.
Hartford, CT 06152
Phone: (614)823-7500
Website: http://www.cigna.com
Jeanne E. McCarthy, President

★ 16753 ★ CIGNA HealthCare of Pennsylvania Inc.
CIGNA Corp.
900 Cottage Grove Rd.
Hartford, CT 06152
Phone: (302)797-3700
Website: http://www.cigna.com
Vincent J. Sobocinski, President

★ 16754 ★ CIGNA HealthCare of St. Louis, Inc.
CIGNA Corp.
900 Cottage Grove Rd.
Hartford, CT 06152
Phone: (314)726-7792
Website: http://www.cigna.com
Paul Bergsteinsson, Vice President

★ 16755 ★ CIGNA HealthCare of South Carolina Inc.
CIGNA Corp.
900 Cottage Grove Rd.
Hartford, CT 06152
Free: 800-962-8811 **Fax:** (803)720-7970
Website: http://www.cigna.com
Catherine N. Ferry, President

★ 16756 ★ CIGNA HealthCare of Tennessee Inc.
CIGNA Corp.
900 Cottage Grove Rd.
Hartford, CT 06152
Phone: (615)595-3000
Website: http://www.cigna.com
John R. Bruce, President

★ 16757 ★ CIGNA HealthCare of Texas Inc.
CIGNA Corp.
900 Cottage Grove Rd.
Hartford, CT 06152
Phone: (713)552-7802
Website: http://www.cigna.com
Kenneth S. Malcolmson, President

★ 16758 ★ CIGNA HealthCare of Utah Inc.
CIGNA Corp.
900 Cottage Grove Rd.
Hartford, CT 06152
Phone: (801)265-2777
Website: http://www.cigna.com
Robert A. Immitt, President

★ 16759 ★ CIGNA HealthCare of Virginia Inc.
CIGNA Corp.
900 Cottage Grove Rd.
Hartford, CT 06152
Phone: (804)267-5100
Website: http://www.cigna.com
Gregory S. Bowman, President

★ 16760 ★ CIGNA Insurance Group, Inc.
CIGNA Corp.
900 Cottage Grove Rd.
Hartford, CT 06152
Phone: (603)225-5077
Website: http://www.cigna.com
Brian D. Wells, President

★ 16761 ★ CIGNA Insurance Services Co.
CIGNA Corp.
900 Cottage Grove Rd.
Bloomfield, CT 06002
Free: 800-962-8811
Website: http://www.cigna.com
Catherine N. Ferry, President

★ 16762 ★ CIGNA Life Insurance Co.
CIGNA Corp.
900 Cottage Grove Rd., S-330
Bloomfield, CT 06002
Phone: (860)226-6000
Website: http://www.cigna.com
Thomas C. Jones, President

★ 16763 ★ CIGNA Life Insurance Co. of New York
CIGNA Corp.
900 Cottage Grove Rd., S-330
Bloomfield, CT 06002
Phone: (212)618-5757 **Fax:** (212)618-5759
Website: http://www.cigna.com
Robert H. Brickweg, President

★ 16764 ★ CIGNA Worldwide Insurance Co.
CIGNA Corp.
PO Box 15050
Wilmington, DE 19850
Phone: (302)479-6617 **Fax:** (302)479-4430
Website: http://www.cigna.com
Nick Amin, President

★ 16765 ★ Cimarron Health Plan Inc.
Health Care Horizons
7801 Academy NE, Ste. 205
Albuquerque, NM 87109
Phone: (505)342-4660 **Fax:** (505)342-4711
Website: http://www.cimarronhealthplan.com

★ 16766 ★ Cincinnati Equitable Life Insurance Co.
Cincinnati Equitable Companies, Inc.
PO Box 3428
Cincinnati, OH 45202-3428
Phone: (513)621-1826 **Fax:** (513)621-4531
James W. Ketring, CEO & Pres

★ 16767 ★ The Cincinnati Life Insurance Co.
Cincinnati Financial Corp.
PO Box 145496
Cincinnati, OH 45250-5496
Phone: (513)870-2000 **Fax:** (513)603-5500
Website: http://www.cinfin.com
David H. Popplewell, President
John J. Schiff, Jr., CEO

★ 16768 ★ Citicorp Life Insurance Co.
Citigroup
307 W 7th St., Ste. 400
Fort Worth, TX 76102
Phone: (860)277-0111
George C. Kokulis, CEO & Pres

★ 16769 ★ Citizens Accident and Health Insurance Co.
Protective Life Corp.
2801 Hwy. 280 S
Birmingham, AL 35223
Phone: (847)948-8988 **Fax:** (847)948-1186
Website: http://www.protective.com
Steven A. Schultz, CEO & Chm Bd

★ 16770 ★ Citizens Fidelity Insurance Co.
PO Box 25440
Little Rock, AR 72221-5440
Phone: (501)228-5134 **Fax:** (501)223-0181
George W. Booker, II, President

★ 16771 ★ Citizens Insurance Co. of America
Citizens, Inc. Group
PO Box 149151
Austin, TX 78714-9151
Phone: (512)837-7100 **Fax:** (512)836-9785
Website: http://www.citizensinc.com
Rick D. Riley, CEO & Chm Bd

★ 16772 ★ Citizens Security Life Insurance Co.
Citizens Financial Group
PO Box 436149
Louisville, KY 40253-6149
Phone: (502)244-2420 **Fax:** (502)244-2439
Website: http://www.citizenssecuritylife.com
Lane Hersman, President
Robert N. Greenwood, Senior VP

★ 16773 ★ Clarica Life Insurance Co.
Sun Life Financial Group
227 King St. S
Waterloo, ON, Canada N2J 4C5
Phone: (519)888-3900 **Fax:** (519)888-3899
Website: http://www.clarica.com
Robert M. Astley, CEO & Pres

★ 16774 ★ Clarica Life Insurance Co. of the U.S.
Sun Life Financial Group
13890 Bishop's Dr., Ste. 300
Brookfield, WI 53008-0503
Phone: (701)237-5700
Website: http://www.clarica.com
Bruce Crozier, CEO & Pres

★ 16775 ★ Clarica Life Reinsurance Co.
Sun Life Financial Group
13890 Bishop's Dr., Ste. 300
Brookfield, WI 53008-0503
Phone: (416)947-2601 **Fax:** (416)947-2660
Website: http://www.clarica.com
James R. Smith, CEO & Pres

★ 16776 ★ Classic Life Assurance Co.
Life of the South Group
100 W Bay St.
Jacksonville, FL 32202-3806
Phone: (904)350-9660 **Free:** 800-888-2738
Fax: (904)354-4525
Website: http://www.life-south.com
Kenneth N. Hamil, President

★ 16777 ★ CM Assurance Co.
MassMutual Financial Group
1295 State St.
Springfield, MA 01111
Phone: (413)788-8411
Website: http://www.massmutual.com
Lawrence V. Burkett, Jr., CEO & Pres

★ 16778 ★ CM Benefit Insurance Co.
MassMutual Financial Group
1295 State St.
Springfield, MA 01111
Phone: (413)788-8411
Website: http://www.massmutual.com
Lawrence V. Burkett, Jr., CEO & Pres

★ 16779 ★ CNA Group Life Assurance Co.
CNA Insurance Group
CNA Plaza
Chicago, IL 60685
Phone: (312)822-5000 **Fax:** (312)822-4671
Website: http://www.cna.com
Bernard L. Hengesbaugh, President
Joseph R. Herman, Senior VP
Frmly: American Continental Life Insurance Co.

★ 16780 ★ Colonial American Life Insurance Co.
United Security Assurance Group
673 Cherry Ln.
Souderton, PA 18964
Phone: (215)723-3044 **Fax:** (215)723-8036
Website: http://www.usa-cal.com
Ronald A. Landes, President

★ 16781 ★ Colonial Life and Accident Insurance Co.
UnumProvident Corp.
1 Fountain Sq.
Chattanooga, TN 37402-1330
Phone: (803)798-7000 **Fax:** (803)772-0251
Website: http://www.unumprovident.com
Robert O. Best, CEO & Pres
J. Harold Chandler, Chairman of the Board

★ 16782 ★ Colonial Life Insurance Co. of Texas
PO Box 2543
Fort Worth, TX 76113-2543
Phone: (817)390-2350 **Fax:** (817)390-2209
Website: http://colonialinsurance.com
E. A. DuBose, President

★ 16783 ★ Colonial Security Life Insurance Co.
PO Box 191029
Dallas, TX 75219-1029
Phone: (214)252-0313 **Fax:** (214)252-0312
Website: http://www.gibgroup.com
Cecil A. Nettle, President

★ 16784 ★ Colorado Access
501 S Cherry St., Ste. 700
Denver, CO 80246
Phone: (303)355-6707
Website: http://www.coaccess.com

★ 16785 ★ Colorado Bankers Life Insurance Co.
Health Care Service Corp.
5990 Greenwood Plaza Blvd.
Greenwood Village, CO 80111
Phone: (303)220-8500 **Fax:** (303)220-8056
Website: http://www.cblnet.com
David Pavletich, President

★ 16786 ★ Colorado Dental Service, Inc.
PO Box 5468
Denver, CO 80217-5468
Phone: (303)741-9300
Kathryn A. Paul, President

★ 16787 ★ Columbia United Providers Inc.
19120 SE 34th St., Ste. 201
Vancouver, WA 98683
Phone: (360)449-8861

★ 16788 ★ Columbia Universal Life Insurance Co.
Allstate Financial Group
3100 Sanders Rd.
Northbrook, IL 60062
Phone: (847)402-5000
Website: http://www.allstate.com
Thomas J. Wilson, II, CEO & Chm Bd

★ 16789 ★ Columbian Family Life Insurance Co.
Columbian Financial Group
PO Box 1381
Binghamton, NY 13902-1381
Phone: (607)724-2472 **Fax:** (607)724-6180
Website: http://www.cfglife.com
Thomas E. Rattmann, CEO & Chm Bd

★ 16790 ★ Columbian Life Insurance Co.
Columbian Financial Group
PO Box 1381
Binghamton, NY 13902-1381
Phone: (607)724-2472 **Fax:** (607)724-6180
Website: http://www.cfglife.com
Thomas E. Rattmann, CEO & Chm Bd

★ 16791 ★ Columbian Mutual Life Insurance Co.
Columbian Financial Group
PO Box 1381
Binghamton, NY 13902-1381
Phone: (607)724-2472 **Fax:** (607)724-6180
Website: http://www.cfglife.com
Thomas E. Rattmann, CEO & Chm Bd

★ 16792 ★ Columbus Life Insurance Co.
Western & Southern Financial Group
400 Broadway
Cincinnati, OH 45202
Phone: (513)361-6700 **Fax:** (513)361-6888
Website: http://www.columbuslife.com
Lawrence Lee Grypp, CEO & Pres

★ 16793 ★ Comanche County Hospital Authority
3811 W Gore Blvd., Ste. 10
PO Box 129
Lawton, OK 73502
Phone: (580)357-6684
Website: http://www.memorialhealthsource.com

★ 16794 ★ Combined Insurance Co. of America
Combined Specialty A & H Group
Aon Ctr., 5th Fl.
200 E Randolph Dr.
Chicago, IL 60601
Phone: (312)381-1000 **Fax:** (312)381-0118
Richard M. Ravin, CEO & Chm Bd

★ 16795 ★ Combined Life Insurance Co. of New York
Combined Specialty A & H Group
11 British American Blvd.
Latham, NY 12110
Phone: (518)220-9333 **Fax:** (518)381-0118
Richard M. Ravin, President

★ 16796 ★ Combined Underwriters Life Insurance Co.
Citizens Inc. Group
PO Box 149151
Austin, TX 78714-9151
Phone: (512)837-7100 **Fax:** (512)836-9785
Gary C. Cole, President

★ 16797 ★ Commencement Bay Life Insurance Co.
PO Box 21267
Seattle, WA 98111-3267
Phone: (206)464-5536
Robert Scott Kuecker, President

★ 16798 ★ Commerce National Insurance Co.
PO Box 1187
Starkville, MS 39760
Phone: (770)763-1560
Thomas J. Prince, Jr., President

★ 16799 ★ Commercial Bankers Life Insurance Co.
PO Box 6144
Fishers, IN 46038
Phone: (317)501-0952
John Smith Milliken, President

★ 16800 ★ Commercial Travelers Mutual Insurance Co.
Commercial Travelers Mutual Group
70 Genesee St.
Utica, NY 13502-3502
Phone: (315)797-5200 **Fax:** (315)797-3198
Website: http://www.commercialtravelers.com
Herbert E. Trevvett, CEO & Pres
John B. Stetson, Chairman of the Board

★ 16801 ★ Commonwealth Dealers Life Insurance Co.
8001 W Broad St.
Richmond, VA 23294
Phone: (804)270-9494 **Fax:** (804)270-7474
Richard G. Barkhouser, Chairman of the Board
Mark Albert, President

★ 16802 ★ Community Bank Life & Health Insurance Co.
PO Box 20210
Hot Springs, AR 71903
Phone: (865)970-7500
Richard G. Trammell, President

★ 16803 ★ Community Care Behavioral Health
1 Chatham Ctr., Ste. 700
112 Washington Pl.
Pittsburgh, PA 15219
Phone: (412)454-2120
Website: http://www.ccbh.com

★ 16804 ★ Community Choice Michigan
2369 Woodlake Dr., Ste. 200
Okemos, MI 48864
Phone: (517)349-5288

★ 16805 ★ Community First Health Plans Inc.
Bexar County Hospital District
4801 NW Loop 410, Ste. 1000
San Antonio, TX 78229
Phone: (210)227-2347

★ 16806 ★ Community Health Choice Inc.
2525 Holly Hall
Houston, TX 77054
Phone: (713)746-6999

★ 16807 ★ Community Health Group
740 Bay Blvd.
Chula Vista, CA 91910
Phone: (619)422-0422

★ 16808 ★ Community Health Plan
Bldg. A9, East 2nd Fl.
1000 S Fremont Ave.
Alhambra, CA 91803
Phone: (213)240-7775

★ 16809 ★ Community Health Plan
Heartland Health
137 N Belt Hwy.
Saint Joseph, MO 64506
Phone: (816)271-1247
Lowell C. Kruse, President

★ 16810 ★ Community Health Plan of the Rockies, Inc.
400 S Colorado Blvd., Ste. 300
Denver, CO 80246-1238
Free: 800-935-3220
Website: http://www.chpr.com

★ 16811 ★ Community Insurance Co.
Anthem Inc.
4361 Irwin Simpson Rd.
Mason, OH 45040
Phone: (513)872-8100 **Fax:** (513)336-2155
Website: http://www.anthem-inc.com
Keith R. Faller, President

★ 16812 ★ CommunityCare HMO Inc.
218 W 6th St.
Tulsa, OK 74119
Phone: (918)594-5200

★ 16813 ★ CommunityCare Life and Health Insurance Co.
218 W 6th St.
Tulsa, OK 74119
Phone: (918)594-5295
Richard Wesley Todd, President

★ 16814 ★ Companion Life Insurance Co.
Blue Cross & Blue Shield of South Carolina Group
2501 Faraway Dr.
PO Box 100102
Columbia, SC 29202-3102
Phone: (803)735-1251 **Fax:** (803)735-0736
Website: http://www.companionlife.com
M. Edward Sellers, Chairman of the Board

★ 16815 ★ Companion Life Insurance Co.
Mutual of Omaha Group
Mutual of Omaha Plaza
Omaha, NE 68175
Phone: (402)342-7600
Randall C. Horn, President

★ 16816 ★ CompBenefits Insurance Co.
110 Wild Basin Rd., Ste. 370
Austin, TX 78746
Phone: (770)998-8936
Phyllis Adele Klock, President

★ 16817 ★ CompCare Health Services Insurance Corp.
Cobalt Corp.
20855 Watertown Rd., Ste. 140
Waukesha, WI 53186
Phone: (262)785-7830
Website: http://www.bluecrosswisconsin.com

★ 16818 ★ Concert Health Plan Insurance Co.
2425 W 22nd St., Ste. 209
Oak Brook, IL 60523
Phone: (630)990-1090

★ 16819 ★ Concord Heritage Life Insurance Co.
Allstate Financial Group
3100 Sanders Rd.
Northbrook, IL 60062
Phone: (603)224-7746 **Fax:** (603)225-6027
Website: http://www.allstate.com
Charles R. Morehead, Chairman of the Board

★ 16820 ★ Concord National Life Insurance Co.
3003 E 98th St., Ste. 107
Indianapolis, IN 46280
Phone: (312)332-0430
Charles R. Royal, President

★ 16821 ★ Condeaux Life Insurance Co.
2929 N 44th St., Ste. 120
Phoenix, AZ 85018
Phone: (305)253-2244
Floyd G. Denison, President

★ 16822 ★ Congress Life Insurance Co.
Banc One Insurance Group
111 E Wisconsin Ave., Ste. 1250
Milwaukee, WI 53202
Phone: (414)765-3454 **Fax:** (414)765-7185
Glen J. Mileskо, CEO & Pres

★ 16823 ★ ConnectiCare Inc.
30 Batterson Park Rd.
Farmington, CT 06032-2574
Phone: (860)674-5700

★ 16824 ★ Connecticut General Life Insurance Co.
CIGNA Corp.
900 Cottage Grove Rd., S-330
Bloomfield, CT 06002
Phone: (860)226-6000
Website: http://www.cigna.com
Thomas C. Jones, President

★ 16825 ★ Connecticut Life Insurance & Annuity Corp.
4700 E Thomas Rd., Ste. 204
Phoenix, AZ 85018
Phone: (602)952-6761 **Fax:** (602)549-6200
Frederick S. Townsend, Jr., President

★ 16826 ★ Conseco Annuity Assurance Co.
Conseco Insurance Group
11815 N Pennsylvania St.
Carmel, IN 46032
Phone: (317)817-4000 **Fax:** (317)817-2161
Website: http://www.conseco.com
Elizabeth C. Georgakopoulos, President

★ 16827 ★ Conseco Direct Life Insurance Co.
Conseco Insurance Group
11815 N Pennsylvania St.
Carmel, IN 46032
Phone: (215)928-8000 **Fax:** (215)928-6492
Website: http://www.conseco.com
Robert F. Vickery, President

★ 16828 ★ Conseco Health Insurance Co.
Conseco Insurance Group
11815 N Pennsylvania St.
Carmel, IN 46032
Phone: (317)817-4300 **Fax:** (317)817-2161
Website: http://www.conseco.com
Elizabeth C. Georgakopoulos, President

★ 16829 ★ Conseco Life Insurance Co.
Conseco Insurance Group
11815 N Pennsylvania St.
Carmel, IN 46032-4570
Phone: (317)817-6400 **Fax:** (317)817-2161
Website: http://www.conseco.com
Elizabeth C. Georgakopoulos, President

★ 16830 ★ Conseco Life Insurance Co. of New York
Conseco Insurance Group
11815 N Pennsylvania St.
Carmel, IN 46032
Phone: (914)398-4405 **Fax:** (914)817-2161
Website: http://www.conseco.com
Elizabeth C. Georgakopoulos, President

★ 16831 ★ Conseco Life Insurance Co. of Texas
Conseco Insurance Group
11815 N Pennsylvania St.
Carmel, IN 46032
Phone: (317)817-3700 **Fax:** (317)817-2161
Website: http://www.conseco.com
Elizabeth C. Georgakopoulos, President

★ 16832 ★ Conseco Medical Insurance Co.
Conseco Insurance Group
11815 N Pennsylvania St.
Carmel, IN 46032
Phone: (815)987-5000 **Fax:** (317)817-2161
Website: http://www.conseco.com
William J. Shea, President

★ 16833 ★ Conseco Senior Health Insurance Co.
Conseco Insurance Group
11815 N Pennsylvania St.
Carmel, IN 46032
Phone: (317)817-3700 **Fax:** (317)817-2161
Website: http://www.conseco.com
Elizabeth C. Georgakopoulos, President

★ 16834 ★ Conseco Variable Insurance Co.
Conseco Insurance Group
11815 N Pennsylvania St.
Carmel, IN 46032
Phone: (317)817-3700 **Fax:** (317)817-2161
Website: http://www.conseco.com
Elizabeth C. Georgakopoulos, President

★ 16835 ★ Consolidated General Life Insurance Co.
Titus Group
2817 Maple Ave.
Dallas, TX 75201
Phone: (214)871-0332 **Fax:** (214)871-0334
Gary Dobbie, President

★ 16836 ★ Constitution Life Insurance Co.
Universal American Financial Corp.
600 Courtland St.
Orlando, FL 32804
Phone: (407)628-1776 **Fax:** (407)628-4227
Gary W. Bryant, CEO & Pres

★ 16837 ★ Consumer Life Insurance Co.
111 Westminster St.
Providence, RI 02903
Phone: (401)278-6189 **Fax:** (401)278-3761
Donald F. Armstrong, President

★ 16838 ★ Consumers Life Insurance Co.
PO Box 26
Camp Hill, PA 17001-0026
Phone: (717)730-6306
James C. Robertson, President

★ 16839 ★ Continental American Insurance Co.
PO Box 427
Columbia, SC 29202
Phone: (803)256-6265 **Fax:** (803)779-4406
D. Christian Goodall, President

★ 16840 ★ Continental Assurance Co.
CNA Insurance Group
CNA Plaza, 22 South
Chicago, IL 60685
Phone: (312)822-5000 **Fax:** (312)822-6419
Website: http://www.cna.com
Bernard L. Hengesbaugh, CEO & Chm Bd

★ 16841 ★ Continental General Insurance Co.
Ceres Group
PO Box 247007
Omaha, NE 68114
Phone: (402)397-3200 **Fax:** (402)397-2836
Website: http://www.continentalgeneral.com
Mark A. Nielsen, President
Charles E. Miller, Exec VP

★ 16842 ★ Continental Life Insurance Co.
Burlen Corp.
8049 W Chester Pike
Upper Darby, PA 19082-1317
Phone: (610)853-2100 **Fax:** (610)853-2107
Walter H. Lenhard, President

★ 16843 ★ Continental Life Insurance Co. of Brentwood, Tennessee
PO Box 1188
Brentwood, TN 37027
Phone: (615)377-1300 **Fax:** (615)373-0272
Website: http://www.cont-life.com
Roger S. Baskin, President

★ 16844 ★ Continental Life Insurance Co. of South Carolina
3830 Forest Dr., Ste. 202
PO Box 6138
Columbia, SC 29260-6138
Phone: (803)782-4947 **Fax:** (803)782-4949
Frank L. Graham, Chairman of the Board

★ 16845 ★ Contra Costa Health Plan
20 Allen St.
Martinez, CA 94553
Phone: (510)313-6004

★ 16846 ★ Cook Children's Health Plan
801 7th Ave.
PO Box 2488
Fort Worth, TX 76101-2488
Phone: (817)334-2247
Website: http://www.chp.org

★ 16847 ★ Cooperativa de Seguros de Vida de Puerto Rico
PO Box 363428
San Juan, PR 00936-3428
Phone: (787)751-5656 **Fax:** (787)281-6327
Website: http://www.cosvi.com
Carlos Fernandez, President

★ 16848 ★ Cooperative Life Insurance Co.
PO Box 5206
Pine Bluff, AR 71611
Phone: (870)534-3134
Adam B. Robinson, President

★ 16849 ★ Coordinated Care Corp. Indiana, Inc.
Centene Corp.
7711 Carondelet Ave., Ste. 800
Saint Louis, MO 63105
Phone: (314)725-4477
Website: http://www.centene.com

★ 16850 ★ Coordinated Health Partners Inc.
Blue Cross & Blue Shield of Rhode Island
15 LaSalle Sq.
Providence, RI 02903
Phone: (401)459-5500
Website: http://www.bcbsri.org

★ 16851 ★ Cornhusker Life Insurance Co.
PO Box 95023
Lincoln, NE 68509
Phone: (402)475-1079
A. Loy Todd, Jr., President

★ 16852 ★ Corporate Health Insurance Co.
Aetna Inc. Group
151 Farmington Ave., MC 64
Hartford, CT 06156-0417
Phone: (215)628-4800 **Fax:** (215)283-6790
Felicia F. Norwood, President

★ 16853 ★ Cosmopolitan Life Insurance Co.
2800 Percy Machin Dr.
North Little Rock, AR 72114
Phone: (501)753-1910
Stephen Whitwell, President

★ 16854 ★ Cotton States Life Insurance Co.
Cotton States Group
244 Perimeter Ctr. Pkwy. NE
Atlanta, GA 30346
Phone: (770)391-8600 **Fax:** (770)391-8710
Website: http://www.cottonstatesinsurance.com
J. Ridley Howard, CEO & Pres

★ 16855 ★ Country Investors Life Assurance Co.
Country Insurance & Financial Services
PO Box 2000
Bloomington, IL 61702-2000
Phone: (309)821-3000 **Fax:** (309)821-3538
Website: http://www.countryfinancial.com
Ronald R. Warfield, President

★ 16856 ★ Country Life Insurance Co.
Country Insurance & Financial Services
PO Box 2000
Bloomington, IL 61702-2000
Phone: (309)821-3000 **Fax:** (309)821-3538
Website: http://www.countryfinancial.com
Ronald R. Warfield, President
John D. Blackburn, CEO

★ 16857 ★ Country Medical Plans, Inc.
Country Insurance & Financial Services
PO Box 2000
Bloomington, IL 61702-2000
Phone: (309)821-3000 **Fax:** (309)821-3538
Website: http://www.countryfinancial.com
Ronald R. Warfield, President

★ 16858 ★ Coventry Carelink Insurance Co. of Maryland
1302 Concourse Dr., Ste. 202
Linthicum, MD 21090
Phone: (419)850-9060
Robert B. Haldeman, President

★ 16859 ★ Coventry Health Care of the Carolinas Inc.
Coventry Health Care Inc.
6330 Quadrangle Dr., Ste. 500
Chapel Hill, NC 27514-9872
Free: 800-935-7284
Website: http://www.cvty.com

★ 16860 ★ Coventry Health Care of Delaware Inc.
Coventry Health Care Inc.
2751 Centerville Rd., Ste. 400
Wilmington, DE 19808-1627
Phone: (302)995-6100
Website: http://www.cvty.com

★ 16861 ★ Coventry Health Care of Georgia Inc.
Coventry Health Care Inc.
1100 Circle 75 Pkwy., Ste. 1400
Atlanta, GA 30339
Phone: (678)202-2100
Website: http://www.cvty.com

★ 16862 ★ Coventry Health Care of Iowa Inc.
Coventry Health Care Inc.
4600 Westown Pkwy., Regency 6, Ste. 200
West Des Moines, IA 50266
Phone: (515)225-1234
Website: http://www.cvty.com

★ 16863 ★ Coventry Health Care of Kansas Inc.
Coventry Health Care Inc.
1001 E 101st Terrace, Ste. 300
Kansas City, MO 64131
Phone: (816)941-3030
Website: http://www.cvty.com

★ 16864 ★ Coventry Health Care of Louisiana Inc.
Coventry Health Care Inc.
2424 Edenborn Ave., Ste. 350
Metairie, LA 70001
Phone: (504)834-0840
Website: http://www.cvty.com

★ 16865 ★ Coventry Health Care of Nebraska Inc.
Coventry Health Care Inc.
13305 Birch St., Ste. 100
Omaha, NE 68154
Phone: (402)498-9030
Website: http://www.cvty.com

★ 16866 ★ Coventry Health and Life Insurance Co.
6705 Rockledge Dr., 10th Fl.
Bethesda, MD 20817
Phone: (301)581-5631 **Free:** 800-743-7421
Dale B. Wolf, President

★ 16867 ★ Cox Health Systems Insurance Co.
3525 S National, Ste. 205
Springfield, MO 65807
Phone: (417)269-2970
Gary G. Jacobs, President

★ 16868 ★ CPIC Life Insurance Co.
Blue Shield of California Group
PO Box 7725
San Francisco, CA 94120-7725
Phone: (415)229-5703 **Fax:** (415)229-5744
Website: http://www.cpiclife.com
Debra E. Bowles, CEO & Pres

★ 16869 ★ Croatian Fraternal Union of America
100 Delaney Dr.
Pittsburgh, PA 15235
Phone: (412)351-3909 **Fax:** (412)823-1594
Bernard M. Luketich, President

★ 16870 ★ Crocker Life Insurance Co.
1220 Concord Ave.
Concord, CA 94520
Phone: (515)557-8414
Timothy J. King, President

★ 16871 ★ CSA Fraternal Life
PO Box 3039
Oak Brook, IL 60522-3039
Phone: (630)472-0500 **Fax:** (630)472-1100
Website: http://www.csafraternallife.org
Vera A. Wilt, President

★ 16872 ★ CUNA Mutual Insurance Society
CUNA Mutual Group
PO Box 391
Madison, WI 53701-0391
Phone: (608)238-5851 **Fax:** (608)238-0830
Website: http://www.cunamutual.com
Michael B. Kitchen, CEO & Pres

★ 16873 ★ CUNA Mutual Life Insurance Co.
CUNA Mutual Group
PO Box 391
Madison, WI 53701-0391
Phone: (319)352-4090 **Fax:** (319)352-1611
Website: http://www.cunamutual.com
Michael B. Kitchen, CEO & Pres

★ 16874 ★ Dallas General Life Insurance Co.
Dallas General Group
PO Box 131080
Dallas, TX 75313
Phone: (214)880-0808 **Fax:** (214)880-0920
Richard C. Murphy, President

★ 16875 ★ Davis Vision of Michigan Inc.
Highmark Inc.
159 Express St.
Plainview, NY 11803
Phone: (516)932-9500
George F. Grode, Chairman of the Board

★ 16876 ★ Dayton Area Health Plan
1 S Main St.
Dayton, OH 45402
Phone: (937)224-3300

★ 16877 ★ Dean Health Plan Inc.
Dean Health System/SSM Health Care
1277 Deming Way
Madison, WI 53717
Phone: (608)836-1400
Website: http://www.deanhealth.com

★ 16878 ★ Delaware American Life Insurance Co.
American International Group
PO Box 667
Wilmington, DE 19899
Phone: (302)594-2000 **Fax:** (302)654-5436
Gerald W. Wyndorf, CEO & Pres
Robinson K. Nottingham, Chairman of the Board

★ 16879 ★ Delmarv, a Health Plan Inc.
CareFirst of Maryland Inc.
10455 Mill Run Circle
Owings Mills, MD 21117-5559
Phone: (410)822-7223

★ 16880 ★ Delta Life & Annuity Co.
AmerUs Group
555 S Kansas Ave.
Topeka, KS 66603-3404
Phone: (785)232-6945 **Fax:** (785)232-3534
Website: http://www.deltalife.com
Mark V. Heitz, CEO & Pres

★ 16881 ★ Delta Life Insurance Co.
Atlantic American/Delta Group
4370 Peachtree Rd. NE
Atlanta, GA 30319-3000
Phone: (404)231-2111 **Fax:** (404)231-2123
J. Mack Robinson, President

★ 16882 ★ Dennis Life Insurance Co.
PO Box 795
Shawnee Mission, KS 66201
Phone: (913)432-6400
Larry L. Van Tuyl, President

★ 16883 ★ Dental Service Corp. of North Dakota
Noridian Mutual Insurance Co.
4510 13th Ave. SW
Fargo, ND 58121-0001
Phone: (701)282-1100
Robert B. Carlson, President

★ 16884 ★ DentCare Delivery Systems Inc.
60 Charles Lindbergh Blvd.
Uniondale, NY 11553
Phone: (516)794-3000

★ 16885 ★ Dentegra Inc., Florida
Fortis Inc.
3595 Grandview Pkwy., Ste. 150
Birmingham, AL 35243
Phone: (205)909-6000
Michael J. Peninger, President

★ 16886 ★ Dentegra Inc., Kentucky
Fortis Inc.
3595 Grandview Pkwy., Ste. 150
Birmingham, AL 35243
Phone: (205)909-6000
Michael J. Peninger, President

★ 16887 ★ Denticare of Arkansas Inc.
Fortis Inc.
3595 Grandview Pkwy., Ste. 150
Birmingham, AL 35243
Phone: (205)909-6000
Michael J. Peninger, President

★ 16888 ★ Denticare of Oklahoma Inc.
Fortis Inc.
3595 Grandview Pkwy., Ste. 150
Birmingham, AL 35243
Phone: (205)909-6000
Michael J. Peninger, President

★ 16889 ★ Deseret Mutual Insurance Co.
PO Box 45530
Salt Lake City, UT 84145
Phone: (801)578-5854
Michael J. Stapley, President
Frmly: Deseret Mutual Benefit Association.

★ 16890 ★ Destiny Health Insurance Co.
1211 W 22nd St., Ste. 305
Oak Brook, IL 60523
Phone: (630)590-4200
Kenneth J. Linde, President

★ 16891 ★ Direct Life Insurance Co.
Direct General
1281 Murfreesboro Rd.
Nashville, TN 37217-2432
Phone: (615)365-3605 **Fax:** (615)366-3722
Jacqueline C. Adair, President

★ 16892 ★ Directors Life Assurance Co.
PO Box 20428
Oklahoma City, OK 73120
Phone: (405)842-1234 **Fax:** (405)842-4998
Bob C. Lamirand, President

★ 16893 ★ Dixie Life Insurance Co. Inc.
PO Box 69
Bogalusa, LA 70429-0069
Phone: (504)735-1710
Charles J. D. Gerrets, III, President

★ 16894 ★ Dixie National Life Insurance Co.
Standard Management Group
10689 N Pennsylvania St.
Indianapolis, IN 46280
Phone: (317)574-6200 **Fax:** (317)574-6227
Website: http://www.smancorp.com
Raymond J. Ohlson, CEO & Chm Bd

★ 16895 ★ DOBCO Life Insurance Co.
American Road Insurance Group
1 American Rd.
Dearborn, MI 48121-6027
Phone: (313)322-7287 **Fax:** (313)323-9479
J. M. Moritz, President

★ 16896 ★ Doctors Health Plan
DHP Holdings
3104 Croasdaile Dr., Ste. 300
Durham, NC 27705
Phone: (919)383-4175
George C. Stokes, President

★ 16897 ★ The Doctors' Life Insurance Co.
Doctors' Co. Insurance Group
185 Greenwood Rd.
Napa, CA 94558-0900
Phone: (707)226-0100 **Fax:** (707)226-0180
Website: http://www.thedoctors.com
Manuel S. Puebla, President

★ 16898 ★ Dorsey Life Insurance Co.
PO Box 431
Marlin, TX 76661
Phone: (254)803-2586
Robert D. Dorsey, President

★ 16899 ★ Eastern Vision Service Plan
Vision Services Group
3333 Quality Dr.
Rancho Cordova, CA 95670
Phone: (916)851-5000 **Fax:** (916)858-5388
Roger J. Valine, President

★ 16900 ★ Educators Life Insurance Co. of America
Horace Mann Group
1 Horace Mann Plaza
Springfield, IL 62715
Phone: (217)789-2500 **Fax:** (217)535-7117
Website: http://www.horacemann.com
Louis G. Lower, II, CEO & Pres

★ 16901 ★ Educators Mutual Insurance Association
852 E Arrowhead Ln.
Murray, UT 84107-5298
Phone: (801)262-7476
Rolando I. Galano, President

★ 16902 ★ Educators Mutual Life Insurance Co.
Educators Mutual
PO Box 83149
Lancaster, PA 17608-3149
Phone: (717)391-5703 **Fax:** (717)393-7014
Website: http://www.emlife.com
Alex T. Schneebacher, Jr., CEO & Pres

★ 16903 ★ Emphesys Insurance Co.
Humana Inc.
PO Box 740036
Louisville, KY 40201-7436
Phone: (502)580-1000
Website: http://www.humana.com
Michael B. McCallister, CEO & Pres

★ 16904 ★ Emphesys Wisconsin Insurance Co.
Humana Inc.
PO Box 740036
Louisville, KY 40201-7436
Phone: (920)336-1100
Website: http://www.humana.com
Michael B. McCallister, CEO & Pres

★ 16905 ★ Empire Blue Cross and Blue Shield
Empire Blue Cross and Blue Shield Group
11 West 42nd St.
New York, NY 10036
Phone: (212)476-1000
Michael A. Stocker, MD, President

★ 16906 ★ Empire Fidelity Investments Life Insurance Co.
Fidelity Investments Group
PO Box 3767
New York, NY 10008-3767
Phone: (212)804-4470 **Fax:** (212)809-8984
Rodney R. Rohda, CEO & Chm Bd

★ 16907 ★ Empire General Life Assurance Corp.
Protective Life Corp.
2801 Hwy. 280 S
Birmingham, AL 35223
Phone: (205)879-9230 **Fax:** (205)868-3270
Website: http://www.protective.com
Douglas K. Adam, President

★ 16908 ★ Empire HealthChoice Assurance Inc.
Empire Blue Cross & Blue Shield Group
11 West 42nd St.
New York, NY 10036
Phone: (212)476-1000 **Fax:** (212)476-1694
Michael A. Stocker, MD, CEO

★ 16909 ★ Empire HealthChoice Inc.
Empire Blue Cross and Blue Shield Group
11 Corporate Woods Blvd.
Albany, NY 12211
Phone: (212)476-1000
Website: http://www.empirehealthcare.com
Philip Briggs, Chairman of the Board

★ 16910 ★ Empire HealthChoice Inc. (HMO)
Empire Blue Cross and Blue Shield Group
11 W 42nd St.
New York, NY 10036
Phone: (212)476-1000 **Fax:** (212)476-1281
Website: http://www.empireblue.com

★ 16911 ★ Employees Life Co. (Mutual)
916 Sherwood Dr.
Lake Bluff, IL 60044-2285
Phone: (847)295-6000 **Fax:** (847)295-1145
Website: http://www.elcoins.com
William D. Bruce, President
Edmund J. Kulpins, Exec VP

★ 16912 ★ Employees Life Insurance Co.
9311 San Pedro, Ste. 550
San Antonio, TX 78216
Phone: (210)321-7361 **Fax:** (210)525-1247
Website: http://www.swbc.com
Karen L. Ware, President

★ 16913 ★ Employers Life Insurance Co.
333 S Pine St.
PO Box 6305
Spartanburg, SC 29304
Phone: (864)573-8653
William Worthy, President

★ 16914 ★ Employers Modern Life Co.
EMC Insurance Companies
PO Box 712
Des Moines, IA 50303-0712
Phone: (515)280-2511 **Fax:** (515)284-1599
Website: http://www.emlins.com
Alan D. Huisinga, President

★ 16915 ★ Employers Reassurance Corp.
Employers Re Group
PO Box 2981
Shawnee Mission, KS 66201-1381
Phone: (913)676-5950 **Fax:** (913)676-6216
Website: http://www.ercgroup.com
John E. Tiller, President

★ 16916 ★ Enterprise Life Insurance Co.
Enterprise Financial Group
PO Box 167667
Irving, TX 75016-7667
Phone: (972)751-5544 **Fax:** (972)445-8380
Website: http://www.efgcompanies.com
Michael Boyd, President

★ 16917 ★ The EPIC Life Insurance Co.
Wisconsin Physicians Service Group
PO Box 14196
Madison, WI 53714-0196
Phone: (608)221-6882 **Fax:** (608)223-2159
Website: http://www.epiclife.com
James R. Riordan, President

★ 16918 ★ The Equitable of Colorado, Inc.
Equitable Group
1290 6th Ave., 16th Fl.
New York, NY 10104
Phone: (212)554-1234 **Fax:** (212)707-1805
Website: http://www.axa-financial.com
Christopher M. Condron, CEO & Chm Bd

★ 16919 ★ The Equitable Life Assurance Society of the United States
Equitable Group
1290 6th Ave., 16th Fl.
New York, NY 10104
Phone: (212)554-1234 **Fax:** (212)707-1805
Website: http://www.axa-financial.com
Christopher M. Condron, CEO & Chm Bd

★ 16920 ★ Equitable Life and Casualty Insurance Co.
PO Box 2460
Salt Lake City, UT 84110
Phone: (801)579-3400 **Fax:** (801)579-3790
Website: http://www.equilife.com
E. Rod Ross, CEO & Chm Bd

★ 16921 ★ Equitable Life Insurance Co. of Iowa
ING Group
5780 Powers Ferry Rd. NW
Atlanta, GA 30327
Phone: (515)698-7000 **Fax:** (515)698-6973
Chris D. Schreier, President

★ 16922 ★ Equitable Reserve Association
PO Box 448
Neenah, WI 54957-0448
Phone: (920)722-1574 **Fax:** (920)725-2869
Website: http://www.equitablereserve.com
Robert E. Miller, President

★ 16923 ★ EquiTrust Life Insurance Co.
Farm Bureau Group of Iowa
5400 University Ave.
West Des Moines, IA 50266-5997
Phone: (515)225-5400 **Fax:** (515)225-5604
Website: http://www.fbfs.com
Craig A. Lang, President

★ 16924 ★ ERC Life Reinsurance Corp.
Employers Re Group
PO Box 29175
Overland Park, KS 66201-9175
Phone: (913)676-5950 **Fax:** (913)676-6216
Website: http://www.ercgroup.com
John E. Tiller, President

★ 16925 ★ Erie Family Life Insurance Co.
Erie Insurance Group
100 Erie Insurance Pl.
Erie, PA 16530
Phone: (814)870-2000 **Fax:** (814)870-3126
Website: http://www.erieinsurance.com
Stephen A. Milne, CEO & Pres

★ 16926 ★ Escude Life Insurance Co.
200 Leglise St.
PO Box 429
Mansura, LA 71350
Phone: (318)964-2441

★ 16927 ★ Evangeline Life Insurance Co. Inc.
PO Box 13098
New Iberia, LA 70562-3098
Phone: (318)364-1721
Charles J. D. Gerrets, III, President

★ 16928 ★ Excalibur Insurance Corp.
Citizens, Inc. Group
400 E Anderson Ln.
Austin, TX 78752
Phone: (512)837-7100 **Fax:** (512)836-9785
Rick D. Riley, President

★ 16929 ★ Excellus Health Plan, Inc.
Excellus Inc.
165 Court St.
Rochester, NY 14647
Phone: (585)454-1700 **Fax:** (585)238-4400
Website: http://www.excellus.com
David H. Klein, President

★ 16930 ★ Exclusive Healthcare Inc.
Mutual of Omaha Group
Mutual of Omaha Plaza
Omaha, NE 68175
Phone: (402)342-7600
Daniel P. Neary, President

★ 16931 ★ Fairlane Life Insurance Co.
American Road Insurance Group
1 American Rd.
Dearborn, MI 48121-6027
Phone: (313)322-7287 **Fax:** (313)323-9479
J. M. Moritz, President

★ 16932 ★ Fallon Community Health Plan Inc.
Fallon Foundation
10 Chestnut St.
Worcester, MA 01608-2810
Phone: (508)799-2100 **Fax:** (508)831-1137
Website: http://www.fchp.org

★ 16933 ★ Fallon Health & Life Assurance Co.
10 Chestnut St.
Worcester, MA 01608
Phone: (508)368-9475
James J. Egan, III, President

★ 16934 ★ Family Benefit Life Insurance Co.
PO Box 665
Jefferson City, MO 65102
Phone: (573)636-3181 **Fax:** (573)634-7381
Ross A. Walquist, President

★ 16935 ★ Family Financial Life Insurance Co.
PO Box 19685
New Orleans, LA 70179-0685
Phone: (504)456-0101 **Fax:** (504)456-7324
Jack P. Panno, President

★ 16936 ★ Family Guaranty Life Insurance Co.
PO Box 681389
Franklin, TN 37068-1389
Phone: (615)790-0464 **Fax:** (615)790-9962
John A. Hackney, President

★ 16937 ★ Family Health Plan Inc.
Farley Health Care Corp.
2200 Jefferson Ave., 6th Fl.
Toledo, OH 43624
Phone: (419)241-6501

★ 16938 ★ Family Heritage Life Co. of America
3 Summit Park Dr.
PO Box 31420
Cleveland, OH 44131-0420
Phone: (216)520-2800
Howard L. Lewis, President

★ 16939 ★ Family Insurance Corp.
Citigroup
307 W 7th St., Ste. 400
Fort Worth, TX 76102
Phone: (817)348-7500
Darrell J. Gambero, President

★ 16940 ★ Family Liberty Life Insurance Co.
PO Box 1199
Texarkana, TX 75504
Phone: (903)794-3714
Thomas Fuqua, Jr., President

★ 16941 ★ Family Life Insurance Co.
FIC Insurance Group
6500 River Place Blvd., Bldg. 1
Austin, TX 78730
Phone: (512)404-5000 **Fax:** (512)404-5051
Website: http://www.ficgroup.com
Roy F. Mitte, CEO & Chm Bd

★ 16942 ★ Family Life Insurance Co. of America
PO Box 535304
Grand Prairie, TX 75053-5304
Phone: (713)467-8811
Susan Pahler Jarrell, President

★ 16943 ★ Family Security Life Insurance Co., Inc.
PO Box 1226
Natchez, MS 39120-1226
Phone: (601)442-4041
Charles M. Laird, President

★ 16944 ★ Family Service Life Insurance Co.
Guardian Life
7 Hanover St.
New York, NY 10004-2616
Phone: (212)598-8000 **Free:** 800-538-6203
Fax: (212)919-2910
Website: http://www.glic.com
Joseph D. Sargent, Chairman of the Board

★ 16945 ★ Farm Bureau Life Insurance Co.
Farm Bureau Group of Iowa
5400 University Ave.
West Des Moines, IA 50266-5997
Phone: (515)225-5400 **Fax:** (515)225-5604
Website: http://www.fbfs.com
Craig A. Lang, President

★ 16946 ★ Farm Bureau Life Insurance Co. of Michigan
Michigan Farm Bureau Group
PO Box 30200
Lansing, MI 48909
Phone: (517)323-7000 **Fax:** (517)323-6574
Website: http://www.farmbureauinsurance-mi.com
Wayne H. Wood, President

★ 16947 ★ Farm Bureau Life Insurance Co. of Missouri
Missouri Farm Bureau Services
PO Box 658
Jefferson City, MO 65102-0658
Phone: (573)893-1400 **Fax:** (573)893-1540
Website: http://www.fb.com/mofb/
Charles E. Kruse, President
R. Jay Plattner, Vice President

★ 16948 ★ Farm Family Life Insurance Co.
American National Group
PO Box 656
Albany, NY 12201-0656
Phone: (518)431-5000 **Fax:** (518)431-5979
Philip P. Weber, CEO & Pres
Clark W. Hinsdale, III, Chairman of the Board

★ 16949 ★ Farmers New World Life Insurance Co.
Zurich Insurance Group
3003 77th Ave. SE
Mercer Island, WA 98040-2890
Phone: (206)232-8400 **Fax:** (206)236-6645
Website: http://www.farmersinsurance.com
C. Paul Patsis, President

★ 16950 ★ Farmers and Ranchers Life Insurance Co.
Oklahoma State Union Farmers Education & Cooperative Union
PO Box 25968
Oklahoma City, OK 73125
Phone: (405)603-1102
Raymond L. Wulf, President

★ 16951 ★ Farmers and Traders Life Insurance Co.
PO Box 1056
Syracuse, NY 13201-1056
Phone: (315)471-5656 **Fax:** (315)472-3109
Website: http://www.ftlife.com
William R. Hess, CEO & Pres
Terence M. Mawhinney, Exec VP

★ 16952 ★ Federal Home Life Insurance Co.
GE Financial Assurance Group
6604 W Broad St., 5th Fl.
Richmond, VA 23230
Phone: (804)845-0911
Website: http://www.gefinancialassurance.com
Leon E. Roday, CEO & Pres

★ 16953 ★ Federal Kemper Life Assurance Co.
Zurich Insurance Group
1600 McConnor Pkwy.
Schaumburg, IL 60196
Phone: (847)874-4000 **Fax:** (847)874-5643
Website: http://www.zurichlifeus.com
Martin D. Feinstein, Chairman of the Board
Gale K. Caruso, CEO & Pres

★ 16954 ★ Federal Life Insurance Co. (Mutual)
3750 W Deerfield Rd.
Riverwoods, IL 60015
Phone: (847)520-1900
Joseph D. Austin, President

★ 16955 ★ Federated Life Insurance Co.
Federated Mutual Group
121 E Park Sq.
Owatonna, MN 55060-3046
Phone: (507)455-5200 **Fax:** (507)455-5145
Website: http://www.federatedinsurance.com
A. T. Annexstad, CEO & Pres

★ 16956 ★ Fidelity and Guaranty Life Insurance Co.
Old Mutual US Life Holdings Inc.
PO Box 1137
Baltimore, MD 21203-1137
Phone: (410)895-0100 **Fax:** (410)895-0132
Website: http://www.fglife.com
Harry N. Stout, CEO & Pres
Guy V. Barker, Chairman of the Board

★ 16957 ★ Fidelity and Guaranty Life Insurance Co. of New York
Old Mutual U.S. Life Holdings Inc.
PO Box 1137
Baltimore, MD 21203-1137
Phone: (914)251-2362 **Fax:** (914)251-1183
Website: http://www.fglife.com
James R. Morrison, President
Frmly: Thomas Jefferson Life Insurance Co.

★ 16958 ★ Fidelity Investments Life Insurance Co.
Fidelity Investments Group
82 Devonshire St., R27A
Boston, MA 02109-3104
Phone: (617)563-4395 **Fax:** (617)692-5435
Rodney R. Rohda, CEO & Pres

★ 16959 ★ Fidelity Life Association A Mutual Legal Reserve Co.
Zurich Insurance Group
1600 McConnor Pkwy.
Schaumburg, IL 60196-6801
Phone: (847)874-4000 **Fax:** (847)874-5643
Website: http://www.zurichlifeus.com
Gale K. Caruso, CEO & Pres

★ 16960 ★ Fidelity Life Insurance Co.
250 King of Prussia Rd.
Radnor, PA 19087
Phone: (610)964-7245
William S. Taylor, Jr., President

★ 16961 ★ Fidelity Security Life Insurance Co.
Fidelity Security Group
3130 Broadway
Kansas City, MO 64111-2452
Phone: (816)756-1060 **Fax:** (816)968-0585
Website: http://www.fslins.com
Richard F. Jones, President

★ 16962 ★ Fiduciary Insurance Co. of America
Guardian Group
7 Hanover Sq.
New York, NY 10004-2616
Phone: (212)598-8000
Website: http://www.fiduciaryinsurance.com
Joseph D. Sargent, President

★ 16963 ★ Financial American Life Insurance Co.
5900 Monona Dr., Ste. 100
Madison, WI 53716
Phone: (608)222-9986 **Fax:** (608)222-9941
Website: http://www.famli.com
Patricia Farrell, President

★ 16964 ★ Financial Assurance Life Insurance Co.
Americo Life Group
PO Box 13487
Kansas City, MO 64199-3487
Phone: (816)391-2000 **Fax:** (816)391-2083
Website: http://www.americo.com
Gary L. Muller, CEO & Pres

★ 16965 ★ Financial Benefit Life Insurance Co.
AmerUs Group
PO Box 3502
Topeka, KS 66601-3502
Phone: (785)232-6945 **Fax:** (785)232-3534
Mark V. Heitz, CEO & Pres

★ 16966 ★ Financial Cooperative Life Insurance Co.
PO Box 8007
Redwood City, CA 94065
Phone: (650)508-0300

★ 16967 ★ Financial Life Insurance Co. of Georgia
PO Box 4148, MC 505
Atlanta, GA 30302
Phone: (704)374-2017
Robert Steven Kniejski, President

★ 16968 ★ First Alliance Insurance Co.
2285 Executive Dr., Ste. 308
Lexington, KY 40505
Phone: (859)299-7656
Michael Fink, President

★ 16969 ★ First Allmerica Financial Life Insurance Co.
Allmerica Financial Group
440 Lincoln St.
Worcester, MA 01653
Phone: (508)855-1000 **Fax:** (508)853-6332
Website: http://www.allmerica.com
John F. O'Brien, CEO & Pres

★ 16970 ★ First Ameritas Life Insurance Corp. of New York
Ameritas Acacia Group
400 Rella Blvd., Ste. 304
Suffern, NY 10901
Phone: (845)357-3816

Website: http://www.firstameritas.com
Mitchell F. Politzer, CEO & Pres

★ 16971 ★ First Amtenn Life Insurance Co.
PO Box 50355
Atlanta, GA 30339-2111
Phone: (770)763-2452
Prodyodth Kumar Cahatterjee, President

★ 16972 ★ First Assurance Life of America
LDS Group
PO Box 83480
Baton Rouge, LA 70884-3480
Phone: (225)769-9923 **Fax:** (225)767-7656
Website: http://www.theldsgroup.com
Dick S. Taylor, President

★ 16973 ★ First AUSA Life Insurance Co.
AEGON USA, Inc.
4333 Edgewood Rd. NE
Cedar Rapids, IA 52499
Phone: (319)398-8511 **Fax:** (319)369-2210
Patrick S. Baird, President

★ 16974 ★ First Care, Inc.
10455 Mill Run Cir.
Owings Mills, MD 21117
Phone: (410)998-7011
David Wolf, President

★ 16975 ★ First Catholic Slovak Ladies Association of the U.S.A.
24950 Chagrin Blvd.
Cleveland, OH 44122-5634
Free: 800-464-4642 **Fax:** 800-464-9260
Website: http://www.fcsla.com
Mary Ann Sabol Johanek, President

★ 16976 ★ First Catholic Slovak Union of the U.S.A. and Canada
6611 Rockside Rd.
Independence, OH 44131
Phone: (216)642-9406 **Fax:** (216)642-4310
Thomas M. Hricik, President

★ 16977 ★ First Central National Life Insurance Co. of New York
Household Insurance Group
200 Somerset Corporate Blvd., Ste. 100
Bridgewater, NJ 08807
Phone: (212)564-1740 **Free:** 800-627-7282
Daniel R. O'Brien, CEO & Pres

★ 16978 ★ First Choice Health Plan Inc.
601 Union St., Ste. 1100
Seattle, WA 98101
Phone: (206)292-8255
Website: http://www.fchn.com

★ 16979 ★ First Citicorp Life Insurance Co.
Citigroup
307 W 7th St., Ste. 400
Fort Worth, TX 76102
Phone: (212)615-7201
George C. Kokulis, CEO & Pres

★ 16980 ★ First Colony Life Insurance Co.
GE Financial Assurance Group
700 Main St.
Lynchburg, VA 24504
Phone: (804)845-0911
Website: http://www.firstcolonylife.com
George R. Zippel, President

★ 16981 ★ First Columbine Life Insurance Co.
ING Group
5780 Powers Ferry Rd. NW
Atlanta, GA 30327
Phone: (303)860-1290
Gregory G. McGreevey, President

★ 16982 ★ First Command Life Insurance Co.
3700 S Stonebridge Dr.
McKinney, TX 75070
Phone: (972)569-3258 **Fax:** (972)569-3728
Howard M. Crump, President
Frmly: Bankers & Farmers Life Insurance Co.

★ 16983 ★ First Commonwealth Insurance Co.
444 N Wells, Ste. 600
Chicago, IL 60610
Phone: (312)644-1800
David Mulligan, President

★ 16984 ★ First Continental Life and Accident Insurance Co.
Wasatch Crest Group Inc.
PO Box 27008
Salt Lake City, UT 84127-0008
Phone: (801)972-7555 **Fax:** (801)972-7545
John A. Igoe, President

★ 16985 ★ First Dimension Life Insurance Co.
PO Box 487
Stillwater, OK 74076
Phone: (405)372-4951
Bill Bernhardt, Jr., President

★ 16986 ★ First Dominion Mutual Life Insurance Co.
1011 Boulder Springs Dr.
Richmond, VA 23225
Phone: (512)404-6555

★ 16987 ★ First Fortis Life Insurance Co.
Fortis, Inc. Group
PO Box 3209
Syracuse, NY 13220
Phone: (315)451-0066 **Fax:** (315)453-2343
Website: http://www.fortis.com
Robert B. Pollock, President

★ 16988 ★ First Golden American Life Insurance Co. of New York
ING Group
5780 Powers Ferry Rd. NW
Atlanta, GA 30327
Phone: (516)682-8700
Website: http://ingvariableannuities.com
Stephen J. Preston, President

★ 16989 ★ First Great-West Life & Annuity Insurance Co.
Great-West Life Group
8515 E Orchard Rd.
Greenwood Village, CO 80111
Phone: (518)437-1816 **Fax:** (518)437-1817
Website: http://www.gwla.com
William T. McCallum, CEO & Pres

★ 16990 ★ First Guaranty Insurance Co.
PO Box 848
Ashdown, AR 71822-0848
Phone: (870)898-5191
Robert William Eichelberger, President

★ 16991 ★ First Health Life & Health Insurance Co.
First Health Group Corp.
3200 Highland Ave.
Downers Grove, IL 60515-1282
Phone: (630)737-7900 **Fax:** (630)737-7855
Edward L. Wristen, President

★ 16992 ★ First Investors Life Insurance Co.
95 Wall St.
New York, NY 10005
Phone: (212)858-8200 **Fax:** (212)858-8205
Website: http://www.firstinvestorslife.com
William H. Drinkwater, President
Glenn O. Head, Chairman of the Board

★ 16993 ★ First Landmark Life Insurance Co.
PO Box 249
Wilmington, DE 19899
Phone: (302)429-4900
Martin Oliner, President

★ 16994 ★ First Life American Corp.
1303 SW 1st American Pl.
Topeka, KS 66604
Phone: (785)267-7077
Rick Meyer, President

★ 16995 ★ First M & F Insurance Co.
PO Box 520
Kosciusko, MS 39090
Phone: (651)451-6205
Hugh Potts, Jr., President

★ 16996 ★ First Medical Health Plan Inc.
Union Plaza Bldg., Ste. 18B
San Juan, PR 00918
Phone: (787)622-0777

★ 16997 ★ First MetLife Investors Insurance Co.
Metropolitan Life and Affiliated Cos.
1 MetLife Plaza, Area 7B
Long Island City, NY 11101
Phone: (949)717-6536
Website: http://www.cova.com
Gregory P. Brakovich, President
Frmly: First Cova Life Insurance Co.

★ 16998 ★ First National Indemnity Life Insurance Co.
Campbell Centre II, Ste. 1900
8150 N Central Expy.
Dallas, TX 75206
Phone: (214)365-1361
Anna Elizabeth Dolak, President

★ 16999 ★ First National Life Insurance Co. of America
PO Box 11316
Birmingham, AL 35202-1316
Phone: (205)942-2112 **Fax:** (205)941-1716
John A. Hackney, CEO & Pres

★ 17000 ★ First National Life Insurance Co. of the USA
3600 S 48th St.
Lincoln, NE 68506
Phone: (402)483-1776 **Fax:** (402)483-2341
Kenneth D. Tenhulzen, President

★ 17001 ★ First Penn-Pacific Life Insurance Co.
Lincoln National Corp.
1300 S Clinton St.
Fort Wayne, IN 46802-3518
Phone: (847)466-8000
Website: http://www.firstpenn.com
John H. Gotta, President

★ 17002 ★ First Plan of Minnesota
409 17th Ave.
Two Harbors, MN 55616
Phone: (218)834-7207 **Fax:** (218)834-6215
Website: http://www.firstplan.org
Milton Larson, Chairman of the Board

★ 17003 ★ First Priority Life Insurance Co.
19 N Main St.
Wilkes Barre, PA 18711
Phone: (570)829-6137
Thomas Ward, President

★ 17004 ★ The First Pyramid Life Insurance Co. of America
Arkansas Blue Cross & Blue Shield Group
PO Box 1151
Little Rock, AR 72203-1151
Phone: (501)378-5628 **Fax:** (501)378-5633
Robert L. Shoptaw, President

★ 17005 ★ First Rehabilitation Life Insurance Co. of America
600 Northern Blvd.
Great Neck, NY 11021-5202
Phone: (516)829-8100 **Fax:** (516)829-8211
Website: http://www.firstrehab.com
John Baldwin, President

★ 17006 ★ First Reliance Standard Life Insurance Co.
Reliance Standard Life Group
2001 Market St., Ste. 1500
Philadelphia, PA 19103
Phone: (212)303-8400 **Fax:** (212)303-8437
Website: http://www.rsli.com
Lawrence E. Daurelle, CEO & Pres

★ 17007 ★ First SAFECO National Life Insurance Co. of New York
SAFECO Life Group
PO Box 34690
Seattle, WA 98124-1690
Phone: (425)376-8000 **Fax:** (425)376-5818
Website: http://www.safeco.com
Randall H. Talbot, President

★ 17008 ★ First Security Benefit Life Insurance & Annuity Co. of New York
Security Benefit Group
70 W Red Oak Ln.
White Plains, NY 10604
Phone: (914)697-4748 **Fax:** (914)697-4912
Website: http://securitybenefit.com
Kris A. Robbins, CEO & Pres

★ 17009 ★ First Standard Security Insurance Co.
Independence Holding Group
485 Madison Ave.
New York, NY 10022-5872
Phone: (212)355-4141 **Fax:** (212)754-3346
Alex Giordano, President

★ 17010 ★ First SunAmerica Life Insurance Co.
American International Group
1 SunAmerica Ctr.
Los Angeles, CA 90067-6022
Phone: (310)772-6090 **Fax:** (310)772-6635
Website: http://www.sunamerica.com
Jay S. Wintrob, President

★ 17011 ★ First United American Life Insurance Co.
Torchmark Corp.
PO Box 3125
Syracuse, NY 13220
Phone: (315)451-2544
Mark S. McAndrew, CEO & Pres

★ 17012 ★ First Unum Life Insurance Co.
UnumProvident Corp.
1 Fountain Sq.
Chattanooga, TN 37402-1330
Phone: (914)524-4000 **Fax:** (914)524-4058
Website: http://www.unumprovident.com
James H. Chandler, CEO & Chm Bd

★ 17013 ★ First Variable Life Insurance Co.
Protective Life Corp.
2801 Hwy. 280 S
Birmingham, AL 35223
Phone: (205)879-9230 **Fax:** (205)423-5595
Website: http://www.firstvariable.com
Jim E. Massengale, President

★ 17014 ★ First Virginia Life Insurance Co.
6400 Arlington Blvd.
Falls Church, VA 22042-2336
Phone: (703)241-4426 **Fax:** (703)241-3576
Shirley C. Beavers, Jr., CEO & Pres

★ 17015 ★ FirstGuard Health Plan Inc.
Models Cities Health Corp.
4001 Blue Pkwy.
Kansas City, MO 64130
Phone: (816)922-7250
Website: http://www.firstguard.com

★ 17016 ★ FirstReturn Insurance Co., Inc.
93 Worcester St.
Wellesley, MA 02481
Phone: (781)263-6000
Bruce M. Bullen, President

★ 17017 ★ Five Star Life Insurance Co.
909 N Washington St.
Alexandria, VA 22314
Free: 800-776-2322 **Fax:** (703)549-0593
Website: http://www.afba.com
Craig S. Piers, President

★ 17018 ★ Florida Combined Life Insurance Co.
Blue Cross & Blue Shield of Florida Group
4800 Deerwood Campus Pkwy., DCC 1-6
Jacksonville, FL 32246
Phone: (904)828-7826 **Fax:** (904)730-7861
Walter T. Liptak, President

★ 17019 ★ Florida Health Care Plan Inc.
1340 Ridgewood Ave.
Holly Hill, FL 32117
Phone: (386)676-7100 **Fax:** (386)676-7196
Website: http://www.floridahealthcares.com

★ 17020 ★ Florida 1st Health Plans Inc.
Mid-Florida Medical Services Inc.
3425 Lake Alfred Rd.
PO Box 9126
Winter Haven, FL 33883-9126
Phone: (863)293-0785

★ 17021 ★ Forethought Life Assurance Co.
Forethought Group
Forethought Ctr.
Batesville, IN 47006-9170
Phone: (812)934-7139 **Fax:** (812)934-8564
Website: http://www.forethought.com
Stephen R. Lang, CEO & Chm Bd

★ 17022 ★ Fort Dearborn Life Insurance Co.
Health Care Service Corp.
300 E Randolph St.
Chicago, IL 60601-5099
Phone: (312)653-6500 **Fax:** (312)938-6652
Website: http://www.fdl-life.com
Larry J. Newsom, CEO & Pres

★ 17023 ★ Fort Wayne Health & Casualty Insurance Co.
Swiss Re Group
1700 Magnavox Way
PO Box 7808
Fort Wayne, IN 46801-7808
Phone: (260)455-2000 **Fax:** (260)455-4120
Website: http://www.lnrc.com
Lawrence T. Rowland, President

★ 17024 ★ Fortis Benefits Insurance Co.
Fortis, Inc. Group
PO Box 419052
Kansas City, MO 64141-6052
Phone: (651)361-4456 **Fax:** (651)361-5356
Website: http://www.fortisbenefis.us.fortis.com
Robert B. Pollock, CEO & Pres

★ 17025 ★ Fortis Insurance Co.
Fortis, Inc. Group
PO Box 3050
Milwaukee, WI 53201-3050
Phone: (414)271-3011 **Fax:** (414)224-0472
Website: http://www.fortishealth.com
Benjamin M. Cutler, II, CEO & Pres

★ 17026 ★ Foundation Life Insurance Co. of Arkansas
109 N 6th St.
Fort Smith, AR 72901
Phone: (479)785-1714
Bennie B. Westphal, President

★ 17027 ★ Frandisco Life Insurance Co.
213 E Tugalo St.
Toccoa, GA 30577
Phone: (706)886-7571
Benjamin Cheek, III, President

★ 17028 ★ Franklin Life Insurance Co.
American International Group
1 Franklin Sq.
Springfield, IL 62713-0001
Phone: (217)528-2011 **Fax:** (217)528-3960
Website: http://www.thefranklin.com
Donald W. Britton, President

★ 17029 ★ Franklin Protective Life Insurance Co.
PO Box 681389
Franklin, TN 37068-1389

Phone: (615)790-0464 **Fax:** (615)790-9962
John A. Hackney, President

★ 17030 ★ Free State Health Plan Inc.
CareFirst of Maryland Inc.
10455 Mill Run Circle
Owings Mills, MD 21117
Phone: (410)581-3000
Patrick J. Mitchell, CEO & Chm Bd

★ 17031 ★ Freedom Life Insurance Co. of America
Ascent Assurance, Inc.
110 W 7th St., Ste. 300
Fort Worth, TX 76102
Phone: (817)878-3300 **Fax:** (817)878-3672
Website: http://www.ascentassurance.com
Patrick J. Mitchell, CEO & Pres

★ 17032 ★ Fremont Life Insurance Co.
Fremont General Corp.
3070 Bristol St., Ste. 600
Costa Mesa, CA 92626
Phone: (714)429-2610 **Fax:** (714)429-2690
Louis J. Rampino, CEO & Pres

★ 17033 ★ Fringe Benefit Life Insurance Co.
2901 Morton St.
Fort Worth, TX 76107
Phone: (817)885-8223
Kelly B. Keller, President

★ 17034 ★ Frontier Life Insurance Co.
1601 Rio Grande St., Ste. 420
Austin, TX 78701
Phone: (512)236-1936
Gregory J. Weber, President

★ 17035 ★ Funeral Directors Life Insurance Co.
Funeral Directors Group
PO Box 5649
Abilene, TX 79606
Phone: (915)695-3412 **Fax:** (915)695-7840
Website: http://www.funeraldirectorslife.com
B. Kris Seale, President

★ 17036 ★ Futural Life Insurance Co.
2700 N 3rd St.
Phoenix, AZ 85004
Phone: (602)200-6900
Robert L. Terrell, President

★ 17037 ★ Garden State Life Insurance Co.
American National Group
1 Moody Plz., 17th Fl.
Galveston, TX 77550
Phone: (281)538-1037 **Fax:** (281)538-3705
Website: http://wwww.gardenstatelife.com
Scott K. Luchesi, CEO & Pres

★ 17038 ★ Gateway Health Plan Inc.
Gateway Health Plan LP
2 Chatham Ctr., Ste. 500
Pittsburgh, PA 15219
Phone: (412)255-4678

★ 17039 ★ GE Capital Life Assurance Co. of New York
GE Financial Assurance Group
6604 W Broad St.
Richmond, VA 23230
Phone: (212)672-4299
Website: http://www.gefinancialassurance.com
Cheryl C. Whaley, CEO & Pres

★ 17040 ★ GE Group Life Assurance Co.
GE Financial Assurance Group
6604 W Broad St.
Richmond, VA 23230
Phone: (860)737-1000
Website: http://www.ge.com
Marcia I. Cantor-Grable, President

★ 17041 ★ GE Life and Annuity Assurance Co.
GE Financial Assurance Group
6604 W Broad St., 5th Fl.
Richmond, VA 23230
Phone: (804)662-2400
Website: http://www.gelifeandannuity.com
Pamela S. Schutz, CEO & Chm Bd

★ 17042 ★ Geisinger Health Plan
Geisinger Health System Foundation
100 N Academy Ave.
Danville, PA 17822
Phone: (570)271-8760
Website: http://www.thehealthplan.com

★ 17043 ★ Geisinger Indemnity Insurance Co.
100 N Academy Ave.
Danville, PA 17822-3051
Phone: (570)271-8761 **Free:** 800-631-1656
Website: http://www.thehealthplan.com
Glenn D. Steele, Jr., CEO & Chm Bd

★ 17044 ★ Gem Insurance Co.
Health Net Inc.
21281 Burbank Blvd., Bldg. B3
Woodland Hills, CA 91367
Phone: (818)676-8256 **Fax:** (818)676-6521
Website: http://www.healthnet.com
David W. Anderson, President

★ 17045 ★ General American Life Insurance Co.
Metropolitan Life and Affiliated Cos.
700 Market St.
Saint Louis, MO 63101
Phone: (314)843-8700 **Fax:** (314)444-0486
Website: http://www.genamerica.com
Kevin C. Eichner, CEO & Pres

★ 17046 ★ General & Cologne Life Re of America
Berkshire Hathaway Group
695 E Main St.
Stamford, CT 06904-0300
Phone: (203)352-3000
Website: http://www.gcr.com
Thomas M. West, CEO & Chm Bd

★ 17047 ★ General Electric Capital Assurance Co.
GE Financial Assurance Group
6604 W Broad St.
Richmond, VA 23230
Phone: (804)662-2400 **Free:** 800-344-2914
Website: http://www.gefinancialassurance.com
Geoffrey S. Stiff, CEO & Pres

★ 17048 ★ General Fidelity Life Insurance Co.
BankAmerica Group
201 N Tryon St.
NC1-022-19-02
Charlotte, NC 28255
Phone: (704)386-8814 **Fax:** (619)515-1427
Dean A. Purvis, President

★ 17049 ★ General Life Insurance Co.
Metropolitan Life and Affiliated Cos.
901 Congress Ave.
Austin, TX 78714
Phone: (618)659-9510 **Fax:** (618)659-0310
Website: http://www.generalife.com
John E. Petersen, President

★ 17050 ★ Genesis Health Plan of Ohio, Inc.
Catholic HealthCare Partners
205 W 20th St., Ste. A510
Lorain, OH 44052
Phone: (440)244-2060

★ 17051 ★ Geneva Life Insurance Co.
55 S Harding St.
Indianapolis, IN 46222
Phone: (317)634-6190
John V. Loudermilk, President

★ 17052 ★ The George Washington University Health Plan Inc.
George Washington University
4550 Montgomery Ave., Ste. 800
Bethesda, MD 20814
Phone: (301)941-2000

★ 17053 ★ Gerber Life Insurance Co.
1311 Mamaroneck Ave.
White Plains, NY 10605
Phone: (914)272-4000 **Fax:** (914)272-4099
Website: http://www.gerberlife.com
Ronald J. Masiero, President

★ 17054 ★ Gerling Global Life Reinsurance Co.
Gerling Group Consolidated
480 University Ave.
Toronto, ON, Canada M5G 1V6
Phone: (416)598-4677 **Fax:** (416)598-3901
Website: http://www2.gerling.com/ggreinter
Gaetano Geretto, CEO & Pres

★ 17055 ★ Germania Life Insurance Co.
Germania Mutual Group
PO Box 645
Brenham, TX 77834
Phone: (979)836-5224 **Fax:** (979)277-1900
Website: http://www.germania-ins.com
David C. Sommer, President

★ 17056 ★ Gertrude Geddes Willis Life Insurance Co.
PO Box 53272
New Orleans, LA 70153
Phone: (504)522-2525
Joseph O. Misshoure, Jr., President

★ 17057 ★ GHI HMO Select Inc.
Group Health Inc.
25 Barbarosa Ln.
Kingston, NY 12401
Phone: (845)340-2200
Website: http://www.ghihmo.com

★ 17058 ★ GHS Health Maintenance Organization
Blue Cross & Blue Shield of Oklahoma Group
1400 S Boston
Tulsa, OK 74119
Phone: (918)561-9900 **Fax:** (918)592-0611
Website: http://www.bcbsok.com

★ 17059 ★ Gleaner Life Insurance Society
PO Box 1894
Adrian, MI 49221-7894
Phone: (517)263-2244 **Fax:** (517)265-7745
Website: http://www.gleanerlife.com
Michael J. Wade, President

★ 17060 ★ Glenbrook Life and Annuity Co.
Allstate Financial Group
3100 Sanders Rd.
Northbrook, IL 60062
Phone: (847)402-5000
Website: http://www.allstate.com
Thomas J. Wilson, II, CEO & Pres

★ 17061 ★ Globe Life and Accident Insurance Co.
Torchmark Corp.
Globe Life Ctr.
Oklahoma City, OK 73184
Phone: (405)270-1400 **Fax:** (405)270-1496
Website: http://www.globelifeins.com
Mark S. McAndrew, CEO & Pres

★ 17062 ★ GMHP Health Insurance Ltd.
177 Chalan Pasaher
Tamuning, GU 96911
Phone: (671)472-4647

★ 17063 ★ Golden American Life Insurance Co.
ING Group
5780 Powers Ferry Rd. NW
Atlanta, GA 30327
Phone: (610)425-3400 **Free:** 800-366-0066
Fax: (610)425-3857
Website: http://www.ingvariableannuities.com
Chris D. Schreier, President

★ 17064 ★ Golden Circle Life Insurance Co.
39 Jackson Ave.
PO Box 293
Brownsville, TN 38012
Phone: (901)772-9283

★ 17065 ★ Golden Rule Insurance Co.
Golden Rule Group
7440 Woodland Dr.
Indianapolis, IN 46278-1719
Phone: (618)943-8000 **Fax:** (618)943-8031
Website: http://www.goldenrule.com
John M. Whelan, CEO & Pres
Therese A. Rooney, Chairman of the Board

★ 17066 ★ Golden Security Life Insurance Co.
PO Box 23
Memphis, TN 38101
Phone: (901)544-2111 **Fax:** (901)544-2337
Thomas Kinser, President

★ 17067 ★ Golden State Mutual Life Insurance Co.
PO Box 512332
Los Angeles, CA 90051-0332
Phone: (213)731-1131 **Fax:** (213)732-2139
Website: http://www.gsmlife.com
Larkin Teasley, President

★ 17068 ★ Good Health HMO Inc.
Blue Cross & Blue Shield of Kansas City
2301 Main St.
PO Box 413163
Kansas City, MO 64108
Phone: (816)395-2222
Website: http://www.bcbskc.com

★ 17069 ★ Good Samaritan Life Insurance Co.
PO Box 833879
Richardson, TX 75083-3879
Phone: (972)699-2770 **Fax:** (972)699-2788
Juan G. Fuentes, Jr., President
Frmly: East Funeral Benefit Insurance Co.

★ 17070 ★ Government Personnel Mutual Life Insurance Co.
PO Box 659567
San Antonio, TX 78265-9567
Phone: (210)357-2222 **Fax:** (210)357-6722
Website: http://www.gpmlife.com
Peter J. Hennessey, III, President

★ 17071 ★ Grange Life Insurance Co.
Grange Mutual Casualty Group
650 S Front St.
PO Box 1218
Columbus, OH 43216-1212
Phone: (614)445-2900 **Fax:** (614)445-2619
Website: http://www.grangeinsurance.com
Philip H. Urban, CEO

★ 17072 ★ Grant Life Insurance Co.
PO Box 1896
Marion, IN 46952
Phone: (260)428-7082
James C. Marcuccilli, President

★ 17073 ★ Graphics Arts Benefit Corp.
11414 Livingston Rd.
Fort Washington, MD 20744-5146
Phone: (202)682-3001
Gerard J. McGeehan, Jr., President

★ 17074 ★ Great American Life Assurance Co.
American Financial Group
PO Box 5420
Cincinnati, OH 45201-5420
Phone: (513)357-3300 **Fax:** (513)357-3397
Website: http://www.gafri.com
Charles R. Scheper, CEO & Pres

★ 17075 ★ Great American Life Assurance Co. of Puerto Rico, Inc.
American Financial Group
PO Box 363786
San Juan, PR 00936-3786
Phone: (787)758-4888 **Fax:** (787)766-1985
Arturo Carrion, President

★ 17076 ★ Great American Life Insurance Co.
American Financial Group
PO Box 5420
Cincinnati, OH 45201-5420
Phone: (513)357-3300 **Fax:** (513)357-3399
Website: http://www.gafri.com
Charles R. Scheper, CEO & Pres

★ 17077 ★ Great American Life Insurance Co. of New York
American Financial Group
PO Box 21029
New York, NY 10129-1029
Phone: (212)306-5000
Website: http://www.gafri.com
Charles R. Scheper, President

★ 17078 ★ Great Atlantic Life Insurance Co.
2090 Palm Beach Lakes Blvd.
West Palm Beach, FL 33409
Phone: (561)683-0202 **Fax:** (561)689-3829
Patricia B. Dean, President

★ 17079 ★ Great Central Life Insurance Co.
PO Box 687
Oakdale, LA 71463
Phone: (318)335-0500
Howard J. Rush, Sr., President

★ 17080 ★ Great Fidelity Life Insurance Co.
American Underwriters Life Group
PO Box 9510
Wichita, KS 67277
Phone: (316)794-2200 **Fax:** (316)794-8470
Website: http://www.iai-online.com
R. Kell Hawkins, Chairman of the Board

★ 17081 ★ Great Lakes Delta Insurance Co.
PO Box 30416
Lansing, MI 48909-7916
Phone: (517)349-6000
C. Richard Seitz, President

★ 17082 ★ Great Lakes Health Plan Inc.
17117 W 9th Mile Rd., Ste. 1600
Southfield, MI 48075
Phone: (248)559-5656
Website: http://www.glhp.com

★ 17083 ★ Great Midwest Life Insurance Co.
PO Box 15808
Del City, OK 73115
Phone: (405)677-0781
Charles L. Smith, President

★ 17084 ★ Great Plains Reinsurance Co.
201 N Central Ave.
Phoenix, AZ 85073-3300
Free: 800-332-5455
Barrett A. Toan, President

★ 17085 ★ Great Republic Life Insurance Co.
1900 W Nickerson St., Ste. 200
Seattle, WA 98119-1650
Phone: (206)285-1422 **Fax:** (206)282-5865
Patricia D. Pritchett, President

★ 17086 ★ Great Southeastern Life Insurance Co.
2929 N 44th St., Ste. 120
Phoenix, AZ 85018
Phone: (602)994-5813 **Free:** 800-888-2738
David A. Siegel, President

★ 17087 ★ Great Southern Life Insurance Co.
Americo Life Group
PO Box 13487
Kansas City, MO 64199-3487
Phone: (214)954-8100 **Fax:** (214)954-8220
Website: http://www.americo.com
Gary L. Muller, CEO & Pres

★ 17088 ★ Great-West Life and Annuity Insurance Co.
Great-West Life Group
8515 E Orchard Rd.
Greenwood Village, CO 80111

Phone: (303)737-3000 Fax: (303)689-4321
Website: http://www.gwl.com
William T. McCallum, CEO & Pres

★ 17089 ★ The Great-West Life Assurance Co.
Great-West Life Group
100 Osborne St. N
Winnipeg, MB, Canada R3C 3A5
Phone: (204)946-1190 Fax: (204)946-4060
Website: http://www.gwl.ca
Raymond McFeetors, CEO & Pres

★ 17090 ★ Great Western Insurance Co.
Great Western Group
PO Box 3428
Ogden, UT 84409-1428
Phone: (801)621-5688 Fax: (801)621-5835
Website: http://www.gwic.com
John E. Lindquist, President

★ 17091 ★ Great Western Life Insurance Co.
Great Western Group
PO Box 3428
Ogden, UT 84409-1428
Phone: (801)621-5688 Fax: (801)621-5835
John E. Lindquist, President

★ 17092 ★ Greater Beneficial Union of Pittsburgh
4254 Clairton Blvd.
Pittsburgh, PA 15227-3394
Phone: (412)884-5100 Free: 800-765-4428
Fax: (412)884-9815
Website: http://www.gbu.org
James D. Reagan, Chairman of the Board

★ 17093 ★ Greater Georgia Life Insurance Co.
WellPoint Health Networks Inc.
PO Box 4445
Atlanta, GA 30302
Phone: (678)443-5200 Fax: (678)443-5209
Website: http://www.bcbsga.com
Frederick Raach, President

★ 17094 ★ Greek Catholic Union of the USA
5400 Tuscarawas Rd.
Beaver, PA 15009-9513
Phone: (724)495-3400 Fax: (724)495-3421
Website: http://www.gcuusa.com
Michael I. Roman, President

★ 17095 ★ Gregg Insurance Co.
PO Box 1850
Jonesboro, AR 72403-1850
Phone: (870)935-5566
Maxine S. Gregg, President

★ 17096 ★ Group Health Cooperative of Eau Claire
PO Box 3217
Eau Claire, WI 54702
Phone: (715)552-4300 Fax: (715)836-7683
Website: http://www.group-health.com

★ 17097 ★ Group Health Cooperative of Puget Sound
521 Wall St.
Seattle, WA 98121
Phone: (206)448-5528
Website: http://www.ghc.org

★ 17098 ★ Group Health Cooperative of South Central Wisconsin
8202 Excelsior Dr.
Madison, WI 53717
Phone: (608)251-4156
Website: http://www.ghc-hmo.com

★ 17099 ★ Group Health Inc.
441 9th Ave.
New York, NY 10001
Phone: (212)615-0000
Frank J. Branchini, President

★ 17100 ★ Group Health Options
Group Health Cooperative of Puget Sound
521 Wall St.
Seattle, WA 98121
Phone: (206)448-2965
Maureen P. McLaughlin, President

★ 17101 ★ Group Health Plan Inc.
Coventry Health Care Inc.
111 Corporate Office Dr., Ste. 400
Earth City, MO 63045
Phone: (314)506-1700
Website: http://www.cvty.com

★ 17102 ★ Group Health Plan Inc.
HealthPartners Inc.
8100 34th Ave. S
Minneapolis, MN 55440-1309
Phone: (952)883-6000 Fax: (952)883-6500

★ 17103 ★ Group Health Service of Oklahoma
Blue Cross & Blue Shield of Oklahoma Group
PO Box 3283
Tulsa, OK 74102-3283
Phone: (918)560-3500 Fax: (918)592-9399
Website: http://www.bcbsok.com
Ronald F. King, CEO & Pres

★ 17104 ★ Group Hospitalization and Medical Services
550 12th St. SW
Washington, DC 20065
Phone: (202)479-8000
William L. Jews, President

★ 17105 ★ Guarantee Reserve Life Insurance Co.
Ilona Financial Group, Inc.
530 River Oaks W
Calumet City, IL 60409
Phone: (708)868-4232 Fax: (708)891-8886
Website: http://www.grli.com
Steven Weiss, President

★ 17106 ★ Guarantee Security Life Insurance Co. of Arizona
Guarantee Trust Group
1275 Milwaukee Ave.
Glenview, IL 60025-2489
Phone: (602)952-6761 Fax: (847)699-0636
Richard S. Holson, Jr., President

★ 17107 ★ Guarantee Trust Life Insurance Co.
Guarantee Trust Group
1275 Milwaukee Ave.
Glenview, IL 60025-2489
Phone: (847)699-0600 Fax: (847)460-2963
Website: http://www.gtlic.com
Richard S. Holson, III, CEO & Pres

★ 17108 ★ Guaranty Income Life Insurance Co.
PO Box 2231
Baton Rouge, LA 70821-2231
Phone: (225)383-0355 Fax: (225)383-0047
Website: http://www.gilico.com
John H. Lancaster, President

★ 17109 ★ Guaranty Reassurance Corp.
4190 Belfort Rd., Ste. 200
Jacksonville, FL 32216
Phone: (904)279-9310
Martin C. Eltrich, Jr., President

★ 17110 ★ The Guardian Insurance & Annuity Co., Inc.
Guardian Life
7 Hanover Sq.
New York, NY 10004-2616
Phone: (212)598-8000 Fax: (212)598-7034
Website: http://www.glic.com
Joseph D. Sargent, CEO & Pres

★ 17111 ★ The Guardian Life Insurance Co. of America
Guardian Life
7 Hanover Sq.
New York, NY 10004-2616
Phone: (212)919-2910 Fax: (212)598-8815
Website: http://www.glic.com
Joseph D. Sargent, CEO & Chm Bd
Dennis J. Manning, President

★ 17112 ★ GuideOne Life Insurance Co.
GuideOne Life Group
1111 Ashworth Rd.
West Des Moines, IA 50265-3538
Phone: (515)267-5000 Fax: (515)267-5546
Website: http://www.guideone.com
James D. Wallace, CEO & Chm Bd

★ 17113 ★ Gulf Guaranty Life Insurance Co.
Gulf Guaranty Group
PO Box 12409
Jackson, MS 39236-2409
Phone: (601)981-4920 Fax: (601)981-3402
Richard C. Robertson, President

★ 17114 ★ Gulf States Life Insurance Co., Inc.
PO Box 753
Opelousas, LA 70570
Phone: (337)942-5691
Bobby Dupre, President

★ 17115 ★ Gulfco Life Insurance Co.
Protective Life Corp.
2801 Hwy. 280 S
Birmingham, AL 35223
Phone: (318)253-7564 Fax: (318)253-4903
Roland G. Anderson, President

★ 17116 ★ Gunderson Lutheran Health Plan Inc.
1836 South Ave.
La Crosse, WI 54601
Phone: (608)782-7300

★ 17117 ★ Hallmark Life Insurance Co.
Westward Insurance Group
PO Box 6025
Lakewood, CA 90714
Phone: (562)420-6103 Fax: (562)425-7869
James H. Smith, President

★ 17118 ★ Hannover Life Reassurance Co. of America
Hannover Rueckversicherungs AG
800 N Magnolia Ave., Ste. 1400
Orlando, FL 32803-3268
Phone: (407)649-8411 **Fax:** (407)648-1468
Website: http://www.hlramerica.com
Peter R. Schaefer, CEO & Pres

★ 17119 ★ Harleysville Life Insurance Co.
Harleysville Insurance Companies
355 Maple Ave.
Harleysville, PA 19438-2297
Phone: (215)256-5000 **Fax:** (215)256-5457
Website: http://www.harleysvillelife.com
Wayne D. Butz, President
Walter R. Bateman, II, CEO & Chm Bd

★ 17120 ★ Harmony Health Plan of Illinois Inc.
Harmony Health Systems Inc.
125 S Wacker Dr., Ste. 2900
Chicago, IL 60606
Phone: (312)630-2025

★ 17121 ★ Harrison Life Insurance Co.
2510 14th St.
PO Box 4019
Gulfport, MS 39502
Phone: (770)763-1560
Charles A. Webb, Jr., President

★ 17122 ★ Hart Life Insurance Co.
Hartford Life, Inc.
PO Box 2999
Hartford, CT 06104-2999
Phone: (860)525-8555 **Fax:** (860)843-5568
Website: http://www.thehartford.com
Thomas M. Marra, President

★ 17123 ★ Hartford International Life Reassurance Corp.
Hartford Life, Inc.
PO Box 2999
Hartford, CT 06104-2999
Phone: (860)525-8555 **Fax:** (860)843-5568
Website: http://www.thehartford.com
Thomas M. Marra, President

★ 17124 ★ Hartford Life and Accident Insurance Co.
Hartford Life, Inc.
PO Box 2999
Hartford, CT 06104-2999
Phone: (860)525-8555 **Fax:** (860)843-5568
Website: http://www.thehartford.com
Thomas M. Marra, President

★ 17125 ★ Hartford Life & Annuity Insurance Co.
Hartford Life, Inc.
PO Box 2999
Hartford, CT 06104-2999
Phone: (860)525-8555 **Fax:** (860)843-5568
Website: http://www.thehartford.com
Thomas M. Marra, President

★ 17126 ★ Hartford Life Insurance Co.
Hartford Life, Inc.
PO Box 2999
Hartford, CT 06104-2999
Phone: (860)525-8555 **Fax:** (860)843-5568
Website: http://www.thehartford.com
Thomas M. Marra, President

★ 17127 ★ Harvard Pilgrim Health Care of New England Inc.
Harvard Pilgrim Health Care Group
93 Worcester St.
Wellesley, MA 02481-9181
Phone: (781)263-6000
Charles D. Baker, President

★ 17128 ★ Hawaii Management Alliance Association
737 Bishop St., Ste. 1200
Honolulu, HI 96813
Phone: (808)591-0088
Arnold M. Baptiste, Jr., President

★ 17129 ★ Hawaii Medical Service Association
PO Box 860
Honolulu, HI 96808
Phone: (808)948-5274
Robert P. Hiam, CEO & Pres

★ 17130 ★ Hawkeye Life Insurance Group Inc.
1111 Office Park Rd.
West Des Moines, IA 50265
Free: 800-323-4747

★ 17131 ★ Hawthorn Life Insurance Co.
PO Box 234
Carthage, TX 75633
Phone: (972)699-2700
Charlie Allison, President

★ 17132 ★ HCC Life Insurance Co.
HCC Insurance Group
13403 Northwest Fwy.
Houston, TX 77040-6094
Phone: (713)996-1200 **Fax:** (713)462-4210
Website: http://www.hcch.com
Benjamin D. Wilcox, CEO & Pres

★ 17133 ★ HCSC Insurance Services Co.
Health Care Service Corp.
300 E Randolph St.
Chicago, IL 60601-5099
Phone: (312)653-6361 **Fax:** (314)525-8519
Brian R. Van Vlierbergen, President

★ 17134 ★ Health Alliance Medical Plans
102 E Main St.
Urbana, IL 61801
Phone: (217)383-8203 **Free:** 800-851-3379
Fax: (217)337-8093
Website: http://www.healthalliance.org
Jeffrey C. Ingrum, President

★ 17135 ★ Health Alliance Plan of Michigan
Henry Ford Health System
2850 W Grand Blvd.
Detroit, MI 48202
Phone: (313)872-8100
Website: http://www.hapcorp.org

★ 17136 ★ Health Care Service Corp. A Mutual Legal Reserve Co.
300 E Randolph St.
Chicago, IL 60601-5099
Phone: (312)653-6000 **Fax:** (312)540-0544
Website: http://www.bcbsil.com
Raymond F. McCaskey, CEO & Pres

★ 17137 ★ Health First Health Plans
Health First Inc.
8247 Devereaux Dr., Ste. 103
Melbourne, FL 32940
Phone: (321)434-5600 **Fax:** (321)752-1129
Website: http://www.health-first.org
Jerry Senne, President

★ 17138 ★ Health Insurance Corp. of Alabama
2055 E South Blvd., Ste. 1000
PO Box 24430
Montgomery, AL 36124
Phone: (334)273-4217

★ 17139 ★ Health Insurance Exchange, A Mutual Co.
PO Box 16444
Jackson, MS 39236-6444
Phone: (601)368-3223
Sam W. Cameron, President

★ 17140 ★ Health Insurance Plan of Greater New York
HIP Group of Health Plans
7 W 34th St.
New York, NY 10001
Phone: (212)630-5000 **Fax:** (212)630-8210
Website: http://www.hipusa.com

★ 17141 ★ Health Net of Arizona Inc.
Health Net Inc.
21650 Oxnard St., 25th Fl.
Woodland Hills, CA 91367
Phone: (520)721-1122

★ 17142 ★ Health Net of California Inc.
Health Net Inc.
21650 Oxnard St., 25th Fl.
Woodland Hills, CA 91367
Phone: (818)676-6775
Christopher P. Wing, CEO & Pres

★ 17143 ★ Health Net of Connecticut Inc.
Health Net Inc.
1 Far Mill Crossing
PO Box 904
Shelton, CT 06484-0944
Phone: (203)402-4200
Website: http://www.health.net
George H. Rubin, MD, Chairman of the Board

★ 17144 ★ Health Net HMO Inc.
Health Net Management Inc.
44 Vantage Way, Ste. 300
Nashville, TN 37228-1513
Phone: (615)291-7000

★ 17145 ★ Health Net Insurance of Connecticut Inc.
Health Net Inc.
1 Far Mill Crossing
PO Box 904
Shelton, CT 06484-0944
Phone: (203)402-4200 **Fax:** (203)402-7073
Website: http://www.health.net
Barry W. Averill, President

★ 17146 ★ Health Net Insurance of New York Inc.
Health Net Inc.
1 Far Mill Crossing
PO Box 904
Shelton, CT 06484-0944
Phone: (203)402-4200
Website: http://www.health.net

★ 17147 ★ Health Net Life Insurance Co.
Health Net Inc.
21281 Burbank Blvd., Bldg. B3
Woodland Hills, CA 91367
Phone: (818)676-8256 **Fax:** (818)676-6521
Website: http://www.healthnet.com
Christopher P. Wing, CEO & Chm Bd

★ 17148 ★ Health Net of New Jersey Inc.
Health Net Inc.
1 Far Mill Crossing
PO Box 904
Shelton, CT 06484-0944
Phone: (203)402-4200
Website: http://www.health.net
Barry W. Averill, President

★ 17149 ★ Health Net of New York Inc.
Health Net Inc.
1 Far Mill Crossing
PO Box 904
Shelton, CT 06484-0944
Phone: (203)381-6400 **Fax:** (203)225-4038
Website: http://www.health.net
Anju Sikka, MD, Chairman of the Board

★ 17150 ★ Health Net of Pennsylvania Inc.
Health Net Inc.
21650 Oxnard St., 25th Fl.
Woodland Hills, CA 91367
Phone: (215)209-6300
Website: http://www.health.net
Joseph R. Singer, MD, President

★ 17151 ★ Health Net Plan of Oregon Inc.
Health Net Inc.
12901 SE 97th Ave.
PO Box 286
Clackamas, OR 97015-0286
Phone: (503)802-7000
Website: http://www.health.net
Stephen D. Lynch, President

★ 17152 ★ Health New England Inc.
1 Monarch Pl., Ste. 1500
Springfield, MA 01144
Phone: (413)787-4000
Website: http://www.hne.com
Peter F. Straley, President

★ 17153 ★ Health Options Inc.
Blue Cross & Blue Shield of Florida
4800 Deerwood Campus Pkwy., DCC 1-6
Jacksonville, FL 32246
Phone: (904)791-6111 **Fax:** (904)905-4177
Website: http://www.bcbsfl.com
Robert I. Lufrano, President

★ 17154 ★ Health Partners of Philadelphia Inc.
833 Chestnut St., Ste. 900
Philadelphia, PA 19107
Phone: (215)849-9606

★ 17155 ★ Health Plan of Nevada Inc.
2720 N Tenaya Way
PO Box 15645
Las Vegas, NV 89114-5645
Phone: (702)242-7703 **Fax:** (702)242-7937
Website: http://www.sierrahealth.com
Jonathon W. Bunker, President

★ 17156 ★ Health Plan of the Redwoods
3033 Cleveland Ave.
Santa Rosa, CA 95403
Phone: (707)544-2273

★ 17157 ★ Health Plan of San Diego
1550 W Fremont St., Ste. 200
Stockton, CA 95203-2643
Phone: (209)939-3500

★ 17158 ★ Health Plan of Texas
110 N College, Ste. 900
Tyler, TX 75702
Phone: (903)531-4447

★ 17159 ★ Health Plan of the Upper Ohio Valley Inc.
52160 National Rd.
Saint Clairsville, OH 43950
Phone: (740)695-3585

★ 17160 ★ Health Plus of Louisiana Inc.
Willis-Knighton Medical Center
2751 Albert L. Bicknell Dr., Ste. 2B
Shreveport, LA 71103
Phone: (318)632-8800

★ 17161 ★ Health Tradition Health Plan
PO Box 188
La Crosse, WI 54602-0188
Phone: (608)781-9692

★ 17162 ★ Health Ventures Network
Delta Dental Plan of Minnesota Group
3560 Delta Dental Dr.
Eagan, MN 55122-3166
Phone: (651)406-5900 **Fax:** (651)406-5900
Michael F. Walsh, President

★ 17163 ★ HealthCare Oklahoma Inc.
WellCor America Inc.
3050 Northwest Expy., Ste. 140
Oklahoma City, OK 73112
Phone: (405)951-4700
Al Walker, CEO & Pres

★ 17164 ★ HealthCare USA of Missouri LLC
Coventry Health Care Inc.
10 S Broadway, Ste. 1200
Saint Louis, MO 63102
Phone: (314)241-5300

★ 17165 ★ HealthGuard of Lancaster Inc.
Highmark Inc.
280 Granite Run Dr., Ste. 105
Lancaster, PA 17601-6810
Phone: (717)560-9049

★ 17166 ★ HealthGuard Services of Washington
322 N Commercial St., Ste. 300
Bellingham, WA 98225
Phone: (360)647-3849
Howard W. Kriz, President

★ 17167 ★ HealthKeepers Inc.
Trigon Healthcare Inc.
2220 Edward Holland Dr.
Richmond, VA 23230
Phone: (804)354-3479
Website: http://www.trigon.com
Thomas G. Snead, Jr., Chairman of the Board

★ 17168 ★ HealthLink HMO Inc.
WellPoint Health Networks Inc.
12443 Olive Blvd.
Saint Louis, MO 63141
Phone: (314)923-4831
David T. Ott, President

★ 17169 ★ HealthNet Inc.
Mid-America Health Partners
2 Pershing Sq.
Kansas City, MO 64108
Phone: (816)221-8400

★ 17170 ★ HealthNow NY Inc.
1901 Main St.
Buffalo, NY 14208
Phone: (716)887-6900
Thomas P. Hartnett, CEO & Pres

★ 17171 ★ HealthPartners Inc.
8100 34th Ave. S
Minneapolis, MN 55440
Phone: (952)883-6000 **Fax:** (952)883-6500
Website: http://www.healthpartners.com

★ 17172 ★ HealthPlan Southeast Inc.
Health Enterprises Inc.
3520 Thomasville Rd., Ste. 200
Tallahassee, FL 32308
Phone: (850)668-3000

★ 17173 ★ HealthPlus of Michigan Inc.
2050 S Linden Rd.
Flint, MI 48532
Free: 800-332-9161

★ 17174 ★ Healthy Alliance Life Insurance Co.
WellPoint Health Networks Inc.
1831 Chestnut St.
Saint Louis, MO 63103-2275
Phone: (314)923-4444
John A. O'Rourke, CEO & Chm Bd

★ 17175 ★ Heartland Health Plan of Oklahoma
100 N Broadway, Ste. 1400
Oklahoma City, OK 73102-8601
Phone: (405)239-2234

★ 17176 ★ Heritage Health Group Hospital Service Corp.
110 N College St., Ste. 900
Tyler, TX 75702
Phone: (903)531-4447
O. Edwin McClusky, MD, President

★ 17177 ★ Heritage Life Insurance Co.
GE Financial Assurance Group
500 Virginia Dr.
Fort Washington, PA 19034
Phone: (267)468-2000 **Fax:** (267)468-3401
Kathryn V. Marinello, President

★ 17178 ★ Heritage Provider Network Inc.
18107 Sherman Way, Ste. 100
Reseda, CA 91335
Phone: (818)654-3455

★ 17179 ★ Higginbotham Burial Insurance Co.
PO Box 686
Walnut Ridge, AR 72476
Phone: (870)932-8306
Mary Jo Higginbotham, President

★ 17180 ★ Highmark Inc.
Highmark Inc. Group
1800 Center St.
Camp Hill, PA 17011
Phone: (412)255-7000 **Fax:** (412)544-8112

Website: http://www.highmark.com
John S. Brouse, CEO & Pres

★ 17181 ★ Highmark Life Insurance Co.
Highmark Inc. Group
PO Box 535061
Pittsburgh, PA 15253-5061
Phone: (860)550-6000 **Fax:** (860)550-6885
Website: http://www.highmarklife.com
Dennis M. Kubit, President

★ 17182 ★ Highmark Life Insurance Co. of New York
Highmark Inc. Group
PO Box 535061
Pittsburgh, PA 15253-5061
Free: 800-235-6753 **Fax:** (212)921-0539
Website: http://www.highmarklife.com
Dennis M. Kubit, President

★ 17183 ★ HIP Insurance Co. of New York
HIP Group of Health Plans
7 W 34th St.
New York, NY 10010
Phone: (212)630-5000 **Fax:** (212)630-8290
Website: http://www.hipusa.com
Leslie Strassberg, President

★ 17184 ★ HMO Blue
Blue Cross and Blue Shield of Massachusetts Inc.
401 Park Dr.
Boston, MA 02215
Phone: (617)246-5000

★ 17185 ★ HMO Colorado Inc.
Anthem Inc.
120 Monument Cir.
Indianapolis, IN 46204
Phone: (303)831-2131
Website: http://www.anthem.com

★ 17186 ★ HMO Illinois
Health Care Service Corp.
300 E Randolph St.
Chicago, IL 60601
Phone: (312)653-6000 **Fax:** (312)540-0544
Website: http://www.bcbsil.com
Raymond F. McCaskey, President

★ 17187 ★ HMO Louisiana Inc.
Louisiana Health Services Group
5525 Reitz Ave.
Baton Rouge, LA 70809-3802
Phone: (225)295-3307

★ 17188 ★ HMO Maine
Anthem Inc.
120 Monument Cir.
Indianapolis, IN 46204
Phone: (207)822-7000
Website: http://www.anthem.com

★ 17189 ★ HMO Minnesota
Aware Integrated Inc.
3535 Blue Cross Rd.
Eagan, MN 55122
Phone: (651)662-1668 **Fax:** (651)662-2164
Website: http://www.bluecrossmn.com
George Émslie, Chairman of the Board

★ 17190 ★ HMO Missouri Inc.
WellPoint Health Networks Inc.
1831 Chestnut St.
Saint Louis, MO 63103
Phone: (314)923-4831
John A. O'Rourke, CEO & Chm Bd

★ 17191 ★ HMO New Mexico
Health Care Service Corp.
12800 Indian School Rd. NE
Albuquerque, NM 87112
Phone: (505)291-3500
Norman P. Becker, CEO & Pres

★ 17192 ★ HMO of Northeastern Pennsylvania
Blue Cross of NE Pennsylvania
19 N Main St.
Wilkes Barre, PA 18711
Free: 800-432-8015 **Fax:** (570)200-6866
Website: http://www.bcnepa.com

★ 17193 ★ HMO Partners Inc.
AR Blue Cross and Blue Shield and Baptist Health
26 Corporate Hill Dr.
Little Rock, AR 72205-4538
Phone: (501)221-1800
David F. Bridges, President

★ 17194 ★ Holy Family Society of the USA
PO Box 2909
Joliet, IL 60434
Phone: (815)725-5880 **Fax:** (815)725-0105
Robert M. Kochevar, President

★ 17195 ★ Home Owners Life Insurance Co.
Old Republic Insurance Group
307 N Michigan Ave.
Chicago, IL 60601
Phone: (312)346-8100
Aldo C. Zucaro, CEO & Chm Bd
Paul D. Adams, Senior VP

★ 17196 ★ Homeshield Insurance Co.
Homeshield Insurance Group
501 NW Grand Blvd., Ste. 365
PO Box 18223
Oklahoma City, OK 73154-0223
Phone: (405)236-2640 **Fax:** (405)767-7217
Gary R. Peterson, President

★ 17197 ★ Homesteaders Life Co.
PO Box 1756
Des Moines, IA 50306-1756
Phone: (515)288-7481 **Fax:** (515)246-9874
Website: http://www.homesteaderslife.com
Graham J. Cook, CEO & Chm Bd

★ 17198 ★ Hometown Health Plan
Health Group
100 Lillian Gish Blvd., Ste. 301
Massillon, OH 44647
Phone: (330)834-2200

★ 17199 ★ Hometown Health Plan
Washoe Health System Inc.
400 S Wells Ave.
Reno, NV 89502
Phone: (775)982-3000

★ 17200 ★ Hoosier Motor Mutual Insurance Co.
PO Box 88505
Indianapolis, IN 46208-0505
Phone: (317)923-1500 **Fax:** (317)925-4710
Terry R. Farias, CEO & Pres

★ 17201 ★ Horace Mann Life Insurance Co.
Horace Mann Group
1 Horace Mann Plz.
Springfield, IL 62715
Phone: (217)789-2500 **Fax:** (217)535-7117
Website: http://www.horacemann.com
Louis G. Lower, II, CEO & Pres

★ 17202 ★ Horizon Healthcare of New Jersey Inc.
Horizon Healthcare Services Inc.
3 Penn Plaza E
Newark, NJ 07105
Phone: (973)466-8600

★ 17203 ★ Hospital Service Association of Northeastern Pennsylvania
Blue Cross of NE Pennsylvania
19 N Main St.
Wilkes Barre, PA 18711
Free: 800-432-8015
Website: http://www.bcnepa.com
Denise S. Cesare, CEO & Pres

★ 17204 ★ Household Life Insurance Co.
Household Insurance Group
200 Somerset Corporate Blvd., Ste. 100
Bridgewater, NJ 08807
Free: 800-627-7282 **Fax:** (908)203-4229
Daniel R. O'Brien, CEO & Pres

★ 17205 ★ Household Life Insurance Co. of Arizona
Household Insurance Group
200 Somerset Corporate Blvd., Ste. 100
Bridgewater, NJ 08807
Free: 800-627-7282 **Fax:** (908)203-4229
Daniel R. O'Brien, President

★ 17206 ★ Household Life Insurance Co. of Delaware
Household Insurance Group
200 Somerset Corporate Blvd.
Bridgewater, NJ 08807
Free: 800-627-7282 **Fax:** (908)203-4229
Daniel R. O'Brien, CEO & Pres

★ 17207 ★ Houston National Life Insurance Co.
Fortis, Inc. Group
PO Box 3050
Milwaukee, WI 53201-3050
Phone: (414)271-3011 **Fax:** (414)224-0472
Website: http://www.fortishealth.com
Benjamin M. Cutler, II, CEO & Pres

★ 17208 ★ Humana Employers Health Plan of Georgia Inc.
Humana Inc.
500 W Main St.
PO Box 740036
Louisville, KY 40201-7436
Phone: (770)393-9226
Michael B. McCallister, President

★ 17209 ★ Humana Health Insurance Co. of Florida, Inc.
Humana Inc.
PO Box 740036
Louisville, KY 40201-7436
Phone: (904)296-7908 **Fax:** (502)580-4089
Website: http://www.humana.com
Michael B. McCallister, CEO & Pres

★ 17210 ★ Humana Health Plan Inc.
Humana Inc.
201 W Main St.
PO Box 740036
Louisville, KY 40201-7436
Phone: (502)580-8352
Website: http://www.humana.com
Michael B. McCallister, CEO & Pres

★ 17211 ★ Humana Health Plan of Ohio Inc.
Humana Inc.
PO Box 740036
Louisville, KY 40201-7436
Phone: (513)784-5320
Website: http://www.humana.com
Michael B. McCallister, CEO & Pres

★ 17212 ★ Humana Health Plan of Texas Inc.
Humana Inc.
PO Box 740036
Louisville, KY 40201-7436
Phone: (210)617-1708
Website: http://www.humana.com
Michael B. McCallister, CEO & Pres

★ 17213 ★ Humana Health Plans of Puerto Rico Inc.
Humana Inc.
500 W Main St.
Louisville, KY 40202
Phone: (787)282-7900 **Fax:** (787)282-6290
Website: http://www.humana.com
Victor S. Gutierrez, CEO & Pres

★ 17214 ★ Humana Insurance Co.
Humana Inc.
PO Box 740036
Louisville, KY 40201-7436
Phone: (920)336-1100 **Fax:** (920)336-2338
Website: http://www.humana.com
Michael B. McCallister, CEO & Pres

★ 17215 ★ Humana Insurance Co. of Kentucky
Humana Inc.
PO Box 740036
Louisville, KY 40201-7346
Phone: (502)580-1000
Website: http://www.humana.com
Michael B. McCallister, CEO & Pres

★ 17216 ★ Humana Insurance of Puerto Rico, Inc.
Humana Inc.
500 W Main St.
Louisville, KY 40202
Phone: (787)282-7900 **Fax:** (787)282-6290
Victor S. Gutierrez, MD, President

★ 17217 ★ Humana Medical Plan Inc.
Humana Inc.
500 W Main St.
PO Box 740036
Louisville, KY 40201-7436
Phone: (305)626-5616
Michael B. McCallister, CEO & Pres

★ 17218 ★ Humana Wisconsin Health Organization Insurance Corp.
Humana Inc.
500 W Main St.
PO Box 740036
Louisville, KY 40201-7436
Phone: (414)223-3300
Website: http://www.humana.com
Michael B. McCallister, CEO & Pres

★ 17219 ★ HumanaDental Insurance Co.
Humana Inc.
PO Box 740036
Louisville, KY 40201-7436
Phone: (502)580-1000
Gerald L. Ganoni, President

★ 17220 ★ IBA Health and Life Assurance Co.
PO Box 51100
Kalamazoo, MI 49005-1100
Phone: (616)341-7289
Terrance Allen Newmyer, President

★ 17221 ★ IBC Life Insurance Co.
PO Box 1359
Laredo, TX 78040
Phone: (956)722-7611
Dennis Nixon, President

★ 17222 ★ IdeaLife Insurance Co.
Berkshire Hathaway Group
695 E Main St.
Stamford, CT 06904-0300
Phone: (203)352-3000
Website: http://www.egr.com
Thomas M. West, CEO & Chm Bd

★ 17223 ★ IDS Life Insurance Co.
American Express Financial Corp.
227 AXP Financial Ctr.
Minneapolis, MN 55474
Phone: (612)671-3131 **Fax:** (612)671-7543
Website: http://www.americanexpress.com
Timothy V. Bechtold, President

★ 17224 ★ IDS Life Insurance Co. of New York
American Express Financial Corp.
227 AXP Financial Ctr.
Minneapolis, MN 55474
Phone: (518)869-8613 **Fax:** (518)869-8753
Website: http://www.americanexpress.com
Timothy V. Bechtold, President

★ 17225 ★ IHC Benefit Assurance Co., Inc.
IHC, Inc.
4646 Lake Park Blvd.
Salt Lake City, UT 84120-8212
Phone: (801)442-5000
Website: http://www.ihc.com/healthplans/
William H. Nelson, President

★ 17226 ★ IHC Health Plans Inc.
IHC Inc.
4646 Lake Park Blvd.
Salt Lake City, UT 84120-8212
Phone: (801)442-5000 **Fax:** (801)442-4331

★ 17227 ★ Illinois Annuity and Insurance Co.
AmerUs Group
PO Box 7149
Indianapolis, IN 46207-7149
Phone: (317)927-6500 **Fax:** (317)927-3511
Website: http://www.ilannuity.com
Garrett P. Ryan, President

★ 17228 ★ Illinois Mutual Life Insurance Co.
300 SW Adams St.
Peoria, IL 61634
Phone: (309)674-8255 **Fax:** (309)674-8637
Website: http://www.illinoismutual.com
Michael A. McCord, President
W. E. Palmatier, Senior VP

★ 17229 ★ Imperial Life Insurance Co.
PO Box 3375
Little Rock, AR 72202
Phone: (501)228-2700
Robert W. Howeth, President

★ 17230 ★ Independence Life & Annuity Co.
Sun Life Financial Group
1 Sun Life Executive Park
Wellesley Hills, MA 02481
Phone: (781)237-6030
Website: http://www.websaver.com
James A. McNulty, III, President

★ 17231 ★ Independent Health Association
511 Farber Lakes Dr.
Buffalo, NY 14221
Phone: (716)631-3001

★ 17232 ★ Independent Health Benefits Corp.
511 Farber Lakes Dr.
Buffalo, NY 14221
Phone: (716)631-3001
Frank Colantuono, Chairman of the Board

★ 17233 ★ Independent Order of Foresters
Independent Order of Foresters Group
789 Don Mills Rd.
Toronto, ON, Canada M3C 1T9
Phone: (416)429-3000 **Fax:** (416)467-2526
Website: http://www.foresters.biz
Michael J. White, CEO & Pres

★ 17234 ★ Independent State Life Insurance Co.
Columbia Insurance Group
PO Box 618
Columbia, MO 65205
Phone: (573)474-6193 **Fax:** (573)474-5865
Robert J. Wagner, President

★ 17235 ★ Indiana Vision Services Inc.
Vision Service Plan
3333 Quality Dr.
Rancho Cordova, CA 95670
Phone: (916)851-5000
Roger J. Valine, President

★ 17236 ★ Indianapolis Life Insurance Co.
AmerUs Group
PO Box 1230
Indianapolis, IN 46206-1230
Phone: (317)927-6500 **Fax:** (317)927-3393
Website: http://www.indianapolislife.com
Gary R. McPhail, CEO & Pres

★ 17237 ★ Individual Assurance Co., Life, Health & Accident
Individual Assurance Group
1600 Oak St.
Kansas City, MO 64108-1406
Phone: (816)842-8842 **Fax:** (816)218-1391
Michael M. Strickland, President
Robert E. Stroud, Chairman of the Board

★ 17238 ★ ING Insurance Co. of America
ING Group
5780 Powers Ferry Rd. NW
Atlanta, GA 30327
Phone: (860)273-0123
Thomas J. McInerney, President
Shaun P. Matthews, V Chm Bd

Frmly: Aetna Insurance Co. of America, Connecticut.

★ 17239 ★ ING Life Insurance and Annuity Co.
ING Group
151 Farmington Ave.
Hartford, CT 06156
Phone: (860)273-0123 **Fax:** (860)273-6348
Thomas J. McInerney, President

★ 17240 ★ Inland Empire Health Plan
303 E Vanderbilt Way, Ste. 400
San Bernardino, CA 92408
Phone: (909)890-2010 **Fax:** (909)890-2019
Website: http://www.iehp.org

★ 17241 ★ Inreco International Reinsurance Co.
Pan-American Life Group
PO Box 52201
New Orleans, LA 70152-2201
Phone: (504)566-1300 **Fax:** (504)566-3950
Jan S. Jobe, President
Frmly: International Reinsurance Co.

★ 17242 ★ Institutional Founders Life Insurance Co.
Sammons Financial Group
1 Midland Plaza
Sioux Falls, SD 57193-0001
Phone: (312)648-7600 **Fax:** (312)648-7787
Website: http://www.nacolah.com
Michael M. Masterson, CEO & Chm Bd

★ 17243 ★ Insurance Investors Life Insurance Co.
National Life Group
1300 W Mockingbird Ln.
Dallas, TX 75247-4921
Phone: (214)638-9206 **Fax:** (214)638-9140
Wade H. Mayo, President

★ 17244 ★ Integrity Life Insurance Co.
Western & Southern Financial Group
515 W Market St.
Louisville, KY 40202-3319
Phone: (502)582-7900 **Fax:** (502)582-7903
John R. Lindholm, President

★ 17245 ★ Inter-County Hospitalization Plan, Inc.
Independence Blue Cross Group
720 Blair Mill Rd.
Horsham, PA 19044-2244
Phone: (215)657-8900
George W. Gannon, President

★ 17246 ★ Inter-State Assurance Co.
Protective Life Corp.
2801 Hwy. 280 S
Birmingham, AL 35223
Phone: (205)879-9230
Website: http://www.iaclink.com
Jimmy E. Massengale, President

★ 17247 ★ Inter Valley Health Plan Inc.
300 S Park Ave.
PO Box 6002
Pomona, CA 91769
Phone: (909)623-6333

★ 17248 ★ International American Life Insurance Co.
PO Box 982005
Fort Worth, TX 76182-8005
Phone: (817)284-4888

★ 17249 ★ International Financial Services Life Insurance Co.
PO Box 681389
Franklin, TN 37068-1389
Phone: (615)790-0464 **Fax:** (615)790-9962
John A. Hackney, President

★ 17250 ★ Interstate Bankers Life Insurance Co.
Interstate Bankers Financial Corp.
8501 W Higgins Rd., Ste. 710
Chicago, IL 60631
Phone: (773)693-3930 **Fax:** (773)693-3278
John J. Chiaro, President

★ 17251 ★ Intramerica Life Insurance Co.
Allstate Financial Group
3100 Sanders Rd.
Northbrook, IL 60062
Phone: (847)402-5000
Website: http://www.allstate.com
Thomas J. Wilson, II, CEO & Pres

★ 17252 ★ Investors Consolidated Insurance Co.
Central United Group
Wortham Tower, 6th Fl.
2727 Allen Pkwy.
Houston, TX 77019-2115
Phone: (713)529-0045 **Fax:** (713)529-9425
Website: http://www.culins.com
David W. Harris, President

★ 17253 ★ Investors Growth Life Insurance Co.
PO Box 196
Stillwater, MN 55082-0196
Phone: (651)439-7098 **Fax:** (651)439-0200
Mark L. Desch, President

★ 17254 ★ Investors Guaranty Life Insurance Co.
Oxford Health Plans Inc.
48 Monroe Turnpike
Trumbull, CT 06611
Phone: (203)459-6000
Charles G. Berg, President

★ 17255 ★ Investors Heritage Life Insurance Co.
PO Box 717
Frankfort, KY 40602-0717
Phone: (502)223-2361 **Fax:** (502)875-7084
Website: http://www.investorsheritage.com
Harry Lee Waterfield, II, CEO & Chm Bd

★ 17256 ★ Investors Insurance Corp.
SCOR Life US Group
PO Box 56050
Jacksonville, FL 32241-6050
Phone: (904)260-6990 **Fax:** (904)268-0684
Website: http://www.scor.com
Romain Durand, President

★ 17257 ★ Investors Life Insurance Co. of Indiana
FIC Insurance Group
6500 River Place Blvd., Bldg. 1
Austin, TX 78730
Phone: (512)404-5000 **Fax:** (512)404-5051
Website: http://www.ficgroup.com
Roy F. Mitte, CEO & Chm Bd

★ 17258 ★ Investors Life Insurance Co. of North America
FIC Insurance Group
6500 River Place Blvd., Bldg. 1
Austin, TX 78730-1113
Phone: (512)404-5000 **Fax:** (512)404-5051
Website: http://www.ficgroup.com
Roy F. Mitte, CEO & Chm Bd

★ 17259 ★ Investors Partner Life Insurance Co.
John Hancock Financial Services Group
PO Box 717
Boston, MA 02117-0717
Phone: (617)572-6000 **Fax:** (617)572-6698
Website: http://www.jhancock.com
Michele G. Van Leer, President

★ 17260 ★ Island Care
Queen's Health Management Corp.
500 Ala Moana Blvd., Ste. 2-200
Honolulu, HI 96813
Phone: (808)532-7500

★ 17261 ★ IU Health Plan Inc.
3901 W 86th St., Ste. 230
Indianapolis, IN 46268
Phone: (317)871-8812 **Fax:** (317)871-8833
Website: http://www.iuhp.com

★ 17262 ★ J. C. Penney Life Insurance Co.
AEGON USA, Inc.
2700 W Plano Pkwy., No. 3C
Plano, TX 75075-8200
Phone: (972)881-6000 **Fax:** (972)881-6976
Marilyn Carp, President

★ 17263 ★ Jackson Griffin Insurance Co.
PO Box 577
Newport, AR 72112-0577
Phone: (870)523-5822
Jan Maris, President

★ 17264 ★ Jackson National Life Insurance Co.
Jackson National Group
1 Corporate Way
Lansing, MI 48951
Phone: (517)381-5500 **Fax:** (517)706-5524
Website: http://www.jnl.com
Clark P. Manning, CEO & Chm Bd

★ 17265 ★ Jackson National Life Insurance Co. of New York
Jackson National Group
1 Corporate Way
Lansing, MI 48951
Phone: (517)381-5500
Website: http://www.jnl.com
Clark P. Manning, CEO & Chm Bd

★ 17266 ★ Jacksonville Life Insurance Co.
PO Box 951
Jacksonville, TX 75766
Phone: (770)763-1560
Jeff Austin, Jr., President

★ 17267 ★ Jamestown Life Insurance Co.
GE Financial Assurance Group
6604 W Broad St.
Richmond, VA 23230
Phone: (804)845-0911 **Free:** 888-325-5433
Website: http://www.gefinancialassurance.com
Frank T. Gencarelli, President

★ 17268 ★ Jeff Davis Mortuary Benefit Association
PO Box 782
Jennings, LA 70546
Phone: (337)824-2395
Dorothy M. Bryan, President

★ 17269 ★ Jefferson Life Insurance Co.
Dallas General Group
PO Box 749008
Dallas, TX 75201
Phone: (214)808-0808 **Fax:** (214)340-6114
Richard C. Murphy, President

★ 17270 ★ Jefferson Pilot Financial Insurance Co.
Jefferson-Pilot Corp.
100 N Greene St.
Greensboro, NC 27401
Phone: (603)226-5000
Website: http://www.jpfinancial.com
Kenneth C. Mlekush, President

★ 17271 ★ Jefferson-Pilot Life Insurance Co.
Jefferson-Pilot Corp.
PO Box 21008
Greensboro, NC 27420
Phone: (336)691-3000 **Fax:** (336)691-3938
Website: http://www.jpfinancial.com
Kenneth C. Mlekush, President

★ 17272 ★ Jefferson Pilot LifeAmerica Insurance Co.
Jefferson-Pilot Corp.
100 N Greene St.
Greensboro, NC 27401
Phone: (603)226-5000
Website: http://www.jpfinancial.com
Kenneth C. Mlekush, President

★ 17273 ★ Jefferson Standard Life Insurance Co.
Jefferson-Pilot Corp.
PO Box 21008
Greensboro, NC 27420
Phone: (336)691-3000 **Fax:** (336)691-3258
Kenneth C. Mlekush, President

★ 17274 ★ JMIC Life Insurance Co.
JMIC Life Group
500 NW 12th Ave.
Deerfield Beach, FL 33442
Phone: (954)429-2150 **Fax:** (954)429-2660
Website: http://www.jmfamily.com
Lou R. Feagles, President

★ 17275 ★ John Alden Life Insurance Co.
Fortis, Inc. Group
PO Box 3050
Milwaukee, WI 53201-3050
Phone: (414)271-3011 **Fax:** (414)224-0472
Website: http://www.fortishealth.com
Benjamin M. Cutler, II, CEO & Pres
David McDonough, Exec VP

★ 17276 ★ John Deere Health Plan Inc.
John Deere Health Care Inc.
1300 River Dr.
Moline, IL 61265
Phone: (309)765-1200

★ 17277 ★ John Hancock Life Insurance Co.
John Hancock Financial Services Group
PO Box 111
Boston, MA 02117-0111
Phone: (617)572-6000
Website: http://www.jhancock.com
David D'Alessandro, CEO & Chm Bd

★ 17278 ★ John Hancock Variable Life Insurance Co.
John Hancock Financial Services Group
PO Box 717
Boston, MA 02117-0717
Phone: (617)572-6000 **Fax:** (617)572-6698
Website: http://www.jhancock.com
Michele G. Van Leer, President

★ 17279 ★ Jordan Funeral and Insurance Co., Inc.
PO Box 610
Centre, AL 35960
Phone: (256)927-5870

★ 17280 ★ Kaiser Foundation Health Plan of Colorado
Kaiser Foundation Group of Health Plans
10350 E Dakota Ave.
Denver, CO 80231-1314
Phone: (303)344-7287

★ 17281 ★ Kaiser Foundation Health Plan of Georgia Inc.
Kaiser Foundation Group of Health Plans
3495 Piedmont Rd. NE, Bldg. 9
Atlanta, GA 30305-1736
Phone: (404)364-7000

★ 17282 ★ Kaiser Foundation Health Plan Inc.
Kaiser Foundation Group of Health Plans
1 Kaiser Plaza
Ordway Blvd.
Oakland, CA 94612
Phone: (510)271-5910

★ 17283 ★ Kaiser Foundation Health Plan of Kansas City Inc.
Kaiser Foundation Group of Health Plans
10561 Barkley, Ste. 500
Overland Park, KS 66212
Phone: (913)967-4600

★ 17284 ★ Kaiser Foundation Health Plan of the Mid-Atlantic States Inc.
Kaiser Foundation Group of Health Plans
2101 E Jefferson St.
Rockville, MD 20852
Phone: (301)816-6683

★ 17285 ★ Kaiser Foundation Health Plan of the Northwest
Kaiser Foundation Group of Health Plans
500 NE Multnomah St., Ste. 100
Portland, OR 97232-2099
Phone: (503)813-2800

★ 17286 ★ Kaiser Foundation Health Plan of Ohio
Kaiser Foundation Group of Health Plans
1 Kaiser Plaza
Ordway Blvd.
Oakland, CA 94612
Phone: (510)271-5910

★ 17287 ★ Kaiser Permanente Health Alternatives
Kaiser Foundation Group of Health Plans
500 NE Multnomah St.
Portland, OR 97232-2099
Phone: (503)813-2502
Barbara A. West, President

★ 17288 ★ Kaiser Permanente Insurance Co.
1 Kaiser Plaza, Ste. 25-B
Oakland, CA 94612
Phone: (510)271-2343
John A. Price, President

★ 17289 ★ Kanawha Insurance Co.
PO Box 610
Lancaster, SC 29721-0610
Phone: (803)283-5300 **Fax:** (803)283-5313
Website: http://www.kanawha.com
Stanley D. Johnson, CEO & Chm Bd

★ 17290 ★ Kansas City Life Insurance Co.
Kansas City Life Group
PO Box 219139
Kansas City, MO 64121-9139
Phone: (816)753-7000 **Fax:** (816)753-4902
Website: http://www.kclife.com
R. Philip Bixby, CEO & Pres

★ 17291 ★ Kapi'olani Health Hawaii
55 Merchant St., 26th Fl.
Honolulu, HI 96813
Phone: (808)535-7234

★ 17292 ★ Kemper Investors Life Insurance Co.
Zurich Insurance Group
1600 McConnor Pkwy.
Schaumburg, IL 60196
Phone: (847)550-5500 **Fax:** (847)874-5643
Website: http://www.zurichlifeus.com
Gale K. Caruso, CEO & Pres

★ 17293 ★ Kentucky Funeral Directors Life Insurance Co.
Funeral Directors Group
108 St. James Ct., Ste. 101
Frankfort, KY 40601-8486
Phone: (502)226-4921 **Fax:** (502)226-4922
Website: http://www.kfdlic.com
Billy K. Seale, President

★ 17294 ★ Kentucky Home Life Insurance Co.
NGL Insurance Group
PO Box 1191
Madison, WI 53701-1191
Phone: (608)257-5611 **Fax:** (608)257-4308
Website: http://www.nationalguardian.com/khl.html
J. D. Larson, President

★ 17295 ★ Keyport Benefit Life Insurance Co.
Sun Life Financial Group
1 Sun Life Executive Park
Wellesley Hills, MA 02481
Phone: (781)237-6030 **Free:** 800-367-3653
James A. McNulty, III, President

★ 17296 ★ Keyport Life Insurance Co.
Sun Life Financial Group
1 Sun Life Executive Park
Wellesley Hills, MA 02481
Phone: (781)237-6030

Website: http://www.keyport.com
James A. McNulty, III, President

★ 17297 ★ Keystone Health Plan Central Inc.
Highmark Inc./Capital Blue Cross
300 Corporate Ctr. Dr.
Camp Hill, PA 17011
Phone: (717)763-3458

★ 17298 ★ Keystone Health Plan East Inc.
Independence Blue Cross
1901 Market St.
Philadelphia, PA 19101
Phone: (215)241-2001

★ 17299 ★ Keystone Health Plan West Inc.
Highmark Inc.
120 5th Ave., 5th Ave. Pl.
Pittsburgh, PA 15222
Phone: (412)544-8852 **Fax:** (412)544-8112
Website: http://www.highmark.com
James M. Klingensmith, Chairman of the Board

★ 17300 ★ Keystone State Life Insurance Co.
Allstate Financial Group
3100 Sanders Rd.
Northbrook, IL 60062
Phone: (847)402-5000 **Fax:** (215)591-0453
Website: http://www.allstate.com
Thomas J. Wilson, II, CEO & Chm Bd

★ 17301 ★ Kilpatrick Life Insurance Co. of Louisiana
PO Box 88
Shreveport, LA 71161
Phone: (318)222-0555
Virginia K. Shehee, President

★ 17302 ★ Knights of Columbus
PO Box 1670
New Haven, CT 06507-0901
Phone: (203)772-2130 **Fax:** (203)865-2310
Website: http://www.kofc.org
Carl A. Anderson, President

★ 17303 ★ KPS Health Plans
PO Box 339
Bremerton, WA 98337
Phone: (360)377-5576
Elizabeth A. Gilje, President

★ 17304 ★ Lafayette Life Insurance Co.
PO Box 7007
Lafayette, IN 47903-7007
Phone: (765)477-7411 **Fax:** (765)477-3321
Website: http://www.llic.com
Robert J. Gibbons, CEO & Chm Bd
Thomas K. Gross, Exec VP

★ 17305 ★ LaFourche Life Insurance Co.
PO Box 246
Raceland, LA 70394
Phone: (504)537-7537
Charles J. D. Gerrets, President

★ 17306 ★ Landcar Life Insurance Co.
9350 South 150 East, Ste. 1000
Sandy, UT 84070
Phone: (801)563-4153
Karen G. Miller, President

★ 17307 ★ Landmark Life Insurance Co.
PO Box 40
Brownwood, TX 76804-0040
Phone: (915)646-6579 **Fax:** (915)646-3688
Website: http://www.landmarklife.com
Thomas A. Munson, President

★ 17308 ★ Laurel Life Insurance Co.
Vesta Insurance Group
PO Box 52121
Phoenix, AZ 85072-2121
Phone: (602)957-0778 **Fax:** (602)224-6884
Wayne A. Schreck, President
Kenneth W. Phillips, Chairman of the Board

★ 17309 ★ Leaders Life Insurance Co.
PO Box 35768
Tulsa, OK 74153
Phone: (918)254-0200 **Fax:** (918)252-1441
Website: http://www.leaderslife.com
Burt B. Holmes, President

★ 17310 ★ Leafre Reinsurance Co.
224 W 35th St., 11th Fl.
New York, NY 10001-2507
Phone: (212)967-8600
Robert J. Leaf, President

★ 17311 ★ Lewer Life Insurance Co.
PO Box 32395
Kansas City, MO 64171-5395
Phone: (816)753-4390 **Fax:** (816)561-6840
Website: http://www.lewer.com
D. C. Lewer, CEO & Chm Bd

★ 17312 ★ Lewis Life Insurance Co.
512 E Bowie
Marshall, TX 75670
Phone: (903)935-5556
J. W. Reeves, President

★ 17313 ★ Liberty Bankers Life Insurance Co.
NCMIC Life Insurance Group
1452 29th St., Ste. 102
West Des Moines, IA 50266
Phone: (414)540-0628 **Free:** 800-745-4927
Fax: (414)540-0752
Patrick E. McNerney, President

★ 17314 ★ Liberty Life Assurance Co. of Boston
Liberty Mutual Insurance Cos.
100 Liberty Way
Dover, NH 03820-1525
Phone: (617)357-9500 **Fax:** (617)482-4761
Edmund F. Kelly, CEO & Chm Bd

★ 17315 ★ Liberty Life Insurance Co.
RBC Insurance Group
PO Box 789
Greenville, SC 29602-0789
Phone: (864)609-8111 **Fax:** (864)609-4768
Website: http://www.libertylife.com
Robert E. Evans, President
H. Neel Hipp, Chairman of the Board

★ 17316 ★ Liberty National Life Insurance Co.
Torchmark Corp.
PO Box 2612
Birmingham, AL 35202
Phone: (205)325-2722 **Fax:** (205)325-2502
Website: http://www.libnat.com
Anthony L. McWhorter, CEO & Pres
Vurl Duce, Exec VP

★ 17317 ★ Liberty Union Life Assurance Co.
30775 Barrington Ave.
Madison Heights, MI 48071
Phone: (248)583-7123 **Fax:** (248)583-4647
Christopher T. Mazur, President

★ 17318 ★ Life of America Insurance Co.
Life of America Group
8200 Brookriver Dr., Ste. 600N
Dallas, TX 75247-4069
Phone: (214)631-6310 **Fax:** (214)688-7475
Joseph S. Meziere, President

★ 17319 ★ Life Assurance Co. of America
2215 York Rd., Ste. 106
Oak Brook, IL 60523
Phone: (630)571-2100
Anthony C. Borcich, President

★ 17320 ★ Life Assurance Co. Inc.
PO Box 20667
Oklahoma City, OK 73156
Phone: (405)810-1111 **Fax:** (405)810-1122
Website: http://www.lacinc.com
Denny S. Baze, President

★ 17321 ★ Life and Health Insurance Co. of America
Life & Health Group
220 W Germantown Pike
Plymouth Meeting, PA 19462
Phone: (610)940-1477 **Fax:** (610)940-1478
Melvyn K. Miller, President

★ 17322 ★ Life Insurance Co. of Alabama
PO Box 349
Gadsden, AL 35901
Phone: (256)543-2022 **Fax:** (256)549-0070
Website: http://www.licoa.com
Clarence W. Daugette, III, President
Florence T. Daugette, Chairman of the Board

★ 17323 ★ Life Insurance Co. of Boston and New York
Boston Mutual Group
21 E 40th St., 3rd Fl.
New York, NY 10016-0501
Phone: (212)684-2000 **Fax:** (212)231-6080
Website: http://lifeofboston.com
Paul E. Petry, President

★ 17324 ★ Life Insurance Co. of Georgia
ING Group
5780 Powers Ferry Rd. NW
Atlanta, GA 30327
Phone: (770)980-5100 **Fax:** (770)980-5800
James D. Thompson, President
Stephen M. Christopher, Chairman of the Board

★ 17325 ★ Life Insurance Co. of Louisiana
PO Box 1803
Shreveport, LA 71166
Phone: (318)221-0646 **Fax:** (318)429-0599
George D. Nelson, President

★ 17326 ★ Life Insurance Co. of Mississippi
Fortis, Inc. Group
715 S Pear Orchard Rd., Ste. 400
Ridgeland, MS 39157
Phone: (601)978-6732 **Fax:** (601)978-6756
Website: http://www.msdiversified.com
Charles H. Shamburger, III, President

★ 17327 ★ Life Insurance Co. of North America
CIGNA Corp.
900 Cottage Grove Rd., S-330
Bloomfield, CT 06002
Phone: (215)761-1000 **Fax:** (215)761-5606
Website: http://www.cigna.com
Michael W. Bell, President

★ 17328 ★ Life Insurance Co. of the Southwest
National Life Group
PO Box 569080
Dallas, TX 75356-9080
Phone: (214)638-7100 **Fax:** (214)638-9140
Wade H. Mayo, CEO & Pres
Carl J. Lutz, Senior VP

★ 17329 ★ Life Investors Insurance Co. of America
AEGON USA, Inc.
4333 Edgewood Rd. NE
Cedar Rapids, IA 52499
Phone: (319)398-8511 **Fax:** (319)398-2218
Rex B. Eno, Chairman of the Board

★ 17330 ★ Life of Maryland, Inc.
Baltimore Life Group
10075 Red Run Blvd.
Owings Mills, MD 21117-6050
Phone: (410)581-6600 **Fax:** (410)581-6612
Website: http://www.baltlife.com
L. John Pearson, CEO & Chm Bd

★ 17331 ★ Life Protection Insurance Co.
Titus Group
2817 Maple Ave.
Dallas, TX 75201
Phone: (214)871-0332 **Fax:** (214)871-0334
Gary A. Dobbie, President

★ 17332 ★ Life of the South Insurance Co.
Life of the South Group
100 W Bay St.
Jacksonville, FL 32202
Phone: (912)350-9660 **Fax:** (912)354-4525
Website: http://www.life-south.com
Loyd L. Shaw, President

★ 17333 ★ Lifecare Assurance Co.
PO Box 4243
Woodland Hills, CA 91365-4243
Phone: (818)867-2226 **Fax:** (818)887-4595
Website: http://www.lifecareassurance.com
James M. Glickman, CEO & Pres

★ 17334 ★ Lifeguard Inc.
Lifeguard Inc. Group
2840 Junction Ave.
PO Box 5506
San Jose, CA 95150
Phone: (408)432-3699 **Fax:** (408)383-4209
Website: http://www.lifeguard.com
Mark G. Hyde, President

★ 17335 ★ Lifeguard Life Insurance Co.
Lifeguard Inc. Group
2840 Junction Ave.
San Jose, CA 95134
Phone: (408)432-3699 **Fax:** (408)383-4209
Website: http://www.lifeguard.com
Mark G. Hyde, President

★ 17336 ★ Lifeline Underwriters Life Insurance Co.
Citizens Inc. Group
400 E Anderson Ln.
PO Box 149151
Austin, TX 78714-9151
Phone: (512)837-7100 **Fax:** (512)836-9785
Gary C. Cole, President

★ 17337 ★ LifeRe Insurance Co.
PO Box 792070
San Antonio, TX 78279-2070
Phone: (210)357-1000 **Fax:** (210)357-1020
Website: http://www.lifere.net
James C. Black, Jr., President

★ 17338 ★ LifeUSA Insurance Co.
Allianz Insurance Group
5701 Golden Hills Dr.
PO Box 1344
Minneapolis, MN 55440-1344
Phone: (763)765-6500 **Fax:** (763)765-6657
Website: http://www.allianzlife.com
Robert W. MacDonald, Chairman of the Board
Charles M. Kavitsky, President

★ 17339 ★ Lifewise, A Premera Health Plan, Inc.
Premera Group
7001 220th St. SW, Bldg. 2
Mountlake Terrace, WA 98043-2124
Phone: (503)295-6707 **Fax:** (503)295-1943
Mark Charpentier, CEO & Pres

★ 17340 ★ Lincoln Benefit Life Co.
Allstate Financial Group
2940 S 84th St.
Lincoln, NE 68506-4142
Free: 800-525-9287 **Fax:** (402)479-7393
Website: http://www.allstate.com
B. Eugene Wraith, President

★ 17341 ★ Lincoln Direct Life Insurance Co.
Lincoln Insurance Group
PO Box 82448
Lincoln, NE 68501-2448
Phone: (402)423-7191 **Fax:** (402)423-7197
Website: http://www.lincolndirectlife.com
Thomas D. Potter, CEO & Chm Bd

★ 17342 ★ Lincoln Heritage Life Insurance Co.
4343 E Camelback Rd.
Phoenix, AZ 85018
Phone: (602)957-1650 **Fax:** (602)840-9765
Website: http://www.lhlic.com
Thomas A. Londen, President

★ 17343 ★ Lincoln Life & Annuity Co. of New York
Lincoln National Corp.
100 Madison St., Ste. 1860
Syracuse, NY 13202-2802
Phone: (315)428-8400 **Fax:** (315)428-8419
Website: http://www.lincolnlife-ny.com
Lorry J. Stensrud, President

★ 17344 ★ Lincoln Memorial Life Insurance Co.
PO Box 160050
Austin, TX 78716-0050
Phone: (512)328-0075 **Free:** 800-283-8840
Randall K. Sutton, President

★ 17345 ★ Lincoln Mutual Life and Casualty Insurance Co.
PO Box 1918
Fargo, ND 58107-1918
Phone: (701)282-1807 **Fax:** (701)282-1840
Website: http://www.lml.com
John S. Koltes, President
Michael B. Unhjem, Chairman of the Board

★ 17346 ★ The Lincoln National Life Insurance Co.
Lincoln National Corp.
1300 S Clinton St.
Fort Wayne, IN 46802
Phone: (260)455-2000 **Fax:** (260)455-4140
Website: http://www.lfg.com
Jon A. Boscia, President

★ 17347 ★ Lincoln National Reassurance Co.
Swiss Reinsurance Group
1700 Magnavox Way
Fort Wayne, IN 46804
Phone: (260)455-2000 **Fax:** (260)455-4120
Website: http://www.lnrc.com
Lawrence T. Rowland, President

★ 17348 ★ Locomotive Engineers and Conductors Mutual Protection Association
535 Griswold, Ste. 1210
Detroit, MI 48226-3689
Free: 800-514-0010

★ 17349 ★ London Life Reinsurance Co.
Great-West Life Group
PO Box 1120
Blue Bell, PA 19422-0319
Phone: (215)542-7200 **Fax:** (215)542-1295
Monica M. Hainer, CEO & Pres

★ 17350 ★ London Pacific Life & Annuity Co.
3101 Poplarwood Ct.
Raleigh, NC 27604
Phone: (919)790-2243 **Free:** 800-827-5177
Fax: (919)981-2797
Website: http://www.londonpacific.com
George C. Nicholson, President

★ 17351 ★ Louisiana Health Service & Indemnity Co.
Louisiana Health Services Group
PO Box 98029
Baton Rouge, LA 70898-9029
Phone: (504)295-3307
Kathryn M. Sullivan, President

★ 17352 ★ Lovelace Health Systems
CIGNA Corp.
900 Cottage Grove Rd.
Bloomfield, CT 06002
Phone: (505)262-7075
Website: http://www.cigna.com
Mark T. Bertolini, President

★ 17353 ★ Loyal American Life Insurance Co.
American Financial Group
PO Box 5418
Cincinnati, OH 45201-5418
Phone: (513)412-2200 **Free:** 800-633-6752
Fax: (513)412-2817
Website: http://www.gafri.com
Charles R. Scheper, CEO & Pres
Robert A. Adams, Chairman of the Board

★ 17354 ★ Loyal Christian Benefit Association
PO Box 13005
Erie, PA 16514-1305
Phone: (814)453-4331 **Fax:** (814)453-3211
Website: http://www.lcba.com
Jacqueline J. Sobania-Robison, President

★ 17355 ★ Lutheran Brotherhood
Thrivent Financial for Lutherans Group
625 4th Ave. S
Minneapolis, MN 55415
Phone: (612)340-7000 **Fax:** (612)340-7373
Website: http://www.thrivent.com
Robert P. Gandrud, Chairman of the Board
Bruce J. Nicholson, President

★ 17356 ★ Lutheran Brotherhood Variable Insurance Products Co.
Thrivent Financial for Lutherans Group
625 4th Ave. S
Minneapolis, MN 55415
Phone: (612)340-7000 **Fax:** (612)340-7373
Website: http://www.thrivent.com
Bruce J. Nicholson, CEO & Chm Bd

★ 17357 ★ Lyndon Life Insurance Co.
XL Capital Group
20 N Martindale Rd., Ste. 200
Schaumburg, IL 60173
Phone: (847)517-2990
James E. Hohmann, President

★ 17358 ★ M-Care Inc.
University of Michigan
2301 Commonwealth Blvd.
Ann Arbor, MI 48105
Phone: (734)747-8700 **Fax:** (734)747-7152
Website: http://www.mcare.org

★ 17359 ★ M. D. Individual Practice Association Inc.
Mid Atlantic Medical Services Inc.
4 Taft Ct.
Rockville, MD 20850
Phone: (301)762-8205

★ 17360 ★ M Life Insurance Co.
1290 Broadway
Denver, CO 80203
Phone: (503)232-6960
Fred H. Jonske, President

★ 17361 ★ M-Plan Inc.
Clarian Health Partners Inc.
8802 N Meridian St., Ste. 100
Indianapolis, IN 46260
Phone: (317)571-5300

★ 17362 ★ Madison National Life Insurance Co. Inc.
Independence Holding Group
PO Box 5008
Madison, WI 53705-0008
Phone: (608)238-2691 **Fax:** (608)238-7028
Website: http://www.madisonlife.com
Larry R. Graber, President

★ 17363 ★ Magna Insurance Co.
PO Box 19685
New Orleans, LA 70179-0685
Phone: (504)456-0101 **Fax:** (504)456-7324
Alan W. Kennebeck, Chairman of the Board

★ 17364 ★ Maine Dental Service Corp.
1 Delta Dr.
Concord, NH 03302-2002
Phone: (603)233-1000
Thomas Raffio, President

★ 17365 ★ Maine Partners Health Plan Inc.
Anthem Inc.
2 Gannett Dr.
South Portland, ME 04106
Phone: (207)822-7000
Roger T. Pezzuti, MD, Chairman of the Board

★ 17366 ★ Majestic Life Insurance Co.
1125 N Clairborne Ave.
New Orleans, LA 70116
Phone: (504)525-0375
Cecilia H. Robert, President

★ 17367 ★ MAMSI Life and Health Insurance Co.
Mid Atlantic Medical Services Inc. Group
4 Taft Ct.
Rockville, MD 20850
Phone: (301)762-8205 **Fax:** (301)762-0658
Thomas P. Barbera, CEO & Pres
Mark D. Groban, Chairman of the Board

★ 17368 ★ Managed Health Services Insurance Corp.
Centene Corp.
7711 Carondelet Ave., Ste. 600
Saint Louis, MO 63105
Phone: (314)725-4706

★ 17369 ★ Manhattan Life Insurance Co.
Central United Group
2727 Allen Pkwy., Ste. 500
Houston, TX 77019-2115
Phone: (212)582-2819 **Fax:** (860)298-9538
Daniel J. George, President

★ 17370 ★ Manhattan National Life Insurance Co.
Conseco Insurance Group
11815 N Pennsylvania St.
Carmel, IN 46032
Phone: (317)817-4600 **Fax:** (317)817-2161
Website: http://www.conseco.com
Elizabeth C. Georgakopoulos, President

★ 17371 ★ The Manufacturers Life Insurance Co.
Manulife Financial Group
200 Bloor St. E
Toronto, ON, Canada M4W 1E5
Phone: (416)926-3000 **Fax:** (416)926-5454
Website: http://www.manulife.com
Dominic F. D'Alessandro, CEO & Pres

★ 17372 ★ The Manufacturers Life Insurance Co. of America
Manulife Financial Group
200 Bloor St. E
Toronto, ON, Canada M4W 1E5
Phone: (416)926-0100 **Fax:** (416)926-5699
Website: http://www.manulife.com
Donald A. Guloien, President

★ 17373 ★ The Manufacturers Life Insurance Co. of New York
Manulife Financial Group
100 Summit Lake Dr., 2nd Fl.
Valhalla, NY 10595
Phone: (914)773-0708 **Fax:** (914)773-0709
Website: http://www.manulife.com
John D. Gallagher, President

★ 17374 ★ The Manufacturers Life Insurance Co. of North America
Manulife Financial Group
500 Boylston St., Ste. 400
Boston, MA 02116-3739
Phone: (416)926-0100 **Fax:** (416)926-6150
Website: http://www.manulife.com
James R. Boyle, President

★ 17375 ★ The Manufacturers Life Insurance Co. (USA)
Manulife Financial Group
200 Bloor St. E
Toronto, ON, Canada M4W 1E5
Phone: (617)854-4300 **Free:** 800-827-8603
Website: http://www.manulife.com
John DesPrez, III, President

★ 17376 ★ Manulife Reinsurance Corp. (USA)
Manulife Financial Group
38500 Woodward Ave.
Bloomfield Hills, MI 48304
Phone: (416)926-0100 **Fax:** (416)926-5454
Website: http://www.manulife.com
Steven Mannik, President

★ 17377 ★ Marquette Indemnity and Life Insurance Co.
1000 Des Peres Rd., Ste. 350
Saint Louis, MO 63131
Phone: (314)909-9100 **Fax:** (314)909-9157
Thomas J. Conley, President

★ 17378 ★ Marquette National Life Insurance Co.
Universal American Financial Corp.
600 Courtland St.
Orlando, FL 32804
Phone: (407)628-1776 **Fax:** (407)628-4227
Gary W. Bryant, CEO & Pres

★ 17379 ★ Massachusetts Mutual Life Insurance Co.
MassMutual Financial Group
1295 State St.
Springfield, MA 01111
Phone: (413)788-8411
Website: http://www.massmutual.com
Robert J. O'Connell, CEO & Chm Bd

★ 17380 ★ Massachusetts Vision Service Plan
Vision Service Plan
3333 Quality Dr.
Rancho Cordova, CA 95670
Phone: (916)851-5000 **Fax:** (916)858-5388
Roger J. Valine, President

★ 17381 ★ Matthew Thornton Health Plan
Anthem Inc.
120 Monument Cir.
Indianapolis, IN 46204
Phone: (603)695-7000
Website: http://www.anthem.com
Larry C. Glasscock, Chairman of the Board

★ 17382 ★ Maxicare Life and Health Insurance Co.
Maxicare Health Plans, Inc.
1149 S Broadway St., Ste. 910
Los Angeles, CA 90015
Phone: (213)765-2000 **Fax:** (213)765-2684
Website: http://www.maxicare.com
Susan M. Blais, President

★ 17383 ★ Mayflower National Life Insurance Co.
Alderwoods Group Inc.
1055 St. Charles Ave., Ste. 600
New Orleans, LA 70130
Phone: (504)561-7700 **Fax:** (504)561-7740
Website: http://www.mayflowernational.com
Aaron P. Shipper, CEO & Chm Bd

★ 17384 ★ Mayo Health Plan Inc.
4168 Southpoint Pkwy., Ste. 102
Jacksonville, FL 32216
Phone: (904)279-2646

★ 17385 ★ McDonald Life Insurance Co.
PO Box 702567
Dallas, TX 75370
Phone: (512)479-9901
Fredrick E. McDonald, III, President

★ 17386 ★ McKinley Life Insurance Co.
Aultman Health Foundation
2600 6th St. SW
Canton, OH 44710
Phone: (330)438-6360 **Fax:** (330)438-2911
Rick L. Haines, President

★ 17387 ★ MCS Health Management Options Inc.
Medical Card System Inc.
255 Ponce de Leon Ave., Ste. 203
Hato Rey, PR 00917
Phone: (787)758-2500

★ 17388 ★ MCS Life Insurance Co.
PO Box 193310
San Juan, PR 00919-3310
Phone: (787)758-2500

★ 17389 ★ MDNY Healthcare Inc.
1 Huntington Quadrangle
Melville, NY 11747
Phone: (516)454-1900

★ 17390 ★ MedAmerica Insurance Co.
Excellus Inc. Group
165 Court St.
Rochester, NY 14647
Phone: (585)238-4209
Website: http://www.medamericaltc.com
Howard Berman, President

★ 17391 ★ MedAmerica Insurance Co. of New York
Excellus Inc. Group
165 Court St.
Rochester, NY 14647
Phone: (585)238-4209
Website: http://www.yourlongtermcare.com
Christopher D. Perna, President

★ 17392 ★ Medco Containment Insurance Co. of New Jersey
Medco Containment Group
100 Parsons Pond Dr., Bldg. F3
Franklin Lakes, NJ 07417-2603
Phone: (201)269-3400 **Fax:** (201)269-1108
Richard T. Clark, President

★ 17393 ★ Medco Containment Insurance Co. of New York
Medco Containment Group
110 Clifton Corporate Pkwy.
Clifton Park, NY 12065
Phone: (212)878-7876 **Free:** 800-248-2268
Fax: 800-364-9603
Richard T. Clark, President

★ 17394 ★ Medco Containment Life Insurance Co.
Medco Containment Group
100 Parsons Pond Dr., Bldg. F3
Franklin Lakes, NJ 07417-2603
Phone: (201)269-3400 **Fax:** (201)269-1108
Richard T. Clark, President

★ 17395 ★ Medica Health Plans
Allina Health System
PO Box 9310
Minneapolis, MN 55440
Phone: (952)992-3635

★ 17396 ★ Medica Insurance Co.
Allina Health System
PO Box 1459
Minneapolis, MN 55440-1459
Phone: (952)992-2058
Jane E. Rollinson, President

★ 17397 ★ Medical Associates Health Plan Inc.
Medical Associates Clinic PC
700 Locust St., Ste. 230
PO Box 5002
Dubuque, IA 52004-5002
Phone: (319)556-8070

★ 17398 ★ Medical Benefits Mutual Life Insurance Co.
PO Box 1009
Newark, OH 43058-1009
Phone: (740)522-7324 **Fax:** (740)522-7484
Website: http://www.medben.com
Douglas J. Freeman, President

★ 17399 ★ Medical Health Insuring Corp. of Ohio
Medical Mutual of Ohio Group
2060 E 9th St.
Cleveland, OH 44115-1355
Phone: (216)687-7000

★ 17400 ★ Medical Life Insurance Co.
Health Care Service Corp.
1220 Huron Rd.
Cleveland, OH 44115-1700
Phone: (216)687-6800 **Fax:** (216)522-8702
Website: http://www.med-life.com
Larry J. Newsom, CEO & Chm Bd

★ 17401 ★ Medical Savings Insurance Co.
5835 W 74th St.
Indianapolis, IN 46278-1757
Phone: (317)329-8222 **Fax:** (317)329-3080
Website: http://www.medicalsavings.com
Randal E. Suttles, President

★ 17402 ★ Medico Life Insurance Co.
Mutual Protective Group
PO Box 3477
Omaha, NE 68103
Phone: (402)391-6900 **Fax:** (402)391-6489
Website: http://www.mutprot.com
Arthur C. Larson, CEO & Chm Bd

★ 17403 ★ MedSpan Health Options Inc.
Oxford Health Plans Inc.
48 Monroe Turnpike
Trumbull, CT 06611
Phone: (860)616-2200
Kevin W. Kelly, President

★ 17404 ★ The MEGA Life and Health Insurance Co.
United Insurance Cos., Inc. Group
4001 McEwen Dr., Ste. 200
Dallas, TX 75244
Phone: (972)392-6700 **Fax:** (972)392-6778
Website: http://www.uici.net
Phillip J. Myhra, CEO & Pres

★ 17405 ★ Melancon Life Insurance Co.
PO Box 100
Carencro, LA 70520
Phone: (337)235-3315
Gerald Melancon, President

★ 17406 ★ Mellon Life Insurance Co.
1 Mellon Bank Ctr., Rm. 4905
Pittsburgh, PA 15258
Phone: (412)234-6398 **Fax:** (412)236-6715
Kenneth J. Schweiger, President

★ 17407 ★ Member Service Life Insurance Co.
Blue Cross & Blue Shield of Oklahoma Group
1400 S Boston
Tulsa, OK 74119
Phone: (918)560-3200 **Fax:** (918)560-3223
Ronald F. King, CEO & Chm Bd

★ 17408 ★ MEMBERS Life Insurance Co.
CUNA Mutual Group
PO Box 391
Madison, WI 53701-0391
Phone: (608)238-5851 **Fax:** (608)238-0830
Website: http://www.cunamutual.com
Michael B. Kitchen, CEO & Pres

★ 17409 ★ Memorial Insurance Co. of America
PO Box 505
Blytheville, AR 72316
Phone: (870)763-0713

★ 17410 ★ Memorial Service Life Insurance Co.
PO Box 160090
Austin, TX 78716-0090
Phone: (512)328-0075
Randall K. Sutton, President

★ 17411 ★ Memphis Managed Care Corp.
Memphis and UT Medical Group Inc.
1407 Union Ave.
Memphis, TN 38104
Phone: (901)725-7100

★ 17412 ★ Menlo Life Insurance Co.
Fremont General Corp.
3070 Bristol St., Ste. 600
Costa Mesa, CA 92626
Phone: (714)429-2610 **Fax:** (714)429-2690
Mary-Lou Ann Misrahy, CEO & Pres

★ 17413 ★ Mercy Health Plans of Missouri Inc.
425 S Woods Mill Rd.
Chesterfield, MO 63017
Phone: (314)214-8100

★ 17414 ★ Mercycare Insurance Co.
PO Box 2770
Janesville, WI 53547-2770
Free: 800-752-3431
Javon R. Bea, President

★ 17415 ★ **Merit Life Insurance Co.**
American International Group
PO Box 39
Evansville, IN 47701-0039
Phone: (812)424-8031 **Fax:** (812)468-5549
Website: http://www.agfinance.com
Frederick W. Geissinger, CEO & Chm Bd

★ 17416 ★ **Merrill Lynch Insurance Group Inc.**
425 W Capitol Ave., Ste. 1800
Little Rock, AR 72201

★ 17417 ★ **Merrill Lynch Life Insurance Co.**
Merrill Lynch Insurance Group Inc.
PO Box 9061
Princeton, NJ 08543-9061
Phone: (609)627-3700 **Fax:** (609)627-3877
Nikos K. Kardassis, CEO & Pres

★ 17418 ★ **Methodist Care Inc.**
WellPoint Health Networks Inc.
2 Greenway Plaza, Ste. 500
Houston, TX 77046
Phone: (713)479-4100 **Fax:** (713)479-4269
Website: http://www.methodistcare.com
Albert R. Zimmerli, President

★ 17419 ★ **Methodist Health Insurance Co.**
WellPoint Health Networks Inc.
2 Greenway Plaza, Ste. 500
Houston, TX 77046
Phone: (713)479-4100 **Fax:** (713)479-4269
Website: http://www.methodistcare.com
Albert R. Zimmerli, CEO

★ 17420 ★ **MetLife Investors Insurance Co.**
Metropolitan Life and Affiliated Companies
700 Market St.
Saint Louis, MO 63101
Phone: (630)368-6215 **Fax:** (630)368-6240
Website: http://www.cova.com
Gregory P. Brakovich, President

★ 17421 ★ **MetLife Investors Insurance Co. of California**
Metropolitan Life and Affiliated Cos.
4100 Newport Pl. Dr., Ste. 840
Newport Beach, CA 92660
Phone: (630)368-6215 **Fax:** (630)368-6240
Website: http://www.cova.com
Gregory P. Brakovich, President
Frmly: Cova Financial Life Insurance Co.

★ 17422 ★ **MetLife Investors USA Insurance Co.**
Metropolitan Life and Affiliated Companies
222 Delaware Ave., Ste. 900
Wilmington, DE 19899
Phone: (813)801-2100 **Fax:** (813)870-8035
Website: http://www.securityfirstgroup.com
Richard C. Pearson, President

★ 17423 ★ **MetLife Security Insurance Co. of Louisiana**
Metropolitan Life and Affiliated Cos.
2121 Airline Dr., Ste. 203
Metairie, LA 70001
Phone: (212)578-2211 **Fax:** (918)252-8721
Stanley J. Talbi, CEO & Chm Bd

★ 17424 ★ **Metropolitan Health Plan**
Hennepin County
822 S 3rd St., Ste. 140
Minneapolis, MN 55415
Phone: (612)347-3353 **Fax:** (612)904-4329
Website: http://www.co.hennepin.mn.us/mhp/mhp.html

★ 17425 ★ **Metropolitan Insurance & Annuity Co.**
Metropolitan Life and Affiliated Cos.
220 Continental Dr., Ste. 212
Newark, DE 19713
Phone: (212)578-2211 **Fax:** (212)578-7298
Gary A. Beller, CEO & Chm Bd

★ 17426 ★ **Metropolitan Life Insurance Co.**
Metropolitan Life and Affiliated Cos.
1 MetLife Plaza, Area 7B
Long Island City, NY 11101
Phone: (212)578-2211 **Fax:** (212)578-7298
Website: http://www.metlife.com
Robert H. Benmosche, CEO & Chm Bd

★ 17427 ★ **Metropolitan Tower Life Insurance Co.**
Metropolitan Life and Affiliated Cos.
220 Continental Dr., Ste. 212
Newark, DE 19713
Phone: (212)578-2211 **Fax:** (212)578-7298
Gary A. Beller, CEO & Chm Bd

★ 17428 ★ **MHN Reinsurance Co. of Arizona**
Health Net Inc.
1600 Los Gamos Dr., Ste. 300
San Rafael, CA 94903
Phone: (415)491-7565
Jeffrey J. Bairstow, President

★ 17429 ★ **MIC Life Insurance Corp.**
Motors Insurance Group
300 Galleria Officentre
Southfield, MI 48034
Phone: (313)556-5000 **Fax:** (313)974-5616
William B. Noll, President

★ 17430 ★ **Michigan Dental Plan, Inc.**
G-2503 S Linden Rd.
Flint, MI 48532
Phone: (810)733-8255
William J. Nicholson, President

★ 17431 ★ **Michigan Eyecare Associates Inc.**
23409 Michigan Ave.
Dearborn, MI 48124
Phone: (313)565-5000 **Fax:** (313)562-3000

★ 17432 ★ **Mid-America Credit Life Assurance Co.**
PO Box 30416
Lansing, MI 48909-7916
Phone: (414)574-6836
Glen J. Milesko, President

★ 17433 ★ **Mid-American Century Life Insurance Co.**
813 W Stadium Blvd.
Jefferson City, MO 65109
Phone: (573)659-8545
Harold D. Woodward, President

★ 17434 ★ **Mid-Atlantic Vision Service Plan, Inc.**
Vision Service Plan
3333 Quality Dr.
Rancho Cordova, CA 95670
Phone: (916)851-5000 **Fax:** (916)858-5388
Roger J. Valine, President

★ 17435 ★ **Mid-Continent Life Insurance Co.**
1400 Classen Dr.
PO Box 18637
Oklahoma City, OK 73154
Phone: (405)522-4618 **Fax:** (405)523-3840

★ 17436 ★ **Mid-South Insurance Co.**
World Insurance Co.
PO Box 3160
Omaha, NE 68103-0160
Phone: (910)822-1020 **Fax:** (910)822-1212
Website: http://www.trigon.com
T. D. Eilers, President

★ 17437 ★ **Mid-West National Life Insurance Co. of Tennessee**
United Insurance Cos., Inc. Group
4001 McEwen Dr., Ste. 200
Dallas, TX 75244
Phone: (972)392-6700 **Fax:** (972)392-6778
Website: http://www.uici.net
Phillip J. Myhra, CEO & Pres

★ 17438 ★ **MidAmerica Life Insurance Co.**
World Insurance Co.
PO Box 3160
Omaha, NE 68103-0160
Phone: (402)496-8000 **Fax:** (402)496-8040
T. D. Eilers, President

★ 17439 ★ **Midland Life Insurance Co.**
Swiss Reinsurance Group
969 High Ridge Rd.
Stamford, CT 06905
Phone: (614)228-2001
Website: http://www.themidland.com
Ihor W. Hron, CEO & Pres

★ 17440 ★ **Midland National Life Insurance Co.**
Sammons Financial Group
1 Midland Plaza
Sioux Falls, SD 57193-0001
Phone: (605)335-5700 **Fax:** (605)373-8558
Website: http://www.mnlife.com
Michael M. Masterson, CEO & Chm Bd

★ 17441 ★ **Midwest Health Plan Inc.**
Midwest-HC Inc.
5050 Schaefer Rd.
Dearborn, MI 48126
Phone: (313)581-3700

★ 17442 ★ **Midwest Security Life Insurance Co.**
2700 Midwest Dr.
Onalaska, WI 54650-8764
Phone: (608)783-7130 **Fax:** (608)783-8585
Website: http://www.midwestsecurity.com
Ronald W. Houser, President

★ 17443 ★ **Midwestern Dental Plans Inc.**
5050 Schaefer Rd.
Dearborn, MI 48126
Phone: (313)582-0745
Melvin Feiler, President

★ 17444 ★ Midwestern United Life Insurance Co.
ING Group
5780 Powers Ferry Rd. NW
Atlanta, GA 30327
Phone: (303)860-1290 **Fax:** (303)860-2679
Chris D. Schreier, President

★ 17445 ★ MII Life, Inc.
Aware Integrated, Inc.
PO Box 64560
Saint Paul, MN 55164-0193
Phone: (651)662-8441 **Fax:** (651)662-6316
Website: http://www.miilife.com
Christopher L. Aasland, CEO & Pres

★ 17446 ★ Mililani Life Insurance Co.
38 S Kukui St.
Honolulu, HI 96813
Phone: (808)532-3002

★ 17447 ★ MIMLIC Life Insurance Co.
Minnesota Mutual Group
400 Robert St. N
Saint Paul, MN 55101
Phone: (651)665-3500 **Fax:** (651)665-4488
Website: http://www.minnesotamutual.com
Paul W. Anderson, President

★ 17448 ★ Ministers Life Insurance Co.
Minnesota Mutual Group
400 Robert St. N
Saint Paul, MN 55101
Phone: (651)665-3500 **Fax:** (651)665-4488
Website: http://www.minnesotamutual.com
Robert L. Senkler, CEO & Chm Bd

★ 17449 ★ Minnesota Life Insurance Co.
Minnesota Mutual Group
400 Robert St. N
Saint Paul, MN 55101
Phone: (651)665-3500 **Fax:** (651)665-4488
Website: http://www.minnesotamutual.com
Robert L. Senkler, CEO & Chm Bd

★ 17450 ★ Mission Life Insurance Co. of America
2121 Sage Rd., Ste. 200
Houston, TX 77056
Phone: (713)984-1517 **Fax:** (713)984-0215
Website: http://www.missionlife.com
Michael R. Earthman, President

★ 17451 ★ Missouri Care Plan
217 University Hall
Columbia, MO 65212
Phone: (573)441-2100

★ 17452 ★ Missouri Valley Life & Health Insurance Co.
PO Box 419169
Kansas City, MO 64141-6169
Phone: (816)395-2750
John W. Kennedy, President

★ 17453 ★ ML Life Insurance Co. of New York
Merrill Lynch Insurance Group, Inc.
7 Roszel Rd.
Princeton, NJ 08540
Phone: (609)627-3700 **Fax:** (609)627-3877
Nikos K. Kardassis, CEO & Pres

★ 17454 ★ MMA Insurance Co.
PO Box 483
Goshen, IN 46527
Phone: (574)533-9511
Howard L. Brenneman, Contact

★ 17455 ★ MML Bay State Life Insurance Co.
MassMutual Financial Group
1295 State St.
Springfield, MA 01111
Phone: (413)788-8411
Website: http://www.massmutual.com
Robert J. O'Connell, CEO & Pres

★ 17456 ★ Modern Life Insurance Co. of Arizona, Inc.
American Modern Insurance Group
PO Box 5323
Cincinnati, OH 45201-5323
Phone: (513)943-7200 **Fax:** (513)943-7201
Website: http://www.midlandcompany.com
John W. Hayden, CEO & Chm Bd

★ 17457 ★ Modern Woodmen of America
1701 1st Ave.
Rock Island, IL 61201-8779
Phone: (309)786-6481 **Fax:** (309)793-5507
Website: http://www.modern-woodmen.org
Clyde C. Schoeck, President

★ 17458 ★ Molina Healthcare of Utah Inc.
Molina Healthcare Inc.
2120 South 1300 East, Ste. 303
Salt Lake City, UT 84106
Phone: (801)486-1664

★ 17459 ★ Molina Healthcare of Washington Inc.
Molina Healthcare Inc.
2331 130th Ave. NE, Ste. 200
Bellevue, WA 98009
Phone: (425)869-3500

★ 17460 ★ Molina Medical Centers
1 Golden Shore Dr.
Long Beach, CA 90802
Phone: (562)435-3666

★ 17461 ★ Monarch Life Insurance Co.
Regal Reinsurance Group
1 Monarch Pl.
Springfield, MA 01133
Phone: (413)784-2000 **Fax:** (413)784-6408
Kevin J. McAdoo, President
Stephan A. Frentzos, Senior VP

★ 17462 ★ Monitor Life Insurance Co. of New York
Commercial Travelers Mutual Group
70 Genesee St.
Utica, NY 13502-3502
Phone: (315)797-5200 **Fax:** (315)797-3198
Website: http://www.monitorlife.com
Donald E. Joslin, CEO & Pres

★ 17463 ★ Montana Benefits and Life Co.
PO Box 548
Kalispell, MT 59903
Phone: (406)751-3333

★ 17464 ★ Monumental Life Insurance Co.
AEGON USA, Inc.
2 E Chase St.
Baltimore, MD 21202
Phone: (410)685-2900 **Fax:** (410)347-8686
Henry G. Hagan, CEO & Pres

★ 17465 ★ MONY Life Insurance Co.
MONY Group
1740 Broadway at 55th St.
New York, NY 10019-4386
Phone: (212)708-2000 **Fax:** (212)708-2104
Website: http://www.mony.com
Samuel J. Foti, President

★ 17466 ★ MONY Life Insurance Co. of America
MONY Group
1740 Broadway
New York, NY 10019-4386
Phone: (212)708-2000 **Fax:** (212)708-2104
Website: http://www.mony.com
Samuel J. Foti, President

★ 17467 ★ Mothe Life Insurance Co.
PO Box 2128
Gretna, LA 70056
Phone: (504)398-0777
Charles Gerrets, III, President

★ 17468 ★ Motorists Life Insurance Co.
Motorists Insurance Group
471 E Broad St.
Columbus, OH 43215-3861
Phone: (614)225-8358 **Fax:** (614)225-8365
Website: http://motoristslife.com
John J. Bishop, CEO & Pres

★ 17469 ★ Mount Carmel Health Plan Inc.
Mount Carmel Health System
495 Cooper Rd., Ste. 200
Westerville, OH 43081
Phone: (614)898-8750

★ 17470 ★ Mountain Life Insurance Co.
PO Box 240
Alcoa, TN 37701-0240
Phone: (865)970-2800 **Fax:** (865)970-2885
Website: http://www.mountainlife.com
Daniel J. McPherson, CEO & Chm Bd

★ 17471 ★ Mountain State Blue Cross & Blue Shield, Inc.
Highmark Inc.
PO Box 1948
Parkersburg, WV 26102
Phone: (304)424-9813 **Fax:** (304)424-7704
Website: http://www.msbcbs.com
Gregory K. Smith, President

★ 17472 ★ MS Diversified Life Insurance Co.
Fortis, Inc. Group
260 Interstate Cir. NW
Atlanta, GA 30339
Phone: (601)978-6732 **Fax:** (601)978-6709
Website: http://www.msdiversified.com
Adam D. Lamnin, President

★ 17473 ★ MS Life Insurance Co.
Fortis, Inc. Group
260 Interstate Cir. NW
Atlanta, GA 30339
Phone: (601)978-6732 **Fax:** (601)978-6709
Website: http://www.msdiversified.com
John E. Gough, President

★ 17474 ★ MSC Life Insurance Co.
Premera Group
3900 E Sprague
Spokane, WA 99202
Phone: (509)536-4700 **Fax:** (509)536-2857
Steve Melton, President

★ 17475 ★ MTL Insurance Co.
1200 Jorie Blvd.
Oak Brook, IL 60523-2218
Phone: (630)990-1000 **Fax:** (630)990-7083
Website: http://www.mutualtrust.com
Gary L. Eisenbarth, CEO & Pres

★ 17476 ★ MTM Life Insurance Co.
PO Box 14000
San Antonio, TX 78214
Phone: (214)342-0400
Robert D. Tips, President

★ 17477 ★ Mulhearn Protective Insurance Co.
PO Box 1411
Monroe, LA 71210
Phone: (318)329-0141
Peter G. Mulhearn, Sr., CEO & Pres

★ 17478 ★ Munich American Reassurance Co.
Munich Reinsurance Group
PO Box 3210
Atlanta, GA 30302-3210
Phone: (770)350-3200 **Fax:** (770)350-3300
Website: http://www.marclife.com
David M. Holland, CEO & Pres
D. Raymond Riddle, Chairman of the Board

★ 17479 ★ Municipal Insurance Co. of America
721 Dundee Ave.
Elgin, IL 60120-3822
Phone: (847)695-1400 **Fax:** (847)695-1244
Noa W. Horner, President
Jean M. Barry, CEO & Chm Bd

★ 17480 ★ Mutual of America Life Insurance Co.
320 Park Ave.
New York, NY 10022
Phone: (212)224-1600 **Fax:** (212)224-2520
Thomas J. Moran, CEO & Pres

★ 17481 ★ Mutual of Detroit Insurance Co.
333 Plymouth Rd.
Plymouth, MI 48170-0500
Phone: (734)453-8500 **Fax:** (734)453-2610
J. M. Love, CEO & Pres

★ 17482 ★ Mutual of Omaha Insurance Co.
Mutual of Omaha Group
Mutual of Omaha Plaza
Omaha, NE 68175
Phone: (402)342-7600 **Fax:** (402)351-2775
Website: http://www.mutualofomaha.com
John A. Sturgeon, President
John W. Weekly, CEO & Chm Bd

★ 17483 ★ Mutual Protective Insurance Co.
Mutual Protective Group
PO Box 3477
Omaha, NE 68103
Phone: (402)391-6900 **Fax:** (402)391-6489
Website: http://www.mutprot.com
George W. Egermayer, Jr., President

★ 17484 ★ Mutual Savings Life Insurance Co.
Primesco, Inc.
PO Box 2222
Decatur, AL 35609-2222
Phone: (256)552-7011 **Fax:** (256)552-7284
C. Larimore Whitaker, CEO & Chm Bd
Walter J. Hughes, Exec VP

★ 17485 ★ Mutual Service Life Insurance Co.
Mutual Service Group
PO Box 64035
Saint Paul, MN 55164
Phone: (651)631-7000 **Fax:** (651)639-5400
Website: http://www.msi-insurance.com
John D. Blackburn, President

★ 17486 ★ MVP Health Plan
MVP Group
625 State St.
Schenectady, NY 12305
Phone: (518)370-4793

★ 17487 ★ MVP Health Services Corp.
MVP Group
625 State St.
Schenectady, NY 12301
Phone: (518)370-4793
David W. Oliker, President

★ 17488 ★ NAP Life Insurance Co.
3755 Capital of Texas Hwy. S, Ste. 148
Austin, TX 78704-6600
Phone: (512)462-2728
Edgar A. Brown, Jr., President

★ 17489 ★ National Affiliated Investors Life Insurance Co.
PO Box 12190
Alexandria, LA 71315-2190
Phone: (318)473-4355 **Fax:** (318)442-3318
Edward J. Birrane, President

★ 17490 ★ National Benefit Life Insurance Co.
Citigroup
307 W 7th St., Ste. 400
Fort Worth, TX 76102
Phone: (212)615-7500 **Fax:** (212)615-7308
Raul Rivera, CEO & Chm Bd

★ 17491 ★ National Capital Life Insurance Co.
Alderwoods Group Inc.
1055 St. Charles Ave., Ste. 600
New Orleans, LA 70130
Phone: (504)561-7700 **Fax:** (504)561-7740
Website: http://www.mayflowernational.com
Aaron P. Shipper, President

★ 17492 ★ National City Life Insurance Co.
2700 N 3rd St., Ste. 2000
Phoenix, AZ 85004
Phone: (602)200-6900
Thomas J. Cook, President

★ 17493 ★ National Family Care Life Insurance Co.
13530 Inwood Rd.
Dallas, TX 75244
Phone: (972)387-8553
Clyde W. Tullis, President

★ 17494 ★ National Farm Life Insurance Co.
PO Box 1486
Fort Worth, TX 76101-1486
Phone: (817)451-9550 **Fax:** (814)451-6358
Website: http://www.nflic.com
Ronald G. Downing, President

★ 17495 ★ National Farmers Union Life Insurance Co.
Americo Life Group
PO Box 13487
Kansas City, MO 64199-3487
Phone: (816)391-2000 **Fax:** (816)391-2083
Website: http://www.americo.com
Gary L. Muller, CEO & Pres

★ 17496 ★ National Financial Insurance Co.
Ascent Assurance, Inc.
110 W 7th St., Ste. 300
Fort Worth, TX 76102
Phone: (817)878-3300 **Fax:** (817)878-3672
Website: http://www.ascentassurance.com
Patrick J. Mitchell, CEO & Chm Bd

★ 17497 ★ National Foot Care Program Inc.
17117 W 9 Mile Rd., Ste. 1050
Southfield, MI 48075
Phone: (248)559-2579
Website: http://www.nationalfootcare.com
William Hoffman, President

★ 17498 ★ National Foundation Life Insurance Co.
Ascent Assurance, Inc.
110 W 7th St., Ste. 300
Fort Worth, TX 76102
Phone: (817)878-3300 **Fax:** (817)878-3672
Website: http://www.assentassurance.com
Patrick J. Mitchell, CEO & Chm Bd

★ 17499 ★ National Guardian Life Insurance Co.
NGL Insurance Group
PO Box 1191
Madison, WI 53701-1191
Phone: (608)257-5611 **Fax:** (608)257-4308
Website: http://www.nglic.com
J. D. Larson, CEO & Pres

★ 17500 ★ National Health Insurance Co.
National Health Corp.
PO Box 619999
Dallas, TX 75261-9999
Phone: (817)640-1900 **Fax:** (817)640-3443
Website: http://www.nhic.com
G. Scott Smith, CEO & Pres

★ 17501 ★ National Heritage Insurance Co.
5400 Legacy Dr., H1-4D-34
Plano, TX 75024
Phone: (972)605-5998
Kimber L. McMann, President

★ 17502 ★ National Home Life and Accident Insurance Co.
PO Box 279
Beech Grove, IN 46107
Phone: (410)515-8603

★ 17503 ★ National Income Life Insurance Co.
Torchmark Corp.
PO Box 3125
Syracuse, NY 13220
Phone: (315)451-2544
Website: http://www.torchmarkcorp.com
Mark S. McAndrew, CEO & Pres

★ 17504 ★ National Insurance Co. of Wisconsin, Inc.
250 S Executive Dr.
Brookfield, WI 53005
Phone: (262)785-9995 **Fax:** (262)785-9269
Website: http://www.nicw.com
Bruce A. Miller, President

★ 17505 ★ National Integrity Life Insurance Co.
Western & Southern Financial Group
15 Matthews St., Ste. 200
Goshen, NY 10924
Phone: (914)615-1018 **Fax:** (212)973-2231
John R. Lindholm, President

★ 17506 ★ The National Life & Accident Insurance Co.
American International Group
PO Box 39
Evansville, IN 47701
Phone: (812)424-8031 **Fax:** (812)468-5549
Website: http://www.agfinance.com
Frederick W. Geissinger, CEO & Chm Bd

★ 17507 ★ National Life Insurance Co.
National Financial Group
PO Box 366107
San Juan, PR 00936-6107
Phone: (787)758-8080 **Fax:** (787)756-7360
Website: http://www.nalicpr.com
Carlos M. Benitez, Jr., CEO & Chm Bd

★ 17508 ★ National Life Insurance Co.
National Life Group
1 National Life Dr.
Montpelier, VT 05604
Phone: (802)229-3333 **Fax:** (802)229-9281
Website: http://www.nationallife.com
Thomas H. MacLeay, CEO & Chm Bd

★ 17509 ★ National Masonic Provident Association
632 N Park St.
Columbus, OH 43215
Phone: (614)228-5130
Thomas G. Luffy, President

★ 17510 ★ National Med Inc.
Tenet HealthSystem Hospitals Inc.
1005 W Orangeburg Ave., Ste. B
Modesto, CA 95350
Phone: (209)527-3350

★ 17511 ★ National Mutual Benefit
6522 Grand Teton Plaza
Madison, WI 53719
Phone: (608)833-1936 **Fax:** (608)833-8714
Website: http://www.nmbfrat.org
George F. Yanna, CEO & Pres

★ 17512 ★ National Mutual Life Insurance Co.
10800 E Washington St., Ste. 201
Indianapolis, IN 46229
Phone: (317)396-3751
Bruce W. Buchnan, President

★ 17513 ★ National Partners Group Life Insurance Co.
11815 N Pennsylvania St.
Carmel, IN 46032-4572
Phone: (317)817-6100
Warren Steinborn, President

★ 17514 ★ National Safety Life Insurance Co.
Philanthropic Companies
401 Plymouth Rd., Ste. 100
Plymouth Meeting, PA 19462
Phone: (610)684-2400 **Fax:** (610)684-2480
Website: http://www.thephilanthropic.com
Richard E. Bauer, President

★ 17515 ★ National Security Insurance Co.
National Security Group, Inc.
661 E Davis St.
Elba, AL 36323
Phone: (334)897-2273 **Fax:** (334)897-5694
Website: http://www.nationalsecuritygroup.com
William L. Brunson, Jr., President
Mickey L. Murdock, Senior VP

★ 17516 ★ National Security Life and Annuity Co.
100 Court St.
PO Box 1625
Binghamton, NY 13902-1625
Phone: 877-446-3060 **Fax:** (607)724-1607
Daniel J. Fischer, President
Frmly: First ING Life Insurance Co. of New York.

★ 17517 ★ National States Insurance Co.
1830 Craig Park Ct.
Saint Louis, MO 63146-6925
Phone: (314)878-0101 **Fax:** (314)878-8118
Thomas R. Green, President

★ 17518 ★ National Teachers Associates Life Insurance Co.
PO Box 802207
Dallas, TX 75380-2207
Phone: (972)532-2100 **Fax:** (972)532-2194
Website: http://www.ntalife.com
Raymond J. Martin, Jr., CEO & Pres

★ 17519 ★ National Travelers Life Co.
National Travelers Group
5700 Westown Pkwy.
West Des Moines, IA 50266-8221
Phone: (515)221-0101 **Fax:** (515)327-5711
Website: http://www.nationaltravelerslife.com
Melvin L. Rambo, President
Maynard J. Axtell, Chairman of the Board

★ 17520 ★ National Western Life Insurance Co.
850 E Anderson Ln.
Austin, TX 78752-1602
Phone: (512)836-1010 **Fax:** (512)719-8511
Website: http://www.nationalwesternlife.com
Ross R. Moody, President
Robert L. Moody, CEO & Chm Bd

★ 17521 ★ NationalCare Insurance Co.
Unitrin, Inc.
6100 NW Grand Blvd.
Oklahoma City, OK 73118
Phone: (405)848-7931 **Fax:** (405)843-3850
Website: http://www.unitrin.com
Roger W. Cole, President

★ 17522 ★ NationsBanc Insurance Co., Inc.
BankAmerica Group
201 N Tryon St., NC1-022-19-02
Charlotte, NC 28255
Phone: (704)388-7764 **Fax:** (704)386-0810
Dean A. Purvis, President

★ 17523 ★ Nationwide Life and Annuity Insurance Co.
Nationwide Group
1 Nationwide Plaza
Columbus, OH 43215-2220
Free: 800-882-2822
Website: http://www.nationwidefinancial.com
Joseph J. Gasper, President

★ 17524 ★ Nationwide Life Insurance Co.
Nationwide Group
1 Nationwide Plaza
Columbus, OH 43215-2220
Phone: (614)249-7111 **Fax:** (614)249-6590
Website: http://www.nationwidefinancial.com
Joseph J. Gasper, President

★ 17525 ★ Neighborhood Health Partnership Inc.
John Alden Services and Dimension PHO
7600 Corporate Ctr. Dr.
PO Box 025680
Miami, FL 33126
Phone: (305)715-2200

★ 17526 ★ Neighborhood Health Plans of Rhode Island Inc.
50 Holden St.
Providence, RI 02908
Phone: (401)459-6000

★ 17527 ★ Netcare Life and Health Insurance Co.
424 W Obrein Dr., Ste. 107
Hagatna, GU 96910
Phone: (671)472-3610
Kurt S. Moylan, President

★ 17528 ★ Network Health Insurance Corp.
Affinity Health System
1570 Midway Pl.
PO Box 120
Menasha, WI 54952
Phone: (920)720-1452
Website: http://www.networkhealth.com
Tim D. Temperly, President

★ 17529 ★ Network Health Plan of Wisconsin Inc.
Affinity Health System
1570 Midway Pl.
Menasha, WI 54952
Phone: (920)720-1200
Michael D. Wolff, President

★ 17530 ★ NevadaCare Inc.
Health Management Solutions Inc.
10600 W Charleston Blvd.
Las Vegas, NV 89135-1014
Phone: (702)304-5500 **Fax:** (702)474-7168

★ 17531 ★ New England Life Insurance Co.
Metropolitan Life and Affiliated Cos.
501 Boylston St.
Boston, MA 02117
Phone: (617)578-2000 **Fax:** (617)578-6459

Website: http://www.nefn.com
James M. Benson, CEO & Chm Bd

★ 17532 ★ New England Pension & Annuity Co.
Metropolitan Life and Affiliated Cos.
1209 Orange St.
Wilmington, DE 19801
Phone: (617)578-2000 **Fax:** (617)578-6459
Website: http://www.nefn.com
Mary Ann Brown, CEO & Chm Bd

★ 17533 ★ New Era Life Insurance Co.
New Era Group
200 Westlake Park Blvd., Ste. 1200
Houston, TX 77079-2663
Phone: (281)368-7200 **Fax:** (281)368-7286
Bill S. Chen, President

★ 17534 ★ New Era Life Insurance Co. of the Midwest
New Era Group
200 Westlake Park Blvd., Ste. 1200
Houston, TX 77079-2663
Phone: (281)368-7200 **Fax:** (281)368-7286
Bill S. Chen, President

★ 17535 ★ New South Life Insurance Co.
PO Box 1139
Jackson, MS 39201
Phone: (662)746-9129
James W. Covington, President

★ 17536 ★ New York Life Agents Reinsurance Co.
2999 N 44th St., Ste. 250
Phoenix, AZ 85018
Phone: (602)266-1166
Joe A. Shapiro, President

★ 17537 ★ New York Life & Health Insurance Co.
Aetna Inc. Group
151 Farmington Ave.
MC 64
Hartford, CT 06156-0417
Free: 800-872-3862
Alan M. Bennett, President

★ 17538 ★ New York Life Insurance & Annuity Corp.
New York Life Group
51 Madison Ave.
New York, NY 10010
Phone: (212)576-7000 **Fax:** (212)447-4272
Website: http://www.newyorklife.com
Frederick J. Sievert, President

★ 17539 ★ New York Life Insurance Co.
New York Life Group
51 Madison Ave.
New York, NY 10010
Phone: (212)576-7000 **Fax:** (212)447-4272
Website: http://www.newyorklife.com
Seymour Sternberg, CEO & Chm Bd

★ 17540 ★ NGL American Life Insurance Co.
NGL Insurance Group
PO Box 1031
Madison, WI 53701-1031
Phone: (608)257-5612 **Fax:** (608)257-2136
Website: http://www.nationalguardian.com/nglamerican.html
J. D. Larson, President

★ 17541 ★ Nippon Life Insurance Co. of America
450 Lexington Ave., Ste. 3200
New York, NY 10017
Phone: (212)682-3000 **Fax:** (212)682-3002
Website: http://www.nlia.com
Koichi Toyomaru, CEO & Pres

★ 17542 ★ Noridian Mutual Insurance Co.
Noridian Mutual Insurance Group
4510 13th Ave. SW
Fargo, ND 58121-0001
Phone: (701)282-1100 **Fax:** (701)282-1866
Website: http://www.noridian.com
Michael B. Unhjem, CEO & Pres

★ 17543 ★ North American Co. for Life and Health Insurance
Sammons Financial Group
1 Midland Plaza
Sioux Falls, SD 57193-0001
Phone: (312)648-7600 **Fax:** (312)648-7787
Website: http://www.nacolah.com
Michael M. Masterson, CEO & Chm Bd

★ 17544 ★ North American Co. for Life and Health Insurance of New York
Sammons Financial Group
1 Midland Plaza
Sioux Falls, SD 57193-0001
Phone: (516)228-8899 **Fax:** (516)228-7087
Website: http://www.nacolah.com
Michael M. Masterson, CEO & Chm Bd

★ 17545 ★ North American Insurance Co.
AMERCO Group
2721 N Central Ave.
Phoenix, AZ 85004
Phone: (608)662-1232 **Fax:** (608)662-1220
Website: http://www.nains.com
Mark A. Haydukovich, CEO & Pres

★ 17546 ★ North American Life Insurance Co. of Texas
1250 S Capitol of Texas Hwy., Bldg. 3, No. 150
Austin, TX 78746
Phone: (281)592-3311

★ 17547 ★ North American National Life Insurance Co.
North American National Life Group
6535 S Dayton St., Ste. 1100
Greenwood Village, CO 80111
Phone: (303)790-2090
John Ridings Lee, Sr., President

★ 17548 ★ North American National Reinsurance Co.
North American National Life Group
6535 S Dayton St.
Greenwood Village, CO 80111
Phone: (303)790-2090
John R. Lee, Sr., President

★ 17549 ★ North Carolina Mutual Life Insurance Co.
411 W Chapel Hill St.
Durham, NC 27701-3616
Phone: (919)682-9201 **Fax:** (919)683-1694
Website: http://www.ncmutuallife.com
Bert Collins, CEO & Pres
Nathan T. Garrett, Chairman of the Board

★ 17550 ★ North Central Life Insurance Co.
American International Group
3600 Rte. 66
Neptune, NJ 07754
Phone: (651)227-8000 **Fax:** (651)292-1830
William M. Keeler, CEO

★ 17551 ★ North Coast Life Insurance Co.
PO Box 1445
Spokane, WA 99210-1445
Phone: (509)838-4235 **Fax:** (509)747-8569
Website: http://www.nclife.com
C. Robert Ogden, President

★ 17552 ★ Northbrook Life Insurance Co.
Allstate Financial Group
3100 Sanders Rd.
Northbrook, IL 60062
Phone: (847)402-5000
Website: http://www.allstate.com
Thomas J. Wilson, II, CEO

★ 17553 ★ Northeast United Life Insurance Co.
30 Clarksville St.
Paris, TX 75460
Phone: (817)608-0619
P. Gene Roden, President

★ 17554 ★ Northern Life Insurance Co.
ING Group
5780 Powers Ferry Rd. NW
Atlanta, GA 30327
Phone: (206)292-1111 **Fax:** 800-531-5025
Website: http://www.northernlifetsa.com
Thomas J. McInerney, CEO & Pres
J. G. Turner, Chairman of the Board

★ 17555 ★ Northern National Life Insurance Co. of Rhode Island
1 Home Loan Plaza, Ste. 3
Warwick, RI 02886-1765
Phone: (401)739-8800

★ 17556 ★ Northstar Life Insurance Co.
Minnesota Mutual Group
400 Robert St. N
Saint Paul, MN 55101
Phone: (716)832-8678 **Fax:** (651)665-4488
Website: http://www.minnesotamutual.com
Robert E. Hunstad, CEO & Pres

★ 17557 ★ Northwestern Long Term Care Insurance Co.
Northwestern Mutual Group
720 E Wisconsin Ave.
Milwaukee, WI 53202
Phone: (414)271-1444 **Fax:** (414)665-2507
Website: http://www.northwesternmutual.com
Edward J. Zore, CEO & Pres

★ 17558 ★ The Northwestern Mutual Life Insurance Co.
Northwestern Mutual Group
720 E Wisconsin Ave.
Milwaukee, WI 53202-4797
Phone: (414)271-1444 **Fax:** (414)665-2507
Website: http://www.northwesternmutual.com
James D. Ericson, Chairman of the Board
Edward J. Zore, CEO & Pres

★ 17559 ★ Nutmeg Life Insurance Co.
Hartford Life, Inc.
200 Hopmeadow St.
Simsbury, CT 06089

Phone: (860)525-8555 **Fax:** (860)843-5568
Website: http://www.thehartford.com
Thomas M. Marra, President

★ 17560 ★ NYLIFE Insurance Co. of Arizona
New York Life Group
51 Madison Ave.
New York, NY 10010
Phone: (212)576-7000 **Fax:** (212)576-8192
Website: http://www.newyorklife.com
Frederick J. Sievert, President

★ 17561 ★ The Oath, a Health Plan for Alabama Inc.
2 Perimeter Park S, Ste. 200W
Birmingham, AL 35243
Phone: (205)968-1000

★ 17562 ★ Occidental Life Insurance Co. of North Carolina
American Amicable Group
PO Box 2595
Waco, TX 76702-2595
Phone: (254)297-2775 **Fax:** (254)297-2784
Website: http://www.occidentallife.com
S. Lanny Peavy, President

★ 17563 ★ ODS Health Plan, Inc.
Oregon Dental Service Group
601 SW 2nd Ave.
Portland, OR 97204
Phone: (503)228-6554 **Fax:** (503)948-5557
Website: http://www.odshp.com
Robert G. Gootee, President

★ 17564 ★ Ohio Motorists Life Insurance Co.
PO Box 6150
Cleveland, OH 44101
Phone: (216)606-6312 **Fax:** (216)606-6371
Peter C. Ohlheiser, President

★ 17565 ★ Ohio National Life Assurance Corp.
Ohio National Life Group
4 Financial Way
Cincinnati, OH 45242
Phone: (513)794-6100 **Fax:** (513)794-4519
Website: http://www.ohionatl.com
David B. O'Maley, CEO & Chm Bd

★ 17566 ★ The Ohio National Life Insurance Co.
Ohio National Life Group
PO Box 237
Cincinnati, OH 45201
Phone: (513)794-6100 **Fax:** (513)794-4519
Website: http://www.ohionatl.com
David B. O'Maley, CEO & Chm Bd

★ 17567 ★ The Ohio State Life Insurance Co.
Americo Life Group
PO Box 13487
Kansas City, MO 64199-3487
Phone: (816)391-2000 **Fax:** (816)391-2083
Website: http://www.americo.com
Gary L. Muller, CEO & Pres

★ 17568 ★ OhioHealth Group HMO Inc.
OhioHealth Group Ltd.
300 E Wilson Bridge Rd., Ste. 200
Worthington, OH 43085-2339
Phone: (614)566-0123

★ 17569 ★ Old American Insurance Co.
Kansas City Life Group
PO Box 218573
Kansas City, MO 64121-8573
Phone: (816)753-4900 **Fax:** (816)753-4914
Website: http://www.oaic.com
Walter E. Bixby, President

★ 17570 ★ Old Dominion Life Insurance Co.
Shenandoah Life Group
2301 Brambleton Ave. SW
Roanoke, VA 24015
Phone: (540)985-4400 **Fax:** (540)985-4444
Robert W. Clark, President

★ 17571 ★ The Old Line Life Insurance Co. of America
American International Group
PO Box 401
Milwaukee, WI 53201-0401
Phone: (414)286-1500 **Fax:** (414)286-1550
Donald W. Britton, President

★ 17572 ★ Old Reliance Insurance Co.
PO Box 13150
Phoenix, AZ 85002-3150
Phone: (602)604-9181 **Fax:** (602)604-9171
Richard J. Lawson, President

★ 17573 ★ Old Republic Life Insurance Co.
Old Republic Insurance Group
307 N Michigan Ave.
Chicago, IL 60601
Phone: (312)346-8100
A. C. Zucaro, CEO & Chm Bd
Paul D. Adams, Senior VP

★ 17574 ★ Old South Life Insurance Co.
PO Box 159
Jonesboro, LA 71251-0159
Phone: (318)628-3985
Larry L. Price, President

★ 17575 ★ Old Spartan Life Insurance Co. Inc.
PO Box 811
Spartanburg, SC 29304-0811
Phone: (864)582-8195
Albert R. Biggs, President

★ 17576 ★ Old Standard Life Insurance Co.
Metropolitan Mortgage Group
PO Box 45419
Boise, ID 83711
Phone: (208)376-8260 **Fax:** (208)375-8307
Clayton Rudd, President

★ 17577 ★ Old Surety Life Insurance Co.
PO Box 54407
Oklahoma City, OK 73154
Phone: (405)523-2112 **Fax:** (405)524-4011
Dale L. Phillips, President
Carl R. Gibson, Chairman of the Board

★ 17578 ★ Old United Life Insurance Co.
Old United Group
PO Box 795
Shawnee Mission, KS 66201
Phone: (913)432-6400
Cecil L. Van Tuyl, President

★ 17579 ★ Old United Reinsurance Co.
Old United Group
PO Box 795
Shawnee Mission, KS 66201
Phone: (913)432-6400
Cecil L. Van Tuyl, President

★ 17580 ★ Old West Annuity & Life Insurance Co.
Metropolitan Mortgage Group
PO Box 45419
Boise, ID 83711
Phone: (208)376-8260 **Fax:** (208)375-8307
Clayton Rudd, President

★ 17581 ★ Omaha Life Insurance Co.
PO Box 2879
Omaha, NE 68103-2879
Phone: (402)398-3701
Richard L. Guffey, President

★ 17582 ★ Omega Reinsurance Corp.
Metropolitan Life and Affiliated Companies
2929 N 44th St., Ste. 120
Phoenix, AZ 85018
Phone: (617)578-2000
Thomas W. Moore, President

★ 17583 ★ Omnia Life Insurance Co.
Old Mutual US Life Holdings Inc.
12900 Metcalf Ave., Ste. 200
Overland Park, KS 66213
Phone: (913)402-2300
John P. Clifford, President

★ 17584 ★ Omnicare Health Plan
United American HealthCare of LA Inc.
1155 Brewery Park, Ste. 200
Detroit, MI 48207-7944
Phone: (313)393-4510
Harcourt G. Harris, MD, Chairman of the Board

★ 17585 ★ Omnicare Health Plan Inc.
United American HealthCare Corp.
1991 Corporate Ave., 4th Fl.
Memphis, TN 38132
Phone: (901)346-0064

★ 17586 ★ One Health Plan of California Inc.
One Benefits Inc.
8515 E Orchard Rd.
Greenwood Village, CO 80111
Phone: (818)539-0984 **Fax:** (818)545-7591
Jackie James, President

★ 17587 ★ One Health Plan of Colorado Inc.
One Benefits Inc.
8525 E Orchard Rd.
Greenwood Village, CO 80111
Phone: (303)773-0046 **Fax:** (303)773-0938
Christine A. Miller, President

★ 17588 ★ One Health Plan of Georgia Inc.
One Benefits Inc.
245 Perimeter Ctr. Pkwy., 7th Fl.
Atlanta, GA 30346
Phone: (770)290-7000 **Fax:** (770)290-7022
David E. Record, Jr., President

★ 17589 ★ One Health Plan of Illinois Inc.
One Benefits Inc.
6250 River Rd., No. 3030
Rosemont, IL 60018
Phone: (847)518-0490 **Fax:** (847)518-8865
Karen A. Smith, President

★ 17590 ★ One Health Plan of Texas Inc.
One Benefits Inc.
8525 E Orchard Rd.
Greenwood Village, CO 80111
Phone: (972)813-7000 **Fax:** (214)363-9785
Wally H. Gomaa, President

★ 17591 ★ Optima Health Plan
Sentara Health System
6015 Poplar Hall
Norfolk, VA 23502
Phone: (757)552-7220

★ 17592 ★ Optimum Choice of the Carolinas Inc.
Mid Atlantic Medical Services Inc.
4 Taft Ct.
Rockville, MD 20850
Phone: (301)762-8205

★ 17593 ★ Optimum Choice Inc.
Mid Atlantic Medical Services Inc.
4 Taft Ct.
Rockville, MD 20850
Phone: (301)762-8205

★ 17594 ★ Optimum Re Insurance Co.
Optimum Re Group
PO Box 660010
Dallas, TX 75266-0010
Phone: (214)528-2020 **Fax:** (214)528-2777
Website: http://www.optimumre.com
Mario Georgiev, President

★ 17595 ★ The Order of the Sons of Hermann in Texas
PO Box 1941
San Antonio, TX 78297
Phone: (210)226-9261 **Fax:** (210)226-3055
Website: http://www.texashermannsons.org
Leroy Muehlstein, CEO & Pres

★ 17596 ★ The Order of United Commercial Travelers of America
632 N Park St.
Columbus, OH 43215
Phone: (614)228-3276 **Fax:** (614)228-1898
Website: http://www.uct.org
John A. Engel, President

★ 17597 ★ Oregon Dental Service
Oregon Dental Service Group
601 SW 2nd Ave.
Portland, OR 97204
Phone: (503)228-6554 **Fax:** (503)948-5557
Website: http://www.odshp.com
Robert G. Gootee, President

★ 17598 ★ Orion Life Insurance Co.
1209 Orange St.
Wilmington, DE 19801
Phone: (314)595-3746
Dennis P. Moody, President

★ 17599 ★ OSF Health Plans Inc.
7915 N Hale Ave., Ste. D
Peoria, IL 61615
Phone: (309)677-8342

★ 17600 ★ Oshsner Health Plan
1 Galleria Blvd., Ste. 850
Metairie, LA 70001
Phone: (504)836-6600 **Fax:** (504)836-6566
Website: http://www.ohpnow.com

★ 17601 ★ Ouachita Life Insurance Co.
Southern Pioneer Group
PO Box 8006
Little Rock, AR 72203
Phone: (501)374-5715
Website: http://www.southern-pioneer.com
Ben R. Hyneman, President

★ 17602 ★ Owens-Brumley Funeral Insurance Co.
PO Box 1980
Wichita Falls, TX 76307
Phone: (940)766-4321

★ 17603 ★ Oxford Health Insurance, Inc.
Oxford Health Plans, Inc.
48 Monroe Turnpike
Trumbull, CT 06611
Phone: (203)459-6000
Website: http://www.oxfordhealth.com
Charles G. Berg, President

★ 17604 ★ Oxford Health Plans (CT) Inc.
Oxford Health Plans Inc.
48 Monroe Turnpike
Trumbull, CT 06611
Phone: (203)459-6000
Website: http://www.oxfordhealth.com
Charles M. Schneider, President

★ 17605 ★ Oxford Health Plans (NJ) Inc.
Oxford Health Plans Inc.
48 Monroe Turnpike
Trumbull, CT 06611
Phone: (203)459-6000
Website: http://www.oxfordhealth.com
Norman C. Payson, MD, President

★ 17606 ★ Oxford Health Plans (NY) Inc.
Oxford Health Plans Inc.
48 Monroe Turnpike
Trumbull, CT 06611
Phone: (203)852-1442
Website: http://www.oxfordhealth.com
Charles M. Schneider, President

★ 17607 ★ Oxford Life Insurance Co.
AMERCO Group
2721 N Central Ave.
Phoenix, AZ 85004
Phone: (602)263-6666 **Fax:** (602)277-5901
Website: http://www.oxfordlife.com
Mark A. Haydukovich, President

★ 17608 ★ Ozark National Life Insurance Co.
PO Box 15688
Kansas City, MO 64106-0688
Phone: (816)842-6300 **Fax:** (816)842-8373
Website: http://www.ozark-national.com
Charles N. Sharpe, President
S. Alan Weber, Exec VP

★ 17609 ★ Ozark National Life Insurance Co.
10201 W Markham St.
Little Rock, AR 72205-2182
Phone: (501)227-4444
John P. Jones, President

★ 17610 ★ PacifCare Health Insurance Co. of Micronesia
231 Guerrero Dr.
Tamuning, GU 96911
Phone: (671)646-6956

★ 17611 ★ Pacific Beacon Life Reassurance Inc.
AAA Life Group
745 Fort St., Ste. 800
Honolulu, HI 96813
Phone: (808)585-3533
James R. Pouliot, President

★ 17612 ★ Pacific Century Life Insurance Corp.
2700 N 3rd St., Ste. 200
Phoenix, AZ 85004
Phone: (602)200-6900
Corinne Jebhardt, President

★ 17613 ★ Pacific Guardian Life Insurance Co., Ltd.
Meiji Life Group
1440 Kapiolani Blvd.
Honolulu, HI 96814-3846
Phone: (808)955-2236 **Fax:** (808)942-1290
Website: http://www.pacificguardian.com
Yoji Nakamura, CEO & Pres
Alan M. Goda, Chairman of the Board

★ 17614 ★ Pacific Life & Accident Insurance Co.
Swiss Reinsurance Group
175 King St.
Armonk, NY 10504
Phone: 877-794-7773 **Fax:** (914)828-7835
Chris C. Stroup, CEO & Pres

★ 17615 ★ Pacific Life & Annuity Co.
Pacific Life Group
700 Newport Ctr. Dr.
Newport Beach, CA 92660
Phone: (949)219-3011 **Fax:** (949)760-6810
Website: http://www.pacificlifeandannuity.com
Thomas C. Sutton, CEO & Chm Bd

★ 17616 ★ Pacific Life Insurance Co.
Pacific Life Group
700 Newport Ctr. Dr.
Newport Beach, CA 92660
Phone: (949)219-3011 **Fax:** (949)760-6810
Website: http://www.pacificlife.com
Glenn S. Schafer, President

★ 17617 ★ Pacific Union Assurance Co.
American International Group
PO Box 667
Wilmington, DE 19899
Phone: (302)594-2000 **Fax:** (302)654-5436
Gerald W. Wyndorf, CEO & Pres

★ 17618 ★ Pacific Visioncare, Washington, Inc.
2517 NE Kresky Ave.
Chehalis, WA 98532
Phone: (360)748-8632
Debbie J. Eldredge, President

★ 17619 ★ PacifiCare of Arizona Inc.
PacifiCare Health Systems Inc.
3110 Lake Ctr. Dr., LC05-308
Santa Ana, CA 92704
Phone: (602)244-8200
Website: http://www.pacificare.com
Ace M. Hodgin, Jr., President

★ 17620 ★ PacifiCare Behavioral Health of California Inc.
PacifiCare Health Systems Inc.
5995 Plaza Dr.
Cypress, CA 90630
Phone: (714)952-1121
Brad Bowlus, Chairman of the Board

★ 17621 ★ PacifiCare of California Inc.
PacifiCare Health Systems Inc.
5995 Plaza Dr.
Cypress, CA 90630
Phone: (714)952-1121 **Fax:** (714)226-3914
Website: http://www.pacificare.com
Brad Bowlus, Chairman of the Board

★ 17622 ★ PacifiCare of Colorado Inc.
PacifiCare Health Systems Inc.
3120 Lake Ctr. Dr.
Santa Ana, CA 92704
Phone: (303)220-5800
Website: http://www.pacificare.com
Val C. Dean, MD, President

★ 17623 ★ PacifiCare Dental
PacifiCare Health Systems Inc.
2099 S State College Blvd., Ste. 500
PO Box 66033
Anaheim, CA 92816
Phone: (714)704-9494
James G. Stumpfel, President

★ 17624 ★ PacifiCare Life Assurance Co.
PacifiCare Health Systems Inc.
3100 W Lake Ctr. Dr.
Mail Stop LC03-381
Santa Ana, CA 92704
Phone: (714)825-5379 **Free:** 800-204-6629
Fax: (949)348-5610
Website: http://www.pacificare.com
Ronald M. Davis, President

★ 17625 ★ PacifiCare Life and Health Insurance Co.
PacifiCare Health Systems Inc.
3100 W Lake Ctr. Dr.
Mail Stop LC03-381
Santa Ana, CA 92704
Phone: (714)825-5379 **Free:** 800-204-6629
Fax: (949)348-5610
Website: http://www.pacificare.com
Ronald M. Davis, President

★ 17626 ★ PacifiCare Life Insurance Co.
PacifiCare Health Systems Inc.
3100 W Lake Ctr. Dr.
Mail Stop LC03-381
Santa Ana, CA 92704
Phone: (714)825-3300 **Free:** 800-204-6629
Website: http://www.pacificare.com
Ronald M. Davis, President

★ 17627 ★ PacifiCare of Nevada Inc.
PacifiCare Health Systems Inc.
3120 Lake Ctr. Dr.
Santa Ana, CA 92704
Phone: (702)269-7500
Website: http://www.pacificare.com
Harold B. Coats, President

★ 17628 ★ PacifiCare of Oklahoma Inc.
PacifiCare Health Systems Inc.
7666 E 61st St.
Tulsa, OK 74133
Phone: (918)459-1100 **Fax:** (918)459-1450
Website: http://www.pacificare.com
Bradford A. Bowlus, Chairman of the Board

★ 17629 ★ PacifiCare of Oregon Inc.
PacifiCare Health Systems Inc.
3110 Lake Ctr. Dr., LC05-308
Santa Ana, CA 92704
Phone: (503)603-7355 **Fax:** (503)603-7123
Website: http://www.pacificare.com
Donald E. Costa, President

★ 17630 ★ PacifiCare of Texas Inc.
PacifiCare Health Systems Inc.
3110 Lake Ctr. Dr., LC05-308
Santa Ana, CA 92704
Phone: (972)866-1693
Website: http://www.pacificare.com
James Cassity, President

★ 17631 ★ PacifiCare of Washington
PacifiCare Health Systems Inc.
7525 SE 24th St., Ste. 200
PO Box 9005
Mercer Island, WA 98040
Phone: (206)230-7400 **Fax:** (206)232-3099
Website: http://www.pacificare.com
Donald E. Costa, President

★ 17632 ★ Pan-American Assurance Co.
Pan-American Life Group
PO Box 53372
New Orleans, LA 70153-3372
Phone: (504)566-1300 **Fax:** (504)566-3950
Jan S. Jobe, CEO & Pres

★ 17633 ★ Pan-American Life Insurance Co.
Pan-American Life Group
PO Box 60219
New Orleans, LA 70160-0219
Phone: (504)566-1300 **Fax:** (504)566-3950
Website: http://www.wewill4u.com
Jan S. Jobe, CEO & Pres

★ 17634 ★ Paragon Life Insurance Co.
Metropolitan Life and Affiliated Cos.
100 S Brentwood Blvd.
Saint Louis, MO 63105
Phone: (314)862-2211 **Fax:** (314)862-5171
Website: http://www.paragonlife.com
Anthony F. Trani, CEO & Pres

★ 17635 ★ Paramount Care Inc.
ProMedica Insurance Corp.
1901 Indian Wood Cir.
Maumee, OH 43537
Phone: (419)887-2500
John C. Randolph, President

★ 17636 ★ Paramount Care of Michigan
ProMedica Insurance Corp.
PO Box 928
Toledo, OH 43697-0928
Phone: (313)241-5998
Website: http://www.paramounthealthcare.com
John C. Randolph, President

★ 17637 ★ Paramount Security Life Insurance Co.
1524 Irving Pl.
Shreveport, LA 71101
Phone: (318)222-9489
Charles J. Stamper, President

★ 17638 ★ Park Avenue Life Insurance Co.
Guardian Life Group
7 Hanover Sq.
New York, NY 10004-2616
Phone: (212)598-8000
Website: http://www.glic.com
Peter L. Hutchings, President

★ 17639 ★ Parkland Community Health Plan Inc.
6300 Harry Hines, Ste. 300
Dallas, TX 75235
Phone: (214)590-0966 **Fax:** (214)590-4840

★ 17640 ★ Partners National Health Plans of Indiana Inc.
100 E Wayne St., Ste. 502
South Bend, IN 46601
Phone: (219)233-4899

★ 17641 ★ Partners National Health Plans of North Carolina Inc.
Blue Cross & Blue Shield of N. Carolina
2085 Frontis Plaza Blvd.
Winston-Salem, NC 27103
Phone: (336)760-4822

★ 17642 ★ Pathmark Assurance Co.
Ameritas Acacia Group
PO Box 81889
Lincoln, NE 68501
Phone: (402)467-1122 **Fax:** (402)465-6100
Website: http://www.ameritasacacia.com
David C. Moore, President

★ 17643 ★ Patriot Life Insurance Co.
110 Free St.
Portland, ME 04101
Phone: (207)822-5920
Robert G. Schatz, President

★ 17644 ★ The Paul Revere Life Insurance Co.
UnumProvident Corp.
1 Fountain Sq.
Chattanooga, TN 37402-1330
Phone: (423)755-1011 **Fax:** (423)642-4260
Website: http://www.unumprovident.com
J. Harold Chandler, CEO & Chm Bd

★ 17645 ★ The Paul Revere Variable Annuity Insurance Co.
UnumProvident Corp.
1 Fountain Sq.
Chattanooga, TN 37402-1330
Phone: (423)755-1011 **Fax:** (423)642-4260
Website: http://www.unumprovident.com
J. Harold Chandler, CEO & Chm Bd

★ 17646 ★ Pekin Financial Life Insurance Co.
Pekin Insurance Group
2505 Court St.
Pekin, IL 61558
Phone: (309)346-1161 **Fax:** (309)346-8512
Website: http://www.pekininsurance.com
Robert W. Scheffler, CEO & Chm Bd

★ 17647 ★ Pekin Life Insurance Co.
Pekin Insurance Group
2505 Court St.
Pekin, IL 61558-0001
Phone: (309)346-1161 **Fax:** (309)346-8512
Website: http://www.pekininsurance.com
Robert W. Scheffler, CEO & Chm Bd
Ronnie Fry, Senior VP

★ 17648 ★ Pellerin Life Insurance Co.
PO Box 130
Breaux Bridge, LA 70517-0130
Phone: (337)332-2111
Frank E. Pellerin, President

★ 17649 ★ PEMCO Life Insurance Co.
PEMCO Insurance Companies
325 Eastlake Ave. E
Seattle, WA 98109-5466
Phone: (206)628-4290 **Fax:** (206)628-8718
Website: http://www.pemco.com
Stan W. McNaughton, President

★ 17650 ★ Peninsula Health Care Inc.
Trigon Healthcare Inc.
606 Denbigh Blvd., Ste. 500
Newport News, VA 23608
Phone: (757)875-5760
Website: http://www.trigon.com
Richard J. Pearce, Chairman of the Board

★ 17651 ★ Peninsular Life Insurance Co.
Universal American Financial Corp.
600 Courtland St.
Orlando, FL 32804
Phone: (407)628-1776 **Fax:** (407)628-4227
Gary W. Bryant, President

★ 17652 ★ Penn Insurance and Annuity Co.
Penn Mutual Group
600 Dresher Rd.
Horsham, PA 19044
Phone: (215)956-9177 **Fax:** (215)956-8145
Website: http://www.penmutual.com
Daniel J. Toran, President

★ 17653 ★ The Penn Mutual Life Insurance Co.
Penn Mutual Group
600 Dresher Rd.
Horsham, PA 19044
Phone: (215)956-8000 **Fax:** (215)956-8145
Website: http://www.pennmutual.com
Daniel J. Toran, President
Robert E. Chappell, CEO & Chm Bd

★ 17654 ★ Penn Treaty Network America Insurance Co.
Penn Treaty American Corp.
3440 Lehigh St.
Allentown, PA 18103-7001
Phone: (610)965-2222 **Fax:** (610)967-4616
Website: http://www.penntreaty.com
Irving Levit, CEO & Chm Bd

★ 17655 ★ Pennsylvania Dental Service Corp.
Dentegra Group Inc.
1 Delta Dr.
Mechanicsburg, PA 17055
Phone: (717)766-8500
Gary D. Radine, President

★ 17656 ★ Pennsylvania Life Insurance Co.
Universal American Financial Corp.
600 Courtland St.
Orlando, FL 32804
Phone: (407)628-1776 **Fax:** (407)628-3647
William E. Wehner, Jr., President

★ 17657 ★ Pension Life Insurance Co. of America
AEGON USA, Inc.
200 Moores Rd.
Frazer, PA 19355
Phone: (610)648-5000 **Fax:** (610)648-5326
Paul Reaburn, President

★ 17658 ★ Peoples Benefit Life Insurance Co.
AEGON USA, Inc.
4333 Edgewood Rd. NE
Cedar Rapids, IA 52499
Phone: (319)398-8511
Marilyn Carp, President

★ 17659 ★ Peoples Savings Life Insurance Co.
PO Box 729
Alexander City, AL 35010
Phone: (904)384-1204

★ 17660 ★ Performance Life of America
LDS Group
PO Box 83480
Baton Rouge, LA 70884-3480
Phone: (225)769-9923 **Fax:** (225)767-7656
Website: http://www.theldsgroup.com
Dick S. Taylor, President

★ 17661 ★ PersonalCare Insurance of Illinois, Inc.
PersonalCare Health Management Inc.
2110 Fox Dr.
Champaign, IL 61820
Phone: (217)366-1226 **Fax:** (217)366-5580
Website: http://www.personalcarehmo.com
David L. Line, CEO & Pres

★ 17662 ★ The Pharmacists Life Insurance Co.
Pharmacists Insurance Group
PO Box 370
Algona, IA 50511
Phone: (515)295-2461 **Fax:** (515)295-3261
Website: http://www.phmic.com
Kirk M. Hayes, Chairman of the Board

★ 17663 ★ Philadelphia American Life Insurance Co.
New Era Group
200 Westlake Park Blvd.
Houston, TX 77079-2663
Phone: (281)368-7200
Bill S. Chen, CEO & Pres

★ 17664 ★ Philadelphia-United Life Insurance Co.
Philadelphia-United Insurance Cos.
150 Monument Rd., Ste. 600
Bala Cynwyd, PA 19004
Phone: (610)660-6600 **Fax:** (610)660-6604
Robert B. Ries, President
Chester B. Radecki, Vice President

★ 17665 ★ Philanthropic Mutual Life Insurance Co.
Philanthropic Companies
401 Plymouth Rd., Ste. 100
Plymouth Meeting, PA 19462
Phone: (610)684-2400 **Fax:** (610)684-2480
Website: http://www.thephilanthropic.com
Richard E. Bauer, President

★ 17666 ★ PHL Variable Insurance Co.
Phoenix Life Group
1 American Row
Hartford, CT 06115
Phone: (860)403-1000
Website: http://www.phoenix.wm.com
Simon Yeh-Cheng Tan, President

★ 17667 ★ PHN-HMO Inc.
Preferred Health Network of Maryland
1099 Winterson Rd.
Linthicum, MD 21090-2216
Phone: (410)850-7461

★ 17668 ★ Phoenix Life and Annuity Co.
Phoenix Life Group
1 American Row
Hartford, CT 06115
Phone: (860)403-1000
Website: http://www.phoenixwm.com
Simon Y. Tan, President

★ 17669 ★ Phoenix Life Insurance Co.
Phoenix Life Group
1 American Row
Hartford, CT 06115
Phone: (518)479-8000
Website: http://www.phoenixwm.com
Dona D. Young, President
Frmly: Phoenix Home Life Mutual Insurance Co.

★ 17670 ★ Phoenix Life & Reassurance Co. of New York
Phoenix Life Group
1 American Row
Hartford, CT 06115
Phone: (518)479-8000
Website: http://www.phoenixwm.com
David R. Pellerin, President

★ 17671 ★ Phoenix National Insurance Co.
Phoenix Life Group
1 American Row
Hartford, CT 06115
Phone: (860)403-1000
Website: http://www.phoenixwm.com
Gina C. O'Connell, President

★ 17672 ★ PHP Insurance Plan Inc.
Prevea Health Services Inc.
PO Box 11625
Green Bay, WI 54307-1625
Phone: (715)845-5211

★ 17673 ★ Physicians Benefits Trust Life Insurance Co.
20 N Michigan Ave., Ste. 700
Chicago, IL 60602
Phone: (217)363-0170 **Free:** 888-471-4741
Donald A. Udstuen, President

★ 17674 ★ Physicians Health Plan of Mid-Michigan
Sparrow Health System
825 Centennial Way
Lansing, MI 48917-9277
Phone: (517)327-0640

★ 17675 ★ Physicians Health Plan of Northern Indiana Inc.
8101 W Jefferson Blvd.
Fort Wayne, IN 46804
Phone: (219)432-6690 **Fax:** (219)432-0493

★ 17676 ★ Physicians Healthcare Plans Inc.
1410 N Westshore Blvd., Ste. 200
Tampa, FL 33607
Phone: (813)273-7474 **Fax:** (813)829-8308
Website: http://www.php.com

★ 17677 ★ Physicians Life Insurance Co.
Physicians Mutual Group
2600 Dodge St.
Omaha, NE 68131
Phone: (402)633-1000 **Fax:** (402)633-1096
Website: http://www.pmic.com
Robert A. Reed, President

★ 17678 ★ Physicians Mutual Insurance Co.
Physicians Mutual Group
2600 Dodge St.
Omaha, NE 68131
Phone: (402)633-1000 **Fax:** (402)633-1096
Website: http://www.physiciansmutual.com
Robert A. Reed, CEO & Pres

★ 17679 ★ Physicians Plus Insurance Corp.
22 E Mifflin St.
Madison, WI 53703
Phone: (608)282-8900

★ 17680 ★ Piedmont Insurance Co.
PO Box 979
Marion, SC 29571
Phone: (803)423-5541
Jones T. Hunter, Jr., President

★ 17681 ★ Pioneer American Insurance Co.
American Amicable Group
PO Box 240
Waco, TX 76703-0240
Phone: (254)297-2776 **Fax:** (254)297-2784
Website: http://www.pioneeramerican.com
S. Lanny Peavy, CEO & Pres

★ 17682 ★ Pioneer Life Insurance Co.
Conseco Insurance Group
11815 N Pennsylvania St.
Carmel, IN 46032
Phone: (317)817-4800 **Fax:** (317)817-2161
Website: http://www.conseco.com
Elizabeth C. Georgakopoulos, President

★ 17683 ★ Pioneer Mutual Life Insurance Co.
American United Life Group
PO Box 2546
Fargo, ND 58108-2546
Phone: (701)277-2300 **Fax:** (701)277-2234
Website: http://www.pmlife.com
Douglas C. Oksendahl, CEO & Pres

★ 17684 ★ Pioneer Security Life Insurance Co.
American Amicable Group
PO Box 2550
Waco, TX 76702-2550
Phone: (254)297-2778 **Fax:** (254)297-2784
Website: http://www.pioneersecuritylife.com
S. Lanny Peavy, CEO & Pres

★ 17685 ★ Plateau Insurance Co.
Plateau Group, Inc.
PO Box 7001
Crossville, TN 38557-7001
Phone: (931)484-8411 **Fax:** (931)484-0692
Website: http://www.plateaugroup.com
William D. Williams, CEO & Pres

★ 17686 ★ Polish Roman Catholic Union of America
984 Milwaukee Ave.
Chicago, IL 60622-4101
Phone: (773)782-2600 **Fax:** (773)278-4595
Website: http://www.prcua.org
Wallace M. Ozog, President

★ 17687 ★ Port-O-Call Life Insurance Co.
3131 Olive St.
Pine Bluff, AR 71603
Phone: (870)535-2885
Henry F. Trotter, Jr., President

★ 17688 ★ Preferred Assurance Co. Inc.
259 Monroe Ave.
Rochester, NY 14607
Phone: (585)325-3920
John Urban, President

★ 17689 ★ Preferred Health
Calle Maximo Alomar 1167 Urb.
San Agustin
San Juan, PR 00924
Phone: (787)641-1500 **Fax:** (787)758-1508
Website: http://www.preferredhealthplan.com

★ 17690 ★ Preferred Health Northwest, Inc.
Regence Group
PO Box 1271
Portland, OR 97207-1271
Phone: (503)225-5221 **Fax:** (503)225-6755
Website: http://www.or.regence.com
Mark B. Ganz, President

★ 17691 ★ Preferred Health Partnership of Tennessee Inc.
PHP Companies Inc.
1420 Centerpoint Blvd.
Knoxville, TN 37932
Phone: (423)470-7470

★ 17692 ★ Preferred Health Systems Inc.
Blue Cross & Blue Shield of South Carolina
I-20 E at Alpine Rd.
Columbia, SC 29219
Phone: (803)788-0222
Website: http://www.southcarolinablues.com
Thomas G. Faulds, President

★ 17693 ★ Preferred Health Systems Insurance Co.
8535 E 21st St. N
Wichita, KS 67206
Phone: (316)609-2345 **Fax:** (316)609-2346
Website: http://www.phsystems.com
Marlon R. Dauner, President

★ 17694 ★ Preferred Life Insurance Co. of New York
Allianz Insurance Group
152 W 57th St., 18th Fl.
New York, NY 10019
Phone: (212)586-7733 **Fax:** (212)586-6949
Website: http://www.allianzlife.com
Charles M. Kavitsky, CEO & Chm Bd

★ 17695 ★ Preferred Medical Plan
4950 SW 8th St.
Coral Gables, FL 33134
Phone: (305)447-8373

★ 17696 ★ Preferred Plus of Kansas Inc.
Preferred Health System Inc.
8535 E 21st N
Wichita, KS 67206
Phone: (316)609-2345

★ 17697 ★ Preferred Security Life Insurance Co.
PO Box 5357
Dallas, TX 75208
Phone: (214)941-9592
Rhonda Hughes, President

★ 17698 ★ PreferredOne Community Health Plan
Fairview Health System & North Memorial Health Center
6105 Golden Hills Dr.
Golden Valley, MN 55416
Phone: (763)847-4000

★ 17699 ★ Premier Access Insurance Co.
Access Dental Plan
555 University Ave., Ste. 182
Sacramento, CA 95825
Phone: (916)920-2500
Reza Abbaszadeh, President

★ 17700 ★ Premier Behavioral Systems of Tennessee LLC
222 2nd Ave. N, Ste. 220
Nashville, TN 37201
Phone: (615)313-4400

★ 17701 ★ Premier Health Inc.
Blue Cross & Blue Shield of Kansas
419 W 29th St.
Topeka, KS 66611
Phone: (785)291-8700
John W. Knack, CEO & Chm Bd

★ 17702 ★ Premier Medical Insurance Group, Inc.
Dean Health System/SSM Health Care
1277 Deming Way
Madison, WI 53717
Phone: (608)836-1400
John A. Turcott, President

★ 17703 ★ Preneed Reinsurance Co. of America
NGL Insurance Group
2 E Gilman St.
PO Box 1191
Madison, WI 53701-1191
Phone: (608)257-5612
John D. Larson, CEO & Pres

★ 17704 ★ Presbyterian Health Plan Inc.
Presbyterian Network Inc.
2301 Buena Vista SE
Albuquerque, NM 87106
Phone: (505)923-5700
Website: http://www.phs.org

★ 17705 ★ Preservation Life Insurance Co.
3401 W Truman Blvd., Ste. 100-A
Jefferson City, MO 65109
Phone: (573)635-8492
John W. McCulloch, President
Frmly: OakRe Life Insurance Co.

★ 17706 ★ Presidential Life Insurance Co.
Presidential Life Corp.
69 Lydecker St.
Nyack, NY 10960
Phone: (845)358-2300 **Fax:** (845)353-0273
Website: http://www.presidentiallife.com
Donald Barnes, President

★ 17707 ★ Primary Health Network Inc.
PO Box 191050
Boise, ID 83712
Phone: (208)344-1811
Elden R. Mitchell, President

★ 17708 ★ PrimeHealth of Alabama Inc.
USA Foundation
1400 University Blvd. S
Mobile, AL 36609
Phone: (334)342-0022

★ 17709 ★ Primerica Life Insurance Co.
Citigroup
307 W 7th St., Ste. 400
Fort Worth, TX 76102
Phone: (770)381-1000 **Fax:** (770)564-6279
Website: http://www.primerica.com
Jeffrey S. Fendler, President

★ 17710 ★ Primetime Medical Insurance Co.
Aultman Health Foundation
PO Box 6910
Canton, OH 44706-0910
Phone: (330)438-6360
Rick L. Haines, President

★ 17711 ★ Princeton Reinsurance Co.
201 N Central Ave.
Phoenix, AZ 85073
Phone: (952)945-3579
Dolores G. Fiabane, President

★ 17712 ★ Principal Life Insurance Co.
Principal Financial Group
711 High St.
Des Moines, IA 50392-2300
Phone: (515)247-5111 **Fax:** (515)247-5930
Website: http://www.principal.com
J. Barry Griswell, CEO & Chm Bd

★ 17713 ★ Priority Health
Spectrum Health Corp. and Holland Hospital
1231 E Beltline NE
Grand Rapids, MI 49525
Free: 800-942-0954
Website: http://www.priority-health.com

★ 17714 ★ Priority Health Care Inc.
Trigon Healthcare Inc.
2220 Edward Holland Dr.
Richmond, VA 23230
Phone: (804)354-3479
Website: http://www.trigon.com
Thomas G. Snead, Jr., Chairman of the Board

★ 17715 ★ Private Medical-Care Inc.
Dentegra Group Inc.
100 1st St.
San Francisco, CA 94105
Phone: (562)924-8311 **Fax:** (562)924-8039
Website: http://www.deltadentalca.org
William T. Ward, Chairman of the Board

★ 17716 ★ Professional Insurance Co.
GE Financial Assurance Group
6604 W Broad St.
Richmond, VA 23230
Free: 800-730-6484
Website: http://www.gefinancialassurance.com
Marcia Cantor-Grable, President

★ 17717 ★ Professional Life and Casualty Co.
20 N Wacker Dr., Ste. 3110
Chicago, IL 60606
Phone: (312)220-0655 **Fax:** (312)220-0882
Paul F. Nord, MD, President
Robert Bruce, Chairman of the Board

★ 17718 ★ Programmed Life Insurance Co.
6535 S Dayton St., Ste. 1100
Greenwood Village, CO 80111
Phone: (303)790-2090
Website: http://www.conseco.com
Gregory J. Richards, President

★ 17719 ★ Progressive American Life Insurance Co.
Progressive Corp.
6300 Wilson Mills Rd., W33
Mayfield Village, OH 44143-2182
Phone: (440)461-5000 **Fax:** (440)446-7168
Website: http://www.progressive.com
Peter B. Lewis, Chairman of the Board
Charles C. Boucherle, President

★ 17720 ★ Protected Home Mutual Life Insurance Co.
30 E State St.
Sharon, PA 16146-1767
Phone: (724)981-1520 **Fax:** (724)981-0199
Website: http://www.protectedlife.com
Leonard S. Miller, CEO & Pres
Raymond E. Burckart, Senior VP

★ 17721 ★ Protective Dental Care Inc.
Fortis Inc.
3595 Grandview Pkwy., Ste. 150
Birmingham, AL 35243
Phone: (205)909-6000
Michael J. Peninger, CEO

★ 17722 ★ Protective Dentalcare of New Jersey Inc.
Fortis Inc.
3595 Grandview Pkwy., Ste. 150
Birmingham, AL 35243
Phone: (205)909-6000
Michael J. Peninger, CEO

★ 17723 ★ Protective Industrial Insurance Co. of Alabama
Protective Industrial of Alabama Group
PO Box 2744
Birmingham, AL 35202-2744
Phone: (205)323-5256 **Fax:** (205)251-7614
James C. Harrison, President

★ 17724 ★ Protective Life & Annuity Insurance Co.
Protective Life Corp.
2801 Hwy. 280 S
Birmingham, AL 35223
Phone: (205)879-9230 **Fax:** (205)868-3270
Website: http://www.protective.com
Wayne E. Stuenkel, President

★ 17725 ★ Protective Life Insurance Co.
Protective Life Corp.
2801 Hwy. 280 S
Birmingham, AL 35223
Phone: (205)879-9230 **Fax:** (205)868-3270
Website: http://www.protective.com
John D. Johns, CEO & Pres
Drayton Nabers, Jr., Chairman of the Board

★ 17726 ★ Protective Life Insurance Co. of Kentucky
Protective Life Corp.
2801 Hwy. 280 S
Birmingham, AL 35223
Phone: (205)879-9230
Website: http://www.protective.com
Steven A. Schultz, President

★ 17727 ★ Protective Life Insurance Co. of Ohio
Protective Life Corp.
2801 Hwy. 280 S
Birmingham, AL 35223
Phone: (205)879-9230
Steven A. Schultz, President

★ 17728 ★ Providence Health Plan
Providence Health Group
3601 SW Murray Blvd., Ste. 10
Beaverton, OR 97005
Phone: (503)215-3215

★ 17729 ★ Provident American Insurance Co.
PO Box 679005
Dallas, TX 75367-9005
Phone: (214)696-9091 **Fax:** (214)696-1681
Website: http://www.providentamerican.com
James E. Ludlum, III, President

★ 17730 ★ Provident American Life & Health Insurance Co.
Ceres Group Inc.
17800 Royalton Rd.
Strongsville, OH 44136-5197
Phone: (440)572-2400 **Fax:** (440)878-3600
Anthony J. Pino, President

★ 17731 ★ Provident Indemnity Life Insurance Co.
PO Box 511
Norristown, PA 19404-0511
Phone: (610)278-5482 **Fax:** (610)279-1486
Alvin H. Clemens, President

★ 17732 ★ Provident Life and Accident Insurance Co.
UnumProvident Corp.
1 Fountain Sq.
Chattanooga, TN 37402-1330
Phone: (423)755-1011 **Fax:** (423)642-4260
Website: http://www.unumprovident.com
J. Harold Chandler, CEO & Chm Bd

★ 17733 ★ Provident Life and Casualty Insurance Co.
UnumProvident Corp.
1 Fountain Sq.
Chattanooga, TN 37402-1330
Phone: (423)755-1011 **Fax:** (423)642-4260
Website: http://www.unumprovident.com
J. Harold Chandler, CEO & Chm Bd

★ 17734 ★ Provident Mutual International Life Insurance Co.
Provident Mutual Life Group
PO Box 15750
Wilmington, DE 19850-5750
Phone: (610)407-1717
Website: http://www.providentmutual.com
Robert W. Kloss, CEO & Pres

★ 17735 ★ Provident Mutual Life & Annuity Co. of America
Provident Mutual Life Group
PO Box 15760
Wilmington, DE 19850-5750
Phone: (610)407-1717 **Fax:** (610)407-1438
Website: http://www.providentmutual.com
Robert W. Kloss, President

★ 17736 ★ Provident Mutual Life Insurance Co.
Provident Mutual Life Group
PO Box 1717
Valley Forge, PA 19482-1717
Phone: (610)407-1717 **Fax:** (610)407-1438
Website: http://www.providentmutual.com
Robert W. Kloss, CEO & Chm Bd

★ 17737 ★ Pruco Life Insurance Co.
Prudential of America Group
213 Washington St.
Newark, NJ 07102-2992
Phone: (973)802-6000 **Free:** 877-301-1212
Fax: (973)367-8204
Vivian L. Banta, President

★ 17738 ★ Pruco Life Insurance Co. of New Jersey
Prudential of America Group
213 Washington St.
Newark, NJ 07102-2992
Phone: (973)802-6000 **Fax:** (973)367-8204
Vivian L. Banta, President

★ 17739 ★ Prudential Dental Maintenance Organization Inc.
Aetna Inc.
2777 Stemmons Fwy., Ste. 400
Dallas, TX 75207
Free: 800-872-3862
Scott A. Schnuckle, President

★ 17740 ★ Prudential Health Care Plan of California Inc.
Aetna Inc.
980 Jolly Rd.
Blue Bell, PA 19422
Phone: (818)712-5046
Website: http://www.aetnaushc.com

★ 17741 ★ Prudential Health Care Plan of Georgia Inc.
Aetna Inc.
980 Jolly Rd.
Blue Bell, PA 19422
Free: 800-872-3862
Website: http://www.aetnaushc.com
Joseph T. Blanford, III, President

★ 17742 ★ Prudential Health Care Plan Inc.
Aetna Inc.
980 Jolly Rd.
Blue Bell, PA 19422
Free: 800-872-3862
Website: http://www.aetnaushc.com
John W. Coyle, President

★ 17743 ★ The Prudential Insurance Co. of America
Prudential of America Group
213 Washington St., 9th Fl.
Newark, NJ 07102-2992
Phone: (973)802-6000 **Fax:** (973)367-8204
Website: http://www.prudential.com
Arthur F. Ryan, CEO & Chm Bd

★ 17744 ★ Prudential Select Life Insurance Co. of America
Prudential of America Group
213 Washington St.
Newark, NJ 07102-2992
Phone: (973)802-6000
Vivian L. Banta, President

★ 17745 ★ Public Health Trust of Dade County
1801 NW 9th Ave., Ste. 700
Miami, FL 33136
Phone: (305)578-3700

★ 17746 ★ Puerto Rican-American Life Insurance Co.
PO Box 70297
San Juan, PR 00936
Phone: (787)753-6161 **Fax:** (787)758-7409
Website: http://www.praico.com
Juan A. Terrassa, CEO & Chm Bd

★ 17747 ★ Pupil Benefits Plan Inc.
126 Saratoga Rd.
Glenville, NY 12302
Phone: (518)399-0510
Michael Picciano, President

★ 17748 ★ Pyramid Life Insurance Co.
Ceres Group Inc.
17800 Royalton Rd.
Strongsville, OH 44136
Phone: (913)722-1110 **Fax:** (913)722-3567
Website: http://www.pyramidlife.com
Mark A. Nielsen, President
Peter W. Nauert, Chairman of the Board

★ 17749 ★ QCA Health Plan Inc.
Tenet HealthSystem Hospitals Inc.
10800 Financial Centre Pkwy., Ste. 540
Little Rock, AR 72211
Phone: (501)228-7111

★ 17750 ★ QCC Insurance Co.
1901 Market St., 42nd Fl.
Philadelphia, PA 19103-1480
Phone: (215)241-2529
G. Fred DiBona, Jr., President

★ 17751 ★ QualChoice Health Plan, Inc.
University Hospitals Health System, Inc.
6000 Parkland Blvd.
Cleveland, OH 44124
Phone: (440)460-0093 **Fax:** (440)460-4000
Website: http://www.qchp.com
Thomas A. Sullivan, President

★ 17752 ★ QualChoice of North Carolina Inc.
North Carolina Baptist Hospital
100 Kimel Forest Dr.
Winston-Salem, NC 27103
Phone: (336)716-0900

★ 17753 ★ Rabenhorst Life Insurance Co.
PO Box 2666
Baton Rouge, LA 70821
Phone: (225)387-0171
David L. Rabenhorst, President

★ 17754 ★ Reassure America Life Insurance Co.
Swiss Reinsurance Group
175 King St.
Armonk, NY 10504
Phone: (217)291-2000 **Fax:** (217)245-1922
Website: http://www.swissre.com
Chris C. Stroup, CEO & Pres

★ 17755 ★ Regal Life of America Insurance Co.
PO Box 982005
Fort Worth, TX 76182-8005
Phone: (817)284-4888
Frank M. Croy, President

★ 17756 ★ Regal Life Insurance Co. ALS
704 Quince Orchard Rd., Ste. 310
Gaithersburg, MD 20878
Phone: (301)948-9000 **Fax:** (301)948-4753
Website: http://www.bankersins.com
Lloyd Yavener, President

★ 17757 ★ Regal Reinsurance Co.
Regal Reinsurance Group
1 Monarch Pl.
Springfield, MA 01133
Phone: (413)784-2000 **Fax:** (413)784-6408
Kevin J. McAdoo, President

★ 17758 ★ Regence Life & Health Insurance Co.
Regence Group
PO Box 1271/MS E3-A
Portland, OR 97207-1271
Phone: (503)225-6048 **Fax:** (503)276-1893
John Nicklo, CEO & Pres

★ 17759 ★ Regence Northwest Health
Regence Group
PO Box 21267
Seattle, WA 98111-3267
Phone: (509)525-5220
Mary O. McWilliams, President

★ 17760 ★ Reinsurance Co. of Missouri, Inc.
Metropolitan Life and Affiliated Companies
1370 Timberlake Manor Pkwy.
Chesterfield, MO 63017-6039
Phone: (636)736-7368
David B. Atkinson, CEO & Pres

★ 17761 ★ Reliable Life Insurance Co.
718 Jackson St.
PO Box 1157
Mobile, AL 36633
Phone: (318)387-1000

★ 17762 ★ The Reliable Life Insurance Co.
Unitrin, Inc.
231 W Lockwood Ave.
Webster Groves, MO 63119-2327
Phone: (314)968-4900 **Fax:** (314)968-6778
Website: http://www.unitrin.com
Don M. Royster, Sr., President
Donald G. Southwell, Chairman of the Board

★ 17763 ★ The Reliable Life Insurance Co. of Texas
Unitrin, Inc.
1 E Wacker Dr.
Chicago, IL 60601
Phone: (817)295-7205
Website: http://www.unitrin.com
Don M. Royster, Sr., President

★ 17764 ★ Reliable Service Insurance Co.
PO Box 1157
Monroe, AL 71210
Phone: (318)387-1000

★ 17765 ★ Reliance Life Insurance Co.
Reliance
3 Parkway
Philadelphia, PA 19102
Phone: (215)864-4000
Robert E. Haberle, President

★ 17766 ★ Reliance Standard Life Insurance Co.
Reliance Standard Life Group
2001 Market St., Ste. 1500
Philadelphia, PA 19103
Phone: (267)256-3500 **Fax:** (267)256-3522
Website: http://www.rsli.com
Lawrence E. Daurelle, CEO & Pres
Robert Rosenkranz, Chairman of the Board

★ 17767 ★ Reliance Standard Life Insurance Co. of Texas
Reliance Standard Life Group
2001 Market St., Ste. 1500
Philadelphia, PA 19103
Phone: (267)256-3500 **Fax:** (267)256-3522
Website: http://www.rsli.com
Lawrence E. Daurelle, CEO & Pres

★ 17768 ★ ReliaStar Life Insurance Co.
ING Group
5780 Powers Ferry Rd. NW
Atlanta, GA 30327
Phone: (612)372-5432
Website: http://www.reliastar.com
Chris D. Schreier, President

★ 17769 ★ ReliaStar Life Insurance Co. of New York
ING Group
1000 Woodbury Rd., Ste. 102
Woodbury, NY 11797
Phone: (516)682-8700
James R. Gelder, CEO & Pres

★ 17770 ★ Renaissance Health Plan
EHN Holdings Inc.
1100 Superior Ave.
Cleveland, OH 44114
Phone: (216)902-7562

★ 17771 ★ Renaissance Life & Health Insurance Co.
PO Box 30416
Lansing, MI 48909-7916
Phone: (517)349-6000

★ 17772 ★ Republic American Life Insurance Co.
Life of America Group
8200 Brookriver Dr., Ste. 600N
Dallas, TX 75247-4069
Phone: (214)631-6310 **Fax:** (214)688-7475
Joseph S. Meziere, President

★ 17773 ★ Republic-Vanguard Life Insurance Co.
SCOR Life US Group
15305 Dallas Pkwy., Ste. 700
Addison, TX 75001
Phone: (972)560-9500 **Fax:** (972)560-9535
Website: http://www.scor.com
Yves I. Corcos, CEO

★ 17774 ★ Reserve National Insurance Co.
Unitrin, Inc.
6100 NW Grand Blvd.
Oklahoma City, OK 73118
Phone: (405)848-7931 **Fax:** (405)842-0499
Website: http://www.unitrin.com
Roger W. Cole, President
Joe Cole, Exec VP

★ 17775 ★ Resource Life Insurance Co.
Combined Specialty A & H Group
Aon Ctr., 5th Fl.
200 E Randolph Dr.
Chicago, IL 60601
Phone: (312)381-1000 **Fax:** (312)381-0118
Steven E. Lippai, President

★ 17776 ★ RGA Reinsurance Co.
RGA Group
1370 Timberlake Manor Pkwy.
Chesterfield, MO 63017-6039
Phone: (636)736-7000 **Fax:** (636)736-7155
Website: http://www.rgare.com
David B. Atkinson, CEO & Pres

★ 17777 ★ Rhodes Life Insurance Co. of Louisiana, Inc.
1716 N Claiborne Ave.
New Orleans, LA 70116
Phone: (504)943-6621
D. Joan Brown, President

★ 17778 ★ RightChoice Insurance Co.
WellPoint Health Networks Inc.
1831 Chestnut St.
Saint Louis, MO 63103-2275
Phone: (314)923-4444 **Fax:** (314)923-8958
Website: http://www.abcbs.com
John A. O'Rourke, CEO & Chm Bd

★ 17779 ★ Rochester Area Health Maintenance Organization Inc.
Preferred Care Inc.
259 Monroe Ave.
Rochester, NY 14607
Phone: (716)325-3920

★ 17780 ★ Rockford Health Plans, Inc.
3401 Perryville Rd.
Rockford, IL 61114
Phone: (815)971-5845
Edward A. Pattrozzi, President

★ 17781 ★ Rocky Mountain Health Maintenance Organization Inc.
Rocky Mountain HealthCare Options Inc.
2775 Crossroads Blvd.
Grand Junction, CO 81506
Phone: (970)244-7760

★ 17782 ★ Rocky Mountain HealthCare Options, Inc.
PO Box 10600
Grand Junction, CO 81502-5600
Phone: (970)244-7760
John P. Hopkins, President

★ 17783 ★ Rocky Mountain Hospital & Medical Service
Anthem Inc.
700 Broadway
Denver, CO 80273-0002
Phone: (303)831-2131
Website: http://www.anthem-inc.com
Larry C. Glasscock, CEO & Pres

★ 17784 ★ Rooney Life Insurance Co.
Golden Rule Group
7440 Woodland Dr.
Indianapolis, IN 46278-1719
Phone: (317)297-4123 **Fax:** (317)298-0875
Therese A. Rooney, CEO & Chm Bd

★ 17785 ★ Royal Neighbors of America
230 16th St.
Rock Island, IL 61201
Phone: (309)788-4561 **Fax:** (309)788-4936
Website: http://www.royalneighbors.org
Karen E. Anagnos, President

★ 17786 ★ Royal State National Insurance Co., Ltd.
819 S Beretania St., Ste. 100
Honolulu, HI 96813
Phone: (808)539-1600 **Fax:** (808)523-3803
Lilia Yu-Lum, CEO & Pres

★ 17787 ★ Ruffin & Jarrett Insurance Co.
PO Box 164867
Little Rock, AR 72216
Phone: (501)375-2403
Eunice Reed, President

★ 17788 ★ Rushmore Life Insurance Co.
North American National Life Group
6535 S Dayton St., Ste. 1100
Greenwood Village, CO 80111
Phone: (303)790-2090
Website: http://www.rushmark.com
John R. Lee, Sr., President

★ 17789 ★ Rushmore National Life Insurance Co.
Fortis, Inc. Group
PO Box 1320
Rapid City, SD 57709-1320
Phone: (605)719-0999 **Free:** 800-810-9046
Fax: (605)719-0853
John E. Wade, President

★ 17790 ★ Sabine Life Insurance Co.
PO Box 119
Many, LA 71449-0119
Phone: (318)256-2812
Floyd Josseph Giblin, President

★ 17791 ★ SAFECO Life Insurance Co.
SAFECO Life Group
PO Box 34690
Seattle, WA 98124-1690
Phone: (425)376-8000 **Fax:** (425)376-5818
Website: http://www.safeco.com
Randall H. Talbot, President
Roger Eigsti, Chairman of the Board

★ 17792 ★ SAFECO National Life Insurance Co.
SAFECO Life Group
PO Box 34690
Seattle, WA 98124-1690
Phone: (425)376-8000 **Fax:** (425)376-5818
Website: http://www.safeco.com
Randall H. Talbot, President

★ 17793 ★ SafeHealth Life Insurance Co.
PO Box 30930
Laguna Hills, CA 92654-0930
Phone: (949)425-4531

★ 17794 ★ Sage Life Assurance of America Inc.
300 Atlantic St., Ste. 302
Stamford, CT 06901

Phone: (203)602-6500 Fax: (203)324-6173
Website: http://www.sagelife.com
Robin I. Marsden, CEO & Pres

★ 17795 ★ Saint Mary's HealthFirst Inc.
Saint Mary's Managed Care Corp.
1155 W 4th St., Ste. 216
Reno, NV 89503
Phone: (775)829-6000

★ 17796 ★ St. Mary's Preferred Health Insurance Co.
1155 W 4th St., Ste. 121
Reno, NV 89506
Phone: (775)770-6229
Stanley I. Thompson, President

★ 17797 ★ San Mateo Health Commission
701 Gateway Blvd., Ste. 400
South San Francisco, CA 94080
Phone: (650)616-0050

★ 17798 ★ Savings Bank Life Insurance Co.
111 Founders Plz., Ste.601
East Hartford, CT 06108-8309
Phone: (860)291-2000 **Fax:** (860)291-2036
Website: http://www.sblict.com
Peter L. Tedone, CEO & Pres
Duncan C. Stoddard, Chairman of the Board

★ 17799 ★ Savings Bank Life Insurance Co. of Massachusetts
PO Box 4046
Woburn, MA 01888-9973
Phone: (781)938-3500 **Fax:** (781)938-6574
Website: http://www.sbli.com
Robert K. Sheridan, CEO & Pres

★ 17800 ★ SBLI USA Financial Services Life Insurance Co., Inc.
SBLI USA Group
PO Box 1050
Newark, NJ 07101
Free: 877-725-4375
Website: http://www.sbliusa.com
Vikki L. Pryor, CEO & Pres

★ 17801 ★ SBLI USA Mutual Life Insurance Co., Inc.
SBLI USA Group
460 W 34th St., Ste. 800
New York, NY 10001-2320
Phone: (212)356-0300 **Fax:** (212)624-0746
Website: http://www.sbliusa.com
Vikki L. Pryor, CEO & Pres

★ 17802 ★ Schoen Life Insurance Co.
PO Box 19263
New Orleans, LA 70179
Phone: (504)486-7212
Charles J. D. Gerrets, III, President

★ 17803 ★ SCOR Life U.S. Re Insurance Co.
SCOR Life US Group
15305 Dallas Pkwy., Ste. 700
Addison, TX 75001
Phone: (972)560-9500 **Fax:** (972)560-9535
Website: http://www.scor.com
Yves I. Corcos, CEO

★ 17804 ★ Scott Life Insurance Co.
201 N Central Ave., Ste. 3300
Phoenix, AZ 85073
Phone: (515)557-7036
Steve R. Wagner, President

★ 17805 ★ Scott & White Group Hospital Service Corp.
Scott & White Health Plan
2401 S 31 St.
Temple, TX 76508
Phone: (254)298-3001
Alfred B. Knight, MD, President

★ 17806 ★ Scott & White Health Plan
Scott & White Health Plan Group
2401 S 31st St.
Temple, TX 76508
Phone: (254)298-3000

★ 17807 ★ Scottish Re (U.S.) Inc.
Scottish Annuity and Life Group
15800 John J. Delaney Dr., Ste. 200
Charlotte, NC 28277
Phone: (704)542-9192 **Fax:** (704)542-5744
Website: http://www.scottishre.com
Oscar R. Scofield, President

★ 17808 ★ Sears Life Insurance Co.
10255 W Higgins Rd.
Rosemont, IL 60018
Phone: (847)375-8001 **Fax:** (847)824-3428
Timothy E. Devereux, Jr., President

★ 17809 ★ SEB Trygg (USA) Assurance Ltd.
2999 N 44th St., Ste. 250
Phoenix, AZ 85018
Phone: (602)200-6900
Anders G. Mossberg, President

★ 17810 ★ Security Alliance Insurance Co.
PO Box 9494
Springfield, MO 65801
Phone: (573)659-8545
Rebecca J. Rhoden, President

★ 17811 ★ Security Benefit Life Insurance Co.
Security Benefit Group
700 SW Harrison St.
Topeka, KS 66636-0001
Phone: (785)431-3000 **Fax:** (785)438-3223
Website: http://www.securitybenefit.com
Kris A. Robbins, CEO & Pres
Howard R. Fricke, Chairman of the Board

★ 17812 ★ Security-Connecticut Life Insurance Co.
ING Group
5780 Powers Ferry Rd. NW
Atlanta, GA 30327
Phone: (612)372-5432
Website: http://www.ingsecuritylife.com
James R. Gelder, CEO & Pres
Richard R. Crowl, Senior VP

★ 17813 ★ Security Equity Life Insurance Co.
Metropolitan Life and Affiliated Cos.
1 MetLife Plaza, Area 7-B
Long Island City, NY 11101
Phone: (914)273-1290 **Fax:** (914)273-1586
William C. Thather, President

★ 17814 ★ Security Financial Life Insurance Co.
PO Box 82248
Lincoln, NE 68501-2248
Phone: (402)434-9500 **Fax:** (402)434-9599
Website: http://www.secmut.com
Thomas E. Henning, CEO & Pres

★ 17815 ★ Security General Life Insurance Co.
American Fidelity Group
PO Box 25360
Oklahoma City, OK 73125-0360
Phone: (405)523-2000 **Fax:** (405)416-7879
Website: http://www.afadvantage.com
William E. Durrett, President

★ 17816 ★ Security Health Plan of Wisconsin Inc.
Marshfield Clinic
1515 St. Joseph Ave.
PO Box 8000
Marshfield, WI 54449
Phone: (715)221-9555 **Fax:** (715)221-9500
Website: http://www.securityhealth.org

★ 17817 ★ Security Life of Denver Insurance Co.
ING Group
1290 Broadway
Denver, CO 80203
Phone: (303)860-1290 **Fax:** (303)860-2679
Chris D. Schreier, President

★ 17818 ★ Security Life Insurance Co. of America
10901 Red Circle Dr.
Minnetonka, MN 55343-9137
Phone: (952)544-2121 **Fax:** (952)945-3419
Website: http://www.securitylife.com
Susan J. Albrecht, President
J. Stephen Beckman, CEO & Pres

★ 17819 ★ Security Mutual Life Insurance Co. of New York
PO Box 1625
Binghamton, NY 13902-1625
Phone: (607)723-3551 **Fax:** (607)724-1607
Website: http://www.smlny.com
Bruce W. Boyea, CEO & Chm Bd

★ 17820 ★ Security National Life Insurance Co.
Security National Life Group
PO Box 57220
Salt Lake City, UT 84157-0220
Phone: (801)264-1060 **Fax:** (801)265-9882
George R. Quist, President

★ 17821 ★ Security Plan Life Insurance Co.
Alderwoods Group Inc.
205 Railroad Ave.
Donaldsonville, LA 70346
Phone: (225)473-8654 **Fax:** (225)473-6966
Website: http://www.mayflowernational.com
Stephen J. Smith, President

★ 17822 ★ Seguros De Vida Triple-S, Inc.
Triple-S Management Corp.
GPO Box 70314
San Juan, PR 00936-8314
Phone: (787)792-0909 **Fax:** (787)277-6077
Website: http://www.ssspr.com
Roberto O. Morales, President

★ 17823 ★ Select Health of South Carolina Inc.
Select Holding Inc.
7410 Northside Dr., Ste. 100
Charleston, SC 29420
Phone: (843)569-1759

★ 17824 ★ SelectCare HMO Inc.
SelectCare Inc.
2401 W Big Beaver Rd., Ste. 700
Troy, MI 48084
Phone: (248)637-5300

★ 17825 ★ Selected Funeral & Life Insurance Co.
PO Box 6040
Hot Springs, AR 71901
Phone: (501)624-2172
Courtney C. Crouch, Jr., President

★ 17826 ★ Senate Insurance Co.
United Community Insurance Group
5150 Trail Lake Dr.
Fort Worth, TX 76133
Phone: (817)263-0016
David S. Baggett, CEO & Pres

★ 17827 ★ Senate National Life Insurance Co.
United Community Insurance Group
5150 Trail Lake Dr.
Fort Worth, TX 76133
Phone: (817)263-0016 **Fax:** (817)263-0042
David S. Baggett, CEO & Pres

★ 17828 ★ Senior American Life Insurance Co.
AF & L Group
1800 St. Rd.
Warrington, PA 18976
Phone: (215)918-0515 **Fax:** (215)918-0467
Website: http://www.aflltc.com
Aloysius J. Abel, III, President

★ 17829 ★ Senior Life Insurance Co.
PO Box 2447
Thomasville, GA 31799-2447
Phone: (229)228-6936
Dale Ronald Powell, President

★ 17830 ★ Sentara Health Plans Inc.
4417 Corporation Ln.
Virginia Beach, VA 23462
Phone: (757)552-7220
Michael M. Dudley, President

★ 17831 ★ Sentinel American Life Insurance Co.
Guardian Life Group
7 Hanover Sq.
New York, NY 10004-2616
Phone: (212)598-8000 **Free:** 800-538-6203
Fax: (212)919-2910
Website: http://www.glic.com
Peter L. Hutchings, President

★ 17832 ★ Sentinel Security Life Insurance Co.
2121 S State St.
Salt Lake City, UT 84115
Phone: (801)484-8514 **Fax:** (801)484-2459
Website: http://www.sentinellife.org
Thomas W. Bartlett, CEO & Pres

★ 17833 ★ Sentry Life Insurance Co.
Sentry Insurance Group
1800 N Point Dr.
Stevens Point, WI 54481
Phone: (715)346-6000 **Fax:** (715)346-7516
Website: http://www.sentry.com
Dale R. Schuh, Chairman of the Board
Wallace D. Taylor, President

★ 17834 ★ Sentry Life Insurance Co. of New York
Sentry Insurance Group
220 Salina Meadows Pkwy., Ste. 255
PO Box 4944
Syracuse, NY 13221
Phone: (315)453-6308 **Fax:** (315)453-3017
Website: http://www.sentry.com
Harold A. Rice, President

★ 17835 ★ Servco Life Insurance Co.
PO Box 41194
Houston, TX 77241-1194
Phone: (713)580-3080 **Fax:** (713)580-5080
Gregory W. Kraft, President

★ 17836 ★ Service Life & Casualty Insurance Co.
Service Insurance Group
PO Box 26800
Austin, TX 78755-0800
Phone: (512)343-0600 **Fax:** (512)343-8673
Website: http://www.serviceinsurancegroup.com
Terry Williams, President

★ 17837 ★ Servus Life Insurance Co.
Hartford Life, Inc.
PO Box 2999
Hartford, CT 06104-2999
Phone: (860)843-5867 **Fax:** (860)843-5568
Website: http://www.thehartford.com
Thomas M. Marra, President

★ 17838 ★ Seton Health Plan Inc.
Seton Healthcare Network
305 E Huntland Dr., Ste. 200
Austin, TX 78752
Phone: (512)323-1953

★ 17839 ★ Settlers Life Insurance Co.
NGL Insurance Group
PO Box 8600
Bristol, VA 24203-8600
Phone: (540)645-4300 **Fax:** (540)645-4399
Website: http://www.settlerslife.com
John D. Larson, President

★ 17840 ★ SHA LLC
Covenant Health System
12940 Research Blvd.
Austin, TX 78750
Phone: (515)257-6001

★ 17841 ★ Sharp Health Plan
San Diego Hospital Association
9325 Sky Park Ct.
San Diego, CA 92123
Phone: (858)637-6550

★ 17842 ★ Shelter Life Insurance Co.
Shelter Insurance Companies
1817 W Broadway
Columbia, MO 65218-0001
Phone: (573)445-8441 **Fax:** (573)446-7318
Website: http://www.shelterins.com
J. Donald Duello, CEO & Pres

★ 17843 ★ Shenandoah Life Insurance Co.
Shenandoah Life Group
2301 Brambleton Ave. SW
Roanoke, VA 24015
Phone: (540)985-4400 **Fax:** (540)857-5910
Website: http://www.shenlife.com
Robert W. Clark, CEO & Pres

★ 17844 ★ Sheridan Life Insurance Co.
Wichita National Life Group
PO Box 1709
Lawton, OK 73502
Phone: (580)353-5776 **Fax:** (580)353-6482
Randall Gilliland, President

★ 17845 ★ Sierra Health and Life Insurance Co., Inc.
Sierra Health Services Group
PO Box 14396
Las Vegas, NV 89114-4396
Phone: (702)243-8528 **Fax:** (702)233-0397
Website: http://www.sierrahealth.com
Jonathon W. Bunker, President

★ 17846 ★ Sierra Pacific Life Insurance Co.
Merchant Hall and Co., Inc.
PO Box 2430
Napa, CA 94558-0242
Phone: (707)255-6800 **Fax:** (707)255-2144
Website: http://www.sierrapacificins.com
Robert D. Robertson, President

★ 17847 ★ Signature Life Insurance Co. of America
905 LaHarpe Blvd.
PO Box 3437
Little Rock, AR 72203-3437
Phone: (501)372-3355

★ 17848 ★ Sioux Valley Health Plan
Sioux Valley Hospital & Health System
1200 N West Ave.
Sioux Falls, SD 57104-1335
Phone: (605)357-6868

★ 17849 ★ Sloans Lake Health Insurance Co.
5570 DTC Pkwy.
Englewood, CO 80111
Phone: (303)804-8229

★ 17850 ★ Sloans Lake Health Plan Inc.
1355 S Colorado Blvd., Ste. 902
Denver, CO 80222
Phone: (303)691-2200

★ 17851 ★ Slovene National Benefit Society
247 W Allegheny Rd.
Imperial, PA 15126
Phone: (724)695-1100 **Fax:** (724)695-1555
Website: http://www.snpj.com
Joseph C. Evanish, President

★ 17852 ★ Smith Burial & Life Insurance Co.
310 Church St.
Stamps, AR 71860
Phone: (870)246-4563

★ 17853 ★ South Dakota State Medical Holding Co., Inc.
1323 S Minnesota Ave.
Sioux Falls, SD 57105

Phone: (605)334-4000 Fax: (605)336-0270
Website: http://www.dakotacare.com

★ 17854 ★ Southeast Family Life Insurance Co.
JMIC Life Group
500 NW 12th Ave.
Deerfield Beach, FL 33442
Phone: (954)429-2333 **Fax:** (954)429-2660
Website: http://www.jmfamily.com
Louis R. Feagles, President

★ 17855 ★ Southern Capital Life Insurance Co.
Southern Farm Bureau Group
PO Box 78
Jackson, MS 39205
Phone: (601)981-7422 **Fax:** (601)981-9894
Website: http://www.sfbli.com
Carl B. Loop, Jr., President

★ 17856 ★ Southern Farm Bureau Life Insurance Co.
Southern Farm Bureau Group
PO Box 78
Jackson, MS 39205
Phone: (601)981-7422 **Fax:** (601)981-9894
Website: http://www.sfbli.com
Carl B. Loop, Jr., President
Bobby P. Waters, Exec VP

★ 17857 ★ Southern Fidelity Life Insurance Co.
310 Church St.
Stamps, AR 71860
Phone: (870)246-4563

★ 17858 ★ Southern Financial Life Insurance Co.
516 Lakeview Rd., Villa 2
Clearwater, FL 33756
Phone: (727)442-4084 **Fax:** (727)445-1860
David N. Wakely, President

★ 17859 ★ Southern Financial Life Insurance Co.
Life of the South Group
100 W Bay St.
Jacksonville, FL 32202-3806
Phone: (904)350-9660 **Fax:** (904)354-4525
Website: http://www.life-south.com
Kenneth N. Hamil, President

★ 17860 ★ Southern Health Services Inc.
Coventry Health Care Inc.
9881 Mayland Dr.
Richmond, VA 23233
Phone: (804)747-3700

★ 17861 ★ Southern Life & Health Insurance Co.
PO Box 55975
Birmingham, AL 35255-5975
Phone: (205)414-3000 **Fax:** (205)414-3027
Larry R. Graber, President

★ 17862 ★ Southern National Life Insurance Co., Inc.
Louisiana Health Services Group
PO Box 98044
Baton Rouge, LA 70898-9044
Phone: (225)295-2583
Kathryn M. Sullivan, President

★ 17863 ★ Southern Pioneer Life Insurance Co.
Southern Pioneer Group
PO Box 30
Trumann, AR 72472
Phone: (870)483-6355 **Fax:** (870)483-6328
Website: http://www.southern-pioneer.com
Ben R. Hyneman, President

★ 17864 ★ Southern Protective Life Insurance Co.
1725 Memorial Park Dr.
Jacksonville, FL 32204-4117
Phone: (904)354-1069 **Fax:** (904)355-8046
Walter A. McRae, Jr., President

★ 17865 ★ Southern Security Life Insurance Co.
Security National Life Group
PO Box 958402
Lake Mary, FL 32795-8402
Phone: (407)321-7113 **Fax:** (407)323-9701
George R. Quist, President

★ 17866 ★ Southern Security Life Insurance Co., Inc.
PO Box 250
Kosciusko, MS 39090
Phone: (662)289-4113
Harold B. Nowell, Jr., President

★ 17867 ★ Southland Life Insurance Co.
ING Group
5780 Powers Ferry Rd. NW
Atlanta, GA 30327
Phone: (770)980-5100 **Fax:** (770)980-6590
Website: http://www.southlandlife.com
Chris D. Schreier, President

★ 17868 ★ Southland National Insurance Corp.
Collateral Investment Group
1812 University Blvd.
Tuscaloosa, AL 35401
Phone: (205)345-7410 **Fax:** (205)343-9013
Website: http://www.sninscorp.com
Dennis E. Painter, CEO & Pres

★ 17869 ★ Southwest Credit Life Inc.
PO Box 1377
Gallup, NM 87305
Phone: (505)722-6621
Patrick J. Gurley, President

★ 17870 ★ Southwest Home Life Insurance Co.
2414 N Akard, Ste. 500
PO Box 130930
Dallas, TX 75313-0808
Phone: (214)880-0808 **Fax:** (214)742-9103
Richard Camp Murphy, President

★ 17871 ★ Southwest Life and Health Insurance Co.
Covenant Health System
12940 Research Blvd.
Austin, TX 78750-3203
Phone: (512)257-6001 **Fax:** (512)257-6037
Website: http://www.firstcare.com
Charles L. Walker, President

★ 17872 ★ Southwest Service Life Insurance Co.
PO Box 982005
Fort Worth, TX 76182-8005
Phone: (817)284-4888

★ 17873 ★ Southwest Texas HMO Inc.
Health Care Service Corp.
901 S Central Expy.
Richardson, TX 75080
Phone: (972)766-6900
Patricia A. Hemingway Hall, President

★ 17874 ★ Southwestern Life Insurance Co.
Swiss Reinsurance Group
969 High Ridge Rd.
Stamford, CT 06905
Phone: (214)954-7111 **Fax:** (214)954-7008
Website: http://www.swlins.com
Chris C. Stroup, CEO & Pres

★ 17875 ★ Spectera Insurance Co., Inc.
UnitedHealth Inc.
2811 Lord Baltimore Dr.
Baltimore, MD 21244
Phone: (410)265-6033 **Fax:** (301)265-5013
Laurence A. Manchio, President

★ 17876 ★ Spectera Insurance Co., Inc.
UnitedHealth Inc.
2811 Lord Baltimore Dr.
Baltimore, MD 21244
Phone: (410)265-6033
Laurence A. Manchio, President

★ 17877 ★ SPJST
PO Box 100
Temple, TX 76503
Phone: (254)773-1575 **Fax:** (254)774-7447
Website: http://www.spjst.com
Howard B. Leshikar, President

★ 17878 ★ Standard American Life & Annuity Co.
3801 W 50th St.
Minneapolis, MN 55410-2071
Phone: (612)920-3357
Richard J. Zierden, President

★ 17879 ★ Standard Insurance Co.
StanCorp Financial Group
1100 SW 6th Ave.
Portland, OR 97204
Phone: (503)321-7000 **Fax:** (503)478-5037
Website: http://www.standard.com
Ronald E. Timpe, CEO & Chm Bd

★ 17880 ★ Standard Life and Accident Insurance Co.
American National Group
1 Moody Plz., 17th Fl.
Galveston, TX 77550-7999
Phone: (409)763-4661 **Fax:** (409)766-6663
Website: http://www.slaico.com
G. Richard Ferdinandtsen, CEO & Chm Bd

★ 17881 ★ Standard Life & Casualty Insurance Co.
PO Box 1514
Fort Mill, SC 29716
Phone: (803)548-3657
John F. Piercey, President

★ 17882 ★ Standard Life Insurance Co. of Indiana
Standard Management Group
10689 N Pennsylvania St.
Indianapolis, IN 46280
Phone: (317)574-6200 **Fax:** (317)574-6227
Website: http://www.smancorp.com
Raymond J. Ohlson, President

★ 17883 ★ The Standard Life Insurance Co. of New York
StanCorp Financial Group
1100 SW 6th Ave.
Portland, OR 97204
Phone: (914)989-4400 **Fax:** 800-378-8361
Website: http://www.standard-ny.com
Douglas T. Maines, CEO & Pres

★ 17884 ★ Standard Security Life Insurance Co. of New York
Independence Holding Group
485 Madison Ave., 14th Fl.
New York, NY 10022-5872
Phone: (212)355-4141 **Fax:** (212)754-3346
Website: http://www.sslicny.com
Rachel Lipari, President
Roy T. K. Thung, CEO & Chm Bd

★ 17885 ★ Starmount Life Insurance Co.
PO Box 14389
Baton Rouge, LA 70898-4389
Phone: (225)926-2888 **Fax:** (225)926-6292
Website: http://www.starmountlife.com
Erich Sternberg, President

★ 17886 ★ State Farm Annuity & Life Insurance Co.
State Farm Group
1 State Farm Plz.
Bloomington, IL 61710
Phone: (309)766-2311 **Fax:** (309)766-0400
Website: http://www.statefarm.com
Edward B. Rust, Jr., President

★ 17887 ★ State Farm Life & Accident Assurance Co.
State Farm Group
1 State Farm Plz.
Bloomington, IL 61710
Phone: (309)766-2311 **Fax:** (309)766-0400
Website: http://www.statefarm.com
Edward B. Rust, Jr., President

★ 17888 ★ State Farm Life Insurance Co.
State Farm Group
1 State Farm Plz.
Bloomington, IL 61710
Phone: (309)766-2311 **Fax:** (309)766-0400
Website: http://www.statefarm.com
Edward B. Rust, Jr., President

★ 17889 ★ State Life Insurance Co.
1 American Sq.
PO Box 406
Indianapolis, IN 46206-0368
Phone: (317)285-1877 **Fax:** (317)285-2380
Website: http://www.statelife.com
Jerry D. Semler, CEO & Chm Bd

★ 17890 ★ State Life Insurance Fund of Wisconsin
PO Box 7873
Madison, WI 53707-7873
Phone: (608)266-0107 **Fax:** (608)266-9935
Website: http://oci.wi.gov/slif.htm
Connie O'Connell, Exec Director

★ 17891 ★ State Mutual Insurance Co.
PO Box 153
Rome, GA 30162-0153
Phone: (706)291-1054 **Fax:** (706)291-9459
Delos H. Yancey, III, CEO & Chm Bd

★ 17892 ★ States General Life Insurance Co.
Vesta Insurance Group
115 W 7th St., Ste. 1205
Fort Worth, TX 76102-7012
Phone: (817)338-4395 **Free:** 800-782-8375
Fax: (817)338-1074
Kenneth W. Phillips, President

★ 17893 ★ States West Life Insurance Co.
Premera Group
7001 220th St. SW, Bldg. 2, MS 222
Mountlake Terrace, WA 98043-2124
Phone: (425)670-4575 **Fax:** (425)670-4485
Website: http://www.stateswestlife.com
Stephen D. Melton, CEO & Pres

★ 17894 ★ Statesman National Life Insurance Co.
4701 W Gate Blvd., No. A-102
Austin, TX 78745-1479
Phone: (713)974-2242 **Fax:** (713)630-7520
John D. Cornett, President

★ 17895 ★ Sterling Investors Life Insurance Co.
1 Progress Plz., Ste. 810
Saint Petersburg, FL 33701
Phone: (727)896-6434 **Fax:** (727)896-1264
Website: http://www.sterlinginvestors.com
Rodney L. Hale, CEO & Pres

★ 17896 ★ Sterling Life Insurance Co.
Combined Specialty A & H Group
Aon Ctr., 5th Fl.
200 E Randolph Dr.
Chicago, IL 60601
Phone: (312)381-1000 **Fax:** (312)381-0118
Steven E. Lippai, CEO & Chm Bd

★ 17897 ★ Stonebridge Insurance Co.
AEGON USA, Inc.
2700 W Plano Pkwy., 3C
Plano, TX 75075-8200
Phone: (972)881-6000 **Fax:** (972)881-6976
Marilyn Carp, President

★ 17898 ★ Sullivan Life Insurance Co.
PO Box 2051
Marshall, TX 75671-2051
Phone: (972)699-2700
Charlie Allison, President

★ 17899 ★ SummaCare Inc.
Summa Health Systems
10 N Main St.
PO Box 3620
Akron, OH 44309-3620
Phone: (330)996-8410
Website: http://www.summacare.com

★ 17900 ★ Summit Insurance Co.
550 Summit Ave., Ste. 101
Troy, OH 45373-3068
Phone: (937)332-8400 **Fax:** (937)339-6901
Website: http://www.summitins.com
Ronald Musilli, CEO & Pres

★ 17901 ★ Sun Life Assurance Co. of Canada
Sun Life Financial Group
150 King St. W
Toronto, ON, Canada M5H 1J9
Phone: (416)979-9966 **Fax:** (416)585-9546
Website: http://www.sunlife.com
Donald A. Stewart, CEO & Chm Bd
C. James Prieur, President

★ 17902 ★ Sun Life Assurance Co. of Canada (U.S.)
Sun Life Financial Group
1 Sun Life Executive Park
Wellesley Hills, MA 02481
Phone: (781)237-6030 **Fax:** (781)239-1682
Website: http://www.sunlife-usa.com
James A. McNulty, III, President

★ 17903 ★ Sun Life Insurance and Annuity Co. of New York
Sun Life Financial Group
1 Sun Life Executive Park
Wellesley Hills, MA 02481
Phone: (212)983-6352 **Fax:** (212)983-6356
Website: http://www.sunlife-usa.com
James A. McNulty, III, President

★ 17904 ★ Sun States Life Insurance Co.
CBD Holdings, Ltd.
500 Stanton-Christiana Rd., 2-OPS-1
Newark, DE 19713
Phone: (302)634-1469
Website: http://www.chase.com
Paul G. Petrylak, President

★ 17905 ★ SunAmerica Life Insurance Co.
American International Group
1 SunAmerica Ctr.
Los Angeles, CA 90067-6022
Phone: (310)772-6000 **Fax:** (310)772-6635
Website: http://www.sunamerica.com
Jay S. Wintrob, President

★ 17906 ★ Sunland Life Insurance Co.
PO Box 191
Cisco, TX 76437
Phone: (254)442-4451 **Fax:** (254)442-3977
Joe J. Cooper, President

★ 17907 ★ Sunset Life Insurance Co. of America
Kansas City Life Group
PO Box 219532
Kansas City, MO 64121-9532
Phone: (816)753-7000 **Fax:** (816)753-1354
Website: http://www.sunsetlife.com
Robert Philip Bixby, President

★ 17908 ★ Suntrust Insurance Co.
101 N 1st Ave., Ste. 2460
Phoenix, AZ 85003
Phone: (602)254-5866
James Aloysius Murphy, President

★ 17909 ★ Surety American Life Insurance Co.
Surety American Group
5845 Onix, Ste. 300
El Paso, TX 79912-5552
Phone: (915)585-0292
George R. Luttrell, President

★ 17910 ★ Surety Life Insurance Co.
Allstate Financial Group
3100 Sanders Rd.
Northbrook, IL 60062
Free: 800-525-9287
Website: http://www.allstate.com
B. Eugene Wraith, President

★ 17911 ★ Surety Mutual Life & Casualty Co.
PO Box 7157
Fargo, ND 58103

Phone: (701)235-6653
Franklyn C. Gokey, President

★ 17912 ★ Sutter Preferred Health & Life Insurance Co.
PO Box 30416
Lansing, MI 48909-7916
Phone: (517)349-6000
C. Richard Seitz, President

★ 17913 ★ Swiss-Am Reassurance Co.
Swiss Reinsurance Group
969 High Ridge Rd.
Stamford, CT 06905
Phone: (203)321-3000 **Fax:** (203)968-0920
Website: http://www.swissre.com
Chris C. Stroup, President

★ 17914 ★ Swiss Re Life & Health America, Inc.
Swiss Reinsurance Group
969 High Ridge Rd.
Stamford, CT 06905
Phone: (203)321-3000 **Fax:** (203)968-0920
Website: http://www.swissre.com
Lawrence T. Rowland, President

★ 17915 ★ Tandy Life Insurance Co.
1800 One Tandy Ctr.
Fort Worth, TX 76102
Phone: (817)415-3739
Leonard Roberts, President

★ 17916 ★ Taylor Life Insurance Co.
PO Box 222
Taylor, TX 76574
Phone: (512)352-9511

★ 17917 ★ Teachers Insurance and Annuity Association of America
TIAA Group
730 3rd Ave.
New York, NY 10017
Phone: (212)490-9000 **Fax:** 800-842-5916
Website: http://www.tiaa-cref.org
John H. Biggs, CEO & Chm Bd

★ 17918 ★ Teachers Protective Mutual Life Insurance Co.
PO Box 597
Lancaster, PA 17608-0597
Phone: (717)394-7156 **Fax:** (717)394-7024
Website: http://www.tpmins.com
D. Edward Young, President

★ 17919 ★ Team Life Insurance Co.
307 W 7th St., Ste. 400
Fort Worth, TX 76102
Phone: (214)630-7160

★ 17920 ★ Templeton Funds Annuity Co.
PO Box 33030
Saint Petersburg, FL 33733-8030
Free: 800-237-0738 **Fax:** (727)299-8750
Kenneth A. Lewis, CEO & Pres

★ 17921 ★ Tenet Choices Inc.
Tenet HealthSystem Hospitals Inc.
200 W Esplanade Ave., Ste. 600
Kenner, LA 70065
Phone: (504)461-9800

★ 17922 ★ Tennessee Coordinated Care Network
Metro Ctr.
210 Athens Way
Nashville, TN 37228-1308
Phone: (615)255-2700
Babajide Bamigboye, MD, Chairman of the Board

★ 17923 ★ Tennessee Farmers Life Insurance Co.
Tennessee Farmers Insurance Group
147 Bear Creek Pike
PO Box 307
Columbia, TN 38402-0307
Phone: (931)388-7872 **Fax:** (615)380-2192
Website: http://www.tennesseefarmers.com
Flavius Barker, President

★ 17924 ★ Tennessee Farmers Life Reassurance Co.
Tennessee Farmers Insurance Group
147 Bear Creek Pike
PO Box 307
Columbia, TN 38402-0307
Phone: (931)388-7872 **Fax:** (931)380-2192
Website: http://www.tennesseefarmers.com
Flavius Barker, President

★ 17925 ★ Tennessee Health Care Network Inc.
Blue Cross & Blue Shield of Tennessee
801 Pine St.
Chattanooga, TN 37402
Phone: (423)755-5600 **Fax:** (423)752-8331
Website: http://www.bcbst.com

★ 17926 ★ Tennessee Life Insurance Co.
Plateau Group, Inc.
PO Box 7001
Crossville, TN 38557-7001
Phone: (931)484-8411 **Fax:** (931)484-0692
William D. Williams, President

★ 17927 ★ Texas Burial Life Insurance Co.
PO Box 341899
Austin, TX 78734
Phone: (512)263-6977
Craig A. Cates, President

★ 17928 ★ Texas Children's Health Plan Inc.
Texas Children's Hospital
1919 S Braeswood, 6th Fl.
PO Box 31011
Houston, TX 77230-1011
Phone: (713)770-2090

★ 17929 ★ Texas Directors Life Insurance Co.
Funeral Directors Group
PO Box 5649
Abilene, TX 79608
Phone: (915)695-3412 **Fax:** (915)695-7840
Website: http://www.funeraldirectorslife.com
B. Kris Seale, President

★ 17930 ★ Texas Imperial Life Insurance Co.
American Capitol Group
PO Box 42813
Houston, TX 77242
Phone: (713)974-2242 **Fax:** (713)953-7920
John D. Cornett, President

★ 17931 ★ Texas International Life Insurance Co.
1810 E Fox Ln.
Fox Point, WI 53217
Phone: (414)351-1400 **Fax:** (414)351-1403
Barbara R. Barrow, President

★ 17932 ★ Texas Life Insurance Co.
Metropolitan Life and Affiliated Cos.
900 Washington Ave.
Waco, TX 76701
Phone: (254)752-6521 **Fax:** (254)754-7629
Website: http://www.texlife.com
Steven T. Cates, CEO & Pres

★ 17933 ★ Texas Savings Life Insurance Co.
Homeshield Insurance Group
515 Congress Ave., Ste. 1500
PO Box 684247
Austin, TX 78768-4247
Phone: (512)479-9901
Gary R. Peterson, President

★ 17934 ★ Texas Security Mutual Life Insurance Co.
9430 Old Katy Rd., Ste. 120
Houston, TX 77055-6341
Phone: (713)827-0484
Wendell A. Klein, President

★ 17935 ★ Texas Service Life Insurance Co.
PO Box 341889
Austin, TX 78734
Phone: (512)263-6977
Susan M. Thomas, President

★ 17936 ★ Texas State Life Insurance Co.
2929 N 44th St., Ste. 120
Phoenix, AZ 85018
Phone: (770)763-1560

★ 17937 ★ Three River Health Plans Inc.
300 Oxford Dr.
Monroeville, PA 15146
Phone: (412)858-4000 **Fax:** (412)858-4060
Website: http://www.threerivershealth.com

★ 17938 ★ Thrivent Financial for Lutherans
Thrivent Financial for Lutherans Group
4321 N Ballard Rd.
Appleton, WI 54919-0001
Phone: (920)734-5721 **Fax:** (920)628-5161
Website: http://www.thrivent.com
John O. Gilbert, Chairman of the Board

★ 17939 ★ TIAA-CREF Life Insurance Co.
TIAA Group
730 3rd Ave.
New York, NY 10017
Free: 888-842-5433 **Fax:** (212)907-3241
Website: http://www.tiaa-cref.org
Bertram L. Scott, CEO & Chm Bd

★ 17940 ★ TJM Life Insurance Co.
PO Box 1001
McKinney, TX 75070-1007
Phone: (972)542-2601
Billy W. Turrentine, President

★ 17941 ★ Total Health Choice Inc.
Total Health Care Inc.
8701 SW 137th Ave., Ste. 200
Miami, FL 33183

Phone: (305)408-5700
Website: http://www.totalhealthchoiceonline.com

★ 17942 ★ Touchpoint Health Plan Inc.
5 Innovation Ct.
Appleton, WI 54912-0507
Phone: (920)735-6300 Fax: (920)831-6716
Website: http://www.thedacare.org

★ 17943 ★ Touchpoint Insurance Co., Inc.
5 Innovation Ct.
Appleton, WI 54912-0507
Phone: (920)735-6300
Jay Fulkerson, President

★ 17944 ★ Tower Life Insurance Co.
310 S St. Mary's St.
San Antonio, TX 78205
Phone: (210)554-4400 Fax: (210)554-4401
James P. Zachry, President

★ 17945 ★ Town & Country Life Insurance Co.
PO Box 11026
Salt Lake City, UT 84147-0026
Phone: (801)363-5227 Fax: (801)363-6157
Henry S. Hemingway, President

★ 17946 ★ Trans City Life Insurance Co.
Trans City
7500 E McDonald Dr., Ste. 700
Scottsdale, AZ 85250-6055
Phone: (480)483-6500 Fax: (480)483-2553
Michael E. Jones, President

★ 17947 ★ Trans-National Life Insurance Co.
4545 Post Oak Pl., Ste. 302
Houston, TX 77027
Phone: (713)622-1080
Charles N. Davis, Jr., President

★ 17948 ★ Trans-Oceanic Life Insurance Co.
PO Box 363467
San Juan, PR 00936-3467
Phone: (787)620-2680 Fax: (787)782-3783
Website: http://www.tolic.com
Madeline Hernandez Urquiza, President
Nicolas Touma-Correa, Chairman of the Board

★ 17949 ★ Trans-Western Life Insurance Co.
20770 Hwy. 281 N, No. 108-604
San Antonio, TX 78258
Phone: (214)342-0400
Robert D. Tips, President

★ 17950 ★ Trans World Assurance Co.
Trans World Assurance Group
885 S El Camino Real
San Mateo, CA 94402
Phone: (650)348-2300 Fax: (650)348-7318
Charles B. Royals, President

★ 17951 ★ TransAm Assurance Co.
Trans World Assurance Group
PO Box 16130
Pensacola, FL 32507
Phone: (850)456-7406 Fax: (850)453-5440
Barbara J. Woodbury, President

★ 17952 ★ Transamerica Assurance Co.
AEGON USA, Inc.
1150 S Olive St.
Los Angeles, CA 90015
Phone: (213)742-3466 Fax: (213)742-2438
Website: http://www.transamerica.com
Daniel E. Jund, CEO & Pres

★ 17953 ★ Transamerica Life Insurance & Annuity Co.
AEGON USA, Inc.
1150 S Olive St.
Los Angeles, CA 90015
Phone: (213)742-3111 Fax: (213)742-2469
Website: http://www.transamerica.com
Larry Norman, President

★ 17954 ★ Transamerica Life Insurance Co.
AEGON USA, Inc.
4333 Edgewood Rd. NE
Cedar Rapids, IA 52499
Phone: (319)398-8511
Larry Norman, President

★ 17955 ★ Transamerica Life Insurance Co. of New York
AEGON USA, Inc.
100 Manhattanville Rd.
Purchase, NY 10577
Phone: (914)701-6000
Website: http://www.transamerica.com
Tom Schlossberg, CEO & Pres

★ 17956 ★ Transamerica Occidental Life Insurance Co.
AEGON USA, Inc.
4333 Edgewood Rd. NE
Cedar Rapids, IA 52499
Phone: (213)742-2111 Fax: (213)742-2469
Website: http://www.transamerica.com
Paul E. Rutledge, III, President

★ 17957 ★ The Travelers Insurance Co., Life Department
Citigroup
307 W 7th St., Ste. 400
Fort Worth, TX 76102
Phone: (860)277-0111
George C. Kokulis, CEO & Pres

★ 17958 ★ The Travelers Life and Annuity Co.
Citigroup
307 W 7th St., Ste. 400
Fort Worth, TX 76102
Phone: (860)277-0111
George C. Kokulis, CEO & Chm Bd

★ 17959 ★ TRH Health Insurance Co.
PO Box 1801
Columbia, TN 38402-1801
Phone: (931)388-7872

★ 17960 ★ Triangle Life Insurance Co.
PO Box 18526
Raleigh, NC 27619
Phone: (919)716-7571
David S. Perry, President

★ 17961 ★ Trigon Health & Life Insurance Co.
Trigon Healthcare Group
2221 Edward Holland Dr.
Richmond, VA 23230
Phone: (804)354-7283 Fax: (804)673-5970
Website: http://www.trigon.com
Thomas G. Snead, Jr., President

★ 17962 ★ Trigon Insurance Co.
Trigon Healthcare Group
2221 Edward Holland Dr.
Richmond, VA 23230
Phone: (804)354-7000
Website: http://www.trigon.com
Thomas G. Snead, Jr., CEO & Chm Bd

★ 17963 ★ Triumphe Life Insurance Co.
Triumphe Insurance Holdings
PO Box 26131
Greensboro, NC 27409
Phone: (336)931-3796 Fax: (336)931-4535
Richard Kahlbaugh, CEO & Pres

★ 17964 ★ Trustmark Insurance Co.
Trustmark Group Inc.
400 Field Dr.
Lake Forest, IL 60045-2581
Phone: (847)615-1500 Fax: (847)615-3910
Website: http://www.trustmarkins.com
James G. Thomas, Jr., CEO & Chm Bd

★ 17965 ★ Trustmark Life Insurance Co.
Trustmark Group Inc.
400 Field Dr.
Lake Forest, IL 60045-2581
Phone: (847)615-1500 Fax: (847)615-3910
Website: http://www.trustmarkins.com
James G. Thomas, Jr., CEO & Chm Bd

★ 17966 ★ Tufts Associated Health Maintenance Organization Inc.
Tufts Associated Health Plans Inc.
333 Wyman St.
Waltham, MA 02451
Phone: (781)466-9400

★ 17967 ★ Twin Life Insurance Co.
PO Box 167667
Irving, TX 75016-7667
Phone: (972)751-5544
Harold Jacobs, President

★ 17968 ★ UBS PaineWebber Life Insurance Co.
PO Box 10
Des Moines, IA 50301
Phone: (515)245-2069 Fax: (515)247-2440
John W. Mulhall, President
Frmly: PaineWebber Life Insurance Co.

★ 17969 ★ UCare Minnesota
2000 Summer St. NE
Minneapolis, MN 55413
Phone: (612)676-6500

★ 17970 ★ UCSD Health Plan
1899 McKee St.
San Diego, CA 92110
Phone: (619)294-3743

★ 17971 ★ UDC Dental California Inc.
Fortis Inc.
3111 Camino Del Rio N, No. 1000
San Diego, CA 92108
Phone: (619)521-5750
Susan A. Dickey, President

★ 17972 ★ UDC Life and Health Insurance Co.
Fortis Inc.
13601 Preston Rd., Ste. 500-E
Dallas, TX 75240
Phone: (972)458-7474 **Fax:** (205)868-3270
Bradley C. Johnson, President

★ 17973 ★ UDC Ohio Inc.
Fortis Inc.
3595 Grandview Pkwy., Ste. 150
Birmingham, AL 35243
Phone: (205)909-6000
Michael J. Peninger, CEO

★ 17974 ★ Ukrainian National Association Inc.
2200 Rte. 10
Parsippany, NJ 07054
Phone: (973)292-9800
Ulana Diachuk, President

★ 17975 ★ ULLICO Life Insurance Co.
ULLICO Group
111 Massachusetts Ave. NW
Washington, DC 20001
Phone: (202)682-0900 **Fax:** (202)682-7997
Website: http://www.ullico.com
Robert A. Georgine, CEO & Chm Bd

★ 17976 ★ UNICARE Health Insurance Co. of the Midwest
WellPoint Health Networks Inc.
4553 La Tienda Dr.
Thousand Oaks, CA 91362
Phone: 877-864-2273
Website: http://www.unicare.com
Leonard D. Schaeffer, President

★ 17977 ★ UNICARE Health Plans of the Midwest Inc.
WellPoint Health Networks Inc.
4553 La Tienda Dr.
Thousand Oaks, CA 91362
Phone: 877-864-2273
Leonard D. Schaeffer, President

★ 17978 ★ UNICARE Life and Health Insurance Co.
WellPoint Health Networks Inc.
1209 Orange St.
Wilmington, DE 19801
Phone: 877-864-2273
Website: http://www.unicare.com
D. Mark Weinberg, President

★ 17979 ★ Unified Life Insurance Co.
Old Mutual US Life Holdings Inc.
7201 W 129th St., Ste. 300
Overland Park, KS 66213
Phone: (913)685-2233 **Fax:** (913)685-2204
Frank M. Neidig, President

★ 17980 ★ Unimerica Insurance Co.
UnitedHealth Inc.
7200 Wisconsin Ave.
Bethesda, MD 20814
Phone: (301)718-7511
Website: http://www.principal.com
Edward Murphy, President

★ 17981 ★ Union Bankers Insurance Co.
Universal American Financial Corp.
600 Courtland St.
Orlando, FL 32804
Phone: (407)628-1776 **Fax:** (407)628-4227
Website: http://www.ubins.com
Gary W. Bryant, CEO & Pres

★ 17982 ★ Union Central Life Insurance Co.
PO Box 40888
Cincinnati, OH 45240
Phone: (513)595-2200 **Fax:** (513)595-2206
Website: http://www.unioncentral.com
John H. Jacobs, CEO & Pres
Stephen R. Hatcher, Exec VP

★ 17983 ★ Union Fidelity Life Insurance Co.
GE Financial Assurance Group
6604 W Broad St.
Richmond, VA 23230
Phone: (267)468-2000
Kathryn V. Marinello, President

★ 17984 ★ Union Health Service Inc.
1634 W Polk St.
Chicago, IL 60612
Phone: (312)829-4224

★ 17985 ★ The Union Labor Life Insurance Co.
ULLICO Group
111 Massachusetts Ave. NW
Washington, DC 20001
Phone: (202)682-0900 **Fax:** (202)682-4911
Website: http://www.ullico.com
Robert A. Georgine, CEO & Chm Bd
James W. Luce, Exec VP

★ 17986 ★ Union Life Insurance Co.
Southern Pioneer Group
216 W Main St.
PO Box 30
Trumann, AR 72472
Phone: (870)483-6355
Benjamin Rowan Hyneman, President

★ 17987 ★ Union National Life Insurance Co.
Unitrin, Inc.
PO Box 3638
Baton Rouge, LA 70821-3638
Phone: (225)927-3430 **Fax:** (225)231-7499
Website: http://www.unitrin.com
Jerry W. Hester, President

★ 17988 ★ Union Savings American Life Insurance Co.
PO Box 820
Gautier, MS 39553
Phone: (228)497-9935
William Higdon, III, President

★ 17989 ★ Union Security Life Insurance Co.
Fortis, Inc. Group
260 Interstate N Cir. NW
Atlanta, GA 30339
Phone: (770)763-1000 **Fax:** (770)859-4403
Website: http://www.assurant.com
R. Kevin Klotz, CEO & Pres

★ 17990 ★ Union Standard of America Life Insurance Co.
ULLICO Group
111 Massachusetts Ave. NW
Washington, DC 20001
Phone: (202)682-0900 **Fax:** (202)682-4911
Website: http://www.ullico.com
Robert A. Georgine, CEO & Chm Bd

★ 17991 ★ United American Insurance Co.
Torchmark Corp.
PO Box 8080
McKinney, TX 75070
Phone: (972)529-5085 **Fax:** (972)569-3282
Website: http://www.unitedamerican.com
Mark S. McAndrew, CEO & Pres

★ 17992 ★ United Assurance Life Insurance Co.
PO Box 982005
Fort Worth, TX 76182-8005
Phone: (817)284-4888
Frank M. Croy, President

★ 17993 ★ United Benefit Life Insurance Co.
Ceres Group
17800 Royalton Rd.
Strongsville, OH 44136
Phone: (440)572-2400 **Fax:** (440)572-8850
Anthony J. Pino, President

★ 17994 ★ United Concordia Dental Plans of California Inc.
Highmark Inc.
4401 Deer Path Rd.
Harrisburg, PA 17110
Phone: (818)710-9400 **Fax:** (818)704-5033
Website: http://www.ucci.com
Thomas A. Dzuryachko, Chairman of the Board

★ 17995 ★ United Concordia Dental Plans Inc.
Highmark Inc.
4401 Deer Path Rd.
Harrisburg, PA 17110
Phone: (410)512-4200 **Fax:** (410)296-4333
Website: http://www.ucci.com
Thomas A. Dzuryachko, CEO & Chm Bd

★ 17996 ★ United Concordia Dental Plans of Kentucky Inc.
Highmark Inc.
4401 Deer Path Rd.
Harrisburg, PA 17110
Phone: (502)897-7711 **Fax:** (502)897-3565
Website: http://www.ucci.com
Thomas A. Dzuryachko, Chairman of the Board

★ 17997 ★ United Concordia Dental Plans of the Midwest (Michigan) Inc.
Highmark Inc.
4401 Deer Path Rd.
Harrisburg, PA 17110
Phone: (248)353-6410 **Fax:** (248)353-0727
Website: http://www.ucci.com
Thomas A. Dzuryachko, Chairman of the Board

★ 17998 ★ United Concordia Dental Plans of Pennsylvania Inc.
Highmark Inc.
4401 Deer Path Rd.
Harrisburg, PA 17110
Phone: (717)260-6800
Website: http://www.ucci.com
Thomas A. Dzuryachko, Chairman of the Board

★ 17999 ★ United Concordia Insurance Co.
Highmark Inc.
4401 Deer Path Rd.
Harrisburg, PA 17110
Phone: (717)260-7081
Website: http://www.ucci.com
Thomas A. Dzuryachko, President

★ 18000 ★ United Concordia Insurance Co. of New York
Highmark Inc.
4401 Deer Path Rd.
Harrisburg, PA 17110
Phone: (717)260-7081
Website: http://www.ucci.com
Thomas A. Dzuryachko, Chairman of the Board

★ 18001 ★ United Concordia Life & Health Insurance Co.
Highmark Inc.
4401 Deer Path Rd.
Harrisburg, PA 17110
Phone: (717)260-6081
Website: http://www.ucci.com
Thomas A. Dzuryachko, President

★ 18002 ★ United Dental Care of Arizona Inc.
Fortis Inc.
3595 Grandview Pkwy., Ste. 150
Birmingham, AL 35243
Phone: (205)909-6000
Michael J. Peninger, CEO

★ 18003 ★ United Dental Care of Colorado Inc.
Fortis Inc.
3595 Grandview Pkwy., Ste. 150
Birmingham, AL 35243
Phone: (205)909-6000
Michael J. Peninger, CEO

★ 18004 ★ United Dental Care of Indiana Inc.
Fortis Inc.
3595 Grandview Pkwy., Ste. 150
Birmingham, AL 35243
Phone: (205)909-6000
Michael J. Peninger, CEO

★ 18005 ★ United Dental Care Insurance Co.
Fortis Inc.
13601 Preston Rd., Ste. 300 E
Dallas, TX 75240
Phone: (972)458-7474 **Fax:** (972)458-7963
Bradley C. Johnson, President

★ 18006 ★ United Dental Care of Michigan Inc.
Fortis Inc.
3595 Grandview Pkwy., Ste. 150
Birmingham, AL 35243
Phone: (205)909-6000
Michael J. Peninger, CEO

★ 18007 ★ United Dental Care of Missouri Inc.
Fortis Inc.
3595 Grandview Pkwy., Ste. 150
Birmingham, AL 35243
Phone: (205)909-6000
Michael J. Peninger, CEO

★ 18008 ★ United Dental Care of Nebraska Inc.
Fortis Inc.
3595 Grandview Pkwy., Ste. 150
Birmingham, AL 35243
Phone: (205)909-6000
Michael J. Peninger, CEO

★ 18009 ★ United Dental Care of New Mexico Inc.
Fortis Inc.
3595 Grandview Pkwy., Ste. 150
Birmingham, AL 35243
Phone: (205)909-6000
Michael J. Peninger, CEO

★ 18010 ★ United Dental Care of Pennsylvania Inc.
Fortis Inc.
3595 Grandview Pkwy., Ste. 150
Birmingham, AL 35243
Phone: (205)909-6000
Michael J. Peninger, CEO

★ 18011 ★ United Dental Care of Texas Inc.
Fortis Inc.
3595 Grandview Pkwy., Ste. 150
Birmingham, AL 35243
Phone: (205)909-6000
Michael J. Peninger, CEO

★ 18012 ★ United Dental Care of Utah Inc.
Fortis Inc.
3595 Grandview Pkwy., Ste. 150
Birmingham, AL 35243
Phone: (205)909-6000
Michael J. Peninger, CEO

★ 18013 ★ United Family Life Insurance Co.
Fortis, Inc. Group
10 Glenlake Pkwy. NE, Ste. 500
Atlanta, GA 30328-3473
Phone: (770)206-6400 **Free:** 800-801-0800
Fax: (770)206-6382
Website: http://www.fortisfamily.com
Robert B. Pollock, CEO & Chm Bd

★ 18014 ★ United Farm Family Life Insurance Co.
Indiana Farm Bureau Group
PO Box 1250
Indianapolis, IN 46206-1250
Phone: (317)692-7200 **Fax:** (317)692-7950
Website: http://www.farmbureau.com
Donald B. Villwock, President
Harry N. Frenchak, Exec VP

★ 18015 ★ United Fidelity Life Insurance Co.
Americo Life Group
PO Box 13487
Kansas City, MO 64199-3487
Phone: (816)391-2000 **Fax:** (816)391-2083
Website: http://www.americo.com
Gary L. Muller, CEO & Pres

★ 18016 ★ United Funeral Benefit Life Insurance Co.
PO Box 831670
Richardson, TX 75083-1670
Phone: (940)699-2700 **Fax:** (940)397-0581
Charlie Allison, President

★ 18017 ★ United Funeral Directors Benefit Life Insurance Co.
PO Box 831670
Richardson, TX 75081
Phone: (469)330-2200
Charlie Allison, President

★ 18018 ★ United Healthcare of Alabama Inc.
UnitedHealth Inc.
9900 Bren Rd. E
MN008-T380
Minnetonka, MN 55343
Phone: (205)977-6300
Website: http://www.unitedhealthgroup.com
John A. Wickens, President

★ 18019 ★ United Healthcare of Arizona Inc.
UnitedHealth Inc.
3141 N 3rd Ave.
Phoenix, AZ 85013
Phone: (602)664-2600
Kenneth A. Burdick, President

★ 18020 ★ United Healthcare of Arkansas Inc.
UnitedHealth Inc.
9900 Bren Rd. E
MN008-T380
Minnetonka, MN 55343
Phone: (501)664-7700
Website: http://www.unitedhealthgroup.com
Jack Wickens, President

★ 18021 ★ United Healthcare of Colorado Inc.
UnitedHealth Inc.
9900 Bren Rd. E
MN008-T380
Minnetonka, MN 55343
Phone: (303)267-4500
Website: http://www.unitedhealthgroup.com
Victor Lazzaro, Jr., President

★ 18022 ★ United Healthcare of Florida Inc.
UnitedHealth Inc.
300 Opus Ctr.
9900 Bren Rd. E
Minnetonka, MN 55343
Phone: (407)428-2302
Website: http://www.unitedhealthgroup.com
Gary L. Schulz, President

★ 18023 ★ United Healthcare of Georgia Inc.
UnitedHealth Inc.
PO Box 1459
Minneapolis, MN 55440-1459
Phone: (952)992-8800
Website: http://www.unitedhealthgroup.com
Teresa L. Kline, President

★ 18024 ★ United Healthcare of Illinois Inc.
UnitedHealth Inc.
9900 Bren Rd. E
MN008-T380
Minnetonka, MN 55343
Phone: (312)424-4600 **Fax:** (312)424-4448
Website: http://www.unitedhealthgroup.com
William P. Whitely, President

★ 18025 ★ United HealthCare Insurance Co.
UnitedHealth Group
450 Columbus Blvd.
Hartford, CT 06103
Phone: 877-832-7734 **Fax:** (612)936-3095
Website: http://www.unitedhealthgroup.com
Ronald B. Colby, CEO & Pres

★ 18026 ★ United HealthCare Insurance Co. of Illinois
UnitedHealth Group
450 Columbus Blvd.
Hartford, CT 06103
Phone: (312)424-4460 **Fax:** (312)424-4448
Website: http://www.unitedhealthgroup.com
Ronald B. Colby, CEO & Chm Bd

★ 18027 ★ United HealthCare Insurance Co. of New York
UnitedHealth Group
PO Box 1459
Minneapolis, MN 55440-1459
Phone: (516)348-5644 **Fax:** (516)348-5927
Website: http://www.unitedhealthgroup.com
Ronald B. Colby, President

★ 18028 ★ United HealthCare Insurance Co. of Ohio
UnitedHealth Group
450 Columbus Blvd.
Hartford, CT 06103
Phone: (614)410-7000 **Fax:** (614)442-6400
Website: http://www.unitedhealthgroup.com
Ronald B. Colby, CEO & Chm Bd

★ 18029 ★ United Healthcare of Kentucky Inc.
UnitedHealth Inc.
9900 Bren Rd. E
MN008-T380
Minnetonka, MN 55343
Phone: (859)260-3600
Website: http://www.unitedhealthgroup.com
Walter W. Wakefield, President

★ 18030 ★ United Healthcare of Louisiana Inc.
UnitedHealth Inc.
9900 Bren Rd. E
MN008-T380
Minnetonka, MN 55343
Phone: (504)849-3510 **Fax:** (504)849-3550
Website: http://www.unitedhealthgroup.com
John A. Wickens, President

★ 18031 ★ United Healthcare of the Mid-Atlantic Inc.
UnitedHealth Inc.
9900 Bren Rd. E
MN008-T380
Minnetonka, MN 55343
Phone: (410)277-6000
Website: http://www.unitedhealthgroup.com
Allan E. Hanssen, CEO

★ 18032 ★ United Healthcare of the Midlands Inc.
UnitedHealth Inc.
9900 Bren Rd. E
MN008-T380
Minnetonka, MN 55343
Phone: (402)445-5000 **Fax:** (402)445-5572
Website: http://www.unitedhealthgroup.com
Kathleen A. Mallatt, President

★ 18033 ★ United Healthcare of the Midwest Inc.
UnitedHealth Inc.
9900 Bren Rd. E
MN008-T380
Minnetonka, MN 55343
Phone: (314)592-7000
Website: http://www.unitedhealthgroup.com
Victor E. Turvey, President

★ 18034 ★ United Healthcare of Mississippi Inc.
UnitedHealth Inc.
9900 Bren Rd. E
MN008-T380
Minnetonka, MN 55343
Phone: (504)849-3510
Website: http://www.unitedhealthgroup.com
John A. Wickens, President

★ 18035 ★ United Healthcare of New England Inc.
UnitedHealth Inc.
9900 Bren Rd. E
MN008-T380
Minnetonka, MN 55343
Phone: (401)737-6900 **Fax:** (401)737-6959
Website: http://www.unitedhealthgroup.com
Elwood B. Fisher, President

★ 18036 ★ United Healthcare of Ohio Inc.
UnitedHealth Inc.
9900 Bren Rd. E
MN008-T380
Minnetonka, MN 55343
Phone: (614)410-7000
Website: http://www.unitedhealthgroup.com
George D. Shafer, CEO & Pres

★ 18037 ★ United Healthcare of Tennessee Inc.
UnitedHealth Inc.
9900 Bren Rd. E
MN008-T380
Minnetonka, MN 55343
Phone: (615)297-9500 **Fax:** (615)297-5467
Website: http://www.unitedhealthgroup.com
John A. Wickens, President

★ 18038 ★ United Healthcare of Texas Inc.
UnitedHealth Inc.
9900 Bren Rd. E
MN008-T380
Minnetonka, MN 55343
Phone: (512)347-2600
Website: http://www.unitedhealthgroup.com
Thomas J. Quirk, President

★ 18039 ★ United Healthcare of Utah
UnitedHealth Inc.
5901 Lincoln Dr.
MN012-N282
Edina, MN 55436-1611
Phone: (801)942-6200 **Fax:** (801)944-0940
Website: http://www.unitedhealthgroup.com
Robert G. Adams, CEO & Chm Bd

★ 18040 ★ United Heartland Life Insurance Co.
Cobalt Corp.
PO Box 2013
Milwaukee, WI 53201-2013
Phone: (262)787-7400 **Fax:** (262)787-7673
Website: http://www.cobaltcorporation.com
Thomas E. Liechty, President

★ 18041 ★ United Heritage Life Insurance Co.
PO Box 7777
Meridian, ID 83680-7777
Phone: (208)493-6100 **Fax:** (208)466-0825
Website: http://www.unitedheritage.com
Dennis L. Johnson, CEO & Pres
Richard E. Hall, Chairman of the Board
Frmly: United Heritage Mutual Life Co.

★ 18042 ★ United Home Life Insurance Co.
Indiana Farm Bureau Group
PO Box 7192
Indianapolis, IN 46207-7192
Phone: (317)692-7979 **Fax:** (317)692-7711
Harry L. Pearson, President
Harry N. Frenchak, CEO

★ 18043 ★ United Insurance Co. of America
Unitrin, Inc.
1 E Wacker Dr.
Chicago, IL 60601
Phone: (312)661-4500 **Fax:** (312)661-3660
Website: http://www.unitrin.com
Don M. Royster, Sr., President

★ 18044 ★ United International Life Insurance Co.
Vesta Insurance Group
115 W 7th St., Ste. 1205
Fort Worth, TX 76102-7012
Phone: (817)338-4395 **Free:** 800-782-8375
Fax: (817)338-1074
Kenneth W. Phillips, President

★ 18045 ★ United Investors Life Insurance Co.
Torchmark Corp.
PO Box 10207
Birmingham, AL 35202-0207
Phone: (205)325-4300 **Fax:** (205)325-2720
Anthony L. McWhorter, CEO & Pres

★ 18046 ★ United Liberty Life Insurance Co.
Citizens Financial Group
PO Box 437249
Louisville, KY 40253-7249
Phone: (502)244-2420 **Fax:** (502)244-2439
Website: http://www.citfin.com
Lane A. Hersman, President

★ 18047 ★ United Life & Annuity Insurance Co.
ING Group
909 Locust St.
Des Moines, IA 50309
Phone: (515)698-7000
Website: http://www.ing.com
Christopher R. Welp, President

★ 18048 ★ United Life Insurance Co.
United Fire and Casualty Group
PO Box 73909
Cedar Rapids, IA 52407-3909
Phone: (319)399-5700 **Fax:** (319)399-5401
Website: http://www.unitedfiregroup.com
John A. Rife, President
John S. McIntyre, Jr., Chairman of the Board

★ 18049 ★ United Mercantile Life Insurance Co.
Surety American Group
5845 Onix, Ste. 300
El Paso, TX 79912-5552
Phone: (915)585-0292 **Fax:** (915)585-9925
George R. Luttrell, President

★ 18050 ★ United National Life Insurance Co. of America
1275 Milwaukee Ave.
Glenview, IL 60025
Phone: (847)803-5252 **Fax:** (847)699-0229
Thomas B. Dunkin, President

★ 18051 ★ United of Omaha Life Insurance Co.
Mutual of Omaha Group
Mutual of Omaha Plaza
Omaha, NE 68175
Phone: (402)342-7600 **Fax:** (402)351-2775
Website: http://www.mutualofomaha.com
John A. Sturgeon, President
John W. Weekly, CEO & Chm Bd

★ 18052 ★ United Security Assurance Co. of Pennsylvania
United Security Assurance Group
PO Box 64477
Souderton, PA 18964-0477
Phone: (215)723-3044 **Fax:** (215)723-8036
Website: http://www.usa-cal.com
Ronald A. Landes, President

★ 18053 ★ United Security Life Insurance Co. of Illinois
American Transit Group
10275 W Higgins Rd.
Rosemont, IL 60018-3864
Phone: (847)298-1400 **Free:** 800-875-4422
Fax: (847)298-1407
Website: http://www.uslofil.com
Edward T. McGettigan, Sr., CEO & Chm Bd

★ 18054 ★ U.S. Financial Life Insurance Co.
MONY Group
PO Box 429560
Cincinnati, OH 45242
Phone: (513)686-2000 **Fax:** (513)686-2270
Website: http://www.usfli.com
Paul P. Aniskovich, CEO & Pres

★ 18055 ★ U.S. Health Insurance Co.
830 Taylor St.
Fort Worth, TX 76102
Phone: (817)877-5861
Randal S. Mitchell, President

★ 18056 ★ U.S. Health and Life Insurance Co.
8220 Irving Rd.
Sterling Heights, MI 48312
Phone: (586)693-4300 **Fax:** (586)693-4835
Anthony Lapiana, CEO & Chm Bd

★ 18057 ★ The United States Life Insurance Co. in the City of New York
American International Group
3600 Rte. 66
Neptune, NJ 07754-1580
Phone: (212)709-6000 **Fax:** (212)709-6241
Rodney O. Martin, Jr., CEO & Chm Bd

★ 18058 ★ United Teacher Associates Insurance Co.
American Financial Group
PO Box 26580
Austin, TX 78755-0580
Phone: (512)451-2224 **Fax:** (512)467-7040
Website: http://www.utaic.com
Billy B. Hill, Jr., President

★ 18059 ★ United Transportation Union Insurance Association
14600 Detroit Ave.
Cleveland, OH 44107
Phone: (216)228-9400 **Fax:** (216)228-0411
Website: http://www.utuia.org
Byron A. Boyd, Jr., President

★ 18060 ★ United Trust Insurance Co.
450 Riverchase Pkwy. E
Birmingham, AL 35298
Phone: (205)220-6307
Horace L. Jones, President

★ 18061 ★ United Western Life Insurance Co.
3636 Executive Ctr. Dr., Ste. G22
PO Box 684247
Austin, TX 78768-4247
Phone: (512)338-4397
David W. Mann, President

★ 18062 ★ United Wisconsin Life Insurance Co.
American Medical Security Group, Inc.
PO Box 19032
Green Bay, WI 54313
Phone: (920)661-6020 **Free:** 800-232-5432
Fax: (920)661-2132
Website: http://www.amchoices.com
Samuel V. Miller, CEO & Chm Bd

★ 18063 ★ United World Life Insurance Co.
Mutual of Omaha Group
Mutual of Omaha Plaza
Omaha, NE 68175
Phone: (402)342-7600 **Fax:** (402)351-2775
Website: http://www.mutualofomaha.com
John A. Sturgeon, President

★ 18064 ★ UnitedHealthcare of New Jersey Inc.
UnitedHealth Inc.
9900 Bren Rd. E
MN008-T380
Minnetonka, MN 55343
Phone: (212)216-6400
Website: http://www.unitedhealthgroup.com
Amy K. Knapp, President

★ 18065 ★ UnitedHealthcare of New York Inc.
UnitedHealth Inc.
300 Opus Ctr.
9900 Bren Rd. E
Minnetonka, MN 55343
Phone: (212)216-6400
Website: http://www.unitedhealthgroup.com
Amy K. Knapp, President

★ 18066 ★ UnitedHealthcare of North Carolina Inc.
UnitedHealth Inc.
9900 Bren Rd. E
MN008-T380
Minnetonka, MN 55343
Phone: (336)282-0900 **Fax:** (336)288-5206
Website: http://www.unitedhealthgroup.com
Frank R. Mascia, CEO & Pres

★ 18067 ★ UnitedHealthcare of Upstate New York Inc.
UnitedHealth Inc.
300 Opus Ctr.
9900 Bren Rd. E
MN008-T380
Minnetonka, MN 55343
Phone: (315)433-5700
Website: http://www.unitedhealthgroup.com
Amy K. Knapp, President

★ 18068 ★ UnitedHealthcare of Wisconsin Inc.
UnitedHealth Inc.
9900 Bren Rd. E
MN008-T380
Minnetonka, MN 55343
Phone: (414)443-4000
Website: http://www.unitedhealthgroup.com
William D. Felsing, President

★ 18069 ★ Unity Dental Service Plan
363 Rte. 48 W
Fairfield, NJ 07004
Phone: (973)276-4900
Robert H. Dubman, President

★ 18070 ★ Unity Financial Life Insurance Co.
11311 Cornell Park Dr., Ste. 200
Cincinnati, OH 45242
Phone: (315)448-7000 **Fax:** (315)448-7002
Website: http://www.unity-life.com
Patrick A. Mannion, Chairman of the Board

★ 18071 ★ Unity Health Plans Insurance Corp.
Cobalt Corp.
840 Carolina St.
Sauk City, WI 53583
Phone: (608)643-2491 **Fax:** (608)643-2564
Website: http://www.cobaltcorporation.com
Jane Barnett, Chairman of the Board

★ 18072 ★ Unity Mutual Life Insurance Co.
1 Unity Plaza at Franklin Sq.
Syracuse, NY 13250-5000
Phone: (315)448-7000 **Fax:** (315)448-7100
Website: http://www.unity-life.com
Patrick A. Mannion, CEO & Pres
John F. X. Mannion, Chairman of the Board

★ 18073 ★ Univantage Insurance Co.
392 East 6400 South
Murray, UT 84107
Phone: (801)288-8000 **Fax:** (801)288-8111
Lane A. Summerhays, President

★ 18074 ★ Universal Care
1600 E Hill St.
Signal Hill, CA 90806
Phone: (310)424-6200
Website: http://www.universalcare.com
Howard E. Davis, President

★ 18075 ★ Universal Fidelity Life Insurance Co.
2211 N Highway 81
Duncan, OK 73533
Phone: (580)255-8530 **Fax:** (580)255-0951
Jimmie L. Gray, President
Steven R. Hague, Chairman of the Board

★ 18076 ★ Universal Guaranty Life Insurance Co.
United Trust, Inc. Group
PO Box 5147
Springfield, IL 62705-5147
Phone: (217)241-6300
Randall L. Attkisson, President

★ 18077 ★ Universal Life Insurance Co.
PO Box 2145
San Juan, PR 00922-2145
Phone: (787)706-7337 **Fax:** (787)782-0692
Website: http://www.universalpr.com
Ramon L. Galanes, President

★ 18078 ★ Universal Life Insurance Co.
Protective Industrial of Alabama Group
2300 11th Ave. N
PO Box 2744
Birmingham, AL 35202
Phone: (205)323-5256
James C. Harrison, Sr., President

★ 18079 ★ Universal Underwriters Life Insurance Co.
Zurich Insurance Group
7045 College Blvd.
Overland Park, KS 66211
Phone: (913)339-1000 **Fax:** (913)469-3725
Stephen R. Smith, CEO & Pres
J. J. Amore, Chairman of the Board

★ 18080 ★ Universe Life Insurance Co.
PO Box 538
Lewiston, ID 83501
Phone: (208)799-9000 **Fax:** (208)746-8159
Paul D. Durant, II, President

★ 18081 ★ University Health Alliance
700 Bishop St., Ste. 300
Honolulu, HI 96813
Phone: (808)532-4000 **Fax:** (808)522-8895
Website: http://www.uhahealth.com
Max G. Botticelli, MD, CEO

★ 18082 ★ University Health Care Inc.
305 W Broadway Ave., 3rd Fl.
Louisville, KY 40202
Phone: (502)852-5872

★ 18083 ★ University Health Plans Inc.
University of Medicine and Dentistry NJ
550 Broad St., 17th Fl.
Newark, NJ 07102
Phone: (973)623-8700

★ 18084 ★ Unum Life Insurance Co. of America
UnumProvident Corp.
1 Fountain Sq.
Chattanooga, TN 37402-1330
Phone: (207)575-2211
Website: http://www.unumprovident.com
James H. Chandler, CEO & Pres

★ 18085 ★ UPMC Health Benefits Inc.
UPMC Health System Inc.
112 Washington Pl.
Pittsburgh, PA 15221
Phone: (412)434-1200
Patricia A. Liebman, CEO

★ 18086 ★ UPMC Health Plan Inc.
UPMC Health System Inc.
112 Washington Pl., 8th Fl.
Pittsburgh, PA 15219
Phone: (412)434-1200
Patricia A. Liebman, CEO

★ 18087 ★ USA Life One Insurance Co. of Indiana
227 E Main St.
PO Box 312
Crawfordsville, IN 47933
Phone: (765)362-4500
Roger W. Smith, President

★ 18088 ★ USAA Life Insurance Co.
USAA Life Group
9800 Fredericksburg Rd.
San Antonio, TX 78288
Phone: (210)498-8000 **Fax:** (210)498-4624
Website: http://www.usaa.com
James M. Middleton, CEO & Pres

★ 18089 ★ USAA Life Insurance Co. of New York
USAA Life Group
9800 Fredericksburg Rd.
San Antonio, TX 78288
Phone: (210)498-8000 **Fax:** (210)498-4624
Website: http://www.usaa.com
James M. Middleton, President

★ 18090 ★ USAble Life
Arkansas Blue Cross & Blue Shield Group
PO Box 1650
Little Rock, AR 72203-1650
Phone: (501)375-7200 **Fax:** (501)378-3381
James B. House, CEO & Pres

★ 18091 ★ USG Annuity & Life Co.
ING Group
PO Box 617
Des Moines, IA 50303-0617
Phone: (515)698-7000 **Fax:** (515)698-6973
Chris D. Schreier, President

★ 18092 ★ USLIFE Credit Life Insurance Co. of Arizona
American International Group
1000 Woodfield Rd.
Schaumburg, IL 60173-4793
Phone: (847)517-6000 **Fax:** (847)517-6005
Donald W. Britton, President

★ 18093 ★ Utica National Life Insurance Co.
Utica National Group
PO Box 6576
Utica, NY 13503
Phone: (315)734-2000 **Fax:** (315)734-2941
Website: http://www.uticanational.com
David C. Cunningham, President

★ 18094 ★ UTMB Health Plans Inc.
700 University Blvd.
Galveston, TX 77550
Phone: (409)797-8000

★ 18095 ★ Valley Baptist Health Plan Inc.
Valley Baptist Medical Development Corp.
2005 Ed Carey Dr.
Harlingen, TX 78550
Phone: (956)389-2273
Karen K. Pederson, President

★ 18096 ★ Valley Forge Life Insurance Co.
CNA Insurance Group
CNA Plz., 22 S
Chicago, IL 60685
Phone: (312)822-5000 **Fax:** (312)822-6419
Website: http://www.cna.com
Thomas F. Taylor, Exec VP
Bernard L. Hengesbaugh, CEO & Chm Bd

★ 18097 ★ Valley Group Hospital Service Corp.
2005 Ed Carey Dr.
Harlingen, TX 78550
Phone: (956)389-2273

★ 18098 ★ Valley Health Plan Inc.
Cobalt Corp.
401 W Michigan St.
Milwaukee, WI 53203
Phone: (414)226-5000 **Fax:** (715)836-1298
Website: http://www.cobaltcorporation.com
Thomas Hefty, CEO

★ 18099 ★ Value Behavioral Health of Pennsylvania
240 Corporate Blvd.
Norfolk, VA 23502
Phone: (757)459-5446
Ronald I. Dozoretz, MD, President

★ 18100 ★ ValueOptions of Texas Inc.
FHC Health Systems Inc.
240 Corporate Blvd.
Norfolk, VA 23502
Phone: (757)459-5100

★ 18101 ★ The Variable Annuity Life Insurance Co.
American International Group
PO Box 3206
Houston, TX 77253-3206
Phone: (713)522-1111 **Fax:** (713)831-4940
Website: http://www.valic.com
John A. Graf, CEO

★ 18102 ★ Venture Life Insurance Co.
PO Box 26800
Austin, TX 78755-0800
Phone: (512)343-0600 **Fax:** (512)343-8673
Glen R. Pollard, President

★ 18103 ★ Vermont Health Plan LLC
Blue Cross & Blue Shield of Vermont
445 Industrial Ln.
Berlin, VT 05602
Phone: (802)223-6131

★ 18104 ★ Versant Life Insurance Co.
LDS Group
PO Box 84410
Baton Rouge, LA 70884-4410
Phone: (225)769-9923 **Fax:** (225)767-7656
Dick S. Taylor, President

★ 18105 ★ Veterans Life Insurance Co.
AEGON USA, Inc.
20 Moores Rd.
Frazer, PA 19355
Phone: (610)648-5000 **Fax:** (610)648-5326
Brian A. Smith, President

★ 18106 ★ Victory Health Plan Inc.
Windsor Health Group
215 Centerview Dr., Ste. 300
Brentwood, TN 37027
Phone: (615)782-7800
Website: http://www.vhptn.com

★ 18107 ★ Virginia Premier Health Plan
UHS Managed Care Inc.
600 E Broad St., Ste. 400
Richmond, VA 23219
Phone: (804)819-5151

★ 18108 ★ Vision Benefits of America
300 Weyman Plz., Ste. 400
Pittsburgh, PA 15236-1588
Michael S. Gissin, President

★ 18109 ★ Vision Care of Oregon, Inc.
Vision Service Plan
3333 Quality Dr.
Rancho Cordova, CA 95670
Phone: (916)851-5000 **Fax:** (916)858-5388
Roger J. Valine, President

★ 18110 ★ Vision Service Plan of Idaho, Inc.
Vision Service Plan
3333 Quality Dr.
Rancho Cordova, CA 95670
Phone: (916)851-5000 **Fax:** (916)858-5388
Roger J. Valine, President

★ 18111 ★ Vision Service Plan, Inc.
Vision Service Plan
3333 Quality Dr.
Rancho Cordova, CA 95670
Phone: (916)851-5000 **Fax:** (916)858-5388
Roger J. Valine, President

★ 18112 ★ Vision Service Plan Insurance Co.—Connecticut
Vision Service Plan
3333 Quality Dr.
Rancho Cordova, CA 95670
Phone: (916)851-5000 **Fax:** (916)858-5388
Website: http://www.vsp.com
Roger J. Valine, President

★ 18113 ★ Vision Service Plan Insurance Co.—Missouri
Vision Service Plan
3333 Quality Dr.
Rancho Cordova, CA 95670
Phone: (916)851-5000
Roger J. Valine, President

★ 18114 ★ Vision Service Plan of Ohio
Vision Service Plan
3333 Quality Dr.
Rancho Cordova, CA 95670
Phone: (916)851-5000 **Fax:** (916)858-5388
Roger J. Valine, President

★ 18115 ★ Vision Service Plan of Washington
Vision Service Plan
3333 Quality Dr.
Rancho Cordova, CA 95670
Phone: (916)851-5000 **Fax:** (916)858-5388
Roger J. Valine, President

★ 18116 ★ Vision Services Plan, Inc., Oklahoma
Vision Service Plan
3333 Quality Dr.
Rancho Cordova, CA 95670
Phone: (916)851-5000 **Fax:** (916)858-5388
Roger J. Valine, President

★ 18117 ★ Vista Health Plan Inc.
Vista Service Corp.
7801 N Interstate Hwy. 35
Austin, TX 78753
Phone: (512)433-1000

★ 18118 ★ Vista Insurance Plan
300 S Park Rd.
Hollywood, FL 33021
Phone: (954)962-3008

★ 18119 ★ Vista Life Insurance Co.
American Road Insurance Group
PO Box 6027
Dearborn, MI 48121-6027
Phone: (313)322-7287 **Fax:** (313)323-9479
J. M. Moritz, President

★ 18120 ★ Viva Health Inc.
Triton Health Systems LLC
1400 21st Pl S
Birmingham, AL 35205
Phone: (205)939-1718

★ 18121 ★ Volunteer State Health Plan Inc.
Blue Cross & Blue Shield of Tennessee
801 Pine St.
Chattanooga, TN 37402-2555
Phone: (423)755-5600 **Fax:** (423)752-8331
Website: http://www.bcbst.com

★ 18122 ★ Voyager Life and Health Insurance Co.
Fortis, Inc. Group
260 Interstate Cir. NW
Atlanta, GA 30339
Phone: (770)763-1000
Thomas E. McCraw, President

★ 18123 ★ Voyager Life Insurance Co.
Fortis, Inc. Group
260 Interstate Cir. NW
Atlanta, GA 30339
Phone: (817)390-1700 **Fax:** (817)390-1029
Rudi K. Klotz, President

★ 18124 ★ Vytra Health Plans Long Island Inc.
HIP Group of Health Plans
Corporate Ctr.
395 N Service Rd.
Melville, NY 11747-3127
Phone: (516)694-4000

★ 18125 ★ Vytra Health Services Inc.
HIP Group of Health Plans
395 N Service Rd.
Melville, NY 11747
Phone: (631)694-4000
Thomas J. McAteer, Jr., President

★ 18126 ★ Washington Dental Service
PO Box 75688
Seattle, WA 98125-0688
Phone: (206)522-1300 **Fax:** (206)528-2399
Website: http://www.deltadentalwa.com
James S. Garrison, President

★ 18127 ★ Washington National Insurance Co.
Conseco Insurance Group
11815 N Pennsylvania St.
Carmel, IN 46032
Phone: (317)817-6100 **Fax:** (317)817-2161
Website: http://www.conseco.com
Elizabeth C. Georgakopoulos, President
Stephen C. Hilbert, Chairman of the Board

★ 18128 ★ Washington Security Life Insurance Co.
1511 Christy Dr.
Jefferson City, MO 65101
Phone: (847)615-9255

★ 18129 ★ Wateree Life Insurance Co.
PO Box 29
Columbia, SC 29202
Phone: (803)733-2620
Jay C. Case, President

★ 18130 ★ Watts Health Foundation Inc.
Watts Health Systems Inc.
3405 W Imperial Hwy.
Inglewood, CA 90303
Phone: (310)671-3465
Clyde W. Oden, President

★ 18131 ★ WEA Insurance Corp.
PO Box 7338
Madison, WI 53707-7338
Phone: (608)276-4000 **Fax:** (608)276-9119
Website: http://www.weatrust.com
Alan J. Jacobs, President

★ 18132 ★ Welborn Clinic
421 Chestnut St.
Evansville, IN 47713
Phone: (812)426-9884

★ 18133 ★ Welch State Life Insurance Co.
PO Box 1712
Longview, TX 75606
Phone: (903)633-6700

★ 18134 ★ Well Care HMO Inc.
6800 N Dale Mabry Hwy., Ste. 209-211
Tampa, FL 33614
Phone: (813)290-6209

★ 18135 ★ WellCare of New York Inc.
WellCare Management Group Inc.
280 Broadway, 3rd Fl.
Newburgh, NY 12550
Phone: (813)290-6200

★ 18136 ★ WellChoice Insurance of New Jersey Inc.
Empire Blue Cross & Blue Shield Group
11 W 42nd St.
New York, NY 10036
Phone: (212)476-1000 **Fax:** (212)476-1281
Website: http://www.empireblue.com
Michael A. Stocker, MD, Chairman of the Board

★ 18137 ★ Wellington Life Insurance Co.
2929 N 44th St., Ste. 120
Phoenix, AZ 85018
Phone: (787)892-5784
Ronald I. Dozoretz, President

★ 18138 ★ Wellmark Community Insurance, Inc.
Wellmark Group
636 Grand Ave.
Des Moines, IA 50309-2565
Phone: (515)245-4500 **Fax:** (515)248-5617
Website: http://www.wellmark.com
John D. Forsyth, President

★ 18139 ★ Wellmark Health Plan of Iowa Inc.
Wellmark Inc.
636 Grand Ave.
Des Moines, IA 50309-2565
Phone: (515)245-4500 **Fax:** (515)248-5617
Peter W. Roberts, President

★ 18140 ★ Wellmark, Inc.
Wellmark Group
636 Grand Ave.
Des Moines, IA 50309
Phone: (515)245-4500 **Fax:** (515)248-5617
Website: http://www.wellmark.com
John D. Forsyth, CEO & Chm Bd

★ 18141 ★ Wellmark of South Dakota, Inc.
Wellmark Group
1601 W Madison St.
Sioux Falls, SD 57104
Phone: (605)361-5800 **Fax:** (605)361-5898
Website: http://www.wellmark.com
Philip M. Davis, President

★ 18142 ★ The Wellness Plan
2875 W Grand Blvd.
Detroit, MI 48202
Phone: (313)875-4200

★ 18143 ★ WellPath Select Inc.
Coventry Health Care Inc.
6330 Quadrangle Dr., Ste. 500
Chapel Hill, NC 27514-9872
Phone: (919)493-1210

★ 18144 ★ West Coast Life Insurance Co.
Protective Life Corp.
2801 Hwy. 280 S
Birmingham, AL 35223
Phone: (415)591-8200 **Fax:** (415)433-1372
Website: http://www.westcoastlife.com
John D. Johns, President
Drayton Nabers, Chairman of the Board

★ 18145 ★ Western American Life Insurance Co.
Insmark Group
PO Box 833879
Richardson, TX 75083-3879
Phone: (972)699-2770 **Fax:** (972)699-2788
William H. Lewis, Jr., President

★ 18146 ★ Western Diversified Life Insurance Co.
777 Front St.
San Diego, CA 92101
Phone: (619)578-2000
Website: http://www.protective.com
George T. DeVries, III, President

★ 18147 ★ Western Family Life Insurance Co.
2333 State St., Ste. 300
Carlsbad, CA 92008
Phone: (760)730-0130 **Fax:** (760)730-0197
Richard A. McMahan, President

★ 18148 ★ Western Fraternal Life Association
1900 1st Ave. NE
Cedar Rapids, IA 52402-5372
Phone: (319)363-2653 **Fax:** (319)363-8806
Website: http://www.wflains.com
Philip J. Torticill, President

★ 18149 ★ Western General Life Insurance Co.
3636 Executive Center Dr., Ste. G22
PO Box 684247
Austin, TX 78768-4247
Phone: (512)479-9901
James R. Cravens, Jr., President

★ 18150 ★ Western Health Advantage
1331 Garden Hwy., Ste. 100
Sacramento, CA 95833
Phone: (916)563-3180

★ 18151 ★ Western Hemisphere Life Insurance Co.
CBD Holdings, Ltd.
500 Stanton-Christiana Rd., 2-OPS-1
Newark, DE 19713
Phone: (302)634-1469
Website: http://www.chase.com
Paul G. Petrylak, President

★ 18152 ★ Western Mutual Insurance Co.
PO Box 572450
Murray, UT 84157-2450
Phone: (801)263-8000 **Fax:** (801)263-1247
Website: http://www.wpma.com
David T. Leo, President

★ 18153 ★ Western Reserve Life Assurance Co. of Ohio
AEGON USA, Inc.
570 Carillon Pkwy.
Saint Petersburg, FL 33716
Phone: (727)299-1800 **Fax:** (727)299-1834
Jerome C. Vahl, President

★ 18154 ★ Western Security Life Insurance Co.
Dentegra Group Inc.
PO Box 7161
Indianapolis, IN 46207-7161
Phone: (317)927-6500 **Fax:** (317)927-6507
Website: http://www.indianapolislife.com
Marc D. Novotney, President

★ 18155 ★ Western-Southern Life Assurance Co.
Western & Southern Financial Group
400 Broadway
Cincinnati, OH 45202
Phone: (513)629-1800 **Fax:** (513)629-1871
John F. Barrett, CEO & Pres

★ 18156 ★ Western United Life Assurance Co.
Metropolitan Mortgage Group
PO Box 428
Spokane, WA 99210-0428
Phone: (509)227-7500 **Fax:** (509)227-7759
Website: http://www.wula.com
John Van Engelen, President

★ 18157 ★ Westhrift Life Insurance Co.
101 N 1st Ave., Ste. 2460
Phoenix, AZ 85003
Phone: (602)254-5866
Stephen M. Locko, President

★ 18158 ★ Westport Life Insurance Co.
Individual Assurance Group
1600 Oak St.
Kansas City, MO 64108-1406
Phone: (816)842-8842 **Fax:** (816)842-1567
Robert E. Stroud, President

★ 18159 ★ Westward Life Insurance Co.
Westward Insurance Group
PO Box 6025
Lakewood, CA 90714-6025
Phone: (562)420-6103 **Fax:** (562)425-7869
James H. Smith, President

★ 18160 ★ Westwood Life Insurance Co.
GE Financial Assurance Group
6604 W Broad St.
Richmond, VA 23230
Phone: (267)468-2000
Kathryn V. Marinello, President

★ 18161 ★ White River Valley Insurance Co.
Citizens Fidelity Group
PO Box 2576
Batesville, AR 72503
Phone: (870)793-4161
Mark A. Faith, President

★ 18162 ★ Wichita National Life Insurance Co.
Wichita National Life Group
PO Box 1709
Lawton, OK 73502
Phone: (580)353-5776 **Fax:** (580)353-6482
Randall B. Gilliland, President
Ronnie Denham, Vice President

★ 18163 ★ William Penn Association
709 Brighton Rd.
Pittsburgh, PA 15233-1821
Phone: (412)231-2979 **Fax:** (412)231-8535
George S. Charles, Jr., President

★ 18164 ★ William Penn Life Insurance Co. of New York
Legal & General America, Inc.
1701 Research Blvd.
Rockville, MD 20850
Phone: (516)794-3700 **Fax:** (301)279-4178
Website: http://www.lgamerica.com
Joseph M. Sullivan, President
David S. Lenaburg, CEO & Chm Bd

★ 18165 ★ Williams Progressive Life and Accident Insurance Co.
348 S Academy St.
PO Box 898
Opelousas, LA 70571-0898
Phone: (318)948-8238

★ 18166 ★ Windsor Life Insurance Co.
Optimum Re Group
PO Box 660010
Dallas, TX 75266-0010
Phone: (214)559-0850 **Fax:** (214)528-9862
Website: http://www.windsorlifeinsuranceco.com
Mike Simard, President

★ 18167 ★ Winnfield Life Insurance Co.
PO Box 816
Natchitoches, LA 71458
Phone: (318)352-8346
Larry G. Lenius, President

★ 18168 ★ Wisconsin Auto & Truck Dealers Insurance Co.
PO Box 5345
Madison, WI 53705-0345
Phone: (608)251-5577

★ 18169 ★ Wisconsin Physicians Service Insurance Corp.
Wisconsin Physicians Service Group
1717 W Broadway
Madison, WI 53713-1895
Phone: (608)221-4711
Website: http://www.wpsic.com
James R. Riordan, President

★ 18170 ★ Wisconsin Vision Service Plan, Inc.
Vision Service Plan
3333 Quality Dr.
Rancho Cordova, CA 95670
Phone: (916)851-5000 **Fax:** (916)858-5388
Roger J. Valine, President

★ 18171 ★ Woman's Life Insurance Society
PO Box 5020
Port Huron, MI 48061-5020
Phone: (810)985-5191 **Fax:** (810)985-6970
Website: http://www.womanslifeins.com
Janice U. Whipple, President

★ 18172 ★ Women's Life Insurance Co. of America
PO Box 535304
San Antonio, TX 78279-1070
Phone: (713)467-8811
Meryl Grantham Crosbie, President

★ 18173 ★ Wonder State Life Insurance Co.
Southern Pioneer Group
216 W Main St.
Trumann, AR 72472
Phone: (870)483-6355 **Fax:** (870)483-6328
Benjamin R. Hyneman, President

★ 18174 ★ Woodmen Accident and Life Co.
Lincoln Insurance Group
PO Box 82288
Lincoln, NE 68501-2288
Phone: (402)476-6500 **Fax:** (402)437-4395
Website: http://www.walco.com
Thomas D. Potter, CEO & Pres

★ 18175 ★ Woodmen of the World and/or Assured Life Association
PO Box 266000
Highlands Ranch, CO 80163-6000
Phone: (303)792-9777 **Fax:** (303)792-9793
Website: http://www.denverwoodmen.com
David E. Wilson, President

★ 18176 ★ Woodmen of the World Life Insurance Society and/or Omaha Woodmen Life Insurance Society
1700 Farnam St.
Omaha, NE 68102
Phone: (402)342-1890 **Fax:** (402)449-7732
Website: http://www.woodmen.com
James L. Mounce, President

★ 18177 ★ Workmen's Benefit Fund of the United States of America
99 N Broadway
Hicksville, NY 11801-2905
Phone: (516)938-6060 **Fax:** (516)938-6882
John Z. Sebastian, President

★ 18178 ★ Workmen's Life Insurance Co.
Workmen's Insurance Companies
PO Box 54845
Los Angeles, CA 90054-0845
Phone: (213)747-6492 **Fax:** (213)747-4699
Robert J. Sharp, President

★ 18179 ★ World Insurance Co.
World Insurance Co. Group
PO Box 3160
Omaha, NE 68103-0160
Phone: (402)496-8000 **Fax:** (402)496-8040
Website: http://worldinsco.com
T. D. Eilers, President

★ 18180 ★ World Service Life Insurance Co.
Citigroup
307 W 7th St., Ste. 400
Fort Worth, TX 76102
Phone: (817)348-7559 **Free:** 800-316-5607
Fax: (817)348-7596
Peter B. Dahlberg, President

★ 18181 ★ Xantus Healthplan of Tennessee Inc.
3401 W End Ave., Ste. 470
Nashville, TN 37203
Phone: (615)298-3666

★ 18182 ★ Zale Life Insurance Co.
Zale Group
PO Box 152762, MS 5A9
Irving, TX 75015-2762
Phone: (972)580-4080 **Fax:** (972)580-5198
Sue E. Gove, President

★ 18183 ★ Zurich Kemper Life Insurance Co. of New York
Zurich Insurance Group
1600 McConnor Pkwy.
Schaumburg, IL 60196-6801
Phone: (847)874-4000 **Fax:** (847)874-5643
Website: http://www.zurichlifeus.com
Gale K. Caruso, CEO & Pres

★ 18184 ★ Zurich Life Insurance Co. of America
Zurich Insurance Group
1600 McConnor Pkwy.
Schaumburg, IL 60196
Phone: (847)874-4000 **Fax:** (847)874-5643
Website: http://www.zurichlifeus.com
Gale K. Caruso, President

Chapter 12
Managed Health Care Organizations

Listed in this chapter are five types of managed health care organizations: (1) Health Maintenance Organizations (HMOs), (2) Preferred Provider Organizations (PPOs), (3) Point-of-Service (POS) Plans, (4) Specialty HMOs, and (5) Specialty PPOs. Within each category, entries are arranged by the states they serve, then by organization names within states. Consult the "User's Guide" located at the front of the directory for additional information.

Health Maintenance Organizations (HMOs)

Alabama

★ 18185 ★ Health Insurance Corp. of Alabama
HMO Plan
2055 E South Blvd.
Montgomery, AL 36111-0010
Phone: (334)288-2100 **Fax:** (334)286-5602
Randall Hoover, CEO

★ 18186 ★ The Oath, A Health Plan for Alabama
HMO Plan
Two Perimeter Park S, Ste. 200W
Birmingham, AL 35242
Phone: (205)968-1000 **Free:** 800-888-7647
Fax: (205)968-2277
Website: http://www.healthpartners.com
John Davis, President

★ 18187 ★ PrimeHealth
HMO Plan
1400 University Blvd. S
Mobile, AL 36609-2999
Phone: (251)342-0022 **Free:** 800-928-7716
Fax: (251)342-1176
Website: http://www.primehealthonline.com
Kathryn Parks, CEO

★ 18188 ★ United Healthcare of Alabama, Inc.
HMO Plan
PO Box 830637
Birmingham, AL 35255
Phone: (205)977-6300 **Free:** 800-345-1520
Fax: (205)977-6537
Website: http://www.uhc.com
William W. McGuire, MD, Chairman of the Board

★ 18189 ★ Viva Health, Inc.
HMO Plan
1401 21st St. S
Birmingham, AL 35205
Phone: (205)939-1718 **Fax:** (205)939-1748
Brad Rollow, CEO

Arizona

★ 18190 ★ Aetna Inc—Arizona
HMO Plan
7720 N 16th St., Ste. 400
Phoenix, AZ 85020
Phone: (602)427-2200 **Fax:** (602)427-2176
Website: http://www.aetna.com
John W. Rowe, MD, Chairman of the Board

★ 18191 ★ Blue Cross Blue Shield of Arizona
Blue Choice (HMO)
PO Box 13466
Phoenix, AZ 85062-3466
Phone: (602)864-4613 **Free:** 800-232-2345
Fax: (602)864-4184
Website: http://www.bcbaz.com
Robert B. Bulla, Chairman of the Board

★ 18192 ★ Blue Cross Blue Shield of Arizona
Blue Select (HMO)
PO Box 13466
Phoenix, AZ 85062-3466
Phone: (602)864-4613 **Free:** 800-232-2345
Fax: (602)864-4184
Website: http://www.bcbaz.com
Robert B. Bulla, Chairman of the Board

★ 18193 ★ CIGNA HealthCare of Arizona
HMO Plan
7225 N Mona Lisa Rd.
Tucson, AZ 85741
Phone: (520)571-0111 **Fax:** (520)575-4950
Website: http://www.cigna.com/healthcare/hs/ar.html
Frank Benedetto, Contact

★ 18194 ★ CIGNA Healthcare of Arizona
HMO Plan
11001 N Black Canyon Hwy., No. 400
Phoenix, AZ 85029-4754
Phone: (602)942-4462 **Fax:** (602)371-2625
Website: http://www.cigna.com
Edward Handway, CEO

★ 18195 ★ Evercare Select
3141 N Third Ave., Ste. 100
Phoenix, AZ 85013
Phone: (602)331-5100 **Free:** 800-293-3740
Fax: (502)331-5199
Website: http://www.lifemarkcorp.com
Rhonda Brede, President

★ 18196 ★ Health Net of Arizona
HMO Plan
930 N Finance Ctr. Dr, Ste. 100
Tucson, AZ 85710
Phone: (520)721-1122 **Free:** 800-289-2818
Fax: (520)290-7585
Website: http://www.az.health.net
Mark El-Tawil, President

★ 18197 ★ Humana Health Plan, Inc.
HMO Plan
2710 E Camelback Rd.
Phoenix, AZ 85016-3245
Phone: (602)553-2000 **Free:** 800-288-6442
Fax: (602)381-4389
Website: http://www.humana.com
William J. Howard, CEO & Pres

★ 18198 ★ Maricopa Managed Care Systems
HMO Plan
2502 E University Dr., Ste. 125
Phoenix, AZ 85034
Phone: (602)344-8703 **Free:** 800-582-8686
Fax: (602)342-8933
Linda Mushkatel, CEO

★ 18199 ★ Mayo Health Plan Arizona
HMO Plan
13400 E Shea Blvd.
Scottsdale, AZ 85259
Phone: (480)515-6296 **Free:** 800-335-6296
Fax: (507)284-1963
Website: http://www.mayo.ivi.com
Nancy Lashutka, Contact

★ 18200 ★ Medisun
13632 N 99th Ave
Sun City, AZ 85351
Phone: (623)974-7430 **Fax:** (623)974-7439
Website: http://www.sunhealth.org
Leland Peterson, CEO

★ 18201 ★ Mercy Care Plan
HMO Plan
PO Box 25009
Phoenix, AZ 85002-5009
Phone: (602)248-0800 **Free:** 800-624-3879
Fax: (602)351-2303
Website: http://www.schn.com
Stan Aronovitch, CEO

★ 18202 ★ One Health Plan of Arizona
HMO Plan
3131 E Camelback Rd., Ste. 240
Phoenix, AZ 85016
Phone: (602)667-9537 **Fax:** (602)508-8972
Website: http://www.onehealthplan.com
Roger Stinton, Contact

★ 18203 ★ PacifiCare of Arizona
HMO Plan
PO Box 52078
Phoenix, AZ 85072
Phone: (602)244-8200 **Free:** 800-221-2462
Fax: (602)681-7000
Website: http://www.pacificare.com
Rick Badger, President

★ 18204 ★ Phoenix Health Plan
HMO Plan
2700 N 3rd St., Ste. 3000
Phoenix, AZ 85004
Phone: (602)824-3700 **Free:** 800-747-7997
Fax: (602)824-3857

Website: http://www.phxmemorialhospital.com
Nancy Novick, CEO

★ 18205 ★ Pima Health Care System
HMO Plan
5055 E Broadway, Ste. 200
Tucson, AZ 85711-3640
Phone: (520)512-5500 **Free:** 800-423-3801
Fax: (520)745-6386
Karen Fields, CEO

★ 18206 ★ United HealthCare of Arizona, Inc.
Choice (HMO)
3141 N 3rd Ave.
Phoenix, AZ 85013
Phone: (602)664-5000 **Free:** 800-442-4119
Fax: (602)664-2732
Website: http://www.unitedhealthcare.com
William W. McGuire, MD, Chairman of the Board

★ 18207 ★ University Family Care
575 E River Rd.
Tucson, AZ 85704
Phone: (520)795-3500 **Fax:** (520)690-2480
Website: http://www.azumc.com
Gloria Reynolds, CEO

Arkansas

★ 18208 ★ Health Advantage
HMO Plan
26 Corporate Hill Dr.
Little Rock, AR 72205
Phone: (501)221-1800 **Fax:** (501)221-7103
Website: http://www.healthadvantage-hmo.com
David Frank Bridges, CEO

★ 18209 ★ Healthlink of Arkansas Inc.
HMO Plan
3901 McCain Park Dr, Ste. 201
North Little Rock, AR 72116-7849
Phone: (501)771-2111 **Fax:** (501)771-1936
Website: http://www.healthlink.com
Brett Kirkman, Contact

★ 18210 ★ HMO Partners Inc
HMO Plan
26 Corporate Hill Dr.
Little Rock, AR 72205-4538
Phone: (501)221-1800 **Fax:** (501)228-8716
Website: http://www.arkbluecross.com
David Frank Bridges, CEO

★ 18211 ★ QCA Health Plan, Inc.
HMO Plan
10800 Financial Center Pkwy., Ste. 450
Little Rock, AR 72211
Phone: (501)228-7111 **Fax:** (501)801-2959
Francis Browning, CEO

★ 18212 ★ United HealthCare of Arkansas
HMO Plan
415 N McKinley, Ste. 820
Little Rock, AR 72205
Phone: (501)664-7700 **Free:** 800-678-3176
Fax: (501)664-7768
Website: http://www.uhc.com
John A. Wickens, President

California

★ 18213 ★ Aetna Inc.—California
HMO Plan
2409 Comino Ramon
San Ramon, CA 94583
Phone: (925)543-9000 **Fax:** (925)543-9010
Website: http://www.aetna.com
John W. Rowe, MD, Chairman of the Board

★ 18214 ★ Aetna Inc.—California
HMO Plan
5800 Canoga Ave.
Woodland Hills, CA 91367
Phone: (818)992-2000 **Free:** 800-553-2952
Fax: (818)593-7108
Website: http://www.aetna.com
John W. Rowe, MD, Chairman of the Board

★ 18215 ★ Aetna Inc.—California
HMO Plan
1200 W 7th St., Ste. 400
Los Angeles, CA 90017
Phone: (310)955-3100 **Fax:** (310)955-3185
Website: http://www.aetna.com
John W. Rowe, MD, Chairman of the Board

★ 18216 ★ Alameda Alliance for Health
HMO Plan
1240 S Loop Rd.
Alameda, CA 94502
Phone: (510)747-4500 **Fax:** (510)747-4502
Irena Ibarra, CEO

★ 18217 ★ Care 1st Health Plan
HMO Plan
1000 Fremont Ave., Bldg. A-11, U-22
Alhambra, CA 91803
Phone: (626)299-4299 **Fax:** (626)458-0415
S. R. Wong, Chairman of the Board

★ 18218 ★ Cedars-Sinai Provider Plan LLC
633 W Fifth St., Ste. 4000
Los Angeles, CA 90071
Phone: (213)891-8762

★ 18219 ★ Chinese Community Health Plan
HMO Plan
170 Columbus Ave., Ste. 210
San Francisco, CA 94133-4851
Phone: (415)397-3190 **Fax:** (415)397-6140
Website: http://www.cchphmo.com
Richard Loos, CEO

★ 18220 ★ CIGNA HealthCare of California
HMO Plan
400 N Brand Blvd., Ste. 500
Glendale, CA 91203
Phone: (818)500-6262 **Free:** 800-344-7421
Fax: (818)500-6480
Website: http://www.cigna.com/healthcare
Bud Volberding, President

★ 18221 ★ CIGNA Healthcare of California, Inc. - San Diego
HMO Plan
3131 Camino Del Rio N, Ste. 900
San Diego, CA 92108
Phone: (619)641-5400 **Free:** 800-368-2471
Fax: (619)641-5499
Website: http://www.cigna.com
Bud Volberding, CEO

★ 18222 ★ Community Health Group
HMO Plan
740 Bay Blvd., 2nd Fl.
Chula Vista, CA 91910
Phone: (619)422-0422 **Free:** 800-640-4662
Fax: (619)422-5930
Website: http://www.chgsd.com
Norma Diaz, CEO

★ 18223 ★ Community Health Plan
HMO Plan
1000 S Fremont Ave., Bldg. A-9 East 2nd Fl., Unit 4
Alhambra, CA 91803
Phone: (626)299-5300 **Fax:** (626)458-6761
Website: http://www.dhs.co.la.ca.us
Pauline Rodriguez, Contact

★ 18224 ★ Contra Costa Health Plan
HMO Plan
595 Center Ave., Ste. 100
Martinez, CA 94553
Phone: (925)313-6000 **Fax:** (925)313-6002
Website: http://www.cchealth.org
Milton Camhi, CEO

★ 18225 ★ Great West Life
HMO Plan
101 N Brand Blvd., Ste 1950
Glendale, CA 91203
Phone: (818)247-9102 **Free:** 800-877-9102
Fax: (818)247-3033
Website: http://www.onehealthplan.com
Gary Smith, Contact

★ 18226 ★ Great West Life
HMO Plan
3480 Buskirk Ave., Ste. 350
Pleasant Hill, CA 94523
Phone: (925)938-7788 **Fax:** (925)210-0975
Website: http://www.onehealthplan.com
Vicki Mahoney, Contact

★ 18227 ★ Health Net of California
HMO Plan
21281 Burbank Blvd.
Woodland Hills, CA 91367
Phone: (818)676-6775 **Free:** 800-522-0088
Fax: (818)676-6982
Website: http://www.healthnet.com
Jennifer M. Gutzmore, MD, Contact

★ 18228 ★ Health Net, Inc. - Corporate Headquarters
Health Net HMO
21650 Oxnard St.
Woodland Hills, CA 91367
Phone: (818)676-6775 **Free:** 800-474-6676
Fax: (818)676-7315
Website: http://www.health.net
Jay M. Gellert, CEO

★ 18229 ★ Health Plan of the Redwoods
HMO Plan
3033 Cleveland Ave.
Santa Rosa, CA 95403
Phone: (707)544-2273 **Free:** 800-248-2070
Fax: (707)525-4261
Website: http://www.hrp.org
Katie Pierce, Chairman of the Board

★ 18230 ★ Health Plan of San Joaquin
HMO Plan
1550 W Fremont St., Ste. 200
Stockton, CA 95203
Phone: (209)939-3500 **Fax:** (209)939-3535
Website: http://www.hpsj.com
Terry Mack, CEO

★ 18231 ★ Health Plan of San Mateo
HMO Plan
701 Gateway Blvd., Ste. 400
South San Francisco, CA 94080
Phone: (650)616-0050 **Free:** 800-750-4776
Fax: (650)616-0060
Michael Murray, CEO

★ 18232 ★ Heritage Provider Network, Inc.
18107 Sherman Way, Ste. 100
Reseda, CA 91335
Phone: (818)654-3455
Richard Merkin, CEO

★ 18233 ★ Inland Empire Health Plan
HMO Plan
303 E Vanderbilt Way, Ste. 400
San Bernardino, CA 92408
Phone: (909)890-2000 **Fax:** (909)890-2019
Website: http://www.iehp.org
Richard Bruno, CEO

★ 18234 ★ Inter Valley Health Plan
HMO Plan
PO Box 6002
Pomona, CA 91769-6002
Phone: (909)623-6333 **Free:** 800-255-6882
Fax: (909)622-2907
Website: http://www.ivhp.com
Richard Kirkendall, PhD, Chairman of the Board

★ 18235 ★ Kaiser Foundation Health Plan of Northern California
HMO Plan
1950 Franklin St.
Oakland, CA 94612
Phone: (510)987-1000 **Fax:** (510)987-4178
Website: http://www.kaiserpermanente.org
George Halvorson, CEO

★ 18236 ★ Kaiser Foundation Health Plan of Southern California
393 E Walnut St.
Pasadena, CA 91188
Phone: (626)405-5534 **Fax:** (626)405-3176
Website: http://www.kaiserparmanente.org
George Halvorson, CEO

★ 18237 ★ Kaiser Permanente
Kaiser Foundation Health Plan (HMO)
One Kaiser Plaza
Oakland, CA 94612
Phone: (510)271-5934 **Fax:** (510)271-5820
Website: http://www.kaiserpermanente.org
George Halvorson, Chairman of the Board

★ 18238 ★ Kern Family Health Care
HMO Plan
1600 Norris Rd.
Bakersfield, CA 93308
Phone: (661)391-4000 **Free:** 800-391-2000
Fax: (661)391-4106
Carol Sorrell, CEO

★ 18239 ★ LA Care Health Plan
HMO Plan
555 W 5th St., 18th Fl.
Los Angeles, CA 90013-3036
Phone: (213)694-1250 **Free:** 888-452-2273
Fax: (213)694-1249
Website: http://lacare.org
Robert E. Tranquada, Chairman of the Board

★ 18240 ★ Lakewood Health Plan, Inc.
HMO Plan
4909 Lakewood Blvd., Ste. 200
Lakewood, CA 90712
Phone: (562)602-1563 **Fax:** (562)531-0937
Website: http://www.lhpipa.com
David Neer, MD, JD, Contact

★ 18241 ★ Lifeguard, Inc.
HMO Plan
PO Box 5506
San Jose, CA 95150-5506
Phone: (408)943-9400 **Free:** 800-995-0380
Fax: (408)432-3695
Website: http://www.lifeguard.com
Mark Hyde, CEO

★ 18242 ★ Mendocino and Lake Counties Foundation for Medical Care
PPO Plan
PO Box 1030
Ukiah, CA 95482-4355
Phone: (707)462-7607 **Fax:** (707)462-1206
Robert Faulk, CEO

★ 18243 ★ Molina
HMO Plan
1 Golden Shore Dr.
Long Beach, CA 90802
Phone: (562)435-3666 **Free:** 800-526-8196
Fax: (562)437-1335
Website: http://www.molinahealthcare.com
Joseph M. Molina, MD, Chairman of the Board

★ 18244 ★ One Health Plan of California
HMO Plan
655 N Central Ave., No. 1900
Glendale, CA 91203-1441
Phone: (818)539-1900 **Fax:** (818)545-9238
Website: http://www.onehealthplan.com
Jackie James, President

★ 18245 ★ Orange Prevention & Treatment Integrated
PO Box 11033
Orange, CA 92856
Phone: (714)246-8400 **Fax:** (714)246-8492
Website: http://www.caloptima.org
Mary Dewane, CEO

★ 18246 ★ Pacific IPA
HMO Plan
430 S Garfield Ave., No. 301
Alhambra, CA 91801
Phone: (626)281-3400 **Free:** 888-888-PIPA
Fax: (626)281-0444
Peter Lindbion, CEO

★ 18247 ★ PacifiCare of California
HMO Plan
5701 Katella Ave.
Cypress, CA 90630-5028
Phone: (714)952-1121 **Free:** 800-624-8822
Fax: (714)226-3996
Website: http://www.pacificare.com
Howard G. Phanstiel, CEO

★ 18248 ★ Pacificare Health Systems - Corporate Headquarters
HMO Plan
PO Box 25186
Santa Ana, CA 92799-5186
Phone: (714)952-1121 **Free:** 800-624-8822
Fax: (714)825-2201
Website: http://www.pacificare.com
Howard G. Phanstiel, CEO

★ 18249 ★ Partnership Healthplan of California
HMO Plan
360 Campus Lane, Ste. 100
Suisun City, CA 94585
Phone: (707)863-4100 **Free:** 800-863-4155
Fax: (707)863-4117
Website: http://www.partnershiphp.org
Jack Horn, CEO

★ 18250 ★ Primecare Medical Network
HMO Plan
3281 E Guasti Rd., 7th Fl.
Ontario, CA 91761
Phone: (909)605-8000 **Free:** 800-864-7500
Fax: (909)605-8031
Rene Moret, CEO

★ 18251 ★ San Francisco Health Plan
HMO Plan
568 Howard St., 5th Fl.
San Francisco, CA 94105
Phone: (415)547-7800 **Free:** 800-288-5555
Fax: (415)547-7824
Website: http://www.sfhp.org
Jean Frasier, CEO

★ 18252 ★ Santa Clara County Health Authority
Santa Clara Family Health Plan (HMO)
210 E Hacienda Ave.
Campbell, CA 95008
Phone: (408)376-2000 **Free:** 800-260-2055
Fax: (408)874-1955
Leona Butler, CEO

★ 18253 ★ Santa Cruz - Monterey Managed Medical Care Commission
375 Encinal St., Ste. A
Santa Cruz, CA 95060
Phone: (831)457-3850 **Fax:** (831)466-4310
Alan McKay, CEO

★ 18254 ★ Sante Community Physicians
HMO Plan
1180 E Shaw Ave., Ste. 101
Fresno, CA 93710
Phone: (559)228-5400 **Free:** 800-652-2900
Fax: (559)224-2046
Scott Wells, CEO

★ 18255 ★ SCAN Health Plan
HMO Plan
3800 Kilroy Airport Way, No. 100
Long Beach, CA 90806
Phone: (562)989-5100 **Free:** 800-247-5091
Fax: (562)989-5200
Website: http://www.scanhealthplan.com
Sam Ervin, CEO & Pres

★ 18256 ★ Scripps Clinic Health Plan Services, Inc.
10666 N Torrey Pines Rd.
La Jolla, CA 92037
Phone: (858)784-5961 **Fax:** (858)784-5837
Mark Reynolds, CEO

★ 18257 ★ Sharp Health Plan
HMO Plan
9325 Sky Park Court, Ste. 300
San Diego, CA 92123
Phone: (858)637-6500 **Free:** 800-359-2002
Fax: (858)637-6504
Website: http://www.sharp.com
B. Kathlyn Mead, CEO & Pres

★ 18258 ★ UHP Healthcare
United Health Plan HMO
34650 Imperial Hwy.
Inglewood, CA 90303
Phone: (310)671-3465 **Fax:** (310)673-9176
Website: http://www.whs.com
Frank Stevens, CEO

★ 18259 ★ United Healthcare of Oregon
180 E Ocean Blvd., Ste. 500
Long Beach, CA 90802

Phone: (562)951-6400 **Free:** 800-325-6651
Fax: (562)951-6885
Website: http://www.uhc.com
Emery Dameron, CEO

★ 18260 ★ Universal Care
HMO Plan
1600 E Hill St.
Signal Hill, CA 90806
Phone: (562)424-6200 **Free:** 800-635-6668
Fax: (562)595-0872
Howard Davis, CEO

★ 18261 ★ University of California - San Diego
HMO Plan
1899 McKee St.
San Diego, CA 92110
Phone: (619)543-5916
Marsha Killian, Contact

★ 18262 ★ Valley Health Plan
HMO Plan
2325 Emborg Lane, Ste. 290
San Jose, CA 95128
Phone: (408)885-4760 **Fax:** (408)885-5926
Greg Price, CEO

★ 18263 ★ Ventura County Health Care Plan
HMO Plan
2323 Knoll Dr., Ste. 417
Ventura, CA 93003
Phone: (805)677-8787 **Free:** 800-600-8247
Fax: (805)677-5179
Larry Keller, CEO

★ 18264 ★ WellPoint Health Networks, Inc. - Corporate Headquarters
HMO Plan
One WellPoint Way
Thousand Oaks, CA 91362
Phone: (818)703-4000 **Fax:** (805)557-6872
Website: http://www.wellpoint.com
Leonard Schaeffer, CEO & Chm Bd

★ 18265 ★ Western Health Advantage
HMO Plan
1331 Garden Hwy., Ste. 100
Sacramento, CA 95833
Phone: (916)563-3180 **Free:** 888-227-5942
Fax: (916)563-3182
Garry Maisel, CEO

Colorado

★ 18266 ★ Aetna Inc. - Colorado
HMO Plan
4643 S Ulster St., Ste. 1000
Denver, CO 80237
Phone: (303)796-6100 **Free:** 800-481-3841
Fax: (303)796-6183
Website: http://www.aetna.com
John W. Rowe, CEO

★ 18267 ★ Aetna Inc. - Colorado
HMO Plan
6430 S Fiddlers Green Cir., No. 200
Englewood, CO 80111
Phone: (303)793-2500 **Fax:** (303)793-2510
Website: http://www.aetna.com
John W. Rowe, CEO

★ 18268 ★ Antero Health Plans Inc.
6455 S Yosemite St.
Greenwood Village, CO 80111
Phone: (303)714-3542 **Fax:** (303)714-3990
Richard Rivers, CEO

★ 18269 ★ CIGNA HealthCare of Colorado
HMO Plan
3900 E Mexico Ave., Ste. 1100
Denver, CO 80210
Phone: (303)782-1500 **Free:** 800-832-3211
Fax: (303)782-1577
Website: http://www.cigna.com
Daryl Edmonds, CEO

★ 18270 ★ Colorado Access
HMO Plan
PO Box 17470
Denver, CO 80217-0470
Phone: (303)333-8900 **Free:** 800-511-5010
Fax: (303)755-2896
Website: http://www.coaccess.com
Don Hall, CEO

★ 18271 ★ Community Health Plan of the Rockies, Inc.
HMO Plan
400 S Colorado Blvd., Ste. 300
Denver, CO 80246
Phone: (303)355-3220 **Free:** 800-935-3220
Fax: (303)355-3224
Website: http://www.healthquotes.com/chpr.htm
Lawrence Rachmel, CEO

★ 18272 ★ Denver Health Medical Plan
HMO Plan
777 Bannock St.
Denver, CO 80204
Phone: (303)436-7726 **Fax:** (303)436-3885
Doug Clinkscales, CEO

★ 18273 ★ Great West Life Annuity Insurance Co.
HMO Plan
PO Box 1700
Denver, CO 80201
Phone: (303)737-3000 **Fax:** (303)737-3198
Website: http://www.gwla.com
William McCallum, CEO

★ 18274 ★ Great-West/One Health Plan
HMO Plan
8505 E Orchard Rd.
Greenwood Village, CO 80111
Phone: (303)737-3000 **Fax:** (303)737-3405
Website: http://www.onehealthplan.com
William T. McCallum, CEO & Pres

★ 18275 ★ HMO Health Plans Inc.
95 W First Ave.
Monte Vista, CO 81144
Phone: (719)852-4055 **Fax:** (719)852-3481
Cynthia Palmer, CEO

★ 18276 ★ Kaiser Foundation Health Plan of Colorado
HMO Plan
10350 E Dakota Ave.
Denver, CO 80231
Phone: (303)344-7200 **Fax:** (303)344-7956
Website: http://www.kaiserpermanente.org
Christopher Brinkley, CEO

★ 18277 ★ Kaiser Permanente
HMO Plan
2500 S Havana St.
Aurora, CO 80014
Phone: (303)338-3700 **Free:** 800-632-9700
Fax: (303)338-3797
Website: http://www.kaiserpermanente.org
Christopher Binkley, CEO

★ 18278 ★ One Health Plan of Colorado
HMO Plan
8525 E Orchard Rd., No. 3
Greenwood Village, CO 80111-5002
Phone: (303)305-1000 **Fax:** (303)737-3198
Website: http://www.onehealthplan.com
Chris Miller, President

★ 18279 ★ PacifiCare of Colorado
HMO Plan
6455 S Yosemite
Englewood, CO 80111
Phone: (303)220-5800 **Free:** 800-877-6685
Fax: (303)714-3999
Website: http://www.pacificare.com
Jeffrey Folick, Chairman of the Board
Program(s): Chiropractic, Dental, Home Care, Inpatient SNF, Long-Term Care, Pharmaceutical Mail Order, Podiatry, Psychiatric, Behavioral Health, Physical Therapy, Transplant, Vision, Wellness.

★ 18280 ★ Rocky Mountain HMO
HMO Plan
2775 Crossroads Blvd.
Grand Junction, CO 81506
Phone: (970)244-7760 **Free:** 800-843-0719
Fax: (970)244-7880
Website: http://www.rmhmo.org
John Hopkins, CEO

★ 18281 ★ Sloan's Lake Health Plan
HMO Plan
1355 S Colorado Blvd., Ste. 902
Denver, CO 80222
Phone: (303)753-7537 **Free:** 800-457-2345
Fax: (303)504-4321
Website: http://www.sloanslake.com
Blair Tikker, CEO

★ 18282 ★ United HealthCare of Colorado
HMO Plan
8051 E Maplewood Ave., Ste. 300
Englewood, CO 80111
Phone: (303)267-3300 **Free:** 800-518-3344
Fax: (303)267-3599
Website: http://www.uhc.com
Victor Lazzaro, Jr., CEO & Pres

Connecticut

★ 18283 ★ Aetna, Inc. - Corporate Headquarters
HMO Plan
151 Farmington Ave.
Hartford, CT 06156-1000
Phone: (860)273-0123 **Free:** 800-225-2949
Fax: (860)636-4513
Website: http://www.aetna.com
John W. Rowe, CEO & Chm Bd

★ 18284 ★ Aetna US Healthcare of New England
HMO Plan
1000 Middle St.
Middletown, CT 06457-3342
Phone: (860)273-0123 **Fax:** (860)273-6872
Website: http://www.aetna.com
John W. Rowe, MD, Chairman of the Board

★ 18285 ★ CIGNA HealthCare of Connecticut, Inc.
HMO Plan
900 Cottage Grove Rd., A-118
Hartford, CT 06152-1118

Phone: (860)769-2300 **Free:** 800-345-9458
Fax: (860)769-2398
Website: http://www.cigna.com
Kirk Weimer, CEO

★ 18286 ★ Community Health Network of Connecticut, Inc.
290 Pratt St.
Meriden, CT 06450
Phone: (203)237-4000 **Fax:** (203)634-8411
Website: http://www.chnct.org
Silvia Kelly, CEO

★ 18287 ★ ConnectiCare, Inc.
HMO Plan
30 Batterson Park Rd.
Farmington, CT 06032
Phone: (860)674-5700 **Free:** 800-251-7722
Fax: (860)674-2011
Website: http://www.connecticare.com
Marcel Gamache, CEO & Pres

★ 18288 ★ Health Net - Connecticut
HMO Plan
PO Box 904
Shelton, CT 06484-0914
Phone: (203)402-4200 **Free:** 800-848-4747
Fax: (203)225-4000
Website: http://www.health.net
Barry Averill, CEO & Pres

★ 18289 ★ Health Net Inc. — Northeast Corporate Headquarters
HMO Plan
PO Box 904
Shelton, CT 06484-0944
Phone: (203)402-4200 **Free:** 800-848-4747
Fax: (203)225-4000
Website: http://www.health.net
Barry Averill, CEO & Pres

★ 18290 ★ MedSpan, Inc.
HMO Plan
225 Asylum St., 11th Fl.
Hartford, CT 06103
Phone: (860)616-2200 **Fax:** (860)616-2540
Website: http://www.medspan.com
Kevin Kelly, President

★ 18291 ★ Oxford Health Plans - Connecticut
HMO Plan
PO Box 7081
Bridgeport, CT 06601-7081
Free: 800-444-6222 **Fax:** (203)851-1491
Website: http://www.oxhp.com
Norman Payson, MD, CEO & Chm Bd

★ 18292 ★ Oxford Health Plans, Inc. - Corporate Headquarters
HMO Plan
48 Monroe Turnpike
Trumbull, CT 06611
Free: 800-889-7658 **Fax:** (203)459-6464
Website: http://www.oxhp.com
Norman Payson, MD, CEO & Chm Bd

★ 18293 ★ Yale University Health Plan
HMO Plan
17 Hillhouse Ave.
New Haven, CT 06520
Phone: (203)432-0076 **Fax:** (203)432-7289
Website: http://www.yale.edu/uhs
Paul Genecin, MD, CEO

Delaware

★ 18294 ★ Aetna Inc. - Delaware
HMO Plan
650 Naamans Rd.
Claymont, DE 19703
Phone: (302)793-1520 **Fax:** (302)798-1877
Website: http://www.aetna.com
John W. Rowe, MD, Chairman of the Board

★ 18295 ★ AmeriHealth Insurance Co.
HMO Plan
919 N Market St., Mellon Ctr. Ste. 1200
Wilmington, DE 19801-3021
Phone: (302)777-6400 **Free:** 800-899-4373
Fax: (302)777-6444
Richard Neeson, Contact

★ 18296 ★ Christiana Care Health Plans, Inc.
HMO Plan
11 Reads Way
New Castle, DE 19720
Phone: (302)327-7650 **Free:** 800-362-4214
Fax: (302)327-7711
Website: http://www.christianacare.org
Ken Bates, CEO

★ 18297 ★ CIGNA HealthCare of Delaware Valley
HMO Plan
PO Box 15408
Wilmington, DE 19850-5408
Phone: (302)477-3700 **Free:** 800-320-0251
Fax: (302)477-3708
Website: http://www.cigna.com
Vincent Sobocinski, Contact

★ 18298 ★ Coventry Health Care Inc.—Delaware, Inc.
HMO Plan
2751 Centerville Rd., Ste. 400
Wilmington, DE 19808
Phone: (302)995-6100 **Free:** 800-833-7423
Fax: (302)998-7085
Website: http://www.chcde.com
Ron Chaffin, CEO & Pres

District of Columbia

★ 18299 ★ Advantage Health Inc.
PO Box 5939
Washington, DC 20016
Phone: (301)636-9840 **Fax:** (301)636-9870
Elliot Wolff, CEO

★ 18300 ★ Amerigroup - District of Columbia
514 10th St., 6th Fl.
Washington, DC 20004
Phone: (202)793-8100 **Fax:** (202)783-8207
Website: http://www.amerigrouporp.com
James Thompson, CEO

★ 18301 ★ Capital Community Health Plan
750 First St. NE, Ste. 1120
Washington, DC 20002
Phone: (202)408-0460 **Fax:** (202)408-0881
Tamara Smith, CEO

★ 18302 ★ DC Chartered Health Plan, Inc.
HMO Plan
820 1st St. NE, Ste. LL100
Washington, DC 20002-4205
Phone: (202)408-4710 **Free:** 800-799-4710
Fax: (202)408-4730
Website: http://www.chartered-health.com
Dr. Charles Bowles, Jr., Chairman of the Board

Florida

★ 18303 ★ Aetna Inc. - Florida
HMO Plan
5100 W Lemon St., Ste. 218
Tampa, FL 33609
Phone: (813)261-9630 **Fax:** (813)636-0658
Website: http://www.aetna.com
John W. Rowe, MD, Chairman of the Board

★ 18304 ★ Aetna Inc. - Jacksonville
HMO Plan
1200 Riverplace Blvd., Ste. 701
Jacksonville, FL 32207
Phone: (904)346-5800 **Fax:** (904)346-5888
Website: http://www.aetna.com
John W. Rowe, MD, Chairman of the Board

★ 18305 ★ Aetna Inc. - Plantation
HMO Plan
8201 Peters Rd.
Plantation, FL 33324
Phone: (954)382-8100 **Fax:** (954)424-4448
Website: http://www.aetna.com
John W. Rowe, MD, Chairman of the Board

★ 18306 ★ Aetna Inc. - Tampa
HMO Plan
5100 W Lemon St., Ste. 218
Tampa, FL 33609
Phone: (813)261-9630 **Free:** 800-232-2385
Fax: (813)636-0658
Website: http://www.aetna.com
John W. Rowe, MD, Chairman of the Board

★ 18307 ★ America's Health Choice Medical Plans, Inc.
1175 S US Hwy. 1
Vero Beach, FL 32962
Phone: (561)794-0030 **Fax:** (561)794-0023
Walter H. Janke, President

★ 18308 ★ Av-Med Health Plan - Gainesville
HMO Plan
PO Box 749
Gainesville, FL 32602
Phone: (352)372-8400 **Free:** 800-346-0231
Fax: (352)337-8888
Website: http://www.avmed.com
Robert Hudson, CEO

★ 18309 ★ Av-Med Health Plan - Jacksonville
HMO Plan
1300 Riverplace Blvd., No. 200-201
Jacksonville, FL 32207-9054
Phone: (904)858-1300 **Fax:** (904)858-1335
Website: http://www.avmed.com
Robert Hudson, CEO

★ 18310 ★ Av-Med Health Plan - Miami
HMO Plan
9400 S Dadeland Blvd.
Miami, FL 33156
Phone: (305)671-5437 **Free:** 800-432-6676
Fax: (305)671-4764
Website: http://www.avmed.com
Robert Hudson, CEO

★ 18311 ★ Av-Med Health Plan - Orlando
HMO Plan
541 S Orlando Ave., Ste. 205
Maitland, FL 32751

Phone: (407)539-0007 **Fax:** (407)975-1623
Website: http://www.avmed.com
Robert Hudson, CEO

★ 18312 ★ Av-Med Health Plan - Tampa
HMO Plan
1511 N Westshore Blvd., Ste. 700
Tampa, FL 33607
Phone: (813)281-5650 **Free:** 800-257-2273
Fax: (813)281-0659
Website: http://www.avmed.com
Douglas Cooper, CEO

★ 18313 ★ Beacon Health Plans
HMO Plan
PO Box 459012
Sunrise, FL 33345
Phone: (305)460-2000 **Fax:** (305)774-2617
Website: http://www.beaconhealth.com
Wilfredo Gonzalez, President

★ 18314 ★ Capital Health Plan
HMO Plan
2140 Centerville Pl.
Tallahassee, FL 32308-4300
Phone: (850)383-3333 **Free:** 800-390-1434
Fax: (850)383-3497
Website: http://www.capitalhealth.com
John Hogan, CEO

★ 18315 ★ CIGNA HealthCare of Florida
HMO Plan
1580 Sawgrass Corp. Pkwy., Ste 200
Sunrise, FL 33323
Phone: (954)693-7500 **Fax:** (954)693-7540
Website: http://www.cigna.com
William Taylor, CEO

★ 18316 ★ CIGNA HealthCare of Florida
HMO Plan
5404 Cypress Center Dr.
Tampa, FL 33609
Phone: (813)281-1000 **Free:** 800-942-2471
Fax: (813)289-0363
Website: http://www.cigna.com
Andrew Crooks, CEO & Pres

★ 18317 ★ Florida Health Care Plan, Inc.
HMO Plan
1340 Ridgewood Ave.
Holly Hill, FL 32117
Phone: (386)676-7110 **Free:** 800-352-9824
Fax: (386)676-7119
Edward Simpson, Jr., CEO

★ 18318 ★ Foundation Health, A Florida Health Plan
HMO Plan
1340 Concord Terrace
Sunrise, FL 33323
Phone: (954)858-3000 **Free:** 800-422-7335
Fax: (954)846-0331
Website: http://www.fhfl.com
Robert Berzing, CEO

★ 18319 ★ Great West Life - Florida
HMO Plan
110 E Broward Blvd., Ste. 750
Fort Lauderdale, FL 33301
Phone: (954)463-2720 **Fax:** (954)463-2750
Website: http://www.onehealthplan.com
Tracy Carter, Contact

★ 18320 ★ Health First Health Plans, Inc.
HMO Plan
8247 Devereaux Dr., Ste. 103
Melbourne, FL 32940-7955
Phone: (321)434-5600 **Free:** 800-716-7737
Fax: (321)752-1129
Website: http://www.health-first.org
Jerry Senne, CEO

★ 18321 ★ Health Plan Southeast, Inc.
HMO Plan
PO Box 13700
Tallahassee, FL 32317-3700
Phone: (850)668-3000 **Free:** 800-833-2169
Fax: (850)668-3133
Website: http://www.hpse.com
Robert Wychulis, CEO

★ 18322 ★ Healthease of Florida Inc.
6800 N Dale Mabry Hwy., No. 270
Tampa, FL 33614
Phone: (813)290-6219 **Free:** 800-610-4466
Fax: (813)290-6294
Rupesh Shah, CEO

★ 18323 ★ Healthy Palm Beaches, Inc.
HMO Plan
324 Datura St., Ste. 401
West Palm Beach, FL 33401
Phone: (561)659-1270 **Fax:** (561)659-4620
Website: http://www.hcdphc.org
Dwight Chenette, CEO

★ 18324 ★ Humana Health Care Plans of Orlando
HMO Plan
PO Box 9148000
Longwood, FL 32779
Phone: (407)661-6000 **Fax:** (407)661-6414
Website: http://www.humana.com/orlando/home.html
Michael B. McCallister, President

★ 18325 ★ Humana Health Plan - Jacksonville
HMO Plan
76 S Laura St., 16th Fl.
Jacksonville, FL 32202
Phone: (904)376-1100 **Free:** 800-945-7703
Fax: (904)376-2370
Website: http://www.humana.com
David A. Jones, Chairman of the Board

★ 18326 ★ Humana Medical Plan - Daytona
HMO Plan
135 Executive Circle
Daytona Beach, FL 32114
Phone: (386)676-1800 **Free:** 800-320-9565
Fax: (386)676-1806
Website: http://www.humana.com
David A. Jones, Chairman of the Board

★ 18327 ★ Humana Medical Plan - Tampa
HMO Plan
5401 W Kennedy Blvd.
Tampa, FL 33609
Phone: (813)286-8829 **Fax:** (813)207-0995
Website: http://www.humana.com
David A. Jones, Chairman of the Board

★ 18328 ★ Humana Medical Plans, Inc.
HMO Plan
3501 SW 160th Ave.
Miramar, FL 33027
Phone: (305)621-5499 **Free:** 800-442-5555
Fax: (305)626-5297
Website: http://www.humana.com
David A. Jones, Chairman of the Board

★ 18329 ★ Jackson Memorial Health Plan
1801 NW 9th Ave., Ste. 700
Miami, FL 33129-2610
Phone: (305)575-3700 **Free:** 800-721-2993
Fax: (305)545-5212
Website: http://www.um-jmh.org
Joseph Rogers, CEO

★ 18330 ★ Neighborhood Health Partnership
HMO Plan
7600 Corporate Dr.
Miami, FL 33126
Phone: (305)715-2200 **Free:** 800-873-7474
Fax: (305)715-4306
Website: http://jalden.com
Joseph Papa, CEO

★ 18331 ★ One Health Plan of Florida
HMO Plan
7650 Courtney Campbell Csy, Ste. 850
Tampa, FL 33607
Phone: (813)207-0216 **Free:** 800-533-0919
Fax: (813)207-0613
Website: http://www.onehealthplan.com
Susan Griffin, Contact

★ 18332 ★ Physicians Healthcare Plans, Inc.
HMO Plan
1410 N Westshore Blvd., Ste. 200
Tampa, FL 33607
Phone: (813)273-7474 **Free:** 800-873-7474
Fax: (813)829-6302
Michael Fernandez, CEO

★ 18333 ★ Preferred Medical Plan, Inc.
HMO Plan
4950 SW 8th St.
Coral Gables, FL 33134
Phone: (305)648-4000 **Fax:** (305)447-4959
Website: http://www.preferredmedicalplan.com
Tamara Meyerson, CEO

★ 18334 ★ Total Health Choice, Inc.
HMO Plan
PO Box 830010
Miami, FL 33283-0010
Phone: (305)408-5700 **Free:** 800-887-6888
Fax: (305)408-5710
Kenneth G. Rimmer, CEO

★ 18335 ★ United HealthCare of Florida, Inc.
HMO Plan
7077 Bonneval Rd., Ste. 103
Jacksonville, FL 32216
Phone: (904)296-1332 **Free:** 800-250-6178
Fax: (904)296-2649
Website: http://www.uhc.com
Matthew Davies, CEO

★ 18336 ★ United HealthCare of Florida, Inc.
HMO Plan
13621 NW 12th St.
Sunrise, FL 33323
Phone: (954)858-4000 **Fax:** (954)858-3815
Website: http://www.uhc.com
Michael Muchnicki, CEO

★ 18337 ★ United HealthCare of Florida, Inc.
HMO Plan
9009 Corporate Lake Dr.
Tampa, FL 33624
Phone: (813)890-4500 **Free:** 800-595-0440
Fax: (813)357-5079

Website: http://www.uhc.com
Ken L. Hoverman, CEO

★ 18338 ★ United HealthCare of Florida, Inc. - Orlando
HMO Plan
800 N Magnolia Ave., Ste. 600
Orlando, FL 32803
Phone: (407)872-1000 **Free:** 800-899-6500
Fax: (407)423-2232
Website: http://www.uhc.com
Matthew Davies, CEO

★ 18339 ★ Vista Health Plan Inc.
HMO Plan
300 S Park Rd.
Hollywood, FL 33021
Free: 800-422-7335 **Fax:** (954)986-6013
Joe Berding, CEO

★ 18340 ★ Well Care HMO, Inc.
HMO Plan
6800 N Dale Mabry Hwy., Ste. 270-299
Tampa, FL 33614
Phone: (813)290-6219 **Free:** 800-610-4466
Fax: (813)290-6294
Rupesh Shah, CEO

Georgia

★ 18341 ★ Aetna Inc. - Georgia
HMO Plan
11675 Great Oaks Way
Alpharetta, GA 30022
Phone: (770)346-4300 **Free:** 800-353-5980
Fax: (770)346-2157
Website: http://www.aetna.com
John W. Rowe, Chairman of the Board

★ 18342 ★ Athens Area Health Plan Select, Inc.
HMO Plan
295 W Clayton St.
Athens, GA 30601
Phone: (706)549-0549 **Free:** 800-293-6260
Fax: (706)549-8004
Website: http://www.aahps.com
Larry Webb, President

★ 18343 ★ CIGNA and Ace USA
HMO Plan
100 Peachtree St. NW, Ste. 800
Atlanta, GA 30303
Phone: (404)681-7690 **Free:** 800-542-0301
Fax: (404)681-6636
James Boone, President

★ 18344 ★ CIGNA HealthCare of Georgia
HMO Plan
100 Peachtree St., Ste. 800
Atlanta, GA 30303
Phone: (404)681-7000 **Fax:** (404)681-7031
Website: http://www.cigna.com
Robert Youngk, CEO

★ 18345 ★ Coventry Health Care Inc. - Georgia, Inc.
HMO Plan
1100 Circle 75 Pkwy., Ste. 1400
Atlanta, GA 30339
Phone: (678)202-2100 **Free:** 800-470-2004
Fax: (678)202-2196
Website: http://www.cvty.com
Thomas A. Davis, CEO

★ 18346 ★ Humana Health Plans of Georgia
HMO Plan
900 Ashwood Pkwy., Ste. 400
Atlanta, GA 30338
Phone: (770)393-9226 **Free:** 800-234-3486
Fax: (770)393-2845
Website: http://www.humana.com/georgia/home.html
Karen Hornsby, Contact

★ 18347 ★ Kaiser Foundation Health Plan of Georgia, Inc.
HMO Plan
3495 Piedmont Rd. NE, Bldg. 9
Atlanta, GA 30305-1736
Phone: (404)364-7000 **Fax:** (404)364-4791
Website: http://www.kaiserpermanante.org
Carolyn Kenny, CEO

★ 18348 ★ One Health Plan of Georgia, Inc.
HMO Plan
245 Perimeter Ctr. Pkwy., 7th Fl.
Atlanta, GA 30346
Phone: (770)290-7000 **Free:** 800-511-3899
Fax: (770)290-7022
Website: http://www.onehealthplan.com
David Record, CEO

★ 18349 ★ United HealthCare of Georgia
HMO Plan
2970 Clairmont Rd., Ste. 300
Atlanta, GA 30329-1634
Phone: (404)982-8800 **Free:** 800-842-6219
Fax: (404)320-8351
Website: http://www.uhc.com
Teresa Kline, CEO

Guam

★ 18350 ★ Guam Memorial Health Plan
HMO Plan
177 A Chalan Pasaherv St. A
Tamuning, GU 96911
Phone: (671)647-4647 **Fax:** (671)646-1036
Website: http://www.gmha.org
Frank Rosario, CEO

★ 18351 ★ Health Maintenance Life, Inc.
HMO Plan
231 Guerrero Dr.
Tamuning, GU 96931
Phone: (671)646-6956 **Fax:** (671)647-3520
Mary Kleschen, MD, Contact

★ 18352 ★ PacifiCare Asia Pacific
HMO Plan
PO Box 6578
Tamuning, GU 96931
Phone: (671)646-6956 **Fax:** (671)646-6923
Website: http://www.pacificare.com
Mary Kleschen, MD, Contact

Hawaii

★ 18353 ★ Kaiser Permanente Health Plan
HMO Plan
711 Kapiolani Blvd.
Honolulu, HI 96813-5249
Phone: (808)597-5955 **Fax:** (808)983-4989
Bruce Behnke, Contact

★ 18354 ★ Kapi'olani
55 Merchant St.
Honolulu, HI 96813
Phone: (808)535-7401 **Free:** 800-363-6512
Fax: (808)535-7251
Website: http://www.kapiolani.org
Roger Drue, CEO

★ 18355 ★ Queen's Island Care
HMO Plan
500 Ala Moana Blvd., Ste. 200
Honolulu, HI 96813
Phone: (808)522-7560 **Fax:** (808)522-7561
Paul Yamashita, CEO

Idaho

★ 18356 ★ Group Health Northwest
HMO Plan
2010 N Lakewood Dr.
Coeur D'Arlene, ID 83814-2635
Phone: (208)664-5174 **Free:** 800-497-2210
Fax: (208)664-9315
Website: http://www.ghc.org
Cheryl Scott, CEO

★ 18357 ★ Primary Health Plan
HMO Plan
800 Park Blvd., Ste. 760
Boise, ID 83712
Phone: (208)344-1811 **Free:** 800-688-5008
Fax: (208)344-4262
Website: http://www.primaryhealth.com
Elden Mitchell, CEO & Pres

Illinois

★ 18358 ★ Aetna Inc. - Illinois
HMO Plan
100 N Riverside Plaza, 20th Fl.
Chicago, IL 60606-1518
Phone: (312)928-3000 **Free:** 800-627-5039
Fax: (312)928-3232
Website: http://www.aetna.com
John W. Rowe, MD, Chairman of the Board

★ 18359 ★ Amerigroup Illinois
HMO Plan
211 W Wacker Dr., Ste. 1350
Chicago, IL 60606
Phone: (312)214-0400 **Fax:** (312)214-0424
Website: http://www.amerigroupcorp.com
Dr. Dwight Jones, MD, CEO

★ 18360 ★ CIGNA Healthcare of Illinois, Inc.
HMO Plan
525 W Monroe St., Ste. 1800
Chicago, IL 60661-3629
Phone: (312)648-2460 **Free:** 800-541-7526
Fax: (312)648-3617
Website: http://www.cigna.com
Bert Wagner, CEO

★ 18361 ★ Great West Life
6250 River Rd., Ste. 10-100
Rosemont, IL 60018
Phone: (847)292-0024 **Fax:** (847)292-0015
Website: http://www.onehealthplan.com
Scott Burnett, Contact

★ 18362 ★ Harmony Health Plan
HMO Plan
125 S Wacker Dr., Ste. 2900
Chicago, IL 60606-4420
Phone: (312)516-4900 **Free:** 888-684-2026
Fax: (312)630-2022
Website: http://www.harmonyhpi.com
John Blank, CEO

★ 18363 ★ Health Alliance Medical Plans - Corporate Headquarters
HMO Plan
102 E Main St.
Urbana, IL 61801
Phone: (217)337-8000 **Free:** 800-851-3379
Fax: (217)337-8093
Website: http://www.hapcorp.org
Jeffery Ingrum, MD, CEO

★ 18364 ★ Healthcare Service Corp. - Corporate Headquarters
HMO Plan
300 E Randolph St.
Chicago, IL 60601-5099
Phone: (312)653-6000 **Fax:** (312)819-1220
Website: http://www.bcbsil.com
Raymond McCaskey, CEO

★ 18365 ★ Humana Health Care Plans of Illinois
HMO Plan
30 S Wacker Dr., Ste. 3100
Chicago, IL 60606
Phone: (312)441-9111 **Free:** 800-852-9556
Fax: (312)441-5901
Website: http://www.humana.com/Illinois/home.html
David Jones, Chairman of the Board

★ 18366 ★ John Deere Health
HMO Plan
7210 N Villa Lake Dr.
Peoria, IL 61614
Phone: (309)689-4630 **Free:** 800-224-6599
Fax: (309)689-3165
Website: http://www.johndeerehealth.com
Richard L. Bartsh, MD, President

★ 18367 ★ John Deere Health - Corporate Headquarters
HMO Plan
1300 River Dr., Ste. 200
Moline, IL 61265
Phone: (309)765-1200 **Fax:** (309)748-1322
Website: http://www.johndeerehealth.com
Richard L. Bartsh, MD, President

★ 18368 ★ OSF Health Plans
HMO Plan
7915 N Hale Ave., Ste. D
Peoria, IL 61615-2047
Phone: (309)677-8200 **Fax:** (309)677-8338
Website: http://www.osfhealthplans.com
Kevin Schoeplein, CEO

★ 18369 ★ Personal Care
HMO Plan
2110 Fox Dr.
Champaign, IL 61820
Phone: (217)366-1226 **Free:** 800-366-6730
Fax: (217)366-5410
David Line, CEO

★ 18370 ★ Rockford Health Plans, Inc.
HMO Plan
3401 N Perryville Rd.
Rockford, IL 61114
Phone: (815)971-1000 **Free:** 800-331-0424
Fax: (815)654-5188
Website: http://www.rockfordhealthplans.com
Edward Pattarozzi, CEO & Pres

★ 18371 ★ UniCare
HMO Plan
233 S Wacker Dr., Ste. 3900
Chicago, IL 60606
Phone: (312)234-7000 **Free:** 888-234-7747
Fax: (312)234-8001
Website: http://www.rushpru.com
Sandra Van Trease, CEO

★ 18372 ★ Union Health Service, Inc.
HMO Plan
1634 W Polk St.
Chicago, IL 60612
Phone: (312)829-4224 **Fax:** (312)423-4326
Leon Wolin, President

★ 18373 ★ United HealthCare of Illinois, Inc.
HMO Plan
233 N Michigan Ave.
Chicago, IL 60601
Phone: (312)424-4460 **Fax:** (312)424-4905
Website: http://www.uhc.com
William Moeller, CEO

★ 18374 ★ United HealthCare of Illinois, Inc.
Premier (HMO)
233 N Michigan Ave.
Chicago, IL 60601
Phone: (312)424-4460 **Fax:** (312)424-4905
Website: http://www.uhc.com
William Moeller, CEO

★ 18375 ★ United HealthCare of Illinois, Inc.
Select (HMO)
233 N Michigan Ave.
Chicago, IL 60601
Phone: (312)424-4460 **Fax:** (312)424-4905
Website: http://www.uhc.com
William Moeller, CEO

Indiana

★ 18376 ★ Advantage Health Plan Inc.
11555 N Meridian St., Ste. 240
Carmel, IN 46032
Phone: (317)573-2700 **Free:** 877-903-2237
Fax: (317)580-8009
Website: http://www.advantageplan.com
Vincent Caponi, Chairman of the Board

★ 18377 ★ Aetna Inc. - Indiana
HMO Plan
8425 Woodfield Crossing Blvd.
Indianapolis, IN 46240
Phone: (317)815-4300 **Free:** 800-382-3209
Fax: (317)815-4397
Website: http://www.aetna.com
John W. Rowe, MD, Chairman of the Board

★ 18378 ★ Arnett Health Plans
HMO Plan
PO Box 6108
Lafayette, IN 47903
Phone: (765)448-7701 **Fax:** (765)448-7700
Website: http://www.arnettplans.com
James Brunnemer, CEO

★ 18379 ★ Cigna Healthcare of Indiana
HMO Plan
429 N Pennsylvania, Ste. 301
Indianapolis, IN 46204
Phone: (317)615-1200 **Free:** 800-276-0363
Fax: (317)615-1301
Website: http://www.cigna.com
Mary Brandt, CEO

★ 18380 ★ Humana, Inc. - Indiana
HMO Plan
8500 Keystone Crossing, Ste. 470
Indianapolis, IN 46240-1438
Phone: (317)722-2075 **Free:** 800-444-9137
Fax: (317)722-2088
Website: http://www.humana.com
David A. Jones, Chairman of the Board

★ 18381 ★ IU Health Plan
HMO Plan
3901 W 86th St., Ste. 230
Indianapolis, IN 46268
Phone: (317)871-8811 **Fax:** (317)871-8833
Website: http://www.iuhp.com
Kim Singleton, President

★ 18382 ★ M Plan, Inc.
HMO Plan
8802 N Meridian St., Ste. 100
Indianapolis, IN 46260-5371
Phone: (317)571-5300 **Free:** 800-878-8802
Fax: (317)571-5306
Website: http://www.mplan.com
Alex Slabosky, CEO & Pres

★ 18383 ★ Managed Care Services
HMO Plan
3000 Coliseum Blvd. E, Ste. 100
Fort Wayne, IN 46805
Phone: (260)373-9000 **Free:** 800-666-4449
Fax: (260)373-9005
Website: http://www.parkview.com
Barbara Clayton, Contact

★ 18384 ★ Managed Health Services Indiana Inc.
HMO Plan
1099 N Meridian St., Ste., 400
Indianapolis, IN 46204
Phone: (317)684-9478 **Free:** 800-944-9661
Fax: (317)684-0297
Website: http://www.cenlene.com
Rita Johnson-Mills, CEO

★ 18385 ★ Partners National Health Plans of Indiana, Inc.
HMO Plan
100 E Wayne St., Ste. 302
South Bend, IN 46601
Phone: (260)233-4899 **Free:** 800-876-2655
Fax: (260)234-7484
Website: http://www.partnersindiana.com
Bruce Greenberg, CEO

★ 18386 ★ Physicians Health Plan of Northern Indiana
HMO Plan
8101 W Jefferson Blvd.
Fort Wayne, IN 46804-4163
Phone: (260)432-6690 **Free:** 800-982-6257
Fax: (260)432-0493
Website: http://www.phpni.com
Jay Gilbert, CEO

★ 18387 ★ Southeastern Indiana Health Organization, Inc.
HMO Plan
PO Box 1787
Columbus, IN 47202-1787
Phone: (812)378-7000 **Fax:** (812)348-4592
Website: http://www.siho.org
David Barker, CEO & Pres

★ 18388 ★ Suburban Health Organization
HMO Plan
2780 Waterfront Pkwy. E Dr., No. 300
Indianapolis, IN 46214
Phone: (317)692-5222 **Fax:** (317)692-5233
Julie Carmichael, CEO

★ 18389 ★ Welborn Health Plans
HMO Plan
421 Chestnut St.
Evansville, IN 47713-1337
Phone: (812)426-6600 **Free:** 800-521-0265
Fax: (812)426-9874
Website: http://www.welbornclinic.com
David Christeson, MD, Chairman of the Board

Iowa

★ 18390 ★ Coventry Health Care Inc. - Iowa
HMO Plan
4600 Westown Pkwy., Ste. 200
West Des Moines, IA 50266-1099
Phone: (515)225-1234 **Free:** 800-257-4692
Fax: (515)223-9239
Website: http://www.chciowa.com
Michael Teachaut, CEO

★ 18391 ★ Iowa Health Solutions
HMO Plan
2550 Middle Rd., Ste. 405
Bettendorf, IA 52722
Phone: (563)359-8999 **Fax:** (563)359-9034
Website: http://www.iowahealthsolutions.com
James Dyer, Chairman of the Board

★ 18392 ★ John Deere Health
HMO Plan
1660 Embassy W Dr., Ste. 150
Dubuque, IA 52002
Phone: (319)588-2831 **Free:** 800-224-6597
Fax: (319)588-2920
Website: http://www.johndeerehealth.com
Richard L. Bartsh, MD, President

★ 18393 ★ John Deere Health
HMO Plan
PO Box 9000
Waterloo, IA 50704
Phone: (319)291-3291 **Free:** 800-224-6596
Fax: (319)291-7838
Website: http://www.johndeerehealth.com
Richard L. Bartsh, MD, President

★ 18394 ★ John Deere Health
HMO Plan
4201 W Towne Pkwy., Ste. 325
West Des Moines, IA 50266-6720
Phone: (515)327-2000 **Free:** 800-373-5050
Fax: (515)327-1128
Website: http://www.johndeerehealth.com
Richard L. Bartsh, MD, CEO

★ 18395 ★ John Deere Health
HMO Plan
635 E Pennsylvania Ave.
Ottumwa, IA 52501
Phone: (515)682-9751 **Free:** 800-224-6578
Fax: (515)682-8751
Website: http://www.johndeerehealth.com
Richard L. Bartsh, MD, President

★ 18396 ★ John Deere Health Care
HMO Plan
1845 51st St. NE
Cedar Rapids, IA 52402
Phone: (319)378-5200 **Free:** 800-373-9811
Fax: (319)378-0566
Website: http://www.johndeerehealth.com
Richard L. Bartsh, MD, President

★ 18397 ★ Medical Associates Health Plans
HMO Plan
700 Locust St., Ste. 230
Dubuque, IA 52004
Phone: (563)556-8070 **Free:** 800-747-8900
Fax: (563)556-5134
Website: http://www.mahealthcare.com
Alan Avery, CEO

★ 18398 ★ Mercy Health Network
HMO Plan
1100 6th Ave., Ste. 201
West Des Moines, IA 50266-6735
Phone: (515)643-5300 **Fax:** (515)643-5350
Website: http://www.mercydubuque.com
Dave Vellinga, CEO

★ 18399 ★ SecureCare of Iowa
HMO Plan
11141 Aurora Ave.
Des Moines, IA 50322
Free: 888-881-8820 **Fax:** (515)331-7848
Don Burrows, CEO

★ 18400 ★ Wellmark, Inc. - Corporate Headquarters
HMO Plan
636 Grand Ave.
Des Moines, IA 50309-2565
Phone: (515)245-4500 **Fax:** (515)245-5090
Website: http://www.wellmark.com
John Forsyth, CEO & Chm Bd

Kansas

★ 18401 ★ CIGNA Health Plan of Kansas/Missouri
HMO Plan
7400 W 110th St., Ste. 600
Overland Park, KS 66210
Phone: (913)451-9389 **Fax:** (913)451-0974
Website: http://www.cigna.com
Rick Grizzle, Contact

★ 18402 ★ Coventry Health Care Inc. - Wichita
HMO Plan
8301 E 21st St. N, No. 300
Wichita, KS 67206
Phone: (316)634-1222 **Free:** 800-664-9251
Fax: (316)634-1266
Website: http://www.cvty.com
Jan Stallmeyer, CEO

★ 18403 ★ Great West Life
82 Corp Woods
10851 Maslin 200
Overland Park, KS 66210
Phone: (913)491-9436 **Fax:** (913)491-9417
Website: http://www.onehealthplan.com
Greg Watkins, Contact

★ 18404 ★ One Health Plan of Kansas/Missouri
8575 W 110th, Ste. 108
Overland Park, KS 66210
Phone: (913)451-0101 **Free:** 800-218-7723
Fax: (913)317-8824
Website: http://www.onehealthplan.com
William T. McCallum, CEO

★ 18405 ★ Preferred Health Systems
HMO Plan
8535 E 21st St. N
Wichita, KS 67206
Phone: (316)609-2345 **Free:** 800-990-0345
Fax: (316)609-2346
Website: http://www.phsystems.com
Marlon Dauner, CEO & Pres

★ 18406 ★ United HealthCare of the Midwest, Inc.
HMO Plan
9393 W 110th St., Bldg. 51, No. 300
Overland Park, KS 66210-2002
Phone: (913)663-6500 **Free:** 800-340-9716
Fax: (913)663-6549
Website: http://www.uhc.com
William Tracy, CEO

Kentucky

★ 18407 ★ Aetna Inc. - Kentucky
HMO Plan
305 N Hurstbourne Pkwy., Ste. 100
Louisville, KY 40222-5146
Phone: (502)423-6240 **Fax:** (502)339-7639
Website: http://www.aetna.com
John W. Rowe, Chairman of the Board

★ 18408 ★ Bluegrass Family Health, Inc.
HMO Plan
651 Perimeter Dr., Ste. 300
Lexington, KY 40517
Phone: (859)269-4475 **Fax:** (859)269-6447
Website: http://www.bgfh.com
James Fritz, CEO & Pres

★ 18409 ★ CHA Health
HMO Plan
300 W Vine St.
Lexington, KY 40503
Phone: (859)271-5055 **Free:** 800-457-5683
Fax: (859)232-8557
Website: http://www.cha.com
Mark Birdwhistell, CEO

★ 18410 ★ CIGNA Healthcare of Kentucky
HMO Plan
5111 Commerce Crossing Dr.
Louisville, KY 40229
Phone: (502)753-2341 **Free:** 800-808-1534
Fax: (502)753-2365
Website: http://www.cigna.com
Robert Bruce, CEO

★ 18411 ★ Commonwealth Health Plan
300 W Vine St.
Lexington, KY 40507
Phone: (859)232-8686 **Free:** 800-457-5683
Fax: (859)232-8557
Website: http://www.cha-health.com
Mark Birdwhistle, CEO

★ 18412 ★ Humana Health Care Plans of Lexington
HMO Plan
500 W Main St.
Lexington, KY 40507
Phone: (859)263-1400 **Free:** 800-221-8390
Fax: (859)263-1488
Website: http://www.humana.com/lexington/home.html
Michael McCallister, CEO & Pres

★ 18413 ★ Humana Health Care Plans of San Antonio
HMO Plan
500 W Main St.
Louisville, KY 40201-1438
Phone: (210)617-1000 **Fax:** (210)615-0090
Website: http://www.humana.com
David A. Jones, Chairman of the Board

★ 18414 ★ Humana Health Plan - Kentucky
HMO Plan
500 W Main St.
Louisville, KY 40202
Phone: (502)580-1860 **Fax:** (502)580-3127
Website: http://www.humana.com
Michael McCallister, CEO & Pres

★ 18415 ★ Humana Inc. - Corporate Headquarters
HMO Plan
PO Box 740036
Louisville, KY 40201-7436
Phone: (502)580-1860 **Fax:** (502)580-3127
Website: http://www.humana.com
David Jones, Chairman of the Board

★ 18416 ★ Humana, Inc. - Ohio
HMO Plan
500 W Main St.
Louisville, KY 40201-1438
Phone: (502)784-5200 **Fax:** (502)543-7158
Website: http://www.humana.com
Michael McCallister, CEO & Pres

★ 18417 ★ Humana, Inc. - Oklahoma
HMO Plan
500 W Main St.
Louisville, KY 40201
Phone: (502)580-5804 **Fax:** (502)580-8528
Website: http://www.humana.com
Michael McCallister, CEO & Pres

★ 18418 ★ Humana, Inc. - Tennessee
HMO Plan
PO Box 740036
Louisville, KY 40201-1438
Phone: (901)685-8351 **Free:** 800-283-8510
Fax: (901)685-0194
Website: http://www.humana.com
Michael McCallister, CEO & Pres

★ 18419 ★ Humana, Inc. - Virginia
HMO Plan
PO Box 740036
Louisville, KY 40201-1438
Phone: (502)580-1860 **Fax:** (502)580-3127
Website: http://www.humana.com
Michael McCallister, CEO & Pres

★ 18420 ★ Humana Military Service, Inc.
HMO Plan
500 W Main St.
Louisville, KY 40201
Phone: (502)580-5804 **Fax:** (502)580-8528
Website: http://www.humana.com
David Jones, Chairman of the Board

★ 18421 ★ United HealthCare of Kentucky, Inc.
HMO Plan
2424 Harrodsburg Rd.
Lexington, KY 40504-3329
Phone: (859)296-6000 **Fax:** (859)224-3732
Website: http://www.uhc.com
Charles Price, CEO

★ 18422 ★ University Health Care, Inc.
571 S Floyd St., Ste. 423
Louisville, KY 40202
Phone: (502)852-5872 **Free:** 800-578-0603
Fax: (502)852-7741
Robert Slaton, EDD, CEO

Louisiana

★ 18423 ★ Aetna US Healthcare - Louisiana
HMO Plan
3900 N Causeway Blvd., Ste. 410
Metairie, LA 70002-7283
Phone: (504)830-5600 **Free:** 800-685-4857
Fax: (504)837-6571
Website: http://www.aetna.com
John W. Rowe, Chairman of the Board

★ 18424 ★ AmCare Health Plans of Louisiana
HMO Plan
5353 Essen Ln., Ste. 450
Baton Rouge, LA 70809
Phone: (225)763-5300 **Free:** 800-772-2995
Fax: (225)763-6211
Website: http://www.amcarehealthplans.com
Thomas Lucksinger, CEO

★ 18425 ★ CIGNA HealthCare of Louisiana
HMO Plan
4354 S Sherwood Forest, No. 240
Baton Rouge, LA 70816
Phone: (225)295-2800 **Fax:** (225)295-2888
Website: http://www.cigna.com
Sharon Oliver, CEO

★ 18426 ★ CIGNA Healthcare of Louisiana, Inc.
HMO Plan
3838 N Causeway Blvd., No. 2850
Metairie, LA 70002
Free: 800-832-3211 **Fax:** (504)831-7499
Website: http://www.cigna.com
Patrick Welch, President

★ 18427 ★ Coventry Health Care Inc. - Louisiana
HMO Plan
2424 Edenborn Ave., Ste. 350
Metairie, LA 70001
Phone: (504)834-0840 **Free:** 800-341-6613
Fax: (504)834-2694
Website: http://www.cvty.com
Keith Benoit, Sr., CEO

★ 18428 ★ Health Plus of Louisiana, Inc.
HMO Plan
2751 Albert L. Bicknell Dr., 2B
Shreveport, LA 71103
Phone: (318)212-8800 **Free:** 800-331-5055
Fax: (318)212-4095
Website: http://www.wkmc.com
James K. Elrod, Chairman of the Board

★ 18429 ★ HMO Louisiana, Inc.
HMO Plan
5525 Reitz Ave.
Baton Rouge, LA 70898-9024
Phone: (225)295-3307 **Free:** 800-376-7741
Fax: (225)295-2054
Website: http://www.bcbsla.com
Richard Atkins, Chairman of the Board

★ 18430 ★ Ochsner Health Plan
Kid's First (HMO)
One Galleria Blvd., Ste. 850
Metairie, LA 70001
Phone: (504)836-6600 **Free:** 888-882-9806
Fax: (504)836-6688
Website: http://www.ohp-louisiana.com
Terry Schilling, CEO

★ 18431 ★ Ochsner Health Plan
Total Health Choice & Total Health Plan (HMO)
One Galleria Blvd., Ste. 850
Metairie, LA 70001
Phone: (504)836-6600 **Free:** 888-882-9806
Fax: (504)836-6688
Website: http://www.ohp-louisiana.com
Terry Schilling, CEO

★ 18432 ★ Ochsner Health Plan
Total Health One (HMO)
One Galleria Blvd., Ste. 850
Metairie, LA 70001
Phone: (504)836-6600 **Free:** 888-882-9806
Fax: (504)836-6688
Website: http://www.ohp-louisiana.com
Terry Schilling, CEO

★ 18433 ★ SMA Health Plan, Inc.
HMO Plan
1555 Poydres
New Orleans, LA 70112
Phone: (504)837-7374 **Free:** 800-259-7370
Fax: (504)837-7115
Website: http://www.sma.net
Robert Gormley, MD, Contact

★ 18434 ★ Tenet Choices, Inc.
HMO Plan
200 W Esplanade Ave., Ste. 600
Kenner, LA 70065
Phone: (504)461-9800 **Free:** 800-631-8443
Fax: (504)464-1015
Reynold J. Jennings, President

★ 18435 ★ United HealthCare of Louisiana, Inc.
HMO Plan
3838 N Causeway Blvd., Ste. 2100
Metairie, LA 70009
Phone: (504)849-3510 **Free:** 800-864-4799
Fax: (504)849-3551
Website: http://www.uhc.com
Sam Patterson, CEO

★ 18436 ★ Vantage Health Plan, Inc.
HMO Plan
909 N 18th St., Ste. 201
Monroe, LA 71201
Phone: (318)361-0900 **Free:** 888-823-1910
Fax: (318)361-2159
Patrick Jones, MD, CEO

Maine

★ 18437 ★ Aetna Inc. - Maine
HMO Plan
One Monument Sq., 5th Fl.
Portland, ME 04101
Phone: (207)879-1995 **Fax:** (207)879-7951
Website: http://www.aetna.com
John W. Rowe, MD, Chairman of the Board

★ 18438 ★ Cigna Healthcare of Maine, Inc.
HMO Plan
2 Stonewood Dr.
Freeport, ME 04032-0447
Phone: (207)865-5000 **Free:** 800-642-5551
Fax: (207)865-5633
Website: http://www.cigna.com/healthcare/hs/me.html
Richard White, CEO & Pres

★ 18439 ★ Maine Partners Health Plan
HMO Plan
2 Gannett Dr.
South Portland, ME 04106-6911
Phone: (207)822-7000 **Fax:** (207)822-7350
Website: http://www.mainebluecross.com
Jim Parker, Contact

Maryland

★ 18440 ★ Aetna Inc. - DE, MD, DC
HMO Plan
1302 Concourse Dr., Ste. 402
Linthicum, MD 21090
Phone: (410)691-1080 **Free:** 800-328-8742
Fax: (410)691-1198
Website: http://www.aetna.com
John W. Rowe, Chairman of the Board

★ 18441 ★ Amerigroup Maryland, Inc.
857 Elkridge Landing Rd.
Linthicum, MD 21090
Phone: (410)859-5800 **Fax:** (410)981-4070
Website: http://www.amerigroupcorp.com
Don Gilmore, CEO

★ 18442 ★ BCE Emergis - California
HMO Plan
2273 Research Blvd.
Rockville, MD 20850
Phone: (301)548-1000 **Free:** 800-248-7744
Fax: (301)296-5020
Francois Cole, CEO & Pres

★ 18443 ★ CIGNA Healthcare Mid-Atlantic
HMO Plan
9700 Patuxent Woods Dr.
Columbia, MD 21046
Phone: (410)720-5800 **Free:** 800-541-7526
Fax: (410)720-5860
Website: http://www.cigna.com/healthcare/hs/md.html
Matt Manders, CEO

★ 18444 ★ Coventry Health Care, Inc. - Corporate Headquarters
HMO Plan
6705 Rockledge Dr., Ste. 900
Bethesda, MD 20817
Phone: (301)581-0600 **Fax:** (301)493-0700
Website: http://www.cvty.com
Allen Wise, CEO

★ 18445 ★ Delmarva Health Plan, Inc.
HMO Plan
10455 Mill Run Circle
Owings Mills, MD 21117
Phone: (410)822-7223 **Free:** 800-334-3427
Fax: (410)822-8152
William Jews, MD, CEO & Pres

★ 18446 ★ Freestate Health Plan
HMO Plan
10455 Mill Run Circle
Owings Mills, MD 21117
Phone: (410)654-8670 **Free:** 800-445-6036
Fax: (410)528-7013
Website: http://www.carefirst.com
William Jews, CEO & Pres

★ 18447 ★ Great West life
HMO Plan
14504 Green View Dr., Ste. 400
Laurel, MD 20708
Phone: (301)497-1700 **Fax:** (301)494-8066
Website: http://www.onehealthplan.com
William T. McCallum, CEO

★ 18448 ★ Kaiser Foundation Health Plan - Mid-Atlantic States
HMO Plan
2101 E Jefferson St.
Rockville, MD 20849
Phone: (301)816-2474 **Free:** 800-368-5784
Fax: (301)816-7491
Website: http://www.kpne.org
Marilyn Kowamura, CEO

★ 18449 ★ MD-Individual Practice Association, Inc. (MD IPA)
HMO Plan
4 Taft Court
Rockville, MD 20850
Phone: (301)838-5645 **Free:** 800-544-2853
Fax: (301)545-5388
Website: http://www.mamsi.com
Thomas Barbera, CEO & Pres

★ 18450 ★ Mid Atlantic Medical Services, Inc. (MAMSI)
HMO Plan
4 Taft Court
Rockville, MD 20850
Phone: (301)762-8205 **Fax:** (301)738-1230
Website: http://www.mamsi.com
Thomas Barbera, CEO & Pres

★ 18451 ★ Optimum Choice, Inc.
HMO Plan
4 Taft Court
Rockville, MD 20850
Phone: (301)360-8040 **Free:** 800-331-2102
Fax: (301)545-5393
Website: http://www.mamsi.com
Thomas Barbera, CEO

★ 18452 ★ Preferred Health Network
HMO Plan
1099 Winterson Rd.
Linthicum, MD 21090
Phone: (410)850-7461 **Free:** 800-422-1996
Fax: (410)855-8840
Website: http://www.preferredhealthnetwork.com
Pat Leininger, CEO

★ 18453 ★ Sheppard Pratt Health Plan
HMO Plan
PO Box 1470
Rockville, MD 20849
Phone: (410)938-3200 **Free:** 800-881-2279
Fax: (410)938-4099
Website: http://www.sheppardpratt.org
Steven Sharfstein, MD, CEO

★ 18454 ★ Total Health Care, Inc.
HMO Plan
1501 Division St.
Baltimore, MD 21217
Phone: (410)383-8300 **Fax:** (410)728-4412
Dennis Cherot, CEO

★ 18455 ★ United HealthCare of the Mid-Atlantic, Inc.
HMO Plan
6300 Security Blvd.
Baltimore, MD 21207
Phone: (410)277-6000 **Fax:** (410)277-6661
Website: http://www.uhc.com
Bob Fleshner, CEO

Massachusetts

★ 18456 ★ Aetna Inc. - Massachusetts
HMO Plan
400-1 Totten Pond Rd.
Waltham, MA 02451
Phone: (781)902-3800 **Free:** 800-448-8742
Fax: (781)902-3854
Website: http://www.aetna.com
John W. Rowe, MD, Chairman of the Board

★ 18457 ★ Bridgewater Goddard Park Medical Associates
HMO Plan
110 Liberty
Brockton, MA 02301
Phone: (508)586-3600 **Fax:** (508)894-0412
Debra Wilson, CEO

★ 18458 ★ CIGNA Healthcare of Massachusetts
HMO Plan
3 Newton Executive Pkwy.
Newton, MA 02462
Phone: (617)630-4300 **Fax:** (617)630-4380
Website: http://www.cigna.com
Imre Toth, MD, Contact

★ 18459 ★ CIGNA Healthcare of Massachusetts
HMO Plan
100 Front St., Ste. 300
Worcester, MA 01608-1449
Phone: (508)798-8667 **Free:** 800-922-8380
Fax: (508)849-4299
Website: http://www.cigna.com
Linda Dwyer, CEO

★ 18460 ★ Fallon Community Health Plan
HMO Plan
10 Chestnut St.
Worcester, MA 01608-2810
Phone: (508)799-2100 **Free:** 800-283-2556
Fax: (508)797-4387
Website: http://www.fchp.org
Robert Cavanaugh, MD, Chairman of the Board

★ 18461 ★ Great West
HMO Plan
One Apple Hill Dr., Ste. 104
Natick, MA 01760-2072
Free: 800-733-2750 **Fax:** (508)650-9598
Website: http://www.onehealthplan.com
John Kelley, Contact

★ 18462 ★ Harvard Pilgrim Health Care - Corporate Headquarters
HMO Plan
93 Worchester St.
Wellesley, MA 02481
Phone: (781)263-6000 **Free:** 800-742-8326
Fax: (617)509-2515
Website: http://www.harvardpilgrim.org
Charles Baker, CEO & Pres

★ 18463 ★ Health New England
HMO Plan
One Monarch Place
Springfield, MA 01144-1006
Phone: (413)787-4000 **Free:** 800-842-4464
Fax: (413)734-3356
Website: http://www.healthnewengland.com
Peter F. Straley, CEO & Pres

★ 18464 ★ MIT Health Plan
HMO Plan
77 Massachusetts Ave.
Cambridge, MA 02139
Phone: (617)253-1322 **Fax:** (617)253-6558
Website: http://www.web.mit.edu
Annette Jacobs, CEO

★ 18465 ★ Neighborhood Health Plan, Inc.
HMO Plan
253 Summer St.
Boston, MA 02210
Phone: (617)772-5500 **Free:** 800-433-5556
Fax: (617)772-5513
Website: http://www.nhp.org
James Hooley, CEO & Pres

★ 18466 ★ Tufts Health Plan
HMO Plan
333 Wyman St.
Waltham, MA 02454
Phone: (781)466-9400 **Free:** 800-394-3993
Website: http://www.tufts-healthplan.com
Harris Berman, MD, CEO

Michigan

★ 18467 ★ Botsford Health Plan
HMO Plan
28050 Grand River
Farmington, MI 48336
Free: 800-479-5122 **Fax:** (248)356-1382
Website: http://www.botsfordsystem.com
Ronald Szumski, CEO & Pres

★ 18468 ★ Cape Health Plan
HMO Plan
26711 Northwestern Hwy., Ste. 300
Southfield, MI 48034
Phone: (248)386-3000 **Free:** 888-354-2273
Fax: (248)945-9149
Website: http://www.capehealth.com
Susan Sarin, CEO

★ 18469 ★ Care Choices HMO
34605 Twelve Mile Rd.
Farmington Hills, MI 48331
Phone: (248)489-6203 **Free:** 800-852-9780
Fax: (248)489-6280
Website: http://www.carechoices.com
William R. Alvin, CEO & Pres

★ 18470 ★ Community Care Plan
HMO Plan
2100 Raybrook SE, Ste. 203
Grand Rapids, MI 49546
Phone: (616)252-4590 **Free:** 800-807-5244
Fax: (616)252-4552
Website: http://www.communitycareplan.org
Keith Sherwood, Contact

★ 18471 ★ Community Choice Michigan
HMO Plan
2369 Woodlake Dr.
Okemos, MI 48864
Phone: (517)349-9922 **Free:** 800-390-7102
Fax: (517)349-5343
Website: http://www.ccmhmo.org
Richard Nowakowski, CEO

★ 18472 ★ Community Health Plan
DBA Ultimed HMO of Michigan
2401 20th St.
Detroit, MI 48216
Phone: (313)961-1717 **Free:** 800-242-7955
Fax: (313)961-9660
Website: http://www.ultimed-hmo.com
Harley Brown, CEO & Chm Bd

★ 18473 ★ Grand Valley Health Plan
HMO Plan
829 Forest Hill Ave. SE
Grand Rapids, MI 49546-3697
Phone: (616)949-2410 **Fax:** (616)949-4978
Website: http://www.gvhpchoosewell.com
Roland Palmer, CEO

★ 18474 ★ Great Lakes Health Plan
17117 W Nine Mile Rd., Ste. 1600
Southfield, MI 48075-2127
Phone: (248)559-5656 **Fax:** (248)559-4640
Website: http://www.glhp.com
Bryan L. Schefman, CEO & Pres

★ 18475 ★ Health Alliance Plan
HMO Plan
2850 W Grand Blvd.
Detroit, MI 48202
Phone: (313)872-8100 **Free:** 800-422-4641
Website: http://www.hapcorp.org
Cleve Killingsworth, CEO & Pres

★ 18476 ★ Health Plan of Michigan
HMO Plan
17515 W Nine Mile Rd., Ste. 650
Southfield, MI 48075
Phone: (248)557-3700 **Free:** 888-437-0606
Fax: (248)569-4702
Website: http://www.hpmich.com
David Cotton, MD, President

★ 18477 ★ Health Plus of Michigan, Inc.
HMO Plan
PO Box 1700
Flint, MI 48501-1700
Phone: (810)230-2000 **Free:** 800-332-9161
Fax: (810)230-2208
Website: http://www.healthplus.com
Paul Fuhs, PhD, CEO & Pres

★ 18478 ★ Henry Ford Health System
HMO Plan
1 Ford Place
Detroit, MI 48202-2608
Phone: (313)916-2600 **Fax:** (313)874-4730
Website: http://www.henryford.com
Gail Warden, CEO

★ 18479 ★ M-CARE, Inc.
HMO Plan
2301 Commonwealth Blvd.
Ann Arbor, MI 48105
Phone: (734)747-8700 **Free:** 800-658-8878
Fax: (734)998-1253
Website: http://www.mcare.org
Zelda Geyer-Sylvia, CEO

★ 18480 ★ McLaren Health Plan
PO Box 1511
Flint, MI 48501-1511
Free: 888-327-0671 **Fax:** 877-502-1567
Website: http://www.mclaren.org
Kathy Kendall, CEO

★ 18481 ★ Midwest Health Plan
5050 Schaefer Rd.
Dearborn, MI 48126
Phone: (313)581-3700 **Free:** 888-654-2200
Fax: (313)581-2780
Website: http://www.midwesthealthplan.com
Mark B. Saffer, President

★ 18482 ★ Molina Healthcare of Michigan Inc.
100 W Big Beaver Rd., Ste. 600
Troy, MI 48084
Phone: (248)925-1700 **Free:** 888-898-7969
Fax: (248)925-1709
Website: http://www.molinahealthcare.com
Joseph M. Molina, MD, Chairman of the Board

★ 18483 ★ OmniCare Health Plan
HMO Plan
1155 Brewery Park Blvd.
Detroit, MI 48207-9998
Phone: (313)259-4000 **Fax:** (313)393-7944
Website: http://www.ochptn.com
Gregory Moses, Jr., CEO

★ 18484 ★ Paramount Care of Michigan
106 Park Place
Dundee, MI 48131
Free: 888-241-5604 **Fax:** (734)529-8896
Website: http://www.paramountcareofmichigan.com
John Charles Randolph, CEO

★ 18485 ★ Physician Health Plan of Southwest Michigan
HMO Plan
PO Box 51100
Kalamazoo, MI 49005-1100
Phone: (616)341-7200 **Fax:** (616)341-6864
Website: http://www.phcares.com
David Kibbe, CEO

★ 18486 ★ Physicians Health Plan, Inc.
HMO Plan
PO Box 30377
Lansing, MI 48909-7877
Phone: (517)364-8400 **Free:** 800-661-8299
Fax: (517)364-8280
Website: http://www.phpmm.org
Olga Dazzo, CEO

★ 18487 ★ Physicians Health Plan of South Michigan, Inc.
HMO Plan
PO Box 4055
Jackson, MI 49204
Phone: (517)782-7154 **Fax:** (517)782-4512
Jerry Grannan, CEO

★ 18488 ★ Priority Health
HMO Plan
1231 E Beltline NE
Grand Rapids, MI 49525
Phone: (616)942-0954 **Free:** 800-942-0954
Fax: (616)942-5651
Website: http://www.priority-health.com
Kimberly Horn, CEO

★ 18489 ★ Pro-Care Health Plan
3956 Mt. Elliot
Detroit, MI 48207
Phone: (313)925-4607 **Fax:** (313)925-0472
Augustine Kole-James, MD, CEO

★ 18490 ★ Total Health Care, Inc.
HMO Plan
3011 W Grand Blvd., Ste. 1600
Detroit, MI 48202
Phone: (313)871-2000 **Fax:** (313)871-6400
Kenneth Rimmer, CEO

★ 18491 ★ Upper Peninsula Health Plan
HMO Plan
228 W Washington St.
Marquette, MI 49855
Phone: (906)225-7500 **Free:** 888-904-7526
Fax: (906)225-7690
William Streur, CEO

★ 18492 ★ The Wellness Plan
HMO Plan
2875 W Grand Blvd.
Detroit, MI 48202
Phone: (313)875-4200 **Free:** 800-680-9355
Fax: (313)875-5670
Isadore King, CEO

Minnesota

★ 18493 ★ First Plan of Minnesota
First Plan HMO
1601 London Rd.
Duluth, MN 55812
Phone: (218)834-7207 **Free:** 800-635-4159
Fax: (218)834-6215
Website: http://www.firstplan.org
Milt Larson, Chairman of the Board

★ 18494 ★ Medica
HMO Plan
PO Box 9310
Minneapolis, MN 55440-1587
Phone: (952)992-2900 **Fax:** (952)992-3554
Website: http://www.medica.com
David Strand, President

★ 18495 ★ Metropolitan Health Plan
HMO Plan
822 S Third St., Ste. 140
Minneapolis, MN 55415-1289
Phone: (612)347-8557 **Fax:** (612)904-4493
Website: http://www.co.hennepin.mn.us/mhp/mhp.html
Jeff Spartz, CEO

★ 18496 ★ One Health Plan of Minnestota, Inc.
900 Second Ave. S, Ste. 250
Minneapolis, MN 55402
Phone: (612)332-3590 **Free:** 888-612-2957
Fax: (612)332-3589
Website: http://www.onehealthplan.com
Wally Gomaa, President

★ 18497 ★ Preferred One
HMO Plan
6150 Golden Hills Dr.
Golden Valley, MN 55416
Phone: (763)847-4000 **Fax:** (763)847-4010
Website: http://www.preferredone.com
Marcus Merz, CEO

★ 18498 ★ Ucare Minnesota
HMO Plan
PO Box 52
Minneapolis, MN 55413
Phone: (612)676-6840 **Free:** 800-203-7225
Fax: (612)676-6501
Website: http://www.ucare.org
Nancy Feldman, CEO

★ 18499 ★ United Health Group - Corporate Headquarters
HMO Plan
9900 Bren Rd. E
Opus Center
Minnetonka, MN 55343
Phone: (952)936-1300 **Fax:** (952)936-0044
Website: http://www.uhc.com
William McGuire, MD, CEO & Pres

Mississippi

★ 18500 ★ Family Health Care Plus
HMO Plan
PO Box 54268
Pearl, MS 39288-4268
Phone: (601)825-7280 **Free:** 800-323-1999
Fax: (601)825-8130
Margaret Gray, DPA, CEO

★ 18501 ★ Mississippi Select Health Care
HMO Plan
14110 Airport Rd., Ste. 100
Gulfport, MS 39503
Phone: (228)865-0514 **Free:** 800-847-6621
Fax: (228)865-0550
Website: http://www.hmhs.com
Thomas Wicklund, CEO

★ 18502 ★ Physicians Plus Baptist & St. Dominic, Inc.
HMO Plan
969 Lakeland Dr.
Jackson, MS 39216
Phone: (601)364-6843 **Fax:** (601)364-6854
Sr. Mary Dorothea Sondgeroth, CEO

★ 18503 ★ United HealthCare of Mississippi, Inc.
HMO Plan
800 Woodlands Pkwy., Ste. 102
Ridgeland, MS 39157
Free: 800-264-3639 **Fax:** (601)957-1306
Website: http://www.uhc.com
Robert J. Sheehy, CEO

Missouri

★ 18504 ★ Aetna Inc. - Missouri
HMO Plan
2 Cityplace Dr., Ste. 300
Saint Louis, MO 63141
Phone: (314)567-6660 **Fax:** (314)567-3627
Website: http://www.aetna.com
John W. Rowe, Chairman of the Board

★ 18505 ★ CIGNA HealthCare of Missouri
HMO Plan
1 N Brentwood Blvd.
Clayton, MO 63105
Phone: (314)726-7850 **Free:** 800-832-3211
Fax: (314)726-7819
Website: http://www.cigna.com
James Young, President

★ 18506 ★ Community Care Plus
HMO Plan
5615 Pershing Ave.
Saint Louis, MO 63112
Phone: (314)454-1100 **Fax:** (314)361-7250
Jerry Linder, CEO & Pres

★ 18507 ★ Community Health Plan
HMO Plan
137 N Belt Hwy.
Saint Joseph, MO 64506
Phone: (816)271-1247 **Free:** 800-990-9247
Fax: (816)271-1266
Lowell Kruse, CEO

★ 18508 ★ Coventry Health Care, Inc. - Kansas City
HMO Plan
1001 E 101st Terrace, Ste. 300
Kansas City, MO 64131
Phone: (816)941-3030 **Free:** 800-969-3343
Fax: (816)941-8516
Website: http://www.cvty.com
Jan Stallmeyer, CEO & Pres

★ 18509 ★ Cox Health Systems HMO, Inc.
HMO Plan
PO Box 5750
Springfield, MO 65801-5720
Phone: (417)269-2900 **Free:** 800-205-7665
Fax: (417)269-2925
Website: http://www.coxhealthplans.com
Gary Jacobs, President

★ 18510 ★ Family Health Partners
HMO Plan
215 W Pershing Rd., 6th Fl.
Kansas City, MO 64108
Phone: (816)855-1888 **Free:** 800-347-9363
Fax: (816)842-2326
Website: http://www.fhp.org
Jo Stueve, President

★ 18511 ★ First Guard Health Plan
HMO Plan
3801 Blue Parkway
Kansas City, MO 64130
Phone: (816)922-7200 **Free:** 888-828-5698
Fax: (816)922-7251
Joy Wheeler, CEO

★ 18512 ★ Group Health Plan
HMO Plan
111 Corporate Office Dr., No. 400
Earth City, MO 63045
Phone: (314)506-1700 **Free:** 800-743-3901
Fax: (314)209-8225
Website: http://www.ghp.com
Charles R. Stark, CEO & Pres

★ 18513 ★ Healthcare USA of Missouri LLC
10 S Broadway, No. 1200
Saint Louis, MO 63102-1712
Phone: (314)241-5300 **Free:** 800-213-7792
Fax: (314)241-8010
Claudia Bjerre, President

★ 18514 ★ HealthLink, Inc.
HMO Plan
12443 Olive Blvd.
Saint Louis, MO 63141
Phone: (314)989-6000 **Free:** 800-624-2356
Website: http://www.healthlink.com
David T. Ott, CEO & Pres

★ 18515 ★ HealthLink, Inc. - Corporate Headquarters
HMO Plan
12443 Olive Blvd.
Saint Louis, MO 63141
Phone: (314)989-6000 **Fax:** (314)989-6620
Website: http://www.healthlink.com
David T. Ott, CEO & Pres

★ 18516 ★ Mercy Health Plans of Missouri, Inc.
HMO Plan
425 S Old Woods Mill Rd., No. 100
Chesterfield, MO 63017
Phone: (314)214-8100 **Free:** 800-830-1918
Fax: (314)214-8101
Website: http://www.mercyhealthplans.com
Tom Kelly, CEO

★ 18517 ★ Mid America Health
HMO Plan
8321 Parkway
Kansas City, MO 64114
Phone: (816)221-8400 **Free:** 800-468-1442
Fax: (816)221-7709
Website: http://www.healthnet.com
George Pagels, MD, CEO

★ 18518 ★ One Health Plan of Kansas/ Missouri
622 Emerson Rd., Ste. 220
Saint Louis, MO 63141-6708

Phone: (314)994-7205 **Free:** 877-994-7205
Fax: (314)994-7270
Website: http://www.onehealthplan.com
William T. McCallum, CEO

★ 18519 ★ Total Healthcare
2301 Main St.
Kansas City, MO 64108
Phone: (816)395-2222 **Fax:** (816)802-3959
Tom Bowser, CEO

★ 18520 ★ TriSource Health Care
2301 Main St.
Kansas City, MO 64108
Phone: (816)395-2222 **Fax:** (816)802-4451
Tom Bowser, CEO

★ 18521 ★ United HealthCare of the Midwest, Inc.
HMO Plan
PO Box 2560
Maryland Heights, MO 63043-8560
Phone: (314)592-7000 **Free:** 800-535-9291
Fax: (314)592-7650
Website: http://www.uhc.com
Victor Turvey, CEO & Pres

Montana

★ 18522 ★ New West Health Plan
40 W 14th St., Ste. 3
Helena, MT 59601
Phone: (406)457-2200 **Fax:** (406)457-2299
Website: http://www.newwesthealth.com
Nicholas Wolter, MD, President

Nebraska

★ 18523 ★ Coventry Health Care of Nebraska, Inc.
HMO Plan
PO Box 54120
Omaha, NE 68154-9210
Phone: (402)498-9030 **Free:** 800-471-0240
Fax: (402)498-9706
Website: http://www.cvty.com
Rick Cochran, CEO

★ 18524 ★ Mutual of Omaha - HMO
HMO Plan
Mutual of Omaha Plaza
Omaha, NE 68175
Phone: (402)342-7600 **Free:** 800-228-0286
Fax: (402)351-2775
Website: http://www.mutualofomaha.com
John Weekly, Chairman of the Board

★ 18525 ★ Mutual of Omaha of South Dakota and Community Health Plus HMO, Inc.
HMO Plan
Mutual of Omaha Plaza
Omaha, NE 68175
Phone: (402)342-7600 **Free:** 800-228-0286
Fax: (402)351-2775
Website: http://www.mutualofomaha.com
John Weekly, CEO

★ 18526 ★ United HealthCare of the Midlands, Inc.
HMO Plan
2717 N 118th Circle
Omaha, NE 68164-9672
Phone: (402)445-5000 **Free:** 800-284-0626
Fax: (402)445-5575
Website: http://www.uhc.com
John Braasch, President

Nevada

★ 18527 ★ Aetna Inc. - Nevada
HMO Plan
4040 S Eastern Ave., Ste. 240
Las Vegas, NV 89119
Phone: (702)650-8200 **Fax:** (702)650-8256
Website: http://www.aetna.com
John W. Rowe, Chairman of the Board

★ 18528 ★ Health Plan of Nevada, Inc.
HMO Plan
PO Box 15645
Las Vegas, NV 89114-5645
Phone: (702)242-7216 **Free:** 800-777-1840
Fax: (702)242-0376
Website: http://www.sierrahealth.com
Jonathan Bunker, President

★ 18529 ★ HMO Nevada
HMO Plan
6900 Westcliff Dr., Ste. 600
Las Vegas, NV 89145
Phone: (702)228-2583 **Free:** 800-438-5270
Fax: (702)228-1259
Website: http://www.anthem-inc.com
Tony Pointer, CEO

★ 18530 ★ Hometown Health Plan
HMO Plan
400 S Wells Ave.
Reno, NV 89502
Phone: (775)982-3000 **Fax:** (775)982-3220
Website: http://www.hometownhealth.com
Jim Miller, CEO

★ 18531 ★ Nevada Care, Inc.
HMO Plan
10600 W Charleston Blvd.
Las Vegas, NV 89102-2320
Phone: (702)474-7241 **Fax:** (702)474-7592
Website: http://www.nevadacare.com
Keith Beagle, President

★ 18532 ★ PacifiCare of Nevada
HMO Plan
700 E Warm Springs Rd.
Las Vegas, NV 89119-4323
Phone: (702)269-7500 **Free:** 800-826-4347
Fax: (702)269-2649
Website: http://www.pacificare.com
Bard Coats, MD, CEO

★ 18533 ★ Saint Mary's Health First
HMO Plan
235 W 6th St.
Reno, NV 89502
Phone: (775)770-6060 **Fax:** (775)770-6253
Don Kowitz, CEO

★ 18534 ★ Sierra Health Services, Inc. - Corporate Headquarters
HMO Plan
PO Box 15645
Las Vegas, NV 89114-5645
Phone: (702)242-7000 **Fax:** (702)242-7915
Website: http://www.sierrahealth.com
Anthony Marlon, MD, CEO & Chm Bd

New Hampshire

★ 18535 ★ CIGNA Healthcare New Hampshire
HMO Plan
PO Box 2041
Concord, NH 03302-2041
Phone: (603)225-5077 **Free:** 800-531-3121
Fax: (603)229-2978
Website: http://www.cigna.com
Brian Wells, CEO & Pres

★ 18536 ★ Matthew Thornton Health Plan
HMO Plan
3000 Guffs Fall Rd.
Manchester, NH 03111
Phone: (603)695-7000 **Free:** 800-874-7122
Fax: (603)695-7002
Website: http://www.mthp.com
Gray Somers, CEO

New Jersey

★ 18537 ★ Aetna Inc. - New Jersey
HMO Plan
8000 Mid Atlantic Dr., Ste. 100N
Mount Laurel, NJ 08054
Phone: (856)222-5560 **Fax:** (856)727-8490
Website: http://www.aetna.com
John W. Rowe, MD, Chairman of the Board

★ 18538 ★ Aetna Inc. - New Jersey
HMO Plan
55 Lane Rd.
Fairfield, NJ 07004
Phone: (973)575-5600 **Free:** 800-852-0629
Fax: (973)244-3990
Website: http://www.aetna.com
John W. Rowe, Chairman of the Board

★ 18539 ★ Americaid New Jersey, Inc.
HMO Plan
399 Thornall St., 9th Fl.
Edison, NJ 08818
Phone: (732)452-6000 **Fax:** (732)906-2037
Website: http://www.amerigroupcorp.com
Norine Yukon, CEO

★ 18540 ★ AmeriChoice of New Jersey
HMO Plan
PO Box 200098
Newark, NJ 07102-0304
Phone: (973)297-5500 **Free:** 800-941-4647
Fax: (973)297-5599
Website: http://www.americhoice.com
Anthony Welters, CEO

★ 18541 ★ AmeriHealth Insurance Co. - New Jersey North
HMO Plan
485 Rt. 1 S, 3rd Fl., Bldg. C
Iselin, NJ 08830
Phone: (732)726-6700 **Fax:** (732)726-6753
Website: http://www.amerihealth.com
Dan Pedriani, CEO

★ 18542 ★ AmeriHealth Insurance Co. - New Jersey South
HMO Plan
8000 Midlantic Dr., Ste. 333
Mount Laurel, NJ 08054-1560
Phone: (856)778-6500 **Free:** 800-454-7651
Fax: (856)778-6550
Website: http://www.amerihealth.com
G. Fred DiBona, Jr., CEO

★ 18543 ★ AtlantiCare Health Plans, Inc.
HMO Plan
6727 Delilah Rd.
Egg Harbor Township, NJ 08234
Free: 800-272-5995 **Fax:** (609)407-2013
Website: http://www.atlanticare.org
Patricia Koeling, CEO

★ 18544 ★ CIGNA Healthcare of New York and New Jersey
HMO Plan
499 Washington Blvd.
Jersey City, NJ 07310
Phone: (201)533-7000 **Fax:** (201)533-7164
Website: http://www.cigna.com
Kurt Weimer, CEO & Pres

★ 18545 ★ Great West Life
HMO Plan
1 Centennial Ave.
Piscataway, NJ 08855-6870
Phone: (732)980-8777 **Fax:** 888-604-2201
Website: http://www.onehealthplan.com
Matt Kenyon, Contact

★ 18546 ★ Health Net - New Jersey
HMO Plan
3501 Hwy. 66
Neptune, NJ 07753
Phone: (732)643-7400 **Free:** 800-848-4747
Fax: (732)918-6991
Website: http://www.health.net
Barry Averill, CEO

★ 18547 ★ Horizon Mercy
HMO Plan
433 Market St., Ste. 102
Camden, NJ 08102
Phone: (856)962-9393 **Free:** 800-682-9092
Fax: (856)962-8282
Website: http://www.horizon-mercy.com
Delvet Miller, CEO

★ 18548 ★ One Health Plan of Massachusetts
HMO Plan
1 Centennial Ave.
Piscataway, NJ 08855
Phone: (781)622-2400 **Fax:** (781)622-1462
Website: http://www.onehealthplan.com
Randall Cook, Contact

★ 18549 ★ One Health Plan of New Jersey, Inc.
HMO Plan
One Centennial Ave.
Piscataway, NJ 08854
Phone: (732)980-8623 **Free:** 800-644-9175
Fax: (732)980-8598
Website: http://www.onehealthplan.com
Daniel Dragalin, MD, Contact

★ 18550 ★ Oxford Health Plans of New Jersey, Inc.
HMO Plan
111 Wood Ave. S, Ste. 2
Iselin, NJ 08830
Phone: (203)459-6000 **Free:** 800-889-4694
Fax: (732)623-1900
Website: http://www.oxhp.com
Norman Payson, MD, CEO & Chm Bd

★ 18551 ★ QualCare, Inc.
HMO Plan
242 Old New Brunswick Rd.
Piscataway, NJ 08854-3754
Phone: (732)562-0833 **Free:** 800-992-6613
Fax: (732)562-2833
Annette Catino, CEO

★ 18552 ★ University Health Plans, Inc.
HMO Plan
550 Broad St.
Newark, NJ 07102-4599
Phone: (973)623-8700 **Free:** 800-TRI-UHP1
Fax: (973)623-3635
Website: http://www.uhpnet.com
Alexander H. McLean, CEO & Pres

New Mexico

★ 18553 ★ Cimarron Health Plan
HMO Plan
7801 Academy NE, Bldg. Ste. 2
Albuquerque, NM 87109
Phone: (505)342-4660 **Free:** 800-792-3174
Fax: (505)798-7380
Website: http://www.cimarron.com
Robertos Talamantes, MD, Chairman of the Board

★ 18554 ★ HMO New Mexico, Inc.
HMO Plan
12800 Indian School Rd. NE
Albuquerque, NM 87112
Phone: (505)291-6945 **Fax:** (505)816-3600
Website: http://www.bcbsnm.com
Norman Becker, CEO

★ 18555 ★ Lovelace Health Plan
HMO Plan
4101 Central NE
Albuquerque, NM 87110
Phone: (505)262-7363 **Fax:** (505)262-7545
Website: http://www.lovelace.com
Martin Hickey, MD, CEO

★ 18556 ★ Presbyterian Health Plan
HMO Plan
PO Box 27489
Albuquerque, NM 87125-7489
Phone: (505)923-5700 **Free:** 800-356-2884
Fax: (505)923-5277
Website: http://www.phs.org
Jim Hinton, Chairman of the Board

New York

★ 18557 ★ ABC Health Plan
16 E 16th St.
New York, NY 10003
Phone: (212)633-0815 **Free:** 800-298-2420
Fax: (212)627-2958
Audrey Brahamsha, Contact

★ 18558 ★ Aetna Inc. - New York
HMO Plan
2700 Westchester Ave.
Purchase, NY 10577
Phone: (914)251-0600 **Fax:** (914)251-1537
Website: http://www.aetna.com
John W. Rowe, MD, Chairman of the Board

★ 18559 ★ Aetna Inc. - New York
HMO Plan
333 Earle Ovington Blvd., Ste. 502
Uniondale, NY 11553
Phone: (516)794-6565 **Free:** 800-322-8742
Fax: (516)794-2389
Website: http://www.aetna.com
John W. Rowe, MD, Chairman of the Board

★ 18560 ★ Affinity Health Plan
One Fordham Plaza
Bronx, NY 10458
Phone: (718)733-4747 **Fax:** (718)733-4750
Website: http://www.affinityplan.org
Maura Bluestone, CEO

★ 18561 ★ AmeriChoice of New York
HMO Plan
7 Hanover Sq., 5th Fl.
New York, NY 10004
Phone: (212)509-5999 **Fax:** (212)509-1929
Thelma Dugson, CEO

★ 18562 ★ AmeriHealth Health Plan, Inc.
HMO Plan
100 Clearbrook Rd.
Elmsford, NY 10523
Phone: (914)784-2900 **Free:** 800-473-4161
Fax: (914)592-4171
Website: http://www.amerihealth.com
Fred Debona, CEO

★ 18563 ★ Buffalo Community Health Inc.
205 Park Club Ln.
Buffalo, NY 14221-5239
Phone: (716)847-1480 **Fax:** (716)857-4667
Website: http://www.univerahealthcare.org
Valerie Rosenhock, CEO

★ 18564 ★ Capital District Physicians Health Plan, Inc.
HMO Plan
1223 Washington Ave.
Albany, NY 12206
Phone: (518)641-3000 **Free:** 800-993-7299
Fax: (518)641-3507
Website: http://www.cdphp.com
William Cromie, MD, CEO

★ 18565 ★ CarePlus Health Plan
HMO Plan
360 W 31st St., Fl. 5
New York, NY 10001
Phone: (212)563-5570 **Fax:** (212)563-5975
Website: http://www.careplus.net
Karen Ajmani, CEO

★ 18566 ★ CenterCare
HMO Plan
555 W 57th St., 18th Fl.
New York, NY 10019-2925
Phone: (212)293-9200 **Fax:** (212)293-9297
Website: http://www.centercare.org
Julio Bellber, CEO

★ 18567 ★ Community Choice Health Plan of Westchester, Inc.
HMO Plan
30 S Broadway, No. 4
Yonkers, NY 10701-3712
Phone: (914)377-0710 **Fax:** (914)337-0727
Website: http://www.ahcahp.org
Lynda Gray, CEO

★ 18568 ★ Community Premier Plus, Inc.
534 W 135th St.
New York, NY 10031
Phone: (212)491-2333 **Free:** 800-867-5885
Fax: (212)491-2315
Harris Lampert, MD, CEO & Pres

★ 18569 ★ Fidelis Care New York
HMO Plan
95-25 Queens Blvd.
Rego Park, NY 11374
Phone: (718)896-6500 **Free:** 888-343-3547
Fax: (718)896-1920
Website: http://www.fideliscareny.com
Mark Lane, CEO

★ 18570 ★ GHI HMO Select, Inc.
HMO Plan
PO Box 4332
Kingston, NY 12402
Phone: (845)340-2300 **Free:** 877-244-4466
Fax: (914)334-8940
Website: http://www.ghi.com
Frank Branchini, CEO

★ 18571 ★ Group Health Inc.
441 Ninth Ave.
New York, NY 10001-1681
Phone: (212)615-0000 **Fax:** (212)563-8553
Website: http://www.ghi.com
Frank J. Branchini, CEO

★ 18572 ★ Guardian Life Insurance Co. of America
HMO Plan
7 Hanover St.
New York, NY 10004
Phone: (212)598-8000 **Fax:** (212)919-2423
Website: http://www.glic.com
Joseph Dudley Sargent, CEO

★ 18573 ★ Health Net - New York
399 Knollwood Rd., No. 212
White Plains, NY 10603-1914
Phone: 888-747-4090 **Free:** 800-848-4747
Fax: (914)682-5692
Website: http://www.health.net
Barry Averill, CEO

★ 18574 ★ Health Services Medical Corp.
HMO Plan
82787 Willett Pkwy.
Baldwinsville, NY 13027
Phone: (315)638-2133 **Free:** 800-388-3264
Fax: (315)638-6338
Website: http://www.phphmo.com
Frederick Yanni, Chairman of the Board

★ 18575 ★ HealthFirst
25 Broadway, 9th Fl.
New York, NY 10004
Phone: (212)801-1502 **Fax:** (212)801-1771
Website: http://www.healthfirst.org
Paul Dickstein, CEO

★ 18576 ★ HealthPlus
HMO Plan
241 37th St.
Brooklyn, NY 11232
Phone: (718)745-0030 **Fax:** (718)745-1180
Website: http://www.healthplus-ny.com
Thomas Early, CEO

★ 18577 ★ HIP Health Plan of New York
HMO Plan
7 W 34th St.
New York, NY 10001
Phone: (212)630-5000 **Free:** 800-447-8255
Fax: (212)630-8290
Website: http://www.hipusa.com
Anthony Watson, CEO & Chm Bd

★ 18578 ★ Independent Health
HMO Plan
511 Farber Lakes Dr.
Buffalo, NY 14221
Free: 800-486-5840 **Fax:** (716)635-3838
Frank Colantuono, CEO

★ 18579 ★ Independent Health Association, Inc.
HMO Plan
511 Farber Lakes Dr.
Buffalo, NY 14221
Phone: (716)631-3001 **Free:** 800-247-1466
Fax: (716)631-0430
Website: http://www.independenthealth.com
Frank Colantuono, CEO

★ 18580 ★ MagnaCare
HMO Plan
825 E Gate Blvd., Ste. 200
Garden City, NY 11530
Phone: (516)227-6900 **Fax:** (516)227-6967
Website: http://www.pcms-magnacare.com
Anthony Bacchi, MD, CEO

★ 18581 ★ MDNY Healthcare, Inc.
HMO Plan
1 Huntington Quadrangle, Ste. 4C01
Melville, NY 11747
Phone: (631)454-1900 **Free:** 800-707-6369
Fax: (631)454-1915
Website: http://www.mdny.com
Salvatore Cavatella, MD, CEO

★ 18582 ★ MetroPlus Health Plan
HMO Plan
11 W 42nd St., 2nd Fl.
New York, NY 10036-8002
Phone: (212)597-8600 **Fax:** (212)597-8666
Barbara Radin, Contact

★ 18583 ★ MVP Health Plan, Inc.
HMO Plan
625 State St.
Schenectady, NY 12305
Phone: (518)370-4793 **Free:** 800-777-4793
Fax: (518)386-7869
Website: http://www.mvphealthplan.com
David W. Oliker, CEO

★ 18584 ★ New York Hospital Community Health Plan
HMO Plan
527 3rd Ave., Box 303
New York, NY 10016
Phone: (212)297-5514 **Fax:** (212)297-5923
Emilio Carillo, MD,MPH, CEO

★ 18585 ★ One Health Plan of New York
475 Park Ave. S, 23rd Fl.
New York, NY 10016
Phone: (212)685-5999 **Fax:** (212)685-6446
Website: http://www.onehealthplan.com
Jane Florek, Contact

★ 18586 ★ Oxford Health Plans of New York, Inc.
HMO Plan
1133 Ave. of the Americas
New York, NY 10036
Phone: (212)805-3400 **Free:** 800-444-6222
Fax: (212)805-6671
Website: http://www.oxhp.com
Norman Payson, MD, CEO & Chm Bd

★ 18587 ★ Preferred Care/Rochester HMO
HMO Plan
259 Monroe Ave.
Rochester, NY 14607-3699
Phone: (585)325-3920 **Free:** 800-933-3920
Fax: (585)327-2298
Website: http://www.preferredcare.org
John Urban, CEO

★ 18588 ★ St. Barnabas Community Health Plan
HMO Plan
2595 Webster Ave.
Bronx, NY 10458
Phone: (718)960-3991 **Free:** 800-652-1332
Fax: (718)960-3652
Wendy Rodriguez, Chairman of the Board

★ 18589 ★ United HealthCare of New York Metropolitan
HMO Plan
Two Penn Plaza, 7th Fl.
New York, NY 10121-1097
Phone: (212)216-6400 **Fax:** (212)216-6591
Website: http://www.uhc.com
Amy Knapp, CEO

★ 18590 ★ United HealthCare of Upstate New York
HMO Plan
5015 Campuswood Dr., Ste. 303
East Syracuse, NY 13057
Phone: (315)433-5700 **Fax:** (315)433-5826
Website: http://www.uhc.com
Jay Fisher, CEO

★ 18591 ★ Univera Health Care
205 Park Club Ln.
Buffalo, NY 14221-5239
Phone: (716)847-0881 **Free:** 800-644-4580
Fax: (716)847-1257
Website: http://www.univerahealthcare.org
Arthur R. Goshin, MD, CEO

★ 18592 ★ Univera Health Care - Corporate Headquarters
205 Park Club Ln.
Buffalo, NY 14221-5239
Phone: (716)847-0881 **Free:** 800-644-4580
Fax: (716)847-1257
Website: http://www.univerahealthcare.org
Arthur R. Goshin, MD, CEO

★ 18593 ★ Univera Healthcare Central New York
HMO Plan
8278 Willett Pkwy.
Baldwinsville, NY 13027
Phone: (315)635-1222 **Fax:** (315)638-6338
Website: http://www.universalhealthcare.org
Arthur R. Goshin, MD, CEO

★ 18594 ★ Univera Healthcare of Western New York
HMO Plan
205 Park Club Ln.
Buffalo, NY 14221-5239
Phone: (716)847-0881 **Free:** 800-628-8451
Fax: (716)847-1257
Website: http://www.univerahealthcare.org
Arthur Goshin, MD, CEO & Pres

★ 18595 ★ Vytra Healthcare
HMO Plan
395 N Service Rd.
Melville, NY 11747
Phone: (631)694-4000 **Free:** 800-406-0806
Fax: (631)719-7619
Website: http://www.vytra.com
Thomas McAteer, CEO

★ 18596 ★ WellCare of New York, Inc.
HMO Plan
PO Box 1652
Newburgh, NY 12551-1652
Free: 800-288-5441
Website: http://www.wellcare.com
Kiran Patel, MD, CEO

★ 18597 ★ Westchester Prepaid Health Services Plan, Inc.
HMO Plan
303 S Broadway, Ste. 321
Tarrytown, NY 10591
Phone: (914)631-1611 **Fax:** (914)631-1615
Georganne Chapin, CEO

North Carolina

★ 18598 ★ Aetna Inc. of the Carolinas
HMO Plan
128 S Tryon, Ste. 2000
Charlotte, NC 28202
Phone: (704)379-6700 **Fax:** (704)379-7502
Website: http://www.aetna.com
John W. Rowe, Chairman of the Board

★ 18599 ★ Aetna Inc. - North Carolina
HMO Plan
2701 Coltsgate Rd., Ste. 100
Charlotte, NC 28211
Phone: (704)379-6700 **Free:** 800-643-3609
Fax: (704)379-1729
Website: http://www.aetna.com
John W. Rowe, MD, Chairman of the Board

★ 18600 ★ CIGNA Healthcare of North Carolina
HMO Plan
200 Regency Executive Dr.
Charlotte, NC 28217
Phone: (704)586-0708 **Free:** 800-235-5707
Fax: (704)556-5840
Website: http://www.cigna.com
Steve White, CEO

★ 18601 ★ CIGNA Healthcare of North Carolina
HMO Plan
701 Corporate Center Dr.
Raleigh, NC 27607
Phone: (919)854-7000 **Free:** 800-849-9300
Fax: (919)854-7102
Website: http://www.cigna.com
Steve White, President

★ 18602 ★ Coventry Health Care Inc. - Carolinas
HMO Plan
2815 Coliseum Ctr. Dr., Ste. 550
Charlotte, NC 28217
Phone: (704)357-1421 **Free:** 800-470-4523
Fax: (704)357-3164
Website: http://www.cvty.com
Tracy Baker, CEO

★ 18603 ★ Doctors Health Plan, Inc.
HMO Plan
PO Box 15940
Durham, NC 27705
Phone: (919)383-4175 **Free:** 800-476-2303
Fax: (919)383-3286
Website: http://www.dhpcares.com
Erin Molitot, Contact

★ 18604 ★ One Health Plan of North Carolina, Inc.
HMO Plan
6000 Fairview Rd., Ste. 500
Charlotte, NC 28210
Phone: (704)552-9642 **Free:** 800-663-8081
Fax: (704)556-2149
Website: http://www.onehealthplan.com
William T. McCallum, CEO

★ 18605 ★ PARTNERS National Health Plans of North Carolina, Inc.
HMO Plan
PO Box 24907
Winston-Salem, NC 27114-4907
Phone: (336)760-4822 **Free:** 800-942-5695
Fax: (336)760-3198
Website: http://www.partnershealth.com
Jim Broderick, CEO

★ 18606 ★ QualChoice of North Carolina, Inc.
HMO Plan
PO Box 340
Winston-Salem, NC 27102-0340
Phone: (336)716-0900 **Free:** 800-816-8117
Fax: (336)716-0920
Website: http://www.bgsm.edu/qualchoice
David Patterson, CEO

★ 18607 ★ United HealthCare of North Carolina, Inc.
HMO Plan
3803 N Elm St.
Greensboro, NC 27455
Phone: (336)282-0900 **Free:** 800-772-1180
Fax: (336)545-5099
Website: http://www.uhc.com
Frank Mascia, CEO

★ 18608 ★ WellPath of Carolina, Inc.
HMO Plan
6330 Quadrangle Dr., Ste. 500
Chapel Hill, NC 27514
Phone: (919)493-1210 **Free:** 800-935-7284
Fax: (919)419-3871
Website: http://www.wellpathchp.com
Tracy H. Baker, CEO

North Dakota

★ 18609 ★ Heart of America HMO
HMO Plan
810 S Main Ave.
Rugby, ND 58368
Phone: (701)776-5848 **Fax:** (701)776-5425
Website: http://www.hamc.com
Philip Sedo, MD, Contact

Ohio

★ 18610 ★ Aetna Inc. - Ohio
HMO Plan
205 W 4th St., Ste. 1000
Cincinnati, OH 45202
Phone: (513)579-3385 **Free:** 800-230-3241
Fax: (513)579-3316
Website: http://www.aetna.com
John W. Rowe, MD, Chairman of the Board

★ 18611 ★ Aetna Inc. - Ohio
HMO Plan
4059 Kinross Lakes Pkwy.
Richfield, OH 44286
Phone: (330)659-8000 **Free:** 800-458-3940
Fax: (330)659-8034
Website: http://www.aetna.com
John W. Rowe, MD, Chairman of the Board

★ 18612 ★ AultCare
HMO Plan
2600 6th St. SW
Canton, OH 44710-1799
Phone: (330)438-6390 **Free:** 800-344-8858
Fax: (330)454-7845
Website: http://www.aultcare.com
Rick Haines, CEO

★ 18613 ★ CareSource
1 S Main St., Ste. 440
Dayton, OH 45402
Phone: (937)224-3300 **Free:** 888-825-9297
Fax: (937)224-2272
Website: http://www.care-source.com
Pamela B. Morris, CEO

★ 18614 ★ CHN MCO
HMO Plan
6000 West Creek, Ste. 20
Independence, OH 44131
Phone: (216)986-1100 **Fax:** (216)328-7551
Website: http://www.chnetwork.com
Martin Hauser, CEO

★ 18615 ★ ChoiceCare/Humana
HMO Plan
655 Eden Park Dr., Ste. 400
Cincinnati, OH 45202-6056
Phone: (513)784-5200 **Free:** 800-543-7158
Fax: (513)784-5345
Website: http://www.choicecare.com
Larry Savage, CEO & Pres

★ 18616 ★ CIGNA HealthCare of Ohio, Inc.
HMO Plan
5005 Rockside Rd., Ste. 700
Cleveland, OH 44131
Phone: (216)642-2920 **Free:** 800-647-7748
Fax: (216)642-2990
Website: http://www.cigna.com
Jeanne McCarthy, President

★ 18617 ★ CIGNA PPO of Ohio
HMO Plan
7 W 7th St., Ste. 1402
Cincinnati, OH 45202-2417
Phone: (513)629-2640 **Fax:** (513)629-2639
Website: http://www.cigna.com
Ed Hanway, CEO

★ 18618 ★ Community Choice/ Community Preferred Plan
HMO Plan
1351 William H. Taft Rd.
Cincinnati, OH 45206
Phone: (513)872-8100 **Fax:** (513)336-2021
Website: http://www.anthem-inc.com
Larry Glasscock, CEO

★ 18619 ★ Family Health Plan
HMO Plan
2200 Jefferson Ave.
Toledo, OH 43624
Phone: (419)251-6501 **Free:** 800-231-8274
Fax: (419)246-0236
Thomas Beaty, CEO

★ 18620 ★ Great West
HMO Plan
445 Hutchinson Ave., Ste. 240
Columbus, OH 43235
Phone: (614)848-5369 **Fax:** (614)848-3593
Website: http://www.onehealthplan.com
Jack West, Chairman of the Board

★ 18621 ★ Health Plan of the Upper Ohio Valley
HMO Plan
52160 National Rd. E
Saint Clairsville, OH 43950
Phone: (740)695-3585 **Free:** 800-624-6961
Fax: (740)695-5297
Website: http://www.healthplan.org
Phil Wright, CEO

★ 18622 ★ HMO Health Ohio (Cleveland)
HMO Plan
2060 E 9th St.
Cleveland, OH 44115-1355
Phone: (216)687-7685 **Free:** 800-700-2583
Fax: (216)687-7274
Kent Clapp, CEO

★ 18623 ★ Hometown Health Network
HMO Plan
100 Lillian Gish Blvd., Ste. 301
Massillon, OH 44647
Phone: (330)837-6880 **Free:** 800-426-9013
Fax: (330)837-6869
Website: http://www.hometownhealth.com
William Epling, President

★ 18624 ★ Kaiser Permanente Foundation Health Plan of Ohio, Inc.
HMO Plan
1001 Lakeside Ave., Ste. 1200
Cleveland, OH 44114
Phone: (216)621-5600 **Free:** 800-524-7371
Fax: (216)623-8776
Website: http://www.kaiperm.org
Ronald Copeland, MD, CEO

★ 18625 ★ Medical Mutual of Ohio
HMO Plan
2060 E 9th St.
Cleveland, OH 44115
Phone: (216)687-7000 **Free:** 800-782-3651
Fax: (419)473-6033
Website: http://www.mmoh.com
Kent Clapp, CEO & Pres

★ 18626 ★ Mount Carmel Healthplan, Inc.
HMO Plan
495 Cooper Rd., Ste. 200
Westerville, OH 43081
Phone: (614)898-8750 **Free:** 800-255-0726
Fax: (614)898-8587
Website: http://www.medigold.com
Mark Richardson, CEO

★ 18627 ★ Nationwide Health Plans
HMO Plan
5525 Park Center Circle
Dublin, OH 43017-3685
Phone: (614)854-3001 **Free:** 800-826-9017
Fax: (614)854-3648
Website: http://www.nationwide-health.com
Joe SanFilippo, CEO

★ 18628 ★ One Health Plan of Ohio, Inc.
HMO Plan
24950 Country Club Blvd., Ste. 400
North Olmsted, OH 44070
Phone: (440)716-1777 **Free:** 800-644-9335
Fax: (440)716-1221
Website: http://www.onehealthplan.com
William McCallum, CEO

★ 18629 ★ Paramount Health Care Plan
HMO Plan
1901 Indian Wood Cr.
Maumee, OH 43537-4068
Phone: (419)887-2500 **Free:** 800-462-3589
Fax: (419)887-2530
Website: http://www.promedica.org
John Randolph, CEO

★ 18630 ★ QualChoice
HMO Plan
6000 Parkland Blvd.
Cleveland, OH 44124
Phone: (440)460-0093 **Free:** 800-208-1232
Fax: (440)460-4005
Website: http://www.qchp.com
Thomas Sullivan, CEO

★ 18631 ★ SummaCare, Inc.
HMO Plan
PO Box 3620
Akron, OH 44309-3620
Phone: (330)996-8410 **Free:** 800-996-8411
Fax: (330)996-8454
Website: http://www.summacare.com
Martin Hanser, CEO

★ 18632 ★ Super Med
HMO Plan
2060 E 9th St.
Cleveland, OH 44115-1355
Phone: (216)687-7685 **Free:** 800-700-2583
Fax: (216)687-7274
Website: http://www.mmoh.com
Kent Clapp, CEO

★ 18633 ★ United HealthCare of Ohio, Inc.
HMO Plan
9200 Worthington Rd.
Westerville, OH 43082
Phone: (614)410-7000 **Free:** 888-328-8835
Fax: (614)410-1011
Website: http://www.uhc.com
Brett Baby, CEO

★ 18634 ★ United Healthcare of Ohio Inc. - Cleveland
13775 E 9th St., Ste. 700
Cleveland, OH 44114
Free: 800-225-7951
Website: http://www.uhc.com
Ken Hoverman, CEO

★ 18635 ★ United HealthCare of Ohio, Inc. - Dayton/Cincinnati
HMO Plan
9050 Centre Pointe Dr., Ste. 400
West Chester, OH 45069
Free: 877-832-7734 **Fax:** (937)439-8999
Website: http://www.uhc.com
Tom Brady, CEO

★ 18636 ★ Vantage Health Plan
HMO Plan
4602 Timber Commons Dr.
Sandusky, OH 44870
Phone: (419)621-9858 **Free:** 800-878-4394
Fax: (419)621-9859
Website: http://www.vantagehealthplan.com
Dr. Shukirk, CEO

Oklahoma

★ 18637 ★ Aetna Inc. - Oklahoma
HMO Plan
4013 NW Expressway, Ste. 300
Oklahoma City, OK 73116
Phone: (405)879-1780 **Fax:** (405)475-6500
Website: http://www.aetna.com
John W. Rowe, MD, CEO

★ 18638 ★ Aetna Inc. - Tulsa
HMO Plan
7912 E 31st Ct., Ste. 300
Tulsa, OK 74145-1339
Phone: (918)624-4700 **Free:** 800-435-8310
Fax: (918)627-9759
Website: http://www.aetna.com
John W. Rowe, Chairman of the Board

★ 18639 ★ AmCare Health Plans of Oklahoma
HMO Plan
4100 Perimeter Center, Ste. 200
Oklahoma City, OK 73112
Phone: (405)917-8401 **Fax:** (405)917-8499
Website: http://www.amcarehealthplans.com
Thomas Lucksinger, CEO

★ 18640 ★ Bluelincs HMO
HMO Plan
1400 S Boston
Tulsa, OK 74119-3618
Phone: (918)561-9900 **Fax:** (918)592-0611
Ronald King, CEO

★ 18641 ★ Bluelincs HMO
HMO Plan
3401 NW 63rd.
Oklahoma City, OK 73116
Fax: (405)841-9778
Ronald King, CEO

★ 18642 ★ CommunityCare Managed Healthcare Plans of Oklahoma, Inc.
HMO Plan
PO Box 3249
Tulsa, OK 74101
Phone: (918)594-5200 **Free:** 800-278-7563
Fax: (918)594-5260
Website: http://www.ccmhp.com
Richard Todd, CEO & Pres

★ 18643 ★ Heartland Health Plan of Oklahoma
HMO Plan
100 N Broadway, Ste. 1400
Oklahoma City, OK 73102
Phone: (405)239-2234 **Free:** 800-492-7639
Fax: (405)552-6596
Website: http://www.okhealthcenter.com
Sally Venator, CEO

★ 18644 ★ PacifiCare of Oklahoma, Inc.
HMO Plan
7666 E 61st St., Ste. 500
Tulsa, OK 74133
Phone: (918)459-1100 **Fax:** (918)459-1452
Website: http://www.pacificare.com
Dan Comrie, Contact

★ 18645 ★ Prime Advantage Health Plan
PO Box 129
Lawton, OK 73502
Phone: (580)357-6684 **Fax:** (580)250-6546
Tanya Case, CEO

★ 18646 ★ Unicare Health Plans of Oklahoma
47 NE 23rd St.
Oklahoma City, OK 73105
Phone: (405)419-1400 **Fax:** (405)524-4807
Daniel Sorrels, CEO

★ 18647 ★ Wellcor America
HMO Plan
3503 NW 63, Ste. 304
Oklahoma City, OK 73116
Phone: (405)843-9551 **Free:** 800-535-2244
Fax: (405)843-0956
Martin Sholder, CEO

Oregon

★ 18648 ★ Cascade East Health Plans, Inc.
645 W Orchard Ave.
Hermiston, OR 97838
Phone: (541)567-5555 **Free:** (866)577-2347
Fax: (541)567-5577
Website: http://www.gshealth.org
Dennis Burke, CEO & Pres

★ 18649 ★ Health Net Health Plan of Oregon, Inc.
12901 SE 97th Ave.
Clackamas, OR 97015
Phone: (503)802-7000 **Free:** 888-802-7001
Fax: (503)802-7136
Website: http://www.qualmed.com
Stephen Lynch, CEO

★ 18650 ★ Kaiser Foundation Health Plan Northwest
HMO Plan
500 NE Multnomah St., Ste. 100
Portland, OR 97232-1191
Phone: (503)813-2800 **Fax:** (503)813-4967
Website: http://www.kaipermanente.org
Allan J. Weiland, MD, Contact

★ 18651 ★ Lane Oregon Health Plans
HMO Plan
PO Box 11740
Eugene, OR 97440
Phone: (541)485-2155 **Fax:** (541)485-0737
Website: http://www.lipa.net
Terry Coplin, CEO

★ 18652 ★ One Health Plan of Oregon, Inc.
HMO Plan
1800 SW First Ave., Ste. 230
Portland, OR 97201
Phone: (503)222-3014 **Fax:** (503)222-3253
Website: http://www.onehealthplan.com
Sara Mason, Contact

★ 18653 ★ PacifiCare of Oregon
HMO Plan
5 Centerpointe Dr., Ste. 600
Lake Oswego, OR 97035-8650
Phone: (503)603-7355 **Free:** 800-922-1444
Fax: (503)603-7377
Website: http://www.pacificare.com
Donald E. Costa, CEO

★ 18654 ★ Providence Health Plans
HMO Plan
3601 SW Murray Blvd.
Beaverton, OR 97005
Free: 800-826-7218 **Fax:** (503)574-8600
Website: http://www.providence.org
Russ Danielson, CEO

★ 18655 ★ Regence HMO Oregon
HMO Plan
100 SW Market
Portland, OR 97201
Phone: (503)364-4868 **Free:** 800-452-7278
Fax: (503)225-4848
Website: http://www.regence.com
Richard L. Woolworth, Chairman of the Board

Pennsylvania

★ 18656 ★ Aetna Inc. of Central and Eastern Pennsylvania
HMO Plan
2201 Renaissance Blvd.
Norristown, PA 19406
Phone: (484)322-2000 **Fax:** (484)322-6437
Website: http://www.aetna.com
John W. Rowe, MD, Chairman of the Board

★ 18657 ★ Aetna Inc. - Corporate Headquarters
HMO Plan
PO Box 1109
Blue Bell, PA 19422-1109
Phone: (215)775-4800 **Free:** 800-872-3862
Fax: (215)775-6401
Website: http://www.aetna.com
John W. Rowe, MD, Chairman of the Board

★ 18658 ★ Aetna Inc. - Pennsylvania
HMO Plan
5313 Campbell's Run Rd.
Pittsburgh, PA 15205-2758
Phone: (412)788-0500 **Fax:** (412)788-5067
Website: http://www.aetna.com
John W. Rowe, MD, Chairman of the Board

★ 18659 ★ Aetna Inc. - Pennsylvania Region
HMO Plan
PO Box 1109
Blue Bell, PA 19422-1109
Phone: (215)775-4800 **Fax:** (215)775-6401
Website: http://www.aetna.com
John W. Rowe, MD, Chairman of the Board

★ 18660 ★ Berkshire Health Plan
HMO Plan
50 Commerce Ct.
Wyomissing, PA 19610
Phone: (610)372-8044 **Fax:** (610)371-0310
Website: http://www.bhp.org
Charles Wills, President

★ 18661 ★ Berkshire Health Plan/Medicus Resource Management
HMO Plan
50 Commerce Ct.
Wyomissing, PA 19610
Phone: (610)372-8044 **Fax:** (610)371-0310
Website: http://www.bhp.org
Charles Wills, President

★ 18662 ★ CIGNA Healthcare - Corporate Headquarters
HMO Plan
One Liberty Pl.
1650 Market St.
Philadelphia, PA 19192-1550
Phone: (215)761-1000 **Fax:** (215)761-5517
Website: http://www.cigna.com
H. Edward Hanway, CEO
Program(s): Chiropractic, Dental, Home Care, Inpatient SNF, Long-Term Care, Pharmaceutical Mail Order, Podiatry, Psychiatric, Transplant, Vision, Wellness, Workers' Compensation.

★ 18663 ★ Coordinated Health Systems
HMO Plan
2775 Schoenersville Rd.
Bethlehem, PA 18017
Phone: (610)861-8111 **Fax:** (610)807-0366
Website: http://www.chs4health
Emil DiLorio, MD, CEO

★ 18664 ★ Gateway Health Plan, Inc.
HMO Plan
Two Chatham Center, Ste. 500
Pittsburgh, PA 15219-3427
Phone: (412)255-4640 **Free:** 800-392-1147
Fax: (412)255-4334
Website: http://www.gatewayhealthplan.com
Michael Blackwood, CEO & Pres

★ 18665 ★ Geisinger Health Plan
HMO Plan
100 N Academy Ave.
Danville, PA 17822-3020
Phone: (717)271-8760 **Free:** 800-631-1656
Fax: (717)271-5218
Website: http://www.thehealthplan.edu
Dr. Glen Steele, Jr., CEO
Program(s): Chiropractic, Home Care, Inpatient SNF, Pharmaceutical Mail Order, Podiatry, Psychiatric, Behavioral Health, Physical Therapy, Transplant, Vision, Wellness.

★ 18666 ★ Health Net - Pennsylvania
1835 Market St.
Philadelphia, PA 19103
Free: 800-848-4747 **Fax:** (732)918-6991
Website: http://www.health.net
Barry Averill, CEO

★ 18667 ★ Health Net - Pennsylvania
1065 Hwy 315, Ste. 201
Wilkes Barre, PA 18701
Free: 800-848-4747 **Fax:** (732)918-6991
Website: http://www.health.net
Barry Averill, CEO

★ 18668 ★ Health Partners
HMO Plan
833 E Chestnut St., Ste. 900
Philadelphia, PA 19107
Phone: (215)849-9606 **Free:** 800-533-0784
Fax: (215)849-9636
Website: http://www.healthpart.com
Robert Tremain, CEO

★ 18669 ★ HealthAmerica of Central Pennsylvania
HMO Plan
2575 Interstate Dr.
Harrisburg, PA 17110
Phone: (717)540-4260 **Free:** 800-788-6445
Fax: (717)541-5739
Website: http://www.healthamerica.cvty.com
Francis Soistman, Jr., CEO

★ 18670 ★ HealthAmerica Pennsylvania, Inc. - Western Region
HMO Plan
5 Gateway Center
Pittsburgh, PA 15222
Phone: (412)553-7522 **Free:** 800-735-4404
Fax: (412)553-7523
Website: http://www.healthamerica.cvty.com
Francis Soistman, Jr., CEO

★ 18671 ★ Healthcare Management Alternatives Health Plan
HMO Plan
100 Penn Sq. E, Ste. 900
Philadelphia, PA 19107
Phone: (215)832-4500 **Free:** 800-321-4462
Fax: (215)832-4619
Website: http://www.americhoice.com
Chris Paterson, MD, CEO

★ 18672 ★ HealthGuard of Lancaster
HMO Plan
280 Granite Run Dr.
Lancaster, PA 17601-6810
Phone: (717)560-9049 **Free:** 800-822-0350
Fax: (717)581-4580
Website: http://www.hguard.com
James Godfrey, President

★ 18673 ★ Keystone Health Plan Central
HMO Plan
PO Box 898812
Camp Hill, PA 17089-8812
Phone: (717)302-0200 **Free:** 800-622-2843
Fax: (717)302-0591
Joseph Pfister, CEO

★ 18674 ★ Keystone Health Plan East Inc.
HMO Plan
1901 Market St.
Philadelphia, PA 19103
Phone: (215)241-2001 **Free:** 800-227-3114
Fax: (215)241-2017
Website: http://www.khpe.com
G. Fred DiBona, CEO & Pres

★ 18675 ★ Keystone Mercy Health Plan
HMO Plan
200 Stevens Dr.
Philadelphia, PA 19113
Phone: (215)937-8493 **Fax:** (215)937-5363
Website: http://www.mercyhealth.org/keystone.html
Daniel Hilferty, CEO

★ 18676 ★ New Alliance Health Plan
HMO Plan
1700 Peach St., Ste. 244
Erie, PA 16501
Phone: (814)878-1700 **Free:** 800-255-4281
Fax: (814)452-4358
Website: http://www.newalliancehealth.com
Joseph Prischak, Chairman of the Board

★ 18677 ★ One Health Plan of Pennsylvania, Inc.
HMO Plan
8 Penn Center
1628 JFK Blvd., Ste. 1010
Philadelphia, PA 19103
Phone: (215)832-3400 **Free:** 800-303-4635
Fax: (215)832-3441
Website: http://www.onehealthplan.com
Dan Dragalin, MD, President

★ 18678 ★ PhilCare Health Systems HMO
2000 Market St., 6th Fl.
Philadelphia, PA 19103
Phone: (215)564-4061 **Free:** 800-371-6664
Fax: (215)557-4469
Website: http://www.tylerhospital.com
Gary Walker, CEO

★ 18679 ★ Three River Health Plans
HMO Plan
300 Oxford Dr.
Monroeville, PA 15146
Phone: (412)858-4000 **Free:** 800-414-9025
Fax: (412)858-4060
Warren Carmichael, CEO

★ 18680 ★ UPMC Health Plan - University of Pittsburgh Medical Center
HMO Plan
1 Chatham Center
112 Washington Pl.
Pittsburgh, PA 15219
Phone: (412)434-1200 **Fax:** (412)454-7711
Website: http://www.upmc.edu/upmchealthplan
Patricia Liebman, CEO

Puerto Rico

★ 18681 ★ Humana, Inc./PCA - Puerto Rico
HMO Plan
383 FD Roosevelt, 3rd Fl.
San Juan, PR 00918-2131
Phone: (787)282-7900 **Free:** 800-314-3121
Fax: (787)282-6277
Website: http://www.humana.com
Drayton Nabers, Jr., CEO

★ 18682 ★ Triple-S, Inc.
HMO Plan
PO Box 363628
San Juan, PR 00936-3628
Phone: (787)749-4949 **Fax:** (787)749-4193
Website: http://www.ssspr.com
Arturo Delahongra, Contact

★ 18683 ★ United Healthcare Plans of Puerto Rico, Inc.
PO Box 364864
San Juan, PR 00936-4864
Phone: (809)782-7005
Website: http://www.unitedhealthcare.com
William W. McGuire, MD, CEO & Pres

Rhode Island

★ 18684 ★ Coordinated Health Partners, Inc.
HMO Plan
15 LaSalle Sq.
Providence, RI 02903-4138
Phone: (401)459-5992 **Free:** 800-564-0888
Fax: (401)459-5568
Lynne Urbani, CEO & Pres

★ 18685 ★ Neighborhood Health Plan of Rhode Island, Inc.
HMO Plan
50 Holden St., Ste. 200
Providence, RI 02908
Phone: (401)459-6000 **Fax:** (401)459-6175
Website: http://www.nhpri.org
Christopher Koller, CEO

★ 18686 ★ United Health Plans of New England
475 Kilvert St.
Warwick, RI 02886-1392
Phone: (401)737-6900 **Free:** 800-447-1245
Fax: (401)732-7210
Website: http://www.uhc.com
Bud Fisher, CEO

South Carolina

★ 18687 ★ CIGNA Healthcare of South Carolina
HMO Plan
259 Commonwealth, Ste. 110
Greenville, SC 29615-4847
Phone: (864)234-7768 **Free:** 800-949-0325
Fax: (864)297-1389
Website: http://www.cigna.com
Ed Hanaway, CEO

★ 18688 ★ Companion Healthcare Corp.
HMO Plan
4101 Percical Rd.
Columbia, SC 29223
Phone: (803)786-8466 **Free:** 800-327-3183
Fax: (803)714-6461
Website: http://www.companionhealthcare.com
Ed Sails, CEO

★ 18689 ★ Select Health of South Carolina, Inc.
HMO Plan
7410 Northside Dr., Ste. 100
North Charleston, SC 29420
Phone: (843)569-1759 **Fax:** (843)569-0702
Michael Jernigan, CEO

South Dakota

★ 18690 ★ Avera Health Plans, Inc.
HMO Plan
3900 W Avera Dr., Ste. 200
Sioux Falls, SD 57108
Phone: (605)322-4500 **Fax:** (605)322-4535
Website: http://www.avera.org
Jean Reed, CEO & Pres

★ 18691 ★ DakotaCare
HMO Plan
1323 S Minnesota Ave.
Sioux Falls, SD 57105-0685
Phone: (605)334-4000 **Free:** 800-325-5598
Fax: (605)336-0270
Website: http://www.dakotacare.com
Paul Jensen, CEO
Program(s): Chiropractic, Home Care, Podiatry, Psychiatric, Behavioral Health, Physical Therapy, Transplant, Vision, Wellness.

★ 18692 ★ Sioux Valley Health Plan
HMO Plan
1200 N West Ave.
Sioux Falls, SD 57104
Phone: (605)328-6868 **Fax:** (605)328-6811
Ruth Krystopolski, CEO

Tennessee

★ 18693 ★ Aetna Inc. - Tennessee
HMO Plan
1801 W End Ave., Ste. 500
Palmer Plaza
Nashville, TN 37203
Phone: (615)322-1600 **Fax:** (615)322-1646
Website: http://www.aetna.com
John W. Rowe, MD, Chairman of the Board

★ 18694 ★ Aetna Inc. - Tennessee
HMO Plan
3150 Lenox Park Blvd., Ste. 110
Memphis, TN 38118
Phone: (901)541-9400 **Fax:** (901)541-9343
Website: http://www.aetna.com
John W. Rowe, MD, Chairman of the Board

★ 18695 ★ Baptist Health Services Group
HMO Plan
6750 Poplar Ave., Ste. 301
Memphis, TN 38138-7445
Phone: (901)759-5000 **Fax:** (901)759-5001
Website: http://www.bmhcc.org
David Elliot, CEO

★ 18696 ★ Cariten Healthcare
HMO Plan
1420 Centerpoint Blvd.
Knoxville, TN 37932
Phone: (865)470-7470 **Free:** 800-793-1495
Fax: (865)670-7255
Website: http://www.cariten.com
Lance Hunsinger, CEO & Pres

★ 18697 ★ CIGNA Healthcare of Tennessee, Inc.
HMO Plan
6555 Quince Rd., Ste. 215
Memphis, TN 38119
Free: 800-832-3211 **Fax:** (901)758-5110
Website: http://www.cigna.com
William Pastore, CEO

★ 18698 ★ CIGNA Healthcare of Tennessee Inc.
HMO Plan
1000 Corporate Center Dr.
Franklin, TN 37067
Phone: (423)296-2065 **Free:** 800-492-2224
Fax: (615)595-3590
Website: http://www.cigna.com
David Mathis, Contact

★ 18699 ★ Health Choice LLC
HMO Plan
1000 Brookfield, 2nd Fl.
Memphis, TN 38104
Phone: (901)821-6700 **Free:** 800-328-2579
Fax: (901)821-6751
Website: http://www.healthchoice.org
William Breen, Jr., CEO

★ 18700 ★ Health Springs
HMO Plan
44 Vantage Way, Ste. 300
Nashville, TN 37228
Phone: (615)291-7000 **Fax:** (615)291-7011
Website: http://www.myhealthspring.com
Herbert A. Fritch, CEO

★ 18701 ★ HealthNow
HMO Plan
5959 Park Ave.
Memphis, TN 38119
Phone: (901)765-3190 **Fax:** (901)765-3179
Dave Archer, CEO

★ 18702 ★ John Deere Health
HMO Plan
57213 Noah Reid Rd., Ste. I
Chattanooga, TN 37404
Phone: (423)499-0673 **Free:** 800-224-6601
Fax: (423)954-9907
Website: http://www.johndeerehealth.com
Richard L. Bartsh, MD, President

★ 18703 ★ John Deere Health
HMO Plan
408 N Cedar Bluff Rd., Ste. 400
Knoxville, TN 37923
Phone: (865)690-5572 **Free:** 800-209-0034
Fax: (865)690-2741
Website: http://www.johndeerehealth.com
Richard L. Bartsh, MD, President

★ 18704 ★ John Deere Health Care
HMO Plan
2578 E Stone Dr., Ste. A
Kingsport, TN 37660-4203
Phone: (423)378-5122 **Free:** 800-224-6602
Fax: (423)378-4752
Website: http://www.johndeerehealth.com
Richard L. Bartsh, MD, President

★ 18705 ★ Memphis Managed Care
1407 Union Ave., Ste. 1100
Memphis, TN 38104
Phone: (901)725-7100 **Free:** 800-473-6523
Fax: (901)725-2846
Al King, CEO

★ 18706 ★ OmniCare Health Plan - Tennessee
HMO Plan
1991 Corporate Ave., 4th Fl.
Memphis, TN 38132
Phone: (901)346-0064 **Free:** 800-346-0034
Fax: (901)346-1032
Website: http://www.ochptn.com
Osbie Howard, CEO

★ 18707 ★ One Health Plan of Tennessee, Inc.
HMO Plan
3100 W End Ave., Ste. 600
Nashville, TN 37203
Phone: (615)269-6983 **Fax:** (615)269-5889
Website: http://www.onehealthplan.com
David Record, President

★ 18708 ★ PHP Companies, Inc.
HMO Plan
1420 Centerpoint Blvd.
Knoxville, TN 37932
Phone: (865)470-7470 **Free:** 800-747-0008
Fax: (865)470-7485
Tony Stezia, CEO

★ 18709 ★ Tennessee Health Care Network, Inc.
HMO Plan
801 Pine St.
Chattanooga, TN 37402
Phone: (423)763-3130 **Fax:** (423)752-8331
Vickie Gregg, CEO

★ 18710 ★ TLC Family Care Health Plan
HMO Plan
1407 Union Ave., Ste. 1100
Memphis, TN 38104
Phone: (901)725-7100 **Free:** 800-473-6523
Fax: (901)725-3817
Website: http://www.mmcc-tlc.com
Al King, CEO

★ 18711 ★ United HealthCare of Tennessee, Inc.
HMO Plan
10 Cadillac Dr.
Brentwood, TN 37027
Phone: (615)372-3622 **Free:** 800-695-1273
Fax: (615)372-3640
Website: http://www.uhc.com
C. Brian Shipp, CEO

★ 18712 ★ Xantus Health Plan of Tennessee
HMO Plan
3401 W End Ave., Ste. 470
Nashville, TN 37203-1069
Phone: (615)298-3666 **Free:** 800-730-2299
Fax: (615)460-9918
Website: http://www.xantuscorp.com
Richard Sandstrom, CEO

Texas

★ 18713 ★ Aetna Inc. - Austin
HMO Plan
7700 Chevy Chase Dr., Ste. 500
Austin, TX 78752
Phone: (512)323-0440 **Fax:** (512)465-5441
Website: http://www.aetna.com
John W. Rowe, MD, Chairman of the Board

★ 18714 ★ Aetna Inc. - El Paso
HMO Plan
100 N Stanton, Ste. 1301
El Paso, TX 79901-1448
Phone: (915)532-0700 **Fax:** (915)532-0342
Website: http://www.aetna.com
John W. Rowe, MD, Chairman of the Board

★ 18715 ★ Aetna Inc. - Houston
HMO Plan
3 Greenway Plaza, MS G-201
Houston, TX 77046
Phone: (713)350-2260 **Free:** 800-876-7778
Fax: (713)350-2920
Website: http://www.aetna.com
John W. Rowe, MD, Chairman of the Board

★ 18716 ★ Aetna Inc. of North Texas
HMO Plan
2777 Stemmons Frwy.
Dallas, TX 75207
Phone: (214)200-8000 **Free:** 800-992-7947
Fax: (214)200-8580
Website: http://www.aetna.com
John W. Rowe, MD, Chairman of the Board

★ 18717 ★ AmCare Health Plans of Texas
HMO Plan
3411 Richmond Ave., Ste. 500
Houston, TX 77046-3409
Phone: (713)985-4100 **Free:** 800-782-8373
Fax: (713)985-4101
Website: http://www.amcarehealthplans.com
Thomas Lucksinger, CEO

★ 18718 ★ AmCareCo, Inc. - Corporate Headquarters
HMO Plan
3411 Richmond Ave., Ste. 500
Houston, TX 77046-3409
Phone: (713)985-4100 **Free:** 800-782-8373
Fax: (713)985-4101
Website: http://www.amcarehealthplans.com
Thomas Lucksinger, CEO

★ 18719 ★ Americaid Texas, Inc.
HMO Plan
1200 E Copeland Rd., Ste. 200
Arlington, TX 76011-4936
Phone: (817)861-7700 **Free:** 800-839-6275
Fax: (817)548-7125
Website: http://www.amerigroupcorp.com
James Donovan, Jr., CEO

★ 18720 ★ AmeriHealth of Texas, Inc.
HMO Plan
3411 Richmond, Ste. 500
Houston, TX 77046-3401
Phone: (713)985-4100 **Free:** 800-888-2442
Fax: (713)985-4101
Website: http://www.amerihealth.com
Thomas S. Lucksinger, CEO

★ 18721 ★ Amil Intenational
HMO Plan
9229 Waterford Center Blvd., Ste. 500
Austin, TX 78758
Phone: (512)349-4050 **Free:** 888-247-2645
Fax: (512)349-4329
Website: http://www.amiltx.com
Marco Santos, CEO

★ 18722 ★ CIGNA Healthcare of North Texas
HMO Plan
6600 E Campus Circle Dr., Ste. 400
Irving, TX 75063
Phone: (972)263-2718 **Free:** 800-772-4462
Fax: (972)582-7618
Website: http://www.cigna.com
Ken Malcomson, CEO

★ 18723 ★ CIGNA Healthcare of Texas, Inc.
HMO Plan
2 Riverway, Ste. 1200
Houston, TX 77056
Phone: (713)552-7600 **Free:** 800-772-4462
Fax: (713)552-7699
Website: http://www.cigna.com
Pat Stewart, CEO

★ 18724 ★ Community First Health Plans, Inc.
HMO Plan
4801 NW Loop 410, Ste. 1000
San Antonio, TX 78229
Free: 800-434-2347 **Fax:** (210)358-6039
Website: http://www.cfhp.com
Johnny E. Lovejoy, II, Chairman of the Board

★ 18725 ★ Community Health Choice, Inc.
HMO Plan
2636 S Loop West
Houston, TX 77054
Phone: (713)746-6999 **Fax:** (713)566-4365
Glen Johnson, CEO

★ 18726 ★ Cooks Childrens Health Plan
HMO Plan
801 7th St.
Fort Worth, TX 76104-2796
Phone: (817)885-4000 **Free:** 800-964-2247
Fax: (817)885-1437
Website: http://www.cookchildrens.org
John Grigson, President

★ 18727 ★ Driscoll Children's Health Plan
HMO Plan
3455 S Alameda
Corpus Christi, TX 78411
Phone: (361)694-6780 **Fax:** (361)851-6889
Website: http://www.drisollchildrens.org
Charles Carroll, CEO & Pres

★ 18728 ★ El Paso First Health Plans, Inc.
2501 N Mesa
El Paso, TX 79902
Phone: (915)532-3778 **Free:** 877-532-3778
Fax: (915)532-2877
Website: http://www.ep1st.com
David Rodriguez, CEO & Pres

★ 18729 ★ Family Healthcare Centers, Inc.
UTMB Healthcare Systems
301 University Blvd.
Galveston, TX 77555-0116
Phone: (409)797-8010 **Fax:** (409)737-7091
Kent Norman, CEO

★ 18730 ★ Fortis Health - Texas
16775 Addison Rd., Ste. 500
Addison, TX 75001
Free: 800-262-5388 **Fax:** (214)258-1102
Website: http://www.fortisbenefitsdental.com
Michael Hawkins, MD, Contact

★ 18731 ★ Great West
HMO Plan
4807 Spice Woods Spring, Ste. 200
Austin, TX 78759
Phone: (512)345-3565 **Fax:** (512)345-4964
Website: http://www.onehealthplan.com
Steve Quenville, Contact

★ 18732 ★ HealthPlan of Texas, Inc. - Heritage Health Plan
HMO Plan
110 N College, Ste. 900
Tyler, TX 75702
Phone: (903)531-4447 **Fax:** (903)531-5770
Paul Christman, CEO

★ 18733 ★ Humana Health Care Plans of Corpus Christi
HMO Plan
802 N Carancahua, Ste. 1700
Corpus Christi, TX 78470
Phone: (361)866-2239 **Fax:** (361)866-2299
Website: http://www.humana.com/corpuschristi/home.html
David Jones, Chairman of the Board

★ 18734 ★ Humana Health Care Plans of Dallas
HMO Plan
8111 LBJ Freeway., Ste. 1500
Dallas, TX 75251
Phone: (972)643-1600 **Free:** 800-651-9079
Fax: (972)437-9243
Website: http://www.humana.com/dallas/home.html
David A. Jones, Chairman of the Board

★ 18735 ★ Humana Health Care Plans of Houston
HMO Plan
1980 Post Oak Blvd., Ste. 1900
Houston, TX 77056
Phone: (713)622-6639 **Fax:** (713)622-6649
Website: http://www.humana.com/houston/home.html
Ken Janda, CEO & Pres

★ 18736 ★ Humana Health Plan of Austin
HMO Plan
1221 S Mopac Blvd., Ste. 200
Austin, TX 78746
Phone: (512)338-6100 **Free:** 800-234-7912
Fax: (512)338-6137
Website: http://www.humana.com/austin/austin.html
David Jones, Chairman of the Board

★ 18737 ★ Methodist Care
HMO Plan
2 Greenway Plaza, Ste. 500
Houston, TX 77046
Phone: (713)479-4100 **Fax:** (713)479-4269
Website: http://www.methodistcare.com
Stephen Nesbitt, DO, Contact

★ 18738 ★ One Health Plan of Texas
HMO Plan
8310 Capitol of Texas Hwy. N, Ste. 340
Austin, TX 78731
Phone: (512)342-1706 **Fax:** (512)795-2105
Website: http://www.onehealthplan.com
Wally Gomaa, CEO

★ 18739 ★ One Health Plan of Texas
HMO Plan
1360 Post Oak Blvd., Ste. 2050
Houston, TX 77056
Phone: (713)629-4465 **Fax:** (713)626-2350
Website: http://www.onehealthplan.com
Wally Gomaa, President

★ 18740 ★ One Health Plan of Texas - Dallas
HMO Plan
8350 N Central Expwy., Ste. M1000
Dallas, TX 75206
Phone: (972)813-7000 **Free:** 800-866-3136
Fax: (214)363-9785
Website: http://www.onehealthplan.com
Wally Gomaa, CEO

★ 18741 ★ Pacificare
HMO Plan
1800 W Loop South, Ste. 350
Houston, TX 77027
Free: 800-825-9355 **Fax:** (713)993-3295
Website: http://www.pacificare.com
Ron Davis, CEO

★ 18742 ★ Pacificare of Texas - Arlington
HMO Plan
601 Ryan Plaza Dr., Ste. 156
Arlington, TX 76011
Phone: (817)299-3400 **Free:** 800-356-5152
Fax: (817)299-5872
George Becker, CEO

★ 18743 ★ PacifiCare of Texas - Dallas
HMO Plan
5001 LBJ Fwy., Ste. 600
Dallas, TX 75244-6130
Phone: (972)866-1693 **Free:** 800-297-9355
Fax: (972)866-1970
Website: http://www.pacificare.com
George Becker, CEO

★ 18744 ★ PacifiCare of Texas Inc.
HMO Plan
5001 LBJ Fwy., Ste. 600
Dallas, TX 75244
Free: 800-825-9355 **Fax:** (972)866-1658
Website: http://www.pacificare.com
Ron Davis, CEO

★ 18745 ★ Parkland Community Health Plan, Inc.
HMO Plan
6300 Harry Hines Blvd., Ste. 300
Dallas, TX 75235
Phone: (214)590-4571 **Fax:** (214)590-4840
Website: http://www.pchp.org
Ron Anderson, MD, CEO & Pres

★ 18746 ★ Scott and White Health Plan
HMO Plan
2401 S 31st St.
Temple, TX 76508-0001
Phone: (254)298-3000 **Free:** 800-321-7947
Fax: (254)298-3385
Website: http://www.sw.org
Alfred Knight, MD, President

★ 18747 ★ Seton Health Plan, Inc.
HMO Plan
305 E Huntland Dr.
Austin, TX 78752
Phone: (512)324-4200 **Free:** 800-749-7404
Fax: (512)324-1952
Website: http://www.seton.net
John Evler, III, CEO

★ 18748 ★ Southwest Health Alliance (SHA LLC)
HMO Plan
12940 Research Blvd.
Austin, TX 78750
Phone: (512)257-6000 **Free:** 800-365-1051
Fax: (512)257-6037
Website: http://www.first.com
Keith Lundien, CEO

★ 18749 ★ Superior Health Plan, Inc.
HMO Plan
823 Congress Ave., Ste. 600
Austin, TX 78701
Phone: (512)482-9559 **Free:** 800-208-9007
Fax: (512)482-9779
Website: http://www.cenlene.com
Chris Bowers, CEO

★ 18750 ★ Texas Children's Health Plan, Inc.
HMO Plan
1919 S Braeswood Blvd.
Houston, TX 77030
Phone: (832)824-2600 **Free:** 800-990-8247
Fax: (832)825-2686
Christopher Born, CEO

★ 18751 ★ United HealthCare of Texas, Inc. - Dallas
HMO Plan
5800 Granite Pkwy., No. 900
Plano, TX 75024
Phone: (469)633-8500 **Free:** 800-635-4418
Fax: (469)633-8805
Website: http://www.uhc.com
Thomas Quirk, CEO

★ 18752 ★ United HealthCare of Texas, Inc. - Houston
HMO Plan
2000 W Loop S, Ste. 700
Houston, TX 77027-3416
Phone: (713)296-4800 **Fax:** (713)961-4431
Website: http://www.uhc.com
Steve C. Walli, CEO

★ 18753 ★ United HealthCare of Texas, Inc. - San Antonio
HMO Plan
8401 Datapoint Dr., Ste. 175
San Antonio, TX 78229
Phone: (210)617-6850 **Fax:** (210)617-6868
Website: http://www.uch.com
Thomas Quirk, CEO
Program(s): Chiropractic, Dental, Home Care, Inpatient SNF, Pharmaceutical Mail Order, Podiatry, Psychiatric, Behavioral Health, Physical Therapy, Transplant, Vision, Wellness.

★ 18754 ★ Valley Health Plans
HMO Plan
2005 Ed Carey Dr.
Harlingen, TX 78550
Phone: (956)389-2273 **Free:** 800-422-4400
Fax: (956)389-2281
Website: http://www.vbmc.org
Karen Pederson, CEO

Utah

★ 18755 ★ Altius Health Plans
HMO Plans
10421 S Jordan Gateway, Ste. 400
South Jordan, UT 84095
Phone: (801)355-1234 **Free:** 800-365-1334
Fax: (801)323-6100
Website: http://www.altiushealthplans.com
Larry Hancock, CEO

★ 18756 ★ CIGNA Health Plan of Utah, Inc.
HMO Plan
5295 South 320 West, Ste. 280
Salt Lake City, UT 84107
Phone: (801)265-2777 **Free:** 800-245-2471
Fax: (801)261-5349
Website: http://www.cigna.com
Robert Immitt, CEO & Pres

★ 18757 ★ Deseret Healthcare
HMO Plan
PO Box 45530
Salt Lake City, UT 84145-0530
Phone: (801)578-5600 **Free:** 800-777-3622
Fax: (801)578-5905
Website: http://www.dmba.com
Michael Stapley, CEO

★ 18758 ★ Healthwise
HMO Plan
PO Box 30804
Salt Lake City, UT 84130-0804
Free: 800-662-3398 **Fax:** (801)333-6552
John Ruch, CEO

★ 18759 ★ HMO Blue
HMO Plan
PO Box 30270
Salt Lake City, UT 84130
Phone: (801)333-2583 **Free:** 800-662-0876
Fax: (801)333-6552
Website: http://www.ut.regence.com
John Ruch, CEO

★ 18760 ★ IHC Health Plans, Inc.
HMO Plan
4646 W Lake Park Blvd.
Salt Lake City, UT 84120
Phone: (801)442-5000 **Free:** 800-538-5038
Fax: (801)442-5183
Website: http://www.ihc.com
Richard J. Galbraith, Chairman of the Board

★ 18761 ★ Molina Healthcare of Utah, Inc.
7 Union Park Center, Ste. 200
Midvale, UT 84047
Phone: (801)858-0400 **Fax:** (801)858-0409
Website: http://www.molinahealthcare.com
Joseph M. Molina, MD, Chairman of the Board

★ 18762 ★ United HealthCare of Utah, Inc.
HMO Plan
PO Box 71409
Salt Lake City, UT 84171-0409
Free: 800-624-2942 **Fax:** (801)947-0459
Website: http://www.uhc.com
Annette Herman, CEO

Virginia

★ 18763 ★ Aetna Health Plans of Mid-Atlantic
HMO Plan
7600 A Leesburg Pike
Falls Church, VA 22043
Phone: (703)903-7100 **Fax:** (703)903-0316
Website: http://www.aetna.com
John W. Rowe, MD, Chairman of the Board

★ 18764 ★ Aetna Inc. - Virginia
HMO Plan
1000 Boulders Pkwy.
Richmond, VA 23225
Phone: (804)323-0900 **Free:** 800-323-0467
Website: http://www.aetna.com
John W. Rowe, MD, CEO & Chm Bd

★ 18765 ★ Amerigroup Corp.
4425 Corporation Ln.
Virginia Beach, VA 23462
Phone: (757)518-3671
Website: http://www.amerigroupcorp.com
Jeffrey L. McWaters, CEO & Chm Bd

★ 18766 ★ Carilion Health Plans, Inc.
HMO Plan
110 Campbell Ave., Ste. 107
Roanoke, VA 24011
Phone: (540)857-5200 **Free:** 800-856-5206
Fax: (540)857-5343
Website: http://www.carilionhealthplans.com
Carolyn Chrisman, CEO

★ 18767 ★ CIGNA Healthcare of Virginia
HMO Plan
7501 Boulders View Dr., Ste 500
Richmond, VA 23294
Phone: (757)463-8606 **Fax:** (757)463-8606
Website: http://www.cigna.com
Matt Manders, CEO

★ 18768 ★ CIGNA HealthCare of Virginia, Inc. - Richmond
HMO Plan
PO Box 31353
Richmond, VA 23294-1353
Phone: (804)267-5100 **Free:** 800-533-1708
Fax: (804)267-5062
Website: http://www.cigna.com
Matt Manders, CEO

★ 18769 ★ One Health Plan of Virginia, Inc.
10400 Eaton Pl., Ste. 430
Fairfax, VA 22030
Phone: (703)279-7800 **Free:** 888-241-8614
Fax: (703)279-7821
Website: http://www.onehealthplan.com
Douglas Ford, Contact

★ 18770 ★ Optima Health Plan, Inc.
HMO Plan
4417 Corporation Lane
Virginia Beach, VA 23462-3162
Phone: (757)552-7400 **Fax:** (757)687-6031
Website: http://www.optimahealth.com
Michael Dudley, President

★ 18771 ★ Priority Health Care
HMO Plan
621 Lynnhaven Pkwy.
Virginia Beach, VA 23452-7330
Phone: (757)463-4600 **Fax:** (757)463-7172
John Coyle, President

★ 18772 ★ QualChoice of Virginia Health Plan
HMO Plan
1000 Research Park Blvd.
Charlottesville, VA 22911
Phone: (434)975-1212 **Free:** 800-975-1213
Fax: (434)975-1414
Cosby Davis, CEO

★ 18773 ★ Southern Health Services, Inc.
HMO Plan
9881 Mayland Dr.
Richmond, VA 23233-1458
Phone: (804)747-3700 **Free:** 800-424-0077
Fax: (804)762-9349
Website: http://www.southernhealth.com
Cosby Davis, CEO

★ 18774 ★ United HealthCare of Virginia
HMO Plan
9020 Stony Point Pkwy., Ste. 400
Richmond, VA 23235
Phone: (804)267-5200 **Free:** 888-286-4908
Fax: (804)267-5285
Website: http://www.uhc.com
James Carney, MD, Contact

★ 18775 ★ Virginia Premier Health Plans
PO Box 5307
Richmond, VA 23220-0307
Phone: (804)819-5151 **Fax:** (804)819-5187
James S. Parrott, CEO

Washington

★ 18776 ★ Aetna Inc. - Washington HMO Plan
601 Union Square, Ste. 800
Seattle, WA 98101
Phone: (206)701-8000 **Fax:** (206)701-8125
Website: http://www.aetna.com
John W. Rowe, MD, Chairman of the Board

★ 18777 ★ Aetna Inc. - Washington HMO Plan
600 University St., Ste. 1400
Seattle, WA 98101-1158
Phone: (206)710-1100 **Free:** 800-654-3250
Fax: (206)701-1125
Website: http://www.aetna.com
John W. Rowe, MD, CEO & Chm Bd

★ 18778 ★ Columbia United Providers
19120 SE 34th St., Ste. 201
Vancouver, WA 98683
Phone: (360)891-1520 **Free:** 800-315-7862
Fax: (360)449-8881
Website: http://www.wa.gov
Erin Glynn, CEO

★ 18779 ★ Community Health Plan of Washington
HMO Plan
720 Olive Way, Ste. 300
Seattle, WA 98101-1866
Phone: (206)521-8833 **Free:** 800-440-1561
Fax: (206)521-8834
Website: http://www.chpw.org
Casandra Undlin, CEO

★ 18780 ★ First Choice Healthplan
HMO Plan
601 Union St., Ste. 1100
Seattle, WA 98101-1838
Phone: (206)292-8255 **Fax:** (206)624-4953
Website: http://www.fchn.com
Gary Gannaway, CEO
Program(s): Dental, Inpatient SNF, Podiatry.

★ 18781 ★ Group Health Cooperative
HMO Plan
PO Box 204
Spokane, WA 99210
Phone: (509)838-9100 **Free:** 800-497-2210
Fax: (509)458-0368
Website: http://www.ghnw.org
Jack Dutzar, MD, Contact

★ 18782 ★ Group Health Cooperative of Puget Sound
HMO Plan
521 Wall St.
Seattle, WA 98121
Phone: (206)448-5528 **Free:** 800-442-4062
Fax: (206)448-5105
Website: http://www.ghc.org
Cheryl Scott, CEO

★ 18783 ★ HealthPlus
HMO Plan
PO Box 2113
Seattle, WA 98111-2113
Phone: (425)670-4700 **Fax:** (425)670-5922
Website: http://www.healthplus.com
Gubby Barlow, CEO

★ 18784 ★ Kitsap Physicians Service
HMO Plan
PO Box 339
Bremerton, WA 98337
Phone: (360)377-5576 **Free:** 800-552-7114
Fax: (360)478-2632
Website: http://www.kpshealthplans.com
Elizabeth Gilje, CEO & Pres

★ 18785 ★ Molina Healthcare of Washington, Inc.
HMO Plan
PO Box 1469
Bothell, WA 98041-1469
Phone: (425)424-1100 **Free:** 800-869-7175
Fax: (425)424-1132
Website: http://www.molinamedical.com
Joseph M. Molina, MD, Chairman of the Board

★ 18786 ★ PacifiCare of Washington
HMO Plan
7525 SE 24th St.
Mercer Island, WA 98040
Phone: (206)236-2500 **Free:** 800-722-9666
Fax: (206)230-7496
Website: http://www.pacificare.com
Chris Wing, President

West Virginia

★ 18787 ★ Carelink
HMO Plan
887 National Rd.
Wheeling, WV 26003
Phone: (304)234-5100 **Free:** 800-519-3368
Fax: (304)234-5119
Website: http://www.chccarelink.com
Ted Cheatham, CEO

★ 18788 ★ Carelink Health Plans
HMO Plan
500 Virginia St., Ste. 400
Charleston, WV 25301
Phone: (304)348-2970 **Fax:** (304)561-6985
Website: http://www.camcare.com
Ted Cheatham, CEO

Wisconsin

★ 18789 ★ Atrium Health Plan
HMO Plan
2215 Vine St., Ste. E
Hudson, WI 54016
Phone: (715)386-6886 **Fax:** (715)386-8326
Website: http://www.atriumhealthplan.com
Greg Larsen, President

★ 18790 ★ Cobalt Corp.
HMO Plan
401 W Michigan St.
Milwaukee, WI 53203
Phone: (414)226-6600 **Fax:** (414)226-6279
Website: http://www.cobaltcorporation.com
Thomas Hefty, Chairman of the Board

★ 18791 ★ CompCare Health Services Insurance Corp.
HMO Plan
401 W Michigan Ave.
Milwaukee, WI 53203
Phone: (414)226-6600 **Free:** 800-242-7312
Fax: (262)814-4890
Website: http://www.bcbsuw.org
Michael Bernstein, President

★ 18792 ★ Dean Health Plan, Inc.
HMO Plan
PO Box 56099
Madison, WI 53705-9399
Phone: (608)836-1400 **Free:** 800-356-7344
Fax: (608)836-9620
Website: http://www.deancare.com
Robert Palmer, CEO & Pres

★ 18793 ★ Doral Dental USA
12121 N Corporate Pkwy.
Mequon, WI 53092
Phone: (262)241-7140 **Free:** 800-417-7140
Fax: (262)241-7366
Website: http://www.doral.com
Gregory J. Borca, CEO

★ 18794 ★ Group Health Cooperative of Eau Claire
HMO Plan
2503 N Hillcrest Pkwy.
Altoona, WI 54720-2602
Phone: (715)836-8552 **Fax:** (715)836-7683
Website: http://www.ghc.org
Peter Farrow, CEO

★ 18795 ★ Group Health Cooperative of South Central Wisconsin
HMO Plan
PO Box 44971
Madison, WI 53744-4971
Phone: (608)251-4156 **Free:** 800-605-4327
Fax: (608)257-3842
Website: http://www.ghc-hmo.com
Larry Zanoni, CEO

★ 18796 ★ Gundersen Lutheran Health Plan
HMO Plan
1836 South Ave.
La Crosse, WI 54601
Phone: (608)775-8000 **Free:** 800-370-9718
Fax: (608)775-8042
Patrick Killeen, CEO

★ 18797 ★ Health Tradition Health Plans
HMO Plan
PO Box 188
La Crosse, WI 54602-0188
Phone: (608)783-9507 **Free:** 800-545-8499
Fax: (608)781-9653
Steven M. Kunes, CEO

★ 18798 ★ Humana CareNetwork, Inc.
HMO Plan
PO Box 12359
Milwaukee, WI 53212-0359
Phone: (414)223-3300 **Fax:** (414)223-0184
Website: http://www.humana.com
Michael B. McCallister, CEO & Pres

★ 18799 ★ Humana Employers Health Insurance
HMO Plan
1100 Employers Blvd.
Green Bay, WI 54344
Phone: (920)337-5233 **Free:** 800-558-4444
Fax: (920)337-8129
Kathy Augustian-Hinkfuss, CEO

★ 18800 ★ MercyCare Health Plan, Inc.
HMO Plan
PO Box 2770
Janesville, WI 53547-2770
Phone: (608)752-3431 **Free:** 800-752-3431
Fax: (608)752-3751
Website: http://www.mercyhealthsystem.org
Javon Bea, CEO

★ 18801 ★ Network Health Plan of Wisconsin
HMO Plan
1165 Appleton Rd.
Menasha, WI 54952
Phone: (920)727-0100 **Fax:** (929)720-1756
Website: http://www.networkhealth.com
Michael Wolff, CEO

★ 18802 ★ Physicians Plus Insurance Corp.
HMO Plan
22 E Mifflin St., No. 200
Madison, WI 53703-4220
Phone: (608)282-8900 **Fax:** (608)282-8365
Website: http://www.pplusic.com
Martin Preizler, CEO

★ 18803 ★ Prevea Health Plan
HMO Plan
PO Box 11625
Green Bay, WI 54307-1625
Phone: (920)490-6900 **Free:** 888-711-1444
Fax: (920)490-6943
Website: http://www.prevea.com
Mark Minsloff, CEO

★ 18804 ★ Security Health Plan of Wisconsin, Inc.
HMO Plan
1515 St. Joseph Ave.
Marshfield, WI 54449-5703
Phone: (715)387-5621 **Free:** 800-472-2363
Fax: (715)221-9500
John Smiley, CEO

★ 18805 ★ TouchPoint Health Plan
HMO Plan
PO Box 507
Appleton, WI 54912-0507
Phone: (920)735-6440 **Free:** 800-735-6305
Fax: (920)831-6886
Website: http://www.thedacare.org
Jay Fulkerson, CEO

★ 18806 ★ United HealthCare of Wisconsin
HMO Plan
10701 W Research Dr.
Milwaukee, WI 53226
Phone: (414)443-4710 **Free:** 800-879-0071
Fax: (414)443-4750
Website: http://www.uhc.com
William Felsing, CEO

★ 18807 ★ United Healthcare of Wisconsin, Inc.
HMO Plan
10701 W Research Dr.
Milwaukee, WI 53226
Phone: (414)443-4000 **Free:** 800-879-0071
Fax: (414)443-4750
William Felsing, CEO

★ 18808 ★ Unity Health Plans
HMO Plan
840 Carolina St.
Sauk City, WI 53583-1374
Phone: (608)643-2491 **Free:** 800-362-3308
Fax: (608)643-2564
Tery Bolz, CEO

★ 18809 ★ Valley Health Plan
HMO Plan
PO Box 3128
Eau Claire, WI 54702
Phone: (715)832-3235 **Free:** 800-472-5411
Fax: (715)836-1298
Website: http://www.valley.uwz.com
Norman L. Keller, President

★ 18810 ★ Wausau Benefits, Inc.
HMO Plan
PO Box 8017
Wausau, WI 54402-8017
Phone: (715)845-8582 **Free:** 800-435-4401
Fax: (715)843-3613
Website: http://www.libertymutual.com
Fred Moore, President

★ 18811 ★ Wausau Insurance Co.
HMO Plan
PO Box 1060
Eau Claire, WI 54702-1060
Phone: (715)835-6174 **Free:** 800-835-6174
Fax: (715)838-0220
John Laehn, CEO

★ 18812 ★ Wisconsin Physicians Service Insurance Co.
HMO Plan
PO Box 8190
Madison, WI 53708-8190
Phone: (608)221-4711 **Fax:** (608)223-3603
James R. Riordan, CEO

Wyoming

★ 18813 ★ WIN Health Partners
HMO Plan
2515 Warren Ave., Ste. 504
Cheyenne, WY 82001
Phone: (307)638-7700 **Fax:** (307)663-7701
Beth Wasson, CEO

Preferred Provider Organizations (PPOs)

Alabama

★ 18814 ★ Aetna Inc.—Alabama Inc.
PPO Plan
3000 Riverside Galleria, Ste. 780
Birmingham, AL 35244
Phone: (205)985-3550 **Fax:** (205)985-3316
Website: http://www.aetna.com
John W. Rowe, CEO

★ 18815 ★ CIGNA Healthcare Plans of Alabama
PPO Plan
10 Inverness Center Pkwy., No. 230
Birmingham, AL 35242
Phone: (205)991-1005 **Fax:** (205)995-8511
Website: http://www.cigna.com
Robert A. Yungk, CEO

★ 18816 ★ Gulf Coast Regional PAC
PPO Plan
6801 Airport Blvd., Ste. D435
Mobile, AL 36608
Phone: (251)639-0188 **Fax:** (251)639-2029
Phillip Madonia, MD, CEO

★ 18817 ★ Gulf Health Plans PPO, Inc.
PPO Plan
2559 Emogene St.
Mobile, AL 36606
Phone: (251)470-0207 **Fax:** (251)450-3307
Website: http://www.mimc.com
Kerry D. Goff, President

★ 18818 ★ Healthchoice
3500 Blue Lake Dr., Ste. 215
Birmingham, AL 35243
Phone: (205)715-4801 **Fax:** (205)715-4802
Scott Sheedy, CEO

★ 18819 ★ Preferred Health Alliance, Inc.
PPO Plan
300 Corporate Pkwy., Ste. 3
Birmingham, AL 35242
Phone: (205)969-1155 **Fax:** (205)969-1199
W. Hal Shepherd, CEO & Pres

★ 18820 ★ Premier Health Plans - Alabama
PPO Plan
PO Box 18788
Huntsville, AL 35804
Phone: (256)864-4100 **Fax:** (256)864-4401
Doris Anderson, CEO

★ 18821 ★ United Healthcare of Alabama, Inc.
PPO Plan
PO Box 830637
Birmingham, AL 35255
Phone: (205)977-6300 **Free:** 800-345-1520
Fax: (205)977-6537
Website: http://www.uhc.com
William W. McGuire, MD, Chairman of the Board

Arizona

★ 18822 ★ Aetna Inc—Arizona
PPO Plan
7720 N 16th St., Ste. 400
Phoenix, AZ 85020
Phone: (602)427-2200 **Fax:** (602)427-2176
Website: http://www.aetna.com
John W. Rowe, MD, Chairman of the Board

★ 18823 ★ Arizona Foundation for Medical Care
PPO Plan
326 E Coronado Rd.
Phoenix, AZ 85004
Phone: (602)252-4042 **Free:** 800-624-4277
Fax: (602)256-7816
Website: http://www.azfmc.com
Anthony D. Mitten, JD, CEO

★ 18824 ★ Arizona Medical Network
PPO Plan
1600 W Broadway, Ste. 385
Tempe, AZ 85282
Phone: (480)921-8941 **Free:** 800-448-3585
Fax: 888-567-5230
Mark Dyer, CEO

★ 18825 ★ Arizona Preferred Provider
6464 E Grant Rd.
Tucson, AZ 85715-3819
Phone: (520)298-5297 **Fax:** (520)296-7948
Dwight Babcock, CEO

★ 18826 ★ Avesis, Inc.
PPO Plan
3724 N 3rd St., Ste. 300
Phoenix, AZ 85012
Phone: (602)241-3400 **Free:** 800-522-0258
Fax: (602)240-9101
Alan S. Cohen, President

★ 18827 ★ Blue Cross Blue Shield of Arizona
Blue Preferred (PPO)
PO Box 13466
Phoenix, AZ 85062-3466
Phone: (602)864-4613 **Free:** 800-232-2345
Fax: (602)864-4184
Website: http://www.bcbaz.com
Robert B. Bulla, Chairman of the Board

★ 18828 ★ CIGNA HealthCare of Arizona
PPO Plan
7225 N Mona Lisa Rd.
Tucson, AZ 85741
Phone: (520)571-0111 **Fax:** (520)575-4950
Website: http://www.cigna.com/healthcare/hs/ar.html
Frank Benedetto, Contact

★ 18829 ★ CIGNA Healthcare of Arizona
PPO Plan
11001 N Black Canyon Hwy., No. 400
Phoenix, AZ 85029-4754
Phone: (602)942-4462 **Fax:** (602)371-2625
Website: http://www.cigna.com
Edward Handway, CEO

★ 18830 ★ Health Net of Arizona
PPO Plan
930 N Finance Ctr. Dr, Ste. 100
Tucson, AZ 85710
Phone: (520)721-1122 **Free:** 800-289-2818
Fax: (520)290-7585
Website: http://www.az.health.net
Mark El-Tawil, President

★ 18831 ★ Humana Health Care Plans of Arizona
PPO Plan
2710 E Camelback Rd.
Phoenix, AZ 85016-3245
Phone: (602)553-2000 **Free:** 800-288-6442
Fax: (602)381-4389
Website: http://www.humana.com
William J. Howard, CEO & Pres

★ 18832 ★ One Health Plan of Arizona, Inc.
PPO Plan
3131 E Camelback Rd., Ste. 240
Phoenix, AZ 85016
Phone: (602)667-9527 **Fax:** (602)508-8972
Website: http://www.onehealthplan.com
Roger Stinton, Contact

★ 18833 ★ PacifiCare of Arizona
PPO Plan
PO Box 52078
Phoenix, AZ 85072
Phone: (602)244-8200 **Free:** 800-221-2462
Fax: (602)681-7000
Website: http://www.pacificare.com
Rick Badger, President

★ 18834 ★ United HealthCare of Arizona, Inc.
PPO Plan
3141 N 3rd Ave.
Phoenix, AZ 85013
Phone: (602)664-5000 **Free:** 800-442-4119
Fax: (602)664-2732
Website: http://www.unitedhealthcare.com
William W. McGuire, MD, Chairman of the Board

★ 18835 ★ USA Managed Care Organization
PPO Plan
7301 N 16th St., Ste. 201
Phoenix, AZ 85020
Phone: (602)371-3880 **Free:** 800-872-0020
Fax: (602)861-2805
Website: http://www.usamco.com
George Bogle, CEO

Arkansas

★ 18836 ★ Aetna Inc.—Arkansas
PPO Plan
10810 Executive Center Dr., No. 402
Little Rock, AR 72211-3525
Phone: (501)227-7776 **Free:** 800-821-8787
Fax: (501)227-0581
Website: http://www.aetna.com
John W. Rowe, Chairman of the Board

★ 18837 ★ Arkansas Managed Care Organization
PPO Plan
10 Corporate Hill Dr., Ste. 200
Little Rock, AR 72205
Phone: (501)225-8470 **Free:** 800-278-8470
Fax: (501)225-7954
Website: http://www.amcoppo.com
Janell Mason, CEO

★ 18838 ★ CIGNA Healthcare - Arkansas
PPO Plan
333 Executive Court, Ste. 301
Little Rock, AR 72205
Phone: (501)227-7222 **Free:** 800-301-0303
Fax: (501)221-0677
Website: http://www.cigna.com
Bob Bruce, CEO

★ 18839 ★ Gibraltar
1406 Cantrall Rd.
Little Rock, AR 72201
Phone: (501)374-7755 **Free:** 800-648-4642
Fax: (501)374-4033
Website: http://www.gibralterins.com
M. Kelly Woolridge, President

★ 18840 ★ Healthlink of Arkansas Inc.
PPO Plan
3901 McCain Park Dr, Ste. 201
North Little Rock, AR 72116-7849
Phone: (501)771-2111 **Fax:** (501)771-1936
Website: http://www.healthlink.com
Brett Kirkman, Contact

★ 18841 ★ Novasys Health Network
PPO Plan
10801 Executive Center Dr., No. 305
Little Rock, AR 72211
Phone: (501)219-4444 **Fax:** (501)219-4455
John Glassford, CEO

★ 18842 ★ United HealthCare Insurance Co.
PPO Plan
415 N McKinley, Ste. 820
Little Rock, AR 72205
Phone: (501)664-7700 **Free:** 800-678-3176
Fax: (501)664-7768
Website: http://www.uhc.com
John A. Wickens, President

California

★ 18843 ★ Admar Corp.
PO Box 1049
Santa Ana, CA 92705
Phone: (714)953-9600 **Free:** 800-422-0294
Fax: (714)953-9060
Website: http://www.admarinc.com
Edward Evans, President

★ 18844 ★ Aetna Inc.—California
PPO Plan
2409 Comino Ramon
San Ramon, CA 94583
Phone: (925)543-9000 **Fax:** (925)543-9010
Website: http://www.aetna.com
John W. Rowe, MD, Chairman of the Board

★ 18845 ★ Aetna Inc.—California
PPO Plan
1200 W 7th St., Ste. 400
Los Angeles, CA 90017
Phone: (310)955-3100 **Fax:** (310)955-3185
Website: http://www.aetna.com
John W. Rowe, MD, Chairman of the Board

★ 18846 ★ Aetna Inc.—California
PPO Plan
5800 Canoga Ave.
Woodland Hills, CA 91367
Phone: (818)992-2000 **Free:** 800-553-2952
Fax: (818)593-7108
Website: http://www.aetna.com
John W. Rowe, MD, Chairman of the Board

★ 18847 ★ American Life and Health Insurance Co.
PPO Plan
27725 Santa Margarita Pkwy., No. 220
Mission Viejo, CA 92691-6707
Phone: (949)380-0233 **Free:** 800-338-7634
Fax: (949)859-2815
Jane Hannabach, President

★ 18848 ★ Beech Street - Alaska
PPO Plan
25500 Commercentre Dr.
Lake Forest, CA 92630
Phone: (949)639-3800 **Free:** 800-987-7292
Fax: (949)639-3880
Website: http://www.beechstreet.com
William Fickling, Jr., Chairman of the Board

★ 18849 ★ Beech Street - Arizona
PPO Plan
25500 Commercentre Dr.
Lake Forest, CA 92630
Phone: (949)639-3800 **Free:** 800-987-7292
Fax: (949)639-3880
Website: http://www.beechstreet.com
William Fickling, Jr., Chairman of the Board

★ 18850 ★ Beech Street - California
PPO Plan
25500 Commercentre Dr.
Lake Forest, CA 92630
Phone: (949)639-3800 **Free:** 800-987-7292
Fax: (949)639-3880
Website: http://www.beechstreet.com
William Fickling, Jr., Chairman of the Board
Program(s): Chiropractic, Home Care, Inpatient SNF, Long-Term Care, Podiatry, Psychiatric, Behavioral Health, Transplant, Workers' Compensation, Alternative Medicine.

★ 18851 ★ Beech Street - Colorado
PPO Plan
25500 Commercentre Dr.
Lake Forest, CA 92630
Phone: (949)639-3800 **Free:** 800-987-7292
Fax: (949)639-3880
Website: http://www.beechstreet.com
William Fickling, Jr., Chairman of the Board
Program(s): Chiropractic, Home Care, Inpatient SNF, Long-Term Care, Podiatry, Psychiatric, Behavioral Health, Transplant, Workers' Compensation, Alternative Medicine.

★ 18852 ★ Beech Street Corp. - Corporate Headquarters
PPO Plan
25500 Commercentre Dr.
Lake Forest, CA 92630
Phone: (949)672-1000 **Free:** 800-877-1666
Fax: (949)672-1111
Website: http://www.beechstreet.com
William Fickling, Jr., Chairman of the Board
Program(s): Chiropractic, Home Care, Inpatient SNF, Long-Term Care, Podiatry, Psychiatric, Behavioral Health, Transplant, Workers' Compensation, Alternative Medicine.

★ 18853 ★ Beech Street - Hawaii
PPO Plan
25500 Commercentre Dr.
Lake Forest, CA 92630
Phone: (949)639-3800 **Free:** 800-987-7292
Fax: (949)639-3880
Website: http://www.beechstreet.com
William Fickling, Jr., Chairman of the Board

★ 18854 ★ Beech Street - Idaho
PPO Plan
25500 Commercentre Dr.
Lake Forest, CA 92630
Phone: (949)639-3800 **Free:** 800-987-7292
Fax: (949)639-3880
Website: http://www.beechstreet.com
William Fickling, Jr., Chairman of the Board

★ 18855 ★ Beech Street - Montana
PPO Plan
25500 Commercentre Dr.
Lake Forest, CA 92630
Phone: (949)639-3800 **Free:** 800-987-7292
Fax: (949)639-3880
Website: http://www.beechstreet.com
William A. Fickling, Jr., Chairman of the Board

★ 18856 ★ Beech Street - Nevada
PPO Plan
25500 Commercentre Dr.
Lake Forest, CA 92630
Phone: (949)639-3800 **Free:** 800-987-7292
Fax: (949)639-3880
Website: http://www.beechstreet.com
William Fickling, Jr., Chairman of the Board

★ 18857 ★ Beech Street - New Mexico
PPO Plan
25500 Commercentre Dr.
Lake Forest, CA 92630
Phone: (949)639-3800 **Free:** 800-987-7292
Fax: (949)639-3880
Website: http://www.beechstreet.com
William Fickling, Jr., Chairman of the Board

★ 18858 ★ Beech Street - Oklahoma
PPO Plan
25500 Commercentre Dr.
Lake Forest, CA 92630
Phone: (949)639-3800 **Free:** 800-987-7292
Fax: (949)639-3880
Website: http://www.beechstreet.com
William Fickling, Jr., Chairman of the Board

★ 18859 ★ Beech Street - Oregon
PPO Plan
25500 Commerccentre Dr.
Lake Forest, CA 92630
Phone: (949)639-3800 **Free:** 800-987-7292
Fax: (949)639-3880
Website: http://www.beechstreet.com
William Fickling, Jr., Chairman of the Board

★ 18860 ★ Beech Street - Texas
PPO Plan
25500 Commercentre Dr.
Lake Forest, CA 92630
Phone: (949)639-3800 **Free:** 800-987-7292
Fax: (949)639-3880
Website: http://www.beechstreet.com
William Fickling, Jr., Chairman of the Board

★ 18861 ★ Beech Street - Utah
PPO Plan
25500 Commercentre Dr.
Lake Forest, CA 92630
Phone: (949)639-3800 **Free:** 800-987-7292
Fax: (949)639-3880
Website: http://www.beechstreet.com
William Fickling, Jr., Chairman of the Board

★ 18862 ★ Beech Street - Washington
PPO Plan
25500 Commercentre Dr.
Lake Forest, CA 92630
Phone: (949)639-3800 **Free:** 800-987-7292
Fax: (949)639-3880
Website: http://www.beechstreet.com
William Fickling, Jr., Chairman of the Board

★ 18863 ★ Beech Street - Wyoming
PPO Plan
25500 Commerccentre Dr.
Lake Forest, CA 92630
Phone: (949)639-3800 **Free:** 800-987-7292
Fax: (949)639-3880
Website: http://www.beechstreet.com
William Fickling, Jr., Chairman of the Board

★ 18864 ★ CCN - Alaska
PPO Plan
5251 Viewridge Ct.
San Diego, CA 92123
Phone: (858)278-2273 **Free:** 800-247-2898
Fax: (858)278-8621
Website: http://www.ccnusa.com
Patrick G. Dills, President

★ 18865 ★ CCN - Arizona
PPO Plan
5251 Viewridge Ct.
San Diego, CA 92123
Phone: (858)278-2273 **Free:** 800-247-2898
Fax: (858)278-8621
Website: http://www.ccnusa.com
Patrick G. Dills, CEO & Pres

★ 18866 ★ CCN - California
PPO Plan
5251 Viewridge Ct.
San Diego, CA 92123
Phone: (858)278-2273 **Free:** 800-247-2898
Fax: (858)278-1262
Website: http://www.ccnusa.com
Patrick G. Dills, President

★ 18867 ★ CCN - Corporate Headquarters
PPO Plan
5251 Viewridge Court
San Diego, CA 92123
Phone: (858)278-2273 **Free:** 800-247-2898
Fax: (858)278-8621
Website: http://www.ccnusa.com
Patrick G. Dills, CEO & Pres

★ 18868 ★ CCN - Hawaii
PPO Plan
5251 Viewridge Ct.
San Diego, CA 92123
Phone: (858)278-2273 **Free:** 800-247-2898
Fax: (858)278-8621
Website: http://www.ccnusa.com
Patrick Dills, President

★ 18869 ★ CCN - Nevada
PPO Plan
5251 Viewridge Ct.
San Diego, CA 92123
Phone: (858)278-2273 **Free:** 800-247-2898
Fax: (858)278-8621
Website: http://www.ccnusa.com
Patrick G. Dills, President

★ 18870 ★ CCN - New Mexico
PPO Plan
5251 Viewridge Ct.
San Diego, CA 92123
Phone: (858)278-2273 **Free:** 800-247-2898
Fax: (858)278-8621
Website: http://www.ccnusa.com
Patrick G. Dills, CEO & Chm Bd

★ 18871 ★ CCN - Oregon
PPO Plan
5251 Viewridge Ct.
San Diego, CA 92123
Phone: (858)278-2273 **Free:** 800-247-2898
Fax: (858)278-8621
Website: http://www.ccnusa.com
Patrick G. Dills, President

★ 18872 ★ CCN - Washington
PPO Plan
5251 Viewridge Ct.
San Diego, CA 92123
Phone: (858)278-2273 **Free:** 800-247-2898
Fax: (858)278-8621
Website: http://www.ccnusa.com
Patrick G. Dills, President

★ 18873 ★ ChiroSource - Corporate Headquarters
PPO Plan
PO Box 130
Clayton, CA 94517
Phone: (925)672-5333 **Free:** 800-680-9997
Fax: (925)672-6657
Website: http://www.chirosource.com
Ronald S. Cataldo, DC, CEO & Pres
Program(s): Chiropractic; worker's compensation.

★ 18874 ★ CIGNA HealthCare of California
PPO Plan
400 N Brand Blvd., Ste. 500
Glendale, CA 91203
Phone: (818)500-6262 **Free:** 800-344-7421
Fax: (818)500-6480
Website: http://www.cigna.com/healthcare
Bud Volberding, President

★ 18875 ★ Coastal HealthCare Administrators
PPO Plan
19040 Portola Dr.
Salinas, CA 93908
Phone: (831)455-1833 **Fax:** (831)455-2310
Debi Hardwick, CEO & Pres

★ 18876 ★ Corvel Corp.
PPO Plan
2010 Main St., Ste. 1020
Irvine, CA 92614
Phone: (949)851-1473 **Free:** 888-726-7835
Fax: (949)851-1469
Website: http://www.corvel.com
Gordon Clemons, CEO

★ 18877 ★ First Health - California PPO Plan
750 Riverpoint Dr.
West Sacramento, CA 95605
Phone: (916)374-4600 **Free:** 800-937-6824
Fax: (916)374-4634
Ed Wristen, CEO

★ 18878 ★ Great West Life PPO Plan
3480 Buskirk Ave., Ste. 350
Pleasant Hill, CA 94523
Phone: (925)938-7788 **Fax:** (925)210-0975
Website: http://www.onehealthplan.com
Vicki Mahoney, Contact

★ 18879 ★ Great West Life PPO Plan
101 N Brand Blvd., Ste 1950
Glendale, CA 91203
Phone: (818)247-9102 **Free:** 800-877-9102
Fax: (818)247-3033
Website: http://www.onehealthplan.com
Gary Smith, Contact

★ 18880 ★ Health Management Center PPO Plan
7755 Center Ave., Ste. 1000
Huntington Beach, CA 92647
Phone: (714)898-8311 **Free:** 800-260-6076
Fax: (714)934-5555
Bob Ellis, Contact

★ 18881 ★ Health Net Health Net PPO
21650 Oxnard St.
Woodland Hills, CA 91367
Phone: (818)676-6775 **Free:** 800-474-6676
Fax: (818)676-7315
Website: http://www.health.net
Jay M. Gellert, CEO

★ 18882 ★ Health Net of California PPO Plan
21281 Burbank Blvd.
Woodland Hills, CA 91367
Phone: (818)676-6775 **Free:** 800-522-0088
Fax: (818)676-6982
Website: http://www.healthnet.com
Jennifer M. Gutzmore, MD, Contact

★ 18883 ★ Interplan Corp. PPO Plan
2575 Grand Canal Blvd., 2nd Fl.
Stockton, CA 95207
Phone: (209)473-0811 **Fax:** (209)473-0863
Daniel Sheehy, President

★ 18884 ★ Kern Foundation Preferred Provider Organization (PPO)
333 Palmer Dr., Ste. 200
Bakersfield, CA 93309
Phone: (661)327-0770 **Fax:** (661)327-5129
Website: http://www.kernfmc.com
Carolyn Temple, CEO

★ 18885 ★ Lifeguard, Inc. PPO Plan
PO Box 5506
San Jose, CA 95150-5506
Phone: (408)943-9400 **Free:** 800-995-0380
Fax: (408)432-3695
Website: http://www.lifeguard.com
Mark Hyde, CEO

★ 18886 ★ One Health Plan of California PPO Plan
655 N Central Ave., No. 1900
Glendale, CA 91203-1441
Phone: (818)539-1900 **Fax:** (818)545-9238
Website: http://www.onehealthplan.com
Jackie James, President

★ 18887 ★ Orange County PPO
300 S Flower St.
Orange, CA 92868
Phone: (714)978-5048 **Fax:** (714)634-9655
Website: http://www.cfmcnet.org
Elizabeth Ciaccio, CEO

★ 18888 ★ Pacific Foundation for Medical Care PPO Plan
3033 Cleveland Ave.
Santa Rosa, CA 95403
Phone: (707)544-2010 **Fax:** (707)544-0312
Website: http://www.pfmc.org
John Nacol, CEO

★ 18889 ★ Pacific Health Alliance PPO Plan
1350 Old Bayshore Hwy., No. 560
Burlingame, CA 94010
Phone: (650)375-5800 **Fax:** (650)375-5820
Lawrence Cappel, PhD, CEO

★ 18890 ★ Pacific IPA PPO Plan
430 S Garfield Ave., No. 301
Alhambra, CA 91801
Phone: (626)281-3400 **Free:** 888-888-PIPA
Fax: (626)281-0444
Peter Lindbion, CEO

★ 18891 ★ Pacific Life and Annuity Co.
PO Box 2890
Newport Beach, CA 92658
Free: 800-733-7020 **Fax:** (949)219-5301
Website: http://www.pacificlifeandannuity.com
Thomas Sutton, CEO

★ 18892 ★ PacifiCare of California PPO Plan
5701 Katella Ave.
Cypress, CA 90630-5028
Phone: (714)952-1121 **Free:** 800-624-8822
Fax: (714)226-3996
Website: http://www.pacificare.com
Howard G. Phanstiel, CEO

★ 18893 ★ Pacificare Health Systems - Corporate Headquarters PPO Plan
PO Box 25186
Santa Ana, CA 92799-5186
Phone: (714)952-1121 **Free:** 800-624-8822
Fax: (714)825-2201
Website: http://www.pacificare.com
Howard G. Phanstiel, CEO

★ 18894 ★ Physicians Foundation for Medical Care PPO Plan
PO Box 5760
San Jose, CA 95150-5760
Phone: (408)248-9400 **Fax:** (408)248-9419
Jim Reikes, CEO

★ 18895 ★ PPO Next
301 E Ocean Blvd., Ste. 900
Long Beach, CA 90802
Free: 800-253-4360 **Fax:** (562)308-7320
Website: http://www.healthstarinc.com
Stephen Carder, CEO

★ 18896 ★ Primary Provider Management Co., Inc.
2525 Camino Del Rio S, Ste. 300
San Diego, CA 92108
Phone: (858)297-8704 **Fax:** (619)297-7839
Jay Zybelman, President

★ 18897 ★ Progressive Administrative Resources PPO Plan
PO Box 850
Agoura Hills, CA 91376
Free: 800-995-4310 **Fax:** (818)707-9182
Wayne Foff, CEO

★ 18898 ★ Riverside County Foundation for Medical Care
3993 Jurupa Ave.
Riverside, CA 92506
Phone: (909)686-9049 **Fax:** (909)686-1692
Website: http://www.cfmcnet.org
Dolores Green, CEO

★ 18899 ★ San Joaquin Foundation PPO PPO Plan
PO Box 779
Stockton, CA 95201
Phone: (209)951-5762 **Fax:** (209)728-0646
Boyd Thompson, Contact

★ 18900 ★ Silver State Medical Administrators
2755 Bristal st., Ste. 250
Costa Mesa, CA 92626
Phone: (714)549-7052 **Fax:** (714)549-4816

★ 18901 ★ Smile Saver
2787 Bristol St., Ste. 3200
Costa Mesa, CA 92626
Phone: (714)429-0200 **Free:** 800-445-8119
Fax: (714)429-1261
Mark Johnson, CEO
Program(s): Dental, Vision.

★ 18902 ★ South Bay Independent Physicians Medical Group, Inc. PPO Plan
3480 Torrance Blvd., Ste. 220
Torrance, CA 90503
Phone: (310)543-8805 **Fax:** (310)543-8811
William Averill, MD, Chairman of the Board

★ 18903 ★ Stanislaus Medical Society PPO Plan
PO Box 576007
Modesto, CA 95357-6007
Phone: (209)527-1704 **Fax:** (209)527-5861
Gary Padovani, MD, President

★ 18904 ★ UniCare Life and Health UniCare/Cost Care (PPO)
One WellPoint Way
Thousand Oaks, CA 91362
Phone: (818)703-4000 **Free:** 800-336-2290
Fax: (805)557-6872
Website: http://www.unicare.com
Leonard Schaeffer, CEO

★ 18905 ★ United Healthcare of Oregon
180 E Ocean Blvd., Ste. 500
Long Beach, CA 90802
Phone: (562)951-6400 **Free:** 800-325-6651
Fax: (562)951-6885

Website: http://www.uhc.com
Emery Dameron, CEO

★ 18906 ★ Universal Care
PPO Plan
1600 E Hill St.
Signal Hill, CA 90806
Phone: (562)424-6200 **Free:** 800-635-6668
Fax: (562)595-0872
Howard Davis, CEO

★ 18907 ★ Ventura Foundation for Medical Care
PPO Plan
330 N Wood Rd., Ste. D
Camarillo, CA 93010
Phone: (805)383-9740 **Free:** 800-232-9043
Fax: (805)482-5561
Website: http://www.menet.org
Richard Michel, CEO

★ 18908 ★ WellPoint Health Networks, Inc. - Corporate Headquarters
PPO Plan
One WellPoint Way
Thousand Oaks, CA 91362
Phone: (818)703-4000 **Fax:** (805)557-6872
Website: http://www.wellpoint.com
Leonard Schaeffer, CEO & Chm Bd

Colorado

★ 18909 ★ Aetna Inc. - Colorado
PPO Plan
6430 S Fiddlers Green Cir., No. 200
Englewood, CO 80111
Phone: (303)793-2500 **Fax:** (303)793-2510
Website: http://www.aetna.com
John W. Rowe, CEO

★ 18910 ★ CIGNA HealthCare of Colorado
PPO Plan
3900 E Mexico Ave., Ste. 1100
Denver, CO 80210
Phone: (303)782-1500 **Free:** 800-832-3211
Fax: (303)782-1577
Website: http://www.cigna.com
Daryl Edmonds, CEO

★ 18911 ★ Exempla Healthcare LLC
PPO Plan
600 Grant St., Ste. 700
Denver, CO 80203-3525
Phone: (303)813-5000 **Fax:** (303)813-5001
Website: http://www.exempla.org
Jeffrey Selburg, CEO & Pres

★ 18912 ★ Great West Life Annuity Insurance Co.
PPO Plan
PO Box 1700
Denver, CO 80201
Phone: (303)737-3000 **Fax:** (303)737-3198
Website: http://www.gwla.com
William McCallum, CEO

★ 18913 ★ Great-West/One Health Plan
PPO Plan
8505 E Orchard Rd.
Greenwood Village, CO 80111
Phone: (303)737-3000 **Fax:** (303)737-3405
Website: http://www.onehealthplan.com
William T. McCallum, CEO & Pres

★ 18914 ★ Mountain Medical Affiliates
PPO Plan
5889 S Greenwood Plaza Blvd., Ste. 200
Greenwood Village, CO 80111
Phone: (303)290-9696 **Free:** 800-647-1856
Fax: (303)770-5005
Website: http://www.mma-bp.com
Robert Ruiz-Moss, CEO & Pres

★ 18915 ★ New England Financial
PPO Plan
8505 E Orchard Rd.
Greenwood Village, CO 80111
Phone: (303)737-3000 **Fax:** (303)737-3198
Website: http://www.nefn.com
William McCallum, CEO

★ 18916 ★ One Health Plan of Colorado
PPO Plan
8525 E Orchard Rd., No. 3
Greenwood Village, CO 80111-5002
Phone: (303)305-1000 **Fax:** (303)737-3198
Website: http://www.onehealthplan.com
Chris Miller, President

★ 18917 ★ PacifiCare of Colorado
PPO Plan
6455 S Yosemite
Englewood, CO 80111
Phone: (303)220-5800 **Free:** 800-877-6685
Fax: (303)714-3999
Website: http://www.pacificare.com
Jeffrey Folick, Chairman of the Board
Program(s): Chiropractic, Dental, Home Care, Inpatient SNF, Long-Term Care, Pharmaceutical Mail Order, Podiatry, Psychiatric, Behavioral Health, Physical Therapy, Transplant, Vision, Wellness.

★ 18918 ★ Pueblo Health Care
PPO Plan
400 W 16th St.
Pueblo, CO 81003
Phone: (719)584-4371 **Fax:** (719)584-4038
Michael Baxter, CEO

★ 18919 ★ Sloan's Lake Health Plan
PPO Plan
1355 S Colorado Blvd., Ste. 902
Denver, CO 80222
Phone: (303)753-7537 **Free:** 800-457-2345
Fax: (303)504-4321
Website: http://www.sloanslake.com
Blair Tikker, CEO

★ 18920 ★ United HealthCare of Colorado
PPO Plan
8051 E Maplewood Ave., Ste. 300
Englewood, CO 80111
Phone: (303)267-3300 **Free:** 800-518-3344
Fax: (303)267-3599
Website: http://www.uhc.com
Victor Lazzaro, Jr., CEO & Pres

Connecticut

★ 18921 ★ Aetna, Inc. - Corporate Headquarters
PPO Plan
151 Farmington Ave.
Hartford, CT 06156-1000
Phone: (860)273-0123 **Free:** 800-225-2949
Fax: (860)636-4513
Website: http://www.aetna.com
John W. Rowe, CEO & Chm Bd

★ 18922 ★ Aetna US Healthcare of New England
PPO Plan
1000 Middle St.
Middletown, CT 06457-3342
Phone: (860)273-0123 **Fax:** (860)273-6872
Website: http://www.aetna.com
John W. Rowe, MD, Chairman of the Board

★ 18923 ★ CIGNA HealthCare of Connecticut
PPO Plan
900 Cottage Grove Rd., A-118
Hartford, CT 06152-1118
Phone: (860)769-2300 **Free:** 800-345-9458
Fax: (860)769-2398
Website: http://www.cigna.com
Kirk Weimer, CEO

★ 18924 ★ GE Financial
PPO Plan
100 Bright Meadow Blvd.
Enfield, CT 06082
Free: 800-451-2513 **Fax:** (860)403-1306
Website: http://www.gefn.com
Robert W. Fiondella, CEO

★ 18925 ★ Health Net - Connecticut
PPO Plan
PO Box 904
Shelton, CT 06484-0914
Phone: (203)402-4200 **Free:** 800-848-4747
Fax: (203)225-4000
Website: http://www.health.net
Barry Averill, CEO & Pres

★ 18926 ★ Health Net Inc. - Northeast Corporate Headquarters
PPO Plan
PO Box 904
Shelton, CT 06484-0944
Phone: (203)402-4200 **Free:** 800-848-4747
Fax: (203)225-4000
Website: http://www.health.net
Barry Averill, CEO & Pres

★ 18927 ★ MedSpan, Inc.
PPO Plan
225 Asylum St., 11th Fl.
Hartford, CT 06103
Phone: (860)616-2200 **Fax:** (860)616-2540
Website: http://www.medspan.com
Kevin Kelly, President

★ 18928 ★ Northeast Health Direct LLC
PPO Plan
PO Box 435
Marlborough, CT 06447
Phone: (860)295-8261 **Free:** 800-423-6619
Fax: (860)295-8679
Website: http://www.ne-directhealth.com
F. Bernard Forand, President

★ 18929 ★ Oxford Health Plans, Inc. - Corporate Headquarters
PPO Plan
48 Monroe Turnpike
Trumbull, CT 06611
Free: 800-889-7658 **Fax:** (203)459-6464
Website: http://www.oxhp.com
Norman Payson, MD, CEO & Chm Bd

Delaware

★ 18930 ★ Aetna Inc. - Delaware
PPO Plan
650 Naamans Rd.
Claymont, DE 19703

Phone: (302)793-1520 **Fax:** (302)798-1877
Website: http://www.aetna.com
John W. Rowe, MD, Chairman of the Board

★ 18931 ★ AmeriHealth Insurance Co.
PPO Plan
919 N Market St., Mellon Ctr. Ste. 1200
Wilmington, DE 19801-3021
Phone: (302)777-6400 **Free:** 800-899-4373
Fax: (302)777-6444
Richard Neeson, Contact

★ 18932 ★ Christiana Care Health Plans, Inc.
PPO Plan
11 Reads Way
New Castle, DE 19720
Phone: (302)327-7650 **Free:** 800-362-4214
Fax: (302)327-7711
Website: http://www.christianacare.org
Ken Bates, CEO

★ 18933 ★ CIGNA HealthCare of Delaware Valley
PPO Plan
PO Box 15408
Wilmington, DE 19850-5408
Phone: (302)477-3700 **Free:** 800-320-0251
Fax: (302)477-3708
Website: http://www.cigna.com
Vincent Sobocinski, Contact

★ 18934 ★ Coventry Health Care Inc.—Delaware, Inc.
PPO Plan
2751 Centerville Rd., Ste. 400
Wilmington, DE 19808
Phone: (302)995-6100 **Free:** 800-833-7423
Fax: (302)998-7085
Website: http://www.chcde.com
Ron Chaffin, CEO & Pres

Florida

★ 18935 ★ Accountable Health Plans of America, Inc. - Florida
PPO Plan
555 Winderley Place, Ste. 410
Maitland, FL 32751
Free: 800-498-8741 **Fax:** (407)660-9696
Walter Vinson, Contact

★ 18936 ★ Accountable Health Plans of America, Inc. - Florida
PPO Plan
4014 Gunn Hwy., Ste 180
Tampa, FL 33624
Phone: (813)962-4222 **Free:** 800-943-6869
Fax: (813)962-2595
Walter Vinson, Contact

★ 18937 ★ Aetna Inc. - Florida
PPO Plan
5100 W Lemon St., Ste. 218
Tampa, FL 33609
Phone: (813)261-9630 **Fax:** (813)636-0658
Website: http://www.aetna.com
John W. Rowe, MD, Chairman of the Board

★ 18938 ★ Aetna Inc. - Jacksonville
PPO Plan
1200 Riverplace Blvd., Ste. 701
Jacksonville, FL 32207
Phone: (904)346-5800 **Fax:** (904)346-5888
Website: http://www.aetna.com
John W. Rowe, MD, Chairman of the Board

★ 18939 ★ Aetna Inc. - Plantation
PPO Plan
8201 Peters Rd.
Plantation, FL 33324
Phone: (954)382-8100 **Fax:** (954)424-4448
Website: http://www.aetna.com
John W. Rowe, MD, Chairman of the Board

★ 18940 ★ Aetna Inc. - Tampa
PPO Plan
5100 W Lemon St., Ste. 218
Tampa, FL 33609
Phone: (813)261-9630 **Free:** 800-232-2385
Fax: (813)636-0658
Website: http://www.aetna.com
John W. Rowe, MD, Chairman of the Board

★ 18941 ★ All Florida PPO, Inc.
PPO Plan
351 S Cypress Rd., Ste. 303
Pompano Beach, FL 33060
Phone: (954)946-5183 **Free:** 800-831-9710
Fax: (954)946-0978
Reg Watkins, CEO & Pres

★ 18942 ★ AnciCare PPO, Inc.
3700 Lakeside Dr., Ste. 401
Miramar, FL 33027
Phone: (954)441-7600 **Free:** 800-414-4674
Fax: (954)441-0398
Website: http://www.ancicare.com
Michael Cabrera, CEO & Pres

★ 18943 ★ BayCare Health Network
PPO Plan
380 Parkplace Blvd., Ste. 200
Clearwater, FL 33759
Phone: (727)799-3335 **Free:** 800-524-1553
Fax: (727)726-8801
John Vretas, CEO

★ 18944 ★ BCE Emergis
9950 Princess Palm Ave., Ste. 220
Tampa, FL 33619
Phone: (813)621-8099 **Free:** 800-927-7783
Fax: (813)621-3488
Website: http://www.flhealth.com
Nancy Connaway, President

★ 18945 ★ CCN - Alabama
PPO Plan
1507 N Falkenburg Rd.
Tampa, FL 33619
Phone: (813)663-3700 **Free:** 800-633-8033
Fax: (813)620-4973
Website: http://www.ccnusa.com
Patrick G. Dills, President

★ 18946 ★ CCN - Arkansas
PPO Plan
1507 N Falkenburg Rd.
Tampa, FL 33619
Phone: (813)663-3700 **Free:** 800-633-8033
Fax: (858)620-4973
Website: http://www.ccnusa.com
Patrick G. Dills, President

★ 18947 ★ CCN - Connecticut
PPO Plan
1507 N Falkenburg Rd.
Tampa, FL 33619
Phone: (813)663-3700 **Free:** 800-633-8033
Fax: (813)620-4973
Website: http://www.ccnusa.com
Patrick G. Dills, President

★ 18948 ★ CCN - Delaware
PPO Plan
1507 N Falkenburg Rd.
Tampa, FL 33619
Phone: (813)663-3700 **Free:** 800-633-8033
Fax: (813)620-4973
Website: http://www.ccnusa.com
Patrick G. Dills, President

★ 18949 ★ CCN - District of Columbia
PPO Plan
1507 N Falkenburg Rd.
Tampa, FL 33619
Phone: (813)663-3700 **Free:** 800-633-8033
Fax: (813)620-4973
Website: http://www.ccnusa.com
Patrick G. Dills, President

★ 18950 ★ CCN - Florida
PPO Plan
1507 N Falkenburg Rd.
Tampa, FL 33619
Phone: (813)663-3700 **Free:** 800-633-8033
Fax: (813)620-4973
Website: http://www.ccnusa.com
Patrick G. Dills, President

★ 18951 ★ CCN - Georgia
PPO Plan
1507 N Falkenburg Rd.
Tampa, FL 33619
Phone: (813)663-3700 **Free:** 800-633-8033
Fax: (813)620-4973
Website: http://www.ccnusa.com
Patrick G. Dills, President

★ 18952 ★ CCN - Kentucky
PPO Plan
1507 N Falkenburg Rd.
Tampa, FL 33619
Phone: (813)663-3700 **Free:** 800-633-8033
Fax: (813)620-4973
Website: http://www.ccnusa.com
Patrick G. Dills, President

★ 18953 ★ CCN - Louisiana
PPO Plan
1507 N Falkenburg Rd.
Tampa, FL 33619
Phone: (813)663-3700 **Free:** 800-633-8033
Fax: (813)620-4973
Website: http://www.ccnusa.com
Patrick G. Dills, President

★ 18954 ★ CCN - Maryland
PPO Plan
1507 N Falkenburg Rd.
Tampa, FL 33619
Phone: (813)663-3700 **Free:** 800-633-8033
Fax: (813)620-4973
Website: http://www.ccnusa.com
Patrick G. Dills, President

★ 18955 ★ CCN - Massachusetts
PPO Plan
1507 N Falkenburg Rd.
Tampa, FL 33619
Phone: (813)663-3700 **Free:** 800-633-8033
Fax: (813)620-4973
Website: http://www.ccnusa.com
Patrick G. Dills, President

★ 18956 ★ CCN - Mississippi
PPO Plan
1507 N Falkenburg Rd.
Tampa, FL 33619
Phone: (813)663-3700 **Free:** 800-633-8033
Fax: (813)620-4973

Website: http://www.ccnusa.com
Patrick G. Dills, President

★ 18957 ★ CCN - New Hampshire
PPO Plan
1507 N Falkenburg Rd.
Tampa, FL 33619
Phone: (813)663-3700 **Free:** 800-633-8033
Fax: (813)620-4973
Website: http://www.ccnusa.com
Patrick G. Dills, President

★ 18958 ★ CCN - New Jersey
PPO Plan
1507 N Falkenburg Rd.
Tampa, FL 33619
Phone: (813)663-3700 **Free:** 800-633-8033
Fax: (813)620-4973
Website: http://www.ccnusa.com
Patrick G. Dills, President

★ 18959 ★ CCN - New York
PPO Plan
1507 N Falkenburg Rd.
Tampa, FL 33619
Phone: (813)663-3700 **Free:** 800-633-8033
Fax: (813)620-4973
Website: http://www.ccnusa.com
Patrick G. Dills, President

★ 18960 ★ CCN - North Carolina
PPO Plan
1507 N Falkenburg Rd.
Tampa, FL 33619
Phone: (813)663-3700 **Free:** 800-633-8033
Fax: (813)620-4973
Website: http://www.ccnusa.com
Patrick G. Dills, President

★ 18961 ★ CCN - Pennsylvania
PPO Plan
1507 N Falkenburg Rd.
Tampa, FL 33619
Phone: (813)663-3700 **Free:** 800-633-8033
Fax: (813)620-4973
Website: http://www.ccnusa.com
Patrick G. Dills, President

★ 18962 ★ CCN - Rhode Island
PPO Plan
1507 N Falkenburg Rd.
Tampa, FL 33619
Phone: (813)663-3700 **Free:** 800-633-8033
Fax: (813)620-4973
Website: http://www.ccnusa.com
Patrick G. Dills, President

★ 18963 ★ CCN - South Carolina
PPO Plan
1507 N Falkenburg Rd.
Tampa, FL 33619
Phone: (813)663-3700 **Free:** 800-633-8033
Fax: (813)620-4973
Website: http://www.ccnusa.com
Patrick G. Dills, President

★ 18964 ★ CCN - Tennessee
PPO Plan
1507 N Falkenburg Rd.
Tampa, FL 33619
Phone: (813)663-3700 **Free:** 800-633-8033
Fax: (813)620-4973
Website: http://www.ccnusa.com
Patrick G. Dills, President

★ 18965 ★ CCN - Vermont
PPO Plan
1507 N Falkenburg Rd.
Tampa, FL 33619
Phone: (813)663-3700 **Free:** 800-633-8033
Fax: (813)620-4973
Website: http://www.ccnusa.com
Patrick G. Dills, President

★ 18966 ★ CCN - Virginia
PPO Plan
1507 N Falkenburg Rd.
Tampa, FL 33619
Phone: (813)663-3700 **Free:** 800-633-8033
Fax: (813)620-4973
Website: http://www.ccnusa.com
Patrick G. Dills, President

★ 18967 ★ CCN - West Virginia
PPO Plan
1507 N Falkenburg Rd.
Tampa, FL 33619
Phone: (813)663-3700 **Free:** 800-633-8033
Fax: (813)620-4973
Website: http://www.ccnusa.com
Patrick G. Dills, President

★ 18968 ★ CIGNA HealthCare of Florida
PPO Plan
1580 Sawgrass Corp. Pkwy., Ste 200
Sunrise, FL 33323
Phone: (954)693-7500 **Fax:** (954)693-7540
Website: http://www.cigna.com
William Taylor, CEO

★ 18969 ★ CIGNA HealthCare of Florida
PPO Plan
5404 Cypress Center Dr.
Tampa, FL 33609
Phone: (813)281-1000 **Free:** 800-942-2471
Fax: (813)289-0363
Website: http://www.cigna.com
Andrew Crooks, CEO & Pres

★ 18970 ★ Dimension Health
PPO Plan
15500 New Barn Rd., Ste. 101
Miami Lakes, FL 33014
Phone: (305)823-7664 **Free:** 800-483-4992
Fax: (305)818-8814
Charles Lindgren, CEO & Pres

★ 18971 ★ Fortis Health - Florida
PPO Plan
7300 Corporate Center Dr.
Miami, FL 33126
Phone: (305)715-2000 **Free:** 800-435-7969
Fax: (305)715-3220
Ben Cutler, CEO

★ 18972 ★ Foundation Health, A Florida Health Plan
PPO Plan
1340 Concord Terrace
Sunrise, FL 33323
Phone: (954)858-3000 **Free:** 800-422-7335
Fax: (954)846-0331
Website: http://www.fhfl.com
Robert Berzing, CEO

★ 18973 ★ Great West Life - Florida
PPO Plan
110 E Broward Blvd., Ste. 750
Fort Lauderdale, FL 33301
Phone: (954)463-2720 **Fax:** (954)463-2750
Website: http://www.onehealthplan.com
Tracy Carter, Contact

★ 18974 ★ Humana Health Care Plans of Orlando
PPO Plan
PO Box 9148000
Longwood, FL 32779
Phone: (407)661-6000 **Fax:** (407)661-6414
Website: http://www.humana.com/orlando/home.html
Michael B. McCallister, President

★ 18975 ★ Humana Health Plan - Jacksonville
PPO Plan
76 S Laura St., 16th Fl.
Jacksonville, FL 32202
Phone: (904)376-1100 **Free:** 800-945-7703
Fax: (904)376-2370
Website: http://www.humana.com
David A. Jones, Chairman of the Board

★ 18976 ★ Humana Medical Plan - Daytona
PPO Plan
135 Executive Circle
Daytona Beach, FL 32114
Phone: (386)676-1800 **Free:** 800-320-9565
Fax: (386)676-1806
Website: http://www.humana.com
David A. Jones, Chairman of the Board

★ 18977 ★ Humana Medical Plans, Inc.
PPO Plan
3501 SW 160th Ave.
Miramar, FL 33027
Phone: (305)621-5499 **Free:** 800-442-5555
Fax: (305)626-5297
Website: http://www.humana.com
David A. Jones, Chairman of the Board

★ 18978 ★ Kemper National Services Preferred Providers
PPO Plan
1601 SW 80th Terrace
Plantation, FL 33324-4036
Phone: (954)452-4000 **Free:** 800-726-8898
Fax: (954)452-4059
Website: http://www.kemperinsurance.com
David Patterson, CEO

★ 18979 ★ Lower Keys MedicalCenter
PPO Plan
PO Box 9107
Key West, FL 33041-9107
Phone: (305)294-5531 **Fax:** (305)294-8065
Ron Beerman, CEO

★ 18980 ★ One Health Plan of Florida
PPO Plan
7650 Courtney Campbell Csy, Ste. 850
Tampa, FL 33607
Phone: (813)207-0216 **Free:** 800-533-0919
Fax: (813)207-0613
Website: http://www.onehealthplan.com
Susan Griffin, Contact

★ 18981 ★ United HealthCare of Florida
PPO Plan
13621 NW 12th St.
Sunrise, FL 33323
Phone: (954)858-4000 **Fax:** (954)858-3815
Website: http://www.uhc.com
Michael Muchnicki, CEO

★ 18982 ★ United HealthCare of Florida, Inc.
PPO Plan
9009 Corporate Lake Dr.
Tampa, FL 33624

Phone: (813)890-4500 **Free:** 800-595-0440
Fax: (813)357-5079
Website: http://www.uhc.com
Ken L. Hoverman, CEO

★ 18983 ★ United HealthCare of Florida, Inc.
PPO Plan
7077 Bonneval Rd., Ste. 103
Jacksonville, FL 32216
Phone: (904)296-1332 **Free:** 800-250-6178
Fax: (904)296-2649
Website: http://www.uhc.com
Matthew Davies, CEO

★ 18984 ★ Vista Health Plan Inc.
PPO Plan
300 S Park Rd.
Hollywood, FL 33021
Free: 800-422-7335 **Fax:** (954)986-6013
Joe Berding, CEO

★ 18985 ★ Volusia Health Network
PPO Plan
400 N Clyde Morris Blvd.
Daytona Beach, FL 32114-3414
Phone: (386)258-4896 **Fax:** (386)253-2756
James Foster, Contact

Georgia

★ 18986 ★ Aetna Inc. - Georgia
PPO Plan
11675 Great Oaks Way
Alpharetta, GA 30022
Phone: (770)346-4300 **Free:** 800-353-5980
Fax: (770)346-2157
Website: http://www.aetna.com
John W. Rowe, Chairman of the Board

★ 18987 ★ Beech Street - Arkansas
PPO Plan
3460 Preston Ridge Rd., Ste. 300
Alpharetta, GA 30005
Phone: (770)346-0520 **Free:** 800-655-1855
Fax: (770)346-0506
Website: http://www.beechstreet.com
William Fickling, Jr., Chairman of the Board

★ 18988 ★ Beech Street - Delaware
PPO Plan
3460 Preston Ridge Rd., Ste. 300
Alpharetta, GA 30005
Phone: (770)346-0520 **Fax:** (770)346-0506
Website: http://www.beechstreet.com
William Fickling, Jr., Chairman of the Board

★ 18989 ★ Beech Street - District of Columbia
PPO Plan
3460 Preston Ridge Rd., Ste. 300
Alpharetta, GA 30005
Phone: (770)346-0520 **Fax:** (770)346-0506
Website: http://www.beechstreet.com
William Fickling, Jr., Chairman of the Board

★ 18990 ★ Beech Street - Florida
PPO Plan
3460 Preston Ridge Rd., Ste. 300
Alpharetta, GA 30005
Phone: (770)346-0520 **Free:** 800-655-1855
Fax: (770)346-0506
Website: http://www.beechstreet.com
William Fickling, Jr., Chairman of the Board
Program(s): Chiropractic, Home Care, Inpatient SNF, Long-Term Care, Podiatry, Psychiatric, Behavioral Health, Transplant, Workers' Compensation, Alternative Medicine.

★ 18991 ★ Beech Street - Georgia
PPO Plan
3460 Preston Ridge Rd., Ste. 300
Alpharetta, GA 30005
Phone: (770)346-0520 **Free:** 800-655-1855
Fax: (770)346-0506
Website: http://www.beechstreet.com
William Fickling, Jr., CEO & Chm Bd

★ 18992 ★ Beech Street - Kentucky
PPO Plan
3460 Preston Ridge Rd., Ste. 300
Alpharetta, GA 30005
Phone: (770)346-0520 **Free:** 800-655-1855
Fax: (770)346-0506
Website: http://www.beechstreet.com
William Fickling, Jr., Chairman of the Board

★ 18993 ★ Beech Street - Louisiana
PPO Plan
3460 Preston Ridge Rd., Ste. 300
Alpharetta, GA 30005
Phone: (770)346-0520 **Free:** 800-655-1855
Fax: (770)346-0506
Website: http://www.beechstreet.com
William Fickling, Jr., Chairman of the Board

★ 18994 ★ Beech Street - Maryland
PPO Plan
3460 Preston Ridge Rd., Ste. 300
Alpharetta, GA 30005
Phone: (770)346-0520 **Free:** 800-655-1855
Fax: (770)346-0506
Website: http://www.beechstreet.com
William Hale, CEO & Pres

★ 18995 ★ Beech Street - Mississippi
PPO Plan
3460 Preston Ridge Rd., Ste. 300
Alpharetta, GA 30005
Phone: (770)346-0520 **Free:** 800-655-1855
Fax: (770)346-0506
Website: http://www.beechstreet.com
William Fickling, Jr., Chairman of the Board

★ 18996 ★ Beech Street - North Carolina
PPO Plan
3460 Preston Ridge Rd., Ste. 300
Alpharetta, GA 30005
Phone: (770)346-0520 **Free:** 800-655-1855
Fax: (770)346-0506
Website: http://www.beechstreet.com
William Fickling, Jr., CEO & Chm Bd

★ 18997 ★ Beech Street - Puerto Rico
PPO Plan
3460 Preston Ridge Rd., Ste. 300
Alpharetta, GA 30005
Phone: (770)346-0520 **Free:** 800-655-1855
Fax: (770)346-0506
Website: http://www.beechstreet.com
William Fickling, Jr., Chairman of the Board

★ 18998 ★ Beech Street - South Carolina
PPO Plan
3460 Preston Ridge Rd., Ste. 300
Alpharetta, GA 30005
Phone: (770)346-0520 **Free:** 800-655-1855
Fax: (770)346-0506
Website: http://www.beechstreet.com
William Fickling, Jr., Chairman of the Board

★ 18999 ★ Beech Street - Tennessee
PPO Plan
3460 Preston Ridge Rd., Ste. 300
Alpharetta, GA 30005
Phone: (770)346-0520 **Free:** 800-655-1855
Fax: (770)346-0506
Website: http://www.beechstreet.com
William Fickling, Jr., CEO & Chm Bd

★ 19000 ★ Beech Street - West Virginia
PPO Plan
3460 Preston Ridge Rd., Ste. 300
Alpharetta, GA 30005
Phone: (770)346-0520 **Free:** 800-655-1855
Fax: (770)346-0506
Website: http://www.beechstreet.com
William Fickling, Jr., Chairman of the Board

★ 19001 ★ CIGNA HealthCare of Georgia
PPO Plan
100 Peachtree St., Ste. 800
Atlanta, GA 30303
Phone: (404)681-7000 **Fax:** (404)681-7031
Website: http://www.cigna.com
Robert Youngk, CEO

★ 19002 ★ Coalition America, Inc.
PPO Plan
4151 Ashford Dunwoody Rd., No. 615
Atlanta, GA 30319
Phone: (404)459-7201 **Fax:** (404)459-6645
Website: http://www.coalitionamerica.com
Sean Smith, CEO
Program(s): Chiropractic, Dental, Home Care, Inpatient SNF, Long-Term Care, Pharmaceutical Mail Order, Podiatry, Psychiatric, Behavioral Health, Physical Therapy, Transplant, Vision, Wellness, Workers' Compensation, Other Benefits.

★ 19003 ★ Columbus Physician Association
PPO Plan
6501 Veterans Pkwy., Bldg. 3
Columbus, GA 31901
Phone: (706)322-8999 **Fax:** (706)324-7524
William J. Shellem, CEO

★ 19004 ★ Coventry Health Care Inc. - Georgia, Inc.
PPO Plan
1100 Circle 75 Pkwy., Ste. 1400
Atlanta, GA 30339
Phone: (678)202-2100 **Free:** 800-470-2004
Fax: (678)202-2196
Website: http://www.cvty.com
Thomas A. Davis, CEO

★ 19005 ★ Evergreen Medical Group LLC
PO Box 790
Columbus, GA 31902
Phone: (706)660-6175 **Fax:** (706)660-6515
Website: http://www.evergreenhealthplan.com
Mike Hill, CEO

★ 19006 ★ Healthcare Preferred & Southcare PPO
1100 Circle 75 Pkwy, Ste. 1400
Atlanta, GA 30339
Phone: (678)202-2100 **Free:** 800-470-2004
Fax: (678)202-2193
Website: http://www.southcareppo.com
Tom Davis, CEO

★ 19007 ★ Humana Health Plans of Georgia
PPO Plan
900 Ashwood Pkwy., Ste. 400
Atlanta, GA 30338
Phone: (770)393-9226 **Free:** 800-234-3486
Fax: (770)393-2845
Website: http://www.humana.com/georgia/home.html
Karen Hornsby, Contact

★ 19008 ★ One Health Plan of Georgia, Inc.
PPO Plan
245 Perimeter Ctr. Pkwy., 7th Fl.
Atlanta, GA 30346
Phone: (770)290-7000 **Free:** 800-511-3899
Fax: (770)290-7022
Website: http://www.onehealthplan.com
David Record, CEO

★ 19009 ★ Phoebe Health Partners
PPO Plan
PO Box 1828
Albany, GA 31701
Phone: (229)312-8061 **Fax:** (229)312-8068
Website: http://www.ppmh.org
Pat Sumner, CEO

★ 19010 ★ Preferred Plan
PPO Plan
4 Executive Park E, Ste. 325
Atlanta, GA 30329
Free: 800-662-5665 **Fax:** (404)325-7906
Website: http://www.preferredplan.com
Rick Zwzenak, Contact

★ 19011 ★ Private Healthcare Systems - Georgia
PPO Plan
5600 New Northside Dr., Ste. 700
Atlanta, GA 30328
Phone: (770)818-9048 **Free:** 800-253-4417
Fax: (770)818-9101
Website: http://www.phcs.com
Joseph Driscoll, CEO & Pres

★ 19012 ★ Secure Health Plans of Georgia, LLC
PPO Plan
PO Box 4088
Macon, GA 31210
Phone: (478)314-2400 **Free:** 800-648-7563
Fax: (478)738-9596
Website: http://www.shpg.com
George Israel, CEO

★ 19013 ★ South Georgia Health Partners
PO Box 7410
Tifton, GA 31793
Free: 800-486-0868 **Fax:** (229)387-1156
Website: http://www.sghp.com
C. Frank Riley, CEO

★ 19014 ★ United HealthCare of Georgia
PPO Plan
2970 Clairmont Rd., Ste. 300
Atlanta, GA 30329-1634
Phone: (404)982-8800 **Free:** 800-842-6219
Fax: (404)320-8351
Website: http://www.uhc.com
Teresa Kline, CEO

Hawaii

★ 19015 ★ Queen's Health Care Plan
PPO Plan
2 Waterfront Plaza, Ste. 200
Honolulu, HI 96813-4988
Phone: (808)522-7500 **Fax:** (808)242-6788
Nate Nygaard, CEO

Idaho

★ 19016 ★ Primary Health Plan
PPO Plan
800 Park Blvd., Ste. 760
Boise, ID 83712
Phone: (208)344-1811 **Free:** 800-688-5008
Fax: (208)344-4262
Website: http://www.primaryhealth.com
Elden Mitchell, CEO & Pres

Illinois

★ 19017 ★ Aetna Inc. - Illinois
PPO Plan
100 N Riverside Plaza, 20th Fl.
Chicago, IL 60606-1518
Phone: (312)928-3000 **Free:** 800-627-5039
Fax: (312)928-3232
Website: http://www.aetna.com
John W. Rowe, MD, Chairman of the Board

★ 19018 ★ Beech Street - Illinois
PPO Plan
Two Trans Am Plaza, Ste. 400
Oakbrook Terrace, IL 60181
Phone: (630)705-8560 **Free:** 800-772-2844
Fax: (630)705-1414
Website: http://www.beechstreet.comm
William Fickling, Jr., Chairman of the Board

★ 19019 ★ Beech Street - Indiana
PPO Plan
Two Trans Am Plaza, Ste. 400
Oakbrook Terrace, IL 60181
Phone: (630)705-8560 **Free:** 800-772-2844
Fax: (630)705-1414
Website: http://www.beechstreet.com
William Fickling, Jr., Chairman of the Board

★ 19020 ★ Beech Street - Kansas
PPO Plan
Two Trans Am Plaza, Ste. 400
Oakbrook Terrace, IL 60181
Phone: (630)705-8560 **Free:** 800-772-2844
Fax: (630)705-1414
Website: http://www.beechstreet.com
William Fickling, Jr., Chairman of the Board

★ 19021 ★ Beech Street - Michigan
PPO Plan
Two Trans Am Plaza, Ste. 400
Oakbrook Terrace, IL 60181
Phone: (630)705-8560 **Free:** 800-772-2844
Fax: (630)705-1414
Website: http://www.beechstreet.com
William Fickling, Jr., Chairman of the Board

★ 19022 ★ Beech Street - Minnesota
PPO Plan
Two Trans Am Plaza, Ste. 400
Oakbrook Terrace, IL 60181
Phone: (630)705-8560 **Free:** 800-772-2844
Fax: (630)705-1414
Website: http://www.beechstreet.com
William Fickling, Jr., Chairman of the Board

★ 19023 ★ Beech Street - Missouri
PPO Plan
Two Trans Am Plaza, Ste. 400
Oakbrook Terrace, IL 60181
Phone: (630)705-8560 **Free:** 800-772-2844
Fax: (630)705-1414
Website: http://www.beechstreet.com
William Fickling, Jr., Chairman of the Board

★ 19024 ★ Beech Street - Nebraska
PPO Plan
Two Trans Am Plaza, Ste. 400
Oakbrook Terrace, IL 60181
Phone: (630)705-8560 **Free:** 800-772-2844
Fax: (630)705-1414
Website: http://www.beechstreet.com
William Fickling, Jr., Chairman of the Board

★ 19025 ★ Beech Street - Ohio
PPO Plan
Two Trans Am Plaza, Ste. 400
Oakbrook Terrace, IL 60181
Phone: (630)705-8560 **Free:** 800-772-2844
Fax: (630)705-1414
Website: http://www.beechstreet.com
William Fickling, Jr., Chairman of the Board

★ 19026 ★ Beech Street - South Dakota
PPO Plan
Two Trans Am Plaza, Ste. 400
Oakbrook Terrace, IL 60181
Phone: (630)705-8560 **Fax:** (630)705-1414
Website: http://www.beechstreet.com
William Fickling, Jr., Chairman of the Board

★ 19027 ★ Beech Street - Wisconsin
PPO Plan
Two Trans Am Plaza, Ste. 400
Oakbrook Terrace, IL 60181
Phone: (630)750-8560 **Free:** 800-772-2844
Fax: (630)705-1414
Website: http://www.beechstreet.com
William Fickling, Jr., Chairman of the Board

★ 19028 ★ First Care of Illinois
1444 N Farnsworth Ave., No. 202
Aurora, IL 60505
Gwen Bruns, CEO

★ 19029 ★ First Health Group Corp.
3200 Highland Ave.
Downers Grove, IL 60515
Phone: (630)737-7900 **Free:** 800-455-1425
Fax: (630)737-7856
Website: http://www.firsthealth.com
Edward L. Wristen, CEO & Pres

★ 19030 ★ GE Financial Assurance/ Partnership Marketing Group
PPO Plan
200 N Martingale Rd.
Schaumburg, IL 60173-2096
Phone: (847)605-3000 **Free:** 800-277-8484
Fax: (847)605-7256
Website: http://www.thesignaturegroup.com
Kathy Marinello, CEO

★ 19031 ★ Great West Life
6250 River Rd., Ste. 10-100
Rosemont, IL 60018
Phone: (847)292-0024 **Fax:** (847)292-0015
Website: http://www.onehealthplan.com
Scott Burnett, Contact

★ 19032 ★ Health Alliance Medical Plans - Corporate Headquarters
PPO Plan
102 E Main St.
Urbana, IL 61801
Phone: (217)337-8000 **Free:** 800-851-3379
Fax: (217)337-8093
Website: http://www.hapcorp.org
Jeffery Ingrum, MD, CEO

★ 19033 ★ Health Dynamics Inc.
204 17th St.
Wilmette, IL 60091
Phone: (847)920-9052
Joseph N. Mohr, CEO

★ 19034 ★ Health Marketing, Inc.
PPO Plan
940 W Adams St., Ste. 102
Chicago, IL 60607
Phone: (312)432-0800 **Fax:** (312)432-0898

Website: http://www.healthmarketing.com
Charles Baygood, CEO & Pres

★ 19035 ★ Health Plus
PPO Plan
5409 N Knoxville Ave.
Peoria, IL 61614
Phone: (309)689-8600 **Fax:** (309)689-8601
Website: http://www.healthpluspeoria.org
Philip Walker, II, CEO & Pres

★ 19036 ★ Healthcare Service Corp. - Corporate Headquarters
PPO Plan
300 E Randolph St.
Chicago, IL 60601-5099
Phone: (312)653-6000 **Fax:** (312)819-1220
Website: http://www.bcbsil.com
Raymond McCaskey, CEO

★ 19037 ★ Humana Health Care Plans of Illinois
PPO Plan
30 S Wacker Dr., Ste. 3100
Chicago, IL 60606
Phone: (312)441-9111 **Free:** 800-852-9556
Fax: (312)441-5901
Website: http://www.humana.com/Illinois/hcme.html
David Jones, Chairman of the Board

★ 19038 ★ Personal Care
PPO Plan
2110 Fox Dr.
Champaign, IL 61820
Phone: (217)366-1226 **Free:** 800-366-6730
Fax: (217)366-5410
David Line, CEO

★ 19039 ★ PPONext - Ohio
8745 W Higgins Rd., Ste. 300
Chicago, IL 60631
Free: 888-446-6098 **Fax:** (216)642-0161
Website: http://www.healthstarinc.com
Steve Carder, President

★ 19040 ★ Preferred Podiatry Group
425 Huehl Rd.
Northbrook, IL 60062
Phone: (847)504-5000 **Free:** 800-654-3772
Fax: (847)504-5015
Sanford Mason, MD, CEO

★ 19041 ★ Quincy Health Care Management Inc.
PPO Plan
1246 Broadway
Quincy, IL 62301
Phone: (217)222-9157 **Free:** 800-637-7100
Fax: (217)222-1732
Website: http://www.riverguestnetwork.com
Karen J. Brown, Contact

★ 19042 ★ Rockford Health Plans, Inc.
PPO Plan
3401 N Perryville Rd.
Rockford, IL 61114
Phone: (815)971-1000 **Free:** 800-331-0424
Fax: (815)654-5188
Website: http://www.rockfordhealthplans.com
Edward Pattarozzi, CEO & Pres

★ 19043 ★ Trustmark Insurance Co.
400 Field Dr.
Lake Forest, IL 60045
Phone: (847)615-1500 **Fax:** (847)615-3907
J. Grover Thomas, Jr., CEO

★ 19044 ★ UniCare
PPO Plan
233 S Wacker Dr., Ste. 3900
Chicago, IL 60606
Phone: (312)234-7000 **Free:** 888-234-7747
Fax: (312)234-8001
Website: http://www.rushpru.com
Sandra Van Trease, CEO

★ 19045 ★ United HealthCare of Illinois, Inc.
PPO Plan
233 N Michigan Ave.
Chicago, IL 60601
Phone: (312)424-4460 **Fax:** (312)424-4905
Website: http://www.uhc.com
William Moeller, CEO

Indiana

★ 19046 ★ Aetna Inc. - Indiana
PPO Plan
8425 Woodfield Crossing Blvd.
Indianapolis, IN 46240
Phone: (317)815-4300 **Free:** 800-382-3209
Fax: (317)815-4397
Website: http://www.aetna.com
John W. Rowe, MD, Chairman of the Board

★ 19047 ★ Aetna Inc. - Indiana
PPO Plan
9365 Counselors Row, Ste. 110
Indianapolis, IN 46240
Phone: (317)815-4300 **Fax:** (317)815-4317
Website: http://www.aetna.com
John W. Rowe, Chairman of the Board

★ 19048 ★ Arnett Health Plans
PPO Plan
PO Box 6108
Lafayette, IN 47903
Phone: (765)448-7701 **Fax:** (765)448-7700
Website: http://www.arnettplans.com
James Brunnemer, CEO

★ 19049 ★ Cigna Healthcare of Indiana
PPO Plan
429 N Pennsylvania, Ste. 301
Indianapolis, IN 46204
Phone: (317)615-1200 **Free:** 800-276-0363
Fax: (317)615-1301
Website: http://www.cigna.com
Mary Brandt, CEO

★ 19050 ★ Community Health Alliance
328 N Michigan, Ste. 200
South Bend, IN 46601
Phone: (574)284-1820 **Fax:** (574)284-1825
Website: http://www.chanetwork.com
Diane Maas, CEO

★ 19051 ★ Corvel Corp.
PPO Plan
450 E 96th St., Ste. 340
Indianapolis, IN 46240
Phone: (317)816-6996 **Free:** 800-959-7958
Fax: (317)816-6990
Website: http://www.corvel.com
Rhonda Moran, CEO

★ 19052 ★ Deaconess Health Partners
PPO Plan
600 Mary St.
Evansville, IN 47747-0002
Phone: (812)450-7265 **Free:** 800-374-8993
Fax: (812)450-2030
Website: http://www.deaconess.com
Joyce Hudson, CEO

★ 19053 ★ Encore Health Network
PPO Plan
8802 N Meridian, Ste. 100
Indianapolis, IN 46260
Phone: (317)705-3280 **Free:** 888-446-5584
Fax: (317)705-3281
Website: http://www.encorehealthnetwork.com
Mark A. Hochstetler, MD, CEO

★ 19054 ★ Health Resources, Inc.
PO Box 15660
Evansville, IN 47716-0660
Phone: (812)424-1444 **Free:** 800-727-1444
Fax: (812)424-2096
Website: http://www.hri-dro.com
Edward Fritz, DDS, Chairman of the Board
Program(s): Dental.

★ 19055 ★ Humana, Inc. - Indiana
PPO Plan
8500 Keystone Crossing, Ste. 470
Indianapolis, IN 46240-1438
Phone: (317)722-2075 **Free:** 800-444-9137
Fax: (317)722-2088
Website: http://www.humana.com
David A. Jones, Chairman of the Board

★ 19056 ★ Indiana Health Network
8330 Allison Pointe Tr.
Indianapolis, IN 46250
Phone: (317)284-7171 **Free:** 888-446-6670
Fax: (317)284-7080
Website: http://www.ihnppo.com
Larry Dust, CEO

★ 19057 ★ Indiana Pro Health Network
PPO Plan
8180 Clearvista Pkwy., Ste. 230
Indianapolis, IN 46256
Free: 800-344-8672 **Fax:** (317)588-7470
William Corley, CEO

★ 19058 ★ Individualized Care Management, Inc.
PPO Plan
PO Box 6298
Lafayette, IN 47905-6298
Phone: (765)448-1864 **Free:** 800-278-0327
Fax: (765)447-8335
Website: http://www.icmcorporate.com
Ann Roberts, CEO

★ 19059 ★ Lutheran Preferred
PPO Plan
7950 W Jefferson Blvd.
Fort Wayne, IN 46804
Phone: 800-444-2001 **Free:** 800-258-0974
Fax: (219)435-6940
Website: http://www.lutheranpreferred.com
Thomas Miller, CEO

★ 19060 ★ Managed Care Services
PPO Plan
3000 Coliseum Blvd. E, Ste. 100
Fort Wayne, IN 46805
Phone: (260)373-9000 **Free:** 800-666-4449
Fax: (260)373-9005
Website: http://www.parkview.com
Barbara Clayton, Contact

★ 19061 ★ Partners National Health Plans of Indiana, Inc.
PPO Plan
100 E Wayne St., Ste. 302
South Bend, IN 46601
Phone: (260)233-4899 **Free:** 800-876-2655
Fax: (260)234-7484

Website: http://www.partnersindiana.com
Bruce Greenberg, CEO

★ 19062 ★ PNI
PPO Plan
PO Box 11328
South Bend, IN 46634
Phone: (574)233-9014 **Free:** 800-622-5398
Fax: (574)232-9003
Website: http://www.partnersindiana.com
Bruce Greenberg, CEO

★ 19063 ★ Precision Health Network LLC
1155 W Third St.
Bloomington, IN 47404
Phone: (812)330-8003 **Free:** 800-608-8444
Fax: (812)330-2392
Website: http://www.phn-in.com
Michael Bishop, CEO

★ 19064 ★ Sagamore Health Network, Inc.
PPO Plan
11555 N Meridian St., Ste. 400
Carmel, IN 46032
Free: 800-382-8414 **Fax:** (317)573-2946
Website: http://www.sagamorehn.com
Greg Yust, CEO

★ 19065 ★ St. Mary's Managed Care Services
PPO Plan
2330 Lynch Rd., Ste. 100
Evansville, IN 47711
Phone: (812)485-7990 **Fax:** (812)485-7995
Kiishor Bhatt, Contact

★ 19066 ★ Select Circle Health Plan
PPO Plan
1512 White River Blvd.
Muncie, IN 47303
Phone: (765)286-2150 **Fax:** (765)286-4375
Karen Popovich, CEO

★ 19067 ★ Signature Care, Inc.
PPO Plan
3000 Coliseum Blvd. E, Ste. 100
Fort Wayne, IN 46805
Phone: (260)373-9000 **Free:** 800-666-4449
Fax: (260)496-4110
Website: http://www.signaturecareppo.com
Michelle Lobe, Contact

★ 19068 ★ Southeastern Indiana Health Organization, Inc.
PPO Plan
PO Box 1787
Columbus, IN 47202-1787
Phone: (812)378-7000 **Fax:** (812)348-4592
Website: http://www.siho.org
David Barker, CEO & Pres

Iowa

★ 19069 ★ Advantage Health Plan
PPO Plan
736 Federal St.
Davenport, IA 52803
Phone: (563)324-2547 **Free:** 800-386-7150
Fax: (563)324-2606
Website: http://www.cha-advantage.com
Amir Arbisser, MD, CEO

★ 19070 ★ American Republic Insurance Co.
PO Box 1
Des Moines, IA 50334
Phone: (515)245-2000 **Free:** 800-247-2190
Fax: (515)245-2305
Website: http://www.aric.om
Michael E. Abbott, CEO

★ 19071 ★ Corvel Corp.
PPO Plan
1701 48th St., Ste. 275
West Des Moines, IA 50266
Phone: (515)225-9668 **Free:** 800-929-1160
Fax: (515)225-9772
Website: http://www.corvel.com
Gordon Clemons, CEO

★ 19072 ★ Coventry Health Care Inc. - Iowa
PPO Plan
4600 Westown Pkwy., Ste. 200
West Des Moines, IA 50266-1099
Phone: (515)225-1234 **Free:** 800-257-4692
Fax: (515)223-9239
Website: http://www.chciowa.com
Michael Teachaut, CEO

★ 19073 ★ Foundation for Medical Care/ Encompass
PPO Plan
6000 Westown Pkwy., Ste. 350E
West Des Moines, IA 50266-7771
Phone: (515)223-2900 **Free:** 800-383-2856
Fax: (515)223-2990
Website: http://www.encompass.com
Fred Ferree, CEO
Program(s): Chiropractic, Home Care, Inpatient SNF, Long-Term Care, Pharmaceutical Mail Order, Psychiatric, Transplant, Wellness, Workers' Compensation.

★ 19074 ★ Principal Life Insurance Co. - Oregon
711 High St.
Des Moines, IA 50392
Phone: (515)247-5111 **Free:** 800-986-3343
Fax: (515)248-2499
Barry Griswold, CEO

★ 19075 ★ Priority Health Network
PPO Plan
625 S Gilbert St., Ste. 2
Iowa City, IA 52245
Phone: (319)339-3992 **Free:** 800-358-2767
Fax: (319)339-3973
Website: http://www.mercyic.com

★ 19076 ★ SecureCare of Iowa
PPO Plan
11141 Aurora Ave.
Des Moines, IA 50322
Free: 888-881-8820 **Fax:** (515)331-7848
Don Burrows, CEO

★ 19077 ★ Wellmark, Inc. - Corporate Headquarters
PPO Plan
636 Grand Ave.
Des Moines, IA 50309-2565
Phone: (515)245-4500 **Fax:** (515)245-5090
Website: http://www.wellmark.com
John Forsyth, CEO & Chm Bd

Kansas

★ 19078 ★ CIGNA HealthCare of Kansas/ Missouri
PPO Plan
7400 W 110th St., Ste. 600
Overland Park, KS 66210
Phone: (913)451-9389 **Fax:** (913)451-0974
Website: http://www.cigna.com
Rick Grizzle, Contact

★ 19079 ★ Coventry Health Care Inc. - Wichita
PPO Plan
8301 E 21st St. N, No. 300
Wichita, KS 67206
Phone: (316)634-1222 **Free:** 800-664-9251
Fax: (316)634-1266
Website: http://www.cvty.com
Jan Stallmeyer, CEO

★ 19080 ★ Great West Life
82 Corp Woods
10851 Maslin 200
Overland Park, KS 66210
Phone: (913)491-9436 **Fax:** (913)491-9417
Website: http://www.onehealthplan.com
Greg Watkins, Contact

★ 19081 ★ One Health Plan of Kansas/ Missouri
8575 W 110th, Ste. 108
Overland Park, KS 66210
Phone: (913)451-0101 **Free:** 800-218-7723
Fax: (913)317-8824
Website: http://www.onehealthplan.com
William T. McCallum, CEO

★ 19082 ★ Preferred Health Professionals
PPO Plan
12920 Metcalf Ave., Ste. 200
Overland Park, KS 66213-2620
Phone: (913)685-6300 **Free:** 800-544-3014
Fax: (913)685-6355
John Kennedy, Chairman of the Board

★ 19083 ★ Preferred Health Systems
PPO Plan
8535 E 21st St. N
Wichita, KS 67206
Phone: (316)609-2345 **Free:** 800-990-0345
Fax: (316)609-2346
Website: http://www.phsystems.com
Marlon Dauner, CEO & Pres

★ 19084 ★ United HealthCare of the Midwest, Inc.
PPO Plan
9393 W 110th St., Bldg. 51, No. 300
Overland Park, KS 66210-2002
Phone: (913)663-6500 **Free:** 800-340-9716
Fax: (913)663-6549
Website: http://www.uhc.com
William Tracy, CEO

★ 19085 ★ Via Christie Medical Management
PPO Plan
3 Medical Center Circle, Ste. A
Pittsburg, KS 66762
Phone: (620)235-0390 **Fax:** (620)235-0364
Clark Stevens, Contact

★ 19086 ★ WPPA, Inc.
PPO Plan
1102 S Hillside
Wichita, KS 67211-4004
Phone: (316)683-4111 **Free:** 800-801-9772
Fax: (316)683-6255
Website: http://www.wppainc.com
Serena Lubbers, Contact

Kentucky

★ 19087 ★ Aetna Inc. - Kentucky
PPO Plan
305 N Hurstbourne Pkwy., Ste. 100
Louisville, KY 40222-5146
Phone: (502)423-6240 **Fax:** (502)339-7639
Website: http://www.aetna.com
John W. Rowe, Chairman of the Board

★ 19088 ★ Bluegrass Family Health, Inc.
PPO Plan
651 Perimeter Dr., Ste. 300
Lexington, KY 40517
Phone: (859)269-4475 **Fax:** (859)269-6447
Website: http://www.bgfh.com
James Fritz, CEO & Pres

★ 19089 ★ Center Care Community Health Plans
Center Care PPO
1225 Fairway St.
Bowling Green, KY 42103
Phone: (270)745-1517 **Free:** 800-972-7038
Fax: (270)796-2106
Website: http://www.centercare.com
Teresa Wilson, Contact

★ 19090 ★ CIGNA Healthcare of Kentucky
PPO Plan
5111 Commerce Crossing Dr.
Louisville, KY 40229
Phone: (502)753-2341 **Free:** 800-808-1534
Fax: (502)753-2365
Website: http://www.cigna.com
Robert Bruce, CEO

★ 19091 ★ Commonwealth Health Plan
300 W Vine St.
Lexington, KY 40507
Phone: (859)232-8686 **Free:** 800-457-5683
Fax: (859)232-8557
Website: http://www.cha-health.com
Mark Birdwhistle, CEO

★ 19092 ★ Humana Health Care Plans of Kansas & Missouri
PPO Plan
500 W Main St.
Louisville, KY 40201-1438
Phone: (816)941-8900 **Free:** 800-842-6188
Fax: (816)941-0879
Website: http://www.humana.com/kansascity/home.html
Michael McCallister, CEO

★ 19093 ★ Humana Health Care Plans of Lexington
PPO Plan
500 W Main St.
Lexington, KY 40507
Phone: (859)263-1400 **Free:** 800-221-8390
Fax: (859)263-1488
Website: http://www.humana.com/lexington/home.html
Michael McCallister, CEO & Pres

★ 19094 ★ Humana Health Care Plans of San Antonio
PPO Plan
500 W Main St.
Louisville, KY 40201-1438
Phone: (210)617-1000 **Fax:** (210)615-0090
Website: http://www.humana.com
David A. Jones, Chairman of the Board

★ 19095 ★ Humana Health Plan - Kentucky
PPO Plan
500 W Main St.
Louisville, KY 40202
Phone: (502)580-1860 **Fax:** (502)580-3127
Website: http://www.humana.com
Michael McCallister, CEO

★ 19096 ★ Humana, Inc. - Alabama
PPO Plan
500 W Main St.
Louisville, KY 40201-1438
Phone: (502)580-1000 **Fax:** (502)580-3127
Website: http://www.humana.com
David Jones, Chairman of the Board

★ 19097 ★ Humana, Inc. - Alaska
PPO Plan
PO Box 740036
Louisville, KY 40201-7436
Phone: (502)580-1550 **Fax:** (502)580-8528
Website: http://www.humana.com
David Jones, Chairman of the Board

★ 19098 ★ Humana, Inc. - Arkansas
PPO Plan
500 W Main St.
Louisville, KY 40201-1438
Phone: (502)580-1000 **Fax:** (502)580-4106
Website: http://www.humana.com
David Jones, Chairman of the Board

★ 19099 ★ Humana, Inc. - California
PPO Plan
PO Box 740036
Louisville, KY 40201-7436
Phone: (502)580-5005 **Fax:** (502)580-8528
Website: http://www.humana.com
Michael B. McCallister, Chairman of the Board

★ 19100 ★ Humana, Inc. - Colorado
PPO Plan
PO Box 740036
Louisville, KY 40201-7436
Phone: (303)694-1044 **Free:** 800-825-7496
Fax: (303)694-1105
Website: http://www.humana.com
David Jones, Chairman of the Board

★ 19101 ★ Humana Inc. - Corporate Headquarters
PPO Plan
PO Box 740036
Louisville, KY 40201-7436
Phone: (502)580-1860 **Fax:** (502)580-3127
Website: http://www.humana.com
David Jones, Chairman of the Board

★ 19102 ★ Humana, Inc. - District of Columbia
PPO Plan
PO Box 740036
Louisville, KY 40201-7436
Phone: (502)580-5005 **Fax:** (502)580-8528
Website: http://www.humana.com
David Jones, Chairman of the Board

★ 19103 ★ Humana, Inc. - Iowa
PPO Plan
PO Box 740036
Louisville, KY 40201-7436
Phone: (502)580-5005 **Fax:** (502)580-8528
Website: http://www.humana.com
David A. Jones, Chairman of the Board

★ 19104 ★ Humana, Inc. - Louisiana
PPO Plan
500 W Main St.
Louisville, KY 40201
Phone: (502)580-5804 **Fax:** (502)980-8528
Website: http://www.humana.com
David Jones, Chairman of the Board

★ 19105 ★ Humana, Inc. - Maryland
PPO Plan
PO Box 740036
Louisville, KY 40202-1438
Phone: (502)580-5005 **Fax:** (502)580-8528
Website: http://www.humana.com
Michael McCallister, CEO & Pres

★ 19106 ★ Humana, Inc. - Michigan
PPO Plan
PO Box 740036
Louisville, KY 40202-1438
Phone: (248)680-8920 **Fax:** (248)680-8897
Website: http://www.humana.com
Michael McCallister, CEO & Pres

★ 19107 ★ Humana, Inc. - Mississippi
PPO Plan
500 W Main
Louisville, KY 40201
Phone: (502)580-5804 **Fax:** (502)980-8528
Website: http://www.humana.com
Michael McCallister, CEO & Pres

★ 19108 ★ Humana, Inc. - Nebraska
PPO Plan
PO Box 740036
Louisville, KY 40201-7436
Phone: (502)580-5005 **Fax:** (502)580-8528
Website: http://www.humana.com
Michael McCallister, CEO & Pres

★ 19109 ★ Humana, Inc. - New Mexico
PPO Plan
500 W Main St.
Louisville, KY 40201
Phone: (502)580-5804 **Fax:** (502)980-8528
Website: http://www.humana.com
Michael McCallister, CEO & Pres

★ 19110 ★ Humana, Inc. - North Carolina
PPO Plan
500 W Main St.
Louisville, KY 40201
Phone: (704)643-0400 **Free:** 800-234-9761
Fax: (704)643-0306
Website: http://www.humana.com
Michael McCallister, CEO

★ 19111 ★ Humana, Inc. - North Dakota
PPO Plan
500 W Main St.
Louisville, KY 40201
Phone: (502)580-5804 **Fax:** (502)980-8528
Website: http://www.humana.com
Michael McCallister, CEO & Pres

★ 19112 ★ Humana, Inc. - Ohio
PPO Plan
500 W Main St.
Louisville, KY 40201-1438
Phone: (502)784-5200 **Fax:** (502)543-7158
Website: http://www.humana.com
Michael McCallister, CEO & Pres

★ 19113 ★ Humana, Inc. - Oklahoma
PPO Plan
500 W Main St.
Louisville, KY 40201
Phone: (502)580-5804 **Fax:** (502)580-8528

Website: http://www.humana.com
Michael McCallister, CEO & Pres

★ 19114 ★ Humana, Inc. - South Carolina
PO Box 740036
Louisville, KY 40201-7436
Phone: (502)580-1550 **Fax:** (502)580-8528
Website: http://www.humana.com
David Jones, Chairman of the Board

★ 19115 ★ Humana, Inc. - South Dakota
PPO Plan
500 W Main St.
Louisville, KY 40201
Phone: (502)580-5804 **Fax:** (502)980-8528
Website: http://www.humana.com
Michael McCallister, CEO & Pres

★ 19116 ★ Humana, Inc. - Tennessee
PPO Plan
PO Box 740036
Louisville, KY 40201-1438
Phone: (901)685-8351 **Free:** 800-283-8510
Fax: (901)685-0194
Website: http://www.humana.com
Michael McCallister, CEO & Pres

★ 19117 ★ Humana, Inc. - Utah
PPO Plan
500 W Main St.
Louisville, KY 40201
Phone: (502)580-5804 **Fax:** (502)980-8528
Website: http://www.humana.com
Michael McCallister, CEO & Pres

★ 19118 ★ Humana, Inc. - Virginia
PPO Plan
PO Box 740036
Louisville, KY 40201-1438
Phone: (502)580-1860 **Fax:** (502)580-3127
Website: http://www.humana.com
Michael McCallister, CEO & Pres

★ 19119 ★ Humana, Inc. - Washington
PPO Plan
500 W Main St.
Louisville, KY 40201
Phone: (502)580-5804 **Fax:** (502)980-8528
Website: http://www.humana.com
Michael McCallister, CEO & Pres

★ 19120 ★ Humana, Inc. - West Virginia
PPO Plan
500 W Main St.
Louisville, KY 40201
Phone: (502)580-5804 **Fax:** (502)980-8528
Website: http://www.humana.com
Michael McCallister, CEO & Pres

★ 19121 ★ Humana, Inc. - Wyoming
PPO Plan
500 W Main St.
Louisville, KY 40201
Phone: (502)580-5804 **Fax:** (502)980-8528
Website: http://www.humana.com
Michael McCallister, CEO & Pres

★ 19122 ★ Humana Military Service, Inc.
PPO Plan
500 W Main St.
Louisville, KY 40201
Phone: (502)580-5804 **Fax:** (502)580-8528
Website: http://www.humana.com
David Jones, Chairman of the Board

★ 19123 ★ United HealthCare of Kentucky, Inc.
PPO Plan
2424 Harrodsburg Rd.
Lexington, KY 40504-3329
Phone: (859)296-6000 **Fax:** (859)224-3732
Website: http://www.uhc.com
Charles Price, CEO

Louisiana

★ 19124 ★ Aetna US Healthcare - Arkansas
PPO Plan
3900 N Causeway Blvd., Ste. 410
Metairie, LA 70002-7283
Phone: (504)830-5600 **Free:** 800-685-4857
Fax: (504)837-6571
Website: http://www.aetna.com
John W. Rowe, Chairman of the Board

★ 19125 ★ AmCare Health Plans of Louisiana
PPO Plan
5353 Essen Ln., Ste. 450
Baton Rouge, LA 70809
Phone: (225)763-5300 **Free:** 800-772-2995
Fax: (225)763-6211
Website: http://www.amcarehealthplans.com
Thomas Lucksinger, CEO

★ 19126 ★ American LifeCare Corporate Headquarters
PPO Plan
650 Poydras St., Ste. 1150
New Orleans, LA 70130-6131
Phone: (504)561-0600 **Fax:** (504)679-0150
Website: http://www.americanlifecare.com
Edward Michael Reggie, Chairman of the Board

★ 19127 ★ CIGNA HealthCare of Louisiana, Inc.
PPO Plan
3838 N Causeway Blvd., No. 2850
Metairie, LA 70002
Free: 800-832-3211 **Fax:** (504)831-7499
Website: http://www.cigna.com
Patrick Welch, President

★ 19128 ★ Coventry Health Care Inc. - Louisiana
PPO Plan
2424 Edenborn Ave., Ste. 350
Metairie, LA 70001
Phone: (504)834-0840 **Free:** 800-341-6613
Fax: (504)834-2694
Website: http://www.cvty.com
Keith Benoit, Sr., CEO

★ 19129 ★ FARA Healthcare Management
PPO Plan
2360 Fifth Ave.
Mandeville, LA 70471
Phone: (985)624-8383 **Free:** 800-259-8388
Fax: (985)624-8489
Website: http://www.fara.com
Reed Bell, CEO

★ 19130 ★ Med-Comp USA
PPO Plan
2901 N Causeway Blvd., Ste. 202
Metairie, LA 70002
Phone: (504)832-4106 **Fax:** (504)835-1079
Website: http://www.medcompusa.com
Michael McCrossen, CEO

★ 19131 ★ SMA Health Plan, Inc.
PPO Plan
1555 Poydres
New Orleans, LA 70112
Phone: (504)837-7374 **Free:** 800-259-7370
Fax: (504)837-7115
Website: http://www.sma.net
Robert Gormley, MD, Contact

★ 19132 ★ United HealthCare of Louisiana, Inc.
PPO Plan
3838 N Causeway Blvd., Ste. 2100
Metairie, LA 70009
Phone: (504)849-3510 **Free:** 800-864-4799
Fax: (504)849-3551
Website: http://www.uhc.com
Sam Patterson, CEO

★ 19133 ★ Universal Health Network - Louisiana
PPO Plan
800 Virtue St., Ste. 211
Chalmette, LA 70043
Phone: (504)620-7004 **Free:** 877-537-7556
Fax: (504)620-7001
Website: http://www.universalhealthnet.com
Robert Danforth, CEO

★ 19134 ★ Vantage Health Plan, Inc.
PPO Plan
909 N 18th St., Ste. 201
Monroe, LA 71201
Phone: (318)361-0900 **Free:** 888-823-1910
Fax: (318)361-2159
Patrick Jones, MD, CEO

Maine

★ 19135 ★ Aetna Inc. - Maine
PPO Plan
One Monument Sq., 5th Fl.
Portland, ME 04101
Phone: (207)879-1995 **Fax:** (207)879-7951
Website: http://www.aetna.com
John W. Rowe, MD, Chairman of the Board

★ 19136 ★ Cigna Healthcare of Maine, Inc.
PPO Plan
2 Stonewood Dr.
Freeport, ME 04032-0447
Phone: (207)865-5000 **Free:** 800-642-5551
Fax: (207)865-5633
Website: http://www.cigna.com/healthcare/hs/me.html
Richard White, CEO & Pres

★ 19137 ★ Martins Point Health Care
PPO Plan
PO Box 9746
Portland, ME 04104-5040
Phone: (207)774-5801 **Fax:** (207)828-2446
Website: http://www.martinspoint.org
David Howes, MD, CEO

★ 19138 ★ Medical Network, Inc.
PPO Plan
59 Middle St., 3rd Fl.
Portland, ME 04101
Phone: (207)773-5116 **Free:** 800-556-1144
Fax: (207)773-1739
Website: http://www.mainemednet.com
Vincent Furey, Jr., CEO

★ 19139 ★ One Health Plan of Maine, Inc.
PPO Plan
100 Foden Rd. E, Ste. 202
South Portland, ME 04106
Phone: (207)828-5084 **Fax:** (207)828-4672
Website: http://www.onehealthplan.com
William Schulz, Contact

Maryland

★ 19140 ★ Aetna Inc. - DE, MD, DC
PPO Plan
1302 Concourse Dr., Ste. 402
Linthicum, MD 21090
Phone: (410)691-1080 **Free:** 800-328-8742
Fax: (410)691-1198
Website: http://www.aetna.com
John W. Rowe, Chairman of the Board

★ 19141 ★ Alliance PPO LLC
PPO Plan
4 Taft Court
Rockville, MD 20850
Free: 800-331-2102 **Fax:** (301)545-5388
Website: http://www.mamsi.com
Mark Groban, MD, Chairman of the Board

★ 19142 ★ BCE Emergis - California
PPO Plan
2273 Research Blvd.
Rockville, MD 20850
Phone: (301)548-1000 **Free:** 800-248-7744
Fax: (301)296-5020
Francois Cole, CEO & Pres

★ 19143 ★ BCE Emergis Corp.
2273 Research Blvd.
Rockville, MD 20850
Free: 800-247-3155 **Fax:** (301)548-8828
Website: http://www.emergis.com/ehealth
Francois Cote, CEO & Pres

★ 19144 ★ CIGNA Healthcare Mid-Atlantic
PPO Plan
9700 Patuxent Woods Dr.
Columbia, MD 21046
Phone: (410)720-5800 **Free:** 800-541-7526
Fax: (410)720-5860
Website: http://www.cigna.com/healthcare/hs/md.html
Matt Manders, CEO

★ 19145 ★ Coventry Health Care, Inc. - Corporate Headquarters
PPO Plan
6705 Rockledge Dr., Ste. 900
Bethesda, MD 20817
Phone: (301)581-0600 **Fax:** (301)493-0700
Website: http://www.cvty.com
Allen Wise, CEO

★ 19146 ★ Fidelity Benefit Administrators Inc.
201 International Cir., 4th Fl.
Hunt Valley, MD 21030
Phone: (410)329-0900 **Fax:** (410)329-1011
Website: http://www.hc2000.com
Thomas J. Knox, CEO & Pres

★ 19147 ★ Great West Life
PPO Plan
14504 Green View Dr., Ste. 400
Laurel, MD 20708
Phone: (301)497-1700 **Fax:** (301)494-8066
Website: http://www.onehealthplan.com
William T. McCallum, CEO

★ 19148 ★ MD-Individual Practice Association, Inc. (MD IPA)
PPO Plan
4 Taft Court
Rockville, MD 20850
Phone: (301)838-5645 **Free:** 800-544-2853
Fax: (301)545-5388
Website: http://www.mamsi.com
Thomas Barbera, CEO & Pres

★ 19149 ★ Mid Atlantic Medical Services, Inc. (MAMSI)
PPO Plan
4 Taft Court
Rockville, MD 20850
Phone: (301)762-8205 **Fax:** (301)738-1230
Website: http://www.mamsi.com
Thomas Barbera, CEO & Pres

★ 19150 ★ Sheppard Pratt Health Plan
PPO Plan
PO Box 1470
Rockville, MD 20849
Phone: (410)938-3200 **Free:** 800-881-2279
Fax: (410)938-4099
Website: http://www.sheppardpratt.org
Steven Sharfstein, MD, CEO

★ 19151 ★ United HealthCare of the Mid Atlantic
PPO Plan
6300 Security Blvd.
Baltimore, MD 21207
Phone: (410)277-6000 **Fax:** (410)277-6661
Website: http://www.uhc.com
Bob Fleshner, CEO

★ 19152 ★ United Payors and United Providers
PPO Plan
2273 Research Blvd.
Rockville, MD 20850
Phone: (301)548-1000 **Free:** 800-247-4144
Fax: (301)548-8828
Website: http://www.upup.com
Faye Baggiano, MD, CEO

Massachusetts

★ 19153 ★ CIGNA Healthcare of Massachusetts
PPO Plan
3 Newton Executive Pkwy.
Newton, MA 02462
Phone: (617)630-4300 **Fax:** (617)630-4380
Website: http://www.cigna.com
Imre Toth, MD, Contact

★ 19154 ★ CIGNA Healthcare of Massachusetts
PPO Plan
100 Front St., Ste. 300
Worcester, MA 01608-1449
Phone: (508)798-8667 **Free:** 800-922-8380
Fax: (508)849-4299
Website: http://www.cigna.com
Linda Dwyer, CEO

★ 19155 ★ First All America Financial
PPO Plan
440 Lincoln St.
Worcester, MA 01653
Phone: (508)855-1000 **Free:** 800-634-8647
Fax: (508)853-6202
Website: http://www.allamerica.com
Jack O'Brien, CEO

★ 19156 ★ Freedom Care, Inc.
PPO Plan
100 Front St., Ste. 600
Worcester, MA 01615
Phone: (508)752-2480 **Free:** 800-343-7674
Fax: (508)754-9664
William Briedenbach, President

★ 19157 ★ Great West
PPO Plan
One Apple Hill Dr., Ste. 104
Natick, MA 01760-2072
Free: 800-733-2750 **Fax:** (508)650-9598
Website: http://www.onehealthplan.com
John Kelley, Contact

★ 19158 ★ Harvard Pilgrim Health Care - Corporate Headquarters
PPO Plan
93 Worchester St.
Wellesley, MA 02481
Phone: (781)263-6000 **Free:** 800-742-8326
Fax: (617)509-2515
Website: http://www.harvardpilgrim.org
Charles Baker, CEO & Pres

★ 19159 ★ Healthcare Value Management Inc.
100 River Ridge Dr.
Norwood, MA 02062
Phone: (781)762-5511 **Fax:** (781)762-5318
Website: http://www.hcum.com
Charles Donahue, Jr., President

★ 19160 ★ New England Financial - Corporate Headquarters
PPO Plan
501 Boylston St.
Boston, MA 02116-3700
Phone: (617)578-2000 **Free:** 800-388-4000
Fax: (617)578-3088
Website: http://www.nefn.com
James Benson, CEO & Pres

★ 19161 ★ Pioneer Health
PPO Plan
330 Whitney Ave.
Holyoke, MA 01040-6600
Phone: (413)534-3200 **Fax:** (413)534-0687
Website: http://www.pioneerhealth.com
Bruce Suchy, President

★ 19162 ★ Private Healthcare Systems - California
PPO Plan
1100 Winter St.
Waltham, MA 02451
Phone: (949)476-9816 **Free:** 800-253-4417
Fax: (949)476-0650
Website: http://www.phcs.com
Joseph Driscoll, CEO & Pres

★ 19163 ★ Private Healthcare Systems - Corporate Headquarters
PPO Plan
1100 Winter St.
Waltham, MA 02451
Phone: (781)895-7500 **Free:** 800-253-4417
Fax: (781)895-3477
Website: http://www.phcs.com
Joseph Driscoll, CEO & Pres

★ 19164 ★ Private Healthcare Systems - Florida
PPO Plan
1100 Winter St.
Waltham, MA 02451

Phone: (781)895-7500 **Free:** 800-253-4417
Fax: (781)895-3477
Website: http://www.phcs.com
Barbara Dailey, Contact

★ 19165 ★ Private Healthcare Systems - Illinois
PPO Plan
1100 Winter St.
Waltham, MA 02451
Phone: (847)292-6700 **Free:** 800-253-4417
Fax: (781)292-6736
Website: http://www.phcs.com
Joseph Driscoll, Contact

★ 19166 ★ Private Healthcare Systems - Michigan
PPO Plan
1100 Winter St.
Waltham, MA 02451
Phone: (781)895-7500 **Free:** 800-253-4417
Fax: (781)895-3477
Website: http://www.phcs.com
Joseph Driscoll, CEO & Pres

★ 19167 ★ Private Healthcare Systems - Missouri
PPO Plan
1100 Winter St.
Waltham, MA 02451
Phone: (816)221-4455 **Free:** 800-253-4417
Fax: (816)221-4466
Website: http://www.phcs.com
Joseph Driscoll, CEO & Pres

★ 19168 ★ Private Healthcare Systems - New Jersey
PPO Plan
1100 Winter St.
Waltham, MA 02451
Phone: (201)909-8803 **Free:** 800-253-4417
Fax: (201)909-0260
Website: http://www.phcs.com
Joseph Driscoll, CEO & Pres

★ 19169 ★ Private Healthcare Systems - New York
PPO Plan
1100 Winter St.
Waltham, MA 02451
Phone: (781)895-7500 **Free:** 800-253-4417
Fax: (781)895-3477
Website: http://www.phcs.com
Joseph Driscoll, CEO & Pres

★ 19170 ★ Private Healthcare Systems - Ohio
PPO Plan
1100 Winter St.
Waltham, MA 02451
Phone: (781)895-7500 **Free:** 800-253-4417
Fax: (781)895-3477
Website: http://www.phcs.com
Joseph Driscoll, CEO & Pres

★ 19171 ★ Private Healthcare Systems - Tennessee
PPO Plan
1100 Winter St.
Waltham, MA 02451
Phone: (781)895-7500 **Free:** 800-253-4417
Fax: (781)895-3477
Website: http://www.phcs.com
Joseph Driscoll, CEO & Pres

★ 19172 ★ Private Healthcare Systems - Texas
PPO Plan
1100 Winter St.
Waltham, MA 02451
Phone: (781)895-7500 **Free:** 800-253-4417
Fax: (781)895-3477
Website: http://www.phcs.com
Joseph Driscoll, CEO & Pres

★ 19173 ★ Private Healthcare Systems - Virginia
PPO Plan
1100 Winter St.
Waltham, MA 02451
Phone: (781)895-7500 **Free:** 800-253-4417
Fax: (781)895-3477
Website: http://www.phcs.com
Joseph Driscoll, CEO & Pres

★ 19174 ★ Private Healthcare Systems - Washington
PPO Plan
1100 Winter St.
Waltham, MA 02451
Phone: (781)895-7500 **Free:** 800-253-4417
Fax: (781)895-3477
Website: http://www.phcs.com
Joseph Driscoll, CEO & Pres

★ 19175 ★ Tufts Health Plan
PPO Plan
333 Wyman St.
Waltham, MA 02454
Phone: (781)466-9400 **Free:** 800-394-3993
Website: http://www.tufts-healthplan.com
Harris Berman, MD, CEO

Michigan

★ 19176 ★ Care Choices HMO
PPO Plan
34605 Twelve Mile Rd.
Farmington Hills, MI 48331
Phone: (248)489-6203 **Free:** 800-852-9780
Fax: (248)489-6280
Website: http://www.carechoices.com
William R. Alvin, CEO & Pres

★ 19177 ★ ConnectCare
PPO Plan
4009 Orchard Dr., Ste. 3021
Midland, MI 48640
Phone: (989)839-1615 **Fax:** (989)839-1626
Website: http://www.connectcare.com
Brian Rodgers, CEO & Pres

★ 19178 ★ Health Alliance Plan
PPO Plan
2850 W Grand Blvd.
Detroit, MI 48202
Phone: (313)872-8100 **Free:** 800-422-4641
Website: http://www.hapcorp.org
Cleve Killingsworth, CEO & Pres

★ 19179 ★ Health Care Exchange Limited Co.
32290 5 Mile Rd.
Livonia, MI 48154
Phone: (734)452-2500 **Fax:** (734)452-2501
Website: http://www.dentemax.com
Kenneth R. Dallafior, CEO
Program(s): Dental.

★ 19180 ★ Henry Ford Health System
PPO Plan
1 Ford Place
Detroit, MI 48202-2608
Phone: (313)916-2600 **Fax:** (313)874-4730
Website: http://www.henryford.com
Gail Warden, CEO

★ 19181 ★ IBA Health Plan
PPO Plan
106 Farmers Alley, Ste. 300
Kalamazoo, MI 49005-1100
Phone: (616)341-7200 **Fax:** (616)341-6864
Website: http://www.phpcares.com
David Kibbe, CEO

★ 19182 ★ Physicians Health Plan of South Michigan
PPO Plan
PO Box 4055
Jackson, MI 49204
Phone: (517)782-7154 **Fax:** (517)782-4512
Jerry Grannan, CEO

★ 19183 ★ Preferred Provider Organization of Michigan (PPOM)
PPO Plan
28588 Northwestern Hwy.
Southfield, MI 48034-8318
Phone: (248)357-7766 **Free:** 800-878-7766
Fax: (248)357-2418
Website: http://www.ppom.com
Jeff Connolly, CEO

★ 19184 ★ Priority Health
PPO Plan
1231 E Beltline NE
Grand Rapids, MI 49525
Phone: (616)942-0954 **Free:** 800-942-0954
Fax: (616)942-5651
Website: http://www.priority-health.com
Kimberly Horn, CEO

★ 19185 ★ ProAmerica Managed Care
PPO Plan
975 Spaulding Ave. SE
Grand Rapids, MI 49546
Phone: (616)942-8628 **Fax:** (616)942-1602
Website: http://www.proamerica.com
Susan Isrleson, Vice President

Minnesota

★ 19186 ★ Allianz Life Insurance Co. of America
PPO Plan
5701 Golden Hills, Dr.
Minneapolis, MN 55416-1297
Phone: (763)765-6500 **Free:** 800-328-5600
Fax: (763)765-6657
Website: http://www.allianzlife.com
Bob MacDonald, CEO

★ 19187 ★ Healtheast Care, Inc.
PPO Plan
1690 University Ave., Ste. 370
Saint Paul, MN 55104
Phone: (651)232-5070 **Fax:** (651)232-5069
Website: http://www.healtheast.org
Robert Moravec, MD, Contact

★ 19188 ★ HealthPartners Inc.
PPO Plan
PO Box 1309
Minneapolis, MN 55440-1309
Phone: (952)883-6000 **Free:** 888-470-4470
Fax: (952)883-5380
Website: http://www.healthpartners.com
Mary Brainerd, CEO & Pres

★ 19189 ★ Medica
PPO Plan
PO Box 9310
Minneapolis, MN 55440-1587
Phone: (952)992-2900 **Fax:** (952)992-3554
Website: http://www.medica.com
David Strand, President

★ 19190 ★ Preferred One
PPO Plan
6150 Golden Hills Dr.
Golden Valley, MN 55416
Phone: (763)847-4000 **Fax:** (763)847-4010
Website: http://www.preferredone.com
Marcus Merz, CEO

★ 19191 ★ United Health Group - Corporate Headquarters
PPO Plan
9900 Bren Rd. E
Opus Center
Minnetonka, MN 55343
Phone: (952)936-1300 **Fax:** (952)936-0044
Website: http://www.uhc.com
William McGuire, MD, CEO & Pres

Mississippi

★ 19192 ★ American Lifecare
1675 Lakeland Dr., Ste. 550
Jackson, MS 39216
Phone: (601)713-1930 **Free:** 877-460-0352
Fax: (601)713-1931
Website: http://www.americanlifecare.com
Ed Michael Reggie, Chairman of the Board

★ 19193 ★ Mississippi Select Health Care
PPO Plan
14110 Airport Rd., Ste. 100
Gulfport, MS 39503
Phone: (228)865-0514 **Free:** 800-847-6621
Fax: (228)865-0550
Website: http://www.hmhs.com
Thomas Wicklund, CEO

★ 19194 ★ United HealthCare of Mississippi
PPO Plan
800 Woodlands Pkwy., Ste. 102
Ridgeland, MS 39157
Free: 800-264-3639 **Fax:** (601)957-1306
Website: http://www.uhc.com
Robert J. Sheehy, CEO

Missouri

★ 19195 ★ Aetna Inc. - Misssouri
PPO Plan
2 Cityplace Dr., Ste. 300
Saint Louis, MO 63141
Phone: (314)567-6660 **Fax:** (314)567-3627
Website: http://www.aetna.com
John W. Rowe, Chairman of the Board

★ 19196 ★ American Health Care Alliance
PPO Plan
9229 Ward Pkwy., Ste. 300
Kansas City, MO 64114
Phone: (816)523-7799 **Fax:** (816)523-1098
Website: http://www.aha.ppo.net
Ed Cosler, CEO

★ 19197 ★ Cigna Healthcare of Missouri
PPO Plan
1 N Brentwood Blvd.
Clayton, MO 63105
Phone: (314)726-7850 **Free:** 800-832-3211
Fax: (314)726-7819
Website: http://www.cigna.com
James Young, President

★ 19198 ★ Coventry Health Care, Inc. - Kansas City
PPO Plan
1001 E 101st Terrace, Ste. 300
Kansas City, MO 64131
Phone: (816)941-3030 **Free:** 800-969-3343
Fax: (816)941-8516
Website: http://www.cvty.com
Jan Stallmeyer, CEO & Pres

★ 19199 ★ General American Life Insurance Co. - Corporate Headquarters
PPO Plan
13045 Tesson Ferry Rd.
Saint Louis, MO 63128
Phone: (314)843-8700
Website: http://www.genam.com
Warren Winer, President

★ 19200 ★ Great West
622 Emerson Rd., Ste. 250
Saint Louis, MO 63144
Phone: (314)569-3232 **Fax:** (314)569-2022
Website: http://www.onehealthplan.com
Greg Watkins, Contact

★ 19201 ★ HealthLink, Inc.
PPO Plan
12443 Olive Blvd.
Saint Louis, MO 63141
Phone: (314)989-6000 **Free:** 800-624-2356
Website: http://www.healthlink.com
David T. Ott, CEO & Pres

★ 19202 ★ HealthLink, Inc. - Corporate Headquarters
PPO Plan
12443 Olive Blvd.
Saint Louis, MO 63141
Phone: (314)989-6000 **Fax:** (314)989-6620
Website: http://www.healthlink.com
David T. Ott, CEO & Pres

★ 19203 ★ Mid America Health
PPO Plan
8321 Parkway
Kansas City, MO 64114
Phone: (816)221-8400 **Free:** 800-468-1442
Fax: (816)221-7709
Website: http://www.healthnet.com
George Pagels, MD, CEO

★ 19204 ★ PPO USA, Inc.
310 NE Mulberry
Lees Summit, MO 64086
Free: 877-477-6872
Website: http://www.ppousa.com
Joseph Witkowski, CEO

★ 19205 ★ United HealthCare of the Midwest, Inc.
PPO Plan
PO Box 2560
Maryland Heights, MO 63043-8560
Phone: (314)592-7000 **Free:** 800-535-9291
Fax: (314)592-7650
Website: http://www.uhc.com
Victor Turvey, CEO & Pres

Nebraska

★ 19206 ★ Midlands Choice
PPO Plan
8420 W Dodge Rd., Ste. 210
Omaha, NE 68114
Phone: (402)390-8233 **Free:** 800-605-8259
Fax: (402)390-8239
Website: http://www.midlandschoice.com
Ralph Morocco, CEO

★ 19207 ★ Mutual of Omaha - Corporate Headquarters
PPO Plan
Mutual of Omaha Plaza
Omaha, NE 68175
Phone: (402)342-7600 **Free:** 800-228-0286
Fax: (402)351-2775
Website: http://www.mutualofomaha.com
John Weekly, Chairman of the Board

★ 19208 ★ United HealthCare of the Midlands, Inc.
PPO Plan
2717 N 118th Circle
Omaha, NE 68164-9672
Phone: (402)445-5000 **Free:** 800-284-0626
Fax: (402)445-5575
Website: http://www.uhc.com
John Braasch, President

★ 19209 ★ United of Omaha Life Insurance Co. - Oregon
Mutual of Omaha Plz.
Omaha, NE 68175
Phone: (402)344-7600 **Fax:** (402)351-2775
Website: http://www.mutualofomaha.com
John Weekly, CEO

Nevada

★ 19210 ★ Hometown Health Plan
PPO Plan
400 S Wells Ave.
Reno, NV 89502
Phone: (775)982-3000 **Fax:** (775)982-3220
Website: http://www.hometownhealth.com
Jim Miller, CEO

★ 19211 ★ Horizon Health
PPO Plan
5440 W Sahara Ave., Ste. 106
Las Vegas, NV 89146
Phone: (702)367-2222 **Free:** 800-884-6875
Fax: (702)247-4758
Website: http://www.horizonhealthppo.com
Marcy Platt, Contact

★ 19212 ★ Managed Care Consultants, Inc.
PPO Plan
311 N Pecos Rd., Ste 100
Henderson, NV 89074
Phone: (702)792-2944 **Free:** 800-748-6842
Fax: (702)451-7307
Website: http://www.mccnevada.com
Joe Lawrence, CEO

★ 19213 ★ Nevada Care, Inc.
PPO Plan
10600 W Charleston Blvd.
Las Vegas, NV 89102-2320
Phone: (702)474-7241 **Fax:** (702)474-7592
Website: http://www.nevadacare.com
Keith Beagle, President

★ 19214 ★ **Nevada Preferred Professionals**
PPO Plan
4170 S Dacator Blvd., A-8
Las Vegas, NV 89103
Phone: (702)384-3366 **Free:** 888-288-0677
Fax: (702)384-9781
Website: http://www.nvpp.com
Robert W. Danforth, Contact

★ 19215 ★ **PacifiCare of Nevada**
PPO Plan
700 E Warm Springs Rd.
Las Vegas, NV 89119-4323
Phone: (702)269-7500 **Free:** 800-826-4347
Fax: (702)269-2649
Website: http://www.pacificare.com
Bard Coats, MD, CEO

★ 19216 ★ **Saint Mary's Health First**
PPO Plan
235 W 6th St.
Reno, NV 89502
Phone: (775)770-6060 **Fax:** (775)770-6253
Don Kowitz, CEO

★ 19217 ★ **Sierra Health Services, Inc. - Corporate Headquarters**
PPO Plan
PO Box 15645
Las Vegas, NV 89114-5645
Phone: (702)242-7000 **Fax:** (702)242-7915
Website: http://www.sierrahealth.com
Anthony Marlon, MD, CEO & Chm Bd

★ 19218 ★ **Universal Health Network - Corporate Headquarters**
PPO Plan
PO Box 30007
Reno, NV 89520-3007
Phone: (775)356-1159 **Free:** 800-776-6959
Fax: (775)356-5746
Website: http://www.universalhealthnet.com
Robert Danforth, CEO

★ 19219 ★ **Universal Health Network - Corporate Headquarters**
PPO Plan
PO Box 30007
Reno, NV 89520-3007
Phone: (775)356-1159 **Free:** 800-776-6959
Fax: (775)356-5746
Website: http://www.universalhealthnet.com
Robert Danforth, CEO

New Hampshire

★ 19220 ★ **CIGNA Healthcare New Hampshire**
PPO Plan
PO Box 2041
Concord, NH 03302-2041
Phone: (603)225-5077 **Free:** 800-531-3121
Fax: (603)229-2978
Website: http://www.cigna.com
Brian Wells, CEO & Pres

New Jersey

★ 19221 ★ **Aetna Inc. - New Jersey**
PPO Plan
8000 Mid Atlantic Dr., Ste. 100N
Mount Laurel, NJ 08054
Phone: (856)222-5560 **Fax:** (856)727-8490
Website: http://www.aetna.com
John W. Rowe, MD, Chairman of the Board

★ 19222 ★ **Aetna Inc. - New Jersey**
PPO Plan
55 Lane Rd.
Fairfield, NJ 07004
Phone: (973)575-5600 **Free:** 800-852-0629
Fax: (973)244-3990
Website: http://www.aetna.com
John W. Rowe, Chairman of the Board

★ 19223 ★ **Alta Health & Life Insurance**
PPO Plan
One Centennial Ave.
Piscataway, NJ 08855-1326
Phone: (732)980-4000 **Free:** 800-221-3231
Fax: (732)357-2893
Website: http://www.ahlic.com
James White, President

★ 19224 ★ **AmeriHealth Insurance Co. - New Jersey North**
PPO Plan
485 Rt. 1 S, 3rd Fl., Bldg. C
Iselin, NJ 08830
Phone: (732)726-6700 **Fax:** (732)726-6753
Website: http://www.amerihealth.com
Dan Pedriani, CEO

★ 19225 ★ **AmeriHealth Insurance Co. - New Jersey South**
PPO Plan
8000 Midlantic Dr., Ste. 333
Mount Laurel, NJ 08054-1560
Phone: (856)778-6500 **Free:** 800-454-7651
Fax: (856)778-6550
Website: http://www.amerihealth.com
G. Fred DiBona, Jr., CEO

★ 19226 ★ **AtlantiCare Health Plans, Inc.**
PPO Plan
6727 Delilah Rd.
Egg Harbor Township, NJ 08234
Free: 800-272-5995 **Fax:** (609)407-2013
Website: http://www.atlanticare.org
Patricia Koeling, CEO

★ 19227 ★ **Beech Street MediChoice**
PPO Plan
1240 Sussex Turnpike
Randolph, NJ 07869
Phone: (973)895-2244 **Free:** 800-640-6708
Fax: (973)895-2266
Website: http://www.beechstreet.com
William Fickling, Jr., Chairman of the Board

★ 19228 ★ **CIGNA Healthcare of New York and New Jersey**
PPO Plan
499 Washington Blvd.
Jersey City, NJ 07310
Phone: (201)533-7000 **Fax:** (201)533-7164
Website: http://www.cigna.com
Kurt Weimer, CEO & Pres

★ 19229 ★ **Consumer Health Network**
PPO Plan
1 Cragwood Rd., 3rd Fl.
South Plainfield, NJ 07080
Phone: (908)222-9300 **Free:** 800-225-4246
Fax: (908)222-7506
Website: http://www.chnnetwork.com
Leonard Weinman, CEO & Pres

★ 19230 ★ **Family Choice Health Alliance**
PPO Plan
401 Hackensack Ave.
Hackensack, NJ 07601-6411
Phone: (201)487-6002 **Free:** 800-732-7892
Fax: (201)487-1116
Andrew Baker, CEO

★ 19231 ★ **Great West Life**
PPO Plan
1 Centennial Ave.
Piscataway, NJ 08855-6870
Phone: (732)980-8777 **Fax:** 888-604-2201
Website: http://www.onehealthplan.com
Matt Kenyon, Contact

★ 19232 ★ **MagNet, Inc.**
PPO Plan
65 Willowbrook Blvd.
Wayne, NJ 07470
Phone: (973)890-4657 **Fax:** (973)890-1434
Website: http://www.pcms-magnacare.com
Don Tribus, CEO

★ 19233 ★ **Medical Resource**
PPO Plan
5 Eve Dr., Ste. 120
Marlton, NJ 08053
Phone: (856)988-1910 **Free:** 800-543-5260
Fax: (856)983-0435
Website: http://www.medicalres.com
Beverly McCullough, Contact

★ 19234 ★ **One Health Plan of Massachusetts**
PPO Plan
1 Centennial Ave.
Piscataway, NJ 08855
Phone: (781)622-2400 **Fax:** (781)622-1462
Website: http://www.onehealthplan.com
Randall Cook, Contact

★ 19235 ★ **Oxford Health Plans of New Jersey, Inc.**
PPO Plan
111 Wood Ave. S, Ste. 2
Iselin, NJ 08830
Phone: (203)459-6000 **Free:** 800-889-4694
Fax: (732)623-1900
Website: http://www.oxhp.com
Norman Payson, MD, CEO & Chm Bd

★ 19236 ★ **QualCare, Inc.**
PPO Plan
242 Old New Brunswick Rd.
Piscataway, NJ 08854-3754
Phone: (732)562-0833 **Free:** 800-992-6613
Fax: (732)562-2833
Annette Catino, CEO

★ 19237 ★ **University Health Plans, Inc.**
PPO Plan
550 Broad St.
Newark, NJ 07102-4599
Phone: (973)623-8700 **Free:** 800-TRI-UHP1
Fax: (973)623-3635
Website: http://www.uhpnet.com
Alexander H. McLean, CEO & Pres

★ 19238 ★ **US Life Care/American General Assurance**
PPO Plan
3600 Rt. 66
Neptune, NJ 07754-1580
Phone: (732)922-7000 **Free:** 800-346-7692
Fax: (732)922-7604
William Keeler, CEO

New Mexico

★ 19239 ★ Lovelace Health Plan
PPO Plan
4101 Central NE
Albuquerque, NM 87110
Phone: (505)262-7363 **Fax:** (505)262-7545
Website: http://www.lovelace.com
Martin Hickey, MD, CEO

★ 19240 ★ Presbyterian Health Plan
PPO Plan
PO Box 27489
Albuquerque, NM 87125-7489
Phone: (505)923-5700 **Free:** 800-356-2884
Fax: (505)923-5277
Website: http://www.phs.org
Jim Hinton, Chairman of the Board

New York

★ 19241 ★ Aetna Inc. - New York
PPO Plan
2700 Westchester Ave.
Purchase, NY 10577
Phone: (914)251-0600 **Fax:** (914)251-1537
Website: http://www.aetna.com
John W. Rowe, MD, Chairman of the Board

★ 19242 ★ Aetna Inc. - New York
PPO Plan
333 Earle Ovington Blvd., Ste. 502
Uniondale, NY 11553
Phone: (516)794-6565 **Free:** 800-322-8742
Fax: (516)794-2389
Website: http://www.aetna.com
John W. Rowe, MD, Chairman of the Board

★ 19243 ★ Anthem Health Network
PPO Plan
PO Box 140724
Staten Island, NY 10314
Phone: (718)370-5380 **Free:** 800-455-0294
Fax: 800-370-6098
Website: http://www.anthemhealth.com
Carmine Morano, CEO

★ 19244 ★ Beech Street - Maine
PPO Plan
24 W 40th St., 16th Fl.
New York, NY 10018
Phone: (646)366-0870 **Free:** 800-777-1444
Fax: (646)366-1636
Website: http://www.beechstreet.com
William Fickling, Jr., Chairman of the Board

★ 19245 ★ Beech Street - Massachusetts
PPO Plan
24 W 40th St., 16th Fl.
New York, NY 10018
Phone: (646)366-0870 **Free:** 800-777-1444
Fax: (646)366-1636
Website: http://www.beechstreet.com
William Fickling, Jr., Chairman of the Board

★ 19246 ★ Beech Street - New Hampshire
PPO Plan
24 W 40th St., 16th Fl.
New York, NY 10018
Phone: (646)366-0870 **Free:** 800-777-1444
Fax: (646)366-1636
Website: http://www.beechstreet.com
William Fickling, Jr., Chairman of the Board

★ 19247 ★ Beech Street - New Jersey
PPO Plan
24 W 40th St., 16th Fl.
New York, NY 10018
Phone: (646)366-0870 **Free:** 800-777-1444
Fax: (646)366-1636
Website: http://www.beechstreet.com
William Fickling, Jr., Chairman of the Board

★ 19248 ★ Beech Street - New York
PPO Plan
24 W 40th St., 16th Fl.
New York, NY 10018
Phone: (646)366-0870 **Free:** 800-777-1444
Fax: (646)366-1636
Website: http://www.beechstreet.com
William Fickling, Jr., Chairman of the Board

★ 19249 ★ Beech Street - Pennsylvania
PPO Plan
24 W 40th St., 16th Fl.
New York, NY 10018
Phone: (646)366-0870 **Free:** 800-777-1444
Fax: (646)366-1636
Website: http://www.beechstreet.com
William Fickling, Jr., Chairman of the Board

★ 19250 ★ Beech Street - Rhode Island
PPO Plan
24 W 40th St., 16th Fl.
New York, NY 10018
Phone: (646)366-0870 **Free:** 800-777-1444
Fax: (646)366-1636
Website: http://www.beechstreet.com
William Fickling, Jr., Chairman of the Board

★ 19251 ★ Beech Street - Vermont
PPO Plan
24 W 40th St., 16th Fl.
New York, NY 10018
Phone: (646)366-0870 **Free:** 800-777-1444
Fax: (646)366-1636
Website: http://www.beechstreet.com
William Fickling, Jr., Chairman of the Board

★ 19252 ★ Finger Lakes Community Care Network
PPO Plan
350 Parrish St.
Canandaigua, NY 14424
Phone: (585)396-6460 **Fax:** (585)396-6674
Website: http://www.thomsonhealth.com
Virginia Tyler Homsy, CEO

★ 19253 ★ First Great West
PO Box 1607
Pearl River, NY 10965
Free: 800-736-0700 **Fax:** 888-490-8194
Website: http://www.onehealthplan.com
Matt Kenyon, Contact

★ 19254 ★ Guardian Life Insurance Co. of America
PPO Plan
7 Hanover St.
New York, NY 10004
Phone: (212)598-8000 **Fax:** (212)919-2423
Website: http://www.glic.com
Joseph Dudley Sargent, CEO

★ 19255 ★ HealthFirst
25 Broadway, 9th Fl.
New York, NY 10004
Phone: (212)801-1502 **Fax:** (212)801-1771
Website: http://www.healthfirst.org
Paul Dickstein, CEO

★ 19256 ★ Independent Health Association, Inc.
PPO Plan
511 Farber Lakes Dr.
Buffalo, NY 14221
Phone: (716)631-3001 **Free:** 800-247-1466
Fax: (716)631-0430
Website: http://www.independenthealth.com
Frank Colantuono, CEO

★ 19257 ★ MagnaCare
PPO Plan
825 E Gate Blvd., Ste. 200
Garden City, NY 11530
Phone: (516)227-6900 **Fax:** (516)227-6967
Website: http://www.pcms-magnacare.com
Anthony Bacchi, MD, CEO

★ 19258 ★ MultiPlan, Inc. - Corporate Headquarters
PPO Plan
115 Fifth Ave., 7th Fl.
New York, NY 10003-1004
Phone: (212)780-2000 **Free:** 800-677-1098
Fax: (212)780-0410
Website: http://www.multiplan.com
Donald Rubin, Chairman of the Board
Program(s): Chiropractic, Home Care, Inpatient SNF, Long-Term Care, Podiatry, Psychiatric, Behavioral Health, Physical Therapy, Transplant, Vision, Wellness.

★ 19259 ★ National Health Plan
PPO Plan
11 Penn Plaza, Ste. 310
New York, NY 10001
Phone: (212)279-3232 **Free:** 800-647-2677
Fax: (212)629-0749
Alvin Konigsberg, CEO

★ 19260 ★ North American Preferred
PPO Plan
PO Box 9501
Amherst, NY 14226
Phone: (716)446-5500 **Free:** 800-828-6922
Fax: (716)319-5732
Website: http://www.nahp.com
Ronald Zoeller, CEO & Pres

★ 19261 ★ Oxford Health Plans of New York, Inc.
PPO Plan
1133 Ave. of the Americas
New York, NY 10036
Phone: (212)805-3400 **Free:** 800-444-6222
Fax: (212)805-6671
Website: http://www.oxhp.com
Norman Payson, MD, CEO & Chm Bd

★ 19262 ★ Plan Vista Solutions
419 E Main St.
Middletown, NY 10940
Phone: (845)343-1600 **Free:** 800-863-3320
Fax: (845)343-6113
Website: http://www.planvista.com
Jeffrey Markle, President

★ 19263 ★ United HealthCare of New York Metropolitan
PPO Plan
Two Penn Plaza, 7th Fl.
New York, NY 10121-1097
Phone: (212)216-6400 **Fax:** (212)216-6591
Website: http://www.uhc.com
Amy Knapp, CEO

★ 19264 ★ Univera Health Care - Corporate Headquarters
205 Park Club Ln.
Buffalo, NY 14221-5239
Phone: (716)847-0881 **Free:** 800-644-4580
Fax: (716)847-1257
Website: http://www.univerahealthcare.org
Arthur R. Goshin, MD, CEO

★ 19265 ★ USI Administrators
1 Huntington Quadrangle, Ste. 4N
Melville, NY 11747
Phone: (516)775-5420 **Free:** 800-831-7783
Fax: (631)694-5540
Website: http://www.selectpro.com
James M. Pennington, CEO

★ 19266 ★ Vytra Healthcare
PPO Plan
395 N Service Rd.
Melville, NY 11747
Phone: (631)694-4000 **Free:** 800-406-0806
Fax: (631)719-7619
Website: http://www.vytra.com
Thomas McAteer, CEO

North Carolina

★ 19267 ★ Aetna Inc. of the Carolinas
PPO Plan
128 S Tryon, Ste. 2000
Charlotte, NC 28202
Phone: (704)379-6700 **Fax:** (704)379-7502
Website: http://www.aetna.com
John W. Rowe, Chairman of the Board

★ 19268 ★ Atlantic Integrated Health, Inc.
PPO Plan
1315 S Glenburnie Rd., Ste. D3
New Bern, NC 28562
Phone: (252)514-0057 **Fax:** (252)514-0750
Website: http://www.aihine.com
James Smackhouse, MD, Chairman of the Board

★ 19269 ★ CIGNA Healthcare of North Carolina
PPO Plan
200 Regency Executive Dr.
Charlotte, NC 28217
Phone: (704)586-0708 **Free:** 800-235-5707
Fax: (704)556-5840
Website: http://www.cigna.com
Steve White, CEO

★ 19270 ★ Coventry Health Care Inc. - Carolinas
PPO Plan
2815 Coliseum Ctr. Dr., Ste. 550
Charlotte, NC 28217
Phone: (704)357-1421 **Free:** 800-470-4523
Fax: (704)357-3164
Website: http://www.cvty.com
Tracy Baker, CEO

★ 19271 ★ Duke Health Direct
3100 Tower Blvd., Ste 600, Box 80
Durham, NC 27707
Phone: (919)419-5016 **Fax:** (919)493-9159
Website: http://www.dukehealthdirect.com
Joseph Vincoli, Contact

★ 19272 ★ Health Care Savings, Inc.
PPO Plan
4530 Park Rd., Ste. 110
Charlotte, NC 28209
Phone: (704)527-6261 **Free:** 800-833-8464
Fax: (704)527-0677
Website: http://www.healthcaresavings.com
Lawrence Cutchin, MD, CEO & Pres

★ 19273 ★ Health Care Savings, Inc.
PPO Plan
222 N Person St., 2nd Fl.
Raleigh, NC 27607
Phone: (919)828-1789 **Free:** 800-331-2877
Fax: (919)828-1720
Lawrence Cutchin, MD, CEO

★ 19274 ★ MedCost, LLC
PPO Plan
PO Box 25347
Winston-Salem, NC 27114
Phone: (336)760-3090 **Fax:** (336)774-4291
Website: http://www.medcost.com
William Ketner, CEO

★ 19275 ★ Mountain Health Care
PPO Plan
2 Hendersonville Rd., Ste. C
Asheville, NC 28803
Phone: (828)259-9110 **Free:** 800-245-1965
Fax: (828)259-9543
Website: http://www.mountainhealthcare.com
Ellen Wells, CEO

★ 19276 ★ One Health Plan of North Carolina, Inc.
PPO Plan
6000 Fairview Rd., Ste. 500
Charlotte, NC 28210
Phone: (704)552-9642 **Free:** 800-663-8081
Fax: (704)556-2149
Website: http://www.onehealthplan.com
William T. McCallum, CEO

★ 19277 ★ Spectrum Comp Works
PPO Plan
2621 Spring Forest Rd., Ste. 101
Raleigh, NC 27616
Phone: (919)875-1414 **Fax:** (919)875-0811
Robert Morrell, MD, Chairman of the Board

★ 19278 ★ WellPath of Carolina, Inc.
PPO Plan
6330 Quadrangle Dr., Ste. 500
Chapel Hill, NC 27514
Phone: (919)493-1210 **Free:** 800-935-7284
Fax: (919)419-3871
Website: http://www.wellpathchp.com
Tracy H. Baker, CEO

Ohio

★ 19279 ★ Aetna Inc. - Ohio
PPO Plan
205 W 4th St., Ste. 1000
Cincinnati, OH 45202
Phone: (513)579-3385 **Free:** 800-230-3241
Fax: (513)579-3316
Website: http://www.aetna.com
John W. Rowe, MD, Chairman of the Board

★ 19280 ★ AultCare
PPO Plan
2600 6th St. SW
Canton, OH 44710-1799
Phone: (330)438-6390 **Free:** 800-344-8858
Fax: (330)454-7845
Website: http://www.aultcare.com
Rick Haines, CEO

★ 19281 ★ Central Benefits Mutual Insurance Co.
PPO Plan
PO Box 16526
Columbus, OH 43216
Phone: (614)797-5200 **Free:** 800-333-5711
Fax: (614)797-5265
Website: http://www.centralbenefits.com
John Reinhardt, Jr., CEO

★ 19282 ★ CHN MCO
PPO Plan
6000 West Creek, Ste. 20
Independence, OH 44131
Phone: (216)986-1100 **Fax:** (216)328-7551
Website: http://www.chnetwork.com
Martin Hauser, CEO

★ 19283 ★ ChoiceCare/Humana
PPO Plan
655 Eden Park Dr., Ste. 400
Cincinnati, OH 45202-6056
Phone: (513)784-5200 **Free:** 800-543-7158
Fax: (513)784-5345
Website: http://www.choicecare.com
Larry Savage, CEO & Pres

★ 19284 ★ CIGNA HealthCare of Ohio, Inc.
PPO Plan
5005 Rockside Rd., Ste. 700
Cleveland, OH 44131
Phone: (216)642-2920 **Free:** 800-647-7748
Fax: (216)642-2990
Website: http://www.cigna.com
Jeanne McCarthy, President

★ 19285 ★ CIGNA HealthCare of Ohio, Inc.
PPO Plan
3700 Corporate Dr.
Columbus, OH 43231
Phone: (614)823-7500 **Free:** 800-542-7526
Fax: (614)823-7776
Website: http://www.cigna.com
Jeanne McCarthy, President

★ 19286 ★ CIGNA PPO of Ohio
PPO Plan
7 W 7th St., Ste. 1402
Cincinnati, OH 45202-2417
Phone: (513)629-2640 **Fax:** (513)629-2639
Website: http://www.cigna.com
Ed Hanway, CEO

★ 19287 ★ Community Choice/ Community Preferred Plan
PPO Plan
1351 William H. Taft Rd.
Cincinnati, OH 45206
Phone: (513)872-8100 **Fax:** (513)336-2021
Website: http://www.anthem-inc.com
Larry Glasscock, CEO

★ 19288 ★ Cooperative Health Network
PPO Plan
PO Box 2790
Toledo, OH 43606
Phone: (419)578-8009 **Fax:** (419)259-6001
Website: http://www.chnppo.com
Patrick R. Hylant, CEO

★ 19289 ★ Creative Health Plans
Stratford Pl.
4301 Darrow Rd.
Stow, OH 44224
Phone: (330)686-7030 **Free:** 800-266-5896
Fax: (330)686-7031

Website: http://www.creativehealthplans.com
Arthur W. Chandler, Chairman of the Board

★ 19290 ★ DirectCare America, Inc.
PPO Plan
4301 Darrow Rd.
Strafford Pl.
Stow, OH 44224
Phone: (330)686-7030 **Free:** 800-266-5896
Fax: (330)686-7031
Website: http://www.directcareamerica.com
Arthur Chandler, Chairman of the Board

★ 19291 ★ Emerald Health Network, Inc.
PPO Plan
11499 Chester Rd.
Cincinnati, OH 45246
Phone: (216)479-2030 **Free:** 800-683-6830
Fax: (216)479-2039
Website: http://www.emeraldhealth.com
Burt Bundgus, Chairman of the Board

★ 19292 ★ Emerald PPO, Inc.
PPO Plan
1100 Superior Ave., 16th Fl.
Cleveland, OH 44114
Phone: (216)479-2030 **Free:** 800-683-6830
Fax: (216)479-2039
Website: http://www.emeraldhealth.com
Peter R. Osenar, CEO & Pres

★ 19293 ★ EMH Regional Health Care System
PPO Plan
630 E River St.
Elyria, OH 44035-5902
Phone: (440)329-7500 **Fax:** (440)329-7507
Website: http://www.emh-healthcare.org
Kevin Martin, CEO

★ 19294 ★ Flora Health Network
PPO Plan
4511 Rockside Rd., Ste. 320
Cleveland, OH 44131
Phone: (216)464-8090 **Free:** 800-966-0200
Fax: (216)642-9644
Website: http://www.floramidwest.com
Jeff Connolly, CEO

★ 19295 ★ Great West
PPO Plan
445 Hutchinson Ave., Ste. 240
Columbus, OH 43235
Phone: (614)848-5369 **Fax:** (614)848-3593
Website: http://www.onehealthplan.com
Jack West, Chairman of the Board

★ 19296 ★ Health Design Plus
PPO Plan
1755 Georgetown Rd.
Hudson, OH 44236
Phone: (330)656-1072 **Free:** 800-877-5843
Fax: (330)656-9387
Website: http://www.hdplus.com
M. Ruth Coleman, CEO

★ 19297 ★ Health Payors Organization Ltd.
4301 Darrow Rd.
Stow, OH 44224
Phone: (330)686-7040 **Free:** 800-337-3677
Fax: (330)686-7041
Website: http://www.hpoltd.com
Arthur W. Chandler, Chairman of the Board

★ 19298 ★ Hometown Health Network
PPO Plan
100 Lillian Gish Blvd., Ste. 301
Massillon, OH 44647
Phone: (330)837-6880 **Free:** 800-426-9013
Fax: (330)837-6869
Website: http://www.hometownhealth.com
William Epling, President

★ 19299 ★ Integra Group
16 Triangle Park Dr., Ste. 1600
Cincinnati, OH 45246
Phone: (513)326-5600 **Free:** 800-424-8384
Fax: (513)326-5614
Kathleen J. Lutz, President

★ 19300 ★ John Alden Life
PPO Plan
5500 Glendon Ct.
Dublin, OH 43017
Phone: (614)764-9300 **Free:** 800-366-6762
Fax: (614)798-2023
Website: http://www.us.fortis.com
Ben Cutler, CEO

★ 19301 ★ Medical Mutual of Ohio
PPO Plan
2060 E 9th St.
Cleveland, OH 44115
Phone: (216)687-7000 **Free:** 800-782-3651
Fax: (419)473-6033
Website: http://www.mmoh.com
Kent Clapp, CEO & Pres

★ 19302 ★ Nationwide Health Plans
PPO Plan
5525 Park Center Circle
Dublin, OH 43017-3685
Phone: (614)854-3001 **Free:** 800-826-9017
Fax: (614)854-3648
Website: http://www.nationwide-health.com
Joe SanFilippo, CEO

★ 19303 ★ Ohio Health Choice
PPO Plan
PO Box 93538
Cleveland, OH 44101
Phone: (440)250-4700 **Free:** 800-554-0027
Fax: (440)250-9872
Website: http://www.ohiohealthchoice.com
Joanie Mason, CEO

★ 19304 ★ Ohio State University Managed Health Care Systems, Inc.
PPO Plan
1375 Perry St., Ste. 40, 6th Fl.
Columbus, OH 43201
Phone: (614)293-2054 **Free:** 800-447-5836
Fax: (614)293-2297
Website: http://www.osumhcs.com
Fred Sanfilippo, MD,PhD, President

★ 19305 ★ One Health Plan of Ohio
PPO Plan
24950 Country Club Blvd., Ste. 400
North Olmsted, OH 44070
Phone: (440)716-1777 **Free:** 800-644-9335
Fax: (440)716-1221
Website: http://www.onehealthplan.com
William McCallum, CEO

★ 19306 ★ Paramount Health Care Plan
PPO Plan
1901 Indian Wood Cr.
Maumee, OH 43537-4068
Phone: (419)887-2500 **Free:** 800-462-3589
Fax: (419)887-2530
Website: http://www.promedica.org
John Randolph, CEO

★ 19307 ★ Primary Health Services, Inc.
PPO Plan
4301 Darrow Rd.
Stratford Pl.
Stow, OH 44224
Phone: (330)686-7050 **Free:** 800-266-5896
Fax: (330)686-7031
Website: http://www.primaryhealthservices.com
Arthur Chandler, Chairman of the Board

★ 19308 ★ QualChoice
PPO Plan
6000 Parkland Blvd.
Cleveland, OH 44124
Phone: (440)460-0093 **Free:** 800-208-1232
Fax: (440)460-4005
Website: http://www.qchp.com
Thomas Sullivan, CEO

★ 19309 ★ SummaCare, Inc.
PPO Plan
PO Box 3620
Akron, OH 44309-3620
Phone: (330)996-8410 **Free:** 800-996-8411
Fax: (330)996-8454
Website: http://www.summacare.com
Martin Hanser, CEO

★ 19310 ★ Superien Health Network, Inc.
Stratford Pl.
4301 Darrow Rd.
Stow, OH 44224
Phone: (330)689-7025 **Free:** 888-315-6045
Fax: (330)686-7087
Website: http://www.superienhealthnetwork.com
Arthur W. Chandler, Chairman of the Board

★ 19311 ★ United HealthCare of Ohio, Inc.
PPO Plan
9200 Worthington Rd.
Westerville, OH 43082
Phone: (614)410-7000 **Free:** 883-328-8835
Fax: (614)410-1011
Website: http://www.uhc.com
Brett Baby, CEO

★ 19312 ★ United Healthcare of Ohio Inc. - Cleveland
13775 E 9th St., Ste. 700
Cleveland, OH 44114
Free: 800-225-7951
Website: http://www.uhc.com
Ken Hoverman, CEO

★ 19313 ★ United HealthCare of Ohio, Inc. - Dayton/Cincinnati
PPO Plan
9050 Centre Pointe Dr., Ste. 400
West Chester, OH 45069
Free: 877-832-7734 **Fax:** (937)439-8999
Website: http://www.uhc.com
Tom Brady, CEO

★ 19314 ★ Universal Preferred Health Network
PPO Plan
110 Boggs Ln., Ste. 460
Cincinnati, OH 45246
Phone: (513)772-3933 **Free:** 800-766-8746
Fax: (513)772-9174
Richard Rostowsky, CEO

★ 19315 ★ Vantage Health Plan
PPO Plan
4602 Timber Commons Dr.
Sandusky, OH 44870

Phone: (419)621-9858 **Free:** 800-878-4394
Fax: (419)621-9859
Website: http://www.vantagehealthplan.com
Dr. Shukirk, CEO

Oklahoma

★ 19316 ★ Aetna Inc. - Tulsa
PPO Plan
7912 E 31st Ct., Ste. 300
Tulsa, OK 74145-1339
Phone: (918)624-4700 **Free:** 800-435-8310
Fax: (918)627-9759
Website: http://www.aetna.com
John W. Rowe, Chairman of the Board

★ 19317 ★ CIGNA HealthCare of Oklahoma
PPO Plan
4110 Perimeter Center Dr., Ste. 240
Oklahoma City, OK 73112
Phone: (405)943-7711 **Free:** 800-959-8232
Fax: (405)946-9568
Website: http://www.cigna.com
Rick Grizzle, Contact

★ 19318 ★ CommunityCare Managed Healthcare Plans of Oklahoma, Inc.
PPO Plan
PO Box 3249
Tulsa, OK 74101
Phone: (918)594-5200 **Free:** 800-278-7563
Fax: (918)594-5260
Website: http://www.ccmhp.com
Richard Todd, CEO & Pres

★ 19319 ★ PPO Oklahoma, Inc.
PPO Plan
3503 NW 63rd St., Ste. 304
Oklahoma City, OK 73116
Phone: (405)843-9551 **Fax:** (405)843-0956
Website: http://www.ppooklahoma.com
Martin Sholder, CEO

Oregon

★ 19320 ★ Health Net Health Plan of Oregon, Inc.
12901 SE 97th Ave.
Clackamas, OR 97015
Phone: (503)802-7000 **Free:** 888-802-7001
Fax: (503)802-7136
Website: http://www.qualmed.com
Stephen Lynch, CEO

★ 19321 ★ Lifewise, A Premera Health Plan
3020 SW 4th Ave., Ste. 1000
Portland, OR 97201
Phone: (503)295-6707 **Fax:** (503)279-5295
Website: http://www.premera.com
Mark Charpentier, CEO

★ 19322 ★ Managed HealthCare Northwest, Inc. (MHN)
PPO Plan
1120 NW 20th Ave., No. 200
Portland, OR 97209-1539
Phone: (503)413-5800 **Free:** 800-648-6356
Fax: (503)413-5801
Website: http://www.mhninc.com
Dolores Russell, CEO & Pres

★ 19323 ★ ODS Health Plan
PPO Plan
601 SW 2nd Ave.
Portland, OR 97204
Phone: (503)228-6554 **Fax:** (503)948-5558
Website: http://www.odshp.com
Robert Gootee, CEO

★ 19324 ★ One Health Plan of Oregon, Inc.
PPO Plan
1800 SW First Ave., Ste. 230
Portland, OR 97201
Phone: (503)222-3014 **Fax:** (503)222-3253
Website: http://www.onehealthplan.com
Sara Mason, Contact

★ 19325 ★ Pacific Source Health Plans
PPO Plan
250 Country Club Rd.
Eugene, OR 97401-0068
Phone: (541)686-1242 **Free:** 800-624-6052
Fax: (541)485-0915
Website: http://www.pacificsource.com
Robert Loomis, MD, Contact

★ 19326 ★ Providence Health Plans
PPO Plan
3601 SW Murray Blvd.
Beaverton, OR 97005
Free: 800-826-7218 **Fax:** (503)574-8600
Website: http://www.providence.org
Russ Danielson, CEO

★ 19327 ★ Regence HMO Oregon
PPO Plan
100 SW Market
Portland, OR 97201
Phone: (503)364-4868 **Free:** 800-452-7278
Fax: (503)225-4848
Website: http://www.regence.com
Richard L. Woolworth, Chairman of the Board

Pennsylvania

★ 19328 ★ Aetna Inc. of Central and Eastern Pennsylvania
PPO Plan
2201 Renaissance Blvd.
Norristown, PA 19406
Phone: (484)322-2000 **Fax:** (484)322-6437
Website: http://www.aetna.com
John W. Rowe, MD, Chairman of the Board

★ 19329 ★ Aetna Inc. - Corporate Headquarters
PPO Plan
PO Box 1109
Blue Bell, PA 19422-1109
Phone: (215)775-4800 **Free:** 800-872-3862
Fax: (215)775-6401
Website: http://www.aetna.com
John W. Rowe, MD, Chairman of the Board

★ 19330 ★ Aetna Inc. - Pennsylvania
PPO Plan
5313 Campbell's Run Rd.
Pittsburgh, PA 15205-2758
Phone: (412)788-0500 **Fax:** (412)788-5067
Website: http://www.aetna.com
John W. Rowe, MD, Chairman of the Board

★ 19331 ★ Aetna Inc. - Pennsylvania Region
PPO Plan
PO Box 1109
Blue Bell, PA 19422-1109
Phone: (215)775-4800 **Fax:** (215)775-6401
Website: http://www.aetna.com
John W. Rowe, MD, Chairman of the Board

★ 19332 ★ Alliance Health Plan
PPO Plan
PO Box 7507
Lancaster, PA 17604
Phone: (717)291-8416 **Fax:** (717)391-7833
Website: http://www.ahp-ppo.com
Larry W. Rodabauch, CEO

★ 19333 ★ Berkshire Health Plan/Medicus Resource Management
PPO Plan
50 Commerce Ct.
Wyomissing, PA 19610
Phone: (610)372-8044 **Fax:** (610)371-0310
Website: http://www.bhp.org
Charles Wills, President

★ 19334 ★ Blue Ridge Health Network
PPO Plan
1900 W End Ave.
Pottsville, PA 17901
Phone: (570)628-2236 **Free:** 800-730-0134
Fax: (570)628-1880
Website: http://www.blueridgehealthnetwork.com
Robert Jones, President

★ 19335 ★ Bucks County Physician Hospital Alliance
PPO Plan
595 W State St.
Doylestown, PA 18901
Phone: (215)345-2119 **Fax:** (215)345-2633
Website: http://www.bcpha.com
Sherri Putnam, CEO

★ 19336 ★ Central Susquehanna Healthcare
PPO Plan
1 Hospital Dr.
Lewisburg, PA 17837
Phone: (570)522-2748 **Fax:** (570)522-4072
Website: http://www.cshpnetwork.com
Marcia Cooney, Contact

★ 19337 ★ CIGNA Healthcare - Corporate Headquarters
PPO Plan
One Liberty Pl.
1650 Market St.
Philadelphia, PA 19192-1550
Phone: (215)761-1000 **Fax:** (215)761-5517
Website: http://www.cigna.com
H. Edward Hanway, CEO
Program(s): Chiropractic, Dental, Home Care, Inpatient SNF, Long-Term Care, Pharmaceutical Mail Order, Podiatry, Psychiatric, Transplant, Vision, Wellness, Workers' Compensation.

★ 19338 ★ Clear-Care Corp. - Corporate Headquarters
PPO Plan
1229 S 2nd St.
Clearfield, PA 16830
Phone: (814)765-0221 **Fax:** (814)765-3011
Website: http://www.clearcarecorp.com
S. Maureen Rafferty, President

★ 19339 ★ Clear-Choice Corp.
PPO Plan
PO Box 1442
Clearfield, PA 16830
Phone: (814)765-0221 **Fax:** (814)765-3011
Website: http://www.clearcarecorp.com
James P. Davidson, MD, Chairman of the Board

★ 19340 ★ Coordinated Health Systems
PPO Plan
2775 Schoenersville Rd.
Bethlehem, PA 18017
Phone: (610)861-8111 **Fax:** (610)807-0366
Website: http://www.chs4health
Emil DiLorio, MD, CEO

★ 19341 ★ Crawford Health Plan
PPO Plan
PO Box 455
Meadville, PA 16335
Phone: (814)333-5247 **Fax:** (814)333-5244
Website: http://www.mmchs.org
Anthony Defail, CEO

★ 19342 ★ Devon Health Services, Inc.
PPO Plan
1100 1st Ave.
King of Prussia, PA 19406
Phone: (610)265-8000 **Free:** 800-431-2273
Fax: (610)768-4509
Website: http://www.devonhealth.com
John Bennett, MD, CEO

★ 19343 ★ Eastern Pennsylvania Health Network
PPO Plan
65 E Elizabeth Ave., Ste. 410
Bethlehem, PA 18018
Phone: (610)954-3577 **Free:** 800-422-7340
Fax: (610)954-6500
Website: http://www.ephn.com
Anne Baum, Contact

★ 19344 ★ Geisinger Health Plan
PPO Plan
100 N Academy Ave.
Danville, PA 17822-3020
Phone: (717)271-8760 **Free:** 800-631-1656
Fax: (717)271-5218
Website: http://www.thehealthplan.edu
Dr. Glen Steele, Jr., CEO
Program(s): Chiropractic, Home Care, Inpatient SNF, Pharmaceutical Mail Order, Podiatry, Psychiatric, Behavioral Health, Physical Therapy, Transplant, Vision, Wellness.

★ 19345 ★ HealthAmerica of Central Pennsylvania
PPO Plan
2575 Interstate Dr.
Harrisburg, PA 17110
Phone: (717)540-4260 **Free:** 800-788-6445
Fax: (717)541-5739
Website: http://www.healthamerica.cvty.com
Francis Soistman, Jr., CEO

★ 19346 ★ HealthAmerica Pennsylvania, Inc. - Western Region
PPO Plan
5 Gateway Center
Pittsburgh, PA 15222
Phone: (412)553-7522 **Free:** 800-735-4404
Fax: (412)553-7523
Website: http://www.healthamerica.cvty.com
Francis Soistman, Jr., CEO

★ 19347 ★ Integra, Inc.
PPO Plan
1060 1st Ave., Ste. 410
King of Prussia, PA 19406
Phone: (610)992-2600 **Free:** 800-544-3573
Fax: (610)992-7046
Website: http://www.integra-ease.com
Gregory Santore, CEO

★ 19348 ★ Intergroup Services Corp.
PPO Plan
101 Lindenwood Dr., Ste. 150
Malvern, PA 19355
Phone: (610)640-0646 **Free:** 800-537-9389
Fax: (610)647-5383
Website: http://www.igs-ppo.com
G. Martin Dudley, CEO

★ 19349 ★ Keystone Health Plan East Inc.
PPO Plan
1901 Market St.
Philadelphia, PA 19103
Phone: (215)241-2001 **Free:** 800-227-3114
Fax: (215)241-2017
Website: http://www.khpe.com
G. Fred DiBona, CEO & Pres

★ 19350 ★ Mercer First Choice
PPO Plan
740 E State St.
Sharon, PA 16146
Phone: (724)983-3801 **Fax:** (724)983-3958
Wayne Johnston, CEO

★ 19351 ★ Mercy Workcare
PPO Plan
2821 Island Ave., Ste. 147
Philadelphia, PA 19153
Phone: (215)365-4606 **Fax:** (215)863-2368
Website: http://www.mercyhealth.org
Elizabeth Genovese-Stone, MD, Contact

★ 19352 ★ Metro Health Plan
PPO Plan
223 4th Ave.
1100 Benedum T. Bldg.
Pittsburgh, PA 15222
Phone: (412)355-5009 **Fax:** (412)355-5094
Robert E. Hagan, Jr., CEO

★ 19353 ★ Mid-Atlantic Managed Care Organization of Pennsylvania, Inc.
PPO Plan
PO Box 1060
Gettysburg, PA 17325
Phone: (717)334-9247 **Free:** 800-497-4474
Fax: (717)334-9167
Ronald Pack, CLU, CEO & Pres

★ 19354 ★ New Alliance Health Plan
PPO Plan
1700 Peach St., Ste. 244
Erie, PA 16501
Phone: (814)878-1700 **Free:** 800-255-4281
Fax: (814)452-4358
Website: http://www.newalliancehealth.com
Joseph Prischak, Chairman of the Board

★ 19355 ★ One Health Plan of Pennsylvania, Inc.
PPO Plan
8 Penn Center
1628 JFK Blvd., Ste. 1010
Philadelphia, PA 19103
Phone: (215)832-3400 **Free:** 800-303-4635
Fax: (215)832-3441
Website: http://www.onehealthplan.com
Dan Dragalin, MD, President

★ 19356 ★ Penn Highlands Health Plan
PPO Plan
1086 Franklin St.
Johnstown, PA 15905
Phone: (814)536-7525 **Fax:** (814)533-1544
Website: http://www.conemaugh.org
Jack Lipomi, President

★ 19357 ★ Preferred Care, Inc.
PPO Plan
6 Neshaminy Interplex, Ste. 205
Trevose, PA 19053
Phone: (215)639-6208 **Fax:** (215)639-2674
Richard Matthew, President

★ 19358 ★ Preferred Health Care
PPO Plan
PO Box 4824
Lancaster, PA 17604
Phone: (717)560-9290 **Fax:** (717)560-2312
Website: http://www.phcunity.com
Cynthia Smith, CEO

★ 19359 ★ Preferred Healthcare Systems, Inc.
PPO Plan
620 Howard Ave.
Altoona, PA 16601
Phone: (814)949-3099 **Free:** 800-238-9900
Fax: (814)949-3166
Website: http://www.phsppo.com
Joseph Fromknecht, Contact

★ 19360 ★ Primesource Health Network
PPO Plan
409 S 2nd St., Ste. 2C
Harrisburg, PA 17104
Phone: (717)230-3400 **Fax:** (717)230-3411
Robin Scherer, Contact

★ 19361 ★ SelectCare Access Corp.
PPO Plan
820 Parish St.
Pittsburgh, PA 15220
Phone: (412)922-0780 **Fax:** (412)922-3071
Phyllis Shehab, CEO

★ 19362 ★ South Central Preferred
PPO Plan
1803 Mt. Rose Ave., Ste. B5
York, PA 17403
Phone: (717)851-6800 **Free:** 800-842-1768
Fax: (717)851-6775
Charles Chodroff, MD, CEO

★ 19363 ★ Susquehanna Health Care
109 N Mulberry St.
Berwick, PA 18603-4706
Phone: (570)759-1702 **Fax:** (570)759-2559
William Cusatis, CEO & Pres
Program(s): Home Care, Inpatient SNF, Pharmaceutical Mail Order, Podiatry, Psychiatric, Behavioral Health, Physical Therapy, Transplant, Wellness.

★ 19364 ★ United Behavioral Health
100 E Penn Sq., Ste. 400
Philadelphia, PA 19107
Phone: (215)557-6126
Website: http://www.uhc.com
Saul Feldman, CEO

★ 19365 ★ Valley Preferred
PPO Plan
2166 S 12th St., Ste. 401
Allentown, PA 18103-4799
Phone: (610)402-7485 **Free:** 800-955-6620
Fax: (610)402-7439
John Jaffe, MD, Chairman of the Board

★ 19366 ★ Valuscript PSAO
PO Box 2448
Altoona, PA 16603
Phone: (814)944-9316 **Fax:** (814)944-9553
John Letizia, CEO

Puerto Rico

★ 19367 ★ Humana, Inc./PCA - Puerto Rico
PPO Plan
383 FD Roosevelt, 3rd Fl.
San Juan, PR 00918-2131
Phone: (787)282-7900 **Free:** 800-314-3121
Fax: (787)282-6277
Website: http://www.humana.com
Drayton Nabers, Jr., CEO

Rhode Island

★ 19368 ★ United Health Plans of New England
475 Kilvert St.
Warwick, RI 02886-1392
Phone: (401)737-6900 **Free:** 800-447-1245
Fax: (401)732-7210
Website: http://www.uhc.com
Bud Fisher, CEO

South Carolina

★ 19369 ★ Companion Healthcare Corp.
PPO Plan
4101 Percical Rd.
Columbia, SC 29223
Phone: (803)786-8466 **Free:** 800-327-3183
Fax: (803)714-6461
Website: http://www.companionhealthcare.com
Ed Sails, CEO

★ 19370 ★ Kanawha HealthCare Solutions
PPO Plan
PO Box 610
Lancaster, SC 29721-0610
Phone: (803)283-5300 **Free:** 800-822-1274
Fax: (803)283-5410
Website: http://www.khsonline.com
Stan Johnson, CEO

★ 19371 ★ Physicians Care Network
PPO Plan
PO Box 101111
Columbia, SC 29211
Phone: (803)750-7028 **Free:** 888-327-1021
Fax: (803)771-9474
Website: http://www.scmanet.org
William Mahon, CEO

★ 19372 ★ St. Francis Optimum Health Network
PPO Plan
86 A Villa Rd.
Greenville, SC 29615
Phone: (864)213-4989 **Fax:** (864)213-4928
Website: http://www.st.francishealth.com
Steve Poole, CEO

South Dakota

★ 19373 ★ Araz Great Plains
PPO Plan
2900 E 26th St., Ste. 305
Sioux Falls, SD 57103
Phone: (605)330-9010 **Fax:** (605)330-4196
Website: http://www.araz.com
M. Nazie Eftekhari, CEO

★ 19374 ★ First Choice of the Midwest, Inc.
PPO Plan
PO Box 5078
Sioux Falls, SD 57103
Phone: (605)332-5955 **Fax:** (605)332-5953
Website: http://www.1choicem.com
Mike Hagert, CEO

Tennessee

★ 19375 ★ Aetna US Healthcare - Tennessee
PPO Plan
1801 W End Ave., Ste. 500
Palmer Plaza
Nashville, TN 37203
Phone: (615)322-1600 **Fax:** (615)322-1646
Website: http://www.aetna.com
John W. Rowe, MD, Chairman of the Board

★ 19376 ★ Baptist Health Services Group
PPO Plan
6750 Poplar Ave., Ste. 301
Memphis, TN 38138-7445
Phone: (901)759-5000 **Fax:** (901)759-5001
Website: http://www.bmhcc.org
David Elliot, CEO

★ 19377 ★ Baptist Health Services Group
PPO Plan
6750 Poplar Ave., Ste. 301
Memphis, TN 38138-7445
Phone: (901)759-5000 **Fax:** (901)759-5001
Website: http://www.bmhcc.org
David Elliot, CEO

★ 19378 ★ Cariten Healthcare
PPO Plan
1420 Centerpoint Blvd.
Knoxville, TN 37932
Phone: (865)470-7470 **Free:** 800-793-1495
Fax: (865)670-7255
Website: http://www.cariten.com
Lance Hunsinger, CEO & Pres

★ 19379 ★ CIGNA HealthCare of Tennessee, Inc.
PPO Plan
6555 Quince Rd., Ste. 215
Memphis, TN 38119
Free: 800-832-3211 **Fax:** (901)758-5110
Website: http://www.cigna.com
William Pastore, CEO

★ 19380 ★ Focus Healthcare Management, Inc.
PPO Plan
720 Cool Springs Blvd., Ste. 300
Franklin, TN 37067
Phone: (615)778-4000 **Fax:** (615)778-0915
Website: http://www.focus-ppo.com
Thomas Cox, CEO & Pres

★ 19381 ★ Health Choice, LLC
PPO Plan
1000 Brookfield, 2nd Fl.
Memphis, TN 38104
Phone: (901)821-6700 **Free:** 800-328-2579
Fax: (901)821-6751
Website: http://www.healthchoice.org
William Breen, Jr., CEO

★ 19382 ★ Health Springs
PPO Plan
44 Vantage Way, Ste. 300
Nashville, TN 37228
Phone: (615)291-7000 **Fax:** (615)291-7011
Website: http://www.myhealthspring.com
Herbert A. Fritch, CEO

★ 19383 ★ HealthNow
PPO Plan
5959 Park Ave.
Memphis, TN 38119
Phone: (901)765-3190 **Fax:** (901)765-3179
Dave Archer, CEO

★ 19384 ★ Initial Group, Inc.
PPO Plan
PO Box 3818
Knoxville, TN 37927-3818
Phone: (865)546-1893 **Free:** 800-858-3203
Fax: (865)546-2126
Website: http://www.intitialgroup.com
Lisa Wear, CEO

★ 19385 ★ PHP Companies, Inc.
PPO Plan
1420 Centerpoint Blvd.
Knoxville, TN 37932
Phone: (865)470-7470 **Free:** 800-747-0008
Fax: (865)470-7485
Tony Stezia, CEO

★ 19386 ★ Signature Health Alliance
PPO Plan
618 Church St., Ste. 301
Nashville, TN 37219
Phone: (615)251-4674 **Free:** 800-264-3060
Fax: (615)251-1782
Website: http://www.signaturehealth.com
Barbara Dowl, President

★ 19387 ★ Tennessee Healthcare LLC.
1620 Westgate Circle, Ste. 225
Brentwood, TN 37027
Phone: (615)301-4500 **Fax:** (615)301-4501
Tom McElroy, President

★ 19388 ★ United HealthCare of Tennessee, Inc.
PPO Plan
10 Cadillac Dr.
Brentwood, TN 37027
Phone: (615)372-3622 **Free:** 800-695-1273
Fax: (615)372-3640
Website: http://www.uhc.com
C. Brian Shipp, CEO

Texas

★ 19389 ★ Accountable Health Plans of America
PPO Plan
600 Six Flags Dr., Ste. 200
Arlington, TX 76011
Phone: (817)633-8335 **Free:** 800-613-1124
Fax: (817)640-1009
Website: http://ww.ahppo.com
Lovie Pollinger, CEO

★ 19390 ★ Aetna Inc. - Austin
PPO Plan
7700 Chevy Chase Dr., Ste. 500
Austin, TX 78752
Phone: (512)323-0440 **Fax:** (512)465-5441
Website: http://www.aetna.com
John W. Rowe, MD, Chairman of the Board

★ 19391 ★ Aetna Inc. - El Paso
PPO Plan
100 N Stanton, Ste. 1301
El Paso, TX 79901-1448
Phone: (915)532-0700 **Fax:** (915)532-0342
Website: http://www.aetna.com
John W. Rowe, MD, Chairman of the Board

★ 19392 ★ Aetna Inc. - Houston
PPO Plan
3 Greenway Plaza, MS G-201
Houston, TX 77046
Phone: (713)350-2260 **Free:** 800-876-7778
Fax: (713)350-2920
Website: http://www.aetna.com
John W. Rowe, MD, Chairman of the Board

★ 19393 ★ Aetna Inc. of North Texas
PPO Plan
2777 Stemmons Frwy.
Dallas, TX 75207
Phone: (214)200-8000 **Free:** 800-992-7947
Fax: (214)200-8580
Website: http://www.aetna.com
John W. Rowe, MD, Chairman of the Bcard

★ 19394 ★ Alliance Regional Health Network
PO Box 51980
Amarillo, TX 79159-1980
Phone: (806)351-5151 **Free:** 800-687-8007
Fax: (806)351-5159
Website: http://www.nwtexashealthcare.com
Scott Carlisle, Contact

★ 19395 ★ AmCareCo, Inc. - Corporate Headquarters
PPO Plan
3411 Richmond Ave., Ste. 500
Houston, TX 77046-3409
Phone: (713)985-4100 **Free:** 800-782-8373
Fax: (713)985-4101
Website: http://www.amcarehealthplans.com
Thomas Lucksinger, CEO

★ 19396 ★ American National Insurance Co.
PPO Plan
1 Moody Plaza
Galveston, TX 77550
Phone: (409)763-4661 **Free:** 800-899-6808
Fax: (409)766-6663
Website: http://www.anico.com
Robert Moody, CEO

★ 19397 ★ American Preferred Provider Organization LLC
PO Box 6008
Arlington, TX 76011
Free: 877-233-3372 **Fax:** (817)633-4557
Website: http://www.ahcp.org

★ 19398 ★ Brazos Valley Health Network
PPO Plan
3201 Pine Ave.
Waco, TX 76710
Phone: (254)202-5320 **Fax:** (254)202-5310
Website: http://www.hillcrest.net
Mike Burchardt, CEO

★ 19399 ★ CCN - Colorado
PPO Plan
5501 LBJ Fwy., Ste 1200-1201
Dallas, TX 75240
Phone: (972)387-0100 **Free:** 877-366-3415
Fax: (972)387-1076
Website: http://www.ccnusa.com
Patrick G. Dills, President

★ 19400 ★ CCN - Idaho
PPO Plan
5501 LBJ Fwy., Ste. 1200-1201
Dallas, TX 75240
Phone: (972)387-0100 **Free:** 877-366-3415
Fax: (972)387-1076
Website: http://www.ccnusa.com
Patrick G. Dills, President

★ 19401 ★ CCN - Illinois
PPO Plan
5501 LBJ Fwy., Ste. 1200-1201
Dallas, TX 75240
Phone: (972)387-0100 **Free:** 877-366-3415
Fax: (972)387-1076
Website: http://www.ccnusa.com
Patrick G. Dills, President

★ 19402 ★ CCN - Indiana
PPO Plan
5501 LBJ Fwy., Ste. 1200-1201
Dallas, TX 75240
Phone: (972)387-0100 **Free:** 877-366-3415
Fax: (972)387-1076
Website: http://www.ccnusa.com
Patrick G. Dills, President

★ 19403 ★ CCN - Iowa
PPO Plan
5501 LBJ Fwy., Ste. 1200-1201
Dallas, TX 75240
Phone: (972)387-0100 **Free:** 877-366-3415
Fax: (972)387-1076
Website: http://www.ccnusa.com
Patrick G. Dills, President

★ 19404 ★ CCN - Kansas
PPO Plan
5501 LBJ Fwy., Ste. 1200-1201
Dallas, TX 75240
Phone: (972)387-0100 **Free:** 877-366-3415
Fax: (972)387-1076
Website: http://www.ccnusa.com
Patrick G. Dills, President

★ 19405 ★ CCN - Michigan
PPO Plan
5501 LBJ Fwy., Ste. 1200-1201
Dallas, TX 75240
Phone: (972)387-0100 **Free:** 877-366-3415
Fax: (972)387-1076
Website: http://www.ccnusa.com
Patrick G. Dills, President

★ 19406 ★ CCN - Minnesota
PPO Plan
5501 LBJ Fwy., Ste 1200-1201
Dallas, TX 75240
Phone: (972)387-0100 **Free:** 877-366-3415
Fax: (972)387-1076
Website: http://www.ccnusa.com
Patrick G. Dills, President

★ 19407 ★ CCN - Missouri
PPO Plan
5501 LBJ Fwy., Ste. 1200-1201
Dallas, TX 75240
Phone: (972)387-0100 **Free:** 877-366-3415
Fax: (972)387-1076
Website: http://www.ccnusa.com
Patrick G. Dills, President

★ 19408 ★ CCN - Ohio
PPO Plan
5501 LBJ Fwy., Ste. 1200-1201
Dallas, TX 75240
Phone: (972)387-0100 **Free:** 877-366-3415
Fax: (972)387-1076
Website: http://www.ccnusa.com
Patrick G. Dills, President

★ 19409 ★ CCN - Oklahoma
PPO Plan
5501 LBJ Fwy., Ste. 1200-1201
Dallas, TX 75240
Phone: (972)387-0100 **Free:** 877-366-3415
Fax: (972)387-1076
Website: http://www.ccnusa.com
Patrick G. Dills, President

★ 19410 ★ CCN - Regional
PPO Plan
3625 W Raw Ln., Ste. 150
Irving, TX 75063
Phone: 800-231-2254 **Free:** 877-366-3415
Website: http://www.ccnusa.com
Patrick G. Dills, President

★ 19411 ★ CCN - Texas
PPO Plan
3625 W Raw Ln., Ste. 150
Irving, TX 75063
Phone: 800-231-2254 **Free:** 877-366-3415
Website: http://www.ccnusa.com
Patrick G. Dills, President

★ 19412 ★ CCN - Utah
PPO Plan
5501 LBJ Fwy., Ste. 1200-1201
Dallas, TX 75240
Phone: (972)387-0100 **Free:** 877-366-3415
Fax: (972)387-1076
Website: http://www.ccnusa.com
Patrick G. Dills, President

★ 19413 ★ CCN - Wisconsin
PPO Plan
5501 LBJ Fwy., Ste. 1200-1201
Dallas, TX 75240
Phone: (972)387-0100 **Free:** 877-366-3415
Fax: (972)387-1076
Website: http://www.ccnusa.com
Patrick G. Dills, President

★ 19414 ★ CCN - Wyoming
PPO Plan
5501 LBJ Fwy., Ste. 1200-1201
Dallas, TX 75240
Phone: (972)387-0100 **Free:** 877-366-3415
Fax: (972)387-1076
Website: http://www.ccnusa.com
Patrick G. Dills, President

★ 19415 ★ CIGNA Healthcare of North Texas
PPO Plan
6600 E Campus Circle Dr., Ste. 400
Irving, TX 75063
Phone: (972)263-2718 **Free:** 800-772-4462
Fax: (972)582-7618
Website: http://www.cigna.com
Ken Malcomson, CEO

★ 19416 ★ CIGNA Healthcare of Texas, Inc.
PPO Plan
2 Riverway, Ste. 1200
Houston, TX 77056
Phone: (713)552-7600 **Free:** 800-772-4462
Fax: (713)552-7699
Website: http://www.cigna.com
Pat Stewart, CEO

★ 19417 ★ Corphealth, Inc.
1300 Summit, Ste. 600
Fort Worth, TX 76102
Phone: (817)332-2519 **Fax:** (817)335-9100
Website: http://www.corphealth.com
Patrick D. Gotcher, CEO

★ 19418 ★ Forte-Compkey
PPO Plan
7600 Chevy Chase Dr., Ste. 400
Austin, TX 78752
Phone: (512)371-8100 **Free:** 800-580-4567
Fax: (512)371-0327
Ronald Luke, CEO

★ 19419 ★ Fortis Health - Texas
16775 Addison Rd., Ste. 500
Addison, TX 75001
Free: 800-262-5388 **Fax:** (214)258-1102
Website: http://www.fortisbenefitsdental.com
Michael Hawkins, MD, Contact

★ 19420 ★ Galaxy Health Network
PO Box 2014725
Arlington, TX 76006-1425
Phone: (817)633-5822 **Fax:** (817)633-5729
Website: http://www.galaxyhealth.net
Ernie Parks, CEO

★ 19421 ★ Great West
PPO Plan
4807 Spice Woods Spring, Ste. 200
Austin, TX 78759
Phone: (512)345-3565 **Fax:** (512)345-4964
Website: http://www.onehealthplan.com
Steve Quenville, Contact

★ 19422 ★ HAS Premier Providers, Inc.
PPO Plan
100 Glenborough, Ste. 450
Houston, TX 77067-3610
Phone: (281)873-8682 **Free:** 800-749-2714
Fax: (281)872-4669
Website: http://www.hasonline.com
Steve Gaven, CEO

★ 19423 ★ Healthcare Partners of East Texas, Inc.
PPO Plan
PO Box 2749
Longview, TX 75606
Phone: (903)238-8845 **Free:** 800-362-3041
Fax: (903)757-6204
Website: http://www.hpet.org
Joy McGee-Cory, CEO & Pres

★ 19424 ★ Humana Health Care Plans of Corpus Christi
PPO Plan
802 N Carancahua, Ste. 1700
Corpus Christi, TX 78470
Phone: (361)866-2239 **Fax:** (361)866-2299
Website: http://www.humana.com/corpuschristi/home.html
David Jones, Chairman of the Board

★ 19425 ★ Humana Health Care Plans of Dallas
PPO Plan
8111 LBJ Freeway., Ste. 1500
Dallas, TX 75251
Phone: (972)643-1600 **Free:** 800-651-9079
Fax: (972)437-9243
Website: http://www.humana.com/dallas/home.html
David A. Jones, Chairman of the Board

★ 19426 ★ Humana Health Care Plans of Houston
PPO Plan
1980 Post Oak Blvd., Ste. 1900
Houston, TX 77056
Phone: (713)622-6639 **Fax:** (713)622-6649
Website: http://www.humana.com/houston/home.html
Ken Janda, CEO & Pres

★ 19427 ★ Humana Health Plan of Austin
PPO Plan
1221 S Mopac Blvd., Ste. 200
Austin, TX 78746
Phone: (512)338-6100 **Free:** 800-234-7912
Fax: (512)338-6137
Website: http://www.humana.com/austin/austin.html
David Jones, Chairman of the Board

★ 19428 ★ Medical Care Referral Group
PPO Plan
4100 Rio Bravo, Ste. 211
El Paso, TX 79902-1010
Phone: (915)532-2100 **Fax:** (915)532-1772
Website: http://www.mcrg.net
Lorri Halow, CEO

★ 19429 ★ Mega Life & Health Insurance Co.
4001 McEwen, Ste. 200
Dallas, TX 75244
Phone: (972)392-6700 **Free:** 800-767-0700
Fax: (972)392-6721
Website: http://www.vici.net
Greg Metz, CEO

★ 19430 ★ National HealthCare Alliance, Inc.
PPO Plan
770 S Post Oak Ln., Ste. 445
Houston, TX 77056
Phone: (713)888-1902 **Free:** 800-759-3118
Fax: (713)888-1986
Website: http://www.nhausa.com
Robert Woolfolk, CEO
Program(s): Chiropractic, Dental, Home Care, Inpatient SNF, Pharmaceutical Mail Order, Podiatry, Psychiatric, Behavioral Health, Physical Therapy, Transplant, Vision, Wellness, Workers' Compensation.

★ 19431 ★ North Texas Healthcare Network
PPO Plan
5601 N McArthur Blvd., Ste. 300
Irving, TX 75038
Phone: (972)751-2300 **Free:** 800-444-3995
Fax: (972)751-2415
Website: http://www.nthn.com
Robert Brown, CEO & Pres

★ 19432 ★ One Health Plan of Texas
PPO Plan
8310 Capitol of Texas Hwy. N, Ste. 340
Austin, TX 78731
Phone: (512)342-1706 **Fax:** (512)795-2105
Website: http://www.onehealthplan.com
Wally Gomaa, CEO

★ 19433 ★ One Health Plan of Texas - Dallas
PPO Plan
8350 N Central Expwy., Ste. M1000
Dallas, TX 75206
Phone: (972)813-7000 **Free:** 800-866-3136
Fax: (214)363-9785
Website: http://www.onehealthplan.com
Wally Gomaa, CEO

★ 19434 ★ Pacificare of Texas - Dallas
PPO Plan
5001 LBJ Fwy., Ste. 600
Dallas, TX 75244-6130
Phone: (972)866-1693 **Free:** 800-297-9355
Fax: (972)866-1970
Website: http://www.pacificare.com
George Becker, CEO

★ 19435 ★ PPONext
8225 King George, Ste. 300
Dallas, TX 75354
Phone: 800-860-6381 **Free:** 888-446-6098
Fax: (214)267-3345
Website: http://www.mdcl.com
Barbara Rodin, CEO

★ 19436 ★ Provider Networks of America
PPO Plan
4100 International Plaza, Ste. 400
Fort Worth, TX 76109
Phone: (817)735-8293 **Fax:** (817)735-8293
Website: http://www.providernetworks.com
Allen Rafeh, MD, CEO

★ 19437 ★ Seton Health Plan
PPO Plan
305 E Huntland Dr.
Austin, TX 78752
Phone: (512)324-4200 **Free:** 800-749-7404
Fax: (512)324-1952
Website: http://www.seton.net
John Evler, III, CEO

★ 19438 ★ Southwest Health Alliance (SHA LLC)
PPO Plan
12940 Research Blvd.
Austin, TX 78750
Phone: (512)257-6000 **Free:** 800-365-1051
Fax: (512)257-6037
Website: http://www.first.com
Keith Lundien, CEO

★ 19439 ★ Texas True Choice
5000 Legacy Dr., Ste 190
Plano, TX 75024
Free: 800-683-4856 **Fax:** (972)739-6614
Website: http://www.benplan.com
Michael Wilson, CEO

★ 19440 ★ UniCare Life and Health Insurance Co., Inc.
PPO Plan
11200 Westheimer Rd., Ste. 700
Houston, TX 77042
Phone: (281)914-3525 **Free:** 888-697-3790
Fax: (713)917-8175
Jeff Kamil, Contact

★ 19441 ★ United HealthCare of Texas, Inc. - Houston
PPO Plan
2000 W Loop S, Ste. 700
Houston, TX 77027-3416
Phone: (713)296-4800 **Fax:** (713)961-4431
Website: http://www.uhc.com
Steve C. Walli, CEO

★ 19442 ★ United HealthCare of Texas, Inc. - San Antonio
PPO Plan
8401 Datapoint Dr., Ste. 175
San Antonio, TX 78229
Phone: (210)617-6850 **Fax:** (210)617-6868
Website: http://www.uch.com
Thomas Quirk, CEO
Program(s): Chiropractic, Dental, Home Care, Inpatient SNF, Pharmaceutical Mail Order, Podiatry, Psychiatric, Behavioral Health, Physical Therapy, Transplant, Vision, Wellness.

Utah

★ 19443 ★ Altius Health Plans
PPO Plans
10421 S Jordan Gateway, Ste. 400
South Jordan, UT 84095
Phone: (801)355-1234 **Free:** 800-365-1334
Fax: (801)323-6100
Website: http://www.altiushealthplans.com
Larry Hancock, CEO

★ 19444 ★ CIGNA Health Plan of Utah, Inc.
PPO Plan
5295 South 320 West, Ste. 280
Salt Lake City, UT 84107
Phone: (801)265-2777 **Free:** 800-245-2471
Fax: (801)261-5349
Website: http://www.cigna.com
Robert Immitt, CEO & Pres

★ 19445 ★ Deseret Healthcare
PPO Plan
PO Box 45530
Salt Lake City, UT 84145-0530
Phone: (801)578-5600 **Free:** 800-777-3622
Fax: (801)578-5905
Website: http://www.dmba.com
Michael Stapley, CEO

★ 19446 ★ Educators Health Care
PPO Plan
852 E Arrowhead Ln.
Murray, UT 84107-6399
Phone: (801)262-7476 **Free:** 800-662-5850
Fax: (801)269-9734
Rolando Galano, CEO

★ 19447 ★ IHC Health Plans, Inc.
PPO Plan
4646 W Lake Park Blvd.
Salt Lake City, UT 84120
Phone: (801)442-5000 **Free:** 800-538-5038
Fax: (801)442-5183
Website: http://www.ihc.com
Richard J. Galbraith, Chairman of the Board

★ 19448 ★ United HealthCare of Utah, Inc.
PPO Plan
PO Box 71409
Salt Lake City, UT 84171-0409
Free: 800-624-2942 **Fax:** (801)947-0459
Website: http://www.uhc.com
Annette Herman, CEO

★ 19449 ★ Utah Public Employees Health Program
PPO Plan
560 East 200 South
Salt Lake City, UT 84102
Phone: (801)366-7555 **Fax:** (801)366-7596
Linn Baker, CEO

★ 19450 ★ ValuCare
PPO Plan
PO Box 25956
Salt Lake City, UT 84130
Phone: (801)333-2310 **Free:** 800-245-0026
Fax: (801)333-6523
John Ruch, CEO

Vermont

★ 19451 ★ CIGNA Managed Care Network of Northern New England
PPO Plan
30 Main St., Ste. 130
Burlington, VT 05401
Phone: (802)865-6309 **Fax:** (802)658-9212
Website: http://www.cigna.com
Linda Johnson, CEO

Virginia

★ 19452 ★ Aetna Health Plans of Mid-Atlantic
PPO Plan
7600 A Leesburg Pike
Falls Church, VA 22043
Phone: (703)903-7100 **Fax:** (703)903-0316
Website: http://www.aetna.com
John W. Rowe, MD, Chairman of the Board

★ 19453 ★ Aetna Inc. - Virginia
PPO Plan
1000 Boulders Pkwy.
Richmond, VA 23225
Phone: (804)323-0900 **Free:** 800-323-0467
Website: http://www.aetna.com
John W. Rowe, MD, CEO & Chm Bd

★ 19454 ★ Alexander Randolph, Inc.
8500 Leesburg Pike, Ste. 314
Vienna, VA 22182
Phone: (703)734-1507 **Fax:** (703)556-9264
Website: http://www.alexrand.com
Don Swabe, CEO

★ 19455 ★ Carilion Health Plans, Inc.
PPO Plan
110 Campbell Ave., Ste. 107
Roanoke, VA 24011
Phone: (540)857-5200 **Free:** 800-856-5206
Fax: (540)857-5343
Website: http://www.carilionhealthplans.com
Carolyn Chrisman, CEO

★ 19456 ★ CIGNA Healthcare of Virginia, Inc. - Richmond
PPO Plan
PO Box 31353
Richmond, VA 23294-1353
Phone: (804)267-5100 **Free:** 800-533-1708
Fax: (804)267-5062
Website: http://www.cigna.com
Matt Manders, CEO

★ 19457 ★ National Capital PPO
PPO Plan
6850 Versar Center, Ste. 420
Springfield, VA 22151
Phone: (703)914-5650 **Free:** 800-272-5911
Fax: (703)914-5685
Website: http://www.ncppo.com
Fredric Garner, MD, Contact

★ 19458 ★ Optima Health Plan, Inc.
PPO Plan
4417 Corporation Lane
Virginia Beach, VA 23462-3162
Phone: (757)552-7400 **Fax:** (757)687-6031
Website: http://www.optimahealth.com
Michael Dudley, President

★ 19459 ★ Southern Health Services, Inc.
PPO Plan
9881 Mayland Dr.
Richmond, VA 23233-1458
Phone: (804)747-3700 **Free:** 800-424-0077
Fax: (804)762-9349
Website: http://www.southernhealth.com
Cosby Davis, CEO

★ 19460 ★ United HealthCare of Virginia
PPO Plan
9020 Stony Point Pkwy., Ste. 400
Richmond, VA 23235
Phone: (804)267-5200 **Free:** 888-286-4908
Fax: (804)267-5285
Website: http://www.uhc.com
James Carney, MD, Contact

★ 19461 ★ ValueOptions - Corporate Headquarters
PPO Plan
3110 Fairview Park Dr. S
Falls Church, VA 22042
Phone: (703)205-7000 **Free:** 800-236-4648
Fax: (703)205-6505
Website: http://www.valueoptions.com
Ronald Dozoretz, Chairman of the Board

★ 19462 ★ Virginia Health Network, Inc.
PPO Plan
7400 Beaufont Springs Dr.
Richmond, VA 23225
Phone: (804)320-3837 **Free:** 800-989-3837
Fax: (804)320-5984
James Brittain, President

Washington

★ 19463 ★ Aetna Inc. - Washington
PPO Plan
601 Union Square, Ste. 800
Seattle, WA 98101
Phone: (206)701-8000 **Fax:** (206)701-8125
Website: http://www.aetna.com
John W. Rowe, MD, Chairman of the Board

★ 19464 ★ Aetna Inc. - Washington
PPO Plan
600 University St., Ste. 1400
Seattle, WA 98101-1158
Phone: (206)710-1100 **Free:** 800-654-3250
Fax: (206)701-1125
Website: http://www.aetna.com
John W. Rowe, MD, CEO & Chm Bd

★ 19465 ★ First Choice Health Network
PPO Plan
601 Union St., Ste. 1100
Seattle, WA 98101-1838
Phone: (206)292-8255 **Fax:** (206)624-4953
Website: http://www.fchn.com
Gary Gannaway, CEO
Program(s): Dental, Inpatient SNF, Podiatry.

★ 19466 ★ Kitsap Physicians Service
PPO Plan
PO Box 339
Bremerton, WA 98337
Phone: (360)377-5576 **Free:** 800-552-7114
Fax: (360)478-2632
Website: http://www.kpshealthplans.com
Elizabeth Gilje, CEO & Pres

★ 19467 ★ Northwest One
PPO Plan
1101 First St., No. 400
Snohomish, WA 98290
Phone: (360)862-1411 **Free:** 800-799-8933
Fax: (360)862-1562
Paul Glover, Chairman of the Board

★ 19468 ★ One Health Plan of Washington, Inc.
PPO Plan
3005 112th Ave. NE, Corp. Camp E
Bellevue, WA 98004
Phone: (425)827-2282 **Free:** 800-332-0151
Fax: (425)827-2466
Website: http://www.onehealthplan.com
Teresa Davis, Contact

★ 19469 ★ United Northwest Services
PPO Plan
1121 N Argonne Rd., Ste. 200
Spokane, WA 99212-2699
Phone: (509)928-2569 **Free:** 800-245-6024
Fax: (509)926-3056
Mary O. McWilliams, CEO

West Virginia

★ 19470 ★ Aetna Inc. - West Virginia
PPO Plan
121 Washington St. E
Charleston, WV 25301
Phone: (304)346-5322 **Fax:** (304)346-5327
Website: http://www.aetna.com
John W. Rowe, MD, Chairman of the Board

★ 19471 ★ Carelink
PPO Plan
887 National Rd.
Wheeling, WV 26003
Phone: (304)234-5100 **Free:** 800-519-3368
Fax: (304)234-5119
Website: http://www.chccarelink.com
Ted Cheatham, CEO

★ 19472 ★ Carelink Health Plans
PPO Plan
500 Virginia St., Ste. 400
Charleston, WV 25301
Phone: (304)348-2970 **Fax:** (304)561-6985
Website: http://www.camcare.com
Ted Cheatham, CEO

Wisconsin

★ 19473 ★ Accountable Health Plans of America, Inc. - Corporate Headquarters
PPO Plan
2831 N Grandview Blvd.
Pewaukee, WI 53072
Phone: (262)544-5337 **Free:** 800-308-3344
Fax: (262)544-9320
Walter Vinson, CEO

★ 19474 ★ Accountable Health Plans of America, Inc. - Wisconsin
PPO Plan
PO Box 810
Pewaukee, WI 53072
Free: 800-308-3344 **Fax:** (262)544-9320
Walter Vinson, CEO

★ 19475 ★ Aetna Inc. - Wisconsin
PPO Plan
2675 N Mayfair Rd., Ste. 600
Milwaukee, WI 53226
Phone: (414)266-9700 **Fax:** (414)266-9705
Website: http://www.aetna.com
John W. Rowe, MD, Chairman of the Board

★ 19476 ★ AHC
PPO Plan
PO Box 981
Brookfield, WI 53008-0981
Phone: (262)879-0100 **Free:** 800-952-8661
Fax: (262)879-0876
Website: http://www.ahcppo.com
Richard Blomquist, CEO & Pres

★ 19477 ★ Cobalt Corp.
PPO Plan
401 W Michigan St.
Milwaukee, WI 53203
Phone: (414)226-6600 **Fax:** (414)226-6279
Website: http://www.cobaltcorporation.com
Thomas Hefty, Chairman of the Board

★ 19478 ★ CompCare Health Services Insurance Corp.
PPO Plan
401 W Michigan Ave.
Milwaukee, WI 53203
Phone: (414)226-6600 **Free:** 800-242-7312
Fax: (262)814-4890
Website: http://www.bcbsuw.org
Michael Bernstein, President

★ 19479 ★ EBC Review
PPO Plan
9275 N 49th St., Ste. 300
Milwaukee, WI 53223
Phone: (414)365-4600 **Fax:** (414)365-4610
Website: http://www.ebc-tpa.com
Bruce Flunker, CEO

★ 19480 ★ Fortis Health - Corporate Headquarters
PPO Plan
PO Box 624
Milwaukee, WI 53201-0624
Phone: (414)299-8026 **Fax:** (414)224-0472
Website: http://www.us.fortis.com
Ben Cutler, CEO

★ 19481 ★ Fortis Health - Oregon
501 W Michigan
Milwaukee, WI 53203
Phone: (414)271-3011 **Fax:** (414)224-0472
Website: http://www.us.fortis.com
Ben Cutler, CEO

★ 19482 ★ Health Care Network of Wisconsin
PPO Plan
250 Bishops Way, Ste. 300
Brookfield, WI 53005-5957
Phone: (262)784-0223 **Free:** 800-451-2577
Fax: (262)796-9084
Website: http://www.wppn.com
James Wrocklage, CEO

★ 19483 ★ Humana CareNetwork, Inc.
PPO Plan
PO Box 12359
Milwaukee, WI 53212-0359
Phone: (414)223-3300 **Fax:** (414)223-0184
Website: http://www.humana.com
Michael B. McCallister, CEO & Pres

★ 19484 ★ Network Health Plan of Wisconsin
PPO Plan
1165 Appleton Rd.
Menasha, WI 54952
Phone: (920)727-0100 **Fax:** (929)720-1756
Website: http://www.networkhealth.com
Michael Wolff, CEO

★ 19485 ★ Prevea Health Plan
PPO Plan
PO Box 11625
Green Bay, WI 54307-1625
Phone: (920)490-6900 **Free:** 888-711-1444
Fax: (920)490-6943
Website: http://www.prevea.com
Mark Minsloff, CEO

★ 19486 ★ Sentry Insurance
PPO Plan
1800 N Point Dr.
Stevens Point, WI 54481
Phone: (715)346-6000 **Fax:** (715)346-6363
Dale Schuh, CEO

★ 19487 ★ TouchPoint Health Plan
PPO Plan
PO Box 507
Appleton, WI 54912-0507
Phone: (920)735-6440 **Free:** 800-735-6305
Fax: (920)831-6886
Website: http://www.thedacare.org
Jay Fulkerson, CEO

★ 19488 ★ United Healthcare of Wisconsin, Inc.
PPO Plan
10701 W Research Dr.
Milwaukee, WI 53226
Phone: (414)443-4000 **Free:** 800-879-0071
Fax: (414)443-4750
William Felsing, CEO

★ 19489 ★ Wausau Benefits, Inc.
PPO Plan
PO Box 8017
Wausau, WI 54402-8017
Phone: (715)845-8582 **Free:** 800-435-4401
Fax: (715)843-3613
Website: http://www.libertymutual.com
Fred Moore, President

★ 19490 ★ Wausau Insurance Co.
PPO Plan
PO Box 1060
Eau Claire, WI 54702-1060
Phone: (715)835-6174 **Free:** 800-835-6174
Fax: (715)838-0220
John Laehn, CEO

★ 19491 ★ Wausau Preferred Health Plan
PPO Plan
PO Box 245037
Milwaukee, WI 53224-9537
Phone: (414)577-2100 **Free:** 800-242-0472
Fax: (414)577-2437
Website: http://www.wausau.com
Christopher Drayna, MD, Contact

★ 19492 ★ Wisconsin Physicians Services Insurance Co.
PPO Plan
PO Box 8190
Madison, WI 53708-8190
Phone: (608)221-4711 **Fax:** (608)223-3603
James R. Riordan, CEO

Wyoming

★ 19493 ★ WIN Health Partners
PPO Plan
2515 Warren Ave., Ste. 504
Cheyenne, WY 82001
Phone: (307)638-7700 **Fax:** (307)663-7701
Beth Wasson, CEO

Point-of-Service (POS) Plans

Alabama

★ 19494 ★ Aetna Inc.—Alabama Inc.
POS Plan
3000 Riverside Galleria, Ste. 780
Birmingham, AL 35244
Phone: (205)985-3550 **Fax:** (205)985-3316
Website: http://www.aetna.com
John W. Rowe, MD, CEO

★ 19495 ★ CIGNA Healthcare Plans of Alabama
POS Plan
10 Inverness Center Pkwy., No. 230
Birmingham, AL 35242
Phone: (205)991-1005 **Fax:** (205)995-8511
Website: http://www.cigna.com
Robert A. Yungk, CEO

★ 19496 ★ The Oath, A Health Plan for Alabama
POS Plan
Two Perimeter Park S, Ste. 200W
Birmingham, AL 35242
Phone: (205)968-1000 **Free:** 800-888-7647
Fax: (205)968-2277
Website: http://www.healthpartners.com
John Davis, President

★ 19497 ★ PrimeHealth
POS Plan
1400 University Blvd. S
Mobile, AL 36609-2999
Phone: (251)342-0022 **Free:** 800-928-7716
Fax: (251)342-1176
Website: http://www.primehealthonline.com
Kathryn Parks, CEO

★ 19498 ★ United Concordia Co., Inc. - Alabama
POS Plan
400 Vestavia Pkwy, Ste. 205
Birmingham, AL 35216
Free: 800-554-6155 **Fax:** (205)822-1653
Website: http://www.ucci.com
Thomas A. Dzuryachko, CEO
Program(s): Dental.

★ 19499 ★ United Healthcare of Alabama, Inc.
POS Plan
PO Box 830637
Birmingham, AL 35255
Phone: (205)977-6300 **Free:** 800-345-1520
Fax: (205)977-6537
Website: http://www.uhc.com
William W. McGuire, MD, Chairman of the Board

Arizona

★ 19500 ★ Aetna Inc—Arizona
POS Plan
7720 N 16th St., Ste. 400
Phoenix, AZ 85020
Phone: (602)427-2200 **Fax:** (602)427-2176
Website: http://www.aetna.com
John W. Rowe, MD, Chairman of the Board

★ 19501 ★ Arizona Foundation for Medical Care
326 E Coronado
Phoenix, AZ 85004
Phone: (602)252-4042 **Free:** 800-624-4277
Fax: (602)256-7816
Website: http://www.azfmc.com
Anthony D. Mitten, JD, CEO

★ 19502 ★ Catalina Behavioral Health Services
POS Plan
2400 N Central Ave., Ste. 203A
Phoenix, AZ 85004
Phone: (602)452-1200 **Free:** 800-977-0281
Fax: (602)257-1644
Karen Smith-Hagman, CEO
Program(s): Behavioral health; psychiatric.

★ 19503 ★ CIGNA HealthCare of Arizona
POS Plan
7225 N Mona Lisa Rd.
Tucson, AZ 85741
Phone: (520)571-0111 **Fax:** (520)575-4950
Website: http://www.cigna.com/healthcare/hs/ar.html
Frank Benedetto, Contact

★ 19504 ★ CIGNA Healthcare of Arizona
POS Plan
11001 N Black Canyon Hwy., No. 400
Phoenix, AZ 85029-4754
Phone: (602)942-4462 **Fax:** (602)371-2625
Website: http://www.cigna.com
Edward Handway, CEO

★ 19505 ★ Health Net of Arizona
POS Plan
930 N Finance Ctr. Dr, Ste. 100
Tucson, AZ 85710
Phone: (520)721-1122 **Free:** 800-289-2818
Fax: (520)290-7585
Website: http://www.az.health.net
Mark El-Tawil, President

★ 19506 ★ Humana Health Care Plans of Arizona
POS Plan
2710 E Camelback Rd.
Phoenix, AZ 85016-3245
Phone: (602)553-2000 **Free:** 800-288-6442
Fax: (602)381-4389
Website: http://www.humana.com
William J. Howard, CEO & Pres

★ 19507 ★ One Health Plan of Arizona
POS Plan
3131 E Camelback Rd., Ste. 240
Phoenix, AZ 85016
Phone: (602)667-9537 **Fax:** (602)508-8972
Website: http://www.onehealthplan.com
Roger Stinton, Contact

★ 19508 ★ PacifiCare of Arizona
Secure Horizons (POS)
PO Box 52078
Phoenix, AZ 85072
Phone: (602)244-8200 **Free:** 800-221-2462
Fax: (602)681-7000
Website: http://www.pacificare.com
Rick Badger, President

★ 19509 ★ United Concordia Co., Inc. - Arizona
POS Plan
2198 Camelback Rd., Ste. 260
Phoenix, AZ 85016
Phone: (717)260-7500 **Free:** 800-322-0366
Fax: (717)612-4996
Website: http://www.ucci.com
Thomas Dzuryachko, CEO

★ 19510 ★ United HealthCare of Arizona, Inc.
POS Plan
3141 N 3rd Ave.
Phoenix, AZ 85013
Phone: (602)664-5000 **Free:** 800-442-4119
Fax: (602)664-2732
Website: http://www.unitedhealthcare.com
William W. McGuire, MD, Chairman of the Board

Arkansas

★ 19511 ★ Aetna Inc.—Arkansas
POS Plan
10810 Executive Center Dr., No. 402
Little Rock, AR 72211-3525
Phone: (501)227-7776 **Free:** 800-821-8787
Fax: (501)227-0581
Website: http://www.aetna.com
John W. Rowe, Chairman of the Board

★ 19512 ★ Health Advantage
POS Plan
26 Corporate Hill Dr.
Little Rock, AR 72205
Phone: (501)221-1800 **Fax:** (501)221-7103
Website: http://www.healthadvantage-hmo.com
David Frank Bridges, CEO

★ 19513 ★ United HealthCare of Arkansas
POS Plan
415 N McKinley, Ste. 820
Little Rock, AR 72205
Phone: (501)664-7700 **Free:** 800-678-3176
Fax: (501)664-7768
Website: http://www.uhc.com
John A. Wickens, President

California

★ 19514 ★ Aetna Inc.—California
POS Plan
2409 Comino Ramon
San Ramon, CA 94583
Phone: (925)543-9000 **Fax:** (925)543-9010
Website: http://www.aetna.com
John W. Rowe, MD, Chairman of the Board

★ 19515 ★ Aetna Inc.—California
POS Plan
1200 W 7th St., Ste. 400
Los Angeles, CA 90017
Phone: (310)955-3100 **Fax:** (310)955-3185
Website: http://www.aetna.com
John W. Rowe, MD, Chairman of the Board

★ 19516 ★ Aetna Inc.—California
POS Plan
5800 Canoga Ave.
Woodland Hills, CA 91367
Phone: (818)992-2000 **Free:** 800-553-2952
Fax: (818)593-7108
Website: http://www.aetna.com
John W. Rowe, MD, Chairman of the Board

★ 19517 ★ CCN - Alaska
POS Plan
5251 Viewridge Ct.
San Diego, CA 92123
Phone: (858)278-2273 **Free:** 800-247-2898
Fax: (858)278-8621
Website: http://www.ccnusa.com
Patrick G. Dills, President

★ 19518 ★ CCN - Arizona
POS Plan
5251 Viewridge Ct.
San Diego, CA 92123
Phone: (858)278-2273 **Free:** 800-247-2898
Fax: (858)278-8621
Website: http://www.ccnusa.com
Patrick G. Dills, CEO & Pres

★ 19519 ★ CCN - California
POS Plan
5251 Viewridge Ct.
San Diego, CA 92123
Phone: (858)278-2273 **Free:** 800-247-2898
Fax: (858)278-1262
Website: http://www.ccnusa.com
Patrick G. Dills, President

★ 19520 ★ CCN - Florida
POS Plan
1507 N Falkenburg Rd.
Tampa, CA 33619
Phone: (813)663-3700 **Free:** 800-633-8033
Fax: (813)620-4973
Website: http://www.ccnusa.com
Patrick G. Dills, President

★ 19521 ★ CCN - Hawaii
POS Plan
5251 Viewridge Ct.
San Diego, CA 92123
Phone: (858)278-2273 **Free:** 800-247-2898
Fax: (858)278-8621
Website: http://www.ccnusa.com
Patrick Dills, President

★ 19522 ★ CCN - Nevada
POS Plan
5251 Viewridge Ct.
San Diego, CA 92123
Phone: (858)278-2273 **Free:** 800-247-2898
Fax: (858)278-8621
Website: http://www.ccnusa.com
Patrick G. Dills, President

★ 19523 ★ CCN - New Mexico
POS Plan
5251 Viewridge Ct.
San Diego, CA 92123
Phone: (858)278-2273 **Free:** 800-247-2898
Fax: (858)278-8621
Website: http://www.ccnusa.com
Patrick G. Dills, CEO & Chm Bd

★ 19524 ★ CCN - Oregon
POS Plan
5251 Viewridge Ct.
San Diego, CA 92123
Phone: (858)278-2273 **Free:** 800-247-2898
Fax: (858)278-8621
Website: http://www.ccnusa.com
Patrick G. Dills, President

★ 19525 ★ CCN - Washington
POS Plan
5251 Viewridge Ct.
San Diego, CA 92123
Phone: (858)278-2273 **Free:** 800-247-2898
Fax: (858)278-8621
Website: http://www.ccnusa.com
Patrick G. Dills, President

★ 19526 ★ Chirosource - Corporate Headquarters
POS Plan
PO Box 130
Clayton, CA 94517
Phone: (925)672-5333 **Free:** 800-680-9997
Fax: (925)672-6657
Website: http://www.chirosource.com
Ronald S. Cataldo, DC, CEO & Pres
Program(s): Chiropractic; worker's compensation.

★ 19527 ★ CIGNA Healthcare of California
POS Plan
400 N Brand Blvd., Ste. 500
Glendale, CA 91203
Phone: (818)500-6262 **Free:** 800-344-7421
Fax: (818)500-6480
Website: http://www.cigna.com/healthcare
Bud Volberding, President

★ 19528 ★ CIGNA HealthCare California, Inc. - San Diego
POS Plan
3131 Camino Del Rio N, Ste. 900
San Diego, CA 92108
Phone: (619)641-5400 **Free:** 800-368-2471
Fax: (619)641-5499
Website: http://www.cigna.com
Bud Volberding, CEO

★ 19529 ★ Great West Life
POS Plan
3480 Buskirk Ave., Ste. 350
Pleasant Hill, CA 94523
Phone: (925)938-7788 **Fax:** (925)210-0975
Website: http://www.onehealthplan.com
Vicki Mahoney, Contact

★ 19530 ★ Health Net of California
POS Plan
21281 Burbank Blvd.
Woodland Hills, CA 91367
Phone: (818)676-6775 **Free:** 800-522-0088
Fax: (818)676-6982
Website: http://www.healthnet.com
Jennifer M. Gutzmore, MD, Contact

★ 19531 ★ Health Net, Inc. - Corporate Headquarters
Health Net POS
21650 Oxnard St.
Woodland Hills, CA 91367
Phone: (818)676-6775 **Free:** 800-474-6676
Fax: (818)676-7315
Website: http://www.health.net
Jay M. Gellert, CEO

★ 19532 ★ Landmark Healthcare, Inc.
POS Plan
1750 Howe Ave., Ste. 300
Sacramento, CA 95825
Phone: (916)646-3477 **Fax:** (916)929-8350
Website: http://www.landmarkhealthcare.com
Joseph Kleigner, CEO
Program(s): Chiropractic, Alternative Medicine.

★ 19533 ★ Lifeguard, Inc.
POS Plan
PO Box 5506
San Jose, CA 95150-5506
Phone: (408)943-9400 **Free:** 800-995-0380
Fax: (408)432-3695
Website: http://www.lifeguard.com
Mark Hyde, CEO

★ 19534 ★ Managed Health Network
POS Plan
1600 Los Gamos Dr., Ste. 300
San Rafael, CA 94903
Phone: (415)491-7200 **Free:** 800-327-7526
Fax: (415)472-8187
Website: http://www.mhn.com
Robert Fusco, Contact
Program(s): Psychiatric, Behavioral Health.

★ 19535 ★ MRA/Managed Care Solutions
POS Plan
901 Elm Ave.
Long Beach, CA 90813
Phone: (562)437-4331 **Free:** 800-832-4975
Fax: (562)437-7721
Website: http://www.go2mra.com
Victoria Fullerton, CEO

★ 19536 ★ One Health Plan of California
POS Plan
655 N Central Ave., No. 1900
Glendale, CA 91203-1441
Phone: (818)539-1900 **Fax:** (818)545-9238
Website: http://www.onehealthplan.com
Jackie James, President

★ 19537 ★ Pacificare Behavioral Health
POS Plan
23046 Avenida de la Carlota, Ste. 700
Laguna Hills, CA 92653
Phone: (949)859-7971 **Fax:** (949)859-9824
Website: http://www.pacificare.com
Jerome Vaccaro, MD, CEO

★ 19538 ★ Pacificare of California
POS Plan
5701 Katella Ave.
Cypress, CA 90630-5028
Phone: (714)952-1121 **Free:** 800-624-8822
Fax: (714)226-3996
Website: http://www.pacificare.com
Howard G. Phanstiel, CEO

★ 19539 ★ Pacificare Health Systems - Corporate Headquarters
POS Plan
PO Box 25186
Santa Ana, CA 92799-5186
Phone: (714)952-1121 **Free:** 800-624-8822
Fax: (714)825-2201
Website: http://www.pacificare.com
Howard G. Phanstiel, CEO

★ 19540 ★ PMI Dental Health Plan
POS Plan
12898 Towne Center Dr.
Artesia, CA 90703
Phone: (562)924-8311 **Free:** 800-422-4234
Fax: (562)924-8039
Website: http://www.deltadentalca.org
Belinda Martinez, CEO

★ 19541 ★ Progressive Administrative Resources
POS Plan
PO Box 850
Agoura Hills, CA 91376
Free: 800-995-4310 **Fax:** (818)707-9182
Wayne Foff, CEO

★ 19542 ★ South Bay Independent Physicians Medical Group, Inc.
POS Plan
3480 Torrance Blvd., Ste. 220
Torrance, CA 90503
Phone: (310)543-8805 **Fax:** (310)543-8811
William Averill, MD, Chairman of the Board

★ 19543 ★ United Behavioral Health
POS Plan
425 Market St., 27th Fl.
San Francisco, CA 94105
Phone: (415)547-5000 **Fax:** (415)547-6100
Website: http://www.unitedbehavioralhealth.com
Saul Feldman, MD, CEO

★ 19544 ★ United Concordia Co., Inc. - California
POS Plan
21700 Oxnard, Ste. 500
Woodland Hills, CA 91367-3642
Phone: (717)731-2532 **Free:** 800-876-6432
Fax: (717)972-0410
Website: http://www.ucci.com
Thomas Dzuryachko, Chairman of the Board
Program(s): Dental.

★ 19545 ★ United Healthcare of Oregon
POS Plan
180 E Ocean Blvd., Ste. 500
Long Beach, CA 90802
Phone: (562)951-6400 **Free:** 800-325-6651
Fax: (562)951-6885
Website: http://www.uhc.com
Emery Dameron, CEO

★ 19546 ★ WellPoint Health Networks, Inc. - Corporate Headquarters
POS Plan
One WellPoint Way
Thousand Oaks, CA 91362
Phone: (818)703-4000 **Fax:** (805)557-6872
Website: http://www.wellpoint.com
Leonard Schaeffer, CEO & Chm Bd

Colorado

★ 19547 ★ Aetna Inc. - Colorado
POS Plan
6430 S Fiddlers Green Cir. No. 200
Englewood, CO 80111
Phone: (303)793-2500 **Fax:** (303)793-2510
Website: http://www.aetna.com
John W. Rowe, CEO

★ 19548 ★ Aetna Inc. - Colorado
POS Plan
4643 S Ulster St., Ste. 1000
Denver, CO 80237
Phone: (303)796-6100 **Free:** 800-481-3841
Fax: (303)796-6183
Website: http://www.aetna.com
John W. Rowe, CEO

★ 19549 ★ CIGNA HealthCare of Colorado
POS Plan
3900 E Mexico Ave., Ste. 1100
Denver, CO 80210
Phone: (303)782-1500 **Free:** 800-832-3211
Fax: (303)782-1577
Website: http://www.cigna.com
Daryl Edmonds, CEO

★ 19550 ★ Great West Life Annuity Insurance Co.
POS Plan
PO Box 1700
Denver, CO 80201
Phone: (303)737-3000 **Fax:** (303)737-3198
Website: http://www.gwla.com
William McCallum, CEO

★ 19551 ★ Great-West/One Health Plan
POS Plan
8505 E Orchard Rd.
Greenwood Village, CO 80111
Phone: (303)737-3000 **Fax:** (303)737-3405
Website: http://www.onehealthplan.com
William T. McCallum, CEO & Pres

★ 19552 ★ Kaiser Permanente
POS Plan
2500 S Havana St.
Aurora, CO 80014
Phone: (303)338-3700 **Free:** 800-632-9700
Fax: (303)338-3797
Website: http://www.kaiserpermanente.org
Christopher Binkley, CEO

★ 19553 ★ New England Financial
POS Plan
8505 E Orchard Rd.
Greenwood Village, CO 80111
Phone: (303)737-3000 **Fax:** (303)737-3198
Website: http://www.nefn.com
William McCallum, CEO

★ 19554 ★ One Health Plan of Colorado
POS Plan
8525 E Orchard Rd., No. 3
Greenwood Village, CO 80111-5002
Phone: (303)305-1000 **Fax:** (303)737-3198
Website: http://www.onehealthplan.com
Chris Miller, President

★ 19555 ★ PacifiCare of Colorado
POS Plan
6455 S Yosemite
Englewood, CO 80111
Phone: (303)220-5800 **Free:** 800-877-6685
Fax: (303)714-3999
Website: http://www.pacificare.com
Jeffrey Folick, Chairman of the Board
Program(s): Chiropractic, Dental, Home Care, Inpatient SNF, Long-Term Care, Pharmaceutical Mail Order, Podiatry, Psychiatric, Behavioral Health, Physical Therapy, Transplant, Vision, Wellness.

★ 19556 ★ Rocky Mountain HMO
POS Plan
2775 Crossroads Blvd.
Grand Junction, CO 81506
Phone: (970)244-7760 **Free:** 800-843-0719
Fax: (970)244-7880
Website: http://www.rmhmo.org
John Hopkins, CEO

★ 19557 ★ Sloan's Lake Health Plan
POS Plan
1355 S Colorado Blvd., Ste. 902
Denver, CO 80222
Phone: (303)753-7537 **Free:** 800-457-2345
Fax: (303)504-4321
Website: http://www.sloanslake.com
Blair Tikker, CEO

★ 19558 ★ United HealthCare of Colorado
POS Plan
8051 E Maplewood Ave., Ste. 300
Englewood, CO 80111
Phone: (303)267-3300 **Free:** 800-518-3344
Fax: (303)267-3599
Website: http://www.uhc.com
Victor Lazzaro, Jr., CEO & Pres

Connecticut

★ 19559 ★ Aetna, Inc. - Corporate Headquarters
POS Plan
151 Farmington Ave.
Hartford, CT 06156-1000
Phone: (860)273-0123 **Free:** 800-225-2949
Fax: (860)636-4513
Website: http://www.aetna.com
John W. Rowe, CEO & Chm Bd

★ 19560 ★ Aetna US Healthcare of New England
POS Plan
1000 Middle St.
Middletown, CT 06457-3342
Phone: (860)273-0123 **Fax:** (860)273-6872
Website: http://www.aetna.com
John W. Rowe, MD, Chairman of the Board

★ 19561 ★ CIGNA HealthCare of Connecticut, Inc.
POS Plan
900 Cottage Grove Rd., A-118
Hartford, CT 06152-1118
Phone: (860)769-2300 **Free:** 800-345-9458
Fax: (860)769-2398
Website: http://www.cigna.com
Kirk Weimer, CEO

★ 19562 ★ GE Financial
POS Plan
100 Bright Meadow Blvd.
Enfield, CT 06082
Free: 800-451-2513 **Fax:** (860)403-1306
Website: http://www.gefn.com
Robert W. Fiondella, CEO

★ 19563 ★ Health Net - Connecticut
POS Plan
PO Box 904
Shelton, CT 06484-0914
Phone: (203)402-4200 **Free:** 800-848-4747
Fax: (203)225-4000
Website: http://www.health.net
Barry Averill, CEO & Pres

★ 19564 ★ Health Net Inc. - Northeast Corporate Headquarters
POS Plan
PO Box 904
Shelton, CT 06484-0944
Phone: (203)402-4200 **Free:** 800-848-4747
Fax: (203)225-4000
Website: http://www.health.net
Barry Averill, CEO & Pres

★ 19565 ★ Oxford Health Plans - Connecticut
POS Plan
PO Box 7081
Bridgeport, CT 06601-7081
Free: 800-444-6222 **Fax:** (203)851-1491
Website: http://www.oxhp.com
Norman Payson, MD, CEO & Chm Bd

Delaware

★ 19566 ★ Aetna Inc. - Delaware
POS Plan
650 Naamans Rd.
Claymont, DE 19703
Phone: (302)793-1520 **Fax:** (302)798-1877
Website: http://www.aetna.com
John W. Rowe, MD, Chairman of the Board

★ 19567 ★ AmeriHealth Insurance Co.
POS Plan
919 N Market St., Mellon Ctr. Ste. 1200
Wilmington, DE 19801-3021
Phone: (302)777-6400 **Free:** 800-899-4373
Fax: (302)777-6444
Richard Neeson, Contact

★ 19568 ★ Christiana Care Health Plans, Inc.
POS Plan
11 Reads Way
New Castle, DE 19720

Phone: (302)327-7650 **Free:** 800-362-4214
Fax: (302)327-7711
Website: http://www.christianacare.org
Ken Bates, CEO

★ 19569 ★ CIGNA HealthCare of Delaware Valley
POS Plan
PO Box 15408
Wilmington, DE 19850-5408
Phone: (302)477-3700 **Free:** 800-320-0251
Fax: (302)477-3708
Website: http://www.cigna.com
Vincent Sobocinski, Contact

★ 19570 ★ Coventry Health Care Inc.—Delaware, Inc.
POS Plan
2751 Centerville Rd., Ste. 400
Wilmington, DE 19808
Phone: (302)995-6100 **Free:** 800-833-7423
Fax: (302)998-7085
Website: http://www.chcde.com
Ron Chaffin, CEO & Pres

Florida

★ 19571 ★ Aetna Inc. - Altamonte Springs
385 Douglas Ave.
Altamonte Springs, FL 32714
Free: 800-225-9451 **Fax:** (407)618-2511
Website: http://www.aetna.com
John W. Rowe, Chairman of the Board

★ 19572 ★ Aetna Inc. - Florida
POS Plan
5100 W Lemon St., Ste. 218
Tampa, FL 33609
Phone: (813)261-9630 **Fax:** (813)636-0658
Website: http://www.aetna.com
John W. Rowe, MD, Chairman of the Board

★ 19573 ★ Aetna Inc. - Jacksonville
POS Plan
1200 Riverplace Blvd., Ste. 701
Jacksonville, FL 32207
Phone: (904)346-5800 **Fax:** (904)346-5888
Website: http://www.aetna.com
John W. Rowe, MD, Chairman of the Board

★ 19574 ★ Aetna Inc. - Plantation
POS Plan
8201 Peters Rd.
Plantation, FL 33324
Phone: (954)382-8100 **Fax:** (954)424-4448
Website: http://www.aetna.com
John W. Rowe, MD, Chairman of the Board

★ 19575 ★ Av-Med Health Plan - Jacksonville
POS Plan
1300 Riverplace Blvd., No. 200-201
Jacksonville, FL 32207-9054
Phone: (904)858-1300 **Fax:** (904)858-1335
Website: http://www.avmed.com
Robert Hudson, CEO

★ 19576 ★ Av-Med Health Plan - Orlando
POS Plan
541 S Orlando Ave., Ste. 205
Maitland, FL 32751
Phone: (407)539-0007 **Fax:** (407)975-1623
Website: http://www.avmed.com
Robert Hudson, CEO

★ 19577 ★ Av-Med Health Plan - Tampa
POS Plan
1511 N Westshore Blvd., Ste. 700
Tampa, FL 33607
Phone: (813)281-5650 **Free:** 800-257-2273
Fax: (813)281-0659
Website: http://www.avmed.com
Douglas Cooper, CEO

★ 19578 ★ Beacon Health Plans
POS Plan
PO Box 459012
Sunrise, FL 33345
Phone: (305)460-2000 **Fax:** (305)774-2617
Website: http://www.beaconhealth.com
Wilfredo Gonzalez, President

★ 19579 ★ CCN - Alabama
POS Plan
1507 N Falkenburg Rd.
Tampa, FL 33619
Phone: (813)663-3700 **Free:** 800-633-8033
Fax: (813)620-4973
Website: http://www.ccnusa.com
Patrick G. Dills, President

★ 19580 ★ CCN - Arkansas
POS Plan
1507 N Falkenburg Rd.
Tampa, FL 33619
Phone: (813)663-3700 **Free:** 800-633-8033
Fax: (858)620-4973
Website: http://www.ccnusa.com
Patrick G. Dills, President

★ 19581 ★ CCN - Connecticut
POS Plan
1507 N Falkenburg Rd.
Tampa, FL 33619
Phone: (813)663-3700 **Free:** 800-633-8033
Fax: (813)620-4973
Website: http://www.ccnusa.com
Patrick G. Dills, President

★ 19582 ★ CCN - Delaware
POS Plan
1507 N Falkenburg Rd.
Tampa, FL 33619
Phone: (813)663-3700 **Free:** 800-633-8033
Fax: (813)620-4973
Website: http://www.ccnusa.com
Patrick G. Dills, President

★ 19583 ★ CCN - District of Columbia
POS Plan
1507 N Falkenburg Rd.
Tampa, FL 33619
Phone: (813)663-3700 **Free:** 800-633-8033
Fax: (813)620-4973
Website: http://www.ccnusa.com
Patrick G. Dills, President

★ 19584 ★ CCN - Georgia
POS Plan
1507 N Falkenburg Rd.
Tampa, FL 33619
Phone: (813)663-3700 **Free:** 800-633-8033
Fax: (813)620-4973
Website: http://www.ccnusa.com
Patrick G. Dills, President

★ 19585 ★ CCN - Kentucky
POS Plan
1507 N Falkenburg Rd.
Tampa, FL 33619
Phone: (813)663-3700 **Free:** 800-633-8033
Fax: (813)620-4973
Website: http://www.ccnusa.com
Patrick G. Dills, President

★ 19586 ★ CCN - Louisiana
POS Plan
1507 N Falkenburg Rd.
Tampa, FL 33619
Phone: (813)663-3700 **Free:** 800-633-8033
Fax: (813)620-4973
Website: http://www.ccnusa.com
Patrick G. Dills, President

★ 19587 ★ CCN - Maryland
POS Plan
1507 N Falkenburg Rd.
Tampa, FL 33619
Phone: (813)663-3700 **Free:** 800-633-8033
Fax: (813)620-4973
Website: http://www.ccnusa.com
Patrick G. Dills, President

★ 19588 ★ CCN - Massachusetts
POS Plan
1507 N Falkenburg Rd.
Tampa, FL 33619
Phone: (813)663-3700 **Free:** 800-633-8033
Fax: (813)620-4973
Website: http://www.ccnusa.com
Patrick G. Dills, President

★ 19589 ★ CCN - Mississippi
POS Plan
1507 N Falkenburg Rd.
Tampa, FL 33619
Phone: (813)663-3700 **Free:** 800-633-8033
Fax: (813)620-4973
Website: http://www.ccnusa.com
Patrick G. Dills, President

★ 19590 ★ CCN - New Hampshire
POS Plan
1507 N Falkenburg Rd.
Tampa, FL 33619
Phone: (813)663-3700 **Free:** 800-633-8033
Fax: (813)620-4973
Website: http://www.ccnusa.com
Patrick G. Dills, President

★ 19591 ★ CCN - New Jersey
POS Plan
1507 N Falkenburg Rd.
Tampa, FL 33619
Phone: (813)663-3700 **Free:** 800-633-8033
Fax: (813)620-4973
Website: http://www.ccnusa.com
Patrick G. Dills, President

★ 19592 ★ CCN - New York
POS Plan
1507 N Falkenburg Rd.
Tampa, FL 33619
Phone: (813)663-3700 **Free:** 800-633-8033
Fax: (813)620-4973
Website: http://www.ccnusa.com
Patrick G. Dills, President

★ 19593 ★ CCN - North Carolina
POS Plan
1507 N Falkenburg Rd.
Tampa, FL 33619
Phone: (813)663-3700 **Free:** 800-633-8033
Fax: (813)620-4973
Website: http://www.ccnusa.com
Patrick G. Dills, President

★ 19594 ★ CCN - Pennsylvania
POS Plan
1507 N Falkenburg Rd.
Tampa, FL 33619
Phone: (813)663-3700 **Free:** 800-633-8033
Fax: (813)620-4973

Website: http://www.ccnusa.com
Patrick G. Dills, President

★ 19595 ★ CCN - Rhode Island
POS Plan
1507 N Falkenburg Rd.
Tampa, FL 33619
Phone: (813)663-3700 **Free:** 800-633-8033
Fax: (813)620-4973
Website: http://www.ccnusa.com
Patrick G. Dills, President

★ 19596 ★ CCN - South Carolina
POS Plan
1507 N Falkenburg Rd.
Tampa, FL 33619
Phone: (813)663-3700 **Free:** 800-633-8033
Fax: (813)620-4973
Website: http://www.ccnusa.com
Patrick G. Dills, President

★ 19597 ★ CCN - Tennessee
POS Plan
1507 N Falkenburg Rd.
Tampa, FL 33619
Phone: (813)663-3700 **Free:** 800-633-8033
Fax: (813)620-4973
Website: http://www.ccnusa.com
Patrick G. Dills, President

★ 19598 ★ CCN - Vermont
POS Plan
1507 N Falkenburg Rd.
Tampa, FL 33619
Phone: (813)663-3700 **Free:** 800-633-8033
Fax: (813)620-4973
Website: http://www.ccnusa.com
Patrick G. Dills, President

★ 19599 ★ CCN - Virginia
POS Plan
1507 N Falkenburg Rd.
Tampa, FL 33619
Phone: (813)663-3700 **Free:** 800-633-8033
Fax: (813)620-4973
Website: http://www.ccnusa.com
Patrick G. Dills, President

★ 19600 ★ CCN - West Virginia
POS Plan
1507 N Falkenburg Rd.
Tampa, FL 33619
Phone: (813)663-3700 **Free:** 800-633-8033
Fax: (813)620-4973
Website: http://www.ccnusa.com
Patrick G. Dills, President

★ 19601 ★ CIGNA HealthCare of Florida
POS Plan
5404 Cypress Center Dr.
Tampa, FL 33609
Phone: (813)281-1000 **Free:** 800-942-2471
Fax: (813)289-0363
Website: http://www.cigna.com
Andrew Crooks, CEO & Pres

★ 19602 ★ CIGNA HealthCare of Florida
POS Plan
1580 Sawgrass Corp. Pkwy., Ste 200
Sunrise, FL 33323
Phone: (954)693-7500 **Fax:** (954)693-7540
Website: http://www.cigna.com
William Taylor, CEO

★ 19603 ★ Foundation Health, A Florida Health Plan
POS Plan
1340 Concord Terrace
Sunrise, FL 33323
Phone: (954)858-3000 **Free:** 800-422-7335
Fax: (954)846-0331
Website: http://www.fhfl.com
Robert Berzing, CEO

★ 19604 ★ Humana Health Care Plans of Orlando
POS Plan
PO Box 9148000
Longwood, FL 32779
Phone: (407)661-6000 **Fax:** (407)661-6414
Website: http://www.humana.com/orlando/home.html
Michael B. McCallister, President

★ 19605 ★ Humana Health Plan - Jacksonville
POS Plan
76 S Laura St., 16th Fl.
Jacksonville, FL 32202
Phone: (904)376-1100 **Free:** 800-945-7703
Fax: (904)376-2370
Website: http://www.humana.com
David A. Jones, Chairman of the Board

★ 19606 ★ Humana Medical Plans, Inc.
POS Plan
3501 SW 160th Ave.
Miramar, FL 33027
Phone: (305)621-5499 **Free:** 800-442-5555
Fax: (305)626-5297
Website: http://www.humana.com
David A. Jones, Chairman of the Board

★ 19607 ★ One Health Plan of Florida
POS Plan
7650 Courtney Campbell Csy, Ste. 850
Tampa, FL 33607
Phone: (813)207-0216 **Free:** 800-533-0919
Fax: (813)207-0613
Website: http://www.onehealthplan.com
Susan Griffin, Contact

★ 19608 ★ Physicians Healthcare Plans, Inc.
POS Plan
1410 N Westshore Blvd., Ste. 200
Tampa, FL 33607
Phone: (813)273-7474 **Free:** 800-873-7474
Fax: (813)829-6302
Michael Fernandez, CEO

★ 19609 ★ United Concordia Co., Inc. - Florida
POS Plan
601 Cleveland St., Ste. 415
Clearwater, FL 33755
Phone: (727)441-8585 **Free:** 800-322-0366
Fax: (727)441-6090
Website: http://www.ucci.com
Thomas Dzuryachko, CEO
Program(s): Dental.

★ 19610 ★ United HealthCare of Florida, Inc.
POS Plan
9009 Corporate Lake Dr.
Tampa, FL 33624
Phone: (813)890-4500 **Free:** 800-595-0440
Fax: (813)357-5079
Website: http://www.uhc.com
Ken L. Hoverman, CEO

★ 19611 ★ United HealthCare of Florida, Inc.
POS Plan
13621 NW 12th St.
Sunrise, FL 33323
Phone: (954)858-4000 **Fax:** (954)858-3815
Website: http://www.uhc.com
Michael Muchnicki, CEO

★ 19612 ★ Vista Health Plan Inc.
POS Plan
300 S Park Rd.
Hollywood, FL 33021
Free: 800-422-7335 **Fax:** (954)986-6013
Joe Berding, CEO

Georgia

★ 19613 ★ Aetna Inc. - Georgia
POS Plan
11675 Great Oaks Way
Alpharetta, GA 30022
Phone: (770)346-4300 **Free:** 800-353-5980
Fax: (770)346-2157
Website: http://www.aetna.com
John W. Rowe, Chairman of the Board

★ 19614 ★ Athens Area Health Plan Select, Inc.
POS Plan
295 W Clayton St.
Athens, GA 30601
Phone: (706)549-0549 **Free:** 800-293-6260
Fax: (706)549-8004
Website: http://www.aahps.com
Larry Webb, President

★ 19615 ★ CIGNA HealthCare of Georgia
POS Plan
100 Peachtree St., Ste. 800
Atlanta, GA 30303
Phone: (404)681-7000 **Fax:** (404)681-7031
Website: http://www.cigna.com
Robert Youngk, CEO

★ 19616 ★ Coventry Health Care Inc. - Georgia, Inc.
POS Plan
1100 Circle 75 Pkwy., Ste. 1400
Atlanta, GA 30339
Phone: (678)202-2100 **Free:** 800-470-2004
Fax: (678)202-2196
Website: http://www.cvty.com
Thomas A. Davis, CEO

★ 19617 ★ Humana Health Plans of Georgia
POS Plan
900 Ashwood Pkwy., Ste. 400
Atlanta, GA 30338
Phone: (770)393-9226 **Free:** 800-234-3486
Fax: (770)393-2845
Website: http://www.humana.com/georgia/home.html
Karen Hornsby, Contact

★ 19618 ★ Kaiser Foundation Health Plan of Georgia
POS Plan
3495 Piedmont Rd. NE, Bldg. 9
Atlanta, GA 30305-1736
Phone: (404)364-7000 **Fax:** (404)364-4791
Website: http://www.kaiserpermanante.org
Carolyn Kenny, CEO

★ 19619 ★ Magellan Behavioral Health of Georgia
POS Plan
125 Plantation Center Dr.
Macon, GA 31210
Free: 800-458-2740 **Fax:** (410)953-2426
Website: http://www.magellanhealth.com
Henry T. Harbin, MD, Chairman of the Board

★ 19620 ★ One Health Plan of Georgia, Inc.
POS Plan
245 Perimeter Ctr. Pkwy., 7th Fl.
Atlanta, GA 30346
Phone: (770)290-7000 **Free:** 800-511-3899
Fax: (770)290-7022
Website: http://www.onehealthplan.com
David Record, CEO

★ 19621 ★ Private Healthcare Systems - Georgia
POS Plan
5600 New Northside Dr., Ste. 700
Atlanta, GA 30328
Phone: (770)818-9048 **Free:** 800-253-4417
Fax: (770)818-9101
Website: http://www.phcs.com
Joseph Driscoll, CEO & Pres

★ 19622 ★ Secure Health Plans of Georgia, LLC
POS Plan
PO Box 4088
Macon, GA 31210
Phone: (478)314-2400 **Free:** 800-648-7563
Fax: (478)738-9596
Website: http://www.shpg.com
George Israel, CEO

★ 19623 ★ United HealthCare of Georgia
POS Plan
2970 Clairmont Rd., Ste. 300
Atlanta, GA 30329-1634
Phone: (404)982-8800 **Free:** 800-842-6219
Fax: (404)320-8351
Website: http://www.uhc.com
Teresa Kline, CEO

Idaho

★ 19624 ★ Group Health Northwest
POS Plan
2010 N Lakewood Dr.
Coeur D'Arlene, ID 83814-2635
Phone: (208)664-5174 **Free:** 800-497-2210
Fax: (208)664-9315
Website: http://www.ghc.org
Cheryl Scott, CEO

★ 19625 ★ Primary Health Plan
POS Plan
800 Park Blvd., Ste. 760
Boise, ID 83712
Phone: (208)344-1811 **Free:** 800-688-5008
Fax: (208)344-4262
Website: http://www.primaryhealth.com
Elden Mitchell, CEO & Pres

Illinois

★ 19626 ★ Aetna Inc. - Illinois
POS Plan
100 N Riverside Plaza, 20th Fl.
Chicago, IL 60606-1518
Phone: (312)928-3000 **Free:** 800-627-5039
Fax: (312)928-3232
Website: http://www.aetna.com
John W. Rowe, MD, Chairman of the Board

★ 19627 ★ CIGNA Healthcare of Illinois, Inc.
POS Plan
525 W Monroe St., Ste. 1800
Chicago, IL 60661-3629
Phone: (312)648-2460 **Free:** 800-541-7526
Fax: (312)648-3617
Website: http://www.cigna.com
Bert Wagner, CEO

★ 19628 ★ Delta Dental Plan of Illinois
POS Plan
801 Ogden Ave.
Lisle, IL 60532
Phone: (630)964-2400 **Free:** 800-331-0538
Fax: (630)964-2596
Website: http://www.deltadentalil.com
Robert Dennison, DMD, CEO & Pres

★ 19629 ★ Health Alliance Medical Plans - Corporate Headquarters
POS Plan
102 E Main St.
Urbana, IL 61801
Phone: (217)337-8000 **Free:** 800-851-3379
Fax: (217)337-8093
Website: http://www.hapcorp.org
Jeffery Ingrum, MD, CEO

★ 19630 ★ Health Plus
POS Plan
5409 N Knoxville Ave.
Peoria, IL 61614
Phone: (309)689-8600 **Fax:** (309)689-8601
Website: http://www.healthpluspeoria.org
Philip Walker, II, CEO & Pres

★ 19631 ★ Healthcare Service Corp. - Corporate Headquarters
POS Plan
300 E Randolph St.
Chicago, IL 60601-5099
Phone: (312)653-6000 **Fax:** (312)819-1220
Website: http://www.bcbsil.com
Raymond McCaskey, CEO

★ 19632 ★ Humana Health Care Plans of Illinois
POS Plan
30 S Wacker Dr., Ste. 3100
Chicago, IL 60606
Phone: (312)441-9111 **Free:** 800-852-9556
Fax: (312)441-5901
Website: http://www.humana.com/Illinois/home.html
David Jones, Chairman of the Board

★ 19633 ★ John Deere Health
POS Plan
7210 N Villa Lake Dr.
Peoria, IL 61614
Phone: (309)689-4630 **Free:** 800-224-6599
Fax: (309)689-3165
Website: http://www.johndeerehealth.com
Richard L. Bartsh, MD, President

★ 19634 ★ John Deere Health - Corporate Headquarters
POS Plan
1300 River Dr., Ste. 200
Moline, IL 61265
Phone: (309)765-1200 **Fax:** (309)748-1322
Website: http://www.johndeerehealth.com
Richard L. Bartsh, MD, President

★ 19635 ★ OSF Health Plans
POS Plan
7915 N Hale Ave., Ste. D
Peoria, IL 61615-2047
Phone: (309)677-8200 **Fax:** (309)677-8338
Website: http://www.osfhealthplans.com
Kevin Schoeplein, CEO

★ 19636 ★ Personal Care
POS Plan
2110 Fox Dr.
Champaign, IL 61820
Phone: (217)366-1226 **Free:** 800-366-6730
Fax: (217)366-5410
David Line, CEO

★ 19637 ★ PPONext - Ohio
8745 W Higgins Rd., Ste. 300
Chicago, IL 60631
Free: 888-446-6098 **Fax:** (216)642-0161
Website: http://www.healthstarinc.com
Steve Carder, President

★ 19638 ★ Quincy Health Care Management Inc.
POS Plan
1246 Broadway
Quincy, IL 62301
Phone: (217)222-9157 **Free:** 800-637-7100
Fax: (217)222-1732
Website: http://www.riverguestnetwork.com
Karen J. Brown, Contact

★ 19639 ★ Rockford Health Plans, Inc.
POS Plan
3401 N Perryville Rd.
Rockford, IL 61114
Phone: (815)971-1000 **Free:** 800-331-0424
Fax: (815)654-5188
Website: http://www.rockfordhealthplans.com
Edward Pattarozzi, CEO & Pres

★ 19640 ★ UniCare
POS Plan
233 S Wacker Dr., Ste. 3900
Chicago, IL 60606
Phone: (312)234-7000 **Free:** 888-234-7747
Fax: (312)234-8001
Website: http://www.rushpru.com
Sandra Van Trease, CEO

★ 19641 ★ Unicare Inc.
POS Plan
8420 W Bryn Mawr, Ste. 700
Chicago, IL 60631
Phone: (847)843-2200 **Free:** 800-949-5449
Fax: 888-788-5526
Charles Mitchell, Contact

★ 19642 ★ United HealthCare of Illinois, Inc.
POS Plan
233 N Michigan Ave.
Chicago, IL 60601
Phone: (312)424-4460 **Fax:** (312)424-4905
Website: http://www.uhc.com
William Moeller, CEO

Indiana

★ 19643 ★ Advantage Health Plan Inc.
11555 N Meridian St., Ste. 240
Carmel, IN 46032
Phone: (317)573-2700 **Free:** 877-903-2237
Fax: (317)580-8009
Website: http://www.advantageplan.com
Vincent Caponi, Chairman of the Board

★ 19644 ★ Aetna Inc. - Indiana
POS Plan
8425 Woodfield Crossing Blvd.
Indianapolis, IN 46240

Phone: (317)815-4300 Free: 800-382-3209
Fax: (317)815-4397
Website: http://www.aetna.com
John W. Rowe, MD, Chairman of the Board

★ 19645 ★ Aetna Inc. - Indiana
POS Plan
9365 Counselors Row, Ste. 110
Indianapolis, IN 46240
Phone: (317)815-4300 Fax: (317)815-4317
Website: http://www.aetna.com
John W. Rowe, Chairman of the Board

★ 19646 ★ Arnett Health Plans
POS Plan
PO Box 6108
Lafayette, IN 47903
Phone: (765)448-7701 Fax: (765)448-7700
Website: http://www.arnettplans.com
James Brunnemer, CEO

★ 19647 ★ CIGNA Healthcare of Indiana
POS Plan
429 N Pennsylvania, Ste. 301
Indianapolis, IN 46204
Phone: (317)615-1200 Free: 800-276-0363
Fax: (317)615-1301
Website: http://www.cigna.com
Mary Brandt, CEO

★ 19648 ★ Deaconess Health Plans
POS Plan
600 Mary St.
Evansville, IN 47747-0002
Phone: (812)450-7265 Free: 800-374-8993
Fax: (812)450-2030
Website: http://www.deaconess.com
Joyce Hudson, CEO

★ 19649 ★ IU Health Plan
POS Plan
3901 W 86th St., Ste. 230
Indianapolis, IN 46268
Phone: (317)871-8811 Fax: (317)371-8833
Website: http://www.iuhp.com
Kim Singleton, President

★ 19650 ★ Lutheran Preferred
POS Plan
7950 W Jefferson Blvd.
Fort Wayne, IN 46804
Phone: 800-444-2001 Free: 800-258-0974
Fax: (219)435-6940
Website: http://www.lutheranpreferred.com
Thomas Miller, CEO

★ 19651 ★ M Plan, Inc.
POS Plan
8802 N Meridian St., Ste. 100
Indianapolis, IN 46260-5371
Phone: (317)571-5300 Free: 800-878-8802
Fax: (317)571-5306
Website: http://www.mplan.com
Alex Slabosky, CEO & Pres

★ 19652 ★ Partners National Health Plans of Indiana, Inc.
POS Plan
100 E Wayne St., Ste. 302
South Bend, IN 46601
Phone: (260)233-4899 Free: 800-876-2655
Fax: (260)234-7484
Website: http://www.partnersindiana.com
Bruce Greenberg, CEO

★ 19653 ★ Physicians Health Plan of Northern Indiana
POS Plan
8101 W Jefferson Blvd.
Fort Wayne, IN 46804-4163
Phone: (260)432-6690 Free: 800-982-6257
Fax: (260)432-0493
Website: http://www.phpni.com
Jay Gilbert, CEO

★ 19654 ★ Southeastern Indiana Health Organization, Inc.
POS Plan
PO Box 1787
Columbus, IN 47202-1787
Phone: (812)378-7000 Fax: (812)348-4592
Website: http://www.siho.org
David Barker, CEO & Pres

★ 19655 ★ Welborn Health Plans
POS Plan
421 Chestnut St.
Evansville, IN 47713-1337
Phone: (812)426-6600 Free: 800-521-0265
Fax: (812)426-9874
Website: http://www.welbornclinic.com
David Christeson, MD, Chairman of the Board

Iowa

★ 19656 ★ Coventry Health Care Inc. - Iowa
POS Plan
4600 Westown Pkwy., Ste. 200
West Des Moines, IA 50266-1099
Phone: (515)225-1234 Free: 800-257-4692
Fax: (515)223-9239
Website: http://www.chciowa.com
Michael Teachaut, CEO

★ 19657 ★ Foundation for Medical Care/ Encompass
POS Plan
6000 Westown Pkwy., Ste. 350E
West Des Moines, IA 50266-7771
Phone: (515)223-2900 Free: 800-383-2856
Fax: (515)223-2990
Website: http://www.encompass.com
Fred Ferree, CEO
Program(s): Chiropractic, Home Care, Inpatient SNF, Long-Term Care, Pharmaceutical Mail Order, Psychiatric, Transplant, Wellness, Workers' Compensation.

★ 19658 ★ John Deere Health
POS Plan
4201 W Towne Pkwy., Ste. 325
West Des Moines, IA 50266-6720
Phone: (515)327-2000 Free: 800-373-5050
Fax: (515)327-1128
Website: http://www.johndeerehealth.com
Richard L. Bartsh, MD, President

★ 19659 ★ John Deere Health
POS Plan
635 E Pennsylvania Ave.
Ottumwa, IA 52501
Phone: (515)682-9751 Free: 800-224-6578
Fax: (515)682-8751
Website: http://www.johndeerehealth.com
Richard L. Bartsh, MD, President

★ 19660 ★ John Deere Health
POS Plan
PO Box 9000
Waterloo, IA 50704
Phone: (319)291-3291 Free: 800-224-6596
Fax: (319)291-7838
Website: http://www.johndeerehealth.com
Richard L. Bartsh, MD, President

★ 19661 ★ John Deere Health
POS Plan
1660 Embassy W Dr., Ste. 150
Dubuque, IA 52002
Phone: (319)588-2831 Free: 800-224-6597
Fax: (319)588-2920
Website: http://www.johndeerehealth.com
Richard L. Bartsh, MD, President

★ 19662 ★ John Deere Health
POS Plan
1845 51st St. NE
Cedar Rapids, IA 52402
Phone: (319)378-5200 Free: 800-373-9811
Fax: (319)378-0566
Website: http://www.johndeerehealth.com
Richard L. Bartsh, MD, President

★ 19663 ★ Medical Associates Health Plans
POS Plan
700 Locust St., Ste. 230
Dubuque, IA 52004
Phone: (563)556-8070 Free: 800-747-8900
Fax: (563)556-5134
Website: http://www.mahealthcare.com
Alan Avery, CEO

★ 19664 ★ Wellmark, Inc. - Corporate Headquarters
POS Plan
636 Grand Ave.
Des Moines, IA 50309-2565
Phone: (515)245-4500 Fax: (515)245-5090
Website: http://www.wellmark.com
John Forsyth, CEO & Chm Bd

Kansas

★ 19665 ★ CIGNA HealthCare of Kansas/ Missouri
POS Plan
7400 W 110th St., Ste. 600
Overland Park, KS 66210
Phone: (913)451-9389 Fax: (913)451-0974
Website: http://www.cigna.com
Rick Grizzle, Contact

★ 19666 ★ Coventry Health Care Inc. - Wichita
POS Plan
8301 E 21st St. N, No. 300
Wichita, KS 67206
Phone: (316)634-1222 Free: 800-664-9251
Fax: (316)634-1266
Website: http://www.cvty.com
Jan Stallmeyer, CEO

★ 19667 ★ Preferred Health Systems
POS Plan
8535 E 21st St. N
Wichita, KS 67206
Phone: (316)609-2345 Free: 800-990-0345
Fax: (316)609-2346
Website: http://www.phsystems.com
Marlon Dauner, CEO & Pres

★ 19668 ★ Spectrum Vision Systems, Inc.
POS Plan
7101 College Blvd., Ste. 520
Overland Park, KS 66210
Phone: (913)451-1672 Free: 800-635-7874
Fax: (913)451-1704
Paul Disser, CEO

★ 19669 ★ United HealthCare of the Midwest, Inc.
POS Plan
9393 W 110th St., Bldg. 51, No. 300
Overland Park, KS 66210-2002
Phone: (913)663-6500 **Free:** 800-340-9716
Fax: (913)663-6549
Website: http://www.uhc.com
William Tracy, CEO

★ 19670 ★ WPPA, Inc.
POS Plan
1102 S Hillside
Wichita, KS 67211-4004
Phone: (316)683-4111 **Free:** 800-801-9772
Fax: (316)683-6255
Website: http://www.wppainc.com
Serena Lubbers, Contact

Kentucky

★ 19671 ★ Aetna Inc. - Kentucky
POS Plan
305 N Hurstbourne Pkwy., Ste. 100
Louisville, KY 40222-5146
Phone: (502)423-6240 **Fax:** (502)339-7639
Website: http://www.aetna.com
John W. Rowe, Chairman of the Board

★ 19672 ★ Bluegrass Family Health, Inc.
POS Plan
651 Perimeter Dr., Ste. 300
Lexington, KY 40517
Phone: (859)269-4475 **Fax:** (859)269-6447
Website: http://www.bgfh.com
James Fritz, CEO & Pres

★ 19673 ★ Center Care Community Health Plans
POS Plan
1225 Fairway St.
Bowling Green, KY 42103
Phone: (270)745-1517 **Free:** 800-972-7038
Fax: (270)796-2106
Website: http://www.centercare.com
Teresa Wilson, Contact

★ 19674 ★ CHA Health
POS Plan
300 W Vine St.
Lexington, KY 40503
Phone: (859)271-5055 **Free:** 800-457-5683
Fax: (859)232-8557
Website: http://www.cha.com
Mark Birdwhistell, CEO

★ 19675 ★ CIGNA Healthcare of Kentucky
POS Plan
5111 Commerce Crossing Dr.
Louisville, KY 40229
Phone: (502)753-2341 **Free:** 800-808-1534
Fax: (502)753-2365
Website: http://www.cigna.com
Robert Bruce, CEO

★ 19676 ★ Commonwealth Health Plan
300 W Vine St.
Lexington, KY 40507
Phone: (859)232-8686 **Free:** 800-457-5683
Fax: (859)232-8557
Website: http://www.cha-health.com
Mark Birdwhistle, CEO

★ 19677 ★ Humana Health Care Plans of Kansas & Missouri
POS Plan
500 W Main St.
Louisville, KY 40201-1438
Phone: (816)941-8900 **Free:** 800-842-6188
Fax: (816)941-0879
Website: http://www.humana.com/kansascity/home.html
Michael McCallister, CEO

★ 19678 ★ Humana Health Care Plans of Lexington
POS Plan
500 W Main St.
Lexington, KY 40507
Phone: (859)263-1400 **Free:** 800-221-8390
Fax: (859)263-1488
Website: http://www.humana.com/lexington/home.html
Michael McCallister, CEO & Pres

★ 19679 ★ Humana Health Care Plans of San Antonio
POS Plan
500 W Main St.
Louisville, KY 40201-1438
Phone: (210)617-1000 **Fax:** (210)615-0090
Website: http://www.humana.com
David A. Jones, Chairman of the Board

★ 19680 ★ Humana Health Plan - Kentucky
POS Plan
500 W Main St.
Louisville, KY 40202
Phone: (502)580-1860 **Fax:** (502)580-3127
Website: http://www.humana.com
Michael McCallister, CEO

★ 19681 ★ Humana, Inc. - Alabama
POS Plan
500 W Main St.
Louisville, KY 40201-1438
Phone: (502)580-1000 **Fax:** (502)580-3127
Website: http://www.humana.com
David Jones, Chairman of the Board

★ 19682 ★ Humana, Inc. - Arkansas
POS Plan
500 W Main St.
Louisville, KY 40201-1438
Phone: (502)580-1000 **Fax:** (502)580-4106
Website: http://www.humana.com
David Jones, Chairman of the Board

★ 19683 ★ Humana Inc. - Corporate Headquarters
POS Plan
PO Box 740036
Louisville, KY 40201-7436
Phone: (502)580-1860 **Fax:** (502)580-3127
Website: http://www.humana.com
David Jones, Chairman of the Board

★ 19684 ★ Humana, Inc. - Ohio
POS Plan
500 W Main St.
Louisville, KY 40201-1438
Phone: (502)784-5200 **Fax:** (502)543-7158
Website: http://www.humana.com
Michael McCallister, CEO & Pres

★ 19685 ★ Humana, Inc. - Virginia
POS Plan
PO Box 740036
Louisville, KY 40201-1438
Phone: (502)580-1860 **Fax:** (502)580-3127
Website: http://www.humana.com
Michael McCallister, CEO & Pres

★ 19686 ★ Humana Military Service, Inc.
POS Plan
500 W Main St.
Louisville, KY 40201
Phone: (502)580-5804 **Fax:** (502)580-8528
Website: http://www.humana.com
David Jones, Chairman of the Board

★ 19687 ★ United Concordia Co., Inc. - Kentucky
POS Plan
4010 Dupont Cir., Ste. L-03
Louisville, KY 40207
Phone: (717)731-2532 **Free:** 800-568-6432
Fax: (717)972-0410
Website: http://www.ucci.com
Thomas Dzuryachko, CEO
Program(s): Dental.

★ 19688 ★ United HealthCare of Kentucky, Inc.
POS Plan
2424 Harrodsburg Rd.
Lexington, KY 40504-3329
Phone: (859)296-6000 **Fax:** (859)224-3732
Website: http://www.uhc.com
Charles Price, CEO

Louisiana

★ 19689 ★ Aetna Inc. - Arkansas
POS Plan
3900 N Causeway Blvd., Ste. 410
Metairie, LA 70002-7283
Phone: (504)830-5600 **Free:** 800-685-4857
Fax: (504)837-6571
Website: http://www.aetna.com
John W. Rowe, Chairman of the Board

★ 19690 ★ Aetna Inc. - Louisiana
POS Plan
3900 N Causeway Blvd., Ste. 410
Metairie, LA 70002-7283
Phone: (504)830-5600 **Free:** 800-685-4857
Fax: (504)837-6571
Website: http://www.aetna.com
John W. Rowe, Chairman of the Board

★ 19691 ★ AmCare Health Plans of Louisiana
POS Plan
5353 Essen Ln., Ste. 450
Baton Rouge, LA 70809
Phone: (225)763-5300 **Free:** 800-772-2995
Fax: (225)763-6211
Website: http://www.amcarehealthplans.com
Thomas Lucksinger, CEO

★ 19692 ★ American LifeCare Corporate Headquarters
POS Plan
650 Poydras St., Ste. 1150
New Orleans, LA 70130-6131
Phone: (504)561-0600 **Fax:** (504)679-0150
Website: http://www.americanlifecare.com
Edward Michael Reggie, Chairman of the Board

★ 19693 ★ Coventry Health Care Inc. - Louisiana
POS Plan
2424 Edenborn Ave., Ste. 350
Metairie, LA 70001
Phone: (504)834-0840 **Free:** 800-341-6613
Fax: (504)834-2694

Website: http://www.cvty.com
Keith Benoit, Sr., CEO

★ 19694 ★ FARA Healthcare Management
POS Plan
2360 Fifth Ave.
Mandeville, LA 70471
Phone: (985)624-8383 **Free:** 800-259-8388
Fax: (985)624-8489
Website: http://www.fara.com
Reed Bell, CEO

★ 19695 ★ Health Plus of Louisiana, Inc.
POS Plan
2751 Albert L. Bicknell Dr., 2B
Shreveport, LA 71103
Phone: (318)212-8800 **Free:** 800-331-5055
Fax: (318)212-4095
Website: http://www.wkmc.com
James K. Elrod, Chairman of the Board

★ 19696 ★ HMO Louisiana, Inc.
POS Plan
5525 Reitz Ave.
Baton Rouge, LA 70898-9024
Phone: (225)295-3307 **Free:** 800-376-7741
Fax: (225)295-2054
Website: http://www.bcbsla.com
Richard Atkins, Chairman of the Board

★ 19697 ★ Ochsner Health Plan
Total Health Choice & Total Health Plus (POS)
One Galleria Blvd., Ste. 850
Metairie, LA 70001
Phone: (504)836-6600 **Free:** 888-882-9806
Fax: (504)836-6688
Website: http://www.ohp-louisiana.com
Terry Schilling, CEO

★ 19698 ★ SMA Health Plan, Inc.
POS Plan
1555 Poydres
New Orleans, LA 70112
Phone: (504)837-7374 **Free:** 800-259-7370
Fax: (504)837-7115
Website: http://www.sma.net
Robert Gormley, MD, Contact

★ 19699 ★ Tulane Preferred Health Plan
POS Plan
1430 Tulane Ave., TW3
New Orleans, LA 70112
Free: 800-708-2470 **Fax:** (504)988-7757
Steven Wallin, CEO

★ 19700 ★ United HealthCare of Louisiana, Inc.
POS Plan
3838 N Causeway Blvd., Ste. 2100
Metairie, LA 70009
Phone: (504)849-3510 **Free:** 800-864-4799
Fax: (504)849-3551
Website: http://www.uhc.com
Sam Patterson, CEO

Maine

★ 19701 ★ Aetna Inc. - Maine
POS Plan
One Monument Sq., 5th Fl.
Portland, ME 04101
Phone: (207)879-1995 **Fax:** (207)879-7951
Website: http://www.aetna.com
John W. Rowe, MD, Chairman of the Board

★ 19702 ★ Cigna Healthcare of Maine, Inc.
POS Plan
2 Stonewood Dr.
Freeport, ME 04032-0447
Phone: (207)865-5000 **Free:** 800-642-5551
Fax: (207)865-5633
Website: http://www.cigna.com/healthcare/hs/me.html
Richard White, CEO & Pres

Maryland

★ 19703 ★ Aetna Inc. - DE, MD, DC
POS Plan
1302 Concourse Dr., Ste. 402
Linthicum, MD 21090
Phone: (410)691-1080 **Free:** 800-328-8742
Fax: (410)691-1198
Website: http://www.aetna.com
John W. Rowe, Chairman of the Board

★ 19704 ★ APS Healthcare Inc.
POS Plan
6705 Rockledge Dr., Ste. 200
Bethesda, MD 20817
Phone: (301)571-0633 **Free:** 800-305-3720
Website: http://www.apscare.com
Ken Kessler, MD, CEO & Chm Bd

★ 19705 ★ BCE Emergis - California
POS Plan
2273 Research Blvd.
Rockville, MD 20850
Phone: (301)548-1000 **Free:** 800-248-7744
Fax: (301)296-5020
Francois Cole, CEO & Pres

★ 19706 ★ CIGNA Healthcare Mid-Atlantic
POS Plan
9700 Patuxent Woods Dr.
Columbia, MD 21046
Phone: (410)720-5800 **Free:** 800-541-7526
Fax: (410)720-5860
Website: http://www.cigna.com/healthcare/hs/md.html
Matt Manders, CEO

★ 19707 ★ Coventry Health Care, Inc. - Corporate Headquarters
POS Plan
6705 Rockledge Dr., Ste. 900
Bethesda, MD 20817
Phone: (301)581-0600 **Fax:** (301)493-0700
Website: http://www.cvty.com
Allen Wise, CEO

★ 19708 ★ Delmarva Health Care Plan, Inc.
POS Plan
10455 Mill Run Circle
Owings Mills, MD 21117
Phone: (410)822-7223 **Free:** 800-334-3427
Fax: (410)822-8152
William Jews, CEO & Pres

★ 19709 ★ Dental Benefit Providers, Inc. - Corporate Headquarters
POS Plan
7200 Wisconsin Ave., Ste. 800
Bethesda, MD 20814
Phone: (301)654-6900 **Free:** 800-445-9090
Fax: (301)986-7965
Website: http://www.dbp.com
Edward Murphy, CEO

★ 19710 ★ Freestate Health Plan
POS Plan
10455 Mill Run Circle
Owings Mills, MD 21117
Phone: (410)654-8670 **Free:** 800-445-6036
Fax: (410)528-7013
Website: http://www.carefirst.com
William Jews, CEO & Pres

★ 19711 ★ Kaiser Foundation Health Plan - Mid-Atlantic States
POS Plan
2101 E Jefferson St.
Rockville, MD 20849
Phone: (301)816-2474 **Free:** 800-368-5784
Fax: (301)816-7491
Website: http://www.kpne.org
Marilyn Kowamura, CEO

★ 19712 ★ Magellan Health Services
POS Plan
6950 Columbia Gateway Dr.
Columbia, MD 21046
Phone: (410)953-1000 **Free:** 800-458-2740
Fax: (410)953-5200
Website: http://www.magellanhealth.com
Henry T. Harbin, MD, Chairman of the Board
Program(s): Behavioral Health.

★ 19713 ★ Mid Atlantic Medical Services, Inc. (MAMSI)
POS Plan
4 Taft Court
Rockville, MD 20850
Phone: (301)762-8205 **Fax:** (301)738-1230
Website: http://www.mamsi.com
Thomas Barbera, CEO & Pres

★ 19714 ★ Sheppard Pratt Health Plan
POS Plan
PO Box 1470
Rockville, MD 20849
Phone: (410)938-3200 **Free:** 800-881-2279
Fax: (410)938-4099
Website: http://www.sheppardpratt.org
Steven Sharfstein, MD, CEO

★ 19715 ★ United Concordia Co., Inc. - Maryland
POS Plan
1220 B E Joppa Rd., Ste. 421
Towson, MD 21286-5811
Free: 800-272-8865 **Fax:** (410)296-4367
Website: http://www.ucci.com
Thomas Dzuryachko, CEO
Program(s): Dental.

★ 19716 ★ United HealthCare of the Mid Atlantic
POS Plan
6300 Security Blvd.
Baltimore, MD 21207
Phone: (410)277-6000 **Fax:** (410)277-6661
Website: http://www.uhc.com
Bob Fleshner, CEO

Massachusetts

★ 19717 ★ CIGNA Healthcare of Massachusetts
POS Plan
3 Newton Executive Pkwy.
Newton, MA 02462
Phone: (617)630-4300 **Fax:** (617)630-4380
Website: http://www.cigna.com
Imre Toth, MD, Contact

★ 19718 ★ CIGNA Healthcare of Massachusetts
POS Plan
100 Front St., Ste. 300
Worcester, MA 01608-1449
Phone: (508)798-8667 **Free:** 800-922-8380
Fax: (508)849-4299
Website: http://www.cigna.com
Linda Dwyer, CEO

★ 19719 ★ Fallon Community Health Plan
Fallon Flex (POS)
10 Chestnut St.
Worcester, MA 01608-2810
Phone: (508)799-2100 **Free:** 800-283-2556
Fax: (508)797-4387
Website: http://www.fchp.org
Robert Cavanaugh, MD, Chairman of the Board

★ 19720 ★ First All America Financial
POS Plan
440 Lincoln St.
Worcester, MA 01653
Phone: (508)855-1000 **Free:** 800-634-8647
Fax: (508)853-6202
Website: http://www.allamerica.com
Jack O'Brien, CEO

★ 19721 ★ Harvard Pilgrim Health Care - Corporate Headquarters
POS Plan
93 Worchester St.
Wellesley, MA 02481
Phone: (781)263-6000 **Free:** 800-742-8326
Fax: (617)509-2515
Website: http://www.harvardpilgrim.org
Charles Baker, CEO & Pres

★ 19722 ★ Health New England
POS Plan
One Monarch Place
Springfield, MA 01144-1006
Phone: (413)787-4000 **Free:** 800-842-4464
Fax: (413)734-3356
Website: http://www.healthnewengland.com
Peter F. Straley, CEO & Pres

★ 19723 ★ Private Healthcare Systems - California
POS Plan
1100 Winter St.
Waltham, MA 02451
Phone: (949)476-9816 **Free:** 800-253-4417
Fax: (949)476-0650
Website: http://www.phcs.com
Joseph Driscoll, CEO & Pres

★ 19724 ★ Private Healthcare Systems - Corporate Headquarters
POS Plan
1100 Winter St.
Waltham, MA 02451
Phone: (781)895-7500 **Free:** 800-253-4417
Fax: (781)895-3477
Website: http://www.phcs.com
Joseph Driscoll, CEO & Pres

★ 19725 ★ Private Healthcare Systems - Florida
POS Plan
1100 Winter St.
Waltham, MA 02451
Phone: (781)895-7500 **Free:** 800-253-4417
Fax: (781)895-3477
Website: http://www.phcs.com
Barbara Dailey, Contact

★ 19726 ★ Private Healthcare Systems - Illinois
POS Plan
1100 Winter St.
Waltham, MA 02451
Phone: (847)292-6700 **Free:** 800-253-4417
Fax: (781)292-6736
Website: http://www.phcs.com
Joseph Driscoll, Contact

★ 19727 ★ Private Healthcare Systems - Michigan
POS Plan
1100 Winter St.
Waltham, MA 02451
Phone: (781)895-7500 **Free:** 800-253-4417
Fax: (781)895-3477
Website: http://www.phcs.com
Joseph Driscoll, CEO & Pres

★ 19728 ★ Private Healthcare Systems - Missouri
POS Plan
1100 Winter St.
Waltham, MA 02451
Phone: (816)221-4455 **Free:** 800-253-4417
Fax: (816)221-4466
Website: http://www.phcs.com
Joseph Driscoll, CEO & Pres

★ 19729 ★ Private Healthcare Systems - New Jersey
POS Plan
1100 Winter St.
Waltham, MA 02451
Phone: (201)909-8803 **Free:** 800-253-4417
Fax: (201)909-0260
Website: http://www.phcs.com
Joseph Driscoll, CEO & Pres

★ 19730 ★ Private Healthcare Systems - New York
POS Plan
1100 Winter St.
Waltham, MA 02451
Phone: (781)895-7500 **Free:** 800-253-4417
Fax: (781)895-3477
Website: http://www.phcs.com
Joseph Driscoll, CEO & Pres

★ 19731 ★ Private Healthcare Systems - Ohio
POS Plan
1100 Winter St.
Waltham, MA 02451
Phone: (781)895-7500 **Free:** 800-253-4417
Fax: (781)895-3477
Website: http://www.phcs.com
Joseph Driscoll, CEO & Pres

★ 19732 ★ Private Healthcare Systems - Tennessee
POS Plan
1100 Winter St.
Waltham, MA 02451
Phone: (781)895-7500 **Free:** 800-253-4417
Fax: (781)895-3477
Website: http://www.phcs.com
Joseph Driscoll, CEO & Pres

★ 19733 ★ Private Healthcare Systems - Texas
POS Plan
1100 Winter St.
Waltham, MA 02451
Phone: (781)895-7500 **Free:** 800-253-4417
Fax: (781)895-3477
Website: http://www.phcs.com
Joseph Driscoll, CEO & Pres

★ 19734 ★ Private Healthcare Systems - Virginia
POS Plan
1100 Winter St.
Waltham, MA 02451
Phone: (781)895-7500 **Free:** 800-253-4417
Fax: (781)895-3477
Website: http://www.phcs.com
Joseph Driscoll, CEO & Pres

★ 19735 ★ Private Healthcare Systems - Washington
POS Plan
1100 Winter St.
Waltham, MA 02451
Phone: (781)895-7500 **Free:** 800-253-4417
Fax: (781)895-3477
Website: http://www.phcs.com
Joseph Driscoll, CEO & Pres

★ 19736 ★ Tufts Health Plan
POS Plan
333 Wyman St.
Waltham, MA 02454
Phone: (781)466-9400 **Free:** 800-394-3993
Website: http://www.tufts-healthplan.com
Harris Berman, MD, CEO

Michigan

★ 19737 ★ ConnectCare
POS Plan
4009 Orchard Dr., Ste. 3021
Midland, MI 48640
Phone: (989)839-1615 **Fax:** (989)839-1626
Website: http://www.connectcare.com
Brian Rodgers, CEO & Pres

★ 19738 ★ Health Alliance Plan
POS Plan
2850 W Grand Blvd.
Detroit, MI 48202
Phone: (313)872-8100 **Free:** 800-422-4641
Website: http://www.hapcorp.org
Cleve Killingsworth, CEO & Pres

★ 19739 ★ Health Care Exchange Limited Co.
POS Plan
32290 5 Mile Rd.
Livonia, MI 48154
Phone: (734)452-2500 **Fax:** (734)452-2501
Website: http://www.dentemax.com
Kenneth R. Dallafior, CEO
Program(s): Dental.

★ 19740 ★ Health Plus of Michigan, Inc.
POS Plan
PO Box 1700
Flint, MI 48501-1700
Phone: (810)230-2000 **Free:** 800-332-9161
Fax: (810)230-2208
Website: http://www.healthplus.com
Paul Fuhs, PhD, CEO & Pres

★ 19741 ★ Henry Ford Health System
POS Plan
1 Ford Place
Detroit, MI 48202-2608
Phone: (313)916-2600 **Fax:** (313)874-4730
Website: http://www.henryford.com
Gail Warden, CEO

★ 19742 ★ M-CARE, Inc.
POS Plan
2301 Commonwealth Blvd.
Ann Arbor, MI 48105

Phone: (734)747-8700 **Free:** 800-658-8878
Fax: (734)998-1253
Website: http://www.mcare.org
Zelda Geyer-Sylvia, CEO

★ 19743 ★ OmniCare Health Plan
POS Plan
1155 Brewery Park Blvd.
Detroit, MI 48207-9998
Phone: (313)259-4000 **Fax:** (313)393-7944
Website: http://www.ochptn.com
Gregory Moses, Jr., CEO

★ 19744 ★ Physician Health Plan of Southwest Michigan
POS Plan
PO Box 51100
Kalamazoo, MI 49005-1100
Phone: (616)341-7200 **Fax:** (616)341-6864
Website: http://www.phcares.com
David Kibbe, CEO

★ 19745 ★ Physicians Health Plan of South Michigan
POS Plan
PO Box 4055
Jackson, MI 49204
Phone: (517)782-7154 **Fax:** (517)782-4512
Jerry Grannan, CEO

★ 19746 ★ Priority Health
POS Plan
1231 E Beltline NE
Grand Rapids, MI 49525
Phone: (616)942-0954 **Free:** 800-942-0954
Fax: (616)942-5651
Website: http://www.priority-health.com
Kimberly Horn, CEO

★ 19747 ★ United Concordia Co., Inc. - Michigan
POS Plan
2000 Town Center, Ste. 2200
Southfield, MI 48075
Phone: (717)731-2532 **Free:** 800-944-6432
Fax: (248)304-2708
Website: http://www.ucci.com
Thomas Dzuryachko, CEO
Program(s): Dental.

Minnesota

★ 19748 ★ The Araz Group - Corporate Headquarters
POS Plan
8500 Normandale Lake Blvd.
Bloomington, MN 55437-3800
Phone: (952)896-1200 **Free:** 800-444-3005
Fax: (952)896-4888
Website: http://www.araz.com
Amir Eftekhari, CEO
Program(s): Chiropractic, Pharmaceutical Mail Order, Behavioral Health, Psychiatric, Wellness, Workers' Compensation.

★ 19749 ★ First Plan of Minnesota
POS Plan
1601 London Rd.
Duluth, MN 55812
Phone: (218)834-7207 **Free:** 800-635-4159
Fax: (218)834-6215
Website: http://www.firstplan.org
Milt Larson, Chairman of the Board

★ 19750 ★ Medica
POS Plan
PO Box 9310
Minneapolis, MN 55440-1587
Phone: (952)992-2900 **Fax:** (952)992-3554
Website: http://www.medica.com
David Strand, President

★ 19751 ★ United Health Group - Corporate Headquarters
POS Plan
9900 Bren Rd. E
Opus Center
Minnetonka, MN 55343
Phone: (952)936-1300 **Fax:** (952)936-0044
Website: http://www.uhc.com
William McGuire, MD, CEO & Pres

Mississippi

★ 19752 ★ Mississippi Select Health Care
POS Plan
14110 Airport Rd., Ste. 100
Gulfport, MS 39503
Phone: (228)865-0514 **Free:** 800-847-6621
Fax: (228)865-0550
Website: http://www.hmhs.com
Thomas Wicklund, CEO

★ 19753 ★ United HealthCare of Mississippi
POS Plan
800 Woodlands Pkwy., Ste. 102
Ridgeland, MS 39157
Free: 800-264-3639 **Fax:** (601)957-1306
Website: http://www.uhc.com
Robert J. Sheehy, CEO

Missouri

★ 19754 ★ Aetna Inc. - Missouri
POS Plan
2 Cityplace Dr., Ste. 300
Saint Louis, MO 63141
Phone: (314)567-6660 **Fax:** (314)567-3627
Website: http://www.aetna.com
John W. Rowe, Chairman of the Board

★ 19755 ★ Aetna Inc. - Missouri
POS Plan
2 Cityplace Dr., Ste. 300
Saint Louis, MO 63141
Phone: (314)567-6660 **Fax:** (314)567-3627
Website: http://www.aetna.com
John W. Rowe, Chairman of the Board

★ 19756 ★ Cigna Healthcare of Missouri
POS Plan
1 N Brentwood Blvd.
Clayton, MO 63105
Phone: (314)726-7850 **Free:** 800-832-3211
Fax: (314)726-7819
Website: http://www.cigna.com
James Young, President

★ 19757 ★ Community Health Plan
POS Plan
137 N Belt Hwy.
Saint Joseph, MO 64506
Phone: (816)271-1247 **Free:** 800-990-9247
Fax: (816)271-1266
Lowell Kruse, CEO

★ 19758 ★ Coventry Health Care, Inc. - Kansas City
POS Plan
1001 E 101st Terrace, Ste. 300
Kansas City, MO 64131
Phone: (816)941-3030 **Free:** 800-969-3343
Fax: (816)941-8516
Website: http://www.cvty.com
Jan Stallmeyer, CEO & Pres

★ 19759 ★ Cox Health Systems HMO, Inc.
POS Plan
PO Box 5750
Springfield, MO 65801-5720
Phone: (417)269-2900 **Free:** 800-205-7665
Fax: (417)269-2925
Website: http://www.coxhealthplans.com
Gary Jacobs, President

★ 19760 ★ First Guard Health Plan
POS Plan
3801 Blue Parkway
Kansas City, MO 64130
Phone: (816)922-7200 **Free:** 888-828-5698
Fax: (816)922-7251
Joy Wheeler, CEO

★ 19761 ★ General American Life Insurance Co. - Corporate Headquarters
POS Plan
13045 Tesson Ferry Rd.
Saint Louis, MO 63128
Phone: (314)843-8700
Website: http://www.genam.com
Warren Winer, President

★ 19762 ★ Group Health Plan
POS Plan
111 Corporate Office Dr., No. 400
Earth City, MO 63045
Phone: (314)506-1700 **Free:** 800-743-3901
Fax: (314)209-8225
Website: http://www.ghp.com
Charles R. Stark, CEO & Pres

★ 19763 ★ HealthLink, Inc. - Corporate Headquarters
POS Plan
12443 Olive Blvd.
Saint Louis, MO 63141
Phone: (314)989-6000 **Fax:** (314)989-6620
Website: http://www.healthlink.com
David T. Ott, CEO & Pres

★ 19764 ★ Mercy Health Plan of Missouri, Inc.
POS Plan
425 S Old Woods Mill Rd., No. 100
Chesterfield, MO 63017
Phone: (314)214-8100 **Free:** 800-830-1918
Fax: (314)214-8101
Website: http://www.mercyhealthplans.com
Tom Kelly, CEO

★ 19765 ★ United Concordia Co., Inc. - Missouri
POS Plan
390 South Woods Mill Rd., Ste. 175
Chesterfield, MO 63017
Phone: (717)731-2532 **Free:** 800-374-6432
Fax: (314)205-9601
Website: http://www.ucci.com
Thomas A. Dzuryacko, CEO
Program(s): Dental.

★ 19766 ★ United HealthCare of the Midwest, Inc.
POS Plan
PO Box 2560
Maryland Heights, MO 63043-8560
Phone: (314)592-7000 **Free:** 800-535-9291
Fax: (314)592-7650

Website: http://www.uhc.com
Victor Turvey, CEO & Pres

Montana

★ 19767 ★ Employee Benefit Management Services, Inc.
POS Plan
PO Box 21367
Billings, MT 59104-1367
Phone: (406)245-3575 **Free:** 800-777-3575
Fax: (406)652-5380
Website: http://www.ebmtpa.com
Rick Larson, President
Program(s): Chiropractic, Dental, Home Care, Inpatient SNF, Long-Term Care, Pharmaceutical Mail Order, Podiatry, Psychiatric, Transplant, Vision, Wellness.

Nebraska

★ 19768 ★ Coventry Health Care of Nebraska, Inc.
POS Plan
PO Box 54120
Omaha, NE 68154-9210
Phone: (402)498-9030 **Free:** 800-471-0240
Fax: (402)498-9706
Website: http://www.cvty.com
Rick Cochran, CEO

★ 19769 ★ Mutual of Omaha of South Dakota and Community Health Plus HMO, Inc.
POS plan
Mutual of Omaha Plaza
Omaha, NE 68175
Phone: (402)342-7600 **Free:** 800-228-0286
Fax: (402)351-2775
Website: http://www.mutualofomaha.com
John Weekly, CEO

★ 19770 ★ United HealthCare of the Midlands, Inc.
POS Plan
2717 N 118th Circle
Omaha, NE 68164-9672
Phone: (402)445-5000 **Free:** 800-284-0626
Fax: (402)445-5575
Website: http://www.uhc.com
John Braasch, President

Nevada

★ 19771 ★ Behavioral Healthcare Options, Inc.
POS Plan
2801 S Valley View, Ste. 6
Las Vegas, NV 89102
Phone: (702)364-1484 **Free:** 800-873-2246
Fax: (702)364-1771
Website: http://www.sierrahealth.com
Michael Adams, CEO

★ 19772 ★ Managed Care Consultants, Inc.
POS Plan
311 N Pecos Rd., Ste 100
Henderson, NV 89074
Phone: (702)792-2944 **Free:** 800-748-6842
Fax: (702)451-7307
Website: http://www.mccnevada.com
Joe Lawrence, CEO

★ 19773 ★ Nevada Care, Inc.
POS Plan
10600 W Charleston Blvd.
Las Vegas, NV 89102-2320
Phone: (702)474-7241 **Fax:** (702)474-7592
Website: http://www.nevadacare.com
Keith Beagle, President

★ 19774 ★ Sierra Health Services, Inc. - Corporate Headquarters
POS Plan
PO Box 15645
Las Vegas, NV 89114-5645
Phone: (702)242-7000 **Fax:** (702)242-7915
Website: http://www.sierrahealth.com
Anthony Marlon, MD, CEO & Chm Bd

New Hampshire

★ 19775 ★ CIGNA Healthcare New Hampshire
POS Plan
PO Box 2041
Concord, NH 03302-2041
Phone: (603)225-5077 **Free:** 800-531-3121
Fax: (603)229-2978
Website: http://www.cigna.com
Brian Wells, CEO & Pres

★ 19776 ★ Matthew Thornton Health Plan
POS Plan
3000 Guffs Fall Rd.
Manchester, NH 03111
Phone: (603)695-7000 **Free:** 800-874-7122
Fax: (603)695-7002
Website: http://www.mthp.com
Gray Somers, CEO

New Jersey

★ 19777 ★ Aetna Inc. - New Jersey
POS Plan
8000 Mid Atlantic Dr., Ste. 100N
Mount Laurel, NJ 08054
Phone: (856)222-5560 **Fax:** (856)727-8490
Website: http://www.aetna.com
John W. Rowe, MD, Chairman of the Board

★ 19778 ★ Aetna Inc. - New Jersey
POS Plan
55 Lane Rd.
Fairfield, NJ 07004
Phone: (973)575-5600 **Free:** 800-852-0629
Fax: (973)244-3990
Website: http://www.aetna.com
John W. Rowe, Chairman of the Board

★ 19779 ★ Alta Health & Life Insurance
POS Plan
One Centennial Ave.
Piscataway, NJ 08855-1326
Phone: (732)980-4000 **Free:** 800-221-3231
Fax: (732)357-2893
Website: http://www.ahlic.com
James White, President

★ 19780 ★ AmeriHealth Insurance Co. - New Jersey North
POS Plan
485 Rt. 1 S, 3rd Fl., Bldg. C
Iselin, NJ 08830
Phone: (732)726-6700 **Fax:** (732)726-6753
Website: http://www.amerihealth.com
Dan Pedriani, CEO

★ 19781 ★ AmeriHealth Insurance Co. - New Jersey South
POS Plan
8000 Midlantic Dr., Ste. 333
Mount Laurel, NJ 08054-1560
Phone: (856)778-6500 **Free:** 800-454-7651
Fax: (856)778-6550
Website: http://www.amerihealth.com
G. Fred DiBona, Jr., CEO

★ 19782 ★ Beech Street MediChoice
POS Plan
1240 Sussex Turnpike
Randolph, NJ 07869
Phone: (973)895-2244 **Free:** 800-640-6708
Fax: (973)895-2266
Website: http://www.beechstreet.com
William Fickling, Jr., Chairman of the Board

★ 19783 ★ CIGNA Healthcare of New York and New Jersey
POS Plan
499 Washington Blvd.
Jersey City, NJ 07310
Phone: (201)533-7000 **Fax:** (201)533-7164
Website: http://www.cigna.com
Kurt Weimer, CEO & Pres

★ 19784 ★ Health Net - New Jersey
POS Plan
3501 Hwy. 66
Neptune, NJ 07753
Phone: (732)643-7400 **Free:** 800-848-4747
Fax: (732)918-6991
Website: http://www.health.net
Barry Averill, CEO

★ 19785 ★ One Health Plan of Massachusetts
POS Plan
1 Centennial Ave.
Piscataway, NJ 08855
Phone: (781)622-2400 **Fax:** (781)622-1462
Website: http://www.onehealthplan.com
Randall Cook, Contact

★ 19786 ★ Oxford Health Plans of New Jersey, Inc.
POS Plan
111 Wood Ave. S, Ste. 2
Iselin, NJ 08830
Phone: (203)459-6000 **Free:** 800-889-4694
Fax: (732)623-1900
Website: http://www.oxhp.com
Norman Payson, MD, CEO & Chm Bd

★ 19787 ★ University Health Plans, Inc.
POS Plan
550 Broad St.
Newark, NJ 07102-4599
Phone: (973)623-8700 **Free:** 800-TRI-UHP1
Fax: (973)623-3635
Website: http://www.uhpnet.com
Alexander H. McLean, CEO & Pres

New Mexico

★ 19788 ★ Cimarron Health Plan
POS Plan
7801 Academy NE, Bldg. Ste. 2
Albuquerque, NM 87109
Phone: (505)342-4660 **Free:** 800-792-3174
Fax: (505)798-7380
Website: http://www.cimarron.com
Robertos Talamantes, MD, Chairman of the Board

★ 19789 ★ Fortis Benefits Dental - New Mexico
POS Plan
1128 Pennsylvania St. NE, Ste. 210
Albuquerque, NM 87110
Phone: (505)266-7709 **Free:** 800-269-5415
Fax: (505)265-3576
Website: http://www.fortisbenefitsdental.com
Debra Rush, CEO

★ 19790 ★ HMO New Mexico, Inc.
POS Plan
12800 Indian School Rd. NE
Albuquerque, NM 87112
Phone: (505)291-6945 **Fax:** (505)816-3600
Website: http://www.bcbsnm.com
Norman Becker, CEO

★ 19791 ★ Lovelace Health Plan
POS Plan
4101 Central NE
Albuquerque, NM 87110
Phone: (505)262-7363 **Fax:** (505)262-7545
Website: http://www.lovelace.com
Martin Hickey, MD, CEO

★ 19792 ★ Presbyterian Health Plan
POS Plan
PO Box 27489
Albuquerque, NM 87125-7489
Phone: (505)923-5700 **Free:** 800-356-2884
Fax: (505)923-5277
Website: http://www.phs.org
Jim Hinton, Chairman of the Board

New York

★ 19793 ★ Aetna Inc. - New York
POS Plan
2700 Westchester Ave.
Purchase, NY 10577
Phone: (914)251-0600 **Fax:** (914)251-1537
Website: http://www.aetna.com
John W. Rowe, MD, Chairman of the Board

★ 19794 ★ Dentcare Delivery Systems, Inc.
POS Plan
60 Charles Lindbergh Blvd.
Uniondale, NY 11553
Phone: (516)542-2200 **Free:** 800-468-0608
Fax: (516)794-3186
Website: http://www.healthplex.com
John Forte, Contact

★ 19795 ★ GHI HMO Select, Inc.
POS Plan
PO Box 4332
Kingston, NY 12402
Phone: (845)340-2300 **Free:** 877-244-4466
Fax: (914)334-8940
Website: http://www.ghi.com
Frank Branchini, CEO

★ 19796 ★ Guardian Life Insurance Co. of America
POS Plan
7 Hanover St.
New York, NY 10004
Phone: (212)598-8000 **Fax:** (212)919-2423
Website: http://www.glic.com
Joseph Dudley Sargent, CEO

★ 19797 ★ Health Net - New York
399 Knollwood Rd., No. 212
White Plains, NY 10603-1914
Phone: 888-747-4090 **Free:** 800-848-4747
Fax: (914)682-5692
Website: http://www.health.net
Barry Averill, CEO

★ 19798 ★ Health Services Medical Corp.
POS Plan
82787 Willett Pkwy.
Baldwinsville, NY 13027
Phone: (315)638-2133 **Free:** 800-388-3264
Fax: (315)638-6338
Website: http://www.phphmo.com
Frederick Yanni, Chairman of the Board

★ 19799 ★ HealthPlex, Inc.
POS Plan
60 Charles Lindbergh Blvd.
Uniondale, NY 11553
Phone: (516)542-2200 **Free:** 800-468-0608
Fax: (516)227-1143
Website: http://www.healthplex.com
John Forte, Chairman of the Board
Program(s): Dental.

★ 19800 ★ HIP Health Plan of New York
POS Plan
7 W 34th St.
New York, NY 10001
Phone: (212)630-5000 **Free:** 800-447-8255
Fax: (212)630-8290
Website: http://www.hipusa.com
Anthony Watson, CEO & Chm Bd

★ 19801 ★ Independent Health Association, Inc.
POS Plan
511 Farber Lakes Dr.
Buffalo, NY 14221
Phone: (716)631-3001 **Free:** 800-247-1466
Fax: (716)631-0430
Website: http://www.independenthealth.com
Frank Colantuono, CEO

★ 19802 ★ MagnaCare
POS Plan
825 E Gate Blvd., Ste. 200
Garden City, NY 11530
Phone: (516)227-6900 **Fax:** (516)227-6967
Website: http://www.pcms-magnacare.com
Anthony Bacchi, MD, CEO

★ 19803 ★ MVP Health Plan, Inc.
POS Plan
625 State St.
Schenectady, NY 12305
Phone: (518)370-4793 **Free:** 800-777-4793
Fax: (518)386-7869
Website: http://www.mvphealthplan.com
David W. Oliker, CEO

★ 19804 ★ National Health Plan
POS Plan
11 Penn Plaza, Ste. 310
New York, NY 10001
Phone: (212)279-3232 **Free:** 800-647-2677
Fax: (212)629-0749
Alvin Konigsberg, CEO

★ 19805 ★ North American Preferred
POS Plan
PO Box 9501
Amherst, NY 14226
Phone: (716)446-5500 **Free:** 800-828-6922
Fax: (716)319-5732
Website: http://www.nahp.com
Ronald Zoeller, CEO & Pres

★ 19806 ★ Oxford Health Plans of New York, Inc.
POS Plan
1133 Ave. of the Americas
New York, NY 10036
Phone: (212)805-3400 **Free:** 800-444-6222
Fax: (212)805-6671
Website: http://www.oxhp.com
Norman Payson, MD, CEO & Chm Bd

★ 19807 ★ Preferred Care/Rochester HMO
POS Plan
259 Monroe Ave.
Rochester, NY 14607-3699
Phone: (585)325-3920 **Free:** 800-933-3920
Fax: (585)327-2298
Website: http://www.preferredcare.org
John Urban, CEO

★ 19808 ★ United Concordia Co., Inc. - New York
POS Plan
159 Express St.
Plainview, NY 11803
Phone: (516)827-6720 **Fax:** (516)827-6618
Website: http://www.ucci.com
Thomas A. Dzuryachko, CEO

★ 19809 ★ United HealthCare of New York Metropolitan
POS Plan
Two Penn Plaza, 7th Fl.
New York, NY 10121-1097
Phone: (212)216-6400 **Fax:** (212)216-6591
Website: http://www.uhc.com
Amy Knapp, CEO

★ 19810 ★ United HealthCare Upstate New York
POS Plan
5015 Campuswood Dr., Ste. 303
East Syracuse, NY 13057
Phone: (315)433-5700 **Fax:** (315)433-5826
Website: http://www.uhc.com
Jay Fisher, CEO

★ 19811 ★ Univera Health Care
205 Park Club Ln.
Buffalo, NY 14221-5239
Phone: (716)847-0881 **Free:** 800-644-4580
Fax: (716)847-1257
Website: http://www.univerahealthcare.org
Arthur R. Goshin, MD, CEO

★ 19812 ★ Univera Health Care - Corporate Headquarters
205 Park Club Ln.
Buffalo, NY 14221-5239
Phone: (716)847-0881 **Free:** 800-644-4580
Fax: (716)847-1257
Website: http://www.univerahealthcare.org
Arthur R. Goshin, MD, CEO

★ 19813 ★ Univera Healthcare Central New York
POS Plan
8278 Willett Pkwy.
Baldwinsville, NY 13027
Phone: (315)635-1222 **Fax:** (315)638-6338
Website: http://www.universalhealthcare.org
Arthur R. Goshin, MD, CEO

★ 19814 ★ Vytra Healthcare
POS Plan
395 N Service Rd.
Melville, NY 11747
Phone: (631)694-4000 **Free:** 800-406-0806
Fax: (631)719-7619
Website: http://www.vytra.com
Thomas McAteer, CEO

North Carolina

★ 19815 ★ Aetna Inc. of the Carolinas
POS Plan
128 S Tryon, Ste. 2000
Charlotte, NC 28202

Phone: (704)379-6700 **Fax:** (704)379-7502
Website: http://www.aetna.com
John W. Rowe, Chairman of the Board

★ 19816 ★ Aetna Inc. - North Carolina
POS Plan
2701 Coltsgate Rd., Ste. 100
Charlotte, NC 28211
Phone: (704)379-6700 **Free:** 800-643-3609
Fax: (704)379-1729
Website: http://www.aetna.com
John W. Rowe, MD, Chairman of the Board

★ 19817 ★ CIGNA Healthcare of North Carolina
POS Plan
200 Regency Executive Dr.
Charlotte, NC 28217
Phone: (704)586-0708 **Free:** 800-235-5707
Fax: (704)556-5840
Website: http://www.cigna.com
Steve White, CEO

★ 19818 ★ CIGNA Healthcare of North Carolina
POS Plan
701 Corporate Center Dr.
Raleigh, NC 27607
Phone: (919)854-7000 **Free:** 800-849-9300
Fax: (919)854-7102
Website: http://www.cigna.com
Steve White, President

★ 19819 ★ Coventry Health Care Inc. - Carolinas
POS Plan
2815 Coliseum Ctr. Dr., Ste. 550
Charlotte, NC 28217
Phone: (704)357-1421 **Free:** 800-470-4523
Fax: (704)357-3164
Website: http://www.cvty.com
Tracy Baker, CEO

★ 19820 ★ Doctors Health Plan, Inc.
POS Plan
PO Box 15940
Durham, NC 27705
Phone: (919)383-4175 **Free:** 800-476-2303
Fax: (919)383-3286
Website: http://www.dhpcares.com
Erin Molitot, Contact

★ 19821 ★ One Health Plan of North Carolina, Inc.
POS Plan
6000 Fairview Rd., Ste. 500
Charlotte, NC 28210
Phone: (704)552-9642 **Free:** 800-663-8081
Fax: (704)556-2149
Website: http://www.onehealthplan.com
William T. McCallum, CEO

★ 19822 ★ PARTNERS National Health Plans of North Carolina, Inc.
POS Plan
PO Box 24907
Winston-Salem, NC 27114-4907
Phone: (336)760-4822 **Free:** 800-942-5695
Fax: (336)760-3198
Website: http://www.partnershealth.com
Jim Broderick, CEO

★ 19823 ★ QualChoice of North Carolina, Inc.
POS Plan
PO Box 340
Winston-Salem, NC 27102-0340
Phone: (336)716-0900 **Free:** 800-816-8117
Fax: (336)716-0920
Website: http://www.bgsm.edu/qualchoice
David Patterson, CEO

★ 19824 ★ WellPath of Carolina, Inc.
POS Plan
6330 Quadrangle Dr., Ste. 500
Chapel Hill, NC 27514
Phone: (919)493-1210 **Free:** 800-935-7284
Fax: (919)419-3871
Website: http://www.wellpathchp.com
Tracy H. Baker, CEO

Ohio

★ 19825 ★ Aetna Inc. - Ohio
POS Plan
205 W 4th St., Ste. 1000
Cincinnati, OH 45202
Phone: (513)579-3385 **Free:** 800-230-3241
Fax: (513)579-3316
Website: http://www.aetna.com
John W. Rowe, MD, Chairman of the Board

★ 19826 ★ Aetna Inc. - Ohio
POS Plan
4059 Kinross Lakes Pkwy.
Richfield, OH 44286
Phone: (330)659-8000 **Free:** 800-458-3940
Fax: (330)659-8034
Website: http://www.aetna.com
John W. Rowe, MD, Chairman of the Board

★ 19827 ★ CHN MCO
POS Plan
6000 West Creek, Ste. 20
Independence, OH 44131
Phone: (216)986-1100 **Fax:** (216)328-7551
Website: http://www.chnetwork.com
Martin Hauser, CEO

★ 19828 ★ ChoiceCare/Humana
POS Plan
655 Eden Park Dr., Ste. 400
Cincinnati, OH 45202-6056
Phone: (513)784-5200 **Free:** 800-543-7158
Fax: (513)784-5345
Website: http://www.choicecare.com
Larry Savage, CEO & Pres

★ 19829 ★ CIGNA Healthcare of Ohio, Inc.
POS Plan
3700 Corporate Dr.
Columbus, OH 43231
Phone: (614)823-7500 **Free:** 800-542-7526
Fax: (614)823-7776
Website: http://www.cigna.com
Jeanne McCarthy, President

★ 19830 ★ CIGNA Healthcare of Ohio, Inc.
POS Plan
5005 Rockside Rd., Ste. 700
Cleveland, OH 44131
Phone: (216)642-2920 **Free:** 800-647-7748
Fax: (216)642-2990
Website: http://www.cigna.com
Jeanne McCarthy, President

★ 19831 ★ CIGNA PPO of Ohio
POS Plan
7 W 7th St., Ste. 1402
Cincinnati, OH 45202-2417
Phone: (513)629-2640 **Fax:** (513)629-2639
Website: http://www.cigna.com
Ed Hanway, CEO

★ 19832 ★ Community Choice/ Community Preferred Plan
POS Plan
1351 William H. Taft Rd.
Cincinnati, OH 45206
Phone: (513)872-8100 **Fax:** (513)336-2021
Website: http://www.anthem-inc.com
Larry Glasscock, CEO

★ 19833 ★ DirectCare America, Inc.
POS Plan
4301 Darrow Rd.
Strafford Pl.
Stow, OH 44224
Phone: (330)686-7030 **Free:** 800-266-5896
Fax: (330)686-7031
Website: http://www.directcareamerica.com
Arthur Chandler, Chairman of the Board

★ 19834 ★ Hometown Health Network
POS Plan
100 Lillian Gish Blvd., Ste. 301
Massillon, OH 44647
Phone: (330)837-6880 **Free:** 800-426-9013
Fax: (330)837-6869
Website: http://www.hometownhealth.com
William Epling, President

★ 19835 ★ Kaiser Permanente Foundation Health Plan of Ohio, Inc.
POS Plan
1001 Lakeside Ave., Ste. 1200
Cleveland, OH 44114
Phone: (216)621-5600 **Free:** 800-524-7371
Fax: (216)623-8776
Website: http://www.kaiperm.org
Ronald Copeland, MD, CEO

★ 19836 ★ Medical Mutual of Ohio
POS Plan
2060 E 9th St.
Cleveland, OH 44115
Phone: (216)687-7000 **Free:** 800-782-3651
Fax: (419)473-6033
Website: http://www.mmoh.com
Kent Clapp, CEO & Pres

★ 19837 ★ Nationwide Health Plans
POS Plan
5525 Park Center Circle
Dublin, OH 43017-3685
Phone: (614)854-3001 **Free:** 800-826-9017
Fax: (614)854-3648
Website: http://www.nationwide-health.com
Joe SanFilippo, CEO

★ 19838 ★ Ohio Health Choice
POS Plan
PO Box 93538
Cleveland, OH 44101
Phone: (440)250-4700 **Free:** 800-554-0027
Fax: (440)250-9872
Website: http://www.ohiohealthchoice.com
Joanie Mason, CEO

★ 19839 ★ One Health Plan of Ohio
POS Plan
24950 Country Club Blvd., Ste. 400
North Olmsted, OH 44070
Phone: (440)716-1777 **Free:** 800-644-9335
Fax: (440)716-1221
Website: http://www.onehealthplan.com
William McCallum, CEO

★ 19840 ★ Paramount Health Care Plan
POS Plan
1901 Indian Wood Cr.
Maumee, OH 43537-4068

Phone: (419)887-2500 **Free:** 800-462-3589
Fax: (419)887-2530
Website: http://www.promedica.org
John Randolph, CEO

★ 19841 ★ Primary Health Services, Inc.
POS Plan
4301 Darrow Rd.
Stratford Pl.
Stow, OH 44224
Phone: (330)686-7050 **Free:** 800-266-5896
Fax: (330)686-7031
Website: http://www.primaryhealthservices.com
Arthur Chandler, Chairman of the Board

★ 19842 ★ QualChoice
POS Plan
6000 Parkland Blvd.
Cleveland, OH 44124
Phone: (440)460-0093 **Free:** 800-208-1232
Fax: (440)460-4005
Website: http://www.qchp.com
Thomas Sullivan, CEO

★ 19843 ★ SummaCare, Inc.
POS Plan
PO Box 3620
Akron, OH 44309-3620
Phone: (330)996-8410 **Free:** 800-996-8411
Fax: (330)996-8454
Website: http://www.summacare.com
Martin Hanser, CEO

★ 19844 ★ United Healthcare of Ohio Inc. - Cleveland
13775 E 9th St., Ste. 700
Cleveland, OH 44114
Free: 800-225-7951
Website: http://www.uhc.com
Ken Hoverman, CEO

★ 19845 ★ United HealthCare of Ohio, Inc. - Dayton/Cincinnati
POS Plan
9050 Centre Pointe Dr., Ste. 400
West Chester, OH 45069
Free: 877-832-7734 **Fax:** (937)439-8999
Website: http://www.uhc.com
Tom Brady, CEO

Oklahoma

★ 19846 ★ Aetna Inc. - Oklahoma
POS Plan
4013 NW Expressway, Ste. 300
Oklahoma City, OK 73116
Phone: (405)879-1780 **Fax:** (405)475-6500
Website: http://www.aetna.com
John W. Rowe, MD, CEO

★ 19847 ★ Aetna Inc. - Tulsa
POS Plan
7912 E 31st Ct., Ste. 300
Tulsa, OK 74145-1339
Phone: (918)624-4700 **Free:** 800-435-8310
Fax: (918)627-9759
Website: http://www.aetna.com
John W. Rowe, Chairman of the Board

★ 19848 ★ CIGNA Healthcare of Oklahoma
POS Plan
4110 Perimeter Center Dr., Ste. 240
Oklahoma City, OK 73112
Phone: (405)943-7711 **Free:** 800-959-8232
Fax: (405)946-9568
Website: http://www.cigna.com
Rick Grizzle, Contact

★ 19849 ★ CommunityCare Managed Healthcare Plans of Oklahoma, Inc.
POS Plan
PO Box 3249
Tulsa, OK 74101
Phone: (918)594-5200 **Free:** 800-278-7563
Fax: (918)594-5260
Website: http://www.ccmhp.com
Richard Todd, CEO & Pres

Oregon

★ 19850 ★ Cascade East Health Plans, Inc.
645 W Orchard Ave.
Hermiston, OR 97838
Phone: (541)567-5555 **Free:** (866)577-2347
Fax: (541)567-5577
Website: http://www.gshealth.org
Dennis Burke, CEO & Pres

★ 19851 ★ Health Net Health Plan of Oregon, Inc.
12901 SE 97th Ave.
Clackamas, OR 97015
Phone: (503)802-7000 **Free:** 888-802-7001
Fax: (503)802-7136
Website: http://www.qualmed.com
Stephen Lynch, CEO

★ 19852 ★ ODS Health Plan
POS Plan
601 SW 2nd Ave.
Portland, OR 97204
Phone: (503)228-6554 **Fax:** (503)948-5558
Website: http://www.odshp.com
Robert Gootee, CEO

★ 19853 ★ One Health Plan of Oregon, Inc.
POS Plan
1800 SW First Ave., Ste. 230
Portland, OR 97201
Phone: (503)222-3014 **Fax:** (503)222-3253
Website: http://www.onehealthplan.com
Sara Mason, Contact

★ 19854 ★ Providence Health Plans
POS Plan
3601 SW Murray Blvd.
Beaverton, OR 97005
Free: 800-826-7218 **Fax:** (503)574-8600
Website: http://www.providence.org
Russ Danielson, CEO

★ 19855 ★ Regence HMO Oregon
POS Plan
100 SW Market
Portland, OR 97201
Phone: (503)364-4868 **Free:** 800-452-7278
Fax: (503)225-4848
Website: http://www.regence.com
Richard L. Woolworth, Chairman of the Board

Pennsylvania

★ 19856 ★ Aetna Inc. of Central and Eastern Pennsylvania
POS Plan
2201 Renaissance Blvd.
Norristown, PA 19406
Phone: (484)322-2000 **Fax:** (484)322-6437
Website: http://www.aetna.com
John W. Rowe, MD, Chairman of the Board

★ 19857 ★ Aetna Inc. - Corporate Headquarters
POS Plan
PO Box 1109
Blue Bell, PA 19422-1109
Phone: (215)775-4800 **Free:** 800-872-3862
Fax: (215)775-6401
Website: http://www.aetna.com
John W. Rowe, MD, Chairman of the Board

★ 19858 ★ Aetna Inc. - Pennsylvania
POS Plan
5313 Campbell's Run Rd.
Pittsburgh, PA 15205-2758
Phone: (412)788-0500 **Fax:** (412)788-5067
Website: http://www.aetna.com
John W. Rowe, MD, Chairman of the Board

★ 19859 ★ Aetna Inc. - Pennsylvania Region
POS Plan
PO Box 1109
Blue Bell, PA 19422-1109
Phone: (215)775-4800 **Fax:** (215)775-6401
Website: http://www.aetna.com
John W. Rowe, MD, Chairman of the Board

★ 19860 ★ Alignis Healthcare - Corporate Headquarters
100 Mattsonford Rd., Bldg 5, No. 445
Radnor, PA 19087
Phone: (610)688-3700 **Free:** 800-863-2932
Fax: (610)688-1765
Jack D. Williams, CEO

★ 19861 ★ Berkshire Health Plan/Medicus Resource Management
POS Plan
50 Commerce Ct.
Wyomissing, PA 19610
Phone: (610)372-8044 **Fax:** (610)371-0310
Website: http://www.bhp.org
Charles Wills, President

★ 19862 ★ Berkshire Health Plan/Medicus Resource Management
POS Plan
50 Commerce Ct.
Wyomissing, PA 19610
Phone: (610)372-8044 **Fax:** (610)371-0310
Website: http://www.bhp.org
Charles Wills, President

★ 19863 ★ CIGNA Healthcare - Corporate Headquarters
POS Plan
One Liberty Pl.
1650 Market St.
Philadelphia, PA 19192-1550
Phone: (215)761-1000 **Fax:** (215)761-5517
Website: http://www.cigna.com
H. Edward Hanway, CEO
Program(s): Chiropractic, Dental, Home Care, Inpatient SNF, Long-Term Care, Pharmaceutical Mail Order, Podiatry, Psychiatric, Transplant, Vision, Wellness, Workers' Compensation.

★ 19864 ★ Eastern Pennsylvania Health Network
POS Plan
65 E Elizabeth Ave., Ste. 410
Bethlehem, PA 18018
Phone: (610)954-3577 **Free:** 800-422-7340
Fax: (610)954-6500
Website: http://www.ephn.com
Anne Baum, Contact

★ 19865 ★ **Geisinger Health Plan**
100 N Academy Ave.
Danville, PA 17822-3020
Phone: (717)271-8760 **Free:** 800-631-1656
Fax: (717)271-5218
Website: http://www.thehealthplan.edu
Dr. Glen Steele, Jr., CEO
Program(s): Chiropractic, Home Care, Inpatient SNF, Pharmaceutical Mail Order, Podiatry, Psychiatric, Behavioral Health, Physical Therapy, Transplant, Vision, Wellness.

★ 19866 ★ **HealthAmerica of Central Pennsylvania**
POS Plan
2575 Interstate Dr.
Harrisburg, PA 17110
Phone: (717)540-4260 **Free:** 800-788-6445
Fax: (717)541-5739
Website: http://www.healthamerica.cvty.com
Francis Soistman, Jr., CEO

★ 19867 ★ **HealthAmerica Pennsylvania, Inc. - Western Region**
POS Plan
5 Gateway Center
Pittsburgh, PA 15222
Phone: (412)553-7522 **Free:** 800-735-4404
Fax: (412)553-7523
Website: http://www.healthamerica.cvty.com
Francis Soistman, Jr., CEO

★ 19868 ★ **Healthguard of Lancaster**
POS Plan
280 Granite Run Dr.
Lancaster, PA 17601-6810
Phone: (717)560-9049 **Free:** 800-822-0350
Fax: (717)581-4580
Website: http://www.hguard.com
James Godfrey, President

★ 19869 ★ **Integra, Inc.**
POS Plan
1060 1st Ave., Ste. 410
King of Prussia, PA 19406
Phone: (610)992-2600 **Free:** 800-544-3573
Fax: (610)992-7046
Website: http://www.integra-ease.com
Gregory Santore, CEO

★ 19870 ★ **Keystone Health Plan East Inc.**
POS Plan
1901 Market St.
Philadelphia, PA 19103
Phone: (215)241-2001 **Free:** 800-227-3114
Fax: (215)241-2017
Website: http://www.khpe.com
G. Fred DiBona, CEO & Pres

★ 19871 ★ **New Alliance Health Plan**
POS Plan
1700 Peach St., Ste. 244
Erie, PA 16501
Phone: (814)878-1700 **Free:** 800-255-4281
Fax: (814)452-4358
Website: http://www.newalliancehealth.com
Joseph Prischak, Chairman of the Board

★ 19872 ★ **One Health Plan of Pennsylvania, Inc.**
POS Plan
8 Penn Center
1628 JFK Blvd., Ste. 1010
Philadelphia, PA 19103
Phone: (215)832-3400 **Free:** 800-303-4635
Fax: (215)832-3441
Website: http://www.onehealthplan.com
Dan Dragalin, MD, President

★ 19873 ★ **Penn Highlands Health Plan**
POS Plan
1086 Franklin St.
Johnstown, PA 15905
Phone: (814)536-7525 **Fax:** (814)533-1544
Website: http://www.conemaugh.org
Jack Lipomi, President

★ 19874 ★ **United Behavioral Health**
100 E Penn Sq., Ste. 400
Philadelphia, PA 19107
Phone: (215)557-6126
Website: http://www.uhc.com
Saul Feldman, CEO

★ 19875 ★ **United Concordia Co., Inc. - Corporate Headquarters**
POS Plan
4401 Deer Path Rd.
Harrisburg, PA 17110
Phone: (717)360-6800 **Free:** 800-972-4191
Fax: (717)612-4996
Website: http://www.ucci.com
Thomas Dzuryachko, CEO
Program(s): Dental.

★ 19876 ★ **United Concordia Co., Inc. - Pennsylvania**
4401 Deer Path Rd.
Harrisburg, PA 17110
Phone: (717)360-6800 **Free:** 800-972-4191
Fax: (717)612-4996
Website: http://www.ucci.com
Thomas A. Dzuryachko, CEO

★ 19877 ★ **United Concordia Co., Inc. - Pennsylvania**
175 Pine St.
Williamsport, PA 17701
Phone: (570)321-5124 **Fax:** (570)321-5199
Website: http://www.ucci.com
Thomas A. Dzuryachko, CEO

★ 19878 ★ **UPMC Health Plan - University of Pittsburgh Medical Center**
POS Plan
1 Chatham Center
112 Washington Pl.
Pittsburgh, PA 15219
Phone: (412)434-1200 **Fax:** (412)454-7711
Website: http://www.upmc.edu/upmchealthplan
Patricia Liebman, CEO

Puerto Rico

★ 19879 ★ **Medical Card System**
POS Plan
255 Ponce De Leon Ave., Ste. 1600
Hato Rey, PR 00917
Phone: (787)758-2500 **Fax:** (787)250-0380
Website: http://www.mcs.com
Felipe Benedit, CEO
Program(s): Chiropractic, Dental, Pharmaceutical Mail Order, Podiatry, Psychiatric, Behavioral Health, Vision.

Rhode Island

★ 19880 ★ **Coordinated Health Partners, Inc.**
POS Plan
15 LaSalle Sq.
Providence, RI 02903-4138
Phone: (401)459-5992 **Free:** 800-564-0888
Fax: (401)459-5568
Lynne Urbani, CEO & Pres

★ 19881 ★ **United Health Plans of New England**
475 Kilvert St.
Warwick, RI 02886-1392
Phone: (401)737-6900 **Free:** 800-447-1245
Fax: (401)732-7210
Website: http://www.uhc.com
Bud Fisher, CEO

South Carolina

★ 19882 ★ **Kanawha HealthCare Solutions**
POS Plan
PO Box 610
Lancaster, SC 29721-0610
Phone: (803)283-5300 **Free:** 800-822-1274
Fax: (803)283-5410
Website: http://www.khsonline.com
Stan Johnson, CEO

South Dakota

★ 19883 ★ **Avera Health Plans, Inc.**
POS Plan
3900 W Avera Dr., Ste. 200
Sioux Falls, SD 57108
Phone: (605)322-4500 **Fax:** (605)322-4535
Website: http://www.avera.org
Jean Reed, CEO & Pres

★ 19884 ★ **DakotaCare**
POS Plan
1323 S Minnesota Ave.
Sioux Falls, SD 57105-0685
Phone: (605)334-4000 **Free:** 800-325-5598
Fax: (605)336-0270
Website: http://www.dakotacare.com
Paul Jensen, CEO
Program(s): Chiropractic, Home Care, Podiatry, Psychiatric, Behavioral Health, Physical Therapy, Transplant, Vision, Wellness.

Tennessee

★ 19885 ★ **Aetna Inc. - Tennessee**
POS Plan
3150 Lenox Park Blvd., Ste. 110
Memphis, TN 38118
Phone: (901)541-9400 **Fax:** (901)541-9343
Website: http://www.aetna.com
John W. Rowe, MD, Chairman of the Board

★ 19886 ★ **Aetna US Healthcare - Tennessee**
POS Plan
1801 W End Ave., Ste. 500
Palmer Plaza
Nashville, TN 37203
Phone: (615)322-1600 **Fax:** (615)322-1646
Website: http://www.aetna.com
John W. Rowe, MD, Chairman of the Board

★ 19887 ★ **Baptist Health Services Group**
POS Plan
6750 Poplar Ave., Ste. 301
Memphis, TN 38138-7445
Phone: (901)759-5000 **Fax:** (901)759-5001
Website: http://www.bmhcc.org
David Elliot, CEO

★ 19888 ★ **Cariten Healthcare**
1420 Centerpoint Blvd.
Knoxville, TN 37932
Phone: (865)470-7470 **Free:** 800-793-1495
Fax: (865)670-7255
Website: http://www.cariten.com
Lance Hunsinger, CEO & Pres

★ 19889 ★ Cigna Healthcare of Tennessee
POS Plan
6555 Quince Rd., Ste. 215
Memphis, TN 38119
Free: 800-832-3211 **Fax:** (901)758-5110
Website: http://www.cigna.com
William Pastore, CEO

★ 19890 ★ CIGNA Healthcare of Tennessee, Inc.
POS Plan
1000 Corporate Center Dr.
Franklin, TN 37067
Phone: (423)296-2065 **Free:** 800-492-2224
Fax: (615)595-3590
Website: http://www.cigna.com
David Mathis, Contact

★ 19891 ★ Health Springs
POS Plan
44 Vantage Way, Ste. 300
Nashville, TN 37228
Phone: (615)291-7000 **Fax:** (615)291-7011
Website: http://www.myhealthspring.com
Herbert A. Fritch, CEO

★ 19892 ★ Initial Group
POS Plan
PO Box 3818
Knoxville, TN 37927-3818
Phone: (865)546-1893 **Free:** 800-858-3203
Fax: (865)546-2126
Website: http://www.intitialgroup.com
Lisa Wear, CEO

★ 19893 ★ John Deere Health
POS Plan
57213 Noah Reid Rd., Ste. I
Chattanooga, TN 37404
Phone: (423)499-0673 **Free:** 800-224-6601
Fax: (423)954-9907
Website: http://www.johndeerehealth.com
Richard L. Bartsh, MD, President

★ 19894 ★ John Deere Health
POS Plan
408 N Cedar Bluff Rd., Ste. 400
Knoxville, TN 37923
Phone: (865)690-5572 **Free:** 800-209-0034
Fax: (865)690-2741
Website: http://www.johndeerehealth.com
Richard L. Bartsh, MD, President

★ 19895 ★ John Deere Health Care
POS Plan
2578 E Stone Dr., Ste. A
Kingsport, TN 37660-4203
Phone: (423)378-5122 **Free:** 800-224-6602
Fax: (423)378-4752
Website: http://www.johndeerehealth.com
Richard L. Bartsh, MD, President

★ 19896 ★ PHP Companies, Inc.
POS Plan
1420 Centerpoint Blvd.
Knoxville, TN 37932
Phone: (865)470-7470 **Free:** 800-747-0008
Fax: (865)470-7485
Tony Stezia, CEO

★ 19897 ★ United HealthCare of Tennessee, Inc.
POS Plan
10 Cadillac Dr.
Brentwood, TN 37027
Phone: (615)372-3622 **Free:** 800-695-1273
Fax: (615)372-3640
Website: http://www.uhc.com
C. Brian Shipp, CEO

★ 19898 ★ Xantus Health Plan of Tennessee, Inc.
POS Plan
3401 W End Ave., Ste. 470
Nashville, TN 37203-1069
Phone: (615)298-3666 **Free:** 800-730-2299
Fax: (615)460-9918
Website: http://www.xantuscorp.com
Richard Sandstrom, CEO

Texas

★ 19899 ★ Aetna Inc. - Austin
POS Plan
7700 Chevy Chase Dr., Ste. 500
Austin, TX 78752
Phone: (512)323-0440 **Fax:** (512)465-5441
Website: http://www.aetna.com
John W. Rowe, MD, Chairman of the Board

★ 19900 ★ Aetna Inc. - El Paso
POS Plan
100 N Stanton, Ste. 1301
El Paso, TX 79901-1448
Phone: (915)532-0700 **Fax:** (915)532-0342
Website: http://www.aetna.com
John W. Rowe, MD, Chairman of the Board

★ 19901 ★ Aetna Inc. - Houston
POS Plan
3 Greenway Plaza, MS G-201
Houston, TX 77046
Phone: (713)350-2260 **Free:** 800-876-7778
Fax: (713)350-2920
Website: http://www.aetna.com
John W. Rowe, MD, Chairman of the Board

★ 19902 ★ Aetna Inc. of North Texas
POS Plan
2777 Stemmons Frwy.
Dallas, TX 75207
Phone: (214)200-8000 **Free:** 800-992-7947
Fax: (214)200-8580
Website: http://www.aetna.com
John W. Rowe, MD, Chairman of the Board

★ 19903 ★ CCN - Colorado
POS Plan
5501 LBJ Fwy., Ste 1200-1201
Dallas, TX 75240
Phone: (972)387-0100 **Free:** 877-366-3415
Fax: (972)387-1076
Website: http://www.ccnusa.com
Patrick G. Dills, President

★ 19904 ★ CCN - Idaho
POS Plan
5501 LBJ Fwy., Ste. 1200-1201
Dallas, TX 75240
Phone: (972)387-0100 **Free:** 877-366-3415
Fax: (972)387-1076
Website: http://www.ccnusa.com
Patrick G. Dills, President

★ 19905 ★ CCN - Illinois
POS Plan
5501 LBJ Fwy., Ste. 1200-1201
Dallas, TX 75240
Phone: (972)387-0100 **Free:** 877-366-3415
Fax: (972)387-1076
Website: http://www.ccnusa.com
Patrick G. Dills, President

★ 19906 ★ CCN - Indiana
POS Plan
5501 LBJ Fwy., Ste. 1200-1201
Dallas, TX 75240
Phone: (972)387-0100 **Free:** 877-366-3415
Fax: (972)387-1076
Website: http://www.ccnusa.com
Patrick G. Dills, President

★ 19907 ★ CCN - Iowa
POS Plan
5501 LBJ Fwy., Ste. 1200-1201
Dallas, TX 75240
Phone: (972)387-0100 **Free:** 877-366-3415
Fax: (972)387-1076
Website: http://www.ccnusa.com
Patrick G. Dills, President

★ 19908 ★ CCN - Kansas
POS Plan
5501 LBJ Fwy., Ste. 1200-1201
Dallas, TX 75240
Phone: (972)387-0100 **Free:** 877-366-3415
Fax: (972)387-1076
Website: http://www.ccnusa.com
Patrick G. Dills, President

★ 19909 ★ CCN - Michigan
POS Plan
5501 LBJ Fwy., Ste. 1200-1201
Dallas, TX 75240
Phone: (972)387-0100 **Free:** 877-366-3415
Fax: (972)387-1076
Website: http://www.ccnusa.com
Patrick G. Dills, President

★ 19910 ★ CCN - Minnesota
POS Plan
5501 LBJ Fwy., Ste 1200-1201
Dallas, TX 75240
Phone: (972)387-0100 **Free:** 877-366-3415
Fax: (972)387-1076
Website: http://www.ccnusa.com
Patrick G. Dills, President

★ 19911 ★ CCN - Missouri
POS Plan
5501 LBJ Fwy., Ste. 1200-1201
Dallas, TX 75240
Phone: (972)387-0100 **Free:** 877-366-3415
Fax: (972)387-1076
Website: http://www.ccnusa.com
Patrick G. Dills, President

★ 19912 ★ CCN - Ohio
POS Plan
5501 LBJ Fwy., Ste. 1200-1201
Dallas, TX 75240
Phone: (972)387-0100 **Free:** 877-366-3415
Fax: (972)387-1076
Website: http://www.ccnusa.com
Patrick G. Dills, President

★ 19913 ★ CCN - Oklahoma
POS Plan
5501 LBJ Fwy., Ste. 1200-1201
Dallas, TX 75240
Phone: (972)387-0100 **Free:** 877-366-3415
Fax: (972)387-1076
Website: http://www.ccnusa.com
Patrick G. Dills, President

★ 19914 ★ CCN - Regional
POS Plan
3625 W Raw Ln., Ste. 150
Irving, TX 75063
Phone: 800-231-2254 **Free:** 877-366-3415
Website: http://www.ccnusa.com
Patrick G. Dills, President

★ 19915 ★ CCN - Texas
POS Plan
3625 W Raw Ln., Ste. 150
Irving, TX 75063
Phone: 800-231-2254 **Free:** 877-366-3415
Website: http://www.ccnusa.com
Patrick G. Dills, President

★ 19916 ★ CCN - Utah
POS Plan
5501 LBJ Fwy., Ste. 1200-1201
Dallas, TX 75240
Phone: (972)387-0100 **Free:** 877-366-3415
Fax: (972)387-1076
Website: http://www.ccnusa.com
Patrick G. Dills, President

★ 19917 ★ CCN - Wisconsin
POS Plan
5501 LBJ Fwy., Ste. 1200-1201
Dallas, TX 75240
Phone: (972)387-0100 **Free:** 877-366-3415
Fax: (972)387-1076
Website: http://www.ccnusa.com
Patrick G. Dills, President

★ 19918 ★ CCN - Wyoming
POS Plan
5501 LBJ Fwy., Ste. 1200-1201
Dallas, TX 75240
Phone: (972)387-0100 **Free:** 877-366-3415
Fax: (972)387-1076
Website: http://www.ccnusa.com
Patrick G. Dills, President

★ 19919 ★ Fortis Health - Texas
16775 Addison Rd., Ste. 500
Addison, TX 75001
Free: 800-262-5388 **Fax:** (214)258-1102
Website: http://www.fortisbenefitsdental.com
Michael Hawkins, MD, Contact

★ 19920 ★ Medical Care Referral Group
POS Plan
4100 Rio Bravo, Ste. 211
El Paso, TX 79902-1010
Phone: (915)532-2100 **Fax:** (915)532-1772
Website: http://www.mcrg.net
Lorri Halow, CEO

★ 19921 ★ National Health Care Alliance
POS Plan
770 S Post Oak Ln., Ste. 445
Houston, TX 77056
Phone: (713)888-1902 **Free:** 800-759-3118
Fax: (713)888-1986
Website: http://www.nhausa.com
Robert Woolfolk, CEO
Program(s): Chiropractic, Dental, Home Care, Inpatient SNF, Pharmaceutical Mail Order, Podiatry, Psychiatric, Behavioral Health, Physical Therapy, Transplant, Vision, Wellness, Workers' Compensation.

★ 19922 ★ North Texas Healthcare Network
POS Plan
5601 N McArthur Blvd., Ste. 300
Irving, TX 75038
Phone: (972)751-2300 **Free:** 800-444-3995
Fax: (972)751-2415
Website: http://www.nthn.com
Robert Brown, CEO & Pres

★ 19923 ★ One Health Plan of Texas
POS Plan
8310 Capitol of Texas Hwy. N, Ste. 340
Austin, TX 78731
Phone: (512)342-1706 **Fax:** (512)795-2105
Website: http://www.onehealthplan.com
Wally Gomaa, CEO

★ 19924 ★ One Health Plan of Texas - Dallas
POS Plan
8350 N Central Expwy., Ste. M1000
Dallas, TX 75206
Phone: (972)813-7000 **Free:** 800-866-3136
Fax: (214)363-9785
Website: http://www.onehealthplan.com
Wally Gomaa, CEO

★ 19925 ★ Pacificare
POS Plan
1800 W Loop South, Ste. 350
Houston, TX 77027
Free: 800-825-9355 **Fax:** (713)993-3295
Website: http://www.pacificare.com
Ron Davis, CEO

★ 19926 ★ PacifiCare of Texas Inc.
POS Plan
5001 LBJ Fwy., Ste. 600
Dallas, TX 75244
Free: 800-825-9355 **Fax:** (972)866-1658
Website: http://www.pacificare.com
Ron Davis, CEO

★ 19927 ★ Provider Networks of America
POS Plan
4100 International Plaza, Ste. 400
Fort Worth, TX 76109
Phone: (817)735-8293 **Fax:** (817)735-8293
Website: http://www.providernetworks.com
Allen Rafeh, MD, CEO

★ 19928 ★ Seton Health Plan
POS Plan
305 E Huntland Dr.
Austin, TX 78752
Phone: (512)324-4200 **Free:** 800-749-7404
Fax: (512)324-1952
Website: http://www.seton.net
John Evler, III, CEO

★ 19929 ★ United Concordia Co., Inc. - Texas
POS Plan
8214 Westchester Dr.
Dallas, TX 75225
Phone: (214)378-6410 **Fax:** (214)378-6306
Website: http://www.ucci.com
Thomas Dzuryachko, CEO
Program(s): Dental.

★ 19930 ★ United HealthCare of Texas, Inc. - Houston
POS Plan
2000 W Loop S, Ste. 700
Houston, TX 77027-3416
Phone: (713)296-4800 **Fax:** (713)961-4431
Website: http://www.uhc.com
Steve C. Walli, CEO

★ 19931 ★ United HealthCare of Texas, Inc. - San Antonio
POS Plan
8401 Datapoint Dr., Ste. 175
San Antonio, TX 78229
Phone: (210)617-6850 **Fax:** (210)617-6868
Website: http://www.uch.com
Thomas Quirk, CEO
Program(s): Chiropractic, Dental, Home Care, Inpatient SNF, Pharmaceutical Mail Order, Podiatry, Psychiatric, Behavioral Health, Physical Therapy, Transplant, Vision, Wellness.

Utah

★ 19932 ★ Altius Health Plans
POS Plans
10421 S Jordan Gateway, Ste. 400
South Jordan, UT 84095
Phone: (801)355-1234 **Free:** 800-365-1334
Fax: (801)323-6100
Website: http://www.altiushealthplans.com
Larry Hancock, CEO

★ 19933 ★ IHC Health Plans, Inc.
POS Plan
4646 W Lake Park Blvd.
Salt Lake City, UT 84120
Phone: (801)442-5000 **Free:** 800-538-5038
Fax: (801)442-5183
Website: http://www.ihc.com
Richard J. Galbraith, Chairman of the Board

★ 19934 ★ United HealthCare of Utah, Inc.
POS Plan
PO Box 71409
Salt Lake City, UT 84171-0409
Free: 800-624-2942 **Fax:** (801)947-0459
Website: http://www.uhc.com
Annette Herman, CEO

Vermont

★ 19935 ★ CIGNA Managed Care Network of Northern New England
POS Plan
30 Main St., Ste. 130
Burlington, VT 05401
Phone: (802)865-6309 **Fax:** (802)658-9212
Website: http://www.cigna.com
Linda Johnson, CEO

Virginia

★ 19936 ★ Aetna Health Plans of Mid-Atlantic
POS Plan
7600 A Leesburg Pike
Falls Church, VA 22043
Phone: (703)903-7100 **Fax:** (703)903-0316
Website: http://www.aetna.com
John W. Rowe, MD, Chairman of the Board

★ 19937 ★ Carilion Health Plans, Inc.
POS Plan
110 Campbell Ave., Ste. 107
Roanoke, VA 24011
Phone: (540)857-5200 **Free:** 800-856-5206
Fax: (540)857-5343
Website: http://www.carilionhealthplans.com
Carolyn Chrisman, CEO

★ 19938 ★ CIGNA Healthcare of Virginia, Inc. - Richmond
POS Plan
PO Box 31353
Richmond, VA 23294-1353
Phone: (804)267-5100 **Free:** 800-533-1708
Fax: (804)267-5062
Website: http://www.cigna.com
Matt Manders, CEO

★ 19939 ★ Optima Health Plan, Inc.
POS Plan
4417 Corporation Lane
Virginia Beach, VA 23462-3162
Phone: (757)552-7400 **Fax:** (757)687-6031
Website: http://www.optimahealth.com
Michael Dudley, President

★ 19940 ★ QualChoice of Virginia Health Plan
POS Plan
1000 Research Park Blvd.
Charlottesville, VA 22911
Phone: (434)975-1212 **Free:** 800-975-1213
Fax: (434)975-1414
Cosby Davis, CEO

★ 19941 ★ Southern Health Services, Inc.
POS Plan
9881 Mayland Dr.
Richmond, VA 23233-1458
Phone: (804)747-3700 **Free:** 800-424-0077
Fax: (804)762-9349
Website: http://www.southernhealth.com
Cosby Davis, CEO

★ 19942 ★ United Concordia Co., Inc. - Virginia
POS Plan
4860 Cox Rd., Ste. 200
Glen Allen, VA 23060
Free: 800-454-3224 **Fax:** (804)217-8368
Website: http://www.ucci.com
Thomas Dzuryacko, Contact
Program(s): Dental.

★ 19943 ★ United HealthCare of Virginia
POS Plan
9020 Stony Point Pkwy., Ste. 400
Richmond, VA 23235
Phone: (804)267-5200 **Free:** 888-286-4908
Fax: (804)267-5285
Website: http://www.uhc.com
James Carney, MD, Contact

★ 19944 ★ ValueOptions - Corporate Headquarters
POS Plan
3110 Fairview Park Dr. S
Falls Church, VA 22042
Phone: (703)205-7000 **Free:** 800-236-4648
Fax: (703)205-6505
Website: http://www.valueoptions.com
Ronald Dozoretz, Chairman of the Board

★ 19945 ★ Virginia Health Network
POS Plan
7400 Beaufont Springs Dr.
Richmond, VA 23225
Phone: (804)320-3837 **Free:** 800-989-3837
Fax: (804)320-5984
James Brittain, President

Washington

★ 19946 ★ Aetna Inc. - Washington
POS Plan
601 Union Square, Ste. 800
Seattle, WA 98101
Phone: (206)701-8000 **Fax:** (206)701-8125
Website: http://www.aetna.com
John W. Rowe, MD, Chairman of the Board

★ 19947 ★ Group Health Cooperative
POS Plan
PO Box 204
Spokane, WA 99210
Phone: (509)838-9100 **Free:** 800-497-2210
Fax: (509)458-0368
Website: http://www.ghnw.org
Jack Dutzar, MD, Contact

★ 19948 ★ Group Health Cooperative of Puget Sound
POS Plan
521 Wall St.
Seattle, WA 98121
Phone: (206)448-5528 **Free:** 800-442-4062
Fax: (206)448-5105
Website: http://www.ghc.org
Cheryl Scott, CEO

★ 19949 ★ Molina Healthcare of Washington, Inc.
POS Plan
PO Box 1469
Bothell, WA 98041-1469
Phone: (425)424-1100 **Free:** 800-869-7175
Fax: (425)424-1132
Website: http://www.molinamedical.com
Joseph M. Molina, MD, Chairman of the Board

★ 19950 ★ One Health Plan of Washington, Inc.
POS Plan
3005 112th Ave. NE, Corp. Camp E
Bellevue, WA 98004
Phone: (425)827-2282 **Free:** 800-332-0151
Fax: (425)827-2466
Website: http://www.onehealthplan.com
Teresa Davis, Contact

★ 19951 ★ Options Health Care, Inc.
POS Plan
521 Wall St.
Seattle, WA 98121
Phone: (206)901-6200 **Free:** 800-542-6312
Fax: (206)287-2557
Website: http://www.ghc.org
Cheryl Scott, CEO

★ 19952 ★ PacifiCare of Washington
POS Plan
7525 SE 24th St.
Mercer Island, WA 98040
Phone: (206)236-2500 **Free:** 800-722-9666
Fax: (206)230-7496
Website: http://www.pacificare.com
Chris Wing, President

★ 19953 ★ United Concordia Co., Inc. - Washington
POS Plan
2200 Sixth Ave., Ste. 620
Seattle, WA 98121
Free: 888-245-8224 **Fax:** (206)728-2740
Website: http://www.ucci.com
Thomas Dzuryacko, CEO
Program(s): Dental.

West Virginia

★ 19954 ★ Aetna Inc. - West Virginia
POS Plan
121 Washington St. E
Charleston, WV 25301
Phone: (304)346-5322 **Fax:** (304)346-5327
Website: http://www.aetna.com
John W. Rowe, MD, Chairman of the Board

★ 19955 ★ Carelink
POS Plan
887 National Rd.
Wheeling, WV 26003
Phone: (304)234-5100 **Free:** 800-519-3368
Fax: (304)234-5119
Website: http://www.chccarelink.com
Ted Cheatham, CEO

★ 19956 ★ Carelink Health Plans
POS Plan
500 Virginia St., Ste. 400
Charleston, WV 25301
Phone: (304)348-2970 **Fax:** (304)561-6985
Website: http://www.camcare.com
Ted Cheatham, CEO

Wisconsin

★ 19957 ★ Aetna Inc. - Wisconsin
POS Plan
2675 N Mayfair Rd., Ste. 600
Milwaukee, WI 53226
Phone: (414)266-9700 **Fax:** (414)266-9705
Website: http://www.aetna.com
John W. Rowe, MD, Chairman of the Board

★ 19958 ★ Cobalt Corp.
POS Plan
401 W Michigan St.
Milwaukee, WI 53203
Phone: (414)226-6600 **Fax:** (414)226-6279
Website: http://www.cobaltcorporation.com
Thomas Hefty, Chairman of the Board

★ 19959 ★ Dean Health Plan, Inc.
POS Plan
PO Box 56099
Madison, WI 53705-9399
Phone: (608)836-1400 **Free:** 800-356-7344
Fax: (608)836-9620
Website: http://www.deancare.com
Robert Palmer, CEO & Pres

★ 19960 ★ EBC Review
POS Plan
9275 N 49th St., Ste. 300
Milwaukee, WI 53223
Phone: (414)365-4600 **Fax:** (414)365-4610
Website: http://www.ebc-tpa.com
Bruce Flunker, CEO

★ 19961 ★ Gundersen Lutheran Health Plan, Inc.
POS Plan
1836 South Ave.
La Crosse, WI 54601
Phone: (608)775-8000 **Free:** 800-370-9718
Fax: (608)775-8042
Patrick Killeen, CEO

★ 19962 ★ Health Care Network of Wisconsin
POS Plan
250 Bishops Way, Ste. 300
Brookfield, WI 53005-5957
Phone: (262)784-0223 **Free:** 800-451-2577
Fax: (262)796-9084
Website: http://www.wppn.com
James Wrocklage, CEO

★ 19963 ★ Health Tradition Health Plans
POS Plan
PO Box 188
La Crosse, WI 54602-0188
Phone: (608)783-9507 **Free:** 800-545-8499
Fax: (608)781-9653
Steven M. Kunes, CEO

★ 19964 ★ MercyCare Health Plan, Inc.
POS Plan
PO Box 2770
Janesville, WI 53547-2770
Phone: (608)752-3431 **Free:** 800-752-3431
Fax: (608)752-3751
Website: http://www.mercyhealthsystem.org
Javon Bea, CEO

★ 19965 ★ Network Health Plan of Wisconsin
POS Plan
1165 Appleton Rd.
Menasha, WI 54952
Phone: (920)727-0100 **Fax:** (929)720-1756
Website: http://www.networkhealth.com
Michael Wolff, CEO

★ 19966 ★ Prevea Health Plan
POS Plan
PO Box 11625
Green Bay, WI 54307-1625
Phone: (920)490-6900 **Free:** 888-711-1444
Fax: (920)490-6943
Website: http://www.prevea.com
Mark Minsloff, CEO

★ 19967 ★ United Healthcare of Wisconsin, Inc.
POS Plan
10701 W Research Dr.
Milwaukee, WI 53226
Phone: (414)443-4000 **Free:** 800-879-0071
Fax: (414)443-4750
William Felsing, CEO

★ 19968 ★ Unity Health Plans
POS Plan
840 Carolina St.
Sauk City, WI 53583-1374
Phone: (608)643-2491 **Free:** 800-362-3308
Fax: (608)643-2564
Tery Bolz, CEO

★ 19969 ★ Wausau Benefits, Inc.
POS Plan
PO Box 8017
Wausau, WI 54402-8017
Phone: (715)845-8582 **Free:** 800-435-4401
Fax: (715)843-3613
Website: http://www.libertymutual.com
Fred Moore, President

★ 19970 ★ Wausau Preferred Health Plan
POS Plan
PO Box 245037
Milwaukee, WI 53224-9537
Phone: (414)577-2100 **Free:** 800-242-0472
Fax: (414)577-2437
Website: http://www.wausau.com
Christopher Drayna, MD, Contact

★ 19971 ★ Wisconsin Physicians Services Insurance Co.
POS Plan
PO Box 8190
Madison, WI 53708-8190
Phone: (608)221-4711 **Fax:** (608)223-3603
James R. Riordan, CEO

Wyoming

★ 19972 ★ WIN Health Partners
POS Plan
2515 Warren Ave., Ste. 504
Cheyenne, WY 82001
Phone: (307)638-7700 **Fax:** (307)663-7701
Beth Wasson, CEO

Specialty HMOs

Alabama

★ 19973 ★ Fortis Benefits Dental - Alabama
3595 Grandview Pkwy.
Birmingham, AL 35243
Free: 800-262-5388 **Fax:** (205)868-3010
Website: http://www.fortisbenefitsdental.com
Peter Barnett, President

★ 19974 ★ United Concordia Co., Inc. - Alabama
400 Vestavia Pkwy, Ste. 205
Birmingham, AL 35216
Free: 800-554-6155 **Fax:** (205)822-1653
Website: http://www.ucci.com
Thomas A. Dzuryachko, CEO
Program(s): Dental.

Arizona

★ 19975 ★ Catalina Behavioral Health Services, Inc.
2400 N Central Ave., Ste. 203A
Phoenix, AZ 85004
Phone: (602)452-1200 **Free:** 800-977-0281
Fax: (602)257-1644
Karen Smith-Hagman, CEO
Program(s): Behavioral health; psychiatric.

★ 19976 ★ CIGNA Medical Group
7600 N 15th St., No. 185
Phoenix, AZ 85020-4324
Phone: (602)678-3000 **Free:** 800-367-1037
Fax: (602)678-3068
Website: http://www.cigna.com/dental
Michael Hudson, CEO
Program(s): Dental.

★ 19977 ★ Employers Dental Services, Inc.
4747 N 7th St., No. 300
Phoenix, AZ 85014-3656
Phone: (602)266-3424 **Free:** 800-722-9772
Fax: (602)266-3704
Don Altman, Contact

★ 19978 ★ Fortis Benefits Dental - Arizona
1702 E Highland Ave., Ste. 110
Phoenix, AZ 85016
Phone: (602)604-1123 **Free:** 800-233-0881
Fax: (602)263-0187
Website: http://www.fortisbenefitsdental.com
Danny L. Bentley, CEO

★ 19979 ★ Total Dental Administrators Health Plan
5353 N 16th St., No. 120
Phoenix, AZ 85016
Phone: (602)266-1995 **Free:** 888-422-1995
Fax: (602)266-1948
Website: http://www.totaldentaladmin.com
Nelson P. Leatherwood, CEO & Pres

★ 19980 ★ United Concordia Co., Inc. - Arizona
HMO Plan
2198 Camelback Rd., Ste. 260
Phoenix, AZ 85016
Phone: (717)260-7500 **Free:** 800-322-0366
Fax: (717)612-4996
Website: http://www.ucci.com
Thomas Dzuryachko, CEO

★ 19981 ★ Vision Service Plan of Arizona
2111 E Highland Ave., Ste. B160
Phoenix, AZ 85016
Fax: (602)956-3679
Website: http://www.vsp.com
Roger Baline, CEO

Arkansas

★ 19982 ★ Comp Benefits
614 Center St.
Little Rock, AR 72201-4214
Phone: (501)376-0544 **Free:** 800-633-1262
Fax: (501)371-3820
Website: http://www.compdent.com
Phillis A. Klock, President

California

★ 19983 ★ Access Dental Services
555 University Ave., Ste. 182
Sacramento, CA 95825
Phone: (916)922-5000 **Free:** 800-757-6453
Fax: (916)646-9000
Reza Abbaszadeh, DDS, CEO

★ 19984 ★ Aetna, Inc. - California
HMO Plan
1200 W 7th St., Ste. 400
Los Angeles, CA 90017
Phone: (310)935-3100 **Fax:** (310)955-3185
Website: http://www.aetnaushc.com
John W. Rowe, MD, Chairman of the Board

★ 19985 ★ Aetna Inc.—Dental Care of California Inc.
2409 Comino Ramon
San Ramon, CA 94583
Phone: (925)543-9000 **Fax:** (925)543-9010
Website: http://www.aetna.com
John W. Rowe, MD, Chairman of the Board

★ 19986 ★ American Healthguard Corp.
30 E Santa Clara, Ste. D
Arcadia, CA 91006
Phone: (626)821-5500 **Free:** 800-727-6453
Fax: (626)821-5514
David Kutner, CEO
Program(s): Dental.

★ 19987 ★ Ameritas Managed Dental Plan, Inc.
151 Kalmus Dr., Ste. J3
Costa Mesa, CA 92626-5988
Phone: (714)437-5966 **Free:** 800-336-6661
Fax: (714)437-5967
Website: http://www.yourdentalsolutions.com
Sherry Hobbs, President

★ 19988 ★ California Benefits Dental Plan
3611 S Harbor Blvd., Ste. 150
Santa Ana, CA 92704-6928
Phone: (714)540-4255 **Free:** 800-350-3999
Fax: (714)540-4754
Valerie A. Clark, CEO

★ 19989 ★ California Dental Network
1971 E 4th St., Ste. 184
Santa Ana, CA 92705
Phone: (714)479-0777
Stephen R. Casey, CEO & Pres

★ 19990 ★ Century Dental Plan
117 S Los Robles
Pasadena, CA 91101
Phone: (626)585-9544 **Fax:** (626)584-1987

Website: http://www.centurydental.com
David S. Campbell, CEO

★ 19991 ★ Chirosave Health Plan
3833 Atlantic Ave.
Long Beach, CA 90807
Phone: (562)595-8164 **Free:** 800-526-4470
Fax: (562)426-5352
J. Rodney Shelley, DC, CEO
Program(s): Chiropractic.

★ 19992 ★ ChiroSource - Corporate Headquarters
PO Box 130
Clayton, CA 94517
Phone: (925)672-5333 **Free:** 800-680-9997
Fax: (925)672-6657
Website: http://www.chirosource.com
Ronald S. Cataldo, DC, CEO & Pres
Program(s): Chiropractic; worker's compensation.

★ 19993 ★ CIGNA Behavioral Health, Inc.
450 N Brand Blvd., Ste. 500
Glendale, CA 91203
Phone: (818)551-2200 **Free:** 800-234-3596
Fax: (818)551-2786
Website: http://www.mcc-care.com
Susan Urbanski, CEO

★ 19994 ★ CIGNA Dental Health of California, Inc.
5990 Sepulveda Blvd., Ste. 500
Van Nuys, CA 91411
Phone: (818)756-2900 **Free:** 800-367-1037
Fax: (818)756-2997
Website: http://www.cigna.com/dental
Susan Klarner, CEO

★ 19995 ★ CIGNA Dental Health of New Mexico
PO Box 2125
Glendale, CA 91209-2125
Phone: (818)546-5000 **Free:** 800-367-1037
Fax: (818)546-5110
Website: http://www.cigna.com/dental
Susan Klarner, CEO

★ 19996 ★ Community Dental Services
PO Box 92009
Los Angeles, CA 90009
Phone: (949)756-5476 **Fax:** (714)708-5399
Mary Ellen Hardin, CEO

★ 19997 ★ Consumer Health Inc.
201 E Sandpointe, Ste. 200
Santa Ana, CA 92707
Phone: (714)668-1300 **Free:** 800-347-6453
Fax: (714)668-9422
Website: http:/www.brightnow.com
Steven C. Bilt, CEO & Pres

★ 19998 ★ Dedicated Dental Systems
3990 Ming Ave.
Bakersfield, CA 93309
Phone: (661)397-5513 **Fax:** (661)397-2888
Arthur Kaiser, DDS, CEO

★ 19999 ★ Dental Associates of Torrance
21229 Hawthorne Blvd.
Torrance, CA 90503
Phone: (310)792-5600 **Fax:** (310)792-5628
Theresa Reyoso, CEO

★ 20000 ★ Dental Health Services
3833 Atlantic Ave.
Long Beach, CA 90807-3505
Phone: (562)595-6000 **Fax:** (562)424-0150
Godfrey Pernell, CEO

★ 20001 ★ Eyecare Service Plan, Inc.
100 Corporate Point, Ste. 285
Culver City, CA 90230
Phone: (310)242-6200 **Fax:** (310)242-6222
Paige Sanders, CEO

★ 20002 ★ Eyexam of California, Inc.
170 Newport Center Dr., Ste. 130
Newport Beach, CA 92660
Phone: (949)718-1431 **Fax:** (949)718-1432
Yvon Wagner, CEO

★ 20003 ★ For Eyes Vision Plan, Inc.
2112 Shattuck Ave.
Berkeley, CA 94704
Phone: (510)843-3200 **Fax:** (510)843-2597
Fred Hjerpe, MD, CEO & Pres

★ 20004 ★ Fortis Benefits Dental - California
450 B St., Ste. 880
San Diego, CA 92101
Phone: (619)236-9595 **Fax:** (619)236-8151
Website: http://www.fortisbenefitsdental.com
Susan A. Dickey, President

★ 20005 ★ Golden West Dental & Vision
888 W Ventura Blvd.
Camarillo, CA 93010
Phone: (805)987-8941 **Free:** 800-995-4124
Fax: (805)987-6110
Website: http://www.goldenwestdental.com
Chris Kamen, DDS, CEO

★ 20006 ★ Health Net Dental, Inc. HMO Plan
125 Technology Dr., Ste. 100
Irvine, CA 92618
Phone: (949)790-3400 **Free:** 800-999-2848
Fax: (949)790-3452
Website: http://www.dv.healthnet.com
David Anderson, President

★ 20007 ★ Health Net Vision Inc. HMO Plan
125 Tehnology Dr., Ste. 100
Irvine, CA 92618
Phone: (949)790-3400 **Free:** 800-443-4994
Fax: (949)790-3452
Website: http://www.dv.healthnet.com
David Anderson, CEO

★ 20008 ★ Healthdent of California, Inc.
3840 Rosin Ct., Ste 190
Sacramento, CA 95834
Phone: (916)486-0749 **Free:** 800-937-3400
Fax: (916)922-5630
Mohander Narala, DDS, CEO
Program(s): Dental.

★ 20009 ★ Holman Professional Counseling Centers
21050 Vanowen St.
Canoga Park, CA 91303
Phone: (818)704-1444 **Fax:** (818)704-4252
Website: http://www.holmangroup.com
Ron Holman, CEO

★ 20010 ★ Human Affairs International of California
300 Continental Blvd., Ste. 240
El Segundo, CA 90245
Phone: (310)726-7000 **Fax:** (310)726-7104
Flora Vivaldo, CEO
Program(s): Psychiatric, Behavioral Health, Wellness.

★ 20011 ★ Integrated Insights
9370 Sky Park Ct., Ste. 140
San Diego, CA 92123
Phone: (858)571-1698 **Free:** 800-342-8111
Fax: 888-285-2207
Website: http://www.hhr.com
Stephen Heidel, MD, CEO

★ 20012 ★ Landmark Healthcare, Inc.
1750 Howe Ave., Ste. 300
Sacramento, CA 95825
Phone: (916)646-3477 **Fax:** (916)929-8350
Website: http://www.landmarkhealthcare.com
Joseph Kleigner, CEO
Program(s): Chiropractic, Alternative Medicine.

★ 20013 ★ Liberty Dental Plan of California
3636 Birch St., Ste. 250
Newport Beach, CA 92660
Phone: (949)223-0007 **Free:** (999)703-6999
Fax: (949)223-0011
Website: http://www.libertydentalplan.com
Amir Neshat, DDS, CEO & Pres

★ 20014 ★ Managed Dental Care
6200 Canoga Ave., Ste. 100
Woodland Hills, CA 91367
Phone: (818)598-6599 **Free:** 800-273-3330
Fax: (818)347-7302
Candee Bolye, CEO

★ 20015 ★ Managed Health Network
1600 Los Gamos Dr., Ste. 300
San Rafael, CA 94903
Phone: (415)491-7200 **Free:** 800-327-7526
Fax: (415)472-8187
Website: http://www.mhn.com
Robert Fusco, Contact
Program(s): Psychiatric, Behavioral Health.

★ 20016 ★ Medical Eye Services, Inc.
PO Box 93033
Long Beach, CA 90809
Phone: (562)425-9528 **Free:** 800-877-6372
Fax: (562)496-4768
Website: http://www.mesvision.com
Robert Bjorkquist, CEO

★ 20017 ★ Newport Dental Plan
201 E Sandpointe, Ste. 200
Santa Ana, CA 92707
Phone: (714)668-1300 **Free:** 800-347-6453
Fax: (714)668-9422
Website: http://www.brightnow.com
Steven C. Bilt, CEO & Pres

★ 20018 ★ On Lok Senior Health Services
1333 Bush St.
San Francisco, CA 94109-5611
Phone: (415)292-8888 **Free:** 888-886-6565
Fax: (415)292-8745
Website: http://www.onlok.org
Claudio Tarchi, Chairman of the Board
Program(s): Dental, Home Care, Inpatient SNF, Long-Term Care, Podiatry, Physical Therapy, Vision, Alternative Medicine.

★ 20019 ★ Pacific Dental Benefits Inc.
1390 Willow Poss Rd., No. 800
Concord, CA 94520
Phone: (925)363-6000 **Free:** 800-999-3367
Fax: (925)363-6099
John Gaebel, DDS, CEO & Pres

★ 20020 ★ Pacificare Behavioral Health
23046 Avenida de la Carlota, Ste. 700
Laguna Hills, CA 92653
Phone: (949)859-7971 **Fax:** (949)859-9824
Website: http://www.pacificare.com
Jerome Vaccaro, MD, CEO

★ 20021 ★ Pacificare Dental and Vision
3110 Lake Center Dr.
Santa Ana, CA 92704
Free: 800-622-6388 **Fax:** (714)513-6381
Website: http://www.pacificare.com
James Stumpfel, CEO

★ 20022 ★ Pearle Visioncare Inc.
6727 Flanders Dr., Ste. 104
San Diego, CA 92121
Free: 800-843-6706
Website: http://www.pearlevision.com
Debbie Hyde-Duby, President

★ 20023 ★ PMI Dental Health Plan
12898 Towne Center Dr.
Artesia, CA 90703
Phone: (562)924-8311 **Free:** 800-422-4234
Fax: (562)924-8039
Website: http://www.deltadentalca.org
Belinda Martinez, CEO

★ 20024 ★ Procare Eye Exam, Inc.
2345 W Foot Hill Blvd., No. 2
Upland, CA 91786
Phone: (909)920-5008 **Free:** 877-477-6227
Fax: (909)932-0062
Sandra Mandre, CEO

★ 20025 ★ Safeguard Health Plans, Inc.
95 Enterprise
Aliso Viejo, CA 92656-2601
Phone: (949)425-4300 **Free:** 800-204-0463
Fax: (949)425-4308
James Buncher, CEO
Program(s): Dental, vision.

★ 20026 ★ Smile Saver
2787 Bristol St., Ste. 3200
Costa Mesa, CA 92626
Phone: (714)429-0200 **Free:** 800-445-8119
Fax: (714)429-1261
Mark Johnson, CEO
Program(s): Dental, Vision.

★ 20027 ★ Smile Saver Dental Plan
30851 W Agoura Rd., No. 300
Agoura Hills, CA 91301
Phone: (818)706-6600 **Free:** 800-333-9561
Fax: (818)706-6697
Website: http://www.smilesaver.com
Lou Morales, President
Program(s): Dental, Vision.

★ 20028 ★ United Behavioral Health (UBH)
425 Market St., 27th Fl.
San Francisco, CA 94105
Phone: (415)547-5000 **Fax:** (415)547-6100
Website: http://www.unitedbehavioralhealth.com
Saul Feldman, MD, CEO

★ 20029 ★ United Concordia Co., Inc. - California
21700 Oxnard, Ste. 500
Woodland Hills, CA 91367-3642
Phone: (717)731-2532 **Free:** 800-876-6432
Fax: (717)972-0410
Website: http://www.ucci.com
Thomas Dzuryachko, Chairman of the Board
Program(s): Dental.

★ 20030 ★ Valueoptions of California Inc.
340 Golden Shore
Long Beach, CA 90802
Phone: (562)951-6001 **Fax:** (562)951-6130
Julie Larson, CEO

★ 20031 ★ Vision First Eye Care Inc.
1937-A Tully Rd.
San Jose, CA 95122
Phone: (408)923-0400
James K. Eu, President

★ 20032 ★ Vision Plan of America
3255 Wilshire Blvd., Ste. 1610
Los Angeles, CA 90010
Phone: (213)384-2600 **Free:** 800-400-4872
Fax: (213)384-0084
Website: http://www.visionplanofamerica.com
Stuart Needleman, OD, CEO

★ 20033 ★ Vision Service Plan
3333 Quality Dr.
Rancho Cordova, CA 95670
Phone: (916)851-5000 **Free:** 800-852-7600
Fax: (916)858-5329
Website: http://www.vsp.com
Roger Valine, CEO & Pres

★ 20034 ★ Visioncare of California
9663 Tierra Grande, Ste. 203
San Diego, CA 92121
Phone: (858)831-9322 **Fax:** (858)831-0225
Nick Shashati, MD, CEO

★ 20035 ★ Western Dental Services
530 S Main St.
Orange, CA 92863
Phone: (714)480-3000 **Free:** 800-417-4444
Fax: (714)480-3001
David Joe, CEO

Colorado

★ 20036 ★ Behavioral Healthcare, Inc.
6801 S Yosemite St., Ste. 100
Englewood, CO 80112
Phone: (303)617-2701 **Fax:** (303)889-4808
Randy Stith, CEO

★ 20037 ★ Colorado Health Networks
665 Southpointe Ct., Ste. 200
Colorado Springs, CO 80906
Phone: (719)538-1430 **Free:** 800-804-5040
Fax: (719)538-1433
Website: http://www.valueoptions.com
Stephen Holsenbeck, MD, CEO
Program(s):

★ 20038 ★ Fortis Benefits Dental - Colorado
5350 S Roslyn St., Ste. 450
Greenwood Village, CO 80111
Phone: (303)796-7990 **Free:** 800-759-7985
Fax: (303)796-2769
Website: http://www.fortisbenefitsdental.com
Peter Barnett, President

★ 20039 ★ Pacificare of Colorado
6455 S Yosemite
Englewood, CO 80111
Phone: (303)220-5800 **Free:** 800-877-6685
Fax: (303)714-3999
Website: http://www.pacificare.com
Jeffrey Folick, Chairman of the Board
Program(s): Chiropractic, Dental, Home Care, Inpatient SNF, Long-Term Care, Pharmaceutical Mail Order, Podiatry, Psychiatric, Behavioral Health, Physical Therapy, Transplant, Vision, Wellness.

Connecticut

★ 20040 ★ Cigna Behavioral Health, Inc.
900 Cottage Grove Rd.
Hartford, CT 06152-2317
Free: 800-873-7904 **Fax:** (860)226-5650
Website: http://www.mcc-care.com
Keith Dixon, CEO

Florida

★ 20041 ★ CIGNA Dental Health of Colorado
PO Box 189060
Plantation, FL 33318
Phone: (954)423-5800 **Fax:** (954)423-5490
Website: http://www.cigna.com/dental
Benjamin Hynes, CEO

★ 20042 ★ CIGNA Dental Health of Delaware, Inc.
PO Box 189060
Plantation, FL 33318-9060
Phone: (954)423-5800 **Free:** 800-367-1037
Fax: (954)423-5499
Website: http://www.cigna.com/dental
Benjamin Haynes, CEO

★ 20043 ★ CIGNA Dental Health of Florida
PO Box 189060
Plantation, FL 33318-9060
Phone: (954)423-5800 **Free:** 800-367-1037
Fax: (954)423-5491
Website: http://www.cigna.com/dental
Sam Westover, CEO

★ 20044 ★ CIGNA Dental Health Inc. - Corp. Headquarters
PO Box 189060
Plantation, FL 33318-9060
Phone: (954)423-5800 **Free:** 800-367-1037
Fax: (954)423-5491
Website: http://www.cigna.com/dental
Sam Westover, CEO

★ 20045 ★ CIGNA Dental Health of Kansas, Inc.
PO Box 189060
Plantation, FL 33318-9060
Phone: (954)423-5800 **Free:** 800-367-1037
Fax: (954)423-5490
Website: http://www.cigna.com/dental
Benjamin Haynes, CEO

★ 20046 ★ CIGNA Dental Health of Maryland, Inc.
PO Box 189060
Plantation, FL 33318-9060
Phone: (954)423-5800 **Free:** 800-367-1037
Fax: (954)423-5499
Website: http://www.cigna.com/dental
Benjamin Haynes, CEO

★ 20047 ★ CIGNA Dental Health of North Carolina, Inc.
PO Box 189060
Plantation, FL 33318-9060
Phone: (954)423-5800 **Free:** 800-367-1037
Fax: (954)423-5491
Website: http://www.cigna.com/dental
Randee Lehrer, CEO

★ 20048 ★ CIGNA Dental Health of Ohio, Inc.
PO Box 189060
Plantation, FL 33324

Phone: (954)423-5800 **Free:** 800-367-1037
Fax: (954)423-5491
Website: http://www.cigna.com/dental
Kevin Tylus, Chairman of the Board

★ 20049 ★ Comprehensive Behavioral Care, Inc.
200 S Hoover Blvd., Bldg. 219, No. 200
Tampa, FL 33609
Phone: (813)288-4808 **Fax:** (813)288-4844
Mary Jane Johnson, CEO

★ 20050 ★ Fortis Benefits Dental - Florida
3550 Buschwood Pk. Dr.
Tampa, FL 33618
Phone: (813)932-4777 **Free:** 800-943-9644
Fax: (813)933-8411
Website: http://www.fortisbenefitsdental.com
Jerry W. DeFoor, CEO

★ 20051 ★ Fortis Benefits Dental - Georgia
80 Johnson Ferry Rd., Ste. 450
Atlanta, FL 30342
Phone: (770)455-8860 **Free:** 800-876-6728
Fax: (770)455-3610
Website: http://www.fortisbenefitsdental.com
Peter Barnett, President

★ 20052 ★ United Concordia Co., Inc. - Florida
HMO Plan
601 Cleveland St., Ste. 415
Clearwater, FL 33755
Phone: (727)441-8585 **Free:** 800-322-0366
Fax: (727)441-6090
Website: http://www.ucci.com
Thomas Dzuryachko, CEO
Program(s): Dental.

Georgia

★ 20053 ★ Comp Benefits Corp. - Corporate Headquarters
100 Mansell Ct. E, Ste. 400
Roswell, GA 30076
Phone: (770)998-8936 **Free:** 800-633-1262
Fax: (770)998-6871
Website: http://www.compbenefits.com
Phyllis A. Klock, President

★ 20054 ★ Magellan Behavioral Health of Georgia
HMO Plan
125 Plantation Center Dr.
Macon, GA 31210
Free: 800-458-2740 **Fax:** (410)953-2426
Website: http://www.magellanhealth.com
Henry T. Harbin, MD, Chairman of the Board

Idaho

★ 20055 ★ Columbia Dental of Idaho, Inc.
8950 W Emerald St., Ste. 108
Boise, ID 83704
Phone: 877-329-7965 **Free:** 800-603-1738
Fax: (208)672-8684
Website: http://www.denkor.com
Eugene Stourtes, CEO

Illinois

★ 20056 ★ Delta Dental Plan of Illinois
HMO Plan
801 Ogden Ave.
Lisle, IL 60532
Phone: (630)964-2400 **Free:** 800-331-0538
Fax: (630)964-2596
Website: http://www.deltadentalil.com
Robert Dennison, DMD, CEO & Pres

★ 20057 ★ Dental Network of America
2 Trans Am Plaza Dr., Ste. 500
Oakbrook Terrace, IL 60181
Phone: (630)691-1133 **Free:** 800-323-6840
Fax: (630)495-0575
Website: http://www.dnoa.com
Harold Firfer, DDS, CEO

★ 20058 ★ First Commonwealth
444 N Wells, Ste. 600
Chicago, IL 60610
Phone: (312)644-1800 **Free:** 800-788-3384
Fax: (312)832-0065
Website: http://www.fcwi.net
David Mulligan, CEO & Pres
Program(s): Dental.

★ 20059 ★ Fortis Benefits Dental - Illinois
450 E Devon Ave.
Itasca, IL 60143
Phone: (630)227-0225 **Free:** 888-773-4220
Fax: (630)227-0231
Website: http://www.fortisbenefitsdental.com
Danny L. Bentley, CEO

★ 20060 ★ Unicare Inc.
HMO Plan
8420 W Bryn Mawr, Ste. 700
Chicago, IL 60631
Phone: (847)843-2200 **Free:** 800-949-5449
Fax: 888-788-5526
Charles Mitchell, Contact

★ 20061 ★ United Concordia Co., Inc. - Illinois
246 E Janata Blvd
Lombard, IL 60148
Phone: (630)629-2471 **Fax:** (630)693-4688
Website: http://www.ucci.com
Thomas Dzuryachko, CEO
Program(s): Dental.

Indiana

★ 20062 ★ Health Resources, Inc.
PO Box 15660
Evansville, IN 47716-0660
Phone: (812)424-1444 **Free:** 800-727-1444
Fax: (812)424-2096
Website: http://www.hri-dro.com
Edward Fritz, DDS, Chairman of the Board
Program(s): Dental.

★ 20063 ★ Managed Health Services Indiana Inc.
HMO Plan
1099 N Meridian St., Ste., 400
Indianapolis, IN 46204
Phone: (317)684-9478 **Free:** 800-944-9661
Fax: (317)684-0297
Website: http://www.cenlene.com
Rita Johnson-Mills, CEO

Iowa

★ 20064 ★ Iowa Health Solutions
2550 Middle Rd., Ste. 405
Bettendorf, IA 52722
Phone: (563)359-8999 **Fax:** (563)359-9034
Website: http://www.iowahealthsolutions.com
James Dyer, Chairman of the Board

Kentucky

★ 20065 ★ Humana, Inc. - Alabama HMO Plan
500 W Main St.
Louisville, KY 40201-1438
Phone: (502)580-1860 **Fax:** (502)580-3127
Website: http://www.humana.com
David Jones, Chairman of the Board

★ 20066 ★ Humana, Inc. - Arkansas HMO Plan
500 W Main St.
Louisville, KY 40201-1438
Phone: (502)580-1000 **Fax:** (502)580-4106
Website: http://www.humana.com
David Jones, Chairman of the Board

★ 20067 ★ Humana, Inc. - Colorado HMO Plan
PO Box 740036
Louisville, KY 40201-7436
Phone: (303)694-1044 **Free:** 800-825-7496
Fax: (303)694-1105
Website: http://www.humana.com
David Jones, Chairman of the Board

★ 20068 ★ United Concordia Co., Inc. - Kentucky
4010 Dupont Cir., Ste. L-03
Louisville, KY 40207
Phone: (717)731-2532 **Free:** 800-568-6432
Fax: (717)972-0410
Website: http://www.ucci.com
Thomas Dzuryachko, CEO
Program(s): Dental.

Maryland

★ 20069 ★ APS Healthcare Inc.
HMO Plan
6705 Rockledge Dr., Ste. 200
Bethesda, MD 20817
Phone: (301)571-0633 **Free:** 800-305-3720
Website: http://www.apscare.com
Ken Kessler, MD, CEO & Chm Bd

★ 20070 ★ Consumer Dental Care Co.
HMO Plan
4061 Powder Mill Rd., No. 325
Beltsville, MD 20705
Phone: (301)937-4447 **Free:** 800-879-0288
Fax: (301)937-0245
Website: http://www.consumerdentalcare.com
Dr. Steven Keller, CEO

★ 20071 ★ Dental Benefit Providers, Inc. - Corporate Headquarters
7200 Wisconsin Ave., Ste. 800
Bethesda, MD 20814
Phone: (301)654-6900 **Free:** 800-445-9090
Fax: (301)986-7965
Website: http://www.dbp.com
Edward Murphy, CEO

★ 20072 ★ Magellan Health Services
HMO Plan
6950 Columbia Gateway Dr.
Columbia, MD 21046
Phone: (410)953-1000 **Free:** 800-458-2740
Fax: (410)953-5200
Website: http://www.magellanhealth.com
Henry T. Harbin, MD, Chairman of the Board
Program(s): Behavioral Health.

★ 20073 ★ Podiatric Care Management
218 N Charles St., Ste. 101
Baltimore, MD 21201

Phone: (410)539-4282 **Fax:** (410)727-4350
Michael Sherman, DPM, CEO

★ 20074 ★ United Concordia Co., Inc. - Maryland
1220 B E Joppa Rd., Ste. 421
Towson, MD 21286-5811
Free: 800-272-8865 **Fax:** (410)296-4367
Website: http://www.ucci.com
Thomas Dzuryachko, CEO
Program(s): Dental.

Massachusetts

★ 20075 ★ Community Medical Alliance
253 Summer St.
Boston, MA 02210
Phone: (617)423-0040 **Fax:** (617)772-5519
Jim Hooley, CEO

★ 20076 ★ ManagedComp
10 Presidential Way
Woburn, MA 01801
Free: 800-832-1600 **Fax:** (781)938-2003
Website: http://www.managedcomp.com
Jon Gice, President

Michigan

★ 20077 ★ CO/OP Optical Services, Inc.
2424 E 8 Mile Rd.
Detroit, MI 48234-1010
Phone: (313)366-5100 **Fax:** (313)366-2246
Patrick Korth, CEO

★ 20078 ★ Comprehensive Behavioral Care, Inc.
1750 S Telegraph, Ste. 106
Bloomfield Hills, MI 48302
Phone: (248)332-8718 **Free:** 800-688-6885
Fax: (248)332-4522
Website: http://www.comprehensivecare.com
Michelle Brochu, CEO

★ 20079 ★ Dencap Dental Plans
45 E Milwaukee
Detroit, MI 48202
Phone: (313)972-1400 **Free:** 800-875-2400
Fax: (313)972-4662
Website: http://www.dencap.com
Joseph Lentine, CEO

★ 20080 ★ Fortis Benefits Dental - Michigan
3001 W Big Beaver Rd., Ste. 330
Troy, MI 48084
Phone: (248)649-4410 **Free:** 800-262-5388
Fax: (214)258-1100
Website: http://www.fortisbenefitsdental.com
Peter Barnett, President

★ 20081 ★ Golden Dental Plans, Inc.
29377 Hoover Rd.
Warren, MI 48093-3475
Free: 800-451-5918 **Fax:** (586)573-8720
Website: http://www.goldendentalplans.com
Ed Petersmarck, CEO

★ 20082 ★ Midwestern Dental Plans, Inc.
5050 Schaefer Rd.
Dearborn, MI 48126-3221
Phone: (313)582-8150 **Free:** 800-544-6374
Fax: (313)582-6015
John Morgan, Vice President

★ 20083 ★ S V S Visions, Inc.
140 Macomb St.
Mount Clemens, MI 48043-5651
Phone: (586)468-7612 **Free:** 800-225-3095
Fax: (586)468-7682
Ronald Dooley, CEO

★ 20084 ★ United Concordia Co., Inc. - Michigan
2000 Town Center, Ste. 2200
Southfield, MI 48075
Phone: (717)731-2532 **Free:** 800-944-6432
Fax: (248)304-2708
Website: http://www.ucci.com
Thomas Dzuryachko, CEO
Program(s): Dental.

Missouri

★ 20085 ★ United Concordia Co., Inc. - Missouri
390 South Woods Mill Rd., Ste. 175
Chesterfield, MO 63017
Phone: (717)731-2532 **Free:** 800-374-6432
Fax: (314)205-9601
Website: http://www.ucci.com
Thomas A. Dzuryacko, CEO
Program(s): Dental.

Montana

★ 20086 ★ APS Healthcare Northwest, Inc.
HMO Plan
PO Box 16090
Missoula, MT 59806-6090
Phone: (406)327-7000 **Free:** 800-390-9150
Fax: (406)327-7786
Website: http://www.apscare.com
Ken Kessler, MD, CEO & Chm Bd

Nevada

★ 20087 ★ Behavioral Healthcare Options, Inc.
HMO Plan
2801 S Valley View, Ste. 6
Las Vegas, NV 89102
Phone: (702)364-1484 **Free:** 800-873-2246
Fax: (702)364-1771
Website: http://www.sierrahealth.com
Michael Adams, CEO

★ 20088 ★ Nevada Pacific Dental
1432 S Jones Blvd.
Las Vegas, NV 89102-1231
Phone: (702)737-8900 **Free:** 800-926-0925
Fax: (702)259-8381

New Jersey

★ 20089 ★ Dental Group of New Jersey
924 N Wood Ave.
Linden, NJ 07036
Phone: (908)925-6022 **Fax:** (908)925-4416
Richard Lukenda, DMD, CEO

★ 20090 ★ Magellan Behavioral Health
199 Pomerly
Parsippany, NJ 07054
Phone: (973)515-5010 **Fax:** (973)515-2012
Website: http://www.magellanhealth.com
Jay Levin, President

★ 20091 ★ Unity Dental Health Services
1219 Main Ave.
Clifton, NJ 07011
Phone: (973)473-0900 **Free:** 800-722-0948
Fax: (973)772-3989
Daryl Aiken, CEO & Pres

★ 20092 ★ Value Health Care
PO Box 1442
Wall, NJ 07719
Free: 800-516-4343 **Fax:** (732)292-1111
Phyllis MacKelvie, CEO

New Mexico

★ 20093 ★ Fortis Benefits Dental - New Mexico
HMO Plan
1128 Pennsylvania St. NE, Ste. 210
Albuquerque, NM 87110
Phone: (505)266-7709 **Free:** 800-269-5415
Fax: (505)265-3576
Website: http://www.fortisbenefitsdental.com
Debra Rush, CEO

New York

★ 20094 ★ Affinity Health Plan
One Executive Blvd., 2nd Fl.
Yonkers, NY 10701
Phone: (914)476-6000 **Fax:** (914)476-4844
Website: http://www.affinityplan.org
Maura Bluestone, CEO

★ 20095 ★ Dentcare Delivery Systems, Inc.
HMO Plan
60 Charles Lindbergh Blvd.
Uniondale, NY 11553
Phone: (516)542-2200 **Free:** 800-468-0608
Fax: (516)794-3186
Website: http://www.healthplex.com
John Forte, Contact

★ 20096 ★ Elderplan, Inc.
6323 7th Ave.
Brooklyn, NY 11220
Phone: (718)921-7898 **Fax:** (718)630-2565
Website: http://www.elderplan.org
Eli Feldman, CEO
Program(s): Chiropractic, Dental, Home Care, Inpatient SNF, Long-Term Care, Pharmaceutical Mail Order, Podiatry, Psychiatric, Behavioral Health, Physical Therapy, Transplant, Vision, Wellness.

★ 20097 ★ Fortis Benefits Dental
1633 Broadway, Ste. 2020
New York, NY 10019
Phone: (212)246-0200 **Free:** 888-424-0030
Fax: (212)246-5199
Website: http://www.fortisbenefitsdental.com
Danny L. Bentley, CEO

★ 20098 ★ Healthplex, Inc.
60 Charles Lindbergh Blvd.
Uniondale, NY 11553
Phone: (516)542-2200 **Free:** 800-468-0608
Fax: (516)227-1143
Website: http://www.healthplex.com
John Forte, Chairman of the Board
Program(s): Dental.

★ 20099 ★ Neighborhood Health Providers
521 5th Ave.
New York, NY 10175
Phone: (212)808-4775 **Fax:** (212)808-4772
Website: http://www.brookdalehospital.org
Steven Bory, CEO & Pres

★ 20100 ★ New York State Catholic Health Plan, Inc.
95-25 Queens Blvd.
Rego Park, NY 11374
Phone: (718)896-6500 **Free:** 888-343-3547
Fax: (718)896-1920
Website: http://www.fideliscareny.org
Mark L. Lane, CEO
Program(s): Dental, Home Care, Podiatry, Psychiatric, Behavioral Health, Physical Therapy, Transplant, Vision, Wellness.

★ 20101 ★ NMHCRX
HMO Plan
26 Harbor Pk. Dr.
Port Washington, NY 11050
Phone: (516)605-6638 **Free:** 800-251-3883
Fax: (516)605-6981
Website: http://www.nmhcrx.com
Bert Brodsky, Chairman of the Board

★ 20102 ★ NY Compensation Managers Inc.
6250 S Bay Rd.
Syracuse, NY 13220
Phone: (315)699-8475 **Fax:** (315)699-1438
David Francey, CEO

★ 20103 ★ SCHC Total Care, Inc.
PO Box 11507
Syracuse, NY 13218-1507
Phone: (315)476-7921 **Free:** 800-223-7242
Fax: (315)475-1448
Reuben P. Cowart, DDS, CEO
Program(s): Home Care, Podiatry, Psychiatric, Physical Therapy, Transplant, Vision, Wellness.

★ 20104 ★ United Concordia Co., Inc. - New York
HMO Plan
159 Express St.
Plainview, NY 11803
Phone: (516)827-6720 **Fax:** (516)827-6618
Website: http://www.ucci.com
Thomas A. Dzuryachko, CEO

North Carolina

★ 20105 ★ Opticare Health Systems
110 Zebulon Ct.
Rocky Mount, NC 27804
Phone: (252)937-6650 **Free:** 800-334-3937
Fax: (252)451-2182
Website: http://www.opticare-ehn.com
Jason Harrold, CEO

Ohio

★ 20106 ★ Fortis Benefits Dental - Ohio
312 Elm St., Ste. 1500
Cincinnati, OH 45202
Phone: (513)621-1924 **Free:** 800-543-7266
Fax: (513)621-4553
Website: http://www.fortisbenefitsdental.com
Danny L. Bentley, CEO

★ 20107 ★ North America Benefits Network Inc.
19800 Detroit Rd.
Cleveland, OH 44116
Phone: (440)356-8212 **Free:** 800-356-6226
Fax: (440)356-0210
Donald T. Baker, CEO

★ 20108 ★ Superior Dental Care, Inc.
6683 Centerville Business Pkwy.
Dayton, OH 45459
Phone: (937)438-0283 **Free:** 800-762-3159
Fax: (937)438-0288
Rebecca York, CEO

Oklahoma

★ 20109 ★ Fortis Benefits Dental - Oklahoma
7112 S Mingo Rd., Ste 108
Tulsa, OK 74133
Phone: (918)254-9161 **Free:** 888-247-1142
Fax: (918)254-9076
Website: http://www.fortisbenefitsdental.com
Peter Barnett, CEO

★ 20110 ★ Preferred Podiatrists of Oklahoma
3818 N Rockwell St.
Bethany, OK 73008-3350
Phone: (405)787-8820 **Fax:** (405)495-6523
Richard Traczyk, DPM, CEO

Oregon

★ 20111 ★ Columbia Dental of Washington, Inc.
14025 SW Farmington Rd., Ste. 300
Beaverton, OR 97005
Phone: (503)644-6444 **Free:** 800-460-7644
Fax: (503)644-2170
Website: http://www.denkor.com
Eugene Skourtes, CEO

★ 20112 ★ Williamette Dental Group PC
14025 SW Farmington Rd.
Beaverton, OR 97005
Phone: (503)644-6444 **Free:** 800-460-7644
Fax: (503)644-2170
Website: http://www.denkor.com
Steve Petruzelli, CEO

Pennsylvania

★ 20113 ★ Alignis Healthcare - Corporate Headquarters
100 Mattsonford Rd., Bldg 5, No. 445
Radnor, PA 19087
Phone: (610)688-3700 **Free:** 800-863-2932
Fax: (610)688-1765
Jack D. Williams, CEO

★ 20114 ★ Fortis Benefits Dental - Pennsylvania
1 Bala Plz., Ste. 4001
Bala Cynwyd, PA 19004
Free: 800-220-1957 **Fax:** (610)660-8077
Website: http://www.fortisbenefitsdental.com
Danny L. Bentley, CEO

★ 20115 ★ Keystone Health Plan East Inc.
HMO Plan
1901 Market St.
Philadelphia, PA 19103
Phone: (215)241-2001 **Free:** 800-227-3114
Fax: (215)241-2017
Website: http://www.khpe.com
G. Fred DiBona, CEO & Pres

★ 20116 ★ United Concordia Co., Inc. - Corporate Headquarters
HMO Plan
4401 Deer Path Rd.
Harrisburg, PA 17110
Phone: (717)360-6800 **Free:** 800-972-4191
Fax: (717)612-4996
Website: http://www.ucci.com
Thomas Dzuryachko, CEO
Program(s): Dental.

★ 20117 ★ United Concordia Co., Inc. - Pennsylvania
4401 Deer Path Rd.
Harrisburg, PA 17110
Phone: (717)360-6800 **Free:** 800-972-4191
Fax: (717)612-4996
Website: http://www.ucci.com
Thomas A. Dzuryachko, CEO

★ 20118 ★ United Concordia Co., Inc. - Pennsylvania
175 Pine St.
Williamsport, PA 17701
Phone: (570)321-5124 **Fax:** (570)321-5199
Website: http://www.ucci.com
Thomas A. Dzuryachko, CEO

Rhode Island

★ 20119 ★ DMS Dental Plan
1429 Warwick Ave.
Warwick, RI 02888
Phone: (401)463-5116 **Free:** 800-456-8715
Fax: (401)463-6059
Lorin Kinney, CEO

Texas

★ 20120 ★ AECC Total Vision Health Plan of Texas, Inc.
3010 LBJ Freeway, Ste. 240
Dallas, TX 75234
Phone: (972)620-8909 **Free:** 800-268-8847
Fax: (972)620-9484
Bill Henderson, CEO

★ 20121 ★ Aetna Inc. - Dental Plan of Texas
2777 Stemmons Fwy.
Dallas, TX 75207
Phone: (214)200-8000 **Free:** 800-825-7935
Fax: (214)200-8916
Website: http://www.aetna.com
John W. Rowe, MD, Chairman of the Board

★ 20122 ★ Alpha Dental Programs, Inc.
1431 Greenway Dr., Ste. 520
Irving, TX 75038
Phone: (972)580-1616 **Free:** 800-775-0523
Fax: (972)580-1333
Website: http://www.deltadentalins.com
Robert Budd, CEO

★ 20123 ★ Block Vision of Texas, Inc.
14228 Midway, Ste. 213
Dallas, TX 75244
Phone: (972)991-8816 **Free:** 800-914-9795
Fax: (972)991-4704
Andrew Alcorn, CEO

★ 20124 ★ CIGNA Behavioral Health, Inc.
6600 E Campus Circle Dr., Ste 110
Irving, TX 75063
Free: 888-800-8849 **Fax:** (972)465-7001
Website: http://www.mcc-care.com
Keith Dixon, CEO

★ 20125 ★ CIGNA Dental Health of Texas, Inc.
6600 E Campus Circle Dr., Ste. 100
Irving, TX 75063
Free: 800-367-1037 **Fax:** (954)423-5490
Website: http://www.cigna.com/dental
Allen West, CEO

★ 20126 ★ CompBenefits
2929 Briar Park, Ste. 314
Houston, TX 77042
Phone: (713)784-7011 **Free:** 800-950-1071
Fax: (713)784-9440
David Klock, MD, CEO
Program(s): Dental.

★ 20127 ★ Coordinated Care Solutions of Texas, Inc.
1235 N Loop W, Ste 420
Houston, TX 77008
Free: 888-721-9797
Richard M. Hassett, MD, CEO

★ 20128 ★ ECCA - Managed Vision Care, Inc.
11103 West Ave.
San Antonio, TX 78213
Phone: (210)340-3531 **Fax:** (210)524-6587
Website: http://www.ecca.com
Bernie Andrews, CEO

★ 20129 ★ Fortis Benefits Dental - Delaware HMO Plan
16775 Addison Rd., Ste. 5000
Addison, TX 75001
Phone: (972)458-7474 **Free:** 800-262-5388
Fax: (214)258-1100
Website: http://www.fortisbenefitsdental.com
Peter Barnett, President

★ 20130 ★ Fortis Benefits Dental - Indiana
16775 Addison Rd., Ste. 500
Addison, TX 75001
Phone: (317)466-0958 **Free:** 800-262-5388
Fax: (317)291-5188
Website: http://www.fortisbenefitsdental.com
Danny L. Bentley, CEO

★ 20131 ★ Fortis Benefits Dental - Texas
16775 Addison Rd., Ste. 500
Addison, TX 75001
Phone: (214)258-1020 **Free:** 800-442-0911
Fax: (214)258-1100
Website: http://www.fortisbenefitsdental.com
Greg Dowling, Contact

★ 20132 ★ Fortis Benefits Dental - Utah
16775 Addison Rd., Ste. 500
Addison, TX 75001
Phone: (801)263-6473 **Free:** 800-262-5388
Fax: (801)263-8243
Website: http://www.fortisbenefitsdental.com
Danny Bentley, CEO

★ 20133 ★ Horizon Behavioral Services
1500 Waters Ridge Dr.
Lewisville, TX 75057-6011
Free: 888-802-6084 **Fax:** (972)420-8247
Website: http://www.horizoncare.net
James McAtee, CEO

★ 20134 ★ MenningerCare Systems
4006 Belt Line Rd., No. 205
Addison, TX 75001-5831
Phone: (972)588-2400 **Free:** 800-866-7242
Fax: (972)931-1938
Website: http://www.minningercare.com
John Quick, PhD, CEO
Program(s): Behavioral Health.

★ 20135 ★ Metrowest Health Plan, Inc.
1617 Hemphill St.
Fort Worth, TX 76104
Phone: (817)665-5100 **Free:** 888-924-8852
Fax: (817)665-5120
Website: http://www.jpshealthnet.org/metrowest
Jerry Anderson, Contact

★ 20136 ★ Oraquest Dental Plans
12946 Dairy Ashford, Ste. 360
Sugar Land, TX 77478
Phone: (281)313-7170 **Free:** 800-660-6064
Fax: (281)313-7155
Website: http://www.oraquest.com
James Taylor, CEO & Pres

★ 20137 ★ Pearle Vision Managed Care - HMO of Texas, Inc.
2465 Joe Field Rd.
Dallas, TX 75229-3479
Free: 800-267-9894 **Fax:** (972)277-6424
Jim Easter, CEO

★ 20138 ★ Safeguard Health Plans, Inc.
5495 Beltline Rd., No. 155
Dallas, TX 75240-7010
Phone: (972)364-5000 **Free:** 800-880-1800
Fax: (972)364-5015
Jim Buacher, CEO
Program(s): Dental.

★ 20139 ★ Spectra Dental
1445 North Loop West, Ste. 1000
Houston, TX 77008
Phone: (713)861-3231 **Free:** 800-232-0990
Fax: (713)861-0008
Ken Sheldon, CEO

★ 20140 ★ Texas Universities Health Plan
701 Brazos St., Ste. 950
Austin, TX 78701
Phone: (512)481-8847 **Fax:** (512)481-8849
Thomas Wise, CEO

★ 20141 ★ United Concordia Co., Inc. - Texas
8214 Westchester Dr.
Dallas, TX 75225
Phone: (214)378-6410 **Fax:** (214)378-6306
Website: http://www.ucci.com
Thomas Dzuryachko, CEO
Program(s): Dental.

★ 20142 ★ ValueOptions of Texas, Inc.
8710 Freeport Pkwy, Ste. 200
Irving, TX 75063
Phone: (217)492-6107 **Fax:** (214)492-1682
Conway McDaniel, Contact

★ 20143 ★ VHP Dental, Inc.
7801 North Ih 35
Austin, TX 78761
Phone: (512)433-1000 **Free:** 800-852-1040
Fax: (512)433-1827
Paul Tovar, CEO

★ 20144 ★ Vista Health Plan, Inc.
PO Box 15800
Austin, TX 78761-5800
Phone: (512)433-1000 **Free:** 800-852-1040
Fax: (512)433-1827
Paul Tovar, CEO
Program(s): Psychiatric, Behavioral Health.

Utah

★ 20145 ★ Standard Optical
1901 W Parkway Blvd.
Salt Lake City, UT 84119
Phone: (801)886-2020 **Free:** 800-363-0950
Fax: (801)954-0054
Stephen Schubach, CEO

Virginia

★ 20146 ★ CIGNA Behavioral Health, Inc.
7501 Boulder View Dr., Ste. 500
Richmond, VA 23225
Phone: (804)272-1000 **Fax:** (804)272-3011
Website: http://www.mcc-care.com
Matt Manders, CEO

★ 20147 ★ Dominion Dental Services - Corporate Headquarters
110 N Royal St., Ste. 405
Alexandria, VA 22314
Phone: (703)518-5000 **Free:** 888-681-5100
Fax: (703)518-8849
Website: http://www.dominiondental.com
Mitchell McGlynn, CEO & Chm Bd

★ 20148 ★ United Concordia Co., Inc. - Virginia
4860 Cox Rd., Ste. 200
Glen Allen, VA 23060
Free: 800-454-3224 **Fax:** (804)217-8368
Website: http://www.ucci.com
Thomas Dzuryacko, Contact
Program(s): Dental.

Washington

★ 20149 ★ Dental Health Services, Inc.
936 N 34th St., Ste. 208
Seattle, WA 98133
Phone: (206)633-2300 **Free:** 800-248-8108
Fax: (206)624-8755
Gary Pernell, Contact

★ 20150 ★ United Concordia Co., Inc. - Washington
2200 Sixth Ave., Ste. 620
Seattle, WA 98121
Free: 888-245-8224 **Fax:** (206)728-2740
Website: http://www.ucci.com
Thomas Dzuryacko, CEO
Program(s): Dental.

Wisconsin

★ 20151 ★ American WholeHealth Networks, Inc.
PO Box 594
Hartland, WI 53029-0594
Phone: (262)367-3200 **Free:** 800-274-7526
Fax: (262)367-5934
Website: http://www.awhnet.com
Bill Luben, CEO
Program(s): Chiropractic, Pharmaceutical Mail Order, Physical Therapy, Wellness, Alternative Medicine.

★ 20152 ★ Dental Associates Ltd.
11711 W Burleigh St.
Wauwatosa, WI 53222
Phone: (414)771-5000 **Fax:** (414)456-9911
John G. Gonis, MD, Chairman of the Board

★ 20153 ★ Doral Dental USA
12121 N Corporate Pkwy.
Mequon, WI 53092
Phone: (262)241-7140 **Free:** 800-417-7140
Fax: (262)241-7366
Website: http://www.doral.com
Gregory J. Borca, CEO

★ 20154 ★ Eye Care of Wisconsin
8705 N Port Washington Rd.
Milwaukee, WI 53217-2213
Phone: (414)351-3030 **Free:** 800-373-6370
Fax: (414)351-3603
Patrick Cashin, CEO & Chm Bd

★ 20155 ★ Midwest Dental Plan
680 Hehli Way
Mondovi, WI 54755
Phone: (715)926-5050 **Fax:** (715)926-5405
Yvonne Mayberry, CEO

★ 20156 ★ Racine Dental Group
1320 S Green Bay Rd.
Racine, WI 53406
Phone: (262)637-9371 **Fax:** (262)637-3071
Dr. Newton, CEO

★ 20157 ★ Vision Care Network
1421 Washington Ave.
Racine, WI 53403
Phone: (262)637-7494 **Free:** 800-767-8801
Fax: (262)637-7958
Bruce Savin, OD, CEO

★ 20158 ★ Vision Insurance Plan of America, Inc. - Corporate Headquarters
1126 S 70th St., Ste. 101A
West Allis, WI 53214-3151
Phone: (414)475-1875 **Free:** 800-883-5747
Fax: (414)475-1599
Website: http://www.visionplans.com
Thomas Witter, CEO

Specialty PPOs

Alabama

★ 20159 ★ Behavioral Health Systems, Inc.
PO Box 830724
Birmingham, AL 35283-0724
Phone: (205)879-1150 **Free:** 800-245-1150
Fax: (205)879-1178
Website: http://www.bhs-inc.com
Deborah L Stephens, CPA, President

★ 20160 ★ NAMCI Premier PPO
188 Sparkman Dr.
Huntsville, AL 35805
Phone: (256)864-4100 **Fax:** (256)864-4401
Sherree N. Clark, Exec Director
Program(s): Home Care.

★ 20161 ★ United Concordia Co., Inc. - Alabama
400 Vestavia Pkwy, Ste. 205
Birmingham, AL 35216
Free: 800-554-6155 **Fax:** (205)822-1653
Website: http://www.ucci.com
Thomas A. Dzuryachko, CEO
Program(s): Dental.

Arizona

★ 20162 ★ Avesis, Inc.
3724 N 3rd St., Ste. 300
Phoenix, AZ 85012
Phone: (602)241-3400 **Free:** 800-522-0258
Fax: (602)240-9101
Alan S. Cohen, President
Program(s): Chiropractic, Dental, Vision.

★ 20163 ★ Catalina Behavioral Health Services, Inc.
2400 N Central Ave., Ste. 203A
Phoenix, AZ 85004
Phone: (602)452-1200 **Free:** 800-977-0281
Fax: (602)257-1644
Karen Smith-Hagman, CEO
Program(s): Behavioral health; psychiatric.

★ 20164 ★ Chiropractic Arizona Network, Inc.
3625 N 16th St.
Phoenix, AZ 85016
Phone: (602)264-2606 **Fax:** (602)285-0121
David L. Popejoy, CEO
Program(s): Chiropractic.

★ 20165 ★ Outlook Vision Service
40 N Center, No. 104
Mesa, AZ 85201
Phone: (480)461-9001 **Free:** 800-342-7188
Fax: (480)461-9021
Website: http://www.outlookvision.com
Ron Johnson, CEO

★ 20166 ★ Preferred Therapy Providers of America - Corporate Headquarters
5010 E Shea Blvd., Ste. A220
Scottsdale, AZ 85254-4681
Phone: (480)443-3900 **Free:** 800-664-5240
Fax: (480)443-2565
Website: http://www.preferredtherapy.com
Jaxene Hillebert, CEO & Pres

★ 20167 ★ SW Preferred Dental Organization
3625 N 16th St., Ste. 206
Phoenix, AZ 85016-6447
Phone: (602)234-3266 **Fax:** (602)285-0121
David Popejoy, CEO

★ 20168 ★ United Concordia Co., Inc. - Arizona PPO Plan
2198 Camelback Rd., Ste. 260
Phoenix, AZ 85016
Phone: (717)260-7500 **Free:** 800-322-0366
Fax: (717)612-4996
Website: http://www.ucci.com
Thomas Dzuryachko, CEO

California

★ 20169 ★ Access Dental Services
555 University Ave., Ste. 182
Sacramento, CA 95825
Phone: (916)922-5000 **Free:** 800-757-6453
Fax: (916)646-9000
Reza Abbaszadeh, DDS, CEO

★ 20170 ★ Aetna, Inc. - California PPO Plan
1200 W 7th St., Ste. 400
Los Angeles, CA 90017
Phone: (310)935-3100 **Fax:** (310)955-3185
Website: http://www.aetnaushc.com
John W. Rowe, MD, Chairman of the Board

★ 20171 ★ American Dental Network, Inc.
2700 N Main St., Ste. 620
Santa Ana, CA 92705
Free: 800-760-7352 **Fax:** (714)835-5380
Skip Gray, CEO & Pres

★ 20172 ★ ChiroSource - Corporate Headquarters
PO Box 130
Clayton, CA 94517
Phone: (925)672-5333 **Free:** 800-680-9997
Fax: (925)672-6657
Website: http://www.chirosource.com
Ronald S. Cataldo, DC, CEO & Pres
Program(s): Chiropractic; worker's compensation.

★ 20173 ★ Community Dental Services
PO Box 92009
Los Angeles, CA 90009
Phone: (949)756-5476 **Fax:** (714)708-5399
Mary Ellen Hardin, CEO

★ 20174 ★ Dental Health Services
3833 Atlantic Ave.
Long Beach, CA 90807-3505
Phone: (562)595-6000 **Fax:** (562)424-0150
Godfrey Pernell, CEO

★ 20175 ★ Dentistat Insurance Dentists of America PPO Plan
18805 Cox Ave., Ste. 250
Saratoga, CA 95070
Phone: (408)376-3801 **Free:** 800-336-8250
Fax: (408)376-3535
Website: http://www.dentistat.com
Lawrence N. Wallace, MD, Contact

★ 20176 ★ Direct Dental Administrators, Inc.
PO Box 2667
San Anselmo, CA 94979-2667
Free: 877-983-7070 **Fax:** (415)454-9228
John Cunningham, CEO

★ 20177 ★ Eye Med Vision Care
79 Daily Dr., Ste. 207
Camarillo, CA 93010
Phone: (805)445-9894 **Fax:** (805)445-9552
Website: http://www.ecpa.com
Amy Watson, Contact

★ 20178 ★ Golden West Dental & Vision
888 W Ventura Blvd.
Camarillo, CA 93010
Phone: (805)987-8941 **Free:** 800-995-4124
Fax: (805)987-6110
Website: http://www.goldenwestdental.com
Chris Kamen, DDS, CEO

★ 20179 ★ Health Net Dental, Inc. PPO Plan
125 Technology Dr., Ste. 100
Irvine, CA 92618
Phone: (949)790-3400 **Free:** 800-999-2848
Fax: (949)790-3452
Website: http://www.dv.healthnet.com
David Anderson, President

★ 20180 ★ Health Net Vision Inc. PPO Plan
125 Tehnology Dr., Ste. 100
Irvine, CA 92618
Phone: (949)790-3400 **Free:** 800-443-4994
Fax: (949)790-3452
Website: http://www.dv.healthnet.com
David Anderson, CEO

★ 20181 ★ Landmark Healthcare, Inc.
1750 Howe Ave., Ste. 300
Sacramento, CA 95825
Phone: (916)646-3477 **Fax:** (916)929-8350
Website: http://www.landmarkhealthcare.com
Joseph Kleigner, CEO

Program(s): Chiropractic, Alternative Medicine.

★ 20182 ★ Managed Health Network
1600 Los Gamos Dr., Ste. 300
San Rafael, CA 94903
Phone: (415)491-7200 **Free:** 800-327-7526
Fax: (415)472-8187
Website: http://www.mhn.com
Robert Fusco, Contact
Program(s): Psychiatric, Behavioral Health.

★ 20183 ★ MedFocus Radiology Network
2811 Wilshire Blvd., Ste. 900
Santa Monica, CA 90403
Phone: (310)828-4472 **Free:** 800-398-8999
Fax: (310)829-3366
Website: http://www.medfocus.net
Kathy Lewis, CEO
Program(s): Workers' Compensation.

★ 20184 ★ Newport Dental Plan
201 E Sandpointe, Ste. 200
Santa Ana, CA 92707
Phone: (714)668-1300 **Free:** 800-347-6453
Fax: (714)668-9422
Website: http://www.brightnow.com
Steven C. Bilt, CEO & Pres

★ 20185 ★ Pacificare Behavioral Health
23046 Avenida de la Carlota, Ste. 700
Laguna Hills, CA 92653
Phone: (949)859-7971 **Fax:** (949)859-9824
Website: http://www.pacificare.com
Jerome Vaccaro, MD, CEO

★ 20186 ★ Pacificare Dental and Vision
3110 Lake Center Dr.
Santa Ana, CA 92704
Free: 800-622-6388 **Fax:** (714)513-6381
Website: http://www.pacificare.com
James Stumpfel, CEO

★ 20187 ★ Physical Therapy Provider Network - Corporate Headquarters
26635 W Agoura Rd.
Calabasas, CA 91302
Phone: (818)883-7876 **Free:** 800-766-7876
Fax: (818)737-0260
Website: http://www.ptpn.com
Michael Weinper, MPH,PT, CEO

★ 20188 ★ Safeguard Health Plans, Inc.
95 Enterprise
Aliso Viejo, CA 92656-2601
Phone: (949)425-4300 **Free:** 800-204-0463
Fax: (949)425-4308
James Buncher, CEO
Program(s): Dental, vision.

★ 20189 ★ Superior Vision Services, Inc.
24012 Calle de la Plata, Ste. 350
Laguna Hills, CA 92653-7624
Phone: (949)461-3300 **Free:** 800-923-6766
Fax: (949)461-3311
Website: http://www.superiorvision.com
Rick Corbett, CEO

★ 20190 ★ United Behavioral Health (UBH)
425 Market St., 27th Fl.
San Francisco, CA 94105
Phone: (415)547-5000 **Fax:** (415)547-6100
Website: http://www.unitedbehavioralhealth.com
Saul Feldman, MD, CEO

★ 20191 ★ United Concordia Co., Inc. - California
21700 Oxnard, Ste. 500
Woodland Hills, CA 91367-3642
Phone: (717)731-2532 **Free:** 800-876-6432
Fax: (717)972-0410
Website: http://www.ucci.com
Thomas Dzuryachko, Chairman of the Board
Program(s): Dental.

★ 20192 ★ Vision Plan of America
3255 Wilshire Blvd., Ste. 1610
Los Angeles, CA 90010
Phone: (213)384-2600 **Free:** 800-400-4872
Fax: (213)384-0084
Website: http://www.visionplanofaamerica.com
Stuart Needleman, CEO

★ 20193 ★ Vision Service Plan
3333 Quality Dr.
Rancho Cordova, CA 95670
Phone: (916)851-5000 **Free:** 800-852-7600
Fax: (916)858-5329
Website: http://www.vsp.com
Roger Valine, CEO & Pres

Colorado

★ 20194 ★ Alpha Dental Plan of Colorado
609 E Speer Blvd., No. 200
Denver, CO 80203
Phone: (303)744-3007 **Fax:** (303)744-2890
Website: http://www.alphadentalplan.com
Kay McFarland, President

★ 20195 ★ Eye Med Vision Care
10669 Melody Dr.
Northglenn, CO 80234
Free: 877-846-0727 **Fax:** (303)254-6480
Website: http://www.ecpa.com
Peter Barnett, President

★ 20196 ★ Pacificare of Colorado
6455 S Yosemite
Englewood, CO 80111
Phone: (303)220-5800 **Free:** 800-877-6685
Fax: (303)714-3999
Website: http://www.pacificare.com
Jeffrey Folick, Chairman of the Board
Program(s): Chiropractic, Dental, Home Care, Inpatient SNF, Long-Term Care, Pharmaceutical Mail Order, Podiatry, Psychiatric, Behavioral Health, Physical Therapy, Transplant, Vision, Wellness.

★ 20197 ★ Vision Service Plan
1050 17th St., Ste. 1885
Denver, CO 80265
Phone: (303)892-7663 **Fax:** (303)892-7768
Website: http://www.vsp.com
John Alenius, Contact

Connecticut

★ 20198 ★ Berkley Administrators
PO Box 4012
Farmington, CT 06034-4012
Phone: (860)409-2300 **Free:** 800-251-2035
Fax: (860)409-2333
Website: http://www.berkleyrisk.com
Gregory Bickle, President
Program(s): Workers' Compensation.

★ 20199 ★ Connecticut General
900 Cottage Grove Rd.
Bloomfield, CT 06002
Phone: (860)726-6000 **Free:** 888-DEN-TALS
Fax: (860)726-5667
Ed Hanway, CEO
Program(s): Dental.

★ 20200 ★ HealthDirect
PO Box 975
Farmington, CT 06034-0975
Phone: (860)677-2331 **Free:** 800-842-1456
Fax: (860)678-0995
Website: http://www.hdirect.com
William Packer, President
Program(s): Workers' Compensation.

Florida

★ 20201 ★ AnciCare PPO, Inc.
3700 Lakeside Dr., Ste. 401
Miramar, FL 33027
Phone: (954)441-7600 **Free:** 800-414-4674
Fax: (954)441-0398
Website: http://www.ancicare.com
Michael Cabrera, CEO & Pres

★ 20202 ★ CIGNA Dental Health of Colorado
PO Box 189060
Plantation, FL 33318
Phone: (954)423-5800 **Fax:** (954)423-5490
Website: http://www.cigna.com/dental
Benjamin Hynes, CEO

★ 20203 ★ CIGNA Dental Health of New Jersey, Inc.
300 NW 82nd Ave., Ste. 700
Plantation, FL 33318-9060
Phone: (954)423-5800 **Free:** 800-367-1037
Fax: (954)423-5490
Website: http://www.cigna.com/dental
Val Nelimark, DDS, Contact

★ 20204 ★ Global Medical Management
7901 SW 36th St., Ste. 100
Davie, FL 33328-1914
Phone: (954)370-6404 **Free:** 800-682-6065
Fax: (954)370-6301
Website: http://www.gmmusa.com
Martin Smith, CEO & Pres

★ 20205 ★ Horizon Behavioral Health
1035 Greenwood, Ste. 201
Lake Mary, FL 32746
Phone: (407)647-6153 **Free:** 800-400-2606
Fax: (407)915-0050
Website: http://www.horizoncare.net
Linda Latner, CEO

★ 20206 ★ Physical Therapy Provider Network
4800 Linton Blvd., Ste. F-117
Delray Beach, FL 33445
Phone: (561)498-1423 **Fax:** (561)498-7848
Website: http://www.ptpn.com
Linda Zane, CEO

★ 20207 ★ Unipsych Systems
7777 Davie Rd. Ext., Ste 100
Hollywood, FL 33024-2515
Phone: (954)704-8686 **Free:** 800-272-3626
Fax: (954)704-8677
Leo Bradman, CEO

★ 20208 ★ United Concordia Co., Inc. - Florida
601 Cleveland St., Ste. 415
Clearwater, FL 33755
Phone: (727)441-8585 **Free:** 800-322-0366
Fax: (727)441-6090

Website: http://www.ucci.com
Thomas Dzuryachko, CEO
Program(s): Dental.

Georgia

★ 20209 ★ Beech Street - Alabama
3460 Preston Ridge Rd., Ste. 300
Alpharetta, GA 30005
Phone: (770)346-0520 **Free:** 800-655-1855
Fax: (770)346-0506
Website: http://www.beechstreet.com
William Fickling, Jr., Chairman of the Board
Program(s): Chiropractic, Home Care, Inpatient SNF, Long-Term Care, Podiatry, Psychiatric, Behavioral Health, Transplant, Workers' Compensation, Alternative Medicine.

★ 20210 ★ Coalition America, Inc.
4151 Ashford Dunwoody Rd., No. 615
Atlanta, GA 30319
Phone: (404)459-7201 **Fax:** (404)459-6645
Website: http://www.coalitionamerica.com
Sean Smith, CEO
Program(s): Chiropractic, Dental, Home Care, Inpatient SNF, Long-Term Care, Pharmaceutical Mail Order, Podiatry, Psychiatric, Behavioral Health, Physical Therapy, Transplant, Vision, Wellness, Workers' Compensation, Other Benefits.

★ 20211 ★ Comp Benefits Corp. - Corporate Headquarters
100 Mansell Ct. E, Ste. 400
Roswell, GA 30076
Phone: (770)998-8936 **Free:** 800-633-1262
Fax: (770)998-6871
Website: http://www.compbenefits.com
Phyllis A. Klock, President

★ 20212 ★ Comprehensive Health Group, Inc.
5672 Peachtree Pkwy., Ste. F
Norcross, GA 30092
Phone: (770)448-4677 **Free:** 800-669-8682
Fax: (770)448-4749
Website: http://www.chgallied.com
George Spalding, Jr., CPA, CEO
Program(s): Chiropractic, Dental, Pharmaceutical Mail Order, Psychiatric, Physical Therapy, Vision, Wellness, Alternative Medicine.

★ 20213 ★ Magellan Behavioral Health of Georgia
PPO Plan
125 Plantation Center Dr.
Macon, GA 31210
Free: 800-458-2740 **Fax:** (410)953-2426
Website: http://www.magellanhealth.com
Henry T. Harbin, MD, Chairman of the Board

Illinois

★ 20214 ★ Beech Street - North Dakota
Two Trans Am Plaza, Ste. 400
Oakbrook Terrace, IL 60181
Phone: (630)705-8560 **Free:** 800-722-2844
Fax: (630)705-1414
Website: http://www.beechstreet.com
William Fickling, Jr., Chairman of the Board
Program(s): Chiropractic, Home Care, Inpatient SNF, Long-Term Care, Podiatry, Psychiatric, Behavioral Health, Transplant, Workers' Compensation, Alternative Medicine.

★ 20215 ★ Compsych Behavioral Health
NBC Tower, 24th Fl.
Chicago, IL 60611-5506
Phone: (312)595-4000 **Free:** 800-755-3050
Fax: (312)595-3125
Website: http://www.compsych.com
Richard Chaifetz, MD, CEO & Chm Bd

★ 20216 ★ Delta Dental Plan of Illinois
PPO Plan
801 Ogden Ave.
Lisle, IL 60532
Phone: (630)964-2400 **Free:** 800-331-0538
Fax: (630)964-2596
Website: http://www.deltadentalil.com
Robert Dennison, DMD, CEO & Pres

★ 20217 ★ Dental Care of America, Ltd.
482 N Milwaukee Ave.
Wheeling, IL 60090
Phone: (847)520-3390 **Fax:** (847)520-8161
Angelo Lendino, CEO

★ 20218 ★ Dental Network of America
2 Trans Am Plaza Dr., Ste. 500
Oakbrook Terrace, IL 60181
Phone: (630)691-1133 **Free:** 800-323-6840
Fax: (630)495-0575
Website: http://www.dnoa.com
Harold Firfer, DDS, CEO

★ 20219 ★ First Commonwealth
444 N Wells, Ste. 600
Chicago, IL 60610
Phone: (312)644-1800 **Free:** 800-788-3384
Fax: (312)832-0065
Website: http://www.fcwi.net
David Mulligan, CEO & Pres
Program(s): Dental.

★ 20220 ★ GE Financial - Illinois
200 N Martingale Rd.
Schaumburg, IL 60173-2096
Phone: (847)605-3000 **Fax:** (847)605-3096
Website: http://www.gefn.com
Kathy Marinello, CEO

★ 20221 ★ PPONext
8745 W Higgins Rd., Ste. 300
Chicago, IL 60631
Phone: (773)693-7827 **Free:** 800-269-1817
Fax: (773)693-7907
Website: http://www.pponext.com
Barbara Rodin, CEO & Pres

★ 20222 ★ Preferred Plan, Inc.
10600 W Higgins Rd., Ste. 405
Rosemont, IL 60018
Phone: (847)564-0235 **Fax:** (847)296-8197
Robert Curry, CEO
Program(s): Chiropractic, Home Care, Inpatient SNF, Long-Term Care, Podiatry, Psychiatric, Behavioral Health, Physical Therapy, Transplant, Wellness.

★ 20223 ★ Preferred Podiatry Group
425 Huehl Rd.
Northbrook, IL 60062
Phone: (847)504-5000 **Free:** 800-654-3772
Fax: (847)504-5015
Sanford Mason, MD, CEO

★ 20224 ★ Unicare Inc.
PPO Plan
8420 W Bryn Mawr, Ste. 700
Chicago, IL 60631
Phone: (847)843-2200 **Free:** 800-949-5449
Fax: 888-788-5526
Charles Mitchell, Contact

★ 20225 ★ United Concordia Co., Inc. - Illinois
246 E Janata Blvd
Lombard, IL 60148
Phone: (630)629-2471 **Fax:** (630)693-4688
Website: http://www.ucci.com
Thomas Dzuryachko, CEO
Program(s): Dental.

★ 20226 ★ Vision Health Management
2828 S Indiana Ave.
Chicago, IL 60616
Phone: (312)225-6930 **Fax:** (312)791-0187
Robert Johnson, OD, CEO

Indiana

★ 20227 ★ Group Link
PPO Plan
6612 E 75th St, Ste. 200
Indianapolis, IN 46250
Phone: (317)578-7128 **Free:** 888-462-2062
Fax: (317)578-7306
Website: http://www.grouplinktpa.com
Roger Skinner, CEO

Iowa

★ 20228 ★ Foundation for Medical Care/ Encompass
6000 Westown Pkwy., Ste. 350E
West Des Moines, IA 50266-7771
Phone: (515)223-2900 **Free:** 800-383-2856
Fax: (515)223-2990
Website: http://www.encompass.com
Fred Ferree, CEO
Program(s): Chiropractic, Home Care, Inpatient SNF, Long-Term Care, Pharmaceutical Mail Order, Psychiatric, Transplant, Wellness, Workers' Compensation.

★ 20229 ★ Midland's Choice
3535 Southern Hills Dr.
Sioux City, IA 51106
Phone: (712)293-7800 **Free:** 800-682-4376
Fax: (712)293-7809
Website: http://www.midlandschoice.com
Ralph Morroco, CEO
Program(s): Chiropractic, Home Care, Inpatient SNF, Psychiatric, Podiatry, Physical Therapy, Workers' Compensation.

Kansas

★ 20230 ★ Preferred Chiropractic Care
555 N McLean Blvd.
Wichita, KS 67203
Phone: (316)263-7800 **Fax:** (316)263-7814
Website: http://www.pccnetwork.com
Brad Dopps, President

★ 20231 ★ Preferred Mental Health Management
401 E Douglas, 3rd Fl.
Wichita, KS 67202
Phone: (316)262-0444 **Free:** 800-264-7496
Fax: (316)262-0003
Website: http://www.pmhm.com
Les Ruthven, PhD, CEO

Kentucky

★ 20232 ★ American Pharmacy Services Corp.
102 Enterprise Dr.
Frankfort, KY 40601-6514
Phone: (502)695-8899 **Free:** 800-928-2228
Fax: (502)695-9912

Website: http://www.apscnet.com
Ralph Bouvetto, CEO

★ 20233 ★ United Concordia Co., Inc. - Kentucky
4010 Dupont Cir., Ste. L-03
Louisville, KY 40207
Phone: (717)731-2532 **Free:** 800-568-6432
Fax: (717)972-0410
Website: http://www.ucci.com
Thomas Dzuryachko, CEO
Program(s): Dental.

Louisiana

★ 20234 ★ Family Managed Care
5745 Essen Ln., Ste. 100
Baton Rouge, LA 70810
Phone: (225)215-2100 **Free:** (866)615-2100
Fax: (225)215-2170
Website: http://www.calaishealth.com
John W. Chioco, CEO

Maryland

★ 20235 ★ APS Healthcare Inc. PPO Plan
6705 Rockledge Dr., Ste. 200
Bethesda, MD 20817
Phone: (301)571-0633 **Free:** 800-305-3720
Website: http://www.apscare.com
Ken Kessler, MD, CEO & Chm Bd

★ 20236 ★ Consumer Dental Care Co. PPO Plan
4061 Powder Mill Rd., No. 325
Beltsville, MD 20705
Phone: (301)937-4447 **Free:** 800-879-0288
Fax: (301)937-0245
Website: http://www.consumerdentalcare.com
Dr. Steven Keller, CEO

★ 20237 ★ Magellan Health Services
6950 Columbia Gateway Dr.
Columbia, MD 21046
Phone: (410)953-1000 **Free:** 800-458-2740
Fax: (410)953-5200
Website: http://www.magellanhealth.com
Henry T. Harbin, MD, Chairman of the Board
Program(s): Behavioral Health.

★ 20238 ★ United Concordia Co., Inc. - Maryland
1220 B E Joppa Rd., Ste. 421
Towson, MD 21286-5811
Free: 800-272-8865 **Fax:** (410)296-4367
Website: http://www.ucci.com
Thomas Dzuryachko, CEO
Program(s): Dental.

Massachusetts

★ 20239 ★ HMA Behavioral Health Inc.
PO Box 706
Worcester, MA 01613
Phone: (508)757-2290 **Free:** 800-248-9908
Fax: (508)754-3616
Website: http://www.hmabh.com
Paul F. Bellows, Chairman of the Board

★ 20240 ★ Preferred Dental Network (PDN)
300 Congress St.
Quincy, MA 02169
Phone: (617)471-4100 **Fax:** (617)471-6323
Website: http://www.medicalclaimsservice.com
William McKelvey, CEO

Michigan

★ 20241 ★ American Dental Group
300 E Long Lake Rd., Ste. 311
Bloomfield Hills, MI 48304
Phone: (248)203-1100 **Free:** 888-764-5380
Fax: (248)594-6587
Dr. Walter Kynsz, Jr., Chairman of the Board

★ 20242 ★ Comprehensive Behavioral Care, Inc.
1750 S Telegraph, Ste. 106
Bloomfield Hills, MI 48302
Phone: (248)332-8718 **Free:** 800-688-6885
Fax: (248)332-4522
Website: http://www.comprehensivecare.com
Michelle Brochu, CEO

★ 20243 ★ First Optometry Vision Plans, Inc.
655 W 13 Mile Rd.
Madison Heights, MI 48071
Phone: (248)588-9300 **Fax:** (248)588-3355
Website: http://www.optimeyes.com
Donald Borsand, MD, CEO

★ 20244 ★ Health Care Exchange Limited Co.
32290 5 Mile Rd.
Livonia, MI 48154
Phone: (734)452-2500 **Fax:** (734)452-2501
Website: http://www.dentemax.com
Kenneth R. Dallafior, CEO
Program(s): Dental.

★ 20245 ★ National Footcare Program, Inc.
PO Box 760547
Lathrup Village, MI 48076
Phone: (248)559-2579 **Free:** 800-922-1695
Fax: (248)423-1077
Website: http://www.nationalfootcare.com
William Hoffman, CEO

★ 20246 ★ National Rehabilitation Center
17117 W Nine Mile Rd., Ste. 1050
Southfield, MI 48075
Phone: (248)559-2579 **Free:** 800-922-1695
Fax: (248)423-1077
Website: http://www.nationalfootcare.com
William Hoffman, CEO & Pres
Program(s): Physical therapy.

★ 20247 ★ PTPN
496 West Ann Arbor Tr., Ste. 106
Plymouth, MI 48170
Phone: (734)207-5440 **Free:** 800-349-PTPN
Fax: (734)207-5441
Website: http://www.ptpn.com
Bruce Diven, President

★ 20248 ★ United Concordia Co., Inc. - Michigan
2000 Town Center, Ste. 2200
Southfield, MI 48075
Phone: (717)731-2532 **Free:** 800-944-6432
Fax: (248)304-2708
Website: http://www.ucci.com
Thomas Dzuryachko, CEO
Program(s): Dental.

Minnesota

★ 20249 ★ American Chiropractic Network
5700 Smetana Dr., Ste. 300
Minnetonka, MN 55343-9686
Phone: (952)938-6909 **Free:** 800-873-4575
Fax: (952)938-5187
Website: http://www.theacngroup.com
Thomas Allenburg, DC, CEO & Pres

★ 20250 ★ The Araz Group - Corporate Headquarters
8500 Normandale Lake Blvd.
Bloomington, MN 55437-3800
Phone: (952)896-1200 **Free:** 800-444-3005
Fax: (952)896-4888
Website: http://www.araz.com
Amir Eftekhari, CEO
Program(s): Chiropractic, Pharmaceutical Mail Order, Behavioral Health, Psychiatric, Wellness, Workers' Compensation.

★ 20251 ★ Chirocare of Minnesota
5620 Smetana Dr., Ste. 225
Minnetonka, MN 55343
Phone: (952)938-0212 **Fax:** (952)938-5187
Thomas Allenburg, DC, CEO

★ 20252 ★ CIGNA Behavioral Health, Inc. - Corporate Headquarters
11095 Viking Dr., Ste. 350
Eden Prairie, MN 55344
Phone: (952)296-2000 **Free:** 800-433-5768
Fax: (952)996-2579
Website: http://www.cignabehavioral.com
Keith Dixon, CEO

Missouri

★ 20253 ★ Managed Pharmacy Benefits
1100 N Lindbergh Blvd.
Saint Louis, MO 63132
Phone: (314)993-6000 **Free:** 800-585-5051
Fax: (314)872-5500
Website: http://www.mpbrx.com
Kent B. Friedman, CEO

★ 20254 ★ United Concordia Co., Inc. - Missouri
390 South Woods Mill Rd., Ste. 175
Chesterfield, MO 63017
Phone: (717)731-2532 **Free:** 800-374-6432
Fax: (314)205-9601
Website: http://www.ucci.com
Thomas A. Dzuryacko, CEO
Program(s): Dental.

Montana

★ 20255 ★ Employee Benefit Management Services, Inc.
PO Box 21367
Billings, MT 59104-1367
Phone: (406)245-3575 **Free:** 800-777-3575
Fax: (406)652-5380
Website: http://www.ebmtpa.com
Rick Larson, President
Program(s): Chiropractic, Dental, Home Care, Inpatient SNF, Long-Term Care, Pharmaceutical Mail Order, Podiatry, Psychiatric, Transplant, Vision, Wellness.

Nebraska

★ 20256 ★ Ameritas Group Dental PPO Plan
PO Box 81889
Lincoln, NE 68501-1889
Phone: (402)467-1122 **Free:** 800-776-9446
Fax: (402)465-6190
Website: http://www.yourdentalsolutions.com
Lawrence Arth, CEO

Nevada

★ 20257 ★ Behavioral Healthcare Options, Inc.
PPO Plan
2801 S Valley View, Ste. 6
Las Vegas, NV 89102
Phone: (702)364-1484 **Free:** 800-873-2246
Fax: (702)364-1771
Website: http://www.sierrahealth.com
Michael Adams, CEO

★ 20258 ★ PPNM's Mastercare Network
518 Pyramid Way
Sparks, NV 89431-5057
Phone: (775)359-3732 **Fax:** (775)359-0162
Website: http://www.dentsppo.com
Dr. Joseph Evans, MD, CEO
Program(s): Dental.

New Jersey

★ 20259 ★ Hope Resources Providers (HRP)
PO Box 456
Allenwood, NJ 08720
Free: 800-516-4343 **Fax:** (732)292-0620
Barbara Flories, Chairman of the Board
Program(s): Chiropractic, Dental, Home Care, Inpatient SNF, Long-Term Care, Pharmaceutical Mail Order, Podiatry, Psychiatric, Behavioral Health, Transplant, Vision, Wellness, Workers' Compensation.

★ 20260 ★ Merck-Medco Managed Care, LLC
100 Parsons Pond Dr.
Franklin Lakes, NJ 07417
Phone: (201)269-3400 **Free:** 800-248-2268
Website: http://www.merck-medco.com
Richard Clark, CEO

★ 20261 ★ One Call Medical, Inc.
20 Waterview Blvd.
Parsippany, NJ 07054
Phone: (973)257-1000 **Free:** 800-872-2875
Fax: (973)257-0044
Website: http://www.onecallmedical.com
Elizabeth Griggs, Chairman of the Board
Program(s): Workers' Compensation.

★ 20262 ★ Union Labor Life Insurance Co.
700 E Gate Dr., Ste. 115
Mount Laurel, NJ 08054
Phone: (856)727-9200 **Free:** 800-526-6648
Fax: (856)727-3763
Website: http://www.ullico.com
Robert Georgine, CEO
Program(s): Chiropractic, Dental, Home Care, Inpatient SNF, Long-Term Care, Pharmaceutical Mail Order, Podiatry, Psychiatric, Behavioral Health, Physical Therapy, Transplant, Vision, Wellness, Workers' Compensation, Alternative Medicine.

★ 20263 ★ Unity Dental Health Services
1219 Main Ave.
Clifton, NJ 07011
Phone: (973)473-0900 **Free:** 800-722-0948
Fax: (973)772-3989
Daryl Aiken, CEO & Pres

New Mexico

★ 20264 ★ Fortis Benefits Dental - New Mexico
PPO Plan
1128 Pennsylvania St. NE, Ste. 210
Albuquerque, NM 87110
Phone: (505)266-7709 **Free:** 800-269-5415
Fax: (505)265-3576
Website: http://www.fortisbenefitsdental.com
Debra Rush, CEO

New York

★ 20265 ★ Davis Vision
159 Express St.
Plainview, NY 11803
Phone: (516)932-9500 **Free:** 800-328-4728
Fax: (516)932-9770
Website: http://www.davisvision.com
Walt Froh, CEO & Pres

★ 20266 ★ Dentcare Delivery Systems, Inc.
PPO Plan
60 Charles Lindbergh Blvd.
Uniondale, NY 11553
Phone: (516)542-2200 **Free:** 800-468-0608
Fax: (516)794-3186
Website: http://www.healthplex.com
John Forte, Contact

★ 20267 ★ HealthPlex, Inc.
PPO Plan
60 Charles Lindbergh Blvd.
Uniondale, NY 11553
Phone: (516)542-2200 **Free:** 800-468-0608
Fax: (516)227-1143
Website: http://www.healthplex.com
John Forte, Chairman of the Board
Program(s): Dental.

★ 20268 ★ National Dental Consultants Inc.
PO Box 10
Islip, NY 11751
Free: 800-632-3444 **Fax:** (631)581-2772
Charles Silverstien, CEO

★ 20269 ★ New York State Catholic Health Plan, Inc.
95-25 Queens Blvd.
Rego Park, NY 11374
Phone: (718)896-6500 **Free:** 888-343-3547
Fax: (718)896-1920
Website: http://www.fideliscareny.org
Mark L. Lane, CEO
Program(s): Dental, Home Care, Podiatry, Psychiatric, Behavioral Health, Physical Therapy, Transplant, Vision, Wellness.

★ 20270 ★ NMHCRX
PPO Plan
26 Harbor Pk. Dr.
Port Washington, NY 11050
Phone: (516)605-6638 **Free:** 800-251-3883
Fax: (516)605-6981
Website: http://www.nmhcrx.com
Bert Brodsky, Chairman of the Board

★ 20271 ★ United Concordia Co., Inc. - New York
PPO Plan
159 Express St.
Plainview, NY 11803
Phone: (516)827-6720 **Fax:** (516)827-6618
Website: http://www.ucci.com
Thomas A. Dzuryachko, CEO

North Carolina

★ 20272 ★ Fortis Benefits Dental - North Carolina
3700 National Dr.
Raleigh, NC 27612
Phone: (919)787-0125 **Free:** 800-347-1870
Fax: (919)781-0906
Website: http://www.fortisbenefitsdental.com
Jerry DeFoor, Contact

★ 20273 ★ OptiCare Health Systems
PPO Plan
110 Zebulon Ct.
Rocky Mount, NC 27804
Phone: (252)937-6650 **Free:** 800-334-3937
Fax: (252)451-2182
Website: http://www.opticare-ehn.com
Jason Harrold, CEO

Ohio

★ 20274 ★ Corvel Corp.
5555 Airport Hwy., Ste. 145
Toledo, OH 43615
Phone: (419)868-5230 **Free:** 800-952-3462
Fax: (419)865-6841
Website: http://www.corvel.com
Gail Puppos, CEO

★ 20275 ★ EyeMed Vision Care
8600 Governors Hill Dr.
Cincinnati, OH 45249
Free: 888-439-3633 **Fax:** (513)697-3078
Website: http://www.ecpa.com
Cliff Bartow, CEO

★ 20276 ★ Gateway Health Management Services
19800 Detroit Rd.
Cleveland, OH 44116
Phone: (440)356-8223 **Free:** 800-321-4085
Fax: (440)356-0140
Website: http://www.nabn.com
Donald Baker, CEO
Program(s): Chiropractic, Dental, Home Care, Inpatient SNF, Long-Term Care, Pharmaceutical Mail Order, Podiatry, Psychiatric, Behavioral Health, Physical Therapy, Transplant, Vision, Wellness.

★ 20277 ★ Mental Health Provider Systems
5370 S O. M. Center
Willoughby, OH 44094
Phone: (440)975-1552 **Free:** 800-255-6339
Fax: (440)946-4117
Roger Hess, CEO

★ 20278 ★ Ohio Comp Network, Inc.
4301 Darrow Rd.
Stratford Pl.
Stow, OH 44224
Phone: (330)686-7070 **Fax:** (330)686-7071
Website: http://www.ohiocompnetwork.com
Arthur Chandler, Chairman of the Board

Oklahoma

★ 20279 ★ Heritage National Dental Care of Oklahoma
PO Box 472200
Tulsa, OK 74147-2200
Phone: (918)622-0880 **Free:** 800-274-1323
Fax: (918)664-8896
Bradley Frost, President

Oregon

★ 20280 ★ Complementary Healthcare Plans
5319 SW Westgate Dr., Ste. 130
Portland, OR 97221-2430
Phone: (503)203-8333 **Free:** 800-449-9479
Fax: (503)203-5141

Website: http://www.chpnetworks.com
Richard Tilden, Chairman of the Board
Program(s): Chiropractic, Alternative Medicine.

★ 20281 ★ Managed HealthCare Northwest, Inc. (MHN)
PPO Plan
1120 NW 20th Ave., No. 200
Portland, OR 97209-1539
Phone: (503)413-5800 **Free:** 800-648-6356
Fax: (503)413-5801
Website: http://www.mhninc.com
Dolores Russell, CEO & Pres

★ 20282 ★ Northwest Rehab Alliance
11481 SW Hall Blvd., Ste. 201
Portland, OR 97223
Phone: (503)626-7724 **Fax:** 888-224-9578
Website: http://www.nwrehab.com
Ron Anderson, CEO

Pennsylvania

★ 20283 ★ Alignis Healthcare
100 Mattsonford Rd.
Radnor, PA 19087
Phone: (610)688-3700 **Free:** 800-863-2932
Fax: (610)688-1765
Jack D. Williams, CEO

★ 20284 ★ Alignis Healthcare - Corporate Headquarters
100 Mattsonford Rd., Bldg 5, No. 445
Radnor, PA 19087
Phone: (610)688-3700 **Free:** 800-863-2932
Fax: (610)688-1765
Jack D. Williams, CEO

★ 20285 ★ Behavioral Health PC
1229 Scenery Dr.
Mechanicsburg, PA 17055
Phone: (717)796-6550 **Fax:** (717)796-6551
Raymond Klein, CEO

★ 20286 ★ Community Behavioral Healthcare Cooperative of Pennsylvania
2400 Park Dr.
Harrisburg, PA 17110
Phone: (717)545-9741 **Fax:** (717)545-7733
Richard Edley, PhD, CEO

★ 20287 ★ Concentra
700 River Ave., Ste. 400
Pittsburgh, PA 15212
Phone: (412)323-8500 **Fax:** (412)323-8502
Website: http://www.ghc.org
Joseph McCabe, CEO

★ 20288 ★ DentalComp, Inc.
3501 N Front St.
Harrisburg, PA 17110
Phone: (717)221-1026 **Free:** 888-221-1026
Fax: (717)221-1027
Website: http://www.dentalcomp.com
Jofa Kauffman, CEO

★ 20289 ★ Fidelio Insurance Co.
2826 Mt. Carmel Ave.
Glenside, PA 19038
Phone: (215)885-2443 **Fax:** (215)576-5849
Mario Mele, CEO
Program(s): Dental.

★ 20290 ★ Mental Health Consultants
1878 Sugar Bottom Rd.
Furlong, PA 18925
Phone: (215)345-7838 **Fax:** (215)345-8488
Edward Haaz, CEO

★ 20291 ★ Quantum/Employee Assistance Resource
115 E Washington Ave.
Newtown, PA 18940
Phone: (215)968-0844 **Fax:** (215)968-0298
Stephen Lower, CEO
Program(s): Behavioral Health.

★ 20292 ★ Raytel Imaging Network
430 Park Ave., Ste. 102
Collegeville, PA 19426
Phone: (610)831-1112 **Free:** 800-453-0574
Fax: (610)831-1122
Swapan Sen, CEO
Program(s): Diagnostic Imaging.

★ 20293 ★ Susquehanna Health Care
109 N Mulberry St.
Berwick, PA 18603-4706
Phone: (570)759-1702 **Fax:** (570)759-2559
William Cusatis, CEO & Pres
Program(s): Home Care, Inpatient SNF, Pharmaceutical Mail Order, Podiatry, Psychiatric, Behavioral Health, Physical Therapy, Transplant, Wellness.

★ 20294 ★ United Concordia Co., Inc. - Corporate Headquarters
4401 Deer Path Rd.
Harrisburg, PA 17110
Phone: (717)360-6800 **Free:** 800-972-4191
Fax: (717)612-4996
Website: http://www.ucci.com
Thomas Dzuryachko, CEO
Program(s): Dental.

★ 20295 ★ United Concordia Co., Inc. - Pennsylvania
4401 Deer Path Rd.
Harrisburg, PA 17110
Phone: (717)360-6800 **Free:** 800-972-4191
Fax: (717)612-4996
Website: http://www.ucci.com
Thomas A. Dzuryachko, CEO

★ 20296 ★ United Concordia Co., Inc. - Pennsylvania
175 Pine St.
Williamsport, PA 17701
Phone: (570)321-5124 **Fax:** (570)321-5199
Website: http://www.ucci.com
Thomas A. Dzuryachko, CEO

★ 20297 ★ Valley Preferred
PPO Plan
2166 S 12th St., Ste. 401
Allentown, PA 18103-4799
Phone: (610)402-7485 **Free:** 800-955-6620
Fax: (610)402-7439
John Jaffe, MD, Chairman of the Board

Puerto Rico

★ 20298 ★ Medical Card System
255 Ponce De Leon Ave., Ste. 1600
Hato Rey, PR 00917
Phone: (787)758-2500 **Fax:** (787)250-0380
Website: http://www.mcs.com
Felipe Benedit, CEO
Program(s): Chiropractic, Dental, Pharmaceutical Mail Order, Podiatry, Psychiatric, Behavioral Health, Vision.

Tennessee

★ 20299 ★ MedSolutions
730 Cool Springs Blvd., Ste 800
Franklin, TN 37067
Phone: (615)269-3233 **Free:** 800-467-3424
Fax: (615)468-0600
Website: http://www.medsolutions.com
Curt Thorne, CEO

Texas

★ 20300 ★ Aetna Inc. - Dental Plan of Texas
PPO Plan
2777 Stemmons Fwy.
Dallas, TX 75207
Phone: (214)200-8000 **Free:** 800-825-7935
Fax: (214)200-8916
Website: http://www.aetna.com
John W. Rowe, MD, Chairman of the Board

★ 20301 ★ CAREington International
7400 Gaylord Pkwy
Frisco, TX 75034
Phone: (972)661-0411 **Free:** 800-441-0380
Fax: (972)661-0427
Website: http://www.careington
Barbara Flood, CEO
Program(s): Dental.

★ 20302 ★ Corphealth, Inc.
1300 Summit, Ste. 600
Fort Worth, TX 76102
Phone: (817)332-2519 **Fax:** (817)335-9100
Website: http://www.corphealth.com
Patrick D. Gotcher, CEO

★ 20303 ★ Fortis Benefits Dental - Delaware
PPO Plan
16775 Addison Rd., Ste. 5000
Addison, TX 75001
Phone: (972)458-7474 **Free:** 800-262-5388
Fax: (214)258-1100
Website: http://www.fortisbenefitsdental.com
Peter Barnett, President

★ 20304 ★ Horizon Behavioral Services
1500 Waters Ridge Dr.
Lewisville, TX 75057-6011
Free: 888-802-6084 **Fax:** (972)420-8247
Website: http://www.horizoncare.net
James McAtee, CEO

★ 20305 ★ MenningerCare Systems
4006 Belt Line Rd., No. 205
Addison, TX 75001-5831
Phone: (972)588-2400 **Free:** 800-866-7242
Fax: (972)931-1938
Website: http://www.minningercare.com
John Quick, PhD, CEO
Program(s): Behavioral Health.

★ 20306 ★ Plan 21, Inc.
PO Box 744925
Houston, TX 77274-4925
Free: 800-622-7276 **Fax:** (281)621-6560
Joseph Madonia, PhD, CEO
Program(s): Psychiatric, Behavioral Health.

★ 20307 ★ Script Care, Inc.
87 IH 10 N, Ste. 100
Beaumont, TX 77707
Phone: (409)832-3041 **Free:** 800-880-9988
Fax: (409)832-3109
Jim Brown, CEO

Program(s): Pharmaceutical Mail Order, Pharmacy Benefits Management.

★ 20308 ★ Texas Dental Plan
85 NE Loop 410
San Antonio, TX 78216
Phone: (210)979-3940 **Fax:** (210)979-3982
David Klock, CEO

★ 20309 ★ United Concordia Co., Inc. - Texas
8214 Westchester Dr.
Dallas, TX 75225
Phone: (214)378-6410 **Fax:** (214)378-6306
Website: http://www.ucci.com
Thomas Dzuryachko, CEO
Program(s): Dental.

Utah

★ 20310 ★ Magellan Behavioral Health PPO Plan
10150 S Centennial Pkwy.
Sandy, UT 84070
Phone: (801)256-7000 **Free:** 800-424-4047
Fax: (801)256-7664
Website: http://www.magellanhealth.com
Jay J. Levin, President

Virginia

★ 20311 ★ United Concordia Co., Inc. - Virginia
4860 Cox Rd., Ste. 200
Glen Allen, VA 23060
Free: 800-454-3224 **Fax:** (804)217-8368
Website: http://www.ucci.com
Thomas Dzuryacko, Contact
Program(s): Dental.

★ 20312 ★ ValueOptions - Corporate Headquarters
3110 Fairview Park Dr. S
Falls Church, VA 22042
Phone: (703)205-7000 **Free:** 800-236-4648
Fax: (703)205-6505
Website: http://www.valueoptions.com
Ronald Dozoretz, Chairman of the Board

Washington

★ 20313 ★ Dental Health Services, Inc.
936 N 34th St., Ste. 208
Seattle, WA 98133
Phone: (206)633-2300 **Free:** 800-248-8108
Fax: (206)624-8755
Gary Pernell, Contact

★ 20314 ★ First Choice Health Network
601 Union St., Ste. 1100
Seattle, WA 98101-1838
Phone: (206)292-8255 **Fax:** (206)624-4953
Website: http://www.fchn.com
Gary Gannaway, CEO
Program(s): Dental, Inpatient SNF, Podiatry.

★ 20315 ★ United Concordia Co., Inc. - Washington
2200 Sixth Ave., Ste. 620
Seattle, WA 98121
Free: 888-245-8224 **Fax:** (206)728-2740
Website: http://www.ucci.com
Thomas Dzuryacko, CEO
Program(s): Dental.

★ 20316 ★ Washington Dental Service
9706 Fourth Ave. NE
Seattle, WA 98115
Phone: (206)526-7685 **Free:** 800-342-8355
Fax: (206)525-2330
Website: http://www.deltadentalwa.com
James Dwyer, CEO

Wisconsin

★ 20317 ★ American WholeHealth Networks, Inc.
PO Box 594
Hartland, WI 53029-0594
Phone: (262)367-3200 **Free:** 800-274-7526
Fax: (262)367-5934
Website: http://www.awhnet.com
Bill Luben, CEO
Program(s): Chiropractic, Pharmaceutical Mail Order, Physical Therapy, Wellness, Alternative Medicine.

★ 20318 ★ Innovative Resource Group
2514 S 102nd St., Ste. 100
Milwaukee, WI 53227
Phone: (414)327-5197 **Free:** 800-654-5160
Fax: (414)327-0886
Jim Hartert, MD, President

★ 20319 ★ Racine Dental Group
1320 S Green Bay Rd.
Racine, WI 53406
Phone: (262)637-9371 **Fax:** (262)637-3071
Dr. Newton, CEO

Chapter 13
Federal Government Agencies

Entries listed below are arranged alphabetically by agency names. Consult the "User's Guide" located at the front of this directory for additional information.

★ 20320 ★ Architectural and Transportation Barriers Compliance Board
1331 F St. NW, Ste. 1000
Washington, DC 20004-1111
Phone: (202)272-5434
Website: http://www.access-board.gov
Desc: The Board was established to investigate and examine alternative approaches to the architectural, transportation, and attitudinal barriers confronting disabled persons; determine what measures are being taken by federal, state, and local governments and by other public and private agencies to eliminate those barriers; and promote the use of the International Accessibility Symbol in all public facilities that meet the standards prescribed by the Administrator of the General Services Administration Board. **AKA:** Access Board.

★ 20321 ★ Consumer Product Safety Commission
East-West Towers
4330 East-West Hwy.
Bethesda, MD 20814
Phone: (301)504-0580 **Free:** 800-638-CPSC
Website: http://www.cpsc.gov/
Ann Brown, Chairman of the Board
Desc: The purpose of the Consumer Product Safety Commission is to protect the public against unreasonable risks of injury from consumer products; to assist consumers in evaluating the comparative safety of consumer products; to develop uniform safety standards for consumer products and minimize conflicting state and local regulations; and to promote research and investigation into the causes and prevention of product-related deaths, illnesses, and injuries.

★ 20322 ★ Environmental Protection Agency (EPA)
1200 Pennsylvania Ave., NW
Washington, DC 20460-0001
Free: 888-372-8255
Website: http://www.epa.gov/
Christine Todd Whitman, Dir of Admin
Desc: The EPA functions to protect human health and to safeguard the natural environment in cooperation with state and local governments. Its mission is to control and abate pollution in the areas of air, water, solid waste, pesticides, radiation, and toxic substances.

★ 20323 ★ Executive Office of the President
Office of Policy Development
Domestic Policy Council
Director of National AIDS Policy
Eisenhower Executive Office Bldg., Rm. 216
Washington, DC 20502
Phone: (202)456-2216
Sandra Thurman, Director

★ 20324 ★ Federal Mine Safety and Health Review Commission
1730 K St. NW, Ste. 6000
Washington, DC 20006-3867
Phone: (202)653-5625 **Fax:** (202)653-5030
Email: info@fmshrc.gov
Website: http://www.fmshrc.gov
Mary Lu Jordan, Chairman of the Board
Desc: The Commission ensures compliance with occupational safety and health standards in the Nation's surface and underground coal, metal, and nonmetal mines.

★ 20325 ★ Federal Trade Commission (FTC)
600 Pennsylvania Ave. NW
Washington, DC 20580
Phone: (202)326-2222 **Fax:** (202)326-3676
Website: http://www.ftc.gov/
Timothy J. Muris, Chairman of the Board
Desc: The objective of the FTC is to maintain competitive enterprise as the keystone of the American economic system, and to prevent the free enterprise system from being fettered by monopoly or restraints on trade or corrupted by unfair or deceptive trade practices. The Commission is charged with keeping competition both free and fair.

★ 20326 ★ Interagency Committee on Employment of People With Disabilities
Equal Employment Opportunity Commission
Federal Sector Programs
1801 L St., NW, Rm. 5238
Washington, DC 20507
Phone: (202)663-4560 **Fax:** (202)376-6219
Desc: Seeks to identify and eliminate barriers standing in the way of full social and vocational opportunities for physically handicapped, mentally retarded, and mentally restored persons; promotes employment opportunities for the physically and mentally handicapped. **Alt. Contact:** (202)663-4593 (TDD).

★ 20327 ★ National Council on Disability
1331 F St. NW, Ste. 1050
Washington, DC 20004
Phone: (202)272-2004
Website: http://www.ncd.gov
Desc: The Council reviews all laws, programs, and policies of the federal government that affect individuals with disabilities. The Council then makes recommendations to the President, Congress, and federal agencies on these issues. In addition, the Council is studying the availability of health insurance coverage for persons with disabilities and sponsors conferences for families caring for the disabled. **Alt. Contact:** (202)272-2074 (TDD).

★ 20328 ★ Nuclear Regulatory Commission (NRC)
11555 Rockville Pike
Washington, DC 20555
Phone: (301)415-7000
Website: http://www.nrc.gov/
Richard A. Meserve, Chairman of the Board
Desc: The Nuclear Regulatory Commission licenses and regulates the civilian uses of nuclear energy to protect public health and safety and the environment.

★ 20329 ★ Occupational Safety and Health Review Commission
1120 20th St. NW
Washington, DC 20036-3419
Phone: (202)606-5100 **Fax:** (202)606-5050
Website: http://www.oshrc.gov/
Thomasina V. Rogers, Chairman of the Board
Desc: The Commission works to ensure the timely and fair resolution of cases involving the alleged exposure of American workers to unsafe or unhealthy working conditions.

★ 20330 ★ Railroad Retirement Board
844 N Rush St.
Chicago, IL 60611-2092
Phone: (312)751-4776
Website: http://www.rrb.gov/
Cherryl T. Thomas, Chairman of the Board
Desc: The Railroad Retirement Board administers comprehensive retirement-survivor and unemployment-sickness benefit programs for the nation's railroad workers and their families.

★ 20331 ★ Smithsonian Institution
National Museum of American History
Department of the History of Science and Technology
Science, Medicine, and Society Division
14th St. & Constitution Ave. NW
Washington, DC 20560
Phone: (202)357-2700
Desc: Division is concerned with the history of public health and pharmacy, 17th-20th century history of medical and dental technology, and 20th century health sciences.

★ 20332 ★ Tennessee Valley Authority
Health Services
20 E 11th St., EB 8A
Chattanooga, TN 37402-2801
Phone: (423)751-2091
Website: http://www.tva.gov

★ 20333 ★ U.S. Department of Agriculture
Agricultural Research Service (ARS)
5601 Sunnyside Ave., Rm. 1-2250
Beltsville, MD 20705-5128
Phone: (301)504-1638 **Fax:** (301)504-1648
Website: http://www.usda.gov
Desc: The Agricultural Research Service conducts research to develop and transfer solutions to agricultural problems of high national priority. It provides information access and dissemination to ensue high-

quality, safe food and other agricultural products; assess the nutritional needs of Americans; sustain a competitive agricultural economy; enhance the natural resource base and the environment; and provide economic opportunities for rural citizens, communities, and society as a whole.

★ 20334 ★ U.S. Department of Agriculture
Agricultural Research Service (ARS)
National Agricultural Library (NAL)
5601 Sunnyside Ave., Rm. 1-2250
Beltsville, MD 20705-5128
Phone: (301)504-1638 **Fax:** (301)504-1648
Website: http://www.usda.gov

Desc: The National Agricultural Library provides information services over a broad range of agricultural interests to a wide cross-section of users, from research scientists to the general public. The Library assists users through a variety of specialized information centers.

★ 20335 ★ U.S. Department of Agriculture
Animal and Plant Health Inspection Service
Veterinary Services
Legislative and Public Affairs
Washington, DC 20250
Phone: (202)720-2511
Website: http://www.usda.gov

Desc: Animal health officials are responsible for programs to protect and improve the health, quality, and marketability of U.S. animals and animal products. The programs are carried out through cooperative links with States, foreign governments, livestock producers, and other Federal agencies. Service officials exclude, control, and eradicate animal pests and diseases by carrying out eradication and control programs for certain diseases, providing diagnostic services, and gathering and disseminating information regarding animal health in the United States through land, air and ocean ports. They also certify as to the health status of animals and animal products being exported to other countries and respond to animal disease incursions or epidemics which threaten the health status of U.S. livestock and poultry. The service also administers a Federal law intended that all veterinary biological products, whether developed by conventional or new biotechnological procedures, used in the diagnosis, prevention and treatment of animal diseases are safe, pure, potent and effective. The Service regulates firms that manufacture veterinary biological products subject to the act, including licensing the manufacturing establishment and its products, inspecting production facilities and production methods, and testing products under a surveillance program.

★ 20336 ★ U.S. Department of Agriculture
Center for Nutrition Policy and Promotion
1120 20th St. NW, Ste. 200
Washington, DC 20036-3406
Phone: (202)418-2312 **Fax:** (202)208-2321
Website: http://www.cnpp.usda.gov

Desc: The Center for Nutrition Policy and Promotion coordinates nutrition policy in the USDA and provides overall leadership in nutrition education for the American public. It also coordinates with the Department of Health and Human Services in the review, revision, and dissemination of the *Dietary Guidelines for Americans,* the federal government's statement of nutrition policy formed by a consensus of scientific and medical professionals.

★ 20337 ★ U.S. Department of Agriculture
Food and Nutrition Service
3101 Park Center Dr.
Alexandria, VA 22302
Phone: (703)305-2286 **Fax:** (703)305-2420
Website: http://www.usda.gov/fns.htm

Desc: The Food and Nutrition Service, operated in cooperation with states and local governments, administers programs to make food assistance available to people in need. In particular, the service administers Special Nutrition Programs designed to improve the nutrition of children, particularly those from low income families.

★ 20338 ★ U.S. Department of Agriculture
Food Safety and Inspection Service
14th St. & Independence Ave. SW
Washington, DC 20250
Phone: (202)720-7943 **Fax:** (202)720-1843
Website: http://www.usda.gov/agency/fsis/homepage.htm

Desc: The service is responsible for ensuring that meat and poultry products moving in interstate and foreign commerce for human consumption are safe, wholesome, and accurately labeled.

★ 20339 ★ U.S. Department of Commerce
National Institute of Standards and Technology
Office of the Director of Administration
Occupational Health and Safety Division
Washington, DC 20230
Phone: (301)975-6478 **Fax:** (301)926-1630
Email: inquiries@nist.gov
Website: http://www.nist.gov/

★ 20340 ★ U.S. Department of Defense
Department of the Air Force
Air Staff
Surgeon General of the Air Force
1670 Air Force Pentagon
Washington, DC 20330-1670
Phone: (703)697-6061
Website: www.af.mil
Paul K. Carlton, Jr., Surgeon General of the Air Force

Desc: The Surgeon General is part of the Air Staff, independent of the basic staff structure, providing advisory and support services to both the Chief of Staff and the Air Staff. Operating components are: (1) Assistant Surgeon General for Dental Services, (2) Biomedical Sciences Corps, (3) Congressional and Public Affairs, (4) Health Care Studies and Evaluations, (5) Medical Programs and Resources, (6) Medical Support, and (7) Nursing Services.

★ 20341 ★ U.S. Department of Defense
Department of the Army
Army Medical Command (MEDCOM)
Washington, DC 20310
Phone: (703)681-3000
Website: http://www.armymedicine.army.mil/
Lt.Gen. James B. Peake, Director

Desc: The U.S. Army Medical Command provides direction and planning for the Army Medical Department in conjunction with the Office of the Surgeon General. It develops and integrates doctrine, training, leader development, organization, and material for Army health services. MEDCOM also allocates resources and evaluates delivery of services.

★ 20342 ★ U.S. Department of Defense
Department of the Army
Army Staff
Office of the Army Surgeon General
c/o Department of the Army
The Pentagon
Washington, DC 20310
Phone: (703)695-2442
Website: http://www.army.mil/
Lt.Gen. James B. Peake, Surgeon General of the Army

Desc: The office of the Surgeon General manages health services for the Army and, as directed, for other services, agencies, and organizations. Other responsibilities include health standards for Army personnel; health professional education and training; career management for missioned and warrant officer personnel of the Army Medical Department; medical research, material development and test and evaluation; policies concerning health aspects of Army environmental programs and prevention of diseases; and planning, programming, and budgeting for Army-wide health services. Major components of the Office of the Surgeon General include: (1) Dental Services/Dental Corps; (2) Veterinary Services/Veterinary Corps; (3) Army Medical Specialist Corps; (4) Army Nurse Corps; and (5) the Health Facility Planning Agency.

★ 20343 ★ U.S. Department of Defense
Department of the Navy
Bureau of Medicine and Surgery
c/o Department of the Navy
23rd and E Sts. NW
Washington, DC 20372-5120
Phone: (202)762-3701 **Fax:** (202)762-3211
Website: http://www.navy.mil
R.A. Nelson, Chief, Bureau of Medicine and Surgery

Desc: The Bureau directs the provision of medical and dental services for Navy and Marine Corps personnel and their dependants; administers the execution and implementation of contingency support plans and programs to provide effective medical and dental readiness capability; provides professional and technical medical and dental services to the fleet, fleet marine force, and shore activities of the Navy; and ensures cooperation with civil authorities in matters pertaining to public health disasters and other emergencies.

★ 20344 ★ U.S. Department of Defense
Department of the Navy
United States Marine Corps
Office of Health Services
2 Navy Annex
Washington, DC 20380-1775
Phone: (703)614-1034
Website: http://www.usmc.mil/

★ 20345 ★ U.S. Department of Defense
Office of Assistant Secretary of Defense for Health Affairs
The Pentagon
Washington, DC 20301-1155
Phone: (703)545-6700 **Fax:** (703)614-3537
Website: http://www.defenselink.mil/

Desc: Office is responsible for Department of Defense health matters, including preventive medicine; medical readiness; health care delivery; drug and alcohol abuse prevention; and procurement, development, and retention of medical personnel.

★ 20346 ★ U.S. Department of Defense
Office of Assistant Secretary of Defense for Health Affairs
TRICARE Management Activity (TMA)
c/o The Pentagon
Skyline 5, Ste. 810
5111 Leesburg Pike
Falls Church, VA 22041-3206
Phone: (703)681-1730 **Fax:** (703)681-3665
Website: http://www.tricare.osd.mil

Desc: TRICARE was formed from the consolidation of the TRICARE Support Office, the Defense Medical Programs Activity, and the integration of health management program functions formerly located in the Office of the Assistant Secretary of Defense for Health Affairs. The TMA mission is to manage TRICARE; administer and manage the Defense Health Program appropriation; provide operational direction and support to the Uniformed Services in the management and administration of the TRICARE program; and administer CHAMPUS. medical/dental services provided to active duty service members by civilian medical personnel.

★ 20347 ★ U.S. Department of Defense Uniformed Services University of the Health Sciences (USUHS)
4301 Jones Bridge Rd.
Bethesda, MD 20814-4799
Phone: (301)295-3030 **Fax:** (301)295-1960
Website: http://www.usuhs.mil
James A. Zimble, MD, President
Desc: The Uniformed Services University of the Health Sciences was established to educate career-oriented medical officers for the Military Departments and the Public Health Service. The University currently incorporates the F. Edward Hebert School of Medicine and the Graduate School of Nursing.

★ 20348 ★ U.S. Department of Education Office of Special Education and Rehabilitative Services (OSERS)
400 Maryland Ave. SW
Washington, DC 20202
Free: 800-USA-LEARN
Website: http://www.ed.gov/
Desc: The Office of Special Education and Rehabilitative Services provides leadership to ensure that people with disabilities have services, resources, and equal opportunities to learn, work, and live as fully-integrated, contributing members of society. OSERS supports programs that serve millions of disabled children, youth, and adults and that impact on the lives of the nation's 49 million citizens with disabilities. It coordinates the activities of the Office of Special Education Programs, which works to help states provide quality educational opportunities and early-intervention services to help students with disabilities achieve their goals. OSERS' Rehabilitation Services Administration, among other efforts, supports state vocational rehabilitation programs that give disabled people the education, job training, and job placement services they need to gain meaningful employment. OSERS' National Institute on Disability and Rehabilitation Research supports research and technological programs that are crafting blueprints for a barrier-free, inclusive society.

★ 20349 ★ U.S. Department of Energy Office of the Environment, Safety, and Health
1000 Independence Ave. SW
Washington, DC 20585
Phone: (202)586-5000 **Fax:** (202)586-0956
Website: http://www.doe.gov/
Steven C. Cary, Acting Assistant Secretary
Desc: Provides independent oversight of departmental execution of environmental, occupational safety and health, and nuclear/nonnuclear safety and security laws, regulations, and policies; ensures that departmental programs are in compliance with environmental, health, and nuclear/nonnuclear safety protection plans, regulations, and procedures; exercises independent review and approval of environmental impact statements prepared within the Department; and carries out the legal functions of the nuclear safety civil penalty and criminal referral activities.

★ 20350 ★ U.S. Department of Health and Human Services
200 Independence Ave. SW
Washington, DC 20201
Phone: (202)619-0257
Website: http://www.dhhs.gov/
Tommy G. Thompson, Secretary
Desc: The Department of Health and Human Services is the cabinet-level department of the federal executive branch most concerned with people and most involved with the nation's human concerns. The Secretary of HHS advises the President on health, welfare, and income security plans, policies, and programs of the federal government. Principal operating components of the Department include the Administration for Children and Families, the Health Care Financing Administration, the Administration on Aging, the Centers for Disease Control and Prevention, the Food and Drug Administration, and the National Institutes of Health.

★ 20351 ★ U.S. Department of Health and Human Services Administration on Aging (AOA)
330 Independence Ave. SW
Washington, DC 20201
Phone: (202)401-4541 **Fax:** (202)619-3759
Website: http://www.aoa.dhhs.gov/
Desc: The Administration on Aging is the principal agency designated to carry out the provisions of the Older Americans Act of 1965. It is responsible for all issues involving the elderly. The Administration develops policies, plans, and programs designed to promote the welfare of the elderly; promotes their needs by planning programs and developing policy; provides policy, procedural direction, and technical assistance to States and Native American tribal governments.

★ 20352 ★ U.S. Department of Health and Human Services Administration for Children and Families (ACF)
370 L'Enfant Promenade SW
Washington, DC 20447
Phone: (202)401-9200
Website: http://www.acf.dhhs.gov
Desc: The Administration for Children and Families provides national leadership and direction to plan, manage, and coordinate comprehensive support services for vulnerable children and families, Native Americans, people with disabilities, refugees and legalized aliens. The mission of ACF is to promote stability, economic security, responsibility and self-sufficiency. There are seven major program offices: Administration for Children, Youth and Families (ACYF), Administration on Developmental Disabilities, Administration for Native Americans, Office of Family Assistance, Office of Child Support Enforcement, Office of Community Service, and Office of Refugee Resettlement.

★ 20353 ★ U.S. Department of Health and Human Services Administration for Children and Families (ACF) Administration on Children, Youth and Families (ACYF)
370 L'Enfant Promenade SW
Washington, DC 20447
Phone: (202)205-8347
Website: http://www.acf.dhhs.gov/programs/acyf/acyf.htm
Desc: The Administration for Children, Youth, and Families manages State grant and child care programs including programs to increase child abuse prevention and treatment activities and to develop family preservation and family support services; the Head Start program; programs which provide services for runaway and homeless youth and their families; child welfare training programs; and child abuse and neglect research and demonstration programs.

★ 20354 ★ U.S. Department of Health and Human Services Administration for Children and Families (ACF) Administration on Developmental Disabilities (ADD)
370 L'Enfant Promenade SW
Washington, DC 20447
Phone: (202)690-6590
Website: http://www.acf.hhs.gov/programs/add/
Desc: The Administration on Developmental Disabilities (ADD) supports and encourages provision of quality services to persons with developmental disabilities; assists States in increasing the independence, productivity, and community inclusion of all persons with developmental disabilities, through the design and implementation of a comprehensive and continuing State plan; administers the State developmental disabilities councils, the Protection and Advocacy Grant Program, and the discretionary grant programs.

★ 20355 ★ U.S. Department of Health and Human Services Administration for Children and Families (ACF) Administration for Native Americans (ANA)
370 L'Enfant Promenade SW
Washington, DC 20447
Phone: (202)690-7776
Website: http://www.acf.hhs.gov/programs/ana/
Desc: The Administration for Native Americans represents and promotes the goal of developmental, social, economic, and lasting self-sufficiency of American Indians, Alaskan Natives; and Pacific Natives.

★ 20356 ★ U.S. Department of Health and Human Services Agency for Healthcare Research and Quality
2101 E Jefferson St.
Rockville, MD 20852
Phone: (301)594-6662
Email: info@ahrq.gov
Website: http://www.ahrq.gov/
John M. Eisenberg, Director
Desc: The Agency for Healthcare Research and Quality supports research aimed at reducing health-care costs, medical errors, and patient safety concerns, as well as improving the quality and availability of care.

★ 20357 ★ U.S. Department of Health and Human Services Agency for Toxic Substances and Disease Registry
1600 Clifton Rd. NE
Atlanta, GA 30333
Phone: (404)639-0700
Website: http://www.atsdr.cdc.gov
Jeffrey Koplan, Administrator
Desc: The Agency's mission is to prevent exposure and adverse health effects and diminished quality of life associated with exposure to hazardous substances from waste sites, unplanned releases, and other sources of pollution present in the environment.

★ 20358 ★ U.S. Department of Health and Human Services Centers for Disease Control and Prevention (CDCP)
1600 Clifton Rd. NE
Atlanta, GA 30333
Phone: (404)639-3311
Website: http://www.cdc.gov/
Dr. Julie L. Gerberding, Director
Desc: The Centers for Disease Control is charged with protecting the public health of the Nation by providing leadership and direction in the prevention and control of diseases and other preventable conditions and responding to public health emergencies.

★ 20359 ★ U.S. Department of Health and Human Services Centers for Disease Control and Prevention Epidemiology Program Office
1600 Clifton Rd. NE
Atlanta, GA 30333
Phone: (404)639-3311
Website: http://www.cdc.gov/

★ 20360 ★ U.S. Department of Health and Human Services
Centers for Disease Control and Prevention
National Center on Birth Defects and Developmental Disabilities
1600 Clifton Rd. NE
Atlanta, GA 30333
Phone: (404)639-3311
Website: http://www.cdc.gov/ncbddd/

★ 20361 ★ U.S. Department of Health and Human Services
Centers for Disease Control and Prevention
National Center for Chronic Disease Prevention and Health Promotion
1600 Clifton Rd. NE
Atlanta, GA 30333
Phone: (404)639-3311
Website: http://www.cdc.gov/nccdphp/index.htm

★ 20362 ★ U.S. Department of Health and Human Services
Centers for Disease Control and Prevention
National Center for Environmental Health
1600 Clifton Rd. NE
Atlanta, GA 30333
Phone: (404)639-3311 **Fax:** (404)488-7015
Website: http://www.cdc.gov/nceh/default.htm
Richard J. Jackson, MD, Director
Desc: The Center administers national programs that promote a healthy environment and prevent premature death and avoidable illness and disability caused by non-infectious, non-occupational, environmental and related factors.

★ 20363 ★ U.S. Department of Health and Human Services
Centers for Disease Control and Prevention (CDCP)
National Center for Health Statistics (NCHS)
1600 Clifton Rd. NE
Atlanta, GA 30333
Phone: (404)639-3311
Website: http://www.cdc.gov/nchs/
Desc: The NCHS mission is to collect, analyze, and disseminate national health statistics; conduct research in survey and statistical methodology; provide specialized training programs and technical assistance; and coordinate cooperative programs with state, national, and international organizations. NCHS maintains data systems that produce data in the following areas: extent of illness and disability in the population; distribution and normative standards for physiological and nutritional measurements; national vital statistics, including births, deaths, marriages, and divorces; hospital, nursing home, and ambulatory care utilization; health expenditures; family formation, growth, and dissolution; and other major health topics.

★ 20364 ★ U.S. Department of Health and Human Services
Centers for Disease Control and Prevention
National Center for HIV, STD, and TB Prevention
1600 Clifton Rd. NE
Atlanta, GA 30333
Phone: (404)639-3311
Website: http://www.cdc.gov/nchstp/od/nchstp.html

★ 20365 ★ U.S. Department of Health and Human Services
Centers for Disease Control and Prevention
National Center for Infectious Diseases
1600 Clifton Rd. NE
Atlanta, GA 30333
Phone: (404)639-3311 **Fax:** (404)639-3039
Website: http://www.cdc.gov/ncidod/
Desc: The Center for Infectious Diseases coordinates a national program to improve the identification, investigation, diagnosis, prevention, and control of infectious diseases. It maintains programs dealing with AIDS, hospital infections, sexually transmitted diseases, bacterial diseases, host factors, mycotic diseases, parasitic diseases, viral diseases, and vector-borne viral diseases.

★ 20366 ★ U.S. Department of Health and Human Services
Centers for Disease Control and Prevention
National Center for Injury Prevention and Control
1600 Clifton Rd. NE
Atlanta, GA 30333
Phone: (404)639-3311
Website: http://www.cdc.gov/ncipc/ncipchm.htm

★ 20367 ★ U.S. Department of Health and Human Services
Centers for Disease Control and Prevention
National Immunization Program Office
1600 Clifton Rd. NE
Atlanta, GA 30333
Phone: (404)639-3311
Website: http://www.cdc.gov/nip/

★ 20368 ★ U.S. Department of Health and Human Services
Centers for Disease Control and Prevention (CDCP)
National Institute for Occupational Safety and Health (NIOSH)
1600 Clifton Rd. NE
Atlanta, GA 30333
Phone: (404)639-3311
Website: http://www.cdc.gov/niosh/homepage.html
Desc: NIOSH is the primary federal agency engaged in research to eliminate on-the-job hazards to health and safety. Institute is responsible for identifying occupational safety and health hazards, for determining methods to control them, and for recommending federal standards to limit the hazards. Institute is also responsible for administering the X-ray surveillance program for coal miners, and testing and certifying respirators and hazard measuring devices.

★ 20369 ★ U.S. Department of Health and Human Services
Centers for Disease Control and Prevention
Public Health Practice Program Office
1600 Clifton Rd. NE
Atlanta, GA 30333
Phone: (404)639-3311
Website: http://www.phppo.cdc.gov/

★ 20370 ★ U.S. Department of Health and Human Services
Food and Drug Administration (FDA)
5600 Fishers Ln.
Rockville, MD 20857
Phone: (301)443-1544
Website: http://www.fda.gov/
Desc: The mission of the Food and Drug Administration is to ensure that food is safe, pure, and wholesome; human and animal drugs, biological products, and medical devices are safe and effective; and electronic products that emit radiation ar safe. The Administration's major operating components are: (1) the Center for Biologics Evaluation and Research, (2) the Center for Devices and Radiological Health, (3) the Center for Drug Evaluation and Research, (4) the Center for Food Safety and Applied Nutrition, (5) the Center for Veterinary Medicine, and (6) the National Center for Toxicological Research.

★ 20371 ★ U.S. Department of Health and Human Services
Food and Drug Administration
Center for Biologics Evaluation and Research
1401 Rockville Pike, Ste. 200N
Rockville, MD 20852-1448
Phone: (301)827-1800 **Free:** 800-835-4709
Website: http://www.fda.gov/cber
Kathryn C. Zoon, PhD, Director
Desc: The Center regulates biological products, plans and conducts research on both new and old biological products, inspects manufacturers' facilities for compliance with standards, tests products submitted for release, establishes written and physical standards, and approves licensing of manufacturers to produce biological products. The Center plans and conducts research on the preparation, preservation, and safety of blood and blood products, the methods of testing safety, purity, potency, and efficacy of such products for therapeutic use, and the immunological problems concerned with products, testing, and use of diagnostic reagents employed in grouping and typing blood.

★ 20372 ★ U.S. Department of Health and Human Services
Food and Drug Administration
Center for Devices and Radiological Health
1350 Piccard Dr., HFZ-210
Rockville, MD 20850
Phone: (301)827-3990 **Free:** 888-463-6332
Website: http://www.fda.gov/cdrh
David W. Feigal, MD, Director
Desc: The Center develops and carries out a national program designed to control unnecessary exposure of humans to potentially hazardous ionizing and non-ionizing radiation and ensure its safe use. It develops policy and priorities regarding FDA programs relating to the safety, effectiveness, and labeling of medical devises for human use; conducts and electronic product radiation control program; develops regulations, standards, and criteria and recommends changes in FDA legislative authority necessary to protect the public health; and provides scientific and technical support to other components within the FDA and other agencies on matters relating to radiological health and medical devices.

★ 20373 ★ U.S. Department of Health and Human Services
Food and Drug Administration
Center for Drug Evaluation and Research
5600 Fishers Ln.
Rockville, MD 20857
Phone: (301)827-4573
Website: http://www.fda.gov/cder
Janet Woodcock, MD, Director
Desc: Center develops FDA policy with regard to the safety, effectiveness, and labeling of all drugs for human use; reviews and evaluates new drug applications and investigates new drug applications; develops and implements standards for the safety and effectiveness of all over-the-counter drugs; and monitors the quality of marketed drugs through product testing, surveillance, and compliance programs.

★ 20374 ★ U.S. Department of Health and Human Services
Food and Drug Administration
Center for Food Safety and Applied Nutrition
5100 Paint Branch Parkway
College Park, MD 20740-3835
Free: 888-463-6332
Website: http://www.cfsan.fda.gov/
Joseph A. Levitt, Director

Desc: The Center conducts research and develops standards on the composition, quality, nutrition, and safety of foods, food additives, colors, and cosmetics; conducts research designed to improve the detection, prevention, and control of contamination that may be responsible for illness or injury conveyed by foods, colors, and cosmetics; coordinates and evaluates FDA's surveillance and compliance programs relating to foods, color, and cosmetics.

★ 20375 ★ U.S. Department of Health and Human Services
Food and Drug Administration
Center for Veterinary Medicine
7519 Standish Pl.
Rockville, MD 20855
Phone: (301)827-3800
Website: http://www.fda.gov/cvm/default.html
Stephen F. Sundlof, DVM, Director

Desc: The Center develops and conducts programs with respect to the safety and efficacy of veterinary preparations and devices; evaluates proposed use of veterinary preparations for animal safety and efficacy; and evaluates FDA's surveillance and compliance programs relating to veterinary drugs and other veterinary medical matters.

★ 20376 ★ U.S. Department of Health and Human Services
Food and Drug Administration
National Center for Toxicological Research
3900 NC.T.R. Rd.
Jefferson, AR 72079-9502
Phone: (870)543-7130
Website: http://www.fda.gov/nctr
Bernard A. Schwetz, Director

Desc: The Center conducts peer-reviewed scientific research which supports and anticipates FDA current and future regulatory needs. This involves fundamental and applied research specifically designed to define mechanisms of action underlying the toxicity of products regulated by the FDA. The research is aimed at understanding critical biological events in the expression of toxicity and at development methods to improve assessment of human exposure, susceptibility and risk.

★ 20377 ★ U.S. Department of Health and Human Services
Health Care Financing Administration (HCFA)
200 Independence Ave. SW
Washington, DC 20201
Phone: (202)690-6726 **Fax:** (202)690-6262
Website: http://www.hcfa.gov/
Thomas Scully, Dir of Admin

Desc: The Health Care Financing Administration oversees the Medicare program, a federal health insurance program for persons over 65 years of age and certain disabled persons; the Medicaid program, which supplies grants to states to provide medical services to the needy; and related federal medical care quality control staffs.

★ 20378 ★ U.S. Department of Health and Human Services
Health Resources and Services Administration (HRSA)
5600 Fishers Ln.
Rockville, MD 20857
Phone: (301)443-2086
Website: http://www.hrsa.gov

Desc: HRSA is the principle primary health care service agency of the federal government. Its mission is to make essential primary care services accessible to the poor, uninsured, and geographically isolated–populations severely underserved by the private health care system.

★ 20379 ★ U.S. Department of Health and Human Services
Health Resources and Services Administration (HRSA)
Bureau of Health Professions (BHPR)
Parklawn Bldg.
5600 Fishers Ln.
Rockville, MD 20857
Phone: (301)443-1590
Website: http://bhpr.hrsa.gov/
Kerry P. Nesseler, Assoc. Administrator

Desc: The Bureau provides national leadership in coordinating, evaluating, and supporting the development and utilization of the nation's health personnel. To accomplish this goal, the Bureau provides financial aid to health professions students and support for health professions data analysis and research. It provides leadership for promoting equity in access to health services and health careers for the disadvantaged, and provides technical assistance activities for international projects relevant to domestic health personnel problems.

★ 20380 ★ U.S. Department of Health and Human Services
Health Resources and Services Administration (HRSA)
Bureau of Primary Health Care (BPHC)
4350 East West Highway
Bethesda, MD 20814
Phone: (301)594-4100 **Fax:** (301)594-5008
Website: http://bphc.hrsa.gov/
Sam Shekar, MD, Assoc. Administrator

Desc: The Bureau provides national leadership for efforts to increase access to comprehensive preventative and primary health care for underserved and vulnerable populations; provides grants to community, migrant, and school-based health centers, health care for the homeless programs, and public housing primary care programs; and administers the Federal occupational health program of the PHS drug pricing program.

★ 20381 ★ U.S. Department of Health and Human Services
Health Resources and Services Administration
HIV/AIDS Bureau
5600 Fishers Lane
Rockville, MD 20857
Phone: (301)443-3376
Website: http://hab.hrsa.gov/

Desc: The Bureau administers the Ryan White Comprehensive AIDS Resources Emergency (CARE) Act and conducts a wide range of programs which provide primary care and support services to low-income, uninsured, and underinsured individuals and families affected by HIV/AIDS. It also provides HIV emergency relief grants to eligible metropolitan areas, and HIV care grants to States and U.S Territories; funds the AIDS Drug Assistance Program for all States and eligible territories; and supports projects examining economic changes and managed care effects of the Nation's network of HIV/AIDS care delivery.

★ 20382 ★ U.S. Department of Health and Human Services
Health Resources and Services Administration
Maternal and Child Health Bureau
5600 Fishers Ln.
Rockville, MD 20857
Phone: (301)443-2170
Website: http://mchb.hrsa.gov/
Peter C. Van Dyck, MD, Assoc. Administrator

Desc: The Bureau provides national leadership in supporting, identifying, and interpreting national trends and issues relating to the health needs of mothers, infants, children and adolescents, including those with special health care needs.

★ 20383 ★ U.S. Department of Health and Human Services
Indian Health Service (IHS)
5600 Fishers Ln.
Rockville, MD 20857
Phone: (301)443-1083
Website: http://www.ihs.gov/
Michael H. Trujillo, MD, Director

Desc: The Indian Health Service assures a comprehensive health services delivery system for American Indians and Alaska Natives, with sufficient options to provide for maximum tribal involvement in meeting their health needs. The goal of the Service is to raise the health level of the Indian and Alaska Native people to the highest possible level.

★ 20384 ★ U.S. Department of Health and Human Services
National Institutes of Health (NIH)
9000 Rockville Pike
Bethesda, MD 20892
Phone: (301)496-4000
Website: http://www.nih.gov/
Ruth L. Kirschstein, Acting Director

Desc: The National Institutes of Health supports biomedical and behavioral research domestically and abroad, conducts research in its own laboratories and clinics, trains promising young researchers, and promotes acquisition and distribution of medical knowledge. Research activities conducted or supported by NIH will determine the scope and direction of medical treatment and disease prevention in the future. The NIH is comprised of: National Institute on Aging; National Institute of Alcohol Abuse and Alcoholism; National Institute of Allergy and Infectious Diseases; National Institute of Arthritis and Musculoskeletal and Skin Diseases; National Institute of Cancer; National Institute of Child Health and Human Development; Clinical Center; National Institute on Deafness and Other Communication Disorders; National Institute of Dental and Craniofacial Research; National Institute of Diabetes, Digestive and Kidney Diseases; National Institute on Drug Abuse; National Institute of Environmental Health Sciences; Fogarty International Center; National Institute of General Medical Sciences; National Heart, Lung, and Blood Institute; National Human Genome Research Institute; National Library of Medicine; National Institute of Mental Health; National Institute of Neurological Disorders and Stroke; National Institute of Nursing Research; National Eye Institute; National Center for Research Resources; and the Center for Scientific Review.

★ 20385 ★ U.S. Department of Health and Human Services
National Institutes of Health (NIH)
Center for Scientific Review (CSR)
9000 Rockville Pike
Bethesda, MD 20892
Phone: (301)435-1111
Website: http://www.csr.nih.gov

Desc: The Center receives and assigns applications for peer reviews to scientific review groups whose members hold advanced degrees and are established investigators in the extramural community. After review, applications are referred to funding components for potential award. The Center develops and implements innovative, flexible ways to conduct referral and review for all aspects of science.

★ 20386 ★ U.S. Department of Health and Human Services
National Institutes of Health
Clinical Center
9000 Rockville Pike
Bethesda, MD 20892
Phone: (301)496-3227
Website: http://www.cc.nih.gov/
John I. Gallin, Director
Desc: The Center is designed to bring scientists working in the Center's laboratories into proximity with clinicians caring for patients, so that they may collaborate on problems of mutual concern.

★ 20387 ★ U.S. Department of Health and Human Services
National Institutes of Health (NIH)
Fogarty International Center (FIC)
9000 Rockville Pike
Bethesda, MD 20892
Phone: (301)496-2075 **Fax:** (301)594-1211
Website: http://www.nih.gov/fic/
Gerald T. Keusch, Director
Desc: The center is dedicated to advancing health of the people of the United States and other nations through international scientific cooperation. In pursuit of its mission, the Center fosters biomedical research partnership between U.S. scientists and foreign counterparts through grants, fellowships, and international agreements, and provides leadership in international science policy and research strategies.

★ 20388 ★ U.S. Department of Health and Human Services
National Institutes of Health (NIH)
National Center for Complimentary and Alternative Medicine (NCCAM)
9000 Rockville Pike
Bethesda, MD 20892
Phone: (301)435-5042
Website: http://www.nccam.nih.gov
Desc: The Center works to prevent and alleviate human suffering by stimulating, developing, conducting, and supporting research on complimentary and alternative medicine. Research training programs develop skilled investigators necessary to conduct rigorous and relevant research to determine which complimentary and alternative medicine practices work, which do not, and why.

★ 20389 ★ U.S. Department of Health and Human Services
National Institutes of Health (NIH)
National Center for Research Resources (NCRR)
9000 Rockville Pike
Bethesda, MD 20892
Phone: (301)435-0888
Website: http://www.ncrr.nih.gov/
Judith L. Vaitukaitis, MD, Director
Desc: The NCRR supports the development of technologies to enable sophisticated research; creates and supports a broad range of sophisticated multi-disciplinary research facilities for basic, clinical, and animal research; and supports development for minority-serving institutions which award doctoral degrees in health-related sciences. Programs include supporting biorepositories with companion web-based databases for a wide range of organisms.

★ 20390 ★ U.S. Department of Health and Human Services
National Institutes of Health (NIH)
National Eye Institute (NEI)
9000 Rockville Pike
Bethesda, MD 20892
Phone: (301)496-2234 **Fax:** (301)496-9970
Website: http://www.nei.nih.gov/
Paul A. Sieving, Director
Desc: The Institute conducts, fosters, and supports research on the causes, natural history, prevention, diagnosis and treatment of disorders of the eye and visual system; directs the National Eye Health Education Program; provides research grants and individual and institutional research training awards; works in cooperation and collaboration with voluntary organizations and other institutions engaged in research and training in the special health problems of the blind; and collects and disseminates information on research and findings.

★ 20391 ★ U.S. Department of Health and Human Services
National Institutes of Health (NIH)
National Heart, Lung, and Blood Institute (NHLBI)
9000 Rockville Pike
Bethesda, MD 20892
Phone: (301)496-2411 **Fax:** (301)402-0818
Website: http://www.nhlbi.nih.gov
Claude J.M. Lenfant, MD, Director
Desc: NHLBI provides leadership for a national program in diseases of the heart, blood vessels, blood, lungs; sleep disorders; and blood resources. It conducts, fosters, and supports an integrated and coordinated program of basic research, clinical investigations and trials, and observational studies.

★ 20392 ★ U.S. Department of Health and Human Services
National Institutes of Health
National Human Genome Research Institute
9000 Rockville Rd.
Bethesda, MD 20892
Phone: (301)496-0844
Website: http://www.nhgri.nih.gov/
Francis S. Collins, MD, Director
Desc: The Center formulates research goals and long-range plans to accomplish the mission of the human genome project, including the study of ethical, legal, and social implications of human genome research. It supports and administers research and research training programs in human genome research including chromosome mapping, DNA sequencing, database development, and technology development for genome research; provides coordination of genome research and with industry and academia; and conducts research on human genetic disease.

★ 20393 ★ U.S. Department of Health and Human Services
National Institutes of Health (NIH)
National Institute on Aging (NIA)
9000 Rockville Pike
Bethesda, MD 20892
Phone: (301)496-1752
Website: http://www.nih.gov/nia/
Richard J. Hodes, MD, Director
Desc: The Institute conducts and supports biomedical and behavioral research to increase the knowledge of the aging process and associated physical, psychological, and social factors resulting from advanced age. Alzheimer's Disease, health and retirement, menopause, and fraility are among the areas of special concern.

★ 20394 ★ U.S. Department of Health and Human Services
National Institutes of Health (NIH)
National Institute on Alcohol Abuse and Alcoholism (NIAAA)
9000 Rockville Pike
Bethesda, MD 20892
Phone: (301)443-3885
Website: http://www.niaaa.nih.gov/
Enoch Gordis, MD, Director
Desc: The Institute conducts and supports biomedical and behavioral research, in order to provide science-based approaches to the prevention and treatment of alcohol abuse and alcoholism. It provides a national focus for the Federal effort to increase knowledge and disseminate research findings to the scientific community, health care system ,and the public.

★ 20395 ★ U.S. Department of Health and Human Services
National Institutes of Health (NIH)
National Institute of Allergy and Infectious Diseases (NIAID)
9000 Rockville Pike
Bethesda, MD 20892
Phone: (301)496-5717 **Fax:** (301)496-4409
Website: http://www.niaid.nih.gov/
Anthony S. Fauci, MD, Director
Desc: NIAID conducts and supports research, research training, and clinical evaluations on the causes, treatment and prevention of a wide variety of infectious, allergic, and immunologic diseases. Areas of special emphasis include AIDS; asthma and allergic diseases; immunologic diseases; transplantation; emerging and reemerging infectious diseases; sexually transmitted diseases; enteric diseases such as hepatitis; food-borne diseases; influenza and other respiratory infections; malaria and other parasitic diseases; and tuberculosis.

★ 20396 ★ U.S. Department of Health and Human Services
National Institutes of Health (NIH)
National Institute of Arthritis and Musculoskeletal and Skin Diseases (NIAMS)
9000 Rockville Pike
Bethesda, MD 20892
Phone: (301)496-4353
Website: http://www.nih.gov/niams/
Steven I. Katz, MD, Director
Desc: The Institute supports research into the causes, treatment, and prevention of arthritis and musculoskeletal and skin diseases; the training of basic and clinical scientists to carry out this research; and the dissemination of information on research progress in these diseases.

★ 20397 ★ U.S. Department of Health and Human Services
National Institutes of Health (NIH)
National Institute of Cancer (NIC)
9000 Rockville Pike
Bethesda, MD 20892
Phone: (301)435-3848 **Free:** 800-422-6237
Website: http://www.cancer.gov
Richard Klausner, MD, Director
Desc: NIC has developed a national cancer program to expand existing scientific knowledge on cancer cause and prevention, as well as on the diagnosis, treatment, and rehabilitation of cancer patients. Research activities cover a broad spectrum encompassing basic biological, clinical, prevention, and behavioral research.

★ 20398 ★ U.S. Department of Health and Human Services
National Institutes of Health (NIH)
National Institute of Child Health and Human Development (NICHD)
9000 Rockville Pike
Bethesda, MD 20892
Phone: (301)496-5133 **Fax:** (301)402-1104
Website: http://www.nichd.nih.gov/
Duane F. Alexander, MD, Director
Desc: The Institute conducts and supports biomedical and behavioral research on child health and maternal health; sudden infant death syndrome (SIDS); pediatric, maternal, and adolescent AIDS; the reproductive process; problems of human development; mental retardation and developmental disabilities; family structure; and the dynamics of human population.

★ 20399 ★ U.S. Department of Health and Human Services
National Institutes of Health (NIH)
National Institute on Deafness and Other Communication Disorders (NIDCD)
9000 Rockville Pike
Bethesda, MD 20892
Phone: (301)496-7243
Website: http://www.nidcd.nih.gov
James F. Battey, Jr., Director
Desc: NIDCD conducts and supports biomedical and behavioral research and research training on normal mechanisms as well as diseases and disorders of hearing, balance, smell, taste, voice, speech, and language through a deiversity of research performed in its own laboratories; a program of research grants, individual and institutional research training awards, career development awards, center grants, and contracts to public and private research institutions and organizations.

★ 20400 ★ U.S. Department of Health and Human Services
National Institutes of Health (NIH)
National Institute of Dental and Craniofacial Research (NIDR)
9000 Rockville Pike
Bethesda, MD 20892
Phone: (301)496-4261
Website: http://www.nidr.nih.gov/
Lawrence A. Tabak, Director
Desc: The Institute supports and conducts clinical and laboratory research into the causes, prevention, diagnosis, and treatment of oral diseases and conditions.

★ 20401 ★ U.S. Department of Health and Human Services
National Institutes of Health (NIH)
National Institute of Diabetes, Digestive and Kidney Diseases (NIDDK)
9000 Rockville Pike
Bethesda, MD 20892
Phone: (301)496-3583
Website: http://www.niddk.nih.gov/
Allen M. Spiegel, Director
Desc: The Institute conducts, fosters, and supports basic and clinical research into the causes, prevention, diagnosis, and treatment of diabetes, endocrine and metabolic diseases, digestive diseases and nutrition, kidney and urologic diseases, and blood diseases. It provides research grants and individual and institutional research training awards, and conducts and supports epidemiological and clinical studies on selected populations in the United States.

★ 20402 ★ U.S. Department of Health and Human Services
National Institutes of Health (NIH)
National Institute on Drug Abuse (NIDA)
9000 Rockville Pike
Bethesda, MD 20892
Phone: (301)443-1124
Website: http://www.nida.nih.gov/
Kenneth Olden, Director
Desc: The Institute's mission is to lead the Nation in bringing the power of science to bear on drug abuse and addiction, through the strategic support and conduct of research across a broad range of disciplines, and the rapid and effective dissemination and use of the results of that research to significantly improve drug abuse and addiction prevention, treatment, and policy.

★ 20403 ★ U.S. Department of Health and Human Services
National Institutes of Health (NIH)
National Institute of Environmental Health Sciences (NIEHS)
PO Box 12233
Research Triangle Park, NC 27709
Phone: (919)541-3211
Website: http://www.niehs.nih.gov/
Desc: NIEHS seeks to reduce the burden of human illness and dysfunction by understanding the elements of environmental exposures, human susceptibility, and time and how these elements interrelate. The mission is achieved through multidisciplinary biomedical research programs, prevention and intervention efforts, and communication strategies that encompass training, education, technology transfer, and community outreach.

★ 20404 ★ U.S. Department of Health and Human Services
National Institutes of Health (NIH)
National Institute of General Medical Sciences (NIGMS)
9000 Rockville Pike
Bethesda, MD 20892
Phone: (301)496-7301 **Fax:** (301)402-0156
Website: http://www.nih.gov/nigms/
Marvin Cassman, Director
Desc: NIGMS supports research and research training in basic biomedical sciences. Institute activities range from cell biology to genetics to pharmacology and systemic response to trauma and anesthesia.

★ 20405 ★ U.S. Department of Health and Human Services
National Institutes of Health (NIH)
National Institute of Mental Health (HIMH)
9000 Rockville Pike
Bethesda, MD 20892
Phone: (301)443-3673 **Fax:** (301)443-0008
Website: http://www.nimh.nih.gov/
Steven E. Hyman, MD, Director
Desc: The Institute supports and conducts fundamental research in neuroscience, genetics, molecular biology, and behavior as the foundation of an extensive clinical research portfolio which seeks to expand and refine treatments available for illnesses such as schizophrenia; depressive disorders; severe anxiety; childhood mental disorders; and other mental disorders. It supports research on treatment outcomes in actual practice settings, including primary care settings and seeks to establish a sound scientific basis for the prevention of mental illness.

★ 20406 ★ U.S. Department of Health and Human Services
National Institutes of Health (NIH)
National Institute of Nursing Research (NINR)
9000 Rockville Pike
Bethesda, MD 20892
Phone: (301)496-0207
Website: http://www.nih.gov.ninr/
Patricia A. Grady, Director
Desc: The Institute provides leadership for nursing research, supports and conducts research and training, and disseminates information to build a scientific base for nursing practice and patient care and to promote health and ameliorate the effects of illness on the American people.

★ 20407 ★ U.S. Department of Health and Human Services
National Institutes of Health (NIH)
National Library of Medicine (NLM)
9000 Rockville Pike
Bethesda, MD 20892
Phone: (301)496-6308
Website: http://www.nlm.nih.gov/
Donald A.B. Lindberg, MD, Director
Desc: The National Library of Medicine is the Nation's primary medical information source and is authorized to provide medical library services and online bibliographic search capabilities to public and private agencies, organizations, institutions, and individuals. It sponsors and conducts research and development in biomedical communications, in such areas as telemedicine, expert systems, and advanced medical imaging projects.

★ 20408 ★ U.S. Department of Health and Human Services
Office of Public Health and Science (OPHS)
5600 Fishers Ln.
Rockville, MD 20857
Phone: (301)443-3921
Desc: The Office ensures that the Department conducts broad-based public health assessments designed to anticipate future public health issues and problems and devises and implements appropriate interventions and evaluations to maintain, sustain, and improve the health of the Nation; provides assistance in managing the implementation and coordination of Secretarial decisions for PHS operating divisions and coordination of population-based health, clinical prevention services, and science initiatives that cut across operating divisions; provides presentations to foreign governments and multilateral agencies on international health issues; and provides direction and policy oversight, through the Surgeon General, for the Public Health Service Commissioned Corps.

★ 20409 ★ U.S. Department of Health and Human Services
Office of Public Health and Science
Office of the Assistant Secretary for Health and Surgeon General
200 Independence Ave. SW
Washington, DC 20201
Phone: (202)619-0257
Website: http://www.dhhs.gov
Eve E. Slater, MD, Assistant Secretary for Health
Desc: The Office consists of general and special staff offices that support the Assistant Secretary for Health in planning and directing the activities of the Public Health Service. Components include the Office of the Surgeon General, the Office of Disease Prevention and Health Promotion, the Office of Health Communications, the Office of Health Operations, the Office of Health Planning and Evaluation, the Office of Intergovernmental Affairs, and the Office of Population Affairs. Also under the administration of the Assistant Secretary for Health are the President's Council on Physical Fitness and Sports and a major operating center, the Agency for Health Care Policy and Research.

★ 20410 ★ U.S. Department of Health and Human Services
Substance Abuse and Mental Health Services Administration (SAMHSA)
5600 Fishers Ln.
Rockville, MD 20857
Phone: (301)443-4797
Website: http://www.samhsa.gov/
Joseph H. Autry, Acting Administrator
Desc: The mission of SAMHSA is to ensure that knowledge, based on science and state-of-the-art

practice is effectively used for the prevention and treatment of addictive and mental disorders. Major components include: Center for Substance Abuse Prevention , Center for Substance Abuse Treatment, and the Center for Mental Health Services.

★ 20411 ★ U.S. Department of Health and Human Services
Substance Abuse and Mental Health Services Administration
Center for Mental Health Services
5600 Fishers Lane
Rockville, MD 20857
Phone: (301)443-0001
Website: http://www.samhsa.gov/centers/cmhs/cmhs.html
Gail P. Hutchings, Director

Desc: The Center provides national leadership to promote the improved state of mental health and the rehabilitation of people with mental disorders and others affected. The Center administers grants, contracts, and cooperative agreements which support the development and application of new knowledge in the health care field; supports activities to improve management of mental health care; collects data on the various forms of mental illness; cooperates with other Federal components to coordinate disaster assistance, community response, and other mental health emergency services as a consequence of national disasters; and collaborates with the alcohol, drug abuse, and mental health institutes on services research issues.

★ 20412 ★ U.S. Department of Health and Human Services
Substance Abuse and Mental Health Services Administration
Center for Substance Abuse Prevention
5600 Fishers Lane
Rockville, MD 20857
Phone: (301)443-0365
Website: http://www.samhsa.gov/centers/csap/csap.html
Ruth Sanchez-Way, PhD, Director

Desc: The Center provides a national focus for the federal effort to prevent alcohol and other drug abuse. To this end, it develops and reviews policy; administers grants; helps disseminate research findings; and supports training for substance abuse practitioners.

★ 20413 ★ U.S. Department of Health and Human Services
Substance Abuse and Mental Health Services Administration
Center for Substance Abuse Treatment
5600 Fishers Lane
Rockville, MD 20857
Phone: (301)443-8956
Website: http://www.samhsa.gov/centers/csat2002/csat_frame.html
H. Westley Clarke, MD, Director

Desc: The principal function of the Center is to provide national leadership for the federal effort to enhance approaches and provide resources to ensure provision of services and programs focusing on the treatment of substance abuse and the co-occurring physical and/or psychiatric conditions.

★ 20414 ★ U.S. Department of Justice
Bureau of Prisons
Health Services Division
320 1st St. NW
Washington, DC 20534
Phone: (202)307-3198 **Free:** 888-317-8455
Website: http://www.bop.gov
Kathleen M. Hawk Sawyer, Director

Desc: The Health Services Division has oversight responsibility for all medical and psychiatric programs; environmental and occupational health services; food and nutrition services; and farm operations.

★ 20415 ★ U.S. Department of Labor
Bureau of Labor Statistics
Office of Compensation and Working Conditions
Office of Safety, Health, and Working Conditions
2 Massachusetts Ave. NW
Washington, DC 20212
Phone: (202)691-5200

Desc: Office compiles occupational safety and health statistics; and makes grants to states and other local agencies to assist in the development and administration of programs dealing with occupational safety and health statistics. Office maintains the nationwide employer record keeping system on job-related injuries and illnesses, conducts the annual survey based on these records, analyzes the results, and compiles supplementary statistics from other sources. Office also implements the Supplementary Data System (SDS), by which states provide additional information on occupational accidents and exposures from workers' compensation records in order to give a more accurate definition of occupational safety and health problems, associated characteristics, and possible action indicators. In addition, Office examines selected types of work injuries in order to develop a detailed profile of characteristics associated with data from questionnaires completed by injured workers.

★ 20416 ★ U.S. Department of Labor
Mine Safety and Health Administration (MSHA)
4015 Wilson Blvd., Ste. 601
Arlington, VA 22203
Phone: (703)235-1452 **Fax:** (703)235-1563

Desc: The Mine Safety and Health Administration develops and promulgates mandatory safety and health standards; ensures compliance with such standards; assesses civil penalties for violations; investigates accidents; cooperates with and provides assistance to the states in the development of effective state mine safety and health programs; improves and expands training programs in cooperation with the states and the mining industry; and in coordination with the Department of Health and Human Services and the Department of the Interior, contributes to the improvement and expansion of mine safety and health research and development. All of these activities are aimed at preventing and reducing mine accidents and occupational diseases in the mining industry.

★ 20417 ★ U.S. Department of Labor
Occupational Safety and Health Administration (OSHA)
200 Constitution Ave. NW
Washington, DC 20210
Phone: (202)693-1999

Desc: The Occupational Safety and Health Administration sets and enforces workplace safety and health standards and assists employers in complying with these standards. The Administration has a four-fold focus: firm and fair enforcement of safety and health rules; partnership with States running their own OSHA-approved programs and with employers and employees interested in developing effective workplace safety and health programs; efficient promulgation of new rules that are clear and easy to understand and follow; and increased outreach and training to help employers and employees eliminate safety and health standards.

★ 20418 ★ U.S. Department of State
Office of Medical Services
2201 C St. NW
Washington, DC 20520
Phone: (202)663-1748
Website: http://www.state.gov/

Desc: The Office develops, manages, and staffs a worldwide primary health care system for U.S. citizen employees and their eligible dependents residing abroad. The Office approves and monitors the medical evacuation of patients, conducts pre-employment and in-service physical examinations, and provides clinical referral and advisory services. The Office also provides for emergency medical response in the event of a crisis at an overseas post.

★ 20419 ★ U.S. Department of Transportation
Federal Aviation Administration (FAA)
Associate Administrator for Regulation and Certification
Office of Aerospace Medicine
800 Independence Ave. SW
Washington, DC 20591
Phone: (202)366-4000
Website: http://www.cami.jccbi.gov/
Thomas A. Hart, Asst. Admin. for Reg. and Cert.

Desc: The Office is responsible for the medical certification of all airmen. It maintains the Civil Aeromedical Institute at the FAA Aeronautical Center in Oklahoma City.

★ 20420 ★ U.S. Department of Veterans Affairs
Veterans Benefits Administration
Vocational Rehabilitation Service
810 Vermont Ave. NW
Washington, DC 20420
Phone: (202)273-4800
Website: http://www.va.gov/
Joseph Thompson, Under Secretary for Benefits

Desc: The Vocational Rehabilitation Service is responsible for outreach, motivation, evaluation, counseling, training, employment, and other rehabilitation services to disabled veterans; evaluation, counseling, and miscellaneous services to veterans and service persons and other VA education programs; evaluation, counseling, education and miscellaneous services to sons, daughters and spouses of totally and permanently disabled veterans and to surviving orphans, widows, or widowers of certain deceased veterans, including rehabilitation services to to certain handicapped dependents,; affirmative action activities; and vocational training and rehabilitation to children with spina bifida who are children of Vietnam veterans.

★ 20421 ★ U.S. Department of Veterans Affairs
Veterans Health Administration
810 Vermont Ave. NW
Washington, DC 20420
Phone: (202)273-4800
Website: http://www.va.gov/

Desc: The Veterans Health Administration (formerly Health Services and Research Administration) provides hospital, nursing home and domiciliary care, and outpatient medical and dental care to eligible veterans of military service in the Armed Forces. It operates medical centers, domiciliaries, clinics, and nursing home units in the U.S., the Commonwealth of Puerto Rico, and the Republic of the Philippines, and provides for similar care under VA auspices in non-VA hospitals and community nursing homes, and for visits by veterans to non-VA physicians and dentists for outpatient treatment. Under the Civilian Health and Medical Program, dependents of certain veterans are provided with medical care supplied by non-VA institutions and physicians. The Administration conducts both individual medical and health-care delivery research projects and multi-hospital research programs. It assists in the education of physicians and dentists, and with training of many other health care professionals through affiliations with educational institutions and organizations.

★ 20422 ★ U.S. Library of Congress
National Library Service for the Blind and Physically Handicapped
1291 Taylor St. NW
Washington, DC 20542-4960
Phone: (202)707-5100

Desc: Talking and braille books and magazines are distributed through 142 regional and subregional libraries to blind and physically handicapped residents of the U.S. and its territories.

★ 20423 ★ U.S. Social Security Administration (SSA)

6401 Security Blvd.
Baltimore, MD 21235
Phone: (410)965-1234 **Fax:** (410)966-1463
Website: http://www.ssa.gov/
William A. Halter, Contact

Desc: The Social Security Administration manages the Nation's social insurance program, consisting of retirement, survivors, and disability insurance programs. It also administer the Supplemental Security Income program for the aged, blind and disabled. The Administration is responsible for studying the problems of poverty and economic insecurity among Americans and making recommendations on effective methods of solving these problems through social insurance. The Administration also assigns Social Security numbers to U.S citizens and maintains earnings records for workers under their Social Security numbers.

Chapter 14
Federal Domestic Assistance Programs

Entries in this chapter are arranged alphabetically by agency and program names. For additional information, consult the "User's Guide" located at the front of this directory.

★ 20424 ★ Office of Personnel Management
Employment Service
Diversity Office
Federal Employment for Individuals with Disabilities
1900 E St. NW, Rm. 2445
Washington, DC 20415
Phone: (202)606-1059
Website: http://www.opm.gov
Armando E. Rodriguez, Director

Cat. No: 27.005 **Objectives:** To encourage federal agencies to provide assistance to persons with disabilities, including disabled veterans, in obtaining and retaining federal employment. **Assist. Types:** Federal employment. **Applicant Eligibility:** Persons who qualify under the definitions of being "disabled" under title 29, Rehabilitation Act of 1973, as amended. **Beneficiary Eligibility:** Persons with physical, cognitive, or mental disabilities.

★ 20425 ★ Office of Technical and Information Services
Architectural and Transportation Barriers Compliance Board
1331 F St. NW, Ste. 1000
Washington, DC 20004-1111
Phone: (202)272-5434 **Free:** 800-872-2253
Fax: (202)272-5447
Email: info@access-board.gov
Website: http://www.access-board.gov

Cat. No: 88.001 **Objectives:** To enforce federal laws requiring accessibility for persons with disabilities in certain federally funded buildings and facilities throughout the Nation; set guidelines and requirements for accessibility standards prescribed by federal agencies under the Americans with Disabilities Act, Telecommunications Act, and the Architectural Barriers Act; provide technical assistance to organizations and agencies, and individuals requesting help in explaining the guidelines and requirements and in solving accessible design and construction problems; conduct research to determine appropriate specifications for accessibility. **Assist. Types:** Dissemination of technical information. **Applicant Eligibility:** Requests for information may be made by the general public as well as all agencies of Federal, State, and local government. **Beneficiary Eligibility:** General public, all levels of government and private organizations.

★ 20426 ★ U.S. Department of Agriculture
Agricultural Research Service
National Agricultural Library
Beltsville, MD 20705-2351
Phone: (301)504-6780
Website: http://www.nal.usda.gov

Cat. No: 10.700 **Objectives:** To serve as the nation's chief agricultural information resource by providing agricultural information products and services through traditional library functions and through modern electronic dissemination to agencies of the USDA, public organizations, and individuals. **Assist. Types:** Dissemination of technical information. **Applicant Eligibility:** Individuals, state and local governments, educational organizations, research societies, business and industry, including those located in the U.S. territories. **Beneficiary Eligibility:** Same as Applicant Eligibility.

★ 20427 ★ U.S. Department of Agriculture
Cooperative State Research, Education, and Extension Service
Animal Health and Disease Research
Washington, DC 20250
Phone: (202)401-4329 **Fax:** (202)401-4888
Email: wwagner@reeusda.gov
Website: http://www.reeusda.gov

Cat. No: 10.207 **Objectives:** To support animal health and disease research at eligible schools and colleges of veterinary medicine and state agricultural experiment stations whose purpose is to improve the health and productivity of food animals and horses through effective prevention, control, or treatment of disease; reduce losses from transportation and other hazards; and protect human health through control of animal diseases transmissible to people. **Assist. Types:** formula grants. **Applicant Eligibility:** Eligibility is restricted to the following public nonprofit institutions demonstrating capacity in animal and disease research: (1)Schools and Colleges of Veterinary Medicine; (2) State Agricultural Experiment Stations. **Beneficiary Eligibility:** Same as Applicant Eligibility.

★ 20428 ★ U.S. Department of Agriculture
Food and Nutrition Service
Child Nutrition Division
Child and Adult Care Food Program
3101 Park Center Dr., Rm. 1017
Alexandria, VA 22302
Phone: (703)305-2590 **Fax:** (703)305-2879
Website: http://www.fns.usda.gov/cnd
Stanley C. Garnett, Director

Cat. No: 10.558 **Objectives:** To assist states, through grants-in-aid and other means, to initiate and maintain nonprofit food service programs for children and elderly or impaired adults in non-residential day care facilities. **Assist. Types:** Formula grants. **Applicant Eligibility:** The state or U.S. Territory agency applies for and signs an annual agreement to receive federal funds for disbursement. Where the state does not administer the program, institutions may receive funds directly from USDA. **Beneficiary Eligibility:** Public and nonprofit private organizations.

★ 20429 ★ U.S. Department of Agriculture
Food and Nutrition Service
Child Nutrition Division
National School Lunch Program
3101 Park Center Dr., Rm. 1017
Alexandria, VA 22302
Phone: (703)305-2590
Website: http://www.fns.usda.gov/cnd
Stanley C. Garnett, Director

Cat. No: 10.555 **Objectives:** To assist states, through cash grants and food donations, in making the school lunch program available to school students and to encourage the domestic consumption of nutritious agricultural commodities. **Assist. Types:** Formula grants. **Applicant Eligibility:** State and U.S. territory agencies; public and nonprofit private schools of high school grade and under; public and nonprofit private residential child care institutions, except Job Corps Centers; residential summer camps that participate in the Summer Food Service Program for children; and private foster homes. Schools and residential child care institutions desiring to participate must agree to operate a nonprofit food service that is available to all children regardless of race, sex, color, national origin, age, or disability. **Beneficiary Eligibility:** All students enrolled in schools where the lunch program is operating may participate.

★ 20430 ★ U.S. Department of Agriculture
Food and Nutrition Service
Child Nutrition Division
School Breakfast Program
3101 Park Center Dr., Rm. 1017
Alexandria, VA 22302
Phone: (703)305-2590
Website: http://www.fns.usda.gov/cnd
Stanley C. Garnett, Director

Cat. No: 10.553 **Objectives:** To assist states in providing nutritious breakfasts for school students, through cash grants and food donations. **Assist. Types:** Formula grants. **Applicant Eligibility:** State and U.S. Territory agencies; public and nonprofit private schools of high school grade and under; public and nonprofit private residential child care institutions, except Job Corps Centers; residential summer camps that participate in the Summer Food Service Program for children; and private foster homes. Schools desiring to participate must agree to operate a nonprofit breakfast program that is available to all children regardless of race, sex, color, national origin, age, or disability. **Beneficiary Eligibility:** All students attending schools where the breakfast program is operating may participate.

★ 20431 ★ U.S. Department of Agriculture
Food and Nutrition Service
Child Nutrition Division
Special Milk Program for Children
3101 Park Center Dr., Rm. 1017
Alexandria, VA 22302
Phone: (703)305-2590
Website: http://www.fns.usda.gov/cnd
Stanley C. Garnett, Director

Cat. No: 10.556 **Objectives:** To provide subsidies to schools and institutions to encourage the consumption of fluid milk by children. **Assist. Types:** Formula grants. **Applicant Eligibility:** Any state or U.S. territory, public and nonprofit private school, or child care institution of high school grade or under, except Job Corps Centers, may participate in the Special Milk Program upon request if it does not participate in a meal service program authorized under the National School Lunch Act or the Child Nutrition Act of 1966. **Beneficiary Eligibility:** All students attending schools and institutions in which the Special Milk Program is in operation may participate in the program.

★ 20432 ★ U.S. Department of Agriculture
Food and Nutrition Service
Child Nutrition Division
State Administrative Expenses for Child Nutrition
3101 Park Center Dr., Rm. 1008
Alexandria, VA 22302
Phone: (703)305-2590
Website: http://www.fns.usda.gov/cnd
Stanley C. Garnett, Director

Cat. No: 10.560 **Objectives:** To provide each state agency with funds for its administrative expenses in supervising and giving technical assistance to local schools, school districts, and institutions in their conduct of child nutrition programs. State agencies that administer the distribution of USDA donated commodities to schools or child or adult care institutions are also provided with state administrative expense funds. **Assist. Types:** Formula grants. **Applicant Eligibility:** State agencies responsible for the conduct of child nutrition programs, and agencies responsible for the distribution of USDA donated commodities to schools or child or adult care institutions, including agencies in the U.S. territories. **Beneficiary Eligibility:** Same as Applicant Eligibility.

★ 20433 ★ U.S. Department of Agriculture
Food and Nutrition Service
Food Distribution Division
Commodity Supplemental Food Program
3101 Park Center Dr., Rm. 517
Alexandria, VA 22302
Phone: (703)305-2680 **Fax:** (703)305-2420
Website: http://www.fns.usda.gov/fncs
Les Johnson, Director

Cat. No: 10.565 **Objectives:** To improve the health and nutritional status of low income pregnant, postpartum, and breastfeeding women; infants and children up to age of 6; and elderly persons through the donation of supplemental foods. **Assist. Types:** Sale, exchange, or donation of property and goods; formula grants. **Applicant Eligibility:** Agreements are made between the Department and the state agency, or an Indian tribe, band, or group recognized by the Department of the Interior for the administration of the program, and between the Department, the state agency, and distributing agency for the distribution of commodities to eligible persons. **Beneficiary Eligibility:** To be eligible for program benefits, each applicant must be: (a) Categorically eligible as an infant; child up to age 6; pregnant, postpartum or breastfeeding woman; or elderly person 60 years of age or older, residing in an area where the program operates; (b) income eligible under existing federal, state, or local food, health, or welfare programs for low-income persons; elderly must have an annual income at or below 130 percent of federal poverty income guidelines; and (c), at state agency discretion, at nutritional risk as determined by a competent health professional at the local agency.

★ 20434 ★ U.S. Department of Agriculture
Food and Nutrition Service
Food Stamp Program
Nutrition Assistance for Puerto Rico
3101 Park Center Dr., Rm. 710
Alexandria, VA 22302
Phone: (703)305-2026
Website: http://www.fns.usda.gov
Bonny O'Neil, Acting Deputy Administrator

Cat. No: 10.566 **Objectives:** A cash grant alternative to the Food Stamp program to improve diets of needy persons residing in the Commonwealth of Puerto Rico. **Assist. Types:** Direct payments for specified use. **Applicant Eligibility:** The Commonwealth of Puerto Rico alone is eligible. **Beneficiary Eligibility:** Low income individuals and families are eligible for benefits.

★ 20435 ★ U.S. Department of Agriculture
Food and Nutrition Service
Supplemental Food Programs Division
Nutrition Program for Women, Infants, and Children
3101 Park Center Dr., Rm. 517
Alexandria, VA 22302
Phone: (703)305-2746 **Fax:** (703)305-2196
Website: http://www.fns.usda.gov
Patricia Daniels, Director

Cat. No: 10.557 **Objectives:** To provide, at no cost, supplemental nutritious foods, nutrition education, and referrals to health care to low income pregnant, breastfeeding, and postpartum women; infants; and children to age five determined to be at nutritional risk. **Assist. Types:** Formula grants. **Applicant Eligibility:** A local agency is eligible to apply to locally deliver the serivces of the WIC program provided: (1) it serves a population of low-income women, infants, and children at nutritional risk; (2) it is a public or private nonprofit health or human service agency. All local agencies must apply through the responsible state or U.S. territory agency. **Beneficiary Eligibility:** Pregnant, postpartum, or breastfeeding women; infants; and children up to 5 years of age which meet specific requirements.

★ 20436 ★ U.S. Department of Defense
Army Medical Research and Material Command
Military Medical Research and Development
Attn: MCMR-ACQ-BA
Fort Detrick
Frederick, MD 21702-5012
Phone: (301)619-7216 **Fax:** (301)619-2937
Email: craig-lebo@ftdetrick-ccmail.army.mil
Website: http://mrmc-www.army.mil

Cat. No: 12.420 **Objectives:** To reduce illness and injury aquired by U.S. military personnel on the battlefield through basic and applied medical research executed largely through grants and contracts with civilian educational and research institutions. **Assist. Types:** Project grants. **Applicant Eligibility:** Applicants must be a public, nonprofit institution/organization, other public institution/organization, private not-profit institution/organization, specialized group, or quasi-public nonprofit institution/organization. **Beneficiary Eligibility:** Beneficiaries are relatively independent investigators associated with an applicant organization.

★ 20437 ★ U.S. Department of Education
Office of Elementary and Secondary Education
Safe and Drug-Free Schools Program
Safe and Drug-Free Schools and Communities—National Programs
400 Maryland Ave. SW
Portals Bldg., Rm. 603
Washington, DC 20202-6123
Phone: (202)260-3954
Website: http://www.ed.gov/offices/oese/sdfs
William Modzeleski, Contact

Cat. No: 84.184 **Objectives:** To enhance the Nation's efforts to prevent the illegal use of drugs and violence among, and promote safety and discipline for, students at all educational levels. **Assist. Types:** Project grants (contracts); project grants (cooperative agreements); project grants (discretionery). **Applicant Eligibility:** Public and private nonprofit organizations, and individuals. **Beneficiary Eligibility:** Institutions of higher educations, SEAS, LEAS, and nonprofits will benefit, as will students, teachers, and parents.

★ 20438 ★ U.S. Department of Education
Office of Elementary and Secondary Education
Safe and Drug-Free Schools Program
Safe and Drug-Free Schools and Communities—State Grants Program
400 Maryland Ave. SW, Rm. 3E314
Washington, DC 20202-6123
Phone: (202)401-3354
Website: http://www.ed.gov/offices/oese/sdfs/
Robert Alexander, Contact

Cat. No: 84.186 A&B **Objectives:** To support programs to meet the National Education Goal that, by the year 2000, every school in the United States will be free of drugs, violence, and the unauthorized presence of firearms and alcohol. To offer a disciplined environment conducive to learning by preventing violence in and around schools and strengthening programs that prevent the illegal use of alcohol, tobacco, and drugs. **Assist. Types:** Formula grants. **Applicant Eligibility:** State Governors; SEAs, Guam, American Samoa, the Virgin Islands, and the Commonwealth of the Northern Mariana Islands may apply. **Beneficiary Eligibility:** Governors' offices, SEAs, LEAs, Insular Areas, Tribal governments, and other public and private nonprofit organizations (including parent groups, community action agencies, and other community-based organizations), American Indians and Native Hawaiians, and students and teachers in public and private schools in each state.

★ 20439 ★ U.S. Department of Education
Office of Special Education and Rehabilitation Services
Centers for Independent Living
Switzer Bldg.
330 C St. SW
Washington, DC 20202-2575
Phone: (202)205-8292
Website: http://www.ed.gov/offices/osers/rsa/pgms/cil.html
Brenda Bacergeay, Contact

Cat. No: 84.132 **Objectives:** To provide independent living services to individuals with severe disabilities to assist them to function more independently in family and community settings, by developing and supporting a statewide network of centers for independent living. **Assist. Types:** Project grants (contracts). **Applicant Eligibility:** The principal eligible applicants are the private, nonprofit agencies that received funding directly or through subgrants or contracts under the Centers for Independent Living program in fiscal year 1992. If funds remain available after all principal eligible applicants have been funded, other centers for independent living (as defined in Section 702 of the Rehabilitation Act) and state agencies may receive funding based on satisfactory applications (including territories and outlying areas). **Beneficiary Eligibility:** Individuals with significant physical, mental, cognitive, or sensor impairments whose abilities to function independently in the families or communities or whose abilities to obtain, maintain, or advance in employment is substantially limited. Eligibility shall not be based on the presence of any one or more specific severe disabilities.

★ 20440 ★ U.S. Department of Education
Office of Special Education and Rehabilitation Services
Grants for Infants and Families with Disabilities
400 Maryland Ave. SW
Washington, DC 20202
Phone: (202)205-5547
Email: ruth.ryder@ed.gov
Website: htpp://www.ed.gov/offices/osers/osep/
Ruth Ryder, Contact

Cat. No: 84.181 **Objectives:** To assist each state and territory to develop a state-wide comprehensive, coordinated, multidisciplinary, interagency system to provide early intervention services for infants and toddlers with disabilities and their families. **Assist. Types:** Formula grants. **Applicant Eligibility:** The 50 states, the District of Columbia, Puerto Rico, U.S. Territories, and the Secretary of the Interior may apply. **Beneficiary Eligibility:** Disabled infants and toddlers and their families.

★ 20441 ★ U.S. Department of Education Office of Special Education and Rehabilitation Services Office of Program Operations Independent Living—State Grants

330 C St. SW
Washington, DC 20202-2741
Phone: (202)205-9362
Website: http://www.ed.gov/offices/osers/rsa/pgms/il-state-grants.html
James Billy, Contact

Cat. No: 84.169 **Objectives:** To assist states to promote a philosophy of independent living including a philosophy of consumer control, peer support, self-help, self-determination, equal access, and individual and system advocacy, in order to maximize the leadership, empowerment, independence, and productivity of indivivuals with disabilities, and the integration and full inclusion of individuals with disabilities into the mainstream American society, by providing financial assistance for providing, expanding, and improving the provision of independent living services. **Assist. Types:** Formula grants. **Applicant Eligibility:** State agencies (including territories) designated as the state unit to administer the state's independent living rehabilitation services program may apply. **Beneficiary Eligibility:** Eligibility is based upon: (1) the presence of a severe physical or mental impairment; (2) the presence of a severe limitation in ability to function independently in the family or community or to engage or continue in employment; and (3) a reasonable expectation that services will assist the individual to improve ability to function independently in the family or community or to engage in or continue in employment.

★ 20442 ★ U.S. Department of Education Office of Special Education and Rehabilitation Services Rehabilitation Long-Term Training

400 Maryland SW
Washington, DC 20202-2649
Phone: (202)205-8926
Email: RSA_Training@ed.gov
Website: http://www.ed.gov/offices/OSERS/RSA/PGMS/rt.html
Tim Muzzio, Contact

Cat. No: 84.129 **Objectives:** To support projects to increase the numbers and improve the skills of personnel trained in providing vocational rehabilitation services to individuals with disabilities in areas targeted as having personnel shortages. **Assist. Types:** Project grants (contracts). **Applicant Eligibility:** State vocational rehabilitation agencies (including territories/possessions), and other public or nonprofit agencies and organizations, including institutions of higher education. **Beneficiary Eligibility:** Individuals preparing for employment in the field of rehabilitation of individuals with disabilities.

★ 20443 ★ U.S. Department of Education Office of Special Education and Rehabilitation Services Rehabilitation Services—Client Assistance Program

600 Independence Ave. SW
Washington, DC 20202
Phone: (202)205-8719
Email: roseann_eshbach@ed.gov
RoseAnn Ashby, Contact

Cat. No: 84.161 **Objectives:** (1) To provide assistance in informing and advising clients and client applicants of available benefits under the Rehabilitation Act; (2) to assist and advocate for clients and client applicants in their relationships with projects, programs, and services provided under this act, including assistance and advocacy in pursuing legal, administrative and other appropriate remedies; (3) to provide information on available services under the Act and Title 1 of the Americans with Disabilities Act to any individual with disabilities in the state. **Assist. Types:** Formula grants. **Applicant Eligibility:** States and territories (through the Governor) are eligible for awards. **Beneficiary Eligibility:** Clients and client applicants receiving services or interested in seeking assistance under the Rehabilitation Act of 1973 will benefit.

★ 20444 ★ U.S. Department of Education Office of Special Education and Rehabilitation Services Rehabilitation Services—Independent Living Services for Older Individuals who are Blind

400 Maryland SW, Rm. 3327
Washington, DC 20202-2741
Phone: (202)205-9320
Website: http://www.ed.gov/offices/osers/rsa/pgms/il-older-blind.html
Edna Johnson, Contact

Cat. No: 84.177 **Objectives:** To provide independent living services to individuals aged fifty-five or older who are blind, whose severe visual impairments make competitive employment extremely difficult to attain but for whom independent living in their own homes and communities is feasible. **Assist. Types:** Project grants. **Applicant Eligibility:** Any state agencies (including territories/possessions designated by the state as a state agency) authorized to provide rehabilitation services to blind individuals. **Beneficiary Eligibility:** Individuals aged 55 or older with severe visual impairments.

★ 20445 ★ U.S. Department of Education Office of Special Education and Rehabilitation Services Rehabilitation Services—Service Projects

330 C St. SW, Rm. 3228
Washington, DC 20202
Phone: (202)205-8435
Website: http://www.ed.gov/offices/osers/rsa
Mary Chambers, Contact

Cat. No: 84.128 **Objectives:** To provide discretionary grant funds to state vocational rehabilitation agencies and public nonprofit organizations for special projects and demonstrations which hold promise of expanding and otherwise improving services to individuals with disabilities over and above those provided by the Basic Support Program administered by states. **Assist. Types:** Project grants. **Applicant Eligibility:** Recreational projects are awarded to states, public agencies and nonprofit organizations. Grants cannot be made directly to individuals. Migratory worker projects are funded by grants to state vocational rehabilitation agencies (including territories/possessions) and to nonprofit and local agencies in collaboration with the state agencies. **Beneficiary Eligibility:** Individuals with physical, mental, or emotional disabilities which result in a handicap to employment; emphasis is on those with the most severe disabilities.

★ 20446 ★ U.S. Department of Education Office of Special Education and Rehabilitation Services Rehabilitation Services—Vocational Rehabilitation Grants to States

400 Maryland Ave. SW
Washington, DC 20202
Phone: (202)205-8719
Email: RoseAnn_Ashby@ed.gov
Website: http://www.ed.gov/offices/osers/osep/rsa/pgms/bvrs.html
RoseAnn Ashby, Contact

Cat. No: 84.126 **Objectives:** To assist states in operating comprehensive, coordinated, effective, efficient, and accountable programs of vocational rehabilitation; to assess, plan, develop, and provide vocational rehabilitation services for individuals with disabilities, consistent with their strengths, resources, priorities, concerns, abilities, and capabilities so they may prepare for and engage in competitive employment. **Assist. Types:** Formula grants. **Applicant Eligibility:** State agencies (including territories/possessions) designated as the sole state agency to administer the vocational rehabilitation program. **Beneficiary Eligibility:** Eligibility for vocational rehabilitation services is based on the presence of a physical and/or mental impairment, which for such an individual constitutes or results in a substantial impediment to employment, and the need for vocational rehabilitation services that may be expected to benefit the individual in terms of employment outcome.

★ 20447 ★ U.S. Department of Education Office of Special Education and Rehabilitation Services Rehabilitation Short-Term Training

400 Maryland Ave. SW
Washington, DC 20202-2649
Free: 800-USA-LEARN **Fax:** (202)401-0689
Email: rsa_training@ed.gov
Website: http://www.ed.gov/offices/osers/rsa/pgms/rt.html
Timothy Muzzio, Contact

Cat. No: 84.246 **Objectives:** To support special seminars, institutes, workshops, and other short-term courses in technical matters relating to the delivery of vocational, medical, social, and psychological services. **Assist. Types:** Project grants (contracts). **Applicant Eligibility:** State vocational rehabilitation agencies (including territories/possessions), and other public or nonprofit agencies and organizations, including institutions of higher education. **Beneficiary Eligibility:** Individuals preparing for or employed in positions relating to the rehabilitation of individuals with disabilities.

★ 20448 ★ U.S. Department of Education Office of Special Education and Rehabilitation Services Special Education—Preschool Grants

400 Maryland Ave. SW
Washington, DC 20202
Phone: (202)205-9097
Website: http://www.ed.gov/offices/osers/osep/
Nancy Treusch, Contact

Cat. No: 84.173 **Objectives:** To provide grants to states to assist them in providing a free appropriate public education to preschool disabled children aged three to five years. **Assist. Types:** Formula grants. **Applicant Eligibility:** State education agencies in the 50 States, District of Columbia, and Puerto Rico. **Beneficiary Eligibility:** Three through five-year-old children, and (at the State's option) two-year-old children that will reach age 3 during the school year, having mental retardation, hearing impairments, including deafness, speech or language impairments, visual impairments, including blindness, serious emotional disturbance, orthopedic impairments, autism, traumatic brain injury, other health impairments or developmental delays that require special education and related services.

★ 20449 ★ U.S. Department of Education Office of Special Education and Rehabilitation Services Special Education—Technology and Media Services for Individuals with Disabilities

400 Maryland Ave. SW
Washington, DC 20202
Phone: (202)205-8883
Jeffrey Payne, Contact

Cat. No: 84.327 **Objectives:** To promote the development, demonstration, and utilization of technology; support educational media activities designed to be of educational value to children with disabilities and other specified media-related activities; and support for some captioning, video description, and cultural activities. **Assist. Types:** Project grants, project grants (cooperative agreements), project grants (contracts). **Applicant Eligibility:** Profit and nonprofit public and private agencies, organizations, or institutions. **Beneficiary Eligibility:** Individuals with disabilities.

★ 20450 ★ U.S. Department of Education Office of Special Education and Rehabilitation Services Supported Employment Services for Individuals with Severe Disabilities
400 Maryland Ave. SW
Washington, DC 20202-2574
Phone: (202)205-8719
Website: http://www.ed.gov/offices/osers/rsa/pgms/supported-employment.html
RoseAnn Ashby, Contact

Cat. No: 84.187 **Objectives:** To provide grants for time limited services leading to supported employment for individuals with the most severe disabilities to enable such individuals to achieve the employment outcome of supported employment. **Assist. Types:** Formula grants. **Applicant Eligibility:** State vocational rehabilitation agencies (including territories and possessions) designated in the state plan to administer the Vocational Rehabilitation Program. **Beneficiary Eligibility:** Individuals with the most severe disabilities whose ability or potential to engage in a training program leading to supported employment and has been determined by evaluating rehabilitation potential. In addition, individuals must need extended services in order to perform competitive work and have the ability to work in a supported employment setting.

★ 20451 ★ U.S. Department of Education Office of Special Education and Rehabilitation Services Training Interpreters for Individuals who are Deaf and Individuals who are Deaf-Blind
400 Maryland Ave. SW
Washington, DC 20202-2736
Phone: (202)205-9393 **Fax:** (202)205-9340
Website: http://www.ed.gov/offices/osers/rsa/gfms/rt/catinter.html
Mary Lovely, Contact

Cat. No: 84.160 **Objectives:** To support projects to increase the numbers and improve the skills of manual, tactile, oral, and cued speech interpreters providing services to individuals wha are deaf and individuals who are deaf-blind. **Assist. Types:** Project grants (contracts). **Applicant Eligibility:** Public or private nonprofit agencies and organizations, including institutions of higher education. **Beneficiary Eligibility:** Individuals preparing for employment as interpreters for individuals who are deaf and individuals who are deaf-blind who are presently serving as interpreters and wish to maintain or raise the level of their skills, and persons who will receive the services of interpreters.

★ 20452 ★ U.S. Department of Education Office of Special Education and Rehabilitative Services National Institute on Disability and Rehabilitation Research
400 Maryland Ave. SW
Washington, DC 20202-2572
Phone: (202)205-5880 **Fax:** (202)205-5479
Website: http://www.ed.gov/offices/osers/rsa/nidrr
Donna Nangle, Contact
Ellen Blasiotti, Contact

Cat. No: 84.133 **Objectives:** To support and coordinate research and its utilization to improve the lives of people of all ages with physical and mental disabilities, especially persons with severe disabilities through: (1) identifying and eliminating causes and consequences of disability; (2) maximizing the health, physical and emotional status of persons with disabilities and their functional ability, self-sufficiency, self-development, and personal autonomy; (3) preventing or minimizing personal and family, physical, mental, social, educational, vocational and economic effects of disability; and (4) reducing and eliminating physical, social, educational, vocational and environmental barriers to permit access to services and assistance and to use their abilities in daily life. **Assist. Types:** Project grants; project grants (contracts); project grants (cooperative agreements); project grants (fellowships). **Applicant Eligibility:** Grants and cooperative agreements may be made to and contracts with states, public, private, or nonprofit agencies and organizations and institutions of higher education, and Indian tribes and tribal organizations for research projects and specialized research activities related to the rehabilitation of individuals with disabilities; fellowships may be awarded to individuals. **Beneficiary Eligibility:** Individuals with disabilities of all ages.

★ 20453 ★ U.S. Department of Education Office of Special Education and Rehabilitative Services Special Education—Grants to States
400 Maryland Ave. SW
Washington, DC 20202
Phone: (202)205-5547
Email: Ruth.Ryder@ed.gov
Website: http://www.ed.gov/offices/osers/osep/index.html
Ruth Ryder, Contact

Cat. No: 84.027 **Objectives:** To provide grants to states to assist them in providing a free appropriate public education to all children with disabilities. **Assist. Types:** Formula grants. **Applicant Eligibility:** State education agencies in the 50 States, District of Columbia, Puerto Rico, American Samoa, Commonwealth of the Northern Mariana Islands, Guam, and Virgin Islands may apply to the Department of Education for participation in the Part B, IDEA program. The Department of the Interior, Bureau of Indian Affairs receives 1.226 percent of the total amount available to states. Local education agencies apply to their state educational agency for funds. **Beneficiary Eligibility:** Children and youth with disabilities.

★ 20454 ★ U.S. Department of Health and Human Services Administration for Children and Families Administration on Developmental Disabilities Developmental Disabilities Basic Support and Advocacy Grants
370 L'Enfant Promenade SW
Washington, DC 20447
Phone: (202)690-5962
Website: http://www.acf.dhhs.gov/programs/add
Ray Sanchez, Contact

Cat. No: 93.630 **Objectives:** To enable individuals with developmental disabilities to become independent, productive, integrated and included into their communities. Funding under these programs is to assist states in the development of a plan for a comprehensive and coordinated system of services and other activites to enhance the lives of individuals with developemtnal disabilities and their families to their maximum potential, and to support a system which protects the legal and human rights of individuals with developemtnal disabilities. **Assist. Types:** Formula grants. **Applicant Eligibility:** State grant agencies are the designated state agencies of the respective states, the District of Columbia, Puerto Rico, the Virgin Islands, Guam, the Northern Mariana Islands, American Samoa, and the Republic of Palau. Under the basic developmental disabilities program, the designated state agency must not provide or pay for services to persons with developmental disabilities, unless it has held such designation continuously since June 30, 1988. The state can only receive funding under the basic developmental disabilities program if it is also participating in the protection and advocacy program. **Beneficiary Eligibility:** Eligible beneficiaries of these two programs must be persons with developmental disabilities. Developmental disability is defined here as a severe chronic disability of persons 5 years old or older, that is attributable to mental or physical or combination of impairments, that is manifested before age 22, that is likely to continue indefinitely, that results in substantial functional limitations in three or more of the seven major life activities (self-care, receptive and expressive language, learning, mobility, self-direction, capacity for independent living, and economic self-sufficiency), and that reflects a person's lifelong need for services. Infants and children under age 5 are included if they have a developmental delay or condition with a high probability of resulting in developmental disabilities if services are not provided. provided.

★ 20455 ★ U.S. Department of Health and Human Services Administration for Children and Families Administration on Developmental Disabilities Developmental Disabilities—Projects of National Significance
370 L'Enfant Promenade SW
Washington, DC 20447
Phone: (202)690-7693 **Fax:** (202)690-6904
Website: http://www.acf.dhhs.gov/programs/add
Leola Brooks, Contact

Cat. No: 93.631 **Objectives:** To provide grants and contracts for projects of national significance to increase and support the independence, productivity, integration, and inclusion into the community of individuals with developmental disabilities. **Assist. Types:** Project grants; project grants (contracts). **Applicant Eligibility:** Any state, local, public, or private nonprofit organization or agency may apply. **Beneficiary Eligibility:** Same as applicant eligibility.

★ 20456 ★ U.S. Department of Health and Human Services Administration for Children and Families Administration on Developmental Disabilities University Centers for Excellence in Developmental Disabilities Education, Research, and Service
370 L'Enfant Promenade SW
Washington, DC 20447
Phone: (202)690-7693 **Fax:** (202)690-6904
Email: lbrooks@acf.dhhs.gov
Website: http://www.acf.dhhs.gov/programs/add
Leola Brooks, Contact

Cat. No: 93.632 **Objectives:** To defray the cost of administration and operation of programs that: provide interdisciplinary training for personnel concerned with developmental disabilities; demonstrate community service activities which include training and technical assistance and may include direct services, e.g., family support, individual support, personal assistance services, educational, vocational, clinical, health, and prevention; disseminate findings related to the provision of services to researchers and government agencies; and generate information on the need for further service-related research. **Assist. Types:** Project grants. **Applicant Eligibility:** A public or nonprofit entity which is associated with, or is an integral part of a college or university and which provides at least: interdisciplinary training; demonstration of exemplary services, technical assistance, and dissemination of findings. **Beneficiary Eligibility:** Persons of all ages with developmental disabilities attributable to a mental and/or physical impairment, their families, and personnel and trainees providing services to them.

★ 20457 ★ U.S. Department of Health and Human Services Administration for Children and Families Children's Bureau Child Abuse and Neglect State Grants
330 C St. SW
Washington, DC 20447
Phone: (202)205-2629

Website: http://www.acf.dhhs.gov/progrmas/cb
Geraldine Neal, Contact

Cat. No: 93.669 **Objectives:** To assist states in the support and improvement of their child protective services systems. **Assist. Types:** Formula grants. **Applicant Eligibility:** States and the District of Columbia, Puerto Rico, Guam, the Virgin Islands, American Samoa, the Republic of Palau, and the Commonwealth of the Northern Mariana Islands. **Beneficiary Eligibility:** Abused or neglected children and their families.

★ 20458 ★ U.S. Department of Health and Human Services
Administration for Children and Families
Children's Bureau
Child Welfare Services—State Grants
PO Box 1182
Washington, DC 20013
Phone: (202)401-2779
Website: http://www.acf.dhhs.gov/programs/cb
Marianne Rufty, Contact

Cat. No: 93.645 **Objectives:** To establish, extend, and strengthen child welfare services provided by state and local public welfare agencies to enable children to remain in their own homes, or, where that is impossible, to provide alternate permanent homes for them. **Assist. Types:** Formula grants. **Applicant Eligibility:** Any single state agency in the United States, the District of Columbia, Puerto Rico, the Northern Marianas, the Virgin Islands, Guam, and American Samoa. **Beneficiary Eligibility:** Any families and children in need of child welfare services.

★ 20459 ★ U.S. Department of Health and Human Services
Administration for Children and Families
Children's Bureau
Child Welfare Services—Training Grants
330 C St. SW
Washington, DC 20447
Phone: (202)205-8405
Website: http://www.acf.dhhs.gov/programs/cb
Marva P. Benjamin, Contact

Cat. No: 93.648 **Objectives:** To develop and maintain an adequate supply of qualified and trained personnel for the child welfare field, and to improve educational programs and resources for preparing personnel for this field. **Assist. Types:** Project grants. **Applicant Eligibility:** Accredited institutions of higher learning. **Beneficiary Eligibility:** Same as applicant eligibility.

★ 20460 ★ U.S. Department of Health and Human Services
Administration for Children and Families
Children's Bureau
Promoting Safe and Stable Families
330 C St. SW
Washington, DC 20447
Phone: (202)401-2779
Website: http://www.acf.dhhs.gov/programs/cb
Marianne Rufty, Contact

Cat. No: 93.556 **Objectives:** To fund community-based family support services that promote the safety and well-being of children and families by enhancing family functioning and child development; to fund family preservation programs that serve families at risk or in crisis, including the following services: reunification or adoption services, preplacement/preventive services, follow-up services after return of child from foster care, respite care, and improved parenting skills; to fund time-limited family reunification services to facilitate the reunification of the child safely and appropriately within a timely fashion; and to fund adoption promotion and support services designed to encourage more adoption, out of the foster care system, when adoptions promote the best interests of children. **Assist. Types:** Formula grants. **Applicant Eligibility:** States, territories and certain Indian tribes are eligible applicants. **Beneficiary Eligibility:** Families and children who need and would benefit from services to assist them to stabilize their lives, strengthen family functioning, prevent out-of-home placement of children, enhance child development, increase competence in parenting abilities, facilitate timely reunification of the child, and promote appropriate adoptions.

★ 20461 ★ U.S. Department of Health and Human Services
Administration for Children and Families
Head Start Bureau
Head Start
330 C St. SW
Washington, DC 20447
Phone: (202)205-8572
Website: http://www.acf.dhhs.gov/programs.hsb

Cat. No: 93.600 **Objectives:** To provide comprehensive health, educational, nutritional, social and other services primarily to economically disadvantaged preschool children, including Indian children on federally-recognized reservations, and children of migratory workers and their families; and to involve parents in activities with their children so that the children will attain overall social competence. **Assist. Types:** Project grants. **Applicant Eligibility:** Any local government, federally-recognized Indian tribe, or public or private nonprofit agency which meets the requirements may apply for a grant. Grantee agencies may subcontract with other child-serving agencies to provide services to Head Start children. **Beneficiary Eligibility:** Head Start programs are for children from birth up to the age when the child enters the school system. No less than 10 percent of the total enrollment opportunities in each Head Start program shall be available for children with disabilities.

★ 20462 ★ U.S. Department of Health and Human Services
Administration for Children and Families
Mental Retardation—President's Committee on Mental Retardation
Washington, DC 20447
Phone: (202)619-0634 **Fax:** (202)205-9519
Website: http://www.acf.dhhs.gov/programs/pcmr

Cat. No: 93.613 **Objectives:** To advise and assist the President on all matters pertaining to mental retardation; study national, state and local efforts; help coordinate federal activities; facilitate communication between federal, state and local agencies; inform the public about mental retardation; and mobilize support for related activities. **Assist. Types:** Dissemination of technical information. **Applicant Eligibility:** General public. **Beneficiary Eligibility:** General public.

★ 20463 ★ U.S. Department of Health and Human Services
Administration for Children and Families
Office of Community Services
Family Violence Prevention and Services/ Grants for Battered Women's Shelters—Discretionary Grants
370 L'Enfant Promenade SW
Washington, DC 20447
Phone: (202)401-5529
Website: http://www.acf.dhhs.gov/programs/ocs
William Riley, Contact

Cat. No: 93.592 **Objectives:** To fund a wide range of discretionary activities for the purpose of preventing family violence; protecting victims and their dependents; improving the design, delivery, and coordination of services to address family violence; gathering information on the incidence of family violence; and increasing knowledge and understanding of the issue through research, demonstration, and evaluation projects. **Assist. Types:** Project grants. **Applicant Eligibility:** Depending on the purpose of the project and the statutory requirements, an applicant may be a public agency, a private agency (for profit or nonprofit), a federally-recognized Indian tribe, an Alaska Native Village, or nonprofit Alaska Native Regional Corporation. **Beneficiary Eligibility:** These discretionary grants will benefit victims of family violence, their dependents, families, other interested persons, and the general public.

★ 20464 ★ U.S. Department of Health and Human Services
Administration for Children and Families
Office of Community Services
Family Violence Prevention and Services/ Grants for Battered Women's Shelters—Grants to State Domestic Violence Coalitions
370 L'Enfant Promenade SW
Washington, DC 20447
Phone: (202)401-5529
Website: http://www.acf.dhhs.gov/programs/ocs
William Riley, Contact

Cat. No: 93.591 **Objectives:** To further the purposes of domestic violence intervention and prevention through a range of direct and coordinated activities. **Assist. Types:** Formula grants. **Applicant Eligibility:** To be eligible for a grant under this section, and entity shall be a statewide nonprofit state domestic violence coalition. **Beneficiary Eligibility:** This program will benefit victims of domestic violence, their children and other dependents, their families, and other persons affected by such violence including friends, relatives, and the general public.

★ 20465 ★ U.S. Department of Health and Human Services
Administration for Children and Families
Office of Community Services
Family Violence Prevention and Services/ Grants for Battered Women's Shelters—Grants to States and Indian Tribes
370 L'Enfant Promenade SW, 5th Fl.
Washington, DC 20447
Phone: (202)401-5529
Website: http://www.acf.dhhs.gov/programs/ocs
William Riley, Contact

Cat. No: 93.671 **Objectives:** To assist states and Indian tribes in the prevention of family violence and to provide immediate shelter and related assistance for victims of family violence and their dependents. **Assist. Types:** Formula grants. **Applicant Eligibility:** The 50 States, the District of Columbia, the Commonwealth of Puerto Rico, Guam, American Samoa, the Virgin Islands, the Northern Mariana Islands, Palau, and certain federally-recognized Indian Tribes. **Beneficiary Eligibility:** Victims of family violence and their dependents.

★ 20466 ★ U.S. Department of Health and Human Services
Administration for Children and Families
Office of Community Services
Social Services Block Grant
370 L'Enfant Promenade SW
Washington, DC 20447
Phone: (202)401-2333
Website: http://www.acf.dhhs.gov/programs/ocs/ssbg
Margaret Washnitzer, Contact

Cat. No: 93.667 **Objectives:** To enable each state to furnish social services best suited to the needs of the individuals residing in the state. Federal block grant funds may be used to provide services directed toward one of the following five goals specified in the law: (1) to prevent, reduce, or eliminate dependency; (2) to achieve or maintain self-sufficiency; (3) to prevent neglect, abuse, or exploitation of children and adults; (4) to prevent or reduce inappropriate institutional care; and (5) to secure admission or referral for institutional care when other forms of care are not appropriate. **Assist. Types:** Formula grants. **Applicant Eligibility:** The 50 states, the District of Columbia, Puerto Rico, Guam, the Virgin Islands, the Commonwealth of the Northern Mariana Islands, and American Samoa. **Beneficiary Eligibility:** Under Title XX, each eligible jurisdiction determines the services that will be provided and the individuals that will be eligible to receive services.

★ 20467 ★ U.S. Department of Health and Human Services
Administration for Children and Families
Office of Planning, Research and Evaluation
Social Services Research and Demonstration
370 L'Enfant Promenade SW, 7th Fl.
Washington, DC 20447
Phone: (202)205-4829 **Fax:** (202)205-3598
Email: KJagannathan@ACF.DHHS.GOV
Website: http://www.acf.dhhs.gov/programs/ocs
Dr. K.A. Jagannathan, Contact

Cat. No: 93.647 **Objectives:** To promote the ability of families to be financially self-sufficient, and to promote the healthy development and greater social well-being of children and families. **Assist. Types:** Project grants; project grants (cooperative agreements and contracts). **Applicant Eligibility:** Grants and cooperative agreements may be made to or with governmental entities, colleges, universities, nonprofit and for-profit organizations. Contracts may be awarded to nonprofit or for-profit organizations. Grants or cooperative agreements cannot be made directly to individuals. **Beneficiary Eligibility:** Low-income individuals, children, youth, families, individuals with developmental disabilities, and Native Americans. Native Americans.

★ 20468 ★ U.S. Department of Health and Human Services
Administration for Children and Families
Office of Refugee Resettlement
Refugee and Entrant Assistance—Wilson/ Fish Programs
370 L'Enfant Promenade SW, 6th Fl.
Washington, DC 20447
Phone: (202)401-4558
Website: http://www.acf.dhhs.gov/programs/orr
Barbara Chesnik, Contact

Cat. No: 93.583 **Objectives:** To develop alternative projects which promote early employment of refugees, including Amerasian immigrants and Cuban and Haitian entrants. States, voluntary resettlement agencies, and other resettlement organizations may develop innovative approaches for the provision of refugee cash and medical assistance, social services, and case management otherwise available through the State-administered program. Wilson/Fish demonstration projects typically emphasize one or more of the following elements: preclusion of otherwise eligible refugees for public assistance; elimination or modification of work disincentives; creation of a front-loaded service system which provides intensive services to refugees in the early months after arrival; and integration of case management, cash assistance, and employment services. **Assist. Types:** Project grants. **Applicant Eligibility:** States, voluntary resettlement agencies, and other refugee resettlement organizations may apply to initiate an alternative program. No separate funding is appropriated for Wilson/Fish demonstration projects. Funds are drawn instead from funds earmarked for refugee cash and medical assistance grants and social services allocations for the state-administered program according to ORR projections. **Beneficiary Eligibility:** Same as applicant eligibility.

★ 20469 ★ U.S. Department of Health and Human Services
Agency for Health Care Policy and Research
National Research Service Awards—Health Services Research Training
2101 E Jefferson St., Ste. 601
Rockville, MD 20852
Phone: (301)594-1449
Website: http://www.ahrq.gov
Al Deal, Contact

Cat. No: 93.225 **Objectives:** To provide predoctoral and postdoctoral training opportunities in health services research. Individual fellowships will be awarded directly to applicants for postdoctoral research training. Domestic institutions will also be awarded grants to enhance predoctoral and postdoctoral training programs and provide support to trainees selected by them. **Assist. Types:** Project grants. **Applicant Eligibility:** Domestic public or private nonprofit organizations or institutions may apply for training grants. State or local governments and U.S. territories are eligible. Profit-making organizations are not eligible. Individual applicants for fellowships must have received a doctoral degree. All persons supported as fellows or trainees must be citizens of the United States, or have been lawfully admitted for permanent residence. **Beneficiary Eligibility:** Same as applicant eligibility.

★ 20470 ★ U.S. Department of Health and Human Services
Agency for Healthcare Research and Quality
Research on Healthcare Costs, Quality and Outcomes
2101 E Jefferson St., Ste. 601
Rockville, MD 20852
Phone: (301)594-1447
Website: http://www.ahrq.gov
Mable L. Lam, Contact

Cat. No: 93.226 **Objectives:** To support health services research to create new knowledge and better understanding of the process by which health services are made available, and how they may be provided more efficiently and effectively. **Assist. Types:** Project grants. **Applicant Eligibility:** Federal, state or local government agencies; federally-recognized Indian tribal governments; U.S. territories; sponsored organizations; non-government organizations; minority groups; specialized groups; public or private institutions of higher education; and other public or nonprofit private agencies, institutions, or organizations. Research project grants may also be awarded to individuals. Profit-making organizations are not eligible for these grants. **Beneficiary Eligibility:** Same as Applicant Eligibility.

★ 20471 ★ U.S. Department of Health and Human Services
Agency for Toxic Substances and Disease Registry
Division of Health Studies
Human Health Studies—Applied Research and Development
1600 Clifton Rd. NE
Mail Stop E-31
Atlanta, GA 30333
Phone: (404)498-0546 **Fax:** (404)498-0077
Email: mmf2@cdc.gov
Website: http://www.atsdr.cdc.gov
Mrs. Maggie Warren, Contact

Cat. No: 93.206 **Objectives:** To solicit scientific proposals designed to answer public health questions arising from situations commonly encountered at hazardous waste sites. The objective of this research program is to fill gaps in knowledge regarding human health effects of hazardous substances identified during the conduct of ATSDR's health assessments, consultations, toxological profiles, and health studies, including but not limited to health conditions prioritized by the ATSDR. The Agency for Toxic Substances and Disease Registry (ATSDR) Priority Health Conditions are (in alphabetical order): (1) Birth Defects and Reproductive Disorders. (2) Cancers (selected anatomic sites); (3) Immune Function Disorders; (4) Kidney Dysfunction; (5) Liver Dysfunction; (6) Lung and Respiratory Diseases; and (7) Neurotoxic Disorders. **Assist. Types:** Project grants. **Applicant Eligibility:** Eligible applicants are State health departments and the District of Columbia, the Commonwealth of Puerto Rico, the Virgin Islands, Guam, the Federated States of Micronesia, the Republic of the Marshall Islands, the Republic of Palau, the Northern Mariana Islands, American Samoa, the political subdivisions thereof, which may include State universities, State colleges, and State research institutions, and federally-recognized Indian tribal governments. **Beneficiary Eligibility:** Federal, State, local, other public institutions/organizations, federally-recognized Indian tribal governments, U.S. Territories/possessions, and the general public in their ability to address potential health problems related to environmental exposures and adverse health outcomes.

★ 20472 ★ U.S. Department of Health and Human Services
Agency for Toxic Substances and Disease Registry
Division of Health Studies
Surveillance of Hazardous Substance Emergency Events
1600 Clifton Rd. NE
Mail Stop E-31
Atlanta, GA 30333
Phone: (404)498-0546 **Fax:** (404)498-0058
Email: mmf2@cdc.gov
Website: http://www.atsdr.cdc.gov
Maggie Warren, Contact

Cat. No: 93.204 **Objectives:** To assist State health departments in developing a state-based surveillance system for monitoring hazardous substance emergency events. This surveillance system will allow the state health department to better understand the public health impact of hazardous substance emergencies by developing, implementing, and evaluating a state-based surveillance system. **Assist. Types:** Project grants. **Applicant Eligibility:** The official public health departments of the States and the District of Columbia, the Commonwealth of Puerto Rico, the Virgin Islands, Guam, the Federated States of Micronesia, the Republic of the Marshall Islands, the Republic of Palau, the Northern Mariana Islands, and American Samoa and federally-recognized Indian Tribal Governments. **Beneficiary Eligibility:** Federal, state, local, other public institutions/organizations, federally-recognized Indian tribal governments, U.S. Territories/possessions, and the general public.

★ 20473 ★ U.S. Department of Health and Human Services
Center for Substance Abuse Treatment
Division of State and Community Assistance
Block Grants for Prevention and Treatment of Substance Abuse
5600 Fishers Lane
Rockwall II, 8th Fl.
Rockville, MD 20857
Phone: (301)443-7541
Website: http://www.samhsa.gov
H. Rick Sampson, Contact

Cat. No: 93.959 **Objectives:** To provide financial assistance to states and territories to support projects for the development and implementation of prevention, treatment and rehabilitation activities directed to the diseases of alcohol and drug abuse. **Assist. Types:** Formula grants. **Applicant Eligibility:** State and U.S. Territory governments; Indian tribes or tribal organizations. **Beneficiary Eligibility:** Recipients of state and U.S. Territory governments and members of Indian tribes and tribal organizations.

★ 20474 ★ U.S. Department of Health and Human Services
Centers for Disease Control and Prevention
Centers for Disease Control—Investigations and Technical Assistance
2920 Brandywine Rd., Rm. 3000
Atlanta, GA 30341
Phone: (770)488-2700
Website: http://www.cdc.gov
Nealean Austin, Contact

Cat. No: 93.283 **Objectives:** To assist state and local health authorities and other health related organizations in controlling communicable diseases, chronic diseases, and other preventable health conditions. **Assist. Types:** Project grants. **Applicant Eligibility:** States, political subdivisions of states, local health authorities, and organizations with specialized health interests. **Beneficiary Eligibility:** Same as Applicant Eligibility.

★ 20475 ★ U.S. Department of Health and Human Services
Centers for Disease Control and Prevention
Division of HIV/AIDS Prevention
Acquired Immunodeficiency Syndrome Activity
1600 Clifton Rd.
Atlanta, GA 30333
Phone: (404)639-0930
Website: http://www.cdc.gov
Ron Van Duyne, Contact

Cat. No: 93.118 **Objectives:** To develop and implement HIV prevention programs of public information and education. **Assist. Types:** Project grants (cooperative agreements). **Applicant Eligibility:** Public and private organizations, both nonprofit and for-profit (universities, colleges, research institutions, and other public and private organizations); state and local governments, U.S. Territories and possessions; small and minority businesses, and businesses owned by women. **Beneficiary Eligibility:** Official health and education agencies, as well as individuals subject to AIDS.

★ 20476 ★ U.S. Department of Health and Human Services
Centers for Disease Control and Prevention
Immunization Services Division
Immunization Grants
1600 Clifton Rd. NE
Atlanta, GA 30333
Phone: (404)639-8208 **Fax:** (404)639-8627
Email: LAR9@cdc.gov
Website: http://www.cdc.gov
Dr. Lance Rodewald, Director

Cat. No: 93.268 **Objectives:** To assist states and communities in establishing and maintaining preventive health service programs to immunize individuals against vaccine preventable diseases (including measles, rubella, poliomyelitis, diphtheria, pertussis, tetanus, hepatitus b, mumps and haemaphilus influenza type b). **Assist. Types:** Project grants. **Applicant Eligibility:** Any state and in consultation with state health authorities, political subdivisions of states and other public entities. Private individuals and private nonprofit agencies are not eligible. **Beneficiary Eligibility:** Same as Applicant Eligibility.

★ 20477 ★ U.S. Department of Health and Human Services
Centers for Disease Control and Prevention
Injury Prevention and Control Research and State and Community Based Programs
1600 Clifton Rd. NE
Atlanta, GA 30333
Phone: (770)488-4265 **Fax:** (770)488-1662
Email: dph2@cdc.gov
Website: http://www.cdc.gov

Cat. No: 93.136 **Objectives:** Research Grants: (1) To support injury control research on priority issues; (2) to integrate aspects of engineering, public health, behavioral sciences, medicine, and other disciplines in order to prevent and control injuries more effectively; (3) to rigorously apply and evaluate current and new interventions, methods, and strategies that focus on the prevention and control of injuries; (4) to stimulate and support Injury Control Research Centers (ICRC) in academic institutions which will develop a comprehensive and integrated approach to injury control research and training; and (5) to bring the knowledge and expertise of ICRC to bear on the development of effective public health programs for injury control. State and Community Program Grants: (1) to develop and eveluate new methods or to evaluate existing methods and techniques used in injury surveillance by public health agencies; and (2) to develop, expand, or improve injury control programs to reduce morbidity, mortality, severity, disability, and cost from injuries. **Assist. Types:** Project grants; (cooperative agreements). **Applicant Eligibility:** For Injury Prevention and Control Research Projects, Injury Control Research Centers, and Injury Control Research Program Projects: Eligible applicants include any non-profit or for-profit organization. For State and Community Program Grants: Official public health agencies of the States, the District of Columbia, the Federated States of Micronesia, Guam, the Northern Mariana Islands, the Republic of Marshall Islands, and the Republic of Palau. Also eligible are official public health agencies of city or county governments with jurisdictional populations greater than 1,000,000. **Beneficiary Eligibility:** Academic health centers, scientist/researchers, operational public health programs, state and local governments, and public and private organizations involved in injury research. For state grants: State and local health departments.

★ 20478 ★ U.S. Department of Health and Human Services
Centers for Disease Control and Prevention
National Center for Chronic Disease Prevention and Health Promotion
Centers for Research and Demonstration for Health Promotion and Disease Prevention
4770 Buford Hwy., K-30
Atlanta, GA 30333
Phone: (770)488-5395
Website: http://www.cdc.gov/prc

Cat. No: 93.135 **Objectives:** (1) To establish, maintain, and operate academic-based centers for high quality research and demonstration with respect to health promotion and disease prevention; (2) to establish linkages, where applicable, between ongoing, basic research in a wide array of fields and applied research in disease prevention and health promotion; (3) to bring the knowledge and expertise of academic health centers to bear on practical public health problems; (4) to field test and rigorously evaluate more cost-effective methods and strategies for preventing unnecessary illness and promoting good health; and (5) to shorten the time lag between the development of new and proven effective disease prevention and health promotion techniques and their widespread application. **Assist. Types:** Project grants (cooperative agreements). **Applicant Eligibility:** Eligible applicants are schools of medicine, schools of osteopathy, and schools of public health as defined in Section 701(4) of Public Health Service Act. **Beneficiary Eligibility:** Academic health centers, scientist/researchers, operational public health programs, targeted high risk groups, selected demonstration areas, and the general public.

★ 20479 ★ U.S. Department of Health and Human Services
Centers for Disease Control and Prevention
National Center for Chronic Disease Prevention and Health Promotion
Cooperative Agreements for State-Based Diabetes Control Programs and Evaluation of Surveillance Systems
1600 Clifton Rd. NE
Atlanta, GA 30333
Phone: (770)488-5046
Website: http://www.cdc.gov

Cat. No: 93.988 **Objectives:** To implement comprehensive programs which will ensure that persons with diabetes who are at high risk for certain complications of diabetes are identified, entered into the health care system, and receive on-going state-of-the-art preventive care and treatment; and to develop, demonstrate, and evaluate statewide public health surveillance systems for diabetes and its complications. **Assist. Types:** Project grants (cooperative agreements). **Applicant Eligibility:** Official state health agencies of the United States, the District of Columbia, and U.S. Territories. **Beneficiary Eligibility:** Same as Applicant Eligibility.

★ 20480 ★ U.S. Department of Health and Human Services
Centers for Disease Control and Prevention
National Center for Chronic Disease Prevention and Health Promotion
Preventive Health and Health Services Block Grant
4770 Bufford Hwy. NE
Mail Stack K-30
Atlanta, GA 30341-3724
Phone: (770)488-5645
Website: http://www.cdc.gov
Robin J. Forbes, Contact

Cat. No: 93.991 **Objectives:** To provide states with resources to improve the health status of the population of each grantee through: (A) activities leading to the accomplishment of the year 2000 objectives for the nation; (B) rodent control and community-school fluoridation activities; (C) specified emergency medical services excluding most equipment purchases; (D) services for sex offense victims including prevention activities; and (E) for related administration, education, monitoring and evaluation activities. **Assist. Types:** Formula grants. **Applicant Eligibility:** State and territorial governments, the District of Columbia, the Kickapoo Tribe of Kansas and the Sante Sioux Tribe of Nebraska are eligible. **Beneficiary Eligibility:** The general public will benefit from the objectives of this program with special attention to disparately affected populations.

★ 20481 ★ U.S. Department of Health and Human Services
Centers for Disease Control and Prevention
National Center for HIV, STD, and TB Prevention
Preventive Health Services—Sexually Transmitted Diseases Control Grants
1600 Clifton Rd. NE
Atlanta, GA 30333
Phone: (404)639-8260 **Fax:** (404)639-8608
Website: http://www.cdc.gov
Candice Nowicki, Contact

Cat. No: 93.977 **Objectives:** To reduce morbidity and mortality by preventing cases and complications of sexually transmitted diseases. **Assist. Types:** Project grants. **Applicant Eligibility:** Any state or authorized subdivision. **Beneficiary Eligibility:** Same as Applicant Eligibility.

★ 20482 ★ U.S. Department of Health and Human Services
Centers for Disease Control and Prevention
National Center for HIV, STD, and TB Prevention
Preventive Health Services—Sexually Transmitted Diseases Research, Demonstrations, and Public Information and Education Grants
1600 Clifton Rd. NE
Atlanta, GA 30333
Phone: (404)639-8260 **Fax:** (404)639-8608
Website: http://www.cdc.gov
Judith N. Wasserheit, MD, Contact

Cat. No: 93.978 **Objectives:** To develop, improve, apply, and evaluate methods for the prevention and control of syphilis, gonorrhea, chlamydia, and other sexually transmitted diseases (STD) through demonstrations and applied research; to develop, improve, apply, and evaluate methods and strategies for public information and education about syphilis, gonorrhea, and other STD; to support professional (including appropriate allied health personnel) STD education, training, and clinical skills improvement activities. **Assist. Types:** Project grants. **Applicant Eligibility:** Any state, political subdivisions of states, and any other public or private nonprofit institutions. **Beneficiary Eligibility:** Same as Applicant Eligibility.

★ 20483 ★ U.S. Department of Health and Human Services
Centers for Disease Control and Prevention
National Center for HIV, STD and TB Prevention
Project Grants and Cooperative Agreements for Tuberculosis Control Programs
1600 Clifton Rd. NE
Atlanta, GA 30333
Phone: (404)639-8125

Cat. No: 93.116 **Objectives:** To assist state and local health agencies in carrying out tuberculosis control activities designed to prevent transmission of infection and disease. **Assist. Types:** Project grants (cooperative agreements). **Applicant Eligibility:** Official public health agencies of state and local governments, including the District of Columbia and U.S. Territories. **Beneficiary Eligibility:** Same as Applicant Eligibility.

★ 20484 ★ U.S. Department of Health and Human Services
Centers for Disease Control and Prevention
National Institute for Occupational Safety and Health
Occupational Safety and Health—Research Grants
1600 Clifton Rd. NE
Atlanta, GA 30333
Phone: (404)498-2530
Email: RMF2@cdc.gov
Website: http://www.cdc.gov/

Cat. No: 93.262 **Objectives:** To develop knowledge that can be used in preventing occupational diseases and injuries. Small Business Innovation Research (SBIR) objectives are: to stimulate technological innovation; use small business to meet federal research and development needs; increase private sector commercialization of innovations derived from federal research and development; and foster and encourage participation by minority and disadvantaged persons in technological innovation. **Assist. Types:** Project grants. **Applicant Eligibility:** Eligible applicants include profit and nonprofit organizations. Thus, universities, colleges, research institutions, and other public and private organizations, including state and local governments, and small, minority and/or women-owned businesses are eligible. **Beneficiary Eligibility:** Research institutions and agencies, as well as workers affected by occupational hazards.

★ 20485 ★ U.S. Department of Health and Human Services
Centers for Disease Control and Prevention
National Institute for Occupational Safety and Health
Occupational Safety and Health—Training Grants
1600 Clifton Rd.
Atlanta, GA 30333
Phone: (404)498-2537 **Fax:** (404)498-2571
Email: bbk1@cdc.gov
Website: http://www.cdc.gov
Dr. Bernadine Kuchinski, Contact

Cat. No: 93.263 **Objectives:** To develop specialized professional and paraprofessional personnel in occupational safety and health field with training in occupational medicine, occupational health nursing, industrial hygiene, and occupational safety. **Assist. Types:** Project grants. **Applicant Eligibility:** Any public or private educational institution or agency that has demonstrated competency involved in occupational safety and health training at technical, professional, or graduate levels. **Beneficiary Eligibility:** Trainees must be admissible to the grantee institution and must be enrolled in occupational safety and health training programs.

★ 20486 ★ U.S. Department of Health and Human Services
Centers for Medicare and Medicaid Services
Medical Assistance Program
7500 Security Blvd., C4-25-02
Baltimore, MD 21244
Phone: (410)786-3870
Website: http://www.cms.hhs.gov/contracts/

Cat. No: 93.778 **Objectives:** To provide financial assistance to states for payments of medical assistance on behalf of cash assistance recipients, children, pregnant women, and the aged who meet income and resource requirements and other categorically-eligible groups. In certain states that elect to provide such coverage, other medically-needy persons, who, except for income and resources, would be eligible for cash assistance, may be eligible for medical assistance payments under this program. Financial assistance is also provided to states to pay for Medicare premiums, copayments and deductibles of qualified Medicare beneficiaries meeting certain income requirements. **Assist. Types:** Formula grants. **Applicant Eligibility:** State and local welfare agencies must operate under an HHS approved medicaid state plan and comply with all federal regulations governing aid and medical assistance to the needy. **Beneficiary Eligibility:** Needy persons who are over age 65, blind, disabled, members of families with dependent children, low-income children and pregnant women, qualified Medicare beneficiaries and, in some states, persons under age 21 may apply to a state or local welfare agency for medical assistance. Eligibility is determined by the state in accordance with federal regulations.

★ 20487 ★ U.S. Department of Health and Human Services
Centers for Medicare and Medicaid Services
Medicare—Hospital Insurance
6325 Security Blvd., Rm. 311
Baltimore, MD 21207
Phone: (410)965-8050 **Free:** 800-MEDICARE
Website: http://www.cms.hhs.gov/contracts/

Cat. No: 93.773 **Objectives:** To provide hospital insurance protection for covered services to any person 65 or above, to certain disabled persons, and to individuals with chronic renal disease. **Assist. Types:** Direct payments for specified use. **Applicant Eligibility:** Persons age 65 or over and certain disabled persons are eligible for hospital insurance protection. Hospital insurance is also available to persons, 65 or over, not otherwise eligible through payment of a monthly premium. Persons under age 65 who have been entitled for at least 24 months to Social Security disability benefits, or for 29 consecutive months to railroad retirement benefits based on disability, are eligible for hospital insurance benefits. Also, most people who have chronic kidney disease and require dialysis or transplant are eligible. **Beneficiary Eligibility:** Persons age 65 or over and qualified disabled persons.

★ 20488 ★ U.S. Department of Health and Human Services
Food and Drug Administration
Office of Facilities, Acquisition and Central Services
Food and Drug Administration—Research
5630 Fishers Lane, Rm. 2129
Rockville, MD 20857
Phone: (301)827-7160 **Fax:** (301)827-7101
Email: pjones1@oc.fda.gov
Website: http://www.fda.gov
Peggy L. Jones, Contact

Cat. No: 93.103 **Objectives:** To assist profit making organizations, public and other nonprofit institutions, to establish, expand, and improve research demonstration, education, and information dissemination activities concerned with acquired immunodeficiency syndrome (AIDS), poison control, drug hazards, human and veterinary drugs (including drugs for orphan product development), medical devices and diagnostic products, biologics, and radiation emitting devices and materials. Small Business Innovation Research (SBIR) Programs: to stimulate technological innovation; to use small business to meet federal research and development needs; to increase private sector commercialization of innovations derived from federal research and development; and to foster and encourage participation by minority and disadvantagedpersons in technological innovation. **Assist. Types:** Project grants. **Applicant Eligibility:** Awards can be made to any public or private nonprofit university, college, hospital, laboratory, or other institution, including state and local units of government. Commercial and nonprofit organizations are also eligible. **Beneficiary Eligibility:** Colleges, universities, profit-making organizations, nonprofit institutions, and state and local governments.

★ 20489 ★ U.S. Department of Health and Human Services
Health Professions Bureau
Student Assistance Division
Scholarships for Health Professions Students From Disadvantaged Backgrounds
5600 Fishers Ln., Rm. 8-34
Rockville, MD 20857
Phone: (301)443-4776
Website: http://www.hrsa.dhhs.gov/bhpr/dsa/dsa.htm

Cat. No: 93.925 **Objectives:** To make funds available for grants to schools of medicine, nursing, osteopathic medicine, dentistry, pharmacy, podiatric medicine, optometry, veterinary medicine, allied health, or public health, or schools that offer graduate programs in clinical psychology for the purpose of assisting such schools in providing scholarships to individuals from disadvantaged backgrounds who are enrolled (or accepted for enrollment) as full-time students in the schools. **Assist. Types:** Project grants. **Applicant Eligibility:** Accredited public or private nonprofit schools of medicine, nursing, osteopathic medicine, dentistry, pharmacy, podiatric medicine, optometry, veterinary medicine, public health, or allied health, or schools offering graduate programs in clinical psychology. **Beneficiary Eligibility:** Students who are (1) citizens, U.S. nationals, aliens lawfully admitted for permanent residency in the U.S., or U.S. Territories; and (2) accepted for enrollment as full-time students in a health professions school.

★ 20490 ★ U.S. Department of Health and Human Services
Health Resources and Services Administration
Advance Education Nursing Traineeships
5600 Fishers Lane, Rm. 9-36
Rockville, MD 20857
Phone: (301)443-6193 **Fax:** (301)443-8586
Email: mstarbecker@hrsa.gov
Website: http://www.hrsa.gov/bhpr/dn/dn.htm
Marcia Starbecker, Contact

Cat. No: 93.358 **Objectives:** To prepare individuals who have completed basic nursing preparation as nurse educators, public health nurses, nurse midwives, and nurse practitioners, or to serve as clinical nursing specialists for positions in hospitals and related institutions, in public health agencies, in schools of nursing, and in other settings requiring advanced training. **Assist. Types:** Formula grants. **Applicant Eligibility:** Public or private nonprofit entities providing individuals with full-time advanced education, leading to a graduate degree or for nurse-midwifery, a certificate and meeting the purpose of the Professional Nurse Traineeships Grant Program. **Beneficiary Eligibility:** Trainees are selected by participating institutions.

★ 20491 ★ U.S. Department of Health and Human Services
Health Resources and Services Administration
Bureau of Health Professions
Academic Administrative Units in Primary Care
5600 Fishers Lane, Rm. 9A-20
Rockville, MD 20857
Phone: (301)443-1467
Website: http://www.hrsa.gov/bhpr

Cat. No: 93.984 **Objectives:** To assist in establishing, maintaining, or improving family medicine academic administrative units to provide clinical instruction in family medicine in order that these units are comparable in status, faculty and curriculum to those other clinical units at the applying school. **Assist. Types:** Project grants. **Applicant Eligibility:** Accredited public or nonprofit private school of medicine or osteopathic medicine. **Beneficiary Eligibility:** Same as Applicant Eligibility.

★ 20492 ★ U.S. Department of Health and Human Services
Health Resources and Services Administration
Bureau of Health Professions
Basic/Core Area Health Education Centers
5600 Fishers Lane, Rm. 9-105
Rockville, MD 20857
Phone: (301)443-6950
Email: cgleich@hrsa.dhhs.gov
Website: http://www.hrsa.gov/bhpr

Cat. No: 93.824 **Objectives:** To improve the distribution, supply, quality, utilization, and efficiency of health personnel in the health service delivery system, and for the purpose of increasing the regionalization of educational responsibilities of health professional schools. **Assist. Types:** Project grants (cooperative agreements). **Applicant Eligibility:** An accredited public or nonprofit schools of medicine or osteopathy, a consortium of such schools, or the parent institution on behalf of such schools. **Beneficiary Eligibility:** Same as Applicant Eligibility.

★ 20493 ★ U.S. Department of Health and Human Services
Health Resources and Services Administration
Bureau of Health Professions
Centers of Excellence
5600 Fishers Lane, Rm. 8A-09
Rockville, MD 20857
Phone: (301)443-2100 **Fax:** (301)443-4943
Website: http://www.hrsa.gov/bhpr
Sheila Norris, Contact

Cat. No: 93.157 **Objectives:** To strengthen the national capacity to train minority students in the health professions; and to support the health professions schools which train a significant number of minority health professionals. **Assist. Types:** Project grants. **Frmly:** Health Professions Bureau, Disadvantaged Assistance Division, Programs of Excellence in Health Professions Education for Minorities. **Applicant Eligibility:** Schools of medicine, osteopathic medicine, dentistry, and pharmacy, as described under Section 739(h), and as accredited in Section 799(1)(E) of the Act, as well as Historically Black Colleges and Universities, as described in Section 799(1)(A) which received a contract under Section 788B of the Public Health Service Act (Advanced Financial Distress Assistance) for fiscal year 1987 may apply for grants under Section 739 of the Act. As specified in section 739(d)(3), Native American Centers of Excellence, a grant for a Native American Center of Excellence may also be made to a consortium of schools that collectively meet conditions, without regard to whether the schools of the consortium individually meet the conditions. **Beneficiary Eligibility:** Same as Applicant Eligibility.

★ 20494 ★ U.S. Department of Health and Human Services
Health Resources and Services Administration
Bureau of Health Professions
Chiropractic Demonstration Project Grants
5600 Fishers Lane, Rm. 8C-02
Rockville, MD 20857
Phone: (301)443-0908
Website: http://bhpr.hrsa.gov/interdisciplinary/chiro.html

Cat. No: 93.212 **Objectives:** To make grants to and enter into contracts with schools, colleges, and universities of chiropractic for the purpose of carrying out demonstration projects in which chiropractors and physicians collaborate to identify and provide effective treatment for spinal and lower-back conditions. **Assist. Types:** Project grants. **Applicant Eligibility:** Public or private nonprofit schools, colleges, and universities of chiropractic medicine. **Beneficiary Eligibility:** Same as applicant eligibility.

★ 20495 ★ U.S. Department of Health and Human Services
Health Resources and Services Administration
Bureau of Health Professions
Disadvantaged Health Professions Faculty Loan Repayment and Fellowship Program
5600 Fishers Ln., Rm. 8-34
Rockville, MD 20857
Phone: (301)443-4776 **Fax:** (301)443-0846
Email: flrp_info@hrsa.gov
Website: http://www.hrsa.dhhs.gov/bhpr

Cat. No: 93.923 **Objectives:** To attract amd retain disadvantaged health professions faculty members for accredited health professions schools of medicine, nursing, osteopathic medicine, dentistry, pharmacy, podiatric medicine, optometry, veterinary medicine, public health, or a school that offers a graduate program in clinical psychology for at least 2 years and to repay their annual educational loan balance for those years. **Assist. Types:** Direct payments for specified use. **Applicant Eligibility:** Individuals from disadvantaged backgrounds who (1) have a degree in medicine, osteopathic medicine, dentistry, pharmacy, podiatric medicine, optometry, veterinary medicine, nursing, graduate public health, or graduate clinical psychology; (2) are enrolled in an approved graduate training program in medicine, osteopathic medicine, dentistry, or other health profession; or (3) are enrolled as full-time students in accredited institutions described above and in the final course of study or program leading to a degree from the institution; and (4) have not, during the 18 months period preceeding the date which the Secretary receives the request of the individual, been a member of the faculty of any school at any time. **Beneficiary Eligibility:** Individuals who are from disadvantaged backgrounds.

★ 20496 ★ U.S. Department of Health and Human Services
Health Resources and Services Administration
Bureau of Health Professions
Geriatric Education Centers
5600 Fishers Lane, Rm. 8-103
Rockville, MD 20857
Phone: (301)443-6887 **Fax:** (301)443-1164
Website: http://www.hrsa.dhhs.gov/bhpr

Cat. No: 93.969 **Objectives:** To develop regional resource centers focused on strengthening multidisciplinary training of health professionals in geriatric health care. **Assist. Types:** Project grants. **Applicant Eligibility:** Any accredited health professions school or school of allied health, as defined in Section 799(1) or (4) of the Public Health Service Act, any school of nursing, as defined in section 853(2) of the Public Health Service Act; any accredited graduate program in health administration, clinical psychology, clinical social work or marriage and family therapy, as defined in section 799(1) of the Public Health Service Act; or any program for the training of physician assistants, as defined in Section 799(3)(A) of the Public Health Service Act. **Beneficiary Eligibility:** Professional schools, faculty of institutions of higher education, and health practitioners.

★ 20497 ★ U.S. Department of Health and Human Services
Health Resources and Services Administration
Bureau of Health Professions
Geriatric Training for Physicians, Dentists, and Behavioral/Mental Health Professionals
5600 Fishers Lane, Rm. 8C-103
Rockville, MD 20857
Phone: (301)443-6887
Website: http://www.hrsa.gov/bhpr

Cat. No: 93.156 **Objectives:** To assist in the operation of postdoctoral training preparing current and future faculty for leadership roles in geriatric medicine and dentistry. To provide support, including traineeships and fellowships, for geriatric medicine training projects to train physicians and dentists who plan to teach geriatric medicine, geriatric psychiatry, or geriatric dentistry. **Assist. Types:** Project grants. **Applicant Eligibility:** Accredited public or private nonprofit schools of medicine, schools of osteopathy, teaching hospitals, and graduate medical education programs. **Beneficiary Eligibility:** Same as Applicant Eligibility.

★ 20498 ★ U.S. Department of Health and Human Services
Health Resources and Services Administration
Bureau of Health Professions
Grants for Dental Public Health Residency Training
5600 Fishers Lane, Rm. 8C-09
Rockville, MD 20857
Phone: (301)443-6896 **Fax:** (301)443-1164
Website: http://www.hrsa.gov/bhpr/grants.html
Dr. Kathy Hayes, Contact

Cat. No: 93.236 **Objectives:** To promote the post-graduate education of dentists in public health. **Assist. Types:** Project grants. **Applicant Eligibility:** Any accredited public or private school of public health or dentistry. **Beneficiary Eligibility:** Same as Applicant Eligibility.

★ 20499 ★ U.S. Department of Health and Human Services Health Resources and Services Administration Bureau of Health Professions Grants for Faculty Development in Family Medicine
5600 Fishers Lane, Rm. 9A-27
Rockville, MD 20857
Phone: (301)443-1467 **Fax:** (301)443-1945
Website: http://www.hrsa.gov/bhpr
Cat. No: 93.895 **Objectives:** To increase the supply of physician faculty available to teach in family medicine programs and to enhance the pedagogical skills of faculty presently teaching in family medicine. **Assist. Types:** Project grants. **Applicant Eligibility:** Public or nonprofit private hospitals; accredited public or nonprofit schools of medicine or of osteopathy; or public or private nonprofit health or educational institutions. **Beneficiary Eligibility:** Same as Applicant Eligibility.

★ 20500 ★ U.S. Department of Health and Human Services Health Resources and Services Administration Bureau of Health Professions Grants for Preventive Medicine
5600 Fishers Lane, Rm. 8C-09
Rockville, MD 20857
Phone: (301)443-6896 **Fax:** (301)443-1164
Website: http://www.hrsa.gov/bhpr
Ron Merrill, Contact
Cat. No: 93.117 **Objectives:** To promote the postgraduate education of physicians in preventive medicine. **Assist. Types:** Project grants. **Applicant Eligibility:** Any accredited public or private school of medicine, osteopathic medicine, or public health. **Beneficiary Eligibility:** Same as Applicant Eligibility.

★ 20501 ★ U.S. Department of Health and Human Services Health Resources and Services Administration Bureau of Health Professions Grants for Residency Training in General Internal Medicine and General Pediatrics
5600 Fishers Lane, Rm. 9A-27
Rockville, MD 20857
Phone: (301)443-1467 **Fax:** (301)443-1945
Website: http://www.hrsa.dhhs.gov/bhpr
Cat. No: 93.884 **Objectives:** To promote the graduate education of physicians who plan to enter the practice of general internal medicine or general pediatrics. **Assist. Types:** Project grants. **Applicant Eligibility:** An accredited public or private nonprofit school of medicine or osteopathic medicine, or a public or private nonprofit hospital or other entity. **Beneficiary Eligibility:** Same as Applicant Eligibility.

★ 20502 ★ U.S. Department of Health and Human Services Health Resources and Services Administration Bureau of Health Professions Health Administration Traineeships and Special Projects Program
5600 Fishers Lane, Rm. 8C-09
Rockville, MD 20857
Phone: (301)443-6896
Email: tperez@hrsa.dhhs.gov
Website: http://www.hrsa.gov/bhpr
Cat. No: 93.962 **Objectives:** To support eligible students enrolled in accredited graduate programs in health administration, hospital administration, or health policy analysis and planning and to assist in the development or improvement of programs to prepare students for employment with public or nonprofit private entities. **Assist. Types:** Formula grants. **Applicant Eligibility:** Any public or private nonprofit educational entity (excluding accredited schools of public health) offering a graduate program in health administration, hospital administration, or health policy analysis and planning which has been accredited by the Accrediting Commission on Education in Health Services Administration. **Beneficiary Eligibility:** Must be a U.S. citizen or have visa permitting permanent residence, and enrolled in an accredited program in health administration, hospital administration, or health policy analysis and planning.

★ 20503 ★ U.S. Department of Health and Human Services Health Resources and Services Administration Bureau of Health Professions Health Careers Opportunity Program
5600 Fishers Lane, Rm. 8A-09
Rockville, MD 20857
Phone: (301)443-2100 **Fax:** (301)443-5242
Website: http://www.hrsa.gov/bhpr
Cat. No: 93.822 **Objectives:** To identify, recruit, and select individuals from disadvantaged backgrounds for education and training in a health or allied health professions school; facilitate entry of eligible students into such schools; provide counseling or other services designed to assist such individuals to successfully complete their education and training; provide preliminary education for a period prior to entry into the regular course of education, designed to assist students in successfully completing regular courses of education, or refer the appropriate individuals to institutions providing preliminary education; and publicize existing sources of financial aid. **Assist. Types:** Project grants. **Applicant Eligibility:** Health professions schools and public or private nonprofit health or educational entities. **Beneficiary Eligibility:** Disadvantaged individuals and those from families living below economic levels determined by the U.S. Bureau of Census.

★ 20504 ★ U.S. Department of Health and Human Services Health Resources and Services Administration Bureau of Health Professions Health Education Assistance Loans
5600 Fishers Lane, Rm. 8-37
Rockville, MD 20857
Phone: (301)443-1540 **Fax:** (301)594-6911
Website: http://www.hrsa.gov/bhpr
Cat. No: 93.108 **Objectives:** To authorize loans for educational expenses available from eligible lenders. Loans are made to students enrolled in eligible health professions educational programs at participating institutions. **Assist. Types:** Guaranteed/insured loans. **Applicant Eligibility:** Generally, any U.S. citizen, National, or person lawfully admitted to the United States for permanent residence, who is enrolled on a full-time basis at an eligible health professions school. **Beneficiary Eligibility:** Same as Applicant Eligibility.

★ 20505 ★ U.S. Department of Health and Human Services Health Resources and Services Administration Bureau of Health Professions Health Professions Student Loans, Including Primary Care Loans/Loans for Disadvantaged Students
5600 Fishers Lane, Rm. 8-34
Rockville, MD 20857
Phone: (301)443-4776
Website: http://www.hrsa.dhhs.gov/bhpr/dsa/dsa.htm
Cat. No: 93.342 **Objectives:** To increase educational opportunities for students in need of financial assistance to pursue a course of study in specified health professions by providing long-term, low interest loans. **Assist. Types:** Direct loans. **Applicant Eligibility:** Any accredited public or other nonprofit private school of medicine, dentistry, osteopathy, optometry, podiatry, pharmacy, or veterinary medicine which provides a course of study leading to a Doctoral or equivalent degree, located in a state, District of Columbia, or Puerto Rico. **Beneficiary Eligibility:** Any student enrolled or accepted for enrollment in a school, as above, and pursuing a course of study which constitutes a full-time academic workload leading to a degree.

★ 20506 ★ U.S. Department of Health and Human Services Health Resources and Services Administration Bureau of Health Professions Model State-Supported Area Health Education Centers
5600 Fishers Ln., Rm. 9-105
Rockville, MD 20857
Phone: (301)443-6950
Email: cgleich@hrsa.dhhs.gov
Website: http://www.hrsa.gov/bhpr
Cat. No: 93.107 **Objectives:** To provide assistance for the cost of operating the area health education centers program and for carrying out activities in specified areas. **Assist. Types:** Project grants (cooperative agreements). **Applicant Eligibility:** Accredited schools of medicine or osteopathic medicine that are operating an area health education center program and are not receiving federal assistance under the parent program, section 746(a)(1). **Beneficiary Eligibility:** Same as Applicant Eligibility.

★ 20507 ★ U.S. Department of Health and Human Services Health Resources and Services Administration Bureau of Health Professions National Health Service Corps Scholarship Program
4350 East-West Hwy., 10th Fl.
Bethesda, MD 20814
Phone: (301)594-4410
Website: http://www.hrsa.gov
Cat. No: 93.288 **Objectives:** To provide service-obligated scholarships to health professions students to assure an adequate supply of physicians, dentists, certified nurse midwives, certified nurse practitioners, and physician assistants in Health Professional Shortage Areas of the U.S.A.; and, if needed by the National Health Service Corps, an adequate supply of other health professionals. **Assist. Types:** Project grants. **Applicant Eligibility:** At the time of award, the applicant must be a U.S. citizen or national and enrolled or accepted for enrollment in an accredited U.S. school. **Beneficiary Eligibility:** The grantee is the beneficiary.

★ 20508 ★ U.S. Department of Health and Human Services Health Resources and Services Administration Bureau of Health Professions Nurse Anesthetist Traineeships
5600 Fishers Lane, Rm. 9-36
Rockville, MD 20857
Phone: (301)443-5763 **Fax:** (301)443-8586
Email: mstarbecker@hrsa.gov
Website: http://www.hrsa.gov/bhpr/dn/dn.htm
Marcia Starbecker, Contact
Cat. No: 93.124 **Objectives:** To provide traineeships for full-time study in accredited training programs for registered nurses who have completed 12 months of study in nurse anesthetist training programs. **Assist. Types:** Project grants. **Applicant Eligibility:** Public and private nonprofit institutions providing nurse anesthetist training. **Beneficiary Eligibility:** A candidate must be a citizen of the United States or have been lawfully admitted for permanent residence; be enrolled full-time in a participating nurse anesthetist education program; have successfully completed 12 months of

the nurse anesthetist training program; and demonstrate financial need, as determined by the institution.

★ 20509 ★ U.S. Department of Health and Human Services
Health Resources and Services Administration
Bureau of Health Professions
Nursing Student Loans
5600 Fishers Lane, Rm. 8-34
Rockville, MD 20857
Phone: (301)443-4776
Website: http://www.hrsa.dhhs.gov/bhpr/dsa/dsa.htm

Cat. No: 93.364 **Objectives:** To assist students in need of financial assistance to pursue a course of study in professional nursing education by providing long-term, low-interest loans. **Assist. Types:** Direct loans. **Applicant Eligibility:** All accredited public and nonprofit private schools of nursing that prepare students for practice as registered or graduate nurses, and that do not discriminate against students because of race, color, origin, sex, or handicapping conditions. **Beneficiary Eligibility:** Nursing students.

★ 20510 ★ U.S. Department of Health and Human Services
Health Resources and Services Administration
Bureau of Health Professions
Physician Assistant Training in Primary Care
5600 Fishers Lane, Rm. 9A-27
Rockville, MD 20857
Phone: (301)443-1467
Website: http://www.hrsa.gov/bhpr

Cat. No: 93.886 **Objectives:** To enable public or nonprofit private health or educational entities to meet the cost of projects to plan, develop, and operate programs for the training of physician's assistants. **Assist. Types:** Project grants. **Applicant Eligibility:** State and local government entity, or nonprofit private health or educational institution. **Beneficiary Eligibility:** Same as Applicant Eligibility.

★ 20511 ★ U.S. Department of Health and Human Services
Health Resources and Services Administration
Bureau of Health Professions
Predoctoral Training in Primary Care
5600 Fishers Lane, Rm. 9A-27
Rockville, MD 20857
Phone: (301)443-1467
Email: bball@hrsa.dhhs.gov
Website: http://www.hrsa.gov/bhpr
Brenda Williamson, Contact

Cat. No: 93.896 **Objectives:** To assist schools of medicine and osteopathy in meeting the costs of projects to plan, develop, and operate professional predoctoral training programs in the field of family medicine. **Assist. Types:** Project grants. **Applicant Eligibility:** Any accredited nonprofit school of medicine or osteopathy. **Beneficiary Eligibility:** Same as Applicant Eligibility.

★ 20512 ★ U.S. Department of Health and Human Services
Health Resources and Services Administration
Bureau of Health Professions
Public Health Traineeships
5600 Fishers Lane, Rm. 8C-09
Rockville, MD 20857
Phone: (301)443-6896
Website: http://www.hrsa.gov/bhpr

Cat. No: 93.964 **Objectives:** To support traineeships for students in graduate educational programs in accredited schools of public health and to other public or nonprofit private institutions accredited for the provision of graduate or specialized training in public health which offer graduate programs in public health fields with a severe shortage, including: (1) biostatistics, (2) epidemiology; planning or health policy analysis and planning; (3) environmental health; (4) toxicology; and (5) public health nutrition. **Assist. Types:** Formula grants. **Applicant Eligibility:** Accredited schools of public health and other accredited public or nonprofit private institutions. **Beneficiary Eligibility:** (1) Trainees must be United States Citizens or noncitizen nationals having in their possession a visa permitting permanent residence in the United States; (2) trainees must be pursuing a graduate degree in an accredited school of public health or enrolled in an eligible program; (3) for grants awarded on the basis of a formula, all trainees must meet the admission requirements specified in the application and those of the institution.

★ 20513 ★ U.S. Department of Health and Human Services
Health Resources and Services Administration
Bureau of Health Professions
Residencies and Advanced Education in the General Practice of Dentistry
5600 Fishers Lane, Rm. 8C-09
Rockville, MD 20857
Phone: (301)443-6896
Website: http://www.hrsa.gov/bhpr

Cat. No: 93.897 **Objectives:** To assist schools of dentistry and institutions conducting post-graduate dental training in defraying the costs of projects to plan, develop, and operate an approved residency or advanced educational program in the general practice of dentistry. **Assist. Types:** Project grants. **Applicant Eligibility:** Public or private nonprofit school of dentistry or accredited post-graduate dental training institution located in the U.S. or U.S. Territories. **Beneficiary Eligibility:** Same as Applicant Eligibility.

★ 20514 ★ U.S. Department of Health and Human Services
Health Resources and Services Administration
Bureau of Primary Health Care
Grants for State Loan Repayment
4350 East-West Hwy., 10th Fl.
Bethesda, MD 20814
Phone: (301)594-4400 **Free:** 800-435-6464
Fax: (301)594-4981
Website: http://www.hrsa.gov
Susan Salter, Contact

Cat. No: 93.165 **Objectives:** To assist states in operating programs for the repayment of educational loans for health professionals in return for their practice in health professional shortage areas (HPSAs) to increase the availability of primary care in HPSAs. **Assist. Types:** Project grants. **Applicant Eligibility:** Any state. **Beneficiary Eligibility:** State governments will benefit by securing health professions manpower for health professional shortage areas in states. This program will also benefit those whose loans would be repaid for service under the state program.

★ 20515 ★ U.S. Department of Health and Human Services
Health Resources and Services Administration
Bureau of Primary Health Care
Hansen's Disease National Ambulatory Care Program
4350 East-West Hwy., 11th Fl.
Bethesda, MD 20814
Phone: (301)594-4235
Website: http://www.bphc.hrsa.gov/nhdp

Cat. No: 93.215 **Objectives:** To provide screening and testing of contacts of patients diagnosed with Hansen's disease, and to provide ambulatory care and treatment services to any person diagnosed with Hansen's disease who needs and requests care and treatment for that disease; and such care that may be provided without charge. **Assist. Types:** Project grants. **Applicant Eligibility:** Existing Hansen's Disease Centers. **Beneficiary Eligibility:** Patients and contacts of patients diagnosed with Hansen's disease.

★ 20516 ★ U.S. Department of Health and Human Services
Health Resources and Services Administration
Bureau of Primary Health Care
National Health Service Corps Loan Repayment Program
4350 East-West Hwy., 10th Fl.
Bethesda, MD 20814
Phone: (301)594-4400 **Free:** 800-435-6464
Website: http://bhpr.hrsa.gov/nhsc

Cat. No: 93.162 **Objectives:** To help assure an adequate supply of trained health professionals for the National Health Service Corps (NHSC) by providing for the repayment of educational loans for participants who agree (by written contract) to serve an applicabale period of time in a health manpower shortage area. **Assist. Types:** Project grants. **Applicant Eligibility:** Individuals who are: (1) U.S. citizens; (2) enrolled as full-time students in the final year of study in an accredited health profession education institution; or (3) possess a health professions degree and are either enrolled in post-graduate health professions training or are in professional practice. **Beneficiary Eligibility:** Full-time students of medicine, dentistry, or nursing; prospective or currently commissioned officers in the Regular or Reserve Corps of the United States Public Health Service; and eligible civilians in the National Health Service Corps.

★ 20517 ★ U.S. Department of Health and Human Services
Health Resources and Services Administration
Bureau of Primary Health Care
Technical and Non-Financial Assistance to Health Centers and National Health Service Corps Delivery Sites
4350 East-West Hwy., 3rd Fl.
Bethesda, MD 20814
Phone: (301)594-4488
Website: http://www.hrsa.gov

Cat. No: 93.129 **Objectives:** To provide assistance to health centers and NHSC delivery sites in the following areas: (1) collaborative activities on state or regional levels; (2) involvement of state agencies in assuring primary care to medically underserved populations; (3) development of shared servicesand joint purchasing arrangements; (4) provision of, or arrangement for, training, assessment of community health center needs, expertise in dealing with the homeless, public housing, farm workers, children, rural health, and other special populations, and management and maximization of non-federal resources; and (5) expanding the health center network and ensuring high quality in health centers. **Assist. Types:** Project grants. **Applicant Eligibility:** Eligible applicants are private nonprofit entities, including previously existing and newly established state and regional primary care associations. **Beneficiary Eligibility:** Medically-underserved populations.

★ 20518 ★ U.S. Department of Health and Human Services
Health Resources and Services Administration
Community and Migrant Health Division
Community Health Centers
4350 East-West Hwy., 7th Fl.
Bethesda, MD 20814
Phone: (301)594-4300
Website: http://www.bphc.hrsa.gov

Cat. No: 93.224 **Objectives:** To support the development and operation of community health centers which provide primary health services, supplemental health services, and environmental health services to medically underserved populations. **Assist. Types:** Project grants. **Applicant Eligibility:** Public or nonprofit private agencies, institutions, or organizations and a limited number of state and local governments. **Beneficiary Eligibility:** Population groups in medically underserved areas.

★ 20519 ★ U.S. Department of Health and Human Services
Health Resources and Services Administration
Division of Facilities Compliance and Recovery
Project Grants for Renovation or Construction of Health Care Facilities
5600 Fishers Lane, Rm. 10C-16
Rockville, MD 20857
Phone: (301)443-5656
Email: dfcrcomm@hrsa.gov
Website: http://www.hrsa.gov/osp
Eulas Dortch, Contact

Cat. No: 93.887 **Objectives:** To assure that obligated health care facilities provide free or reduced cost medical services to those persons who are uninsured and underinsured and meet eligibility criteria. **Assist. Types:** Project grants. **Applicant Eligibility:** Public or nonprofit entities. **Beneficiary Eligibility:** Public or other nonprofit entities which provide non-acute health care.

★ 20520 ★ U.S. Department of Health and Human Services
Health Resources and Services Administration
Division of State and Community Health
Maternal and Child Health Services Block Grant to the States
5600 Fishers Lane, Rm. 18-31
Rockville, MD 20857
Phone: (301)443-2204 **Fax:** (301)443-9354
Website: http://www.mchb.hrsa.gov/osch.htm

Cat. No: 93.994 **Objectives:** To enable states to maintain and strengthen their leadership in planning, promoting, coordinating, and evaluating health care for pregnant women, mothers, infants and children, and children with special health care needs in providing health services for mothers and children who do not have access to adequate health care. **Assist. Types:** Formula grants. **Applicant Eligibility:** Limited to states and insular areas. **Beneficiary Eligibility:** Mothers, infants and children, and children with special health care needs, particularly of low income families.

★ 20521 ★ U.S. Department of Health and Human Services
Health Resources and Services Administration
Division of Transplantation
Grants to Increase Organ Donation
5600 Fishers Lane, Rm. 7C-22
Rockville, MD 20857
Phone: (301)443-7577 **Fax:** (301)594-6095
Email: lwegman@hrsa.dhhs.gov
Website: http://www.hrsa.gov

Cat. No: 93.134 **Objectives:** To manage the Organ Procurement and Transplantation Network (OPTN), the Scientific Registry of Transplant Recipients (SRTR), and the Marrow Donor Registry. Promotes public and professional education programs to increase organ donation in the United States, including implementation of the Clinton Administration's National Organ and Tissue Donation Initiative. **Applicant Eligibility:** None. **Beneficiary Eligibility:** All organ/tissue and marrow transplant recipients.

★ 20522 ★ U.S. Department of Health and Human Services
Health Resources and Services Administration
HIV/AIDS Bureau
AIDS Education and Training Centers
5600 Fishers Lane, Rm. 7-29
Rockville, MD 20857
Phone: (301)443-6364 **Fax:** (301)443-9887
Website: http://www.hrsa.gov

Cat. No: 93.145 **Objectives:** To: (1) provide education and training to primary care providers and others on the treatment and prevention of acquired immune deficiency syndrome (AIDS), in collaboration with health professions schools, local hospitals, and health departments; (2) provide updates of new and timely information about HIV infection to primary and secondary health care providers; and (3) serve as the support system for area health professions through AIDS Hotlines, clearinghouses, and referral activities. **Assist. Types:** Project grants (cooperative agreements). **Applicant Eligibility:** Public and private nonprofit entities and schools and academic health science centers. **Beneficiary Eligibility:** Primary health care personnel.

★ 20523 ★ U.S. Department of Health and Human Services
Health Resources and Services Administration
HIV/AIDS Bureau
Coordinated Services and Access to Research for Women, Children, and Youth
5600 Fishers Lane, Rm. 7-47
Rockville, MD 20857
Phone: (301)443-9051
Website: http://www.hrsa.gov

Cat. No: 93.153 **Objectives:** To support, improve, and expand the system of comprehensive care services for children, youth, women, and families who are infected with or infected by human immune deficiency (HIV) and acquired immune deficiency syndrom (AIDS) and to link comprehensive care systems with clinical research. **Assist. Types:** Project grants. **Applicant Eligibility:** All public and private entities, nonprofit and for-profit. Proof of nonprofit status is required for nonprofit organizations. **Beneficiary Eligibility:** Women, adolescents, and children with HIV/AIDS, or who are at risk of contracting HIV/AIDS.

★ 20524 ★ U.S. Department of Health and Human Services
Health Resources and Services Administration
HIV/AIDS Bureau
Grants to Provide Outpatient Early Intervention Services with Respect to HIV Disease
5600 Fishers Ln., Rm. 7A-30
Rockville, MD 20857
Phone: (301)443-0735
Website: http://www.hrsa.gov
Lois Eldred, Director

Cat. No: 93.918 **Objectives:** To increase the capacity of entities that provide comprehensive primary care services to persons with Human Immunodeficiency Virus (HIV) infection, or who are at-risk of infection, and to offer more early intervention services. The services will include increased counseling and testing, partner involvement in risk reduction, transmission prevention, appropriate primary care diagnostic and treatment services, and, as needed, case-management to ensure that individual service needs are met. **Assist. Types:** Project grants. **Frmly:** U.S. Department of Health and Human Services, Primary Health Care Care Bureau, Programs Bureau for Special Populations Division. **Applicant Eligibility:** Eligible applicants are public and private nonprofit entities that are: migrant health centers under Section 330g of the Public Health Service Act or community health centers under Section 330 of the Public Health Service Act; family planning grantees under Section 1001 of the Public Health Service Act other than states; comprehensive hemophilia diagnostic and treatment centers; federally-qualified health centers under Section 1905(1)(B) of the Social Security Act; or a public or private nonprofit entity that provides comprehensive primary care services to populations at-risk of HIV disease. **Beneficiary Eligibility:** Persons infected with HIV or who are at high risk of HIV infection.

★ 20525 ★ U.S. Department of Health and Human Services
Health Resources and Services Administration
HIV/AIDS Bureau
HIV Care Formula Grants
5600 Fishers Ln., Rm. 7A-55
Rockville, MD 20857
Phone: (301)443-6745
Website: http://www.hrsa.gov

Cat. No: 93.917 **Objectives:** To enable states to improve the quality, availability and organization of health care and support services for individuals and families with Human Immunodeficiency Virus (HIV) disease. **Assist. Types:** Formula grants. **Applicant Eligibility:** All 50 state of the United States, the District of Columbia and U.S. Territories (and possessions) of the United States. **Beneficiary Eligibility:** Individuals and families with HIV disease.

★ 20526 ★ U.S. Department of Health and Human Services
Health Resources and Services Administration
HIV/AIDS Bureau
HIV Emergency Relief Project Grants
5600 Fishers Ln., Rm. 7A-55
Rockville, MD 20857
Phone: (301)443-6745
Website: http://www.hrsa.gov

Cat. No: 93.914 **Objectives:** To provide emergency assistance to localities that are disproportionately affected by the Human Immunodeficiency Virus (HIV) epidemic and to make financial assistance available to states and other public or private nonprofit entities to provide for the development, organization, coordination and operation of more effective and cost efficient systems for the delivery of essential services to individuals and families with HIV disease. **Assist. Types:** Project grants. **Applicant Eligibility:** Metropolitan areas reporting more than 2,000 cases of AIDS as of March 31, 1993, as defined in the Centers for Disease Control HIV Surveillance Report, include: Atlanta, Georgia; Baltimore, Maryland; Boston, Massachusetts; Chicago, Illinois; Dallas, Texas; Ft. Lauderdale, Florida; Houston, Texas; Los Angeles, California; Miami, Florida; New York, New York; Newark, New Jersey; Oakland, California; Philadelphia, Pennsylvania; San Diego, California; San Francisco, California; San Juan, Puerto Rico; Washington, DC.; Orange County, California; Nassau/Suffolk Counties, New York; Detroit, Michigan; Seattle, Washington; New Orleans, Louisiana; and Tampa/St. Petersburg, Florida; Ponce, Puerto Rico; Patterson, New Jersey; Denver, Colorado; Kansas City, Missouri; New Haven, Connecticut; Orange County, Florida; Phoenix, Arizona; San Bernardino, California; St. Louis, Missouri; West Palm Beach, Florida; Jacksonville, Florida; Austin, Texas; San Antonio, Texas; and Portland Oregon. Metropolitan areas that have a per capita indicence of reported AIDS cases of 0.0025, as defined by the Centers for Disease Control HIV Surveillance Report, include Jersey City, New Jersey, Ponce, Puerto Rico; Caguas, Puerto Rico; Dutchess County, New York; Vineland, New Jersey; Santa Rosa, California. **Beneficiary Eligibility:** Individuals and families with HIV disease.

★ 20527 ★ U.S. Department of Health and Human Services
Health Resources and Services Administration
HIV/AIDS Bureau
Ryan White HIV / AIDS Dental Reimbursements
5600 Fishers Ln., Rm. 7A-21
Rockville, MD 20857
Phone: (301)443-1434

Cat. No: 93.924 **Objectives:** To compensate dental schools and postdoctoral dental education programs for unreimbursed costs they have incurred in providing oral health services to human immunodeficiency virus or acquired immunodeficiency syndrome (HIV/AIDS) patients. **Assist. Types:** Direct payments for specified use. **Applicant Eligibility:** Public or private nonprofit schools of dentistry or accredited post-graduate dental training programs, located in the 50 United States, the District of Columbia, and U.S. Territories. **Beneficiary Eligibility:** Any public or private nonprofit school of dentistry or accredited post-graduate dental institution.

★ 20528 ★ U.S. Department of Health and Human Services
Health Resources and Services Administration
Maternal and Child Health Bureau
Maternal and Child Health Federal Consolidated Programs
5600 Fishers Lane, Rm. 18-05
Rockville, MD 20857
Phone: (301)443-2170
Website: http://www.hrsa.gov

Cat. No: 93.110 **Objectives:** To carry out special projects of regional and national significance; conduct training, and research; conduct genetic disease testing, counseling, and information development and dissemination programs; and support comprehensive hemophilia diagnostic and treatment centers. **Assist. Types:** Project grants. **Applicant Eligibility:** Training grants may be made to public or private nonprofit institutions of higher learning. Research grants may be made to public or private nonprofit institutions of higher learning, and public or private nonprofit agencies and organizations engaged in research, or in Maternal and Child Health or Children with Special Health Care Needs programs. Any public or private entity is eligible for hemophilia and genetics grants and special projects grants. **Beneficiary Eligibility:** For training grants: (1) trainees in the maternal and child health professions; and (2) mothers and children who receive services through training programs. For research grants: public or private nonprofit agencies and organizations engaged in research or in maternal and child health or children with special health care needs programs. For hemophilia, genetics and special projects: (1) public or private agencies, organizations and institutions; and (2) mothers and children, and persons with hemophilia (any age), who receive services through the programs.

★ 20529 ★ U.S. Department of Health and Human Services
Health Resources and Services Administration
Migrant Health Branch
Health Centers Grants for Migrant and Seasonal Farmworkers
4350 East-West Hwy., 7th Fl.
Bethesda, MD 20814
Phone: (301)594-4160
Email: amata@hrsa.gov
Website: http://www.hrsa.gov
Benjamin Flores, Contact

Cat. No: 93.246 **Objectives:** To support the development and operation of migrant health centers and projects which provide primary health care services, supplemental health services, and environmental health services which are accessible to migrant and seasonal agricultural farm workers and their families as they move and work. **Assist. Types:** Project grants. **Applicant Eligibility:** Any public or nonprofit private entity. **Beneficiary Eligibility:** Migratory agricultural workers, seasonal agricultural workers, and members of their families.

★ 20530 ★ U.S. Department of Health and Human Services
Health Resources and Services Administration
Office of Rural Health Policy
Development and Coordination of Rural Health Services
5600 Fishers Lane, Rm. 9A-55
Rockville, MD 20857
Phone: (301)443-0835 **Fax:** (301)443-2803
Website: http://www.ruralhealth.hrsa.gov

Cat. No: 93.223 **Objectives:** To develop and disseminate information to assist rural communities and rural health care organization in developing and coordinating rural health care services. Sources of information include, but are not limited to, Federal and State agencies working in rural health care, health publications, research reports, and reports from national health care associations. **Assist. Types:** Projects grants (cooperative agreements). **Applicant Eligibility:** Nonprofit private organizations that represent national, State and local health constituencies. The applicant must represent State and local constituency groups who are interested in and committed to improvements in rural health care. **Beneficiary Eligibility:** Underserved populations in rural areas and rural health care providerswishing to expand their services. Rural health care advocacy groups and their constituents.

★ 20531 ★ U.S. Department of Health and Human Services
Health Resources and Services Administration
Office of Rural Health Policy
Grants to States for Operation of Offices of Rural Health
5600 Fishers Ln., Rm. 9A-55
Rockville, MD 20857
Phone: (301)443-0835
Website: http://www.ruralhealth.hrsa.gov

Cat. No: 93.913 **Objectives:** To improve health care in rural areas through the establishment of state offices of rural health. **Assist. Types:** Project grants. **Applicant Eligibility:** The 50 states. **Beneficiary Eligibility:** Underserved populations in rural areas; facilities and services in rural areas.

★ 20532 ★ U.S. Department of Health and Human Services
Health Resources and Services Administration
Office of Rural Health Policy
Rural Health Outreach and Rural Network Development Program
5600 Fishers Ln., Rm. 9A-55
Rockville, MD 20857
Phone: (301)443-7529 **Fax:** (301)443-2803
Website: http://www.hrsa.gov/oa.html

Cat. No: 93.912 **Objectives:** To enable services to be provided to rural populations that are not receiving them; to enhance service capacity or expand service area(s), thus, increasing the number of individuals and families receiving services; to facilitate integration and coordination of services in or among rural communities; and to enhance linkages, integration and cooperation among the various entities eligible to receive grants. **Assist. Types:** Project grants. **Applicant Eligibility:** Not-for-profit, public or private entities located in a non-metropolitan statistical area or a rural area within selected large MSAS are eligible to apply for grant funds. **Beneficiary Eligibility:** Medically underserved populations in rural areas will receive expanded services in rural communities where they did not previously exist.

★ 20533 ★ U.S. Department of Health and Human Services
Health Resources and Services Administration
Office of Rural Health Policy
Rural Health Research Centers
5600 Fishers Lane, Rm. 9A-55
Rockville, MD 20857
Phone: (301)443-0835 **Fax:** (301)443-2803
Website: http://www.ruralhealth.hrsa.gov
Joan Van Nostrand, Contact

CAT 93.155 **Objectives:** To support the operation of rural health research cneters to provide an information base and policy analysis capability on the full range of rural health services issues, including financing, recruitment, and retention of health professionals, access to care, and rural delivery systems. **Assist. Types:** Project grants. **Applicant Eligibility:** All public and private entities, nonprofit and for profit, are eligible to apply. **Beneficiary Eligibility:** Health care personnel, health research personnel, and the general public.

★ 20534 ★ U.S. Department of Health and Human Services
Health Resources and Services Administration
Office of Rural Health Policy
Rural Telemedicine Grants
5600 Fishers Lane, Rm. 11A-16
Rockville, MD 20857
Phone: (301)443-1293
Website: http://www.telehealth.hrsa.gov

Cat. No: 93.211 **Objectives:** To demonstrate and collect information on the feasibility, costs, appropriateness, and acceptability (to practitioners and patients) of telemedicine for improving access to health services for rural residents and reducing the isolation of rural practitioners and to demonstrate how telemedicine can be used as an effective tool for the development of integrated systems of health care for rural areas. **Assist. Types:** Project grants. **Applicant Eligibility:** Nonprofit public (non-federal) or private entities, non-profit or for profit, that can provide a wide range of medical specialty consultation services on a 24-hour basis to rural sites using telecommunications. **Beneficiary Eligibility:** Rural health care providers, patients, and rural communities.

★ 20535 ★ U.S. Department of Health and Human Services
Health Resources and Services Administration
Primary Care Services—Resource Coordination and Development
5600 Fishers Lane, Rm. 9-105
Rockville, MD 20857
Phone: (301)443-1648
Website: http://www.hrsa.gov

Cat. No: 93.130 **Objectives:** To coordinate local, state, and federal resources contributing to primary care service delivery in the state to meet the needs of medically-underserved populations through health centers and other community-based providers of comprehensive primary care, and the retention, recruitment, and oversight of the health professions for medically underserved populations. **Assist. Types:** Project grants. **Applicant Eligibility:** Cooperative agreements will be made to a state, state agency, or other statewide public or nonprofit entity that operates solely within one state. **Beneficiary Eligibility:** Same as Applicant Eligibility.

★ 20536 ★ U.S. Department of Health and Human Services
Health Resources and Services Administration
Primary Health Care Bureau
Health Center Grants for Homeless Populations
4350 East-West Hwy., 9th Fl.
Bethesda, MD 20814

Phone: (301)594-4430
Website: http://www.hrsa.gov

Cat. No: 93.151 **Objectives:** To award grants for the purpose of enabling grantees, directly or through contracts, to provide for the delivery of primary health services and substance abuse (alcohol and/or illicit drugs) services to homeless individuals including homeless children. **Assist. Types:** Prcject grants. **Applicant Eligibility:** Nonprofit private organizations and public entities, including state and local government agencies. **Beneficiary Eligibility:** Homeless individuals including children, elderly persons, handicapped persons, families with children, Native Americans, and veterans.

★ 20537 ★ U.S. Department of Health and Human Services
Indian Health Service
Division of Acquisitions and Grants Management
Health Professions Recruitment Program for Indians

801 Thompson Ave., Ste. 120
Rockville, MD 20852
Phone: (301)443-5204
Website: http://www.ihs.gov

Cat. No: 93.970 **Objectives:** To identify American Indians and native Alaskans with a potential for education or training in the health professions, and to encourage and assist them in enrolling in health or allied health professional schools; and to increase the number of nurses, nurse mid-wives, and nurse practitioners who deliver health care services to American Indians and native Alaskans. **Assist. Types:** Project grants; project grants (cooperative agreements). **Applicant Eligibility:** Public or private nonprofit health or educational entities or Indian tribes or tribal organizations. **Beneficiary Eligibility:** Preference is given to applicants in the following order of priority: (1) Indian tribes, (2) tribal organizations, (3) urban Indian organizations and other Indian health organizations, (4) other public or nonprofit health or educational entities.

★ 20538 ★ U.S. Department of Health and Human Services
Indian Health Service
Division of Acquisitions and Grants Management
Indian Health Service—Health Management Development Program

801 Thompson Ave., Ste. 120
Rockville, MD 20852
Phone: (301)443-5204
Website: http://www.ihs.gov

Cat. No: 93.228 **Objectives:** To improve the quality of the health of American Indians and native Alaskans by providing a full range of curative, preventive, and rehabilitative health services; and to increase the capability of American Indians and native Alaskans to manage their own health programs. **Assist. Types:** Project grants. **Applicant Eligibility:** Federally recognized tribes and tribal organizations. **Beneficiary Eligibility:** Generally, individuals who are members of an eligible applicant tribe, band, group, or village.

★ 20539 ★ U.S. Department of Health and Human Services
Indian Health Service
IHS Scholarship Program
Health Professions Pregraduate Scholarship Program for Indians

801 Thompson Ave., Ste. 120
Rockville, MD 20852
Phone: (301)443-6197
Website: http://www.ihs.gov

Cat. No: 93.123 **Objectives:** To provide scholarships to American Indians and native Alaskans for the purpose of completing pregraduate education leading to a baccalaureate degree only in the following areas: (1) Pre-Medicine: priority as follows: senior, junior, sophomore, freshman; (2) Pre-Dentistry: priority as follows: senior, junior, sophomore, freshman. **Assist. Types:** Project grants. **Applicant Eligibility:** Individuals of American Indian or native Alaskan descent, who have successfully completed high school or equivalency, and have been accepted for enrollment in an accredited pregraduate program in a health profession. **Beneficiary Eligibility:** Same as Applicant Eligibility.

★ 20540 ★ U.S. Department of Health and Human Services
Indian Health Service
IHS Scholarship Program
Health Professions Preparatory Scholarship Program for Indians

801 Thompson Ave., Ste. 120
Rockville, MD 20852
Phone: (301)443-6197
Website: http://www.ihs.gov

Cat. No: 93.971 **Objectives:** To make scholarship grants to American Indians and natives of Alaska for the purpose of completing compensatory pre-professional education to enable the recipient to qualify for enrollment or re-enrollment in a health professions school or curriculum. **Assist. Types:** Project grants. **Applicant Eligibility:** Individuals of American Indian or native Alaskan descent who have successfully completed high school education or high school equivalency. **Beneficiary Eligibility:** Same as Applicant Eligibility.

★ 20541 ★ U.S. Department of Health and Human Services
Indian Health Service
IHS Scholarship Program
Health Professions Scholarship Program

801 Thompson Ave., Ste. 120
Rockville, MD 20852
Phone: (301)443-6197
Website: http://www.ihs.gov

Cat. No: 93.972 **Objectives:** To provide scholarships to American Indians and Native Alaskans at health professions schools in order to obtain health professionals to serve Indians. **Assist. Types:** Project grants. **Applicant Eligibility:** Individuals of American native Indian or Alaskan descent are eligible. **Beneficiary Eligibility:** Individuals of American native Indian or Alaskan descent; full-time students of medicine or other health professions; prospective or currently commissioned officers in the Regular or Reserve Corps of the Public Health Services; and eligible civilians of the Indian Health Service.

★ 20542 ★ U.S. Department of Health and Human Services
Indian Health Service
IHS Scholarship Program
Matching Grants for Health Professions Scholarships to Indian Tribes

801 Thompson Ave., Ste. 120
Rockville, MD 20852
Phone: (301)443-5204
Website: http://www.ihs.gov

Cat. No: 93.219 **Objectives:** To provide scholarships to Indians for health professions education through Indian tribes and tribal organizations. **Assist. Types:** Project grants. **Applicant Eligibility:** An federally-recognized Indian tribe or tribal organization is eligible to aply for a grant. **Beneficiary Eligibility:** Members of a federally-recognized Indian tribe or tribal organization.

★ 20543 ★ U.S. Department of Health and Human Services
Indian Health Service
Loan Repayment Program
Indian Health Service Educational Loan Repayment

801 Thompson Ave., Ste. 120
Rockville, MD 20852
Phone: (301)443-3396
Email: cahhaitt@smtp.ihs.gov
Website: http://www.ihs.gov

Cat. No: 93.164 **Objectives:** To help insure an adequate supply of trained health professionals for Indian Health Service (IHS) facilities by providing for the repayment of educational loans for participants who agree (by written contract) to serve an applicable period of time at a facility IHS has designated as a Priority Site or in a designated specialty at a site with an appropriate position. **Assist. Types:** Project grants. **Applicant Eligibility:** (1) Individuals who (a) are enrolled as full-time students in the final year of a course of study or program leading to a degree in allopathic or osteopathic medicine, dentistry, or other health profession in a state; (b) are enrolled in an approved graduate training program in allopathic or osteopathic medicine, dentistry, or other health profession; (c) have a degree in allopathic or osteopathic medicine, dentistry, or other health profession and have completed an approved graduate training program and have a current and valid license to practice such health profession in a state; (2) be eligible for appointment as a commissioned officer in the regular or reserve corps of the Public HealthService or are eligible for selection for civilian service in the IHS; or be an employee of a tribal health program or urban Indian Health program funded under Title V of Public Law 94-437 and its amendments; (3) submit an application to participate in the Loan Repayment Program, and (4) sign and submit to the Secretary for Health and Human Services, at the time of such application, a written contract agreeing to accept repayment of educational loans and to serve for the applicable period of service in a retention/recruitment site as determined by the Secretary. **Beneficiary Eligibility:** Health professionals who have unpaid educational loans.

★ 20544 ★ U.S. Department of Health and Human Services
Indian Health Service
Office of Tribal Self-Governance
Tribal Self-Governance Demonstration Program: Planning and Negotiation Cooperative Agreements and IHS Compacts

801 Thompson Ave., Ste. 240
Rockville, MD 20852
Phone: (301)443-7821 **Fax:** (301)443-1050
Website: http://www.ihs.gov

Cat. No: 93.210 **Objectives:** The Self-Governance Demonstration Program (SGDP) was established by the Congress as a demonstration project. The Planning and Negotiation Cooperative Agreement Program is authorized by Title III of the Indian Self-Determination and Education Assistance Act, Public Law (P.L.) 93-638, as amended. The purpose of the program is to award cooperative agreements that provide planning or negotiation resources to tribes interested in participating as prescribed by Public Law 96-502, the Single Audit Act of 1984, for the previous 3 yers that contain no significant or material audit exceptions. For each fiscal year, an additional 30 tribes may be eligible for selection to participate in the SGDP. **Beneficiary Eligibility:** Indian tribes.

★ 20545 ★ U.S. Department of Health and Human Services
National Institues of Health
Fogarty International Center
Minority International Research Training Grant in the Biomedical and Behavioral Sciences

NIH Bldg. 31, Rm. B2C32
9000 Rockville Pike
Bethesda, MD 20892-2220
Phone: (301)496-1653
Website: http://www.nih.gov/fic
Dr. Barbara Sina, Contact

Cat. No: 93.106 **Objectives:** To enable qualified minority undergraduate students, graduate students and faculty members to participate in international biomedical and behavioral research programs; to acquaint minority students and scientists with the full range of career opportunities in biomedical and behavioral research; to strengthen teaching programs at U.S. institutions; and to strengthen ties with research institutes abroad. **Assist. Types:** Project grants. **Applicant Eligibility:** Two or four year domestic schools, colleges or universities may apply or consortiums comprised of the two or four year schools, colleges or universities. **Beneficiary Eligibility:** African American, Hispanic American, Native American, and Pacific Islander undergraduate and graduate students and faculty members.

★ 20546 ★ U.S. Department of Health and Human Services
National Institues of Health
National Center for Research Resources
Biomedical Technology
6705 Rockledge Dr., Rm. 6160
Bethesda, MD 20892-7965
Phone: (301)435-0755
Website: http://www.nih.gov

Cat. No: 93.371 **Objectives:** To assist academic, nonprofit organizations in the development, use, and dissemination of innovative technologies useful for the advance of biomedical science. **Assist. Types:** Project grants. **Applicant Eligibility:** Institutions of higher education, hospitals, and other institutions and organizations with programs of biomedical research. **Beneficiary Eligibility:** Scientists at any nonprofit or for-profit organization or institution engaged in biomedical research.

★ 20547 ★ U.S. Department of Health and Human Services
National Institues of Health
National Center for Research Resources
Comparative Medicine
6705 Rockledge Dr., Rm. 6168
Bethesda, MD 20892-7965
Phone: (301)435-0744 **Fax:** (301)480-3819
Email: LeoW@ep.ncrr.nik.gov
Website: http://www.hhs.gov
Leo A. Whitehair, Director

Cat. No: 93.306 **Objectives:** To support resource projects that enable biomedical scientists to use animals effectively in research on human health problems. **Assist. Types:** Project grants. **Applicant Eligibility:** Institutions of higher education, hospitals, and other institutions and organizations seeking to establish, continue, or enlarge programs consistent with the objectives of the program. **Beneficiary Eligibility:** Investigators at for-profit and nonprofit hospitals, institutions of higher education, and other research institutions and organizations.

★ 20548 ★ U.S. Department of Health and Human Services
National Institues of Health
National Eye Institute
Vision Research
6120 Executive Blvd., Rm. 350
Bethesda, MD 20892
Phone: (301)451-2020
Website: http://www.nei.nih.gov

Cat. No: 93.867 **Objectives:** Supports vision research projects that address the leading causes of blindness and impaired vision in the U.S., including retinal deseases, corneal diseases, cataract, glaucoma, strabismuss, and amblyopia. Seeks to increase understanding of the normal development and function of the visual system; to understand the causes of, and better diagnose, prevent, and treat sight-threatening conditions; and to enhance the rehabilitation and training or individuals who are blind or partially-sighted. **Assist. Types:** Project grants. **Applicant Eligibility:** Research grant and cooperative agreement proposals eligible for support are those concerned with laboratory and clinical research on the causes, diagnosis, and prevention of retinal and choroidal diseases. Universities, colleges, hospitals, laboratories, federal institutions, state and local units of government, nonprofit or for-profit domestic institutions, including small businesses, are eligible to make application for research grants, cooperative agreements, and career development awards. Foreign institutions may apply for research grants only. NRSAs are provided for predoctoral and postdoctoral research training. Individual NRSAs may be made for applicants who hold a professional or scientific degree. **Beneficiary Eligibility:** Any nonprofit or for-profit organization, company, or institution engaged in research to protect and improve the visual health of the nation.

★ 20549 ★ U.S. Department of Health and Human Services
National Institues of Health
National Heart, Lung, and Blood Institute
Blood Diseases and Resources Research
6701 Rockledge Dr., Rm. 10160
Bethesda, MD 20892
Phone: (301)435-0080
Website: http://www.nhlbi.nih.gov

Cat. No: 93.839 **Objectives:** To foster research for the prevention and improved diagnosis and treatment of blood diseases; to promote research for improving the availability, safety, and use of blood products; and to develop new scientists for blood disease research. **Assist. Types:** Project grants; project grants (cooperative agreements). **Applicant Eligibility:** Any nonprofit organization engaged in biomedical research. Institutions or companies organized for profit may apply for grants and contracts, with the exception of NRS awards. An individual may apply for a NRS award or, in some cases, may qualify for a research grant if he has adequate facilities in which to perform the research. **Beneficiary Eligibility:** Any nonprofit or for-profit organization, company, or institution engaged in biomedical research.

★ 20550 ★ U.S. Department of Health and Human Services
National Institues of Health
National Institute of Dental and Craniofacial Research
Oral Diseases and Disorders Research
NIH Bldg. 45, Rm. 4AN-12
Bethesda, MD 20892
Phone: (301)594-7711 **Fax:** (301)480-8319
Website: http://www.nidr.nih.gov

Cat. No: 93.121 **Objectives:** To obtain improved information on the early diagnosis etiology and prevention of dental caries; develop improved restorative materials and devices, including dental implants, for the repair of damaged oral structures; develop new knowledge on the etiology, pathology, diagnosis, treatment, and prevention of periodontal and oral soft tissue diseases, the oral manifestations of AIDS, herpes simplex and candida albicans infections, and diseases of the tooth pulp; develop new knowledge of relationships between nutritional factors and oral health and of the benefits and risks of fluoride regimens in disease prevention; and improve the understanding of the role of salivary secretions in the prevention of oral disease; to conduct research on the cause, prevention, and treatment of cleft lip/palate, other craniofacial birth defects, malocclusion of the teeth and jaws, and disfigurements acquired through accidents and surgery to reduce their impact; to determine the vepidemiology pathogenesis, etiology, prevention and management of acute and chronic dental orificial pain conditions in order to develop more effective means of prevention, diagnosis, and treatment; to study normal and impaired oral-motor and oral-sensory function; and to determine how behavioral or social factors influence disease risks, prevention, diagnosis, and dental treatment. **Assist. Types:** Project grants. **Applicant Eligibility:** Grants: Scientists at universities, hospitals, laboratories, other public or private nonprofit and for-profit institutions. **Beneficiary Eligibility:** Any nonprofit or for-profit organization, company or institution engaged in biomedical research.

★ 20551 ★ U.S. Department of Health and Human Services
National Institues of Health
National Institute of Mental Health
Mental Health Research Career/Scientist Development Awards
6001 Executive Blvd., Rm. 6122
Bethesda, MD 20892
Phone: (301)443-3563
Website: http://www.nih.gov

Cat. No: 93.281 **Objectives:** To provide support for research relating to the problems of mental illness and mental health, to raise the level of competence, and to increase the number of individuals engaged in such research via special levels of National Institute of Mental Health support. **Assist. Types:** Project grants. **Applicant Eligibility:** Awards are made to appropriate research centers, medical schools, departments of psychiatry, non-medical academic departments, psychiatric hospitals or hospitals with psychiatric services, community mental health centers, biomedical research institutes, and department of behavioral science on behalf of individuals who need the opportunity to realize research potentials. **Beneficiary Eligibility:** Public and private profit or nonprofit organizations.

★ 20552 ★ U.S. Department of Health and Human Services
National Institues of Health
Fogarty International Center
International Cooperative Biodiversity Groups Program
31 Center Dr., MSC 2220
Bethesda, MD 20892-2220
Phone: (301)496-1653
Website: http://www.nih.gov
Dr. Joshua Rosenthal, Contact

Cat. No: 93.168 **Objectives:** (1) Discover, isolate, and evaluate preclinically, agents from natural sources to treat or prevent cancer, infectious diseases including AIDS, cardiovascular diseases, mental disorders, and other diseases or medical conditions of primary concern to developing countries. (2) Undertake inventories of biological diversity and develop collection practices compatible with conserving bio-diversity, and produce documentation of all collected material in the form of museum catalogues, published works, and/or databases, reporting specific locality and all features of biology relevant to standard botanical and zoological collections; assure accessibility of inventory data to all individuals, including those not associated with the International Cooperatavie Biodiversity Groups (ICBG), by housing catalogues and databases in public institutions (such as universities and national museums) and, when databases are kept on computer systems in private institutions, by including in publications specific references to these databases. (3) Support research training targeted toward the needs of the developing country or other countries represented within the Group and related to the scope of work of the Request for Applications (RFA), and to augment field experience and training of U.S. scientists in areas of knowledge unique to the developing country. **Assist. Types:** Project grants. **Applicant Eligibility:** Public and private nonprofit institutions, Governments, and their agencies, and foreign institutions are eligible to participate. **Beneficiary Eligibility:** At least one of the associate programs must be located in a developing country.

★ 20553 ★ U.S. Department of Health and Human Services
National Institues of Health
National Cancer Institute
Cancer Biology Research
6130 Executive Blvd., EPN-5000
Bethesda, MD 20892
Phone: (301)435-5255
Website: http://www.nih.gov

Cat. No: 93.396 **Objectives:** To provide fundamental information on the cause and nature of cancer in man with the expectation that this will result in better methods of prevention, detection, diagnosis, and treatment of neoplastic diseases. **Assist. Types:** Project grants (cooperative agreements). **Applicant Eligibility:** University, college, hospital, public agency, nonprofit research institution, or for-profit organization. **Beneficiary Eligibility:** Any nonprofit or for-profit organization, company, or institution engaged in biomedical research.

★ 20554 ★ U.S. Department of Health and Human Services
National Institutes of Health
National Cancer Institute
Cancer Cause and Prevention Research
6130 Executive Blvd., EPN 5113B
Bethesda, MD 20892
Phone: (301)496-9600
Website: http://www.nih.gov

Cat. No: 93.393 **Objectives:** To identify those factors which cause cancer in man, and to develop mechanisms for preventing cancer. **Lang(s):** Spanish. **Assist. Types:** Project grants (cooperative agreements). **Applicant Eligibility:** University, college, hospital, public agency, nonprofit research institution or for-profit organization. **Beneficiary Eligibility:** Any nonprofit or for-profit organization, company, or institution engaged in biomedical research on cancer.

★ 20555 ★ U.S. Department of Health and Human Services
National Institutes of Health
National Cancer Institute
Cancer Centers Support Grants
6116 Executive Blvd., Ste. 700
Bethesda, MD 20892
Phone: (301)496-8531
Website: http://www.nih.gov

Cat. No: 93.397 **Objectives:** To provide an organizational focus and stimulus for the highest quality cancer research that promotes interdisciplinary cancer research aimed toward the ultimate goal of reducing cancer incidence, mortality, and morbidity. **Assist. Types:** Project grants. **Applicant Eligibility:** The awardee will be a university, college, hospital, public agency, nonprofit research institution or for-profit organization that submits an application and receives a grant for support of research by a named principal investigator. **Beneficiary Eligibility:** Any nonprofit or for-profit organization, company, or institution engaged in biomedical research.

★ 20556 ★ U.S. Department of Health and Human Services
National Institutes of Health
National Cancer Institute
Cancer Control
6130 Evecutive Blvd., MSC 7309
Rockville, MD 20852
Phone: (301)496-6616
Email: bk76p@nih.gov
Website: http://www.nih.gov

Cat. No: 93.399 **Objectives:** To reduce cancer incidence, morbidity, and mortality through research on interventions and applications of this research. Primary emphasis is on the inclusion of a cancer control intervention in any proposed study. **Assist. Types:** Project grants (cooperative agreements). **Applicant Eligibility:** University, college, hospital, public agency, nonprofit research institution or for-profit organization. **Beneficiary Eligibility:** Same as Applicant Eligibility.

★ 20557 ★ U.S. Department of Health and Human Services
National Institutes of Health
National Cancer Institute
Cancer Detection and Diagnosis Research
6130 Executive Blvd., EPN-6035A
Bethesda, MD 20892
Phone: (301)496-8639
Website: http://www.nih.gov

Cat. No: 93.394 **Objectives:** To improve screening and early detection strategies and to develop accurate diagnostic techniques and methods for predicting the course of disease in cancer patients. **Assist. Types:** Project grants (cooperative agreements). **Applicant Eligibility:** University, college, hospital, public agency, nonprofit research institution or organization, or for-profit organization. **Beneficiary Eligibility:** Any nonprofit or for-profit organization, company, or institution engaged in biomedical research.

★ 20558 ★ U.S. Department of Health and Human Services
National Institutes of Health
National Cancer Institute
Cancer Research Manpower
6116 Executive Blvd., Rm. 7019
Bethesda, MD 20892
Phone: (301)496-8580
Website: http://www.nih.gov

Cat. No: 93.398 **Objectives:** To make available grant support for profit and nonprofit institutions interested in providing biomedical training opportunities for individuals interested in careers in basic and clinical research to support important areas of the National Cancer Program. **Assist. Types:** Project grants. **Applicant Eligibility:** University, college, hospital, public agency, or nonprofit research institution for institutional grants, and individuals for fellowships. **Beneficiary Eligibility:** Same as Applicant Eligibility.

★ 20559 ★ U.S. Department of Health and Human Services
National Institutes of Health
National Cancer Institute
Cancer Treatment Research
NIH Bldg. 31, Rm. 3A44
9000 Rockville Pike
Bethesda, MD 20892-2440
Phone: (301)496-4291 **Fax:** (301)496-0826
Email: wittes@nih.gov
Website: http://www.nci.nih.gov

Cat. No: 93.395 **Objectives:** To develop the means to diagnose accurately and cure as many cancer patients as possible and to control the disease in those patients who are not cured. **Assist. Types:** Grants and cooperative agents. **Applicant Eligibility:** University, college, hospital, public agency, nonprofit research institution or for-profit organization. **Beneficiary Eligibility:** Any nonprofit or for-profit organization, company, or institution engaged in biomedical research.

★ 20560 ★ U.S. Department of Health and Human Services
National Institutes of Health
National Center for Complementary and Alternative Medicine
Research and Training in Complementary and Alternative Medicine
6707 Democracy Blvd., Ste. 401
Bethesda, MD 20892-5475
Phone: (301)496-4792 **Free:** 888-644-6226
Fax: (301)402-4741
Website: http://www.alt.od.nih.gov

Cat. No: 93.213 **Objectives:** To evaluate alternative or unconventional medical treatments. **Assist. Types:** Project grants. **Applicant Eligibility:** The awardee will be either a university, college, hospital, public agency, nonprofit research institutions, or for-profit organization that submits an application and receives a grant or cooperative agreement for support of research by a named principal investigator. For those Investigators who will submit proposals for training areas outside of conventional medicine such as acupuncture, chiropractic, or homeopathy can be included. **Beneficiary Eligibility:** Any nonprofit or for-profit organization, company, or institution engaged in biomedical research.

★ 20561 ★ U.S. Department of Health and Human Services
National Institutes of Health
National Center for Research Resources
Clinical Research
6705 Rockledge Dr., Rm. 6120
MSC-7965
Bethesda, MD 20892-7965
Phone: (301)435-0790 **Fax:** (301)480-3661
Website: http://www.ncrr.nih.gov
Inese Z. Beitins, MD, Director

Cat. No: 93.333 **Objectives:** To create and sustain specialized institutional resources in which clinical investigators can observe and study human physiology and disease/disorder, as well as study and treat disease with innovative approaches. **Assist. Types:** Project grants. **Applicant Eligibility:** Medical Schools, research hospitals, and other institutions capable of carrying out well-designed studies in any pre-clinical or clinical science involving human beings as research subjects. **Beneficiary Eligibility:** Biomedical investigators at any nonprofit or for-profit organization, company, or institution engaged in biomedical research.

★ 20562 ★ U.S. Department of Health and Human Services
National Institutes of Health
National Center for Research Resources
Research Infrastructure
6705 Rockledge Dr., Rm. 6136
Bethesda, MD 20892-7965
Phone: (301)435-0788
Website: http://www.nih.gov

Cat. No: 93.389 **Objectives:** To expand the national capability for research in the health sciences by: (1) assisting predominantly minority institutions that offer doctoral degrees in health professions and/or related health sciences; and (2) enhancing significantly the capacity for the conduct of biomedical and/or behavioral research at such minority institutions by strengthening their research environment. **Assist. Types:** Project grants. **Applicant Eligibility:** An institution must have more than 50 percent minority enrollment, award an M.D., a D.D.S., or D.V.M., or other doctoral degree in the health professions and/or a Ph.D. in the sciences related to health. **Beneficiary Eligibility:** Institutions described above and the faculty and students of such institutions.

★ 20563 ★ U.S. Department of Health and Human Services
National Institutes of Health
National Heart, Lung, and Blood Institute
Heart and Vascular Diseases Research
6701 Rockledge Dr., Rm. 9170
Bethesda, MD 20892
Phone: (301)435-0466
Website: http://www.nih.gov

Cat. No: 93.837 **Objectives:** To foster research and prevention, education, and control activities related to heart and vascular diseases, and to develop young scientific investigators in these areas. **Assist. Types:** Project grants; project grants (cooperative agreements). **Applicant Eligibility:** Any nonprofit organization engaged in biomedical research. Institutions or companies organized for profit may apply for grants with the exception of NRS awards. An individual may apply for a NRS award or, in some cases, for a research grant if adequate facilities in which to perform the research are available. **Beneficiary Eligibility:** Any nonprofit or for-profit organization, company, or institution engaged in biomedical research.

★ 20564 ★ U.S. Department of Health and Human Services
National Institutes of Health
National Heart, Lung, and Blood Institute
Lung Diseases Research
6701 Rockledge Dr., Rm. 10122
Bethesda, MD 20892

Phone: (301)435-0233 **Fax:** (301)480-3547
Website: http://www.nhlbi.nih.gov

Cat. No: 93.838 **Objectives:** To use available knowledge and technology to solve specific disease problems of the lungs; to promote further studies on the structure and function of the lung; and to achieve improvement in prevention and treatment of lung diseases. **Assist. Types:** Project grants (cooperative agreements). **Applicant Eligibility:** Any nonprofit organization engaged in biomedical research. Institutions or companies organized for profit may apply for grants and contracts, with the exception of NRS awards. An individual may apply for a NRS award or, in some cases, may qualify for a research grant if adequate facilities in which to perform the research are available. **Beneficiary Eligibility:** Any nonprofit or for-profit organization, company, or institution engaged in biomedical research.

★ 20565 ★ U.S. Department of Health and Human Services
National Institutes of Health
National Institute on Aging
Aging Research
7201 Wisconsin Ave., Rm. 2C231
Bethesda, MD 20892
Phone: (301)496-4996 **Fax:** (301)402-0010
Website: http://www.nia.nih.gov

Cat. No: 93.866 **Objectives:** To encourage biomedical, social, and behavioral research and research training directed toward greater understanding of the aging process and the diseases, special problems, and needs of people as they age. **Assist. Types:** Project grants. **Applicant Eligibility:** Grants are awarded to: universities; colleges; medical, dental, and nursing schools; schools of public health; laboratories; hospitals; state and local health departments; other public or private institutions, both profit and nonprofit; and individuals. National Research Service Awards may be made for postdoctoral training to applicants who hold a professional or scientific degree. **Beneficiary Eligibility:** Any nonprofit or for-profit organization, company, or institution engaged in biomedical research.

★ 20566 ★ U.S. Department of Health and Human Services
National Institutes of Health
National Institute on Alcohol Abuse and Alcoholism
Alcohol National Research Service Awards for Research Training
6000 Executive Blvd., Rm. 402
Rockville, MD 20852
Phone: (301)443-2530
Website: http://www.nih.gov

Cat. No: 93.272 **Objectives:** To assure the maintenance of an adequate supply of well-trained alcohol researchers through the provision of both individual fellowships and grants to training institutions for support of training at both the predoctoral and postdoctoral levels. Awards are made for training in clinical research, treatment assessment research, problems of health promotion and alcoholism prevention, and basic biological and behavioral processes applicable to alcohol research. **Assist. Types:** Project grants. **Applicant Eligibility:** Domestic public or private nonprofit organizations may apply for training grants. The applicant institution must have, or be able to develop, the staff and facilities to provide the proposed research training in an environment suitable for performing high quality work. An applicant for individual predoctoral support must have completed 2 or more years of graduate work and be enrolled in a doctoral degree program. A postdoctoral applicant must have received a doctoral degree. **Beneficiary Eligibility:** Individuals; public and private nonprofit organizations.

★ 20567 ★ U.S. Department of Health and Human Services
National Institutes of Health
National Institute on Alcohol Abuse and Alcoholism
Alcohol Research and Career Development Awards for Scientists and Clinicians
6000 Executive Blvd., Rm. 402
Rockville, MD 20852
Phone: (301)443-2530
Website: http://www.nih.gov

Cat. No: 93.271 **Objectives:** To provide support for increased research experience relating to the problems of alcohol abuse and alcoholism prevention, treatment, and rehabilitation; to raise the level of competence; and to increase the number of individuals engaged in such research. **Assist. Types:** Project grants. **Applicant Eligibility:** Mentored Research Scientist Devlopment Awards, Mentored Clinical Scientist Development Awards, Independent Scientist Awards, Senior Scientist Awards, and Academic Career Awards for Clinical faculty are made to appropriate research centers; medical schools, departments of psychiatry, non-medical academic departments, psychiatric hospitals or hospitals with psychiatric services, community mental health centers, biomedical research institutes, and departments of behavioral science on behalf of individuals who need the opportunity to realize research potentials. **Beneficiary Eligibility:** Public and private profit or nonprofit organizations.

★ 20568 ★ U.S. Department of Health and Human Services
National Institutes of Health
National Institute on Alcohol Abuse and Alcoholism
Alcohol Research Center Grants
6000 Executive Blvd., Rm. 402
Rockville, MD 20852
Phone: (301)443-2351
Website: http://www.nih.gov

Cat. No: 93.891 **Objectives:** To provide long-term support for a concerted and multi-disciplinary research effort into the problems of alcohol use and alcoholism by coordinating the activities of investigators from biomedical, behavioral, and social science disciplines around a basic research theme. An alcohol research center is expected to realize its greater potential for contributing to the basic store of knowledge about alcohol and alcoholism and to become a significant regional and national source. **Assist. Types:** Project grants. **Applicant Eligibility:** State and local governments, any domestic (non-federal) public or nonprofit private institution may apply for a center grant. The proposed center must be affiliated with an institution, such as a university, medical center, or research center, that has the resources to sustain a long-term coordinated research program around a central theme related to problems of alcohol use and alcoholism. An applicant institution must demonstrate the ability to attract high quality scientists from biomedical, behavioral, and social science disciplines who are willing to make a long-term commitment to alcohol research. In addition, the applicant must assure that alcoholism related research and clinical training opportunities will be available. **Beneficiary Eligibility:** Public and private nonprofit organizations.

★ 20569 ★ U.S. Department of Health and Human Services
National Institutes of Health
National Institute on Alcohol Abuse and Alcoholism
Alcohol Research Programs
6000 Executive Blvd., Rm. 402
Rockville, MD 20852
Phone: (301)443-2530
Website: http://www.nih.gov

Cat. No: 93.273 **Objectives:** To develop a sound fundamental knowledge base which can be applied to the development of improved methods of treatment and more effective strategies for preventing alcoholism and alcohol-related problems. The National Institute on Alcohol Abuse and Alcoholism (NIAAA) supports research in a broad range of discipline and subject areas related to biomedical and genetic factors, psychological and environmental factors, and alcohol-related problems and medical disorders. **Assist. Types:** Project grants (cooperative agreements). **Applicant Eligibility:** Public or private profit and nonprofit agencies, including state, local, or regional government agencies, universities, colleges, hospitals, academic or research institutions. **Beneficiary Eligibility:** Same as Applicant Eligibility.

★ 20570 ★ U.S. Department of Health and Human Services
National Institutes of Health
National Institute of Allergy and Infectious Diseases
Allergy, Immunology, and Transplantation Research
Solar Bldg., Rm. 3C20
9000 Rockville Pike
Bethesda, MD 20892
Phone: (301)496-7291
Website: http://www.nih.gov

Cat. No: 93.855 **Objectives:** To assist public and private nonprofit institutions and individuals to establish, expand, and improve biomedical research and research training in allergical and immunological diseases and related areas; to assist public, private and commercial institutions to conduct developmental research; to produce and test research materials; and to provide research services as required by the agency for research progress in allergical and immunological diseases. **Assist. Types:** Project grants. **Applicant Eligibility:** Universities, colleges, hospitals, laboratories, and other public or private nonprofit domestic institutions, including state and local units of government, and individuals. For-profit organizations are also eligible, with the exception of NRSA and BRSG programs. **Beneficiary Eligibility:** Any nonprofit or for-profit organization, company, or institution engaged in biomedical research.

★ 20571 ★ U.S. Department of Health and Human Services
National Institutes of Health
National Institute of Allergy and Infectious Diseases
Microbiology and Infectious Diseases Research
Solar Bldg., Rm. 3C20
9000 Rockville Pike
Bethesda, MD 20892
Phone: (301)496-7291
Website: http://www.nih.gov

Cat. No: 93.856 **Objectives:** To support research related to microbiology and infectious diseases with the broad aim of improving health by controlling disease caused by infectious or parasitic agents. **Assist. Types:** Project grants. **Applicant Eligibility:** Universities, colleges, hospitals, laboratories and other public or private nonprofit domestic institutions, including state and local units of government, and individuals. For-profit organizations are also eligible, with the exception of NRSA and BRSG programs. **Beneficiary Eligibility:** Any nonprofit or for-profit organization, company, or institution engaged in biomedical research.

★ 20572 ★ U.S. Department of Health and Human Services
National Institutes of Health
National Institute of Arthritis, and Musculoskeletal and Skin Diseases
Arthritis, Musculoskeletal and Skin Diseases Research
Natcher Bldg., Rm. 5AS-13F
45 Center Dr., MSC 6500
Bethesda, MD 20892-6500
Phone: (301)594-2463

Website: http://www.nih.gov/niams

Cat. No: 93.846 **Objectives:** To support research relevant to arthrities, muscoloskeletal and skin diseases, the National Institute of Arthritis and Musculoskeletel and skin diseases (NIAMS) supports research training and basic and clinical investigations including epidemiology and clinical trials in each of the following program areas: Arthrities, Muscle Biology, Muscoskeletal Diseases, and Skin Diseases. The Centers Program supports large programs in arthritis and muscoskeletal and skin disease. **Assist. Types:** Project grants. **Applicant Eligibility:** Research grants are awarded to individuals, and public and private institutions, both nonprofit and for-profit, who propose to establish, expand, and improve research activities in health sciences and realated fields. National Research Service Awards are to individuals. Nonprofit domestic organizations may apply for the Institutional National Research Service grant. **Beneficiary Eligibility:** Same as Applicant Eligibility.

★ 20573 ★ U.S. Department of Health and Human Services
National Institutes of Health
National Institute of Child Health and Human Development
Contraception and Infertility Research Loan Repayment Program

9000 Rockville Pike
Bethesda, MD 20892
Phone: (301)496-6515 **Fax:** (301)496-0962
Email: ld38p@mih.gov
Website: http://nichd.nih.gov/cpr-rs/repayment-program.html

Cat. No: 93.209 **Objectives:** The CIR-LRP is designed to provide an incentive for health professionals to work in areas of reproductive research directly related to contraceptive development and/or infertility diagnosis and treatment by providing assistance in repaying educational loans for individuals. **Assist. Types:** Direct payments for specified use. **Applicant Eligibility:** Qualified health and allied professionals including, but not limited to, physicians, scientists, nurses and physician assistants, as well as graduate students and postgraduate research fellows training in the health professions. **Beneficiary Eligibility:** Assistance in the form of loan repayments will be made to qualified health professionals (including graduate students) who are participants in the CIR-LRP.

★ 20574 ★ U.S. Department of Health and Human Services
National Institutes of Health
National Institute of Child Health and Human Development
Population Research

NIH Rm. 8B07
9000 Rockville Pike
Bethesda, MD 20892
Phone: (301)496-1101
Website: http://www.nichd.nih.gov

Cat. No: 93.864 **Objectives:** To seek solutions to the fundamental problems of the reproductive processes, to strive to develop and evaluate safer and more effective contraceptives, and works to understand how population structure and change affect the health and well-being of individuals and society. **Assist. Types:** Project grants. **Applicant Eligibility:** Grants are made to universities; colleges; medical, dental, and nursing schools; schools of public health; laboratories; hospitals; state and local health departments; other for-profit public or private institutions; and individuals. National Research Service Awards provide support for academic and research training only, in health and health-related areas which are periodically specified by National Institutes of Health. Domestic organizations may apply for the Institutional NRSA grant. **Beneficiary Eligibility:** Any nonprofit or for-profit organization, company, or institution engaged in biomedical research.

★ 20575 ★ U.S. Department of Health and Human Services
National Institutes of Health
National Institute of Diabetes and Digestive and Kidney Diseases
Diabetes, Endocrinology and Metabolism Research

NIH Bldg. 31, Rm. 9A16
31 Center Dr., MSC 2560
Bethesda, MD 20892-2560
Phone: (301)496-7348
Email: eastmand@extra.niddk.nih.gov
Website: http://www.niddk.nih.gov

Cat. No: 93.847 **Objectives:** To encourage basic and clinical biomedical research and research training for a greater understanding of diabetes and the underlying mechanisms that cause diabetes and related complications. To support extramural basic laboratory research and clinical investigations and to provide postdoctoral biomedical research training for individuals interested in careers in health sciences and fields related to these programs. **Assist. Types:** Project grants. **Applicant Eligibility:** Research grants are awarded to individuals, and public and private institutions, both nonprofit and for-profit, who propose to establish, expand, and improve research activities in health sciences and related fields. National Research Service Awards are given to individuals. Nonprofit domestic organizations may apply for the institutional National Research Service grant. **Beneficiary Eligibility:** Same as Applicant Eligibility.

★ 20576 ★ U.S. Department of Health and Human Services
National Institutes of Health
National Institute of Diabetes and Digestive and Kidney Diseases
Digestive Diseases and Nutrition Research

31 Center Dr., No. 9A23
Bethesda, MD 20892-2560
Phone: (301)496-1333
Website: http://www.niddk.nih.gov

Cat. No: 93.848 **Objectives:** To extramurally support basic laboratory research and clinical investigations and to provide postdoctoral biomedical research training for individuals interested in careers in health sciences and fields related to these programs. **Assist. Types:** Project grants. **Applicant Eligibility:** Research grants are awarded to individuals, and public and private institutions, both nonprofit and for-profit, who propose to establish, expand, and improve research activities in health sciences and related fields. National Research Service Awards are given to individuals. Nonprofit domestic organizations may apply for the institutional National Research Service grant. **Beneficiary Eligibility:** Same as Applicant Eligibility.

★ 20577 ★ U.S. Department of Health and Human Services
National Institutes of Health
National Institute of Diabetes and Digestive and Kidney Diseases
Kidney Diseases, Urology and Hematology Research

NIH Bldg. 31, Rm. 9A17
9000 Rockville Pike
Bethesda, MD 20892
Phone: (301)496-6325
Website: http://www.niddk.nih.gov
Josephine Briggs, Director

Cat. No: 93.849 **Objectives:** To extramurally support basic laboratory research and clinical investigations and to provide postdoctoral biomedical research training for individuals interested in careers in health sciences and fields related to these programs. **Assist. Types:** Project grants. **Applicant Eligibility:** Research grants are awarded to individuals, and public and private institutions, both nonprofit and for-profit, who propose to establish, expand, and improve research activities in health sciences and related fields. National Research Service Awards are given to individuals. Nonprofit domestic organizations may apply for the institutional National Research Service grant. **Beneficiary Eligibility:** Same as Applicant Eligibility.

★ 20578 ★ U.S. Department of Health and Human Services
National Institutes of Health
National Institute on Drug Abuse
Career Development Awards

6001 Executive Blvd, Rm. 4282, MSC 9555
Bethesda, MD 20892
Phone: (301)443-1887
Website: http://www.nida.nih.gov

Cat. No: 93.277 **Objectives:** To provide support for research relating to the problems of and drug abuse and addiction, to raise the level of competence, and to increase the number of individuals engaged in such research via special levels of National Institute on Drug Abuse (NIDA) support. **Assist. Types:** Project grants. **Applicant Eligibility:** Awards are made to appropriate research centers, medical schools, departments of psychiatry, non-medical academic departments, psychiatric hospitals or hospitals with psychiatric services, community mental health centers, biomedical research institutes, and departments of behavioral science on behalf of individuals who need the opportunity to realize research potentials. **Beneficiary Eligibility:** Public and private profit or nonprofit organizations.

★ 20579 ★ U.S. Department of Health and Human Services
National Institutes of Health
National Institute on Drug Abuse
Drug Abuse National Research Service Awards for Research Training

6001 Executive Blvd., Rm 4282
Bethesda, MD 20892-9555
Phone: (301)443-1887 **Fax:** (301)594-6043
Website: http://www.nih.gov

Cat. No: 93.278 **Objectives:** To provide high quality training in the drug abuse field including: (1) basic and applied studies in all of the life sciences relevant to drug abuse; (2) research on behavioral and societal factors and the epidemiology of drug use and abuse; and (3) special training in experimental design methodology. The National Institute on Drug Abuse (NIDA) research program consists of training grants to institutions and fellowships to individuals at both the predoctoral and postdoctoral level. These grants and awards are directed toward young scientists just beginning their research careers. **Assist. Types:** Project grants. **Applicant Eligibility:** Applicants for training grants must be a domestic public or nonprofit private organization. An applicant for individual predoctoral support must have completed 2 or more years of graduate work and be enrolled in a doctoral degree program. A postdoctoral applicant must have received a doctoral degree. **Beneficiary Eligibility:** Individuals and public and private nonprofit organizations.

★ 20580 ★ U.S. Department of Health and Human Services
National Institutes of Health
National Institute on Drug Abuse
Drug Abuse Research Programs

6001 Executive Blvd., Rm. 4282, MSC 9555
Bethesda, MD 20892-9555
Phone: (301)443-1887 **Fax:** (301)594-6043
Website: http://www.nih.nida.gov

Cat. No: 93.279 **Objectives:** To develop new knowledge and approaches to the epidemiology, etiology, diagnosis, treatment, control, and prevention of narcotic addiction, intravenous (IV)-related AIDS, and drug abuse through basic, clinical, and applied research, investigations, experiments, and studies. **Assist. Types:** Project grants (cooperative agreements). **Applicant Eligibility:** Public or private profit and nonprofit agencies, including state, local, or regional government agencies, universities, colleges, hospitals, and academic or research institutions. **Beneficiary**

Eligibility: Public or private profit and nonprofit organizations.

★ 20581 ★ U.S. Department of Health and Human Services
National Institutes of Health
National Institute of Environmental Health Sciences
Applied Toxicological Research and Testing
PO Box 12233
Research Triangle Park, NC 27709
Phone: (919)541-7628
Website: http://www.cdc.gov

Cat. No: 93.114 **Objectives:** To develop scientific information about potentially toxic and hazardous chemicals by concentrating on toxicological research, testing and test development, and validation efforts. **Assist. Types:** Project grants. **Applicant Eligibility:** Universities, colleges, hospitals, state or local governments, nonprofit research institutions or for-profit organizations may receive a grant for support of research by a named principal investigator. **Beneficiary Eligibility:** Any nonprofit or for-profit organization, company, or institution engaged in biomedical research.

★ 20582 ★ U.S. Department of Health and Human Services
National Institutes of Health
National Institute of Environmental Health Sciences
Biological Response to Environmental Health Hazards
PO Box 12233
Research Triangle Park, NC 27709
Phone: (919)541-7634
Website: http://www.cdc.gov

Cat. No: 93.113 **Objectives:** To focus on understanding how chemical and physical agents cause pathological changes in molecules, cells, tissues and organs and become manifested as respiratory disease; neurological, behavioral, and developmental abnormalities, cancer, and other disorders. **Assist. Types:** Project grants. **Applicant Eligibility:** Universities, colleges, hospitals, state or local governments, nonprofit research institutions, or for-profit organizations may receive a grant for support of research by a named principal investigator. **Beneficiary Eligibility:** Any nonprofit or for-profit organization, company, or institution engaged in biomedical research.

★ 20583 ★ U.S. Department of Health and Human Services
National Institutes of Health
National Institute of Environmental Health Sciences
Biometry and Risk Estimation—Health Risks from Environmental Exposures
PO Box 12233
Research Triangle Park, NC 27709
Phone: (919)541-7628
Website: http://www.cdc.gov

Cat. No: 93.115 **Objectives:** To conduct a broad-scale effort in biometry and risk estimation. Most of the research conducted by the National Institute of Environmental Health Sciences (NIEHS) in statistics, biomathematics, epidemiology, and risk estimation is directed towards estimating probable health risks of cancer, reproductive and neurological effects, and other adverse effects from various environmental hazards. **Assist. Types:** Project grants. **Applicant Eligibility:** Universities, colleges, hospitals, state or local governments, nonprofit research institutions, or for-profit organizations may receive a grant for support of research by a named principal investigator. **Beneficiary Eligibility:** Any nonprofit or for-profit organization, company, or institution engaged in biomedical research.

★ 20584 ★ U.S. Department of Health and Human Services
National Institutes of Health
National Institute of Environmental Health Sciences
NIEHS Hazardous Waste Worker Health and Safety Training
PO Box 12233
Research Triangle Park, NC 27709
Phone: (919)541-0797
Website: http://www.nih.gov

Cat. No: 93.142 **Objectives:** To provide grant support for the development and administration of training programs consisting of classroom and practical health and safety training of hazardous waste workers and their supervisors, who are engaged in activities related to hazardous waste removal, containment, transportation, or emergency response. To assist organizations in the development of institutional competency to provide appropriate training and education to hazardous waste workers. **Assist. Types:** Project grants. **Applicant Eligibility:** Any public or private nonprofit entity providing worker health and safety education and training. **Beneficiary Eligibility:** Same as Applicant Eligibility.

★ 20585 ★ U.S. Department of Health and Human Services
National Institutes of Health
National Institute of Environmental Health Sciences
NIEHS Superfund Hazardous Substances—Basic Research and Education
PO Box 12233
Research Triangle Park, NC 27709
Phone: (919)541-0797
Website: http://www.nih.gov

Cat. No: 93.143 **Objectives:** To establish and support an innovative program of basic research and training consisting of multi-project, interdisciplinary efforts which may include each of the following: (1) advance techniques for the detection, assessment, and evaluation of the effects of hazardous substances on humans; (2) methods to assess the risks to human health presented by hazardous substances; and (3) methods and technologies to detect hazardous substances in the environment, and basic biological, chemical, and physical methods to reduce the amount and toxicity of hazardous substances. **Assist. Types:** Project grants. **Applicant Eligibility:** An accredited institution of higher education, as defined in the Higher Education Act, 20 USC (annotated) 3381, may submit an application and receive a grant for support of research by a named principal investigator. **Beneficiary Eligibility:** Any accredited institution of higher education engaged in biomedical research and/or engineering and ecological research.

★ 20586 ★ U.S. Department of Health and Human Services
National Institutes of Health
National Institute of Environmental Health Sciences
Resource and Manpower Development in the Environmental Health Sciences
PO Box 12233
Research Triangle Park, NC 27709
Phone: (919)541-7634
Website: http://www.nih.gov

Cat. No: 93.894 **Objectives:** To provide long-term stable support for broadly based multidisciplinary research and training on environmental health problems in Environmental Health Sciences Centers (EHS Centers), and Marine and Freshwater Biomedical Sciences Centers (MFBS Centers). **Assist. Types:** Project grants. **Applicant Eligibility:** Centers: A university-based, nonprofit research institution, or for-profit organization whose proposed research program covers activities ranging from very basic research to the actual application of research results in the prevention and control of environmental health problems. National Research Service Awards: Nonprofit domestic organizations may apply for the institutional NRS grant. Individual NRS awardees must be nominated and sponsored by a public or nonprofit private institution having staff and facilities appropriate to the proposed research training program. **Beneficiary Eligibility:** Same as Applicant Eligibility.

★ 20587 ★ U.S. Department of Health and Human Services
National Institutes of Health
National Institute of General Medical Sciences
Cell Biology and Biophysics Research
Natcher Bldg., Rm. 2AS-13D
45 Center Dr., MSC 6200
Bethesda, MD 20892-6500
Phone: (301)594-0828
Website: http://www.nigms.nih.gov

Cat. No: 93.821 **Objectives:** To support studies aimed at understanding the structure and function of cells. The long-range goal is to find ways to prevent, treat, and cure diseases that result from disturbed or abnormal cell activity. The division also supports studies that encourage the development of antiviral drugs, for the treatment of AIDS. **Assist. Types:** Project grants. **Applicant Eligibility:** Research projects: Any public or private for-profit or nonprofit university, college, hospital, laboratory, or other institution, including state and local units of government, or to any individual and, through the Small Business Innovation Research Program, to qualifying small businesses. Non-federal public and private nonprofit domestic organizations may apply for an institutional National Research Service Award. Individual National Research Service awardees must be nominated and sponsored by a public or nonprofit private institution having staff and facilities appropriate to the proposed research training program. **Beneficiary Eligibility:** Any nonprofit or for-profit organization, company, or institution engaged in biomedical research.

★ 20588 ★ U.S. Department of Health and Human Services
National Institutes of Health
National Institute of General Medical Sciences
Genetics and Developmental Biology Research and Research Training
45 Center Dr., Rm. 2AS-25
Bethesda, MD 20892-6200
Phone: (301)594-0943 **Fax:** (301)480-2228
Email: greenbej@nigms.nih.gov
Website: http://www.nigms.nih.gov

Cat. No: 93.862 **Objectives:** To support studies aimed at gaining a better understanding of the fundamental mechanisms of inheritance and development. These studies are expected to eventually lead to the diagnosis, prevention, therapy, and cure of human genetic and developmental disorders. **Assist. Types:** Project grants. **Applicant Eligibility:** Research projects: Any public or private for-profit or nonprofit university, college, hospital, laboratory, or other institution, including state and local unites of government, or any individual and, through the Small Business Innovation Research Program, qualified small businesses. National Research Service Awards are available to individuals and to nonfederal public and private nonprofit domestic organizations. **Beneficiary Eligibility:** Any nonprofit or for-profit organization, company, or institution engaged in biomedical research.

★ 20589 ★ U.S. Department of Health and Human Services
National Institutes of Health
National Institute of General Medical Sciences
Minority Access to Research Careers
45 Center Dr., Rm. 2AS-37H
Bethesda, MD 20892-6200
Phone: (301)594-3900

Website: http://www.nigms.nih.gov/about-nigms/more.htmlmarc

Cat. No: 93.880 **Objectives:** To assist minority institutions to train greater numbers of scientists and teachers in health related fields, and increase the number of minority students who can compete successfully for entry into graduate programs which lead to the Ph.D. degree or M.D.-Ph.D. degree in biomedical science fields. **Assist. Types:** Project grants. **Applicant Eligibility:** Any nonfederal, public or private nonprofit, 4-year university or college, with substantial enrollment of ethnic minority students, may apply for the institutional National Research Service Awards. Individual National Research Service awardees must be nominated and sponsored by a public or nonprofit private institution having staff and facilities appropriate to the proposed research training program. **Beneficiary Eligibility:** Same as Applicant Eligibility.

★ 20590 ★ U.S. Department of Health and Human Services
National Institutes of Health
National Institute of General Medical Sciences
Minority Biomedical Research Support
45 Center Dr., Rm. 2AS-37H
Bethesda, MD 20892-6200
Phone: (301)594-3900
Website: http://www.nigms.nih.gov

Cat. No: 93.375 **Objectives:** To address the lack of representation of minorities in biomedical research by increasing the pool of minorities pursuing research careers. **Assist. Types:** Project grants. **Applicant Eligibility:** (1) Four-year colleges, universities, and health professional schools with over 50 percent minority enrollment; (2) four-year institutions with significant but not necessarily over 50 percent minority enrollment, provided they have a history of encouragement and assistance to minorities; (3) two-year colleges with 50 percent minority enrollment; (4) Indian tribes which have a recognized governing body and perform substantial governmental functions; or (5) Alaskan Regional Corporations, as defined in the Alaska Native Claims Settlement Act. **Beneficiary Eligibility:** Minority students and faculty, and investigators at eligible institutions.

★ 20591 ★ U.S. Department of Health and Human Services
National Institutes of Health
National Institute General Medical Sciences
Pharmacology, Physiology, and Biological Chemistry Research
45 Center Dr., MSC 6200
Bethesda, MD 20892-6200
Phone: (301)496-7301 **Fax:** (301)402-0224
Website: http://www.nigms.nih.gov

Cat. No: 93.859 **Objectives:** To support research in the areas of chemistry, biochemistry, pharmacology, physiology, and biotechnology. The results of these studies improve our understanding of how the body works and pave the way for the discovery and development of new drugs. **Assist. Types:** Project grants. **Applicant Eligibility:** Research projects: Awards can be made to any public or private nonprofit university, college, hospital, laboratory, or other institution, including state and local units of government, qualifying small businesses (through the Small Business Innovation Research Program) and to individuals. Nonfederal public and private nonprofit domestic organizations may apply for an institutional National Research Service Award. Individual National Research Service awardees must be nominated and sponsored by a public or nonprofit private institution having staff and facilities appropriate to the proposed research training program. **Beneficiary Eligibility:** Any nonprofit or for-profit organization, company, or institution engaged in biomedical research.

★ 20592 ★ U.S. Department of Health and Human Services
National Institutes of Health
National Institute of General Medical Sciences
Special Minority Initiatives
45 Center Dr. MSC 6200
Bethesda, MD 20892
Phone: (301)594-0943
Website: http://www.nigms.nih.gov/about=nigms/more.htmlspecial

Cat. No: 93.960 **Objectives:** To increase the number of minority students trained to pursue careers in biomedical research through the use of National Research Service Awards, institutional education programs and conferences. **Assist. Types:** Project grants. **Applicant Eligibility:** Students who are U.S. citizens, noncitizen nationals, or permanent residents from ethnic/racial groups that are underrepresented in research in the biomedical sciences in the United States. Individual NRSA awardees must be nominated and sponsored by a public or nonprofit private institution having staff and facilities appropriate to the proposed research training program. Conference grant applications may be submitted by public, private or nonprofit agencies or organizations including state and local government agencies, universities, colleges, and academic or research institutions. **Beneficiary Eligibility:** Individuals with public, private, profit or nonprofit organizations.

★ 20593 ★ U.S. Department of Health and Human Services
National Institutes of Health
National Institute of Mental Health
Mental Health National Research Service Awards for Research Training
6001 Executive Blvd., Rm. 6122
Bethesda, MD 20892
Phone: (301)443-3563
Website: http://www.nih.gov

Cat. No: 93.282 **Objectives:** To assure a continuing and adequate supply of well-trained personnel who are able to conduct research on mental health problems. The program provides training grants to institutions and fellowships to individuals at both the predoctoral and postdoctoral levels. In addition, there are special programs targeted toward minorities. Awards are made for training in the areas of: basic biomedical, clinical, and behavioral research; the epidemiology of mental disorders; the etiology, description, diagnosis and pathogenesis of mental disorders; treatment development, assessment and evaluation; public health intervention and prevention approaches; and programs designed to increase the supply of minority mental health research scientists trained to work in the above areas. **Assist. Types:** Project grants. **Applicant Eligibility:** For a training grant, an institution must be a domestic public or nonprofit private organization. An applicant for individual predoctoral support must have completed 2 or more years of graduate work and be enrolled in a doctoral degree program. A postdoctoral applicant must have received a doctoral degree. An institution applying for a MARC Honors Undergraduate Program Award must be a 4-year college, university, or health professional school whose student enrollment is drawn substantially from one or more of the following ethnic groups: American Indians or Alaskan Natives; Asian or Pacific Islanders; Black, not of Hispanic origin; and Hispanic. MARC Faculty Fellows must be a full-time faculty member at a 4-year college, university or health professional institution whose student enrollment is drawn substantially from ethnic minority groups. **Beneficiary Eligibility:** Individuals and nonprofit organizations.

★ 20594 ★ U.S. Department of Health and Human Services
National Institutes of Health
National Institute of Mental Health
Mental Health Research Grants
6001 Executive Blvd., Rm. 7204
Bethesda, MD 20892-9645
Phone: (301)443-3563 **Fax:** (301)443-1731
Website: http://www.nimh.nih.gov

Cat. No: 93.242 **Objectives:** To increase knowledge and improve research methods on mental and behavioral disorders; to generate information regarding basic biological and behavioral disorders; to generate information regarding basic biological and behavioral processes underlying these disorders and the maintenance of mental health; and to improve mental health services. **Assist. Types:** Project grants (cooperative agreements). **Applicant Eligibility:** Public, private, profit, or nonprofit agencies, (including state and local government agencies); eligible federal agencies; universities; colleges; hospitals; and academic or research institutions. **Beneficiary Eligibility:** Public, private, profit or nonprofit organizations.

★ 20595 ★ U.S. Department of Health and Human Services
National Institutes of Health
National Institute of Nursing Research
Nursing Research
NIH Bldg. 45, Rm. 3AN12
9000 Rockville Pike, MSC 6300
Bethesda, MD 20892
Phone: (301)594-6906 **Fax:** (301)480-8260
Website: http://www.nih.gov/ninr

Cat. No: 93.361 **Objectives:** To support nursing research and research training related to patient care, the promotion of health, the prevention of disease, the mitigation of the effects of acute and chronic illnesses and disabilities, the clinical practice environment in which health care is provided, and the influence of practice on outcomes of care. **Assist. Types:** Project grants. **Applicant Eligibility:** Research grants: Any corporation, public or private institution or agency, or other legal entity, either nonprofit or for-profit, may apply. NRSAs (Individual): An applicant must be a registered professional nurse with either a baccalaureate and/or master's degree in nursing or a related field and must be a citizen of the United States or lawfully admitted for permanent residence. **Beneficiary Eligibility:** Individuals and public or private institutions.

★ 20596 ★ U.S. Department of Health and Human Services
National Institutes of Health
National Library of Medicine
Medical Library Assistance
NIH Bldg. 38, Rm. 2E17B
9000 Rockville Pike
Bethesda, MD 20894
Phone: (301)496-6221
Email: custserv@nlm.nih.gov
Website: http://www.nlm.nih.gov

Cat. No: 93.879 **Objectives:** To improve health information services by providing funds to train professional personnel; strengthen library and information services; plan and develop advanced information networks; support biomedical publications; and conduct research in medical informatics and related services. **Assist. Types:** Project grants. **Applicant Eligibility:** For Information Access Grants: any public or private nonprofit institution which maintains or plans to establish a library and information services to clientele in the health professions. For Information System Grants: Any not for profit institution or organization whose primary function is the acqusition, preservation, dissemination, and/or processing of information related to the health sciences. For Scientific Publications Grants: appropriate public or private nonprofit institution of higher education may apply in behalf of the principal investigator on the project, and, individuals may apply directly. For Research Grants: institutions or organizations with research capabilities in health information fields or in medical informatics Training Grants may be made to non-federal public and nonprofit private institutions. **Beneficiary Eligibility:** Any organization, company, institution, or individual with a need for health science information.

★ 20597 ★ U.S. Department of Health and Human Services
National Institutes of Health
NIH Loan Repayment Programs
Clinical Research Loan Repayment Program for Individuals from Disadvantaged Backgrounds
2 Center Dr., Rm. 2E24
Bethesda, MD 20892
Free: (866)849-4047 **Fax:** (866)849-4046
Website: http://lrp.nih.gov

Cat. No: 93.220 **Objectives:** To recruit and retain individuals from disadvantaged backgrounds to conduct clinical research at the national Institutes of Health (NIH) by providing for the repayment of educational loans for participants with substantial amounts of educational debt relative to income, who agree by written contract to engage in clinical research as employees of the NIH for a minimum two-year period. **Assist. Types:** Project grants. **Applicant Eligibility:** Eligible applicants must (1) be citizens, nationals, or permanent residents of the United States; (2) have a M.D., PH.D., D.O., D.D.S., D.M.D., B.S.N./A.D.N., R.N., or an equivalent degree; (3) come from a disadvantaged background as determined by the Secretary of Health and Human Services; (4) have qualified educational debt, which results from governmental or commercial loans obtained to support their undergraduate and/or graduate education, in excess of 20 percent of their annual NIH salary on the program eligibility date; (5) be appointed under any temporary or permanent emplotment mechanism, so long as their employment has the potential to las a minimum of 2 yers; (6) are not eligible to participate in the LRP if they have an existing service obligation to Federal, State, or other entities, until such obligation is discharged or unless it is deferred during the period of program service; (7) submit an application to participate in the LRP; and (8) sign and sumit to the Secretary of Health and Human Services, at the time of agreeing to accept repayment of educational loans, a contract agreeing to engage in clinical research as an employee of the NIH for a minimum of 2 years. **Beneficiary Eligibility:** Clinical researchers who have unpaid educational loans.

★ 20598 ★ U.S. Department of Health and Human Services
National Institutes of Health
NIH Loan Repayment and Scholarship Programs
Undergraduate Scholarship Program for Individuals from Disadvantaged Backgrounds
2 Center Dr., Rm. 2E24
Bethesda, MD 20892-9121
Free: 800-528-7689 **Fax:** (301)480-5481
Website: http://ugsp.info.nih.gov

Cat. No: 93.187 **Objectives:** To provide service-conditioned scholarships to individuals from disadvantaged backgrounds who agree to pursue undergraduate education at accredited institutions. Individuals must pursue a course of academic study which prepares them for professions needed by the National Institutes of Health (NIH). **Assist. Types:** Project grants. **Applicant Eligibility:** An eligible applicant must be (1) a U.S. citizen, national, or permanent resident; (2) enrolled or accepted for enrollment as a full-time student at an accredited Undergraduate institution of higher education; (3) from a disadvantaged background as determined by the Secretary of Health and Human Services; (4) in good academic standing with his/her educational institution; (5) submit an application to participate in the Undergraduate Scholarship (UGS) Program; (6) agree to serve as full-time NIH employee for not less than 10 consecutive weeks of each year during which the individual is attending the educational institution and receiving a shcolarship; (7) agree to serve as a full-time NIH employee for 12 months for each academic year during which the scholarship was provided, not later than 60 days after obtaining his or her academic degree, unless a service deferment is granted. **Beneficiary Eligibility:** Undergraduate students from disadvantaged backgrounds pursuing academic programs supporting professions needed by the NIH.

★ 20599 ★ U.S. Department of Health and Human Services
National Institutes of Health
Office of Extramural Research
Academic Research Enhancement Award
6701 Rockledge Dr.
Bethesda, MD 20892-7965
Phone: (301)435-2689
Website: http://www.nih.gov/grants/funding.area.htm

Cat. No: 93.390 **Objectives:** To develop the research environment of educational institutions that are not major participants in National Institutes of Health (NIH) extramural research programs, through Academic Research Enhancement Awards (AREA). **Assist. Types:** Project grants. **Applicant Eligibility:** (1) Educational institutions granting baccalaureate and higher degrees in the health sciences except those that received NIH research grants totaling more than $2 million per year in 4 or more years of the last 7 years; and (2) faculty members of such institutions who will not have an active NIH research grant at the time of award of an AREA grant. **Beneficiary Eligibility:** Institutions as described above and the faculty and students of such institutions.

★ 20600 ★ U.S. Department of Health and Human Services
National Institutes of Health
Office of Intramural Affairs
Intramural Research Training Award
NIH Bldg. 1, Rm. 140
9000 Rockville Pike
Bethesda, MD 20892
Phone: (301)496-4920
Website: http://www.nih.gov

Cat. No: 93.140 **Objectives:** To provide advanced training and practical research experience to physicians and doctoral-level investigators who are at the beginning stages of their professional research careers. **Assist. Types:** Project grants. **Applicant Eligibility:** Individuals only. **Beneficiary Eligibility:** Program participants.

★ 20601 ★ U.S. Department of Health and Human Services
Office of Disease Prevention and Health Promotion
National Health Promotion
200 Independence Ave. SW, Rm. 738G
Washington, DC 20201
Phone: (202)205-8611
Website: http://www.health.gov/healthypeople

Cat. No: 93.990 **Objectives:** To engage national membership organizations from various sectors as a means of expanding and coordinating health promotion efforts. To promote the development, implementation and coordination of programs that promote good health habits and programs that are designed to prevent disease and disability. **Assist. Types:** Project grants (cooperative agreements). **Applicant Eligibility:** Public or private nonprofit organizations. **Beneficiary Eligibility:** General public.

★ 20602 ★ U.S. Department of Health and Human Services
Office of Population Affairs
Adolescent Family Life—Demonstration Projects
4350 East-West Hwy., Ste. 200
Bethesda, MD 20814
Phone: (301)594-4004 **Fax:** (301)594-5981
Email: psheeran@osophs.dhhs.gov
Website: http://www.opa.osophs.dhhs.gov

Cat. No: 93.995 **Objectives:** To promote abstinence from premarital sexual relations through provision of age-appropriate education on sexuality and decision-making skills as the most effective method of preventing adolescent pregnancy and avoiding sexually transmitted diseases; and to establish innovative, comprehensive, and integrated approaches to the delivery of care services for pregnant adolescents, with primary emphasis on unmarried adolescents who are seventeen years of age and under and for adolescent parents. **Assist. Types:** Project grants. **Applicant Eligibility:** Public (including city, county, regional, and state government) organizations, and private nonprofit organizations. **Beneficiary Eligibility:** For prevention services: non-pregnant adolescents and their families. For care services: pregnant adolescents, infants, adolescent parents, and their families.

★ 20603 ★ U.S. Department of Health and Human Services
Office of Population Affairs
Office of Adolescent Pregnancy Programs
Adolescent Family Life Research Grants
4330 East-West Hwy., Ste. 200
Bethesda, MD 20814
Phone: (301)594-4008 **Fax:** (301)594-5980
Email: opa@osophs.dhhs.gov
Website: http://www.hhs.gov/progorg/opa
Eugenia Eckard, Director

Cat. No: 93.111 **Objectives:** To encourage and support research projects and dissemination activities concerning the societal causes and consequences of adolescent premarital sexual relations, contraceptive use, pregnancy and child rearing; and to determine ways to alleviate, eliminate, or resolve negative consequences of adolescent premarital sexual relations or childbearing for parents, children and their families. **Assist. Types:** Project grants. **Applicant Eligibility:** State and local governments; private organizations (nonprofit and profit); institutions of higher education. **Beneficiary Eligibility:** Non-pregnant adolescents, pregnant adolescents, adolescent parents, and their families.

★ 20604 ★ U.S. Department of Health and Human Services
Office of Population Affairs
Office of Family Planning
Family Planning—Personnel Training
4350 East-West Hwy., Ste. 200
Bethesda, MD 20814
Phone: (301)594-4008
George Jones, Contact

Cat. No: 93.260 **Objectives:** To provide job specific training for personnel to improve the delivery of family planning services. **Assist. Types:** Project grants. **Applicant Eligibility:** Any public entity or nonprofit private entity located in the United States and U.S. Territories. **Beneficiary Eligibility:** Personnel delivering family planning services in Title X projects.

★ 20605 ★ U.S. Department of Health and Human Services
Office of Population Affairs
Office of Family Planning
Family Planning—Service Delivery Improvement Research Grants
4350 East-West Hwy., Ste. 200
Bethesda, MD 20814
Phone: (301)594-4008 **Fax:** (301)594-5980
Email: opa@osophs.dhhs.gov
Website: htpp://www.opa.osophs.dhhs.gov

Cat. No: 93.974 **Objectives:** To promote service delivery improvement through research studies, and application of knowledge. **Assist. Types:** Project grants. **Applicant Eligibility:** Any public or private nonprofit entity located in the United States and U.S. Territories. **Beneficiary Eligibility:** All levels of government and nonprofit entities responsible for the efficient and effective delivery of family planning services; providers and recipients of family planning services; and the general public.

★ 20606 ★ U.S. Department of Health and Human Services
Office of Population Affairs
Office of Family Planning
Family Planning—Services
4350 East-West Hwy., Ste. 200
Bethesda, MD 20814
Phone: (301)594-4008
Website: http://www.opa.osophs.dhhs.gov
Susan B. Moskosky, Contact

Cat. No: 93.217 **Objectives:** To provide educational, counseling, comprehensive medical and social services necessary to enable individuals to freely determine the number and spacing of their children, and by so doing, helping to reduce maternal and infant mortality and promote the health of mothers and children. **Assist. Types:** Project grants. **Applicant Eligibility:** Any city, county, local, regional, and state governments, or nonprofit private entity located in the United States and U.S. Territories. **Beneficiary Eligibility:** Persons who desire family planning services and who would not otherwise have access to them.

★ 20607 ★ U.S. Department of Health and Human Services
Office of Public Health and Science
Office of Minority Health
Bilingual/Bicultural Service Demonstration Grants
5515 Security Ln., Ste. 1000
Rockville, MD 20852
Phone: (301)594-0769
Website: http://www.omhrc.gov

Cat. No: 93.105 **Objectives:** To provide support to minority community-based healthcare facilities to improve the ability of health care professionals to deliver linguistically and culturally competent health services to limited English-proficient populations. **Assist. Types:** Project grants. **Applicant Eligibility:** Public and private nonprofit minority community-based organizations or health care facilities. **Beneficiary Eligibility:** Members of the minority groups whose native language is other than English: Asian/Pacific Islanders, Hispanics, Native Americans, Alaska natives, Native Hawaiians, people from the Caribbean Basin, or a subgroup of any of these groups.

★ 20608 ★ U.S. Department of Health and Human Services
Office of Public Health and Science
Office of Minority Health
Community Programs to Improve Minority Health Grant Program
Rockwall II Blgd., Ste. 1000
5515 Security Ln.
Rockville, MD 20852
Phone: (301)594-0769
Website: http://www.omhrc.gov
Cynthia H. Amis, Director
Carolyn A. Williams, Grants Management Officer

Cat. No: 93.137 **Objectives:** To support minority community health coalitions to develop, implement, and conduct demonstration projects which coordinate integrated community-based screening and outreach services, and include linkages for access and treatment to minorities in high-risk, low-income communities. **Assist. Types:** Project grants. **Applicant Eligibility:** Public and private nonprofit organizations. **Beneficiary Eligibility:** Asian/Pacific Islanders, Blacks, Hispanics, Latinos, Native Americans, Alaska natives, or a subgroup of any of these groups.

★ 20609 ★ U.S. Department of Health and Human Services
Office of the Secretary, Office of Inspector General
Office of Investigations
State Medicaid Fraud Control Units
330 Independence Ave. SW, Rm. 5228
Washington, DC 20201
Phone: (202)619-3557 **Fax:** (202)401-0502
Website: http://www.dhhs.gov/progorg/oig

Cat. No: 93.775 **Objectives:** To control provider fraud in the states' Medicaid program. **Assist. Types:** Formula grants. **Applicant Eligibility:** A single identifiable entity of the state government which the Secretary certifies (and annually re-certifies) as meeting the requirements of 1903(a)(6), 1903(b)(3) and 1903(q) of the Social Security Act (42CFR, Part 1007) regarding location, function and and procedure. **Beneficiary Eligibility:** State governments.

★ 20610 ★ U.S. Department of Health and Human Services
Primary Health Care Bureau
Community and Migrant Health Division
Coal Miners Respiratory Impairment Treatment Clinics and Services
4350 East-West Hwy., 7th Fl.
Bethesda, MD 20814
Phone: (301)594-4420
Website: http://www.bphc.hrsa.gov

Cat. No: 93.965 **Objectives:** (1) To develop high quality, patient-oriented, integrated systems of care which assure access to and continuity of appropriate primary, secondary, and tertiary care with maximum use of existing resources; (2) to emphasize patient and family member education to maximize the patient's ability for self-care; and, (3) to minimize the effects of respiratory and pulmonary impairments in coal miners. **Assist. Types:** Project grants. **Applicant Eligibility:** State and local government agencies; private nonprofit agencies. **Beneficiary Eligibility:** Coal workers with respiratory and pulmonary impairments.

★ 20611 ★ U.S. Department of Health and Human Services
Public Health Service
Agency for Toxic Substances and Disease Registry
Health Program for Toxic Substances and Disease Registry
1600 Clifton Rd. NE, Rm. 3726
Atlanta, GA 30333
Phone: (404)639-0700
Website: http://www.atsdr.cdc.gov

Cat. No: 93.161 **Objectives:** To work closely with state, local, and other federal agencies to reduce or eliminate illness, disability, and death resulting from exposure of the public and workers to toxic substances at spill and waste disposal sites. **Assist. Types:** Project grants; project grants (cooperative agreements). **Applicant Eligibility:** States, political subdivisions of states, state universities, state colleges, state research institutions, state hospitals, and state and local health departments, National organizations, and Federally-recognized Indian tribal governments. **Beneficiary Eligibility:** The general public and particularly individuals and families who reside around or near hazardous waste sites.

★ 20612 ★ U.S. Department of Health and Human Services
Public Health Service
Office of the Assistant Secretary for Health
President's Council on Physical Fitness and Sports
200 Independence SW, Rm. 738H
Washington, DC 20201
Phone: (202)690-9000 **Fax:** (202)690-5211
Website: http://www.fitness.gov

Cat. No: 93.289 **Objectives:** To promote physical fitness for Americans of all ages by encouraging the development, implementation and improvement of physical fitness and sports programs. **Assist. Types:** Provision of specialized services; advisory services and counseling; dissemination of technical information; training. **Applicant Eligibility:** General public. **Beneficiary Eligibility:** General public.

★ 20613 ★ U.S. Department of Health and Human Services
Public Health Services
Office of the Assistant Secretary for Health
Public Health and Social Services Emergency Fund
5600 Fishers Lane
Rockville, MD 20857
Phone: (301)443-3846
Website: http://www.hhs.gov

Cat. No: 93.003 **Objectives:** To provide supplemental funding for public health and social service emergencies created by Tropical Storm Alberto and other natural disasters. **Assist. Types:** Project grants. **Applicant Eligibility:** Federal agencies, State and local governments, and other service providers in areas impacted by Tropical Storm Alberto, or other natural disasters. **Beneficiary Eligibility:** Individuals, families, Federal, State and local government agencies.

★ 20614 ★ U.S. Department of Health and Human Services
Social Security Administration
Office of Public Inquiries
Social Security—Disability Insurance
6401 Security Blvd., Rm. 4100
Baltimore, MD 21235
Phone: (410)965-2736
Website: http://www.ssa.gov

Cat. No: 96.001 **Objectives:** To replace part of the earnings lost because of a physical or mental impairment severe enough to prevent a person from working. **Assist. Types:** Direct payments with unrestricted use; direct payments for specified use. **Applicant Eligibility:** A disabled worker under age 65 is eligible for Social Security disability benefits if he has worked for a sufficient period of time under Social Security to be insured. **Beneficiary Eligibility:** Same as Applicant Eligibility.

★ 20615 ★ U.S. Department of Health and Human Services
Social Security Administration
Office of Public Inquiries
Special Benefits for Disabled Coal Miners
6401 Security Blvd., Rm. 4100
Baltimore, MD 21235
Phone: (410)965-2736
Website: http://www.ssa.gov

Cat. No: 96.005 **Objectives:** To pay benefits to coal miners who have become disabled due to pneumoconiosis (black lung disease or other chronic lung disease arising from coal mine employment), and their dependents or survivors. **Assist. Types:** Direct payments with unrestricted use. **Applicant Eligibility:** In order to become entitled, the miner must have become "disabled" from black lung or another chronic lung disease arising from coal mine employment and have already applied for benefits. Widow(er)s of coal miners whose deaths or disability at the time of death resulted from black lung or other chronic lung disease arising from coal mine employment are also eligible for benefits, as are other categories of beneficiaries. **Beneficiary Eligibility:** Disabled coal miners and their eligible dependents or survivors.

★ 20616 ★ U.S. Department of Health and Human Services
Substance Abuse and Mental Health Services Administration
Center for Mental Health Services
Block Grants for Community Mental Health Services
5600 Fishers Ln., Rm. 15C-26
Rockville, MD 20857
Phone: (301)443-4257
Website: http://www.samhsa.gov

Cat. No: 93.958 **Objectives:** To provide financial assistance to states and territories to enable them to carry out the state's plan for providing comprehensive community mental health services to adults with a serious mental illness and to children with a serious emotional disturbance; evaluate programs and services carried out under the plan; and conduct planning, administration and educational activities related to providing services under the plan. **Assist. Types:** Formula grants. **Applicant Eligibility:** State and U.S. Territory governments. **Beneficiary Eligibility:** State and U.S. Territory government recipients.

★ 20617 ★ U.S. Department of Health and Human Services
Substance Abuse and Mental Health Services Administration
Center for Mental Health Services
Comprehensive Community Mental Health Services for Children with Serious Emotional Disturbances
5600 Fishers Ln., Rm. 18-49
Rockville, MD 20857
Phone: (301)443-1333 **Fax:** (301)443-3693
Email: gdecarol@samhsa.gov
Website: http://www.samhsa.gov
Gary DeCarolis, Contact

Cat. No: 93.104 **Objectives:** To provide community-based systems of care for children and adolescents with a serious emotional disturbance and their families. **Assist. Types:** Project grants. **Applicant Eligibility:** States, political subdivisions of a state such as county or local governments, and federally-recognized Indian tribal governments. **Beneficiary Eligibility:** Children under age 22 with a diagnosed serious emotional disturbance, serious behavioral disorder, or serious mental disorder.

★ 20618 ★ U.S. Department of Health and Human Services
Substance Abuse and Mental Health Services Administration
Center for Mental Health Services
Mental Health Clinical and AIDS Service-Related Training Grants
5600 Fishers Lane, Rm. 15C-18
Rockville, MD 20857
Phone: (301)443-5850
Website: http://www.samhsa.gov
Anne Mathews-Younes, Contact

Cat. No: 93.244 **Objectives:** (1) Institutions Clinical Training Grants: To encourage mental health specialists to work in areas and settings where severe shortages exist; to increase the number of qualified minority personnel in the mental health professions, and the number of mental health personnel trained to deal with the special problems of children, adolescents, the elderly, the seriously mentally ill, and rural populations; and to assure that the skills and knowledge of mental health personnel are appropriate to the needs of those they serve; (2) State Human Resource Development (HRD) Grants: To assist State mental health authorities in the development of human resources. **Assist. Types:** Project grants. **Applicant Eligibility:** Grants are awarded to public or private nonprofit institutions and organizations, and to state and local government agencies for training relevant to mental health service priorities in the mental health disciplines of psychiatry, psychology, social work, psychiatric nursing, marriage and family therapy and in specialized areas of high priority and need such as state manpower development projects; and for state mental health agencies to plan, implement, and evaluate systems for mental health services manpower development. Trainees in psychology, psychiatry, psychiatric nursing, social work, or marriage and family therapy unless training program is of limited duration or experimental nature, will be subject to payback requirements of Section 303 of the PHS Act. **Beneficiary Eligibility:** Trainee stipends may be awarded only to citizens or nationals of the United States, or to persons lawfully admitted for permanent residence.

★ 20619 ★ U.S. Department of Health and Human Services
Substance Abuse and Mental Health Services Administration
Center for Mental Health Services
Mental Health Disaster Assistance and Emergency Mental Health
5600 Fishers Lane, Rm. 16C-26
Rockville, MD 20857
Phone: (301)443-4735 **Fax:** (301)443-8040
Website: http://www.samhsa.gov
Mary Elizabeth Nelson, MSW, Contact

Cat. No: 93.982 **Objectives:** Provision of supplemental emergency mental health counseling to individuals affected by major disasters, including the training of volunteers to provide such counseling. **Assist. Types:** Project grants. **Applicant Eligibility:** Applicants may be state or local non-profit agencies as recommended by the state governor and accepted by the Secretary. **Beneficiary Eligibility:** Individuals who were victims of major disasters.

★ 20620 ★ U.S. Department of Health and Human Services
Substance Abuse and Mental Health Services Administration
Center for Mental Health Services
Protection and Advocacy for Individuals with Mental Illness
5600 Fishers Lane, Rm. 15C-26
Rockville, MD 20857
Phone: (301)443-3667 **Fax:** (301)594-0091
Email: karmstro@samhsa.gov
Website: http://www.samhsa.gov
Karen S. Armstrong, Contact

Cat. No: 93.138 **Objectives:** To enable the expansion of the Protection and Advocacy system established in each state to: (1) protect and advocate the rights of mentally ill individuals and (2) investigate incidents of abuse and neglect of mentally ill individuals if the incidents are reported to the system or if there is probable cause to believe that the incidents occurred. **Assist. Types:** Formula grants. **Applicant Eligibility:** State and local government agencies, public or private organizations designated by the Governor as systems to protect and advocate the rights of persons with developmental disabilities in that state. **Beneficiary Eligibility:** Mentally ill individuals are eligible while they are inpatients or residents in facilities rendering care or treatment, and for 90 days following discharge from such facilities.

★ 20621 ★ U.S. Department of Health and Human Services
Substance Abuse and Mental Health Services Administration
Center for Substance Abuse Treatment
Demonstration Cooperative Agreements for Development and Implementation of Criminal Justice Treatment Networks
5600 Fishers Ln., 7th Fl.
Rockville, MD 20857
Phone: (301)443-6533 **Fax:** (301)443-3543
Website: http://www.samhsa.gov
Nicholas Demos, Contact

Cat. No: 93.229 **Objectives:** To fund integrated criminal justice treatment networks made up of a consortium of criminal justice, substance abuse treatment, primary health and mental health care, and allied social services and job placement agencies in the following three offender populations: Adult Female Offenders, Juvenile Justice Populations and Adult Male Offenders. **Assist. Types:** Project grants. **Applicant Eligibility:** Applicant Eligibility for this program is limited to State Alcohol and Drug Abuse Agency which applies on behalf of a consortium of relevant State and local officials, and public and nonprofit private entities who provide or have jurisdiction over providing treatment for substance abuse to individuals under criminal justice supervision. **Beneficiary Eligibility:** Male and female adult and juvenile offenders with substance abuse and related health problems.

★ 20622 ★ U.S. Department of Health and Human Services
Substance Abuse and Mental Health Services Administration
Division of Knowledge Development and System Change
Projects for Assistance in Transition from Homelessness
5600 Fishers Lane, Rm.11C-05
Rockville, MD 20857
Phone: (301)443-4456
Website: http://sss.samhsa.gov

Cat. No: 93.150 **Objectives:** To provide financial assistance to states to support services for individuals who are suffering from serious mental illness; serious mental illness and substance abuse; and are homeless or at imminent risk of becoming homeless. Programs and activities include: (1) outreach services; (2) screening and diagnostic treatment services; (3) habilitation and rehabilitation services; (4) community mental health services; (5) alcohol or drug treatment services; (6) staff training; (7) case management services; (8) supportive and supervisory services in residential settings; (9) referrals for primary health services, job training, education services, and relevant housing services; and (10) prescribed set of housing services. **Assist. Types:** Formula grants. **Applicant Eligibility:** State governments, District of Columbia, Guam, American Samoa, the Commonwealths of Puerto Rico, and the Northern Mariana Islands, and the Virgin Islands. **Beneficiary Eligibility:** Individuals who are suffering from serious mental illness; serious mental illness and substance abuse; and are homeless or are at imminent risk of becoming homeless.

★ 20623 ★ U.S. Department of Housing and Urban Development
Office for Housing—Federal Housing Administration
Mortgage Insurance—Hospitals
451 Seventh St. SW, Rm. 9224
Washington, DC 20410
Phone: (202)708-0599 **Free:** 877-263-0763
Email: roger_E._miller@hud.gov
Website: http://www.hud.gov/offices/hsg/hosp/hsphospi.cfm

Cat. No: 14.128 **Objectives:** To make possible the financing of hospitals. **Assist. Types:** Guaranteed/insured loans. **Applicant Eligibility:** Hospitals licensed or regulated by the state, municipality, or other political subdivision. At least 50 percent of the care must be for general acute patients. **Beneficiary Eligibility:** Persons needing the services of these hospitals are eligible to benefit by using the facilities covered under an insured mortgage.

★ 20624 ★ U.S. Department of Housing and Urban Development
Office of Insured Multifamily Housing Development
Policies and Procedures Division
Mortgage Insurance—Nursing Homes, Intermediate Care Facilities, and Board and Care Homes and Assisted Living Facilities
451 Seventh St. SW, Rm. 6142
Washington, DC 20410
Phone: (202)708-2556
Website: http://www.hud.gov/fha/mfh/fhamfbus.html

Cat. No: 14.129 **Objectives:** To make possible financing for construction or rehabilitation of nursing homes, intermediate care facilities, and board and care homes and assisted living facilities, to allow purchase or financing with or without repairs of projects currently insured by HUD, but not requiring insurance to install fire safety equipment. **Assist. Types:** Guaranteed/insured loans. **Applicant Eligibility:** Eligible mortgagors, including investors, builders, developers, public entities, and private nonprofit corporations or associations licensed or regulated by the state for the accommodation of convalescents and persons requiring skilled nursing or intermediate care. **Beneficiary**

Eligibility: Patients requiring skilled nursing, custodial care, and assistance with activities of daily living are eligible to live in a structure whose mortgage is insured under the program.

★ 20625 ★ U.S. Department of Housing and Urban Development
Office of Insured Multifamily Housing Development
Policies and Procedures Division
Supplemental Loan Insurance—Multifamily Rental Housing

451 Seventh St. SW, Rm. 6142
Washington, DC 20410
Phone: (202)708-2556
Website: http://www.hud.gov/fha/mfh/fhamfbus.html

Cat. No: 14.151 **Objectives:** To finance repairs, additions and improvements to multifamily projects, group practice facilities, hospitals, or nursing homes insured by HUD or held by HUD. Major movable equipment for insured nursing homes, group practice facilities or hospitals may be covered by a mortgage under this program. **Assist. Types:** Guaranteed/insured loans. **Applicant Eligibility:** Owners of a multifamily project or facility subject to a mortgage insured by HUD or held by HUD. **Beneficiary Eligibility:** Individuals/families and owners of multifamily projects.

★ 20626 ★ U.S. Department of Housing and Urban Development
Office of Multifamily Housing Programs
Office of Business Products
Supportive Housing for the Elderly

451 Seventh St. SW, Rm. 6138
Washington, DC 20410
Phone: (202)708-2866 **Fax:** (202)708-3104
Website: http://www.hud.gov/
Aretha Williams, Mgr

Cat. No: 14.157 **Objectives:** To expand the supply of housing with supportive services for the elderly. **Assist. Types:** Project grants. **Frmly:** Office of Elderly and Assisted Housing, Assisted Elderly and Handicapped Housing Division. **Applicant Eligibility:** Private nonprofit corporations and consumer cooperatives. Public bodies and their instrumentalities are not eligible. **Beneficiary Eligibility:** Beneficiaries of housing developed under this program must be elderly (62 years of age or older) with low-income status.

★ 20627 ★ U.S. Department of Labor
Employment Standards Administration
Office of Workers' Compensation Programs
Coal Mine Workers' Compensation

200 Constitution Ave. NW, C3520
Washington, DC 20210
Phone: (202)693-0046 **Fax:** (202)693-1395
Website: http://www.dol.gov

Cat. No: 17.307 **Objectives:** To provide benefits to coal miners who have become totally disabled due to coal workers' pneumoconiosis (CWP), and to widows and other surviving dependents of miners who have died of this disease. **Assist. Types:** Direct payments with unrestricted use. **Applicant Eligibility:** The miners (including some workers involved in coal transportation in and around mines and coal mine construction workers) must have worked in the Nation's coal mines or a coal preparation facility and become "totally disabled" (as defined in the Act) from coal workers' pneumoconiosis. The applicant may be able to work in areas other than coal mines and still be eligible for benefits. Widows and other surviving dependents of coal miners whose death resulted from coal workers' pneumoconiosis are also eligible for benefits with earnings offsets applicable to certain classes of dependents. **Beneficiary Eligibility:** Disabled coal miners, widows, and other surviving dependents of the deceased.

★ 20628 ★ U.S. Department of Labor
Mine Safety and Health Administration
Educational Policy and Development Directorate
Mine Health and Safety Grants

4015 Wilson Blvd., Rm. 529
Arlington, VA 22203
Phone: (703)235-1515
Website: http://www.msha.gov

Cat. No: 17.600 **Objectives:** To assist states in developing and enforcing effective mine health and safety laws and regulations, to improve state workmen's compensation and occupational disease laws and programs, and to promote federal-state coordination and cooperation in improving health and safety conditions. **Assist. Types:** Project grants. **Applicant Eligibility:** Any mining state of the United States through its mine inspection or safety agency. **Beneficiary Eligibility:** States.

★ 20629 ★ U.S. Department of Labor
Mine Safety and Health Administration
Office of Educational Policy and Development
Mine Health and Safety Counseling and Technical Assistance

4015 Wilson Blvd., Rm. 927
Arlington, VA 22203-1954
Phone: (703)235-1580 **Fax:** (703)235-9899
Website: http://www.msha.gov

Cat. No: 17.601 **Objectives:** To improve conditions of health and safety in and around coal, metal, and nonmetallic mines and mineral facilities through technical advice, special studies, investigations, development of state mine health and safety programs, and inspections with enforcement authority. **Assist. Types:** Advisory services and counseling; dissemination of technical information. **Applicant Eligibility:** Any state, organization or person interested in employing healthful and safe mine or mineral industry working conditions. **Beneficiary Eligibility:** States, organizations, individuals.

★ 20630 ★ U.S. Department of Labor
Mine Safety and Health Administration
Office of Educational Policy and Development
Mine Health and Safety Education and Training

4015 Wilson Blvd., Rm. 529
Arlington, VA 22203
Phone: (703)235-1515
Website: http://www.msha.gov

Cat. No: 17.602 **Objectives:** To provide technical training for Federal mine inspectors and representatives of the mining industry. **Assist. Types:** Training. **Applicant Eligibility:** Any mine operator or miner or their agent can request training or training materials. **Beneficiary Eligibility:** Mine operators, miners or their agent, organizations and individuals.

★ 20631 ★ U.S. Department of Labor
Office of the Assistant Secretary for Veterans' Employment and Training
Office of Veterans' Employment, Reemployment, and Training
Disabled Veterans Outreach Program

200 Constitution Ave. NW, Rm. S-1316
Washington, DC 20210
Phone: (202)693-4701
Website: http://www.dol.gov/dol/vets

Cat. No: 17.801 **Objectives:** To provide job and job training opportunities for disabled and other veterans through contacts with employers; promote and develop on-the-job training and apprenticeship and other on-the-job training positions within VA programs; provide outreach to veterans through all community agencies and organizations; provide assistance to community-based groups and organizations and appropriate grantees under other federal and federally funded employment and training programs; provide outreach assistance to local employment service offices; develop linkages with other agencies to promote maximum employment opportunities for veterans; promote entry-level and career job opportunities for veterans; and to provide job placement, counseling, testing, job referral to eligible veterans, especially disabled veterans of the Vietnam-era. **Assist. Types:** Formula grants. **Applicant Eligibility:** State Employment Security Agencies designated under Section 4 of the Wagner Peyser Act, as amended. **Beneficiary Eligibility:** Veterans.

★ 20632 ★ U.S. Department of Veterans Affairs
Veterans Benefits Administration
Office of Chief Benefits Director
Specially Adapted Housing for Disabled Veterans

810 Vermont Ave. NW, Rm. 520
Washington, DC 20420
Phone: (202)273-7355 **Fax:** (202)275-3523
Email: lgybbixl@vba.va.gov
Website: http://www.va.gov

Cat. No: 64.106 **Objectives:** To assist certain severely disabled veterans in acquiring suitable housing units, with special fixtures and facilities made necessary by the nature of the veterans' disabilities. **Assist. Types:** Direct payments for specified use. **Applicant Eligibility:** Veterans with permanent, total and compensable disabilities based on service after April 20, 1898. **Beneficiary Eligibility:** Permanently and totally disabled veterans.

★ 20633 ★ U.S. Department of Veterans Affairs
Veterans Benefits Administration
Vocational Rehabilitation Service
Vocational Rehabilitation for Disabled Veterans

810 Vermont Ave. NW, Rm. 501
Washington, DC 20420
Phone: (202)273-7419 **Fax:** (202)275-5636
Email: vrccgraf@vba.va.gov
Website: http://www.va.gov

Cat. No: 64.116 **Objectives:** To provide all services and assistance necessary to enable service-disabled veterans and service persons hospitalized pending discharge to achieve maximum independence in daily living and, to the maximum extent feasible, to become employable and to obtain and maintain suitable employment. **Assist. Types:** Direct payments with unrestricted use; direct payments for specified use; direct loans; advisory services and counseling. **Applicant Eligibility:** Veterans of World War II and later service with a service-connected disability or disabilities rated at least 20 percent compensable and certain hospitalized servicepersons pending discharge or release from service if VA determines the servicepersons will likely receive at least a 20 percent rating and they need vocational rehabilitation because of an employment handicap. A veteran, but not a service member, with a 10 percent compensable disability may be eligible if the veteran has a serious employment handicap. **Beneficiary Eligibility:** Same as Applicant Eligibility.

★ 20634 ★ U.S. Department of Veterans Affairs
Veterans Health Administration
Geriatrics and Extended Care Healthcare Group
Veterans Home Based Primary Care

810 Vermont Ave. NW, Rm. 1078
Washington, DC 20420
Phone: (202)273-8540
Website: http://www.va.gov

Cat. No: 64.022 **Objectives:** To provide individual medical, nursing, social and rehabilitative services to eligible veterans in their home environment by VA hospital staff. **Assist. Types:** Provision of specialized services. **Applicant Eligibility:** The veteran must require intermittent skilled nursing care and related medical services for a protracted period of time. Medical determination as to need for home health services will be made by a VA hospital physician. **Beneficiary Eligibility:** Same as Applicant Eligibility.

★ 20635 ★ U.S. Department of Veterans Affairs
Veterans Health Administration
Geriatrics and Extended Care Strategic Health Care
Veterans Nursing Home Care
810 Vermont Ave. NW
Washington, DC 20420
Phone: (202)273-8544 **Fax:** (202)273-9131
Website: http://www.va.gov

Cat. No: 64.010 **Objectives:** To accommodate eligible veterans who are not acutely ill and not in need of hospital care, but who require skilled nursing care, related medical services, supportive personal care, and individual adjustment services (including social, diversional, recreational and spiritual activities and opportunities) in a homelike atmosphere. **Assist. Types:** Provision of specialized services. **Applicant Eligibility:** The need for placement in a nursing home is based upon medical and nursing care considerations. The eligible veteran should require skilled nursing supervision, observation and care by an interdisciplinary team, and/or long term rehabilitative programs and supportive health services found only in a hospital based nursing home program. **Beneficiary Eligibility:** Veterans meeting certain criteria for VA hospitalization.

★ 20636 ★ U.S. Department of Veterans Affairs
Veterans Health Administration
Geriatrics and Extended Care Strategic Healthcare Group
Grants to States for Construction of State Home Facilities
810 Vermont Ave., NW, Rm. 1076
Washington, DC 20420
Phone: (202)273-8536 **Fax:** (202)273-9131
Website: http://www.va.gov

Cat. No: 64.005 **Objectives:** To assist states to construct state home facilities for furnishing domiciliary or nursing home care to veterans, and to expand, remodel, or alter existing buildings for furnishing domiciliary, nursing home, hospital or adult day health care to veterans in state homes. **Assist. Types:** Project grants. **Applicant Eligibility:** Any state may apply after assuring that the assisted facility will be maintained and operated by the state and will be used primarily for veterans. **Beneficiary Eligibility:** Veterans meeting VA and state admission criteria.

★ 20637 ★ U.S. Department of Veterans Affairs
Veterans Health Administration
Geriatrics and Extended Care Strategic Healthcare Group
Veterans Domiciliary Care
810 Vermont Ave. NW
Washington, DC 20420
Phone: (202)273-8543 **Fax:** (202)273-9131
Email: richard.olson@mail.va.gov
Website: http://www.va.gov

Cat. No: 64.008 **Objectives:** To provide the least intensive level of VA inpatient care for ambulatory veterans disabled by age or illness who are not in need of more acute hospitalization and who do not need the skilled nursing services provided in nursing homes. To rehabilitate the veteran in anticipation of his/her return to the community in a self-sustaining and independent or semi-independent living situation or to assist the veteran to reach his/her optimal level of functioning in a protective environment. **Assist. Types:** Provision of specialized services. **Applicant Eligibility:** Veterans of the various military services who were discharged for a disability or are in receipt of disability compensation and suffering from a permanent disability, have no adequate means of support, are incapacitated from earning a living and meet certain other requirements. Veterans with nonservice-connected disabilities that incapacitate them from earning a living, but which are not so severe as to require hospitalization, are also eligible if they are unable to defray the expense of domiciliary care and if they meet certain other requirements for care in a domiciliary. **Beneficiary Eligibility:** Disabled veterans meeting the above requirements.

★ 20638 ★ U.S. Department of Veterans Affairs
Veterans Health Administration
Geriatrics and Extended Care Strategic Healthcare Group
Veterans State Domiciliary Care
810 Vermont Ave. NW
Washington, DC 20420
Phone: (202)273-8538
Website: http://www.va.gov

Cat. No: 64.014 **Objectives:** To provide financial assistance to states furnishing domiciliary care to eligible veterans in state veterans' homes which meet the standards prescribed by the Secretary of Veterans Affairs. **Assist. Types:** Formula grants. **Applicant Eligibility:** Applicant is any state which operates a designated facility to furnish domiciliary care primarily for veterans. **Beneficiary Eligibility:** A veteran eligible for care in a VA facility needing domiciliary care and meeting certain conditions.

★ 20639 ★ U.S. Department of Veterans Affairs
Veterans Health Administration
Geriatrics and Extended Care Strategic Healthcare Group
Veterans State Hospital Care
810 Vermont Ave. NW
Washington, DC 20420
Phone: (202)273-8538
Website: http://www.va.gov

Cat. No: 64.016 **Objectives:** To provide financial assistance to states furnishing hospital care to eligible veterans in state veterans' homes which meet the standards prescribed by the Secretary of Veterans Affairs. **Assist. Types:** Formula grants. **Applicant Eligibility:** Applicant is any state which operates a designated facility to furnish hospital care primarily for veterans. **Beneficiary Eligibility:** A veteran eligible for care in a VA facility needing hospital care and meeting certain conditions.

★ 20640 ★ U.S. Department of Veterans Affairs
Veterans Health Administration
Geriatrics and Extended Care Strategic Healthcare Group
Veterans State Nursing Home Care
810 Vermont Ave. NW
Washington, DC 20420
Phone: (202)273-8538
Website: http://www.va.gov

Cat. No: 64.015 **Objectives:** To provide financial assistance to states furnishing nursing home care to veterans in state veterans' homes which meet the standards prescribed by the Secretary of Veterans Affairs. **Assist. Types:** Formula grants. **Applicant Eligibility:** Applicant is any state which operates a designated facility to furnish nursing home care primarily for veterans. **Beneficiary Eligibility:** A veteran eligible for care in a VA facility needing nursing home care and meeting certain conditions.

★ 20641 ★ U.S. Department of Veterans Affairs
Veterans Health Administration
Medical Sharing Office
Sharing Specialized Medical Resources
810 Vermont Ave. NW
Washington, DC 20420
Phone: (202)273-8406
Website: http://www.va.gov

Cat. No: 64.018 **Objectives:** To receive and share the most advanced medical techniques; to secure the use of specialized medical resources which otherwise might not be feasibly available to the VA; and to provide services to the community through specialized medical resources which are not being utilized to their maximum effectiveness within the VA. **Assist. Types:** Provision of specialized services. **Applicant Eligibility:** For sharing of medical resources: medical schools, medical installations having hospital facilities, hospitals, clinics and blood and organ banks. **Beneficiary Eligibility:** Patients of VA medical facilities or patients of medical installations having hospital facilities, hospitals, medical schools, clinics, and blood and organ banks.

★ 20642 ★ U.S. Department of Veterans Affairs
Veterans Health Administration
Pharmacy Benefits Management
Veterans Prescription Service
810 Vermont Ave. NW, Rm. 119
Washington, DC 20420
Phone: (202)273-8429
Website: http://www.va.gov

Cat. No: 64.012 **Objectives:** To provide eligible veterans and certain dependents and survivors of veterans with prescription drugs and expendable prosthetic medical supplies from Veterans Administration pharmacies upon presentation of prescription(s) from a licensed physician. **Assist. Types:** Sale, exchange, or donation of property and goods. **Applicant Eligibility:** Veterans meeting specific conditions. **Beneficiary Eligibility:** Same as Applicant Eligibility.

★ 20643 ★ U.S. Department of Veterans Affairs
Veterans Health Administration
Prosthetic and Sensory Aids Strategic Health Care Group
Veterans Prodthetic Appliances
810 Vermont Ave. NW, Rm. 1064
Washington, DC 20420
Phone: (202)273-8515 **Fax:** (202)273-9110
Website: http://www.va.gov

Cat. No: 64.013 **Objectives:** To provide, through purchase and/or fabrication, prosthetic and related appliances, equipment, and services to disabled veterans so that they may live and work as productive citizens. **Assist. Types:** Sale, exchange, or donation of property and goods. **Applicant Eligibility:** Any disabled veteran or an authorized representative on his behalf, meeting certain criteria, may apply for prosthetic appliances or services. **Beneficiary Eligibility:** Disabled veterans.

★ 20644 ★ U.S. Department of Veterans Affairs
Veterans Health Administration
Rehabilitation Strategic Healthcare Group
Blind Rehabilitation Centers
810 Vermont Ave. NW, Rm. 1071
Washington, DC 20420
Phone: (202)273-8481 **Fax:** (202)273-7603
Website: http://www.va.gov

Cat. No: 64.007 **Objectives:** To provide personal and social adjustment programs, and medical or health-related services for eligible blind veterans at selected VA hospitals maintaining blind rehabilitation centers. **Assist. Types:** Provision of specialized services. **Applicant Eligibility:** Any blind veteran who meets specific requirements for admission to a VA hospital. **Beneficiary Eligibility:** All blind veterans. **Program(s):** The Blind Rehabilitation Center Program; THe Blind Rehabilitation Clinic Program; Research and Clinical Evaluation Programs.

★ 20645 ★ U.S. Department of Veterans Affairs
Veterans Health Administration
Veterans Dental Care
810 Vermont Ave. NW
Washington, DC 20420
Phone: (202)273-8303
Website: http://www.va.gov

Cat. No: 64.011 **Objectives:** To provide medical and dental services, medicines, and medical supplies to eligible veterans on an outpatient basis. **Assist. Types:** Provision of specialized services. **Applicant Eligibility:** Any veteran whose condition or status meets specific requirements. **Beneficiary Eligibility:** Same as Applicant Eligibility.

★ 20646 ★ U.S. Department of Veterans Affairs
Veterans Health Administration
Veterans Medical Care Benefits
810 Vermont Ave. NW, Rm. 1075H
Washington, DC 20420
Phone: (202)273-8302
Website: http://www.va.gov

Cat. No: 64.009 **Objectives:** To provide inpatient, medical, surgical, and neuropsychiatric care and related medical and dental services to eligible veterans. **Assist. Types:** Provision of specialized services. **Applicant Eligibility:** Any veteran who meets specific requirements. In certain cases, spouses or children of veterans may be provided hospital care through the Civilian Health and Medical Program, Veterans Administration (CHAMPVA). **Beneficiary Eligibility:** There are 2 groups of veteran eligibility (mandatory and discretionary) for VA hospital care. The VA has an obligation to provide hospital care to veterans within one group (mandatory) and is permitted to furnish care on a resource-available basis to veterans in the other group (discretionary).

★ 20647 ★ U.S. Library of Congress National Library Service for the Blind and Physically Handicapped
Books for the Blind and Physically Handicapped
1291 Taylor St. NW
Washington, DC 20542
Phone: (202)707-5100 **Free:** 800-424-8567
Email: nls@loc.gov
Website: http://www.loc.gov/nls

Cat. No: 42.001 **Objectives:** To provide library service to the blind and physically handicapped residents of the United States and its territories, and to American citizens living abroad. **Assist. Types:** Use of property, facilities, and equipment. **Applicant Eligibility:** An applicant must provide a certificate, from a competent authority, of his inability to read or manipulate conventional printed material. **Beneficiary Eligibility:** Blind and physically handicapped residents of the United States and its territories, and American citizens living abroad.

Chapter 15
State Government Agencies

Entries in this chapter are listed alphabetically by states within 27 subject categories. For additional information, consult the "User's Guide" located at the front of the directory.

Aging

★ 20648 ★ Alabama Department of Senior Services
770 Washington Ave. RSA Plaza Ste. 470
Montgomery, AL 36130
Phone: (334)242-5743 **Free:** 877-425-2243
Fax: (334)242-5594
Email: ageline@adss.state.al.us
Website: http://www.adss.state.al.us/
Melissa Mauser Galvin, Director
Frmly: Alabama Commission on Aging.

★ 20649 ★ Alaska Department of Administration
Division of Senior Services
Alaska Commission on Aging
PO Box 110209
Juneau, AK 99811-0209
Phone: (907)465-3250 **Fax:** (907)465-4716
Email: bob_taylor@admin.state.ak.us
Website: http://www.alaskaaging.org/
Bob Taylor, PhD, Director

★ 20650 ★ American Samoa Territorial Administration on Aging
Government of American Samoa
Pago Pago, American Samoa 96799
Phone: (684)633-2207 **Fax:** (684)633-2533
Website: http://www.aoa.gov/aoa/pages/state.html
Fa'oalatia Siatu'u, Director

★ 20651 ★ Arizona Department of Economic Security
Aging and Adult Administration
1789 W Jefferson St., Site Code 950A
Phoenix, AZ 85007
Phone: (602)542-4446 **Fax:** (602)542-6575
Email: askdesaaa@mail.de.state.az.us
Website: http://www.de.state.az.us/links/aaa/

★ 20652 ★ Arkansas Department of Human Services
Division of Aging and Adult Services
1417 Donaghey Plaza South, 7th and Main Sts.
PO Box 1437, Slot S-530
Little Rock, AR 72203-1437
Phone: (501)682-2441 **Fax:** (501)682-8155
Email: herb.sanderson@mail.state.ar.us
Website: http://www.state.ar.us/dhs/aging/
Herb Sanderson, Director

★ 20653 ★ California Department of Aging
1600 K St.
Sacramento, CA 95814
Phone: (916)322-3887 **Fax:** (916)324-4989
Email: Webmaster@aging.ca.gov
Website: http://www.aging.state.ca.us/

★ 20654 ★ D.C. Office on Aging
441 4th St., NW, Ste. 900 South
Washington, DC 20001
Phone: (202)724-5622 **Fax:** (202)724-4979
Website: http://www.ftc.gov/bcp/conline/states/dc.htm

★ 20655 ★ Delaware Department of Health and Social Services
Delaware Division of Services for Aging and Adults with Physical Disabilities
Admin. Bldg, First Floor Annex, 1901 N Dupont Hwy.
New Castle, DE 19720
Phone: (302)255-9390 **Free:** 800-223-9074
Fax: (302)255-4445
Email: dsaapdinfo@state.de.us
Website: http://www.dsaapd.com/index.htm
Carolee Burton Kunz, Director

★ 20656 ★ Department of Public Health & Social Services
Division of Senior Citizens
PO Box 2816
Hagatna, GU 96932
Phone: (671)475-0263 **Fax:** (671)477-2930
Email: tommyt@mail.gov.gu
Website: http://www.dphss.govguam.net/dsc/srd/srdindex.htm
Dennis G. Rodriguez, Director

★ 20657 ★ Florida Department of Elder Affairs
4040 Esplanade Way
Tallahassee, FL 32399-7000
Phone: (850)414-2000 **Free:** 800-963-5337
Fax: (850)414-2002
Email: information@elderaffairs.org
Website: http://elderaffairs.state.fl.us/doea/ea.html
Terry F. White, Secretary

★ 20658 ★ Georgia Department of Human Resources
Division of Aging Services
2 Peachtree St. NW, Ste. 9-385
Atlanta, GA 30303-3142
Phone: (404)657-5258 **Fax:** (404)657-5285
Website: http://www.state.ga.us/Departments/dhr/aging.html

★ 20659 ★ Hawaii Executive Office on Aging
250 S Hotel St., Rm 406
Honolulu, HI 96813-2831
Phone: (808)586-0100 **Fax:** (808)586-0185
Email: eoa@mail.health.state.hi.us
Website: http://www2.state.hi.us/eoa/
Marilyn R. Seely, Director

★ 20660 ★ Idaho Commission on Aging
3380 Americana Terrace, Ste. 120
Boise, ID 83706
Phone: (208)334-3833 **Free:** 877-471-2777
Fax: (208)334-3033
Email: senglesby@icoa.state.id.us
Website: http://www2.state.id.us/icoa
Y. Sue Englesby, Contact

★ 20661 ★ Illinois Department on Aging
421 E Capitol Ave., Ste. 100
Springfield, IL 62701
Phone: (217)785-3356 **Free:** 800-252-8966
Fax: (217)785-4477
Email: ilsenior@aging.state.il.us
Website: http://www.state.il.us/aging/
Margo E. Schreiber, Director
Alt. Contact: Chicago Office, 312-814-2630.

★ 20662 ★ Indiana Family and Social Services Administration
Bureau of Aging & In-Home Services
PO Box 7083, MS-21
Indianapolis, IN 46207-7083
Phone: (317)232-7000 **Free:** 800-986-3505
Fax: (317)232-7867
Email: dlewers@fssa.state.in.us
Website: http://www.in.gov/fssa/elderly/aging/index.html
Deborah Lewers, Contact

★ 20663 ★ Iowa Department of Elder Affairs
Clemens Bldg., 3rd Fl.
200 10th St.
Des Moines, IA 50309-3609
Phone: (515)242-3333 **Fax:** (515)242-3300
Email: Sherry.James@dea.state.ia.us
Website: http://www.state.ia.us/elderaffairs/
Mark A. Haverland, Director

★ 20664 ★ Kansas Department on Aging
New England Bldg.
503 S Kansas Ave.
Topeka, KS 66603-3404
Phone: (785)296-4986 **Free:** 800-432-3535
Fax: (785)296-0256
Email: wwwmail@aging.state.ks.us
Website: http://www.k4s.org/kdoa/
Connie Hubbell, Director

★ 20665 ★ Kentucky Cabinet for Health Services
Office of Aging Services
275 E Main St., 5-C
Frankfort, KY 40621
Phone: (502)564-6930 **Fax:** (502)564-4595
Website: http://chs.state.ky.us/aging/
Jerry Whitley, Director

★ 20666 ★ Maine Bureau of Elder and Adult Services
Department of Human Services
11 State House Station
442 Civic Center Dr.
Augusta, ME 04333
Phone: (207)287-9200 **Free:** 800-262-2232
Fax: (207)287-9229
Email: webmaster.beas@state.me.us
Website: http://www.state.me.us/dhs/beas

★ 20667 ★ Maryland Department of Aging
301 W Preston St., Ste 1007
Baltimore, MD 21201
Phone: (410)767-1100 **Free:** 800-243-3425
Fax: (410)333-7943
Email: ptc@mail.ooa.state.md.us
Website: http://www.mdoa.state.md.us/
Sue Fryer Ward, Director

★ 20668 ★ Michigan Office of Services to the Aging
7109 West Saginaw, First Floor
PO Box 30676
Lansing, MI 48909-8176
Phone: (517)373-8230 **Fax:** (517)373-4092
Website: http://www.miseniors.net/
Lynn Alexander, Director

★ 20669 ★ Minnesota Board on Aging
444 Lafayette Rd. North
Saint Paul, MN 55155-3843
Phone: (651)296-2770 **Free:** 800-882-6262
Fax: (651)297-7855
Email: mba@state.mn.us
Website: http://www.mnaging.org/
Jim Varpness, Director

★ 20670 ★ Missouri Department of Health and Senior Services
PO Box 570
Jefferson City, MO 65102
Phone: (573)751-6400 **Free:** 800-235-5503
Fax: (573)751-6041
Email: info@dhss.state.mo.us
Website: http://www.dhss.state.mo.us/
Jerry Simon, Director

★ 20671 ★ Montana Senior and Long Term Care Division
Department of Public Health & Human Services
111 North Sanders, Rm. 210
Helena, MT 59604
Phone: (406)444-4077 **Free:** 800-332-2272
Fax: (406)444-7743
Email: mhanshew@state.mt.us
Website: http://www.dphhs.state.mt.us/sltc
Mike Hanshew, Director

★ 20672 ★ Nebraska Health and Human Services
Division of Aging and Disability Services
State Unit on Aging
PO Box 95044
301 Centennial Mall South, 5th Floor
Lincoln, NE 68509-5044
Phone: (402)471-4623 **Free:** 800-942-7830
Fax: (402)471-4619
Email: joann.weis@hhss.state.ne.us
Website: http://www.hhs.state.ne.us/ags/agsindex.htm
Joann Weis, Contact

★ 20673 ★ Nevada Division for Aging Services
3100 West Sahara Ave., Ste. 103
Las Vegas, NV 89102
Phone: (702)486-3545 **Fax:** (702)486-3572
Email: dasvegas@aging.state.nv.us
Website: http://www.nvaging.net/
Mary Liveratti, Director

★ 20674 ★ New Hampshire Department of Health and Human Services
Division of Elderly and Adult Services
129 Pleasant St.
Concord, NH 03301-3857
Phone: (603)271-4680 **Free:** 800-351-1888
Fax: (603)271-4643
Website: http://www.dhhs.state.nh.us/DHHS/DEAS/default.htm

★ 20675 ★ New Jersey Division of Senior Affairs
PO Box 807
Trenton, NJ 08625-0807
Phone: (609)943-3437 **Free:** 800-792-8820
Fax: (609)588-3601
Website: http://www.state.nj.us/health/senior/sraffair.htm
Nancy Day, Director

★ 20676 ★ New Mexico State Agency on Aging
228 E Palace Ave.
Santa Fe, NM 87501
Phone: (505)827-7640 **Free:** 800-432-2080
Fax: (505)827-7649
Email: nmaoa@state.nm.us
Website: http://www.nmaging.state.nm.us/
Michelle Lujan Grisham, Director

★ 20677 ★ New York State Office for the Aging
112 State St., Room 710
Albany, NY 12207-2069
Phone: (518)447-7179 **Free:** 800-342-9871
Fax: (518)447-7188
Website: http://aging.state.ny.us/index.htm
Patricia P. Pine, Ph.D, Director

★ 20678 ★ North Carolina Division of Aging
693 Palmer Dr.
2101 Mail Service Ctr.
Raleigh, NC 27699-2101
Phone: (919)733-3983 **Fax:** (919)733-0443
Email: karen.gottovi@ncmail.net
Website: http://www.dhhs.state.nc.us/aging/home.htm
Karen E. Gottovi, Director

★ 20679 ★ North Dakota Department of Human Services
Aging Services Division
600 S 2nd St., Ste. 1C
Bismarck, ND 58504-5729
Phone: (701)328-8910 **Free:** 800-451-8693
Fax: (701)328-8989
Email: dhsaging@state.nd.us
Website: http://lnotes.state.nd.us/dhs/dhsweb.nsf/ServicePages/AgingServices
Linda Wright, Director

★ 20680 ★ Office of Adult and Veterans Services
Division of Aging and Adult Services
1575 Sherman St., Ground Floor
Denver, CO 80203
Phone: (303)866-2800 **Fax:** (303)866-2696
Email: viola.mcneace@state.co.us
Website: http://www.cdhs.state.co.us/oss/aas/index1.html
Rita Barreras, Director

★ 20681 ★ Ohio Department of Aging
50 W Broad St., 9th Fl.
Columbus, OH 43215-3363
Phone: (614)466-5500 **Free:** 800-282-1206
Fax: (614)466-5741
Email: ODAMAIL@age.state.oh.us
Website: http://www.state.oh.us/age/
Joan W. Lawrence, Director

★ 20682 ★ Oregon Department of Human Resources
Seniors & People with Disabilities Division
500 Summer St. NE, EO2
Salem, OR 97301-1073
Phone: (503)945-5811 **Free:** 800-282-8096
Fax: (503)373-7823
Email: sdsd.info@state.or.us
Website: http://www.sdsd.hr.state.or.us/
Lydia Lissman, Director

★ 20683 ★ Pennsylvania Department of Aging
555 Walnut St., 5th Fl.
Harrisburg, PA 17101-1919
Phone: (717)783-1550 **Free:** 800-225-7223
Fax: (717)783-6842
Email: aging@state.pa.us
Website: http://www.aging.state.pa.us/
Larissa B. Johnson, Contact

★ 20684 ★ Puerto Rico Governor's Office of Elderly Affairs
PO Box 50063 Old San Juan Station
Call Box 50063
San Juan, PR 00902
Phone: (787)721-5710 **Fax:** (787)721-6510
Email: thooker@ban-gate.aoa.dhhs.gov
Website: http://www.aoa.dhhs.gov/RegionsI-II/stpr.htm
Ruby Rodriguez Ramirez, MHSA, Director

★ 20685 ★ Rhode Island Department of Elderly Affairs
160 Pine St.
Providence, RI 02903
Phone: (401)222-2858 **Fax:** (401)222-1490
Email: larry@dea.state.ri.us
Website: http://www.dea.state.ri.us/
Barbara Rayner, Director

★ 20686 ★ South Carolina Department of Health and Human Services
Office of Senior and Long Term Care Service
PO Box 8206
Columbia, SC 29202-8206
Phone: (803)898-2500 **Fax:** (803)898-4515
Email: adams@dhhs.state.sc.us
Website: http://www.dhhs.state.sc.us/offices/long_term_care/ltcindex.htm
Elizabeth M. Fuller, Director

★ 20687 ★ South Dakota Department of Social Services
Office of Adult Services and Aging
Richard F. Kneip Bldg.
700 Governors Dr.
Pierre, SD 57501-2291
Phone: (605)773-3656 **Free:** (866)854-5465
Fax: (605)773-6834
Email: asaging@dss.state.sd.us
Website: http://www.state.sd.us/social/ASA/index.htm
Gail Ferris, Dir of Admin

★ 20688 ★ State of Connecticut Department of Social Services
Elderly Services Division
25 Sigourney St.
Hartford, CT 06106
Phone: (860)424-5233 **Free:** 800-443-9946
Fax: (860)424-4966
Website: http://www.ctelderlyservices.state.ct.us/
Christine M. Lewis, Director

★ 20689 ★ Tennessee Commission on Aging & Disability
Andrew Jackson Bldg.
500 Deaderick St., 9th Fl.
Nashville, TN 37243-0860
Phone: (615)741-2056 **Fax:** (615)741-3309
Email: ldunn5@mail.state.tn.us
Website: http://www.state.tn.us/comaging/
James S. Whaley, Director

★ 20690 ★ Texas Department on Aging
4900 N Lamar Blvd., 4th Fl.
PO Box 12786
Austin, TX 78711
Phone: (512)424-6840 **Fax:** (512)424-6890
Email: Mary.Sapp@tdoa.state.tx.us
Website: http://www.tdoa.state.tx.us/
Mary Sapp, Director

★ 20691 ★ US Virgin Islands Department of Human Services
Senior Citizens Division
Knud Hansen Complex, Bldg. A 1303
Hospital Ground
St. Thomas, VI 00802
Phone: (340)774-0930 **Fax:** (340)774-3466
Email: humanservices@usvi.org
Website: http://www.usvi.org/humanservices/index.html
Ms. Sedonie Halbert, Director

★ 20692 ★ Utah Division of Aging and Adult Services
120 N 200 West, Rm. 325
Salt Lake City, UT 84103
Phone: (801)538-3910 **Fax:** (801)538-4395
Email: DAAS@utah.gov
Website: http://www.hsdaas.state.ut.us/

★ 20693 ★ Vermont Department of Aging and Disabilities
Waterbury Complex
103 S Main St.
Waterbury, VT 05671-2301
Phone: (802)241-2400 **Fax:** (802)241-2325
Email: webmaster@dad.state.vt.us
Website: http://www.dad.state.vt.us
Patrick Flood, Director

★ 20694 ★ Virginia Department for the Aging
1600 Forest Ave., Ste. 102
Richmond, VA 23229
Phone: (804)662-9333 **Free:** 800-552-3402
Fax: (804)662-9354
Email: aging@vdh.state.va.us
Website: http://www.aging.state.va.us/
Jay W. DeBoer, J.D., Director

★ 20695 ★ Washington Department of Social and Health Services
Aging and Adult Services Administration
PO Box 45040
Olympia, WA 98504-5050
Phone: (360)725-2310 **Free:** 800-422-3263
Fax: (360)438-8633
Email: wongma@dshs.wa.gov
Website: http://www.aasa.dshs.wa.gov/
Kathy Leitch, Director

★ 20696 ★ West Virginia Bureau of Senior Services
Holly Grove, Bldg. 10
1900 Kanawha Blvd. E
Charleston, WV 25305-0160
Phone: (304)558-3317 **Fax:** (304)558-0004
Email: astottlemyer@boss.state.wv.us
Website: http://www.state.wv.us/seniorservices/
Ann M. Stottlemyer, Director

★ 20697 ★ Wyoming Department of Health
Aging Division
259B North Bldg.
6101 Yellowstone Rd.
Cheyenne, WY 82002
Phone: (307)777-7986 **Free:** 800-442-2766
Fax: (307)777-5340
Email: cnoon@state.wy.us
Website: http://wdhfs.state.wy.us/aging/index.htm
Colleen Noon, Contact

AIDS

★ 20698 ★ Alabama Department of Public Health
HIV / AIDS Division
RSA Tower
201 Monroe St., Ste. 1450
PO Box 303017
Montgomery, AL 36130-3017
Phone: (334)206-5364 **Fax:** (334)206-2092
Website: http://www.adph.org/aids/
Jane B. Cheeks, JD, Director

★ 20699 ★ Alaska Department of Health and Social Services
Public Health Division
Epidemiology Section
3601 C St., Ste. 540
PO Box 240249
Anchorage, AK 99524-0249
Phone: (907)269-8000 **Free:** 800-478-0084
Fax: (907)562-7802
Email: epiweb@epi.hss.state.ak.us
Website: http://www.epi.hss.state.ak.us/

★ 20700 ★ Arizona Department of Health Services
Office of Infectious Diseases
Offices of HIV / STD Services
3815 N Black Canyon Hwy.
Phoenix, AZ 85015
Phone: (602)230-5932 **Fax:** (602)263-4943
Email: webmaster@hs.state.az.us
Website: http://www.hs.state.az.us/edc/hivpage.html
Christopher Brown, MBA, Director

★ 20701 ★ California Health and Welfare Agency
Health Services Department
Office of AIDS
611 N 7th St., Ste. A
Sacramento, CA 95814-0208
Phone: (916)445-0553 **Fax:** (916)323-4642
Email: adarr@dhs.ca.gov
Website: http://www.dhs.cahwnet.gov/org/ps/ooa/ooaindex.htm

★ 20702 ★ Connecticut Department of Public Health
Bureau of Community Health
AIDS Division
410 Capitol Ave.
PO Box 340308
Hartford, CT 06134-0308
Phone: (860)509-7801 **Free:** 800-509-7900
Fax: (860)509-7853
Email: webmaster.dph@po.state.ct.us
Website: http://www.dph.state.ct.us/BCH/AIDS/HPAIDS.html
Rosa M. Biaggi, MPH, Director

★ 20703 ★ Delaware Department of Health and Social Services
Division of Public Health
Disease Prevention and Control
HIV / AIDS Epidemiology Program
Jesse Cooper Bldg.
Federal & Water St.
PO Box 637
Dover, DE 19903
Phone: (302)739-2354 **Fax:** (302)739-6659
Email: dhsinfo@state.de.us
Website: http://www.delaware-epi.org/aids1.htm

★ 20704 ★ Florida Department of Health
Health & Human Services
Bureau of HIV / AIDS
4052 Bald Cypress Way, Bin A09
Tallahassee, FL 32399-1715
Phone: (850)245-4444
Email: health@doh.state.fl.us
Website: http://www9.myflorida.com/aids/index.html
Tom Liberti, Director

★ 20705 ★ Georgia Department of Human Resources
Public Health Division
Epidemiology Branch
HIV/STD Epidemiology Unit
2 Peachtree St. NW
Atlanta, GA 30303-3186
Phone: (404)657-2588
Email: gaepinfo@dhr.state.ga.us
Website: http://www.ph.dhr.state.ga.us/epi/aidsunit.shtml
John F. Beltrami, MD, Director

★ 20706 ★ Hawaii Department of Health
Health Resources Adminstration
STD / AIDS Prevention Branch
3627 Kilauea Ave., Room 306
Honolulu, HI 96816
Phone: (808)733-9010 **Fax:** (808)733-9015
Website: http://www.state.hi.us/health/resource/comm_dis/std_aids/index.html
Peter M. Whiticar, Director

★ 20707 ★ Illinois Department of Public Health
Office of Health Protection
AIDS Activities Section
525 W Jefferson St., 2nd Fl.
Springfield, IL 62761-0001
Phone: (217)782-3984 **Fax:** (217)524-0802
Email: thughes@idph.state.il.us
Website: http://www.idph.state.il.us/about/ohp.htm
Tom Hughes, Director

★ 20708 ★ Iowa Department of Public Health
Bureau of Disease Prevention
HIV / AIDS Program
Lucas State Office Bldg.
321 E 12th St.
Des Moines, IA 50319-0075
Phone: (515)242-5838 **Fax:** (515)281-4958
Email: pyoung@idph.state.ia.us
Website: http://www.idph.state.ia.us/fch/inf_dis/hivaids.htm
Patricia Young, Director

★ 20709 ★ Kansas Department of Health and Environment
Division of Health
HIV - STD Section
1000 SW Jackson, Ste. 210
Topeka, KS 66612-1274
Phone: (785)296-6173 **Fax:** (785)296-4197
Email: kmilhon@kdhe.state.ks.us
Website: http://www.kdhe.state.ks.us/hiv-std/index.html
Karl Milhon, Director

★ 20710 ★ Louisiana Department of Health and Hospitals
Office of Public Health
HIV / AIDS Services
234 Loyola Ave., 5th Floor
New Orleans, LA 70112
Phone: (504)568-7474 **Fax:** (504)568-7044
Email: hivweb@dhh.state.la.us
Website: http://www.dhh.state.la.us/OPH/hivstd/Default.htm
Beth Scalco, Director

★ 20711 ★ Maine Department of Human Services
Health Bureau
Disease Control Division
11 State House Station
Augusta, ME 04333
Phone: (207)287-6448 **Fax:** (207)287-3498
Email: sallylou.patterson@state.me.us
Website: http://www.state.me.us/dhs/boh/ddc/HIV_STD.htm
Sally-Lou Patterson, Director

★ 20712 ★ Massachusetts Executive Office of Health and Human Services
Public Health Department
HIV / AIDS Bureau
250 Washington St., 3d Fl.
Boston, MA 02108
Phone: (617)624-5300 **Fax:** (617)624-5399
Email: dph.info@state.ma.us
Website: http://www.state.ma.us/dph/aids/hivaids.htm
Jean Flatley McGuire, PhD, Director

★ 20713 ★ Michigan Department of Community Health
HIV / AIDS - STD Division
Ste. 300
2479 Woodlake Circle
Okemos, MI 48864
Phone: (517)241-5900 **Fax:** (517)241-5911
Email: arias@state.mi.us
Website: http://www.mdch.state.mi.us/dch/hiv_aids.htm
James K. Haveman, Jr., Director

★ 20714 ★ Minnesota Department of Health
STD and HIV Section
717 Delaware St. SE
PO Box 64975
Saint Paul, MN 55164-0975
Phone: (651)215-5800 **Fax:** (651)623-5743
Email: jan.wiehle@health.state.mn.us
Website: http://www.health.state.mn.us/divs/dpc/aids-std/aids-std.htm
Jan Wiehle, Contact

★ 20715 ★ Missouri Department of Health & Senior Services
Section of STD / HIV
930 Wildwood Dr.
PO Box 570
Jefferson City, MO 65102-0570
Phone: (573)751-6439 **Free:** 800-392-0272
Fax: (573)751-6447
Email: info@dhss.state.mo.us
Website: http://www.health.state.mo.us/sshapcs/SSHAPCS.html

★ 20716 ★ Montana Department of Public Health and Human Services
Health Policy and Services Division
Disease Prevention & Control
STD / AIDS Program
1400 Broadway
PO Box 202951
Helena, MT 59620-2951
Phone: (406)444-9028 **Fax:** (406)444-6842
Email: bdeitle@state.mt.us
Website: http://www.dphhs.state.mt.us/hpsd/pubheal/disease/stdhiv/index.htm
Bruce Deitle, Director

★ 20717 ★ Nebraska Department of Health and Human Services
Health Promotion and Disease Prevention
Communicable Disease Section
HIV Prevention Program
301 Centennial Mall S
PO Box 94817
Lincoln, NE 68509-4817
Phone: (402)471-9098 **Free:** 800-782-2437
Fax: (402)471-0382
Email: charles.housman@hhss.state.ne.us
Website: http://www.hhs.state.ne.us/dpc/HIV.htm
Dan Cillessen, Director

★ 20718 ★ New Hampshire Department of Health and Human Services
Office of Community & Public Health
HIV Prevention Program
6 Hazen Dr.
Concord, NH 03301
Phone: (603)271-4502 **Free:** 800-852-3345
Fax: (603)271-4934
Website: http://www.dhhs.state.nh.us/DHHS/HIVPREVENTION/default.htm/

★ 20719 ★ North Carolina Department of Health and Human Services
HIV / STD Prevention & Care Branch
1902 Mail Service Ctr.
Raleigh, NC 27699-1902
Phone: (919)733-7301 **Fax:** (919)733-1020
Email: betsy.school@ncmail.net
Website: http://www.schs.state.nc.us/epi/hiv/

★ 20720 ★ North Dakota Department of Health
Disease Control Division
HIV / AIDS Section
AIDS Program
600 E Boulevard, 2nd Fl.
Bismarck, ND 58505-0200
Phone: (701)328-2378 **Free:** 800-472-2180
Fax: (701)328-2499
Email: kmongeon@state.nd.us
Website: http://www.health.state.nd.us/ndhd/prevent/disease/hiv
Karin Mongeon, Director

★ 20721 ★ Ohio Department of Health
Prevention Division
AIDS Client Resources Section
246 N High St.
PO Box 118
Columbus, OH 43216-0118
Phone: (614)466-6374 **Fax:** (614)564-2432
Email: BCHSSD@gw.odh.state.oh.us
Website: http://www.odh.state.oh.us/ODHPrograms/AIDS/aids1.htm

★ 20722 ★ Oklahoma Department of Health
Personal Health Services
HIV / STD Services
1000 NE 10th St.
Oklahoma City, OK 73117
Phone: (405)271-4636 **Free:** 800-535-2437
Fax: (405)271-3431
Email: michelgg@health.state.ok.us
Website: http://www.health.state.ok.us/PROGRAM/hivstd/index.html
Michelle Green-Gilbert, Contact

★ 20723 ★ Oregon Department of Human Resources
Public Health Services
Sexually Transmitted Diseases Program
800 NE Oregon St.
Portland, OR 97232
Phone: (503)731-4026 **Fax:** (503)731-4608
Email: janet.j.karius@state.or.us
Website: http://www.ohd.hr.state.or.us/std/welcome.htm
Jan Karius, Director

★ 20724 ★ Pennsylvania Department of Health
Public Health Programs
HIV and AIDS Programs
Health and Welfare Bldg.
PO Box 90
Harrisburg, PA 17108
Phone: (717)783-0479 **Free:** 877-724-3258
Fax: (717)772-6959
Email: webmaster@health.state.pa.us
Website: http://www.health.state.pa.us/php/HIV/default.htm

★ 20725 ★ South Carolina Department of Health and Environmental Control
Bureau of Disease Control
STD HIV Program
Mills/Jarrett Comples
PO Box 101106
Columbia, SC 29211-0106
Phone: (803)898-0749 **Free:** 800-277-0873
Email: Kettinld@Columb60.dhec.state.sc.us
Website: http://www.scdhec.net/hs/diseasecont/disease.htm
Lynda Kettinger, Director

★ 20726 ★ South Dakota Department of Health
Disease Prevention
HIV / AIDS Program
615 E 4th St.
Pierre, SD 57501
Phone: (605)773-3737 **Free:** 800-592-1861
Fax: (605)773-5509
Email: DOH.INFO@state.sd.us
Website: http://www.state.sd.us/doh/Disease/index.htm

★ 20727 ★ Tennessee Department of Health
AIDS Program
Cordell Hull Bldg.
435 5th Ave. N
Nashville, TN 37247-5281
Phone: (615)741-3111 **Free:** 800-525-2437
Fax: (615)741-2491
Email: DDenton@mail.state.tn.us
Website: http://www.state.tn.us/health/

★ 20728 ★ Texas Department of Health
HIV / STD Prevention Bureau
1100 W 49th St.
Austin, TX 78756-3199

Phone: (512)490-2505 **Free:** 888-963-7111
Fax: (512)458-9368
Email: hivstd.infoline@tdh.state.tx.us
Website: http://www.tdh.state.tx.us/hivstd/default.htm

★ 20729 ★ Utah Department of Health
Bureau of Communicable Disease Control
HIV and AIDS Bureau
288 N 1460 W
PO Box 142105
Salt Lake City, UT 84114-2105
Phone: (801)538-6096 **Fax:** (801)538-9913
Email: tgarrett@doh.state.ut.us
Website: http://www.health.state.ut.us/els/hivaids/index.html

★ 20730 ★ Vermont Department of Health
HIV / AIDS Program
108 Cherry St.
PO Box 70
Burlington, VT 05402-0070
Phone: (802)863-7245 **Free:** 800-244-7639
Fax: (802)863-7314
Email: webkeeper@vdh.state.vt.us
Website: http://www.state.vt.us/health/_hs/aids/aids.htm

★ 20731 ★ Virginia Department of Health
Division of HIV / STD
1500 E Main St., Rm.112
PO Box 2448
Richmond, VA 23218
Phone: (804)786-6267 **Free:** 800-533-4148
Fax: (804)225-3517
Email: lbranch@vdh.state.va.us
Website: http://www.vdh.state.va.us/std/index.htm
Casey Riley, Director

★ 20732 ★ Washington Department of Health
Community and Family Health Services Division
HIV Client Services
PO Box 47841
Olympia, WA 98504-7841
Phone: (360)236-3426 **Free:** 800-272-2437
Fax: (360)664-2616
Email: Darren.Layman@doh.wa.gov
Website: http://www.doh.wa.gov/cfh/HIV_AIDS/Client_Svcs/default.htm
Darren Layman, Contact

★ 20733 ★ West Virginia Department of Health and Human Resources
Bureau for Public Health
Division of Surveillance and Disease Control
AIDS Program
350 Capitol St., Rm. 125
Charleston, WV 25301-3715
Phone: (304)558-2950 **Free:** 800-642-8244
Fax: (304)558-6335
Email: lorettahaddy@wvdhhr.org
Website: http://www.wvdhhr.org/bph/oehp/sdc/aids.htm
Loretta Haddy, Contact

★ 20734 ★ Wisconsin Department of Health and Family Services
Public Health
Communicable Disease Program
AIDS / HIV Program
1 W Wilson St
Madison, WI 53702
Phone: (608)266-1865 **Fax:** (608)264-6078
Email: webmaildph@dhfs.state.wi.us
Website: http://www.dhfs.state.wi.us/aids-hiv/index.htm

★ 20735 ★ Wyoming Department of Health
HIV / AIDS / Hepatitis Program
Hathaway Bldg., 4th Fl.
Cheyenne, WY 82002
Phone: (307)777-5932 **Fax:** (307)777-7382
Email: srente@state.wy.us
Website: http://wdhfs.state.wy.us/AIDS/
Sharon G. Renter, MS, Director

Blind

★ 20736 ★ Alabama Department of Rehabilitation Services
2129 E South Blvd.
PO Box 11586
Montgomery, AL 36116-2455
Phone: (334)281-8780 **Free:** 800-441-7607
Fax: (334)281-1973
Email: webinfo@rehab.state.al.us
Website: http://www.rehab.state.al.us/
Steve Shivers, Director

★ 20737 ★ Alaska Department of Labor and Workforce Development
Vocational Rehabilitation Division
801 W 10th St., Ste. A
Juneau, AK 99801-1894
Phone: (907)465-2814 **Free:** 800-478-2815
Fax: (907)465-2856
Email: anne_knight@labor.state.ak.us
Website: http://www.labor.state.ak.us/dvr/home.htm
Duane French, Director

★ 20738 ★ Arkansas Department of Human Services
Division of Services for the Blind
522 Main St.
PO Box 3237
Little Rock, AR 72203
Phone: (501)682-5463 **Free:** 800-960-9270
Fax: (501)682-0366
Email: charlie.cain@mail.state.ar.us
Website: http://www.state.ar.us/dhs/dsb/index.html
James C. Hudson, Director

★ 20739 ★ Blind Industries and Services of Maryland
2901 Strickland St.
Baltimore, MD 21223-2796
Phone: (410)233-4567 **Free:** 888-322-4567
Fax: (410)233-0544
Email: dors@msde.state.md.us
Website: http://www.bism.com/

★ 20740 ★ California Health and Welfare Agency
Rehabilitation Department
PO Box 944222
2000 Evergreen St.
Sacramento, CA 95815
Phone: (916)263-8981 **Fax:** (916)327-4567
Email: suggest@rehab.cahwnet.gov
Website: http://www.rehab.ca.gov/

★ 20741 ★ Colorado Department of Human Services
Division of Vocational Rehabilitation
2211 West Evans, Bldg. B
Denver, CO 80223
Phone: (720)884-1234 **Fax:** (720)884-1213
Email: debbie.powell@state.co.us
Website: http://www.cdhs.state.co.us/ods/dvr/index.html
Diana Huerta, Director

★ 20742 ★ Connecticut Board of Education and Services for the Blind
184 Windsor Ave.
Windsor, CT 06095
Phone: (860)602-4000 **Free:** 800-842-4510
Fax: (860)602-4020
Email: besb@po.state.ct.us
Website: http://www.besb.state.ct.us/
Donna Balaski, Director

★ 20743 ★ Delaware Department of Health and Social Services
Visually Impaired Division
Biggs Bldg.
1901 N DuPont Hwy.
New Castle, DE 19720
Phone: (302)255-9800 **Fax:** (302)255-4441
Email: dhssinfo@state.de.us
Website: http://www.state.de.us/dhss/dvi/dvihome.htm
Harry B. Hill, III, Director

★ 20744 ★ Florida Department of Labor and Employment Security
Division of Blind Services
Douglas Bldg.
2551 Executive Center Circle W, Ste. 200
Tallahassee, FL 32399
Phone: (850)487-1260 **Free:** 800-342-1330
Fax: (850)487-1804
Email: craig_kiser@dbs.doe.state.fl.us
Website: http://www.state.fl.us/dbs/
Craig Kiser, Director
Frmly: Florida Department of Education, Blind Services Division. **Program(s):** Talking Book Program; Children and Families Program; Independent Living Adult Program; Rehabilitation Center for the Blind; Business Enterprise Program; Vocational Rehabilitation Program.

★ 20745 ★ Hawaii Department of Human Services
Vocational Rehabilitation and Blind Services Division
601 Kamokila Blvd., Rm. 515
Kapolei, HI 96707
Phone: (808)692-7719 **Fax:** (808)692-7727
Website: http://www.state.hi.us/dhs/
Neil Shim, Director

★ 20746 ★ Idaho Commission for the Blind and Visually Impaired
341 W Washington St.
PO Box 83720
Boise, ID 83720-0012
Phone: (208)334-3220 **Free:** 800-542-8688
Fax: (208)334-2963
Email: dard@icbvi.state.id.us
Website: http://www.icbvi.state.id.us/
Dana Ard, Contact

★ 20747 ★ Illinois Department of Human Services
Aid to the Aged, Blind, or Disabled
100 S Grand Ave. E
Springfield, IL 62762
Phone: (217)557-1564 **Free:** 800-252-8635
Fax: (217)557-2112
Email: nsanchez@dhs.state.il.us
Website: http://www.state.il.us/agency/dhs/aabdnp.html

★ 20748 ★ Iowa Department for the Blind
524 4th St.
Des Moines, IA 50309-2364
Phone: (515)281-1333 **Free:** 800-362-2587
Fax: (515)281-1263
Email: harris.allen@blind.state.ia.us

Website: http://www.blind.state.ia.us/
Allen Harris, Director

★ 20749 ★ Kansas Department of Social and Rehabilitation Services
Rehabilitation Services Division
915 SW Harrison St.
Topeka, KS 66612
Phone: (785)267-5301 **Fax:** (785)296-2173
Website: http://www.srskansas.org/
Dale L. Barnum, Director

★ 20750 ★ Kentucky Department for the Blind
Blind Department
209 St. Clair St.
PO Box 757
Frankfort, KY 40602-0757
Phone: (502)564-4754 **Free:** 877-592-5463
Fax: (502)564-2951
Email: wayne.thompson@mail.state.ky.us
Website: http://kyblind.state.ky.us/

★ 20751 ★ Louisiana Department of Social Services
Rehabilitation Services Division
8225 Florida Blvd.
Baton Rouge, LA 70806
Phone: (225)925-4131 **Free:** 800-737-2958
Fax: (225)925-4484
Email: webmaster@dss.state.la.us
Website: http://www.dss.state.la.us/offlrs/index.htm
James Wallace, Director

★ 20752 ★ Maine Department of Labor
Rehabilitation Services Bureau
Blind and Visually Impaired Division
150 State House Station
Augusta, ME 04333-0150
Phone: (207)624-5950 **Free:** 800-698-4440
Fax: (207)624-5980
Email: Webmaster.BRS@state.me.us
Website: http://www.state.me.us/rehab/

★ 20753 ★ Massachusetts Commission for the Blind
88 Kingston St.
Boston, MA 02111
Phone: (617)727-5550 **Free:** 800-392-6450
Fax: (617)727-5960
Email: david.jansen@state.ma.us
Website: http://www.state.ma.us/mcb/
David Govostes, Director

★ 20754 ★ Michigan Commission for the Blind
201 N Washington Sq.
PO Box 30652
Lansing, MI 48909
Phone: (517)373-6425 **Free:** 800-292-4200
Fax: (517)335-5140
Website: http://www.mfia.state.mi.us/mcb/
Patrick D. Cannon, Director

★ 20755 ★ Minnesota Department of Economic Security
State Services for the Blind
390 N Robert St. Fifth Floor
Saint Paul, MN 55101
Phone: (651)296-1822 **Free:** 800-652-9000
Email: belsey@ngwmail.des.state.mn.us
Website: http://www.mnworkforcecenter.org/burgundy/ssb.htm
Bonnie Elsey, Contact

★ 20756 ★ Mississippi Department of Rehabilitation Services
1281 Hwy. 51 N
PO Box 1698
Jackson, MS 39215-1698
Phone: (601)853-5100 **Free:** 800-443-1000
Fax: (601)853-5205
Email: bmcmillan@mdrs.state.ms.us
Website: http://www.mdrs.state.ms.us/
H.S. McMillan, Director

★ 20757 ★ Missouri Department of Social Services
Family Services Division
Rehabilitation Services for the Blind
3418 Knipp
PO Box 88
Jefferson City, MO 65103-0088
Phone: (573)751-4249 **Free:** 800-592-6004
Fax: (573)751-4984
Email: mgiboney@mail.state.mo.us
Website: http://www.dss.state.mo.us/dfs/rehab/rehab.htm

★ 20758 ★ Montana Disability Services Division
Vocational Rehabilitation Programs
111 N Sanders, Ste. 307
PO Box 4210
Helena, MT 59604-4210
Phone: (406)444-2590 **Free:** 877-296-1197
Fax: (406)444-3632
Email: jmathews@state.mt.gov
Website: http://www.dphhs.state.mt.us/dsd/govt_programs/vrp/index.htm

★ 20759 ★ Nebraska Department of Health and Human Services
Rehabilitation Services for the Visually Impaired
PO Box 95044
Lincoln, NE 68509-5044
Phone: (402)471-2306 **Fax:** (402)471-0820
Email: hhss_system_information@hhss.state.ne.us
Website: http://www.hhs.state.ne.us/vii/viiindex.htm

★ 20760 ★ Nevada Department of Employment, Training and Rehabilitation
Rehabilitation Division
Bureau of Services to the Blind and Visually Impaired
505 E King St., Rm. 505
Carson City, NV 89701
Phone: (775)684-4244
Email: detrbsb@nvdetr.org
Website: http://detr.state.nv.us/rehab/reh_bvi.htm

★ 20761 ★ New Hampshire Bureau of Adult Education
Division of Adult Learning and Rehabilitation
101 Pleasant St.
Concord, NH 03301
Phone: (603)271-6698 **Free:** 800-299-1647
Fax: (603)271-1114
Email: jchaput@ed.state.nh.us
Website: http://www.ed.state.nh.us/adulted/adult.htm
Jeanne Chaput, Contact

★ 20762 ★ New Jersey Department of Human Services
Commission for the Blind and Visually Impaired
153 Halsey St.
PO Box 47017
Newark, NJ 07102
Phone: (973)648-2324 **Fax:** (973)648-7364
Website: http://www.state.nj.us/humanservices/cbvi/index.html
Jamie Casabianca Hilton, Director

★ 20763 ★ New Mexico Commission for the Blind
PERA Bldg., Rm. 553
Santa Fe, NM 87501
Phone: (505)827-4479 **Free:** 888-513-7968
Fax: (505)827-4475
Email: greg.trapp@state.nm.us
Website: http://www.state.nm.us/cftb/
Greg Trapp, Director

★ 20764 ★ New York State Department of Social Services
Blind and Visually Handicapped Commission
40 N Pearl St.
155 Washington Ave.
Albany, NY 12243
Phone: (518)473-1675 **Fax:** (518)473-9255
Email: cbvh@dfa.state.ny.us
Website: http://www.ocfs.state.ny.us/main/cbvh/default.htm
John A. Johnson, Director

★ 20765 ★ North Carolina Department of Health and Human Services
Divison of Services for the Blind
2601 Mail Service Ctr.
309 Ashe Ave. - Fisher Bldg.
Raleigh, NC 27699-2601
Phone: (919)733-9822 **Fax:** (919)733-9769
Email: john.deluca@ncmail.net
Website: http://www.dhhs.state.nc.us/dsb/
John DeLuca, Director

★ 20766 ★ North Dakota Department of Human Services
Disability Services Division
600 S Second St.
Bismarck, ND 58504-5729
Phone: (701)328-8930 **Free:** 800-755-8529
Fax: (701)328-8969
Email: dhsds@state.nd.us
Website: http://lnotes.state.nd.us/dhs/dhsweb.nsf/ServicePages/DisabilityServices

★ 20767 ★ Ohio Rehabilitation Services Commission
Services for the Visually Impaired Bureau
400 E Campus View Blvd., SW3A
Columbus, OH 43235-4604
Phone: (614)438-1255 **Free:** 800-282-4536
Fax: (614)438-1257
Email: RSC_wac@rscnet.al.state.oh.us
Website: http://www.state.oh.us/rsc/VR_Services/BSVI/bsvi.html
William A. Casto, II, Director

★ 20768 ★ Oklahoma Department of Rehabilitation Services
Visual Services Bureau
3535 NW 58th St., Ste. 500
Oklahoma City, OK 73112-4815
Phone: (405)951-3400 **Free:** 800-845-8476
Fax: (405)951-3529
Email: drspiowm@onenet.net
Website: http://www.okrehab.org/

★ 20769 ★ Oregon Commission for the Blind
535 SE 12th Ave.
Portland, OR 97214
Phone: (503)731-3221 **Free:** 888-202-5463
Fax: (503)731-3230
Email: ocbmail@state.or.us
Website: http://www.cfb.state.or.us

★ 20770 ★ Pennsylvania Department of Public Welfare
Blindness and Visual Services Bureau
2923 N 7th St.
Harrisburg, PA 17102
Phone: (717)787-7500
Website: http://www.aging.state.pa.us/aging/cwp/view.asp?a=277&Q=176872

★ 20771 ★ Rhode Island Department of Human Services
Office of Rehabilitation Services
Services for the Blind and Visually Impaired
40 Fountain St.
Providence, RI 02903
Phone: (401)222-2300 **Free:** 800-752-8088
Fax: (401)222-1328
Website: http://www.ors.state.ri.us/sbvipage.htm

★ 20772 ★ South Carolina Commission for the Blind
1430 Confederate Ave.
PO Box 79
Columbia, SC 29202
Phone: (803)898-8800 **Free:** 800-922-2222
Fax: (803)898-8800
Email: publicinfo@sccb.state.sc.us
Website: http://www.sccb.state.sc.us/

★ 20773 ★ South Dakota Department of Human Services
Services to the Blind and Visually Impaired Division
Hillsview Plaza, E Hwy 34
500 E Capitol Ave.
Pierre, SD 57501-5070
Phone: (605)773-5990 **Fax:** (605)773-5483
Email: jeff.kisecker@state.sd.us
Website: http://www.state.sd.us/dhs/sbvi/
Gaye Mattke, Director

★ 20774 ★ Tennessee Department of Human Services
Rehabilitation Services Division
Services for the Blind and Visually Impaired
400 Deaderick St.
Citizens Plaza Bldg, 11th Floor
Nashville, TN 37248-6200
Phone: (615)313-4914 **Fax:** (615)741-4165
Email: lgallon@mail.state.tn.us
Website: http://www.state.tn.us/humanserv/vis-home.html

★ 20775 ★ Texas Commission for the Blind
4800 N Lamar Blvd., Ste. 340
PO Box 12866
Austin, TX 78756-3178
Phone: (512)459-2500 **Free:** 800-252-5204
Fax: (512)377-0685
Email: judy.adams@tcb.state.tx.us
Website: http://www.tcb.state.tx.us/

★ 20776 ★ Vermont Agency of Human Services
Aging and Disabilities Department
Blind and Visually Impaired Division
Osgood Bldg.
103 S Main St.
Waterbury, VT 05671-2304
Phone: (802)241-2210 **Fax:** (802)241-3359
Email: fredj@dad.state.vt.us
Website: http://www.dad.state.vt.us/dbvi/
Fred Jones, Director

★ 20777 ★ Virgin Islands Department of Human Services
Disabilities and Rehabilitation Services Division
Knud Hansen Complex, Bldg. A 1303
Hospital Ground
St. Thomas, VI 00802
Phone: (340)774-0930 **Fax:** (340)774-3466
Email: humanservices@usvi.org
Website: http://www.usvi.org/humanservices/index.html

★ 20778 ★ Virginia Office of Health and Human Resources
Department for the Blind and Visually Impaired
397 Azalea Ave.
Richmond, VA 23227
Phone: (804)371-3353 **Free:** 800-622-2155
Fax: (804)371-3351
Email: bowmanja@dbvi.state.va.us
Website: http://www.vdbvi.org//
Joseph A. Bowman, Director

★ 20779 ★ Washington State Department of Services for the Blind
402 Legion Way SE, Ste. 100
PO Box 40933
Olympia, WA 98504-0933
Phone: (360)586-1224 **Free:** 800-552-7103
Fax: (360)586-7627
Email: dsb_info@listserv.wa.gov
Website: http://www.wa.gov/dsb/

★ 20780 ★ West Virginia State Board of Rehabilitation
Rehabilitation Services Division
State Capitol Complex
PO Box 50890
Charleston, WV 25305-0890
Phone: (304)766-4799 **Free:** 800-642-8207
Fax: (304)766-4905
Email: penneyh@mail.drs.state.wv.us
Website: http://www.wvdrs.org/
Janice Holland, Director

★ 20781 ★ Wisconsin Department of Workforce Development
Vocational Rehabilitation Division
2917 International Ln., Ste. 300
PO Box 7852
Madison, WI 53707-7852
Phone: (608)243-5600 **Free:** 800-442-3477
Fax: (608)243-5680
Email: charlene.dwyer@dwd.state.wi.us
Website: http://www.dwd.state.wi.us/dvr/
Charlene Dwyer, Director

★ 20782 ★ Wyoming Department of Employment
Vocational Rehabilitation Division
1100 Herschler Bldg.
122 W 25th St.
Cheyenne, WY 82002
Phone: (307)777-7389 **Fax:** (307)777-5939
Email: jmcint@state.wy.us
Website: http://wydoe.state.wy.us/doe.asp?ID=5
Gary W. Child, Director

Dental Boards

★ 20783 ★ Alaska State Board of Dental Examiners
PO Box 110806
Juneau, AK 99811-0806
Phone: (907)465-2542 **Fax:** (907)465-2974
Email: wanda_fleming@dced.state.ak.us
Website: http://www.dced.state.ak.us/occ/pden.htm
Ms. Wanda Fleming, Contact

★ 20784 ★ Arkansas State Board of Dental Examiners
101 E Capitol, Ste. 111
Little Rock, AR 72201
Phone: (501)682-2085 **Fax:** (501)682-3543
Email: judith.rickard@mail.state.ar.us
Website: http://www.asbde.org
Ms. Judith Rickard, Director

★ 20785 ★ Board of Dental Examiners, Inc.
North East Regional Board of Dental Examiners, Inc. (NERB)
8484 Georgia Ave., Ste. 900
Silver Spring, MD 20910
Phone: (301)563-3300 **Fax:** (301)563-3307
Website: http://www.nerb.org/
Jack Feldesman, Director

★ 20786 ★ Central Regional Dental Testing Service, Inc.
CRDTS
1725 SW Gage Blvd.
Topeka, KS 66604-3333
Phone: (785)273-0380 **Fax:** (785)273-5015
Email: info@crdts.org
Website: http://www.crdts.org/
Ted Carter, Director

★ 20787 ★ Colorado State Board of Dental Examiners
1560 Broadway, Ste. 1310
Denver, CO 80202
Phone: (303)894-7758 **Fax:** (303)894-7764
Email: Dental@dora.state.co.us
Website: http://www.dora.state.co.us/dental
Karen Brumley, Director

★ 20788 ★ Florida Board of Dentistry
4042 Bald Cypress Way, Bin A13
Tallahassee, FL 32399-1721
Phone: (850)245-4333 **Fax:** (850)921-5389
Email: Sue_Foster@doh.state.fl.us
Website: http://www9.myflorida.com/mqa/dentistry/dn_home.html
Sue Foster, Director

★ 20789 ★ Georgia Board of Dentistry
237 Coliseum Dr.
Macon, GA 31217-3858
Phone: (478)207-1680
Email: tathomas@sos.state.ga.us
Website: http://www.sos.state.ga.us/plb/dentistry/
Tachunta Thomas, Director

★ 20790 ★ Hawaii State Board of Dental Examiners
1010 Richards St.
PO Box 3469
DCCA-PVL
ATTN: DENTAL
Honolulu, HI 96801
Phone: (808)586-3000
Email: dental@dcca.state.hi.us
Website: http://www.state.hi.us/dcca/pvl/areas_dentist.html
Mr. James Kobashigawa, Director

★ 20791 ★ Idaho State Board of Dentistry
708 ½ W Franklin St.
PO Box 83720
Boise, ID 83720-0021
Phone: (208)334-2369 **Fax:** (208)334-3247
Email: smiller@isbd.state.id.us

Website: http://www2.state.id.us/isbd/
Michael Sheeley, Director

★ 20792 ★ Indiana State Board of Dentistry
Health Professions Bureau
402 W Washington, Rm. W041
Indianapolis, IN 46204
Phone: (317)234-2057 **Fax:** (317)233-4236
Email: stansinsin@hpb.state.in.us
Website: http://www.in.gov/hpb/boards/isbd/
Rosendo L. Tansinsin, Director

★ 20793 ★ Iowa Board of Dental Examiners
400 SW 8th St., Ste. D
Des Moines, IA 50309-4687
Phone: (515)281-5157 **Fax:** (515)281-7969
Email: ibde@bon.state.ia.us
Website: http://www.iowaccess.org/dentalboard/
Mrs. Constance L. Price, Director

★ 20794 ★ Kentucky Board of Dentistry
10101 Linn Station Rd., Ste. 540
Louisville, KY 40223
Phone: (502)423-0573 **Fax:** (502)423-1239
Website: http://dentistry.state.ky.us/
Mr. Gary Munsie, Director

★ 20795 ★ Louisiana State Board of Dentistry
365 Canal St., Ste. 2680
New Orleans, LA 70130
Phone: (504)568-8574 **Fax:** (504)568-8598
Email: bogden@lsbd.org
Website: http://www.lsbd.org/
C. Barry Ogden, Esq., Director

★ 20796 ★ Maine Board of Dental Examiners
143 State House Station
Two Bangor St.
Augusta, ME 04333-0143
Phone: (207)287-3333 **Fax:** (207)287-8140
Email: anita.c.merrow@state.me.us
Website: http://www.licenseverification.com/medental/
Anita C. Merrow, Contact

★ 20797 ★ Maryland State Board of Dental Examiners
Benjamin Rush Bldg.
Spring Grove State Hospital
55 Wade Ave.
Baltimore, MD 21228
Phone: (410)402-8501 **Fax:** (410)402-8505
Website: www.dhmh.state.md.us/dental/
Kim Mayer, Director

★ 20798 ★ Massachusetts Board of Registration in Dentistry
239 Causeway St., Ste. 500
Boston, MA 02114
Phone: (617)727-3074 **Fax:** (617)727-2197
Email: REG.Webmaster@state.ma.us
Website: http://www.state.ma.us/reg/boards/dn/default.htm
Patricia Ramsay, Director

★ 20799 ★ Michigan Board of Dentistry
Department of Consumer/Industry Services
PO Box 30670
Lansing, MI 48909
Phone: (517)335-0918 **Fax:** (517)373-2179
Email: bhserinfo@cis.state.mi.us
Website: http://www.cis.state.mi.us/bhser/lic/boards/bdden.htm

★ 20800 ★ Mississippi State Board of Dental Examiners
600 E Amite St.
Jackson, MS 39201-2801
Phone: (601)944-9622 **Fax:** (601)944-9624
Email: dental@msbde.state.ms.us
Website: http://www.msbde.state.ms.us/
Ms. Leah Diane Howell, Director

★ 20801 ★ Missouri Dental Board
3605 Missouri Blvd.
PO Box 1367
Jefferson City, MO 65102
Phone: (573)751-0040 **Fax:** (573)751-8216
Email: dental@mail.state.mo.us
Website: http://www.ecodev.state.mo.us/pr/
Sharlene Rimiller, Director

★ 20802 ★ Montana Board of Dentistry
301 S Park, 4th Fl.
PO Box 200513
Helena, MT 59620-0513
Phone: (406)841-2390 **Fax:** (406)841-2305
Email: dlibsdden@state.mt.us
Website: http://www.discoveringmontana.com/dli/bsd/license/bsd_boards/den_board/board_page.htm
Ms. Sharon McCullough, Director

★ 20803 ★ Nebraska Board of Examiners in Dentistry
Credentialing Division
PO Box 94986
301 Centennial Mall South, 3rd Fl.
Lincoln, NE 68509-4986
Phone: (402)471-2115 **Fax:** (402)471-3577
Email: Marie.Mcclatchey@hhss.state.ne.us
Website: http://www.hhs.state.ne.us/crl/crlindex.htm
Ms. Helen Meeks, Director

★ 20804 ★ Nevada Board of Dental Examiners
2295-B Renaissance Dr.
Las Vegas, NV 89119
Phone: (702)486-7044 **Free:** 800-337-3926
Fax: (702)486-7046
Email: nsbde@govmail.state.nv.us
Website: http://www.nvdentalboard.org/
Ms. VaLonne S. Harmon, Director

★ 20805 ★ New Hampshire Board of Dental Examiners
2 Industrial Park Dr.
Concord, NH 03301-8520
Phone: (603)271-4561 **Fax:** (603)271-6702
Website: http://webster.state.nh.us/dental/
Dr. Raymond J. Jarvis, Secretary

★ 20806 ★ New Jersey State Board of Dentistry
124 Halsey St.
PO Box 45005
Newark, NJ 07101
Phone: (973)504-6405 **Fax:** (973)273-8075
Email: askconsumeraffairs@dca.lps.state.nj.us
Website: http://www.state.nj.us/lps/ca/medical.htmden3
Kevin Earle, Exec Director

★ 20807 ★ New Mexico Board of Dental Health Care
2055 Pacheco St., Ste. 400
Santa Fe, NM 87504
Phone: (505)476-7125 **Fax:** (505)476-7126
Email: Cynthia.Salazar@state.nm.us
Website: http://www.rld.state.nm.us/b&c/dental/index.htm
Ms. Cynthia Salazar, Contact

★ 20808 ★ New York State Education Dept
Office of the Professions
Board of Dentistry
Office of the Professions
State Education Bldg., 2nd Fl.
89 Washington Ave.
Albany, NY 12234
Phone: (518)474-3817 **Fax:** (518)473-6995
Email: dentbd@mail.nysed.gov
Website: http://www.op.nysed.gov/dent.htm

★ 20809 ★ North Carolina State Board of Dental Examiners
15100 Weston Pkwy, Ste. 101
Cary, NC 27513
Phone: (919)678-8223 **Fax:** (919)678-8472
Email: info@ncdentalboard.org
Website: http://www.ncdentalboard.org
David D. Cashwell, Director

★ 20810 ★ North Dakota State Board of Dental Examiners
PO Box 7246
Bismarck, ND 58507-7246
Phone: (701)258-8600 **Fax:** (701)224-9824
Email: ndsbde@aptnd.com
Website: http://www.nddentalboard.org/
Dr. Wayne Mattern, DDS, Director

★ 20811 ★ Ohio State Dental Board
77 S High St.
Columbus, OH 43266-0306
Phone: (614)466-2580 **Fax:** (614)752-8995
Website: http://www.state.oh.us/den/
Lili C. Reitz, Esq., Director

★ 20812 ★ Oklahoma Board of Dentistry
201 NE 23th Terrace Ste. 2
Oklahoma City, OK 73105
Phone: (405)524-9037 **Fax:** (405)524-2223
Email: dentist@oklaosf.state.ok.us
Website: http://www.state.ok.us/~dentist/
Ms. Linda Campbell, CPM, Director

★ 20813 ★ Oregon Board of Dentistry
1515 SW 5th Ave., Ste. 602
Portland, OR 97201-5451
Phone: (503)229-5520 **Fax:** (503)229-6606
Email: information@oregondentistry.org
Website: http://www.oregondentistry.org/
Ms. Jo Ann L. Bones, Director

★ 20814 ★ Pennsylvania State Board of Dentistry
PO Box 2649
Harrisburg, PA 17105-2649
Phone: (717)783-7162 **Fax:** (717)787-7769
Email: dentistr@pados.state.pa.us
Website: http://www.dos.state.pa.us/bpoa/cwp/view.asp?a=1104&q=432687
Lisa M. Burns, Director

★ 20815 ★ Rhode Island State Board of Examiners in Dentistry
3 Capitol Hill , Rm. 404
Providence, RI 02908
Phone: (401)222-2151 **Fax:** (401)222-1272
Email: GailG@doh.state.ri.us
Website: http://www.health.state.ri.us/hsr/dental.htm
Gail Giuliano, Contact

★ 20816 ★ South Carolina State Board of Dentistry
PO Box 11329
Kingstree Bldg.
110 Centerview Dr.
Columbia, SC 29211
Phone: (803)896-4599 **Fax:** (803)896-4596

Email: joness@mail.llr.state.sc.us
Website: http://www.llr.state.sc.us/POL/Dentistry/Default.htm
Mr. Rion Alvey, Contact

★ 20817 ★ South Dakota State Board of Dentistry
PO Box 1037
Pierre, SD 57501-1037
Phone: (605)224-1282 **Fax:** (605)224-7426
Email: sdsbd@dtgnet.com
Website: http://www.state.sd.us/dcr/dentistry/denthom.htm
Mr. Steve Willard, Secretary

★ 20818 ★ Southern Regional Testing Agency, Inc.
SRTA
303 34th St., Ste. 7
Virginia Beach, VA 23451
Phone: (757)428-1003 **Fax:** (757)437-4507
Website: http://www.srta.org/

★ 20819 ★ State of California Department of Consumer Affairs
Dental Board of California
1432 Howe Ave., Ste. 85B
Sacramento, CA 95825
Phone: (916)263-2300 **Fax:** (916)263-2140
Website: http://www.dca.ca.gov/r_r/dentalbd.htm

★ 20820 ★ Tennessee Board of Dentistry
425 5th Ave. N
Cordell Hull Bldg., 1st Fl.
Nashville, TN 37247-1010
Phone: (615)532-5073 **Free:** 888-310-4650
Fax: (615)532-5369
Website: http://170.142.76.180/bmf-bin/BMFprofgen.pl
Denise Moran, Director

★ 20821 ★ Texas State Board of Dental Examiners
333 Guadalupe, Ste. 800, Tower 3
Austin, TX 78701
Phone: (512)463-6400 **Free:** 800-821-3205
Fax: (512)463-7452
Email: webmaster@tsbde.state.tx.us
Website: http://www.tsbde.state.tx.us/Default.htm
Jeffry Hill, Director

★ 20822 ★ Utah Board of Dentists and Dental Hygienists
Division of Occupational and Professional Licencing
160 E 300 South
PO Box 146741
Salt Lake City, UT 84114
Phone: (801)530-6628 **Free:** (866)275-3675
Fax: (801)530-6511
Email: dtjones@br.state.ut.us
Website: http://www.dopl.utah.gov/

★ 20823 ★ Vermont Board of Dental Examiners
26 Terrace St., Drawer 09
Montpelier, VT 05609-1106
Phone: (802)828-2390 **Fax:** (802)828-2465
Website: http://www.nerb.org/stateboards.htm
Diane W. Lafaille, Secretary

★ 20824 ★ Virgin Islands Board of Dental Examiners
Roy Lester Schneider Hospital
48 Sugar Estate
St Thomas, VI 00802
Phone: (340)774-0117 **Fax:** (340)777-4001
Email: webmaster@usvi.org
Website: http://www.usvi.org/health/

★ 20825 ★ Virginia Board of Dentistry
6606 W Broad St., 4th Fl.
Richmond, VA 23230-1717
Phone: (804)662-9906 **Free:** 800-533-1560
Fax: (804)662-7246
Email: denbd@dhp.state.va.us
Website: http://www.dhp.state.va.us/dentistry/default.htm
Ms. Sandra Reen, Director

★ 20826 ★ Washington Dental Health Care
Health Professions Quality Assurance Commission
1112 SE Quince St.
PO Box 47860
Olympia, WA 98504-7860
Phone: (360)236-4700 **Fax:** (360)236-4818
Email: hpqa.csc@doh.wa.gov
Website: https://www2.wa.gov/doh/hpqa-licensing/HPS3/Dental/default.htm
Ms. Lisa Anderson, Contact

★ 20827 ★ West Virginia Board of Dental Examiners
PO Drawer 1459
Beckley, WV 25802-1459
Phone: (304)252-8266 **Fax:** (304)252-2779
Email: perryle@wvnvm.wvnet.edu
Website: http://www.state.wv.us/bep/lmi/license/LICOCCMS.HTMdentist

★ 20828 ★ Western Regional Examining Board (WREB)
9201 N 25 Ave, Ste. 185
Phoenix, AZ 85021
Phone: (602)944-3315 **Fax:** (602)371-8131
Email: generalinfo@wreb.org
Website: http://www.wreb.org/

★ 20829 ★ Wisconsin Dentistry Examining Board
Department of Regulation and Licensing
1400 E Washington Ave.
PO Box 8935
Madison, WI 53708-8935
Phone: (608)261-7083 **Fax:** (608)267-0644
Email: web@drl.state.wi.us
Website: http://badger.state.wi.us/agencies/drl/Regulation/applicant_information/dod087.html

Dental Health

★ 20830 ★ Arizona Department of Health Services
Family Health and Community Services Division
Oral Health Office
1740 W Adams Room 10
Phoenix, AZ 85007
Phone: (602)542-1866 **Fax:** (602)542-2936
Website: http://www.hs.state.az.us/cfhs/ooh/

★ 20831 ★ California Health and Welfare Agency
Health Services Department
Chronic Disease and Injury Control Branch
Office of Oral Health
601 N 7th St., MS-725
PO Box 942732
Sacramento, CA 94234-7320
Phone: (916)322-4933 **Fax:** (916)324-7764
Website: http://www.dhs.ca.gov/ps/cdic/cdcb/Medicine/OralHealth/index.htm

★ 20832 ★ Connecticut Department of Public Health
Community Health Bureau
Oral Health Program
410 Capitol Ave.
PO Box 340308
Hartford, CT 06134-0308
Phone: (860)509-7655 **Fax:** (860)509-7717
Email: webmaster.dph@po.state.ct.us
Website: http://www.state.ct.us/dph/BCH/HPBCH.HTML
Dr. Ardell Wilson, Director

★ 20833 ★ Delaware Department of Health and Social Services
Public Health Division
Community Health Care Access Section
Dental Health Program
Jesse Cooper Bldg.
Federal & Water St.
PO Box 637
Dover, DE 19903
Phone: (302)739-4787 **Fax:** (302)739-6653
Email: dhssinfo@state.de.us
Website: http://www.state.de.us/dhss/dph/chca/hsd_dental.htm

★ 20834 ★ Georgia Department of Human Resources
Public Health Division
Oral Health Section
2 Peachtree St. NW
Atlanta, GA 30303-3186
Phone: (404)657-2571 **Fax:** (404)657-2715
Email: GDPHINFO@dhr.state.ga.us
Website: http://www.ph.dhr.state.ga.us/programs/oral/index.shtml

★ 20835 ★ Hawaii Department of Health
Health Resources Administration
Dental Health Division
Lanakila Health Ctr.
1700 Lanakila Ave.
Honolulu, HI 96817
Phone: (808)832-5700 **Fax:** (808)832-5722
Email: mhkgreer@mail.health.state.hi.us
Website: http://www.state.hi.us/health/resource/dental/index.html
Mark Greer, DMD, Director

★ 20836 ★ Idaho Department of Health and Welfare
Division of Health
Health Promotions Bureau
Oral Health Program
Pete T. Cenarrusa Bldg. 1st Fl. W
450 W State St.
PO Box 83720
Boise, ID 83720-0036
Phone: (208)334-5964 **Free:** 800-926-2588
Fax: (208)334-6573
Email: garzac@idhw.state.id.us
Website: http://www2.state.id.us/dhw/hwgd_www/contentlist.htmlHealth
Catarina Garza, Contact

★ 20837 ★ Illinois Department of Public Health
Office of Health and Wellness
Division of Oral Health
535 W Jefferson St., 2nd Fl.
Springfield, IL 62761
Phone: (217)782-4977 **Fax:** (217)782-3987
Email: mailus@idph.state.il.us
Website: http://www.idph.state.il.us/HealthWellness/oralhlth/home.htm

★ 20838 ★ Iowa Department of Public Health
Family and Community Health Division
Dental Health Bureau
Lucas State Office Bldg.
321 E 12th St.
Des Moines, IA 50319-0075
Phone: (515)281-3733 **Fax:** (515)281-4958
Email: webmaster@idph.state.ia.us
Website: http://www.idph.state.ia.us/fch/dh.htm
Stephen C. Gleason, Director

★ 20839 ★ Kansas Department of Health and Environment
Health Division
Local and Rural Health Systems Bureau
Dental Program
1000 SW Jackson, Ste. 340
Topeka, KS 66612-1365
Phone: (785)296-1200 **Fax:** (785)368-1231
Email: rmorriss@kdhe.state.ks.us
Website: http://www.kdhe.state.ks.us/olrh/
Richard Morrissey, Director

★ 20840 ★ Kentucky Health Services Cabinet
Public Health Department
Maternal and Child Health Services Division
Oral Health Program
275 E Main St.
Frankfort, KY 40621
Phone: (502)564-3246 **Fax:** (502)564-6533
Website: http://publichealth.state.ky.us/dental.htm
Dr. James Curtis Cecil, III, Director

★ 20841 ★ Louisiana Department of Health and Hospitals
Office of Public Health
Maternal and Child Health Division
Oral Health Section
1100 Florida Ave. Box 510
New Orleans, LA 70119
Phone: (504)670-2738 **Fax:** (504)670-2746
Email: koertlin@dhh.state.la.us
Website: http://www.dhh.state.la.us/OPH/mch.htm
Karen M. Oertling, RDH, Director

★ 20842 ★ Maine Department of Human Services
Community and Family Health Division
Oral Health Program
11 State House Station
Key Plaza
286 Water St.
Augusta, ME 04333
Phone: (207)287-3267 **Fax:** (207)287-9058
Email: Judith.a.feinstein@state.me.us
Website: http://www.state.me.us/dhs/bohdcfh/odh/index2.htm
Judith Feinstein, Director

★ 20843 ★ Massachusetts Department of Public Health
Bureau of Family and Community Health
Office of Oral Health
250 Washington St., 5th Fl.
Boston, MA 02108-4619
Phone: (617)624-5943 **Fax:** (617)624-6062
Email: mary.foley@state.ma.us
Website: http://www.state.ma.us/dph/bfch/ooh/index.htm
Mary E. Foley, RDH, Director

★ 20844 ★ Michigan Community Health Department
Child and Family Services Bureau
Oral Health Program
3423 N Martin Luther King, Jr. Blvd.
PO Box 30195
Lansing, MI 48909
Phone: (517)335-9371 **Fax:** (517)335-8560
Email: tallmanjac@state.mi.us
Website: http://www.mdch.state.mi.us/dch/clcf/fch_12.asp
Jackie Tallman, Contact

★ 20845 ★ Missouri Department of Health
Maternal, Child, and Family Health Division
Dental Health Bureau
930 Wildwood
PO Box 570
Jefferson City, MO 65102
Phone: (573)751-6247 **Fax:** (573)751-6041
Email: info@mail.health.state.mo.us
Website: http://www.health.state.mo.us/AbouttheDepartment/DS9.htmldental

★ 20846 ★ Nebraska Department of Health and Human Services
Health Promotion and Disease Prevention
Dental Health Division
301 Centennial Mall S, 3rd Fl.
PO Box 95007
Lincoln, NE 68509-5007
Phone: (402)471-0166 **Fax:** (402)471-0820
Email: kim.mcfarland@hhss.state.ne.us
Website: http://www.hhs.state.ne.us/deh/dehindex.htm
Kim McFarland, Contact

★ 20847 ★ New Hampshire Department of Health and Human Services
Public Health Services Division
Board of Dental Examiners
2 Industrial Park Dr.
Concord, NH 03301-8520
Phone: (603)271-4561 **Fax:** (603)271-6702
Website: http://webster.state.nh.us/dental/
Raymond J. Jarvis, Director

★ 20848 ★ North Carolina Department of Health, and Human Services
Public Health Division
Community Health Division
Oral Health
1910 Mail Service Ctr.
Raleigh, NC 27699-1910
Phone: (919)733-3853 **Fax:** (919)733-4688
Email: rick.mumford@ncmail.net
Website: http://www.communityhealth.dhhs.state.nc.us/dental/
Rick Mumford, Director

★ 20849 ★ Ohio Department of Health
Family and Community Health Services Division
Oral Health Services Bureau
246 N High St.
PO Box 118
Columbus, OH 43216-0118
Phone: (614)466-4180 **Fax:** (614)564-2421
Email: BOHS@gw.odh.state.oh.us
Website: http://www.odh.state.oh.us/ODHPrograms/ORAL/Oral1.htm
Mark D. Siegal, D.D.S., Director

★ 20850 ★ Oklahoma State Department of Health
Personal Health Services
Dental Health Service
1000 NE 10th St.
Room 712
Oklahoma City, OK 73117
Phone: (405)271-5502 **Fax:** (405)271-3431
Website: http://www.health.state.ok.us/PROGRAM/dental/index.html

★ 20851 ★ Oregon Department of Human Resources
Health Division
Dental Health Section
Portland State Office Bldg.
800 NE Oregon St.
Portland, OR 97232
Phone: (503)731-4021 **Fax:** (503)731-4091
Email: h.whitney.payne@state.or.us
Website: http://www.ohd.hr.state.or.us/dental/welcome.htm
H. Whitney Payne, DDS, Director

★ 20852 ★ Pennsylvania Department of Health
Chronic Diseases and Injury Prevention Bureau
Oral Health Program
Health and Welfare Bldg.
PO Box 90
Harrisburg, PA 17108
Phone: (717)783-1760 **Fax:** (717)783-5498
Email: ngardner@state.pa.us
Website: http://www.ohd.hr.state.or.us/dental/welcome.htm
Neil Gardner, DDS, Director

★ 20853 ★ Rhode Island Department of Health
Dental Health Division
3 Capitol Hill, Rm 408
Providence, RI 02908
Phone: (401)222-1171 **Fax:** (401)222-4415
Email: MaureenR@doh.state.ri.us
Website: http://www.healthri.org/disease/primarycare/oralhealth/home.htm

★ 20854 ★ South Dakota Department of Health
Health Promotion Division
Dental Program
600 E Capitol
Pierre, SD 57501-2536
Phone: (605)773-3361 **Free:** 800-738-2301
Fax: (605)773-5509
Email: DOH.INFO@state.sd.us
Website: http://www.state.sd.us/doh/Disease2/index.htm

★ 20855 ★ Tennessee Department of Health
Oral Health Services Division
Cordell Hull Bldg., 5th Fl.
425 5th Ave. N
Nashville, TN 37247
Phone: (615)741-7213 **Fax:** (615)741-1063
Email: Diane.Denton@state.tn.us
Website: http://www2.state.tn.us/health/oralhealth/
Diane Denton, Contact

★ 20856 ★ Texas Department of Health
Dental Health Bureau
1100 W 49th St.
Austin, TX 78756-3199
Phone: (512)458-7323 **Fax:** (512)458-7358
Email: dental@tdh.state.tx.us
Website: http://www.tdh.state.tx.us/dental/default.htm
Jerry Felkner, DDS, Director

★ 20857 ★ Virgin Islands Department of Health
Dental Health Services
St. Thomas Hospital
48 Sugar Estate
Charlotte Amalie, VI 00802
Phone: (340)774-0117 **Fax:** (340)777-4001
Website: http://www.usvi.org/health/index.html

★ 20858 ★ Virginia Office of Health and Human Resources
Health Department
Dental Health Division
1500 E Main St.
Rm. 136
Richmond, VA 23219
Phone: (804)786-3556 **Fax:** (804)371-4004
Email: kday@vdh.state.va.us
Website: http://www.vahealth.org/teeth/index.htm
Karen C. Day, DDS, Director

★ 20859 ★ West Virginia Department of Health and Human Resources
Public Health Bureau
Maternal and Child Health Office
Oral Health Division
350 Capitol St.
Charleston, WV 25301-3712
Phone: (304)558-1117 **Fax:** (304)558-2183
Website: http://www.wvdhhr.org/bph/maternal.htm
Kay Medley, Contact

★ 20860 ★ Wisconsin Department of Health and Family Services
Health Division
Public Health Bureau
Oral Health Program
1 W Wilson St.
PO Box 2659
Madison, WI 53707-2659
Phone: (608)266-5152 **Fax:** (608)267-2832
Email: lemaywr@dhfs.state.wi.us
Website: http://www.dhfs.state.wi.us/health/Oral_Health/
Dr. Warren LeMay, Director

★ 20861 ★ Wyoming Department of Health
Public Health Division
Dental Health Services
Hathaway Bldg., 4th Fl.
Cheyenne, WY 82002
Phone: (307)777-7945 **Fax:** (307)777-3617
Email: cmeyer@state.wy.us
Website: http://wdhfs.state.wy.us/dcfh/
Charlie Meyer, Director

Developmental Disabilities

★ 20862 ★ Alabama Department of Mental Health and Mental Retardation
RSA Union
100 N Union St., Ste. 518
Montgomery, AL 36130-1410
Phone: (334)242-3147 **Fax:** (334)242-0684
Website: http://www.mh.state.al.us/
Kathy E. Sawyer, Director

★ 20863 ★ Alaska Department of Health and Social Services
Mental Health and Developmental Disabilities Division
350 Main St., Ste. 217
PO Box 110620
Juneau, AK 99811-0620
Phone: (907)465-3370 **Free:** 800-465-4828
Fax: (907)465-2668
Email: DMHDD_Webmaster@health.state.ak.us
Website: http://www.hss.state.ak.us/dmhdd/
Leonard Abel, Contact
Karl Brimner, Director

★ 20864 ★ Arkansas Department of Human Services
Developmental Disabilities Services Division
Donaghey Plaza N
PO Box 1437, Slot N503
Little Rock, AR 72203-1437
Phone: (501)682-8665 **Fax:** (501)682-8380
Website: http://www.state.ar.us/dhs/ddds/index.html
David Fray, Director

★ 20865 ★ California Health and Welfare Agency
Developmental Services Department
PO Box 944202
Sacramento, CA 94244-2020
Phone: (916)654-1690 **Fax:** (916)654-2167
Email: ddsweb@dds.ca.gov
Website: http://www.dds.cahwnet.gov

★ 20866 ★ Colorado Department of Human Services
Developmental Disabilities Division
3824 W Princeton Cir.
Denver, CO 80236
Phone: (303)866-7450 **Fax:** (303)866-7470
Website: http://www.cdhs.state.co.us/ohr/dds/DDS_center.html
Kerry O. Stern, Director

★ 20867 ★ Connecticut Department of Mental Retardation
460 Capitol Ave.
Hartford, CT 06106
Phone: (860)418-6000 **Fax:** (860)418-6001
Email: dmrct.co@po.state.ct.us
Website: http://www.dmr.state.ct.us/
Peter H. O'Meara, Director

★ 20868 ★ Delaware Department of Health and Social Services
Mental Retardation Division
Jesse Cooper Bldg.
417 Federal St.
Dover, DE 19901
Phone: (302)739-4452 **Fax:** (302)739-6652
Email: dhssinfo@state.de.us
Website: http://www.state.de.us/dhss/dmr/dmrhome.htm
Marianne Smith, Director

★ 20869 ★ Indiana Family and Social Services Administration
Disability, Aging and Rehabilitative Services Division
Developmental Disability Services Bureau
402 W Washington St.
PO Box 7083
Indianapolis, IN 46207-7083
Phone: (317)232-7842 **Free:** 800-545-2320
Fax: (317)233-2320
Website: http://www.state.in.us/fssa/servicedisabl/ddars/bdds.html

★ 20870 ★ Iowa Department of Human Services
Mental Health, Mental Retardation and Developmental Disabilities Division
Department of Human Services
1305 E Walnut
Des Moines, IA 50319-0114
Phone: (515)281-8472 **Fax:** (515)281-8512
Email: jchesni@dhs.state.ia.us
Website: http://www.dhs.state.ia.us/mhdd/
Jim Chesnik, Contact

★ 20871 ★ Louisiana Department of Health and Hospitals
Citizens with Developmental Disabilities Office
1201 Capitol Access Rd.
PO Box 3117
Baton Rouge, LA 70821-3117
Phone: (225)342-0095 **Fax:** (225)342-8823
Email: Webmaster@dhh.state.la.us
Website: http://www.dhh.state.la.us/OCDD/index.htm
Raymond A. Jetson, Secretary

★ 20872 ★ Maryland Department of Health and Mental Hygiene
Developmental Disabilities Administration
201 W Preston St., 4th Fl.
Baltimore, MD 21201
Phone: (410)767-5600 **Fax:** (410)767-6489
Email: ddaweb@dhmh.state.md.us
Website: http://www.dhmh.state.md.us/dda_md/
Diane K. Coughlin, Director

★ 20873 ★ Massachusetts Executive Office of Health and Human Services
Mental Retardation Services Department
500 Harrison Ave.
Boston, MA 02118
Phone: (617)727-5608 **Fax:** (617)624-7577
Email: info@dmr.state.ma.us
Website: http://www.dmr.state.ma.us/

★ 20874 ★ Michigan Community Health Department
Behavioral Health Services
Developmental Disabilities Council
Lewis Cass Bldg.
Lansing, MI 48913
Phone: (517)334-6123 **Fax:** (517)334-7353
Email: vanhornr@michigan.gov
Website: http://www.michigan.gov/mdch/

★ 20875 ★ Minnesota Department of Human Services
Health and Continuing Care Strategies
Developmental Disabilities Division
444 Lafayette Rd. N
Saint Paul, MN 55155
Phone: (651)296-3933 **Fax:** (651)297-4692
Email: dhs.webmaster@state.mn.us
Website: http://www.dhs.state.mn.us/contcare/default.htm

★ 20876 ★ Mississippi Department of Mental Health
Mental Retardation Bureau
1101 Robert E Lee Bldg.
239 N Lamar St.
Jackson, MS 39201
Phone: (601)359-1288 **Fax:** (601)359-6295
Email: kfeisel@msdmh.org
Website: http://www.dmh.state.ms.us/
Albert R. Hendrix, PhD, Director

★ 20877 ★ Montana Department of Public Health and Human Services
Disability Services Division
111 N Sanders
PO Box 4210
Helena, MT 59604-4210
Phone: (406)444-2590 **Free:** 877-296-1197
Fax: (406)444-3632
Email: jmathews@state.mt.gov
Website: http://www.dphhs.state.mt.us/divisions/dsd/dsd.htm
Joe Mathews, Director

★ 20878 ★ New Jersey Department of Human Services
Developmental Disabilities Division
50 E State St.
PO Box 726
Trenton, NJ 08625-0726
Phone: (609)292-3742 **Free:** 800-832-9173
Fax: (609)292-6610
Email: dmhsmail@dhs.state.nj.us
Website: http://www.state.nj.us/humanservices/dhspwd1.html
James W. Smith, Director

★ 20879 ★ North Carolina Department of Health and Human Services
Mental Health, Developmental Disabilities and Substance Abuse Services Division
Developmental Disabilities Services
3006 Mail Service Ctr.
325 N Salisbury
Raleigh, NC 27699-3006
Phone: (919)733-3654 **Fax:** (919)733-9455
Email: contactdmh@ncmail.net
Website: http://www.dhhs.state.nc.us/mhddsas/
Stan Slawinski, PhD, Director

★ 20880 ★ North Dakota Department of Human Services
Disability Services
600 S Second St.
Bismarck, ND 58504-5729
Phone: (701)328-8930 **Free:** 800-755-8529
Fax: (701)328-8969
Email: dhsds@state.nd.us
Website: http://lnotes.state.nd.us/dhs/dhsweb.nsf/ServicePages/DisabilityServices

★ 20881 ★ Oklahoma Department of Human Services
Developmental Disability Services Division
2400 N Lincoln Blvd.
PO Box 25352
Oklahoma City, OK 73125
Phone: (405)521-6267 **Fax:** (405)522-3037
Email: James.Nicholson@okdhs.org
Website: http://www.okdhs.org/ddsd/
Jim Nicholson, Director

★ 20882 ★ Oregon Department of Human Resources
Mental Health and Developmental Disabilities Services Division
Developmental Disabilities Services Office
2575 Bittern St. NE
Salem, OR 97309
Phone: (503)945-9774 **Fax:** (503)373-7274
Email: dhrinfo@state.or.us
Website: http://oddsweb.mhd.hr.state.or.us/

★ 20883 ★ Pennsylvania Department of Public Welfare
Mental Retardation Office
PO Box 2675
Health & Welfare Bldg., Rm. 512
Harrisburg, PA 17105-2675
Phone: (717)787-3700 **Fax:** (717)772-2062
Website: http://www.dpw.state.pa.us/omr/dpwmr.asp

★ 20884 ★ Rhode Island Department of Mental Health, Retardation and Hospitals
Developmental Disabilities Division
14 Harrington Rd.
Cranston, RI 02920
Phone: (401)462-3234 **Fax:** (401)462-6636
Email: lkahn@mhrh.state.ri.us
Website: http://www.mhrh.state.ri.us/developmental_disabilities.htm
Lynda D. Kahn, Director

★ 20885 ★ South Carolina Department of Disabilities and Special Needs
3440 Harden St. Ext.
PO Box 4706
Columbia, SC 29240
Phone: (803)898-9600 **Free:** 888-376-4636
Fax: (803)898-9653
Email: DDSNweb@ddsn.state.sc.us
Website: http://www.state.sc.us/ddsn
Stan Butkus, Director

★ 20886 ★ Tennessee Department of Mental Health and Mental Retardation
Mental Retardation Services Division
425 Fifth Ave. N
Cordell Hull Bldg.
Nashville, TN 37243
Phone: (615)532-6500 **Fax:** (615)532-6514
Email: martha.robinson@state.tn.us
Website: http://www.state.tn.us/mental/
Elizabeth Rukeyser, Director

★ 20887 ★ Texas Department of Mental Health and Mental Retardation
Mental Retardation Facilities Division
909 W 45th St.
PO Box 12668
Austin, TX 78711-2668
Phone: (512)454-3761 **Free:** 800-252-8154
Fax: (512)206-4560
Email: Webmaster@mhmr.state.tx.us
Website: http://www.mhmr.state.tx.us/
Karen F. Hale, Director

★ 20888 ★ Vermont Agency of Human Services
Developmental and Mental Health Services Department
Mental Retardation Programs Division
Weeks Bldg.
103 S Main St.
Waterbury, VT 05671-1601
Phone: (802)241-2610 **Fax:** (802)241-1129
Email: webmaster@ddmhs.state.vt.us
Website: http://www.state.vt.us/dmh
Susan W. Besio, PhD, Contact

★ 20889 ★ Virginia Office of Health and Human Resources
Mental Health, Retardation and Substance Abuse Services Department
Mental Retardation Division
PO Box 1797
Richmond, VA 23218
Phone: (804)371-3921 **Free:** 800-451-5544
Fax: (804)371-6638
Email: bbrenzovich@dmhmrsas.state.va.us
Website: http://www.dmhmrsas.state.va.us/
James Reinhard, MD, Contact

★ 20890 ★ Wyoming Department of Health
Developmental Disabilities Division
Herschler Bldg., 1st Fl. W
122 W 25th St.
Cheyenne, WY 82002
Phone: (307)777-7115 **Fax:** (307)777-6047
Email: ddmail@state.wy.us
Website: http://ddd.state.wy.us/
Robert T. Clabby, II, Director

Emergency Medical Services

★ 20891 ★ Alaska Department of Health and Social Services
Public Health Division
Community Health and Emergency Medical Services Section
410 Willoughby St., Rm. 109
PO Box 110616
Juneau, AK 99811-0616
Phone: (907)465-3027 **Fax:** (907)465-4101
Email: Mark_Johnson@health.state.ak.us
Website: http://www.chems.alaska.gov/
Mark S. Johnson, Director

★ 20892 ★ Arizona Department of Health Services
Office of Emergency Medical Services
1651 E Morten
Phoenix, AZ 85020
Phone: (602)861-0708 **Free:** 800-200-8523
Fax: (602)861-9812
Email: jcrume@hs.state.az.us
Website: http://www.hs.state.az.us/bems/index.htm
Judi Crume, RN,PhD, Director

★ 20893 ★ Connecticut Department of Public Health
Emergency Medical Services Office
410 Capitol Ave.
PO Box 340308
Hartford, CT 06134-0308
Phone: (860)509-7975 **Fax:** (860)509-7987
Email: webmaster.dph@po.state.ct.us
Website: http://www.state.ct.us/dph/DPH_Main/About_DPH/oems/oems.htm
Mark C. N. Libby, R.N., Director

★ 20894 ★ DOH/Office of Emergency Health and Medical Services
Emergency Health and Medical Services
825 N Capitol St., NE, Rm. 4177
Washington, DC 20002
Phone: (202)442-9111 **Fax:** (202)442-4812
Website: http://www.dchealth.com/ehms/welcome.htm

★ 20895 ★ Florida Department of Health
Bureau of Emergency Medical Services
4052 Esplanade Way, 3rd Fl.
Tallahassee, FL 32311-1738
Phone: (850)245-4440 **Fax:** (850)921-8162
Email: EMSCHR@doh.state.fl.us
Website: http://www.doh.state.fl.us/workforce/ems1/index.html
Charles Bement, Director

★ 20896 ★ Georgia Department of Human Resources
Division of Public Health
Office of Emergency Medical Services
Skyland Ctr., Lower Level
2600 Skyland Dr.
Atlanta, GA 30319
Phone: (404)679-0547 **Fax:** (404)679-0526
Email: gdphinfo@dhr.state.ga.us
Website: http://www.ph.dhr.state.ga.us/programs/ems/index.shtml
R. Keith Wages, Director

★ 20897 ★ Guam Office of Emergency Medical Services
Department of Public Health and Social Services
PO Box 2816
Agana, GU 96932

Phone: (671)735-7303 **Fax:** (671)734-5910
Christine Gyulavics-Reyes, Director

★ 20898 ★ Hawaii State Department of Health
Emergency Medical Services & Injury Prevention System
3627 Kilauea Ave., Rm. 102
Honolulu, HI 96816-2317
Phone: (808)733-9210 **Fax:** (808)733-8332
Email: emss@camhmis.health.state.hi.us
Website: http://www.hawaii.gov/health/resource/ems/
Donna Maiava, Director

★ 20899 ★ Idaho Department of Health and Welfare
Emergency Medical Services Bureau
3092 Elder St.
Boise, ID 83705
Phone: (208)334-4000 **Free:** 800-926-2588
Fax: (208)334-4015
Email: IdahoEMS@idhw.state.id.us
Website: http://www2.state.id.us/dhw/ems/home.htm
Dia Gainor, Director

★ 20900 ★ Illinois Department of Public Health
Emergency Medical Services Division
525 W Jefferson St.
Springfield, IL 62761
Phone: (217)785-2080 **Fax:** (217)785-0253
Email: info@ilems.com
Website: http://www.ilems.com/
Leslee Stein-Spencer, Director

★ 20901 ★ Indiana Emergency Medical Services Commission
302 W Washington, Rm. E208 IGCS
Indianapolis, IN 46204-2258
Phone: (317)232-3980 **Fax:** (317)232-3895
Email: mgarvey@sema.state.in.us
Website: http://www.state.in.us/sema/ems.html

★ 20902 ★ Iowa Department of Public Health
Emergency Medical Services
401 SW 7th St., Ste. D
Des Moines, IA 50309
Phone: (515)281-3239 **Free:** 800-728-3367
Fax: (515)281-4958
Website: http://idph.state.ia.us/pa/ems/default.htm
Timothy D. Peterson, MD, Director

★ 20903 ★ Kansas Board of Emergency Medical Services
109 SW 6th Ave.
Topeka, KS 66603-3826
Phone: (785)296-7296 **Fax:** (785)296-6212
Email: emsdl@ink.org
Website: http://www.ksbems.org/
David Lake, Contact

★ 20904 ★ Kentucky Department for Public Health
Division of Adult and Child Health
Emergency Medical Services Branch
275 E Main St., HS1E-F
Frankfort, KY 40621-0001
Phone: (502)564-8963 **Fax:** (502)564-4687
Email: kbems@mail.state.ky.us
Website: http://www.kbems.org/
Brian Bishop, Director

★ 20905 ★ Louisiana Department of Health and Hospitals
Public Health Services Office
Emergency Medical Services Bureau
1201 Capitol Access Rd.
PO Box 94215
Baton Rouge, LA 70804
Phone: (225)342-4881 **Fax:** (225)342-4419
Website: http://www.dhh.state.la.us/OPH/ems.htm
Nancy Bourgeois, Director

★ 20906 ★ Maine Emergency Medical Services
16 Edison Dr.
Augusta, ME 04330
Phone: (207)287-3953 **Fax:** (207)287-6251
Email: Maine.EMS@state.me.us
Website: http://www.state.me.us/dps/ems/
Jay Bradshaw, Director

★ 20907 ★ Maryland Institute for Emergency Medical Services Systems
653 W Pratt St.
Baltimore, MD 21201-1536
Phone: (410)706-5074 **Fax:** (410)706-4768
Email: jbrown@miemss.org
Website: http://miemss.umaryland.edu/Home.htm
Robert Bass, MD, Director

★ 20908 ★ Massachusetts Department of Public Health
Office of Emergency Medical Services
56 Roland St.
Boston, MA 02129
Phone: (617)284-8300 **Fax:** (617)284-8350
Website: http://www.state.ma.us/dph/oems/oems.htm
Louise Goyette, Director

★ 20909 ★ Michigan Department of Public Health
Emergency Medical Services Division
525 W Ottawa St.
PO Box 30664
Lansing, MI 48909
Phone: (517)241-3020
Email: johnfhubin@michigan.gov
Website: http://www.cis.state.mi.us/bhs/ems/home.htm
John Hubinger, Director

★ 20910 ★ Minnesota Emergency Medical Services Regulatory Board
Emergency Medical Services Section
University Park Plaza
2829 University Ave. SE, Ste. 310
Minneapolis, MN 55414-3250
Phone: (612)627-6000 **Fax:** (612)627-5442
Email: EMSRB.Webmaster@state.mn.us
Website: http://www.emsrb.state.mn.us
Mary Hedges, Director

★ 20911 ★ Mississippi State Department of Health
Emergency Medical Services
570 E Woodrow Wilson, Annex Bldg 3rd Fl.
Jackson, MS 39215-1700
Phone: (601)576-7366 **Fax:** (601)576-7373
Website: http://www.msdh.state.ms.us/ems/index.htm
Jim Craig, Director

★ 20912 ★ Missouri Department of Health
Emergency Medical Services Bureau
PO Box 570
912 Wildwood
Jefferson City, MO 65109
Phone: (573)751-6356 **Fax:** (573)751-6348
Email: info@mail.health.state.mo.us
Website: http://www.health.state.mo.us/EMS/index.html
Steve Hise, DIR, Contact

★ 20913 ★ Montana Department of Health and Environmental Sciences
Emergency Medical Services Bureau
Cogswell Bldg., Rm.C204
1400 Broadway
PO Box 202951
Helena, MT 59620
Phone: (406)444-3895 **Fax:** (406)444-1814
Email: jdetienne@state.mt.us
Website: http://www.dphhs.state.mt.us/hpsd/pubheal/healsafe/ems/index.htm
Ken Leighton-Boster, Director

★ 20914 ★ Nebraska Division of Emergency Medical Services
301 Centennial Mall S, 3rd Fl.
PO Box 95007
Lincoln, NE 68509-5007
Phone: (402)471-3578 **Fax:** (402)471-6446
Email: Doug.Fuller@hhss.state.ne.us
Website: http://www.hhs.state.ne.us/ems/emsindex.htm
Doug Fuller, Contact

★ 20915 ★ New Hampshire Bureau of Emergency Medical Services
10 Hazen Dr.
Concord, NH 03305-0003
Phone: (603)271-4568 **Fax:** (603)271-4567
Email: sprentiss@safety.state.nh.us
Website: http://webster.state.nh.us/safety/ems/
Suzanne Prentiss, Director

★ 20916 ★ North Carolina Office of Emergency Medical Services
701 Barbour Dr.
Raleigh, NC 27603-2008
Phone: (919)855-3935 **Fax:** (919)733-7021
Email: drexdal.pratt@ncmail.net
Website: http://facility-services.state.nc.us/EMS/ems.htm
Drexdal Pratt, Director

★ 20917 ★ North Dakota Department of Health
Emergency Health Services Division
600 E Boulevard Ave.
Bismarck, ND 58505-0200
Phone: (701)328-2388 **Fax:** (701)328-1890
Email: dehs@state.nd.us
Website: http://www.health.state.nd.us/ndhd/resource/dehs/dehs.htm
Timothy W. Wiedrich, Director

★ 20918 ★ Ohio Department of Public Safety
Division of Emergency Medical Services
1970 W Broad St.
PO Box 182073
Columbus, OH 43218-2073
Phone: (614)466-9447 **Free:** 800-233-0785
Fax: (614)466-9461
Email: ltiberi@dps.state.oh.us
Website: http://www.state.oh.us/odps/division/ems/ems_local/default.htm
Laura Ludwig Tiberi, Director

★ 20919 ★ Oklahoma State Department of Health
Emergency Medical Services
1000 NE 10th St., Rm. 1104
Oklahoma City, OK 73117
Phone: (405)271-4027 **Fax:** (405)271-3442
Email: webmaster@health.state.ok.us

Website: http://www.health.state.ok.us/program/ems/index.html
Eddie Manley, Director

★ 20920 ★ Oregon Department of Human Resources
Emergency Medical Services and Systems
800 NE Oregon St., Ste. 607
Portland State Office Bldg.
Portland, OR 97232
Phone: (503)731-4011 **Fax:** (503)731-4077
Email: j.chin@state.or.us
Website: http://www.ohd.hr.state.or.us/ems/welcome.htm
Jonathan Chin, Director

★ 20921 ★ Pennsylvania Division of Emergency Medical Services
Health and Welfare Bldg., Rm. 1033
PO Box 90
Harrisburg, PA 17108
Phone: (717)787-8741 **Fax:** (717)772-0910
Email: ptrimble@health.state.pa.us
Website: http://www.health.state.pa.us/HPA/EMS/DEFAULT.HTM
Margaret E. Trimble, Director

★ 20922 ★ Rhode Island Department of Health
Emergency Medical Services Division
3 Capitol Hill, Rm. 404
Providence, RI 02908-5097
Phone: (401)222-2231 **Fax:** (401)222-6548
Email: peterl@doh.state.ri.us
Website: http://www.health.state.ri.us
Peter Leary, Director

★ 20923 ★ South Dakota Department of Health
Emergency Medical Services Program
600 E Capitol
Pierre, SD 57501-2536
Phone: (605)773-4031 **Free:** 800-738-2301
Fax: (605)773-5904
Email: bob.graff@state.sd.us
Website: http://www.state.sd.us/doh/EMS/index.htm
Robert Graff, Director

★ 20924 ★ Tennessee Department of Health
Manpower and Facilities Bureau
Emergency Medical Services Division
Cordell Hull Bldg., 1st Fl.
425 Fifth Ave. N
Nashville, TN 37247-0701
Phone: (615)741-2584 **Free:** 888-310-4650
Fax: (615)741-4217
Email: DDenton@mail.state.tn.us
Website: www2.state.tn.us/health/ems/
Joseph B. Phillips, Director

★ 20925 ★ Texas Department of Health
Bureau of Emergency Management
EMS Services
1100 49th St.
Austin, TX 78756-3199
Phone: (512)834-6700 **Fax:** (512)834-6736
Email: emsinfo@tdh.state.tx.us
Website: http://www.tdh.state.tx.us/hcqs/ems/emshome.htm
Jim Arnold, Director

★ 20926 ★ Vermont Department of Health
Emergency Medical Services Division
108 Cherry St.
PO Box 70
Burlington, VT 05402-0070
Phone: (802)863-7310 **Free:** 800-244-0911
Fax: (802)863-7577
Email: vtems@vdh.state.vt.us
Website: http://www.state.vt.us/health/ems/
W. Dan Manz, Director

★ 20927 ★ Virginia State Department of Health
Emergency Medical Services Division
1538 E Parham Rd.
Richmond, VA 23228
Phone: (804)371-3500 **Free:** 800-523-6019
Fax: (804)371-3543
Email: gbrown@vdh.state.va.us
Website: http://www.vdh.state.va.us/oems/index.asp
Gary Brown, Director

★ 20928 ★ Washington Department of Health
Office of Emergency Medical and Trauma Prevention
1112 Quince St.
PO Box 47853
Olympia, WA 98504-7853
Phone: (360)705-6700 **Free:** 800-525-0127
Fax: (360)705-6706
Email: marquita.schlender@doh.wa.gov
Website: http://www.doh.wa.gov/hsqa/emtp/default.htm

★ 20929 ★ Wisconsin Division of Health
Emergency Medical Services
1 W Wilson St.
Madison, WI 53702
Phone: (608)266-1865 **Fax:** (608)261-6392
Email: webmaildph@dhfs.state.wi.us
Website: http://www.dhfs.state.wi.us/DPH_EMSIP/index.htm
Jon Morgan, Contact

★ 20930 ★ Wyoming State
Preventative Health and Safety Division
Emergency Medical Services Program
Hathaway Bldg. 4th Floor
Cheyenne, WY 82002
Phone: (307)777-7955 **Free:** 888-228-8996
Fax: (307)777-5639
Email: EMSWebmaster@state.wy.us
Website: http://wdhfs.state.wy.us/ems/
Jimm Murray, Contact

Environmental Health

★ 20931 ★ Alaska Department of Environmental Conservation
Environmental Health Division
555 Cordova St.
Anchorage, AK 99501
Phone: (907)269-7500 **Fax:** (907)269-7600
Email: Kristin_Ryan@envircon.state.ak.us
Website: http://www.state.ak.us/dec/deh/
Kristin Ryan, Contact

★ 20932 ★ Arizona Department of Health Services
Disease Control Services Bureau
Environmental Health Office
3815 N Black Canyon Hwy.
Phoenix, AZ 85015
Phone: (602)230-5948 **Fax:** (602)230-5933
Email: whumble@hs.state.az.us
Website: http://www.hs.state.az.us/phs/oeh/index.htm

★ 20933 ★ California Health and Human Services Agency
Department of Health Services
Division of Environmental and Occupational Disease Control
1515 Clay St., Ste. 1700
Oakland, CA 94612
Phone: (510)622-4500 **Fax:** (510)622-4505
Email: mlee@dhs.ca.gov
Website: http://www.dhs.ca.gov/ps/deodc/

★ 20934 ★ Colorado Public Health and Environment Department
Environment Office
4300 Cherry Creek Dr. S
Denver, CO 80246-1530
Phone: (303)692-2035 **Fax:** (303)782-4969
Email: cdphe.information@state.co.us
Website: http://www.cdphe.state.co.us/environ.asp

★ 20935 ★ Delaware Department of Health and Social Services
Public Health Division
Health Systems Protection Branch
Jesse Cooper Bldg.
Federal & Water St.
PO Box 637
Dover, DE 19903-0637
Phone: (302)739-4731 **Fax:** (302)739-3839
Email: dhssinfo@state.de.us
Website: http://www.state.de.us/dhss/dph/hsp.htm
Kevin E. Charles, Director

★ 20936 ★ Florida Department of Health
Health Program Office
Environmental Health Services Office
4052 Bald Cypress Way, Bin No. A08
Tallahassee, FL 32399-1709
Phone: (850)245-4250
Email: EnvironmentalHealth@doh.state.fl.us
Website: http://www.doh.state.fl.us/

★ 20937 ★ Georgia Department of Human Resources
Public Health Division
Environmental Health Section
2 Peachtree St. NW
Atlanta, GA 30303-3186
Phone: (404)657-6534 **Fax:** (404)657-2715
Email: gdphinfo@dhr.state.ga.us
Website: http://www.ph.dhr.state.ga.us/programs/environmental/index.shtml

★ 20938 ★ Hawaii Department of Health
Environmental Health Administration
919 Ala Moana Blvd.
Honolulu, HI 96814
Phone: (808)586-4424 **Fax:** (808)586-4444
Website: http://www.state.hi.us/health/about/enviro.html
Gary Gill, Director

★ 20939 ★ Idaho Department of Health and Welfare
Health Division
Bureau of Environmental Health and Safety
PO Box 83720
450 W State St.
Boise, ID 83720-0036
Phone: (208)334-0606 **Fax:** (208)334-6581
Email: behs@idhw.state.id.us
Website: http://www2.state.id.us/dhw/BEHS/index.htm
Maura Mack, PhD, Director

★ 20940 ★ Illinois Department of Public Health
Health Protection Office
Environmental Health Division
535 W Jefferson St.
Springfield, IL 62761
Phone: (217)782-4977 **Fax:** (217)782-3987
Email: mailus@idph.state.il.us
Website: http://www.idph.state.il.us/envhealth/eh-home.htm
John R. Lumpkin, MD, Director

★ 20941 ★ Kansas Department of Health and Environment
Environment Division
1000 SW Jackson, Ste. 420
Topeka, KS 66612-1367
Phone: (785)296-1535 **Fax:** (785)296-8464
Email: rhammers@kdhe.state.ks.us
Website: http://www.kdhe.state.ks.us/environment/index.html
Ronald Hammerschmidt, PhD, Director

★ 20942 ★ Louisiana Department of Health and Hospitals
Public Health Office
Center for Environmental Health
6867 Bluebonnet Rd.
Baton Rouge, LA 70810
Phone: (225)763-3590 **Fax:** (225)763-5552
Email: cnenweb@dhh.state.la.us
Website: http://www.oph.dhh.state.la.us/
Bobby Savoie, Director

★ 20943 ★ Maine Department of Human Services
Health Bureau
Disease Control Division
Environmental Health Unit
11 State House Station
286 Water St.
Augusta, ME 04333
Phone: (207)287-3201 **Fax:** (207)287-9058
Email: Philip.W.Haines@state.me.us
Website: http://janus.state.me.us/dhs/boh/index.htm
Philip W. Haines, Contact

★ 20944 ★ Maryland Department of Health and Mental Hygiene
Environmental Health Office
201 W Preston St., 3rd Floor
Baltimore, MD 21210
Phone: (410)767-6941 **Fax:** (410)333-7392
Email: matique@dhmh.state.md.us
Website: http://mdpublichealth.org/oeh/index.html
Mahboobuddin M. Atique, MBBS, Director

★ 20945 ★ Massachusetts Executive Office of Health and Human Services
Public Health Department
Bureau of Environmental Health Assessment
250 Washington St., 7th Fl.
Boston, MA 02108
Phone: (617)624-5757 **Fax:** (617)624-5777
Email: dph.info@state.ma.us
Website: http://www.state.ma.us/dph/beha/beha.htm
Suzanne K. Condon, Director

★ 20946 ★ Minnesota Department of Health
Health Protection Bureau
Environmental Health in Minnesota
PO Box 64975
Saint Paul, MN 55164-0975
Phone: (651)215-5800
Email: ehweb@health.state.mn.us
Website: http://www.health.state.mn.us/divs/eh/index.html

★ 20947 ★ Mississippi Department of Health
General Environmental Services
PO Box 1700
Jackson, MS 39215
Phone: (601)576-7690 **Fax:** (601)576-7632
Email: lstrayer@msdh.state.ms.us
Website: http://www.msdh.state.ms.us/sanitation/index.htm
Lydia Strayer, Contact

★ 20948 ★ New Jersey Department of Health and Senior Services
Consumer and Environmental Health Services
PO Box 369
Trenton, NJ 08625-0369
Phone: (609)588-3120 **Fax:** (609)588-7431
Email: james.brownlee@doh.state.nj.us
Website: http://www.state.nj.us/health/eoh/cehsweb/
James A. Brownlee, Director

★ 20949 ★ New Mexico Department of Environment
Harold S Runnels Bldg
1190 St. Francis Dr.
Santa Fe, NM 87505-4182
Phone: (505)827-2855 **Free:** 800-219-6157
Fax: (505)827-2836
Email: Peter_Maggiore@nmenv.state.nm.us
Website: http://www.nmenv.state.nm.us/
Peter Maggiore, Director

★ 20950 ★ North Dakota Department of Health
Environmental Health Section
1200 Missouri Ave.
PO Box 5520
Bismarck, ND 58506-5520
Phone: (701)328-5150 **Fax:** (701)328-5200
Email: dglatt@state.nd.us
Website: http://www.health.state.nd.us/ndhd/environ/
Dave Glatt, Director

★ 20951 ★ Oklahoma Department of Health
Health Promotion and Policy Analysis
Environmental Health Education
1000 NE 10th St., Rm. 1106
Oklahoma City, OK 73117
Phone: (405)271-3950 **Fax:** (405)271-3431
Email: sharonkt@ionet.net
Website: http://www.health.state.ok.us/PROGRAM/envhlth/index.html
Sharon Montgomery, Director

★ 20952 ★ Oregon Department of Human Resources
Health Division
Environment and Health Systems Office
Portland State Office Bldg., Ste. 640
800 NE Oregon St.
Portland, OR 97232
Phone: (503)731-4009 **Fax:** (503)731-3184
Email: thomas.w.johnson@state.or.us
Website: http://www.ohd.hr.state.or.us/cehs/welcome.htm
Thomas W. Johnson, Director

★ 20953 ★ Rhode Island Department of Health
Environmental Health Services Office
235 Promenade St.
Providence, RI 02908-5767
Phone: (401)222-6800 **Fax:** (401)222-6953
Email: tepstein@dem.state.ri.us
Website: http://www.state.ri.us/dem/
Jan H. Reitsma, Director

★ 20954 ★ South Carolina Department of Health and Environmental Control
Health Services Office
Environmental Health Bureau
2600 Bull St.
Columbia, SC 29201
Phone: (803)896-0647
Email: sheridwd@columb72.dhec.state.sc.us
Website: http://www.scdhec.net/hs/envhlth/envhlth.htm
Wally Sheridan, Contact

★ 20955 ★ Texas Department of Health
Environmental Health Bureau
1100 W 49th St.
Austin, TX 78756-3199
Phone: (512)834-6640 **Fax:** (512)834-6707
Email: claren.kotrla@tdh.state.tx.us
Website: http://www.tdh.state.tx.us/beh/default.htm
Claren Kotrla, Director

★ 20956 ★ Washington Department of Health
Environmental Health Programs
PO Box 47820
Olympia, WA 98504-7820
Phone: (360)236-3000 **Free:** 800-525-0127
Fax: (360)236-2250
Email: teresa.lohr@doh.wa.gov
Website: http://www.doh.wa.gov/ehp/default.htm
Teresa Lohr, Contact

★ 20957 ★ West Virginia Department of Health and Human Resources
Public Health Bureau
Environmental Health Services Office
815 Quarrier St., Ste. 418
Charleston, WV 25301-2616
Phone: (304)558-2981 **Fax:** (304)558-1291
Email: delzey@wvdhhr.org
Website: http://www.wvdhhr.org/oehs/
Barbara S. Taylor, Director

★ 20958 ★ Wyoming Department of Agriculture
Consumer Health Services
2219 Carey Ave.
Cheyenne, WY 82002-0100
Phone: (307)777-7321 **Fax:** (307)777-6593
Email: lleis@state.wy.us
Website: http://wyagric.state.wy.us/CHS/chs.html
Laurie Leis, Director

Funeral Service Examining Boards

★ 20959 ★ Alaska Division of Occupational Licensing
Mortuary Science Section
PO Box 110806
Juneau, AK 99811-0806
Phone: (907)465-2695 **Fax:** (907)465-2974
Email: p.j._gingras@dced.state.ak.us
Website: http://www.dced.state.ak.us/occ/pmor.htm
P. J. Gingras, Contact

★ 20960 ★ Arizona State Board of Funeral Directors and Embalmers
1400 W Washington, Ste. 230
Phoenix, AZ 85007
Phone: (602)542-3095 **Fax:** (602)542-3095
Website: http://www.mmimarketing.com/afda/statebrd.htm
Rudy Thomas, Director

★ 20961 ★ Arkansas State Board of Embalmers and Funeral Directors
101 E Capitol, Ste. 113
Little Rock, AR 72201
Phone: (501)682-0574 **Fax:** (501)682-0575
Email: fdemb@mail.state.ar.us
Website: http://www.state.ar.us/fdemb/
Rachel McGrew, Contact

★ 20962 ★ Board of Embalmers and Funeral Directors of Ohio
77 S High St., 16th Fl.
Columbus, OH 43266-0313
Phone: (614)466-4252 **Fax:** (614)728-6825
Website: http://www.state.oh.us/fun

★ 20963 ★ California Department of Consumer Affairs
Cemetery and Funeral Bureau
400 R St.
Sacramento, CA 95814
Phone: (916)322-7737 **Free:** 800-952-5210
Website: http://www.dca.ca.gov/cemetery/

★ 20964 ★ Colorado Funeral Service Board
7583 E Araphahoe Ct., No. 2100
Englewood, CO 80112-1361
Phone: (303)694-4728 **Fax:** (303)694-4869
Email: mail@cofda.org
Website: http://www.cofda.org/
Scott Moser, MSP, Contact

★ 20965 ★ Delaware State Board of Funeral Services
Cannon Bldg., Ste. 203
861 Silver Lake Blvd.
Dover, DE 19904-2467
Phone: (302)744-4506 **Fax:** (302)739-2711
Email: smiccio@state.de.us
Website: http://professionallicensing.state.de.us/boards/funeralservices/index.shtml
Susan Miccio, Contact

★ 20966 ★ District of Columbia Board of Funeral Directors
Occupational and Professional Licensing Administration
DC Board of Funeral Directors
941 North Capitol St. NE
Washington, DC 20002
Phone: (202)442-4461 **Fax:** (202)442-8390
Website: http://dcra.dc.gov/about/index_bpla_funeral.shtm

★ 20967 ★ Florida Board of Funeral Directors and Embalmers
1940 N Monroe St., Ste. 426
Tallahassee, FL 32399-0754
Phone: (904)488-8690 **Fax:** (904)922-2918
Website: http://www.state.fl.us/dbpr/prof/fd_index.shtml
Sherry Landrum, Director

★ 20968 ★ Georgia State Examining Boards
237 Coliseum Dr.
Macon, GA 31217-3858
Phone: (478)207-1460
Website: http://www.sos.state.ga.us/ebd/
Mollie Fleeman, Director

★ 20969 ★ Hawaii Department of Health
Sanitation Branch
591 Ala Moana
Honolulu, HI 96813
Phone: (808)586-4700 **Fax:** (808)586-4729
Website: http://www.state.hi.us/health/eh/sanitation/index.htm

★ 20970 ★ Idaho Occupational Licensing Bureau
Owyhee Plaza
1109 Main St., Ste. 220
Boise, ID 83702
Phone: (208)334-3233 **Fax:** (208)334-3945
Email: ibol@ibol.state.id.us
Website: http://www2.state.id.us/ibol/
Rayola Jacobson, Contact

★ 20971 ★ Illinois Department of Professional Regulation
Professional Services Section
320 W Washington St.
Springfield, IL 62786
Phone: (217)785-0800 **Fax:** (217)782-7645
Website: http://www.dpr.state.il.us

★ 20972 ★ Indiana Funeral Service Board
302 W Washington, Rm. E034
Indianapolis, IN 46204-2700
Phone: (317)232-2980 **Fax:** (317)232-2312
Website: http://www.state.in.us/pla/funeral/index.html

★ 20973 ★ Iowa Board of Mortuary Science
Iowa Department of Public Health
Lucas State Office Bldg., 5th Fl.
321 E 12th St.
Des Moines, IA 50319-0075
Phone: (515)281-4287 **Fax:** (515)281-3121
Email: mbledsoe@idph.state.ia.us
Website: http://www.iowaccess.org/idph_pl/mortuary/index.html

★ 20974 ★ Kansas State Board of Mortuary Arts
700 SW Jackson, Ste. 904
Topeka, KS 66603-3733
Phone: (785)296-3980 **Fax:** (785)296-0891
Email: boma1@ink.org
Website: http://www.ink.org/public/ksbma/

★ 20975 ★ Kentucky State Board of Embalmers & Funeral Directors
7025 W Hwy. 22, Ste. 7
PO Box 324
Crestwood, KY 40014
Phone: (502)241-3918

★ 20976 ★ Louisiana State Board of Embalmers & Funeral Directors
3500 N Causeway Blvd., Ste. 1232
Metairie, LA 70002
Phone: (504)838-5109 **Fax:** (504)838-5112
Email: labefd@ix.netcom.com
Website: http://www.dhh.state.la.us/boards.htm
Dawn Scardino, Director

★ 20977 ★ Maine Board of Funeral Service
35 State House Station
Augusta, ME 04333-0035
Phone: (207)624-8623 **Fax:** (207)624-8637
Email: elaine.m.thibodeau@state.me.us
Website: http://www.state.me.us/pfr/olr/categories/cat19.htm
Elaine M. Thibodeau, Contact

★ 20978 ★ Maryland State Board of Morticians
Department of Health and Mental Hygiene
4201 Patterson Ave.
Room 315
Baltimore, MD 21215
Phone: (410)764-4792 **Fax:** (410)358-6571
Email: groninge@dhmh.state.md.us
Website: http://www.dhmh.state.md.us/bom/
Elizabeth Groninger, Contact

★ 20979 ★ Massachusetts Board of Funeral Service
239 Causeway St., Ste. 500
Boston, MA 02114
Phone: (617)727-1718 **Fax:** (617)727-2197
Email: kim.m.scully@state.ma.us
Website: http://www.state.ma.us/reg/boards/em/default.htm
Kim Scully, Contact

★ 20980 ★ Michigan Department of Commerce
Board of Examiners in Mortuary Science
PO Box 30004
Lansing, MI 48909
Phone: (517)373-1820 **Fax:** (517)373-2129
Email: bcsinfo@michigan.gov
Website: http://www.michigan.gov/cis/

★ 20981 ★ Minnesota Mortuary Science Section
121 E 7th Pl., Ste. 400
PO Box 64975
Saint Paul, MN 55164-0975
Phone: (651)282-3829 **Fax:** (651)282-3839
Email: david.benke@health.state.mn.us
Website: http://www.health.state.mn.us/divs/hpsc/mortsci/mortsci.htm
David Benke, Contact

★ 20982 ★ Mississippi State Board of Funeral Service
7 Riverbend Place, Ste. A
Flowood, MS 39208
Phone: (601)932-1973 **Fax:** (601)932-1901
Email: funeral_board@msbfs.state.ms.us
Website: http://www.msfuneralboard.com/
Dolores K. Kenney, Director

★ 20983 ★ Missouri State Board of Funeral Directors & Embalmers
3605 Missouri Blvd.
PO Box 423
Jefferson City, MO 65102
Phone: (573)751-0813 **Fax:** (573)751-1155
Email: embalmer@mail.state.mo.us
Website: http://www.ecodev.state.mo.us/pr/embalm/
Patricia A. Handly, Director

★ 20984 ★ Montana Board of Funeral Service
301 S Park, 4th Fl.
PO Box 200513
Helena, MT 59620-0513
Phone: (406)841-2393
Email: compolfnr@mt.gov
Website: http://commerce.state.mt.us/LICENSE/pol/pol_boards/fnr_board/board_page.htm
Cheryl Smith, Contact

★ 20985 ★ Nebraska Department of Health and Human Services
Credentialing Division
301 Centennial Mall South 3rd Flr.
PO Box 94986
Lincoln, NE 68509-4986
Phone: (402)471-2115 **Fax:** (402)471-3577
Email: Marie.McClatchey@hhss.state.ne.us
Website: http://www.hhs.state.ne.us/crl/crlindex.htm
Mary McClatchey, Contact

★ 20986 ★ Nevada State Board of Funeral Directors and Embalmers
4894 Lone Mountain Rd. Ste. 186
Las Vegas, NV 89130
Phone: (702)646-6860
Website: http://www.state.nv.us/funeral/

★ 20987 ★ New Hampshire Board of Registration of Funeral Directors and Embalmers
Health and Welfare Bldg.
6 Hazen Dr.
Concord, NH 03301-6527
Phone: (603)271-4648 **Fax:** (603)271-3447
Email: funeralbd@dhhs.state.nh.us
Website: http://webster.state.nh.us/funeral/
Robert J. Diluzio, Sr., Director

★ 20988 ★ New Jersey State Board of Mortuary Science
Board of Mortuary Science
PO Box 45009
Newark, NJ 07101
Phone: (973)504-6425
Email: askconsumeraffairs@smtp.lps.state.nj.us
Website: http://www.state.nj.us/lps/ca/nonmed.htmmort7
Paul Brush, Director

★ 20989 ★ New Mexico State Board of Thanatopractice
2055 Pacheco St., Ste. 400
Santa Fe, NM 87504
Phone: (505)476-7090 **Fax:** (505)476-7095
Email: FuneralBoard@state.nm.us
Website: http://www.rld.state.nm.us/b&c/thanato/index.htm

★ 20990 ★ New York State Department of Health
Funeral Directing Bureau
Empire State Plaza
Corning Tower
Albany, NY 12237-0681
Phone: (518)474-7354
Website: http://www.health.state.ny.us
Claudia Hutton, Director

★ 20991 ★ North Carolina Board of Mortuary Science
2321 Crabtree Blvd., Ste. 100
PO Box 27368
Raleigh, NC 27611-7368
Phone: (919)733-9380 **Free:** 800-862-0636
Fax: (919)733-8271
Email: aritter@ncbms.org
Website: http://www.ncbms.org/
Andrew Ritter, Director

★ 20992 ★ North Dakota Board of Funeral Service
PO Box 633
Devils Lake, ND 58301
Phone: (701)662-2511
Website: http://www.governor.state.nd.us/boards/boards-query.asp?Board_ID=42
Rodger E. Haugen, Contact
Frmly: North Dakota Board of Embalmers.

★ 20993 ★ Oklahoma State Board of Embalmers and Funeral Directors
4545 N Lincoln Blvd., Ste. 175
Oklahoma City, OK 73105
Phone: (405)522-1790 **Fax:** (405)522-1797
Email: info@okfuneral.com
Website: http://www.state.ok.us/~embalm/index.htm
Terry McEnany, Director

★ 20994 ★ Oregon State Mortuary and Cemetery Board
State Office Bldg., Ste. 430
800 NE Oregon St., Box 19
Portland, OR 97232-2162
Phone: (503)731-4040 **Fax:** (503)731-4494
Website: http://bluebook.state.or.us/state/executive/Mortuary_Cemetary/mortuary_cemetary_home.htm
Carla G. Knapp, Contact

★ 20995 ★ Pennsylvania State Board of Funeral and Funeral Directors
PO Box 2649
Harrisburg, PA 17105-2649
Phone: (717)783-3397 **Fax:** (717)783-7769
Email: funeral@pados.dos.state.pa.us
Website: http://www.nfda.org/careers/licensing/pa.html

★ 20996 ★ Rhode Island Division of Professional Regulation
State Health Department
3 Capital Hill, Rm. 104
Providence, RI 02908
Phone: (401)222-6015 **Fax:** (401)222-1272
Email: DonW@doh.state.ri.us
Website: http://www.health.state.ri.us/hsr/professions_reg.htm
Donald C. Williams, Contact

★ 20997 ★ South Carolina State Board of Funeral Service
Department of Labor, Licensing & Regulation
Koger Office Park
Kingstree Bldg.
110 Centerview Dr., Ste. 104
PO Box 11329
Columbia, SC 29211
Phone: (803)896-4496 **Fax:** (803)896-4484
Email: bryantr@mail.llr.state.sc.us
Website: http://www.llr.state.sc.us/POL/Funeral/Default.htm
Dwight Hayes, Contact

★ 20998 ★ South Dakota State Board of Funeral Service
135 E Illinois
PO Box 214
Spearfish, SD 57783
Phone: (605)642-1600 **Fax:** (605)642-1756
Email: proflic@rushmore.com
Website: http://www.state.sd.us/dcr/funeral/funhom.htm
Carol Tellinghuisen, Contact

★ 20999 ★ Tennessee Board of Funeral Directors and Embalmers
Davy Crockett Tower
500 James Robertson Pkwy., 2nd Fl.
Nashville, TN 37243-1149
Phone: (615)741-5062 **Fax:** (615)532-1903
Email: bteague@mail.state.tn.us
Arthur Giles, Director

★ 21000 ★ Texas Funeral Service Commission
510 S Congress, Ste. 206
PO Box 12217
Austin, TX 78704-7222
Phone: (512)936-2474 **Free:** 888-667-4881
Email: general@tfsc.state.tx.us
Website: http://www.tfsc.state.tx.us/

★ 21001 ★ Utah Department of Professional Licensing
160 E 300 S
PO Box 146701
Salt Lake City, UT 84114-6701
Phone: (801)530-6628 **Fax:** (801)530-6511
Email: gbowen@br.state.ut.us
Website: http://www.commerce.state.ut.us/dopl/dopl1.htm
Gary Bowen, Director

★ 21002 ★ Vermont Board of Funeral Service
Office of Professional Regulation
109 State St.
Montpelier, VT 05609-1106
Phone: (802)828-3228 **Fax:** (802)828-2496
Email: dbacon@sec.state.vt.us
Website: http://www.vtprofessionals.org/funeral/
Judith Churchill, Contact

★ 21003 ★ Virginia Board of Funeral Directors
Department of Health Professions
6606 W Broad St., 4th Fl.
Richmond, VA 23230-1717
Phone: (804)662-9907 **Free:** 800-533-1560
Fax: (804)662-9523
Email: fanbd@dhp.state.va.us
Website: http://www.dhp.state.va.us/fun/default.htm
Elizabeth Y. Tisdale, Contact

★ 21004 ★ Washington Funeral and Cemetery Office
Business & Professional Divisions
PO Box 9012
Olympia, WA 98507-9012
Phone: (360)664-1555 **Fax:** (360)586-4414
Email: Funerals@dol.wa.gov
Website: http://www.wa.gov/dol/bpd/funfront.htm

★ 21005 ★ West Virginia Board of Funeral Directors and Embalmers
179 Summers St., Ste. 305
Charleston, WV 25301
Phone: (304)558-0302
Email: perryle@wvnvm.wvnet.edu
Website: http://www.state.wv.us/bep/lmi/license/LICOCCMS.HTMfuneral

★ 21006 ★ Wisconsin Funeral Directors Examining Board
Department of Regulation and Licensing
1400 E Washington Ave.
PO Box 8935
Madison, WI 53708-8935
Phone: (608)266-5511
Email: dorl@drl.state.wi.us
Website: http://www.drl.state.wi.us/Regulation/applicant_information/dod278.html

★ 21007 ★ Wyoming State Board of Embalming
2020 Carey Ave., Ste. 201
Cheyenne, WY 82002
Phone: (307)777-7788 **Fax:** (307)777-3508
Email: vskora@state.wy.us
Website: http://www.state.wy.us/governor/boards/bdlist.html
Veronica Skoranski, Contact

Health Planning & Development

★ 21008 ★ Alabama Health Planning and Development Agency
100 N Union St, Ste. 870
PO Box 303025
Montgomery, AL 36130-3025
Phone: (334)242-4103 **Fax:** (334)242-4113
Email: info@shpda.state.al.us

Website: http://shpda.state.al.us/

★ 21009 ★ Arizona Department of Health Services
Planning Office
1740 W Adams St.
Phoenix, AZ 85007
Phone: (602)542-1000 **Fax:** (602)542-1062
Website: http://www.hs.state.az.us/

★ 21010 ★ Arkansas Department of Health
Planning Bureau
4815 W Markham
Little Rock, AR 72205
Phone: (501)661-2238 **Fax:** (501)661-2414
Website: http://health.state.ar.us

★ 21011 ★ California Health and Welfare Agency
Statewide Health Planning and Development Office
1600 9th St., Ste. 435
Sacramento, CA 95814
Phone: (916)654-1499 **Fax:** (916)653-2854
Website: http://www.oshpd.cahwnet.gov/

★ 21012 ★ Colorado Department of Human Services
Health Care Policy and Financing Division
Health Plans Operations
1575 Sherman St.
Denver, CO 80203-1714
Phone: (303)866-2993 **Fax:** (303)866-4411
Email: diane.rodriguez@state.co.us
Website: http://www.chcpf.state.co.us/index.html
Karen Reinertson, Contact

★ 21013 ★ Connecticut Department of Public Health
Policy, Planning, and Evaluation Office
Health Information Systems
410 Capitol Ave.
PO Box 340308
Hartford, CT 06134-0308
Phone: (860)509-7163 **Fax:** (860)509-7160
Email: webmaster.dph@po.state.ct.us
Website: http://www.state.ct.us/dph/OPPE/hphis.htm
Daniel J. Saviano, Director

★ 21014 ★ Delaware Department of Health and Social Services
Management Services Division
1901 N DuPont Hwy.
New Castle, DE 19720
Phone: (302)577-4515 **Fax:** (302)577-4539
Email: dhssinfo@state.de.us
Website: http://www.state.de.us/dhss/dms/dmshome.htm
Valencia L. Beaty, Director

★ 21015 ★ Florida Agency Health Care Administration
Fort Knox Executive Center, Bldg. 3
2727 Mahan Dr.
Tallahassee, FL 32308-5407
Free: 888-419-3456
Email: ahca@fdhc.state.fl.us
Website: http://www.fdhc.state.fl.us/

★ 21016 ★ Georgia Department of Community Health
Division of Health Planning
2 Peachtree St. NW
Atlanta, GA 30303
Phone: (404)656-0655 **Fax:** (404)656-0654
Website: http://www.communityhealth.state.ga.us/
Valerie Hepburn, Contact

★ 21017 ★ Hawaii Department of Health
Hawaii State Health Planning and Development Agency
1177 Alakea St. Rm.402
Honolulu, HI 96813
Phone: (808)587-0788 **Fax:** (808)587-0783
Email: shpda@health.state.hi.us
Website: http://www.state.hi.us/health/shpda/

★ 21018 ★ Idaho Department of Health and Welfare
Bureau of Vital Records and Health Statistics
450 W State St.
PO Box 83720
Boise, ID 83720-0036
Phone: (208)334-5976 **Free:** 800-926-2588
Fax: (208)334-6558
Website: http://www2.state.id.us/dhw/index.htm
Jane Smith, Contact

★ 21019 ★ Illinois Department of Public Health
Epidemiology and Health Systems Development Office
525 W Jefferson St., 2nd Fl.
Springfield, IL 62761
Phone: (217)785-2040 **Fax:** (217)785-4308
Email: mrichard@idph.state.il.us
Website: http://www.idph.state.il.us/about/epistudies.htm
Margaret Richards, PhD, Contact

★ 21020 ★ Indiana Department of Health
Health and Planning Division
2 N Meridian St.
Indianapolis, IN 46204
Phone: (317)233-1325
Website: http://www.state.in.us/isdh/

★ 21021 ★ Iowa Department of Public Health
Division of Administration and Regulatory Affairs
Lucas State Office Bldg.
321 E 12th St.
Des Moines, IA 50319-0075
Phone: (515)281-5787
Email: webmaster@idph.state.ia.us
Website: http://www.idph.state.ia.us/ar.htm
David Fries, Contact

★ 21022 ★ Kansas Department of Health and Environment
Health Division
Charles Curtis State Office Bldg.
1000 SW Jackson, suite 300
Topeka, KS 66612-1365
Phone: (785)296-1343 **Fax:** (785)296-1562
Email: info@kdhe.state.ks.us
Website: http://www.kdhe.state.ks.us/health/
J. Michael Moser, MD, Director

★ 21023 ★ Kentucky Families and Children Cabinet
Health Planning and Certification Office
275 E Main St.
Frankfort, KY 40621
Phone: (502)564-7130 **Fax:** (502)564-3866
Email: dean.crawford@mail.state.ky.us
Website: http://cfc.state.ky.us/

★ 21024 ★ Louisiana Department of Health and Hospitals
Division of Community Health
Health Resources Management Bureau
1201 Capitol Access Rd.
PO Box 629
Baton Rouge, LA 70821-0629
Phone: (504)342-9513 **Fax:** (504)342-8098
Email: ophweb@.dhh.state.la.us
Website: http://www.dhh.state.la.us/OPH/resmgt.htm

★ 21025 ★ Maryland Department of Health and Mental Hygiene
Health Care Commission
4201 Patterson Ave., 5th Fl.
Baltimore, MD 21215
Phone: (410)764-3460 **Free:** 877-245-1762
Fax: (410)358-1236
Email: webmaster@mhcc.state.md.us
Website: http://www.mhcc.state.md.us/
Barbara McLean, Director

★ 21026 ★ Massachusetts Executive Office of Health and Human Services
Public Health Department
Policy and Planning Office
250 Washington St.
Boston, MA 02108-4619
Phone: (617)624-6000
Email: dph.info@state.ma.us
Website: http://www.state.ma.us/dph/dphhome.htm

★ 21027 ★ Michigan Community Health Department
Policy and Legal Affairs
Health Legislation and Policy Development
Lewis Cass Bldg., 6th Fl.
320 S Walnut St.
Lansing, MI 48913
Phone: (517)373-3500
Email: arias@.mi.gov
Website: http://www.mdch.state.mi.us/
Carol Isaacs, Contact

★ 21028 ★ Mississippi Department of Health
Health Regulation Office
Health Planning and Resource Development Division
PO Box 1700
570 Woodrow Wilson Blvd.
Jackson, MS 39215-1700
Phone: (601)576-7874 **Fax:** (601)576-7530
Email: harmstrong@msdh.state.ms.us
Website: http://www.msdh.state.ms.us/planning/index.htm

★ 21029 ★ Missouri Department of Health and Senior Services
Director's Office
920 Wildwood Dr.
PO Box 570
Jefferson City, MO 65102
Phone: (573)751-6001 **Fax:** (573)751-6041
Email: info@mail.health.state.mo.us
Website: http://www.health.state.mo.us/AbouttheDepartment/DS3.html

★ 21030 ★ Montana Department of Public Health and Human Services
Health Policy and Services Division
1400 Broadway
PO Box 202951
Helena, MT 59620
Phone: (406)444-4540 **Fax:** (406)444-1861
Email: dphhstech@state.mt.gov

Website: http://www.dphhs.state.mt.us/divisions/hps/hps_phone.htm
Maggie Bullock, Contact

★ 21031 ★ Nebraska Department of Health and Human Services
Health Policy and Service Planning
PO Box 95007
301 Centennial Mall S
Lincoln, NE 68509
Phone: (402)471-9433 **Free:** 800-254-4202
Fax: (402)471-9449
Email: hhsinfo@www.hhs.state.ne.us
Website: http://www.hhs.state.ne.us/poc/pocindex.htm
Chris Peterson, Contact

★ 21032 ★ Nevada Department of Human Resources
Health Division
Health Planning Bureau
505 E King St., Rm. 102
Carson City, NV 89701
Phone: (775)684-4218 **Fax:** (775)684-4156
Email: oitsupport@nvhd.state.nv.us
Website: http://www.state.nv.us/health/

★ 21033 ★ New Hampshire Department of Health and Human Services
Public Health Services Division
Health Services Planning and Review Bureau
129 Pleasant St.
Concord, NH 03301
Phone: (603)271-4606 **Fax:** (603)271-4141
Website: http://www.dhhs.state.nh.us

★ 21034 ★ New Jersey Department of Health
Health Care Systems Analysis Division
John Fitch Plaza
PO Box 360
Trenton, NJ 08625-0360
Phone: (609)984-3939
Website: www.state.nj.us/health/hcsa/hcsadmin.htm
Marilyn Dahl, Contact

★ 21035 ★ New Mexico Health Policy Commission
2055 S Pacheco St., Ste. 200
Santa Fe, NM 87505
Phone: (505)424-3200
Email: hpcwebteam@hpc.state.nm.us
Website: http://hpc.state.nm.us/

★ 21036 ★ North Carolina Department of Health and Human Services
Facility Services Division
State Medical Facilities Planning Section
701 Barbour Dr.
2714 Mail Service Ctr.
Raleigh, NC 27699-2714
Phone: (919)855-3865 **Fax:** (919)715-4413
Website: http://facility-services.state.nc.us/planpage.htm

★ 21037 ★ North Dakota Department of Health
Administrative Services Section
Health Information Systems Division
600 E Boulevard Ave.
Bismarck, ND 58505-0200
Phone: (701)328-2392 **Fax:** (701)328-4727
Website: http://www.health.state.nd.us/ndhd/admin/index.htm
Arvy Smith, Contact

★ 21038 ★ The Office for Oregon Health Plan Policy and Research
255 Capitol St. NE, 5th Fl.
Salem, OR 97310
Phone: (503)378-2422 **Free:** 800-359-9517
Fax: (503)378-5511
Email: dhr.info@state.or.us
Website: http://www.ohppr.state.or.us
John Santa, MD, Director

★ 21039 ★ Oklahoma Department of Health
Health Promotion and Policy Analysis Office
Health Planning
1000 NE 10th St., Rm. 1106
Oklahoma City, OK 73117
Phone: (405)271-1685
Email: philiph@health.state.ok.us
Website: http://www.health.state.ok.us/PROGRAM/planning/index.html

★ 21040 ★ Pennsylvania Department of Health
Quality Assurance
Health Care Financing Bureau
PO Box 90
Health and Welfare Bldg.
Harrisburg, PA 17108
Phone: (717)787-5193 **Free:** 888-466-2787
Fax: (717)705-0947
Email: webmaster@health.state.pa.us
Website: http://www.health.state.pa.us/QA/HMO/default.htm

★ 21041 ★ South Carolina Environmental Control
State Health Plan
2600 Bull St.
Columbia, SC 29201
Phone: (803)898-3432
Email: WhitesAN@Columb54.dhec.state.sc.us
Website: http://www.scdhec.net/Health_Reg/hrshp.htm

★ 21042 ★ South Dakota Department of Health
Policy and External Affairs Office
600 E Capitol
Pierre, SD 57501-2536
Phone: (605)773-3361 **Free:** 800-738-2301
Email: DOH.INFO@state.sd.us
Website: http://www.state.sd.us/doh/
Doneen Hollingsworth, Contact

★ 21043 ★ State Health Planning and Development Agency
825 N Capitol St. NE
Washington, DC 20002
Phone: (202)442-5875
Website: http://www.dchealth.com/shpda

★ 21044 ★ Tennessee Department of Health
TennCare
729 Church St.
Nashville, TN 37243
Phone: (615)532-7542 **Free:** 800-669-1851
Fax: (615)741-0213
Email: ssharpe@mail.state.tn.us
Website: http://www.state.tn.us/tenncare/
Mark Reynolds, Director

★ 21045 ★ Texas Department of Health
Health Data and Policy Analysis Bureau
1100 W 49th St.
Austin, TX 78756-3199
Phone: (512)458-7111 **Free:** 888-963-7111
Website: http://www.tdh.state.tx.us/data.htm

★ 21046 ★ Vermont Agency of Human Services
Social and Rehabilitation Services Department
Planning and Evaluation Division
103 S Main St.
State Complex
Waterbury, VT 05671-2401
Phone: (802)241-2100 **Fax:** (802)241-2980
Email: webmaster@srs.state.vt.us
Website: http://www.state.vt.us/srs

★ 21047 ★ Virginia Office of Health and Human Resources
Medical Assistance Services Department
Policy and Budget Division
600 E Broad St., Ste. 1300
Richmond, VA 23219
Phone: (804)371-7561 **Fax:** (804)786-0729
Email: jsmith@dmas.state.va.us
Website: http://www.cns.state.va.us/dmas/

★ 21048 ★ Washington State Health Care Authority
676 Woodland Sq. Loop SE
PO Box 42682
Olympia, WA 98504-2682
Phone: (360)923-2600
Email: adminwww@hca.wa.gov
Website: http://www.wa.gov/hca/

★ 21049 ★ Wisconsin Department of Health and Family Services
Health Division
Management and Policy Office
PO Box 7850
Madison, WI 53707-7850
Phone: (608)266-6954
Website: http://www.dhfs.state.wi.us/aboutdhfs/dmt/dmt.htm
Sue Reinardy, Contact

Hospital Licensure

★ 21050 ★ Alaska Department of Health and Social Services
Medical Assistance Division
Health Facilities Licensing and Certification Office
4730 Business Park Blvd., Ste. 18
Anchorage, AK 99503
Phone: (907)334-2483 **Fax:** (907)561-3011
Email: shelby_larsen@health.state.ak.us
Website: http://www.hss.state.ak.us/dma/HFLC.HTM
Shelby Larsen, Contact

★ 21051 ★ Arizona Department of Health Services
Health Care Licensure Office
1647 E Morten Ave., Ste. 240
Phoenix, AZ 85020
Phone: (602)674-4340 **Fax:** (602)861-0463
Email: jhaaske@hs.state.az.us
Website: http://www.hs.state.az.us/als/index.html

★ 21052 ★ Arkansas Department of Health
Health Resources Bureau
Health Facility Services and Systems Division
5800 W Tenth St. Ste. 400
Little Rock, AR 72204
Phone: (501)661-2201
Website: http://health.state.ar.us

★ 21053 ★ California Health and Welfare Agency
Health Services Department
Licensing and Certification Division
7801 Folsom Blvd., Ste. 200
PO Box 942732
Sacramento, CA 95826
Phone: (916)229-3400 **Free:** 800-554-0354
Fax: (916)229-3465
Website: http://www.dhs.ca.gov/lnc/index.htm

★ 21054 ★ Colorado Public Health and Environment Department
Health Office
Health Facilities Division
4300 Cherry Creek Dr. S
Denver, CO 80246-1530
Phone: (303)692-2800
Email: health.facilities@state.co.us
Website: http://www.cdphe.state.co.us/hf/

★ 21055 ★ Connecticut Department of Public Health
Regulatory Services Bureau
Health Systems Regulation Division
410 Capitol Ave.
PO Box 340308
Hartford, CT 06134-0308
Phone: (860)509-7406 **Fax:** (860)509-7539
Email: webmaster.dph@po.state.ct.us
Website: http://www.state.ct.us/dph/DPH_Main/About_DPH/brs/brs.htm
Cynthia Denne, Contact

★ 21056 ★ District of Columbia Department of Consumer and Regulatory Affairs
Service Facility Regulations Administration
Health Facility Division
941 N Capital St. NE, Rm. 1100
Washington, DC 20002
Phone: (202)442-4400
Website: http://dcra.dc.gov/main.shtm

★ 21057 ★ Florida Department of Health
Licensure and Certification Office
4052 Bald Cypress Way, Bin A00
Tallahassee, FL 32399
Phone: (850)245-4443
Email: health@doh.state.fl.us
Website: http://www.doh.state.fl.us/

★ 21058 ★ Georgia Department of Human Resources
Regulatory Services Office
Health Care Section
2 Peachtree St. NW,
Atlanta, GA 30303
Phone: (404)657-5550 **Fax:** (404)657-8934
Email: mapalli@dhr.state.ga.us
Website: http://www2.state.ga.us/departments/dhr/ors/orshcs.htm

★ 21059 ★ Hawaii Department of Health
Office of Health Care Assurance
601 Kamokila Blvd.
Rm. 395
Kapolei, HI 96707
Phone: (808)586-4080 **Fax:** (808)586-4444
Email: webmail@health.hi.us
Website: http://www.state.hi.us/health/about/dohphn01.htm
Helen Yoshimi, Contact

★ 21060 ★ Idaho Department of Health and Welfare
Medicaid Division
Facility Standards Bureau
450 West State St.
Boise, ID 83720-0036
Phone: (208)334-6626
Website: http://www2.state.id.us/dhw/FacilStandards/bfs_index.htm
Debra Ransom, Director

★ 21061 ★ Illinois Department of Public Health
Health Care Regulation Office
Health Care Facilities and Programs Division
Hospital Licensing Section
525 W Jefferson St., 5th Fl.
Springfield, IL 62761
Phone: (217)782-2913 **Fax:** (217)524-6292
Email: bbell@idph.state.il.us
Website: http://www.idph.state.il.us/about/ohcr.htm

★ 21062 ★ Indiana Department of Health
Acute Care Division
2 N Meridian St.
Indianapolis, IN 46204
Phone: (317)233-1325
Website: http://www.state.in.us/isdh/regsvcs/acc/acute.htm

★ 21063 ★ Iowa Department of Inspections and Appeals
Health Facilities Division
Lucas State Office Bldg.
321 E 12th St.
Des Moines, IA 50319-0001
Phone: (515)281-4115
Email: mtooman@dia.state.ia.us
Website: http://www.dia-hfd.state.ia.us/
Marvin L. Tooman, Director

★ 21064 ★ Kansas Department of Health and Environment
Health Division
Adult and Child Care Facilities Bureau
Hospital Program
1000 SW Jackson St., Ste. 330
Topeka, KS 66612
Phone: (785)296-1240 **Fax:** (785)296-1266
Email: healthfacilities@kdhe.state.ks.us
Website: http://www.kdhe.state.ks.us/bhfr/

★ 21065 ★ Kentucky Health Services Cabinet
Inspector General Office
Community Health Services Division
275 E Main St, 5E-A
Frankfort, KY 40621
Phone: (502)564-2800 **Fax:** (502)564-6546
Website: http://chs.state.ky.us/oig/community/
Floyd B. Parrish, Director

★ 21066 ★ Louisiana Department of Health and Hospitals
Health Standards Section
Licensing and Certification Division
PO Box 3767
Baton Rouge, LA 70821-3767
Phone: (225)342-0415 **Fax:** (225)342-5292
Email: ldeaton@dhh.state.la.us
Website: http://www.dhh.state.la.us/boards.htm
Lisa M. Deaton, Contact

★ 21067 ★ Maine Department of Human Services
Medical Services Bureau
Licensing and Certification Division
11 State House Station
35 Anthony Ave
Augusta, ME 04333-0011
Phone: (207)624-5443 **Fax:** (207)624-5378
Email: lou.dorogi@state.me.us
Website: http://www.state.me.us/bms/
Lou Dorogi, Director

★ 21068 ★ Maryland Department of Health and Mental Hygiene
Office of Health Care Quality
Spring Grove Hospital Center
Bland Bryant Bldg.
55 Wade Ave.
Catonsville, MD 21228
Phone: (410)402-8000
Email: ohcqweb@dhmh.state.md.us
Website: http://www.dhmh.state.md.us/ohcq/

★ 21069 ★ Massachusetts Executive Office of Health and Human Services
Public Health Department
Health Care Quality Division
10 W St, 5th Fl.
Boston, MA 02111
Phone: (617)753-8000 **Fax:** (617)753-8125
Email: paul.l.dreyer@state.ma.us
Website: http://www.state.ma.us/dph/hcqskel.htm
Paul Dreyer, Director

★ 21070 ★ Michigan Department of Consumer and Industry Services
Commercial Services Bureau
Licensing Division
PO Box 30018
Lansing, MI 48909
Phone: (517)241-9223 **Fax:** (517)241-9280
Email: bcsinfo@cis.state.mi.us
Website: http://www.cis.state.mi.us/bcs/licdiv.htm
Jean Boven, Director

★ 21071 ★ Minnesota Department of Health
Health Systems and Special Populations Bureau
Facility and Provider Compliance Division
PO Box 64975
Saint Paul, MN 55164-0975
Phone: (651)215-5800
Email: fpcmail@mdh-fpc.health.state.mn.us
Website: http://www.health.state.mn.us/divs/fpc/fpc.html

★ 21072 ★ Mississippi Department of Health
Health Regulation Office
Licensure Division
570 Woodrow Wilson Blvd. Ste. 200
PO Box 1700
Jackson, MS 39216
Phone: (601)576-7300 **Fax:** (601)576-7225
Email: vphipps@msdh.state.ms.us
Website: http://www.msdh.state.ms.us/licensure/index.htm

★ 21073 ★ Missouri Department of Health
Health Standards and Licensure Division
Hospital Licensing and Certification Bureau
930 Wildwood
PO Box 570
Jefferson City, MO 65102
Phone: (573)751-6271 **Fax:** (573)526-3621
Email: info@mail.health.state.mo.us

Website: http://www.health.state.mo.us/AbouttheDepartment/DS6.html

★ 21074 ★ Montana Department of Public Health and Human Services
Health Facilities Division
2401 Colonial Dr.
PO Box 202953
Helena, MT 59620-2953
Phone: (406)444-2037 **Fax:** (406)444-1742
Email: ddavis@state.mt.gov
Website: http://www.dphhs.state.mt.us/divisions/qad/qad_phone.htm
Mary Dalton, Director

★ 21075 ★ Nebraska Department of Health and Human Services
Environmental Health
Health Facilities Licensure Division
301 Centennial Mall S
PO Box 95007
Lincoln, NE 68509-5044
Phone: (402)471-0179 **Fax:** (402)471-0555
Email: hmeeks@doh.state.ne.us
Website: http://www.hhs.state.ne.us/enh/enhindex.htm
Helen Meeks, Contact

★ 21076 ★ Nevada Department of Human Resources
Health Division
Licensure and Certification Bureau
1550 E College Parkway, St.158
Carson City, NV 89706
Phone: (775)687-4475 **Fax:** (775)687-6588
Website: http://www.state.nv.us/health/
Luana Ritch, Contact

★ 21077 ★ New Hampshire Department of Health and Human Services
Public Health Services Division
Health Facilities Administration Bureau
129 Pleasant St.
Concord, NH 03301-3857
Phone: (603)271-4592 **Fax:** (603)271-4968
Website: http://www.dhhs.state.nh.us

★ 21078 ★ New Jersey Department of Health
Health Facilities Evaluation and Licensing Division
Licensing, Certification, and Standards Office
120 S Stockton St.
PO Box 367
Trenton, NJ 08625-0367
Phone: (609)633-9051 **Free:** 800-792-9770
Fax: (609)633-9087
Email: ltc@doh.state.nj.us
Website: http://www.state.nj.us/health/ltc/

★ 21079 ★ New Mexico Department of Health
Public Health Division
Licensing and Certification Bureau
2040 S Pacheco St. 2nd Flr., Rm 413
Santa Fe, NM 87505
Phone: (505)476-9025 **Fax:** (505)476-9053
Website: http://www.health.state.nm.us/dhi/HFLC.htm

★ 21080 ★ North Carolina Department of Health and Human Services
Facility Services Division
2706 Mail Service Ctr.
2701 Mail Service Ctr.
Raleigh, NC 27699-2701
Phone: (919)733-2342 **Free:** 800-624-3004
Fax: (919)733-2757
Email: Michelle.Penny@ncmail.net
Website: http://facility-services.state.nc.us/
Lynda McDaniel, Director

★ 21081 ★ North Dakota Department of Health
Health Resources Section
Health Facilities Division
600 E Boulevard, Department 301
Bismarck, ND 58505-0200
Phone: (701)328-2352 **Fax:** (701)328-1890
Email: ajohnson@state.nd.us
Website: http://www.health.state.nd.us/ndhd/resource/facilities/about/
Allen Johnson, Director

★ 21082 ★ Ohio Department of Health
Quality Assurance Division
Regulatory Compliance Bureau
246 N High St.
PO Box 118
Columbus, OH 43216-0118
Phone: (614)644-6220 **Fax:** (614)752-4157
Email: BRC@gw.odh.state.oh.us
Website: http://www.odh.state.oh.us/
Alan Curtis, Director

★ 21083 ★ Oklahoma Department of Health
Special Health Services
Medical and Facilities Services
1000 NE 10th St.
Rm. 1114
Oklahoma City, OK 73117-1299
Phone: (405)271-6576 **Fax:** (405)271-1308
Email: Medicalfacilities@health.state.ok.us
Website: http://www.health.state.ok.us/PROGRAM/medfac/index.html

★ 21084 ★ Oregon Department of Human Resources
Health Division
Health Care Licensure and Certification Section
Portland State Office Bldg.
800 NE Oregon St.
Portland, OR 97232
Phone: (503)731-4013 **Fax:** (503)731-3184
Website: http://www.ohd.hr.state.or.us/hclc/welcome.htm
Kathleen Smail, Contact

★ 21085 ★ Pennsylvania Department of Health
Quality Assurance Bureau
PO Box 90
Health and Welfare Bldg.
Harrisburg, PA 17108
Free: 877-724-3258
Email: webmaster@health.state.pa.us
Website: http://www.health.state.pa.us/qa/
Richard Lee, Contact

★ 21086 ★ Rhode Island Department of Health
Health Services Regulations Office
Facilities Regulations Division
3 Capitol Hill, Rm. 306
Providence, RI 02908
Phone: (401)222-2566 **Free:** 800-745-5555
Website: http://www.health.state.ri.us/hsr/facreg/facreg.htm

★ 21087 ★ South Carolina Department of Health and Environmental Control
Health Services Office
Health Facilities Regulation Bureau
2600 Bull St.
PO Box 101106
Columbia, SC 29211-1708
Phone: (803)545-4663 **Fax:** (803)545-4212
Website: http://www.scdhec.net/hr

★ 21088 ★ South Dakota Department of Health
Licensure and Certification Program
615 E 4th St.
Pierre, SD 57501
Phone: (605)773-3356 **Fax:** (605)773-6667
Email: DOH.INFO@doh.state.sd.us
Website: http://www.state.sd.us/doh/Facility/index.htm

★ 21089 ★ Tennessee Department of Health
Manpower and Facilities Bureau
Health Care Facilities Division
Cordell Hull Bldg., 1st Fl.
425 5th Ave., N
Nashville, TN 37247-0508
Phone: (615)741-7221
Email: Diane.Denton@state.tn.us
Website: http://www2.state.tn.us/health/HCF/

★ 21090 ★ Texas Department of Health
Bureau of Licensing and Compliance
Health Facility Licensing and Compliance Division
1100 W 49th St.
Austin, TX 78756
Phone: (512)834-6650 **Fax:** (512)834-6653
Email: infohflc@tdh.state.tx.us
Website: http://www.tdh.state.tx.us/hfc/hfc-web.htm
Nance Stearman, Director

★ 21091 ★ Utah Department of Health
Health Systems Improvement Division
Health Facilities and Child Care Licensing Bureau
288 N 1460 W
PO Box 142003
Salt Lake City, UT 84114-2003
Phone: (801)538-6152 **Free:** 888-287-3704
Fax: (801)538-6325
Email: mbentley@doh.state.ut.us
Website: http://www.health.state.ut.us/hsi/hfl/
Debra Wynkoop, Contact

★ 21092 ★ Vermont Agency of Human Services
Health Department
Medical Care Regulation Division
108 Cherry St.
PO Box 70
Burlington, VT 05402-0070
Phone: (802)863-7200 **Fax:** (802)865-7754
Email: Webkeeper@.vdh.state.vt.us
Website: http://www.healthyvermonters.info/

★ 21093 ★ Virginia Office of Health and Human Resources
Health Department
Center for Quality Health Care Services and Consumer Protection
3600 W Broad St., St. 216
Richmond, VA 23230
Phone: (804)367-2106 **Free:** 800-955-1819
Fax: (804)367-2804
Website: http://www.vdh.state.va.us/quality/default.htm

★ 21094 ★ Washington Department of Health
Facility and Services Licensing Division
PO Box 47852
Olympia, WA 98504-7852
Phone: (360)705-6652 **Fax:** (360)705-6654
Website: http://www.doh.wa.gov/hsqa/fsl/default.htm

★ 21095 ★ West Virginia Department of Health and Human Resources
Public Health Bureau
Health Facility Licensure and Certification Office
350 Capitol St.
Room 206
Charleston, WV 25301
Phone: (304)558-0050
Email: RobWest@wvdhhr.org
Website: http://www.wvdhhr.org/ohflac/default.htm
John Wilkinson, Director

★ 21096 ★ Wisconsin Department of Health and Family Services
Health Division
Quality Compliance Bureau
PO Box 7851
Madison, WI 53707-7851
Phone: (608)266-0554
Email: webmaster@dhfs.state.wi.us
Website: http://www.dhfs.state.wi.us/aboutdhfs/DSL/dsl.htm
Sinikka McCabe, Contact

Maternal & Child Health

★ 21097 ★ Alabama Department of Public Health
Family Health Services Bureau
RSA Tower
201 Monroe St. Ste 1350
PO Box 303017
Montgomery, AL 36104
Phone: (334)206-5661 **Fax:** (334)206-2950
Email: webmaster@www.alapubhealth.org
Website: http://www.alapubhealth.org

★ 21098 ★ Alaska Department of Health and Social Services
Public Health Division
Maternal and Child Family Health Section
3601 C St., Ste. 934
PO Box 240249
Anchorage, AK 99524-0249
Phone: (907)269-3400 **Free:** 800-799-7570
Fax: (907)269-3465
Email: pam_muth@health.state.ak.us
Website: http://www.hss.state.ak.us/dph/mcfh/SectionMCFH.htm

★ 21099 ★ Arizona Department of Health Services
Family Health and Community Services Division
Women and Children's Health Office
2927 N35th Ave, Ste. 300
Phoenix, AZ 85017
Phone: (602)364-1400 **Fax:** (602)364-1494
Website: http://www.hs.state.az.us/cfhs/owch/

★ 21100 ★ California Health and Welfare Agency
Health Services Department
Maternal and Child Health Branch
714 P St., Rm. 750
Sacramento, CA 95814
Phone: (916)657-1347
Website: http://www.dhs.cahwnet.gov/org/pcfh/mchb/mchbindex.htm

★ 21101 ★ Colorado Public Health and Environment Department
Health Office
Division of Prevention and Intervention Services for Children and Youth
4300 Cherry Creek Dr. S A-4
Denver, CO 80246
Phone: (303)692-2310
Website: http://www.cdphe.state.co.us/fc/fchom.asp

★ 21102 ★ Connecticut Department of Public Health
Community Health Bureau
Child Adolescent Health Division
Hartford, CT
Phone: (860)509-8066 **Fax:** (860)509-7720
Email: webmaster.dph@po.state.ct.us
Website: http://www.state.ct.us/dph/BCH/Family%20Health/HPFamHS.html
Beth Weinstein, M.P.H., Contact

★ 21103 ★ Delaware Department of Health and Social Services
Public Health Division
Family Health Services
Jesse Cooper Bldg.
417 Federal St.
PO Box 637
Dover, DE 19903
Phone: (302)739-4787 **Fax:** (302)739-6653
Email: dhssinfo@state.de.us
Website: http://www.state.de.us/dhss/dph/chca/fhs_index.html

★ 21104 ★ District of Columbia Department of Health
Office of Maternal and Child Health
825 N Capitol St. NE, 3rd Fl.
Washington, DC 20002
Phone: (202)442-5925 **Fax:** (202)442-4947
Website: http://www.dchealth.com/mch

★ 21105 ★ Georgia Department of Community Health
Division of Medical Assistance
Maternal and Child Health Division
2 Peachtree St. NW
Atlanta, GA 30303
Phone: (404)656-4507
Website: http://www.communityhealth.state.ga.us/

★ 21106 ★ Hawaii Department of Health
Health Resources Administration
Family Health Services Division
Maternal and Child Health Branch
741 Sunset Ave.
Honolulu, HI 96816
Phone: (808)733-9022 **Fax:** (808)733-9068
Website: http://www.state.hi.us/health/about/resources.html
Momi Kamau, Director

★ 21107 ★ Idaho Department of Health and Welfare
Health Division
Maternal and Child Health Bureau
PO Box 83720
707 N Armitage Pl.
Boise, ID 83704-0825
Phone: (208)327-8595 **Fax:** (208)334-6581
Website: http://www2.state.id.us/dhw/hwgd_www/contentlist.htmlHealth

★ 21108 ★ Indiana Department of Health
Maternal and Child Health Services Division
2 N Meridian
Indianapolis, IN 46204
Phone: (317)233-1262 **Fax:** (317)233-1299
Email: jganser@isdh.state.in.us
Website: http://www.state.in.us/isdh/programs/mch/index2.htm
Judith A. Ganser, MD, Director

★ 21109 ★ Iowa Department of Public Health
Family and Community Health Division
Maternal and Child Health Section
Lucas State Office Bldg., 3rd Fl.
321 E 12th St.
Des Moines, IA 50319-0075
Phone: (515)242-6388 **Fax:** (515)242-6384
Email: webmaster@idph.state.ia.us
Website: http://idph.state.ia.us/fch/fam_serv/mhs.htm
Janet L. Peterson, Contact

★ 21110 ★ Kansas Department of Health and Environment
Health Division
Family Health Bureau
1000 SW Jackson St., Ste. 220
Topeka, KS 66612-1274
Phone: (785)291-3368 **Fax:** (785)296-6553
Email: lkenney@kdhe.state.ks.us
Website: http://www.kdhe.state.ks.us/bcyf/index.html
Linda Kenney, Director

★ 21111 ★ Kentucky Health Services Cabinet
Health Services Department
Maternal and Child Health Services Division
275 E Main St.
Frankfort, KY 40621
Phone: (502)564-9538 **Fax:** (502)564-7091
Website: http://chs.state.ky.us/

★ 21112 ★ Louisiana Department of Health and Hospitals
Public Health Office
Health Services Programs
Maternal and Child Health Section
325 Loyola Ave.
PO Box 60630
New Orleans, LA 70160
Phone: (504)568-5073 **Fax:** (504)568-8162
Email: ophwebmaster@dhhmail.dhh.state.la.us
Website: http://www.dhh.state.la.us/OPH/mch.htm

★ 21113 ★ Maine Department of Human Services
Health Bureau
Maternal and Child Health Division
11 State House Station
157 Capitol St.
Augusta, ME 04333
Phone: (207)287-8016
Email: Cheryl.M.DiCara@state.me.us
Website: http://janus.state.me.us/dhs/boh/
Marcie Sanders, Contact

★ 21114 ★ Massachusetts Executive Office of Health and Human Services
Public Health Department
Family Health Services Division
250 Washington St. 5th Floor
Boston, MA 02108-4619
Phone: (617)624-6060 **Fax:** (617)624-6062
Website: http://www.state.ma.us/dph/bfch/index.htm
Sally Fogerty, Contact

★ 21115 ★ Minnesota Department of Health
Maternal and Child Health Section
717 Delaware St. SE
PO Box 64975
Minneapolis, MN 55414
Phone: (651)281-9888
Email: fh@kids.health.state.mn.us
Website: http://www.health.state.mn.us/divs/fh/fh.html

★ 21116 ★ Mississippi Department of Health
Health Services Bureau
WIC Services
570 E Woodrow Wilson Blvd.
PO Box 1700
Jackson, MS 39215
Phone: (601)576-7100 **Fax:** (601)576-7070
Email: cjordan@msdh.state.ms.us
Website: http://www.msdh.state.ms.us/osho/fldsvcs/Centrllk.htm
Curtis Jordan, Contact

★ 21117 ★ Missouri Department of Health
Maternal, Child and Family Health Division
930 Wildwood
PO Box 570
Jefferson City, MO 65102
Phone: (573)751-8394 **Fax:** (573)751-6041
Email: info@mail.health.state.mo.us
Website: http://www.health.state.mo.us/AbouttheDepartment/DS9.html

★ 21118 ★ Montana Department of Public Health and Human Services
Child and Family Services Division
1400 Broadway
PO Box 8005
Helena, MT 59604-8005
Phone: (406)444-5900 **Fax:** (406)444-5956
Email: cfsd@state.mt.us
Website: http://www.dphhs.state.mt.us/divisions/cfs/cfs.htm
Chuck Hunter, Director

★ 21119 ★ Nebraska Department of Health and Human Services
Health Promotion and Disease Prevention
Office of Family Health
301 Centennial Mall S
PO Box 95044
Lincoln, NE 68509-5044
Phone: (402)471-2907
Email: family.health@hhs.state.ne.us
Website: http://www.hhs.state.ne.us/hpe/hpeindex.htm
Paula Eurek, Director

★ 21120 ★ Nevada Department of Human Resources
Health Division
Family Health Service
505 E King St.
Carson City, NV 89701
Phone: (775)684-4285
Website: http://health2k.state.nv.us/BFHS/index.htm

★ 21121 ★ New Hampshire Department of Health and Human Services
Public Health Services Division
Maternal and Child Health Bureau
129 Pleasant St.
Concord, NH 03301-6527
Phone: (603)271-4517 **Fax:** (603)271-3827
Website: http://www.dhhs.state.nh.us/

★ 21122 ★ New Jersey Department of Health
Family Health Services Division
Maternal and Child Health Services
E State St.
PO Box 364
Trenton, NJ 08625-0364
Phone: (609)292-4043 **Fax:** (609)292-9599
Email: cfa@doh.state.nj.us
Website: http://www.state.nj.us/health/fhs/chshome.htm
Celeste Andriot Wood, Director

★ 21123 ★ New Mexico Department of Health
Public Health Division
Maternal and Child Health Bureau
1190 St. Francis Dr.
Santa Fe, NM 87502-6110
Phone: (505)476-8586 **Free:** 877-696-1472
Fax: (505)476-8512
Website: http://www.health.state.nm.us/

★ 21124 ★ North Carolina Department of Health, and Human Services
Public Health Division
Women's and Children's Health
1916 Mail Service Ctr.
Raleigh, NC 27699-1916
Phone: (919)715-7937 **Fax:** (919)715-3925
Email: WCH.Info@ncmail.net
Website: http://wch.dhhs.state.nc.us/

★ 21125 ★ North Dakota Department of Health
Preventive Health Section
Maternal and Child Health Division
600 E Boulevard Ave.
Bismarck, ND 58505-0200
Phone: (701)328-2493 **Fax:** (701)328-1412
Email: sanseth@state.nd.us
Website: http://www.health.state.nd.us/ndhd/prevent/mch/
Sandra Anseth, Director

★ 21126 ★ Oklahoma Department of Health
Personal Health Services
Maternal and Child Health Services
1000 NE 10th St., Rm. 506
Oklahoma City, OK 73117
Phone: (405)271-4477
Website: http://www.health.state.ok.us/PROGRAM/mchs/index.html

★ 21127 ★ Oregon Department of Human Resources
Health Division
Child and Family Health Center
Portland State Office Bldg.
800 NE Oregon St.
Portland, OR 97232
Phone: (503)731-4000
Email: ohd.info@state.or.us
Website: http://www.ohd.hr.state.or.us/ccfh/welcome.htm

★ 21128 ★ Rhode Island Department of Health
Family Health Office
3 Capitol Hill, Rm. 302
Providence, RI 02908
Phone: (401)222-2312 **Free:** 800-942-7434
Fax: (401)222-1442
Email: library@health.state.ri.us
Website: http://www.health.state.ri.us/yhd07.htm

★ 21129 ★ South Carolina Department of Health and Environmental Control
Health Services Office
Maternal and Child Health Bureau
2600 Bull St.
PO Box 101106
Columbia, SC 29211-0106
Phone: (803)898-0773
Email: kyleja@dhec.state.sc.us
Website: http://www.scdhec.net/hs/mch/mch.htm

★ 21130 ★ South Dakota Department of Health
Maternal and Child Health Program
615 E Fourth St.
Pierre, SD 57501-1700
Phone: (605)773-3737 **Free:** 800-738-2301
Email: DOH.INFO@state.sd.us
Website: http://www.state.sd.us/doh/Famhlth/index.htm

★ 21131 ★ Tennessee Department of Health
Health Services Bureau
Maternal and Children's Health Section
Cordell Hull Bldg., 5th Fl.
425 5th Ave. North
Nashville, TN 37247-0101
Phone: (615)741-7353 **Fax:** (615)741-1063
Email: DDenton@mail.state.tn.us
Website: http://www.state.tn.us/health/

★ 21132 ★ Vermont Agency of Human Services
Health Department
Maternal and Child Health Bureau
1193 North Ave, Ste. 1
Burlington, VT 05401-2749
Phone: (802)863-7323 **Fax:** (802)863-7571
Website: http://www.state.vt.us/health/
Jan Campbell, Contact

★ 21133 ★ Virginia Office of Health and Human Resources
Health Department
Women and Infants Health Division
1500 E Main St., Rm. 132
Richmond, VA 23219
Phone: (804)786-5420 **Free:** 888-942-3663
Website: http://www.vahealth.org/wic/

★ 21134 ★ Washington Department of Health
Community and Family Health Services Division
New Market Industrial Campus
Bldg. 10
PO Box 47835
Olympia, WA 98504-7835
Phone: (360)236-3505
Email: glenda.moore@doh.wa.gov
Website: http://www.doh.wa.gov/Org/org.htmCommunity

★ 21135 ★ West Virginia Department of Health and Human Resources
Public Health Bureau
Bureau for Children and Families
350 Capitol St.
Room 730
Charleston, WV 25305-3711
Email: michaelpack@wvdhhr.org
Website: http://www.wvdhhr.org/bcf/
Fred Boothe, Contact

★ 21136 ★ Wisconsin Department of Health and Family Services
Division of Public Health
Family Health Program
Maternal and Child Health Section
1 W Wilson St.
PO Box 2659
Madison, WI 53702
Phone: (608)267-3561 **Free:** 800-722-2295
Email: uttecsm@dhfs.state.wi.us
Website: http://www.dhfs.state.wi.us/aboutdhfs/dph/dph.htm
Susan Uttech, Contact

★ 21137 ★ Wyoming Department of Health
Public Health Division
Maternal and Child Health Services
Hathaway Bldg., 4th Fl.
Cheyenne, WY 82002
Phone: (307)777-6004 **Fax:** (307)777-3617
Email: pshera@state.wy.us
Website: http://wdhfs.state.wy.us/dcfh/
Jimm Murray, Contact

Medicaid

★ 21138 ★ Alabama Medicaid Agency
501 Dexter Ave.
PO Box 5624
Montgomery, AL 36103-5624
Phone: (334)242-5000 **Fax:** (334)242-5097
Email: webmaster@www.medicaid.state.al.us
Website: http://www.medicaid.state.al.us

★ 21139 ★ Alaska Department of Health and Social Services
Public Health Division
Division of Medical Assistance
PO Box 110660
Juneau, AK 99811-0610
Phone: (907)465-3355 **Fax:** (907)465-2204
Email: bob_labbe@health.state.ak.us
Website: http://www.hss.state.ak.us/dma/table.htm
Bob Labbe, Director

★ 21140 ★ Arizona Health Care Cost Containment System
Medicaid Program
801 E Jefferson St.
Phoenix, AZ 85034
Phone: (602)417-4000
Email: flopez@ahcccs.state.az.us
Website: http://www.ahcccs.state.az.us/

★ 21141 ★ Arkansas Department of Human Services
Medical Services Division
Donaghey Plaza S
PO Box 1437, Slot 1100
Little Rock, AR 72203-1437
Phone: (501)682-8292 **Fax:** (501)682-1197
Website: http://www.medicaid.state.ar.us/
Ray Hanley, Contact

★ 21142 ★ Colorado Department of Human Services
Health Care Policy and Financing Division
Medicaid Management Information System
1575 Sherman St.
Denver, CO 80203-1714
Email: comments@www.state.co.us
Website: http://www.chcpf.state.co.us/index.html

★ 21143 ★ Connecticut Department of Social Services
Medical Assistance
Medicaid Program
25 Sigourney St.
Hartford, CT 06105-5033
Phone: (860)424-5126 **Free:** 800-842-1508
Fax: (860)951-9544
Email: pgr.dss@po.state.ct.us
Website: http://www.dss.state.ct.us/svcs/medical.htm

★ 21144 ★ Delaware Department of Health and Social Services
Social Services Division
Medicaid Unit
Lewis Bldg.
1901 N DuPont Hwy.
New Castle, DE 19720
Free: 800-372-2022 **Fax:** (302)255-9500
Email: dhssinfo@state.de.us
Website: http://www.state.de.us/dhss/dss/dsshome.htm, Sr.

★ 21145 ★ Florida Agency for Health Care Administration
Medicaid Office
2727 Mahan Dr., Mail Stop 8
Tallahassee, FL 32308
Phone: (850)488-3560 **Free:** 888-419-3456
Fax: (850)488-2520
Website: http://www.fdhc.state.fl.us/Medicaid/index.shtml
Bob Sharpe, Contact

★ 21146 ★ Georgia Department of Community Health
Division of Medical Assistance
2 Peachtree St. NW
Atlanta, GA 30303
Phone: (404)651-8681
Website: http://www.communityhealth.state.ga.us/
Mark Trail, Contact

★ 21147 ★ Idaho Department of Health and Welfare
Medicaid Division
450 W State St., 5th Floor
PO Box 83720
Boise, ID 83720-0036
Phone: (208)334-5747 **Fax:** (208)334-6558
Website: http://www2.state.id.us/dhw/medicaid/index.htm
Joe Brunson, Director

★ 21148 ★ Illinois Department of Public Aid
Medical Programs Division
201 S Grand Ave. E
Springfield, IL 62763-0001
Phone: (217)782-2570 **Fax:** (217)782-5672
Email: aidd2372@mail.idpa.state.il.us
Website: http://WWW.STATE.il.us/dpa/html/medical_news.htm

★ 21149 ★ Indiana Family and Social Services Administration
Medicaid Policy and Planning Office
402 W Washington St.
PO Box 7083
Indianapolis, IN 46207-7083
Phone: (317)233-4455 **Free:** 800-457-4584
Fax: (317)233-4693
Website: http://www.in.gov/fssa/
Melanie Bella, Contact

★ 21150 ★ Iowa Department of Human Services
Medical Services Division
Medicaid Program
Hoover State Office Bldg.
1305 E Walnut
Des Moines, IA 50319
Phone: (515)281-8621 **Free:** 800-972-2017
Email: fdhs@dhs.state.ia.us
Website: http://www.dhs.state.ia.us/dhsphone.asp

★ 21151 ★ Kansas Department of Social and Rehabilitation Services
Adult Medical Services Commission
Docking State Office Bldg.
915 SW Harrison St., Rm 603N
Topeka, KS 66612
Phone: (785)296-3959
Email: libby@srsexec.wpo.state.ks.us
Website: http://www.srskansas.org/srsadult-comm.html
Ann Koci, Contact

★ 21152 ★ Kentucky Health Services Cabinet
Medicaid Services Department
275 E Main St, 6th Floor
Frankfort, KY 40621
Phone: (502)564-4321 **Fax:** (502)564-0509
Email: chs.dmsweb@mail.state.ky.us
Website: http://chs.state.ky.us/dms/

★ 21153 ★ Louisiana Department of Health and Hospitals
Health Services Financing Bureau
1201 Capitol Access Rd.
PO Box 91030
Baton Rouge, LA 70821-9030
Phone: (225)342-5774 **Fax:** (225)342-3893
Email: medweb@dhhmail.dhh.state.la.us
Website: http://www.dhh.state.la.us/medicaid/index.htm

★ 21154 ★ Maine Department of Human Services
Medical Services Bureau
Policy and Provider Services Division
Medicaid Program
442 Civic Center Dr.
11 State House Station
Augusta, ME 04333-0011
Phone: (207)287-3094 **Free:** 800-321-5557
Email: Sandy.Goldman@state.me.us
Website: http://www.state.me.us/bms/bmshome.htm
Sandy Goldman, Director

★ 21155 ★ Massachusetts Executive Office of Health and Human Services
Medical Assistance Division
1 Ashburton Place, rm 1109
Boston, MA 02108
Phone: (617)727-7600 **Fax:** (617)727-5134
Email: contactdma@nt.dma.state.ma.us
Website: http://www.state.ma.us/dma/

★ 21156 ★ Michigan Community Health Department
Health Programs Administration
Medicaid Operations Bureau
320 South Walnut St.
Lewis Cass Bldg., 6th Floor
Lansing, MI 48913
Phone: (517)373-3500
Email: barriep@michigan.gov
Website: http://www.michigan.gov/mdch

★ 21157 ★ Minnesota Department of Human Services
Health and Continuing Care Strategies Division
Medicaid Program
444 Lafayette Rd. N
Saint Paul, MN 55155
Phone: (651)296-8517 **Free:** 800-657-3659
Fax: (651)297-3230
Email: dhs.webmaster@state.mn.us
Website: http://www.dhs.state.mn.us/hlthcare/asstprog/mmap.htm

★ 21158 ★ Mississippi Office of the Governor
Medicaid Division
239 N Lamar St.
801 Robert E Lee Bldg.
Jackson, MS 39201-1399
Phone: (601)359-6050 **Free:** 800-421-2408
Fax: (601)359-6048
Email: webmaster@medicaid.state.ms.us
Website: http://www.dom.state.ms.us/
Rica Lewis-Payton, Director

★ 21159 ★ Missouri Department of Social Services
Medical Services Division
615 Howerton Ct.
PO Box 6500
Jefferson City, MO 65102-6500
Phone: (573)751-3425 **Fax:** (573)751-6564
Email: webmaster@mail.medicaid.state.mo.us
Website: http://www.dss.state.mo.us/dms/index.htm

★ 21160 ★ Nebraska Department of Health and Human Services
Medicaid Division
301 Centennial Mall S
PO Box 95026
Lincoln, NE 68509-5026
Phone: (402)471-9567 **Fax:** (402)471-9449
Email: hhs_system_information@hhs.state.ne.us
Website: http://www.hhs.state.ne.us/med/medindex.htm
Bob Seiffert, Director

★ 21161 ★ Nevada Department of Human Resources
Welfare Division
Medicaid Program
1470 E College Parkway
Carson City, NV 89706
Phone: (775)684-0500
Email: sallsip@welfare.state.nv.us
Website: http://welfare.state.nv.us/

★ 21162 ★ New Hampshire Department of Health and Human Services
Office of Health Planning and Medicaid
Medical Services Bureau
129 Pleasant St.
Concord, NH 03301
Phone: (603)271-5254 **Free:** 800-852-3345
Fax: (603)271-8431
Website: http://www.dhhs.state.nh.us/DHHS/ContactDirectory/default.htm

★ 21163 ★ New Jersey Department of Human Services
Medical Assistance and Health Services Division
Quakerbridge Plaza
PO Box 712
Trenton, NJ 08625-0712
Phone: (609)588-2600 **Free:** 800-356-1561
Fax: (609)588-3583
Email: webmaster@dhs.state.nj.us
Website: http://www.state.nj.us/humanservices/dmahs/index.html

★ 21164 ★ New Mexico Department of Human Services
Medical Assistance Division
PO Box 2348
Santa Fe, NM 87504-2348
Phone: (505)827-3100 **Free:** 888-997-2583
Fax: (505)827-3185
Website: http://www.state.nm.us/hsd/mad/Index.html

★ 21165 ★ New York State Department of Health
Office of Continuing Care
New York State Partnership for Long-Term Care
1 Commerce Plaza
Room 726
99 Washington Ave.
Albany, NY 12260
Phone: (518)473-8083 **Free:** 888-697-7582
Email: pltc@health.state.ny.us
Website: http://www.nyspltc.org/about/index.html

★ 21166 ★ North Carolina Department of Health and Human Services
Medical Assistance Division
1985 Umstead Dr.
2501 Mail Service Ctr.
Raleigh, NC 27699-2501
Phone: (919)857-4011 **Fax:** (919)733-6608
Website: http://www.dhhs.state.nc.us/docs/division.htm
Nina Yeager, Director

★ 21167 ★ North Dakota Department of Human Services
Medical Services Division
600 E Boulevard Ave.
Department 325
Bismarck, ND 58505-0250
Phone: (701)328-2321 **Free:** 800-755-2604
Fax: (701)328-1544
Email: dhsmed@.state.nd.us
Website: http://lnotes.state.nd.us/dhs/dhsweb.nsf/ServicePages/MedicalServices

★ 21168 ★ Ohio Department of Job and Family Services
Medicaid Bureau
30 E Broad St., 31st Fl.
Columbus, OH 43215
Phone: (614)644-0140
Website: http://www.state.oh.us/odjfs/ohp/index.stm
Frmly: Ohio Department of Human Services.

★ 21169 ★ Oklahoma Health Care Authority
4545 N Lincoln Blvd., Ste. 124
Oklahoma City, OK 73105
Phone: (405)522-7300
Website: http://www.ohca.state.ok.us/

★ 21170 ★ Oregon Department of Human Resources
Medical Assistance Program Office
500 Summer St. NE E37
Salem, OR 97301-1079
Phone: (503)945-5772 **Free:** 800-527-5772
Email: dhr.info@state.or.us
Website: http://www.omap.hr.state.or.us/

★ 21171 ★ Pennsylvania Department of Public Welfare
Medical Assistance Office
PO Box 2675
Health & Welfare Bldg., Rm. 515
Harrisburg, PA 17105-2675
Phone: (717)787-1870
Website: http://www.dpw.state.pa.us/omap/dpwomap.asp

★ 21172 ★ Rhode Island Department of Human Services
Medical Services Division
600 New London Ave.
Cranston, RI 02920
Phone: (401)462-6500 **Fax:** (401)464-6504
Website: http://www.dhs.state.ri.us/

★ 21173 ★ South Carolina Health and Human Services Department
Health Services Bureau
Medicaid Program
1801 Main St.
PO Box 8206
Columbia, SC 29202-8206
Phone: (803)898-2640 **Fax:** (803)898-4515
Email: Adams@dhhs.state.sc.us
Website: http://www.state.sc.us/dhhs/

★ 21174 ★ South Dakota Department of Social Services
Program Management Division
Medical Services Office
700 Governors Dr.
Pierre, SD 57501
Phone: (605)773-3495 **Fax:** (605)773-5246
Email: Medicaid@dss.state.sd.us
Website: http://www.state.sd.us/social/medicaid/index.htm

★ 21175 ★ Tennessee Department of Health
Tenncare Division
729 Church St.
Nashville, TN 37243
Phone: (615)532-7542 **Free:** 800-669-1851
Fax: (615)741-0882
Email: you@yours.gov
Website: http://www.state.tn.us/tenncare/
Lola Potter, Contact

★ 21176 ★ Texas Department of Health
Health Care Financing Division
Medicaid Managed Care Bureau
1100 W 49th St.
Austin, TX 78756-3199
Phone: (512)338-6508 **Free:** 888-963-7111
Email: susan.milam@tdh.state.tx.us
Website: http://www.tdh.state.tx.us/hcf/mcstart.htm
Susan Milan, PhD, Director

★ 21177 ★ Utah Department of Health
Health Care Financing Division
Medicaid Policy and Planning Bureau
288 N 1460 W
PO Box 143106
Salt Lake City, UT 84114-3106
Phone: (801)538-6406 **Free:** 800-662-9651
Fax: (801)538-6412
Email: gsix@utah.gov
Website: http://www.health.state.ut.us/medicaid/index.html
Michael Deily, Director

★ 21178 ★ Vermont Agency of Human Services
Prevention, Assistance, Transition and Health Access Department
Health Access Office
103 S Main St.
Waterbury, VT 05671
Phone: (802)241-2880 **Free:** 800-529-4060
Fax: (802)241-2897
Email: WebMaster@wpath.state.vt.us
Website: http://www.dpath.state.vt.us/

★ 21179 ★ Virginia Office of Health and Human Resources
Medical Assistance Services Department
600 E Broad St., Ste. 1300
Richmond, VA 23219
Phone: (804)786-4231
Email: webmaster@dmas.state.va.us
Website: http://165.176.249.159/

★ 21180 ★ Washington Department of Social and Health Services
Medical Assistance Administration
617 8th Ave SE
PO Box 45100
Olympia, WA 98504-5100
Free: 800-562-3022
Website: http://fortress.wa.gov/dshs/maa/

★ 21181 ★ West Virginia Department of Health and Human Resources
Medical Services Bureau
350 Capitol St., Rm. 251
Charleston, WV 25301-3706
Phone: (304)926-1703 **Fax:** (304)558-1451
Email: medcomm@wvdhhr.org
Website: http://www.wvdhhr.org/bms/
Nancy Atkins, Director

★ 21182 ★ Wisconsin Department of Health and Family Services
Health Division
Health Care Financing Bureau
PO Box 309
Madison, WI 53701-0309
Phone: (608)266-2522
Email: webmaster@dhfs.state.wi.us
Website: http://www.dhfs.state.wi.us/aboutdhfs/DHCF/dhcf.htm
Peggy Handrich, Contact

★ 21183 ★ Wyoming Department of Health
Health Care Financing Division
Minimum Medical Program
Hathaway Bldg., 4th Fl.
6101 Yellowstone Rd.
Cheyenne, WY 82002
Phone: (307)777-6004 **Fax:** (307)777-3617
Email: molson@state.wy.us
Website: http://wdhfs.state.wy.us/dcfh/
Mary Olson, Contact

Medical Boards

★ 21184 ★ Alabama State Board of Medical Examiners
848 Washington Ave.
PO Box 946
Montgomery, AL 36101-0946
Phone: (334)242-4116 **Fax:** (334)242-4155
Email: bme@albme.org
Website: http://www.albme.org/

★ 21185 ★ Arizona State Board of Medical Examiners
9545 E Doubletree Ranch Rd.
Scottsdale, AZ 85258-5539
Phone: (480)551-2700 **Free:** 877-255-2212
Website: http://www.bomex.org/index.htm

★ 21186 ★ Arkansas State Medical Board
2100 Riverfront Dr.
Little Rock, AR 72202
Phone: (501)296-1802 **Fax:** (501)296-1805
Email: office@armedicalboard.org
Website: http://www.armedicalboard.org/

★ 21187 ★ Bureau of Health Services
Michigan Board of Medicine
PO Box 30670
Lansing, MI 48909
Phone: (517)335-0918 **Fax:** (517)241-2635
Email: bhserinfo@cis.state.mi.us
Website: http://www.michigan.gov/cis/

★ 21188 ★ California Medical Board
1426 Howe Ave. Ste. 54
Sacramento, CA 95825-3236
Phone: (916)263-2382
Email: Webmaster@medbd.ca.gov
Website: http://www.medbd.ca.gov/

★ 21189 ★ Colorado State Board of Medical Examiners
1560 Broadway, Ste. 1300
Denver, CO 80202
Phone: (303)894-7690 **Fax:** (303)894-7692
Email: medical@dora.state.co.us
Website: http://www.dora.state.co.us/Medical/
Susan Miller, Contact

★ 21190 ★ Connecticut Department of Public Health
Physician Licensure
PO Box 340308
410 Capitol Ave., MS No. 12APP
Hartford, CT 06134-0308
Phone: (860)509-7563
Website: http://www.ct-clic.com/detail.asp?code=1759

★ 21191 ★ Delaware Board of Medical Practice
Cannon Bldg., Ste. 203
861 Silver Lake Blvd.
Dover, DE 19904
Phone: (302)744-4520 **Fax:** (302)739-2711
Email: gfranzolino@.state.de.us
Website: http://www.professionallicensing.state.de.us/boards/
Gayle Franzolino, Contact

★ 21192 ★ District of Columbia Board of Medicine
825 North Capital St, NE, 2nd Fl
Washington, DC 20002
Phone: (202)442-4777 **Fax:** (202)442-9431
Website: http://dchealth.dc.gov/index.asp

★ 21193 ★ Florida Board of Medicine
4052 Bald Cypress Way, Bin C03
Tallahassee, FL 32399-3253
Phone: (850)245-4131 **Fax:** (850)488-9325
Email: MQA_medicine@doh.state.fl.us
Website: http://www9.myflorida.com/Mqa/medical/me_home.html

★ 21194 ★ Georgia Composite State Board of Medical Examiners
2 Peachtree St.
Atlanta, GA 30303
Phone: (404)656-3913
Website: http://www.sos.state.ga.us/ebd-medical/default.htm
Karen Mason, Contact

★ 21195 ★ Hawaii Board of Medical Examiners
Department of Commerce & Consumer Affairs
DCCA-PVL
PO Box 3469
Honolulu, HI 96801
Phone: (808)586-2708
Email: medical@dcca.state.hi.us
Website: http://www.state.hi.us/dcca/pvl/areas_medical.html
Constance Cabral-Makanani, Contact

★ 21196 ★ Idaho State Board of Medicine
1755 Westgate Dr.
PO Box 83720
Boise, ID 83720-0058
Phone: (208)327-7000 **Fax:** (208)327-7005
Email: info@bom.state.id.us
Website: http://www.bom.state.id.us/

★ 21197 ★ Illinois Department of Professional Regulation
Board of Medicine (Licensing)
320 W Washington St.
Springfield, IL 62786
Phone: (217)785-0800 **Fax:** (217)782-7645
Website: http://www.dpr.state.il.us

★ 21198 ★ Indiana Health Professions Bureau
Medical Licensing Board
402 W Washington St., Rm. W041
Indianapolis, IN 46204
Phone: (317)234-2060 **Fax:** (317)233-4236
Email: hpb3@hpb.state.in.us
Website: http://www.in.gov/hpb/boards/mlbi/
Angela Smith-Jones, Director

★ 21199 ★ Iowa State Board of Medical Examiners
400 SW 8th St., Ste. C
Des Moines, IA 50309-4686
Phone: (515)242-6039 **Fax:** (515)242-5908
Email: ann.mowery@ibme.state.ia.us
Website: http://www.docboard.org/ia/ia_home.htm
Ann E. Mowery, PhD, Director

★ 21200 ★ Kansas Board of Healing Arts
235 SW Topeka Blvd.
Topeka, KS 66603-3068
Phone: (785)296-7413 **Fax:** (785)296-0852
Email: Healer3@ink.org
Website: http://www.ksbha.org/

★ 21201 ★ Kentucky Board of Medical Licensure
310 Whittington Pkwy, Ste 1B
Louisville, KY 40222-4916
Phone: (502)429-8046 **Fax:** (502)429-9923
Email: kbml@mail.state.ky.us
Website: http://www.state.ky.us/agencies/kbml/

★ 21202 ★ Louisiana State Board of Medical Examiners
630 Camp St.
PO Box 30250
New Orleans, LA 70190-0250
Phone: (504)568-6820 **Fax:** (504)599-0503
Email: lsbmever@lsbme.org
Website: http://www.lsbme.org/

★ 21203 ★ Maine Board of Licensure in Medicine
137 State House Station
1 Bangor St.
Augusta, ME 04333-0137
Phone: (207)287-3601
Website: http://www.docboard.org/me/me_home.htm
Randal Manning, Director

★ 21204 ★ Maryland Board of Physician Quality Assurance
4201 Patterson Ave.
Baltimore, MD 21215-0095
Phone: (410)764-4777 **Free:** 800-492-6836
Fax: (410)358-2252
Email: bpqa@erols.com
Website: http://www.bpqa.state.md.us/

★ 21205 ★ Massachusetts Board of Registration in Medicine
10 W St., 3rd Fl.
Boston, MA 02111
Phone: (617)727-3086 **Fax:** (617)451-9568
Email: webmaster@massmedboard.org
Website: http://www.massmedboard.org/

★ 21206 ★ Minnesota Board of Medical Practice
2829 University Ave. SE, Ste. 400
Minneapolis, MN 55414-3246
Phone: (612)617-2130 **Free:** 800-657-3709
Fax: (612)617-2166
Email: medical.board@state.mn.us
Website: http://www.bmp.state.mn.us/

★ 21207 ★ Mississippi State Board of Medical Licensure
1867 Crane Ridge Dr., Ste. 200-B
PO Box 9268
Jackson, MS 39286-9268
Phone: (601)987-3079 **Fax:** (601)987-4159
Email: mboard@msbml.state.ms.us
Website: http://www.msbml.state.ms.us/

★ 21208 ★ Missouri State Board of Registration for the Healing Arts
3605 Missouri Blvd.
PO Box 4
Jefferson City, MO 65102
Phone: (573)751-0098 **Fax:** (573)751-3166
Email: healarts@mail.state.mo.us
Website: http://www.ecodev.state.mo.us/pr/healarts/
Tina Steinman, Director

★ 21209 ★ Nebraska Department of Health and Human Services
PO Box 95044
Lincoln, NE 68509-5044
Phone: (402)471-2306 **Fax:** (402)471-3577
Email: hhs_system_information@hhs.state.ne.us
Website: http://www.hhs.state.ne.us/

★ 21210 ★ Nevada State Board of Medical Examiners
1105 Terminal Way, Ste. 301
PO Box 7238
Reno, NV 89510
Phone: (775)688-2559 **Fax:** (775)688-2321
Email: nsbme@govmail.state.nv.us
Website: http://www.state.nv.us/medical/

★ 21211 ★ New Hampshire Board of Medicine
2 Industrial Park Dr., Ste. 8
Concord, NH 03301-8520
Phone: (603)271-1203
Website: http://www.state.nh.us/medicine/index.html
Cynthia Cooper, President

★ 21212 ★ New Jersey Department of Law and Public Safety
New Jersey State Board of Medical Examiners
PO Box 183
Trenton, NJ 08625-0183
Phone: (609)826-7100
Website: http://www.state.nj.us/lps/ca/medical.htmbme5
William Roeder, Director

★ 21213 ★ New Mexico State Board of Medical Examiners
Lamy Bldg., 2nd Fl.
491 Old Santa Fe Trail
Santa Fe, NM 87501
Phone: (505)827-5022 **Free:** 800-945-5845
Fax: (505)827-7377
Website: http://www.state.nm.us/nmbme/

★ 21214 ★ New York State Board for Medicine Licensing
Office of the Professions
State Education Bldg., 2nd Fl.
Albany, NY 12234
Phone: (518)474-3817 **Fax:** (518)486-4846
Email: medbd@mail.nysed.gov
Website: http://www.op.nysed.gov/med.htm
Thomas J. Monahan, Contact

★ 21215 ★ New York State Department of Health
New York State Board for Professional Medical Conduct (Discipline)
433 River St. ste. 303
Troy, NY 12180
Phone: (518)402-0855 **Free:** 800-663-6114
Fax: (518)402-0866
Email: nyhealth@health.state.ny.us
Website: http://www.health.state.ny.us/
Dennis Graziano, Contact

★ 21216 ★ North Carolina Medical Board
1201 Front St, ste.100
Raleigh, NC 27609-7533
Phone: (919)326-1100 **Free:** 800-253-9653
Fax: (919)326-1130
Email: public.affairs@ncmedboard.org
Website: http://www.ncmedboard.org/
Shannon Kingston, Contact

★ 21217 ★ North Dakota State Board of Medical Examiners
418 E Broadway, Ste. 12
City Center Plaza
Bismarck, ND 58501
Phone: (701)328-6500 **Fax:** (701)328-6505
Website: http://www.ndbomex.com/
Rolf P. Sletten, J.D., Contact

★ 21218 ★ Ohio State Medical Board
77 S High St., 17th Fl.
Columbus, OH 43215-6127
Phone: (614)466-3934 **Free:** 800-554-7717
Fax: (614)728-5946
Website: http://www.state.oh.us/med/

★ 21219 ★ Oklahoma State Board of Medical Licensure and Supervision
5104 N Francis, Ste. C
PO Box 18256
Oklahoma City, OK 73154-0256
Phone: (405)848-6841 **Free:** 800-381-4519
Fax: (405)848-8240
Email: executive@osbmls.state.ok.us
Website: http://www.osbmls.state.ok.us

★ 21220 ★ Oregon Board of Medical Examiners
1500 SW 1st Ave., Ste. 620
Portland, OR 97201-5826
Phone: (503)229-5770 **Free:** 877-254-6263
Fax: (503)229-6543
Email: bme.info@state.or.us
Website: http://www.bme.state.or.us/

★ 21221 ★ Pennsylvania State Board of Medicine
PO Box 2649
Harrisburg, PA 17105-2649
Phone: (717)783-1400 **Fax:** (717)787-7769
Email: medicine@pados.dos.state.pa.us
Website: http://www.dos.state.pa.us/bpoa/cwp/view.asp?a=1104&q=432799

★ 21222 ★ Puerto Rico Board of Medical Examiners
Call Box 13969
San Juan, PR 00908
Phone: (787)782-8989 **Fax:** (787)782-8733

★ 21223 ★ Rhode Island Board of Medical Licensure and Discipline
Department of Health
3 Capitol Hill, Room 205
Providence, RI 02908
Phone: (401)222-3855 **Fax:** (401)222-2158
Website: http://www.docboard.org/ri/main.htm

★ 21224 ★ South Carolina Department of Labor, Licensing and Regulation
Board of Medical Examiners
Synergy Business Park
Kingstree Bldg.
110 Centerview Dr., Ste. 202
PO Box 11289
Columbia, SC 29211-1289
Phone: (803)896-4500 **Fax:** (803)896-4515
Email: medboard@mail.llr.state.sc.us
Website: http://www.llr.state.sc.us/POL/Medical/Default.htm

★ 21225 ★ South Dakota State Board of Medical and Osteopathic Examiners
1323 S Minnesota Ave.
Sioux Falls, SD 57105
Phone: (605)334-8343 **Fax:** (605)336-0270
Email: kachenba@sdsma.org
Website: http://www.state.sd.us/dcr/medical/medhom.htm
Paul Jensen, Contact

★ 21226 ★ Tennessee State Board of Medical Examiners
Cordell Hull Bldg., 3rd Fl.
425 Fifth Ave. N
Nashville, TN 37247
Phone: (615)532-3202 **Free:** 888-310-4650
Fax: (615)532-5369
Email: DDenton@mail.state.tn.us
Website: http://170.142.76.180/bmf-bin/BMFprofgen.pl

★ 21227 ★ Texas State Board of Medical Examiners
333 Guadaloupe, Tower 3, Ste. 610
PO Box 2018
Austin, TX 78701
Phone: (512)305-7010 **Free:** 800-248-4062
Fax: (512)305-7008
Website: http://www.tsbme.state.tx.us/

★ 21228 ★ Utah Department of Commerce
Div. of Occupational & Professional Licensure
160 E 300 S, 4th Fl.
PO Box 146741
Salt Lake City, UT 84114-6741
Phone: (801)530-6628 **Free:** 888-275-3675
Fax: (801)530-6511
Email: commerce@br.state.ut.us
Website: http://www.commerce.state.ut.us/dopl/dopl1.htm

★ 21229 ★ Vermont Board of Medical Practice
109 State St.
Montpelier, VT 05609-1106
Phone: (802)828-2673 **Fax:** (802)828-5450
Email: gloria.hurd@medbd.state.vt.us
Website: http://www.docboard.org/vt/vermont.htm
Gloria Hurd, Contact

★ 21230 ★ Virgin Islands Board of Medical Examiners
Virgin Islands Department of Health
48 Sugar Estate
St Thomas, VI 00802
Phone: (340)774-0117 **Fax:** (340)777-4001
Lydia Scott, Contact

★ 21231 ★ Virginia Board of Medicine
6606 W Broad St., 4th Fl.
Richmond, VA 23230-1717
Phone: (804)662-9908 **Free:** 800-533-1560
Fax: (804)662-9517
Email: medbd@dhp.state.va.us
Website: http://www.dhp.state.va.us/medicine/default.htm
William L. Harp, MD, Contact

★ 21232 ★ Washington State Department of Health
Health Professions Quality Assurance
1300 SE Quince St.
PO Box 47860
Olympia, WA 98504-7860
Phone: (360)236-4700 **Fax:** (360)586-4818
Email: glenda.moore@doh.wa.gov
Website: http://www.doh.wa.gov/Medical/default.htm

★ 21233 ★ West Virginia State Board of Medicine
101 Dee Dr.
Charleston, WV 25311
Phone: (304)558-2921 **Fax:** (304)558-2084
Email: crystalwvbom@citynet.net
Website: http://www.wvdhhr.org/wvbom/
Ronald D. Walton, Contact

★ 21234 ★ Wisconsin Medical Examining Board
Department of Regulation & Licensing
1400 E Washington Ave., Rm. 173
PO Box 8935
Madison, WI 53708-8935
Email: web@drl.state.wi.us
Website: http://www.drl.state.wi.us/

★ 21235 ★ Wyoming Board of Medicine
Colony Bldg., 2nd Fl.
211 W 19th St.
Cheyenne, WY 82002
Phone: (307)778-7053 **Free:** 800-438-5784
Fax: (307)778-2069
Email: wyomedical@wyomedicalboard.org
Website: http://wyomedboard.state.wy.us/

Mental Health

★ 21236 ★ Alabama Department of Mental Health and Mental Retardation
RSA Union
100 N Union St., Ste. 518
Montgomery, AL 36130-1410
Phone: (334)242-3107 **Fax:** (334)242-0684
Website: http://www.mh.state.al.us/
Kathy Sawyer, Director

★ 21237 ★ Alaska Department of Health and Social Services
Mental Health and Developmental Disabilities Division
350 Main St., Rm. 217
PO Box 110620
Juneau, AK 99811-0620
Phone: (907)465-3370 **Free:** 800-465-4828
Fax: (907)465-2668
Email: dmhdd_webmaster@health.state.ak.us
Website: http://www.hss.state.ak.us/dmhdd/
Leonard Abel, Contact

★ 21238 ★ Arizona Department of Health Services
Behavioral Health Services Division
2122 E Highland
Phoenix, AZ 85016
Phone: (602)381-8999 **Fax:** (602)553-9140
Email: csmallw@hs.state.az.us
Website: http://www.hs.state.az.us/bhs/home.htm

★ 21239 ★ Arkansas Department of Human Services
Mental Health Services Division
4313 W Markham
Little Rock, AR 72205
Phone: (501)686-9164 **Fax:** (501)686-9182
Email: sheila.duncan@mail.state.ar.us
Website: http://www.state.ar.us/dhs/dmhs/
Sheila Duncan, Contact

★ 21240 ★ California Health and Welfare Agency
Mental Health Department
1600 9th St., Rm. 151
Sacramento, CA 95814
Phone: (916)654-2309 **Free:** 800-896-2512
Fax: (916)654-3198
Email: webmastr@dmhhq.state.ca.us
Website: http://www.dmh.cahwnet.gov/

★ 21241 ★ Colorado Department of Human Services
Mental Health Division
3824 W Princeton Cir.
Denver, CO 80236
Phone: (303)866-7400 **Fax:** (303)866-7428
Email: debbie.kupfer@state.co.us
Website: http://www.cdhs.state.co.us/ohr/mhs/index.html

★ 21242 ★ Connecticut Department of Mental Health and Addiction Services
Mental Health Services
410 Capitol Ave., 4th Fl.
PO Box 341431
Hartford, CT 06134
Phone: (860)418-7000 **Free:** 800-446-7348
Website: http://www.dmhas.state.ct.us/

★ 21243 ★ Delaware Department of Health and Social Services
Alcoholism, Drug Abuse, and Mental Health Division
1901 N Dupont Hwy.
New Castle, DE 19720
Phone: (302)255-9399 **Fax:** (302)577-4486
Email: dhssinfo@state.de.us
Website: http://www.state.de.us/dhss/dadamh/dmhhome.htm
Renata J. Henry, Director

★ 21244 ★ District of Columbia Department of Human Services
Mental Health Commission
2700 Martin Luther King Ave., SE
Washington, DC 20032
Phone: (202)673-7440 **Free:** 800-793-4357
Website: http://dc.gov/contact/index.htm

★ 21245 ★ Florida Department of Children and Families
Alcohol, Drug Abuse and Mental Health Office
1317 Winewood Blvd.
Tallahassee, FL 32399-0700
Phone: (850)487-2920
Website: http://www.state.fl.us/cf_web/adm/

★ 21246 ★ Georgia Department of Human Resources
Mental Health, Mental Retardation and Substance Abuse Division
2 Peachtree St. NW
Atlanta, GA 30303-3142
Phone: (404)657-2272 **Fax:** (404)657-2256
Email: irmcilvaine@dhr.state.ga.us
Website: http://www2.state.ga.us/departments/dhr/mhmrsa/index.html

★ 21247 ★ Hawaii Department of Health
Behavioral Health Administration
1250 Punchbowl St.
Honolulu, HI 96813
Phone: (808)586-4400 **Fax:** (808)586-4444
Website: http://www.state.hi.us/health/about/behavior.html
Anita Swanson, Director

★ 21248 ★ Idaho Department of Health and Welfare
Family and Community Services Division
Mental Health Bureau
1720 Westgate Dr. Ste.s A-D
PO Box 83720
Boise, ID 83720-0026
Phone: (208)334-0800 **Free:** 800-600-6474
Fax: (208)334-0828
Email: connorc@idhw.state.id.us
Website: http://www2.state.id.us/dhw/mentalhealth/index.htm
Kathy Tidwell, Contact

★ 21249 ★ Illinois Department of Human Services
Office of Developmental Disabilities
100 S Grand Ave.
Springfield, IL 62762-0002
Phone: (217)524-0260 **Free:** 800-843-6154
Email: nsanchez@dhs.state.il.us
Website: http://www.state.il.us/agency/dhs/ddnp.html

★ 21250 ★ Indiana Family and Social Services Administration
Mental Health Division
Office of Communications
402 W Washington St.
PO Box 7083
Indianapolis, IN 46207-7083
Phone: (317)232-7800 **Free:** 800-901-1133
Fax: (317)233-4693
Website: http://www.ai.org/fssa/dmh/index.html
Janet Corson, Director

★ 21251 ★ Iowa Department of Human Services
Mental Health, Mental Retardation and Developmental Disabilities Division
Hoover State Office Bldg.
1305 E Walnut
Des Moines, IA 50319-0114
Phone: (515)281-8472 **Free:** 800-972-2017
Fax: (515)281-8512
Email: jchesni@dhs.state.ia.us
Website: http://www.dhs.state.ia.us/HomePages/DHS/MIandDD.htm
Jim Chesnik, Contact

★ 21252 ★ Kansas Department of Social and Rehabilitation Services
Mental Health and Development Disabilities Division
915 SW Harrison
Topeka, KS 66612
Phone: (785)296-3959 **Free:** 888-582-3759
Fax: (785)296-2173
Website: http://www.srskansas.org/hcp/mhsatr/mhsatr.htm

★ 21253 ★ Kentucky Health Services Cabinet
Mental Health and Mental Retardation Department
100 Fair Oaks Ln.
Frankfort, KY 40621
Phone: (502)564-4448 **Fax:** (502)564-3844
Email: BruceW.Scott@mail.state.ky.us
Website: http://dmhmrs.chr.state.ky.us/MH/
Bruce W. Scott, Director

★ 21254 ★ Louisiana Department of Health and Hospitals
Mental Health Office
Louisiana Office of Mental Health
PO Box 4049, Bin 12
Baton Rouge, LA 70821
Phone: (225)342-2540 **Fax:** (225)342-5066
Email: vroyal@dhh.state.la.us
Website: http://www.dhh.state.la.us/OMH/index.htm

★ 21255 ★ Maine Department of Mental Health and Mental Retardation
Mental Health Division
40 State House Station
Augusta, ME 04333-0040
Phone: (207)287-4200 **Fax:** (207)287-4268
Email: Lynn.F.Duby@state.me.us
Website: http://www.state.me.us/dmhmrsa/mhservices/MHservices.htm
Lynn F. Duby, Director

★ 21256 ★ Maryland Department of Health and Mental Hygiene
Mental Hygiene Administration
Spring Grove Hospital Center
55 Wave Ave.
Dix Bldg.
Catonsville, MD 21228
Phone: (410)402-8300 **Free:** 800-888-1965
Fax: (410)402-8301
Website: http://www.dhmh.state.md.us/mha/

★ 21257 ★ Massachusetts Executive Office of Health and Human Services
Mental Health Department
25 Staniford St.
Boston, MA 02114
Phone: (617)727-5600 **Free:** 800-221-0053
Fax: (617)727-4350
Email: richard.copp@state.ma.us
Website: http://www.state.ma.us/eohhs/agencies/dmh.htm
Marylou Sudders, Contact

★ 21258 ★ Michigan Department of Community Health
Lewis Cass Bldg., 6th Fl.
320 S Walnut
Lansing, MI 48913
Phone: (517)373-3500 **Fax:** (517)335-3090
Email: arias@state.mi.us
Website: http://www.mdch.state.mi.us/
James K. Haveman, Contact

★ 21259 ★ Minnesota Department of Human Services
Health and Continuing Care Strategies
Mental Health Services Division
444 Lafayette Rd. N
Saint Paul, MN 55155
Phone: (651)297-3933
Email: dhs.webmaster@state.mn.us
Website: http://www.dhs.state.mn.us/contcare/mhhome.htm

★ 21260 ★ Mississippi Department of Mental Health
1101 Robert E Lee Bldg.
239 N Lamar St.
Jackson, MS 39201
Phone: (601)359-1288 **Free:** 877-210-8513
Fax: (601)359-6295
Website: http://www.dmh.state.ms.us/
Albert R. Hendrix, PhD, Director

★ 21261 ★ Missouri Department of Mental Health
Mental Health Administration Office
1706 E Elm St.
PO Box 687
Jefferson City, MO 65102
Phone: (573)751-4122 **Free:** 800-364-9687
Fax: (573)751-8224
Email: dmhmail@mail.dmh.state.mo.us
Website: http://www.modmh.state.mo.us/cps/cps.html

★ 21262 ★ Montana Department of Public Health and Human Services
Mental Health Division
1400 Broadway
PO Box 202951
Helena, MT 59620
Phone: (406)444-2706 **Fax:** (406)444-4435
Email: rpoulsen@state.mt.gov
Website: http://www.dphhs.state.mt.us/hot/mhap.htm
Randy Poulsen, Contact

★ 21263 ★ Nebraska Department of Health and Human Services
Community Mental Health Division
PO Box 95044
Lincoln, NE 68509
Phone: (402)471-2306
Website: http://www.hhs.state.ne.us/beh/mh/mh.htm

★ 21264 ★ Nevada Department of Human Resources
Mental Health and Developmental Services Division
505 E King St., Rm. 602
Carson City, NV 89701-3790
Phone: (775)684-5943 **Fax:** (775)684-5966
Email: mhds@govmail.state.nv.us
Website: http://mhds.state.nv.us/
Carlos Brandenburg, PhD, Contact

★ 21265 ★ New Hampshire Department of Health and Human Services
Office of Family Services
Community Mental Health Division
6 Hazen Dr.
Concord, NH 03301-5404
Phone: (603)271-4638 **Fax:** (603)271-8705
Website: http://www.dhhs.state.nh.us/

★ 21266 ★ New Jersey Department of Human Services
Mental Health Services Division
50 E State St.
PO Box 727
3535 Quackerbridge Rd.
Trenton, NJ 08625-0727
Phone: (609)777-0702 **Free:** 800-382-6717
Fax: (609)777-0835
Email: dmhsmail@dhs.state.nj.us
Website: http://www.state.nj.us/humanservices/DMHS/index.html
Alan Kaufman, Director

★ 21267 ★ New Mexico Department of Health
Mental Health Division
Harold Runnels Bldg.
1190 St. Francis Dr.
Suite North 3200
Santa Fe, NM 87503
Phone: (505)827-2601 **Free:** 800-962-8963
Website: http://www.health.state.nm.us/bhsd/bhsdonline

★ 21268 ★ New York State Office of Mental Health
44 Holland Ave.
Albany, NY 12229
Phone: (518)474-4403 **Free:** 800-597-8481
Fax: (518)474-2149
Email: webadmin@omh.state.ny.us
Website: http://www.omh.state.ny.us/

★ 21269 ★ North Carolina Department of Health and Human Services
Mental Health, Developmental Disabilities and Substance Abuse Services Division
3014 Mail Service Center
325 N Salisbury
Raleigh, NC 27699-3014
Phone: (919)571-4980 **Fax:** (919)571-4984
Email: susan.m.kelley@ncmail.net
Website: http://www.dhhs.state.nc.us/mhddsas/
Don Willis, Contact

★ 21270 ★ North Dakota Department of Human Services
Mental Health and Substance Abuse Services
Mental Health Issues
600 S Second St., Ste 1D
Bismarck, ND 58504
Phone: (701)328-8940 **Free:** 800-755-2719
Fax: (701)328-8969
Email: solunj@state.nd.us

Website: http://lnotes.state.nd.us/dhs/dhsweb.nsf/ServicePages/MentalHealthandSubstanceAbuseServices

★ 21271 ★ Ohio Department of Mental Health
30 E Broad St., 8th Fl.
Columbus, OH 43266-0414
Phone: (614)466-2596
Email: swankd@mhmail.mh.state.oh.us
Website: http://www.mh.state.oh.us

★ 21272 ★ Oklahoma Department of Mental Health
1200 NE 13th St.
PO Box 53277
Oklahoma City, OK 73152
Phone: (405)522-3908
Website: http://www.odmhsas.org/

★ 21273 ★ Oregon Department of Human Resources
Mental Health and Developmental Disabilities Services Division
Mental Health Services Office
2575 Bittern St. NE
PO Box 14250
Salem, OR 97309-0740
Phone: (503)945-9700 **Fax:** (503)373-7327
Email: karen.wickizer@mail.mhd.hr.state.or.us
Website: http://omhs.mhd.hr.state.or.us/

★ 21274 ★ Pennsylvania Department of Public Welfare
Mental Health Office
PO Box 2675
333 Health & Welfare Bldg., Rm. 502
Harrisburg, PA 17105
Phone: (717)787-6443 **Fax:** (717)787-5394
Website: http://www.dpw.state.pa.us/omhsas/dpwmh.asp

★ 21275 ★ Rhode Island Department of Mental Health, Retardation and Hospitals
Integrated Mental Health Services
14 Harrington Rd.
Cranston, RI 02920
Phone: (401)462-3201 **Fax:** (401)462-3204
Website: http://www.mhrh.state.ri.us/Mental%20Health.htm

★ 21276 ★ South Carolina Department of Mental Health
2414 Bull St.
Columbia, SC 29202
Phone: (803)898-8581
Email: webmaster@dmh.state.sc.us
Website: http://www.state.sc.us/dmh/

★ 21277 ★ South Dakota Department of Human Services
Mental Health Division
Hillsview Plaza, E Hwy 34
500 E Capitol
Pierre, SD 57501-5070
Phone: (605)773-5991 **Fax:** (605)773-7076
Email: infoMH@dhs.state.sd.us
Website: http://www.state.sd.us/dhs/dmh/index.htm

★ 21278 ★ Tennessee Department of Mental Health and Mental Retardation
Mental Health Services Division
425 Fifth Ave. N
Cordell Hull Bldg. 3rd Fl.
Nashville, TN 37243
Phone: (615)532-6767
Email: mrobinson2@mail.state.tn.us
Website: http://www.state.tn.us/mental/mhs.html

★ 21279 ★ Texas Department of Mental Health and Mental Retardation
Mental Health Division
909 W 45th St.
PO Box 12668
Austin, TX 78711-2668
Phone: (512)454-3761
Email: ellen.hurst@mhmr.state.tx.us
Website: http://www.mhmr.state.tx.us/
Karen F. Hale, Director

★ 21280 ★ Utah Department of Human Services
Mental Health Division
120 N 200 W, Ste. 415
PO Box 142200
Salt Lake City, UT 84144-2200
Phone: (801)538-4270 **Fax:** (801)538-9892
Email: jchilton@hs.state.ut.us
Website: http://www.hsmh.state.ut.us/

★ 21281 ★ Vermont Agency of Human Services
Developmental and Mental Health Services Department
Mental Health Division
Weeks Bldg.
103 S Main St.
Waterbury, VT 05671-1601
Phone: (802)241-2610 **Fax:** (802)241-1129
Email: webmaster@ddmhs.state.vt.us
Website: http://www.state.vt.us/dmh

★ 21282 ★ Virginia Office of Health and Human Resources
Mental Health, Retardation and Substance Abuse Services Department
Mental Health Services Division
109 Governor St.
Richmond, VA 23219
Phone: (804)786-4837 **Free:** 800-451-5544
Fax: (804)786-9621
Email: bbrenzovich@dmhmrsas.state.va.us
Website: http://www.dmhmrsas.state.va.us/

★ 21283 ★ Washington Department of Social and Health Services
Health and Rehabilitative Services Office
Mental Health Division
PO Box 45130
Olympia, WA 98504-5130
Phone: (360)902-8070 **Free:** 888-713-6010
Fax: (360)902-0809
Website: http://www.wa.gov/dshs/hrsa/hrsa3ov.htmlMHD

★ 21284 ★ West Virginia Department of Health and Human Resources
Community Support Bureau
Office of Behavioral Health Services Division
350 Capitol St., Rm. 350
Charleston, WV 25301-3702
Phone: (304)558-0627 **Fax:** (304)558-1008
Email: obhs@wvdhhr.org
Website: http://www.wvdhhr.org/obhs/mhcr.htm

★ 21285 ★ Wisconsin Department of Health and Family Services
Supportive Living Division
Community Mental Health Bureau
1 W Wilson St., Rm 433
PO Box 7851
Madison, WI 53707-7851
Phone: (608)267-7792 **Fax:** (608)267-7793
Email: webmaster@dhfs.state.wi.us
Website: http://www.dhfs.state.wi.us/MH_BCMH/index.htm

Nursing Boards

★ 21286 ★ Alabama Board of Nursing
RSA Plaza
770 Washington Ave., Ste. 250
PO Box 3900
Montgomery, AL 36130-3900
Phone: (205)242-4060 **Fax:** (205)242-4360
Email: abn@abn.state.al.us
Website: http://www.abn.state.al.us/

★ 21287 ★ Alaska Board of Nursing Licensing
PO Box 110806
Juneau, AK 99811-0806
Phone: (907)269-8161 **Fax:** (907)269-8196
Email: dorothy_fulton@dced.state.ak.us
Website: http://www.dced.state.ak.us/occ/pnur.htm
Dorothy Fulton, Contact

★ 21288 ★ Arizona Board of Nursing
1651 E Morten Ave., Ste. 150
Phoenix, AZ 85020-4313
Phone: (602)331-8111 **Fax:** (602)906-9365
Email: arizona@azbn.org
Website: http://www.state.az.us/bn

★ 21289 ★ Arkansas State Board of Nursing
University Tower Bldg.
1123 S University, Ste. 800
Little Rock, AR 72204-1619
Phone: (501)686-2700 **Fax:** (501)686-2714
Website: http://www.state.ar.us/nurse/

★ 21290 ★ Board of Nurse Examiners for the State of Texas
333 Guadalupe Ste. 3-460
PO Box 430
Austin, TX 78767
Phone: (512)305-7400 **Fax:** (512)305-7401
Email: webmaster@bne.state.tx.us
Website: http://www.bne.state.tx.us/
Katherine A. Thomas, Director

★ 21291 ★ California Board of Registered Nursing
400 R St., Ste 4030
PO Box 944210
Sacramento, CA 94244-2100
Phone: (916)322-3350 **Fax:** (916)327-4402
Email: webmasterbrn@dca.ca.gov
Website: http://www.rn.ca.gov/

★ 21292 ★ California Board of Registered Nursing
400 R St., Ste. 4030
PO Box 944210
Sacramento, CA 94244-2100
Phone: (916)322-3350 **Fax:** (916)327-4402
Website: http://www.rn.ca.gov/

★ 21293 ★ Colorado Board of Nursing
1560 Broadway, Ste. 880
Denver, CO 80202
Phone: (303)894-2430
Email: Webmaster@dora.state.co.us
Website: http://www.dora.state.co.us/nursing/
Patricia F. Uris, PhD, 180ChiropractChiropractic

★ 21294 ★ Commonwealth of Puerto Rico
Board of Nurse Examiners
800 Roberto H. Todd Ave.
Room 202, Stop 18
Santurce, PR 00908
Phone: (787)725-7506 **Fax:** (787)725-7903
Magda Bouet, Contact

★ 21295 ★ Delaware Board of Nursing
Cannon Bldg., Ste. 203
861 Silver Lake Blvd.
PO Box 1401
Dover, DE 19903-1401
Phone: (302)739-4522 **Fax:** (302)739-2711

★ 21296 ★ DHS Connecticut Board of Examiners for Nursing
410 Capitol Ave. MS No. 12APP
PO Box 340308
Hartford, CT 06134
Phone: (860)509-7624 **Fax:** (860)509-7553
Email: donna.winiarski@po.state.ct.us
Website: http://www.state.ct.us/dph/
Dorothy Pacyna, RN, Contact

★ 21297 ★ District of Columbia Board of Nursing
825 N Capitol St, NE, 2nd Fl.
Washington, DC 20002
Phone: (202)442-4776 **Fax:** (202)442-9431
Website: http://www.dchealth.com/

★ 21298 ★ Florida State Board of Nursing
4052 Bald Cypress Way, BIN CO2
Tallahassee, FL 32399
Phone: (850)488-0595 **Fax:** (850)245-4172
Email: MQA_Nursing@doh.state.fl.us
Website: http://www.doh.state.fl.us/mqa/nursing/rnhome.htm
Ruth R. Stiehl, PhD, Director

★ 21299 ★ Georgia Board of Nursing
237 Coliseum Dr.
Macon, GA 31217-3858
Phone: (478)207-1620 **Fax:** (478)207-1633
Email: sacamp@sos.state.ga.us
Website: http://www.sos.state.ga.us/ebd-rn/
Shirley A. Camp, RN, Director

★ 21300 ★ Georgia State Board of Licensed Practical Nurses
237 Coliseum Dr.
Macon, GA 31217-3858
Email: rtmathis@sos.state.ga.us
Website: http://www.sos.state.ga.us/ebd-lpn/
Jacqueline Hightower, Director

★ 21301 ★ Guam Board of Nurse Examiners
PO Box 2816
Agana, GU 96910
Phone: (671)475-0251 **Fax:** (671)477-4733
Margarita Bautista-Gay, Director

★ 21302 ★ Idaho Board of Nursing
280 N 8th St., Ste. 210
PO Box 83720
Boise, ID 83720
Phone: (208)334-3110 **Fax:** (208)334-3262
Email: lcoley@ibn.state.id.us
Website: http://www2.state.id.us/ibn/ibnhome.htm

★ 21303 ★ Illinois Department of Professional Regulation
Board of Nursing
320 W Washington St.
Springfield, IL 62786
Phone: (217)785-0800 **Fax:** (217)782-7645
Website: http://www.dpr.state.il.us/WHO/nurs.cfm

★ 21304 ★ Indiana State Board of Nursing
State Board of Nursing
402 W Washington St., Rm. W041
Indianapolis, IN 46204
Phone: (317)234-2043
Email: dlafollette@hpb.state.in.us
Website: http://www.state.in.us/hpb/isbn/
Kristen Kelley, Director

★ 21305 ★ Iowa Board of Nursing
River Point Business Park
400 SW 8th St., Ste. B
Des Moines, IA 50309-4685
Phone: (515)281-3255 **Fax:** (515)281-4825
Website: http://www.iowaccess.org/nursing/

★ 21306 ★ Kansas State Board of Nursing
Landon State Office Bldg.
900 SW Jackson, Rm. 551-S
Topeka, KS 66612-1230
Phone: (785)296-4929 **Fax:** (785)296-3929
Email: mary.blubaugh@ksbn.state.ks.us
Website: http://www.ksbn.org/
Mary Blubaugh, R.N., Contact

★ 21307 ★ Kentucky State Board of Nursing
312 Wittington Parkway, Ste. 300
Louisville, KY 40222-5172
Phone: (502)329-7000 **Free:** 800-305-2042
Fax: (502)329-7011
Email: KBNWebmaster@mail.state.ky.us
Website: http://www.kbn.state.ky.us/

★ 21308 ★ Louisiana State Board of Nursing
3510 N Causeway Blvd., Ste. 501
Metairie, LA 70002
Phone: (504)838-5332 **Fax:** (504)838-5349
Email: morvantb@lsbn.state.la.us
Website: http://www.dhh.state.la.us/boards.HTM
Barbara Morvent, Director

★ 21309 ★ Louisiana State Board of Practical Nurse Examiners
3421 N Causeway Blvd., Ste. 203
Metairie, LA 70002
Phone: (504)838-5791 **Fax:** (504)838-5279
Email: claire@lsbpne.com
Website: http://www.dhh.state.la.us/boards.htm
Claire Doody Glavilano, RN, Contact

★ 21310 ★ Maine State Board of Nursing
24 Stone St.
158 State House Station
Augusta, ME 04333
Phone: (207)287-1133 **Fax:** (207)287-1149
Email: myra.a.broadway@state.me.us
Website: http://www.state.me.us/nursingbd/

★ 21311 ★ Maryland Board of Nursing
4140 Patterson Ave.
Baltimore, MD 21215-2299
Phone: (410)585-1900 **Free:** 888-202-9861
Email: wayne48@erols.com
Website: http://www.dhmh.state.md.us/mbn/

★ 21312 ★ Massachusetts Board of Registration in Nursing
239 Causeway St., Ste. 500
Boston, MA 02114
Phone: (617)727-9961
Email: gerald.galvin@state.ma.us
Website: http://www.state.ma.us/reg/boards/rn/default.htm
Theresa Bonanno, Director

★ 21313 ★ Michigan Board of Nursing
PO Box 30670
Lansing, MI 48909-8170
Phone: (517)335-0918 **Fax:** (517)373-2179
Email: bhserinfo@cis.state.mi.us
Website: http://www.cis.state.mi.us/bhser/lic/boards/bdnurse.htm
Margaret Hedlund, Contact

★ 21314 ★ Minnesota Board of Nursing
2829 University Ave. SE, Ste. 500
Minneapolis, MN 55414-3253
Phone: (612)617-2270 **Free:** 888-234-2690
Fax: (612)617-2190
Email: nursing.board@state.mn.us
Website: http://www.nursingboard.state.mn.us/

★ 21315 ★ Mississippi Board of Nursing
1935 Lakeland Dr., Ste. B
Jackson, MS 39216
Phone: (601)987-4188 **Fax:** (601)364-2352
Email: info@msbn.state.ms.us
Website: http://www.msbn.state.ms.us/webtest/

★ 21316 ★ Missouri State Board of Nursing
3605 Missouri Blvd.
PO Box 656
Jefferson City, MO 65102
Phone: (573)751-0681 **Fax:** (573)751-0075
Email: nursing@mail.state.mo.us
Website: http://www.ecodev.state.mo.us/pr/nursing
Calvina Thomas, PhD, Director

★ 21317 ★ Montana State Board of Nursing
301 S Park Ave. 4th Fl.
PO Box 200513
Helena, MT 59620-0513
Phone: (406)841-2340 **Fax:** (406)841-2343
Email: compolnur@state.mt.us
Website: http://commerce.state.mt.us/LICENSE/pol/pol_boards/nur_board/board_page.htm
Barb Swehla, Director

★ 21318 ★ Nebraska Board of Nursing
Bureau of Examining Boards
301 Centennial Mall South
PO Box 94986
Lincoln, NE 68509-4986
Phone: (402)471-4376 **Fax:** (402)471-3577
Email: Charlene.Kelly@hhss.state.ne.us
Website: http://www.hhs.state.ne.us/crl/crlindex.htm
Charlene Kelly, Contact

★ 21319 ★ Nevada State Board of Nursing
1755 E Plumb Ln., Ste. 260
Reno, NV 89502
Phone: (775)688-2620 **Free:** 800-746-3980
Fax: (775)688-2628
Email: nsbnreno@govmail.state.nv.us
Website: http://www.state.nv.us/boards/nsbn/

★ 21320 ★ New Hampshire Board of Nursing
79 Regional Dr., Bldg. B
Concord, NH 03302-3898
Phone: (603)271-6599

Website: http://www.state.nh.us/nursing/
Cynthia Gray, R.N., Contact

★ 21321 ★ New Jersey Board of Nursing
124 Halsey St., 6th Fl.
PO Box 45010
Newark, NJ 07101
Phone: (973)504-6430
Email: askconsumeraffairs@smtp.lps.state.nj.us
Website: http://www.state.nj.us/lps/ca/medical.htmnur6
Patricia A. Polansky, Director

★ 21322 ★ New Mexico Board of Nursing
4206 Louisiana NE, Ste. A
Albuquerque, NM 87109
Phone: (505)841-8340 **Fax:** (505)841-8347
Email: boardofnursing@state.nm.us
Website: http://www.state.nm.us/nursing/

★ 21323 ★ New York State Board of Nursing
Office of the Professions
State Education Bldg., 2nd Fl.
89 Washington Ave.
Albany, NY 12234
Phone: (518)474-3817
Email: op4info@mail.nysed.gov
Website: http://www.op.nysed.gov/nurse.htm
Barbara Zittel, Contact

★ 21324 ★ North Carolina Board of Nursing
PO Box 2129
3724 National Dr., Ste. 201
Raleigh, NC 27602-2129
Phone: (919)782-3211 **Fax:** (919)781-9461
Email: email@ncbon.com
Website: http://www.ncbon.com/

★ 21325 ★ North Dakota Board of Nursing
919 S 7th St., Ste. 504
Bismarck, ND 58504-5881
Phone: (701)328-9778 **Fax:** (701)328-9785
Email: ckalanek@ndbon.org
Website: http://www.ndbon.org/
Constance B. Kalanek, Contact

★ 21326 ★ Ohio Board of Nursing
77 S High St., Ste. 400
Columbus, OH 43215-3412
Phone: (614)466-3947
Email: board@nur.state.oh.us
Website: http://www.state.oh.us/nur/

★ 21327 ★ Oklahoma Board of Nursing Registration and Education
2915 N Classen Blvd., Ste. 524
Oklahoma City, OK 73106
Phone: (405)962-1800 **Fax:** (405)962-1821
Email: obnwebmaster@nursing.state.ok.us
Website: http://www.youroklahoma.com/nursing/
Kim Glazier, Director

★ 21328 ★ Oregon State Board of Nursing
800 NE Oregon St., Ste. 465
Portland, OR 97232-2162
Phone: (503)731-4745 **Fax:** (503)731-4755
Email: oregon.bn.info@state.or.us
Website: http://www.osbn.state.or.us/

★ 21329 ★ Pennsylvania State Board of Nursing
PO Box 2649
124 Pine St.
Harrisburg, PA 17105-2649
Phone: (717)783-7142 **Fax:** (717)783-0822
Email: nursing@pados.dos.state.pa.us
Website: http://www.dos.state.pa.us/bpoa/nurbd/mainpage.htm
Joan Bouchard, Contact

★ 21330 ★ Rhode Island Board of Nursing
105 Cannon Health Bldg.
3 Capitol Hill, Rm. 105
Providence, RI 02908
Phone: (401)222-5700 **Fax:** (401)222-3352
Email: CharlieA@doh.state.ri.us
Website: http://www.health.state.ri.us/hsr/nurses.htm
Charles Alexandre, Director

★ 21331 ★ South Dakota Board of Nursing
4300 S Louise Ave., Ste. C1
Sioux Falls, SD 57106
Phone: (605)362-2760 **Fax:** (605)362-2768
Email: carey.duffy@state.sd.us
Website: http://www.state.sd.us/dcr/nursing/nurshom.htm
Diana Vander Woude, Contact

★ 21332 ★ State Board of Nursing for South Carolina
Koger Office Park
Kingstree Bldg.
110 Centerview Dr., Ste. 202
PO Box 12367
Columbia, SC 29210
Phone: (803)896-4550 **Fax:** (803)896-4525
Email: spiresp@mail.llr.state.sc.us
Website: http://www.llr.state.sc.us/POL/Nursing/Default.htm
Pam Spires, Contact

★ 21333 ★ State of Hawaii Board of Nursing
PO Box 3469
DCCA-PVL
Honolulu, HI 96801
Phone: (808)586-2695 **Fax:** (808)586-2689
Email: nursing@dcca.state.hi.us
Website: http://www.state.hi.us/dcca/pvl/areas_nurse.html
Kathleen Yokouchi-Tokumoto, Contact

★ 21334 ★ Tennessee State Board of Nursing
Cordell Hull Bldg., 3rd Fl.
425 Fifth Ave. N
Nashville, TN 37247
Phone: (615)532-3202 **Free:** 888-310-4650
Email: DDenton@state.tn.us
Website: http://www2.state.tn.us/health/Boards/Nursing/index.htm
Elizabeth Cole, Contact

★ 21335 ★ Texas Board of Vocational Nurse Examiners
333 Guadalupe St., Ste. 3-400
Austin, TX 78701
Phone: (512)305-8100 **Free:** 800-821-3205
Fax: (512)305-8101
Email: info@bvne.state.tx.us
Website: http://www.bvne.state.tx.us/
Geneva Harvey, Director

★ 21336 ★ Utah Department of Occupational and Professional Licensing
Utah State Board of Nursing
160 E 300 South, 4th floor
Salt Lake City, UT 84111
Phone: (801)530-6628 **Fax:** (801)530-6511
Email: lduke@br.state.ut.us
Website: http://www.dopl.utah.gov/licensing/nurse.html
Laura Poe, Director

★ 21337 ★ Vermont State Board of Nursing
109 State St.
Montpelier, VT 05609-1106
Phone: (802)828-2396 **Fax:** (802)828-2484
Email: aristau@sec.state.vt.us
Website: http://www.vtprofessionals.org/opr1/nurses/
Anita Ristau, Director

★ 21338 ★ Virgin Islands Board of Nurse Licensure
Plot No. 3, Kongens Gade
Veterans Dr. Sta.
St Thomas, VI 00803
Phone: (340)776-7397 **Fax:** (340)777-4003
Winifred Garfield, Contact

★ 21339 ★ Virginia State Board of Nursing
6606 W Broad St., 4th Fl.
Richmond, VA 23230-1717
Phone: (804)662-9909 **Fax:** (804)662-9512
Email: nursebd@dhp.state.va.us
Website: http://www.dhp.state.va.us/nursing/default.htm
Nancy K. Durrett, Director

★ 21340 ★ Washington State Health Care Professions Quality Assurance Nursing Care Quality Commission
1300 SE Quince St.
PO Box 1099
Olympia, WA 98504-7864
Phone: (360)236-4700 **Fax:** (360)236-4738
Email: hpqa.csc@doh.wa.gov
Website: http://www.doh.wa.gov/Nursing
Paula Meyer, Director

★ 21341 ★ West Virginia Board of Examiners for Licensed Practical Nurses
101 Dee Dr.
Charleston, WV 25311
Phone: (304)558-3572 **Free:** 877-558-LPNS
Fax: (304)558-4367
Email: lpnboard@state.wv.us
Website: http://www.lpnboard.state.wv.us/
Lanette Anderson, Contact

★ 21342 ★ West Virginia Board of Examiners for Registered Nurses
101 Dee Dr.
Charleston, WV 25311
Phone: (304)558-3596 **Fax:** (304)558-3666
Email: westvirginiarn@ncsbn.org
Website: http://www.state.wv.us/nurses/rn/
Laura Rhodes, Director

★ 21343 ★ Wisconsin Board of Nursing
1400 E Washington Ave.
PO Box 8935
Madison, WI 53708-8935
Phone: (608)266-0145 **Fax:** (608)261-7083
Email: web@drl.state.wi.us
Website: http://www.drl.state.wi.us/
Kimberly Nania, Director

★ 21344 ★ Wyoming State Board of Nursing
2020 Carey Ave., Ste. 110
Cheyenne, WY 82001
Phone: (307)777-7601 **Fax:** (307)777-3519
Email: ckoski@state.wy.us
Website: http://nursing.state.wy.us/
Cheryl L. Koski, Contact

Nursing Home Administrator Examining Boards

★ 21345 ★ Alabama State Board of Examiners for Nursing Home Administrators
4156 Carmichael Rd.
Montgomery, AL 36106
Phone: (334)271-6214
Email: KMagdon@anha.org
Website: http://www.alboenha.state.al.us/

★ 21346 ★ Alaska Board of Nursing Home Administrators
PO Box 110806
Juneau, AK 99811-0806
Phone: (907)465-2695 **Fax:** (907)465-2974
Email: p.j._gingras@dced.state.ak.us
Website: http://www.dced.state.ak.us/occ/pnha.htm

★ 21347 ★ Arizona Board of Examiners for Nursing Care Institution Administrators
1400 W Washington, Ste. 230
Phoenix, AZ 85007
Phone: (602)542-3095 **Fax:** (602)542-3093
Website: http://www.revenue.state.az.us/609/nursing-care.htm
Frances Goetzinger-Amendt, Contact

★ 21348 ★ Arkansas Department of Human Services
Medical Services Division
Long Term Care Office
Nursing Home Certification and Licensure Section
PO Box 1437, Slot 1100
Little Rock, AR 72203-1437
Phone: (501)682-8424 **Fax:** (501)682-6171
Email: OLTC.@mail.state.ar.us
Website: http://www.medicaid.state.ar.us/Arkansas-Medicaid/DMSUnits/OLTC/LTCmain.htm

★ 21349 ★ California Board of Examiners of Nursing Home Administrators
1800 Third St., Ste. 162
PO Box 942732
Sacramento, CA 94234-7320
Phone: (916)323-6838 **Free:** 800-236-9747
Website: http://www.dca.ca.gov/r_r/nurseho1.htm

★ 21350 ★ Colorado Board of Examiners of Nursing Home Administrators
1560 Broadwawy, Ste. 1310
Denver, CO 80202
Phone: (303)894-7760 **Fax:** (303)894-7764
Email: NHA@dora.state.co.us
Website: http://www.dora.state.co.us/Nursing-Home-Administrators/

★ 21351 ★ Connecticut Department of Public Health
Regulatory Services Bureau
Health Systems Regulation Division
410 Capitol Ave.
PO Box 340308
Hartford, CT 06134-0308
Phone: (860)509-7406 **Fax:** (860)509-7539
Email: webmaster.dph@po.state.ct.us
Website: http://www.state.ct.us/dph/DPH_Main/About_DPH/brs/brs.htm
Cynthia Denne, Director

★ 21352 ★ Delaware State Board of Examiners of Nursing Home Administrators
Cannon Bldg, Ste. 203
861 Silver Lake Blvd.
Dover, DE 19904-2467
Phone: (302)739-4505 **Fax:** (302)739-2711
Email: dspruill@state.de.us
Website: http://professionallicensing.state.de.us/boards/nursinghomeadmin/index.shtm
Dana Spruill, Contact

★ 21353 ★ District of Columbia Health Regulation Administration
Health Care Facilities Division
825 N Capitol St. NE
Washington, DC 20002
Phone: (202)442-5888
Website: http://www.dchealth.com/hra/services.htm

★ 21354 ★ Florida Board of Nursing Home Administrators
4052 Bald Cypress Way, Bin C-04
PO Box 6330
Tallahassee, FL 32399-3254
Phone: (850)245-4292
Email: nqa_nursinghomeadmin@doh.state.fl.us
Website: http://www.doh.state.fl.us/mqa/nurshome/nha_home.html

★ 21355 ★ Georgia State Professional Licensing Boards Division
Board of Examiners for Nursing Home Administrators
237 Coliseum Dr.
Macon, GA 31217-3858
Phone: (478)207-1670 **Fax:** (478)207-1676
Website: http://www.sos.state.ga.us/plb/contact.htm/

★ 21356 ★ Hawaii Board of Examiners of Nursing Home Administrators
1010 Richards St.
DCCA-PVL, Attn NHA
PO Box 3469
Honolulu, HI 96801
Phone: (808)586-3000
Email: nursing_home@dcca.state.hi.us
Website: http://www.state.hi.us/dcca/pvl/areas_nursing_home.html
Kathleen Yokouchi-Tokumoto, Contact

★ 21357 ★ Idaho Bureau of Occupational Licenses
Nursing Home Administrator Examining Board
Owyhee Plaza, 2nd Fl.
1109 Main St., Ste. 220
Boise, ID 83702-5642
Phone: (208)334-3233 **Fax:** (208)334-3945
Email: bhetrick@ibol.state.id.us
Website: http://www2.state.id.us/ibol/nha.htm
Budd Hetrick, Contact

★ 21358 ★ Illinois Department of Professional Regulation
Nursing Home Administrators Licensing and Disciplinary Board
320 W Washington St.
Springfield, IL 62786
Phone: (217)785-0800 **Fax:** (217)782-7645
Website: http://www.dpr.state.il.us
Leonard Sherman, Director

★ 21359 ★ Indiana Health Professions Bureau
Board of Health Facility Administrators
402 W Washington, Rm. 041
Indianapolis, IN 46204
Phone: (317)232-2960 **Fax:** (317)234-2051
Email: hpb6@hpb.state.in.us
Website: http://www.in.gov/hpb/
Tonja Thompson, Director

★ 21360 ★ Iowa State Board of Examiners for Nursing Home Administrators
Lucas State Office Bldg, 5th floor
321 E 12th St.
Des Moines, IA 50319-0075
Phone: (515)242-6385 **Fax:** (515)281-3121
Email: sdozier@idph.state.ia.us
Website: http://www.iowaccess.org/idph_pl/nursing_home/index.html

★ 21361 ★ Kansas Health Occupations Credentialing
Board of Adult Care Home Administrators
1000 SW Jackson, Ste. 330
Topeka, KS 66612-1365
Phone: (785)296-0061 **Fax:** (785)296-3075
Email: bnesbitt@kdhe.state.ks.us
Website: http://www.kdhe.state.ks.us/hoc/index.html
Brenda Nesbitt, Contact

★ 21362 ★ Kentucky Board of Licensure for Nursing Home Administrators
PO Box 1360
Frankfort, KY 40602
Phone: (502)564-3296 **Fax:** (502)564-4818
Email: Barbara.Sudduth@mail.state.ky.us
Website: http://www.state.ky.us/agencies/finance/occupations/nursinghomeadmin
Barbara Sudduth, Contact

★ 21363 ★ Louisiana State Board of Examiners for Nursing Facility Administrators
5615 Corporate Blvd., Ste. 8D
Baton Rouge, LA 70808
Phone: (225)922-0009 **Fax:** (225)922-0006
Email: 103736.1436@compuserve.com
Website: http://www.dhh.state.la.us/boards.HTM
C. Kemp Wright, Director

★ 21364 ★ Maine Nursing Home Administrator Licensing Board
35 State House Station
Augusta, ME 04333-0035
Phone: (207)624-8420 **Fax:** (207)624-8637
Email: elaine.m.thibodeau@state.me.us
Website: http://www.state.me.us/pfr/olr/categories/cat27.htm
Elaine Thibodeau, Contact

★ 21365 ★ Maryland Board of Examiners for Nursing Home Administrators
4201 Patterson Ave.
Baltimore, MD 21215-2299
Phone: (410)764-4750 **Fax:** (410)358-9187
Email: hannigap@dhmh.state.md.us
Website: http://www.dhmh.state.md.us/bonha/

★ 21366 ★ Massachusetts Board of Registration for Nursing Home Administrators
239 Causeway St., Ste. 500
Boston, MA 02114
Phone: (617)727-9925 **Fax:** (617)727-2197
Email: stephen.j.nemmers@state.ma.us
Website: http://www.state.ma.us/reg/boards/nh/default.htm
Stephen Nemmers, PhD, Director

★ 21367 ★ Michigan Bureau of Health Services
Board of Nursing Home Administrators
PO Box 30670
Lansing, MI 48909
Phone: (517)335-0918 **Fax:** (517)373-2179
Email: bhserinfo@cis.state.mi.us
Website: http://www.cis.state.mi.us/bcs/nha/home.htm

★ 21368 ★ Minnesota Board of Examiners for Nursing Home Administrators
2829 University Ave. SE, Ste. 440
Minneapolis, MN 55414-3245
Phone: (612)617-2117 **Fax:** (612)617-2119
Email: BENHA@state.mn.us
Website: http://www.benha.state.mn.us/
Randy Snyder, Director

★ 21369 ★ Mississippi State Board of Nursing Home Administrators
1400 Lakeover Rd., Ste. 120
Jackson, MS 39213
Phone: (601)364-2310 **Fax:** (601)364-2306
Email: cwalker@bnha.state.ms.us
Website: http://www.bnha.state.ms.us/
Cathy Walker, Director

★ 21370 ★ Montana Board of Nursing Home Administrators
Arcade Bldg, Lower Level
111 North Jackson
PO Box 200513
Helena, MT 59620
Phone: (406)444-3561 **Fax:** (406)444-1667
Pamela Bragg, Contact

★ 21371 ★ Nebraska Health and Human Services Regulation and Licensing Credentialing Division
Board of Examiners of Nursing Home Administration
301 Centennial Mall South, 3rd floor
PO Box 94986
Lincoln, NE 68509-4986
Phone: (402)471-2115 **Fax:** (402)471-3577
Email: marie.mcclatchey@hhss.state.ne.us
Website: http://www.hhs.state.ne.us/crl/crlindex.htm
Helen Meeks, Contact

★ 21372 ★ New Jersey Department of Health and Senior Services
Long Term Care Systems
New Jersey Nursing Home Administrators Licensing Board
PO Box 367
120 S Stockton St.
Trenton, NJ 08625-0367
Phone: (609)633-9051 **Fax:** (609)633-9087
Email: ltc@doh.state.nj.us
Website: http://www.state.nj.us/health/ltc/nhalb.htm

★ 21373 ★ New Mexico Board of Nursing Home Administrators
2055 Pacheco St., Ste. 400
Santa Fe, NM 87504
Phone: (505)476-7122 **Fax:** (505)827-7095
Email: NursingHomeAdminBd@state.nm.us
Website: http://www.rld.state.nm.us/b&c/nhab/index.htm
Carmen E. Payne, Contact

★ 21374 ★ New York State Department of Health - Office of Continuing Care
Bureau of Professional Credentialing
Board of Examiners of Nursing Home Administrators
161 Delaware Ave.
Delmar, NY 12054
Phone: (518)478-1060 **Fax:** (518)478-1058
Email: nyhealth@health.state.ny.us
Website: http://www.health.state.ny.us/nysdoh/provider/nhadmin/instructions.htm

★ 21375 ★ North Carolina State Board of Examiners for Nursing Home Administrators
3733 National Dr., Ste. 228
Raleigh, NC 27612
Phone: (919)571-4164 **Fax:** (919)571-4166
Email: ncbenha@mindspring.com
Website: http://www.ncbenha.org/
Jane A. Baker, Director

★ 21376 ★ North Dakota Board of Examiners for Nursing Home Administrators
1900 N 11th St.
Bismarck, ND 58501-1914
Phone: (701)222-4867 **Fax:** (701)223-0977
Email: hermanb@btigate.com
Website: http://www.governor.state.nd.us/boards/boards-query.asp?Board_ID=73
Bev Herman, Contact

★ 21377 ★ Ohio Board of Examiners for Nursing Home Administrators
246 N High St, 1st floor
PO Box 118
Columbus, OH 43216-0118
Phone: (614)466-5114 **Fax:** (614)466-0271
Email: dandrews@gw.odh.state.oh.us
Website: http://www.ohiobenha.org/
Douglas R. Andrews, Contact

★ 21378 ★ Oklahoma State Department of Health
Home Care Administrator Registry
1000 NE 10th, Rm. 1109
Oklahoma City, OK 73117
Phone: (405)271-4093
Website: http://www.health.state.ok.us/PROGRAM/hcar/index.html

★ 21379 ★ Oregon Board of Examiners of Nursing Home Administrators
Portland State Office Bldg., Ste. 407C
800 NE Oregon, Ste. 21
Portland, OR 97232
Phone: (503)731-4046 **Fax:** (503)731-4207
Email: barbara.orazio@state.or.us
Barbara Orazio, Contact

★ 21380 ★ Pennsylvania State Board of Examiners of Nursing Home Administrators
PO Box 2649
Harrisburg, PA 17105-2649
Phone: (717)783-7155 **Fax:** (717)787-7769
Email: nha@pados.dos.state.pa.us
Website: http://www.dos.state.pa.us/bpoa/cwp/view.asp?a=1104&q=432855

★ 21381 ★ Rhode Island Health Services Regulation Division
Board of Examiners for Nursing Home Administrators
3 Capitol Hill, Rm 105
Providence, RI 02908-5097
Phone: (401)222-5888 **Fax:** (401)222-3352
Email: PaulaM@doh.state.ri.us
Website: http://www.health.state.ri.us/hsr/nh_admin.htm
Paula Morrissey, Contact

★ 21382 ★ South Carolina Board of Long Term Health Care Administrators
Koger Office Park
Kingstree Bldg.
110 Centerview Dr., Ste. 202
PO Box 11329
Columbia, SC 29211-1329
Phone: (803)896-4544 **Fax:** (803)896-4555
Email: welbornd@mail.llr.state.sc.edu
Website: http://www.llr.state.sc.us/POL/LongTermHealthCare/Default.htm
Dana Welborn, Contact

★ 21383 ★ South Dakota Board of Examiners for Nursing Home Administrators
PO Box 632
Sioux Falls, SD 57101-0632
Phone: (605)331-5040 **Fax:** (605)331-2043
Email: sdnha@uswestmail.net
Website: http://www.state.sd.us/dcr/nursinghome/nurhom-h.htm
Joyce Vos, Contact

★ 21384 ★ Tennessee Board of Examiners for Nursing Home Administrators
Cordell Hull Bldg., 1st Fl.
425 Fifth Ave. N
Nashville, TN 37247-1010
Phone: (615)532-5155 **Free:** 888-310-4650
Fax: (615)532-5369
Website: http://www2.state.tn.us/health/Boards/NHA/index.htm
Harold Walker, Contact

★ 21385 ★ Texas Department of Human Services
Nursing Facility Administrator Advisory Committee
701 W 51st St.
PO Box 149030
Austin, TX 78714
Free: 888-834-7406
Email: credential@dhs.state.tx.us
Website: http://www.dhs.state.tx.us/programs/ltc/credentialing/

★ 21386 ★ Utah Board of Nursing Home Administrator Licensure
160 E 300 S, 4th Fl.
PO Box 146741
Salt Lake City, UT 84114-6741
Phone: (801)530-6254 **Free:** (866)275-3675
Fax: (801)530-6511
Website: http://www.dopl.utah.gov/

★ 21387 ★ Vermont Board of Examiners of Nursing Home Administrators
26 Terrace St.
Drawer 09
Montpelier, VT 05609-1101
Phone: (802)828-2453 **Fax:** (802)828-2496
Email: bashford@sec.state.vt.us
Website: http://vtprofessionals.org/opr1/nursing_homes/
Bob Ashford, Contact

★ 21388 ★ Virginia Board of Nursing Home Administrators
6606 W Broad St., 4th Fl.
Richmond, VA 23230-1717
Phone: (804)662-7457 **Free:** 800-533-1560
Fax: (804)662-7246
Email: denbd@dhp.state.va.us

Website: http://www.dhp.state.va.us/nha/default.htm
Sandra Reen, Director

★ 21389 ★ Washington State Department of Health
Health Professions Quality Assurance Board for Nursing Home Administrators
1300 SE Quince St.
PO Box 47860
Olympia, WA 98504-7860
Phone: (360)236-4700 **Fax:** (360)236-4818
Email: hpqa.csc@doh.wa.gov
Website: https://wws2.wa.gov/doh/hpqa-licensing/HPS3/Nursing_Home_Admin/default.htm

★ 21390 ★ West Virginia Nursing Home Administrator Board
5303 Kensington Dr.
Cross Lanes, WV 25313
Phone: (304)759-0722
Website: http://www.state.wv.us/bep/lmi/license/LI-COCCMS.HTMnursing home administrator

★ 21391 ★ Wisconsin Regulation and Licensing Department
Nursing Home Administrators Examining Board
1400 East Washington Ave.
PO Box 8935
Madison, WI 53708-8935
Phone: (608)266-5511 **Fax:** (608)267-3816
Email: web@drl.state.wi.us
Website: http://www.drl.state.wi.us./Regulation/applicant_information/dod036.html

★ 21392 ★ Wyoming State Board of Nursing Home Administrators
1116 Logan Ave., Rm. 106
Cheyenne, WY 82002
Phone: (307)432-0465 **Fax:** (307)432-0492
Email: vspire@state.wy.us
Website: http://soswy.state.wy.us/director/ag-bd/n-home.htm
Vicki L. Spires, Contact

Occupational Health

★ 21393 ★ Alabama Department of Labor
Occupational Injury Statistics and Fatality Data Division
100 N Union St.
Montgomery, AL 36130
Phone: (334)242-3460 **Fax:** (334)240-3417
Email: jbarnhart@email.state.al.us
Website: http://www.alalabor.state.al.us/
James Barnhart, Director

★ 21394 ★ Alaska Department of Labor
Labor Standards and Safety Division
Occupational Safety and Health Section
PO Box 21149
Juneau, AK 99802-1149
Phone: (907)465-4855 **Fax:** (907)465-3584
Website: http://www.labor.state.ak.us/lss/osh-home.htm

★ 21395 ★ Arizona Industrial Commission
Occupational Safety and Health Division
800 W Washington, 2nd Fl.
Phoenix, AZ 85007
Phone: (602)542-5795 **Fax:** (602)542-1614
Email: webmaster@ica.state.az.us
Website: http://www.ica.state.az.us/
Darin Perkins, Contact

★ 21396 ★ Arkansas Department of Labor
Safety Division
10421 W Markham
Little Rock, AR 72205
Phone: (501)682-4522 **Fax:** (501)682-4535
Email: clark.thomas@osha.gov
Website: http://www.accessarkansas.org/labor/divisions/safety_p1.html
Clark Thomas, Contact

★ 21397 ★ California Department of Industrial Relations
Occupational Safety and Health Division
455 Golden Gate Ave., 10th Fl.
San Francisco, CA 94102
Phone: (415)703-5100 **Fax:** (415)703-5135
Email: InfoCons@dir.ca.gov
Website: http://www.dir.ca.gov/dosh/dosh1.html

★ 21398 ★ Colorado Department of Personnel
General Support Services
Risk Management Division
1313 Sherman St, Rm 114
Denver, CO 80203
Phone: (303)866-3848 **Free:** 800-268-8092
Fax: (303)894-2409
Email: benefits.risk@state.co.us
Website: http://www.state.co.us/gov_dir/gss/hr/risk/riskindex.htm

★ 21399 ★ Connecticut Department of Labor
Occupational Safety and Health Division
38 Wolcott Hill Rd.
Wethersfield, CT 06109
Phone: (860)566-4550 **Fax:** (860)566-6916
Website: http://www.ctdol.state.ct.us/osha/osha.htm
Donald A. Heckler, Director

★ 21400 ★ Delaware Department of Labor
Industrial Affairs Division
Occupational Safety and Health Administration
4425 N Market St, 3rd floor
PO Box 8902
Wilmington, DE 19802
Phone: (302)761-8200
Email: ttrznadel@state.de.us
Website: http://www.delawareworks.com/divisions/industaffairs/occu.safety.htm
Traci Trznadel, Contact

★ 21401 ★ District of Columbia Department of Employment Services
Labor Standards Office
Occupational Safety and Health Office
77 P St. NE
Washington, DC 20002
Phone: (202)671-1800
Website: http://does.ci.washington.dc.us/home/contact.shtm

★ 21402 ★ Hawaii Department of Labor and Industrial Relations
Occupational Safety and Health Branch
Keelikolani Bldg.
830 Punchbowl St., Rm. 423
Honolulu, HI 96813
Phone: (808)586-9100 **Fax:** (808)586-9104
Website: http://www.state.hi.us/dlir/hiosh/

★ 21403 ★ Idaho Department of Labor and Industrial Services
Safety Division
317 W Main St.
Boise, ID 83735-0060
Phone: (208)334-3570 **Fax:** (208)334-6300
Email: WWW@labor.state.id.us
Website: http://www.labor.state.id.us/

★ 21404 ★ Illinois Department of Labor
Public Safety Division
1 W Old State Capitol Plaza, Rm. 300
Springfield, IL 62701-1293
Phone: (217)782-9386
Website: http://www.state.il.us/agency/idol/
Robert M. Healey, Director

★ 21405 ★ Indiana Department of Labor
Safety, Education and Training Bureau
402 W Washington, Rm. W195
Indianapolis, IN 46204
Phone: (317)232-2688 **Fax:** (317)233-3790
Email: mstillman@dol.state.in.us
Website: http://www.state.in.us/labor/busets/buset.html

★ 21406 ★ Kansas Department of Human Resources
Labor-Management Relations and Employment Standards Division
Industrial Safety and Health Section
800 SW Jackson, Ste. 600
Topeka, KS 66612-1227
Phone: (785)296-4386 **Free:** 800-332-0353
Email: astanton@hr.state.ks.us
Website: http://www.hr.state.ks.us/wc/html/wcish.htm

★ 21407 ★ Kentucky Labor Cabinet
Occupational Safety and Health Review Commission
4 Mill Creek Pk.
Milville Rd.
Frankfort, KY 40601-9427
Phone: (502)573-6892 **Fax:** (502)573-4619
Email: george.kilbourne@mail.state.ky.us
Website: http://www.state.ky.us/agencies/labor/rchome.htm

★ 21408 ★ Louisiana Department of Labor
Worker's Compensation Office
Health and Safety Division
1001 N 23 St.
PO Box 94094
Baton Rouge, LA 70804-9094
Phone: (225)342-3111
Email: os@ldol.state.la.us
Website: http://www.ldol.state.la.us/

★ 21409 ★ Maine Department of Labor
Labor Standards Bureau
Safety Division
45 State House Station
Augusta, ME 04333-0045
Phone: (207)624-6400 **Fax:** (207)624-6449
Email: dave.e.wacker@state.me.us
Website: http://janus.state.me.us/labor/worksafe.htm
Michael V. Frett, Director

★ 21410 ★ Maryland Department of Licensing and Regulation
Labor and Industry Division
Occupational Safety and Health Section
1100 N Eutaw St., Rm. 208
Baltimore, MD 21201
Phone: (410)767-7233 **Fax:** (410)767-2003
Email: dli@dllr.state.md.us
Website: http://www.dllr.state.md.us/labor/mosh.html

★ 21411 ★ Massachusetts Department of Labor and Workforce Development
Division of Occupational Safety
OSHA Consultation Division
1001 Watertown St.
West Newton, MA 02465
Phone: (617)969-7177 **Fax:** (617)727-4581
Email: joe.lamalva@state.ma.us
Website: http://www.state.ma.us/dos/Consult/Consult.htm

★ 21412 ★ Michigan Department of Consumer and Industry Services
Bureau of Safety and Regulation
Occupational Health Division
7150 Harris Dr.
PO Box 30649
Lansing, MI 48909-8149
Phone: (517)322-1608 **Free:** 800-866-4674
Email: bsrinfo@cis.state.mi.us
Website: http://www.cis.state.mi.us/bsr/divisions/occ/home.htm

★ 21413 ★ Minnesota Department of Labor and Industry
Work Place Services Division
OSHA Consultation Unit
443 Lafayette Rd. N
Saint Paul, MN 55155
Phone: (651)284-5050 **Free:** 877-470-6742
Email: OSHA.Compliance@state.mn.us
Website: http://www.doli.state.mn.us/mnosha.html

★ 21414 ★ Mississippi Department of Health
Occupational Safety and Health Compliance
Mississippi State Univ.
Center for Safety and Health
106 Crosspark Dr., Suite C
Pearl, MS 39208
Phone: (601)939-2047 **Fax:** (601)939-6742
Email: kelly.tucker@ms-c-jackson.osha.gov
Website: http://www.msstate.edu/dept/csh/

★ 21415 ★ Missouri Department of Labor and Industrial Relations
Labor Standards Division
On-site Safety and Health Consultation Program
3315 W Truman Blvd.
PO Box 449
Jefferson City, MO 65102-0504
Phone: (573)751-3403 **Free:** 800-475-2130
Fax: (573)751-3721
Email: RSimmons@dolir.state.mo.us
Website: http://www.dolir.state.mo.us/ls/onsite/index.html
Robert Simmons, Director

★ 21416 ★ Montana Department of Labor and Industry
Employment Relations Division
Safety Bureau
PO Box 1728
Helena, MT 59624
Phone: (406)444-6401 **Fax:** (406)444-4140
Email: jmaloney@mt.gov
Website: http://erd.dli.state.mt.us/SB/page2.html

★ 21417 ★ Nebraska Department of Labor
Safety Division
301 Centennial Mall S
PO Box 95024
Lincoln, NE 68509-5024
Phone: (402)471-2239 **Free:** 800-582-7076
Website: http://www.dol.state.ne.us/nwd/center.cfm?PRICAT=1&SUBCAT=1D
Gary I. Hirsh, Director

★ 21418 ★ Nevada Department of Business and Industry
Industrial Relations Division
Occupational Safety and Health Enforcement Section
1301 N Green Valley Pkwy., Ste. 200
Henderson, NV 89014
Phone: (702)486-9044 **Fax:** (702)990-0358
Email: jwiles@govmail.state.nv.us
Website: http://dirweb.state.nv.us/oshes.htm
L. Tom Czehowski, Director

★ 21419 ★ New Hampshire Department of Labor
Inspection Division
Safety Office
95 Pleasant St.
PO Box 2230
Concord, NH 03301-3836
Phone: (603)271-6850
Website: http://www.state.nh.us/dol/dol-st/index.html
Cynthia Flynn, Contact

★ 21420 ★ New Jersey Department of Health
Environmental and Occupational Health Services
Occupational Health Services Office
PO Box 360
John Fitch Plaza
Trenton, NJ 08625-0369
Phone: (609)984-1863 **Fax:** (609)984-2779
Email: koleary@doh.state.nj.us
Website: http://www.state.nj.us/health/eoh/odisweb/
Kathleen O'Leary, Contact

★ 21421 ★ New Mexico Department Environment
Environmental Protection Division
Occupational Health and Safety Bureau
Harold S Runnels Bldg
1190 St. Francis Dr.
Santa Fe, NM 87502-0110
Phone: (505)827-2855 **Free:** 800-219-6157
Email: melanie_montoya@nmenv.state.nm.us
Website: http://www.nmenv.state.nm.us/Ohsb/oshahome.htm

★ 21422 ★ New York State Department of Labor
Occupational Safety and Health Division
W Averill Harriman Campus
Rm. 522 Bldg. 12
Albany, NY 12240
Phone: (518)457-1125 **Fax:** (518)457-1167
Website: http://www.labor.state.ny.us/business_ny/employer_responsibilities/safety/shdists.htm
Richard Cucolo, Director

★ 21423 ★ North Carolina Department of Labor
Occupational Safety and Health Review Board
4 W Edenton St., Ste. 105
Raleigh, NC 27603-3432
Phone: (919)733-3589
Email: lkafel@mail.dol.state.nc.us
Website: http://www.dol.state.nc.us/osha/osh.htm

★ 21424 ★ North Dakota Department of Loss Prevention
Worker's Compensation Bureau
500 E Front Ave.
Bismarck, ND 58504-5685
Phone: (701)328-3800 **Free:** 800-777-5033
Email: ndworkerscomp@wcb.state.nd.us
Website: http://www.ndworkerscomp.com/

★ 21425 ★ Ohio Department of Health
Prevention Division
Bureau of Health Promotion and Risk Reduction
246 N High St.
PO Box 118
Columbus, OH 43216
Phone: (614)466-2144
Email: webmaster@gw.odh.state.oh.us
Website: http://www.odh.state.oh.us/
Frank Bright, Director

★ 21426 ★ Oklahoma Department of Labor
OSHA Consultation Division
4001 N Lincoln Blvd.
Oklahoma City, OK 73105-5212
Phone: (405)528-1500 **Free:** 888-269-5353
Fax: (405)528-5751
Email: labor.info@oklaosf.state.ok.us
Website: http://www.state.ok.us/~okdol/osha/index.htm

★ 21427 ★ Oregon Consumer and Business Services Department
Occupational Safety and Health Division
350 Winter St., NE
Rm. 430
Salem, OR 97301-3882
Phone: (503)378-3272 **Free:** 800-922-2689
Fax: (503)947-7461
Email: tia.m.howell@state.or.us
Website: http://www.cbs.state.or.us/osha/

★ 21428 ★ Pennsylvania Department of Labor and Industry
Occupational and Industrial Safety Bureau
Labor and Industry Bldg.
7th & Forster St.
Harrisburg, PA 17121
Phone: (717)787-3323 **Fax:** (717)783-5225
Website: http://www.li.state.pa.us/bois/index.html

★ 21429 ★ Rhode Island Department of Labor and Training
Workforce Regulation and Safety Division
Occupational Safety and Health Administration
Center General Complex
1511 Pontiac Ave.
Cranston, RI 02910
Phone: (401)462-8580
Email: mmadonna@dlt.state.ri.us
Website: http://www.dlt.state.ri.us/

★ 21430 ★ South Carolina Department of Labor, Licensing, and Regulation
Occupational Safety and Health Division
110 Centerview Dr.
Columbia, SC 29210
Phone: (803)734-9599 **Fax:** (803)734-9741
Email: scovp@mail.llr.state.sc.us
Website: http://www.llr.state.sc.us/scovp/index.asp?file=ovpform.htm

★ 21431 ★ South Dakota Department of Health
Health Systems Development and Regulation Division
600 E Capitol
Pierre, SD 57501-2536
Phone: (605)773-3364 **Free:** 800-738-2301
Email: DOH.INFO@state.sd.us

Website: http://www.state.sd.us/doh/programs.htm

★ 21432 ★ Tennessee Department of Labor
Occupational Safety and Health Division
Andrew Johnson Tower, 3rd floor
710 James Robertson Pkwy.
Nashville, TN 37243
Phone: (615)741-2793 **Free:** 800-249-8510
Fax: (615)253-1623
Email: steve.hawkins@state.tn.us
Website: http://www.state.tn.us/labor-wfd/tosha.html
John Winkler, Contact

★ 21433 ★ Texas Department of Health
Toxic Substances Control Division
Industrial Hygiene Branch
1100 W 49th St.
Austin, TX 78756
Phone: (512)834-6600 **Fax:** (512)834-6644
Email: ih@tdh.state.tx.us
Website: http://www.tdh.state.tx.us/beh/ih/

★ 21434 ★ USF Safety Florida Consultation Program
Safety Division
4003 East Fowler Ave
Tampa, FL 33617
Phone: (813)974-9962
Email: cvespi@hsc.usf.edu
Website: http://www.safetyflorida.usf.edu/
Charlene Vespi, Contact

★ 21435 ★ Utah Labor Commission
OSHA Division
160 E 300 S, 3rd Fl.
PO Box 146600
Salt Lake City, UT 84114-6600
Phone: (801)530-6901
Email: nanderson@utah.gov
Website: http://www.uosh.utah.gov/
Larry Patrick, Contact

★ 21436 ★ Vermont Department of Labor and Industry
Occupational Safety and Health Administration
National Life Bldg.
Drawer 20
Montpelier, VT 05620-3401
Phone: (802)828-2765 **Fax:** (802)828-2195
Email: voshainfo@labind.state.vt.us
Website: http://www.state.vt.us/labind/vosha.htm
Robert McLeod, Director

★ 21437 ★ Virginia Department of Labor and Industry
Occupational Health Compliance Division
Powers Taylor Bldg.
13 S 13th St.
Richmond, VA 23219
Phone: (804)786-0574
Email: hcompliance@doli.state.va.us
Website: http://www.dli.state.va.us/programs/safety.htm

★ 21438 ★ Washington Department of Labor and Industries
Consultation and Compliance Services Division
PO Box 44648
Olympia, WA 98504
Phone: (360)902-5588
Website: http://www.wa.gov/lni/scs/

★ 21439 ★ West Virginia Department of Health and Human Resources
Public Health Bureau
Environmental Health Office
Radiation, Toxic, and Indoor Air Quality Division
815 Quarrier St., Ste. 418
Charleston, WV 25301
Phone: (304)558-2981 **Fax:** (304)558-1289
Email: rcurtis@wvdhhr.org
Website: http://www.wvdhhr.org/oehs/rtia.html
Randy C. Curtis, Director

★ 21440 ★ Wisconsin Department of Commerce
Safety and Buildings Division
201 W Washington Ave.
4th floor
Madison, WI 53703
Phone: (608)266-3151
Email: ttaylor@commerce.state.wi.us
Website: http://www.commerce.state.wi.us/SB/SB-HomePage.html

★ 21441 ★ Wyoming Department of Employment
Workers Safety and Compensation Division
1510 E Pershing Blvd.
122 W 25th St.
Cheyenne, WY 82002
Phone: (307)777-7159 **Fax:** (307)777-5946
Email: kmckin1@state.wy.us
Website: http://wydoe.state.wy.us/doe.asp?ID=9
Kathleen McKinna, Contact

Optometry Boards

★ 21442 ★ Alabama State Board of Optometry
1431 Second Ave.
PO Box 448
Bessemer, AL 35020
Phone: (205)481-9993 **Fax:** (205)481-9959
Email: fwallace@al-optometry.org
Website: http://www.al-optometry.org
Dr. Fred Wallace, Contact

★ 21443 ★ Alaska Board of Examiners in Optometry
PO Box 110806
Juneau, AK 99811-0806
Phone: (907)465-2580 **Fax:** (907)465-2974
Email: steve_snyder@dced.state.ak.us
Website: http://www.dced.state.ak.us/occ/popt.htm
Steve Snyder, Contact

★ 21444 ★ Arizona State Board of Optometry
1400 W Washington, Ste. 230
Phoenix, AZ 85007
Phone: (602)542-3095
Email: jconfer@webmail.state.az.us
Website: http://www.asbo.state.az.us/

★ 21445 ★ Arkansas Board of Examiners in Optometry
407 N Elm
Searcy, AR 72143
Phone: (501)268-4351 **Fax:** (501)268-5631
Email: bjsmall@cei.net
Website: http://www.state.ar.us/opt/arkopt.html
Robert Smalling, Director

★ 21446 ★ California Board of Optometry
400 R St., Ste. 4090
Sacramento, CA 95814
Phone: (916)323-8720 **Free:** 800-547-4576
Fax: (916)445-8711
Email: boardemail@optometry.ca.gov
Website: http://www.optometry.ca.gov/

★ 21447 ★ Colorado Board of Examiners in Optometry
1560 Broadway, Rm. 1310
Denver, CO 80202
Phone: (303)894-7751
Email: optometry@dora.state.co.us
Website: http://www.dora.state.co.us/Optometry/
Susan Warren, Contact

★ 21448 ★ Connecticut Board of Examiners in Optometry
410 Capitol Ave.
PO Box 340308
MS 12APP
Hartford, CT 06134-0308
Phone: (860)509-7562
Website: http://www.ct-clic.com/detail.asp?code=1750

★ 21449 ★ Delaware Board of Examiners in Optometry
Cannon Bldg., Ste. 203
861 Silver Lake Blvd.
PO Box 1401
Dover, DE 19904
Phone: (302)739-4512 **Fax:** (302)739-2711
Email: jyoumans@state.de.us
Website: http://professionallicensing.state.de.us/boards/optometry/index.shtml
Jane Youmans, Contact

★ 21450 ★ District of Columbia Board of Optometry
825 North Capitol St., NE
2nd floor
Washington, DC 20002
Phone: (202)442-4775 **Fax:** (202)442-9431
Website: http://dchealth.dc.gov/prof_license/services/boards_main_action.asp?

★ 21451 ★ Florida Board of Optometry
4052 Bald Cypress Way, Bin C-07
PO Box 6330
Tallahassee, FL 32314-6330
Phone: (850)245-4355 **Fax:** (850)922-8876
Email: mqa_optometry@doh.state.fl.us
Website: http://www9.myflorida.com/mqa/optometry/op_home.html

★ 21452 ★ Georgia State Board of Examiners in Optometry
237 Coliseum Dr.
Macon, GA 31217-3858
Phone: (478)207-1686
Email: rfthompson@sos.state.ga.us
Website: http://www.sos.state.ga.us/ebd-optometry/
Anita Martin, Director

★ 21453 ★ Hawaii Board of Examiners in Optometry
1010 Richards St.
DCCA-PVL
PO Box 3469
Honolulu, HI 96801
Phone: (808)587-3295
Website: http://www.state.hi.us/dcca/pvl/areas_optometry.html

★ 21454 ★ Idaho State Optometry Board
Owyhee Plaza, 2nd Fl.
1109 Main St., Ste. 220
Boise, ID 83702-5642
Phone: (208)334-3233 **Fax:** (208)334-3945
Email: drandall@ibol.state.id.us
Website: http://www2.state.id.us/ibol/opt.htm

★ 21455 ★ Illinois Optometry Examining Committee
320 W Washington, 3rd. Fl.
Springfield, IL 62786
Phone: (217)782-8556 **Fax:** (217)782-7645
Website: http://www.dpr.state.il.us/

★ 21456 ★ Indiana Optometry Board
402 Washington St., Rm. W041
Indianapolis, IN 46204
Phone: (317)234-2054 **Fax:** (317)233-4236
Email: hpb8@hpb.state.in.us
Website: http://www.in.gov/hpb/boards/iob/
Cindy Vaught, Director

★ 21457 ★ Iowa Board of Optometry Examiners
Lucas State Office Bldg., 5th Fl.
321 E 12th St.
Des Moines, IA 50319-0075
Phone: (515)242-6385 **Fax:** (515)281-3121
Email: scook@idph.state.ia.us
Website: http://www.iowaccess.org/idph_pl/optometry/index.html

★ 21458 ★ Kansas Board of Optometry Examiners
3111 W 6th St.
Lawrence, KS 66049
Phone: (785)296-0824
Email: kssbeo@terraworld.net

★ 21459 ★ Kentucky Board of Optometric Examiners
301 E Main St., Ste. 850
Lexington, KY 40507
Phone: (859)246-2744 **Fax:** (859)246-2746
Email: KyOptometry@mail.state.ky.us
Website: http://optometry.state.ky.us/

★ 21460 ★ Louisiana State Board of Optometric Examiners
115B N 13th St.
PO Box 555
Oakdale, LA 71463
Phone: (318)335-2989 **Fax:** (318)335-4090
Email: Webmaster@dhhmail.dhh.state.la.us
Website: http://www.dhh.state.la.us/boards.HTM
Dr. James Sandifer, Contact

★ 21461 ★ Maine Board of Registration and Examination in Optometry
113 State House Station
Augusta, ME 04333-0035
Phone: (207)624-8691 **Fax:** (207)624-8692
Email: susan.a.giampetruzzi@state.me.us
Website: http://www.state.me.us/pfr/auxboards/opthome.htm

★ 21462 ★ Maryland Board of Examiners in Optometry
4201 Patterson Ave.
Baltimore, MD 21215-2299
Phone: (410)764-4710 **Fax:** (410)358-2906
Email: optometry@dhmh.state.md.us
Website: http://mdoptometryboard.org/
Patricia Bennett, Contact

★ 21463 ★ Massachusetts Board of Registration in Optometry
239 Causeway St., Ste. 500
Boston, MA 02114
Phone: (617)727-3093 **Fax:** (617)727-2669
Email: gladys.m.clifton@state.ma.us
Website: http://www.state.ma.us/reg/boards/op/default.htm
Gladys Clifton, Contact

★ 21464 ★ Michigan State Board of Optometry Examiners
PO Box 30670
Lansing, MI 48909-8170
Phone: (517)335-0918 **Fax:** (517)373-2179
Email: bhserinfo@cis.state.mi.us
Website: http://www.cis.state.mi.us/bhser/lic/boards/bdopt.htm

★ 21465 ★ Minnesota State Board of Optometry
2829 University Ave. SE, Ste. 550
Minneapolis, MN 55414
Phone: (612)617-2173 **Free:** 800-627-3529
Fax: (612)617-2174
Email: lmi@ngwmail.des.state.mn.us
Website: http://www.mnworkforcecenter.org/lmi/lic_occ/optometr.htm
Laurie Mickelson, Contact

★ 21466 ★ Mississippi State Board of Optometry
PO Box 12370
Jackson, MS 39236-2370
Phone: (601)853-4338 **Fax:** (601)853-0336
Dr. Beverly Limbaugh, Contact

★ 21467 ★ Missouri State Board of Optometry
3605 Missouri Blvd.
PO Box 1335
Jefferson City, MO 65102-0423
Phone: (573)751-0814 **Fax:** (573)751-8216
Email: optom@mail.state.mo.us
Website: http://www.ecodev.state.mo.us/pr/optom/
Sharlene Rimiller, Contact

★ 21468 ★ Montana Board of Optometry
301 S Park, 4th Fl.
PO Box 200513
Helena, MT 59620-0513
Phone: (406)841-2395 **Fax:** (406)841-2305
Email: compolopt@state.mt.gov
Website: http://www.discoveringmontana.com/dli/bsd/license/contact_us.htm
Linda Grief, Contact

★ 21469 ★ Nebraska Board of Examiners in Optometry
PO Box 94986
Lincoln, NE 68509-4986
Phone: (402)471-2118 **Fax:** (402)471-3577
Email: Becky.Wisell@hhss.state.ne.us
Website: http://www.hhs.state.ne.us/crl/crlindex.htm
Becky Wisell, Contact

★ 21470 ★ Nevada Board of Optometry
PO Box 1824
Carson City, NV 89702
Phone: (775)883-8367 **Fax:** (775)883-1938
Email: kennedy@govmail.state.nv.us
Website: http://www.state.nv.us/optometry/

★ 21471 ★ New Hampshire Board of Registration in Optometry
2 Industrial Park Dr., Ste. 8
Concord, NH 03301-8520
Phone: (603)271-2428 **Fax:** (603)271-6702
Website: http://webster.state.nh.us/optometry/
Penny Taylor, Director

★ 21472 ★ New Jersey Board of Optometrists
PO Box 45012
Newark, NJ 07101
Phone: (973)504-6411 **Fax:** (973)648-3536
Email: askconsumeraffairs@smtp.lps.state.nj.us
Website: http://www.state.nj.us/lps/ca/medical.htmopt9
Susan Gartland, Director

★ 21473 ★ New Mexico Board of Examiners in Optometry
2055 Pacheco St., Ste. 400
Santa Fe, NM 87504
Phone: (505)476-7121
Email: OptometryBd@state.nm.us
Website: http://www.rld.state.nm.us/b&c/optometry/index.htm
Carmen E. Payne, Contact

★ 21474 ★ New York State Board of Optometry
Office of the Professions
State Education Bldg., 2nd Fl.
Albany, NY 12234
Phone: (518)474-3817
Email: optombd@mail.nysed.gov
Website: http://www.op.nysed.gov/optom.htm
Peter Ferguson, Contact

★ 21475 ★ North Carolina State Board of Examiners in Optometry
109 N Graham St.
Wallace, NC 28466
Phone: (910)285-3160 **Fax:** (910)285-4546
Email: ncsbeo@duplin.net
Website: http://www.ncoptometry.org/
John D. Robinson, Director

★ 21476 ★ North Dakota State Board of Optometry
341 1st St. E
Dickinson, ND 58601
Phone: (701)483-9141 **Fax:** (701)483-9501
Email: ndsbopt@dickinson.ctctel.com
Website: http://home.ctctel.com/ndsbopt/

★ 21477 ★ Ohio State Board of Optometry
77 S High St., 16th Fl.
Columbus, OH 43215-6108
Phone: (614)466-5115 **Free:** 888-565-3044
Fax: (614)644-3937
Email: Optometry.Board@exchange.state.oh.us
Website: http://www.state.oh.us/opt
Nancy L. Ott, Contact

★ 21478 ★ Oklahoma State Board of Examiners in Optometry
6912 E Reno, Ste. 302
Oklahoma City, OK 73110
Phone: (405)733-7836 **Fax:** (405)741-3060
Website: http://www.state.ok.us/~optometry/
Dr. Russell Laverty, Director

★ 21479 ★ Oregon Board of Optometry
3218 Pringle Rd. SE, Ste.270
Salem, OR 97302-6306
Phone: (503)373-7721 **Fax:** (503)378-3616
Email: David.PLUNKETT@state.or.us
Website: http://www.obo.state.or.us/
David W. Plunkett, Contact

★ 21480 ★ Pennsylvania State Board of Optometry
PO Box 2649
Harrisburg, PA 17105-2649
Phone: (717)783-7155 **Fax:** (717)787-7769
Email: optometr@pados.dos.state.pa.us
Website: http://www.dos.state.pa.us/bpoa/optbd/mainpage.htm
Deb Smith, Contact

★ 21481 ★ Puerto Rico Board of Examiners in Optometry
Call Box 10200
Santurce, PR 00908-0200
Phone: (787)725-8161 **Fax:** (787)725-7903

★ 21482 ★ Rhode Island State Board of Optometry
3 Capitol Hill, Rm. 104
Providence, RI 02908
Phone: (401)222-2827 **Fax:** (401)222-1272
Email: RussellS@doh.state.ri.us
Website: http://www.health.state.ri.us/hsr/optom.htm
Russell Spaight, Contact

★ 21483 ★ South Carolina Board of Examiners in Optometry
Kingstree Bldg.
110 Centerview Dr
PO Box 11329
Columbia, SC 29210
Phone: (803)896-4679 **Fax:** (803)896-4719
Email: combsa@mail.llr.state.sc.us
Website: http://www.llr.state.sc.us/POL/Optometry/Default.htm

★ 21484 ★ South Dakota Board of Optometry
PO Box 370
Sturgis, SD 57785-0370
Phone: (605)347-2136 **Fax:** (605)347-5823
Email: sdoptbd_99@yahoo.com
Website: http://www.state.sd.us/dcr/optometry/optom-ho.htm
Dr. Daniel A. Watson, Contact

★ 21485 ★ Tennessee State Board of Optometry
Cordell Hull Bldg., 3rd Fl.
425 Fifth Ave. N
Nashville, TN 37247
Phone: (615)532-3202 **Free:** 888-310-4650
Email: DDenton@mail.state.tn.us
Website: http://170.142.76.180/bmf-bin/BMFprofgen.pl

★ 21486 ★ Texas Optometry Board
333 Guadalupe St., Ste. 2-420
Austin, TX 78701
Phone: (512)305-8500
Email: lois.ewald@mail.capnet.state.tx.us
Website: http://www.tob.state.tx.us/
Lois Ewald, Contact

★ 21487 ★ Utah Division of Occupational and Professional Licensing
Utah Optometry Board
160 E 300 S
PO Box 146741
Salt Lake City, UT 84114-6741
Phone: (801)530-6621 **Fax:** (801)530-6511
Website: http://www.commerce.utah.gov/opl/index.html
Lynn Bernhard, Contact

★ 21488 ★ Vermont Board of Optometry
26 Terrace St.
Drawer 09
Montpelier, VT 05609-1101
Phone: (802)828-2373 **Fax:** (802)828-2465
Email: patkins@sec.state.vt.us
Website: http://vtprofessionals.org/opr1/optometrists/
Peggy Atkins, Contact

★ 21489 ★ Virgin Islands Board of Optometrical Examiners
Roy Lester Schneider Hospital
48 Sugar Estate
St Thomas, VI 00802
Phone: (340)774-0117 **Fax:** (340)777-4001
Lydia Scott, Contact

★ 21490 ★ Virginia Board of Optometry
6606 W Broad St., 4th Fl.
Richmond, VA 23230-1717
Phone: (804)662-9910 **Free:** 800-533-1560
Fax: (804)662-7098
Email: optbd@dhp.state.va.us
Website: http://www.dhp.state.va.us/optometry/default.htm
Elizabeth A. Carter, Director

★ 21491 ★ Washington State Optometry Board
1300 SE Quince St.
PO Box 47860
Olympia, WA 98504-7860
Phone: (360)236-4700 **Fax:** (360)236-4818
Website: http://www.doh.wa.gov/hsqa/hpqad/Optometry/default.htm
Ben H. Wong, Contact

★ 21492 ★ West Virginia Board of Optometry
101 Michael St.
Clarksburg, WV 26301-3937
Phone: (304)627-2106
Website: http://www.state.wv.us/bep/lmi/license/LICOCCMS.HTMoptometrist

★ 21493 ★ Wisconsin Optometry Examining Board
1400 E Washington Ave.
PO Box 8935
Madison, WI 53708-8935
Phone: (608)266-0145 **Fax:** (608)267-0644
Email: dorl@drl.state.wi.us
Website: http://www.drl.state.wi.us/Regulation/applicant_information/dod272.html

★ 21494 ★ Wyoming State Board of Optometric Examiners
2020 Carey Ave., Ste. 201
Cheyenne, WY 82002
Phone: (307)777-3507
Website: http://www.state.wy.us/governor/boards/bdlist.html
Nanette M. Brown, Contact

Osteopathic Medical Boards

★ 21495 ★ Alabama State Board of Medical Examiners
848 Washington Ave.
PO Box 946
Montgomery, AL 36101-0946
Phone: (334)242-4116 **Fax:** (334)242-4155
Email: bmedixon@mindspring.com
Website: http://www.albme.org/

★ 21496 ★ Alaska State Medical Board
PO Box 110806
Juneau, AK 99811-0806
Phone: (907)269-8163 **Fax:** (907)269-8196
Email: leslie_abel@dced.state.ak.us
Website: http://www.commerce.state.ak.us/occ/pmed.htm

★ 21497 ★ Arizona Board of Osteopathic Examiners in Medicine and Surgery
9535 E Doubletree Ranch Rd.
Scottsdale, AZ 85258
Phone: (480)657-7703 **Fax:** (480)657-7715
Email: information@azosteoboard.org
Website: http://www.azosteoboard.org/
Ann Marie Berger, Director

★ 21498 ★ Arkansas State Medical Board
2100 Riverfront Dr., Ste. 200
Little Rock, AR 72202
Phone: (501)296-1802 **Fax:** (501)296-1805
Email: office@armedicalboard.org
Website: http://www.armedicalboard.org/

★ 21499 ★ Colorado State Board of Medical Examiners
1560 Broadway, Ste. 1300
Denver, CO 80202
Phone: (303)894-7690 **Fax:** (303)894-7692
Email: medical@dora.state.co.us
Website: http://www.dora.state.co.us/Medical/
Susan Miller, Contact

★ 21500 ★ Connecticut State Board of Medical Quality Assurance
410 Capitol Ave.
Hartford, CT 06134
Phone: (860)509-7579 **Fax:** (860)509-8457
Email: webmaster.dph@po.state.ct.us
Website: http://www.state.ct.us/dph/

★ 21501 ★ Delaware Board of Medical Practice
Cannon Bldg, Ste. 203
861 Silver Lake Blvd.
PO Box 1401
Dover, DE 19903
Phone: (302)739-4522 **Fax:** (302)739-2711

★ 21502 ★ District of Columbia Board of Medicine
825 North Capital St, NE, 2nd Fl
Washington, DC 20002
Phone: (202)442-9200 **Fax:** (202)442-9431
Email: dchealth@dc.gov
Website: http://dchealth.dc.gov/index.asp

★ 21503 ★ Florida Board of Osteopathic Medicine
4052 Bald Cypress Way, Bin C-06
Tallahassee, FL 32399-1753
Phone: (850)245-4161 **Fax:** (850)487-9874
Email: Christy_Robinson@doh.state.fl.us
Website: http://www.doh.state.fl.us/mqa/osteopath/oshome.htm
Karen Eaton, Director

★ 21504 ★ Georgia Composite State Board of Medical Examiners
2 Peachtree St.,NW, 10th St.
Atlanta, GA 30303
Phone: (404)656-3913 **Fax:** (404)656-9723
Email: GCox@dma.state.ga.us
Website: http://www.medicalboard.state.ga.us
Karen Mason, Contact

★ 21505 ★ Hawaii Board of Osteopathic Examiners
Department of Commerce & Consumer Affairs
DCCA-PVL
PO Box 3469
Honolulu, HI 96801

Phone: (808)586-2698 **Fax:** (808)586-2874
Website: http://www.state.hi.us/dcca/pvl/areas_medical.html

★ 21506 ★ Idaho State Board of Medicine
1755 Westgate Dr.
PO Box 83720
Boise, ID 83720
Phone: (208)327-7000 **Fax:** (208)327-7005
Email: info@bom.state.id.us
Website: http://www.bom.state.id.us/

★ 21507 ★ Illinois Department of Professional Regulation
Medical Licensing Board
Board of Osteopathic Medicine
320 W Washington St.
Springfield, IL 62786
Phone: (217)785-0800 **Fax:** (217)524-2169
Website: http://www.dpr.state.il.us/WHO/med.cfm

★ 21508 ★ Indiana Health Professions Bureau
Board of Osteopathic Medicine
402 W Washington, Rm. 041
Indianapolis, IN 46204
Phone: (317)232-2960 **Fax:** (317)233-4236
Website: http://www.in.gov/hpb/contact/index.html

★ 21509 ★ Iowa State Board of Medical Examiners
400 SW 8th St., Ste. C
Des Moines, IA 50309-4686
Phone: (515)281-5171 **Fax:** (515)242-5908
Email: amowery@bon.state.ia.us
Website: http://www.docboard.org/ia/ia_home.htm
Ann E. Mowery, PhD, Director

★ 21510 ★ Kansas Board of Healing Arts
235 SW Topeka Blvd.
Topeka, KS 66603-3068
Phone: (785)296-7413 **Fax:** (785)296-0852
Email: Healer3@ink.org
Website: http://www.ksbha.org/

★ 21511 ★ Kentucky Board of Medical Licensure
310 Whittington Pkwy, Ste 1B
310 Whittington Pkwy., Ste 1B
Louisville, KY 40222
Phone: (502)429-8046 **Fax:** (502)429-9923
Email: kbml@mail.state.ky.us
Website: http://www.state.ky.us/agencies/kbml/

★ 21512 ★ Louisiana State Board of Medical Examiners
630 Camp St.
PO Box 30250
New Orleans, LA 70190-0250
Phone: (504)568-6820 **Fax:** (504)599-0503
Email: lsbmever@lsbme.org
Website: http://www.lsbme.org/

★ 21513 ★ Maine Board of Osteopathic Licensure
142 State House Station
2 Bangor St.
Augusta, ME 04333-0142
Phone: (207)287-2480
Email: susan.e.strout@state.me.us
Website: http://www.docboard.org/me-osteo/

★ 21514 ★ Maryland Board of Physician Quality Assurance
4201 Patterson Ave.
Baltimore, MD 21215-0095
Phone: (410)764-4777 **Free:** 800-492-6836
Fax: (410)358-2252
Email: bpqa@erols.com
Website: http://www.bpqa.state.md.us/

★ 21515 ★ Massachusetts Board of Registration in Medicine
10 West St. 3rd Fl.
Boston, MA 02111
Phone: (617)727-3086 **Fax:** (617)451-9568
Email: webmaster@massmedboard.org
Website: http://www.massmedboard.org./

★ 21516 ★ Michigan Board of Osteopathic Medicine and Surgery
PO Box 30670
Lansing, MI 48909-8170
Phone: (517)335-0918 **Fax:** (517)373-2179
Email: bhserinfo@cis.state.mi.us
Website: http://www.michigan.gov/cis

★ 21517 ★ Minnesota Board of Medical Practice
2829 University Ave. SE
Ste. 400
Minneapolis, MN 55414-3246
Phone: (612)617-2130 **Free:** 800-657-3709
Fax: (612)617-2166
Email: medical.board@state.mn.us
Website: http://www.bmp.state.mn.us/

★ 21518 ★ Mississippi State Board of Medical Licensure
1867 Crane Ridge Dr.
Ste. 200-B
PO Box 9268
Jackson, MS 39286-9268
Phone: (601)987-3079 **Fax:** (601)987-4159
Email: mboard@msbml.state.ms.us
Website: http://www.msbml.state.ms.us/

★ 21519 ★ Missouri State Board of Registration for the Healing Arts
3605 Missouri Blvd.
PO Box 4
Jefferson City, MO 65102
Phone: (573)751-0098 **Fax:** (573)751-3166
Email: healarts@mail.state.mo.us
Website: http://www.ecodev.state.mo.us/pr/healarts/
Tina Steinman, Director

★ 21520 ★ Montana Board of Medical Examiners
301 S Park, 4th Fl.
PO Box 200513
Helena, MT 59620-0513
Phone: (406)841-2360 **Fax:** (406)841-2363
Email: dlibsdmed@state.mt.us
Website: http://www.discoveringmontana.com/dli/bsd/license/hc_licensing_boards.htm
Jeanne Worsech, Director

★ 21521 ★ Nebraska Department of Health and Human Services
State Board of Examiners in Medicine and Surgery
PO Box 94986
Lincoln, NE 68509-4986
Phone: (402)471-2118 **Fax:** (402)471-3577
Email: Becky.Wisell@hhss.state.ne.us
Website: http://www.hhs.state.ne.us/crl/msh.htm
Becky Wisell, Contact

★ 21522 ★ Nevada State Board of Osteopathic Medicine
2860 E Flamingo Rd., Ste. G
Las Vegas, NV 89121
Phone: (702)732-2147 **Fax:** (702)732-2079
Website: http://www.osteo.state.nv.us
Larry Tarno, Director

★ 21523 ★ New Hampshire Board of Registration in Medicine
2 Industrial Park Dr., Ste. 8
Concord, NH 03301-8520
Phone: (603)271-1203 **Fax:** (603)271-6702
Website: http://webster.state.nh.us/medicine/

★ 21524 ★ New Jersey State Board of Medical Examiners
PO Box 183
Trenton, NJ 08625-0183
Phone: (609)826-7100 **Fax:** (609)826-7117
Website: http://www.state.nj.us/lps/ca/medical.htmbme5
William Roeder, Director

★ 21525 ★ New Mexico Board of Osteopathic Medical Examiners
92055 Pacheco St., Ste. 400
PO Box 25101
Santa Fe, NM 87504
Phone: (505)476-7120 **Fax:** (505)476-7095
Email: OsteoBoard@state.nm.us
Website: http://www.rld.state.nm.us/b&c/osteopathic_examiners_board.htm

★ 21526 ★ New York State Board for Medicine
Office of the Professions
State Education Bldg., 2nd Fl.
Albany, NY 12234
Phone: (518)474-3817 **Fax:** (518)486-4846
Email: medbd@mail.nysed.gov
Website: http://www.op.nysed.gov/med.htm
Thomas J. Monahan, Contact

★ 21527 ★ North Carolina Board of Medical Examiners
1201 Front St, Ste. 100
Raleigh, NC 27609-7533
Phone: (919)326-1100 **Fax:** (919)326-1130
Email: public.affairs@ncmedboard.org
Website: http://www.ncmedboard.org/

★ 21528 ★ North Dakota State Board of Medical Examiners
418 E Broadway, Ste. 12
Bismarck, ND 58501
Phone: (701)328-6500 **Fax:** (701)328-6505
Website: http://www.ndbomex.com/
Rolf P. Sletten, J.D., Contact

★ 21529 ★ Ohio State Medical Board
77 S High St., 17th Fl.
Columbus, OH 43215-6127
Phone: (614)466-3934 **Free:** 800-554-7717
Fax: (614)728-5946
Website: http://www.state.oh.us/med/

★ 21530 ★ Oklahoma Board of Osteopathic Examiners
4848 N Lincoln Blvd., Ste. 100
Oklahoma City, OK 73105-3335
Phone: (405)528-8625 **Fax:** (405)557-0653
Website: http://www.docboard.org/ok/ok.htm
Paul F. Benien, Director

★ 21531 ★ Oregon Board of Medical Examiners
1500 SW 1st Ave., Ste. 620
Portland, OR 97201
Phone: (503)229-5770 **Free:** 877-254-6263
Fax: (503)229-6543
Email: bme.info@state.or.us
Website: http://www.bme.state.or.us

★ **21532** ★ **Osteopathic Medical Board of California**
2720 Gateway Oaks Dr, Ste 350
Sacramento, CA 95833
Phone: (916)263-3100
Linda J. Bergmann, Director

★ **21533** ★ **Pennsylvania State Board of Osteopathic Medicine**
PO Box 2649
Harrisburg, PA 17105-2649
Phone: (717)783-4858 **Fax:** (717)787-7769
Website: http://www.dos.state.pa.us
Gina K. Bittner, Contact

★ **21534** ★ **Puerto Rico Board of Medical Examiners**
Call Box 13969
San Juan, PR 00908
Phone: (787)792-8949 **Fax:** (787)792-4436
Pablo Valentin-Torres, Director

★ **21535** ★ **Rhode Island Board of Medical Licensure and Discipline**
3 Capitol Hill, Rm. 205
Providence, RI 02908-5097
Phone: (401)222-3855 **Fax:** (401)222-2158
Website: http://www.docboard.org/ri/main.htm

★ **21536** ★ **South Carolina Board of Medical Examiners**
Synergy Business Park
Kingstree Bldg.
110 Centerview Dr., Ste. 202
PO Box 11289
Columbia, SC 29211-1289
Phone: (803)896-4500 **Fax:** (803)896-4515
Email: medboard@mail.llr.state.sc.us
Website: http://www.llr.state.sc.us/POL/Medical/Default.htm

★ **21537** ★ **South Dakota State Board of Medical and Osteopathic Examiners**
1323 S Minnesota Ave.
Sioux Falls, SD 57105
Phone: (605)334-8343 **Fax:** (605)336-0270
Email: jphalen@sdsma.org
Website: http://www.state.sd.us/dcr/medical/medhom.htm
Paul Jensen, Contact

★ **21538** ★ **Tennessee State Board of Osteopathic Examiners**
Cordell Hull Bldg., 3rd Fl.
425 Fifth Ave. N
Nashville, TN 37247-1010
Phone: (615)532-3202 **Free:** 888-310-4650
Fax: (615)253-4484
Email: DDenton@mail.state.tn.us
Website: http://www.fsmb.org/
Rosemarie Otto, Contact

★ **21539** ★ **Texas State Board of Medical Examiners**
333 Guadalupe St., Tower 3, Ste. 610
PO Box 2018
Austin, TX 78768-2018
Phone: (512)305-7010 **Free:** 800-248-4062
Fax: (512)463-9416
Website: http://www.tsbme.state.tx.us/

★ **21540** ★ **Utah Physicians Licensing Board**
Board of Osteopathic Medicine
160 E 300 S, 4th Fl.
PO Box 146741
Salt Lake City, UT 84114
Phone: (801)530-6628 **Fax:** (801)530-6511
Email: lduke@br.state.ut.us
Website: http://www.dopl.utah.gov/
Diana Baker, Contact

★ **21541** ★ **Vermont Board of Osteopathic Physicians and Surgeons**
26 Terrace St.
Drawer 09
Montpelier, VT 05609-1106
Phone: (802)828-2373 **Fax:** (802)828-2465
Email: patkins@sec.state.vt.us
Website: http://www.sec.state.vt.us
Peggy Atkins, Contact

★ **21542** ★ **Virgin Islands Board of Medical Examiners**
Department of Health
48 Sugar Estate
St Thomas, VI 00802
Phone: (340)774-0117 **Fax:** (340)777-4001
Lydia Scott, Contact

★ **21543** ★ **Virginia Board of Medicine**
6606 W Broad St., 4th Fl.
Richmond, VA 23230-1717
Phone: (804)662-9908 **Free:** 800-533-1560
Fax: (804)662-9517
Email: medbd@dhp.state.va.us
Website: http://www.dhp.state.va.us/medicine/default.htm
William L. Harp, MD, Director

★ **21544** ★ **Washington State Board of Osteopathic Medicine and Surgery**
Department of Health
Health Professions Quality Assurance
1112 SE Quince St.
PO Box 47870
Olympia, WA 98504-7870
Phone: (360)236-4943 **Fax:** (360)236-2406
Email: hpqa.csc@doh.wa.gov
Website: http://www.doh.wa.gov
Robert Nicoloff, Director

★ **21545** ★ **West Virginia Board of Osteopathy**
334 Penco Rd.
Weirton, WV 26062
Phone: (304)723-4638 **Fax:** (304)723-6723
Email: bdosteo@mail.wvnet.edu
Website: http://www.state.wv.us/bdosteo/
Cheryl Schreiber, Contact

★ **21546** ★ **Wisconsin Medical Examining Board**
1400 E Washington Ave., Rm. 178
PO Box 8935
Madison, WI 53708-8935
Phone: (608)266-2112 **Fax:** (608)261-7083
Email: web@drl.state.wi.us
Website: http://www.drl.state.wi.us/
Deanna Zychomski, Director

★ **21547** ★ **Wyoming Medical Examiners Board**
211 W 19th St., 2nd Fl.
Cheyenne, WY 82002
Phone: (307)778-7053 **Free:** 800-438-5784
Fax: (307)778-2069
Email: wyomedical@wyomedicalboard.org
Website: http://wyomedboard.state.wy.us/
Carole Shotwell, Contact

Pharmacy Boards

★ **21548** ★ **Alabama State Board of Pharmacy**
1 Perimeter Park S, Ste. 425 S
Birmingham, AL 35243
Phone: (205)967-0130 **Fax:** (205)967-1009
Email: jmoore@albop.com
Website: http://www.albop.com
Jerry Moore, Director

★ **21549** ★ **Arizona State Board of Pharmacy**
4425 W Olive Ave, Ste 140
Glendale, AZ 85302
Phone: (623)463-2727 **Fax:** (623)934-0583
Email: vsevilla@azsbp.com
Website: http://www.pharmacy.state.az.us/
Llyn. A. Lloyd, Director

★ **21550** ★ **Arkansas State Board of Pharmacy**
101 E Capitol, Ste. 218
Little Rock, AR 72201
Phone: (501)682-0190 **Fax:** (501)682-0195
Email: Charlie.campbell@mail.state.ar.us
Website: http://www.state.ar.us/asbp/
Charles S. Campbell, Director

★ **21551** ★ **California State Board of Pharmacy**
400 R St., Ste. 4070
Sacramento, CA 95814
Phone: (916)445-5014 **Fax:** (916)327-6308
Email: rxwebmaster@dca.ca.gov
Website: http://www.pharmacy.ca.gov/
John Jones, Director

★ **21552** ★ **CareMed Chicago**
322 S Green St. Ste. 300
Chicago, IL 60607
Phone: (312)738-8622 **Fax:** (312)738-0317
Email: caremed@caremedchicago.com
Website: http://www.caremedchicago.com/

★ **21553** ★ **Colorado State Board of Pharmacy**
1560 Broadway, Ste. 1310
Denver, CO 80202
Phone: (303)894-7750 **Fax:** (303)894-7764
Email: Pharmacy@dora.state.co.us
Website: http://www.dora.state.co.us/pharmacy/
Susan L. Warren, Contact

★ **21554** ★ **Delaware Department of Administrative Services**
Division of Professional Regulation
Delaware State Board of Pharmacy
Jesse Cooper Bldg, Room 205
PO Box 637
Dover, DE 19903
Phone: (302)739-4547 **Fax:** (302)739-3071
Email: grbunting@state.de.us
Website: http://professionallicensing.state.de.us/boards/pharmacy/index.shtml
Gradella Bunting, Contact

★ **21555** ★ **Department of Consumer Protection**
License Services Division
Connecticut Commission of Pharmacy
165 Capitol Ave.
Hartford, CT 06106
Phone: (860)713-6065 **Fax:** (860)713-7239
Email: drug.control@po.state.ct.us
Website: http://www.dcp.state.ct.us/licensing/drug.htm

★ 21556 ★ District of Columbia Board of Pharmacy
825 N Capitol St, NE, room 2224
Washington, DC 20002
Phone: (202)442-4775 **Fax:** (202)442-9431
Graphelia Ramseur, Contact

★ 21557 ★ Georgia State Board of Pharmacy
237 Coliseum Dr.
Macon, GA 31217-3858
Phone: (678)207-1686 **Fax:** (678)207-1363
Email: rfthompson@sos.state.ga.us
Website: http://www.sos.state.ga.us/plb/
Anita O. Martin, Director

★ 21558 ★ Hawaii State Board of Pharmacy
1010 Richards St.
PO Box 3469
DCCA-PVL
ATT: PHAR
Honolulu, HI 96801
Phone: (808)586-2694
Email: pharmacy@dcca.state.hi.us
Website: http://www.state.hi.us/dcca/pvl/areas_pharmacy.html
Lee Ann Teshima, Contact

★ 21559 ★ Idaho Board of Pharmacy
3380 Americana Terrace., Ste. 320
PO Box 83720
Boise, ID 83720-0067
Phone: (208)334-2356 **Fax:** (208)334-3536
Website: http://www.accessidaho.org/bop/contact/contact.html
Richard Mick Markuson, Director

★ 21560 ★ Illinois Department of Professional Regulation
Board of Pharmacy
320 W Washington St.
Springfield, IL 62786
Phone: (217)785-0800 **Fax:** (217)782-7645
Website: http://www.dpr.state.il.us/WHO/phar.asp
John Rose, Director

★ 21561 ★ Indiana Board of Pharmacy
Health Professions Bureau
402 W Washington St., Rm. 041
Indianapolis, IN 46204
Phone: (317)232-2960 **Fax:** (317)233-4236
Email: mboone@hpb.state.in.us
Website: http://www.in.gov/hpb/
888-333-7515 Donna S. Wall, Director

★ 21562 ★ Iowa Board of Pharmacy Examiners
400 SW Eighth St., Ste. E
Des Moines, IA 50309-4688
Phone: (515)281-5944 **Fax:** (515)281-4609
Email: lloyd.jessen@ibpe.state.ia.us
Website: http://www.iowaccess.org/ibpe/
Lloyd K. Jessen, Director

★ 21563 ★ Kansas State Board of Pharmacy
900 SW Jackson, Rm. 513
Topeka, KS 66612-1231
Phone: (785)296-4056 **Free:** 888-RX-BOARD
Fax: (785)296-8420
Email: pharmacy@ink.org
Website: http://www.ink.org/public/pharmacy/
Jim Kinderknecht, R.Ph., Contact

★ 21564 ★ Kentucky Board of Pharmacy
23 Millcreek Park
Frankfort, KY 40601-9230
Phone: (502)573-1580 **Fax:** (502)573-1582
Website: http://www.state.ky.us/boards/pharmacy/

★ 21565 ★ Louisiana Board of Pharmacy
5615 Corporate Blvd., Ste. 8E
Baton Rouge, LA 70808-2537
Phone: (225)925-6496
Email: labp@labp.com
Website: http://www.labp.com/
Howard B. Bolton, Director

★ 21566 ★ Maine Board of Commissioners of Pharmacy
Department of Professional & Financial Regulation
Division of Licensing & Enforcement
35 State House Station
Augusta, ME 04333
Phone: (207)624-8500 **Fax:** (207)624-8690
Email: jeri.l.betts@state.me.us
Website: http://www.state.me.us/pfr/olr/index.htm
Jeri L. Betts, Contact

★ 21567 ★ Maryland Board of Pharmacy
4201 Patterson Ave.
Baltimore, MD 21215-2299
Phone: (410)764-4755 **Free:** 800-542-4964
Fax: (410)358-6207
Email: md_pharmacy_board@yahoo.com
Website: http://www.dhmh.state.md.us/pharmacyboard/
LaVerne G. Naesea, Director

★ 21568 ★ Massachusetts Board of Registration in Pharmacy
239 Causeway St., Ste. 500
Boston, MA 02114
Phone: (617)727-3074 **Fax:** (617)727-2197
Email: charles.r.young@state.ma.us
Website: http://www.state.ma.us/reg/boards/ph/default.htm
Charles Young, Director

★ 21569 ★ Michigan Board of Pharmacy
PO Box 30670
Lansing, MI 48909-8170
Phone: (517)335-0918 **Fax:** (517)373-2179
Email: bhserinfo@cis.state.mi.us
Website: http://www.cis.state.mi.us/bhser/lic/boards/bdpharm.htm

★ 21570 ★ Minnesota Board of Pharmacy
2829 University Ave. SE, Ste. 530
Minneapolis, MN 55414
Phone: (612)617-2201 **Fax:** (612)617-2212
Email: David.Holmstrom@state.mn.us
Website: http://www.phcybrd.state.mn.us/mn_home.htm
David E. Holmstrom, Director

★ 21571 ★ Mississippi State Board of Pharmacy
PO Box 24507
Jackson, MS 39225-4507
Phone: (601)354-6750 **Fax:** (601)354-6071
Email: cwilliams@mbp.state.ms.us
Website: http://www.mbp.state.ms.us/
Leland "Mac" McDivitt, Director

★ 21572 ★ Missouri Board of Pharmacy
3605 Missouri Blvd.
PO Box 625
Jefferson City, MO 65102
Phone: (573)751-0091 **Fax:** (573)526-3464
Email: pharmacy@mail.state.mo.us
Website: http://www.ded.state.mo.us/regulatorylicensing/
Kevin E. Kinkade, Director

★ 21573 ★ Montana Department of Labor and Industry
Business Standards Division
Montana Board of Pharmacy
301 S Park, 4th Fl.
Helena, MT 59602
Phone: (406)841-2355 **Fax:** (406)841-2305
Email: compolpha@state.mt.us
Website: http://www.discoveringmontana.com/dli/bsd/license/bsd_boards/pha_board/board_page.htm
Rebecca Deschamps, Contact

★ 21574 ★ Nebraska Department of HHS Regulation and Licensure
Nebraska Board of Examiners in Pharmacy
PO Box 95007
Lincoln, NE 68509-5007
Phone: (402)471-4923
Email: hhs_system_information@hhss.state.ne.us
Website: http://www.hhs.state.ne.us/crl/crlindex.htm
Helen Meeks, Contact

★ 21575 ★ Nevada State Board of Pharmacy
555 Double Eagle Court, Ste. 1100
Reno, NV 89511-8991
Phone: (775)850-1440 **Free:** 800-364-2081
Fax: (775)850-1444
Email: pharmacy@govmail.state.nv.us
Website: http://glsuitewww.glsuite.com/nvbopweb/
Larry Pinson, Director

★ 21576 ★ New Hampshire Board of Pharmacy
57 Regional Dr.
Concord, NH 03301-8518
Phone: (603)271-2350 **Fax:** (603)271-2856
Email: nhpharmacy@nhsa.state.nh.us
Website: http://www.state.nh.us/pharmacy/
Paul G. Boisseau, Contact

★ 21577 ★ New Jersey State Board of Pharmacy
PO Box 45013
Newark, NJ 07101
Phone: (973)504-6450
Email: askconsumeraffairs@dca.lps.state.nj.us
Website: http://www.state.nj.us/lps/ca/medical.htmpharm11
Debra Whipple, Director

★ 21578 ★ New Mexico Board of Pharmacy
1650 University Blvd. NE, Ste. 400B
Albuquerque, NM 87102
Phone: (505)841-9102 **Free:** 800-565-9102
Fax: (505)841-9113
Email: pharmacy.board@state.nm.us
Website: http://www.state.nm.us/pharmacy/
Jerry Montoya, Director

★ 21579 ★ New York Board of Pharmacy
State Education Bldg.
Office of the Professions, 2nd Fl.
89 Washington Ave.
Albany, NY 12234
Phone: (518)474-3817 **Fax:** (518)473-6995
Email: pharmbd@mail.nysed.gov
Website: http://www.op.nysed.gov/pharm.htm
Lawrence H. Mokhiber, Contact

★ 21580 ★ North Carolina Board of Pharmacy
Carrboro Plaza
PO Box 459
Carrboro, NC 27510
Phone: (919)942-4454 **Fax:** (919)967-5757
Email: drw@ncbop.org

Website: http://www.ncbop.org/
David R. Work, Director

★ 21581 ★ North Dakota State Board of Pharmacy
405 E Broadway Ave., Rm. 300
PO Box 1354
Bismarck, ND 58502-1354
Phone: (701)328-9535 **Fax:** (701)328-9312
Email: ndboph@btinet.com
Website: http://www.governor.state.nd.us/boards/boards-query.asp?Board_ID=81
Howard C. Anderson, R.Ph, Director

★ 21582 ★ Ohio State Board of Pharmacy
77 S High St., 17th Fl.
Columbus, OH 43215-6126
Phone: (614)466-4143 **Free:** 800-750-0750
Fax: (614)752-4836
Email: exec@bop.state.oh.us
Website: http://www.state.oh.us/pharmacy
William T. Winsley, Director

★ 21583 ★ Oklahoma State Board of Pharmacy
4545 Lincoln Blvd., Ste. 112
Oklahoma City, OK 73105-3488
Phone: (405)521-3815 **Fax:** (405)521-3758
Email: pharmacy@oklaosf.state.ok.us
Website: http://www.state.ok.us/~pharmacy/
Bryan H. Potter, D.Ph., Director

★ 21584 ★ Oregon State Board of Pharmacy
State Office Bldg., Ste. 425
800 NE Oregon St., No. 9
Portland, OR 97232
Phone: (503)731-4032 **Fax:** (503)731-4067
Email: gary.a.schnabel@state.or.us
Website: http://www.pharmacy.state.or.us/
Gary A. Schnabel, Director

★ 21585 ★ Pennsylvania State Board of Pharmacy
PO Box 2649
Harrisburg, PA 17105-2649
Phone: (717)783-7156 **Fax:** (717)787-7769
Email: pharmacy@pados.dos.state.pa.us
Website: http://www.dos.state.pa.us/bpoa/cwp/view.asp?a=1104&q=432995

★ 21586 ★ Puerto Rico Board of Pharmacy
Department of Health
Board of Pharmacy
800 Avenida Robert T. Todd
Office No. 201, Stop No. 18
Call Box 10200
Santurce, PR 00908
Phone: (787)725-8161
Magda Bouet, Director

★ 21587 ★ Rhode Island Board of Pharmacy
Department of Health
Division of Drug Control
3 Capitol Hill, Rm. 205
Providence, RI 02908-5097
Phone: (401)222-2837 **Fax:** (401)222-2158
Email: dianet@doh.state.ri.us
Website: http://www.health.state.ri.us/hsr/pharmacy.htm
Diane Tellier, Contact

★ 21588 ★ South Carolina Board of Pharmacy
PO Box 11927
Columbia, SC 29211-1927
Phone: (803)896-4700 **Fax:** (803)896-4596
Email: funderbm@mail.llr.state.sc.us
Website: http://www.llr.state.sc.us/POL/Pharmacy/Default.htm
Lee Ann Bundrick, Contact

★ 21589 ★ South Dakota State Board of Pharmacy
4305 S Louise Ave., Ste. 104
Sioux Falls, SD 57106
Phone: (605)362-2737 **Fax:** (605)362-2738
Email: dennis.jones@state.sd.us
Website: http://www.state.sd.us/dcr/pharmacy/pharm-ho.htm
David L. Volk, Secretary

★ 21590 ★ Tennessee Board of Pharmacy
Davy Crockett Tower
500 James Robertson Pkwy., 2nd Fl.
Nashville, TN 37243-1149
Phone: (615)741-2718 **Fax:** (615)741-2722
Email: klynch@mail.state.tn.us
Website: http://www.state.tn.us/commerce/pharmacy/index.htm
Kendall M. Lynch, Director

★ 21591 ★ Texas State Board of Pharmacy
333 Guadalupe St., Tower 3, Ste. 600
Austin, TX 78701-3942
Phone: (512)305-8000 **Fax:** (512)305-8082
Email: geninfo@tsbp.state.tx.us
Website: http://www.tsbp.state.tx.us/
Gay Dodson, Director

★ 21592 ★ Utah Board of Pharmacy
160 E 300 S, 4th Fl.
PO Box 146741
Salt Lake City, UT 84145-0805
Phone: (801)530-6633 **Fax:** (801)530-6511
Email: dtjones@br.state.ut.us

★ 21593 ★ Vermont Board of Pharmacy Office of Professional Regulation
109 State St.
Montpelier, VT 05609-1106
Phone: (802)828-2875
Email: cpreston@sec.state.vt.us
Website: http://www.vtprofessionals.org/pharmacists/
Carla Preston, Secretary

★ 21594 ★ Virgin Islands Board of Pharmacy
Department of Health
Roy L. Schneider Hospital
48 Sugar Estate
St Thomas, VI 00802
Phone: (340)774-0117 **Fax:** (340)777-4001
Lydia T. Scott, Director

★ 21595 ★ Virginia Board of Pharmacy
6606 W Broad St., 4th Fl.
Richmond, VA 23230-1717
Phone: (804)662-9911 **Free:** 800-533-1560
Fax: (804)662-9313
Email: pharmbd@dhp.state.va.us
Website: http://www.dhp.state.va.us/pharmacy/default.htm
Elizabeth Scott Russell, Director

★ 21596 ★ Washington State Board of Pharmacy
1300 SE Quince St.
PO Box 47863
Olympia, WA 98504-7863
Phone: (360)236-4825 **Fax:** (360)586-4359
Website: http://www.doh.wa.gov/Pharmacy/default.htm
Donald H. Williams, Director

★ 21597 ★ West Virginia Board of Pharmacy
232 Capitol St.
Charleston, WV 25301
Phone: (304)558-0558 **Fax:** (304)558-0572
Email: bpayne@wvbop.com
Website: http://www.wvbop.com/wvbop/25301/default.htm
William T. Douglas, Jr., Contact

★ 21598 ★ Wisconsin Pharmacy Examining Board
1400 E Washington Ave.
PO Box 8935
Madison, WI 53708-8935
Phone: (608)266-2811 **Fax:** (608)267-0644
Email: dorl@drl.state.wi.us
Website: http://badger.state.wi.us/agencies/drl/Regulation/applicant_information/dod270.html

★ 21599 ★ Wyoming State Board of Pharmacy
1720 S Poplar St., Ste. 4
Casper, WY 82601
Phone: (307)234-0294 **Fax:** (307)234-7226
Email: wypharmbd@wercs.com
Website: http://pharmacyboard.state.wy.us/
James T. Carder, Contact

Podiatry Boards

★ 21600 ★ Alabama State Board of Podiatric Medicine
13 Innisbrook Ln
Birmingham, AL 35242
Phone: (205)995-8537 **Fax:** (205)595-8537
Email: AlPodBoard@aol.com
Website: http://members.aol.com/alpodboard/index.html
Gail Clark, Contact

★ 21601 ★ Alaska State Medical Board
PO Box 110806
Juneau, AK 99811-0806
Phone: (907)269-8163 **Fax:** (907)269-8196
Email: leslie_gallant@dced.state.ak.us
Website: http://www.dced.state.ak.us/occ/pmed.htm
Leslie A. Gallant, Contact

★ 21602 ★ Arizona State Board of Podiatry Examiners
1400 W Washington, Ste. 230
Phoenix, AZ 85007
Phone: (602)542-3095
Website: http://www.revenue.state.az.us/609/licensingguide.htmPROFESSION

★ 21603 ★ Arkansas State Podiatry Examining Board
2001 Georgia Ave.
Little Rock, AR 72207-5014
Phone: (501)664-3668

★ 21604 ★ California Board of Podiatric Medicine
1420 Howe Ave., Ste. 8
Sacramento, CA 95825-3229
Phone: (916)263-2647 **Fax:** (916)263-2651
Email: bpm@dca.ca.gov
Website: http://www.dca.ca.gov/bpm/index.html
James Rathlesberger, Contact

★ 21605 ★ Colorado Podiatry Board
1560 Broadway, Ste. 1545
Denver, CO 80202
Phone: (303)894-2464 **Fax:** (303)894-7885
Email: podiatrists@dora.state.co.us
Website: http://www.dora.state.co.us/Podiatrists/
Kevin D. Heupel, Contact

★ 21606 ★ Connecticut Board of Podiatry Licensure
410 Capitol Ave.
PO Box 340308
Hartford, CT 06134-0308
Phone: (860)509-7562
Website: http://www.ct-clic.com/detail.asp?code=1763

★ 21607 ★ District of Columbia Board of Podiatry
825 N Capital St NE, 2nd floor
Washington, DC 20002
Phone: (202)442-4778 **Fax:** (202)442-9431
Website: http://dchealth.dc.gov/prof_license/services/boards_main.asp

★ 21608 ★ Florida Board of Podiatric Medicine
4052 Bald Cypress Way, Bin C-07
Tallahassee, FL 32399-3257
Phone: (850)245-4355 **Fax:** (850)922-8876
Email: mqa_podiatry@doh.state.fl.us
Website: http://www.doh.state.fl.us/mqa/index.html
Joe Baker, Jr., DIR

★ 21609 ★ Georgia State Board of Podiatry
237 Coliseum Dr.
Macon, GA 31217-3858
Phone: (478)207-1686 **Fax:** (478)207-1363
Email: rfthompson@sos.state.ga.us
Website: http://www.sos.state.ga.us/plb/
Anita O. Martin, Director

★ 21610 ★ Hawaii Board of Podiatric Medicine
DCCA-PVL
PO Box 3469
Honolulu, HI 96801
Phone: (808)586-2708
Email: medical@dcca.state.hi.us
Website: http://www.state.hi.us/dcca/pvl/areas_medical.html
Constance Cabral-Makanani, Director

★ 21611 ★ Idaho State Board of Podiatry
Bureau of Occupational Licenses
1109 Main St., Ste. 220
Boise, ID 83702-5642
Phone: (208)334-3233 **Fax:** (208)334-3945
Email: csimpson@ibol.state.id.us
Website: http://www2.state.id.us/ibol/pod.htm

★ 21612 ★ Illinois Department of Professional Regulation
Podiatry Examining Committee
320 W Washington St.
Springfield, IL 62786
Phone: (217)785-0800 **Fax:** (217)782-7645
Website: http://www.dpr.state.il.us

★ 21613 ★ Indiana Health Professions Bureau
Board Podiatric Medicine
402 W Washington, Rm. W041
Indianapolis, IN 46204-2739
Phone: (317)234-2064
Email: hpb5@hpb.state.in.us
Website: http://www.in.gov/hpb/boards/bpm/
Wade A. Lowhorn, Director

★ 21614 ★ Iowa Bureau of Professional Licensing
Iowa Board of Podiatry Examiners
Lucas State Office Bldg., 5th Fl.
321 E 12th St.
Des Moines, IA 50319-0075
Phone: (515)242-6385 **Fax:** (515)281-3121
Email: jmanning@idph.state.ia.us
Website: http://www.iowaccess.org/idph_pl/podiatry/index.html

★ 21615 ★ Kansas Board of Healing Arts
235 SW Topeka Blvd.
Topeka, KS 66603-3068
Phone: (785)296-7413 **Fax:** (785)296-0852
Email: Healer3@ink.org
Website: http://www.ksbha.org/

★ 21616 ★ Kentucky Board of Podiatry
906B S 12th St.
Murray, KY 42071-2947
Phone: (270)759-0007

★ 21617 ★ Louisiana State Board of Medical Examiners
630 Camp St.
PO Box 30250
New Orleans, LA 70190-0250
Phone: (504)568-6820 **Fax:** (504)599-0503
Email: lsbmever@lsbme.org
Website: http://www.lsbme.org/

★ 21618 ★ Maine Office of Licensing and Registration
Board of Podiatric Examiners
35 State House Station
Augusta, ME 04333-0035
Phone: (207)624-8626 **Fax:** (207)624-8637
Email: diane.l.staples@state.me.us
Website: http://www.state.me.us/pfr/olr/categories/cat33.htm

★ 21619 ★ Maryland Board of Podiatric Medicine Examiners
4201 Patterson Ave.
Baltimore, MD 21215-2299
Phone: (301)764-4785 **Fax:** (410)740-8692
Website: http://www.cmeonline.com/state/maryland.html

★ 21620 ★ Massachusetts Board of Examiners in Podiatry
239 Causeway St., Ste. 500
Boston, MA 02114
Phone: (617)727-4499 **Fax:** (617)727-2197
Email: hansy.noel@state.ma.us
Website: http://www.magnet.state.ma.us/reg/boards/pd/default.htm

★ 21621 ★ Michigan Consumer and Industry Services
Bureau of Health
Board of Podiatric Medicine and Surgery
PO Box 30670
Lansing, MI 48909-8170
Phone: (517)335-0918 **Fax:** (517)373-2179
Email: bhserinfo@cis.state.mi.us
Website: http://www.michigan.gov/cis/

★ 21622 ★ Minnesota Board of Podiatric Medicine
2829 University Ave. SE, Ste. 430
Minneapolis, MN 55414-3246
Phone: (612)617-2200
Website: http://www.mnworkforcecenter.org/lmi/lic_occ/podiatri.htm
Joan Benesh, Director

★ 21623 ★ Mississippi State Board of Medical Licensure
PO Box 9268
Jackson, MS 39286-9268
Phone: (601)987-3079 **Fax:** (601)987-4159
Email: mboard@msbml.state.ms.us
Website: http://www.msbml.state.ms.us/

★ 21624 ★ Missouri State Board of Podiatric Medicine
3605 Missouri Blvd.
PO Box 423
Jefferson City, MO 65102
Phone: (573)751-0873 **Fax:** (573)751-1155
Email: podiatry@mail.state.mo.us
Website: http://www.ecodev.state.mo.us/pr/podiatry/
Patricia A. Handly, Director

★ 21625 ★ Montana Department of Labor and Industry
Business Standards Division
Health Care Licensing Bureau
301 S Park
Room 430
Helena, MT 59602
Phone: (406)841-2300 **Fax:** (406)841-2305
Email: vmanuel@state.mt.us
Website: http://www.discoveringmontana.com/dli/bsd/license/licensing_boards.htm

★ 21626 ★ Nebraska Department of Health and Human Services
Regulation and Licensure
Credentialing Division
PO Box 94986
Lincoln, NE 68509-4986
Phone: (402)471-2115 **Fax:** (402)471-3577
Email: marie.mcclatchey@hhs.state.ne.us
Website: http://www.hhs.state.ne.us/reg/regindex.htm

★ 21627 ★ Nevada State Board of Podiatric Medicine
PO Box 12215
Reno, NV 89510-2215
Phone: (775)789-2605
Website: http://podiatry.state.nv.us/

★ 21628 ★ New Hampshire Board of Registration in Podiatry
2 Industrial Park Dr.
Ste. 8
Concord, NH 03301
Phone: (603)271-1203 **Fax:** (603)271-6702
Website: http://webster.state.nh.us/podiatry/
Brian Fradette, Director

★ 21629 ★ New Jersey State Board of Medical Examiners
PO Box 183
Trenton, NJ 08625-0183
Phone: (609)826-7100
Website: www.state.nj.us/lps/ca/medical.htmbme5
William Roeder, Director

★ 21630 ★ New Mexico Board of Podiatric Medicine
2055 Pacheco St., Ste. 300
Santa Fe, NM 87504
Phone: (505)476-7096

Email: PodiatryBoard@state.nm.us
Website: http://www.rld.state.nm.us/b&c/podiatry_board.htm

★ 21631 ★ New York State Board of Podiatry
Office of the Professions
State Education Bldg., 2nd Fl.
Albany, NY 12234
Phone: (518)474-3817 **Fax:** (518)474-1449
Email: podbd@mail.nysed.gov
Website: http://www.op.nysed.gov/pod.htm

★ 21632 ★ North Carolina Board of Podiatry Examiners
1500 Sunday Dr.
Ste. 102
Raleigh, NC 27607
Phone: (919)561-5583 **Fax:** (919)787-4916
Email: info@ncbpe.org
Website: http://www.ncbpe.org/

★ 21633 ★ North Dakota Board of Registry in Podiatry
PO Box 400
Bismarck, ND 58502-0400
Phone: (701)223-2890 **Fax:** (701)223-7865
Website: http://www.governor.state.nd.us/boards/boards_query.asp?Board_id=84
Gary R. Thune, Director

★ 21634 ★ Ohio State Medical Board
77 S High St., 17th Fl.
Columbus, OH 43266-0315
Phone: (614)466-3934 **Free:** 800-554-7717
Fax: (614)728-5946
Website: http://www.state.oh.us/med/

★ 21635 ★ Oklahoma Board of Medical Licensure and Supervision
Board of Podiatry
5104 N Francis, Ste. C
PO Box 18256
Oklahoma City, OK 73154-0256
Phone: (405)848-6841 **Fax:** (405)848-8240

★ 21636 ★ Oregon Board of Medical Examiners
1500 SW 1st Ave., Ste. 620
Portland, OR 97201
Phone: (503)229-5770 **Free:** 877-254-6263
Fax: (503)229-6543
Email: bme.info@state.or.us
Website: http://www.bme.state.or.us

★ 21637 ★ Pennsylvania State Board of Podiatry
PO Box 2649
Harrisburg, PA 17105-2649
Phone: (717)783-4858 **Fax:** (717)787-7769
Email: podiatry@pados.state.pa.us
Website: http://www.dos.state.pa.us/bpoa/site/default.asp

★ 21638 ★ Puerto Rico Board of Podiatry Examiners
Call Box 10200
San Juan, PR 00908-0200
Phone: (787)725-8161 **Fax:** (787)725-7903

★ 21639 ★ Rhode Island Podiatry Board
3 Capitol Hill, Rm. 104
Providence, RI 02908
Phone: (401)222-2827 **Fax:** (401)222-1272
Email: RussellS@doh.state.ri.us
Website: http://www.healthri.org/hsr/professions/podiat.htm
Russell Spaight, Contact

★ 21640 ★ South Carolina Board of Podiatric Medicine
Synergy Business Park
Kingstree Bldg.
110 Centerview Dr, suite 202
PO Box 11289
Columbia, SC 29211-1289
Phone: (803)896-4685 **Fax:** (803)896-4515
Email: podiatry@mail.llr.state.sc.us
Website: http://www.llr.state.sc.us/POL/Podiatry/Default.htm
John Volmer, Contact

★ 21641 ★ South Dakota Board of Podiatry
135 E Illinois, Ste. 214
Spearfish, SD 57783
Phone: (605)642-1600 **Fax:** (605)642-1756
Email: proflic@rushmore.com
Website: http://www.state.sd.us/dcr/podiatry/pod-home.htm
Carol Tellinghuisen, Contact

★ 21642 ★ Tennessee State Board of Registration in Podiatry
Cordell Hull Bldg., 1st Fl.
425 Fifth Ave. N
Nashville, TN 37247-1010
Phone: (615)532-3202
Website: http://www.tennesseeanytime.org

★ 21643 ★ Texas State Board of Podiatric Medical Examiners
333 Guadalupe St., Ste 2-320
PO Box 12216
Austin, TX 78711-2216
Phone: (512)305-7000 **Fax:** (512)305-7003
Email: allen.hymans@foot.tx.state.us
Website: http://www.foot.state.tx.us/
Allen Hymans, Contact

★ 21644 ★ Utah Division of Occupational and Professional Licensing
160 E 300 S, 4th Fl.
PO Box 146741
Salt Lake City, UT 84114-6741
Phone: (801)530-6628 **Fax:** (801)530-6511
Website: http://www.dopl.utah.gov/directory.html

★ 21645 ★ Vermont Board of Medical Practice
109 State St.
Montpelier, VT 05609-1106
Phone: (802)828-2673 **Fax:** (802)828-5450
Email: gloria.hurd@medbd.state.vt.us
Website: http://www.docboard.org/vt/vermont.htm
Gloria Hurd, Director

★ 21646 ★ Virginia Department of Health Professions
Virginia Board of Medicine
6606 W Broad St., 4th Fl.
Richmond, VA 23230-1717
Phone: (804)662-9908 **Fax:** (804)662-9517
Email: medbd@dhp.state.va.us
Website: http://www.dhp.state.va.us/medicine/default.htm/
William L. Harp, MD, Director

★ 21647 ★ Washington State Department of Health
Health Professions Quality Assurance
Washington State Podiatric Medical Board
1300 SE Quince St.
PO Box 47860
Olympia, WA 98504-7860
Phone: (360)236-4700 **Fax:** (360)236-4818
Email: hpqa.csc@doh.wa.gov
Website: https://wws2.wa.gov/doh/hpqa-licensing/HPS7/Podiatry/default.htm

★ 21648 ★ West Virginia State Board of Medicine
101 Dee Dr.
Charleston, WV 25311
Phone: (304)558-2921 **Fax:** (304)558-2084
Email: ronaldwalton@wvdhhr.org
Website: http://www.wvdhhr.org/wvbom/
Ronald D. Walton, Director

★ 21649 ★ Wisconsin Department of Regulation and Licensing
Wisconsin Podiatry Examining Board
1400 E Washington Ave.
PO Box 8935
Madison, WI 53708-8935
Phone: (608)266-2811
Email: web@drl.state.wi.us
Website: http://badger.state.wi.us/agencies/drl/Regulation/applicant_information/dod135.html

★ 21650 ★ Wyoming Board of Registration in Podiatry
2020 Carey Ave., Ste. 201
Cheyenne, WY 82002
Phone: (307)777-3507 **Fax:** (307)777-3508
Website: http://www.state.wy.us/governor/boards/bdlist.asp
Nanette M. Brown, Contact

Public Health

★ 21651 ★ Arizona Department of Health Services
1740 W Adams St.
Phoenix, AZ 85007
Phone: (602)542-1001 **Fax:** (602)542-0883
Email: webmaster@hs.state.az.us
Website: http://www.hs.state.az.us/
Catherine Eden, Director

★ 21652 ★ Arkansas Department of Health
4815 W Markham
PO Box 3278
Little Rock, AR 72205
Phone: (501)661-2000 **Fax:** (501)671-1450
Website: http://www.healthyarkansas.com
Fay Boozman, Director
Alt. Contact: Second office location: 5800 W. 10th St., Little Rock, AR 72204.

★ 21653 ★ California Department of Health Services
Office of Public Affairs
714 P St, Room 1350
Sacramento, CA 95814
Phone: (916)445-4171 **Fax:** (916)657-0240
Website: http://www.dhs.cahwnet.gov/

★ 21654 ★ Colorado Public Health and Environment Department
Health Office
4300 Cherry Creek Dr. S
Denver, CO 80246-1530
Phone: (303)692-2100 **Fax:** (303)782-0095
Email: cdphe.information@state.co.us
Website: http://www.cdphe.state.co.us/health-h.asp

★ 21655 ★ Connecticut Department of Public Health
410 Capitol Ave.
PO Box 340308
Hartford, CT 06134-0308
Phone: (860)509-8000 **Fax:** (860)509-7227
Email: webmaster.dph@po.state.ct.us
Website: http://www.state.ct.us/dph/
Joxel Garcia, MD, Contact

★ 21656 ★ Delaware Department of Health and Social Services
Public Health Division
Jesse Cooper Bldg.
Federal & Water Sts.
PO Box 637
Dover, DE 19903
Phone: (302)739-4701 **Fax:** (302)739-6659
Email: dhssinfo@state.de.us
Website: http://www.state.de.us/dhss/dph/dphhome.htm
Dr. Ulder Jane Tillman, Director

★ 21657 ★ District of Columbia Department of Health
Office of the Director
825 N Capitol St. NE
Washington, DC 20002
Phone: (202)442-5999 **Fax:** (202)442-4788
Website: http://www.dchealth.dc.gov

★ 21658 ★ Florida Department of Health
4052 Bald Cypress Way, Bin A00
Tallahassee, FL 32399-1701
Phone: (850)245-4443
Email: health@doh.state.fl.us
Website: http://www.doh.state.fl.us/

★ 21659 ★ Georgia Department of Human Resources
Division of Public Health
2 Peachtree St. NW
Atlanta, GA 30303-3186
Phone: (404)657-2700
Email: gdphinfo@dhr.state.ga.us
Website: http://health.state.ga.us/

★ 21660 ★ Hawaii Department of Health
1250 Punchbowl St.
Honolulu, HI 96813
Phone: (808)586-4400 **Fax:** (808)586-4444
Email: webmail@mail.health.state.hi.us
Website: http://www.state.hi.us/health/
Bruce Anderson, PhD, Director

★ 21661 ★ Idaho Department of Health and Welfare
Health Division
Pete T. Cenarrusa Bldg. 4th Fl.
450 W State St.
PO Box 83720
Boise, ID 83720-0036
Phone: (208)334-5945
Email: dhwinfor@idhw.state.id.us
Website: http://www2.state.id.us/dhw/index.htm
Richard H. Schultz, Contact

★ 21662 ★ Illinois Department of Public Health
535 W Jefferson St.
Springfield, IL 62761
Phone: (217)782-4977 **Fax:** (217)782-3987
Email: mailus@idph.state.il.us
Website: http://www.idph.state.il.us/
John R. Lumpkin, MD, Director

★ 21663 ★ Indiana State Department of Health
2 N Meridian St.
Indianapolis, IN 46204
Phone: (317)233-1325
Email: webmaster@ai.org
Website: http://www.state.in.us/doh/
Gregory A. Wilson, MD, Director

★ 21664 ★ Iowa Department of Public Health
Lucas State Office Bldg.
321 E 12th St.
Des Moines, IA 50319-0075
Phone: (515)281-5787
Email: webmaster@idph.state.ia.us
Website: http://idph.state.ia.us/
Stephen C. Gleason, Director

★ 21665 ★ Kansas Department of Health and Environment
Health Division
1000 SW Jackson, ste.300
Topeka, KS 66612-1365
Phone: (785)296-1343 **Fax:** (785)296-1562
Website: http://www.kdhe.state.ks.us/health/
Michael Moser, MD, Director

★ 21666 ★ Kentucky Health Services Cabinet
Department for Public Health
275 E Main St.
Frankfort, KY 40621
Phone: (502)564-3970 **Fax:** (502)564-9377
Email: dphwebsite@mail.state.ky.us
Website: http://publichealth.state.ky.us/
Rice C. Leach, MD, Director

★ 21667 ★ Louisiana Department of Health and Hospitals
Public Health Services Office
Metropolitan Regional Office
1001 Howard Ave., Ste. 100A
New Orleans, LA 70113
Phone: (504)599-0100 **Free:** 800-256-4609
Fax: (504)599-0200
Website: http://www.dhh.state.la.us/OPH/Regions/reg1.htm

★ 21668 ★ Louisiana Public Health Agency
Acadian Regional Office
Brandywine III, Ste. 100
825 Kaliste Saloom Rd.
Lafayette, LA 70508
Phone: (318)262-5311 **Fax:** (318)262-5237
Website: http://www.dhh.state.la.us/OPH/Regions/reg4.htm

★ 21669 ★ Louisiana Public Health Agency
Capitol Regional Office
1772 Wooddale Blvd.
Baton Rouge, LA 70806
Phone: (504)925-7200 **Fax:** (504)925-7245
Website: http://www.dhh.state.la.us/OPH/Regions/reg2.htm

★ 21670 ★ Louisiana Public Health Agency
Region III Office
206 E 3rd
Thibodaux, LA 70301
Phone: (504)447-0916 **Fax:** (504)447-0920
Website: http://www.dhh.state.la.us/OPH/Regions/reg3.htm

★ 21671 ★ Louisiana Public Health Authority
Central Regional Office
1500 Lee St.
PO Box 8199
Alexandria, LA 71306-1199
Phone: (318)487-5262 **Fax:** (318)487-5338
Website: http://www.dhh.state.la.us/OPH/Regions/reg6.htm

★ 21672 ★ Louisiana Public Health Authority
Northeast Regional Office
2913 Betin St.
PO Box 6118
Monroe, LA 71211-6118
Phone: (318)362-5211 **Fax:** (318)362-3163
Website: http://www.dhh.state.la.us/OPH/Regions/reg8.htm

★ 21673 ★ Louisiana Public Health Authority
Northwest Regional Office
1525 Fairfield Ave., Rm. 569
Shreveport, LA 71101-4388
Phone: (318)676-7489 **Fax:** (318)676-7560
Website: http://www.dhh.state.la.us/OPH/Regions/reg7.htm

★ 21674 ★ Louisiana Public Health Authority
Southeast Regional Office
520 Old Spanish Tr., Ste. 100
Slidell, LA 70458
Phone: (504)646-6459 **Fax:** (504)646-6476
Website: http://www.dhh.state.la.us/OPH/Regions/reg9.htm

★ 21675 ★ Lousiana Public Health Authority
Southwest Regional Office
4240 Senator J. Bennett Johnston Ave.
Lake Charles, LA 70615
Phone: (318)491-2040 **Fax:** (318)491-2041
Website: http://www.dhh.state.la.us/OPH/Regions/reg5.htm

★ 21676 ★ Maine Bureau of Health
11 State House Station
157 Capitol St.
Augusta, ME 04333
Phone: (207)287-8016
Email: marcie.sanders@state.me.us
Website: http://www.state.me.us/dhs/boh/index.htm
Lani Graham, MD, Director

★ 21677 ★ Maine Department of Human Services
Health Bureau
11 State House Station
157 Capitol St.
Augusta, ME 04333
Phone: (207)287-8016
Email: kerry.bagley@state.me.us
Website: http://janus.state.me.us/dhs/boh/index.htm
Marcie Sanders, MD, Contact

★ 21678 ★ Maryland Department of Health and Mental Hygiene
Community and Public Health Administration
201 W Preston St., 3rd Fl.
Baltimore, MD 21201
Phone: (410)767-5300
Email: webmaster@dhmh.state.md.us
Website: http://mdpublichealth.org/
Georges C. Benjamin, Contact

★ 21679 ★ Massachusetts Department of Public Health
250 Washington St.
Boston, MA 02108-4619
Phone: (617)624-6000
Email: dph.info@state.ma.us
Website: http://www.state.ma.us/dph/
Howard Koh, MD, Director

★ 21680 ★ Michigan Department of Community Health
Lewis Cass Bldg., 6th Fl.
320 S Walnut St.
Lansing, MI 48913
Phone: (517)373-3500 **Fax:** (517)335-3090
Email: arias@state.mi.us
Website: http://www.mdch.state.mi.us/

★ 21681 ★ Minnesota Department of Health
717 Delaware St. SE
PO Box 64975
Minneapolis, MN 55440-9441
Phone: (651)215-5800 **Fax:** (651)623-5043
Email: library@health.state.mn.us
Website: http://www.health.state.mn.us/

★ 21682 ★ Mississippi State Department of Health
State Board of Health Bldg.
570 E Woodrow Wilson
PO Box 1700
Jackson, MS 39215-1700
Phone: (601)576-7400 **Fax:** (601)576-7364
Email: info@msdh.state.ms.us
Website: http://www.msdh.state.ms.us/

★ 21683 ★ Mississippi State Department of Health
Public Health Statistics
571 Stadium Dr.
PO Box 1700
Jackson, MS 39215-1700
Phone: (601)576-7960 **Fax:** (601)576-7505
Website: http://www.msdh.state.ms.us/phs/index.htm

★ 21684 ★ Missouri Department of Health
920-930 Wildwood Dr.
PO Box 570
Jefferson City, MO 65102-0570
Phone: (573)751-6400 **Fax:** (573)751-6010
Email: info@mail.health.state.mo.us
Website: http://www.health.state.mo.us/
Maureen Dempsey, MD, Director

★ 21685 ★ Montana Department of Public Health and Human Services
Health Policy and Services Division
Cogswell Bldg.
1400 Broadway
PO Box 202951
Helena, MT 59620
Phone: (406)444-4540 **Fax:** (406)444-1861
Email: nellery@state.mt.gov
Website: http://www.dphhs.state.mt.us/divisions/hps/hps_phone.htm
Maggie Bullock, Contact

★ 21686 ★ Nebraska Department of Health and Human Services
Department of Services
PO Box 95044
Lincoln, NE 68509-5044
Phone: (402)471-2306
Email: hhsinfo@www.hhs.state.ne.us
Website: http://www.hhs.state.ne.us/svc/svcindex.htm
Ron Ross, Director

★ 21687 ★ Nevada State Health Division
Administrative Office
505 E King St., Rm. 201
Carson City, NV 89701
Phone: (775)684-4200 **Fax:** (775)684-4211
Website: http://www.state.nv.us/health/

★ 21688 ★ New Hampshire Department of Health and Human Services
Office of Administration
129 Pleasant St.
Concord, NH 03301-3857
Phone: (603)271-4814 **Fax:** (603)271-5590
Website: http://www.dhhs.state.nh.us/

★ 21689 ★ New Jersey Department of Health and Senior Services
John Fitch Plaza
PO Box 360
Trenton, NJ 08625-0360
Phone: (609)292-7837
Website: http://www.state.nj.us/health/
Christine Grant, Director

★ 21690 ★ New Mexico Department of Health
Public Health Division
Harold Runnels Bldg.
1190 St. Francis Dr.
Santa Fe, NM 87504
Phone: (505)827-2613
Website: http://www.health.state.nm.us/

★ 21691 ★ New York State Department of Health
Corning Tower
Empire State Plaza
Albany, NY 12237
Phone: (518)474-2011
Email: nyhealth@health.state.ny.us
Website: http://www.health.state.ny.us/
Maryellen Jacobson, Secretary

★ 21692 ★ North Carolina Department of Health and Human Services
Health Director's Office
Adams Bldg.
101 Blair Dr.
2001 Mail Service Ctr.
Raleigh, NC 27699-2001
Phone: (919)733-4534 **Free:** 800-662-7030
Fax: (919)715-4645
Website: http://www.dhhs.state.nc.us/docs/divinfo/secretary.htm
Carmen Hooker Odom, MD, Secretary

★ 21693 ★ North Dakota Department of Health
600 E Boulevard Ave.
Bismarck, ND 58505-0200
Phone: (701)328-2372 **Fax:** (701)328-4727
Email: ajohnson@state.nd.us
Website: http://www.health.state.nd.us/
Terry Dwelle, Director

★ 21694 ★ Ohio Department of Health
246 N High St.
PO Box 118
Columbus, OH 43215
Phone: (614)466-3543 **Fax:** (614)644-0085
Website: http://www.odh.state.oh.us/
J. Nick Baird, Director

★ 21695 ★ Oklahoma State Department of Health
1000 NE 10th St.
Oklahoma City, OK 73117
Phone: (405)271-5600
Email: webmaster@health.state.ok.us
Website: http://www.health.state.ok.us/
Leslie M. Beitsch, MD, Director

★ 21696 ★ Oregon Department of Human Resources
Health Division
Portland State Office Bldg.
800 NE Oregon St., No. 21
Portland, OR 97232
Phone: (503)731-4000
Email: ohd.info@state.or.us
Website: http://www.ohd.hr.state.or.us/
Martin Wasserman, Director

★ 21697 ★ Pennsylvania Department of Health
Health and Welfare Bldg.
PO Box 90
Harrisburg, PA 17108
Phone: (717)787-6436
Email: webmaster@health.state.pa.us
Website: http://www.health.state.pa.us/
Robert Zimmerman, Director

★ 21698 ★ Rhode Island Department of Health
3 Capitol Hill
Providence, RI 02908
Phone: (401)222-2231 **Free:** 800-745-5555
Fax: (401)222-6548
Email: library@health.state.ri.us
Website: http://www.health.state.ri.us/
Patricia A. Nolan, MD, Director

★ 21699 ★ South Carolina Department of Health and Environmental Control
Health Services Office
2600 Bull St.
PO Box 101106
Columbia, SC 29211-0106
Phone: (803)898-3432
Website: http://www.scdhec.net/hs/

★ 21700 ★ South Dakota Department of Health
Health Bldg.
600 E Capitol
Pierre, SD 57501-2536
Phone: (605)773-3361 **Free:** 800-738-2301
Email: DOH.INFO@state.sd.us
Website: http://www.state.sd.us/doh/
Doneen Hollingsworth, Secretary

★ 21701 ★ Tennessee Department of Health
Health Statistics and Information
Cordell Hull Bldg., 4th Fl.
425 5th Ave. N
Nashville, TN 37247-5262
Phone: (615)741-1954 **Fax:** (615)532-7904
Email: DDenton@mail.state.tn.us
Website: http://www.state.tn.us/health/statistics/

★ 21702 ★ Texas Department of Health
1100 W 49th St.
Austin, TX 78756-3199
Phone: (512)458-7111 **Free:** 888-963-7111
Email: webmaster@tdh.state.tx.us
Website: http://www.tdh.texas.gov/

★ 21703 ★ Utah Department of Health
PO Box 1010
Salt Lake City, UT 84114-1010
Phone: (801)538-6101
Email: pwightma@doh.state.ut.us
Website: http://www.health.state.ut.us/

★ 21704 ★ Vermont Department of Health
108 Cherry St.
PO Box 70
Burlington, VT 05402-0070
Phone: (802)863-7200 **Fax:** (802)865-7754
Email: webkeeper@vdh.state.vt.us
Website: http://www.healthyvermonters.info/

★ 21705 ★ Virgin Islands Department of Health
St. Thomas Hospital
48 Sugar Estate
Charlotte Amalie, VI 00802
Phone: (340)774-0117 **Fax:** (340)777-4001
Website: http://www.usvi.org/health/index.html

★ 21706 ★ Virginia Office of Health and Human Resources
Health Department
Main St. Station
1500 E Main St., Ste. 214
Richmond, VA 23219
Phone: (804)786-3561
Email: rnash@vdh.state.va.us
Website: http://www.vdh.state.va.us/
Robert B. Stroube, MD, Director

★ 21707 ★ Washington State Department of Health
1112 SE Quince St.
PO Box 47890
Olympia, WA 98504-7890
Phone: (360)236-4010 **Free:** 800-525-0127
Email: doh.webmaster@doh.wa.gov
Website: http://www.doh.wa.gov/
Mary Selecky, Director

★ 21708 ★ West Virginia Department of Health and Human Resources
Public Health Bureau
350 Capitol St., Rm. 702
Charleston, WV 25301-3712
Phone: (304)558-2971 **Fax:** (304)558-1035
Website: http://www.wvdhhr.org/bph/
Henry G. Taylor, MD, Director

★ 21709 ★ Wisconsin Department of Health and Family Services
Public Health Division
PO Box 2659
Madison, WI 53701-2659
Phone: (608)266-1251 **Fax:** (608)267-2832
Email: webmaster@dhfs.state.wi.us
Website: http://www.dhfs.state.wi.us/aboutdhfs/dph/dphservs.htm
John Chapin, Director

★ 21710 ★ Wyoming Department of Health
Public Health Division
117 Hathaway Bldg.
Cheyenne, WY 82002
Phone: (307)777-7656 **Fax:** (307)777-7327
Email: wdh@state.wy.us
Website: http://wdhfs.state.wy.us/WDH/
Garry L. McKee, PhD, Director

Rehabilitation

★ 21711 ★ Alabama Department of Rehabilitation Services
2129 E S Blvd.
Montgomery, AL 36116
Phone: (334)281-8780 **Free:** 800-441-7607
Fax: (334)281-1973
Email: webinfo@rehab.state.al.us
Website: http://www.rehab.state.al.us/
Steve Shivers, Director

★ 21712 ★ Alaska Department of Labor and Workforce Development
Vocational Rehabilitation Division
801 W 10th St., Ste. 1A
Juneau, AK 99801-1894
Phone: (907)465-2814 **Free:** 800-478-2815
Fax: (907)465-2856
Email: Vikki_Parson@labor.state.ak.us
Website: http://www.labor.state.ak.us/dvr/home.htm
Duane French, Director

★ 21713 ★ Arizona Department of Economic Security
Employment and Rehabilitation Services Division
Rehabilitation Services Administration
Site Code 733A
PO Box 6123
Phoenix, AZ 85005
Phone: (602)542-3871 **Fax:** (602)542-6474
Email: azrsa@cirs.org
Website: http://www.de.state.az.us/links/economic/webpage/page6.html

★ 21714 ★ Arkansas Department of Education
Rehabilitation Services Division
1616 Brookwood Dr.
Little Rock, AR 72203
Phone: (501)296-1600 **Free:** 800-330-0632
Fax: (501)296-1655
Website: http://www.ark.org/ars/

★ 21715 ★ California Health and Welfare Agency
Rehabilitation Department
PO Box 944222
Sacramento, CA 94244-2220
Phone: (916)263-8681 **Fax:** (916)327-4567
Email: suggest@rehab.cahwnet.gov
Website: http://www.rehab.ca.gov/

★ 21716 ★ Colorado Department of Human Services
Rehabilitation Services Division
2211 West Evans, Bldg. B
Denver, CO 80223
Phone: (720)884-1234 **Fax:** (720)884-1213
Email: debbie.powell@state.co.us
Website: http://www.cdhs.state.co.us/ods/dvr/index.html
Diana Huerta, Director

★ 21717 ★ Connecticut Department of Social Services
Rehabilitation Services Bureau
25 Sigourney St.
Hartford, CT 06105-5033
Phone: (860)424-4848 **Free:** 800-842-1508
Email: brs.dss@po.state.ct.us
Website: http://www.dss.state.ct.us/svcs/rehab.htm

★ 21718 ★ Delaware Department of Labor
Vocational Rehabilitation Division
4425 N Market St.
P.O.Box 9969
Wilmington, DE 19801
Phone: (302)761-8275 **Fax:** (302)761-6611
Email: dlabor@state.de.us
Website: http://www.delawareworks.com/divisions/dvr/welcome.htm
Andrea S. Guest, Director

★ 21719 ★ Florida Department of Labor and Employment Security
Vocational Rehabilitation Division
2002 Old St. Augustine Rd., Bldg. A
Tallahassee, FL 32399-0696
Phone: (850)488-6210 **Free:** 800-451-4327
Fax: (850)921-7215
Website: http://www.rehabworks.org/

★ 21720 ★ Georgia Department of Human Resources
Rehabilitation Services Division
2 Peachtree St. NW, Ste. 376-S
Atlanta, GA 30303
Phone: (404)206-6000 **Fax:** (404)206-6011
Email: defennel@dhr.state.ga.us
Website: http://www.vocrehabga.org/

★ 21721 ★ Idaho Board of Education
Vocational Education Division
650 W State St., Rm. 324
PO Box 83720
Boise, ID 83720-0095
Phone: (208)334-3216 **Fax:** (208)334-2365
Email: bmoench@pte.state.id.us
Website: http://www.pte.state.id.us/
Dr. Mike Rush, Director

★ 21722 ★ Illinois Department of Human Services
Rehabilitation Services Bureau
100 S Grand Ave. East 3rd Flr.
PO Box 19429
Springfield, IL 62762
Phone: (217)785-0234 **Free:** 800-225-3607
Fax: (217)558-4270
Email: ors@dhs.state.il.us
Website: http://WWW.STATE.il.us/agency/dhs/rsnp.html
Carl Suter, Director

★ 21723 ★ Indiana Family and Social Services Administration
Disability, Aging and Rehabilitative Services Division
402 W Washington St.
PO Box 7083
Indianapolis, IN 46207-7083
Phone: (317)232-1147 **Free:** 800-545-7763
Fax: (317)233-4693
Email: webmaster@ai.org
Website: http://www.state.in.us/fssa/HTML/PROGRAMS/2b.html

★ 21724 ★ Iowa Department of Education
Vocational Rehabilitation Division
510 E 12th St.
Des Moines, IA 50319
Phone: (515)281-6731 **Free:** 800-532-1486
Fax: (515)281-4703
Email: dcarlson@dvrs.state.ia.us
Dwight R. Carlson, Director

★ 21725 ★ Kansas Department of Social and Rehabilitation Services
Rehabilitation Services Division
915 SW Harrison St.
Topeka, KS 66612
Phone: (785)296-3959 **Fax:** (785)296-2173
Website: http://www.srskansas.org/ISD.htm

★ 21726 ★ Kentucky Workforce Development Cabinet
Vocational Rehabilitation Department
209 St. Clair St., 2d Fl.
Frankfort, KY 40601
Phone: (502)564-4440 **Free:** 800-372-7172
Fax: (502)564-6742
Email: wfd.vocrehab@mail.state.ky.us

Website: http://kydvr.state.ky.us/

★ 21727 ★ Louisiana Department of Social Services
Rehabilitation Services Division
8225 Florida Blvd.
PO Box 94371
Baton Rouge, LA 70806
Phone: (225)725-4131 **Free:** 800-737-2958
Fax: (225)925-4484
Email: webmaster@dss.state.la.us
Website: http://www.dss.state.la.us/offlrs/index.htm
Ed Barras, Contact

★ 21728 ★ Maine Department of Labor
Rehabilitation Services Office
150 State House Station
Augusta, ME 04333-0150
Phone: (207)624-5950 **Fax:** (207)624-5980
Email: John.G.Shattuck@state.me.us
Website: http://janus.state.me.us/labor/brs/vr.htm

★ 21729 ★ Maryland Department of Education
Vocational Rehabilitation Division
2301 Argonne Dr.
Baltimore, MD 21218-1696
Phone: (410)554-9385 **Fax:** (410)554-9412
Email: dors@msde.state.md.us
Website: http://www.dors.state.md.us/voc_rehab.html

★ 21730 ★ Massachusetts Rehabilitation Commission
Fort Point Pl. Ste. 600
27 Wormwood St.
Boston, MA 02210-1616
Phone: (617)204-3600 **Free:** 800-245-6543
Fax: (617)727-1354
Email: Robert.Donahue@mrc.state.ma.us
Website: http://www.magnet.state.ma.us/mrc/mrc.htm

★ 21731 ★ Michigan Jobs Commission
Rehabilitation Services Division
The Open Door Employment & Disability Network
608 W Allegan
PO Box 30010
Lansing, MI 48909
Phone: (517)373-3390 **Free:** 800-605-6722
Fax: (517)373-0565
Website: http://www.mrs.mjc.state.mi.us/

★ 21732 ★ Minnesota Economic Security Department
Rehabilitation Services Division
390 N Robert St.
Saint Paul, MN 55101
Phone: (651)296-5616 **Free:** 800-328-9095
Email: Howard.Glad@state.mn.us
Website: http://www.mnworkforcecenter.org/burgundy/rehab.htm
Howard Glad, Contact

★ 21733 ★ Mississippi Department of Rehabilitation Services
1281 Hwy. 51 N
Madison, MS 39110
Phone: (601)853-5100 **Free:** 800-443-1000
Fax: (601)853-5205
Email: bmcmillan@mdrs.state.ms.us
Website: http://www.mdrs.state.ms.us/
H.S. McMillan, Director

★ 21734 ★ Missouri Department of Elementary and Secondary Education
Vocational Rehabilitation Division
3024 Dupont Cir.
Jefferson City, MO 65109-0525
Phone: (573)751-3251 **Free:** 877-222-8963
Fax: (573)751-1441
Email: kkendle@movr.dese.state.mo.us
Website: http://www.dese.state.mo.us/divvocrehab/

★ 21735 ★ Montana Department of Public Health and Human Services
Vocational Rehabilitation Program
111 N Sanders, Ste. 307
PO Box 4210
Helena, MT 59604-4210
Phone: (406)444-2590 **Free:** 877-296-1197
Fax: (406)444-3632
Email: jmathews@state.mt.gov
Website: http://www.dphhs.state.mt.us/dsd/govt_programs/vrp/index.htm

★ 21736 ★ Nebraska Department of Education
Rehabilitation Services Division
301 Centennial Mall S
PO Box 94987
Lincoln, NE 68509-4987
Phone: (402)471-6329 **Free:** 800-472-3382
Fax: (402)471-0117
Email: a_sumner@vocrehab.state.ne.us
Website: http://www.vocrehab.state.ne.us/
Frank C. Lloyd, Director

★ 21737 ★ Nevada Department of Employment Training and Rehabilitation
Rehabilitation Division
Vocational Rehabilitation Bureau
505 E King St., Rm. 501
Carson City, NV 89701-3704
Phone: (775)684-4070 **Fax:** (775)684-4161
Email: detrinfo@govmail.state.nv.us
Website: http://detr.state.nv.us/rehab/reh_vorh.htm

★ 21738 ★ New Hampshire Department of Education
Vocational Rehabilitation Bureau
78 Regional Dr., Bldg.2
Concord, NH 03301
Phone: (603)271-3471 **Free:** 800-299-1647
Fax: (603)271-7095
Email: jchaput@ed.state.nh.us
Website: http://www.ed.state.nh.us/adulted/adult.htm
Paul K. Leather, Director

★ 21739 ★ New Jersey Department of Labor
Vocational Rehabilitation Services Division
135 E State St.
PO Box 398
Trenton, NJ 08625-0398
Phone: (609)292-5987 **Fax:** (609)292-8347
Email: dvradmin@dol.state.nj.us
Website: http://www.state.nj.us/labor/dvrs/dvr.html
Thomas G. Jennings, Director

★ 21740 ★ New Mexico Department of Education
Vocational Rehabilitation Division
435-D St. Michaels Dr., Bldg. D
Santa Fe, NM 87505
Phone: (505)954-8500 **Free:** 800-224-7005
Fax: (505)954-8562
Email: afox@state.nm.us
Website: http://www.state.nm.us/dvr/
Amber Fox, Contact

★ 21741 ★ New York State Department of Education
Developmental Disabilities Planning Council
155 Washington Ave., 2nd Fl.
Albany, NY 12210
Phone: (518)486-7505 **Free:** 800-395-3372
Fax: (518)402-3505
Email: ddpc@ddpc.state.ny.us
Website: http://www.ddpc.state.ny.us/

★ 21742 ★ North Carolina Department of Health and Human Services
Vocational Rehabilitation Services Division
805 Ruggles Dr.
2801 Mail Service Ctr.
Raleigh, NC 27603-2038
Phone: (919)733-3364 **Fax:** (919)733-7968
Email: dvr.information@ncmail.net
Website: http://dvr.dhhs.state.nc.us/
Bob Philbeck, Director

★ 21743 ★ North Dakota Department of Human Services
Disability Services
600 S Second St.
Bismarck, ND 58504-5729
Phone: (701)328-8930 **Free:** 800-755-8529
Fax: (701)328-8969
Email: soperc@state.nd.us
Website: http://lnotes.state.nd.us/dhs/dhsweb.nsf/ServicePages/DisabilityServices

★ 21744 ★ Ohio Rehabilitation Services Commission
Vocational Rehabilitation Bureau
400 E Campus View Blvd., SW3C
Columbus, OH 43235-4604
Phone: (614)438-1250 **Free:** 800-282-4536
Fax: (614)438-1257
Email: beverly.jennings@rsc.state.oh.us
Website: http://www.state.oh.us/rsc/VR_Services/BVR/bvr.html
June K. Gutterman, Director

★ 21745 ★ Oklahoma Department of Rehabilitation Services
Rehabilitative Services Bureau
3535 NW 58th St., Ste 500
Oklahoma City, OK 73112
Phone: (405)951-3400 **Free:** 800-845-8476
Fax: (405)951-3259
Website: http://www.okrehab.org/

★ 21746 ★ Oregon Department of Human Resources
Vocational Rehabilitation Division
500 Summer St., NE
E87
Salem, OR 97301-1120
Phone: (503)945-5880 **Fax:** (503)947-5010
Email: dhr.info@state.or.us
Website: http://vrdweb.hr.state.or.us/

★ 21747 ★ Pennsylvania Department of Labor and Industry
Vocational Rehabilitation Office
909 Green St.
Harrisburg, PA 17102
Phone: (717)787-5244 **Free:** 800-442-6351
Email: ovr@dli.state.pa.us
Website: http://www.dli.state.pa.us/landi/cwp/view.asp?a=128&Q=168255

★ 21748 ★ Puerto Rico Department of Social Services
Vocational Rehabilitation Administration
PO Box 191118
San Juan, PR 00919-1118
Phone: (787)729-0160 **Fax:** (787)728-8070
Email: webmaster@govpr.org
Website: http://fortaleza.govpr.org/

★ 21749 ★ Rhode Island Department of Human Services
Community Services
Vocatonal Rehabilitation Services
40 Fountain St.
Providence, RI 02903
Phone: (401)421-7005 **Fax:** (401)222-3574
Website: http://www.ors.state.ri.us/vocpage.htm

★ 21750 ★ South Carolina Department of Vocational Rehabilitation
1410 Boston Ave.
PO Box 15
West Columbia, SC 29171
Phone: (803)896-6504 **Fax:** (803)896-6529
Email: info@scvrd.state.sc.us
Website: http://www.scvrd.net
Larry Bryant, Director

★ 21751 ★ South Dakota Department of Human Services
Rehabilitation Services Division
Hillsview Plaza, E Hwy 34
500 E Capitol
Pierre, SD 57501-5070
Phone: (605)773-3195 **Fax:** (605)773-5483
Email: eric.weiss@state.sd.us
Website: http://www.state.sd.us/dhs/drs/
Grady Kickul, Director

★ 21752 ★ Tennessee Department of Human Services
Rehabilitation Services Division
400 Deaderick St.
15th floor
Nashville, TN 37248-0060
Phone: (615)313-4714 **Fax:** (615)741-4165
Website: http://www.state.tn.us/humanserv/
Carl Brown, Contact

★ 21753 ★ Texas Rehabilitation Commission
4900 N Lamar Blvd.
Austin, TX 78751
Phone: (512)424-4000 **Free:** 800-628-5115
Website: http://www.rehab.state.tx.us/
Vernon Arrell, Director

★ 21754 ★ Utah Rehabilitation Office
Rehabilitation Services Division
250 E 500 S
Salt Lake City, UT 84111
Phone: (801)538-7530 **Fax:** (801)538-7522
Website: http://www.usor.state.ut.us/

★ 21755 ★ Vermont Agency of Human Services
Social and Rehabilitation Services Department
Vocational Rehabilitation Division
Planning and Evaluation Division
103 S Main St.
Waterbury, VT 05671-2401
Phone: (802)241-2131 **Fax:** (802)241-2407
Email: webmaster@srs.state.vt.us
Website: http://www.state.vt.us/srs
Don Mandelkorn, Director

★ 21756 ★ Virgin Islands Department of Human Services
Disabilities and Rehabilitation Services Division
Roy Lester Schneider Hospital
Knud Hansen Complex, Bldg. A 1303
Hospital Ground
St. Thomas, VI 00802
Phone: (340)774-0930 **Fax:** (340)774-3466
Email: humanservices@usvi.org
Website: http://www.usvi.org/humanservices/index.html

★ 21757 ★ Virginia Office of Health and Human Resources
Rehabilitative Services Department
8004 Franklin Farms Dr.
PO Box K300
Richmond, VA 23288
Phone: (804)662-7000 **Free:** 800-552-5019
Fax: (804)662-9140
Email: drs@drs.state.va.us
Website: http://www.vadrs.org/

★ 21758 ★ Washington Department of Social and Health Services
Health and Rehabilitative Services Office
Vocational Rehabilitation Division
PO Box 45340
Olympia, WA 98504-5060
Phone: (360)438-8000 **Free:** 800-637-5627
Fax: (360)438-8007
Website: http://www1.dshs.wa.gov/dvr/index.htm

★ 21759 ★ West Virginia State Board of Education and the Arts
Rehabilitation Services Division
State Capitol Complex
PO Box 50890
Charleston, WV 25305-0890
Phone: (304)766-4600 **Free:** 800-642-8207
Fax: (304)766-4905
Email: penneyh@mail.drs.state.wv.us
Website: http://www.wvdrs.org/
Janice Holland, Director

★ 21760 ★ Wisconsin Department of Workforce Development
Vocational Rehabilitation Division
2917 International Ln., Ste. 300
PO Box 7852
Madison, WI 53707-7852
Phone: (608)243-5600 **Free:** 800-442-3477
Fax: (608)243-5680
Email: dwddvr@dwd.state.wi.us
Website: http://www.dwd.state.wi.us/dvr/

★ 21761 ★ Wyoming Department of Employment
Vocational Rehabilitation Division
1100 Herschler Bldg.
122 W 25th St.
Cheyenne, WY 82002
Phone: (307)777-7389 **Fax:** (307)777-5939
Email: jmcint@state.wy.us
Website: http://wydoe.state.wy.us/doe.asp?ID=5
Gary W. Child, Director

Substance Abuse

★ 21762 ★ Alabama Department of Mental Health and Mental Retardation
Substance Abuse Services Division
100 N Union St.
PO Box 301410
Montgomery, AL 36130-1410
Phone: (334)242-3107
Website: http://www.mh.state.al.us/services/sa/samain.html
John Houston, Contact

★ 21763 ★ Alaska Department of Health and Social Services
Alcoholism and Drug Abuse Division
240 Main St., Ste. 701
PO Box 110607
Juneau, AK 99811-0607
Phone: (907)465-2071 **Free:** 800-478-2072
Fax: (907)465-2185
Website: http://www.hss.state.ak.us/dada/
Carl Lewis, Contact

★ 21764 ★ Arizona Department of Health Services
Behavioral Health Services Division
Substance Abuse Office
2122 E Highland
Phoenix, AZ 85016
Phone: (602)381-8999 **Fax:** (602)553-9143
Email: cdye@hs.state.az.us
Website: http://www.hs.state.az.us/bhs/bsagmh.htm

★ 21765 ★ Arkansas Department of Health
Alcohol and Drug Abuse Prevention Division
4815 W Markham
Little Rock, AR 72205
Phone: (501)280-4500 **Fax:** (501)280-4519
Website: http://health.state.ar.us/
Tommie J. Waters, Contact

★ 21766 ★ California Health and Welfare Agency
Alcohol and Drug Programs Department
1700 K St.
Sacramento, CA 95814
Phone: (916)445-1943
Website: http://www.adp.cahwnet.gov

★ 21767 ★ Colorado Department of Human Services
Alcohol and Drug Abuse Division
4055 S Lowell Blvd.
Denver, CO 80236
Phone: (303)866-7480 **Fax:** (303)866-7481
Email: randall.deyle@state.co.us
Website: http://www.cdhs.state.co.us/ohr/adad/index.html
Janet Wood, Director

★ 21768 ★ Connecticut Department of Mental Health and Addiction Services
Addiction Services
410 Capitol Ave., 4th Fl.
PO Box 341431
Hartford, CT 06134
Phone: (860)418-7000 **Free:** 800-446-7348
Website: http://www.dmhas.state.ct.us/

★ 21769 ★ Delaware Department of Health and Social Services
Alcoholism, Drug Abuse, and Mental Health Division
1901 N Dupont Hwy.
New Castle, DE 19720
Phone: (302)255-9247 **Fax:** (302)255-4427
Email: dhssinfo@state.de.us
Website: http://www.state.de.us/dhss/dadamh/dmhhome.htm
Renata J. Henry, Director

★ 21770 ★ District of Columbia Department of Human Services
Public Health Commission
Alcohol and Drug Abuse Administration
1300 1st St., NE
Washington, DC 20002
Phone: (202)727-9393 **Fax:** (202)727-0092
Website: http://www.dchealth.com/welcome.htm

★ 21771 ★ Florida Department of Children and Families
Human Services Program Office
Alcohol, Drug Abuse and Mental Health Office
1317 Winewood Blvd. Bldg. 6 Room 300
Tallahassee, FL 32399-0700
Phone: (850)487-2920
Website: http://www5.myflorida.com/cf_web/myflorida2/healthhuman/ddp/

★ 21772 ★ Georgia Department of Human Resources
Mental Health, Developmental Disabilities, Addictive Diseases
Alcohol and Drug Abuse Services Office
2 Peachtree St., NW
Atlanta, GA 30303
Phone: (404)657-2272 **Fax:** (404)657-2107
Email: xwiggins@dmh.dhr.state.ga.us
Website: http://www2.state.ga.us/departments/dhr/mhmrsa.html

★ 21773 ★ Hawaii Department of Health
Behavioral Health Administration
Alcohol and Drug Abuse Division
601 Kamokila Blvd.
Kapolei, HI 96707
Phone: (808)692-7506
Website: http://www.state.hi.us/health/resource/drug_abuse.html
Elaine J. Wilson, Director

★ 21774 ★ Idaho Department of Health and Welfare
Family and Community Services Division
Substance Abuse Bureau
450 W State St., 5th Fl.
PO Box 83720
Boise, ID 83720-0036
Phone: (208)334-5593 **Free:** 800-926-2588
Fax: (208)334-6699
Email: connorc@idhw.state.id.us
Website: http://www2.state.id.us/dhw/mentalhealth/index.htm
Pharis Stanger, Contact

★ 21775 ★ Indiana Family and Social Services Administration
Addiction Services Division
Division of Mental Health
402 W Washington St., Rm. W353
Indianapolis, IN 46204-2739
Phone: (317)232-7939 **Free:** 800-901-1133
Fax: (317)233-3472
Website: http://www.ai.org/fssa/dmh/index.html
Janet Corson, Director

★ 21776 ★ Iowa Department of Public Health
Substance Abuse and Health Promotion Division
Lucas State Office Bldg.
321 E 12th St.
Des Moines, IA 50319
Phone: (515)281-4417
Email: webmaster@idph.state.ia.us
Website: http://idph.state.ia.us/SA.HTM

★ 21777 ★ Kansas Department of Social and Rehabilitation Services
Alcohol and Drug Abuse Services
915 SW Harrison St.
Topeka, KS 66612
Phone: (785)296-3271
Website: http://www.srskansas.org/hcp/mhsatr/mhsatr.htm
Janet Schalansky, Contact

★ 21778 ★ Kentucky Health Services Cabinet
Mental Health and Mental Retardation Department
Substance Abuse Division
100 Fair Oaks Ln, 4E-D
Frankfort, KY 40621-0001
Phone: (502)564-2880 **Fax:** (502)564-7152
Email: webmaster@rdmc.org
Website: http://dmhmrs.chr.state.ky.us/SA/

★ 21779 ★ Louisiana Department of Health and Hospitals
Louisiana Office for Addictive Disorders
1201 Capitol Access Rd.
PO Box 2790, Bin 18
Baton Rouge, LA 70821-2790
Phone: (225)342-6717 **Fax:** (225)342-3875
Email: webmaster@dhh.state.la.us
Website: http://www.dhh.state.la.us/OADA/index.htm

★ 21780 ★ Maine Office of the Governor
Substance Abuse Office
159 State House Station
A.M.H.I. Complex, Marquardt Buidling
Augusta, ME 04333-0159
Phone: (207)287-2595 **Fax:** (207)287-4334
Email: kimberly.johnson@state.me.us
Website: http://www.state.me.us/dmhmrsa/osa/
Kimberly Johnson, Contact

★ 21781 ★ Maryland Department of Health and Mental Hygiene
Alcohol and Drug Abuse Administration
55 Wade Ave.
Catonsville, MD 21228
Phone: (410)402-8600 **Fax:** (410)402-8601
Email: adaainfo@dhmh.state.md.us
Website: http://maryland-adaa.org/
Peter F. Luongo, PhD, Director

★ 21782 ★ Massachusetts Executive Office of Health and Human Services
Public Health Department
Substance Abuse Services Bureau
250 Washington St., 3rd Fl.
Boston, MA 02108
Phone: (617)624-5111 **Fax:** (617)624-5185
Email: BSAS.questions@state.ma.us
Website: http://www.state.ma.us/dph/bsas/bsas.htm
Deborah Klein Walker, Director

★ 21783 ★ Michigan Community Health Department
Drug Control and Substance Abuse Services Office
Lewis Cass Bldg, 6th floor
320 S Walnut St.
Lansing, MI 48913
Phone: (517)373-3500 **Fax:** (517)335-2671
Email: yaldooc@michigan.gov
Website: http://www.michigan.gov/mdch/
Craig Yaldoo, Director

★ 21784 ★ Minnesota Department of Human Services
Health and Continuing Care Strategies
Chemical Health Division
444 Lafayette Rd. N
Saint Paul, MN 55155
Phone: (651)582-1832
Email: dhs.info@state.mn.us
Website: http://www.dhs.state.mn.us/contcare/default.htm

★ 21785 ★ Missouri Department of Mental Health
Alcohol and Drug Abuse Division
1706 E Elm St.
PO Box 687
Jefferson City, MO 65102
Phone: (573)751-4942
Email: dmhmail@mail.dmh.state.mo.us
Website: http://www.modmh.state.mo.us/ada/index.html
Michael Couty, Director

★ 21786 ★ Montana Department of Public Health and Human Services
Addictive and Mental Disorders Division
PO Box 202905
PO Box 202951
Helena, MT 59620-2905
Phone: (406)444-3964 **Fax:** (406)444-4435
Email: daanderson@state.mt.gov
Website: http://www.dphhs.state.mt.us/divisions/amd/amd.htm
Dan Anderson, Director

★ 21787 ★ Nebraska Department of Health and Human Services
Mental Health, Substance Abuse and Addiction Services Office
PO Box 98925
Lincoln, NE 68509-8925
Phone: (402)479-5166
Email: hhsinfo@www.hhs.state.ne.us
Website: http://www.hhs.state.ne.us/sua/beh_sua.htm
Ron Sorensen, Director

★ 21788 ★ Nevada Department of Employment Training and Rehabilitation
Rehabilitation Division
Alcohol and Drug Abuse Bureau
500 E 3rd St.
Carson City, NV 89713-0021
Phone: (775)687-4790
Email: detrvr@nvdetr.org
Website: http://detr.state.nv.us/rehab/reh%5Fgen.htm

★ 21789 ★ New Hampshire Department of Health and Human Services
Alcohol & Drug Abuse Prevention & Recovery Division
105 Pleasant St.
Concord, NH 03301-3857
Phone: (603)271-6100 **Fax:** (603)271-6116
Website: http://www.dhhs.state.nh.us/

★ 21790 ★ New Jersey Department of Health
Addiction Services Division
120 S Stockton St.
PO Box 362
Trenton, NJ 08625-0362
Phone: (609)984-0895
Email: tpb@doh.state.nj.us
Website: http://www.state.nj.us/health/as/addsrvs.htm
Theodore P. Bucon, Director

★ 21791 ★ New Mexico Department of Health
Behavioral Health Services Division
Harold Runnels Bldg.
1190 S St. Francis Dr.
PO Box 26110
Santa Fe, NM 87502-6110
Phone: (505)827-2601 **Free:** 800-362-2013
Email: pbrown@health.state.nm.us
Website: http://www.health.state.nm.us/

★ 21792 ★ New York State Office of Alcohol and Substance Abuse Services
1450 Western Ave.
Albany, NY 12203-3526
Phone: (518)473-3460
Email: info@oasas.state.ny.us
Website: http://www.oasas.state.ny.us/

★ 21793 ★ North Carolina Department of Health and Human Services
Mental Health, Developmental Disabilities and Substance Abuse Services Division
Substance Abuse Services Section
3007 Mail Service Ctr.
325 N Salisbury St.
Raleigh, NC 27699-3007
Phone: (919)733-4670 **Fax:** (919)733-9455
Email: jo.yarbrough@ncmail.net
Website: http://www.dhhs.state.nc.us/mhddsas/
Jo Yarbrough, Contact

★ 21794 ★ North Dakota Department of Human Services
Mental Health and Substance Abuse Services
Alcoholism and Drug Abuse Issues
600 S Second St., Ste 1E
Bismarck, ND 58504
Phone: (701)328-8920 **Free:** 800-642-6042
Fax: (701)328-8979
Email: soerhk@state.nd.us
Website: http://lnotes.state.nd.us/dhs/dhsweb.nsf/88f6de947ec9f2778625663c006afc52/83f8cbc7e20b76398625666d007f3b73?OpenDocument

★ 21795 ★ Ohio Department of Alcohol and Drug Addiction Services
280 N High St., 12th Fl.
Columbus, OH 43215-2537
Phone: (614)466-3445 **Fax:** (614)752-8645
Email: general@ada.state.oh.us
Website: http://www.state.oh.us/ada/odada.htm
Luceille Fleming, Director

★ 21796 ★ Oklahoma Department of Mental Health
Substance Abuse Services
1200 NE 13th St.
PO Box 53277
Oklahoma City, OK 73152-3277
Phone: (405)522-3908
Email: rbrown@odmhsas.org
Website: http://www.odmhsas.org/subab.htm
Terry Cline, PhD, Director

★ 21797 ★ Oregon Department of Human Resources
Alcohol and Drug Abuse Programs Office
500 Summer St. NE, E86
Salem, OR 97301-1118
Phone: (503)945-5763 **Fax:** (503)378-8467
Email: oadap.info@state.or.us
Website: http://www.oadap.hr.state.or.us/
Ann Brand, PhD, Director

★ 21798 ★ Pennsylvania Department of Health
Health Promotion, Disease and Substance Abuse Prevention
Drug and Alcohol Programs Bureau
Health and Welfare Bldg.
PO Box 90
Harrisburg, PA 17108
Phone: (717)783-8200
Email: webmaster@health.state.pa.us
Website: http://www.health.state.pa.us/PHP/SCA/default.htm

★ 21799 ★ Rhode Island Division of Behavioral Healthcare
Substance Abuse Treatment and Prevention Services
14 Harrington Rd.
Cranston, RI 02920
Phone: (401)462-2338 **Fax:** (401)462-6078
Website: http://www.mhrh.state.ri.us/Behavioral_Health.htm
Craig S. Stenning, Director

★ 21800 ★ South Carolina Department of Alcohol and Other Drug Abuse Services
101 Business Park Blvd.
Columbia, SC 29203-9498
Phone: (803)896-5555 **Fax:** (803)896-5557
Email: lgrant@daodas.state.sc.us
Website: http://www.daodas.state.sc.us./web/
Wendell Price, Director

★ 21801 ★ South Dakota Department of Human Services
Alcohol and Drug Abuse Division
Hillsview Plaza, E Hwy 34
c/o 500 E Capitol
Pierre, SD 57501
Phone: (605)773-3123 **Fax:** (605)773-7076
Email: infodada@dhs.state.sd.us
Website: http://www.state.sd.us/dhs/ADA/index.htm
Gilbert Sudbeck, Director

★ 21802 ★ Tennessee Department of Health
Alcohol and Drug Abuse Services Bureau
Cordell Hull Bldg.
425 5th Ave. N
Nashville, TN 37247-4401
Phone: (615)741-1921 **Fax:** (615)532-2419
Website: http://www2.state.tn.us/health/A&D/information.htm

★ 21803 ★ Texas Commission on Alcohol and Drug Abuse
9001 N IH 35, Ste. 105
PO Box 80529
Austin, TX 78708
Phone: (512)349-6600 **Free:** 800-832-9623
Email: contact@tcada.state.tx.us
Website: http://www.tcada.state.tx.us/

★ 21804 ★ Utah Department of Human Services
Substance Abuse Division
120 N 200 W, Rm. 201
PO Box 45500
Salt Lake City, UT 84103
Phone: (801)538-3939 **Fax:** (801)538-4696
Website: http://www.hsdsa.state.ut.us/

★ 21805 ★ Vermont Agency of Human Services
Alcohol and Drug Abuse Programs Division
108 Cherry St.
PO Box 70
Burlington, VT 05402-0070
Phone: (802)651-1550 **Fax:** (802)651-1573
Email: vtadap@vdh.state.vt.us
Website: http://www.state.vt.us/adap/
Marcia LaPlante, Director

★ 21806 ★ Virginia Office of Health and Human Resources
Mental Health, Retardation and Substance Abuse Services Department
Substance Abuse Services Division
PO Box 1797
Richmond, VA 23218
Phone: (804)786-3906 **Fax:** (804)371-0091
Email: rjohnson@dmhmrsas.state.va.us
Website: http://www.dmhmrsas.state.va.us/
Robert L. Johnson, Contact

★ 21807 ★ Washington Department of Social and Health Services
Health and Rehabilitative Services Office
Alcohol and Substance Abuse Division
PO Box 45130
Olympia, WA 98504-5130
Free: 877-301-4557
Email: askdshs@dshs.wa.gov
Website: http://www.wa.gov/dshs/hrsa/hrsa3ov.html

★ 21808 ★ West Virginia Department of Health and Human Resources
Community Support Bureau
Behavioral Health Services Office
Alcoholism and Drug Abuse Division
350 Capitol St., Rm. 350
Charleston, WV 25301-3702
Phone: (304)558-4224 **Fax:** (304)558-1008
Email: stevemason@wvdhhr.org
Website: http://www.wvdhhr.org/obhs/
Steve Mason, Director

★ 21809 ★ Wisconsin Department of Health and Family Services
Supportive Living Division
Substance Abuse Bureau
1 Wilson St., Rm. 434
Madison, WI 53702
Phone: (608)266-0040
Email: langkj@dhfs.state.wi.us
Website: http://www.dhfs.state.wi.us/substabuse/index.htm
Keith Lang, Contact

★ 21810 ★ Wyoming Department of Health
Behavioral Health Community Programs Division
Substance Abuse Division
2424 Pioneer Ave., Ste. 306
Cheyenne, WY 82002
Free: 800-535-4006 **Fax:** (307)777-7006
Email: info@state.wy.us
Website: http://substanceabuse.state.wy.us/
Diane Galloway, PhD, Director

Veterinarians

★ 21811 ★ Alabama Department of Agriculture and Industries
State Veterinarian
PO Box 3336
Montgomery, AL 36107
Phone: (334)240-7255 **Fax:** (334)223-7352
Email: stvet@agi.state.al.us
Website: http://www.agi.state.al.us/ANIMAL.htm
Dr. Tony Frazier, Contact
Dr. J. Lee Alley, Contact

★ 21812 ★ Alaska Department of Environmental Conservation
Environmental Health Division
State Veterinarian
500 S Alaska St.
Animal Industries Program
Palmer, AK 99645
Phone: (907)745-3236 **Fax:** (907)745-8125
Email: bgore@envircon.state.ak.us
Website: http://www.state.ak.us/dec/deh/animal/home.htm
Bert Gore, Contact

★ 21813 ★ Arizona Department of Agriculture
Animal Services Division
State Veterinarian
1688 W Adams
Phoenix, AZ 85007
Phone: (602)542-4293 **Fax:** (602)542-4290
Email: statevet@agric.state.az.us
Website: http://agriculture.state.az.us/ASD/state_vet.htm
Dr. R.D. Willer, DIR

★ 21814 ★ Arkansas Livestock and Poultry Commission
State Veterinarian
1 Natural Resources Dr.
PO Box 5497
Little Rock, AR 72205
Phone: (501)224-2836
Website: http://www.arlpc.org/stats.asp

★ 21815 ★ California Department of Food and Agriculture
Animal Industry Division
Animal Health Bureau
1220 N St., Rm. A-114
PO Box 942871
Sacramento, CA 95814
Phone: (916)654-0881 **Fax:** (916)653-4249
Email: ahbfeedback@cdfa.ca.gov
Website: http://www.cdfa.ca.gov/
Richard Breitmeyer, Director

★ 21816 ★ Colorado Department of Agriculture
Animal Industry Division
State Veterinarian
700 Kipling St., Ste. 4000
Lakewood, CO 80215-5894
Phone: (303)239-4158 **Fax:** (303)239-4164
Email: comments@ag.state.co.us
Website: http://www.ag.state.co.us/animals/bureau.html
Dr. John Maulsby, DVM, Contact

★ 21817 ★ Connecticut Department of Agriculture
State Veterinarian
State Office Bldg., Rm. 283
765 Asylum Ave.
Hartford, CT 06105
Phone: (860)713-2504 **Fax:** (860)713-2514
Email: ctdeptag@po.state.ct.us
Website: http://www.state.ct.us/doag/regsinsp/livestok.htm
Mary Jane Liss, D.V.M., Contact

★ 21818 ★ Delaware Department of Agriculture
Poultry and Animal Health Section
2320 S DuPont Hwy.
Dover, DE 19901-5515
Phone: (302)698-4500 **Fax:** (302)697-6287
Email: wes@dda.state.de.us
Website: http://www.state.de.us/deptagri/poultryah/index.htm

★ 21819 ★ Florida Department of Agriculture and Consumer Services
Animal Industry Division
State Veterinarian
Nathan Mayo Bldg., Rm. 335
407 S Calhoun St.
Tallahassee, FL 32399-0800
Phone: (850)410-0900 **Fax:** (850)410-0907
Email: coffmal@doacs.state.fl.us
Website: http://doacs.state.fl.us/ai/ai.html
Leroy M. Coffman, Contact

★ 21820 ★ Georgia Department of Agriculture
Animal Industry Division
State Veterinarian
19 Martin Luther King Jr. Dr. SW Room 106
Atlanta, GA 30334
Phone: (404)656-3671 **Fax:** (404)657-1357
Email: lbrooks@agr.state.ga.us
Website: http://www.agr.state.ga.us/html/animal_industry.html
Lee M. Meyers, Director

★ 21821 ★ Idaho Department of Agriculture
Animal Industries Division
Animal Health Bureau
2270 Old Penitentiary Rd.
PO Box 790
Boise, ID 83701
Phone: (208)332-8534 **Fax:** (208)334-2170
Email: pmamer@agri.state.id.us
Website: http://www.agri.state.id.us/animal/vet_services.htm
Christina Morrison, DVM, Contact

★ 21822 ★ Illinois Department of Agriculture
Animal Health Bureau
State Fairgrounds
PO Box 19281
Springfield, IL 62794-9281
Phone: (217)782-4944 **Free:** 800-273-4763
Fax: (217)524-7702
Email: pio@agr084r1.state.il.us
Website: http://www.agr.state.il.us/ahwf.html

★ 21823 ★ Iowa Department of Agriculture
Regulatory Division
Animal Health Bureau
Wallace Bldg.
Des Moines, IA 50319
Phone: (515)281-8615
Email: John.Schiltz@idals.state.ia.us
Website: http://www2.state.ia.us/agriculture/regulatory.html
Dr. John Schiltz, Contact

★ 21824 ★ Kansas Department of Animal Health
708 SW Jackson
Topeka, KS 66603-3714
Phone: (785)296-2326 **Fax:** (785)296-1765
Website: http://www.ink.org/public/kahd/

★ 21825 ★ Kentucky Department of Agriculture
Division of Animal Health
State Veterinarian
100 Fair Oaks Ln., Ste. 252
Frankfort, KY 40601
Phone: (502)564-3956 **Fax:** (502)564-7852
Email: don.notter@kyagr.com
Website: http://www.state.ky.us/agencies/agr/statevet.htm
Don Notter, DVM, Director

★ 21826 ★ Louisiana Deparment of Agriculture
Office of Animal Health Services
State Veterinarian
PO Box 1951
Baton Rouge, LA 70821-1951
Phone: (225)925-3980 **Fax:** (225)925-4103
Email: maxwel_l@ldaf.state.la.us
Website: http://www.ldaf.state.la.us
Maxwell A. Lea, DVM, Director

★ 21827 ★ Maine Department of Agriculture, Food and Rural Resources
Veterinary Services Division
28 State House Station Deering Bldg.
AMHI Complex
Augusta, ME 04333-0028
Phone: (207)287-3701
Email: Donald.E.Hoenig@state.me.us
Website: http://janus.state.me.us/agriculture/animals/homepage.htm
Donald E. Hoenig, VMD, Contact

★ 21828 ★ Maryland Department of Agriculture
Food Safety Consumer Services Office
Animal Health Division
50 Harry S Truman Pkwy.
Annapolis, MD 21401-7080
Phone: (410)841-5810 **Fax:** (410)841-4914
Email: olsonre@mda.state.md.us
Website: http://www.mda.state.md.us/geninfo/genera4.htm
Roger Olson, DVM, Director

★ 21829 ★ Massachusetts Executive Office of Environmental Affairs
Food and Agriculture Department
Animal Health Bureau
251 Causeway St., Ste. 500
Boston, MA 02114-2151
Phone: (617)626-1795
Email: esther.wegman@state.ma.us
Website: http://www.massdfa.org/animalhealth/index.htm
Fred Mach, Director

★ 21830 ★ Michigan Department of Agriculture
Animal Industry Division
State Veterinarian
PO Box 30017
Lansing, MI 48909
Phone: (517)373-1077 **Free:** 800-292-3939
Fax: (517)373-6015
Email: mda-info@michigan.gov
Website: http://www.michigan.gov/mda
Joan M. Arnold, Director

★ 21831 ★ Minnesota Board of Animal Health
90 W Plato Blvd
Saint Paul, MN 55107
Phone: (651)296-2942 **Fax:** (651)296-7417
Email: bill.hartmann@bah.state.mn.us
Website: http://www.bah.state.mn.us/
Bill Hartmann, DVM, Director

★ 21832 ★ Mississippi Department of Agriculture and Commerce
Animal Health Board
State Veterinarian
121 N Jefferson
PO Box 3889
Jackson, MS 39207
Phone: (601)359-1170 **Free:** 888-646-8731
Fax: (601)359-1177
Email: jimw@mdac.state.ms.us
Website: http://www.mbah.state.ms.us/
James A. Watson, DVM, Director

★ 21833 ★ Missouri Department of Agriculture
Animal Health Division and State Veterinarian
PO Box 630
Jefferson City, MO 65102
Phone: (573)751-3377 **Fax:** (573)751-6919
Email: taylor.woods@mail.state.mo.us
Website: http://www.mda.state.mo.us/i4.htm
Taylor Woods, DVM, Director

★ 21834 ★ Montana Department of Livestock
Animal Health Division
PO Box 202001
Helena, MT 59620-2001
Phone: (406)444-2043 **Fax:** (406)444-1929
Email: agertonson@state.mt.gov
Website: http://agr.state.mt.us/
Dr. Arnold Gertonson, Contact

★ 21835 ★ Nebraska Department of Agriculture
Animal Industry
State Veterinarian
301 Centennial Mall S
PO Box 94787
Lincoln, NE 68509-4787
Phone: (402)471-2351 **Fax:** (402)471-6893
Email: larrylw@agr.state.ne.us
Website: http://www.agr.state.ne.us/division/bai/bai.htm
Larry Williams, DVM, Director

★ 21836 ★ Nevada Department of Business and Industry
Agriculture Division
Animal Industry Bureau
State Veterinarian
350 Capitol Hill Ave.
Reno, NV 89502
Phone: (702)688-1180 **Fax:** (702)688-1178
Email: dthain@govmail.state.nv.us
Website: http://agri.state.nv.us/indexa.htm
David Thain, DVM, Contact

★ 21837 ★ New Hampshire Department of Agriculture
Animal Industry Division
State Veterinarian
PO Box 2042.
Concord, NH 03302
Phone: (603)271-2404 **Fax:** (603)271-1109
Email: cwmcginnis@agr.state.nh.us
Website: http://www.state.nh.us/agric/anin.html
Clifford W. McGinnis, DVM, Director

★ 21838 ★ New Jersey Department of Agriculture
Animal Health Division
John Fitch Plaza
PO Box 330
Trenton, NJ 08625-0330
Phone: (609)292-3965 **Fax:** (609)633-2550
Email: ernest.zirkle@ag.state.nj.us
Website: http://www.state.nj.us/agriculture/animal.htm
Ernest Zirkle, DVM, Director

★ 21839 ★ New Mexico Livestock Board
State Veterinarian
300 San Mateo NE, Ste. 1000
Albuquerque, NM 87108-1500
Phone: (505)841-6161 **Fax:** (505)841-6160
Steven England, DVM, Contact

★ 21840 ★ New York Department of Agriculture and Markets
Animal Industry Division
State Veterinarian
1 Winners Circle
Albany, NY 12235
Phone: (518)457-3502 **Fax:** (518)457-7773
Email: huntleyj@nysnet.net
Website: http://www.agmkt.state.ny.us/
John Huntley, DVM, Director

★ 21841 ★ North Carolina Department of Agriculture
Veterinary Division
2 W Edenton St., Rm. 472
PO Box 26026
Raleigh, NC 27611
Phone: (919)733-7601 **Fax:** (919)733-6431
Email: Joe.Web@ncmail.net
Website: http://www.agr.state.nc.us/vet/
David Marshall, DVM, Director

★ 21842 ★ North Dakota Board of Animal Health
600 E Boulevard Ave., 6th Fl.
Bismarck, ND 58505-0020
Phone: (701)328-2654 **Fax:** (701)328-4567
Email: lschuler@state.nd.us
Website: http://www.state.nd.us/agr/
Larry A. Schuler, D.V.M., Director

★ 21843 ★ Ohio Department of Agriculture
Animal Industry Division
State Veterinarian
8995 E Main St.
Bldg. 6
Reynoldsburg, OH 43068
Phone: (614)728-6220 **Fax:** (614)728-6310
Email: agri@odant.agri.state.oh.us
Website: http://www.state.oh.us/agr/AnimalIndustry-Div.html
Dr. R. David Glauer, Director

★ 21844 ★ Oklahoma Department of Agriculture
Animal Industry Division
State Veterinarian
2800 N Lincoln Blvd.
Oklahoma City, OK 73152
Phone: (405)522-6131 **Fax:** (405)522-0756
Email: bhealey@oda.state.ok.us
Website: http://www.oda.state.ok.us/aind.htm
Burke L. Healey, DVM, Contact

★ 21845 ★ Oregon Department of Agriculture
State Veterinarian
635 Capitol St. NE
Salem, OR 97301-2532
Phone: (503)986-4680
Email: csorrels@oda.state.or.us
Website: http://www.oda.state.or.us/Livestock_Health_ID/animal_health/ah_main.html
Andrew Clark, D.V.M., Director

★ 21846 ★ Pennsylvania Department of Agriculture
Animal Industry Bureau
State Veterinarian
2301 N Cameron St.
Harrisburg, PA 17110-9408
Phone: (717)783-6677
Website: http://www.pda.state.pa.us/

★ 21847 ★ Rhode Island Department of Environmental Management
Agriculture Division
Animal Health Section
235 Promenade St.
Providence, RI 02908-5767
Phone: (401)222-2781 **Fax:** (401)222-6047
Website: http://www.state.ri.us/dem/org/agric.htm

★ 21848 ★ South Carolina State Veterinarian
PO Box 102406
Columbia, SC 29224-2406
Phone: (803)788-2260 **Fax:** (803)788-8058
Email: jbryn@clemson.edu
Dr. Jones W. Bryan, Director

★ 21849 ★ South Dakota Animal Industry Board
State Veterinarian
411 S Fort St.
Pierre, SD 57501-4503
Phone: (605)773-3321 **Fax:** (605)773-5459
Email: Dr.Holland@state.sd.us
Website: http://www.state.sd.us/doa/boards.htm
Sam D. Holland, Contact

★ 21850 ★ Tennessee Department of Agriculture
Animal Industries Division
State Veterinarian
Ellington Agricultural Ctr.
PO Box 40627
Nashville, TN 37204
Phone: (615)837-5120 **Fax:** (615)837-5335
Email: twomack@mail.state.tn.us
Website: http://www.state.tn.us/agriculture/regulate/regulat2.html
Ron Wilson, D.V.M., Director

★ 21851 ★ Texas Animal Health Commission
2105 Kramer Ln.
PO Box 12966
Austin, TX 78711
Phone: (512)719-0700 **Free:** 800-550-8242
Fax: (512)719-0719
Email: comments@tahc.state.tx.us
Website: http://www.tahc.state.tx.us/
Linda M. Logan, D.V.M., Director

★ 21852 ★ Utah Department of Agriculture
Animal Health Division, State Veterinarian
350 N Redwood Rd.
PO Box 146500
Salt Lake City, UT 84114-6500
Phone: (801)538-7162 **Fax:** (801)538-7169
Email: agmain.erogers@email.state.ut.us
Website: http://www.ag.state.ut.us/divisns/animind/animalmp.htm
Dr. Earl Rogers, Director

★ 21853 ★ Vermont Department of Agriculture
State Veterinarian
116 State St.
Drawer 20
Montpelier, VT 05620-2901
Phone: (802)828-2421 **Fax:** (802)828-2361
Email: vtstatvet@aol.com
Website: http://www.state.vt.us/agric/animal.htm
Todd Johnson, D.V.M., Director

★ 21854 ★ Virgin Islands Department of Economic Development and Agriculture
Veterinary Services Division
Estate Lower Love, Kingshill
St Croix, VI 00850
Phone: (340)778-0997 **Fax:** (340)778-3101
Email: agriculture@usvi.org
Website: http://www.usvi.org/agriculture/index.html

★ 21855 ★ Virginia Office of Commerce and Trade
Agriculture and Consumer Services Department
Animal Health Division
1100 Bank St., Rm. 220
PO Box 1163
Richmond, VA 23218
Phone: (804)786-2483 **Free:** 800-786-2373
Fax: (804)371-2380
Email: cowhite@vdacs.state.va.us
Website: http://www.vdacs.state.va.us/animals/index.html

★ 21856 ★ Washington Department of Agriculture
Food Safety and Animal Health Division
State Veterinarian
PO Box 42577
Olympia, WA 98504-2577
Phone: (360)902-1878 **Fax:** (360)902-2087
Email: ahealth@agr.wa.gov
Website: http://www.wa.gov/agr/FoodAnimal/AnimalHealth/default.htm
Dr. Robert W. Mead, Director

★ 21857 ★ West Virginia Department of Agriculture
Animal Health Division
1900 Kanawha Blvd. E
Charleston, WV 25305
Phone: (304)558-2214 **Fax:** (304)558-2231
Email: lthomas@ag.state.wv.us
Website: http://www.state.wv.us/agriculture/Departments_Descriptions/Animal_Health_Division/animal_health_division.html
Dr. Lewis Thomas, Director

★ 21858 ★ Wisconsin Department of Agriculture, Trade and Consumer Protection
Animal Health Division
ATTN: Interstate
PO Box 8911
Madison, WI 53708-8911
Phone: (608)224-4872 **Fax:** (608)224-4871
Email: datcp_web@wheel.datcp.state.wi.us
Website: http://datcp.state.wi.us/static/ah/

★ 21859 ★ Wyoming Livestock Board
State Veterinarian
2020 Carey Ave., 4th Fl.
Cheyenne, WY 82002-0051
Phone: (307)777-7515 **Fax:** (307)777-6561
Email: jlogan1@state.wy.us
Website: http://wlsb.state.wy.us/
Jim Logan, D.V.M., Director

Vital Statistics

★ 21860 ★ Alabama Department of Public Health
Health Statistics Center
Quality Assurance Division
PO Box 5618
Montgomery, AL 36103-5618
Phone: (334)206-5418 **Fax:** (334)206-2733
Website: http://www.alapubhealth.org/

★ 21861 ★ Alaska Department of Health and Social Services
Public Health Division
Vital Statistics Section
PO Box 110675
Juneau, AK 99811-0675
Phone: (907)465-3392 **Fax:** (907)465-3618
Website: http://www.hss.state.ak.us/dph/bvs/
Al Zangri, Director

★ 21862 ★ Arizona Department of Health Services
Vital Records Office
1740 West Adams St.
Phoenix, AZ 85007
Phone: (602)542-1216 **Fax:** (602)542-2940
Email: webmaster@hs.state.az.us
Website: http://www.hs.state.az.us/plan/ohpes.htm

★ 21863 ★ Arkansas Department of Health
Health Resources Bureau
Vital Records Division
4815 W Markham, Slot 44
Little Rock, AR 72205-3867
Phone: (501)661-2371
Website: http://www.healthyarkansas.com/services/services_ts2_all.htmlVital
Sharon Leinbach, Contact

★ 21864 ★ California Health and Welfare Agency
Health Services Department
Vital Records Branch
304 S St.
PO Box 730241
Sacramento, CA 94244-0241
Phone: (916)445-2684
Website: http://www.dhs.cahwnet.gov/org/hisp/chs/chsindex.htm

★ 21865 ★ Colorado Public Health and Environment Department
Administration and Support Office
Health Statistics and Vital Records Division
4300 Cherry Creek Dr. S
Denver, CO 80246-1530
Phone: (303)692-2160 **Fax:** (303)691-7704
Email: health.statistics@state.co.us
Website: http://www.cdphe.state.co.us/hs/hsshom.asp

★ 21866 ★ Connecticut Department of Public Health
Policy, Planning, and Evaluation Office
Vital Records Division
410 Capitol Ave.
PO Box 340308
MS 11VRS
Hartford, CT 06134-0308
Phone: (860)509-7163 **Fax:** (860)509-7160
Email: angela.kasek@po.state.ct.us
Website: http://www.state.ct.us/dph/OPPE/hpvital.htm
Daniel J. Savino, Director

★ 21867 ★ Delaware Department of Health and Social Services
Public Health Division
Office of Vital Statistics
PO Box 637
Dover, DE 19903
Phone: (302)739-4721 **Fax:** (302)736-1862
Email: dhssinfo@state.de.us
Website: http://www.state.de.us/dhss/dph/vs.htm

★ 21868 ★ District of Columbia Department of Human Services
State Center for Health Statistics
Vital Records Branch
825 N Capitol St. NE
First Floor
Washington, DC 20002
Phone: (202)442-9009 **Fax:** (202)442-4833
Website: http://www.dchealth.com/vitalrecords.htm

★ 21869 ★ Florida Department of Health and Rehabilitative Services
Vital Records & Statistics Office
PO Box 210
Jacksonville, FL 32231-0042
Phone: (904)359-6900 **Fax:** (904)359-6931
Email: vitalstats@doh.state.fl.us
Website: http://www9.myflorida.com/planning_eval/phstats/index.html
Ken T. Jones, Contact

★ 21870 ★ Georgia Department of Human Resources
Public Health Division
Vital Records Office
2600 Skyland Dr, NE
Atlanta, GA 30319-3640
Phone: (404)679-4701
Email: gdphinfo@dhr.state.ga.us
Website: http://www.ph.dhr.state.ga.us/programs/vitalrecords/index.shtml

★ 21871 ★ Hawaii Department of Health
Health Status Monitoring Office
Vital Records Section
1250 Punchbowl St., Rm. 103
PO Box 3378
Honolulu, HI 96801
Phone: (808)586-4400 **Fax:** (808)586-4444
Email: vr-info@mail.health.state.hi.us
Website: http://www.state.hi.us/health/records/index.html

★ 21872 ★ Idaho Department of Health and Welfare
Health Division
Vital Records and Health Statistics Bureau
Pete T. Cenarrusa Bldg. 1st Fl.
450 W State St.
PO Box 83720
Boise, ID 83720-0036
Phone: (208)334-5500 **Fax:** (208)334-6558
Email: dhwinfo@idhw.state.id.us
Website: http://www2.state.id.us/dhw/hwgd_www/contentlist.htmlVitalStats
Davalee Leavitt, Contact

★ 21873 ★ Illinois Department of Public Health
Finance and Administration Office
Vital Records Division
605 W Jefferson St.
Springfield, IL 62702-5097
Phone: (217)782-6554 **Fax:** (217)523-2648
Email: mailus@idph.state.il.us
Website: http://www.idph.state.il.us/vital/vitalhome.htm

★ 21874 ★ Indiana Department of Health
Public Health Statistics Division
2 N Meridian St.
Indianapolis, IN 46204
Phone: (317)233-2700 **Fax:** (317)233-7210
Website: http://www.state.in.us/isdh/bdcertifs/birth_and_death_certificates.htm

★ 21875 ★ Iowa Department of Public Health
Planning and Administration Division
Vital Records Bureau
Lucas State Office Bldg.
321 E 12th St.
Des Moines, IA 50319-0075
Phone: (515)281-4944
Email: webmaster@idph.state.ia.us
Website: http://idph.state.ia.us/pa/vr.htm

★ 21876 ★ Kansas Department of Health and Environment
Health and Environment Statistics Division
Vital Statistics Office
1000 SW Jackson, Ste. 120
Topeka, KS 66612-2221
Phone: (785)296-1400 **Fax:** (785)296-8075
Email: Vital.Records@kdhe.state.ks.us
Website: http://www.kdhe.state.ks.us/vital/
Gabriel Faimon, Director

★ 21877 ★ Kentucky Health Services Cabinet
Department for Public Health
Vital Statistics Division
275 E Main St, 1E-A
Frankfort, KY 40621
Phone: (502)564-4212 **Fax:** (502)227-0032
Website: http://publichealth.state.ky.us/vital.htm

★ 21878 ★ Louisiana Department of Health and Hospitals
Health Information Division
Vital Records Registry
PO Box 60630
New Orleans, LA 70160
Phone: (504)568-8353 **Fax:** (504)568-6909
Email: vitalweb@dhh.state.la.us
Website: http://oph.dhh.state.la.us/recordsstatistics/vitalrecords/

★ 21879 ★ Maine Department of Human Services
Research and Vital Statistics Division
11 State House Station
221 State St
Augusta, ME 04333-0011
Phone: (207)287-3181
Email: lorraine.wilson@state.me.us
Website: http://janus.state.me.us/dhs/welcome.htm

★ 21880 ★ Maryland Department of Health and Mental Hygiene
Health Services Analysis and Evaluation Administration
201 W Preston St., 5th Fl.
Baltimore, MD 21201
Phone: (410)767-5806 **Fax:** (410)767-6489
Email: corddrym@dhmh.state.md.us
Website: http://www.dhmh.state.md.us/hsaea/

★ 21881 ★ Massachusetts Executive Office of Health and Human Services
Public Health Department
Vital Records and Statistics Division
150 Mt. Vernon St., 1st Fl.
Dorchester, MA 02125-3105
Phone: (617)740-2600
Email: jean.lorusso@state.ma.us
Website: http://www.state.ma.us/dph/rvr.htm

★ 21882 ★ Michigan Community Health Department
State Registrar and Health Statistics Center
3423 N Martin Luther King Blvd.
PO Box 30691
Lansing, MI 48909
Phone: (517)335-8677 **Fax:** (517)335-9513
Email: Humphrysk@state.mi.us
Website: http://www.mdch.state.mi.us/PHA/OSR/index.htm

★ 21883 ★ Minnesota Department of Health
Center for Health Statistics
Vital Records Section
717 Delaware St. SE
PO Box 9441
Minneapolis, MN 55440-9441
Phone: (612)676-5120
Email: chs1@health.state.mn.us
Website: http://www.health.state.mn.us/divs/chs/data/bd_1.htm

★ 21884 ★ Mississippi Department of Health
Community Health Services Office
Vital Statistics Division
571 Stadium Dr.
PO Box 1700
Jackson, MS 39215-1700
Phone: (601)576-7960 **Fax:** (601)576-7505
Email: vrinfo@msdh.state.ms.us
Website: http://www.msdh.state.ms.us/phs/index.htm

★ 21885 ★ Missouri Department of Health
Health Information Management and Epidemiology Center
Vital Records Bureau
930 Wildwood Dr.
PO Box 570
Jefferson City, MO 65102
Phone: (573)751-6381
Email: info@mail.health.state.mo.us
Website: http://www.health.state.mo.us/BirthAndDeathRecords/BirthAndDeathRecords.html

★ 21886 ★ Montana Department of Public Health and Human Services
Vital Records and Statistics Bureau
PO Box 4210
111 N Sanders
Helena, MT 59604-4210
Phone: (406)444-1756 **Fax:** (406)444-1803
Email: kferlicka@state.mt.us
Website: http://www.dphhs.state.mt.us/divisions/otd/vital_stats.htm
Bruce Schwartz, Contact

★ 21887 ★ Nebraska Department of Health and Human Services
Vital Records Office
Nebraska Department of HHS Finance and Support
Vital Records
PO Box 95065
Lincoln, NE 68509-5065
Phone: (402)471-2871 **Fax:** (402)471-0383
Email: Vitalrecords@hhss.state.ne.us
Website: http://www.hhs.state.ne.us/ced/cedindex.htm

★ 21888 ★ Nevada Department of Human Resources
Health Division
Vital Records Bureau
505 E King St.
Rm. 102
Carson City, NV 89701
Phone: (775)684-4242 **Fax:** (775)684-4156
Website: http://www.state.nv.us/health/

★ 21889 ★ New Hampshire Department of Health and Human Services
Public Health Services Division
Vital Records and Health Statistics Bureau
6 Hazen Dr.
Concord, NH 03301
Phone: (603)271-4650 **Free:** 800-852-3345
Fax: (603)271-3447
Email: vitalrecords@dhhs.state.nh.us
Website: http://www.dhhs.state.nh.us/

★ 21890 ★ New Jersey Department of Health
Health Care Systems Analysis Division
Center for Health Statistics
PO Box 360
Trenton, NJ 08625-0360
Phone: (609)984-6702 **Fax:** (609)984-7633
Email: chs@doh.state.nj.us
Website: http://www.state.nj.us/health/chs/
Katherine Hempstead, Director

★ 21891 ★ New Mexico Department of Health
Public Health Division
Vital Statistics Section
1105 St. Francis Dr.
1190 St. Francis Dr.
Santa Fe, NM 87505
Phone: (505)827-0121
Website: http://dohewbs2.health.state.nm.us/VitalRec/

★ 21892 ★ North Carolina Department of Health and Human Services
North Carolina Center for Health Statistics
Vital Records Section
1903 Mail Service Ctr.
Raleigh, NC 27699-1903
Phone: (919)733-3526
Email: SCHS.Info@ncmail.net
Website: http://www.schs.state.nc.us/SCHS/about/branches/vital.html

★ 21893 ★ North Dakota Department of Health
Administrative Services Section
Vital Records Division
600 E Boulevard Ave.
Bismarck, ND 58505-0200
Phone: (701)328-2360 **Fax:** (701)328-1850
Email: vitalrec@state.nd.us
Website: http://www.health.state.nd.us/ndhd/admin/vital/
Beverly Wittmann, Director

★ 21894 ★ Oklahoma Department of Health
Administrative Services
Vital Records Division
1000 NE 10th St.
Rm. 111
Oklahoma City, OK 73117
Phone: (405)271-4040
Website: http://www.health.state.ok.us/PROGRAM/vital/index.html

★ 21895 ★ Oregon Department of Human Resources
Health Division
Vital Statistics Section
Portland State Office Bldg.
800 NE Oregon St., Ste. 215
PO Box 14050
Portland, OR 97293-0050
Phone: (503)731-4109
Website: http://www.ohd.hr.state.or.us/chs/welcome.htm
Jennifer Woodward, Contact

★ 21896 ★ Pennsylvania Department of Health
Public Health Assessment
Vital Records Division
101 S Mercer St.
PO Box 1528
New Castle, PA 16103-1528
Phone: (717)783-2548 **Fax:** (724)772-3258
Email: webmaster@health.state.pa.us
Website: http://www.health.state.pa.us/hpa/Stats/vital/

★ 21897 ★ Rhode Island Department of Health
Management Services
Vital Record Division
3 Capitol Hill, Rm. 101
Providence, RI 02908
Phone: (401)222-2811
Email: library@health.state.ri.us
Website: http://www.health.state.ri.us/yhd05.htm

★ 21898 ★ South Carolina Department of Health and Environmental Control
Vital Records and Public Health Statistics Office
2600 Bull St.
Columbia, SC 29201
Phone: (803)898-3630 **Fax:** (803)799-0301
Email: goodinj@columb20.dhec.state.sc.us
Website: http://www.scdhec.net/vr/index.htm

★ 21899 ★ South Dakota Department of Health
Vital Records Program
600 E Capitol
Pierre, SD 57501-2536
Phone: (605)773-4961
Email: DOH.INFO@state.sd.us
Website: http://www.state.sd.us/doh/VitalRec/index.htm

★ 21900 ★ Tennessee Department of Health
Administrative Services Bureau
Health Statistics Division
Vital Records Section
Central Services Bldg.
421 5th Ave. N, 1st Fl.
Nashville, TN 37247-0460
Phone: (615)741-1763 **Fax:** (615)741-9860
Email: DDenton@mail.state.tn.us
Website: http://www2.state.tn.us/health/vr/

★ 21901 ★ Texas Department of Health
Vital Statistics Bureau
1100 W 49th St.
PO Box 12040
Austin, TX 78711-2040
Phone: (512)458-7111 **Free:** 888-963-7111
Fax: (512)458-7233
Email: register@tdh.state.tx.us
Website: http://www.tdh.state.tx.us/bvs/default.htm

★ 21902 ★ Utah Department of Health
Health Statistics and Vital Records Bureau
288 N 1460 W
PO Box 141012
Salt Lake City, UT 84114-1012
Phone: (801)538-6105
Email: vrequest@doh.state.ut.us
Website: http://www.health.state.ut.us/bvr/

★ 21903 ★ Vermont Agency of Human Services
Health Department
Public Health, Analysis and Policy Division
Vital Records Unit
108 Cherry St.
PO Box 70
Burlington, VT 05402-0070
Phone: (802)863-7275 **Free:** 800-439-5008
Fax: (802)828-3710
Website: http://www.state.vt.us/health/_hs/vitals/records/vitalrecords.htm

★ 21904 ★ Virginia Office of Health and Human Resources
Health Department
Vital Records Office
PO Box 1000
Richmond, VA 23218-1000
Phone: (804)662-6200
Email: lwhitaker@vdh.state.va.us
Website: http://www.vdh.state.va.us/vitalrec/f_08.htm
Deborah Little-Bowser, Director

★ 21905 ★ Washington Department of Health
Health Statistics Center
1112 SE Quince St.
PO Box 47890
Olympia, WA 98504-7890
Phone: (360)236-4300
Email: glenda.moore@doh.wa.gov
Website: http://www.doh.wa.gov/EHSPHL/CHS/cert.htm

★ 21906 ★ West Virginia Department of Health and Human Resources
Public Health Bureau
Epidemiology and Health Promotion Office
Health Statistics Division
350 Capitol St., Rm. 165
Charleston, WV 25301-3715
Phone: (304)558-9100
Email: danchristy@wvdhhr.org
Website: http://www.wvdhhr.org/bph/oehp/hsc/hschome.htm

★ 21907 ★ Wisconsin Department of Health and Family Services
Health Division
Vital Statistics Office
PO Box 309
Madison, WI 53701-0309
Phone: (608)266-1371 **Fax:** (608)261-4971
Email: VitalRecords@dhfs.state.wi.us
Website: http://www.dhfs.state.wi.us/VitalRecords/index.htm

★ 21908 ★ Wyoming Department of Health
Preventive Health and Safety Division
Vital Records Section
Hathaway Bldg., 4th Fl.
Cheyenne, WY 82002
Phone: (307)777-7591
Email: cmccaf@missc.state.wy.us
Website: http://wdhfs.state.wy.us/vital_records/index.htm
Lucinda McCaffrey, Director

Chapter 16
University-Related & Other Nonprofit Research Centers

Entries listed below are arranged alphabetically by research center name. See the "User's Guide" at the front of this directory for additional information.

★ 21909 ★ Aaron Diamond AIDS Research Center
455 1st Ave., 7th Fl.
New York, NY 10016
Phone: (212)448-5000 **Fax:** (212)725-1126
Website: http://www.adarc.org
David D. Ho, MD, Dir.
Activities/Fields: Pathogenesis of HIV-1 in vivo, maternal-fetal transmission of HIV-1, antibody responses to HIV and vaccine development, mechanism of HIV entry into CD4+ and CD4- cells, anti-HIV therapeutics and viral resistance, search for the causative agent of HIV-negative cases of immunodeficiency, cellular immune responses to HIV-1 in the pathogenesis of AIDS, cellular immune responses to HIV-1 in vaccine development, development of the scid mouse model for HIV studies, receptors for human retroviruses (HIV and HTLV), assembly of HIV virion, function of accessory genes of HIV, interaction of HIV envelope with the cellular receptor, mechanism of viral entry, and mapping of the functional determinants of HIV envelope glycoprotein.

★ 21910 ★ Abbott Northwestern Hospital David F. Hickok Memorial Cancer Research Laboratory
800 E 28th St.
Minneapolis, MN 55407
Phone: (612)863-4339 **Fax:** (612)863-4936
Email: editor@epress.com
Website: http://www.msi.umn.edu/Projects/mg90601/anwhome.html
Lester F. Harris, PhD, Sci. Dir.
Activities/Fields: Breast cancer.

★ 21911 ★ Abilene Christian University Voice Institute of West Texas
Box 28058
Abilene, TX 79699-8048
Phone: (915)674-2074 **Fax:** (915)674-2552
Email: ashbyj@acu.edu
Website: http://www.acu.edu/academics/cas/comm_disorders/voiceinstitute.html
Jon Ashby, PhD, Co-Dir.
Activities/Fields: Human voice, and evaluation, diagnosis, and treatment of voice disorders.

★ 21912 ★ Academy for Educational Development Center for AIDS and Community Health
1825 Connecticut Ave. NW
Washington, DC 20009-5721
Phone: (202)884-8862 **Fax:** (202)884-8474
Email: coach@aed.org
Website: http://www.healthstrategies.org
Frank Beadle de Palomo, Dir.
Activities/Fields: Needs assessment, intervention effectiveness, process evaluation. **Frmly:** Center for Community-Based Health Strategies.

★ 21913 ★ Academy of Pharmaceutical Research and Science
American Pharmaceutical Association
2215 Constitution Ave. NW
Washington, DC 20037-2985
Phone: (202)628-4410 **Free:** 800-237-2742
Fax: (202)628-0443
Email: mrotholz@aphanet.org
Website: http://www.aphanet.org
Mitchel C. Rothholz, Contact
Activities/Fields: Pharmaceuticals, focusing on quality measurement, development of practice-based research, and outcomes research in the broadcast sense.

★ 21914 ★ Ackerman Institute for the Family
149 E 78th St.
New York, NY 10021-0405
Phone: (212)879-4900 **Fax:** (212)744-0206
Email: ackerman@ackerman.org
Website: http://www.ackerman.org
Peter Steinglass, MD, Exec. Dir.
Activities/Fields: Cancer and other chronic illnesses, catastrophic illness, AIDS/AIDS-Related Complex (ARC), school problems, women's issues, family violence, stressful life events, family life cycle issues, family factors in psychiatric disorders, alcoholism, and drug abuse.

★ 21915 ★ Addiction Research and Treatment Corp.
22 Chapel St.
Brooklyn, NY 11201
Phone: (718)260-2917 **Fax:** (718)522-3186
Email: lbrown@artcny.org
Dr. Lawrence S. Brown, Jr., Sr. VP
Activities/Fields: Alcohol and drug addiction, including studies on alcoholism among those addicted to opiates, immunological parameters of drug abuse, stress among patients and staff, and the relationship of patterns of drug abuse and sexual practices to the frequency of human immunodeficiency virus (HIV) infection (exposure to AIDS virus). Conducts clinical trials of drugs for drug abuse and the treatment of HIV disease.

★ 21916 ★ Adelphi University Human Performance Laboratory
Woodruff Hall
South Ave.
Garden City, NY 11530
Phone: (516)877-4276 **Fax:** (516)877-4274
Email: otto@adelphi.edu
Dr. Robert Otto, Dir.
Activities/Fields: Human performance as it relates to exercise.

★ 21917 ★ Adelphi University Hy Weinberg Center for Communication Disorders
PO Box 701
Garden City, NY 11530-4299
Phone: (516)877-4850 **Fax:** (516)877-4865
Email: soman@adelphi.edu
Dr. Bonnie Soman, Dir.
Activities/Fields: Speech-language pathology and audiology, and speech and hearing disorders.

★ 21918 ★ Advanced Medical Research Foundation, Inc.
333 Longwood Ave.
Boston, MA 02115-5711
Phone: (617)278-1800 **Fax:** (617)264-2400
Email: amrf333@msn.com
Nile L. Albright, MD, Pres.
Activities/Fields: Medical and cancer research and science education.

★ 21919 ★ African Medical and Research Foundation, U.S.A.
19 W 44th St., Rm. 710
New York, NY 10036
Phone: (212)768-2440 **Fax:** (212)768-4230
Email: amrefusa@amrefusa.org
Website: http://www.amref.org/
Lisa Meadowcraft, Exec. Dir.
Activities/Fields: The spread and prevention of AIDS, malaria, and hydatid disease. Also creates health care & training models used by developing countries worldwide.

★ 21920 ★ Aging Research Institute
217 SE 8th St.
Topeka, KS 66603-3906
Phone: (785)233-7443 **Fax:** (785)233-9471
Email: jrgrace@kahsa.org
Website: http://www.kahsa.org
John R. Grace, Dir.
Activities/Fields: Managed care and nursing facilities, staff recruitment and retention, worker safety in nursing homes.

★ 21921 ★ Agnes Barr Chase Surgical Research Foundation
Parkinson Pavilion, 4th Fl.
Department of Surgery
Temple University
Broad & Ontario Sts.
Philadelphia, PA 19140
Phone: (215)707-5080 **Fax:** (215)707-1915
Email: jrudy@vm.temple.edu
Dr. Daniel T. Dempsey, Chm., Dept. of Surgery
Activities/Fields: Provides support for research in the Department of Surgery, with emphasis on the specialities of gastrointestinal, vascular, and cardio-thoracic surgery.

★ 21922 ★ AIDS Research Consortium of Atlanta, Inc.
131 Ponce de Leon Ave. NE, Ste. 130
Atlanta, GA 30308-1962
Phone: (404)876-2317 **Fax:** (404)872-1701
Email: arca@aidsresearchatlanta.org
Website: http://www.aidsresearchatlanta.org
Melanie Thompson, MD, Prin. Investigator
Activities/Fields: HIV clinical trials and epidemiology.

★ 21923 ★ Albany Medical College Pediatric Pulmonary and Cystic Fibrosis Care, Research and Teaching Center
47 New Scotland Ave., Mail Code A112
Albany, NY 12208
Phone: (518)262-6880 **Fax:** (518)262-6884
Email: kaslovr@mail.amc.edu
Robert Kaslovsky, MD, Dir.
Activities/Fields: Cystic fibrosis, asthma clinical studies of patients. **Frmly:** Cystic Fibrosis Care Research and Teaching Center.

★ 21924 ★ Albert Einstein Center for Synchrotron Biosciences
Department of Biochemistry & Biophysics
Albert Einstein College of Medicine
Yeshiva University
1300 Morris Park Ave.
Bronx, NY 10461
Phone: (718)430-4136 **Fax:** (718)430-8587
Email: mrc@aecom.yu.edu
Website: http://www.aecom.yu.edu/home/csb/
Mark Chance, PhD, Dir.
Activities/Fields: Biological structure and function at the molecular level using synchrotron radiation, such as studies of protein and RNA folding, protein-protein interactions, structures of the active sites of metalloproteins, and macromolecular crystallography. **Pub:** *PRT Newsletter.* • *Technical Notes.* **Frmly:** Biostructures Participating Research Team.

★ 21925 ★ Albert Einstein College of Medicine
Albert Einstein Cancer Research Center
Chanin Bldg., Rm. 209
1300 Morris Park Ave.
Bronx, NY 10461
Phone: (718)430-2302 **Fax:** (718)430-8550
Email: igoldman@aecom.yu.edu
Website: http://www.aecom.yu.edu/cancer
I. David Goldman, MD, Dir.
Activities/Fields: Encompass basic studies in immuno-oncology, signaling, regulation of tumor motility and invasion, tumor suppressor genes, and membrane molecular biology. These are disease-focused programs or working groups in the areas of Colon Cancer, Lung and Aerodigestive Cancers, and the Biology of Hematopoietic and Lymphoid Cancers. The Experimental Therapeutics program encompasses drug design and development, along with Phase I-III clinical trials. The Cancer Epidemiology program focuses on breast cancer, other solid tumors, and cancers associated with human papilloma virus infections.

★ 21926 ★ Albert Einstein College of Medicine
General Clinical Research Center
Jack and Pearl Resnick Campus
Forchheimer Bldg., Rm. G47
1300 Morris Park Ave.
Bronx, NY 10461
Phone: (718)430-8800 **Fax:** (718)430-8998
Email: shamoon@aecom.yu.edu
Website: http://gcrcweb.aecom.yu.edu/gcrc
Harry Shamoon, MD, Prog. Dir.
Activities/Fields: Major areas of investigation include cancer, diabetes, gastrointestinal disorders, hematology, immunology. liver disease and renal disease.

★ 21927 ★ Albert Einstein College of Medicine
Marion Bessin Liver Research Center
Ullman Bldg., Rm. 625
1300 Morris Park Ave.
Bronx, NY 10461
Phone: (718)430-2098 **Fax:** (718)430-8975
Email: shafritz@aecom.yu.edu
Website: http://www.aecom.yu.edu/liver
Dr. David A. Shafritz, Dir.
Activities/Fields: Mechanisms of liver cell injury and repair, gene regulation, membrane structure/function, cirrhosis, genetic diseases, heavy metal toxicity, cellular growth control, liver progenitor cells, livery cell transplanation, somatic gene therapy, hepatitis virus infection, chronic liver diseases, and hepatic carcinogenesis.

★ 21928 ★ Alberta Cancer Board
Edmonton Radiopharmaceutical Centre
11560 University Ave.
Edmonton, AB, Canada T6G 1Z2
Phone: (780)432-8970 **Fax:** (780)432-8411
Email: dougabra@cancerboard.ab.ca
D.N. Abrams, Dir.
Activities/Fields: Radiopharmaceutical development, including brain blood flow tracers and tumor markers.

★ 21929 ★ Alberta Centre for Active Living
11759 Groat Rd., 3rd Fl.
Edmonton, AB, Canada T5M 3K6
Phone: (780)427-6949 **Fax:** (780)455-2092
Email: active.living@ualberta.ca
Website: http://www.centre4activeliving.ca
Judith Moodie, Dir.
Activities/Fields: Physical activity in Alberta, Canada. **Pub:** *Research Update Bulletin*, quarterly. • *WellSpring*, quarterly. **Frmly:** Alberta Centre for Well-Being.

★ 21930 ★ Alberta Children's Hospital Research Centre
Medical Genetics Group
1820 Richmond Rd. SW
Calgary, AB, Canada T2T 5C7
Phone: (403)229-7373 **Fax:** (403)543-9100
Email: lsiewsin@ucalgary.ca
Website: http://www.ucalgary.ca/UofC/faculties/medicine/medgenetics/index.htm
Dr. Floyd Snyder, Hd.
Activities/Fields: Genetics, including mammalian developmental genetics, genetic control of meiosis, gene mapping and linkage, population genetics, genetic susceptibility to multifactorial inherited disorders such as insulin-dependent diabetes mellitus, use of recombinant DNA methods in clinical medicine, syndrome identification, congenital anomaly surveillance and epidemiology, chromosomal abnormalities in human sperm and eggs, asymmetry, metacarpophalangeal pattern profile studies, regulatory and genetic aspects of nucleotide metabolism, molecular characterization of inherited enzyme abnormalities, and MSAFP - Down Syndrome screen. **Pub:** *Bulletin of the Hereditary Diseases Program of Alberta*, quarterly.

★ 21931 ★ Allergy Research Foundation
11620 Wilshire Blvd., No. 200-210
Los Angeles, CA 90025
Phone: (310)312-5050 **Fax:** (310)575-9292
Email: joncorren@hotmail.com
Jonathan Corren, MD, Dir.
Activities/Fields: Allergies, asthma, urticaria.

★ 21932 ★ ALS Forbes Norris Research Center
2324 Sacramento St., Ste. 111
San Francisco, CA 94115
Phone: (415)923-3604 **Fax:** (415)673-5184
Email: smithsc@sutterhealth.org
Schell Smith, Clinic Coord.
Activities/Fields: Neuromuscular diseases, including Amyotrophic Lateral Sclerosis (Lou Gehrig's Disease).

★ 21933 ★ AMC Cancer Research Center and Foundation
1600 Pierce St.
Denver, CO 80214
Phone: (303)233-6501 **Free:** 800-321-1557
Fax: (303)239-3400
Email: draper@amc.org
Website: http://www.amc.org
Carolyn Draper, Pres.
Activities/Fields: Cancer prevention and control, focusing on early diagnosis, nutrition, chemoprevention, metabolic epidemiology, and intervention trials in human populations, particularly women and underserved populations. Promotes the application of knowledge to reduce cancer incidence and mortality rates.

★ 21934 ★ American Academy of Pediatrics
Division of Health Policy Research
141 NW Point Blvd.
Elk Grove Village, IL 60009-0927
Phone: (847)434-4000 **Fax:** (847)434-8000
Email: byudkowsky@aap.org
Website: http://www.aap.org
Beth K. Yudkowsky, Dir.
Activities/Fields: Organization, financing, and delivery of child health care, including studies on third-party payment programs, health care for low-income and high-risk children, office practices, the distribution of pediatricians, evaluations of pediatric programs, health workforce, and practice parameters/guidelines development. **Pub:** *Newsletter.* **Frmly:** Department of Research.

★ 21935 ★ American Academy of Tropical Medicine and Surgery
16126 E Warren
PO Box 24224
Detroit, MI 48224-0224
Phone: (313)882-0641 **Fax:** (313)882-0979
Dr. Ben Allie, Chm.
Activities/Fields: Tropical diseases, including diarrhea and ankle edema, and evaluation of disease spectrum. **Pub:** *Journal of the American Academy of Tropical Medicine and Surgery.*

★ 21936 ★ American Association for Cancer Research
615 Chestnut St., 17th Fl.
Philadelphia, PA 19106-4404
Phone: (215)440-9300 **Fax:** (215)440-9313
Email: foti@aacr.org
Website: http://www.aacr.org
Margaret Foti, Contact
Activities/Fields: Cancer, focusing on observation, problems, and new significant research.

★ 21937 ★ American Association for Dental Research
1619 Duke St.
Alexandria, VA 22314
Phone: (703)548-0066 **Fax:** (703)548-1883
Email: research@iadr.org
Website: http://www.dentalresearch.org
Activities/Fields: Promotes the advancement of multidisciplinary research of the oral cavity, the adjacent structures, and their relation to the body as a whole. American Association for Dental Research (AADR) supports research fellows and trainees. **Pub:** *Advances in Dental Research*, occasionally. • *Critical Reviews in Oral Biology and Medicine*, bimonthly. • *Journal of Dental Research*, monthly.

★ 21938 ★ American Association on Mental Retardation
444 North Capitol St. NW, Ste. 846
Washington, DC 20001-1512
Phone: (202)387-1968 **Free:** 800-424-3688
Fax: (202)387-2193
Email: dcroser@aamr.org
Website: http://www.aamr.org/index.shtml
M. Doreen Croser, Exec. Dir.
Activities/Fields: Mental retardation, including studies on programmatic aspects of service to persons with mental retardation in residential facilities and community-based settings. Prevention, behavioral, family support, employment, education and health are other areas of research and programmatic concern. **Pub:** *American Journal on Mental Retardation*, bimonthly. • *Mental Retardation*, bimonthly. • *Monographs.* • *News & Notes*, bimonthly.

★ 21939 ★ American Association for the Study of Liver Diseases
1729 King St., Ste. 200
Alexandria, VA 22314-2720
Phone: (703)299-9766 **Fax:** (703)299-9622
Email: scathcart@aasld.org
Website: http://www.aasld.org
Sherrie Cathcart, Contact
Activities/Fields: Liver disease and hepatic research.

★ 21940 ★ American Brain Tumor Association
2720 River Rd., Ste. 146
Des Plaines, IL 60018
Phone: (847)827-9910 **Free:** 800-886-2282
Fax: (847)827-9918
Email: info@abta.org
Website: http://www.abta.org
Naomi Berkowitz, Exec. Dir.
Activities/Fields: Elimination of brain tumors and meeting the needs of brain tumor patients and their families. **Pub:** *The Message Line Newsletter*, 3/year.

★ 21941 ★ American College of Apothecaries Research and Education Foundation
2830 Summer Oaks Dr.
Bartlett, TN 38184-3811
Phone: (901)383-8119 **Fax:** (901)383-8882
Email: acainfo@acainfo.org
Website: http://www.acainfo.org
D.C. Huffman, Jr., Exec. Dir.
Activities/Fields: Three-fold objective of the Foundation is to promote public welfare through development of services in institutions providing health care, encourage and conduct research to improve health care and education, and encourage health care practitioners to improve the quality and availability of their services.

★ 21942 ★ American Council on Science and Health
1995 Broadway, 2nd Fl.
New York, NY 10023-5860
Phone: (212)362-7044 **Fax:** (212)362-4919
Email: acsh@acsh.org
Website: http://www.acsh.org
Dr. Elizabeth M. Whelan, Pres.
Activities/Fields: Relationship between human health and chemicals, foods, nutrition, lifestyle factors, including cigarette smoking, the environment and human health. Activities include studies on animal-to-man extrapolation in laboratory testing, smoking cessation, Lyme disease, Reye's syndrome, hay fever, microwave ovens, infant mortality, life expectancy, AIDS, and automobile occupant restraint systems. **Pub:** *Media Update.* • *Priorities Quarterly Magazine.*

★ 21943 ★ American Federation for Aging Research
70 W 40th St., 11th Fl.
New York, NY 10018
Phone: (212)703-9977 **Free:** 888-582-2327
Fax: (212)997-0330
Email: info@afar.org
Website: http://www.afar.org
Hadley C. Ford, Ch.
Activities/Fields: Aging and associated diseases. **Pub:** *Newsletter*, semiannually.

★ 21944 ★ American Federation for Medical Research
900 Cummings Center, Ste. 221-U
Beverly, MA 01915
Phone: (978)927-8330 **Fax:** (978)524-8890
Email: afmr@prri.com
Website: http://www.afmr.org
Kevin D. O'Brien, Pres.
Activities/Fields: Clinical and laboratory medicine, including cardiovascular, dermatology, endocrinology, gastroenterology, genetics, hematology, immunology and connective tissue, infectious disease, metabolism, neoplastic disease, patient care, pulmonary, renal, and electrolytes. **Pub:** *Journal of Investigative Medicine*, bimonthly.

★ 21945 ★ American Foundation for Aging Research
Biochemistry Department
North Carolina State University
Campus Box 7622
Raleigh, NC 27695-7622
Phone: (919)515-5679 **Fax:** (919)515-2047
Email: afar_office@ncsu.edu
Website: http://www4.ncsu.edu/unity/users/a/agris/afar/afar.htm
Paul F. Agris, Contact
Activities/Fields: Age-related diseases and the biology of aging, focusing on modern biological, genetic, biochemical, and biophysical techniques and approaches to the problems of age-associated diseases and the understanding of aging. **Pub:** *Newsletter*, quarterly.

★ 21946 ★ American Headache Society (AHS)
19 Mantua Rd.
Mount Royal, NJ 08061
Phone: (856)423-0043 **Fax:** (856)423-0082
Email: ahshq@talley.com
Website: http://www.ahsnet.org
Linda McGillicuddy, Contact
Activities/Fields: Headache and head pain. **Pub:** *Headache - The Journal of Head and Face Pain*, 10/year. **Frmly:** American Association for the Study of Headache.

★ 21947 ★ American Hearing Research Foundation
8 S Michigan Ave., Ste. 814
Chicago, IL 60603-4539
Phone: (312)726-9670 **Fax:** (312)726-9695
Email: blederer@american-hearing.org
Website: http://www.american-hearing.org
William L. Lederer, Contact
Activities/Fields: Deafness and hearing disorders, focusing on medical research, education, and public information.

★ 21948 ★ American Institute for Cancer Research (AICR)
1759 R St. NW
Washington, DC 20009
Phone: (202)328-7744 **Free:** 800-843-8114
Fax: (202)328-7226
Email: aicrweb@aicr.org
Website: http://www.aicr.org
Glen Weldon, Contact
Activities/Fields: Provides grants to universities and nonprofit institutions on the role of diet and nutrition in the prevention and adjuvant treatment of cancer. **Pub:** *AICR Newsletter*, quarterly. • *Cancer Resource for cancer patients.* • *Children's newsletter.* • *Meal Planning Reference Book for Dietians.*

★ 21949 ★ American Italian Cancer Foundation
112 E 71st St., Ste. 2B
New York, NY 10021-4121
Phone: (212)628-9090 **Fax:** (212)517-6089
Email: aicf@aicfonline.org
Website: http://www.aicfonline.org
Daniele Bodini, Ch.
Activities/Fields: Cancer prevention and treatment.

★ 21950 ★ American Medical Association Center for Health Policy Research
515 N State St.
Chicago, IL 60610
Phone: (312)464-5387 **Fax:** (312)464-5849
Email: david_emmons@ama-assn.org
Website: http://www.ama-assn.org
David W. Emmons, PhD, Dir.
Activities/Fields: Physician practice arrangements, medical practice costs and reimbursement, antitrust issues, competitiveness of insurance markets, and health system reform. **Pub:** *Physician*, annually. • *Socioeconomic Statistics*, semiannually.

★ 21951 ★ American Society for the Advancement of Anesthesia in Dentistry
6 E Union Ave.
Bound Brook, NJ 08805
Phone: (732)469-9050 **Fax:** (732)271-1985
Website: http://sedation4dentists.com
Dr. David Crystal, Exec. Sec.
Activities/Fields: Anesthesia in dentistry, including the study of sedation and its relation to physiologic sleep and the use of sedatives in dentistry. **Pub:** *Pain Control in Dentistry Journal*, semiannually.

★ 21952 ★ American Society for Bone and Mineral Research
2025 M St. NW, Ste. 800
Washington, DC 20036-3309
Phone: (202)367-1161 **Fax:** (202)367-2161
Email: asbmr@dc.sba.com
Website: http://www.asbmr.org
Joan R. Goldberg, Exec. Dir.
Activities/Fields: Bone, and mineral diseases, focusing on the prevention of osteoporosis. **Pub:** *Journal of Bone and Mineal Research.* • *Primer on Metabolic Bone Diseases and Disorders of Mineral Metabolism.*

★ 21953 ★ American Sudden Infant Death Syndrome Institute
2480 Windy Hill Rd., Ste. 380
Marietta, GA 30067
Phone: (770)612-1030 **Free:** 800-232-SIDS
Fax: (770)612-8277
Email: prevent@sids.org
Website: http://www.sids.org
Alfred Steinschneider, MD, Pres.
Activities/Fields: Sudden Infant Death Syndrome (SIDS), commonly known as crib death, including the search for abnormalities in SIDS victims, study of normal and abnormal infant control mechanisms, pregnancy-related factors, identification of infants at risk, effectiveness of preventive measures, effect of SIDS on families, and effect of preventive measures on families. **Pub:** *Towards an Understanding of SIDS.*

★ 21954 ★ American Type Culture Collection
National Stem Cell Resource
10801 University Blvd.
Manassas, VA 20110-2209
Phone: (703)365-2739 **Fax:** (703)365-2730
Email: rhay@atcc.org
Robert J. Hay, PhD, Prin. Investigator
Activities/Fields: Characterization of nonhuman embryonal stem cells, and lineage- or tissue-specific neonatally derived stem cells from a variety of species with regard to germline chimerism, marker expression, differentiative potential, transfectability, selective agent sensitivity and vector suitability.

★ 21955 ★ American Type Culture Collection
Yeast Genetic Research Resource Center
10801 University Blvd.
Manassas, VA 20110-2209
Phone: (703)365-2742 **Free:** 800-638-6597
Fax: (703)365-2730
Email: sjong@atcc.org
Dr. Shung-Chang Jong, Prin. Investigator
Activities/Fields: Yeast genetic genomic and molecular biology materials.

★ 21956 ★ American University
National Center for Health Fitness
Nebraska Hall, Lower Level
4400 Massachusetts Ave. NW
Washington, DC 20016-8037
Phone: (202)885-6275 **Fax:** (202)885-6288
Email: dhfaa@american.edu
Website: http://www.american.edu/healthpromotion
Dr. Robert C. Karch, Exec. Dir.
Activities/Fields: Worksite health promotion programs, focusing on costs, benefits, and cost-effectiveness, and including international health promotion and special populations.

★ 21957 ★ Anderson Orthopaedic Research Institute
PO Box 7088
Alexandria, VA 22307
Phone: (703)619-4411 **Fax:** (703)799-5982
Email: research@aori.org
Website: http://www.aori.org
Dr. Charles A. Engh, Sr., Med. Dir.
Activities/Fields: Orthopaedics, focusing on total joint replacements.

★ 21958 ★ Andrews-Reiter Epilepsy Research Program
1103 Sonoma Ave.
Santa Rosa, CA 95405-4517
Phone: (707)578-8985 **Fax:** (707)528-1086
Email: djandrews@neteze.com
Website: http://andrewsreiter.com
Donna J. Andrews, PhD, Dir.
Activities/Fields: Behavioral approach to self-control of seizures; adjunctive therapy and medications. **Pub:** *Books, papers.*

★ 21959 ★ Antioch University
Center for Research on Psychological Practice (CROPP)
Graduate School
40 Avon St.
Keene, NH 03431
Phone: (603)357-3122 **Fax:** (603)357-0718
Email: james_fauth@antiochne.edu
Website: http://www.antiochne.edu/prospects/cp/psydcrpp.html
James Fauth, PhD, Dir.
Activities/Fields: Educational aspects of doctoral training in clinical psychology, especially applied clinical research skills and the associated administrative, consultative, and policy-creation roles of doctoral level psychologists. Areas of research include program evaluation and quality assurance issues, such as needs assessment, outcome and satisfaction research, cost-benefit analysis, policy analysis, and other topics relevant to mental health service management; public welfare issues such as treatment access, utilization, and outcome for underserved, rural, low socioeconomic, and minority populations; development of novel treatment and delivery systems; and methodological issues including the assessment and development of methods and measure appropriate for practice research.

★ 21960 ★ Aoki Diabetes Research Institute
1935 Stockton Blvd.
Sacramento, CA 95816
Phone: (916)455-2374 **Fax:** (916)455-3734
Website: http://www.adri.org
Thomas T. Aoki, MD, Dir. of Res.
Activities/Fields: Metabolic diseases, including diabetes mellitus. Current projects include clinical investigations in the treatment of Type I and II diabetic patients.

★ 21961 ★ Arizona Disease Control Research Commission
1616 W Adams, Ste. B-25
Phoenix, AZ 85007
Phone: (602)542-1028 **Fax:** (602)542-6380
Email: adcrc1@getnet.net
Website: http://www.adcrc.com
Dawn C. Schroeder, Exec. Dir.
Activities/Fields: Medical, behavioral, preventive and health policy.

★ 21962 ★ Arizona Health Services Department
Public Health Services
Epidemiology and Disease Control
3815 N Black Canyon Hwy.
Phoenix, AZ 85015
Phone: (602)230-5808 **Fax:** (602)230-5818
Email: lbland@hs.state.az.us
Website: http://www.hs.state.az.us/phs/edc/
Lee A. Bland, Bur. Ch.
Activities/Fields: Epidemiology and disease control.

★ 21963 ★ Arizona Health Services Department
Public Health Services
Epidemiology and Disease Control
Chronic Disease Epidemiology Office
1740 W Adams, Rm. 410
Phoenix, AZ 85007
Phone: (602)542-7333 **Fax:** (602)542-1289
Email: rporter@hs.state.az.us
Richard Porter, Ch.
Activities/Fields: Chronic disease.

★ 21964 ★ Arizona Health Services Department
Public Health Services
Epidemiology and Disease Control
Office of Environmental Health
3815 N Black Canyon Hwy.
Phoenix, AZ 85015
Phone: (602)230-5948 **Fax:** (602)230-5933
Email: lbland@hs.state.az.us
Website: http://www.hs.state.az.us/phs/oeh/
Lee A. Bland, Bur. Ch.
Activities/Fields: Environmental health.

★ 21965 ★ Arizona Health Services Department
Public Health Services
Epidemiology and Disease Control
Office of Infectious Disease Services Office
3815 N Black Canyon Hwy.
Phoenix, AZ 85015
Phone: (602)230-5820 **Fax:** (602)230-5818
Email: vvaz@hs.state.az.us
Website: http://www.hs.state.az.us/phs/oids/index.htm
Victorio J. Vaz, PhD, Ch.
Activities/Fields: Infectious diseases.

★ 21966 ★ Arizona Health Services Department
Public Health Services
Office of Nutrition and Chronic Disease Prevention Services
2927 N 35th Ave., Ste. 400
Phoenix, AZ 85017
Phone: (602)542-1886 **Fax:** (602)542-1890
Email: mtate@hs.state.az.us
Website: http://www.hs.state.az.us/phs/
Margaret Tate, Off. Ch.
Activities/Fields: Health. **Frmly:** Office of Prevention and Health Promotion.

★ 21967 ★ Arizona Health Services Department
Public Health Services
State Laboratory Services
1520 W Adams
Phoenix, AZ 85007-2698
Phone: (602)542-1188 **Fax:** (602)542-0760
Email: wpress@hs.state.az.us
Wesley Press, Contact
Activities/Fields: State health laboratory.

★ 21968 ★ Arizona Health Services Department
Public Health Services
State Laboratory Services
Environmental and Analytical Chemistry Office
1520 W Adams
Phoenix, AZ 85007-2698
Phone: (602)542-6108 **Fax:** (602)364-0281
Email: padler@hs.state.az.us
Website: http://www.hs.state.az.us
Patricia Adler, Mgr.
Activities/Fields: Environmental and analytical chemistry.

★ 21969 ★ Arizona Health Services Department
Public Health Services
State Laboratory Services
Office of Public Health Microbiology
1520 W Adams
Phoenix, AZ 85007-2698
Phone: (602)542-1188 **Fax:** (602)542-0760
Email: vwaddell@hs.state.az.us
Victor Waddell, Contact
Activities/Fields: Microbiology and environmental microbiology. **Frmly:** Environmental and Clinical Microbiology Office.

★ 21970 ★ Arizona Health Services Department
Public Health Services
State Laboratory Services
Tucson Regional Laboratory
416 W Congress St., Ste. 119
Tucson, AZ 85701
Phone: (520)628-6360 **Fax:** (520)628-6356
Judy Fordyce, Mgr.

Activities/Fields: Public health regional lab.

★ 21971 ★ Arizona State University Biomedical Engineering Laboratories
Department of Bioengineering
College of Engineering
PO Box 879709
Tempe, AZ 85287-3028
Phone: (480)965-3028 **Fax:** (480)727-7624
Email: eric.guilbeau@asu.edu
Website: http://www.eas.asu.edu/~bme
Prof. Eric J. Guilbeau, Chm.

Activities/Fields: Biomechanics and bioinstrumentation, including medical devices, artificial organs, biosensors, analysis of motion, and nuclear imaging. Studies cardiovascular, biochemical, and physiological systems in relation to biomedical engineering. Conducts an industrial associate program, develops F.D.A. protocols, provides industrial development support, and offers continuing medical education. **Pub:** *Proceedings.* • *Transactions.*

★ 21972 ★ Arizona State University Cancer Research Institute
PO Box 872404
Tempe, AZ 85287-2404
Phone: (480)965-3351 **Fax:** (480)965-8558
Email: BPettit@asu.edu
Website: http://www.asu.edu/clas/cancer_research/
Dr. George R. Pettit, Dir.

Activities/Fields: Discovery of new cancer chemotherapeutic drugs for human treatment employing organic chemistry, biochemistry, and biology, including a unique program concerned with isolation, structural identification, and syntheses of naturally occurring anticancer agents from marine animals, plants, and microorganisms.

★ 21973 ★ Arizona State University Exercise and Sport Research Institute
E Bldg.
Exercise Science & Physical Education Department
PO Box 870404
Tempe, AZ 85287-0404
Phone: (480)965-3913 **Fax:** (480)965-8108
Email: landers@asu.edu
Website: http://www.asu.edu/clas/espe/
Dr. Daniel M. Landers, Interim Ch.

Activities/Fields: Exercise, and human movement sport, including exercise physiology, sports psychology, exercise biochemistry, biomechanics, and motor behavior of various populations (children, athletes, elderly, adults). **Frmly:** Human Performance Laboratory.

★ 21974 ★ Arkansas Health Department Alcohol and Drug Abuse Prevention Bureau
5800 W 10th, Ste. 907
Little Rock, AR 72204
Phone: (501)280-4500 **Fax:** (501)280-4532
Email: jhill@healthyarkansas.com
Joe Hill, Dir.

Activities/Fields: Substance abuse prevention.

★ 21975 ★ Arthritis and Immune Disorder Research Centre (AIDRC)
Ontario Cancer Institute/Princess Margaret Hospital
610 University Ave., 16th Fl.
Toronto, ON, Canada M5G 2M9
Phone: (416)946-2924 **Fax:** (416)946-2291
Email: aarc@oci.utoronto.ca
Website: http://www.whri.on.ca/index.html
Dr. Edward Keystone, Contact

Activities/Fields: Arthritis and immune disorders, including musculoskeletal and rheumatic diseases, immunology, endocrine disorders, clinical epidemiology, therapeutic endoscopy, vascular diseases, and community health programs.

★ 21976 ★ Arthritis and Immune Disorder Research Centre Arthritis Community Research and Evaluation Unit (ACREU)
Toronto Western Hospital Research Institute
Main Pavilion, 10th Fl., Rm. 316
399 Bathurst St.
Toronto, ON, Canada M5T 2S8
Phone: (416)603-6269 **Fax:** (416)603-6288
Email: acreu@uhnres.utoronto.ca
Website: http://www.acreu.ca
Linda Rothman, Contact

Activities/Fields: Impact of arthritis on people with arthritis in Ontario; identify gaps and needs in services; and develop and evaluate programs for support, care, and health promotion for people with arthritis and their families. **Pub:** *Working papers.*

★ 21977 ★ Arthur M. Fishberg Research Center in Neurobiology
Mt. Sinai School of Medicine, Box 1065
1 Gustave Levy Pl.
New York, NY 10029
Phone: (212)659-5985 **Fax:** (212)849-2510
Email: john.morrison@mssm.edu
Website: http://www.mssm.edu/neurobio/
John H. Morrison, PhD, Dir.

Activities/Fields: Neurobiological systems in humans and mammals, emphasizing aging research. Specific interests include the neuroendocrinology of stress, reproduction and metabolism, the molecular biology of Alzheimer's disease, schizophrenia, and other neurological/psychiatric diseases, and growth factors and growth factor receptor gene expression in the central nervous system.

★ 21978 ★ Association of American Cancer Institutes
Iroquois Bldg., Ste. 305
200 Lothrop St.
Pittsburgh, PA 15213
Phone: (412)647-2076 **Fax:** (412)647-3659
Email: stewartbd@msx.upmc.edu
Website: http://www.aaci-cancer.org
Barbara Duffy Stewart, Exec. Dir.

Activities/Fields: Causes, nature, prevention, treatment, and rehabilitation of cancer.

★ 21979 ★ Association of International Health Researchers
2665 Pleasant Valley Rd.
Mobile, AL 36606
Phone: (334)473-3946
Email: roykadel@mobis.com
Dr. Roy E. Kadel, Contact

Activities/Fields: International health research, focusing on quality, education, techniques and methodologies.

★ 21980 ★ Association for Research of Childhood Cancer
PO Box 251
Buffalo, NY 14225-0251
Phone: (716)681-4433
Website: http://www.arocc.org
Ann O'Donnell, Pres.

Activities/Fields: Pediatric cancer, focusing on funding, expanding, and continuing of research centers. Also provides seed money for pilot projects in cancer research.

★ 21981 ★ Association for Research in Nervous and Mental Disease
Well Medical College
1300 York Ave., Box 171
New York, NY 10021
Phone: (570)839-0296 **Fax:** (570)839-0297
Email: amgooder@med.cornell.edu
Jack D. Barchas, MD, Ch.

Activities/Fields: Neurology, neurosurgery, and psychiatry.

★ 21982 ★ Association for Research in Otolaryngology, Inc. (ARO)
19 Mantua Rd.
Mount Royal, NJ 08061
Phone: (856)423-0041 **Fax:** (856)423-3420
Email: headquarters@aro.org
Website: http://www.aro.org
Tom Sims, Exec. Dir.

Activities/Fields: Basic science and clinical problems associated with hearing, speech, the sense of balance, smell, taste, and diseases of the head and neck. **Pub:** *ARO News*, semiannually. Newsletter. • *Book of Abstracts*, annually. Book. • *JARO Journal of the Association for Research in Otolaryngology*, quarterly.

★ 21983 ★ Atlanta Research and Education Foundation, Inc.
1670 Clairmont Rd., 151F
Decatur, GA 30033-4004
Phone: (404)728-4856 **Fax:** (404)235-3061
Email: aref@mindspring.com
Website: http://www.atlaref.org
Antonio Laracuente, Exec. Dir.

Activities/Fields: Cardiology, pulmonary medicine, HIV/AIDS, infectious diseases, rehabilitation, and cancer,

★ 21984 ★ Atlantic Centre of Excellence for Women's Health (ACEWH)
5940 South St.
PO Box 3070
Halifax, NS, Canada B3J 3G9
Phone: (902)470-6725 **Free:** 888-658-1112
Fax: (902)470-6752
Email: acewh@dal.ca
Website: http://www.medicine.dal.ca/research/organization.htm
Carol Amaratunga, Exec. Dir.

Activities/Fields: Health concerns of Canadian women. **Pub:** *Articles and papers.* • *Newsletters.* • *Reports.*

★ 21985 ★ Augusta Biomedical Research Corp.
PO Box 3134
Augusta, GA 30914-3134
Phone: (706)823-2238 **Fax:** (706)823-3949
Delores H. Vasquez, Exec. Dir.

Activities/Fields: Alzheimer's disease, strokes, cardiology, infectious diseases, gastrointerology, surgery, schizophrenia, neurology, mental health, substance abuse, and Parkinson's Disease.

★ 21986 ★ Aurora Mental Health Research Institute
14301 E Hampden Ave.
Aurora, CO 80014
Phone: (303)617-2300 **Fax:** (303)617-2397
Dr. Randy C. Stith, Ch. Admin.

Activities/Fields: Community-based mental health services and the support systems they require. Provides technical assistance to private and public agencies with special emphasis on person-machine issues relating to microcomputer and mainframe computers.

★ 21987 ★ Autism Research Institute
4182 Adams Ave.
San Diego, CA 92116
Phone: (619)281-7165 **Fax:** (619)563-6840
Website: http://www.autismresearchinstitute.com
Dr. Bernard Rimland, Dir.

Activities/Fields: Causes and treatment of severe behavior disorders in children, particularly autism. Conducts computerized analyses of its diagnostic reports on individual children with severe behavior disorders, and studies the relationship between nutrition and learning and behavior disorders. Serves as an international clearinghouse of information on autism, disseminating information to parents, researchers, hospitals, schools, and professional practitioners. **Pub:** *Autism Research Review International*, quarterly. **Frmly:** Institute for Child Behavior Research.

★ 21988 ★ Axion Research Foundation, Inc.
100 Deepwood Dr.
Hamden, CT 06517
Phone: (203)773-9300 **Fax:** (203)776-2893
Email: bus.manager@axion.org
Dr. D.E. Redmond, Jr., Dir.
Activities/Fields: Neural transplantation, neural imaging, Parkinson's disease, stem cells, and primate visual development.

★ 21989 ★ Ball State University Human Performance Laboratory
Muncie, IN 47306
Phone: (765)285-1158 **Fax:** (765)285-8596
Email: hpl@bsu.edu
Website: http://www.bsu.edu/hpl
Dr. Scott Trappe, Dir.
Activities/Fields: Human performance, including studies on effects of physical training on skeletal muscular metabolism, strength development, aging, research, biomechanics, youth fitness and health, nutritional studies, endocrine mechanisms (e.g. GH), fluid replacement during and following acute dehydration, muscle glycogen utilization during prolonged exertion, and swimming research.

★ 21990 ★ Ball State University Public Health Entomology Laboratory
2000 University Ave.
Muncie, IN 47306
Phone: (765)285-1504 **Fax:** (765)285-3210
Email: rpinger@bsu.edu
Website: http://www.bsu.edu/physiology-health/phel.html
Dr. Robert R. Pinger, Dir.
Activities/Fields: Ticks and tick-borne diseases in Indiana, and other insects affecting human and animal health. Projects include a Rocky Mountain spotted fever and lyme disease tick testing program funded by the Indiana State Department of Health. Provides identification of insects of public health importance. **Pub:** *Pamphlets.*

★ 21991 ★ Baltimore Headache Institute
Johns Hopkins at Green Spring Station
Foxleigh Bldg., Ste. 165
2330 W Joppa Rd.
Lutherville, MD 21093
Phone: (410)583-7171 **Fax:** (410)583-7173
Email: bmondell@jhmi.edu
Dr. Brian Mondell, Med. Dir.
Activities/Fields: Treatment of migraine, muscle contraction, and cluster headaches.

★ 21992 ★ Barbara Ann Karmanos Cancer Institute
4100 John R
Detroit, MI 48201
Phone: (313)966-7170 **Free:** 800-527-6266
Fax: (313)966-7173
Email: ruckdeschel@karmanos.org
Website: http://www.karmanos.org
John C. Ruckdeschel, MD, Pres.
Activities/Fields: Treatment, diagnosis, and prevention of cancer. **Pub:** *Karmanos*, weekly. **Frmly:** Detroit Institute for Cancer Research, Michigan Cancer Foundation.

★ 21993 ★ Barbara Davis Center for Childhood Diabetes
4200 E 9th Ave., Box B140
Denver, CO 80262
Phone: (303)315-8796 **Fax:** (303)315-4124
Email: marian.rewers@uchsc.edu
Website: http://www.uchsc.edu/misc/diabetes/bdc.html
Dr. Marian J. Rewers, Clin. Dir.
Activities/Fields: Diabetes in children and young adults, including immunogenetics, islet cell development and transplantation, complications, and clinical trials of prevention and new treatments in type 1 diabetes and type 2 diabetes in children. **Pub:** *Research papers.*

★ 21994 ★ Barrow Neurological Institute
St. Joseph's Hospital & Medical Center
350 W Thomas Rd.
Phoenix, AZ 85013
Phone: (602)406-3000 **Fax:** (602)406-7167
Email: mholt@chw.edu
Website: http://www.thebni.com
Michael Holt, Contact
Activities/Fields: Neurosciences.

★ 21995 ★ Bassett Healthcare Research Institute
1 Atwell Rd.
Cooperstown, NY 13326
Phone: (607)547-3048 **Fax:** (607)547-3061
Email: research.institute@bassett.org
Allan Green, PhD, Dir.
Activities/Fields: Basic, clinical, and population studies in the following areas: obesity; biochemistry of serum albumin; molecular biology of autoimmune diseases; experimental pathology of cancer; immunology and antigen processing; cardiovascular epidemiology; rural health education; neuroendocrine regulation of breast cancer; nutrition; health care delivery systems; and gut hormones.

★ 21996 ★ Bastyr University Bastyr University AIDS Research Center (BUARC)
Bastyr University Research Institute
14500 Juanita Dr. NE
Kenmore, WA 98028
Phone: (425)602-3165 **Fax:** (425)602-3079
Email: buri@bastyr.edu
Website: http://www.bastyr.edu/research/buarc/
Leanna J. Standish, PhD, Dir.
Activities/Fields: Alternative medical treatments for HIV/AIDS.

★ 21997 ★ Bastyr University Bastyr University Cancer Research Center (BUCRC)
14500 Juanita Dr. NE
Kenmore, WA 98028
Phone: (425)823-1300 **Fax:** (425)823-6222
Email: buri@bastyr.edu
Website: http://www.bastyr.edu/research/bucrc/
Leanna J. Standish, PhD, Res. Dir.
Activities/Fields: Natural medical therapies for treatment and prevention of cancer.

★ 21998 ★ Baton Rouge Regional Tumor Registry
4950 Essen Ln.
Baton Rouge, LA 70809
Phone: (225)767-0430 **Fax:** (225)215-1356
Email: gayd@marybird.com
Gay Duke, Dir.
Activities/Fields: Provides a base of statistical information of cancer incidence in the Baton Rouge area and serves as a useful tool for physicians investigating the success rates of various forms of cancer treatment. Conducts specialized studies in conjunction with the American Cancer Society, National Cancer Institute, and the American College of Surgeons. **Pub:** *Annual Report.* • *Louisiana Tumor Registry.*

★ 21999 ★ Battelle Memorial Institute Centers for Public Health Research and Evaluation (CPHRE)
505 King Ave.
Columbus, OH 43201
Phone: (614)424-6424
Email: solutions@battelle.org
Website: http://www.battelle.org/hhs/cphre/default.stm
Activities/Fields: Health and its determinants, particularly social and behavioral risk assessment and environmental and occupational risk assessment.

★ 22000 ★ Bay Area Tumor Institute
400 30th St., Ste. 301
Oakland, CA 94609-3305
Phone: (510)465-8570 **Fax:** (510)465-8588
Email: bsiegel@bati.org
Website: http://www.bati.org
Barry B. Siegel, Pres.
Activities/Fields: Phase 2 and phase 3 clinical drug trials for cancer therapy.

★ 22001 ★ Baylor College of Medicine Alzheimer's Disease Research Center (ADRC)
6550 Fannin St., 1801
Houston, TX 77030
Phone: (713)798-6660 **Fax:** (713)798-5326
Email: mkenan@bcm.tmc.edu
Website: http://www.bcm.tmc.edu/neurol/struct/adrc/adrc1.html
Rachelle S. Doody, MD, Dir.
Activities/Fields: Alzheimer's Disease.

★ 22002 ★ Baylor College of Medicine Baylor DNA Diagnostic Laboratory
Department of Molecular & Human Genetics
1 Baylor Plz., Rm. 210D
Houston, TX 77030
Phone: (713)798-6536 **Fax:** (713)798-6584
Email: dnalb@bcm.tmc.edu
Website: http://www.bcmgeneticlabs.org/dnadiagnostic.htm
Dr. Benjamin Roa, Dir.
Activities/Fields: DNA-based testing for diagnosis, including carrier detection, prenatal diagnosis of more than 35 genetic diseases, densitometric detection of deletion and duplication mutations, estimations of carrier risk for cystic fibrosis, and rapid diagnosis of Duchenne muscular dystrophy with the multiplex amplication assay.

★ 22003 ★ Baylor College of Medicine Biochemical Genetics Laboratory
1 Baylor Plz., NAB 2015
Houston, TX 77030
Phone: (713)798-4982 **Free:** 800-246-2436
Fax: (713)798-8937
Email: bioc@bcm.tmc.edu
Website: http://www.bcmgeneticlabs.org
William E. O'Brien, PhD, Dir.
Activities/Fields: Diagnosing and monitoring patients with inborn errors of metabolism.

★ 22004 ★ Baylor College of Medicine Center for Allergy and Immunological Disorders
Feigin Center, 4th Fl.
1102 Bates, Ste. 450
Houston, TX 77030
Phone: (832)824-1319 **Fax:** (832)825-1260
Email: wshearer@bcm.tmc.edu
Website: http://www.bcm.tmc.edu/cfar
William T. Shearer, MD, Ch.
Activities/Fields: Allergy and immunological disorders, including basic and clinical projects in cancer immunology, immunoreconstitution of immunodeficient children, immunoregulation of cellular and humoral immune responses, immune complex diseases,

immunotherapy of neoplastic diseases, pulmonary immunology, rheumatic diseases, allergic diseases of children, and AIDS. Facilities available for specialty training of pre- and postdoctoral students on either a research or clinical level.

★ 22005 ★ Baylor College of Medicine Center for Cell and Gene Therapy

Methodist Hospital, Ste. 1100
Houston, TX 77030-2399
Phone: (832)824-4663 **Fax:** (832)825-4668
Email: mbrenner@bcm.tmc.edu
Website: http://www.bcm.tmc.edu/catalog/center_for_cell_and_gene_thera.html
Malcolm K. Brenner, MD, Dir.

Activities/Fields: Correction of hereditary and acquired disorders in humans by delivery of therapeutic genes or cells in patients. Five major areas of research in gene therapy have been targeted: genetic disorders, heart disease, infectious diseases, cancer, and neurological disorders.

★ 22006 ★ Baylor College of Medicine Center for Medical Ethics and Health Policy

1 Baylor Plz.
Houston, TX 77030
Phone: (713)798-6290 **Fax:** (713)798-5678
Email: bbrody@bcm.tmc.edu
Dr. Baruch Brody, Dir.

Activities/Fields: Priorities for health care services, methods of funding health care services, and social controls on health care service, including studies on ethics in clinical decision making and value issues in controlling the cost of medicine. **Pub:** *News Bulletin*, semimonthly.

★ 22007 ★ Baylor College of Medicine Center for Population Research and Studies in Reproduction

Department of Molecular and Cellular Biology
1 Baylor Plz.
Houston, TX 77030
Phone: (713)798-6200 **Fax:** (713)790-1275
Email: berto@bcm.tmc.edu
Dr. Bert W. O'Malley, Dir.

Activities/Fields: Human reproduction, including studies on mechanism of hormone action, male reproduction, steroid regulation and protein synthesis, spermatogenesis, reproductive endocrinology, nucleic acid chemistry and genetic expression, steroid hormonal receptors, physical chemistry, cell proliferation and regulation, biochemistry of chromatin, ribonucleic acid, deoxyribonucleic acid, and cell biology.

★ 22008 ★ Baylor College of Medicine Center for Research on Women with Disabilities (CROWD)

3440 Richmond Ave., Ste. B
Houston, TX 77046
Phone: (713)960-0505 **Free:** 800-442-7693
Fax: (713)961-3555
Email: crowd@bcm.tmc.edu
Website: http://www.bcm.tmc.edu/crowd/
Margaret A. Nosek, PhD, Exec. Dir.

Activities/Fields: Specific problems effecting women with disabilities, particularly such issues as health, aging, civil rights, abuse, and independent living.

★ 22009 ★ Baylor College of Medicine Children's Nutrition Research Center

1100 Bates St.
Houston, TX 77030
Phone: (713)798-7971 **Fax:** (713)798-7098
Email: cnrc@bcm.tmc.edu
Website: http://www.bcm.tmc.edu/cnrc/
Dr. Dennis M. Bier, Dir.

Activities/Fields: Nutrition of infants, children, and pregnant and lactating women. Reseach also focuses on nutrient-gene interactions, and cell, developmental, and plant biology. **Frmly:** Child Health Research Center.

★ 22010 ★ Baylor College of Medicine Cullen Eye Institute

6565 Fannin St., NC-205
Houston, TX 77030
Phone: (713)798-5940 **Fax:** (713)798-4364
Email: ophthalmology@bcm.tmc.edu
Website: http://www.bcm.tmc.edu/ophth/
Dr. Dan B. Jones, Chm.

Activities/Fields: Restoring vision and preventing blindness through a better understanding of the structure, function, and diseases of the eye. Current areas of study include retina research, retinitis pigmentosa, amblyopia, ocular infections, corneal transplantation, genetic diseases of the eye, ocular trauma, cataract, glaucoma, ocular tumors, optic neuritis, laser treatment, vision processing, ocular surface disorders.

★ 22011 ★ Baylor College of Medicine Department of Molecular and Human Genetics

1 Baylor Plz., Rm. T619
Houston, TX 77030
Phone: (713)798-4795 **Fax:** (713)798-7773
Email: genetics@bcm.tmc.edu
Website: http://www.imgen.bcm.tmc.edu/molgen/
Dr. Arthur L. Beaudet, Chm.

Activities/Fields: Genetics including human genome sequencing, mouse genome sequencing, gene replacement therapy, gene expression, structure of human chromosome, gene mapping, cell protein synthesis, recombinant DNA techniques, teratology, dysmorphology, clinical cytogenetics, somatic gene transfer, human lipid storage diseases, molecular biology of immune development and human immunodeficiencies, DNA repair and replication, molecular genetics of heritable eye diseases, prenatal diagnosis of congenital malformations and characterization of families of transgenic mice that show mutant phenotypes. Also coordinates research and patient services in the field of molecular genetics. **Frmly:** Institute for Molecular Genetics.

★ 22012 ★ Baylor College of Medicine Epilepsy Research Center

1 Baylor Plz.
Houston, TX 77030
Phone: (713)790-3109 **Fax:** (713)793-1574
Dr. Peter Kellaway, Dir.

Activities/Fields: Epilepsy research (as related to human patients) in the following areas: clinical research on neurophysiological, pharmacological, and ontogenetic aspects of epilepsy; design and application of computer-based systems to improve EEG detection, characterization, and quantification of the epileptic process in the brain; fundamental studies employing in-vitro brain slice technique to the elucidation of membrane and synaptic mechanisms in epileptogenesis and the mechanisms of action of anticonvulsant and convulsant agents; and developmental neurogenetics of epilepsy.

★ 22013 ★ Baylor College of Medicine General Clinical Research Center

MC 1-3420
Texas Children's Hospital and The Methodist Hospital
TXWT 10041
Houston, TX 77030
Phone: (832)826-1079 **Fax:** (832)825-1061
Email: dbier@bcm.tmc.edu
Dr. Dennis M. Bier, Prog. Dir.

Activities/Fields: Cardiology, endocrinology, gastroenterology, genetics, infectious diseases, pulmonary system, pharmacology, immunology, hematology, rheumatology, and renal disease, including studies on ventricular dysrhythmias, hypopituitarism, bile acid metabolism, argininemia, HIV, and renal tubular acidosis.

★ 22014 ★ Baylor College of Medicine Herbert J. Frensley Center for Imaging Research

1 Baylor Plz.
Department of Radiology
Houston, TX 77030
Phone: (713)798-5146 **Fax:** (713)798-5745
Email: lhayman@bcm.tmc.edu
Dr. L. Anne Hayman, Dir.

Activities/Fields: Magnetic resonance imaging and spectroscopy of brain and muscle in normal and altered states (human experimental animal models, excised samples), the development of novel diagnostic imaging applications, and functional magnetic resonance imaging of normal cognitive function following brain injury in psychiatric conditions.

★ 22015 ★ Baylor College of Medicine Jerry Lewis Neuromuscular Disease Research Center

6501 Fannin St., Ste. NB302
Houston, TX 77030
Phone: (713)798-4072 **Fax:** (713)798-3854
Email: sappel@bcm.tmc.edu
Stanley H. Appel, MD, Dir.

Activities/Fields: Biochemistry, molecular genetics, and physiology of skeletal muscle and motor nerves, including biochemical, physiological, morphological, and genetic techniques to define and compare basic properties of skeletal muscle and neuromuscular disorders. Applies these approaches to animal models of human neuromuscular disease and to cultured muscle and nerve cells from normal and affected people.

★ 22016 ★ Baylor College of Medicine Kleberg Cytogenetics Laboratory

1 Baylor Plz., Rm. 15E
Houston, TX 77030
Phone: (713)798-4984 **Fax:** (713)798-3157
Email: kcl@bcm.tmc.edu
Website: http://www.bcmgeneticlabs.org/klebergcytogenetics.htm
Sau Wai Cheung, PhD, Dir.

Activities/Fields: High-resolution chromosome analysis and development of molecular diagnostic methods for cytogenetic disorders and chromosomal studies.

★ 22017 ★ Baylor College of Medicine Maternal Fetal Medicine

Smith Tower, Ste. 901
6550 Fannin
Houston, TX 77030
Phone: (713)798-7593 **Fax:** (713)798-6956
Email: lwilkins@bcm.tmc.edu
Dr. Isabelle Wilkins, Dir.

Activities/Fields: Prenatal diagnosis by ultrasonography, amniocentesis, and fetal blood sampling, chorionic villi sampling, longitudinal fetal growth, and pre/post-conceptual counseling. Conducts evaluation of intrauterine growth retardation in at-risk patients on prospective basis. **Pub:** *Annual Report of Department of Obstetrics/Gynecology*. **Frmly:** Prenatal Diagnostic Center.

★ 22018 ★ Baylor College of Medicine Mental Retardation Research Center

Mail Stop BCM 225
1 Baylor Plaza, T809
Houston, TX 77030
Phone: (713)798-7353 **Fax:** (713)798-8704
Email: hzoghbi@bcm.tmc.edu
Website: http://mrrc.bcm.tmc.edu
Huda Y. Zoghbi, MD, Dir.

Activities/Fields: Mental retardation and its prevention. Research includes Rett syndrome, epilepsy, Angelman and Prader-Willi syndrome, gene therapy, human X chromosome, cytomegalovirus infection, group b streptococci, chondrodysplasia punctata, and spinocerebellar ataxia, Fragile X Syndrome, Aicardi Syndrome, HIV infection, metabolic disorders, Incontinentia Pigmenti, Williams Syndrome, Retinal degeneration and neuropathies.

★ 22019 ★ Baylor College of Medicine Methodist DeBakey Heart Center
6550 Fannin
Houston, TX 77030
Free: (866)332-2539
Website: http://www.methodisthealth.com/heartcenter
Dr. Michael E. DeBakey, Ch. Surgeon
Activities/Fields: Atherosclerosis with an emphasis on lipoprotein structure and function and cholesterol metabolism; cardiovascular studies on calcium metabolism, fatty acid metabolism, and cellular ultrastructure; cardiology and cardiovascular surgery, including therapeutic intervention in heart failure, ischemic cardiomyopathy, and role of complement in myocardial infarction; transplantation; and hypertension studies that focus on aldosteronerenin ratio antihypertensive agents. Community outreach studies include control of blood pressure, diabetes, and diet modification. **Pub:** *The DeBakey Health Letter.* **Frmly:** Cardiovascular Research and Training Center; National Heart and Blood Vessel Research and Demonstration Center.

★ 22020 ★ Baylor College of Medicine Meyer Center for Developmental Pediatrics
MC 1530
6621 Fannin St.
Houston, TX 77030
Phone: (832)822-3400 **Fax:** (832)825-3399
Dr. Cherry Sellers-Vinson, Actg. Dir.
Activities/Fields: Developmentally disabled, developmental pediatrics, learning disabilities, low-birth-weight infants, maternal medications, cytomegalo inclusion virus, congenital rubella syndrome, neonatal intracranial hemorrhage, outcome prematurity, and attention deficit/hyperactivity disorder. **Frmly:** Child Development Clinics.

★ 22021 ★ Baylor College of Medicine Roy M. and Phyllis Gough Huffington Center on Aging
1 Baylor Plz., M320
Houston, TX 77030
Phone: (713)798-5804 **Fax:** (713)798-6688
Email: rsmith@bcm.tmc.edu
Website: http://www.hcoa.org
Roy G. Smith, PhD, Dir.
Activities/Fields: Cell and molecular biology of aging, cardiovascular disease, and ethics in long-term care.

★ 22022 ★ Baylor College of Medicine Sleep Disorders and Research Center
2002 Holcombe Blvd., 6C344
Houston, TX 77030
Phone: (713)794-7563 **Fax:** (713)794-7563
Email: maxh@bcm.tmc.edu
Max Hirshkowitz, Dir.
Activities/Fields: Neuropsychopharmacology of sleep, sleep disorders and erectile dysfunction.

★ 22023 ★ Baylor College of Medicine Speech and Language Center
6501 Fannin St., Ste. NB302
Houston, TX 77030
Phone: (713)798-7415 **Fax:** (713)798-6417
Email: davidr@bcm.tmc.edu
Dr. David Rosenfield, Dir.
Activities/Fields: Speech motor control system, including stuttering, voice problems, motor control, and digital signal and acoustic processing. **Pub:** *Annual Report.* • *Neuro/Speech Newsletter.* **Frmly:** Stuttering Center and Speech Motor Control Laboratory.

★ 22024 ★ Baylor College of Medicine Three-Dimensional Electron Microscopy of Macromolecules
McLean Department of Biochemistry & Molecular Biology
1 Baylor Plz.
Houston, TX 77030
Phone: (713)798-6985 **Fax:** (713)798-1625
Email: wah@bcm.tmc.edu
Website: http://ncmi.bcm.tmc.edu
Wah Chiu, PhD, Prin. Investigator
Activities/Fields: Application of electron cryomicroscopy to the determination of three-dimensional structures of biological macromolecular assemblies at high resolution.

★ 22025 ★ Baylor University Baylor Research Institute
3434 Live Oak St., No. 125
Dallas, TX 75204-6134
Phone: (214)820-2687 **Fax:** (214)820-4952
Website: http://www.baylorhealth.com/specialtycenters/bri/more_about_bri.htm
Brenda Russell, VP
Activities/Fields: Biomedicine, including digestive diseases, oncology, photobiology, organ transplants, muscle physiology, and metabolic diseases. **Pub:** *Baylor Proceedings*, quarterly. Proceedings.

★ 22026 ★ Baylor University Medical Center Baylor-Tom Landry Sport and Wellness Science Lab
411 N Washington, Ste. 3000
Dallas, TX 75246
Phone: (214)820-1513 **Fax:** (214)820-1682
Email: dg.mcbrayer@baylordallas.edu
Darvin G. McBrayer, Coord.
Activities/Fields: Sports/fitness science, including body composition, basal metabolism, exercise physiology, nutrition and biochemistry for athletes and non-athletes. **Frmly:** Human Performance Center.

★ 22027 ★ Baylor University Medical Center Blood and Bone Marrow Transplant Program
3535 Worth St., Ste. 500
Dallas, TX 75246
Phone: (214)820-2610 **Fax:** (214)820-7346
Email: jw.fay@baylorhealth.edu
Joseph W. Fay, MD, Dir.
Activities/Fields: Bone marrow transplantation research in leukemia/lymphoma studies, including graft-vs-host disease, evaluation of immune recovery post transplant, evaluation of growth factors in transplantation, and applications of molecular biology/gene rearrangement in marrow transplantation, and dendritic cell transplantation.

★ 22028 ★ Benign Essential Blepharospasm Research Foundation, Inc. (BEBRF)
637 N 7th St.
PO Box 12468
Beaumont, TX 77726-2468
Phone: (409)832-0788 **Fax:** (409)832-0890
Email: bebrf@ih2000.net
Website: http://www.blepharospasm.org/
Mary Lou Thompson, Pres.
Activities/Fields: Benign Essential Blepharospasm/Meige (BEB/M) Syndrome and related disorders and infirmities of the facial musculature. BEB/M is an involuntary, uncontrollable spastic contraction of the eyelids and other facial musculature. **Pub:** *Newsletter*, bimonthly.

★ 22029 ★ Bernard W. Gimbel Multiple Sclerosis Comprehensive Care Center (MSCCC)
Holy Name Hospital
718 Teaneck Rd.
Teaneck, NJ 07666
Phone: (201)837-0727 **Fax:** (201)837-8504
Mary Ann Picone, MD, Dir.
Activities/Fields: Treatment and modalities for the relief of symptoms associated with multiple sclerosis, as well as improvement in overall functioning, prevention of worsening of the disease, and promotion of maximal independence. **Pub:** *MSCC Centerpiece Newsletter*, quarterly. Newsletter.

★ 22030 ★ Beth Israel Medical Center General Clinical Research Center
Feldberg & Gryzmish Bldgs., 8th Fl., East Campus
330 Brookline Ave.
Boston, MA 02215
Phone: (617)667-4269 **Fax:** (617)667-5953
Email: mbeck1@caregroup.harvard.edu
Website: http://research.caregroup.org/gcrc
Steven Freedman, MD, Prog. Dir.
Activities/Fields: Biomedicine, cardiology, endocrinology, gastroenterology, gerontology, hematology, nephrology, neurology, nutrition, obstetrics, pulmonary physiology, psychiatry, and surgery.

★ 22031 ★ Biomedical Research Foundation of Northwest Louisiana
1505 Kings Hwy.
Shreveport, LA 71103
Phone: (318)675-4100 **Free:** 800-685-1152
Fax: (318)675-4120
Email: jsharp@biomed.org
Website: http://www.biomed.org
Jack Sharp, Pres.
Activities/Fields: Cardiovascular disease, neurobiology, stroke, medical imaging, medical information. **Pub:** *Annual report.* • *President's Report*, quarterly.

★ 22032 ★ Biomedical Research Institute
12111 Parklawn Dr.
Rockville, MD 20852
Phone: (301)881-3300 **Fax:** (301)881-7640
Email: biomed@afbr-bri.com
Website: http://www.afbr-bri.com
Dr. James L. Leef, Dir.
Activities/Fields: Conducts research on malaria and schistosomiasis, manages a low temperature repository, and performs large scale freeze-drying.

★ 22033 ★ Blanchette Rockefeller Neurosciences Institute
PO Box 9301
Morgantown, WV 26506
Phone: (304)293-3962
Website: http://www.brni.org/body.htm
Dr. Fred Butcher, Interim Exec. Dir.
Activities/Fields: Neurodegenerative diseases and other cognitive disorders, particularly those involving learning and memory; mood disorders, such as depression, anxiety, and schizophrenia; epilepsy; central nervous system injury; post-traumatic stress disorder; and other areas of fundamental neuroscience and neural disorders, including auditory and visual processing, particularly in relation to language development.

★ 22034 ★ The Blood Center
PO Box 2178
Milwaukee, WI 53201-2178
Phone: (414)933-5000 **Fax:** (414)937-6284
Email: cmmiller@bcsew.edu
Website: http://www.bloodctrwise.org
John W. Adamson, MD, Exec. VP/Res.
Activities/Fields: Blood-related research in the areas of platelets, hemostasis/thrombosis, immunogenetics, vascular biology, stem cell biology, and transfusion

medicine. Major activities include the collection and distribution of blood and blood products, basic research, clinical laboratory testing, and bone marrow donor recruitment. **Pub:** *Annual report.*

★ 22035 ★ Blood and Marrow Transplant Laboratory
Children's Hospital of Orange County
455 S Main St.
Orange, CA 92868
Phone: (714)289-4060 **Fax:** (714)639-5907
Dr. Leonard Sender, Medical Dir.

Activities/Fields: Bone marrow immunology experiments, including tumor purging using chemotherapy and monoclonal antibodies, molecular detection of minimal residual disease, purification of hematopoietic stem cells, and purging and cultivation of bone marrow. Also studies umbilical cord blood harvesting, storage, and expansion; and T-cell depletion for unrelated bone marrow transplantation. **Frmly:** Bone Marrow Transplant Laboratory.

★ 22036 ★ Boston Biomedical Research Institute (BBRI)
64 Grove St.
Watertown, MA 02472-2829
Phone: (617)658-7700
Email: morgan@bbri.org
Website: http://www.bbri.org
Dr. Kathleen Morgan, Contact

Activities/Fields: Biological and medical sciences, including fundamental biomedical studies on cell metabolism, developmental biology, gene regulation, recombinant DNA, monoclonal antibodies, intercellular matrix biology, muscle diseases, connective tissue diseases, and muscular dystrophy. **Pub:** *Messenger Newsletter*, semiannually. **Frmly:** Institute of Biological and Medical Sciences.

★ 22037 ★ Boston Comprehensive Sickle Cell Center
FGH Bldg., 2nd Fl.
Boston Medical Center
820 Harrison Ave.
Boston, MA 02118
Phone: (617)414-5727 **Fax:** (617)414-5739
Email: msteinberg@medicine.bu.edu
Dr. Martin H. Steinberg, Co-Dir.

Activities/Fields: Sickle cell trait and sickle cell anemia/disease, including molecular, cellular, tissue, and organ studies. Investigates glucose 6-phosphate dehydrogenase deficiency, coagulation and carbomylation of hemoglobin S, anti-sickling compounds, red cell membrane alterations, fetal jeopardy, fetal hemoglobin synthesis, cardiac manifestations, lung function, and infection. Conducts ultrastructural and clinical studies and seeks to translate basic and clinical research to improved health care at the community level. **Pub:** *Educational Booklets.*

★ 22038 ★ Boston University Alzheimer's Disease Center (ADC)
GRECC Program (182B)
Bedford VAMC
200 Springs Rd.
Bedford, MA 01730
Phone: (781)687-2632 **Fax:** (781)687-3515
Email: nkowall@bu.edu
Neil William Kowall, MD, Dir.

Activities/Fields: Alzheimer's Disease.

★ 22039 ★ Boston University Cancer Research Center (CRC)
715 Albany St., K-703
Boston, MA 02118
Phone: (617)638-8265 **Fax:** (617)638-6518
Email: sfenness@bu.edu
Website: http://www.bumc.bu.edu/Departments/HomeMain.asp?DepartmentID=109
Salli Fennessey, Contact

Activities/Fields: Cancer, including cellular and molecular biology, receptors, carcinogenesis, immunology, toxicology, molecular genetics, nucleic acid damage and repair, mechanism of action of chemotherapeutic agents, and new approaches to cancer treatment. Affiliated hospitals provide a wide variety of specialized approaches to clinical management of cancer, including surgery, radiation therapy, chemotherapy, and immunotherapy. Patients entered on local, regional, and national treatment protocols. **Frmly:** Hubert H. Humphrey Cancer Research Center.

★ 22040 ★ Boston University Center for Anxiety and Related Disorders (CARD)
Kenmore Sq.
648 Beacon St., 6th Fl.
Boston, MA 02215
Phone: (617)353-9610 **Fax:** (617)353-9609
Email: dhbarlow@bu.edu
Website: http://www.bu.edu/anxiety/adult.html
David H. Barlow, PhD, Dir.

Activities/Fields: Anxiety disorders in adults and children, including generalized anxiety disorder, panic disorder, agoraphobia, obsessive-compulsive disorder, social phobia, depression, and various sexual-function disorders.

★ 22041 ★ Boston University Center for Human Genetics
715 Albany St.
Boston, MA 02118-2394
Phone: (617)638-7083 **Fax:** (617)638-7092
Email: amilunsk@bu.edu
Website: http://www.bumc.bu.edu/Departments/HomeMain.asp?DepartmentID=118
Aubrey Milunsky, MD, Dir.

Activities/Fields: Routine and specialized chromosome studies, prenatal diagnosis of genetic disorders, molecular genetic (DNA) analysis for diagnosis and carrier detection, maternal serum quadruple screening, biochemical genetic studies, cancer cytogenetics, paternity testing with DNA analysis, and genetic counseling and birth defects evaluation.

★ 22042 ★ Boston University Center for Rehabilitation Effectiveness (CRE)
Sargent College of Health & Rehabilitation Sciences
635 Commonwealth Ave., 6th Fl.
Boston, MA 02215-1605
Phone: (617)353-3277 **Fax:** (617)358-1355
Email: pandres@bu.edu
Website: http://www.bu.edu/cre/
Patricia Andres, Mgr.

Activities/Fields: Rehabilitative care and its effectiveness across the lifespan, specifically studies on human performance, motor learning and physiological processes underlying clinical improvements; investigations of psychosocial and interpersonal factors affecting rehabilitation outcome; evaluation of rehabilitation protocols on all types of facilities; etc. **Pub:** *Technical manuals.*

★ 22043 ★ Boston University General Clinical Research Center
East Newton Campus, Evans 8
Boston Medical Ctr.
715 Albany St., E-860
Boston, MA 02118
Phone: (617)414-1960 **Fax:** (617)414-1969
Email: jkopp@bu.edu
Website: http://www.bumc.bu.edu/Departments/HomeMain.asp?DepartmentID=291
Janice Kopp, Admin.

Activities/Fields: Cardiovascular disease, collagen vascular disease, diabetes, gastrointestinal disease, nephrology, pediatrics, dermatology, AIDS, psoraisis, amyloidosis, and drug abuse.

★ 22044 ★ Boston University Harold Goodglass Aphasia Research Center
Sch. of Med.
DVAMC, 12A
150 S Huntington Ave.
Boston, MA 02130-4817
Phone: (617)232-9500 **Fax:** (617)522-4786
Email: malbert@bu.edu
Website: http://www.bu.edu/aphasia
Dr. Martin L. Albert, Dir.

Activities/Fields: Cognitive and language impairment following brain damage and closely related topics in psycholinguistics, cognitive science, and behavioral neuroscience. **Frmly:** Aphasia Research Center.

★ 22045 ★ Boston University Hearing Research Center (HRC)
Department of Biomedical Engineering
44 Cummington St.
Boston, MA 02215
Phone: (617)353-4342 **Fax:** (617)353-6766
Email: colburn@bu.edu
Website: http://www.bu.edu/hrc/
H. Steven Colburn, PhD, Dir.

Activities/Fields: Auditory processing in order to understand hearing in both normal and impaired auditory systems. Research focuses on anatomical studies of the cochlea and brainstem, measurements of mechanical properties of cochlear structures, single-unit and multi-unit recordings up to the level of the inferior colliculus, and measurements of auditory evoked potentials and otoacoustic emissions, as well as measurements of hearing abilities of human listeners with and without hearing impairments.

★ 22046 ★ Boston University Hearing Research Center Auditory Neurophysiology Laboratory
Biomedical Engineering Department
44 Cummington St.
Boston, MA 02215
Phone: (617)353-2817 **Fax:** (617)353-6766
Email: hfv@enga.bu.edu
Website: http://www.bu.edu/hrc/research.html
Herbert F. Voigt, Dir.

Activities/Fields: Neuronal circuitry of the cochlear nucleus, particularly the dorsal cochlear nucleus, focusing on functional interactions of neurons and extracellular and intracellular recording and marking studies of neurons in the cochlear nucleus.

★ 22047 ★ Boston University Hearing Research Center Binaural Hearing Laboratory
Biomedical Engineering
44 Cummington St.
Boston, MA 02215
Phone: (617)353-4342 **Fax:** (617)353-6766
Email: colburn@bu.edu
Website: http://www.bu.edu/hrc/research.html
H. Steven Colburn, Dir.

Activities/Fields: Binaural interaction, including phenomena such as sound localization for which monaural processing also plays a major role. The goal of these studies is an integrated understanding of binaural interaction and its role in human sound perception including the interpretation of acoustic cues in complex sound environments.

★ 22048 ★ Boston University Hearing Research Center CNS Psychoacoustics Laboratory
Cognitive & Neural Systems
677 Beacon St., Rm. 311
Boston, MA 02215
Phone: (617)353-5764
Email: shinn@cns.bu.edu
Website: http://www.bu.edu/hrc/research.html
Barbara G. Shinn-Cunningham, Dir.

Activities/Fields: Spatial hearing, learning and plasticity in spatial perception, and quantitative analysis and modeling of human perception and performance.

★ 22049 ★ Boston University Hearing Research Center Cochlear Biophysics Laboratory
Biomedical Engineering
44 Cummington St.
Boston, MA 02215
Phone: (617)353-4343
Email: dcm@bu.edu
Website: http://www.bu.edu/hrc/research.html
David C. Mountain, Contact
Activities/Fields: Mechanisms responsible for the mechanical sensitivity and frequency selectivity of the mammalian cochlea and the measurement and interpretation of electric fields produced by electrically excitable tissues with the major focus being the auditory system.

★ 22050 ★ Boston University Hearing Research Center Knowledge-Based Signal Processing Group
Electrical & Computer Engineering
44 Cummington St.
Boston, MA 02215
Phone: (617)353-4461
Email: hamid@engc.bu.edu
Website: http://www.bu.edu/hrc/research.html
S. Hamid Nawab, Dir.
Activities/Fields: Integration of signal processing and signal understanding technologies and their application to robotic hearing and assisting devices for the hearing impaired.

★ 22051 ★ Boston University Hearing Research Center Laboratory of Cellular and Molecular Hearing Research
BUMC Anatomy & Neurobiology
80 E Concord St.
Boston, MA 02215
Phone: (617)638-4530 **Fax:** (617)638-4531
Email: dcotanche@cajal-1.bu.edu
Website: http://www.bu.edu/hrc/research.html
Douglas A. Cotanche, Dir.
Activities/Fields: Factors which regulate the growth of hair cells in the cochlea during normal embryonic development and in regeneration following noise-induced trauma.

★ 22052 ★ Boston University Hearing Research Center Psychoacoustics Laboratory
Communication Disorders
635 Commonwealth Ave.
Boston, MA 02215
Phone: (617)353-5640 **Fax:** (617)353-7500
Email: gkidd@acs.bu.edu
Website: http://www.bu.edu/hrc/research.html
Gerald Kidd, Jr., Dir.
Activities/Fields: Auditory perception of listeners with normal hearing and listeners with sensorineural hearing loss.

★ 22053 ★ Boston University Hearing Research Center Speech Perception Laboratory
Communication Disorders
635 Commonwealth Ave.
Boston, MA 02215
Phone: (617)353-1983 **Fax:** (617)353-5074
Email: matthies@bu.edu
Website: http://www.bu.edu/hrc/research.html
Melanie L. Matthies, Dir.
Activities/Fields: Perception of a wide range of speech stimuli. Work includes quantifying the changes of the speech of persons who have lost their hearing through neurofibromatosis. It also includes analyzing the speech of subjects who were previously deafened and have received cochlear implants which allows them to improve their speech.

★ 22054 ★ Boston University Laboratory of Neuropsychology
715 Albany St., L-815
Boston, MA 02118
Phone: (617)638-4803 **Fax:** (617)638-4806
Email: hcr@acs.bu.edu
Prof. Marlene Oscar Berman, PhD, Ch.
Activities/Fields: Alcoholism, aphasia, apraxia, dementia, memory disorders, autism, schizophrenia, dyslexia, normal brain function and behavior, and psychopharmacology. Projects emphasize the relationship between brain structure and brain function, especially as related to human neurological disorders. **Pub:** *Bostonia Magazine*, quarterly. • *News & Notes*, monthly. • *Research Reports Quarterly.*

★ 22055 ★ Boston University Mass Spectrometry Resource for Biology and Medicine
Departments of Biochemistry & Biophysics
School of Medicine
715 Albany St., R-806
Boston, MA 02118-2526
Phone: (617)638-6490 **Fax:** (617)638-6491
Email: cecmsms@bu.edu
Website: http://www.bumc.bu.edu/Departments/HomeMain.asp?DepartmentID=354
Catherine E. Costello, PhD, Prin. Investigator
Activities/Fields: High-sensitivity structural determinations and analyses of biological compounds, especially glycoconjugates, oligosaccharides, and proteins; structure-activity studies related to proteins; structure-activity studies related to immunology, carcinogenesis, developmental biology, parasitology and infectious diseases, tissue implantation and rejection; biophysical properties of carbohydrates and glycoconjugates; carbohydrate and amino acid sequence determinations of glycoproteins and proteins; structure elucidation of unusual residues and posttranslational modifications; characterization of oligonucleotides and metal complexes such as imaging agents.

★ 22056 ★ Boston University Neuromuscular Research Center
19 Deerfield St., 4th Fl.
Boston, MA 02215
Phone: (617)353-9757 **Fax:** (617)353-5737
Email: ddwong@bu.edu
Website: http://nmrc.bu.edu
Dr. Carlo J. De Luca, Dir.
Activities/Fields: Motor control, including motor unit firing during sustained isometric contractions, synchronization evaluation, synchronization across muscles, and modeling of force production in the muscle; low back pain, including normative database study of back muscle function, EMG parameters of lumbar back muscles, development of test protocols related to the befavior of back mucles, and muscle performance in the back analysis system compared to lifting tasks; posture and movement, etc. The center is organized into the following components: Motor Unit Lab, Muscle Fatigue Lab, Injury Analysis and Prevention Lab, Motion Analysis Lab, Motor Control Lab, Electrophysiology Lab, Electromyography Lab, Signal Processing Lab and Design Lab. **Pub:** *Annual Activity Report.*

★ 22057 ★ Boston University Neuromuscular Research Center Design Laboratory
19 Deerfield St., 4th Fl.
Boston, MA 02215
Phone: (617)358-0724 **Fax:** (617)353-5737
Email: dgilmore@bu.edu
Website: http://nmrc.bu.edu/labs/dl/index.html
L. Donald Gilmore, Supvr.
Activities/Fields: Develops instrumentation for other NMRC laboratories. Electronic hardware and software technologies, used in the investigation of neuromuscular performance, are designed for eventual implementation into the clinical environment. Several devices, including specialized electrodes for detecting and anlyzing the surface electromyographic signal, have been developed here.

★ 22058 ★ Boston University Neuromuscular Research Center Electromyography Laboratory
19 Deerfield St., 4th Fl.
Boston, MA 02215
Phone: (617)353-9757 **Fax:** (617)353-5737
Email: webmaster@nmrc.edu
Website: http://nmrc.bu.edu
Dr. Carlo J. DeLuca, Dir.
Activities/Fields: Techniques for the detection and analysis of EMG data such as study of the use of innovative electrodes' geometry and comparison of their performance to assess functional activities in ergonomics and risk factors.

★ 22059 ★ Boston University NeuroMuscular Research Center Electrophysiology Laboratory
19 Deerfield St., 4th Fl.
Boston, MA 02215
Phone: (617)358-0718 **Fax:** (617)353-5737
Email: sroy@bu.edu
Website: http://nmrc.bu.edu/labs/epl
Dr. Serge Roy, Supv.
Activities/Fields: In vitro studies of isolated muscles of rats to compare muscle physiology/morphology to the electrical signals produced during muscle contraction. Aims to further the development of surface electromyography (EMG) as a means of assessing human muscle function and fatigue.

★ 22060 ★ Boston University Neuromuscular Research Center Injury Analysis and Prevention Laboratory
19 Deerfield St., 4th Fl.
Boston, MA 02215
Phone: (617)353-9638 **Fax:** (617)353-5737
Email: loddsson@bu.edu
Website: http://nmrc.bu.edu
Dr. Lars I.E. Oddsson, Supvr.
Activities/Fields: Injury mechanism related to postural control during slips and falls, as well as lifting and other types of manual load handling. Biomechanical, neurophysiological, electrophysiological, and epidemiological tools are used to develop a better understanding of mechanisms causing injury, thus increasing the possibility of developing successful preventive measures.

★ 22061 ★ Boston University Neuromuscular Research Center Motor Control Laboratory
19 Deerfield St., 4th Fl.
Boston, MA 02215
Phone: (617)358-0719 **Fax:** (617)353-5737
Email: webmaster@nmrc.edu
Website: http://nmrc.bu.edu
Dr. Gerald L. Gottlieb, Supvr.
Activities/Fields: Voluntary control of human limbs, particularly the determinants of movement which are higher motor centers, reflex mechanism, and muscle properties. Both normal motor control and the behavior of patients with diverse movement disorders are explored.

★ 22062 ★ Boston University NeuroMuscular Research Center Motor Unit Laboratory
19 Deerfield St., 4th Fl.
Boston, MA 02215
Phone: (617)353-9756 **Fax:** (617)353-5737
Email: cjd@bu.edu

Website: http://nmrc.bu.edu/labs/mul
Dr. Carlo J. De Luca, Dir.
Activities/Fields: Investigates how the brain and spinal cord control the activation of muscle cells to produce muscle force. Seeks to examine muscle fiber discharge history in detail, to better understand the physiological rules that regulate muscle contractions, and to improve the ability of the neurologist to categorize and quantify neurological dysfunction.

★ 22063 ★ Boston University NeuroMuscular Research Center Muscle Fatigue Laboratory
19 Deerfield St., 4th Fl.
Boston, MA 02215
Phone: (617)353-0718 **Fax:** (617)353-5737
Email: sroy@bu.edu
Website: http://nmrc.bu.edu/labs/mfl
Dr. Serge Roy, Supv.
Activities/Fields: Use of advanced signal processing techniques for the analysis of electromyographic signals, especially techniques for the analysis of nonstationary surface EMG data, to estimate localized muscle fatigue during static and dynamic contractions.

★ 22064 ★ Boston University Neuromuscular Research Center Signal Processing Laboratory
19 Deerfield St., 4th Fl.
Boston, MA 02215
Phone: (617)358-0715 **Fax:** (617)353-5737
Email: webmaster@nmrc.bu.edu
Website: http://nmrc.bu.edu
Prof. Paolo Bonato, Res. Asst.
Activities/Fields: Use of advanced signal processing techniques for the analysis of electromyographic signals, especially the development of techniques for the analysis of nonstationary surface EMG data.

★ 22065 ★ Boston University Pulmonary Center
Sch. of Medicine
715 Albany St., R-304
Boston, MA 02118
Phone: (617)638-4860 **Fax:** (617)536-8093
Email: mwilliams@lung.bumc.bu.edu
Website: http://www.bupulmonary.org
Mary C. Williams, PhD, Assoc. Dir.
Activities/Fields: Development of an integrated approach to the cell and molecular biology of lung cells.

★ 22066 ★ Boys Town National Research Hospital Center for Hereditary Communication Disorders
555 N 30th St.
Omaha, NE 68131
Phone: (402)498-6556 **Free:** 800-320-1171
Fax: (402)498-6331
William J. Kimberling, Dir.
Activities/Fields: Genetic communication disorders, with emphasis on hearing loss, including Usher Syndrome, recessive non-syndromic hearing loss, dominant progressive hearing loss, branchio-oto-renal syndrome, and hypopigmentation and hearing loss.

★ 22067 ★ Brain-Body Institute (BBI)
St. Joseph's Healthcare Hamilton
50 Charlton Ave. E
Hamilton, ON, Canada L8N 4A6
Phone: (905)522-4941
Email: jbienens@email.stjosham.on.ca
Dr. John Bienenstock, Dir.
Activities/Fields: Relationship between the brain, the nervous system, and bodily disorders, especially the interaction and impact of environmental factors, including stress, early life experiences and early microbial exposure on the brain and nervous system.

★ 22068 ★ Brain Imaging and Analysis Center (BIAC)
PO Box 3918
Durham, NC 27710
Phone: (919)681-9337 **Fax:** (919)681-7033
Email: info@biac.duke.edu
Website: http://www.biac.duke.edu/research/
Gregory McCarthy, PhD, Dir.
Activities/Fields: Functional properties of the human brain by incorporating state-of-the-art research techniques into studies of cognitive processing. Researchers investigate the organization of visual cortex, the cortical control of attention, brain circuits involved with learning and memory. **Pub:** *Papers.*

★ 22069 ★ Brain Research Foundation
5812 S Ellis Ave., Rm. J-141, MC 7112
Chicago, IL 60637
Phone: (773)834-6750 **Fax:** (773)834-6751
Email: info@brainresearchfdn.org
Website: http://www.brainresearchfdn.org
Terre A. Sharma, PhD, Exec. Dir.
Activities/Fields: Provides support for research projects, new equipment, and scientific education in neurology, psychiatry, neurobiology, neurosurgery, and pharmacology/physiology at the Brain Research Institute of the University of Chicago. **Pub:** *Annual Audit. • Annual Report. • Brain Waves Newsletter*, quarterly.

★ 22070 ★ Brandeis University Ashton Graybiel Spatial Orientation Laboratory
Mail Stop 033
415 South St.
Waltham, MA 02454
Phone: (781)736-2033 **Fax:** (781)736-2031
Email: lackner@brandeis.edu
Website: http://graybiel.cc.brandeis.edu/
James R. Lackner, Dir.
Activities/Fields: Human spatial orientation, effects of gravity on vestibulo-ocular reflex, the role of vestibular and cervical sensory and motor activity in hand movement control, oculomotor stability, and effects of different G levels. Also studies human sensorimotor adaptation to unusual force environments.

★ 22071 ★ Brandeis University Council on Health Care Economics and Policy
Schneider Institute for Health Policy
Heller School for Social Policy & Management, MS 035
Waltham, MA 02454-9110
Phone: (781)736-3807 **Fax:** (781)736-3306
Email: shactman@brandeis.edu
Website: http://sihp.brandeis.edu/council/
David Shactman, Dir.
Activities/Fields: Critical issues generated by health system change and the economic impact of such changes. **Pub:** *Journal articles. • Papers.*

★ 22072 ★ Brandeis University Nathan and Toby Starr Center for Mental Retardation
MS 035
Heller School for Social Policy & Management
PO Box 549110
Waltham, MA 02454
Phone: (781)736-3832 **Fax:** (781)736-3864
Email: krauss@brandeis.edu
Website: http://heller.brandies.edu/starr.asp
Marty Wyngaarden Krauss, Dir.
Activities/Fields: Impact on families of lifelong caregiving for a member with mental retardation, the impact of early intervention services on children and families, health care systems for children with special health care needs, and organizational and policy issues in the expansion of community based services for persons with disabilities.

★ 22073 ★ Brandeis University Schneider Institute for Health Policy
Mail Stop 035
Heller School for Social Policy and Management
PO Box 549110
Waltham, MA 02454-9110
Phone: (781)736-3900 **Fax:** (781)736-3928
Email: wallack@brandeis.edu
Website: http://www.heller.brandeis.edu/sihp.asp
Stanley S. Wallack, PhD, Exec. Dir.
Activities/Fields: Health services research and policy analysis, focusing on the design, development, implementation, and evaluation of innovative financing and delivery systems. Specific areas of research include establishing and implementing national health care expenditure limits, all-payer payment systems, an Alcohol and Drug Services Survey, the changing trends of substance abuse, financing and reimbursement of drug abuse treatment programs, and long-term care for the elderly, including home care services for the disabled elderly and cost effective models and standards for assisted living. Operates the Center for Health Policy Analysis and Research; Health Policy Center; Bigel Institute for Health Policy.

★ 22074 ★ Bridgewater State College Human Performance Lab
Bridgewater, MA 02325
Phone: (508)531-1200 **Fax:** (508)531-1717
Email: rhaslam@bridgew.edu
Dr. Robert Haslam, Dir.
Activities/Fields: Exercise physiology, including metabolic responses to exercise, blood flow responses to exercise, prediction of athlete success, and police and fire fighter fitness.

★ 22075 ★ Brigham and Women's Hospital Asthma and Allergic Diseases Cooperative Research Center
Smith Bldg., 6th Fl.
1 Jimmy Fund Way
Boston, MA 02115
Phone: (617)525-1300 **Fax:** (617)525-1310
Email: fausten@rics.bwh.harvard.edu
K. Frank Austen, MD, Contact
Activities/Fields: Clinical areas include allergy, clinical immunology, rheumatology, immunodermatology, and pre-clinical areas include mast cell biology, biology of human peripheral blood, leukocytes including eosinophils, neutrophils and monocytes, arachidonic acid metabolism by the 5-lipoxygenase pathway, and complement biology.

★ 22076 ★ Brigham and Women's Hospital Center for Neurologic Diseases
77 Ave., Louis Pasteur HIM 730
Boston, MA 02115-5817
Phone: (617)525-5300 **Fax:** (617)525-5252
Email: hweiner@rics.bwh.harvard.edu
Dr. Howard L. Weiner, Co-Dir.
Activities/Fields: Human autoimmune diseases, including T-cell immunology, T-cell interactions and regulations by cytokines. Also studies immunoregulatory T-cell abnormalities in multiple sclerosis and other autoimmune diseases, and investigations of mechanisms of immunologic tolerance in humans.

★ 22077 ★ Brigham and Women's Hospital Channing Laboratory
181 Longwood Ave.
Boston, MA 02115
Phone: (617)525-2270 **Fax:** (617)731-1541
Email: dennis_kasper@hms.harvard.edu
Website: http://www.channing.harvard.edu
Dr. Dennis Kasper, Dir.
Activities/Fields: Infectious diseases and population-based medicine.

★ 22078 ★ Brigham and Women's Hospital
Diagnostic Molecular Biology Laboratory
75 Francis St.
Boston, MA 02115
Phone: (617)732-7446 **Fax:** (617)732-7449
Email: jsklar@rics.bwh.harvard.edu
Dr. Jeffrey Sklar, Dir.

Activities/Fields: Molecular biology, human genetics, and molecular oncology, including nucleic acid analysis for the diagnosis of cancer, inherited conditions, and infectious disorders.

★ 22079 ★ Brigham and Women's Hospital
General Clinical Research Center
221 Longwood Ave., 2nd Fl.
Boston, MA 02115
Phone: (617)732-5661 **Fax:** (617)732-5764
Email: gwilliams@partners.org
Dr. Gordon Williams, Prog. Dir.

Activities/Fields: Support facility for clinical investigation of diseases in humans.

★ 22080 ★ Brigham and Women's Hospital
Neuroimaging Analysis Center
Department of Radiology
75 Francis St.
Boston, MA 02115
Phone: (617)732-7692 **Fax:** (617)582-6033
Email: kikinis@bwh.harvard.edu
Website: http://www.spl.harvard.edu
Ron Kikinis, MD, Prin. Investigator

Activities/Fields: Image processing and analysis techniques for basic and clinical neurosciences.

★ 22081 ★ Brigham and Women's Hospital
Robert B. Brigham Multipurpose Arthritis and Musculoskeletal Diseases Center
75 Francis St.
Boston, MA 02115
Phone: (617)732-5356 **Fax:** (617)732-5505
Email: jnkatz@partners.org
Dr. Jeffrey N. Katz, Dir.

Activities/Fields: Rheumatic disease, including technology assessment, policy studies, the relationship between clinical practice, outcome, and efficiency, and psychological, social, and economic factors. Also studies clinimetrics and epidemiology of rheumatic disease, Lyme disease, Carpal Tunnel Syndrome, spinal stenosis, doctor-patient communication, and SLE risk factors.

★ 22082 ★ Brigham Young University
Cancer Research Center
S125 Eyring Science Center
Provo, UT 84602-4629
Phone: (801)378-3913 **Fax:** (801)378-5474
Email: cancer_research@byu.edu
Website: http://cancerresearch.byu.edu
Daniel L. Simmons, PhD, Dir.

Activities/Fields: Chemistry and biochemistry of nucleic acids and their derivatives as potential medicinal agents, including synthesis of antiviral and antitumor agents, detection of carcinogenic materials in the environment, isolation and study of antitumor agents from natural products, and study of the biochemical mechanism of action of various antitumor agents. **Pub:** *The Cancer Chronicle*, bimonthly.

★ 22083 ★ Brigham Young University
Human Performance Research Center
116 RB
Provo, UT 84602
Phone: (801)422-1285 **Fax:** (801)422-0555
Email: ken_knight@byu.edu
Website: http://www.byu.edu/chhp/infos.htmlresearch
Dr. Ken Knight, Contact

Activities/Fields: Exercise physiology, including studies of cardiovascular changes due to exercise, energy cost of various types of exercise, and body composition changes due to exercise.

★ 22084 ★ British Columbia Cancer Agency
British Columbia Cancer Research Centre
Suite 400, East Tower
555 West 12th Ave.
Vancouver, BC, Canada V5Z 3X7
Phone: (604)877-6000 **Fax:** (604)877-6146
Email: vling@bccancer.bc.ca
Website: http://www.bccancer.bc.ca/research
Dr. Victor Ling, VP, Res.

Activities/Fields: Maintains eight departments for cancer research: Advanced Therapeutics - developing and testing new and more effective treatments for cancer. Cancer Control Research - working to understand the risk factors of cancer and developing cancer prevention strategies. Cancer Endocrinology - finding new treatments for endocrine-related cancers, such as prostate cancer. Cancer Genetics and developmental Biology (Centre for Intergrated Genomics) - a specialty lab for identifying genomic changes and the signalling and metabolic pathways associated with tumour development. Cancer Imaging - Focusing on developing new technology for early detection and localization of cancer and pre-cancerous lesions. Genome Sequence Centre- A high-throughput genomic science centre dedicated to cancer research. Medical Biophysics - Making inroads into understanding cancer biology and the practical aspects of radiotherapy and related treatments. Terry Fox Lab - Developing new technology for diagnosis and treatment of cancers of the blood and lymphatic system, and new understanding of the control of cell growth and differentiation, aging and gene regulation. **Pub:** *Annual Report*.

★ 22085 ★ British Columbia Cancer Agency
British Columbia Cancer Research Centre
Department of Cancer Endocrinology
200 - 601 W Broadway
Vancouver, BC, Canada V5Z 4C2
Phone: (604)877-6040 **Fax:** (604)877-6161
Email: schou@bccancer.bc.ca
Website: http://www.bccancer.bc.ca

Activities/Fields: Molecular basis of early progression of prostate cancer to androgen independence, and early detection of primary and metastatic disease. New therapies under development include Intermittent Androgen Suppression (IAS) and peptide memetics to prevent lygand independent activation of the androgen receptor. The experimental Nb2 node lymphoma is also maintained for studies on the mitogenic properties of prolactin and growth hormone.

★ 22086 ★ British Columbia Cancer Agency
British Columbia Cancer Research Centre
Medical Biophysics Department
601 W 10th Ave.
Vancouver, BC, Canada V5Z 1L3
Phone: (604)877-6010 **Fax:** (604)877-6002
Email: rdurand@bccancer.bc.ca
Website: http://www.bccrc.ca/mb/
Dr. R.E. Durand, Hd.

Activities/Fields: Laboratory and clinical studies on control of cancer, particularly radiation therapy and adjuncts to radiation therapy, including radiosensitizers and chemotherapy. Also conducts basic studies of tumor growth, angiogenesis mutagenesis and radiation damage mechanisms.

★ 22087 ★ British Columbia Cancer Agency
British Columbia Cancer Research Centre
Terry Fox Laboratory for Hematology/Oncology
601 W 10th Ave.
Vancouver, BC, Canada V5Z 1L3
Phone: (604)877-6070 **Fax:** (604)877-0712
Email: aeaves@bccancer.bc.ca
Website: http://www.bccrc.ca/tfl/index.html
Dr. Allen C. Eaves, Dir.

Activities/Fields: Hematology and oncology, particularly the regulation of growth and differentiation in normal and malignant hemopoiesis and lymphopoiesis. Research activities focus on studies of hemopoietic progenitors, bone marrow transplantation, gene therapy, aging, cell adhesion, metastasis, growth factors and receptors, and signal transduction mechanisms.

★ 22088 ★ British Columbia Children's Hospital
Children's and Women's Health Centre of British Columbia
980 W 28th Ave.
CMMT Bldg., Rm. 2092
Vancouver, BC, Canada V5Z 4H4
Phone: (604)875-3602 **Fax:** (604)875-3601
Email: dkalousek@cw.bc.ca
Prof. Dagmar K. Kalousek, Dir.

Activities/Fields: Chromosomal mosaicism and its effect on human intrauterine development, specifically the correlation between chromosomal complement of placenta and intrauterine development of the fetus.

★ 22089 ★ British Columbia Research Institute for Children's and Women's Health
Centre for Community Health and Health Evaluation Research (CCHHER)
L408, 4480 Oak St.
Vancouver, BC, Canada V6H 3V4
Phone: (604)875-3687 **Fax:** (604)875-3569
Email: barmstrong@cw.bc.ca
Dr. Robert Armstrong, Co-Dir.

Activities/Fields: Factors that influence and support the healthy development of children and youth and the use and development of scientific methods to measure the effectiveness of health policy, practices and technologies.

★ 22090 ★ Brooklyn College of City University of New York
Applied Vision Institute (AVI)
William James Hall, Rm. 4311
Department of Psychology
2900 Bedford Ave.
Brooklyn, NY 11210-2889
Phone: (718)951-5033
Email: louiseh@brooklyn.cuny.edu
Dr. Louise Hainline, Co-Dir.

Activities/Fields: Adult vision.

★ 22091 ★ Brooklyn College of City University of New York
Infant Study Center
Department of Psychology
2900 Bedford Ave.
Brooklyn, NY 11210
Phone: (718)951-5033 **Fax:** (718)951-4825
Email: louiseh@brooklyn.cuny.edu
Dr. Louise Hainline, Dir.

Activities/Fields: Human vision and normal and abnormal visual development; visual development in infancy, including studies of acuity, pattern perception, color vision, eye movement control, and perception of complex events; behavioral studies of visual attention and use of information in medical images in adults. Assessment procedures utilize photo-refraction methods, visual-evoked response techniques, and electrophysiological studies of dyslexia.

★ 22092 ★ Brooklyn College of City University of New York Speech and Hearing Center
Boylan Hall, Rm. 4400
Brooklyn, NY 11210
Phone: (718)951-5186 **Fax:** (718)951-4363
Email: pbottino@brooklyn.cuny.edu
Patti Bottino, Contact
Activities/Fields: Normal communications and communication disorders, including studies of speech, language, and hearing.

★ 22093 ★ Brown University Center for Alcohol and Addiction Studies
PO Box G - BH
Providence, RI 02912
Phone: (401)444-1800 **Fax:** (401)444-1850
Email: caas@brown.edu
Website: http://www.caas.brown.edu
Peter M. Monti, PhD, Dir.
Activities/Fields: Alcohol and addiction studies, including an individual's relationship to alcohol and the effectiveness of community reinforcement on treatment, the relationship between smoking and drinking among alcoholics, matching treatment focus to dysfunction, social skills treatment of cocaine abusers, cue exposure and social skills treatment for alcoholics, deterring preadolescent drug and AIDS-risky behavior, time dynamics of alcohol treatment outcome, treatment research validation and extension program, substance abuse prevention program for Native American youth, hospital intervention services, and health-care policy. **Pub:** *Digest of Addiction Theory and Application*, monthly.

★ 22094 ★ Brown University Institute for Brain and Neural Systems (IBNS)
PO Box 1843
Providence, RI 02912
Phone: (401)863-2585 **Fax:** (401)863-3494
Email: info@cns.brown.edu
Website: http://www.physics.brown.edu/research/cns/cnspage.html
Leon N. Cooper, Dir.
Activities/Fields: Brain function and neural systems.

★ 22095 ★ Brown University International Health Institute
Box G-B495
171 Meeting St.
Providence, RI 02912
Phone: (401)863-1186 **Fax:** (401)863-1243
Email: Stephen_McGarvey@brown.edu
Website: http://bms.brown.edu/IHI/
Stephen McGarvey, Dir.
Activities/Fields: Health problems of developing nations, including HIV/AIDS, cardiovascular disease, parasites and nutrition.

★ 22096 ★ Buck Institute
8001 Redwood Blvd.
Novato, CA 94945
Phone: (415)209-2000 **Fax:** (415)899-1810
Website: http://www.buckinstitute.org/
Dale E. Bredesen, MD, Pres. /CEO
Activities/Fields: The aging process and age-associated diseases.

★ 22097 ★ Bucknell University Immunobiology Research Laboratory
Department of Biology
Lewisburg, PA 17837
Phone: (570)577-1135 **Fax:** (570)577-3537
Email: pearson@bucknell.edu
Website: http://www.bucknell.edu
Dr. David D. Pearson, Dir.
Activities/Fields: Autoimmune diseases, particularly the causes of rheumatoid arthritis and type I diabetes. Studies techniques to detect the disease, including protein blotting on nitro-cellulose, binding of oligosaccharides to lectins, enzyme-linked immunoabsorbent assay tests, and the relationships between fat metabolism and the immune response with possible involvement of leptin. Also studies methods to detect small quantities of antibodies secreted from single cells and a small number of immunoassays in developmental stages for small amounts of proteins.

★ 22098 ★ Bureau of Legal Dentistry (BLD)
146 2355 East Mall
Vancouver, BC, Canada V6T 1Z4
Phone: (604)822-8822 **Fax:** (604)822-8884
Email: boldlab@unixg.ubc.ca
Website: http://www.boldlab.org/
Dr. David Sweet, Dir.
Activities/Fields: Dental DNA, including the recovery of DNA from teeth, oral structures and bones; bite mark wound healing; etc.

★ 22099 ★ Burnham Institute
10901 N Torrey Pines Rd.
La Jolla, CA 92037
Phone: (858)646-3132 **Fax:** (858)646-3199
Email: info@burnham.org
Website: http://www.burnham.org/
John Reed, MD, Pres. /CEO
Activities/Fields: Cell adhesion and extracellular matrix, neurobiology, glycobiology, gene regulation, oncogene and tumor suppressor gene, apoptosis and cell death, degenerative disease research and aging, and bioinformatics and biological complexity. **Pub:** *Annual Report.*

★ 22100 ★ Burzynski Research Institute
9432 Old Katy Rd., Ste. 200
Houston, TX 77055
Phone: (713)335-5697 **Fax:** (713)335-5699
Email: info@burzynskiclinic.com
Website: http://www.cancermed.com
Dr. Stanislaw R. Burzynski, Founder
Activities/Fields: Antineoplastons A 10 and AS21 in the treatment of cancer. Antineoplastons are peptides and amino acid derivatives that are apoptosis inducers, working at the level of p53 tumor suppressor genes and ras oncogenes. The role of antineoplastons A10 and AS21 in reversing the methylation of promotor sequences and the acetylation of histones to retard the aging process.

★ 22101 ★ California Institute for Medical Research
2260 Clove Dr.
San Jose, CA 95128
Phone: (408)998-4554 **Fax:** (408)998-2723
Email: admin@cimr.org
Website: http://cimr.org
Pat Barnett, Oper. Dir.
Activities/Fields: Medical research, including infectious diseases, stroke, analytical tools for pharmacokinetic study of anticoagulant drugs, neurological disorders, tumor biology, and AIDS. Drugs useful in the treatment of heart diseases.

★ 22102 ★ California Pacific Medical Center Research Institute
2200 Webster St., Rm. 514
San Francisco, CA 94115
Phone: (415)600-1601 **Fax:** (415)600-1753
Email: dfielder@cooper.cpmc.org
Website: http://www.cpmc.org
David R. Fielder, VP, Res.
Activities/Fields: Medical sciences, including basic clinical research on heart and lung disease, organ transplantation, neurology, laboratory medicine, cancer, arthritis, neonatology, gene therapy (non-viral), complementary medicine, and gastroenterology. **Pub:** *California Pacific Currents*. **Frmly:** Medical Research Institute of San Francisco.

★ 22103 ★ Canadian Bacterial Diseases Network
Heritage Medical Research Bldg., Rm. 282
3300 Hospital Dr. NW
Calgary, AB, Canada T2N 4N1
Phone: (403)220-2562 **Fax:** (403)283-5241
Email: woods@acs.uca/gary.ca
Website: http://www.cbdn.ca
Dr. Peter Singer, Dir.
Activities/Fields: Bacterial diseases of humans, animals, fish, and plants. Eight program areas include: antibiotics, including structure/activity relationships at the molecular level, mechanisms of antibiotic resistance, and outer membrane permeability; intracellular bacteria, adherence, and macrophages; live attenuated and subcellular vaccines, including novel attenuated strains as vaccine carriers, outer membrane proteins as carriers for peptide epitopes, and vaccine projects on human and fish pathogens; diagnostics, including analysis of DNA sequences, monoclonal antibodies, and other methods for use as diagnostic agents for Chlamydia, Pseudomonas, Salmonella, Campylobacter, Anaerobes, toxins, beta-lactamases, Neisseria, Yersinia, Bordetella, and major fish, animal, and plant pathogens; fish vaccines and diagnostics; toxins, including toxic shock syndrome, pertussis toxin, and Pasteurella haemolytica toxin; helicobacter, including mechanisms of ineffectivenss of antibiotics, molecular biology and genetics, and surface molecule studies; and sexually transmitted diseases, including molecular biology of surface antigens and molecular typing methods.

★ 22104 ★ Canadian Fitness and Lifestyle Research Institute
201-185 Somerset W
Ottawa, ON, Canada K2P 0J2
Phone: (613)233-5528 **Fax:** (613)233-5536
Email: info@cflri.ca
Website: http://www.cflri.ca/
Activities/Fields: Population fitness levels, recreation habits, and link between physical activity and other life-style patterns of Canadians; benefits and costs of a physically active lifestyle. **Pub:** *The Research File*, 3/year. **Frmly:** Canada Fitness Survey.

★ 22105 ★ Canadian Genetic Diseases Network
NCE Bldg.
2150 Western Pky., Ste. 201
Vancouver, BC, Canada V6T 1V6
Phone: (604)221-7300 **Fax:** (604)221-0778
Email: info@cgdn.generes.ca
Website: http://www.cgdn.generes.ca/
Dr. Ron Woznow, Dir.
Activities/Fields: Genetic causes of diseases, including myotonic dystrophy, Huntington's disease, and Wilson's disease; genetic predisposition to cancer, including colerectal cancer, tuberculosis, and diabetes; carrier screening and mutation and distribution in populations, including cystic fibrosis, cleft palate, thalassemia, and ricketts; cost effective diagnostic testing, including retinoblastoma and alkaline phosphatase definciency; biochemical genetics and models of disease, including Huntington's disease, Tay Sachs, lipoprotein lipase deficiency, retinal myopathies, and metabolic diseases; and new therapy trials, including muscular dystrophy and DNA modification strategies.

★ 22106 ★ Canadian Institute of Child Health (CICH)
384 Bank St., Ste. 300
Ottawa, ON, Canada K2P 1Y4
Phone: (613)230-8838 **Fax:** (613)230-6654
Email: cich@cich.ca
Website: http://www.cich.ca
Judith Erola, Ch.
Activities/Fields: Improving the health and well-being of children and youth in Canada. The objectives to

accomplish this vision include monitoring the health and well-being of children and youth; improving the health and well-being of mothers and infants; creating safe, supportive, nurturing environments for children; and encouraging cooperation between consumers, professionals, industry and government agencies to ensure a better life for Canadian children. **Pub:** *Annual Report.* • *Child Health Newsletter*, quarterly. • *The Health of Canada's Children: A CICH Profile.* • *Our Promise to Children.*

★ 22107 ★ Canadian Institute for Health Information (CIHI)
377 Dalhousie St., Ste. 200
Ottawa, ON, Canada K1N 9N8
Phone: (613)241-7860 **Fax:** (613)241-8120
Email: communications@cihi.ca
Website: http://secure.cihi.ca/
Richard Alvarez, Pres. /CEO
Activities/Fields: Health of Canadians and the Canadian health care system. **Pub:** *Reports.*

★ 22108 ★ Canadian Institutes of Health Research Group in Matrix Dynamics
Medical Science Bldg.
University of Toronto
Fitzgerald Bldg.
150 College St.
Toronto, ON, Canada M5S 3E2
Phone: (416)978-6681 **Fax:** (416)978-5956
Email: christopher.mcculloch@utoronto.ca
Website: http://www.cihrmatrix.ca/indexhtml.html
Christopher A. McCulloch, Dir.
Activities/Fields: Structure and function of periodontal tissues (tooth supporting apparatus), regulation of cell activity, and relationships to periodontal disease and tooth implants.

★ 22109 ★ Canadian Network of Toxicology Centres (CNTC)
Bovey Bldg.
Gordon St.
Guelph, ON, Canada N1G 2W1
Phone: (519)837-3320 **Fax:** (519)837-3861
Email: lritter@tox.uoguelph.ca
Website: http://www.mite-rn.org
Dr. Len Ritter, Exec. Dir.
Activities/Fields: Toxicology, including risk assessment and epidemiology, environmental concerns, carcinogenesis and genetics, teratology, metabolism and pharmacokinetics, pathology, and analytical chemistry. **Pub:** *CNTC/RCCT News Brief.* • *Metals in the Environment News.*

★ 22110 ★ Canadian Stroke Network (CSN)
451 Smyth Rd.
Ottawa, ON, Canada K1H 8M5
Phone: (613)562-5800 **Fax:** (613)562-5631
Email: robin@conadianstrokenetwork.ca
Website: http://www.canadianstrokenetwork.ca
Robin Millbank, Contact
Activities/Fields: Stroke, new treatment plans and medical technologies for stroke, and the creation of policies that will benefit Canada as a whole.

★ 22111 ★ Cancer Biotherapy Research Group (CBRG)
PO Box 680757
Franklin, TN 37068-0757
Phone: (615)791-6393 **Fax:** (615)791-4719
Email: cbrg_cancer@compuserve.com
Website: http://www.cbrg.org
Rosalie A. Crispin, Exec. Dir.
Activities/Fields: Clinical cancer research, focusing on the treatment of solid cancer tumors in adults and the use of biologicals and biological response modifiers alone or in combination with other treatment modalities. **Pub:** *NBSG Newsletter*, biennially. **Frmly:** National Biotherapy Study Group.

★ 22112 ★ Cancer Care Ontario
620 University Ave.
Toronto, ON, Canada M5G 2L7
Phone: (416)971-9800 **Fax:** (416)971-6888
Email: lina.barattin@cancercare.on.ca
Website: http://www.cancercare.on.ca
Dr. Lina Barattin, Contact
Activities/Fields: Cancer prevention, early detection, diagnosis, treatment, and supportive care. Supports basic and clinical scientists at eight Regional Cancer Centers throughout Ontario and in the Division of Preventive Oncology. **Pub:** *Cancer Care.* • *Publications on cancer incidence and mortality.* **Frmly:** Ontario Cancer Treatment and Research Foundation.

★ 22113 ★ Cancer Care Ontario London Regional Cancer Centre
790 Commissioners Rd. E
London, ON, Canada N6A 4L6
Phone: (519)685-8600 **Fax:** (519)685-8614
Email: research@lrcc.on.ca
Website: http://www.lrcc.on.ca/
Dr. James Koropatnick, Dir.
Activities/Fields: Molecular biology of cancer, with emphasis on tumor metastasis and progression and on drug resistance studies; molecular endocrinology, with emphasis on intracellular transportation of steroid hormones; and steroid receptors in breast cancer. Studies include physics and radiation oncology, including 3-D imaging, brachytherapy, portal imaging, and clinical trials. Medical oncology research program focuses on bone marrow transplantation, biological response modifiers, and dose intensity.

★ 22114 ★ Cancer and Leukemia Group B
208 S LaSalle St., Ste. 2000
Chicago, IL 60604-1104
Phone: (773)702-9171 **Fax:** (312)345-0117
Website: http://www.calgb.org/
Richard L. Schilsky, MD, Gp. Chm.
Activities/Fields: Cooperative group conducting therapeutic multi-modal, multi-institutional, randomized cancer clinical trials primarily in seven disease areas: leukemia, lymphoma, breast, gastrointestinal, genitourinary, respiratory and melanoma. Aims to increase the number of cases brought under complete remission from cancer by increasing knowledge of the disease process and appropriate treatments. Affiliated with several pathology, immunology, and cytogenetic laboratories.

★ 22115 ★ Cancer Research Center
3501 Berrywood Dr.
Columbia, MO 65201
Phone: (573)875-2255 **Fax:** (573)443-1202
Email: eisenstarkA@missouri.edu
Website: http://www.cancerresearchcenter.org
Dr. Abraham Eisenstark, Sci. Dir.
Activities/Fields: Basic oncology and studies in immunology, microbiology, protein biochemistry, bioengineering, carcinogenesis, and cancer detection. Specific studies include biochemical markers for early detection of cancer cells, environmental carcinogenesis, and oxidative cellular damage. **Pub:** *The Mirror*, quarterly.

★ 22116 ★ Cancer Research Foundation
PO Box 0493
Chicago, IL 60690-0493
Phone: (312)630-0055 **Fax:** (312)630-0075
Email: crf@cancerresearchfdn.org
Website: http://www.cancerresearchfdn.org
Merle Goldblatt Cohen, Pres.
Activities/Fields: Funds laboratory and clinical cancer research at Chicago universities and medical schools. **Pub:** *Annual Report.* • *Newsletters.*

★ 22117 ★ Cancer Research Institute, Inc.
681 5th Ave.
New York, NY 10022
Phone: (212)688-7515 **Free:** 800-992-2623
Fax: (212)832-9376
Email: info@cancerresearch.org
Website: http://www.cancerresearch.org
Carlos A. Ferrer, Chm.
Activities/Fields: Supports research projects in fundamental immunology and cancer immunology that seek to develop cancer therapies based on the immune system. **Pub:** *Annual Report.* • *Cancer and the Immune System: The Vital Connection.* • *The Cancer Research Institute Help Book: What to Do If Cancer Strikes.* • *Prostate cancer and melanoma brochures.*

★ 22118 ★ Cancer Research Laboratory
Children's Hospital of Orange County
455 S Main St.
Orange, CA 92868
Phone: (714)532-8548 **Fax:** (714)639-5907
Email: lenniesen@aol.com
Dr. Leonard Sender, Medical Dir.
Activities/Fields: Experimental hematopoiesis, tumor vaccines. **Frmly:** Pediatric Cancer Research Laboratory.

★ 22119 ★ Cancer Resource Center
4600 Valley Rd., Ste. 336
Lincoln, NE 68510
Phone: (402)483-2827 **Free:** 800-487-8786
Fax: (402)483-2882
Email: kmadcharo@lmef.org
Website: http://www.lmef.org
Kelly Madcharo, Dir.
Activities/Fields: Oncology, especially pathology and radiotherapy, and drug studies for pharmaceutical companies. **Frmly:** Lincoln Cancer Center.

★ 22120 ★ CancerCare Manitoba
675 McDermot Ave.
Winnipeg, MB, Canada R3E 0V9
Phone: (204)787-2241 **Fax:** (204)787-1184
Email: brent.schacter@cancercare.mb.ca
Website: http://www.cancercare.mb.ca
Dr. Brent A. Schacter, Pres. /CEO
Activities/Fields: Cancer treatment and research, including radiation oncology, psychosocial oncology, surgical oncology, hematology, medical oncology, pediatric oncology, gynecologic oncology, medical physics, epidemiology, biostatistics, molecular biology, biochemical pharmacology, and immunology. Clinical trial research in association with NSABP, NCIC, CCSG. **Pub:** *Annual Report.*

★ 22121 ★ Carcinoid Cancer Foundation, Inc.
333 Mamaroneck Ave., No. 492
White Plains, NY 10605
Phone: (212)722-3132 **Free:** 888-722-3132
Fax: (212)831-3031
Email: monwarner@earthlink.net
Website: http://www.carcinoid.org
Monica Warner, Res. Coord.
Activities/Fields: Carcinoid tumors, carcinoid syndrome, and other related neuroendocrine tumors.

★ 22122 ★ Carleton University Centre for Memory Assessment and Research (CMAR)
B531 Loeb
1125 Colonel By Dr.
Ottawa, ON, Canada K1S 5B6
Phone: (613)520-2659
Email: tom_tombaugh@carleton.ca
Tommy N. Tombaugh, Dir.
Activities/Fields: Testing and assessment for anyone experiencing memory problems due to illness, aging,

injury, or neurological damage; encourages and facilitates research, as well as develops tests for assessing memory and intellectual abilities; and serves as an educational facility and research center focusing on memory illnesses and cognitive rehabilitation.

★ 22123 ★ Carnegie Mellon University
Bone Tissue Engineering Center (BTEC)
125 Smith Hall
5000 Forbes Ave.
Pittsburgh, PA 15213
Phone: (412)268-7211 **Fax:** (412)268-8641
Email: hollinger@cs.cmu.edu
Website: http://www.btec.cmu.edu/reFramed/main/mainPage.html
Jeffrey O. Hollinger, PhD, Dir.
Activities/Fields: Molecular basis for bone formation and wound healing, and the application of this knowledge to engineer tissues using therapeutic systems of biomaterials, cells and signaling molecules.

★ 22124 ★ Carnegie Mellon University
High Performance Computing for Biomedical Research
Mellon Institute Bldg.
4400 5th Ave.
Pittsburgh, PA 15213
Phone: (412)268-4960 **Fax:** (412)268-5832
Email: roskies@psc.edu
Website: http://www.psc.edu/biomed/biomed.html
Ralph Z. Roskies, PhD, Prin. Investigator
Activities/Fields: Biomedical computer programs for access to high-performance computing resources; bioinformatics, structural biology, computational genomics and proteomics, computational neuroscience, computational pathology, and scientific visualization.

★ 22125 ★ Case Western Reserve University
Bolton-Brush Growth Study Center
Bolton Dental Bldg.
School of Dentistry
2123 Abington Rd.
Cleveland, OH 44106-4905
Phone: (216)368-6715 **Fax:** (216)368-3204
Email: mgh4@po.cwru.edu
Website: http://www.cwru.edu/dental/bbgsc/homepage.html
Dr. B. Holly Broadbent, Jr., Dir.
Activities/Fields: Investigations into the growth and development of dentition, face and cranium, and roentgenographic studies of the epiphyses of the human body. Conducts an ongoing study of longitudinal cephalometric radiographs and dental casts.

★ 22126 ★ Case Western Reserve University
Center for Human Genetics
Lakeside Bldg. 1500
University Hospitals of Cleveland
11100 Euclid Ave.
Cleveland, OH 44106-9959
Phone: (216)844-3936 **Fax:** (216)844-7497
Email: glw2@po.cwru.edu
Website: http://genetics.cwru.edu/cfhg.html
Georgia Wiesner, MD, Clin. Dir.
Activities/Fields: Human genetics, clinical genetics, molecular genetics, and cytogenetics. **Frmly:** Genetics Center.

★ 22127 ★ Case Western Reserve University
Center for Inherited Disorders of Energy Metabolism (CIDEM)
Department of Pediatrics, Rm. 4010
Rainbow Babies and Childrens Hospital
11100 Euclid Ave.
Cleveland, OH 44106-6004
Phone: (216)844-1286 **Fax:** (216)844-8005
Email: cidem@po.cwru.edu
Website: http://www.cwru.edu/med/CIDEM/cidem.htm
Dr. Douglas Kerr, Dir.
Activities/Fields: Defects of human energy metabolism, focusing on diagnosis and management. Emphasis is on disorders of pyruvate fatty acid oxidation, and mitochondrial function, including pyruvate metabolism, oxidative phosphorylation, and fatty acid oxidation.

★ 22128 ★ Case Western Reserve University
Cystic Fibrosis and Pediatric Pulmonary Center
Rainbow Babies & Childrens Hospital, Rm. 3001
11100 Euclid Ave.
Cleveland, OH 44106
Phone: (216)844-3267 **Fax:** (216)844-5916
Email: mwk3@po.cwru.edu
Michael W. Konstan, Dir.
Activities/Fields: Cystic fibrosis and pulmonary physiology in children, including basic and clinical studies on evolution and pathology of pulmonary lesion in cystic fibrosis, abnormal mucous secretions of patients with cystic fibrosis, developmental biology of the lung, pulmonary physiology, treatment of chronic obstructive pulmonary disease, intracellular signalling, electrolyte transport and membrane permeability of intestinal, sweat, and respiratory epithelial and individual cells and membrane biopotentials, gene therapy of pulmonary diseases, and inflammation in the cystic fibrosis lung. Asthma studies include basic cell biology of airways and studies of therapeutic regimens for safety and efficacy. Seeks to develop a comprehensive therapeutic regimen for cystic fibrosis.

★ 22129 ★ Case Western Reserve University
Department of Epidemiology and Biostatistics
Human Genetic Analysis Resource
2500 MetroHealth Dr.
Cleveland, OH 44109-1998
Phone: (216)778-3863 **Fax:** (216)778-3280
Email: sage@darwin.cwru.edu
Website: http://darwin.cwru.edu/index.html
Robert Elston, PhD, Dir.
Activities/Fields: Identification and chromosome mapping of genes involved in common diseases that may be primarily environmentally-influenced, as well as the genes underlying rarer monogenic diseases with much smaller environmental influence. Research focuses on theoretical development of statistical methods for analysis of family data, especially to detect and identify genetic components that underlie disease susceptibility. **Pub:** *SAGE Advice*. Newsletter.

★ 22130 ★ Case Western Reserve University
General Clinical Research Center
11100 Euclid Ave.
Cleveland, OH 44106
Phone: (216)844-4902 **Fax:** (216)844-1522
Email: jpd@po.cwru.edu
Website: http://gcrc.meds.cwru.edu
Nathan A. Berger, MD, Prin. Investigator
Activities/Fields: Clinical investigations in humans, including specific, carefully planned studies of illnesses of voluntarily participating adult and pediatric patients. **Frmly:** Metabolic Research Unit.

★ 22131 ★ Case Western Reserve University
Health Systems Management Center
443 Peter B. Lewis Bldg.
Westherhead School of Management
10900 Euclid Ave.
Cleveland, OH 44106-7235
Phone: (216)368-6403 **Fax:** (216)368-6861
Email: bxp4@po.cwru.edu
Website: http://weatherhead.cwru.edu/hsmc/
Barbara J. Bolek, Dir.
Activities/Fields: Health systems management, including health care finance, clinical decision analysis, computer information systems in health care, the physician as manager, and quality and cost in health care. **Pub:** *HSMC Working Papers*.

★ 22132 ★ Case Western Reserve University
Institute of Pathology
2085 Adelbert Rd.
Cleveland, OH 44106
Phone: (216)368-2480 **Fax:** (216)368-0495
Email: pathology@po.cwru.edu
Website: http://www.cwru.edu/med/pathology
Dr. George Perry, Interim Ch.
Activities/Fields: Immunology, immunopathology, aging, cell biology, neurodegenerative disease, and oncology.

★ 22133 ★ Case Western Reserve University
Neural Engineering Center
Wickenden 147
Cleveland, OH 44106
Phone: (216)368-2960 **Fax:** (216)368-4872
Email: dxd6@po.cwru.edu
Website: http://nec.cwru.edu
Dr. Dominique M. Durand, Dir.
Activities/Fields: Function of the nervous system, development of methods to restore damaged neurological function, and creation of artificial systems by integrating physical, chemical, mathematical and engineering tools. **Frmly:** Applied Neural Control Laboratory.

★ 22134 ★ Case Western Reserve University
Northeast Ohio Multipurpose Arthritis Center
3609 Park East, Ste. 307N
Beachwood, OH 44122
Phone: (216)844-3211 **Fax:** (216)844-5172
Email: rolliemoskowitz@aol.com
Dr. Roland W. Moskowitz, Dir.
Activities/Fields: The causes, diagnosis, and treatment of arthritis, including biochemistry and pathophysiology of joints in osteoarthritis, models of degenerative joint disease and inflammatory arthritis, immunologic disorders such as systemic lupus erythematosus and rheumatoid arthritis, disorders of the spine, genetic control of arthritis disorders, and juvenile arthritis. Orthopedic studies include bioengineering, joint replacement, transplant surgery, and bone metabolism. Also investigates community health systems, including self care needs of the elderly, legal needs of patients with chronic illness such as rheumatoid arthritis, and patients' perceived needs for community services.

★ 22135 ★ Case Western Reserve University
Skeletal Research Center
Department of Biology
2080 Adelbert Rd.
Cleveland, OH 44106-7080
Phone: (216)368-3562 **Fax:** (216)368-4077
Email: ddb9@po.cwru.edu
Arnold I. Caplan, PhD, Dir.
Activities/Fields: Tissue engineered regeneration and clinical aspects of skeletal tissue, includi cartilage, bones, tendons, and ligaments.

★ 22136 ★ Case Western Reserve University
University Center on Aging and Health
10900 Euclid Ave.
Cleveland, OH 44106-7131
Phone: (216)368-2692 **Fax:** (216)368-6389
Email: mlw4@po.cwru.edu
Dr. May L. Wykle, Dir.

Activities/Fields: Conducts, supports, and facilitates research at the University Center on Aging and Health, including the effects of stress and strains, and elderly physical health on persons over 65 years of age. Emphasizes prevention, diagnosis, treatment, management of illness or disability, and service utilization of care giver. **Pub:** *Newsletter*, annually.

★ 22137 ★ Case Western Reserve University University Memory and Aging Center
Fairhill Center
12200 Fairhill Rd.
Cleveland, OH 44120
Phone: (216)844-6422 **Free:** 800-252-5048
Fax: (216)844-6446
Email: kxh26@po.cwru.edu
Website: http://www.ohioalzcenter.org
Karl Herrup, PhD, Dir.

Activities/Fields: Long term studies of persons with memory problems, Alzheimer's disease, caregiver studies, and clinical studies to develop effective treatments for memory disorders. Research focuses on animal models, mechanisms of nerve cell death in dementia and the role of inflammation in neurodegenerative disease. **Pub:** *ADAD Newsletter*, quarterly. **Frmly:** University Alzheimer Center.

★ 22138 ★ Center for Advanced Biotechnology and Medicine
679 Hoes Ln.
Piscataway, NJ 08854-5638
Phone: (732)235-5300 **Fax:** (732)235-5318
Email: shatkin@cabm.rutgers.edu
Website: http://www.cabm.rutgers.edu
Prof. Aaron J. Shatkin, PhD, Dir.

Activities/Fields: Cell and developmental biology, molecular pharmacology, molecular genetics, and structural biology. Collaborates with biopharmaceutical firms in New Jersey on technology transfer and research and development.

★ 22139 ★ Center for Allergy and Immunology Research
Rush Medical College
1725 W Harrison, Ste. 117
Chicago, IL 60612
Phone: (312)942-6296 **Fax:** (312)563-2201
Email: jmoy@rush.edu
James N. Moy, MD, Contact

Activities/Fields: Allergy, asthma, basic immunology, and product testing, including therapeutic agent evaluation, allergenic extract developments, immunodeficiency, adverse food reaction pathogensis, Samter Syndrome etiology and pathogenesis, urticaria/angiodema etiology, laboratory assay development, and hypogammaglobulinemia treatment. **Frmly:** Allergy/Immunology Service.

★ 22140 ★ Center for Basic Research in Digestive Diseases
Guggenheim 17
Mayo Clinic
Rochester, MN 55905
Phone: (507)284-0686 **Fax:** (507)284-0762
Email: gores.gregory@mayo.edu
Dr. Gregory J. Gores, Dir.

Activities/Fields: Cell biology, focusing on molecular and biochemical mechanisms of secretion in digestive tissues.

★ 22141 ★ Center for Biological Timing
Gilmer Hall, Rm. 285
Department of Biology
University of Virginia
PO Box 400328
Charlottesville, VA 22904-4328
Phone: (434)982-4501 **Fax:** (434)982-5626
Email: clock@virginia.edu
Website: http://vprweb.eservices.virginia.edu/cbtdocs/index.html
Dr. Gene D. Block, Dir.

Activities/Fields: Problems of biological timing within the nervous and endocrine systems. Specific studies include cellular mechanisms within the neuroendocrine system, environmental control of reproductive cycles, neural basis of rhythmic motor behaviors, and circadian rhythmicity. **Frmly:** Biodynamics Institute.

★ 22142 ★ Center for Biomedical Research
Population Council
1230 York Ave.
New York, NY 10021
Phone: (212)327-8717 **Fax:** (212)327-7678
Email: e-johansson@popcbr.rockefeller.edu
Dr. Elof Johansson, Contact

Activities/Fields: Physiology of human reproduction, especially the male reproductive system, including studies on gametogenesis, sperm ultrastructure, steroid receptors, hormone action, and testicular function. Contraceptive development includes studies on subdermal implants, the contraceptive ring, the levonorgestrel-releasing intrauterine device, and a male hormonal contraceptive. Health issues research relates to current and potential contraceptive methods, hormone replacement therapy, and microbicides that prevent sexually transmitted diseases.

★ 22143 ★ Center for Blood Research
800 Huntington Ave.
Boston, MA 02115
Phone: (617)731-6470 **Fax:** (617)278-3493
Email: lanner@cbr.med.harvard.edu
Website: http://cbr.med.harvard.edu/indexa.html
Michael Lanner, Exec. VP

Activities/Fields: Human blood, including multidisciplinary studies on heart disease, diabetes, cancer, AIDS, hemophilia, sickle cell anemia, mental illness, hepatitis, Rh factor in pregnancy, serum proteins, blood collection methods, preservation of formed elements, methods of plasma fractionation, and characterization of plasma components.

★ 22144 ★ Center for Cardiovascular Biomaterials (CCB)
Department of Biomedical Engineering
Case Western Reserve University
10900 Euclid Ave.
Cleveland, OH 44106-7207
Phone: (216)368-3005 **Fax:** (216)368-4969
Email: rxm4@po.cwru.edu
Website: http://www.case.cwru.edu/research/inter.html
Roger Marchant, Dir.

Activities/Fields: Biomaterials, tissue engineering and biomimetic nanotechnologies for use in cardiovascular implants and drug delivery. Services include nanoscale analysis, blood and tissue biocompatibility evaluations.

★ 22145 ★ Center for Complex Infectious Diseases (CCID)
3328 Stevens Ave., 2nd Fl.
Rosemead, CA 91770
Phone: (626)572-7288 **Fax:** (626)572-9288
Email: ccidlab@hotmail.com
Website: http://www.ccid.org/
Dr. John Martin, Contact

Activities/Fields: Nature, origin, disease associations, modes of transmission, methods of diagnosis and responses to therapy of complex infectious diseases. **Pub:** *Articles*. • *Lab reports*.

★ 22146 ★ Center for Crystallographic Research
Roswell Park Cancer Institute
Elm & Carlton Sts.
Buffalo, NY 14263
Phone: (716)845-3135 **Fax:** (716)845-8899
Email: sekwen.hui@roswellpark.org
Dr. Sek Wen Hui, Dir.

Activities/Fields: Conformational studies of nucleotides, peptides, and carbohydrates to determine interatomic arrangements in biological substances using nuclear magnetic resonance and electron spin resonance. Research is oriented to the field of cancer.

★ 22147 ★ Center for Emergency Medicine of Western Pennsylvania
230 McKee Pl., Ste. 500
Pittsburgh, PA 15213
Phone: (412)647-5300 **Fax:** (412)647-4670
Email: carusoar@msx.upmc.edu
Website: http://www.centerem.com
Dr. James J. Menegazzi, Res. Dir.

Activities/Fields: Systems, therapy, and techniques involved in the delivery of emergency care, including monitoring and evaluation of field care, personnel training and performance, and patient outcome. Sample projects include study of resuscitation from cardiac arrest, endobronchial drug delivery, pediatric ventilation alternatives, surgical versus percutaneous cricothyrotomy, techniques used for the transport of the seriously ill or injured, and alternative methods of emergency airway management, including transillumination methods of intubation and translaryngeal jet ventilation.

★ 22148 ★ Center for Health Care Strategies
1009 Lenox Dr., Ste. 204
Lawrenceville, NJ 08648
Phone: (609)895-8101 **Fax:** (609)895-9648
Email: sas@chcs.org
Website: http://www.chcs.org
Stephen A. Somers, Pres.

Activities/Fields: Development and implementation of effective health and social policy for all Americans.

★ 22149 ★ Center for Health Management Research
CB 357660
Department of Health Services
1959 NE Pacific St., Rm. H660
Seattle, WA 98195-7660
Phone: (206)616-6158 **Fax:** (206)675-1745
Email: chmr@u.washington.edu
Website: http://depts.washington.edu/chmr/about_contact.htm
Douglas A. Conrad, PhD, Dir.

Activities/Fields: New ways to organize and manage patient care, physical-organization relations, and implementation of new approaches to managing quality.

★ 22150 ★ Center for Health and Social Policy
847 25th Ave.
San Francisco, CA 94121
Phone: (415)386-3260 **Fax:** (415)386-1535
Email: sisaacs@chsp.org
Website: http://www.chsp.org/Contact_Us/contact_us.html
Stephen L. Isaacs, Pres.

Activities/Fields: Health and the social and economic factors that affect it, focusing on reproductive health, health reform, and civil society. **Pub:** *Articles*.

★ 22151 ★ Center for Hip and Knee Surgery
JRSI Foundation, Inc.
St. Francis Hospital
1199 Hadley Rd.
Mooresville, IN 46158
Phone: (317)831-2273 **Fax:** (317)831-9347
Email: arobertson@yahoo.com
Website: http://www.hipandkneesurgery.com
Amy Robertson, RN, Dir.

Activities/Fields: Total joint replacement surgery, arthritis surgery, reconstructive joint surgery, sports medicine, physical therapy, and foot, ankle, and shoulder surgery.

★ 22152 ★ Center for Human Nutrition, Inc.
502 S 44th St., Rm. 3007
Omaha, NE 68105
Phone: (402)559-5500 **Fax:** (402)559-7302
Email: chn_icsn@unmc.edu
Dr. Ann Grandjean, Exec. Dir.
Activities/Fields: Basic and clinical nutrition studies, clinical trials, intervention studies, and post marketing studies.

★ 22153 ★ Center for Human Services
7200 Wisconsin Ave., Ste. 600
Bethesda, MD 20814-4811
Phone: (301)654-8338 **Fax:** (301)941-8427
Email: dnicholas@urc-chs.com
Website: http://www.urc-chs.com
Dr. David Nicholas, Dir.
Activities/Fields: Applies quality assurance methods in health care settings around the world and conducts comparative studies of quality assessment, quality assurance costs, and quality relationship. **Pub:** *QA Brief.*

★ 22154 ★ Center for the Improvement of Human Functioning International, Inc.
3100 N Hillside Ave.
Wichita, KS 67219
Phone: (316)682-3100 **Fax:** (316)682-5054
Email: staff@brightspot.org
Website: http://www.brightspot.org
Hugh Riordan, MD, Dir.
Activities/Fields: Human genetic variability and its effects on body chemistry, health and disease, and diagnosis and treatment, especially cancer. Also investigates the measurement of naturally occurring low-energy emission from the human body and effects of extracorporeal subtle energies. **Frmly:** Olive W. Garvey Center for the Improvement of Human Functioning Inc.

★ 22155 ★ Center for Intelligent Biomedical Devices and Musculoskeletal Systems
Brown Hall, Rm. 330A
Colorado School of Mines
1610 Illinois St.
Golden, CO 80401
Phone: (303)384-2032 **Fax:** (303)384-2212
Email: sjackson@mines.edu
Website: http://egweb.mines.edu/ibdms
Dr. Rahmat A. Shoureshi, Dir.
Activities/Fields: Advances in biomedical devices and musculoskeletal systems to enhance the quality of life for citizens with disabilities and reduce health care costs. Areas of interest include smart implants for hips and knees, enhanced mobility, and musculoskeletal systems stimulus.

★ 22156 ★ Center for Medical Consumers
130 MacDougall St.
New York, NY 10012-5030
Phone: (212)674-7105 **Fax:** (212)674-7100
Email: medconsumers@earthlink.net
Website: http://www.medicalconsumers.org
Arthur Levin, Dir.
Activities/Fields: Mainstream and alternative medical treatments. **Pub:** *HEALTHFACTS*, monthly.

★ 22157 ★ Center for Molecular Medicine and Immunology
520 Belleville Ave.
Belleville, NJ 07109
Phone: (973)844-7000 **Fax:** (973)844-7020
Email: dgoldenberg@gscancer.org
Dr. David M. Goldenberg, Pres.
Activities/Fields: Molecular immunology, nuclear medicine, immunobiology, and molecular genetics. Seeks to advance cancer detection techniques and translate them into methods of treatment and control.

★ 22158 ★ Center for Neurochemistry
Nathan S Kline Institute for Psychiatric Research
140 Old Orangeburg Rd.
Orangeburg, NY 10962
Phone: (845)398-5530 **Fax:** (845)398-5531
Email: Lajtha@nki.rfmh.org
Laura Berlanga, Contact
Activities/Fields: Brain protein and peptide metabolism, chronic drug effects, properties of brain receptors, blood-brain barrier, and effects of addictive drugs. **Frmly:** New York State Research Institute for Neurochemistry & Drug Addiction.

★ 22159 ★ Center for Neurodevelopmental Studies, Inc.
5430 W Glenn Dr.
Glendale, AZ 85301-2628
Phone: (623)915-0345 **Fax:** (623)937-5425
Email: cns@netwrx.com
Website: http://web1.cirs.org/homepage/cns
Lorna Jean King, Dir.
Activities/Fields: Effective treatment methods for autism and developmental disabilities and standardizing measures for evaluating adult sensory/motor functions (the Stepping Test, Vertical Writing Test, and Object Manipulation Speed Test). Collects data on specific responses of developmentally delayed children to various types of sensory stimulation. Evaluates the effectiveness of senory-integrative intervention for pre-school children at risk for learning disabilities.

★ 22160 ★ Center for Neurologic Study
9850 Genesee Ave., Ste. 320
La Jolla, CA 92037
Phone: (858)455-5463 **Fax:** (858)455-1713
Email: cns@cts.com
Website: http://www.cnsonline.org
Richard A. Smith, MD, Dir.
Activities/Fields: Neuropharmacology and experimental treatment of neurologic diseases. **Pub:** *Handbook of Amyotrophic Lateral Sclerosis.*

★ 22161 ★ Center for Radiation Therapy
MC 9006
5758 S Maryland Ave.
Chicago, IL 60637
Phone: (773)702-0817 **Fax:** (773)834-7233
Email: rrw@rover.bsd.uchicago.edu
Ralph Weichselbaum, MD, Ch.
Activities/Fields: Cancer and treatment, including studies in radiation oncology, radiation biology, chemotherapy, and oncology information systems.

★ 22162 ★ Center for Research on Population and Security
PO Box 13067
Research Triangle Park, NC 27709
Phone: (919)933-7491 **Fax:** (919)933-0348
Email: mumford@population-security.org
Website: http://population-security.org/intro.htm
Stephen D. Mumford, Pres.
Activities/Fields: Population growth control, contraceptive method research, including international clinical trial technical support, and the relationship between population growth and national and global security.

★ 22163 ★ Center for Research on Services for Severe Mental Illness
Hampton House
624 N Broadway, No. 482
Baltimore, MD 21205-1996
Phone: (410)955-3625 **Fax:** (410)614-9152
Email: dsteinwa@jhsph.edu
Website: http://www.jhsph.edu/~c-smi
Dr. Donald M. Steinwachs, Dir.
Activities/Fields: Issues of organization and finance of services for persons with severe mental illnesses (SMI) and their impact on utilization, quality of care, patient outcomes, and costs. The goals of the Center are to develop further, refine and validate methods (including quality of care criteria) to assure the appropriate match between patient needs and services that can lead to the best outcomes for persons with SMI, and to develop guidelines for the financing and organization of care that meet cost and effectiveness criteria and that take into account variations in patient needs, available resources, and community, social support, and family characteristics. The specific aims of the center are directed at four policy relevant areas; (1) to assess the impact of the course of severe mental illnesses, and their associated problems, on service needs and patterns of treatment; (2) to assess the effectiveness and costs of alternative treatment approaches for persons with SMI which are based on treatment models with established efficacy or accepted practice, and develop and test quality of care criteria for matching treatment needs to services for patients with severe mental illnesses; (3) to examine the role of financing mechanisms as a means to encourage efficiency, assure access to appropriate care for the SMI, and provide incentives for enhancing patient outcomes, including dimensions of mental status, physical status, adequacy of living arrangements, and quality of life; and (4) to examine alternative organizational and system approaches for managing resources, coordinating services to persons with SMI, and evaluating their impact on utilization, housing, general medical care, and resources including income support and payment for treatment and related services. **Frmly:** Center on the Organization and Financing of Care for the Severely Mentally Ill.

★ 22164 ★ Center on State Systems and Employment
Institute for Community Inclusion
Children's Hospital
300 Longwood Ave.
Boston, MA 02115
Phone: (617)355-6506 **Fax:** (617)739-5853
Email: ici@tch.harvard.edu
Website: http://www.childrenshospital.org/ici/rrtc
William E. Kiernan, PhD, Dir.
Activities/Fields: How state agencies provide employment supports to people with disabilities and access to postsecondary education. **Frmly:** Center on Promoting Employment.

★ 22165 ★ Center for the Study of Aging, Inc.
706 Madison Ave.
Albany, NY 12208-3604
Phone: (518)465-6927 **Fax:** (518)462-1339
Email: iapaas@aol.com
Website: http://www.centerforthestudyofaging.org
Sara Harris, Exec. Dir.
Activities/Fields: Social and medical research on aging, including physical activity and aging, housing for the elderly, geriatric cardiology, nutrition, mental health, oral history, public policy, caregiving, prevention, rural aging, and respite care for the frail elderly. **Pub:** *Lifelong Health and Fitness Newsletter*, quarterly.

★ 22166 ★ Center for the Study of Hepatitis C
1230 York Ave.
New York, NY 10021
Free: (866)672-4372
Email: info@hepccenter.org
Website: http://www.hepccenter.org/
Ira Jacobson, MD, Med. Dir.
Activities/Fields: Hepatitis C infection and its associated liver disease.

★ 22167 ★ Center for Study of Multiple Birth
333 E Superior St., Ste. 464
Chicago, IL 60611
Phone: (312)926-7498 **Fax:** (312)926-7780
Email: lgk396@northwestern.edu
Website: http://www.multiplebirth.com
Dr. Louis G. Keith, Contact
Activities/Fields: Multiple birth, twin gestation, twin pregnancy diagnosis, and twin care. Research is aimed at decreasing the high infant mortality rate involved in multiple births.

★ 22168 ★ Center for the Study of Rochester's Health
University of Rochester
601 Elmwood Ave., Box 644
Rochester, NY 14642
Phone: (716)275-6423 **Fax:** (716)756-7761
Email: cfre@son.rochester.edu
Website: http://www.urmc.rochester.edu/URMC/csrh/
Dr. Nancy M. Bennett, Dir.
Activities/Fields: Analysis of community-level data to determine opportunities for intervention, evaluation of community interventions and identification of effective community health practices and multidisciplinary collaborative medicine and public health projects.

★ 22169 ★ Center for Studying Health System Change (HSC)
600 Maryland Ave. SW, No. 550
Washington, DC 20024
Phone: (202)484-5261 **Fax:** (202)484-9258
Email: hscinfo@hschange.org
Website: http://www.hschange.com/
Paul B. Ginsburg, PhD, Pres.
Activities/Fields: U.S. health care system.

★ 22170 ★ Center for Thanatology Research
391 Atlantic Ave.
Brooklyn, NY 11217-1701
Phone: (718)858-3026 **Fax:** (718)852-1846
Email: rhalporn@pipeline.com
Website: http://www.thanatology.org
Roberta Halporn, Dir.
Activities/Fields: Aging, dying, death, bereavement, and gravestone studies. **Pub:** *Advances in Thanatology.* • *Archives of the Foundation of Thanatology.*

★ 22171 ★ Central Institute for the Deaf
4560 Clayton Ave.
Saint Louis, MO 63110
Phone: (314)977-0000 **Free:** 877-444-4574
Fax: (314)977-0025
Email: clark@claycorp.com
Website: http://www.cid.wustl.edu
Robert G. Clark, Exec. Dir.
Activities/Fields: Auditory communication and its disorders, including studies of hearing function, auditory physiology, sensory neuroscience, auditory biophysics and biomechanics, effects of noise, and regeneration in the auditory nervous system. Also performs clinical studies of speech and linguistics, communication in infants and the elderly, characteristics of deaf speech, evaluation of cochlear implants in children, aural rehabilitation, psychosocial therapy, and audiology. Also engineers, designs, and evaluates instruments to evaluate and/or assist the deaf and the hard-of-hearing, and develops multimedia network communication systems with special applications for the deaf community.

★ 22172 ★ Central Institute for the Deaf Center for Childhood Deafness and Adult Aural Rehabilitation
4560 Clayton Rd.
Saint Louis, MO 63110
Phone: (314)977-0156 **Fax:** (314)977-0024
Email: murray@cid.wustl.edu
Website: http://www.cid.wustl.edu/research/ccdaar/intro.htm
Nancy Tye-Murray, PhD, Hd.
Activities/Fields: Problems confronted by hearing-impaired children and adults, including education, use of sensory aids, speech and language acquisition, and communication development, improved telecommunications for the hearing impaired, and the effects of noise on hearing.

★ 22173 ★ Central Institute for the Deaf Fay and Carl Simons Center for Biology of Hearing and Deafness
4560 Clayton Ave.
Saint Louis, MO 63110
Phone: (314)977-0260 **Fax:** (314)977-0030
Email: rbaird@cid.wustl.edu
Website: http://www.cid.wustl.edu/research/fcscbhd/intro.htm
Richard Baird, PhD, Dir.
Activities/Fields: Sensory loss and recovery in the inner ear, with a particular emphasis on increasing understanding of the cellular and molecular mechanisms that may lead to sensory rescue, repair or regeneration. Ongoing research includes studies of inner ear development; age-related, noise-induced, and drug-induced hearing loss; cell proliferation, migraton, and differentiation; neuronal innervation; and auditory and vestibular function.

★ 22174 ★ Centre for Addiction and Mental Health (CAMH)
33 Russell St.
Toronto, ON, Canada M5S 2S1
Phone: (416)535-8501
Email: public_affairs@camh.net
Website: http://www.camh.net/
Dr. Paul Garfinkel, Pres. /CEO
Activities/Fields: Mental illness and addiction. The research initiatives integrate addiction and mental health research from neuroscience, clinical research and social policy and prevention perspectives. **Pub:** *The Guide to the Centre for Addiction and Mental Health.*

★ 22175 ★ Centre for Addiction and Mental Health Clarke Division
33 Russell St.
Toronto, ON, Canada M5T 2S1
Phone: (416)535-8501
Email: public_affairs@camh.net
Website: http://www.camh.net
Dr. Paul Garfinkel, Pres. /CEO
Activities/Fields: Addiction and mental health. Studies include use and effects of alcohol, tobacco, and other drugs, with concentration in proevention and health promotion, drug and alcoholism treatment; socio-behavioral, medical, bio-behavioral, and biochemical research; and program evaluation. Develops and evaluates effectiveness of different treatment methods. Epidemiological studies of alcohol and drug use among general population and sub-groups. Effective strategies for prevention and early intervention, as well as behavioral, psychological, physical, and social/environmental factors that contribute to abuse. Problem gambling. Mental health research and treatment, such as group therapy, crisis management, stress managment, nutritional counselling, case management, living skills, training, therapeutic recreation and relapse prevention. Gender identity, anger managment, mood disorders, neurological impairment, concurrent disorders, developmental handicaps, and psychosocial intervention. **Frmly:** Addiction and Mental Health Services Corp.; Clarke Institute of Psychiatry Division.

★ 22176 ★ Centre for Cancer Therapeutics
Ottawa Regional Cancer Centre
503 Smyth Rd.
Ottawa, ON, Canada K1H 1C4
Phone: (613)737-7700 **Fax:** (613)247-3524
Email: mcburney@med.uottawa.ca
Website: http://www.ohri.ca/programs/cancer_therapeutics/default.asp
Michael W. McBurney, PhD, Res. Dir.
Activities/Fields: Basic biology of cancer cells, and innovative cancer therapies that will exploit their weaknesses.

★ 22177 ★ Centre for Community Child Health Research
4480 Oak St., Rm. L-408
Vancouver, BC, Canada V6H 3V4
Phone: (604)875-3570 **Fax:** (604)875-3569
Email: png@cw.bc.ca
Dr. Robert Armstrong, Dir.
Activities/Fields: Factors that influence and support the healthy development of children and youth and the use and development of scientific methods to measure the effectiveness of health policy, practices, and technologies. **Frmly:** Centre for Community Health and Health Evaluation Research.

★ 22178 ★ Centre for Community Child Health Research British Columbia Injury Research and Prevention Unit (BCIRPU)
L-408-4480 Oak St.
Vancouver, BC, Canada V6H 3V4
Phone: (604)875-3776 **Fax:** (604)875-3569
Email: praina@cw.bc.ca
Website: http://www.injuryresearch.bc.ca/
Parminder Raina, PhD, Dir.
Activities/Fields: Injury reduction and prevention.

★ 22179 ★ Centre for Integrated Genomics (CIG)
Biotechnology Laboratory
University of British Columbia
6174 University Blvd., No. 237
Vancouver, BC, Canada V6T 1Z3
Phone: (604)822-4838 **Fax:** (604)822-2114
Email: biotech@interchange.ubc.ca
Website: http://www.cigenomics.bc.ca/eng/home.shtml
Dr. Doug Kilburn, Co-Dir.
Activities/Fields: Structural and functional genomics as they relate to cancer and the identification of genes involved in, or responsible for, oncogenesis and tumor progression. Although cancer research is the main focus of the center, applying genome science to problems in the basic life sciences and biotechnology is also a consideration.

★ 22180 ★ Centre for Rural and Northern Health Research (CRaNHR)
Health Sciences N
955 Oliver Rd.
Thunder Bay, ON, Canada P7B 5E1
Phone: (807)343-2136
Email: cranhr@flash.lakeheadu.ca
Website: http://flash.lakeheadu.ca/~cranhr/
Bruce Minore, PhD, Dir.
Activities/Fields: Issues affecting the health of rural and northern residents, including Aboriginal populations, children and youth, the elderly and women.

★ 22181 ★ Cerebral Blood Flow Laboratories (CBF Labs)
Veterans Administration Medical Center, Bldg. 110, Rm. 225
2002 Holcombe Blvd.
Houston, TX 77030
Phone: (713)795-5807 **Fax:** (713)794-7583
Email: jmeyer@bcm.tmc.edu
John S. Meyer, MD, Dir.
Activities/Fields: Measurement of CT morphological changes and cerebral blood flow; cerebrovascular disorders; aging, Alzheimer's and ischemic vascular dementias and responses to medical, surgical, phar-

macological, and behavioral treatment; prevention, diagnosis, and treatment of stroke and migraine; cerebral blood flow control and cerebral metabolism; neuropharmacology and physiology; aging; dementia; transient ischemic attacks; and risk factors for stroke. **Pub:** *Books, monographs.* • *Peer-reviewed journal articles.* **Frmly:** Baylor Center for Cerebrovascular Research.

★ 22182 ★ Charles R. Drew University of Medicine and Science
Hypertension Research Center
1621 E 120th St., MP 11
Los Angeles, CA 90059
Phone: (310)668-3177 **Fax:** (323)563-4924
Email: haward@cdrew.edu
Harry Ward, MD, Dir.
Activities/Fields: Epidemiology, causes, and treatment of high blood pressure in blacks. Analyzes twin studies to assess genetic and environmental factors in blood pressure variations. Conducts cross-cultural studies in Barbados and Nigeria.

★ 22183 ★ Chicago Institute of Neurosurgery and Neuroresearch
4501 N Winchester Ave.
Chicago, IL 60614
Phone: (773)250-0500 **Fax:** (773)250-0497
Website: http://www.cinn.org
Dr. Leonard Cerullo, Dir.
Activities/Fields: Molecular glycobiology of brain tumors, glycosyltransferase, molecular biology, and ddrt-pcr-based gene discovery.

★ 22184 ★ Chicago Medical School
H.M. Bligh Cancer Research Laboratories
3333 Green Bay Rd.
North Chicago, IL 60064
Phone: (847)578-3230 **Fax:** (847)578-3349
Email: kimy@finchcms.edu
Prof. Yoon Burn Kim, MD, Actg. Dir.
Activities/Fields: Human cancer research, especially breast and lung cancer. Research activities include early immuno-detection of carcinomas, and active use of T/Tn antigen vaccine to prevent recurrence of advanced breast carcinoma.

★ 22185 ★ Child Health Research Center
Newborn Medicine
Children's Hospital
300 Longwood Ave.
Boston, MA 02115
Phone: (617)355-6366 **Fax:** (617)355-7677
Email: merton.bernfield@tch.harvard.edu
Dr. Merton Bernfield, Co-Dir.
Activities/Fields: Child health, particularly developmental biology.

★ 22186 ★ Child Policy Research Center
Children's Hospital Medical Center
3333 Burnet Ave., ML 7014
Cincinnati, OH 45229
Phone: (513)636-0180 **Fax:** (513)636-0171
Email: cprc@cchmc.org
Website: http://www.cprc-chmc.uc.edu
Dr. Edward F. Donovan, Dir.
Activities/Fields: Children's well-being in regards to health issues, services, and outcomes. **Frmly:** Child Health Statistics Center.

★ 22187 ★ Children's Center for Cancer and Blood Disorders
Richland Memorial Hospital
University of South Carolina School of Medicine
7 Richland Medical Pk., Ste. 203
Columbia, SC 29203
Phone: (803)434-3533 **Fax:** (803)434-3094
Email: ronnie.neuberg@palmettohealth.org
Dr. Ronnie W. Neuberg, Dir.
Activities/Fields: Causes, treatments, and prevention of childhood cancer.

★ 22188 ★ Children's Heart and Health Institute of Texas
PO Box 3966
Corpus Christi, TX 78463
Phone: (361)887-4505 **Fax:** (361)887-0539
Laura Berlanga, CEO
Activities/Fields: Pediatric cardiology. Projects include investigations of the prevalence of developmental disabilities and heart disease risk factors in various counties, coronary disease among Hispanic children, arterial sclerotic heart disease, hypertension, and prevention.

★ 22189 ★ Children's Hospital of Alabama
Southeast Child Safety Institute
1600 7th Ave. S
Birmingham, AL 35233
Phone: (205)939-9720 **Fax:** (205)939-9245
Email: bill.king@chsys.org
Website: http://secsi.chsys.org
Dr. Bill King, Dir.
Activities/Fields: Poisonings, including studies on prescription drug ingestions in preschool age children, research on adolescent parasuicides, and epidemiology of childhood trauma. Provides statewide poison control. **Pub:** *Poison Bulletin*, quarterly.

★ 22190 ★ Children's Hospital (Boston)
General Clinical Research Center
300 Longwood Ave., 7 East
Boston, MA 02115
Phone: (617)355-7541 **Fax:** (617)264-9896
Email: kristine.jordan@tch.harvard.edu
Kristine Jordan, Admin. Mgr.
Activities/Fields: Protocols in bone marrow transplantation, immunodeficiencies, pediatric endocrinology, bone and mineral metabolism, pediatric hematology, neuroimmunology, oncology, and pediatric gastroenterology. **Pub:** *Grand Rounds*, occasionally.

★ 22191 ★ Children's Hospital and Health Center
Center for Pediatric Clinical Research
3020 Children's Way, MC 5105
San Diego, CA 92123-4282
Phone: (858)966-8047 **Fax:** (858)966-8048
Email: lgordon@chsd.org
Website: http://www.chsd.org/body.cfm?id=494
Lauren Gordon, Contact
Activities/Fields: Pharmaceuticals and medical devices for children.

★ 22192 ★ Children's Hospital and Medical Center
Cystic Fibrosis Research Center
Mail Stop 3D-2
4800 Sand Point Way NE
PO Box C5371
Seattle, WA 98105
Phone: (206)987-2024 **Fax:** (206)987-2639
Dr. Bonnie W. Ramsey, Dir.
Activities/Fields: Cystic fibrosis, particularly cardiopulmonary and infectious disease-related pathophysiology, gene therapy, and evaluation of treatment of patients with cystic fibrosis and cardiorespiratory diseases, including clinically oriented research on lung mechanics, and sputum microbiology.

★ 22193 ★ Children's Hospital Medical Center of Cincinnati
General Clinical Research Center
3333 Burnet Ave.
Cincinnati, OH 45229-3039
Phone: (513)636-4273 **Free:** 800-344-2462
Fax: (513)636-4695
Email: andrea.smirh@chmcc.org
Website: http://www.cincinnatichildrens.org/research/research_cores/general_clinical_research_center/default.htm
Andrea Smith, Mgr.
Activities/Fields: Pediatrics, including studies of congenital and acquired diseases of the gastrointestinal tract, pancreas, and liver, cholestatic liver disease, hepatic storage diseases, and cystic fibrosis. Other studies include growth, diabetes mellitus, hypertension, child and adult bone disease (including rickets and osteoporosis), and insulin sensitivity.

★ 22194 ★ Children's Hospital Oakland Research Institute (CHORI)
5700 Martin Luther King Jr. Way
Oakland, CA 94609
Phone: (510)450-7600 **Fax:** (510)450-7910
Email: blubin@chori.org
Website: http://www.chori.org
Dr. Bertram Lubin, Med. Res. Dir.
Activities/Fields: Biomedical sciences, especially pediatric diseases but also cancer, cardiovascular disease, and aging. **Pub:** *Research News*, quarterly.

★ 22195 ★ Children's Hospital of Philadelphia
Comprehensive Sickle Cell Center
34th St. & Civic Center Blvd.
Philadelphia, PA 19104
Phone: (215)590-3423 **Fax:** (215)590-2499
Email: ohene-frempong@email.chop.edu
Website: http://www.chop.edu/consumer/jsp/division/generic.jsp?id=70459
Kwaku Ohene-Frempong, MD, Dir.
Activities/Fields: Sickle cell disease.

★ 22196 ★ Children's Hospital of Philadelphia
General Clinical Research Center
Abramson Research Center
34th St. & Civic Ctr.
Philadelphia, PA 19104
Phone: (215)590-6359 **Fax:** (215)590-7544
Email: adamson@mail.med.upenn.edu
Dr. Peter Adamson, Actg. Prog. Dir.
Activities/Fields: Biomedicine, allergy and immunology, cardiology, diabetes endocrinology, gastroenterology, gene therapy, genetics, hematology, infectious disease, metabolism, neonatology, neurology, nutrition, and oncology.

★ 22197 ★ Children's Hospital of Pittsburgh
Cystic Fibrosis Research Center
3705 5th Ave.
Pittsburgh, PA 15213
Phone: (412)692-5630 **Fax:** (412)692-6645
Email: davido@pitt.edu
David M. Orenstein, MD, Dir.
Activities/Fields: Cystic fibrosis and related diseases, including pediatric pulmonary and pediatric gastrointestinal diseases. Also studies pediatric exercise physiology, and lung cellular immunology.

★ 22198 ★ Children's Hospital of Pittsburgh
General Clinical Research Center
3705 5th Ave.
Pittsburgh, PA 15213
Phone: (412)692-6565 **Fax:** (412)692-6783
Dr. Silva Arslanian, Dir.
Activities/Fields: Biomedicine, allergy and immunology, endocrinology, hematology and oncology, infectious disease, metabolism, nutrition, otolaryngology, pulmonology, pharmacology, transplantation surgery, gastroenterology, and diabetes mellitus.

★ 22199 ★ Children's Hospital of Pittsburgh
Molecular Diagnostics Lab
Pathology Department, B120
1056 E 19th Ave.
Denver, CO 80218
Phone: (303)837-2725 **Fax:** (303)831-4112
Email: wei.qi@tchden.org
Qi Wei, PhD, Supvr.

Activities/Fields: Research and testing for genetic diseases, focusing on cancer. DNA diagno stics testing services include both major and minor breakpoint cluster region (BCR) rearrangments; pre-B cell ALL t(1;19) PCR analysis; Y DNA PCR and probe analysis; retinoblastoma gene deletion and linkage analysis; Wilms' tumor gene deletion analysis; and DNA and RNA isolation for special studies. Research efforts, both basic and applied, are focused on mechanisms of carcinogenesis, emphasizing the development of sensitive methods and techniques for the early (pre-clinical) detection of cancer; measuring biological (genetic) damage induced by human exposure to toxic agents; and determining genetic markers of diagnostic and prognostic value in the clinical care of cancer patients.

★ 22200 ★ Children's Hospital Research Center
3020 Children's Way, MC 5074
San Diego, CA 92123
Phone: (858)576-5934 **Fax:** (858)966-8589
Email: mbenedict@chsd.org
Michael Benedict, Exec. Dir.

Activities/Fields: Causes and prevention of childhood diseases, including studies in diagnostic techniques and methods, neurosciences, autism, language development, sudden infant death syndrome, and industrial technology.

★ 22201 ★ Children's Leukemia Research Association
585 Stewart Ave., Ste. 18
Garden City, NY 11530
Phone: (516)222-1944 **Fax:** (516)222-0457
Email: clra@erols.com
Website: http://www.childrensleukemia.org
Allan D. Weinberg, Exec. Dir.

Activities/Fields: Leukemia research and public awareness of the disease.

★ 22202 ★ Children's Memorial Hospital
Cystic Fibrosis Research Center
2300 N Children's Plz., Box 43
Northwestern University
Chicago, IL 60614
Phone: (773)880-4382 **Fax:** (773)880-6300
Email: smccolley@northwestern.edu
Dr. Susanna McColley, Dir.

Activities/Fields: Cystic fibrosis, particularly airways inflammation, exercise, psychosocial issues, fat absorption, outcomes research, nutrition, and epidemiology. **Pub:** *Cystic Fibrosis Center News*, quarterly.

★ 22203 ★ Children's Research Institute (Columbus, OH)
700 Children's Dr.
Columbus, OH 43205
Phone: (614)722-2700 **Fax:** (614)722-2716
Email: pjohnson@chi.osu.edu
Website: http://www.childrenscolumbus.org
Phil Johnson, Pres.

Activities/Fields: Molecular retrovirology, gene transfer, molecular genetics, vaccine development, vascular and cellular biology, children's cancer chemotherapy, cancer immunology, gastroenterology, infectious diseases, pathology, surgery, virology, metabolic disorders, cystic fibrosis, pulmonology, pharmacology/toxicology, cardiology, neonatology, pediatrics, and clinical problems of infancy and childhood. **Pub:** *Annual Report.* **Frmly:** Children's Hospital Research Foundation (Columbus, OH).

★ 22204 ★ Child's Health Hospital Research Centre
1820 Richmond Rd. SW
Calgary, AB, Canada T2T 5C7
Phone: (403)229-7241 **Fax:** (403)543-9111
Dr. R. Brent Scott, Dir.

Activities/Fields: Centre houses two research groups: the Medical Genetics Research Group which conducts research on genetic epidemiology, genetic linkage, molecular genetics, human sperm chromosome analysis, experimental mammalian teratology, developmental genetics, cytogenetics, and birth defects; and the Behavioural Research Group with programs in childhood conditions such as hyperactivity, diet and behavior, learning disorders, and stress-related disorders. Research and development of diagnostic services in biochemical genetics, cytogenetic and molecular genetics are supported through the Alberta Hereditary Diseases Program and are integrated in the Centre. Also sponsors pediatric research in respirology, gastroenterology, vision research, infectious diseases, neonatology, and other allied health disciplines. **Pub:** *Alberta Children's Hospital Research Centre Annual Reports.* • *Bulletin of the Alberta Hereditary Diseases Program*, quarterly. **Frmly:** Kinsmen Pediatric Research Centre.

★ 22205 ★ Christine M. Kleinert Institute for Hand and Microsurgery, Inc.
225 Abraham Flexner Way, Ste. 850
Louisville, KY 40202
Phone: (502)562-0312 **Fax:** (502)562-0326
Email: fellowship@cmki.org
Website: http://www.cmki.org
Tina McMongal, Coord.

Activities/Fields: Upper extremity care, including nerve compression conditions and carpal tunnel syndrome; nerve regeneration; biomechanical studies; replanted and transplanted tissue and the most effective ways of increasing survival and function; and hand and microsurgery techniques, including anatomical studies.

★ 22206 ★ CIIT Centers for Health Research
6 Davis Dr., Box 12137
Research Triangle Park, NC 27709-2137
Phone: (919)558-1200
Email: CIITinfo@ciit.org
Website: http://www.ciit.org/
Bob Nellis, Contact

Activities/Fields: Potential adverse effects of chemicals, pharmaceuticals, and consumer products on human health. Research is structured into four programs: Chemical Carcinogenesis Program; Endocrine, Reproductive and Developmental Toxicology Program; Neurotoxicology Program; and Respiratory Toxicology Program. **Pub:** *Articles.* • *CIIT Activities Newsletter*, monthly. • *CIIT Annual Report.*

★ 22207 ★ Cincinnati Center for Developmental Disorders
Pavilion Bldg.
3333 Burnet Ave.
Cincinnati, OH 45229-3039
Phone: (513)636-8383 **Fax:** (513)636-7361
Email: sonya.oppenheimer@cchmc.org
Dr. Sonya Oppenheimer, Dir.

Activities/Fields: Prevention, early detection, and improved methods of therapy and management of developmental disabilities. Also studies genetics, learning disabilities, and birth defects. **Pub:** *Developments, Newsletter*, quarterly.

★ 22208 ★ Cincinnati Children's Research Foundation
3333 Burnet Ave.
Cincinnati, OH 45229-3039
Phone: (513)636-4588 **Fax:** (513)636-0345
Email: thomas.boat@cchmc.org
Website: http://www.chmcc.org/chrf.html
Thomas F. Boat, MD, Dir.

Activities/Fields: Development biology, molecular and cell biology, biochemistry, physiology, microbiology, pathology, and clinical investigations of infancy and childhood, and animal models of childhood illnesses. Research activities are carried out in the divisions of adolescent medicine, allergy/immunology, general pediatrics, development biology, cardiology, molecular cardiovascular biology, clinical pharmacology, critical care medicine, emergency medicine, endocrinology, gastroenterology, hematology-oncology, experimental hematology, human genetics, immunobiology, infectious disease, developmental disabilities, molecular cardiovascular biology, neonatology, nephrology, neurology, pathology, child psychology, child psychiatry, pulmonary biology, pulmonary medicine, radiology, rheumatology, surgery, health policy and clinical effectiveness; the veterinary services division provides care and maintenance of laboratory animals. **Frmly:** Children's Hospital Research Foundation.

★ 22209 ★ Cincinnati Sports Medicine Research and Education Foundation
Deaconess Hospital
311 Straight St.
Cincinnati, OH 45219
Phone: (513)559-2818 **Fax:** (513)475-5263
Email: sbwestin@csmref.org
Website: http://www.cincinnatisportsmed.com
Frank R. Noyes, MD, Dir.

Activities/Fields: Orthopedic and sports medicine with emphasis on clinical problems and surgical treatment. Areas of interest include rehabilitation protocols; autograft revision knee ligament reconstruction; meniscal allografts; osteochondral autograft transfer; carticel, posterior cruciate and posterolateral reconstruction; biomechanics of the knee and shoulder; and gait analysis.

★ 22210 ★ City College of City University of New York
Center for the Study of the Cellular and Molecular Basis of Development
City College Science Bldg., Rm. 501
138th St. & Convent Ave.
New York, NY 10031
Phone: (212)650-8300 **Fax:** (212)650-7989
Email: jerry@scisun.sci.ccny.cuny.edu
Dr. Jerry Guyden, Dir.

Activities/Fields: Molecular biology, including biomolecular structure and function, gene expression and regulation, cellular and organismic function, and neurobiology.

★ 22211 ★ City of Hope
National Medical Center and Beckman Research Institute
1500 E Duarte Rd.
Duarte, CA 91010
Phone: (626)359-8111 **Fax:** (626)930-5394
Website: http://www.cityofhope.org
Theodore G. Krontiris, MD, Exec. VP

Activities/Fields: Biology, including cell biology, molecular biology, developmental biology; molecular genetics; molecular immunology; gene regulation; and theoretical biology; immunology; molecular medicine; virology; information sciences; hematology research; radiation research, including radioimmunotherapy; surgical research; experimental therapeutics diabetes research.

★ 22212 ★ City of Hope
National Medical Center and Beckman Research Institute
Department of Nursing Research and Education
1500 E Duarte Rd.
Duarte, CA 91010
Phone: (626)301-2346 **Fax:** (626)301-8941
Email: mgrant@coh.org
Marcia Grant, Dir.

Activities/Fields: Clinical nursing, including nursing administration, nursing education, delivery of nursing services, nursing organization, and the relationship of patient problems to nursing. Research focuses on quality of life, pain and symptom management, improving nursing attitudes and skills in caring for patients and their families, and reducing complications and side effects of therapy and patient psychological distresses associated with therapeutic and diagnostic procedures.

★ 22213 ★ City of Hope National Medical Center and Beckman Research Institute Division of Biology

1450 E Duarte Rd.
Duarte, CA 91010
Phone: (626)359-8111 **Fax:** (626)930-5486
Website: http://www.cityofhope.org
Jack P. Suzar, Ch.

Activities/Fields: Molecular mechanisms of living systems. Research activities are carried out in Departments of Biology, Molecular Biochemistry, Molecular Genetics, and Theoretical Biology. Department of Biology focuses on dynamic and temporal properties of cell growth and proliferation as it is manifested in cultured cells and intact organisms, including cellular clocks, circadian rhythms, and chemical oscillators; mammalian genes and gene control mechanisms and defining the biological function of postreplication DNA modifications that occur in mammalian cells; the mechanisms of gene repression and its relationship to DNA replication time; the role of amino acid sequence in determining protein function and folding patterns; mammalian chromosome inactivation mechanisms; mutational generation and repair mechanisms; genetic imprinting; and embryonic stem cell biology. Department of Molecular Biochemistry studies the use of synthetic oligodeoxyribonucleotides in the study of human disease, including diagnosis of genetic disease and the analysis of bone marrow transplant patients; the role of genetically engineered antibodies for cancer therapy; the biological function of nucleic acids studied by chemical synthesis; genetic mechanisms of imprinting; and isolation and characterization of genes important to immune function and cancer. Department of Molecular Genetics examines gene expression sequence requirements in eukaryotic systems, diagnosis of viral diseases (including HIV and HCMV), biochemistry of RNA splicing, catalytic RNA function and applications in HIV infection and cancer, control of gene expression, isolation of biologically active pure insulin and insulin-like growth factor receptors, mitochondrial-nuclear interactions and mitochondrial biogenesis, and homologous DNA recombinations. Theoretical Biology examines origins of genetic information and patterns in coding regions of gene families.

★ 22214 ★ City of Hope National Medical Center and Beckman Research Institute Division of Neurosciences

1450 E Duarte Rd.
Duarte, CA 91010
Phone: (626)301-8188 **Fax:** (626)301-8948
Email: mbarish@coh.org
Website: http://bricoh.coh.org
Dr. Michael E. Barish, Ch.

Activities/Fields: The Division is composed of 9 research sections studying cell biology, cellular neurochemistry, cellular neurophysiology, developmental neurobiology, membrane biochemistry, molecular biology and genetics, neuroanatomy and ultrastructure, neurobiochemistry, neuroendocrinology, neuropharmacology, neurophysiology, and receptor physiology. Specific studies include the embryonic development of spinal cord neurons; identification, localization, and functions of neuroactive peptides; molecular and functional studies of transmembrane ion channels; the functional relationship between molecular chemical events and electrical excitability of neuronal elements; interactions between neurotransmitter receptor molecules of the membrane with synaptic proteins; developmental and molecular biological processes involved in the function of cholinergic neurons in normal and animal models of Alzheimer's disease; mechanisms of solute transport localized membranes and the effect of lipid components on operation of transport systems; developmental specificity of the formation of neuronal connections; and molecular genetic studies of Alzheimer's disease.

★ 22215 ★ City of Hope National Medical Center and Beckman Research Institute Strategic Program for Innovative Research in AIDS Therapy

Virology & Infectious Diseases/Department of Pediatrics
1500 E Duarte Rd.
Duarte, CA 91010
Phone: (626)301-8436 **Fax:** (626)301-8458
Email: jzaia@coh.org
Dr. John A. Zaia, Prin. Investigator

Activities/Fields: Developmental gene therapy in the treatment of AIDS, including development and delivery of antiviral DNA and RNA; and pathogenesis and treatment of cytomegalovirus infection; and development of CMV vaccine.

★ 22216 ★ Cleveland Clinic Foundation Lerner Research Institute

9500 Euclid Ave.
Cleveland, OH 44195
Phone: (216)444-3900 **Fax:** (216)444-3279
Email: fraserm@ccf.org
Website: http://www.lri.ccf.org/
Paul E. DiCorleto, PhD, Chm.

Activities/Fields: Molecular biology; structure and function in regulation of viral and cellular genes and (proto)oncogenes, and interferon signaling mechanisms; cancer biology and genetics, including Wilms' tumor, cellular gene regulation, transgenic models, and use of newly patented 2-5A antisense technology; cell biology, including vessel wall pathophysiology, lipoprotein oxidation, regulation of gene expression and intracellular signaling pathways. Studies also include immunology, biologic response modifiers in tumor growth and regression, chemokines, nitric oxide synthase; neurosciences emphasizing cellular and genetic mechanisms in multiple sclerosis, effects of AIDS; epilepsy; neuronal signaling in cardiovascular neurobiology and diagnostic methods in cerebrovascular disease and hypertrophy, studies of lipoprotein(a), computerized modeling of protein structures, G-proteins, and study of the basis of hypertension; biomedical engineering, including musculoskeletal biology, imaging research, biomaterials and biocompatibility, and total artificial heart and heart assist devices; and biostatistics and epidemiology. **Pub:** *Annual report.* • *Notations*, bimonthly. Newsletter.

★ 22217 ★ Cleveland FES Center

11000 Cedar Ave., Ste. 230
Cleveland, OH 44106-3052
Phone: (216)231-3257 **Free:** 800-666-2353
Fax: (216)231-3258
Email: info@fesc.org
Website: http://feswww.fes.cwru.edu/
P. Hunter Peckham, PhD, Dir.

Activities/Fields: Functional electrical stimulation (FES) in the restoration of muscle control or sensory function, particularly in the areas of lower and upper extremity deficits, scoliosis, spasticity, respiratory insufficiency, and bladder function. Studies focus on computer-controlled and implanted FES systems for paraplegic and quadraplegic users, persons with hemiplegia due to cerebral trauma or stroke, and persons with spinal cord injuries. **Pub:** *FES Update Newsletter*, semiannually. **Frmly:** Rehabilitation Engineering Center.

★ 22218 ★ Cleveland Hearing and Speech Center

11206 Euclid Ave.
Cleveland, OH 44106-1798
Phone: (216)231-8787 **Fax:** (216)231-7141
Email: bphenri@chsc.org
Website: http://www.chsc.org
Bernard P. Henri, PhD, Exec. Dir.

Activities/Fields: Speech, language, and hearing disorders; speech production in patients with Parkinson's Disease; and managed care, financial incentives and clinical decision making. **Frmly:** Cleveland Association for the Hard of Hearing.

★ 22219 ★ Clinical Research Foundation

212 Church Ave., Ste. A
Chula Vista, CA 91910-2703
Phone: (619)420-8696 **Free:** 800-900-0489
Fax: (619)420-6915
Email: tanaka@cts.com
Website: http://www.terrytanakadds.com
Naomi Tanaka, Exec. Dir.

Activities/Fields: Head, neck and temporomandibular joint (TMJ) diagnosis, treatment and management; anatomy, radiography, and other therapies; restorative dentistry. **Pub:** *TMD and Restorative Dentistry.*

★ 22220 ★ Clinical Research Institute of Montreal

110 Pine Ave. W
Montreal, QC, Canada H2W 1R7
Phone: (514)987-5500 **Fax:** (514)987-5789
Email: guindoy@mailhost.ircm.qc.ca
Website: http://www.ircm.qc.ca
Dr. Yvan Guindon, CEO/Sci. Dir.

Activities/Fields: Causes, mechanisms, and more effective treatments of diseases in many fields of medicine, including research on hypertension, neurobiology and behavior, hyperlipidemias and atherosclerosis, proteins and peptides hormones, lipid metabolism, biomedical engineering, molecular biology, immunology, molecular genetics, bioethics, reproduction, chemical biology and polypeptides, hematopoiesis and leukemia, cancer, and bio-organic chemistry. **Pub:** *Annual Report.* • *Scientific Brochure*, biennially.

★ 22221 ★ College of Staten Island of City University of New York Program in Neuroscience

Bldg. 6-S, Rm. 229
Staten Island, NY 10314
Phone: (718)982-3950 **Fax:** (718)982-3953
Dr. Ekkehart Trenkner, Mng. Dir.

Activities/Fields: Developmental neurobiology and neurochemistry, and synaptic plasticity, focusing on the regulation and adaptation of neural function, utilizing brain slices, neural cell lines, primary CNS neurons grown in culture, aging and development and neuropathological processes (Alzheimer's and genetic diseases). **Frmly:** Center for Developmental Neuroscience and Developmental Disabilities.

★ 22222 ★ Colorado Cancer Research Program

2253 S Oneida, 3rd Fl, Ste. B
Denver, CO 80224-2522
Phone: (303)777-2663 **Free:** 888-785-6789
Fax: (303)777-2642
Email: ccrp@co-cancerresearch.org
Website: http://www.co-cancerresearch.org
Eduardo R. Pajon, MD, Prin. Investigator

Activities/Fields: Cancer and clinical oncology.

★ 22223 ★ Colorado Neurological Institute (CNI)

701 E Hampden Ave., Ste. 330
Englewood, CO 80110
Phone: (303)788-4010 **Fax:** (303)788-5469
Email: jbriles@thecni.org
Website: http://thecni.org/research.htm
Gary D. VanderArk, MD, Pres.

Activities/Fields: Neurological diseases, including Parkinson's disease, Huntington's disease and other movement disorders, epilepsy, brain tumors, spinal cord injuries, head trauma, hearing disorders, stroke, Lou Gehrig's disease, sleep disorders, migraines, neuromuscular disorders.

★ 22224 ★ Colorado Neurological Institute
CNI Brain Tumor Program
701 E Hampden Ave., Ste. 160
Englewood, CO 80110
Phone: (303)806-7420
Email: jbriles@thecni.org
Website: http://thecni.org/braintumor/
Edward B. Arenson, MD, Co-Dir.
Activities/Fields: Photodynamic therapy for the treatment of brain tumors.

★ 22225 ★ Colorado Neurological Institute
CNI Rocky Mountain Cochlear Implant Center
799 E Hampden Ave., Ste. 510
Englewood, CO 80110
Phone: (303)788-7880 **Fax:** (303)788-7884
Email: jbriles@thecni.org
Website: http://thecni.org/hearing/
Dr. David C. Kelsall, Dir.
Activities/Fields: Cochlear implant devices.

★ 22226 ★ Colorado State University
Center for Environmental Toxicology and Technology
Foothills Campus
Fort Collins, CO 80523-1680
Phone: (970)491-8522 **Fax:** (970)491-8304
Email: imonum@colostate.edu
Website: http://www.cvmbs.colostate.edu/enhealth/cett/
Dr. Raymond S.H. Yang, Dir.
Activities/Fields: Hazards associated with environmental exposure to chemical and physical agents, focusing on complex chemical mixtures and chemical-radiation interaction. Also studies growth, reproduction, immune function, physiologically based pharmacokinetics, genetic and molecular markers of disease, and ecotoxicology and bioremediation, focusing on hazardous waste mixtures. **Frmly:** Collaborative Radiological Health Laboratory.

★ 22227 ★ Colorado State University
Colorado Injury Control Research Center (CICRC)
Department of Environmental Health
College of Veterinary Medicine and Biomedical Sciences
Environmental Health Bldg.
Fort Collins, CO 80523-1676
Phone: (970)491-0670 **Fax:** (970)491-1032
Email: loranns@colostate.edu
Website: http://www.cvmbs.colostate.edu/EnHealth/CICRC
Dr. Lorann Stallones, Dir.
Activities/Fields: Acute care, rehabilitation, prevention, and epidemiology in injury control and prevention of injuries in the Rocky Mountain Region.

★ 22228 ★ Colorado State University
Human Performance Laboratory
Department of Health & Exercise Science
Fort Collins, CO 80523
Phone: (970)491-3847 **Fax:** (970)491-7677
Email: israel@cahs.colostate.edu
Dr. Richard Gay Israel, Exec. Dir.
Activities/Fields: Human performance, body composition, metabolism, nutrition and sports performance, and exercise physiology.

★ 22229 ★ Colorado State University
Hypo-Hyperbaric Chamber Facility
College of Veterinary Medicine & Biomedical Sciences
1601 Campus Delivery
Fort Collins, CO 80523
Phone: (970)491-6187 **Fax:** (970)491-7569
Email: alan.tucker@colostate.edu
Website: http://www.cvmbs.colostate.edu/cvmbs/hypo.html
Dr. Alan Tucker, Dir.
Activities/Fields: High altitude physiology, altitude illness, pulmonary hypertension, human performance at various altitudes, hyperbaric physiology, and human and animal studies.

★ 22230 ★ Colorado State University
Institute for Rural Environmental Health
College of Veterinary Medicine & Biomedical Sciences
Fort Collins, CO 80523-1601
Phone: (970)491-7051 **Fax:** (970)491-2250
Email: cvmbsweb@colostate.edu
Website: http://www.cvmbs.colostate.edu/cvmbs/reh.html
Dr. John Reif, Dir.
Activities/Fields: Environmental toxicology, hazardous waste disposal, environmental epidemiology, health risk assessment, comparative human and animal health, and occupational health.

★ 22231 ★ Colorado State University
Macromolecular Resources
Department of Biochemistry, 355 MRB
Fort Collins, CO 80523
Phone: 800-491-0424 **Free:** 800-4DNA-FAX
Fax: (970)491-0239
Email: pwryan@lamar.colostate.edu
Website: http://mmr.bmb.colostate.edu/
Philip W. Ryan, PhD, Dir.
Activities/Fields: Produces custom oligonucleotides for DNA researchers and custom peptides. Also offers mass spectrometry, protein sequencing and DNA sequencing services.

★ 22232 ★ Colorado State University
Program in Molecular, Cellular, and Integrative Neurosciences
Biomedical Sciences Department
Anatomy/Neurobiology Station
1617 Campus Directory
Fort Collins, CO 80523-1617
Phone: (970)491-0425 **Fax:** (970)491-7907
Email: jbamburg@lamar.colostate.edu
Website: http://cvmbs.colostate.edu/mcin
Dr. James R. Bamburg, Dir.
Activities/Fields: Cellular, molecular and integrative approaches to neuroscience, focusing on basic components of the nervous system's development repair, and function largely through studies of cultured neurons, brain slices, and animals. Also investigation of the role of amino acid neurotransmitters in development and aging, structure and function of voltage and ligand gated ion channels, mechanisms of taste reception, basis of circadian rhythms, mechanisms of synaptic function, and regulation of gene expression in early development.

★ 22233 ★ Columbia-Presbyterian Medical Center
Columbia Genome Center
630 W 168 St.
New York, NY 10032-3784
Phone: (212)305-3440 **Fax:** (212)305-1191
Email: ise1@columbia.edu
I.S. Edelman, MD, Dir.
Activities/Fields: DNA and human disease conditions in chromosome 13. The center contains six laboratory sections: Molecular Genetics, Physical mapping, DNA sequencing, Cancer Genetics, Genomic Informatics, and Molecular Bioinformatics.

★ 22234 ★ Columbia-Presbyterian Medical Center
Gertrude H. Sergievsky Center
630 W 168 St.
New York, NY 10032
Phone: (212)305-2515 **Fax:** (212)305-2426
Email: rpm2@columbia.edu
Website: http://cpmcnet.columbia.edu/dept/sergievsky
Dr. Richard Mayeux, Dir.
Activities/Fields: Developmental disorders of the nervous system that affect humans from conception until death, including epilepsy, Parkinson's Disease, essential tremor, and Alzheimer's Disease and other age-related brain diseases.

★ 22235 ★ Columbia-Presbyterian Medical Center
Naomi Berrie Diabetes Center
1150 St. Nicholas Ave.
New York, NY 10032
Phone: (212)304-5494 **Fax:** (212)304-5493
Email: diabetes@columbia.edu
Website: http://cpmcnet.columbia.edu/dept/diabetes
Robin S. Goland, MD, Dir.
Activities/Fields: Biologic basis of diabetes, the prevention of Type 1 and Type 2 diabetes and diabetic complications.

★ 22236 ★ Columbia-Presbyterian Medical Center
Neurological Institute
710 W 168th St.
New York, NY 10032-3784
Phone: (212)305-6489 **Fax:** (212)305-6978
Email: tap2@columbia.edu
Website: http://www.neuroinstitute.org
Timothy A. Pedley, MD, Chm., Neurology Dept.
Activities/Fields: Neurology, neuropathology, neurophysiology, neurological surgery, dystonia, Parkinson's and Alzheimer's diseases, muscular dystrophy, amyotrophic lateral sclerosis (Lou Gehrig's disease), multiple sclerosis, and epilepsy, including basic and clinical studies on function and disease of the nervous system and treatment of nervous diseases and surgical conditions of the brain and nervous system.

★ 22237 ★ Columbia-Presbyterian Medical Center
Richard and Hinda Rosenthal Center for Complementary and Alternative Medicine
Department of Rehabilitative Medicine
College of Physicians & Surgeons
Columbia University
630 W 168 St., Box 75
New York, NY 10032
Phone: (212)543-9542 **Fax:** (212)543-2845
Website: http://cpmcnet.columbia.edu/dept/rosenthal/
Fredi Kronenberg, PhD, Dir.
Activities/Fields: Complementary and alternative medicine, especially regarding effectiveness, safety and mechanisms of action. Research focuses on botanical medicine and traditional medicine systems.

★ 22238 ★ Columbia University
Artificial Organs Research Laboratory
Department of Chemical Engineering
814 Mudd Bldg., MC 4721
New York, NY 10027
Phone: (212)854-4448 **Fax:** (212)854-3054
Email: leonard@columbia.edu
Website: http://www.columbia.edu/~leonard
Prof. Edward F. Leonard, Dir.
Activities/Fields: Engineering and technical solutions for problems associated with extracorporeal circulation, cardiovascular implants, and artificial organs. Also studies blood-biomaterial interactions, extracorporeal immunotherapies, and photochemical reactions to transform cells and inactivate viruses.

★ 22239 ★ Columbia University
Biochemistry and Molecular Biophysics Laboratory
630 W 168th St.
New York, NY 10032
Phone: (212)305-3669 **Fax:** (212)305-7932
Email: dih1@columbia.edu
Website: http://cpmcnet.columbia.edu/dept/gsas/biochem
Dr. David Hirsh, Chr.
Activities/Fields: Biochemistry, molecular biology, biophysics, and biochemical genetics, including X-ray diffraction studies of biological macromolecules, structure and function of membrane receptors and transport proteins, computer studies of protein and nucleic acid structure and function, NMR spectroscopy, neutron and electron diffraction, enzymology, regulation of transcription and translation in prokaryotic and eukaryotic cells, molecular virology, genomic and cDNA cloning in prokaryotes and eukaryotes, recombinant DNA technology, gene transfer and somatic-cell genetics, DNA sequencing, in vitro site-specific mutagenesis of cloned DNA, the role of oncogenes in neoplasia, control of gene expression in development, role of growth factors, regulation of oxygen transport by hemoglobin, hormonal regulation of ion transport, immunochemical properties of membrane antigens, structure and composition of synaptic components, metabolism of neurotransmitters, neurotoxic proteins and protein hormones, and chemical carcinogenesis.

★ 22240 ★ Columbia University
Center for AIDS Research
School of Nursing
630 W 168th St.
New York, NY 10032
Phone: (212)305-5756 **Fax:** (212)305-6937
Email: jka8@columbia.edu
Website: http://cpmcnet.columbia.edu/dept/nursing/institute-centers/aids-research.html
Joyce K. Anastasi, PhD, Dir.
Activities/Fields: Health promotion, disease prevention, symptom management and quality of life for individuals with AIDS. **Pub:** *Journal articles.*

★ 22241 ★ Columbia University
Center for CAM Research in Aging and Women's Health
College of Physicians & Surgeons
630 W 168th St., Box 75
New York, NY 10032
Phone: (212)342-0101 **Fax:** (212)342-0100
Website: http://www.rosenthal.hs.columbia.edu
Fredi Kronenberg, PhD, Dir.
Activities/Fields: Dietary and herbal treatments in postmenopausal women.

★ 22242 ★ Columbia University
Center for Environmental Health in Northern Manhattan
Mailman School of Public Health
701 W 168th St.
New York, NY 10032
Phone: (212)305-1996 **Fax:** (212)305-5328
Email: RPS1@columbia.edu
Website: http://www.niehs.nih.gov/centers/center/colctr.htm
Regina M. Santella, PhD, Dir.
Activities/Fields: Diseases due to, or exacerbated by, hazardous urban ecosystems, particularly neurotoxicology and neurodegenerative diseases; pulmonary disorders, especially asthma; and cancer. The neighborhoods of Northern Manhattan (Harlem and Washington Heights) typify this problem in that their outdoor and indoor environments provide excessive opportunity for exposure to air pollutants and allergens, lead, asbestos, and indoor residues of insecticides.

★ 22243 ★ Columbia University
Center for Health Promotion
Box 114
Teachers College
New York, NY 10027
Phone: (212)678-3960 **Fax:** (212)678-8259
Email: jpa1@columbia.edu
John P. Allegrante, PhD, Dir.
Activities/Fields: Health promotion and disease prevention, focusing on the effects on health of personal behavior and lifestyle, including physical activity and fitness, nutrition, alcohol and other drugs; mental health and mental disorders violent and abusive behavior; and how educational and community-based programs can be used to improve health and prevent premature death and disability throughout the human life span through schools, patient care, workplace, and other community settings.

★ 22244 ★ Columbia University
Center for Molecular Therapeutics (CMT)
Department of Pharmacology
630 W 168th St.
New York, NY 10032
Phone: (212)305-8754 **Fax:** (212)305-8351
Email: mrr1@columbia.edu
Website: http://cpmcnet.columbia.edu/dept/cmt/
Michael Rosen, MD, Contact
Activities/Fields: Strategies, drugs, and devices for delivery of health care.

★ 22245 ★ Columbia University
Center for Opportunities and Outcomes for People with Disabilities
525 W 120th St., Box 223
New York, NY 10027-6698
Phone: (212)678-3076
Email: oopd@columbia.edu
Website: http://www.tc.columbia.edu/centers/oopd/aboutus.htm
Linda Hickson, PhD, Dir.
Activities/Fields: Quality of life for people with disabilities, especially regarding independence and self-determination; eliminating negative outcomes often associated with disability; and exploring disability-related issues of culturally and ethnically diverse groups, including women and minorities. **Pub:** *O&O Newsletters.*

★ 22246 ★ Columbia University
Center for Parkinson's Disease and Other Movement Disorders
Neurological Institute
710 W 168th St., 3rd Fl.
New York, NY 10032
Phone: (212)305-5779 **Fax:** (212)305-1304
Email: fahn@movdis.cis.columbia.edu
Website: http://cpmcnet.columbia.edu/dept/neurology/movdis/
Stanley Fahn, MD, Dir.
Activities/Fields: Phenomenology, pharmacology, myoclonus, treatment, and genetics of Parkinson's disease and other movement disorders. Research activities focus on dystonia, Parkinsonism, tremor, dyskinesia, chorea, and tics. **Frmly:** Dystonia Clinical Research Center.

★ 22247 ★ Columbia University
Center for Radiological Research
630 W 168th St.
New York, NY 10032
Phone: (212)305-5660 **Fax:** (212)305-3229
Email: ejh1@columbia.edu
Website: http://crr-cu.org
Dr. Eric J. Hall, Dir.
Activities/Fields: Human and rodent cell transformation assay systems at the cellular and molecular levels. **Pub:** *Annual report.*

★ 22248 ★ Columbia University
Center for Reproductive Sciences
630 W 168th St.
New York, NY 10032
Phone: (212)305-2304 **Fax:** (212)305-3869
Dr. Rogerio A. Lobo, Dir.
Activities/Fields: Biology of reproduction, including neuroendocrinology, male and female gametogenesis, reproductive endocrinology, genetics, perinatology, angiogenesis, and reproductive oncology.

★ 22249 ★ Columbia University
Center for the Study of Society and Medicine
College of Physicians & Surgeons
630 W 168th St.
New York, NY 10032
Phone: (212)305-4184 **Fax:** (212)305-6416
Email: djr5@columbia.edu
Website: http://www.societyandmedicine.org
Dr. David J. Rothman, Dir.
Activities/Fields: Issues that arise in clinical and research settings, including studies in bioethics and health policy, bioethics and medical decision-making, social policy, analyses of the social history of patienthood.

★ 22250 ★ Columbia University
Clinical Research Center for Muscular Dystrophy
Department of Neurology, 4-420
College of Physicians & Surgeons
630 W 168th St.
New York, NY 10032
Phone: (212)305-1664 **Fax:** (212)305-3986
Email: sd12@columbia.edu
Salvatore DiMauro, MD, Co-Dir.
Activities/Fields: Molecular genetics and hereditary neuromuscular diseases, particularly metabolic myopathies. Conducts molecular genetic, biochemical, and morphological studies of muscle.

★ 22251 ★ Columbia University
Comprehensive Sickle Cell Center
College of Physicians & Surgeons
630 W 168th St.
New York, NY 10032
Phone: (212)305-6531 **Fax:** (212)305-8408
Email: sp23@columbia.edu
Dr. Sergio Piomelli, Dir.
Activities/Fields: Sickle cell disease.

★ 22252 ★ Columbia University
Cystic Fibrosis Referral Center for Susceptibility and Synergy Studies
650 W 168th St., BB4-427
New York, NY 10032
Phone: (212)305-9446 **Fax:** (212)305-9491
Email: synergy@columbia.edu
Website: http://cpmcnet.columbia.edu/dept/synergy/
Lisa Saiman, MD, Dir.
Activities/Fields: Multiply-resistant organisms isolated from cystic fibrosis patients. **Pub:** *Reports.*

★ 22253 ★ Columbia University
Edward S. Harkness Eye Institute
Columbia-Presbyterian Medical Center
635 W 165th St., Rm. 218
New York, NY 10032-3784
Phone: (212)305-2725 **Fax:** (212)305-5962
Email: sc434@columbia.edu
Website: http://cpmcnet.columbia.edu/dept/eye
Stanley Chang, MD, Chm.
Activities/Fields: Ophthalmology, including excimer lasers, new pulsed infrared lasers, pathologyphysiology and surgical management of orbitopathy, topical and depot corticosteroids in the treatment of post-cataract cystoid macular edema, glaucoma, endothelial growth factors for wound healing in animal models, and

effects of diabetes mellitus upon the retinal microvasculature.

★ 22254 ★ Columbia University Eye Radiation and Environmental Research Laboratory
Columbia-Presbyterian Medical Center
630 W 168th St., Rm. 212
New York, NY 10032-3784
Phone: (212)305-6748 **Fax:** (212)305-6749
Email: bvw1@columbia.edu
Website: http://cpmcnet.columbia.edu/dept/eye/rad
Dr. Basil Worgul, Dir.
Activities/Fields: Assessment of the eye lens following exposure to exogenous agents or systemically applied compounds; drugs suspected of cataractotoxicity or being tested for anticataractogenic potential, cellular mechanisms of radiation cataract, cataractogenesis, the effects of heavy particles on ocular tissue, and potential risks to the eyes of astronauts during extended manned flight in the hostile radiational environment of space. Also directing the Ukrainian/American Chernobyl ocular study. **Pub:** *Scientific papers*, bimonthly.

★ 22255 ★ Columbia University Harlem Center for Health Promotion and Disease Prevention
Harlem Hospital Center
506 Lenox Ave., NNR 524
New York, NY 10037
Phone: (212)939-4150 **Fax:** (212)939-4144
Email: nr9@columbia.edu
Dr. Alwyn Cohall, Dir.
Activities/Fields: Assessment of health status and examination of risk factors in the Harlem community, to reduce excess mortality and morbidity.

★ 22256 ★ Columbia University Herbert Irving Comprehensive Cancer Center
622 W 168th St.
New York, NY 10032
Phone: (212)305-9327 **Fax:** (212)305-7846
Email: kha4@columbia.edu
Website: http://www.ccc.columbia.edu/
Karen Antman, MD, Dir.
Activities/Fields: Molecular tumor virology, oncogenes, molecular and clinical genetics, biophysics, cell biology, basic mechanisms of carcinogenesis, molecular epidemiology, biochemistry, endocrinology, developmental biology, cancer epidemiology, sociomedical sciences, occupational health, and biostatistics and data management. **Frmly:** Columbia Presbyterian Cancer Center.

★ 22257 ★ Columbia University Institute for Cancer Genetics (ICG)
Russ Berrie Pavilion
1150 St. Nicholas Ave.
New York, NY 10032
Phone: (212)851-5273 **Fax:** (212)851-5256
Website: http://icg.cpmc.columbia.edu/
Riccardo Dalla-Favera, MD, Dir.
Activities/Fields: Molecular mechanisms and pathogenesis of cancer.

★ 22258 ★ Columbia University Institute of Human Nutrition
College of Physicians & Surgeons
630 W 168th St.
New York, NY 10032
Phone: (212)305-4808 **Fax:** (212)305-3079
Email: rjd20@columbia.edu
Website: http://cpmcnet.columbia.edu/dept/ihn/
Richard J. Deckelbaum, MD, Dir.
Activities/Fields: Atherosclerosis, lipoprotein-receptor-cell interaction; lipid emulsion metabolism; free fatty acids and cell lipid metabolism; basic retinoid and vitamin A physiology, biochemistry, and molecular biology; food and nutrition policy and law; intestinal ion transport mechanisms; enteric nervous system; human lipoprotein metabolism; lipolytic enzymes and endothelial cell biology; atherosclerosis; mineral metabolism and toxicology; carbohydrate and lipid metabolism, obesity, diabetes mellitus, food intake regulation; calcium metabolism; vascular cell biology; pathogenesis of thrombosis; regulation of intracellular cholesterol metabolism; endocytic pathways in macrophages; cholestryl ester transfer; protein structure/function and mutagenesis; regulation of gene expression; molecular nutrition; molecular mechanisms of carcinogenesis. **Frmly:** Institute of Nutrition Sciences.

★ 22259 ★ Columbia University Irving Center for Clinical Research
Columbia-Presbyterian Medical Center
622 W 168th St., PH-10
New York, NY 10032
Phone: (212)305-2071 **Fax:** (212)305-3213
Email: hng1@columbia.edu
Dr. Henry N. Ginsberg, Prog. Dir.
Activities/Fields: Multidisciplinary studies of human disease and clinical pharmacology. Areas include arrhythmia control, heart failure, atherosclerosis, nutrition, metabolism, clinical pharmacology, dermatology, endocrinology, hypertension, immunology, mineral metabolism and skeletal disease, neuromuscular disease, physiology, pulmonary disease, pulmonary physiology, reproductive research studies, neurology (including dementia, stroke, and seizure disorders), oncology, AIDS/infectious disease, geriatrics, epidemiology, and substance abuse.

★ 22260 ★ Columbia University Molecular Genetics Laboratory
1051 Riverside Dr.
New York, NY 10032
Phone: (212)543-5868 **Fax:** (212)543-6211
Email: jak8@columia.edu
Dr. James Knowles, Dir.
Activities/Fields: Human molecular genetics, including genetic and physical mapping of human chromosomes, and the mapping and characterization of human disease genes.

★ 22261 ★ Columbia University Molecular Urology Laboratory
College of Physicians and Surgeons
Department of Urology
161 Fort Washington, 11th Fl.
New York, NY 10032
Phone: (212)305-5727 **Fax:** (212)305-1564
Email: rb46@colombia.edu
Dr. Ralph Buttyan, Dir.
Activities/Fields: Molecular biology, focusing on prostate cancer, bladder disease, renal disease, erectile dysfunction, and cell death research.

★ 22262 ★ Columbia University New York Obesity Research Center
St. Luke's-Roosevelt Hospital
1090 Amsterdam Ave., 14th Fl.
New York, NY 10025
Phone: (212)523-4196 **Fax:** (212)523-3416
Email: fxp1@columbia.edu
Website: http://cpmcnet.columbia.edu/dept/obesectr/NYORC/
Dr. F. Xavier Pi-Sunyer, Dir.
Activities/Fields: Obesity, including molecular genetics, regulation of food intake, nutrient uptake and oxidation, body composition, stable isotope methodology, exercise physiology, diabetes, and insulin resistance.

★ 22263 ★ Columbia University Retina Research Laboratory
Columbia-Presbyterian Medical Center
635 W 165th St.
New York, NY 10032-3784
Phone: (212)305-5688 **Fax:** (212)305-9087
Email: pg10@columbia.edu
Peter Gouras, MD, Dir.
Activities/Fields: Retinal transplantation, biochemical markers for vitamin A metabolism in cultured human retinal epithelial cells, and gene insertion technology.

★ 22264 ★ Columbia University Stroud Center for Geriatrics and Gerontology
100 Haven Ave., Tower 3-30F
New York, NY 10032
Phone: (212)781-0600 **Fax:** (212)795-7696
Email: bjg1@columbia.edu
Dr. Barry Gurland, Dir.
Activities/Fields: Methodological, epidemiological and clinical research in geriatrics/gerontology and long-term care. Specific studies are directed toward mental disorders, psychosocial problems, and funtional impairments of the elderly. The Center has developed model projects using a comprehensive assessment instrument that has been refined for use in various settings. The Center is also active in cross-national research with a collaborating group in London. **Frmly:** Long-Term Care Gerontology Center.

★ 22265 ★ Columbia University Taub Institute for Research on Alzheimer's Disease and the Aging Brain
College of Physicians & Surgeons
630 W 168th St., P&S Box 16
New York, NY 10032
Phone: (212)305-1818 **Fax:** (212)342-2849
Email: taubinstitute@columbia.edu
Website: http://www.alzheimercenter.org
Michael L. Shelanski, MD, Co-Dir.
Activities/Fields: Alzheimer's disease and elderly care. Serves as a resource for tissue, cells, and DNA from Alzheimer's disease and control patients. Areas of research include epidemiology, cell biology, genetics, and aging. **Pub:** *ADRC Newsletter*, semiannually. **Frmly:** Alzheimer's Disease Research Center.

★ 22266 ★ Comprehensive Sickle Cell Center (Cincinnati, OH)
Children's Hospital Medical Center
3333 Burnet Ave.
Cincinnati, OH 45229
Phone: (513)636-4541 **Free:** 800-344-2462
Fax: (513)636-5562
Email: clint.joiner@CHMCC.org
Dr. Clinton Joiner, Dir.
Activities/Fields: Sickle cell disease, including molecular, cellular, tissue, and organ studies. Conducts clinical trials and seeks to translate research to improved health care.

★ 22267 ★ Concordia University (Montreal, QC, Canada) Centre for Research in Human Development (CRHD)
7141 Sherbrooke St W
Montreal, QC, Canada H4B 1R6
Phone: (514)848-2240 **Fax:** (514)848-2815
Email: lserbin@vax2.concordia.ca
Website: http://www-psychology.concordia.ca/department/graduate/res-cen.html
Dr. Lisa Serbin, Dir.
Activities/Fields: Psychological development across the human life-span, focusing on normal social and cognitive development; atypical developmental patterns; and the study of competence in elderly populations. Specific fields of study include developmental, clinical, cognitive and social psychology; education; applied statistics; medicine; pediatrics; and gerontology. **Pub:** *Research Bulletins*, monthly.

★ 22268 ★ Concordia University (Montreal, QC, Canada)
Centre for Studies in Behavioral Neurobiology
Department of Psychology
1455 de Maisonneuve Blvd. W
Montreal, QC, Canada H3G 1M8
Phone: (514)848-2200 **Fax:** (514)848-2817
Email: info@csbn.concordia.ca
Website: http://csbn.concordia.ca/
Peter Shizgal, PhD, Dir.
Activities/Fields: Research addresses the mechanisms that marshall behavior to meet biological needs. Principal topics of study include the neural, hormonal, and psychological processes that maintain homeostasis and ensure successful reproduction as well as the disruption of these processes that leads to drug dependence, obesity, and sexual dysfunction. Research considers three principal themes: reward, motivation, and plasticity. All three combine behavioral measurement methods with techniques in molecular, cellular, and systems neuroscience.

★ 22269 ★ Concordia University (Montreal, QC, Canada)
Concordia Vision Laboratory
Drummond Science Bldg., Rm. 413
Department of Psychology
7141 Sherbrooke St. W
Montreal, QC, Canada H4B 1R6
Phone: (514)848-2212 **Fax:** (514)848-4545
Email: vgrunau@vax2.concordia.ca
Website: http://psychology.concordia.ca/department/CVLab/CVLab.html
Michael von Grünau, Contact
Activities/Fields: Visual texture encoding and segmentation, motion detection, segregation and integration, early encoding of form, simple- and contingent-aftereffects, face perception symmetry, and vection.

★ 22270 ★ Connecticut Eye Bank and Visual Research Foundation, Inc.
100 Grand St.
New Britain, CT 06052
Phone: (860)224-5550 **Free:** 800-355-5520
Fax: (860)224-5720
Email: mrineh@aol.com
Website: http://www.cteyebank.org
Michael J. Rinehart, Pres. /CEO
Activities/Fields: Production of eye material for use in corneal transplantation surgery, surgical study, and for research on blindness. Projects include the Vision Immunology Program, a study of how the eye defends against disease.

★ 22271 ★ Connecticut Hospital Association
110 Barnes Rd.
Wallingford, CT 06492-0090
Phone: (203)265-7611 **Fax:** (203)284-9318
Email: jackson@chime.org
Website: http://www.chime.org
Jennifer Jackson, Pres.
Activities/Fields: Hospital industry, including hospital administration, manpower development and training, quality of care, shared services and facilities, financial reimbursement, ancillary service utilization, and mental health planning.

★ 22272 ★ Consortial Center for Chiropractic Research
741 Brady St.
Davenport, IA 52803
Phone: (319)884-5162 **Fax:** (319)884-5227
Email: info@c3r.org
Website: http://www.c3r.org
William C. Meeker, VP,Res.
Activities/Fields: Potential effectiveness and validity of chiropractic health care.

★ 22273 ★ Contraceptive Research and Development Program (CONRAD)
1611 N Kent St., Ste. 806
Arlington, VA 22209
Phone: (703)524-4744 **Fax:** (703)524-4770
Email: info@conrad.org
Website: http://www.conrad.org
Henry L. Gabelnick, PhD, Dir.
Activities/Fields: Improvement of contraception methods and reproductive health, especially for use in developing countries; further development of contraceptive choices for women and men and to help prevent the transmission of HIV/AIDS and other sexually transmitted diseases (STDs).

★ 22274 ★ Cooper Institute for Aerobics Research
12330 Preston Rd.
Dallas, TX 75230
Phone: (972)341-3200 **Free:** 800-635-7050
Fax: (972)341-3227
Email: courses@cooperinst.org
Website: http://www.cooperinst.org
Dr. Steven N. Blair, Pres. /CEO
Activities/Fields: Cardiovascular disease, stress management, women's health, exercise physiology, health promotion, nutrition, youth fitness, hypertension, aging, and epidemiology. Using data from the affiliated Cooper Clinic, the Institute conducts the Aerobics Center Longitudinal Study, which monitors 25,000 subjects over their lifetime to study the effects of exercise and health habits on death and disability rates from chronic diseases.

★ 22275 ★ Coriell Institute for Medical Research
403 Haddon Ave.
Camden, NJ 08103
Phone: (856)757-4820 **Fax:** (856)964-0254
Email: dabeck@umdnj.edu
Website: http://cimr.umdnj.edu
David P. Beck, PhD, Pres.
Activities/Fields: Cell and molecular biology, microbiology, genetics, aging, cancer and cancer immunology, tumor virology, antibodies, genetic disorders, vascular disorders, infectious diseases and virus/chromosome relationships, environmental mutagenesis, and genetic probes. Studies utilization of cells grown in tissue culture for isolation and characterization of tumor cell antigens, viruses, genetic abnormalities, tumor viruses, and chromosomes. **Pub:** *Biennial Report.* • *Discover.* • *Newsletter*, quarterly.

★ 22276 ★ Cornell University
Brain Trauma Foundation
523 E 72nd St., 8th Fl.
New York, NY 10021
Phone: (212)772-0608 **Fax:** (212)772-0357
Email: info@braintrauma.org
Website: http://www.braintrauma.org/
Pamela Drexel, Exec. Dir.
Activities/Fields: Investigates the pathophysiology of traumatic brain injury, uses an in vitro human glial cell culture model of injury to study brain derived inflammatory mediators, and performs ventricular cerebrospinal fluid analysis in human patients. Established physiological model for post traumatic raised intracranial preserve analysis. **Frmly:** Aitken Neuroscience Center.

★ 22277 ★ Cornell University
Cornell Gerontology Research Institute (CGRI)
MVR Hall
Ithaca, NY 14853
Phone: (607)255-8086 **Fax:** (607)254-2903
Email: kap6@cornell.edu
Website: http://www.blcc.cornell.edu/cagri/
Karl Pillemer, Dir.
Activities/Fields: Social integration of older Americans. **Pub:** *CAGRI Newsletter.*

★ 22278 ★ Cornell University
Cornell Theory Center Biomedical Resource
Frank H.T. Rhodes Hall
Ithaca, NY 14853-3801
Phone: (607)254-8686 **Fax:** (607)254-8888
Website: http://www.tc.cornell.edu/reports/NIH/resource
Dr. Thomas F. Coleman, Prin. Investigator
Activities/Fields: Theoretical developments, the design of computational algorithms, and applications to biomedical problems, particularly protein structure determination and simulations of protein dynamics.

★ 22279 ★ Cornell University
Division of Hypertension
New York Hospital-Cornell Medical Center
520 E 70th St.
New York, NY 10021
Phone: (212)746-2210 **Fax:** (212)746-8277
Email: paugust@med.cornell.edu
Phyllis August, MD, Ch.
Activities/Fields: Research into causation, diagnosis, and treatment of hypertension and related disorders of the heart, kidneys, and adrenal glands. Research also includes pathogenesis and treatment of heart attacks, congestive heart failure, renal failure, and stroke. **Frmly:** Hypertension and Cardiovascular Center.

★ 22280 ★ Cornell University
General Clinical Research Center—Children
525 E 68th St., Rm. P-629
New York, NY 10021-4885
Phone: (212)746-3450
Dr. Patricia J. Grardiea, Interim Prog. Dir.
Activities/Fields: Major areas of investigation include cardiology, endocrinology, genetic diseases, hematology, infectious diseases, metabolism, and neurology.

★ 22281 ★ Cornell University
Health Benefits Research Unit
575 Lexington Ave., 4th Fl.
New York, NY 10022
Phone: (212)572-0794 **Fax:** (212)572-0789
Dr. Eugene G. McCarthy, Dir.
Activities/Fields: Health benefits, including a study on whether physicians offering a second opinion concurred with the original recommendation for elective surgery and a program to identify and direct patients to ambulatory surgical facilities. Arranges appointments between patients and approximately 28,000 board certified surgeons throughout the U.S.

★ 22282 ★ Cornell University
Laboratory for Drug Delivery and Tissue Engineering
120 Olin Hall
School of Chemical Engineering
Ithaca, NY 14850
Phone: (607)255-2657 **Fax:** (607)255-1136
Email: saltzman@cheme.cornell.edu
Website: http://www.cheme.cornell.edu/~saltzman/index.html
Prof. W. Mark Saltzman, Dir.
Activities/Fields: Economical, transportable, and accessible new methods for disease prevention through the delivery of drugs, proteins, and genes and tissue engineering. **Pub:** *Papers.*

★ 22283 ★ Cornell University
Laboratory of Pediatric Critical Care
525 68th St., Rm. M508
New York, NY 10021
Phone: (212)746-3056 **Fax:** (212)746-8332
Email: hmushay@med.cornell.edu
Dr. H. Michael Ushay, Dir.
Activities/Fields: Adrenergic receptor pharmacology, including receptor-related events at the cellular and

molecular levels, and molecular biology of acute lung injury.

★ 22284 ★ Cornell University Pregnancy and Newborn Research Laboratory
T9-020 Veterinary Research Tower
Ithaca, NY 14853
Phone: (607)253-3082 **Fax:** (607)253-3455
Email: pwn1@cornell.edu
Peter W. Nathanielsz, Dir.
Activities/Fields: Development of the animal fetus and newborn for application in human development. **Pub:** *Five-year report.*

★ 22285 ★ Cornell University Weill Medical College General Clinical Research Center
1300 York Ave., Rm. Baker 2006
New York, NY 10021
Phone: (212)746-4745 **Fax:** (212)746-8922
Email: jimperat@mail.med.cornell.edu
Dr. Julianne Imperato-McGinley, Prog. Dir.
Activities/Fields: Cancer prevention, cardiovascular diseases, dermatology, diabetes and metabolism, digestive diseases, endocrinology, gene therapy, hematology, immunology and infectious diseases, neurology and neuroscience, oncology, pharmacology, and psychiatry.

★ 22286 ★ Cornell University Winifred Masterson Burke Medical Research Institute, Inc. Dementia Research Service
785 Mamaroneck Ave.
White Plains, NY 10605
Phone: (914)597-2351 **Fax:** (914)597-2757
Email: jpblass@mail.med.cornell.edu
Dr. John P. Blass, Dir.
Activities/Fields: Clinical and basic studies in genetic, metabolic and nutritional aspects of degenerative diseases of the nervous system, especially Alzheimer's disease. Also studies of the role of reactive oxygen species.

★ 22287 ★ Council for Affordable Health Insurance (CAHI)
112 S West St., Ste. 400
Alexandria, VA 22314
Phone: (703)836-6200 **Fax:** (703)836-6550
Email: mail@cahi.org
Website: http://www.cahi.org
Dr. Merrill Matthews, Jr., Dir.
Activities/Fields: Free market solutions to America's health care challenges. **Pub:** *Reports.*

★ 22288 ★ Craig Center for Spinal Cord Injury Research (CRES)
Research Department
Craig Hospital
3425 S Clarkson St.
Englewood, CO 80110
Phone: (303)789-8204 **Fax:** (303)789-8441
Email: gale@craighospital.org
Gale Whiteneck, PhD, Dir.
Activities/Fields: Spinal cord injuries.

★ 22289 ★ Creighton University Cardiac Center
3006 Webster St.
Omaha, NE 68131
Phone: (402)280-4566 **Fax:** (402)280-4938
Email: smm@cardiac.creighton.edu
Dr. Mohiuddin, Med. Dir.
Activities/Fields: Cardiology, including drug research, medical care, valvular diseases, invasive and noninvasive treatment techniques, electrocardiogram tests, pacemakers, implants, and ventricular assist devices.

★ 22290 ★ Creighton University Center for Allergy, Asthma, and Immunology
2500 California Plz.
Omaha, NE 68178
Phone: (402)280-2940 **Fax:** (402)280-1843
Email: cclase@creighton.edu
Website: http://medicine.creighton.edu/allergy/homepage.html
Robert G. Townley, MD, Ch.
Activities/Fields: Multidisciplinary research in asthma, allergic rhinitis, allergic diseases, clinical and basic immunology, clinical and basic pharmacology and physiology, airway reactivity in patients with asthma, and allergies. Laboratory research consists of studies of human lung, eosinophils, mast cells, lymphocytes, and platelets to correlate adrenergic and cholinergic receptors and receptor mechanisms; and role of pro-inflamatory cytokines, leukotrienes and platelet activating factor on airway reactivity and in asthma and animal models of asthma. Focuses on mechanisms of immediate hypersensitivity and the late allergic reaction. **Pub:** *Allergy Principles & Practice*, quadrennially.

★ 22291 ★ Cross Cancer Institute (CCI) Alberta Breast Cancer Program
11560 University Ave.
Edmonton, AB, Canada T6G 1Z2
Phone: (780)432-8320 **Fax:** (780)432-8425
Email: carolcas@cancerboard.ab.ca
Website: http://www.albertabreast.com/cci/
Dr. Carol E. Cass, Assoc. Dir.
Activities/Fields: Molecular oncology, medical physics and biophysics, radiation and solid tumor biology, tumor immunobiology, and experimental radiotherapy and chemotherapy.

★ 22292 ★ Cross Cultural Health Care Program (CCHCP)
270 S Hanford St., Ste. 100
Seattle, WA 98134
Phone: (206)860-0329 **Fax:** (206)860-0334
Website: http://www.xculture.org/
Activities/Fields: Cultural competency in health and human services, focusing on organizational practices. Research focuses on services provided to non-mainstream, limited English-speaking populations in the Seattle area.

★ 22293 ★ CTRC Research Foundation
14960 Omicron Dr.
San Antonio, TX 78245-3217
Phone: (210)677-3800 **Fax:** (210)677-0058
Email: jcole@saci.org
Website: http://www.ctrc.saci.org
John F. Cole, PhD, COO
Activities/Fields: Prevention and cure of cancer in adults, emphasizing the development of new anticancer agents, and includes xenograft models, angiogenic models, Alzet pump infusion model, molecular targets/biomarker analysis, proteomic analysis, immunohistochemistry, ELISA and other enzyme assays, cell cycle distribution in relation to drug-cell interactions, drug resistance and programmed cell death. **Pub:** *Investigational New Drugs*, quarterly. **Frmly:** Cancer Therapy and Research Center.

★ 22294 ★ CTRC Research Foundation Institute for Drug Development
14960 Omicron Dr.
San Antonio, TX 78245-3217
Phone: (210)677-3800 **Fax:** (210)677-0058
Email: jcole@idd.org
Website: http://www.idd.org
John F. Cole, PhD, COO
Activities/Fields: Anticancer drug discovery and development, including xenograft models, angiogenic models, Alzet pump infusion model, molecular targets/biomarker analysis, proteomic analysis, immunohistochemistry, ELISA and other enzyme assays, cell cycle distribution in relation to drug-cell interactions, drug resistance and programmed cell death. Clinical Investigations Section researches new drugs as they are first introduced into humans, and examines the pharmacokinetic profile of new drugs in a GLP setting. tubulin and topoisomerase I and II; measurement of telomerase activity; growth inhibitory activity of cancer cells from biopsy tissue; and cell cycle distribution in relation to drug-cell interactions, drug resistance, and programmed cell death. Clinical Investigations Section researches new drugs as they are first introduced into humans, and examines the pharmacokinetic profile of new drugs.

★ 22295 ★ Cystic Fibrosis Center (Portland, OR)
Pediatric Pulmonary Division, CDRCP
707 SW Gaines Rd.
Portland, OR 97201
Phone: (503)494-8023 **Fax:** (503)494-8898
Email: wallm@ohsu.edu
Dr. Michael Wall, Dir.
Activities/Fields: Cystic fibrosis, including laboratory and clinical studies of molecular abnormalities in cystic fibrosis and lyses of pulmonary mucus.

★ 22296 ★ Cystic Fibrosis Foundation
6931 Arlington Rd., Ste. 200
Bethesda, MD 20814
Phone: (301)951-4422 **Free:** 800-344-4823
Fax: (301)951-6378
Email: info@cff.org
Website: http://www.cff.org
Robert Beall, PhD, Pres. /CEO
Activities/Fields: Causes and treatment of cystic fibrosis. The Research Development Program involves a network of research centers supported by the Foundation; also supports many care centers thoughout the United States. **Pub:** *Annual Report.* • *Commitment*, quarterly.

★ 22297 ★ Dalhousie University Atlantic Health Promotion Research Centre (AHPRC)
6090 University Ave.
Halifax, NS, Canada B3H 3J5
Phone: (902)494-2240 **Fax:** (902)494-3594
Email: ahprc@dal.ca
Website: http://www.medicine.dal.ca/ahprc
Renee F. Lyons, Dir.
Activities/Fields: Physical, mental, social, and spiritual health of individuals and communities by increasing control over health issues by combining personal choice and social responsibility, and contributes to the health and well being of Atlantic Canadians, health policy, rural health, food security, and quality of life. **Pub:** *General Guidelines for Health Promotion Research Proposals.* • *Health Promotion Atlantic Newsletter*, 3/year. • *What a Difference 8 Years Can Make: Accomplishments of the Atlantic Health Promotion Research Centre.*

★ 22298 ★ Dalhousie University Atlantic Health and Wellness Institute (AHWI)
West End Mall, Ste. 14
6960 Mumford Rd.
Halifax, NS, Canada B3L 4P1
Phone: (902)482-2494 **Fax:** (902)482-2501
Email: health@ahwi.org
Website: http://www.ahwi.org
Dr. Lydia Makrides, Dir.
Activities/Fields: The roles of lifestyle, nutritional, cultural, emotional and economic factors in the development and progression of coronary heart disease. While the center has research projects touching on all these areas, it is particularly interested in the role of exercise. **Pub:** *Newsletters.*

★ 22299 ★ Dalhousie University Atlantic Research Centre
5849 University Ave., Rm. C-302
Halifax, NS, Canada B3H 4H7
Phone: (902)494-7066 **Fax:** (902)494-1394
Email: david.byers@dal.ca
Website: http://www.medicine.dal.ca/arc/
Dr. David M. Byers, Dir.
Activities/Fields: Biochemistry, molecular and cell biology of lipids and membranes, and relationship to human disease processes.

★ 22300 ★ Dalhousie University Ear and Auditory Research Laboratory
Sir Charles Tupper Bldg., Rm. 13L
Department of Anatomy & Neurobiology Surgery
5859 University Ave.
Halifax, NS, Canada B3H 4H7
Phone: (902)494-6375 **Fax:** (902)494-1212
Website: http://www.medicine.dal.ca/ear-lab/introduction.htm
Dr. Manohar Bance, Dir.
Activities/Fields: Middle ear microanatomy, pathophysiology, micromechanics, surgical reconstruction; finite element modeling; middle ear hearing mechanics; innovative hearing technologies; and auditory recordings.

★ 22301 ★ Dalhousie University Population Health Research Unit (PHRU)
Department of Community Health & Epidemiology
Faculty of Medicine
5849 University Ave.
Halifax, NS, Canada B3H 4H7
Phone: (902)494-3860 **Fax:** (902)494-1597
Email: george.kephart@dal.ca
Website: http://www.medicine.dal.ca/che/phru/
George Kephart, Dir.
Activities/Fields: Health and social sciences, particularly population health, health services utilization and their interrelationships.

★ 22302 ★ Dana-Farber Cancer Institute
44 Binney St.
Boston, MA 02115
Phone: (617)632-4266 **Fax:** (617)632-2161
Email: edward_benz@dfci.harvard.edu
Website: http://www.dana-farber.net
Dr. Edward J. Benz, Jr., Pres.
Activities/Fields: Medical oncology, cancer pharmacology, pediatric oncology, cell growth and regulation, cancer genetics, human retrovirology, tumor immunology and virology, immunogenetics, lymphocyte biology, biostatistics and epidemiology, molecular carcinogenesis, biochemical pharmacology, neoplastic disease mechanisms, structural molecular biology, membrane immunochemistry, cancer control, tumor virus genetics, immunopathology, gene regulation, eukaryotic transcription, molecular biology, molecular genetics, molecular immunology, molecular immunobiology, medicine, gynecologic oncology, oncodiagnostic radiology and nuclear medicine, radiotherapy, and surgical oncology. **Pub:** *Scientific Report*, biennially. **Frmly:** Children's Cancer Research Foundation; Sidney Farber Cancer Institute.

★ 22303 ★ Dana-Farber Cancer Institute Department of Biostatistical Science
44 Binney St.
Boston, MA 02115
Phone: (617)632-3012 **Fax:** (617)632-2444
Email: biostatistics@jimmy.harvard.edu
Website: http://biowww.dfci.harvard.edu/
Dr. David P. Harrington, Ch.
Activities/Fields: Organized into the laboratories of biostatistics and computing, which carry on a multifaceted program combining independent research, collaboration, and consulting in quantitative methods as they apply to cancer research. Project areas include methodological research in statistics, mathematical models in chronic disease epidemiology, bioinformatics, statistical computing, and applied probability and database research. Conducts multi-institutional cancer clinical trials.

★ 22304 ★ Dana-Farber Cancer Institute Department of Cancer Immunology and AIDS
44 Binney St.
Boston, MA 02115
Phone: (617)632-3348 **Fax:** (617)632-4630
Email: harvey_cantor@dfci.harvard.edu
Harvey Cantor, Ch.
Activities/Fields: T-cell development and function.

★ 22305 ★ Dartmouth College Biomedical NMR Research Center
Department of Radiology, HB 7786
Dartmouth Medical School
Hanover, NH 03755
Phone: (603)650-1677 **Fax:** (603)650-1717
Email: Jeffrey.F.Dunn@dartmouth.edu
Website: http://www.dartmouth.edu/www/dms/nmrbrl/body.htm
Dr. Jeff Dunn, Dir.
Activities/Fields: Metabolic disorders, especially those disorders linked to hypoxia and oxygen utilization.

★ 22306 ★ Dartmouth College Center for Evaluative Clinical Sciences
Dartmouth Medical Sch.
7251 Strasenburgh
Hanover, NH 03755-3863
Phone: (603)650-6552 **Fax:** (603)650-6525
Email: cecsweb@dartmouth.edu
Website: http://www.dartmouth.edu/dms/cecs/
John E. Wennberg, MD, Dir.
Activities/Fields: Evaluative clinical science and health care delivery, including medical care epidemiology, health policy, health behavior, efficacy of medical procedures, quality of medical and surgical care, distribution of health care resources, medical interventions and consequences for patients, care at the end of life, distribution of health care resources across hospital market areas, geriatric health, and sociology of medical organizations.

★ 22307 ★ Dartmouth College Electron Paramagnetic Resonance Center for the Study of Viable Systems
Department of Radiology
Medical School
7785 Vail, Rm. 702
Hanover, NH 03755
Phone: (603)650-1955 **Fax:** (603)650-1717
Email: harold.swartz@dartmouth.edu
Website: http://www.dartmouth.edu/~eprctr/
Harold M. Swartz, MD, Prin. Investigator
Activities/Fields: Development and application of techniques that make it feasible to carry out well-resolved EPR spectroscopy in fully functional living systems, especially living animals (with or without anesthesia) but also viable cells.

★ 22308 ★ Dartmouth College Sleep Disorders Center
Dartmouth Hitchcock Medical Center
1 Medical Center Dr.
Lebanon, NH 03756
Phone: (603)650-7534 **Fax:** (603)650-7820
Email: michael.j.sateia@dartmouth.edu
Dr. Michael Sateia, Dir.
Activities/Fields: Sleep disorders, sleep apnea due to obesity, hypersomnolence, parasomnias, and insomnia.

★ 22309 ★ Deaconess Billings Clinic Research Division
1045 N 30th St.
Billings, MT 59101
Phone: (406)255-8470 **Free:** 800-996-2663
Fax: (406)255-8479
Email: research@billingsclinic.org
Website: http://www.billingsclinic.com/frontpage/default.htm
Howard R. Knapp, MD, Exec. Dir.
Activities/Fields: Regulation of bone remodeling, arthritis, hormone replacement therapy, infectious diseases in man, hepatitis-C, diabetes, pneumonia, hypertension, and hyperlipidemia.

★ 22310 ★ Deafness Research Foundation
1050 17th St. NW, Ste. 701
Washington, DC 20036
Phone: (202)289-5850 **Free:** 800-829-5934
Fax: (202)293-1805
Email: drf@drf.org
Website: http://www.drf.org
Susan M. Greco, Exec. Dir.
Activities/Fields: Causes and treatment of deafness and other serious ear disorders, including studies of implants, deafness in the young and the elderly, middle ear infections, Meniere's disease, tinnitus (ringing in the ears), excessive noise, hair cell regeneration, genetics, and otoacoustic emissions. **Pub:** *Hearing Health Magazine*, quarterly.

★ 22311 ★ Deep South Center for Occupational Health and Safety
School of Public Health
University of Alabama at Birmingham
1530 3rd Ave. S
Birmingham, AL 35294-0022
Phone: (205)934-7178 **Fax:** (205)975-7179
Email: dsc@uab.edu
Website: http://www.uab.edu/dsc
R. Kent Oestenstad, PhD, Dir.
Activities/Fields: Health and safety of workers.

★ 22312 ★ Detroit Institute of Ophthalmology
15415 E Jefferson Ave.
Grosse Pointe Park, MI 48230-1328
Phone: (313)824-4710 **Fax:** (313)822-4233
Website: http://www.brophy.com/dio
Dr. Philip C. Hessburg, Pres.
Activities/Fields: Ophthalmology, low vision rehabilitation, and studies related to the relationship between vision and the operation of motorized vehicles.

★ 22313 ★ Diabetes Education and Research Center
Franklin Medical Bldg.
829 Spruce St., Ste. 302
Philadelphia, PA 19107
Phone: (215)829-3426 **Fax:** (215)829-5807
Email: webmaster@diabeteseducationandresearchcenter.org
Website: http://www.diabeteseducationandresearchcenter.org
Dr. Theodore G. Duncan, Dir.
Activities/Fields: Diabetes, including the effects of oral diabetic medication, hypertension as an indicator of diabetes, and drug trials.

★ 22314 ★ Disaster Relief and Emergency Medical Services Project (DREAMS)
3139 TAMU
459 Blocker Bldg.
College Station, TX 77843-3139
Phone: (979)458-1135 **Fax:** (979)862-3983
Email: joan@academy.tamu.edu
Website: http://academy.tamu.edu/dreams/
Joan F. Tatge, Contact
Activities/Fields: Enhancement of emergency medical care, particularly in remote areas where medical attention is not readily available through the use of

emerging medical, scientific and telecommunications technologies.

★ 22315 ★ Doheny Eye Institute
1450 San Pablo St.
Los Angeles, CA 90033
Phone: (323)442-7100 **Fax:** (323)442-6688
Email: sryan@hsc.usc.edu
Website: http://www.usc.edu/hsc/doheny
Stephen J. Ryan, MD, Pres.
Activities/Fields: Eyebank, medical clinic group, tonography, electrophysiology, laser surgery center, contact lenses and ocular research facilities for experimental pathology, tissue culture, molecular biology, specialized microscopy, and biostatistics. **Pub:** *Annual Report.* • *Postscript Alumni Newsletter*, biennially. • *Update Newsletter*, quarterly.

★ 22316 ★ Donald Guthrie Foundation for Education and Research
1 Guthrie Sq.
Sayre, PA 18840
Phone: (570)882-4624 **Free:** 888-448-8474
Fax: (570)882-4643
Email: aronstam@ghs.guthrie.org
Website: http://www.guthrie.org/AboutGuthrie/Research/
Dr. Robert Aronstam, Sci. Dir.
Activities/Fields: Cell communication and signal transduction and clinical research in immunology, virology, cancer biology, lung cancer, and neuroscience. **Pub:** *Guthrie Medical Journal*, quarterly.

★ 22317 ★ Douglas Hospital Research Centre
6875 La Salle Blvd.
Verdun, QC, Canada H4H 1R3
Phone: (514)761-6131 **Fax:** (514)762-3033
Email: quirem@douglas.mcgill.ca
Website: http://www.mcgill.ca/douglas
Dr. Rémi Quirion, Sci. Dir.
Activities/Fields: Mental health, including aging, psychoneuroendocrinology, cognitive measurements, and behavior; Alzheimer's disease, incorporating animal models, neurochemistry, and trials of nootropic drugs; depression and its biological markers, with clinical trials of new antidepressants; schizophrenia and alcoholism, including neurochemical studies and new treatment methods; violence neurobiological studies and new treatment methods; social psychiatry and epidemiology; and eating disorders. **Pub:** *Annual report.*

★ 22318 ★ Drexel University Center for Neurosciences Research
College of Medicine
Allegheny General Hospital, South Tower, 8th Fl.
320 E North Ave.
Pittsburgh, PA 15212
Phone: (412)359-3235 **Fax:** (412)359-4499
Email: rubin@wpahs.org
Robert T. Rubin, MD, Dir.
Activities/Fields: Psychobiology of depression, aging. **Frmly:** Neurosciences Research Center.

★ 22319 ★ Dry Eye and Tear Research Center
Department of Ophthalmology
Regions Hospital
640 Jackson St.
Saint Paul, MN 55101
Phone: (651)221-8745 **Fax:** (651)292-4040
Email: j.d.nelson@healthpartners.com
J. Daniel Nelson, MD, Dir.
Activities/Fields: Basic and clinical studies of dry eye and tearing disorders, focusing on ocular surface diseases, the effects of chemicals and nutrients on corneal epithelium, and the role of hormones in the development of dry eye states.

★ 22320 ★ Duke University Anxiety and Traumatic Stress Program
Medical Center, Box 3812
Durham, NC 27710
Phone: (919)684-2880 **Fax:** (919)684-8866
Email: tolme@duke.edu
Dr. Jonathan Davidson, Prog. Dir.
Activities/Fields: Activities focus on diagnosis and treatment of anxiety disorders, including panic disorder, agoraphobia, social phobias, Post-Traumatic Stress Disorder (PTSD), obsessive-compulsive disorder (OCD), and generalized anxiety, as well as complementary and alteractive medicine.

★ 22321 ★ Duke University Behavioral Medicine Research Center
Duke Medical Center
PO Box 3926
Durham, NC 27710
Phone: (919)684-3863 **Fax:** (919)681-8960
Email: redfordw@acpub.duke.edu
Dr. Redford Williams, Dir.
Activities/Fields: Behavior, including emotional stress and personality factors as they affect physical diseases with emphasis on coronary disease and cancer. Uses epidemiological and experimental approaches.

★ 22322 ★ Duke University Center for Cellular and Biosurface Engineering (CBE)
Box 90281
Durham, NC 27708
Phone: (919)660-5452 **Fax:** (919)684-4488
Email: dkatz@acpub.duke.edu
Website: http://bme-www.mc.duke.edu/Research/Cellsurf/
David F. Katz, PhD, Dir.
Activities/Fields: Biotechnology, especially protein engineering, cellular engineering, and biosurface engineering.

★ 22323 ★ Duke University Center for Emerging Cardiovascular Technologies (CECT)
B237 Levine Science Research Center
PO Box 90295
Durham, NC 27708-0295
Phone: (919)660-5137 **Fax:** (919)684-8886
Email: mhr@acpub.duke.edu
Website: http://cect.egr.duke.edu
Olaf T. von Ramm, PhD, Dir.
Activities/Fields: Cardiovascular devices and technologies, including biosensors, implantable defibrillators, real-time 3-D ultrasound imaging equipment, custom integrated electronics, and systems design and simulation. Facilitates technology transfer and promotes interaction between engineering students and industrial investigators.

★ 22324 ★ Duke University Center for Human Genetics (CHG)
DUMC Box 3445
Durham, NC 27710
Phone: (919)684-2063 **Free:** 800-283-4316
Fax: (919)684-0900
Email: center@chg.mc.duke.edu
Website: http://wwwchg.duhs.duke.edu
Margaret A. Pericak-Vance, PhD, Dir.
Activities/Fields: Genetic and epidemiologic basis of human disease, both rare and common.

★ 22325 ★ Duke University Center for Hyperbaric Medicine and Environmental Physiology
Duke Medical Center
PO Box 3823
Durham, NC 27710
Phone: (919)684-6726 **Fax:** (919)684-6002
Website: http://hyperbaric.mc.duke.edu
Dr. Peter B. Bennet, Sr., Dir.
Activities/Fields: Hypobaric and hyperbaric medicine and physiology, including studies of how increased hydrostatic pressure affects cells, tissues, organs, and intact organisms; studies of morphological and metabolic effects of oxygen pressures; clinical investigations of use of hyperbaric oxygen therapy; study of effects of pressure on respiratory and cardiovascular systems and thermal homeostasis; and investigations of causes, mechanisms, and prevention of effects of decompression sickness.

★ 22326 ★ Duke University Center for In Vivo Microscopy
Department of Radiology
CB 3302
Durham, NC 27710
Phone: (919)684-7755 **Fax:** (919)684-7158
Email: gaj@orion.mc.duke.edu
Website: http://wwwcivm.mc.duke.edu
G. Allan Johnson, PhD, Dir.
Activities/Fields: Magnetic resonance microscopy, imaging of disease models, drug discovery and validation, pulmonary imaging, toxicology testing and evaluation in live animals, and in vivo histology and microscopy.

★ 22327 ★ Duke University Center for the Study of Aging and Human Development
Medical Center
PO Box 3003
Durham, NC 27710
Phone: (919)660-7500 **Fax:** (919)684-8569
Email: ray00004@mc.duke.edu
Website: http://www.geri.duke.edu
Harvey Jay Cohen, MD, Dir.
Activities/Fields: Human and animal physiology, immunology, neuroendocrinology, pharmacology, carcinogenesis, enzyme biochemistry, free radical effects, membrane and receptor function, bone metabolism and osteoporosis, central nervous system structure and function, Alzheimer's disease, dementia, cognitive processes, psychometrics, human personality and behavior, family structure and intergenerational relationships, social factors and illness, epidemiology of aging and chronic illness, stress and coping, cell growth and differentiation, signal transduction, and the demographics and economics of aging populations. The Aging Center coordinates research, training, and clinical services in aging for the University. The Division of Geriatrics focuses research on the basic and clinical aspects of aging, emphasizing neoplasia, bone and musculoskeletal disorders and rehabilitation involved, immunology, cardiovascular diseases, cerebrovascular disease/dementia, enzymatic and cellular basis for aging, and health services delivery for the aged. **Pub:** *Center Report*, quarterly. • *Long Term Care Advances.*

★ 22328 ★ Duke University Center for the Study of Medical Ethics and Humanities
108 Seeley G. Mudd Bldg., DUMC 3040
Durham, NC 27710
Phone: (919)668-9000 **Fax:** (919)668-1789
Email: csmeh@mc.duke.edu
Website: http://csmeh.mc.duke.edu/home.html
Jeremy Sugarman, MD, Dir.
Activities/Fields: Medical ethics and the humanities.

★ 22329 ★ Duke University Children's Environmental Health Initiative (CEHI)
Box 90328
Levine Sciences Research Bldg., Rm. A132
Nicholas School of the Environment & Earth Sciences
Durham, NC 27708-0328
Phone: (919)613-8137 **Free:** (866)264-7891
Fax: (919)684-8741

Email: cehi@env.duke.edu
Website: http://www.env.duke.edu/cehi/about/about.htm
Marie Lynn Miranda, PhD, Dir.
Activities/Fields: Environmental threats facing children today.

★ 22330 ★ Duke University
Comprehensive Sickle Cell Center
Medical Center
Box 3939
Durham, NC 27710
Phone: (919)684-6464 **Fax:** (919)681-6174
Email: telen002@mc.duke.edu
Marilyn J. Telen, MD, Dir.
Activities/Fields: Sickle cell disease, including molecular, cellular, tissue, and organ studies. Conducts clinical trials. Seeks to translate basic and clinical research to improved health care at the community level.

★ 22331 ★ Duke University
Division of Pediatric Hematology Oncology
PO Box 2916
Durham, NC 27710
Phone: (919)684-3401 **Fax:** (919)681-7950
Email: rosof001@mc.duke.edu
Dr. Philip Rosoff, Div. Ch.
Activities/Fields: Clinical trials of new cancer therapies for children. Special interests include neuro-oncology and bone marrow transplantation. **Frmly:** Pediatric Oncology Consortium.

★ 22332 ★ Duke University
Duke Center for the Advanced Study of Epilepsy
401 Bryan Res. Bldg.
Res. Dr.
Box 3676
Durham, NC 27710
Phone: (919)684-4241 **Fax:** (919)684-8219
Dr. James O. McNamara, Dir.
Activities/Fields: Clinical and experimental approaches to limbic epilepsy. Current projects include studies of early gene expression in the kindling model of epilepsy, mechanisms of development of Ammon's horn sclerosis, microphysiology of limbic seizures, and role of excitatory amino acids and their receptors in limbic epilepsy.

★ 22333 ★ Duke University
Duke Center for Cerebrovascular Disease
Box 3651
Duke University Medical Center
Durham, NC 27710
Phone: (919)684-3801
Email: golds004@mc.duke.edu
Website: http://stroke.mc.duke.edu/
Larry B. Goldstein, MD, Dir.
Activities/Fields: Molecular biology, neuropharmacology, neurophysiology, developmental neurobiology, receptor biology, cell biology and behavioral recovery.

★ 22334 ★ Duke University
Duke Center for Clinical Health Policy Research (CCHPR)
First Union Tower
2200 W Main St., Ste. 230
Durham, NC 27705
Phone: (919)286-3399 **Fax:** (919)286-5601
Email: match001@mc.duke.edu
Website: http://www.clinpol.mc.duke.edu/About/about.html
David B. Matchar, MD, Dir.
Activities/Fields: Clinical health policy from its development using evidence-based approaches to strategies for optimal implementation.

★ 22335 ★ Duke University
Duke Center for Integrative Medicine (DCIM)
DUMC Box 3022
Durham, NC 27710
Phone: (919)660-6826 **Free:** (866)313-0959
Fax: (919)681-0380
Website: http://dukehealth.org/health_services/integrative_medicine.asp
Tracy W. Gaudet, MD, Dir.
Activities/Fields: Integrative medicine, which combines the best of conventional Western medicine with mind-body-spirit approaches to health, and with complementary techniques (such as acupuncture and herbalism) that have proven efficacy.

★ 22336 ★ Duke University
Duke Comprehensive Cancer Center
Medical Center
PO Box 3843
Durham, NC 27710
Phone: (919)684-3377 **Fax:** (919)684-5653
Website: http://www.cancer.duke.edu/
Dr. Darell D. Bigner, Dir.
Activities/Fields: Prevention, detection, diagnosis, and treatment of cancer, including multidisciplinary studies in cellular and molecular biology, chemical and environmental carcinogenesis, ultrastructure, cell genetics, virology, tumor immunology, epidemiology, and biostatistics. Conducts clinical investigations. **Pub:** *Annual Progress Report.* • *Cancer Patient Support Program.* • *Duke Cancer Center Notes,* quarterly. • *Melanoma.* • *Newsletters on Pediatric Brain Tumors.* • *Recreation Therapy.*

★ 22337 ★ Duke University
Eye Center
PO Box 3802
Durham, NC 27710
Phone: (919)684-5846 **Fax:** (919)681-6343
Email: epste001@mc.duke.edu
Website: http://www.dukeeye.org
David Epstein, MD, Ch.
Activities/Fields: Eye disorders, with special focus on retinal detachment, corneal diseases, and proliferative diabetic retinopathy.

★ 22338 ★ Duke University
Frank Hawkins Kenan Plastic Surgery Research Laboratories
Medical Center
016 Research Park 4
PO Box 3906
Durham, NC 27710
Phone: (919)684-3929 **Fax:** (919)681-2670
Email: klitz@acpub.duke.edu
Website: http://www.duke.edu/~klitz
Prof. Bruce Klitzman, Sr. Dir.
Activities/Fields: Microvascular physiology, tissue engineering, plastic surgery, including wound healing monitoring tissue viability, thrombolytic therapy, preservation of organs, and biocompatibility of synthetic vascular grafts (prostheses). Also conducts studies on microcirculation, skin cancer, and aging skin. **Frmly:** Plastic Surgery Research Laboratories.

★ 22339 ★ Duke University
General Clinical Research Center
Medical Center
368 Jones Bldg.
PO Box 3068
Durham, NC 27710
Phone: (919)684-6263 **Fax:** (919)684-8676
Email: marke001@mc.duke.edu
Website: http://igg1.mc.duke.edu/Gaveston/
Dr. M. Louise Markert, Prog. Dir.
Activities/Fields: Multidisciplinary, clinical research into the cause, progression, prevention, control, and cure of human disease. Sample projects have studied immunodeficiency diseases, Alzheimer's disease, food allergy, X-linked hypophosphatemic rickets, and cardiovascular disease. **Frmly:** Rankin Clinical Research Unit.

★ 22340 ★ Duke University
Institute on Care at the End of Life
023 New Divinity Bldg.
Divinity School
Durham, NC 27708
Phone: (919)660-3553 **Fax:** (919)660-3544
Email: iceol@duke.edu
Website: http://www.iceol.duke.edu
Keith G. Meador, MD, Dir.
Activities/Fields: Care of the dying and their families, with an emphasis on underserved and diverse populations with varied religious and spiritual practices regarding the issue of dying.

★ 22341 ★ Duke University
Joseph and Kathleen Bryan Alzheimer's Disease Research Center
2200 W Main St., Ste. A230
Durham, NC 27705
Phone: (919)416-5380 **Free:** (866)444-2372
Fax: (919)286-3406
Email: desduke@duke.edu
Website: http://adrc.mc.duke.edu/
Donald E. Schmechel, MD, Dir.
Activities/Fields: Diagnosis, management, and treatment of Alzheimer's Disease.

★ 22342 ★ Duke University
Occupational Mental Health Programs
Medical Center
PO Box 3834
Durham, NC 27712
Phone: (919)286-1244 **Free:** 800-336-3853
Fax: (919)286-1121
Dr. Judith Holder, Dir.
Activities/Fields: Occupational mental health, including managed mental health care, employee assistance programs, and mental health outcome research. **Frmly:** Career Assessment and Development Laboratory.

★ 22343 ★ Duke University
Pediatric Asthma and Allergic Disease Center
Medical Center
PO Box 2898
Durham, NC 27710
Phone: (919)684-2922 **Fax:** (919)681-7979
Email: buckl003@mc.duke.edu
Rebecca H. Buckley, Div. Ch.
Activities/Fields: As a unit of NIAID, the Center seeks to integrate the concepts of immunology, genetics, biochemistry, and pharmacology into clinical investigations of patients with asthma and allergic diseases. Specific projects include studies on immunoregulation in atopic eczema and in vitro studies of human immunoglobulin E (IgE) synthesis, including lymphocyte phenotypes and their function in humans with allergic diseases and excessively high IgE antibody production. Functional studies include proliferative responses, in vitro IgE production and the effects of various cytokines on it, and epidermal T cell interactions in atopic dermatitis.

★ 22344 ★ Duke University
Pediatric Cardiac Catheterization Laboratory
Pediatric Cardiology
DUMC 3090
Medical Center, Rm. 7607 DHN
Durham, NC 27710
Phone: (919)684-3574 **Fax:** (919)681-5903
Dr. John F. Rhodes, Jr., Med. Dir.
Activities/Fields: Pediatric cardiology, including development of catheter-delivered devices to treat congenital heart disease.

★ 22345 ★ Duke University Pediatric Rheumatoid Clinic
Duke Medical Center, Box 3212
Durham, NC 27710
Phone: (919)684-6575 **Fax:** (919)684-6616
Email: schan001@mc.duke.edu
Dr. Laura Schanberg, Contact
Activities/Fields: Clinical and laboratory pediatric rheumatology and immunology. **Frmly:** Arthritis Pediatric Research Center.

★ 22346 ★ Duke University Preuss Laboratory for Brain Tumor Research
Medical Center
Research Dr., 177 MSRB
PO Box 3156
Durham, NC 27710
Phone: (919)684-5018 **Fax:** (919)684-6458
Email: bigne001@mc.duke.edu
Dr. Darell D. Bigner, Dir.
Activities/Fields: Brain tumors.

★ 22347 ★ Duke University Program on the Medical Encounter and Palliative Care
VA Medical Center (152)
508 Fulton St.
Durham, NC 27705
Phone: (919)286-6936 **Fax:** (919)416-5838
Email: jtulsky@duke.edu
Website: http://hsrd.Durham.med.va.gov/pmepc/default.htm
Dr. James Tulsky, Dir.
Activities/Fields: Improvement of patient-provider communication and the quality of end-of-life care, including care planning, pain management in seriously ill patients, and psychosocial and spiritual needs of dying patients.

★ 22348 ★ Duke University Udall Parkinson's Disease Research Center of Excellence (PDRCE)
DUMC Box 2903
Durham, NC 27710
Phone: (919)681-5696 **Fax:** (919)681-7894
Email: udall@chg.mc.duhs.edu
Website: http://wwwchg.mc.duke.edu/udall
Jeffery M. Vance, MD, Dir.
Activities/Fields: Cause and cure for Parkinson's disease.

★ 22349 ★ Duluth Clinic Education and Research Foundation
400 E 3rd St.
Duluth, MN 55805-1951
Phone: (218)725-3139 **Fax:** (218)727-7258
Email: jdwyer@smdc.org
Website: http://www.smdc.org
James M. Dwyer, Dir.
Activities/Fields: Parkinson's disease, cancer, heart, stroke, and other medical issues. **Pub:** *Health Strides.*

★ 22350 ★ Dwight David Eisenhower Army Medical Center Department of Clinical Investigation
Bldg. 300
Fort Gordon, GA 30905-5650
Phone: (706)787-4273 **Fax:** (706)787-5216
Email: kent.plowman@se.amedd.army.mil
Website: http://www.ddeamc.amedd.army.mil/clinical/investigation/clin_inv.htm
Col. Kent M. Plowman, Ch.
Activities/Fields: Osteomyelitis in rat tibias, fibroblast attachment to teeth, periodontal implants, pharmacotherapy in burns, hormonal influence of bone growth, synthetic bone grafting materials, wound healing, and markers for malignancy. **Pub:** *Annual Progress Report.*

★ 22351 ★ Dyslexia Research Institute
5746 Centerville Rd.
Tallahassee, FL 32308-2899
Phone: (850)893-2216 **Fax:** (850)893-2440
Email: dri@talstar.com
Website: http://www.dyslexia-add.org
Dr. Patricia K. Hardman, Dir.
Activities/Fields: Dyslexia and attention deficit disorders, including educational techniques, teacher training, diagnostic procedures, biochemistry, allergies, and links alcoholism and eye movement.

★ 22352 ★ Dystonia Medical Research Foundation
1 E Wacker Dr., Ste. 2430
Chicago, IL 60601-1905
Phone: (312)755-0198 **Free:** 800-377-3978
Fax: (312)803-0138
Email: dystonia@dystonia-foundation.org
Website: http://www.dystonia-foundation.org/
Dr. Mahlon R. DeLong, Sci. Dir.
Activities/Fields: Causes and treatment of generalized dystonia, spasmodic torticollis, writer's cramp, blepharospasm, oromandibular dystonia, Meige's disease, and laryngeal dystonia. **Pub:** *Brochures.* • *Manuals.* • *Newsletter*, quarterly.

★ 22353 ★ Dystrophic Epidermolysis Bullosa Research Association of America
5 W 36th St., Rm. 404
New York, NY 10018
Phone: (212)868-1573
Email: staff@debra.org
Website: http://www.debra.org
Martin I. Hassner, Exec. Dir.
Activities/Fields: Epidermolysis Bullosa patients and their families. (Epidermolysis Bullosa represents a group of inherited disorders of the skin characterized by formation of blisters resulting from the most minimal trauma.). **Pub:** *EB Current*, 3/year.

★ 22354 ★ Ear Research Foundation
1901 Floyd St.
Sarasota, FL 34239
Phone: (941)366-1148 **Fax:** (941)365-2269
Email: hsilverste@aol.com
Website: http://www.earsinus.org/frame_intro.htm
Dr. Herbert Silverstein, Pres.
Activities/Fields: Meniere's disease, acoustic neuroma, benign positional vertigo, laser-assisted otological surgery for inner- and middle-ear disorders, cholesteatoma in children, cochlear implants, and vestibular rehabilitation.

★ 22355 ★ East Carolina University Biomechanics Laboratory
251 Sports Medicine Bldg.
Greenville, NC 27858
Phone: (252)328-4564 **Fax:** (252)328-4689
Email: hortobagyit@mail.ecu.edu
Website: http://www.ecu.edu/exss/biomechanics/biomechanics.htm
Tibor Hortobagyi, PhD, Contact
Activities/Fields: Biomechanics of human movement.

★ 22356 ★ East Carolina University Center on Aging
Physician's Quadrangle, Bldg. N
Greenville, NC 27858
Phone: (919)816-2793
Email: mitchellj@mail.ecu.edu
Website: http://www.ecu.edu/aging/
Dr. Jim Mitchell, Dir.
Activities/Fields: Aging issues, including racial and geographical variation in health and long-term care needs, the regional impact of retirement migration, the management of drug costs, the awareness and use of healthcare services, the impact of Medicare/Medicaid eligibility on medical care.

★ 22357 ★ East Carolina University Center for Health Services Research and Development (CHSR&D)
Physician Quadrangle, Bldg. N
Greenville, NC 27858-4354
Phone: (252)744-2785 **Fax:** (252)744-3259
Email: mansfieldc@mail.ecu.edu
Website: http://www.chsrd.med.ecu.edu
Christopher J. Mansfield, PhD, Dir.
Activities/Fields: Health care needs of rural North Carolina, including understanding epidemiology; the organization, finance, and delivery of health services; patient-provider interaction; professional workforce issues; and the effectiveness of clinical practices. **Pub:** *Eastern Carolina Health Care Atlas.* • *Physicians Directory.*

★ 22358 ★ East Carolina University Office of Research and Scholarship
Rivers Bldg., Rm. 215
School of Nursing
Greenville, NC 27858-4353
Phone: (252)328-4325 **Fax:** (252)328-2168
Email: engelkem@mail.ecu.edu
Website: http://www.ecu.edu
Dr. Martha Engelke, Interim Assoc. Dean, Res.
Activities/Fields: Basic and applied nursing research, including symptom management, women's health care, and rural health. **Pub:** *Research Pulsations Newsletter*, bimonthly.

★ 22359 ★ Eastern Cooperative Oncology Group (ECOG)
900 Commonwealth Ave.
Boston, MA 02215-1204
Phone: (617)632-3610 **Fax:** (617)632-2990
Website: http://www.ecog.org
Dr. Robert Comis, Chm.
Activities/Fields: Multidisciplinary cancer trials, including treatment, biologic and basic research, and cancer control and prevention. **Pub:** *Newsletter*, semiannually.

★ 22360 ★ Eastern Virginia Medical School
Thomas R. Lee Center for Ocular Pharmacology
PO Box 1980
Norfolk, VA 23501
Phone: (757)446-5732 **Fax:** (757)624-2270
Email: williams@borg.evms.edu
Website: http://www.evms.edu/ocular-pharm/index.html
Patricia B. Williams, PhD, Dir.
Activities/Fields: Chronic and blinding diseases of the eye, especially glaucoma.

★ 22361 ★ Eaton-Peabody Laboratory of Auditory Physiology
Massachusetts Eye & Ear Infirmary
243 Charles St.
Boston, MA 02114
Phone: (617)573-3745 **Fax:** (617)720-4408
M. Charles Liberman, PhD, Dir.
Activities/Fields: Vertebrate auditory system and auditory information processing, including feedback control systems in normal and pathologic hearing. Approaches include anatomical, physiological, functional imaging, pharmacological, chemical and molecular biological studies of animal models as well as human subjects.

★ 22362 ★ Edward Dana Mitchell Surgical Research Laboratory
956 Court, G228
Department of Surgery
University of Tennessee
Memphis, TN 38163
Phone: (901)448-8370 **Fax:** (901)448-7306

Email: tfabian@utmem.edu
Dr. Timothy Fabian, Dir.

Activities/Fields: Surgery, transplantation, sepsis, shock, nutrition, hepatic dysfunction, and gut immunology.

★ 22363 ★ Eleanor Roosevelt Institute
1899 Gaylord St.
Denver, CO 80206-1210
Phone: (303)336-5600 **Fax:** (303)333-8423
Email: davepatt@eri.uchsc.edu
Website: http://www-eri.uchsc.edu
David Patterson, PhD, Pres.

Activities/Fields: Biochemistry and mammalian genetics. Investigates human and other mammalian cell systems, biosynthetic pathways of purines and pyrimidines, biochemical structure and function of cell surface membranes, cytogenetics, cancer genetics, genetic biochemistry, mutagenesis, carcinogenesis, down syndrome, Lou Gehrig's disease (ALS), and arthritis. Results of studies applied to problems in malignancy, birth defects, and other diseases.

★ 22364 ★ Emory-Georgia Tech Biomedical Technology Research Center
Parker H. Petit Institute for Bioengineering & Bioscience
Georgia Institute of Technology
315 Ferst Dr., Ste. 1126
Atlanta, GA 30332-0535
Phone: (404)894-2768 **Fax:** (404)894-4243
Website: http://www.ibb.gatech.edu
Dr. Robert M. Nerem, Dir.

Activities/Fields: Cardiovascular mechanics, corneal mechanics, medical imaging, biomedical artificial intelligence, biomedical instrumentation, vascular biology, tissue engineering, telemedicine. **Pub:** *Newsletter*, 3/year.

★ 22365 ★ Emory University Cardiac Catheterization Laboratory
1364 Clifton Rd. NE, Ste. C430
Atlanta, GA 30322
Phone: (404)712-7034 **Free:** 800-434-3278
Fax: (404)727-3377
Jane C. Wilson, Mgr., Invasive Cardiology

Activities/Fields: Cardiovascular hemodynamics and coronary circulation.

★ 22366 ★ Emory University Center for Cell and Molecular Signaling
School of Medicine
1648 Pierce Dr.
Atlanta, GA 30322
Phone: (404)727-7421 **Fax:** (404)727-0329
Email: deaton@emory.edu
Website: http://www.emory.edu/WHSC/MED/CCMS/
Douglas C. Eaton, PhD, Dir.

Activities/Fields: Cellular signaling or cellular signal transduction, which is the process by which cells recognize external events and respond to the events with appropriate changes within the cell.

★ 22367 ★ Emory University Center on Complementary and Alternative Medicine in Neurodegenerative Diseases
Department of Neurology
School of Medicine
1639 Pierce Dr., Ste. 6000
Atlanta, GA 30322
Phone: (404)727-3818 **Fax:** (404)727-3157
Email: medmrd@emory.edu
Website: http://nccam.nih.gov/training/centers/descriptions.htm
Dr. Mahlon R. DeLong, Dir.

Activities/Fields: Complementary and alternative treatments for neurodegenerative diseases such as Parkinson's, Alzheimer's, Huntington's disease, multiple sclerosis, stroke.

★ 22368 ★ Emory University Center for Injury Control
1518 Clifton Rd., Ste. 230
Atlanta, GA 30322
Phone: (404)727-9977 **Fax:** (404)727-8744
Email: kellerma@sph.emory.edu
Website: http://www.sph.emory.edu/CIC/index.html
Arthur L. Kellermann, MD, Dir.

Activities/Fields: Prevention and control of injuries, especially the reduction of death and disability due to injury.

★ 22369 ★ Emory University Center for Research on Complementary and Alternative Medicine in Neurodegenerative Diseases
Department of Neurology
School of Medicine
1639 Pierce Dr.
Atlanta, GA 30322
Phone: (404)712-4801 **Fax:** (404)712-5895
Email: swolf@emory.edu
Website: http://www.emory.edu/WHSC/MED/NEUROLOGY/CAM/index.html
Dr. Mahlon R. DeLong, Dir.

Activities/Fields: Interventions that are complementary to traditional medical approaches that preserve or enhance function and quality of life among individuals with neurodegenerative disorders.

★ 22370 ★ Emory University Cystic Fibrosis Care, Teaching and Research Center
1547 Clifton Rd. NE
Atlanta, GA 30322
Phone: (404)727-5728 **Fax:** (404)727-4828
Email: dcaplan@emory.edu
Dr. Daniel B. Caplan, Dir.

Activities/Fields: Cystic fibrosis and respiratory and gastrointestinal diseases of children.

★ 22371 ★ Emory University Emory Alzheimer's Disease Center (ADC)
Wesley Woods Health Center, 2nd Fl.
1841 Clifton Rd.
Atlanta, GA 30329
Phone: (404)728-6950
Email: emoryadc@emory.edu
Website: http://www.emory.edu/WHSC/MED/ADC/
Allan Levey, MD, Dir.

Activities/Fields: Alzheimer's disease.

★ 22372 ★ Emory University Emory Eye Center
Emory Clinic, Bldg. B
1365B Clifton Rd. NE
Atlanta, GA 30322
Phone: (404)778-4456 **Fax:** (404)778-5128
Email: ophttma@emory.edu
Website: http://www.emory.edu/EYE_CENTER/emory_welcome_frame.html
Dr. Thomas M. Aaberg, Sr., Dir.

Activities/Fields: Prevention, diagnosis and treatment of eye diseases. **Pub:** *Molecular Vision Web journal.*

★ 22373 ★ Emory University Emory Eye Center Division of Ophthalmic Research
School of Medicine
1365-B Clifton Rd. NE, Bldg. B
Atlanta, GA 30322
Phone: (404)778-4140 **Fax:** (404)778-4143
Email: ophthfe@emory.edu
Website: http://www.emory.edu/EYE_CENTER
Dr. Henry F. Edelhauser, Dir.

Activities/Fields: Various biochemical, pathobiochemical, physiological, and pathophysiological aspects of fundamental causes of blindness-producing diseases, especially cataract, glaucoma, retinal detachment, diabetes, and diabetic vasculopathy. Maintains strong clinical liaison in research programming.

★ 22374 ★ Emory University Emory Vaccine Research Center
954 Gatewood Rd.
Atlanta, GA 30322
Phone: (404)712-2692 **Fax:** (404)727-3108
Website: http://www.emory.edu/WHSC/YERKES/VRC/
Rafi Ahmed, PhD, Dir.

Activities/Fields: Immunology and vaccines, especially new technologies to prevent AIDS, tuberculosis, malaria, influenza, and respiratory illnesses.

★ 22375 ★ Emory University General Clinical Research Center
School of Medicine
1364 Clifton Rd., Ste. GG23
Atlanta, GA 30322
Phone: (404)712-4722 **Fax:** (404)727-5563
Email: medlsp@emory.edu
Website: http://www.emory.edu/WHSC/MED/RESEARCH/GCRC/
Lawrence S. Phillips, MD, Prog. Dir.

Activities/Fields: Disorders of amino acid, and protein metabolism; branch-chain ketoacid abnormalities; mitochondrial myopathies; clinical nutrition; energy metabolism; metabolic consequences of diabetes and obesity; effects of low protein diets and blood pressure control on the progression of renal disease; and growth disorders. **Frmly:** W. Dean Warren Clinical Research Center.

★ 22376 ★ Emory University Georgia Center for Cancer Statistics
Rollins School of Public Health
1518 Clifton Rd.
Atlanta, GA 30322
Phone: (404)727-3069 **Fax:** (404)727-7261
Website: http://www.sph.emory.edu/GCCS/

Activities/Fields: Serves as a cancer registry for five counties of metropolitan Atlanta and ten rural counties in central Georgia. Seeks to monitor the incidence of cancer in a geographically defined population, identify groups with unusual risks of cancer, monitor oncologic practices within the community, assess the survival experience of cancer patients, and provide a resource for epidemiological and biostatistical studies and training. Studies racial differences in cancer survival, cancers especially prevalent among blacks, passive exposure to cigarette smoke and risk of lung cancer, exposure to agent orange and risk of lymphoma and soft tissue sarcoma, risk factors for selected uterine malignancies, barriers to the early detection of cervical cancer, and viral infection and T-cell leukemias. **Frmly:** Atlanta Cancer Surveillance Center.

★ 22377 ★ Emory University Laboratory for Sleep, Aging, and Chronobiology
Department of Neurology
Medical School
1821 Clifton Rd.
Atlanta, GA 30329
Phone: (404)728-4752 **Fax:** (404)728-4756
Email: dbliwis@emory.edu
Dr. Donald L. Bliwise, Dir.

Activities/Fields: Neurophysiological studies of sleep.

★ 22378 ★ Emory University Winship Cancer Institute
1365 Clifton Rd. NE, Ste. B4100
Atlanta, GA 30322
Phone: (404)778-5180 **Fax:** (404)778-5016
Email: jonathan_simons@emoryhealthcare.org

Website: http://www.emory.edu/WHSC/WCI
Dr. Jonathan W. Simons, Ch.

Activities/Fields: A university-based cancer center coordinating multidisciplinary basic and clinical cancer research, improving methods of treatment, diagnosis, and prevention, training health professionals, and transferring cancer knowledge to surrounding communities.

★ 22379 ★ Emory University
Yerkes National Primate Research Center
954 Gatewood Rd. NE
Atlanta, GA 30329
Phone: (404)727-7732 **Fax:** (404)727-3108
Email: yerkes-info@rmy.emory.edu
Website: http://www.emory.edu/WHSC/YERKES/
Dr. Stuart Zola, Dir.

Activities/Fields: Vaccines for AIDS and malaria; treatments for cocaine addiction, parkinsons's disease and cardiovascular disease. Other research programs include cognitive development and decline, childhood visual defects, organ transplant rejection and social behaviors of primates. **Frmly:** Yale Laboratories of Primate Biology.

★ 22380 ★ Environmental Health Service
Rancho Los Amigos Med. Center
Med. Science Bldg., Rm. 51
7601 E Imperial Hwy.
Downey, CA 90242
Phone: (562)401-7561 **Fax:** (562)803-6883
Email: hgong@dhs.co.la.ca.us
Dr. Henry Gong, Jr., Contact

Activities/Fields: Drug studies of patients with asthma or COPD; air pollution, including effects of ozone on healthy subjects and patients with mild asthma; physiological and cellular responses to acute exposures to ozone, sulfur dioxide, nitrogen dioxide, carbon monoxide, and particulates; health effects of acid aerosols; pharmaceutical drugs; and development of field study programs, including in-home method for self-testing and lung function performance using research quality instrumentation and personal computers, and documentation of typical hourly and daily activity to assess potential effects of air pollution on those activities.

★ 22381 ★ Environmental and Occupational Health Sciences Institute (EOHSI)
170 Frelinghuysen Rd.
Piscataway, NJ 08854
Phone: (732)445-0200 **Fax:** (732)455-0131
Email: info@eohsi.rutgers.edu
Website: http://www.eohsi.rutgers.edu
Deborah A. Cory-Slechta, PhD, Exec. Dir.

Activities/Fields: Toxicology, public education and risk communication, occupational health, exposure measurement and assessment, environmental health, and environmental policy. Studies the basic mechanisms by which environmental exposures harm the body, investigates methods for measuring and reducing exposure and improving health including clinical evaulation of individuals potentially affected adversely by environmental agents, and develops and analyzes ways to communicate information. **Pub:** *EOHSI Newsletter.*

★ 22382 ★ Environmental and Occupational Health Sciences Institute
Ozone Research Center
170 Frelinghuysen Rd.
PO Box 1179
Piscataway, NJ 08854
Phone: (732)445-0200
Email: panosg@fidelio.rutgers.edu
Website: http://www.ccl.rutgers.edu/orc/index.html
Dr. Panos G. Georgopoulos, Dir.

Activities/Fields: Causes, dynamics, and effects of photochemical air pollution (smog), focusing on issues and air quality problems affecting the Northeastern United States and in particular New Jersey, especially the enhancement of the scientific understanding of photochemical air pollution and associated human exposures and health effects and to provide the necessary scientific rationale for developing and implementing efficient air quality management strategies.

★ 22383 ★ EPG Research Foundation, Inc.
111 E Shore Rd.
Manhasset, NY 11030-2922
Phone: (516)365-1288 **Fax:** (516)365-7522
Email: epglabs@igc.org
Dr. J.L. Logan, Dir.

Activities/Fields: Molecular biology.

★ 22384 ★ Eye Institute of New Jersey
New Jersey Medical School
90 Bergen St., 6th Fl.
Newark, NJ 07103-2499
Phone: (973)972-2050 **Fax:** (973)972-7986
Email: heinrige@umdnj.edu
George F. Heinrich, MD, Pres.

Activities/Fields: Ophthalmology, including the cornea, the retina, uveitis, glaucoma, pediatric ophthalmology, age related macular degeneration, and neuro-ophthalmology.

★ 22385 ★ Falor Division of Surgical Research
Summa Health System/Akron City Hospital
525 E Market St.
Akron, OH 44309
Phone: (330)375-3693 **Fax:** (330)375-4648
Email: schmidts@summa-health.org
Dr. Steven Schmidt, Dir.

Activities/Fields: Vascular cells, focusing on cell and molecular biology, hyperplasia, and wound healing. **Frmly:** Vascular Research Laboratory.

★ 22386 ★ Family Health International (FHI)
PO Box 13950
Research Triangle Park, NC 27709
Phone: (919)544-7040 **Fax:** (919)544-7261
Email: brobinson@fhi.org
Website: http://www.fhi.org
Dr. Willard Cates, Jr., Pres.

Activities/Fields: New contraceptive technology, contraceptive acceptability, contraceptive effectiveness and safety, breast-feeding practices, maternal/child health, demography, interventions to reduce the transmission of sexually transmitted diseases and AIDS, economics of family planning and financing of AIDS programming,and infectious diseases, including malaria. Operates the Implementing AIDS Prevention and Care (IMPACT) Project, which seeks to support the local capacity of developing countries to prevent and control HIV. **Pub:** *Network Newsletter*, quarterly.

★ 22387 ★ Fertility Research Foundation
877 Park Ave.
New York, NY 10021
Phone: (212)744-5500 **Fax:** (212)744-6536
Email: frfbaby@msn.com
Website: http://www.frfbaby.com
Dr. Masood Khatamee, Exec. Dir.

Activities/Fields: Fertility and human reproduction, including studies on microsurgery, fertilization, fallopian tube transplant, artificial embryonation, education and prevention of human infertility, in vitro fertilization gender planning, therapeutic donor insemination, and counselling. **Pub:** *Infertility Journal.*

★ 22388 ★ Fitzpatrick Oncology Center
Champlain Valley Physicians Hospital
75 Beekman St.
Plattsburgh, NY 12901
Phone: (518)562-7100 **Fax:** (518)562-7531
Kathy Bracero, Dir.

Activities/Fields: Oncological clinical research.

★ 22389 ★ Florida Atlantic University Center for Complex Systems and Brain Sciences
777 Glades Rd.
Boca Raton, FL 33431
Phone: (561)297-2230 **Fax:** (561)297-3634
Email: kelso@walt.ccs.fau.edu
Website: http://www.ccs.fau.edu
J.A. Scott Kelso, Dir.

Activities/Fields: Multidisciplinary studies of complex biological systems, focusing on coordination between neural processes and their resultant behaviors on cognitive, neural, and biophysical levels. Contains four major research facilities: Human Brain and Behavior Laboratories, including functional magnetic resonance imaging; Theoretical (Computational) Neuroscience Laboratory; Basic Neuroscience Research Laboratories, which includes neural growth and development, neurophysiology, neuroanatomy, and cellular biophysics; Coordination Dynamics Laboratory. Houses National Training Program in Complex Systems and Brain Sciences for pre- and postdoctoral fellows.

★ 22390 ★ Florida Hospital Cancer Institute
Clinical and Research Laboratories
2501 N Orange Ave., Ste. 786
Orlando, FL 32804
Phone: (407)303-2440 **Fax:** (407)303-2441
Email: john.francis@flhosp.org
Website: http://www.fhci-labs.com
Dr. John L. Francis, Dir.

Activities/Fields: Cell biology, cancer metastasis, anticoagulants, hemostasis and thrombosis.

★ 22391 ★ Florida Ophthalmic Institute
7106 NW 11th Pl., Ste. B
Gainesville, FL 32605-3192
Phone: (352)331-2020 **Fax:** (352)331-2019
Email: afn22025@afn.org
Website: http://www.see.yourmd.com
Dr. Norman S. Levy, Dir.

Activities/Fields: Understanding and treatment of human ocular diseases, including glaucoma and external ocular pathology.

★ 22392 ★ Florida State University Center for Prevention and Early Intervention Policy
1339 E Lafayette St.
Tallahassee, FL 32301
Phone: (850)922-1300 **Fax:** (850)922-1352
Email: mgraham@mailer.fsu.edu
Website: http://www.cpeip.fsu.edu
Dr. Mimi A. Graham, Dir.

Activities/Fields: Child care, infant mental health, teen parents, violence prevention.

★ 22393 ★ Florida State University Sensory Research Institute
B-340, NHMFL
1800 E Paul Dirac Dr.
Tallahassee, FL 32306-2741
Phone: (850)644-2637 **Fax:** (850)645-3295
Email: fsusri@psy.fsu.edu
Website: http://www.psy.fsu.edu/~fsusri/welcome.html
Dr. James C. Walker, Dir.

Activities/Fields: Human and animal sensory response to airborne chemicals.

★ 22394 ★ The Forsyth Institute
140 The Fenway
Boston, MA 02115-3799
Phone: (617)262-5200 **Fax:** (617)262-4021
Email: dpdepaola@forsyth.org
Website: http://www.forsyth.org
Dr. Dominick P. DePaola, Pres. /CEO

Activities/Fields: Physical, biomedical, and clinical sciences pertinent to field of oral biology. Seeks to obtain a better understanding of normal and diseased structures of the oral cavity and its related parts, including bioadhesion, molecular genetics, immunology, biomineralization, clinical trials, cytokine biology, periodontology, electron microscopy, nutrition, and craniofocial growth and development. Conducts research into the cause, cure and prevention of dental caries, periodontal diseases, oral cancer, oral and facial deformities and oral manifestations of other diseases.

★ 22395 ★ Foundation for Advanced Cancer Studies, Inc.
333 Briarwood Ave. SE
Grand Rapids, MI 49506-1739
Email: michelle.reed@vai.org
Website: http://www.facsi.org
Dr. G. Vande Woude, Pres.

Activities/Fields: Basic cancer research, focusing on the rapid dissemination of new research information to scientists, clinicians, and the public.

★ 22396 ★ Foundation for Blood Research
69 US Rte. 1
PO Box 190
Scarborough, ME 04070-0190
Phone: (207)883-4131 **Free:** 800-639-8605
Fax: (207)883-1527
Email: fbrinfo@fbr.org
Website: http://www.fbr.org
Robert F. Ritchie, MD, Pres.

Activities/Fields: Health science education, epidemiology, genetics, immunology, oncology, perinatalogy, rheumatology, prenatal diagnosis, and cancer. Immunochemical analysis of human blood and other body fluids is performed and coupled with epidemiological data both for research on and for use in computer applications in disease diagnosis. Also performs clinical testing. **Pub:** *AFP Office Update Newsletter*, quarterly. • *Clinical Genetics Newsletter*, quarterly. • *Genetics Digest Newsletter*, 5/year. • *Proceedings of Scarborough Meetings*, periodically. • *RDL Newsletter*, quarterly.

★ 22397 ★ Foundation for Chiropractic Education and Research
1330 Beacon St., Ste. 315
Brookline, MA 02446-3202
Phone: (617)734-3397 **Free:** 888-690-1378
Fax: (617)734-0989
Email: rosnerfcer@aol.com
Website: http://www.fcer.org
Anthony Rosner, PhD, Dir.,Res. & Educ.

Activities/Fields: Chiropractic medicine. Research areas include biomechanical studies of the spine and related soft tissue structures; the relationship between spine and body functions; the effects of manipulation upon various body functions; clinical traits of spinal manipulation; the effectiveness of manipulation for various conditions; reliability of various chiropractic analytical and diagnostic procedures; the various instrumentations used in chiropractic; and surveys of utilization of chiropractic treatment and epidemiological and sociological studies. **Pub:** *Chiropractic Healthways Pamphlet Series.* • *This Week in Chiropractic Advance.*

★ 22398 ★ Foundation for Hand Research and Education
8501 Harcourt Rd.
PO Box 80434
Indianapolis, IN 46280-0434
Phone: (317)471-4313 **Fax:** (317)876-0462
Email: foundation@indianahandcenter.com
Website: http://www.indianahandcenter.com/foundation.html
Elaine Skopelja, Mgr.

Activities/Fields: Upper extremity surgery and rehabilitation. **Pub:** *Indiana Hand Center Newsletter*, quarterly.

★ 22399 ★ Fox Chase Cancer Center
7701 Burholme Ave.
Philadelphia, PA 19111
Phone: (215)728-6900 **Free:** 888-369-2427
Fax: (215)728-2594
Email: rc_young@fccc.edu
Website: http://www.fccc.edu
Robert C. Young, MD, Pres.

Activities/Fields: Cancer, including biomolecular structure and function, cellular and developmental biology, immunobiology, molecular oncology, virology, medical oncology, nursing research, imaging and spectroscopy, pathology, pharmacology, therapeutic radiology, surgical oncology, behavioral research, epidemiology and biostatistics. **Pub:** *President's Report.* • *Scientific Report*, annually.

★ 22400 ★ Framingham Heart Study
5 Thurber St.
Framingham, MA 01702
Phone: (508)872-6562 **Fax:** (508)626-1262
Email: sandra@fram.nhlbi.nih.gov
Website: http://framingham.com/heart/
Daniel Levy, MD, Dir.

Activities/Fields: Constitutional and conditioning factors in atherosclerotic, hypertensive, and cardiovascular diseases based on a long-term study of a section of the population of Framingham, Massachusetts. There were 5209 men and women who originally participated in the study, begun in 1948, and subsequent studies have focused on 5124 descendents and spouses of descendents in the second generation. One hundred families of its third and fourth generations are also under study.

★ 22401 ★ Fred Hutchinson Cancer Research Center
1100 Fairview Ave. N
PO Box 19024
Seattle, WA 98109-1024
Phone: (206)667-5000 **Free:** 800-4-CANCER
Fax: (206)667-5268
Email: lhartwel@fhcrc.org
Website: http://www.fhcrc.org
Dr. Leland Hartwell, Dir.

Activities/Fields: Cancer, including basic, clinical, and public health sciences. Research programs include basic science, human biology, human immunogenetics, marrow transplantation, organ systems, pain and toxicity, pediatric oncology, transplantation biology, biostatistics, cancer biology, cancer prevention research, and epidemiology.

★ 22402 ★ Friends Research Institute
505 Baltimore Ave.
PO Box 10676
Baltimore, MD 21285
Phone: (410)823-5116 **Fax:** (410)823-5131
Email: fri@friendsresearch.org
Website: http://www.friendsresearch.org
Patrick F. Bogan, Exec. Dir.

Activities/Fields: Studies drug addiction to provide statistical documentation of its relation to crime, effectiveness of addiction treatment programs, and HIV as a result of lifestyle. Also conducts pharmaceutical and medical research. **Pub:** *Newsletter.* **Frmly:** Friends Medical Science Research Center, Inc.

★ 22403 ★ Frontier Science and Technology Research Foundation
1244 Boylston St.
Chestnut Hill, MA 02467
Phone: (617)632-2000 **Fax:** (617)632-2001
Email: fstrf@fstrf.org
Website: http://www.fstrf.org
Dr. Marvin Zelen, Contact

Activities/Fields: Conducts joint research projects with cooperative clinical trial groups and other organizations. Provides biostatistical support and collaboration, data management and processing, project management, and administrative support to researchers.

★ 22404 ★ Gage Occupational and Environmental Health Unit
St. Michael's Hospital
30 Bond St.
Toronto, ON, Canada M5B 1W8
Phone: (416)867-7470 **Fax:** (416)867-3673
Email: stulacj@smh.toronto.on.ca
Website: http://www.utoronto.ca/occmed/
Dr. Linn Holness, Dir.

Activities/Fields: Lung problems related to asthma, bronchitis, and occupational and environmental pollution. Areas of interest include development of more effective treatment for adult asthmatics, connection between asthma and air pollution, acute effects of second-hand tobacco smoke on asthmatics and other people, predictability of asthma outcome, occupational asthma, effects of indoor environments on human comfort and health, and environmental sensitivity. Contact dermatitis, areas of interest include causation, workplace studies, deprostic methods and outcomes, particularly related to return to work and quality of life.

★ 22405 ★ Gamble Program for Clinical Studies
Children's Hospital Medical Center, ML 6014
3333 Burnet Ave., H1
Cincinnati, OH 45229-3039
Phone: (513)636-4578 **Fax:** (513)636-7682
Email: david.bernstein@cchmc.org
David Bernstein, MD, Dir.

Activities/Fields: Virology and immunology, including studies on rubella and rubella vaccines, anti-influenza agents, basic virology of influenza, herpes virus latency, role of complement in sickle cell disease and burn wounds, and basic and clinical studies on rotaviruses, hepatitis, and human immunodeficiency virus. **Frmly:** Christ Hospital Institute of Medical Research; James N. Gamble Institute of Medical Research at the Children's Hospital.

★ 22406 ★ Garden State Cancer Center John P. Caufield Technology Extension Center for Investigational Cancer Treatment
520 Belleville Ave.
Belleville, NJ 07109
Phone: (973)844-7000 **Fax:** (973)844-7020
Email: gscancer@att.net
Dr. David M. Goldenberg, Dir.

Activities/Fields: Develops and provides new and more effective technologies for the early detection, diagnosis, and treatment of cancer; facilitates the transfer of investigational, diagnostic and treatment methods to New Jersey practitioners and hospitals; provides minority populations with access to state-of-the-art cancer protocols and treatment within their own community.

★ 22407 ★ General Clinical Research Center
Medicine SL-90
1430 Tulane Ave.
New Orleans, LA 70112
Phone: (504)585-4000 **Fax:** (504)585-4045
Email: lerclpha@tulane.edu
Website: http://gcrc.tulane.edu
Juan J.L. Lertora, MD, Prog. Dir.

Activities/Fields: Major areas of investigation include AIDS immunosuppression, cardiac diseases, clinical immunology and allergy, gastroenterology and hepatic diseases, neuroendocrinology, oncology and renal diseases.

★ 22408 ★ Genome Sequencing Center
CB 8501
Washington University School of Medicine
4444 Forest Park Blvd.
Saint Louis, MO 63108
Phone: (314)286-1800 **Fax:** (314)286-1810
Email: rwilson@watson.wustl.edu
Website: http://genome.wustl.edu/
Richard K. Wilson, PhD, Dir.
Activities/Fields: Genome mapping and sequencing, technology development, and informatics.

★ 22409 ★ George Washington University Biostatistics Center
6110 Executive Blvd., Ste. 750
Rockville, MD 20852
Phone: (301)881-9260 **Fax:** (301)881-3742
Email: fowler@biostat.bsc.gwu.edu
Website: http://biostat.bsc.gwu.edu
Sarah Fowler, Dir.
Activities/Fields: Biostatistics, focusing on data management and analysis for medical research projects.

★ 22410 ★ George Washington University Center for Health Services Research and Policy
Department of Health Policy
School of Public Health & Health Services
2021 K St. NW, Ste. 800
Washington, DC 20006
Phone: (202)296-6922 **Fax:** (202)296-0025
Email: info@gwhealthpolicy.org
Website: http://www.gwhealthpolicy.org/
Sara Rosenbaum, JD, Dir.
Activities/Fields: Emerging issues in federal health law and policy and the impact of changing federal policies on states, communities, and the health care system. **Pub:** *Journal articles.* • *Manuscripts.* • *Research reports.*

★ 22411 ★ George Washington University Center for Virology, Immunology and Infectious Disease Research
Children's National Medical Center
111 Michigan Ave. NW
Washington, DC 20010-2978
Phone: (202)884-3981 **Fax:** (202)884-3985
Email: chhollan@cnmc.org
Dr. Christie A. Holland, Dir.
Activities/Fields: Virologic and immunologic problems relating to infectious diseases and vaccine development, hospital acquired nosocomial infections.

★ 22412 ★ George Washington University Lipid Research Clinic
908 New Hampshire Ave. NW, Ste. 500
Washington, DC 20037
Phone: (202)872-3700 **Fax:** (202)659-8627
Judith Hsia, Dir.
Activities/Fields: Clinical trials of cholesterol and prevention of heart disease, including cholesterol lowering food and fibers, products, and medication. Also studies cholesterol lowering in senior citizens and trials of postmenopausal hormone replacement and heart disease risk factors in women.

★ 22413 ★ Georgetown University Center for Drug Development Sciences
Department of Pharmacology
Georgetown University Medical Center
Med-Dent Bldg., Rm. NE405
3900 Reservoir Rd. NW
Washington, DC 20007
Phone: (202)687-1618 **Fax:** (202)687-0193
Email: sawlerj@gunet.georgetown.edu
Website: http://www.dml.georgetown.edu/depts/pharmacology/cdds/
Carl C. Peck, MD, Dir.
Activities/Fields: Improvement of clinical evaluation of drugs in development.

★ 22414 ★ Georgetown University Center for Sight
Medical Center, 7th Fl.
3800 Reservoir Rd. NW
Washington, DC 20007
Phone: (202)444-4448
Dr. Howard Cupples, Ch.
Activities/Fields: Effectiveness, outcomes, and utilization of eye care; epidemiology of eye care delivery; functional status and utility assessment. Research includes outcomes of cataract, glaucoma, diabetic eye disease, and barrier reduction related to eye care use. **Frmly:** Worthen Center for Eye Research.

★ 22415 ★ Georgetown University Division of Comparative Medicine
3950 Reservoir Rd. NW, Rm. G05
Washington, DC 20007
Phone: (202)687-2488 **Fax:** (202)687-6256
Stephen P. Schiffer, DVM, Dir.
Activities/Fields: Medical sciences, with particular reference to surgical aspects, including basic studies of tissue transplantation, neuroscience, techniques of extracorporeal circulation, magnetic resonance imaging (MRI) techniques, and technique of perfusion of orbital artery and heart/lung transplantation. Also designs and develops valvular devices and other cardiac instrumentation and evaluates vascular prosthetic devices. **Frmly:** Surgical Research Laboratory; Research Resources Facility.

★ 22416 ★ Georgetown University Imaging Science and Information Systems Research Center
Medical Center, Department of Radiology
Georgetown University Medical Center
2115 Wisconsin Ave. NW, Ste. 603
Washington, DC 20007
Phone: (202)687-5990 **Fax:** (202)784-3479
Email: cleary@isis.imac.georgetown.edu
Website: http://www.isis.georgetown.edu
Kevin R. Cleary, PhD, Dir.
Activities/Fields: Health care improvement through innovations in computers, communication, imaging and information technologies.

★ 22417 ★ Georgetown University Institute for Reproductive Health (IRH)
4301 Connecticut Ave., Ste. 310
Washington, DC 20008
Phone: (202)687-1392 **Fax:** (202)537-7450
Website: http://www.irh.org/
Victoria H. Jennings, PhD, Prin. Investigator
Activities/Fields: Reproductive health care, especially natural family planning (NFP) and fertility awareness (FA) practices.

★ 22418 ★ Georgetown University International Center for Interdisciplinary Studies of Immunology
Kober-Cogan Bldg., Rm. 318
3800 Reservoir Rd. NW
Washington, DC 20057
Phone: (202)687-8227 **Fax:** (202)784-3597
Email: bellantj@georgetown.edu
Website: http://www.immunologycenter.org
Dr. Joseph A. Bellanti, Dir.
Activities/Fields: Immunobiology, immunochemistry, immunogenetics, immunopharmacology, and immunopathology, including the clinical disciplines of allergy and immunology, infectious diseases, respiratory diseases, and disorders of immune regulation. The center's program emphasizes pediatrics. **Frmly:** Center for Interdisciplinary Research on Immunologic Diseases.

★ 22419 ★ Georgetown University Kennedy Institute of Ethics
Box 571212
Washington, DC 20057-1212
Phone: (202)687-8099 **Fax:** (202)687-8089
Email: kicourse@georgetown.edu
Website: http://www.georgetown.edu/research/kie/
Dr. Madison Powers, Dir.
Activities/Fields: Social and ethical issues in biomedical sciences, such as resource allocation in health care, human experimentation, genetic engineering, euthanasia, death and dying, reproductive technologies, physician-patient relations, in vitro fertilization, abortion, research cloning, and organ transplantation. Also researches other fields of applied ethics, such as international relations, government, law, journalism, business, and technology policy. **Pub:** *Bibliography of Bioethics*, annually. • *Bioethics Thesaurus*, annually. • *Encyclopedia of Bioethics.* • *International Directory of Bioethics Organizations.* • *Kennedy Institute of Ethics Journal.* • *New Titles in Bioethics*, quarterly. • *Scope Notes.* • *Searching BIOETHICSLINE.* **Frmly:** Joseph and Rose Kennedy Institute for the Study of Human Reproduction and Bioethics.

★ 22420 ★ Georgetown University Sleep Disorders Center
Main Bldg., Rm. 5411
3800 Reservoir Rd. NW
Washington, DC 20007
Phone: (202)444-3610 **Fax:** (202)444-2920
Dr. Richard Waldhorn, Jr., Dir.
Activities/Fields: Treatment techniques for sleep apnea using nasal continuous positive airway pressure, evaluation of people with nocturnal hypoxia and possible correlates to memory impairment, sleep disturbances in geriatric populations, and psychiatric studies dealing with the presence of depression in people with schizophrenia. Other concentrations include monitoring of epilepsy patients and studies of sudden infant death syndrome.

★ 22421 ★ Georgia Institute of Technology Center for Assistive Technology and Environmental Access (CATEA)
College of Architecture
490 10th St. NW
Atlanta, GA 30332-0156
Phone: (404)894-4960 **Free:** 800-726-9119
Fax: (404)894-9320
Email: hunter.ramseur@arch.gatech.edu
Website: http://www.catea.org/
Joseph A. Koncelik, Dir.
Activities/Fields: Develops procedures to help persons with disabilities. Coordinates research and services related to rehabilitation technology within the University System of Georgia. **Pub:** *Newsletter*, quarterly. **Frmly:** Center for Rehabilitation Technology.

★ 22422 ★ Georgia Institute of Technology Parker H. Petit Institute for Bioengineering and Bioscience
315 Ferst Dr., Ste. 1106
Atlanta, GA 30332-0363
Phone: (404)894-2768 **Fax:** (404)894-2291
Email: robert.nerem@ibb.gatech.edu/flash_index.html
Website: http://www.ibb.gatech.edu
Dr. Robert M. Nerem, Dir.
Activities/Fields: Biomechanics research, including biaxial mechanical properties in tissue, biomechanical design, cardiovascular fluid mechanics, cellular engineering and non-invasive blood flow measurement; tissue engineering; and bioelectrical research, including electromagnetic systems for measuring the electrical properties of tissue, medical device/systems for diagnostic and therapeutic applications, and the applications of either air- or wire-coupled electromagnetic energy to stimulate biofunction; rehabilitation research, which entails developing orthotic devices for patients with lower body dysfunction, evaluating functional electrostimulation, and observance of the parvocellular division of the red nucleus for analyzing movement control; and computer applications re-

search, which involves signal processing, image processing, and visualization, medical informatics, and simulation techniques to assist in making decisions regarding diagnostic and therapeutic strategies.

★ 22423 ★ Georgia Regional Spinal Cord Injury Care System
Shepherd Center Inc.
2020 Peachtree Rd. NW
Atlanta, GA 30309-1402
Phone: (404)350-2020 **Fax:** (404)355-1826
Website: http://www.shepherd.org/shepherdhomepage.nsf/Pages/ProgramsSCI?OpenDocument
Herndon Murray, MD, Contact
Activities/Fields: Spinal cord injuries and paralyzing neuromuscular diseases. **Pub:** *MS Review.* • *Shepherd Clinical Review Newsletter.* • *Spinal Column magazine.* • *Spineline.*

★ 22424 ★ Georgia Southern University Center for Rural Health and Research
PO Box 8148
Statesboro, GA 30460-8148
Phone: (912)681-0260 **Fax:** (912)486-7553
W. Kent Guion, MD, Dir.
Activities/Fields: Rural health in Georgia. Currently conducting a census of programs promoting well-being of children and families in the state and a study of the impact of social suport on the well being of HIV/AIDS patients.

★ 22425 ★ Georgia State University Center for Brain Sciences and Health (CBH)
University Plaza
Atlanta, GA 30303
Phone: (404)463-9611
Website: http://www.gsu.edu/~wwwcbh/
Dr. H. Elliott Albers, Dir.
Activities/Fields: Brain injury; obesity, eating disorders and energy balance; aggression/ violence; sleep and attention disorders.

★ 22426 ★ Georgia State University Viral Immunology Center National B Virus Resource Laboratory
PO Box 4118
Atlanta, GA 30302-4118
Phone: (404)651-0808 **Fax:** (404)651-0814
Email: bvirus@gsu.edu
Website: http://www.gsu.edu/bvirus
Julia K. Hilliard, PhD, Dir.
Activities/Fields: B-virus infections, basic pathogenesis mechanisms of this and other neurotropic herpesviruses, control and prevention strategies. It provides rapid virological and serological analyses and collaborates in studies of Herpes virus simiae and B-virus infections in humans and nonhuman primates, particularly macaques. Also investigating new animal models of herpesvirus disease, antiviral testing and epidemiological analyses of alpha-herpes virus by biochemical, immunological and molecular biological approaches; development of recombinant reagents; identification of effective antiviral strategies and design of putative vaccines; elucidation of host-virus interactions during pathogenesis; collaborative identification and exploration of putative alpha-herpes viruses not previously described.

★ 22427 ★ Georgia Tech/Emory Center for the Engineering of Living Tissues (GTEC)
Parker H. Petit Institute for Bioengineering & Bioscience
315 Ferst Dr.
Atlanta, GA 30332-0363
Phone: (404)385-0216 **Fax:** (404)894-2291
Email: robert.nerem@ibb.gatech.edu
Website: http://www.gtec.gatech.edu
Dr. Robert M. Nerem, Dir.
Activities/Fields: Development of biological substitutes incorporating living cells and synthetic or natural materials to foster tissue regeneration and/or remodeling for the purpose of repair, replacement, or enhancement of tissue function. **Pub:** *Research reports.*

★ 22428 ★ Geraldine Brush Cancer Research Institute
California Pacific Medical Center
Sterm Bldg.
2330 Clay St.
San Francisco, CA 94115
Phone: (415)600-1728 **Fax:** (415)561-1390
Email: nml@cooper.cpmc.org
Dr. Nancy M. Lee, Assoc. Dir.
Activities/Fields: Advanced molecular and cellular biology studies of human cancer. Special emphasis on breast cancer.

★ 22429 ★ Gladstone Institute of Cardiovascular Disease
PO Box 419100
San Francisco, CA 94141-9100
Phone: (415)826-7500 **Fax:** (415)285-5632
Email: rmahley@gladstone.ucsf.edu
Website: http://www.gladstone.ucsf.edu/gladstone/site/gicd/
Robert W. Mahley, MD, Dir.
Activities/Fields: Lipoprotein metabolism and biochemistry, cell biology and arterial wall metabolism, molecular biology, and clinical nutrition and metabolism, including studies of the molecular structures of various liproteins and their function in transporting blood cholesterol, the relationship of diet to cholesterol levels, and the role of platelets and white blood cells in thrombosis and atherosclerosis. **Pub:** *Gladstone Focus Newsletter.* Newsletter. • *SPIN.*

★ 22430 ★ Gladstone Institute of Virology and Immunology
PO Box 419100
San Francisco, CA 94141-9100
Phone: (415)826-7500 **Fax:** (415)826-1817
Email: wgreene@gladstone.ucsf.edu
Website: http://www.gladstone.ucsf.edu/gladstone/site/givi/
Dr. Warner C. Greene, Dir.
Activities/Fields: Human virology and immunology with a focus on HIV and AIDS. **Pub:** *Annual Report.* • *Focus*, quarterly.

★ 22431 ★ Glaucoma Laser Trabeculoplasty Study
Associated Vision Consultants
29275 Northwestern Hwy., Ste. 200
Southfield, MI 48034-5744
Phone: (248)353-1750 **Fax:** (248)353-7645
Email: mnc@avc2020.com
Website: http://www.avc2020.com
Marshall N. Cyrlin, MD, Dir.
Activities/Fields: Glaucoma pharmaceuticals, laser and surgery treatments.

★ 22432 ★ Glaucoma Research Foundation
490 Post St., Ste. 1427
San Francisco, CA 94102-1305
Phone: (415)986-3162 **Free:** 800-826-6693
Fax: (415)986-3763
Email: info@glaucoma.org
Website: http://www.glaucoma.org
Tom Brunner, Pres. /CEO
Activities/Fields: Glaucoma. **Pub:** *Childhood Glaucoma.* • *Gleams Newsletter*, quarterly. Newsletter. • *Understanding and Living with Glaucoma.*

★ 22433 ★ Good Samaritan Hospital Heart Institute
1225 Wilshire Blvd.
Los Angeles, CA 90017-2395
Phone: (213)977-4040 **Fax:** (213)977-4107
Email: rkloner@goodsam.org
Dr. Robert A. Kloner, Dir.
Activities/Fields: Myocardial biochemistry, myocardial infarction, effects of toxins on the heart, clinical hypertension trials, and lipid trials. **Pub:** *Scientific and clinical papers.*

★ 22434 ★ Grand Valley State University Human Performance Laboratory
132 Fieldhouse
Allendale, MI 49401
Phone: (313)895-3228 **Fax:** (313)895-3232
Email: scottj@gvsu.edu
James R. Scott, Coord.
Activities/Fields: Human performance studies, including elite athlete performance profiles (wrestlers), functional electro-stimulation exercise with quadriplegic participants, and faculty/staff fitness and lifestyle assessments.

★ 22435 ★ Great Lakes Regional Center for AIDS Research
North Bldg.
3220 School of Information
University of Michigan
1075 Beal Ave.
Ann Arbor, MI 48109-2112
Phone: (734)764-6132 **Fax:** (734)647-8045
Email: steasley@umich.edu
Website: http://www.greatlakescfar.org/index.html
Stephanie Teasley, PhD, Collaboratory Dir.
Activities/Fields: Acquired immune deficiency syndrome in adults, molecular virology of human immunodeficiency virus (HIV), and experimental therapy of HIV. **Frmly:** Northwestern University; Comprehensive AIDS Center.

★ 22436 ★ Group in Protein Structure and Function
University of Alberta
Department of Biochemistry
4-74 Medical Sciences Bldg.
Edmonton, AB, Canada T6G 2H7
Phone: (780)492-0087 **Fax:** (780)492-0886
Email: brian.sykes@ualberta.ca
Website: http://www.pence.ualberta.ca/mrc/main.html
Dr. B.D. Sykes, Dir.
Activities/Fields: Protein structure and function.

★ 22437 ★ Guardians of Hydrocephalus Research Foundation (GHRF)
2618 Ave. Z
Brooklyn, NY 11235-2023
Phone: (718)743-4473 **Fax:** (718)743-1171
Email: ghrf2618@aol.com
Website: http://ghrf.homestead.com/ghrf.html
Michael Fischetti, Chm.
Activities/Fields: Hydrocephalics and their families, health care professionals, and other concerned individuals. Seeks to find the cause and cure of hydrocephalus which is the buildup of cerebrospinal fluid in the brain cavity, and can cause brain damage or death if untreated. **Pub:** *GUARDIANews*, quarterly. Newsletter.

★ 22438 ★ H.L. Snyder Medical Research Institute
1407 Wheat Rd.
Winfield, KS 67156
Phone: (316)221-4080 **Fax:** (316)221-2684
Email: tsmith@snydermri.com
Website: http://www.snydermri.org
Dr. Jeffrey V. May, Exec. Dir.
Activities/Fields: Biochemical and molecular biological studies of diseases, especially cancer. Develops clinical assays for early cancer detection.

★ 22439 ★ H. Lee Moffitt Cancer Center and Research Institute
12902 Magnolia Dr.
Tampa, FL 33612-9497
Phone: (813)972-4673 **Free:** 888-663-3488
Fax: (813)972-3919
Website: http://www.moffitt.usf.edu
William Dalton, MD, CEO
Activities/Fields: Basic, clinical, and cancer control programs in immunology, molecular oncology, experimental therapeutics, genetic immunotherapy, behavioral oncology, cancer prevention, tobacco intervention, digital medical imaging. Conducts clinical programs in all disease sites, including breast; thoracic oncology, cutaneous, and bone marrow transplantation, etc. **Pub:** *Cancer Control*, quarterly. • *Lifetime Choices*, 3/year. • *Today's Tomorrows*, quarterly.

★ 22440 ★ Hahnemannian Research Center, Inc.
18818 Teller Ave., Ste. 230
Irvine, CA 92612
Phone: (949)852-9038 **Fax:** (949)852-1353
Email: laiushshm@aol.com
Website: http://www.hahnemannian.com
Kattunilathu Oommen George, MD, Pres.
Activities/Fields: Homeopathic medicine and education, including biochemical analysis, micronutrition, Mother Tincture development, structural and degenerative studies, and deficiency detection (electromagnetic disturbances) with attention given to the emotional, mental, and physical aspects. **Pub:** *Hahnemannian Quarterly Publication.*

★ 22441 ★ Hamilton Regional Cancer Center
699 Concession St.
Hamilton, ON, Canada L8V 5C2
Phone: (905)387-9495 **Fax:** (905)575-6323
Email: george.browman@hrcc.on.ca
Dr. George Browman, CEO
Activities/Fields: Basic research focusing on tumor cell signalling and experimental therapeutics and clinical trials and supportive care research in cancer. Translational research focusing on new therapeutics from basic to clinical is highly encouraged.

★ 22442 ★ Harlan/Missouri University Mutant Mouse Regional Resource Center
Harlan Sprague Dawley, Inc.
298 S Carroll Rd.
Indianapolis, IN 46229
Phone: (317)894-7521 **Fax:** (317)894-4473
Email: rjrussell@harlan.com
Robert J. Russell, DVM, Prin. Investigator
Activities/Fields: Cryobiology focusing on improving methods for cryopreservation and banking of mouse spermatozoa and ovarian tissue; health monitoring, focusing on developing novel antemortem techniques for detection of microbial pathogens.

★ 22443 ★ Harvard Brain Tissue Resource Center
McLean Hospital
115 Mill St.
Belmont, MA 02478-9106
Phone: (617)855-2401 **Free:** 800-272-4622
Fax: (617)855-3199
Email: btrc@mclean.harvard.edu
Website: http://www.mcleanhospital.org/research/braintissue.html
Francine M. Benes, MD, Contact
Activities/Fields: Provides tissues to the neuroscience community for studies of movement disorders, major psychoses, and dementia. **Frmly:** Brain Tissue Resource Center.

★ 22444 ★ Harvard Thorndike Laboratory
330 Brookline Ave.
Boston, MA 02215
Phone: (617)667-3020 **Fax:** (617)667-1615
Email: jmorgan@bidmc.harvard.edu
Dr. James P. Morgan, Dir.
Activities/Fields: Effects of drugs and disease on cardiac hypertrophy and failure; cardiovascular effects of drug abuse. Specific areas of research include cardiac and vasculary pharmacology, physiology, and biochemistry.

★ 22445 ★ Harvard University Berman-Gund Laboratory for the Study of Retinal Degenerations
Massachusetts Eye & Ear Infirmary
243 Charles St.
Boston, MA 02114
Phone: (617)573-3600 **Fax:** (617)573-3216
Eliot L. Berson, MD, Dir.
Activities/Fields: Effects of nutrition and light on the retina, gene detection of different forms of retinitis pigmentosa and gene therapy for animal models of hereditary retinal degenerations, human age-related macular degeneration.

★ 22446 ★ Harvard University Center for Biostatistics in AIDS Research
Harvard School of Public Health
651 Huntington Ave.
Boston, MA 02115
Phone: (617)432-2814 **Fax:** (617)432-2843
Email: andersen@sdac.harvard.edu
Dr. Janet Andersen, Exec. Dir.
Activities/Fields: Treatments for persons infected with HIV. **Frmly:** Statistical Data and Analysis Center.

★ 22447 ★ Harvard University Center for Health Communication
Harvard School of Public Health
677 Huntington Ave.
Boston, MA 02115
Phone: (617)432-1038 **Fax:** (617)731-8184
Email: tmendoza@hsph.harvard.edu
Website: http://www.hsph.harvard.edu/chc
Jay A. Winsten, PhD, Dir.
Activities/Fields: Contributions of mass communication to healthy behavior changes and policy. **Pub:** *World Health News.*

★ 22448 ★ Harvard University Center for Health and the Global Environment
Harvard Medical School
333 Longwood Ave., No. 640
Boston, MA 02115
Phone: (617)432-0493 **Fax:** (617)432-2595
Email: chge@hms.harvard.edu
Website: http://www.med.harvard.edu/chge
Eric Chivian, MD, Dir.
Activities/Fields: Human health consequences of global environmental change and the protection of the environment.

★ 22449 ★ Harvard University Center for Quality of Care Research and Education (QCARE)
677 Huntington Ave.
Boston, MA 02115
Phone: (617)432-2027 **Fax:** (617)432-3199
Email: qcare@hsph.harvard.edu
Website: http://www.hsph.harvard.edu/qcare
Dr. R. Heather Palmer, Dir.
Activities/Fields: Clinical performance measures for application in a wide range of health care delivery settings.

★ 22450 ★ Harvard University Division of Health Policy Research and Education
180 Longwood Ave.
Boston, MA 02115
Phone: (617)432-1325 **Fax:** (617)432-3503
Email: newhouse@hcp.med.harvard.edu
Dr. Joseph Newhouse, Dir.
Activities/Fields: Coordinates health policy resources throughout the University, including suggestion of new research initiatives, stimulation of educational activities, coordination of research and educational efforts, promotion of multidisciplinary analysis of complex health policy issues, and dissemination of health policy findings. **Pub:** *Annual Report.*

★ 22451 ★ Harvard University Harvard AIDS Institute
651 Huntington Ave.
Boston, MA 02115
Phone: (617)432-4400 **Fax:** (617)432-4545
Email: hai@hsph.harvard.edu
Website: http://www.aids.harvard.edu
Dr. Richard Marlink, Exec. Dir.
Activities/Fields: HIV-1 subtype C, the subtype predominant in Africa, and development of a vaccine to counter this particular strain.

★ 22452 ★ Harvard University Harvard Center for Cancer Prevention
Harvard School of Public Health
665 Huntington Ave., Bldg. 2, Rm. 105
Boston, MA 02115
Phone: (617)432-0038 **Fax:** (617)432-1722
Email: hccp@hsph.harvard.edu
Website: http://www.hsph.harvard.edu/cancer/index.html
David J. Hunter, MD, Dir.
Activities/Fields: Cancer prevention. **Pub:** *Newsletter*, bimonthly.

★ 22453 ★ Harvard University Harvard Eating Disorders Center (HEDC)
WACC 725
15 Parkman St.
Boston, MA 02114
Phone: (617)236-7766
Email: info@hedc.org
Website: http://www.hedc.org/
David B. Herzog, MD, Pres.
Activities/Fields: Eating disorders, their detection, treatment, and prevention. **Pub:** *Newsletter*, annually.

★ 22454 ★ Harvard University Harvard Education and Research Center
Occupational Health Program
School of Public Health
665 Huntington Ave.
Boston, MA 02115
Phone: (617)432-1260 **Fax:** (617)432-3441
Email: dchris@hohp.harvard.edu
Website: http://www.hsph.harvard.edu/erc/
David C. Christiani, Dir.
Activities/Fields: Cause and prevention of the leading work-related safety and health problems.

★ 22455 ★ Harvard University Harvard NIEHS Center for Environmental Health
665 Huntington Ave.
Boston, MA 02115
Phone: (617)432-1272 **Fax:** (617)277-2382
Email: brain@hsph.harvard.edu
Website: http://www.hsph.harvard.edu/kresge
Prof. Joseph D. Brain, Dir.
Activities/Fields: Environmental health, including interdisciplinary studies on effects and control of air pollutants, occupational health and medicine, environmental and respiratory physiology, radiation biology, toxicology and air sampling, exposure/dose assessment, water microbiology, and personnel protection. **Pub:** *Annual report.* **Frmly:** Kresge Center for Environmental Health.

★ 22456 ★ Harvard University Howe Laboratory of Ophthalmology
Massachusetts Eye & Ear Infirmary
243 Charles St.
Boston, MA 02114
Phone: (617)573-3963 **Fax:** (617)573-4290
Website: http://www.howelaboratory.harvard.edu
Frederick A. Jakobiec, Actg. Dir.
Activities/Fields: Programs to study development, structure, function, and malfunction of the mammalian visual system. Current investigations focus on mechanisms of retinal functioning, development, and degeneration; ocular tumors; glaucoma; corneal wound healing; and ocular inflammatory diseases.

★ 22457 ★ Harvard University Laboratory for Cell and Molecular Biology
Burl Bldg., 5th Fl.
Department of Medicine
New England Deaconess Hospital
185 Pilgrim Rd.
Boston, MA 02215
Phone: (617)632-9982 **Fax:** (617)632-9992
Dr. Arthur J. Sytkowski, Dir.
Activities/Fields: Biology of blood cell production, control mechanisms involved in normal cell growth and development, and identification of factors responsible for malignant transformation and neoplastic or cancerous growth. Ongoing studies include identifying the structural and functional properties of the erythropoietin molecule and the mechanisms of interaction with its receptor on the cell surface, identifying the role of cellular oncogenes in blood cell growth and differentiation, characterizing erythropoietin early response genes, and investigating gene therapy and erythroid burst promoting activity. Studies have direct applications to clinical syndromes accompanied by disordered blood cell production, leukemia, lymphoma, and cancer.

★ 22458 ★ Harvard University Laboratory of Immunology
Harvard Medical Sch.
200 Longwood Ave., 5th Fl., D-530
Boston, MA 02115
Phone: (617)432-1978 **Fax:** (617)432-2789
Email: martin_dorf@hms.harvard.edu
Dr. Martin Dorf, Dir.
Activities/Fields: Indentification of chemokines and their receptors. Applications to autoimmunity.

★ 22459 ★ Harvard University Motion Analysis Laboratory
Harvard Medical School
125 Nashua St.
Boston, MA 02114
Phone: (617)573-2745 **Fax:** (617)573-2769
Email: pbonato@partners.org
Website: http://www.hmcnet.harvard.edu/pmr/
Prof. Paolo Bonato, Contact
Activities/Fields: Human movement, including dynamics and kinematics, with emphasis on the neural control and biomechanics of posture and locomotion.

★ 22460 ★ Harvard University New England Regional Primate Research Center
1 Pine Hill Dr.
PO Box 9102
Southborough, MA 01772-9102
Phone: (508)624-8042 **Fax:** (508)624-8190
Website: http://www.hms.harvard.edu/nerprc/
Dr. Ronald C. Desrosiers, Dir.
Activities/Fields: Diseases of simian primates, as they relate to clinical and comparative pathology, behavioral biology, immunology, molecular virology, microbiology, viral oncology, nutrition, and primatology.

★ 22461 ★ Harvard University Prevention Research Center on Nutrition and Physical Activity
677 Huntington Ave.
Boston, MA 02115
Phone: (617)432-1135 **Fax:** (617)432-3755
Email: sgortmak@hsph.harvard.edu
Steven Gortmaker, Prin. Investigator
Activities/Fields: Public health issues, especially behaviors that place Americans at risk for chronic diseases and conditions. Of particular concern is the improvement in quality of life for special populations, including the young, elderly, racial ethnic populations, and the underserved.

★ 22462 ★ Harvey W. Peters Research Center for the Study of Parkinson's Disease and Disorders of the Central Nervous System
Davidson Hall
Department of Chemistry
Virginia Polytechnic Institute and State University
Blacksburg, VA 24061-0212
Phone: (540)231-8200 **Fax:** (540)231-8890
Prof. James F. Wolfe, Co-Dir.
Activities/Fields: Molecular mechanisms of xenobiotic metabolism, and chemically-induced neurodegenerative processes, focusing on Parkinson's disease and epileptic disorders.

★ 22463 ★ Haskins Laboratories
270 Crown St.
New Haven, CT 06511-6695
Phone: (203)865-6163 **Fax:** (203)865-8963
Email: haskins@haskins.yale.edu
Website: http://www.haskins.yale.edu
Dr. Carol A. Fowler, Pres. /Dir.
Activities/Fields: Speech production and perception by humans and computers, motor control, and reading.

★ 22464 ★ Hauptman-Woodward Medical Research Institute, Inc.
73 High St.
Buffalo, NY 14203-1196
Phone: (716)856-9600 **Fax:** (716)852-6086
Email: hauptman@hwi.buffalo.edu
Website: http://www.hwi.buffalo.edu
Herbert A. Hauptman, PhD, Pres.
Activities/Fields: Molecular endocrinology to determine molecular structures of biologically important small and macromolecular compounds, to correlate the structures with their biological activities, and to elucidate the mechanism of hormone biosynthesis. Also has programs in space- and ground-based crystal growth and phasing methods in macromolecular structure determination. Specific interests include structural biology and molecular endocrinology. molecular level. **Pub:** *Structures Newsletter*, quarterly. **Frmly:** Medical Foundation of Buffalo Inc.

★ 22465 ★ Hawaii Heptachlor Research and Education Foundation
c/o Sherry P. Broder
841 Bishop St., Ste. 800
Honolulu, HI 96813
Phone: (808)531-1411 **Fax:** (808)561-8411
Email: hhref@lava.net
Website: http://www.lava.net/~hhref
Dr. Willis Butler, Pres.
Activities/Fields: Sponsors and supports medical research and medical treatment programs, including research on the effects of pesticides and other toxic substances on humans, and methods and treatment of medical problems caused by exposure to such substances. Current research projects include a medical monitoring program, which will examine the health effects of chronic exposure of Oahu's residents to Heptachlor in dairy products. Other projects sponsored by the Foundation include Induction of Parkinsonian Syndrome by Heptachlor and a feasibility study on the long-term health effects in women of exposure to chlorinated hydrocarbon insecticides.

★ 22466 ★ Head and Neck Center
2157 Main St.
Buffalo, NY 14214
Phone: (716)862-1900 **Fax:** (716)862-1899
Website: http://www.sisters-buffalo.org/home/cancer/headneck/
Patrick J. Wiles, Pres. /CEO
Activities/Fields: Basic and clinical studies on head and neck cancer, especially in the areas of wound healing, bone regeneration, and biomaterials. **Frmly:** Center of Excellence in Otolaryncology.

★ 22467 ★ Health Effects Institute (HEI)
Charlestown Navy Yard
120 2nd Ave.
Boston, MA 02129-4533
Phone: (617)886-9330 **Fax:** (617)886-9335
Email: dgreenbaum@healtheffects.org
Website: http://www.healtheffects.org/index.html
Daniel S. Greenbaum, Pres.
Activities/Fields: Health effects of pollutants from motor vehicles and from other sources in the environment. **Pub:** *Annual report.* • *Newsletter*, quarterly. • *Research reports.* • *Special reports.*

★ 22468 ★ Health Research and Educational Trust of New Jersey
760 Alexander Rd.
Princeton, NJ 08543-0001
Phone: (609)275-4145 **Fax:** (609)275-4228
Email: fvali@njha.com
Website: http://www.njha.com
Valerie Sellers, Sr. VP, Health Plan. & Res.
Activities/Fields: Health services in New Jersey. Topics explored include access to primary healthcare, domestic violence, parenting education, child abuse prevention, breast cancer, newborn screening.

★ 22469 ★ Health Research, Inc.
1 University Pl.
Rensselaer, NY 12144-3455
Phone: (518)431-1200 **Fax:** (518)431-1234
Website: http://www.hrinet.org
Dawn Cox, Dir.
Activities/Fields: Public health and cancer, including basic and clinical research in cause and treatment of cancer and related malignancies; environmental studies to determine long-range health hazards of pesticides, industrial discharge, and radioactive and sewage wastes; and detection and prevention of infectious diseases, including AIDS and tuberculosis. Also studies rehabilitation, biology, immunology, hematology, virology, chemistry, toxicology, and environment.

★ 22470 ★ Heart Disease Research Foundation
50 Court St.
Brooklyn, NY 11201
Phone: (718)649-6210 **Fax:** (718)649-6210
Beatrice Peters, Pres.
Activities/Fields: Early diagnosis, prevention, and treatment of cardiovascular diseases and related medical and social problems. Studies include the effects of acupuncture and electro-therapeutics on blood chemistry and the cardiovascular system and clinical approaches of these methods directed toward the treatment of abnormal brain circulation and blood pressure and lower extremity circulatory disturbances.

★ 22471 ★ Heart Institute of Spokane
122 W 7th Ave., Ste. 230
Spokane, WA 99204-2340
Phone: (509)625-3020 **Fax:** (509)625-3025
Email: ktuttle@this.org
Website: http://www.this.org
Katherine R. Tuttle, MD, Dir.

Activities/Fields: Heart and vascular diseases, focusing on renal diseases. Pub: *Newsletter.*

★ 22472 ★ Heart Research Foundation of Sacramento
3900 J St.
Sacramento, CA 95819
Phone: (916)456-3365 **Fax:** (916)452-7579
Email: hrfsac@hrfsac.org
Website: http://www.hrfsac.org
Patti Gantenbein, Exec. Dir.
Activities/Fields: Clinical and pathological studies of atherosclerosis and coronary, myocardial, and conduction system morphology. **Pub:** *Inflammatory Atherosclerosis: Nature of the Injurious Agent.*

★ 22473 ★ Heart and Stroke Foundation of British Columbia and Yukon
1212 W Broadway
Vancouver, BC, Canada V6H 3V2
Phone: (604)736-4404 **Fax:** (604)736-8732
Email: info@hsf.ca
Website: http://www.heartandstroke.ca
Bobbe Wood, Exec. Dir.
Activities/Fields: Provides research support in the form of personnel awards and grants-in-aid for studies on heart disease and stroke. Fellowships provide salary support for young scientists just beginning a career in research. Grants-in-aid finance research projects of an experienced and salaried professional or university faculty member, paying for such things as equipment, expendables (glassware and chemicals), and technical assistance. A limited number of Heart and Stroke Foundation research traineeships are available to highly qualified graduate students enrolled in a PhD program and who are undertaking full-time research training in the cardiovascular or cerebrovascular fields.

★ 22474 ★ Heart and Stroke Foundation of Canada
222 Queen St., Ste. 1402
Ottawa, ON, Canada K1P 5V9
Phone: (613)569-4361 **Fax:** (613)569-3278
Email: astephen@hsf.ca
Website: http://www.hsf.ca/research
Alison M. Stephen, Dir.
Activities/Fields: Provides grants for research in cardiovascular and cerebrovascular diseases, particularly the elucidation of fundamental laws and the development of materials, devices, systems, or methods useful in treating stroke, heart attack, hypertension, and effects of smoking. **Frmly:** Canadian Heart and Stroke Foundation.

★ 22475 ★ Heart and Stroke Foundation of Newfoundland and Labrador
169-173 Water St.
PO Box 5819
Saint John's, NL, Canada A1C 5X3
Phone: (709)753-8521 **Free:** 888-473-4636
Fax: (709)753-3117
Website: http://ww1.heartandstroke.ca/
Stephen Browne, Exec. Dir.
Activities/Fields: Causes of and cures for cardiovascular and cerebrovascular disease.

★ 22476 ★ Heart and Stroke Foundation of Nova Scotia
5523 Spring Garden Rd., Ste. 204
Halifax, NS, Canada B3J 3T1
Phone: (902)423-7530 **Fax:** (902)492-1464
Website: http://ww2.heartandstroke.ca/
J.E. Fraser, Exec. Dir.
Activities/Fields: Cardiovascular and cerebrovascular basic and clinical research, including educational and behavioral science approaches to cardiovascular health. **Pub:** *Research Directory.* **Frmly:** Nova Scotia Heart Foundation.

★ 22477 ★ Heimlich Institute
311 Straight St.
Cincinnati, OH 45219
Phone: (513)559-2391 **Fax:** (513)559-2403
Email: heimlich@lglou.com
Website: http://www.heimlichinstitute.org
Henry J. Heimlich, MD, Pres.
Activities/Fields: Malaria therapy for cancer and Lyme disease, rehabilitation of swallowing, and transtracheal oxygen therapy for chronic lung diseases, including oxygen-dependent emphysema, black lung, cystic fibrosis, and interstitial fibrosis. Developments include Heimlich Maneuver for choking and drowning, Heimlich chest drainage valve, Heimlich Micro-Trach, and Heimlich operation for esophageal replacement. **Pub:** *Newsletter.* **Frmly:** Dysphagia Foundation.

★ 22478 ★ Heineman Medical Research
PO Box 32861
Charlotte, NC 28232-2861
Phone: (704)355-3200 **Fax:** (704)355-1435
Website: http://www.heineman.org
Francis Robicsek, MD, Pres.
Activities/Fields: Diseases of heart, lungs, and great vessels, with special interest in organ preservation, electrophysiology, and laser applications to arrhythmias and vascular diseases. **Pub:** *Bulletin of Cardiopulmonary Disease.* • *Heineman Report.*

★ 22479 ★ Hektoen Institute for Medical Research
2100 W Harrison St.
Chicago, IL 60612-9982
Phone: (312)738-3100 **Fax:** (312)738-3102
Email: LabHektoen@aol.com
Website: http://www.themeasurementgroup.com/edcpage/hektoen.html
Peter Friedell, MD, Chm.
Activities/Fields: Medicine and surgery, including laboratory and clinical studies in cancer metabolism, kidney disease, virology, hematology, microbiology, bacteriology, endocrinology, pediatric cardiology, neurology, immunology, pathology, gastroenterology, orthopedic surgery, congenital heart diseases, infectious diseases, and hypertension. Specific investigations include treatment of cancer by new modalities, incidence of perinatal mortality and effect of neonatal care, metabolic aspects of renal disease, cell surface alterations in cancer and their effects on metastasis, effects of different hormones in breast carcinoma, influence of hormone receptors on several varieties of soft tissue sarcomas and malignant melanomas, and the immunological aspects of prostatic cancer. **Pub:** *Biennial Report.*

★ 22480 ★ Helen Hayes Hospital Center for Neural Recovery and Rehabilitation Research
Rte. 9W
West Haverstraw, NY 10993-1195
Phone: (845)786-4859 **Fax:** (845)786-4875
Email: scharfmanh@helenhayeshosp.org
Helen E. Scharfman, PhD, Dir.
Activities/Fields: Epilepsy, brain injury, neuroendocrinology, spinal cord injury, neurobiology. Degenerative neurological disorders such as Huntington's and Alzheimer's diseases are also investigated. **Pub:** *Scientific Journals*, 3/year. **Frmly:** Neurology Research Center.

★ 22481 ★ Helen Hayes Hospital Regional Bone Center
Rte. 9W
West Haverstraw, NY 10993
Phone: (845)786-4839 **Free:** 888-707-3422
Fax: (845)786-4878
Email: dempster@helenhayeshosp.org
Website: http://www.helenhayeshospital.org/research.htmregional
David W. Dempster, PhD, Dir.
Activities/Fields: Bone and calcium metabolism, including pathophysiology of bone and clinical research on the pathogenesis and treatment of diseases such as osteoporosis, primary hyperparathyroidism, and Paget's disease. Conducts calciotropic hormone assays, bone biopsies and histomorphometry.

★ 22482 ★ Helen Keller Worldwide
352 Park Ave. S, 12th Fl.
New York, NY 10010-1709
Phone: (212)532-0544 **Free:** 877-535-5374
Fax: (212)791-7590
Email: info@hkworld.org
Website: http://www.hkworld.org
John M. Palmer, Pres.
Activities/Fields: Etiology, prevalence, incidence, and treatment of xerophthalmia (nutritional blindness), trachoma, cataract, onchocerciasis (river blindness), and other eye diseases in developing nations. Research and technical assistance conducted in Bangladesh, Brazil, Burkina Faso, Cambodia, Cameroon, China, Cote d'Ivoire, Ghana, Indonesia, Mali, Mexico, Morocco, Mozambique, Nepal, Niger, Nigeria, The Philippines, South Africa, Tanzania, United States, and Vietnam. **Pub:** *Annual report.* **Frmly:** American Foundation for the Overseas Blind.

★ 22483 ★ Helicon Foundation
4622 Santa Fe St.
San Diego, CA 92109
Phone: (858)272-3884 **Free:** 888-726-8698
Fax: (858)272-1621
Email: cathomas@ix.netcom.com
Dr. Charles A. Thomas, Jr., Pres.
Activities/Fields: Basic biological research in biochemistry, molecular biology, and genetics, including studies on oxidative damage to cellular DNA, structure of chromosomal telomeres, chromatin structure, and role of lipids in radical formation. Seeks to define the biochemical basis of disease prevention through antioxidant diagnostics.

★ 22484 ★ Henry Ford Hospital Sleep Disorders Center
2799 W Grand Blvd., CFP3
Detroit, MI 48202
Phone: (313)916-4417 **Fax:** (313)916-5150
Thomas Roth, PhD, Dir.
Activities/Fields: Psychopharmacology of sleep, daytime sleepiness, and sleep disorders, including sleep-related apnea.

★ 22485 ★ The Heuga Center
27 Main St., Ste. 303
PO Box 491
Edwards, CO 81632-0491
Phone: (970)926-1290 **Free:** 800-367-3101
Fax: (970)926-1295
Email: info@heuga.org
Website: http://www.heuga.org
Brian Hutchinson, Pres. /CEO
Activities/Fields: Improvement of the quality of life for those with multiple sclerosis (MS) and other potentially debilitating neurological disorders. Focuses on the effects of goal-oriented exercise on the fitness of those with MS.

★ 22486 ★ Hipple Cancer Research Center
4100 S Kettering Blvd.
Dayton, OH 45439
Phone: (937)293-8508 **Free:** (866)447-7538
Fax: (937)293-7652
Email: hipple@hipple.org
Website: http://www.hipple.org/mission.htm
Hans J. Berkel, MD, Pres. /CEO
Activities/Fields: Cancer prevention and control. **Pub:** *Newsletter.*

★ 22487 ★ HIV Center for Clinical and Behavioral Studies
New York State Psychiatric Institute
1051 Riverside Dr., Unit 15
New York, NY 10032
Phone: (212)543-5969 **Fax:** (212)543-6003
Email: ehrharda@child.cpmc.columbia.edu
Website: http://www.hivcenternyc.org
Anke A. Ehrhardt, PhD, Dir.
Activities/Fields: Investigates high risk sexual behaviors leading to HIV infection among heterosexual adults (especially women), adolescents, and gay men. Studies include prevention among depressed adolescent girls and gay and lesbian adolescents, development of interventions aimed at heterosexual women and men, serodiscordant male couples, and homeless mentally ill men and women. Methods development and quality assurance proceed in the domains of psychosocial and qualitative assessment, psychosexual assessment, biostatistics, data management, and epidemiology. Conducts programs in community liaison, media-based interventions and education, and ethical, legal, and policy issues. **Pub:** *Bibliography.*

★ 22488 ★ Hollins Communications Research Institute
PO Box 9737
Roanoke, VA 24020-1737
Phone: (540)265-5650 **Fax:** (540)265-0386
Email: admhcri@rbnet.com
Website: http://www.stuttering.org
Ronald L. Webster, PhD, Dir.
Activities/Fields: Basic features of stuttering, behaviorally-based stuttering therapy, and variables that modify speech fluency in people who stutter and fluent speakers.

★ 22489 ★ Holos Institutes of Health
5607 S 222nd Rd.
Fair Grove, MO 65648
Phone: (417)267-2900 **Fax:** (417)267-3102
Email: orme@normshealy.net
C. Norman Shealy, MD, Pres.
Activities/Fields: Clinical studies in holistic medicine with emphasis on neurochemical profiles and management of biochemical aspects of pain and stress. **Frmly:** Shealy Institutes of Health.

★ 22490 ★ Homeopathic Council for Research and Education
50 Park Ave.
New York, NY 10016
Phone: (212)684-2290 **Fax:** (212)684-4694
William Bergman, MD, Contact
Activities/Fields: Homeopathy, focusing on research and education.

★ 22491 ★ Hope Heart Institute
1710 E Jefferson St.
Seattle, WA 98122
Phone: (206)903-2001 **Fax:** (206)903-2144
Email: info@hopeheart.org
Website: http://www.hopeheart.org
Davis B. Fox, Contact
Activities/Fields: Prevention and treatment of cardiovascular disease. The institute has three research divisions: Basic Sciences, Translational Sciences, and Community Public Health. Basic Sciences is primarily studies of vascular biology, angiogenesis and cell and molecular biology of the vascular extracellular matrix. Translational Sciences include cardiovascular gene therapy and tissue engineering, as well as cardioneurology. Community Public Health includes general public education and prevention programs on cardiovascular disease, through outreach and research and multicultural settings. Major research projects include understanding angiogenesis (the growth of new blood vessels), extracellular matrix deposition (the formation of the blood vessel plaques), new techniques for developing blood vessels and heart patches out of a person's own cells, wound healing, and education research in underserved communities. **Pub:** *Booklets.* • *Brochures.* • *Hope Health Newsletter.* • *Medical journals.* • *Take Heart Newsletter.* • *Videos.*

★ 22492 ★ Hospital for Joint Diseases Orthopaedic Institute Geriatric Hip Fracture Research Group
301 E 17th St.
New York, NY 10003
Phone: (212)598-6106 **Fax:** (212)598-6793
Email: gina.aharonoff@med.nyu.edu
Joseph D. Zuckerman, MD, Dir.
Activities/Fields: Hip fracture patients and their recovery after surgery.

★ 22493 ★ Hospital for Joint Diseases Orthopaedic Institute Musculoskeletal Research Center
301 E 17th St., 15th Fl.
New York, NY 10003
Phone: (212)598-6567 **Fax:** (212)598-6096
Email: pedicesare@aol.com
Paul Di Cesare, MD, Dir.
Activities/Fields: Prevention and treatment of musculoskeletal diseases, including basic studies of biological and synthetic biomaterials, biomechanics, kinematics, mathematical modeling, arthritis, and cartilage repair, and gene therapy.

★ 22494 ★ Hospital for Joint Diseases Orthopaedic Institute Shoulder Institute and Research Group
301 E 17th St.
New York, NY 10003
Phone: (212)598-6498 **Fax:** (212)598-6096
Website: http://www.med.nyu.edu/ortho/research5.htmlshoulder
Frances Cuomo, MD, Dir.
Activities/Fields: Shoulder disorders, including the effect of osteoarthritis and instability on proprioceptive ability, strength recovery following rotator cuff repair, operative vs. nonoperative treatment of type II distal clavicle fractures, and recovery of strength and propriaception after two different capsulorrhaphy procedures.

★ 22495 ★ Hospital for Sick Children Research Institute
555 University Ave.
Toronto, ON, Canada M5G 1X8
Phone: (416)813-6350 **Fax:** (416)813-4931
Email: buchwald@sickkids.on.ca
Website: http://www.sickkids.on.ca
Dr. Manuel Buchwald, Dir.
Activities/Fields: Basic and clinical research focused on improving, understanding, preventing, treating and curing children's diseases. Six disciplinary research programs: genetics and genomic biology; structural biology and biochemistry; cell biology; developmental biology; integrative biology; population health sciences. Six interdisciplinary research programs: brain and behavior; cancer and blood; cardiovascular; infection, immunity, injury and repair; lung biology; metabolism. Interdisciplinary research groups focused on specific challenges: cystic fibrosis, lung gene therapy. **Pub:** *Annual Report.*

★ 22496 ★ Hospital for Special Surgery Fannie E. Rippel Flow Cytometry Core Facility
Belaire Bldg., Rm. 705
525 E 71st St.
New York, NY 10021
Phone: (212)606-1925 **Fax:** (212)774-2337
Email: rudchenkos@hss.edu
Website: http://www.hss.edu/htdoc/research/flow/index.asp
Sergei Rudchenko, Dir.
Activities/Fields: Flow cytometry: multiparameter cell sorting and cellular analysis. **Pub:** *HSS Flow Core Newsletter.*

★ 22497 ★ Hospital for Special Surgery Research Division
535 E 70th St.
New York, NY 10021
Phone: (212)774-2394 **Fax:** (212)774-2301
Email: grassiah@hss.edu
Website: http://www.hss.edu
Vincent L. Grassia, Jr., VP, Res. Admin.
Activities/Fields: Orthopedics and rheumatic diseases, including studies on bone, cartilage, connective tissues, immune system, and related areas of musculoskeletal disease. **Pub:** *Discovery to Recovery.* • *HSS Development Office.* **Frmly:** Philip D. Wilson Research Foundation.

★ 22498 ★ Hospital for Special Surgery Research Division Biomechanics and Biomaterials Section
535 E 70th St.
New York, NY 10021
Phone: (212)606-1093 **Fax:** (212)606-1490
Email: wrightt@hss.edu
Website: http://www.hss.edu/
Timothy Wright, PhD, Sect. Hd.
Activities/Fields: Application of principles of mechanics and materials science in order to understand and treat orthopedic problems.

★ 22499 ★ Hospital for Special Surgery Research Division Laboratory for Soft Tissues Research
535 E 70th St.
New York, NY 10021
Phone: (212)606-1178 **Fax:** (212)772-6389
Email: torzilli@hss.edu
Peter A. Torzilli, PhD, Contact
Activities/Fields: Connective soft tissues, such as cartilage, ligament, tendon, meniscus, and how they relate.

★ 22500 ★ Hospital for Special Surgery Research Division Mineralized Tissues Research Section
535 E 70th St.
New York, NY 10021
Phone: (212)606-1459 **Fax:** (212)472-5331
Email: boskeya@hss.edu
Website: http://www.hss.edu
Adele L. Boskey, PhD, Lab. Hd.
Activities/Fields: Mechanisms of calcification and mineralized tissue remodeling, calcium handling by cells, cell and molecular biology of diseases of calcified tissues (including osteoporosis and osteogenesis imperfecta), IR imaging of connective tissues, and fiber optic probe for cartilage evaluation.

★ 22501 ★ House Ear Institute
2100 W 3rd St.
Los Angeles, CA 90057
Phone: (213)483-4431 **Fax:** (213)483-8789
Email: webmaster@hei.org
Website: http://www.hei.org
James D. Boswell, CEO
Activities/Fields: Cause, treatment, and prevention of hearing and balance disorders, including investigations on cochlear implants and auditory prostheses, electrophysiology, electron microscopy, anatomy, cellular and molecular biology, and psychoacoustics. **Pub:** *Annual Report.* • *The Review,* 3/year. **Frmly:** Ear Research Institute.

★ 22502 ★ Houston Advanced Research Center DNA Technology Laboratory
4800 Research Forest Dr.
The Woodlands, TX 77381
Phone: (281)363-7947 **Fax:** (281)363-7935
Email: dao@harc.edu
Website: http://www.harc.edu/dna/
Dr. Dat D. Dao, Dir.

Activities/Fields: Development and application of DNA technologies, especially applications of genosensor technology, which are miniaturized DNA chips that can quickly analyze genetic alterations.

★ 22503 ★ Houston Ear Research Foundation
7737 Southwest Fwy., Ste. 630
Houston, TX 77074
Phone: (713)771-9966 **Free:** 800-843-0807
Fax: (713)771-0546
Email: jangil@hern.org
Jan Gilden, Exec. Dir.
Activities/Fields: Aims to improve health care and education for deaf and hearing-impaired children. Provides funds for follow-up testing for recipients of cochlear implants. **Pub:** *Newsletter*, annually.

★ 22504 ★ Howard Hughes Medical Institute
4000 Jones Bridge Rd.
Chevy Chase, MD 20815-6789
Phone: (301)215-8500 **Fax:** (301)215-8863
Website: http://www.hhmi.org
Thomas R. Cech, PhD, Pres.
Activities/Fields: Molecular biology, especially genetics, immunology, cell biology, structural biology, neuroscience, and computational biology. Conducts research with scientists and staff at over 70 academic medical centers, universities and other research organizations. **Pub:** *Annual report.* • *H HMImagazine*, quarterly.

★ 22505 ★ Howard University Cancer Center
2041 Georgia Ave. NW
Washington, DC 20060
Phone: (202)806-7697 **Fax:** (202)462-8928
Email: ladams-campbell@howard.edu
Website: http://www.med.howard.edu/hucc/
Dr. Lucille Adams-Campbell, Dir.
Activities/Fields: Multidisciplinary genomic research of African-Americans. Basic research includes molecular biology of cancer, mechanisms of metastases, tumor immunology, pharmacology of antineoplastic drugs, clinical chemotherapeutic research, pilot studies for the treatment of various neoplasms, and radiotherapeutic research, including intraoperative radiation therapy, hyperthermia, and combined modality therapy. Epidemiological research includes nutrition, cancer treatment effectiveness and various studies on the medically underserved targeted participants. Purpose is to better understand the biomedical significance of genomic variability underlying susceptability and/or resistance to common, chronic debilitating diseases and disorders using breast cancer as a prototype.

★ 22506 ★ Howard University Center for Sickle Cell Disease
2121 Georgia Ave. NW
Washington, DC 20059
Phone: (202)806-7930 **Fax:** (202)806-4517
Dr. Oswaldo Castro, Dir.
Activities/Fields: Sickle cell disease, including basic and clinical investigations of its nature, causes, effects, and potential control. Develops and implements high quality total care for victims of the disease. Develops and evaluates methods of prevention through screening for sickle and other abnormal hemoglobins and participates in the Mid-Atlantic Regional Genetic Counseling Program. **Pub:** *Annual Report.*

★ 22507 ★ Howard University Child Development Center
Department of Pediatrics & Child Health
College of Medicine
525 Bryant St. NW, Ste. 100-B
Washington, DC 20059
Phone: (202)806-6973 **Fax:** (202)806-7940
Sheila J. Moseend, Dir.
Activities/Fields: Child development and handicapping conditions of childhood, including interdisciplinary studies in pediatrics, neurology, genetics, psychology, speech pathology, and infant development.

★ 22508 ★ Howard University General Clinical Research Center
Howard University Hospital, 4th Fl., West
2041 Georgia Ave. NW
Washington, DC 20060
Phone: (202)865-7272 **Fax:** (202)865-1933
Email: orandall@howard.edu
Website: http://www.gcrc.howard.edu
Otelio S. Randall, MD, Prog. Dir.
Activities/Fields: Major areas of investigation include cardiovascular diseases, dermatology, endocrinology, genetic disorders, geriatrics and gerontology, infectious diseases, metabolism, hyperlipidemia and obesity, neurology and nutrition. **Pub:** *GCRC Newsletter*, quarterly.

★ 22509 ★ Human Performance International (HPI)
402-1228 Hamilton St.
Vancouver, BC, Canada V6B 6L2
Phone: (604)684-6192 **Fax:** (604)684-6194
Email: info@humanperformance.ca
Website: http://www.humanperformance.ca
Dr. Dan Q. Marisi, Dir.
Activities/Fields: Biomechanical, physiological, and psychological and medical factors affecting human performance during competitive racing and other athletic activities, such as the influence of body heat on cardiovascular stress.

★ 22510 ★ Hunter College of City University of New York Center for Study of Gene Structure and Function
695 Park Ave.
New York, NY 10021
Phone: (212)772-5170 **Fax:** (212)772-5466
Email: dottin@genectr.hunter.cuny.edu
Website: http://sonhouse.hunter.cuny.edu/genecenter/
Robert Dottin, Dir.
Activities/Fields: Structure of proteins and nucleic acids by X-ray diffraction and molecular modeling, the characterization of protein-protein interactions involved in signal transduction, and the investigation of mechanisms that regulate neuron functioning and regeneration.

★ 22511 ★ Huntington Medical Research Institutes
734 Fairmount Ave.
Pasadena, CA 91105
Phone: (626)397-5851 **Fax:** (626)397-5857
Email: dougmc@hmri.org
Website: http://www.hmri.org
Douglas B. McCreery, PhD, Dir.
Activities/Fields: Electronic neural prosthetic device development; biology of nitric oxide; prostate and breast cancer; cell biology; moleculor genetics; neural proteomics; drug development; medical applications of magnetic resonance using protons, phosphorous, fluorine, and nitrogen; magnetoencephalography and brain mapping in epilespy. **Pub:** *Newsletter*, quarterly.

★ 22512 ★ Huntington's Disease Center Without Walls
Molecular Neurogenetics Unit
Massachusetts General Hospital East, Bldg. 149, Rm. 6214
13th St.
Charlestown, MA 02129-2060
Phone: (617)726-5724 **Fax:** (617)726-5735
Email: gusella@helix.mgh.harvard.edu
Website: http://www.mgh.harvard.edu/depts/molneur/mnu.htm
Dr. James F. Gusella, Dir.
Activities/Fields: Huntington's Disease (HD), including protein abnormalities in the HD brain and their relationship to neuronal loss, neuropathological examination of autopsy brain sections, location and measurement of chemical messengers, neuropsychological tests evaluating deficits in memory and cognitive functioning, social and psychological impact of HD on families, medications increasing levels of chemical messengers in the brain, DNA studies to determine the HD gene, and peptide localization in the nerve cells.

★ 22513 ★ Illinois Institute of Technology Pritzker Institute of Biomedical Science and Engineering
10 W 32nd St.
Chicago, IL 60616
Phone: (312)567-5324 **Fax:** (312)567-5707
Email: turitto@iit.edu
Website: http://www.iit.edu/~bme
Dr. Vincent Turitto, Dir.
Activities/Fields: Cell and tissue engineering, neuroengineering, medical imaging and biomaterials. **Pub:** *Annual Report of Research.* **Frmly:** Pritzker Institute of Medical Engineering.

★ 22514 ★ Illinois Institute of Technology Research Laboratory in Human Biomechanics
MMAE Department
10 W 32nd St.
Chicago, IL 60616-3793
Phone: (312)567-3179 **Fax:** (312)567-7230
Email: meade@iit.edu
Dr. Kevin Meade, Contact
Activities/Fields: Computer-aided biomechanical engineering and lower extremity neuromuscular engineering, including the use of force transducer arrays.

★ 22515 ★ Illinois Oncology Research Association
900 Main St., Ste. 780
Peoria, IL 61602
Phone: (309)671-5180 **Free:** 800-793-2262
Fax: (309)672-4138
Email: research@ohaci.com
Website: http://www.ohaci.com/research/research.htm
Activities/Fields: Cancer treatment and control, including chemotherapy, immunotherapy, hormonal therapy, and radiation therapy.

★ 22516 ★ Imaging Research Center
Cincinnati Children's Hospital Medical Center
3333 Burnet Ave.
Cincinnati, OH 45229-3039
Phone: (513)636-8574 **Fax:** (513)636-8145
Email: william.ball@chmcc.org
Website: http://www.cincinnatichildrens.org/default.htm
Dr. William S. Ball, Jr., Dir.
Activities/Fields: Diagnostic imaging technologies related to the diagnosis and treatment of diseases in children and young adults.

★ 22517 ★ Indiana University Bowen Research Center
Long Hospital, 2nd Fl.
1110 W Michigan St.
Indianapolis, IN 46202
Phone: (317)278-0300
Email: diallen@iupui.edu
Website: http://www.bowenresearchcenter.iupui.edu/bowen3.htm
Debbie Allen, MD, Dir.

Activities/Fields: Quality-of-life issues, lifestyle changes to prevent disease; health care costs, access to healthcare services for rural and underserved populations.

★ 22518 ★ Indiana University Center for Aging Research (CAR)
The Regenstrief Institute
1050 Wilshire Blvd.
Indianapolis, IN 46202
Phone: (317)630-7200 **Fax:** (317)287-3798
Email: ccallahan@regenstrief.org
Website: http://iucar.iu.edu/
Christopher M. Callahan, MD, Dir.
Activities/Fields: Aging, improvement of quality of life for older adults, how to disseminate health information to older adults and enhance self-care behaviors.

★ 22519 ★ Indiana University Center for Alzheimer's Disease and Related Disorders
550 N University Blvd., Ste. 3124
Indianapolis, IN 46202
Phone: (317)274-4333 **Fax:** (317)274-1497
Website: http://www.indiana.edu/~rugs/ctrdir/cadrnd.html
Ann-Marie Hake, MD, Co-Dir.
Activities/Fields: Alzeheimer Disease and related neuropsychiatric disorders characterized by memory loss and mood disorders in the older adult. **Frmly:** Alzheimer Disease Center and Related Neuropsychiatric Disorders.

★ 22520 ★ Indiana University General Clinical Research Center
550 N University Blvd.
Indianapolis, IN 46202
Phone: (317)274-4356 **Fax:** (317)274-7346
Email: mpeacock@iupui.edu
Website: http://www.gcrc.iupui.edu
Dr. Munro Peacock, Dir.
Activities/Fields: AIDS, alcohol, amyloidosis, bone disease, cancer, cardiology, diabetes, gene therapy, genetics, hypertension, infectious disease, metabolism, neonatalogy, neurology, pharmacology, psychiatry, and transplantation.

★ 22521 ★ Indiana University Herman B. Wells Center for Pediatric Research
Sch. of Medicine
702 Barnhill Dr., Rm. 2600
Indianapolis, IN 46202
Phone: (317)274-8900 **Fax:** (317)274-9906
Email: tnoonan@iupui.edu
Website: http://www.iupui.edu/~wellsctr/
Dr. Mary Dinauer, Dir.
Activities/Fields: Hematology and oncology, cell biology of polarized cells (including the blood-brain barrier), protein sorting in eukaryotic cells, bone marrow transplantation, clinical oncology research, pediatric oncology, DNA repair, gene therapy, developmental biology of neuroblastoma, gene transfer into stem cells, tumor immunology, clinical aspects of childhood acute myelogenous leukemia, the role of protein phosphorylation in control of cell proliferation and differentiation, clinical aspects and molecular biology of neutrophil disorders, neurooncology, late effects of CNS therapy, clinical aspects of supportive care of oncology patients, therapy for neuroblastoma, clinical use of hemotopoietic growth factors, secondary leukemias, clinical aspects of hemostasis, molecular biology of myeloid-specific gene expression, cancer biogenesis using neuroblastoma as a model, and molecular biology of nuclear retinoic acid receptors in myeloid leukemia, neuroblastoma cells, endocrinology, neonatology, pulmonary, cardiovascular development.

★ 22522 ★ Indiana University Mid-America Adolescent Sexually Transmitted Disease Cooperative Research Center
1120 South Dr.
Indianapolis, IN 46202
Phone: (317)274-1427 **Free:** 800-274-4862
Email: dporr@iupui.edu
Donald Orr, MD, Dir.
Activities/Fields: Chlamydia trachomatous, papilloma virus, gonorrhea and HIV, as well as opportunistic diseases such as pneumocystis pneumonia; genital ulcers, including herpes; and drug-resistant strains of gonorrhea.

★ 22523 ★ Indiana University Neuropsychology Research Section
702 Barnhill Dr., Rm. 1773
Indianapolis, IN 46202
Phone: (317)274-7327 **Fax:** (317)274-1337
Email: dkareken@iupui.edu
Dr. David A. Kareken, Dir.
Activities/Fields: Brain-behavior relationships as measured by functional brain imaging and neuropsychological measurement and as affected by neurologic disease and pharmacologic therapies.

★ 22524 ★ Indiana University Bloomington Borish Center for Ophthalmic Research (BCOR)
800 E Atwater Ave.
Bloomington, IN 47405-3680
Phone: (812)855-4093 **Fax:** (812)855-5417
Email: sonip@indiana.edu
Website: http://www.opt.indiana.edu/bcor/index.htm
P. Sarita Soni, Co-Dir.
Activities/Fields: Visual disorders, ocular pathologies, and systemic disease that affect the eye and its adnexia. Recent studies include contact lens comparison trials, extended wear contact lens trial, and decreasing dryness in contact lenses, collaborative longitudinal evaluation of keratoconus, teens and contact lenses, and development of confocal microscopy.

★ 22525 ★ Indiana University Bloomington Center on Aging and Aged
2805 E 10th St.
Bloomington, IN 47408-2698
Phone: (812)855-0815 **Fax:** (812)855-6194
Email: hawkinsb@indiana.edu
Website: http://www.indiana.edu/~caa/
Barbara Hawkins, Dir.
Activities/Fields: Gerontology, including developmentally disabled, handicapped, minorities, rural-isolated, and mainstream aging populations.

★ 22526 ★ Indiana University Bloomington Center for Genomics and Bioinformatics (CGB)
1001 E 3rd St.
Bloomington, IN 47405-3700
Phone: (812)855-6877 **Fax:** (812)856-9340
Email: cherbas@indiana.edu
Website: http://cgb.indiana.edu/
Peter Cherbas, Dir.
Activities/Fields: Genomics and bioinformatics.

★ 22527 ★ Indiana University Bloomington Howard Hughes Medical Institute Research Laboratory
Jordan Hall, Rm. A507
Bloomington, IN 47405
Phone: (812)855-3033 **Fax:** (812)855-2577
Email: kaufman@bio.indiana.edu
Thomas C. Kaufman, Dir.
Activities/Fields: Understanding the genetic basis of the developmental program of higher organisms. Efforts focus on the homeotic genes that play a crucial role in the development of the fruit fly Drosphilia melanogaster.

★ 22528 ★ Indiana University—Northwest Northwest Center for Medical Education
School of Medicine
3400 Broadway
Gary, IN 46403
Phone: (219)980-6556 **Fax:** (219)980-6566
Email: wbaldwin@iun.edu
Website: http://shaw.medlib.iupui.edu/nwcme/nwcme.html
William W. Baldwin, PhD, Dir.
Activities/Fields: Diabetes, mitochondria enzymes, lymphocyte activation microvessels, corneal innervation, autonomic nervous system, blood coagulation, neuroglialneuron interactions, membrane-bound transport enzymes, erthrocyte membrane skeletal proteins, avian musculoskeletal funtional morphology, bacterial growth, immunoglobulin molecular biology.

★ 22529 ★ Indiana University-Purdue University at Indianapolis Center for Bioethics (IUCB)
1481 W 10th St., Ste. CB-112
Indianapolis, IN 46202
Phone: (317)554-0148 **Fax:** (317)554-0122
Email: emeslin@iupui.edu
Website: http://www.bioethics.iu.edu/about.html
Eric M. Meslin, PhD, Dir.
Activities/Fields: Bioethics.

★ 22530 ★ Indiana University-Purdue University at Indianapolis Center for Enhancing Quality of Life in Chronic Illness (CEQL)
School of Nursing
1111 Middle Dr., NU 337B
Indianapolis, IN 46202-5107
Phone: (317)278-0511 **Fax:** (317)278-2021
Email: joausti@iupui.edu
Website: http://nursing.iupui.edu/Research/
Joan K. Austin, Contact
Activities/Fields: Improvement in the health-related quality of life in persons with chronic conditions across the life span. **Pub:** *Newsletter.*

★ 22531 ★ Indiana University-Purdue University at Indianapolis Cystic Fibrosis and Pediatric Pulmonary Clinic
702 Barnhill Dr., Rm. 4270
Indianapolis, IN 46202-5225
Phone: (317)274-5652 **Fax:** (317)274-5791
Email: heigen@iupui.edu
Howard Eigen, MD, Dir.
Activities/Fields: Cystic fibrosis and chronic lung diseases, including clinical studies of pediatric pulmonary, gastrointestinal, genetic problems, and lung inflammation.

★ 22532 ★ Indiana University-Purdue University at Indianapolis De Vault Otologic Research Laboratory
Riley 044
Indianapolis, IN 46202
Phone: (317)274-4915 **Fax:** (317)274-4949
Email: kkirk@iupui.edu
Website: http://www.indiana.edu/~rugs/ctrdir/dvorl.html
Karen Iler Kirk, Dir.
Activities/Fields: Benefit of different sensory aids to hearing-impaired children, specifically changes in speech production, speech perception, language, cognitive skills after cochlear implants.

★ 22533 ★ Indiana University-Purdue University at Indianapolis
Diabetes Research and Training Center
250 University Blvd., Ste. 122
Indianapolis, IN 46202
Phone: (317)630-6375 **Fax:** (317)278-0900
Website: http://www.indiana.edu/~rugs/ctrdir/drtc.html
Dr. David G. Marrerro, Dir.
Activities/Fields: Diabetes mellitus treatment and prevention.

★ 22534 ★ Indiana University-Purdue University at Indianapolis
Hackney Dermatology Research Laboratory
975 W Walnut St., Rm. 349
Indianapolis, IN 46202
Phone: (317)274-7115 **Fax:** (317)278-2815
Email: dspanda@iupui.edu
Website: http://mypage.iu.edu/~dspanda
Dr. Dan F. Spandau, Dir.
Activities/Fields: Skin diseases, including skin cancer and psoriasis and the genetic changes that occur with these conditions. Wound healing and the aging of skin are also studied.

★ 22535 ★ Indiana University-Purdue University at Indianapolis
Human Performance and Biomechanics Laboratory
901 W New York St.
Indianapolis, IN 46202
Phone: (317)274-0608 **Fax:** (317)278-2041
Email: amikesky@iupui.edu
Website: http://www.indiana.edu/~rugs/ctrdir/hpmbl.html
Dr. Alan E. Mikesky, Dir.
Activities/Fields: Sports medicine and biomechanics.

★ 22536 ★ Indiana University-Purdue University at Indianapolis
Hypertension Research Center
541 Clinical Dr., Rm. 423
Indianapolis, IN 46202-5111
Phone: (317)274-8153 **Fax:** (317)278-0673
Email: mweinbe@iupui.edu
Dr. Myron H. Weinberger, Dir.
Activities/Fields: Hypertension, including a broad-based, multidisciplinary research program of clinical studies involving genetics of hypertension, pathophysiology of hypertension with plasma renin suppression, role of renin and aldosterone in toxemia of pregnancy, causes of childhood hypertension, and role of renin and aldosterone in heart failure. Also studies myocardial metabolism and cyclic AMP system in spontaneously hypertensive rats, role of sympathetic nervous system in human experimental forms of hypertension, control of renin release in vitro and of renal sodium handling, role of sodium in blood pressure, sodium restriction in the treatment of hypertension, and role of calcium and potassium in blood pressure. **Frmly:** Specialized Center for Research in Hypertension.

★ 22537 ★ Indiana University-Purdue University at Indianapolis
Indiana AIDS Clinical Trials Unit
550 N University Blvd., No. 5550
Indianapolis, IN 46202
Phone: (317)274-8456 **Free:** 800-421-3316
Fax: (317)274-1876
Email: actg.indiana@fstrf.org
Website: http://www.iupui.edu/it/indyactu/index.html
Joseph Wheat, Prin. Investigator
Activities/Fields: AIDS treatment, including an antiretroviral approach; treatment and prevention of AIDS complications, including pneumocystis, pneumonia, cryptococcal meningitis, histoplasmosis, cytomegalovirus infection, Kaposi's sarcoma, and dementia.

★ 22538 ★ Indiana University-Purdue University at Indianapolis
Indiana Alzheimer Disease Center
School of Medicine
635 Barnhill Dr., MS-A142
Indianapolis, IN 46202-5120
Phone: (317)274-7818 **Fax:** (317)278-2018
Email: bghetti@iupui.edu
Website: http://www.pathology.iupui.edu/ad/default.htm
Bernardino Ghetti, MD, Dir.
Activities/Fields: Causes, diagnosis, treatment, and genetics of Alzheimer's Disease.

★ 22539 ★ Indiana University-Purdue University at Indianapolis
Institute of Action Research for Community Health
1111 Middle Dr., Rm. 236
Indianapolis, IN 46202
Phone: (317)274-3319 **Fax:** (317)274-2285
Email: citynet@iupui.edu
Website: http://www.iupui.edu/~citynet/cnet.html
Dr. Beverly Flynn, Dir.
Activities/Fields: Community health issues in Indiana as well as nationally and internationally.

★ 22540 ★ Indiana University-Purdue University at Indianapolis
Mead Johnson Mass Spectrometry Laboratory
RR 208
Indianapolis, IN 46202
Phone: (317)274-4715 **Fax:** (317)274-2065
Email: sdenne@iupui.edu
Website: http://www.indiana.edu/~rugs/ctrdir/mjmsl.html
Scott C. Denne, MD, Dir.
Activities/Fields: Nutrition and metabolism, including fetal, neonatal, and adult protein and glucose metabolism; infant and adult energy expenditure and body composition; human muscle metabolism and exercise; and diabetes.

★ 22541 ★ Indiana University-Purdue University at Indianapolis
Multipurpose Arthritis and Musculoskeletal Diseases Center
1110 W Michigan, Rm. 545
Indianapolis, IN 46202-5103
Phone: (317)274-4225 **Fax:** (317)274-7792
Email: rgrau@iupui.edu
Dr. Rafael Grau, Dir.
Activities/Fields: Basic and clinical research related to rheumatic diseases. Activities are structured in two major areas: a Biomedical Component and an Epidemiology, Education, and Health Services Research Component. **Pub:** *Newsletter*, 3/year. **Frmly:** Specialized Center of Research in Osteoarthritis.

★ 22542 ★ Indiana University-Purdue University at Indianapolis
Oral Health Research Institute
415 Lansing St.
Indianapolis, IN 46202-2876
Phone: (317)274-8822 **Fax:** (317)274-5425
Email: dzero@iupui.edu
Website: http://134.68.72.125/depts/ohri/default.htm
Domenick Zero, DDS, Dir.
Activities/Fields: Etiology, early detection, and prevention of dental caries and periodontal disease; biocompatibility of dental materials. Investigates preventive measures concentrated on fluorides and antimicrobial agents, including a wide variety of in vitro test procedures, research on a number of animal models for determining safety and therapeutic potential, and human clinical investigations of safety and efficacy.

★ 22543 ★ Indiana University-Purdue University at Indianapolis
Oral Health Research Institute Bioresearch Facility
415 N Lansing St.
Indianapolis, IN 46202-2876
Phone: (317)274-1151 **Fax:** (317)274-5425
Email: jwarrick@iupui.edu
Website: http://www.iusd.iupui.edu/depts/OHRI/Bioresearch.htm
Janice M. Warrick, Dir.
Activities/Fields: Biomechanics, biomaterials, musculoskeletal research, polymers with therapeutic potential, and new dental restorative materials. **Frmly:** Biomechanics and Biomaterials Research Center.

★ 22544 ★ Indiana University-Purdue University at Indianapolis
Performing Arts Medicine Program
Indiana University Medical Center
1110 W Michigan St., L0545
Indianapolis, IN 46202
Phone: (317)274-4225
Email: kbrandt@iupui.edu
Website: http://medicine.iupui.edu/perart.html
Dr. Kenneth D. Brandt, Dir.
Activities/Fields: Performance-related health problems of musicians, dancers, and other performers.

★ 22545 ★ Indiana University-Purdue University at Indianapolis
Pharmacology Research Laboratory
Medical Science Bldg., Rm. A-414
School of Medicine
635 Barnhill Dr.
Indianapolis, IN 46202-5120
Phone: (317)274-7844 **Fax:** (317)274-7714
Email: pharmtox@iupui.edu
Website: http://www.iupui.edu/~pharmtox/rsch/index.htm
Dr. Henry R. Besch, Jr., Chm.
Activities/Fields: Cardiovascular pharmacology, molecular toxicology, drug metabolism, cyclic AMP, membrane biophysics, cancer chemotherapy and cardiac glycosides, and antiarrythmics, including studies on metabolism of transplanted tumors, structure activity relations of cardiac glycosides, and ryanodine analogs.

★ 22546 ★ Indiana University-Purdue University at Indianapolis
Riley Child and Adolescent Psychiatry Clinic
702 Barnhill Dr., Rm. 4300
Indianapolis, IN 46202-5200
Phone: (317)274-8162 **Fax:** (317)278-0609
Email: cmcdougl@iupui.edu
Christopher J. McDougle, MD, Dir.
Activities/Fields: Clinical phenomenology, neurobiology and psychopharmacology of autistic and related pervasive developmental disorders, obsessive-compulsive and chronic tic disorders, attention-deficit and other disruptive behavior disorders, and mood disorders. **Frmly:** Riley Child Guidance Clinic.

★ 22547 ★ Institute for Applied Laser Surgery
2 Bala Plz., Ste. PL-13
Bala Cynwyd, PA 19004
Phone: (610)667-4080 **Fax:** (610)667-2748
Dr. Ronald A. Kirschner, Dir.
Activities/Fields: Surgical applications of lasers and laser-related accessory development. Activities include development of new procedures in cardiovascular, peripheral vascular, cutaneeur, plastic, urologic, gynocologic, orthopedic surgery, and endoscopic surgery. **Pub:** *Newsletter*. **Frmly:** Medical Laser Technology Center.

★ 22548 ★ Institute for Cancer and Blood Diseases
MS412
Hahnemann University
Broad & Vine Sts.
Philadelphia, PA 19102
Phone: (215)762-7026 **Fax:** (215)762-8857
Dr. Isadore Brodsky, Ch.
Activities/Fields: Basic research program with possible clinical trials in the following areas: interferon, oncogenesis, differentiation, molecular biology, viral oncogenesis, immunology, cell biology, and cytogenesis, autoimmune diseases. **Frmly:** Herbert L. Orlowitz Institute for Cancer and Blood Diseases.

★ 22549 ★ Institute for Cancer and Blood Research
150 N Robertson Blvd., Ste. 316
Beverly Hills, CA 90211
Phone: (310)657-4706 **Fax:** (310)657-2185
Dr. Howard R. Bierman, Sci. Dir.
Activities/Fields: Biochemical regulation of cell growth and control of leukocyte maturation in leukemias, including clinical studies to isolate and purify substances that stimulate cell division and maintain normal maturation of neoplastic cells; ultrastructural immunolocalization of novel protein products in myeloid leukemias; prediagnostic detection of cancer, oncogenes, and products for antioncogenes; detailed computer analysis of predictive-oriented data acquired from healthy subjects and patients with neoplastic disease; investigation of tumor diathesis, including preclinical diagnosis of multiple primary neoplasms and studies of families to define increased susceptibility to develop neoplasms; and continuing studies of dermatoglyphics, predictive profiles, and other genetic markers as they relate to neoplasia.

★ 22550 ★ Institute for Cancer Prevention
1 Dana Rd.
Valhalla, NY 10595
Phone: (914)789-7158
Email: dnixon@ifcp.us
Website: http://www.ifcp.us
Daniel W. Nixon, MD, Pres.
Activities/Fields: Improves methods of prevention of cancer and other diseases, trains health professionals, and teaches the public how to reduce risk factors of disease. Conducts collaborative laboratory studies with hospitals in cellular and molecular biology, chemical and environmental carcinogenesis, cell genetics, and the nutritional aspects of disease. **Pub:** *Preventive Medicine*, monthly. **Frmly:** American Health Foundation.

★ 22551 ★ Institute for Cancer Prevention
Naylor Dana Institute for Disease Prevention
1 Dana Rd.
Valhalla, NY 10595
Phone: (914)592-2600 **Fax:** (914)592-6317
Email: jbraley@ifcp.us
Joanne Braley, Libn.
Activities/Fields: Medicine, science, and social science, focusing on cancer, smoking and health, nutrition, and biology and chemistry.

★ 22552 ★ Institute for Cancer Research
Fox Chase Cancer Center
7701 Burholme Ave.
Philadelphia, PA 19111
Phone: (215)728-2490 **Fax:** (215)728-2778
Email: am_skalka@fccc.edu
Website: http://www.fccc.edu
Dr. Anna Marie Skalka, Dir.
Activities/Fields: Causes, nature, diagnosis, and treatment of cancer, including studies in cellular, molecular, and developmental biology, immunology, molecular oncology, structural biology, and virology. **Pub:** *Scientific Report*, annually.

★ 22553 ★ Institute for Clinical Evaluative Sciences (ICES)
2075 Bayview Ave., Rm. G106
Toronto, ON, Canada M4N 3M5
Phone: (416)480-4055 **Fax:** (416)480-6048
Email: info@ices.on.ca
Website: http://www.ices.on.ca/
Dr. Andreas Laupacis, Pres. /CEO
Activities/Fields: Effectiveness, quality, equity and efficiency of health care in Ontario. **Pub:** *ICES Practice Atlas series.* • *Newsletters.* • *Technical papers.*

★ 22554 ★ Institute for Clinical Research, Inc.
PO Box 29545
Washington, DC 20017-0745
Phone: (202)462-6820 **Fax:** (202)462-2006
Email: jpzoch@med.ua.gov
Steven Singh, Chm.
Activities/Fields: Hypertension, cardiology, infectious diseases, and oncology.

★ 22555 ★ Institute for Clinical Science, Inc.
301 S East St., Ste. 3A
Philadelphia, PA 19106
Phone: (215)829-7068 **Fax:** (215)829-3094
Email: sundermanjr@aol.com
Dr. F. William Sunderman, Jr., Pres. /Dir.
Activities/Fields: Anatomic and clinical pathology, including studies in metal carcinogenesis and toxicology. **Pub:** *Annals of Clinical and Laboratory Science.* • *Procedures Manual for the Institute's Applied Seminars.*

★ 22556 ★ Institute for Community Inclusion
Children's Hospital
300 Longwood Ave.
Boston, MA 02115
Phone: (617)355-6000 **Fax:** (617)355-7940
Email: william.kiernan@umb.edu
Website: http://www.communityinclusion.org
William E. Kiernan, PhD, Dir.
Activities/Fields: Etiology of mental retardation, the impact of AIDS in adult populations, the development of employment opportunities for people with disabilties using natural supports, the development of supports for infants at risk, development of a managed care design for children with complex medical needs served in community settings, and clinical investigation of issues of autism and related behavior in community settings. **Pub:** *Institute Briefs.*

★ 22557 ★ Institute of Critical Care Medicine
1695 N Sunrise Way, Bldg. 3
Palm Springs, CA 92262
Phone: (760)323-6867 **Fax:** (760)323-6167
Email: weilm@911research.com
Website: http://www.911research.org
Dr. Max Harry Weil, Pres.
Activities/Fields: Critically ill patients, especially those in coronary care, intensive care, concentrated care, post anaesthesia recovery, and emergency services, suffering from heart attacks, accidents, postsurgical complications, overwhelming infections, blood loss, trauma, central nervous system injury, circulatory shock, burns, and shock from a variety of causes. Interdisciplinary studies focus on critical care medicine, automation of bedside equipment, computer application to bedside medicine, hospital environment, cardiopulmonary resuscitation, physiological instrumentation, and ethical studies of patient care. **Pub:** *Newsletters.*

★ 22558 ★ Institute of Developmental Neuroscience and Aging
301 University Blvd., UTMB
Galveston, TX 77555-0652
Phone: (409)772-3667 **Fax:** (409)772-8028
Email: regino.perez-polo@utmb.edu
Dr. Regino Perez-Polo, Pres.
Activities/Fields: Developmental neuroscience and aging, focusing on establishing neuroscience programs in developing and third world countries.

★ 22559 ★ The Institute for Genomic Research (TIGR)
9712 Medical Center Dr.
Rockville, MD 20850
Phone: (301)838-0200 **Fax:** (301)838-0208
Email: cmfraser@tigr.org
Website: http://www.tigr.org
Claire M. Fraser, PhD, Pres.
Activities/Fields: Structural, functional and comparative analysis of genomes and gene products from a wide variety of organisms including viruses, eubacteria (both pathogens and non-pathogens), archaea (the so-called third domain of life), and eukaryotes (plants, animals, fungi and protists such as the malarial parasite).

★ 22560 ★ Institute of Health Economics
10405 Jasper Ave., No. 1200
Edmonton, AB, Canada T5J 3N4
Phone: (780)448-4881 **Fax:** (780)448-0018
Email: webmaster@ihe.ab.ca
Website: http://www.ihe.ca
Donna Angus, Dir. Commun. & Res. Transfer
Activities/Fields: Health and pharmaceutical economic, outcome and policy research. **Pub:** *IHE News.*

★ 22561 ★ Institute for Health Freedom (IHF)
1825 I St. NW, Ste. 400
Washington, DC 20006
Phone: (202)429-6610 **Fax:** (202)861-1973
Email: feedback@forhealthfreedom.org
Website: http://forhealthfreedom.org/
Sue A. Blevins, Pres.
Activities/Fields: Issues of personal health choice regarding providers and treatment. **Pub:** *Health Freedom Watch Newsletter*, bimonthly. • *Research papers.*

★ 22562 ★ Institute for Jewish Medical Ethics
645 14th Ave.
San Francisco, CA 94118
Phone: (415)752-7333 **Fax:** (415)752-5851
Email: ijmeaa@flash.net
Website: http://www.ijme.org/
Miriam Real, Contact
Activities/Fields: Jewish principles of medical ethics, including Jewish law and human and animal experimentation, physician compassion for the patient, artificial insemination, in-vitro fertilization, surrogate motherhood and abortion, allocation of health care resources, organ transplantation (with emphasis on kidney and developments in Israel), and the right to die.

★ 22563 ★ Institute for Metabolic Research
3508 Market St., Ste. 420
Philadelphia, PA 19104
Phone: (215)222-1818 **Fax:** (215)222-5325
Email: drmpcohen@aol.com
Dr. Margo P. Cohen, Dir.
Activities/Fields: Metabolic effects, diagnosis, and management of diabetes mellitus and other metabolic diseases. Studies include the biochemistry and metabolism of glomerular and retinal microvascular basement membranes; role of polyol pathway in complications of diabetes; structure/function effects of nonenzymatic glycosylation of proteins; measurement of

glycohemoglobin and glycoalbumin in biologic samples by immunologic methods; identification and purification of islet cell antigens.

★ 22564 ★ Institute of Noetic Sciences
101 San Antonio Rd.
Petaluma, CA 94952
Phone: (707)775-3500 **Fax:** (707)781-7420
Email: schlitz@noetic.org
Website: http://www.noetic.org
Dr. Marilyn Schlitz, Res. Dir.

Activities/Fields: Nature and potential of the human mind and consciousness, particularly in the areas of exceptional human abilities, the mind/body link and healing, the role of intentionality, positive global change, and creative altruism. **Pub:** *Audiotapes, videotapes.* • *Connections*, 3/year. • *Noetic Sciences Book.* • *Noetic Sciences Review*, 3/year. • *Special reports*, periodically.

★ 22565 ★ Institute for Psychoanalysis
122 S Michigan, Ste. 1300
Chicago, IL 60603-6107
Phone: (312)922-7474 **Fax:** (312)922-5656
Email: admin@chicagoanalysis.org
Website: http://www.chicagoanalysis.org
Dr. Jerome A. Winer, Dir.

Activities/Fields: Psychoanalysis, psychosomatic medicine, psychiatry, and related behavioral sciences. Topics of interest include parent loss, mourning, and stuttering. **Pub:** *Annual of Pychoanalysis.* • *Classics in Psychoanalysis.* • *Emotions and Behavior Monographs.*

★ 22566 ★ Institute for Quantitative Biomedical Research (QB3)
227 Hildebrand Hall, Ste. 3220
University of California at Berkeley
Berkeley, CA 94720-3220
Phone: (510)643-0167 **Fax:** (510)643-5029
Website: http://www.qb3.org/
Marvin Cassman, PhD, Exec. Dir.

Activities/Fields: Understanding biological systems at all levels of complexity, from atoms and protein molecules to cells, tissue, organs and the entire organism, integrating the disciplines of mathematics, physics, chemistry, and engineering.

★ 22567 ★ The Institute for Rehabilitation and Research (TIRR)
1333 Moursund Ave.
Houston, TX 77030-3405
Phone: (713)799-5000 **Free:** 800-447-3422
Fax: (713)799-7095
Website: http://www.tirr.org
Louisa F. Adelung, Pres.

Activities/Fields: Clinical neurophysiologic, neuroendocrinologic, psychoecologic, and exercise tolerance studies of patients with severe spinal cord injuries; development and assessment of mechanical and electronic assistive devices for neurologically impaired individuals; research and technical developments concerned with the effects of pressure on human tissue; provision of personal assistance for persons with severe physical disabilities; and program evaluations to improve services for persons with head injury, amputation, or spinal cord injury. **Pub:** *TIRR Research Projects Guide.*

★ 22568 ★ The Institute for Rehabilitation and Research Independent Living Research Utilization (ILRU)
2323 S Shepherd, Ste. 1000
Houston, TX 77019
Phone: (713)520-0232 **Fax:** (713)520-5785
Email: ilru@ilru.org
Website: http://www.ilru.org/ilru-projects_2.html
Lex Frieden, PhD, Dir.

Activities/Fields: Strategies for developing and implementing techniques for providing high quality consumer-directed services; addressing the independent living needs of persons who may be unserved or under-served because of barriers related to culture, language, disability type, geographic locale, or other distinguishing factors; and preparing individuals to work in independent living service and advocacy settings. **Pub:** *Monographs.* • *Newsletter*, bimonthly. • *Technical report series.*

★ 22569 ★ Institute for the Study and Treatment of Endometriosis
2425 W 22nd St., Ste. 102
Oak Brook, IL 60523
Phone: (630)954-0054 **Fax:** (630)954-0064
Email: wpdmowski@oakbrookfertility.com
Website: http://www.endometriosisinstitute.com
W. Paul Dmowski, MD, Dir.

Activities/Fields: Elucidation of pathophysiology of endometriosis, identification of new diagnostic tests and development of new treatment methods.

★ 22570 ★ Institute for Systems Biology (ISB)
1441 N 34th St.
Seattle, WA 98103-8904
Phone: (206)732-1201 **Fax:** (206)732-1254
Email: lhood@systemsbiology.org
Website: http://www.systemsbiology.org/
Dr. Leroy Hood, Pres.

Activities/Fields: Study of genes and proteins, especially how genomic DNA, mRNA, proteins, functional proteins, informational pathways and informational networks work together. The goal is to predict and prevent disease.

★ 22571 ★ Institute for Urban Family Health
16 E 16th St.
New York, NY 10003
Phone: (212)633-0800 **Fax:** (212)691-4610
Email: info@institute2000.org
Website: http://www.institute2000.org/
Neil Calman, MD, Pres.

Activities/Fields: Primary health care delivery and primary care education.

★ 22572 ★ Institute for Work and Health
481 University Ave., Ste. 800
Toronto, ON, Canada M5G 2E9
Phone: (416)927-2027 **Fax:** (416)927-4167
Email: info@iwh.on.ca
Website: http://www.iwh.on.ca/
Lorna Marsden, Ch.

Activities/Fields: Underlying factors contributing to workplace health and disability, evaluation of designated Ontario rehabilitation facilities, and provision of pertinent and timely information on workplace health and rehabilitation to health care workers and stakeholders. **Pub:** *Newsletter.*

★ 22573 ★ Institutes for Achievement of Human Potential
8801 Stenton Ave.
Wyndmoor, PA 19038-8397
Phone: (215)233-2050 **Fax:** (215)233-9312
Email: institutes@iahp.org
Website: http://www.iahp.org
Janet Doman, Dir.

Activities/Fields: Methods of treating severely brain-injured children, including investigations of effects of programs of sensory inputs individually designed according to each child's growth, as well as functional gains and effects of nutrition in enhancing children's response to therapeutic programs. Studies effects of applying similar environmental enrichment and neurological organization programs to non-disabled children of preschool age. **Pub:** *The Institute Report*, quarterly.
Frmly: Rehabilitation Center of Philadelphia.

★ 22574 ★ Inter-University Centre for Toxicology (CIRTOX)
Department Biological Sciences
Universite of Quebec at Montreal
PO Box 8888, Downtown Sta.
Montreal, QC, Canada H3C 3P8
Phone: (514)987-3000 **Fax:** (514)987-4647
Email: chevalier.gaston@uqam.ca
Joseph Zayed, PhD, Dir.

Activities/Fields: Biological detection of environmental contaminants in living organisms, characterization of harmful effects of potentially toxic chemicals, and development of diagnostic tests and methods for evaluating toxicity.

★ 22575 ★ International Anesthesia Research Society
2 Summit Park Dr., Ste. 140
Cleveland, OH 44131-2571
Phone: (216)642-1124 **Fax:** (216)642-1127
Email: iarshq@iars.org
Website: http://www.iars.org
Anne F. Maggiore, Exec. Dir.

Activities/Fields: Anesthesiology, focusing on progress and research in all phases of this subject. **Pub:** *Anesthesia and Analgesia*, monthly. Journal.

★ 22576 ★ International Association for Dental Research
Craniofacial Biology Group
Department of Biomedical Sciences
Baylor College of Dentistry
3302 Gaston Ave.
Dallas, TX 75246
Phone: (214)828-8277 **Fax:** (214)828-8951
Email: pdechow@tambcd.edu
Website: http://www.craniofacialbiology.com
Dr. Paul C. Dechow, Pres.

Activities/Fields: Craniofacial biology, including anthropology, teratology, pharmacology, orthodontics, pedodontics, genetics, cellular biology, anatomy, pediatrics, and neurology. **Pub:** *Newsletter*, semiannually.

★ 22577 ★ International Association for the Study of Pain
909 NE 43rd St., Ste. 306
Seattle, WA 98105-6020
Phone: (206)547-6409 **Fax:** (206)547-1703
Email: iaspdesk@juno.com
Website: http://www.iasp-pain.org
Louisa E. Jones, Exec. Off.

Activities/Fields: Pain mechanisms and syndromes, focusing on patients with acute and chronic pain. **Pub:** *Clinical newsletter*, 3/year. • *Newsletter*, bimonthly. • *PAIN Journal*, monthly.

★ 22578 ★ International Center for Aquatic Research
1 Olympic Plz.
Colorado Springs, CO 80909
Phone: (719)866-4578 **Fax:** (719)578-4669
Email: cwielgus@usa-swimming.org
Website: http://www.usa-swimming.org
Chuck Wielgus, Exec. Dir.

Activities/Fields: Human performance studies, including training methodology, exercise biochemistry, physiology of performance, muscle strength/power and conditioning, motion and computer analysis, and sports psychology. **Pub:** *Coaching Development Series.* • *IBM compatible software on Human Performance Programs.* • *Nutrition Logbook and Analysis.* • *Performance Profiles of Developing and Elite Swimmers.* • *Sports Medicine Informational Pamphlets: Volumes One and Two.* Pamphlet. • *Sports Participation and Excercise Induced Asthma.* • *Stretching and Warmup Techniques.* • *Training Agenda.* • *Training Methodology.* • *Winning Spirit Instructional Series.*

★ 22579 ★ International Center for Hearing and Speech Research
52 Lomb Memorial Dr.
Rochester, NY 14623
Phone: (585)475-6403 **Fax:** (585)475-6677
Email: rxf1389@ritvax.isc.rit.edu
Dr. Robert Frisina, Sr., Dir.
Activities/Fields: Prevention, early detection, diagnosis, and treatment of people with hearing and speech impairments.

★ 22580 ★ International Council of Motorsport Sciences
3905 Vincennes Rd., Ste. 303
Indianapolis, IN 46268
Phone: (317)471-3596 **Fax:** (317)471-3508
Email: icmsin@aol.com
Website: http://motorsportsafety.org
Jon Potter, Exec. Dir.
Activities/Fields: Enhancement of performance and safety in automobile racing, including the physical and psychological aspects of race performance as well as the role of diet, exercise, and mental preparation in performance. **Frmly:** Motor Sport Research Council.

★ 22581 ★ International Institute for the Advancement of Medicine (IIAM)
1232 Mid-Valley Dr.
Jessup, PA 18434-1823
Phone: (570)496-3400 **Fax:** (570)343-6993
Email: gina_smith@iiam.org
Website: http://www.iiam.org
Gina Dunne Smith, PhD, Dir.,Prof. Svcs.
Activities/Fields: Acquisition and placement of non-transplantable human organs (including liver, lung, pancreas, heart, intestine, kidneys) and tissue for medical research, education and therapeutic development; research placement with ongoing studies involved with diabetes, asthma, allergies, emphysema, cancer, novel drug development, drug-drug interactions, metabolism/toxicology studies, hepatitis, heart disease, and more; serological testing for infectious disease provided for all donor tissue; fresh/frozen tissue available; slices, microsomes, hepatocytes, subcellular fractions; anatomical tissue.

★ 22582 ★ Iowa Oncology Research Association
1223 Center St., Ste. 19
Des Moines, IA 50309-1014
Phone: (515)244-7586 **Free:** 888-244-6061
Fax: (515)244-3037
Email: sherrijr@iora.org
Website: http://www.iora.org
Sherri Rickabaugh, Admin.
Activities/Fields: Clinical cancer studies, including new chemotherapy agents and radiation therapy techniques.

★ 22583 ★ Iowa State University of Science and Technology Bessey Microscopy Facility
Bessey Hall, Rm. 1
Ames, IA 50011-1020
Phone: (515)294-8635 **Fax:** (515)294-1337
Email: hth@iastate.edu
Website: http://www.biotech.iastate.edu/facilities/BMF/
Prof. Harry T. Horner, Dir.
Activities/Fields: Applications of microscopy in areas of biology, biomedicine, botany, agronomy, animal science, biotechnology, and engineering.

★ 22584 ★ Iowa's Center for Agricultural Safety and Health (ICASH)
124 IREH
100 Oakdale Campus
University of Iowa
Iowa City, IA 52242-5000
Phone: (319)335-4190 **Fax:** (319)335-4225
Email: kelley-donham@uiowa.edu
Website: http://www.public-health.uiowa.edu/ICASH/index.html
Kelley J. Donham, DVM, Dir.
Activities/Fields: Health and safety of Iowa's farm families, farm workers, and the agricultural community. Priority areas include provision of agricultural health and safety services, prevention of tractor injuries, prevention of injuries and illnesses in farm youth, prevention of illnesses among producers working in livestock confinement operations, and surveillance of farm injuries and illnesses. **Pub:** *Annual report.* • *Newsletter*, quarterly.

★ 22585 ★ Irvington Institute for Immunological Research
245 5th Ave., Rm. 2101
New York, NY 10016-8728
Phone: (212)576-1005 **Fax:** (212)576-1006
Email: irving1@ix.netcom.com
Website: http://www.irvingtoninstitute.org
Kerry W. Walsh, Exec. Dir.
Activities/Fields: Diseases and dysfunctions involving the immune system, including AIDS, cancer, diabetes, rheumatoid arthritis, allergies, organ rejection, and systemic lupus erythematosus. **Pub:** *Irvington Institute Newsletter*, quarterly. Newsletter.

★ 22586 ★ Jackson Laboratory
600 Main St.
Bar Harbor, ME 04609-1500
Phone: (207)288-6000 **Free:** 800-422-6423
Fax: (207)288-6150
Email: pubinfo@jax.org
Website: http://www.jax.org
Richard Woychik, PhD, Dir.
Activities/Fields: Formal genetics, molecular genetics, developmental genetics, physiological genetics, immunology, cell biology, and biochemistry as related to cancer, diabetes, anemias, other human diseases, as well as normal growth and development. Annually produces 2,000,000 genetically standardized mutant and inbred mice strains for its own research staff and research workers throughout the world. Five major areas of research include, Cancers, development and aging-related, immune system and blood disorders, neurological and sensory disorders, and metabolic diseases. **Pub:** *Animal Health & Genetic Quality Control Report*, quarterly. • *Annual Report.* • *Handbook of Genetically Standardized JAX Mice.* • *Inside the Jackson Laboratory*, 3/year. • *Scientific Report.*

★ 22587 ★ Jackson Laboratory Cryopreservation of Murine Germplasm
600 Main St.
Bar Harbor, ME 04609-1500
Phone: (207)288-6373 **Fax:** (207)288-6005
Email: lem@jax.org
Website: http://www.jax.org
Larry E. Mobraaten, PhD, Prin. Investigator
Activities/Fields: Cryopreservation of mouse embryos and spermatozoa.

★ 22588 ★ Jackson Laboratory Induced Mutant Resource
600 Main St.
Bar Harbor, ME 04609
Phone: (207)288-6223 **Fax:** (207)288-6149
Email: mtd@jax.org
Website: http://www.jax.org
Muriel T. Davisson, PhD, Contact
Activities/Fields: Imports, establishes on defined genetic background and phenotypically characterizes transgenic, targeted mutation and induced (e.g., ENU mutagenesis) mutation mice; develops sperm cryopreservation methodology, assisted reproduction technology, high throughput genotyping and speed congeic methodology.

★ 22589 ★ Jackson Laboratory Mouse Mutant Resource
600 Main St.
Bar Harbor, ME 04609
Phone: (207)288-6223 **Fax:** (207)288-6149
Email: mtd@jax.org
Website: http://www.jax.org/resources/index.html
Muriel T. Davisson, PhD, Contact
Activities/Fields: Identifies, characterizes, and genetically maps new inherited endocrine, neurological, immunological, skeletal, and other mutations of the laboratory mouse.

★ 22590 ★ Jacobs Institute of Women's Health
409 12th St. SW
Washington, DC 20024-2188
Phone: (202)863-4990 **Fax:** (202)488-4229
Email: rlipner@acog.org
Website: http://www.jiwh.org
Robyn Lipner, Exec. Dir.
Activities/Fields: Women's health care issues, focusing on the interaction of medical and social systems. **Pub:** *InTouch*, quarterly. Newsletter. • *Women's Health Issues*, bimonthly. Journal.

★ 22591 ★ James Madison University Auditory Research Laboratory
1016 Health & Human Services Bldg., MSC 4304
Harrisonburg, VA 22807
Phone: (540)568-7930 **Fax:** (540)568-8077
Email: ryalsbm@cisat.jmu.edu
Website: http://www.csd.jmu.edu/arl/arl-fr5.html
Dr. Brenda M. Ryals, Prin. Investigator
Activities/Fields: Plasticity, or the ability to accommodate change, in the auditory system. The laboratory is especially concerned with plasticity as it impacts the system's response to cochlear injury and hair cell regeneration.

★ 22592 ★ James Madison University Health Communication Institute (HCI)
School of Communication Studies
Harrisonburg, VA 22807
Phone: (540)568-6228
Email: gabbaras@jmu.edu
Website: http://web.jmu.edu/healthcom/history.html
Dr. Anne Gabbard-Alley, Dir.
Activities/Fields: Health communication. **Pub:** *Newsletter*, quarterly. • *Papers.*

★ 22593 ★ Jeanette Kennelly Kroch Center for Twin Studies
Prentice Pavilion
Northwestern Memorial Hospital
333 E Superior St., Rm. 161
Chicago, IL 60611
Phone: (312)926-7519 **Fax:** (312)926-0367
Email: apeacema@nmh.org
Website: http://www.nmh.org/maternity
Alan M. Peaceman, MD, Dir.
Activities/Fields: Multiple births. Conducts ultrasound and genetic research for the early detection of identical or fraternal twins; longitudinal ultrasound studies to determine normal growth patterns in multiple-birth pregnancies; clinical studies of methods to prevent premature labor and delivery, which result in low-birthweight twins; and studies related to specific aspects of twin development, such as speech patterns.

★ 22594 ★ Jerome H. Holland Laboratory
American Red Cross
15601 Crabbs Branch Way
Rockville, MD 20855
Phone: (301)738-0600 **Fax:** (301)738-0553
Dr. Judy Hautala, Dir.
Activities/Fields: Blood cells, blood proteins, cytokines, receptors, blood services technology, tissue biology, epidemiology of transfusion-transmitted dis-

eases, plasma derivatives, adhesion factors, angiogenesis, inflammation. Conducts basic and applied research and development for the Biomedical Services Division of the American Red Cross. **Pub:** *R&D Annual Report*. Annual report. **Frmly:** American Red Cross National Headquarters Lab.

★ 22595 ★ John L. McClellan Memorial Veterans' Hospital
Research Office
4300 W 7th St.
Little Rock, AR 72205
Phone: (501)257-4816 **Fax:** (501)257-4821
Email: dunnsarahl@uams.edu
Philip A. Kern, MD, Dir.
Activities/Fields: Biomedicine, including studies of Histoplasmosis, the molecular biology of aging, molecular biology of tuberculosis and other mycobacterial diseases, molecular biology of diabetes, hyperthermia effects on tumors, anti-tumor drugs, nephrology. Also conducts clinical studies in cardiology, stroke, infectious diseases, prostate cancer, and aneurysms. Rehabilitation Research and Development, particularly research on falling in the elderly; and Health Services Research and Development Field Program for Mental Health, including schizophrenia management, stroke outcomes management, and protein-energy undernutrition among elderly patients.

★ 22596 ★ John P. Robarts Research Institute
Centre for Transplant Research and Development (CTRD)
100 Perth Dr., Rm. 4-34
PO Box 5015
London, ON, Canada N6A 5K8
Phone: (519)663-5777 **Fax:** (519)663-3299
Email: dlilley@robarts.ca
Website: http://www.ctrd-transplant.com/
Anthony M. Jevnikar, MD, Co-Dir.
Activities/Fields: New solutions to the shortage of organ donors and better methods to control the immune response to transplanted organs.

★ 22597 ★ John P. Robarts Research Institute
Diabetes Research Centre
100 Perth Dr.
PO Box 5015
London, ON, Canada N5A 5K8
Phone: (519)663-5777 **Fax:** (519)663-3299
Email: bsingh@uwo.ca
Website: http://www.diabetes-research.org/
Dr. Bhagirath Singh, Co-Dir.
Activities/Fields: New therapies for the prevention and cure of Type I Diabetes.

★ 22598 ★ John P. Robarts Research Institute
Imaging Research Laboratories
100 Perth Dr.
PO Box 5015
London, ON, Canada N6A 5K8
Phone: (519)663-3833 **Fax:** (519)663-3900
Email: afenster@imaging.robarts.ca
Website: http://www.irus.rri.on.ca/
Dr. Aaron Fenster, Dir.
Activities/Fields: Medical imaging systems and techniques, including diagnostic X-rays, computed tomography, ultrasound, and magnetic resonance imaging. Develops new diagnostic imaging systems and techniques focusing on vascular imaging research, three dimensional image processing and display, multimodality display, image guided surgery and therapy, prostate and breast cancer.

★ 22599 ★ John P. Robarts Research Institute
Imaging Research Laboratories
Centre for Vascular Imaging Research
100 Perth Dr.
PO Box 5015
London, ON, Canada N5A 5K8
Phone: (519)663-3462 **Fax:** (519)663-3078
Email: brutt@imaging.robarts.ca
Website: http://www.imaging.robarts.ca/cvir/
Brian K. Rutt, PhD, Sci. Dir.
Activities/Fields: Advanced vascular imaging technology.

★ 22600 ★ John P. Robarts Research Institute
London Clinical Trials Research Group
100 Perth Dr.
PO Box 5015
London, ON, Canada N6A 5K8
Phone: (519)663-3400 **Fax:** (519)663-3807
Email: lctrg@lctrg.com
Website: http://www.lctrg.com
Dr. Brian Feagan, Dir.
Activities/Fields: Evaluates new medications and treatments in a variety of medical fields. Provides biostatistics and data coordination for national and international trials.

★ 22601 ★ Johns Hopkins Bayview Medical Center
General Clinical Research Center
B3NW, Rm. 310
4940 Eastern Ave.
Baltimore, MD 21224
Phone: (410)550-1850 **Fax:** (410)550-1227
Email: pouyang@jhmi.edu
Website: http://www.jhbmc.jhu.edu/gcrc/gcrc.html
Pamela Ouyang, MD, Prog. Dir.
Activities/Fields: Major areas of investigation include aging and cardiovascular diseases.

★ 22602 ★ Johns Hopkins University
Adolescent Idiopathic Scoliosis Laboratory (AIS)
Ross Bldg., Rm. 232
720 Rutland Ave.
Baltimore, MD 21205
Phone: (410)614-3717 **Fax:** (410)502-6414
Email: bmarosy@jhmi.edu
Website: http://www.med.jhu.edu/ais/
Dr. Nancy H. Miller, Contact
Activities/Fields: Genetics of adolescent idiopathic scoliosis, a condition characterized by a lateral curvature of the spine.

★ 22603 ★ Johns Hopkins University
Alzheimer's Disease Research Center
558 Ross Research Bldg.
School of Medicine
720 Rutland Ave.
Baltimore, MD 21205-2196
Phone: (410)955-5632 **Fax:** (410)955-9777
Email: adrc@jhmi.edu
Website: http://www.alzresearch.org
Dr. Donald L. Price, Dir.
Activities/Fields: Alzheimer's disease, including basic and applied studies of cognitive symptons and psychiatric problems. **Pub:** *Family Guidelines Series.*

★ 22604 ★ Johns Hopkins University
Asthma and Allergy Center
5501 Hopkins Bayview Cir.
Baltimore, MD 21224-6801
Phone: (410)550-2101 **Fax:** (410)550-3666
Website: http://www.hopkins-allergy.org/
Dr. Lawrence M. Lichtenstein, Dir.
Activities/Fields: Allergic diseases and individuals with allergic diseases, pulmonary diseases and individuals with pulmonary diseases, and diseases involving inflammation and immunological processes.

★ 22605 ★ Johns Hopkins University
Autoimmune Disease Research Center
Ross Bldg., Rm. 659
720 Rutland Ave.
Baltimore, MD 21205
Phone: (410)955-0330 **Fax:** (410)955-0105
Email: nrrose@jhsph.edu
Website: http://autoimmune.pathology.jhmi.edu/
Noel R. Rose, MD, Dir.
Activities/Fields: Diagnosis, treatment and prevention of autoimmune diseases. **Pub:** *Articles.* • *The Autoimmune Diseases textbook.*

★ 22606 ★ Johns Hopkins University
Baltimore Huntington's Disease Center
Meyer, 2-181
Johns Hopkins Hospital
600 N Wolfe St.
Baltimore, MD 21287-7281
Phone: (410)955-2398 **Fax:** (410)955-8233
Email: dpollard@jhmi.edu
Dr. Christopher A. Ross, Dir.
Activities/Fields: Huntington's Disease (HD), a hereditary brain disorder and the gene which carries it. Both clinical and basic research programs are conducted by faculty from Johns Hopkins Medical Institutions, Departments of Psychiatry, Neurology, Pathology, Biomedical Engineering, Neuroradiology, Pharmacology, Neuroscience, Biostatistics, and Genetics. **Pub:** *A Physicians Guide to the Management of Huntington's Disease.*

★ 22607 ★ Johns Hopkins University
Behavioral Pharmacology Research Unit
Johns Hopkins Bayview Campus
5510 Nathan Shock Dr.
Baltimore, MD 21224-6823
Phone: (410)550-1686 **Fax:** (410)550-0030
Email: bigelow@jhmi.edu
Website: http://bpru.med.jhu.edu
George E. Bigelow, PhD, Sci. Dir.
Activities/Fields: Human behavioral pharmacology of substance abuse and dependence, including clinical studies on abuse liability assessment, performance effects, and applied treatment interventions for opioids (analgesics) and narcotics, sedatives, anxiolytics, alcohol, tobacco, nicotine, caffeine, and cocaine.

★ 22608 ★ Johns Hopkins University
Bill and Melinda Gates Institute for Population and Reproductive Health
Department of Population & Family Health Sciences
Bloomberg School of Public Health
615 N Wolfe St., W4503
Baltimore, MD 21205-2179
Phone: (410)955-2232 **Fax:** (410)955-0792
Email: gates@jhsph.edu
Website: http://www.jhsph.edu/GatesInstitute/index.html
Amy Tsui, PhD, Dir.
Activities/Fields: Reproductive health issues, including sustainable contraceptive service delivery systems and practice, successful integration of reproductive health services, community support and protection of reproductive outcomes.

★ 22609 ★ Johns Hopkins University
Biomechanics Research Laboratory
Department of Orthopaedic Surgery
720 Rutland Ave.
Baltimore, MD 21205-2196
Phone: (410)502-6416 **Fax:** (410)502-6414
Email: echao@jhmi.edu
Website: http://www.biomech.jhu.edu
Dr. Edmund Y.S. Chao, Dir.

Activities/Fields: Orthopedic concerns and the application of engineering principles to the better treatment and care of patients.

★ 22610 ★ Johns Hopkins University Biomedical Instrumentation Laboratory
Department of Biomedical Engineering
School of Medicine
720 Rutland Ave.
Baltimore, MD 21205
Phone: (410)955-0077 **Fax:** (410)955-0549
Email: nthakor@bme.jhu.edu
Website: http://www.bme.jhu.edu/~nthakor/Lab/
Nitish V. Thakor, PhD, Contact
Activities/Fields: Medical instrumentation, signal analysis, and computer modeling and simulation to develop novel diagnostic and therapeutic technologies for cardiovascular diseases and neurological injury.

★ 22611 ★ Johns Hopkins University Biomedical Optics Laboratory
Ross Research Bldg., Rm. 724
Department of Biomedical Engineering
Sch. of Medicine
720 Rutland Ave.
Baltimore, MD 21205
Phone: (410)614-2528 **Fax:** (410)955-0549
Email: skuo@bme.jhu.edu
Website: http://www.bme.jhu.edu/~skuo/Lab/
Scot C. Kuo, Prin. Investigator
Activities/Fields: Optical tools (optical tweezers, optical rheometry, video-enhanced optical microscopy, fluorescence microscopy, digital image processing); cell mechanics (non-invasive, real-time monitoring of cell mechanics during chemotaxis, cell crawling, granule secretion, and mitosis); microtubule-based motility (kinesin force generation, single-molecule assays, genetic engineering, organelle transport, chromosome movement); and collaborations (electromotility of outer hair cells, chromosome movement, biological rheology, and mechanics of biological materials).

★ 22612 ★ Johns Hopkins University Bipolar Pedigree Collection
Affective Disorders Section
Department of Psychiatry & Behavioral Sciences
600 N Wolfe St., Meyer 3-181
Baltimore, MD 21287-7381
Phone: (410)614-1017 **Fax:** (410)955-0152
Email: moods@jhu.edu
Dr. J. Raymond DePaulo, Jr., Prin. Investigator
Activities/Fields: Genetics of bipolar disorder (manic-depressive illness), involving families in which someone is suffering from this condition.

★ 22613 ★ Johns Hopkins University Cardiac Bioelectric Systems Laboratory
Traylor Research Bldg., 7th Fl.
Department of Biomedical Engineering
School of Medicine
720 Rutland Ave.
Baltimore, MD 21205
Phone: (410)955-9603 **Fax:** (410)955-0549
Email: ltung@bme.jhu.edu
Website: http://www.bme.jhu.edu/~ltung/CBS_Lab/
Leslie Tung, PhD, Dir.
Activities/Fields: Electrical properties of the heart, in particular as they relate at the cellular and multicellular levels to defibrillation and arrhythmia.

★ 22614 ★ Johns Hopkins University Center for Adolescent Health Promotion and Disease Prevention
Bloomberg School of Public Health
2007 E Monument St.
Baltimore, MD 21205
Phone: (410)614-3953 **Fax:** (410)614-3956
Email: calexand@jhsph.edu
Website: http://www.jhsph.edu/hao/cah/ceninfo.htm
Dr. Cheryl Alexander, Dir.
Activities/Fields: Health needs of adolescents, including developmental transitions which serve as opportunities for community-based health promotion interventions; interventions to modify risk-taking behaviors; interventions which involve the family, school, and community settings; and dissemination of adolescent health information to practitioners and policy makers.

★ 22615 ★ Johns Hopkins University Center for Alternatives to Animal Testing
School of Hygiene & Public Health
111 Market Pl., Ste. 840
Baltimore, MD 21202-6709
Phone: (410)233-1692 **Fax:** (410)223-1603
Email: caat@jhsph.edu
Website: http://caat.jhsph.edu
Dr. Alan M. Goldberg, Dir.
Activities/Fields: Fosters development of scientifically acceptable in vitro and other alternatives to animal testing for use in development and safety evaluation of commercial and therapeutic products. Catalyzes validation of alternative methods. **Pub:** *Alternative Methods in Toxicology Book Series.* Book. • *Newsletter.* • *Technical Report Series.*

★ 22616 ★ Johns Hopkins University Center for American Indian and Alaskan Native Health
School of Public Health
621 N Washington St.
Baltimore, MD 21205
Phone: (410)955-6931 **Fax:** (410)955-2010
Website: http://ih.jhsph.edu/cnah/mission.htm
Mathuram Santosham, MD, Dir.
Activities/Fields: Health and well being of American Indians and Alaskan Natives.

★ 22617 ★ Johns Hopkins University Center for Cancer Complementary Medicine
1830 E Monument.
Baltimore, MD 21287
Phone: (410)955-2130 **Fax:** (410)955-8172
Email: adobs@jhu.edu
Adrian S. Dobs, MD, Prin. Investigator
Activities/Fields: Complementary and alternative medicine (CAM) modalities for cancer.

★ 22618 ★ Johns Hopkins University Center for Civilian Biodefense Studies
Candler Bldg., Ste. 850
111 Market Pl.
Baltimore, MD 21202
Phone: (410)223-1667 **Fax:** (410)223-1665
Website: http://www.hopkins-biodefense.org
D.A. Henderson, MD, Dir.
Activities/Fields: Medical and public health threats posed by biological weapons, their expected clinical manifestations, available treatment strategies, epidemiology, and potential methods of prophylaxis.

★ 22619 ★ Johns Hopkins University Center for Clinical Trials
615 N Wolfe St., Rm. 5010
Baltimore, MD 21205
Phone: (410)955-8175 **Fax:** (410)955-0932
Email: cctmail@jhsph.edu
Website: http://www.jhsph.edu/Research/Centers/CCT/
Curtis L. Meinert, PhD, Dir.
Activities/Fields: Design, conduct, and analysis of clinical medical trials; analysis of longitudinal data and other methods of analyzing results from trials; publication process; and the language and nomenclature of clinical trials.

★ 22620 ★ Johns Hopkins University Center for Communication Programs
111 Market Pl., Ste. 310
Baltimore, MD 21202-4024
Phone: (410)659-6300 **Fax:** (410)659-6266
Email: ccp@jhuccp.org
Website: http://www.jhuccp.org
Jane Bertrand, PhD, Dir.
Activities/Fields: Behavior change communication in the areas of family health, reproductive health, maternal and child health, and AIDS/STD prevention. Develops communication programs using mass media, interpersonal communication/counseling, advocacy, and community mobilization. Uses behavioral, attitudinal, and other social science research techniques to enhance and document the impact of communication on family planning and related health behavior. **Pub:** *Communication Impact.* Newsletter. • *Field reports.* • *Population reports*, quarterly. • *Working papers.*

★ 22621 ★ Johns Hopkins University Center for Computational Medicine and Biology
Department of Biomedical Engineering
710 Traylor Research Bldg.
720 Rutland Ave.
Baltimore, MD 21205
Phone: (410)614-6685 **Fax:** (410)614-8796
Email: ccmb@bme.jhu.edu
Website: http://www.bme.jhu.edu/ccmb/
Prof. Raimond L. Winslow, Co-Dir.
Activities/Fields: Understanding the integrative function in biological systems, including human, through development and application of computational models, and the application of these models to the design of novel therapeutics.

★ 22622 ★ Johns Hopkins University Center for Computational Medicine and Biology Computational Modeling Group
Department of Biomedical Engineering
School of Medicine
720 Rutland Ave.
Baltimore, MD 21205
Phone: (410)614-6685 **Fax:** (410)614-8796
Email: ccmb@bme.jhu.edu
Website: http://www.cmbl.jhu.edu/
Prof. Raimond L. Winslow, Dir.
Activities/Fields: Understanding the origins of cardiac arrhythmias through the use of biophysically detailed computer models.

★ 22623 ★ Johns Hopkins University Center for Craniofacial Development and Disorders (CCDD)
Children's Medical & Surgical Center, Rm. 1004
John Hopkins Hospital
600 N Wolfe St.
Baltimore, MD 21287-3914
Phone: (410)955-0484 **Fax:** (410)955-0484
Email: ejabs@jhem.jhmi.edu
Website: http://www.hopkinsmedicine.org/craniofacial/Home/Index.cfm
Ethylin Wang Jabs, MD, Dir.
Activities/Fields: Normal and abnormal craniofacial development. **Pub:** *Articles.*

★ 22624 ★ Johns Hopkins University Center for Hereditary Eye Diseases
Maumenee Bldg., Rm. 517
Wilmer Ophthalmological Institute
600 N Wolfe St.
Baltimore, MD 21287-9237
Phone: (410)955-5214 **Fax:** (410)614-4363
Email: jhched@jhmi.edu
Dr. Irene H. Maumenee, Dir.
Activities/Fields: Studies of molecular mechanisms underlying genetic eye diseases. Emphasis on diagnosis and management of common as well as rare

genetic eye diseases, and the prevention of vision loss through early medical or surgical intervention.

★ 22625 ★ Johns Hopkins University Center for Human Nutrition
School of Hygiene & Public Health
615 N Wolfe St.
Baltimore, MD 21205
Phone: (410)614-4070 **Fax:** (410)955-0196
Email: caballero@jhu.edu
Website: http://www.jhsph.edu/Research/Centers/Nutrition
Dr. Benjamin Caballero, Dir.
Activities/Fields: The role of nutrition in health and disease and the development of new ways to apply that knowledge to improve the health of people, including maternal and child nutrition, obesity and chronic diseases, micronutrient deficiencies, and nutrient metabolism.

★ 22626 ★ Johns Hopkins University Center for Immunization Research
Hampton House, Rm. 217A
Johns Hopkins School of Public Health
624 N Broadway
Baltimore, MD 21205-1901
Phone: (410)614-5960 **Fax:** (410)502-6898
Email: dburke@jhsph.edu
Website: http://ih.jhsph.edu/cir/
Dr. Donald Burke, Dir.
Activities/Fields: Influenza, parainfluenza, respiratory syncytial virus, AIDS, and rotavirus vaccines, hepatitis B, immunoglobulins, and antiviral drug efficacy studies. Uses volunteers 18 years of age or older for vaccine studies and children from the ages of 1 month to 48 months for pediatric vaccine studies.

★ 22627 ★ Johns Hopkins University Center for Inherited Disease Research
Triad Technology Center
333 Cassell Dr., Ste. 2000
Baltimore, MD 21224
Website: http://www.cidr.jhmi.edu/
Dr. David Valle, Prin. Investigator
Activities/Fields: Provides genotyping and statistical genetics services for investigators seeking to identify genes that contribute to human disease, primarily on multifactorial hereditary disease.

★ 22628 ★ Johns Hopkins University Center for Inherited Neurovascular Diseases (CIND)
Meyer 5-181
Johns Hopkins Hospital
600 N Wolfe St.
Baltimore, MD 21287
Phone: (410)955-1099 **Fax:** (410)955-9126
Email: hrich@jhmi.edu
Website: http://www.cind.org
Heather Rich, Contact
Activities/Fields: Genetic forms of neurovascular diseases, especially determining which genes are responsible for selected forms of neurovascular disease.

★ 22629 ★ Johns Hopkins University Center for Laryngeal and Voice Disorders
Department of Otolaryngology-Head & Neck Surgery
601 N Caroline St.
Baltimore, MD 21287
Phone: (410)955-1654
Website: http://www.med.jhu.edu/voice/
Paul W. Flint, MD, Dir.
Activities/Fields: Diagnostic and therapeutic protocols for laryngeal and voice disorders.

★ 22630 ★ Johns Hopkins University Center for a Livable Future (CLF)
Bloomberg School of Public Health
615 N Wolfe St., Ste. W8503
Baltimore, MD 21205
Phone: (410)502-7578 **Fax:** (410)502-7579
Email: clf@jhsph.edu
Website: http://www.jhsph.edu/Environment
Robert S. Lawrence, MD, Dir.
Activities/Fields: Interconnections among diet, health, food production, the environment, population and equity for the world's inhabitants. **Pub:** *CLF report. • Position statements. • Scientific papers.*

★ 22631 ★ Johns Hopkins University Center for Osteonecrosis Research and Education
The Good Samaritan Professional Bldg., Rm. 201
Department of Orthopaedic Surgery
School of Medicine
5601 Loch Raven Blvd.
Baltimore, MD 21239
Phone: (410)532-5906 **Fax:** (410)532-5908
Email: dhunger@mail.jhmi.edu
Website: http://www.med.jhu.edu/avncenter/
Lynne C. Jones, PhD, Dir.
Activities/Fields: Etiology, pathogenesis, diagnosis and treatment of osteonecrosis.

★ 22632 ★ Johns Hopkins University Center in Urban Environmental Health
Department of Environmental Health Sciences
School of Hygiene & Public Health Sciences
615 N Wolfe St.
Baltimore, MD 21205
Phone: (410)955-3720 **Fax:** (410)955-9334
Email: jgroopma@jhsph.edu
Website: http://www.niehs.nih.gov/centers/center/jhpctr.htm
John Groopman, PhD, Dir.
Activities/Fields: Identification of environmental exposures and susceptibility factors that alone or together increase the risk of illness for people living in urban environments and to use these findings to develop prevention strategies to improve public health.

★ 22633 ★ Johns Hopkins University Child Health Research Center
600 N Wolfe St., CMSC 2-116
Baltimore, MD 21287
Phone: (410)955-5976 **Fax:** (410)955-9850
Email: gdover@jhmi.edu
Dr. George Dover, Dir.
Activities/Fields: Applies molecular biology techniques to the diagnosis, treatment, and prevention of genetic and acquired hematologic disorders in children. Activities focus on developing techniques to analyze genes and gene products, especially those required for normal development.

★ 22634 ★ Johns Hopkins University Cystic Fibrosis Research Center
Department of Physiology
School of Medicine
725 N Wolfe St.
Baltimore, MD 21205
Phone: (410)955-7166 **Fax:** (410)955-0461
Email: wguggino@jhmi.edu
Website: http://www.johnshopkinscfresearch.org/
Dr. William B. Guggino, Dir.
Activities/Fields: Cystic fibrosis and related fields, including epithelial cell transport, molecular genetics, respiratory cell biology, and biochemistry.

★ 22635 ★ Johns Hopkins University Dana Center for Preventive Ophthalmology
Wilmer 129
Wilmer Eye Institute
600 N Wolfe St.
Baltimore, MD 21287-9019
Phone: (410)955-2777 **Fax:** (410)955-2542
Email: hquigley@jhmi.edu
Website: http://www.wilmer.jhu.edu/research/dana1.htm
Harry A. Quigley, MD, Dir.
Activities/Fields: Aims to identify eye disorders amenable to intervention and to develop intervention strategies. Studies concentrate on cataract and glaucoma, including the role of ultraviolet light in the development of cataract, evaluation of new techniques for diagnosing glaucoma at its earlier stages, and why black Americans develop glaucoma nine times more frequently than white Americans. Other studies focus on diet and measles and other infections as causes of blindness in Asia and Africa, including the effectiveness of periodic, massive dosing with vitamin A, vitamin A fortification of commonly consumed foods, nutritional education to reduce eye disorders caused by vitamin A deficiency in c hildren, and vitamin A in relation to childhood morbidity and mortality; infrequent washing of the face as a cause of trachoma in such water-poor nations as Mexico; and evaluation of the safety and efficacy of drugs used to combat river blindness or onchocerciasis.

★ 22636 ★ Johns Hopkins University Division of Comparative Medicine
600 N Wolfe St.
Baltimore, MD 21287
Phone: (410)955-9770 **Fax:** (410)287-2953
Email: jclement@jhmi.edu
Website: http://www.hopkinsmedicine.org/comparativemedicine
Dr. Janice E. Clements, Dir.
Activities/Fields: Comparative pathology, laboratory animal medicine, retrovirus biology, transgenic biology, infectious diseases, and oncology. Research activities focus on naturally occurring diseases of animals as models of human disease, molecular biology and pathogenesis of lentiviral infections, aquatic toxicology, and benign prostatic hyperplasia.

★ 22637 ★ Johns Hopkins University Education and Research Center for Occupational Safety and Health
Bloomberg School of Public Health
615 N Wolfe St., Rm. W7041
Baltimore, MD 21205-2179
Phone: (410)955-0423 **Fax:** (410)614-4986
Email: dzerbe@jhsph.edu
Website: http://www.jhsph.edu/~c-erc/
Diane Zerbe, Dir.
Activities/Fields: Occupational and environmental safety and health.

★ 22638 ★ Johns Hopkins University Epilepsy Research Laboratory (ERL)
Meyer 2-147
Department of Neurology
School of Medicine
600 N Wolfe St.
Baltimore, MD 21287
Website: http://erl.neuro.jhmi.edu
Prof. Piotr J. Franaszczuk, PhD, Contact
Activities/Fields: Epilepsy, including the localization of seizure onset in patients, analysis of dynamics of seizure spread in time and space, modeling of seizure dynamics and propagation, and detection of nonstationary signals.

★ 22639 ★ Johns Hopkins University General Clinical Research Center
Osler
Johns Hopkins Hospital
600 N Wolfe St.
Baltimore, MD 21205
Phone: (410)614-2717 **Fax:** (410)955-0801
Email: csaudek@jhu.edu
Website: http://www.hopkinsmedicine.org/gcrc
Christopher D. Saudek, MD, Prog. Dir.

Activities/Fields: Major areas of investigation include anesthesiology, cardiology, clinical pharmacology, emergency medicine, endocrinology, gene therapy, genetic diseases, geriatrics and gerontology, hematology, hypertension, infectious diseases, liver diseases, musculoskeletal disorders, neonatal medicine, nephrology, neurology, nutrition, oncology, psychiatry and behavioral sciences, pulmonary diseases and sleep studies.

★ 22640 ★ Johns Hopkins University Health Services Research and Development Center
624 N Broadway, Rm. 482
Baltimore, MD 21205-1996
Phone: (410)955-3625 **Fax:** (410)614-9152
Email: dsteinwa@jhsph.edu
Dr. Donald M. Steinwachs, Dir.
Activities/Fields: Conducts health services research, including studies on the following: determinants of health outcomes; the impacts of alternative health care systems on cost and quality; effective strategies for health promotion and disease prevention; and methods of meeting the needs of high risk populations such as the poor, elderly, mentally ill, disabled, and children. Research is conducted using experimental (randomized controlled trials) or nonexperimental methods, and relies to varying degrees on primary data sources obtained through interviews and observation and secondary data sources obtained from management information systems, financial reports, and existing regional and national data sources and surveys.

★ 22641 ★ Johns Hopkins University Hopkins Center on the Demography of Aging (HCDA)
615 N Wolfe St., Rm. W4027
Baltimore, MD 21205
Phone: (410)955-7803 **Fax:** (410)955-0792
Email: agingctr@jhsph.edu
Website: http://www.jhsph.edu/Research/Centers/Aging
Constance A. Nathanson, PhD, Co-Ch.
Activities/Fields: Demography of aging. **Pub:** *NOAH - News on Aging at Hopkins Newsletter*, quarterly.

★ 22642 ★ Johns Hopkins University Institute for Global Tobacco Control
School of Public Health
615 N Wolfe St.
Baltimore, MD 21205
Phone: (410)614-5378 **Fax:** (410)955-0863
Email: jsamet@jhsph.edu
Website: http://www.jhsph.edu/~o-gtc/
Dr. Jonathan M. Samet, Dir.
Activities/Fields: Prevention of death and disease from tobacco use around the world.

★ 22643 ★ Johns Hopkins University Institute for Vaccine Safety (IVS)
School of Public Health
615 N Wolfe St., Ste. 5515
Baltimore, MD 21205-2179
Email: info@vaccinesafety.edu
Website: http://www.vaccinesafety.edu
Neal A. Halsey, MD, Dir.
Activities/Fields: Vaccine safety issues. **Pub:** *Newsletter*, quarterly.

★ 22644 ★ Johns Hopkins University Johns Hopkins Center for Injury Research and Policy
Department of Health Policy & Management
School of Hygiene & Public Health
624 N Broadway, Rm. 548
Baltimore, MD 21205-1996
Phone: (410)614-4026 **Fax:** (410)614-2797
Website: http://www.jhsph.edu/Research/Centers/CIRP
Ellen MacKenzie, Dir.
Activities/Fields: Adolescent drowning and poisoning, alcohol related injuries, aviation safety, childhood injuries, fall injuries in nursing homes, financing trauma care and rehabilitation, homicide and suicide, injuries from firearms, injuries in developing countries, injury sequelae and rehabilitation, injury severity scoring, injury surveillance systems, mathematical models of response to impact, motor vehicle related injuries, occupational injuries, and elderly and highway safety. Develops injury interventions, evaluates legal interventions, examines preventive measures, and evaluates trauma care. **Frmly:** Injury Prevention Center.

★ 22645 ★ Johns Hopkins University Johns Hopkins Thyroid Tumor Center
Johns Hopkins Hospital
1830 E Monument St., Ste. 333
Baltimore, MD 21287-0003
Phone: (410)955-3663 **Fax:** (410)955-8172
Email: ladenson@jhmi.edu
Paul W. Ladenson, MD, Dir.
Activities/Fields: Causes and treatment of thyroid cancer.

★ 22646 ★ Johns Hopkins University Kathryn and Alan C. Greenberg Center for Skeletal Dysplasias
Blalock 1012
600 N Wolfe St.
Baltimore, MD 21287-4922
Phone: (410)614-0977 **Fax:** (410)614-2522
Website: http://www.med.jhu.edu/Greenberg.Center/Greenbrg.htm
Victor McKusick, MD, Dir.
Activities/Fields: Skeletal dysplasias, especially dwarfism.

★ 22647 ★ Johns Hopkins University Laboratory for Computational Motor Control
416 Traylor Bldg.
Department of Biomedical Engineering
School of Medicine
720 Rutland Ave.
Baltimore, MD 21205-2195
Phone: (410)614-3424 **Fax:** (410)614-9890
Email: reza@bme.jhu.edu
Website: http://www.bme.jhu.edu/~reza/research_page.html
Dr. Reza Shadmehr, Contact
Activities/Fields: The brain and how it controls movements of the arm, particularly how does the brain learn this control; how is the information represented; what parts of the brain are involved in storing the representation and does this change with time; and can damage to the brain affect the ability to learn control. **Frmly:** Laboratory for Human Motor Learning.

★ 22648 ★ Johns Hopkins University Lipid Research Atherosclerosis Unit
550 North Broadway, Ste. 308
Baltimore, MD 21205
Phone: (410)614-0972 **Fax:** (410)955-1276
Email: pkwitero@jhmi.edu
Dr. Peter Kwiterovich, Contact
Activities/Fields: Lipids, lipoproteins, apolipoproteins, atherosclerosis, genetics, coronary artery diseases, and basic serum proteins.

★ 22649 ★ Johns Hopkins University Medical Imaging Laboratory
Departments of Biomedical Engineering & Radiology
School of Medicine
720 Rutland Ave.
Baltimore, MD 21205
Phone: (410)502-6958 **Fax:** (410)955-0549
Activities/Fields: Development of new imaging techniques and advanced applications of existing techniques to solve problems in medicine and biology.

★ 22650 ★ Johns Hopkins University Middle Atlantic Mass Spectrometry Laboratory
B-7 Biophysics Bldg.
725 N Wolfe St.
Baltimore, MD 21205
Phone: (410)955-3022 **Fax:** (410)955-3420
Email: rcotter@jhmi.edu
Website: http://www.med.jhu.edu/mams
Prof. Robert J. Cotter, Dir.
Activities/Fields: Kratos CONCEPT 1H high resolution mass spectrometer, a UV-laser desorption mass spectrometer and a Bio-Ion plasma desorption mass spectrometer as a collaborative resource for researchers from the University, from other academic institutions, or from industry and government laboratories who have need of special instrumentation and assistance in mass spectral measurement, sample preparation, chemical derivatization, and interpretation of spectra. The facility emphasizes analysis of ions of high mass (greater than 2,000 amu) and analysis of nonvolatile compounds. The high resolution mass spectrometer is equipped with an inhomogeneous high mass magnet and interfaced to a DS-90 data system, based upon the Data General Eclipse S-120 CPU with 256K MOS memory. The Laboratory also conducts in-house research focusing on the development of new instrumentation and instrumental techniques for mass spectral measurement.

★ 22651 ★ Johns Hopkins University National Institute for the Study, Prevention, and Treatment of Sexual Trauma
104 E Biddle St.
Baltimore, MD 21202
Phone: (410)955-4150 **Fax:** (410)539-1664
Email: berlinf@aol.com
Website: http://www.fredberlin.com
Dr. Fred S. Berlin, Dir.
Activities/Fields: Biological correlates and treatment of sexual disorders, including pedophilia, sadism, transvestism, voyeurism, exhibitionism, compulsive rape, and other psychosexual disorders. Analyzes and evaluates antiandrogenic and counseling treatment of sex offenders, including the effects of the synthetic progestin, Depo-Provera. **Frmly:** Johns Hopkins Hospital Sexual Disorders Clinic.

★ 22652 ★ Johns Hopkins University National Policy Center for Children with Special Health Care Needs (CSHCN)
Department of Population & Family Health Sciences
School of Public Health
624 N Broadway
Baltimore, MD 21205
Phone: (410)614-5553
Email: cshcn@jhsph.edu
Website: http://www.jhsph.edu/centers/cshcn/
Janis Lambert Connallon, Contact
Activities/Fields: Systems of care for children with special health care needs and their families. **Pub:** *Fact sheets.*

★ 22653 ★ Johns Hopkins University Office of Psychohormonal Research
1235 E Monument St., Ste. LL20
Baltimore, MD 21202
Phone: (410)955-3740
Email: jmoney@mail.jhu.edu
Dr. John Money, Dir.
Activities/Fields: Longitudinal psychohormonal research studies of patients with diverse endocrine, genital, and sexological syndromes, related to clinical psychoendocrinology, clinical sexology, gender identity/role (G-I/R), abuse-dwarfism (Kaspar Hauser syndrome), and Munchausen syndrome by proxy.

★ 22654 ★ Johns Hopkins University Parkinson's Disease Research Center (PDRC)
Carnegie 214
600 N Wolfe St.
Baltimore, MD 21287
Phone: (410)614-3359 **Fax:** (410)614-9568
Website: http://www.hopkinsmedicine.org/parkinsons/
Dr. Ted M. Dawson, Dir.
Activities/Fields: Cause and treatment of Parkinson's Disease.

★ 22655 ★ Johns Hopkins University Phoebe R. Berman Bioethics Institute
Hampton House 352
624 N Broadway
Baltimore, MD 21205-1996
Phone: (410)955-3018 **Fax:** (410)614-9567
Email: bioethic@jhsph.edu
Website: http://www.med.jhu.edu/bioethics_institute
Ruth R. Faden, PhD, Exec. Dir.
Activities/Fields: Moral and policy issues in biomedical science, health care, and health policy, and the development of thoughtful solutions for the benefit of society.

★ 22656 ★ Johns Hopkins University Physiological Mechanics and Transport Laboratory
Department of Biomedical Engineering
School of Medicine
720 Rutland Ave.
611 Traylor Research Bldg.
Baltimore, MD 21205
Phone: (410)955-6419 **Fax:** (410)614-8796
Email: apopel@jhu.edu
Website: http://www.bme.jhu.edu/~apopel/PMTL.html
Prof. Aleksander S. Popel, PhD, Contact
Activities/Fields: Mechanics and regulation of blood flow, oxygen transport to tissue, blood flow and molecular transport in the cerebral circulation, and the mechanics and electromotility of the cochlear outer hair cell.

★ 22657 ★ Johns Hopkins University Polymeric Biomaterials Laboratory
729 Ross Bldg.
Department of Biomedical Engineering
School of Medicine
Baltimore, MD 21205
Phone: (410)955-0075 **Fax:** (410)955-0549
Email: kleong@bme.jhu.edu
Dr. Kam W. Leong, Prin. Investigator
Activities/Fields: Application of synthetic and biological polymers to drug delivery, gene therapy, and tissue engineering, particularly controlled delivery of cytokines and cytokine genes for cancer immunotherapy, particulate HIV vaccine design, combinative gene and drug therapy of cystic fibrosis; and synthesis of new biodegradable poly(phosphoesters) for drug-carrier and tissue scaffold applications.

★ 22658 ★ Johns Hopkins University Primary Care Policy Center for Underserved Populations (PCPC)
452 Hampton House
Department of Health Policy and Management
624 N Broadway
Baltimore, MD 21205
Phone: (410)955-9725 **Fax:** (410)614-9046
Email: bstarfie@jhsph.edu
Website: http://www.jhsph.edu/hao/pcpc/
Dr. Barbara Starfield, Dir.
Activities/Fields: Organization, financing, and mode of delivery for primary care to underserved and vulnerable populations. **Pub:** *White papers.*

★ 22659 ★ Johns Hopkins University Research and Training Center for Hearing and Balance Auditory Anatomy and Physiology Laboratory
Traylor Bldg., Rm. 510
School of Medicine
720 Rutland Ave.
Baltimore, MD 21205
Phone: (410)955-4543 **Fax:** (410)614-4748
Email: dryugo@bme.jhu.edu
Website: http://www.bme.jhu.edu/labs/chb/labs/ap_aud.html
David K. Ryugo, Prin. Investigator
Activities/Fields: Identified cell populations, their synaptic connections, and revealing features of their signaling capabilities.

★ 22660 ★ Johns Hopkins University Research and Training Center for Hearing and Balance Auditory Neurophysiology Laboratory
Ross Research Bldg., Rm. 424
Department of Biomedical Engineering
Sch. of Medicine
720 Rutland Ave.
Baltimore, MD 21205
Phone: (410)614-4547 **Fax:** (410)614-9599
Email: xwang@bme.jhu.edu
Website: http://www.bme.jhu.edu/~xwang/lab.html
Xiaoqin Wang, PhD, Prin. Investigator
Activities/Fields: Auditory neurophysiology.

★ 22661 ★ Johns Hopkins University Research and Training Center for Hearing and Balance Laboratory of Vestibular Neurophysiology
Johns Hopkins Outpatient Center, Rm. 6253
601 N Caroline St.
Baltimore, MD 21287
Phone: (410)955-3403 **Fax:** (410)955-0035
Email: lminor@jhmi.edu
Website: http://www.bme.jhu.edu/labs/chb/labs/neurophys.html
Dr. Lloyd B. Minor, Dir.
Activities/Fields: Neurophysiological mechanisms that control vestibulo-ocular reflexes; development of new diagnostic and treatment modalities applicable to patients with vestibular disorders. **Pub:** *Working papers.*

★ 22662 ★ Johns Hopkins University Research and Training Center for Hearing and Balance Neural Encoding Laboratory
505 Traylor Bldg.
Sch. of Medicine
720 Rutland Ave.
Baltimore, MD 21205
Phone: (410)955-3162 **Fax:** (410)955-1299
Email: eyoung@bme.jhu.edu
Website: http://www.bme.jhu.edu/labs/chb/labs/neural_enc.html
Eric D. Young, PhD, Prin. Investigator
Activities/Fields: Representation and processing of complex stimuli in the auditory system.

★ 22663 ★ Johns Hopkins University Retinal Degenerations Research Center
Maumenee, Rm. 519
Wilmer Ophthalmological Institute
600 N Wolfe St.
Baltimore, MD 21287-9257
Phone: (410)955-7589 **Fax:** (410)955-0749
Email: radler@jhmi.edu
Website: http://www.wilmer.jhu.edu
Dr. Ruben Adler, Dir.
Activities/Fields: Biochemistry of essential constituents of the retina and its adjacent tissues and potential interactions among them as related to retinitis pigmentosa and other retinal degenerations. **Frmly:** Michael M. Wynn Center for the Study of Retinal Degenerations.

★ 22664 ★ Johns Hopkins University Retinal Vascular Center
Maumenee Bldg., Rm. 713
Wilmer Eye Insitute
601 N Wolfe St.
Baltimore, MD 21287-9275
Phone: (410)955-7411 **Fax:** (410)614-1683
Email: aschachat@jhmi.edu
Website: http://www.wilmer.jhu.edu
Dr. Andrew Schachat, Dir.
Activities/Fields: Focuses on halting the progression of a variety of retinal-damaging disorders, including macular degeneration, diabetic retinopathy, and eye tumors. Studies the use of lasers in treating retinal, vascular, and macular disorders and explores the underlying causes of retinal, blood vessel, pigment epithelial, and photoreceptor diseases.

★ 22665 ★ Johns Hopkins University Risk Sciences and Public Policy Institute
615 N Wolfe St., Rm. W6033
Baltimore, MD 21205-2179
Phone: (443)287-5325 **Fax:** (410)955-0863
Email: rwhite@jhsph.edu
Website: http://www.jhsph.edu/Research/Centers/rsppi
Ronald White, Dep. Dir.
Activities/Fields: Interpretation, synthesis, and organization of scientific information for analysis risk; evaluation of the implications of risk assessments for alternative management decisions; and evaluation of risk management outcomes for public health. **Pub:** *Newsletter.*

★ 22666 ★ Johns Hopkins University Robert Packard Center for ALS Research
Department of Neurobiology
600 N Wolfe St.
Baltimore, MD 21287
Phone: (410)502-7677 **Fax:** (410)955-0672
Email: alscenter@jhmi.edu
Website: http://www.hopkinsmedicine.org/alscenter/index.cfm
Jeffrey Rothstein, MD, Med. Dir.
Activities/Fields: Cause, prevention and treatment of amyotrophic lateral sclerosis (ALS).

★ 22667 ★ Johns Hopkins University Sensory Communication and Microsystems Laboratory
223 Latrobe Hall
3400 N Charles St.
Baltimore, MD 21218-2686
Phone: (410)516-8361 **Fax:** (410)516-8313
Email: andreou@jhu.edu
Website: http://olympus.ece.jhu.edu/
Andreas G. Andreou, Gp. Ldr.
Activities/Fields: Sensory microsystems performing tasks such as vision and audition. Research focuses on new technologies and devices, mixed analog/digital circuits, architecture, and algorithms.

★ 22668 ★ Johns Hopkins University Sidney Kimmel Comprehensive Cancer Center
The Harry & Jeanette Weinberg Bldg.
401 N Broadway
Baltimore, MD 21231-2410
Phone: (410)955-8964 **Fax:** (410)955-6787
Email: abeloma@jhmi.edu
Martin D. Abeloff, MD, Dir.
Activities/Fields: Cancer and related disorders, with bone marrow transplantation, cancer biology, medical oncology, pediatric oncology, pharmacology and experimental therapeutics, and radiological sciences. Activities emphasize the application of new knowledge

to management of patients with cancer and prevention of neoplastic diseases and their complications, with major aim of the several complementary research programs of the Center being an increased understanding of human neoplasia and more effective clinical management. **Pub:** *Promise and Progress Magazine*, annually. • *Scientific Report*, biennially. **Frmly:** Oncology Center.

★ 22669 ★ Johns Hopkins University Sleep Disorders Center
Asthma & Allergy Center
Johns Hopkins Bayview Medical Center
5501 Hopkins Bayview Cir.
Baltimore, MD 21224
Phone: (410)550-0571 **Fax:** (410)550-3374
Email: aschwar2@jhmi.edu
Allen Schwartz, MD, Dir.

Activities/Fields: Sleep-related disorders. Studies focus on disorders of daytime hypersomnolence, including narcolepsy, periodic leg movements, psychiatric illness, and sleep apnea; disorder-causing insomnia, psychiatric illness, shift work, and sleep apnea; and disruptive sleep patterns, loud snoring, nocturnal seizures, nocturnal terrors, and sleep walking. Also investigates male erectile impotence, using sleep recordings as a diagnostic tool.

★ 22670 ★ Johns Hopkins University STD Research Group
Ross Bldg., Rm. 1159
School of Medicine
720 Rutland Ave.
Baltimore, MD 21205
Phone: (410)955-7636 **Fax:** (410)614-9775
Email: jzenilma@welchlink.welch.jhu.edu
Website: http://www.med.jhu.edu/jhustd/
Jonathan M. Zenilman, MD, Dir.

Activities/Fields: Edidemiology, prevention and behavioral aspects of sexually transmitted diseases (STDs), and establishing rapid and reliable testing and diagnoses of STDs.

★ 22671 ★ Johns Hopkins University Vascular Bioengineering Laboratory
Department of Biomedical Engineering
School of Medicine
720 Rutland Ave.
619 Traylor
Baltimore, MD 21205
Phone: (410)614-2951 **Fax:** (410)614-8796
Email: ralevria@bme.jhu.edu
Website: http://www.bme.jhu.edu/~thuang/lab/lab.html
B. Rita Alevriadou, PhD, Prin. Investigator

Activities/Fields: Fluid mechanics; thrombosis/atherosclerosis; vascular cell biology; and cell and tissue engineering.

★ 22672 ★ Johns Hopkins University Welch Center for Prevention, Epidemiology, and Clinical Research
2024 E Monument St., Ste. 2-600
Baltimore, MD 21205-2223
Phone: (410)955-6953 **Fax:** (410)955-0476
Email: npowe@jhmi.edu
Website: http://www.med.jhu.edu/welchcenter/
Neil R. Powe, MD, Dir.

Activities/Fields: Etiology of disease and disability in populations, through observational epidemiology, randomized controlled trials, and effectiveness outcomes research. Also responsible for the generation and dissemination of knowledge required for prevention of disease and disability.

★ 22673 ★ Johns Hopkins University Wilmer Ophthalmological Institute
Retinal Vascular Service
600 N Wolfe St.
Baltimore, MD 21287-9278
Phone: (410)955-6846 **Fax:** (410)955-0675
Email: mgoldbrg@gwgatel.jhmi.jhu.edu
Website: http://www.wilmer.jhu.edu
Morton F. Goldberg, MD, Chm.

Activities/Fields: Ophthalmology, including studies of macular degeneration, diabetic retinopathy, cataracts and the cornea, ocular immunology, uveitis (inflammatory eye diseases), retinal-damaging disorders, retinal degenerations, glaucoma, preventive ophthalmology, strabismus (misaligned or crossed eyes), double vision, amblyopia (reduced vision in one eye), hereditary eye diseases, neuroophthalmology, oculomotor functions, correlation of changes in the structure and form of eye tissue with symptoms of illness, development of new technology and techniques to study visual function disorders, development of new optical aids for the visually handicapped, immunohistochemical analysis of the blood retina barrier, retinal gene expression, genetics of eye diseases, molecular biology of eye development, molecular biology of glaucoma, and retinal pigment epithelium (RPE).

★ 22674 ★ Johns Hopkins University Women's and Children's Health Policy Center (WCHPC)
615 N Wolfe St.
Baltimore, MD 21205
Phone: (410)502-5443 **Fax:** (410)502-5831
Email: hgrason@jhsph.edu
Website: http://www.jhsph.edu/wchpc
Holly Grason, Contact

Activities/Fields: Health system reforms impacting the health of women, children, and adolescents. **Pub:** *Research and technical resource briefs.*

★ 22675 ★ Johns Hopkins University Zanvyl Krieger Mind/Brain Institute
Krieger Hall, Rm. 338
3400 N Charles St.
Baltimore, MD 21218
Phone: (410)516-8640 **Fax:** (410)516-8648
Email: kenneth.johnson@jhu.edu
Website: http://www.mb.jhu.edu
Dr. Kenneth Johnson, Prin. Investigator

Activities/Fields: Fundamental activities of the human mind, including learning and the use of language, initiation of action and perception, and nervous system plasticity and regeneration. Attempts to address the basic questions of how consciousness is possible and how mind and brain are related.

★ 22676 ★ Joint Division of Newborn Medicine
Medical Center
600 S 42nd St.
Omaha, NE 68198-1205
Phone: (402)559-6750 **Fax:** (402)559-7341
Dr. Terence Cazh, Dir.

Activities/Fields: Cell and molecular basis of cerebral ischemia, ontogency of C3 complement in human lung, and physiologic and pharmacodynamic evaluation of infants on ECMO therapy. Conducts clinical trials of two types of high frequency ventilation. Participating in clinical trials of Infasurf, a fetal calf surfactant. **Frmly:** Neonatology Research Laboratory.

★ 22677 ★ Joint Program in Biomedical Engineering
University of Texas Southwestern Medical Center at Dallas
5323 Harry Hines Blvd.
Dallas, TX 75390-9058
Phone: (214)648-2503 **Fax:** (214)648-2991
Email: bme@utsouthwestern.edu
Website: http://www.swmed.edu/home_pages/bme/index_frame2.html
Prof. Peter P. Antich, PhD, Ch.

Activities/Fields: Biomedical engineering, including studies in molecular engineering, computational biology, magnetic resonance, gamma and ultrasound image analysis, orthopedics, human performance, biocompatible materials, biomechanics, artificial organs, biosensors, soft tissue biomechanics, neurological signal acquisition and analysis, recombinant DNA technology, human genome project and gene therapy. **Pub:** *BME Information Brochure.* • *BME Student Activity Reports.* • *Internship Brochure.*

★ 22678 ★ Jones Institute for Reproductive Medicine
601 Colley Ave.
Norfolk, VA 23507
Phone: (757)446-7100 **Free:** 800-515-6637
Fax: (757)876-6317
Website: http://www.jonesinstitute.org
Dr. William Gibbons, Chm.

Activities/Fields: Human reproduction, including studies of reproductive physiology during the hours and days surrounding fertilization, fertilization process, gametogenesis, neuroendocrinology, ovarian follicular development, gene expression, reproductive toxicology, endocrine control of menstrual cycle, andrology, reproductive immunology, and cancer.

★ 22679 ★ Joslin Diabetes Center
1 Joslin Pl.
Boston, MA 02215
Phone: (617)732-2400 **Fax:** (617)732-2487
Website: http://www.joslin.harvard.edu/
Dr. C. Ronald Kahn, Pres.

Activities/Fields: Diabetes mellitus, including investigations on chemical composition of basement membrane, physiological control of glucose metabolism, neonatal and fetal growth and metabolism, cellular and molecular mechanisms of insulin action, vascular cell biology, ultrastructure of beta cell, pancreatic islets, muscle perfusion, experimental diabetes in animals, immunologic aspects of diabetes, diabetic eye disease, and epidemiology of diabetes. Conducts clinical studies of early stages of diabetic state, treatment, and prevention of diabetes and its complications, especially of a vascular nature, with emphasis on diabetic retinopathy. **Pub:** *Annual report.* • *Joslin Camp Calendar.* • *Joslin Magazine*, quarterly.

★ 22680 ★ Kaiser Foundation Hospitals Oregon Center for Complementary and Alternative Medicine Research in Craniofacial Disorders
Center for Health Research
3800 N Interstate Ave.
Portland, OR 97227
Phone: (503)335-6734 **Fax:** (503)335-2424
Email: nancy.vuckovic@kpchr.org
Nancy Vuckovic, PhD, Prin. Investigator

Activities/Fields: Potential, effectiveness, acceptability, and effects of complementary and alternative medical practices in reference to craniofacial disorders.

★ 22681 ★ Kaiser Permanente Center for Health Research
3800 N Interstate Ave.
Portland, OR 97227-1098
Phone: (503)335-2400 **Fax:** (503)335-2424
Email: mary.durham@kpchr.org
Website: http://www.kpchr.org/
Mary L. Durham, PhD, Dir.

Activities/Fields: Organization, financing, costs and quality of medical care in an HMO; mental health; medical informatics; patient safety; health behavior interventions; epidemiology; effectiveness of alternative therapies and services; nutrition; genetics; dental research; and biometry and research methods. **Pub:** *Annual Report.* • *The Chronicle*, 3/year. Newsletter. • *Current Studies*, annually. Brochure.

★ 22682 ★ Kaiser Permanente Medical Care Program Division of Research
3505 Broadway
Oakland, CA 94611-5714
Phone: (510)891-3400 **Fax:** (510)450-2073
Email: jvs@dor.kaiser.org

Website: http://www.dor.kaiser.org
Dr. Joseph V. Selby, Dir.

Activities/Fields: Epidemiology, biometrics and biostatistics, technology assessment, health services research, and health education research and evaluation. Supports clinical research in medical centers.

★ 22683 ★ Kansas City Clinical Oncology Program
6601 Rockhill Rd.
Kansas City, MO 64131
Phone: (816)823-0555 **Fax:** (816)823-0563
Email: kccop@kccop.org
Website: http://www.kccop.org
Leslie Herst, Exec. Dir.

Activities/Fields: Oncological clinical trials.

★ 22684 ★ Kansas State University Center for Basic Cancer Research
1 Chalmers Hall
Manhattan, KS 66506-3901
Phone: (785)532-6705 **Fax:** (785)532-6707
Website: http://www.ksu.edu/cancer.center
Dr. Robin Denell, Dir.

Activities/Fields: Cancer autonomy and metastasis; tumor initiation, promotion, and progression; chemotherapeutic compounds; growth regulation, the immune system, and other cellular interactions; and oncogene expression. **Pub:** *Accepting a Challenge Magazine.* • *A Day with Dr. Waddle (children's workbook on cancer).*

★ 22685 ★ Kansas State University University Biochemistry Facility
Willard Hall, Rm. 104
Department of Biochemistry
Manhattan, KS 66506-3702
Phone: (785)532-6121 **Fax:** (785)532-7278
Email: cxhedg@ksu.edu
Website: http://www.ksu.edu/bchem/
Dr. Michael Kanost, Dept. Hd.

Activities/Fields: Biochemistry research, including protein sequencing, peptide sequencing, and oligonucleotide synthesis.

★ 22686 ★ Kellogg Cancer Care Center (KCCC)
Evanston Northwestern Health Care
2650 Ridge Ave.
Evanston, IL 60201
Phone: (847)570-2110 **Free:** 888-909-5222
Fax: (847)570-2905
Email: J.Kmandeicar@nwu.edu
Website: http://www.enh.org
Dr. Janardan Dinkar Khandekar, Dir.

Activities/Fields: Treatment and diagnosis of cancer, including phase 1 and 2 studies, evaluation of new drug protocols, and brain tumor studies. Basic and clinical research also includes studies of breast, head and neck, lung, bladder, and pancreatic cancers, blood clotting and fibrinolytic mechanisms in tumor patients, thromboembolic problems in cancer patients, pituitary tumor surgery, immunology/virology, microbiology, hematology, clinical biochemistry, pharmacology, diagnosis by fine needle aspiration techniques, oncogens, medical oncology, and psychiatry. Also conducts studies in flow cytometry and magnetic resonance imaging and spectroscopy. **Frmly:** Evanston Cancer Care Center.

★ 22687 ★ Kennedy Krieger Institute
707 N Broadway
Baltimore, MD 21205
Phone: (410)502-9483 **Fax:** (410)502-9524
Email: goldstein@kennedykrieger.org
Website: http://www.kennedykrieger.org
Dr. Gary W. Goldstein, Pres.

Activities/Fields: Pediatric rehabilitation evaluation, treatment, and research, including interdisciplinary studies in genetics, biochemistry, toxicology, neurochemistry, metabolic diseases, speech and hearing, pharmacology, behavioral sciences, and special education. Major emphasis is placed on physical rehabilitation, effectiveness of drug support, behavior modification, evaluation of neurological disorders in children, and developing and testing training techniques.

★ 22688 ★ Kennedy Krieger Institute Blood-Brain Barrier Laboratory
707 N Broadway
Baltimore, MD 21205
Phone: (443)923-9300 **Free:** 888-554-2080
Fax: (443)923-9317
Email: goldstein@kennedykrieger.org
Dr. Gary W. Goldstein, Dir.

Activities/Fields: Molecular aspects of brain microvessel differentiation, cell-cell signaling, second messengers, and transport systems. Investigates the effects of lead poisoning.

★ 22689 ★ Kent State University Exercise Physiology Lab
162 Gym Annex
School of Exercise, Leisure & Sport
Kent, OH 44242
Phone: (330)672-2857 **Fax:** (330)672-2250
Email: eglickma@kent.edu
Dr. Ellen Glickman, Contact

Activities/Fields: Exercise physiology, body composition, and physical fitness, including studies of protein metabolism and exercise, cardiovascular/respiratory responses during exercise in heat and cold, an neuromuscular integration/biomechanics, and psychosocial reactivity to behavioral stressors. **Frmly:** Applied Physiology Research Laboratory.

★ 22690 ★ Kent State University Speech and Hearing Clinic
A104 Music & Speech Bldg.
Kent, OH 44242
Phone: (330)672-2672 **Fax:** (330)672-2643
Email: csommer@kent. edu
Carol Sommer, Dir.

Activities/Fields: Speech pathology and audiology, including staff specialties in infant, children's, and adult languages, stuttering, phonology, aural rehabilitation, and hearing aids.

★ 22691 ★ Kentucky Cancer Program
2365 Harrodsburg Rd., Ste. A230
Lexington, KY 40504-3381
Phone: (859)219-0772 **Fax:** (859)219-0548
Email: dka@kcp.uky.edu
Website: http://www.kcr.uky.edu/kcp/
Debra Armstrong, Dir.

Activities/Fields: Cancer control. Collects and disseminates information leading to improved prevention, diagnosis, and treatment of cancer. Serves communities throughout the Commonwealth through identified intermediaries, working through District Cancer Councils and community cancer coalitions. The Cancer Control Program developed the computerized Kentucky Cancer Registry (KCR), and has recently been designated a SEER site to which Kentucky hospitals are legislatively mandated to report cancer incidence. Supports a community-based research component to evaluate cancer control efforts of joint interventions and information dissemination. **Pub:** *CHOICES.* • *For Your Peace of Mind Video.* • *KCR Cancer Incidence Report.* • *Literacy Curriculum for Breast and Cervical Cancer.* • *Pathfinder.* • *Research Findings.* • *Woman Talk, a video about cervical health.*

★ 22692 ★ King James Medical Laboratory/Omegatech
24700 Center Ridge Rd.
Cleveland, OH 44145
Free: 800-437-1404 **Fax:** (440)835-2177
Email: headquarters@kingjamesomegatech-lab.com
Website: http://www.kingjamesomegatech-lab.com
Dr. Raymond J. Shamberger, Dir.

Activities/Fields: Nutrition and trace elements, including role of dietary thiamine, serum enzyme activities, synthesis and utilization of creatine, effect of zinc supplement, and sorption from the gut. **Frmly:** Preventive Medicine Research Center of Cleveland.

★ 22693 ★ Krannert Institute of Cardiology
1800 N Capitol Ave.
Indianapolis, IN 46202
Phone: (317)962-0555 **Fax:** (317)962-0568
Email: dzipes@iupui.edu
Douglas Zipes, Dir.

Activities/Fields: Basic and clinical electrophysiology, cardiac membrane biology, echocardiography, vascular biology, exercise physiology, heart failure, interventional cardiology, and cardiovascular transgenics. **Pub:** *Cardiac Electrophysiology: From Cell to Bedside*, quadrennially. • *Heart Disease textbook*, quadrennially. • *Journal of the American Society of Echocardiography*, bimonthly. • *Journal of Cardiovascular Electrophysiology*, monthly.

★ 22694 ★ La Jolla Institute for Allergy and Immunology
10355 Science Center Dr.
San Diego, CA 92121
Phone: (858)558-3500 **Fax:** (858)558-3525
Website: http://www.liai.org
Dr. Howard Grey, Pres.

Activities/Fields: Increased knowledge of the immune system including the study of the regulatory mechanisms involved in the onset and maintenance of immune response, and the development of new, more sophisticated and precise strategies and/or therapies for managing various immunological and allergic disorders.

★ 22695 ★ La Jolla Institute for Molecular Medicine
4570 Executive Dr., Ste. 100
San Diego, CA 92121
Phone: (858)587-8788 **Fax:** (858)587-6742
Email: moubre@ljimm.org
Website: http://www.ljimm.org/
Dr. Mario A. Bourdon, Sci. Dir.

Activities/Fields: Cause and cures of cancer, immune diseases and genetic disorders.

★ 22696 ★ La Rabida Children's Hospital and Research Center
E 65th St. at Lake Michigan
Chicago, IL 60649
Phone: (773)363-6700 **Fax:** (773)363-7160
Email: info@larabida.org
Website: http://www.larabida.org
Edem Ekwo, MD, Dir.

Activities/Fields: Economic, educational, cultural, and medical effects of childhood chronic illness and disability on families and society. Areas of research include patterns of health care financing, medically complex children, community-based service systems, and the nature of family constellations, including the tracking of child development in family contexts, and intervention studies.

★ 22697 ★ Laban/Bartenieff Institute of Movement Studies, Inc.
520 8th Ave., Ste. 304, 3rd Fl.
New York, NY 10018
Phone: (212)643-8888 **Fax:** (212)643-8388
Email: limsnyc@aol.com
Website: http://www.limsonline.org
Kristine Lindahl, Dir. of Educ.

Activities/Fields: Perception, description, and analysis of human movement for applications in dance and theater, physical therapy, psychotherapy, nonverbal communication, management consulting, anthropology, and fitness and sports training. The Institute's mission is to further the studies of the principles of movement formulated by Rudolf Laban (1879-1958), an Austro-Hungarian dancer, choreographer, and philosopher, and Irmgard Bartenieff (1900-1981), who applied her Laban training to physical therapy, dance therapy, anthropology, and dance. **Pub:** *Movement Studies Journal.* • *Newsletter.*

★ 22698 ★ Laboratory for Research on the Neuroscience of Autism (RNA)
8110 La Jolla Shores Dr., Ste. 201
La Jolla, CA 92037
Phone: (858)551-7925 **Fax:** (858)551-7931
Email: ecourchesne@ucsd.edu
Eric Courchesne, PhD, Dir.
Activities/Fields: Neurophysiological and neuroanatomical basis for autism, including the functional role of the cerebellum in cognition, the brain bases of selective attention, and the neuropsychological consequences of stroke. **Frmly:** Autism and Brain Development Research Laboratory.

★ 22699 ★ Laboratory of Signal Transduction
Memorial Sloan-Kettering Cancer Center
1275 York Ave., Box 254
New York, NY 10021
Phone: (212)639-8573 **Fax:** (212)794-4342
Email: rkolesnick@ski.mskcc.org
Dr. Richard Kolesnick, Prin. Investigator
Activities/Fields: Signal transduction for cytokines and hormones, including tumor necrosis factor-alpha, interleukin-1, and activin.

★ 22700 ★ Laboratory of Tumor Antigen Immunochemistry
Memorial Sloan-Kettering Cancer Center
1275 York Ave.
New York, NY 10021
Phone: (212)639-8613 **Fax:** (646)422-2189
Dr. Thomas Kelly, Dir.
Activities/Fields: Monoclonal antibodies and carbohydrate antigens. **Frmly:** Laboratory of Human Cancer Immunology.

★ 22701 ★ Lahey Clinic Foundation
41 Mall Rd.
Burlington, MA 01805
Phone: (781)744-5100 **Fax:** (781)744-8999
Website: http://www.lahey.org
Dr. David Barett, Dir.
Activities/Fields: Medical, surgical, and radiological techniques, with special emphasis on clinical applications, including studies on high and mega voltage radiation, treatment of cancer with drugs and immunotherapy, cancer cell kinetics, electronic measurement of bacterial growth, pancreatic and renal transplantation, cardiac surgery, diagnostic radiology, amino acid absorption, treatment of pancreatitis, and hospital and prolonged storage by freezing of blood for transfusion. Maintains a clinic for patient care and application of research results and an educational division for postgraduate medical training and residency, both at the clinic and at local hospitals and medical schools. **Pub:** *Lahey Clinic Foundation Bulletin*, quarterly.

★ 22702 ★ Lakehead University Northern Educational Centre for Aging and Health (NECAH)
Health Sciences N
955 Oliver Rd.
Thunder Bay, ON, Canada P7B 5E1
Phone: (807)343-2126 **Fax:** (807)343-2104
Email: necah@lakeheadu.ca
Website: http://www.lakeheadu.ca/~necahwww/
Michael Stones, PhD, Dir.
Activities/Fields: The aging process and its relationship to health and well-being.

★ 22703 ★ Lancaster Cleft Palate Clinic
223 N Lime St.
Lancaster, PA 17602
Phone: (717)396-7415 **Fax:** (717)396-7409
Email: relong@lha.org
Dr. Ross E. Long, Jr., Dir.
Activities/Fields: Plastic surgery, dentistry, orthodontics, prosthodontics, craniofacial morphology, speech, hearing, otolaryngology, genetics, and behavioral science, particularly in regard to children with craniofacial anomalies. Conducts interdisciplinary study of problems of oral/facial growth, orthognathic surgery, and communicative disorders. **Frmly:** H.K. Cooper Clinic.

★ 22704 ★ Lankenau Institute for Medical Research (LIMR)
100 Lancaster Ave.
Wynnewood, PA 19096
Phone: (610)645-3475 **Fax:** (610)645-8533
Email: cristofalov@mlhs.org
Website: http://www.mainlinehealth.org/limr/
Vincent J. Cristofalo, PhD, Pres. /CEO
Activities/Fields: Biological mechanisms of aging and the diseases associated with it, including but not limited to cancer, cardiovascular disease, osteoporosis and age-related neurodegenerative disorders. The focus of this research is to improve the health and quality of life for all, with particular emphasis on older persons. **Pub:** *Abstracts.* • *Newsletters.* • *Papers.*

★ 22705 ★ Laval University Cancer Research Centre
Hotel-Dieu de Quebec
9 McMahon
Quebec, QC, Canada G1R 2J6
Phone: (418)691-5281 **Fax:** (418)691-5439
Email: Luc.Belanger@crhdq.ulaval.ca
Dr. Luc Belanger, Sci. Dir.
Activities/Fields: Cellular and molecular mechanisms relating differentiation and cancer, including genomic organization and molecular regulation of fetoprotein, histones, metallothionein, oncogenes, cytochromes P-450 and developmental tyrosine kinase genes, developmental genes in embryonic stem cell mice, structure of active versus inactive chromatin, nature of neoplastic liver cell progenitors, role of growth factor-cell interactions in tissue growth, differentiation and neoplasia, cell surface markers of bladder cancer, hormone receptors, mechanisms of ribosomal transcription, action of DNA intercalating drugs, carcinogen activation, mutagenesis, DNA repair, signal transductors, and cancer genes therapy. Also conducts research and development activities in clinical oncology, cancer epidemiology and psycho-oncology. Serves as a reference center for flow cytometry, hormone receptor measurements, confocal microscopy, and genetic probes in cancer.

★ 22706 ★ Laval University Cardiopulmonary Institute
2725 Chemin Ste. Foy
Sainte Foy, QC, Canada G1V 4G5
Phone: (418)656-5977 **Fax:** (418)656-4602
Email: denis.richard@phs.ulaval.ca
Denis Richard, PhD, Dir.
Activities/Fields: All major fields of cardiopulmonary diseases, and obesity and energetic metabolism. **Pub:** *Publications and Absracts (200/year).*

★ 22707 ★ Laval University Division of Kinesiology
Department of Social Science et Preventive Medicine
Faculty of Medicine
PEPS Rm. 2142
Quebec, QC, Canada G1K 7P4
Phone: (418)656-7831 **Fax:** (418)656-3044
Email: louis.perusse@kin.msp.ulaval.ca
Louis Perusse, Dir.
Activities/Fields: Genetic and molecular basis of obesity and its co-morbidities. Genetics of performance and adaptation to exercise training. Research focuses on the quantification of heritability levels and the identification of genes and molecular markers through association and linkage analyses.

★ 22708 ★ Laval University Health Services Research Group
Pavillon des Sciences de l'administration
Cite universitaire
Sainte Foy, QC, Canada G1K 7P4
Phone: (418)656-3503 **Fax:** (418)656-2624
Prof. Clermont Begin, Contact
Activities/Fields: Health care organizations, including planning, financing, decision making, information systems, evaluation of health policies, socio-political aspects of organization and evaluation of health services.

★ 22709 ★ Laval University Human Nutrition Research Group
Pavillon Paul-Comtois
Sainte Foy, QC, Canada G1K 7P4
Phone: (418)656-2131 **Fax:** (418)656-3353
Email: helene.jacques@aln.ulaval.ca
Helene Jacques, Dir.
Activities/Fields: Nutrient bioavailability: mechanisms and metabolic impact.

★ 22710 ★ Laval University Infectious Disease Research Centre
2705, blvd. Laurier
Sainte Foy, QC, Canada G1V 4G2
Phone: (418)654-2705 **Fax:** (418)654-2715
Email: michel.g.bergeron@crchul.ulaval.ca
Website: http://www.cri.crchul.ulaval.ca
Michel G. Bergeron, Dir.
Activities/Fields: Molecular basis of action of antimicrobial agents and the mechanisms involved in the microbial resistance against these agents. Develops new transportation vehicles of antimicrobials in bacteria, parasites, and viruses; works on metabolic particularities of parasites; develops new diagnostic kits for quick detection of bacterial and viral infections; and works on new vaccines. Studies AIDS, treatments for HIV-infected patients, and the immunological, pharmacodynamic, and psychosocial factors controlling HIV infections.

★ 22711 ★ Laval University Joseph Rheaume Laboratory
Pavillon Paul-Comtois
Quebec, QC, Canada G1K 7P4
Phone: (418)656-2315 **Fax:** (418)656-3353
Email: laurent.savoie@nhc.ulaval.ca
Laurent Savoie, Dir.
Activities/Fields: Nutrient bioavailability, the effect of food proteins on mineral bioavailability in vitro and in vivo, and kinetics and forms of amino acids at various levels of blood circulation.

★ 22712 ★ Laval University Laboratory of Experimental Tissue Engineering
Hopital du Saint-Sacrement, Research Centre
1050 Chemin Ste.-Foy
Quebec, QC, Canada G1S 4L8
Phone: (418)682-7663 **Fax:** (418)682-8000
Email: Lucie.Germain@chg.ulaval.ca
Website: http://www.fmed.ulaval.ca/loex
Dr. Francois A. Auger, Dir.
Activities/Fields: Clinical and experimental human tissue engineering (blood vessel, skin, musculoskeletal, bronchial, ocular), including tissue transplantation and developing applications for living tissue equivalents such as percutaneous absorption, toxicology, and wound healing.

★ 22713 ★ Laval University
Medical and Environmental Research Group
Philosophy Department
Pavillon Felix Antoine Savard
Quebec, QC, Canada G1K 7P4
Phone: (418)656-2244 **Fax:** (418)656-7267
Marie-Helene Parizeau, Dir.

Activities/Fields: Bioethics, human experimentation, ethical committees, education in ehtics for health professionals.

★ 22714 ★ Laval University
Medical Research Centre
2705 Blvd. Laurier
Sainte Foy, QC, Canada G1V 4G2
Phone: (418)654-2296 **Fax:** (418)654-2735
Email: fernand.labrie@crchul.ulaval.ca
Dr. Fernand Labrie, Hd.

Activities/Fields: Family medicine, rheumatology and immunology, infectious diseases, health and environment, genetics and molecular medicine, ontogeny and reproduction, molecular endocrinology, hypertension, diabetes, lipids, ophthalmology, pediatrics, hormonal bioregulation, and public health.

★ 22715 ★ Laval University
Medical Research Centre
Diabetes Research Group
2705 Blvd. Laurier
Sainte Foy, QC, Canada G1V 4G2
Phone: (418)654-2741 **Fax:** (418)654-2792
Email: andre.nadeau@crchul.ulaval.ca
Andre Nadeau, Dir.

Activities/Fields: The relationship between physical activity and diabetes, and the identification of factors responsible for the increased level of cardiac mortality in diabetes patients. Participation in clinical trials on new therapeutic agents for diabetes mellitus.

★ 22716 ★ Laval University
Medical Research Centre
Family Medicine Research Group
2705 Blvd. Bay-tree
Sainte Foy, QC, Canada G1V 4G2
Phone: (418)654-2701 **Fax:** (418)654-2138
Email: lucie.baillargeon@crchul.ulaval.ca
Lucie Baillargeon, Dir.

Activities/Fields: Causes of, and therapeutic alternatives to, overuse of hypnotic and anxiolytic drugs; family physicians treatment of patients who are facing domestic violence; evaluation of validity of international prostatic symptoms scale; physicians knowledge of diabetic retinopathy; risk of severe perineal tears in relation to median episiotomy; clinical trials on antibiotherapy for various infectious diseases; and smoking cessation.

★ 22717 ★ Laval University
Medical Research Centre
Human Genetics Unit
2705 Blvd. Laurier
Sainte Foy, QC, Canada G1V 4G2
Phone: (418)654-2244 **Fax:** (418)654-2714
Email: sec.drs@crchul.hlaval.ca
Website: http://www.crchul.ulaval.ca/crchul/en/centre/default_pres.htm
Jack Puymirat, MD, Dir.

Activities/Fields: Molecular mechanisms controlling genetic expression; thyroid hormones and central nervous system development; molecular genetics of myotonic dystrophy; implication of cytoskeletal and nucleoskeletal proteins in morphonogenetic and differentiation processes; molecular genetics of Charcot-Marie-Tooth disease; control of cell cycle; gene therapy; myoblasts transplantation for Duchenne's disease, Myotonia congenita, and genetic testing.

★ 22718 ★ Laval University
Medical Research Centre
Lipid Research Centre
2705 Blvd. Laurier, TR-93
Sainte Foy, QC, Canada G1V 4G2
Phone: (418)654-2244 **Fax:** (418)654-2714
Email: pierre.julien@crchul.ulaval.ca
Website: http://www.crchul.ulaval.ca/crchul/fr/default.asp
Pierre Julien, PhD, Dir.

Activities/Fields: Pharmacological studies on hypolipidemic agents, lipoproteins, apoproteins, LDL receptors, lipoprotein lipase and hepatic lipase activity, abdominal and visceral obesity, metabolism and genetic polymorphism, nutritional studies on polysaturated and omega fatty acids, and epidemiology of ischemic heart disease in the region of Quebec City.

★ 22719 ★ Laval University
Medical Research Centre
Oncology and Molecular Endocrinology Research Center
2705 Blvd. Laurier
Sainte Foy, QC, Canada G1V 4G2
Phone: (418)654-2244 **Fax:** (418)654-2714
Email: fernand.labrie@crchul.ulaval.ca
Website: http://www.crchul.ulaval.ca
Dr. Fernand Labrie, Dir.

Activities/Fields: Prostate and other hormone-sensitive cancers, strategies for early screening for prostate cancer, mechanisms regulating C-19 steroid formation by adrenal glands, characterization of effects of steroid sex hormones, adrenal hormone effects on brain dopaminergic systems, molecular mechanisms responsible for the expression of genes in specific tissues and their extinction in others, cloning and characterization of enzymes implicated in steroidogenesis, hormonal control of growth factors, polyamine biosynthesis in human breast cancer, and regulation of the expression of enzymes involved in steroidogenesis in placenta and adrenal glands. **Pub:** *Scientific (400/year).* **Frmly:** Molecular Endocrinology Research Group.

★ 22720 ★ Laval University
Medical Research Centre
Ophthalmology Research Group
2705 Blvd. Laurier
Sainte Foy, QC, Canada G1V 4G2
Phone: (418)654-2105 **Fax:** (418)654-2131
Email: groupe.ophtalmo@crchul.ulaval.ca
Dr. Alain Rousseau, Dir.

Activities/Fields: Laser corneal surgery, ocular melanoma, corneal wound healing and corneal transplantation, retinal pigment epethelium, genetics in melanoma glaucoma, and liver metastases from melanoma.

★ 22721 ★ Laval University
Molecular Microbiology and Protein Engineering Group
Departemente de Biologie Medicale
4142 Pavillon Charles-Eugene-Marchand
Faculte de Medecine
Sainte Foy, QC, Canada G1K 7P4
Phone: (418)656-2131 **Fax:** (418)656-7176
Email: rclevesq@rsvs.ulaval.ca
Roger C. Levesque, Dir.

Activities/Fields: Structure-function analysis of B-lactamases, dihydrofolate reductase and superoxide dismutase in pathogenic microorganisms. Studies also include molecular genetics, phylogeny, and evolution of multiresistant transposons, and sequencing pseudomonas genome.

★ 22722 ★ Laval University
Research Centre on the Biology of Reproduction
Cite Universite
Sainte Foy, QC, Canada G1K 7P4
Phone: (418)656-5229 **Fax:** (418)654-3766
Website: http://www.crbr.ulaval.ca
Marc-Andre Sirard, PhD, Dir.

Activities/Fields: Physiological, cellular, and molecular factors leading to the production of viable embryos, male infertility and contraception, sexual differentiation, implantation and the maintenance of pregnancy. Focuses on the development and applications of new reproductive techniques for domestic animals and humans. **Frmly:** Ontogeny and Reproduction Research Group.

★ 22723 ★ Laval University
Research Group in Oral Ecology
Pavillon de Medecine Dentair
Quebec, QC, Canada G1K 7P4
Phone: (418)656-2131 **Fax:** (418)656-2861
Email: greb@greb.ulaval.ca
Website: http://www.greb.ulaval.ca
Daniel Grenier, Info. Off.

Activities/Fields: Studies the biological equilibrium between host and microorganism, including prevention of microbial diseases of the mouth, early identification of high-risk subjects, and outcome predictions of elaborate and frequently expensive curative treatments.

★ 22724 ★ Laval University
Research Unit in Nephrology
Hotel-Dieu de Quebec Research Centre
11, Cote du Palais
Quebec, QC, Canada G1R 2J6
Phone: (418)525-4444 **Fax:** (418)691-5562
Email: marcel.lebel@crhdq.ulaval.ca
Dr. Marcel Lebel, Dir.

Activities/Fields: Pathogenesis of high blood pressure and renal diseases.

★ 22725 ★ Laval University
Robert Giffard Research Centre
2601, de la Canardiere
Beauport, QC, Canada G1J 2G3
Phone: (418)663-5741 **Fax:** (418)663-9540
Email: michel.maziade@psa.ulaval.ca
Website: http://www.crulrg.ulaval.ca
Michel Maziade, Dir.

Activities/Fields: Fundamental, clinical and epidemiological studies. Alzheimer's disease, bipolar disorder, schizophrenia, autism, other neurological disorders; mapping of characterization of genes involved in schizophrenia and depression; evaluation of mental health services, care delivery and care organization.

★ 22726 ★ Laval University
Saint-Francois-d'Assise Hospital Research Centre
10, Rue de l'Espinay
Quebec, QC, Canada G1L 3L5
Phone: (418)525-4461 **Fax:** (418)525-4481
Email: Jean-Claude.Forest@bcx.ulaval.ca
Website: http://www.crsfa.ulaval.ca
Dr. Jean-Claude Forest, Dir.

Activities/Fields: Reproductive endocrinology, perinatalogy, human genetics, biomaterials, magnetic resonance, and biotechnology.

★ 22727 ★ Laval University
Saint-Francois-d'Assise Hospital Research Centre
Reproductive Endocrinology Unit
10, Rue de l'Espinay
Quebec, QC, Canada G1L 3L5
Phone: (418)525-4461 **Fax:** (418)525-4481
Email: andre.lemay@ogy.ulaval.ca
Website: http://www.crsfa.ulaval.ca
Dr. André Lemay, Ch.

Activities/Fields: New medical treatments of acne and hirstism (polycystic ovarian diseaese PCO), new modalities of hormonal replacement therapy for menopause, and basic research on growth and immune factors implicated in endometriosis.

★ 22728 ★ Laval University Saint-Sacrement Hospital Research Centre
1401, 18e Rue
Quebec, QC, Canada G1J 1Z4
Phone: (418)649-5593 **Fax:** (418)649-5910
Email: suzanne.dupuis@cha.quebec.qc.ca
Website: http://www.crcha.qc.ca
Dr. François A. Auger, Dir.
Activities/Fields: Epidemiology and public health, experimental organogenesis, hematology, and clinical research in gynecology, obstetrics, respiratory diseases, traumatology, gastr-enterology, cardiology and breast cancer.

★ 22729 ★ Laval University Saint-Sacrement Hospital Research Centre
Unite de Recherche en Sante des Populations
1050 Chemin Ste-Foy
Quebec, QC, Canada G1S 4L8
Phone: (418)682-7390 **Fax:** (418)682-7949
Email: jocelyne.moisan@pha.ulaval.ca
Jocelyne Moisan, Dir.
Activities/Fields: Population health research, cancer, infectious diseases, environmental and work related diseases, drug utilisation; biostatistics, and mathematical modelling. Research programs include clinical trials, cohort and case-control studies.

★ 22730 ★ Lawrence Berkeley National Laboratory
Center for Functional Imaging
Mail Stop 55-121
1 Cyclotron Rd.
Berkeley, CA 94720
Phone: (510)486-5435 **Fax:** (510)486-4768
Email: tfbudinger@lbl.gov
Website: http://cfi.lbl.gov
Dr. Thomas F. Budinger, Hd.
Activities/Fields: Researches medicine and radiation biophysics, emphasizing imaging instrumentation and radiopharmaceuticals development, and the diagnosis of human diseases. Develops imaging instrumentation and computer programs for the study of brain and heart disease in conjunction with new pharmaceuticals. **Pub:** *Annual Report.* • *Progress Reports.*

★ 22731 ★ Lawrence Berkeley National Laboratory
Life Sciences Division
1 Cyclotron Rd.
Berkeley, CA 94720
Phone: (510)486-4365 **Fax:** (510)486-5586
Email: mjbissell@lbl.gov
Website: http://www.lbl.gov/lifesciences/
Mina J. Bissell, PhD, Div. Dir.
Activities/Fields: Human Genome Project; mutagenesis and carcinogenesis, emphasizing DNA repair and recombination; mechanisms of tissue-specific gene expression, focusing on mammary gland cells and hemopoiesis; structural biology, concentrating on the three-dimensional structure of integral membrane proteins; and radiobiology, stressing molecular and cellular mechanisms and the risks associated with radiation as an environmental hazard.

★ 22732 ★ Lawrence Livermore National Laboratory
Resource for Biomedical Accelerator Mass Spectrometry
7000 E Ave.
PO Box 808, L-452
Livermore, CA 94551-0808
Phone: (925)423-8152 **Fax:** (925)422-2282
Email: turteltaub2@llnl.gov
Website: http://www.llnl.gov/bioams/
Kenneth W. Turteltaub, PhD, Prin. Investigator
Activities/Fields: New methods and instrumentation for the use of accelerator mass spectrometry in biomedical research.

★ 22733 ★ Lawson Health Research Institute
St. Joseph's Healthe Centre
University of Western Ontario
268 Grosvenor St.
London, ON, Canada N6A 4V2
Phone: (519)646-6005 **Fax:** (519)646-6110
Email: dhill@lri.sjhc.london.on.ca
Website: http://www.lhrionhealth.ca
Dr. David J. Hill, Sci. Dir. /VP,Res.
Activities/Fields: Maternal and newborn health issues, including prematurity and low birth weight; imaging, particularly the improvement of medical diagnosis through use of imaging techniques and understanding the effects of magnetic fields; molecular medicine, especially regarding diabetes and lung biology; musculoskeletal system, including muscles, joints, and wounds; rehabilitation and geriatrics, especially unique approaches to all aspects of management of spinal cord injury and physical mental health of the elderlu; urology; and gastroenterology, vascular biology, transplant, neuroscience, advanced surgical techniques, mental health. **Pub:** *Probe Newsletter.* Newsletter. **Frmly:** Lawson Research Institute.

★ 22734 ★ Legacy Clinical Research and Technology Center
1225 NE 2nd Ave.
Portland, OR 97208-3950
Phone: (503)413-2491 **Fax:** (503)413-4942
Email: tmelarag@lhs.org
Website: http://www.legacyhealth.org
Dr. Anthony J. Melaragno, Res. Ch.
Activities/Fields: Cardiology, biomechanics, neonatalogy, trauma, burns, infectious diseases, neurobiology, pediatric/adult diabetes, ophthalmology, neurology, transplantation, neuromuscular physiology, neurootology. **Frmly:** Emanuel Research Center.

★ 22735 ★ Lexington Clinic Foundation for Medical Education and Research Inc.
1221 S Broadway St.
Lexington, KY 40504
Phone: (859)258-4000
Michael Fitzgerald, MD, Pres.
Activities/Fields: Cancer therapy, muscle physiology and athletic injury, diabetes, and cardiac surgery.

★ 22736 ★ Lighthouse International Arlene R. Gordon Research Institute
111 E 59th St.
New York, NY 10022
Phone: (212)821-9200 **Free:** 800-829-0500
Email: research@lighthouse.org
Website: http://www.lighthouse.org
Amy Horowitz, Sr. VP, Res.
Activities/Fields: Physical, functional, and psychological consequences of vision impairment. Vision research areas include helping individuals with low vision maximize their remaining vision, understanding how best to assess visual function, and devising ways of modifying environments for the safety and comfort of people who are visually impaired. Social research areas include the effects of visual impairment on the ability of people of all ages to function, the processes of adaption to a vision loss, and the social and psychological characteristics that influence adaptive and rehabilitation outcomes. **Pub:** *Lighthouse Research Monograph and Technical Series.*

★ 22737 ★ Little People's Research Fund, Inc.
80 Sister Pierre Dr.
Towson, MD 21204
Phone: (410)494-0055 **Free:** 800-232-5773
Fax: (410)494-0062
Email: lprf@lprf.org
Website: http://www.lprf.org
Charles McElwee, Exec. Dir.
Activities/Fields: Orthopedic disabilities associated with skeletal dysplasia (also known as dwarfism), including child development from adolescence and into adulthood and new surgical procedures. **Pub:** *Newsletter*, semiannually.

★ 22738 ★ Loma Linda University Cancer Institute
11185 Mountain View Ave., Ste. 155B
PO Box 2000
Loma Linda, CA 92354
Phone: (909)588-3391 **Fax:** (909)558-3428
Email: aburk@ahs.llumc.edu
Website: http://www.llu.edu/llu/ci/
James M. Slater, MD, Dir.
Activities/Fields: Cancer prevention and treatment, specifically molecular genetics, neurosciences, and cancer cell and molecular biology and their relationships to cancer; and translating basic science findings into clinical applications.

★ 22739 ★ Loma Linda University Center for Pain Management
11406 Loma Linda Dr.
Loma Linda, CA 92354
Phone: (909)558-6211 **Fax:** (909)558-6212
Email: lreynolds@som.llu.edu
Website: http://www.llu.edu/lluhc/pain/index.html
Lowell Reynolds, MD, Dir.
Activities/Fields: Analgesic medications and pain alleviating devices. Areas of focus include postoperative pain, arthritis, neuropathy, cancer pain, headaches, and low back pain, etc.

★ 22740 ★ Loma Linda University Center for Spiritual Life and Wholeness
Coleman Pavillion, Ste. 11121R
Loma Linda, CA 92350
Phone: (909)558-1000 **Fax:** (909)558-0336
Email: innerweave@som.llu.edu
Website: http://www.llu.edu/llu/wholeness/index.html
Wil Alexander, PhD, Dir.
Activities/Fields: Bio-psycho-social-spiritual connections in the healing, health, wholeness, and restoration of ill human beings.

★ 22741 ★ Loma Linda University Peterson Tribology Laboratory
250 E Caroline St., Ste. H
San Bernardino, CA 92408
Phone: (909)824-0578 **Fax:** (909)824-8493
Email: iclarke@som.llu.edu
Website: http://www.llu.edu/llu/tribology/
Dr. Ian C. Clarke, Dir.
Activities/Fields: Longevity issues involved with total joint prosthesis. **Pub:** *Journal articles.*

★ 22742 ★ Loma Linda VA Medical Center
Sleep Disorders Center
11201 Benton St., 111P Sleep
Loma Linda, CA 92357
Phone: (909)422-3130 **Fax:** (909)777-3214
Email: ralph.downey@med.va.gov
Dr. Ralph Downey, III, Dir.
Activities/Fields: Sleep disorders, including sleep apnea, insomnia, and narcolepsy.

★ 22743 ★ Long Island Jewish Medical Center
Nuclear Medicine Division
270-05 76th Ave.
New Hyde Park, NY 11040
Phone: (718)470-7080 **Fax:** (718)470-9247
Email: palestro@lij.edu
Christopher Palestro, MD, Dir.

Activities/Fields: Applications of radioisotopes to clinical medicine. The Division is especially concerned with research on new applications, including instrumentation, and in use of isotopes in study of metabolic processes and infection.

★ 22744 ★ Los Amigos Research and Education Institute, Inc.
PO Box 3500, Los Amigos Sta.
Downey, CA 90242
Phone: (562)401-8111 **Fax:** (562)803-5569
Email: julial@larei.org
Julia F. LaPlount, Admin. Off.
Activities/Fields: Clinical medicine, including multidisciplinary study of severe chronic disabilities in pulmonary and respiratory functions, cardiology, spinal cord injury, orthopedic disabilities, environmental health, stroke, pathokinesiology, liver disease, neuromuscular stimulation and control, rehabilitation of severely disabled persons, cerebral palsy, problem amputations, arthritis, and diabetes. Treats effects of atmospheric pollutants on human lung function, investigates possible causes of Alzheimer's disease, and explores new methods and procedures for care and treatment of gerontology patients.

★ 22745 ★ Los Amigos Research and Education Institute Inc.
Rehabilitation Engineering Research Center on Spinal Cord Injury
PO Box 3500
Downey, CA 90242
Phone: (562)401-8111 **Fax:** (562)803-5569
Website: http://www.ncddr.org/cgi-bin/mysql/nidrrprofiles.cgi?showproj=H133E020732&location =projabstract
Samuel Landsberger, ScD, Prin. Investigator
Activities/Fields: Improvement in the lives of individuals with spinal cord injury through new technologies and the dissemination of information to this population.

★ 22746 ★ Louisiana Health and Hospitals Department
Research and Development
1201 Capitol Access Rd.
Baton Rouge, LA 70821-2870
Phone: (225)342-2964 **Fax:** (225)342-0080
Email: hrobinso@dhh.state.la.us
Helene Robinson, Actg. Dir.
Activities/Fields: Health, hospitals.

★ 22747 ★ Louisiana State University
Human Development Center
School of Allied Health Professions
1100 Florida Ave., Bldg. 138
New Orleans, LA 70119-2799
Phone: (504)942-8380 **Fax:** (504)942-8305
Email: rcrow@lsuhsc.edu
Website: http://www.hdc.lsumc.edu/
Robert E. Crow, PhD, Dir.
Activities/Fields: Developmental disabilities, including educational technology, curriculum research, and integrated basic and applied behavioral interventions. Operates as a University Affiliated Program for interdisciplinary training, research, and dissemination.

★ 22748 ★ Louisiana State University
Kresge Hearing Research Laboratory of the South
533 Bolivar St., 5th Fl.
New Orleans, LA 70112
Phone: (504)568-4785 **Fax:** (504)568-4460
Email: rbobbin@lsuhsc.edu
Website: http://www.kresgelab.org
Dr. Richard P. Bobbin, Dir.
Activities/Fields: Auditory research, pharmacology, anatomy, psychophysics, molecular genetics, and audiology, including studies on cochlear implants, auditory evoked potentials, ultra-high frequency hearing, effects of hearing impairments on brain structure, temporal order in hearing, auditory processing of frequency-varying signals, perceptual skills in learning-disabled children, speech perception, cochlear emissions, auditory neuropathy, and the role of chemical elements in hearing. **Frmly:** Communication Sciences Laboratory.

★ 22749 ★ Louisiana State University
Pennington Biomedical Research Center
6400 Perkins Rd.
Baton Rouge, LA 70808-4124
Phone: (225)763-2500 **Fax:** (225)763-2525
Website: http://www.pbrc.edu
Claude Bouchard, PhD, Exec. Dir.
Activities/Fields: Nutritional physiology and metabolism, molecular and cellular nutrition, nutrition and behavior, nutritional epidemiology, neurobiology, taste physiology, clinical physchology, biostatistics, and metabolic studies. **Pub:** *Inside Pennington Newsletter.* • *Pennington Nutrition Series.*

★ 22750 ★ Louisiana State University Health Sciences Center
Eye Center
2020 Gravier St., Ste. B
New Orleans, LA 70112
Phone: (504)412-1200 **Fax:** (504)412-1315
Email: dbergs@lsuhsc.edu
Website: http://www.lsu-eye.lsumc.edu/
Dr. Donald R. Bergsma, Chm.
Activities/Fields: Ophthalmology, including lasers in ophthalmology, ocular surgery techniques, biomaterials and drug delivery, graft rejection, neurobiology and neurochemisty, and viral infection, latency, and treatment.

★ 22751 ★ Louisiana State University Medical Center
Neuroscience Center of Excellence
2020 Gravier St., Ste. D
New Orleans, LA 70112
Phone: (504)599-0909 **Fax:** (504)568-5801
Email: nbazan@lsumc.edu
Website: http://www.neuroscience.lsumc.edu
Dr. Nicolas G. Bazan, Dir.
Activities/Fields: Interdisciplinary unit studying clinical and basic neuroscience.

★ 22752 ★ Louisiana State University in Shreveport
Genetics Section of Pediatrics
Medical Center
1501 Kings Hwy.
Shreveport, LA 71130
Phone: (318)675-6083 **Fax:** (318)675-6089
Email: tthurm@lsuhsc.edu
T.F. Thurmon, MD, Dir.
Activities/Fields: Clinical applications of genetics, biochemical genetics, and cytogenetics. Studies include chromatographic diagnostic techniques, heredity of dysmorphic syndromes, and chromosome aberrations in cancer. **Frmly:** Birth Defects Center.

★ 22753 ★ Louisiana Tech University
Center for Biomedical Engineering and Rehabilitation Science
PO Box 3185
Ruston, LA 71272
Phone: (318)257-4562 **Fax:** (318)255-4175
Email: cybers@coes.latech.edu
Website: http://www.cybers.latech.edu
Dr. Charles J. Robinson, Jr., Dir.
Activities/Fields: Studies conditions leading to disabilities (systems physiology), develops and applies technology to assist disabled people, and develops expert systems in systems physiology and rehabilitation services. **Frmly:** Center for Rehabilitation Science and Biomedical Engineering.

★ 22754 ★ Lovelace Respiratory Research Institute
2425 Ridgecrest Dr. SE
Albuquerque, NM 87108-5127
Phone: (505)348-9400 **Fax:** (505)348-8542
Email: rrubin@lrri.org
Website: http://www.lrri.org
Dr. Robert W. Rubin, Pres. /CEO
Activities/Fields: Respiratory disease (primarily asthma and cancer), respiratory pharmaceuticals, inhalation drug delivery, inhalation toxicology, aerosol science, animal models of human respiratory disease, and health risks from inhaled materials in the workplace, home, and general environment. **Pub:** *Gift of Breath*, quarterly. **Frmly:** Lovelace Medical Foundation; The Lovelace Institutes.

★ 22755 ★ Loyola University Chicago
Burn and Shock Trauma Institute
Bldg. 110, 4th Fl.
Loyola University Medical Center
Maywood, IL 60153
Phone: (708)327-2400 **Fax:** (708)327-2813
Email: rgamell@luc.edu
Richard L. Gamelli, MD, Dir.
Activities/Fields: Body responses to injury and post-injury sequelae of infection, metabolic change, alteration in host defense, and wound healing. Clinical research in care and management of injury victims, injury analysis and prevention, etiology, epidemiology, cost, rehabilitation, and outcome of trauma.

★ 22756 ★ Loyola University Chicago
Heart Transplant and Heart Failure Program
2160 S 1st Ave.
Maywood, IL 60153
Phone: (708)216-4810 **Fax:** (708)327-2770
Dr. Barbara Pisani, Actg. Dir.
Activities/Fields: Cardiac transplantation and immunology, including allograft rejection, vascular diseases, and transplant tolerance.

★ 22757 ★ Loyola University Chicago
Neiswanger Institute for Bioethics and Health Policy
Stritch School of Medicine, Bldg. 120, Rm. 280
2160 S 1st Ave.
Maywood, IL 60153
Fax: (708)327-9209
Email: tmorri3@lumc.edu
Website: http://www.meddean.luc.edu/ssom/depts/bioethics/
Mark Kuczewski, PhD, Dir.
Activities/Fields: Bioethics and health policy.

★ 22758 ★ Loyola University Chicago
Parmly Hearing Institute
6525 N Sheridan Rd.
Chicago, IL 60626
Phone: (773)508-2710 **Fax:** (773)508-2719
Email: rfay@luc.edu
Website: http://www.parmly.luc.edu
Dr. Richard R. Fay, Dir.
Activities/Fields: Psychophysics, physiology, and anatomy of audition and investigation of sensory/perceptual processes, including studies on relations among sense/organ action, anatomy and physiology of afferent nervous system, cerebral sensory mechanisms, psychophysical characteristics of auditory system, application of theory of signal detectability to psychophysics, and detection and recognition of auditory signals in noise. **Pub:** *Parmly Hearing Institute Annual report.*

★ 22759 ★ Macula Foundation, Inc.
Manhattan Eye, Ear & Throat Hospital, 8th Fl.
210 E 64th St.
New York, NY 10021

Phone: (212)605-3777 **Free:** 800-622-8524
Fax: (212)605-3795
Email: foundation@retinalresearch.org
Website: http://www.macula.org/foundation/foundation.html
Lawrence A. Yannuzzi, MD, Pres.

Activities/Fields: Macular diseases, including epidemiologic, immunologic, biochemical, and clinical therapeutic studies. **Frmly:** Retinal Research Fund.

★ 22760 ★ Maharishi University of Management
Center for Natural Medicine and Prevention
1000 N 4th St.
Fairfield, IA 52557
Phone: (641)472-1110 **Free:** 800-369-6480
Fax: (641)472-1179
Email: rschneid@mum.edu
Website: http://www.mum.edu/cnmp/index.html
Robert H. Schneider, MD, Dir.

Activities/Fields: Prevention and treatment of major chronic illnesses. **Frmly:** Center for Health and Aging Studies.

★ 22761 ★ Mailman Research Center
115 Mill St.
Belmont, MA 02478
Phone: (617)855-3227 **Fax:** (617)855-3670
Email: cohenb@mclean.harvard.edu
Website: http://www.research.mclean.org
Bruce M. Cohen, PhD, Pres.

Activities/Fields: Neuropharmacology, neurochemistry, neuropathology, molecular neurogenetics, neuroregeneration, and molecular neurobiology with emphasis on psychiatric neurosciences.

★ 22762 ★ Maine Medical Center Research Institute (MMCRI)
81 Research Dr.
Scarborough, ME 04074-7205
Phone: (207)885-8100 **Fax:** (207)885-8110
Website: http://www.mmcri.org
Dr. Ken Ault, Assoc. VP, Res. Dir.

Activities/Fields: Laboratory, clinical, and epidemiologic research on molecular genetics, hematology, infectious diseases, endocrinology, cardiology and nephrology. **Pub:** *Inquiry Newsletter.*

★ 22763 ★ Maisonneuve-Rosemont Hospital Research Centre
5415 de l'Assomption Blvd.
Montreal, QC, Canada H1T 2M4
Phone: (514)252-3400 **Fax:** (514)252-3430
Email: bonnarda@hmr.gc.ca
Website: http://www.guybernier.com
Dr. Alain Bonnardeaux, Dir.

Activities/Fields: Reproductive biology, including epididymal maturation, acrosome reaction, fertilization, and implantation; immunology, including bone marrow transplantation, transplantation of encapsulated cells, DNA repair, lymphocyte function and ontogeny, immunogenetics, and cytokines; hypertension, including angiotensinogen gene; calcium metabolism; kidney physiology; cancer, including prostate and leukemias; nuclear medicine; and neurology, including cerebrovascular diseases and aphasia.

★ 22764 ★ Mallory Institute of Pathology Foundation
784 Massachusetts Ave.
Boston, MA 02118
Phone: (617)414-5314 **Fax:** (617)414-5315
Dr. Leonard S. Gottlieb, Dir.

Activities/Fields: Experimental medicine and pathology, with particular reference to cardiovascular diseases, gastrointestinal diseases, liver and kidney diseases, pulmonary diseases, hematopathology, nutritional pathology, immunopathology, environmental pathology, and oncology.

★ 22765 ★ Margaret S. Mahler Psychiatric Research Foundation
254 Kent Rd.
Wynnewood, PA 19096
Phone: (610)645-5524 **Fax:** (610)645-5524
Email: wsingletarymd@aol.com
Dr. William M. Singletary, Pres.

Activities/Fields: Issues related to child development, education for parenting, and prevention and early intervention.

★ 22766 ★ Marquette University
Rehabilitation Engineering Research Center on Accessible Medical Instrumentation
Department of Biomedical Engineering
PO Box 1881
Milwaukee, WI 53201
Phone: (414)288-3375 **Fax:** (414)288-7938
Email: jack.winter@marquette.edu
Website: http://www.ncddr.org/rpp/techaf/techdfdw/rerc/
Jack Winters, PhD, Prin. Investigator

Activities/Fields: Access to and utilization of healthcare instrumentation and services by individuals with disabilities and employment in the healthcare professions by individuals with disabilities.

★ 22767 ★ Marshall University
Robert C. Byrd Center for Rural Health
1600 Medical Center Dr., Ste. 1400
Huntington, WV 25701-3655
Phone: (304)691-1198 **Fax:** (304)691-1183
Email: walkerrb@marshall.edu
Website: http://crh.marshall.edu/
Robert Walker, MD, Dir.

Activities/Fields: Rural health problems. Also guides predoctoral and postdoctoral research on rural health, rural geriatrics, and prevention in rural populations.

★ 22768 ★ Marshfield Medical Research Foundation
1000 N Oak Ave.
Marshfield, WI 54449-5790
Phone: (715)387-5241 **Free:** 800-782-8581
Fax: (715)389-3131
Email: calwelm@mmrf.mfldclin.edu
Website: http://research.marshfieldclinic.org
Michael D. Caldwell, MD, Dir.

Activities/Fields: Diagnosis and treatment of human disease, including basic and/or applied studies on respiratory disease, human angiotensinogen and renin in hypertension, infertility, human genome mapping, epidemiology and biostatistics, clinical drug trials, searching for tumor suppressor genes, research in infectious disease and vaccine development, zoonotic illness and food safety, genetic epidemiology and pharmacogenomics. Operates the Center for Medical Genetics, which conducts mammalian genotyping; the National Farm Medicine Center, which is designed to improve the quality of life; the Center for Personalized Medicine, which conducts research in genetic epidemiology and pharmacogenetics; and the Epidemiological Research Center which conducts population-based studies using a 80,000-patient study cohort. **Pub:** *Clinical Medicine and Research.*

★ 22769 ★ Mary Bird Perkins Cancer Center
4950 Essen Ln.
Baton Rouge, LA 70809
Phone: (225)767-0847 **Fax:** (225)766-0218
Email: infor@marybird.com
Website: http://www.marybird.org
Todd D. Stevens, Pres. /CEO

Activities/Fields: Radiation treatment, including participation in national clinical trials of the Radiation Therapy Oncology Group and the Southwest Oncology Group, as well as pharmaceutical and in-house studies.

★ 22770 ★ Maryland Long-Term Care Project
Department of Epidemiology & Preventive Medicine
University of Maryland
660 W Redwood St., Ste. 200
Baltimore, MD 21201
Phone: (410)706-3553 **Fax:** (410)706-4433
Email: jmagazin@epi.umaryland.edu
Website: http://gerontology.umaryland.edu/long-term.html
Jay Magaziner, PhD, Ldr.

Activities/Fields: Health of persons in nursing homes, including nursing home acquired infections, the incidence of antibiotic use, the beliefs underlying caregivers' decision to institutionalize a family member, the prevalence of dementia, the relationship of dementia to health, the provision of special care to residents with dementia, the relationship between the structure and process of care to health outcomes for all residents, the prevalence of osteoporosis and its relationship to subsequent fractures; use of hip pads to prevent fractures, restorative care programs, and the educational/training needs of nursing home personnel.

★ 22771 ★ Maryland Medical Research Institute
600 Wyndhurst Ave.
Baltimore, MD 21210-2425
Phone: (410)435-4200 **Fax:** (410)323-8622
Email: postmaster@mmri.org
Website: http://www.mmri.org
Dr. Michael Terrin, Pres. /COO

Activities/Fields: Data gathering, analysis, and design for large-scale clinical trials and epidemiological studies in medical areas such as heart disease, cancer, blood disease, septicemia, AIDS, surgical treatment and laser therapy, and in retinal diseases, and the effects of diet on health status. **Pub:** *Controlled Clinical Trials,* quarterly.

★ 22772 ★ Masonic Medical Research Laboratory (MMRL)
2150 Bleecker St.
Utica, NY 13501
Phone: (315)735-2217 **Fax:** (315)735-5648
Email: ca@mmrl.edu
Website: http://www.mmrl.edu
Dr. Charles Antzelevitch, Exec. Dir.

Activities/Fields: Electrophysiology, molecukar biology and molecular genetics with emphasis on cardiac arrhythmias, ischemic heart disease and forms of sudden death including sudden infant death syndrom (SIDS).

★ 22773 ★ Massachusetts Alzheimer's Disease Research Center
WACC 830
Massachusetts General Hospital
15 Parkman St.
Boston, MA 02114
Phone: (617)726-1728 **Fax:** (617)726-4101
Email: growdon@helix.mgh.edu
Website: http://neuro-www2.mgh.harvard.edu/adrc_home/main.html
John H. Growdon, MD, Prog. Dir.

Activities/Fields: Coordinates research on Alzheimer's disease, including memory loss, dementia, neuropathology, neuropsychology, neurochemistry, and investigational drug studies. Projects focus on biochemical studies on the abnormal proteins that accumulate in the brains of Alzheimer's patients, possible genetic markers or familial traits, anatomical and neurotransmitter abnormalities, and clinical studies of behavior and neuropharmacology.

★ 22774 ★ Massachusetts General Hospital
Center for Functional Neuroimaging Technologies
149 13th St., Rm. 2301
Charlestown, MA 02129
Phone: (617)724-7139 **Fax:** (617)726-7422
Email: bruce@nmr.mgh.harvard.edu
Website: http://www.nmr.mgh.harvard.edu/CFNT
Bruce R. Rosen, MD, Prin. Investigator
Activities/Fields: Understanding of the human brain in health and disease through the development and dissemination of innovative multimodal magnetic resonance based neuroimaging techniques and technologies.

★ 22775 ★ Massachusetts General Hospital
Diabetes Center
50 Staniford St., Ste. 340
Boston, MA 02114-2517
Phone: (617)726-1847 **Fax:** (617)726-1871
Email: nathan@gcrc.mgh.harvard.edu
Dr. David M. Nathan, Prin. Investigator
Activities/Fields: Diabetes research, including clinical trials.

★ 22776 ★ Massachusetts General Hospital
Harvard Cutaneous Biology Research Center
Massachusetts General Hospital East, Bldg. 149
Charlestown, MA 02129
Phone: (617)726-4425 **Fax:** (617)724-9394
Email: john.parrish@cbrc2.mgh.harvard.edu
Website: http://www.mgh.harvard.edu/cbrc
Dr. John Parrish, Dir.
Activities/Fields: Dermatology, including photobiology of skin, including photoimmunology, photoaging, free radical biology and photoprotection; pigment cell biology; growth and differentiation of epidermis, hair and nails, and keratin biochemistry; immunology, allergy, inflammation, and modifiers of host response; physical properties of skin, including water content, percutaneous transport of chemicals, and optical properties; physiology and pharmacology of the skin; and biology of dermis and dermal-epidermal junction and their constituents.

★ 22777 ★ Massachusetts General Hospital
Mallinckrodt General Clinical Research Center
55 Fruit St., WHT 13
Boston, MA 02114-2696
Phone: (617)726-4272 **Fax:** (617)724-3299
Email: ebandrews@partners.org
Website: http://www.mgh.harvard.edu/GCRC
Edwin B. Andrews, Admin. Mgr.
Activities/Fields: The Center's major areas of investigation are aging, diabetes, endocrinology, gastroenterology, genetic diseases, infectious diseases, neuroendocrinology, neurology, neuropsychiatry, oncology, pediatrics, psychiatry, reproductive endocrinology and gynecology and rheumatology.

★ 22778 ★ Massachusetts General Hospital
Reproductive Endocrine Unit
BHX-5
55 Fruit St.
Boston, MA 02114
Phone: (617)724-3038 **Fax:** (617)726-5357
Website: http://www.massgeneral.org/reproendo/
William F. Crowley, MD, Ch.
Activities/Fields: Reproductive endocrinology, focusing on local regulators of gonadal physiology and characterization and regulation of posttransitional processing of inhibin subunits using a variety of techniques, including protein purification and characterization and molecular biology.

★ 22779 ★ Massachusetts General Hospital for Children
Pediatric Pulmonary Unit
55 Fruit St., VBKBA 015
Boston, MA 02114
Phone: (617)726-5576
Email: kinane@helix.mgh.harvard.edu
Bernard Kinane, Contact
Activities/Fields: Sudden infant death, the role of mast cells and eosinophils in asthma and the regulation of lung development.

★ 22780 ★ Massachusetts General Hospital East
Cancer Center
13th St., Bldg. 149
Charlestown, MA 02129
Phone: (617)726-5610 **Fax:** (617)726-5637
Email: isselbacher@helix.mgh.harvard.edu
Kurt Isselbacher, MD, Dir.
Activities/Fields: Cell cycle regulation and cancer genetics, including breast, colon, and melanoma, and metastasis.

★ 22781 ★ Massachusetts Health Data Consortium
460 Totten Pond Rd., Ste. 385
Waltham, MA 02451
Phone: (781)890-6040 **Fax:** (781)768-2510
Email: estone@mahealthdata.org
Website: http://www.mahealthdata.org
Elliot M. Stone, Exec. Dir. /CEO
Activities/Fields: Health services research, including studies of hospitals, patient and physician databases, and discharged patients since 1978. **Pub:** *Datagram.* • *Health Data News*, quarterly. • *Public Meeting Report*, annually. • *Webmasters Digest.*

★ 22782 ★ Massachusetts Institute of Technology
BioInstrumentation Laboratory
77 Massachusetts Ave., Rm. 3-147
Cambridge, MA 02139
Phone: (617)253-4763 **Fax:** (617)252-1849
Email: ihunter@mit.edu
Website: http://biorobotics.mit.edu/
Prof. Ian W. Hunter, Dir.
Activities/Fields: Creation of novel and sophisticated instrumentation with bio-medical and other life science applications.

★ 22783 ★ Massachusetts Institute of Technology
Biotechnology Resource Center for Research in Lasers and Medicine
Bldg. 6, Rm. 014
NCRR
77 Massachusetts Ave.
Cambridge, MA 02139-4307
Phone: (617)253-5377 **Fax:** (617)253-4513
Dr. Ramachandra R. Dasari, Contact
Activities/Fields: Spectral diagnostics for tissue types, which can lead to real-time diagnosis of diseased tissue; and studies laser tissue damage and ablation, as a function of wavelength and the dependence on the optical and thermal properties of the tissue. Research includes development of the portable spectrometer for laser-induced fluorescence studies for use in a clinical setting and use of Raman spectroscopy techniques for diagnosing tissue characteristics.

★ 22784 ★ Massachusetts Institute of Technology
Center for Biological and Computational Learning
Department of Brain & Cognitive Science
77 Massachusetts Ave.
Cambridge, MA 02139-4307
Phone: (617)253-7403 **Fax:** (617)253-2964
Email: tp@ai.mit.edu
Website: http://www.ai.mit.edu/projects/cbcl/web-homepage/web-homepage.html
Tomaso Poggio, PhD, Co-Dir.
Activities/Fields: Investigates mathematics of statistical learning, its engineering applications and the mechanisms of biological information processing. Studies focus on machine and human learning, vision, object recognition, bioinformatics, information search and retrieval.

★ 22785 ★ Massachusetts Institute of Technology
Center for Biomedical Engineering (CBE)
77 Massachusetts Ave., Rm. 56-341
Cambridge, MA 02139
Phone: (617)258-8949 **Fax:** (617)258-0204
Email: cbe-www@mit.edu
Website: http://web.mit.edu/cbe/www/
Prof. Alan Grodzinsky, Dir.
Activities/Fields: Molecular medicine, including molecular engineering, cell and tissue engineering, and physiological systems engineering.

★ 22786 ★ Massachusetts Institute of Technology
Center for Cancer Research
40 Ames St., E-17-110
Cambridge, MA 02139
Phone: (617)253-6403 **Fax:** (617)252-1891
Email: hollyc@mit.edu
Website: http://web.mit.edu/ccr
Dr. Richard Hynes, Dir.
Activities/Fields: Cancer biology, emphasizing molecular biology, genetics, cell biology, developmental biology, and immunology. Specific areas of research include split genes and RNA splicing, cloning oncogenes and tumor suppressor genes from human tumors, T-cell receptors, integrin receptors and cell adhesion, mechanisms, used by tumor cells to evade chemotherapy, gene identification for myotonic dystrophy, Huntington's disease, and Wilm's tumor, the generation of various strains of mutant mice, biochemical mechanisms controlling RNA transcription and splicing, HIV gene studies, cytotoxic and helper T lymphocytes, lymphocyte antigen-specific receptors, molecular mechanisms of antigen presentation, cell surface proteins and cellular adhesion and migration, and cytoskeletal proteins and cell motility and shape.

★ 22787 ★ Massachusetts Institute of Technology
Center for Magnetic Resonance
Francis Bitter Magnet Laboratory
170 Albany St., NW14-3218
Cambridge, MA 02139
Phone: (617)253-5478 **Fax:** (617)253-5405
Email: rgg@mit.edu
Dr. Robert G. Griffin, Dir.
Activities/Fields: Biological molecules (liquid- or solid-state), viral particles, cells, intact tissues, etc. Research includes natural and model membrane structure, dynamics, function, phase diagrams, phase transitions, and solid-state studies of amino acids, peptides, and bone; protein conformation and interactions, e.g., insulin, NMR microscopy; dynamics of energy metabolism in tumors, skeletal muscle, cells, animal brain and heart, and human eye lens; and DNA structure and dynamics.

★ 22788 ★ Massachusetts Institute of Technology
Environmental Health Sciences Center
77 Massachusetts Ave., 16-743B
Cambridge, MA 02139
Phone: (617)258-7813 **Fax:** (617)253-8099
Email: lsamson@mit.edu
Website: http://www.niehs.nih.gov/centers/center/mit-ctr.htm
Leona D. Samson, PhD, Dir.
Activities/Fields: Causes and mechanisms of genetic changes that lead to human disease. The center's primary hypothesis is that a significant fraction of the point mutations and other genetic changes in the human body are caused by exposure to environmental chemicals or radiation.

★ 22789 ★ Massachusetts Institute of Technology
Eric P. and Evelyn E. Newman Laboratory for Biomechanics and Human Rehabilitation
77 Massachusetts Ave., Rm. 3-146
Cambridge, MA 02139
Phone: (617)253-2277 **Fax:** (617)258-7018
Email: neville@mit.edu
Prof. Neville Hogan, Dir.
Activities/Fields: Amputation prostheses, normal and pathological human neuromuscular systems, and diagnosis and therapy of muscular, skeletal, and joint malfunctions using an engineering approach. Studies include cybernetic limb and sensory prostheses, mobility aids for the blind, suppression of tremor, functional electrical stimulation, instrumentation for and kinematic studies of human movement, synovial joint mechanics, pathogenesis of osteoarthritis, biomechanics of the hip, knee, and ankle, musculoskeletal models for pathological diagnosis, and computer-aided surgical simulation. **Pub:** *Bibliography.* • *Excerpt from the Department of Mechanical Engineering Triennial Report.* **Frmly:** Laboratory for Human Mechanics and Rehabilitation.

★ 22790 ★ Massachusetts Institute of Technology
General Clinical Research Center
Bldg. E17-445
77 Massachusetts Ave.
Cambridge, MA 02142
Phone: (617)253-3091 **Fax:** (617)253-6882
Email: dick@mit.edu
Website: http://web.mit.edu/crc/www
Dr. Richard J. Wurtman, Prog. Dir.
Activities/Fields: Normal human metabolism, physiology, and behavior, including studies on hormones, fates of deuterated amino acids, behavioral and neuroendocrine effect of foods (carbohydrate, protein, and caffeine), effects of drugs on memory and other behaviors, and endocrine and metabolic effects on aging. Also studies human diseases such as obesity, Alzheimer's disease, brain injury, Parkinson's disease, use of brain imaging techniques to follow metabolic events, and infectious diseases (HIV).

★ 22791 ★ Massachusetts Institute of Technology
Laboratory of Neuroendocrine Regulation
Bldg. E25-604
Cambridge, MA 02139
Phone: (617)253-6731 **Fax:** (617)253-6882
Email: dick@mit.edu
Dr. Richard J. Wurtman, Dir.
Activities/Fields: Pineal gland and effects of drugs, nutrients, and hormones on brain neurotransmitters and behavior. Specific studies include utilization of choline for acetylcholine and membrane phosphatidylcholine synthesis in cultured neuroblastoma cells and in rat brain; neurotransmitter receptors and second messengers that modulate these two syntheses; interactions of precursor availability (tyrosine and tryptophan) and firing frequency in controlling neurotransmitter (catecholamines and serotonin) release from superfused rat brain slices; effects of tyrosine on catecholamine release from isolated retina; effects of supplemental tyrosine on capacity to withstand stress, sustain motor activity, and perform complex tasks; control of melatonin secretion in rats; mechanisms by which melatonin acts on neurons and induces sleep; aberrant patterns of melatonin secretion in aging and human diseases; effects of macronutrients (carbohydrates and proteins) on brain serotonin synthesis; involvement of serotoninergic neurons in appetite, mood, pain sensitivity, and various appetitive diseases; selective effects of serotoninergic drugs on nutrient selection; Alzheimer's disease; control of APP metabolism by neurotransmitters; and brain phospholipid synthesis; production and maintenance of sleep in humans by melatonin; use of CDP-Choline to treat brain injury or stroke.

★ 22792 ★ Massachusetts Institute of Technology
Laser Biomedical Research Center
77 Massachusetts Ave.
Cambridge, MA 02139
Phone: (617)253-7700 **Fax:** (617)253-4513
Email: msfeld@mit.edu
Dr. Michael S. Feld, Dir.
Activities/Fields: Lasers, medicine, and diagnosis of disease. Development of new methods for real-time spectroscopic identification of tissue types and conditions from the studies of fluorescence, scattering and reflection. Raman spectroscopy studies yield biochemical composition of the tissue. Interferometry and phase dispersion microscopy can detect sub-wavelength changes. Conducts time-resolved picosecond studies in tissue and other biological systems. Pursues collaborative research with researchers from outside institutions and provides facilities to outside scientists and physicians nationwide. **Pub:** *Annual report.* • *The Spectrograph Newsletter.*

★ 22793 ★ Massachusetts Institute of Technology
McGovern Institute for Brain Research
Bldg. E25-435
77 Massachusetts Ave.
Cambridge, MA 02139
Phone: (617)452-2507 **Fax:** (617)452-4119
Email: mcgovern@mit.edu
Website: http://web.mit.edu/mcgovern/
Phillip A. Sharp, Dir.
Activities/Fields: Biological basis of all higher brain function in humans. By determining how the brain works, from the level of gene expression in individual neurons to the interrelationships between complex neural networks, the institute's efforts will work towards improving human health, discovering the basis of learning and recognition, and enhancing education and communication.

★ 22794 ★ Massachusetts Institute of Technology
Program on the Pharmaceutical Industry (POPI)
Bldg. E56-390
Sloan Sch. of Management
38 Memorial Dr.
Cambridge, MA 02139-4307
Phone: (617)253-5194 **Fax:** (617)253-3033
Email: popi-www@mit.edu
Website: http://web.mit.edu/popi/
Stan N. Finkelstein, MD, Dir.
Activities/Fields: Competitiveness, performance, and productivity in the pharmaceutical field.

★ 22795 ★ Matheny Institute for Research in Developmental Disabilities
Matheny School & Hospital
PO Box 339
Peapack, NJ 07977
Phone: (908)234-0011 **Fax:** (908)234-0963
Email: research@matheny.org
Website: http://www.matheny.org
Kenneth Robey, PhD, Dir.
Activities/Fields: Neurodevelopmental disorders such as cerebral palsy, spina bifida, muscular dystrophy, and Lesch-Nyhan Disease; and the improvement of the lives of those with developmental disabilities. **Pub:** *Matheny Bulletin*, quarterly.

★ 22796 ★ Matrix Research Institute
Research Employment, Training and Rehabilitation Services for People with Mental Illness
Robert Morris Bldg., 10th Fl.
100 N 17th St.
Philadelphia, PA 19103
Phone: (215)569-2240 **Fax:** (215)569-2806
Email: pkpmri@aol.com
Daniel Raudenbush, PhD, Dir.
Activities/Fields: Employment needs of persons with serious psychiatric disabilities, specifically improving access to the Social Security Work Incentives; evaluating alternatives to rehabilitation systems; improving access to employment services; women and work; a multicultural perspective on rehabilitation; the nature of the employer/employee relationship; long-term career paths of persons with serious mental illness; costs of employment services; and the impact of managed care on employment services. **Pub:** *Training manuals and educational materials.*

★ 22797 ★ Mayo Biomedical Imaging Resource
Mayo Clinic
200 1st St. SW
Rochester, MN 55905
Phone: (507)284-4937 **Fax:** (507)284-1632
Email: rar@mayo.edu
Website: http://www.mayo.edu/bir
Richard A. Robb, PhD, Dir.
Activities/Fields: Provides expertise and technology related to biomedical imaging, scientific visualization, computer graphics, computer workstations, and computer networks. Through professional consultation, advanced software and hardware systems, and technical support, investigators use the Resource for ongoing research studies, ad hoc projects, feasibility testing, and/or development of applications and systems to be subsequently installed in the user's library. Provides services in six major categories: consultation on biomedical imaging and scientific visualization problems, needs and applications; software packages (ANALYZE) for interactive display and quantitative analysis of multimodality, and multidimensional biomedical images; drop-in center containing several computer workstations connected to a powerful network providing image processing software and computer graphics hardware; hardware systems, including design and configuration of both standard and customized workstations for biomedical image processing; network support for connectivity to the Resource and/or within the investigative laboratory; and training and education in the use of Resource facilities and in biomedical imaging, scientific visualization and computer science.

★ 22798 ★ Mayo Clinic Cancer Center
200 1st St. SW
Rochester, MN 55905
Phone: (507)284-2511 **Fax:** (507)284-0161
Email: prendergast@mayo.edu
Website: http://www.mayoclinic.org/cancercenter-rst/
Dr. Franklyn G. Prendergast, Dir.
Activities/Fields: Broad-based cancer research program ranging from basic and clinical science to clinical studies on prevention, detection, diagnosis, and treatment of cancer. Participates as a comprehensive cancer center for conducting research, improving methods of treatment, diagnosis, and prevention, training health professionals, and transferring cancer knowledge to surrounding communities in National Cancer Institute's nationwide coordination program, established under National Cancer Act of 1971.

★ 22799 ★ Mayo Clinic and Foundation Allergic Diseases Research Laboratory
200 1st St. SW
Rochester, MN 55905
Phone: (507)284-2511 **Fax:** (507)284-0161
Website: http://www.mayoclinic.org/rochester/

Activities/Fields: Causes, prevention, and management of allergic diseases such as asthma, allergies, contact hypersensitivity, immune deficiencies and infection, and autoimmune disorders plus related studies of fundamental immune mechanisms involving immune cells, antibodies, genetic factors, and immune regulatory systems. Projects focus on functions of the eosinophilic leukocyte, immunotherapy of patients with pollen allergies, and clinical studies of passive immunotherapy in patients allergic to honeybee stings who fail to respond to venom immunotherapy and who are members of beekeeping families.

★ 22800 ★ Mayo Clinic and Foundation Alzheimer's Disease Research Center (ADRC)
41st St. Professional Bldg.
Rochester, MN 55905
Phone: (507)284-1324 **Fax:** (507)284-4074
Email: mayoadc@may.edu
Website: http://www.mayo.edu/research/alzheimers_center/
Ronald Petersen, MD, Dir.

Activities/Fields: Alzheimer's Disease. **Pub:** *Coping Newsletter*, quarterly.

★ 22801 ★ Mayo Clinic and Foundation General Clinical Research Center
St. Mary's Hospital
1216 2nd St. SW
Rochester, MN 55902
Phone: (507)255-6122 **Fax:** (507)255-7445
Email: andresen@mayo.edu
Dr. K.S. Nair, Contact

Activities/Fields: Allergy, endocrinology, gastrointestinal disease, lipid disorders, osteoporosis, pediatrics, pharmacology, renal disease, surgery, cardiovascular disease, oncology, neurology, hypertension, and nutrition.

★ 22802 ★ McGill University Anesthesia Research Department
McIntyre Medical Science Bldg.
3655 Promenade Sir William Osler
Montreal, QC, Canada H3G 1Y6
Phone: (514)398-3493
Email: bushnell@med.mcgill.ca
Dr. Datherine M. Bushnell, Dir.

Activities/Fields: Physiology, neurochemistry, and pharmacology of synaptic mechanisms and effects of anoxia and anaesthetic drugs in the central nervous system.

★ 22803 ★ McGill University Artificial Cells and Organs Research Centre
3655 Drummond St.
Montreal, QC, Canada H3G 1Y6
Phone: (514)398-3512 **Fax:** (514)398-4983
Email: artcell@med.mcgill.ca
Website: http://www.medicine.mcgill.ca/artcell/
Prof. T.M.S. Chang, Dir.

Activities/Fields: Interdisciplinary research using biotechnology, biochemistry, chemical engineering, medicine, enzyme engineering, and chemistry on projects concerning artificial cells, blood substitutes from cross-linked hemoglobin and encapsulated hemoglobin, oral therapy for kidney failure, detoxifier, immobilized enzymes, cells, including genetically engineered cells, hemoperfusion, microencapsulation, nanoencapsulation, enzyme replacement therapy, drug carriers, and biomaterials. **Pub:** *Artificial Cells, Blood Substitutes and Immobilization Biotechnology*. Journal. • *International Journal*. Journal.

★ 22804 ★ McGill University Centre for Indigenous Peoples' Nutrition and Environment (CINE)
21,111 Lakeshore Rd.
Sainte Anne de Bellevue, QC, Canada H9X 3V9
Phone: (514)398-7544 **Fax:** (514)398-1020
Email: cine@cine.mcgill.ca
Website: http://www.cine.mcgill.ca/
Dr. Timothy Johns, Dir.

Activities/Fields: Integrity of the traditional food systems of the Aboriginal peoples of Canada, particularly food selection in relation to environment and culture, determination of nutrient and contaminant content in traditional foods and how food use relates to nutrition and health. **Pub:** *Newsletters*. • *Posters*. • *Reports*. • *Videos*.

★ 22805 ★ McGill University Centre for Medicine, Ethics, and Law
3690 Peel St.
Montreal, QC, Canada H3A 1W9
Phone: (514)398-7400 **Fax:** (514)398-4668
Email: margaret.somerville@mcgill.ca
M.A. Somerville, Dir.

Activities/Fields: Social and policy issues which have medical, ethical, and legal dimensions, including medical research, reproductive technology, aging, population, AIDS, euthanasia, genetics, and biotechnology.

★ 22806 ★ McGill University Centre for Nonlinear Dynamics in Physiology and Medicine
McIntyre Medical Science Bldg.
3655 Drummond St.
Montreal, QC, Canada H3G 1Y6
Phone: (514)398-4336 **Fax:** (514)398-7452
Email: mackey@cnd.mcgill.ca
Website: http://www.cnd.mcgill.ca
Michael C. Mackey, Dir.

Activities/Fields: Understanding the origin of dynamic behavior in health and disease, focusing on cyclical hematopoiesis, neurological tremor, and cardiac arythmias.

★ 22807 ★ McGill University Centre for Research on Endocrine Mechanisms
687 Pine Ave. W, Rm. L2-05
Montreal, QC, Canada H3A 1A1
Phone: (514)842-1231 **Fax:** (514)849-3681
Email: yogesh.patel@mcgill.ca
Dr. Yogesh C. Patel, Dir.

Activities/Fields: Endocrinology; molecular biology of peptide hormones and their receptors; molecular pharmacology of G protein coupled receptors; proliferative and anti-proliferative cell signaling; apoptosis; neuropeptides in brain, gut, pancreas, and immune system; peptide hormones and development; prostaglandins and metabolites of arachedonic acid. **Frmly:** Centre for Endocrine Studies.

★ 22808 ★ McGill University Centre for Research in Neuroscience
Montreal General Hospital Research Institute
1650 Cedar Ave.
Montreal, QC, Canada H3G 1A4
Phone: (514)937-6011 **Fax:** (514)934-8250
Email: pierre.drapeau@mcgill.ca
Website: http://www.mcgill.ca/mgh/
Dr. Pierre Drapeau, Dir.

Activities/Fields: Studies in neuroscience, particularly in cellular and molecular approaches to the nervous system with emphasis on neural development, regeneration, and neuroendocrine function. Research methodologies include recombinant DNA and classical neuroanatomical and electrophysiological techniques.

★ 22809 ★ McGill University Centre for Studies in Aging
Douglas Hospital
6825 La Salle Blvd.
Verdun, QC, Canada H4H 1R3
Phone: (514)766-2010 **Fax:** (514)888-4050
Email: jpoiri@pobxo.mcgill.ca
Website: http://www.mcgill.ca/mcsa
Dr. Judes Poirier, Dir.

Activities/Fields: Alzheimer's disease, including diagnostic methods, drug trials, brain banking, and genetic studies; Parkinson's disease; autonomous nervous dysfunction in aging; cellular models of aging; community health and epidemiology; bioethics; nutrition in aging; and social gerontology. **Pub:** *Geronto-McGill Newsletter*.

★ 22810 ★ McGill University Centre for the Study of Host Resistance
Montreal General Hospital
1650 Cedar Ave., Rm. A6.149
Montreal, QC, Canada H3G 1A4
Phone: (514)934-1934 **Fax:** (514)933-7146
Email: emil.skamene@muhc.mcgill.ca
Website: http://www.mcgill.ca/hostres
Dr. Emil Skamene, Dir.

Activities/Fields: Genetic regulation of host susceptibility and resistance in diseases of adulthood, including cancer, tuberculosis, malaria, and other infectious diseases.

★ 22811 ★ McGill University Clinical Trials Research Group (CTRG)
Biomedical Ethics Unit
3647 Peel St.
Montreal, QC, Canada H3A 1X1
Phone: (514)398-6945
Email: kathleen.glass@mcgill.ca
Website: http://www.mcgill.ca/ctrg/
Prof. Kathleen Cranley Glass, Contact

Activities/Fields: Ethical and legal issues in the design, review, and implementation of clinical trials.

★ 22812 ★ McGill University Division of Transplantation
687 Ave. des Pins Ouest
Montreal, QC, Canada H3A 1A1
Phone: (514)843-1649 **Fax:** (514)843-1708
Email: rolf.loertscher@mcgill.ca
Rolf Loertscher, MD, Dir.

Activities/Fields: Performs joint clinical trials in organ transplantation, conducts autoimmunity and other immunobiology/immunogenetics studies, formulates public policy objectives regarding organ grafting, examines the ethical and legal aspects of transplantation and allocation of scarce resources, and evaluates the cost-effectiveness of transplantation programs. Develops computer expert systms for medical diagnosis and medical education. Also centralizes patient data and results of McGill Teaching Hospital programs, serves as an administrative clearinghouse for patient samples and data, and facilitates interaction among the basic science laboratories at the University's Medical School.

★ 22813 ★ McGill University Institute of Parasitology
MacDonald Campus
21111 Lakeshore Rd.
Sainte Anne de Bellevue, QC, Canada H9X 3V9
Phone: (514)398-7722 **Fax:** (514)398-7857
Email: grad_sec@parasit.lan.mcgill.ca
Website: http://www.mcgill.ca/parasitology/
Dr. Terry Spithill, Dir.

Activities/Fields: Epidemiology, ecology, biochemistry, neurophysiology, immunology, population and molecular genetics and molecular biology of parasites. Research includes experimental studies on the relationships and interactions between parasite and host. **Pub:** *Research Reports*. • *Scientific journals peer-reviewed*.

★ 22814 ★ McGill University
Laboratory of Neurotoxicology
Montreal Neurological Institute
3801 University St.
Montreal, QC, Canada H3A 2B4
Phone: (514)398-8509 **Fax:** (514)398-1509
Email: mddm@musica.mcgill.ca
Dr. Heather Durham, Contact
Activities/Fields: Neurodegenerative diseases, neurotoxicology, and neurobiology; the biological basis of motor neuron diseases; cell culture models of motor neuron diseases, including amyotrophic lateral sclerosis and toxic neuropathies; and therapy of motor neuron diseases.

★ 22815 ★ McGill University
Lady Davis Institute for Medical Research
3755 Chemin de la Cote-Sainte-Catherine
Montreal, QC, Canada H3T 1E2
Phone: (514)340-8260 **Fax:** (514)340-7502
Email: wainberg@ldi.jgh.mcgill.ca
Website: http://www.jgh.ca/research/ldi/index.html
Mark A. Wainberg, MD, Dir.
Activities/Fields: AIDS, Aging, Cognitive Neuroscience, Molecular Oncology, Pharmacology of Cancer, Endocrinology and Metabolism, Human Genetics, Iron Metabolism, Cardiovascular Diseases, Clinical Epidemiology, Health Services Research, Psychosocial Aspects of Illness. **Pub:** *Annual Scientific Activity Report.*

★ 22816 ★ McGill University
Lady Davis Institute for Medical Research
McGill AIDS Centre
3755 Chemin de la Cote-Sainte-Catherine, Rm 318
Montreal, QC, Canada H3T 1E2
Phone: (514)340-8260 **Fax:** (514)340-7502
Email: wainberg@ldi.jgh.mcgill.ca
Mark A. Wainberg, MD, Dir.
Activities/Fields: Promotes research on all aspects of HIV/AIDS, the development of new drugs, treatments, and vaccines for HIV/AIDS, as well as the development of comprehensive cost-effective models of care and treatment for HIV infection and AIDS. Sponsors basic, clinical, epidemiological, preventive, and psychosocial studies of HIV/AIDS. Topics include residential drug abuse treatment models for AIDS prevention, immune response in AIDS, regulation of interferon gene expression, HIV-1 resistance to AZT and other drugs, Canadian women and HIV, HIV prevention through peer intervention among youth, assessment of social support for patients with HIV/AIDS, knowledge of HIV/AIDS among daycare workers and parents, and personal strivings and levels of self-determination in predicting adjustments in AIDS. **Pub:** *Newsletter*, quarterly.

★ 22817 ★ McGill University
McConnell Brain Imaging Centre
3801 University St.
Montreal, QC, Canada H3A 2B4
Phone: (514)398-8925 **Fax:** (514)398-8948
Email: doug@mrs.mni.mcgill.ca
Website: http://www.bic.mni.mcgill.ca/bic_welcome.html
Douglas Arnold, PhD, Contact
Activities/Fields: Investigates cerebral function using positron emission tomography (PET) and magnetic resonance imaging (MRI) on healthy volunteers and patients with brain tumors, epilepsy, movement disorders, and other acute and chronic neurological illnesses. Research areas include radiochemistry, imaging physics, mapping of cognitive functions in the brain, kinetic analysis, and modeling of biological systems. **Pub:** *NeuroPIL Bulletin*, monthly.

★ 22818 ★ McGill University
McGill Cancer Centre
McIntyre Medical Sciences Bldg.
3655 Promenade Sir-William Osler
Montreal, QC, Canada H3G 1Y6
Phone: (514)398-3535 **Fax:** (514)398-6769
Email: tremblay@med.mcgill.ca
Website: http://www.medserv.mcgill.ca/cancer
Dr. Michel L. Tremblay, Dir.
Activities/Fields: Cancer, including molecular biology of human and murine carcinoembryonic antigen, family nature and regulation of mammalian origins of DNA replication, molecular biology of dominant and recessive oncogenes, cancer related cellular surface sugar-containing molecules, and molecular basis of spatial differentiation in mice and its aberration in tumors.

★ 22819 ★ McGill University
McGill Centre for the Study of Reproduction
Department of Obstetrics & Gynecology
Woman's Pavilion, Royal Victoria Hospital
687 Pine Ave. W
Montreal, QC, Canada H3A 1A1
Phone: (514)842-1231 **Fax:** (514)843-1662
Email: beryl.rodrigues@muhc.mcgill.ca
Beryl Rodriguez, Exec. Sec.
Activities/Fields: Reproduction, including gametogenesis, fertilization, fetal development, pregnancy, parturition, and structure and function of the brain/pituitary/gonadal axis andbrain/pituitary/testicular/epididymal axis. Activities include studies of oogenesis, assisted reproductive technology (IVF), follicle development, genomic imprinting, testicular and epididmal physiology, reproductive toxicology, fetal growth, reproductive neuroscience. **Pub:** *Annual Report.*

★ 22820 ★ McGill University
McGill Centre for Translational Research in Cancer
Clinical Research Unit
3755 Cote Ste. Catherine Rd.
Montreal, QC, Canada H3T 1E2
Phone: (514)340-8222
Email: wmiller@ldi.jgh.mcgill.ca
Website: http://www.mctrc.org/en/Default.htm
Wilson Miller, MD, Dir.
Activities/Fields: Novel cancer therapeutics, including pharmacokinetics/dynamics.

★ 22821 ★ McGill University
McGill Nutrition and Food Science Centre
Royal Victoria Hospital
687 Pine Ave. W, Rm. H6.61
Montreal, QC, Canada H3A 1A1
Phone: (514)843-1665 **Fax:** (514)843-1706
Email: errol.marliss@muhc.mcgill.ca
Dr. Errol B. Marliss, Dir.
Activities/Fields: Promotes clinical and basic research in nutrition and food science.

★ 22822 ★ McGill University
Meakins-Christie Laboratories
3626 St. Urbain St.
Montreal, QC, Canada H2X 2P2
Phone: (514)398-3864 **Fax:** (514)398-7483
Email: james.martin@mcgill.ca
Website: http://www.meakins.mcgill.ca/meakins/
Dr. James G. Martin, Dir.
Activities/Fields: Respiratory physiology and physiopathology, including studies on control of breathing, respiratory mechanics, respiratory muscle fatigue, electromyography, lung morphology and biochemistry, airway dynamics, smooth muscle growth and contractive signalling, eicosanoids, T-lymphocytes, allergic inflammation.

★ 22823 ★ McGill University
Medical Physics Unit
Montreal General Hospital
1650 Cedar Ave., Rm. L5-109
Montreal, QC, Canada H3G 1A4
Phone: (514)934-8052 **Fax:** (514)934-8229
Email: epodgorsak@medphys.mcgill.ca
Website: http://www.medphys.mcgill.ca
Prof. Ervin B. Podgorsak, Dir.
Activities/Fields: Medical imaging, including resonant cavity imaging, filter functions (computer tomography), positron emission tomography, nuclear magnetic resonance imaging, and electronic processing. Other studies include physical aspects of radiation oncology and radiation dosimetry, radiosurgery, radiation hazards and protection, physical aspects of nuclear cardiology, and dosimetry in diagnostic radiology.

★ 22824 ★ McGill University
Montreal Children's Hospital Research Institute
2300 Tupper St.
Montreal, QC, Canada H3H 1P3
Phone: (514)934-4300 **Fax:** (514)934-4331
Roy Gravel, Dir.
Activities/Fields: Basic, clinical,and epidemiologic research into various disorders affecting infants and children, including diabetes, prematurity cystic fibrosis, abnormal growth, learning disabilities, hyperactivity, and genetic diseases.

★ 22825 ★ McGill University
Montreal Neurological Institute
3801 University St., Rm. 636
Montreal, QC, Canada H3A 2B4
Phone: (514)398-1903 **Fax:** (514)398-8248
Email: director@mni.lan.mcgill.ca
Website: http://www.mni.mcgill.ca
Dr. David R. Colman, Dir.
Activities/Fields: Organic aspects of the nervous system, including studies in molecular neurobiology, neuroanatomy, cerebrovascular disease, neurochemistry, epilepsy, neurogenetics, neuroimaging, neuroimmunology, movement disorders, neuromuscular research, neuro-oncology, neuropharmacology, and neuropsychology. **Pub:** *Annual Report.* • *Neuro Magazine.*

★ 22826 ★ McGill University
Montreal Neurological Institute
Brain Tumour Research Centre
Neuro Development Office
3801 University St.
Montreal, QC, Canada H3A 2B4
Phone: (514)398-1958 **Fax:** (514)398-8072
Website: http://www.mni.mcgill.ca/brain.htm
Dr. David Kaplan, Res. Dir.
Activities/Fields: Causes and treatment of brain tumors.

★ 22827 ★ McGill University
Montreal Neurological Institute
Complex Neural Systems Research Unit
3801 University St.
Montreal, QC, Canada H3A 2B4
Phone: (514)398-1913 **Fax:** (514)398-5871
Email: barbara.jones@mcgill.ca
Dr. Barbara E. Jones, Coord.
Activities/Fields: Neurobiology. **Frmly:** Neurobiology Unit.

★ 22828 ★ McGill University
Montreal Neurological Institute
Neuromuscular Research Group
3801 University St.
Montreal, QC, Canada H3A 2B4
Phone: (514)398-6644 **Fax:** (514)398-8310
Email: mcgk@musica.mcgill.ca
Website: http://www.mcgill.ca/mni/index.html
Dr. George Karpati, Coord.
Activities/Fields: Neuromuscular research, including molecular genetics, muscle biochemistry, muscle metabolism, neurotoxicology, neuropathology, neurophysiology, cytochemistry, and magnetic resonance spectroscopy. Research focuses on gene therapy for muscle and motor neurons, coordinated expression of genes coding for myofibrillar molecules during differentiation and denervation, use of transgenic mice, cell adhesion molecules and molecular mechanisms of

myoblast fusion in vitro, molecular biology of muscle mitochondria (especially in mitochondrial diseases), microscopic and biochemical cytoskeletal alterations in neurons pertaining to diseases such as amyotrophic lateral sclerosis and toxic neuropathies, in vivo magnetic resonance spectroscopy of neuromuscular diseases, comprehensive multidisciplinary investigation of complex neuromuscular diseases, and gene therapy for dystrophin deficiency states, and malignant brain tumors.

★ 22829 ★ McGill University
Spinal Cord Research Group
McIntyre Medical Sciences Bldg., Rm. 1242
3655 Drummond St.
Montreal, QC, Canada H3G 1Y6
Email: ydk@pinalcord.mcgill.ca
Website: http://www.spinalcord.mcgill.ca/
Yves De Koninck, PhD, Prin. Investigator
Activities/Fields: Structural and functional aspects of the dorsal horn of the mammalian spinal cord. Research interests include neurotrophic factor therapy, neuronal plasticity in basic pharmacology and biophysics of synaptic transmission.

★ 22830 ★ McGill University Health Centre (MUHC)
Montreal Chest Institute Research Centre
3650 St. Urbain St.
Montreal, QC, Canada H2X 2P4
Phone: (514)849-5201 **Fax:** (514)843-2095
Email: patrice.vaillancourt@mcgill.ca
Dr. James G. Martin, Dir.
Activities/Fields: Respiratory medicine, focusing on chronic obstructive pulmonary diseases (COPD). Research also includes structure-function, physiology, pharmacology, rehabilitation, environment, body surface motion, asthma, cystic fibrosis, and airway hyperresponsiveness.

★ 22831 ★ McGill University Health Centre
Research Institute
Clinical Research Centre
1650 Cedar Ave., Ste. D13 173
Montreal, QC, Canada H3G 1A4
Phone: (514)934-1934 **Fax:** (514)934-8338
Email: muhc.crc@mcgill.ca
Website: http://www.mcgill.ca/muhc-ri
Dr. Phil Gold, Exec. Dir.
Activities/Fields: All therapeutic areas of medicine.

★ 22832 ★ McLaughlin Research Institute for Biomedical Sciences
1520 23rd St. S
Great Falls, MT 59405-4900
Phone: (406)452-6208 **Fax:** (406)454-6019
Email: davec@po.mri.montana.edu
Website: http://www.montana.edu/wwwmri
Dr. George A. Carlson, Dir.
Activities/Fields: Genetics, immunogenetics, and cancer immunology, including studies of mouse histocompatibility genes and antigens, immunoregulatory gene family diversity and divergence, genetic basis of susceptibility to transmissible neurodegenerative disease, and mitotic recombination in mammalian cells. **Pub:** *Annual Report.* • *Newsletter,* 3/year.

★ 22833 ★ McMaster University
Centre for Electrophotonic Materials and Devices (CEMD)
1280 Main St. W
Hamilton, ON, Canada L8S 4L8
Phone: (905)525-9140 **Fax:** (905)527-8409
Email: cemd@mcmaster.ca
Website: http://www.eng.mcmaster.ca/cemd/
Dr. Doug M. Bruce, Contact
Activities/Fields: Neurosciences, cardiovascular system, mineralization, confocal microscopy, and analytical electron microscopy. Facility is used by many research groups.

★ 22834 ★ McMaster University
Centre for Evaluation of Medicines (CEM)
Faculty of Health Sciences
St. Joseph's Hospital
105 Main St. E, P1
Hamilton, ON, Canada L8N 1G6
Phone: (905)522-1155 **Fax:** (905)521-6136
Email: levinem@mcmaster.ca
Website: http://www.fhs.mcmaster.ca/ceb/acts/cem.htm
Mitchell Levine, Dir.
Activities/Fields: Improved drug therapy.

★ 22835 ★ McMaster University
Centre for Health Economics and Policy Analysis (CHEPA)
Facility of Health Sciences
1200 Main St. W
Hamilton, ON, Canada L8N 3Z5
Phone: (905)525-9140 **Fax:** (905)546-5211
Email: hutchb@fhs.mcmaster.ca
Brian Hutchison, Actg. Dir.
Activities/Fields: Health economics and health policy analysis, including organization, funding, and delivery of health care; the evaluation of health care programs and technologies; the measurement of health at the individual and population level; the determinants of population health; and the processes of health policy making. **Pub:** *CHSPA Working Papers Series,* quarterly.

★ 22836 ★ McMaster University
Father Sean O'Sullivan Research Centre (FSORC)
St. Joseph's Hospital
50 Charlton Ave. E
Hamilton, ON, Canada L8N 4A6
Phone: (289)522-6115 **Fax:** (289)521-6136
Email: smacleod@stjosham.on.ca
Website: http://www.stjosham.on.ca/fsorc/default.htm
Stuart Macleod, Dir.
Activities/Fields: Chest and lung diseases; surgical outcomes; geriatrics, with particular emphasis on drugs in the elderly, the management of incontinence, and treatment of musculoskeletal diseases; women's health; sexually transmitted diseases; mental health.

★ 22837 ★ McMaster University
Health Information Research Unit
1200 Main St. W, Rm. 3H7
Hamilton, ON, Canada L8N 3Z5
Phone: (905)525-9140 **Fax:** (905)546-0401
Website: http://hiru.mcmaster.ca/main.htm
Dr. Alex Jadad, Ch.
Activities/Fields: Workplace disability, particularly the factors that contribute to it; disability treatment, and ways to ensure optimal recovery and a safe return to work. **Pub:** *Newsletter.*

★ 22838 ★ McMaster University
Institute for Molecular Biology and Medicine
Antimicrobial Research Centre (ARC)
Health Sciences Centre, Rm. 4H29
1200 Main St. W
Hamilton, ON, Canada L8N 3Z5
Phone: (905)525-9140 **Fax:** (905)522-9033
Email: kushl@mcmaster.ca
Website: http://www.fhs.mcmaster.ca/arc/
Lisa Kush, Contact
Activities/Fields: Microbial diseases, particularly by those caused by antibiotic-resistant pathogens.

★ 22839 ★ McMaster University
Institute for Molecular Biology and Medicine
Centre for Gene Therapeutics
Health Science Centre
1200 Main St. W
Hamilton, ON, Canada L8N 3Z5
Phone: (905)525-9140 **Fax:** (905)522-6750
Email: bramsonj@mcmaster.ca
Website: http://www.fhs.mcmaster.ca/cgt/
Dr. Jonathan Bramson, Contact
Activities/Fields: Delivery of genes as therapeutic agents in the treatment of human and animal disease. The center focuses on developing novel cures for cancer, inflammatory diseases, and infectious diseases.

★ 22840 ★ McMaster University
Intestinal Disease Research Program (IDRP)
Health Sciences Centre, Rm. 3N5C
1200 Main St. W
Hamilton, ON, Canada L8N 3Z5
Phone: (905)525-9140 **Fax:** (905)522-3454
Email: idrp@mcmaster.ca
Website: http://www.fhs.mcmaster.ca/idrp/
Dr. Mary Perdue, Dir.
Activities/Fields: Intestinal diseases, especially within the following themes: immunophysiology, enteric infection, mucosal immunology, gut-brain interactions, physiology, pharmacology.

★ 22841 ★ McMaster University
McMaster Research Centre for the Promotion of Women's Health (MRCPOWH)
1280 Main St. W, TSH-726
Hamilton, ON, Canada L8S 4M2
Email: ahmedm@mcmail.cis.mcmaster.ca
Website: http://www.mcmaster.ca/mrcpowh/
Dr. Maroussia Hajdukowski-Ahmed, Co-Ch.
Activities/Fields: Women's health promotion. Main areas of research include the impact of work, paid and unpaid, inside the home and outside the home, on women's health; work/health in specific populations of women, e.g. women with disabilities, immigrant women, seniors; the effectiveness of individual coping strategies, and collective social change in promoting women's health; the effectiveness of action-based and participatory research as a community health-promotion strategy.

★ 22842 ★ McMaster University
R. Samuel McLaughlin Centre for Research and Education in Aging and Health
Chedoke Campus, Bldg. 74
1200 Main St. W
Hamilton, ON, Canada L8N 3Z5
Phone: (905)521-2100 **Fax:** (905)318-6556
Email: horvat@mcmaster.ca
Website: http://www.fhs.mcmaster.ca/mcah
Dr. A. Papaioannou, Co-Dir.
Activities/Fields: Health promotion and disease prevention, focusing on health promotion and disease prevention for seniors in the practices of family physicans; aging brain, focusing on dementia, risk factors for dementia, and the impact on caregiver health; aging, mobility and participation, focusing on ways to keep seniors active so they may order their own lives; and pharmacology and therapeutics, focusing on finding ways to reduce polypharmacy. **Pub:** *Quarterly Newsletter.*

★ 22843 ★ McMaster University
Supportive Cancer Care Research Unit (SCCR)
Hamilton Regional Cancer Centre
699 Concession St., Level 3-62
Hamilton, ON, Canada L8V 5C2
Phone: (905)387-9711 **Fax:** (905)575-6308

Email: bainbrd@mcmaster.ca
Website: http://www-fhs.mcmaster.ca/slru/sccru/index.html
Dr. Daryl Bainbridge, Contact
Activities/Fields: Supportive care services provided to cancer patients. Research focuses on three main areas: information exchange, quality of supportive care and evaluation and use of new cancer therapies.

★ 22844 ★ McMaster University System-Linked Research Unit on Health and Social Service Utilization (SLRU)
Faculty of Health Sciences, HSC 3N46
Hamilton, ON, Canada L8N 3Z5
Phone: (905)525-9140 **Fax:** (905)528-5099
Email: browneg@mcmaster.ca
Website: http://www-fhs.mcmaster.ca/slru/welcome.htm
Gina Browne, PhD, Dir.
Activities/Fields: Effects and financial costs of innovative intersectoral, comprehensive health services for vulnerable populations in two regions of Ontario, Canada. **Pub:** *Working papers.*

★ 22845 ★ MCP Hahnemann University of the Health Sciences Computer Vision Center for Vertebrate Brain Mapping
Department of Biology & Anatomy
2900 Queen Ln.
Philadelphia, PA 19129
Phone: (215)991-8410 **Fax:** (215)843-9367
Email: nissanov@drexel.edu
Dr. Jonathan Nissanov, Dir.
Activities/Fields: Algorithms for use in basic biological research with emphasis on the methodological needs of nurobiology, with the overall emphasis on quantitative imaging. Current research projects include artificial intelligence techniques for pattern recognition and automated parcellation of brain structures; quantificaion techniques for analysis of microautoradiograms; correction methods for the differential H-3 quenching between white- and gray-matter; and development of new quantitative descriptors of distribution. **Frmly:** Autoradiographic Image Processing Center.

★ 22846 ★ MCP Hahnemann University of the Health Sciences Institute for Cardiovascular Research
Allegheny General Hospital
320 E North Ave.
Pittsburgh, PA 15212
Phone: (412)359-8255
Stephen F. Vatner, MD, Dir.
Activities/Fields: Cardiovascular disease.

★ 22847 ★ Meadowbrook Medical Education and Research Foundation, Inc.
2201 Hempstead Tpke.
East Meadow, NY 11554-1859
Phone: (516)572-6724 **Fax:** (516)572-4660
Gary E. Bie, Exec. Sec. /Treas.
Activities/Fields: Clinical drugs studies.

★ 22848 ★ Medical College of Georgia Alzheimer's Research Center for Clinical and Basic Research
Department of Pharmacology & Toxicology
Augusta, GA 30912-2300
Phone: (706)721-6355 **Fax:** (706)721-9861
Email: jbuccafu@mail.mcg.edu
Website: http://www.mcg.edu/centers/alz
Dr. Jerry J. Buccafusco, Dir.
Activities/Fields: Multidisciplinary research on all aspects of Alzheimer's disease, including new therapeutic approaches, diagnostic procedures, and basic studies of etiology.

★ 22849 ★ Medical College of Georgia Center for Clinical Investigation
1521 Pope Ave., FF-1001
Augusta, GA 30912-3152
Phone: (706)721-9680 **Fax:** (706)721-9557
Email: amulloy@mcg.edu
Anthony L. Mulloy, PhD, Dir.
Activities/Fields: Pharmaceutical agents and medical devices.

★ 22850 ★ Medical College of Georgia Center for Nursing Research
Jennings Wing, EB-201
School of Nursing
Augusta, GA 30912
Phone: (706)721-3162 **Fax:** (706)721-7049
Email: gbennett@mail.mcg.edu
Website: http://www.mcg.edu/SON/CNR/
Gerald Bennett, PhD, Dir.
Activities/Fields: Cognitive functioning and control in institutionalized elderly; asthma; family, health risk, and lifestyle change; learning with computer-aided education (CAE) equipment, and computer-aided instruction (CAI); and cancer and rehabilitation nursing, rural health, self-esteem, and abuse and homeless issues. **Pub:** *Informer.*

★ 22851 ★ Medical College of Georgia Georgia Prevention Institute (GPI)
HS-1640
Augusta, GA 30912-3710
Phone: (706)721-4534 **Fax:** (706)721-7150
Email: ftreiber@mail.mcg.edu
Website: http://www.mcg.edu/institutes/gpi
Dr. Frank A. Treiber, Dir.
Activities/Fields: Health promotion and disease prevention, mainly in youth, particularly pediatric antecedents of cardiovascular and metabolic disease that are ordinarily manifested in the adult years.

★ 22852 ★ Medical College of Georgia Sickle Cell Center
AC 1004
Augusta, GA 30912-3128
Phone: (706)721-9640 **Fax:** (706)721-9637
Email: akutlar@mail.mcg.edu
Dr. Abdullah Kutlar, Dir.
Activities/Fields: Hemoglobinopathy detection, identification, and characterization, including studies of factors determining severity of sickle cell anemia in adults and the young child, cardiac evaluation of children with sickle cell anemia, thalassemia in association with sickle cell syndromes, biochemical studies in sickle cell anemia and related disorders with special emphasis on heterogeneity of Hb F, immunological identification, DNA gene mapping of hemoglobin variants, nucleotide sequence, and thalassemia genes, and characterization of hemoglobin variants.

★ 22853 ★ Medical College of Georgia Vascular Biology Center (VBC)
1120 15th St.
Augusta, GA 30912-2500
Phone: (706)721-6338 **Fax:** (706)721-9799
Email: jcatrava@mcg.edu
Website: http://www.mcg.edu/Centers/VBC
John D. Catravas, PhD, Dir.
Activities/Fields: Cellular and integrated vascular function under normal and pathologic conditions in order to elucidate specific homeostatic vascular functions, as well as the pathogenesis, diagnosis and treatment of vascular disease. **Pub:** *Vascular Pharmacology*, monthly.

★ 22854 ★ Medical College of Ohio Cancer Research Division
Department of Pathology, HE 202
3055 Arlington Ave.
Toledo, OH 43614-5806
Phone: (419)383-4918 **Fax:** (419)383-3089
Email: hschut@mco.edu
Dr. Herman A.J. Schut, Contact
Activities/Fields: Cancer, including chemical carcinogenesis, chemoprevention, molecular biology, toxicology, and tissue culture. Specific research includes oncogene activation and suppressor gene inactivation in cancer, inhibition of cancer by dietary components, and regulation of tumor promotion.

★ 22855 ★ Medical College of Wisconsin Biophysics Research Institute
8701 Watertown Plank Rd.
Milwaukee, WI 53226-0509
Phone: (414)456-4035 **Fax:** (414)456-6512
Email: balarama@mcw.edu
Dr. Balaraman Kalyanaraman, Dir.
Activities/Fields: Biophysics, with emphasis on functional magnetic resonance imaging and electron spin resonance.

★ 22856 ★ Medical College of Wisconsin Cancer Center
8701 Watertown Plank Rd.
Milwaukee, WI 53226
Phone: (414)805-4455 **Fax:** (414)805-6396
Email: bcampbel@mcw.edu
Website: http://www.mcw.edu/cancercenter/
Bruce H. Campbell, MD, Interim Dir.
Activities/Fields: Experimental Therapy program focuses on developing new agents and strategies for the treatment of cancer, including photodynamic therapy; understanding cell resistance, focusing on glutathione, iron metabolism and nitric oxide; and limiting the toxicity and side effects of cancer treatment, focusing on gastrointestinal effects and chronic renal damage caused by radiation therapy; Cancer Biologyand Molecular Genetics Program studies regulatory mechanisms at the structural, cellular and molecular levels in the following areas: regulation of cell growth and orcogenesis, development, virology and viral transformation, and molecular diagnostics; Cancer Prevention and Control Program conducts several multi-year studies in behavioral interventions are on-going in the areas of environmental hazards (pesticides and cancer risk), smoking cessation interventions, skin cancer prevention education, early screening education and nutrition education; research interest in quality of life issues in the areas of pediatric, breast and head/neck cancers; and studies in chemotherapeutic agents in cancer prevention; Bone Marrow Transplantation/Immunology Program conducts ongoing studies in T-cell depletion, cytokines, graft-vs-host disease; autologous, allogenic, and unrelated donor therapies; lymphocyte infusion; International Bone Marrow Transplant Registry.

★ 22857 ★ Medical College of Wisconsin Center for AIDS Intervention Research (CAIR)
2071 North Summit Ave.
Milwaukee, WI 53202
Phone: (414)456-7700 **Fax:** (414)287-4206
Website: http://www.cair.mcw.edu/
Dr. Jeffrey Kelly, Contact
Activities/Fields: New intervention strategies to prevent HIV infection in populations vulnerable to the disease, including inner-city women, homeless men and women, gay men, youth at risk, and chronic mentally ill adults.

★ 22858 ★ Medical College of Wisconsin Center for the Study of Bioethics
8701 Watertown Plank Rd.
Milwaukee, WI 53226
Phone: (414)456-8498 **Fax:** (414)456-6511
Email: rshapiro@mcw.edu
Website: http://www.mcw.edu/bioethics/
Robyn Shapiro, JD, Dir.
Activities/Fields: Ethics studies, with special emphasis on AIDS, abortion, drug testing, euthanasia, fetal rights, genetics, technology assessment and alloca-

tion of resources, and multicultural approaches to bioethics. **Pub:** *Bioethics Bullentin*, biennially.

★ 22859 ★ Medical College of Wisconsin Cystic Fibrosis Research Center

Specialty Clinic
Milwaukee Children's Hospital of Wisconsin
9000 W Wisconsin Ave., MS 777A, Ste. 223
Milwaukee, WI 53201
Phone: (414)266-6731 **Fax:** (414)266-6742
Email: splain@mcw.edu
Dr. M.L. Splaingard, Dir.

Activities/Fields: Cystic fibrosis, chest impedance measurements, and newborn screening studies. Provides patient care as a service to referring physicians and instruction for small groups of medical students from the College.

★ 22860 ★ Medical College of Wisconsin Free Radical Research Center

Biophysics Research Institute
8701 Watertown Plank Rd.
Milwaukee, WI 53226-0509
Phone: (414)456-4035 **Fax:** (414)456-6512
Email: balarama@mcw.edu
Website: http://www.mcw.edu/frrc/
Dr. Balaraman Kalyanaraman, Dir.

Activities/Fields: Free radicals and their role in disease and prevention, action of antioxidants in human disease.

★ 22861 ★ Medical College of Wisconsin Froedtert and Medical College Eye Institute

925 N 87th St.
Milwaukee, WI 53226
Phone: (414)456-7915 **Fax:** (414)456-6563
Email: dheuer@mcw.edu
Website: http://www.mcw.edu/ophthalmology
Dr. Dale Heuer, Dir.

Activities/Fields: Ophthalmology, including anterior segment reconstruction, cataract, color vision, corneal and external eye diseases, genetics, glaucoma, ocular oncology, ophthalmic pathology, ophthalmic reconstructive surgery, orbital diseases, neuro-ophthalmology, refractive surgery, strabismus and pediatric ophthalmology, visual rehabilitation and vitreoretinal diseases.

★ 22862 ★ Medical College of Wisconsin General Clinical Research Center

9200 W Wisconsin Ave.
Milwaukee, WI 53226
Phone: (414)805-7325 **Fax:** (414)805-7330
Email: gsonnen@mcw.edu
Website: http://www.mcw.edu/gcrc/
Gabriele E. Sonnenberg, MD, Prog. Dir.

Activities/Fields: Physiology and pathophysiology of disease in areas of metabolism, endocrinology, gastroenterology, kidney, central nervous system, connective tissues, hematopietic system, and bone, respiratory, and cardiovascular disorders.

★ 22863 ★ Medical College of Wisconsin Health Policy Institute (HPI)

8701 Watertown Plank Rd.
Milwaukee, WI 53226
Phone: (414)456-8762 **Fax:** (414)456-6529
Website: http://www.mcw.edu/html/body_ov_-hpi.html
Dr. Richard A. Cooper, Dir.

Activities/Fields: Health care policies and issues, including bioethics, health services, epidemiology, and biostatistics.

★ 22864 ★ Medical College of Wisconsin Human and Molecular Genetic Center

8701 Watertown Plank Rd.
Milwaukee, WI 53226
Phone: (414)456-4887 **Fax:** (414)456-6516
Email: jacob@mcw.edu
Website: http://hmgc.mcw.edu
Dr. Howard J. Jacob, Dir.

Activities/Fields: Identification of the genes involved in multifactorial diseases, such as cancer, cardiovascular disease, obesity, insulin dependent diabetes mellitus, and non-insulin dependent diabetes. **Frmly:** Laboratory for Genetics Research.

★ 22865 ★ Medical and Health Research Association of New York City, Inc. (MHRA)

40 Worth St., Ste. 720
New York, NY 10013
Phone: (212)285-0220 **Fax:** (212)385-0565
Email: erautenberg@mhra.org
Website: http://www.mhra.org
Ellen Rautenberg, Pres. /CEO

Activities/Fields: Obstetrics, gynecology, midwifery, nursing, prenatal care and diagnoses, maternity care, infant care, infant mortality, pediatric care, family planning, childhood immunizations, health and HIV education, and nutrition for persons living in New York City. **Pub:** *MHRA News*, semiannually. Newsletter.

★ 22866 ★ Medical Research Modernization Committee

3200 Morley Rd.
Shaker Heights, OH 44122
Phone: (216)283-6702 **Fax:** (216)283-6702
Email: stkaufman@mindspring.com
Website: http://www.mrmcmed.org/
Stephen R. Kaufman, MD, Contact

Activities/Fields: Research modalities, focusing on their medical and scientific merits in order to identify outdated research methods and promote reliable and efficient methods. **Pub:** *Perspectives on Medical Research*, occasionally. Monograph.

★ 22867 ★ Medical Technology and Practice Patterns Institute, Inc.

4733 Bethesda Ave., Ste. 510
Bethesda, MD 20814
Phone: (301)652-4005 **Fax:** (301)652-8335
Email: info@mtppi.org
Website: http://www.mtppi.org
Dennis J. Cotter, Pres.

Activities/Fields: New and emerging health-care technologies and their implications for local, national, and international policy. Research efforts fall into three broad areas: Health Services Research, encompassing patient outcomes, pharmacoeconomics, quality-of-life assessments, and cost-effectiveness analyses; International Activities, including conducting surveys of health technology assessment activities worldwide technology assessment modeling, and sponsorship of workshops and seminars on health policy issues; and Special Programs, encompassing health-facility planning, vaccine research and development, and educational outreach. Technologies studied include magnetic resonance imaging, extracorporeal shockwave lithotripsy, endocardial electrical stimulation, implantable cardiac defibrillators, percutaneous transluminal coronary angioplasty, percutaneous lithotripsy, heart transplantation, ambulatory blood pressure monitoring, total parenteral nutrition, liver transplantation, bone marrow transplantation, and dialysis treatment for end-stage renal disease. **Pub:** *Diagnostic Imaging and Child Abuse.* • *Direct and Indirect Costs of Diabetes.* • *Implications of NAFTA for Trade in Health Care Technology.* • *Rational Use of Health Technologies.* • *Reports on various health technologies.*

★ 22868 ★ Medical University of South Carolina

Department of Pediatrics
Division of Genetics and Developmental Pediatrics
The Vince Moseley Center
135 Rutledge Ave., 395
Charleston, SC 29425
Phone: (843)876-1516 **Fax:** (843)876-1518
Email: pais@musc.edu
Dr. G. Shashida Pai, Dir.

Activities/Fields: Genetic disorders and diseases; learning problems and communication disorders research, including attention deficit disorder, spina bifida, autism, chronic disease and adjustment. **Frmly:** Vince Moseley Center for Children with Developmental Disabilities.

★ 22869 ★ Medical University of South Carolina

General Clinical Research Center
96 Jonathan Lucas St., Ste. 213
PO Box 250609
Charleston, SC 29425
Phone: (843)792-3256 **Fax:** (843)792-2601
Email: keyl@musc.edu
Website: http://www.gcrc.musc.edu
Dr. L. Lyndon Key, Jr., Prog. Dir.

Activities/Fields: Bone and mineral metabolism, cardiology, diabetes, endocrinology, gastroenterology, hypertension, nutrition, obstetrics and gynecology, oncology, hematology, pharmacology, pulmonary medicine, and rheumatology and immunology. Provides medical scientists with the opportunity for clinical research in all aspects of biomedicine. **Pub:** *Annual Report to National Institute of Health.*

★ 22870 ★ Medical University of South Carolina

Institute of Human Values in Health Care
96 Jonathan Lucas St., Ste. 409
PO Box 250612
Charleston, SC 29425
Phone: (843)792-5278 **Fax:** (843)792-8286
Email: values@musc.edu
Website: http://www.values.musc.edu/
Robert M. Sade, MD, Dir.

Activities/Fields: Relationship of human values to the development of health policy, legislation, and systems of delivery of patient care. Specific areas of interest encompass such topics as physician-assisted suicide, the interaction of clinical ethics with managed care, the relation of law enforcement to drug use in pregnancy and ethical issues in gene technology. **Pub:** *Newsletter.* • *Surveys.*

★ 22871 ★ Medical University of South Carolina

Interdisciplinary Program in Cell and Molecular Pharmacology and Experimental Therapeutics
171 Ashley Ave., BSB 303
PO Box 25055
Charleston, SC 29425
Phone: (843)792-2471 **Fax:** (843)792-2475
Email: margolhs@musc.edu
Website: http://www2.musc.edu/pharm/pharm.html
Dr. Harry Margolius, Chm.

Activities/Fields: Pharmacology, toxicology, molecular genetics and structural biology, including structure-function studies of proteins for primary sequence, posttranslational modifications, and characterization of the binding site of ligands; investigations of molecular design; and studies on cellular and molecular processes that control systemic arterial pressure, especially arachidonate metabolism, neurotransmitters, drug disposition and drug toxicity. Conducts studies of excitation-contraction coupling, excitation-secretion coupling, and water transport and regulation in cells and membrane mechanisms by norepinephrine, arachidonic acid metabolites, kallikrein-kinins, atrial peptides, and antihypertensive drugs. Also conducts studies of isolated cells, cell fragments, and isolated membranes, as well as studies on volunteer patients with hypertension, shock, and other cardiovascular-renal abnormalities.

★ 22872 ★ Medical University of South Carolina
Marine Biomedicine and Environmental Sciences Center
221 Ft. Johnson Rd.
Charleston, SC 29412
Phone: (843)762-5530 **Fax:** (843)762-5535
Email: lacyer@musc.edu
Website: http://www.musc.edu/mbes/home.htm
Dr. Eric R. Lacy, Dir.
Activities/Fields: Marine organisms and their cells as models, particularly in toxicology, immunology, pathology, parasitology, and microbiology studies; marine genomics and proteomics.

★ 22873 ★ Medical University of South Carolina
Molecular Morphology and Imaging Core
644 Basic Science Bldg.
Department of Cell Biology & Anatomy
173 Ashley Ave.
Charleston, SC 29425-2204
Phone: (843)792-3756 **Fax:** (843)792-0664
Email: truskt@musc.edu
Website: http://mmi.musc.edu
Thomas C. Trusk, PhD, Dir.
Activities/Fields: Cell biology and cellular and molecular influences on cardiovascular development.

★ 22874 ★ Medical University of South Carolina
Storm Eye Institute
167 Ashley Ave.
Charleston, SC 29425
Phone: (843)792-3758 **Fax:** (843)792-1723
Email: crossonc@musc.edu
Dr. Craig Crosson, Res. Dir.
Activities/Fields: Causes of blinding diseases and development of new treatments to prevent or ameliorate disease progression, including targeting macular degeneration, diabetic retinopathy, glaucoma, cataract and refractive surgery.

★ 22875 ★ Meharry Medical College
Center on Tropical Diseases
Division of Sponsored Research
1005 D.B. Todd Blvd.
Nashville, TN 37208
Phone: (615)327-6193 **Fax:** (615)327-5621
Dr. George C. Hill, Contact
Activities/Fields: Molecular, biochemical, and immunological aspects of tropical disease. Specific research includes studies on African trypanosomiasis, Chagas' disease, schistosomiasis, malaria, and leprosy. **Pub:** *Tropical Diseases Newsletter.* Newsletter.

★ 22876 ★ Meharry Medical College
Clinical Research Center
1005 D.B. Todd Blvd.
Nashville, TN 37208
Phone: (615)327-6353 **Fax:** (615)327-5835
Email: dgrandison@mmc.edu
Dr. David Grandison, Dir.
Activities/Fields: Clinical research, including pulmonary studies, AIDS, sickle cell disease, hypertension, body composition, coronary artery disease, infectious diseases, and oncology.

★ 22877 ★ Melpomene Institute for Women's Health Research
1010 University Ave.
Saint Paul, MN 55104
Phone: (651)642-1951 **Fax:** (651)642-1871
Email: health@melpomene.org
Website: http://www.melpomene.org
Judy Mahle Lutter, Ch.
Activities/Fields: Physically active women and girls, including effects of exercise on menstruation, pregnancy, adolescent girls, self-esteem and physical activity, menopause, body image, osteoporosis, stress and aging, children's introduction to physical activity. **Pub:** *The Bodywise Woman.* • *Breast Cancer: A Handbook.* • *A Guide for Physically Active Women.* • *Level Playing Fields.* • *Melpomene Journal*, 3/year. • *Of Heroes Hopes.* • *Reliable Information about Physical Activity and Health.*

★ 22878 ★ Memorial Sloan-Kettering Cancer Center
1275 York Ave.
New York, NY 10021
Phone: (212)639-2000 **Fax:** (212)639-5850
Email: varmus@mskcc.org
Website: http://www.mskcc.org
Dr. Harold Varmus, Lab Hd.
Activities/Fields: Molecular biology, cell biology and genetics, cellular biochemistry and biophysics, immunology, and molecular pharmacology and therapeutics. Aims to advance the understanding of the nature and fundamental causes of cancer and improve the means available for its prevention, diagnosis, and treatment. **Pub:** *Annual Report.* • *Center Newsletter.* • *Memorial Sloan-Kettering Cancer Center Research and Educational Programs.*

★ 22879 ★ Memorial University of Newfoundland
Centre for Offshore and Remote Medicine (MEDICOR)
Health Science Centre
Saint John's, NL, Canada A1B 3V6
Phone: (709)777-6433 **Fax:** (709)777-6746
Email: kledez@mun.ca
Website: http://www.med.mun.ca/medicor
Dale Decker, Contact
Activities/Fields: Petroleum related offshore health and safety, telemedicine and teleconferencing, hypermedic medicine, occupational medicine, and hypothermia, survival, immersion suits, hyperbaric medicine, and marine research.

★ 22880 ★ Methodist Health Care System
Sid W. Richardson Institute for Preventive Medicine
6550 Fannin St., SM583
Houston, TX 77030
Phone: (713)790-6450 **Fax:** (713)793-1269
Email: cathyeaster@tmh.tmc.edu
Website: http://www.methodisthealth.com/ipm
Cathy Easter DeBusk, Contact
Activities/Fields: Analyzes health insurance claims and employee absentee data to evaluate various preventive medicine programs, evaluates the effect of smoking cessation on the occurrence of chronic lung disease, compares different program approaches taken in cardiac rehabilitation (exercise versus comprehensive approaches), and studies depression in patients with heart disease and their spouses. **Pub:** *The Journal.*

★ 22881 ★ Methodist Research Institute
1701 N Senate Blvd.
PO Box 1367
Indianapolis, IN 46206
Phone: (317)962-3554 **Fax:** (317)962-5954
Email: gzaloga@clarian.org
Website: http://mri.clarian.com
Gary P. Zaloga, MD, Med. Dir.
Activities/Fields: Pharmaceutical and device clinical trials, experimental cell research, cell signalling, ion channel physiology, immunology. Other research involves heart, kidney, lung, pancreas, and liver transplants; biliary and renal extracorporeal shock wave lithotripsy; and clot lysis programs. **Pub:** *Journal of Hemato-therapy & Stem Cell Research*, monthly.

★ 22882 ★ MGMA Center for Research
104 Inverness Ter. E
Englewood, CO 80112-5306
Phone: (303)397-7879 **Fax:** (303)397-1827
Email: research@mgma.com
Website: http://www.mgma.com/research
Dr. Terry Hammons, VP
Activities/Fields: Health services, health economics, patient safety, new management technologies, tools for effective and efficient administration of healthcare organizations, and outcomes research. **Pub:** *Medical Group Management Journal*, bimonthly. **Frmly:** Center for Research in Ambulatory Health Care Administration.

★ 22883 ★ Miami Children's Hospital Research Institute
3100 SW 62nd Ave.
Miami, FL 33155
Phone: (305)663-8542 **Free:** 800-533-1792
Fax: (305)663-2461
Email: stuart.horowitz@mch.com
Website: http://www.mch.com/doctors_caregivers/research/contact.htm
Stuart Horowitz, MD, Dir.
Activities/Fields: Genetic vectoring, nutrition, hematology/oncology, immunology, forensic DNA identity, cardiac surgery, critical care physiology, nephrology. **Pub:** *International Journal of Pediatrics.*

★ 22884 ★ Miami Heart Research Institute
801 Arthur Godfrey Rd., 5th Fl.
Miami Beach, FL 33140
Phone: (305)674-3020 **Fax:** (305)535-3642
Email: mhri@miamiheartresearch.org
Website: http://www.miamiheartresearch.org
Kathleen DuCasse, CEO
Activities/Fields: Cardiovascular disease, including tracking genetic cardiovascular abnormalities, sudden cardiac death, emergency response resuscitation techniques, stress reduction techniques as well as hypertension and cholesterol studies. **Pub:** *Heartbeats Newsletter.*

★ 22885 ★ Miami Jewish Home and Hospital for the Aged
Stein Gerontological Institute, Inc.
5200 NE 2nd Ave.
Miami, FL 33137-2706
Phone: (305)762-1465 **Fax:** (305)762-1445
Email: bernieroos@cs.com
Website: http://www.gate.net/~sgi
Dr. Bernard A. Roos, Dir.
Activities/Fields: Promotes greater independence for the disabled through technology.

★ 22886 ★ Michael Fund/International Foundation for Genetic Research
4371 Northern Pike
Monroeville, PA 15146
Phone: (412)374-0111
Email: tengel@bellatlantic.net
Website: http://www.michaelfund.org
Randy Engel, Contact
Activities/Fields: Down's Syndrome and related genetic disorders with a pro-life philosophy, focusing on funding, prevention, cure or reducing the effects of Down's Syndrome. Also opposes abortion of the unborn, including deliberate euthanasia of children and adults with birth defects. **Pub:** *Friends of the Michael Fund Newsletter.*

★ 22887 ★ Michael Reese Hospital and Medical Center
Singer Pavillion
2959 S Cottage Grove
Chicago, IL 60616
Phone: (312)791-3800 **Fax:** (312)791-3927
Dr. Valentin Berman, Dir.
Activities/Fields: Mental health and mental illness, its etiology, treatment, and prevention, including psychiatry, psychophysiology, clinical psychology, and neurophysiology. Studies ego functions, schizophrenia, the modal adolescent, normal and disturbed adolescents,

family dynamics, and comparison of scales of manifest anxiety. Conducts biological and clinical investigations of affective disorder in children and adolescents; patterns of self-image in normal, delinquent, and disturbed adolescents; and the psychosomatic aspects of juvenile diabetes.

★ 22888 ★ Michigan Public Health Institute (MPHI)
2436 Woodlake Cir., Ste. 300
Okemos, MI 48864
Phone: (517)324-8300 **Fax:** (517)381-0260
Email: central@mphi.org
Website: http://www.mphi.org/
Jeffrey R. Taylor, PhD, Exec. Dir.
Activities/Fields: Public health issues, including disease prevention.

★ 22889 ★ Michigan State University Carcinogenesis Laboratory College of Osteopathic Medicine
Food Safety & Toxicology Bldg., 3rd Fl.
East Lansing, MI 48824
Phone: (517)353-7785 **Fax:** (517)353-9004
Email: maher@msu.edu
Website: http://www.com.msu.edu/carcino/
Prof. Veronica M. Maher, PhD, Co-Dir.
Activities/Fields: Carcinogenesis, including research in cellular and molecular biology, mutagenesis, mammalian cell DNA repair, and homologous recombination. **Pub:** *Monographs.* • *Newsletter*, occasionally. • *Papers.*

★ 22890 ★ Michigan State University Center for Biological Modeling
502B Biochemistry Bldg.
East Lansing, MI 48824-1319
Phone: (517)432-9895 **Fax:** (517)353-9334
Email: cbm@msu.edu
Website: http://biomodel.msu.edu/
Leslie A. Kuhn, Dir.
Activities/Fields: Modeling of biological processes, particularly protein folding, biomolecular catalysis, the spread of disease, rational development of drugs, and the evolution of organisms and molecules.

★ 22891 ★ Michigan State University Institute of International Health
B-301 West Fee Hall
East Lansing, MI 48824-1315
Phone: (517)353-8992 **Fax:** (517)355-1894
Email: petropou@msu.edu
Website: http://www.msu.edu/unit/iih
Dr. Evangelos A. Petropoulos, Dir.
Activities/Fields: World health problems, including overseas health studies. Specific projects include: the Training and Research on Environmental and Occupational Health in the Balkans project focusing on Bulgaria; Minority International Research Training (MIRT), for undergraduate, graduate, and professional level minority students and faculty in biomedical and behavioral research in 12 research sites in nine countries; the Medical Informatics Training in Malawi project; and the Environmental Sciences Training in Japan project. The IIH has conducted research and training on schistosomiasis with Egyptians scientists and worked on the management and prevention of cardiovascular diseases in Bulgaria and has helped develop country background information on health in Sub-Saharan Africa for the World Bank. **Pub:** *Newsletter*, bimonthly.

★ 22892 ★ Michigan State University Laboratory for Comparative Orthopaedic Research (LCOR)
Department of Small Animal Clinical Sciences
G-387 Veterinary Medical Center
East Lansing, MI 48824-1314
Phone: (517)353-8964 **Fax:** (517)353-8980
Email: arnoczky@cvm.msu.edu
Website: http://www.cvm.msu.edu/lcor/descript.htm
Dr. Steven P. Arnoczky, Dir.
Activities/Fields: Musculoskeletal system of humans and animals. The laboratory focuses its research on sports related injuries such as the repair and reconstruction of ligamentous and meniscal injuries of the knee. **Pub:** *Newsletter.*

★ 22893 ★ Michigan State University Office of Medical Education Research and Development (OMERAD)
East Fee Hall, Rm. A-217
College of Human Medicine
East Lansing, MI 48824-1316
Phone: (517)353-7791 **Fax:** (517)353-8926
Email: ander113@msu.edu
Website: http://www.omerad.msu.edu
William A. Anderson, PhD, Dir.
Activities/Fields: Medical education research and development, including program evaluation and performance assessment, faculty development, and the application of technology to improve instruction. Utilizes an interdisciplinary faculty representing the fields of psychology, socialogy, statistics, and education. **Pub:** *Medical Education Online*, quarterly. • *Outcomes Report*, annually. • *Vital Signs*, semiannually. Newsletter.

★ 22894 ★ Microsurgical Transplantation Research Foundation
Davies Medical Center, Ste. 140 North
45 Castro St.
San Francisco, CA 94114
Phone: (415)565-6136 **Fax:** (415)864-1654
Email: gbuncke@buncke.org
Website: http://www.buncke.org
Dr. Gregory Buncke, Dir.
Activities/Fields: Physiological and technical outcomes of microvascular replantation and transplantation; reconstructive microsurgery, and hand surgery; cryopreservation of tissues; hyperbaric oxygen therapy; and tissue oximetry with ischemia/perfusion injury.

★ 22895 ★ Mid-Missouri Mental Health Center
3 Hospital Dr.
Columbia, MO 65201-5296
Phone: (573)884-1300 **Fax:** (573)884-1010
Website: http://www.modmh.state.mo.us/mid_mo/index.htm
Dennis R. Canote, CEO
Activities/Fields: Mental health issues among children and adolscents, including epidemiology of psychiatric disorders, family violence, violence among adolescents, and outcome studies.

★ 22896 ★ Middle Tennessee Research Institute
1310 24th Av. S, Rm. F-201
Nashville, TN 37212-2637
Phone: (615)327-0938 **Fax:** (615)329-1520
Website: http://www.mtri.org
Gary Linn, Dir.
Activities/Fields: Medical clinical trials. **Frmly:** Nashville Research Institute, Inc.

★ 22897 ★ Midwest Biomedical Research Foundation
4801 E Linwood Blvd., Ste. 103
Kansas City, MO 64128-2226
Phone: (816)921-8311 **Fax:** (816)922-4712
Email: kimberly.collins@med.va.gov
Website: http://www.midwestbiomed.org
Kimberly Collins, Exec. Dir.
Activities/Fields: Clinical studies, focusing on improving treatments and cures of health problems prevalent among veteran patients and the general population.

★ 22898 ★ Midwest Ear Institute, Inc.
4200 Pennsylvania Ave., Ste. 100
Kansas City, MO 64111
Phone: (816)932-1660 **Fax:** (816)932-1675
Email: tstohs@mei-kc.org
Website: http://www.mei-kc.org
Teresa Stohs, Exec. Dir.
Activities/Fields: Auditory prostheses.

★ 22899 ★ Midwest Heart Research Foundation
2340 Highland Ave., Ste. 310
Lombard, IL 60148
Phone: (630)932-2165 **Fax:** (630)268-9609
Email: lbarr@midwestheart.com
Lawrence A. Barr, MD, Med. Dir.
Activities/Fields: Cardiovascular medicine clinical research. **Pub:** *Medical Journal.* • *Proceedings.*

★ 22900 ★ Milwaukee School of Engineering Electrical Engineering and Biomedical Science
1025 N Broadway
Milwaukee, WI 53202-3109
Phone: (414)277-7331 **Fax:** (414)277-7465
Email: canino@msoe.edu
Prof. Vincent R. Canino, PhD, Dir.
Activities/Fields: Biomedical instrumentation systems, including the design and evaluation of extracorporeal perfusion instrumentation.

★ 22901 ★ Minneapolis Heart Institute Foundation
920 E 28th St., Ste. 100
Minneapolis, MN 55407
Phone: (612)863-3833 **Free:** 877-800-2729
Fax: (612)863-3801
Email: fordwbell@aol.com
Website: http://www.mplsheartfoundation.org/
Ford Watson Bell, DVM, Pres.
Activities/Fields: Clinical cardiovascular studies with emphasis on cardiac death in the young.

★ 22902 ★ Minneapolis Medical Research Foundation
600 HFA Bldg.
914 S 8th St.
Minneapolis, MN 55404
Phone: (612)347-7680 **Fax:** (612)337-7189
Email: info@mmrf.org
Website: http://www.mmrf.org
Mary Bergaas, VP/COO
Activities/Fields: Medicine, surgery, pediatrics, neurology, urology, renal transplant, endocrinology, nephrology, dialysis, hyperbaric medicine, program evaluation and outcomes research, addiction, traumatic brain injury, international medicine, oncology, cardiology, orthopaedics, tobacco dependence, sleep disorders, AIDS, Alzheimer's disease, and trauma. **Pub:** *Research Connections.*

★ 22903 ★ Minnesota Center for Health Care Ethics
601 25th Ave. S
Minneapolis, MN 55454
Phone: (612)690-7895 **Fax:** (612)690-7774
Karen G. Gervais, PhD, Dir.
Activities/Fields: Diverse faith and cultural perspectives, end-of-life decision making, health care reform, emerging technologies. **Pub:** *Ethical Challenges in Managed Care: A Casebook.* • *Healing by Heart: Clinical & Ethical Case Stories of Hmong Families and Western Providers Summer 2003.* • *A Role Playing Exercise in Managed Care Decision Making.*

★ 22904 ★ Minot State University North Dakota Center for Persons with Disabilities (NDCPD)
500 University Ave. W
Minot, ND 58707
Phone: (701)858-3580 **Free:** 800-233-1737
Fax: (701)858-3483
Email: ndcpd@minotstateu.edu
Website: http://www.ndcpd.org
Dr. M. Bryce Fifield, Exec. Dir.
Activities/Fields: Independence, productivity, integration, and inclusion of people who have disabilities.

★ 22905 ★ Mississippi State University Rehabilitation Research and Training Center on Blindness and Low Vision
PO Box 6189
Mississippi State, MS 39762-6189
Phone: (662)325-2001 **Free:** 800-675-7782
Fax: (662)325-8989
Email: rrtc@colled.msstate.edu
Website: http://www.blind.msstate.edu
Dr. J. Elton Moore, Dir.
Activities/Fields: Career development intervention strategies for people who are blind or severely visually impaired; employment aspects of blindness and low vision.

★ 22906 ★ Mitretek Systems Health Information Technology Institute (HITI)
3150 Fairview Park Dr.
Falls Church, VA 22042
Phone: (703)610-2450 **Fax:** (703)610-2453
Email: hiti@mitretek.org
Website: http://hitiweb.mitretek.org/
Mary Harlow, Dir.
Activities/Fields: Accessible, affordable, and appropriate health care.

★ 22907 ★ Molecular Genetics Laboratory
Davis, 2069
Cedars-Sinai Medical Center
110 George Burns Rd.
Los Angeles, CA 90048
Phone: (310)423-7627 **Fax:** (310)423-0302
Email: julie.korenberg@cshs.org
Website: http://www.csmc.edu/genetics/korenberg/korenberg.html
Dr. Julie Korenberg, Contact
Activities/Fields: Human genome analysis and novel applications; primate evolutionary mechanisms; molecular basis of cognition; genetic origins of congenital heart disease; Down Syndrome; Wiliams Syndrome; DNA isolation and diagnostics, including Southern blotting, libraryscreening, subcloning, probe growth, and preparation. **Frmly:** Molecular Diagnostics Laboratory.

★ 22908 ★ Monell Chemical Senses Center
3500 Market St.
Philadelphia, PA 19104-3308
Phone: (215)898-6666 **Fax:** (215)898-2084
Email: beauchamp@monell.org
Website: http://www.monell.org
Dr. Gary K. Beauchamp, Dir.
Activities/Fields: Mechanisms and functions of the chemical senses (taste, smell) and chemesthesis, chemical irritation, including studies in the areas of biochemistry, biophysics, endocrinology, physiology, ethology, neurology, behavior, genetics, psychophysics, nutrition, organic chemistry, chemical ecology, and zoology. Research relates to solutions of problems in nutrition, environmental odors, reproduction, disease diagnosis, expansion of world food supply, and alternative means of vertebrate pest control. Projects focus on biochemistry of receptor mechanisms, sensory qualities of food, role of early diet in shaping food preferences, relationship between chemosensory function and nutritional and disease states, role of body volatiles in disease diagnosis, methods of altering salt preference, role of taste and smell in food utilization, effect of aging on taste and smell, information processing in taste and smell, diagnosis and treatment of taste and smell disorders, and genetic influence on production and detection of chemostimulants. **Pub:** *The Monell Connection Newsletter.*

★ 22909 ★ Monell-Jefferson Taste and Smell Research Center
925 Chestnut St., 6th Fl.
Philadelphia, PA 19107
Phone: (215)955-5652 **Fax:** (215)923-4532
Email: clinic@monell.org
Website: http://www.monell.org
Beverly J. Cowart, PhD, Clin. Dir.
Activities/Fields: Smell and taste disorders using a multidisciplinary approach (psychophysical, biophysical, medical, and dental).

★ 22910 ★ Montreal Cancer Institute
1560 Sherbrooke St. E
Montreal, QC, Canada H2L 4M1
Phone: (514)890-8213 **Fax:** (514)412-7591
Email: info@icm.qc.ca
Website: http://www.icm.qc.ca
Maral Tersakian, Dir.
Activities/Fields: Viral carcinogenesis, molecular biology, genetic engineering, biochemical changes associated with neoplastic transformation, epidemiology of cancer, and clinical pharmacology.

★ 22911 ★ Morehouse College Prevention Research Center
Center for Public Health Practice
School of Medicine
777 Cleveland Ave., Ste. 410
Atlanta, GA 30310
Phone: (404)752-1624 **Fax:** (404)752-1160
Email: danielb@msm.edu
Daniel Blumenthal, MD, Prin. Investigator
Activities/Fields: Public health issues, especially behaviors that place Americans at risk for chronic diseases and conditions. Of particular concern is the improvement in quality of life for special populations, including the young, elderly, racial ethnic populations, and the underserved.

★ 22912 ★ Mount Sinai Hospital Samuel Lunenfeld Research Institute
600 University Ave.
Toronto, ON, Canada M5G 1X5
Phone: (416)586-4800 **Fax:** (416)586-8857
Email: pawson/rossant@mshri.on.ca
Website: http://www.mshri.on.ca
Dr. Tony Pawson, Interim Co-Dir.
Activities/Fields: Cancer biology, cell biology, clinical epidemiology, endocrinology, hemopoiesis, musculoskeletal diseases, bone mineral metabolism, genetics, developmental biology, immunology, perinatology, neurobiology, physiology, molecular biology, bioinformatics, proteomics, biochemistry, gastroenterology, respiratory research, and hearing research. **Pub:** *Annual Report.* • *Scientific Report.* **Frmly:** Mount Sinai Hospital Research Institute.

★ 22913 ★ Mount Sinai School of Medicine of City University of New York Alzheimer's Disease Research Center
Department of Psychiatry, Box 1230
1 Gustave Levy Pl.
New York, NY 10029
Phone: (718)584-9000 **Fax:** (718)933-2121
Email: mary.sano@mssm.edu
Website: http://www.mssm.edu
Mary Sano, PhD, Contact
Activities/Fields: Etiology, diagnosis, and treatment of Alzheimer's disease and related dementias. Clinical studies include trials of new drugs and biological markers and longitudinal follow-up studies. An active autopsy network obtains brain material from Alzheimer patients.

★ 22914 ★ Mount Sinai School of Medicine of City University of New York Brookdale Center for Molecular Biology
1 Gustave Levy Pl., Box 1020
New York, NY 10029-6574
Phone: (212)241-4272 **Fax:** (212)860-9279
Email: paul.wassarman@mssm.edu
Dr. Paul Wassarman, Dir.
Activities/Fields: Molecular biology and medicine, including molecular neurobiology; developmental molecular biology; receptor and channel structure, function, and regulation; hormone, oncogene, and growth factor actions; the molecular and genetic basis of disease; cytokine action; and control of gene transcription.

★ 22915 ★ Mount Sinai School of Medicine of City University of New York Center for Anatomy and Functional Morphology
1 Gustave L. Levy Pl.
New York, NY 10029
Phone: (212)241-5622 **Fax:** (212)860-1174
Email: jeffrey.laitman@mssm.edu
Website: http://www.mssm.edu/cellbio/
Jeffrey T. Laitman, PhD, Contact
Activities/Fields: Fundamental cellular processes and therapeutic application of these discoveries. Research is carried out on molecules, cells, and organisms.

★ 22916 ★ Mount Sinai School of Medicine of City University of New York Computational Neurobiology and Imaging Center (CNIC)
1 Gustave L. Levy Pl.
New York, NY 10029
Phone: (212)241-5018
Email: susan@camelot.mssm.edu
Website: http://www.mssm.edu/cnic/
Susan L. Weane, PhD, Contact
Activities/Fields: Relationships between neural function and structure at levels ranging from the molecular and cellular, through network organization of the brain.

★ 22917 ★ Mount Sinai School of Medicine of City University of New York General Clinical Research Center
1184 5th Ave., 2nd Fl.
New York, NY 10029
Phone: (212)241-6045 **Fax:** (212)348-5811
Email: vivan.mitroupoulou@mssm.edu
Website: http://www.mssm.edu/gcrc/
Dr. Hugh A. Sampson, Prog. Dir.
Activities/Fields: Nature and treatment of human diseases through clinical investigation, in the following disciplines: Endocrinology: the role of insulin in ovarian dysfunction; ethnic factors influencing bone mass in women, Genetic Diseases: investigation of molecular and phenotypic expressions of Fabry and Gaucher diseases, therapy of metabolic genetic diseases, Geriatrics: drug metabolism - advanced glycation end products (AGEs) in diabetes, Hematology: growth and development in children with hemophilia; betaglobin disorders, Internal medicine: vasodialator response in heart failure; effect of lowering cholestrol in thrombotic factors; lead mobilization during pregnancy and lactation in young urban women, Neurology: therapy of parkinsonism, myoclomus, dysautonomia, seizure disorders; peptide-T in HIV patients, Pediatrics: immunopathogenetic mechanisms of food hypersensitivity in children with atopic dermatitis; cow-milk induced hypersensitivities; peanut hypersensitivity, Psychiatry:

the role of cholinergic neurotransmitters in Alzheimer's disease; neuroendocrine and cognitive correlates in schizophrenia and schizophrenia spectrum disorders; compulsive, impulsive and anxiety disorders; autistic spectrum disorders; post traumatic stress disorder (PTSD); self injurious behavior; and major depression.

★ 22918 ★ Mount Sinai School of Medicine of City University of New York
Vision Research Center in Ophthalmology
1 Gustave L. Levy Pl., Box 1183
New York, NY 10029
Phone: (212)241-6249 **Fax:** (212)289-1799
Email: oscar.candia@mssm.edu
Website: http://www.mssm.edu/ophth/
Dr. Oscar A. Candia, Dir.
Activities/Fields: Ophthalmology.

★ 22919 ★ Mount Sinai Spinal Cord Injury Model System
1 Gustave Levy Pl., Box 1240
New York, NY 10029-6574
Phone: (212)659-9369 **Fax:** (212)348-5901
Email: marcel.dijkers@mssm.edu
Website: http://www.mssm.edu/rehab/spinal/
Marcel Dijkers, PhD, Dir. of Res.
Activities/Fields: Spinal cord injuries.

★ 22920 ★ Mountain States Tumor Institute, Inc.
100 E Idaho
Boise, ID 83712-6241
Phone: (208)381-3132 **Fax:** (208)381-3124
Email: bradyj@slrmc.org
Sharon Frelleson, Clin. Res. Coord.
Activities/Fields: Adult and pediatric oncology clinical trials.

★ 22921 ★ Nathan S. Kline Institute for Psychiatric Research
140 Old Orangeburg Rd.
Orangeburg, NY 10962
Phone: (845)398-5500 **Fax:** (845)398-5510
Website: http://www.rfmh.org/nki/
Robert Cancro, MD, Dir.
Activities/Fields: Mental illness, including multidisciplinary studies on its etiology, epidemiology, treatment, and control; computer sciences, emphasizing clinical and administrative services; and biochemical, genetic, physiological, neurochemical, and psychopharmacological research. Collaborates in research with investigators from other institutions and many countries. Consists of nine divisions: information sciences, statistical sciences and epidemiology, molecular biology, clinical research, analytical psychopharmacology, neurochemistry, neurophysiology, geriatric physchiatry, MICA, and research support.

★ 22922 ★ National Alliance for Research on Schizophrenia and Depression (NARSAD)
60 Cutter Mill Rd., Ste. 404
Great Neck, NY 11021
Phone: (516)829-5576 **Free:** 800-829-8289
Fax: (516)487-6930
Email: amoran@narsad.org
Website: http://www.narsad.org
Audra L. Moran, Dir., Res. Grants Prog.
Activities/Fields: Causes, cure, treatments, and prevention of severe mental illnesses, primarily schizophrenia and depression. Emphasizes biomedical studies of brain diseases. Awards research grants and supports university-based research centers. **Pub:** *NARSAD Research Newsletter.*

★ 22923 ★ National Association for Biomedical Research
818 Connecticut Ave. NW, Ste. 200
Washington, DC 20006
Phone: (202)857-0540 **Fax:** (202)659-1902
Email: info@nabr.org
Website: http://www.nabr.org
Frankie L. Trull, Pres.
Activities/Fields: Biomedical research, education, and testing, focusing on using laboratory animals for such purposes, monitors and attempts to infulence legislation and regulations on behalf of members dependent on laboratory animals for research and testing.

★ 22924 ★ National Association of State Mental Health Program Directors Research Institute, Inc.
66 Canal Center Plz., Ste. 302
Alexandria, VA 22314
Phone: (703)739-9333 **Fax:** (703)548-9517
Email: noel.mazade@nri-inc.org
Website: http://www.nri-inc.org
Dr. Noel A. Mazade, Exec. Dir.
Activities/Fields: Mental health services and management of state mental health programs. Also compiles data and conducts research activities on various aspects of state mental health agencies financing, staffing, clinical services, and mental health service systems. **Pub:** *Outlook*, periodically.

★ 22925 ★ National Biomedical Research Foundation
3900 Reservoir Rd. NW
PO Box 571414
Washington, DC 20007-1414
Phone: (202)687-2121 **Fax:** (202)687-1662
Email: pirmail@nbrf.georgetown.edu
Website: http://pir.georgetown.edu
Dr. Cathy H. Wu, Dir.
Activities/Fields: Application of computers and electronic technology to medical research, including biomedical picture pattern analysis, biology, biochemistry, origins of life, and computer technology. Specific research projects include studies on automatic chromosome analysis, biomedical instrumentation, computer aid to medical diagnosis, and genetics, evolution, and function of proteins and nucleic acids. **Pub:** *Computers in Biology and Medicine*, bimonthly. • *Journal of Computer Languages*, quarterly. • *Journal of Computerized Medical Imaging & Graphics*, bimonthly. • *Pattern Recognition Journal*, monthly.

★ 22926 ★ National Black Leadership Initiative on Cancer II (NBLIC)
720 Westview Dr., SW
Atlanta, GA 30310
Phone: (404)756-5205
Email: hamilts@msm.edu
Website: http://www.nblic.org
Joyce Q. Sheats, Prog. Dir.
Activities/Fields: Cancer prevention and mortality in the black community.

★ 22927 ★ National Cancer Institute Children's Oncology Group Research Data Center
1600 SW Archer Rd., Rm. M401
Gainesville, FL 32610
Phone: (352)392-5633 **Fax:** (352)392-8725
Email: coginfo@childrensoncologygroup.org
Website: http://www.childrensoncologygroup.org
Dr. Stephen Hunger, Contact
Activities/Fields: Pathobiology of childhood cancers, focusing on control measures and improving treatment outcomes.

★ 22928 ★ National Cancer Institute Georgetown University Vincent T. Lombardi Cancer Center
Main Campus
3800 Reservoir Rd. NW
Washington, DC 20007
Phone: (202)784-4000 **Fax:** (202)687-6402
Website: http://lombardi.georgetown.edu
Richard Pestell, MD, Dir.
Activities/Fields: Prevention, detection, diagnosis, and treatment of cancer, including clinical and basic science activities in all oncologic specialties (surgery, medicine, gynecology, pediatrics, radiology, pathology, urology, and immunology) and basic science studies in pharmacology, biochemistry, radiation biology, virology, molecular genetics, analytic chemistry, flow cytometry, and electron microscopy.

★ 22929 ★ National Cancer Institute University of Vermont Vermont Cancer Center
Health Science Research Facility
149 Beaumont Ave.
Burlington, VT 05405-0075
Phone: (802)656-4414 **Fax:** (802)656-8788
Email: vcc@uvm.edu
Website: http://www.vermontcancer.org
Dr. David W. Yandell, Dir.
Activities/Fields: Cancer, including multidisciplinary programs in clinical research, cancer prevention and control research, genome stability and expression, and cell signaling and growth control. Conducts clinical studies in cancer chemotherapy, surgical oncology, radiotherapy and pediatric hematology-oncology. Trains health professionals and transfers cancer knowledge to surrounding communities as part of NCI's nationwide coordinated program to reduce incidence, morbidity, and mortality of cancer established under National Cancer Act of 1971. **Pub:** *Innovations newsletter*, quarterly.

★ 22930 ★ National Cancer Institute of Canada Clinical Trials Group (CTG)
Queen's University
10 Alcorn Ave., Ste. 200
Toronto, ON, Canada M4V 3B1
Phone: (613)533-6430 **Fax:** (613)533-2941
Email: jpater@ctg.queensu.ca
Website: http://www.ncic.cancer.ca/english/index.html
Dr. J.L. Pater, Dir.
Activities/Fields: Cancer, cancer therapy, and supportive care.

★ 22931 ★ National Center for Infectious Diseases Division of Vector-Borne Infectious Diseases Arbovirus Diseases Branch
PO Box 2087
Fort Collins, CO 80522-2087
Phone: (970)221-6442 **Fax:** (970)266-3544
Dr. John T. Roehrig, Branch Ch.
Activities/Fields: Epidemiology of mosquito and tick-borne viral diseases. Provides consultation and on-site investigations for local, state, national, and international health agencies during arthropod-borne viral disease outbreaks. Conducts a national surveillance of arboviral diseases. **Pub:** *Research Reports.*

★ 22932 ★ National Center for Infectious Diseases Division of Vector-Borne Infectious Diseases Bacterial Zoonosis Branch Plague Section
PO Box 2087
Fort Collins, CO 80522
Phone: (970)221-6400 **Fax:** (970)221-6476

Email: dvbid@cdc.gov
Website: http://www.cdc.gov/ncidod/dvbid/plague/index.htm
Dr. Ken Gage, Ch.

Activities/Fields: Diagnosis, therapy, epidemiology, and control of bubonic plague; maintains a surveillance system in collaboration with state and federal health agencies to detect fluctuations of infection in animal populations; and serves as a WHO Reference Center for plague diagnosis and control. **Pub:** *CDC Surveillance Reports.* • *Reference and Research,* biennially.

★ 22933 ★ National Coalition for Research in Neurological Disorders

1250 24th St. NW, Ste. 300
Washington, DC 20037
Phone: (202)293-5453 **Fax:** (202)466-0585
Email: hoffheimer@aol.com
Website: http://www.brainnet.org
Lawrence S. Hoffheimer, Dir.

Activities/Fields: Neurological research, focusing on funding. Also lobbies for increased funding for training and research.

★ 22934 ★ National Development and Research Institutes, Inc.

71 W 23rd St., 8th Fl.
New York, NY 10010
Phone: (212)845-4400 **Fax:** (212)845-4698
Email: wagoner@ndri.org
Website: http://www.ndri.org
Dr. Fred Streit, Exec. Dir

Activities/Fields: Drug abuse, including evaluations of treatment and prevention programs; AIDS research as it relates to substance abuse; epidemiology of drug abuse; drugs and crime; drug abuse and the criminal justice system; street studies of drug sales, use, and prevention; evaluation and enhancement of AIDS outreach; and intervention services for high-risk adolescents. **Frmly:** Narcotic and Drug Research Inc.

★ 22935 ★ National Disease Research Interchange

1880 John F. Kennedy Blvd., 11th Fl.
Philadelphia, PA 19103
Phone: (215)557-7361 **Free:** 800-222-6374
Fax: (215)557-7154
Email: info@ndri.com
Website: http://www.ndri.com
Lee Ducat, Pres.

Activities/Fields: Procurement, preservation, and distribution of over 100 types of human tissues and organs for medical research. Also coordinates retrieval of pancreatic tissue for the clinical trials of islet cell transplants, a treatment being investigated for insulin-dependent diabetics. **Pub:** *Annual Report.* • *Interchange Newsletter.*

★ 22936 ★ National Eye Research Foundation

910 Skokie Blvd., No. 207A
Northbrook, IL 60062
Phone: (847)564-4652 **Free:** 800-621-2258
Fax: (847)564-0807
Email: nerf@eyemac.com
Website: http://www.nerf.org
Andrew Kim, Contact

Activities/Fields: Vision, focusing on better eye care. Also promotes education relating to the eye care and contact lenses. **Pub:** *Quarterly Research Journal.*

★ 22937 ★ National Farm Medicine Center

1000 N Oak Ave.
Marshfield, WI 54449-5790
Free: 800-662-6900 **Fax:** (715)389-4996
Email: barbara@mcrf.mfldclin.edu
Website: http://research.marshfieldclinic.org/nfmc/
Barbara Lee, PhD, Dir.

Activities/Fields: Agriculture-related health problems, including injury, respiratory diseases, noise-induced hearing loss, migrant health, and cancer. **Pub:** *Progress Report.*

★ 22938 ★ National Foundation for Cancer Research (NFCR)

4600 East West Hwy., Ste. 525
Bethesda, MD 20814
Phone: (301)654-1250 **Free:** 800-321-2873
Fax: (301)654-5824
Email: fcsjr@nfcr.org
Website: http://www.nfcr.org
Franklin Salisbury, Jr., Pres.

Activities/Fields: Contracts with major universities for basic science cancer research in the fields of biophysics, theoretical physics and chemistry, biochemistry, chemistry, and biological sciences. **Pub:** *Annual Scientific Report.* • *NFCR Annual Report.*

★ 22939 ★ National Institute on Aging Gerontology Research Center

5600 Nathan Shock Dr.
Baltimore, MD 21224
Phone: (410)558-8110 **Fax:** (410)558-8137
Email: longod@grc.nia.nih.gov
Dr. Dan L. Longo, Dir.

Activities/Fields: Gerontology research, including molecular genetics, human physiology, neurosciences, cardiovascular, personality, behavioral research, and Alzheimer's disease studies.

★ 22940 ★ National Institute for Fitness and Sport

250 University Blvd.
Indianapolis, IN 46202-5192
Phone: (317)274-3432 **Fax:** (317)274-7408
Website: http://www.nifs.org
Jerry Taylor, Pres.

Activities/Fields: Exercise physiology, sports medicine, and health and fitness education. **Pub:** *NIF Source,* bimonthly. Newsletter.

★ 22941 ★ National Institute for Rehabilitation Engineering

Box 1008
Hewitt, NJ 07421
Phone: (973)853-6585 **Free:** 800-736-2216
Website: http://www.tamu.edu/scom/pres/pres.html
Donald Selwyn, Dir.

Activities/Fields: Invention, design, construction, fitting, and servicing of special devices for individuals with any specific physical disability or combination of disabilities; time/motion analyses; job modification engineering; task-performance mobility; driver training; computer software adapted for people with handicapping conditions. **Frmly:** Rehabilitation Engineering Institute.

★ 22942 ★ National Institute of Transplantation

2200 W 3rd St., Ste. 100
Los Angeles, CA 90057
Phone: (213)413-2779 **Fax:** (213)484-6652
Website: http://www.transplantation.com
Robert Mendez, MD, Dir.

Activities/Fields: Kidney and pancreas transplantation and new approaches to organ transplantation and avoiding organ rejection. **Pub:** *Miracle of Life Newsletter,* quarterly. • *NIT Newsletter,* biennially.

★ 22943 ★ National Jewish Medical and Research Center

1400 Jackson St.
Denver, CO 80206
Phone: (303)388-4461 **Free:** 800-222-5864
Fax: (303)270-2165
Email: taussigl@njc.org
Website: http://www.nationaljewish.org
Lynn M. Taussig, MD, Pres. /CEO

Activities/Fields: Etiology, progression, manifestation, treatment, rehabilitation, and prevention of pulmonary, allergic, and immunologic diseases. Studies encompass cellular and molecular biology. **Pub:** *ARIA (Allergy, Rheumatology, Immunology, Asthma) Newsletter.* • *National Jewish Center Scientific Annual Report.* • *New Directions Newsletter.* **Frmly:** National Jewish Center for Immunology and Respiratory Medicine.

★ 22944 ★ National Psoriasis Foundation

6600 SW 92nd, Ste. 300
Portland, OR 97223
Phone: (503)244-7404 **Free:** 800-723-9166
Fax: (503)245-0626
Email: getinfo@npfusa.org
Website: http://www.psoriasis.org
Gail M. Zimmerman, Pres. /CEO

Activities/Fields: Psoriasis, including investigations into causes, treatment, and cure of this dermatological disease. Provides funds to researchers. Recruits volunteers for FDA-approved clinical studies. Searches for three-generation families whose living members are affected by psoriasis, and refers them to the National Psoriasis Tissue Bank. Disseminates authoritative scientific information about psoriasis to psoriatics, physicians, and other concerned persons. **Pub:** *Annual report.* • *Psoriasis Advance,* bimonthly.

★ 22945 ★ National Resource for Imaging Mass Spectrometry

65 Landsdowne St., Ste. 535
Cambridge, MA 02139
Phone: (617)768-8262 **Fax:** (617)768-8260
Email: cpl@harvard.edu
Website: http://www.nrims.hms.harvard.edu
Claude Lechene, MD, Prin. Investigator

Activities/Fields: Use of stable isotopes and quantitative imaging mass spectrometry in biomedical research.

★ 22946 ★ National Space Biomedical Research Institute (NSBRI)

1 Baylor Plz., NA-425
Houston, TX 77030-3498
Phone: (713)798-7412 **Fax:** (713)798-7413
Email: info@www.nsbri.org
Website: http://www.nsbri.org/
Bobby R. Alford, MD, Ch. /CEO

Activities/Fields: Prevention and solution of health problems related to long-duration space travel and prolonged exposure to microgravity. Byproducts of such research would be treatments for conditions such as osteoporosis, muscle wasting, shift-related sleep disorders and radiation-related conditions. The institute also is researching ways to deliver medical care on long-duration space travel through new technologies and remote-treatment advances.

★ 22947 ★ National Surgical Adjuvant Breast and Bowel Project (NSABP)

East Commons Professional Bldg.
4 Allegheny Center, 5th Fl.
Pittsburgh, PA 15212-5234
Phone: (412)330-4600 **Fax:** (412)330-4660
Email: normanwolmark@nsabp.org
Website: http://www.nsabp.pitt.edu
Dr. Norman Wolmark, Chm.

Activities/Fields: Breast and bowel cancer treatments and breast cancer prevention. Operates in cooperation with over 300 member institutions throughout the U.S., Canada, Puerto Rico, and Australia. **Pub:** *Progress Reports,* semiannually.

★ 22948 ★ Neuro Immuno Therapeutics Research Foundation

8800 Hwy. 9
Inman, SC 29349
Phone: (864)592-2989 **Fax:** (864)592-2990
Email: nitrf@juno.com

Website: http://www.nitrf.org
Dr. H. Hugh Fudenberg, Dir.

Activities/Fields: Immunology, Alzheimer's disease, AIDS, autism, and chronic fatigue syndrome. **Pub:** *Scientific Reference Journal*, occasionally. Journal.

★ 22949 ★ Neuropsychiatric Research Institute
700 1st Ave. S
Fargo, ND 58103
Phone: (701)293-1335 **Fax:** (701)293-3226
Email: mail@nrifargo.com
Website: http://www.nrifargo.com/
James E. Mitchell, MD, Pres.

Activities/Fields: Basic and clinical studies of the central nervous system. Specific applications include eating disorders and stroke. **Pub:** *Newsletter (semiannual).*

★ 22950 ★ The Neurosciences Institute
10640 John Jay Hopkins Dr.
San Diego, CA 92121
Phone: (858)626-2000 **Fax:** (858)626-2099
Email: info@nsi.edu
Website: http://www.nsi.edu
W. Einar Gall, Res. Dir.

Activities/Fields: Promotes conceptual and theoretical progress in understanding the function of the nervous system at all levels, particularly higher functions of the brain (perception, memory, sensation) and their implications in understanding human behavior. A research program for resident Institute Fellows in theoretical neurobiology provides training in methods used to construct neural theories and develops theoretical models of neural systems that are biologically sound and experimentally testable at synaptic, cellular, and network levels. The Institute also conducts a research program in experimental neurobiology. The Institute provides opportunities for visiting scientists to interact in modes that would not ordinarily be possible in their home laboratories. Visiting in small groups or individually for periods from several days to several months, scientists design experiments, discuss research questions with experts in other fields, and share information about recent findings.

★ 22951 ★ New England College of Optometry
Myopia Research Center
424 Beacon St.
Boston, MA 02115
Phone: (617)266-2030 **Fax:** (617)369-0174
Email: heldd@ne-optometry.edu
Website: http://www.ne-optometry.edu/research/default.asp
Richard Held, Res. Dir.

Activities/Fields: Human and animal studies on the development of myopia, resolution limits of human eye, and autoimimune response in diabetes. **Pub:** *Perspectives Magazine*, 3/year.

★ 22952 ★ New England Medical Center Hospitals, Inc.
Center for Cardiovascular Health Services Research
New England Medical Center, Box 63
750 Washington St.
Boston, MA 02111
Phone: (617)636-5009 **Fax:** (617)636-8023
Email: hselker@tufts-nemc.org
Harry P. Selker, MD, Contact

Activities/Fields: Cardiovascular health services, particularly in the development and testing of predictive instruments for acute cardiac ischemia, thrombolytic therapy, and the use of cardiac care units in hospitals.

★ 22953 ★ New England Medical Center Hospitals, Inc.
Division of Clinical Care Research
750 Washington St., Box 63
Boston, MA 02111
Phone: (617)636-5009 **Fax:** (617)636-8023
Email: hselker@tufts-nemc.org
Website: http://www.nemc.org/dccr
Harry P. Selker, MD, Ch.

Activities/Fields: Ongoing research programs in clinical trials in emergency room based cardiovascular health services research, mathematical modeling and statistics, meta-analysis and other evidence-based research methodologies. **Frmly:** Center for Health Services Research and Study Design.

★ 22954 ★ New England Medical Center Hospitals, Inc.
Electromyography Laboratory
Neurology Department EMG, Box 314
750 Washington St.
Boston, MA 02111
Phone: (617)636-5848 **Fax:** (617)636-8199
Dr. William Brown, Dir.

Activities/Fields: Electrical studies of nerves and muscles to aid in the research and diagnosis of muscular dystrophy, amyotrophic lateral sclerosis, and other polyneuropathies.

★ 22955 ★ New England Medical Center Hospitals, Inc.
General Clinical Research Center
750 Washington Ave., Box 831
Boston, MA 02111
Phone: (617)636-6149 **Fax:** (617)636-5506
Email: phibberd@tufts-nemc.org
Website: http://www.nemc.org/gcrc
Dr. Patricia L. Hibberd, Prog. Dir.

Activities/Fields: Biomedicine, including endocrinology and metabolism, hematology, neurology, nutrition, oncology, immunology, and infectious disease.

★ 22956 ★ New Hampshire-Dartmouth Psychiatric Research Center
105 Pleasant St.
Concord, NH 03301
Phone: (603)271-5747 **Fax:** (603)271-5265
Website: http://www.dartmouth.edu/dms/psychrc
Robert E. Drake, MD, Dir.

Activities/Fields: Development of effective services for people with dual psychiatric disorders. Research focuses on cost-effective rehabilitation services; relationships between substance abuse, trauma, and victimization, and HIV risk behaviors; alternative service models for older adults; and models for shared decision making between clients and treatment providers.

★ 22957 ★ New Jersey Health and Senior Services Department
Health Planning and Regulation
Health Care Systems Analysis
Research and Development
225 E State St., 8th Fl.
PO Box 360
Trenton, NJ 08625-0360
Phone: (609)292-9354 **Fax:** (609)292-6523
Email: emmanuel.noggoh@doh.state.nj.us
Emmanuel Noggoh, Dir.

Activities/Fields: Health care.

★ 22958 ★ New Jersey Institute of Technology
Center for Biomedical Engineering
323 Martin Luther King, Jr. Blvd.
Newark, NJ 07102
Phone: (973)596-5271 **Fax:** (973)596-5222
Email: whunter@njit.edu
Website: http://www.njit.edu/bme
William Hunter, Dir.

Activities/Fields: Design of prosthetic devices (including knee and hip joints), biosignal processing, heart rate variability studies, rehabilitation engineering, modelling of the cardiovascular system, assessment of lower back pain, gait analysis, biomaterials engineering, tissue engineering, vision engineering, optimization of work performance, neuromuscular control mechanisms, functional MRI, BioMEMS, transdermal devices, blood coagulation studies.

★ 22959 ★ New Jersey Specialized Center of Research and Training for Bioregenerative Life Support
Foran Hall, Rm. 186
Rutgers University
59 Dudley Rd.
New Brunswick, NJ 08901-8520
Phone: (732)932-8978 **Fax:** (732)932-4882
Email: sauser@aesop.rutgers.edu
Dr. Harry W. Janes, Dir.

Activities/Fields: Problems of human life support associated with long duration space missions and lunar or Mars outposts.

★ 22960 ★ New Mexico Clinical Research and Osteoporosis Center
300 Oak NE
Albuquerque, NM 87106
Phone: (505)855-5525 **Fax:** (505)884-4006
Email: medsitenm@aol.com
Website: http://www.nmbonecare.com
Lance Rudolph, MD, Dir.

Activities/Fields: Health care quality, health promotion, clinical research, and continuing medical education. **Pub:** *Newsletter*, quarterly. **Frmly:** New Mexico Medical Group; Research and Education Foundation.

★ 22961 ★ New York Blood Center, Inc.
Lindsley F. Kimball Research Institute
310 E 67th St.
New York, NY 10021
Phone: (212)570-3034 **Fax:** (212)861-8993
Website: http://www.nybloodcenter.org
Robert L. Jones, MD, Pres.

Activities/Fields: Immunogenetics and immunohematology, epidemiology and virology of AIDS and hepatitis viruses, molecular and cell biology of red blood cells and developing erythroid cells, platelet interactions with coagulation proteins, human genetics, and hematopoietic growth factors. Performs studies of plasma proteins and seeks to develop new plasma derivatives for therapeutic use.

★ 22962 ★ New York Foundation for Otologic Research
920 Park Ave.
New York, NY 10028
Phone: (212)988-3100 **Fax:** (212)517-8699
Email: mideardoc@aol.com
Dr. Alan Austin Scheer, Dir.

Activities/Fields: Unsolved hearing problems, including otosclerosis, nerve deafness, Menieres disease, and other associated problems of dizziness and head noises. Analyzes electrical patterns of sound conduction and studies conduction of sound through the skin and dental nerves.

★ 22963 ★ New York Institute for Medical Research, Inc.
PO Box 832
Nyack, NY 10960
Phone: (845)359-7160 **Fax:** (845)359-3801
Email: nyinstitut@aol.com
Website: http://www.nyinstitute.org
Esin Cig, Exec. Admin.

Activities/Fields: Behavioral, psychophysiological, and psychopharmacological research. Topics of interest include depression in young and elderly patients, dementia, anxiety neurosis, behavior and sleep disorders, and phase I studies on healthy volunteers. The Institute provides evaluation and treatment of selected psychiatric outpatients, such as psychiatric assessments, experimental psychological testing, physical and neurological examinations, clinical and diagnostic EEG, computer analyzed resting and sleep EEG, ECG, and clinical chemistry, including hormonal evaluations. **Pub:** *Newsletter*, occasionally.

★ 22964 ★ New York Medical College Bioethics Institute
101 Administration Bldg.
Valhalla, NY 10595
Phone: (915)594-4060
Email: daniel_sulmasy@nymc.edu
Website: http://www.nymc.edu/bioethics/
Daniel P. Sulmasy, MD, Dir.

Activities/Fields: Bioethics, particularly the moral issues that face health care practitioners and patients.

★ 22965 ★ New York Medical College Institute of Breast Diseases
Munger Pavillion, Rm. G-13
Valhalla, NY 10595
Phone: (914)493-8770 **Fax:** (914)493-1651
Email: zachrau@nymc.edu
Reinhard E. Zachrau, MD, Contact

Activities/Fields: Breast diseases, including skin window reactivity and second primary breast cancer.

★ 22966 ★ New York Medical College Westchester Institute for Human Development (WIHD)
Westchester County Medical Center
Valhalla, NY 10595
Phone: (914)493-8204 **Fax:** (914)493-1973
Email: ansley_bacon@nymc.edu
Website: http://www.nymc.edu/wihd/
Ansley Bacon, PhD, Dir.

Activities/Fields: Enhancement of the quality of life of individuals with or at risk for, disabilities and their families.

★ 22967 ★ New York/New Jersey Occupational Safety and Health Education and Research Center
Department of Community & Preventive Medicine
Mt. Sinai School of Medicine
1 Gustave L. Levy Pl.
PO Box 1057
New York, NY 10029-6574
Phone: (212)241-4804 **Fax:** (212)996-0407
Email: phil.landrigan@mssm.edu
Website: http://www.nynjerc.org/
Philip J. Landrigan, MD, Dir.

Activities/Fields: Occupational health and safety.

★ 22968 ★ New York State Department of Health Wadsworth Center
PO Box 509
Albany, NY 12201-0509
Phone: (518)474-7592 **Fax:** (518)474-3439
Email: sturman@wadsworth.org
Website: http://www.wadsworth.org
Lawrence S. Sturman, PhD, Dir.

Activities/Fields: Biomedical and environmental sciences. Investigators study cell and molecular structure, including molecular assemblies, protein and glycoprotein structure and function, and chromosome dynamics; also, genetics, development and cancer, with studies of developmental and human genetics, developmental neuroscience, genetic factors involved in cancer causation, mechanisms of tumor formation, and development of more effective cancer therapies. Researchers also investigate microbial genomics and pathogenesis, including HIV, nucleic acid dynamics, infectious disease epidemiology, environmental chemistry, and molecular toxicology. Emphasis is placed on emerging scientific disciplines, especially genomics, bioinformatics and nanobiotechnology.

★ 22969 ★ New York State Department of Health Wadsworth Center Resource for the Visualization of Biological Complexity
Empire State Plz.
Albany, NY 12201-0509
Phone: (518)474-7002 **Fax:** (518)486-2191
Email: joachim@wadsworth.org
Website: http://www.wadsworth.org/rvbc
Conly Rieder, PhD, Contact

Activities/Fields: Development of methods for the 3-D visualization of biological systems over a wide range of scales, from macromolecular assemblies to cells and tissues.

★ 22970 ★ New York State Institute for Basic Research in Developmental Disabilities
1050 Forest Hill Rd.
Staten Island, NY 10314-6330
Phone: (718)494-0600 **Fax:** (718)494-0833
Dr. Piotr Kozlowski, Dir.

Activities/Fields: Molecular biology and developmental biochemistry of human development, developmental disabilities, and clinical, behavioral, and developmental psychology of mental retardation, including neuroimmunology, membrane biochemistry, lipid biochemistry, neurotransmitter physiology and pathology, inborn errors of metabolism, blood-brain barrier, and persistent, latent, and unconventional viruses. Focuses on the causes and prevention of developmental disabilities, autism, aging and Alzheimer's disease, Down's syndrome, fragile X syndrome, fetal alcohol syndrome, neurodegenerative diseases, pediatric AIDS and neuroinfectious diseases, environmental neurotoxicology (including alcohol, lead, aluminum, and cocaine), prevention (including vaccines, diagnostic tests, and early intervention), and treatment (including drug evaluation). **Pub:** *Annual Report.*

★ 22971 ★ New York State Psychiatric Institute
1051 Riverside Dr.
New York, NY 10032
Phone: (212)543-5000 **Fax:** (212)543-6012
Email: btw1@columbia.edu
Website: http://www.nyspi.org/
Dr. B. Timothy Wald, Interim Dir.

Activities/Fields: Psychiatry and neurosciences, including basic and clinical studies in biochemistry, psychoneuropharmacology, neuroendocrinology, neurotoxicology, psychosocial sciences, research and clinical psychology, genetics, nosology, psychophysiology, developmental psychobiology, sociology, epidemiology, communication sciences and psychoanalysis. **Pub:** *Annual report.*

★ 22972 ★ New York University Center for Neural Science
4 Washington Pl., Rm. 809
New York, NY 10003
Phone: (212)998-7780 **Fax:** (212)995-4011
Email: sanes@nyu.edu
Website: http://www.cns.nyu.edu
Dan Sanes, Dir.

Activities/Fields: Neural science studies, ranging from molecular and cellular aspects to fully integrated systems and cognitive approaches. Specific research includes cell biological mechanisms underlying plasticity and stability of neurons; new sprout formation by adult mammalian neurons; drive and hedonic mechanisms in the brain and how they interact; use of image analysis procedures to study the functional anatomy of sensorimotor integration in the rat brain; neural processes that generate movements; genetic and molecular manipulations in the fruit fly to study the interplay between plasticity and programming in the nervous system; amino acid regulation of dopamine utilization under basal and stress conditions using a variety of techniques, including in vivo microdialysis; individual neurons in visual perception; magnetic fields accompanying the flow of currents within the brain's neurons; effects of developmental visual disorders on the structure and function of the visual system; problems of color vision using both psychophysical and electrophysical techniques; modeling of the human visual system; identification of the neural systems and cellular mechanisms used by the brain to assign emotional significance to sensory stimuli; the acquisition of color information, fusion of visual information from multiple sources, signal detection theory, and visual calibration; analysis of functional properties of neurons; and mathematical and computational models of complex behaviors.

★ 22973 ★ New York University David B. Kriser Dental Center
345 E 24th St.
New York, NY 10010
Phone: (212)998-9800
Email: louis.terracio@nyu.edu
Website: http://www.nyu.edu/dental
Dr. Louis Terracio, Dir.

Activities/Fields: Dentistry, dental history, and allied health sciences. **Pub:** *Newsletter*, 3/year.

★ 22974 ★ New York University General Clinical Research Center
New York University Medical Center
550 1st Ave., New Bellevue 8E
New York, NY 10016
Phone: (212)263-6479 **Fax:** (212)263-8501
Email: romw01@med.nyu.edu
Website: http://gcrc.med.nyu.edu/gcrc/
Dr. William N. Rom, Prog. Dir.

Activities/Fields: The unit is a hospital within a hospital that allows investigators to observe patients for extended lengths of time. Projects include studies in endocrinology and metabolism, rheumatology, immunology, genetics, hypertension, hematology, neurology, neurosurgery, respiratory medicine, and infectious diseases. Focuses on cancer, AIDS, and tuberculosis research. Maintains a nursing staff and laboratories to facilitate research.

★ 22975 ★ New York University Institute of Environmental Medicine
550 1st Ave.
New York, NY 10016
Phone: (212)263-5280 **Fax:** (845)351-2118
Email: costam@env.med.nyu.edu
Max Costa, PhD, Dir.

Activities/Fields: Toxicology, chemical carcinogenesis, radiation carcinogenesis and dosimetry, respiratory disease and aerosol physiology, environmental pollution and ecology, epidemiology, and biostatistics and biomathematics, including studies on skin, bladder, and lung cancer from environmental sources, environmental hazards to which industrial and community populations are exposed, industrial and environmental health hazards and means for their control, and sources of human exposures to radiation. **Pub:** *Annual Report.* **Frmly:** Institute of Industrial Medicine.

★ 22976 ★ New York University Institute of Reconstructive Plastic Surgery
560 1st Ave.
New York, NY 10016
Phone: (212)263-5209 **Fax:** (212)263-2838
Email: joseph.mccarthy@med.nyu.edu
Joseph G. McCarthy, MD, Dir.

Activities/Fields: Etiology and treatment of craniofacial anomalies, bone physiology, including distraction, computer graphics, microvascular surgery, and wound healing, including studies of cleft lip and cleft palate, jaw deformities, ear malformations, hand injuries, and allied problems.

★ 22977 ★ New York University Jerry Lewis Neuromuscular Disease Center
Department of Rehabilitation Medicine
400 E 34th St., Rm. RG 29
New York, NY 10016
Phone: (212)263-6350 **Fax:** (212)263-5499
Dr. Mathew Lee, Chm.
Activities/Fields: Diagnosis and clinical care of patients disabled by neuromuscular disease.

★ 22978 ★ New York University Kaplan Comprehensive Cancer Center
School of Medicine
550 1st Ave.
New York, NY 10016
Phone: (212)263-6485 **Fax:** (212)263-8210
Email: steven.burakoff@med.nyu.edu
Website: http://www.nyucancerinstitute.org
Dr. Steven J. Burakoff, Dir.
Activities/Fields: Cancer research is carried out in designated program units of cancer epidemiology and prevention, cell interactions, clinical oncology, environmental carcinogenesis, genetic and molecular toxicology, growth regulation, molecular and tumor immunology, and molecular and viral oncology. **Pub:** *Kaplan Center Newsletter*, semiannually.

★ 22979 ★ New York University Medical Rehabilitation Research and Training Center
400 E 34th St.
New York, NY 10016
Phone: (212)263-6105 **Fax:** (212)263-8815
Email: Mathew.Lee@med.nyu.edu
Dr. Mathew Lee, Dir.
Activities/Fields: Rehabilitation for Parkinson's disease, Alzheimer's disease, brain trauma and stroke victims, spinal cord injuries, and comprehensive management of neuromuscular disease. Seeks to identify and validate specific treatment modalities applied to persons disabled by these neuromuscular disorders and to develop and improve new and existing treatment modalities, and to quantify and standardize methods of evaluating disease activity and remission.

★ 22980 ★ New York University Particulate Matter Health Research Center
School of Medicine, Environmental Medicine
57 Old Forge Rd.
Tuxedo, NY 10987
Phone: (845)731-3558 **Fax:** (845)351-5472
Email: lippmann@env.med.nyu.edu
Website: http://charlotte.med.nyu.edu/epa-pm-center/
Morton Lippmann, Dir.
Activities/Fields: Roles of airborne particulate matter in causing health effects.

★ 22981 ★ New York University Rusk Institute of Rehabilitation Medicine
400 E 34th St.
New York, NY 10016
Phone: (212)263-5870 **Fax:** (212)263-8510
Website: http://www.ruskinstitute.org/ri/rusk/homepage_rusk.jsp
Dr. Mathew Lee, Chm.
Activities/Fields: Management of neuromuscular disease, Parkinson's disease, Alzheimer's disease, brain trauma and stroke victims.

★ 22982 ★ New York University Medical Center Head Trauma Program
660 1st Ave.
New York, NY 10016
Phone: (212)263-7156 **Fax:** (212)263-6807
Email: yehuda.ben-yishay@med.nyu.edu
Dr. Yehuda Ben-Yishay, Dir.
Activities/Fields: Young adults suffering from head injuries. Conducts systematic remedial training in attention and concentration, various aspects of perception, perceptual-motor integration (eye-hand integration), and logical reasoning and interpersonal skills. Provides individual and family counseling and prevocational explorations. **Pub:** *Working Approaches to Remediation of Cognitive Deficits in Brain Damaged Persons*, annually.

★ 22983 ★ New York University Medical Center Nathan Kline Institute for Psychiatric Research Center for Alzheimer's Disease Research
140 Old Orangeburg Rd.
Orangeburg, NY 10962
Phone: (845)398-5423 **Fax:** (845)398-5422
Email: nixon@nki.rfmh.org
Website: http://www.rfmh.org/nki
Dr. Ralph Nixon, Dir.
Activities/Fields: Molecular neuroscience and aging, including molecular neurobiology of proteases, signal transduction, neurodegenerative disease, protein/peptide analytical techniques, molecular genetics, vesicle biology, transgenic modeling.

★ 22984 ★ New York University Medical Center William and Sylvia Silberstein Institute for Aging and Dementia
550 1st Ave., Rm. MHL 310
New York, NY 10016
Phone: (212)263-8088 **Fax:** (212)263-6991
Email: steven.ferris@med.nyu.edu
Website: http://aging.med.nyu.edu/
Steven Ferris, PhD, Exec. Dir.
Activities/Fields: Memory problems due to normal aging with cognitive impsirment and dementia; the early diagnosis, causes, and treatment of Alzheimer's disease. **Pub:** *Newsletter*, quarterly. **Frmly:** William and Sylvia Silberstein Aging and Dementia Research Center.

★ 22985 ★ Newark Beth Israel Medical Center Sleep Disorders Center
201 Lyons Ave.
Newark, NJ 07112
Phone: (973)926-6668
Email: mkaretzky@sbhcs.com
Website: http://www.njsleephelp.com/
Dr. Monroe Karetzky, Dir.
Activities/Fields: Sleep abnormalities, including insomnia, snoring, sleep apnea, narcolepsy, sleep-wake schedule disorders, daytime sleepiness, sleepwalking, nocturnal myoclonus, nocturnal asthma/COPD, parasomnias, REM sleep behavior disorders, restless leg syndrome, sleep disorders in the elderly, and sleep disorders in children. **Pub:** *Journal articles.*

★ 22986 ★ Nicholas Institute of Sports Medicine and Athletic Trauma
Department of Orthopedic Surgery
Lenox Hill Hospital
100 E 77th St.
New York, NY 10021
Phone: (212)434-2710 **Fax:** (212)434-2687
Email: mchugh@nismat.org
Website: http://www.nismat.org
Dr. Malacby P. McHugh, Res. Coord.
Activities/Fields: Sports medicine in the areas of orthopedics and trauma, fluid and electrolyte balance, nutrition, endocrinology and physical therapy, cardiology, and biomechanics.

★ 22987 ★ Norris Cotton Cancer Center (NCCC)
Dartmouth-Hitchcock Medical Center
Lebanon, NH 03756
Phone: (603)650-6300 **Free:** 800-639-6918
Fax: (603)650-6333
Email: norris.cotton.cancer.center@dartmouth.edu
Website: http://cancer.dartmouth.edu/about/index.shtml
Mark A. Israel, MD, Contact
Activities/Fields: Clinical treatment trials, including bone marrow transplantation, chemotherapy trials, intraoperative radiation therapy, and monoclonal antibody treatment. Studies are conducted in the areas of tumor immunology, radiobiology, carcinogenesis, cancer epidemiology, cancer control, cytogenetics, tumor endocrinology, molecular genetics, advanced imaging, radiobioloby, cancer risk, and palliative care. Participates as one of a group of regional clinical and nonclinical centers conducting multidisciplinary cancer research, improving methods of treatment, diagnosis, and prevention, training health professionals, and transferring cancer knowledge to surrounding communities.

★ 22988 ★ North Carolina State University North Carolina Ergonomics Resource Center (NCERC)
3701 Neil St.
Raleigh, NC 27607
Phone: (919)515-2052 **Free:** 800-664-3746
Email: goehringer@TheErgonimcsCenter.com
Website: http://www.ncerc.com/
Anita R. Goehringer, Exec. Dir.
Activities/Fields: Ergonomic deficiencies in the workplace.

★ 22989 ★ North Central Cancer Treatment Group
Operations Office
200 1st St. SW
Rochester, MN 55905
Phone: (507)284-5999 **Fax:** (507)284-1902
Website: http://ncctg.mayo.edu
Dr. Michael J. O'Connell, Chm.
Activities/Fields: Cancer research and therapy, including surgery, medical oncology, therapeutic radiology, pathology, and cancer control. Seeks to transfer nationwide cancer research and therapy to patients at the community level. Group maintains a patient base of 7,000 and operates 112 separate research protocols.

★ 22990 ★ North York General Hospital North York Regional Genetics Centre
4001 Leslie St.
Toronto, ON, Canada M2K 1E1
Phone: (416)756-6345 **Fax:** (416)756-6727
Email: pwyatt@nygh.on.ca
Dr. Philip Wyatt, Dir.
Activities/Fields: Clinical genetics, prenatal biology, and chromosomal and metabolic diseases.

★ 22991 ★ Northeastern University Center for Cardiovascular Targeting
205 Mugar Life Sciences Bldg.
Department of Pharmaceutical Sciences
Boston, MA 02115
Phone: (617)373-4203 **Fax:** (617)373-3663
Email: b.khaw@nunet.neu.edu
Website: http://www.neu.edu/top/research3.html
Ban-An Khaw, PhD, Dir.
Activities/Fields: In vivo targeting of myriad cardiovascular-related health problems, such as atherosclerotic lesions, myocardial necrosis, brain infarction and various tumors.

★ 22992 ★ Northern California Cancer Center
32960 Alvarado-Niles Rd., Ste. 600
PO Box 5033
Union City, CA 94587
Phone: (510)429-2500 **Fax:** (510)429-2550
Email: dwest@nccc.org

Website: http://www.nccc.org
Dee W. West, PhD, Actg. Exec. Dir.

Activities/Fields: Conducts multidisciplinary studies in epidemiology and related fields. Also conducts cancer research and demonstration activities (detection, psychosocial, prevention, nutrition) with communities in the Center's service area, focusing on the minority populations and the underserved. **Pub:** *Cancer Calendar*, quarterly. • *Estate Planning Brochure.* • *Highlights.* • *Registry Newsletters.*

★ 22993 ★ Northern California Institute for Research and Education (NCIRE)
4150 Clement St. (151NC)
San Francisco, CA 94121-1545
Phone: (415)750-6954 **Fax:** (415)750-9358
Email: askncire@ncire.org
Website: http://www.ncire.org/
Jack Nagan, CEO

Activities/Fields: New medical treatments and procedures, new drugs, rehabilitation, health services delivery, geriatrics, etc.

★ 22994 ★ Northern California Regional Spinal Cord Injury System
Santa Clara Valley Medical Center
950 S Bascom Ave., Ste. 2011
San Jose, CA 95128
Phone: (408)295-9896 **Free:** 800-352-1956
Fax: (408)295-9913
Email: tamara@tbi-sci.org
Website: http://www.tbi-sci.org/
Dr. Tamara Bushnik, Prin. Investigator

Activities/Fields: Spinal cord injuries. **Pub:** *InterAct newsletter*, semiannually. • *Spinal Cord Injury-For Your Information Resource Directory*, biennially.

★ 22995 ★ Northern New Jersey Spinal Cord Injury System (NNJSCIS)
Kessler Medical Rehabilitation Research & Education Corp.
1199 Pleasant Valley Way
West Orange, NJ 07052
Phone: (973)243-6849 **Free:** 800-248-3221
Fax: (973)324-3527
Email: dtulsky@kmrrec.org
Website: http://www.kmrrec.org/nnjscis
David Tulsky, Contact

Activities/Fields: Spinal cord injuries.

★ 22996 ★ Northwest Woodhaven Center Inc.
2900 Southampton Rd.
Philadelphia, PA 19154
Phone: (215)671-5001 **Fax:** (215)671-7522
Michael Barton, MD, VP

Activities/Fields: Treatment effectiveness, program evaluation, clinical treatment research (medications and behavior modification), and policy research in mental retardation at Woodhaven Center, a University-operated residential program for mentally retarded persons. **Pub:** *Evaluation and Research Technical Report Series.*

★ 22997 ★ Northwestern Health Sciences University Wolfe-Harris Center for Clinical Studies
2501 W 84th St.
Bloomington, MN 55431
Phone: (952)888-4777 **Free:** 800-888-4777
Fax: (952)888-1957
Email: csawyer@nwhealth.edu
Website: http://www.nwhealth.edu/
Charles E. Sawyer, VP

Activities/Fields: Chiropractic clinical research, including ambulatory health care.

★ 22998 ★ Northwestern University Asher Center for the Study and Treatment of Depressive Disorders
Ward Bldg., 9th Fl.
303 E Chicago
Chicago, IL 60611
Phone: (312)908-9380 **Fax:** (312)503-0466
Email: b-mckinney@nwu.edu
Website: http://www.ashercenter.nwu.edu/
Dr. William McKinney, Dir.

Activities/Fields: Depressive disorders, especially the neurobiological processes and mechanisms that underlie their development. Three central themes have been emphasized, including animal models of depression, neurobiological substrates of depressive disorders, and developmental perspectives.

★ 22999 ★ Northwestern University Buehler Center on Aging
750 N Lake Shore Dr., Ste. 601
Chicago, IL 60611-2611
Phone: (312)503-3087 **Fax:** (312)503-5868
Email: miris@nwu.edu
Website: http://www.northwestern.edu/aging/index.htm
Dr. Madelyn Iris, Interim Dir.

Activities/Fields: Gerontology and geriatrics to improve the medical/social/emotional functioning and status of the elderly. **Pub:** *Buehler Center on Aging Quarterly Newsletter.* • *Geriatrics Resource Guide.* • *Monograph series.* • *Videos.*

★ 23000 ★ Northwestern University Center for Reproductive Science
2-171 Hogan Hall
2205 Tech Dr.
Evanston, IL 60208-3520
Phone: (847)491-4464 **Fax:** (847)491-5211
Email: k-mayo@northwestern.edu
Website: http://www.northwestern.edu/center-for-reproductive-science
Kelly E. Mayo, Dir.

Activities/Fields: Reproductive biology, focusing on the regulation of ovarian synthesis and secretion of steroid and peptide hormones on the metabolic pathways and messengers within ovarian structures; regulation of testicular development, secretion of spermatogenesis, and the regulation of synthesis and secretion of the pituitary gonadotropic hormones and prolactin, as well as their actions on the brain, gonads, and breast tissue; and interactions of neural tissue in the brain and spinal cord with the pituitary-gonadal axis.

★ 23001 ★ Northwestern University Center for Sleep and Circadian Biology
Department of Neurobiology & Physiology
2205 Tech Dr., Hogan 2-160
Evanston, IL 60208
Phone: (847)467-6512 **Fax:** (847)467-4065
Email: fturek@northwestern.edu
Website: http://www.northwestern.edu/cscb/
Fred W. Turek, Dir.

Activities/Fields: Circadian rhythms and sleep, including the elucidation of the fundamental mechanisms that underlie circadian dysfunctional for human health, safety and productivity and development of treatments to alleviate symptons of circadian dysfunctions. **Frmly:** Center for Circadian Biology and Medicine.

★ 23002 ★ Northwestern University Cognitive Neurology and Alzheimer's Disease Center (CN-ADC)
320 E Superior St., Searle 11-450
Chicago, IL 60611-3008
Phone: (312)908-9339 **Fax:** (312)908-8789
Email: mmesulam@nwu.edu
Website: http://www.brain.nwu.edu/
Marsel Mesulam, MD, Dir.

Activities/Fields: How the brain coordinates mental functions such as memory, language, attention, and emotion for the benefit of patients with brain diseases that impair cognitive function.

★ 23003 ★ Northwestern University General Clinical Research Center
10E Feinberg
Northwestern Memorial Hospital
251 E Huron St.
Chicago, IL 60611
Phone: (312)503-2539 **Fax:** (312)926-8450
Email: wlowe@northwestern.edu
Website: http://www.feinberg.northwestern.edu/gcrc/
Dr. William L. Lowe, Jr., Prog. Dir.

Activities/Fields: Diabetes insipidus, malabsorption in AIDS, cardiac arrhythmias, effects of diabetes on pregnancy, pituitary tumors, tumoral calcinosis, gastrointestinal malabsorption of carbohydrates and other nutrients, monoclonal antibodies in diagnosis and therapy of cancer, and Phase I and II drug trials. **Pub:** *Annual Report.*

★ 23004 ★ Northwestern University Institute for Bioengineering and Nanoscience in Advanced Medicine (IBNAM)
645 N Michigan Ave., Ste. 1058B
Chicago, IL 60611-3008
Phone: (312)503-0807 **Fax:** (312)503-2482
Email: ibnam@northwestern.edu
Website: http://www.ibnam.northwestern.edu/
Samuel I. Stupp, Dir.

Activities/Fields: Use of bioengineering and nanoscience in medicine, in such areas as self-assembly, tissue engineering, genomics, smart drug delivery, and other new technologies.

★ 23005 ★ Northwestern University Institute for Health Services Research and Policy Studies
339 E Chicago Ave., No. 717
Chicago, IL 60611
Phone: (847)491-5643 **Fax:** (847)491-2202
Email: ihsrps@northwestern.edu
Website: http://www.northwestern.edu/ihsrps
Dr. Peter P. Budetti, Dir.

Activities/Fields: Health services research and policy analysis focusing on the relationship between health care delivery systems and health outcomes, health economics, organization behavior in health, competition in the delivery of health services, physician and institutional incentives. **Pub:** *Working paper series.*

★ 23006 ★ Northwestern University Institute for Neuroscience
320 E Superior St.
Chicago, IL 60611
Phone: (312)503-4300 **Fax:** (312)503-7345
Email: e-mugnaini@northwestern.edu
Website: http://www.northwestern.edu/nuin/
Dr. Enrico Mugnaini, Dir.

Activities/Fields: Sensory neurobiology and psychophysics, neuroendocrinology, biological rhythms, neurobiology of disease, cytoskeleton, motor control mechanisms, cognitive and computational neuroscience, neural development and plasticity, electrophysiology and pharmacology of excitable membranes, stem cells, pain, neuroimmunology and virology, neurodegenerative diseases, neurogengineering. **Pub:** *Newsletter*, annually.

★ 23007 ★ Northwestern University John I. Brewer Trophoblastic Disease Center
Prentice Women's Hospital
333 E Superior, Ste. 420
Chicago, IL 60611
Phone: (312)926-7365 **Fax:** (312)926-2188
Email: jlurain@nmh.org
John R. Lurain, MD, Dir.

Activities/Fields: Pathology, epidemiology, and experimental chemotherapy in patients with trophoblastic diseases; experimental protocols and new chemotherapeutic agents and combinations of agents; pathologic studies of choriocarcinoma and hydatidiform mole; and the effect of oral contraceptive use on the development of gestational trophoblastic diseases.

★ 23008 ★ Northwestern University Kellogg Center for Biotechnology
2001 Sheridan Rd.
Evanston, IL 60208
Phone: (847)467-1454 **Fax:** (847)467-2180
Website: http://www.kellogg.northwestern.edu
Alicia Loffler, Dir.

Activities/Fields: Cooperates with industry on issues of national and international significance. **Pub:** *Biotechnology News*, quarterly.

★ 23009 ★ Northwestern University Multipurpose Arthritis and Musculoskeletal Diseases Center
303 E Chicago Ave., Ward 3-315
Chicago, IL 60611
Phone: (312)503-8003 **Fax:** (312)503-0994
Email: rmp158@northwestern.edu
Dr. Richard M. Pope, Dir.

Activities/Fields: Biomedical, educational, and health services research in the musculoskeletal diseases.

★ 23010 ★ Northwestern University Prosthetics Research Laboratory
345 E Superior St., Rm. 1441
Chicago, IL 60611-4496
Phone: (312)238-6500 **Fax:** (312)238-6510
Email: d-childress@northwestern.edu
Website: http://www.repoc.northwestern.edu/
Dr. Dudley S. Childress, Dir.

Activities/Fields: Improvement of prostheses and orthoses, fitting and manufacturing processes for such devices, and basic understanding of human interactions with systems of these types. **Pub:** *Resource Guide of Prosthetics and Orthotics.*

★ 23011 ★ Northwestern University Rehabilitation Engineering Research Center in Prosthetics and Orthotics
Rehabilitation Institute of Chicago
345 E Superior St., Rm. 1441
Chicago, IL 60611-4496
Phone: (312)238-6500 **Fax:** (312)238-6510
Email: d-childress@northwestern.edu
Dr. Dudley S. Childress, Dir.

Activities/Fields: Improvement of prostheses and orthoses, improved fitting and manufacturing processes for prosthesis/orthosis systems, and improved basic understanding of human interactions with these systems. **Pub:** *Reports.* • *Resource Guide of Prosthetics and Orthotics.*

★ 23012 ★ Northwestern University Robert H. Lurie Comprehensive Cancer Center of Northwestern University
Olson Pavillion, Ste. 8250
303 E Chicago Ave.
Chicago, IL 60611-3008
Phone: (312)908-5250 **Fax:** (312)908-1372
Email: s-rosen@northwestern.edu
Website: http://www.cancer.northwestern.edu
Steven T. Rosen, MD, Dir.

Activities/Fields: The Center has ten established research programs. Basic science programs include Viral Oncogenesis, Tumor Invasion, Metastesis and Angiogenesis; Hormone Action and Signal Transduction in Cancer; and Cancer Genes and Molecular Regulation. Clinical science research is conducted in the areas of Breast Cancer, Prostate Cancer, Hematologic Malignancies, Pediatric Oncology, Cancer Prevention and Control. Coordinates multidisciplinary, basic, and clinical cancer research; seeks improved methods of cancer treatment, diagnosis and prevention; trains health care professionals; and transfers cancer knowledge to surrounding communities. **Pub:** *Community Newsletter.* • *Journal of the Robert H. Lurie Cancer Center of Northwestern University*, semiannually. • *Lurie Cancer Center News and Calendar*, bimonthly.

★ 23013 ★ Northwestern University Samuel Sackett Research Laboratory
676 N St. Clair St., Ste. 200
Chicago, IL 60611
Phone: (312)695-5067 **Fax:** (312)695-5088
Dr. Steven M. Wolinsky, Dir.

Activities/Fields: HIV/AIDS cellular and humoral resistance to infection, viral central nervous system infections, pharmacology of antimicrobial agents, investigation of infectious diarrhea, and natural history of infectious diseases.

★ 23014 ★ Nova Scotia Environmental Health Centre
3064 Lake Thomas Dr.
Fall River, NS, Canada B2T 1K6
Phone: (902)860-3066 **Fax:** (902)860-2046
Email: nsehc@dal.ca
Website: http://www.nsehc.com/
Dr. Roy Fox, Dir.

Activities/Fields: Environmentally-triggered sensitivities, causes, and treatment.

★ 23015 ★ Nursing Effectiveness Utilization and Outcomes Research Unit (NRU)
McMaster University
1200 Main St. W, Rm. 2J40
Hamilton, ON, Canada L8N 3Z5
Phone: (905)525-9140 **Fax:** (905)570-0667
Email: baumanna@mcmaster.ca
Website: http://www.fhs.mcmaster.ca/nru/
Andrea Baumann, PhD, Co-Prin. Investigator

Activities/Fields: Supply, distribution and deployment of nurses and how to enable nurses to meet their responsibilities as a result of restructuring in the health care system; maintenance of quality while realizing funding efficiencies in the health care system. **Pub:** *Annual report.* • *Fact sheets.* • *Reports.* • *Working papers.*

★ 23016 ★ NYCAMH
Bassett Healthcare
1 Atwell Rd.
Cooperstown, NY 13326
Phone: (607)547-6023 **Free:** 800-343-7527
Fax: (607)547-6087
Email: jmay@nycamh.com
Website: http://www.nycamh.com
John J. May, MD, Dir.

Activities/Fields: Studies barn dusts, mites, health needs of agricultural workers in New York, dosimetry on farms, agricultural lung hazards, farm machinery safety, and migrant health. **Pub:** *FARMSAFE: Focus on Agricultural Health.* Video. • *How Safe Are Your Farm Tractors?.* • *Respiratory Hazards in the Farm Environment.* • *Using Personal Protective Equipment on the Farm.* • *What You Should Know About Using Dust/Mist Masks on the Farm.* **Frmly:** New York Center for Agricultural Medicine and Health.

★ 23017 ★ Oakland University Eye Research Institute
422 Dodge Hall
Rochester, MI 48309-4480
Phone: (248)370-2391 **Fax:** (248)370-2006
Email: nharriso@oakland.edu
Website: http://www.otus.oakland.edu/eri/
Nancy Harrison, Exec. Sec.

Activities/Fields: Biochemistry, biophysics, cell biology, physiology, pharmacology, and photobiology. Research focuses on ocular tissues and includes the following topics of interest: molecular genetics of lens proteins, ion transport and radiation damage of the cornea, light damage of the retina, signal transduction in photoreceptors, ocular drug metabolism and detoxification, and experimental models of proliferative vitreoretinopathy, uveoretinitis, cataracts (radiation and oxidation and calcium), and diabetic complications of the eye. **Frmly:** Institute of Biological Sciences.

★ 23018 ★ Ochsner Clinic Foundation
1516 Jefferson Hwy.
New Orleans, LA 70121
Phone: (504)842-3000 **Fax:** (504)842-2152
Email: rre@ochsner.org
Website: http://www.ochsner.org
Richard N. Re, MD, Dir.

Activities/Fields: Hypertension, oncology, cardiovascular research, immunology, orthopedics, renal stones, gastrointestinal physiology (motility and perfusion), depression, and clinical pharmacology. **Frmly:** Alton Ochsner Medical Foundation.

★ 23019 ★ Ohio Cancer Research Associates
50 W Broad St., Ste. 1132
Columbus, OH 43215-3388
Phone: (614)224-1127 **Fax:** (614)224-0654
Email: ocra@ohiocancer.org
Website: http://www.ohiocancer.org
Dennis Zack, Exec. Dir.

Activities/Fields: Cancer "seed money" research projects.

★ 23020 ★ Ohio State University Caligiuri Laboratory
A458 Starling-Loving Hall
320 W 10th Ave.
Columbus, OH 43210
Phone: (614)293-7521 **Fax:** (614)293-7522
Email: caligiuri-1@medctr.osu.edu
Website: http://www.jamesline.com/caligiuri
Michael A. Caligiuri, MD, Dir.

Activities/Fields: Research, patient service, and training through a fellowship program on various aspects of hematology and oncology, including cancer immunology, human cancer genetics, lymphocyte signaling, importance of complement in host defense against malignancy, the role of oxygen radicals in mononuclear effector cells and tumor cell targets, and clinical research in the development, implementation, and assessment of protocols in the treatment of leukemia, lymphoma, bone marrow transplantation, and solid tumors. The training program is designed to provide postdoctoral fellowship experience in the development and performance of clinical and laboratory research projects related to hematology and medical oncology.

★ 23021 ★ Ohio State University Center for Retrovirus Research
1925 Coffey Rd.
Columbus, OH 43210-1093
Phone: (614)292-7317 **Fax:** (614)292-6473
Email: mathes.2@osu.edu
Website: http://www.vet.ohio-state.edu/docs/retrovirus/index.html
Dr. Lawrence Mathes, Dir.

Activities/Fields: Animal and human retroviruses, including HIV in humans, feline immunodeficiency virus, equine infectious anemia, and leukemia virus of cats. **Pub:** *Newsletter*, quarterly.

★ 23022 ★ Ohio State University Clinical Pharmacology Division
Graves Hall, Rm. 5084
College of Medicine
333 W 10th Ave.
Columbus, OH 43210-1239
Phone: (614)292-8600 **Fax:** (614)292-4253
Email: apseloff.1@osu.edu

Website: http://www.med.ohio-state.edu/pharm/clinical
Dr. Glen Apseloff, Dir.
Activities/Fields: Clinical drug studies.

★ 23023 ★ Ohio State University Comprehensive Cancer Center
A455 Starling-Loving Hall
220 W 10th Ave.
Columbus, OH 43210
Phone: (614)293-7518 **Free:** 800-293-5066
Fax: (614)293-7520
Website: http://www.jamesline.com
Clara D. Bloomfield, MD, Dir.
Activities/Fields: Carcinogenesis, cancer chemoprevention, cancer control, immunology, developmental therapeutics, hormones and cancer, molecular biology, RNA oncogenic virus, neuro-oncology, head and neck oncology, urologic oncology, and pediatric oncology. Investigations also cover bone marrow transplantation, biochemistry and genetics, breast cancer, clinical trials, and pharmacology and toxicology. **Pub:** *Scientific Report*, biennially.

★ 23024 ★ Ohio State University Division of Infectious Diseases
410 W 10th Ave.
Columbus, OH 43210
Phone: (614)293-8732 **Fax:** (614)293-5240
Dr. Larry Schlesinger, Dir.
Activities/Fields: Pathogenesis, prophylaxis, therapy, pathology, serology of infectious diseases (including Legionnaire's disease, herpes infections, acquired immune deficiency syndrome, and other opportunistic infections), and extensive in vitro and clinical evaluations of antimicrobial agents.

★ 23025 ★ Ohio State University Division of Otologic Research
4331 University Hospitals Clinic
456 W 10th Ave.
Columbus, OH 43210
Phone: (614)293-8103 **Fax:** (614)293-5506
Email: demaria.2@osu.edu
Dr. Thomas F. DeMaria, Dir.
Activities/Fields: Otology, including animal models for otitis media, acoustic trauma, morphological studies on the inner ear, and immunologic investigations of the middle and inner ear. Also studies the development of animal models for studying middle ear infection using microbiological, immunologic, morphologic and molecular biological methods, temporal bone histopathology (human and animal), electron microscopy of auditory and vestibular systems, pathogenesis of otitis media, and sensory transduction mechanism. **Frmly:** Ear Research Group.

★ 23026 ★ Ohio State University Division of Pulmonary and Critical Care Medicine
201 Heart & Lung Research Institute
Department of Internal Medicine
473 W 12th Ave.
Columbus, OH 43210-1228
Phone: (614)293-4925 **Fax:** (614)293-4799
Website: http://www.intmed.med.ohio-state.edu/pulmo/pulmonary_homepage.htm
Mark D. Wewers, MD, Dir.
Activities/Fields: Mechanisms of allergic, immunologic, and inflammatory diseases, including ventilatory control and respiratory failure, inflammatory mechanisms in adult respiratory distress syndrome, cystic fibrosis, emphysema, staging and therapy of pulmonary neoplasms, respiratory distress in HIV, and occupational lung diseases. Collaborates with the departments of physiology and exercise physiology and with the cardiopulmonary unit of the School of Veterinary Medicine at the University.

★ 23027 ★ Ohio State University Dorothy M. Davis Heart and Lung Research Institute
473 W 12th Ave.
Columbus, OH 43210-1252
Phone: (614)247-7766 **Fax:** (614)247-7799
Email: HLRI@medctr.osu.edu
Website: http://heartlung.osu.edu
Mark D. Wewers, MD, Interim Dir.
Activities/Fields: Development of novel strategies to cure patients affected with heart and lung diseases and to prevent such diseases from developing in individuals at risk.

★ 23028 ★ Ohio State University General Clinical Research Center
N 1105 Doan Hall
410 W 10th Ave.
Columbus, OH 43210
Phone: (614)293-8775 **Fax:** (614)293-3796
Email: malarkey-1@medctr.osu.edu
Dr. William Malarkey, Dir.
Activities/Fields: Diabetes, heart disease, endocrine and metabolic disorders, nutrition, neuroendocrine tumors, osteoporosis, cancer, eating disorders, affective disorders and depression, and renal disease.

★ 23029 ★ Ohio State University George C. Paffenbarger Dental Research Laboratory
Postle Hall
College of Dentistry
305 W 12th Ave.
Columbus, OH 43210-1267
Phone: (614)292-0941 **Fax:** (614)292-9422
Email: rosenstiel.1@osu.edu
Website: http://www.dent.ohio-state.edu
Dr. Stephen F. Rosenstiel, Dir.
Activities/Fields: Dental bio-materials engineering. Currently studying dental polymers, maxillo-facial polymer synthesis, and optical properties of esthetic biomaterials.

★ 23030 ★ Ohio State University Laboratory Animal Center
6089 Godown Rd.
Columbus, OH 43235
Phone: (614)292-8541 **Fax:** (614)292-9282
Email: stone.4@osu.edu
Douglas Stone, DVM, Assoc. Dir.
Activities/Fields: Supports University biomedical research activities of all laboratory animals, quarantining of all nonhuman primates and other species depending upon the nature of the study, and long-term housing of nonhuman primates, canines, swine, and other species. Serves as a teaching resource for the College of Veterinary Medicine.

★ 23031 ★ Ohio State University Laboratory of Psychobiology
Townsend Hall, Rm. 48
1885 Neil Ave.
Columbus, OH 43210
Phone: (614)292-1749 **Fax:** (614)292-4537
Email: berntson.2@osu.edu
Dr. Gary G. Berntson, Contact
Activities/Fields: Psychobiology and comparative psychology, including studies on recovery of function after brain damage, psychopharmacology, psychophysiology, developmental processes, and animal cognition. **Frmly:** Laboratory of Comparative and Physiological Psychology.

★ 23032 ★ Ohio State University Nisonger Center for Mental Retardation and Developmental Disabilities
1581 Dodd Dr.
Columbus, OH 43210-1257
Phone: (614)292-9844 **Fax:** (614)292-3727
Email: reiss.7@osu.edu
Website: http://nisonger.osu.edu
Steven Reiss, PhD, Dir.
Activities/Fields: Developmental disabilities, psychometric assessment, rehabilitation engineering, psychopathology, psychopharmacology, adults and aging, and family studies. Special attention given to applied research related to mental retardation and development and implementation of training programs to prepare professional personnel to work with the developmentally disabled. Provides early childhood classes for developmentally disabled preschoolers and offers information services to clients, students, staff, and faculty. **Pub:** *Project Med Booklet.*

★ 23033 ★ Ohio State University Transplant Sciences Laboratories
355 Means Hall
1654 Upham Dr.
Columbus, OH 43210
Phone: (614)293-3212 **Fax:** (614)293-4541
Email: orosz-1@medctr.osu.edu
Website: http://surgery.osu.edu
Dr. Charles Orosz, Dir.
Activities/Fields: Transplantation related immunobiology, inflammation, clinical histocompatibility testing and post-transplant immunologic monitoring, clinical and experimental immunosuppression, and application of complexity theory to immunology, including agent-based computer simulation of immune behavior. **Frmly:** Therapeutic Immunology Laboratories.

★ 23034 ★ Ohio Valley Tissue and Skin Center
2939 Vernon Pl.
Cincinnati, OH 45219
Phone: (513)558-6400 **Free:** 800-558-5004
Fax: (513)558-6440
Website: http://www.ovtsc.org
Edward C. Robb, Exec. Dir.
Activities/Fields: Human tissue, skin and bones.

★ 23035 ★ Okanagan University College Centre for Population and Health Services Research
Okanagan University College
3333 College Way
Kelowna, BC, Canada V1V 1V7
Fax: (250)762-5445
Email: ekrupa@ouc.bc.ca
Website: http://www.cphsr.org
Eugene Krupa, Dir.
Activities/Fields: Health services, economics, and outcomes relevant to the health of the population of the Okanagan region of British Columbia, Canada.

★ 23036 ★ Oklahoma Medical Research Foundation
825 NE 13th St.
Oklahoma City, OK 73104-5046
Phone: (405)271-6673 **Free:** 800-522-0211
Fax: (405)271-7510
Email: Don-Capra@omrf.ouhsc.edu
Website: http://www.omrf.ouhsc.edu
J. Donald Capra, MD, Pres.
Activities/Fields: Arthritis and Immunology, including lupus, rheumatoid arthritis, and scleroderma; Cardiovascular Biology, including heart attack, blood diseases, stroke, and septic shock; Children's Diseases, including cancer, leukemia, genetic disorders, and cystic fibrosis; Clincial Pharmacology, including FDA drug trials for hypertension, cholesterol, asthma, and others; Development Biology, including genetic disorders, Down's syndrome, and obesity; Free Radical Biology and Aging, including Alzheimer's disease, Parkinson's disease, and stroke; Immunobiology and Cancer, including leukemia, Hogkins' disease, lymphoma, and breast cancer; Molecular and Cell Biology, including ALS, muscular dystrophy, multiple sclerosis, and new antibiotics; Molecular Immunogenetics, including diabetes, AIDS, and immune system disorders; and Protein Studies, including AIDS, HIV, diabetes, and ulcers. **Pub:** *Findings Newsletter.*

★ 23037 ★ Oklahoma Medical Research Foundation
Arthritis/Immunology Research Program
825 NE 13th St.
Oklahoma City, OK 73104
Phone: (405)271-7766 **Fax:** (405)271-4110
Email: john-harley@omrf.ouhsc.edu
John Harley, MD, Ch.
Activities/Fields: Molecular aspects of systemic autoimmunity.

★ 23038 ★ Oklahoma Medical Research Foundation
Cardiovascular Biology Research Program
825 NE 13th St.
Oklahoma City, OK 73104-5046
Phone: (405)271-6673 **Free:** 800-522-0211
Fax: (405)271-3980
Email: jdonald-capra@omrf.ouhsc.edu
Website: http://www.omrf.ouhsc.edu/OMRF/Research/15/Program.asp
J. Donald Capra, MD, Pres.
Activities/Fields: Cardiovascular disease, especially blood clotting and inflammatory aspects of vascular diseases; structure determination of blood coagulation enzymes and design of inhibitors; regulation of inflammation by the coagulation system and the impact of inflammation on coagulation; mechanisms by which autoimmune diseases modulate blood coagulation and vascular function; septic shock; and the mechanisms of leukocyte binding to vascular endothelium. Gene deletion and transgenic approaches are designed to identify targets for therapeutic intervention.

★ 23039 ★ Oklahoma Medical Research Foundation
Clinical Pharmacology Research Program
825 NE 13th St.
Oklahoma City, OK 73104
Phone: (405)271-6673 **Fax:** (405)271-3980
Email: carl-manion@omrf.ouhsc.edu
Website: http://www.omrf.org/OMRF/Research/17/Program.asp
Carl V. Manion, MD, Contact
Activities/Fields: Effects of medicines given to treat the heart, lungs and liver.

★ 23040 ★ Oklahoma Medical Research Foundation
Crystallography Research Program
825 NE 13th St.
Oklahoma City, OK 73104
Phone: (405)271-1672 **Fax:** (405)271-7953
Email: allen-edmundson@omrf.ouhsc.edu
Website: http://www.omrf.org/OMRF/Research/04/Welcome.asp
Allen B. Edmundson, PhD, Prog. Hd.
Activities/Fields: Structure and function of protein molecules.

★ 23041 ★ Oklahoma Medical Research Foundation
Developmental Biology Research Program
825 NE 13th St.
Oklahoma City, OK 73104
Phone: (405)271-6673 **Fax:** (405)271-3980
Email: ute-hochgeschwender@omrf.ouhsc.edu
Website: http://www.omrf.org/OMRF/Research/10/Program.asp
Ute Hochgeschwender, MD, Contact
Activities/Fields: Molecular basis of growth and differentiation, using the mouse as a model organism. Of particular interest are the processes of neural differentiation and brain development, as well as the tissue-specific regulation of gene expression and the relative stability of the genome to mutation and DNA recombination.

★ 23042 ★ Oklahoma Medical Research Foundation
Free Radical Biology and Aging Research Program
825 NE 13th St.
Oklahoma City, OK 73104
Phone: (405)271-6673 **Fax:** (405)271-3980
Email: robert-floyd@omrf.ouhsc.edu
Website: http://www.omrf.org/OMRF/Research/13/Program.asp
Robert A. Floyd, PhD, Prog. Hd.
Activities/Fields: Mechanistic basis of aging as well as several diseases of aging including neurodegenerative diseases, cardiovascular disease, cancer and diabetes. Much of the research involves the action of reactive oxygen and nitric oxide species and free radical aspects of signal transduction.

★ 23043 ★ Oklahoma Medical Research Foundation
Functional Proteomics Laboratory
825 NE 13th St.
Oklahoma City, OK 73104
Phone: (405)271-6673 **Fax:** (405)271-3980
Email: xin-li-lin@omrf.ouhsc.edu
Website: http://www.omrf.org/omrf/information/sr2001/functionalproteomics.asp
Xinli Lin, Prog. Hd.
Activities/Fields: Structural genomics and functional proteomics.

★ 23044 ★ Oklahoma Medical Research Foundation
Immunobiology and Cancer Research Program
825 NE 13th St.
Oklahoma City, OK 73104-5046
Phone: (405)271-6673 **Fax:** (405)271-3980
Email: paul-kincade@omrf.ouhsc.edu
Website: http://www.omrf.ouhsc.edu/omrf/research/14
Paul W. Kincade, PhD, Prog. Hd.
Activities/Fields: Mechanisms for regulation of B lymphocyte production in lymphopoietic tissues, including cytokines, hormones, and cell adhesion molecules.

★ 23045 ★ Oklahoma Medical Research Foundation
Lipid and Lipoprotein Laboratory
825 NE 13th St.
Oklahoma City, OK 73104
Phone: (405)271-7703 **Fax:** (405)271-8575
Email: hamptonk@omrf.ouhsc.edu
Dr. Petar Alaupovic, Contact
Activities/Fields: Chemistry and metabolism of plasma lipid transport, pathophysiology and treatment of dyslipoproteinemias, and model systems of atherosclerosis, including studies on the chemistry and interaction of lipoprotein particles, formation and lipolytic degradation of lipoprotein particles, dietary and drug treatment of dyslipoproteinemias, and determination of apolipoprotein profiles in dyslipoproteinemias.

★ 23046 ★ Oklahoma Medical Research Foundation
Molecular Immunogenetics Research Program
825 NE 13th St.
Oklahoma City, OK 73104
Phone: (405)271-6673 **Fax:** (405)271-7510
Email: donald-capra@omrf.ouhsc.edu
Website: http://www.omrf.org/OMRF/Research/05/CapraJD.asp
J. Donald Capra, MD, Prog. Hd.
Activities/Fields: Molecular mechanisms of the immune system.

★ 23047 ★ Oklahoma Medical Research Foundation
Protein Studies Program
825 NE 13th St.
Oklahoma City, OK 73104
Phone: (405)271-7291 **Fax:** (405)271-7249
Email: jordan-tang@omrf.ouhsc.edu
Dr. Jordan Tang, Hd.
Activities/Fields: Alzheimer's Disease, especially regarding protein structure and function, including cloning, expression and mutagenesis of protease genes, mechanisms of proteases, proteolysis by lysosomal enzymes, and streptokinase interaction with plasminogen fibrinolysis.

★ 23048 ★ Oklahoma State University Microbiology and Molecular Genetics
307 Life Sciences East
Stillwater, OK 74078-9947
Phone: (405)744-6243 **Fax:** (405)744-6790
Email: nirmal@okstate.edu
Website: http://microbiology.okstate.edu
Moses Vijayakumar, PhD, Dept. Hd.
Activities/Fields: Production and characterization of hybridomas and monoclonal antibodies and production of polyclonal antiserum. **Frmly:** Hybridoma Center for Agricultural and Biological Sciences.

★ 23049 ★ Olive View-UCLA Medical Center Foundation
14445 Olive View Dr., Cottage J
Sylmar, CA 91342-1495
Phone: (818)364-3686 **Fax:** (818)364-4584
Email: ovinfo@earthlink.net
Website: http://www.oliveviewfoundation.org
Beverly Froelich, Exec. Dir.
Activities/Fields: Community based needs assessments.

★ 23050 ★ Ontario Cancer Institute/ Princess Margaret Hospital
610 University Ave.
Toronto, ON, Canada M5G 2M9
Phone: (416)946-2000 **Fax:** (416)340-2967
Website: http://www.ocipmh.org
Dr. Alan Hudson, CEO
Activities/Fields: Cancer research, including studies on mechanisms regulating cellular growth and differentiation (with emphasis on the hemopoietic system), cellular and molecular immunology (particularly mechanisms involved in immune-recognition), molecular structure (including physical and molecular biological approaches to macromolecular structure and interactions), experimental therapy (including radiobiology and chemotherapy), clinical physics and epidemiology (including research in preventative oncology, quality of life, and clinical trials methodology). Participates in local, national, and international trials, including studies of all sites and types of malignancies, imaging techniques, and therapeutic trials. **Pub:** *Annual Report.*

★ 23051 ★ Oral and Maxillofacial Surgery Foundation
9700 W Bryn Mawr Ave.
Rosemont, IL 60018-5701
Phone: (847)678-6200 **Free:** 800-822-6637
Fax: (847)678-6286
Email: omsf@aaoms.org
Website: http://www.omsfoundation.org
Dr. James F. Kelly, Exec. Dir.
Activities/Fields: Oral and maxillofacial surgery focusing on providing fellowships and grants to both residents and investigators and financial support of other special projects and activities. **Pub:** *American Association of Maxillofacial Surgeons Today.* • *Foundation Insight.* Newsletter. • *Foundation Torch.* • *Journal of Oral and Maxillofacial Surgery.*

★ 23052 ★ Oregon Health and Science University
Biochemical Genetics Laboratory
Department of Molecular & Medical Genetics
3181 SW Sam Jackson Pk. Rd., MP 350
Portland, OR 97201
Phone: (503)494-5400 **Fax:** (503)494-7645
Email: gibsonm@ohsu.edu
K. Michael Gibson, PhD, Dir.
Activities/Fields: Inborn errors of metabolism and mitochondrial myopathies.

★ 23053 ★ Oregon Health and Science University
Center for Ethics in Health Care
3181 SW Sam Jackson Park Rd., UHN-86
Portland, OR 97201-3098
Phone: (503)494-1260
Email: ehtics@ohsu.edu
Website: http://www.ohsu.edu/ethics
Dr. Susan W. Tolle, Dir.
Activities/Fields: Ethics in contemporary health care, including end-of-life care.

★ 23054 ★ Oregon Health and Science University
Center for Research on Occupational and Environmental Toxicology (CROET)
3181 SW Sam Jackson Pk. Rd., L606
Portland, OR 97201-3098
Phone: (503)494-4273 **Fax:** (503)494-4278
Email: spencer@ohsu.edu
Website: http://www.ohsu.edu/croet
Dr. Peter S. Spencer, Dir.
Activities/Fields: Adverse effects of occupational and environmental chemicals on the human nervous system; region-specific surveillance of the use, dissemination and release of occupational chemicals and identification, analysis and categorization of all types of chemicals that may perturb normal neurological function; collaborative research on the exposure pathways and chemical fate of environmental pollutants, and their contact, entry and distribution in human subjects; field-based investigations epidemiological studies on human populations at risk for cancer, neurodegenerative diseases and stress-related disorders that impair workplace performance; studies on the health impact of xenobiotics incorporating, when possible, biological markers of susceptibility exposure and effect, including neurobehavioral (and other) screening batteries for the detection of early, reversible abnormalities in brain function; development of wild-type and transgenic animals as models to investigate the consequences of an environmental-chemical induced genomic and proteomic change and cytotoxicity in the central and peripheral nervous system; studies on the molecular and cellular mechanisms underlying the adverse effects of chemicals on the nervous system during development, in the adult and the aged; development of models to assess the physiological and morphology of neural circuits, including signal transduction, and their responses to chemical attack; investigations into the chronic and delayed actions of chemical substances, the genetic basis for susceptibility to chemical toxicity, and the role of occupational and environmental chemical outreach activities to disseminate information regarding the effects of exposure to occupational and environmental chemicals and current research at the center.

★ 23055 ★ Oregon Health and Science University
Center on Self-Determination
3608 SE Powell Blvd.
Portland, OR 97202
Phone: (503)232-9154 **Free:** 800-410-7069
Fax: (503)232-6423
Email: powersl@ohsu.edu
Website: http://cdrc.ohsu.edu/selfdetermination/
Laurie Powers, PhD, Co-Dir.
Activities/Fields: Identification, development, validation on and communication of policies and practices that promote the self-determination of people with and without disabilities. **Pub:** *Educational materials.*

★ 23056 ★ Oregon Health and Science University
Center for Women's Health
Baird Hall, Rm. 1036
3181 SW Sam Jackson Park Rd., L466
Portland, OR 97239
Phone: (503)494-0515
Email: cwh@ohsu.edu
Website: http://www.ohsu.edu/women/
Dr. Joanna Cain, Dir.
Activities/Fields: Gender-based biology.

★ 23057 ★ Oregon Health and Science University
Child Development and Rehabilitation Center (CDRC)
PO Box 574
Portland, OR 97207
Phone: (503)494-8364 **Fax:** (503)494-6868
Email: oidd@ohsu.edu
Website: http://www.ohsu.edu/cdrc/
Gloria Krahn, PhD, Exec. Dir.
Activities/Fields: Empowerment of individuals with developmental disabilities to improve the quality of their lives by developing, enhancing and sustaining culturally sensitive areas of support systems which function across the entire life span and include all domains of daily life.

★ 23058 ★ Oregon Health and Science University
DMSO Research Laboratory
3181 SW Sam Jackson Pk. Rd., L225
Portland, OR 97201
Phone: (503)494-8474 **Fax:** (503)494-5352
Email: jacobs@ohsu.edu
Website: http://www.dmso.org
Stanley W. Jacob, MD, Hd.
Activities/Fields: Pharmacological properties of dimethyl sulfoxide (DMSO). Provides staff consultants in clinical and basic research relevant to pharmacological activity of dimethyl sulfoxide.

★ 23059 ★ Oregon Health and Science University
General Clinical Research Center
3181 SW Sam Jackson Pk. Rd., CR107
Portland, OR 97201-3098
Phone: (503)494-7601 **Fax:** (503)494-0165
Email: pillowe@ohsu.edu
Website: http://www.ohsu.edu/gcrc/
Eric Orwoll, MD, Prog. Dir.
Activities/Fields: Cardiovascular disease, collagen vascular disease and immunology, endocrinology, hematology, hypertension, metabolism, neurology, oncology, pediatric nephrology, pharmacology, psychiatry, renal disease, and rheumatology. Testing services include steroid receptor analysis, membrane receptor analysis, radioimmunoassay, and spectrophotometric analyses.

★ 23060 ★ Oregon Health and Science University
Heart Research Center
3181 SW Sam Jackson Pk. Rd., L-464
Portland, OR 97201-3098
Phone: (503)494-2382 **Fax:** (503)494-4352
Email: thornbur@ohsu.edu
Website: http://www.ohsu.edu/chrc/
Kent L. Thornburg, PhD, Dir.
Activities/Fields: Broad-based heart research, including the link between fetal heart development and adult heart disease. **Pub:** *Heart Developments*, periodically. Newsletter. • *Heart Sounds*, semiannually.

★ 23061 ★ Oregon Health and Science University
Neurological Sciences Institute
West Campus
505 NW 185th Ave.
Beaverton, OR 97006
Phone: (503)418-2500 **Fax:** (503)418-2501
Website: http://www.ohsu.edu/nsi/
Paul J. Cordo, PhD, Dir.
Activities/Fields: Structure and function of the nervous system, from the level of the molecule to the level of the brain and sensory organs. Research focuses on balance and dizziness disorders, Alzheimer's and Parkinson's diseases, stroke, memory loss, multiple sclerosis, blindness, as well as a number of other neurological disorders. **Pub:** *Annual Report.* • *NSI Newsletter.*

★ 23062 ★ Oregon Health and Science University
Oregon Aging and Alzheimer's Disease Center (OADC)
Department of Neurology, CR131
3181 SW Sam Jackson Park Rd.
Portland, OR 97201-3098
Phone: (503)494-6976 **Fax:** (503)494-7499
Email: kaye@ohsu.edu
Website: http://www.ohsu.edu/som-alzheimers/
Dr. Jeffrey Kaye, Dir.
Activities/Fields: Alzheimer's Disease and related disorders.

★ 23063 ★ Oregon Health and Science University
Oregon Cancer Institute (OCI)
CR 145
3181 SW Sam Jackson Park Rd.
Portland, OR 97201-3098
Phone: (503)494-1617 **Fax:** (503)494-7096
Email: cancer@ohsu.edu
Website: http://www.ohsu.edu/oci/
Dr. Grover C. Bagby, Jr., Dir.
Activities/Fields: Prevention, treatment, diagnosis and control of cancer by identifying the specific pathophysiologically significant molecular defects in cancer cells.

★ 23064 ★ Oregon Health and Science University
Oregon Cancer Institute Leukemia Center
Mail Code UHN73A
3181 SW Sam Jackson Park Rd.
Portland, OR 97201-3098
Phone: (503)494-5058
Email: leukemia@ohsu.edu
Website: http://www.ohsuhealth.com/providers/fad_clinic_pre.asp?ClinicID=1000078&ps=P
Brian J. Druker, MD, Dir.
Activities/Fields: Hematological disorders with a focus on Chronic Myelogenous Leukemia (CML).

★ 23065 ★ Oregon Health and Science University
Oregon Center for Complementary and Alternative Medicine in Neurological Disorders
3181 SW Sam Jackson Park Rd.
Portland, OR 97239
Phone: (503)494-9519 **Fax:** (503)494-9520
Email: orcamind@ohsu.edu
Website: http://www.ohsu.edu/orccamind
Barry S. Oken, MD, Dir.
Activities/Fields: The use of CAM therapies as treatments for neurodegenerative and demyelinating diseases.

★ 23066 ★ Oregon Health and Science University
Oregon Hearing Research Center
3181 SW Sam Jackson Pk. Rd.
Portland, OR 97201-3098
Phone: (503)494-8032 **Free:** 800-222-6478
Fax: (503)494-5656
Email: ohrc@ohsu.edu
Website: http://www.ohsu.edu/ohrc/
Alfred L. Nuttall, PhD, Dir.
Activities/Fields: Hearing problems, including clinical studies of ototoxicity, vestibular physiology, noise damage, anatomy of the ear, tinnitus, and interactions between various insults to the ear, through a multiple attack utilizing electrophysiological measures, behavioral measures, histological evaluations, and human psychophysics. **Frmly:** Kresge Hearing Research Laboratory.

★ 23067 ★ Oregon Health and Science University
Oregon Regional Primate Research Center
505 NW 185th Ave.
Beaverton, OR 97006
Phone: (503)645-1141 **Fax:** (503)690-5532
Email: smithsu@ohsu.edu
Website: http://onprc.ohsu.edu/
Dr. M. Susan Smith, PhD, Dir.
Activities/Fields: Nonhuman primates, particularly reproductive biology, neuroscience, and experimental pathology. Specific projects include studies on the events that control fertility in primates, causes and control of premature labor, mechanisms of steroid action, and factors affecting neural differentiation, function and plasticity. Other projects seek to understand physiological mechanisms involved in atherosclerosis and immune deficiency diseases. Provides research facilities for staff and collaborative scientists.

★ 23068 ★ Oregon Health and Science University
Portland Alcohol Research Center (PARC)
VA Medical Center, R&D 12
Portland, OR 97239
Phone: (503)220-8262 **Fax:** (503)721-1029
Email: rutledgm@ohsu.edu
Website: http://www.ohsu.edu/parc
Dr. John Crabbe, Dir.
Activities/Fields: Genetics of neuroadaptation to ethanol, specifically how the brain adapts to alcohol, and mapping the genes underlying alcoholism risk.

★ 23069 ★ Oregon Health and Science University
Transplant and Immunogenetics Laboratory
2611 SW 3rd, Ste. 360
Portland, OR 97201
Phone: (503)494-8394 **Fax:** (503)494-7695
Email: normand@ohsu.edu
Douglas Norman, MD, Dir.
Activities/Fields: Human immunobiology of organ transplantation.

★ 23070 ★ Oregon Health and Science University
Vollum Institute
3181 SW Sam Jackson Pk. Rd., L474
Portland, OR 97239-3098
Phone: (503)494-5453 **Fax:** (503)494-4590
Email: goodmanr@ohsu.edu
Website: http://www.ohsu.edu/vollum
Dr. Richard H. Goodman, Dir.
Activities/Fields: Molecular biology, protein chemistry, virology, and immunology of the endocrine system and brain and nervous system. Also conducts studies in electrophysiology and pharmacology. **Pub:** *Biennial Report.*

★ 23071 ★ Oregon Institute of Science and Medicine
2251 Dick George Rd.
Cave Junction, OR 97523-9622
Phone: (541)592-4142 **Fax:** (541)592-2597
Email: art@oism.org
Website: http://www.oism.org
Arthur B. Robinson, PhD, Pres.
Activities/Fields: Protein chemistry, molecular biology, nutrition and preventive medicine, and medical diagnostic techniques.

★ 23072 ★ Oregon State University
Environmental Health Sciences Center
1011 ALS
Corvallis, OR 97331-7302
Phone: (541)737-8820 **Fax:** (541)737-4371
Email: joe.beckman@oregonstate.edu
Website: http://www.ehsc.orst.edu
Joe Beckman, PhD, Contact
Activities/Fields: Provides and stimulates coordinated multidisciplinary research to assess the impact of environmental chemicals on human health and to predict associated short- and long-term effects. Specific research draws upon capabilities of faculty, staff, and graduate students in chemistry, biochemistry, agricultural chemistry, biology, food science, fisheries and wildlife, veterinary medicine, pharmacology, toxicology, immunology, and statistics. Focal areas include toxicology of environmental chemicals and naturally occurring toxins, cellular and biochemical toxicology, carcinogenesis of environmental chemicals, mechanisms of toxicity, genetic toxicology, immunotoxicology, mass spectrometry, statistical studies, and analysis of enumerative data related to environmental health research.

★ 23073 ★ Oregon State University
Linus Pauling Institute (LPI)
571 Weniger Hall
Corvallis, OR 97331
Phone: (541)737-5075 **Fax:** (541)737-5077
Email: lpi@oregonstate.edu
Website: http://oregonstate.edu/dept/lpi/
Balz Frei, Dir.
Activities/Fields: Function and role of micronutrients, vitamins, and phytochemicals in promoting optimum health and preventing and treating disease; and the role of oxidative stress and antioxidants in human health and disease. **Pub:** *Newsletter*, semiannually.

★ 23074 ★ Orentreich Foundation for the Advancement of Science, Inc.
Biomedical Research Station
855 Rte. 301
Cold Spring, NY 10516
Phone: (845)265-4200 **Fax:** (845)265-4210
Email: ofas1@juno.com
Rozlyn Krajcik, Asst. Dir.
Activities/Fields: Dermatology, aging, endocrinology, and serum markers for human diseases. **Pub:** *Report of the Director.*

★ 23075 ★ Orthodontic Education and Research Foundation
3320 Rutger
Saint Louis, MO 63104
Phone: (314)577-8189 **Fax:** (314)268-5673
Email: moscalb@slu.edu
Becky Moscal, Contact
Activities/Fields: Orthodontics, focusing on research and education.

★ 23076 ★ Orthopaedic Research Institute
929 N St. Francis
Wichita, KS 67214-3882
Phone: (316)268-5454 **Fax:** (316)291-4998
Email: ori@via-christi.org
David A. McQueen, Pres.
Activities/Fields: Design, development, and testing of orthopaedic implants, materials, and instruments. Specific areas of research include artificial replacement joints, absorbable pins and rods for surgically stabilizing bone fractures, devices for the fusion of severely compromised knees, applying a metal foam to orthopaedic implants for tissue attachment, improving external frames for controlling grossly unstable fractures of the pelvis, and combining absorbable glass fibers and plastics for composite implants in the human body. **Pub:** *Orthopaedic Technology Brief*, occasionally.

★ 23077 ★ Orthopedic Biomechanics Institute
5848 S Fashion Blvd.
Murray, UT 84107
Phone: (801)314-4030 **Fax:** (801)314-4015
Benjamin Ellis, Dir.
Activities/Fields: Orthopedic biomechanics and sports injuries.

★ 23078 ★ Orthopedic Research Society
6300 N River Rd., Ste. 727
Rosemont, IL 60018
Phone: (847)698-1625 **Fax:** (847)823-4921
Email: ors@aaos.org
Website: http://www.ors.org
Brenda Welborn, Exec. Dir.
Activities/Fields: Orthopedic surgery and research.

★ 23079 ★ OSHTECH Inc.
400 York St., Ste. 100
London, ON, Canada N6B 3N2
Phone: (519)642-1122 **Fax:** (519)542-0331
Email: oshtech@oshtechinc.com
Website: http://www.oshtechinc.com
Dr. Peter Pityn, Contact
Activities/Fields: Occupational health and safety, residential and office air quality, ergonomics, inhalational studies, and occupational hygiene, analytical methods development. **Pub:** *Reports.* **Frmly:** Occupational Health and Safety Resource Centre.

★ 23080 ★ Ottawa Health Research Institute (OHRI)
725 Parkdale Ave.
Ottawa, ON, Canada K1Y 4E9
Phone: (613)761-4395 **Fax:** (613)761-4920
Email: info@ohri.ca
Website: http://www.ohri.ca/
Dr. Ronald G. Worton, CEO/Sci. Dir.
Activities/Fields: Health and disease, particularly increasing understanding what is happening at the molecular and cellular level in complex disease states, and best practices in the delivery of health care.

★ 23081 ★ Ottawa Heart Institute Research Corp.
40 Ruskin St.
Ottawa, ON, Canada K1Y 4W7
Phone: (613)761-4585 **Fax:** (613)761-4214
Email: jirvine@ottawaheart.ca
Website: http://www.ottawaheart.ca
D. Joe Irvine, Pres.
Activities/Fields: Cardiac diseases, emphasizing arteriosclerosis research and dyslipidemia, hypertension, cell and molecular biology of the heart, vascular biology, pharmacology, medical devices, artificial hearts, clinical trials and prevention and rehabilitation.

★ 23082 ★ Ottawa Regional Cancer Center
503 Smyth Rd.
Ottawa, ON, Canada K1H 1C4
Phone: (613)737-7700
Website: http://www.orcc.on.ca/
Hartley Stern, MD, CEO
Activities/Fields: Improvement in cancer patient care, extending survival, and ultimately curing patients

of their cancer by means of innovative cancer therapies. Other programs investigate the basic biology of cancer cells as well as the application of radiation in cancer therapy.

★ 23083 ★ Pacific Health Research Institute
Thomas Sq. Ctr.
846 S Hotel St., Ste. 303
Honolulu, HI 96813
Phone: (808)524-4411 **Fax:** (808)524-5559
Email: vshamba@phri.hawaii-health.com
Website: http://www.phrihawaii.org
Dr. J. David Curb, CEO/Med. Dir.
Activities/Fields: Health services and clinical research, including breast cancer, hypertension, osteoporosis, diabetes, heart attacks, drug studies, effects of chemical exposure, and cost-effectiveness analysis. Specific studies focus on risk factors associated with breast cancer, methods of delaying or preventing postmenopausal osteoporosis, isolated systolic hypertension among the elderly, outcomes research, leprosy, interactive videodiscs, geriatrics, and prostate, lung, colorectal, and ovarian cancer screening. Participates in a statewide consortium of hospitals to address quality and cost of care. Hawaii MEDTEP (Medical Treatment Effectiveness Program) Research Center, outcomes research with a focus on minority populations. **Frmly:** Straub Medical Research Institute.

★ 23084 ★ Pacific Institute for Research and Evaluation
Decision Sciences Institute
120 Wayland Ave., Ste. 7
Providence, RI 02906
Phone: (401)751-1314 **Fax:** (401)751-1592
Email: dwight@pire.org
Website: http://www.pire.org/centers/DSI.asp
Robert Stout, PhD, Dir.
Activities/Fields: Decision-making in areas such as long-term cost-effectiveness of alcohol treatment, impact of addictions and mental health treatment on general medical care, and managed care.

★ 23085 ★ Pacific Institute for Research and Evaluation
PIRE Chapel Hill Center
1229 E Franklin St., 2nd Fl.
Chapel Hill, NC 27514
Phone: (919)967-8998 **Fax:** (919)968-1498
Email: jester@pire.org
Website: http://www.pire.org/centers/ChapelHill.asp
Janet Jester, Contact
Activities/Fields: Design and implementation of innovative program evaluation and needs assessment studies, and epidemiological research relating to public health issues.

★ 23086 ★ Pacific Northwest Research Institute
720 Broadway
Seattle, WA 98122
Phone: (206)726-1200 **Fax:** (206)726-1217
Email: donations@pnri.org
Website: http://www.pnri.org
R. Paul Robertson, MD, CEO/Sci. Dir.
Activities/Fields: Medical sciences, including Type I and II diabetes, pancreas and islet transplantation, environmental biochemistry, membrane biochemistry, biochemical oncology, molecular epidemiology, and cell and molecular biology.

★ 23087 ★ Pacific Vascular Research Foundation
3627 Sacramento St.
San Francisco, CA 94118
Phone: (415)771-3541 **Fax:** (415)771-3902
Email: info@pvrf.org
Website: http://www.pvrf.org
Juli L. Weiss, PhD, Dir.
Activities/Fields: Issues related to vascular health and diseases and initiatives that promote public awareness and education about vascular diseases.

★ 23088 ★ Packard Children's Hospital at Stanford
Rehabilitation Technology Center
1010 Corporation Way
Palo Alto, CA 94303
Phone: (650)237-9200 **Fax:** (650)237-9204
Email: re.hzo@lpch.stanford.edu
Website: http://www-med.stanford.edu/lpch/rec/
Hugh O'Neill, Actg. Dir.
Activities/Fields: Rehabilitation technology, emphasizing speech aids, prosthetics, orthotics, seating, mobility, and worksite accommodation for people with disabilities.

★ 23089 ★ Palo Alto Institute of Molecular Medicine
2462 Wyandotte St.
Mountain View, CA 94043
Phone: (650)694-1420 **Fax:** (650)694-7717
Email: paimm@netgate.net
Website: http://www.paimm.org
Dr. James W. Larrick, Dir.
Activities/Fields: Cellular and molecular biology, cancer, and immunoinflammatory diseases.

★ 23090 ★ Palo Alto Medical Foundation
795 El Camino Real
Palo Alto, CA 94301
Phone: (650)321-4121 **Fax:** (650)853-5702
Website: http://www.pamf.org
David Druker, MD, Pres. /CEO
Activities/Fields: Basic and clinical biomedical research.

★ 23091 ★ Paralyzed Veterans of America
Spinal Cord Research Foundation (SCRF)
801 18th St. NW
Washington, DC 20006-3517
Phone: (202)416-7651 **Free:** 800-424-8200
Fax: (202)416-7641
Email: foundations@pva.org
Website: http://www.pva.org/NEWPVASITE/research%20&%20education/scrf/scrf.htm
Activities/Fields: Clinical, psychosocial, and technological aspects of spinal cord injury or dysfunction.

★ 23092 ★ Parker Hughes Cancer Center
2699 Patton Rd.
Roseville, MN 55113
Phone: (651)796-5400
Email: info@parkerhughes.org
Website: http://www.ih.org/
Fatih M. Uckun, MD, Med. Dir.
Activities/Fields: Cancer treatments, especially the development of new, effective anti-cancer drugs.

★ 23093 ★ Parkinson's Institute
1170 Morse Ave.
Sunnyvale, CA 94089-1605
Phone: (408)734-2800 **Free:** 800-786-2958
Fax: (408)734-8522
Website: http://www.parkinsonsinstitute.org
Dr. J. William Langston, CEO
Activities/Fields: Cause and cure of movement disorders, identification of better treatment and diagnostic tools, and development of prevention strategies.

★ 23094 ★ Parkinson's and Movement Disorder Institute (PMDI)
9940 Talbert Ave., Ste. 204
Fountain Valley, CA 92708
Phone: (714)378-5062 **Fax:** (714)378-5061
Email: dtruong@pmdi.org
Website: http://www.pmdi.org/pmdi.html
Dr. Daniel D. Truong, Contact
Activities/Fields: Parkinson's disease and movement disorders such as dystonia, myoclonus, tremor, and chorea.

★ 23095 ★ Pediatric Clinical Trials International
555 S 18th St., Ste. 6E
Columbus, OH 43205
Phone: (614)722-4453 **Fax:** (614)722-2663
Email: wentzelg@pedcti.com
Website: http://www.pedcti.com
Belinda Pinyerd, PhD, Oper. Dir.
Activities/Fields: Childhood illnesses, pharmacology, metabolic and infectious diseases, drug metabolism in children, and endocrine disorders of children. **Frmly:** Children's Hospital Clinical Studies Center.

★ 23096 ★ Pediatric Oncology Group
Operations Office
645 N Michigan Ave., Ste. 910
Chicago, IL 60611
Phone: (312)482-9944 **Fax:** (312)482-9460
Website: http://www.pog.ufl.edu/publ/org.htm
Dr. Sharon B. Murphy, Hd.
Activities/Fields: Investigations of childhood cancers. Provides a national cooperative mechanism to promote new treatment methods through comparison of patients who receive different treatments.

★ 23097 ★ Pennsylvania College of Optometry
Cornea and Specialty Contact Lens Service (CASCLS)
1200 W Godfrey Ave.
Philadelphia, PA 19141
Phone: (215)276-6000 **Fax:** (215)276-6101
Email: joel@pco.edu
Dr. Joel A. Silbert, Ch.
Activities/Fields: Progression of the corneal warpage syndrome known as keratoconus; cornea and contact lenses studies, including testing lenses and lens care products for various manufacturers. The study on keratoconus, known as the Collaborative Longitudinal Evaluation of Keratoconus, is funded by the National Eye Institute.

★ 23098 ★ Pennsylvania College of Optometry
Glaucoma Research Center
1200 W Godfrey Ave.
Philadelphia, PA 19141
Phone: (215)276-6000 **Fax:** (215)276-6101
Email: rbennett@pco.edu
G. Richard Bennett, OD, Dir.
Activities/Fields: Determining whether patients with ocular hypertension (elevated eye pressure but without glaucoma) benefit over the longer term from medical management of their pressure. This study, known as the Ocular Hypertension Treatment Study, is funded by the National Eye Institute for eight years.

★ 23099 ★ Pennsylvania College of Optometry
Hafter Family Light and Laser Institute
Old York Rd. & Township Line Rd.
Philadelphia, PA 19141
Phone: (215)780-1427 **Fax:** (215)780-1325
Email: felix@pco.edu
Dr. Felix M. Barker, Dir.
Activities/Fields: Corneal and retinal light damage effects, especially from short wavelength energy sources; ocular photosensitization; laser effects; excimer laser studies, including corneal wound healing in normal and diabetic individuals; glaucoma; myopia; keratoconus.

★ 23100 ★ Pennsylvania College of Optometry
Institute for the Visually Impaired (IVI)
8360 Old York Rd.
Elkins Park, PA 19027
Phone: (215)780-1400 **Fax:** (215)780-1336
Email: nancy@pco.edu
Audrey J. Smith, Exec. Dir.
Activities/Fields: Partial sight or low vision, including rehabilitation teaching, and low vision rehabilitation, orientation, and mobility.

★ 23101 ★ Pennsylvania Department of Health
Bureau of Epidemiology
Health & Welfare Bldg., Rm. 933
Harrisburg, PA 17108
Phone: (717)783-4677 **Fax:** (717)772-6975
Joel Hersh, Dir.
Activities/Fields: Disease control and incidences in populations for the purposes of intervention. Specific programs include: communicable disease epidemiology, environmental health assessment, HIV/AIDS epidemiology, cancer epidemiology, and chronic disease epidemiology.

★ 23102 ★ Pennsylvania Department of Health
Bureau of Laboratories
110 Pickering Way
Lionville, PA 19353
Phone: (610)280-3464 **Fax:** (610)450-1932
Email: bkleger@state.pa.us
Bruce Kleger, Dir.
Activities/Fields: Public health issues.

★ 23103 ★ Pennsylvania State University
Artificial Heart Research Project
Milton S Hershey Medical Center
500 University Dr.
Hershey, PA 17033
Phone: (717)531-6301 **Fax:** (717)531-4464
Email: grosenberg@psu.edu
Website: http://www.hmc.psu.edu
Gerson Rosenberg, PhD, Dir.
Activities/Fields: Development of an implantable, long-term, motor-driven left ventricular assist pump, an implantable, pneumatically-driven total artificial heart, and an implantable, motor-driven electric artificial heart, including all aspects of design of implantable blood pumps, implantable energy convertors, bench testing and evaluation, and animal implantation studies.

★ 23104 ★ Pennsylvania State University
BioBehavioral Health Studies Laboratory
315 E Health & Human Development
Department of Biobehavioral Health
University Park, PA 16802
Phone: (814)865-8813 **Fax:** (814)863-7525
Email: lxk18@psu.edu
Website: http://bbh.hhdev.psu.edu/labs/bbhsl/
Dr. Laura Cousino Klein, Dir.
Activities/Fields: Individual differences in the biobehavioral effects of stress. Research focuses on the effects of stress on appetite behaviors (i.e., cigarette smoking, eating); sex differences in neuroendocrine, immunological, and behavioral responses to stress; and developmental influences on biobehavioral stress responses.

★ 23105 ★ Pennsylvania State University
Biomechanics Laboratory
39 Recreation Hall
University Park, PA 16802
Phone: (814)865-3445 **Fax:** (814)865-2440
Email: vxz1@psu.edu
Website: http://www.psu.edu/dept/biomechanics
Dr. Vladimir Zatisiorsky, Dir.
Activities/Fields: Human movement, including scientific study and analysis of human motion as observed in sports, industry, and activities of daily living. Analyzes gymnastics, diving, cross-country skiing, swimming, and other sports through use of high-speed video, force measuring devices, and online computer techniques. Studies of elite athletes in Olympic and world championships are conducted with support of U.S. Olympic Committee and the Medical Commission of the International Olympic Committee. Testing, evaluation, and development of sports equipment and playground surface materials are also conducted.

★ 23106 ★ Pennsylvania State University
Center for Locomotion Studies
Recreation Bldg., Rm. 29
University Park, PA 16802-2002
Phone: (814)865-1972 **Fax:** (814)863-4755
Email: celos@psu.edu
Website: http://www.celos.psu.edu
Neil A. Sharkey, PhD, Interim Dir.
Activities/Fields: Gait analysis and foot mechanics with particular emphasis on diabetic patients, children with cerebral palsy, and the elderly; elucidation of the pathogenesis of osteoporosis, including genetic control, and development of preventative interventions; development of computer modeling tools for selection of cerebral palsy patients who are likely to benefit from specific interventions and providing rationales for new measures to correct the mechanics of walking disrupted by cerebral palsy; the nature and causes of locomotor pathologies. **Pub:** *The Foot in Diabetes: A Bibliography.*

★ 23107 ★ Pennsylvania State University
Center for Sports Medicine
1850 E Park Ave., Ste. 112
State College, PA 16803
Phone: (814)865-3566 **Fax:** (814)865-7803
Email: wsebastianell@psu.edu
Dr. Wayne Sebastianelli, Dir.
Activities/Fields: Physiology of human performance, sports conditioning, and the role of exercise in the prevention and rehabilitation of sports injuries. Areas of investigation include molecular biology, physiology, biomechanics, locomotion studies, nutrition, bioengineering, and epidemiology.

★ 23108 ★ Pennsylvania State University
Children's Eating Laboratory (CEL)
S-110 Henderson Bldg.
University Park, PA 16802
Phone: (814)863-9972 **Fax:** (814)865-7307
Email: llb15@psu.edu
Website: http://www.psu.edu/dept/kidseatinglab/
Dr. Leann L. Birch, Dir.
Activities/Fields: Development of children's eating behaviors, including food preferences, food selection, and regulation of meal size.

★ 23109 ★ Pennsylvania State University
Doctors Kienle Center for Humanistic Medicine
Milton S Hershey Medical Center
500 University Dr.
Hershey, PA 17033-0850
Phone: (717)531-8778 **Fax:** (717)531-3894
Email: dhufford@psu.edu
David J. Hufford, PhD, Dir.
Activities/Fields: Developing programs in humanistic medicine, including medical curriculum concerning the patients experience of care, phenomonology of care, and human diversity and medicine.

★ 23110 ★ Pennsylvania State University
Gastrointestinal Psychophysiology Laboratory
535 Moore Bldg.
Department of Psychology
University Park, PA 16802
Phone: (814)865-6218
Email: rs3@psu.edu
Website: http://psych.la.psu.edu/egglab/egg.htm
Robert M. Stern, PhD, Dir.
Activities/Fields: Psychophysiology of the gastrointestinal system in people suffering from gastrointestinal and eating disorders and those who do not.

★ 23111 ★ Pennsylvania State University
General Clinical Research Center
Milton S Hershey Medical Center
Box 850, Mail Code H147
Hershey, PA 17033
Phone: (717)531-5154 **Free:** 800-336-2591
Fax: (717)531-3836
Email: lsinoway@psu.edu
Website: http://www.hmc.psu.edu/gcrc
Lawrence I. Sinoway, MD, Prog. Dir.
Activities/Fields: Major areas of investigation include cardiovascular metabolic responses, diabetes and metabolism, gastrointestinal research, pediatric metabolism, pulmonary metabolic responses, sleep-related metabolic responses and women's health.

★ 23112 ★ Pennsylvania State University
Gerontology Center
S-105 Henderson Bldg.
University Park, PA 16802
Phone: (814)865-1710 **Fax:** (814)863-9423
Email: gero@psu.edu
Website: http://geron.psu.edu
Dr. K. Warner Schaie, Dir.
Activities/Fields: Aging, including cognition in aging, developmental methodology, family and informal supports, human services for the elderly, caregiving, urinary incontinence, and the use of pharmaceutical products. **Pub:** *Annual preprint/reprint catalog*, biennially. • *Newsletter*, biennially.

★ 23113 ★ Pennsylvania State University
Laboratory for the Study of Human Ingestive Behavior
226 Henderson Bldg.
State College, PA 16803
Phone: (814)863-8482 **Fax:** (814)863-8574
Email: bjr4@psu.edu
Website: http://nutrition.hhdev.psu.edu/foodlab/miss_obj/
Dr. Barbara Jean Rolls, Dir.
Activities/Fields: Human eating behavior in a variety of populations and settings, especially how human food intake is regulated in different populations (i.e. lean versus obese; male versus female; young versus elderly).

★ 23114 ★ Pennsylvania State University
Motor Control Laboratory
Recreational Bldg., 20
State College, PA 16801
Phone: (814)863-4424 **Fax:** (814)863-4424
Email: mll11@psu.edu
Website: http://www.personal.psu.edu/faculty/m/l/mll11/mcl.html
Prof. Mark L. Latash, PhD, Dir.
Activities/Fields: Multi-joint limb movements, postural control, multi-limb coordination; changes in movement and posture coordination with age; and neurological disorders. **Pub:** *Refereed publications.*

★ 23115 ★ Pennsylvania State University
Movement Neuroscience Laboratory
27 REC Bldg.
University Park, PA 16802
Phone: (814)863-7938 **Fax:** (814)865-1275
Email: rls45@psu.edu
Website: http://www.personal.psu.edu/rls45
Robert L. Sainburg, PhD, Dir.
Activities/Fields: Neural mechanisms underlying control of multijoint reaching movements in humans, specifically, the roles of proprioception and vision in

planning and executing reaching movements, and the neural foundations of handedness.

★ 23116 ★ Pennsylvania State University Noll Physiological Research Center
129 Noll Laboratory Bldg.
University Park, PA 16802-6900
Phone: (814)865-3453 **Fax:** (814)865-4602
Email: paf4@psu.edu
Website: http://www.noll.psu.edu/
Dr. Peter A. Farrell, Dir.
Activities/Fields: Metabolic adaptations to stress, biology of aging, and environmental and exercise physiology. Studies the effects of aging, physical inactivity, nutritional status, and heat, cold, and altitude stress on muscle metabolism and function, thermoregulation and cardiovascular control, reproduction, function and carbohydrate, insulin, and protein metabolism. **Frmly:** Laboratory for Human Performance Research.

★ 23117 ★ Pennsylvania State University Noll Physiological Research Center General Clinical Research Center (GCRC)
112 Elmore Research Wing
University Park, PA 16802-6501
Phone: (814)865-4302 **Fax:** (814)865-0351
Email: gcrc@psu.edu
Website: http://www.gcrc.psu.edu/
Jan Ulbrecht, MD, Assoc. Prog. Dir.
Activities/Fields: Pathogenic mechanisms of disease and strategies for health promotion and disease prevention.

★ 23118 ★ Pennsylvania State University Vascular Health Interventions Laboratory
315 Health & Human Development Bldg. E
Department of Biobehavioral Health
University Park, PA 16802
Phone: (814)863-0176 **Fax:** (814)863-7525
Email: sgw2@psu.edu
Website: http://bbh.hhdev.psu.edu/labs/westlab/
Prof. Sheila G. West, PhD, Dir.
Activities/Fields: Changes in cardiovascular responses to psychological stress after dietary interventions. The ultimate goal is to allow new interventions to be tested for their effects on multiple coronary risk markers simultaneously, in order to aid in the design of new functional foods and new dietary regimens for patients with cardiovascular problems.

★ 23119 ★ Philadelphia Biomedical Research Institute
100 Ross & Royal Rds.
King of Prussia, PA 19406
Phone: (610)962-0615 **Fax:** (610)962-0614
Email: stohnishi@aol.com
Website: http://members.aol.com/stohnishi/phila_biomed/sickle.htm
S. Tsuyoshi Ohnishi, PhD, Dir.
Activities/Fields: Mechanisms, methods of diagnosis, and pharmacological treatment of membrane-linked diseases through investigation of structure-function relationship in normal and abnormal biological membranes. Studies focus on the nutritional means to manage sickle cell anemia. **Pub:** *Arzneimittel Forschung/Drug Research.* • *Brain Research.* • *Cancer Letters.* • *Free Radicals in Biology and Medicine.* • *Prostaglandins Leucotrienes and Essential Fatty Acids.*

★ 23120 ★ Physical Medicine Research Foundation (PMRF)
856 Homer St., Ste. 204
Vancouver, BC, Canada V6B 2W5
Phone: (604)684-4148 **Fax:** (604)684-6247
Email: pmrf@icpro.org
Website: http://www.icpro.org/index2.htm
Activities/Fields: Reduction of disability and impairment from soft tissue injuries.

★ 23121 ★ Pittsburgh Adolescent Alcohol Research Center (PAARC)
3811 O'Hara St.
Pittsburgh, PA 15213
Phone: (412)624-2636 **Fax:** (412)624-0850
Email: clarkdb@msx.upmc.edu
Website: http://www.pitt.edu/~paarc/paarc.html
Dr. Duncan B. Clark, Dir.
Activities/Fields: Adolescent alcohol abuse and dependence, including biobehavioral manifestations. **Pub:** *Newsletter.*

★ 23122 ★ PKD Foundation
4901 Main St., Ste. 200
Kansas City, MO 64112-2634
Phone: (816)931-2600 **Free:** 800-753-2873
Fax: (816)931-8655
Email: pkdcure@pkdcure.org
Website: http://www.pkdcure.org
Dave Switzer, Mktg. /PR Dir.
Activities/Fields: Treatment and cure of polycystic kidney disease (PKD). Activities include identification of gene defect responsible for PKD, analysis of abnormal cell and cyst growth, and analysis of kidney function and progressive kidney failure. **Pub:** *The Family and ADPKD: A Guide for Children and Parents.* • *Health Tips for Living with PKD.* • *PKD Patients Manual "Your Child, Your Family and ARPKD".* • *PKD Progress Newsletter.* • *Q&A on PKD.* **Frmly:** Polycystic Kidney Research Foundation.

★ 23123 ★ Plastic Surgery Research Council (Hanover, NH)
45 Lyme Rd., Ste. 304
Hanover, NH 03755
Phone: (603)643-2325 **Fax:** (603)643-1444
Email: psrc@sover.net
Website: http://www.ps-rc.org
Catherin B. Foss, Contact
Activities/Fields: Plastic surgery.

★ 23124 ★ Plastic Surgery Research Council (Pittsburgh, PA)
Scaife Hall, 666
University of Pittsburgh Medical Center
3550 Terrace St.
Pittsburgh, PA 15261
Phone: (412)648-8100 **Fax:** (412)648-1987
Email: mandersek@upmc.edu
Dr. Ernest K. Manders, Dir.
Activities/Fields: Tissue engineering.

★ 23125 ★ Plattsburgh State University of New York Auditory Research Laboratory
107 Beaumont Hall
Plattsburgh, NY 12901
Phone: (518)564-7700 **Fax:** (518)564-7827
Email: hamernrp@plattsburgh.edu
Website: http://www.plattsburgh.edu/arl/
Dr. Roger P. Hamernik, Dir.
Activities/Fields: Pathology of hearing associated with noise, drugs, congenital birth defects, and disease processes.

★ 23126 ★ Polytechnical School of Montreal Research Group in Biomechanics and Biomaterials
Institut de genie biomedical
PO Box 6079, Downtown Sta.
Montreal, QC, Canada H3C 3A7
Phone: (514)340-4711 **Fax:** (514)340-4611
Email: yahia@grbb.polymtl.ca
Website: http://www.grbb.polymtl.ca
L'Hocine Yahia, Dir.
Activities/Fields: Biomechanical behavior of the musculoskeletal system, including the following: modelling of the behavior of human joints and biological tissues; graphic representation of biological structures; biomechanics and microstructure of biological tissues and artificial substitutes; computer-aided design and manufacturing of orthopedic and rehabilitation devices; and stress analysis of knee implants.

★ 23127 ★ Pope Paul VI Institute for the Study of Human Reproduction, Inc.
6901 Mercy Rd.
Omaha, NE 68106-2604
Phone: (402)390-6600 **Fax:** (402)390-9851
Email: popepaul@popepaulvi.com
Website: http://www.popepaulvi.com
Dr. Thomas W. Hilgers, Dir.
Activities/Fields: Human reproduction and Down's Syndrome.

★ 23128 ★ Population Council
1 Dag Hammarskjold Plz.
New York, NY 10017
Phone: (212)339-0500 **Fax:** (212)755-6052
Email: pubinfo@popcouncil.org
Website: http://www.popcouncil.org
Linda G. Martin, Pres.
Activities/Fields: Biomedical, social science, and public health research. Analyzes demographic trends; conducts biomedical research to understand human reproductive physiology more fully, leading to development of new contraceptives and reproductive health products; works with public and private agencies to promote client-centered reproductive health services of high quality; helps governments design and implement population and development policies; communicates the results of research in the population field; and helps build research capacities in developing countries. **Pub:** *Annual report.* • *Fact books,* quarterly. • *Newsletter,* bimonthly. • *Population and Development Review,* quarterly. • *Studies in Family Planning,* bimonthly.

★ 23129 ★ Portland VA Research Foundation, Inc.
PO Box 69539
Portland, OR 97201-0539
Phone: (503)273-5228 **Fax:** (503)402-2866
Email: david.hickam@med.va.gov
David Hickam, MD, Pres.
Activities/Fields: Medicine and medical research.

★ 23130 ★ Precision Chiropractic Research Society
3462 Windsor Ct.
Costa Mesa, CA 92626
Phone: (714)641-4700
A.C. Fulkerson, Pres.
Activities/Fields: Spinal problems and treatment, including an investigation of the relationship between the cure for headaches and spinal adjustment. Also studies Duchenne muscular dystrophy.

★ 23131 ★ Preventive Medicine Institute
428 E 72nd St.
New York, NY 10021-4601
Phone: (212)794-4900 **Fax:** (212)794-4959
Email: osborne@strang.org
Website: http://www.strang.org
Dr. Michael P. Osborne, Pres.
Activities/Fields: Breast, colon, prostate, and other cancers and nutrition. **Pub:** *Newsletter,* semiannually.

★ 23132 ★ Preventive Medicine Research Institute
900 Bridgeway
Sausalito, CA 94965
Phone: (415)332-2525 **Fax:** (415)332-5730
Email: ebpett@aol.com
Website: http://www.pmri.org
Dean Ornish, MD, Pres. /Dir.
Activities/Fields: Prevention and treatment of heart disease and other chronic diseases and lifestyle risk factors through modification of diet, exercise, and

relaxation techniques such as yoga, meditation, and visualization.

★ 23133 ★ Primate Foundation of Arizona
PO Box 20027
Mesa, AZ 85277-0027
Phone: (480)832-3780 **Fax:** (480)830-7039
Email: jopfa@qwest.net
Jo Fritz, Prin. Investigator
Activities/Fields: Improvement in the captive management of chimpanzees. **Pub:** *Newsletter*, quarterly.

★ 23134 ★ Princess Margaret Hospital Prostate Centre
610 University Ave., 4th Fl.
Toronto, ON, Canada M5G 2M9
Phone: (416)946-2100 **Fax:** (416)598-9997
Email: john.trachtenberg@utoronto.ca
Website: http://www.prostatecanada.net
John Trachtenberg, MD, Dir.
Activities/Fields: Prostatic disease.

★ 23135 ★ Princeton University Center for the Study of Brain, Mind, and Behavior (CSBMB)
Green Hall
Princeton, NJ 08544
Phone: (609)258-2696 **Fax:** (609)258-2549
Email: jdc@princeton.edu
Website: http://www.csbmb.princeton.edu/
Prof. Jonathan D. Cohen, Dir.
Activities/Fields: Relationship of brain and mind. The specific focus of research is on the neural bases of higher mental functions; that is, the brain mechanisms by which memory, thought and action are integrated and controlled by higher level goals, and modulated by states of arousal, motivation, and emotion.

★ 23136 ★ Princeton University Cutaneous Communication Laboratory
Green Hall
Psychology Department
Princeton, NJ 08544-1010
Phone: (609)258-5277 **Fax:** (609)258-1113
Email: rcholewi@princeton.edu
Website: http://www.princeton.edu/~pucclabs
Dr. Roger W. Cholewiak, Prin. Investigator
Activities/Fields: Sensory psychophysiology and experimental psychology, including experimental investigations in all phases of cutaneous sensitivity with special reference to utilization of data in communication systems, under conditions of sensory handicap, or when other sensory modalities are overloaded. Research includes studies of pattern recognition and discrimination with psychophysical procedures and scaling techniques, including multidimensional designs; more elementary dimensions of tactile experience; and the interrelations of various dimensions of touch.

★ 23137 ★ Princeton University Lewis-Sigler Institute for Integrative Genomics
119B Lewis Thomas Laboratories
Princeton, NJ 08544
Phone: (609)258-3731 **Fax:** (609)258-7070
Email: genomics@princeton.edu
Website: http://www.genomics.princeton.edu/
David Botstein, Dir.
Activities/Fields: Biology in a post genomic era, particularly an understanding of how biological systems organize and integrate complex processes.

★ 23138 ★ Productive Rehabilitation Institute of Dallas for Ergonomics (PRIDE)
5701 Maple, Ste. 100
Dallas, TX 75235
Phone: (214)351-6600 **Fax:** (214)351-6453
Email: prode@airmail.net
Website: http://www.pridedallas.com
Robert J. Gatchel, PhD, Dir.
Activities/Fields: Ergonomics. Projects focus on utilizing physical exercise for rehabilitating chronic back problems. Patients use gym and spa equipment, participate in aerobics, and mimic job-related conditions such as crawling through pipes, moving equipment on assembly lines, driving four-wheelers, crawling around on building skeletons, and jumping up and onto a moving platform. **Pub:** *Functional Restoration*, quarterly.

★ 23139 ★ Project Hope Center for Health Affairs
7500 Old Georgetown Rd., Ste. 600
Bethesda, MD 20814-6133
Phone: (301)656-7401 **Fax:** (301)654-0629
Email: mberk@projecthope.org
Website: http://www.projecthope.org/CHA/
Marc L. Berk, PhD, Dir.
Activities/Fields: U.S. and foreign health systems, especially financing, care for vulnerable populations, quality of care. **Pub:** *CHA News.* • *Meeting proceedings.* • *Policy analysis briefs.* • *Research reports.*

★ 23140 ★ Prosthetics Research Study
675 S Lane St., Ste. 100
Seattle, WA 98104-2942
Phone: (206)903-8136 **Fax:** (206)903-8141
Email: dgsmith@u.washington.edu
Website: http://www.prs-research.org
Douglas G. Smith, MD, Dir.
Activities/Fields: Wound healing and limb viability, prosthesis research and development, mobility aids and artificial limbs, functional electrical physiological response, pain control, neuromuscular assist devices, electrical osteogenesis, mechanical engineering and automated fabrication of prosthetic components and mobility aids, and amputation surgery and post-surgical management.

★ 23141 ★ Protein Engineering Network (PENCE)
750 Heritage Medical Research Centre
University of Alberta
Edmonton, AB, Canada T6G 2S2
Phone: (780)492-8851 **Fax:** (780)492-6995
Email: info@pence.ca
Website: http://www.pence.ca
Steve Withers, CEO & Sci. Dir.
Activities/Fields: Research focuses on both discovery and development of proteins, peptides, glycopeptides and bioinformatics for applications as products or services for medical, veterinary and industry applications. **Pub:** *Pence News.* Newsletter.

★ 23142 ★ Providence Ambulatory Center
5050 NE Hoyt St., Ste. 540
Portland, OR 97213
Phone: (503)215-6258 **Fax:** (503)215-6857
Email: david.gilbert@providence.org
David N. Gilbert, MD, Dir.
Activities/Fields: Clinical and basic investigations in cancer immunology, cardiovascular diseases, infectious diseases, and diabetes and metabolism. **Pub:** *Annual Report.*

★ 23143 ★ Psychiatric Research Institute
1100 N St. Francis, Ste. 200
Wichita, KS 67214-2878
Phone: (316)291-4774 **Fax:** (316)291-7704
Website: http://www.pri-research.org
Dr. W. Dale Horst, Admin. Dir.
Activities/Fields: Clinical drug testing for depression in adults and children, Alzheimer's disease, schizophrenia (inpatient and outpatient), centralized anxiety disorder, panic disorder, antiobesity, and pharmacokinetic drug testing.

★ 23144 ★ Public Citizen Health Research Group
1600 20th St. NW
Washington, DC 20009
Phone: (202)588-1000 **Fax:** (202)588-7796
Website: http://www.citizen.org/hrg
Sidney M. Wolfe, MD, Dir.
Activities/Fields: Health care delivery, workplace safety and health, drug regulation, food additives, medical device safety, and environmental influences on health. Conducts consumer advocacy and lobbying on health matters and monitors the enforcement of health and safety legislation. **Pub:** *Health Letter*, monthly. • *Health Research Group List of Publications*, annually. • *Worst Pills, Best Bills.* • *Worst Pills Best Pills News*, monthly.

★ 23145 ★ Public Health Centre
2400 D'Estimauville St.
Beauport, QC, Canada G1E 7G9
Phone: (418)666-7000 **Fax:** (418)666-2776
Michel Vezina, Dir.
Activities/Fields: Operational research, including effectiveness of interventions of sexual behavior of seropositive individuals; psychological stress of homosexual AIDS patients; and studies on organochlorinated contaminants.

★ 23146 ★ Public Health Institute
2001 Addison St., 2nd Fl.
Berkeley, CA 94704-1103
Phone: (510)644-8200 **Fax:** (510)644-9319
Email: dssofaer@phi.org
Website: http://www.phi.org
Joseph M. Hafey, Pres. /CEO
Activities/Fields: Conducts research on a broad range of public health issues, including drug and alcohol problems, occupational health, diet and nutrition, maternal and child health, violence, reproductive health, genetics, and lead poisoning prevention. **Frmly:** California Public Health Foundation.

★ 23147 ★ Public Health Research Institute
c/o International Center for Public Health
225 Warren St.
Newark, NJ 07103-3535
Phone: (973)854-3100 **Fax:** (973)854-3101
Email: lmw@phri.org
Website: http://www.phri.org
Lewis M. Weinstein, Pres.
Activities/Fields: Biomedical research with a focus on infectious diseases and public health issues. **Pub:** *Annual report.* • *Symposium proceedings.*

★ 23148 ★ Public Responsibility in Medicine and Research
132 Boylston St., 4th Fl.
Boston, MA 02116
Phone: (617)423-4112 **Fax:** (617)423-1185
Email: info@primr.org
Website: http://www.primr.org
Joan Rachlin, Exec. Dir.
Activities/Fields: Medical research, focusing on education of public responsibility and regulation of research. **Pub:** *Conference proceedings.* • *Educational Materials.* • *IRB/IACUC Mailing Lists.*

★ 23149 ★ Purdue University Botanical Center for Age-Related Diseases
Stone Hall
West Lafayette, IN 47907
Phone: (765)494-8237 **Fax:** (765)494-0674
Email: weavercm@cfs.purdue.edu
Website: http://fn.cfs.purdue.edu/bot/
Connie M. Weaver, PhD, Prin. Investigator
Activities/Fields: Health effects of polyphenols, a diverse group of chemical components widely distributed in plants, including soy, grapes, green tea, and

several herbs. Research is focused on heart disease and cancer, and to two leading causes of diminished quality of life, osteoporosis and cognitive decline.

★ 23150 ★ Purdue University Cancer Center
Life Science Research Bldg.
1524 Hansen
West Lafayette, IN 47907-1524
Phone: (765)494-9129 **Fax:** (765)494-9193
Website: http://www.cancer.purdue.edu
Richard F. Borch, MD, Dir.
Activities/Fields: Experimental therapeutics and diagnostics, structural biology, cell growth and differentiation. **Pub:** *Annual report.*

★ 23151 ★ Purdue University Center for Paralysis Research
408 S University St.
West Lafayette, IN 47907-2096
Phone: (765)494-7600 **Fax:** (765)494-7605
Email: cpr@purdue.edu
Website: http://www.vet.purdue.edu/cpr
Dr. Richard Borgens, Dir.
Activities/Fields: Treatments for spinal cord injury, focusing on recruitment of spared pathways in the spinal cord through the use of 4-Aminopyridine (4-AP), reconnection and regeneration of severely damaged nerve pathways through the use of oscillating electrical fields and treatment with injectable polymers that seak damaged cells, and replacement of spinal cord using enteric neuron transplantation.

★ 23152 ★ Purdue University Center for Pharmaceutical Processing Research (CPPR)
1336 Robert E Heine Pharmacy Bldg.
Department of Industrial & Physical Pharmacy
West Lafayette, IN 47907-1336
Phone: (765)494-1401 **Fax:** (765)494-6545
Email: slnail@pharmacy.purdue.edu
Website: http://www.pharmacy.purdue.edu/~nsf/
Steven L. Nail, Dir.
Activities/Fields: Pharmaceutical processing.

★ 23153 ★ Queens College of City University of New York Augmentative Communication Center
Linguistics & Communication Disorders Department
65-30 Kissena Blvd.
Flushing, NY 11367-1597
Phone: (718)997-2940 **Fax:** (718)997-2935
Email: arlene_kraat@qc.edu
Dr. Arlene Kraat, Dir.
Activities/Fields: Severe speech and language disabilities, including treatment methods of augmentative and alternative communication (AAC) modes. AAC enhances communication through the use of signs, symbolic gestures, language boards, and computerized communication devices.

★ 23154 ★ Queens College of City University of New York Speech and Hearing Center
Gertz Bldg.
65-30 Kissena Blvd.
Flushing, NY 11367-1597
Phone: (718)997-2932 **Fax:** (718)997-2935
Dr. Joel Stark, Dir.
Activities/Fields: Communicative disorders in children and adults, focusing on testing and treatment.

★ 23155 ★ Queen's University at Kingston Cancer Research Laboratories (QCRL)
Botterell Hall, 3rd Fl.
Kingston, ON, Canada K7L 3N6
Phone: (613)533-2778 **Fax:** (613)533-6830
Email: deeleyr@post.queensu.ca
Website: http://meds-ss10.meds.queensu.ca/medicine/crl/
Roger G. Deeley, PhD, Dir.
Activities/Fields: Cancer biology, including drug resistance and metabolism; tumor progression; and the regulation of cell growth, proliferation and differentiation.

★ 23156 ★ Queen's University at Kingston Cytogenetics and DNA Research Laboratory
Ongwanada
191 Portsmouth Ave.
Kingston, ON, Canada K7M 8A6
Phone: (613)548-4417 **Fax:** (613)548-8135
Email: ong@kos.net
Website: http://www.ongwanada.com/research.html
Jeanette J.A. Holden, PhD, Dir.
Activities/Fields: Cytogenetics, DNA markers, linkage studies, fragile-X syndrome, X-linked mental retardation, x-linked hydrocephalus, Down's syndrome, autism, affective disorders, schizophrenia, melanoma, and chromosome instability.

★ 23157 ★ Queen's University at Kingston Human Mobility Research Centre
Syl & Molly Apps Research Centre
Kingston General Hospital
Kingston, ON, Canada K7L 3N6
Phone: (613)548-2430 **Fax:** (613)549-2529
Email: alden@post.queensu.ca
Website: http://me.queensu.ca/hmrc/
Dr. Marg Alden, Dir.
Activities/Fields: Mechanism of musculoskeletal diseases and disorders i.e. the causes, the prevention, and the treatment of bone and joint disorders caused by arthritis, osteoporosis, and injury. **Frmly:** Clinical Mechanics Group.

★ 23158 ★ R.A. Cowley Shock Trauma Center
University of Maryland Shock Trauma Center
22 S Greene St.
Baltimore, MD 21201
Phone: (410)328-8667 **Fax:** (410)328-8925
Website: http://www.umm.edu/shocktrauma/
Thomas Scalea, MD, Dir.
Activities/Fields: Clinical research on resuscitation and treatment of critically ill and severely injured. Crash injury research studies focus on automotive safety and design based on in-depth engineering analysis of automotive crashes. Emerging technologies such as telemedicine initiatives, blood substitute studies, and biomechanics and clinical aspects of orthopedic injuries are also explored.

★ 23159 ★ Radiation Oncology Research and Development Center
3990 John R
Detroit, MI 48201
Phone: (313)745-9191 **Fax:** (313)745-2341
Email: foremanu@karmanos.org
Website: http://www.roc.wayne.edu
Dr. Jeffery Forman, Dir.
Activities/Fields: Radiation therapy, cancer research, medical information systems, three-dimensional imaging, neutron therapy, radiosurgery, brachytherapy, clinical protocols, and unsealed source therapy.

★ 23160 ★ Ranawat Orthopedic Research Foundation, Inc.
William Black Hall, 11th Fl.
Lenox Hill Hospital
130 E 77th St.
New York, NY 10021-1803
Phone: (212)434-4700 **Fax:** (212)628-4782
Email: csranawat@mindspring.com
Website: http://www.totaljoint.com
Chitranjan S. Ranawat, MD, Dir.
Activities/Fields: Materials and methods related to total hip and knee replacement surgery.

★ 23161 ★ Rancho Rehabilitation Engineering Program
Los Amigos Research & Education Institute, Inc.
7503 Bonita St.
Downey, CA 90242
Phone: (562)401-7994 **Fax:** (562)803-6117
Website: http://www.ranchorep.org
Dr. Donald McNeal, Co-Dir.
Activities/Fields: Develops appropriate technology and assessment procedures in the field of rehabilitation engineering and assures their availability to individuals with physical disabilities.

★ 23162 ★ RAND Center for Employer-Sponsored Health and Pension Benefits
1200 S Hayes St.
Arlington, VA 22202-5050
Phone: (703)413-1100 **Fax:** (703)413-8111
Email: jar@rand.org
Website: http://www.rand.org/health/dol/
Jeannette Rogowski, Dir.
Activities/Fields: Employee benefits. **Pub:** *Conference papers.*

★ 23163 ★ RAND Center for Healthcare and the Internet
1700 Main St.
Santa Monica, CA 90407
Phone: (310)393-0411 **Fax:** (310)451-7025
Email: spranca@rand.org
Website: http://www.rand.org/health/internet.html
Mark Spranca, PhD, Dir.
Activities/Fields: Understanding and developing the potential of the Internet and related technologies to improve the healthcare system.

★ 23164 ★ RAND Center for the Study of Aging
1700 Main St.
PO Box 2138
Santa Monica, CA 90407-2138
Phone: (310)393-0411 **Fax:** (310)451-6923
Email: mhurd@rand.org
Website: http://www.rand.org/labor/aging/
Michael D. Hurd, Dir.
Activities/Fields: Relationships among institutional and socioeconomic factors, health, and financial well-being among the elderly. **Pub:** *Reports.*

★ 23165 ★ Rat Resource and Research Center
University of Missouri—Columbia
Columbia, MO 65211
Phone: (573)884-9469 **Fax:** (573)884-7521
Email: critserj@missouri.edu
Website: http://www.radil.missouri.edu/rrrc
John K. Critser, PhD, Prin. Investigator
Activities/Fields: Rats as animal models, particularly development of efficacious methods for nuclear transfer in the rat; development of efficient methods for genome resource banking and strain/stock reconstitution, including ovarian tissue preservation and transplantation in combination with artificial insemination with cryopreserved spermatozoa; and improved methods for health monitoring of rats using molecular diagnostics and environmental monitoring.

★ 23166 ★ Rees-Stealy Research Foundation
2001 4th Ave.
San Diego, CA 92101
Phone: (619)235-8744 **Fax:** (619)235-8745
Dr. Phillip Gausewitz, Dir.

Activities/Fields: Basic cardiac research involving cardio myocyte contractility studies. Research includes the analysis of recording heart cell function, utilizing the video camera technique of living motion using electronic devices for computer transfer, heart cell preparation, and cell culture.

★ 23167 ★ Regenstrief Institute for Health Care Research
1050 Wishard Blvd.
Indianapolis, IN 46202
Phone: (317)630-7070 **Fax:** (317)630-2466
Email: cmcdonald@regenstrief.org
Website: http://www.regenstrief.org
Dr. Clement McDonald, Dir.
Activities/Fields: Health care, including use of computers in health care delivery, and use of engineering and computer techniques to improve medical diagnosis and therapy.

★ 23168 ★ Rehabilitation Engineering Research Center on Wheelchair Transportation Safety
5044 Forbes Tower
School of Health & Rehabilitation
University of Pittsburgh
Pittsburgh, PA 15260
Phone: (412)383-6595
Email: ginaber@pitt.edu
Website: http://www.rercwts.pitt.edu/
Gina E. Bertocci, PhD, Dir.
Activities/Fields: Safety of wheelchair users who remain seated in their wheelchairs while using public and private motor vehicles.

★ 23169 ★ Rehabilitation Institute of Chicago
345 E Superior, Ste. 1406
Chicago, IL 60611
Phone: (312)238-3919 **Fax:** (312)238-2208
Email: w-rymer@northwestern.edu
Website: http://www.smpp.nwu.edu
Dr. William Z. Rymer, Res. Dir.
Activities/Fields: Rehabilitation medicine, brain trauma, stroke, atherosclerosis, neuromuscular diseases, applied neurophysiology, deep venous thrombosis, spinal cord injury, arthritis, prosthetics/orthotics, rehabilitation nursing, allied health, and communicative disorders.

★ 23170 ★ Rehabilitation Institute of Michigan
261 Mack Ave.
Detroit, MI 48201
Phone: (313)745-9735 **Fax:** (313)745-2240
Email: mwayland@dmc.org
Website: http://www.rimrehab.org/rim/
Dr. Marilyn Wayland, Dir.
Activities/Fields: Physical medicine and rehabilitation medicine, including electromyography, rehabilitation engineering, neuropsychology, measures of rehabilitation outcome, and methods of evaluation and treatment of patients with closed head injuries, spinal cord injuries, cerebrovascular accidents, and other diagnoses. **Pub:** *Research report*, annually. • *Thinking Cap.*

★ 23171 ★ Rehabilitation Research and Training Center on Aging With a Disability
Rancho Los Amigos National Rehabilitation Center
7601 E Imperial Hwy., Bldg. 800-W
Downey, CA 90242
Phone: (562)401-7402 **Fax:** (562)401-7011
Email: gracefg@agingwithdisability.org
Website: http://www.agingwithdisability.org
Bryan Kemp, PhD, Dir.
Activities/Fields: Problems people face as they age with disabilities, including those who are post-polio, have rheumatoid arthritis, cerebral palsy, or have suffered a stroke. **Pub:** *Fact Sheet: Aging with a Disability Instrument Development.* • *A Life Course Perspective: Aging with Long-Term Disability.* • *A Research Perspective: Next Steps in Bridging the Gap Between Aging and Disability.* • *Resource List: Wellness, Self-Care, Exercise and Aging with Disability.*

★ 23172 ★ Reproductive Toxicology Center
7831 Woodmont Ave., Ste. 375
Bethesda, MD 20814-6030
Phone: (301)620-8690
Email: reprotox@reprotox.org
Website: http://reprotox.org
Anthony Scialli, MD, Dir.
Activities/Fields: Effects of the chemical and physical environment on human fertility, pregnancy, and development.

★ 23173 ★ Research Center for Alcoholic Liver and Pancreatic Diseases
1333 San Pablo St., MMR, 4th Fl.
Los Angeles, CA 90089-9141
Phone: (323)442-3121 **Fax:** (323)442-3126
Email: htsukamo@hsc.usc.edu
Website: http://www.usc.edu/schools/medicine/research/alcohol_center/
Hide Tsukamoto, PhD, Dir.
Activities/Fields: Mechanisms by which ethanol sensitizes and primes the liver and pancreas to diseases. **Pub:** *Papers.*

★ 23174 ★ Research Center on Managed Care for Psychiatric Disorders
10920 Wilshire Blvd., Ste. 300
Los Angeles, CA 90024-6505
Phone: (310)794-3725 **Fax:** (310)794-3724
Email: punzalan@ucla.edu
Kenneth Wells, MD, Dir.
Activities/Fields: Managed care for vulnerable populations with psychiatric disorders. **Pub:** *Working papers series.*

★ 23175 ★ Research and Development Institute
PO Box 351
Sycamore, IL 60178-2738
Phone: (815)895-3078 **Fax:** (815)895-2448
Email: gkapper@niu.edu
Dr. Gaylen G. Kapperman, Dir.
Activities/Fields: Rehabilitation and education for disabled persons, with emphasis on blindness and visual impairment.

★ 23176 ★ Research Institute of Kansas
2600 N Woodlawn
Wichita, KS 67220
Phone: (316)858-2598 **Fax:** (316)858-2521
Email: lterry@galichia.com
Activities/Fields: Pharmaceutic drug and device studies.

★ 23177 ★ Research Institute of Palo Alto Medical Foundation
Ames Bldg.
795 El Camino Real
Palo Alto, CA 94301
Phone: (650)326-8120 **Fax:** (650)329-9114
Email: ohearnk@pamfri.org
Website: http://www.pamf.org
Dr. Allen D. Cooper, Dir.
Activities/Fields: Clinical and general medical sciences, including immunology, infectious diseases, health services research, cardiac physiology, metabolism, atherosclerosis, and cancer cell biology. **Pub:** *News*, quarterly. **Frmly:** Palo Alto Medical Research Foundation.

★ 23178 ★ Research to Prevent Blindness
645 Madison Ave., 21st Fl.
New York, NY 10022-1010
Phone: (212)752-4333 **Free:** 800-621-0026
Fax: (212)688-6231
Email: tfurlong@rpbusa.org
Website: http://www.rpbusa.org/hc2/index.asp
James V. Romano, PhD, Contact
Activities/Fields: Blinding eye-diseases, focusing on causes, prevention, and treatment. **Pub:** *Eye Research Newsletter.* • *Report*, annually. • *Research reports.* • *Visual Acuity/Macular Degeneration Test Card.* Brochure.

★ 23179 ★ Research Resource for Complex Physiologic Signals
Department of Medicine
Beth Israel Deaconess Medical Center
330 Brookline Ave.
Boston, MA 02215
Phone: (617)667-4267 **Fax:** (617)667-7268
Email: ary@astro.bidmc.harvard.edu
Website: http://www.physionet.org
Ary L. Goldberger, MD, Prin. Investigator
Activities/Fields: Complex physiologic signals.

★ 23180 ★ Research and Training Center on Community Integration of Individuals With Traumatic Brain Injury
Mount Sinai Medical Center
1 Gustave L Levy Pl., Box 1240
New York, NY 10029
Phone: (212)241-5152 **Free:** 888-241-5152
Fax: (212)241-0137
Email: teresa.ashman@mssm.edu
Website: http://www.mssm.edu/tbinet/
Dr. Wayne Gordon, Prin. Investigator
Activities/Fields: Community integration of traumatic brain injury (TBI) survivors, including increasing understanding of how TBI affects community integration, developing new models of community integration, and treating cognitive/behavioral disorders that most affect the TBI survivor's functioning within the community. **Pub:** *Consumer reports.* • *TBI-NET.* • *Tools for Community Living: A Handbook for Survivors of Traumatic Brain Injury.*

★ 23181 ★ Research and Training Center on Managed Care and Disability (RTC-MC&D)
6858 Old Dominion Dr., Ste. 250
McLean, VA 22101
Phone: (703)448-6155 **Fax:** (703)442-9015
Website: http://www.cessi.net/contracts/dps/nrhrc_rtcmcd.html
Bonnie O'Day, PhD, Contact
Activities/Fields: Delivery of quality health care to people with disabilities, particularly the impact of alternative managed care arrangements on the provision of acute care services for working-age people with disabilities.

★ 23182 ★ Respiratory Pathogens Research Unit
Department of Molecular Virology & Microbiology
Texas Medical Center
1 Baylor Plz., Rm. 205 A
Houston, TX 77030
Phone: (713)798-4474 **Fax:** (713)798-7375
Email: rcouch@bcm.tmc.edu
Robert B. Couch, MD, Dir.
Activities/Fields: Multidisciplinary studies of acute respiratory diseases in humans and animals, including bacteriologic, virologic, and immunologic studies and vaccine and evaluations.

★ 23183 ★ Retina Foundation of the Southwest (RFSW)
9900 N Central Expy., Ste. 400
Dallas, TX 75231
Phone: (214)363-3911 **Fax:** (214)363-4538
Email: rfsw@retinafoundation.org
Website: http://www.retinafoundation.org/aboutRFSW.htm
David G. Birch, PhD, Res. Dir.
Activities/Fields: Understanding, treatment, and prevention of blinding eye diseases.

★ 23184 ★ Rice University Institute of Biosciences and Bioengineering
W 100 George Brown Hall
6100 Main St.
Houston, TX 77005-1892
Phone: (713)527-6034 **Fax:** (713)285-5154
Email: ibb@rice.edu
Website: http://www.bioc.rice.edu/Institute/IBB/
Dr. Larry V. McIntire, Ch.
Activities/Fields: Application of engineering skills to problems in biology and medicine, including cellular and tissue engineering, studies on circulation assistance devices, cardiovascular tissue mechanics, blood proteins, effects of physical forces on various components of blood, fluid mechanics and transport processes related to cardiovascular system, hematologic complications with prostheses, rheology, fluid mechanics of blood and blood flow, tissue culture reactor evaluation, biochemical reactor engineering, applications of artificial intelligence in bioreactor control and dynamics, plant cell bioreactors, bioseparation systems, and development of in vitro methods for studying cellular mechanisms of thrombosis and atherogenesis.

★ 23185 ★ Riverside Research Institute
156 William St., 9th Fl.
New York, NY 10038-2609
Phone: (212)502-1725 **Fax:** (212)502-1729
Website: http://www.rri-usa.org
Activities/Fields: Biomedical ultrasound, electromagnetic scattering and interactions, photonic systems, signal processing, image processing, radar, military systems, intelligence, surveillance, reconnaissance, and computer modeling of physical processes in ultrasound and electromagneticism.

★ 23186 ★ Robarts Research Institute
100 Perth Dr.
PO Box 5015
London, ON, Canada N6A 5K8
Phone: (519)663-5777 **Fax:** (519)663-3789
Email: info@robarts.ca
Website: http://www.roberts.ca
Dr. Mark J. Poznansky, Pres. /CEO
Activities/Fields: Cardiovascular sciences, immunology, neuroscience, imaging, clinical trials, and molecular virology. Research is conducted into major causes of death and disability such as stroke, heart disease, Alzheimer's, organ failure, and diabetes, with the goal to develop new treatments and cures as a result of advances in genetic medicine and diagnostic imaging techniques. **Pub:** *Annual Report.*

★ 23187 ★ Rockburn Institute
6581 Belmont Woods Rd.
Elkridge, MD 21075
Phone: (410)796-4554 **Fax:** (410)796-3173
Dale N. Schumacher, MD, Pres.
Activities/Fields: Health care services and effective and efficient management of health care institutions.

★ 23188 ★ Rockefeller University Fisher Center for Research on Alzheimer's Disease
1230 York Ave.
New York, NY 10021
Phone: (212)327-8780 **Fax:** (212)327-7746
Email: greengd@mail.rockefeller.edu
Website: http://www.rockefeller.edu/graduate/cenzach.htm
Prof. Paul Greengard, Dir.
Activities/Fields: Alzheimer's disease, including how brain cells process the amyloid precursor phosphoprotein (APP) leading to the production of b-amlyoid, a major component of the plaques that are a hallmark of Alzheimer's disease.

★ 23189 ★ Rockefeller University General Clinical Research Center
Rockefeller University Hospital, Box 178
1230 York Ave.
New York, NY 10021-6399
Phone: (212)327-7730 **Fax:** (212)327-8232
Email: kruegej@mail.rockefeller.edu
Website: http://clinfo.rockefeller.edu
James G. Krueger, MD, Dir.
Activities/Fields: Chronic immune disorders, dermatology, gastrointestinal motility, lipid metabolism, metabolic disorders, medical biochemistry, cystic fibrostic, AIDS, tuberculosis, neurological disorders, and obesity and nutrition.

★ 23190 ★ Rockefeller University Laboratory of Bacteriology, Pathogenesis and Immunology
1230 York Ave., DWB 800
New York, NY 10021-6399
Phone: (212)327-8157 **Fax:** (212)327-8960
Email: vas@mail.rockefeller.edu
Dr. Vincent A. Fischetti, Dir.
Activities/Fields: Investigates the parastic mechanisms used by pathogenic bacteria, especially streptococci and neisseria. Also studies the derangements of the human immune system which lead to chronic diseases such as rheumatic fever and glomerulonephritis as a result of infection with streptococci.

★ 23191 ★ Rockefeller University Laboratory of Biochemical Genetics and Metabolism
1230 York Ave.
PO Box 179
New York, NY 10021
Phone: (212)327-7700 **Fax:** (212)327-7165
Email: breslow@rockefeller.edu
Prof. Jan L. Breslow, MD, Contact
Activities/Fields: Human genetic susceptibility to atherosclerosis, especially the molecular genetics and clincial significance of the apolipoproteins, a group of proteins that coat the lipoprotein particles and determine their metabolism.

★ 23192 ★ Rockefeller University Laboratory of the Biology of Addictive Diseases
1230 York Ave.
New York, NY 10021-6399
Phone: (212)327-8000 **Fax:** (212)327-8574
Email: kreek@rockvax.rockefeller.edu
Website: http://www.rockefeller.edu
Dr. Mary Jeanne Kreek, Hd.
Activities/Fields: Biological basis of opiate, alcohol, and cocaine addiction; the biological correlates of addictive disease, including the physiological and pharmacological effects of chronic drug use; and the medical complications of drug use, especially hepatitis B and C, hepatitis delta, and human immunodeficiency viral infections. Other areas include molecular neurobiology and human molecular genetics of the addictive diseases with special attention on the role of the endogenous opioid system in these disorders, including cocaine dependency and alcoholism, as well as opiate addition; and the role of the endogenous opioids and the specific opioid receptors in the addictive diseases and in normal and abnormal physiology of the neuroendocrine and gastrointestinal systems.

★ 23193 ★ Rockefeller University Laboratory of Cellular Physiology and Immunology
1230 York Ave.
New York, NY 10021-6399
Phone: (212)327-7763 **Fax:** (212)327-8875
Email: steinm@mail.rockefeller.edu
Dr. Ralph Steinman, Contact
Activities/Fields: Functional properties of eukaryotic cells and their role in physiologic and pathologic events. Using the tools of immunology, cell biology, and biochemistry, the Lab studies problems of inflammation, the immune response, and host defense against parasites and tumor cells.

★ 23194 ★ Rockefeller University Laboratory of Clinical Microbiology and Immunology
1230 York Ave., Box 255
New York, NY 10021
Phone: (212)327-8155 **Fax:** (212)327-7579
Email: zabrisk@mail.rockefeller.edu
Dr. John B. Zabriskie, Dir.
Activities/Fields: Microbe-induced autoimmunity and human genetics, including molecular biology emphasizing eukaryotic systems, protein chemistry, and immunology.

★ 23195 ★ Rockefeller University Laboratory of Human Genetics and Hematology
1230 York Ave.
New York, NY 10021
Phone: (212)327-8862 **Fax:** (212)327-8262
Email: auerbac@mail.rockefeller.edu
Website: http://www.rockefeller.edu/labheads/auerbach/auerbach.html
Arleen D. Auerbach, Dir.
Activities/Fields: Fanconi anemia (FA), an autosomal recessive disorder characterized clinically by progressive pancytopenia, variable skeletal and other congenital abnormalities, predisposition to malignancy, particularly acute myelogenous leukemia (AML), prenatal diagnosis of FA, and identification of genes that cause FA.

★ 23196 ★ Rockefeller University Laboratory for Investigative Dermatology
1230 York Ave.
New York, NY 10021-6399
Phone: (212)327-8333 **Fax:** (212)327-8232
Email: kruegej@mail.rockefeller.edu
James G. Krueger, MD, Contact
Activities/Fields: A variety of skin conditions, including the biology of epithelial cells and the study of psoriasis.

★ 23197 ★ Rockefeller University Laboratory of Metabolism-Pharmacology
1230 York Ave.
New York, NY 10021-6399
Phone: (212)327-8494 **Fax:** (212)327-8690
Email: kappas@mail.rockefeller.edu
Dr. Attallah Kappas, Hd.
Activities/Fields: Regulation of heme biosynthesis and heme catabolism as affected by those genetic and environmental factors that have major influences on the oxidative metabolism of drugs, hormones, and environmental chemicals in liver and other tissues.

★ 23198 ★ Rockefeller University Laboratory of Neuroendocrinology
1230 York Ave.
PO Box 165
New York, NY 10021-6399
Phone: (212)327-8624 **Fax:** (212)327-8634
Email: mcewen@rockvax.rockefeller.edu
Dr. Bruce S. McEwen, Hd.
Activities/Fields: Seeks to locate brain sites and understand the mechanisms by which hormones pro-

mote neural plasticity and thereby alter endocrine function, behavior, neurological states, and mood. Also studies the influence of gonadal and adrenal hormones on aging in the brain.

★ 23199 ★ Rockefeller University National Resource for Mass Spectrometry of Biological Macro-Molecules
1230 York Ave.
New York, NY 10021
Phone: (212)327-8849 **Fax:** (212)327-7547
Email: chait@rockfeller.edu
Dr. Brian T. Chait, Dir.
Activities/Fields: Application of mass spectrometry to biomedical problems.

★ 23200 ★ Rockefeller University Starr Center for Human Genetics
1230 York Ave.
New York, NY 10021
Phone: (212)327-8000 **Free:** 888-920-9100
Fax: (212)327-7373
Email: friedj@rockvax.rockefeller.edu
Website: http://www.rockefeller.edu/graduate/censtarr.htm
Dr. Jeffrey M. Friedman, Dir.
Activities/Fields: Genetic analysis of human disease and biology, including heart disease, obesity, diabetes, schizophrenia, hearing loss, obsessive-compulsive disorder, and addictive disorders.

★ 23201 ★ Rocky Mountain Clinical Research, Inc.
29 Rogers Ct.
Golden, CO 80401-6515
Phone: (303)279-1550 **Fax:** (303)278-2602
Email: gailrmcr@aol.com
Gail Danhour, Exec. Dir.
Activities/Fields: Medical research, clinical drug trials, and the development of new diagnostic techniques. **Frmly:** Rocky Mountain Heart Research Institute Inc.; Rocky Mountain Assoc., Inc.

★ 23202 ★ Rocky Mountain Research Institute
PO Box 190149
Boise, ID 83719
Email: farner@micron.net
Website: http://www.ufoinfo.com/organizations/usa_idaho.html
Activities/Fields: Anomalous experiences, unexplained phenomena, unidentified flying objects.

★ 23203 ★ Roger Williams Hospital Roger Williams Cancer Center
Roger Williams Medical Center
825 Chalkstone Ave.
Providence, RI 02908
Phone: (401)456-6565 **Fax:** (401)456-6793
Email: sharpel@rwmc.org
Sharon Harpel, Contact
Activities/Fields: Cellular immunotherapy of tumors, stem cell plasticity, molecular biology of breast and prostate cancer, molecular regulation of myelopoiesis, clinical stem cell transplantation, and cancer prevention and early detection.

★ 23204 ★ Rolf Institute of Structural Integration
205 Canyon Blvd.
Boulder, CO 80302
Phone: (303)449-5903 **Free:** 800-530-8875
Fax: (303)449-5978
Email: ifo@rolf.org
Website: http://www.rolf.org
Lorraine Lombard, Contact
Activities/Fields: Rolfing (registered trademark) technique of connective tissue manipulation and its effect on integration of human physical structure and physical, emotional, and psychological functioning, including studies on human imbalance and its correction and/or improvement by a technique for reordering of the body to bring its major segments, head, shoulders, thorax, pelvis, and legs, toward a vertical alignment. **Pub:** *ROLF Lines*.

★ 23205 ★ Roosevelt Warm Springs Institute for Rehabilitation
PO Box 1000
Warm Springs, GA 31830-0268
Phone: (706)655-5616 **Fax:** (706)655-5630
Email: evprather@dhr.state.ga.us
Website: http://www.rooseveltrehab.org
Evelyn Prather, Res. Spec.
Activities/Fields: Clinical aspects of rehabilitation, marketing, administration, and product development. **Pub:** *Research Brief*, annually. • *The Spirit Newsletter*, quarterly.

★ 23206 ★ Rosenstiel Basic Medical Sciences Research Center
Brandeis University
415 South St.
Waltham, MA 02454
Phone: (781)736-2400 **Fax:** (781)736-2405
Email: petsko@brandeis.edu
Website: http://www.rose.brandeis.edu/
Dr. Gregory Petsko, Dir.
Activities/Fields: Genetics and molecular biology, biochemistry, structural biology, protein crytallography, microbiology, biophysics, and cellular immunology.

★ 23207 ★ Roswell Park Cancer Institute
Elm & Carlton Sts.
Buffalo, NY 14263
Phone: (716)845-2300 **Free:** 800-685-6825
Fax: (716)845-8261
Email: askrpci@roswellpark.org
Website: http://www.roswellpark.org
Activities/Fields: Genetics, biophysical therapies, immunology, experimental therapeutics,and epidemiology of cancer, including the clinical application of recent findings in cancer research and the effectiveness of surgery, chemotherapy, and radiation in cancer therapy. Research program includes work in drug development, pharmacokinetics, crystallography, photodynamic therapy, and biological response modifiers. **Pub:** *Annual Scientific Report*. • *Cancer Report*. • *Monday Morning Oncology Update*. • *Roswellness*.

★ 23208 ★ Roswell Park Cancer Institute Laboratory of Flow Cytometry
Elm & Carlton Sts.
Buffalo, NY 14263
Phone: (716)845-8471 **Fax:** (716)845-8806
Email: flow@attglobal.net
Website: http://rpciflowcytometry.com
Dr. Carleton Stewart, Dir.
Activities/Fields: Licensed reference laboratory for the classification by immunophenotyping of leukemias and lymphomas, monitoring of transplant patients, and evaluation of DNA in solid tumors. Also uses multiparameter flow cytometry to study normal myeloid cell differentiation and the development of molecular phenotyping. Provides clinical research support for protocols that require specific immunophenotyping follow-up to monitor the progress of therapy and develops new tests to improve cancer management. **Pub:** *Annual Report*, annually.

★ 23209 ★ Roswell Park Cancer Institute Transgenic Facility
Elm & Carlton Sts.
Buffalo, NY 14263
Phone: (716)845-5843 **Fax:** (716)845-5908
Email: paul.soloway@roswellpark.org
Kenneth Gross, PhD, Co-Dir.
Activities/Fields: Transgenics, including genome modification.

★ 23210 ★ Royal Ottawa Health Care Group Institute of Mental Health Research (IMHR)
Royal Ottawa Hospital, LG 2044
1145 Carling Ave.
Ottawa, ON, Canada K1Z 7K4
Phone: (613)722-6521 **Fax:** (613)722-5871
Email: imhr@rohcg.on.ca
Zul Merali, PhD, Dir. Gen.
Activities/Fields: Biopsychosocial research into the major psychiatric disorders, including schizophrenia, affective disorders, and anxiety disorders. Other areas of interest are geriatrics, forensics, addictions, and children's mental health.

★ 23211 ★ RTI International Division for Health Economics Research
411 Waverley Oaks Rd., Ste. 330
Waltham, MA 02452-8414
Phone: (781)788-8100 **Fax:** (781)788-8101
Email: inso@her-cher.org
Website: http://www.her-cher.org
Dr. Janet B. Mitchell, Pres.
Activities/Fields: Health economics, including alternative ways of reimbursing capital under the Medicare prospective payment system, access to care, physician payment, hospital costs, black-white treatment differences, and cost-effectiveness of technology.

★ 23212 ★ Rumbaugh-Goodwin Institute for Cancer Research Inc.
1850 NW 69th Ave., Ste. 5
Plantation, FL 33313
Phone: (954)587-9020 **Fax:** (954)321-5311
Email: mike@gicr.com
Website: http://guide.labanimal.com/guide/companyd.jsp?b=3080
Michael J. Dauphinee, PhD, Dir.
Activities/Fields: Biological sciences using specific pathogen-free animals to develop human tumor xenograft models to improve cancer therapy by drug synergism, immunotherapy and improved delivery of treatment modalities. Studies cover hybridoma technology and application, tumor therapy, immunohistochemistry, hemopoietic and tumor stem cell growth (promotion and inhibition), and tumor behavior in immunosuppressed animals. Research services include preclinical trials for anticancer agents, monoclonal antibody production in mouse ascites or in vitro and downstream processing. Maintains laboratories in biochemistry, immunology, immunohistochemistry, flow cytometry, molecular biology, and cell culture. **Frmly:** Germfree Life Research Center; Goodwin Institute for Cancer Research.

★ 23213 ★ Rural Center for AIDS/STD Prevention (RCAP)
801 E 7th St.
Bloomington, IN 47405-3085
Phone: (812)855-1718 **Free:** 800-566-8644
Fax: (812)855-3717
Email: aids@indiana.edu
Website: http://www.indiana.edu/~aids/
William L. Yarber, Dir.
Activities/Fields: AIDS, HIV, and STD prevention in rural areas.

★ 23214 ★ Rush University Biological Rhythms Research Laboratory
Rush-Presbyterian-St. Luke's Medical Center
1645 W Jackson Blvd., Ste. 425
Chicago, IL 60612
Phone: (312)850-7788 **Fax:** (312)850-7707
Email: ceastman@rush.edu
Charmane Eastman, PhD, Dir.
Activities/Fields: Human circadian rhythms, focusing on the use of bright light, and melatonin for adaptation to night shift work, and jet-lag.

★ 23215 ★ Rush University Bone Marrow Transplant Center
Rush-Presbyterian-St. Luke's Medical Center
1725 W Harrison St., Ste. 809
Chicago, IL 60612
Phone: (312)942-3049 **Fax:** (312)733-1590
Email: hklingem@rush.edu
Website: http://www.bone-marrow-transplant.org
Dr. Hans Klingemann, Dir.
Activities/Fields: Bone marrow transplantation in the treatment of leukemia, malignant lymphoma, myeloma, breast cancer, and graft-versus host disease in allogenic bone marrow transplantation.

★ 23216 ★ Rush University Center for Health Management Studies
Rush-Presbyterian-St. Luke's Medical Center
1700 W Van Burren St., Rm. 126-B
Chicago, IL 60612
Phone: (312)942-5402 **Fax:** (312)942-3833
Email: rush_hsm@rush.edu
Website: http://www.rushu.rush.edu
Dr. Denise Oleske, Dir.
Activities/Fields: Health care organizations, including studies in organization and administration, organizational behavior, research design and statistics, cost containment, health economics, health care financial management, quantitative methods and epidemiology, long-term care, and information systems. **Pub:** *Annual Report.* • *Working Paper Series*, semiannually.

★ 23217 ★ Rush University Center for SIDS Research and Disorders of Respiratory Control in Infancy and Childhood
Rush-Presbyterian-St. Luke's Medical Center
1653 W Congress Pky.
Chicago, IL 60612
Phone: (312)942-2723 **Fax:** (312)942-3087
Email: dweese@rush.edu
Dr. Debra E. Weese-Mayer, Dir.
Activities/Fields: Sudden infant death syndrome (SIDS) research, including monitoring high-risk infants for apnea, congenital central hypoventilation syndrome, genetic characterization of congenital central hypoventilation syndrome, and the effect of prenatal cocaine (throughout gestation) on development and function of the autonomic neurosystem.

★ 23218 ★ Rush University Center for Suicide Research and Prevention
Rush-Presbyterian-St. Luke's Medical Center
600 S Paulina, Ste. 529
Chicago, IL 60612
Phone: (312)942-3351 **Fax:** (312)942-6876
Email: dclark@rush.edu
David C. Clark, PhD, Dir.
Activities/Fields: Suicidal behavior, including epidemiological and prevention research.

★ 23219 ★ Rush University Multiple Sclerosis Center
1725 W Harrison St., Ste. 309
Chicago, IL 60612
Phone: (312)942-8011 **Fax:** (312)942-2253
Dusan Stefoski, MD, Dir.
Activities/Fields: Multiple sclerosis, including understanding of nerve impulse conduction in both normal and pathologic states and pathophysiology of conduction in multiple sclerosis and allied demyelinating conditions, improving conduction in diseased nerves by pharmacologic therapy, and development of a detailed molecular model of the organization of the ion-specific channels of the nerve membrane. Patient studies include programs in neuroactive drugs, thermolability phenomena, analysis of individual's psychological stresses and the resulting coping mechanisms, and the effect of disease on children of patients and the overall family unit.

★ 23220 ★ Rush University Pediatric Critical Care Research Center
Rush-Presbyterian-St. Luke's Medical Center
1653 W Congress Pky.
Chicago, IL 60612
Phone: (312)942-6194 **Fax:** (312)942-4370
Email: sbarnes@rush.edu
Dr. Steven Barnes, Res. Dir.
Activities/Fields: Pediatric patients, analgesia (for pain relief), sedation, broncholitis, neonatal tetanus in Nigeria.

★ 23221 ★ Rush University Rush Alzheimer's Disease Center
8 North
710 S Paulina
Chicago, IL 60612
Phone: (312)942-4463 **Fax:** (312)942-4154
Email: dbennett@rush.edu
Dr. David Bennett, Dir.
Activities/Fields: Alzheimer's disease, including causes, treatment, and cure. Conducts clinical trials of new drug treatments and analyzes potential risk factors in the development of Alzheimer's disease.

★ 23222 ★ Rush University Rush Arthritis and Orthopedics Institute
1725 W Harrison St., Ste. 1055
Chicago, IL 60612
Phone: (312)563-2420 **Fax:** (312)243-7707
Email: arth-orth-institute@rush.edu
Website: http://www.rush.edu/arthritis/
Dr. Jorge O. Galante, Dir.
Activities/Fields: Osteoarthritis and cartilage physiology, inflammatory joint disease, joint replacement, low back pain, orthopedic oncology (musculoskeletal tumors), sports medicine, and scoliosis.

★ 23223 ★ Rush University Rush Arthritis and Orthopedics Institute Center for Clinical Studies
1725 W Harrison St., Ste. 1017
Chicago, IL 60612-3824
Phone: (312)942-2167 **Fax:** (312)563-2267
Email: ccs@rush.edu
Website: http://www.rush.edu
Dr. Joel A. Block, Dir.
Activities/Fields: New treatments and therapies for arthritis and related conditions.

★ 23224 ★ Rush University Rush Cancer Institute
Professional Bldg. I, Ste. 809
Rush-Presbyterian-St. Luke's Medical Center
1725 W Harrison St.
Chicago, IL 60612
Phone: (312)563-2190 **Free:** 800-224-7874
Fax: (312)455-9635
Email: jhylton@rush.edu
John Hylton, Admin.
Activities/Fields: Cancer, including biochemistry, immunology surveillance, virology, lymphomal leukemia, and psychosocial studies. Participates in the National Cancer Institute's nationwide program for coordinating multidisciplinary basic and clincial cancer research, improving methods of treatment, diagnosis, and prevention, training health professionals, and transferring cancer knowledge to surrounding communities. **Pub:** *Rush Center Institute Newsletter.*

★ 23225 ★ Rush University Rush Heart Institute
Rush-Presbyterian-St. Luke's Medical Center
1725 W Harrison, Ste. 1159
Chicago, IL 60612
Phone: (312)563-2230 **Free:** 800-942-4144
Fax: (312)733-1221
Email: rusheart@rush.edu
Website: http://www.rush.edu/patients/heart/index.html
Dr. James E. Calvin, Dir. of Cardiology
Activities/Fields: Medical cardiovascular research, including cardiac and vascular physiology and cardiovascular surgery, including open heart procedures and major aortic replacement surgery.

★ 23226 ★ Rush University Rush Institute for Healthy Aging
1645 W Jackson Blvd., Ste. 675
Chicago, IL 60612
Phone: (312)942-3350 **Fax:** (312)942-2861
Email: denis_evans@rush.edu
Dr. Denis A. Evans, Co-Dir.
Activities/Fields: Epidemiology of Alzheimer's disease, community-based studies of Alzheimer's disease and other common problems of older persons, physical functions among older persons, and statistical methods in aging research.

★ 23227 ★ Rush University Rush Institute for Mental Well-Being
1720 W Polk St.
Chicago, IL 60612
Phone: (312)942-4000 **Fax:** (312)942-3113
Website: http://www.rush.edu/patients/mental/
Dr. Jan Fawcett, Dir.
Activities/Fields: Clinical treatment of depression and related disorders, including alcoholism, anxiety disorders, and psychoses; treatment for damages caused by such disorders, including social and work impairment, recurrent episodes, and suicides; methods for prevention of depression and related disorders; and stress management techniques.

★ 23228 ★ Rush University Rush Neuroscience Institute
Rush-Presbyterian-St. Luke's Medical Center
1725 W Harrison St.
Chicago, IL 60612
Phone: (312)942-8729 **Fax:** (312)942-2380
Email: jfox@rush.edu
Dr. Jacob H. Fox, Chm.
Activities/Fields: Alzheimer's disease, Parkinson's disease, and stroke, including community-based studies, clinical investigations, and laboratory investigations using brain tissue and animal experimentation. Studies also focus on development of new drugs to improve symptoms of multiple sclerosis.

★ 23229 ★ Rutgers University Bureau of Biological Research
FAS Division of Life Science - Nelson Biological Laboratorie
604 Allison Rd.
Piscataway, NJ 08854-8082
Phone: (732)445-3972 **Fax:** (732)445-6370
Email: martin@biology.rutgers.edu
Charles Martin, Dir.
Activities/Fields: Neurobiology and physiology, cell and developmental biology, molecular biology, biomoleculer structure, biochemistry.

★ 23230 ★ Rutgers University Cell and Cell Products Fermentation Facility
Waksman Institute
190 Frelinghuysen Rd.
Piscataway, NJ 08855-8020
Phone: (732)445-2925 **Fax:** (732)445-5735
Email: callanan@mbcl.rutgers.edu
Website: http://mbclserver.rutgers.edu/ferment/
Kenneth R. Callanan, Mgr.
Activities/Fields: Cell fermentation and production of primary and secondary metabolites such as recombinant proteins, hormones, enzymes, regulatory proteins, and antiviral, antibacterial, and antifungal compounds.

★ 23231 ★ Rutgers University Center of Alcohol Studies
607 Allison Rd.
Piscataway, NJ 08854-8001
Phone: (732)445-2190 **Fax:** (732)445-3500
Email: chrouse@rci.rutgers.edu
Website: http://www.rci.rutgers.edu/~cas2
Robert J. Pandina, PhD, Dir.

Activities/Fields: Causes and treatment of alcoholism and drug abuse, diverse actions of alcohol and other drugs on the body, means to prevent alcohol and other drug misuse, and the incidence and prevalence of normal and problem alcohol consumption in the U.S. and the world, including human enzyme systems important in alcohol metabolism, development of tolerance and physical dependence on alcohol, and hormonal changes. **Pub:** *Journal of Studies on Alcohol*, bimonthly. • *Monographs of the Rutgers Center of Alcohol Studies.* • *National Institute of Alcohol Abuse and Alcoholism-Rutgers University Center of Alcohol Studies (NIAAA-RUCAS) Treatment Series.*

★ 23232 ★ Rutgers University Center for Molecular and Behavioral Neuroscience
197 University Ave.
Newark, NJ 07102
Phone: (973)353-1080 **Fax:** (973)353-1760
Email: tallal@axon.rutgers.edu
Website: http://www.cmbn.rutgers.edu/
Dr. Paula Tallal, Co-Dir.

Activities/Fields: Molecular and behavioral neuroscience research for applications to behavioral dysfunctions in humans. Serves as a technology transfer unit between the University and industry.

★ 23233 ★ Rutgers University Center for Research on the Organization and Financing of Care for the Severely Mentally Ill
30 College Ave.
New Brunswick, NJ 08901-1293
Phone: (732)932-8415 **Fax:** (732)932-6872
Email: mechanic@rci.rutgers.edu
Website: http://www.ihhcpar.rutgers.edu/
Dr. David Mechanic, Dir.

Activities/Fields: Mental health services and policy in the state and nationally. Research agenda includes mental health and mental health policy; barriers to successful patient outcomes following hospitalization; economic mental consequences of mental illness; facilitating appropriate housing for the severely mentally ill; insurance coverage for young mentally ill adults; improving general medical care for the severely mentally ill; impact of mental health services under managed care; mental health aspects of the AIDS epidemic; psychiatric care in general hospitals; relationships between the general medical and the specialty psychiatric sectors; relationships between minority families and the public mental health system; service elements and the quality of functioning among the chronically mentally ill; study of post-World War II mental health policy; trends in children's mental health services; depression among the elderly; using managed care to improve mental health services; improving compliance to antipsychotic medications; the impact of the deinstitutionalization on communities; diversion programs for individuals with a mental illness who are in the criminal justice system; and cultural issues in mental health treatment.

★ 23234 ★ Rutgers University Center for State Health Policy (CSHP)
317 George St., Ste. 400
New Brunswick, NJ 08901-2008
Phone: (732)932-3105 **Fax:** (732)932-0069
Email: info@cshp.rutgers.edu
Website: http://www.cshp.rutgers.edu/
Joel C. Cantor, Dir.

Activities/Fields: State health policy issues in New Jersey, including long-term care, access to health care, racial and ethnic health disparities, health care performance measurement, pharmaceutical policy. **Pub:** *CSHP News*, quarterly. • *Issue briefs.* • *Reports.*

★ 23235 ★ Rutgers University Institute for Health, Health Care Policy, and Aging Research
30 College Ave.
New Brunswick, NJ 08901-1293
Phone: (732)932-8413 **Fax:** (732)932-6872
Email: caboyer@rci.rutgers.edu
Website: http://www-ihhcpar.rutgers.edu/
Dr. David Mechanic, Dir.

Activities/Fields: Research divisions include and focus on the following activities: the Division of Health studies the impact of stress on emotional states and health and risk behaviors and how these latter factors influence the immune system and morbidity and mortality, and studies how stress and emotional states affect symptom appraisal and the decision to use health care; the Division of Health Care Policy analyzes the health and cost outcomes of the current allocation of health and resources, with emphasis on preventive care and chronic illnesses; analyses the evolution of managed care and its impact on patient outcomes, medical professions and utilization of services; examines trust relationships among consumers and physicians and managed care organizations; the Division on Aging measures income inequality, investigates the role of instrumental and social support as buffers against stress and chronic illness, and identifies predictors of poor self-assessments of health among the elderly; the AIDS Policy Research Group measures health care utilization and cost among patients with HIV illness; the Center for Research on the Organization and Financing of Care for the Severely Mentally Ill provides a structure for interdisciplinary research and training on mental health services and policy for persons with severe and persistent mental illness and examines the human services and family support systems that shape outcomes for patients and their families. Multi-investigator research teams work in the areas of successful community living, organization and financing incentives in treatment programs, service systems integration, and managed care and rationing; the Center for State Health Policy is a recent initiative established to create a formal capacity within the university for policy analysis, research, training, facilitation, and consultation on state health policy. The center informs, supports, and stimulates sound and creative state health policy in New Jersey and around the nation.

★ 23236 ★ Rutgers University Institute for Health, Health Care Policy, and Aging Research Division on Aging AIDS Policy Research Group
30 College Ave.
New Brunswick, NJ 08901-1293
Phone: (732)932-8579 **Fax:** (732)932-6872
Email: scrystal@rci.rutgers.edu
Website: http://www.ihhcpar.rutgers.edu
Stephen Crystal, PhD, Dir.

Activities/Fields: Social and behavioral research on AIDS, focusing on policy issues and applying social science methodology to the planning and evaluation of programs and policies designed to meet public health objectives. Specific areas of research include HIV health services, long-term care, social networks, mental health programs, the social context of health-related behavior in Hispanic and black subcultures, health cognition and health belief systems, legal aspects of serving endangered and high-risk populations, and cost of care and services utilization studies. Special areas of emphasis include quality of life and long-term care for the elderly, intervention-focused behavioral science research, increasing patient-provider communication, furthering methods of research in health services field, adherence and access to prescription drugs and medical care, social and behavioral AIDS research, and mental health issues in relation to previous areas listed.

★ 23237 ★ Rutgers University Laboratory for Cancer Research
Department of Chemical Biology
College of Pharmacy
164 Frelinghuysen Rd.
Piscataway, NJ 08854-8020
Phone: (732)445-3400 **Fax:** (732)445-0687
Email: aconney@rci.rutgers.edu
Website: http://pharmacy.rutgers.edu/lcr/
Prof. Allan H. Conney, Dir.

Activities/Fields: Mechanisms of chemical carcinogenesis and mutagenesis; mechanisms of inhibition of carcinogenesis; factors influencing the metabolism and action of drugs, carcinogens, environmental chemicals and steroid hormones; regulation and biological significance of multiple cytochromes P-450; drug interactions; induced synthesis of microsomal enzymes.

★ 23238 ★ Sacro Occipital Research Society International
605 Central Ave. E
Winter Haven, FL 33880
Phone: (863)293-7789 **Free:** 888-245-1011
Fax: (863)293-5838
Email: cbinyon@kc.rr.com
Website: http://www.sorsi.com
Bernice Johnson, Pres.

Activities/Fields: Chiropractic studies, focusing on the sacro occipital area of the brain.

★ 23239 ★ Saginaw Valley State University Genetic Research Laboratory
7400 Bay Rd.
University Center, MI 48710
Phone: (989)790-4358 **Fax:** (989)790-2717
Email: cfp@svsu.edu
Website: http://www.svsu.edu/biology/
Dr. Charles F. Pelzer, Hd.

Activities/Fields: Molecular genetics, emphasizing electrophoresis and Southern Blots of human DNA, isoelectric focusing of blood proteins in health and disease such as breast cancer, and biochemical genetics of red cell isozymes in the mouse. Performs restriction fragment length polymorphism (RFLP) analysis to help map human chromosone number 10 and Southern blotting to identify tumor suppressor genes.

★ 23240 ★ St. Boniface General Hospital Research Centre
351 Tache Ave.
Winnipeg, MB, Canada R2H 2A6
Phone: (204)235-3206 **Fax:** (204)235-0793
Email: admin_office@sbrc.ca
Website: http://www.sbrc.ca/
Dr. John Foerster, Res. Dir.

Activities/Fields: Cardiovascular sciences, magnetic resonance imaging and spectroscopy, and the degenerative disorders associated with aging, such as senile dementias.

★ 23241 ★ St. Clare's Hospital and Health Center Spellman Center for HIV-Related Disease
415 W 51st St.
New York, NY 10019
Phone: (212)459-8130 **Fax:** (212)459-8353
Debbie Kane, Dir.

Activities/Fields: Clinical drug trials, including immune modulators, anti-retrovirals, prophylactic therapies for infections, DDI, and granulocyte-macrophage colony-stimulating activity factors.

★ 23242 ★ St. Francis Hospital (Brookville, NY) DeMatteis Center for Education and Research
Northern Blvd.
Brookville, NY 11545

Phone: (516)629-2000 **Fax:** (516)629-2113
Website: http://www.stfrancisheartcenter.com/preventive/index.html
Dr. Yadon Arad, Dir.
Activities/Fields: Heart studies, focusing on drugs and diet in reversing coronary heart disease; lipid metabolism; diabetes; steroid hormones.

★ 23243 ★ St. Francis Hospital (Tulsa, OK)
Natalie Warren Bryant Cancer Center
Warren Cancer Research Foundation
6151 S Yale, Ste. B103
Tulsa, OK 74136
Phone: (918)491-5878 **Fax:** (918)494-1527
Email: jblockhart@surgassoc.com
Dr. James Lockhart, Prin. Investigator
Activities/Fields: Bone marrow transplants, medical oncology, radiotherapy, pathology, and surgery. Conducts clinical trials.

★ 23244 ★ St. Francis Xavier University Comparative Biomechanics Research Laboratory
Biology Department
PO Box 5000
Antigonish, NS, Canada B2G 2W5
Phone: (902)867-5116 **Fax:** (902)867-2368
Email: edemont@stfx.ca
Website: http://www.stfx.ca/people/edemont/biomechanics-lab.html
M. Edwin DeMont, Dir.
Activities/Fields: Biological fluid dynamics and biomaterials.

★ 23245 ★ St. Joseph's Hospital
Firestone Institute of Respiratory Health
50 Charlton Ave. E
Hamilton, ON, Canada L8N 4A6
Phone: (905)522-1155
Email: dmartins@email.stjosham.on.ca
Website: http://www.stjosham.on.ca/firestone/index.htm
Dr. Dwayne Martins, Dir.
Activities/Fields: Respiratory diseases, including asthma, emphysema, chronic obstructive pulmonary disease, tuberculosis and other respiratory ailments.

★ 23246 ★ St. Jude Children's Research Hospital
332 N Lauderdale
Memphis, TN 38105-2794
Phone: (901)495-3300 **Free:** (866)278-5833
Fax: (901)495-3103
Website: http://www.stjude.org
Arthur W. Nienhuis, MD, Dir.
Activities/Fields: Pediatric studies in hematology, oncology, infectious diseases, diagnostic imaging, pharmaceutical sciences, behavioral medicine, and pathology; biomedical studies in biochemistry, immunology, molecular pharmacology, genetics and tumor cell biology, biostatistics, structural biology, surgery, developmental neurobiology, clinical informatics, and radiation oncology. **Pub:** *Annual Report.* • *Scientific Report*, semiannually. • *St Jude Rounds Newsletter for Pediatricians*, quarterly.

★ 23247 ★ St. Jude Children's Research Hospital
Department of Molecular Pharmacology
332 N Lauderdale
Memphis, TN 38105-2729
Phone: (901)495-3440 **Fax:** (901)495-4290
Email: peter.haughton@stjude.org
Website: http://www.stjude.org/molecular-pharmacology
Dr. Peter Houghton, Chm.
Activities/Fields: Human tumor xenografts, experimental chemotherapy, selectivity of drug action in in vivo, cytostasis and cytotoxicity, colon carcinoma and rhabdomyosarcoma, thymidylate synthase, molecular events controlling cell death, and relationships between genes involved in cell cycle control and sensitivity to chemotherapy.

★ 23248 ★ St. Louis University Center for Health Care Ethics
Health Science Center
3545 Lafayette Ave.
Saint Louis, MO 63104
Phone: (314)977-6660 **Fax:** (314)977-5150
Email: magill@slu.edu
Website: http://www.slu.edu/centers/chce
Prof. Gerard Magill, PhD, Dir.
Activities/Fields: Issues in health care ethics, including human genomics, stem cell research, organ transplants, end of life concerns, organizational ethics in health care, empirical research in health ethics. **Pub:** *Health Care Ethics USA Electronic Journal*, quarterly.

★ 23249 ★ St. Louis University Institute for Molecular Virology
3681 Park Ave.
Saint Louis, MO 63110
Phone: (314)577-8403 **Fax:** (314)577-8406
Email: green@slu.edu
Dr. Maurice Green, Chm.
Activities/Fields: Molecular biology, virology, cell biology, oncology, and AIDS, including structure and function of human viruses and mechanism of virus replication and cell transformation by ribonucleic and deoxyribose acid tumor viruses.

★ 23250 ★ St. Louis University Prevention Research Center
School of Public Health
3545 Lafayette Ave., 300
Saint Louis, MO 63104-1314
Phone: (314)977-8110 **Fax:** (314)977-3234
Email: brownson@slu.edu
Website: http://www.cdc.gov/prc/centers-stlouis.htm
Ross C. Brownson, PhD, Prin. Investigator
Activities/Fields: Public health issues, especially behaviors that place Americans at risk for chronic diseases and conditions. Of particular concern is the improvement in quality of life for special populations, including the young, elderly, racial ethnic populations, and the underserved.

★ 23251 ★ St. Louis University Theodore Cooper Surgical Research Institute
Department of Surgery
1402 S Grand Blvd.
Saint Louis, MO 63104
Phone: (314)577-8561 **Fax:** (314)268-5180
Email: smithp2@slu.edu
Dr. Gregory S. Smith, Dir.
Activities/Fields: Gastrointestinal and hepatic physiology, bioartificial liver, myocardial revascularization, drug metabolism, pharmacokinetics, toxicokinetics, organ transplantation and preservation, cardiac assist and replacement, myocardial preservation and pulmonary function, islet cell transplantation, immunology/nutrition, shock and multiple organ failure, neuropharmacology, transplantation immunogenetics, image guided surgery, and molecular biology. **Pub:** *Research Prospectus*, annually. • *SRI Insights*, quarterly. **Frmly:** Vallee Willman Surgical Research Institute; Institute of Experimental Surgery.

★ 23252 ★ St. Luke's-Roosevelt Hospital Center
James P. Mara Center for Lung Disease
1000 10th Ave., Ste. 3A55
New York, NY 10019
Phone: (212)523-5471 **Fax:** (212)523-8426
Email: ltartell@chpnet.org
Website: http://www.bethisraelny.org/directory/lung-site/
Activities/Fields: Airway biology, lung vascular permeability, chronic obstructive lung disease, pulmonary emphysema, asthma.

★ 23253 ★ Salk Institute for Biological Studies
PO Box 85800
San Diego, CA 92186-5800
Phone: (858)453-4100 **Fax:** (858)552-8285
Email: murphy@salk.edu
Website: http://www.salk.edu
Richard Murphy, Pres.
Activities/Fields: Cellular and molecular biology and neuroscience with particular emphasis on cancer, molecular genetics, tumor virology, reproductive biology, neurobiology, neuroendocrinology, growth control, prebiotic chemistry, and neurotransmitter/neuroreceptor structure and function; research aimed toward the discovery of cause, prevention, control, and cure of disease. **Pub:** *Newsletters.* • *Research Reports.*

★ 23254 ★ Salk Institute for Biological Studies
Cancer Center
PO Box 85800
San Diego, CA 92186-5800
Phone: (858)453-4100 **Fax:** (858)457-4765
Email: eckhart@salk.edu
Website: http://www.salk.edu
Dr. Walter Eckhart, Dir.
Activities/Fields: Participates as one of a group of selected nonclinical cancer centers in National Cancer Institute's nationwide program for coordinating multidisciplinary basic and clinical cancer research, improving methods of treatment, diagnosis, and prevention, training health professionals, and transferring cancer knowledge to surrounding communities, established under National Cancer Act of 1971. Areas of research include molecular biology, molecular genetics, cell biology, and developmental biology. Conducts basic research into mechanisms of cell regulation and growth control. **Frmly:** Armand Hammer Center for Cancer Biology.

★ 23255 ★ Salk Institute for Biological Studies
Computational Neurobiology Laboratory (CNL)
10010 N Torrey Pines Rd.
La Jolla, CA 92037
Phone: (858)453-4100
Email: terry@salk.edu
Website: http://www.cnl.salk.edu/
Dr. Terrence Sejnowski, Contact
Activities/Fields: Computational resources of the brain from the biophysical to the systems levels. The central issues being addressed are how dendrites integrate synaptic signals in neurons, how networks of neurons generate dynamical patterns of activity, how sensory information is represented in the cerebral cortex, how memory representations are formed and consolidated during sleep and how visuo-motor transformations are adaptively organized. **Pub:** *Annual report.* • *Papers.*

★ 23256 ★ San Diego State University Interwork Institute
Center for Pacific Studies
3590 Camino Del Rio N
San Diego, CA 92108-5313
Phone: (619)594-0139
Email: kgaleai@interwork.sdsu.edu
Website: http://interwork.sdsu.edu/
Kenneth Galeai, PhD, Contact
Activities/Fields: Improvement of the quality of rehabilitation services for persons with disabilities, especially to assure culturally relevant rehabilitation systems; to expand capacity building through research and training activities; to expand, improve and implement effective use of rehabilitation database systems; and to promote assistive technology. Research fo-

cuses on meeting the needs of Pacific Islanders with disabilities in Hawaii, Palau, Micronesia, the Marshall Islands, Guam, the Northern Marianas, and American Samoa.

★ 23257 ★ San Francisco Heart Institute
1900 Sullivan Ave.
Daly City, CA 94015
Phone: (650)991-6358 **Fax:** (650)755-7315
Email: richardshaw@dochs.org
Website: http://www.sfhi.com
Richard E. Shaw, PhD, Dir. Res. & Oper.
Activities/Fields: Analysis of success, complications, and long-term outcome of coronary angioplasty and cardiac surgery; technological advances applied to angioplasty, including balloons, lasers, and coronary stents; transdermal therapies in treatment of hypertension; and atherectomy (rotational and directional) research.

★ 23258 ★ San Francisco State University Center for Biomedical Laboratory Science
1600 Holloway Ave.
San Francisco, CA 94132
Phone: (415)338-1696 **Fax:** (415)338-7747
Email: lblackwo@sfsu.edu
Website: http://www.sfsu.edu/~cbls
Dr. Linda Blackwood, Actg. Dir.
Activities/Fields: Clinical chemistry, immunology, microbiology, hematology, and virology. **Frmly:** Center for Advanced Medical Technology.

★ 23259 ★ Sansum Medical Research Institute
2219 Bath St.
Santa Barbara, CA 93105
Phone: (805)682-7638 **Fax:** (805)682-3332
Email: ljovanovic@sansum.org
Website: http://www.sansum.org
Lois Jovanovic, MD, Dir.
Activities/Fields: Diabetes mellitus, immunology, cancer, gastrointestinal disorders and physiology.

★ 23260 ★ Saskatchewan Cancer Agency Cancer Research Unit
20 Campus Dr.
Saskatoon, SK, Canada S7N 4H4
Phone: (306)655-2778 **Fax:** (306)655-2635
Email: scarlsen@scf.sk.ca
Dr. S.A. Carlsen, Exec. Dir.
Activities/Fields: Basic cancer research, including elucidation of the properties of signal transduction, oncogene expression, tumor metastasis, drug sensitivity, and genetic engineering of novel biological reagents for tumor diagnosis and therapy.

★ 23261 ★ Saskatchewan Population Health and Evaluation Research Unit (SPHERU)
University of Regina
Regina, SK, Canada S4S 0A2
Phone: (306)585-5674 **Fax:** (306)585-5694
Email: spheru@regina.ca
Website: http://www.uregina.ca/spheru/
George W. Maslany, PhD, Assoc. Dir.
Activities/Fields: Population health determinants. Major research program areas are economic and environmental globalization, governance, and health; community environment as a health determinant; multiple roles, gender and health; and determinants of healthy childhood development. **Pub:** *Annual review.*

★ 23262 ★ Schepens Eye Research Institute
20 Staniford St.
Boston, MA 02114-2500
Phone: (617)912-0100 **Fax:** (617)912-0101
Email: geninfo@vision.eri.harvard.edu
Website: http://www.eri.harvard.edu
Dr. J. Wayne Streilein, Pres.
Activities/Fields: Retina, vitreous, cornea, glaucoma, immunology, neuroscience, transplantation, physiological optics, biomedical physics, oculartumors, and pharmacology with strong collaboration between clinic and laboratory studies on diseases of the retina and cornea, and on glaucoma. Develops ophthalmic instruments and devices for diagnosis and treatment of eye disease, and for low vision aids. **Pub:** *Sundial*, semiannually. **Frmly:** Retina Foundation; Eye Research Institute of Retina Foundation.

★ 23263 ★ Scripps Research Institute
10550 N Torrey Pines Rd.
La Jolla, CA 92037
Phone: (858)784-1000 **Fax:** (858)784-9899
Email: info@scripps.edu
Website: http://www.scripps.edu
Richard A. Lerner, MD, Pres.
Activities/Fields: Immunology and immunopathology, biochemistry, cell biology, molecular biology, structural biology, oncology, autoimmune diseases, cardiopulmonary diseases, hematology, diabetes and endocrinology, virology, preclinical neuroscience, neuropharmacology, vascular biology, synthetic bioorganic chemistry, biocatalysis and protein design, plant biology, and synthetic and vaccine development. **Pub:** *Scientific report.* **Frmly:** Research Institute of Scripps Clinic.

★ 23264 ★ Scripps Research Institute General Clinical Research Center
10550 N Torrey Pines Rd.
La Jolla, CA 92037
Phone: (858)784-1000
Email: info@scripps.edu
Website: http://gcrc.scripps.edu/
Francis V. Chisari, MD, Div. Hd.
Activities/Fields: Develops and evaluates new and experimental therapeutic procedures, including therapies for cancer, vascular disease, thrombotic disease, sleep disorders, multiple sclerosis, hepatitis, inflammatory bowel disease, asthma, alcoholism and depression, and autoimmune diseases such as rheumatoid arthritis and systemic lupus erythematosus.

★ 23265 ★ Scripps Research Institute Multiscale Modeling Tools for Structural Biology
10550 N Torrey Pines Rd.
La Jolla, CA 92037
Phone: (858)784-8035 **Fax:** (858)784-8688
Email: brooks@scripps.edu
Website: http://mmtsb.scripps.edu
Dr. Charles L. Brooks, III, Prin. Investigator
Activities/Fields: Structural biology, focusing on the development of new and integrated approaches to multiscale modeling, especially large-scale assemblies of nucleic acids and proteins with nucleic acids; development of methods that combine lattice-based dynamic Monte Carlo and all atom molecular dynamics; the study of physical processes involved in and the development of models for the interactions associated with virus assembly; establishment of new tools for the combined treatment of crystallographic and low-resolution structural models from cryo-electron microscopy.

★ 23266 ★ Scripps Research Institute W.M. Keck Autoimmune Diseases Center
10550 N Torrey Pines Rd.
La Jolla, CA 92037
Phone: (858)784-1000 **Fax:** (858)784-2131
Email: jbux@scripps.edu
Dr. Joel Buxbum, Dir.
Activities/Fields: Immunologic studies on the development of allergic disorders, especially aspirin and related drug sensitivities, bisulfite-sensitivity in asthma, and hereditary angioedema. Investigates the role of leukotrienes in the development of allergic disorders and conducts studies on drug-induced lupus reactions and the role specific autoantibodies may play in the development of the disease. Emphasizes immunology and molecular biology of autoimmunity related to lupus, scleroderma, Sjogren's syndrome, dermatomyositis, and polymyositis.

★ 23267 ★ Serological Research Institute (SERI)
3053 Research Dr.
Richmond, CA 94806
Phone: (510)223-7374 **Fax:** (510)222-8887
Email: bwraxall@serological.com
Website: http://www.serological.com/
Brian Wraxall, Exec. Dir.
Activities/Fields: Analyzing blood and other body fluids encountered as evidence in criminal and civil matters, including genetic marker typing in blood and other bodily fluid stains and new or improved methods of analysis of serological evidence.

★ 23268 ★ Sherbrooke University Centre for Study and Valorization of Microbial Diversity
Departement de Biologie
Faculte des Sciences
2500, boul. de l'Universite
Sherbrooke, QC, Canada J1K 2R1
Phone: (819)821-7062 **Fax:** (819)821-8049
Email: rbrzezin@courrier.usherb.ca
Website: http://www.usherb.ca/SCES/BIO/microbio.html
Ryszard Brzezinski, PhD, Contact
Activities/Fields: Molecular biology and genetic engineering of actinomycetes, gene cloning and characterization, development of new cloning vectors. Studies on pathogenesis mechanisms of potato scab. Development of biocontrol agents against plant disease. Development of streptomyces strains for biotechnological product ion of enzymes (xylanase; glucanases, chitosanase). **Frmly:** Actinomycete Biology Research Group.

★ 23269 ★ Sherbrooke University Gerontology and Geriatrics Research Centre
1036 Belvedere S
Sherbrooke, QC, Canada J1H 4C4
Phone: (819)829-7131 **Fax:** (819)829-7141
Email: info@cdrv.ca
Website: http://www.cdrv.ca
Dr. Helene Payette, Dir.
Activities/Fields: Biology of aging, oxidative stress, biosignalisation, rehabilitation, validation of measurement tools and methods, psychological distress, cognitive decline, family caregivers, quality of care, integrated services, Alzheimer's disease, diabetes, nutrition, epidemiology and prevention of functional decline, physical activity, gait and balance, psycho-sociology of aging, sleep disorders, medicine consumption, actualization of potential, psychological and spiritual well-being, abuse and crime issues, road and home safety, and emotion recognition.

★ 23270 ★ Sherbrooke University Group of the Canadian Institutes of Health in the Radiation Sciences
Faculty of Medicine
3001 12th Ave. N
Sherbrooke, QC, Canada J1H 5H3
Phone: (819)346-1110 **Fax:** (819)564-5442
Email: leon.sanche@usherbrooke.ca
Website: http://www.mednuc.usherb.ca
Dr. Leon Sanche, Dir.
Activities/Fields: Identification of the complex sequences of events initiated by the absorption of energy from ionizing radiation in biological material (which ultimately result in transformations at the cellular level), and the development of new types of drugs to enhance the therapeutic and diagnostic efficiency of radiation for the purpose of improving the treatment of human cancer with radio- and phototherapy. **Pub:** *Cahiers de radiobiologie: Aspects physiques, chi-*

miques et biologiques, 3/year. **Frmly:** MRC Group in the Radiation Sciences.

★ 23271 ★ Sherbrooke University Institute of Pharmacology of Sherbrooke
Faculty of Medicine
3001 12 Ave. Nord
Sherbrooke, QC, Canada J1H 5N4
Phone: (819)346-1110 **Fax:** (819)564-5398
Email: p.sirois@courrier.usherb.ca
Website: http://ips.med.usherb.ca/
Prof. Pierre Sirois, Contact
Activities/Fields: Cardiovascular and pulmonary pharmacology, including peptides and lipids, prostaglandins, leukotrienes, angiotensin, bradykinin, and related compounds.

★ 23272 ★ Shriners Burns Institute
815 Market St.
Galveston, TX 77550-2725
Phone: (409)770-6731 **Fax:** (409)770-6919
Email: dherndon@sbi.utmb.edu
David N. Herndon, MD, Ch.
Activities/Fields: Thermal injuries, wound healing, and scar formation, including treatment of burned children, cardiopulmonary complications, microcirculatory changes, nutritional and metabolic status, epidemiology and ideology of burn injuries, host responsiveness to secondary infections, lung injuries, and long term outcomes.

★ 23273 ★ Shriners Hospital for Children (Portland, OR) Research Center
3101 SW Sam Jackson Pk. Rd.
Portland, OR 97201-3095
Phone: (503)221-1537 **Fax:** (503)221-3451
Email: wah@shcc.org
Website: http://www.shcc.org/
Dr. William A. Horton, Res. Dir.
Activities/Fields: Connective tissues, matrix biology, skeletal development.

★ 23274 ★ Shriners Hospital for Children (St. Louis, MO) Center for Metabolic Bone Disease and Molecular Research
2001 S Lindbergh Blvd.
Saint Louis, MO 63131-3597
Phone: (314)432-3600 **Fax:** (314)872-7844
Email: mwhyte@shrinenet.org
Michael P. Whyte, MD, Med. Dir.
Activities/Fields: Metabolic bone diseases and skeletal dysplasias in children, including evaluation of potential medical therapies and analysis of inheritance factors. **Frmly:** Metabolic Research Unit.

★ 23275 ★ Shute Medical Clinic
367 Princess Ave.
London, ON, Canada N6B 2A7
Phone: (519)432-1884 **Fax:** (519)432-1886
Email: shutemedical@lweb.net
Dr. Julian Oates, Contact
Activities/Fields: Total approach to patient care, vitamin dosage response, use of vitamin E for burn treatment, and medicinal use of d-alpha tocopheryl in diabetes, stroke, angina, coronary artery diseases, and intermittent claudication and phlebitis.

★ 23276 ★ Sickle Cell Association of the Texas Gulf Coast
2626 S Loop W, Ste. 245
Houston, TX 77054
Phone: (713)666-0300 **Fax:** (713)666-0217
Email: kbeatty@sicklecell-texas.org
Website: http://www.sicklecell-texas.org
Kenneth G. Beatty, Exec. Dir.
Activities/Fields: Performs laboratory tests to identify persons with sickle cell disease. **Pub:** *Consumer Chronicles*, bimonthly. • *Sickle Cell Anemia Fast Facts.* • *Sickle Scope Newsletter*, quarterly. **Frmly:** Sickle Cell Disease Research Foundation of Texas Inc.

★ 23277 ★ Sidney Kimmel Cancer Center (SKCC)
10835 Altman Row
San Diego, CA 92121
Phone: (858)450-5990 **Fax:** (858)450-3251
Website: http://www.skcc.org/
Albert B. Deisseroth, MD, Pres. /CEO
Activities/Fields: Cancer diagnosis, treatment and prevention, based on understanding the genetic components of cancer which may lead to gene therapy, vaccine therapy and immunotherapy. **Pub:** *SKCC News.*

★ 23278 ★ Sierra Biomedical Research Corp.
1000 Locust St.
Reno, NV 89502-2597
Phone: (775)328-1487 **Fax:** (775)328-1816
Email: joseph.cardillo@med.va.gov
Joseph E. Cardillo, PhD, Contact
Activities/Fields: Biomedical and clinical research.

★ 23279 ★ Simon Fraser University Environmental Physiology Unit
Sch. of Kinesiology
8888 University Dr.
Burnaby, BC, Canada V5A 1S6
Phone: (604)291-3276 **Fax:** (604)291-3040
Email: ablaber@sfu.ca
Website: http://www.sfu.ca/epu
Andrew P. Blaber, Dir.
Activities/Fields: Professional divers response to carbon dioxide and nitrogin narcosis, models of thermoregulatory control, altitude acclimation, decompression sickness, astronaut EVA decompression protocols, health hazard appraisal, design and performance evaluation of underwater breathing apparatus, hyperbaric oxygen toxicity, evaluation of personal flotation devices, hypothermia protection, environmental testing of equipment, and pressure testing of diving equipment.

★ 23280 ★ Smith-Kettlewell Eye Research Institute
2318 Fillmore St.
San Francisco, CA 94115
Phone: (415)345-2000 **Fax:** (415)345-8455
Email: abs@ski.org
Website: http://www.ski.org
Alan B. Scott, MD, Exec. Dir.
Activities/Fields: Visual sciences, oculomotor functioning, and rehabilitation engineering, including long-term study of the surgical and pharmacological treatment of strabismus; development of diagnostic tests for glaucoma, retinitis pigmentosa, diabetic retinopathy, and senile macular degeneration; research on the physiological basis of eye movements; studies in motion detection, pattern perception, and stereopsis; and development and evaluation of sensory aids and devices for the deaf, blind, deaf/blind, and sensory-impaired individuals. **Pub:** *Rehabilitation Engineering Center Annual Report.*

★ 23281 ★ Smith-Kettlewell Rehabilitation Engineering Research Center
2318 Fillmore St.
San Francisco, CA 94115
Phone: (415)345-2110 **Fax:** (415)345-8455
Email: rerc@ski.org
Website: http://www.ski.org/Rehab/
Dr. John A. Brabyn, Dir.
Activities/Fields: Technology for blindness, visual impairment, and multi-sensory loss. **Pub:** *Annual Report.* • *IBM diskette.* • *Smith-Kettlewell Technical File Journal (in braille)*, quarterly.

★ 23282 ★ Social Psychiatry Research Institute
150 E 69th St., No. 2-H
New York, NY 10021
Phone: (212)628-4800 **Fax:** (212)249-8546
Dr. Ari Kiev, Pres.
Activities/Fields: Mental health and psychiatry, including psychopharmacological studies of antidepressant, anti-anxiety, and Alzheimer's medications. Conducts clinical drug trials. Assembles data for the mental health and psychiatric professions.

★ 23283 ★ Society for Epidemiologic Research
Department of Family & Preventive Medicine
375 Chipeta Way, Ste. A
Salt Lake City, UT 84108
Phone: (801)581-7234 **Fax:** (801)587-3353
Email: jlyon@dfpm.utah.edu
Website: http://www.epiresearch.org
Dr. Joseph L. Lyon, Treas.
Activities/Fields: Epidemiology, focusing on research and education. **Pub:** *American Journal of Epidemology.*

★ 23284 ★ Society for Menstrual Cycle Research
10559 N 104th Pl.
Scottsdale, AZ 85258
Phone: (480)451-9731 **Fax:** (480)451-9731
Email: maryannafriederich@msn.com
Website: http://www.pop.psu.edu/smcr
Mary Anna Friederich, MD, Contact
Activities/Fields: Women's menstrual cycles, including endocrinology, genetics, physiology, psychology, medicine, sociology, and research, focusing on menstrual cycle networking and the health needs of women. **Pub:** *Newsletter*, semiannually. • *Proceedings*, biennially.

★ 23285 ★ Society for the Study of Blood
VA Medical
800 Poly Pl.
Brooklyn, NY 11209
Phone: (718)836-6600 **Fax:** (718)630-2822
Email: luhrs.carol@new-york.va.gov
Dr. Carol Luhrs, Contact
Activities/Fields: Hematology, blood groupings, transfusion, physiology, and pathology of blood.

★ 23286 ★ Society for the Study of Reproduction
1619 Monroe St.
Madison, WI 53711-2063
Phone: (608)256-2777 **Fax:** (608)256-4610
Email: ssr@ssr.org
Website: http://www.ssr.org
P. Landis Keyes, Pres.
Activities/Fields: Reproduction, focusing on interdisciplinary communication within the science. **Pub:** *Biology of Reproduction (13/year).* • *Biology of Reproduction Monograph.*

★ 23287 ★ Solomon Park Research Institute
12815 NE 124th St., Ste. L
Kirkland, WA 98034-8313
Phone: (425)650-2020 **Fax:** (425)650-2028
Email: pclapshaw@solomon.org
Website: http://www.solomon.org
Patric A. Clapshaw, PhD, Dir.
Activities/Fields: Amyotrophic lateral sclerosis (ALS), also known as Lou Gehrig's Disease.

★ 23288 ★ South Carolina Health and Environmental Control Department
Health Services Division
Bureau of Environmental Health
2600 Bull St.
Columbia, SC 29201
Phone: (803)896-0646 **Fax:** (803)896-0645
Email: scottrd@dhec.sc.gov
Website: http://www.scdhec.net
Roger D. Scott, Dir.
Activities/Fields: Environmental pollution and its effects.

★ 23289 ★ South Carolina Health and Environmental Control Department
Health Services Division
Bureau of Laboratories
8231 Parklane Rd.
Columbia, SC 29223
Phone: (803)896-0800 **Fax:** (803)896-0983
Email: dowdahe@columb68.dhec.state.sc.us
Website: http://www.scdhec.net/hs/lab/lab.htm
Harold Dowda, PhD, Ch.
Activities/Fields: Health issues. **Pub:** *Bureau of Laboratories Annual Report.*

★ 23290 ★ South Carolina Health and Environmental Control Department
Health Services Division
Bureau of Laboratories
Diagnostic Microbiology Division
8231 Parklane Rd.
Columbia, SC 29223
Phone: (803)896-0965 **Fax:** (803)896-0657
Email: wozniaka@columb68.dhec.state.sc.us
Dr. Arthur Wozniak, Dir.
Activities/Fields: Arboviruses, emerging diseases. **Frmly:** Virology/Serology Division.

★ 23291 ★ South Carolina Health and Environmental Control Department
Health Services Division
Bureau of Laboratories
Division of Clinical Cytology
8231 Parklane Rd.
Columbia, SC 29223
Phone: (803)896-0892 **Fax:** (803)896-0983
Marc S. Busnardo, MD, Dir.
Activities/Fields: Nature of diseases and the changes caused by them.

★ 23292 ★ Southern California Evidence-Based Practice Center (EPC)
1700 Main St.
PO Box 2138
Santa Monica, CA 90407-2138
Phone: (310)393-0411
Email: paul_shekelle@rand.org
Website: http://www.rand.org/health/epc/
Dr. Paul G. Shekelle, Dir.
Activities/Fields: Improving the methods of synthesizing the evidence and technology assessments from reviews of all aspects of health care.

★ 23293 ★ Southern California Research Institute
11914 W Washington Blvd.
Los Angeles, CA 90066
Phone: (310)390-8481 **Fax:** (310)398-6651
Email: mburns5573@aol.com
Website: http://www.scri.org
Dr. Marcelline Burns, Dir.
Activities/Fields: Effects of alcohol and drugs on behavior, including effects of alcohol and drugs on driving.

★ 23294 ★ Southern Illinois University at Carbondale
Center for Alzheimer Disease and Related Disorders (CADRD)
PO Box 19643
Springfield, IL 62794-9643
Phone: (217)545-8249 **Fax:** (217)545-1903
Email: neuro@siumed.edu
Website: http://www.siumed.edu/neuro/cadrd.html
Rodger J. Elble, PhD, Dir.
Activities/Fields: Aging, Alzheimer's Disease, Parkinson's Disease, vascular dementia, and gait disturbances in the elderly.

★ 23295 ★ Southern Illinois University at Carbondale
Center for Rural Health and Social Service Development (CRHSSD)
Office of Economic & Regional Development, MC 6892
Carbondale, IL 62901-6892
Phone: (618)453-1262 **Fax:** (618)453-5040
Email: tessh@siu.edu
Website: http://www.siu.edu/~crhssd/
Tess D. Heiple, PhD, Dir.
Activities/Fields: Health care and social service issues that impact the lives and productivity of the citizens in the state and nation, including alternative service delivery systems and policy alternatives. Studies include rural primary health care, rural safety and health promotion, and rural environmental health.

★ 23296 ★ Southern Louisiana Cystic Fibrosis Clinical Care and Research Center/Pediatric Pulmonary Center
Tulane University
1430 Tulane Ave.
New Orleans, LA 70112
Phone: (504)588-5601 **Fax:** (504)588-5490
Email: shdavis@tulane.edu
Dr. Scott Davis, Dir.
Activities/Fields: Cystic fibrosis, childhood asthma, apnea, sleep disorders and sleep disordered breathing, SIDS, control of breathing in immature mammal models.

★ 23297 ★ Southwest Foundation for Biomedical Research
PO Box 760549
San Antonio, TX 78245-0549
Phone: (210)258-9400 **Fax:** (210)670-3301
Email: fledford@icarus.sfbr.org
Website: http://www.sfbr.org
Dr. Frank F. Ledford, Jr., Pres.
Activities/Fields: Arteriosclerosis, hypertension, cancer, pulmonary disease, aging, genetics, endocrinology, reproductive physiology, virology, neuropharmacology, behavioral science, and organic chemistry. **Pub:** *Annual Report.* • *Progress in Medical Research,* quarterly.

★ 23298 ★ Southwest Foundation for Biomedical Research
Genetics Core Laboratory
Department of Genetics
PO Box 760549
San Antonio, TX 78245-0147
Phone: (210)258-9688 **Fax:** (210)670-3344
Email: scole@darwin.sfbr.org
Website: http://www.sfbr.org
Dr. Shelley Cole, Dir.
Activities/Fields: Molecular genetics of chronic diseases in humans and nonhuman primates. **Frmly:** Molecular Genetics Laboratory.

★ 23299 ★ Southwest Foundation for Biomedical Research
Southwest National Primate Research Center
PO Box 760549
San Antonio, TX 78245-0549
Phone: (210)258-9885 **Fax:** (210)258-9883
Email: stardif@sfbr.org
Website: http://www.sfbr.org/srprc/welcome.html
John L. VandeBerg, PhD, Dir.
Activities/Fields: Nonhuman primate models of human diseases, including common chronic diseases and infectious diseases; genetic and environmental effects on physiological processes and on susceptibility to specific diseases.

★ 23300 ★ Southwest SIDS Research Institute, Inc.
100 Medical Dr.
Lake Jackson, TX 77566-5674
Phone: (979)297-4411 **Free:** 800-245-SIDS
Fax: (979)297-6682
Email: swsids@sat.net
Website: http://www.swsids.hicd.com
Judith A. Henslee, Exec. Dir.
Activities/Fields: Sudden Infant Death Sydrome (SIDS). **Pub:** *Medical articles and abstracts.*

★ 23301 ★ Stanford University
AIDS Clinical Trials Unit
Division of Infectious Diseases, Rm. S-156
Stanford, CA 94305-5107
Phone: (650)723-6231 **Fax:** (650)725-2395
Email: merigan@stanford.edu
Website: http://www-leland.stanford.edu/group/aids/index.html
Dr. Thomas C. Merigan, Dir.
Activities/Fields: Antiviral drug studies, including inhibitors of HIV, HBV, and herpes replication using in vitro and in vivo antiviral models.

★ 23302 ★ Stanford University
Beckman Center for Molecular and Genetic Medicine
Department of Developmental Biology
School of Medicine
279 Campus Dr.
Stanford, CA 94305
Phone: (650)725-7657 **Fax:** (650)725-7739
Email: shapiro@cmgm.stanford.edu
Dr. Lucy Shapiro, Dir.
Activities/Fields: Molecular understanding of critical biological functions and how these are affected by disease, including study of genes related to human disease, development of new diagnostic tests for known and newly recognized diseases, and development of therapies based on gene or cell replacement models.

★ 23303 ★ Stanford University
Center for Advanced Magnetic Resonance Technology
Lucas Magnetic Resonance Spectroscopy & Imaging Center
Schools of Medicine & Engineering
Stanford, CA 94305-5488
Phone: (650)723-7577 **Fax:** (650)723-5795
Email: gary@s-word.stanford.edu
Website: http://www-radiology.stanford.edu/research/RR.html
Gary H. Glover, PhD, Prin. Investigator
Activities/Fields: Development of innovative magnetic resonance techniques for fundamental anatomic, physiologic, and pathophysiologic studies involving animals and humans. Core technology development encompasses these five areas: reconstruction methods, imaging of brain activation, MR spectroscopy and multinuclear imaging, cardiovascular structure and function, and interventional imaging methods.

★ 23304 ★ Stanford University
Center for Biomedical Ethics
701A Welch Rd., Ste. 1105
Palo Alto, CA 94304
Phone: (650)723-5760 **Fax:** (650)725-6131
Email: tar@stanford.edu
Website: http://scbe.stanford.edu
Dr. Tom Raffin, Co-Dir.
Activities/Fields: Scientific and biomedical ethics, focusing on applying ethical reasoning to actual moral problems in the practice of medicine and science; contributing to the national and international discussion of biomedical and scientific issues through research, with a focus on empirical bioethics studies; convening scholars, professionals, and policymakers to debate and propose policy solutions regarding biomedical and scientific ethical issues; and serving as a scholarly resource for the University and the community.

★ 23305 ★ Stanford University
Center of Excellence for the Diagnosis and Treatment of Sleep Disorders
701 Welch Rd., Ste. 2226
Palo Alto, CA 94304
Phone: (650)725-6416 **Fax:** (650)725-7341
Email: dement@stanford.edu
Website: http://www.med.stanford.edu/school/psychiatry/coe/
Dr. William C. Dement, Dir.
Activities/Fields: Sleep disorders, narcolepsy, circadian rhythms, and human sleep.

★ 23306 ★ Stanford University
Center for Health Policy (CHP)
117 Encina Commons
Stanford, CA 94305-6019
Phone: (650)723-1020 **Fax:** (650)723-1919
Email: info@healthpolicy.stanford.edu
Website: http://chppcor.stanford.edu/
Alan M. Garber, Dir.
Activities/Fields: Comparative health care systems and epidemiology, health care financing, health expenditure forecasting, effects of the legal and regulatory environment on medical practices and costs, and managed care and the effects of structural changes in the health care market. **Pub:** *Newsletter.*

★ 23307 ★ Stanford University
Center for Primary Care and Outcomes Research (PCOR)
117 Encina Commons
Stanford, CA 94305-6019
Phone: (650)723-1020 **Fax:** (650)723-1919
Email: info@healthpolicy.stanford.edu
Website: http://chppcor.stanford.edu/
Alan M. Garber, Dir.
Activities/Fields: Clinical practice and public health, including medical technology assessment, advancement of primary care policy and practice, clinical decision making and practice guideline development, and medical outcomes. **Pub:** *Newsletter.*

★ 23308 ★ Stanford University
General Clinical Research Center
300 Pasteur Dr., Unit H1 Wing, Mail Code 5251
Stanford, CA 94305
Phone: (650)724-0921 **Fax:** (650)725-6698
Email: brandy@stanford.edu
Website: http://www.stanford.edu/dept/gcrc
Branimir I. Sikic, MD, Prog. Dir.
Activities/Fields: Clinical research on nutrition, diabetes, growth hormone deficiencies and growth hormone therapies, oncology, monoclonal antibodies, lupus nephritis, epidermolysis bullosa, pharmokinetics of drugs, interferon, infectious diseases, human immunodeficiency virus (HIV), and sleep disorders; physiological and pathophysiological adaptations of prematurely born infants, critically ill term infants, and normal infants. Also focuses on computer modelling of pressure-limited mechanical ventilation, infant heme catabolism, modulation of circadian rhythmicity in preterm infants, treatment of perinatal infectious diseases such as neonatal herpes simplex infection and AIDS, markers of basement membrane disruption, late pulmonary sequelae of BPD, treatment of newborn skin, cystic fibrosis, and extra corporeal membrane oxygenation (ECMO).

★ 23309 ★ Stanford University
Image Guidance Laboratories (IGL)
Department of Neurosurgery
School of Medicine
300 Pasteur Dr., MC No. 5327 at S-008
Stanford, CA 94305-5327
Phone: (650)498-7958 **Fax:** (650)724-4846
Email: info@igl.stanford.edu
Website: http://neurosurgery.stanford.edu/igl/
Prof. Ramin Shahidi, Dir.
Activities/Fields: Surgical navigation techniques and minimally invasive surgical technology. **Pub:** *Papers.*

★ 23310 ★ Stanford University
Laboratory for Transplantation Immunology
Falk Cardiovascular Research Bldg., MS 5407
Department of Cardiothoracic Surgery
School of Medicine
300 Pasteur Dr.
Stanford, CA 94305-5407
Phone: (650)498-6391 **Fax:** (650)498-7854
Email: dborie@stanford.edu
Dominic Borie, Contact
Activities/Fields: Development of compounds to reduce rejection of transplanted organs. Studies focus on small molecules, monoclonal antibodies, and naturally occurring substances.

★ 23311 ★ Stanford University
Liver Transplant Program
750 Welch Rd., Ste. 215
Palo Alto, CA 94304-1509
Phone: (650)725-3360 **Fax:** (650)498-5692
Email: ggarcia@stanford.edu
Dr. Gabriel Garcia, Contact
Activities/Fields: Gastroenterology, focusing on treatment of viral hepatitis. **Frmly:** Gastroenterology Clinic.

★ 23312 ★ Stanford University
National Biocomputation Center
701 Welch Rd., Ste. 1128
Palo Alto, CA 94304
Phone: (650)498-6978 **Fax:** (650)498-5626
Email: kevin@biocomp.stanford.edu
Website: http://biocomp.stanford.edu
Kevin Montgomery, PhD, Tech. Dir.
Activities/Fields: Wireless telemedicine, 3D imaging, visualization, and simulation.

★ 23313 ★ Stanford University
Pain Management Center
300 Pasteur Dr., Rm. A408
Stanford, CA 94305
Phone: (650)723-6238 **Fax:** (650)725-7743
Email: gaeta@stanford.edu
Website: http://paincenter.stanford.edu/main.html
Raymond Gaeta, MD, Dir.
Activities/Fields: Pain mechanisms, actions of analgesic substances, and pharmacokinetic and pharmacodynamic modeling.

★ 23314 ★ Stanford University
Sleep Research Center
701 Welch Rd., Ste. 2226
Palo Alto, CA 94304
Phone: (650)723-5876 **Fax:** (650)725-7341
Website: http://www.med.stanford.edu/school/Psychiatry/scn/score8.html
Dr. William C. Dement, Dir.
Activities/Fields: Sleep, including brain mechanisms which control transitions between sleep and wakefulness, transitions between sleep states, and the circadian timing between those various states. **Frmly:** Center for Research on Sleep and Circadian Rhythm.

★ 23315 ★ Stanford University
Stanford Cardiac Rehabilitation Program
780 Welch Rd., Ste. 106
Palo Alto, CA 94304-5735
Phone: (650)723-6463 **Fax:** (650)723-6798
Email: lisa.shultz@stanford.edu
Robert F. DeBusk, MD, Dir.
Activities/Fields: Recovery from heart attack and coronary heart surgery, systems to facilitate risk factor modification in healthy individuals and patients with heart disease, and systems to enhance the cost-effectiveness of care provided to patients with heart disease. Coordinates random clinical trials in Kaiser foundation hospitals.

★ 23316 ★ Stanford University
Stanford Center for Narcolepsy
Department of Psychiatry & Behavioral Sciences
Stanford University Medical Center/Sleep Research Center
701 B Welch Rd., Rm. 143
Palo Alto, CA 94304-5742
Phone: (650)725-6517 **Fax:** (650)725-4913
Email: mignot@stanford.edu
Website: http://www.med.stanford.edu/school/psychiatry/narcolepsy
Dr. Emmanuel Mignot, Dir.
Activities/Fields: Narcolepsy, from pharmacological treatments for patients to isolating the genes.

★ 23317 ★ Stanford University
Stanford Center for Tuberculosis Research
Division of Infectious Diseases & Geographic Medicine
Stanford University Medical Center, Rm. S143
Stanford, CA 94305-5107
Phone: (650)725-7908 **Fax:** (650)498-7011
Email: peter@molepi.stanford.edu
Website: http://molepi.stanford.edu/tb.www.html
Prof. Peter M. Small, MD, Prin. Investigator
Activities/Fields: Contemporary transmission dynamics and pathogenesis of tuberculosis, using the integration of molecular and conventional epidemiology.

★ 23318 ★ Stanford University
Stanford Human Genome Center
975 California
Palo Alto, CA 94304
Phone: (650)320-5800 **Fax:** (650)320-5801
Email: myers@shgc.stanford.edu
Website: http://shgc.stanford.edu/
Richard Myers, Dir.
Activities/Fields: Construction of high resolution Radiation Hybrid maps of the human genome and the sequencing of large, contiguous genomic relations.

★ 23319 ★ Stanford University
Stanford Medical Informatics (SMI)
MSOB X-215
251 Campus Dr.
Stanford, CA 94305-5479
Phone: (650)723-6979 **Fax:** (650)725-7944
Email: musen@smi.stanford.edu
Website: http://www-camis.stanford.edu/main.html
Prof. Mark A. Musen, MD, Hd.
Activities/Fields: Methods for acquiring, representing, processing, and managing knowledge and data within health care and the biomedical sciences.

★ 23320 ★ Stanford University
Stanford Prevention Research Center
Hoover Pavilion, Rm. N229
211 Quarry Rd.
Stanford, CA 94305-5705
Phone: (650)723-6145 **Fax:** (650)725-6906
Email: fortmann@stanford.edu
Website: http://prevention.stanford.edu
Stephen P. Fortmann, MD, Dir.
Activities/Fields: Prevention and control of chronic disease, alcohol and drug abuse, and injury and death. Stresses a public health or community approach to disease prevention and health promotion and seeks methods to improve the overall level of community health by favorably modifying the environmental and personal factors known to influence chronic disease incidence, including blood pressure, blood cholesterol, cigarette use, nutrition, obesity, physical activity, and stress. **Pub:** *Catalogue available for health promotion materials.* **Frmly:** Center for Research in Disease Prevention; Stanford Heart Disease Prevention Program.

★ 23321 ★ Stanford University
Stanford/VA NIH Alzheimer's Disease Research Center
3801 Miranda Ave. (151Y)
Palo Alto, CA 94304
Phone: (650)852-3287 **Fax:** (650)852-3297
Email: yesavage@stanford.edu
Website: http://www.stanford.edu/~yesavage/ACRC.html
Dr. Jerome Yesavage, Dir.
Activities/Fields: Alzheimer's Disease, especially cognitive changes in older adults.

★ 23322 ★ State University of New York at Binghamton
Institute for Primary and Preventative Health Care
Academic Bldg. B, Rm. 116
PO Box 6000
Binghamton, NY 13902-6000
Phone: (607)777-6086 **Fax:** (607)777-6162
Email: gdjames@binghamton.edu
Website: http://www.binghamton.edu/ipph/abou-tipph.html
Gary D. James, Dir.
Activities/Fields: Causes and consequences of health and disease; implementation, organization, and effectiveness of primary and preventative health care regimens.

★ 23323 ★ State University of New York at Binghamton
Roger L. Kresge Center for Nursing Research
Decker School of Nursing
PO Box 6000
Binghamton, NY 13902-6000
Email: gspencer@binghamton.edu
Website: http://dson.binghamton.edu/kresge.htm
Prof. Gale A. Spencer, PhD, Dir.
Activities/Fields: Health care and nursing science. **Pub:** *Newsletter.*

★ 23324 ★ State University of New York at Buffalo
Center for Anxiety Research
337 Park Hall
Department of Psychology
Buffalo, NY 14260
Phone: (716)645-3550
Email: jgbeck@buffalo.edu
Website: http://pluto.fss.buffalo.edu/jgbeck/MVA/index.html
Dr. Gayle Beck, Contact
Activities/Fields: Assessment and treatment of anxiety disorders. Research interests involve the interaction of cognitive, affective, and physiological processes as these influence the development and maintenance of behavior disorders in adults.

★ 23325 ★ State University of New York at Buffalo
Center for Assistive Technology (CAT)
515 Kimball Tower
Buffalo, NY 14214-3079
Phone: (716)829-3141 **Free:** 800-828-2281
Fax: (716)829-3217
Email: kbeaver@acsu.buffalo.edu
Website: http://cat.buffalo.edu/
Dr. William C. Mann, Dir.
Activities/Fields: Assistive devices for persons with disabilities.

★ 23326 ★ State University of New York at Buffalo
Center for Dental Studies
250 Squire Hall
School of Dental Medicine
Buffalo, NY 14214
Phone: (716)829-3848 **Fax:** (716)837-7623
Email: ciancio@buffalo.edu
Website: http://www.sdm.buffalo.edu/dept.asp?dept=CDS
Dr. Sebastian G. Ciancio, Dir.
Activities/Fields: Dental research, including new product evaluation.

★ 23327 ★ State University of New York at Buffalo
Center of Excellence in Bioinformatics
901 Washington St., Ste. 300
Buffalo, NY 14203-1199
Phone: (716)849-6719 **Fax:** (716)849-6747
Email: bceb@buffalo.edu
Website: http://www.bioinformatics.buffalo.edu
Dr. Jeffrey Skolnick, Dir.
Activities/Fields: Systems biology - what proteins do, how they interact and how drugs to treat diseases can be designed. Research interests include bioinformatics, protein function prediction, protein structure prediction, elucidation of metabolic pathways, development and implementation of algorithms for large-scale computer simulations of proteins.

★ 23328 ★ State University of New York at Buffalo
Center for Hearing and Deafness
215 Parker Hall
3435 Main St.
Buffalo, NY 14214
Phone: (716)829-2001 **Fax:** (716)829-2980
Email: salvi@buffalo.edu
Website: http://wings.buffalo.edu/faculty/research/chd/
Dr. Richard J. Salvi, Hd.
Activities/Fields: Restoring the hearing of the deaf, hearing loss due to loud noises, medication, or age, middle ear infections in children, hearing loss in infants. Studies include hair cell regeneration, drug therapy and otoxic drugs, noise-induced hearing loss, middle ear disease, infant hearing assessment, auditory plasticity, mechanical transduction, age-related hearing loss, and central auditory processing.

★ 23329 ★ State University of New York at Buffalo
Center for Oral Health Research
Foster Hall
3435 Main St.
Buffalo, NY 14214
Phone: (716)829-2854 **Fax:** (716)829-2387
Email: rjgenco@acsu.buffalo.edu
Dr. Robert J. Genco, Chm. /Dir.
Activities/Fields: Laboratory, clinical, and epidemiological investigations of periodontal disease, particularly the etiology, risk factors pathogenesis, and management of this and other chronic bacterial infections; Specific areas of study include microbiology, host response mechanisms, clinical analysis, risk factors, and the development of genetic probes, novel antibiotics, and growth factors as they apply to periodontal diseases. Periodontal disease as a factor in poor diabetic control, cardiovascular disease, respiratory disease and other systemic conditions is also under investigation. **Pub:** *Contemporary Periodontics.* **Frmly:** Periodontal Disease Research Center; Comprehensive Oral Health Research Center of Discovery.

★ 23330 ★ State University of New York at Buffalo
Center for Positron Emission Tomography
105 Parker Hall
Buffalo, NY 14214-3007
Phone: (716)838-5889 **Fax:** (716)838-4918
Email: rea@buffalo.edu
Website: http://www.nucmed.buffalo.edu/cpethm.htm
Dr. Robert E. Ackerhalt, Dir.
Activities/Fields: Neurology, oncology, and cardiology, focusing on the use of Positron Emission Tomography (PET).

★ 23331 ★ State University of New York at Buffalo
Clinical Pharmacokinetics Laboratory
Hochstetter Hall 543
School of Pharmacy
Amherst, NY 14260
Phone: (716)867-0550 **Fax:** (716)838-0756
Email: schentag@buffalo.edu
Dr. Jerome J. Schentag, Dir.
Activities/Fields: Pharmacokinetics and pharmacodynamics of drugs in volunteers and hospitalized patients. Major emphasis on geriatric patients, pharmacology, nutrition, cancer, cardiology, metabolism, and infectious disease states. Other research activities include technology transfer using computer software in the critical care unit and influence of disease states on the pharmacokinetics and pharmacodynamics of drugs. **Pub:** *Research Papers.*

★ 23332 ★ State University of New York at Buffalo
Hearing Research Laboratory
215 Parker Hall
3435 Main St.
Buffalo, NY 14214
Phone: (716)829-2001 **Fax:** (716)829-2980
Email: salvi@acsu.buffalo.edu
Website: http://wings.buffalo.edu/faculty/research/chd
Dr. Richard J. Salvi, Co-Dir.
Activities/Fields: Hearing, including effects of noise, effects of ototoxic drugs, and basic auditory processes. **Pub:** *J. Acoustical Society of America*, 3/year.

★ 23333 ★ State University of New York at Buffalo
Hemodynamics Laboratory
323 Jarvis Hall
Buffalo, NY 14260-4400
Phone: (716)645-2593
Email: scottw@eng.buffalo.edu
Website: http://www.eng.buffalo.edu/Research/Hemo/
Scott H. Woodward, Tech. Dir.
Activities/Fields: Understanding the blood flow through cerebral aneurysms and characterizing the hemodynamic parameters associated with aneurysm formation, growth and rupture.

★ 23334 ★ State University of New York at Buffalo
Infectious and Chronic Disease Center (ICDC)
School of Dental Medicine
Department of Oral Biology
115 Foster Hall

3435 Main St.
Buffalo, NY 14214
Phone: (716)829-2844 **Fax:** (716)829-2387
Email: rjgenco@acsu.buffalo.edu
Dr. Robert J. Genco, Prin. Investigator
Activities/Fields: Interactions of infections, such as periodontal disease, with chronic diseases including heart disease, respiratory disease, and osteoporosis.

★ 23335 ★ State University of New York at Buffalo
Periodontal Disease Clinical Research Center
Foster Hall, Rm. 120
Buffalo, NY 14260
Phone: (716)829-2853 **Fax:** (716)829-2387
Email: rigenco@buffalo.edu
Website: http://www.sdm.buffalo.edu/research/cent_per.html
Dr. Robert J. Genco, Dir.
Activities/Fields: Periodontal disease.

★ 23336 ★ State University of New York at Buffalo
Rehabilitation Engineering Research Center on Universal Design and the Built Environment at Buffalo
378 Hayes Hall
School of Architecture & Planning
Buffalo, NY 14228-2567
Phone: (716)829-3483 **Fax:** (716)829-3861
Email: arced@ap.buffalo.edu
Website: http://www.ncddr.org/cgi-bin/mysql/nidrrprofiles.cgi?showproj=H133E990005&location =projabstract
Edward Steinfeld, Prin. Investigator
Activities/Fields: Universal and ergonomic design of the built environment. **Pub:** *Technical reports.*

★ 23337 ★ State University of New York at Buffalo
Research Institute on Addictions
1021 Main St.
Buffalo, NY 14203-1016
Phone: (716)887-2566 **Fax:** (716)887-2252
Email: connors@ria.buffalo.edu
Website: http://www.ria.buffalo.edu
Gerard J. Connors, PhD, Dir.
Activities/Fields: Etiology, course, treatment, and prevention of alcoholism and substance abuse. Studies the following six aspects of substance abuse: normative patterns; biochemical, physiological, psychological, and social antecedents and consequences; biopsychosocial aspects of consumption in early and middle adulthood; family aspects; alcohol-drug interactions; and treatment and prevention strategies. **Pub:** *RIA Annual Report.* • *RIA Report,* quarterly. **Frmly:** Research Institute on Alcoholism.

★ 23338 ★ State University of New York at Buffalo
Speech-Language and Hearing Clinic
50 Biomedical Education Bldg.
3435 Main St.
Buffalo, NY 14214
Phone: (716)829-3980 **Fax:** (716)829-3974
Email: srobert@acsu.buffalo.edu
Susan T. Roberts, Dir.
Activities/Fields: Audiology, speech and hearing sciences, speech/language pathology, speech perception and acoustics, and augmentative communication. **Pub:** *Journal of Speech and Hearing Disorders.* • *Journal of Speech/Hearing Research.*

★ 23339 ★ State University of New York at Buffalo
Visual Perception Laboratory
Park Hall 189
Department of Psychology
Buffalo, NY 14260
Phone: (716)645-3650
Email: wcswcs@buffalo.edu
Website: http://www.acsu.buffalo.edu/~wcswcs/
William C. Schmidt, Dir.
Activities/Fields: Mechanisms involved in early vision. Topics studied include visual illusions and neuropsychological breakdown.

★ 23340 ★ State University of New York at Buffalo
Witebsky Center for Microbial Pathogenesis and Immunology
243 Biomedical Research Bldg.
Buffalo, NY 14260
Phone: (716)829-2848 **Fax:** (716)829-3534
Website: http://www.smbs.buffalo.edu/wcmpi/
Thomas Melendy, PhD, Dir.
Activities/Fields: Molecular mechanisms of infectious diseases.

★ 23341 ★ State University of New York College at Fredonia
Youngerman Center for Communications Disorders
Thompson Hall
Fredonia, NY 14063
Phone: (716)673-3202 **Fax:** (716)673-3235
Email: nottem@fredonia.edu
Dr. Michele T. Notte, Dir.
Activities/Fields: Community clinic and student training center for speech/language pathology and audiology. Provides facilities and data for faculty engaged in research projects in the areas of audiology, voice and speech science, and language.

★ 23342 ★ State University of New York Health Science Center at Brooklyn
Ambulatory Surgery Unit
450 Clarkson Ave., Box 6
Brooklyn, NY 11203-2012
Phone: (718)780-1350 **Fax:** (718)780-1358
Email: rtwersky@chpnet.org
Rebecca S. Twersky, MD, Dir.
Activities/Fields: Pain assessment in the mentally-challenged patient undergoing ambulatory surgical procedures.

★ 23343 ★ State University of New York Health Science Center at Brooklyn
Diabetes Diagnostic and Research Center
Box 123
450 Clarkson Ave.
Brooklyn, NY 11203
Phone: (718)270-2813 **Fax:** (718)270-3240
Dr. Marianne Banerji, Actg. Dir.
Activities/Fields: Diabetes, endocrinology, immunology and metabolism, nephrology, and carcinoid syndrome. **Frmly:** General Clinical Research Center.

★ 23344 ★ State University of New York Health Science Center at Brooklyn
Infant and Child Learning Center
450 Clarkson Ave., Box 1203
Brooklyn, NY 11203
Phone: (718)270-2598 **Fax:** (718)270-3910
Email: joan.hittelman@downstate.edu
Dr. Joan Hittelman, Exec. Dir. /CEO
Activities/Fields: Infant development, including evaluation of various methods of eye protection in jaundiced newborn infants undergoing phototherapy with respect to behavioral, physiological, and biochemical parameters; studies of the contribution of the neonate's sex to the parent-child interaction, particularly with respect to neonatal eye contact and maternal attitudes toward the baby; and follow-up of high risk infants (infants born weighing less than 1000 grams and infants exposed to the HIV virus).

★ 23345 ★ State University of New York Health Science Center at Brooklyn
Neurodynamic Laboratory
Department of Psychiatry
450 Clarkson Ave., Box 1203
Brooklyn, NY 11203
Phone: (718)270-2024 **Fax:** (718)270-4081
Email: hb@cns.hscbklyn.edu
Dr. Henri Begleiter, Dir.
Activities/Fields: Use of evoked brain potentials to assess central nervous system changes due to alcoholism and drug addiction. **Frmly:** Evoked Potential Laboratory.

★ 23346 ★ State University of New York Health Science Center at Brooklyn
Primate Behavior Laboratory
450 Clarkson Ave., Box 120
Brooklyn, NY 11203
Phone: (718)270-3355 **Fax:** (718)270-3355
Email: lrosenbl@downstate.edu
Dr. Leonard A. Rosenblum, Dir.
Activities/Fields: Normative and experimental studies of the development of bonnet and pigtail macaques and squirrel monkeys, including the development of mother-infant relations and infant social development, environmental factors and social development, psychosocial factors, nonhuman primate sexual behavior, primate models of psychopathology, and experimental studies of environmental enrichment, learning, and perception with computer-mediated video tasks in individual and group settings.

★ 23347 ★ State University of New York Health Science Center at Brooklyn
Research Unit on Communicative Processes
450 Clarkson Ave., Box 88
Brooklyn, NY 11203
Phone: (718)270-3078 **Fax:** (718)270-3017
Dr. Norbert Freedman, Dir.
Activities/Fields: Communicative issues in psychiatric treatment, including doctor-patient interaction, the clinical interview, the psychotherapeutic interview, and the psychoanalytic interview. Objective studies of communicative behavior are also conducted through analysis of language, kinesics, and cognitive processes.

★ 23348 ★ State University of New York Health Science Center at Stony Brook
Center for Photographic Images of Medicine and Health Care
Media Services, Level 3, Rm. 044
Health Science Center
Stony Brook, NY 11794-8030
Phone: (631)444-3228 **Fax:** (631)444-6172
Email: kgebhart@notes.cc.sunysb.edu
Kathleen Gebhart, Dir.
Activities/Fields: Houses 3,000 photographic images of medical practices. Activities include searching historical records and archives for additional photographs. **Pub:** *Illustrated Catalog of the Slide Archive of Historical Medical Photographs at Stony Brook.*

★ 23349 ★ State University of New York Health Science Center at Stony Brook
General Clinical Research Center
12S-136 Stony Brook University Hospital
Stony Brook, NY 11794-7124
Phone: (631)444-6900 **Fax:** (631)444-6930
Email: marie.gelato@stonybrook.edu
Website: http://webster.gcrc.sunysb.edu
Marie C. Gelato, MD, Prog. Dir.
Activities/Fields: Major areas of investigation include aging, diabetes, Dupuytren Disease, Lyme Disease, metabolism, osteoporosis, psychiatry and renal failure.

★ 23350 ★ State University of New York Health Science Center at Stony Brook Institute for Mental Health Research
Department of Psychiatry & Behavioral Science
Stony Brook, NY 11794-8101
Phone: (631)444-2990 **Fax:** (631)444-7534
Website: http://www.uhmc.sunysb.edu:80/psychiatry/
Mark J. Sedler, MD, Actg. Chm.
Activities/Fields: Seeks to determine neurobiological factors in mental illnesses that can be used to aid in the development of improved treatments. Conducts basic neurobiological research and applied clinical studies. Areas of interest include psychopharmacology, molecular neurobiology, child psychopathology, behavioral biology, and behavioral medicine. **Frmly:** Long Island Research Institute.

★ 23351 ★ State University of New York Health Science Center at Stony Brook Osteoporosis Center
26 Research Way, Technology Park
Belle Meade Rd.
Setauket, NY 11733
Phone: (631)444-2663
Email: barry.gruber@stonybrook.edu
Website: http://www.informatics.sunysb.edu/internalmed/osteo/osteo.html
Barry L. Gruber, MD, Dir.
Activities/Fields: Osteoporosis, particularly bone biology.

★ 23352 ★ State University of New York at Stony Brook Center for Biotechnology
Psychology A Bldg., 3rd Fl.
Stony Brook, NY 11794-2580
Phone: (631)632-8521 **Fax:** (631)632-8577
Email: clinton.rubin@sunysb.edu
Website: http://www.biotech.sunysb.edu
Prof. Clinton T. Rubin, PhD, Dir.
Activities/Fields: Medical biotechnology, including molecular and cell biology, medical laboratory technology, drug discovery high-throughput screening, and drug development.

★ 23353 ★ State University of New York at Stony Brook Stony Brook HIV Treatment Development Center
State University of New York Health Science Center, HSC T-15
Stony Brook, NY 11794-8153
Phone: (631)444-1659 **Fax:** (631)444-7518
Email: rsteigb@mail.som.sunysb.edu
Website: http://www.informatics.sunysb.edu/internalmed/AidsHIV/HIVhome.html
Roy T. Steigbigel, MD, Dir.
Activities/Fields: Treatment of HIV infection.

★ 23354 ★ State University of New York Upstate Medical University at Syracuse Center for Bioethics and Humanities (CBH)
725 Irving Ave., Ste. 406
Syracuse, NY 13210
Phone: (315)464-5404 **Fax:** (315)464-5407
Email: cbh@upstate.edu
Website: http://www.upstate.edu/cbh/
Kathy Faber-Langendoen, MD, Dir.
Activities/Fields: Bioethics and the medical humanities. **Pub:** *Bioethics in Brief Newsletter.* • *The Healing Muse Journal*, annually.

★ 23355 ★ State University of New York Upstate Medical University at Syracuse Clinical Research Unit
University Hospital
750 E Adams St., Rm. 8602
Syracuse, NY 13210-2375
Phone: (315)464-9000 **Fax:** (315)464-9011
Email: mosesa@upstate.edu
Website: http://www.upstate.edu/cru
Arnold M. Moses, MD, Dir.
Activities/Fields: Endocrinology, gastroenterology, metabolism, nephrology, oncology, nutrition, and neurology.

★ 23356 ★ State University of New York Upstate Medical University at Syracuse Robert C. Schwartz Cystic Fibrosis Center and Pediatric Pulmonary Center
750 E Adams, 5th Fl., Pediatrics
Syracuse, NY 13210
Phone: (315)464-6323 **Fax:** (315)464-6322
Email: anbarr@mail.upstate.edu
Dr. Ran D. Anbar, Dir.
Activities/Fields: Cystic fibrosis, asthma, and hypnosis, including clinical studies.

★ 23357 ★ Stehlin Foundation for Cancer Research
1315 St. Joseph Pky., Ste. 1818
Houston, TX 77002
Phone: (713)659-1336 **Fax:** (713)659-1503
Website: http://www.stehlin.org
Robert Anderson, Exec. Dir.
Activities/Fields: Tissue culture of human cancers, transplantation of human cancers into athymic mice, experimental chemotherapy of human cancers growing in tissue culture or nude mice, investigation and development of new anticancer drugs, immunology of human cancers, effects of heat on human cancers, development and treatment of breast cancer, relationships between virus and human cancer, rapid screening of anticancer drugs and clinical trials for potential anti-cancer drugs.

★ 23358 ★ Stowers Institute for Medical Research
1000 E 50th St.
Kansas City, MO 64110
Phone: (816)926-4000 **Fax:** (816)444-8644
Email: info@stowers-institute.org
Website: http://www.stowers-institute.org/Splash.asp
Robert E. Krumlauf, PhD, Sci. Dir.
Activities/Fields: Complex genetic systems to unlock the mysteries of disease and find the keys to their causes, treatment and prevention. **Pub:** *The Stowers Report*, quarterly.

★ 23359 ★ Strang Cancer Prevention Center
428 E 72nd St.
New York, NY 10021
Phone: (212)794-4900 **Fax:** (212)396-1244
Email: osborne@strang.org
Website: http://www.strang.org
Dr. Michael P. Osborne, Pres. /CEO
Activities/Fields: Molecular genetics; hormonal carcinogens; evaluation of new preventive agents for colon, breast and prostate cancer. **Pub:** *Progressions Newsletter.* Newsletter.

★ 23360 ★ Sun Health Research Institute Christopher Center for Parkinson's Research
10515 W Santa Fe Dr.
Sun City, AZ 85351
Phone: (623)876-5328 **Fax:** (623)876-5695
Email: jeffrey.joyce@sunhealth.org
Website: http://www.shri.org/parkinson/index.html
Jeffrey N. Joyce, PhD, Sr. Sci.
Activities/Fields: Parkinson's disease, focusing on treatment strategies and basic research on causes.

★ 23361 ★ Sun Health Research Institute L.J. Roberts Center for Alzheimer's Research
10515 W Santa Fe Dr.
Sun City, AZ 85372
Phone: (623)876-5328 **Fax:** (623)876-5461
Website: http://www.shri.org/robertalz/index1.html
Dr. Joseph Rogers, Sr. Sci.
Activities/Fields: Alzheimer's disease causes and prevention. **Frmly:** Alzheimer's Center.

★ 23362 ★ Susan Love MD Breast Cancer Foundation
427 E Carrillo St.
Santa Barbara, CA 93101
Phone: (805)963-2877 **Fax:** (805)565-2246
Email: slovebcf@aol.com
Website: http://www.susanlovemdfoundation.org
Elizabeth Thompson, Exec. Dir.
Activities/Fields: Breast cancer, including methods of detection and treatment, with special emphasis on the intraductal approach. **Frmly:** Santa Barbara Breast Cancer Institute.

★ 23363 ★ Swedish Cancer Institute
1221 Madison St.
Seattle, WA 98104
Phone: (206)386-2323 **Fax:** (206)386-2393
Dr. Todd Barnett, Dir.
Activities/Fields: Cancer, including research, treatment, prevention, pain management, early detection, genetics, and related psychosocial issues. Center also conducts on Phase I-III clinical trials in treatment, prevention, control, and epidemiology of cancer, and investigates methods of instruction in cancer pain management. **Pub:** *Cancer Institute Annual Report.*

★ 23364 ★ Syracuse Cancer Research Institute
600 E Genesee St.
Syracuse, NY 13202
Phone: (315)472-6616
Website: http://www.scri.ngen.com
Joseph Gold, MD, Dir.
Activities/Fields: Cachexia, or weight loss and debilitation as a result of cancer. Specifically studies the drug hydrazine sulfate, a chemical that acts to block the body's chemical machinery which converts lactic acid, amino acids, and other carbon 2-5 molecules to glucose and thus depletes the normal body energy pools; and experimental combinations of chemotherapy with hydrazine sulfate and cytotoxic chemotherapeutic agents, hormones, and recombinant DNA products.

★ 23365 ★ Syracuse University Institute for Sensory Research
621 Skytop Rd.
Syracuse, NY 13244-5290
Phone: (315)443-4164 **Fax:** (315)443-1184
Email: bob_smith@isr.syr.edu
Dr. Robert L. Smith, Dir.
Activities/Fields: Sensory processes (hearing, vision, and touch) and orofacial biomechanics, using an interdisciplinary approach, including psychophysics, neurophysiology, neurochemistry, anatomy, cell biology, physiology, biosimulation, biomaterials, and orofacial biomechanics. **Frmly:** Bioacoustics Laboratory; Laboratory of Sensory Communication.

★ 23366 ★ Taconic Farms Inc. Mutant Mouse Regional Resource Center
273 Hover Ave.
Germantown, NY 12526
Phone: (518)537-5200 **Fax:** (518)537-7287
Email: jgei@taconic.com
Website: http://www.taconic.com
James G. Geistfeld, DVM, Prin. Investigator

Activities/Fields: Value of microarray technology for mutant mice and behavioral phenotyping of mice and behavioral phenotyping.

★ 23367 ★ Tampa Bay Research Institute
10900 Roosevelt Blvd.
Saint Petersburg, FL 33716-2308
Phone: (727)576-6675 **Fax:** (727)577-9862
Email: apelaez@tampabayresearch.org
Website: http://www.tampabayresearch.org
April Palaez, VP

Activities/Fields: Molecular genetics, virology, Hepatitis C, cellular biochemistry, AIDS, gene therapy, cytokines, and cancer. **Pub:** *Newsletter*, quarterly. **Frmly:** Showa University Research Institute.

★ 23368 ★ Temple University Adult Anxiety Clinic of Temple (AACT)
419 Weiss Hall
Department of Psychology
1701 N 13th St.
Philadelphia, PA 19122
Phone: (215)204-1575 **Fax:** (215)204-5184
Email: phobia@blue.temple.edu
Website: http://www.temple.edu/phobia/
Richard G. Heimberg, PhD, Dir.

Activities/Fields: Effectiveness of treatments of social and generalized anxiety.

★ 23369 ★ Temple University Biokinetics Research Laboratory
127 Pearson Hall
Philadelphia, PA 19122
Phone: (215)204-9555 **Fax:** (215)204-4414
Email: cswanik@astro.temple.edu
Dr. C. Buz Swanik, Dir.

Activities/Fields: Exercise physiology, biomechanics, and motor learning, including studies on biochemical adaptations to exercise, muscular strength and endurance, longitudinal effects of regular vigorous physical activity, environmental influences on physical work, metabolism, and perceptual motor behavior.

★ 23370 ★ Temple University Center for Neurovirology and Cancer Biology
BioLife Sciences Bldg., MS 015-96
College of Science & Technology
1900 N 12th St.
Philadelphia, PA 19122
Phone: (215)204-0678 **Fax:** (215)204-0679
Email: kamel.khalili@temple.edu
Website: http://www.temple.edu/cnvcb
Dr. Kamel Khalili, Dir.

Activities/Fields: Neurologic disorders. **Pub:** *Journal of NeuroVirology.*

★ 23371 ★ Temple University Center for Neurovirology and Cancer Biology Laboratory of AIDS Pathogenesis and Molecular Therapeutics
BioLife Sciences Bldg.
College of Science & Technology
1900 N 12th St.
Philadelphia, PA 19122
Phone: (215)204-0605 **Fax:** (215)204-0679
Email: jayrapp@astro.temple.edu
Website: http://www.temple.edu/cnvcb
Dr. Jay F. Rappaport, Prin. Investigator

Activities/Fields: Treatment of viral-induced neurological disorders and brain tumors using a molecular therapeutic strategy featuring RNA and DNA molecules, the molecular pathogenesis of HIV-1 induced neurological disorders, and HIV vaccine development.

★ 23372 ★ Temple University Center for Neurovirology and Cancer Biology Laboratory of Cancer Biology and Intervention
BioLife Sciences Bldg., Rm. 203
College of Science & Technology
1900 N 12th St.
Philadelphia, PA 19122
Phone: (215)204-0620 **Fax:** (215)204-0679
Email: kamel.khalili.reiss@temple.edu
Website: http://www.temple.edu/cnvcb/cancerbio_lab.html
Dr. Kamel Khalili, Dir.

Activities/Fields: Molecular pathways involved in the development of cancer, especially brain cancer.

★ 23373 ★ Temple University Center for Neurovirology and Cancer Biology Laboratory of NeuroAIDS and Gene Therapy
BioLife Sciences Bldg., Rm. 203
College of Science & Technology
1900 N 12th St.
Philadelphia, PA 19122
Phone: (215)204-0678 **Fax:** (215)204-0679
Email: ashohreh@astro.temple.edu
Website: http://www.temple.edu/cnvcb/neuroaids_lab.html
Dr. Shohreh Amini, Prin. Investigator

Activities/Fields: Human immunodeficiency virus (HIV) bacterial antigens.

★ 23374 ★ Temple University Center for Neurovirology and Cancer Biology Laboratory of Neuropathology (LNP)
BioLife Sciences Bldg.
College of Science & Technology
1900 N 12th St., Ste. 240
Philadelphia, PA 19122
Phone: (215)204-0631 **Fax:** (215)204-0679
Email: lvalle@astro.temple.edu
Website: http://www.temple.edu/cnvcb/neuropath_lab.html
Luis Del Valle, MD, Prin. Investigator

Activities/Fields: Viral infection of the brain and the effect of pathobiological alternatives. **Pub:** *Journal of Neurovirology*, bimonthly.

★ 23375 ★ Temple University Center for Neurovirology and Cancer Biology Laboratory of Neurovirology and Neuro-oncology
BioLife Sciences Bldg.
College of Science & Technology
1900 N 12th St.
Philadelphia, PA 19122
Phone: (215)204-0678 **Fax:** (215)204-0679
Email: kamel.khalili@temple.edu
Dr. Kamel Khalili, Dir.

Activities/Fields: Molecular basis for the involvement of the blood-brain barrier in trafficking of inflammatory cells and neurotropic viruses (HIV-1, MHV-4) in the central nervous system, and identification of central nervous system endothelial specific compounds mediating viral infection of the brain.

★ 23376 ★ Temple University Fels Institute for Cancer Research and Molecular Biology
School of Medicine
3307 N Broad St., Rm. 150
Philadelphia, PA 19140
Phone: (215)707-4300 **Fax:** (215)707-4588
Email: reddy@unix.temple.edu
Website: http://medschool.temple.edu/Fels_Institute_for_Cancer_Research/program_general_information.html
E. Premkumar Reddy, Dir.

Activities/Fields: Basic sciences, with emphasis on biochemical, molecular, and genetic aspects of cancer, including molecular biology, cell biology, and biochemistry. **Pub:** *Annual Report.*

★ 23377 ★ Temple University Gait Study Center
School of Podiatric Medicine
8th & Race Sts.
Philadelphia, PA 19107
Phone: (215)625-5366 **Fax:** (215)629-0278
Email: hhillstrom@tuspm.temple.edu
Website: http://podiatry.temple.edu/gaitlab/index.htm
Dr. Howard Hillstrom, Dir.

Activities/Fields: Posture and locomotion studies, focusing on the causes of abnormal gait conditions. Conducts basic and clinical research in biomechanics and biomedical engineering with special emphasis on the lower extremities. Areas of interest include the functional role of in-shoe orthoses and insoles; the role of conservative realignment and innovative therapies to treat osteoarthritis; the etiology and management of neuropathic ulcers in the diabetic foot; and optimization of foot and ankle surgeries and related fixation parameters.

★ 23378 ★ Temple University General Clinical Research Center
3401 N Broad St.
Philadelphia, PA 19140
Phone: (215)707-3086 **Fax:** (215)707-1560
Email: gcrc@bm.temple.edu
Website: http://www.health.temple.edu/tuh/gcrc.html
Guenther Boden, MD, Prog. Dir.

Activities/Fields: Gastroenterology, cardiology, metabolism, nephrology, neurology, AIDS, pulmonary research, and social phobias.

★ 23379 ★ Temple University Institute on Aging
3400 N Broad St.
Philadelphia, PA 19140
Phone: (215)707-4741 **Fax:** (215)707-5174
Website: http://www.temple.edu/aging
Albert J. Finestone, MD, Actg. Dir.

Activities/Fields: Changes in adaptive capabilities during aging, anti-aging effects of dehydroepiandrosterone (DHEA), the influences of characteristics of elderly disabled clients on their experiences in case management, minority/ethnic aging research, and service management and services to the frail elderly. **Frmly:** Aging Research Center.

★ 23380 ★ Temple University Motility Laboratory/Gastroenterology
Parkinson Bldg.
School of Medicine
3401 N Broad St.
Philadelphia, PA 19140
Phone: (215)707-3428 **Fax:** (215)707-2684
Email: hparkman@nimbus.temple.edu
Dr. Robert Fisher, Dir.

Activities/Fields: Neurohumoral control of gastrointestinal motility, including mechanical properties and neuropeptide receptor characteristics of gastrointestinal tract smooth muscle and neurohormonal interactions in gastrointestinal motility; applied clinical research. **Frmly:** Institute of Gastroenterology.

★ 23381 ★ Temple University Motor Development Laboratory
Pearson Hall
Biokinetics Research Laboratory
Philadelphia, PA 19122
Phone: (215)204-1960
Email: mridenou@temple.edu
Dr. Marcella V. Ridenour, Dir.

Activities/Fields: Motor development of infants and young children, including studies on safety of toys, juvenile furniture, cribs, strollers, walkers, high chairs, tricycles and wheeled toys, and playgrounds. Performs biomechanics analysis of infants and young children and evaluations of toys and play equipment through the use of motion pictures.

★ 23382 ★ Temple University Section of Audiology and Auditory Research
Kresge W Bldg., Rm. 302
3440 N Broad St.
Philadelphia, PA 19140
Phone: (215)707-3661 **Fax:** (215)707-8079
Dr. Robert Nozza, Dir.
Activities/Fields: Psychological and physiological acoustics, clinical research in audiology, clinical and basic research in evoked potentials, auditory and vestibular functioning, and human and animal experimentation in otology.

★ 23383 ★ Temple University Sol Sherry Thrombosis Research Center
Old Medical School
3400 N Broad St., Rm. 300
Philadelphia, PA 19140
Phone: (215)707-4665 **Fax:** (215)707-2783
Email: colmanr@vm.temple.edu
Website: http://www.medschool.temple.edu/Sol_Sherry_Thrombosis_Research_Center/
Robert W. Colman, MD, Dir.
Activities/Fields: Thrombotic hemorrhage disorders, biochemistry and molecular biology of blood coagulation, platelet structure and function, and vascular biology and angiogeneses. Clinical studies are conducted. Core laboratories are established for cell culture, monoclonal antibody production, and molecular modeling.

★ 23384 ★ Tennessee Center for the Study and Treatment of Dyslexia
Middle Tennessee State University
200 N Baird Ln.
PO Box 397
Murfreesboro, TN 37132
Phone: (615)494-8880 **Fax:** (615)494-8881
Email: dyslexia@mtsu.edu
Website: http://www.mtsu.edu/~dyslexia
Diane J. Sawyer, PhD, Dir.
Activities/Fields: Dyslexia, focusing on diagnostic services and monitoring the progress of students with dyslexia who are receiving intervention in their schools.

★ 23385 ★ Tennessee State University Institute of Government
CB 140
330 10th Ave. N
Nashville, TN 37203
Phone: (615)963-7241 **Fax:** (615)963-7245
Email: arizzo@tnstate.edu
Website: http://www.tnstate.edu/IOG/instgov.html
Dr. Ann-Marie Rizzo, Dir.
Activities/Fields: Public administration and public services. **Pub:** *The Public Servant*, 3/year. Newsletter.

★ 23386 ★ Terry Beirn Community Programs for Clinical Research on AIDS (CPCRA)
8757 Georgia Ave., 12th Fl.
Silver Spring, MD 20910-3714
Phone: (301)230-9670 **Fax:** (301)230-7190
Email: mdiggins@s-3.com
Website: http://www.cpcra.org/
Meg Diggins, Clinical Sec. Coord.
Activities/Fields: Day-to-day medical management of HIV disease; treatment and therapies for AIDS.

★ 23387 ★ Texas A&M University Alkek Institute of Biosciences and Technology Center for Genome Research
2121 W Holcombe Blvd.
Houston, TX 77030-3303
Phone: (713)677-7651 **Fax:** (713)677-7689
Email: rwells@ibt.tamu.edu
Dr. Robert Wells, Dir.
Activities/Fields: Structure and biology of DNA in living cells and viruses and its role in the developmental expression of genetic information. Specific research areas include cancer and other human genetic diseases, maintenance and stability of chromosome ends, and the processing of information from DNA into functional messenger ribonucleic acid (RNA) for expression into proteins.

★ 23388 ★ Texas A&M University Cardiovascular Research Institute
1114 TAMU
System Health Science Center
College Station, TX 77843-1114
Phone: (979)845-7816 **Fax:** (979)862-4638
Email: granger@tamu.edu
Website: http://mphywww.tamu.edu/cvri.html
Dr. Harris J. Granger, Dir.
Activities/Fields: Applies high technology to analysis of normal and diseased microscopic blood vessels, including studies on bloodflow in both normal and diseased states, basic control and exchange processes in microcirculation, role of microcirculation in hypertension, edema, stroke, and diabetes, computer analysis of microscopic images, cellular and molecular bases of endothelial and vascular smooth muscle functions, and pathobiology of inflammation and ischemic injury. **Frmly:** Microcirculation Research Institute.

★ 23389 ★ Texas A&M University Center for Environmental and Rural Health (CERH)
Department of Veterinary Physiology & Pharmacology
College Station, TX 77843-4466
Phone: (979)845-5993 **Fax:** (979)862-4929
Email: kramos@cvm.tamu.edu
Website: http://www.niehs.nih.gov/centers/center/tam-ctr.htm
Kenneth Ramos, PhD, Dir.
Activities/Fields: Impact of environmental factors on human health and disease in rural communities. **Pub:** *Annual report.*

★ 23390 ★ Texas A&M University Center for Urban and Structural Entomology
Department of Entomology
2475 TAMU
College Station, TX 77843-2475
Phone: (979)845-5855 **Fax:** (979)845-5926
Website: http://urbanentomology.tamu.edu
Dr. Roger Gold, Dir.
Activities/Fields: Urban and public health entomology, focusing on investigations of the parasites and predators of cockroaches.

★ 23391 ★ Texas A&M University Computer-Assisted Medical Diagnostic Imaging Laboratory (CAMDI)
Zachary Engineering Bldg., Rm. 9
Department of Electrical Engineering
College Station, TX 77843-3407
Phone: (979)862-8896
Email: e-dougherty@tamu.edu
Website: http://gsp.tamu.edu/index.htm
Dr. Edward Dougherty, Dir.
Activities/Fields: Medical diagnostic imaging, especially for use in mammography and genomics.

★ 23392 ★ Texas A&M University Institute of Biosciences and Technology
2121 W Holcombe Blvd.
Houston, TX 77030-3303
Phone: (713)677-7777 **Fax:** (713)677-7725
Email: rfinnell@ibt.tamu.edu
Website: http://www.tamu.edu/ibt/ibt.htm
Richard H. Finnell, PhD, Dir.
Activities/Fields: Genome research, mammalian DNA and RNA viruses, eucaryotic gene expression, neurobiology, human nutrition, matrix biology, plant molecular biology, and cancer biology.

★ 23393 ★ Texas A&M University Institute of Ocular Pharmacology
College of Medicine
College Station, TX 77843-1114
Phone: (979)845-2817 **Fax:** (979)845-0699
Email: gchiou@tamu.edu
Dr. George C.Y. Chiou, Dir.
Activities/Fields: Ocular pharmacology (the use of drugs for treating eye disease), including glaucoma, ocular inflamation, retinal degeneration, myopia, and cataract treatment. **Pub:** *Journal of Ocular Pharmacology.* • *Opthalmic Toxicology.*

★ 23394 ★ Texas A&M University Laboratory for Protein and Amino Acid Analysis
Kleberg Center, Rm. 212
Department of Animal Science
College Station, TX 77843-2471
Phone: (979)845-1817 **Fax:** (979)845-6057
Email: g-wu@tamu.edu
Dr. Guoyao Wu, Contact
Activities/Fields: Analysis of amino acids and how they relate to various biochemical systems in fetal and neonatal systems, including Arginine metabolism and its crucial role in nitric oxide synthesis.

★ 23395 ★ Texas A&M University Occupational Health and Safety Institute
Department of Nuclear Engineering
3133 TAMU
College Station, TX 77843-3133
Phone: (979)862-4409 **Fax:** (979)845-6443
Email: j-rock@tamu.edu
Dr. James C. Rock, Dir.
Activities/Fields: Occupational health and safety, with a goal of safe use and disposal of essential hazardous materials and processes. Areas of study include industrial hygiene, health physics, safety engineering, aerosol science, occupational epidemiology, fire protection engineering, product safety engineering, occupational exposure assessment, industrial ventilation, indoor air quality, noise and vibration control, material substitution, electrofiltration, separation sciences, indoor bioaerosols, electrostatic separation for hazardous waste streams, low toxicity product substitution, pulsed power and high energy density plasma physics experiments and applications.

★ 23396 ★ Texas Cancer Data Center
1515 Holcombe Blvd.-573
Houston, TX 77030-4009
Phone: (713)792-2277 **Fax:** (713)794-1951
Email: tcdc@txcancer.org
Website: http://www.txcancer.org
Lewis E. Foxhill, MD, Contact
Activities/Fields: Reduction of human suffering and economic impact of cancer on Texans by the collection of computerized information on cancer resources, services, and statistics.

★ 23397 ★ Texas Health Research Institute (THRI)
6300 W Parker Rd., Ste. 100
Plano, TX 75093
Phone: (972)981-3740 **Fax:** (972)981-3779
Email: georgepearson@texashealth.org

Website: http://www.thri.org
George Pearson, Actg. Pres. /CEO
Activities/Fields: Biomechanical testing/engineering, pre-clinical studies, minimally invasive technologies, clinical trials in general surgery, orthopedics/spine, oncology, interventional cardiology, urology, OB/Gyn, and internal medicine. **Frmly:** Institute for Spine and Biomedical Research.

★ 23398 ★ Texas Heart Institute
6770 Bertner Ave.
PO Box 20345
Houston, TX 77225-0345
Phone: (832)355-4011
Email: dcooley@heart.thi.tmc.edu
Website: http://www.texasheart.org
Denton A. Cooley, MD, Pres.
Activities/Fields: Diseases of the heart and cardiovascular system. Specific areas of study include cardiovascular surgery, including coronary artery bypass surgery, valve replacement, transplantation, and mechanical circulatory support and replacement/assist devices; invasive and non-invasive cardiology, including gene therapy, and molecular biochemistry; cardiovascular anesthesiology and pathology; and biostatistics and epidemiology. **Pub:** *Texas Heart Institute Journal*, quarterly.

★ 23399 ★ Texas Scottish Rite Hospital for Children Research Department
2222 Welborn St.
Dallas, TX 75219
Phone: (214)559-7877 **Fax:** (214)559-7872
Email: richb@tsrh.org
Website: http://www.tsrh.org
Charles E. Johnston, II, Med. Dir.,Res.
Activities/Fields: Treatment of children with orthopedic and neuromuscular disorders: Primary areas of focus are bioengineering and orthopedic biomechanics, including Ilizarov fixators, spine mechanics, spinal implants design and evaluation, and physical properties of bone; and neurophysiology, including gait analysis and muscle strength assessment. Also conducts drug research, studies of innovative care, and application of new technology.

★ 23400 ★ Texas Tech University Tarbox Parkinson's Disease Institute
Health Science Center
3601 4th St., Rm. 3A105
Lubbock, TX 79430
Phone: (806)743-2391 **Fax:** (806)743-5687
Website: http://www.ttuhsc.edu/SOM/Neuropsychiatry/TARBOX.HTM
Activities/Fields: Neurophysical and neuropharmacological studies of the central nervous system of vertebrates as they relate to Parkinson's disease and other neurological disorders.

★ 23401 ★ Thomas Jefferson University Cardeza Foundation for Hematologic Research
1015 Walnut St.
Philadelphia, PA 19107
Phone: (215)955-7786 **Fax:** (215)955-2366
Email: steven.mckenzie@mail.tju.edu
Steven E. McKenzie, MD, Dir.
Activities/Fields: Hematology, especially vascular biology.

★ 23402 ★ Thomas Jefferson University Center for Research in Medical Education and Health Care
Jefferson Medical College
1025 Walnut St., Rm. 119
Philadelphia, PA 19107-5083
Phone: (215)955-8907 **Fax:** (215)923-6939
Email: daniel.louis@mail.tju.edu
Website: http://www.tju.edu/jmc/crmehc
Joseph S. Gonnella, MD, Dir.
Activities/Fields: Medical education process and factors affecting the quality of cost of health care. Medical education research focuses on the following areas: measurement of physician competence; long-term follow-up study of graduates; program evaluation; specialty choice; and refinement of evaluation methods. Health services research focuses on the concept and system of disease staging for classification of severity of illness, cost, and quality of care. **Pub:** *ABSTRACTS: Longitudinal Study of Medical Students and Graduates.* • *Annual Report.*

★ 23403 ★ Thomas Jefferson University Daniel Baugh Institute
Jefferson Alumni Hall
1020 Locust St.
Philadelphia, PA 19107
Phone: (215)503-7820 **Fax:** (215)923-3808
Email: james.schwaber@mail.tju.edu
Dr. James Schwaber, Dir.
Activities/Fields: Developmental biology; reproductive toxicology; biochemical, molecular and genetic mechanisms of birth defects; tissue and embryo culture, molecular biology, and cell biology.

★ 23404 ★ Thomas Jefferson University Jefferson Center for Biomedical Research (JCBR)
700 E Butler Ave.
Doylestown, PA 18901
Phone: (215)489-4947
Email: tim.block@mail.tju.edu
Website: http://www.tju.edu/jcbr/
Timothy Block, PhD, Dir.
Activities/Fields: Transgenic plants and animals, virology, gene therapy, and vaccine production and delivery systems.

★ 23405 ★ Thomas Jefferson University Jefferson Institute of Molecular Medicine
450 BLSB
233 S 10th St.
Philadelphia, PA 19107
Phone: (215)503-5785 **Fax:** (215)503-5788
Email: jouni.uitto@jefferson.edu
Dr. Jouni Uitto, Dir.
Activities/Fields: Biochemistry and molecular medicine.

★ 23406 ★ Thomas Jefferson University Kimmel Cancer Center
1050 Bluemle Life Sciences Bldg.
233 S 10th St.
Philadelphia, PA 19107-6799
Phone: (215)503-4645 **Fax:** (215)923-3528
Email: carlo.croce@mail.tju.edu
Website: http://www.kcc.tju.edu/default.htm
Carlo M. Croce, MD, Dir.
Activities/Fields: Genetics, including molecular genetic analysis of the normal human genome, cytogenetics of aneuploidy syndromes, genetics of the immune system, genetics of collagen and extracellular matrix genes, and molecular genetics of human hematopoietic neoplasias and solid tumors; immunology, including antigen presentation, autoimmunity, B-cell development, cancer immunology, cell growth regulation and differentiation, cellular immunology, cell activation and signal transduction, cytokines, developmental immunology, and immunochemistry; and microbiology and molecular virology, including chemical and antigenic structure of virus particles, viral replication, antiviral agents, regulation of viral gene expression, viral oncogenes, virus-cell interactions, latent virus infections, neurovirology, microbial immunology, microbial pathogenesis, antiparasite vaccine development, cell biology of malaria, and immunobiology of river blindness. **Frmly:** Jefferson Cancer Institute.

★ 23407 ★ Thomas Jefferson University Lupus Center
1015 Chestnut St., Ste. 1520
Philadelphia, PA 19107
Phone: (215)955-8430 **Fax:** (215)923-5828
Email: raphaeldehoratius@mail.tju.edu
Raphael J. DeHoratius, MD, Dir.
Activities/Fields: Systemic lupus erthematosus and autoimmune diseases, including reproductive immunology.

★ 23408 ★ Thomas Jefferson University Malignant Hyperthermia Research Center
8490 Gibbon
Department of Anesthesiology
Jefferson Medical College
111 S 11th St.
Philadelphia, PA 19107
Phone: (215)955-6161 **Fax:** (215)923-5507
Email: carlos.wilkerson@mail.tju.edu
Dr. Carlos Wilkerson, Dir.
Activities/Fields: Malignant hyperthermia, neuromuscular blocking agents, and general anesthetic agents. Studies focus on diagnosis of malignant hyperthermia susceptibility and basic research in mechanisms underlying malignant hyperthermia, anesthetic action, and drug mechanisms.

★ 23409 ★ Thomas Jefferson University Occupational and Environmental Health Sciences Division
Jefferson Medical College
1020 Locust St., Rm. 314-JAH
Philadelphia, PA 19107
Phone: (215)955-8381 **Fax:** (215)955-1275
Email: lance.simpson@mail.tju.edu
Dr. Lance Simpson, Dir.
Activities/Fields: Mechanisms and actions of toxins at the cellular, subcellular, and molecular levels.

★ 23410 ★ Thomas Jefferson University Regional Spinal Cord Injury System of Delaware Valley
132 S 10th St., Ste. 375 Main Bldg.
Philadelphia, PA 19107-5099
Phone: (215)955-6579 **Fax:** (215)955-5152
Email: john.ditunno@mail.tju.edu
Website: http://www.spinalcordcenter.org
Dr. John F. Ditunno, Jr., Proj. Dir.
Activities/Fields: Acute care and rehabilitation for individuals disabled by spinal cord injury, including recovery of upper and lower extremity strength and function and the development of international standards to measure improvements in walking. The center is one of five nationwide participating in a study utilizing body weight-supported ambulation therapy funded by the National Institute of Child Health and Human Development of the National Institutes of Health. The center is also involved in multi-center drug trials and other therapeutic interventions and participates in the collection and storage of training and educational materials for spinal cord injury. **Pub:** *Newsletter.* • *SCI Research Update*, annually.

★ 23411 ★ Thomas Jefferson University Scleroderma and Arthritis Research Center
233 S 10th St.
Philadelphia, PA 19107
Phone: (215)503-5042 **Fax:** (215)923-4649
Email: sergio.jimenez@mail.tju.edu
Dr. Sergio A. Jimenez, Dir.
Activities/Fields: Molecular biology and biochemistry of the connective tissue, pathogenesis of scleroderma and other fibrotic diseases, biological functions of the immune system in health and disease, molecular biology of articular cartilage matrix and heritable diseases of articular cartilage, and identification of gene mutations in human connective tissue diseases and animal models of disease. **Pub:** *Scientific Re-*

search Articles/Scientific Reviews. **Frmly:** Arthritis Clinical Research Center.

★ 23412 ★ Thomas Jefferson University Sleep Disorders Center
Jefferson Medical College
1015 Walnut St., Ste. 316
Philadelphia, PA 19107
Phone: (215)955-6175 **Fax:** (215)955-9783
Email: karl.doghramji@mail.tju.edu
Website: http://www.jeffersonhospital.org/psych/e3front.dll?durki=4263&site=336&return=6680
Karl Doghramji, MD, Dir.
Activities/Fields: Hypnotics, wake-promoting agents, antidepressants, sleep/wake disorders or disorders which may have characteristic sleep markers. Also studies seasonal affective disorder; phototherapy for circadian rhythm disorders; and human sexuality, particularly erectile impotence; sleep apnea syndrome, narcolepsy insomnia, and daytime hypersomnia. Research studies are developed in connection with clinical services and with subject groups recruited for special projects. **Frmly:** Center for the Study of Sleep.

★ 23413 ★ Thompson Cancer Survival Center
1915 White Ave.
Knoxville, TN 37916
Phone: (865)541-1678 **Fax:** (865)541-2823
Website: http://www.thompsoncancer.com
Activities/Fields: Oncology, including phase I, II, and III trials of drug, radiation, or biology therapies and laser treatments. Center comprises the following research departments: Clinical Trials; Laser Photodynamic Therapy; and Bone Marrow Transplant Laboratory.

★ 23414 ★ Tom Baker Cancer Centre
1331 29th St. NW
Calgary, AB, Canada T2N 4N2
Phone: (403)670-1711 **Fax:** (403)283-1651
Email: gavinst@cancerboard.ab.ca
Dr. Gavin C.E. Stuart, Dir.
Activities/Fields: Cancer, concentrating on interleukins, cell and molecular biology, metastasis, oncogenes, immunology of melanoma, and neuroblastoma and small cell lung cancer. Clinical trials focus on cancer therapy, biotherapy, epidemiology, and prevention. **Frmly:** Southern Alberta Cancer Centre.

★ 23415 ★ Toronto Rehabilitation Institute Stroke Rehabilitation Unit
550 University Ave.
Toronto, ON, Canada M5G 2A2
Phone: (416)597-3422 **Fax:** (416)597-1977
Email: hajek@sprint.ca
Dr. V.E. Hajek, Contact
Activities/Fields: Monitors and evaluates aspects of the rehabilitation experience on the Stroke Unit, including patients' response and progress to different therapies and treatments, and to orthotic devices and aids. Also participates in a study of mood disorders and cognitive impairment resulting from stroke.

★ 23416 ★ Torrey Pines Institute for Molecular Studies (TPIMS)
3550 General Atomics Ct.
San Diego, CA 92121-1122
Phone: (858)455-3803 **Fax:** (858)455-3804
Email: houghten@tpims.org
Website: http://www.tpims.org/home.html
Richard A. Houghten, Pres.
Activities/Fields: Treatments for major medical conditions, including multiple sclerosis, AIDS, Alzheimer's disease, pain, heart disease, many types of cancer, and more.

★ 23417 ★ Totts Gap Medical Research Laboratories, Inc.
1430 Totts Gap Rd.
Bangor, PA 18013
Phone: (610)588-0572 **Fax:** (610)588-8452
Email: tottsgap@epix.net
Stewart Wolf, MD, Dir.
Activities/Fields: Neural regulation of visceral function, emphasizing current focus on the cardiovascular system. Specific projects involve the study of the mechanisms of cardiac arrhythmia and sudden death and other aspects of neurocardiology. **Frmly:** Stewart Wolf Medical Research Foundation.

★ 23418 ★ Trauma Foundation
San Francisco General Hospital
San Francisco, CA 94110
Phone: (415)821-8209 **Fax:** (415)282-2563
Email: tf@tf.org
Website: http://www.tf.org
Andrew McGuire, Exec. Dir.
Activities/Fields: Injury and violence prevention, public policy, and epidemiology, including epidemiology of traumatic injuries and health policy research on such issues as fire-safe cigarettes, motorcycle helmets, burn injury prevention, violence prevention, handgun control, and alcohol policy. **Pub:** *Newsletter.* • *Policy papers, briefs, factsheets.*

★ 23419 ★ TraumaLink
3535 TraumaLink, 10th Fl.
34th & Civic Center Dr.
Philadelphia, PA 19104
Phone: (215)590-3118 **Fax:** (215)590-5425
Email: traumalink@email.chop.edu
Website: http://www.chop.edu/consumer/jsp/division/service.jsp?id=27708
Flaura Koplin Winston, MD, Dir.
Activities/Fields: Prevention and treatment of pediatric injury. **Pub:** *Reports.*

★ 23420 ★ Trudeau Institute, Inc.
100 Algonquin Ave.
PO Box 59
Saranac Lake, NY 12983
Phone: (518)891-3080 **Fax:** (518)891-5126
Email: scooper@trudeauinstitute.org
Website: http://www.trudeauinstitute.org
Susan Cooper, Dir., Inst. Advancement
Activities/Fields: Cellular immunology and infectious disease, particularly tuberculosis, influenza, cancer, the opportunistic infections in the AIDS patient and the effects of aging on immunity, vaccines, immune memory, and other immunotherapies. **Pub:** *Annual Report.* • *Focus Newsletter.*

★ 23421 ★ Tufts Center for the Study of Drug Development
Tufts University
192 South St., Ste. 550
Boston, MA 02111
Phone: (617)636-2185 **Fax:** (617)636-2425
Kenneth I. Kaitin, PhD, Dir.
Activities/Fields: Public policy on worldwide drug development and its trends, including study of the impact of drug regulation on pharmaceutical innovation; survey of pharmaceutical firms to determine origin, flow, and fate of new chemical entities (NCEs) and biopharmaceuticals; evaluation of therapeutic significance of marketed drugs; economic analysis of drug development costs; and legal and regulatory issues in drug development and distribution. **Pub:** *Tufts CSDD Impact Report.* **Frmly:** Center for the Study of Drug Development.

★ 23422 ★ Tufts-New England Medical Center Gynecologic Oncology Group (GOG)
Box 232
750 Washington St.
Boston, MA 02111
Phone: (617)636-6058 **Fax:** (617)636-3258
Website: http://www.nemc.org
Kenneth L. Noller, MD, Prin. Investigator
Activities/Fields: Treatment of gynecologic cancer. Evaluates surgical techniques, radiation therapy, and new chemotherapeutic agents. Emphasizes trophoblastic disease and cancers of the uterus, cervix, vulva, and ovaries.

★ 23423 ★ Tufts University Antioxidants Research Laboratory
711 Washington St.
Boston, MA 02111-1524
Phone: (617)556-3333 **Fax:** (617)556-3295
Email: blumberg@hnrc.tufts.edu
Website: http://hnrc.tufts.edu/departments/labs/antioxidants.shtml
Jeffrey B. Blumberg, PhD, Dir.
Activities/Fields: Impact of dietary antioxidants on free radical reactions and changes in oxidative stress status during aging. Understanding how antioxidants reduce oxidative stress and affect the pathogenesis of chronic disease presents opportunities for health promotion and alternative therapeutic modalities for an aging population.

★ 23424 ★ Tufts University Biomedical Engineering Laboratory (BEL)
Halligan Hall
Electrical Engineering & Computer Science Department
Medford, MA 02155
Phone: (617)627-5191 **Fax:** (617)627-3220
Email: vovantoi@eecs.tufts.edu
Website: http://www.cs.tufts.ed/~vanvo/bel.html
Prof. Vo Van Toi, Dir.
Activities/Fields: Design and application of medical devices, particularly ophthalmic instruments.

★ 23425 ★ Tufts University Body Composition Research Program
711 Washington St.
Boston, MA 02111-1524
Phone: (617)556-3162 **Fax:** (617)556-3344
Email: jkehayias@hnrc.tufts.edu
Website: http://hnrc.tufts.edu/departments/labs/comp.shtml
Joseph J. Kehayias, PhD, Dir.
Activities/Fields: Mechanisms leading to the age-related loss of muscle mass and the development of appropriate interventions that will slow down or reverse this decline. Research examines the effect of nutrition on the dynamic interactions between the body's protein, water, fat, and bone and the relationship of these changes to the aging process. It also studies obesity patterns and health status and evaluates the efficacy of anticachexia and antiobesity treatments.

★ 23426 ★ Tufts University Bone Metabolism Laboratory
711 Washington St.
Boston, MA 02111-1524
Phone: (617)556-3064 **Fax:** (617)556-3305
Email: hughesb@hnrc.tufts.edu
Website: http://hnrc.tufts.edu/departments/labs/calcium.shtml
Bess Dawson-Hughes, MD, Dir.
Activities/Fields: Intake requirements for calcium, vitamin D, protein and other nutrients that influence bone health in adult men and women and prevent osteoporosis.

★ 23427 ★ Tufts University Cardiovascular Nutrition Research Program
711 Washington St.
Boston, MA 02111-1524
Phone: (617)556-3127 **Fax:** (617)556-3103
Email: lichtenstein@hnrc.tufts.edu

Website: http://hnrc.tufts.edu/departments/labs/cardio.shtml
Alice H. Lichenstein, Dir.

Activities/Fields: Relationship between diet and cardiovascular disease. Specific emphasis is placed on examining the effect of advancing age on dietary responsiveness, and dietary components that have received less attention in regard to cardiovascular disease risk, such as trans fatty acids, soy protein and isoflavones, sterol/stanol esters and genetically modified/selectively breed oils.

★ 23428 ★ Tufts University
Center for Adaptation Genetics and Drug Resistance
School of Medicine
136 Harrison Ave.
Boston, MA 02111
Phone: (617)636-0458 **Fax:** (617)636-6765
Email: slevy@opal.tufts.edu
Website: http://www.healthsci.tufts.edu/labs/sblevy/home.html
Stuart B. Levy, MD, Dir.

Activities/Fields: Molecular basis of patients' resistance to drugs used to treat infectious diseases and cancer. **Pub:** *Articles.*

★ 23429 ★ Tufts University
Center for Gastroenterology Research on Absorptive and Secretory Processes (GRASP)
750 Washington St., NEMC 842
Boston, MA 02111
Phone: (617)636-5408 **Fax:** (617)636-7783
Email: aplaut_mib@opal.tufts.edu
Website: http://www.graspcenter.org/frontpage.html
Andrew G. Plaut, MD, Dir.

Activities/Fields: Human digestive processes.

★ 23430 ★ Tufts University
Center on Nutrition Communication
Friedman School of Nutrition Science & Policy
68 Harrison Ave., 5th Fl.
Boston, MA 02111
Phone: (617)636-3423 **Fax:** (617)636-2714
Email: jeanne.goldberg@tufts.edu
Website: http://nutcomm.tufts.edu/
Jeanne P. Goldberg, Dir.

Activities/Fields: The ability to influence human behavior regarding nutrition, resulting in healthy lifestyles.

★ 23431 ★ Tufts University
Dietary Assessment Research Program
711 Washington St.
Boston, MA 02111-1524
Phone: (617)556-3351 **Fax:** (617)556-3344
Email: tucker@hnrc.tufts.edu
Website: http://hnrc.tufts.edu/departments/labs/diet.shtml
Katherine L. Tucker, PhD, Dir.

Activities/Fields: Dietary status of population groups; factors associated with differing dietary patterns; and relationships between dietary patterns, nutrient intake, nutrition status and health.

★ 23432 ★ Tufts University
Energy Metabolism Laboratory
711 Washington St.
Boston, MA 02111-1524
Phone: (617)556-3238 **Fax:** (617)556-3234
Email: sroberts@hnrc.tufts.edu
Website: http://hnrc.tufts.edu/departments/labs/energy.shtml
Susan B. Roberts, PhD, Dir.

Activities/Fields: Genetic and environmental factors that determine body composition and energy regulation, as well as quantifying optimal dietary energy requirements. Hormonal and cellular investigations are conducted to identify the underlying metabolic cause of individual differences in body composition and energy regulation.

★ 23433 ★ Tufts University
Laboratory for Nutrition and Vision Research
711 Washington St.
Boston, MA 02111-1524
Phone: (617)556-3155 **Fax:** (617)556-3344
Email: ataylor@hnrc.tufts.edu
Website: http://hnrc.tufts.edu/departments/labs/nutvis.shtml
Allen Taylor, PhD, Ch.

Activities/Fields: Age-related cataract and retinal diseases, such as age-related maculopathy (ARM). Because oxidative stress, particularly to proteins, has been shown to be causally related to these debilities, the laboratory investigates antioxidant vitamins and pharmacological reagents as well as proteolytic enzymes that are involved in the recognition, identification and removal of damaged proteins. The laboratory also seeks to determine nutrients and foods that are associated with diminished risk for cataract and ARM.

★ 23434 ★ Tufts University
Lipid Metabolism Laboratory
711 Washington St.
Boston, MA 02111-1524
Phone: (617)556-3100 **Fax:** (617)556-3103
Email: schaefer@hnrc.tufts.edu
Website: http://hnrc.tufts.edu/departments/labs/lipid.shtml
Ernst J. Schaefer, MD, Dir.

Activities/Fields: Interrelationships between cholesterol, dietary fatty acid, and carbohydrate consumption, lipoprotein metabolism, genetics and aging in the development of cardiovascular disease. Studies focus on identifying lipid and lipoprotein abnormalities and genetic mutations associated with coronary heart disease, stroke, and dementia risk.

★ 23435 ★ Tufts University
Mineral Bioavailability Laboratory
711 Washington St.
Boston, MA 02111-1524
Phone: (617)556-3192 **Fax:** (617)556-3344
Email: rwood@hnrc.tufts.edu
Website: http://hnrc.tufts.edu/departments/labs/bioavailability.shtml
Richard J. Wood, PhD, Dir.

Activities/Fields: Biochemical and physiological basis for age-associated changes in absorption and utilization of minerals and determines the effects of aging on mineral requirements in the elderly. Researches focuses specifically on understanding calcium and iron metabolism in the elderly, as well as the effects of nutrient and hormonal changes on the expression of genes that modulate mineral metabolism.

★ 23436 ★ Tufts University
Molecular Cardiology Research Institute
Tufts-New England Medical Center
750 Washington St., Box 080
Boston, MA 02111
Phone: (617)636-9370 **Fax:** (617)636-1444
Email: mmendelsohn@lifespan.org
Website: http://www.nemc.org/mcri/
Michael E. Mendelsohn, MD, Exec. Dir.

Activities/Fields: Molecular mechanisms of human disease and new strategies for diagnosis and therapy.

★ 23437 ★ Tufts University
Molecular Cardiology Research Institute Molecular Cardiology Research Center (MCRC)
Tufts-New England Medical Center
750 Washington St., Box No. 80
Boston, MA 02111
Phone: (617)636-9370 **Fax:** (617)636-1444
Email: mmendelsohn@lifespan.org
Website: http://www.nemc.org/mcri/MCRC/mcrc.htm
Michael E. Mendelsohn, MD, Dir.

Activities/Fields: Molecular mechanisms that underlie cardiovascular biology and disease.

★ 23438 ★ Tufts University
Neuroscience Laboratory
711 Washington St.
Boston, MA 02111-1524
Phone: (617)556-3178 **Fax:** (617)556-3222
Email: jjoseph@hnrc.tufts.edu
Website: http://hnrc.tufts.edu/departments/labs/neuroscience.shtml
James A. Joseph, PhD, Ch.

Activities/Fields: Factors that increase susceptibility to oxidate stress, with a view toward identifying nutrient antioxidant regimens to restore or prevent the decline of motor and memory functions in the elderly. Research is aimed at determining the membrane and neurotransmitter receptor characteristics that alter calcium homeostasis and increase oxidative stress vulnerability and, ultimately, cell viability in neuronal aging. Studies examine the expression of age-related behavioral deficits using cognitive and motor behavior assessments. The laboratory also investigates the effects of dietary supplementation with fruits and vegetables high in antioxidant activity, as well as other antioxidants, on retarding age-related cellular, neuronal, and behavioral deficits and on neurotransmitter internalization and sensitivity. Experiments are also conducted to ascertain the role of neuronal stimulation in subsequent protection against oxidative stress.

★ 23439 ★ Tufts University
Nutrition and Cancer Biology Laboratory
711 Washington St.
Boston, MA 02111-1524
Phone: (617)556-3130 **Fax:** (617)556-3344
Email: xwang@hnrc.tufts.edu
Website: http://hnrc.tufts.edu/departments/labs/cancerbiology.shtml
Xiang-Dong Wang, MD, Dir.

Activities/Fields: How fruits and vegetables modify molecular and signaling pathways which alter the development of cancers, such as those of the lung, stomach, liver, breast and prostate. This laboratory also examines how this response is modified by other exogenous factors (e.g., tobacco smoking, alcohol, and chemical carcinogen exposure).

★ 23440 ★ Tufts University
Nutrition, Exercise Physiology, and Sarcopenia Laboratory
711 Washington St.
Boston, MA 02111-1524
Phone: (617)556-3081 **Fax:** (617)556-3083
Email: ccastaneda@hnrc.tufts.edu
Website: http://hnrc.tufts.edu/departments/labs/sarcopenia.shtml
Carmen Castaneda-Sceppa, MD, Actg. Dir.

Activities/Fields: Interaction of nutritional, hormonal and immunologic factors in sarcopenia, the loss of muscle mass and function that comes with aging. The laboratory also studies the protein requirements of the elderly and the impact of exercise on chronic degenerative conditions such as heart failure, kidney failure, and arthritis.

★ 23441 ★ Tufts University
Nutrition and Genomics Laboratory
711 Washington St.
Boston, MA 02111-1524
Phone: (617)556-3102 **Fax:** (617)556-3103
Email: ordovas@hnrc.tufts.edu
Website: http://hnrc.tufts.edu/departments/labs/genomics.shtml
Jose M. Ordovas, PhD, Dir.

Activities/Fields: Nutritional status and genotype/phenotype interactions as a means to increase understanding of nutritional requirements and disease susceptibility in human populations.

★ 23442 ★ Tufts University
Nutrition/Infection Unit
Arnold 205
136 Harrison Ave.
Boston, MA 02111
Phone: (617)636-3811 **Fax:** (617)636-3810
Email: med-nutrition-infection@tufts.edu
Website: http://www.tufts.edu/med/nutrition_HIV/
Sherwood L. Gorbach, MD, Dir.
Activities/Fields: Role of nutrition in the lives of people with HIV and other diseases. **Pub:** *NFHL Newsletter.*

★ 23443 ★ Tufts University
Nutritional Epidemiology Program
711 Washington St.
Boston, MA 02111-1524
Phone: (617)556-3322 **Fax:** (617)556-3344
Email: paul@hnrc.tufts.edu
Website: http://hnrc.tufts.edu/departments/labs/epidemiology.shtml
Paul F. Jacques, DSc, Ch.
Activities/Fields: Role of nutrition in healthy aging. The research focuses on identifying the determinants of nutrition status and intake in the elderly, relating nutrition status and intake to measures of health and well-being, and improving methodology for nutrition, dietary assessment and aging research.

★ 23444 ★ Tufts University
Nutritional Immunology Laboratory
711 Washington St.
Boston, MA 02111-1524
Phone: (617)556-3129 **Fax:** (617)556-3224
Email: smeydani@hnrc.tufts.edu
Website: http://hnrc.tufts.edu/departments/labs/immunology.shtml
Simin Nikbin Meydani, PhD, Ch.
Activities/Fields: Role of dietary components and their interactions with other environmental factors in age-associated changes of the immune and inflammatory responses. Research looks to reverse and/or delay the onset of these immunologic and age-related changes by appropriate dietary modifications and to determine the molecular mechanisms by which antioxidant and prooxidant nutrients modulate immune cell functions.

★ 23445 ★ Tufts University
Program in Obesity and Metabolism
711 Washington St.
Boston, MA 02111-1524
Phone: (617)556-3144 **Fax:** (617)556-3224
Email: agreenberg@hnrc.tufts.edu
Website: http://hnrc.tufts.edu/departments/labs/obesity.shtml
Andrew S. Greenberg, MD, Dir.
Activities/Fields: Underlying molecular mechanisms that control fat metabolism and storage in humans by proteins called perilipins.

★ 23446 ★ Tufts University
Tufts Center for Conservation Medicine (CCM)
Bernice Barbour Wildlife Medicine Bldg.
School of Veterinary Medicine
200 Westboro Rd.
North Grafton, MA 01536
Phone: (508)887-4789 **Fax:** (508)839-7946
Website: http://www.tufts.edu/vet/ccm/
Activities/Fields: Effects of human influence on the environment, and in turn on human and animal health.

★ 23447 ★ Tufts University
Vascular Biology Research Program
711 Washington St.
Boston, MA 02111-1524
Phone: (617)556-3126 **Fax:** (617)556-3224
Email: mmeydani@hnrc.tufts.edu
Website: http://hnrc.tufts.edu/departments/labs/vascular.shtml
Mohsen Meydani, PhD, Dir.
Activities/Fields: Role of dietary components, particularly antioxidants and lipids, and oxidative stress and other factors on age-associated changes in vascular function. Studies examine the molecular mechanisms of antioxidants and prooxidants in modulating the interaction of immune and inflammatory cells with other cellular components of the vascular system in the development of atherosclrosis and tumor angiogenesis. Nutrient modification of vascular function is explored using cell-cell interactions, biochemical indices, and molecular markers of oxidative stress at the cellular and whole organism levels.

★ 23448 ★ Tufts University
Vitamin K Research Program
711 Washington St.
Boston, MA 02111-1524
Phone: (617)556-3231 **Fax:** (617)556-3149
Email: sbooth@hnrc.tufts.edu
Website: http://hnrc.tufts.edu/departments/labs/vitamink.shtml
Sarah Booth, PhD, Dir.
Activities/Fields: Dietary requirements for vitamin K in humans during different stages of adult life, and the relationship between vitamin K status and chronic diseases, such as cardiovascular disease and osteoporosis.

★ 23449 ★ Tufts University
Vitamin Metabolism Laboratory
711 Washington St.
Boston, MA 02111-1524
Phone: (617)556-3191 **Fax:** (617)556-3166
Email: jselhub@hnrc.tufts.edu
Website: http://hnrc.tufts.edu/departments/labs/vitamin.shtml
Jacob Selhub, PhD, Ch.
Activities/Fields: Status of folic acid and vitamins B2, B6 and B12 in the elderly, with emphasis on the prevalence of inadequate status. The laboratory examines the relationship of elevated plasma homocysteine levels to inadequate B vitamin intake and status and increased risk for cardiovascular disease, thrombosis and stroke, cognitive dysfunction, and certain cancers. These studies emphasize the dietary requirements and long-term effects of inadequate vitamin status.

★ 23450 ★ Tufts University
Vitamins and Carcinogenesis Laboratory
711 Washington St.
Boston, MA 02111-1524
Phone: (617)556-3194 **Fax:** (617)556-3166
Email: jmason@hnrc.tufts.edu
Website: http://hnrc.tufts.edu/departments/labs/carcinogenesis.shtml
Joel B. Mason, MD, Dir.
Activities/Fields: Role that diet plays in modifying metabolic and genetic pathways that lead to human carcinogenesis and thereby define the means by which cancers can be nutritionally prevented. The program of research emphasizes how these dietary compounds interact with genetic background to modify molecular and signaling pathways which alter the development of cancers and to examine how other exogenous factors, such as tobacco smoking and alcohol consumption, also play a role.

★ 23451 ★ Tulane University
Cancer Center
1430 Tulane Ave., Box SL-68
New Orleans, LA 70112-2699
Phone: (504)585-6060 **Fax:** (504)585-6077
Email: rweiner@tulane.edu
Website: http://www.som.tulane.edu/cancer
Dr. Roy S. Weiner, Dir.
Activities/Fields: Cancer, including AIDS-related cancers, biochemistry, bone marrow transplant, breast cancer, chemotherapy, diet and nutrition, endocrine, environmental carcinogens, epidemiology, eye, ear, nose, and throat, gastro-intestinal cancer, general cancer research, genetics, genito-urinary, gynecological and obstetric, head and neck cancer, hepatocellular cancer, Hodgkin's disease, kidney cancer, leukemia, lung and esophageal cancer, lymphoma, melanoma, myeloma, occupational carcinogens, ophthamology, otolaryngology, ovarian and cervical cancers, pain and anesthesia, pediatric oncology, prevention of cancer, prostate cancer, psych-oncology, racial and ethnic factors, radiation and radiotherapy, skin cancer, surgical oncology, and Wilms' tumor. **Pub:** *Inside the Tulane Cancer Center*, quarterly.

★ 23452 ★ Tulane University
Center for Applied Environmental Public Health (CAEPH)
School of Public Health & Tropical Medicine
1440 Canal St.
New Orleans, LA 70112
Phone: (504)584-1774 **Free:** 800-862-2122
Email: lawhite@tulane.edu
Website: http://www.caeph.tulane.edu/
Dr. LuAnn White, Dir.
Activities/Fields: Occupational and environmental public health. Areas of interest include community-based prevention; childhood lead poisoning; Mississippi River water quality; risk communication, dissemination research and the translation of research for practice.

★ 23453 ★ Tulane University
Center for Infectious Diseases (CID)
J. Bennett Johnston Bldg., 5th Fl.
Tulane University Medical Center
1430 Tulane Ave., SL-71
New Orleans, LA 70112-2699
Phone: (504)584-3552 **Fax:** (504)988-6686
Email: center.infecdis@tulane.edu
Website: http://www.tulane.edu/~cid/
Dr. Donald J. Krogstad, Dir.
Activities/Fields: Emerging and re-emerging infectious diseases, both in the United States and abroad.

★ 23454 ★ Tulane University
Center for International Resource Development
School of Public Health & Tropical Medicine
1440 Canal St., Ste. 2200
New Orleans, LA 70112
Phone: (504)584-3655 **Fax:** (504)584-3653
Email: mock@tulane.edu
Dr. Nancy Mock, Dir.
Activities/Fields: Research and evaluation of international health and development. Center conducts family planning and reproductive health projects in Africa and South and Central America, nutritional epidemiology, family planning impact evaluations worldwide, and health and human resources analysis for Africa.

★ 23455 ★ Tulane University
Clinical Immunology Section
1700 Perdido St., 3rd Fl.
New Orleans, LA 70112
Phone: (504)588-5578 **Fax:** (504)584-3686
Email: malopez@tulane.edu
Prof. Manuel Lopez, MD, Dir.
Activities/Fields: Provides a focus for research into the causes, prevention, and management of diseases such as asthma, allergies, immune deficiencies and infections, and autoimmune disorders, plus related studies of fundamental immune mechanisms involving immune cells, antibodies, genetic factors, and immune regulatory systems, especially as they relate to the lung. Investigates tobacco smoke products as possible allergens, mechanisms of AIDS, and immunologic mechanisms of occupational and environmental lung disease.

★ 23456 ★ Tulane University
Department of Orthopaedic Research
Sch. of Medicine
1430 Tulane Ave., Box SL-32
New Orleans, LA 70112-2699
Phone: (504)588-2273 **Fax:** (504)584-2722
Email: scook2@tulane.edu
Stephen D. Cook, PhD, Dir.
Activities/Fields: Biomaterials, including study of the properties of porous materials and materials-bone interfaces; surface studies of tissue-implant interactions; and corrosion resistance analysis, especially degradation characteristics of materials in an in vivo environment. Conducts histological and microradiographic evaluations of bone and implant composites. **Frmly:** Biomaterials Laboratory.

★ 23457 ★ Tulane University
Environmental Diseases Prevention Research Center
School of Public Health & Tropical Medicine
Tulane Medical Center, TW-43
1430 Tulane Ave.
New Orleans, LA 70112
Phone: (504)584-1774 **Fax:** (504)587-7352
Email: hartley@tulane.edu
Website: http://www.cdc.gov/prc/centers-tulane.htm
William R. Hartley, Prin. Investigator
Activities/Fields: Public health issues, especially behaviors that place Americans at risk for chronic diseases and conditions. Of particular concern is the improvement in quality of life for special populations, including the young, elderly, racial ethnic populations, and the underserved.

★ 23458 ★ Tulane University
Environmental Health Sciences Research Laboratory
Department of Environmental Health Sciences
1440 Canal St., Ste. 2100
New Orleans, LA 70112
Phone: (504)588-5374 **Fax:** (504)584-1726
Email: assafa@tulane.edu
Website: http://www.sph.tulane.edu
Dr. Assaf Abdelghani, Dir.
Activities/Fields: Chemical contaminants in air, water, food and the environment. Areas of interest include, air and water pollution abatement, water quality evaluation and control, environmental health management, bacterial and mammalian cell mutagenesis, toxicology, occupational safety and health, interdisciplinary studies of toxic effects of pesticides on the environment, biological and physical-chemical treatment of industrial waste, environmental toxicology, industrial hygiene, and heavy metal, hazardous waste management.

★ 23459 ★ Tulane University
Gene Therapy Center
1430 Tulane Ave., SL-99
New Orleans, LA 70112
Phone: (504)988-7711 **Fax:** (504)988-7710
Email: d.procko@tulane.edu
Website: http://www.som.tulane.edu/gene_therapy/
Dr. Darwin J. Prockop, Dir.
Activities/Fields: Adult stem cell therapy of bone and cartilage diseases, Parkinson's Disease, brain tumors, and spinal cord injury. **Pub:** *Peer reviewed research reports.*

★ 23460 ★ Tulane University
Tulane Center for Cardiovascular Health
1430 Tulane Ave., Box SL 29
New Orleans, LA 70112
Phone: (504)585-7197 **Fax:** (504)585-7194
Email: berenson@mailhost.tcs.tulane.edu
Website: http://www.tmc.tulane.edu/cardiohealth/
Gerald S. Berenson, MD, Dir.
Activities/Fields: Cardiovascular disease risk factors in children and young adults, including a descriptive epidemiology study (Bogalusa Heart Study), laboratory investigations on the mechanisms of arteriosclerosis, structural studies of proteoglycans, and health education and promotion in elementary school children (Health Ahead/Heart Smart).

★ 23461 ★ Tulane University
Tulane National Primate Research Center
18703 Three Rivers Rd.
Covington, LA 70433
Phone: (985)892-2040 **Fax:** (985)871-6569
Email: alackner@tpc.tulane.edu
Website: http://www2.tulane.edu/primate_center.cfm
Andrew A. Lackner, PhD, Dir.
Activities/Fields: Use of nonhuman primates in biomedical research projects in fields of immunology, infectious diseases, primate medicine, parasitology, primatology, pathology, reproductive physiology, urology, gene therapy and veterinary science. **Frmly:** Delta Regional Primate Research Center.

★ 23462 ★ Tulane University Health Sciences Center
U.S.-Japan Biomedical Research Laboratories
F. Edward Herbert Research Center, Bldg. 30
3705 Main St.
Belle Chasse, LA 70037-3001
Phone: (504)394-7199 **Fax:** (504)394-7169
Email: arimura@tulane.edu
Dr. Akira Arimura, Dir.
Activities/Fields: Neuroendocrinology and neuroscience, particularly in the areas of neuropeptides and immune-neuroendocrine interactions. **Pub:** *Neurendocrinology*, 10/year. • *Neuroscience*, 10/year.

★ 23463 ★ United Cerebral Palsy Research and Educational Foundation
1660 L St. NW, Ste. 700
Washington, DC 20036
Phone: (202)776-0406 **Free:** 800-872-5827
Fax: (202)776-0414
Email: lsmithslade@ucp.org
Website: http://ucp.org
Murray Goldstein, DO, Contact
Activities/Fields: Cerebral palsy, focusing on improving the treatment, management, and functioning of persons with cerebral palsy. **Pub:** *Research Fact Sheets*, monthly.

★ 23464 ★ United States Sports Academy (USSA)
1 Academy Dr.
Daphne, AL 36526
Phone: (251)626-3303 **Fax:** (251)625-1035
Email: academy@.ussa.edu
Website: http://www.ussa.edu
Robert C. Campbell, III, Ch.
Activities/Fields: Sport and sport education in an effort to upgrade sports medicine, sport coaching, sport management, and fitness management, including studies of athletic injuries, body composition of adults, motor performance of youth, physical fitness of adults, ECG abnormalities and changes due to exercise, biomechanical analysis of gross motor skills and three-dimensional gait analysis, product and equipment evaluation and drug use/abuse in sports evaluation and analysis. Research is carried on with local high school athletes, members of the USSA student body, youth involved in the Academy's overseas projects, and selected off-campus program participants. **Pub:** *Sport Supplement*, quarterly. • *USSA Academy News*, quarterly.

★ 23465 ★ University of Akron
Center for Nursing
209 Caroll St., R116
Akron, OH 44325
Phone: (330)972-6968 **Fax:** (330)972-5883
Email: ekinion@uakron.edu
Dr. Elizabeth Kinion, Dir.
Activities/Fields: Nursing outcomes, education and research and the relationship between family influences and health behaviors. Offers health care services to vulnerable individuals and families and provides a clinical laboratory for faculty and students to address patient care and response to care.

★ 23466 ★ University of Akron
Institute for Biomedical Engineering Research
Sidney L. Olson Research Center
260 S Forge St.
Akron, OH 44325-0302
Phone: (330)972-6650 **Fax:** (330)374-8834
Email: srittgers@uakron.edu
Website: http://www.biomed.uakron.edu
Dr. Stanley E. Rittgers, Dir.
Activities/Fields: Biomedical engineering, using and coordinating expertise and resources of biological, medical, engineering, and other scientific disciplines in greater Akron area for conducting research and promoting educational programs at the University, area hospitals, and the College of Medicine. **Pub:** *IBER Update Newsletter*, quarterly.

★ 23467 ★ University of Akron
Institute for Life-Span Development and Gerontology
326 Polsky
Akron, OH 44325-4307
Phone: (330)972-7243 **Fax:** (330)972-5174
Email: hsterns@uakron.edu
Website: http://www.uakron.edu/ilsdg
Dr. Harvey L. Sterns, Dir.
Activities/Fields: Improving older adult cognitive functioning, aging and work, career development, training and retraining adult and older adult workers, mental retardation and aging, gender identity, human development, health and aging, and family and aging. Programs concentrate on aging changes in perception, perceptual style, selective attention, and learning and memory. Other studies focus on performance appraisal and selection of older adult workers. **Pub:** *Continuum Newsletter.*

★ 23468 ★ University of Alabama
Institute for Rural Health Research (IRHR)
Box 870326, Nott Hall
Tuscaloosa, AL 35487-0326
Phone: (205)348-0025 **Free:** 877-363-2247
Email: irhr@cchs.ua.edu
Website: http://irhr.ua.edu/
John C. Higginbotham, PhD, Dir.
Activities/Fields: Health issues that affect people who live in rural areas.

★ 23469 ★ University of Alabama
Speech and Hearing Center
Department of Communicative Disorders, Box 870242
Tuscaloosa, AL 35487-0242
Phone: (205)348-7131 **Fax:** (205)348-1845
Email: ktucker@cd.as.ua.edu
Website: http://www.as.ua.edu/comdis/
Dr. Gerald L. Culton, Chm.
Activities/Fields: Communication disorders, including clinical studies associated with graduate training in speech-language pathology and audiology.

★ 23470 ★ University of Alabama at Birmingham
Alzheimer's Disease Center (ADC)
Sparks Research Bldg., Ste. 454
1720 7th Ave. S
Birmingham, AL 35294-0017
Phone: (205)934-1668 **Fax:** (205)975-7365
Email: adbrain@uab.edu
Website: http://main.uab.edu/show.asp?durki=11627
Lindy E. Harnell, MD, Dir.

Activities/Fields: Alzheimer's disease and related dementias. **Pub:** *Newsletter*, monthly.

★ 23471 ★ University of Alabama at Birmingham
Arthritis and Musculoskeletal Center
Tinsley Harrison Tower, Rm. 429
1900 University Blvd.
Birmingham, AL 35294-0006
Phone: (205)934-5306 **Fax:** (205)934-1564
Email: rpk@uab.edu
Website: http://info.dom.uab.edu/rheum/centers/arthritis.htm
Dr. Robert P. Kimberly, Dir.
Activities/Fields: Arthritis and related rheumatic disorders, including investigations into cause, diagnosis, control, and treatment of arthritis and complications resulting from arthritis and related musculoskeletal disorders. **Pub:** *Arthritis Today Newsletter*, biennially.

★ 23472 ★ University of Alabama at Birmingham
Center for Aging
201 Community Health Services Bldg.
933 S 19th St.
Birmingham, AL 35294-2041
Phone: (205)934-9261 **Fax:** (205)934-7354
Email: rallman@uab.edu
Website: http://www.aging.uab.edu
Richard M. Allman, MD, Dir.
Activities/Fields: Patient-oriented research, social-behavior science, basic science, public policy and health services. **Pub:** *Insight on Aging*.

★ 23473 ★ University of Alabama at Birmingham
Center for Biophysical Sciences and Engineering (CBSE)
MCLM 262
1530 3rd Ave. S
Birmingham, AL 35294-0005
Phone: (205)934-3841 **Fax:** (205)934-2659
Email: delucas@cmc.uab.edu
Website: http://www.cbse.uab.edu/
Lawrence J. DeLucas, PhD, Dir.
Activities/Fields: Structure and function of macromolecules as applied to new drug discovery.

★ 23474 ★ University of Alabama at Birmingham
Center for Health Promotion
Ryals Public Health Bldg.
School of Public
1665 University Blvd., Ste. 227
Birmingham, AL 35294
Phone: (205)934-6020 **Fax:** (205)934-9325
Email: maxm@uab.edu
Website: http://www.uab.edu/chp
Max Michael, MD, Dir.
Activities/Fields: Health promotion and disease prevention for underserved populations in Alabama. The center is divided into several components, including the Behavioral Assessment and Intervention Core, Biopsychosocial Laboratory, Community Core, Dissemination Office, Evaluation Unit, Health Communications Unit, Project Assessment Core, Surveillance Unit, Survey Research Unit, and Training Office. **Pub:** *Center for Health Promotion Newsletter*, 3/year.

★ 23475 ★ University of Alabama at Birmingham
Center for Injury Sciences
KB 120
1922 7th Ave., S
Birmingham, AL 35294-0016
Phone: (205)975-3030 **Fax:** (205)975-3040
Website: http://injuryscience.hs.uab.edu/
Dr. Loring W. Rue, III, Dir.
Activities/Fields: Prevention and treatment of injuries.

★ 23476 ★ University of Alabama at Birmingham
Center for Metabolic Bone Disease (CMBD)
509 Lyons-Harrison Research Bldg.
701 S 19th St.
Birmingham, AL 35294-0007
Phone: (205)934-6666 **Fax:** (205)975-9927
Email: cmbd@path.uab.edu
Website: http://www.path.uab.edu/cmbd
Jay McDonald, MD, Dir.
Activities/Fields: Metabolic bone diseases, including osteoporosis. **Pub:** *Newsletter*.

★ 23477 ★ University of Alabama at Birmingham
Center for Nuclear Imaging Research (CNIR)
School of Medicine
Center for NMR Research and Development
CNIR 106
Birmingham, AL 35294-4470
Phone: (205)934-9450 **Fax:** (205)934-7367
Email: ferry@uab.edu
Website: http://www.cnir.uab.edu/cnir.htm
Gerald M. Pohost, MD, Dir.
Activities/Fields: Application of clinical magnetic resonance methods to biological systems.

★ 23478 ★ University of Alabama at Birmingham
Center for Outcomes and Effectiveness Research and Education (COERE)
MT 412
1530 3rd Ave. S
Birmingham, AL 35294-4410
Phone: (205)934-6838 **Fax:** (205)934-4888
Email: coere@uab.edu
Website: http://www.dopm.uab.edu/coere
Catarina I. Kiefe, PhD, Co-Dir.
Activities/Fields: Analysis of the outcomes and effectiveness of health services that takes patients' experiences, preferences, and values into account.

★ 23479 ★ University of Alabama at Birmingham
Center for Research in Applied Gerontology
Campbell Hall, Ste. 201
Department of Psychology
1300 University Blvd.
Birmingham, AL 35294-1170
Phone: (205)934-3850
Email: kball@uab.edu
Website: http://main.uab.edu/show.asp?durki=6771
Dr. Karlene Ball, Dir.
Activities/Fields: Gerontology, particularly interventions which will allow older individuals to remain independent and to experience a high quality of life. The research of the center is designed to evaluate the ways in which improved visual, attentional and cognitive functions enhance everyday activities, focusing on the area of mobility.

★ 23480 ★ University of Alabama at Birmingham
Center for Research in Oral Biology
845 S 19th St., BBRB 258/5
Birmingham, AL 35294-2170
Phone: (205)934-3470 **Fax:** (205)934-9256
Email: suemich@uab.edu
Dr. Suzanne M. Michalek, Dir.
Activities/Fields: Oral biology, mucosal immunology, and connective tissue biochemistry. **Frmly:** Institute of Dental Research.

★ 23481 ★ University of Alabama at Birmingham
Comprehensive Cancer Center
1824 6th Ave. S
Birmingham, AL 35294-3300
Phone: (205)934-5077 **Free:** 800-822-0933
Fax: (205)975-7428
Email: lobuglio@uab.edu
Website: http://www.ccc.uab.edu/
Dr. Albert F. LoBuglio, Dir.
Activities/Fields: Oncology, involving medicine, dentistry, surgery, bone marrow transplantation, basic science, pathology, radiation oncology, obstetrics and gynecology, virology, biophysics, molecular biology, epidemiology, and pediatrics. Programs concentrate on the molecular biology and molecular genetics of malignant tranformation, (including oncogene and retroviral mechanisms), nature of the transformed membrane, structure of its antigens and their biologic function, and role and interaction of T and B cells in protection against cancer. Also concerned with models for assessment of effect of surgery, immunotherapy and chemotherapy in intact animals, possessing models for myeloma and osteogenic sarcoma, and crystalline and solution biochem istry of anticancer agents. Conducts clinical activities, including investigations into biology and usefulness of certain tumor scanning agents, including monoclonal antibodies, magnetic resonance imaging, and use of new agents for treatment of a wide variety of human tumors. **Pub:** *Cancer Center Magazine*, quarterly. • *Communications Newsletter*, 8/year.

★ 23482 ★ University of Alabama at Birmingham
Comprehensive Sickle Cell Center
1530 3rd Ave. S
Birmingham, AL 35294-0024
Phone: (205)975-2280 **Fax:** (205)975-5264
Email: eskridge@uab.edu
Website: http://main.uab.edu/show.asp?durki=34750
Tim M. Townes, PhD, Dir.
Activities/Fields: Sickle cell disease.

★ 23483 ★ University of Alabama at Birmingham
Division of Clinical Immunology and Rheumatology
Tinsley Harrison Tower, 429A
Birmingham, AL 35294-0006
Phone: (205)934-5306 **Fax:** (205)934-1564
Email: rpk@uab.edu
Website: http://info.dom.uab.edu/rheum/index.htm
Dr. Robert P. Kimberly, Dir.
Activities/Fields: Rheumatic diseases and clinical immunology, including clinical studies on antibody receptor structure and function, glycopeptide chemistry, chemistry and physiology of complement, biochemical and biophysical properties of immunoglobulins, molecular biology of genetic risk factors, and pathophysiology of bone calcification. Conducts laboratory investigations in macromolecular physical chemistry, protein structure, polysaccharide chemistry, and immunology. **Pub:** *Arthritis Today Newsletter*, biennially.

★ 23484 ★ University of Alabama at Birmingham
Gregory Fleming James Cystic Fibrosis Research Center
790 McCallum Bldg.
Birmingham, AL 35294-0005
Phone: (205)934-7210 **Fax:** (205)934-7593
Email: sorscher@uab.edu
Dr. Eric J. Sorscher, Dir.
Activities/Fields: Cystic fibrosis, including electrolyte transport and metabolism, mucin secretion and biochemistry, genetics, regulation of immune mechanisms, membrane traffic regulation, gene therapy, and pharmacologic therapy.

★ 23485 ★ University of Alabama at Birmingham
Injury Control Research Center
Community Health Service Bldg.-19th
CH19 403
Birmingham, AL 35294-2041
Phone: (205)934-7845 **Fax:** (205)975-8143
Email: rfine@uab.edu
Website: http://www.uab.edu/icrc
Russ Fine, PhD, Dir.
Activities/Fields: Rehabilitation and occupationally-related injuries, spinal cord injuries, and traumatic brain injuries, focusing on improving rehabilitation practices and processes to help persons with injuries achieve maximum rehabilitation potential; stimulating local faculty development of prevention, acute-care, rehabilitation, epidemiology, and biomechanics research projects; training health care workers and other practitioners, scientists, and students in the discipline of injury prevention and control; providing technical assistance and disseminate information in support of the nation's injury control agenda; and promoting the explicit incorporation of injury prevention initiatives targeting high-risk populations. Center also conducts multidisciplinary research involving faculty from other areas of the University. **Pub:** *Newsletter.* • *Report*, biennially.

★ 23486 ★ University of Alabama at Birmingham
Kirklin Pain Treatment Center
UAB Medical Ctr.
2000 6th Ave. S, 1st Fl.
Birmingham, AL 35233
Phone: (205)801-8250 **Fax:** (205)801-8253
Dr. Ann Still, Med. Dir.
Activities/Fields: Chronic pain and the management of chronic pain from benign or malignant sources. Also conducts studies on the effectiveness of group outpatient therapy for pain patients and their families and prior physical and/or sexual trauma and its relation to pain. Multimodal therapeutic regimes include behavior therapy, nerve blocks, hypnotherapy, stimulation produced analgesia (transcutaneous electrical nerve stimulation, acupuncture, and deep brain stimulation), biofeedback, and neuroablation. Affiliated with numerous departments and research centers at the University, which allows for patients to be treated according to their specific needs.

★ 23487 ★ University of Alabama at Birmingham
Lister Hill Center for Health Policy
330 Ryals Public Health Bldg.
1665 University Blvd.
Birmingham, AL 35294-0022
Phone: (205)975-8966 **Fax:** (205)934-3347
Email: morrisey@uab.edu
Website: http://www.healthpolicy.uab.edu
Michael A. Morrisey, PhD, Dir.
Activities/Fields: Health policy research, focusing on health care markets and managed care, maternal and child health, management in public health organizations, aging policy, and outcomes research. **Pub:** *Health Policy Abstract*, monthly.

★ 23488 ★ University of Alabama at Birmingham
Liver Center
MCLM Bldg., 2nd Fl.
1900 University Blvd.
Birmingham, AL 35294-0005
Phone: (205)975-9698 **Fax:** (205)975-9777
Email: jbloomer@uab.edu
Website: http://info.dom.uab.edu/gastro/livercenter/LC.html
Joseph R. Bloomer, MD, Dir.
Activities/Fields: Diagnosis and treatment of liver disease and related disorders.

★ 23489 ★ University of Alabama at Birmingham
Model Regional Spinal Cord Injury Care System
Spain Rehab Center, Rm. 529
619 19th St. S
Birmingham, AL 35249-7330
Phone: (205)934-3334 **Fax:** (205)975-4691
Email: jacksona@uab.edu
Website: http://main.uab.edu/show.asp?durki=10712
Amie Jackson, MD, Proj. Dir. & Ch.
Activities/Fields: Rehabilitation needs of those with spinal cord injury (SCI), including urological studies. System objectives include: to deliver and improve comprehensive medical, vocational, and psychosocial rehabilitation services for individuals with SCI; to evaluate both the effectiveness of services and their costs and benefits; to produce new and useful information; to demonstrate and evaluate the application of improved methods and equipment; and to participate in national studies of the benefits of a spinal cord injury service system. **Pub:** *Spinal Cord Injury: Clinical Outcomes.*

★ 23490 ★ University of Alabama at Birmingham
National Spinal Cord Injury Statistical Center
1717 6th Ave. S, Rm. 515
Birmingham, AL 35233-7330
Phone: (205)934-5049 **Fax:** (205)934-2709
Email: nscisc@uab.edu
Website: http://www.spinalcord.uab.edu
Vicki Farris, Contact
Activities/Fields: Data collection, storage, and analyses of national spinal cord injury statistics, submitted by 16 federally sponsored Spinal Cord Injury Care Systems. **Pub:** *Reports.* • *SCI: The Facts and Figures.* Book.

★ 23491 ★ University of Alabama at Birmingham
Nephrology Research and Training Center
647 Tinsley Harrison Tower
Division of Nephrology
1900 University Blvd.
Birmingham, AL 35294-0007
Phone: (205)934-3585 **Fax:** (205)934-1879
Email: dwarnock@uab.edu
Website: http://www.nrtc.uab.edu
David G. Warnock, MD, Dir.
Activities/Fields: Membrane transport, renal tubular transport, acid base physiology, renal hypertension, renal ultrastructure, epithelial ion transport, electron microprobe, erythropoietin, and population studies of genetic factors in hypertension.

★ 23492 ★ University of Alabama at Birmingham
Ob/Gyn Infectious Disease Research Laboratory
Department of Ob/Gyn
618 20th St. S
Birmingham, AL 35249-7333
Phone: (205)934-5271 **Fax:** (205)975-4375
Email: bandrews@uab.campus.mci.net
Dr. William W. Andrews, Dir.
Activities/Fields: Infectious etiologies of preterm labor, premature rupture of membranes, markers for preterm birth, new antimicrobial therapies for postpartum endometritis, the relationship between maternal infection and subsequent neonatal sepsis, and sexually transmitted diseases.

★ 23493 ★ University of Alabama at Birmingham
Parkinson's Disease Center
1225 Jefferson Tower
Birmingham, AL 35294-7340
Phone: (205)934-9100 **Fax:** (205)934-0928
Email: atchison@uab.edu
Website: http://main.uab.edu/show.asp?durki=11026
Paul Atchison, MD, Co-Dir.
Activities/Fields: Investigates Parkinson's disease, catecholamine receptors, genetics, and basal ganglion; and conducts related drug studies.

★ 23494 ★ University of Alabama at Birmingham
Pittman General Clinical Research Center
MEB 907
1530 3rd Ave. S
Birmingham, AL 35294-6909
Phone: (205)934-4852 **Fax:** (205)975-6616
Email: gcrc@uab.edu
Website: http://gcrc.hs.uab.edu
Larry W. Moreland, MD, Prog. Dir.
Activities/Fields: Patient care and laboratory support of clinical investigations for all departments and divisions of the Medical Center, including the Schools of Medicine and Dentistry. Studies are conducted on metabolism, cardiology, hematology, rheumatology, infectious diseases, virology, immunology, pulmonary medicine, renal medicine, gastroenterology, oncology, neurosurgery, AIDS, and the mechanisms of disease.

★ 23495 ★ University of Alabama at Birmingham
Rehabilitation Research and Training Center on Secondary Conditions of Spinal Cord Injury
Department of Physical Medicine & Rehabilitation
Spain Rehab Center
1717 6th Ave. S, Rm. 190
Birmingham, AL 35233-7330
Phone: (205)934-3450 **Fax:** (205)975-4691
Email: richards@uab.edu
Website: http://main.uab.edu/show.asp?durki=8762
J. Scott Richards, PhD, Contact
Activities/Fields: Prevention and treatment of secondary conditions of spinal cord injury (SCI), including urologic, respiratory and pulmonary complications; pain; psycho-social conditions; nutrition; and assessment of secondary conditions. **Pub:** *Pushin' On.*

★ 23496 ★ University of Alabama at Birmingham
Speech and Hearing Sciences Department
CH 20, Rm. 117
1530 3rd Ave. S
Birmingham, AL 35294-2030
Phone: (205)934-4814 **Fax:** (205)934-7438
Email: adamsl@uab.edu
Dr. Larry Adams, Hd.
Activities/Fields: Physiology, aerodynamics, acoustics, and perception of speech. Activities focus on basic physiology and acoustic studies of normal and abnormal speech learning. Experimental populations include hearing impaired, foreign dialect, and oral surgical patients. Specific research includes studies of temporomandibular joint functions and disorders, second-language speech acquisition, deaf speech, and neurogenic communication disorders. **Pub:** *Biocommunication Research Reports*, periodically.

★ 23497 ★ University of Alabama at Birmingham
Traumatic Brain Injury Care System (TBICS)
619 19th St. S, SRC529
Birmingham, AL 35249-7330
Phone: (205)934-3454 **Free:** 800-346-2742
Fax: (205)975-4691
Email: novack@uab.edu
Website: http://main.uab.edu/show.asp?durki=9505
Thomas Novack, PhD, Prin. Investigator
Activities/Fields: Effectiveness of care, rehabilitation, and recovery outcomes for people with traumatic brain injuries. **Pub:** *TBI Research Update.*

★ 23498 ★ University of Alabama at Birmingham
UAB Civitan International Research Center
1719 6th Ave. S
Birmingham, AL 35294-0021
Phone: (205)934-8900 **Fax:** (205)975-6330
Email: info@civmail.circ.uab.edu
Website: http://www.circ.uab.edu
Dr. Michael Friedlander, Dir.
Activities/Fields: Brain development/disorders, developmental disabilities. **Frmly:** Sparks Center.

★ 23499 ★ University of Alabama at Birmingham
Urological Rehabilitation and Research Center
The Kirklin Clinic
UAB Medical Center
2000 6th Ave. S
Birmingham, AL 35249
Phone: (205)934-9999 **Fax:** (205)934-2709
Email: klloyd@uab.edu
Website: http://www.health.uab.edu/show.asp?durki=10551
L. Keith Lloyd, MD, Dir.
Activities/Fields: Urological dysfunctions.

★ 23500 ★ University of Alaska Anchorage
Center for Human Development
2210 ARCA Dr.
Anchorage, AK 99508
Phone: (907)272-8270 **Fax:** (907)274-4802
Email: info@alaskachd.org
Website: http://www.alaskachd.org
Karen Ward, Dir.
Activities/Fields: Improvement in the lives of the disabled.

★ 23501 ★ University of Alaska Anchorage
Institute for Circumpolar Health Studies (ICHS)
3211 Providence Dr., Ste. DPL 404
Anchorage, AK 99508
Phone: (907)786-6575 **Fax:** (907)786-6576
Email: anbls@uaa.alaska.edu
Website: http://ichs.uaa.alaska.edu
Brian Saylor, PhD, Contact
Activities/Fields: Health problems and issues facing Alaskans and other populations in the circumpolar north, including epidemiologic studies of population health problems; studies of health services need, access and utilization; and evaluation of health policy and the effectiveness of new health programs.

★ 23502 ★ University at Albany, State University of New York
Center for Neuroscience Research
Biology 121
1400 Washington Ave.
Albany, NY 12222
Phone: (518)442-4309 **Fax:** (518)442-4767
Email: js213@albany.edu
Website: http://www.albany.edu/neuron/center/
John T. Schmidt, Dir.
Activities/Fields: Nervous system, particularly neuroplasticity, including the development and plasticity of the nervous system and factors that underlie and influence neurodegeneration and/or behavior. The center investigates the formation of synaptic connections in many different animals and examines how neurons make connections, how excess connections are removed, how neurons recover from damage, and how such neural connections modulate or control behavior. These research approaches are relevant for such problems as Alzheimer's Disease, epilepsy, strabismus, amblyopia, amyotrophic lateral sclerosis, Parkinson's disease and jet lag.

★ 23503 ★ University of Alberta
Alberta Peptide Institute
728 Heritage Medical Research Centre
Edmonton, AB, Canada T6G 2S2
Phone: (780)492-2522 **Fax:** (780)492-1473
Email: bob.parker@ualberta.ca
Website: http://www.api.ualberta.ca/
J.M. Robert Parker, Mgr.
Activities/Fields: Peptide synthesis, analysis, and purification, amino acid analysis, sequencing, and mass spectrometry.

★ 23504 ★ University of Alberta
Centre for the Cross-Cultural Study of Health and Healing
347 Old Arts Bldg.
Edmonton, AB, Canada T6G 2E6
Phone: (780)492-0403 **Fax:** (780)492-2715
Email: denise.spitzer@ualberta.ca
Dr. Earle Waugh, Co-Dir.
Activities/Fields: Multicultural health issues, including healing practices and efficacy of traditional healers, and developing a cross-cultural model for understanding similarities and differences among traditional healers; documentation and assessment of alternative healing practices; how societies deal with relationships among traditional, alternative and modern biomedicine; and programs which can best meet the needs of all Canadians, including aboriginals, established ethnic groups, and new immigrants.

★ 23505 ★ University of Alberta
Centre for Health Promotion Studies
5-10 University Extension Centre
8303-112 St.
Edmonton, AB, Canada T6G 2T4
Phone: (780)492-4039 **Fax:** (780)492-9579
Email: kim.raine@ualberta.ca
Website: http://www.chps.ualberta.ca
Dr. Kim Raine, Dir.
Activities/Fields: Health promotion.

★ 23506 ★ University of Alberta
Centre for Studies in Clinical Education (CSCE)
3-48 Corbett Hall
Faculty of Rehabilitation Medicine
Edmonton, AB, Canada T6G 2G4
Phone: (780)492-2903 **Fax:** (780)492-1626
Email: vivien.hollis@ualberta.ca
Vivien Hollis, PhD, Dir.
Activities/Fields: Clinical education, curriculum development, supervisor effectiveness.

★ 23507 ★ University of Alberta
EPICORE (Epidemiology Coordinating and Research) Centre
213 Heritage Medical Research Centre
Division of Cardiology
Edmonton, AB, Canada T6G 2S2
Phone: (780)492-8525 **Free:** 877-876-9888
Fax: (780)492-6059
Email: ross.tsuyuki@ualberta.ca
Website: http://www.epicore.ualberta.ca/
Dr. Ross T. Tsuyuki, Dir.
Activities/Fields: Healthcare practices and patient outcomes, epidemiologic studies.

★ 23508 ★ University of Alberta
Faculty of Pharmacy and Pharmaceutical Sciences
Noujaim Institute for Pharmaceutical Oncology Research
3118 Dentistry/Pharmacy Bldg.
University of Alberta
Edmonton, AB, Canada T6G 2N8
Phone: (780)492-5904 **Fax:** (780)492-8241
Email: gmiller@pharmacy.ualberta.ca
Website: http://www.pharmacy.ualberta.ca/noujaim/About.html
Gerald G. Miller, PhD, Dir.
Activities/Fields: Targeted anticancer therapy and drug delivery.

★ 23509 ★ University of Alberta
Institute for Biomolecular Design (IBD)
3-67 Medical Sciences Bldg.
Edmonton, AB, Canada T6G 2H7
Phone: (780)492-9334 **Fax:** (780)492-9394
Email: mike.ellison@ualberta.ca
Website: http://www.ualberta.ca/~csps/JPPS2(2)/D.Wishart/institute.htm
Michael Ellison, Exec. Dir.
Activities/Fields: Molecular nature of protein structure, function and proteomics and applications in agriculture, the environment, medicine, and biotechnology.

★ 23510 ★ University of Alberta
John Dossetor Health Ethics Centre
5-16 University Extension Centre
Edmonton, AB, Canada T6G 2T4
Phone: (780)492-6676 **Fax:** (780)492-0673
Email: dossetor.centre@ualberta.ca
Website: http://www.ualberta.ca/BIOETHICS/
Paul Byrne, Interim Dir.
Activities/Fields: Ethical and moral issues in the provision of healthcare. **Pub:** *Health Ethics Today.*

★ 23511 ★ University of Alberta
Molecular Biology of Membrane Proteins Research Group (CIHR)
Department of Biochemistry
356 medical sciences bldg
Edmonton, AB, Canada T6G 2H7
Phone: (780)492-4853 **Fax:** (780)492-0886
Email: bernard.lemire@ualberta.ca
Website: http://www.membranegroup.ualberta.ca
Dr. Marek Michalak, Dir.
Activities/Fields: Structure, function and biogenesis of biological membranes and subcellular compartments under normal and pathological conditions.

★ 23512 ★ University of Alberta
Muttart Diabetes Research and Training Centre
458 Heritage Medical Research
Edmonton, AB, Canada T6G 2S2
Phone: (780)492-6855 **Fax:** (780)492-4666
A. Rabinovitch, MD, Co-Dir.
Activities/Fields: Causes, treatment, and prevention of diabetes mellitus in humans and experimental animals. Provides core research laboratory support services. **Pub:** *Annual Reports.*

★ 23513 ★ University of Alberta
Neurochemical Research Unit
MacKenzie Centre
Department of Psychiatry
Edmonton, AB, Canada T6G 2B7
Phone: (780)492-7604 **Fax:** (780)492-6841
Email: glen.baker@ualberta.ca
Prof. G.B. Baker, Co-Dir.
Activities/Fields: Biochemical basis of depression, anxiety disorders and stroke; studies on the mechanisms of action of antidepressants and neuroleptics; neurochemical bases of reward; mechanisms of brain cell death; synthesis and pharmacological testing of potential antidepressants, anxiolytics and neuroprotective drugs; roles of amino acids and neuroactive steroids in the etiology and pharmacotherapy of anxiety disorders; drug metabolism and drug-drug interactions involving cytochrome P450 enzymes.

★ 23514 ★ University of Alberta Perinatal Research Centre (PRC)
220 HMRC
Edmonton, AB, Canada T6G 2S2
Phone: (780)492-2765 **Fax:** (780)492-1308
Email: david.olson@ualberta.ca
Website: http://www.ualberta.ca/PERINATAL/
Dr. David Olson, Dir.

Activities/Fields: Causes and cures of perinatal illness.

★ 23515 ★ University of Alberta Steadward Centre for Personal and Physical Achievement
W1-67 Van Vliet Centre
Edmonton, AB, Canada T6G 2H9
Phone: (780)492-3182 **Fax:** (780)492-7161
Email: info@steadwardcentre.org
Website: http://www.steadwardcentre.org
Dr. Robert D. Steadward, Dir.

Activities/Fields: Fitness, sport training and conditioning, and motor performance for adults with disabilities. **Frmly:** Rick Hansen Centre.

★ 23516 ★ University of Alberta Surgical-Medical Research Institute
1074 Dentistry Pharmacy Centre
Edmonton, AB, Canada T6G 2N8
Phone: (780)492-3386 **Fax:** (780)492-1627
Email: rrajotte@ualberta.ca
Dr. Ray V. Rajotte, Dir.

Activities/Fields: Institute is composed of multidisciplinary teams carrying out biomedical research. Principal fields of study include: islet transplantation, the immunology of diabetes, glucose regulation studies, experiments for extending the application of laparoscopic surgery and including a minimal access laboratory, and metabolic aspects of organ preservation (liver, heart, small bowel).

★ 23517 ★ University of Arizona Advanced Biotechnology Laboratory
Department of Anesthesiology
1501 N Campbell
Tucson, AZ 85724-5114
Phone: (520)626-5605 **Fax:** (520)626-5596
Email: malan@u.arizona.edu
Website: http://www.ahsc.arizona.edu/anesth/anes_res.shtml
Prof. T. Philip Malan, MD, Contact

Activities/Fields: Pharmacologic clinic research in acute post-operative pain models, including investigational anesthetics and intraoperative and postoperative medications; medications for the treatment of chronic pain in inpatients and outpatients; implementation of advanced technology to anesthesia, including utilization of computers for automation of monitoring and data collection; development of improved anesthesia delivery and monitoring equipment; basic research and development of new monitoring parameters; and ergonomic approaches to anesthesia tasks. **Pub:** *Pain*, quarterly.

★ 23518 ★ University of Arizona Arizona Arthritis Center
1501 N Campbell Ave.
PO Box 245093
Tucson, AZ 85724
Free: 888-285-3047
Email: aac@u.arizona.edu
Website: http://www.arthritis.arizona.edu
David E. Yocum, MD, Dir.

Activities/Fields: Arthritis and related connective and soft tissue diseases. The center is investigating immune system chemicals and the mind and body integrative approach to dealing with such diseases.

★ 23519 ★ University of Arizona Arizona Cancer Center
1515 N Campbell Ave.
PO Box 245024
Tucson, AZ 85724
Phone: (520)626-7925 **Fax:** (520)626-6898
Email: dvonhoff@azcc.arizona.edu
Website: http://www.arizonacancercenter.org
Dr. Daniel D. Von Hoff, Dir.

Activities/Fields: Clinical and laboratory cancer studies, including microarray technology, tumor cell kinetics, clinical pharmacology and pharmacokinetics, new targeted drug development, drug resistance mechanisms, human tumor cloning, markers of cellular activity in malignant tumors, cell and molecular biology, immunology, carcinogenesis, medical imaging, cancer prevention and control, cytogenetics, pain management, stereotactic radiosurgery, bone marrow transplantation, gene therapy, epidemiology, and biostatistics. Clinical studies focus on histological tumor types, staging of disease, tumor kinetics, measurement of tumor burden, and new approaches to chemotherapy. New approaches to biological therapy include developing interleukins, interferons, colony stimulating factors, and tumor vaccines. Ongoing projects focus on developing new cytotoxic derivatives of anticancer drugs and pharmacokinetics in tumor systems. Conducts reversal of clinical drug resistance studies, clinical pharmacology of anticancer drugs research, and drug interaction evaluations. Performs clinical cancer research on patients with all types of tumors, with special competence in treating breast, colon, ovarian, pancreatic, lung, and prostate cancers; melanoma; sarcoma; Hodgkin's disease; lymphoma, including mycosis fungoids; head and neck cancers; and brain tumors. **Pub:** *Annual Report.* • *Newsletter.* • *Scientific Report.* • *Special Interest Periodicals.*

★ 23520 ★ University of Arizona Arizona Emergency Medicine Research Center (AEMRC)
Box 245057
1501 N Campbell Ave.
Tucson, AZ 85724-5057
Phone: (520)626-6312 **Fax:** (520)626-2455
Email: harvey@aemrc.arizona.edu
Website: http://www.aemrc.arizona.edu
Harvey W. Meislin, MD, Dir.

Activities/Fields: Prevention of injuries. Specific areas of research include epidemiology of acute medical and traumatic problems, epidemiology and prevention of injury, pathophysiology of acute illness and injury, characteristics and performance of prehospital emergency medical care systems, and outcome research relating to injuries and traumatic deaths.

★ 23521 ★ University of Arizona Arizona Poison and Drug Information Center
College of Pharmacy
1501 N Campbell Ave., Rm. 1156
Tucson, AZ 85724
Phone: (520)626-6016 **Fax:** (520)626-2720
Email: tong@pharmacy.arizona.edu
Dr. Theodore G. Tong, Dir.

Activities/Fields: Toxicology and psychopharmacology, including studies of relative efficacy of certain antidotes in treatment of various poisonings. Conducts research in drug information, including patent information services, post-marketing surveillances, and adverse drug reactions. **Pub:** *Newsletter*, quarterly.

★ 23522 ★ University of Arizona Arizona Respiratory Center
1501 N Campbell Ave., Ste. 2349
PO Box 245030
Tucson, AZ 85724-5030
Phone: (520)626-6387 **Fax:** (520)626-6623
Email: inquire@respiratory.arizona.edu
Website: http://www.resp-sci.arizona.edu
Fernando D. Martinez, MD, Dir.

Activities/Fields: Causes and modes of development of emphysema, chronic bronchitis and asthma. **Pub:** *Newsletter.*

★ 23523 ★ University of Arizona Center for Gamma-Ray Imaging
Department of Radiology
Arizona Health Sciences Center
PO Box 245067
Tucson, AZ 85724
Phone: (520)626-6815 **Fax:** (520)626-2892
Email: barrett@radiology.arizona.edu
Website: http://gamma.radiology.arizona.edu
Harrison H. Barrett, PhD, Prin. Investigator

Activities/Fields: Gamma-ray imaging instruments with dramatically improved spatial and temporal resolution for use in research in functional genomics, cardiovascular disease, cognitive neuroscience, breast cancer, and surgical tumor detection.

★ 23524 ★ University of Arizona Center for Health Outcomes and PharmacoEconomic Research
College of Pharmacy
Tucson, AZ 85721
Phone: (520)626-4721 **Fax:** (520)626-2023
Email: grizzle@pharmacy.arizona.edu
Website: http://www.pharmacy.arizona.edu
Amy Grizzle, Asst. Dir.

Activities/Fields: Assessment of costs and outcomes associated with the use of pharmaceuticals, including quality of life assessment and pharmacoeconomic analysis (cost-effectiveness and decision analysis). Also focuses on pharmaceutical policy evaluation. **Frmly:** Center for Pharmaceutical Economics.

★ 23525 ★ University of Arizona Center for Phytomedicine Research
College of Pharmacy
1703 E Mabel
PO Box 210207
Tucson, AZ 85721-0207
Phone: (520)626-6775 **Fax:** (520)626-2515
Email: acprx@pharmacy.arizona.edu
Website: http://www.acprx.pharmacy.arizona.edu
Barbara N. Timmermann, PhD, Prin. Investigator

Activities/Fields: Ginger, tumeric, and boswellia, widely used in Ayurvedic medicine for the treatment of inflammatory disease. Ayurveda, a medical system primarily practiced in India, includes diet and herbal remedies, while emphasizing the body, mind, and spirit in disease prevention and treatment. Studies include arthritis and other chronic inflammatory conditions, including respiratory diseases such as asthma. **Pub:** *The Leaf*, quarterly. Newsletter.

★ 23526 ★ University of Arizona National Center for Neurogenic Communication Disorders (NCNCD)
Speech & Hearing Sciences Bldg., Rm. 500
1131 E 2nd St.
Tucson, AZ 85721-0071
Phone: (520)621-1472
Email: hixon@u.arizona.edu
Website: http://cnet.shs.arizona.edu/
Thomas J. Hixon, PhD, Dir.

Activities/Fields: Speech and language disorders caused by diseases of the nervous system. Areas studied include muscular control of speech and voice production, auditory and visual perception of speech, cognition, and the impairment of language function after stroke or as a result of nervous system disease.

★ 23527 ★ University of Arizona Native American Research and Training Center
1642 E Helen
Tucson, AZ 85719
Phone: (520)621-5075 **Fax:** (520)621-9802
Email: lclore@u.arizona.edu

Website: http://www.ahsc.arizona.edu/nartc
Jennie R. Joe, PhD, Dir.

Activities/Fields: Health and rehabilitation of disabled and chronically ill Native Americans. Core areas include the following: needs assessment, service delivery, and evaluation as determined by or in cooperation with the tribal community and empowerment that is sensitive to Indian values and needs. Also studies the impact of government policy on the delivery of health care. Promotes self determination and parity among Native Americans in health and rehabilitation. Serves as a national resource for all North American tribes and Alaska natives. **Pub:** *Books.* • *Dual track videotapes.* • *Reports.*

★ 23528 ★ University of Arizona
Pediatric Center for Complementary and Alternative Medicine
Department of Pediatrics
Health Sciences Center
1501 N Campbell
PO Box 245073
Tucson, AZ 85724-5073
Phone: (520)626-5170 **Fax:** (520)626-7176
Email: kjensen@peds.arizona.edu
Website: http://www.crc.arizona.edu
Dr. Fayez K. Ghishan, Prin. Investigator

Activities/Fields: Integrative approaches in pediatrics to common pediatric problems, including asthma, inflammatory bowel disease, cerebral palsy.

★ 23529 ★ University of Arizona
Sarver Heart Center
1501 N Campbell Ave.
PO Box 245046
Tucson, AZ 85724-5046
Phone: (520)626-7925 **Free:** 800-665-2328
Fax: (520)626-2666
Email: gaewy@aol.com
Website: http://www.heart.arizona.edu
Dr. Gordon A. Ewy, Dir.

Activities/Fields: Multidisciplinary studies of the heart, including basic, preclinical and clinical research. Basic research focuses on cell growth and development, including genetics, biochemistry, and molecular biology; preclinical research focuses on the microvascular, pharmacologic, and physiologic aspects of heart disease; and clinical research focuses on new drugs, techniques, devices, and interventions. Specific areas of study include cardiac elecrtrical instability, molecular biology and genetics, end-stage heart disease (including heart and lung transplantation and the use of mechanical assist devices and the artificial heart), atherosclerotic heart and vascular disease, detection and diagnosis of cardiovascular disorders, congenital heart disorders, microvascular and vascular disorders, heart disease prevention, cardiovascular diseases specific to Hispanics and Native Americans, and cardiovascular diseases in women and the elderly. **Pub:** *Newsletter.*

★ 23530 ★ University of Arizona
Sleep Disorders Center
University Medical Center, Rm. 1338
College of Medicine
Tucson, AZ 85724
Phone: (520)694-6112 **Fax:** (520)694-2515
Stuart F. Quan, MD, Dir.

Activities/Fields: Sleep disorders. Research efforts concentrate on sleep apnea, sudden infant death syndrome, nocturnal penile tumescence, male sexual dysfunction, seizure disorders, insomnia, narcolepsy, and restless leg syndrome.

★ 23531 ★ University of Arizona
Southwest Center for Community Health Promotion
1145 N Campbell
PO Box 210028
Tucson, AZ 85721-0028
Phone: (520)318-7270 **Fax:** (520)326-0435
Email: mlebowit@u.arizona.edu
Michael Lebowitz, PhD, Dir.

Activities/Fields: Public health issues, especially behaviors that place Americans at risk for chronic diseases and conditions. Of particular concern is the improvement in quality of life for special populations, including the young, elderly, racial ethnic populations, and the underserved.

★ 23532 ★ University of Arizona
Southwest Environmental Health Sciences Center (SWEHSC)
Center for Toxicology
College of Pharmacy
1703 E Mabel St.
Tucson, AZ 85721
Phone: (520)626-4488 **Fax:** (520)626-2466
Email: liebler@pharmacy.arizona.edu
Website: http://www.niehs.nih.gov/centers/center/az-ctr.htm
Daniel Liebler, PhD, Dir.

Activities/Fields: Health effects of environmental agents on living organisms. Activity has been grouped into five research cores: cellular processing of chemicals, cell injury, and environmental carcinogenesis and prevention.

★ 23533 ★ University of Arizona
Steele Memorial Children's Research Center
PO Box 245073
Tucson, AZ 85724-5073
Phone: (520)626-6053 **Fax:** (520)626-7176
Email: kvaldes@peds.arizona.edu
Website: http://www.crc.arizona.edu/
Dr. Fayez K. Ghishan, Hd.

Activities/Fields: Causes and cures for childhood illnesses and diseases.

★ 23534 ★ University of Arkansas at Little Rock
Arkansas Children's Hospital Cystic Fibrosis Center
800 Marshall
Little Rock, AR 72202-3591
Phone: (501)320-1018 **Fax:** (501)320-3930
Dr. John L. Caroll, Dir.

Activities/Fields: Cystic fibrosis and related respiratory diseases of children, including aerosol deposition and pulmonary function testing in children.

★ 23535 ★ University of Arkansas at Little Rock
Biomedical Research Center
College of Pharmacy, Slot 522-3
4301 W Markham
Little Rock, AR 72205
Phone: (501)686-6493 **Fax:** (501)686-6057
Email: compadrecesarm@wams.edu
Dr. Cesar Compadre, Dir.

Activities/Fields: Molecular modeling, including protein structure function relationships, toxicity modeling, and pharmocokinetic modeling; anatomical visualization, 3-D animation, and educational development. **Pub:** *Journals.*

★ 23536 ★ University of Arkansas at Little Rock
Partners for Inclusive Communities
Center on Developmental Disabilities
2001 Pershing Cir., Ste. 300
North Little Rock, AR 72114
Phone: (501)682-9900 **Free:** 800-831-4827
Fax: (501)682-9901
Email: swansonmarke@uams.edu
Mark E. Swanson, MD, Dir.

Activities/Fields: Improvement in the life of individuals with disabilities and families of children with disabilities to fully and meaningfully participate in community life. **Frmly:** Center for Research on Teaching and Learning.

★ 23537 ★ University of Arkansas at Little Rock
Rehabilitation Research and Training Center for Persons Who Are Deaf or Hard of Hearing
4601 W Markham
Little Rock, AR 72205
Phone: (501)686-9691 **Fax:** (501)686-9698
Email: DWatson@uark.edu
Website: http://www.uark.edu/depts/rehabres
Dr. Douglas Watson, Dir.

Activities/Fields: Improvement of vocational rehabilitation outcomes for individuals who are deaf or hard of hearing, focusing on improving career preparation, entry, retention, and advancement of these individuals in the workplace. **Frmly:** Research & Training Center on Deafness & Hearing Impairment.

★ 23538 ★ University of Arkansas for Medical Sciences
Alzheimer's Disease Center (ADC)
Donald W Reynolds Department of Geriatrics
4301 W Markham, Slot 811
Little Rock, AR 72205-7199
Phone: (501)526-5751 **Fax:** (501)526-5760
Email: beckcornelia@uams.edu
Website: http://alzheimer.uams.edu
Cornelia M. Beck, PhD, Dir.

Activities/Fields: Causes, treatment and cure of Alzheimer's Disease and other dementias.

★ 23539 ★ University of Arkansas for Medical Sciences
Arkansas Cancer Research Center
4301 W Markham, Slot 623
Little Rock, AR 72205
Phone: (501)686-8300 **Fax:** (501)686-8029
Email: suenjamesy@uams.edu
Website: http://www.acrc.uams.edu
James Suen, MD, Dir.

Activities/Fields: Molecular, cellular, and genetic mechanisms of cancer therapies, including studies in immunology, mechanisms of metastases, radiation enteropathy, cell surface proteases, growth factors and cytokines, angiogenesis, cell genesis and differentiation. Clinical research projects concentrate on hematologic malignancies and solid tumors, including their etiology, epidemiology, and the role of diet; mechanisms of growth; improved methods of diagnosis; responses to new therapies; and patient outreach, education, outcomes, and quality of life.

★ 23540 ★ University of Arkansas for Medical Sciences
Arkansas Center for Birth Defects Research and Prevention
11219 Financial Centre Pky., Ste. 250
Little Rock, AR 72211
Phone: (501)364-5001 **Free:** 877-662-4567
Fax: (501)364-5107
Email: hobbscharlotte@uams.edu
Website: http://arbirthdefectsresearch.uams.edu/
Charlotte A. Hobbs, MD, Co-Dir.

Activities/Fields: Causes of birth defects and a reduction in the economic, social, and psychological impact of birth defects at both state and national levels.

★ 23541 ★ University of Arkansas for Medical Sciences
Arkansas Center for Eye Research
Harvey & Bernice Jones Eye Institute
4301 W Markham St., Slot 523
Little Rock, AR 72205
Phone: (501)686-8293 **Fax:** (501)686-7037
Email: dixrichardd@uams.edu

Website: http://www.uams.edu/jei/acer.htm
Richard D. Dix, PhD, Dir.
Activities/Fields: Understanding the role viruses play in eye disease.

★ 23542 ★ University of Arkansas for Medical Sciences
Arkansas Center for Health Improvement (ACHI)
5800 W 10th St., Ste. 410
Little Rock, AR 72204
Phone: (501)660-7561 **Fax:** (501)660-7577
Email: smithgrichard@uams.edu
Website: http://www.achi.net
Dr. G. Richard Smith, Jr., Dir.
Activities/Fields: Policies that improve the health of the citizens of Arkansas.

★ 23543 ★ University of Arkansas for Medical Sciences
Center for Orthopaedic Research
4301 W Markham St., Slot 644
Little Rock, AR 72205
Phone: (501)526-6110 **Fax:** (501)686-8987
Email: suvalarryj@uams.edu
Website: http://www.cor.uams.edu
Larry J. Suva, PhD, Dir.
Activities/Fields: Prevention and treatment of osteoporosis, arthritis and related disorders.

★ 23544 ★ University of Arkansas for Medical Sciences
Center for Osteoporosis and Metabolic Bone Diseases
Division of Endocrinology & Metabolism
4301 W Markham St., Slot 587
Little Rock, AR 72205
Phone: (501)686-5130 **Fax:** (501)296-1002
Email: manolagas.stavros@uams.edu
Stavros C. Manolagas, MD, Dir.
Activities/Fields: Osteoporosis and its treatment. The focus of the research is to improve the understanding of the pathophysiology of the bone fragility syndrome of osteoporosis, and develop optimal therapies for its treatment.

★ 23545 ★ University of Arkansas for Medical Sciences
Centers for Mental Healthcare Research Center for Outcomes Research and Effectiveness (CORE)
Department of Psychiatry
5800 W 10th St., Ste. 712
Little Rock, AR 72204
Phone: (501)660-7550 **Fax:** (501)660-7543
Email: coreinfo@exchange.uams.edu
Website: http://www.uams.edu/CORE/home.htm
Dr. G. Richard Smith, Jr., Dir.
Activities/Fields: Impact of treatment on the outcomes of health care, particularly while adjusting for prognostic characteristics in a diagnostically similar patient population. **Pub:** *Annual report.*

★ 23546 ★ University of Arkansas for Medical Sciences
Donald W. Reynolds Center on Aging
4301 W Markham, Slot 748
Little Rock, AR 72205
Phone: (501)296-1000 **Free:** 800-942-8267
Email: lipschitzdavida@uams.edu
Website: http://centeronaging.uams.edu/
David A. Lipschitz, MD, Dir.
Activities/Fields: Aging and age-related diseases.

★ 23547 ★ University of Arkansas for Medical Sciences
Myeloma Institute for Research and Therapy
4301 W Markham St., Slot 776
Little Rock, AR 72205
Phone: (501)526-2873 **Fax:** (501)526-2273
Email: barlogiebart@uams.edu
Website: http://myeloma.uams.edu/institute.htm
Bart Barlogie, MD, Dir.
Activities/Fields: Therapies for multiple myeloma and related diseases.

★ 23548 ★ University of Arkansas for Medical Sciences
Myeloma and Transplantation Research Center (MTRC)
4301 W Markham, Slot 776
Little Rock, AR 72205
Phone: (501)686-8250 **Fax:** (501)686-6442
Email: mtrc@exchange.uams.edu
Website: http://myeloma.uams.edu
Guido Tricot, MD, Dir.
Activities/Fields: Treatment of multiple myeloma as well as other hematological malignancies.

★ 23549 ★ University of British Columbia
Biomechanics Laboratory
War Memorial Gymnasium
29 6081 University Blvd.
Vancouver, BC, Canada V6T 1Z1
Phone: (604)822-9192 **Fax:** (604)822-6842
Email: david.sanderson@ubc.ca
Website: http://www.hkin.educ.ubc.ca/biomech/hometop.htm
David J. Sanderson, PhD, Dir.
Activities/Fields: Human motions which are cyclical in nature such as cycling, walking, running and wheelchair propulsion, encompassing amputee, spinal cord injured, and non-injured individuals. The similarities in these movements across individuals reflect the mechanical properties of the musculoskeletal system and that forms the backdrop of the lab's work.

★ 23550 ★ University of British Columbia
The Biomedical Research Centre
2222 Health Science Mall
Vancouver, BC, Canada V6T 1Z3
Phone: (604)822-7810 **Fax:** (604)822-7815
Email: john@brc.ubc.ca
Website: http://www.brc.ubc.ca/
Dr. John W. Schrader, Dir.
Activities/Fields: Structure and function of genes and proteins involved in regulation of the growth and differentiation of cells of the immune system, including growth factors or cytokines, their cell surface receptors, and the intracellular enzymes and other proteins that control cellular growth and function. Research activities lie in the general areas of immunology, cancer, ontogeny, and technology development. Uses gene targeting and transgenic animal techniques to develop novel models of human diseases, and analyzes mechanisms in lymphocyte development, tolerance, and autoimmunity.

★ 23551 ★ University of British Columbia
Biotechnology Laboratory
Wesbrook Bldg., Rm. 237
6174 University Blvd.
Vancouver, BC, Canada V6T 1Z3
Phone: (604)822-4838 **Fax:** (604)822-2114
Email: dcrowe@cmmt.ubc.ca
Website: http://www.biotech.ubc.ca
Dr. Philip Hieter, Dir.
Activities/Fields: Molecular genetics as related to forest, plant, and animal biology and medicine. Interests include process engineering and fermentation studies. **Frmly:** Molecular Genetics Centre.

★ 23552 ★ University of British Columbia
Brain Research Centre
2211 Wesbrook Mall
Vancouver, BC, Canada V6T 2B5
Phone: (604)822-7246 **Fax:** (604)822-0361
Email: info@brain.ubc.ca
Website: http://www.brain.ubc.ca
Dr. Max S. Cynader, Dir.
Activities/Fields: Neuroscience, especially neurodegeneration, multiple sclerosis, schizophrenia and mood disorders, stroke, neurotrauma, and vision.

★ 23553 ★ University of British Columbia
Centre for Disease Control (CDC)
655 W 12th Ave.
Vancouver, BC, Canada V5Z 4R4
Phone: (604)660-2626
Email: robert.brunham@bccdc.ca
Website: http://www.cdc.ubc.ca/noflash/about.html
Dr. Robert C. Brunham, Dir.
Activities/Fields: Surveillance, control, and prevention of communicable disease.

★ 23554 ★ University of British Columbia
Centre for Molecular Medicine and Therapeutics (CMMT)
950 W 28th Ave.
Vancouver, BC, Canada V5Z 4H4
Phone: (604)875-3535 **Fax:** (604)875-3819
Email: info@cmmt.ubc.ca
Website: http://www.cmmt.ubc.ca/main/about.php
Michael Hayden, Dir.
Activities/Fields: Determination and control of genetic susceptibility to disease.

★ 23555 ★ University of British Columbia
G.F. Strong Research Laboratory for Medical Research
Division of Infectious Diseases
2733 Heather St., Rm. 452, Fl. D
Vancouver, BC, Canada V5Z 3J5
Phone: (604)875-4588 **Fax:** (604)875-4013
Email: ethan@interchange.ubc.ca
Dr. Reiner, Dir.
Activities/Fields: Infectious diseases, immunology, toxic shock syndrome, HIV/AIDS, host defense, macrophage cell regulation, tuberculosis, and leishmaniasis.

★ 23556 ★ University of British Columbia
Human Auditory Physiology Laboratory (HAP Lab)
IRC, Rm. B27
School of Audiology & Speech Sciences
Vancouver, BC, Canada V6T 1Z3
Phone: (604)822-7424 **Fax:** (604)822-6569
Email: stapells@audiospeech.ubc.ca
Website: http://www.audiospeech.ubc.ca/haplab/haplab.htm
Dr. David R. Stapells, Dir.
Activities/Fields: Brain mechanisms underlying normal and impaired hearing and language in humans; and the development, refinement, and application of physiological measurement techniques for the identification and assessment of hearing impairment in infants and young children. **Pub:** *Papers.*

★ 23557 ★ University of British Columbia
Institute of Health Promotion Research
Library Processing Centre, Rm. 324
2206 East Mall
Vancouver, BC, Canada V6T 1Z3
Phone: (604)822-2258 **Fax:** (604)822-9210
Email: info@ihpr.ubc.ca
Website: http://www.ihpr.ubc.ca/aboutus.htm
C. James Frankish, Actg. Dir.
Activities/Fields: Social, behavioral, and environmental determinants of health and the factors that predispose, enable, and reinforce individual and collective actions in relation to these determinants.

Research projects include policy analyses, epidemiological study of social and behavioral causes of health and disease or injury, design and evaluation of innovative approaches to bring about change in these factors, and studies of the implementation and diffusion of these innovations by policymakers, institutions, agencies, communities, practitioners, and populations.

★ 23558 ★ University of British Columbia Institute of Hearing Accessibility Research (IHEAR)
5804 Fairview Ave.
Vancouver, BC, Canada V6T 1Z3
Phone: (604)822-9474 **Fax:** (604)822-6569
Email: kathy@audiospeech.ubc.ca
Dr. M. Kathleen Pichora-Fuller, Dir.
Activities/Fields: Problems facing hard-of-hearing people, in order to find appropriate solutions to these problems and to promote hearing accessibility.

★ 23559 ★ University of British Columbia Jack Bell Research Centre
Vancouver Hospital & Health Sciences Centre
2660 Oak St.
Vancouver, BC, Canada V6H 3Z6
Phone: (604)875-5840 **Fax:** (604)875-5684
Email: dmclean@vanhosp.bc.ca
Dr. David McLean, VP, Res.
Activities/Fields: Steroid hormone receptors, cancer chemotherapy, inmunogenetics, kinases, micro-surgical procedures for repairing the bladder and uretha after an injury, and lung hazards in the work place and their effects on workers. Research also focuses on improving patient care, determining causes and treatments of diseases, detecting cancer at an early stage, and improving facilities for specialized surgery.

★ 23560 ★ University of British Columbia Kinsmen Laboratory of Neurological Research
2255 Wesbrook Mall
Graduate Secretary
Room 4830
Vancouver, BC, Canada V6T 1Z3
Phone: (604)822-7375 **Fax:** (604)822-7981
Email: neurosci@interchange.ubc.ca
Website: http://www.interchg.ubc.ca/neurosci/
Dr. Steven Vincent, Hd.
Activities/Fields: Neurological sciences, including studies on behavioral effects of specific brain lesions and/or drugs, central nervous system histochemistry and electron microscopy, Parkinsonism, epilepsy, Alzheimer's disease, dystonia, neurotransmitter systems and behavior, chorea, muscular dystrophy, psychopharmacology, and in vivo brain microdialysis and voltammetry.

★ 23561 ★ University of British Columbia Laboratories of Neurophysiology
Copp Bldg.
Department of Physiology
2146 Health Science Mall
Vancouver, BC, Canada V6T 1Z3
Phone: (604)822-2494 **Fax:** (604)822-6048
Email: info@physiology.ubc.ca
Website: http://www.physiology.ubc.ca
Dr. Kenneth Baimbridge, Dir.
Activities/Fields: Neurophysiology, including studies of basal ganglia, limbic forebrain, spinal cord, mechanisms of synaptic transmission in central nervous system, and amino acids.

★ 23562 ★ University of British Columbia McDonald Research Laboratories
St. Paul's Hospital
1081 Burrard St.
Vancouver, BC, Canada V6Z 1Y6
Phone: (604)682-2344 **Fax:** (604)806-8135
Email: jmcmanus@mrl.ubc.ca
Website: http://www.providencehealthcare.org
Dr. Michael O'Shaughnessy, Dir.
Activities/Fields: Pulmonary, cardiovascular and critical care research, including studies of asthma, chronic obstructive pulmonary disease, and acute lung injury. Areas of study include latent viral infections in the heart, pathology, biochemistry, molecular biology, physiology, immunology, structure and ultrastructure, and toxicology. Cardiovascular research includes studies on inflammatory diseases of the heart and blood vessels, viral injury, persistence and trafficking, cardiac myocyte metabolism, injury and repair, and vascular wall biology. **Pub:** *Annual Report.*

★ 23563 ★ University of British Columbia McDonald Research Laboratories/ iCAPTURE Centre Atherosclerosis Specialty Laboratory
St. Paul's Hospital
Healthy Heart Program
1081 Burrard St., Rm. B-180-1081
Vancouver, BC, Canada V6Z 1Y6
Phone: (604)806-8616 **Fax:** (604)806-8590
Email: jshill@interchange.ubc.ca
Website: http://www.healthyheart.org
Dr. John S. Hill, Dir.
Activities/Fields: Lipids and lipoproteins, lipoprotein metabolism, inherited disorders of lipoprotein metabolism, the enzymes lecithin, cholesterol acyltransferase (LCAT), hepatic lipase (HL), and lipoprotein lipase (LPL); the relationship of genetic polymorphisms and coronary artery disease. Conducts clinical research trials. **Frmly:** Lipid and Lipoprotein Research Laboratory.

★ 23564 ★ University of British Columbia VGH/UBC Eye Care Centre
Department of Ophthalmology
2550 Willow St.
Vancouver, BC, Canada V5Z 3N9
Phone: (604)875-4199 **Fax:** (604)875-4663
Email: jrootman@vanhosp.bc.ca
Dr. Jack Rootman, Hd.
Activities/Fields: Effects of diabetes on the eye with specific emphasis on circulation, electroneurophysiology of the retina, glaucoma epidemiology, visual perception, ocular therapeutics, color vision in ocular diseases, ocular oncology, orbital disease, thyroid orbitopathy, congenital glaucoma, neurophysiology and neuropharmacology of cortical vision, experimental pathology, central nervous system development, neural mechanisms underlying amblyopia and strabismus, computational vision, anatomical connections of the central visual system, molecular biological studies of neurotransmitters, receptors, and growth factors in the visual system.

★ 23565 ★ University of Calgary Cancer Biology Research Group
Health Science Centre
3330 Hospital Dr. NW
Calgary, AB, Canada T2N 4N1
Phone: (403)220-8695 **Fax:** (403)270-0834
Email: karl@ucalgary.ca
Website: http://www.cancer.ucalgary.ca/
Dr. Karl Riabowol, Chm.
Activities/Fields: Cell and molecular biology and their importance in the development and treatment of human cancers, including growth regulation, cell adhesion and metastasis, tumor differentiation, gene expression, cell surface markers, experimental cancer therapy, and relationship of cancer and aging. **Pub:** *Annual Report.*

★ 23566 ★ University of Calgary Cardiovascular Research Group
Health Science Centre
Faculty of Medicine
3330 Hospital Dr. NW
Calgary, AB, Canada T2N 4N1
Phone: (403)220-4525 **Fax:** (403)270-0313
Email: terkeurs@ucalgary.ca
Website: http://www.cvr.ucalgary.ca
Dr. Henk J. Keurs, Contact
Activities/Fields: Clinical and basic cardiac electrophysiology, cardiac mechanics, and heart failure. Research thrusts include: ion channels, electrophysiology, and arrhythmias, focusing on cardiovascular electrophysiology of cardiac and smooth muscle under physiological and pathophysiological conditions; electrical-mechanical coupling, cardiovascular mechanics, and congestive heart failure, emphasizing electrical-mechanical coupling and cardiovascular mechanics under physiological and pathophysiological conditions; and ischemia and interventional cardiology, focusing on coronary ischemia and reperfusion.

★ 23567 ★ University of Calgary Diabetes and Endocrine Research Group
Health Sciences Centre, Rm. 2556
3330 Hospital Dr. NW
Calgary, AB, Canada T2N 4N1
Phone: (403)220-2261 **Fax:** (403)210-8113
Email: dcwlau@ucalgary.ca
Dr. D.C.W. Lau, Dir.
Activities/Fields: Cause, cure and prevention of type I and type II diabetes and obesity from molecular, cellular and clinical approaches. Participates in national and international collaborative research projects.

★ 23568 ★ University of Calgary Gastrointestinal Research Group
Health Science Centre
3330 Hospital Dr. NW
Calgary, AB, Canada T2N 4N1
Phone: (403)220-7611 **Fax:** (403)220-0995
Email: ksharkey@ucalgary.ca
Website: http://www.ucalgary.ca/~girg/
Dr. Keith Sharkey, Ch.
Activities/Fields: Neuroendocrine control of gastrointestinal (GI) function, secretory functions in the GI tract, motility of the biliary tract and intestine, intestinal absorption, membrane physiology, immunology of the GI tract, intestinal inflammation, inflammatory bowel disease, developmental physiology, hepatobiliary disease, hepatic receptors, malnutrition, satiety and appetite control, intestinal adaptation, gut hormone, and splanchnic blood flow.

★ 23569 ★ University of Calgary Health Science Centre Immunology Research Group
3330 Hospital Dr. NW
Calgary, AB, Canada T2N 4N1
Phone: (403)220-8558 **Fax:** (403)283-1267
Email: pkubes@acs.ucalgary.ca
Dr. Paul Kubes, Chm.
Activities/Fields: Characteristics and modulation of immune and inflammatory responses in normal and disease states. **Pub:** *Annual Report.*

★ 23570 ★ University of Calgary Human Performance Laboratory
Faculty of Kinesiology
2500 University Dr. NW
Calgary, AB, Canada T2N 1N4
Phone: (403)220-3436 **Fax:** (403)284-3553
Email: zernicke@ucalgary.ca
Website: http://www.kin.ucalgary.ca
Dr. Ronald Zernicke, Dean
Activities/Fields: Mobility and longevity; biomechanics, including load on the musculoskeletal system, basic muscle mechanics, joint mechanics, lower back biomechanics, orthoses, sport shoes, and sports equipment; exercise physiology, including muscle physiology, limiting factors in performance and biochemistry of high performance; and neuromotor psychology, including studies involving ice hockey video discs and studies of eye movement in sports. **Pub:** *Annual Report.* **Frmly:** Laboratory for Human Performance Studies.

★ 23571 ★ University of Calgary Injury Research Unit
3330 Hospital Dr. NW
Calgary, AB, Canada T2N 2A1
Phone: (403)531-3383 **Fax:** (403)283-2805
Email: vppanlil@ucalgary.ca
Prof. Vladimir P. Panlilio, Contact
Activities/Fields: Conducts multidisciplinary contract studies of motor vehicle accidents. Specific projects include the study of injuries in accidents involving light trucks, vans, and passenger cars; pedestrian injury; protection of children with handicaps in motor vehicles; effectiveness of child car seats; injury scoring; and air cushion restraint systems. **Pub:** *Proceedings of the Canadian Multidisciplinary Road Safety Conferences.* **Frmly:** Multidisciplinary Accident Investigation Unit.

★ 23572 ★ University of Calgary Joint Injury and Arthritis Research Group
Heritage Medical Research Bldg.
3330 Hospital Dr. NW
Calgary, AB, Canada T2N 4N1
Phone: (403)220-8666
Email: rcbray@ucalgary.ca
Website: http://joint.mccaig.ucalgary.ca/jiarg/
Dr. Robert C. Bray, Contact
Activities/Fields: Biological and nonbiological transplants of joints and ligaments and gene therapy of injured tissues, including studies of joint reconstruction, gait analysis, sports medicine and athletic injuries, inherited connective tissue diseases, osteoarthritis and rheumatism.

★ 23573 ★ University of Calgary Lions Sight Centre
Faculty of Medicine
313-4411 16th Ave NW
Calgary, AB, Canada T3B 0M3
Phone: (403)286-3335 **Fax:** (403)286-3316
Email: huangp@cadvision.com
Dr. Peter T. Huang, Dir.
Activities/Fields: Structure, function, molecular genetics, chemistry, and development of vertebrate photoreceptors (rods and cones) and neural retina. Also studies retinal development and regeneration; myopia and regulation of ocular growth; diabetic retinopathy; and molecular genetics of human vision disorders.

★ 23574 ★ University of Calgary McCaig Centre for Joint Injury and Arthritis Research
3330 Hospital Dr. NW
Calgary, AB, Canada T2N 4N1
Phone: (403)220-8666
Email: rcbray@ucalgary.ca
Website: http://joint.mccaig.ucalgary.ca/jiarg/
Dr. Robert C. Bray, Ch.
Activities/Fields: Joint injuries and arthritis. **Pub:** *Annual report.*

★ 23575 ★ University of Calgary Neuroscience Research Group
3330 Hospital Dr. NW
Calgary, AB, Canada T2N 4N1
Phone: (403)220-4472 **Fax:** (403)283-2700
Email: tgiroux@ucalgary.ca
Website: http://www.acs.ucalgary.ca/~neuro/
Dr. Brian Macvicar, Chm.
Activities/Fields: Multidisciplinary group of independently funded researchers investigating various aspects of the nervous system, including hypothalamic mechanisms of thermoregulation, endocrine and autonomic control, axonal transport, nerve regeneration, actions of anesthetics, developmental neurobiology, synaptic circuitry, molluscan neurobiology, neurotransmitter/peptide pharmacology, structure and function of visual system, neuropathological disorders, molecular neurobiology, molecular biology of neurodegenerative disorders, sensory and motor physiology, cerebellar structure and function, and restorative neurology.

★ 23576 ★ University of Calgary Respiratory Research Group
3330 Hospital Dr. NW, Rm. 211
Calgary, AB, Canada T2N 4N1
Phone: (403)210-3816 **Fax:** (403)270-8928
Email: dproud@ucalgary.ca
Website: http://www.ucalgary.ca/~resprg
Dr. David Proud, Ch.
Activities/Fields: Normal and diseased respiratory systems, including mechanics of the respiratory system, muscles of respiration, neural control of breathing, membrane biophysics of smooth muscles. Pathogenesis of asthma and asthma attacks, airway inflammation, Cells of the airway and their response to provocative agents in asthma, lung pathology and occupational lung disease, neonatal lung development and disease, sudden infant death syndrome, surface properties of the alveoli of the lung, and blood flow to, and from, and through the lungs.

★ 23577 ★ University of Calgary Sport Medicine Centre
2500 University Dr. NW
Calgary, AB, Canada T2N 1N4
Phone: (403)220-8232 **Fax:** (403)282-6170
Email: rcjackso@ucalgary.ca
Website: http://www.kin.ucalgary.ca/strc/
Roger Jackson, Dir.
Activities/Fields: Human movement and sport, including anthropometry, athletic therapy, biochemistry, biomechanics, epidemiology, growth and development, nutrition, orthopedics, orthotics, physiology, physiotherapy, and sport medicine.

★ 23578 ★ University of Calgary Thrombosis Research Unit
Foothills Hospital, 601 S Tower
1403 29th St. NW
Calgary, AB, Canada T2N 2T9
Phone: (403)944-8047 **Fax:** (403)270-7891
Email: tru@calgary.ca
Website: http://www.ucalgary.ca/UofC/faculties/medicine/TRU
Dr. Russell Hull, Dir.
Activities/Fields: Diagnosis, prevention, treatment, and management of venous thromboembolism.

★ 23579 ★ University of Calgary Vision and Aging Laboratory
Administration 237
Department of Psychology
2500 University Dr. NW
Calgary, AB, Canada T2N 1N4
Phone: (403)220-4969 **Fax:** (403)282-8249
Email: donkline@ucalgary.ca
Website: http://www.psych.ucalgary.ca/PACE/VA-Lab/
Prof. Donald Kline, PhD, Dir.
Activities/Fields: Aging effects on vision, optical and neural aspects of visual aging, visual aging, human factors & everyday tasks; visual health, refractive surgery, vision change and quality-of-life, visual testing.

★ 23580 ★ University of California at Berkeley Cancer Research Laboratory
447 Life Science Addition
Berkeley, CA 94720-2751
Phone: (510)642-4711 **Fax:** (510)642-5741
Email: jallison@uclink4.berkeley.edu
Website: http://biology.berkeley.edu/crl/
Dr. James P. Allison, Dir.
Activities/Fields: Biology of epithelial neoplasia, with special emphasis on mammary and hepatic cancers; molecular pathogenesis of leukemia; factors involved in transformation of normal cells to neoplastic cells; and mechanism of neoplasia. Also studies production of monoclonal antibodies to cell surface structures altered during neoplastic transformation.

★ 23581 ★ University of California at Berkeley Center for Family and Community Health
140 Warren Hall
Berkeley, CA 94720-7360
Phone: (510)643-7314 **Fax:** (510)643-7316
Email: jmm@uclink.berkeley.edu
Website: http://socrates.berkeley.edu/~sph/CFCH
Joel Moskowitz, PhD, Dir.
Activities/Fields: Health issues such as AIDS; breast, cervical and prostate cancer; cardiovascular disease; alcohol and tobacco use; and the geographic distribution of health problems.

★ 23582 ★ University of California at Berkeley Center for Mental Health Services Research (CMHSR)
2020 Milvia St., Ste. 405
Berkeley, CA 94720-5610
Phone: (510)643-3555 **Fax:** (510)643-3522
Email: snowden@uclink4.berkeley.edu
Website: http://socrates.berkeley.edu/~cmhsr
Dr. Lonnie Snowden, Ch.
Activities/Fields: Organization and financing of care for severely mentally ill persons, including financing and economics, organization of services and systems, and methods and measurement.

★ 23583 ★ University of California at Berkeley Center for Occupational and Environmental Health
School of Public Health
Berkeley, CA 94720-7360
Phone: (510)643-4422 **Fax:** (510)642-5815
Email: llew@uclink4.berkeley.edu
Website: http://coeh.berkeley.edu/
Dr. John R. Balmes, Dir.
Activities/Fields: Occupational medicine, toxicology, industrial hygiene, epidemiology, occupational health nursing, and ergonomics. Specific research includes studies on the causes, diagnosis, and prevention of occupational and environmental injuries and illnesses. **Pub:** *Center for Occupational and Environmental Health Newsletter*, quarterly. **Frmly:** Northern California Occupational Health Center.

★ 23584 ★ University of California at Berkeley Center for Social Services Research Health Research Group
120 Haviland Hall
School of Social Welfare
Berkeley, CA 94720-7400
Phone: (510)642-1899 **Fax:** (510)642-1895
Email: lmidanik@uclink.berkeley.edu
Website: http://cssr.berkeley.edu/health/
Lorraine Midanik, Contact
Activities/Fields: Intersection of health issues and social welfare policy.

★ 23585 ★ University of California at Berkeley Cholesterol, Genetics and Heart Disease Institute
839 Mitten Rd.
Burlingame, CA 94010
Phone: (650)697-4500 **Free:** 800-HEART-89
Fax: (650)697-4501
Email: superko@heartdisease.org
Dr. Robert Superko, Dir.
Activities/Fields: Atherosclerosis and lipidology. **Frmly:** Center for Progressive Atherosclerosis Management.

★ 23586 ★ University of California at Berkeley
Environmental Health Sciences Center
School of Public Health
Berkeley, CA 94720-7360
Phone: (510)642-8770 **Fax:** (510)642-5815
Email: martynts@uclink4.berkeley.edu
Website: http://www.niehs.nih.gov/centers/center/ucb-ctr.htm
Prof. Martyn T. Smith, PhD, Dir.
Activities/Fields: DNA damage and its consequences for health, as well as the causes, mechanisms, and prevention of DNA damage and cancer.

★ 23587 ★ University of California, Davis
AIDS Virus Diagnostic Laboratory
1 Shields Ave.
Davis, CA 95616-8542
Phone: (530)752-8242 **Fax:** (530)752-4816
Email: jcarlson@clb.ucdmc.ucdavis.edu
James R. Carlson, PhD, Dir.
Activities/Fields: Human immunodeficiency virus (HIV) serology, HIV production and purification, bioassays of HIV inactivation, comparative retrovirology, and vaccine development.

★ 23588 ★ University of California, Davis
Allergy-Clinical Immunology Program
Sch. of Medicine, TB 192
1 Shields Ave.
Davis, CA 95616
Phone: (530)752-2884 **Fax:** (530)754-6047
Email: ssteuber@ucdavis.edu
Dr. Suzanne S. Teuber, Dir.
Activities/Fields: Cellular immunology and immunochemistry, especially the immunopathogenesis of systemic rheumatic diseases and autoimmune disorders, and the immunobiology of food allergies.

★ 23589 ★ University of California, Davis
Alzheimer's Disease Center (ADC)
4860 Y St., Ste. 3900
Sacramento, CA 95817
Phone: (916)734-5496 **Fax:** (916)456-9350
Email: wjjagust@lbl.gov
Website: http://alzheimer.ucdavis.edu/
William Jagust, MD, Dir.
Activities/Fields: Causes and potential treatments for Alzheimer's Disease and dementia. **Pub:** *Family Connection Newsletter.*

★ 23590 ★ University of California, Davis
California National Primate Research Center
1 Shields Ave.
Davis, CA 95616-8542
Phone: (530)752-0447 **Fax:** (530)752-2880
Email: crprc@ucdavis.edu
Website: http://www.crprc.ucdavis.edu/index.html
Dr. Andrew G. Hendrickx, Dir.
Activities/Fields: Developmental and reproductive biology, behavioral and neurology, genetics, neurosciences, virology and immunology, infectious diseases, pulmonary and respiratory diseases, primate medicine, and primate pathology. Focuses on preventive medicine for humans through the use of nonhuman primates as animal models in such studies as the effects of toxic compounds, developmental toxicology, metabolic diseases, infectious agents, altered environments, and pharmacokinetics of various drugs. **Pub:** *Annual Progress Report.*

★ 23591 ★ University of California, Davis
Center for Comparative Medicine (CCM)
1 Shields Ave.
Davis, CA 95616
Phone: (530)752-7913 **Fax:** (530)752-7914
Website: http://ccm.ucdavis.edu
Stephen Barthold, PhD, Dir.
Activities/Fields: Persistent infectious diseases common to humans and animals, especially host-agent interactions and intervention strategies.

★ 23592 ★ University of California, Davis
Center for Environmental Health Sciences (CEHS)
1 Shields Ave.
Davis, CA 95616
Phone: (530)752-2732 **Fax:** (530)752-3394
Email: rlmorrison@ucdavis.edu
Website: http://www.envtox.ucdavis.edu/cehs/
Dr. Fumio Matsumura, Dir.
Activities/Fields: Effects of the environment on human health, including human epidemiology, target organ toxicity, biomarkers of exposure, and effects and mechanisms of toxics. **Pub:** *Annual report.* • *Newsletters.*

★ 23593 ★ University of California, Davis
Center for Health and the Environment
1 Shields Ave.
Davis, CA 95616
Phone: (530)752-1340 **Fax:** (530)752-5300
Email: pahunter@ucdavis.edu
Website: http://che.ucdavis.edu/
Dr. Kent E. Pinkerton, Dir.
Activities/Fields: Effect of environmental agents, including chemicals and radiation, on the heath of humans, animals and other organisms. Conducts epidemiologic studies in human populations, and experiments are performed with animals, organisms, cells, and molecules to measure environmental exposures as well as heath outcomes associated with them. Research on the development of agents for population control of humans and wildlife seeks to mitigate the adverse effects of overabundance on the environment. **Pub:** *Research report*, annually. **Frmly:** Institute of Toxicology and Environmental Health.

★ 23594 ★ University of California, Davis
Center for Neuroscience
1544 Newton Ct.
Davis, CA 95616
Phone: (530)757-8708 **Fax:** (530)757-8827
Email: ejones@ucdavis.edu
Website: http://neuroscience.ucdavis.edu/
Edward G. Jones, PhD, Dir.
Activities/Fields: Single-cell recordings; neuronal populations in isolation; human perception, attention, memory, language; and the nature of consciousness.

★ 23595 ★ University of California, Davis
Center for the Study of Environmental Factors in Etiology of Autism
1278 Surge III
1 Shields Ave.
Davis, CA 95616
Phone: (530)752-6696
Email: inpessah@ucdavis.edu
Website: http://es.epa.gov/ncer_abstracts/centers/cecehdpr/01/pessah.html
Prof. Isaac Pessah, PhD, Dir.
Activities/Fields: Environmental risk factors contributing to the incidence and severity of childhood autism.

★ 23596 ★ University of California, Davis
Center for Tissue Regeneration and Repair
Orthopaedic Research Laboratories
4635 2nd Ave., Ste. 2000
Sacramento, CA 95817
Phone: (916)734-3311 **Fax:** (916)734-5750
Email: ahreddi@ucdavis.edu
Website: http://ctrr.ucdmc.ucdavis.edu/
Dr. A. Hari Reddi, Dir.
Activities/Fields: Human tissue regeneration and repair.

★ 23597 ★ University of California, Davis
Clinical Nutrition Research Unit
Division of Clinical Nutrition & Metabolism
TB 156 School of Medicine
Davis, CA 95616
Phone: (530)752-6778 **Fax:** (530)752-3470
Email: chalstead@ucdavis.edu
Dr. Charles Halsted, Dir.
Activities/Fields: Human nutrition in health and disease. Studies focus on the relationship of diet to disease, energy metabolism, and development.

★ 23598 ★ University of California, Davis
Division of Agriculture and Natural Resources
Genetic Resources Conservation Program
1 Shields Ave.
Davis, CA 95616-8602
Phone: (530)754-8501 **Fax:** (530)754-8505
Email: grcp@ucdavis.edu
Website: http://www.grcp.ucdavis.edu
Dr. Patrick E. McGuire, Dir.
Activities/Fields: Facilitates the collection and maintenance of animal, plant, and microbial genetic resources; identifies animal, plant, and microbial genetic resources critical to California and supports their conservation; and develops improved methods and strategies for procuring and maintaining genetic resources.

★ 23599 ★ University of California, Davis
Gastroenterology and Nutrition Center
Pediatric GI
UCD Medical Center
2516 Stockton Blvd., 3rd Fl.
Sacramento, CA 95817
Phone: (916)734-3750 **Fax:** (916)734-4098
Email: michael.haight@ucdmc.ucdavis.edu
Website: http://www.ucdmc.ucdavis.edu
Dr. Michael Haight, Ch., Pediatric Gastroenterology
Activities/Fields: Pediatric nutritional support, and feeding problems in children, Pediatric Short Bowel Syndrome, outcomes and lactation. **Pub:** *Educational booklets, videos.*

★ 23600 ★ University of California, Davis
Genetics Typing Laboratory
Department of Anthropology
209 Young Hall
Davis, CA 95616
Phone: (530)752-6343 **Fax:** (530)752-8885
Email: dgsmith@ucdavis.edu
Website: http://www.anthro.ucdavis.edu/~DGSMITH
Prof. David Glenn Smith, PhD, Prin. Investigator
Activities/Fields: Identification and characterization of previously unknown polymorphisms; the effectiveness of alternative genetic management strategies and the effect of demographic factors on the population/genetic structure of captive groups of primates; identification of marker loci for genes that influence susceptibility to retroviral, B-virus, and other infections; and employment of both ancient and contemporary mitochondrial DNA and microsatellite DNA loci for studies of ancestor-descendant relationships.

★ 23601 ★ University of California, Davis
M.I.N.D. (Medical Investigation of Neurodevelopmental Disorders) Institute
UC Davis Medical Center
4860 Y St., Rm. 3020
Sacramento, CA 95817
Free: 888-883-0961 **Fax:** (916)734-5153
Email: dgamaral@ucdavis.edu
Website: http://mindinstitute.ucdmc.ucdavis.edu
David G. Amaral, PhD, Res. Dir.
Activities/Fields: Neurodevelopmental disorders in children and adults, including autism and autism spectrum disorders; pervasive developmental disorder; cerebral palsy; Fragile X Syndrome; Tourette's Syndrome; mental retardation; attention deficit hyper-

activity disorder; dyslexia; and other learning, developmental delay, and communication disorders.

★ 23602 ★ University of California, Davis Rehabilitation Research and Training Center in Neuromuscular Diseases
Department of Physical Medicine & Rehabilitation, TB 191
School of Medicine
Davis, CA 95616-8655
Phone: (530)752-2903 **Fax:** (530)752-3468
Email: NMDinfo@ucdavis.edu
Website: http://www.rehabinfo.net
Craig McDonald, MD, Dir.
Activities/Fields: Increase of functional capacity, quality of life, and community integration of persons with neuromuscular diseases. Twelve research and/or training projects are organized into four cores: Interventions to Preserve Functional Capacity; Genetic Information and Research; Interventions to Enhance Community Integration; and Training and Information Services. The projects include Management of Muscle Wasting in Neuromuscular Disease; Exercise and Dietary Intervention in Slowly Progressive Neuromuscular Disease; Nutritional Assessment and Intervention in Duchenne Muscular Dystrophy; Exercise-Related Fatigue and Injury in an Animal Model of Muscular Dystrophy; Pain in Neuromuscular Disease: Incidence, Severity and Relationship to Physical Impairment and Disability; Outcome of Lower-Limb Orthotic Intervention in Hereditary and Acquired Neuromuscular Disease; Role of Personal Strivings in the Quality of life and Community Integration of Individuals with Neuromuscular Disorders; Stress and Coping in Children and Adolescents Living with Muscular Dystrophy and other Neuromuscular Diseases; Enhancing Medical Students' Attitudes and Knowledge about Those Who Live with Disabilities; Meeting Information Needs to Enhance the Community Integration of Individuals with Neuromuscular Disease; Risks and Benefits of Genetic Testing in Persons with Hereditary Neuromuscular Disease; and National Clearinghouse of Information on Neuromuscular Disease. **Pub:** *RRTC Newsletter.*

★ 23603 ★ University of California, Irvine Air Pollution Health Effects Laboratory
Department of Community & Environmental Medicine
Irvine, CA 92697-1825
Phone: (949)824-5860 **Fax:** (949)824-4763
Email: rfphalen@uci.edu
Dr. Robert F. Phalen, Dir.
Activities/Fields: Lung development and defenses, particle deposition in the lungs, inhalation exposure to oxidant, fine particulate and acidic aerosol mixtures, inhalation exposure methodology, and environmental and occupational inhalation toxicology, emphasizing particle plus gas mixtures. Also develops and validates mathematical models of inhaled particle deposition. **Pub:** *Scientic Journal Articles.*

★ 23604 ★ University of California, Irvine Beckman Laser Institute
1002 Health Sciences Rd. E
Irvine, CA 92612
Phone: (949)824-4713 **Fax:** (949)824-8413
Email: mberns@laser.bli.uci.edu
Website: http://www.bli.uci.edu
Dr. Michael W. Berns, Dir.
Activities/Fields: Basic research includes genetics, cell biology, spectroscopy, and biophysics. Conducts basic laser studies of cellular functions, including genetic expression, cell motility, and cell membrane behavior; and biophysical studies of thermal, fluorescence, acoustic/mechanical, photochemical, and ionization effects of radiation on biological material. Conducts applied research in cancer detection and treatment; reshaping of cornea with excimer laser, diagnosis (imaging) and treatment of portwine stain birthmarks; application of lasers to women's health problems; and development of medical laser devices. **Pub:** *Beckman Laser Institute News*, quarterly. Newsletter.

★ 23605 ★ University of California, Irvine Brain Imaging Center
109 Irvine Hall
College of Medicine
Irvine, CA 92697-3960
Phone: (949)824-7872 **Fax:** (949)824-9650
Email: jcwu@uci.edu
Joseph C. Wu, MD, Clin. Dir.
Activities/Fields: PET scan analysis of brain functions focusing on mental illness, brain tumors, Alzheimer's disease, near drowning, traumatic brain injury, and aberrant behavior.

★ 23606 ★ University of California, Irvine Cancer Research Institute
236 Sprague Hall
Irvine, CA 92697-3905
Phone: (949)824-5886 **Fax:** (949)824-4023
Email: hyfan@uci.edu
Dr. Hung Fan, Dir.
Activities/Fields: Focuses on immunology, virology, and growth factors, emphasizing basic research in various aspects of cancer. Also conducts studies in other areas central to understanding regulation in eukaryotic cells.

★ 23607 ★ University of California, Irvine Chao Family Comprehensive Cancer Center
101 The City Dr., Bldg. 23
Rte. 81
Orange, CA 92868
Phone: (714)456-6310 **Fax:** (714)456-2240
Email: flmeyske@uci.edu
Dr. Frank L. Meyskens, Jr., Dir.
Activities/Fields: Cancer treatment.

★ 23608 ★ University of California, Irvine Health Promotion Center
School of Social Ecology
Irvine, CA 92697
Phone: (949)824-5047 **Fax:** (949)824-8566
Email: ucihpc@uci.edu
Website: http://www.healthpromotioncenter.uci.edu/
Daniel Stokols, PhD, Co-Dir.
Activities/Fields: Health promotion. Research focuses on comprehensive, integrated approaches to health promotion, especially on workplace-based health promotion. **Pub:** *Newsletter.* • *Technical reports.* • *Wellness Programming Guides.*

★ 23609 ★ University of California, Irvine Herklotz Research Facility Center for the Neurobiology of Learning and Memory
320 Qureshey Research Laboratory
Herklotz Research Facility
Irvine, CA 92697-3800
Phone: (949)824-5401 **Fax:** (949)824-2952
Email: jlmcgaug@uci.edu
Website: http://www.cnlm.uci.edu
Dr. James L. McGaugh, Dir.
Activities/Fields: Neurobiology of learning and memory, including biochemical mechanisms, systems neurophysiology, modulation of memory, cognitive neuropsychology, and neural modeling. **Pub:** *Annual report.* • *Conference proceedings.*

★ 23610 ★ University of California, Irvine Institute for Brain Aging and Dementia
1113 Gillespie Neuroscience Research Facility
Irvine, CA 92697
Phone: (949)824-5847 **Fax:** (949)824-2071
Email: cwcotman@uci.edu
Website: http://www.alz.uci.edu/
Carl W. Cotman, PhD, Dir.
Activities/Fields: Causes of dementia and Alzheimer's Disease.

★ 23611 ★ University of California, Irvine Laser Microbeam and Medical Program (LAMMP)
Beckman Laser Institute Medical Clinic
1002 Health Sciences Rd. E
Irvine, CA 92612
Phone: (949)824-8367 **Fax:** (949)824-6969
Email: tromberg@bli.uci.edu
Website: http://www.bli.uci.edu/lammp/index.html
Dr. Bruce J. Tromberg, Dir.
Activities/Fields: Combines sophisticated methods of microscopy, computational methods, and laser spectroscopy to investigate cellular, genetic, and developmental problems that are related to cancer, heart disease, neurobiology, and other health problems. Focuses on basic and translational research, particularly in the areas of laser-tissue interactions, tissue optics, photodynamic therapy, and functional imaging.

★ 23612 ★ University of California, Irvine Memory Disorders Clinic
Department of Neurology
Irvine, CA 92697
Phone: (949)824-6088 **Fax:** (949)824-2132
Email: astarr@uci.edu
Arnold Starr, MD, Dir.
Activities/Fields: Multidisciplinary approach to diagnosis and treatment of memory disorders, including the development and testing of memory enhancement programs.

★ 23613 ★ University of California, Irvine Reeve-Irvine Research Center
1105 Gillespie Neuroscience Research Facility
Irvine, CA 92697-4292
Phone: (949)824-3993 **Fax:** (949)824-9900
Email: osteward@uci.edu
Website: http://www.reeve.uci.edu
Oswald Steward, PhD, Dir.
Activities/Fields: Injuries to and diseases of the spinal cord that result in paralysis or other loss of neurologic function, with the goal of finding a cure. **Pub:** *Newsletter.* • *Research manuscripts.*

★ 23614 ★ University of California, Irvine Susan Samueli Center for Complementary and Alternative Medicine
College of Medicine
University Tower, Ste. 620
4199 Campus Dr.
Irvine, CA 92612-5850
Phone: (949)824-9278 **Fax:** (949)824-2812
Email: dfelten@uci.edu
Website: http://www.ucihs.uci.edu/com/samueli/
David Felten, MD, Exec. Dir.
Activities/Fields: Use of complementary and alternative medical approaches for maintaining wellness, preventing disease, and treating specific illness.

★ 23615 ★ University of California, Los Angeles Ahmanson/UCLA Adult Congenital Heart Disease Center
Center for the Health Sciences, Rm. 47-123
Departments of Medicine, Pediatrics & Surgery
UCLA School of Medicine
650 Charles E Young Dr. S
Los Angeles, CA 90095-1679
Phone: (310)825-2019 **Fax:** (310)206-9133
Email: achdc@mednet.ucla.edu
Website: http://www.healthcare.ucla.edu/Programs/program.asp?version=1956&programid=288
John S. Child, MD, Dir.
Activities/Fields: Congenital heart disease in adults.

★ 23616 ★ University of California, Los Angeles
Alcohol Research Center
Neuropsychiatric Institute
760 Westwood Plz.
Los Angeles, CA 90024
Phone: (310)825-1891 **Fax:** (310)206-7309
Dr. Ernest P. Noble, Dir.
Activities/Fields: Causes of alcoholism, including genetic predisposition.

★ 23617 ★ University of California, Los Angeles
Alzheimer's Disease Center (ADC)
710 Westwood Plz., Rm. 2238
Los Angeles, CA 90095-1769
Phone: (310)206-5238 **Fax:** (310)206-5287
Email: adc@ucla.edu
Website: http://www.adc.ucla.edu
Dr. Jeffrey Cummings, Dir.
Activities/Fields: Diagnosis, pathophysiology, and treatment of dementing illnesses, such as Alzheimer's disease. **Pub:** *Newsletter*, annually.

★ 23618 ★ University of California, Los Angeles
Biocybernetics Laboratory
4531 Boelter Hall
Computer Science Department
Los Angeles, CA 90095-1596
Phone: (310)825-7482 **Fax:** (310)794-5057
Email: joed@cs.ucla.edu
Website: http://biocyb.cs.ucla.edu/
Prof. Joseph J. DiStefano, III, Dir.
Activities/Fields: Synergistic and methodologic interface between modeling and laboratory experimentation, with a focus on integrated approaches for solving complex biosystem problems from sparse biodata.

★ 23619 ★ University of California, Los Angeles
Brain Research Institute (BRI)
Gonda Goldschmied Neuroscience & Genetics Research Center
Los Angeles, CA 90095-1761
Phone: (310)825-5061 **Fax:** (310)206-5855
Website: http://www.bri.ucla.edu
Allan Tobin, Dir.
Activities/Fields: Brain and central nervous system, including interdisciplinary studies in developmental neurobiology, molecular neurobiology, neuroanatomy, neurobiophysics, neurochemistry, neurocytology, neuroendocrinology, neuroimaging, neuromuscular physiology, neuropathology, neuropharmacology, neurophysiology, behavior, neuroimmunology, and experimental epilepsy. Also conducts research on aging, Alzheimer's Disease, alcohol effects on the central nervous system, cellular neurobiology, neuroendocrinology, and neuromuscular plasticity. **Pub:** *Neuroscience News.*

★ 23620 ★ University of California, Los Angeles
Cardiovascular Research Laboratory
MRLB, Rm. 3645
675 Charles E Young Dr. S
Los Angeles, CA 90095-1760
Phone: (310)825-2554 **Fax:** (310)206-5777
Email: jweiss@mednet.ucla.edu
Website: http://www.heartlab.mednet.ucla.edu
Dr. James N. Weiss, Dir.
Activities/Fields: Cellular and subcellular mechanisms of cardiovascular physiology, including ultrastructure, electrophysiology, mechanics, biochemistry, molecular biology, and molecular genetics.

★ 23621 ★ University of California, Los Angeles
Center for Dietary Supplements Research: Botanicals
10945 LeConte Ave., Ste. 1401
Los Angeles, CA 90095-1406
David Heber, MD, Prin. Investigator
Activities/Fields: Explores potential mechanisms of action of yeast-fermented rice for cholesterol reduction; examines implications for heart disease prevention, green tea extract and soy for inhibition of tumor growth, St. John's wort, an herb used for relieving mild depression; assesses levels of bioactive compounds in several botanicals available as dietary supplements.

★ 23622 ★ University of California, Los Angeles
Center for Health Policy Research
10911 Weyburn Ave., Ste. 300
Los Angeles, CA 90024
Phone: (310)794-0909 **Fax:** (310)794-2686
Email: chpr@ucla.edu
Website: http://www.healthpolicy.ucla.edu
E. Richard Brown, PhD, Dir.
Activities/Fields: Cost-effectiveness of health programs and services and their effects on health of communities and consumers; policy analysis and develops policy tools that address issues of health promotion and disease prevention.

★ 23623 ★ University of California, Los Angeles
Center for Public Health and Disasters
School of Public Health
1145 Gayley Ave., Ste. 304
Los Angeles, CA 90024
Phone: (310)794-0864
Website: http://www.ph.ucla.edu/cphdr/
Steven J. Rottman, MD, Dir.
Activities/Fields: How natural and human generated disasters affect the public's health. **Frmly:** Center for Public Health and Disaster Relief.

★ 23624 ★ University of California, Los Angeles
Center for Sleep Research
Siegel Laboratory
Neurobiology Research 151A3
Department of Psychiatry
North Hills, CA 91343
Phone: (818)891-7711
Email: jsiegel@ucla.edu
Website: http://www.npi.ucla.edu/sleepresearch
Jerry Siegel, PhD, Contact
Activities/Fields: Evolution, function, and disorders of REM sleep.

★ 23625 ★ University of California, Los Angeles
Crump Institute for Molecular Imaging
700 Westwood Blvd.
Los Angeles, CA 90095-1770
Phone: (310)206-8975 **Fax:** (310)209-4655
Email: sgambhir@mednet.ucla.edu
Website: http://www.crump.ucla.edu/
Sanjiv Sam Gambhir, Dir.
Activities/Fields: Biological imaging technologies, including positron emmision tomography; autoradiographic images for in viro and in vitro assays of biochemical and biological process in tissue preparations; fluorescent microscopy to provide images of changing chemical environments in tissue and isolated cell preparations; and image based communication and educational systems using game strategies, expert systems, knowledge navigators, and personal computers.

★ 23626 ★ University of California, Los Angeles
CURE: Digestive Diseases Research Center
Bldg. 115, Rm. 115
VA Greater LA Healthcare Center
11301 Wilshire Blvd.
Los Angeles, CA 90073
Phone: (310)312-9284 **Fax:** (310)268-4963
Email: ytache@ucla.edu
Website: http://www.cure.med.ucla.edu
Yvette Tache, PhD, Dir.
Activities/Fields: Peptic ulcer disease, relationship of Helicobacter pylori infection to ulcers. Etiology and treatment of functional bowel disease, cell proliferation, gastrointestinal neoplasm, and nutritional intestinal absorption. **Frmly:** Center for Ulcer Research and Education.

★ 23627 ★ University of California, Los Angeles
Dental Research Institute
Center for Health Science
PO Box 951668
Los Angeles, CA 90095-1668
Phone: (310)206-6063 **Fax:** (310)267-1072
Email: npark@dent.ucla.edu
Website: http://www.dent.ucla.edu/
Dr. No-Hee Park, Dir.
Activities/Fields: Oral cancer, molecular oncology, viral oncology, molecular mechanisms of periodontal diseases, ultrastructure and cell biology, dental implantology, TMJ disorders and orofacial pain, neuroimmunology, molecular immunology, AIDS/HIV immunology, pain control/pharmacology, biomaterials, and wound repair/keloid tissue formation mechanisms. Also conducts clinical dental science studies. **Pub:** *International Journal of Oral Biology*, quarterly. • *UCLA Dental Research Annual Report.*

★ 23628 ★ University of California, Los Angeles
Duchenne Muscular Dystrophy Research Center (DMDRC)
Life Science Bldg.
621 Charles Young Dr. S
Los Angeles, CA 90095
Fax: (310)825-8489
Email: dmdrc@physci.ucla.edu
Website: http://www.physci.ucla.edu/DMD/
Dr. James Tidball, Dir.
Activities/Fields: Development of treatments for Duchenne muscular dystrophy. Researchers are most interested in understanding the role the immune system plays in this condition.

★ 23629 ★ University of California, Los Angeles
Harbor-UCLA Medical Center
Center for the Study of Inflammatory Bowel Disease
1124 W Carson St., Bldg. N-21
Torrance, CA 90502
Phone: (310)222-2475 **Fax:** (310)212-7837
Email: Veysselein@rei.edu
Viktor E. Eysselein, MD, Ch.
Activities/Fields: Inflammatory bowel disease, particularly the origin, causes, and treatment of ulcerative colitis and Crohn's disease. Conducts related studies in molecular biology, cell biology, and immunology. Performs clinical trials of new drugs.

★ 23630 ★ University of California, Los Angeles
Harbor-UCLA Medical Center
General Clinical Research Center
1000 W Carson St., Box 16
Torrance, CA 90509
Phone: (310)222-2503 **Fax:** (310)533-6972
Email: wang@gcrc.rei.edu

Website: http://gcrc.humc.edu
Dr. Christina Wang, Prog. Dir.

Activities/Fields: Biomedicine, endocrinology, reproductive physiology, gastroenterology, genetics, immunology and infectious disease, nephrology, obstetrics and gynecology, labor and delivery, diabetes, metabolism, oncology, pediatrics, nutrition, psychiatry, neurology, AIDS research and neonatology.

★ 23631 ★ University of California, Los Angeles
Harbor-UCLA Medical Center Research and Education Institute
1124 W Carson St.
Torrance, CA 90502-2006
Phone: (310)222-3601 **Fax:** (310)222-3603
Website: http://www.rei.edu
Gail V. Anderson, MD, Dir.

Activities/Fields: Role of ethnicity (including culture) and biological variables in the mental health of ethnic minority populations. Conducts studies using pharmacokinetic, pharmacodynamic, and pharmacogenetic research techniques to examine ethnic and individual differences in responses to psychotropic drugs.

★ 23632 ★ University of California, Los Angeles
Harbor-UCLA Medical Center Research and Education Institute Center for Vaccine Research
Liu Research Bldg.
1124 W Carson St.
Torrance, CA 90502
Phone: (310)781-3636 **Fax:** (310)972-2962
Email: joelward@ucla.edu
Dr. Joel Ward, Dir.

Activities/Fields: Clinical, epidemiologic, laboratory, and pharmacoeconomic studies of vaccines vaccine preventable diseases (all age groups, normal and high risk populations). Evaluation of mechanisms of immune responses to vaccines. Design and conduct multicenter trials nationally and internationally.

★ 23633 ★ University of California, Los Angeles
Jules Stein Eye Institute
Box 957000
Department of Opthalmology
100 Stein Plz.
Los Angeles, CA 90095-7000
Phone: (310)825-5000 **Fax:** (310)206-7488
Email: mondino@jsei.ucla.edu
Website: http://www.jsei.org/
Bartly J. Mondino, MD, Dir.

Activities/Fields: Research and study in sciences related to vision, care of patients with eye disease, and education in ophthalmology. **Pub:** *Annual report.* • *Clinical Update*, 3/year. Newsletter. • *EYE*, 3/year. Newsletter.

★ 23634 ★ University of California, Los Angeles
Leo G. Rigler Center for Radiological Research
Center for Health Science, Rm. BV-135
Department of Radiology
UCLA Medical Center
Los Angeles, CA 90024
Phone: (310)825-6561
Email: Radiology/riglercenter@medmail3.mednet.ucla.edu
John Robert, Res. Assoc.

Activities/Fields: Radiological science and its application to diagnosis and treatment of catastrophic diseases, involving such techniques as magnetic resonance imaging (MRI), internal radiation management of carcinomatous lesions, vascular occlusion with ferrosilicone in tumor management, and cobalt source gamma irradiation of brain tumors.

★ 23635 ★ University of California, Los Angeles
Marrow and Stem Cell Transplantation Program
Center for Health Science
Los Angeles, CA 90095-1678
Phone: (310)206-5789 **Fax:** (310)206-5511
Email: mterrito@medl.medsch.ucla.edu
Website: http://www.cancer.mednet.ucla.edu/
Mary Territo, MD, Dir.

Activities/Fields: Treatment of leukemia, lymphoma, myeloma, breast cancer, solid tumors, and aplastic anemia. Evaluates the use of bone marrow, cord blood, and stem cell transplantation as treatment for a number of hematologic and malignant diseases. **Frmly:** University of California, Los Angeles - Bone Marrow Transplantation Program.

★ 23636 ★ University of California, Los Angeles
Mental Retardation Research Center
Neuropsychiatric Institute & Hospital
760 Westwood Plz., 68-177 NPI
Los Angeles, CA 90024-1759
Phone: (310)825-9395 **Fax:** (310)206-5061
Email: jdevellis@mednet.ucla.edu
Website: http://www.mrrc.npi.ucla.edu/mrrc/page1.html
Dr. Jean de Vellis, Dir.

Activities/Fields: Mental retardation and related aspects of human development, including interdisciplinary basic and clinical studies on problems in developmental biology, human genetics, neurobiochemistry, neurophysiology, and sociobehavioral categories. Collaborates with other institutes, schools, and departments at the University. **Pub:** *Annual Report.*

★ 23637 ★ University of California, Los Angeles
Neuropsychiatric Institute
760 Westwood Plz.
Los Angeles, CA 90024
Phone: (310)825-0511 **Fax:** (310)825-3942
Website: http://www.npi.ucla.edu
Dr. Peter C. Whybrow, Dir.

Activities/Fields: Genetics, pharmacology, mental retardation; developmental neurobiology; behavioral sciences, including anthropology; biochemistry, neurophysiology, cognitive neuroscience, brain imaging, health services and social policy.

★ 23638 ★ University of California, Los Angeles
Program on Psychosocial Adaptation and the Future
Neuropsychiatric Institute
760 Westwood Plz.
Los Angeles, CA 90095
Phone: (310)825-0463 **Fax:** (310)476-3099
Email: preadapt@ucla.edu
Roderic Gorney, PhD, Dir.

Activities/Fields: Psychosocial and cultural determinants of behavior, including impact of television on adults and the clinical role of the sense of the future in mental illness.

★ 23639 ★ University of California, Los Angeles
Reed Neurological Research Center Laboratory of Neuro Imaging
710 Westwood Plz., Rm. 4-238
Los Angeles, CA 90095-1769
Phone: (310)206-2101 **Fax:** (310)206-5518
Email: toga@loni.ucla.edu
Website: http://www.loni.ucla.edu
Arthur W. Toga, PhD, Dir.

Activities/Fields: Neuroanatomy, neuroimaging, neurophysiology, and neurological diseases.

★ 23640 ★ University of California, Los Angeles
Southern California Education and Research Center
School of Public Health
650 Charles E Young Dr., S
CHS 56-071
Los Angeles, CA 90095-1772
Phone: (310)206-2304 **Fax:** (310)794-9317
Email: whinds@ucla.edu
Website: http://www.ph.ucla.edu/erc
William C. Hinds, ScD, Dir.

Activities/Fields: Occupational and environmental health issues. **Pub:** *Newsletter*, quarterly.

★ 23641 ★ University of California, Los Angeles
Southern California Injury Prevention Research Center
School of Public Health
10911 Weyburn Ave., Ste. 200
Los Angeles, CA 90024-2884
Phone: (310)794-2706 **Fax:** (310)794-0787
Email: jfkraus@ucla.edu
Website: http://www.ph.ucla.edu/sciprc
Jess F. Kraus, PhD, Dir.

Activities/Fields: Intentional and unintentional injuries in the socioeconomically disadvantaged, underserved, and ethnically diverse populations in the Southern California region. Research projects include: work-related injuries in high-risk occupations; risk of motor vehicle crash; injuries to children; injuries and deaths; injuries in the elderly; worksite intervention to reduce work-related assault; earthquake injury and preparedness; expanding methods in injury epidemiology; long-term consequences of brain and spinal cord injuries; violence in contemporary American film.

★ 23642 ★ University of California, Los Angeles
UCLA-DOE Institute of Genomics and Proteomics
201 Boyer Hall, Box 951570
611 Young Dr. E
Los Angeles, CA 90095
Phone: (310)825-3754 **Fax:** (310)206-3914
Email: david@mbi.ucla.edu
Website: http://www.doe-mbi.ucla.edu
Dr. David Eisenberg, Dir.

Activities/Fields: Structural biology and nuclear medicine, including supporting fields of physics, engineering and radiopharmacology. **Frmly:** Laboratory of Structural Biology and Molecular Medicine; Laboratory of Biomedical and Environmental Sciences.

★ 23643 ★ University of California, Los Angeles
UCLA Jonsson Comprehensive Cancer Center
8-684 Factor Bldg.
PO Box 951781
Los Angeles, CA 90095-1781
Phone: (310)825-5268 **Free:** 888-798-0719
Fax: (310)206-5553
Email: kirwin@mednet.ucla.edu
Website: http://www.cancer.mednet.ucla.edu
Dr. Judith C. Gasson, Dir.

Activities/Fields: Cancer, including both basic science research in molecular, cellular, and developmental biology, signal transduction, tumor immunology, and viral and chemical carcinogenesis and clinical/translational research in breast and women's reproductive cancers, hematopoietic malignancies and bone marrow transplantation, prostate oncology, and solid tumor oncology in the following fields: central nervous system, thoracic, gastrointestinal, musculoskeletal, melanoma, and head and neck. Also conducts cancer prevention and control demonstration and research projects under the headings of patients and survivors, and healthy and at-risk populations. Sponsors support groups for cancer patients. **Pub:** *Discoveries*, annually.

★ 23644 ★ University of California, Los Angeles
UCLA/RAND Center for Adolescent Health Promotion
Department of Pediatrics, 12-466 MDCC
Box 951752
10833 Le Conte Ave.
Los Angeles, CA 90095-1752
Phone: (310)206-1954 **Fax:** (310)206-4855
Email: schuster@rand.org
Mark A. Schuster, MD, Dir.
Activities/Fields: Public health issues, especially behaviors that place Americans at risk for chronic diseases and conditions. Of particular concern is the improvement in quality of life for special populations, including the young, elderly, racial ethnic populations, and the underserved.

★ 23645 ★ University of California, Riverside
Biotechnology Impacts Center (BIC)
2113 Batchelor Hall
Riverside, CA 92521
Phone: (909)787-2601 **Fax:** (909)787-4437
Email: norman.ellstrand@ucr.edu
Website: http://genomics.ucr.edu/centers/biotech/index.html
Norman C. Ellstrand, Dir.
Activities/Fields: Potential benefits and consequences of the genomics revolution.

★ 23646 ★ University of California, Riverside
Genomics Institute
2113 Batchelor Hall
900 University Ave.
Riverside, CA 92521
Phone: (909)787-2601 **Fax:** (909)787-4437
Email: michael.clegg@ucr.edu
Website: http://genomics.ucr.edu/
Michael T. Clegg, Dir.
Activities/Fields: Scientific and technical knowledge that will afford economic and social benefits to agriculture, the environment, and human health, thus improving the quality of life. This will be accomplished by making, exploiting, and evaluating the impacts of discoveries in genomics, proteomics, and bioinformatics through focused efforts in insect genomics, plant and microbial genomics, health and environmental genomics, and bioinformatics.

★ 23647 ★ University of California, San Diego
Alzheimer's Disease Research Center
8950 Villa La Jolla Dr., Ste. C129
La Jolla, CA 92037
Phone: (858)622-5800 **Fax:** (858)622-1017
Email: adrc@ucsd.edu
Website: http://adrc.ucsd.edu
Dr. Leon Thal, Dir.
Activities/Fields: Longitudinal research on the clinical and cognitive changes associated with Alzheimer's disease and other dementing illnesses by obtaining epidemiological data, medical histories, analysis of blood and sera, administration of batteries of neuropsychological tests, and neurological examinations of patients. Performs clinical drug trials, research on electrophysiology and neuroimaging studies, evaluations of the effects of caregiving stress on the caregivers, studies of memory and language dysfunction, and the possibility of a genetic or metabolic basis for Alzheimer's disease. Also conducts olfaction studies.

★ 23648 ★ University of California, San Diego
Cartilage Tissue Engineering Laboratory
Department of Bioengineering, Mail Code 0412
9500 Gilman Dr.
La Jolla, CA 92093-0412
Phone: (858)534-0821 **Fax:** (858)534-6896
Email: rsah@ucsd.edu
Website: http://www-bioeng.ucsd.edu/research/research_groups/cte/
Robert L. Sah, MD, Prin. Investigator
Activities/Fields: Biological processes of cartilage growth, aging, degeneration, and repair by examining the relationships between tissue with the ultimate goal of improving clinical treatment, diagnosis, and prevention.

★ 23649 ★ University of California, San Diego
Center for AIDS Research (CFAR)
9500 Gilman Dr., MC 0616
La Jolla, CA 92093-0616
Phone: (858)534-5545 **Fax:** (858)822-1934
Email: csussman@ucsd.edu
Website: http://www.ari.ucsd.edu/cfar/cfar.html
Douglas Richman, MD, Dir.
Activities/Fields: Development of improved vaccines and therapies for HIV infection and associated diseases through the study of molecular pathogenesis and immunopathogenesis of HIV infection and clinical trials of therapies and vaccines. **Pub:** *Newsletter.*

★ 23650 ★ University of California, San Diego
Center for Medicinal Cannabis Research (CMCR)
150 W Washington, 2nd Fl.
San Diego, CA 92103
Phone: (619)543-5024 **Fax:** (619)543-5073
Email: cmcr@ucsd.edu
Website: http://www.cmcr.ucsd.edu/
Igor Grant, MD, Dir.
Activities/Fields: Safety and efficacy of cannabis and cannabis compounds for treating medical conditions.

★ 23651 ★ University of California, San Diego
Center for Transplantation
200 W Arbor Dr.
San Diego, CA 92103-8745
Phone: (619)294-6257
Email: kkrzeminski@ucsd.edu
Website: http://www.health.ucsd.edu/transplant/
Mary Cunanan, Exec. Dir.
Activities/Fields: Immunosuppressive and anti-infection drugs, the development of extra conporeal liver assist technologies, the biology of rejection, organ preservation, and the long-term medical problems of transplant recipients.

★ 23652 ★ University of California, San Diego
Chemosensory Perception Laboratory
Mail Code 0957
9500 Gilman Dr.
La Jolla, CA 92093-0957
Phone: (858)622-5830 **Fax:** (858)458-9417
Email: wcain@ucsd.edu
Website: http://orpheus.ucsd.edu/chemosensorylab/
William S. Cain, PhD, Contact
Activities/Fields: How people perceive chemicals and how chemicals exert short-term effects on people. The laboratory focuses on the workings of the senses of smell and taste, and physiological and psychological consequences of chemical stimulation.

★ 23653 ★ University of California, San Diego
Division of Pulmonary and Critical Care Medicine
9300 Campus Point Dr., MC 7372
La Jolla, CA 92037-1300
Phone: (858)657-7105 **Fax:** (858)657-7144
Email: pdwagner@ucsd.edu
Website: http://medicine.ucsd.edu/pulmonary
Peter D. Wagner, MD, Contact
Activities/Fields: Chronic obstructive pulmonary disease, tuberculosis, acute respiratory failure, including its pathogenesis and management, pulmonary vascular diseases. **Frmly:** Specialized Center of Research in Acute Respiratory Failure.

★ 23654 ★ University of California, San Diego
General Clinical Research Center
UCSD Medical Center, 8203
200 W Arbor Dr.
San Diego, CA 92103-8203
Phone: (619)543-6180 **Fax:** (619)543-5536
Email: mziegler@ucsd.edu
Website: http://gcrc.ucsd.edu
Michael G. Ziegler, MD, Dir.
Activities/Fields: Cardiovascular disease, endocrinology, gastroenterology, genetic disease, immunology, infectious disease, metabolism, neurological disease, oncology, pulmonary medicine, renal disease, reproductive endocrinology, rheumatology, hypertension, and gene therapy.

★ 23655 ★ University of California, San Diego
Hyperbaric Medicine Center
USCD Medical Center
200 W Arbor Dr.
San Diego, CA 92103-8688
Phone: (619)543-6463 **Fax:** (619)543-3115
Email: tneuman@ucsd.edu
Dr. Tom Neuman, Dir.
Activities/Fields: Hyperbaric oxygen therapy, including application in burns, infectious diseases, wound healing, and diving medicine.

★ 23656 ★ University of California, San Diego
Ludwig Institute for Cancer Research Laboratory of Cancer Biology
9500 Gilman Dr.
La Jolla, CA 92093
Phone: (619)534-7802
Email: rkolodner@ucsd.edu
Website: http://ludwig.ucsd.edu/
Dr. Richard Kolodner, Hd.
Activities/Fields: Genetic and biochemical dissection of the processes of DNA recombination and repair.

★ 23657 ★ University of California, San Diego
Ludwig Institute for Cancer Research Laboratory of Cell Biology
9500 Gilman Dr.
La Jolla, CA 92093
Phone: (619)534-7802
Email: dcleveland@ucsd.edu
Website: http://ludwig.ucsd.edu/
Don W. Cleveland, Hd.
Activities/Fields: How chromosomes are faithfully moved into each daughter cell just prior to division, how neurofilaments structure the cytoplasm of neurons, and the use of transgenic mice to investigate mechanisms of motor neuron disease.

★ 23658 ★ University of California, San Diego
Ludwig Institute for Cancer Research Laboratory of Tumor Biology
9500 Gilman Dr.
La Jolla, CA 92093
Phone: (619)534-7802
Email: wcavenee@ucsd.edu
Website: http://ludwig.ucsd.edu/
W.K. Cavenee, Dir.
Activities/Fields: Genetic dissection of human cancer.

★ 23659 ★ University of California, San Diego
Muscle Physiology Laboratory
VA Medical Center, MC 151
3350 La Jolla Village Dr.
San Diego, CA 92161
Phone: (858)552-8585 **Fax:** (858)552-4381
Email: rlieber@ucsd.edu
Website: http://muscle.ucsd.edu/index.html
Richard L. Lieber, Contact
Activities/Fields: Design and plasticity of the neuromuscular system. **Pub:** *Abstracts.* • *Papers.*

★ 23660 ★ University of California, San Diego
Psychopathology and Psychophysiology Research Laboratory
Department of Psychology, 0109
9500 Gilman Dr.
La Jolla, CA 92093-0109
Phone: (619)534-6283 **Fax:** (619)534-7190
Email: bclementz@ucsd.edu
Website: http://psy.ucsd.edu/~sczlab/
Dr. Brett A. Clementz, Prin. Investigator
Activities/Fields: Neuropathology and genetics of schizophrenia and other psychiatric illnesses. Other topics of interest are quantitative genetic analysis of family data and comprehensive symptom evaluation for use in classification. Ongoing projects include similar studies with obsessive compulsive disorder, Tourette's syndrome and bipolar disorder patients.

★ 23661 ★ University of California, San Diego
Raz Laboratory
126 Stein Clinical Research Bldg., MC 0663
9500 Gilman Dr.
La Jolla, CA 92093-0663
Phone: (858)534-5444 **Fax:** (858)534-5399
Email: eraz@ucsd.edu
Website: http://www.raz.ucsd.edu/
Eyal Raz, MD, Prin. Investigator
Activities/Fields: Immunostimulatory DNA sequences, both the basic science of how and why these sequences function and the applied science of how to prevent and treat human disease using their immunologic properties.

★ 23662 ★ University of California, San Diego
Rebecca and John Moores UCSD Cancer Center
9500 Gilman Dr., MC 0658
La Jolla, CA 92093-0658
Phone: (858)822-1222 **Fax:** (858)534-7628
Email: nspencer@ucsd.edu
Website: http://cancer.ucsd.edu
Dr. Gordon N. Gill, Interim Dir.
Activities/Fields: Cancer, including clinical trials, outreach (education, prevention and treatment), and basic/clinical/prevention studies, including cancer biology, cancer genetics, cancer pharmacology, cancer prevention and control, cancer symptom control, translational oncology, and viral malignancy. **Frmly:** University of California, San Diego; Cancer Center.

★ 23663 ★ University of California, San Diego
Resource for Solid-State Nuclear Magnetic Resonance of Proteins
Department of Chemistry & Biochemistry
9500 Gilman Dr., 0307
La Jolla, CA 92093-0307
Phone: (858)822-4820 **Fax:** (858)822-4821
Email: sopella@ucsd.edu
Website: http://chem-faculty.ucsd.edu/opella/resource
Stanley J. Opella, PhD, Prin. Investigator
Activities/Fields: Development and application of solid-state Nuclear Magnetic Resonance (NMR) spectroscopy for structure determination of peptides and proteins.

★ 23664 ★ University of California, San Diego
Sam and Rose Stein Institute for Research on Aging
MC 0664
School of Medicine
9500 Gilman Dr.
La Jolla, CA 92093-0664
Phone: (858)534-6299 **Fax:** (858)534-5475
Email: steininstitute@ucsd.edu
Website: http://sira.ucsd.edu/
Dr. Dennis A. Carson, Dir.
Activities/Fields: Degenerative diseases of later life, including aging and Alzheimer's disease, arthritis, osteoporosis, cardiovascular disease, sleep disorders, genetics, and mind, body, and health relationships. Investigates the relationships between the deterioration of the central nervous system and speech, hearing, and sleep problems; studies the effects of aging on production of hormones; evaluates alternatives to nursing home confinement; investigates immune system deteriorations; and studies the genetic and biochemical basis for long and healthy lifespans and the genetic basis of human diseases of accelerated aging. Also conducts studies of the susceptibility to infections in the elderly, loss of bone minerals, changes in the vascular system and the development of glaucoma. **Pub:** *Healthwise Newsletter*, monthly.

★ 23665 ★ University of California, San Diego
San Diego Supercomputer Center National Biomedical Computation Resource
9500 Gilman Dr.
La Jolla, CA 92093-0505
Phone: (858)534-5079 **Fax:** (858)822-0948
Email: parzberg@sdsc.edu
Website: http://nbcr.sdsc.edu
Peter W. Arzberger, PhD, Prin. Investigator
Activities/Fields: Advanced computational technology, particularly the integration of computational and visualization tools in a transparent, advanced computing environment to enable better access to distributed data, computational resource and instruments; development and deployment of advanced computational tools for modeling, data query, linking of data resources, 3-D image processing, and interactive visualization.

★ 23666 ★ University of California, San Diego
Specialized Center of Research in Molecular Medicine and Atherosclerosis
MC 0682
Department of Medicine
9500 Gilman Dr.
La Jolla, CA 92093-0682
Phone: (858)534-0569 **Fax:** (858)534-2005
Dr. Joseph L. Witztam, Dir.
Activities/Fields: Arteriosclerosis and atherogenesis, including studies of lipoprotein metabolism, oxidation of low density lipoprotein molecules, and molecular basis of arteriosclerosis.

★ 23667 ★ University of California, San Diego
Swartz Center for Computational Neuroscience (SCCN)
Regents Medical Center, Ste. 320
4150 Regents Pk. Row
La Jolla, CA 92037-1417
Phone: (858)458-1927 **Fax:** (858)458-1847
Email: tpjung@ucsd.edu
Website: http://www.sccn.ucsd.edu/
Scott Makeig, Dir.
Activities/Fields: How functional activities in multiple brain areas interact dynamically to support human awareness, creativity and interaction.

★ 23668 ★ University of California, San Diego
Whitaker Institute of Biomedical Engineering
PFBH Rm. 131, MC 0427
9500 Gilman Dr.
La Jolla, CA 92093-0427
Phone: (858)822-2290 **Fax:** (858)822-1160
Email: tmatusov@ucsd.edu
Website: http://www-bioeng.ucsd.edu/wibe/
Dr. Shu Chien, Dir.
Activities/Fields: Biomedical engineering, emphasizing structure-function relationships in normal and pathological tissues and the development of biological substitutes to restore, maintain, or improve tissue functions. Tissue studies focus on the heart, blood, lung, kidney, liver, pancreas, muscle, bone, cartilage, tendon, ligament, skin, nerve, brain, retina, and cochlea. **Frmly:** Institute for Biomedical Engineering.

★ 23669 ★ University of California, San Francisco
AIDS Research Institute (ARI)
CB 0886
74 New Montgomery, Ste. 600
San Francisco, CA 94105
Phone: (415)597-9203 **Fax:** (415)597-9213
Email: ari@psg.ucsf.edu
Website: http://ari.ucsf.edu/
Thomas J. Coates, PhD, Dir.
Activities/Fields: AIDS vaccine, new therapies, transmission dynamics and prevention, AIDS policy and ethics. **Pub:** *ARI Newsletter.*

★ 23670 ★ University of California, San Francisco
Bay Area Perinatal AIDS Center (BAPAC)
1001 Potrero Ave., Ward 6D-33
San Francisco, CA 94110
Phone: (415)206-8919 **Fax:** (415)206-3626
Email: cohand@obgyn.ucsf.edu
Website: http://php.ucsf.edu/research.html
Deborah Cohen, Med. Dir.
Activities/Fields: Strategies to improve maternal health and further reduce perinatal AIDS transmission rates both in the United States and worldwide.

★ 23671 ★ University of California, San Francisco
Bio-organic Biomedical Mass Spectrometry Resource
521 Parnassus, Rm. 1124S
San Francisco, CA 94143-0446
Phone: (415)476-5641 **Fax:** (415)476-0688
Email: alb@itsa.ucsf.edu
Website: http://donatello.ucsf.edu
Prof. Alma L. Burlingame, PhD, Prin. Investigator
Activities/Fields: Mass spectrometric techniques for sequencing peptides and structural characterization of modified proteins and glycoconjugates.

★ 23672 ★ University of California, San Francisco
Brain Tumor Research Center
PO Box 0520
San Francisco, CA 94143-0520
Phone: (415)476-4590 **Fax:** (415)476-9687
Website: http://www.som.ucsf.edu/departments/neuros/neurosurgery_research/BTRC/index.html
Mitchel S. Berger, MD, Ch.
Activities/Fields: Cytotoxic therapies, radiation therapy, and chemotherapy; elucidates the difference between normal brain cells and brain tumor cells; molecular biology of brain tumors.

★ 23673 ★ University of California, San Francisco
California AIDS Research Center (C-ARC)
UCSF Box 0422
Department of Stomatology
San Francisco, CA 94143-0422
Phone: (415)476-5415 **Fax:** (415)476-4204
Email: greenspanj@dentistry.ucsf.edu
Dr. John S. Greenspan, Dir.
Activities/Fields: Understanding the mechanisms by which HIV infection is avoided or slowed and translational studies to understand how to make these findings clinically relevant. The center is organized around 4 research themes: natural immunity resistance to infection, role of CXCR4 signaling in CD8+ T-cell apoptosis during HIV infection, dissecting the molecular basis for virologic but not immunologic failure in HIV-infected patients receiving protease inhibitor therapy, and transmission of drug-resistant HIV-1.

★ 23674 ★ University of California, San Francisco
Cardiovascular Research Institute
505 Parnassus Ave., Box 0130
San Francisco, CA 94143-0130
Fax: (415)476-8173
Email: couglin@cvrimail.ucsf.edu
Website: http://cvri.ucsf.edu/default.html
Dr. Shaun R. Coughlin, Dir.
Activities/Fields: Physiology, biochemistry, pharmacology, cell biology, molecular biology, and immunology of the cardiovascular, pulmonary, respiratory, and renal systems; circulation, respiration, lung development, and metabolism of the fetus and newborn; membrane transduction systems; lipoprotein metabolism; growth factors and atherosclerosis; water and electrolyte transport; physical chemistry of contraction/relaxation of muscle; lung injury and repair; myocardial growth and development; macromolecular conformation; and mathematical analysis of biological systems.

★ 23675 ★ University of California, San Francisco
Cardiovascular Research Institute
Intravascular Ultrasound Laboratory
1347 Moffitt Hospital
505 Parnassus Ave.
San Francisco, CA 94143-0130
Phone: (415)476-1614 **Fax:** (415)476-1020
Email: ports@medicine.ucsf.edu
Website: http://cardiology.ucsf.edu/clinical/ivus
Thomas Ports, MD, Co-Dir.
Activities/Fields: Use of catheter-based ultrasound devices to examine coronary physiology.

★ 23676 ★ University of California, San Francisco
Center for AIDS Prevention Studies (CAPS)
AIDS Research Institute
74 New Montgomery St., Ste. 600
San Francisco, CA 94105
Phone: (415)597-9100 **Fax:** (415)597-9213
Email: tcoates@psg.ucsf.edu
Website: http://www.caps.ucsf.edu/capsweb
Thomas J. Coates, PhD, Dir.
Activities/Fields: Methods to change AIDS high risk behavior. Activities include developing and testing AIDS prevention strategies for at-risk populations, promoting multidisciplinary research on the prevention of HIV disease, funding pilot studies on minority issues in AIDS, and operating the CAPS International Visiting Scholars Program, which brings scholars from Africa, Asia, Eastern Europe, and Latin America to work with CAPS scientists in developing AIDS prevention research protocols. **Pub:** *CAPS Bibliography.* • *Prevention Fact Sheets.*

★ 23677 ★ University of California, San Francisco
Center for Health Improvement and Prevention Studies (CHIPS)
350 Parnassus Ave., Ste. 905
San Francisco, CA 94117
Phone: (415)502-7283 **Fax:** (415)502-7314
Email: chips@itsa.ucsf.edu
Website: http://itsa.ucsf.edu/~chips/
Barbara Gerbert, PhD, Res. Dir.
Activities/Fields: Behavioral risks and patient, provider, and systemic barriers to optimal health care delivery.

★ 23678 ★ University of California, San Francisco
Center for Reproductive Sciences
513 Parnassus Ave., HSW 1656
San Francisco, CA 94143-0556
Phone: (415)476-4295 **Fax:** (415)502-7866
Email: taylorr@obgyn.ucsf.edu
Dr. Robert N. Taylor, Dir.
Activities/Fields: Hormonal regulation of reproductive events at the subcellular, cellular, tissular, and organismic levels. Research projects utilize a variety of species, including domestic and laboratory animals, subhuman primates, and humans. Conducts a multifaceted investigative and training program directed toward studies of the hypothalamic/pituitary/gonadal/target tissue axis and the endocrinologic physiology of pregnancy. **Frmly:** Reproductive Endocrinology Center.

★ 23679 ★ University of California, San Francisco
Comprehensive Cancer Center
Box 0128
San Francisco, CA 94143-0128
Phone: (415)476-2201 **Fax:** (415)502-3179
Email: cceditor@cc.ucsf.edu
Website: http://cc.ucsf.edu/
Frank McCormick, PhD, Dir.
Activities/Fields: Cancer and hematology, endocrinology, fundamental properties of cell membranes, role of interferon and cell-cell interactions in immune response to cancer, surface markers on leukemic cells, role of viruses in cancer, management of breast cancer, factors involved in control of cell proliferation and differentiation, use of liposomes to deliver drug and macromolecules into cells, mechanism of membrane fusion, molecular pharmacology of antineoplastic drugs, and interaction between the coagulation and fibrinolytic systems and cancer cells.

★ 23680 ★ University of California, San Francisco
Dermatology Drug Research Unit
PO Box 1212
515 Spruce
San Francisco, CA 94101
Phone: (415)476-4701 **Fax:** (415)502-4126
Email: jxmkoo@orca.ucsf.edu
John Koo, MD, Dir.
Activities/Fields: Conducts clinical testing of new or existing pharmacologic agents used in the treatment of skin disorders and develops protocols for drug testing. Areas of interest include phototherapy, psoriasis, and psychodermatology.

★ 23681 ★ University of California, San Francisco
Disability Statistics Center
Institute for Health & Aging
3333 California St., Ste. 340
Campus Mail Box 0646
San Francisco, CA 94118
Phone: (415)502-5205 **Fax:** (415)502-5208
Email: laplant@itsa.ucsf.edu
Mitchell P. LaPlante, PhD, Dir.
Activities/Fields: Production and dissemination of statistical information on disability and the status of people with disabilities in society and the establishment and monitoring of indicators on how conditions are changing to meet their health, housing, economic and social needs. **Pub:** *Disability Statistics Abstracts.* • *Disability Statistics Reports.*

★ 23682 ★ University of California, San Francisco
Ernest Gallo Clinic and Research Center
5858 Horton St., Ste. 200
Emeryville, CA 94608
Phone: (510)985-3100 **Fax:** (510)985-3888
Email: ray@itsa.ucsf.edu
Website: http://www.egcrc.org
Dr. Ray White, Dir.
Activities/Fields: Alcoholism, with special emphasis on molecular, cellular, physiological and genetic mechanisms of tolerance, dependence and addiction to ethanol.

★ 23683 ★ University of California, San Francisco
Francis I. Proctor Foundation for Research in Ophthalmology
95 Kirkham St., Box 0944
San Francisco, CA 94143-4419
Phone: (415)476-1441 **Fax:** (415)476-0527
Email: tpms@itsa.ucsf.edu
Todd P. Margolis, MD, Contact
Activities/Fields: Infectious and inflammatory diseases of the eye with particular emphasis on chlamydial infections, trachoma, herpetic eye infections, dry eye conditions, and uveitis.

★ 23684 ★ University of California, San Francisco
General Clinical Research Center—Adults
M1202
505 Parnassus Ave.
San Francisco, CA 94143-0126
Phone: (415)476-9232 **Fax:** (415)476-0986
Email: tierneyc@gcrc.ucsf.edu
Website: http://www.gcrc.ucsf.edu
Joel Palefsky, MD, Prog. Dir.
Activities/Fields: Cardiovascular disease, hypertension, clinical pharmacology, lipid metabolism, nephrology, nutrition, oncology, acid-base physiology, dermatology, infectious diseases, reproductive endocrinology, AIDS, potassium metabolism, osteoporosis, recombinant human hemoglobin, liver disease, aging, psychopharmacology, hereditary fructose intolerance, gene theraphy, and wound healing.

★ 23685 ★ University of California, San Francisco
General Clinical Research Center—Children
Box 0105
M679 Moffitt Hospital
San Francisco, CA 94143
Phone: (415)476-2865 **Fax:** (415)476-3466
Email: warad@peds.ucsf.edu
Diane W. Wara, MD, Prog. Dir.
Activities/Fields: Major areas of investigation include adolescent medicine, biochemistry, endocrinology, genetic diseases, immunology, neonatology, nephrology, nutrition, oncology, pediatric AIDS, pharmacology and radiation therapy.

★ 23686 ★ University of California, San Francisco
George Williams Hooper Foundation
513 Parnassus Ave., HSW1501
San Francisco, CA 94143-0552
Phone: (415)476-5157 **Fax:** (415)476-6185
Email: gracest@itsa.ucsf.edu
Dr. J. Michael Bishop, Dir.
Activities/Fields: Cancer biology; genetics and physiology of mammalian cells and organisms; animal models resembling human cancers; and cell biology,

immunology and the pathogenesis of infectious diseases.

★ 23687 ★ University of California, San Francisco
Gladstone Institute of Neurological Disease (GIND)
PO Box 419100
San Francisco, CA 94141-9100
Phone: (415)695-3819 **Fax:** (415)826-6541
Website: http://gladstone.ucsf.edu/gind/
Lennart Mucke, MD, Dir.
Activities/Fields: Understanding the central nervous system so that rational strategies can be developed to more effectively treat Alzheimer's disease, Huntington's disease, HIV-associated dementia, and stroke.

★ 23688 ★ University of California, San Francisco
Hormone Research Institute
513 Parnassus Ave.
PO Box 0534
San Francisco, CA 94143-0534
Phone: (415)514-1683 **Fax:** (415)564-5813
Email: jbluest@diabetes.ucsf.edu
Dr. Jeffrey Bluestone, Dir.
Activities/Fields: Hormone receptors, gene regulation in endocrine tissue, mechanisms of regulated secretion, glutamic acid decarboxylase in juvenile diabetes, the immunology of Type 1 diabetes, and the development of the endocrine pancreas.

★ 23689 ★ University of California, San Francisco
Immunogenetics and Transplantation Laboratory
Main Hospital, Level B
Davies Medical Center
45 Castro St.
San Francisco, CA 94114
Phone: (415)476-3883 **Fax:** (415)476-0379
Email: baxterlowel@surgery.uscf.edu
Lee Ann Baxter-Lowe, PhD, Dir.
Activities/Fields: Immunogenetics and transplantation, including immunopharmacology of immunosuppressive agents.

★ 23690 ★ University of California, San Francisco
Institute for Health Policy Studies
3333 California St., Ste. 265
San Francisco, CA 94143-0936
Phone: (415)476-4921 **Fax:** (415)476-0705
Email: hluft@itsa.ucsf.edu
Website: http://ihps.ucsf.edu
Harold S. Luft, Dir.
Activities/Fields: Health policy and health services.

★ 23691 ★ University of California, San Francisco
Langley Porter Psychiatric Institute
401 Parnassus Ave.
San Francisco, CA 94143
Phone: (415)476-7000 **Free:** 800-723-7140
Fax: (415)476-7320
Email: cvd@lppi.ucsf.edu
Website: http://psych.ucsf.edu
Craig Van Dyke, MD, Dir.
Activities/Fields: Clinical studies of psychiatric disorders and psychotherapy and basic research studies in psychopharmacology, neurobiology, cellular and molecular biology, behavioral biology, and social sciences.

★ 23692 ★ University of California, San Francisco
Lung Biology Center
CB 0854
San Francisco, CA 94143-0854
Phone: (415)206-5959 **Fax:** (415)206-4123
Email: deans@itsa.ucsf.edu
Website: http://dom.ucsf.edu/lbc/
Dean Sheppard, MD, Dir.
Activities/Fields: Diseases of the lung and airways.

★ 23693 ★ University of California, San Francisco
Magnetic Resonance Laboratory
Department of Pharmaceutical Chemistry
513 Parnassus Ave.
San Francisco, CA 94143-0446
Phone: (415)476-4378 **Fax:** (415)476-0688
Email: james@picasso.ucsf.edu
Website: http://picasso.ucsf.edu/
Prof. Thomas L. James, Ch.
Activities/Fields: Theory and practice of nuclear magnetic resonance and computer modeling studies of proteins and nucleic acids. Performs quantitative determinations of molecular structure in noncrystalline environments using nuclear Overhauser effects and complete relaxation matrix calculations.

★ 23694 ★ University of California, San Francisco
Mass Spectrometry Facility
Department of Pharmaceutical Chemistry
San Francisco, CA 94143
Phone: (415)476-5641 **Fax:** (415)476-0688
Email: alb@itsa.ucsf.edu
Website: http://donatello.ucsf.edu/
Prof. Alma L. Burlingame, PhD, Dir.
Activities/Fields: Molecular identification problems in human health and disease and biological chemistry, including studies in chemical and biochemical structure and mechanism. Conducts investigations of the structure of covalently modified informational biopolymers, drug metabolism, chemical carcinogenesis, signal transduction, proteins in cancer biology, irreversible inhibitors of cytochrome P-450, various genetic diseases, and membrane-bound glycoproteins, such as acetylcholine receptor and esterase, and scrapie glycoprotein. Develops techniques of computerized mass spectrometry. **Pub:** *Annual Report.*

★ 23695 ★ University of California, San Francisco
Multiple Sclerosis Center
350 Parnassus Ave., Ste. 908
San Francisco, CA 94117
Phone: (415)514-1684 **Fax:** (415)514-2443
Website: http://mscenter.ucsf.edu
Douglas S. Goodin, MD, Dir.
Activities/Fields: Cause and treatment of multiple sclerosis.

★ 23696 ★ University of California, San Francisco
Northern California Comprehensive Sickle Cell Center
San Francisco General Hospital
1001 Potrero Ave., Rm. 331, Bldg. 100
San Francisco, CA 94110
Phone: (415)206-5169 **Fax:** (415)206-3071
Email: wmentzer@sfghpeds.ucsf.edu
William C. Mentzer, MD, Dir.
Activities/Fields: Sickle cell disease, including molecular, cellular, tissue, and organ studies. Conducts clinical trials. Seeks to translate research on sickle cell disease to improved health care at the community level.

★ 23697 ★ University of California, San Francisco
Ocular Oncology Research Unit
Beckman Vision Center-Department of Ophthalmology
10 Koret Way, Box 730
San Francisco, CA 94143
Phone: (415)476-0779 **Fax:** (415)502-3230
Joan M. O'Brien, MD, Dir.
Activities/Fields: Molecular biology and immunology of intracolar tumors, new treatment protocols, genetic testing and therapy.

★ 23698 ★ University of California, San Francisco
Oral AIDS Center (OAC)
513 Parnassus Ave.
San Francisco, CA 94143-0422
Phone: (415)476-5415 **Fax:** (415)476-4204
Email: greenspanj@dentistry.ucsf.edu
Website: http://itsa.ucsf.edu/~ucstoma/Oac.htm
Dr. John S. Greenspan, Dir.
Activities/Fields: Oral manifestations of HIV infection.

★ 23699 ★ University of California, San Francisco
Osher Center for Integrative Medicine (OCIM)
1701 Divisadero St., Ste. 150
San Francisco, CA 94115-3010
Phone: (415)353-7700 **Fax:** (415)353-7711
Email: ocim@ocim.ucsf.edu
Website: http://www.ucsf.edu/ocim/
Susan Folkman, PhD, Dir.
Activities/Fields: Integrative medicine which seeks the most effective treatments for patients by combining non-traditional and traditional approaches that address all aspects of their health and wellness: biological, psychological, social, and spiritual.

★ 23700 ★ University of California, San Francisco
Pain Clinical Research Center (PCRC)
1701 Divisadero, Ste. 480
San Francisco, CA 94117
Phone: (415)885-7899 **Fax:** (415)885-7855
Email: mcrwind@itsa.ucsf.edu
Website: http://itsa.ucsf.edu/~pcrc/general.html
Marlene Berro, Contact
Activities/Fields: Neuropathic pain, which is pain from damage to nerves that has occurred from disease processes, viruses, or injury.

★ 23701 ★ University of California, San Francisco
Radiation Oncology Research Laboratory
1855 Folsom, Rm. MCB 200, Box 0806
San Francisco, CA 94103
Phone: (415)476-2461 **Fax:** (415)476-9069
Email: dewey@rorl.ucsf.edu
Dr. Wm. Dewey, Dir.
Activities/Fields: Effects of ionizing radiation and hyperthermia in killing mammalian cells and interfering with cell cycle progression, with emphasis on applying basic concepts to radiation oncology.

★ 23702 ★ University of California, San Francisco
Resource for Biocomputing, Visualization, and Informatics
Computer Graphics Laboratory
San Francisco, CA 94143-0446
Phone: (415)476-2299 **Fax:** (415)502-1755
Email: tef@cgl.ucsf.edu
Website: http://www.cgl.ucsf.edu/
Thomas E. Ferrin, PhD, Prin. Investigator
Activities/Fields: Genomic and molecular recognition problems. Research focuses on three key areas: sequence analysis and bioinformatics, structural informatics, and functional informatics.

★ 23703 ★ University of California, San Francisco
Rosalind Russell Medical Research Center for Arthritis
350 Parnassus Ave., Ste. 600
San Francisco, CA 94117
Phone: (415)476-1141 **Fax:** (415)476-3526
Email: aweiss@itsa.ucsf.edu
Website: http://medicine.ucsf.edu/rheum/russell.shtml
Dr. Arthur Weiss, Contact
Activities/Fields: Arthritis and its probable causes, focusing on on immunology, immunogenetics, and inflammation. Examines health services and policy and educational approaches and methods for arthritis patients and health professionals.

★ 23704 ★ University of California, San Francisco
San Francisco Injury Center
San Francisco General Hospital
Department of Surgery, Ward 3A, Box 0807
1001 Potrero Ave.
San Francisco, CA 94110
Phone: (415)206-4623 **Fax:** (415)206-5950
Email: pknudson@sfghsurg.ucsf.edu
Website: http://www.surgery.ucsf.edu/sfic
M. Margaret Knudson, MD, Dir.
Activities/Fields: Acute trauma care, injury prevention and surveillance.

★ 23705 ★ University of California, San Francisco
Vascular Research Laboratory
Cardiology Division
1347 Moffitt Hospital, Box 0130
San Francisco, CA 94143-0130
Free: 800-827-3478
Email: seivers@medicine.ucsf.edu
Website: http://cardiology.ucsf.edu/research/vascular/
Richard Sievers, Contact
Activities/Fields: Determinants of vascular tone and its role in the genesis of atherosclerotic disease, specifically the effects of sex steroid hormones on the conductance and resistance arterial vasculature in coronary, pulmonary, and systemic circulation.

★ 23706 ★ University of California, San Francisco
W.M. Keck Foundation Center for Integrative Neuroscience
513 Parnassus Ave., Rm. HSE-812, Box 0444
San Francisco, CA 94143-0444
Phone: (415)502-4975 **Fax:** (415)502-4848
Email: keck-info@phy.ucsf.edu
Website: http://www.keck.ucsf.edu/keck/
Dr. Steve Lisberger, Dir.
Activities/Fields: Neurochemistry of pain modulatory systems in the brainstem and spinal cord, using in vivo microdialysis, cytochemistry and high pressure liquid chromotography.

★ 23707 ★ University of California, San Francisco
Wheeler Center for the Neurobiology of Addiction
UCSF Box 0453
San Francisco, CA 94143-0453
Phone: (415)502-4140 **Fax:** (415)476-9386
Email: ucsfcna@itsa.ucsf.edu
Website: http://www.ucsf.edu/cnba/Center
Dr. Howard Fields, Dir.
Activities/Fields: Identification of the neural circuits, molecular targets, and biochemical actions that help drugs of abuse take command of the brain. **Pub:** *Wheeler Center Newsletter.*

★ 23708 ★ University of California, Santa Barbara
Autism Research and Training Center
Phelps Hall, Rm. 1180
Research Office
Graduate School of Education
Santa Barbara, CA 93106-9490
Phone: (805)893-8136 **Fax:** (805)893-2176
Email: koegel@education.ucsb.edu
Website: http://kady.education.ucsb.edu/autism
Robert Koegel, PhD, Dir.
Activities/Fields: Autism, especially education for autistic children; the effect of treatment programs on the child, the child's family and the integration of the child in the school setting and the community; and the development and use of non-aversive treatment for severe problems such as self-injury and aggression, as often seen in autistic children.

★ 23709 ★ University of California, Santa Barbara
Neuroscience Research Institute
Santa Barbara, CA 93106-5060
Phone: (805)893-2659 **Fax:** (805)893-2005
Website: http://www.nri.ucsb.edu
Prof. Stuart C. Feinstein, Interim Dir.
Activities/Fields: Basic biology and medicine, pharmacology, psychology, chemistry, and electrical engineering. Research areas include the genetics, biochemistry, and structural organization of the developing nervous system; the ultrastructure, function (and malfunction) of the retina; the role of ion channels in neuronal function; the structural and enzymatic basis of vesicle function at axonal endings; the role of extracellular matrix in neurodevelopment; and the molecular biology of neurotrophins and their receptors. **Frmly:** Environmental Stress Laboratory; Institute of Environmental Stress.

★ 23710 ★ University of California, Santa Barbara
Neuroscience Research Institute Center for the Study of Neurodegenerative Disorders
Department of Molecular, Cellular & Developmental Biology
Santa Barbara, CA 93106
Phone: (805)893-2659 **Fax:** (805)893-2005
Email: feinstei@lifesci.ucsb.edu
Website: http://www.lifesci.ucsb.edu/~nriweb/CSND/index.html
Prof. Stuart C. Feinstein, Interim Dir.
Activities/Fields: Degeneration of the central nervous system, with the focus on multiple sclerosis, Alzheimer's disease, spinal cord injury, and aging.

★ 23711 ★ University of Central Florida
Center for Discovery of Drugs and Diagnostics (CD3)
12722 Research Pky.
Orlando, FL 32826-3227
Phone: (407)384-2818 **Fax:** (407)384-2062
Email: jgood@mail.ucf.edu
John Goodchild, PhD, Dir.
Activities/Fields: Molecular medicine, leading to the identification of new drugs and diagnostic procedures. Greatest emphasis is placed on preventing and treating diseases of most concern to the citizens of Florida.

★ 23712 ★ University of Chicago
Animal Resources Center
MC 1030
5841 S Maryland Ave.
Chicago, IL 60637-1030
Phone: (773)702-6756 **Fax:** (773)702-9152
Email: glangan@arc-1.bsd.uchicago.edu
Dr. George Langan, Contact
Activities/Fields: Supports research on animals and animal models. **Frmly:** Office of Animal Care; A.J. Carson Animal Research Facility.

★ 23713 ★ University of Chicago
Ben May Institute for Cancer Research
MC 6027
5841 S Maryland Ave.
Chicago, IL 60637
Phone: (773)702-0380 **Fax:** (773)702-4634
Email: mrosner@ben-may.bsd.uchicago.edu
Website: http://ben-may.bsd.uchicago.edu
Dr. Marsha Rosner, Dir.
Activities/Fields: Cancer and hormone-dependent tumors, including cancer of breast and prostate through studies in immunobiology, biochemistry, clinical medicine, experimental pathology, organic chemistry, and physiology on morphology and function of cells.

★ 23714 ★ University of Chicago
BioCARS: A Synchrotron Structural Biology Resource
Bldg. 434B
9700 S Cass Ave.
Argonne, IL 60439
Phone: (630)252-0450
Email: moffat@cars.uchicago.edu
Website: http://cars9.uchicago.edu/biocars/
Keith Moffat, PhD, Prin. Investigator
Activities/Fields: Crystallographic studies of viruses, ribosomes and other complexes with very large unit cells; studies of microcrystals; time-resolved crystallography; and scattering from less-ordered biological systems. In all cases, the goal is to understand basic biological processes in structural terms, a goal fundamental to the pharmaceutical and biotechnology industries as well as to basic science.

★ 23715 ★ University of Chicago
Cancer Research Center
5841 S Maryland Ave., MC 1140
Chicago, IL 60637-1470
Phone: (773)702-6180 **Fax:** (773)702-9311
Email: uccrc@medicine.bsd.uchicago.edu
Website: http://www-uccrc.bsd.uchicago.edu
Nicholas J. Vogelzang, MD, Dir.
Activities/Fields: Cause, prevention, and treatment of cancer, including investigations of gynecologic cancers, lung cancer, head and neck cancer, pediatric cancers, gastro-intestinal cancers, breast cancer, lymphoma, leukemia, autologous bone marrow transplantation. Conducts research in cancer biology, molecular genetics, tumor immunology, developmental therapeutics, clinical research, diagnostics using radiology and radionuclide imaging, radiotherapy, radiation physics, radiation biology, developmental biology, and biochemistry. Major program areas include: molecular biology of cell growth and differentiation, chromosomes and cancer, immunology and cancer, developmental therapeutics, clinical investigations, cancer prevention and control, and advanced medical imaging. Developing programs include cancer prevention, breast cancer and prostate cancer. **Pub:** *Annual scientific report.* • *UCCRC Update.*

★ 23716 ★ University of Chicago
Clinical Nutrition Research Unit
MC 4080
5841 S Maryland Ave.
Chicago, IL 60637
Phone: (773)702-6741 **Fax:** (773)702-6972
Email: jnewton@medicine.bsd.uchicago.edu
Dr. Jeanette Newton-Keith, Dir.
Activities/Fields: Human and clinical nutritional biology, particularly in relation to pregnancy, growth retardation, digestive and cardiovascular diseases, diabetes, and cancer. Conducts vitamin metabolism, lipoprotein, lipid, stable isotope, trace metal, and radioimmunoassay analyses.

★ 23717 ★ University of Chicago
Diabetes Research and Training Center
MC 1027
5841 S Maryland Ave.
Chicago, IL 60637

Phone: (773)702-6217 **Fax:** (773)834-0486
Dr. Donald Steiner, Dir.

Activities/Fields: Etiology and pathogenesis of diabetes mellitus and improvement of care of diabetic patients, including studies on isolation and properties of proinsulin, proglucagon and amylin, isolation and characterization of beta cell plasma membranes, regulation of insulin biosynthesis and secretion, hyperlipidemia in diabetes, tissue culture of islet cells and cell tumors, mechanism of enzymatic conversion of proinsulin to insulin, insulin binding, degradation and action, serum proinsulin and C-peptide levels in normal and diabetic subjects, including studies of insulin of secretion and metabolism. Encourages new endeavors and provides a framework and stimulus for additional collaborative research programs among investigators of different disciplines and backgrounds. Conducts studies into the genetic basis of diabetes and alterations in gene expression in diabetes. Works to define the role of ion channels in insulin secretion.

★ 23718 ★ University of Chicago EM Core Facility for Biological Research

920 E 58th St.
Chicago, IL 60637
Phone: (773)702-1077 **Fax:** (773)834-1094
Email: bob@besvax.uchicago.edu
Website: http://gingi.uchicago.edu
Prof. Bob Joseph, Contact

Activities/Fields: Biomedical research, including cell biology and molecular imaging.

★ 23719 ★ University of Chicago General Clinical Research Center

MC 7100
5841 S Maryland Ave.
Chicago, IL 60637
Phone: (773)702-6227 **Fax:** (773)702-6952
Email: mfavus@medicine.bsd.uchicago.edu
Website: http://gcrc.bsd.uchicago.edu
Murray J. Favus, Dir.

Activities/Fields: Endocrinology, including insulin metabolism in health and disease, evaluation and treatment of hormonal disorders of growth and puberty, and polycystic ovary syndrome; psychiatry, including substance abuse; pharmacology; oncological research chemotherapies in the treatment of malignancies; investigations into human circadian rhythms; and genetics of diabetes, osteoporosis, and asthma.

★ 23720 ★ University of Chicago Inflammatory Bowel Disease Research Center

Department of Medicine, MC 6084
5841 S Maryland Ave.
Chicago, IL 60637-6084
Phone: (773)702-6458 **Fax:** (773)702-2281
Email: echang@medicine.bsd.uchicago.edu
Dr. Eugene B. Chang, Dir.

Activities/Fields: Pathophysiology and treatment of inflammatory bowel diseases, including molecular and cellular immunology, epithelial cell biology, human genetics, inflammation, therapeutic clinical trials, and clinical epidemiology. **Pub:** *IBD Center Newsletter*, quarterly. Newsletter.

★ 23721 ★ University of Chicago Institute for Mind and Biology

940 E 57th St.
Chicago, IL 60637
Phone: (773)702-2579
Email: MKM1@midway.uchicago.edu
Website: http://psychology.uchicago.edu/socpsych
Martha K. McClintock, Dir.

Activities/Fields: Relationship between the mind, the brain and the body in health and disease.

★ 23722 ★ University of Chicago Joseph B. Kirsner Center for the Study of Digestive Diseases

5841 S Maryland Ave.
Chicago, IL 60637
Phone: (773)702-9790 **Fax:** (773)702-2182
Email: bhunt@medicine.bsd.uchicago.edu
Dr. Stephen Hanauer, Dir.

Activities/Fields: Gastroenterology, including colon cancer, inflammatory bowel disease, irritable bowel syndrome, disorders of the esophagus, and pancreatic cancer.

★ 23723 ★ University of Chicago Joseph P. Kennedy, Jr., Mental Retardation Research Center

Children's Hospital, MC 5058
5841 S Maryland Ave.
Chicago, IL 60637
Phone: (773)702-6428 **Fax:** (773)702-9234
Email: nbs0@midway.uchicago.edu
Website: http://peds-www.bsd.uchicago.edu/sections/Kennedy/index.html
Dr. Nancy B. Schwartz, Dir.

Activities/Fields: Mental retardation, emphasizing membrane glycococonjugate structure and synthesis, lysosomes (inborn errors of metabolism), regulation of enzymatic action, protein chemistry, chemistry and metabolism of sphingolipids and other lipids and lipoprotein complexes, carbohydrate chemistry, biology of biochemistry of the extracellular matrix (normal development and inborn errors), collagen gene structure and expression, DNA sequence studies, DNA methylation and chromatin structure, recombinant DNA technology, cell-free translation and transcription in differentiating eukaryotic cells, regulation of gene expression and mRNA regulation during embryonic development, regulation of catecholamine neurotransmitter biosynthesis and secretion, signal transduction pathways in neuronal systems, opioid actions during embryogenesis and opioid signal transduction, muscarinic receptor signal transduction pathways in differentiating neurons, proteoglycan participation in CNS histomorphogenesis, glia phenotypes and the role of protein kinases, electron microscope visualization of specific gene products in differentiating nervous system and cartilage (use of monoclonal antibodies), neurotransmitter receptor structure and function, mechanisms of synapse formation, neurobiology and neuropathology of dopaminergic pathways, regulation of myelination (oligodendrocyte neurobiology), isolation and tissue culture of specialized cells (oligodendrocytes, neurononal aggregates, neuroblastoma x neuron hybrids, chromaffin cells, and chondrocytes), neuroanatomical mapping, mitochondrial function and dysfunction, and neurological, genetic, biological, biochemical, and embryological studies.

★ 23724 ★ University of Chicago Kurt Rossmann Laboratories for Radiologic Image Research

Department of Radiology
5841 S Maryland Ave., M/C 2026
Chicago, IL 60637
Phone: (773)702-6154 **Fax:** (773)702-0371
Email: k-doi@uchicago.edu
Website: http://xray.bsd.uchicago.edu/krl/
Kunio Doi, PhD, Dir.

Activities/Fields: Diagnostic accuracy of radiological imaging techniques and minimization of patient exposure incurred during radiographic examinations.

★ 23725 ★ University of Chicago Liver Study Unit

MC 4076
5841 S Maryland Ave.
Chicago, IL 60637-4076
Phone: (773)702-6145 **Fax:** (773)834-1288
Dr. Stephen Hanauer, Sec. Ch.

Activities/Fields: Role of nutrition in avoiding or managing liver diseases and new therapeutic approaches for treatment of specific liver diseases. Provides comprehensive care for patients with liver diseases, including assessment of severity using noninvasion methods and management of chronic hepatitis patients.

★ 23726 ★ University of Chicago Maclean Center for Clinical Medical Ethics

MC 6098
Department of Medicine
5841 S Maryland Ave.
Chicago, IL 60637-1470
Phone: (773)702-1453 **Fax:** (773)702-0090
Email: msiegler@medicine.bsd.uchicago.edu
Website: http://ethics.bsd.uchicago.edu/
Mark Siegler, MD, Dir.

Activities/Fields: Clinical medical ethics, bioethics, technology assessment, and medical outcomes research.

★ 23727 ★ University of Chicago Perinatal Center

MC 2050
5841 S Maryland Ave.
Chicago, IL 60637
Phone: (773)702-3733 **Fax:** (773)702-1085
Email: mismail@babies.bsd.uchicago.edu
Dr. Mahmoud Ismail, Co-Dir.

Activities/Fields: Fetal-maternal medicine, neonatology, and morbidity and mortality within perinatal medicine.

★ 23728 ★ University of Chicago Visual Sciences Center

5841 S Maryland, MC 2114
Chicago, IL 60637
Phone: (773)702-8888 **Fax:** (773)702-8094
Email: jernest@midway.uchicago.edu
Website: http://ophthalmology.bsd.uchicago.edu
Dr. J. Terry Ernest, Chm., Ophthalmology

Activities/Fields: Ophthalmology, visual physiology and function of the retina, color vision, evoked occipital response, laser and xenon photocoagulation for retinal disease, and pharmacology of the retinal pigment epithelium. Also conducts electron microscopy and visual molecular biology studies. **Frmly:** Eye Research Laboratories.

★ 23729 ★ University of Cincinnati Barrett Cancer Center

234 Goodman St.
Cincinnati, OH 45219
Phone: (513)584-3200
Website: http://www.med.uc.edu/medcente/barrett/Barrett.htm
John C. Winkelmann, MD, Assoc. Dir., Clin. Svcs.

Activities/Fields: Cancer, in conjunction with the National Surgical Adjuvant Breast Project, Southwest Oncology Group, Gynecologic Oncology Group, and Radiation Therapy Oncology Group. Also studies gynecologic oncology, surgical oncology, neurologic oncology, and radiation therapy and radiation oncology. **Pub:** *Annual Reports*. Annual report.

★ 23730 ★ University of Cincinnati Cardio-Vascular Laboratory

University Hospital
234 Goodman Ave.
Cincinnati, OH 45219
Phone: (513)584-5148 **Fax:** (513)584-3515
Email: adkinsb@healthall.com
Wm. Brian Adkins, Contact

Activities/Fields: Computerized vascular research, including ultrasound, instrumentation, and pharmaceutical research.

★ 23731 ★ University of Cincinnati Cardiovascular Research and Education Center
231 Albert B. Sabin Way
Cincinnati, OH 45267-0542
Phone: (513)558-4721 **Fax:** (513)558-3116
Email: jerald.dorn@uc.edu
Dr. Jerald W. Dorn, II, Dir.
Activities/Fields: Cardiology and drug device clinical trials.

★ 23732 ★ University of Cincinnati Center for Environmental Genetics (CEG)
Department of Environmental Health
College of Medicine
3223 Eden Ave.
Cincinnati, OH 45267-0056
Phone: (513)558-3625 **Fax:** (513)558-4617
Email: marshall.anderson@uc.edu
Website: http://www.niehs.nih.gov/centers/center/cin-ctr.htm
Marshall W. Anderson, PhD, Dir.
Activities/Fields: Environmental health sciences, with a focus on the interaction between genes and the environment, especially the impact of genetic diversity on the response of the individual to toxic environmental agents.

★ 23733 ★ University of Cincinnati Center for the Study of Prevalent Neurotoxicants in Children
Children's Hospital of Cincinnati
CH-TCHRF 6527
PO Box 670054
Cincinnati, OH 45267-0054
Fax: (513)636-4402
Email: bruce.lanphear@chmcc.org
Website: http://es.epa.gov/ncer_abstracts/centers/ce-cehdpr/01/lanphear.html
Bruce Lanphear, PhD, Dir.
Activities/Fields: Neurobehavioral effects of childhood exposure to environmental agents including lead, mercury, PCBs, and environmental tobacco smoke.

★ 23734 ★ University of Cincinnati Cincinnati Rheumatic Disease Study Group
231 Bethesda Ave., 670563
Cincinnati, OH 45267
Phone: (513)558-5538
Dr. Michael Luggen, Dir.
Activities/Fields: Rheumatic and allergic diseases, including abnormalities in systemic lupus erythematosus, immunogenetics of connective tissue disease, mechanisms of tolerance and immunomodulation, and asthma pathogenesis autoimmune disease.

★ 23735 ★ University of Cincinnati Division of Epidemiology and Biostatistics
PO Box 670183
Cincinnati, OH 45267-0183
Phone: (513)558-1410 **Fax:** (513)558-4838
Email: charles.buncher@uc.edu
Website: http://www.uc.edu
Dr. C.R. Buncher, Hd.
Activities/Fields: Epidemiologic and biostatistical research, especially in environmental, occupational, and medical fields.

★ 23736 ★ University of Cincinnati Education and Research Center (ERC)
3223 Eden Ave., ML No. 0056
Cincinnati, OH 45267-0056
Phone: (513)558-1749 **Fax:** (513)556-4999
Email: clarkcs@uc.edu
Website: http://www.uc.edu/erc/about_us.htm
Dr. Scott Clark, Dir.
Activities/Fields: Occupational safety and health.

★ 23737 ★ University of Cincinnati Headache Center
Aring Neurology Department
222 Piedmont Ave., Ste. 2300
Cincinnati, OH 45219
Phone: (513)475-8730 **Fax:** (513)475-8033
Dr. Joseph Nicolas, Co-Dir.
Activities/Fields: Migraine headaches.

★ 23738 ★ University of Cincinnati Institute for Health Policy and Health Services Research (IHPHSR)
Mail Location 0840
University of Cincinnati Medical Center
French Bldg. East, Ste. 275
Cincinnati, OH 45267-0840
Phone: (513)558-2756 **Fax:** (513)558-2744
Email: alfred.tuchfarber@uc.edu
Website: http://www.ihphsr.uc.edu
Dr. Alfred Tuchfarber, Dir.
Activities/Fields: Health policy and health services, especially cost effectiveness and outcomes.

★ 23739 ★ University of Cincinnati Institute for Health Policy and Health Services Research Center for Clinical Effectiveness
University of Cincinnati Medical Center
202 Goodman Dr., Ste. 275
Cincinnati, OH 45267-0840
Phone: (513)558-2756 **Fax:** (513)558-2744
Email: alfred.tuchfarber@uc.edu
Dr. Alfred Tuchfarber, Dir.
Activities/Fields: Health-related quality of life, cost effectiveness of diagnostic and treatment strategies, pharmacoeconomics, outcomes, and severity of illness.

★ 23740 ★ University of Cincinnati Noyes-Giannestres Biomechanics Laboratories
2901 Campus Way, Rm. 893
Biomedical Engineering Department, ML 0048
College of Engineering
PO Box 210048
Cincinnati, OH 45221-0048
Phone: (513)556-4171 **Fax:** (513)556-4162
Email: david.butler@uc.edu
David L. Butler, Contact
Activities/Fields: Promotes graduate student involvement in biomechanics research, including functional tissue engineering, human body dynamics, joint mechanics and kinematics, soft tissue mechanics, robotics, ergonomics, mechanical stresses in the work place, and sports medicine. **Frmly:** Center for Biomechanics Studies and Research.

★ 23741 ★ University of Cincinnati Shriners Hospitals for Children—Cincinnati
3229 Burnet Ave.
Cincinnati, OH 45229-3095
Phone: (513)872-6206 **Fax:** (513)872-6999
Glenn D. Warden, MD, Dir.
Activities/Fields: Burns, including nutrition, infection, coverage (autografts/allografts), conversion (topical antimicrobials), pain, scar formation, and care and treatment of children who have suffered from thermal injuries and resulting problems. **Frmly:** Shriners Burns Institute.

★ 23742 ★ University of Colorado B.F. Stolinsky Research Laboratories
4200 E 9th Ave., Campus Box C233
Denver, CO 80262
Phone: (303)315-7301 **Fax:** (303)315-8080
Email: stephen.goodman@uchsc.edu
Stephen I. Goodman, MD, Dir.
Activities/Fields: Biochemical genetics and nutrition. The Laboratories are federally designated as a center for research in mental retardation or related aspects of human development.

★ 23743 ★ University of Colorado Cancer Center
4200 E 9th Ave., B188
Denver, CO 80262
Phone: (303)315-3007 **Fax:** (303)315-3304
Email: paul.bunn@uchsc.edu
Website: http://uch.uchsc.edu/uccc
Dr. Paul A. Bunn, Jr., Dir.
Activities/Fields: Prevention, early detection, and treatment of cancer.

★ 23744 ★ University of Colorado Center for Health Services Research
1355 S Colorado Blvd., Ste. 306
Denver, CO 80222
Phone: (303)756-8350 **Fax:** (303)759-8196
Email: pete.shaughnessy@uchsc.edu
Peter W. Shaughnessy, PhD, Dir.
Activities/Fields: Health services research and health policy research for federal and state governments, foundations, and related organizations, emphasizing general health policy topics and issues in long-term care quality, access, cost and cost effectiveness. Studies emphasize Medicare and Medicaid quality assurance and reimbursement for long-term care providers, including home health agencies, subacute care facilities, swing-bed hospitals, and traditional nursing homes. Studies focus on the collection and analysis of extensive primary and secondary cross-sectional and longitudinal data at the patient and facility levels. Contributes to federal and state policy deliberations on regulatory and reimbursement issues in long-term care, and to clinical practice and decision making (especially in quality assurance.).

★ 23745 ★ University of Colorado Center for Human Nutrition
CB C225
4200 E 9th
Denver, CO 80262
Phone: (303)315-4084
Email: james.hill@uchsc.edu
Website: http://www.uchsc.edu/nutrition/
James O. Hill, PhD, Dir.
Activities/Fields: Obesity and diabetes, developmental aspects of nutrient utilization and function, and micronutrient absorption and bioavailability.

★ 23746 ★ University of Colorado Clinical Mass Spectrometry Research Resource
4200 E 9th Ave.
Denver, CO 80262
Phone: (303)315-7286 **Fax:** (303)315-0080
Email: paul.fennessey@uchsc.edu
Website: http://www.uchsc.edu
Dr. P.V. Fennessey, Co-Dir.
Activities/Fields: Clinical applications of mass spectrometry, including gas chromatograph mass spectrometry, high resolution mass spectrometry, bioactive substances, and application of fast atom bombardment mass spectrometry to biomolecules. Emphasizes methods for synthesis of internal standards for the quantitative analysis of bioactive molecules found in physiological fluids, identification of steroid profiles in patients with biochemical and pathological irregularities, and stable isotope studies for measuring the utilization of important metabolic intermediates in humans.

★ 23747 ★ University of Colorado General Clinical Research Center—Adults
Health Science Center
4200 E 9th Ave., B-141
Denver, CO 80262
Phone: (303)372-8799 **Fax:** (303)372-5866
Email: robert.eckel@uchsc.edu

Website: http://www.uchsc.edu/gcrc
Robert H. Eckel, MD, Prog. Dir.

Activities/Fields: Cardiovascular disease, connective tissue disease, dermatology, endocrinology, gastroenterology, hematology, immunology, metabolism and nutrition, nephrology, neurology, oncology, psychiatry, and pulmonary disease.

★ 23748 ★ University of Colorado General Clinical Research Center—Pediatric
The Children's Hospital
1056 E 19th Ave., Box B-218
Denver, CO 80218
Phone: (303)837-2957 **Fax:** (303)764-8407
Email: sokol.ronald@tchden.org
Website: http://www.uchsc.edu/pedsgcrc/
Ronald J. Sokol, MD, Prog. Dir.

Activities/Fields: Developmental behavior, diabetes mellitus, gastroenterology, genetics, hematology, immunology, infectious disease, metabolism, neonatology, neurology, nephrology, nutrition, and pulmonary physiology.

★ 23749 ★ University of Colorado Immunology Center
Division of Allergy & Clinical Immunology
4200 E 9th Ave., B164
Denver, CO 80262
Phone: (303)315-7601 **Fax:** (303)315-7642
Email: brian.kotzin@uchsc.edu
Dr. Brian L. Kotzin, Dir.

Activities/Fields: Provides a focus for research into the causes, prevention, and management of diseases such as asthma, allergies, systemic lupus erythematosus, rheumatoid arthritis, immune deficiencies and infection, plus related studies of fundamental immune mechanisms involving immune cells, antibodies, genetic factors, and immune regulatory systems. Ongoing studies include investigations of the genetic bais of autoimmunity, T cell activation in immuno-mediated diseases, mast cell activation in allergic and infectious diseases, the effects of benzopyrenes (from tobacco smoke) on T cell function, mechanisms underlying recurrent miscarriages, the role of soluble T cell receptors in contact hypersensitivity, and xenotransplantation of pancreatic islets.

★ 23750 ★ University of Colorado National Center for American Indian and Alaska Native Mental Health Research
Nighthorse Campbell Native Health Bldg.
PO Box 6508, MS F800
Aurora, CO 80045-0508
Phone: (303)724-1453 **Fax:** (303)724-1474
Email: spero.manson@uchsc.edu
Website: http://www.uchsc.edu/sm
Dr. Spero Manson, PhD, Dir.

Activities/Fields: Determination and improvement of the performance characteristics of self-report measures of serious psychological dysfunction and diagnostic interviews for assessing alcohol, drug, and mental (ADM) disorders; establishment of the prevalence and incidence of ADM disorders and related risk factors through descriptive and experimental epidemiological investigations; development and evaluation of methods for detecting and managing ADM disorders presented in human service settings; and examination of the effectiveness of interventions for preventing ADM disorders and promoting well-being. Ongoing studies include the Healthy Ways Project, which studies the behavioral and biomedical epidemiology of HIV/AIDS and STDs in two American Indian tribes and uses this information to design individual and community level preventive interventions; the American Indian Pathways to Abstinence Project, which investigates how problem drinking and abstinence are meaningfully construed and experienced by American Indian men and women; the American Indian Spirituality and Alcohol Project, which explores potential relationships between spirituality/religiousness and concurrent patterns of alcohol use and misuse; the American Indian Child Development and Attachment Project, which examines the impact of maternal attachment status on child attachment status and social-emotional and cognitive developmental progess at 12-14 months; and Native Elders, Dementia, and Family Caregiving Project, which examines family caregiving for older Natives with dementia. **Pub:** *American Indian and Alaska Native Mental Health Research Journal*, 3/year. • *Annual Monograph.*

★ 23751 ★ University of Colorado Rocky Mountain Prevention Research Center
Department of Preventive Medicine & Biometrics, C-245
4200 E 9th Ave.
Denver, CO 80262
Phone: (303)315-6863 **Fax:** (303)315-3183
Email: rmprc@uchsc.edu
Richard F. Hamman, MD, Dir.

Activities/Fields: Public health issues, especially behaviors that place Americans at risk for chronic diseases and conditions. Of particular concern is the improvement in quality of life for special populations, including the young, elderly, racial ethnic populations, and the underserved.

★ 23752 ★ University of Colorado at Boulder Institute for Behavioral Genetics
CB 447
Boulder, CO 80309
Phone: (303)492-7362 **Fax:** (303)492-8063
Email: Toni.Smolen@colorado.edu
Website: http://ibg.colorado.edu
Dr. Toni N. Smolen, Asst. Dir.

Activities/Fields: Application of behavioral genetics to pharmacogenetics, learning disabilities, cognitive development, and vulnerability to drug abuse. Specific interests include genetics of aging, reading disability, genetic and neurobiological correlates of animal behavior, human alcohol studies, and genetic factors in personality and cognitive development of twins and adopted children.

★ 23753 ★ University of Colorado at Boulder Speech, Language, and Hearing Center
Campus Box 409
Boulder, CO 80309
Phone: (303)492-5375 **Fax:** (303)492-3274
Email: susan.moore@colorado.edu
Susan M. Moore, Dir.

Activities/Fields: Evaluation and treatment of speech, language, learning, and hearing disorders. **Frmly:** Communication Disorders Clinic.

★ 23754 ★ University of Colorado—Denver Alcohol Research Center
CB C236
4200 E 9th Ave.
Denver, CO 80262
Phone: (303)315-7076 **Fax:** (303)315-7097
Email: richard.deitrich@uchsc.edu
Dr. Richard A. Deitrich, Sci. Dir.

Activities/Fields: Mechanism of the action of alcohol to determine the ways in which alcohol affects the brain during both acute and chronic periods of intake, including studies on alcohol as a stimulus, different responses elicited by alcohol, and the products of alcohol metabolism. Uses genetic manipulation in animal models to define the acute and chronic affects of alcohol in relation to heredity.

★ 23755 ★ University of Colorado—Denver Center for Human Investment Policy
1445 Market St., Ste. 350
Denver, CO 80202
Phone: (303)820-5631 **Fax:** (303)820-5656
Email: dgarnett@carbon.cudenver.edu
Website: http://www.cudenver.edu/chip/chip.htm
Donna Garnett, Exec. Dir.

Activities/Fields: Ethical and policy issues in health care, including health care for the medically indigent, cost of care, rural health care, medical malpractice costs, prenatal care, public health, euthanasia, and the role of public opinion in policy formation. **Pub:** *FrontLines.*

★ 23756 ★ University of Colorado—Denver Rocky Mountain Taste and Smell Center
Campus Box B-205
4200 E 9th Ave.
Denver, CO 80262-0205
Phone: (303)315-6600 **Fax:** (303)315-8787
Email: bruce.jafek@uchsc.edu
Bruce W. Jafek, MD, Med. Dir.

Activities/Fields: Taste and smell dysfunction, using animal and human models, including ultrastructural change in the sense of smell during post viral states, head trauma, aging and taste dysfunction due to radiation therapy, and drugs.

★ 23757 ★ University of Connecticut A.J. Pappanikou Center for Developmental Disabilities
263 Farmington Ave., MC 6222
Farmington, CT 06030
Phone: (860)679-1500 **Free:** (866)623-1315
Fax: (860)679-1571
Email: bruder@nso1.uchc.edu
Website: http://www.uconnced.org
Mary Beth Bruder, PhD, Dir.

Activities/Fields: Developmental disabilities across the life span, psychosocial developmental needs mainly of children with disabilities, best practices in early intervention, learning opportunities for children in natural environments, assistive technology, employment, health services; addresses needs of persons with disabilities across academic and community settings, focuses on life span. **Pub:** *Monographs.* **Frmly:** Research and Training Center for Pediatric Rehabilitation; Pediatric Research and Training Center.

★ 23758 ★ University of Connecticut Alcohol Research Center
MC-2103
263 Farmington Ave.
Farmington, CT 06030-1410
Phone: (860)679-3423 **Fax:** (860)679-4077
Email: hesselb@psych.uchc.edu
Victor Hesselbrock, PhD, Sci. Dir.,Prod.

Activities/Fields: Genetic, psychiatric, biological, behavioral, and cross-cultural aspects of alcoholism, including alcoholic typologies, treatment matching, familial alcoholism, alcohol dependence syndrome, and early intervention. Activities focus on clinical trials of new psychotherapies and pharmacotherapies, biological responses to alcohol-related stimuli, diagnosis of alcohol dependence, animal studies of neurobiological correlates of alcohol consumption, ASP and family history variables as risk factors in the development of alcohol dependence, and research on treatment services for alcoholics.

★ 23759 ★ University of Connecticut Center for Environmental Health
Department of Animal Science
College of Agriculture & Natural Resources
3636 Horsebarn Rd., Box U-39
Storrs, CT 06269-4039
Phone: (860)486-6073 **Fax:** (860)486-5067
Email: wendy.west@uconn.edu
Website: http://www.sp.uconn.edu/~an226vc/index.html
Dr. Ian C. Hart, Dir.

Activities/Fields: Interdisciplinary studies of environmental health problems of concern to Connecticut, emphasizing carcinogenesis, pesticides, epidemiology and biostatistics, and genetic biomonitoring.

★ 23760 ★ University of Connecticut
Center for Health Fitness
359 Mansfield Rd., Rm. 105
Storrs, CT 06269-2034
Phone: (860)486-2763 **Fax:** (860)486-2776
Email: camaione@uconn.edu
Dr. David N. Camaione, Dir.
Activities/Fields: Biophysical and social sciences, including the complex interaction between physiology and behavioral responses related to physical activity and health. **Pub:** *Brochures.* • *Newsletters.*

★ 23761 ★ University of Connecticut
Center for International Community Health Studies
School of Medicine
263 Farmington Ave.
Farmington, CT 06030-6330
Phone: (860)679-1570 **Fax:** (860)679-5464
Email: schensul@nso2.uchc.edu
Website: http://www.commed.uchc.edu/cichs/default.htm
Stephen L. Schensul, PhD, Dir.
Activities/Fields: The health of underprivileged people in the U.S. and abroad, emphasizing international primary health care and community health, including international health policy, urban health in developing and developed countries, maternal and child health, health programs and problems in Peru, Sri Lanka, Kenya, Mauritius, and Connecticut, effects of economic development on health, and the role of the hospital in the developing world. Facilitates international health research for faculty and graduate students through consultation on grant proposals, networking with international contacts, advocating for researchers within international agencies, and establishing foreign research and educational placements. **Pub:** *Annual Training Program Catalogue.* • *CICHS Connections Newsletter.*

★ 23762 ★ University of Connecticut
Center for Neurological Sciences
University of Connecticut Health Center
263 Farmington Ave., Rm. L4071A
Farmington, CT 06030-3401
Phone: (860)679-2645 **Fax:** (860)679-8766
Email: kent@neuron.uchc.edu
Website: http://www3.uchc.edu/~nsinfo/
D. Kent Morest, MD, Dir.
Activities/Fields: Normal functions and disorders of the nervous system. expression and membrane biogenesis in neurons and glia; gene expression, release, and physiological roles of endogenous opioids; electrophysiology of excitable tissue at the cellular and systems level; development of the heart and the autonomic nervous system; cell culture of neural tissue and neural crest development; stimulus coding, synaptic organization, and development of sensory systems; communicative sciences; structure and function of auditory and gustatory systems; mathematical modeling of neural systems; central nervous system trauma; biology of multiple sclerosis; regeneration and transplantation; biology of epilepsy; and neurobiology of Alzheimer's.

★ 23763 ★ University of Connecticut
Connecticut Chemosensory Clinical Research Center
University of Connecticut Health Center
263 Farmington Ave.
Farmington, CT 06030
Phone: (860)679-1000 **Fax:** (860)679-1856
Email: bonkovsky@unch.edu
Dr. Herbert L. Bonkovsky, Dir.
Activities/Fields: Taste and smell disorders of various etiologies, plus independent research projects studying chemosensory function.

★ 23764 ★ University of Connecticut Health Center
Center for Biomaterials
MC 1615
263 Farmington Ave.
Farmington, CT 06030-1615
Phone: (860)679-3743 **Fax:** (860)679-1370
Email: goldberg@nso1.uchc.edu
Website: http://it.uchc.edu/biomaterials/General.html
A. Jon Goldberg, Dir.
Activities/Fields: Structure, properties, and function of biomaterials, especially material-tissue interfacial behavior for use in restoration, reconstruction, biosensors, and drug delivery systems in the areas of orthopedics, endocrinology, prosthodontics, restorative dentistry, oral surgery, surgery, orthodontics, endodontics and pharmacology.

★ 23765 ★ University of Connecticut Health Center
Center for Biomedical Imaging Technology (CBIT)
263 Farmington Ave.
Farmington, CT 06030-1507
Phone: (860)679-1452
Website: http://www.cbit.uchc.edu/
Leslie M. Loew, PhD, Dir.
Activities/Fields: Diagnostic and cell biological imaging, optoelectronic design, and computer/imaging science.

★ 23766 ★ University of Connecticut Health Center
Center for Microbial Pathogenesis
263 Farmington Ave.
Farmington, CT 06030
Phone: (860)679-8129 **Fax:** (860)679-8130
Email: swikel@up.uchc.edu
Website: http://cmp.uchc.edu/
Stephen Wikel, PhD, Dir.
Activities/Fields: Parasitic strategies which enable microbial pathogens to cause disease.

★ 23767 ★ University of Connecticut Health Center
Center for Vascular Biology (CVB)
Academic Research Bldg., E5052
Department of Physiology
263 Farmington Ave.
Farmington, CT 06030-3501
Phone: (860)679-4128 **Fax:** (860)679-1201
Email: hla@sun.uchc.edu
Website: http://cvb.uchc.edu/
Timothy Hla, PhD, Prin. Investigator
Activities/Fields: Molecular mechanisms of blood vessels in normal physiological conditions and in disease. Research focuses on tumor angiogenesis, signal transduction in endothelial cells, vascular proteomics, post-transcriptional gene expression, vascular developmental biology and cell invasion and metastasis.

★ 23768 ★ University of Connecticut Health Center
General Clinical Research Center
263 Farmington Ave.
Farmington, CT 06030-3805
Phone: (860)679-4145 **Fax:** (860)679-1931
Email: bonkovsky@uchc.edu
Dr. Herbert L. Bonkovsky, Dir.
Activities/Fields: Major areas of investigation include asthma, cardiology, diabetes, endocrinology, genetic diseases, obstetrics and gynecology, oncology, pediatrics, psychiatry and rheumatology.

★ 23769 ★ University of Connecticut Health Center
Health Policy and Primary Care Research Center
263 Farmington Ave., Ste. 260
Farmington, CT 06030-6325
Phone: (860)679-5487 **Fax:** (860)679-5463
Email: bailit@nso1.uch.edu
Website: http://www.commed.uchc.edu/directory/healthpolicy.asp
Dr. Howard Bailit, Dir.
Activities/Fields: Health care, especially community delivery systems, alcohol and addiction services, mental health, dental health.

★ 23770 ★ University of Connecticut Health Center
National Resource for Cell Analysis and Modeling
Center for Biomedical Imaging Technology
Farmington, CT 06030-1507
Email: les@volt.uchc.edu
Website: http://www.nrcam.uchc.edu
Leslie M. Loew, PhD, Prin. Investigator
Activities/Fields: Modeling of cell physiological processes in the context of the actual 3-D structure of individual cells.

★ 23771 ★ University of Connecticut Health Center
Waterborne Disease Center
School of Dental Medicine
263 Farmington Ave.
Farmington, CT 06030-3705
Phone: (860)679-2622 **Fax:** (860)679-2910
Email: drrossomando@waterbornediseases.org
Website: http://www.waterbornediseases.org
Edward Rossomando, DDS, Dir.
Activities/Fields: Global and national health problems caused by waterborne diseases.

★ 23772 ★ University of Delaware
Center for Disabilities Studies
166 Graham Hall
Academy St.
Newark, DE 19716-7355
Phone: (302)831-6974 **Fax:** (302)831-4690
Email: mgm@udel.edu
Website: http://www.udel.edu/chep/cds
Michael Gamel-McCormick, PhD, Dir.
Activities/Fields: Enhancement of the lives of disabled individuals and their families through research, education, and service in the areas of prevention and intervention. **Pub:** *Annual report.* • *delAWARE.*

★ 23773 ★ University of Delaware
Human Performance Laboratory
547 S College Ave.
Newark, DE 19716
Phone: (302)831-8006 **Fax:** (302)831-3693
Email: provost@udel.edu
Michelle Provost-Craig, PhD, Co-Dir.
Activities/Fields: Sports science, biomechanics, excercise physiology, bone density, and elite skaters. **Frmly:** Sports Science Laboratory.

★ 23774 ★ University of Florida
Center for Ambulatory Studies
930 NW 8th Ave.
Gainesville, FL 32601
Phone: (352)375-0607
Dr. Mark Kane Goldstein, Dir.
Activities/Fields: Behavioral and biomedical engineering, including remote monitoring of ambulatory patients and behavioral aspects of chronically ill outpatients, precision measurement of health-related behaviors, and study of simulated breast with lumps for training in breast self-examination for cancer detection.

★ 23775 ★ University of Florida
Center for Drug Discovery
Pharmaceutics Department
College of Pharmacy
J. Hillis Miller Health Center
PO Box 100497
Gainesville, FL 32610-0497
Phone: (352)392-8186 **Fax:** (352)392-8589
Email: bodor@cop.ufl.edu
Website: http://www.cop.ufl.edu/
Prof. Nicholas Bodor, PhD, Exec. Dir.
Activities/Fields: Computer-aided drug design, medicinal chemistry, drug stability and formulation development, drug metabolism and toxicity, retrometabolic drug design. **Frmly:** Center for Drug Design and Delivery.

★ 23776 ★ University of Florida
Center for Environmental and Human Toxicology
College of Veterinary Medicine
PO Box 110885
Gainesville, FL 32611-0885
Phone: (352)392-4700 **Fax:** (352)392-4707
Email: smr@ufl.edu
Website: http://www.floridatox.org
Dr. Stephen M. Roberts, Dir.
Activities/Fields: Environmental and human toxicology.

★ 23777 ★ University of Florida
Center for Exercise Science
25 Florida Gym
Gainesville, FL 32611
Phone: (352)392-9575 **Fax:** (352)392-0316
Email: spowers@hhp.ufl.edu
Website: http://www.hhp.ufl.edu/ess/ces
Scott Powers, PhD, Dir.
Activities/Fields: Fitness as it relates to athletic performance, as well as the general population, including research on biomechanics and skill acquisition; health risk factors; exercise and the lumbar and cervical spine, sports, aging, menopause, diabetes, and athletic performance. **Pub:** *Journal of Cardiopulmonary Rehabilitation.* **Frmly:** Center for Physical and Motor Fitness.

★ 23778 ★ University of Florida
Center for Gerontological Studies
2326 Turlington Hall
PO Box 117335
Gainesville, FL 32611-7335
Phone: (352)392-2116 **Fax:** (352)392-8524
Email: pkricos@csd.ufl.edu
Website: http://www.geron.ufl.edu/
Dr. Patricia Kricos, Dir.
Activities/Fields: Interdisciplinary studies on family economic status, labor force participation and survivorship in life course perspective, alternative living arrangements for older people, political attitudes and policy issues in aging, fall prevention, rehabilitation, nutritional status of elderly, memory fitness and intelligence in adulthood and old age, training needs of counselors and physician assistants, geriatric dentistry, health care for older persons, care giving and demography. **Pub:** *Outlook on Aging: Florida.* • *Pathways to Aging.*

★ 23779 ★ University of Florida
Center for Mammalian Genetics
1600 Archer Rd. SW
PO Box 100245
Gainesville, FL 32611
Phone: (352)392-3054 **Fax:** (352)392-9053
Email: carolc@ufl.edu
Thomas P. Yang, PhD, Dir.
Activities/Fields: Genetic and physical mapping of human disease genes, mutation analysis of human disease genes, gene therapy, somatic genome stability, cytogenetics, clinical genetics and dysmorphology, viral genetics, immunogenetics, neurogenetics, population and evolutionary genetics, and regulation of eukaryotic gene expression.

★ 23780 ★ University of Florida
Center for Neurobiological Sciences
Medical Science, PO Box 100244
Gainesville, FL 32610-0244
Phone: (352)392-3383 **Fax:** (352)392-8347
Email: vierck@mbi.ufl.edu
Dr. Charles Vierck, Jr., Dir.
Activities/Fields: Neurobiological sciences, including neuroanatomy, neurology, neuropsychology, neurophysiology, neurochemistry, neuropharmacology, and neuroendocrinology. Centralizes interdisciplinary communication and research training in neurobiological sciences and coordinates graduate student, postdoctoral, and faculty research in this area at the University.

★ 23781 ★ University of Florida
Center for Neurobiology of Aging
College of Pharmacy
Box 100487, JHMHC
Gainesville, FL 32610
Phone: (352)392-8509 **Fax:** (352)392-9364
Email: meyerlab@grove.ufl.edu
Website: http://www.cop.ufl.edu/centers/cna/cna.htm
Edwin M. Meyer, PhD, Dir.
Activities/Fields: Alzheimer's disease studies, including evaluation of gene expression in Alzheimer's patients and evaluation of complex behaviors, especially memory.

★ 23782 ★ University of Florida
Center for Vision Research
JHMHC
PO Box 100284
Gainesville, FL 32610-0284
Phone: (352)392-3451 **Fax:** (352)392-8554
Email: sherwood@eye1.eye.ufl.edu
Website: http://www.eye.ufl.edu/cenvissc.htm
Mark B. Sherwood, MD, Dir.
Activities/Fields: Electrophysiology of the retina and biochemistry, immunology, molecular genetics, and oncology of ocular diseases.

★ 23783 ★ University of Florida
Claude D. Pepper Center for Research on Oral Health in Aging
JHMHSC
PO Box 100416
Gainesville, FL 32610
Phone: (352)392-6796 **Fax:** (352)846-0588
Email: mheft@dental.ufl.edu
Dr. Marc Heft, Dir.
Activities/Fields: Health services research and basic oral-health functions of the elderly, including the development of periodontal disease, the effects of medications on saliva production, and the effects of aging on the senses.

★ 23784 ★ University of Florida
Computational Neuroengineering Laboratory (CNEL)
Center Dr., Bldg. 33, Rm. NEB486
PO Box 116130
Gainesville, FL 32611
Phone: (352)392-2682 **Fax:** (352)392-0044
Email: principe@cnel.ufl.edu
Website: http://www.cnel.ufl.edu/leftframe1.php
Dr. Jose C. Principe, Dir.
Activities/Fields: Adaptive information processing systems, particularly nonlinear adaptive signal processing, pattern recognition, neuromorphic computation and neurobiologically inspired models and devices. **Pub:** *Dissertations.* • *Papers.* • *Reports.* • *Theses.*

★ 23785 ★ University of Florida
Craniofacial Center
JHMHC
PO Box 100424
Gainesville, FL 32610-0424
Phone: (352)846-0801 **Fax:** (352)846-1539
Email: williams@dental.ufl.edu
Dr. W.N. Williams, Dir.
Activities/Fields: Studies the efficacy of specific surgical, prosthetic, and health-related professional management and therapy procedures in the early treatment of cleft palate and related craniofacial anomalies; prevention of communicative disorders in children from birth to three years; relationship between craniofacial abnormalities, speech, and hearing disorders; studies on craniofacial, cleft lip, and palate surgery; facial growth and disfigurement; psychological effects of craniofacial disfigurement; and the efficacy of a coordinated, interdisciplinary, team approach in health care delivery. Maintains records on clinical research and graduate or professional education within the three colleges. **Pub:** *Communicative Disorders Related to Cleft Lip and Palate.*

★ 23786 ★ University of Florida
Division of Hematology and Medical Oncology
Department of Medicine
College of Medicine
PO Box 100277
Gainesville, FL 32610
Phone: (352)392-3000 **Fax:** (352)392-8530
Website: http://www.medicine.ufl.edu/hemaonc/index.shtml
Dr. William Stratford-May, Div. Ch.
Activities/Fields: Oncology, including medicine, radiotherapy, pathology, and surgery. Focuses on growth regulation of normal and malignant cells.

★ 23787 ★ University of Florida
Florida Center for Health Promotion
PO Box 118211, FLG-23
Gainesville, FL 32611-8211
Phone: (352)392-0583 **Fax:** (352)392-1909
Email: wchen@hhp.ufl.edu
Website: http://www.hhp.ufl.edu/hse/main/flcntrhp.htm
W. William Chen, PhD, Dir.
Activities/Fields: Health promotion strategies for racial, ethnic and cultural groups of all ages.

★ 23788 ★ University of Florida
General Clinical Research Center
1600 SW Archer Rd.
PO Box 100322
Gainesville, FL 32610-0322
Phone: (352)265-8909 **Fax:** (352)265-8910
Email: stacpool@gcrc.ufl.edu
Website: http://www.gcrc.ufl.edu
Dr. Peter W. Stacpoole, Prog. Dir.
Activities/Fields: Allergy, immunology, rheumatology, cardiology, endocrinology, gastroenterology, hematology, metabolism, obstetrics and gynecology, oncology, and surgery.

★ 23789 ★ University of Florida
Health Science Center-Jacksonville Office for Research Affairs
653 1 W 8th St.
Jacksonville, FL 32209
Phone: (904)244-6693 **Fax:** (904)244-6844
Email: teresa.dillinger@jax.ufl.edu
Teresa Dillinger, Dir.
Activities/Fields: Clinical medicine, including cardiology, obstetrics and gynecology, pediatrics, gastroenterology, hematology/oncology, nephrology, neurology, and fetal medicine.

★ 23790 ★ University of Florida Institute for Child Health Policy
5700 SW 34th St., Ste. 323
Gainesville, FL 32608-5367
Phone: (352)392-5904 **Free:** 888-433-1851
Fax: (352)392-8822
Email: saf@ichp.edu
Website: http://www.ichp.edu
Steve A. Freedman, PhD, Exec. Dir.
Activities/Fields: Child health policy and family and child health care delivery issues, including development of an equitable and comprehensive child health policy model for states; development of case management programs for children with special health care needs; development of health care financing strategies, including school enrollment-based health insurance; and comprehensive program development and health services research and evaluation. **Pub:** *Developmental Screening and Family-Centered Care Module. • Florida Children's Medical Services Five Year Plan. • Maternal and Child Health Thesaurus. • Special Care. • Special Children. • SSI Handbook. • SSI Liaison Newsletter. • SSInsights. • Think! A Forum for Ideas on Child Health Policy Newsletter.*

★ 23791 ★ University of Florida Interdisciplinary Center for Biotechnology Research (ICBR)
S Newell Dr.
PO Box 110580
Gainesville, FL 32611-0580
Phone: (352)392-8408 **Fax:** (352)392-8598
Email: schuster@biotech.ufl.edu
Website: http://www.biotech.ufl.edu
Dr. Sheldon M. Schuster, Dir.
Activities/Fields: Biotechnology, including flow cytometric analysis, DNA sequencing, hybridoma technologies, protein microisolation, peptide synthesis, electron microscopy, biological computing, and genetics and reproductive analyses. Research activities include biotechnologies for ecological, evolutionary, and conservation sciences.

★ 23792 ★ University of Florida McKnight Brain Institute
PO Box 100015
Gainesville, FL 32610-0015
Phone: (352)392-0490 **Fax:** (352)846-0185
Email: ufbi@ufbi.ufl.edu
Website: http://www.mbi.ufl.edu/
William G. Luttge, PhD, Exec. Dir.
Activities/Fields: Peripheral Nerve Trauma Research Program, including biomaterials research, peripheral nerve regeneration, and mechanisms and control of pain associated with peripheral nerve trauma; Head Injury Research Program, including injury- and/or stroke-induced problems with memory, language, attention, emotion, motor skills, and epilepsy; molecular, cellular, and immunological mechanisms involved in nerve cell death and injury following stroke or closed head injury; Neurodegenerative Diseases Program, including molecular biologic studies of genetic bases of a variety of neurologic dysfunctions, including neurodegenerative movement disorders, cell biological studies on Batten's disease, and cell biological and MRI studies of laboratory animal models of multiple sclerosis. Additional studies include the underlying causes of Alzheimer's disease; the neurobiological consequences of alcohol and cocaine abuse in both adults and fetuses; and the molecular and cellular mechanisms and the behavioral and neurologic consequences of such viral-induced neurodegenerative diseases as AIDS, polio, and measles.

★ 23793 ★ University of Florida Periodontal Disease Research Center
JHMHC
PO Box 100442
Gainesville, FL 32610-0442
Phone: (352)392-4377 **Fax:** (352)392-2361
Email: macarthur@dental.ufl.edu
Dr. William P. McArthur, Dir.
Activities/Fields: Microbial etiology of destructive periodontal diseases, antibiotic therapy in the treatment of periodontal diseases, mechanisms of bacterial attachment to teeth, bacterial virulence factors in periodontal diseases, and immune response to bacterial antigens. Evaluates risk factors for periodontal disease. Studies statistical models for progression of periodontal disease. Specializes in clinical trials.

★ 23794 ★ University of Florida Radiation Oncology Clinic
Shands Cancer Center
PO Box 100385
Gainesville, FL 32610-0385
Phone: (352)265-0287 **Fax:** (352)265-0546
Email: mendenan@shands.ufl.edu
Website: http://www.med.ufl.edu/radonc
Dr. Nancy Mendenhall, Dept. Ch.
Activities/Fields: Cancer and radiation therapy and treatment.

★ 23795 ★ University of Florida Women's Health Research Center
Box 100171
Gainesville, FL 32610-0171
Phone: (352)392-9000 **Fax:** (352)392-9018
Email: whrc@vpha.health.ufl.edu
Website: http://womenshealth.ufl.edu
Mary Ann Burg, PhD, Dir.
Activities/Fields: Women's health and disease processes. **Frmly:** Center for Research on Women's Health.

★ 23796 ★ University of Georgia Drug Discovery Group
College of Pharmacy
Athens, GA 30602-2352
Phone: (706)542-5379 **Fax:** (706)542-5381
Email: dchu@rx.uga.edu
Website: http://www.rx.uga.edu/main/home/chugroup/
Prof. David C.K. Chu, Contact
Activities/Fields: Design and discovery of compounds for the treatment of various emerging infectious diseases. The main area of research includes the structure-based drug design and synthesis of novel agents against human immunodeficiency virus (HIV), hepatitis B virus (HBV), hepatitis C virus (HCV), and drug resistant bacteria as well as agents against cancer.

★ 23797 ★ University of Georgia Institute on Human Development and Disability (IHDD)
Rivers Crossing Bldg.
College of Family & Consumer Science
850 College Station Rd.
Athens, GA 30602-4806
Phone: (706)542-3457 **Fax:** (706)542-4815
Email: ihddweb@uap.uga.edu
Website: http://www.uap.uga.edu
Zolinda Stoneman, PhD, Dir.
Activities/Fields: Improvement of the quality of life for people with disabilities and their families. **Pub:** *Newsletter.*

★ 23798 ★ University of Georgia Resource Center for Biomedical Complex Carbohydrates
Complex Carbohydrate Research Center
220 Riverbend Rd.
Athens, GA 30602-4712
Phone: (706)542-4404 **Fax:** (706)542-4412
Email: palbersh@ccrc.uga.edu
Website: http://www.ccrc.uga.edu/
Dr. Peter Albersheim, Prin. Investigator
Activities/Fields: Characterization of complex carbohydrates.

★ 23799 ★ University of Guelph Human Nutraceutical Research Unit (HNRU)
J.T. Powell Bldg.
Health & Performance Centre
Guelph, ON, Canada N1G 2W1
Phone: (519)824-4120 **Fax:** (519)821-4007
Email: hnru@uoguelph.ca
Website: http://www.uoguelph.ca/hnru
Julie Conquer, PhD, Dir.
Activities/Fields: Natural health products and value-added novel foods which offer health promotion, performance enhancement, as well as disease prevention and management.

★ 23800 ★ University of Hawaii Cancer Research Center of Hawaii
1236 Lauhala St.
Honolulu, HI 96813
Phone: (808)586-3013 **Fax:** (808)586-3052
Website: http://www.crch.org
Carl-Wilhelm Vogel, MD, Dir.
Activities/Fields: Cancer, with major emphasis in cancer epidemiology, focused on multidisciplinary cancer etiology studies that utilize Hawaii's unique ethnic population distribution for basic and demographic research; basic science, including environmental carcinogenesis, experimental therapeutics, and cell transformation and differentiation; and prevention and control; research, including clinical treatment trials, chemoprevention and other cancer control interventions. **Pub:** *Annual reports. • Newsletters. • Scientific report,* triennially.

★ 23801 ★ University of Hawaii Hawaii AIDS Clinical Research Program
Leahi Hospital
Young Bldg., 6th Fl.
3675 Kilauea Ave.
Honolulu, HI 96816
Phone: (808)737-2751 **Fax:** (808)735-7047
Email: shikuma@hawaii.edu
Cecilia M. Shikuma, MD, Dir.
Activities/Fields: AIDS, HIV, and complications of HIV.

★ 23802 ★ University of Hawaii at Manoa Center on Disability Studies
1776 University Ave., UA 4-6
Honolulu, HI 96822
Phone: (808)956-5011 **Fax:** (808)956-7878
Email: juana@hawaii.edu
Website: http://www.cds.hawaii.edu
Robert A. Stodden, PhD, Exec. Dir.
Activities/Fields: Improvement in the quality of life, inclusion, and empowerment of all persons with disabilities and their families.

★ 23803 ★ University of Hawaii at Manoa Kewalo Marine Laboratory
41 Ahui St.
Honolulu, HI 96813
Phone: (808)539-7300 **Fax:** (808)599-4817
Email: hadfield@hawaii.edu
Website: http://www.kewalo.hawaii.edu/
Dr. Michael G. Hadfield, Dir.
Activities/Fields: Marine biology, including developmental, cellular and molecular biology; and symbiosis and microbiology using marine organisms as experimental models.

★ 23804 ★ University of Hawaii at Manoa Pacific Biomedical Research Center
1993 East-West Rd.
Honolulu, HI 96822
Phone: (808)956-7401 **Fax:** (808)956-4768
Email: director@pbrc.hawaii.edu
Website: http://www.pbrc.hawaii.edu
Dr. Martin D. Rayner, Interim Dir.

Activities/Fields: Cell biology, neuro-behavioral biology, molecular biology, matrix pathobiology, biotechnology, Hawaiian evolutionary and conservation biology, molecular endocrinology, retrovirology (HIV and HTLV-1), infectious diseases, and native Hawaiian health research.

★ 23805 ★ University Hospital of Quebec Pavilion CHUL Research Center Rheumatology and Immunology Research Center
2705 Blvd. Laurier, Rm. T 1-49
Sainte Foy, QC, Canada G1V 4G2
Phone: (418)654-2772 **Fax:** (418)654-2765
Email: sec.crri@crchul.ulaval.ca
Website: http://www.crchul.ulaval.ca/crchul/en/acti/Unite/rhum.htm
Pierre Borgeat, Dir.
Activities/Fields: Tissue damage in rheumatoid arthritis, regulation of leukotriene synthesis, arachidonic acid metabolism, regulation of antibody production, identification of major surface antigens, molecular mechanisms of neutrophil activation, effects of virus-leukocyte interactions on cell functional responses, regulation of apoptosis, MHC class II-mediated cell signaling, and importance of cellular compatibility.

★ 23806 ★ University of Houston Biological Clocks Program
Department of Biology and Biochemistry
Houston, TX 77204-5513
Phone: (713)743-2652 **Fax:** (713)743-2636
Email: phardin@uh.edu
Website: http://www.bchs.uh.edu/research/clocks/
Prof. Paul Hardin, Contact
Activities/Fields: Cellular and molecular clock mechanisms in animal nervous systems, including behavioral, physiological, biochemical, genetic, and molecular studies of invertebrates and vertebrates.

★ 23807 ★ University of Houston Heart and Kidney Institute
SR2, Rm. 460
4800 Calhoun
Houston, TX 77204-5515
Phone: (713)743-1218 **Fax:** (713)743-1232
Email: jandhyala@uh.edu
Dr. B.S. Jandhyala, Dir.
Activities/Fields: Cardiovascular research, including central and peripheral control of the cardiovascular system and renal functions; pharmacology of compounds affecting cardiovascular function, ischemia-reperfusion injury; oxygen free radicals; anti-oxidants; organ protection; hypertension in obesity; and insulin resistance. **Frmly:** Institute for Cardiovascular Studies.

★ 23808 ★ University of Houston Institute for Health Care Marketing
334 Melcher Hall
C.T. Bauer College of Business
Houston, TX 77204-6021
Phone: (713)743-4576 **Fax:** (713)743-4622
Email: partha@uh.edu
Website: http://www.cba.uh.edu/ihcm/index.html
Prof. Partha Krishnamurthy, Dir.
Activities/Fields: Health care marketing and health promotion.

★ 23809 ★ University of Idaho Center on Disabilities and Human Development (CDHD)
129 W 3rd St.
Moscow, ID 83843
Phone: (208)885-3559 **Fax:** (208)885-3628
Email: jfodor@uidaho.edu
Website: http://www.its.uidaho.edu/cdhd/
Julie Fodor, Dir.
Activities/Fields: Improvement of the quality of life for people with developmental disabilities across the age span by promoting their independence, productivity, and participation in integrated community settings.

★ 23810 ★ University of Illinois Health Systems Research
College of Medicine
1601 Parkview Ave.
Rockford, IL 61107
Phone: (815)395-5639 **Fax:** (815)395-5602
Email: joelc@uic.edu
Website: http://www.rockford.uic.edu/HSR/hsr.htm
Joel B. Cowen, Asst. Dean
Activities/Fields: Community health, including multiple sclerosis prevalence, primary care, public health, geriatrics, substance abuse, evaluation of delivery of health services, survey research, focus groups, demographic studies, health care planning, program evaluation, and feasibility studies.

★ 23811 ★ University of Illinois at Chicago Biologic Resource Laboratory
MC 533
1840 W Taylor St.
Chicago, IL 60612-0533
Phone: (312)996-7040 **Fax:** (312)996-8065
Email: btb@uic.edu
Dr. B. Taylor Bennett, Dir.
Activities/Fields: Houses animals and provides research and teaching support involving animal models for Colleges of Medicine, Dentistry, Pharmacy, and Nursing of the University.

★ 23812 ★ University of Illinois at Chicago Botanical Dietary Supplements for Women's Health
809 S Marshfield Ave.
Chicago, IL 60612
Phone: (312)413-9299 **Fax:** (312)413-5894
Email: norman@uic.edu
Website: http://www.uic.edu/pharmacy/research/diet/
Norman R. Farnsworth, PhD, Dir.
Activities/Fields: Ten herbal supplements that have implications for benefit in women's health issues, including therapies for menopause.

★ 23813 ★ University of Illinois at Chicago Center on Emergent Disability
Department of Disability & Human Development, MC 626
College of Health & Human Development Sciences
1640 W Roosevelt Rd.
Chicago, IL 60608
Phone: (312)413-1977 **Fax:** (312)413-4098
Email: Gfujiura@uic.edu
Website: http://www.uic.edu/depts/idhd/ced
Glenn T. Fujiura, PhD, Coord.
Activities/Fields: Impact of major health, social, and economic trends on the manifestation of disability in America.

★ 23814 ★ University of Illinois at Chicago Center on Health Promotion for Persons with Disabilities (CHP)
Department of Disability & Human Development
College of Applied Health Sciences
1919 W Taylor St., Rm. 560
Chicago, IL 60612-7249
Phone: (312)413-9651
Email: dhd@uic.edu
Website: http://www.uic.edu/depts/idhd/chp.htm
Prof. James Rimmer, PhD, Dir.
Activities/Fields: Effects of exercise and health promotion on persons with stroke, diabetes, arthritis, spinal cord injury, and Down syndrome.

★ 23815 ★ University of Illinois at Chicago Center for Health Services Research
MC 275
850 W Jackson Blvd., Ste. 400
Chicago, IL 60607
Phone: (312)413-9816 **Fax:** (312)355-2801
Email: warnecke@uic.edu
Richard B. Warnecke, PhD, Dir.
Activities/Fields: New health care tehnologies, medical informatics, health manpower, observation unit medicine in the hospital emergency room, and performance of preventive through tertiary healthcare delivery at the systems, program, and specific intervention levels. Studies focus on access, appropriateness, acceptibility, cost, safety, availability, effectiveness, benefits, and overall quality of healthcare. Specific topics include clinical decision-making, health information management, psychological and social sciences, and public health policy analysis. **Frmly:** Center for Study of Patient Care and Community Health.

★ 23816 ★ University of Illinois at Chicago Center for Molecular Biology of Oral Diseases
MC 860
801 S Paulina
Chicago, IL 60612-7213
Phone: (312)996-6118 **Fax:** (312)413-1604
Email: donc@vic.edu
Website: http://www.uic.edu/UI-Service/programs/UIC131.html
Dr. Donald A. Chambers, Dir.
Activities/Fields: Molecular biological approaches to pathobiology, including the molecular biology of cell proliferation and differentiation, the molecular basis of hematology, immunobiology and the inflammatory response, and mechanisms of host-microbial interaction.

★ 23817 ★ University of Illinois at Chicago Center for Narcolepsy Research (CNR)
College of Nursing, M/C 802
845 S Damen Ave., Rm. 215
Chicago, IL 60612-7350
Phone: (312)996-5176 **Fax:** (312)996-7008
Email: narcolep@listserv.uic.edu
Website: http://www.uic.edu/depts/cnr/
Dr. Sharon L. Merritt, Dir.
Activities/Fields: Biobehavioral impact of excessive daytime sleepiness on persons and their families.

★ 23818 ★ University of Illinois at Chicago Center for Pharmaceutical Biotechnology
MC 870
Molecular Biology Research Bldg.
College of Pharmacy
900 S Ashland Ave., Rm. 3002
Chicago, IL 60607-7313
Phone: (312)996-0796 **Fax:** (312)413-9303
Email: mjohnson@uic.edu
Website: http://www.uic.edu/pharmacy/research/cphb
Dr. Michael E. Johnson, Dir.
Activities/Fields: Structural and molecular biology focusing on pharmaceutical applications.

★ 23819 ★ University of Illinois at Chicago Center for Research on Health and Aging (CRHA)
Health Research & Policy Centers, M/C 275
850 W Jackson Blvd., Ste. 400
Chicago, IL 60607
Phone: (312)996-1473 **Fax:** (312)996-2703
Email: shughes@uic.edu
Website: http://www.uic.edu/depts/ovcr/hrpc/centers/rha.html
Prof. Susan L. Hughes, Co-Dir.

Activities/Fields: Health issues for older persons, including prevention, health maintenance, and the cost, quality and effectiveness of health care delivery systems such as long-term care and managed care.

★ 23820 ★ University of Illinois at Chicago
Chicago Center for Disability Research
Department of Disability & Human Development
College of Health & Human Development Sciences
1640 W Roosevelt Rd.
Chicago, IL 60608
Phone: (312)355-0550
Email: cg16@uic.edu
Carol J. Gill, PhD, Dir.
Activities/Fields: Disabilities.

★ 23821 ★ University of Illinois at Chicago
Craniofacial Center
811 S Paulina, 1st Fl.
Chicago, IL 60612-7308
Phone: (312)996-7546 **Fax:** (312)413-1157
Email: dreisber@uic.edu
Dr. David J. Reisberg, Dir.
Activities/Fields: Craniofacial biology, growth, and genetics, including mechanisms of cleft palate and psychological and speech development of children with cleft palate and other craniofacial anamolies. **Pub:** *Journal articles.* Journal.

★ 23822 ★ University of Illinois at Chicago
Electroencephalography Laboratory
MC 722
Department of Neurology
1740 W Taylor, 5th Fl., 5 East
Chicago, IL 60612
Phone: (312)996-3865 **Fax:** (312)413-8540
Email: jhughes@uic.edu
Dr. John R. Hughes, Dir.
Activities/Fields: Psychophysiology, including studies on clinical correlates of electroencephalic abnormalities, epilepsy, and organic brain disease.

★ 23823 ★ University of Illinois at Chicago
Great Lakes Center for Occupational and Environmental Safety and Health
School of Public Health
2121 W Taylor St., Rm. 215, M/C 922
Chicago, IL 60612
Phone: (312)996-7887 **Fax:** (312)413-7369
Email: dhryhorc@uic.edu
Website: http://www.uic.edu/sph/glakes/
Daniel Hryhorczuk, MD, Dir.
Activities/Fields: Occupational and environmental safety and health.

★ 23824 ★ University of Illinois at Chicago
Illinois Prevention Research Center
M/C 275
850 W Jackson Blvd., Ste. 400
Chicago, IL 60607
Phone: (312)996-1167 **Fax:** (312)996-2703
Email: slevy@uic.edu
Susan R. Levy, PhD, Prin. Investigator
Activities/Fields: Public health issues, especially behaviors that place Americans at risk for chronic diseases and conditions. Of particular concern is the improvement in quality of life for special populations, including the young, elderly, racial ethnic populations, and the underserved.

★ 23825 ★ University of Illinois at Chicago
Institute for Tuberculosis Research
College of Pharmacy, MC 964
833 S Wood St.
Chicago, IL 60612-7231
Phone: (312)355-1715 **Fax:** (312)355-2693
Email: sgf@uic.edu
Website: http://itr.pharm.uic.edu
Scott G. Franzblau, PhD, Dir.
Activities/Fields: New drugs for tuberculosis, leprosy, and othe mycobacterial diseases, including tetracyclines, dications, efflux pump inhibitors, and natural products from plant and microbial sources. Drug delivery systems for established and experimental drugs are also researched. **Pub:** *Annual Reports.* • *Chicago Symposium Proceedings (1973-82).*

★ 23826 ★ University of Illinois at Chicago
Laboratory for Molecular Biology
MC 567
Department of Biological Science
900 S Ashland
Chicago, IL 60607-7020
Phone: (312)996-0716 **Fax:** (312)413-2691
Email: damorris@uic.edu
Website: http://www.uic.edu/depts/bios/lmb
Don Morrison, Coord.
Activities/Fields: Regulatory mechanisms involving signal transduction pathways and eukaryotic developmental systems.

★ 23827 ★ University of Illinois at Chicago
Lions of Illinois Eye Research Institute
1905 W Taylor St., MC 649
Chicago, IL 60612
Phone: (312)996-6590 **Fax:** (312)996-7770
Email: josepuli@uic.edu
Website: http://www.uic.edu/com/eye/
Prof. Jose S. Pulido, Hd.
Activities/Fields: Diabetic retinopathy, glaucoma, cataracts, macular degeneration, retinitis pigmentosa, corneal biochemistry, molecular biology, and retinal photoreceptors. Houses the clinical trials of the UIC Department of Ophthalmology and Visual Sciences, including the Advanced Glaucoma Intervention Study, Collaborative Ocular Melanoma Study, Herpetic Eye Disease Study, and Retinopathy of Prematurity; research studies of the Applied Physics Laboratory, Lens Biochemistry Laboratory, Ophthalmic Pathology Laboratory, Ocular Molecular Biology Laboratories, Ocular Biochemistry Laboratory, Photoreceptor Research Laboratory, Laboratory of Retinal Physiology and Neurobiology, and Retinal Cell Biology Laboratory. **Pub:** *Annual Report.* • *Eye Facts.* • *Eyewitness News.*

★ 23828 ★ University of Illinois at Chicago
Low Vision Rehabilitation Laboratory
Department of Ophthalmology
1855 W Taylor
Chicago, IL 60612
Phone: (312)996-7179 **Fax:** (312)996-6685
Email: janeszly@uic.edu
Dr. Janet Szlyk, Dir.
Activities/Fields: Physiology of normal and pathologic retinas utilizing computer analyzed digitized images.

★ 23829 ★ University of Illinois at Chicago
Midwest Latino Health, Research, Training, and Policy Center (MLHRC)
Jane Addams College of Social Work
1640 W Roosevelt, Ste. 636
Chicago, IL 60608
Phone: (312)413-1952 **Fax:** (312)996-3212
Email: aida@uic.edu
Website: http://www.uic.edu/jaddams/mlhrc/mlhrc.html
Aida L. Giachello, PhD, Dir.
Activities/Fields: Latino health and health services, in Chicago and throughout the Midwest region.

★ 23830 ★ University of Illinois at Chicago
National Research and Training Center on Psychiatric Disability
104 S Michigan Ave., Ste. 900
Chicago, IL 60603
Phone: (312)422-8180 **Fax:** (312)422-0740
Email: jcook@ripco.com
Website: http://www.psych.uic.edu/uicnrtc
Judith A. Cook, PhD, Dir.
Activities/Fields: Psychiatric disabilities. Activities focus on five core areas that emphasize self-determination for people with psychiatric disabilities, including choice in treatment decision-making, economic self-sufficiency, consumer advocacy under managed care, career development through real jobs and real wages, and strengthening self-determination skills and self-advocacy.

★ 23831 ★ University of Illinois at Chicago
Rehabilitation Engineering Research Center on Recreational Technologies and Exercise Physiology Benefiting Persons with Disabilities
Department of Disability & Human Development
1640 W Roosevelt Rd., Ste. 712
Chicago, IL 60608-6904
Phone: (312)413-9651 **Fax:** (312)355-4058
Email: jrimmer@uic.edu
Website: http://www.ncddr.org/cgi-bin/mysql/nidrrprofiles.cgi?showproj=H133E020715&location =projabstract
James H. Rimmer, PhD, Prin. Investigator
Activities/Fields: Access to recreational opportunities and physical endurance of people with disabilities. The center targets four primary areas: increased access to fitness and recreation environments, interventions to increase physical activity and recreation participation, adherence strategies to reduce physical activity relapse and dropout rates, and randomized clinical trials to evaluate improvements in health and function.

★ 23832 ★ University of Illinois at Chicago
Rehabilitation Research and Training Center on Aging with Developmental Disabilities (RRTCADD)
Department of Disability & Human Development
1640 W Roosevelt Rd.
Chicago, IL 60608-6904
Phone: (312)413-1520 **Free:** 800-996-8845
Fax: (312)996-6942
Email: theller@uic.edu
Website: http://www.uic.edu/orgs/rrtcamr
Tamar Heller, PhD, Dir.
Activities/Fields: How age-related changes in physical and psychological well being affect a person's ability to function in the community; the changing support needs of adults with developmental disabilities and their families as they age; and the effectiveness of innovative public policies and services in addressing later life needs. Research priorities include promoting health and wellness; understanding women's health issues; understanding family, including sibling caregiving roles across residential settings; developing effective approaches that support individuals and their families in making future plans; identifying gaps in age-related health resources and employment; and developing universal design and assistive technology capabilities to maintain employability and enhance functioning in the community. **Pub:** *ADDVANTAGE Newsletter*, semiannually. • *Factsheets.* • *Research and policy briefs.*

★ 23833 ★ University of Illinois at Chicago
Research Resources Center
M/C 937
835 S Wolcott Ave.
Chicago, IL 60612-7341
Phone: (312)996-7600 **Fax:** (312)996-0539
Email: charlieb@uic.edu
Website: http://www.rrc.uic.edu/
Dr. C.E. Brown, Dir.
Activities/Fields: Electronic and mechanical instrumentation, biostatistics, micro and mini computer programming and databases, electron microscopy, confocal microscopy, raman microscopy, electron microprobe, nuclear magnetic resonance spectrometry, micro-imaging, mass spectrometry, X-ray crystallography, flow cytometry, and protein sequencing/peptide synthesis, DNA sequencing, bioinformatics, production and analysis of high-density DNA arrays using gene sets produced by the human genome project, and generation of transgenic and gene-targeted (knockout) mice. **Pub:** *Annual Users Report.*

★ 23834 ★ University of Illinois at Chicago
Surgical Oncology
MC 820
Clinical Science Bldg., MC 820
College of Medicine
840 S Wood St.
Chicago, IL 60612
Phone: (312)996-6666 **Fax:** (312)996-9365
Email: ncornel@uic.edu
Dr. Tapas Das Gupta, Prog. Coord.
Activities/Fields: Tumor biology, including molecular biology and molecular genetics, drug development, chemoprevention, drug resistance, genetic rearrangement, gene regulation, signal transduction, epidemiology prevention, and clinical research. Center specializes in the study of cancers of the head and neck region, breast, esophagus, stomach, small and large bowel, colon and rectum, liver and pancreas, skin, and soft body tissue.

★ 23835 ★ University of Illinois at Urbana-Champaign
Electron Paramagnetic Resonance Research Center
190 Medical Sciences Bldg.
College of Medicine
506 S Mathews Ave.
Urbana, IL 61801
Phone: (217)333-3969 **Fax:** (217)333-8868
Email: ierc@uiuc.edu
Website: http://ierc.scs.uiuc.edu
R. Linn Belford, PhD, Dir.
Activities/Fields: Free radicals and metal ion centers, especially in biological systems; characterization of metalloproteins; development and evaluation of S-band (2-4 GHz) ESE, high-frequency (e.g. 94GHz) EPR, and low-frequency DNP spectrometry; EPR study of paramagnetic contrast agents for magnetic resonance imaging (MRI); research in EPR and ENDOR theory; dynamics in biomolecules; protein folding and unfolding. **Pub:** *EPR Newsletter.*

★ 23836 ★ University of Illinois at Urbana-Champaign
Friend's Children's Environmental Health Center
3808 VMBSB, MC002
2001 S Lincoln
Urbana, IL 61802
Phone: (217)333-6230
Email: schantz@staff.uiuc.edu
Website: http://es.epa.gov/ncer_abstracts/centers/cecehdpr/01/schantz.html
Susan Schantz, PhD, Dir.
Activities/Fields: Impact of exposure to polychlorinated bipbenyls (PCBs) and methyl mercury on cognitive, sensory and motor development of children.

★ 23837 ★ University of Illinois at Urbana-Champaign
Resource for Macromolecular Modeling and Bioinformatics
3147 Beckman Institute
405 N Mathews Ave.
Urbana, IL 61801
Phone: (217)244-1604 **Fax:** (217)244-6078
Email: kschulte@ks.uiuc.edu
Website: http://www.ks.uiuc.edu/
Klaus J. Schulten, PhD, Prin. Investigator
Activities/Fields: Structure and function of biopolymers and biopolymer aggregates by theoretical and computational means and investigation of genomes from different origins.

★ 23838 ★ University of Iowa
Alzheimer's Disease Research Center
Department of Neurology
College of Medicine
200 Hawkins Dr.
Iowa City, IA 52242
Phone: (319)356-4296 **Fax:** (319)356-4505
Email: antonio-damasio@uiowa.edu
Dr. Antonio Damasio, Dir.
Activities/Fields: Alzheimer's disease and related conditions. Departments with participating specialists include anatomy, radiology, pathology, ophthalmology and psychology.

★ 23839 ★ University of Iowa
Birth Defects and Genetic Disorders Unit
Pediatrics, 4181 MERF
Iowa City, IA 52242
Phone: (319)335-6937 **Fax:** (319)335-7588
Email: val-sheffield@uiowa.edu
Dr. Val Sheffield, Dir.
Activities/Fields: Causes, prevention, and treatment of birth defects and genetic disorders. Coordinates University clinical service programs and related educational programs throughout the state of Iowa with afflicted individuals. Service and research fields include biochemical and molecular genetics, teratology, dysmorphology, genetic counseling, management of inborn errors of metabolism, epidemiology of birth defects and genetic screening, and neuromuscular disorders.

★ 23840 ★ University of Iowa
Bone Healing Research Laboratory
Orthopaedic Surgery, 1012 RCP
Iowa City, IA 52242
Phone: (319)356-2466 **Fax:** (319)353-8968
Email: james-nepola@uiowa.edu
Website: http://www.uiowa.edu/~vpr/research/organize/boneheal.htm
James V. Nepola, Co-Dir.
Activities/Fields: Bone healing, including effects of pulsed electromagnetic fields, distraction osteogenesis, synthetic bone graft and vertebral disc materials, and the prevention of osteomyelitis.

★ 23841 ★ University of Iowa
Center for Advanced Drug Development (CADD)
100 Oakdale Campus, Rm. 1 PRL
Iowa City, IA 52242
Phone: (319)335-4096 **Fax:** (319)335-4374
Email: alta-botha@uiowa.edu
Website: http://www.uiowa.edu/~cadd/
Dr. S. Alta Botha, Lab. Dir.
Activities/Fields: New and old drug substances and formulations, particuarly regarding stability indication and validation, preformulation studies, in vitro testing of dosage forms, stability studies, testing on active pharmaceutical ingredients.

★ 23842 ★ University of Iowa
Center for Health Effects of Environmental Contamination (CHEEC)
100 Oakdale Campus, Rm. N202 0H
Iowa City, IA 52242-5000
Phone: (319)335-4550 **Fax:** (319)335-4077
Email: peter-weyer@uiowa.edu
Website: http://www.cheec.uiowa.edu
Peter Weyer, PhD, Dir.
Activities/Fields: Fate and transport of toxic substances in the environment, radon and indoor air contaminants, nonpoint source chemical contamination of water supplies, and epidemiologic studies that relate the occurrence of diseases to contaminant exposure. **Pub:** *Annual Report.* • *Newsletter.* • *Technical Report.*

★ 23843 ★ University of Iowa
Center for International Rural and Environmental Health (CIREH)
120 IREH Bldg.
100 Oakdale Campus
Iowa City, IA 52242-5000
Phone: (319)335-4541 **Fax:** (319)335-2445
Email: rungar@uiowa.edu
Website: http://www.public-health.uiowa.edu/cireh
Dr. Thomas Cook, Dir.
Activities/Fields: Occupational, environmental and public health topics, particularly issues connected to rural and agricultural populations. epidemiology and care models, and the history of medicine science and public health.

★ 23844 ★ University of Iowa
Center for Nursing Classification and Clinical Effectiveness
407 Nursing Bldg.
College of Nursing
Iowa City, IA 52242
Phone: (319)335-7051 **Fax:** (319)335-7082
Email: joanne-dochterman@uiowa.edu
Website: http://ncvhs.hhs.gov/970416w6.htm
Joanne McCloskey Dochterman, Dir.
Activities/Fields: Nursing language classifications. **Pub:** *NIC/NOC Classifications.* • *NIC/NOC Letter*, semiannually.

★ 23845 ★ University of Iowa
Child Health Research Center
Department of Pediatrics
Iowa City, IA 52242
Phone: (319)356-0469 **Fax:** (319)356-4855
Email: frank-morriss@uiowa.edu
Dr. Frank H. Morriss, Jr., Dir.
Activities/Fields: Pediatrics, particularly developmental molecular biology. Activities emphasize the identification and localization of genes on the human genome, investigations of the mechanisms used by specific genes to regulate the synthesis and timing of gene products, and a study on the effects of gene products on the structure and function of developing tissues.

★ 23846 ★ University of Iowa
Cleft Palate Research Center
Otolaryngology, 21200 PFP
200 Hawkins Dr.
Iowa City, IA 52242
Phone: (319)356-2292 **Fax:** (319)356-6739
Email: michael-karnell@uiowa.edu
Michael P. Karnell, Contact
Activities/Fields: Cleft lip and palate and related disorders. Research is focused on maxillofacial growth, surgery, speech pathology, speech physiology, and neuropsychology.

★ 23847 ★ University of Iowa Cochlear Implant Clinical Research Center
Otolaryngology, 21200 PFP
Iowa City, IA 52242
Phone: (319)356-2173 **Fax:** (319)356-3967
Email: bruce-gantz@uiowa.edu
Website: http://www.uiowa.edu/~vpr/research/organize/cochlear.htm
Bruce J. Gantz, Dir.
Activities/Fields: Cochlear implants in deaf children and adults. Research areas include audiology, psychophysics, aural rehabilitation, psychology, electrophysiology, speech production, and music.

★ 23848 ★ University of Iowa Cystic Fibrosis Research Center
Internal Medicine, 500 EMRB
Iowa City, IA 52242
Phone: (319)335-7619
Email: michael-welsh@uiowa.edu
Michael J. Welsh, Dir.
Activities/Fields: Cystic fibrosis. Because cystic fibrosis is caused by gene mutations, the center is especially interested in the development of gene therapy for this disease.

★ 23849 ★ University of Iowa Dental Clinical Research Center
College of Dentistry
Iowa City, IA 52242
Phone: (319)335-7381 **Fax:** (319)335-8895
Email: clark-stanford@uiowa.edu
Website: http://www.uiowa.edu/~ocrdent
Dr. Clark Stanford, Dir.
Activities/Fields: Oral health, including disease processes (caries, periodontal disease, and oral lesions), restorative materials, and preventive techniques and agents. **Frmly:** Center for Clinical Studies.

★ 23850 ★ University of Iowa Dows Institute for Dental Research
Dental Science Bldg.
Iowa City, IA 52242
Phone: (319)335-7388 **Fax:** (319)335-8895
Email: chris-white@uiowa.edu
Website: http://www.dentistry.uiowa.edu
Dr. Christopher A. Squier, Assoc. Dean, Res.
Activities/Fields: Normal and pathological development and ultrastructure of oral soft tissues, cariology, oral microbiology, implant biomaterials and bone. Center for Clinical Studies performs research and testing of new oral health materials, products, and treatment modalities in normal and special populations. Provides supportive environment for investigations contributing to the goal of achieving the maintenance of sound dental health through elimination of major oral diseases.

★ 23851 ★ University of Iowa Environmental Health Sciences Research Center (EHSRC)
Department of Occupational & Environmental Health
Oakdale Campus
Iowa City, IA 52242
Phone: (319)335-4756 **Fax:** (319)335-4006
Email: peter-thorne@uiowa.edu
Website: http://www.public-health.uiowa.edu/ehsrc
Peter S. Thorne, PhD, Dir.
Activities/Fields: Agricultural and rural environmental exposures and their effects on health, particularly environmental cancer, pulmonary biology, and environmental assessment and control. **Pub:** *EHSRC Newsletter*, 3/year. • *Scientific and biomedical.*

★ 23852 ★ University of Iowa Epidemiology of Diabetes Intervention and Complications Study
316 GH
Iowa City, IA 52242
Phone: (319)356-4878 **Fax:** (319)356-3564
Email: william-sivitz@uiowa.edu
Website: http://www.uiowa.edu/~vpr/research/organize/edics.htm
Wm. Sivitz, MD, Co-Dir.
Activities/Fields: Progression of diabetes and the effect of treatment on patients. **Frmly:** Diabetes Research and Programs.

★ 23853 ★ University of Iowa Flow Cytometry Facility
48 EMRB
College of Medicine
Iowa City, IA 52242
Phone: (319)335-8103 **Fax:** (319)335-8049
Email: justin-fishbaugh@uiowa.edu
Website: http://www.medicine.uiowa.edu/flowcytometry
Justin Fishbaugh, Tech. Dir.
Activities/Fields: Cytometry research in the biomedical sciences, including cell biology, cancer biology, immunology, neurology, hepatology, pathology, tumor biology, and genetics.

★ 23854 ★ University of Iowa Free Radical and Radiation Biology Program
Medical Laboratories, Rm. B180
Iowa City, IA 52242
Phone: (319)335-8019 **Fax:** (319)335-8039
Email: larry-oberley@uiowa.edu
Website: http://www.radiology.uiowa.edu/FRRB
Larry W. Oberley, PhD, Dir.
Activities/Fields: Radiation biology, free radical biology, antioxidant enzymes, gene expression, and gene therapy. **Frmly:** Radiation Research Laboratory.

★ 23855 ★ University of Iowa General Clinical Research Center
157 Medical Research Facility
University of Iowa Hospitals
Iowa City, IA 52242
Phone: (319)384-8305 **Fax:** (319)384-8325
Email: william-haynes@uiowa.edu
Website: http://www.medicine.uiowa.edu/gcrc
William A. Haynes, MD, Prog. Dir.
Activities/Fields: Major areas of investigation include cardiology, clinical pharmacology, endocrinology, gastroenterology, infectious diseases, neonatology, nephrology, neurology, nutrition, oncology and hematology, opthalmology, orthopedics, otolaryngology, pediatrics, psychiatry, pulmonary diseases, rheumatology, urology and women's studies.

★ 23856 ★ University of Iowa Gerontological Nursing Interventions Research Center
410 Nursing Bldg.
College of Nursing
Iowa City, IA 52242
Phone: (319)335-7133 **Fax:** (319)353-5535
Email: toni-reimer@uiowa.edu
Website: http://www.nursing.uiowa.edu/gnirc
Dr. Toni Tripp-Reimer, Dir.
Activities/Fields: Nursing intervention in care of the elderly. **Pub:** *Advances in Gerontological Nursing*, annually. • *Iowa Aging News*, quarterly.

★ 23857 ★ University of Iowa Great Plains Center for Agricultural Health
Institute for Rural and Environmental Health
Iowa City, IA 52242-5000
Phone: (319)335-4207 **Free:** 877-611-4971
Fax: (319)335-4290
Email: gpch@mail.public-health.uiowa.edu
Website: http://www.public-health.uiowa.edu/GPCAH/
Dr. Wayne T. Sanderson, Dir.
Activities/Fields: Training of agricultural health professionals; farm safety chapter development; education of health professionals; production of materials; industrial hygiene, including respirator evaluation, anhydrous ammonia, pesticide exposure, composting exposure, and dust reduction studies; toxicology, including organic dust induced lung inflammation, molecular biology methods for bioaerosol exposure assessment, and inhalation toxicology models; ergonomics, including etiology and prevention of carpal tunnel syndrome, and evaluation of assistive technologies; and rural health, including respiratory disease, dermatologic and allergic disease, hearing loss, neurologic disease and mental health, reproductive health outcomes, and the determinants of these disease outcomes in a random sample of farm, rural non-farm and town households in the Keokuk County, Iowa. **Frmly:** Center for Agricultural Disease and Injury Research, Education, and Prevention.

★ 23858 ★ University of Iowa Holden Comprehensive Cancer Center
University of Iowa Hospitals & Clinics
200 Hawkins Dr.
Iowa City, IA 52242-1002
Phone: (319)353-8620 **Free:** 800-237-1225
Fax: (319)353-8988
Email: george-weiner@uiowa.edu
Website: http://www.uihealthcare.com/DeptsClinicalServices/CancerCenter
George J. Weiner, MD, Dir.
Activities/Fields: The Holden is organized into seven research programs including: Cancer Epidemiology; Cellular Activation in Cancer; Experimental Therapeutics; Free Radicals and Membranes; Molecular and Tumor Virology; Molecular Mechanisms of Metastasis, and prostate. **Pub:** *Newsletter.* **Frmly:** Cancer Center.

★ 23859 ★ University of Iowa Hybridoma Facility
EMRB
238 Eckstein Medical Research Bldg.
College of Medicine
Iowa City, IA 52242-1101
Phone: (319)335-8004 **Fax:** (319)335-6718
Email: charles-lovig@uiowa.edu
Dr. Charles Lovig, Contact
Activities/Fields: Provides monoclonal antibodies, tissue cultures, and reagents for cell cultures to individual investigators for their research.

★ 23860 ★ University of Iowa Injury Prevention Research Center
College of Public Health
100 Oakdale Campus, No. 158 IREH
Iowa City, IA 52242-5000
Phone: (319)335-4458 **Fax:** (319)335-4631
Email: john-lundell@uiowa.edu
Website: http://www.public-health.uiowa.edu/iprc
Dr. Craig Zwerling, Dir.
Activities/Fields: Control and prevention of rural injuries in these high risk populations through research, education and training, and public policy targeting especially rural motor vehicle injuries and farm and other occupational injuries. The specific aims of the research projects include examining the rates and risk factors of farm-related injuries among Iowa farmers; evaluating the effectiveness of trauma care in Iowa; and examining driving avoidance behavior in drivers with traumatic brain injuries.

★ 23861 ★ University of Iowa Institute for Rural and Environmental Health
Department of Occupational & Environmental Health
IREH, Oakdale Campus
Iowa City, IA 52242-5000

Phone: (319)335-4415 **Fax:** (319)335-4225
Email: craig-zwerling@uiowa.edu
Dr. Craig Zwerling, Dir.

Activities/Fields: Occupational injury and disease research and prevention and environmental health among farmers, those living in rural areas, and general industry. Conducts multidisciplinary studies of health effects due to modern agricultural and industrial practices, particularly in the areas of agricultural medicine, occupational medicine, industrial hygiene, environmental health, and environmental chemistry. **Frmly:** Institute of Agricultural Medicine and Occupational Health.

★ 23862 ★ University of Iowa
Iowa Cardiovascular Center
616 MRC
College of Medicine
Iowa City, IA 52242-1182
Phone: (319)335-8588 **Fax:** (319)335-6969
Email: francois-abboud@uiowa.edu
Prof. Francois M. Abboud, Dir.

Activities/Fields: Coronary and vascular disease, hypertension, lipid arteriosclerosis, the regulation of circulation in pathological states, neurovascular control, clinical management of lipid disorders, lipoproteins, cerebral blood vessels, occupational and immunologic lung disease, cystic fibrosis, and cardiovascular research training program.

★ 23863 ★ University of Iowa
Iowa Spine Research Center
Biomedical Engineering, 1202 EB
Iowa City, IA 52242
Phone: (319)384-0504 **Fax:** (319)353-7139
Email: malcolm-pope@uiowa.edu
Website: http://www.uiowa.edu/~vpr/research/organize/spine.htm
Malcolm H. Pope, Dir.

Activities/Fields: Causes, prevention, treatment, and rehabilitation of low back pain and other spinal disorders, including ergonomics, biomechanics, outcomes research, and epidemiology.

★ 23864 ★ University of Iowa
James A. Clifton Center for Digestive Diseases
Internal Medicine, 4500 JCP
Iowa City, IA 52242
Phone: (319)356-3127
Email: joel-weinstock@uiowa.edu
Website: http://www.uiowa.edu/~vpr/research/organize/clifton.htm
Joel V. Weinstock, Dir.

Activities/Fields: Diseases and conditions of the digestive system, including nutrition, inflammatory bowel disease, abdominal pain, and liver disease. Other basic medical research areas emphasized are motility, absorption, organ-regeneration, and transplantion.

★ 23865 ★ University of Iowa
Lipid Research Clinic
Westlawn, 2191
Department of Internal Medicine/Preventive Medicine
Iowa City, IA 52242
Phone: (319)384-5030 **Free:** 800-887-6917
Fax: (319)356-6671
Email: helmut-schrott@uiowa.edu
Website: http://www.public-health.uiowa.edu/lipid/
Helmut G. Schrott, MD, Dir.

Activities/Fields: Lipids, including the relationship of cholesterol and other blood lipids to heart disease. Conducts studies on cholesterol reducing effects of lipid lowering drugs. Also studies community cholesterol screening and educational programs for physicians. Awarded a clinical lipid disorders treatment program. Other activities include studies in post-menopausal women (PEPI Trial and HRS Trial) and diabetes studies (DCCT Trial).

★ 23866 ★ University of Iowa
Molecular Analysis Facility
355 EMRB
Iowa City, IA 52242
Phone: (319)335-7956 **Fax:** (319)353-5937
Email: lynn-teesch@uiowa.edu
Website: http://www.medicine.uiowa.edu/maf/
Lynn M. Teesch, Dir.

Activities/Fields: Proteins and peptides, focusing on amino acid composition and sequence, HPLC separations, and equilibrium and kinetic solution spectroscopy, GC-MS, LC-MS, Maldi-Tof MS. **Frmly:** Protein Structure Facility; GC/MC Facility.

★ 23867 ★ University of Iowa
National Center for Voice and Speech
250 Hawkins Dr.
Iowa City, IA 52242
Phone: (319)335-6600 **Fax:** (319)335-8851
Email: ingo-titze@uiowa.edu
Website: http://www.ncvs.org
Ingo R. Titze, PhD, Dir.

Activities/Fields: Protection, rehabilitation, and enhancement of voice and speech, including biomechanic and neurological investigations of the voice and speech mechanisms; normal, pathological and highly trained voices, and surgical techniques for correcting voice disorders.

★ 23868 ★ University of Iowa
National Maternal and Child Health Resource Center
Law, 406 BLB
Iowa City, IA 52242
Phone: (319)335-9073 **Fax:** (319)335-9098
Email: josephine-gittler@uiowa.edu
Website: http://www.uiowa.edu/~vpr/research/organize/maternal.htm
Josephine Gittler, Co-Dir.

Activities/Fields: Organization and financing of maternal and child health services, children in the legal system, and public policy in these areas.

★ 23869 ★ University of Iowa
Orthopaedic Biochemistry and Cell Biology Laboratory
Orthopaedic Surgery, 1182 ML
Iowa City, IA 52242
Phone: (319)335-2595
Email: joseph-buckwalter@uiowa.edu
Website: http://www.uiowa.edu/~vpr/research/organize/orthchem.htm
Joseph A. Buckwalter, Dir.

Activities/Fields: Biochemistry and cell biology of the musculoskeletal system, including proteoglycan biochemistry, age related changes in articular cartilage and intervertebral disc, degeneration and repair of articular cartilage, and synthesis of selected bone proteins.

★ 23870 ★ University of Iowa
Orthopaedic Biomechanics Laboratory
Orthopedic Surgery
2181 Westlawn Bldg.
Iowa City, IA 52242
Phone: (319)335-7528 **Fax:** (319)335-7530
Email: tom-brown@uiowa.edu
Website: http://www.uiowa.edu/~vpr/research/organize/orthmech.htm
Thomas D. Brown, Dir.

Activities/Fields: Mechanics of the musculoskeletal system, including articular joint pathology and estimating forces and stresses in bones, cartilage, muscles, and ligaments, mechanical devices for clinical application in orthopedic surgery, and the relationship between the mechanical environment and tissue and cell responses and their mechanisms.

★ 23871 ★ University of Iowa
Pharmaceutical Service Division
College of Pharmacy
115 S Grand Ave.
Iowa City, IA 52242
Phone: (319)335-8674 **Fax:** (319)335-9418
Email: rolland-poust@uiowa.edu
Website: http://www.uiowa.edu/~pharmser/
Rolland I. Poust, Dir.

Activities/Fields: Drug delivery systems for pharmaceutical investigations, including parenterals, capsules, tablets, liquids, lyophilized products, and dermatologicals, for human clinical trials.

★ 23872 ★ University of Iowa
Public Policy Center
Health Policy Research Program
212 South Quadrangle
Iowa City, IA 52242-1192
Phone: (319)335-6813 **Fax:** (319)335-6801
Email: peter-damiano@uiowa.edu
Website: http://www.uiowa.edu/~ppc/hlth.html
Peter C. Damiano, Dir.

Activities/Fields: Effects of policy initiatives and government activities on the cost, access, and quality of health care.

★ 23873 ★ University of Iowa
State Hygienic Laboratory
102 Oakdale Campus, H101 OH
Iowa City, IA 52242-5002
Phone: (319)335-4500 **Fax:** (319)335-4600
Email: director@uhl.uiowa.edu
Website: http://www.uhl.uiowa.edu
Mary J.R. Gilchrist, PhD, Dir.

Activities/Fields: Virolology, limnology, industrial hygiene, neonatal metabolic and prenatal diseases detection, microbiology, and organic, inorganic, and radiation chemistry. Conducts research and service in all areas relating to the environment and public health, including rapid diagnosis of disease agents by molecular methods and enzyme immunoassay, and monitoring immune status by flow cytometry. Studies the epidemiology of infectious diseases, food quality control, surface and/or groundwater contaminants, radioisotopes in groundwater, airborne contaminants and various contaminants in soil. The Laboratory develops and evaluates test methods for a wide variety of analyses and sample matrices, often to provide data as an aid to the decision and rule making process. **Pub:** *Annual Report.* • *Lab Hotline*, monthly.

★ 23874 ★ University of Kansas
Allergy and Immunology Clinic
3901 Rainbow Blvd.
Kansas City, KS 66160-7317
Phone: (913)588-6009 **Fax:** (913)588-3987
Email: dstechsc@kumc.edu
Dr. Daniel J. Stechschulte, Dir.

Activities/Fields: Studies of the normal mechanism that attract and inhibit the accumulation of WBG (type of defense cells) in the lungs and synovial membranes, clinical trials to evaluate the effectiveness of less toxic drugs in the treatment of systemic lupus erythematosus and rheumatoid arthritis, and studies on the role of mediators in the disease course of asthma.

★ 23875 ★ University of Kansas
Alzheimer's Disease Center (ADC)
G043 Delp Pavilion
3901 Rainbow Blvd.
Kansas City, KS 66160
Phone: (913)588-6981 **Fax:** (913)588-6965
Email: glopez@kumc.edu
Website: http://adc.kumc.edu/
Grisel Lopez, MD, Dir.

Activities/Fields: Causes and treatments for Alzheimer's disease and other dementing illnesses.

★ 23876 ★ University of Kansas Animal Care Unit
B054 Malott
Lawrence, KS 66045
Phone: (785)864-5587 **Fax:** (785)864-5305
Email: acu@ku.edu
Website: http://www.ukans.edu/~acu/acu.html
James F. Bresnahan, DVM, Dir.
Activities/Fields: Provides care to animals used in research, teaching, and public education at the Lawrence campus. Provides animal care, diagnostic, treatment, and necropsy services to control disease conditions and monitor health status of animal colonies. **Pub:** *Handbook for the Use of Animals in Research and Education.*

★ 23877 ★ University of Kansas Biochemical Research Service Laboratory
6037 Malott Hall
Department of Chemistry
1251 Wescoe Hall Dr.
Lawrence, KS 66045
Phone: (785)864-4166 **Fax:** (785)864-5396
Email: malterman@ku.edu
Website: http://anylresc.idl.ukans.edu/BRSL
Mike Alterman, Dir.
Activities/Fields: Primarily a service facility, the Laboratory cultures large quantities of microorganisms, purifies and characterizes enzymes and other biological materials, immobilizes proteins, performs amino acid analyses, bio-mass spectrometry, protein sequence analyses, analytical and preparative HPLC, peptide synthesis, and automated DNA sequencing. **Frmly:** Enzyme Laboratory.

★ 23878 ★ University of Kansas Center on Aging
Kansas University Medical Center
5026 Wescoe Pavillion
3901 Rainbow Blvd.
Kansas City, KS 66160-7117
Phone: (913)588-1203 **Fax:** (913)588-1201
Email: rnudo@kumc.edu
Website: http://www2.kumc.edu/coa
Randolph Nudo, PhD, Dir.
Activities/Fields: Provides support for interdisciplinary research on issues of age and aging.

★ 23879 ★ University of Kansas Center for Drug Delivery Research
Higuchi Biosciences Center
2099 Constant Ave.
Lawrence, KS 66047-2535
Phone: (785)864-5183 **Fax:** (785)864-3578
Email: decedue@ku.edu
Website: http://hbc.ukans.edu
Charles J. Decedue, PhD, Exec. Dir.
Activities/Fields: Basic and applied research on chemically-driven drug delivery systems; physiochemical and biological factors that affect delivery systems; and unstable and insoluble drugs such as anticancer agents, peptides, and proteins.

★ 23880 ★ University of Kansas Center for Environmental and Occupational Health
University of Kansas Medical Center
3901 Rainbow Blvd.
Kansas City, KS 66160-7417
Phone: (913)588-7146 **Fax:** (913)588-7160
Email: wbarkman@kumc.edu
Website: http://www2.kumc.edu/ceoh/
H. William Barkman, MD, Dir.
Activities/Fields: Relationships between human health and hazards in the environment.

★ 23881 ★ University of Kansas Center for Neurobiology and Immunology Research (CNIR)
Higuchi Biosciences Center
2099 Constant Ave.
Lawrence, KS 66047-2535
Phone: (785)864-7339 **Fax:** (785)864-5738
Email: emichaelis@ku.edu
Website: http://www.hbc.ku.edu/
Dr. Elias K. Michaelis, Dir.
Activities/Fields: Neurobiology and immunology, focusing on the problems of chronic, neurodegenerative diseases and immunological disorders. Specific interests include the development of new analytical methods for monitoring nerve cell activity in the brain, exploratory research in the mechanisms of neurodegeneration and the development of new therapeutic strategies based on the use of proteins or oligonucleotides as drug treatments, studies of the regulation of antibody production by immune system cells and the development of new screening procedures for immunotherapeutic agents, designing of new peptide drugs for the control of immune rejection reactions, and new molecular biological tools for recombinant DNA research. **Pub:** *HBC Newsletter*, 3/year.

★ 23882 ★ University of Kansas Division of Nephrology and Hypertension
3901 Rainbow Blvd.
Kansas City, KS 66160-7382
Phone: (913)588-6074 **Fax:** (913)588-3867
Email: ddiederi@kumc.edu
Dennis Diederich, MD, Dir.
Activities/Fields: Laboratory and clinical investigations into kidney physiology, polycystic kidney disease, basement membrane structure and function, kidney stones, acute renal failure, and diuretics. Research methods include tubule microperfusion, amino acid analyses, peptide synthesis, and morphometrics.

★ 23883 ★ University of Kansas Higuchi Biosciences Center (HBC)
2099 Constant Ave.
Lawrence, KS 66047-2535
Phone: (785)864-5183 **Fax:** (785)864-3738
Email: hbc@ku.edu
Website: http://www.hbc.ukans.edu
Dr. Elias K. Michaelis, Dir.
Activities/Fields: Biomedical problems, bioanalytical chemistry, drug delivery systems, neurological science, immunology, combinatorial chemistry, gene delivery, and related biotechnology. **Pub:** *HBC Newsletter*, 3/year. Newsletter.

★ 23884 ★ University of Kansas Higuchi Biosciences Center Center for Bioanalytical Research
2099 Constant Ave.
Lawrence, KS 66047-2535
Phone: (785)864-3996 **Fax:** (785)864-5738
Email: stobaugh@ku.edu
Website: http://www.hbc.ukans.edu
Dr. John F. Stobaugh, Dir.
Activities/Fields: Integration of various aspects of drug design currently directed at several specific diseases such as epilepsy, cancer, heart and lung disease, and various mental disorders. Conducts biomedical and chemical projects in neurotransmitter receptors, ion transport mechanisms, phase transport kinetics, metabolism as a barrier to drug delivery, and development of highly sensitive bioanalytical techniques. **Frmly:** Center for Drug Design; Center for Biomedical Research.

★ 23885 ★ University of Kansas Kansas Cancer Institute
University of Kansas Medical Center, Mail Stop 1027
3901 Rainbow Blvd.
Kansas City, KS 66160-7312
Phone: (913)588-4700 **Fax:** (913)588-4701
Email: agaier@kumc.edu
Website: http://www2.kumc.edu/kci/
Amy E. Gaier, Proj. Dir.
Activities/Fields: Cancer, including interdisciplinary studies on its prevention, detection, and diagnosis. Programs focus on hormonally regulated cancers, chemotherapy, radiation therapy, immunotherapy, surgical therapy, psychosocial rehabilitation of pediatric patients and families, drug development, cellular and molecular biology, chemical and environmental carcinogenesis, tumor immunology, epidemiology, and biostatistics. Also conducts clinical trial investigations.

★ 23886 ★ University of Kansas Laboratory Animal Resources
University of Kansas Medical Center
2010 W 39th St.
Kansas City, KS 66160-7185
Phone: (913)588-7015 **Fax:** (913)588-7277
Email: dpinson@kumc.edu
David M. Pinson, DVM, Dir.
Activities/Fields: Houses and maintains many species of animals required for various facets of biomedical research and for teaching purposes at the University. Supports a wide variety of research projects involving laboratory animals and operates a comprehensive laboratory animal program.

★ 23887 ★ University of Kansas Mental Retardation Research Center (MRRC)
University of Kansas Medical Center
3901 Rainbow Blvd., Mailstop No. 3051
Kansas City, KS 66160
Phone: (913)588-5970 **Fax:** (913)588-5677
Email: psmith@kumc.edu
Website: http://www2.kumc.edu/mrrc
Dr. Peter G. Smith, Dir.
Activities/Fields: Fundamental problems of mental retardation and developmental disabilties, including molecular biology and physiology of pregnancy, neuroendocrinology, fetal development, impaired fetal and infant development, infant language, cognitive development, prenatal and postnatal risk factors, developmental neurobiology and neuroplasticity. Conducts animal models studies concerning pregnancy, early developmental processes, and neurobiological mechanisms involved in motor and sensory functions of the brain and neuropathology of AIDS.

★ 23888 ★ University of Kansas Neurobiology Research Laboratory
VA Medical Center
4801 Linwood Blvd.
Kansas City, MO 64128
Phone: (816)861-4700 **Fax:** (816)922-3375
Email: bfestoff@kumc.edu
Website: http://www.kumc.edu/kcvamc/research/nbrl
Barry W. Festoff, MD, Dir.
Activities/Fields: Development, plasticity, and diseases of the nervous system. Studies focus on synaptic formation and metabolism; roles of serine proteases and inhibitors (serpins); regulation of amyloid precursor protein processing in Alzheimer's disease; and biological markers in head injuries.

★ 23889 ★ University of Kansas University Affiliated Program for Developmental Disabilities
1052 Dole Center
Lawrence, KS 66045
Phone: (785)864-4950 **Fax:** (785)864-5338
Email: schroede@kuhub.cc.ukans.edu
Steve Schroeder, PhD, Dir.
Activities/Fields: Improvement in the lives of persons with disabilities who live in metropolitan and rural eastern Kansas.

★ 23890 ★ University of Kentucky
Center on Drug and Alcohol Research
643 Maxwelton Ct.
Lexington, KY 40506-0350
Phone: (859)257-2355 **Fax:** (859)323-1193
Email: cleukef@uky.edu
Website: http://www.uky.edu/RGS/CDAR/cdar2.htm
Dr. Carl G. Leukefeld, Dir.
Activities/Fields: Biological, social, and psychological aspects of alcohol and drug abuse; and HIV/AIDS. Conducts household and other surveys. **Frmly:** Multidisciplinary Research Center on Drug and Alcohol Abuse.

★ 23891 ★ University of Kentucky
Center for Excellence in Rural Health
100 Airport Gardens Rd.
Hazard, KY 41701
Phone: (606)439-3557 **Fax:** (606)436-8833
Email: jjones3@uky.edu
Website: http://www.mc.uky.edu/ruralhealth
Judy Jones, Dir.
Activities/Fields: Rural health in Kentucky, focusing on health manpower needs, health care delivery, health care policy, and health problems unique to rural populations. Specific areas of study include assessments of new health policy, legislation, and regulation and their impact on rural health delivery, health problems among rural low-income persons and rural population needs in the areas of mental health, substance abuse and prevention. Policy oriented studies include surveys of local attitudes and perceptions of health care, rural and small hospitals, longitudinal study on the impact of rural-based health professions education, and health professionals distribution; and a survey of small businesses in Kentucky and their experiences with health insurance; a survey of physicians and midwives to determine the nature, scope, and future of obstetrical practice; and a household health survey of health needs, perceptions of health status and the health care system, and functional status of the elderly. Participatory action research being conducted in 16 countries which revolves around stimulating rural economics by increasing local health services utilization. **Pub:** *Rural Health Initiative.* Newsletter.

★ 23892 ★ University of Kentucky
Center for Health Services Management and Research
College of Applied Health Professions Bldg., Rms. 102 & 109
121 Washington Ave.
Lexington, KY 40536-0003
Phone: (859)257-6504 **Fax:** (859)257-2454
Email: scutch@pop.uky.edu
Website: http://www.mc.uky.edu/CHSMR
F. Douglas Scutchfield, MD, Dir.
Activities/Fields: Improvement of access to, and the use, quality, accessibility, delivery, organization, financing, and outcomes of health care services and an increase in knowledge and understanding of the structure, processes, and effects of health services for individuals and populations. **Pub:** *Newsletter.* • *White papers.*

★ 23893 ★ University of Kentucky
Center for Minimally Invasive Surgery
Chandler Medical Center
800 Rose St., C-344
Lexington, KY 40536-0293
Phone: (859)323-6278 **Fax:** (859)257-1428
Email: apark@uky.edu
Website: http://www-mis.uky.edu/
Adrian Park, MD, Dir.
Activities/Fields: Surgery using an endoscope and its benefits especially regarding recovery time and economic impact.

★ 23894 ★ University of Kentucky
Center for Pharmaceutical Science and Technology
309 College of Pharmacy Bldg. 0082
Rose St.
Lexington, KY 40536-0082
Phone: (859)323-6899 **Fax:** (859)323-4899
Email: jay@pop.uky.edu
Website: http://www.rgs.uky.edu/ca/infrastructure/centers/cpst.html
Dr. Michael Jay, Dir.
Activities/Fields: Drug product development and evaluation. Provides industrial support through the development and preparation of clinical supplies of drug products under government regulations.

★ 23895 ★ University of Kentucky
Center for Reproductive Medicine
Department of OB/GYN
College of Medicine
AB Chandler Medical Center, Rm. MNC18
Lexington, KY 40536-0293
Phone: (859)323-6166 **Fax:** (859)323-1931
Email: tecurry@pop.uky.edu
Website: http://www.mc.uky.edu/obg/
Prof. Thomas Curry, Dir.
Activities/Fields: Reproductive medicine, including artificial insemination; in-vitro fertilization; interfallopian tube transfer; ovulation; and follicular development.

★ 23896 ★ University of Kentucky
Center for Sensor Technology (CenSeT)
306 Davis Mills Bldg.
800 Rose St.
Lexington, KY 40536-0098
Phone: (859)323-4531 **Fax:** (859)257-5310
Email: censet@pop.uky.edu
Website: http://www.mc.uky.edu/censet/
Greg Gerhardt, PhD, Dir.
Activities/Fields: Design and construction of computer-based microsensor techniques to directly monitor biological signaling of the intact brain in real time. The long-term goal is to develop methods leading to improved health care for individuals with brain disorders.

★ 23897 ★ University of Kentucky
Children's Cancer Study Group
College of Medicine
740 S Limestone, Rm. J-457
Lexington, KY 40536-0284
Phone: (859)323-5694 **Fax:** (859)257-6048
Email: mfgree0@uky.edu
M.F. Greenwood, MD, Dir.
Activities/Fields: Pediatric oncology, including clinical trials and bone marrow transplantation.

★ 23898 ★ University of Kentucky
General Clinical Research Center
University of Kentucky Medical Center, Rm. MN578
800 Rose St.
Lexington, KY 40536-0293
Phone: (859)323-6623 **Fax:** (859)257-9560
Email: nkuku2@uky.edu
Website: http://www.mc.uky.edu/gcrc/
Hartmut Malluche, MD, Prog. Dir.
Activities/Fields: Major areas of investigation include aging, behavioral science, cardiology and biomedical engineering, gastroenterology, infectious diseases, neurology, nutrition, obstetrics and gynecology, oncology, pharmacy, psychiatry, pulmonary disorders and renal diseases.

★ 23899 ★ University of Kentucky
Gill Heart Institute (GHI)
Kentucky Clinic, Rm. L543
Division of Cardiovascular Medicine
740 S Limestone St.
Lexington, KY 40536-0284
Phone: (859)323-5479 **Fax:** (859)323-6475
Website: http://www.mc.uky.edu/ghi/
William T. Abraham, MD, Dir.
Activities/Fields: Atherosclerosis, coronary artery disease and heart failure, especially the mechanisms causing acute onset of these diseases.

★ 23900 ★ University of Kentucky
Lucille Parker Markey Cancer Center
800 Rose St.
Lexington, KY 40536-0093
Phone: (859)257-4500 **Fax:** (859)323-2074
Email: acohen@email.uky.edu
Website: http://www.mc.uky.edu/markey
Dr. Alfred M. Cohen, Dir. /CEO
Activities/Fields: Cancer research, including cancer etiology, cancer prevention and control, tumor immunology, hematologic malignancies, brain, gynecologic, breast, prostate, lung, head and neck and gastrointestinal cancers, experimental therapeutics, molecular biology/genetics/regulation, DNA repair and apoptosis. Core facilities include macromolecular structure, flow cytometry, tissue procurement, clinical research services, NMR spectroscopy/molecular modeling and transgenic mouse construction. **Pub:** *Electronic newsletter*, weekly. • *Program updates*, periodically.

★ 23901 ★ University of Kentucky
Metabolic Research Group (MRG)
919 S Limestone St.
Lexington, KY 40536-9841
Phone: (859)257-4058 **Fax:** (859)257-8410
Email: rlposk0@pop.uky.edu
Website: http://www.mc.uky.edu/nutritionresearch/Default.htm
James W. Anderson, MD, Dir.
Activities/Fields: Metabolic diseases, including diabetes, obesity, atherosclerosis, and high cholesterol.

★ 23902 ★ University of Kentucky
Prevention Research Center
Markey Cancer Center
2365 Harrodsburg Rd., Ste. B100
Lexington, KY 40504-3381
Phone: (859)219-0771 **Fax:** (859)219-0557
Email: swyatt@kcp.uky.edu
Stephen A. Wyatt, MD, Prin. Investigator
Activities/Fields: Public health issues, especially behaviors that place Americans at risk for chronic diseases and conditions. Of particular concern is the improvement in quality of life for special populations, including the young, elderly, racial ethnic populations, and the underserved.

★ 23903 ★ University of Kentucky
Radiation Therapy Oncology Center
UK Medical Center
800 Rose St.
Lexington, KY 40536
Phone: (859)323-6486 **Fax:** (859)257-4931
Email: mohmohi@uky.edu
Mohammed Mohiuddin, MD, Dir.
Activities/Fields: Radiation oncology research, participates in national cooperative group studies, RTOG, SWOG, NSABP, and GOG. Studies brain, bowel, head and neck cancer, and chemotherapy. Conducts research on radiation therapy, cancer treatment using radiation, hyperthermia, and chemotherapy.

★ 23904 ★ University of Kentucky
Sanders-Brown Center on Aging
101 Sanders-Brown Bldg.
Lexington, KY 40536-0230
Phone: (859)257-1412 **Fax:** (859)323-2866
Email: growles@aging.coa.uky.edu
Website: http://www.mc.uky.edu/coa
Graham Rowles, Assoc. Dir.
Activities/Fields: Biology of aging, including studies on aging nervous systems, Alzheimer's disease, stroke, hypertension in the elderly, immunology, geri-

atrics, and social-behavioral science. **Pub:** *Kentucky Atlas of the Elderly.* • *Sounding Board*, quarterly. **Frmly:** Multidisciplinary Center on Gerontology.

★ 23905 ★ University of Kentucky Sanders-Brown Center on Aging Alzheimer's Disease Research Center
101A Sanders-Brown Bldg.
Lexington, KY 40536-0230
Phone: (859)323-6040 **Fax:** (859)323-2866
Email: wmarkesbery@aging.coa.uky.edu
Website: http://www.mc.uky.edu/coa/ADRC/adrc.htm
William R. Markesbery, MD, Dir.
Activities/Fields: Alzheimer's disease, focusing on the cause, treatment, and eventual cure. **Pub:** *ADRC Update*, quarterly. Newsletter. • *Alzheimer's Disease Review.* Journal.

★ 23906 ★ University of Kentucky Sanders-Brown Center on Aging Stroke Program
101 Sanders-Brown Bldg.
800 S Limestone St.
Lexington, KY 40536-0230
Phone: (859)257-5560 **Fax:** (859)257-8990
Email: swillia@uky.edu
Website: http://www.mc.uky.edu/stroke
Dr. L. Creed Pettigrew, Dir.
Activities/Fields: Role of vitamins in stroke prevention and treatment of aphasia and related disorders; use of proteolysis in cerebral ischemia and apolipoprotein E in neuronal cell death.

★ 23907 ★ University of Kentucky Spinal Cord and Brain Injury Research Center (SCoBIRC)
226 Sanders-Brown Bldg.
Chandler Medical Center
800 S Limestone
Lexington, KY 40536-0230
Phone: (859)257-1412 **Fax:** (859)323-2866
Email: jgeddes@uky.edu
Website: http://www.mc.uky.edu/scobirc/default.asp
James W. Geddes, PhD, Dir.
Activities/Fields: Injuries to the spinal cord and brain that result in paralysis or other loss of neurologic function.

★ 23908 ★ University of Kentucky Tobacco and Health Research Institute (THRI)
Cooper & University Drs.
Lexington, KY 40546-0236
Phone: (859)257-5798 **Fax:** (859)323-1077
Email: mdavies@pop.uky.edu
Website: http://www.uky.edu/RGS/THRI/
Maelor Davies, Dir.
Activities/Fields: Application of biotechnology for the development of new crops based on the tobacco plant and the investigation of animal physiology related to the use of tobacco products.

★ 23909 ★ University of Louisiana at Lafayette New Iberia Research Center
4401 W Admiral Doyle Dr.
New Iberia, LA 70560
Phone: (337)482-2411 **Fax:** (318)373-0057
Email: bxs3829@louisiana.edu
Website: http://www.louisiana.edu/Research/NIRC/
Activities/Fields: Human disease research, animal models development, and pharmacology/toxicology research.

★ 23910 ★ University of Louisiana at Monroe Institute of Toxicology
Sugar Hall 306
700 University Ave.
Monroe, LA 71209
Phone: (318)342-1691 **Fax:** (318)342-1686
Email: pymenhendale@ulm.edu
Website: http://rxweb.ulm.edu/pharmacy/Mehendale/lithmpg.htm
Dr. Harihara M. Mehendale, Dir.
Activities/Fields: Molecular mechanisms by which chemicals (both drugs and environmental agents) cause harmful effects.

★ 23911 ★ University of Louisiana at Monroe Louisiana Drug and Poison Information Center
School of Pharmacy, Rm. 152
Monroe, LA 71209
Phone: (318)342-3648 **Fax:** (318)342-1744
Email: pydick@alpha.nlu.edu
Website: http://www.lapcc.org
Dr. Ronald M. Dick, Dir.
Activities/Fields: New poison antidotes, efficacy of current poisoning treatments.

★ 23912 ★ University of Louisville Birth Defects Center
501 S Preston St., Ste. 301
Louisville, KY 40292
Fax: (502)852-8309
Email: greene@louisville.edu
Website: http://www.louisville.edu/hsc/birthdefectscenter/director.htm
Prof. Robert M. Greene, PhD, Dir.
Activities/Fields: Molecular and molecular genetic aspects of embryonic development and congenital malformations. **Pub:** *Newsletter*, quarterly.

★ 23913 ★ University of Louisville Child Evaluation Center
571 S Floyd, Ste. 100
Louisville, KY 40202-3828
Phone: (502)852-5331 **Fax:** (502)852-0955
Email: jhhers01@gwise.louisville.edu
Joseph Herst, MD, Dir.
Activities/Fields: Developmentally disabled and handicapped children in Kentucky. Clinical research is conducted in support of the following clinical, evaluative, and consultative service programs: diagnosis and evaluation, learning disorders, genetics and dysmorphology, genetics testing, education and counseling, genetics laboratory, community clinics and outreach, hyperactive child treatment, infant therapy, behavior modification, diagnostic teaching, pastoral counseling, and cytogenetics laboratory.

★ 23914 ★ University of Louisville Health Promotion and Wellness Center
Crawford Gym
Louisville, KY 40292
Phone: (502)852-5711 **Fax:** (502)852-4534
Email: bryant@louisville.edu
Bryant A. Stamford, PhD, Dir.
Activities/Fields: Performs fitness analyses for county police departments, fire fighters, and commonwealth police. Also studies exercise routines.

★ 23915 ★ University of Louisville Henry Vogt Cancer Research Institute
James Graham Brown Cancer Center
529 S Jackson St., Rm. 430
Louisville, KY 40202-3256
Phone: (502)562-4369 **Fax:** (502)562-4368
Email: caw@bcc.louisville.edu
Website: http://www.bcc.louisville.edu/vogt/
Stephen C. Peiper, MD, Dir.
Activities/Fields: Molecular hematology/oncology, marrow transplantation, horomone receptors, anticancer drug development, molecular carcinogenesis, methods of drug delivery, laser therapy, growth factors, and drug disposition (clinical pharmacy).

★ 23916 ★ University of Louisville Institute for Cellular Therapeutics
570 S Preston St., Ste. 404
Louisville, KY 40202
Phone: (502)453-7823
Email: stilds01@gwise.edu
Website: http://louisville.edu
Suzanne T. Ildstad, MD, Dir.
Activities/Fields: Stem cell biology and bone marrow transplantation to fight disease. **Pub:** *Newsletter*, semiannually.

★ 23917 ★ University of Louisville Institute for Molecular Diversity and Drug Design (IMD3)
Department of Chemistry
Louisville, KY 40292
Phone: (502)852-5979 **Fax:** (502)852-3899
Email: spatola@louisville.edu
Website: http://www.imd3.org/
Dr. Arno F. Spatola, Dir.
Activities/Fields: Drug design, focusing on modern methods of rational and combinatorial lead generation, bioassays, structure optimization, including receptor selectivity, biostability, and pharmacokinetics, as well as process development and including bioinfomatics.

★ 23918 ★ University of Louisville Kentucky Lions Eye Center
301 E Muhammad Ali Blvd.
Louisville, KY 40202
Phone: (502)852-3716 **Fax:** (502)852-4595
Email: hank.kaplan@louisville.edu
Website: http://www.louisville.edu/medschool/ophthalmology
Dr. Henry J. Kaplan, Chm.
Activities/Fields: Visual sciences and eye diseases.

★ 23919 ★ University of Louisville Kidney Disease Program
615 S Preston St.
Louisville, KY 40202
Phone: (502)852-5757 **Fax:** (502)852-7643
Email: garonoff@e-mail.kdp-baptist.louisville.edu
Website: http://www.kdp-baptist.louisville.edu/deptovr.asp
George R. Aronoff, MD, Ch.
Activities/Fields: Kidney disease, focusing on the following areas: proteomics, cellular physiology, second messengers, biological transport, cellular immunology, transplantation, artificial membranes, dialysis, clinical pharmacology, pharmacokinetics, nephrotoxicity, drug metabolism, hypertension, and tissue typing. **Frmly:** Bioengineering Laboratory.

★ 23920 ★ University of Louisville Louisville Twin Study
Child Development Unit
Health Sciences Center
Louisville, KY 40292
Phone: (502)852-5140 **Fax:** (502)852-1093
Activities/Fields: Human behavior genetics, including a longitudinal study of twins and siblings from birth to early adulthood, assessment of temperament and mental development, biomedical studies of twins, and multivariate analyses of their cognitive, pe;ceptual, and motor skills.

★ 23921 ★ University of Maine Albert D. Conley Speech and Hearing Center
5724 Dunn Hall
Orono, ME 04469

Phone: (207)581-2006 **Fax:** (207)581-2060
Email: mboyd@maine.edu
Website: http://www.umaine.edu/comscidis/
Dr. Nancy E. Hall, Contact

Activities/Fields: Vocal development, speech and language disorders of adults and children, including aphasia, voice disorders, acquisition of language by children, stuttering, articulation disorders, apraxia, and interpersonal skills in clinical processes.

★ 23922 ★ University of Manitoba Alcohol and Tobacco Research Unit
MS-740B
Department of Community Health Sciences
820 Sherbrook St.
Winnipeg, MB, Canada R3A 1R9
Phone: (204)787-4514 **Fax:** (204)787-4547
Email: rmurray@hsc.mb.ca
Website: http://www.umanitoba.ca/faculties/medicine/chs/department/alcoh.html
Dr. Robert P. Murray, Contact

Activities/Fields: Health, behavioral, social and economic correlates and consequences of the use of alcohol, tobacco and other drugs consumed for non-therapeutic purposes.

★ 23923 ★ University of Manitoba Centre for Aboriginal Health Research
Department of Community Health Sciences
750 Bannatyne Ave.
Winnipeg, MB, Canada R3E 0W3
Phone: (204)789-3250 **Fax:** (204)975-7783
Email: cahr@umanitoba.ca
Website: http://www.umanitoba.ca/centres/cahr
John D. O'Neil, Dir.

Activities/Fields: Problems relevant to the health of Aboriginal and northern peoples in Canada. **Frmly:** Northern Health Research Unit.

★ 23924 ★ University of Manitoba Diabetes Research and Treatment Centre (DRTC)
Health Sciences Centre, Rm. GB409
820 Sherbrook St.
Room GB409
Winnipeg, MB, Canada R3A 1R9
Phone: (204)787-3381 **Fax:** (204)787-3279
Email: aangel@hsc.mb.ca
Website: http://www.umanitoba.ca/outreach/drtc/
Dr. Aubie Angel, Pres.

Activities/Fields: Diabetes, its treatment and awareness; health promotion, disease prevention.

★ 23925 ★ University of Manitoba Health, Leisure, and Human Performance Research Institute (HLHP)
307 Max Bell Centre
Winnipeg, MB, Canada R3T 2N2
Phone: (204)474-7087 **Fax:** (204)261-4802
Email: gardine2@ms.umanitoba.ca
Website: http://www.umanitoba.ca/faculties/physed/research
Dr. Phillip Gardiner, Dir.

Activities/Fields: Health and Wellness Research Group, Lifespan and Disability Research Group, Exercise and Environmental Medicine Research Group, Leisure and Tourism Research Group, Sport and Human Performance Research Group. **Frmly:** Sport and Exercise Sciences Research Institute.

★ 23926 ★ University of Manitoba Health Sciences Centre Surgical Research Office
Department of Surgery
GE 611-820 Sherbrook St.
Winnipeg, MB, Canada R3A 1R9
Phone: (204)787-3791 **Fax:** (204)787-7143
Email: hunruh@hsc.mb.ca
Dr. Helmut Unruh, Res. Dir.

Activities/Fields: Orthopedics, oncology, gastrointestinal surgery, neurosurgery, respirology, urology, cardiology, and pediatric and general surgery.

★ 23927 ★ University of Manitoba Manitoba Centre for Health Policy and Evaluation (MCHPE)
Department of Community Health Sciences
Faculty of Medicine
S101-750 Bannatyne Ave.
Winnipeg, MB, Canada R3E 0W3
Phone: (204)789-3819 **Fax:** (204)789-3910
Email: DeCoster@cpe.umanitoba.ca
Website: http://www.umanitoba.ca/centres/mchpe/
Noralou Roos, Dir.

Activities/Fields: How health care services are used by Manitobans. It examines patterns of illness in the population, and studies how people use health care services. It also researches the factors that affect health, since there is considerable evidence that many factors influence physical well-being, including income, education, employment, and social status, as well as nutrition, early childhood programs and even highway safety. **Pub:** *Annual report.* • *Newsletter.*

★ 23928 ★ University of Manitoba Manitoba Institute of Cell Biology
675 McDermot Ave.
Winnipeg, MB, Canada R3E 0V9
Phone: (204)787-2155 **Fax:** (204)787-2190
Email: lestera@ms.umanitoba.ca
Website: http://www.umanitoba.ca/institutes/manitoba_institute_cell_biology/

Activities/Fields: Molecular mechanisms of cancer and other diseases, through cell biology, genomics, molecular biology, biochemistry, experimental chemotherapy, and tumor immunology.

★ 23929 ★ University of Manitoba Manitoba Nursing Research Institute
Helen Glass Centre, Room 302
Winnipeg, MB, Canada R3T 2N2
Phone: (204)474-9080 **Fax:** (204)474-7683
Email: nursing_research@umanitoba.ca
Website: http://www.umanitoba.ca/nursing/research/mnri
Prof. Lorna Guse, PhD, Dir.

Activities/Fields: Health outcomes, and surveys of nurses.

★ 23930 ★ University of Manitoba Rheumatic Diseases Research Laboratory
805 John Buhler Research Centre
715 McDermot Ave.
Winnipeg, MB, Canada R3E 3P4
Phone: (204)789-3835 **Fax:** (204)789-3987
Email: jwilkin@cc.umanitoba.ca
Dr. John Wilkins, Sci. Dir.

Activities/Fields: Immunoregulatory abnormalities and inflammation in rheumatic diseases.

★ 23931 ★ University of Manitoba Spinal Cord Research Centre (SCRC)
Faculty of Medicine
436 Basic Medical Science Bldg.
730 William Ave.
Winnipeg, MB, Canada R3E 3J7
Phone: (204)789-3761 **Fax:** (204)789-3930
Email: info@scrc.umanitoba.ca
Website: http://www.scrc.umanitoba.ca/scrc/about.html
Prof. Larry M. Jordan, PhD, Dir.

Activities/Fields: Mechanisms controlling major functional systems in the brain and spinal cord and development of clinical tools for the treatment of injury and diseases affecting these systems.

★ 23932 ★ University of Maryland Biotechnology Institute Medical Biotechnology Center
725 W Lombard St.
Baltimore, MD 21201
Phone: (410)706-8181 **Fax:** (410)706-8184
Email: lederer@umbi.umd.edu
Website: http://www.umbi.umd.edu/~mbc/
W. Jonathon Lederer, MD, Dir.

Activities/Fields: Bioengineering, optical biology, biosensing, neurobiology, genetics molecular and cellular signalling, molecular cardiology, biology of aging, cellular biophysics, muscle biology, protein structure and function.

★ 23933 ★ University of Maryland Center for Alternative Medicine Research on Arthritis
Complementary Medicine Program
School of Medicine
2200 Kernan Dr.
Baltimore, MD 21207-6693
Phone: (410)448-6871 **Fax:** (410)448-6875
Email: bberman@compmed.ummc.edu
Brian M. Berman, MD, Prin. Investigator

Activities/Fields: The potential efficacy, safety, and cost-effectiveness of CAM therapies, including acupuncture treatment for osteoarthritis of the knee, mind/body therapies for fibromyalgia; electroacupuncture on persistent pain and inflammation; and a herbal combination with immunomodulatory properties.

★ 23934 ★ University of Maryland Center on Drugs and Public Policy
School of Pharmacy
100 N Greene St., 6th Fl.
Baltimore, MD 21201-1563
Phone: (410)706-0133 **Fax:** (410)706-5394
Email: fpalumbo@rx.umaryland.edu
Website: http://www.pharmacy.umaryland.edu/cdpp/
Dr. Francis B. Palumbo, JD, Dir.

Activities/Fields: Dug policy, legal and regulatory; drug utilization review; outpatient drug benefits under the OBRA 90; cost effective drug therapies; pharmaceutical care services; health outcomes related to drug therapy; pharmacoepidemiology, pharmacy manpower; the pharmaceutical industry; impact of changes in the organization and financing of health care services; and patient compliance with prescribed drug regimen.

★ 23935 ★ University of Maryland Division of Infectious Diseases
Medical School Teaching Facility
10 S Pine St., Rm. 900
Baltimore, MD 21201
Phone: (410)706-7560 **Fax:** (410)706-8700
Michael Bonnenberg, Hd.

Activities/Fields: Infections in the elderly, including infection from urinary catheterization, epidemiology of nursing home patients, tests of antimicrobial agents, and pharmacokinetics and microbiology using animal models and clinical techniques.

★ 23936 ★ University of Maryland Graduate Program in Molecular and Cell Biology
Microbiology Bldg.
College Park, MD 20742
Phone: (301)405-8422 **Fax:** (301)314-9921
Email: ia1@umail.umd.edu
Website: http://www.life.umd.edu/grad/mocb/index.html
Dr. Ibrahim Z. Ades, Dir.

Activities/Fields: Molecular genetics, cell biology, regulation of gene expression, molecular virology and immunology, membrane biochemistry, photoregulation, cell mobility, signal transduction, host-parasite interactions, transport channels, protein and enzyme and function, and neural processes.

★ 23937 ★ University of Maryland
Lamy Center on Drug Therapy and Aging
515 W Fayette St., 1st Fl.
Baltimore, MD 21201
Phone: (410)706-2434 **Fax:** (410)706-1488
Email: brucestuar@rx.umaryland.edu
Website: http://www.pharmacy.umaryland.edu/lamy
Bruce C. Stuart, PhD, Dir.
Activities/Fields: Geriatrics and gerontology, focusing on drug use in the elderly and the development of artificial intelligence programs in support of optimal drug use. **Pub:** *Eldercare News*, quarterly. Newsletter. **Frmly:** Center for the Study of Pharmacy and Therapeutics for the Elderly.

★ 23938 ★ University of Maryland
Maryland Center for Multiple Sclerosis
Neurology Department
11 S Paca St., 4th Fl.
Baltimore, MD 21201
Phone: (410)328-5605 **Fax:** (410)328-5425
Email: scoates@mdcms.org
Website: http://www.mdcms.org
Kenneth P. Johnson, MD, Dir.
Activities/Fields: Immunologic and virologic research in multiple sclerosis. Also conducts clinical trials of new treatment for multiple sclerosis.

★ 23939 ★ University of Maryland
Maryland Psychiatric Research Center
PO Box 21247
Baltimore, MD 21228-0747
Phone: (410)402-7666 **Fax:** (410)402-7198
Email: wcarpent@mprc.umaryland.edu
Website: http://www.mprc.umaryland.edu
Dr. William T. Carpenter, Jr., Dir.
Activities/Fields: Etiology and treatment of chronic schizophrenia and including assessment of therapeutic efficacy of treatment, design of safer approaches to antipsychotic and other drug treatments, definition of subgroups of patients to permit clinicians to match patients and treatments, design and implementation of experimental treatments. Neuroscience program studies brain mechanisms involved in the causes, manifestations, and treatment of mental illness. Provides clinical and diagnostic services and education for families and patients.

★ 23940 ★ University of Maryland
Maryland Stroke Center
655 W Baltimore St., Rm. 12-006
Baltimore, MD 21201-1559
Phone: (410)706-0414 **Fax:** (410)706-0816
Email: skittner@umaryland.edu
Dr. Steven Kittner, Dir.
Activities/Fields: Stroke in young adults, including genetics of stroke; recovery and neuroplasticity after stroke; acute interventions for stroke and secondary prevention after stroke; telemedicine. **Pub:** *Newsletter*, quarterly. **Frmly:** Clinical Stroke Research Center; Center for the Study of Cerebrovascular Disease and Stroke.

★ 23941 ★ University of Maryland
Medical Biotechnology Center
Institute of Human Virology
725 W Lombard St.
Baltimore, MD 21201
Phone: (410)706-8614 **Fax:** (410)706-1952
Robert C. Gallo, MD, Dir.
Activities/Fields: Chronic viral diseases and virally-linked cancers, specifically HIV/AIDS. **Pub:** *Discovery*, quarterly. • *Journal of Human Virology*, bimonthly.

★ 23942 ★ University of Maryland
Nutrition Laboratory
Henson Center, Rm. 2101
Department of Human Ecology
Princess Anne, MD 21853
Phone: (410)651-6056 **Fax:** (410)651-6207
Email: bwblakely@mail.umes.edu
Dr. Bettie Blakely, Contact
Activities/Fields: Nutrition and metabolism.

★ 23943 ★ University of Maryland
Obesity and Diabetes Research Center
Sch. of Medicine
10 S Pine St., Rm. 6-00MSTF
Baltimore, MD 21201
Phone: (410)706-3168 **Fax:** (410)706-7540
Email: bchansen@aol.com
Dr. Barbara Hansen, Dir.
Activities/Fields: Basic and applied research focusing on the mechanisms underlying the metabolic and endocrine disorders associated with obesity, diabetes and aging. Also studies hypertriglyceridemia, low HDL-cholesterol, hypertension, nephropathy, neuropathy, retinopathy and therapeutic agents for treatment of diabetes.

★ 23944 ★ University of Maryland
Pediatric Sleep Disorder Center
22 S Greene St., Rm. N5W65
Baltimore, MD 21201
Phone: (410)328-3363 **Fax:** (410)328-0645
Email: cblaisdell@peds.umaryland.edu
Dr. Carol Blaisdell, Dir.
Activities/Fields: Sudden Infant Death Syndrome (SIDS), including efforts to detect abnormalities present before or at death, correlation of data from clinical evaluation of infants at risk (especially those suffering from apnea or cyanosis), development of animal models to test hypotheses about the etiology of SIDS, examination of tissues from infants who have died from SIDS and other illnesses, animal studies to determine the relationship of specific tissue abnormalities to cause of death, and the psychological effect of infant death on family members. **Frmly:** Sudden Infant Death Syndrome Institute.

★ 23945 ★ University of Maryland
Pharmacokinetics/Biopharmaceutics Laboratory (PBL)
School of Pharmacy
100 N Penn St., AHB Rm. 540
Baltimore, MD 21201
Phone: (410)706-0884 **Fax:** (410)706-6580
Email: tdowling@rx.umaryland.edu
Website: http://rxsecure.umaryland.edu/research/tdowling/PBL.htm
Prof. Thomas C. Dowling, PhD, Contact
Activities/Fields: Pharmacokinetics, pharmacodynamics, and drug metabolism.

★ 23946 ★ University of Maryland
Women's Health Research Group (WHRG)
Howard Hall, Rm. 100E
Department of Epidemiology & Preventive Medicine
660 W Redwood St.
Baltimore, MD 21201
Phone: (410)706-3251
Email: plangenb@umaryland.edu
Website: http://medschool.umaryland.edu/womenshealth/
Patricia Langenberg, PhD, Dir.
Activities/Fields: Women's health issues, including menopause, hip fracture, breast cancer, osteoporosis, hormone replacement therapy, uterine fibroids, hysterectomy, caregiving, ovarian functioning, genetics, environmental toxins, health promotions, nutrition, and mental health.

★ 23947 ★ University of Maryland at Baltimore
Baltimore Hip Studies
Department of Epidemiology & Preventive Medicine
660 W Redwood St., Ste. 200
Baltimore, MD 21201
Phone: (410)706-3553 **Fax:** (410)706-4433
Email: jmagazin@epi.umaryland.edu
Website: http://gerontology.umaryland.edu/hipstudy.html
Jay Magaziner, PhD, Dir.
Activities/Fields: Recovery from hip fracture, including changes in functional ability, changes in bone mineral density, examination of markers of bone turnover, and the design and evaluation of interventions to enhance recovery from hip fracture.

★ 23948 ★ University of Maryland at Baltimore
Center for Celiac Research (CFCR)
22 S Greene St., Box 140
Baltimore, MD 21201
Phone: (410)706-8021
Email: afasano@peds.umaryland.edu
Website: http://www.celiaccenter.org/
Alessio Fasano, MD, Co-Med. Dir.
Activities/Fields: Celiac disease, including the prevalence of the disease worldwide; pathophysiology, autoimmune mechanisms, inflammatory processes, genetics of the disease; association with other autoimmune diseases; complications including infertility, osteoporosis and malignant transformation; and challenges of the treatment of the disease.

★ 23949 ★ University of Maryland at Baltimore
Center for Fluorescence Spectroscopy
School of Medicine
725 W Lombard St.
Baltimore, MD 21201
Phone: (410)706-8409 **Fax:** (410)706-8408
Email: cfs@cfs.umbi.umd.edu
Website: http://cfs.umbi.umd.edu/cfs
Joseph R. Lakowicz, PhD, Prin. Investigator
Activities/Fields: Fluorescence spectroscopy and its applications to the biological and medical sciences.

★ 23950 ★ University of Maryland at Baltimore
Center for Studies in Reproduction
Bressler Research Laboratory, Rm. 11-019
655 W Baltimore St.
Baltimore, MD 21201
Phone: (410)706-3391 **Fax:** (410)706-5747
Email: ealbrech@umaryland.edu
Website: http://csr.umaryland.edu/
Dr. Eugene D. Albrecht, Dir.
Activities/Fields: Reproductive biology, including reproductive neuroendocrinology and cellular reproductive endocrinology, cellular endocrinology, perinatal endocrinology, fetal-placental development, uterine and ovarian physiology and biochemistry, steroid regulation of cancer, ovarian embryology and physiology, neuroendocrine regulation of peptidergic neurons, neuroendocrinology of prolactin secretion, neuroendocrinology of aging, and cancer research.

★ 23951 ★ University of Maryland at Baltimore
Center for Vaccine Development (CVD)
685 W Baltimore St., Rm. 480
Baltimore, MD 21201-1509
Phone: (410)706-5328 **Fax:** (410)706-6205
Email: cvd@medicine.umaryland.edu
Website: http://medschool.umaryland.edu/CVD/som.html
Myron M. Levine, MD, Dir.
Activities/Fields: Bacterial diseases, parasitic diseases, viral diseases, novel delivery systems, combination vaccines and public health and policy.

★ 23952 ★ University of Maryland at Baltimore
Claude D. Pepper Older Americans Independence Center (UM-OAIC)
VA Medical Center, GRECC 18
10 N Greene St.
Baltimore, MD 21201

Phone: (410)605-7185 **Fax:** (410)705-7913
Email: apgoldbe@umaryland.edu
Website: http://gerontology.umaryland.edu/pepper.html
Andrew P. Goldberg, MD, Prin. Investigator
Activities/Fields: Effects of aggressive risk factor modification in the treatment of disability in older patients with claudication due to peripheral arterial disease (PAD) or congestive heart failure (CHF). The center conducts clinical trials to improve functional independence, reduce cardiovascular risk factors and enrich the lifestyle of such patients. There are also investigations in the pathophysiology and mechanisms by which exercise and diet rehabilitation collectively improve muscular, cardiovascular and metabolic function in older patients with PAD and CHF.

★ 23953 ★ University of Maryland at Baltimore
Geriatric Research, Education, and Clinical Center-Baltimore
Baltimore VA Medical Center, GRECC (BT/GR/18)
10 N Greene St.
Baltimore, MD 21201
Phone: (410)605-7185 **Fax:** (410)605-7913
Email: agoldber@grecc.umaryland.edu
Website: http://www.grecc.umaryland.edu/
Andrew P. Goldberg, MD, Dir.
Activities/Fields: Hormonal regulation of lipoprotein lipid, glucose, adipose metabolism; effects of interdisciplinary exercise and weight loss treatments of risk factors for cardiovascular disease in older people. **Pub:** *Advances in Aging.*

★ 23954 ★ University of Maryland at Baltimore
Greenbaum Cancer Center
22 S Greene St.
Baltimore, MD 21201
Phone: (410)328-7904 **Fax:** (410)328-8667
Website: http://www.umm.edu/cancer
Barry Meisenberg, MD, Dep. Dir.
Activities/Fields: Pharmacology, clinical pharmacology, infectious diseases, molecular biology, pathology, cytogenetics, immunology, electron microscopy, and drug and blood and marrow transplantation and combined modality treatment of cancer patients, with emphasis on acute leukemia, breast cancer, sarcomas, lymphomas, lung cancer, prostate cancer, breast and neck cancers and other solid tumors. Maintains programs in the following areas: the chemotherapeutic approach to cancer therapy and the development of experimental protocols; infectious disease relationship to cancer; cell component therapy and cellular replacement; critical care of cancer patients; angiogenesis; signal transduction; molecular and structure biology; hormonal therapy; biomarkers, viral carcinogenesis; pharmacology and the use of cancer chemotherapeutic agents; anti-cancer drug development; combined modalities treatments, biological treatment; cellular and molecular biology of cancer; supportive care; and pharmacokinetics and pharmacodynamics of antineoplastic agents.

★ 23955 ★ University of Maryland at Baltimore
National Study Center for Trauma and Emergency Medical Systems
School of Medicine
701 W Pratt St., 5th Fl.
Baltimore, MD 21201-1023
Phone: (410)328-5085 **Fax:** (410)328-3699
Email: cmack003@umaryland.edu
Website: http://nsc.umaryland.edu
Colin F. Mackenzie, MD, Dir.
Activities/Fields: Trauma, emergency medicine, and emergency medical systems.

★ 23956 ★ University of Maryland at Baltimore
Organized Research Center in Health Promotion and Disease Prevention
Department of Epidemiology & Preventive Medicine
Howard Hall, Ste. 109
660 W Redwood St.
Baltimore, MD 21201
Phone: (410)706-3450
Email: shavas@epi.umaryland.edu
Dr. Stephen Havas, Co-Dir.
Activities/Fields: Health promotion and disease prevention, especially prevention of cancer, heart disease, and stroke.

★ 23957 ★ University of Maryland, Baltimore County
Center for Health Program Development and Management (CHPDM)
1000 Hilltop Cir.
Baltimore, MD 21250
Phone: (410)455-6854 **Fax:** (410)455-6850
Email: jkaelin@chpdm.umbc.edu
Website: http://www.umbc.edu/chpdm/
John Kaelin, Exec. Dir.
Activities/Fields: Healthcare programs and policies, focusing on improving overall quality and purchaser value.

★ 23958 ★ University of Maryland, Baltimore County
Remote Sensing Signal and Image Processing Laboratory (RSSIPL)
ECS Bldg., Rm. 335
1000 Hilltop Cir.
Baltimore, MD 21250
Phone: (410)455-6583 **Fax:** (410)455-3969
Email: cchang@umbc.edu
Website: http://www.umbc.edu/rssipl/homepage.html
Dr. Chein-I Chang, Dir.
Activities/Fields: Remote sensing image processing, which includes target detection and classification; identification and quantification analysis; medical imaging, which includes breast cancer detection; MRI classification; enhancement and restoration of text and video images including low resolution expansion; text detection and tracking in video frames and automatic pattern recognition, which includes handwritten character recognition and shape analysis. **Pub:** *Conference papers. • Journal articles.*

★ 23959 ★ University of Maryland at College Park
Neuroscience and Cognitive Science Program
2239 Biology/Psychology Bldg.
College of Life Science
College Park, MD 20742
Phone: (301)405-8910 **Fax:** (301)314-9358
Email: nacs@umail.umd.edu
Website: http://www.inform.umd.edu/nacs
Dr. Arthur Popper, Dir.
Activities/Fields: Neurosciences, cognitive neuroscience, and computational neuroscience.

★ 23960 ★ University of Maryland at College Park
Public Health Informatics Research Laboratory (PHI)
Department of Health Education
Valley Dr., Ste. 2387
College Park, MD 20742-2611
Phone: (301)405-2522 **Fax:** (301)405-1654
Email: rg14@umail.umd.edu
Website: http://www.phi.umd.edu
Robert S. Gold, PhD, Dir.
Activities/Fields: Improvement of the health of populations through the appropriate use of technology.

★ 23961 ★ University of Massachusetts
Eunice Kennedy Shriver Center for Mental Retardation, Inc.
Medical School
200 Trapelo Rd.
Waltham, MA 02452-6319
Phone: (781)642-0001 **Fax:** (781)893-5340
Email: shriver.center@umassmed.edu
Website: http://www.umassmed.edu/shriver
Dr. William McIlvane, Dir.
Activities/Fields: Interdisciplinary studies in mental retardation and developmental disabilities, conducted through two research departments: Biomedical Sciences and Psychological Sciences. **Pub:** *Newsletter*, quarterly.

★ 23962 ★ University of Massachusetts at Amherst
Center for Neuroendocrine Studies (CNS)
Tobin Hall
Neuroscience & Behavior Program
135 Hicks Way
Amherst, MA 01003-7720
Phone: (413)545-1524 **Fax:** (413)545-0769
Email: blaustein@cns.umass.edu
Website: http://www.umass.edu/cns/
Prof. Jeffrey D. Blaustein, Dir.
Activities/Fields: Relationships among hormones, the brain, physiology, and behavior, including the relationship of environmental pollutants to reproduction and hormonal response, sexual differentiation of the nervous system and behavior, neuroendocrine control of circadian rhythms, and hormonal regulation of behaviors.

★ 23963 ★ University of Massachusetts at Amherst
Center for Nutrition in Sport and Human Performance (CNSHP)
210 Chenoweth
School of Public Health & Health Sciences
100 Holdsworth Way
Amherst, MA 01003-9282
Phone: (413)545-1076
Email: volpe@nutrition.umass.edu
Website: http://www.umass.edu/cnshp/index.html
Stella L. Volpe, PhD, Dir.
Activities/Fields: Issues at the interface of health, nutrition, and exercise or sport, especially the role of nutrition and exercise through the life span. **Pub:** *Brochure. • Coach's Newsletter.*

★ 23964 ★ University of Massachusetts at Amherst
Center for Research and Education in Women's Health (CREWH)
Arnold House
School of Public Health & Health Services
Amherst, MA 01003
Phone: (413)545-2529 **Fax:** (413)545-6536
Email: stoddard@schoolph.umass.edu
Website: http://www.umass.edu/sphhs/centers/womanh.html
Anne M. Stoddard, Dir.
Activities/Fields: Promotion and improvement of the health of women and girls across their life spans.

★ 23965 ★ University of Massachusetts at Amherst
Northeast Regional Environmental Public Health Center (NREPHC)
Morrill Science Center I, N233
Department of Environmental Health Sciences
School of Public Health & Health Sciences
639 N Pleasant St.
Amherst, MA 01003-9298
Phone: (413)545-3164
Email: edwardc@schoolph.umass.edu
Website: http://www.umass.edu/sphhs/centers/nrephc.html
Edward J. Calabrese, Contact

Activities/Fields: Environmental health, focusing on regional issues of national importance, namely the analysis, assessment, and remediation of contaminated soils and groundwater; and the biological effects of low levels of exposure.

★ 23966 ★ University of Massachusetts Lowell
Center for Health and Disease Research
3 Solomont Way, Ste. 4
Lowell, MA 01854-5125
Phone: (978)934-4501 **Fax:** (978)934-3025
Email: robert.nicolosi@uml.edu
Dr. Robert J. Nicolosi, Dir.
Activities/Fields: Chronic diseases with a focus on the diagnosis, treatment and prevention of heart disease, cancer, and neurodegenerative diseases including Alzheimer's disease. Also develops, evaluates, and assesses whole foods and certain micro nutrients with medical benefits and conventional pharmaceuticals, and medical devices and procedures. **Frmly:** Center for Chronic Disease Control.

★ 23967 ★ University of Massachusetts Lowell
Center for Public Health Research and Health Promotion
3 Solomont Way, Ste. 3
Lowell, MA 01854
Phone: (978)934-4461 **Fax:** (978)934-3006
Email: Barbara_Mawn@uml.edu
Website: http://www.uml.edu/res/misc/health.html
Dr. Barbara Mawn, Co. -Dir.
Activities/Fields: Health professions. **Frmly:** Center for Health Promotion; Center for Health Sciences, Health Promotion, and Public Health.

★ 23968 ★ University of Massachusetts at Worcester
Diabetes-Endocrinology Research Center
Medical School
373 Plantation St., Ste. 218
Worcester, MA 01605
Phone: (508)856-3800 **Fax:** (508)856-4093
Email: aldo.rossini@umassmed.edu
Dr. Aldo A. Rossini, Dir.
Activities/Fields: Diabetes, including autoimmunity of diabetic rats (Biobreeding/Worcester variety), renin secretion of kidney, lipid metabolism, lipid and growth factor receptors, neurotensin calcium metabolism and bone disease steroid action, and steroid receptors. **Pub:** *Annual Report.* • *Highlights.*

★ 23969 ★ University of Medicine and Dentistry of New Jersey
The Cancer Institute of New Jersey
195 Little Albany St.
New Brunswick, NJ 08901
Phone: (732)235-2465 **Free:** 877-864-3627
Fax: (732)235-6949
Website: http://www.cinj.org/
William N. Hait, MD, Dir.
Activities/Fields: Basic, clinical, population and translational cancer. Multidisciplinary programs include bone marrow/stem cell transplant, breast oncology, cancer risk assessment and genetic counseling, gastrointestinal/hepatobiliary oncology, general oncology service, genitourinary oncology, leukemia/lymphoma, melanoma and soft tissue oncology, neuro-oncology, pediatric hematology-oncology, Phase I/developmental therapeutics, symptom management supportive care, and thoracic oncology.

★ 23970 ★ University of Medicine and Dentistry of New Jersey
Center for Childhood Neurotoxicology and Assessment
St. Peters Medical Center
254 Easton Ave.
New Brunswick, NJ 08901
Phone: (732)745-8523 **Fax:** (732)249-6306
Email: glabbort@umdnj.edu
Website: http://es.epa.gov/ncer_abstracts/centers/cecehdpr/01/lambert.html
George Lambert, MD, Dir.
Activities/Fields: Influence of exposure to neurotoxicants on child neurological health and development with autism and related learning disabilities.

★ 23971 ★ University of Medicine and Dentistry of New Jersey
Dental Research Center
University Heights
185 S Orange Ave.
MSB-C-636
Newark, NJ 07103-2400
Phone: (973)972-3728 **Fax:** (973)972-0045
Email: finedh@umdnj.edu
Dr. Daniel H. Fine, Dir.
Activities/Fields: Host-bacterial interactions in infectious diseases, such as periodontal diseases, mucositis, colitis, cloning of virulence genes that enable attachment and penetration of noxious substances; mucus-drug interaction; synthesis, cotranslational, and posttranslational processing of mucus glycoproteins; sulfation; proteoglycans; and intergrins.

★ 23972 ★ University of Medicine and Dentistry of New Jersey
Lyme Disease Center
Medical Education Bldg., 484
1 Robert Wood Johnson Pl.
New Brunswick, NJ 08901
Phone: (732)235-7704 **Fax:** (732)235-7238
Email: sigallh@umdnj.edu
Leonard H. Sigal, MD, Dir.
Activities/Fields: Lyme disease, including epidemiology and clinical manifestations, immunopathogenesis, and the molecular biology of neurologic manifestations.

★ 23973 ★ University of Medicine and Dentistry of New Jersey
Robert Wood Johnson Medical School Clinical Research Center
1 Robert Wood Johnson Pl.
PO Box 19
New Brunswick, NJ 08903-0019
Phone: (732)418-8479 **Fax:** (732)418-8480
Email: gottliab@umdnj.edu
Website: http://rwjms.umdnj.edu/news/
Alice B. Gottlieb, PhD, Dir.
Activities/Fields: Immunology, dermatology, adult and pediatric clinical pharmacology, psoriasis.

★ 23974 ★ University of Medicine and Dentistry of New Jersey
Urology Research Laboratory
185 S Orange Ave., Rm. H516
Newark, NJ 07103-2714
Phone: (973)972-7728 **Fax:** (973)972-3892
Email: huanghf@umdnj.edu
Dr. Hosea F.S. Huang, Ch.
Activities/Fields: Interaction between retinoids and audiogens in the control of prostate cells and its role in prostate cancer. Effects of spinal cord injury on male reproduction and testing regimens to prevent such effects.

★ 23975 ★ University of Memphis
Center for Health Services Research
119 Mccord Hall
Division of Health Administration
Memphis, TN 38152
Phone: (901)678-2794 **Fax:** (901)678-2981
Email: peftzgrl@memphis.edu
Dr. Paul Fitzgerald, Dir.
Activities/Fields: Health services research, including health administration, health utilization and access, health finance, health policy and law, guardianship, medical malpractice, mental health policy and law, health ethics, research methodology in health services research, and health decision making.

★ 23976 ★ University of Memphis
Center for Research Initiatives and Strategies for the Communicatively Impaired (CRISCI)
807 Jefferson Ave.
Memphis, TN 38105
Phone: (901)678-5800 **Fax:** (901)525-1282
Email: mmendel@memphis.edu
Maurice I. Mendel, Dir.
Activities/Fields: Speech and hearing, especially high technology applications to habilitation and rehabilitation of the communicatively impaired. Contributes to master's and doctoral programs in speech and hearing sciences. **Pub:** *Reports.*

★ 23977 ★ University of Miami
Bascom Palmer Eye Institute
Department of Ophthalmology
School of Medicine
900 NW 17th St.
Miami, FL 33136
Phone: (305)326-6000 **Fax:** (305)326-6417
Website: http://www.bascompalmer.org
Dr. Carmen A. Puliafito, Dir.
Activities/Fields: Glaucoma, infectious and external corneal diseases, molecular biology and genetics, neurophysiology, ocular virology, ocular immunology, hereditary retinal diseases with special emphasis on Retinitis Pigmentosa, and ophthalmic applications of lasers and polymers. Also conducts studies to improve the techniques and technology related to patient care and the prevention of blindness.

★ 23978 ★ University of Miami
Bascom Palmer Eye Institute
Ophthalmic Biophysics Center
Department of Ophthalmology
PO Box 016880
Miami, FL 33101-6880
Phone: (305)326-6069 **Fax:** (305)326-6139
Email: jmparel@med.miami.edu
Prof. Jean-Marie Parel, Dir.
Activities/Fields: Development and refinement of ophthalmic devices, including testing and design of the Phaco-Ersatz, a lens substitute for intraocular lenses commonly used after cataract surgery, and the development of an implant to permit the sustained release of small amounts of medication over an extended period of time, as well as several glaucoma shunt-valves devices, a controlled iontophoresis system designed to non-invasively transfer drugs into the eye to avoid systemic side effects, and an artificial cornea. Additional research includes selection of individual lasers for ophthalmic use and testing of two high speed laser cutting systems designed to offer new precision and beam control for delicate surgeries.

★ 23979 ★ University of Miami
Behavioral Medicine Research Center (BMRC)
Department of Psychology
PO Box 248185
Coral Gables, FL 33124
Email: nschneid@miami.edu
Website: http://www.bmrc.miami.edu/
Neil Schneiderman, PhD, Dir.
Activities/Fields: Application of behavioral, psychosocial, and biomedical science knowledge to the prevention, etiology, diagnosis, treatment and rehabilitation of disease and illness.

★ 23980 ★ University of Miami Behavioral Medicine Research Center Center for Psycho-Oncology Research (CPOR)
Behavioral Medicine Research Bldg.
Department of Psychology
PO Box 248185
Coral Gables, FL 33124
Phone: (305)284-4186
Email: mantoni@miami.edu
Website: http://www.bmrc.miami.edu/research/cardiovascular/index.asp
Michael H. Antoni, PhD, Dir.
Activities/Fields: Interrelationships among cognition, emotion, biological processes, and physical health in patients with different forms of cancer including women with breast cancer, older men with prostate cancer, and women at high risk for cervical cancer due to co-infection with Human Immunodeficiency Virus and Human Papillomavirus.

★ 23981 ★ University of Miami Center on Aging and Disabilities
1400 NW 10th Ave., Ste. 601
Miami, FL 33136
Phone: (305)243-6397 **Fax:** (305)243-4804
Email: jsherman@med.miami.edu
Dr. Jean Sherman, Dir.
Activities/Fields: Future care planning for adults with developmental disabilities; pet therapy.

★ 23982 ★ University of Miami Center for Liver Diseases
Division of Hepatology
School of Medicine
1500 NW 12th Ave., No. 1101
Miami, FL 33136
Phone: (305)243-5787
Website: http://www.med.miami.edu/med/hepatology/laboratory.asp
Dr. Eugene R. Schiff, Dir.
Activities/Fields: Diseases of the liver and biliary tract.

★ 23983 ★ University of Miami Center for Tropical and Parasitic Diseases
Medical School
1600 NW 10th Ave.
Miami, FL 33136
Phone: (305)243-3116 **Fax:** (305)243-3888
Email: aager@med.miami.edu
Dr. Arba Ager, Dir.
Activities/Fields: All aspects of malaria, including malaria drug testing in rodents. Also conducts nutritional and chemotherapy research.

★ 23984 ★ University of Miami Cerebral Vascular Disease Research Center
Department of Neurology, D4-5
PO Box 016960
Miami, FL 33101-6960
Phone: (305)243-6449 **Fax:** (305)243-5830
Email: mdginsberg@stroke.med.miami.edu
Dr. Myron D. Ginsberg, Dir.
Activities/Fields: Cerebrovascular physiology, brain metabolism, and pathophysiology of cerebral ischemia/hypoxia, focusing on animal models of focal and global ischemia.

★ 23985 ★ University of Miami Cystic Fibrosis Research Center
PO Box 016820
Miami, FL 33101-6820
Phone: (305)243-6641 **Fax:** (305)243-6708
Email: gpiedimo@med.miami.edu
Dr. Giovanni Piedimonte, Dir.
Activities/Fields: Cystic fibrosis, asthma, pulmonary manifestations of pediatric AIDS, and respiratory diseases of children. Also studies pediatric exercise physiology and sleep and apnea disorders.

★ 23986 ★ University of Miami Diabetes Research Institute
School of Medicine
1450 NW 10th Ave.
Miami, FL 33136
Phone: (305)243-5300 **Fax:** (305)243-4404
Email: ricordi@miami.edu
Website: http://www.drinet.org
Camillo Ricordi, MD, Sci. Dir.
Activities/Fields: Etiology, pathogenesis, and treatment of diabetes mellitus, emphasizing the cure of diabetes through biological replacement strategies, particularly the study of the immunoregulatory defects that result in the destruction of the pancreatic beta cell as well as the transplantation of (allogeneic and/or xenogeneic) pancreatic islets cells in insulin-deficient diabetic animals and humans. Clinical investigations include new intervention studies to prevent progression of latent insulin-dependent diabetes to clinical diseases, and studies of new insulin analogues and evaluation of procedures to quantify high standards for care of patients with diabetes in community-based studies.

★ 23987 ★ University of Miami Ear Institute
PO Box 016960
Miami, FL 33101-6960
Phone: (305)243-4641 **Fax:** (305)243-5552
Email: ftelisch@med.miami.edu
Website: http://ent.med.miami.edu
Dr. Fred. F. Telischi, Dir.
Activities/Fields: Diseases of the ear and other communication disorders, with emphasis on implantable hearing aids and cochlear implants.

★ 23988 ★ University of Miami Institute for the Study of Culture and Nursing
School of Nursing
5801 Red Rd.
Coral Gables, FL 33143
Phone: (305)284-1553 **Fax:** (305)284-5686
Email: swalsh@miami.edu
Dr. S. Walsh, Dir.
Activities/Fields: Clinical nursing, focusing on serving multicultural populations and managing multicultural organizations.

★ 23989 ★ University of Miami Laboratory of Clinical and Applied Physiology
PO Box 248065
Coral Gables, FL 33124-8065
Phone: (305)284-3024 **Fax:** (305)284-5168
Email: aperry@miami.edu
Website: http://www.education.miami.edu
Dr. Arlette Perry, Dir.
Activities/Fields: Kinesiology, muscle cell and cardiovascular physiology, sports nutrition, obesity, electromyography, lipid physiology, exercise biochemistry, and health/exercise prescription. **Pub:** *American Journal of Clinical Nutrition.* • *International Journal of Sports Nutrition.* • *Journal of Applied Physiology.* • *Medicine and Science in Sports and Exercise.* **Frmly:** Human Performance Laboratory.

★ 23990 ★ University of Miami Mailman Center for Child Development
School of Medicine
1601 NW 12th Ave.
Miami, FL 33136
Phone: (305)243-6801 **Fax:** (305)243-5978
Email: darmstrong@miami.edu
Website: http://pediatrics.med.miami.edu/mailman/mailman.htm
F. Daniel Armstrong, PhD, Dir.
Activities/Fields: Developmental disabilities, genetic disorders, sensory disorders, and child behavior and development, including prevention and intervention strategies. **Pub:** *Annual Report.*

★ 23991 ★ University of Miami Marine and Freshwater Biomedical Sciences Center
Rosenstiel Sch. of Marine & Atmospheric Science
4600 Rickenbacker Cswy.
Miami, FL 33149-1098
Phone: (305)361-4738 **Free:** 888-232-8635
Fax: (305)361-4001
Email: pwalsh@rsmas.miami.edu
Website: http://www.rsmas.miami.edu/groups/niehs
Patrick J. Walsh, PhD, Dir.
Activities/Fields: Neurotoxicology, potent marine metabolites present in seafood, a description of a piscine model for human neurofibromatosis, environmental toxicants, fisheries models for hepatic metabolism, and development of sentinel species for xenobiotic evaluation.

★ 23992 ★ University of Miami Miami Project to Cure Paralysis
Mail Locator R-48
School of Medicine
PO Box 016960
Miami, FL 33101-6960
Phone: (305)243-7108 **Free:** 800-782-6387
Fax: (305)243-3913
Email: mpinfo@miamiproject.miami.edu
Website: http://www.themiamiproject.org
Maria Amador, Contact
Activities/Fields: Spinal cord injury (SCI), emphasizing characterization of SCI (magnetic resonance imaging, electron microscopy, experimental models, and electrophysiology); design of effective treatments (molecular neurobiology, neuroprotection, cell therapy, and tissue transplantation); and maximization of function (body weight support gait training, functional electrical stimulation, sexual function/male fertility, and motor-evoked potentials). **Pub:** *The Connection e-newsletter*, monthly. • *The Project Newsletter*, semiannually.

★ 23993 ★ University of Miami Sylvester Comprehensive Cancer Center
School of Medicine
1475 NW 12 Ave., Rm C002
Miami, FL 33136
Phone: (305)243-4918 **Free:** 800-545-2292
Fax: (305)243-4901
Email: wgoodwin@miami.edu
Website: http://www.sylvester.org
Dr. W. Jarrard Goodwin, Dir.
Activities/Fields: Cancer, including clinical investigation related to treatment of cancer, especially solid tumors and malignancies adults; molecular and cell biology as related to causation and pathogenesis of cancer; epidemiological research as related to environmental etiology of cancer in Florida and its prevention; and cellular differentation, cell population kinetics, epidemiology of cancer, viral oncology, and immunology.

★ 23994 ★ University of Miami Touch Research Institutes
Department of Pediatrics
Sch. of Medicine
PO Box 016820
Miami, FL 33101-6820
Phone: (305)243-6781 **Fax:** (305)243-6488
Email: tfield@med.miami.edu
Website: http://www.miami.edu/touch-research
Dr. Tiffany M. Field, Dir.
Activities/Fields: Sense of touch, including the biology of touch in health and development, and the role of touch therapy in medicine and the treatment of disease. Specific research areas include the use of massage in enhancing immune function in AIDS and cancer patients, massage effects on growth in prema-

ture infants, underlying mechanism responsible for the relationship between touch and physical growth and emotional development in infants and children, the role of massage in sports medicine and wound healing, the effects of touch therapy on addictive personalities, pain reduction during invasive medical procedures, and alleviation of skin disorders such as eczema and psoriasis. Studies the effects of touch on persons of all ages. **Pub:** *Touch Research Series.* • *Touchpoints Newsletter.*

★ 23995 ★ University of Miami Toxicology Laboratory
Bldg. B
12500 SW 152 St.
Miami, FL 33177-1411
Phone: (305)232-7020 **Fax:** (305)232-7461
Email: hchipw@aol.com
Chip Walls, Lab. Mgr.
Activities/Fields: Pesticides, air pollutants, carcinogens, and chemicals, with emphasis on biological, agricultural, and environmental samples. **Frmly:** Pesticide Residue, Toxic Waste and Basic Research Analytical Laboratory.

★ 23996 ★ University of Michigan Addiction Research Center
Substance Abuse Div.
Department of Psychiatry
400 E Eisenhower Pky. Ste. 2A
Ann Arbor, MI 48108-0740
Phone: (734)615-6060 **Fax:** (734)615-6085
Email: zuckerra@umich.edu
Website: http://www.med.umich.edu/psych/sub/index.html
Dr. Robert A. Zucker, Dir.
Activities/Fields: Developmental psychopathology and genetics of substance use disorders, alcohol problems among the elderly, etiology and treatment of alcoholism, treatment outcomes and other health services research with alcohol and other substance abusing patients, pharmacotherapy trials, efficacy of brief intervention techniques with alcohol abusing populations. **Frmly:** Alcohol Research Center.

★ 23997 ★ University of Michigan Antiviral Laboratory
4222 School of Dentistry
1011 N University Ave.
Ann Arbor, MI 48109
Phone: (734)763-5579 **Fax:** (734)764-4497
Email: jcdrach@umich.edu
Website: http://www.umich.edu/~websvcs/doughb/bms/people/drach.html
Dr. John C. Drach, PhD, Contact
Activities/Fields: Antiviral drugs, including the discovery of new antiviral drugs, how such drugs act at the genetic, cellular and biochemical level, and how they are metabolized in uninfected and virus-infected cells. Areas of research include viruses, herpes, and AIDS.

★ 23998 ★ University of Michigan Bacteriology Laboratory
3209 Sch. of Dentistry
1101 N University Ave.
Ann Arbor, MI 48109
Phone: (734)764-8386 **Fax:** (734)764-2110
Email: wloesche@umich.edu
Walter J. Loesche, PhD, Dir.
Activities/Fields: Oral bacteria and its role in human tooth decay and periodontal disease. Current studies focus on the development of diagnostic indicators of anaerobic infections in periodontal disease, the treatment of anaerobic infections, and the connection between good dental health, xerostomia, swallowing, cardiovascular disease, and aspiration pneumonia in senior citizens.

★ 23999 ★ University of Michigan Biochemical Engineering Laboratory
3324 H.H. Dow Bldg.
Department of Chemical Engineering
Ann Arbor, MI 48109-2136
Phone: (734)763-5659 **Fax:** (734)764-7453
Email: hywang@engin.umich.edu
Dr. Henry Y. Wang, Dir.
Activities/Fields: Biochemistry and biochemical engineering, including cell culture engineering and scale-up of genetically engineered microbial products and their bioseparation.

★ 24000 ★ University of Michigan Biomaterials Research Center
Department of Biologic & Materials Science
Sch. of Dentistry
1011 N University Ave.
Ann Arbor, MI 48109-1078
Phone: (734)763-9339 **Fax:** (734)647-5293
Email: wjobrien@umich.edu
Dr. William J. O'Brien, Dir.
Activities/Fields: Develops elastomers for dental prostheses and denture liners, polymerceramic composites for dental restorations, and advanced ceramics for crowns and bridges. Also establishes biocompatibility of dental materials. **Frmly:** Specialized Materials Science Research Center.

★ 24001 ★ University of Michigan Biomechanics Research Laboratory (BRL)
3216 G.G. Brown Bldg.
2350 Hayward St.
Ann Arbor, MI 48109-2125
Phone: (734)936-0366 **Fax:** (734)763-9332
Email: jaam@umich.edu
Website: http://www.engin.umich.edu/dept/meam/brl/
Dr. James A. Ashton-Miller, Dir.
Activities/Fields: How the brain coordinates and controls a myriad of muscles in human locomotion and how aging affects that control.

★ 24002 ★ University of Michigan Center for Craniofacial Regeneration
School of Dentistry, Rm. 3323
1101 N University Ave.
Ann Arbor, MI 48109-1078
Phone: (734)763-3388 **Fax:** (734)764-8046
Email: CCRegen@umich.edu
Website: http://www.umich.edu/~cboh
Laurie K. McCauley, DDS, Dir.
Activities/Fields: Mechanisms of development and regeneration of oral and craniofacial tissues, including bones, teeth, and oral mucosa; development of regeneration therapies to restore oral and craniofacial tissues. **Frmly:** Laboratories for Connective Tissue Research; Center for Biorestoration of Oral Health.

★ 24003 ★ University of Michigan Center for Human Growth and Development
300 N Ingalls Bldg., 10th Level
Ann Arbor, MI 48109-0406
Phone: (734)764-2443 **Fax:** (734)936-9288
Email: blozoff@umich.edu
Website: http://www.umich.edu/~chgdwww/
Dr. Betsy Lozoff, Dir.
Activities/Fields: Human growth and development through childhood and adolescence, including interdisciplinary studies on normal and abnormal behavioral, physical, and mental development, focusing especially on the challenges to children who grow up in adverse conditions. **Pub:** *Biennial Report.* • *Craniofacial Growth Monograph Series*, annually.

★ 24004 ★ University of Michigan Center for Neural Communication Technology
Electrical Engineering & Computer Science
1301 Beal Ave.
Ann Arbor, MI 48109-2122
Phone: (734)764-5252 **Fax:** (734)763-8041
Email: dja@eecs.umich.edu
Website: http://www.engin.umich.edu/facility/cnct/
Prof. David J. Anderson, PhD, Dir.
Activities/Fields: Design of silicon substrate multichannel microelectrodes for use in electrophysiology and clinical applications; device fabrication and post processing technologies such as coatings and packaging; use technology such as delivery systems, signal processing, and data handling.

★ 24005 ★ University of Michigan Center for Occupational Health and Safety Engineering (COHSE)
109 S Observatory
Ann Arbor, MI 48109-2029
Phone: (734)936-0757 **Fax:** (734)763-8095
Email: trobins@umich.edu
Website: http://www.engin.umich.edu/dept/ioe/COHSE/
Thomas G. Robins, MD, Dir.
Activities/Fields: Occupational and safety health issues.

★ 24006 ★ University of Michigan Clinical Research Laboratories
1324 Sch. of Dentistry
1011 N University Ave.
Ann Arbor, MI 48109
Phone: (734)764-9148 **Fax:** (734)936-0374
Email: homlay@umich.edu
Dr. Hom-Lay Wang, Dir.
Activities/Fields: Etiology of periodontal diseases, focusing on preventive and surgical methods; determining risk factors to predict and treat periodontal disease; assessment of the effectiveness of specific factors and materials in the regeneration of tissues lost through disease; and assessment of implant materials for optimal osseous integration.

★ 24007 ★ University of Michigan Comprehensive Cancer Center
1500 E Medical Center Dr., CCGC 6-303
Ann Arbor, MI 48109-0944
Phone: (734)647-8904 **Free:** 800-865-1125
Fax: (734)647-9271
Email: mwicha@umich.edu
Website: http://www.cancer.med.umich.edu/
Dr. Max S. Wicha, Dir.
Activities/Fields: Responsible for stimulating interest in cancer and clinical research in cell biology among faculty and students of the University and procurement of funds for support of their research. Funds dispensed on basis of formal applications submitted to the Committee.

★ 24008 ★ University of Michigan Diabetes Research and Training Center
Box 0580
1331 E Ann St., Rm. 5111
Ann Arbor, MI 48109-0580
Phone: (734)763-5730 **Fax:** (734)647-2307
Email: wherman@umich.edu
William H. Herman, MD, Dir.
Activities/Fields: Diabetes, including studies on thematic foci of islet hormone secretion and action and complications of diabetes. **Pub:** *MDRTC Newsletter.*

★ 24009 ★ University of Michigan Division of Nuclear Medicine
University Hospital
1500 E Medical Center Dr., B1G505
Ann Arbor, MI 48109-0028
Phone: (734)936-5388 **Fax:** (734)936-8182

Email: bshulkin@umich.edu
Dr. Barry Shulkin, Contact

Activities/Fields: Diagnosis and treatment of disease using radionuclides and radionuclide-labeled compounds. Develops methods of nuclear medicine procedures.

★ 24010 ★ University of Michigan Electrodiagnostic and Electromyographic Laboratory
1565 Kuehnle
Ann Arbor, MI 48103
Phone: (734)763-3367
Email: sew@umich.edu
Dr. Sven E. Widmalm, Dir.

Activities/Fields: Etiology and treatment of functional disturbances of the masticatory system, including disturbances of the muscles and joints of mastication.

★ 24011 ★ University of Michigan General Clinical Research Center
University Hospital, A7007
PO Box 0108
Ann Arbor, MI 48109-0108
Phone: (734)936-8080 **Fax:** (734)936-4024
Email: jwiley@umich.edu
Website: http://www.med.umich.edu/gcrc/
Dr. John Wiley, Dir.

Activities/Fields: Multicategorical research program geared to research on humans in support of clinical studies at department or subspecialty sectional level throughout the Medical School and the Hospital.

★ 24012 ★ University of Michigan Health Management Research Center
1027 E Huron St.
Ann Arbor, MI 48104-1688
Phone: (734)763-2462 **Fax:** (734)763-2206
Email: dwe@umich.edu
Website: http://www.umich.edu/~hmrc
Dr. D.W. Edington, Dir.

Activities/Fields: Examines the relationships between lifestyle behaviors, quality of life, organizational productivity, and health care costs. **Pub:** *Cost Benefit Analysis*, annually. **Frmly:** Fitness Research Center.

★ 24013 ★ University of Michigan Hypertension Division
Department of Internal Medicine
3918 Taubman Center
1500 E Medical Center Dr.
Ann Arbor, MI 48109-0356
Phone: (734)936-4790 **Fax:** (734)936-8898
Email: aweder@umich.edu
Website: http://www.med.umich.edu/intmed/hypertension
Dr. Alan B. Weder, Div. Ch.

Activities/Fields: Hypertension and hyperlipidemia, including pathophysiology of various forms of human hypertension, epidemiology, mechanism of action of drugs, and improvement of health care delivery.

★ 24014 ★ University of Michigan Immunology Laboratory
4208 School of Dentistry
1011 N University Ave.
Ann Arbor, MI 48109
Phone: (734)647-3912 **Fax:** (734)764-2425
Email: lopatin@umich.edu
Dr. Dennis E. Lopatin, Dir.

Activities/Fields: Aspects of the interactions between the oral microbial flora and the immune system. Studies address humoral immunity to specific oral microorganisms; cellular networks involved in the responses to different classes of antigens; oral factors that create risk for the development of a variety of diseases and negative health consequences such as caries, periodontal disease, aspiration pneumonia, cardiovascular disease, and immunochemical reagents for the identification of specific microorganisms in dental plaque.

★ 24015 ★ University of Michigan Institute of Gerontology
300 N Ingalls
Ann Arbor, MI 48109-2007
Phone: (734)764-3493 **Fax:** (734)936-2116
Email: brcarl@umich.edu
Website: http://www.IOG.umich.edu
Bruce M. Carlson, MD, Dir.

Activities/Fields: Gerontological research studies in the behavioral, biological, clinical, and social sciences and the humanities. **Pub:** *Annual Report.*

★ 24016 ★ University of Michigan Kresge Hearing Research Institute
1301 E Ann St.
Ann Arbor, MI 48109-0506
Phone: (734)764-8110 **Fax:** (734)764-0014
Email: carolet@umich.edu
Website: http://www.med.umich.edu/khri/
Dr. Jochen Schacht, Dir.

Activities/Fields: Auditory physiology and pathology, including studies on the reception, coding and processing of complex speech signals by the auditory system, transduction processes of the inner ear, cochlear blood flow and inner ear metabolism, development of cochlear prostheses and appropriate speech processor schemes, immune mediated hearing loss, the effects of age and environmental stress factors on hearing, biochemistry and motility of hair cells, afferent and efferent transmitters of the inner ear, psychophysics of hearing in normal individuals, immunology and immune systems related to squamous cell carcinoma, mechanisms of sound, localization, molecular biology and genetics of the inner ear, and human genetics (limkage studies).

★ 24017 ★ University of Michigan Kresge Hearing Research Institute Auditory Anatomy Laboratory
1301 E Ann St.
Ann Arbor, MI 48109-0506
Phone: (734)763-0060 **Fax:** (734)764-0014
Email: shuler@umich.edu
Website: http://www.khri.med.umich.edu/research/altschuler_lab/index.htm
Dr. Richard Altschuler, Dir.

Activities/Fields: Protective mechanisms to develop molecular interventions to reduce acquired deafness, such as from noise or ototoxic drugs; central auditory pathways, neurotransmitters, receptors and channels in normal function, how they change as a consequence of deafness and interventions to restore hearing; evaluate the risks of new otologic treatments and devices, including the cochlear prosthesis. **Frmly:** Otopathology Laboratory.

★ 24018 ★ University of Michigan Kresge Hearing Research Institute Auditory Prosthesis Animal Psychophysics Laboratory
Bldg. 0506, Rm. 4010
Ann Arbor, MI 48109-0506
Phone: (734)764-8110 **Fax:** (734)764-0014
Dr. Bryan Pfingst, Dir.

Activities/Fields: Restoration of hearing in profoundly deaf persons. Studies the processing of speech in the brain and encoding of speech in the auditory system, and uses hearing tests with rhesus monkeys, humans, and other animals to design and develop bionic ear implants, also called cochlear prostheses.

★ 24019 ★ University of Michigan Kresge Hearing Research Institute Biochemistry Laboratory
1301 E Ann St.
Ann Arbor, MI 48109-0506
Phone: (734)763-3572 **Fax:** (734)764-0014
Email: schacht@umich.edu
Website: http://www.med.umich.edu/khri/biochem/
Dr. Jochen Schacht, Dir.

Activities/Fields: Cellular and molecular mechanisms of hearing and deafness. Investigates the normal biochemical events that occur in cells of the inner ear when hearing and that are impaired in hearing disorders such as those induced by noise and certain drugs. Studies methods for ameliorating hearing loss.

★ 24020 ★ University of Michigan Kresge Hearing Research Institute Electrophysiology Laboratory
1301 E Ann St.
Ann Arbor, MI 48109-0506
Phone: (734)764-8110 **Fax:** (734)764-0014
Email: ddolan@umich.edu
David F. Dolan, PhD, Dir.

Activities/Fields: Electrical responses to sound in the inner ear. Studies the response of individual receptor cells, or hair cells, of one ear while the other ear is acoustically or electrically stimulated. Also investigates the relationship between hearing loss and hair cell loss.

★ 24021 ★ University of Michigan Kresge Hearing Research Institute Pharmacology Laboratory
1301 E Ann St.
Ann Arbor, MI 48109-0506
Phone: (734)764-8111 **Fax:** (734)764-0014
Email: sbledsoe@umich.edu
Dr. Sanford Bledsoe, Contact

Activities/Fields: Studies the chemical substances (transmitters), used in intercellular communication which mediate the transduction and encoding of sounds from the inner ear to the auditory structures of the brain. Also studies auditory physiology, psychophysics, molecular biology and genetics, clinical investigations of auditory function.

★ 24022 ★ University of Michigan Mental Health Research Institute
205 Zina Pitcher Pl.
Ann Arbor, MI 48109-0720
Phone: (734)764-4235 **Fax:** (734)647-4130
Email: rpfreed@umich.edu
Website: http://www.med.umich.edu/mhri
Ruth P. Freedman, Admin.

Activities/Fields: Biological and behavioral studies relevant to normal and pathological human behavior and treatment of mental illness. Conducts studies on basic biological mechanisms relevant to normal and pathological behavior. Emphasis on neuroscience and biological psychiatry. **Pub:** *MHRI Annual Report*, biennially.

★ 24023 ★ University of Michigan Michigan Alzheimer's Disease Research Center
Department of Neurology, TC 1914
300 N Ingalls, Rm. 3D05
Ann Arbor, MI 48109-0489
Phone: (734)764-2190 **Fax:** (734)936-8967
Email: sacuster@umich.edu
Website: http://www.med.umich.edu/madrc/
Sid Gilman, MD, Ch.

Activities/Fields: Alzheimer's disease and other neurodegenerative diseases associated with dementia, including Dementia with lewy bodies, Parkinson's disease, multiple system atrophy, progressive supranuclear palsy, and olivopontocerebellar atrophy. The effects on the health of caregivers of Alzheimer's disease patients is also studies. **Pub:** *Newsletter*, 3/year. Newsletter.

★ 24024 ★ University of Michigan Michigan Bone Health Study
Department of Epidemiology
School of Public Health
Ann Arbor, MI 48109-2029
Phone: (734)936-3892 **Fax:** (734)763-4552
Mary Fran Sowers, PhD, Chm.
Activities/Fields: Epidemiology of health and disease, including investigation of origins, nature, and interrelations of major chronic disorders, particularly cardiovascular diseases, diabetes, arthritis, chronic respiratory diseases, and cancer. Also studies biological, social, and physical variables of chronic disease, including environmental factors and stresses as observed in families, households, and other subgroups of the population. Focuses on interactions between constitutional/genetic factors and environmental influences. The Tecumseh Community Health Study, a continuing multidisciplinary, multifaceted investigation, has been underway since 1957 in a total community of 10,000 inhabitants, with the aim of identifying disease precursors and indices of susceptibility as early in life as possible, with a view to prevention. **Frmly:** Tecumseh Community Health Study.

★ 24025 ★ University of Michigan Michigan Gastrointestinal Peptide Research Center
6520 MSRB I
1150 W Medical Dr.
Ann Arbor, MI 48109-0682
Phone: (734)647-2942 **Fax:** (734)763-2535
Email: jcole@umich.edu
Website: http://www.med.umich.edu/mgpc
Chung Owyang, MD, Dir.
Activities/Fields: Gastroenterology, including chemistry and biology of gut hormones as they relate to the physiology and pathology of the digestive tract, liver cell differentiation, effect of nutrients on pancreatic endocrine and exocrine secretions, and neuroendocrine modulation of smooth muscle cell function and gut motility. **Frmly:** Gastroenterology Research Laboratory.

★ 24026 ★ University of Michigan Multipurpose Arthritis and Musculoskeletal Diseases Center
3918 Taubman Center, Box 0358
1500 E Medical Center Dr.
Ann Arbor, MI 48109-0358
Phone: (734)936-5566 **Fax:** (734)763-1253
Email: dcox@umich.edu
Website: http://www.research.umich.edu/proposals/proposal_dev/UM_Resources/Arthritis.html
David A. Fox, MD, Dir.
Activities/Fields: HLA-DRB1 allele-specific signaling aberration in rheumatoid arthritis, role of apoptosis in supraspinatus tendinosis, biomarkers of osteoarthritis and their epidemiology, cognitive and neurochemical function in fibromyalgia. Research focuses on biostatistics, flow cytometry, hydridoma, protein and carbohydate strcuture, transgenic animals, biomechanics and image processing, and DNA sequencing. **Pub:** *MAC Mainline Newsletter*, monthly.

★ 24027 ★ University of Michigan Neurobiology Laboratory
6223 School of Dentistry
1101 N University Ave.
Ann Arbor, MI 48109-1078
Phone: (734)763-1080 **Fax:** (734)764-2110
Email: rmbrad@umich.edu
Prof. Robert M. Bradley, Contact
Activities/Fields: Sensory and motor circuits, taste sensation, and associated reflexes, including salivation. Specific areas of study include the sense of taste, focusing on the cellular factors that regulate functional differentiation of salt taste pathways; interrelations between afferent taste input and brainstem control of salivary gland reflexes; and regeneration of peripheral taste nerves through micro-electrode arrays to develop a system from chronic, in vivo study of regenerated sensory nerve fibers.

★ 24028 ★ University of Michigan Neurosurgery Laboratory
Kresge Medical Research Bldg., Rm. 5550
Ann Arbor, MI 48109
Phone: (734)764-1207 **Fax:** (734)763-7322
Email: jhoff@umich.edu
Dr. J.T. Hoff, Dir.
Activities/Fields: Cerebral ischemia, edema, structure and function of central nervous system and its ability to sustain trauma, vascular insufficiency, and brain tumor oncogenesis.

★ 24029 ★ University of Michigan Orthopaedic Research Laboratories
400 N Ingalls Bldg.
Ann Arbor, MI 48109-0486
Phone: (734)763-9674 **Fax:** (734)647-0003
Website: http://www.orl.med.umich.edu/orl/orl.html
Dr. S.A. Goldstein, Dir.
Activities/Fields: Applies principles of engineering to understand the musculoskeletal system, investigates orthopedic clinical problems, and develops prosthetic devices for treatment of arthritis. **Frmly:** Biomechanics Trauma and Sports Medicine Laboratory.

★ 24030 ★ University of Michigan Pediatric Surgery Research Laboratories
F3970 Mott Children's Hospital
Ann Arbor, MI 48109-0245
Phone: (734)764-4151 **Fax:** (734)936-9784
Email: acoran@umich.edu
Arnold G. Coran, MD, Dir.
Activities/Fields: Pediatric surgery, including physiological and biochemical changes during septic and hemorrhagic shock in puppies, physiology and metabolism of patients receiving total parenteral nutrition, physiology of endorectal pull-through operations for Hirschprung's disease in dogs, determination of trace element levels in infants receiving oral feedings or total parenteral nutritional solutions, and bacterial translocation in newborn babies.

★ 24031 ★ University of Michigan Prevention Research Center of Michigan
School of Public Health
109 Observatory
Ann Arbor, MI 48109-2029
Phone: (734)763-5454 **Fax:** (734)763-5455
Email: nmclark@umich.edu
Website: http://www.sph.umich.edu/prc
Noreen Clark, PhD, Prin. Investigator
Activities/Fields: Public health issues, especially behaviors that place Americans at risk for chronic diseases and conditions. Of particular concern is the improvement in quality of life for special populations, including the young, elderly, racial ethnic populations, and the underserved.

★ 24032 ★ University of Michigan Prosthodontic Research Laboratory
1011 N University Ave., Rm. 1064
Ann Arbor, MI 48109-1078
Phone: (734)763-5280 **Fax:** (734)763-3453
Email: merim@umich.edu
Prof. Michael Razzoog, Dir.
Activities/Fields: Measures wear of prosthodontic devices and conducts serial and longitudinal biopsies of bone.

★ 24033 ★ University of Michigan Protein Folding and Stability Research Laboratory
Institute of Gerontology
300 N Ingalls St., Rm. 947
Ann Arbor, MI 48109-2007
Phone: (734)936-7685 **Fax:** (734)936-2116
Email: arigafni@umich.edu
Website: http://www.umich.edu/~protein/
Dr. Ari Gafni, Prin. Investigator
Activities/Fields: Mechanisms of protein folding and stability.

★ 24034 ★ University of Michigan Pulmonary and Critical Care Medicine Division
6301 MSRB 111
1150 W Medical Center Dr.
Ann Arbor, MI 48109-0642
Phone: (734)936-5010 **Fax:** (734)764-4556
Email: gtoews@umich.edu
Website: http://www.med.umich.edu/intmed/pulmonary
Dr. Galen B. Toews, Dir.
Activities/Fields: Pulmonary diseases and critical care, including cell biology, immunology, and biochemistry of lung and heart.

★ 24035 ★ University of Michigan Reproductive Sciences Program
300 N Ingalls Bldg., 11th Fl.
Ann Arbor, MI 48109-0404
Phone: (734)763-0247 **Fax:** (734)936-8620
Email: dlfoster@umich.edu
Website: http://www.umich.edu/~rspwww/
Douglas Foster, Chm.
Activities/Fields: Biological and behavioral aspects of reproduction, including clinical medicine relating to endocrinological disorders; neuroendocrine regulation of reproduction; morphological and functional studies on the hypothalmic-pituitary-gonadal axis; development of novel, nonradioactive analytical techniques; biosensors and on-line feedback control systems; biological signalling and chronobiology; neuroendocrine physiology and psychology; biochemical endrocrinology relevant to steroidogenesis and hormone action; molecular biology and gene expression; reproductive pharmacology; neurophysiological and sensory regulation of behavior; growth regulation; physical activity and its relationship to neuroendocrine function; biochemical, biological, and behavioral correlates of pregnancy; chemistry and immunology of hormones; synthesis, processing, and secretion of cellular products, including gonadotropins and extracellular matrix; calcium/calmodulin actions; and infertility research.

★ 24036 ★ University of Michigan Thoracic Surgery Research Lab
University Medical Center
Ann Arbor, MI 48109
Phone: (734)936-5800 **Fax:** (734)615-2656
Email: morrin@umich.edu
Dr. Mark Orringer, Sec. Hd.
Activities/Fields: Cardiovascular and pulmonary physiology and transplantations, cellular and molecular aspects of allograft rejection and tolerance, molecular genetics of human lung and esophageal cancer, regional ventricular function (using sonomicrometry measurements) in conditions of ischemia, infarction, and reperfusion, neonatal myocardial performance and protection of the neonatal heart during ischemia, and role of cytokines in cardiac and pulmonary injury.

★ 24037 ★ University of Michigan Trauma Burn Center
1500 E Medical Center Dr.
1 C-421-UH
Ann Arbor, MI 48109-0033
Phone: (734)936-9666 **Fax:** (734)936-9657
Email: traumaburn@umich.edu
Website: http://www.traumaburn.org/traumaburn/
Dr. Paul Taheri, Div. Ch.
Activities/Fields: Clinical research, standards review, and vaccine and plasma preparation to combat growth of gram negative organisms in burns. **Pub:** *International Bibliography on Burns.*

★ 24038 ★ University of Michigan
Unit for Laboratory Animal Medicine
018 Animal Research Facility
1301 E Catherine St.
Ann Arbor, MI 48109-0614
Phone: (734)764-0277 **Fax:** (734)936-3235
Email: ulamvets@umich.edu
Website: http://www.ulam.umich.edu
Howard G. Rush, Dir.
Activities/Fields: Biomedical sciences including comparative medicine, laboratory animal medicine, animal models for biomedical research, and proper use and care of laboratory animals. Provides veterinary care for all vertebrate animals used in research and education at the University.

★ 24039 ★ University of Michigan
University of Michigan Model Spinal Cord Injury Care System
University of Michigan Health System
Department of Physical Medicine & Rehabilitation
300 N Ingalls, Rm. NI2A09
Ann Arbor, MI 48109-0491
Phone: (734)763-0971 **Fax:** (734)936-5492
Email: model_sci@umich.edu
Website: http://www.med.umich.edu/pmr/model_sci/
David R. Gater, MD, Co-Dir.
Activities/Fields: Spinal cord injuries. **Pub:** *SCI ACCESS Newsletter*, semiannually.

★ 24040 ★ University of Michigan
Upjohn Center for Clinical Pharmacology
3709 Upjohn Center
School of Medicine
Ann Arbor, MI 48109-0504
Phone: (734)764-5468 **Fax:** (734)763-3438
Email: PLF@umich.edu
Dr. William D. Ensminger, Dir.
Activities/Fields: Clinical pharmacology.

★ 24041 ★ University of Michigan—Flint
Physical Therapy Cumulative Trauma Disorders Laboratory
WSW Bldg., Rm. 1113
Physical Therapy Department
School of Health Professions & Studies
Flint, MI 48502
Phone: (810)762-3373 **Fax:** (810)766-6668
Email: cpfalzer@umich.edu
Website: http://www.flint.umich.edu/departments/pt
Lucinda Pfalzer, PhD, Dir.
Activities/Fields: Cumulative trauma disorders in the workplace, particularly carpal tunnel syndrome. Also studies the biomechanical, lifestyle, psychosocial, and economic factors involved in injury prevention in the work place. **Pub:** *Instructional Video.* • *Practice Video and Booklet.*

★ 24042 ★ University of Minnesota
Biomedical Engineering Institute (BMEI)
MMC 609
420 Delaware St. SE
Minneapolis, MN 55455
Phone: (612)624-8483
Email: bmei@umn.edu
Website: http://www.bmei.umn.edu/contactus.htm
Jeffrey McCullough, MD, Dir.
Activities/Fields: Tissue and cell engineering, biocompatible materials, miniaturization technologies for implantable medical devices and bioanalysis, genomics and diagnostic devices and strategies derived from gene research, diagnostic and therapeutic instruments and devices incorporating advanced information processing, drug and gene delivery systems, and implementation of the mentioned technologies in animal and clinical trials. **Pub:** *Newsflash Newsletter.*

★ 24043 ★ University of Minnesota
Biomedical Genomics Center (BMGC)
Snyder Hall, Rm. 20
1475 Gortner Ave.
Saint Paul, MN 55108
Phone: (612)625-7736 **Fax:** (612)624-2785
Email: agac@umn.edu
Website: http://www.bmgc.umn.edu/about.html
Ashley Haase, Dir.
Activities/Fields: Prevention and treatment of disease in humans and animals. Research focuses on cancer genomics, pharmacogenomics, genomics of complex traits and disease, microbial pathogenomics, immunogenomics, stem cell genomics, structural genomics/proteomics, and genomics and bioethical, social and legal issues.

★ 24044 ★ University of Minnesota
Caenorhabditis Genetics Center
6-160 Jackson Hall
321 Church St., SE
Minneapolis, MN 55455
Phone: (612)625-2265 **Fax:** (612)625-4648
Email: stier@biosci.cbs.umn.edu
Dr. Robert K. Herman, Dir.
Activities/Fields: Acquisition, banking, distribution, and coordination of genetic nomenclature of Caenorhabditis elegans strains maintained for distribution to researchers. **Pub:** *Celegans Genetic Map.* • *Worm Breeder's Gazette.*

★ 24045 ★ University of Minnesota
Center for Computational Genomics and Bioinformatics (CCGB)
650 Children's Rehabilitation Center, MMC 43
420 Delaware St. SE
Minneapolis, MN 55455
Phone: (612)624-3993 **Fax:** (612)626-6069
Email: ernest@ccgb.umn.edu
Website: http://ccgb.umn.edu/info/mission/
Ernest Retzel, PhD, Dir.
Activities/Fields: Computational genomics and bioinformatics. Areas of focus include applied mathematics, algorithm and process development, distributed computing, data mining, visualization, collaboratory development, database infrastructure development, the development of scalable data warehouses and new query languages for genomics, genome biology and protein-related issues.

★ 24046 ★ University of Minnesota
Center for Environment and Health Policy
MNC 807
Mayo Memorial Bldg.
420 Delaware St. SE
Minneapolis, MN 55455
Phone: (612)626-4244 **Fax:** (612)626-0650
Email: ksexton@mail.umn.edu
Ken Sexton, Dir.
Activities/Fields: Center promotes the use of environmental, biological, and social science knowledge in the development of public policies relevant to environmental agents and their effects on the health of people. Center's focus is on applying existing scientific data to analyze environmental risks while considering economic, social, and political implications. Programmatic areas of the Center include risk analysis, risk communication, economic analysis, and legal/regulatory affairs.

★ 24047 ★ University of Minnesota
Center for Infectious Disease Research and Policy (CIDRAP)
Academic Health Center, MMC 263
420 Delaware St. SE
Minneapolis, MN 55455
Phone: (612)626-6770 **Fax:** (612)626-6783
Email: cidrap@umn.edu
Website: http://www.cidrap.umn.edu/cidrap/center/mission/
Michael T. Osterholm, PhD, Dir.
Activities/Fields: Epidemiology, prevention, and control of infectious diseases.

★ 24048 ★ University of Minnesota
Center for Magnetic Resonance Research Nuclear Magnetic Resonance Imaging and Localized Spectroscopy
2021 6th St. SE
Minneapolis, MN 55455
Phone: (612)626-9591 **Fax:** (612)626-2004
Email: kamil@cmrr.umn.edu
Website: http://www.cmrr.umn.edu
Kamil Ugurbil, PhD, Prin. Investigator
Activities/Fields: Development of high-resolution and high-contrast anatomic images of the human brain; functional images of the human brain for sensory and cognitive tasks; localized spectroscopy in humans; adiabatic pulses for imaging and multinuclear spectroscopy; and improved methods for chemical shift imaging, functional imaging, and single voxel localized spectroscopy.

★ 24049 ★ University of Minnesota
Center for Muscle and Muscle Disorders
Medical School, MMC 295
420 Delaware St. SE
Minneapolis, MN 55455-0374
Phone: (612)625-6180 **Fax:** (612)625-7950
Email: johnday@umn.edu
Website: http://www1.umn.edu/cmmd/
John Day, MD, Co-Dir.
Activities/Fields: Muscle function and disorders.

★ 24050 ★ University of Minnesota
Clinical Outcomes Research Center (CORC)
Department of Orthopaedic Surgery
Medical School
420 Delaware St. SE, MMC 492
Minneapolis, MN 55455
Phone: (612)273-7981 **Fax:** (612)626-6032
Email: corc@umn.edu
Website: http://www.hsr.umn.edu/corc/what_is_corc.htm
Marc F. Swiontkowski, MD, Co-Dir.
Activities/Fields: Outcomes of medical care, especially how the variations in the way health care is delivered relates to the outcomes of that care. **Pub:** *Annual report.*

★ 24051 ★ University of Minnesota
Coordinating Centers for Biometric Research
Division of Biostatistics
2221 University Ave. SE, Ste. 200
Minneapolis, MN 55414-3080
Phone: (612)626-8887 **Fax:** (612)626-9054
Email: biostat@ccbr.umn.edu
Website: http://www.biostat.umn.edu
John Connett, Div. Hd.
Activities/Fields: Cancer, AIDS, chronic obstructive pulmonary disease, coronary heart disease, otitis media (ear infection), and hypertension. Research activities include developing new statistical methodology; collaborating on applied projects that influence clinical, public health, and public policy; and applied and methodological research.

★ 24052 ★ University of Minnesota
Cystic Fibrosis Center
University of Minnesota Hospital
420 Delaware St. SE
Minneapolis, MN 55455
Phone: (612)626-4440 **Fax:** (612)624-0696
Email: milla005@tc.umn.edu
Dr. Carlos E. Milla, Dir.
Activities/Fields: Cystic fibrosis, pediatric pulmonary diseases, pulmonary physiology, infant pulmonary function, biochemistry of cystic fibrosis, nutrition, liver disease, inflamation, psychosocial intervention, home

monitoring, heart-lung and lung transplantation, sweat test, bioengineering, biophysics, and physical therapy. Activities include development of high frequency compression therapy. **Pub:** *CF Guidebook*.

★ 24053 ★ University of Minnesota
Dental Research Institute
18-104 Moos Tower
515 Delaware St. SE
Minneapolis, MN 55455
Phone: (612)626-3349 **Fax:** (612)626-7017
Email: dri@tc.umn.edu
Website: http://www1.umn.edu/dri/
Dr. Charles F. Schachtele, Dir.

Activities/Fields: Coordinates research and training proposals, pilot projects funding, space and equipment maintenance, and research faculty recruitment and development.

★ 24054 ★ University of Minnesota
Dental Research Institute
Minnesota Dental Research Center for Biomaterials and Biomechanics
16-212 Moos Health Sciences Tower
Sch. of Dentistry
515 Delaware St. SE
Minneapolis, MN 55455
Phone: (612)625-9636 **Fax:** (612)626-1484
Email: dougl001@tc.umn.edu
Website: http://web.dent.umn.edu
Dr. William Douglas, Dir.

Activities/Fields: Conducts research on the density dependent growth of dental and other bacterial plaques; neural pathways and electronic anaesthesia; and the development of simulated dental wear, including lubrication and friction of dental wear structures, toothbrush biomechanics, and the fracture toughness of dental hard tissues. Program missions include investigation of new evaluative technologies in biomechanics, service evaluation of biomaterials, and the clinical measurement of anatomic change in oral structures.

★ 24055 ★ University of Minnesota
Division of Health Services Research and Policy
Box 729
Mayo Memorial Bldg.
Minneapolis, MN 55455
Phone: (612)624-6151 **Fax:** (612)624-2196
Email: foote003@tc.umn.edu
Website: http://www.hsr.umn.edu
Susan Bartlett Foote, Div. Hd.

Activities/Fields: Long-term care, health insurance, managed health care, patient care outcomes, rural health services, and health policy analysis. **Pub:** *Institute News*, 3/year. • *Research brief*, monthly. **Frmly:** Institute for Health Services Research.

★ 24056 ★ University of Minnesota
Drug Delivery Center
Weaver-Densford Hall
308 Harvard St. SE
Minneapolis, MN 55455
Phone: (612)624-4433 **Fax:** (612)624-4974
Email: grant001@umn.edu
Website: http://www.ahc.umn.edu/ahc_content/colleges/Pharmacy/
Prof. David J.W. Grant, PhD, Dir.

Activities/Fields: Design, development and evaluation of novel systems for the delivery of therapeutic agents.

★ 24057 ★ University of Minnesota
Experimental Surgical Services Laboratories
MMC 220
420 Delaware St. SE
Minneapolis, MN 55455
Phone: (612)625-5914 **Fax:** (612)626-6949
Email: bianc001@tc.umn.edu
Website: http://www.ess-umn.com
Richard Bianco, Dir.

Activities/Fields: Cardiovascular surgery devices and techniques. **Frmly:** Cardiovascular Surgical Research Laboratories.

★ 24058 ★ University of Minnesota
General Clinical Research Center
420 Delaware St. SE, MC 8504
Minneapolis, MN 55455
Phone: (612)626-0476 **Fax:** (612)626-2456
Email: seaqu001@umn.edu
Website: http://www.gcrc.med.umn.edu
Dr. Elizabeth R. Seaquist, Prog. Dir.

Activities/Fields: Human disease, including normal and abnormal physiology and biochemistry in the human being, AIDS, cystic fibrosis, organ transplantation, human growth, carbohydrate metabolism, and a broad range of other medical areas.

★ 24059 ★ University of Minnesota
Hematology, Oncology and Transplantation Division
420 Delaware St. SE, Box 480
Minneapolis, MN 55455
Phone: (612)625-2654 **Fax:** (612)625-6919
Website: http://www.dom.umn.edu/hot
Cheryl Ptacek, Contact

Activities/Fields: Pediatric, surgical, medical, and radiation oncology in the areas of breast cancer, acute leukemia, lung cancer, lymphomas, testicular cancer, ovarian cancer, melanoma, and autologous marrow transplantation. Participates in cooperative group research, investigates local protocol, performs clinical analyses of malignancies. Conducts laboratory studies in signal transduction, gene regulation, biologic markers, cell differentiation, monoclonal antibodies, pharmacokinetics, cytogenetics, and molecular biology of normal and malignant cells. **Pub:** *Masonic Cancer Center News*, quarterly. **Frmly:** Masonic Cancer Center.

★ 24060 ★ University of Minnesota
Hormel Institute
801 16th Ave. NE
Austin, MN 55912
Phone: (507)433-8804 **Fax:** (507)437-9606
Email: zgdong@hi.umn.edu
Website: http://www.hi.umn.edu
Dr. Zigang Dong, Exec. Dir.

Activities/Fields: Biochemistry, molecular and cellular biology, developmental biology, cancer biology, membrane biology. Research related to molecular mechanisms of chemoprevention and chemotherapeutics; molecular mechanisms of cellular signal transduction; role of membrane lipids in heart disease and cancer. **Pub:** *Annual report*.

★ 24061 ★ University of Minnesota
Institute of Human Genetics
420 Delaware St. SE, MMC 206
Minneapolis, MN 55455
Phone: (612)624-9180 **Fax:** (612)626-0623
Email: faras001@umn.edu
Website: http://www.ihg.med.umn.edu/index.html
Dr. Anthony J. Faras, Dir.

Activities/Fields: Human genetics and developmental biology, including biochemical, molecular, and clinical genetics, cytogenetics, metabolism, and genetic counseling. Current research involves tumor viruses; gene transfer; eukaryotic gene regulation; rearrangement and regulation of immunoglobulin genes; molecular genetics of the major histocompatibility complex; genetic defects of human pigment genes; and bone marrow transplantation. **Pub:** *MicroChem News*.

★ 24062 ★ University of Minnesota
KDWB Variety Family Center
University Gateway/McNamara Alumni Center
200 Oak St. SE, Ste. 160
Minneapolis, MN 55455-2002
Phone: (612)626-3087 **Free:** 800-276-8642
Fax: (612)624-0097
Email: kdwb-var@umn.edu
Website: http://www.allaboutkids.umn.edu
Peggy Mann Rinehart, Exec. Dir.

Activities/Fields: Family dynamics and resiliency; self-regulation abilities; physical, emotional, psychological and social health and well-being for children and youth at risk, especially children and youth with disabilities. **Pub:** *Health Issues*. **Frmly:** Institute for Health and Disability; Center for Children with Chronic Illness and Disability.

★ 24063 ★ University of Minnesota
Lillehei Heart Institute
DVCCRC, Rm. 124, MMC 195
Academic Health Center
Medical School
425 E River Rd.
Minneapolis, MN 55455
Phone: (612)625-8988 **Fax:** (612)625-0404
Email: d-mcma@umn.edu
Website: http://www.lhi.umn.edu/
Dr. R. Morton Bolman, III, Exec. Dir.

Activities/Fields: Cardiovascular and respiratory health.

★ 24064 ★ University of Minnesota
Midwest Center for Occupational Health and Safety
School of Public Health
420 Delaware St. SE
Minneapolis, MN 55455
Phone: (612)626-0900 **Fax:** (612)626-4837
Website: http://www1.umn.edu/eoh
Ian A. Greaves, MD, Dir.

Activities/Fields: Occupational health and safety.

★ 24065 ★ University of Minnesota
Minnesota Molecular and Cellular Therapeutics Facility
1900 Fitch Ave.
Saint Paul, MN 55108
Phone: (612)624-8700 **Fax:** (612)624-1777
Email: john.s.coleman-1@tc.umn.edu
Website: http://www.ahc.umn.edu/mmct/
John S. Coleman, Dir.

Activities/Fields: Gene therapy, cell therapy (which involves the purification, expansion and genetic modification of blood and bone marrow cells), biotherapeutics, and educational issues.

★ 24066 ★ University of Minnesota
Minnesota Oral Health Clinical Research Center
17-116 Moos Health Sciences Tower
School of Dentistry
Minneapolis, MN 55455
Phone: (612)626-5722 **Fax:** (612)626-2651
Email: micha002@umn.edu
Website: http://www.dentistry.umn.edu/facultystaff/ohcrc211.html
Dr. Bryan Michalowicz, Contact

Activities/Fields: Dentistry, including materials and restorative sciences, oral facial pain and neuroscience, and caries and periodontal disease.

★ 24067 ★ University of Minnesota
National Teen Pregnancy Prevention Research Center
University Gateway
200 Oak St. SE, Ste. 260
Minneapolis, MN 55455-2002
Phone: (612)624-9111 **Fax:** (612)626-2134
Email: resni001@tc.umn.edu

Website: http://www.cdc.gov/prc/centers-minn.htm
Michael Resnick, PhD, Dir.

Activities/Fields: Public health issues, especially behaviors that place Americans at risk for chronic diseases and conditions. Of particular concern is the improvement in quality of life for special populations, including the young, elderly, racial ethnic populations, and the underserved.

★ 24068 ★ University of Minnesota
Pediatric Bone Marrow Transplantation
420 Delaware St. SE, MMC 366
Minneapolis, MN 55455-0374
Phone: (612)626-2961 **Fax:** (612)626-4074
Email: ramsa001@umn.edu
Website: http://www.peds.umn.edu/divisions/bmt/directory.html
Dr. Norma Ramsay, Dir.

Activities/Fields: Bone marrow transplantation.

★ 24069 ★ University of Minnesota
Rural Health Research Center
Division of Health Services Research & Policy
420 Delaware St. SE, MMC 729
Minneapolis, MN 55455-0392
Phone: (612)624-6151 **Fax:** (612)624-2196
Email: mosco001@umn.edu
Website: http://www.hsr.umn.edu/rhrc/
Ira Moscovice, PhD, Dir./Prin. Investigator

Activities/Fields: Health care needs of rural America, including rural health care financing, rural systems building, outcomes and delivery of care in rural areas. **Pub:** *Working papers.*

★ 24070 ★ University of Minnesota
Stem Cell Institute
515 Delaware St. SE
Minneapolis, MN 55455
Phone: (612)624-3921 **Fax:** (612)624-2436
Email: verfa001@umn.edu
Website: http://www1.umn.edu/stemcell/sci/sup8-6/pg/patch2gar2v2.shtml
Catherine Verfaillie, MD, Dir.

Activities/Fields: Potential of stem cells to improve human and animal health, especially in developing novel therapies for genetic and degenerative disorders.

★ 24071 ★ University of Mississippi
National Center for Natural Products Research (NCNPR)
Thad Cochran Research Center
School of Pharmacy
PO Box 1848
University, MS 38677
Phone: (662)915-1005 **Fax:** (662)915-1006
Email: ncnpr@olemiss.edu
Website: http://www.olemiss.edu/depts/ncnpr/
Dr. Larry Walker, Interim Dir.

Activities/Fields: Discovery and development of natural products for use as pharmaceuticals, dietary supplements, and agrochemicals, and understanding of the biological and chemical properties of medicinal plants. **Pub:** *Newsletter.*

★ 24072 ★ University of Mississippi
Pharmaceutical Marketing and Management Research Program
Waller Lab Complex, Rm. 101
University, MS 38677
Phone: (662)915-5948 **Fax:** (662)915-5262
Email: davidjm@olemiss.edu
Website: http://www.olemiss.edu/depts/rips/pmmrp/
Dr. David J. McCaffrey, III, Interim Coord.

Activities/Fields: Proprietary and inhouse marketing and management studies relating to pharmaceutical products, including formulary decision factors, generic substitution, reimbursement issues, medication compliance and consumer preferences. Conducts mail surveys, telephone interviews, focus groups, internet surveys, consumer reaction panels, and surveys of professionals at national and state meetings.

★ 24073 ★ University of Mississippi
Research Institute of Pharmaceutical Sciences
School of Pharmacy
University, MS 38677-1848
Phone: (662)915-7265 **Fax:** (662)915-5704
Email: wells@olemiss.edu
Website: http://www.olemiss.edu/depts/pharm_school/
Dr. Barbara G. Wells, Dean/Exec. Dir.

Activities/Fields: Discovery and design of important biologically active natural products; health services; toxicology studies on the fate and effects of environmental chemicals; pharmaceutical marketing and management. **Pub:** *Pharmacy Report*, semiannually.

★ 24074 ★ University of Mississippi
Research Institute of Pharmaceutical Sciences
Environmental Toxicology Research Program (ETRP)
University, MS 38677
Phone: (662)915-5759 **Fax:** (662)915-1285
Email: etrp@olemiss.edu
Website: http://www.olemiss.edu/depts/pharmacology/etrp/index.html

Activities/Fields: Identification and resolution of problems related to environmental health issues.

★ 24075 ★ University of Missouri—Columbia
Cosmopolitan International Diabetes Center
Columbia, MO 65212
Phone: (573)882-3818 **Fax:** (573)884-4609
Dr. David W. Gardner, Interim Dir.

Activities/Fields: Hormonal control of lipolysis, glycosylated proteins, and the effect of diabetic control on vascular complications of diabetes.

★ 24076 ★ University of Missouri—Columbia
Cystic Fibrosis Research Center
Health Science Center
Department of Child Health
Columbia, MO 65212
Phone: (573)882-6978 **Fax:** (573)882-2742
Email: konigp@missouri.edu
Peter Konig, MD, Dir.

Activities/Fields: Intracellular control mechanisms of secretion as they relate to cystic fibrosis, secretory mechanisms for water and electroytes in exocrine glands, structure and function of pulmonary glycoproteins in cystic fibrosis and other chronic pulmonary diseases, and therapies for pulmonary disease in cystic fibrosis.

★ 24077 ★ University of Missouri—Columbia
Exercise Physiology Graduate Program
217 Gwynn Hall
Department of Nutritional Sciences
Columbia, MO 65211
Phone: (573)882-4288 **Fax:** (573)882-0185
Email: thomastr@missouri.edu
Website: http://www.missouri.edu/~nutsci/exphy.htm
Tom R. Thomas, PhD, Contact

Activities/Fields: Exercise physiology, including calorie expenditure and different modes of exercise; exercise and blood lipoproteins.

★ 24078 ★ University of Missouri—Columbia
John M. Dalton Cardiovascular Research Center
134 Research Park Dr.
Columbia, MO 65211
Phone: (573)882-7586 **Fax:** (573)884-4232
Email: dalton@missouri.edu
Website: http://www.missouri.edu/~dalton/
Edward H. Blaine, PhD, Dir.

Activities/Fields: Multidisciplinary research in health science and related areas, emphasizing cardiovascular studies.

★ 24079 ★ University of Missouri—Columbia
Missouri Arthritis Rehabilitation Research and Training Center (MARRTC)
130 AP Green, DC 330.00
1 Hospital Dr.
Columbia, MO 65212
Phone: (573)882-6826 **Free:** 800-735-2966
Fax: (573)884-3020
Email: marrtc@health.missouri.edu
Website: http://www.muhealth.org/~arthritis/
Jerry C. Parker, PhD, Prin. Investigator

Activities/Fields: Arthritis and arthritis rehabilitation, including management of depression and disability in rheumatoid arthritis; an exercise self management program for persons with arthritis; impact of managed care on persons with arthritis; a vocational enablement program for persons with arthritis and related musculoskeletal diseases. **Pub:** *Newsletter "Arthritis Newsbreak"*, quarterly.

★ 24080 ★ University of Missouri—Columbia
Missouri Institute of Mental Health
5400 Arsenal St.
Saint Louis, MO 63139-1494
Phone: (314)644-8787 **Fax:** (314)644-8834
Email: weddingd@minh.edu
Website: http://www.mimh.edu
Danny Wedding, PhD, Dir.

Activities/Fields: Mental health policy and ethics, mental health information systems, computer applications for the assessment and treatment of the mentally retarded and mentally ill, outcomes assessments, and mental health program evaluation research. **Frmly:** Missouri Institute of Psychiatry.

★ 24081 ★ University of Missouri—Columbia
Missouri Model Spinal Cord Injury System (MOMSCIS)
Department of Health Psychology
1 Hospital Dr., DC-046.46
Columbia, MO 65212
Phone: (573)882-6271 **Free:** 800-720-6286
Fax: (573)884-7971
Email: momsics@health.missouri.edu
Website: http://www.hsc.missouri.edu/~momscis/
Larry Nossaman, Contact

Activities/Fields: Spinal cord injuries. **Pub:** *The Spinal Series newsletter*, semiannually.

★ 24082 ★ University of Missouri—Columbia
Radiation Oncology Program
Ellis Fischel Cancer Center
115 Business Loop 70 W
Columbia, MO 65203
Phone: (573)882-8644 **Fax:** (573)882-8817
Email: westgates@health.missouri.edu
Steven Westgate, Contact

Activities/Fields: Clinical protocols; national multi-institutional studies for cancer problems.

★ 24083 ★ University of Missouri—Columbia
Research Animal Diagnostic Laboratory
1600 E Rollins
Columbia, MO 65211
Phone: (573)882-5983 **Free:** 800-669-0825
Fax: (573)884-7521
Email: radil@missouri.edu
Website: http://www.radil.missouri.edu
Dr. Lela K. Riley, Dir.
Activities/Fields: Human health research through the use of animals. **Pub:** *Infectious Diseases.*

★ 24084 ★ University of Missouri—Kansas City
Clinical Research Center
650 E 25th St.
Kansas City, MO 64108
Phone: (816)235-2200 **Fax:** (816)235-5472
Email: williamsk@umkc.edu
Karen B. Williams, Dir.
Activities/Fields: Biochemistry, dental biomaterials, radiology, analgesics, and pathology, related to dentistry. Clinical programs include study of anomalies of oral region, hard and soft tissues, prosthodontics, occlusion, durapatite particles, prostaglandins and analgesic inflammation, orthodontics, pedodontics, oral diagnosis, periodontics, bone physiology, dental caries, and related pathoses. **Pub:** *Explorer*, quarterly. **Frmly:** Dental Research Program.

★ 24085 ★ University of Missouri—Kansas City
Laboratory Animal Center
1015 E 50th St.
Kansas City, MO 64110
Phone: (816)235-1681 **Fax:** (816)235-5275
Email: lac@umkc.edu
Bonnie Taylor, Proj. Mgr.
Activities/Fields: Physiology, exploratory surgery, and immunology.

★ 24086 ★ University of Missouri—St. Louis
Center for Neurodynamics
8001 Natural Bridge Rd.
Saint Louis, MO 63121
Phone: (314)516-5015 **Fax:** (314)516-6152
Email: mossf@umsl.edu
Website: http://neurodyn.umsl.edu
Dr. Frank Moss, Dir.
Activities/Fields: Study of the dynamical properties of neurons in the central nervous system.

★ 24087 ★ University of Missouri—St. Louis
Center for Trauma Recovery
Weinman Bldg., Lower Level
Department of Psychology
8001 Natural Bridge Rd.
Saint Louis, MO 63121
Phone: (314)516-6738 **Fax:** (314)516-7233
Email: resick@umsl.edu
Website: http://www.umsl.edu/divisions/artscience/psychology/CVRPResearch.html
Patricia A. Resick, PhD, Dir.
Activities/Fields: Posttraumatic stress disorder (PTSD), its causes and treatments.

★ 24088 ★ University of Montana
Primate Laboratory
Department of Psychology
Missoula, MT 59812-1584
Phone: (406)243-2091 **Fax:** (406)243-6366
Email: pyadp@selway.umt.edu
Website: http://www.cas.umt.edu/psych
Dr. Allen D. Szalda-Petree, Contact
Activities/Fields: Social and learning behaviors of developing monkeys, specifically rhesus monkeys (Macaca mulatta). Also conducts research in the use of computer video tasks to study discrimination learning, foraging behavior, and perceptual motor skills in primates. **Frmly:** Animal Behavior Laboratory.

★ 24089 ★ University of Montana
Research and Training Center on Disability in Rural Communities
52 Corbin Hall
Missoula, MT 59812
Phone: (406)243-5467 **Free:** 888-268-2743
Fax: (406)243-2349
Email: ruraldoc@selway.umt.edu
Website: http://rtc.ruralinstitute.umt.edu/
Tom Seekins, PhD, Dir.
Activities/Fields: Employment and vocational rehabilitation service needs of people with disabilities in rural areas; intervention development to improve employment outcomes; rural self-employment models; rural independent living; improvment of transportation, health care, housing, and accessibility; rural models for prevention of secondary disabilities; disability legislation and American Indian tribes; and alternative models of delivery of rural rehabilitation services. **Pub:** *Newsletter*, quarterly. **Frmly:** Research and Training Center on Rural Rehabilitation Services.

★ 24090 ★ University of Montana
Rural Institute: Center for Excellence in Developmental Disabilities Education, Research, and Service
52 N Corbin Hall
Missoula, MT 59812
Phone: (406)243-5467 **Free:** 800-732-0323
Fax: (406)243-4730
Email: rtvogels@selway.umt.edu
Website: http://www.ruralinstitute.umt.edu
R. Timm Vogelsberg, Dir.
Activities/Fields: Human resources and technical services for rural Americans with disabilities. Studies encompass the areas of employment, housing, transportation, health promotion, secondary conditions, special education, social work, guidance and counseling, physical medicine and rehabilitation, mechanical and rehabilitation engineering, business management, sociology, interpersonal communication, and psychology. **Pub:** *Child Care Plus.* • *Common Threads Newsletter.* • *Research Reports.* • *The Rural Exchange.* • *Transition Topics.* **Frmly:** Institute for Human Resources in Rural America; University Affiliated Rural Institute on Disabilities.

★ 24091 ★ University of Montreal
Biomedical Modeling Research Group (BMRG)
PO Box 6128, Downtown Sta.
Montreal, QC, Canada H3C 3J7
Phone: (514)343-7515 **Fax:** (514)343-6112
Email: roberge@igb.umontreal.ca
Website: http://www.igb.umontreal.ca/GRMB/EngHome.html
Fernard A. Roberge, Dir.
Activities/Fields: Computer simulation and mathematical modeling in cardiac electrophysiology, biomechanics of joints, and characterization of biological tissues by imaging.

★ 24092 ★ University of Montreal
Centre for Occupational Stress and Health
Sch. of Industrial Relations
Montreal, QC, Canada H3C 3J7
Phone: (514)343-7320 **Fax:** (514)343-5764
Dr. Shimon L. Dolan, Dir.
Activities/Fields: Diagnosis and intervention in the field of occupational stress, focusing on stress in police officers, social workers, hospital workers, executive personnel, and workers in other stressful occupations.

★ 24093 ★ University of Montreal
Clinical Research Institute of Montreal
Multidisciplinary Research Group on Hypertension
110 Pine Ave. W
Montreal, QC, Canada H2W 1R7
Phone: (514)987-5528 **Fax:** (514)987-5602
Email: schiffe@ircm.qc.ca
Dr. Ernesto L. Schiffrin, Dir.
Activities/Fields: Biochemistry; molecular biology; cellular physiology; pharmacology and clinical and experimental pathophysiology of hypertension, with an emphasis on the renin-angiotensin system, the neurobiology of hypertension, and the biology of blood vessels and the heart and kidney; the role of vasoactive peptides, particularly angiotensin, endothelin, and the role of endothelium; the effects of antihypertensive treatment on blood vessels of hypertensive patients; and the biochemical, molecular, and genetic determinants of elevated blood pressure and cardiac development and hypertrophy.

★ 24094 ★ University of Montreal
Experimental Neuropsychology Research Group
PO Box 6128, Downtown Sta.
Montreal, QC, Canada H3C 3J7
Phone: (514)343-2341 **Fax:** (514)343-5787
Email: franco.lepore@umontreal.ca
Dr. Franco Lepore, Dir.
Activities/Fields: Neural substrates of sensory-motor integration in animals and humans, focusing on the functional organization of sensory systems (vision, somesthesis, audition) in several animal species, especially monkeys and cats. Behavioral evaluation of humans with normal sensory-motor function (visual perception, visuomotor functions, audition), music perception, and humans with congenital or acquired cerebral damage (agenesis of the corpus callosum, hemispherectomies, and Alzheimer). Also studies various higher level cognition functions, such as language and memory both in normal subjects and neurologically or functionally anamolous subjects.

★ 24095 ★ University of Montreal
Fernand-Seguin Research Centre
Hopital Louis-H.-Lafontaine
7331 Rue Hochelaga
Montreal, QC, Canada H1N 3V2
Phone: (514)251-4015 **Fax:** (514)251-2617
Email: directeur.scientifique@crfs.umontreal.ca
André Lemieux, Dir.
Activities/Fields: Neurochemistry, including drug mechanisms of action; psychopharmacology, including pharmacodynamics and pharmacokinetics of psychoactive drugs; and psychosocial behavioral and clinical evaluations, including the development of psychotherapeutic methods, evaluation of programs, and societal problems.

★ 24096 ★ University of Montreal
Institute of Biomedical Engineering
Faculte de Medicine
PO Box 6128, Downtown Sta.
Montreal, QC, Canada H3C 3J7
Phone: (514)343-6357 **Fax:** (514)343-6112
Email: secretariat@igb.umontreal.ca
Website: http://www.igb.umontreal.ca
Activities/Fields: Cardiac electrophysiology, biomechanics, biomaterials, electrocardiology, biomedical modelling, neuromuscular physiology, medical imaging, medical instrumentati, and clinical engineering. **Pub:** *Annual Report.*

★ 24097 ★ University of Montreal
Interdisciplinary Health Research Group
CP 6128 Succursale Centre-Ville
Montreal, QC, Canada H3C 3J7
Phone: (514)343-6185 **Fax:** (514)343-2207
Email: gris@umontreal.ca

Website: http://www.medsp.umontreal.ca
Paul Lamarche, Dir.

Activities/Fields: Health services, including analysis of health care system, evaluation of interventions, studies of determinants of health in populations, and investigations of methodological and conceptual developments in the field of health services research. Specific projects conducted in areas of curative and preventive practices, global health care, behavior of professionals and organizations, health education, health promotion, and maternal and child health. **Pub:** *RUPTURES*, semiannually.

★ 24098 ★ University of Montreal Membrane Transport Research Group
PO Box 6128, Downtown Sta.
Montreal, QC, Canada H3C 3J7
Phone: (514)343-7924 **Fax:** (514)343-7146
Email: grtm@physio.umontreal.ca
Jean-Yves Lapointe, PhD, Dir.

Activities/Fields: Structure/function relationship of different types of membrane proteins, including ion channels, transporters, cotransporters, receptors, and toxins. Expression in heterologous systems, site-directed mutagenesis, electrophysiology, spectrofluorescence, radiolabeled substrate uptake, immunohistochemistry, computer simulation of atomic model, molecular dynamics, atomic force microscopy. Integrated role of the membrane and its proteins on a variety of physiological functions performed by the kidney, intestine, lung, liver, heart, blood vessels, bone. Studies of genetic diseases related to membrane protein malfunction.

★ 24099 ★ University of Montreal Montreal Heart Institute Research Centre
5000 Belanger St.
Montreal, QC, Canada H1T 1C8
Phone: (514)376-3330 **Fax:** (514)593-2540
Email: nattel@icm.umontreal.ca
Website: http://www.icm-mhi.org/english/default.asp
Dr. Stanley Nattel, Dir.

Activities/Fields: Cardiovascular physiology, pharmacology, molecular biology, and electrophysiology. Develops visualization techniques such as quantitative angiography, numerical angiography, and videodensitometry in echocardiography and nuclear medicine. **Pub:** *Annual Report.*

★ 24100 ★ University of Montreal Neurological Sciences Research Centre
C.P. 6128, succ.
centre-ville
Montreal, QC, Canada H3C 3J7
Phone: (514)343-6366 **Fax:** (514)343-6113
Email: crsn@physio.umontreal.ca
Website: http://www.crsn.umontreal.ca
Dr. Serge Rossignol, Dir.

Activities/Fields: Functions of the nervous system, including sensory motor functions, the cortical and subcortical control of rhythmical movements of the arm and the hand; the sensory motor system; sensory mechanisms concerning pain and plasticity; functional properties and localization of cell ensembles defined by their neurotransmitter in various regions of the brain; and functions of sleep, speech, and aging.

★ 24101 ★ University of Montreal Rehabilitation Institute of Montreal
6300 Darlington Ave.
Montreal, QC, Canada H3S 2J4
Phone: (514)340-2085 **Fax:** (514)340-2091
Email: treeves@ssss.gouv.qc.ca
Website: http://ireadapt.qc.ca
Mindy Levin, Sci. Dir.

Activities/Fields: Biomedical research, focusing on rehabilitation of patients suffering from spinal cord injury, amputation, stroke, and traumatic head injuries; behavioral research, including studies of the physical, psychological, and occupational obstacles that prevent brain-injured persons from being reintegrated into society; and rehabilitation engineering for upper- and lower-limb amputees.

★ 24102 ★ University of Montreal Research Centre, Hospital du Sacre-Coeur
5400 blvd. Gouin W
Montreal, QC, Canada H4J 1C5
Phone: (514)338-2172 **Fax:** (514)338-2694
Email: abastado@crhsc.umontreal.ca
Website: http://www.crhsc.umontreal.ca
Diane Abastado, Dir.

Activities/Fields: Biomedical modelling, pharmacology, and clinical studies of cardiac arrhythmias, with the aim of describing the spatial distribution of cardiac arrhythmias, their relationship to the nervous system, and their treatment by pharmacologic and noninvasive surgical methods. Centre also studies occupational respiratory diseases, biology of asthma, sleep disorders and neuropsychobiology, and molecular genetics of kidney diseases.

★ 24103 ★ University of Montreal Research Group on the Autonomic Nervous System
Department of Physiology/Faculty of Medicine
2900 blvd. Edouard-Montpetit
PO Box 6128, Downtown Sta.
Montreal, QC, Canada H3C 3J7
Phone: (514)343-7562 **Fax:** (514)343-2257
Email: grsna@ere.umontreal.ca
Dr. Jacques de Champlain, Dir.

Activities/Fields: Studies of the autonomic nervous system, focusing on cell and molecular biology of sympathetic neurotransmission, receptors, second messengers, cardiovascular regulation, and clinical research projects in hypertension and cardiac dysfunctions. **Pub:** *Annual Report.* Annual report.

★ 24104 ★ University of Montreal Riviere-des-Prairies Hospital Research Centre
7070 Blvd. Perras
Montreal, QC, Canada H1E 1A4
Phone: (514)323-7260 **Fax:** (514)323-4163
Email: jj.breton.hrdp@ssss.gouv.qc.ca
Dr. Jean-Jacques Breton, Dir.

Activities/Fields: Epidemiology of mental disorders, screening, suicide, autism, sleep disorders. **Pub:** *Journal Articles.*

★ 24105 ★ University of Montreal Sainte-Justine Hospital Research Centre
3175 Chemin de la Cote-Sainte-Catherine
Montreal, QC, Canada H3T 1C5
Phone: (514)345-4691 **Fax:** (514)345-4698
Email: levye@justine.umontreal.ca
Website: http://www.hsj.qc.ca
Emile Levy, Dir.

Activities/Fields: Basic and clinical research in the field of diseases of the mother and child, including cardiology and pulmonary medicine, endocrinology, gastroenterology, nutrition, orthopedics, and epidemiology. Studies also include hematology-oncology, immunology, microbiology, virology, medical genetics, nephrology, and obstetrics. **Pub:** *Annual Report.*

★ 24106 ★ University of Montreal Health Centre Research Centre
3850 Rue Saint-Urbain
Montreal, QC, Canada H2W 1T8
Phone: (514)890-8110 **Fax:** (514)412-7204
Email: hamet@umontreal.ca
Dr. Pavel Hamet, Dir.

Activities/Fields: AIDS, burns and after-effects, cancer and nutrition, cardiovascular diseases and hypertension, diabetes and nutrition, epidemiology, gastroenterology-heptology, hormone signaling and metabolism, imaging, immunology and host defense, medical genetics, respiratory electrophysiology, pulmonary diseases and anesthesia, gene and cellular therapy, including cardiovascular biochemistry, cellular biology of hypertension, experimental surgery, locomotion, microbiology, molecular endocrinology, gene medicine, molecular oncopathology, neurological sciences, nuclear medicine, oncology, pain and health research, clinical pharmacology and pharmacogenetics, pharmacoepidemiology and pharacoeconomics, population health and genetics, rheumatology, toxicology, and transplantation. **Frmly:** Montreal Research Centre, Hotel-Dieu.

★ 24107 ★ University of Nebraska—Lincoln Barkley Memorial Center
Barkley Center, Rm. 301
Lincoln, NE 68583-0738
Phone: (402)472-5496 **Fax:** (402)472-7697
Email: ereiners1@unl.edu
Website: http://www.unl.edu/barkley
John Bernthal, Dir.

Activities/Fields: Communication deficiency and disorder research, including study of brain stem audiometry; fluency, motor speech disorders, phonological, speech perception, language and learning disorders; behavioral impairment; hearing impairment; behavioral disorders and children with behavioral disorders; school violence; augmentative and alternative communication; and use of paraprofessionals in special education.

★ 24108 ★ University of Nebraska—Lincoln Nebraska Center for Virology (NCV)
E249A Beadle
Lincoln, NE 68588-0666
Phone: (402)472-4560
Email: cwood1@unl.edu
Website: http://www.unl.edu/virologycenter/
Dr. Charles Wood, Dir.

Activities/Fields: Infectious agents and the host responses that may lead to pathological changes, especially neuropathogenesis and apoptosis.

★ 24109 ★ University of Nebraska Medical Center Center for Neurovirology and Neurodegenerative Disorders (CNND)
985215 Nebraska Medical Center
Omaha, NE 68198-5215
Phone: (402)559-2797
Email: hegendel@unmc.edu
Website: http://www.unmc.edu/cnnd/
Dr. Howard E. Gendelman, Dir.

Activities/Fields: Neurodegenerative disorders, especially focusing on the concept that the pathophysiological basis for neurodegenerative disorders revolves around brain inflammation and the production of neurotoxic factors by glial cells.

★ 24110 ★ University of Nebraska Medical Center Eppley Institute for Research in Cancer and Allied Diseases
986805 Nebraska Medical Center
Omaha, NE 68198-6805
Phone: (402)559-4090 **Fax:** (402)559-4651
Email: kcowan@unmc.edu
Website: http://www.unmc.edu/Eppley/default.htm
Dr. Kenneth H. Cowan, Dir.

Activities/Fields: Mechanisms, causes, prevention, early diagnosis, and treatment of cancer, including programs in molecular, cellular and structural biology, and developmental therapeutics. **Pub:** *Annual Report.* • *Cancer Update Newsletter.* • *Eppley Facts.* • *Graduate Brochure.* • *Scientific Report.*

★ 24111 ★ University of Nebraska Medical Center
Hattie B. Munroe Center for Human Genetics
985440 Nebraska Medical Center
Omaha, NE 68198-5440
Phone: (402)559-5070 **Fax:** (402)559-9463
Email: wgsanger@unmc.edu
Website: http://www.unmc.edu/services/geneticslab
Warren G. Sanger, PhD, Dir.
Activities/Fields: Research and treatment concentrating in cancer cytogenetics and prenatal diagnosis, including lymphoma, leukemia, and solid tumor research, chromosome changes in response to treatment, diagnostics of chromosome abnormalities, and treatment of prenatal genetic conditions associated with mental retardation and disability.

★ 24112 ★ University of Nebraska Medical Center
Laboratory of Cell Stabilization
984515 Nebraska Medical Center
Department of Obstetrics & Gynecology
Omaha, NE 68198-4515
Phone: (402)559-6162 **Fax:** (402)569-6164
Email: pbturpen@unmc.edu
Website: http://www.unmc.edu/Olson/research/labas.htm
Paula B. Turpen, PhD, Dir.
Activities/Fields: Preservation of cellular information, specifically protein antigens and nucleic acids, for diagnosis and disease progression.

★ 24113 ★ University of Nebraska Medical Center
Molecular Reproductive Endocrinology Laboratory
Department of Obstetrics & Gynecology
Olson Center for Women's Health
600 S 42nd St.
Omaha, NE 68198-4515
Phone: (402)559-6163
Website: http://www.unmc.edu/Olson/research/labmre.htm
Shyamal K. Roy, PhD, Dir.
Activities/Fields: How preantral follicular growth is regulated by the orchestrated actions of pituitary gonadotropins and intraovarian peptide growth factors.

★ 24114 ★ University of Nebraska Medical Center
Munroe-Meyer Institute
985450 Nebraska Medical Center
Omaha, NE 68198-5450
Phone: (402)559-6400 **Free:** 800-65-MEYER
Fax: (402)559-5737
Email: mleibowi@unmc.edu
Website: http://www.unmc.edu/mmi/
Dr. Bruce Buehler, Dir.
Activities/Fields: Problems and needs of children and adults (medical, genetic, or behavioral), including interdisciplinary studies on congenital disorders, dentistry, infant development, language and cognitive disorders, behavioral disorders, and sensory/motor development. Subject populations include families receiving service at the Institute, infants, preschoolers, adolescents, and adults with developmental disabilities. **Pub:** *Annual Report.* **Frmly:** Meyer Rehabilitation Institute.

★ 24115 ★ University of Nebraska Medical Center
Nebraska Center for Rural Health Research
984350 Nebraska Medical Center
Omaha, NE 68198-4350
Phone: (402)559-5260 **Fax:** (402)559-7259
Email: kmueller@unmc.edu
Website: http://www.unmc.edu/rural
Keith J. Mueller, PhD, Dir.
Activities/Fields: Improvement of health care delivery in rural areas.

★ 24116 ★ University of Nebraska Medical Center
Signal Transduction Laboratory
983255 Nebraska Medical Center
Omaha, NE 68198-3255
Website: http://www.unmc.edu/Olson/research/labsig.htm
John S. Davis, PhD, Dir.
Activities/Fields: Cellular and molecular mechanisms that are responsible for relaying the actions of gonadotropins, growth factors, and cytokines in ovarian cells. The laboratory examines novel intracellular signal transduction pathways that govern cell survival and death, cell proliferation, cellular differentiation, gene expression, and steroidogenesis.

★ 24117 ★ University of Nebraska at Omaha
Pediatric Pulmonary and Cystic Fibrosis Research Center
985190 NE Medical Center
Omaha, NE 68198-5190
Phone: (402)559-6275 **Fax:** (402)559-7062
Email: jcolombo@unmc.edu
Dr. John L. Colombo, Dir.
Activities/Fields: Cystic fibrosis, including optimal use of antibiotics and respiratory therapy modalities; optimal use of aerosolized drug therapy; pancreatic function; effects of chronic aspiration, particularly on airway hyperactivity and inflammation; and bronchoalveolar lavage cytology in acute and chronic pediatric diseases.

★ 24118 ★ University of Nevada, Las Vegas
Exercise Physiology Laboratory
Box 3034
4505 Maryland Pky.
Las Vegas, NV 89154-3034
Phone: (702)895-3766 **Fax:** (702)895-4191
Email: golding@ccmail.nevada.edu
Website: http://www.lagolding.com
Dr. Lawrence A. Golding, Dir.
Activities/Fields: Primary function and research emphasis is the study of the biology of exercise. Studies include the physiological effect of both the immediate effect of exercise and the long range effect of physical training, the effect of the environment on physical performance (heat, humidity, cold, altitude, and pollution), the effect of aging on physical performance, and the impact of exercise on the older adult, the effects of drug use and diet supplement on physical performance, and a longitudinal study on the effect of regular exercise on coronary risk factors and aging.

★ 24119 ★ University of Nevada, Reno
Allie M. Lee Cancer Research Laboratory
Department of Biochemistry, Mail Stop 330
Reno, NV 89557
Phone: (775)784-4107 **Fax:** (775)784-1419
Email: ronp@cabnr.unr.edu
Dr. Ronald S. Pardini, Dir.
Activities/Fields: Nutritional intervention in the treatment of cancer with omega-3 fatty acids. Role of dietary fat in regulating tumor growth by altering expression of tumor suppressor genes and oncogenes, pharmacological investigations of natural products for the treatment of cancer.

★ 24120 ★ University of Nevada, Reno
Center of Biomedical Research Excellence (COBRE)
Department of Pharmacology MS/308
School of Medicine
Reno, NV 89557-0046
Phone: (775)784-6956 **Fax:** (775)784-1620
Email: joeh@med.unr.edu
Website: http://www.unr.edu/med/dept/pharmacology/COBRE/Default.htm
Joseph R. Hume, PhD, Dir.
Activities/Fields: Function and role of chloride channel transport proteins in cardiovascular disease.

★ 24121 ★ University of Nevada, Reno
Natural Products Lab
Department of Biochemistry, Mail Stop 330
Reno, NV 89557
Phone: (775)784-4107 **Fax:** (775)784-1419
Email: ronp@cabnr.unr.edu
Dr. Ronald S. Pardini, Dir.
Activities/Fields: Cancer, biochemical pharmacology, and oxidative stress, including investigations of biochemical mechanisms of antitumor drugs and evaluations of the role of oxidative stress in the anticancer activity of drugs.

★ 24122 ★ University of Nevada, Reno
Nutrition Education and Research Program
Redfield Bldg., Mail Stop 153
Sch. of Medicine
Reno, NV 89557
Phone: (775)784-4474 **Fax:** (775)784-4468
Email: sach@unr.edu
Dr. Sachiko T. St. Jeor, Dir.
Activities/Fields: Clinical nutrition.

★ 24123 ★ University of Nevada, Reno
Sanford Center for Aging
Reno, NV 89557
Phone: (775)784-4774 **Fax:** (775)784-1814
Email: weisslj@unr.edu
Website: http://www.unr.edu/hcs/sanford/
Dr. Lawrence J. Weiss, Dir.
Activities/Fields: Aging, especially as it relates to health ecology, nutrition psychology, sociology, nursing, and medicine.

★ 24124 ★ University of New Brunswick
Institute of Biomedical Engineering
PO Box 4400
25 Dineen Dr.
Fredericton, NB, Canada E3B 5A3
Phone: (506)453-4966 **Fax:** (506)453-4827
Email: biomed@unb.ca
Website: http://www.unb.ca/biomed
Dr. Bernard Hudgins, Dir.
Activities/Fields: Interaction of man and modern technology, particularly in health care. Research focuses on developing electronic control systems for artificial limbs, bioelectric signal processing, modeling of human operators and muscle function, applications of electronic instrumentation in orthopedics, medical imaging, ergonomics, exercise physiology, and biomechanics. **Frmly:** Bio-Engineering Institute.

★ 24125 ★ University of New Hampshire
Institute on Disability (IOD)
7 Leavitt Ln., Ste. 101
Durham, NH 03824-3522
Phone: (603)862-4320 **Fax:** (603)862-0555
Email: institute.disability@unh.edu
Website: http://www.iod.unh.edu/
Dr. Jan Nisbet, Dir.
Activities/Fields: Needs of individuals with severe disabilities. **Pub:** *Newsletters.*

★ 24126 ★ University of New Mexico
Artificial Muscle Research Institute (AMRI)
School of Engineering
School of Medicine
Albuquerque, NM 87131
Phone: (505)277-3966 **Fax:** (505)277-1571
Email: amri@unm.edu

Website: http://www.unm.edu/~amri/
Dr. Mohsen Shahinpoor, Dir.
Activities/Fields: Electrically and chemically controlled artificial muscles.

★ 24127 ★ University of New Mexico Cancer Research and Treatment Center
2325 Camino de Salud
Albuquerque, NM 87131
Phone: (505)272-4249 **Fax:** (505)272-6995
Email: lsklar@salud.unm.edu
Website: http://hsc.unm.edu/crtc/
Larry A. Sklar, PhD, Contact
Activities/Fields: Clinical investigations in growth-factor-supplemented high dose chemotherapy, hyperthermia, and various national cooperative group trials; tumor immunology; non-invasive diagnostic technology and development of magnetic resonance imaging; cell surface marker studies in hematopoetic and solid tumors; HPV/cervical cancer; hepatitis virus replication; HTLV-I and II; and cancer in Hispanics and Native Americans. Studies also include biology of natural killer cells and molecular mechanisms of immunosuppression, gene expression, signal transduction, oncogenes, and immune regulation.

★ 24128 ★ University of New Mexico Cancer Research and Treatment Center New Mexico Tumor Registry
2325 Camino de Salud NE
Albuquerque, NM 87131-5306
Phone: (505)272-5541 **Fax:** (505)272-8572
Email: ckey@nmtr.unm.edu
Website: http://hsc.unm.edu/epiccpro/
Dr. Charles R. Key, Co-Dir.
Activities/Fields: Cancer epidemiology, with emphasis on Hispanics and American Indians. Participates in the NCI's SEER (Surveillance Epidemiology and End Results) Program. **Pub:** *New Mexico Tumor Registry Newsletter*, quarterly.

★ 24129 ★ University of New Mexico Center for Health Promotion and Disease Prevention
Surge Bldg., Rm. 251
Health Sciences Center
2701 Frontier NE
Albuquerque, NM 87131-5311
Phone: (505)272-4462 **Fax:** (505)272-4857
Email: smdavis@unm.edu
Sally Davis, PhD, Prin. Investigator
Activities/Fields: Public health issues, especially behaviors that place Americans at risk for chronic diseases and conditions. Of particular concern is the improvement in quality of life for special populations, including the young, elderly, racial ethnic populations, and the underserved.

★ 24130 ★ University of New Mexico Clinical and Magnetic Resonance Research Center
1201 Yale Blvd. NE
Albuquerque, NM 87131-5021
Phone: (505)272-0760 **Fax:** (505)272-4056
Email: cford@salud.unm.edu
Website: http://cmrrc.unm.edu
Dr. Corey C. Ford, Contact
Activities/Fields: Magnetic resonance imaging and spectroscopy, neurology, multiple sclerosis, stroke, traumatic brain surgery, lupus, and schizophrenia. **Frmly:** Center for Non-Invasive Diagnosis.

★ 24131 ★ University of New Mexico Environmental Health Sciences Developmental Center
Internal Medicine, 5-ACC, Rm.5168
Albuquerque, NM 87131-5271
Phone: (505)272-4289 **Fax:** (505)272-4628
Email: nmniehs@salud.unm.edu
Website: http://www.niehs.nih.gov/centers/admin/unm.htm
Scott Burchiel, PhD, Dir.
Activities/Fields: Centers mission is to address the needs and concerns of Southwestern communities of New Mexico and the surrounding areas relating to environmental public health issues. The Center conducts basic and transnational research on regionally-relevant environmental public health issues. The main focus is directed on potential environmental causes of airway inflammation, asthma, cancer, and other environmental diseases.

★ 24132 ★ University of New Mexico General Clinical Research Center
915 Camino de Salud NE, MSC 10-5540
Albuquerque, NM 87131
Phone: (505)272-2366 **Fax:** (505)272-0266
Email: klegoza@salud.unm.edu
Website: http://hsc.unm.edu/gcrc/index.shtml
Selina Keryte, Prog. Mgr.
Activities/Fields: Diabetes, renal diseases, arthritis, premature infants, asthma, depression, hypertension. Provides inpatient, outpatient, and neonatal facilities (including laboratory, dietary, and nursing support) in support of clinical research.

★ 24133 ★ University of North Alabama Occupational and Environmental Health Laboratory
UNA Box 5211
Department of Chemistry & Industrial Hygiene
Florence, AL 35632-0001
Phone: (256)765-4474 **Fax:** (256)765-4958
Email: cefigueroa@una.edu
Dr. Crescente Figueroa, Contact
Activities/Fields: Conducts research in the areas of environmental health, industrial hygiene, and risk assessment.

★ 24134 ★ University of North Carolina at Chapel Hill Bowles Center for Alcohol Studies
CB 7178
Thurston-Bowles Bldg.
Chapel Hill, NC 27599-7178
Phone: (919)966-5678 **Fax:** (919)966-5679
Email: ftcrews@med.unc.edu
Website: http://www.med.unc.edu/alcohol/
Fulton T. Crews, PhD, Dir.
Activities/Fields: Broad range of studies on alcohol effects on brain, liver and fetus. **Pub:** *Centerline Newsletter*. **Frmly:** Center for Alcohol Studies.

★ 24135 ★ University of North Carolina at Chapel Hill Cecil G. Sheps Center for Health Services Research
CB 7590
725 Airport Rd.
Chapel Hill, NC 27599-7590
Phone: (919)966-5011 **Fax:** (919)966-5764
Email: tim_carey@unc.edu
Website: http://www.shepscenter.unc.edu
Timothy S. Carey, MD, Dir.
Activities/Fields: Aging, disability, and long-term care; child health services; health care economics and finance; health care organization; medical practice; mental health and substance abuse services and systems research; health professions and primary care; preventive health services; rural health research; and women's health research. **Pub:** *Consensus in DHHS Region IV: Women and Infant Health Indicators for Planning and Evaluation*. • *North Carolina Health Professions Data Book*. • *North Carolina Health Professions Fact Sheet*.

★ 24136 ★ University of North Carolina at Chapel Hill Cecil G. Sheps Center for Health Services Research North Carolina Rural Health Research and Policy Analysis Program (RHRP)
CB 7590
725 Airport Rd.
Chapel Hill, NC 27599-7590
Phone: (919)966-5541 **Fax:** (919)966-5764
Email: tom_ricketts@unc.edu
Website: http://www.schsr.unc.edu/research_programs/rural_program/rhp.html
Thomas C. Ricketts, PhD, Dir.
Activities/Fields: Rural health services. **Pub:** *Articles*. • *Findings briefs*. • *Reports*. • *Working papers*.

★ 24137 ★ University of North Carolina at Chapel Hill Center for AIDS Research (CFAR)
Lineberger Comprehensive Cancer Center, CB 7295
Chapel Hill, NC 27599
Phone: (919)966-8645
Email: mohr4me@med.unc.edu
Website: http://www.cfar.unc.edu/
Ronald I. Swanstrom, PhD, Dir.
Activities/Fields: Prevention, detection, and treatment of HIV infection.

★ 24138 ★ University of North Carolina at Chapel Hill Center for Environmental Medicine, Asthma, and Lung Biology
CB 7310
104 Mason Farm Rd.
Chapel Hill, NC 27599-7310
Phone: (919)962-0126 **Fax:** (919)966-9863
Email: pwspar@med.unc.edu
Website: http://www.med.unc.edu/envlung/welcome1.htm
Philip A. Bromberg, MD, Sci. Dir.
Activities/Fields: Environmental impacts on human health, including effects of inhaled agents on the respiratory system in diseased and healthy human subjects and on human cell lines and basic and clinical studies in environmental health sciences.

★ 24139 ★ University of North Carolina at Chapel Hill Center for Functional GI and Motility Disorders
CB 7080
Bioinformattics Bldg.
Mason Farm Rd.
Chapel Hill, NC 27599-7080
Phone: (919)966-0144 **Fax:** (919)966-8929
Email: douglas_drossman@med.unc.edu
Website: http://www.med.unc.edu/ibs
Douglas A. Drossman, MD, Co-Dir.
Activities/Fields: Physiological and psychosocial mechanisms underlying functional gastrointestinal and motility disorders, their impact on quality of life and health outcome, and their treatment. **Pub:** *Annual report*. • *Digest Newsletter*, quarterly. • *Educational Brochures*.

★ 24140 ★ University of North Carolina at Chapel Hill Center for Gastrointestinal Biology and Diseases (CGIBD)
CB 7555
Mason Farm Rd., Unit 49
Chapel Hill, NC 27599-7555
Phone: (919)966-1757 **Fax:** (919)966-7592
Email: cgibd@med.unc.edu
Website: http://www.niddk.nih.gov/
Robert Sandler, MD, Co-Dir.

Activities/Fields: Mechanisms of inflammation and fibrosis in the liver and intestine as they relate to inflammatory bowel disease.

★ 24141 ★ University of North Carolina at Chapel Hill
Center for Health Promotion and Disease Prevention
CB 7426
1700 Airport Rd.
Chapel Hill, NC 27599-7400
Phone: (919)966-6035 **Fax:** (919)966-6264
Email: across@unc.edu
Dr. Alan W. Cross, Dir.
Activities/Fields: Health promotion and disease prevention at state, regional, and national levels, focusing on women and minority health, children's health, tobacco and health promotion in the workplace.

★ 24142 ★ University of North Carolina at Chapel Hill
Center for Health Statistics Research (CHSR)
CB 2400
730 Airport Rd., Ste. 107
Chapel Hill, NC 27599-2400
Phone: (919)962-3282 **Fax:** (919)966-2221
Email: chsr@unc.edu
Website: http://www.sph.unc.edu/chsr/about_bottom.htm
Dr. William D. Kalsbeek, Dir.
Activities/Fields: Statistical design and analysis issues tied to research focusing on high-risk populations, especially that which leads to new insights in health promotion and disease prevention.

★ 24143 ★ University of North Carolina at Chapel Hill
Center for Research on Chronic Illness (CRCI)
Carrington Hall, CB 7460
School of Nursing
Chapel Hill, NC 27599
Phone: (919)966-0453 **Fax:** (919)966-0456
Email: crci@unc.edu
Website: http://nursing.unc.edu/crci/
Prof. Joanne S. Harrell, PhD, Dir.
Activities/Fields: Prevention and management of chronic illness in vulnerable people.

★ 24144 ★ University of North Carolina at Chapel Hill
Center for Thrombosis and Hemostasis
CB 7015
School of Medicine
Manning Dr.
Chapel Hill, NC 27599-7015
Phone: (919)966-6011 **Fax:** (919)966-6012
Email: margo_price@med.unc.edu
Website: http://www.med.unc.edu/thromb/
Gilbert C. White, II, MD, Dir.
Activities/Fields: Thrombosis and hemostasis; the genetics and molecular biology of blood coagulation, including recombinant factors VIII and VIIA and the rationale for treatment or prophylaxis of thrombosis and hemorrhage, including research on peptide growth factors, platelets, lipoprotein metabolism, von Willebrand factor, factor VIII, fibrinogen and fibrin assembly, fibronectin, protease inhibitors, heparin and antithrombins, endothelial cell culture, thrombin and prothrombin, and factor IX and its variants, factor X, acute phase reactants, actin filament system, and gene replacement therapy.

★ 24145 ★ University of North Carolina at Chapel Hill
Clinical Nutrition Research Center (CNRC)
2210 McGavran Greenberg
Chapel Hill, NC 27599-7400
Phone: (919)966-3474 **Fax:** (919)966-7216
Email: steven_zeisel@unc.edu
Website: http://www.cnrc.unc.edu/about.htm
Steven Zeisel, Dir.
Activities/Fields: Role of nutrition in health.

★ 24146 ★ University of North Carolina at Chapel Hill
Clinical Research Unit
809 Ruggles Dr.
Raleigh, NC 27603
Phone: (919)733-5227 **Fax:** (919)733-5869
Email: jlieberman@med.unc.edu
Jeffrey Lieberman, MD, Dir.
Activities/Fields: Schizophrenia, including but not limited to treatments dealing with first episode psychosis and treatment for refractory schizophrenia patients.

★ 24147 ★ University of North Carolina at Chapel Hill
Comprehensive Center for Inflammatory Disorders (CCID)
CB 7455
Dental Research Center, Rm. 101
Chapel Hill, NC 27599-7455
Phone: (919)966-1455 **Fax:** (919)966-3683
Email: ccid@dentistry.unc.edu
Website: http://www.dent.unc.edu/research/ccid/
Dr. Patrick Flood, Dir.
Activities/Fields: Mechanisms of oral inflammation and the relationship between inflammation and systemic medical conditions.

★ 24148 ★ University of North Carolina at Chapel Hill
Dental Research Center
CB 7450
Chapel Hill, NC 27599-7450
Phone: (919)966-1538 **Fax:** (919)966-3683
Email: pat_flood@dentistry.unc.edu
Website: http://www.dent.unc.edu/research/drc
Dr. Patrick Flood, Dir.
Activities/Fields: Oral health problems organized into several primary areas: biomaterials research, growth mechanisms, hemostasis research, mechanisms of mineralization, neural mechanisms, biology of extracellular matrices, viral properties and host-pathogen interaction in oral biology, involving both basic and clinical research. Studies problems in oral health related to growth, development, and function of craniofacial region.

★ 24149 ★ University of North Carolina at Chapel Hill
General Clinical Research Center
CB 7600, APCF
101 Manning Dr.
Chapel Hill, NC 27599-7600
Phone: (919)966-1435 **Fax:** (919)966-1576
Email: pbwatkins@med.unc.edu
Website: http://verne.med.unc.edu/home.html
Paul B. Watkins, MD, Dir.
Activities/Fields: Human physiology and pharmacology, including research on growth hormone, hemophilia, AIDS and other sexually transmitted diseases, stress and cardiovascular physiology, cystic fibrosis, drug metabolism and disposition in patients with hepatic and renal dysfunction, glomerular diseases, the neuropsychopharmacologic correlates of depression and other mental illnesses, cancer chemotherapy and immunotherapy, sickle cell anemia and related red blood cell diseases, and cardiac diseases such as congestive failure and arrhythmias.

★ 24150 ★ University of North Carolina at Chapel Hill
Histocompatibility Laboratory
1011 Anderson Pavilion
McLendon Clinical Labs
101 Manning Dr.
Chapel Hill, NC 27514
Phone: (919)966-4057 **Fax:** (919)966-7897
Email: jschmitz@unch.unc.edu
Dr. John Schmitz, Dir.
Activities/Fields: Diseases associated with histocompatibility antigens.

★ 24151 ★ University of North Carolina at Chapel Hill
Injury Prevention Research Center
Bank of America Bldg., Ste. 500
137 E Franklin St., CB 7505
Chapel Hill, NC 27599-7505
Phone: (919)966-2251 **Fax:** (919)966-0466
Email: iprc@unc.edu
Website: http://www.sph.unc.edu/iprc/
Carol W. Runyan, PhD, Dir.
Activities/Fields: Studies the epidemiology, prevention, acute care, and rehabilitation aspects of injuries, including workplace injury, road safety, violence, childhood injury, and program development and evaluation. **Pub:** *IPRC News.*

★ 24152 ★ University of North Carolina at Chapel Hill
Interactive Graphics for Molecular Studies and Microscopy
Sitterson Hall, CB 3175
Chapel Hill, NC 27599-3175
Phone: (919)962-1876 **Fax:** (919)962-1799
Email: rsuper@physics.unc.edu
Website: http://www.cs.unc.edu/research/nano/cismm
Dr. Richard Superfine, Prin. Investigator
Activities/Fields: The development of instruments and interfaces in microscopy so that individual macromolecules, viruses, and cells can be imaged, their properties can be measured, and they can be physically modified.

★ 24153 ★ University of North Carolina at Chapel Hill
Mutant Mouse Regional Resource Center
102 Mason Farm Rd.
Program in Molecular Biology & Biotechnology
Chapel Hill, NC 27599-3280
Phone: (919)962-2145 **Fax:** (919)966-6329
Email: tvdlab@med.unc.edu
Terry A. VanDyke, PhD, Prin. Investigator
Activities/Fields: Mouse models, especially in the areas of development and genomics, cardiovascular, and cancer; development of the ability to efficiently clone mice from somatic cells; development of reporter mouse strains that facilitate rapid phenotyping within particular cell/tissue types.

★ 24154 ★ University of North Carolina at Chapel Hill
National Center for Catastrophic Sports Injury Research
CB 8700
204 Fetzer Gymnasium
Chapel Hill, NC 27599-8700
Phone: (919)962-5171 **Fax:** (919)962-0489
Email: mueller@email.unc.edu
Website: http://www.unc.edu/depts/nccsi
Dr. Frederick O. Mueller, Dir.
Activities/Fields: Fatality and permanent injury in sports, especially football. **Pub:** *Annual Report.*

★ 24155 ★ University of North Carolina at Chapel Hill
Neurodevelopmental Disorders Research Center
CB 3366
7023 Neurosciences Hospital
Chapel Hill, NC 27599-3366
Phone: (919)843-8641 **Fax:** (919)966-8994
Email: joe_piven@med.unc.edu
Website: http://www.fpg.unc.edu/~NDRC/
Joe Piven, MD, Dir.

Activities/Fields: Pathogenesis and treatment of neurodevelopmental disorders.

★ 24156 ★ University of North Carolina at Chapel Hill
Neuroscience Center
Neurosciences Research Bldg., CB 7250
103 Mason Farm Rd.
Chapel Hill, NC 27599-7250
Phone: (919)966-4068 **Fax:** (919)966-1844
Email: william_snider@med.unc.edu
Website: http://www.neuroscience.unc.edu
William D. Snider, MD, Dir.
Activities/Fields: Prevention, diagnosis, and treatment of mental retardation and related aspects of human development utilizing a single disciplinary or interdisciplinary approach. Basic research is targeted at obtaining new knowledge of structure and function of the developing nervous system to be applied to other neurological and psychiatric illness. Studies include childhood autism, childhood hyperactivity with learning disabilities, genetic disorders associated with mental retardation, children whose nervous systems have been damaged by metallic environmental pollutants, and mentally retarded children whose aggressive stereotypic and self-injurious behavior requires that they be institutionalized. **Frmly:** Biological Sciences Research Center; Brain and Development Research Center.

★ 24157 ★ University of North Carolina at Chapel Hill
North Carolina Occupational Safety and Health Education and Research Center (NCERC)
3300 Hwy. 54 West
Chapel Hill, NC 27516-8264
Phone: (919)962-2101 **Free:** 888-235-3320
Fax: (919)966-7579
Email: oshercww@sph.unc.edu
Website: http://www.sph.unc.edu/osherc/
B. Rogers, Dir.
Activities/Fields: Occupational health and safety.

★ 24158 ★ University of North Carolina at Chapel Hill
Thurston Arthritis Research Center
CB 7280
3330 Thurston Bldg.
Chapel Hill, NC 27599-7280
Free: (866)827-2862 **Fax:** (919)966-1739
Email: coaina@med.unc.edu
Website: http://www.med.unc.edu/mac/
Dhaval Patel, MD, Dir.
Activities/Fields: Arthritis and autoimmune diseases. Laboratory research focuses on immunogenetics, immunoregulation, molecular biology, animal models, and complement studies. Non-laboratory research emphasizes social, behavioral, epidemiology, and educational aspects of chronic arthritis. **Frmly:** Multipurpose Arthritis Center.

★ 24159 ★ University of North Carolina at Chapel Hill
UNC Lineberger Comprehensive Cancer Center
CB 7295, Lineberger
School of Medicine
Chapel Hill, NC 27599-7295
Phone: (919)966-3036 **Fax:** (919)966-3015
Email: dgs@med.unc.edu
Website: http://cancer.med.unc.edu
Dr. Dianne Shaw, Contact
Activities/Fields: Cancer cell biology, immunology, molecular carcinogenesis, molecular therapeutics, virology, cancer genetics clinical research, breast cancer, radiobiology and imaging, cancer epidemiology, and cancer prevention and control. **Pub:** *Newsletter.*

★ 24160 ★ University of North Carolina at Greensboro
Institute for Health, Science, and Society (IHSS)
PO Box 26170
Greensboro, NC 27402-6170
Phone: (336)334-4775 **Fax:** (336)334-4794
Email: health_institute@uncg.edu
Website: http://www.uncg.edu/ihs/
Jennifer Kimbrough, Asst. Dir.
Activities/Fields: Health and health care needs, especially child/adolescent health, obesity prevention, alcohol/tobacco prevention, genomic medicine, proteonics. **Pub:** *Guilford County Health Trends 1991-1998.*

★ 24161 ★ University of North Dakota
Center for Rural Health
School of Medicine & Health Sciences
PO Box 9037
Grand Forks, ND 58202-9037
Phone: (701)777-3848 **Fax:** (701)777-6779
Email: mwake@medicine.nodak.edu
Website: http://www.med.und.nodak.edu/depts/rural/
Mary K. Wakefield, PhD, Dir.
Activities/Fields: Rural health issues. **Pub:** *Focus on Rural Health.*

★ 24162 ★ University of North Texas Health Science Center at Fort Worth
Center for Osteoporosis Prevention and Treatment (COPT)
Medical Education Bldg. 1, 2nd Fl.
3500 Camp Bowie Blvd.
Fort Worth, TX 76107
Phone: (817)735-2660
Email: brubin@hsc.unt.edu
Website: http://www.hsc.unt.edu/departments/intmed/osteocenter.htm
Bernard R. Rubin, Med. Dir.
Activities/Fields: Treatment and prevention of postmenopausal osteoporosis, treatment of steroid-induced osteoporosis, and epidemiology of osteoporosis among various ethnic groups.

★ 24163 ★ University of North Texas Health Science Center at Fort Worth
Institute of Forensic Medicine
3500 Camp Bowie Blvd.
Fort Worth, TX 76107-2699
Phone: (817)735-2429 **Fax:** (817)735-2424
Email: lnancy@hsc.unt.edu
Stephen L. Putthoff, DO, Chm.
Activities/Fields: Sudden death due to cardiovascular disease, sudden infant death syndrome, gunshot wounds, blunt and sharp force injuries, and forensic aspects of mass disasters.

★ 24164 ★ University of North Texas Health Science Center at Fort Worth
North Texas Eye Research Institute (NTERI)
3500 Camp Bowie Blvd., ME2-202
Fort Worth, TX 76107
Phone: (817)735-2045 **Fax:** (817)735-2610
Email: pcammara@hsc.unt.edu
Website: http://www.hsc.unt.edu/research/ifd/ntrei/eye_home.asp
Patrick R. Cammarata, PhD, Dir.
Activities/Fields: Eye diseases, including studies on the retina, RPE cells, trophic factors, ocular diabetes, autoimmune diseases, optic nerve regeneration, glaucoma, corneal wound healing, cell death, and aging.

★ 24165 ★ University of North Texas Health Science Center at Fort Worth
Special Projects on Aging
3500 Camp Bowie Blvd.
Fort Worth, TX 76107-2699
Phone: (817)735-5440 **Fax:** (817)735-0483
Email: tfairchi@hsc.unt.edu
Website: http://www.hsc.unt.edu/research/ifd/care/welcome.cfm
Thomas J. Fairchild, PhD, Dir.
Activities/Fields: Biology of aging, including fundamental chemical and molecular biological changes that may cause aging; health promotion in older adults including health programs promoting physical, psychological, and social well being; geriatric care and practice including evaluation of new clinical programs, physical/mental functions, long term care system development focusing on case management, and in-home health screen/assessment of home-bound elderly. **Frmly:** Texas Institute for Research and Education on Aging; Geriatrics Education and Research Institute.

★ 24166 ★ University of Notre Dame
Lobund Laboratory
Notre Dame, IN 46556
Phone: (574)631-7564 **Fax:** (574)631-8583
Email: morris.pollard.3@nd.edu
Dr. Morris Pollard, Dir.
Activities/Fields: Research on prostate cancer including the development and use of model systems to study nutrition and endocrine manipulations for prevention and treatment of the disease; metastasis and angiogenesis.

★ 24167 ★ University of Notre Dame
W.M. Keck Center for Transgene Research (CTR)
229 Nieuwland Science Hall
College of Science
Notre Dame, IN 46556
Phone: (219)631-6375
Website: http://www.nd.edu/~transgen/
Dr. Francis J. Castellino, Dir.
Activities/Fields: Pathophysiological roles of the genes of the blood coagulation, anticoagulation, and fibrinolytic pathways in hemostasis, with associated relevance to embryonic development, vessel wall development, cancer, pulmonary fibrosis, and arteriosclerosis.

★ 24168 ★ University of Oklahoma
Animal Resources
Health Science Center, BMSB 203
PO Box 26901
Oklahoma City, OK 73190
Phone: (405)271-5185 **Fax:** (405)271-2660
Email: gary-white@ouhsc.edu
Gary L. White, DVM, Dir.
Activities/Fields: Biomedical studies in general areas of physiology, pathology, microbiology, surgery, and internal medicine.

★ 24169 ★ University of Oklahoma
Baboon Research Resources
Division of Animal Resources
Health Sciences Center
940 SL Young Blvd., BMSB 203
Oklahoma City, OK 73190
Phone: (405)271-5185 **Fax:** (405)271-2660
Email: gary-white@ouhsc.edu
Gary L. White, DVM, Prin. Investigator
Activities/Fields: Captive baboons.

★ 24170 ★ University of Oklahoma
Keys Speech and Hearing Center
825 Northeast 14th St.
PO Box 26901
Oklahoma City, OK 73104
Phone: (405)271-4214 **Fax:** (405)271-3360
Email: richard-talbott@ouhsc.edu
Dr. Richard Talbott, Dept. Chm.
Activities/Fields: Loudness and acoustic reflex, temporal integration and acoustic reflex, critical bands measured with pulsation pattern psychophysical tech-

nique, sensory scaling, absolute thresholds for frequency modulated signals, bone conduction vibrator calibration, bone conduction speech audiometry, intelligibility of distorted speech, electrocochleography, brain stem auditory-evoked responses, acoustic correlates of abnormal vocal quality, aerodynamics of voice production, phonemic and morphologic studies of language of the communicatively impaired, and assessment of receptive and expressive language abilities.

★ 24171 ★ University of Oklahoma Native American Prevention Research Center
Rogers Bldg., Rm. 532
Health Sciences Center
College of Public Health
800 NE 15th
Oklahoma City, OK 73104
Phone: (405)271-2330 **Fax:** (405)271-6285
Email: everett-rhoades@ouhsc.edu
Everett R. Rhoades, MD, Prin. Investigator
Activities/Fields: Public health issues, especially behaviors that place Americans at risk for chronic diseases and conditions. Of particular concern is the improvement in quality of life for special populations, including the young, elderly, racial ethnic populations, and the underserved.

★ 24172 ★ University of Oklahoma Pulmonary and Cystic Fibrosis Center
Children's Hospital of Oklahoma, Rm. 3B 3314
940 NE 13th St.
Oklahoma City, OK 73104
Phone: (405)271-6390 **Fax:** (405)271-2873
Email: james-royall@ouhsc.edu
James Royall, Dir.
Activities/Fields: Cystic fibrosis and other respiratory diseases of children.

★ 24173 ★ University of Oklahoma Thrombosis and Coagulation Laboratory
Oklahoma University Hospital, Rm. EB 400
PO Box 26307
Oklahoma City, OK 73126
Phone: (405)271-6161 **Fax:** (405)271-3620
William Kern, MD, Dir., Clin. Hematopathology
Activities/Fields: Thrombosis, fibrinolysis, and anticoagulation. Develops clinical assays for protein C and protein S.

★ 24174 ★ University of Oklahoma Health Sciences Center Center for American Indian Health Research
College of Public Health
801 NE 13th St.
PO Box 26901
Oklahoma City, OK 73190
Phone: (405)271-3090
Email: chris-mcglory@ouhsc.edu
Website: http://w3.ouhsc.edu/coph/CophSub/CAIHRtxt.htm
Chris McGlory, Contact
Activities/Fields: Chronic disease, particularly diabetes and cardiovascular disease, health education and promotions, infectious disease, social/behavioral epidemiology, genetic disorders, molecular epidemiology, and injury epidemiology among Native Americans.

★ 24175 ★ University of Oklahoma Health Sciences Center Dean A. McGee Eye Institute
608 Stanton L. Young Blvd.
Oklahoma City, OK 73104-5065
Phone: (405)271-6060 **Fax:** (405)271-4442
Email: david-parke@ouhsc.edu
Website: http://www.dmei.org
Dr. David W. Parke, II, Pres. /CEO
Activities/Fields: Basic and clinical investigation in visual sciences; studies also include retinal biochemistry, molecular biology, and ocular microbiology.

★ 24176 ★ University of Oklahoma Health Sciences Center Dean A. McGee Eye Institute Molecular Pathogenesis of Eye Infection Center (MPEIR)
608 Stanton L. Young Blvd., DMEI 419
Oklahoma City, OK 73104
Phone: (405)271-1084 **Fax:** (405)271-8781
Email: michael-gilmore@ouhsc.edu
Website: http://w3.uokhsc.edu/MPEIR/
Michael S. Gilmore, PhD, Contact
Activities/Fields: Infectious diseases of the eye.

★ 24177 ★ University of Oregon Institute of Neuroscience (ION)
222 Huestis Hall
1425 E 13th Ave.
Eugene, OR 97403-1254
Phone: (541)346-4556 **Fax:** (541)346-4548
Email: roberts@uoneuro.uoregon.edu
Website: http://www.neuro.uoregon.edu
Dr. William Roberts, Dir.
Activities/Fields: Interdisciplinary approaches to basic questions in neuroscience, with particular emphasis on behavior, neurochemistry, neurophysiology, developmental neurobiology, and sensory systems. The Institute is composed of faculty members from the Departments of Biology, Computer Science, Psychology, and Physical Education. **Pub:** *Graduate Studies at the Institute of Neuroscience.*

★ 24178 ★ University of Ottawa Centre for Neuromuscular Disease
Health Sciences Bldg., Rm. 3153
Ottawa, ON, Canada K1N 6N5
Phone: (613)562-5800 **Fax:** (613)562-5434
Email: jasmin@uottawa.ca
Website: http://www.medicine.uottawa.ca/neuromuscular/
Bernard Jasmin, PhD, Dir.
Activities/Fields: Neuromuscular disorders. Although the emphasis is on skeletal muscle, a significant proportion of the research effort is also relevant to several heart conditions and neurological disorders.

★ 24179 ★ University of Ottawa Centre for Research in Biopharmaceuticals (CRB)
Faculty of Medicine, Rm. 4163
451 Smyth Rd.
Ottawa, ON, Canada K1H 8M5
Phone: (613)562-5800 **Fax:** (613)562-5699
Email: crb@uottawa.ca
Website: http://www.crb.uottawa.ca
Dr. Jo-Anne Dillon, Dir.
Activities/Fields: Identification of compounds of biopharmaceutical interest for the treatment of disease.

★ 24180 ★ University of Ottawa Centre for Research on Environmental Microbiology (CREM)
Faculty of Medicine, Rm. 4119
451 Smyth Rd.
Ottawa, ON, Canada K1H 8M5
Phone: (613)562-5800 **Fax:** (613)562-5452
Email: crem@uottawa.ca
Website: http://www.environmental-microbiology.ca/
Dr. Syed A. Sattar, Dir./Prin. Investigator
Activities/Fields: Environmental microbiology as it relates to public health. Some themes are treatment of drinking water, foodborne pathogens, disinfection and sterilization in health care, germicide and antibiotic resistance, biomedical waste treatment.

★ 24181 ★ University of Ottawa Community Health Research Unit (CHRU)
451 Smyth Rd.
Ottawa, ON, Canada K1H 8M5
Phone: (613)562-5800 **Fax:** (613)562-5658
Email: chru@zeus.med.uottawa.ca
Website: http://www.uottawa.ca/academic/med/epid/chru.html
Nancy Edwards, PhD, Dir.
Activities/Fields: Public health practices, including strengthening self-care capacity and action, fostering collective capacity and action, and building supportive environments.

★ 24182 ★ University of Ottawa Eye Institute
501 Smyth Rd., Tower 3
Ottawa, ON, Canada K1H 8L6
Phone: (613)737-8575 **Fax:** (613)737-8836
Email: bjackson@ottawahospital.on.ca
Website: http://www.eyeinstitute.net/
W. Bruce Jackson, Dir.
Activities/Fields: Visual system with emphasis on those visual disorders of major public health concern.

★ 24183 ★ University of Ottawa Heart Institute
40 Ruskin St.
Ottawa, ON, Canada K1Y 4W7
Phone: (613)761-4905 **Fax:** (613)761-5281
Email: aaffairs@ottawaheart.ca
Website: http://www.ottawaheart.ca/
Dr. Yves Maral, Ch. Sci. Off.
Activities/Fields: All aspects of heart disease, including hypertension, cardiovascular devices, genetics of cardiovascular diseases, vascular biology, arrythmia, cardiac surgery, cardiac anesthesia, and prevention and rehabilitation. **Pub:** *Annual report.*

★ 24184 ★ University of Ottawa Institute of Population Health
1 Stewart St.
Ottawa, ON, Canada K1N 6N5
Phone: (613)562-5660 **Fax:** (613)562-5659
Email: jlosos@uottawa.ca
Website: http://www.iph.uottawa.ca/
Joe Losos, MD, Dir.
Activities/Fields: Population health, particularly why some people and communities are healthy and others are not.

★ 24185 ★ University of Ottawa Neurosciences Research Institute
451 Smyth Rd.
Ottawa, ON, Canada K2H 8M5
Phone: (613)562-5800 **Fax:** (613)562-5403
Email: kchaundy@uottawa.ca
Website: http://www.nri.on.ca
K. Chaundy, Contact
Activities/Fields: Neuroprotection, neuronal regeneration and recovery, mechanisms of cell injury, stroke, depression, schizophrenia, and axotomy.

★ 24186 ★ University of Pennsylvania Abramson Cancer Center
Penn Tower, 16th Fl.
3400 Spruce St.
Philadelphia, PA 19104-4283
Phone: (215)662-6065 **Fax:** (215)349-5325
Email: glickjh@mail.med.upenn.edu
Website: http://www.oncolink.org/treatment/matching.cfm
John H. Glick, MD, Dir.
Activities/Fields: Cancer biology, diagnosis, cause, prevention, treatment, control, and rehabilitation, including programs in immunobiology, cell biology, virology, clinical investigations, pediatric oncology, cancer epidemiology, melanoma, stem cell biology and therapeutic breast cancer prevention, neuro-oncology, behavioral sciences and health sciences.

★ 24187 ★ University of Pennsylvania Brain Behavior Laboratory
10 Gates Pavilion
Neuropsychiatry Section
Department of Psychiatry
3400 Spruce St.
Philadelphia, PA 19104-4283
Phone: (215)662-2826 **Fax:** (215)662-7903
Email: raquel@bbl.med.penn.edu
Website: http://www.med.upenn.edu/bbl/
Raquel Gur, PhD, Dir.
Activities/Fields: New techniques for measuring regional brain function in relationship to behavior including cerebral blood flow, and metabolism using positron emmission tomography (PET); and functional MRI (FMRI); anatomic measures using magnetic resonance imaging (MRI), and neuropsychological testing for studying brain behavior relationships. Populations studied include normals (average and talented), psychiatric (schizophrenic, major depression, anxiety disorders, and dementia), and neurologic (stroke or cerebrovascular disease, epilepsy and parkinsonism).

★ 24188 ★ University of Pennsylvania Center for Bioethics
3401 Market St., Ste. 320
Philadelphia, PA 19104-3319
Phone: (215)898-7136 **Fax:** (215)573-3036
Email: caplan@mail.med.upenn.edu
Website: http://www.bioethics.org
Prof. Arthur Caplan, PhD, Dir.
Activities/Fields: Improvement in the practices and delivery of medical care. **Pub:** *PennBioethics*, semiannually.

★ 24189 ★ University of Pennsylvania Center for Cancer Pharmacology
1257 BRB II/III
Philadelphia, PA 19104-6160
Phone: (215)573-9885 **Fax:** (215)573-9889
Email: ian@spirit.gcrc.upenn.edu
Website: http://www.med.upenn.edu/ccp/
Ian A. Blair, Dir.
Activities/Fields: Pharmacologically based strategies for the treatment and prevention of cancer and development of a methodology for assessing cancer risk in human populations.

★ 24190 ★ University of Pennsylvania Center for Clinical Epidemiology and Biostatistics
824 Blockley Hall
Sch. of Medicine
423 Guardian Dr.
Philadelphia, PA 19104-6021
Phone: (215)898-2368 **Fax:** (215)573-5315
Email: bstrom@cceb.med.upenn.edu
Website: http://cceb.med.upenn.edu
Dr. Brian L. Strom, Dir.
Activities/Fields: Epidemiology of disease and risk factors of clinical importance, especially pharamacoepidemiology, molecular epidemiology, cancer, cardiovascular disease, renal disease, women's health, reproductive epidemiology, emergency medicine, injury, and aging. **Frmly:** Clinical Epidemiology Unit.

★ 24191 ★ University of Pennsylvania Center for Cognitive Therapy
Department of Psychiatry
School of Medicine
3535 Market St., 2nd Fl.
Philadelphia, PA 19104-2649
Phone: (215)898-4100 **Fax:** (215)898-1865
Email: psycct@mail.med.upenn.edu
Website: http://www.uphs.upenn.edu/psycct
Cory F. Newman, PhD, Dir.
Activities/Fields: Psychiatric outpatient clinic, engaged in developing different assessment instruments to measure constructs of cognitive theory, extending the cognitive approach to anxiety and other psychiatric disorders, assessing and predicting suicidal risks, studying outpatient populations, and assessing different training models for cognitive therapists. **Pub:** *Center for Cognitive Therapy Newsletter*.

★ 24192 ★ University of Pennsylvania Center for Experimental Therapeutics
153 Johnson Pavilion
3620 Hamilton Walk
Philadelphia, PA 19104-6084
Phone: (215)898-1184 **Fax:** (215)573-9135
Email: garret@spirit.gcrc.upenn.edu
Website: http://www.uphs.upenn.edu/CET/
Garret A. FitzGerald, MD, Dir.
Activities/Fields: Mechanisms of drug action, the genetic and environmental factors which contribute to interindividual differences in drug response in humans, pharmacological probes to uncover mechanisms in physiology and disease.

★ 24193 ★ University of Pennsylvania Center for Health Outcomes and Policy Research
School of Nursing
Nursing Education Bldg.
420 Guardian Dr., Fl. 3R
Philadelphia, PA 19104-6096
Phone: (215)898-5673 **Fax:** (215)573-2062
Email: laiken@nursing.upenn.edu
Website: http://www.nursing.upenn.edu/chopr/
Linda H. Aiken, Dir.
Activities/Fields: Health care and workforce organization, financing, and outcomes; and public policies that influence nursing and health care delivery nationally and internationally.

★ 24194 ★ University of Pennsylvania Center for Human Appearance
Medical Center
Penn Tower Hotel, 10th Fl.
3400 Spruce St.
Philadelphia, PA 19104
Phone: (215)662-7095 **Free:** 800-234-7366
Fax: (215)349-5895
Email: linton.whitaker@uphs.upenn.edu
Dr. Linton A. Whitaker, Dir.
Activities/Fields: Treatment of appearance-related problems, including reconstructive and cosmetic procedures to correct aesthetic and functional problems of the face, body, and extremities resulting from birth defects, traumatic injury, and diseases such as cancer and other tumors. The Center is divided into six patient treatment sections: craniofacial, to correct severe deformities of facial areas above the jaws; dentofacial, to correct dental and bone abnormalities of the lower portion of the face; interface, to improve variations in normal facial form; aging, to correct facial, body, and skin changes caused by the aging process; body contour, to improve the appearance of various areas of the body for both medical and cosmetic reasons; and self-image, to counsel patients with body image problems.

★ 24195 ★ University of Pennsylvania Center for Mental Health Policy and Services Research
3535 Market St., 3rd Fl.
Philadelphia, PA 19104-2648
Phone: (215)662-2886 **Fax:** (215)349-8715
Email: thadley@mail.med.upenn.edu
Website: http://www.uphs.upenn.edu/cmhpsr/
Trevor Hadley, PhD, Dir.
Activities/Fields: Mental health policy and services.

★ 24196 ★ University of Pennsylvania Center for Molecular Studies in Digestive and Liver Disease
Clinical Research Bldg., Ste. 600
School of Medicine
Philadelphia, PA 19104-6140
Phone: (215)573-4264 **Fax:** (215)573-2024
Email: anil2@mail.med.upenn.edu
Website: http://www.uphs.upenn.edu/moleculr/
Dr. Anil K. Rustgi, Dir.
Activities/Fields: Digestive biology, pathobiology, and therapy, specifically the molecular controls of cellular growth and differentiation in digestive organs.

★ 24197 ★ University of Pennsylvania Center for Neurodegenerative Disease Research (CNDR)
Maloney Bldg., 3rd Fl.
Department of Pathology & Laboratory Medicine
3600 Spruce St.
Philadelphia, PA 19104
Phone: (215)662-4708 **Fax:** (215)349-5909
Email: viale@mail.med.upenn.edu
Website: http://www.uphs.upenn.edu/cndr/
Virginia M.-Y. Lee, PhD, Co-Dir.
Activities/Fields: Causes and mechanisms leading to brain dysfunction and degeneration in Alzheimer's disease, Parkinson's disease, motor neuron disease and other less common neurodegenerative disorders that also occur more frequently with advancing age.

★ 24198 ★ University of Pennsylvania Center for Research on Reproduction and Women's Health
1355 Biomedical Research Bldg. II/III
University of Pennsylvania Medical Center
Philadelphia, PA 19104-6142
Phone: (215)898-0147 **Fax:** (215)573-5408
Email: jfs3@mail.med.upenn.edu
Website: http://www.med.upenn.edu/~crrwh/
Dr. Jerome F. Strauss, III, Dir.
Activities/Fields: Human reproduction as it relates to fertility regulation and the diagnosis and treatment of male and female infertility and health issues specific to women.

★ 24199 ★ University of Pennsylvania Center for Sleep and Respiratory Neurobiology (CSRN)
991 Maloney Bldg.
3600 Spruce St.
Philadelphia, PA 19104-4283
Phone: (215)662-3305 **Fax:** (215)662-7749
Email: pack@mail.med.upenn.edu
Website: http://www.uphs.upenn.edu/sleepctr/
Allan I. Pack, MD, Dir.
Activities/Fields: Sleep disorders and the neural control of breathing. **Pub:** *Abstracts*.

★ 24200 ★ University of Pennsylvania Center for the Treatment and Study of Anxiety (CTSA)
3535 Market St., 6th Fl.
Philadelphia, PA 19104
Phone: (215)746-3327 **Fax:** (215)746-3311
Email: ctsa@mail.med.upenn.edu
Website: http://www.med.upenn.edu/ctsa/
Edna B. Foa, PhD, Dir.
Activities/Fields: Therapies for anxiety and stress disorders.

★ 24201 ★ University of Pennsylvania Center for Urban Health Research
School of Nursing
Nursing Education Bldg.
420 Guardian Dr.
Philadelphia, PA 19104
Phone: (215)898-6373 **Fax:** (215)573-9193
Email: jemmott@nursing.upenn.edu
Website: http://www.nursing.upenn.edu/urban/
Dr. Loretta Sweet Jemmott, Dir.
Activities/Fields: Identification of factors that influence health risk-related behaviors and the design of culturally tailored interventions to promote healthy lifestyles, with a focus on AIDS, pregnancy, and violence prevention.

★ 24202 ★ University of Pennsylvania Cerebrovascular Research Center
Stemmler Hall, Rm. 415
3450 Hamilton Walk
Philadelphia, PA 19104-6063
Phone: (215)662-2632 **Fax:** (215)349-5629
Email: reivich@cvrc.med.upenn.edu
Dr. Martin Reivich, Dir.
Activities/Fields: Cerebrovascular research with an emphasis on cerebral circulation and metabolism. Conducts PET, SPECT, MRI, neuropsychologic, and neurologic studies on various brain disorders, including acute stroke, brain tumor, epilepsy, dementia,Parkinson's disease,and schizophrenia. Studies include measurements of regional cerebral blood flow, glucose and oxygen metabolism, blood volume, and neuroreceptor number and affinity. Also conducts basic animal research, including development of blood flow agents for the brain, research on animal models of stroke, and studies on treatment modalities for acute stroke in animal models.

★ 24203 ★ University of Pennsylvania David Mahoney Institute of Neurological Sciences
Stemmler Hall, Ste. 215
Philadelphia, PA 19104-6074
Phone: (215)898-8754
Email: Levitani@mail.med.upenn.edu
Website: http://www.med.upenn.edu/ins/
Dr. Irwin Levitan, Dir.
Activities/Fields: Nervous system, including neuroanatomy, neurobiology, neurochemistry, neuroembryology, neurophysiology, neuropharmacology, physiological psychology, computational neuroscience, cognitive neuroscience, pathophysiology of neurological, and psychiatric diseases. **Pub:** *Newsletter.*

★ 24204 ★ University of Pennsylvania Deafness and Family Communication Center (DFCC)
3535 Market St., 9th Fl.
Philadelphia, PA 19104
Phone: (215)590-7440
Email: dfcc@www.med.upenn.edu
Website: http://www.uphs.upenn.edu/dfcc/
Annie Steinberg, MD, Dir.
Activities/Fields: Impact of deafness on the mental health and well-being of children, adolescents, and their families.

★ 24205 ★ University of Pennsylvania Depression Research Unit
University City Science Center
3535 Market St., 3rd Fl.
Philadelphia, PA 19104-2649
Phone: (215)662-3462 **Fax:** (215)662-6443
Email: jamsterd@mail.med.upenn.edu
Jay D. Amsterdam, MD, Dir.
Activities/Fields: Affective disorders. Research areas include psychopharmacology, particularly development of new antidepressant drugs; clinical neuroendocrinology; and the biochemical causes of major depression.

★ 24206 ★ University of Pennsylvania Eldridge Reeves Johnson Foundation
1005 Stellar-Chance Bldg.
Department of Biochemistry & Biophysics
University of Pennsylvania Medical Center
Philadelphia, PA 19104-6059
Phone: (215)898-8699 **Fax:** (215)573-2235
Email: dutton@mail.med.upenn.edu
Website: http://www.uphs.upenn.edu/~biocbiop/jf/jf.html
P. Leslie Dutton, Dir.
Activities/Fields: Biochemical and biophysical aspects of medicine and biology.

★ 24207 ★ University of Pennsylvania General Clinical Research Center
160 Dulles Bldg.
3400 Spruce St.
Philadelphia, PA 19104-4283
Phone: (215)662-2641 **Fax:** (215)662-2643
Email: garret@spirit.gcrc.upenn.edu
Website: http://www.gcrc.upenn.edu/
Garret A. FitzGerald, MD, Dir.
Activities/Fields: AIDS, cardiovascular research, chemical senses, chronobiology and sleep, dermatology, endocrinology, gene therapy, metabolism, neonatal medicine, neurology, oncology, psychiatry, and women and minority health issues.

★ 24208 ★ University of Pennsylvania Harrison Department of Surgical Research
Margarett M. Clark Laboratories
313 Stemmler Hall
3450 Hamilton Walk
Philadelphia, PA 19104-6070
Phone: (215)898-8081 **Fax:** (215)573-2001
Email: larry.kaiser@uphs.upenn.edu
Website: http://www.uphs.upenn.edu/surgery/res/research.html
Dr. Larry Kaiser, Dir.
Activities/Fields: Cancer, cardiovascular disease, gastrointestinal physiology, shock and surgical bacteriology, nutrition of surgical patients, and surgical specialities, including studies of stomach and duodenum, pancreas, colon, liver, blood flow, hypertension, equilibrium tissue oxygen requirements, tissue oxygen, oxygen supply in shock and shock-like states, chemotherapy, patient antitumor agents, immunology, ultraviolet light in protection against wound infection, transplantation of tissues and organs, and role of electronics in surgical research. **Pub:** *Annual report.*

★ 24209 ★ University of Pennsylvania Health Services Research Unit (HSRU)
Blockley Hall, Rm. 1211
Division of General Internal Medicine
423 Guardian Dr.
Philadelphia, PA 19104-6021
Phone: (215)898-6868 **Fax:** (215)898-0611
Email: hlthsvrs@mail.med.upenn.edu
Website: http://www.uphs.upenn.edu/dgimhsr/
Dr. Henry Glick, Dir.
Activities/Fields: Allocation and appropriate use of health care resources, including cost-effectiveness of new pharmaceuticals, managed care and the physician workforce, and methodology of cost analysis.

★ 24210 ★ University of Pennsylvania Institute on Aging
3615 Chestnut St.
Philadelphia, PA 19104-6006
Phone: (215)898-3163 **Fax:** (215)573-8684
Email: trojanow@mail.med.upenn.edu
Website: http://www.uphs.upenn.edu/aging/
John Q. Trojanowski, MD, Dir.
Activities/Fields: Biomedical and social science research on aging, including cellular mechanisms of aging, Alzheimer's disease, sleep disturbances, arthritis, osteoporosis, population demographics of aging, nursing home quality, organization and structure of life care communities, social security, and social support systems for the aged. **Pub:** *Newsletter*, quarterly. **Frmly:** Center for the Study of Aging.

★ 24211 ★ University of Pennsylvania Institute for Environmental Medicine
1 John Morgan Bldg.
3620 Hamilton Walk
Philadelphia, PA 19104-6068
Phone: (215)898-9100 **Fax:** (215)898-0868
Email: abf@mail.med.upenn.edu
Website: http://www.med.upenn.edu/~ifem
Dr. Aron B. Fisher, Dir.
Activities/Fields: Cellular and molecular biology of lung function with special emphasis on the lung surfactant system, undersea physiology, physiological and toxic effects of oxygen, isobaric gas counterdiffusion, and hyperbaric oxygen therapy. **Pub:** *Research Reports.*

★ 24212 ★ University of Pennsylvania Metabolic Magnetic Resonance Research and Computing Center
Stellar-Chance Laboratories, B1
Department of Radiology
Philadelphia, PA 19104-6100
Phone: (215)898-2044 **Fax:** (215)573-2113
Email: jack@mail.mmrrcc.upenn.edu
Website: http://www.mmrrcc.upenn.edu
John S. Leigh, PhD, Dir.
Activities/Fields: Performs in vivo monitoring of specific metabolites in localized regions of tissues and organs in humans utilizing multinuclear magnetic resonance spectroscopy and metabolic imaging; develops targeted magnetite-based contrast agents for gene therapy and diagnosis; and develops techniques for near infrared optical imaging and spectroscopy in humans. **Pub:** *Newsletter.*

★ 24213 ★ University of Pennsylvania Mood and Anxiety Disorders Section
3535 Market St., Ste. 670
Philadelphia, PA 19104-3309
Phone: (215)898-4301 **Fax:** (215)898-0509
Email: krickels@mail.med.upenn.edu
Dr. Karl Rickels, Dir.
Activities/Fields: Psychopharmacology, including short- and long-term clinical trials on the effects of antidepressive and antianxiety medications. **Frmly:** Psychopharmacology Research Unit.

★ 24214 ★ University of Pennsylvania Penn Diabetes Center
501 Stemmler Hall
36th & Hamilton Walk
Philadelphia, PA 19104-6015
Phone: (215)898-4365 **Fax:** (215)898-2178
Email: lazar@mail.med.upenn.edu
Dr. Mitchell Lazar, Dir.
Activities/Fields: Diabetes. Conducts basic studies on both pancreatic islet cell function and insulin action; evaluates new methods to detect and measure early signs of diabetes affecting the nervous systems, the retina, the vascular system, the heart, and the kidney; performs controlled clinical trials of new diets, drugs, and insulin-administration techniques; defines the nature of genetic susceptibility to diabetes; studies factors that increase the risk of complications in diabetes; and reevaluates the long-term benefits of kidney and pancreas transplants in diabetics. The Center is organized in two components: Core Basic Research Facilities, which supply investigators with special equipment and support, and the Clinical Center for Diabetes Research and Education, which provides the opportunity to perform controlled studies on volunteer ambulatory diabetic patients.

★ 24215 ★ University of Pennsylvania Pennsylvania Muscle Institute
D700 Richards Bldg.
School of Medicine
3700 Hamilton Walk
Philadelphia, PA 19104-6083
Phone: (215)898-4017 **Fax:** (215)898-2653
Email: goldmany@mail.med.upenn.edu
Website: http://www.uphs.upenn.edu/pmi/
Dr. Yale E. Goldman, Dir.
Activities/Fields: Studies muscle tissue as it relates to heart disease using specialized techniques developed by the Institute, including rapid spectroscopic methods for measurement of cytoplasmic ions, electron energy loss analysis, and electron probe X-ray analysis for obtaining compositional information about cells. Serves as a regional interdisciplinary center for collaborative studies on development, molecular orga-

nization, and function of contractile and regulatory proteins and on mechanics, energetics, excitation/contraction coupling mechanism, and intracellular ion movements in cardiac, smooth, and skeletal muscle.

★ 24216 ★ University of Pennsylvania Referral Center for Animal Models of Human Genetic Disease
Rosenthal Bldg., Rm. 307
Veterinary School
3800 Spruce St.
Philadelphia, PA 19104-6051
Phone: (215)898-4852 **Fax:** (215)898-0719
Email: mhaskins@vet.upenn.edu
Dr. Mark Haskins, Prin. Investigator
Activities/Fields: Identification, characterization, evaluation, and dissemination of animal models of human genetic disease, particularly models that occur in domestic animals, with emphasis on hereditary metabolic diseases, hereditary defects in sexual development, congenital malformations, and hereditary diseases of blood. Activities include characterization of mutant genes at the molecular level.

★ 24217 ★ University of Pennsylvania Research Center in Oral Biology
240 S 40th St.
Philadelphia, PA 19104-6002
Phone: (215)898-5959 **Fax:** (215)573-2050
Email: shenker@path.dental.upenn.edu
Dr. Bruce Shenker, Dir.
Activities/Fields: Oral health, including team studies on biochemistry of connective and hard tissues, analyses of structural and functional constituents of oral microbes, and immunobiology of oral tissues and investigation of plaque formation and effect on periodontal tissues. **Pub:** *COHR Newsletter*. **Frmly:** Center for Oral Health Research.

★ 24218 ★ University of Pennsylvania Resource for Magnetic Resonance Research and Optical Research
B1, Stellar-Chance Laboratories
Department of Radiology
422 Curie Blvd.
Philadelphia, PA 19104-6100
Phone: (215)898-9357 **Fax:** (215)573-2113
Email: jack@mail.mmrrcc.upenn.edu
Website: http://www.mmrrcc.upenn.edu
John S. Leigh, PhD, Prin. Investigator
Activities/Fields: Instrumentation, methodologies, and data analysis for in vivo monitoring of specific metabolites in localized regions of tissues and organs in humans, utilizing multinuclear magnetic resonance spectroscopy; and novel spectral functional and perfusion imaging techniques.

★ 24219 ★ University of Pennsylvania Smell and Taste Center
5 Ravdin Bldg.
3400 Spruce St.
Philadelphia, PA 19104
Phone: (215)662-6580 **Fax:** (215)349-5266
Email: doty@mail.med.upenn.edu
Website: http://www.smellandtastecenter.com/
Dr. Richard L. Doty, Dir.
Activities/Fields: Identifies and treats disorders of taste and smell. Develops clinical smell and taste tests, investigates nasal airflow parameters, examines gustatory glucose sensitivity in diabetes and depression, studies MRI-based measures of brain volume changes in olfactory disorders, studies neuroendocrine relations with chemosensory function, conducts behavioral and neurophysiological studies of olfactory and trigeminal function, and studies the pathophysiology of oral sensory abnormalities.

★ 24220 ★ University of Pennsylvania Social Work Mental Health Research Center (SWMHRC)
School of Social Work
3701 Locust Walk
Philadelphia, PA 19104-6214
Phone: (215)573-9688
Email: solomonp@ssw.upenn.edu
Website: http://www.ssw.upenn.edu/SWMHRC/index.htm
Phyllis L. Solomon, PhD, Co-Dir.
Activities/Fields: Mental health services and the social welfare of persons with severe mental illnesses. The center focuses on three areas of intervention: legal, mental health managed care, and mental health and supportive services.

★ 24221 ★ University of Pennsylvania Specialized Center for Research in Hyperbaric Oxygen Therapy
3451 Walnut St., Rm. P221
Philadelphia, PA 19104-6205
Phone: (215)898-9095
Email: sthan@mail.med.upenn.edu
Stephen R. Thom, MD, Prin. Investigator
Activities/Fields: Mechanisms of action, safety and clinical efficacy of hyperbaric oxygen therapy for head and neck tumors, and radiation injury.

★ 24222 ★ University of Pennsylvania Substance Abuse Treatment Unit
Bldg. 7, 116-D
VA Medical Center
28 Woodland Ave.
Philadelphia, PA 19104
Phone: (215)823-5188 **Fax:** (215)823-4248
Wayne Barber, MD, Dir.
Activities/Fields: Alcohol and drug dependence, including research on psychotherapy, endocrine system, alcoholism and schizophrenia, methadone-maintained cocaine abusers, and outpatient versus inpatient detoxification.

★ 24223 ★ University of Pennsylvania Ultrafast Optical Processes Laboratory
231 S 34th St.
Philadelphia, PA 19104-6323
Phone: (215)898-8410 **Fax:** (215)898-0590
Email: hochstra@sas.upenn.edu
Website: http://rlbl.chem.upenn.edu
Prof. Robin M. Hochstrasser, PhD, Prin. Investigator
Activities/Fields: Development of methods for the investigation of rapid structural changes and ultrafast processes in proteins, enzymes, and nucleic acids.

★ 24224 ★ University of Pennsylvania Vision Research Center
143 Anatomy-Chemistry Bldg.
School of Medicine
36th & Hamilton Walk
Philadelphia, PA 19104
Phone: (215)898-6917 **Fax:** (215)573-8093
Email: liebmanp@mail.med.upenn.edu
Website: http://vrc.med.upenn.edu/
Dr. Paul Liebman, Dir.
Activities/Fields: Serves as a branch of the National Eye Institute of the National Institutes of Health to fund eye research projects at the University. Studies concentrate on mechanisms of normal and defective vision, including their molecular, genetic, developmental, electrophysiological, neural, and cognitive aspects.

★ 24225 ★ University of Pennsylvania Weight and Eating Disorders Program
Department of Psychiatry
3535 Market St., Ste. 3108
Philadelphia, PA 19104
Phone: (215)898-7314 **Fax:** (215)898-2878
Email: wadden@mail.med.upenn.edu
Website: http://www.uphs.upenn.edu/~weight
Dr. Thomas A. Wadden, Dir.
Activities/Fields: Obesity, binge eating disorder, bulimia (including behavioral treatments for all). body image, metabolic rate and body fat measures, and predictors of adiposity in infancy.

★ 24226 ★ University of Pennsylvania William Pepper Laboratory
Hospital of University of Pennsylvania
Philadelphia, PA 19104
Phone: (215)662-3435 **Fax:** (215)349-5090
Email: donaldyo@mail.med.upenn.edu
Donald S. Young, MD, Dir.
Activities/Fields: Microbiology, immunology, clinical chemistry, hematology, toxicology, therapeutic drug monitoring characterization and specificity of blood group, characterization and specificity of blood group antibodies, clinical correlation of disturbances of endocrine metabolism, coagulation disorders, and clinical enzymology. Conducts complete histocompatability evaluations, blood component therapy, therapeutic plasma exchange, therapeutic red cell exchange procedures, tumor receptor-site studies, as well as basic research in cancer biology, endocrine biochemistry, and membrane biology.

★ 24227 ★ University of Pittsburgh Alzheimer's Disease Research Center (ADRC)
4 W Montefiore University Hospital
200 Lothrop St.
Pittsburgh, PA 15213-2582
Phone: (412)692-2700 **Fax:** (412)692-2710
Email: dekosky@pitt.edu
Website: http://www.adrc.pitt.edu/index.html-ssi
Steven T. DeKosky, MD, Dir.
Activities/Fields: Alzheimer's Disease and related dementias.

★ 24228 ★ University of Pittsburgh Cancer Institute
Iroquois Bldg., Ste. 206
3600 Forbes Ave.
Pittsburgh, PA 15213
Free: 800-237-4724 **Fax:** (412)624-1936
Email: pci-info@msx.upmc.edu
Website: http://www.upci.upmc.edu
Ronald B. Herberman, MD, Dir.
Activities/Fields: Cancer's causes, course and cure.

★ 24229 ★ University of Pittsburgh Center for Bioethics and Health Law
Medical Arts Bldg., Ste. 300
3708 5th Ave.
Pittsburgh, PA 15213
Phone: (412)647-5700 **Fax:** (412)647-5877
Email: bioethic@pitt.edu
Website: http://www.law.pitt.edu/~bioethic/faculty.htm
Dr. Alan Meisel, Dir.
Activities/Fields: Theoretical and clinical analysis of the complex ethical issues surrounding the health care process from a multidisciplinary perspective. Research areas include ethical issues surrounding the recruitment of patients to cancer chemotherapy clinical trials, effectiveness of required request laws and policies for organ and tissue donation, quality of nursing care provided to patients with AIDS, doctor-patient communication regarding advance directives, doctor-family communication in an intensive care unit, coercion in management of psychiatric patients, and comparison of ethical issues in engineering with medical ethics issues. **Frmly:** Center for Medical Ethics.

★ 24230 ★ University of Pittsburgh Center for Clinical Pharmacology
623 Scaife Hall
Pittsburgh, PA 15213
Phone: (412)648-2380 **Fax:** (412)648-1837
Email: branch@msx.dept-med.pitt.edu

Website: http://www.upmc.edu/ClinPharm/
Robert A. Branch, MD, Dir.
Activities/Fields: Drug development, drug metabolism, drugs in psychiatry, renal pathophysiology, pharmacoepidemiology.

★ 24231 ★ University of Pittsburgh Center for Exercise and Health-Fitness Research
A149B Trees Hall
Pittsburgh, PA 15261
Phone: (412)648-8251 **Fax:** (412)648-7092
Email: rrobert@pitt.edu
Dr. Robert J. Robertson, Dir.
Activities/Fields: Physiology of exercise and work, perception of physical exertion, cardiac rehabilitation, and ergogenic aids, including studies conducted by full-time faculty members and graduate students of the University. **Frmly:** Human Energy Research Laboratory.

★ 24232 ★ University of Pittsburgh Center for Injury Research and Control (CIRCL)
200 Lothrop St., Ste. B400-PUH
Pittsburgh, PA 15213
Phone: (412)648-2600 **Fax:** (412)648-8924
Email: circl@pitt.edu
Website: http://www.circl.pitt.edu
Harold B. Weiss, PhD, Dir.
Activities/Fields: Understanding of injuries and the reduction of their occurrence, severity, and consequences, including traumatic brain injury and spinal cord injury. **Pub:** *Frontlines Newsletter*, quarterly.

★ 24233 ★ University of Pittsburgh Center for Mental Health Services Research (CMHSR)
Cathedral of Learning, Rm. 2217
Pittsburgh, PA 15260
Phone: (412)624-6572 **Fax:** (412)624-1159
Email: cmhsr@pitt.edu
Carol M. Anderson, PhD, Dir.
Activities/Fields: Understanding of individual, community and mental health service systems factors that facilitate or discourage the use of treatment resources; identification of barriers and modification of pathways to mental health care; and adaptation, design, and testing interventions for low income, minority, and other community populations.

★ 24234 ★ University of Pittsburgh Center for Neuroscience
Biomedical Science Tower, E1440
Pittsburgh, PA 15261
Phone: (412)648-9537 **Fax:** (412)648-1441
Email: strickp@pitt.edu
Website: http://cnup.neurobio.pitt.edu/
Dr. Peter L. Strick, Co-Dir.
Activities/Fields: Neuroscience and neural diseases.

★ 24235 ★ University of Pittsburgh Center for Nursing Research
School of Nursing
3500 Victoria St., Rm. 360
Pittsburgh, PA 15261
Phone: (412)624-4854 **Fax:** (412)624-1201
Email: mek1@pitt.edu
Website: http://cnr.nursing.pitt.edu/
Prof. Mary E. Kerr, PhD, Dir.
Activities/Fields: Health care of individuals across the life span, including adolescent health, chronic disorders, critical care, and health care outcomes. **Pub:** *Newsletter*, quarterly.

★ 24236 ★ University of Pittsburgh Center for Research in Chronic Disorders (CRCD)
460 Victoria Bldg.
School of Nursing
3500 Victoria St.
Pittsburgh, PA 15261
Phone: (412)624-7838 **Fax:** (412)624-1508
Email: crcd@pitt.edu
Website: http://crcd.nursing.pitt.edu/
Jaqueline Dunbar-Jacob, PhD, Dir.
Activities/Fields: Chronic disorders, with particular emphasis on quality of life, functional status, cognitive function, and adherence to treatment regimens as they are impacted by and impact management of those disorders. Additionally, the center is interested in the moderating effects of comorbid conditions and sociodemographic characteristics on these four outcomes.

★ 24237 ★ University of Pittsburgh Center for Research on Health Care (CRHC)
UPMC Montefiore, Ste. E820
Pittsburgh, PA 15213
Phone: (412)692-4853 **Fax:** (412)692-4838
Email: ctrrhc@pitt.edu
Website: http://www.pitt.edu/~ctrrhc/
Wishwa N. Kapoor, MD, Dir.
Activities/Fields: Health services.

★ 24238 ★ University of Pittsburgh Center for Research in Reproductive Physiology
Scaife Hall, S 828
Pittsburgh, PA 15261
Phone: (412)648-9281 **Fax:** (412)383-7159
Email: plant1@pitt.edu
Website: http://www.crrp.pitt.edu
Tony M. Plant, PhD, Dir.
Activities/Fields: Neuroendocrine control of reproduction in rhesus monkeys. **Frmly:** Center for Research in Primate Reproduction.

★ 24239 ★ University of Pittsburgh Cleft Palate-Craniofacial Center
School of Dental Medicine
317 Salk Hall
3501 Terrace St.
Pittsburgh, PA 15261
Phone: (412)648-8400 **Free:** 800-408-7390
Fax: (412)648-8404
Email: cleft@cpc.pitt.edu
Website: http://www.cpc.pitt.edu
Dr. Michael Buckley, Dir.
Activities/Fields: Cleft palate, cleft lip, and craniofacial anomalies, including interdisciplinary, basic, clinical, genetic, embryological, and teratology studies. Also studies ear diseases, velopharyngeal valving, laryngeal characteristics and motor control for speech, computer reconstruction of nasal capsule, and anatomy of pharyngeal walls.

★ 24240 ★ University of Pittsburgh General Clinical Research Center
Montefiore University Hospital
200 Lothrop St.
Pittsburgh, PA 15213-2582
Phone: (412)648-6691 **Fax:** (412)648-1837
Email: branch@msx.dept-med.pitt.edu
Robert A. Branch, MD, Prog. Dir.
Activities/Fields: Cardiology, connective tissue disease, diabetes, endocrinology, hematology and oncology, hypertension, infectious disease, pulmonary physiology, nephrology, transplantation, behavioral medicine, psychiatry and women's health.

★ 24241 ★ University of Pittsburgh McGowan Institute for Regenerative Medicine (MIRM)
409 Center for Biotechnology & Bioengineering
300 Technology Dr.
Pittsburgh, PA 15219-3112
Phone: (412)383-9998 **Fax:** (412)383-9460
Email: mirm@pitt.edu
Website: http://www.mirm.pitt.edu/contact.htm
Alan J. Russell, PhD, Dir.
Activities/Fields: Tissue engineering, cellular therapies, biosurgery, and artificial and biohybrid organ devices.

★ 24242 ★ University of Pittsburgh Nutrition Biochemistry Laboratory
503 Parran Hall
Department of Epidemiology
Graduate Sch. of Public Health
Pittsburgh, PA 15261
Phone: (412)624-2020 **Fax:** (412)624-3120
Email: rwe2@pitt.edu
Dr. Rhobert Evans, Dir.
Activities/Fields: Etiology and treatment of chronic diseases, including study of lipids, lipoproteins, osteoporsis, diabetes, hypertension, cancer, and aging.

★ 24243 ★ University of Pittsburgh Safar Center for Resuscitation Research
3434 5th Ave.
Pittsburgh, PA 15260
Phone: (412)383-1900 **Fax:** (412)624-0943
Email: kochanekpm@ccm.upmc.edu
Website: http://www.safar.pitt.edu
Patrick M. Kochanek, MD, Dir.
Activities/Fields: Traumatic brain injury and mechanisms of secondary injury, cardiopulmonary arrest and resuscitation, disaster medicine, and suspended animation. **Pub:** *Annual Report*. **Frmly:** Resuscitation Research Center.

★ 24244 ★ University of Pittsburgh Medical Center Thomas E. Starzl Transplantation Institute
Falk Medical Bldg., 4th Fl.
3601 5th Ave.
Pittsburgh, PA 15213
Phone: (412)648-3200 **Free:** 877-640-6746
Fax: (412)648-3085
Email: sticlinic@msx.upmc.edu
Website: http://www.sti.upmc.edu/Overview/about_sti.htm
John J. Fung, MD, CEO
Activities/Fields: All aspects of the transplantation of organs, including islet cell transplantation, bioartificial organ development, xenotransplantation, immunosuppression, organ preservation, immunobiology of rejection, mechanisms of tolerance and chronic rejection, autoimmunity. **Pub:** *Books*. • *Chapters*. • *Manuscripts*.

★ 24245 ★ University of Pittsburgh Medical Center Western Psychiatric Institute and Clinic
3811 O'Hara St.
Pittsburgh, PA 15213
Phone: (412)624-2100 **Fax:** (412)624-8015
Email: pilkonispa@msx.upmc.edu
Website: http://www.wpic.pitt.edu
Paul A. Pilkonis, PhD, Dir.
Activities/Fields: Advancement of basic and clinical knowledge in psychological, biological, environmental, and social interactions related to mental health and psychiatric care. Conducts research on psychiatric disorders, including depression, manic-depression, schizophrenia, anorexia nervosa, Alzheimer's disease, autism, anxiety, obsessive-compulsive disorders, and borderline disorders. Clinical services are organized around comprehensive treatment modules in the following areas: adolescent and young adult disorders, adult affective disorders, geriatrics, schizophrenia, chemical dependency, and children's services. Clinical

laboratory investigations include studies in clinical pharmacology, neuroendocrinology, psychophysiology, neuropharmacology, neurophysics, molecular neurobiology and genetics, and EEG sleep. Also researches health habits and precursors of medical disease states such as hypertension, diabetes, obesity, effects of drug abuse, and epidemiology of psychiatric disorders.

★ 24246 ★ University of Puerto Rico
Caribbean Primate Research Center
Medical Science Campus
PO Box 1053
Sabana Seca, PR 00952-1053
Phone: (787)784-0322 **Fax:** (787)795-6700
Email: mkessler@coqui.net
Website: http://cprc.rcm.upr.edu/
Dr. Matthew J. Kessler, Interim Dir.
Activities/Fields: General primate behavior and biology with emphasis on sociobiology and diseases of nonhuman primates. The nonhuman primate populations and associated genealogical records make possible an evaluation of genetic, ecological, and social influences on the incidence and progress of disorders of adaptation and enable research to be conducted on control of population growth, evolution of social interaction by family selection, inbreeding potential of confined populations, reproductive behavior, positional behaviors and the development of degenerative joint disease, diabetes, obesity, and macular degeneration. The Center has been active as a site for dissertation research and for long-term, follow-up studies on a collaborative basis with research investigators.

★ 24247 ★ University of Puerto Rico
Puerto Rico Cancer Center
PO Box 365067
San Juan, PR 00936-5067
Phone: (787)763-2443 **Fax:** (787)751-6242
Website: http://rcm-medicine.upr.clu.edu/ccpr/eng/index.htm
Dr. Reynold Lopez Enriquez, Dir.
Activities/Fields: Cancer biology and carcinogenesis, solid-state carcinogenesis, bioactivation of precarcinogens, asbestos carcinogenesis, synthesis of antineoplastic agents, synthesis of radiosensitizers, tumor immunology, dietary factors in carcinogenesis, and radiation. Seeks cancer control through the Center's Cancer Tumor Registry, Detection Program, and public education. Cancer control research involves epidemiology, biostatistics, health management, and economics. **Pub:** *Cancer in Puerto Rico*, annually.

★ 24248 ★ University of Quebec
National Institute for Scientific Research
Armand-Frappier Institute
531, Blvd. des Prairies
Laval, QC, Canada H7V 1B7
Phone: (450)687-5515 **Fax:** (450)686-5566
Email: pierre.talbot@inrs-iaf.uquebec.ca
Website: http://www.inrs-iaf.uquebec.ca
Dr. Pierre Talbot, Dir.
Activities/Fields: Microbiology and immunity, including host-pathogen interactions, functions of regulators of immunity; environmental health, including toxicology and epidemiology; molecular pharmacochemistry, including peptides, natural products, and control of doping in sports.

★ 24249 ★ University of Quebec at Montreal
Centre for Study of Biological Interactions Between Environment and Health (CINBIOSE)
PO Box 8888, Downtown Sta.
Montreal, QC, Canada H3C 3P8
Phone: (514)987-3915 **Fax:** (514)987-6183
Email: leduc.johanne@uqam.ca
Website: http://www.unites.uqam.ca/cinbiose/
Johanne Leduc, Contact
Activities/Fields: Occupational health, ergonomics.

★ 24250 ★ University of Quebec at Montreal
Cognitive Neuroscience Centre
PO Box 8888
Succ. Centre-Ville
Montreal, QC, Canada H3C 3P8
Phone: (514)987-3000 **Fax:** (514)987-8952
Email: cnc@uqam.ca
Website: http://www.er.uqam.ca/nobel/cnc
Henri Cohen, PhD, Dir.
Activities/Fields: Cognitive neuroscience, including frontal dysfunction, movement disorders and cerebral bases of speech, language, attention, and memory. Also performs fMRi, evoked potential modeling and quantitative speech analysis.

★ 24251 ★ University of Quebec at Trois-Rivieres
Departmental Laboratory of Gerontology
PO Box 500
Trois-Rivieres, QC, Canada G9A 5H7
Phone: (819)376-5090 **Fax:** (819)376-5195
Email: sylvie_lapierre@uqtr.ca
Website: http://www.uqtr.ca/psycho/gerontologie/
Sylvie Lapierre, Dir.
Activities/Fields: Gerontology and the elderly, including personal goals, suicidal ideas and behavior, self-actualization and well-being, grief and bereavement, and prevention of osteoporosis, grand-parenthood and the AIDS epidemic, post-traumatic stress disorder.

★ 24252 ★ University of Quebec at Trois-Rivieres
Research Group in Cellular and Molecular Biopathologies
PO Box 500
Trois-Rivieres, QC, Canada G9A 5H7
Phone: (819)376-5011 **Fax:** (819)376-5012
Email: eric_asselin@uqtr.ca
Website: http://www.uqtr.ca
Eric Asselin, PhD, Dir.
Activities/Fields: Fundamental research on the use of artificial membrane systems applied to biophysical and medical problems. Research includes the study of cytoskeleton-membrane interactions, pharmacological use of liposomes, and physiochemical basis of membrane interactions with physiologically active substances. **Frmly:** Research Group in Membrane Biotechnology.

★ 24253 ★ University of Regina
Centre on Aging and Health (CAH)
Department of Psychology
Regina, SK, Canada S4S 0A2
Phone: (306)585-4457 **Fax:** (306)337-2321
Email: thomas.hadjistavropoulos@uregina.ca
Website: http://uregina.ca/hadjistt/centre_index.htm
Thomas Hadjistavropoulos, PhD, Dir.
Activities/Fields: Health and aging issues, especially those related to rural and aboriginal populations.

★ 24254 ★ University of Rhode Island
Cancer Prevention Research Center (CPRC)
2 Chafee Rd.
Kingston, RI 02881
Phone: (401)874-2830
Email: cprc@etal.uri.edu
Website: http://www.uri.edu/research/cprc/
Prof. James O. Prochaska, PhD, Dir.
Activities/Fields: Prevention of cancer, other chronic diseases, and premature death by developing better solutions to the most common killers and cripplers today, namely life-style factors like smoking, substance abuse, high-risk sex, unhealthy diets, and sedentary life styles.

★ 24255 ★ University of Rhode Island
Exercise Science Laboratories
Independence Sq. 2
25 W Independence Way
Kingston, RI 02881
Phone: (401)874-2976 **Fax:** (401)874-5630
Email: manfredi@uri.edu
Thomas Manfredi, PhD, Co-Dir.
Activities/Fields: Physiological profiles of athletic populations, diet and weight loss, aging and exercise. **Frmly:** Human Performance Laboratory.

★ 24256 ★ University of Rochester
Aab Institute of Biomedical Sciences
Center for Cardiovascular Research
School of Medicine & Dentistry
601 Elmwood Ave., Box 679
Rochester, NY 14642
Phone: (716)273-1947 **Fax:** (716)473-1573
Email: bradford_berk@urmc.rochester.edu
Website: http://www.urmc.rochester.edu/Aab/Cardio.htm
Bradford C. Berk, MD, Dir.
Activities/Fields: Pathophysiology of cardiovascular disease. Research focuses on vascular biology; developmental biology; ischemic injury, molecular pharmacology and signal transduction; and genetics of cardiovascular disease.

★ 24257 ★ University of Rochester
Aab Institute of Biomedical Sciences
Center for Human Genetics and Molecular Pediatric Disease (CHGMPD)
School of Medicine & Dentistry
601 Elmwood Ave., Box 703
Rochester, NY 14642
Phone: (585)273-2428 **Fax:** (585)506-0233
Email: richard_insel@urmc.rochester.edu
Website: http://www.urmc.rochester.edu/Aab/geneped/
Richard A. Insel, MD, Dir.
Activities/Fields: Identifying, characterizing, and understanding gene-disease relationships and environmental contributions, defining the molecular basis and pathogenesis of human disease, identifying pathways of gene expression, and elucidating targets and interventions for the prevention and therapy of human disease.

★ 24258 ★ University of Rochester
Aab Institute of Biomedical Sciences
Center for Oral Biology
Medical Center
601 Elmwood Ave.
PO Box 611
Rochester, NY 14642-8611
Phone: (585)275-3441 **Fax:** (585)506-0190
Email: james_melvin@URMC.Rochester.edu
Website: http://www.urmc.rochester.edu/aab/oralbio2/index.html
Dr. James E. Melvin, Dir.
Activities/Fields: Saliva glucosyltransferase interactions on surfaces, polysaccharide metabolism by oral bacteria, base production in dental plaque, regulation of mucous cell secretion, basic and applied microbial physiology, interaction of infectious eukaryotic microorganisms with host defense systems, mechanisms and regulation of fluid and electrolyte secretion, genetic engineering of bacteria and regulation of bacterial gene expression, and biosynthesis, structure, function of mucin-glycoproteins, craniofacial development, transgenic and gene-targeted miue, and role of O-glycosylation in oro-pharyngeal development.

★ 24259 ★ University of Rochester
Aab Institute of Biomedical Sciences
Center for Vaccine Biology and Immunology
601 Elmwood Ave., Box 609
Rochester, NY 14642
Phone: (716)275-9120 **Fax:** (716)273-2452

Email: tim_mosmann@urmc.rochester.edu
Website: http://www.urmc.rochester.edu/Aab/vacc-bio/
Tim Mosmann, PhD, Dir.
Activities/Fields: Vaccines for difficult infectious diseases such as tuberculosis, malaria and AIDS, and creation of new types of vaccines for treating cancer, allergy and autoimmunity.

★ 24260 ★ University of Rochester Center for Future Health (CFH)
PO Box CFH
601 Elmwood Ave.
Rochester, NY 14627-0231
Phone: (585)273-5107 **Fax:** (585)273-2981
Website: http://www.futurehealth.rochester.edu
Prof. Philippe M. Fauchet, Dir.
Activities/Fields: System of affordable, easy to use and integrated smart health technology modules for use by consumers in their homes, including technologies for aging well, healthy skin, pathogen detection and health care support for developing nations and underserved communities.

★ 24261 ★ University of Rochester Center for Visual Science
274 Meliora Hall
Rochester, NY 14627
Phone: (585)275-2459 **Fax:** (585)271-3043
Email: david@cvs.rochester.edu
Website: http://www.cvs.rochester.edu/
Dr. David Williams, Dir.
Activities/Fields: Psychophysical, physiological, computational, anatomical and clinical approaches to visual science.

★ 24262 ★ University of Rochester Eastman Dental Center
Department of Dentistry, Box 683
625 Elmwood Ave.
Rochester, NY 14620-2989
Phone: (716)275-6006 **Fax:** (716)256-3154
Email: cyril_meyerowitz@URMC.Rochester.edu
Website: http://www.urmc.rochester.edu/dentistry
Cyril Meyerowitz, DDS, Dir.
Activities/Fields: Oral diseases, including dental caries, periodontal disease, craniofacial disorders, oral pain and health behavior.

★ 24263 ★ University of Rochester Environmental Health Sciences Center
Medical Center
601 Elmwood Ave.
Rochester, NY 14642
Phone: (585)275-3265 **Fax:** (585)256-2591
Email: deborah_slechta@urmc.rochester.edu
Website: http://www.niehs.nih.gov/centers/center/roc-ctr.htm
Deborah A. Cory-Slechta, PhD, Dir.
Activities/Fields: Understanding of the mechanisms whereby exposures to environmental and occupational agents contribute to human disease and dysfunction. The center operates four research cores. The Neurotoxicology Core focuses on the extent to which toxicants act as risk factors for diseases and dysfunctions of the nervous system, particularly on the interaction between environmental factors and genetic predisposition. The Pulmonary Toxicology Core addresses mechanisms of lung injury and how these are modulated by underlying disease processes. The Protein Modulators of Toxicity Core focuses on the biologically active proteins that critically regulate molecules in normal cells as molecular mechanisms of toxicity. The Osteotoxicology Core addresses the impact of environmental and occupational agents on mineralized tissue, in particular the role of lead in caries in children, and the extent to which lead exposure serves as a risk factor for osteoporosis and related skeletal diseases associated with advanced aging.

★ 24264 ★ University of Rochester General Clinical Research Center
Strong Memorial Hospital, 4th Fl.
601 Elmwood Ave.
Rochester, NY 14642
Phone: (585)275-5295 **Fax:** (585)461-4737
Email: clinfomgr@cln1.medicine.rochester.edu
Website: http://www.urmc.rochester.edu/smd/crc/crcweb.html
John E. Gerich, MD, Prog. Dir.
Activities/Fields: Studies of normal and deranged tissue and organ function in humans, including endocrinology, metabolism, neurology, gastroenterology, immunology, pulmonary disease, cardiology, hematology, psychiatry, dermatology, infectious disease, oncology, and pediatrics. Functions as a resource for Medical Center faculty.

★ 24265 ★ University of Rochester James P. Wilmot Cancer Center
601 Elmwood Ave.
PO Box 704
Rochester, NY 14642
Phone: (585)275-9484 **Fax:** (585)273-1042
Email: richard_fisher@urmc.rochester.edu
Website: http://www.urmc.rochester.edu/cancercenter/index.html
Richard I. Fisher, MD, Dir.
Activities/Fields: Diagnosis and therapy of cancer, with particular emphasis on experimental therapeutics. Conducts laboratory research in biochemical genetics, radiation biology, immunology, endocrine biochemistry, and cancer pharmacology, utilizing animal tumor research, biomathematics/statistics, cell culture, nucleic acid sequencing, and ultrastructure facilities. Participant in five national cooperative groups.

★ 24266 ★ University of Rochester Nephrology Research Program
601 Elmwood Ave.
PO Box 675
Rochester, NY 14642
Phone: (585)275-4517 **Fax:** (585)442-9201
Email: david_bushinsky@urmc.rochester.edu
Dr. David Bushinsky, Dir.
Activities/Fields: Physiological regulation of water and salt excretion, renal potassium handling in vivo and in the isolated perfused kidney, regulation of intrarenal blood flow, fluorescence videomicroscopy studies of inner medullary blood flow, role of nucleosides as regulators of kidney function and hemodynamics, renal microvascular endothelium and epithelial cell cultures, in vivo perfusion of capillaries from the renal microcirculation, pathogenesis of acute renal failure, modulators of renal ischemic injury, and studies of tubular functioning in humans.

★ 24267 ★ University of Rochester Particulate Matter Center
School of Medicine & Dentistry
575 Elmwood Ave.
Rochester, NY 14642
Phone: (585)275-3804 **Fax:** (585)256-2631
Email: gunter_oberdorster@urmc.rochester.edu
Website: http://www2.envmed.rochester.edu/envmed/pmc/indexpmc.html
Gunter Oberdorster, DVM, Dir.
Activities/Fields: Role of airborne particulate matter, especially ultrafine particles, in causing health problems. **Pub:** *Progress reports.*

★ 24268 ★ University of Rochester Resource for the Study of Neural Models of Behavior
734 Computer Science Department
Rochester, NY 14627-0226
Phone: (716)275-3772 **Fax:** (716)461-2018
Email: dana@cs.rochester.edu
Website: http://www.cs.rochester.edu/research/brain
Dana H. Ballard, PhD, Prin. Investigator
Activities/Fields: Monitoring and simulation of behavior in conjunction with relevant neural parameters to extend the capability to monitor behavior in natural situations. Under development are equipment to measure eye movements in freely moving head situations; devices for measuring kinematic state, such as arm and hand movements; devices for producing whole-body accelerations; and anthropomorphic devices to simulate experiments and develop experimental protocols.

★ 24269 ★ University of Rochester Rochester Alzheimer's Disease Center
601 Elmwood Ave., Box 645
Rochester, NY 14642
Phone: (716)275-7704 **Fax:** (716)273-1132
Email: paul_coleman@urmc.rochester.edu
Website: http://www.urmc.rochester.edu/adc/index.html
Paul D. Coleman, PhD, Dir.
Activities/Fields: Alzheimer's Disease.

★ 24270 ★ University of Rochester Rochester Center for Biomedical Ultrasound
Hopeman Bldg., Rm. 203
PO Box 270127
Rochester, NY 14627-0127
Phone: (585)275-9542 **Fax:** (585)273-4919
Email: rcbu@ece.rochester.edu
Website: http://www.ece.rochester.edu/users/rcbu/
Prof. Kevin J. Parker, Dir.
Activities/Fields: Ultrasonic diagnosis, including imaging and Doppler ultrasound; ultrasonic treatment, including diathermy and the treatment of glaucoma and kidney and gall stones ultrasonic biophysics, including acoustic cavitation, generation and detection of ultrasound, tissue characterization, attenuation and scattering, shock fields, and nonlinear sound propagation; and biological effects of ultrasound. Also conducts research to establish safety limits for the use of ultrasound and to discover new applications, including new contrast agents. **Pub:** *Annual report.*

★ 24271 ★ University of Rochester Sleep Research Laboratory
300 Crittenden Blvd.
Rochester, NY 14642
Phone: (585)275-2900 **Fax:** (585)273-3682
Email: michael_perils@urmc.rochester.edu
Website: http://www.urmc.rochester.edu/smd/Psych/SRL/index.html
Dr. Michael L. Perlis, Dir.
Activities/Fields: Sleep and depression, mechanisms underlying the manifestations of sleep disorders, and the neuropsychological effects of sleep abnormalities.

★ 24272 ★ University of Rochester Strong Center for Developmental Disabilities (SCDD)
PO Box 14627
Rochester, NY 14627-0140
Phone: (716)275-4031 **Fax:** (716)275-9492
Email: scdd@cc.urmc.rochester.edu
Website: http://www.urmc.rochester.edu/strong/scdd
Philip W. Davidson, PhD, Exec. Dir.
Activities/Fields: Inclusion of persons with developmental disabilities in their communities and the maximization of their potential for leading independent and productive lives.

★ 24273 ★ University of Rochester Strong Children's Research Center
Medical Center
601 Elmwood Ave.
PO Box 777
Rochester, NY 14642
Phone: (716)275-0414 **Fax:** (716)271-7512
Email: scrc@urmc.rochester.edu
Website: http://www.urmc.rochester.edu/scrc
George J. Schwartz, MD, Dir.

Activities/Fields: Pediatrics. **Pub:** *Newsletter*, quarterly.

★ 24274 ★ University of Saskatchewan Cameco MS Neuroscience Research Centre
Saskatoon City Hospital, Rm. 5800
701 Queen St.
Saskatoon, SK, Canada S7K 0M7
Phone: (306)655-8711 **Fax:** (306)966-8709
Website: http://www.usask.ca/healthsci/cmsnrc
Prof. David J. Schreyer, Dir.
Activities/Fields: Treatment and cure of multiple sclerosis and other neurological disorders.

★ 24275 ★ University of Saskatchewan Institute of Agricultural Rural and Environmental Health
Royal University Hospital,
PO Box 120
103 Hospital Dr.
Saskatoon, SK, Canada S7N 0W8
Phone: (306)966-8286 **Fax:** (306)966-8799
Email: ruggi@sask.usask.ca
Website: http://iareh.usask.ca/
James A. Dosman, MD, Dir.
Activities/Fields: Agricultural health problems, including farm accidents, lung disease, cancer, stress, skin problems, and hearing loss. **Frmly:** Centre for Agricultural Medicine.

★ 24276 ★ University of Saskatchewan Reproductive Biology Research Unit
Royal University Hospital
Department of Obstetrics & Gynecology
College of Medicine
103 Hospital Dr.
Saskatoon, SK, Canada S7N 0W8
Phone: (306)966-8033 **Fax:** (306)966-8040
Email: pierson@erato.usask.ca
Website: http://erato.usask.ca
Dr. Roger A. Pierson, Dir.
Activities/Fields: Mammalian reproduction, emphasizing human reproductive biology, fertility, infertility, contraception, and embryo transfer. Emphasizes basic and applied ovarian physiology, including superovulation. Also studies reproductive ultrasonography, three-dimensional ultrasonography, and computerized image processing. **Pub:** *Annual Report.*

★ 24277 ★ University of Saskatchewan Saskatchewan Stroke Research Centre
Royal University Hospital
Saskatoon, SK, Canada S7N 0W8
Phone: (306)966-7695 **Fax:** (306)966-7685
Email: cardiff@duke.usask.ca
Website: http://www.usask.ca/medicine/ssrc
Dr. J. Kalra, Dir.
Activities/Fields: Treatment and prevention of strokes.

★ 24278 ★ University of Sherbrooke Immunobiology Research Group Clinical Research Center
Faculty of Medicine
3001 N 12 Ave.
Sherbrooke, QC, Canada J1H 5N4
Phone: (819)346-1110 **Fax:** (819)564-5215
Email: mrolaple@courrier.usherb.ca
Dr. Marek Rola-Pleszczynski, Dir.
Activities/Fields: Immunoglobulin gene expression and control, lymphocyte activation pathways and second messangers, stem cell biology, cytokine receptor physiology, structure-function studies of lipid mediator receptors, natural cytotoxicity against tumor cells, ultraviolet-irradiation and immune functions, and immune interactions in atherosclerosis.

★ 24279 ★ University of Sherbrooke Molecular Biology Research Centre RNA Group
Departement de Microbiologie et Infectiologie
Faculte de Medecine
3001 12e Ave. Nord
Sherbrooke, QC, Canada J1H 5N4
Phone: (819)564-5321 **Fax:** (819)564-5392
Benoit Chabot, Contact
Activities/Fields: Gene expression in vitro and in vivo, including the recombination of viral and cellular genes, alternative splicing of RNA, expression and function of transformation genes, replication of telomeres and clinical applications of PCR.

★ 24280 ★ University of South Alabama Comprehensive Sickle Cell Center (SCC)
College of Medicine
307 University Blvd., 2015 MSB
Mobile, AL 36688
Phone: (334)460-7334 **Fax:** (334)460-6604
Email: jhaynes@usouthal.edu
Website: http://www.southalabama.edu/usahealthsystem/sicklecell/
Dr. Johnson Haynes, Jr., Dir.
Activities/Fields: Diagnosis and treatment of sickle cell disease.

★ 24281 ★ University of South Alabama Primate Research Laboratory
Department of Comparative Medicine, MSB 992
College of Medicine
Mobile, AL 36688-0002
Phone: (334)460-6293 **Fax:** (334)460-6286
Email: lwilliam@usouthal.edu
Bob Ricker, Lab. Supv.
Activities/Fields: Primates, especially as animal models of human diseases.

★ 24282 ★ University of South Carolina at Columbia Center for Disability Resources
Department of Pediatrics
School of Medicine
Columbia, SC 29208-0001
Phone: (803)935-5248 **Fax:** (803)935-5059
Website: http://www.cdd.sc.edu
Richard R. Ferrante, PhD, Exec. Dir.
Activities/Fields: Causation and prevention of developmental disabilities and the delivery of family centered approaches for assisting people with developmental disabilities.

★ 24283 ★ University of South Carolina at Columbia Center for Health Promotion and Risk Reduction in Special Populations
Williams-Brice Bldg., No. 56
College of Nursing
Columbia, SC 29208
Phone: (803)777-2861
Email: carolyn.murdaugh@sc.edu
Website: http://www.sc.edu/nursing/center/index.htm
Carolyn Murdaugh, PhD, Dir.
Activities/Fields: Health promotion and health risk reduction in special populations. **Pub:** *Newsletter.*

★ 24284 ★ University of South Carolina at Columbia Prevention Research Center
Arnold School of Public Health
730 Devine St.
Columbia, SC 29208
Phone: (803)777-4253 **Fax:** (803)777-9007
Email: bainsworth@gwm.sc.edu
Website: http://prevention.sph.sc.edu
Barbara Ainsworth, PhD, Prin. Investigator
Activities/Fields: Public health issues, especially behaviors that place Americans at risk for chronic diseases and conditions. Of particular concern is the improvement in quality of life for special populations, including the young, elderly, racial ethnic populations, and the underserved.

★ 24285 ★ University of South Carolina at Columbia South Carolina Rural Health Research Center
220 Stoneridge Dr., Ste. 204
Columbia, SC 29210
Phone: (803)251-6317 **Fax:** (803)251-1836
Email: jprobst@gwm.sc.edu
Website: http://rhr.sph.sc.edu
Dr. Janice C. Probst, Dir.
Activities/Fields: Inequities in health status among the population of the rural U.S. with an emphasis on factors related to socioeconomic status, race and ethnicity, and access to healthcare services.

★ 24286 ★ University of South Florida Center for Community-Based Prevention Marketing
Department of Community & Family Health, MDC 56
College of Public Health
13201 Bruce B. Downs Blvd.
Tampa, FL 33612-3805
Phone: (813)974-4867 **Fax:** (813)974-5172
Email: rmcdermo@hsc.usf.edu
Website: http://www.cdc.gov/prc/centers/southflorida.htm
Robert J. McDermott, PhD, Prin. Investigator
Activities/Fields: Public health issues, especially behaviors that place Americans at risk for chronic diseases and conditions. Of particular concern is the improvement in quality of life for special populations, including the young, elderly, racial ethnic populations, and the underserved.

★ 24287 ★ University of South Florida Center for HIV Education and Research
13301 Bruce B. Downs Blvd.
Tampa, FL 33612
Phone: (813)974-4430 **Fax:** (813)974-8451
Email: knox@fmhi.usf.edu
Website: http://www.fmhi.usf.edu/hiv
Prof. Michael D. Knox, Dir.
Activities/Fields: Treatment of persons infected with HIV, study of HIV risk factors, and AIDS prevention. Provides current AIDS and HIV information to physicians, psychologists, dentists, nurses, and other health care providers.

★ 24288 ★ University of South Florida Florida Prevention Research Center (FPRC)
4809 E Busch Blvd.
Tampa, FL 33617
Phone: (813)971-2119 **Fax:** (813)971-2280
Email: rmcdermo@com1.med.usf.edu
Website: http://www.hsc.usf.edu/prc/index.html
Robert J. McDermott, PhD, Dir.
Activities/Fields: Sustained disease prevention and health promotion, through community-based prevention marketing.

★ 24289 ★ University of South Florida Institute on Aging
13201 Bruce B. Downs Blvd., MDC-56
Tampa, FL 33612-3899
Phone: (813)974-9808 **Fax:** (813)974-7047
Email: nhallfor@hsc.usf.edu
Website: http://www.hsc.usf.edu/ioa/
James A. Mortimer, Dir.
Activities/Fields: Needs and knowledge of senior citizens, especially regarding Alzheimer's disease where researchers contribute to understanding the biological, epidemiological, clinical and social aspects of this illness.

★ 24290 ★ University of South Florida Lawton and Rhea Chiles Center for Healthy Mothers and Babies
College of Public Health
13201 Bruce B. Downs Blvd., MDC 56
Tampa, FL 33612-3805
Phone: (813)974-8888 **Free:** 877-724-2359
Fax: (813)974-8889
Email: llanders@hsc.usf.edu
Website: http://www.chilescenter.org
Dr. Stanley N. Graven, Dir.
Activities/Fields: Pregnancy, infancy, and childhood up to age five. The goal is to determine the most effective strategies, programs and systems for reducing illness and death among mothers and babies, and promoting a healthy, productive lifestyle.

★ 24291 ★ University of South Florida Louis de la Parte Florida Mental Health Institute
13301 Bruce B. Downs Blvd.
Tampa, FL 33612-3807
Phone: (813)974-4602 **Fax:** (813)974-4699
Email: shern@fmhi.usf.edu
Website: http://www.fmhi.usf.edu
Dr. David Shern, Dean
Activities/Fields: Mental health care, including aging and mental health, child and family studies, community mental health, and mental health law and policy. **Pub:** *Journal of Behavioral Health Services and Research*, quarterly. • *Journal of Mental Health and Aging*, quarterly. • *Mental Health Reviews.* **Frmly:** Florida Mental Health Institute.

★ 24292 ★ University of South Florida Research and Training Center for Children's Mental Health
Florida Mental Health Institute
13301 Bruce B. Downs Blvd.
Tampa, FL 33612-3807
Phone: (813)974-4661 **Fax:** (813)974-6257
Email: friedman@mirage.fmhi.usf.edu
Website: http://rtckids.fmhi.usf.edu/
Robert M. Friedman, PhD, Exec. Dir.
Activities/Fields: Strives to strengthen the empirical foundation for effective systems of care through an integrated set of research, training, consultation, and dissemination activities. The Center also seeks to enhance the capacity of the children's mental health field to engage in system development, research, and evaluation activities specifically through training, technical assistance, and dissemination activities. **Pub:** *Data Trends*, weekly.

★ 24293 ★ University of South Florida Roskamp Institute for Research into Neurodegenerative Diseases
3515 E Fletcher Ave.
Tampa, FL 33613
Phone: (813)974-3722 **Fax:** (813)974-3915
Email: roskamp@hsc.usf.edu
Michael Mullan, MD, Dir.
Activities/Fields: Cause of and potential therapies for Alzheimer's disease.

★ 24294 ★ University of South Florida Sunshine Education and Research Center
College of Public Health
13201 Bruce B. Downs Blvd., MDC 56
Tampa, FL 33612-3805
Phone: (813)974-6624 **Fax:** (813)974-7857
Email: dmcclusk@hsc.usf.edu
Website: http://www.hsc.usf.edu/erc/
Dr. Stuart M. Brooks, Dir.
Activities/Fields: Health in the workplace, including prevention of occupational asthma, analysis of repetitive motion injuries and ergonomic controls, management of indoor air quality, function and use of personal protective equipment, occupational infectious diseases including blood-borne pathogens, strategies that integrate the principles of risk analysis and assessment, and cost and quality issues of managed care for workers' compensation programs.

★ 24295 ★ University of Southern California Alfred E. Mann Institute for Biomedical Engineering
1042 W 36th Pl., DRB 101
Los Angeles, CA 90089-1112
Phone: (213)821-1745 **Fax:** (213)821-1120
Email: staudhammer@usc.edu
Website: http://ami.usc.edu/
Peter Staudhammer, PhD, Dir. /COO
Activities/Fields: Biomedical devices and technologies.

★ 24296 ★ University of Southern California Biomedical Simulations Resource (BMSR)
Department of Biomedical Engineering
School of Engineering, OHE 500
3650 McClintock Ave.
Los Angeles, CA 90089-1451
Phone: (213)740-0342 **Fax:** (213)740-0343
Email: vzm@bmsr.usc.edu
Website: http://bmsr.usc.edu
Vasilis Z. Marmarelis, PhD, Prin. Investigator
Activities/Fields: Development of modeling methodologies for nonlinear and nonstationary dynamic systems, sparse-data systems, and biological control systems. Application areas include sensory and neuronal systems, pharmacodynamics, and cardiorespiratory control.

★ 24297 ★ University of Southern California Cardiovascular Care Research
1200 N State St., Rm. 8350
PO Box 305
Los Angeles, CA 90033
Phone: (323)226-7116 **Fax:** (323)226-7458
Email: jhaywood@hsc.usc.edu
Dr. L. Julian Haywood, Dir.
Activities/Fields: Clinical pathophysiology and management of myocardial infarction and other cardiovascular disorders, rhythm disturbances of the heart, computer-based monitoring techniques, vectorcardiography, and related investigations of electrophysiology, with emphasis on noninvasive methods, the use of radioisotopes in nuclear cardiology, and other radiological techniques. **Frmly:** Coronary Care Research.

★ 24298 ★ University of Southern California Center for Craniofacial Molecular Biology
School of Dentistry
2250 Alcazar St., CSA 1003
Los Angeles, CA 90033
Phone: (323)442-3170 **Fax:** (323)442-2981
Email: emiranda@hsc.usc.edu
Website: http://www.usc.edu/hsc/dental/ccmb/index.html
Dr. Charles F. Shuler, Dir.
Activities/Fields: Craniofacial molecular biology, including cleft palate, congenital malformations, myogenesis, and taste and biotechnologies.

★ 24299 ★ University of Southern California Center for Pediatric Health Outcomes Research (C-PHOR)
Children's Hospital of Los Angeles
Department of Pediatrics
Keck School of Medicine
4650 Sunset Blvd., MS No. 71
Los Angeles, CA 90027
Phone: (323)669-5955 **Fax:** (323)671-1800
Website: http://www.usc.edu/hsc/research/cphor/
Tricia Morphew, Proj. Mgr.
Activities/Fields: Quality of care and quality of life of infants, children and youths, particularly the indigent, in the Greater Los Angeles area.

★ 24300 ★ University of Southern California Comprehensive Sickle Cell Center
2025 Zonal Ave., Rm. 304
Los Angeles, CA 90033
Phone: (323)442-1259 **Fax:** (323)442-1255
Email: cagejohn@usc.edu
Dr. Cage S. Johnson, Dir.
Activities/Fields: Sickle cell disease, including studies on molecular biology of red cells, fetal hemoglobin identification, and renal, cardiovascular, and endocrine functions.

★ 24301 ★ University of Southern California Division of Nephrology
1200 N State St., Rm. GNH 4250
Los Angeles, CA 90033
Phone: (323)226-7307 **Fax:** (323)226-5390
Email: campese@hsc.usc.edu
Dr. Vito Campese, Ch.
Activities/Fields: Hypertension, renal disease, hypertension and the progression of renal disese.

★ 24302 ★ University of Southern California Division of Rheumatology and Immunology
2011 Zonal Ave., HMR 711
Los Angeles, CA 90033
Phone: (323)442-1946 **Fax:** (323)442-2874
Email: dhorwitz@hsc.usc.edu
David A. Horwitz, MD, Ch.
Activities/Fields: Pathogensis and treatment of human autoimmune diseases emphasizing systemic lupus erythematosus. The potential of regulatory T cells generated ex-vivo as a therapy for autoimmune diseases, for graft-versus-host disease associated with adoptive immunotherapy, and for the long-term survival or organ grafts.

★ 24303 ★ University of Southern California Environmental Health Sciences Center (SCEHSC)
Bldg. CHP 236
School of Medicine
1540 Alcazar St.
Los Angeles, CA 90033
Phone: (323)442-1096 **Fax:** (323)442-3272
Email: jpeters@hsc.usc.edu
Website: http://www.niehs.nih.gov/centers/center/usc-ctr.htm
John Peters, MD, Dir.
Activities/Fields: Effects of the environment on human health and how personal factors modify response, especially with regard to multiethnic populations of California and the Pacific Rim.

★ 24304 ★ University of Southern California General Clinical Research Center (GCRC)
1200 N State St., Rm. GNH 6602
Los Angeles, CA 90033
Phone: (323)226-4632
Website: http://www.usc.edu/hsc/gcrc/
Joseph P. Van Der Meulen, MD, Prin. Investigator
Activities/Fields: Normal human function, as well as the mechanisms, treatment, and prevention of human disease.

★ 24305 ★ University of Southern California
Hematology, Hematologic Malignancy and Retrovial Research Program
Division of Hematology
1441 Eastlake Ave., Rm. 3468
Los Angeles, CA 90033
Phone: (323)865-3913 **Fax:** (323)865-0060
Email: hornor@hsc.usc.edu
Website: http://www.uscnorris.com
Alexandra Levine, MD, Hd.
Activities/Fields: Hematologic malignancies, including non-Hodgkin's lymphoma, Hodgkin's disease, leukemia and multiple myeloma; bone marrow transplantation program, including state-of-the-art gene therapy and marking program; HIV, and AIDS-related cancers, including lymphoma, Kaposi's sarcoma, and cervical cancer; and immune-based therapy for malignant disease. Other areas include hemostasis, including studies on blood coagulation, platelets, etiology of thrombosis, chemical separation and characterization of blood clotting factors and antibody to blood clotting factors; sickle cell disease and other hemoglobinopathies. **Frmly:** Hematology Research Laboratory.

★ 24306 ★ University of Southern California
Hematopathology Unit
1200 N State St., Rm. 2422
Los Angeles, CA 90033
Phone: (323)226-7064 **Fax:** (323)226-7119
Email: nathwani@hsc.usc.edu
Dr. Bharat N. Nathwani, Ch.
Activities/Fields: Investigates neoplasms of hematopoietic system, molecular biology, and polymerase chain reactions.

★ 24307 ★ University of Southern California
Infectious Disease Research Laboratories
General Research Laboratory, Rm. 2G4
LAC-USC Med. Center
1801 E Marengo
Los Angeles, CA 90033
Phone: (323)226-3825 **Fax:** (323)226-3827
Email: holtom@hsc.usc.edu
Dr. Paul Holtom, Dir.
Activities/Fields: Infectious diseases, bacteriology, and miscellaneous antibiotic trials.

★ 24308 ★ University of Southern California
Institute for Health Promotion and Disease Prevention Research
1000 S Fremont Ave.
Alhambra, CA 91803
Phone: (626)457-4023 **Fax:** (626)457-4044
Email: kobayak@hsc.usc.edu
Website: http://www.usc.edu/go/ipr
C. Anderson Johnson, PhD, Dir.
Activities/Fields: Chronic disease prevention, behavioral epidemiology, obesity prevention, patient compliance, HIV/AIDS, and tobacco, alcohol, and other and drug abuse. Activities focus on research in health promotion and disease prevention, with young people as the principal target. **Pub:** *Technical Reports.* **Frmly:** Health Behavior Research Institute.

★ 24309 ★ University of Southern California
International Twin Study
1441 Eastlake Ave.
Los Angeles, CA 90033
Phone: (323)865-0445 **Fax:** (323)865-0141
Email: tmack@usc.edu
Dr. Thomas Mack, Dir.
Activities/Fields: Epidemiologic investigation of the etiology of various chronic diseases in twins, including cancers (breast, gastrointestinal tract, and melanoma), multiple sclerosis, diabetes, and other chronic diseases.

★ 24310 ★ University of Southern California
John T. Nicoloff General Clinical Research Center
LACUSC Medical Center
1200 N State St., Ward 6800
Los Angeles, CA 90033
Phone: (323)226-4632 **Fax:** (323)226-2796
Email: buchanan@usc.edu
Website: http://www.usc.edu/hsc/gcrc/
Dr. Thomas Buchanan, Prog. Dir.
Activities/Fields: Clinical endocrinology, infectious diseases, cancer, cardiology, rheumatology, neurology, obstetrics and gynecology, surgery, pediatrics, psychiatry, and radiology, including studies on thyroid hormone metabolism, reproductive endocrinology, calcium and bone metabolism, water and electrolyte metabolism, androgen metabolism, obesity, hypertension, diabetes, fasting, and neuromuscular disease. **Pub:** *Annual report.*

★ 24311 ★ University of Southern California
Laboratory of Applied Pharmacokinetics
Clinical Science Center, Rm. 134-B
Keck School of Medicine
2250 Alcazar St.
Los Angeles, CA 90033
Phone: (323)442-1300 **Fax:** (323)442-1302
Email: jelliffe@usc.edu
Website: http://www.usc.edu/hsc/lab_apk
Roger W. Jelliffe, MD, Dir.
Activities/Fields: Designing systems for pharmacokinetic studies and strategies for optimal therapeutic drug monitoring in patients and optimally individualized adaptive control of drug dosage regimens for patients. Activities include development and testing of computer programs for simulation, parameter identification, parametric and nonparametric population pharmacokinetic and pharmacodynamic modeling,and optimal multiple model adaptive control of drug dosage regimens and pharmacokinetic systems in clinical settings; investigation of process and measurement noise in the clinical therapeutic environment; development of software for making population pharmacokinetic models; software for stochastic adaptive control of drug dosage regimens; and development of clinically reliable interfaces and intelligent automated apparatus for delivering complex drug regimens. **Pub:** *Manuscripts.* • *Technical Reports.*

★ 24312 ★ University of Southern California
Laboratory for Developmental Genetics
School of Dentistry
University Park
925 W 34th St., DEN 4264
Los Angeles, CA 90089-0641
Phone: (213)740-1400 **Fax:** (213)740-7560
Email: tjaskoll@hsc.usc.edu
Dr. Tina Jaskoll, Co-Dir.
Activities/Fields: Cellular, molecular, and developmental biology issues associated with craniofacial and salivary gland development, with an emphasis on functional genomics of craniofacial genetics.

★ 24313 ★ University of Southern California
Liver Office
7601 E Imperial Hwy.
Downey, CA 90242
Phone: (562)401-8961 **Fax:** (562)401-7615
Dr. Bruce A. Runyon, Prog. Ch.
Activities/Fields: Liver diseases, including both clinical and basic biochemical and virologic studies of cirrhosis and viral hepatitis.

★ 24314 ★ University of Southern California
Medical Oncology Research Program
1441 Eastlake Ave.
Los Angeles, CA 90033
Phone: (323)865-3963 **Fax:** (323)865-0061
Email: dmoody@hsc.usc.edu
Derek Raghavan, MD, Ch.
Activities/Fields: Medical oncology, chemotherapy, and immunotherapy of cancer. Conducts laboratory and clinical investigations into the biology and treatment of cancer, including studies on innovative treatments, new drugs and biological agents, locoregional therapy such as hyperthermia, and preclinical and clinical pharmacology. Major studies are also conducted in autologous bone marrow transplantation for solid tumors and in biological response modifiers, including interleukin-2 interferons, monoclonal antibodies, and melanoma vaccines.

★ 24315 ★ University of Southern California
Neonatology Research Units
1240 N Mission Rd., Rm. L919
Los Angeles, CA 90033
Phone: (323)226-3409 **Fax:** (323)226-3440
Email: ramanath@usc.edu
Dr. Rangasamy Ramanathan, Dir.
Activities/Fields: Clinical problems of the newborn and premature infant, including studies on neonatal jaundice, phototherapy, nutrition and energy metabolism, body composition, renal function, pulmonary function and assisted ventilation, circulation, Sudden Infant Death Syndrome, biophysical monitoring of neonates, and follow-up of motor/mental performance of high risk infants. Operates in conjunction with the Hospital's newborn service, which delivers and cares for 18,000 infants yearly; investigation of research problems is integrated with clinical care of infants and training program for physicians.

★ 24316 ★ University of Southern California
Norris Comprehensive Cancer Center
1441 Eastlake Ave.
Los Angeles, CA 90089-9181
Phone: (323)865-0816 **Fax:** (323)865-0102
Email: jones_p@ccnt.hsc.usc.edu
Website: http://ccnt.hsc.usc.edu/
Peter A. Jones, PhD, Dir.
Activities/Fields: Multidisciplinary basic, clinical, epidemiological and translational studies in the following program areas: molecular genetics, regulatory biology, developmental therapeutics and clinical trials, cancer epidemeology, cancer control research, gemitourinary cancer, gastrointestinal cancer, breast cancer, and hematologic malignancies/retroviral disease. **Pub:** *Cancer Center Report*, 3/year.

★ 24317 ★ University of Southern California
Resource Center for Medical Ultrasonic Transducer Technology
136 Denny Research Bldg.
Los Angeles, CA 90089-1451
Phone: (213)821-2652 **Fax:** (213)740-0343
Email: kkshung@usc.edu
Dr. K. Kirk Shung, Dir.
Activities/Fields: Very high frequency ultrasonic transducers, arrays and imaging applications.

★ 24318 ★ University of Southern Maine Edmund S. Muskie School of Public Service
Maine Rural Health Research Center (MRHRC)
96 Falmouth St.
PO Box 9300
Portland, ME 04104-9300
Phone: (207)780-4435 **Fax:** (207)780-4417
Email: andyc@usm.maine.edu

Website: http://www.muskie.usm.maine.edu/research/ruralheal/
Andrew F. Coburn, PhD, Dir.

Activities/Fields: Rural health services, with special focus on rural mental health services, institutional and community-based services for rural elders, and private and public health insurance in rural areas. **Pub:** *Research and policy briefs. • Working papers.*

★ 24319 ★ University of Southern Mississippi
Sleep Research Laboratory
Box 5025
Hattiesburg, MS 39406-5025
Phone: (601)266-4611 **Fax:** (601)266-4611
Email: sleep@usm.edu
Website: http://sleep.ep.usm.edu/
John R. Harsh, PhD, Dir.

Activities/Fields: Sleep disorders. **Pub:** *Reports.*

★ 24320 ★ University of Tennessee
Boling Center for Developmental Disabilities (BCDD)
711 Jefferson
Memphis, TN 38105
Phone: (901)448-6511 **Free:** 888-572-2249
Fax: (901)448-7097
Email: fpalmer@utmem.edu
Website: http://www.utmem.edu/bcdd
Frederick B. Palmer, MD, Dir.

Activities/Fields: Independence, productivity, integration, and inclusion of individuals with disabilities and their families in the community. **Pub:** *newsletter.*

★ 24321 ★ University of Tennessee
Center of Excellence in Pediatric Pharmacokinetics and Therapeutics
Pharmacokinetics
St. Jude Children's Research Hospital
332 N Lauderdale
Memphis, TN 38105
Phone: (901)495-4995 **Fax:** (901)525-3125
Email: william.evans@stjude.org
Dr. William E. Evans, Co-Dir.

Activities/Fields: Drug therapy research in children. Seeks to promote and protect children's well-being by minimizing or eliminating pharmaceutical risks. Addresses the child's stage of physical development and rate of metabolism, in addition to body-weight and size, in determining effects of drugs.

★ 24322 ★ University of Tennessee
Division of Cardiovascular Diseases
951 Court Ave.
Memphis, TN 38163
Phone: (901)448-5759 **Fax:** (901)448-8084
Email: ktweber@utmem.edu
Dr. Karl T. Weber, Dir.

Activities/Fields: Cardiovascular system in health and disease, including investigations of hypertension, hemodynamics, echocardiographs, estrogen replacement, and cardiovascular pharmacology.

★ 24323 ★ University of Tennessee
Drug Information Center
875 Monroe, Ste. 109
Memphis, TN 38163
Phone: (901)448-5555 **Fax:** (901)448-5419
Email: namarshi@utmem.edu
Dr. Naseem Amarshi, Dir.

Activities/Fields: Therapeutic and pharmaceutical drugs. Provides therapeutic and pharmaceutic drug information to health care professionals.

★ 24324 ★ University of Tennessee
General Clinical Research Center
777 Washington Ave.
Memphis, TN 38105
Phone: (901)570-3380 **Fax:** (901)448-7608
Email: bsalpert@utmem.edu
Website: http://www.utmem.edu/crc
Bruce Alpert, MD, Dir.

Activities/Fields: Provides general clinical research facilities for controlled inpatient and outpatient studies on human subjects with various disorders, including sickle cell anemia, diabetes mellitus, hyperandrogenism and other endocrine disorders, kidney disease, liver disorders, hypertension, brain tumors, muscular dystrophy, obesity, metabolic bone diseases, psychiatric disorders, osteoporosis, Reye's syndrome, hirsutism, sexual disorders, reproduction problems, thyroid disorders, breast cancer, and leukemia. Also studies the physiology of hypertension and the metabolic effect of exercise. **Pub:** *Annual Report.*

★ 24325 ★ University of Tennessee
Institute Neuroscience
875 Monroe Ave., Rm. 422
Memphis, TN 38163-2194
Phone: (901)448-5956 **Fax:** (901)448-4685
Email: dvsmith@utmem.edu
Website: http://cns.utmem.edu/
Dr. David V. Smith, Dir.

Activities/Fields: General neurosciences, including epilepsy studies; movement disorders (Parkinson's disease, Huntington's disease, and muscular dystrophy); vision studies (retinal disease and central visual pathways malfunction); developmental neurobiology (tissue culture and transplant in the basal ganglia, development of neural circuitry in the central visual system, neurological mutants and chimeras, development of cerebral and cerebellar cortical cytoarchitechtonics, and development of synapses in the retina); neuroendocrinology (control of brain neurotransmitters, temperature regulation in host defense response to infectious agents, and hormonal regulation of neuroeffector mechanisms); neurotransmitter action in the brain (biochemical analysis of neurotransmitters and hormone action, second messenger systems and effect of psychiatric medicine on these systems, and neuropeptide systems involved in pain and stress); and central nervous system control of the cardiovascular system (hypertension and temperature regulation); and sleep mechanisms.

★ 24326 ★ University of Tennessee
Medical Center at Knoxville
Graduate Sch. of Medicine
1924 Alcoa Hwy.
Knoxville, TN 37920-6969
Phone: (865)544-9000 **Fax:** (865)544-6819
Email: mcaudle@utk.edu
Website: http://www.utmedicalcenter.org
Dr. Michael R. Caudle, Dean

Activities/Fields: Hematology, oncology, and the molecular processes of disease, including cellular and humoral immunity, colon cancer and colitis, cytogenetics, experimental and comparative pathology, platelet function, immunobiology, and membrane transport.

★ 24327 ★ University of Tennessee
Memphis Cancer Center
910 Madison Ave., Ste. 917
Memphis, TN 38163
Phone: (901)448-5150 **Fax:** (901)448-5033
Email: hniel@utmem.edu
Harvey B. Niell, MD, Dir.

Activities/Fields: Detection, evaluation, and treatment of cancer, specifically, clinical therapeutic research, cancer drug development, cell growth and regulation, and gene regulation and expression. **Pub:** *Cancer Education Bulletin*, monthly.

★ 24328 ★ University of Tennessee
Molecular Resource Center
Coleman Bldg., Rm. A-130
956 Court Ave.
Memphis, TN 38163
Phone: (901)448-6191 **Fax:** (901)448-8229
Email: mdockter@utmem.edu
Dr. Michael Dockter, Exec. Dir.

Activities/Fields: Function and regulation of genes. Conducts experiments with gene replication and with isolation and manipulation of genetic components, with applications to cancer. Studies include cloning, mapping, probing, and sequencing of genes. **Pub:** *Annual Report.*

★ 24329 ★ University of Tennessee, Knoxville
Children's Mental Health Services Research Center
128 Henson Hall
Knoxville, TN 37996-3332
Phone: (865)974-1707 **Fax:** (865)974-1662
Email: cglisson@utk.edu
Website: http://utcmhsrc.csw.utk.edu/
Dr. Charles Glisson, Dir.

Activities/Fields: Children who are at risk for mental illness, the factors which place them at risk, the quality of the services being provided to them, and the long-term outcomes.

★ 24330 ★ University of Tennessee, Knoxville
Community Health Research Group (CHRG)
Conference Center Bldg., Ste. 309
Knoxville, TN 37996-4133
Phone: (865)974-4511 **Fax:** (865)974-4521
Email: chrg@utk.edu
Website: http://web.utk.edu/~chrg/hit/chrghome.htm
Sandra L. Putnam, PhD, Dir.

Activities/Fields: Social and medical epidemiology and the planning, organization, delivery, financing, and quality of health care, at local, regional and national levels. **Pub:** *Reports.*

★ 24331 ★ University of Tennessee, Knoxville
Experimental Oncology Laboratory
College of Veterinary Medicine
2407 River Dr.
Knoxville, TN 37996
Phone: (865)974-8217 **Fax:** (865)974-5616
Email: hmsch@utk.edu
Dr. Hildegard M. Schuller, Dir.

Activities/Fields: Oncology research, focusing on role of receptor mediated signal transduction pathways, their role in chemical carcinogenesis mechanisms, and exploitation of such pathways for cancer prevention and treatment.

★ 24332 ★ University of Tennessee, Knoxville
Human Immunology and Cancer Program (HICP)
1924 Alcoa Hwy.
Knoxville, TN 37920-6999
Phone: (865)544-9165 **Fax:** (865)544-6865
Email: asolomon@mc.utmck.edu
Website: http://www.utmck.edu/hicp/default.asp
Alan Solomon, MD, Dir.

Activities/Fields: Pathogenesis, diagnosis, and treatment of multiple myeloma and Amyloidosis. **Pub:** *Scientific journals.*

★ 24333 ★ University of Texas
M.D. Anderson Cancer Center
Texas Medical Center
1515 Holcombe Blvd.
Houston, TX 77030
Phone: (713)792-2121 **Free:** 800-392-1611
Website: http://www.mdanderson.org
John Mendelsohn, MD, Mng. Dir.

Activities/Fields: Biochemistry and molecular biology, biomathematics, carcinogenesis, cancer biology, metastasis and angiogenesis; immunology and molecular genetics; clinical research programs in brain tumor, breast cancer, gastrointestinal oncology, gynecological and ovarian cancer, head and neck oncology, leukemia/lymphoma and hematologic malignancies, lung cancer, pediatric oncology, prostate and genitourinary cancer, sarcoma and skin cancer; thematic research programs in bone marrow transplantation, cancer bioimmunotherapy, diagnostic oncology including laboratory medicine, pathology, and nuclear medicine, cancer drug development, gene therapy and molecular therapeutics, radiation oncology and biology, cancer supportive care, and veterinary medicine and surgery; and population-based research programs in behavioral science, clinical cancer prevention and epidemiology. Extensive translational research projects anchor the continuum from basic research to clinical application to improve early detection, diagnostic techniques, multidisciplinary therapy, rehabilitation, and cancer prevention. **Pub:** *OncoLog*, quarterly. • *Reports*, biennially.

★ 24334 ★ University of Texas M.D. Anderson Cancer Center Center for Research on Environmental Disease (CRED)
Science Park Research Division
Park Rd. 1C
PO Box 389
Smithville, TX 78957
Phone: (512)237-9444 **Fax:** (512)237-2990
Email: jdigiovanni@sprd1.mdacc.tmc.edu
Website: http://www.niehs.nih.gov/centers/center/utsctr.htm
John DiGiovanni, PhD, Dir.
Activities/Fields: Mechanisms by which environmental factors may cause or influence human disease and methods for early detection, prevention, and control of environmentally related diseases. **Pub:** *Annual report*. • *Newsletter*.

★ 24335 ★ University of Texas M.D. Anderson Cancer Center Levit Radiologic-Pathologic Institute
1515 Holcombe Blvd.
Houston, TX 77030
Phone: (713)792-6161 **Fax:** (713)792-0812
Email: shildebr@mdanderson.org
Website: http://www.mdanderson.org/departments/LevitRPI/
Stan Hildebrand, Dir.
Activities/Fields: Treatment of cancer patients and the diagnosis and prevention of cancer. Also involved in imaging support for multi-discipinary treatment conferences, electronic publishing, and simplified communication of patient records between referring consulting physicians.

★ 24336 ★ University of Texas at Arlington Center for Hispanic Studies in Nursing and Health
Box 19407
School of Nursing
411 S Nedderman Dr.
Arlington, TX 76019-0407
Phone: (817)272-2776 **Fax:** (817)272-5006
Email: mlbond@uta.edu
Website: http://www.uta.edu/nursing/hispanic.htm
Dr. Mary Lou Bond, Co-Dir.
Activities/Fields: Effects of the Hispanic culture on health and treatment outcomes.

★ 24337 ★ University of Texas at Arlington Center for Nursing Research
PO Box 19407
Arlington, TX 76019
Phone: (817)272-2776 **Fax:** (817)272-5006
Email: clcason@uta.edu
Dr. Carolyn L. Cason, Dir.
Activities/Fields: Hispanic health needs, health promotion and prevention of illness, palliative care, rural health care, nursing care outcomes, and economics of health care delivery.

★ 24338 ★ University of Texas at Arlington Human Performance Institute
PO Box 19180
Arlington, TX 76019-0180
Phone: (817)273-2335
Email: gvk@hpi.uta.edu
Website: http://www-ee.uta.edu/hpi/
Dr. George Kondraske, Dir.
Activities/Fields: Methods of measurement of human performance, including performance theory, human performance conceptual framework, and specialized instrumentation; studies have broad applications in the fields of space, rehabilitation, the military, and industry. Fundamental focus is on the human system-task interface. Projects include development of a computer-automated system to measure basic elements of human performance, testing of both normal and impaired individuals, and the development of methods for automated, objective disability determination. Conducts longitudinal studies of patients to characterize disease history. Also studies human performance in relation to spasmodic dysphonia, athletes, post-polio syndrome, and head injuries. Develops software tools for automated assessment of complex sets of measurements. **Pub:** *Newsletter*, semiannually. • *Progress Report*, annually.

★ 24339 ★ University of Texas at Austin Animal Resources Center
CMC A2500
2701 Speedway
Austin, TX 78705
Phone: (512)471-7534 **Fax:** (512)471-4336
Email: j.fineg@mail.utexas.edu
Website: http://www.utexas.edu/research/arc/
Jerry Fineg, DVM, Dir.
Activities/Fields: Provides a facility for research and housing of research animals. Also involved in diagnostic and procedural manipulation of the animals used in research and teaching elsewhere in the University. Research laboratories are provided for studies in anthropology, biochemistry, pharmaceutics, biomedical engineering, microbiology, nutrition, pharmacology, kienesiology, and zoology.

★ 24340 ★ University of Texas at Austin Biochemical Institute
WEL 5.266B
Austin, TX 78712
Phone: (512)471-1105 **Fax:** (512)471-8696
Email: m.hackert@mail.utexas.edu
Website: http://neon.cm.utexas.edu/bioinst/
Dr. Marvin L. Hackert, Dir.
Activities/Fields: Drug metabolism, mechanism and regulation of protein synthesis, structure, function, and regulation of enzymes and other proteins, nutritional aspects of human disease, and cloning, sequencing, and site specific mutagenesis of genes, their regulation, and repair. **Frmly:** Clayton Foundation Biochemical Institute.

★ 24341 ★ University of Texas at Austin Biomedical Engineering Graduate Program
Engineering Science Bldg., 610
Austin, TX 78712-1084
Phone: (512)471-3604 **Fax:** (512)471-0616
Email: kdiller@mail.utexas.edu
Website: http://www.bme.utexas.edu
Dr. Kenneth R. Diller, Dir.
Activities/Fields: Application of scientific and engineering knowledge to the solution of medical problems. Projects deal with molecular bioengineering, antibiotic synthesis, spectroscopic detection of early cancers, diagnostic applications of tissue fluorescence, image analysis by computer, cryopreservation of organs and tissues, quantitative thermographic imaging, electrosurgical safety, thrombosis on injured vessel and atherosclerotic surfaces and on polymeric biomaterials, pulsatile-flow cardiopulmonary bypass, chromatographic features of polar and nonpolar cardiac glycosides, hyperthermia in cancer therapy, effects of coenzyme Q-10 on cardiac function, biodegradable polymer implants for use in surgery, computer graphics analysis of sport biomechanics, rheology of synovial fluids, robotic surgical lasers, laser-tissue interaction, structure and function of hybrid proteins, and microvascular analysis of burn wounds.

★ 24342 ★ University of Texas at Austin Biomedical Engineering Laser Laboratory (BELL)
Engineering Science Bldg. R20
Austin, TX 78712
Phone: (512)471-1826 **Fax:** (512)471-0616
Email: rylander@mail.utexas.edu
Website: http://www.ece.utexas.edu/bell/
Dr. H. Grady Rylander, III, Contact
Activities/Fields: Use of light in therapeutic and diagnostic medical applications. Research establishing an understanding of the basic (optical, thermal, chemical, physiological, etc.) focuses on phenomena involved in laser-tissue interaction.

★ 24343 ★ University of Texas at Austin Center for Biotechnology
WEL, 4.260C
Austin, TX 78712-1159
Phone: (512)471-3279 **Fax:** (512)471-8696
Email: bkitto@mail.utexas.edu
Barrie Kitto, PhD, Dir.
Activities/Fields: Biotechnology.

★ 24344 ★ University of Texas at Austin Center for Health Promotion Research (CHPR)
School of Nursing
1700 Red River
Austin, TX 78701-1499
Phone: (512)471-9910 **Fax:** (512)471-4673
Email: chpr@mail.nur.utexas.edu
Website: http://www.nur.utexas.edu/CHPR2000/CHPR.html
Alexa Stuifbergen, PhD, Dir.
Activities/Fields: Reduction in health disparities of underserved groups.

★ 24345 ★ University of Texas at Austin Center for Pharmacoeconomic Studies
College of Pharmacy
Austin, TX 78712
Phone: (512)471-2819 **Fax:** (512)471-8762
Email: johnsrud@mail.utexas.edu
Website: http://www.utexas.edu/pharmacy/research/institutes/pharmacoeconomics/index.html
Michael T. Johnsrud, PhD, Assoc. Dir.
Activities/Fields: Impact of pharmaceutical services and products on patients' quality of life and health care outcomes through cost-effectiveness, cost-benefit, cost-utility, and cost-minimization analyses.

★ 24346 ★ University of Texas at Austin Drug Dynamics Institute
College of Pharmacy
Austin, TX 78712-1074
Phone: (512)471-4841 **Fax:** (512)471-2746
Email: mcginity.jw@mail.utexas.edu
James W. McGinity, Dir.
Activities/Fields: Pharmaceutical research, development, and testing, including discovery of new medicinal agents, improvement of drug therapy, mechanisms of drug action, and re-evaluation of marketed products.

★ 24347 ★ University of Texas at Austin Female Sexual Psychophysiology Laboratory
Seay Bldg., 3rd Fl.
108 E Dean Keaton St.
Austin, TX 78712

Phone: (512)232-4805 **Fax:** (512)471-6175
Email: meston@psy.utexas.edu
Website: http://homepage.psy.utexas.edu/homepage/group/MestonLAB/index.htm
Cindy M. Meston, PhD, Dir.
Activities/Fields: Sexual psychophysiology of women.

★ 24348 ★ University of Texas at Austin Laboratory for Artificial Neural Systems
ACES 3.106
Department of Electrical & Computer Engineering
Austin, TX 78712-1084
Phone: (512)471-8980 **Fax:** (512)471-2893
Email: ghosh@ece.utexas.edu
Website: http://www.lans.ece.utexas.edu/
Prof. Joydeep Ghosh, Dir.
Activities/Fields: Artificial neural systems.

★ 24349 ★ University of Texas at Austin Laboratory for the Study of Anxiety Disorders
Seay Psychology Bldg., Ste. 3.122
Department of Psychology
1 University Station
Austin, TX 78712
Phone: (512)404-9308 **Fax:** (512)471-6572
Email: lsad@techlab.com
Website: http://homepage.psy.utexas.edu/homepage/group/telchlab/home.htm
Prof. Michael J. Telch, PhD, Dir.
Activities/Fields: Nature and treatment of anxiety-related disorders, including panic-related disorders; social anxiety; specific phobias such as claustrophobia, spider phobia, and dog phobia; obsessive-compulsive disorder; and generalized anxiety.

★ 24350 ★ University of Texas at Austin Reproductive Biology Laboratory
Section for Integrative Biology
Division of Biological Sciences
Austin, TX 78712
Phone: (512)471-1113 **Fax:** (512)471-6078
Email: crews@mail.utexas.edu
Website: http://uts.cc.utexas.edu/~crewslab/index.html
Dr. David Crews, Dir.
Activities/Fields: Reproductive biology, principally the development and function of sex differences.

★ 24351 ★ University of Texas at Austin Waggoner Center for Alcohol and Addiction Research
2500 Speedway, MBB 1.124
Austin, TX 78712-1095
Phone: (512)232-2514
Email: harris@mail.utexas.edu
Website: http://www.utexas.edu/cons/wcaar/index.html
R. Adron Harris, PhD, Dir.
Activities/Fields: Alcohol and drug dependence, especially defining the molecular actions of alcohol and related drugs on brain signaling systems and understanding the molecular basis of genetic differences in alcohol susceptibility.

★ 24352 ★ University of Texas at Dallas Aging and Memory Research Laboratories
Cognition & Neuroscience
School of Human Development, GR 4.814
Richardson, TX 75083
Phone: (972)883-4933 **Fax:** (972)883-2491
Email: tres@utdallas.edu
Website: http://www.utdallas.edu/~tres/aging_memory.html
Dr. Tres Thompson, Prog. Hd.
Activities/Fields: Cellular mechanisms and changes and how they affect memory during aging.

★ 24353 ★ University of Texas at Dallas Callier Center for Communication Disorders
1966 Inwood Rd.
Dallas, TX 75235-7298
Phone: (214)905-3000 **Fax:** (214)905-3022
Email: roeser@utdallas.edu
Website: http://www.callier.utdallas.edu/
Dr. Ross J. Roeser, Dir.
Activities/Fields: Behavioral, electrophysiological, and anatomical studies of audition; behavioral and electrophysiological studies of normal and disordered speech production and perception; evoked potential and brain mapping; the linguistic and cognitive abilities of persons with aphasia and other neurogenic speech and language impairments; language development of children with chronic otitis media; development and assessment of communicative abilities in children with multiple handicaps; vibrotactile aids; and aural rehabilitation.

★ 24354 ★ University of Texas at Dallas Molecular and Cell Biology Program
Mail Stop FO3.1
PO Box 830688
Richardson, TX 75083-0688
Phone: (972)883-4870 **Fax:** (972)883-2409
Email: sgoodmn@utdallas.edu
Website: http://nsm1.utdallas.edu/bioweb/centers/centers.htm
Dr. Steven R. Goodman, Interim Prog. Hd.
Activities/Fields: Biochemistry, macromolecular physical chemistry, microbial and molecular genetics, and cell biology. **Pub:** *Research Reports.*

★ 24355 ★ University of Texas at El Paso Border Biomedical Research Center (BBRC)
Biology Bldg. 225
El Paso, TX 79968
Phone: (915)747-6850 **Fax:** (915)747-5808
Email: dnatalicio@utep.edu
Website: http://www.utep.edu/biology/bbrc/main.htm
Diana Natalicio, Prin. Investigator
Activities/Fields: Infectious diseases, environmental health, neuroscience and metabolic disorders in the border region of the U.S. and Mexico.

★ 24356 ★ University of Texas Health Center at Tyler Southwest Center for Agricultural Health, Injury Prevention, and Education
11937 US Hwy. 271
Tyler, TX 75708-3154
Website: http://swcenter.uthct.edu/
Arthur L. Frank, MD, Dir.
Activities/Fields: Occupational injuries and diseases among agricultural workers and their families.

★ 24357 ★ University of Texas Health Science Center at San Antonio Center for Environmental Radiation Toxicology
MSC 7889
7703 Floyd Curl Dr.
San Antonio, TX 78229-3900
Phone: (210)567-8025 **Fax:** (210)567-8051
Email: meltz@uthscsa.edu
Martin Meltz, PhD, Dir.
Activities/Fields: Effects of individual and combined exposures to ultrawideband and extremely hight peak power pulsed microwave radiation, ionizing radiation, UV light and chemicals on biological systems. Current investigations focus on a variety of normal and cancerous in vitro cell lines, and human peripheral blood lymphocytes. The endpoints studied include signal transduction mechanisms, protein and gene induction, primary DNA damage and repair, and proteomics. **Frmly:** Center for Basic Research in Radiation Bioeffects.

★ 24358 ★ University of Texas Health Science Center at San Antonio Institute for Biotechnology
15355 Lambda
San Antonio, TX 78245-3207
Phone: (210)567-7200 **Fax:** (210)567-7277
Email: hottle@uthscsa.edu
Website: http://www.molecularmedicine.uthscsa.edu
Dr. Wen-Hwa Lee, Dir. /Ch.
Activities/Fields: Biotechnology and molecular medicine.

★ 24359 ★ University of Texas—Houston Health Science Center Center for Health Policy Studies (CHAMPS)
1200 Herman Pressler, Ste. E-735
Houston, TX 77025
Phone: (713)500-9390 **Fax:** (713)500-9359
Website: http://www.sph.uth.tmc.edu:8052/champs/champs.html
Frank I. Moore, PhD, Dir.
Activities/Fields: Health policy options and program effects, including community health needs assessments in metropolitan counties and underserved regions of Texas; studies concerned with health expenditures and with supply and distribution of the health professions workforce in Texas; program evaluations of teen pregnancy prevention, managed care and community-oriented primary care programs; public health internships in the Lower Rio Grande Valley; and health workforce development in third world countries.

★ 24360 ★ University of Texas—Houston Health Science Center Center for Health Promotion and Prevention Research
School of Public Health
7000 Fannin, 25th Fl.
Houston, TX 77030
Phone: (713)500-9609 **Fax:** (713)500-9602
Email: chppr@sph.uth.tmc.edu
Website: http://www.sph.uth.tmc.edu/chppr
Dr. Stephen H. Kelder, Dir.
Activities/Fields: Health promotion research and development, with emphasis on institutional settings (worksites, medical care facilities, schools, and communities). Studies include the interaction of educational, economic, and environmental influences on health promotion, testing interventions directed toward institutions and individuals, and the innovation, diffusion, and maintenance of health promotion programs. Conducts survey research for monitoring and surveillance of health knowledge, attitudes, opinion, and behavior; evaluates methods and strategies for health care adapted to select populations; provides technical assistance, consultation, and collaboration with agencies, industries, institutions, media, and universities throughout Texas; and helps develop educational materials. **Pub:** *Prevention Research News*, semiannually. Newsletter. **Frmly:** Center for Health Promotion Research and Development.

★ 24361 ★ University of Texas—Houston Health Science Center Center for Society and Population Health
1200 Herman Pressler, RAS E-901
Houston, TX 77030
Phone: (713)500-9485 **Fax:** (713)500-9493
Email: david.low@uth.tmc.edu
Website: http://www.sph.uth.tmc.edu:8052/csph/
Dr. M. David Low, Dir.
Activities/Fields: Improvement in the health of all people, particularly those living in Texas. **Frmly:** Health Policy Institute.

★ 24362 ★ University of Texas—Houston Health Science Center
Genetic Marker Laboratory
School of Public Health
1200 Hermann Pressler, Ste. E-453
Houston, TX 77030
Phone: (713)500-9816 **Fax:** (713)500-0900
Email: eric.boerwinkle@uth.tmc.edu
Dr. Eric Boerwinkle, Dir.
Activities/Fields: Investigates DNA polymorphisms to find genetic bases for diseases, with special emphasis on common chronic diseases such as diabetes and heart disease. Approaches include linkage and pedigree analysis, DNA automated typing, and sequencing.

★ 24363 ★ University of Texas—Houston Health Science Center
Hermann Eye Center
Department of Ophthalmology & Visual Science
6411 Fannin St., Rm. 7024
Houston, TX 77030
Phone: (713)500-0002 **Fax:** (713)500-0682
Richard S. Ruiz, MD, Dir.
Activities/Fields: Cataracts, corneal disease, glaucoma, neuroophthalmology, ophthalmic surgery, pediatric ophthalmology, strabismus, and retinal disease. Additional studies include ocular melanoma, retinitis pigmentosa, diabetes, retinal pigment epithelial transplantation, ischemic optic neuropathy decompression, and pattern electrogram in Alzheimer's disease.

★ 24364 ★ University of Texas—Houston Health Science Center
Houston Biomaterials Research Center
6516 M.D. Anderson Blvd., Rm. 4.109
Houston, TX 77030-3402
Phone: (713)500-4191 **Fax:** (713)500-4372
Email: biomaterials@mail.db.uth.tmc.edu
Website: http://www.db.uth.tmc.edu/Biomaterials/default.htm
John M. Powers, PhD, Dir.
Activities/Fields: Biological, clinical, mechanical, chemical, and physical properties of biomaterials for dental, orthopaedic, craniofacial and other applications.

★ 24365 ★ University of Texas—Houston Health Science Center
Human Genetics Center
School of Public Health
1200 Hermann Pressler, Ste. E-453
Houston, TX 77030
Phone: (713)500-9816 **Fax:** (713)500-0900
Email: eric.boerwinkle@uth.tmc.edu
Dr. Eric Boerwinkle, Dir.
Activities/Fields: Genetic analysis of the common chronic diseases to identify and characterize the genes contributing to morbidity and mortality in most westernized populations. Research involves genetic linkage studies to localize and characterize genes contributing to disease susceptibility. Such information provides the opportunity to better predict the occurrence of disease onset and better understand mechanisms of disease etiology and pathophysiology. The research activities in the Center emphasize the evolutionary origin of disease susceptibility mutations, the genetic analysis of cardiovascular disease risk factors, and chronic disease among the Mexican-American population in South Texas. **Pub:** *Center for Demographic and Population Genetics Reports.*

★ 24366 ★ University of Texas—Houston Health Science Center
Mental Sciences Institute
1300 Moursund Ave.
Houston, TX 77030
Phone: (713)500-2500 **Fax:** (713)500-2530
Email: robert.w.guynn@uth.tmc.edu
Website: http://www.uth.tmc.edu/schools/med/psychiatry/msi/
Dr. Robert Guynn, Dir.
Activities/Fields: Biochemical and behavioral aspects of psychiatric diseases, particularly physiopathology and pharmacology of alcohol and drug addiction, and affective and anxiety disorders. Performs basic and clinical studies in neuroendocrinology, metabolism, behavioral science, disorders, developmental disorders, neurochemistry, psychophysiology, biochemistry, crime and delinquency, and gerontology. **Frmly:** Houston State Psychiatric Institute; Texas Research Institute of Mental Science.

★ 24367 ★ University of Texas—Houston Health Science Center
Neuroscience Research Center (NRC)
Medical School Bldg. 7.046
6431 Fannin
Houston, TX 77030
Phone: (713)500-5540 **Fax:** (713)500-0623
Email: nba-nrc@uth.tmc.edu
Website: http://nba19.med.uth.tmc.edu/nrc/
John H. Byrne, PhD, Dir.
Activities/Fields: Neurobehavioral sciences, particularly understanding, preventing, and treating various neural and behavioral disorders such as: dementias resulting from Alzheimer's Disease and stroke; mental retardation and learning and developmental disabilities; mental illnesses, including schizophrenia and manic-depressive illness; alcoholism and other substance abuse problems; and loss of cognitive functions due to factors such as the aging process and head trauma. **Pub:** *Newsletter.*

★ 24368 ★ University of Texas—Houston Health Science Center
Southwest Center for Occupational and Environmental Health (SWCOEH)
School of Public Health
PO Box 20186
Houston, TX 77225-0186
Phone: (713)500-9440 **Fax:** (713)500-9442
Website: http://www.sph.uth.tmc.edu:8052/swcoeh/SWCOEH.htm
George L. Delclos, MD, Dir.
Activities/Fields: Occupational and environmental health.

★ 24369 ★ University of Texas Medical Branch at Galveston
Asthma and Allergic Diseases Research Center
Division of Allergy & Immunology
Galveston, TX 77555-1083
Phone: (409)772-3411 **Fax:** (409)772-5841
Email: sasur@utmb.edu
Website: http://www2.utmb.edu/asthmacenter/
Sanjiv Sur, MD, Interim Dir.
Activities/Fields: Asthma and allergic diseases, especially the role of eosinophils which constrict airways.

★ 24370 ★ University of Texas Medical Branch at Galveston
Cardiovascular/Thoracic Surgery
6.120 John Sealy Annex
301 University Blvd.
Galveston, TX 77555-0528
Phone: (409)772-1203 **Fax:** (409)772-1421
Email: vconti@utmb.edu
Dr. Vincent R. Conti, Dir.
Activities/Fields: Myocardial metabolism with ischemia using the isolated working rat heart and isolated cardiac mitochondria. Also conducts laboratory and clinical studies of the physiologic effects of cardiopulmonary bypass.

★ 24371 ★ University of Texas Medical Branch at Galveston
Center in Environmental Toxicology
5.138 MR Bldg.
Sealy Center for Molecular Science
Department of Human Biological Genetics & Chemistry
301 University Blvd.
Galveston, TX 77555-1071
Phone: (409)772-2179 **Fax:** (409)772-1790
Email: rslloyd@utmb.edu
Website: http://www.niehs.nih.gov/centers/center/utgctr.htm
R. Stephen Lloyd, PhD, Dir.
Activities/Fields: Effects of environmental factors on the health of a local community, particularly the molecular and cellular factors that influence the onset and severity of asthma, and asthma's relationship to environmental toxicants. **Pub:** *Annual report.*

★ 24372 ★ University of Texas Medical Branch at Galveston
Center for Tropical Diseases
1.116 Keiller Bldg.
Department of Pathology
Galveston, TX 77555-0609
Phone: (409)772-2856
Email: dwalker@utmb.edu
Website: http://www.utmb.edu/ctd/
Dr. David H. Walker, Chm.
Activities/Fields: Tropical emerging and reemerging infectious diseases.

★ 24373 ★ University of Texas Medical Branch at Galveston
Child Health Research Center (CHRC)
Department of Pediatrics
301 University Blvd.
Galveston, TX 77555-0351
Phone: (409)772-1751 **Fax:** (409)772-1761
Email: lstanbe@utmb.edu
Dr. Lawrence Stanberry, Chm.
Activities/Fields: Pediatrics, focusing on applying research in developmental immunology, improving health, and combatting childhhod diseases. **Pub:** *The Growth Chart*, biennially.

★ 24374 ★ University of Texas Medical Branch at Galveston
General Clinical Research Center
301 University Blvd.
Rte. 0264
Galveston, TX 77555-0264
Phone: (409)772-1950 **Fax:** (409)772-8097
Email: dpowell@tmb.edu
Website: http://www.utmb.edu/gcrc/
Dr. Don W. Powell, Prog. Dir.
Activities/Fields: Aging, AIDS, burn injuries, cardiovascular disease, endocrinology, exercise, gastroenterology, geriatrics, gynecology, immunology, infectious diseases, metabolism, nutrition, obstetrics, oncology, ophthalmology, preventive medicine and occupational health, pulmonary diseases, rare diseases, rheumatology, sleep and space medicine.

★ 24375 ★ University of Texas Medical Branch at Galveston
Marine Biomedical Institute
301 University Blvd.
Galveston, TX 77555
Phone: (409)772-2103 **Fax:** (409)772-4687
Email: wdwillis@utmb.edu
Website: http://www.utmb.edu/mbi/
Dr. William D. Willis, Jr., Dir.
Activities/Fields: Studies on problems in comparative neurobiology, marine medicine and biology, and biophysics. **Pub:** *Bulletin.* • *Project Reports.*

★ 24376 ★ University of Texas Medical Branch at Galveston
Sealy Center for Cancer Cell Biology
301 University Blvd.
Galveston, TX 77550-1048
Phone: (409)747-1935 **Fax:** (409)747-1938
Email: afields@utmb.edu
Website: http://www2.utmb.edu/scccb/
Mark Evers, PhD, Interim Dir.
Activities/Fields: Cancer cell biology to reduce incidence, morbidity, and mortality of cancer. **Frmly:** Educational Cancer Research Center; Sealy Center for Oncology and Hematology/Educational Cancer Center.

★ 24377 ★ University of Texas Medical Branch at Galveston
Sealy Center for Molecular Science
5.104 Medical Research Bldg., Rte. 1068
301 University Blvd.
Galveston, TX 77555-1068
Phone: (409)772-3367 **Fax:** (409)772-6334
Email: lpipper@utmb.edu
Website: http://www.scms.utmb.edu/
Dr. E. Brad Thompson, Interim Dir.
Activities/Fields: Molecular biology and biochemistry. Specialized research includes eukaryotic DNA repair; HIV molecular biology, molecular toxicology and oncology, transcription regulation, signal transduction steroids and apoptosis. **Pub:** *Departmental Newsletter*, semiannually.

★ 24378 ★ University of Texas Medical Branch at Galveston
Sealy Center for Structural Biology (SCSB)
5.138 Medical Research Bldg.
Galveston, TX 77555-1055
Phone: (409)772-2281 **Fax:** (409)772-4298
Email: jclee@utmb.edu
Website: http://www.scsb.utmb.edu/
James C. Lee, PhD, Dir.
Activities/Fields: Biomolecular structure. Research focuses on molecular recognition, signal transduction, allosteric regulations, protein folding and drug design.

★ 24379 ★ University of Texas Southwestern Medical Center at Dallas
Alzheimer's Disease Center
Department of Psychiatry
5323 Harry Hines Blvd.
Dallas, TX 75390-9044
Phone: (214)648-4646 **Fax:** (214)648-4660
Email: munro.cullum@utsouthwestern.edu
Dr. Munro Cullum, Dir., Neuropsychology
Activities/Fields: Alzheimer's disease and aging in the brain, focusing on loss of cognitive functions and test measurements including IQ, problem solving, abstract thinking, spatial and dexterity skills, attention and concentration, language function, and memory.

★ 24380 ★ University of Texas Southwestern Medical Center at Dallas
Cancer Immunobiology Center (CIC)
5323 Harry Hines Blvd.
Dallas, TX 75390-8576
Phone: (214)648-1200 **Fax:** (214)649-1252
Email: ellen.vitetta@utsouthwestern.edu
Website: http://www2.utsouthwestern.edu/cic/
Dr. Ellen Vitetta, Dir.
Activities/Fields: Immunologically-based strategies for the diagnosis and therapy of cancer and AIDS.

★ 24381 ★ University of Texas Southwestern Medical Center at Dallas
Cecil H. and Ida Green Center for Reproductive Biology Science
5323 Harry Hines Blvd.
Dallas, TX 75390-9051
Phone: (214)648-6498 **Fax:** (214)648-5087
Email: david.garbers@email.swmed.edu
Website: http://greencenter.swmed.edu
Dr. David Garbers, Dir.
Activities/Fields: Reproductive biology: gametogenesis, fertilization and nuclear transplantation/reprogramming. Provides a link between research in gamete development, fertilization, and reprogramming of the somatic cell nucleus.

★ 24382 ★ University of Texas Southwestern Medical Center at Dallas
Center for Basic Neuroscience
5323 Harry Hines Blvd.
Dallas, TX 75390-9111
Phone: (214)648-1876 **Fax:** (214)648-1879
Email: tsudho@mednet.swmed.edu
Website: http://www2.swmed.edu/cbn/
Prof. Thomas C. Südhof, MD, Dir.
Activities/Fields: Brain functions in health and disease, ranging from the development of the nervous system over studies on fundamental mechanisms of synaptic transmission to investigations of vision and olfaction.

★ 24383 ★ University of Texas Southwestern Medical Center at Dallas
Center for Biomedical Inventions (CBI)
6000 Harry Hines Blvd.
Dallas, TX 75390-9185
Phone: (214)648-1408 **Fax:** (214)648-4156
Email: thomas.kodadek@utsouthwestern.edu
Website: http://cbi.swmed.edu/
Thomas J. Kodadek, Contact
Activities/Fields: Biomedicine, particularly relating to the diagnosis and treatment of cancer and heart disease. Research focuses on chemical synthesis, tissue culture, molecular biology, computation, robotics, and instrument construction.

★ 24384 ★ University of Texas Southwestern Medical Center at Dallas
Center for Developmental Biology (CDB)
5323 Harry Hines Blvd.
Dallas, TX 75390-9133
Phone: (214)648-1951 **Fax:** (214)648-1960
Email: luis.parada@utsouthwestern.edu
Website: http://www2.utsouthwestern.edu/devbio/center_frame.htm
Luis F. Parada, PhD, Dir.
Activities/Fields: Embryonic development, especially intracellular signaling pathways.

★ 24385 ★ University of Texas Southwestern Medical Center at Dallas
Center for Human Nutrition
5323 Harry Hines Blvd.
Dallas, TX 75390
Phone: (214)648-2890 **Fax:** (214)648-4837
Email: scott.grundy@utsouthwestern.edu
Website: http://www2.swmed.edu/humannutrition
Dr. Scott M. Grundy, Dir.
Activities/Fields: Human nutrition. Investigates the preventive effects of vitamins C and E on atherosclerosis.

★ 24386 ★ University of Texas Southwestern Medical Center at Dallas
Center for Immunology
Department of Microbiology
5323 Harry Hines Blvd.
Dallas, TX 75390-9093
Phone: (214)648-7330 **Fax:** (214)648-7331
Email: edward.wakeland@utsouthwestern.edu
Website: http://www.swmed.edu/home_pages/immunology
Prof. Edward K. Wakeland, PhD, Dir.
Activities/Fields: Characterization of animal models of human diseases, with an emphasis on the delineation of molecular mechanisms mediating normal and abnormal immune functions.

★ 24387 ★ University of Texas Southwestern Medical Center at Dallas
Division of Communicative and Vestibular Disorders
Department of Otolaryngology-Head and Neck Surgery
5323 Harry Hines Blvd.
Dallas, TX 75390-9035
Phone: (214)648-8568 **Fax:** (214)648-9122
Email: angela.shoup@utsouthwestern.edu
Website: http://www.swmed.edu
Angela Shoup, PhD, Contact
Activities/Fields: Dizziness, vertigo, gait and balance disorders, inner ear fluid disorders, auditory perception, auditory neurophysiology, and cochlear implants. **Frmly:** Audiovestibular Laboratory.

★ 24388 ★ University of Texas Southwestern Medical Center at Dallas
Eugene McDermott Center for Human Growth and Development
6000 Harry Hines Blvd., 10th Fl., Rm. 10.204
Dallas, TX 75390-8591
Phone: (214)648-1636 **Fax:** (214)648-1666
Email: helen.hobbs@utsouthwestern.edu
Website: http://mcdermott.swmed.edu
Dr. Helen H. Hobbs, Dir.
Activities/Fields: Genetic factors that contribute to human health and disease. The center promotes research in diverse areas including lipid metabolism, atherosclerosis, energy metabolism, chromosomal rearrangements, DNA repair, human growth and development, reproduction, cancer genetics, and biotechnology.

★ 24389 ★ University of Texas Southwestern Medical Center at Dallas
General Clinical Research Center
5323 Harry Hines Blvd.
Dallas, TX 75390-8891
Phone: (214)590-7783 **Fax:** (214)590-4091
Email: khashayar.sakhaee@utsouthwestern.edu
Website: http://crcdec.swmed.edu
Khashayar Sakhaee, MD, Prog. Dir.
Activities/Fields: Calcium metabolism, cardiopulmonary system, endocrinology, liver diseases, lipid disorders, nephrology, neurology, oncology, and pharmacology.

★ 24390 ★ University of Texas Southwestern Medical Center at Dallas
Hamon Center for Basic Research in Cancer
Department of Molecular Biology, MC-9148
5323 Harry Hines Blvd.
Dallas, TX 75390-9148
Phone: (214)648-1187 **Fax:** (214)648-1196
Email: eolson@hamon.swmed.edu
Website: http://hamon.swmed.edu/
Eric Olson, PhD, Ch.
Activities/Fields: Understanding mechanisms that control normal and abnormal cell growth and differentiation during development and disease.

★ 24391 ★ University of Texas Southwestern Medical Center at Dallas
Hamon Center for Therapeutic Oncology Research
6000 Harry Hines Blvd., NB8.206
Dallas, TX 75390-8593
Phone: (214)648-4900 **Fax:** (214)648-4940
Email: brenda.zielke@utsouthwestern.edu
Website: http://www.utsouthwestern.edu/cancer/
Brenda Zielke, Contact
Activities/Fields: Prevention, early detection, diagnosis, prognostic assessment, and treatment of human cancer.

★ 24392 ★ University of Texas Southwestern Medical Center at Dallas Harold C. Simmons Arthritis Research Center
5323 Harry Hines Blvd.
Dallas, TX 75390-8884
Phone: (214)648-9110 **Fax:** (214)648-7995
Email: david.karp@utsouthwestern.edu
Website: http://www.swmed.edu/home_pages/rheumatology
David R. Karp, MD, Interim Dir.
Activities/Fields: Inflammatory arthritis, autoimmune disease.

★ 24393 ★ University of Texas Southwestern Medical Center at Dallas Neuromuscular Treatment Center
Department of Neurology
5323 Harry Hines Blvd.
Dallas, TX 75390-8897
Phone: (214)648-6419 **Fax:** (214)648-9311
Email: gil.wolfe@utsouthwestern.edu
Website: http://neurology.swmed.edu
Gil Wolfe, MD, Dir.
Activities/Fields: Immune-mediated neuromuscular disorders, including myasthenia gravis, inflammatory neuropathy, amyotrophic lateral sclerosis (Lou Gehrig's Disease), spinal muscular atrophy. Activities include clinical therapeutic trials.

★ 24394 ★ University of Texas Southwestern Medical Center at Dallas Sickle Cell Case Management Program
5323 Harry Hines Blvd.
Dallas, TX 75390-9063
Phone: (214)648-8594 **Fax:** (214)648-3122
Email: gbuch2@mednet.swmed.edu
Dr. George Buchanan, Dir.
Activities/Fields: Researches morbidity and mortality of pediatric sickle cell patients.

★ 24395 ★ University of Texas Southwestern Medical Center at Dallas Sleep Disorders Center for Children
Children's Medical Center of Dallas
1935 Motor St.
Dallas, TX 75235-7794
Phone: (214)456-2793 **Fax:** (214)456-8740
Email: john.herman@utsouthwestern.edu
Dr. John Herman, Dir.
Activities/Fields: Studies infants with respiratory problems, children with obstructive sleep apnea, and excessive daytime sleepiness (narcolepsy). Conducts studies of vigilance and related visual evoked potentials.

★ 24396 ★ University of Texas Southwestern Medical Center at Dallas Southwestern Biomedical Magnetic Resonance Facility
Mary Nell & Ralph B. Rogers Magnetic Resonance Center
5801 Forest Park Rd.
Dallas, TX 75235-9085
Phone: (214)648-5886 **Fax:** (214)648-5881
Email: cmallo@mednet.swmed.edu
Website: http://www.swmed.edu/home_pages/rogersmr
Dr. Craig R. Malloy, Prin. Investigator
Activities/Fields: Development and refinement of the use of Nuclear Magnetic Resonance (NMR) isotopomer analysis for the investigation of intermediary metabolism in intact, functioning tissues, and application of these methods to current questions in metabolism; mathematical models to estimate the flux through different metabolic pathways using isotopomer analysis of NMR and/or mass spectroscopy data; techniques and agents for monitoring intercellular actions, particularly sodium, magnesium, and calcium, in perfused tissues and in vivo.

★ 24397 ★ University of Texas Southwestern Medical Center at Dallas Southwestern Magnetic Resonance Facility Mary Nell and Ralph B. Rogers Magnetic Resonance Center
5801 Forest Park Dr.
Dallas, TX 75235-9085
Phone: (214)648-5886 **Fax:** (214)648-5881
Email: jthach@mednet.swmed.edu
Website: http://www2.utsouthwestern.edu/rogersmr/
Dr. Craig R. Malloy, Dir.
Activities/Fields: Magnetic resonance imaging and spectroscopy of analytical samples, perfused organs, and small animals.

★ 24398 ★ University of Toledo Center for Applied Pharmacology
College of Pharmacy
2801 W Bancroft St.
Toledo, OH 43606-3390
Phone: (419)530-2010 **Fax:** (419)530-8407
Email: kbachma@utnet.utoledo.edu
Website: http://www.utoledo.edu/pharmcap/
Kenneth Bachmann, PhD, Contact
Activities/Fields: Relationship between drug disposition and drug dynamics, especially pharmacokinetics and pharmacodynamics in normal healthy subjects and in defined patient groups, bioavailability, pharmacokinetic/pharmacodynamic modeling, population kinetics, and drug interactions. **Pub:** *Reports.*

★ 24399 ★ University of Toledo Center for Drug Design and Development (CD3)
College of Pharmacy
2801 W Bancroft St.
Toledo, OH 43606-3390
Phone: (419)530-4257 **Fax:** (419)530-6110
Website: http://www.utoledo.edu/cd3/
Activities/Fields: Drug therapies and diagnostics.

★ 24400 ★ University of Toronto Centre for Cardiovascular Research
Toronto General Hospital
200 Elizabeth St.
Toronto, ON, Canada M5G 2C4
Phone: (416)340-4790 **Fax:** (416)340-5985
Email: msole@torhosp.toronto.on.ca
Michael J. Sole, MD, Dir.
Activities/Fields: Atherosclerotic cardiovascular disease, myocardial hypertrophy and failure, and arrhythmias and sudden death.

★ 24401 ★ University of Toronto Centre for Cardiovascular Research Cardiac Gene Unit
Department of Laboratory Medicine & Pathobiology
100 College St., Rm. 418A
Toronto, ON, Canada M5G 1L5
Phone: (416)978-8758 **Fax:** (416)978-5650
Email: cliew@rics.bwh.harvard.edu
C.C. Liew, PhD, Dir.
Activities/Fields: Genes that may be associated with cardiovascular disease. **Pub:** *Monographs, papers, and abstracts.*

★ 24402 ★ University of Toronto Centre for Health Promotion
Banting Institute
100 College St., Rm. 207
Toronto, ON, Canada M5G 1L5
Phone: (416)978-1809 **Fax:** (416)971-1365
Email: centre.healthpromotion@utoronto.ca
Website: http://www.utoronto.ca/chp/
Dr. Suzanne Jackson, Actg. Dir.
Activities/Fields: Health promotion, including tobacco research, quality of life issues, health communication, evaluation, best practices in health promotion, health policy, policy development, and workplace health policy. **Pub:** *Centre for Health Promotion Annual Report*, annually. • *The Health Communication Update*, quarterly. • *Information Update*, 3/year.

★ 24403 ★ University of Toronto Centre for Health Promotion Ontario Tobacco Research Unit
33 Russell St.
Toronto, ON, Canada M5S 2S1
Phone: (416)595-6888 **Fax:** (416)595-6068
Email: otru@camh.net
Website: http://www.camh.net/otru
Roberta Ferrence, Dir.
Activities/Fields: Tobacco control, including epidemiology of tobacco use and cessation, tobacco and youth, gender issues in tobacco use, ethnicity and tobacco use, economic factors in tobacco use, tobacco policy attitudes, policy and program evaluation, community interventions, and enviromental tobacco smoke. **Pub:** *Current Abstracts on Tobacco.* • *Directory, literature reviews, special reports, annotated bibliographies, information updates.* • *Working papers.*

★ 24404 ★ University of Toronto Centre for Health Promotion Quality of Life Research Unit
500 University Ave., Suite 914,
Toronto, ON, Canada M5G 1V7
Phone: (416)978-1457 **Fax:** (416)978-4363
Email: quality.oflife@utoronto.ca
Website: http://www.utoronto.ca/qol
Rebecca Renwick, Dir.
Activities/Fields: Quality of life, defined as factors that make living both meaningful and enjoyable, for seniors, adolescents, people with developmental disabilities, persons with physical disabilities, and adults in the general population.

★ 24405 ★ University of Toronto Centre for Research in Neurodegenerative Diseases
Tanz Neuroscience Bldg.
6 Queen's Park Cres. W
Toronto, ON, Canada M5S 3H2
Phone: (416)978-7461 **Fax:** (416)978-1878
Email: crnd.info@utoronto.ca
Website: http://www.utoronto.ca/crnd
Dr. Peter St. George-Hyslop, Interim Dir.
Activities/Fields: Neurodegenerative diseases of the human brain, focusing on the causes of Alzheimer's disease, Amyotrophic Lateral Sclerosis, and other nerve cell defects, the development of effective treatment for patient care, and clinical trials. Specific areas of study include genetic mutation of chromosome 21, protein degeneration of synapses and synaptic vesicles, identification and characterization of the molecular development of the nervous systems, collaborative studies on the aluminum hypothesis for Alzheimer's disease, and the study of motor control and the mechanisms that result in nerve cell degeneration in both the brain and the spinal cord.

★ 24406 ★ University of Toronto Centre for Research in Women's Health (CRWH)
790 Bay St., 7th Fl.
Toronto, ON, Canada M5G 1N8
Phone: (416)351-3732 **Fax:** (416)351-3746
Email: crwh.research@utoronto.ca
Website: http://www.crwh.org/
Dr. Heather Maclean, Dir.
Activities/Fields: Women's health issues, including cancers common in women, pharmacotherapy, reproductive health, violence against women, women's life course, women's mental health. **Pub:** *Annual reports.* • *Newsletters.*

★ 24407 ★ University of Toronto Home and Community Care Evaluation and Research Centre
50 St. George St.
Toronto, ON, Canada M5S 3H4
Phone: (416)978-8369 **Fax:** (416)978-8222
Email: peter.coyte@utoronto.ca
Website: http://www.hcerc.utoronto.ca
Dr. Peter Coyte, Co-Dir.

Activities/Fields: People, technologies, and health care settings. **Pub:** *Annual report.* • *Children and Youth Home Care Newsletter.* • *Newsletter.* • *Working Papers Series.* **Frmly:** Home Care Evaluation and Research Centre.

★ 24408 ★ University of Toronto Hospital Management Research Unit (HMRU)
McMurrich Bldg., 2nd Fl.
Department of Health Policy, Management & Evaluation
Faculty of Medicine
12 Queen's Park Cres. W
Toronto, ON, Canada M5S 1A8
Phone: (416)978-6963 **Fax:** (416)978-6177
Email: healthadmin@utoronto.ca
Website: http://www.utoronto.ca/hpme/hmru/hmru_index.htm
Dr. Louise Lemieux-Charles, Dir.

Activities/Fields: Health services assessment, particularly home care and care for the elderly. **Pub:** *Reports.*

★ 24409 ★ University of Toronto Institute of Medical Science
Medical Science Bldg., Rm. 7213
1 King's College Cir.
Toronto, ON, Canada M5S 1A8
Phone: (416)978-8886 **Fax:** (416)971-2253
Email: dir.medscience@utoronto.ca
Website: http://www.library.utoronto.ca/ims
Dr. Ori D. Rotstein, Dir.

Activities/Fields: Multidisciplinary research in clinical and basic medical science and related fields. Research is focused in three distinct areas: molecular; clinical investigation of whole organ integrative biology, and clinical investigation of quantitative methodological approaches to health outcomes. Studies focus around fields such as cardiovascular sciences, bioethics, membrane biology, respiratory medicine, and psychosomatic medicine. Collaborative programs include: bioethics; cardiovascular sciences; history of medicine; neurosciences; toxicology; and alcohol, tobacco, and other psychoactive substances.

★ 24410 ★ University of Toronto Research Services Unit
Department of Public Health Sciences
Faculty of Medicine
401B McMurruch Blvd.
Toronto, ON, Canada M5S 1A8
Phone: (416)978-5351 **Fax:** (416)978-8299
Email: vartouhi.jazmaji@utoronto.ca
Vartouhi Jazmaji, Dir.

Activities/Fields: Design and analysis of clinical trials and epidemiological studies, including biostatistics, demography, and data management and analysis.

★ 24411 ★ University of Toronto Toronto Western Research Institute University Health Network
399 Bathurst St.
Toronto, ON, Canada M5T 2S8
Phone: (416)603-5030 **Fax:** (416)603-5745
Email: chris.wallace@uhn.on.ca
Dr. M. Christopher Wallace, Dir.

Activities/Fields: Cell and membrane neurobiology, molecular neurobiology, neuroprotection, cognitive and neurophysiological aspects of normal and abnormal limb movement control, normal and pathological eye movement control and visual processing, neuropharmacology, spinal cord injury, neuro-oncology, epilepsy and cerebrovascular disease. **Frmly:** Toronto Hospital Research Institute; Playfair Neuroscience Unit.

★ 24412 ★ University of Tulsa Mary K. Chapman Center for Communicative Disorders
600 S College Ave.
Tulsa, OK 74104-3189
Phone: (918)631-2504 **Fax:** (918)631-3668
Email: karen-patterson@utulsa.edu
Website: http://www.cas.utulsa.edu/commdis/
Karen Patterson, PhD, Contact

Activities/Fields: Communication disorders, including laryngectomy and speech, and language and hearing problems. Also conducts aid tests.

★ 24413 ★ University of Utah Cardiovascular Genetic Research Program
410 Chipeta Way, Rm. 161
Salt Lake City, UT 84108
Phone: (801)581-3888 **Fax:** (801)581-6862
Email: steve@ucvg.med.utah.edu
Website: http://www.cvg.med.utah.edu
Steven C. Hunt, PhD, Co-Dir.

Activities/Fields: Cardiovascular genetics, focusing on the correlations between environment, genetics, and the incidence of early heart disease.

★ 24414 ★ University of Utah Center for Cell Signaling (CCS)
421 Wakara Way, Ste. 360
Salt Lake City, UT 84108
Phone: (801)585-9704 **Fax:** (801)585-6354
Email: nbernshaw@hnu.pharm.utah.edu
Website: http://hnu.pharm.utah.edu/CCS/
Glenn D. Prestwich, PhD, Dir.

Activities/Fields: Molecular mechanisms by which cells communicate in normal conditions and in disease states, in efforts to develop new technologies important to the treatment of cancer, allergy, asthma and inflammation.

★ 24415 ★ University of Utah Center for Controlled Chemical Delivery
Biomedical Polymers Research Bldg., Rm. 205
Salt Lake City, UT 84112
Phone: (801)581-6654 **Fax:** (801)581-7848
Email: rburns@pharm.utah.edu
Dr. Sung Wan Kim, Dir.

Activities/Fields: Controlled drug delivery systems. Specific studies include the following: hydrogel and polymer synthesis, including water-soluble, bioactive, and biodegradable polymers; transdermal drug delivery, including skin immunoreaction and sensitization, irritation mechanism, drug interaction with stratum corneum membranes, physicochemical analysis of drug permeation mechanisms, and design of optimum delivery of matrix or rate-controlling membranes; functional polymers for gastrointestinal drug delivery; polymeric prodrugs and chemical modification of drugs for specific organ targeting or long-term delivery of therapeutic agents; and delivery of peptides and protein drugs.

★ 24416 ★ University of Utah Center for Engineering Design
50 Central Campus Dr., Rm. 2202
Salt Lake City, UT 84112-9208
Phone: (801)581-6499 **Fax:** (801)581-5304
Email: s.jacobsen@ced.utah.edu
Dr. Stephen C. Jacobsen, Dir.

Activities/Fields: Robotic design and control, including teloperated and entertainment robots; actuator technology; touch sensors; micro-electromechanical systems; biomechanics; bioengineering; rehabilitation research, including projects in artificial limb design; and micro pumps and fluid delivery systems. **Frmly:** Center for Biomedical Design.

★ 24417 ★ University of Utah Center for Human Toxicology
20 South 30 East, Rm. 490
Salt Lake City, UT 84112-9457
Phone: (801)581-5117 **Fax:** (801)581-5034
Email: dcrouch@alanine.pham.utah.edu
Dennis Crouch, Co-Dir.

Activities/Fields: Clinical, forensic, and bioanalytical toxicology, including studies in clinical pharmacology and toxicology, drug metabolism, disposition, adverse interactions, alcohol/drugs and driving, proficiency testing, postmortem toxicology, data interpretation, and new chromatographic and mass spectrometry techniques in toxicology.

★ 24418 ★ University of Utah Dixon Laser Institute
155 South 1452 East, No. 405
Salt Lake City, UT 84112-8906
Phone: (801)585-3791 **Fax:** (801)585-5366
Email: vicky@chpc.utah.edu
Dr. Werner Gellerman, Dir.

Activities/Fields: Laser research, including applications of lasers in medicine, industry, and the military. Biomedical studies focus on gastroenterology, cardiology, otolaryngology, obstetrics-gynecology, urology, genetics, microsurgery, dentistry, and photodynamic therapy. In association with the Vanderbildt University Free Electron Laser Lab, the Institute is investigating the development and application of free electron laser technology in medicine and materials science.

★ 24419 ★ University of Utah DNA Diagnostic Laboratory
Center for Advanced Medical Technologies, Rm. 150
729 S Arapeen Dr.
Salt Lake City, UT 84108
Phone: (801)581-8334 **Free:** 888-DNA-MAPS
Fax: (801)585-3876
Email: ken.ward@hsc.utahh.edu
Kenneth Ward, MD, Dir.

Activities/Fields: Gene mapping, genetic diagnosis, preimplantation testing, pregnancy loss, birth defect genes, and preeclampsia genes.

★ 24420 ★ University of Utah Human Performance Research Laboratory
235 Health, Physical Education & Recreation North Bldg.
Salt Lake City, UT 84112
Phone: (801)581-8687 **Fax:** (801)585-3992
Dr. Andrea T. White, Dir.

Activities/Fields: Effects of exercise and environment on muscular, cardiovascular, respiratory, nervous, and thermoregulatory systems of the human body. Programs are conducted on exercise and multiple sclerosis patients, women at risk for osteoporosis, exercise and functional abilities and health benefits.

★ 24421 ★ University of Utah Huntsman General Clinical Research Center
50 N Medical Dr., Rm. 4R210
Salt Lake City, UT 84132
Phone: (801)581-6736 **Fax:** (801)585-1461
Email: jkushner@crc.med.utah.edu
Website: http://crc-gw.med.utah.edu
James P. Kushner, MD, Dir.

Activities/Fields: Provides facilities for School of Medicine faculty conducting clinical investigations in the areas of renal and cardiac failure, cardiac transplantation, genetic diseases, nutrition and cancer, atherosclerosis, diabetes and obesity, psychiatric and neuromuscular disorders, disorders of intermediary metabolism (porphyrins, carbohydrates, lipids, trace elements), diseases of the endocrine system (adrenal, pituitary, gonad, thyroid, and pancreas), infectious disease, and drug therapy of human diseases.

★ 24422 ★ University of Utah Intermountain Cystic Fibrosis Center
School of Medicine
50 N Medical Dr.
Salt Lake City, UT 84132
Phone: (801)581-2410 **Fax:** (801)587-9620
Email: barbara.chatfield@hsc.utah.edu
Website: http://www.med.utah.edu/pulm/cf/
Barbara Chatfield, Pediatrics Dir.

Activities/Fields: Cystic fibrosis and pulmonary disease, including studies electrolyte metabolism in the lung, lung mechanics, clinical studies of new therapies, and antibiotic pharmacology. **Pub:** *CF Informer Newletter*, quarterly.

★ 24423 ★ University of Utah Intermountain Injury Control Research Center (IICRC)
615 Arapeen Dr., Ste. 202
Salt Lake City, UT 84108-1226
Phone: (801)581-6410 **Fax:** (801)581-8686
Email: lenora.olson@hsc.utah.edu
Website: http://iicrc.med.utah.edu/
Lenora Olson, Dir.

Activities/Fields: Reduction in the incidence and severity of injury in the states of Colorado, Montana, North Dakota, South Dakota, Utah, and Wyoming.

★ 24424 ★ University of Utah Nora Eccles Harrison Cardiovascular Research and Training Institute (CVRTI)
95 South 2000 East Back
Salt Lake City, UT 84112-5000
Phone: (801)581-8183 **Fax:** (801)581-3128
Email: info@cvrti.utah.edu
Website: http://www.cvrti.utah.edu/
Dr. Rob MacLeod, Co-Dir.

Activities/Fields: Cardiac electrophysiology, with investigative expertise ranging from the molecular/cellular level to the whole heart. Two other areas of cellular research are intracellular PH regulation and excitation-contraction coupling in cardiac cells.

★ 24425 ★ University of Utah Radiobiology Laboratory
729 Arapeen Dr., Ste. 2334
Salt Lake City, UT 84102-1218
Phone: (801)581-6600 **Fax:** (801)581-7008
Email: scott.miller@hsc.utah.edu
Website: http://www.utah.edu/radiobiology
Dr. Scott C. Miller, Dir.

Activities/Fields: Chemistry, physics, biochemistry, bone sciences, and veterinary aspects and pathology of long-term physiological and biochemical effects of internally deposited radioisotopes. **Pub:** *Research in Radiobiology*, annually. Report.

★ 24426 ★ University of Utah Rocky Mountain Center for Occupational and Environmental Health
75 South 2000 East
Salt Lake City, UT 84112
Phone: (801)581-8719 **Fax:** (801)581-7224
Email: khegmann@rmcoeh.utah.edu
Website: http://www.rmcoeh.utah.edu/
Dr. Kurt Hegmann, Dir.

Activities/Fields: Occupational and environmental health and safety with emphasis on exposure assessment, environmental epidemiology, asbestos-related health problems, musculoskeletal and other injury evaluation and prevention, and ergonomic aspects of the work environment.

★ 24427 ★ University of Vermont Center on Disability and Community Inclusion
101 Cherry St., Ste. 450
Burlington, VT 05401-4439
Phone: (802)656-4031 **Fax:** (802)656-1357
Email: ccloning@zoo.uvm.edu
Website: http://www.uvm.edu/~uapvt/
Chigee Cloninger, Exec. Dir.

Activities/Fields: Independence, inclusion, participation, and personal choice of individuals with disabilities of all ages in all environments.

★ 24428 ★ University of Vermont Clinical Neuroscience Research Unit (CNRU)
UHC Campus, Arnold 6
1 S Prospect St.
Burlington, VT 05401-1195
Phone: (802)847-4560 **Fax:** (802)847-7889
Email: paul.newhouse@uvm.edu
Website: http://www.uvm.edu/~cnru
Paul Newhouse, MD, Dir.

Activities/Fields: Mechanisms, treatment, and amelioration of complex neuropsychiatric disorders. Disorders of particular interest include those that have a behavioral and cognitive component, such as Alzheimer's disease and Parkinson's disease. The center also studies complex neuropsychiatric disorders function after menopause; new pharmaceutical agents for Alzheimer's disease; and depression, post-traumatic stress disorder and anxiety disorders in young and elderly populations.

★ 24429 ★ University of Vermont General Clinical Research Center
111 Colchester Ave.
Burlington, VT 05401
Phone: (802)847-2777 **Fax:** (802)847-5562
Email: richard.galbraith@uvm.edu
Website: http://www.uvm.edu/~gcrc
Dr. Richard A. Galbraith, Dir.

Activities/Fields: Various medical and surgical problems. Provides research facility for individual research studies.

★ 24430 ★ University of Vermont McClure Musculoskeletal Research Center
Stafford Hall, 4th Fl.
Department of Orthopaedic and Rehabilitation
Burlington, VT 05405-0084
Phone: (802)656-2250 **Fax:** (802)656-4247
Email: bruce.beymon@uvm.edu
Website: http://www.uvm.edu/~ortho
Bruce D. Beynnon, PhD, Dir.

Activities/Fields: Occupational and sports injuries and nontraumatic and congenital disorders, including how musculoskeletal structures are injured and how they heal. Research focuses on lower back pain, including studies of vehicle vibration, exercise, and different low back pain treatments; sports medicine, including knee, shoulder, and ankle injuries; scoliosis, including the etiology of idiopathic scoliosis and growth asymmetry research; osteoarthritis; and joint replacement studies.

★ 24431 ★ University of Vermont Office of Health Promotion Research
1 S Prospect St.
Burlington, VT 05401
Phone: (802)656-4187 **Fax:** (802)656-8826
Email: brian.flynn@uvm.edu
Website: http://www.uvm.edu/~ohpr
Dr. Brian S. Flynn, Dir.

Activities/Fields: Health education, smoking prevention (primarily with youth), smoking cessation, particularly with women of child-bearing age; breast screening promotion, breast self-exam education, behavioral/lifestyle change, and alcohol-use prevention in adolescents. **Frmly:** Vermont Lung Center.

★ 24432 ★ University of Victoria Centre on Aging
PO Box 1700, STN CSC
Victoria, BC, Canada V8W 2Y2
Phone: (250)721-6369 **Fax:** (250)721-6499
Email: dfh@uvic.ca
Website: http://www.coag.uvic.ca/
David F. Hultsch, PhD, Dir.

Activities/Fields: Health and wellbeing of the elderly.

★ 24433 ★ University of Victoria Centre for Biomedical Research
PO Box 1700, STN CSC
Victoria, BC, Canada V8W 2Y2
Phone: (250)472-4071 **Fax:** (250)472-4075
Email: bkoop@uvic.ca
Website: http://web.uvic.ca/ceh/index.html
Ben F. Koop, PhD, Dir.

Activities/Fields: Impact and influence of the environment on genetic organization and expression, and the consequences of this impact upon the health and genetic integrity of individuals, populations, and species. **Frmly:** Centre for Environmental Health.

★ 24434 ★ University of Virginia Asthma and Allergic Diseases Center
Division of Asthmas, Allergy & Immunology
University of Virginia Health System
Charlottesville, VA 22908
Phone: (434)924-5917 **Fax:** (434)924-5779
Email: tap2z@virginia.edu
Website: http://www.med.virginia.edu/medicine/clinical/internal/allergy/
Thomas A.E. Platts-Mills, MD, Dir.

Activities/Fields: Allergic and immunologic respiratory and skin diseases, especially asthma, hives, immunodeficiency diseases, respiratory fungal diseases, drug allergies, hay fever, and insect venom sensitivity.

★ 24435 ★ University of Virginia Beirne Carter Center for Immunology Research
Health Science Center
PO Box 801386
Charlottesville, VA 22908-1386
Phone: (434)924-9233 **Fax:** (434)924-1221
Email: lbm6b@galen.med.virginia.edu
Website: http://www.healthsystem.virginia.edu/cic
Dr. Thomas J. Braciale, Dir.

Activities/Fields: Basic and clinical immunology, infectious diseases, cancer, autoimmune diseases, and cell signaling in the immune system. **Pub:** *Annual report.* • *Carter Immunology Center Newsletter.* • *Research and training brochure.*

★ 24436 ★ University of Virginia Cancer Center
Box 800334
Charlottesville, VA 22908-0334
Phone: (434)924-9333 **Free:** 800-251-3627
Fax: (434)982-0049
Email: ba4n@virginia.edu
Website: http://www.med.virginia.edu/medcntr/cancer/home.html
Barry Anderson, Jr., Admin.

Activities/Fields: Cancer.

★ 24437 ★ University of Virginia Cardiovascular Research Center (CVRC)
MR-4 Bldg., 6th Fl.
University of Virginia Health System, Box 801394
Charlottesville, VA 22908
Phone: (434)924-5092 **Fax:** (434)924-2828
Website: http://www.healthsystem.virginia.edu/internet/cvrc/
Brian R. Duling, PhD, Dir.

Activities/Fields: Cardiovascular disease.

★ 24438 ★ University of Virginia Center for Biomedical Ethics
PO Box 800758
Charlottesville, VA 22908
Phone: (434)924-5974 **Fax:** (434)982-3971
Email: jdm8n@virginia.edu
Website: http://www.med.virginia.edu/bioethics
Jonathan D. Moreno, Dir.
Activities/Fields: Identification, analysis, and resolution of ethical problems in health care.

★ 24439 ★ University of Virginia Center for Cell Signaling
Health Science Center
PO Box 800577
Charlottesville, VA 22908
Phone: (434)924-1235 **Fax:** (434)243-2829
Email: signals@virginia.edu
Website: http://hsc.virginia.edu/signals/
David L. Brautigan, PhD, Dir.
Activities/Fields: Molecular biology of cellular signaling processes, including membranes, receptors, transduction, genome-level signals, and molecular structure. **Frmly:** Markey Center.

★ 24440 ★ University of Virginia Center for the Engineering of Wound Prevention and Repair
Box 277, Health Science Center
Department of Biomedical Engineering
School of Engineering & Applied Science
Charlottesville, VA 22908
Phone: (434)924-0270 **Fax:** (434)982-3780
Email: tskalak@virginia.edu
Website: http://yakko.bme.virginia.edu/wound/index.html
Thomas Skalak, Dir.
Activities/Fields: Principles governing mechanical and biological events in chronic skin wounds, to eradicate chronic wounds in hospital settings, to apply these principles to accelerate the repair of acute skin wounds caused by trauma, and to improve therapies for skin flap procedures, intestinal ulcers, and neurological injury.

★ 24441 ★ University of Virginia Center for Improving Minority Health (CIMH)
800729 UVa Health System
Charlottesville, VA 22908
Phone: (434)924-1165 **Fax:** (434)243-2916
Website: http://www.med.virginia.edu/cimh/
Dr. M. Norman Oliver, Dir.
Activities/Fields: Health care delivery, access, and outcomes among minority populations, especially disparities in health care and outcomes.

★ 24442 ★ University of Virginia Center for Research in Contraceptive and Reproductive Health
University of Virginia Health System
PO Box 800732
Charlottesville, VA 22908
Phone: (434)924-1202 **Fax:** (434)982-3912
Email: jch7k@virginia.edu
Website: http://hsc.virginia.edu/medicine/basic-sci/cellbio/crgcv/
John Herr, Dir.
Activities/Fields: Human contraceptive vaccine based upon recombinant DNA techniques for both males and females, male contraceptives based on regulation of spermatogenesis. **Frmly:** Center for Recombinant Gamete Contraceptive Vaccinogens.

★ 24443 ★ University of Virginia Center for Research in Reproduction
UVA Health Sciences Center
PO Box 800391
Charlottesville, VA 22908
Phone: (434)924-1807 **Fax:** (434)982-0701
Website: http://www.med.virginia.edu/medcntr/centers/crr/
Dr. John C. Marshall, Dir.
Activities/Fields: Human reproduction.

★ 24444 ★ University of Virginia Center for Structural Biology (CSB)
Molecular Physiology & Biological Physics
PO Box 800736
Charlottesville, VA 22906-0736
Phone: (434)924-5926 **Fax:** (434)982-1616
Email: aps2n@virginia.edu
Website: http://olenka.med.virginia.edu/newcsb2/Consort.html
Andrew P. Somlyo, Dir.
Activities/Fields: Cellular and macromolecular structure, function and interactions.

★ 24445 ★ University of Virginia Center for the Study of Complementary and Alternative Therapies (CSCAT)
PO Box 800905
Charlottesville, VA 22908-0905
Phone: (434)924-0113 **Fax:** (434)243-9938
Email: cscat@virginia.edu
Website: http://www.healthsystem.virginia.edu/internet/cscat
Ann Gill Taylor, Dir.
Activities/Fields: Complementary and alternative medicine, especially in treating pain.

★ 24446 ★ University of Virginia Center for the Study of Mind and Human Interaction (CSMHI)
PO Box 800657
Charlottesville, VA 22908-0657
Phone: (434)982-1045 **Fax:** (434)982-2524
Email: mind@virginia.edu
Website: http://www.healthsystem.virginia.edu/csmhi
Dr. Lisa Aronson, Dir.
Activities/Fields: Large-group dynamics, including ethnic tension, racism, national identity, terrorism, societal trauma, leader-follower relationships, and other aspects of national and international conflict. **Pub:** *Mind and Human Interaction.*

★ 24447 ★ University of Virginia Center for the Study of Neurodegenerative Diseases (CSND)
Box 801404
No. 186 Gilmer Hall
Charlottesville, VA 22904
Phone: (434)924-8374 **Fax:** (434)924-0370
Email: bennett@virginia.edu
Dr. James P. Bennett, Jr., Dir.
Activities/Fields: Abnormal mitochondrial function and its role in causing neurodegenerative brain diseases. The major hypothesis being examined is that individuals with sporadic forms of Parkinson's and Alzheimer's diseases inherit mitochondria with mutations in the mitochondrial DNA. These mutations lead to reduced activities of enzyme complexes in the electron transport chain and an increased susceptibility to programmed cell death.

★ 24448 ★ University of Virginia Communication Disorders Program
Speech Language Hearing Center
2205 Fountain Ave., Ste. 305
Charlottesville, VA 22903
Phone: (804)924-6351 **Fax:** (804)924-4621
Email: rrr7w@virginia.edu
Website: http://curry.edschool.virginia.edu/commdis/projects/clinic/
Dr. Randall Robbey, Dir.
Activities/Fields: Speech and language pathology, audiology, early detection in infant speech/language/hearing disorders, education of the deaf, and speech and hearing science, including computer applications to communications disorders treatment. Supervises doctoral research in these fields and sponsors meetings of interest to speech and language pathologists, audiologists, and educators of the hearing impaired. **Frmly:** Speech and Hearing Center.

★ 24449 ★ University of Virginia Digestive Health Center of Excellence
Division of GI/Hepatology
PO Box 800708
Charlottesville, VA 22908
Phone: (434)924-2959
Email: fc4q@virginia.edu
Website: http://www.hsc.virginia.edu/internal/digestive-health/home.html
Fabio Cominelli, MD, Dir.
Activities/Fields: Underlying causes of many gastrointestinal diseases. The research program is centered around five themes: mucosal immunology and gut inflammation, gastrointestinal cancer, bacterial/viral-host interactions, epithelial cell and hepatocyte transport, clinical epidemiology and outcomes research.

★ 24450 ★ University of Virginia General Clinical Research Center
School of Medicine
PO Box 800787
Charlottesville, VA 22908
Phone: (434)924-3160 **Fax:** (434)924-2073
Dr. Eugene J. Barrett, Dir.
Activities/Fields: Endocrinology, neurology, surgery, gastroenterology, ophthalmology, cardiology, obstetrics/gynecology, immunology, renal diseases, and ear, nose, and throat studies. Special interests include neuroendocrinology, hypertension, vascular disease, juvenile diabetes mellitus, genetic disorders, fertility disorders, digestive and growth disorders, sleep disorders, asthma and pulmonary disorders, congestive heart failure, arrhythmias, and epilepsy. Personnel are trained in rapid blood sampling and blood processing and a biostatistician is available to assist in research protocol design. Serves as a general clinical center for use by entire faculty of the School for any type of clinical investigation.

★ 24451 ★ University of Virginia International Health Care Worker Safety Center
PO Box 800764
Charlottesville, VA 22903
Phone: (434)924-5159 **Fax:** (434)982-0821
Website: http://www.med.virginia.edu/~epinet/center2.html
Janine Jagger, PhD, Dir.
Activities/Fields: Reduction of occupational exposures to and transmission of bloodborne pathogens to health care workers worldwide. **Pub:** *Advances in Exposure Prevention*, bimonthly.

★ 24452 ★ University of Virginia Molecular Biomechanics Laboratory
Box 800759
Department of Biomedical Engineering
Charlottesville, VA 22908
Phone: (434)243-2740 **Fax:** (434)982-3870
Email: guilford@virginia.edu
Website: http://yakko.bme.virginia.edu/lab/
Prof. William H.O. Guilford, PhD, Dir.
Activities/Fields: Molecular mechanisms by which cells move, and the application of this knowledge to the understanding and treatment of cardiovascular disease.

★ 24453 ★ University of Virginia Myles Thaler Center for AIDS and Human Retrovirus Research
PO Box 800743
Charlottesville, VA 22908
Phone: (434)982-1597 **Fax:** (434)982-1590
Email: thalercenter@virginia.edu

Website: http://www.med.virginia.edu/medcntr/centers/thaler/home.html
Prof. David Rekosh, PhD, Dir.
Activities/Fields: Human retrovirus life cycle, viral regulatory genes, viral assembly and viral entry.

★ 24454 ★ University of Virginia Nephrology Clinical Research Center (NCRC)
Box 800133
Charlottesville, VA 22908
Phone: (434)924-5820 **Fax:** (434)924-1979
Email: ncrc@virginia.edu
Website: http://www.healthsystem.virginia.edu/internet/nephrology/ncrc.cfm
W. Kline Bolton, MD, Contact
Activities/Fields: Kidney disease and related problems, such as hypertension and diabetes; renal insufficiency; end stage renal disease and related problems, such as anemia and hyperparathyroidism; and polycystic kidney disease.

★ 24455 ★ University of Virginia Neuromuscular Center
Department of Neurology
UVA Medical Center
PO Box 800394
Charlottesville, VA 22908
Phone: (434)924-2706 **Fax:** (434)924-9068
Dr. George F. Wooten, Dir.
Activities/Fields: Electrophysiology of dystrophy skeletal muscle fibers, biochemical studies of the properties of normal and dystrophic cells in culture, structure and chromosome linkage of human muscle genes, genetic heterogeneity among the hereditary motor sensory neuropathies, long chain fatty acids in Olivo-Ponto-cerebellar atrophy, the axonal cytoskeleton following IDPN administration, biochemical differences in shrimp claw muscle protein, membrane enzymes involved in muscle regulation, safety margin of neuromuscular transmission in normal and diseased muscle, and the humoral hypothesis in the Eaton-Lambert syndrome. Also conducts clinical research in such neuromuscular diseases as myasthenia gravis, Eaton-Lambert syndrome, Charcot-Marie-tooth disease, and diabetic polyneuropathy.

★ 24456 ★ University of Virginia Southeastern Rural Mental Health Research Center
Health Science Center, Box 800782
Charlottesville, VA 22908-0782
Phone: (434)982-3273 **Fax:** (434)982-3275
Email: srmhrc@virginia.edu
Website: http://minerva.acc.virginia.edu/~srmhrc/
Elizabeth Merwin, Dir.
Activities/Fields: Rural mental health, focusing African-Americans and impoverished mentally ill individuals and their families. Specific area of study include the incidence and prevalence of mental disorders and co-occurring physical health problems, informal and formal care networks and interventions accessed and utilized by rural high risk populations in need of mental health and health service, and the cost and effectiveness of outreach and alternative models linking mental health, social service, and health care providers in the delivery of services to seriously mentally ill adults, the elderly, women, and children.

★ 24457 ★ University of Virginia Surgical Therapeutic Advancement Center (STAC)
MR 4 Bldg., Rm. 3122
University of Virginia Health System
PO Box 801373
Charlottesville, VA 22908-1373
Phone: (434)243-0315 **Fax:** (434)243-0318
Email: uvatac@virginia.edu
William D. Spotnitz, MD, Dir.
Activities/Fields: Development of innovations in the field of surgery to improve the clinical care of patients. **Pub:** *Journal manuscripts.*

★ 24458 ★ University of Virginia Surgical Therapeutic Advancement Center Tissue Adhesive Center
MR 4 Bldg., Rm. 3122
PO Box 801373
Charlottesville, VA 22908-1373
Phone: (434)243-0315 **Fax:** (434)243-0318
Email: uvatac@virginia.edu
William D. Spotnitz, MD, Dir.
Activities/Fields: Tissue adhesives for the clinical care of patients, and especially cellular biology, adhesive strength profiling, and animal modeling.

★ 24459 ★ University of Virginia Vascular Medicine and Preventive Cardiology Unit
UVA Health System, Box 800146
Charlottesville, VA 22908-0146
Phone: (434)924-2765 **Fax:** (434)924-9604
Email: cra2e@virginia.edu
Website: http://www.hsc.virginia.edu/heart
Carlos R. Ayers, MD, Hd.
Activities/Fields: Cardiovascular problems, including hypertension, hyperlipidemia, renal blood flow, renin-angiotension-aldosterone metabolism, catecholamine metabolism, plethysmography, peripheral vascular physiology and disease, and cardiovascular risk reduction. **Frmly:** Virginia Heart Laboratory; Hypertension/Atherosclerosis Unit.

★ 24460 ★ University of Washington Alcohol and Drug Abuse Institute
1107 NE 45th St., Ste. 120
PO Box 354805
Seattle, WA 98105-4631
Phone: (206)543-0937 **Fax:** (206)543-5473
Email: ddonovan@u.washington.edu
Website: http://adai.washington.edu
Dennis M. Donovan, PhD, Dir.
Activities/Fields: Social, clinical, and psychological aspects of alcohol and drug abuse. **Pub:** *ADAI Technical Reports.*

★ 24461 ★ University of Washington Alzheimer's Disease Research Center
1660 S Columbian Way (116 MIRECC)
Seattle, WA 98108
Phone: (206)782-1010 **Free:** 800-317-5382
Fax: (206)768-5456
Email: wamble@u.washington.edu
Website: http://depts.washington.edu/adrcweb/
Molly Wamble, Contact
Activities/Fields: Basic mechanisms underlying the development of adult dementing disorders, with particular attention to heritable susceptibility factors underlying Alzheimer's disease. **Pub:** *Dimensions Newsletter*, quarterly.

★ 24462 ★ University of Washington Center for Child Environmental Health Risks Research (CHC)
Department of Environmental Health
4225 Roosevelt Way NE, No. 100
Seattle, WA 98105-6099
Phone: (206)616-9133 **Fax:** (206)616-4875
Email: chc@u.washington.edu
Website: http://depts.washington.edu/chc/
Thomas Burbacher, PhD, Dep. Dir.
Activities/Fields: Children's susceptibility to pesticides and the ways pesticides affect normal development and learning.

★ 24463 ★ University of Washington Center for Cost and Outcomes Research (CCOR)
Box 358853
Seattle, WA 98195
Phone: (206)543-4943
Email: deyo@u.washington.edu
Website: http://depts.washington.edu/ccor/
Richard A. Deyo, MD, Co-Dir.
Activities/Fields: Cost-effective approaches to improving the health of patients and populations and identification of ways to put these improvements into practice. **Pub:** *Annual report.*

★ 24464 ★ University of Washington Center for Disability Policy and Research (CDPR)
Department of Health Services, Box 358852
School of Public Health & Community Medicine
146 N Canal St., Ste. 313
Seattle, WA 98103-8652
Phone: (206)685-7260 **Fax:** (206)616-3135
Email: cdpr@u.washington.edu
Website: http://depts.washington.edu/cdpr/
Donald Patrick, Co-Dir.
Activities/Fields: Disablement process and disabling conditions, the health needs of people with disabilities, the personal, and the delivery of health and human services to people with disabilities and their families. **Pub:** *Reports.*

★ 24465 ★ University of Washington Center for Health Education and Research (CHER)
901 Boren Ave., Ste. 1100
Seattle, WA 98104
Phone: (206)221-4944 **Fax:** (206)221-4945
Email: marnae@u.washington.edu
Website: http://depts.washington.edu/cherweb/
King K. Holmes, MD, Dir.
Activities/Fields: Health and quality of life of individuals and communities.

★ 24466 ★ University of Washington Center on Human Development and Disability
PO Box 357920
Seattle, WA 98195-7920
Phone: (206)543-2832 **Fax:** (206)543-3417
Email: chdd@u.washington.edu
Website: http://depts.washington.edu/chdd
Michael J. Guralnick, PhD, Dir.
Activities/Fields: Biomedical and behavioral research of human development, including studies in developmental biology, perinatal biology, neurological sciences, psychology, psychiatry, speech and hearing sciences, social work, nursing, and special education. **Pub:** *Outlook*, quarterly. **Frmly:** Child Development and Mental Retardation Center.

★ 24467 ★ University of Washington Center for Videoendoscopic Surgery (CVES)
Department of Surgery, Box 356410
1959 NE Pacific St., Rm. BB-487
Seattle, WA 98195
Phone: (206)685-9076 **Fax:** (206)685-6912
Email: cwesterg@u.washington.edu
Website: http://depts.washington.edu/cves/
Prof. Carlos A. Pellegrini, MD, Dir.
Activities/Fields: Development of new minimally invasive surgical techniques.

★ 24468 ★ University of Washington Center for Women's Health Research (CWHR)
Box 357261
T624 Health Sciences Bldg.
Seattle, WA 98195-7261

Phone: (206)543-1414 **Free:** 877-543-1414
Fax: (206)543-4091
Email: cwhr@u.washington.edu
Website: http://www.uw-cwhr.org
Margaret Heitkemper, Dir.

Activities/Fields: Health of women across the life span. **Pub:** *Newsletter*.

★ 24469 ★ University of Washington Child Health Institute (CHI)

146 N Canal St., Ste. 300
Seattle, WA 98103-8652
Phone: (206)616-9410 **Fax:** (206)543-5318
Email: chiorg@u.washington.edu
Website: http://depts.washington.edu/chiorg/
Dimitri Christakis, Co-Dir.

Activities/Fields: Access, cost-effectiveness, quality and outcomes of health care for children.

★ 24470 ★ University of Washington Children's Hospital and Medical Center Exstrophy of Excellence

4800 Sand Point Way NE
PO Box 5371/CH-78
Seattle, WA 98105
Phone: (206)987-2509 **Fax:** (206)987-3835
Michael Mitchell, MD, Dir.

Activities/Fields: Cloacal or bladder exstrophy in children. **Pub:** *Meeting Reports.*

★ 24471 ★ University of Washington Clinical Nutrition Research Unit

PO Box 356426
Seattle, WA 98195-6426
Phone: (206)543-6166 **Fax:** (206)685-3781
Email: uwcnru@u.washington.edu
Website: http://depts.washington.edu/uwcnru/
Prof. Alan Chait, MD, Dir.

Activities/Fields: Human nutrition in health and disease, including nutritional health maintenance, improved nutritional support of the acutely and chronically ill, assessment of nutritional status, effects of diseased states on nutritional needs, and effects of nutrition on disease states. Conducts research with human subjects and populations. Also basic and animal research.

★ 24472 ★ University of Washington Comprehensive Biology-Exploiting the Yeast Genome

Box 357350
Departments of Genetics, Molecular Biotechnology & Biochemis
Seattle, WA 98195-7360
Phone: (206)543-5345 **Fax:** (206)685-1792
Email: tdavis@u.washington.edu
Website: http://depts.washington.edu/~yeastrc/
Trisha Davis, PhD, Prin. Investigator

Activities/Fields: Analysis of macromolecular interactions using the methods of mass spectrometry, the two-hybrid system, microscopy, and protein structure prediction.

★ 24473 ★ University of Washington Comprehensive Center for Oral Health Research

B-530 HSB, Box 357480
1959 NE Pacific St.
Seattle, WA 98195-7480
Phone: (206)543-5599 **Fax:** (206)685-8024
Email: ccohr@u.washington.edu
Website: http://depts.washington.edu/ccohr
Dr. Timothy DeRouen, Dir.

Activities/Fields: Children's dentistry, caries, innate immunity, etc. **Pub:** *Annual report.* **Frmly:** Research Center in Oral Biology.

★ 24474 ★ University of Washington Department of Bioengineering Simulation Resource in Circulatory Transport, Exchange and Metabolism

Harris Hydraulics Laboratory
PO Box 357962
Seattle, WA 98195
Phone: (206)685-2005 **Fax:** (206)685-3300
Email: jbb@bioeng.washington.edu
Website: http://nsr.bioeng.washington.edu/PLN
James B. Bassingthwaights, Dir.

Activities/Fields: Logical structures for experiment design and analysis, including automating and fitting models to data, assessing the goodness-of-fit, choosing numerical approximations and, in some situations, the form of the model. Studies include estimates of conductances of capillary and cell membranes, volumes of distribution, and regional flows in organs; identification of receptor affinities and metabolic rates in intact organs via various tracer techniques; cell metabolic models, and development of an interactive simulation system that permits formulation of models without programming. Applications include: transport of hydrophilic molecules in microvasculature; simulation analysis for estimation of tracer uptake and depositionin cells, as indicators of regional blood flow and cellular function; use of fractals in describing heterogeneous systems, such as spatial and temporal flow variation. **Pub:** *Newsletter*, semiannually.

★ 24475 ★ University of Washington Developmental Speech Physiology Laboratory

Department of Speech & Hearing Sciences, Box 354875
1417 NE 42nd St.
Seattle, WA 98105-6246
Phone: (206)616-5273 **Fax:** (206)543-1093
Email: camoore@u.washington.edu
Website: http://faculty.washington.edu/spchphys/
Prof. Christopher A. Moore, PhD, Contact

Activities/Fields: Development of articulatory, laryngeal, and respiratory coordination for speech and other oromotor behaviors, including chewing and sucking.

★ 24476 ★ University of Washington Diabetes Endocrinology Research Center

DVA Puget Sound Health Care System
1660 S Columbian Way
PO 358285
Seattle, WA 98108
Phone: (206)764-2688 **Fax:** (206)764-2693
Email: jpp@u.washington.edu
Website: http://depts.washington.edu/diabetes/
Jerry P. Palmer, MD, Dir.

Activities/Fields: Diabetes Mellitus and its complications. Provides biomedical research facilities and services that are not readily available to individual investigators, including light and electron microscopy, recruitment of patient volunteers, radioimmunoassays, skin fibroblast and other cultures. Supports investigators in the field through a pilot and feasability program.

★ 24477 ★ University of Washington Diagnostic Imaging Sciences Center

HSB AA048
Box 357115
1959 Pacific Ave.
Seattle, WA 98195
Phone: (206)685-0457 **Fax:** (206)543-3495
Email: kmarav@u.washington.edu
Dr. Kenneth Maraville, Dir.

Activities/Fields: Diagnostic imaging, including PET, NMR spectroscopy and imaging, nucle ar medicine imaging and therapy, x-ray physics, ultrasound imaging, physiology, including angio-intervention techniques, image processing, and contrast media testing.

★ 24478 ★ University of Washington End of Life Care Research Program

Harborview Medical Center, Box 359762
325 9th Ave.
Seattle, WA 98104
Phone: (206)731-3356 **Fax:** (206)731-8584
Email: jrc@u.washington.edu
Website: http://depts.washington.edu/eolcare/
J. Randall Curtis, Co-Dir.

Activities/Fields: Improvement of end-of-life care, including quality of care and communication about end-of-life care.

★ 24479 ★ University of Washington Engineering Research Center for Engineered Biomaterials

PO Box 351720
Seattle, WA 98195-1720
Phone: (206)685-1005 **Fax:** (206)616-9763
Email: ratner@uweb.engr.washington.edu
Website: http://www.uweb.engr.washington.edu
Dr. Buddy D. Ratner, Dir.

Activities/Fields: Exploitation of specific biological recognition mechanisms in order to develop a new generation of biomaterials for medical implants that will heal in the body in a facile, physiologically normal manner. **Pub:** *Journal of Undergraduate Research in Bioengineering.*

★ 24480 ★ University of Washington Fetal Alcohol and Drug Unit

Department of Psychiatry & Behavioral Sciences
180 Nickerson St., Ste. 309
Seattle, WA 98109
Phone: (206)543-7155 **Fax:** (206)685-2903
Email: astreiss@u.washington.edu
Website: http://depts.washington.edu/fadu/content.html
Prof. Ann P. Streissguth, PhD, Dir.

Activities/Fields: Prevention, intervention and treatment of Fetal Alcohol Syndrome (FAS) and Fetal Alcohol Effects (FAE).

★ 24481 ★ University of Washington General Clinical Research Center

1959 NEPacific St., Rm. SS732
Seattle, WA 98195-6178
Phone: (206)598-4700 **Fax:** (206)598-2890
Email: brunzell@u.washington.edu
Website: http://www.crc.washington.edu
John D. Brunzell, MD, Prog. Dir.

Activities/Fields: Conducts a diversified research program designed to make possible precise, laboratory-type measurements of patients' disease states and their progress under various types of treatment.

★ 24482 ★ University of Washington Genome Center

Fluke Hall, Box 352145
Mason Rd.
Seattle, WA 98195
Phone: (206)685-7366 **Fax:** (206)685-7344
Email: uwgchelp@u.washington.edu
Website: http://www.genome.washington.edu/UWGC/
Maynard Olson, Dir.

Activities/Fields: Mapping of human genomic DNA.

★ 24483 ★ University of Washington Glomerular Disease Research Group

Division of Nephrology
University of Washington Medical Center
Seattle, WA 98195
Phone: (206)543-3695
Email: wgc@u.washington.edu
Website: http://faculty.washington.edu/uwrenal/
Dr. William G. Couser, Co-Prin. Investigator

Activities/Fields: Pathogenesis of glomerular and interstitial diseases using experimental models and cellular and molecular technology.

★ 24484 ★ University of Washington Harborview Injury Prevention and Research Center
325 9th Ave.
PO Box 359960
Seattle, WA 98104
Phone: (206)521-1520 **Fax:** (206)521-1562
Email: navajo@u.washington.edu
Website: http://depts.washington.edu/hiprc/
David C. Grossman, MD, Dir.
Activities/Fields: Injury prevention and the causes, effects and treatment of injuries, including studies in epidemiology, health education, psychology, acute care, biomechanics, rehabilitation.

★ 24485 ★ University of Washington Health Promotion Research Center (HPRC)
School of Public Health & Community Medicine, Box 354804
1107 NE 45th St., Ste. 200
Seattle, WA 98105
Phone: (206)543-2891 **Fax:** (206)543-8841
Email: logerfo@u.washington.edu
Website: http://depts.washington.edu/hprc/
James P. LoGerfo, MD, Dir.
Activities/Fields: Promotion of the health and well-being of Washington state residents, with a focus on older adults.

★ 24486 ★ University of Washington Institute for Risk Analysis and Risk Communication (IRARC)
Department of Environmental Health & Occupational Health Sci
School of Public Health & Community Medicine
4225 Roosevelt Way NE, Ste. 100
Seattle, WA 98105-6099
Phone: (206)543-9394 **Fax:** (206)616-4875
Email: irarc@u.washington.edu
Website: http://depts.washington.edu/irarc/
Elaine M. Faustman, PhD, Dir.
Activities/Fields: Biological risk caused by chemicals.

★ 24487 ★ University of Washington National ESCA and Surface Analysis Center for Biomedical Problems
Departments of Bioengineering and Chemical Engineering
PO Box 351750
Seattle, WA 98195-1750
Phone: (206)685-1229 **Fax:** (206)543-3778
Email: castner@nb.engr.washington.edu
Website: http://www.nb.engr.washington.edu
David G. Castner, PhD, Dir.
Activities/Fields: Surface analysis of biomaterial, polymer, and biological surfaces. Research directed toward integrating electron spectroscopy for chemical analytical tools for biomedical sciences. Provides ESCA and SIMS analysis of organic, metallic, and inorganic materials. Activities focus on understanding the nature of interactions that occur at biological interfaces such as tissue-body fluid, synthetic material-blood, and tooth-saliva. **Pub:** *Photoemissions Newsletter*.

★ 24488 ★ University of Washington Northwest Center for Occupational Health and Safety
Department of Environmental Health, Box 357234
School of Public Health
Seattle, WA 98195-7234
Phone: (206)685-3250 **Fax:** (206)616-2687
Email: mmorgan@u.washington.edu
Prof. Michael Morgan, Dir.
Activities/Fields: Occupational health and safety.

★ 24489 ★ University of Washington Northwest Center for Particulate Air Pollution and Health
Box 354803
1107 NE 45th St., Ste. 355
Seattle, WA 98195-4803
Phone: (206)543-2026 **Fax:** (206)685-3990
Email: jkoenig@u.washington.edu
Website: http://depts.Washington.edu/pmcenter/
Jane Q. Koenig, Dir.
Activities/Fields: Effects on human health of particulate air pollution. **Pub:** *Dust, Smoke & Haze Newsletter*, semiannually.

★ 24490 ★ University of Washington Northwest Regional Spinal Cord Injury System
Department of Rahabilitation Medicine
School of Medicine
Box 356490
Seattle, WA 98195-6490
Phone: (206)543-3600 **Fax:** (206)685-3244
Email: rehab@u.washington.edu
Website: http://depts.washington.edu/rehab/sci/
Dr. Diana D. Cardenas, Proj. Dir.
Activities/Fields: Spinal cord injuries. **Pub:** *Spinal Cord Injury Update Newsletter*, 3/year. Newsletter. • *Staying Healthy After a Spinal Cord Injury (Series of 10 brochures)*. Brochure.

★ 24491 ★ University of Washington Pediatric Epilepsy Research Center (PERC)
HSB RR 705A
Box 356470
1959 NE Pacific Ave.
Seattle, WA 98195-6470
Phone: (206)221-5364 **Fax:** (206)221-5721
Email: perc@u.washington.edu
Philip Schwarzkroin, PhD, Dir.
Activities/Fields: Prevention, control, and cure of pediatric epilepsy.

★ 24492 ★ University of Washington Pharmaceutical Outcomes Research and Policy Program (PORPP)
Box 357630
Health Sciences Bldg., Rm. H375
Department of Pharmacy
Seattle, WA 98195-7630
Phone: (206)543-6788 **Fax:** (206)543-3835
Email: sdsull@u.washington.edu
Website: http://depts.washington.edu/porpp/
Prof. Sean D. Sullivan, PhD, Dir.
Activities/Fields: Effects and use of pharmaceuticals in human populations.

★ 24493 ★ University of Washington Resource Facility for Population Kinetics
Box 352255
Department of Bioengineering
Seattle, WA 98195-2255
Phone: (206)685-3021 **Fax:** (206)543-3081
Email: vicini@u.washington.edu
Website: http://depts.washington.edu/rfpk/
Paolo Vicini, PhD, Prin. Investigator
Activities/Fields: Application of computer modeling in biomedical research, focusing on compartmental population kinetics. Population kinetics is the methodology used to quantify intersubject variability in kinetic studies.

★ 24494 ★ University of Washington Virginia Merrill Bloedel Hearing Research Center
Box 357923
CHDD Bldg., CD176
Seattle, WA 98195-7923
Phone: (206)685-2962 **Fax:** (206)616-1828
Email: bloedel@u.washington.edu
Website: http://depts.washington.edu/hearing/
Dr. George Gates, Contact
Activities/Fields: Hearing, hearing loss, and related communication disorders.

★ 24495 ★ University of Washington Washington Regional Primate Research Center (WaRPRC)
I-421 Health Sciences
Box 357330
Seattle, WA 98195-7330
Phone: (206)543-1430 **Fax:** (206)685-0305
Email: pattir@bart.rprc.washington.edu
William R. Morton, DVM, Dir.
Activities/Fields: Use of nonhuman primates for biomedical research on AIDS, developmental biology, neurobiological and behavioral sciences, cardiovascular physiology, molecular and cell biology, immunology, virology, transplantation and stem cell biology, genomics and primate disease models.

★ 24496 ★ University of Washington WWAMI Rural Health Research Center
Box 354696
Department of Family Medicine
Seattle, WA 98195-4696
Phone: (206)685-0402 **Fax:** (206)616-4768
Email: jhansen@fammed.washington.edu
Website: http://www.fammed.washington.edu/wwamirhrc/
L. Gary Hart, PhD, Dir./Prin. Investigator
Activities/Fields: Rural health care. Research focuses on the training and supply of rural health care providers and content and outcomes of the care they provide; the availability and quality of care for rural women and children, including obstetric and perinatal care; and access to high-quality care for vulnerable and minority rural populations.

★ 24497 ★ University of Waterloo BioTechnology Research Centre
200 University Ave. W
Waterloo, ON, Canada N2L 3G1
Phone: (519)888-4567 **Fax:** (519)746-4979
Email: rllegge@engmail.uwaterloo.ca
Website: http://www.uwaterloo.ca
Dr. R.L. Legge, Exec. Dir.
Activities/Fields: Fundamental and applied R&D, including research in molecular biology, genetics, cell culture, biochemistry, bioorganic and natural products chemistry, enyzmology, molecular modeling, bioreactor and bioprocess development, bioseparations engineering and environmental biotechnology.

★ 24498 ★ University of Waterloo Centre for Applied Health Research
Faculty of Applied Health Science
Burt Matthews Hall
Waterloo, ON, Canada N2L 3G1
Phone: (519)888-4567 **Fax:** (519)746-6776
Email: deanahs@healthy.uwaterloo.ca
Website: http://www.ahs.uwaterloo.ca
Dr. Michael Sharratt, Dean
Activities/Fields: Research conducted through several centers: Murray Alzheimer Research and Education Program; Health Behaviour Research Group; Functional Independence for Seniors; Program Training and Consultation Centre; and Ergonomics and Safety Consulting Services. **Pub:** *CAHR News*.

★ 24499 ★ University of Waterloo Centre for Contact Lens Research
School of Optometry
University of Waterloo
Waterloo, ON, Canada N2L 3G1
Phone: (519)888-4742 **Fax:** (519)884-8769
Email: dfonn@sciborg.uwaterloo.ca
Website: http://www.optometry.uwaterloo.ca/~cclr/
Dr. Desmond Fonn, Dir.

Activities/Fields: All areas related to contact lenses in order to monitor and understand the effects of contact lenses on the eye, the development of methods for evaluating and measuring the reactions to contact lens wear, and the safety and efficacy of pre and post market release of new lens materials and related products.

★ 24500 ★ University of Western Ontario Child Health Research Institute
800 Commissioners Rd. E
London, ON, Canada N6C 2V5
Phone: (519)685-8306 **Fax:** (519)685-8186
Email: vhan@uwo.ca
Website: http://www.chri.org/
Dr. Victor K.M. Han, Sci. Dir.
Activities/Fields: Causes, cures and long term effects of children's diseases and disabilities, and evaluation of new therapies for infants and children.

★ 24501 ★ University of Western Ontario Dementia Study Group
University Hospital
London, ON, Canada N6A 5C1
Phone: (519)663-3035
Harold Merskey, Dir.
Activities/Fields: Clinical, pathological, and neurochemical analyses of normal aging in the human nervous system and in organic senile dementias, especially Alzheimer's disease. Clinical trials.

★ 24502 ★ University of Western Ontario Population and Community Health Unit (PCHU)
245-100 Collip Cir.
London, ON, Canada N6G 4X8
Phone: (519)858-5063 **Fax:** (519)858-5029
Email: pchu@uwo.ca
Website: http://www.uwo.ca/fammed/pchu/index.html
Evelyn Vingilis, PhD, Dir.
Activities/Fields: Population health issues in the communities of Southwestern Ontario, Canada.

★ 24503 ★ University of Wisconsin—Madison Allergy/Asthma Clinical Research Unit
Medical School, K4/952 CSC
600 Highland Ave.
Madison, WI 53792-9988
Phone: (608)262-2804 **Fax:** (608)265-9890
Email: mjb@medicine.wisc.edu
Dr. William W. Busse, Dir.
Activities/Fields: Relationship between viruses and asthma using correlative studies derived from animal models and human experiments. In particular, the effect of virus infections on beta-adrenergic receptor structure, airway mechanics, mediator release from pulmonary alveolar cells, and the late phase reaction are studied. Research also involves characterization of B cell isotype repertoire responses to viral antigens. **Frmly:** Asthma and Allergic Diseases Cooperative Research Center.

★ 24504 ★ University of Wisconsin—Madison Auditory Physiology Research Laboratory
625 Waisman Center
Madison, WI 53706
Phone: (608)263-5928 **Fax:** (608)265-4103
Email: brugge@physiology.wisc.edu
Website: http://www.physiology.wisc.edu/aud/
Dr. John F. Brugge, Contact
Activities/Fields: Auditory research at the systems, cellular, and molecular levels.

★ 24505 ★ University of Wisconsin—Madison Biodynamics Laboratory
2000 Observatory Dr., Rm. 1149
Madison, WI 53706
Phone: (608)263-6308 **Fax:** (608)262-1656
Email: gcartee@education.wisc.edu
Dr. Greg Cartee, Dir.
Activities/Fields: Mechanisms associated with the response and adaptation of humans and animals to exercise and environmental stress, focusing on cardiorespiratory and musculoskeletal systems.

★ 24506 ★ University of Wisconsin—Madison Cardiovascular Research Center (CVRC)
5710 Medical Sciences Center
1300 University Ave.
Madison, WI 53706
Phone: (608)263-2266 **Fax:** (608)265-8745
Email: uwcvrc@cardiovascres.wisc.edu
Website: http://www.cardiovascres.wisc.edu/
Richard L. Moss, PhD, Dir.
Activities/Fields: Diagnosis and treatment of diseases of the heart and blood vessels.

★ 24507 ★ University of Wisconsin—Madison Center for Health Systems Research and Analysis
WARF Bldg., Rm. 1163
610 Walnut St.
Madison, WI 53726
Phone: (608)263-5722 **Fax:** (608)263-4523
Email: davidz@chsra.wisc.edu
Website: http://www.chsra.wisc.edu
Dr. David R. Zimmerman, Dir.
Activities/Fields: Five major research areas: quality assessment and improvement, long term care, public health policy and program evaluation, consumer decision making, and patient education and support.

★ 24508 ★ University of Wisconsin—Madison Center for Human Performance and Risk Analysis (CHPRA)
456 Mechanical Engineering Bldg.
1513 University Ave.
Madison, WI 53706-1572
Phone: (608)263-7456 **Fax:** (608)265-9094
Email: chpra@engr.wisc.edu
Website: http://www.engr.wisc.edu/centers/chpra/
Prof. Vickie M. Bier, Dir.
Activities/Fields: Issues of human performance and the role human performance plays in industrial accidents. **Pub:** *The Human Element Newsletter*, quarterly.

★ 24509 ★ University of Wisconsin—Madison Comprehensive Cancer Center
600 Highland Ave.
Madison, WI 53792-6164
Phone: (608)263-8600 **Free:** 800-622-8922
Fax: (608)263-8613
Website: http://www.cancer.wisc.edu/
George Wilding, MD, Actg. Dir.
Activities/Fields: Biology of cancer, focused on human-oriented problems in cause, prevention, tumor localization, and treatment. Organized into eight collaborative research programs: Cancer Control and Population Sciences; Cancer Genetics; Cell Signaling and Growth Control; Etiology and Chemoprevention; Experimental Therapeutics; Human Cancer Virology; Imaging and Radiation Sciences; Immunology and Immunotherapy. Four of these programs have clinical trial activity and all eight interact closely with fourteen Disease Oriented Multidisciplinary Working Groups. **Pub:** *Annual Report.* • *Newsletter (Advances)*, semiannually.

★ 24510 ★ University of Wisconsin—Madison General Clinical Research Center
600 Highland Ave., D6/6
Madison, WI 53792-6724
Phone: (608)263-6183 **Fax:** (608)265-9225
Email: wwb@medicine.wisc.edu
Website: http://www.medsch.wisc.edu/uwgcrc/index.html
Dr. William W. Busse, Prog. Dir.
Activities/Fields: Major areas of investigation include immunology, oncology, pediatrics, pulmonary medicine, sleep disorders, surgery and whole-body hyperthermia.

★ 24511 ★ University of Wisconsin—Madison HealthEmotions Research Institute
6001 Research Pk. Blvd.
Madison, WI 53719-1176
Phone: (608)263-6161 **Fax:** (608)263-9340
Email: kalin@healthemotions.org
Website: http://www.healthemotions.org
Ned H. Kalin, MD, Dir.
Activities/Fields: Relationships between positive emotions, physiological systems, and health.

★ 24512 ★ University of Wisconsin—Madison Hearing Development Research Laboratory (HDRL)
573 Waisman Center
1500 Highland Ave.
Madison, WI 53705-2280
Phone: (608)263-3270 **Fax:** (608)263-2918
Email: wightman@waisman.wisc.edu
Website: http://www.waisman.wisc.edu/~wightman/
Frederic Wightman, Dir.
Activities/Fields: Mechanisms and processes of human hearing.

★ 24513 ★ University of Wisconsin—Madison Hematology Research Laboratory
Medical Science Center, Rm. 4285
1300 University Ave.
Madison, WI 53706
Phone: (608)262-1576 **Fax:** (608)263-4969
Email: dfmosher@facstaff.wisc.edu
Dr. Deane Mosher, Dir.
Activities/Fields: Biology and biochemistry. Conducts studies on cell cultures, particularly the plasma proteins, fibronectin, vitronectin, and the platelet protein thrombospondin. Characterizes proteins for biomedical applications.

★ 24514 ★ University of Wisconsin—Madison Laboratory of Genetics
445 Henry Mall
Madison, WI 53706
Phone: (608)262-1069 **Fax:** (608)262-2976
Email: mrculber@facstaff.wisc.edu
Website: http://www.genetics.wisc.edu/index.html
Prof. Michael Culbertson, Chm.
Activities/Fields: Genetics, including molecular, human, nematode, population, microbial, behavioral, and plant genetics, cytogenetics, yeast genetics, somatic cells, zebrafish, genomics, and other areas ranging from theoretical genetics to agricultural and medical genetics.

★ 24515 ★ University of Wisconsin—Madison McArdle Laboratory for Cancer Research
Department of Oncology
1400 University Ave.
Madison, WI 53706-1599
Phone: (608)262-7992 **Fax:** (608)262-2824
Email: drinkwater@oncology.wisc.edu

Website: http://www.mcardle.wisc.edu
Dr. Norman R. Drinkwater, Dir.

Activities/Fields: Cellular, developmental, molecular, animal cell, and viral biology; and genetics, biochemistry, and immunology. Emphasizes mechanisms and controls of transcription, translation, and replication in cells and viruses; mechanisms of environmental, chemical, and viral carcinogenesis; and chemistry and metabolism of nucleic acids and proteins.

★ 24516 ★ University of Wisconsin—Madison
Molecular and Environmental Toxicology Center
Enzyme Institute, Rm. 290
1710 University Ave.
Madison, WI 53726-4087
Phone: (608)263-4580 **Fax:** (608)262-5245
Email: jefcoate@facstaff.wisc.edu
Website: http://www.wisc.edu/metc/
Prof. Colin R. Jefcoate, PhD, Dir.

Activities/Fields: Toxicology and problems related to presence of potentially hazardous synthetic and naturally occurring chemicals in the environment, e.g. heavy metals, chlorinated hydrocarbons, pesticides, mycotoxins, and food-borne toxins, including identification, quantification, and toxicologic studies of such chemicals. **Pub:** *Newsletter*, occasionally. **Frmly:** Environmental Toxicology Center.

★ 24517 ★ University of Wisconsin—Madison
National Magnetic Resonance Facility
Biochemistry Addition Bldg., Room 171
Department of Biochemistry
433 Babcock Dr.
Madison, WI 53706-1544
Phone: (608)262-3173 **Fax:** (608)262-3759
Email: markley@nmrfam.wisc.edu
Website: http://www.nmrfam.wisc.edu
John L. Markley, Hd.

Activities/Fields: Structural and conformational analysis of proteins, nucleic acids, carbohydrates, lipids, and other biomolecules; structure-function studies of macromolecular assemblies; noninvasive analysis of the biochemistry or intact cells, tissue, or organs; in vivo investigations of the biochemistry of rats or other small animals; nuclear magnetic resonance (NMR) imaging of small objects. Current core and collaborative projects include: strategies for assigning NMR spectra of proteins; determination of three dimensional (3-D) structures of small proteins and nucleic acids from NMR data; preparation of stable-isotope labeled amino acids and proteins; uses of stable isotopes in multi-dimensional (NMR) studies of proteins; applications of NMR to protein engineering; elucidation of enzyme mechanisms and protein-ligand interactions; application of 2-D and 3-D NMR methodology to the study of cellular biochemistry; computer-aided design of NMR experiments; post-acquisition processing of NMR data; and semi-automated analysis of NMR data from proteins.

★ 24518 ★ University of Wisconsin—Madison
National Primate Research Center
1220 Capitol Ct.
Madison, WI 53715-1299
Phone: (608)263-3500 **Fax:** (608)263-4031
Email: kemnitz@primate.wisc.edu
Website: http://www.primate.wisc.edu
Dr. Joseph W. Kemnitz, Dir.

Activities/Fields: Reproduction and development, immunogenetics and vaccine development, aging and metabolic disorders, neurobiology, women's health. Emphasizes biomedical research and studies on captive and wild primate conservation; rhesus, marmoset, and cynomolgus colonies for research and breeding. **Pub:** *Audio Visual Catalog*, biennially. • *Centerline Newsletter*. • *International Directory of Primatology*, biennially. **Frmly:** Wisconsin Regional Primate Research Center.

★ 24519 ★ University of Wisconsin—Madison
Neuropsychology Laboratory
600 N Highland Ave.
Madison, WI 53792-6180
Phone: (608)263-5430 **Fax:** (608)265-0172
Email: hermann@neurology.wisc.edu
Dr. Bruce Hermann, Dir.

Activities/Fields: Clinical neuropsychology in neuropsychological correlates of epilepsy, cognitive and affective changes in aging, and differential diagnosis of dementia with a view toward cognitive and memory remediation.

★ 24520 ★ University of Wisconsin—Madison
Office of International Health Affairs
1760 MSC
1300 University Ave.
Madison, WI 53706
Phone: (608)263-4150 **Fax:** (608)262-2327
Email: jlladins@facstaff.wisc.edu
Dr. Judith L. Ladinsky, Dir.

Activities/Fields: International health issues. **Pub:** *Newsletter*.

★ 24521 ★ University of Wisconsin—Madison
Pediatric Pulmonary Center
Clinical Science Center, Rm. K4/938
University Hospitals
600 Highland Ave.
Madison, WI 53792
Phone: (608)263-8555 **Fax:** (608)263-0510
Email: cggreen@facstaff.wisc.edu
Website: http://www2.medsch.wisc.edu/childrenshosp/ppc/ppchome.html
Dr. Christopher G. Green, Dir.

Activities/Fields: Cystic fibrosis and other respiratory diseases of children; home care of technology-dependent children.

★ 24522 ★ University of Wisconsin—Madison
Pulmonary and Critical Care Medicine Section
Department of Medicine
600 Highland Ave., K4/930
Madison, WI 53792-9988
Phone: (608)263-3035 **Fax:** (608)263-3746
Dr. James Skatrud, Sect. Hd.

Activities/Fields: Pulmonary physiology, occupational lung disease, and mechanisms of acute lung injury.

★ 24523 ★ University of Wisconsin—Madison
Radioimmunoassay Laboratory
Veterinary Medicine
2015 Linden Dr. W, Rm. 4426
Madison, WI 53706-1102
Phone: (608)263-4908 **Fax:** (608)263-6748
Email: armstroj@svm.vetmed.wisc.edu
Website: http://www.vetmed.wisc.edu/research/radioimmunoassay

Activities/Fields: Performs peptide iodinations and radioimmunoassay tests of endocrinologic samples, including antiserum development and immunocytochemistry, with the potential for development of peptide and protein hormone antisera and purification and labeling of antisera.

★ 24524 ★ University of Wisconsin—Madison
Research Animal Resources Center
Enzyme Institute
1710 University Ave.
Madison, WI 53705
Phone: (608)262-1238 **Fax:** (608)265-2698
Email: parks@rarc.wisc.edu
Website: http://www.rarc.wisc.edu
Christine M. Parks, Dir.

Activities/Fields: Laboratory animal diseases. **Pub:** *Animals Newsletter*.

★ 24525 ★ University of Wisconsin—Madison
State Laboratory of Hygiene
465 Henry Mall
Madison, WI 53706
Phone: (608)262-0322 **Free:** 888-494-4324
Fax: (608)262-3257
Email: rhl@prof.slh.wisc.edu
Website: http://www.slh.wisc.edu/index.shtml
Dr. Ronald H. Laessig, Dir.

Activities/Fields: Bacteriology, cancer cytology, cytogenetics, immunology, industrial hygiene, environmental health, pathology, clinical chemistry, toxicology, and virology, including respiratory and enterovirus infections, a survey of zoonosis in Wisconsin, especially California encephalitis virus, and chromosomal studies in congenital anomalies. **Pub:** *Results*, quarterly. • *Wisconsin State Laboratory of Hygiene Research, Teaching and Outreach Activity Report*, annually.

★ 24526 ★ University of Wisconsin—Madison
State Laboratory of Hygiene Bacteriology/Parasitology
465 Henry Mall
Madison, WI 53706
Free: 800-862-1013 **Fax:** (608)262-3257
Email: rhl@prof.slh.wisc.edu
Website: http://www.slh.wisc.edu/services/clinical/index.html
Dr. Ronald H. Laessig, Dir.

Activities/Fields: Antimicrobial susceptibility studies, enteric serotyping, and culture and identification of fastidious and unusual pathogens. Provides bacteriology laboratory support for outbreak management.

★ 24527 ★ University of Wisconsin—Madison
Trace Research and Development Center
Engineering Centers Bldg., Rm. 2107
1500 Engineering Dr.
Madison, WI 53706
Phone: (608)262-6966
Email: info@trace.wisc.edu
Website: http://www.trace.wisc.edu
Dr. Gregg Vanderheiden, Dir.

Activities/Fields: How to make standard information technologies and telecommunications systems more accessible and usable by people with disabilites. **Pub:** *Annual Report*. • *Trace Resourcebook Series*. **Frmly:** Cerebral Palsy Communication Group.

★ 24528 ★ University of Wisconsin—Madison
Wisconsin Occupational Health Laboratory
PO Box 7996
Madison, WI 53703-7996
Free: 800-446-0403 **Fax:** (608)224-6213
Email: WOHLdirector@mail.slh.wisc.edu
Website: http://www.slh.wisc.edu/wohl/

Activities/Fields: Industrial hygiene. **Pub:** *Reactions Newsletter*. Newsletter.

★ 24529 ★ University of Wisconsin—Milwaukee
Marine and Freshwater Biomedical Sciences Center
600 E Greenfield Ave.
PO Box 413
Milwaukee, WI 53201-0413
Phone: (414)229-5853 **Fax:** (414)229-5427
Email: petering@uwm.edu

Website: http://www.uwm.edu/Dept/MFB
Dr. David Petering, Dir.

Activities/Fields: Aquatic models in biomedicine and comparative toxicology. Studies transformation and metabolism of toxic organic chemicals and metals and investigates genetic, neurobehavioral, and immunological responses of organisms to such chemicals. **Pub:** *Annual report.*

★ 24530 ★ University of Wisconsin—Stout
Research and Training Center on Community Rehabilitation Programs to Improve Employment Outcomes

Stout Vocational Rehabilitation Institute
College of Human Development
Menomonie, WI 54751
Phone: (715)232-1389 **Fax:** (715)232-2251
Email: menz@uwstout.edu
Website: http://www.rtc.uwstout.edu
Dr. Fredrick E. Menz, Dir.

Activities/Fields: Improvement of community-based rehabilitation through vocational transition of people with disabilities from community-based rehabilitation programs into competitive employment.

★ 24531 ★ University of Wyoming
Wyoming Institute for Disabilities (WIND)

PO Box 4298
Laramie, WY 82071-4298
Phone: (307)766-2761
Email: wind.uw@uwyo.edu
Website: http://wind.uwyo.edu
Keith A. Miller, PhD, Exec. Dir.

Activities/Fields: Disabilities, particularly in the area of developmental disabilities.

★ 24532 ★ USDA Agricultural Research Service
Grand Forks Human Nutrition Research Center

2420 2nd Ave. N
PO Box 9034
Grand Forks, ND 58202-9034
Phone: (701)795-8353 **Fax:** (701)795-8395
Email: speters@gfhnrc.ars.usda.gov
Website: http://www.gfhnrc.ars.usda.gov
Dr. Gerald F. Combs, Jr., Dir.

Activities/Fields: Nutritional roles of minerals and other interests in bone, cardiovascular, and brain development, maintenance.

★ 24533 ★ USDA Human Nutrition Research Center on Aging

Tufts University
711 Washington St.
Boston, MA 02111-1524
Phone: (617)556-3335 **Fax:** (617)556-3295
Email: kathleen.cappellano@tufts.edu
Website: http://www.hnrc.tufts.edu
Robert M. Russell, MD, Dir.

Activities/Fields: Investigates the relationship of nutrition to aging, including research programs in nutrient metabolism, nutrient requirements, nutritional epidemiology, functional systems, and drug-nutrient interactions. **Pub:** *HNRC Newsletter,* monthly.

★ 24534 ★ Utah Artificial Heart Institute

803 North 300 West St., Rm. 304 W
Salt Lake City, UT 84103-1414
Phone: (801)323-1122 **Fax:** (801)323-1110
Email: dolsen@uahi.org
Dr. Don B. Olsen, Pres.

Activities/Fields: Cardiac replacement, cardiac assist devices, and artificial organs, including investigations into acute and chronic ventricular assist and total replacement, cardiac valves, total artificial hearts (pneumatic, electrohydraulic, and electromechanical), and associated pathophysiology. Experiments concern the introduction of such devices in sheep and calves.

★ 24535 ★ Utah State University
Center for Persons with Disabilities

6800 Old Main Hill
Logan, UT 84322-6800
Phone: (435)797-1981 **Free:** (866)284-2821
Fax: (435)797-3944
Email: s_rule@cpd2.usu.edu
Website: http://www.cpd.usu.edu
Dr. Sarah Rule, Dir.

Activities/Fields: Developmental disabilities including biomedical research, systems change, assistive technologies, video production, and distance education. **Pub:** *Annual report.* • *CPD News.* • *Parent Newsletter.*

★ 24536 ★ Utah State University
Institute for Antiviral Research

5600 Old Main Hill
Logan, UT 84322-5600
Phone: (435)797-1902 **Fax:** (435)797-3959
Email: rsidwell@cc.usu.edu
Website: http://www.usu.edu/iar/index.html
Dr. Robert W. Sidwell, Dir.

Activities/Fields: Control of viral diseases. **Pub:** *Reports.*

★ 24537 ★ Van Andel Research Institute (VARI)

333 Bostwick NE
Grand Rapids, MI 49503
Phone: (616)234-5000 **Fax:** (616)234-5001
Email: george.vandewoude@vai.org
Website: http://www.vai.org/vari/home.htm
George F. Vande Woude, PhD, Dir.

Activities/Fields: Improvement of human health, especially determination of the causes and treatment of cancer.

★ 24538 ★ Vancouver Hospital and Health Sciences Centre
Prostate Centre

828 West 10th Ave.
Vancouver, BC, Canada V5Z 1L8
Phone: (604)875-4372 **Fax:** (604)875-5684
Email: lgold@interchange.ubc.ca
Website: http://www.research.vhhsc.ca/s/Prostate.asp
Dr. Larry Goldenberg, Dir.

Activities/Fields: Prevention, diagnosis and treatment of prostate cancer, especially surgical techniques, radiotherapy and hormonal therapy.

★ 24539 ★ Vanderbilt University
Autonomic Dysfunction Center

AA-3228 Medical Center N
Nashville, TN 37232-2195
Phone: (615)343-6499 **Fax:** (615)343-8649
Email: david.robertson@mcmail.vanderbilt.edu
Website: http://www.mc.vanderbilt.edu/gcrc/adc
Dr. David Robertson, Dir.

Activities/Fields: Pathophysiology of autonomic disorders and orthostatic hypotension, including dopamine-B-hydroxylase deficiency, a syndrome characterized by congenital absence of norepinephrine and epinephrine, and norepinephrine transporter deficiency. Other areas of research focus on therapeutic modalities for the management of orthostatic intolerance and tachycardia, Shy-Drager syndrome, multiple system atrophy, and baroreflex failure in human subjects.

★ 24540 ★ Vanderbilt University
Center for Clinical and Research Ethics

319 Oxford House
Vanderbilt University Medical Center
Nashville, TN 37232-4350
Phone: (615)936-2686 **Fax:** (615)936-3800
Email: med.ethics@mcmmail.vanderbilt.edu
Website: http://www.mc.vanderbilt.edu/ethics/
Stuart G. Finder, Dir.

Activities/Fields: Moral and ethical issues.

★ 24541 ★ Vanderbilt University
Center for Mental Health Policy

1207 18th Ave. S
Nashville, TN 37212
Phone: (615)322-8435 **Fax:** (615)322-7049
Email: bickman@attglobal.net
Website: http://www.vanderbilt.edu/VIPPS/CMHP/cmhphome.html
Dr. Leonard Bickman, Dir.

Activities/Fields: Evaluation of homeless family programs, effects of family empowerment on children's mental health, patterns of psychiatric hospitalization of children, and evaluation of school mental health services.

★ 24542 ★ Vanderbilt University
Center in Molecular Toxicology

Biochemistry Department
23rd Ave. & Pierce
Nashville, TN 37232-0146
Phone: (615)322-2261 **Fax:** (615)322-3141
Email: info@toxicology.mc.vanderbilt.edu
Website: http://www.toxicology.mc.vanderbilt.edu
Dr. F. Peter Guengerich, Dir.

Activities/Fields: Biochemical and chemical toxicology and carcinogenesis, including enzymatic oxidation and conjugation, oxidative damage, DNA damage and mutagenesis, regulation of gene expression, and neurotoxicology. Service core facilities include mass spectrometry, NMR, cell biology, protein chemistry, and molecular recognition. **Pub:** *Annual report.*

★ 24543 ★ Vanderbilt University
Clinical Nutrition Research Unit

C2104 Medical Center
21st & Garland Ave.
Nashville, TN 37232-2279
Phone: (615)322-7740 **Fax:** (615)343-6229
Email: raymond.burk@vanderbilt.edu
Website: http://www.mc.vanderbilt.edu/nutrition/
Raymond F. Burk, MD, Dir.

Activities/Fields: Mechanisms of body weight and regulation, focusing on exercise and energy expenditure. Metabolism of amino acids, carbohydrates, lipids, minerals, and trace elements. Research also includes molecular nutrition.

★ 24544 ★ Vanderbilt University
Diabetes Research and Training Center

707 Light Hall
Vanderbilt University Medical Center
Nashville, TN 37232-0615
Phone: (615)322-7004 **Fax:** (615)343-0172
Email: daryl.granner@vanderbilt.edu
Website: http://www.mc.vanderbilt.edu/vumc/centers/drtc/
Dr. Daryl K. Granner, Contact

Activities/Fields: Diabetes and diabetes treatment.

★ 24545 ★ Vanderbilt University
Energy Balance Laboratory

Clinical Research Center
21st Ave. S
Nashville, TN 37232-2195
Phone: (615)343-8497 **Fax:** (615)343-6229
Email: kong.chen@vanderbilt.edu
Dr. Kong Chen, Dir.

Activities/Fields: Use of indirect calorimetry to measure energy expenditure, and metabolic rate and physical activities under a variety of conditions, including exercise, dietary intake, and environmental changes. Emphasis is on the identification of determinants of energy expenditure and body weight regulation. Uses hydrostatic weighing, bioelectrical impedance, and other methods to measure body composition.

★ 24546 ★ Vanderbilt University General Clinical Research Center
21st Ave. S
Nashville, TN 37232-2195
Phone: (615)343-6499 **Fax:** (615)343-8649
Email: david.robertson@mcmail.vanderbilt.edu
Website: http://www.mc.vanderbilt.edu./gcrc/
Dr. David Robertson, Dir.
Activities/Fields: Human physiology and diseases, including studies in medicine, neuroscience, molecular biology, pharmacology, hematology, cardiovascular diseases, genetics, obstetrics and gynecology, pediatrics, psychiatry, surgery, and psychology. Activities focus on hypertension, hypotension, arrhythmias, carcinoid syndrome, and disorders of the autonomic nervous system. **Pub:** *Elliot Newman Handbook*.

★ 24547 ★ Vanderbilt University John F. Kennedy Center for Research on Human Development
Box 40
230 Appleton Place
Peabody College
Nashville, TN 37203-5701
Phone: (615)322-8240 **Fax:** (615)322-8236
Email: elaine.bush@mcmail.vanderbilt.edu
Website: http://www.vanderbilt.edu/kennedy
Elaine Sanders-Bush, PhD, Contact
Activities/Fields: Behavioral, biomedical, and educational aspects of mental retardation and other disabilities and child development, including cognitive strategies, social and communicative processes, neural development, neural plasticity. Investigates cognitive modifiability, computer applications to facilitate thinking and learning, normal and abnormal nervous system maturation, perceptual and locomotor behavior, self-injurious behavior, language and social development, development of aggressive behavior, early education of mentally retarded and economically disadvantaged children. **Pub:** *Kennedy Center News*, quarterly. • *Research Project Brochures*. • *TOT Talk*, semiannually.

★ 24548 ★ Vanderbilt University Neuromagnetic Pain Management Project
407 Godchaux Hall
461 21st Ave. S
Nashville, TN 37240
Phone: (615)322-2783 **Fax:** (615)343-3998
Email: sharon.jones@vanderbilt.edu
Website: http://www.mc.vanderbilt.edu/nursing
Sharon Jones, Contact
Activities/Fields: Pain, especially the mechanisms underlying painful conditions and techniques for interrupting pain by altering pain pathways. **Frmly:** Center for Pain Research and Neuromagnetics.

★ 24549 ★ Vanderbilt University S.R. Light Laboratory for Surgical Research
MCN, Rm. CC-2307
Nashville, TN 37232
Phone: (615)322-2096 **Fax:** (615)343-1355
Email: phil.williams@vanderbilt.edu
Website: http://www.mc.vanderbilt.edu/surgery/rsrch-div.htm
Phillip E. Williams, Dir.
Activities/Fields: All phases of medicine involving use of experimental animals. Specific research includes studies of metabolism, particularly mechanisms of stress-related changes in glucose and amino acids; cardiothoracic study of pathophysiology of ischemic myocardium; and renovascular physiology. Also develops new surgical instrumentation and techniques.

★ 24550 ★ Vanderbilt University Vanderbilt Addiction Center (VAC)
Psychiatric Hospital at Vanderbilt
1601 23rd Ave. S
Nashville, TN 37212-8645
Phone: (615)322-3527 **Free:** 800-365-2270
Email: vac.webmail@mcmail.vanderbilt.edu
Website: http://www.mc.vanderbilt.edu/addiction/
Peter R. Martin, MD, Dir.
Activities/Fields: Drug and alcohol dependence, especially genetic-environmental interactions.

★ 24551 ★ Vanderbilt University Vanderbilt Bill Wilkerson Center for Otolaryngology and Communication Sciences (VBWC)
1301 22nd Ave. S, No. 2900
Nashville, TN 37232
Phone: (615)343-7267 **Fax:** (615)322-9725
Email: robert.ossoff@mcmail.vanderbilt.edu
Website: http://www.mc.vanderbilt.edu/VanderbiltBill-WilkersonCenter/
Robert H. Ossoff, Dir.
Activities/Fields: Otolaryngological, communicative and related diseases and disorders. **Pub:** *Research report*, annually.

★ 24552 ★ Vanderbilt University Vanderbilt-Ingram Cancer Center (VICC)
649 Preston Bldg.
Nashville, TN 37232-6838
Phone: (615)936-1782 **Fax:** (615)936-1790
Website: http://www.mc.vanderbilt.edu/vicc/
Harold L. Moses, MD, Dir.
Activities/Fields: Cancer treatment, diagnosis, and prevention.

★ 24553 ★ Very Low Frequency Electron Paramagnetic Resonance Imaging for In Vivo Physiology
Department of Radiation/Cell Oncology, MC1105
University of Chicago
5841 S Maryland Ave.
Chicago, IL 60637
Phone: (773)702-6871 **Fax:** (773)702-5940
Email: h-halpern@uchicago.edu
Howard J. Halpern, MD, Prin. Investigator
Activities/Fields: Development of instrumentation, analysis techniques, spin probes and spin traps, and methodologies for imaging physiologically relevant aspects of tissue fluids, including high-resolution oxygen maps, with very low frequency electron paramagnetic resonance imaging.

★ 24554 ★ Veterans Affairs Medical Center (Birmingham, AL) Research and Development Service
700 S 19th St.
Birmingham, AL 35233
Phone: (205)558-4747 **Fax:** (205)933-4471
Email: warren.blackburn@med.va.gov
Dr. Warren D. Blackburn, Jr., Assoc. Ch. of Staff
Activities/Fields: Cancer, gastroenterology, rheumatology and arthritis, neurology, and spinal cord injury, repair systems, cordiology, nephrology, pulmonary disease, endocrinology, informatics and health services research.

★ 24555 ★ Veterans Affairs Medical Center (Danville, IL) Research and Development Service
1900 E Main St.
Danville, IL 61832
Phone: (217)442-5534 **Fax:** (217)554-4836
Email: mukund.prabhudesai@med.va.gov
Mukund Prabhudesai, MD, R&D Coord.
Activities/Fields: Alcoholism, rehabilitation, psychology, drugs, and nutrition. Also studies health care management and psychiatry.

★ 24556 ★ Veterans Affairs Medical Center (Martinez, CA) Research Administration Office
150 Muir Rd.
Martinez, CA 94553
Phone: (925)372-2484 **Fax:** (925)228-5738
Email: gakaysen@ucdavis.edu
Dr. George Kaysen, Assoc. Ch.
Activities/Fields: Basic and clinical biomedical research.

★ 24557 ★ Veterans Affairs Medical Center (Minneapolis, MN)
1 Veterans Dr.
Minneapolis, MN 55417-2300
Phone: (612)725-2033 **Fax:** (612)725-2093
Email: michael.levitt@med.va.gov
Dr. Michael D. Levitt, Res. Ch.
Activities/Fields: Health services, including cooperative clinical trials, psychiatry, prostate cancer, and kidney disease.

★ 24558 ★ Veterans Affairs Medical Center (Omaha, NE) Research and Development Service
4101 Woolworth Ave.
Omaha, NE 68105
Phone: (402)346-8800 **Fax:** (402)449-0604
Email: nowling.stephan_d@omaha.va.gov
Dr. Lynell W. Klassen, MD, Contact
Activities/Fields: Immunology, infectious disease, oncology, liver disease, diabetes, orthopedics, pulmonary disease, gastroenterology, and endocrinology. Utilizes rats, mice, and rabbits, as animal models.

★ 24559 ★ Veterans Affairs Pittsburgh Health Care System Research Service
University Dr. C
Pittsburgh, PA 15240
Phone: (412)688-6104 **Fax:** (412)688-6945
Email: steven.graham@med.va.gov
Website: http://www.research.vares-pitt.org
Dr. Steven H. Graham, Assoc. Ch. of Staff, Res. Devel.
Activities/Fields: Oncogene expression in colon cancer, immunochemical targeting of tumors, dermatology, vascular surgery, three-dimensional structure of bacterial toxins, and transplantation. Neurosciences studies focus on epilepsy, hypertension, and schizophrenia and rehabilitation.

★ 24560 ★ Veterans Affairs Salt Lake City Health Care System Research Service
500 Foothill Dr.
Salt Lake City, UT 84148
Phone: (801)584-1271 **Fax:** (801)583-9624
Email: marl.lestad@hsc.utah.edu
Mark Lestad, Actg. Admin.
Activities/Fields: Diabetes, cancer, arthritis, aging and alcoholism, stroke and rehabilitation, dermatitis, neuroimmunological diseases, myasthenia gravis, tumors, dementia, laser medicine and surgery, herpes, genetics, cardiology, immunology, basic science, molecular biology, national cooperative drug studies, and rehabilitation research and development of artificial limbs, and clinical outcomes research. **Pub:** *Scientific Journal*, annually. Journal.

★ 24561 ★ Veterans Affairs Sierra Nevada Health Care System Research Service
1000 Locust St.
Reno, NV 89502-2597
Phone: (775)328-1486 **Fax:** (775)328-1816
Dr. Jon Schrage, Res. Dir.
Activities/Fields: Alzheimer's disease, cancer, cardiology, clinical trials of investigational drugs, diabetes, in-utero transplantation of blood-forming cells, pulmonary medicine, stress in employment, health services, nursing, rheumatology, nutrition, and surgery.

★ 24562 ★ Veterans Health Administration
Geriatric Research, Education, and Clinical Center-Ann Arbor
VA Ann Arbor Healthcare System GRECC (11G)
2215 Fuller Rd.
Ann Arbor, MI 48105
Phone: (734)761-7686 **Fax:** (734)761-7489
Email: msupiano@umich.edu
Website: http://www.med.umich.edu/geriatrics_center/grecc
Mark A. Supiano, MD, Dir.
Activities/Fields: Neurosciences, metabolism/nutrition, autonomic function, diabetes, hypertension, oral health, cost and quality of health care.

★ 24563 ★ Veterans Health Administration
Geriatric Research, Education, and Clinical Center-Bedford
VA Medical Center
Bedford, MA 01730
Phone: (781)687-3167 **Fax:** (781)687-3515
Email: nkowall@bu.edu
Neil William Kowall, MD, Dir.
Activities/Fields: Neurosciences/cognitive disorders, dementia.

★ 24564 ★ Veterans Health Administration
Geriatric Research, Education, and Clinical Center-Brockton
VA Medical Center
1400 VFW Pky.
West Roxbury, MA 02132
Phone: (617)323-7700 **Fax:** (617)363-5503
Dr. Mangdhara R. Madineedi, Dir.
Activities/Fields: Metabolism, cardiovascular physiology and pharmacology, genito-urinary conditions, dehydration, cognition, epidemiology.

★ 24565 ★ Veterans Health Administration
Geriatric Research, Education, and Clinical Center-Durham
VA Medical Center
Durham, NC 27705
Phone: (919)286-6932 **Fax:** (919)286-6823
Email: harvey.cohen@duke.edu
Website: http://www.va.gov/seniors/health/grecc/durham.htm
Harvey Jay Cohen, MD, Dir.
Activities/Fields: Neoplasms and aging; cardiovascular disease and aging; cancer; bones, joints and dysmobility; health promotion and disease prevention.

★ 24566 ★ Veterans Health Administration
Geriatric Research, Education and Clinical Center-Gainesville
GRECC, 182
1601 Archer Rd.
Gainesville, FL 32608-1197
Phone: (352)374-6077 **Fax:** (352)374-6142
Email: david.lowenthal@med.va.gov
Website: http://www.med.ufl.edu/pharm/facdata/GRECC
Dr. David T. Lowenthal, Dir. Emeritus
Activities/Fields: Geropharmacology, including mechanisms of drug action, pharmacokinetics, therapeutic uses, drug abuse, polypharmacy and drug compliance as it applies to geriatric patients. Clinical research is conducted in the areas of exercise in the healthy, frail, and elderly, cardiovascular function, and cognitive disorders in the elderly. Basic research is conducted in pharmacologic mechanisms of temperature regulation, obesity, febril response to infections, immunology, and muscle strength.

★ 24567 ★ Veterans Health Administration
Geriatric Research, Education, and Clinical Center-Little Rock
VA Medical Center
Little Rock, AR 72205
Phone: (501)257-5542 **Fax:** (501)257-4531
Website: http://www.littlerockgrecc.org/default.asp
Dennis H. Sullivan, MD, Dir.
Activities/Fields: Cellular and molecular biology of aging; nutrition, exercise and metabolism in the elderly.

★ 24568 ★ Veterans Health Administration
Geriatric Research, Education, and Clinical Center-Los Angeles
VA Medical Center West
Bldg. 220, Rm. 315
11301 Wilshire Blvd., 11G
Los Angeles, CA 90073
Phone: (310)268-4110 **Fax:** (310)268-4842
Email: thahn@ucla.edu
Theodore J. Hahn, MD, Dir.
Activities/Fields: Osteoporosis, immunology and osteoarthritis, health care utilization, rehabilitative medicine.

★ 24569 ★ Veterans Health Administration
Geriatric Research, Education, and Clinical Center-Madison
VA Medical Center
Madison, WI 53705
Phone: (608)262-7089 **Fax:** (608)262-7648
Email: steven.barczi@med.va.gov
Steven Barczi, MD, Actg. Dir.
Activities/Fields: Cancer/immunity/nutrition, swallowing, geriatric oncology, long-term care.

★ 24570 ★ Veterans Health Administration
Geriatric Research, Education, and Clinical Center-Miami
VA Medical Center, 11 GRC
1201 NW 16th St.
Miami, FL 33170
Phone: (305)575-3388 **Fax:** (305)575-3365
Email: broos@miami.edu
Dr. Bernard A. Roos, Dir.
Activities/Fields: Bone and cartilage metabolism, prostate disease, neurodegeneration, osteoporosis and osteoarthritis, Paget's disease, rehabilitation from falls and injuries, biopsychosocial intervention.

★ 24571 ★ Veterans Health Administration
Geriatric Research, Education, and Clinical Center-Minneapolis
VA Medical Center
1 Veterans Dr.
Minneapolis, MN 55417
Phone: (612)725-2051 **Fax:** (612)725-2084
Email: dyske001@umn.edu
Maurice Dysken, MD, Dir.
Activities/Fields: Neurochemistry, pharmacology, Alzheimer's Disease, caregiver education.

★ 24572 ★ Veterans Health Administration
Geriatric Research, Education, and Clinical Center-Palo Alto
Palo Alto Health Care System, Ste. 182B
3801 Miranda Ave.
Palo Alto, CA 94304
Phone: (650)858-3933 **Fax:** (650)496-2505
Email: arhoffman@stanford.edu
Website: http://www.palo-alto.med.va.gov/programs/grecc/grecc.htm
Elizabeth Joyce Freeman, Dir.
Activities/Fields: Endocrinological and metabolic aspects of aging, advanced care directives, family caregiving issues, medication adherence.

★ 24573 ★ Veterans Health Administration
Geriatric Research, Education, and Clinical Center-St. Louis
VA Medical Center, 11G
Jefferson Barracks Dr.
Saint Louis, MO 63125
Phone: (314)894-6510 **Fax:** (314)894-6614
Email: morley@slu.edu
John E. Morley, MD, Dir.
Activities/Fields: Physiology and metabolic concomitants of aging, effects of exercise and nutrition on physiological and metabolic parameters, health care utilization, nursing home care. **Pub:** *Aging Successfully*, 3/year. Newsletter.

★ 24574 ★ Veterans Health Administration
Geriatric Research, Education, and Clinical Center-Salt Lake City
VA Salt Lake City Healthcare System
500 Foothill Dr., GRECC 182
Salt Lake City, UT 84148
Phone: (801)584-2522 **Fax:** (801)583-7338
Email: byron.bair@med.va.gov
Byron Bair, MD, Dir.
Activities/Fields: Fundamental changes during aging which lead to impaired immunity, and increased susceptibility to cancer, depressions in the physiologic status of important organ systems, and decline in brain function.

★ 24575 ★ Veterans Health Administration
Geriatric Research, Education, and Clinical Center-San Antonio
VA Medical Center
San Antonio, TX 78284
Phone: (210)617-5197 **Fax:** (210)617-5312
Email: katz@uthscsa.edu
Michael S. Katz, MD, Dir.
Activities/Fields: Metabolism/endocrinology, nutrition, oral health/dentistry, metabolic diseases, cognitive sensory impairment, health care utilization, long-term care.

★ 24576 ★ Veterans Health Administration
Geriatric Research, Education, and Clinical Center-Seattle
VA Puget Sound HealthCare System
1660 S Columbian Way, S 182 GRECC
Seattle, WA 98108
Phone: (206)764-2308 **Fax:** (206)764-2569
Email: jcsb@u.washington.edu
John Breitner, MD, Dir.
Activities/Fields: Neurobiologic and neuroendocrine aspects of aging and Alzheimer's Disease, metabolic diseases and cognitive sensory impairment, bioethical aspects of medical decision making regarding the elderly.

★ 24577 ★ Veterans Health Administration
Geriatric Research, Education, and Clinical Center-Sepulveda
VA Facility
16111 Plummer (11E)
Sepulveda, CA 91343
Phone: (818)895-9311 **Fax:** (818)895-9519
Email: laurence.rubenstein@med.va.gov
Laurence Z. Rubenstein, MD, Dir.

Activities/Fields: Alzheimer's Disease, molecular biology, endocrinology, falls and mobility problems, long-term care, exercise, pain, sleep, quality of care, cost-effective health care delivery.

★ 24578 ★ Veterans Health Administration
Office of Research and Development Center for Health Care Evaluation (CHCE)
795 Willow Rd. (152-MPD)
Menlo Park, CA 94025
Phone: (650)493-5000
Website: http://www.chce.research.med.va.gov/chce/content/main.htm
Paul G. Barnett, PhD, Dir.
Activities/Fields: Improvement in the organization and delivery of health care services; improvement in diagnostic assessment, screening procedures, and clinical decision making; improvement in treatment for substance use and psychiatric disorders; and improvement in health services research methods.

★ 24579 ★ Veterans Health Administration
Office of Research and Development Center for Health Equity Research and Promotion (CHERP)
VA Pittsburgh Healthcare System
University Dr. C, 11E130-B (130-U)
Pittsburgh, PA 15240
Phone: (412)688-6477 **Fax:** (412)688-6916
Email: mary.walsh3@med.va.gov
Website: http://www.cherp.org
Michael J. Fine, MD, Dir.
Activities/Fields: Health and health care disparities among vulnerable groups of veterans. **Pub:** *Briefs*, quarterly.

★ 24580 ★ Veterans Health Administration
Office of Research and Development Health Services Research and Development Service Center of Excellence
VA Medical Center, 152
3801 Miranda Ave.
Palo Alto, CA 94304
Phone: (650)617-2746 **Fax:** (650)617-2736
Email: janice.beyer@med.va.gov
Website: http://www.chce.research.med.va.gov
John Finney, PhD, Dir.
Activities/Fields: Organization and delivery of health care services; diagnostic assessment, screening, and clinical decision making; evaluation of treatments for substance abuse and psychiatric disorders; health services research methodology. Current project involve improving HIV screening policies; implementing practice guidelines; evaluating the effectiveness and cost-effectiveness of interventions for alcohol abuse, drug abuse, and depression. **Pub:** *Newsletter.*

★ 24581 ★ Veterans Health Administration
Office of Research and Development Rehabilitation Outcomes Research Center
North Florida/South Georgia Veterans Health System Research
Gainesville, FL 32608
Phone: (352)376-1611 **Fax:** (352)271-4540
Email: rorc@med.va.gov
Pamela W. Duncan, PhD, Dir.
Activities/Fields: Structure, process, and outcomes of rehabilitation services for patients with central nervous system damage; emerging therapies and technologies for these same patients.

★ 24582 ★ Veterans Research Foundation
921 NE 13th St.
Oklahoma City, OK 73104-5028
Phone: (405)270-5170 **Fax:** (405)297-5911
Email: debbie_simmons@ouhsc.edu
Deborah J. Simmons, Exec. Dir.
Activities/Fields: Biomedical research for veterans.

★ 24583 ★ Via Christi Research, Inc.
1100 N St. Francis, Ste. 200
Wichita, KS 67214-2878
Phone: (316)291-4900 **Fax:** (316)291-7704
Email: dale_horst@via-christi.org
Website: http://www.viamtec.org
Dr. W. Dale Horst, Dir.
Activities/Fields: Psychiatry; phase I, II, and III clinical drug studies; orthopedic research; biomedical device and materials research and development; technology transfer and product development; hospital operations research; and pharmacoeconomic research. **Frmly:** St. Francis Research Institute, Inc.

★ 24584 ★ Victoria Heart Institute Foundation (VHIF)
315-1900 Richmond Ave.
Victoria, BC, Canada V8R 4R2
Phone: (250)595-1884 **Fax:** (250)595-5367
Email: vhif@vhif.org
Website: http://www.vhif.org/html/about_vhif.htm
Dr. W. Peter Klinke, MD, Dir.
Activities/Fields: Cardiovascular disease.

★ 24585 ★ Virginia Commonwealth University
Clinical Research Center for Periodontal Diseases
Wood Bldg., Rm. 401
Richmond, VA 23298
Phone: (804)828-9185 **Fax:** (804)828-5787
Email: haschenk@vcu.edu
Website: http://www.dentistry.vcu.edu/research/crcpd.htm
Dr. Harvey A. Schenkein, Dir.
Activities/Fields: Periodontal diseases, including bacteriology, immunology, and genetics, to determine causative bacteria and the mechanism and role of genetic factors and host response in pathogenesis in order to devise improved preventive and therapeutic methods.

★ 24586 ★ Virginia Commonwealth University
General Clinical Research Center
PO Box 980155
Richmond, VA 23298
Phone: (804)828-9228 **Fax:** (804)828-5002
Email: clore@hsc.vcu.edu
John N. Clore, MD, Prog. Dir.
Activities/Fields: Endocrinology, gastroenterology, infectious disease, metabolism, neurology, pediatrics, pharmacology, psychiatry, pulmonary physiology, and surgery.

★ 24587 ★ Virginia Commonwealth University
Hepatology Section and Liver Transplant Program
PO Box 980341
Richmond, VA 23298-0711
Phone: (434)828-4060 **Fax:** (434)828-4945
Email: mshiffma@hsc.vcu.edu
Dr. Shiffman, Dir.
Activities/Fields: Anti-viral therapy for chronic viral hepatitis B and C; new treatments for chronic liver disease; complications of chronic liver disease including ascites, variceal hemorrhage, and hepatic encephalopathy; liver transplantation including the development of new immunosupressive therapies.

★ 24588 ★ Virginia Commonwealth University
Massey Cancer Center
401 College St.
PO Box 980037
Richmond, VA 23298-0037
Phone: (804)828-0450 **Fax:** (804)828-8453
Email: ginder@vcu.edu
Website: http://www.vcu.edu/mcc/
Dr. Gordon D. Ginder, Dir.
Activities/Fields: Molecular biology, immunobiology, molecular therapeutics, neurooncology, carcinogenesis, genetics, hematopoiesis, bone marrow transplantation, cancer prevention, and structural biology. Clinical studies include translational research and participation in national cooperative groups. Focuses on decision analysis methodologies for evaluation of cancer treatment outcomes and costs through a Health Sciences Research Program. **Pub:** *Advance*, semiannually. • *In-Advance*, monthly.

★ 24589 ★ Virginia Commonwealth University
Medical Informatics and Technology Applications Consortium (MITAC)
1101 E Marshall St., Ste. 8017
PO Box 980480
Richmond, VA 23298-0480
Phone: (434)827-1020 **Fax:** (434)827-1029
Email: charles.doarn@vcu.edu
Website: http://www.meditac.com/
Charles R. Doarn, Exec. Dir.
Activities/Fields: Medical informatics and health care delivery systems that will revolutionize health care in space and on Earth.

★ 24590 ★ Virginia Commonwealth University
Neurosciences Center
1200 E Broad St.
PO Box 980317
Richmond, VA 23298-0317
Phone: (434)828-6370 **Fax:** (434)828-2501
Website: http://stealth.nsc.vcu.edu/nsc
John D. Ward, MD, Dir.
Activities/Fields: Neurosciences, particularly neuroimaging, neurochemistry, and molecular neurobiology.

★ 24591 ★ Virginia Commonwealth University
Outcomes Research Institute
Virginia Biotechnology Research Park, Biotech One
800 E Leigh St., Ste 115B
PO Box 980219
Richmond, VA 23298-0219
Phone: (434)225-3450 **Fax:** (434)827-0087
Email: rwenzel@hsc.vcu.edu
Website: http://www.trials-outcomes.clt.vcu.edu/outcomes/mission.html
Richard P. Wenzel, MD, Exec. Dir.
Activities/Fields: Delivery of the best medical care with the best possible outcome to patients in a health care system.

★ 24592 ★ Virginia Commonwealth University
Rehabilitation Research and Training Center on Workplace Supports
1314 W Main St.
PO Box 842011
Richmond, VA 23284-2011
Phone: (434)828-1851 **Fax:** (434)828-2193
Website: http://www.worksupport.com/
Paul Wehman, PhD, Dir.
Activities/Fields: Return to work strategies for persons who become disabled while employed; key components of effective disability management programs; financial tax credits to encourage hiring, retention, and advancement of the disabled; the impact of work support interventions on employment and ad-

vancement; employer perceptions of obstacles to hiring and retaining the disabled; and the significance of structural changes in the American economy on people with disabilities. **Pub:** *Newsletter.*

★ 24593 ★ Virginia Commonwealth University
Virginia Center on Aging
Medical College of Virginia Campus
520 N 12th St., Rm. B-25
PO Box 980229
Richmond, VA 23298-0229
Phone: (434)828-1525 **Fax:** (434)828-7905
Email: eansello@hsc.vcu.edu
Website: http://www.vcu.edu/vcoa
Edward F. Ansello, PhD, Dir.
Activities/Fields: Mental and physical health of the elderly, focusing on community-living and health-related factors of aging. Studies include: eldercare responsibilities of employed family caregivers, inter-system cooperation in delivery of human services, impact of aging of adults with developmental disabilities, minority healthcare utilization, caregiving of demented elders, research and documentation project on rural geropharmacy. **Pub:** *AGE In Action Newsletter*, quarterly.

★ 24594 ★ Virginia Commonwealth University
Virginia Commonwealth Regional Spinal Cord Injury System
Medical College of Virginia
Department of Physical Medicine & Rehabilitation
Box 980677
1233 E Marshall St., 4th Fl.
Richmond, VA 23298-0677
Phone: (434)828-4230 **Fax:** (434)828-6340
Email: wmckinle@hsc.vcu.edu
Website: http://www.pmr.vcu.edu/department/faculty/clinical/wmckinley.html
Dr. William O. McKinley, Dir.
Activities/Fields: Spinal cord injuries, including exploration of clinical pathway outcomes across the continuum of care; evaluation of innovative medical issues related to spinal cord injuries; delineation of the incidence of and formulation of management strategies for the rehabilitation of persons with dual diagnosis of spinal cord injuries and traumatic brain injury; and identification of incidences and treatment strategies for individuals with spinal cord injuries and substance abuse.

★ 24595 ★ Virginia Commonwealth University
Virginia Institute for Developmental Disabilities (VIDD)
700 E Franklin St., 10th Fl.
PO Box 843020
Richmond, VA 23284-3020
Phone: (434)828-3876 **Fax:** (434)828-0042
Email: forelove@saturn.vcu.edu
Website: http://www.vcu.edu/vidd
Fred P. Orelove, PhD, Exec. Dir.
Activities/Fields: Independence, productivity, integration, and inclusion of individuals with developmental disabilities.

★ 24596 ★ Virginia Department of Health
Epidemiology Office
1500 E Main St.
PO Box 2448
Richmond, VA 23218
Phone: (804)786-6029 **Fax:** (804)786-1076
Email: jmarr@vdh.state.va.us
Dr. John S. Marr, Dir.
Activities/Fields: Epidemiology.

★ 24597 ★ Virginia Lions Hearing Foundation and Research Center, Inc.
University of Virginia Health System
PO Box 800477
Charlottesville, VA 22908-0477
Phone: (434)296-5466 **Free:** 800-251-3627
Fax: (434)243-6732
Email: grb8b@virginia.edu
Website: http://www.lions24b.org/VLHF/
Gwynn Berkowitz, Admin.
Activities/Fields: Cochlear implants, newborn hearing screening, implantable hearing aids, hair cell regeneration in the cochlea, ototoxicity (drug damage), noise damage, electrical stimulation of auditory nerves. **Pub:** *Eardrum Update*, quarterly.

★ 24598 ★ Virginia Mason Research Center
1201 9th Ave.
Seattle, WA 98101-2795
Phone: (206)583-6525 **Fax:** (206)223-7543
Email: info@vmresearch.org
Website: http://www.vmresearch.org
Dr. Gerald T. Nepom, Dir.
Activities/Fields: Immunology, diabetes and clinical research. **Pub:** *Bulletin of the Virginia Mason Clinic.*

★ 24599 ★ W.M. Keck Center for Computational Biology
Rice University
6100 S Main St.
Houston, TX 77005
Phone: (713)348-8750 **Fax:** (713)348-4659
Email: keckcenter@bioc.rice.edu
Website: http://www.bioc.rice.edu/keck
George N. Phillips, Co-Dir.
Activities/Fields: Biological research, including chemistry and molecular biology of DNA binding, molecular genetics of inborn errors of metabolism, electron crystallography and tomography of macromolecular assemblies, DNA sequence information and human disease, computational neuroscience, parallel computation and language, high resolution NMR spectroscopy of macromolecular structure and dynamics, computation in molecular genetics, computation in image reconstruction and biofluid mechanics, structure and metabolism of lipoproteins, rapid kinetics of hemeprotein-ligand reactions, structure and function of electron transport proteins, nicotonic synaptic transmission in the central nervous system, X-ray crystallography, molecular dynamics of proteins and nucleic acids, a tomic structures and functions of proteins, artificial intelligence, and design and analysis of algorithms. **Pub:** *Keck Center Newsletter.*

★ 24600 ★ W.M. Krogman Center for Research in Child Growth and Development
University of Pennsylvania
4019 Irving St.
Philadelphia, PA 19104-6003
Phone: (215)898-1470 **Fax:** (215)898-5243
Website: http://www.upenn.edu/krogman/krogman.html
Dr. Solomon H. Katz, Dir.
Activities/Fields: Obesity, nutrition, and other health and mental disorders, epidemiology of high blood pressure in adolescents, neuropsychological development, developmental disorders, hypertension, and subclinical lead intoxication and other trace element studies in children. Also establishes norms of physical growth and development of Philadelphia and international children from birth to 17 years of age, including norms for head, face, and jaws (cephalometric and roentgenographic cephalometric), body (height, weight, somatometric size, and proportion of trunk and limbs), and maturation levels (via X-ray films and hand and knee), applied to clinical problems in medicine and dentistry. **Frmly:** Philadelphia Center for Research in Child Growth and Development.

★ 24601 ★ Waisman Center
University of Wisconsin—Madison
1500 Highland Ave.
Madison, WI 53705
Phone: (608)263-5910 **Fax:** (608)263-0529
Email: mseltzer@waisman.wisc.edu
Website: http://www.waisman.wisc.edu
Marsha Mailick Seltzer, PhD, Dir.
Activities/Fields: Individuals with developmental disabilities, including noncompromised infants, children, and adults, as well as nonhuman subjects. Studies focus on genetics, molecular biology, neurochemistry, sensory and perceptual processes, neurophysiology, communication processes, development intervention processes, and biological, behavioral, and social processes across the lifespan. Divided into the following units: Molecular and Genetic Sciences Unit, Sensory and Cognitive Processes Unit, Communication Processes Unit, Social and Affective Processes Unit. **Pub:** *Waisman Center Interactions*, annually. **Frmly:** Harry A. Waisman Center.

★ 24602 ★ Wake Forest University Center for Investigative Neuroscience (CIN)
School of Medicine
Medical Center Blvd.
Winston Salem, NC 27157
Phone: (336)716-0083 **Fax:** (336)716-4480
Email: bestein@wfubmc.edu
Website: http://www.wfubmc.edu/CIN/
Barry E. Stein, PhD, Interim Dir.
Activities/Fields: Diseases of the central nervous system.

★ 24603 ★ Wake Forest University Center for Medical Ultrasound (CMU)
School of Medicine
Medical Center Blvd.
Winston Salem, NC 27157
Phone: (336)716-4505 **Fax:** (336)716-2447
Email: cmu@wfubmc.edu
Website: http://www.wfubmc.edu/research/med_ultra.html
Dr. Frederick W. Kremkau, Dir.
Activities/Fields: Application of ultrasound in medical diagnosis and therapy for better patient care.

★ 24604 ★ Wake Forest University Cerebrovascular Research Center
Department of Neurology
Medical Center Blvd.
Winston Salem, NC 27157-1068
Phone: (336)716-2336 **Fax:** (336)716-5477
Email: jtoole@wfubmc.edu
Dr. James F. Toole, Dir.
Activities/Fields: Cerebrovascular research, including ultrasound, neurological diseases, coronary studies, biostatistics, transient ischemic attack (TIA), comparative medicine in atherosclerosis, neuropsychological evaluation, cerebral circulation, and anatomy/physiology. **Pub:** *Stroke Monitor Newsletter*, quarterly.

★ 24605 ★ Wake Forest University Comparative Medicine Clinical Research Center
School of Medicine
Medical Center Blvd.
Winston Salem, NC 27157-1040
Phone: (336)716-2673 **Fax:** (336)716-6279
Email: rstclair@wfubmc.edu
Website: http://www.wfubmc.edu/research/comp_med.html
Richard W. St. Clair, PhD, Dir.
Activities/Fields: Animal models of human disease studies, including research in heart disease, osteoporosis, women's health, and arteriosclerosis. Also studies relationship between aggression and low cholesterol levels.

★ 24606 ★ Wake Forest University Comprehensive Cancer Center
Medical Center Blvd.
Winston Salem, NC 27157
Phone: (336)716-7971 **Fax:** (336)716-0293
Email: ftorti@wfubmc.edu
Website: http://www.wfubmc.edu/cancer/
Dr. Frank M. Torti, Dir.
Activities/Fields: Cause and therapy of cancer, in a multidisciplinary effort to determine cause of cancer and to develop more effective means of treating malignant disease. **Frmly:** Oncology Research Center.

★ 24607 ★ Wake Forest University Comprehensive Epilepsy Center
Department of Neurology
School of Medicine
Medical Center Blvd.
Winston Salem, NC 27157
Phone: (336)716-0488 **Fax:** (336)716-7548
Email: wbell@wfubmc.edu
William L. Bell, MD, Dir.
Activities/Fields: Epilepsy, especially methods for detecting seizures, epilepsy surgery, psychosocial issues, antiepileptic drugs, etc.

★ 24608 ★ Wake Forest University Epilepsy Education Information Service
Medical Center Blvd.
Winston Salem, NC 27157-1078
Phone: (336)716-2321 **Free:** 800-642-0500
Fax: (336)716-9489
Email: pgibson@wfubmc.edu
Patricia Gibson, Dir.
Activities/Fields: Social and psychological aspects of epilepsy and clinical trials of anti-epileptic medication.

★ 24609 ★ Wake Forest University General Clinical Research Center
Medical Center Blvd.
Winston Salem, NC 27157
Phone: (336)716-9750 **Fax:** (336)716-5055
Email: chmcall@wfubmc.edu
Website: http://www.gcrc.wfubmc.edu
Charles E. McCall, MD, Prog. Dir.
Activities/Fields: Major areas of investigation include anesthesiology, autoimmune diseases, dermatology, endocrinology, gastroenterology, genetics, geriatrics and gerontology, hematology and oncology, hypertension, infectious diseases, nephrology, neurology, obstetrics and gynecology, pediatrics, psychiatry, pulmonary diseases, and women's health.

★ 24610 ★ Wake Forest University Hypertension and Vascular Disease Center
School of Medicine
Medical Center Blvd.
Winston Salem, NC 27157-1032
Phone: (336)716-5819 **Free:** 800-277-8839
Fax: (336)716-6644
Email: cferrari@wfubme.edu
Website: http://www.wfubmc.edu/hypertension
Dr. Carlos Ferrario, Dir.
Activities/Fields: Hypertension and cardiovascular disease. Activities include a clinical hypertension drug trial to treat high blood pressure on individuals 70 years or older and two clinical hypertension drug trials to treat high blood pressure on individuals 21 years or older. **Frmly:** Hypertension Center.

★ 24611 ★ Wake Forest University J. Paul Sticht Center on Aging and Rehabilitation
North Carolina Baptist Hospitals, Inc.
Medical Center Blvd.
Winston Salem, NC 27157
Phone: (336)716-2011 **Fax:** (336)713-8588
Email: mpahor@wfubmc.edu
Website: http://www.wfubmc.edu/sticht
Marco Pahor, MD, Dir.
Activities/Fields: Metabolic and biomedical research in aging and rehabilitation, focusing on physical disabilities and problems in the elderly.

★ 24612 ★ Wake Forest University Lipid Analytic Laboratory
Gray Bldg., Rm. 2063
School of Medicine
Medical Center Blvd.
Winston Salem, NC 27157-1072
Email: rstclair@wfubmc.edu
Website: http://www.wfubmc.edu/or/core31.html
Richard W. St. Clair, PhD, Dir.
Activities/Fields: Provision of standardized plasma lipid and lipoprotein analyses for clinical and research purposes.

★ 24613 ★ Wake Forest University Pain Mechanisms Laboratory
Gray Bldg.
Medical Center Blvd.
Winston Salem, NC 27157
Phone: (336)716-2591 **Fax:** (336)716-3220
Email: eisenach@wfubmc.edu
Website: http://www.wfubmc.edu/painlab/main.html
James C. Eisenach, MD, Dir.
Activities/Fields: Pain and analgesia.

★ 24614 ★ Wake Forest University Women's Health Center of Excellence
Medical Center Blvd.
PO Box 573050
Winston Salem, NC 27157-3050
Phone: (336)713-4220
Website: http://www.wfubmc.edu/women/wc_t_nat-center.html
Sally A. Shumaker, PhD, Dir.
Activities/Fields: Diseases that affect women, delivery of health care services to women, and health education for women. **Pub:** *Newsletter*, monthly.

★ 24615 ★ Walt Disney Memorial Cancer Institute
Cancer Research Division
2501 N Orange Ave., Ste. 786
Orlando, FL 32804
Phone: (407)303-2440 **Fax:** (407)303-2441
Dr. John L. Francis, Dir.
Activities/Fields: Cancer, including cell biology and cell regulation, molecular biology, structural biology and drug design, and hemostasis and thrombosis.

★ 24616 ★ Walther Cancer Institute, Inc.
3202 N Meridian St.
Indianapolis, IN 46208
Phone: (317)921-2040 **Fax:** (317)924-4688
Website: http://www.walther.org
Leonard Betley, Pres. /CEO
Activities/Fields: Treatment, prevention, and cure of cancer and studies on the care of cancer patients and families. **Pub:** *Annual Report.* • *Newsletter*, quarterly. **Frmly:** Walther Medical Research Institute.

★ 24617 ★ Walther Cancer Institute, Inc. Mary Margaret Walther Program for Cancer Care Research
School of Nursing
Indiana University
1111 Middle Dr., Rm. 340
Indianapolis, IN 46202
Phone: (317)274-7563 **Fax:** (317)278-2021
Email: vchampio@iupui.edu
Dr. Victoria L. Champion, Dir.
Activities/Fields: Cancer prevention/control, survivorship, and cancer care delivery, focusing on developing an interdisciplinary effort to conduct behavioral research improving the quality of life for cancer patients and their families. Research addresses the psychological, economic, sociological and spiritual needs of those going through the cancer experience; increasing early detection of cancer and decreasing the occurrence of cancer through individual, family, and community behaviors; and improving the delivery of cost-effective cancer care by health professionals to cancer patients and their families. **Pub:** *Brochures*, annually.

★ 24618 ★ Walther Cancer Institute, Inc. Walther Oncology Center
Indiana University School of Medicine
950 W Walnut St., Rm. 302
Indianapolis, IN 46202-5181
Phone: (317)274-7501 **Fax:** (317)274-7592
Email: hbroxmey@iupui.edu
Website: http://www.iupui.edu/~woc/
Hal E. Broxmeyer, PhD, Sci. Dir.
Activities/Fields: Blood cell and solid tumor studies, including regulation of the production of normal and cancer cells and umbilical cord blood transplantation, growth factors, suppressor molecules, receptors, gene regulation, oncogenes, differentiation, signal transduction, phosphorylation, cell division cycle genes, and protein tyrosine phosphatases.

★ 24619 ★ Washington Home Center for Palliative Care Studies (CPCS)
4200 Wisconsin Ave. NW, 4th Fl.
Washington, DC 20016
Phone: (202)895-2625 **Fax:** (202)966-5410
Email: info@medicaring.org
Website: http://www.medicaring.org
Joanne Lynn, MD, Dir.
Activities/Fields: Management of end-of-life issues, improvement of the practices of health care providers at this time. **Pub:** *Handbook for Mortals.* • *Improving Care for the End of Life: A Sourcebook for Clinicians and Managers.*

★ 24620 ★ Washington Institute for Mental Illness Research and Training
Washington State University Spokane
310 N Riverpoint Blvd.
PO Box 1495
Spokane, WA 99210-1495
Phone: (509)358-7618 **Fax:** (509)358-7619
Email: dyck@wsu.edu
Website: http://www.spokane.wsu.edu/research&service/wimirt/wimirthome.html
Dennis G. Dyck, PhD, Dir.
Activities/Fields: Mental health clinical and services research for persons with severe and persistent mental illness; family and patient psychoeducation and support.

★ 24621 ★ Washington University in St. Louis
Alzheimer's Disease Research Center
4488 Forest Park Ave., Ste. 130
Saint Louis, MO 63108
Phone: (314)286-2881 **Fax:** (314)286-2763
Email: adrc@neuro.wustl.edu
Website: http://www.adrc.wustl.edu
John C. Morris, MD, Dir.
Activities/Fields: Aging and dementia, neurobiology of aging and cognition, Alzheimer's disease and related disorders, and the impact of dementia on the family or caregiver and the community. Studies include clinical research, clinical drug trials, neuropathological (autopsy) studies, genetic and other medical studies of persons with dementia, bench studies, behavioral/social research, and psychometric studies. **Pub:** *Horizons Newsletter.*

★ 24622 ★ Washington University in St. Louis
Atherosclerosis, Nutrition, and Lipid Research Division
660 S Euclid Ave., Campus Box 8127
Saint Louis, MO 63110

Phone: (314)362-7038 **Fax:** (314)747-4477
Email: semenkov@im.wustl.edu
Clay F. Semenkovich, MD, Assoc. Dir.
Activities/Fields: Atherosclerosis and lipid disorders, including research on genetic lipid disorders, atherogenesis and the roles of growth factors, cytokines, and chemically modified oxidized lipoproteins. Uses chemical, molecular, biologic, immunologic and cell culture techniques for studies of lipogenesis, lipoprotein structure and function. Performs clinical trials to determine optimum diagnostic and treatment modalities for dyslipoproteinemias. **Frmly:** Lipid Research Center.

★ 24623 ★ Washington University in St. Louis
Biomedical Research Program
Department of Internal Medicine, CB 8212
660 S Euclid
Saint Louis, MO 63110
Phone: (314)362-5300 **Fax:** (314)362-5306
David Kipnis, MD, Dir.
Activities/Fields: Allocates funds for exploratory and basic research and product development on the proteins, peptides, and other molecules regulating cellular communication and function. Facilitates the exchange of information between individual investigators in the Medical School and Monsanto's scientists.

★ 24624 ★ Washington University in St. Louis
Center for Mental Health Services Research (CMHSR)
CB 1093
Saint Louis, MO 63130-4899
Phone: (314)935-5687 **Fax:** (314)935-7508
Email: cmhsr@gwbmail.wustl.edu
Website: http://gwbweb.wustl.edu/Users/cmhsr/
Enola K. Proctor, PhD, Dir.
Activities/Fields: Mental health services from a variety of care providers, ranging from mental health specialists to family members.

★ 24625 ★ Washington University in St. Louis
Chromalloy American Kidney Center
660 S Euclid, CB 8129
Saint Louis, MO 63110
Phone: (314)362-8231 **Fax:** (314)362-7232
Email: jdelmez@im.wustl.edu
Dr. James Delmez, Dir.
Activities/Fields: Lipid abnormalities in uremia, muscle protein metabolism in uremia, metabolic bone disease in uremia, parathyroid hormone, and vitamin D and aluminum metabolism.

★ 24626 ★ Washington University in St. Louis
Cystic Fibrosis Center
1 Children's Pl.
Saint Louis, MO 63110
Phone: (314)454-2694 **Fax:** (314)454-2515
Email: ferkol_t@kids.wustl.edu
Dr. Thomas Ferkol, Dir.
Activities/Fields: Cystic fibrosis and pulmonary diseases, plus nutrition and malabsorption in relation to cystic fibrosis and liver diseases and effects of mechanisms of inflammatory response in cyctic fibrosis-related diseases. Conducts research on lung transplantation and nutrition in cystic fibrosis, as well as basic studies of immune mechanisms. Provides clinical material to departments of the University engaged in related research and offers educational programs for patients, parents, and professionals.

★ 24627 ★ Washington University in St. Louis
Diabetes Research and Training Center
660 S Euclid Ave., CB 8127
Saint Louis, MO 63110
Phone: (314)362-8680 **Fax:** (314)747-2692
Email: apermutt@im.wustl.edu
Website: http://www.medicine.wustl.edu/drtc
M. Alan Permutt, Dir.
Activities/Fields: Diabetes research, including the causes of diabetes, insulin action, growth factors, and diabetic complications. Promotes biomedical and psychosocial studies of diabetes mellitus by operating core facilities to support established investigators. Core facilities include the Clinical Research Facility, where a patient registry of 500 diabetic patients undergoes clinical evaluation and is available for clinical studies; Radioimmunoassay Facility, which provides assays of insulin and conducts hormone studies; Mass Spectrometry Facility, supporting analytic and metabolic studies requiring mass spectrometry techniques; Animal and Transgenic Core Facility; Morphology Facility; Training and Translation Facility with an Education Center specialized in training professionals for diabetic patient care; Molecular Biology Facility; and Human Pancreatic Islet Facility, which provides human islets for NIH-funded projects.

★ 24628 ★ Washington University in St. Louis
General Clinical Research Center
Barnard Hospital, 4th Fl., Box 8071
Saint Louis, MO 63110
Phone: (314)362-7617 **Fax:** (314)362-7989
Email: pcryer@im.wustl.edu
Website: http://www.ncrr.nih.gov/ncrrprog/clindir/missouri.asp
Dr. Philip E. Cryer, Dir.
Activities/Fields: Provides clinical research facilities for faculty members of the School.

★ 24629 ★ Washington University in St. Louis
Hyperthermia Service
Department of Radiation Oncology
4921 Parkview Pl.
Saint Louis, MO 63110
Phone: (314)362-8503 **Fax:** (314)747-9557
Email: myerson@radonc.wustl.edu
Robert J. Myerson, MD, Ch.
Activities/Fields: Hyperthermia treatment of cancer, simultaneous thermoradiotherapy, and bioassay of predictors of hyperthermic response.

★ 24630 ★ Washington University in St. Louis
Mallinckrodt Institute of Radiology
510 S Kingshighway Blvd.
Saint Louis, MO 63110
Phone: (314)362-8436 **Fax:** (314)362-8399
Email: welchm@mir.wustl.edu
Website: http://www.mir.wustl.edu
Dr. Michael Welch, Contact
Activities/Fields: Radiological diagnostic, treatment, research, and training center including nuclear medicine, radiation oncology, radiation sciences, and diagnostic radiology. The diagnostic radiology division is comprised of seven sections: abdominal, cardiac, chest, computer, musculoskeletal, pediatric, and neuroradiology. Maintains laboratories for research in digital image processing, computer sciences, nuclear medicine, radiation oncology, cancer biology, diagnostic radiology, and magnetic resonance imaging. **Pub:** *Focal Spot*, 3/year.

★ 24631 ★ Washington University in St. Louis
Resource for Biomedical and Bio-organic Mass Spectrometry
1 Brookings Dr.
Saint Louis, MO 63130
Phone: (314)935-4814 **Fax:** (314)935-7484
Email: mgross@wuchem.wustl.edu
Website: http://wunmr.wustl.edu/~msf
Michael L. Gross, PhD, Prin. Investigator
Activities/Fields: Instrument and method development of mass spectrometry; structure determination of peptides, proteins, carcinogen-modified DNA fragments, and lipids; stable isotope tracer and complex lipids.

★ 24632 ★ Washington University in St. Louis
Siteman Cancer Center
Box 8100
660 S Euclid
Saint Louis, MO 63110-1093
Phone: (314)747-7222 **Free:** 800-600-3606
Website: http://www.siteman.wustl.edu/
Timothy J. Eberlein, MD, Dir.
Activities/Fields: Treatment, prevention and control of cancer. Areas of interest include cancer genetics, cellular and developmental biology, tumor immunology, cellular proliferation, hematopoietic development and malignancy, oncologic imaging, clinical and translational research, prevention and control, chemoprevention, developmental therapeutics.

★ 24633 ★ Wayne State University
Bioengineering Center
818 W Hancock St.
Detroit, MI 48202
Phone: (313)577-1344 **Fax:** (313)577-8333
Email: king@rrb.eng.wayne.edu
Dr. Albert I. King, Dir.
Activities/Fields: Automotive and aircraft safety, injury mechanisms, and spinal function, including lower back pain, orthopedic biomechanics, and head injury.

★ 24634 ★ Wayne State University
C.S. Mott Center for Human Growth and Development
275 E Hancock St.
Detroit, MI 48201
Phone: (313)577-1337 **Fax:** (313)577-8554
Email: rsokol@moose.med.wayne.edu
Dr. Robert J. Sokol, Dir.
Activities/Fields: Human growth and development, including causative factors, identification, prevention, and remedy of birth defects. Uses mechanical, chemical, and hormonal devices as well as acceptable social, psychological, ethical, and moral approaches. Identifies environmental pollutants, drugs, infections, and other teratogens responsible for increasing incidence of birth defects and studies the relationships between environmental deterioration, dwindling natural resources, population density, and quality of human existence. Develops and implements population controls. **Pub:** *Annual Report*.

★ 24635 ★ Wayne State University
Center for Health Research
317 Cohn
College of Nursing
5557 Cass Ave.
Detroit, MI 48202-3515
Phone: (313)577-3911 **Fax:** (313)577-5777
Email: m.nies@wayne.edu
Website: http://www.nursing.wayne.edu/
Mary A. Nies, Assoc. Dean, Res.
Activities/Fields: Nursing, urban health, pain reduction, adolescent health, teen pregnancy, aging, chronicity, health education and promotion (e.g. smoking cessation, and physical activity), community health, psychosocial oncology, health behavior, self care, stress and coping, parent/child health, family health, caregivers of aged individuals, drug use, violence and abuse, sleep patterns, risk-taking with respect to teen pregnancy and sexually transmitted diseases (including HIV). Multidisciplinary studies involve health professionals and faculty members from disciplines such as nursing, psychology, sociology, anthropology, medicine, and epidemiology. **Frmly:** Center for Nursing Research.

★ 24636 ★ Wayne State University Center for Healthcare Effectiveness Research (CHER)
121 Shiffman Medical Library
4325 Brush
Detroit, MI 48201
Phone: (313)577-5189 **Fax:** (313)577-1773
Email: mmassana@med.wayne.edu
Website: http://www.med.wayne.edu/cher/open-er.htm
Dr. Mike Massanari, Contact
Activities/Fields: Health care services and their effectiveness.

★ 24637 ★ Wayne State University Center for Molecular Medicine and Genetics
Scott Hall, Rm. 3216
540 E Canfield
Detroit, MI 48201
Phone: (313)577-5323 **Fax:** (313)577-5218
Email: info@genetics.wayne.edu
Website: http://cmmg.biosci.wayne.edu
Dr. Mark Hughes, Dir.
Activities/Fields: Development and differentiation, including studies into meiotic differentiation, cell type-specific gene regulation, protein structure and function, and genome organization and stability; cancer and metastasis, including mapping of cancer genes, induction of carcinogenesis, gene regulation in cancer, and mechanisms of metastasis; human genetics and disease, comprising the genetic cause of Huntington's disease, arthritis and tissue remodeling, and diabetes and insulin action; viral disease, including papilloma viruses in cervical cancer; and gene therapeutics, including fetal gene therapy, and gene therapy for lymphoma and leukemia.

★ 24638 ★ Wayne State University Cystic Fibrosis Care, Teaching and Resource Center
Children's Hospital of Michigan
3901 Beaubien
Detroit, MI 48201
Phone: (313)745-5541 **Fax:** (313)993-2948
Email: dtoder@med.wayne.edu
Debbie Toder, MD, Dir.
Activities/Fields: Cystic fibrosis and pediatric pulmonary diseases. Also participates in multi-centered clinical trials.

★ 24639 ★ Wayne State University Institute of Environmental Health Sciences
2727 2nd Ave., Rm. 4000
Detroit, MI 48201-2654
Phone: (313)577-0100 **Fax:** (313)577-0082
Email: rnovak@wayne.edu
Website: http://www.chemtox.org
Dr. Raymond F. Novak, Dir.
Activities/Fields: Chemical hazards of the environment and industrial workplace, including toxicology of air pollutants, solvents, and heavy metals. Also studies carcinogenesis, metabolic, and hematologic effects resulting from exposure to toxic agents; and molecular and cellular approaches to examine early events in toxicity. **Frmly:** Institute of Chemical Toxicology.

★ 24640 ★ Wayne State University Institute of Maternal-Child Health (IMCH)
Department of Community Medicine
4201 St. Antoine, No. 9D UHC
Detroit, MI 48201
Phone: (313)577-1033
Email: aa2266@wayne.edu
Dr. John B. Waller, Ch.
Activities/Fields: Maternal and child health.

★ 24641 ★ Wayne State University Kresge Eye Institute
4717 St. Antoine
Detroit, MI 48201
Phone: (313)577-8900 **Fax:** (313)577-5482
Email: gabrams@med.wayne.edu
Website: http://www.med.wayne.edu/kresgeeye/
Gary W. Abrams, MD, Chm.
Activities/Fields: Cellular and molecular biology, electron microscopy, electrophysiology, neuro-ophthalmology, ophthalmic pathology, orthoptics, biochemistry of phototransduction in the vertebrate retina, cornea, glaucoma, vitreoretinal, and biochemistry and immunology of the eye.

★ 24642 ★ Wayne State University Laura S. Nye Surgical Research Fund for Desmoid Tumors
Harper Hospital
Department of Surgery
3990 John R
Detroit, MI 48201
Phone: (313)745-8778 **Fax:** (313)745-1873
Email: dfsurg@aol.com
David Fromm, MD, Ch.
Activities/Fields: Desmoid tumor treatment, including photodynamic therapy after excision of tumor.

★ 24643 ★ Wayne State University MR Research Facility
MR Center Concourse E
Harper Hospital
3990 John R
Detroit, MI 48201
Phone: (313)745-1395 **Fax:** (313)745-9182
Email: nmrimaging@aol.com
E. Mark Haacke, PhD, Dir.
Activities/Fields: Evaluates the potential for NMR (nuclear magnetic resonance) spectroscopy and imaging to provide predictors of response to chemotherapeutic drugs.

★ 24644 ★ Wayne State University Pre-Natal/Cancer-Cytogenetics Laboratory
Hutzel Professional Bldg., Ste. 401-412
Department of Pathology
4727 St. Antoine
Detroit, MI 48201
Phone: (313)966-0680 **Fax:** (313)966-0687
Email: sebrahim@med.wayne.edu
Dr. Salah Ebrahim, Dir.
Activities/Fields: Cytogenetics, including studies in the areas of neonatal development and endocrinology. Performs tests on amniotic fluids, CVS, bloods, bone marrows, and solid tissues.

★ 24645 ★ Wayne State University Sickle Cell Center
Children's Hospital of Michigan
3901 Beaubien
Detroit, MI 48201
Phone: (313)745-5613 **Fax:** (313)745-5237
Email: ssarnaik@wayne.med.edu
Dr. S. Sarnaik, Dir.
Activities/Fields: Sickle cell diseases, including clinical trials of new drugs, psychosocial research, and newborn screening and follow-up of infants with sickle cell diseases.

★ 24646 ★ Webb-Waring Institute for Cancer, Aging, and Antioxidant Research
Box C-321
4200 E 9th Ave.
Denver, CO 80262
Phone: (303)315-8231 **Fax:** (303)315-8541
Email: john.repine@uchsc.edu
Website: http://www.uchsc.edu/sm/waring/webpages/
John E. Repine, MD, Pres. /Dir. /CEO
Activities/Fields: Role of oxygen radicals in health and diseases, oxidants and antioxidants, air pollution, basic immunology, biochemistry, genetics, cell biology, pathology, and physiology. **Pub:** *Annual report.* Newsletter. **Frmly:** Webb-Waring Institute for Biomedical Research.

★ 24647 ★ West Virginia University Addiction and Psychiatric Medicine Research Center
RCB Health Sciences
PO Box 9135
Morgantown, WV 26505
Phone: (304)293-6988 **Fax:** (304)293-4693
Email: eglover@hsc.wvu.edu
Website: http://www.apmresearch.com
Elbert D. Glover, PhD, Dir.
Activities/Fields: Addictions, psychiatric conditions, obesity, diabetes. **Frmly:** Tobacco Research Center.

★ 24648 ★ West Virginia University Center for Health Ethics and Law
1195 Health Sciences N
Robert C. Byrd Health Sciences Center
PO Box 9022
Morgantown, WV 26506-9022
Phone: (304)293-7618 **Fax:** (304)293-7442
Email: amoss@hsc.wvu.edu
Website: http://www.hsc.wvu.edu/chel/
Alvin H. Moss, MD, Dir.
Activities/Fields: Health ethics and law.

★ 24649 ★ West Virginia University Center for Rural Emergency Medicine (CREM)
Robert C. Byrd Health Sciences Center
1299 Pineview Dr.
PO Box 9151
Morgantown, WV 26506-9151
Phone: (304)293-6682 **Fax:** (304)293-0265
Email: jwilliams@hfc.wvu.edu
Website: http://www.hsc.wvu.edu/som/crem/
Dr. Janet M. Williams, Dir.
Activities/Fields: Delivery and efficacy of emergency medical care in rural areas, including the etiologies and risk factors associated with emergency care visits and the reduction of morbidity and mortality in rural areas.

★ 24650 ★ West Virginia University Institute of Occupational and Environmental Health
3801 Health Sciences South
School of Medicine
PO Box 9190
Morgantown, WV 26506-9190
Phone: (304)293-3693 **Fax:** (304)293-2629
Email: cmartin@hsc.wvu.edu
Website: http://www.hsc.wvu.edu/ioeh
Edward Doyle, MD, Dir.
Activities/Fields: Occupational and environmental health, including occupational medicine and environmental toxicology. **Pub:** *Occupational Health.*

★ 24651 ★ West Virginia University Mary Babb Randolph Cancer Center
Health Science Center
PO Box 9300
Morgantown, WV 26506
Phone: (304)293-3528 **Fax:** (304)599-1552
Website: http://www.hsc.wvu.edu/mbrcc/
Eddie Reed, MD, Dir.
Activities/Fields: Cancer, especially among residents of West Virginia.

★ 24652 ★ West Virginia University Office of Health Services Research
Health Science Center
PO Box 9190
Morgantown, WV 26506-9190
Phone: (304)293-2601 **Fax:** (304)293-6685
Email: cpollard@hsc.wvu.edu
Cecil Pollard, Dir.

Activities/Fields: Health services research, manpower studies, resource allocation, demography, and computer technology support. **Pub:** *Newsletter*, quarterly.

★ 24653 ★ West Virginia University Prevention Research Center
Robert C. Byrd Health Sciences Center
PO Box 9190
Morgantown, WV 26506-9190
Phone: (304)293-8612 **Fax:** (304)293-8624
Email: gdino@hsc.wvu.edu
Geri A. Dino, PhD, Prin. Investigator

Activities/Fields: Public health issues, especially behaviors that place Americans at risk for chronic diseases and conditions. Of particular concern is the improvement in quality of life for special populations, including the young, elderly, racial ethnic populations, and the underserved.

★ 24654 ★ West Virginia University University Affiliated Center for Developmental Disabilities (UACDD)
955 Hartman Run Rd.
Morgantown, WV 26505
Phone: (304)293-4692 **Fax:** (304)293-7294
Email: adey@hsc.wvu.edu
Ashok S. Dey, Dir.

Activities/Fields: Developmental disabilities, mental retardation (all ages), nutrition, under nutrition, brain development, speech and language development, medical aspects of developmental disabilities, high-risk families, and program evaluation. Graduate research assistants come from various University disciplines to participate in applied research activities. **Pub:** *Quarterly Report.*

★ 24655 ★ West Virginia University West Virginia Poison Center
3110 MacCorkle Ave. SE
Charleston, WV 25304
Phone: (304)347-1212 **Fax:** (304)388-9560
Website: http://www.wvpoisoncenter.org
Elizabeth J. Scharman, Dir.

Activities/Fields: Demographics of poison victims and epidemiology of poisoning. Research is conducted in support of the Center's service program in poison prevention and management.

★ 24656 ★ Western Michigan University Occupational Therapy Teaching Research Clinic
Occupational Therapy Department
1000 Oakland Dr.
Kalamazoo, MI 49008
Phone: (269)387-7271
Email: berit.miller@wmich.edu
Berit Miller, Coord.

Activities/Fields: Occupational therapy and clinical research on developmental disabilities and learning disabilities.

★ 24657 ★ The Western Pennsylvania Hospital Foundation
4818 Liberty Ave.
Pittsburgh, PA 15224
Phone: (412)578-5153 **Fax:** (412)578-4428
Email: bbeisgen@wpahs.org
Website: http://trfn.clpgh.org/wphf/
Arlene Apfel Snyder, Pres.

Activities/Fields: Oncology, infertility, cardiology, genetics, geriatrics, pharmaceutical studies, and other health research. **Pub:** *Outcomes*, semiannually. Newsletter.

★ 24658 ★ Whitehead Institute for Biomedical Research
9 Cambridge Center
Cambridge, MA 02142-1479
Phone: (617)258-5000 **Fax:** (617)258-6294
Email: info@wi.mit.edu
Website: http://www.wi.mit.edu/home.html
Dr. Susan Lindquist, Dir.

Activities/Fields: Cancer, genomics, infectious disease, developmental and cell biology, structural biology, and molecular medicine. **Pub:** *BiologyWeek Newsletter*, weekly. • *Director's Report*, biennially. • *Discovery*, quarterly. • *Research summaries*, annually.

★ 24659 ★ Whittier Institute for Diabetes
9894 Genesee Ave., Ste. 316
La Jolla, CA 92037
Phone: (858)450-1280 **Fax:** (858)626-5680
Email: demichele.john@scrippshealth.org
Website: http://www.whittier.org
John Engle, Pres. /CEO

Activities/Fields: Diabetes and endocrinology research, including islet transplantation, CNS and pituitary function, reproductive biology, growth factor biochemistry, and angiogenesis.

★ 24660 ★ William T. Gossett Parkinson's Disease Center
Department of Neurology
Henry Ford Hospital
2799 W Grand Blvd.
Detroit, MI 48202
Phone: (313)916-7323 **Fax:** (313)916-3014
Email: gorell@neuro.hfh.edu
Jay M. Gorell, MD, Dir.

Activities/Fields: Parkinson's disease and its causes and treatments, including risk factors, cognitive and motor deficits, new medication trials, animal nerve cell investigations, and disordered brain chemistry measurements.

★ 24661 ★ Wills Eye Hospital Research Division
840 Walnut St.
Philadelphia, PA 19107
Phone: (215)928-1060
Email: ldonoson@hslc.org
Dr. Larry A. Donoso, Co-Dir.

Activities/Fields: Vitreoretinal surgery, and vitreoretinal disease management and research. Develops new instrumentation and surgical techniques and ocular application of various laser wavelengths in the various ophthalmic subspecialties in addition to vitreoretinal diseases.

★ 24662 ★ Windsor Regional Hospital Ozad Institute
3901 Connaught Ave.
Windsor, ON, Canada N9C 4H4
Phone: (519)257-5219 **Fax:** (519)257-5215
Email: ozad@wrh.on.ca
Website: http://www.wrchildrenscentre.org/ozadweb/ozadhome.html
John Strang, PhD, Dir.

Activities/Fields: Developmental disabilities in children, focusing on social learning neurodevelopmental disorders, differential diagnosis in neurodevelopmental disorders, outcomes in neurodevelopmental disorders. **Frmly:** Ozad Institute for Developmental Disabilities.

★ 24663 ★ The Wistar Institute
3601 Spruce St.
Philadelphia, PA 19104
Phone: (215)898-7325 **Fax:** (215)573-2097
Email: kaufman@wistar.upenn.edu
Website: http://www.wistar.upenn.edu
Russel Kaufman, MD, Dir. /CEO

Activities/Fields: Gene expression and regulation; immunology; and molecular and cellular oncogenesis. The institute has particular research strengths in the study of gene regulation and function; molecular structures; tumor biology; and mechanisms of inflamation, immunity, and autoimmunity, in addition to its long-standing expertise in virology and vaccine development. **Pub:** *Annual report magazine*, 3/year. **Frmly:** Wistar Institute of Anatomy and Biology.

★ 24664 ★ Wood Hudson Cancer Research Laboratory
931 Isabella St.
Newport, KY 41071-4701
Phone: (859)581-7249 **Fax:** (859)581-2392
Email: woodhdsn@iac.net
Website: http://woodhudson.org
Julia Carter, Pres.

Activities/Fields: Cancer, particularly the study of clinical cases and animal models to learn new methods for diagnosing and treating cancer and the study of environmental causes of cancer. **Pub:** *Abstracts, articles.* • *Newsletter.*

★ 24665 ★ World Life Research Institute
23000 Grand Terrace Rd.
Colton, CA 92324
Phone: (909)825-4773 **Fax:** (909)783-3477
Email: wlri@linklinc.com
Bruce W. Halstead, MD, Dir.

Activities/Fields: Toxicology, medical research, poisonous and venomous marine animals, drugs from the sea, chronic degenerative diseases, marine biotoxicology, and ethnobotany and terrestrial phytochemistry in a search for new drugs from natural resources, especially organic chemical agents derived from plants or animals having application to therapeutic medicine and human nutrition. Maintains extensive foreign contacts in 6,000 regions of the world, particularly underdeveloped areas in Asia and Latin America, in search of new drugs.

★ 24666 ★ World Research Foundation
41 Bell Rock Plz.
Sedona, AZ 86351-8804
Phone: (928)284-3300 **Fax:** (928)284-3530
Email: info@wrf.org
Website: http://www.wrf.org
Steven Ross, PhD, Pres.

Activities/Fields: Encourages and supports scientific research to evaluate the phenomenon of healing as it occurs beyond the boundaries of traditional medicine. Projects at major universities funded by the Center have included the following: the existence of a measurable healing energy, the healing potential of lucid dreaming, the positive effects of self-help groups for persons suffering from catastrophic illness, the therapeutic effects of meditation and imagery as stress reducing factors in elementary school children, suggestion and psychic healing in human surgical patients, good humor and good health, and behavioral approaches to reduce pain and nausea of cancer treatments. **Pub:** *Research Report Series.* • *Research Reporter*, quarterly.

★ 24667 ★ Wright State University Center for Healthy Communities (CHC)
Eugene W Kettering Center
140 E Monument Ave.
Dayton, OH 45402
Phone: (937)775-1114 **Fax:** (937)775-1110
Email: katherine.cauley@wright.edu
Website: http://www.med.wright.edu/CHC/
Kate Cauley, PhD, Dir.

Activities/Fields: Health care needs and problems. **Pub:** *Annual report.* • *Healthy Tomorrows Newsletter.* • *Journal articles.*

★ 24668 ★ Wright State University
Rehabilitation Research and Training Center on Drugs and Disability
Sch. of Medicine
PO Box 927
Dayton, OH 45401-0927
Phone: (937)775-1484 **Fax:** (937)775-1495
Email: sardi@wright.edu
Dennis Moore, EdD, Dir.
Activities/Fields: Substance abuse issues among individuals qualifying for vocational rehabilitation services. **Pub:** *Online newsletter*, 3/year.

★ 24669 ★ Yale University
Boyer Center for Molecular Medicine
School of Medicine
295 Congress Ave., Rm. 109
PO Box 9812
New Haven, CT 06536-0812
Phone: (203)737-2266 **Fax:** (203)737-2267
Email: vincent.marchesi@yale.edu
Website: http://www.info.med.yale.edu/bcmm/
Dr. Vincent Marchesi, Dir.
Activities/Fields: Molecular oncology and medicine, focusing on multicellular oncology and organisms.

★ 24670 ★ Yale University
Child Health Research Center
Department of Pediatrics
PO Box 208081
New Haven, CT 06520
Phone: (203)737-5970 **Fax:** (203)737-5972
Email: scott.rivkees@yale.edu
Scott Rivkees, MD, Dir.
Activities/Fields: Cellular and molecular biological studies of normal development and the ability of the fetus and child to adapt to environmental or genetic influences.

★ 24671 ★ Yale University
General Clinical Research Center—Adults
Yale New Haven Hospital, East Pavilion 10-5
20 York St.
New Haven, CT 06520-8076
Phone: (203)688-4106 **Fax:** (203)688-3100
Website: http://www.info.med.yale.edu/crc/gcrc/
Gerald I. Shulman, PhD, Dir.
Activities/Fields: Endocrinology, gastroenterology, mineral metabolism, oncology, psychology and pharmacology, respiratory psychology, and rheumatology.

★ 24672 ★ Yale University
General Clinical Research Center—Children
7-4 South Pavilion
Yale-New Haven Hospital
20 York St.
New Haven, CT 06504
Phone: (203)785-4648 **Fax:** (203)737-1998
Email: william.tamborlane@yale.edu
Website: http://info.med.yale.edu/crc/welcome.html
Dr. William V. Tamborlane, Jr., Dir.
Activities/Fields: Major areas of investigation include anesthesiology, cardiology, endocrinology, gastrointestinal disorders, genetic diseases, infectious diseases, mineral and bone metabolism, neonatology, neurology, psychiatry and pulmonary diseases.

★ 24673 ★ Yale University
Pediatric Cystic Fibrosis Research Center
Sch. of Medicine
333 Cedar St.
PO Box 208064
New Haven, CT 06520-8064
Phone: (203)785-2480 **Fax:** (203)785-6337
Email: regina.palazzo@yale.edu
Dr. Regina M. Palazzo, Dir.
Activities/Fields: Cystic fibrosis and related respiratory diseases of children, with special emphasis on control of respiration.

★ 24674 ★ Yale University
PVA/EPVA Center for Neuroscience and Regeneration Research
Medical Center, Bldg. 34, 127A
West Haven, CT 06516
Phone: (203)937-3802 **Fax:** (203)937-3801
Email: stephen_waxman@qm.yale.edu
Website: http://info.med.yale.edu/neurol/pva-epva-center
Dr. Stephen G. Waxman, Dir.
Activities/Fields: Basic mechanisms of central nervous system development, function, injury, and functional recovery with a major emphasis on spinal cord dysfunction. Concerns include molecular basis for neurological disorders, nerve cell growth and regeneration, pathophysiology of conduction in injured nerve fibers, regeneration of the central nervous system in mammalian species, and multiple sclerosis as a model for understanding how demyelinated nerve fibers regain their ability to effectively transmit electrical impulses. Areas of expertise of scientific staff include neurocytology, experimental neuropathology, immunology, developmental neuroscience, electrophysiology, biophysics, and molecular biology.

★ 24675 ★ Yale University
Ribicoff Research Facilities of the Connecticut Mental Health Center
34 Park St.
New Haven, CT 06508
Phone: (203)974-7726 **Fax:** (203)974-7724
Email: ronald.duman@yale.edu
Dr. Ronald S. Duman, Dir.
Activities/Fields: Preclinical and clinical studies of the neurobiological basis of severe mental disorders, including depression, anxiety, schizophrenia, and drug addiction. Conducts basic research programs in molecular, biochemical, neurophysiological, neuropharmacological, and behavioral fields. **Pub:** *Yale Psychiatry.*

★ 24676 ★ Yale University
Vision Research Center
Boardman Bldg., Box 208061
330 Cedar St.
PO Box 208061
New Haven, CT 06520-8061
Phone: (203)785-2405 **Fax:** (203)785-7401
Email: Nigel.Daw@yale.edu
Website: http://www.info.med.yale.edu/ophtha/
Nigel W. Daw, Dir.
Activities/Fields: Vision including studies on transduction, transport, myopia, neurobiology of growth and development, glaucoma, and diabetic retinopathy.

★ 24677 ★ Yale University
Yale Cancer Center
333 Cedar St.
PO Box 208028
New Haven, CT 06520-8028
Phone: (203)785-4095 **Fax:** (203)785-4116
Email: vincent.devita@yale.edu
Website: http://www.med.yale.edu/ycc
Dr. Vincent T. DeVita, Jr., Dir.
Activities/Fields: Cell biology, developmental therapeutics, immunology, molecular oncology and development, molecular virology, as well as cancer prevention and control, and cancer genetics. Clinical research programs include therapeutic radiology, ovarian cancer, stem cell biology and transplantation, genetic therapy, medical oncology, breast cancer, and lymphoma. Therapeutic clinical trials are conducted in various disease specific areas. **Pub:** *Cancer Connections.* • *Cancer Genetic Counseling Newsletter.* • *Caring Newsletter*, semiannually. • *Protocols.* • *Yale Cancer Center Referring Physicians Directory.*

★ 24678 ★ Yale University
Yale Liver Center
Department of Medicine
PO Box 208019
New Haven, CT 06520-8019
Phone: (203)785-5279 **Fax:** (203)785-7273
Email: James.boyer@yale.edu
Website: http://livercenter.yale.edu
James L. Boyer, MD, Dir.
Activities/Fields: Liver structure, function, and disease.

★ 24679 ★ Yale University
Yale University-Griffin Hospital Prevention Research Center
Department of Epidemiology & Public Health
School of Medicine
60 College St.
PO Box 208034
New Haven, CT 06520-8034
Phone: (203)785-2867 **Fax:** (203)785-6103
Email: michael.merson@yale.edu
Michael H. Merson, MD, Prin. Investigator
Activities/Fields: Public health issues, especially behaviors that place Americans at risk for chronic diseases and conditions. Of particular concern is the improvement in quality of life for special populations, including the young, elderly, racial ethnic populations, and the underserved.

★ 24680 ★ Yeshiva University
Analytical Imaging Facility
Albert Einstein College of Medicine
Resnick Campus
1300 Morris Park Ave.
Bronx, NY 10461
Phone: (718)430-3547 **Fax:** (718)430-8996
Email: macaluso@aecom.yu.edu
Website: http://www.aecom.yu.edu/aif/welcome.htm
Dr. John Condeelis, Sci. Dir.
Activities/Fields: Analytical imaging for medical studies.

★ 24681 ★ Yeshiva University
Diabetes Research and Training Center
Albert Einstein College of Medicine
1300 Morris Park Ave.
Bronx, NY 10461
Phone: (718)430-2908 **Fax:** (718)430-8557
Email: diabetes@aecom.yu.edu
Website: http://medicine.aecom.yu.edu/diabetes/DRTC.htm
Norman Fleischer, MD, Dir.
Activities/Fields: Development and assessment of interventions focused on both primary and secondary prevention of complications of diabetes. Evaluation of innovative health professional educational materials and research instruments. **Pub:** *Books, papers, education materials.*

★ 24682 ★ Yeshiva University
Institute of Communication Disorders
c/o Montefiore Medical Center
Department ENT, 3rd Fl., Green Pavillion
3400 Bainbridge Ave.
Bronx, NY 10467
Phone: (718)920-2484 **Fax:** (718)405-9014
Email: mfried@montefiore.org
Dr. Marvin Fried, Contact
Activities/Fields: Communicative disorders, including hearing, listening, voice, speech, and language studies; molecular developmental biology; molecular genetics; the synergy of culture and disease; morbidity; genetic studies; and genetics of communication disorders.

★ 24683 ★ Yeshiva University Preventive Intervention Research Center for Child Health
1400 Pelham Pky. S
Bronx, NY 10461
Phone: (718)918-4390 **Fax:** (718)918-5007
Jennifer Hagen, Dir.
Activities/Fields: Children with serious ongoing health problems (infancy through adolescence) and their families and the effect of parental illness on children. Activities include preventive interventions for children with asthma and HIV/AIDS, secondary analyses of large scale data sets on childhood disability, measurement development on chronic conditions, functional status and social support. Also studies the social support of minority mothers of chronically ill youngsters, epidemiology and consequences of serious ongoing health conditions, psychological and social adaptation among children with juvenile rheumatoid arthritis.

★ 24684 ★ Yeshiva University Rose F. Kennedy Center for Research in Mental Retardation and Developmental Disabilities
Albert Einstein College of Medicine
1410 Pelham Pky. S
Bronx, NY 10461
Phone: (718)430-2511 **Fax:** (718)430-8821
Email: dfaber@aecom.yu.edu
Dr. Donald S. Faber, Dir.
Activities/Fields: Mental retardation and other forms of aberrant human development, including biomedical, behavioral, educational, and social studies.

★ 24685 ★ Yeshiva University Sound View-Throgs Neck Community Mental Health Center
2527 Glebe Ave.
Bronx, NY 10461
Phone: (718)904-4400 **Fax:** (718)931-7307
Dr. Thomas Betzler, Exec. Dir.
Activities/Fields: Mental health, mental illness, and recovery from mental illness.

★ 24686 ★ York University Centre for Health Studies (YCHS)
Rm. 214 York Lanes
4700 Keele St.
Toronto, ON, Canada M3J 1P3
Phone: (416)736-5941 **Fax:** (416)736-5986
Email: ychs@yorku.ca
Website: http://www.yorku.ca/ychs/
Marcia Rioux, PhD, Dir.
Activities/Fields: Political economy of health; health policy, institutions and professions; women and health; culture, ethnicity and health; mental and physical fitness; and health and the environment. **Pub:** *Newsletter.*

★ 24687 ★ York University Centre for Vision Research
4700 Keele St.
Room 0009 CSB
North York, ON, Canada M3J 1P3
Phone: (416)736-5659 **Fax:** (416)736-5857
Email: manini@cvr.yorku.ca
Website: http://cvr.yorku.ca
Prof. John K. Tsotsos, Dir.
Activities/Fields: Human and animal vision using psychophysical, physiological and computational procedures, focusing on spatial vision as applied to work in aviation, medicine, and space research.

★ 24688 ★ Zero to Three/National Center for Infants, Toddlers and Families
2000 M St. NW, Ste. 200
Washington, DC 20036
Phone: (202)638-1144 **Fax:** (202)638-0851
Email: order@zerotothree.org
Website: http://www.zerotothree.org
Matthew E. Melmed, Exec. Dir.
Activities/Fields: Parent informational needs (conducted through survey and focus groups) and development of a diagnostic classification system for mental health and development disorders of infants and young children.

Chapter 17
Federal Government Research Agencies, Facilities & Programs

Entries below are arranged alphabetically by agency names. For additional information, consult the "User's Guide" located at the front of this directory.

★ 24689 ★ Consumer Product Safety Commission
Epidemiology and Health Sciences Directorate
4330 East-West Hwy.
Bethesda, MD 20814-4408
Phone: (301)504-0957 **Fax:** (301)504-0124
Website: http://www.cpsc.gov
Dr. Mary Ann Danello, Dir.
Activities/Fields: Determines exposure to hazardous chemicals from consumer products. This includes investigation of children's products; pollutant emissions (both chemical and biological) from structural materials, consumer products, and indoor combustion sources and their impact on indoor air quality; bioavailability and potential for consumer exposure to carcinogenic and other chemical hazard-containing commercial substances; and acute and chemical toxicity of various household products to determine proper precautionary and first aid labeling. Directorate is also responsible for implementation of the Poison Prevention Packaging Act with respect to hazardous household substances, including drugs; and processing requests for exemption from regulations under this Act. Also studies design and effectiveness of child resistant packaging and supports work on physiological modeling and other injury behavior.

★ 24690 ★ Consumer Product Safety Commission
Epidemiology and Health Sciences Directorate
Hazard Analysis Division
4330 East-West Hwy.
Bethesda, MD 20814
Phone: (301)504-0470 **Fax:** (301)504-0081
Email: rroegner@cpsc.gov
Website: http://cpsc.gov
Russ Roegner, PhD, Dir.
Activities/Fields: Analyses of product-related injury data to the Commission and other organizations to guide and support remedial strategy development and decision-making. As a part of this function, Division analysts and statisticians participate in the selection and planning of projects; develop guidelines for investigations and surveys and monitor their progress; compile and analyze data and information available from established Commission projects, other health and safety-oriented organizations, and computer searches of medical, scientific, and technical literature databases; prepare issue-oriented data summaries, reports, and memoranda describing the frequency and severity of injuries and major hazard patterns related to specific types of products; participate in oral briefings of the Commission on the nature and scope of injuries to be addressed by each remedial option considered; participate in the identification of injury reductions related to past Commission actions; and identify emerging hazards through continuous monitoring of injury trends. **Pub:** *Division's Hazard Analyses. • Special Reports.*

★ 24691 ★ Environmental Protection Agency
Office of Research and Development
Office of Health and Environmental Assessment
Human Health Assessment Group
Mail Code 6103
401 M St., SW
Washington, DC 20460
Fax: (202)260-9766
Robert Brenner, Dir.
Activities/Fields: Health assessments for carcinogens, genotoxic agents, and reproductive and developmental toxicants as encountered in environmental exposure scenarios. **Pub:** *Proceedings.*

★ 24692 ★ Independent Agencies
U.S. International Development Cooperation Agency
U.S. Agency for International Development
Bureau for Global Programs, Field Support and Research
((Center for Population, Health and Nutrition)
HIV/AIDS Division — HIV-AIDS)
USAID/G/PHN/HN/HIV-AIDS
Ronald Reagan Bldg.
Washington, DC 20523-1000
Phone: (202)712-4810 **Fax:** (202)216-3524
Website: http://www.usaid.gov/pop_health/aids/
Activities/Fields: Reducing "high risk" sexual behavior; treatment and control of sexually transmitted infections and disearse; and development of surveillance systems to more clearly understand the dynamics of transmission, the impact of the epidemics and the effect of the interventions designed to curtail them.

★ 24693 ★ Legislative, Judicial, and Executive Offices
National Science and Technology Council
Committee on International Science, Engineering, and Technology
Task Force on Emerging Infectious Diseases
Executive Secretariat
CISET Task Force on Emerging Infectious Diseases
2201 C St. NW
Washington, DC 20520
Website: http://www.state.gov/www/global/oes/health/task_force/index.html
Activities/Fields: Supports researchers and regional and international resources to focus on diagnostic reagents for low incidence diseases and identification of rare and unusual diseases. Provides research and training assistance to WHO and other organizations for establishment of guidelines for proper use of antimicrobial drugs and for development of new chemotherapeutic agents; promotes collaborations among U.S. agencies.

★ 24694 ★ National Aeronautics and Space Administration
George C. Marshall Space Flight Center
Space Sciences Laboratory
Space Plasma Physics
Mailcode ES83
Huntsville, AL 35812
Phone: (256)544-5339 **Fax:** (256)544-5244
Email: jim.spann@msfc.nasa.gov
Website: http://science.nasa.gov/ssl/pad/sppb/
James F. Spann, Jr., Contact
Activities/Fields: Physical processes that control the geospace plasma environment and its interaction with both banatural and man-made bodies in space. Emphases are on the plasma that originates in the ionosphere, and its heating in auroral light displays.

★ 24695 ★ National Science Foundation
Directorate for Biological Sciences
Division of Integrative Biology and Neuroscience
Developmental Neuroscience Program
4201 Wilson Blvd., Rm. 685
Arlington, VA 22230
Phone: (703)292-8423 **Fax:** (703)292-9153
Email: hvaessin@nsf.gov
Website: http://www.nsf.gov/bio/ibn/ibnneuro.htmde
Elizabeth B. Bell, Prog. and Tech. Anal.
Activities/Fields: Supports research on the factors that influence the formation, growth, and aging of the nervous system; how neurons and glia differentiate and regenerate; how connections between neurons are formed and maintained; and the interactions of environmental and genetic factors in neural development.

★ 24696 ★ National Science Foundation
Directorate for Biological Sciences
Division of Integrative Biology and Neuroscience
Neuroscience Program
4201 Wilson Blvd., Rm. 685
Arlington, VA 22230
Phone: (703)292-8420 **Fax:** (703)292-9153
Email: slim@nsf.gov
Dr. Soo Siang Lim, Prog. Dir.
Activities/Fields: Neuroscience.

★ 24697 ★ National Science Foundation (NSF)
Directorate for Biological Sciences (BIO)
Division of Molecular and Cellular Biosciences
Ecological and Evolutionary Physiology Program (EEP)
4201 Wilson Blvd.
Rm. 685
Arlington, VA 22230
Phone: (703)292-8421 **Fax:** (703)292-9153
Email: jhayes@nfs.gov

Website: http://www.nsf.gov/bio/ibn/ibnphysio.htmeep
Jack Hayes, Prog. Dir.

Activities/Fields: Ecological or evolutionary morphology, comparative physiology, physiological ecology, and biomechanics of plants, animals, protists, fungi and bacteria. **Frmly:** Regulatory Biology Program; Physiological Processes Program.

★ 24698 ★ National Science Foundation
Directorate for Biological Sciences
Division of Molecular and Cellular Biosciences
Microbial Genetics Program
4201 Wilson Blvd., Rm. 655
Arlington, VA 22230
Phone: (703)292-8439 **Fax:** (703)292-9061
Email: pdennis@nsf.gov
Website: http://www.nsf.gov/bio/mcb/mcbgenetics.htmmg
Patrick P. Dennis, Prog. Dir.

Activities/Fields: Supports research focused on the organization, function, transmission, mutation, regulation, and recombination of genetic information of microorganisms. Other topics supported include gene evolution, genetics of microbial interactions with eukaryotic organisms, and genetics of microbial plasmids and viruses.

★ 24699 ★ National Science Foundation
Directorate for Engineering
Division of Bioengineering and Environmental Systems
4201 Wilson Blvd., Rm. 565
Arlington, VA 22230
Phone: (703)292-7066 **Fax:** (703)292-9098
Email: bhamilton@nsf.gov
Website: http://www.eng.nsf.gov/bes
Bruce K. Hamilton, Div. Dir.

Activities/Fields: Critical engineering systems are those that are essential either because they significantly affect the economic viability and security needs of the nation, or because they are required for maintaining the public infrastructure. Major program areas include: biochemical and biomedical engineering; environmental engineering; research to aid people with disabilities. **Frmly:** (1993) Division of Biological and Environmental Systems; Division of Critical Engineering Systems.

★ 24700 ★ National Science Foundation
Directorate for Engineering
Division of Bioengineering and Environmental Systems
Biochemical Engineering Program
4201 Wilson Blvd., Rm. 565
Arlington, VA 22230
Phone: (703)292-8320 **Fax:** (703)292-9098
Email: fheineke@nsf.gov
Dr. Frederick Heineken, Prog. Dir.

Activities/Fields: Design and development of novel bioreactors, bioseparation systems, and the control of biochemical processes, as well as research aimed at improved utilization of biologically based resources. This includes support for programs in biochemical engineering fundamentals, biomass processing, and food process engineering.

★ 24701 ★ National Science Foundation
Directorate of Engineering
Division of Bioengineering and Environmental Systems
Bioengineering and Aiding Persons with Disabilities Program
4201 Wilson Blvd., Rm. 565
Arlington, VA 22230
Phone: (703)292-7943 **Fax:** (703)292-9098
Email: gdevey@nsf.gov
Gilbert Devey, Prog. Dir.

Activities/Fields: Provides funding for fundamental and applied academic engineering research relevant to medical needs. To qualify for support, investigations should be directed toward engineering research associated with the characterization, restoration, or substitution of human structure, function, or control. Emphasis is on fundamental and applied research with a potential to produce medical-engineering technologies, especially those that could become medically valuable within 10 years. (Normally this medical-oriented research should have such a strong engineering component that direct clinical input to its activities is not required; however, clinicians may supply data or specimens necessary to conduct the engineering effort.). **Frmly:** Bioengineering and Research to Aid the Handicapped Program.

★ 24702 ★ U.S. Department of the Air Force
Wilford Hall USAF Medical Center
Clinical Investigation Facility
ATTN: WHMC/MSR
1255 Wilford Hall Loop
Lackland AFB, TX 78236-5319
Phone: (210)292-7141 **Fax:** (210)292-6053
Email: willard.mollerstrom@lackland.af.mil
Col. Willard Mollerstrom, Comdr.

Activities/Fields: Medical research includes biological, behavioral, and psychological studies. Investigative efforts have contributed to improved disease prevention, diagnosis, and treatment modalities, including: advances in the application of hyperbaric oxygen therapy in a variety of conditions; better biochemical characterization of disease leading to enhanced understanding of underlying mechanisms in a spectrum of non-cancer diseases; improved procedures for cancer chemo-, immuno-, radiotherapy, and surgical techniques; pioneer development of extracorporeal membrane oxygenation, high frequency ventilation, and organ transplantation techniques; and selection of improved dental procedures through critical evaluation of safety and effectiveness.

★ 24703 ★ U.S. Department of Defense
Air Force Materiel Command
Armstrong Laboratory
Division of Biodynamics and Biocommunications
ATTN: AL/CFB
Wright Patterson AFB, OH 45433-7901
Fax: (513)255-2781

Activities/Fields: Conducts a multidisciplinary research and development program to protect man against mechanical force environments, provide him with the best protective equipment, and guarantee his full performance capability. The Division's program includes basic research, exploratory development, advanced development, and operational systems support in the areas of: noise, impact, acceleration, vibration, locomotion, microgravity, pilot performance, aircraft operations, communication effectiveness, aircrew protection, and emergency escape. Activities are carried out in these branches: Bioacoustics and Biocommunications, Vulnerability Assessment, Escape and Impact Protection, and Combined Stress.

★ 24704 ★ U.S. Department of Defense
Air Force Materiel Command
Armstrong Laboratory
Division of Human Engineering
2610 Seventh St., Bldg. 441
Wright Patterson AFB, OH 45433-7901
Phone: (937)255-5227 **Fax:** (937)656-7617
Email: ken.boff@wpafb.af.mil
Dr. Kenneth R. Boff, Chf. Scientist

Activities/Fields: Science and leading edge technology to define human capabilities, vulnerabilities, and effectiveness; train warriors; integrate operators and weapon systems; protect Air Force people; and sustain aerospace operations. **Pub:** *Proceedings.* • *Research Reports.*

★ 24705 ★ U.S. Department of Defense
Air Force Materiel Command
Human Systems Center
Air Force School of Aerospace Medicine
2601 Louis Bauer Dr.
USAFSAM
Brooks AFB Branch, TX 78235
Phone: (210)536-3500 **Fax:** (210)536-2216
Col. Laura Alvarado, Comdr.

Activities/Fields: Science and technology divisions (Clinical Sciences, Crew Technology, and Radiation Sciences); operational support; and aeromedical education and training divisions (Education, Epidemiology, and Hyperbaric Medicine). Technical and Veterinary Sciences provide support. Products and services provided by the USAFSAM impact the USAF in crew protection and performance enhancement; occupational, safety and health by making sure appropriate standards are followed to protect the work force; and medical readiness in combat casualty care and aeromedical evacuation. **Pub:** *Technical Reports.*

★ 24706 ★ U.S. Department of Defense
Army Medical Research and Materiel Command
504 Scott St.
Ft. Detrick
Frederick, MD 21702-5012
Phone: (301)619-7613 **Fax:** (301)619-2982
Brig.Gen. Russell Zajtchuk, Comdr.

Activities/Fields: Solving medical problems of military importance. The program, which is designed to maintain or restore the health of the individual soldier, involves: assessment, prevention, diagnosis, and treatment of infectious diseases that would hamper military operations; disease vector surveillance; combat casualty care and rapid return to duty of injured soldiers; management of maxillofacial injury; assessment and prevention of oral diseases; research in dental materials; studies on health hazards of military materiel; studies on factors limiting soldier effectiveness; medical countermeasures to chemical warfare agents, including pretreatment and antidote drugs, skin decontamination compounds and medical management of chemical casualities. Command has nine major research and development laboratories including Letterman Army Institute of Research; Aeromedical Research Laboratory; Biomedical Research and Development Laboratory; Institute of Dental Research; Institute of Surgical Research; Medical Research Institute of Chemical Defense; Medical Research Institute of Infectious Diseases; Medical Research Institute of Environmental Medicine; and Walter Reed Army Institute of Research. **Pub:** *Technical reports.*

★ 24707 ★ U.S. Department of Defense
Army Medical Research and Materiel Command
Army Aeromedical Research Laboratory
PO Box 620577
Fort Rucker, AL 36362-0577
Phone: (334)255-6907 **Fax:** (334)255-6067
Email: ssc@amedd.army.mil
Website: http://www.usaarl.army.mil
Col. Brian Campbell, Comdr., Contact

Activities/Fields: Health hazards of Army aviation, tactical combat vehicles, and selected weapon systems; assessing stress and fatigue in personnel operating these systems and developing countermeasures; and assisting in the development of criteria upon which to base standards for entry and retention in Army aviation specialties. Principal areas of interest include medical study of visual/auditory functions, man-machine integration, physiological responses to operational environments, impact of continuous operations on individual and crew performance, testing of aeromedical evacuation life support equipment, development of improved means of patient evacuation, and airworthiness.

★ 24708 ★ U.S. Department of Defense
Army Medical Research and Materiel Command
Army Institute of Surgical Research
Ft. Sam Houston, Bldg. 3611
3400 Rawley E Chambers Ave.
San Antonio, TX 78234-6315
Phone: (210)916-2720 **Fax:** (210)227-8502
Col. John B. Holcomb, Comdr. & Dir.

Activities/Fields: Investigation of problems of mechanical and thermal injuries; care of patients with such injuries; education and training of physicians and ancillary medical personnel in the principles of management of injured patients; and investigative studies at both the basic and clinical levels. Principal subject of research (basic and applied) is burn and trauma care, including studies in fluid resuscitation, host resistance, metabolic response, nutrition, leukocyte dysfunction, thyroid hormone kinetics, wound care, surgical infection, inhalation injury, surgical critical care, skin substitutes, and mechanical trauma. **Pub:** *USAISR Anniversary Symposia.* • *USAISR Annual Research Reports.*

★ 24709 ★ U.S. Department of Defense
Army Medical Research and Materiel Command
Army Medical Research Institute of Chemical Defense
Attn: MCMR-UV-RC
3100 Ricketts Point Rd.
Aberdeen Proving Ground, MD 21010-5400
Phone: (410)436-3628 **Fax:** (410)436-1960
Email: mricd.pao@apg.amedd.army.mil
Website: http://usamricd.apgea.army.mil
Col. James A. Romano, Comdr.

Activities/Fields: Medical defense of chemical warfare (CW). This includes basic research on mechanisms of action of CW agents and antidotes to establish a database from which to devise improved methods for the prevention, resuscitation, treatment, and management of chemical casualties; and assistance in the integration of products into the logistical system, doctrine development, and training of medical and nonmedical personnel in the management and prevention of chemical casualties. Basic research is conducted on neuronal, physiologic, and pharmacologic mechanisms of chemical warfare agents and pretreatment and treatment compounds. Applied research is directed toward the development of biomedical models; standardization of methods and procedures; pretreatment and treatment drug screening; biomedical data acquisition; analysis, prediction, and information transfer; toxicological and behavioral effects of sublethal doses of CW agents; tolerance to chronic CW agent exposure; toxicological effects of chemotherapeutics; safety and efficacy of pretreatment compounds; sensory effects of CW agents; vesicant treatment technology; soldier and patient decontamination technology; skin protection technology; skin toxicology; and management and treatment of mass chemical casualties. Research efforts are supplemented by a complementary research and development contract program and by collaboration with USAMRMC sister institutes, other government laboratories, universities, and research efforts with allied countries. **Pub:** *Bioscience review proceedings.* • *Historical Report*, annually. • *Proceedings.* • *Research Reports.*

★ 24710 ★ U.S. Department of Defense
Army Medical Research and Materiel Command
Army Medical Research Institute of Infectious Diseases
Ft. Detrick
1425 Porter St.
Frederick, MD 21702-5011
Phone: (301)619-2833 **Fax:** (301)619-4625
Email: usamriidweb@amedd.army.mil
Website: http://www.usamriid.army.mil
Col. Gerald W. Parker, Comdr.

Activities/Fields: USAMRIID develops vaccines, drugs and diagnostics to protect U.S. forces from biological warfare threats and endemic infectious diseases requiring special containment. The Institute also develops and conducts educational programs on medical management of builogical casualties, and maintains a world-class reference laboratory capability for identification of biological threat agents. While USAMRIID's primary focus in on protecting the military, its research has civilian applications as well. **Pub:** *Conference Proceedings.* • *Research Reports.*

★ 24711 ★ U.S. Department of Defense
Army Medical Research and Materiel Command
Army Research Institute of Environmental Medicine
Bldg. 42, Kansas St.
Natick, MA 01760-5007
Phone: (508)233-4811 **Fax:** (508)233-5298
Website: http://www.usariem.army.mil
Col. Marie Stephens, Contact

Activities/Fields: Effects of temperature, altitude, work, chemical defense, and military nutrition on the soldier's life processes, performance, and health; defining the complex interaction of environmental stress, the body's defenses, and the techniques, equipment, and procedures best calculated to protect the soldier and make the soldier operationally effective; assessing decrements to soldier performance caused by the synergy of environmental extremes and protective measures against chemical agents; and conducting research in the physiology and health effects of Army physical fitness training. In coordination with the U.S. Army Natick Research, Development, and Engineering Center, Institute conducts nutrition research for the Department of Defense Food and Nutrition Research, Development, Testing, and Engineering Program to develop feeding strategies for operational rations and supplements to minimize decrements in the soldier's performance under sustained combat conditions. USARIEM also assists the Natick center in the development of personal clothing and equipment by assessing the physiological impact of these items under all climatic conditions. In addition, Institute acts as a liaison with other federal agencies to develop the research technology base to discharge the Army Surgeon General's responsibilities as DoD executive agent for nutrition. USARIEM also provides technical advice and consultant services to Army commanders, installations, and activities in support of the Army Preventive Medicine Program and, on request, to other federal agencies.

★ 24712 ★ U.S. Department of Defense
Army Medical Research and Materiel Command
Army Research Institute of Environmental Medicine
Military Nutrition and Biochemistry Division
Natick, MA 01760-5007
Phone: (508)233-4194 **Fax:** (508)233-4869
Email: rfrancesconi@natick-ccmail.army.mil
Website: http://www.usariem.army.mil/nbd/milnut.htm
Ralph P. Francesconi, PhD, Chf.

Activities/Fields: Nutrition research, development, testing, evaluation, and engineering support to the Department of Defense Food and Nutrition Research, Development, Test, and Evaluation and Engineering Program; and provides technical assistance to the Surgeon General of the Army on biomedical aspects of nutrition and performance. **Pub:** *Proceedings.* • *Research Reports.*

★ 24713 ★ U.S. Department of Defense
Army Medical Research and Materiel Command
Army Research Institute of Environmental Medicine
Occupational Health and Performance Directorate
Bldg. 42
Natick, MA 01760-5007
Phone: (508)233-4800 **Fax:** (508)233-4195
Email: stephen.allison@na.amedd.army.mil
Dr. Stephen C. Allison, Dir.

Activities/Fields: Interactive effects of environment, nutrition, and the physiologic and psychologic demands of military operations on soldier health and performance. Objectives focus on the identification and quantification of military operational stressors, characterization of dose-response or energy-injury manifestation, development of attenuation or prevention measures, and development of predictive health and performance models. Research activities include: a program on epidemiologic field survey methods and models of environmental operational factors affecting soldier health and performance, designed to identify and relate environmental/operational stressors to soldier health and performance and develop predictive epidemiologic models for field validation; studies on the impact of the environment and sustained operations on military performance, which use military tasks involving specified psychomotor and cognitive skills in laboratory/field experiments to determine task components most influenced by environmental stressors; and assessment of the interactive effects of chemical defense factors and environmental stressors with animal/human performance models in order to evaluate independent and synergistic effects of environmental stressors and chemical defense factors (e.g., agents, antidotes, pretreatments) on performance parameters, determine dose-response relationships, develop attenuation/preventive measures of performance decrements, and develop and validate predictive models. **Frmly:** Occupational Health and Performance Division.

★ 24714 ★ U.S. Department of Defense
Army Medical Research and Materiel Command
Army Research Institute of Environmental Medicine
Thermal and Mountain Medicine Division
Kansas St. Bldg. 42
Natick, MA 01760-5007
Phone: (508)233-5665 **Fax:** (508)233-5298
Email: michael.sawka@na.amedd.army.mil
Dr. Michael Sawka, Dir.

Activities/Fields: Illnesses, injuries, and physiological performance effects associated with exposure to the environmental extremes of heat, cold, and high altitude.

★ 24715 ★ U.S. Department of Defense
Army Medical Research and Materiel Command
Walter Reed Army Institute of Research
Washington, DC 20307-5100
Phone: (202)782-3551 **Fax:** (202)782-3114
Col. E.T. Takafuji, Commander

Activities/Fields: Biologically-active substances such as bacteria, viruses, biological and chemical threat agents, and toxic environmental contaminants; trauma and high-energy (wound infections, traumatic organ failure, blood substitutes, laser injury, and high-power microwaves); and stress and performance (combat psychiatric casualties, and sustained operations). Maintains permanent subordinate laboratories in Thailand, Brazil, Kenya, and Germany. Maintains subordinate detachments collocated with Navy or Air Force at Brooks Air Force Base, TX; Wright Patterson Air Force Base, Dayton, OH; and Bethesda Naval Center, MD.

★ 24716 ★ U.S. Department of Defense Army Medical Research and Materiel Command
Walter Reed Army Institute of Research Biochemistry Division
Steven Sitter Ave.
Washington, DC 20307-5100
Phone: (202)782-3001 **Fax:** (202)782-6304
Website: http://wrair-www.army.mil/divisions.htm
Bhupendra P. Doctor, Dir.
Activities/Fields: Divisional components include the Departments of Biological Chemistry, Applied Biochemistry and Membrane Biochemistry. The Department of Biological Chemistry investigates the use of biological products, such as exogenous cholinesterases, and pharmaceutical products, such as huperzine, as pretreatment drugs for organophosphate exposure. Work also includes studies designed to elucidate the three-dimensional structure of the cholinesterases, the mechannisms of inhibition by reversible nonreversible inhibitors, and the reactivation of cholinesterases by oximes. The Department of Membrane Biochemistry develops liposomes and liposome-adjuvant formulatins, evaluating the immunogenicity of various liposome-adjuvant vaccine formulations, developing method for the manufacture of liposomal vaccines according to current Good Manufacturing Pratices (cGMP) of the U.S. Food and Drug Administration, and using the cGMP methods developed to manufacture liposomal vaccines for use in clinical trials.

★ 24717 ★ U.S. Department of Defense Army Medical Research and Materiel Command
Walter Reed Army Institute of Research Biometrics Division
Washington, DC 20307-5100
Phone: (202)782-3151 **Fax:** (202)782-6950
Lt.Col. John P. Litrio, Dir.
Activities/Fields: Provides automation, biomedical engineering, and biostatistics services and support to all elements of the Institute; manages the WRAIR automation program; and advises and provides consultative services on experimental design, data analysis, data processing, systems engineering, and data communications.

★ 24718 ★ U.S. Department of Defense Army Medical Research and Materiel Command
Walter Reed Army Institute of Research Communicable Diseases and Immunology Division
Bldg. 40, Rm. 2129
Washington, DC 20307-5100
Phone: (202)782-3561 **Fax:** (202)782-0748
Col. Charles H. Hoke, Jr., Dir.
Activities/Fields: Ecology, etiology, pathogenesis, diagnosis, prevention, and therapy of selected diseases of military importance and develop, validate, and apply methods of disease control through the use of immunizing agents (including studies of modification induced in the host by exposure to disease agents); develop methods of production (including actual emergency manufacture) and methods of assaying the biologicals required by the Armed Forces; and provide reference and consultative services on the diagnosis, epidemiology, control, and chemotherapy of infectious diseases of military importance. Divisional components include departments of Bacterial Diseases, Biologics Research, Enteric Infections, Entomology, Immunology, and Virus Disea ses.

★ 24719 ★ U.S. Department of Defense Army Medical Research and Materiel Command
Walter Reed Army Institute of Research Department of Applied Biochemistry
Silver Spring, MD 20910-7500
Phone: (301)319-9987 **Fax:** (301)319-9571
Email: richard.gordon@na.amedd.army.mil
Website: http://wrair-www.army.mil
Richard K. Gordon, PhD, Chf.
Activities/Fields: Develops novel drugs and treatments to treat military diseases or threats and to elucidate the attendant biochemical pharmacology. Focus areas include medical countermeasures for Botulinum Toxin; nerve agent countermeasures advanced anticonvulsants; medical countermeasures to decontaminate troops exposed to chemical warfare agents.

★ 24720 ★ U.S. Department of Defense Army Medical Research and Materiel Command
Walter Reed Army Institute of Research Division of Neurosciences
503 Robert Grant Ave.
Silver Spring, MD 20910
Phone: (301)319-9324 **Fax:** (301)319-9905
Email: michael.russo@na.amedd.army.mil
Lt. Col. Michael Russo, Dir.
Activities/Fields: Pertinent aspects of military medicine that involve the central nervous system. Research is performed to improve neuroprotection and treatment for combat casualty care, operational stress, infectious disease, and defense against biological and chemical threats.

★ 24721 ★ U.S. Department of Defense Army Medical Research and Materiel Command
Walter Reed Army Institute of Research Medical Audio-Visual Services Division
Washington, DC 20307-5100
Fax: (202)782-2136
Imre L. Toth, Dir.
Activities/Fields: Provides medical scientific illustration, medical research photography, motion picture production, and classroom/auditorium support meetings (held at WRAIR) for WRAIR research activities; serves as production agency for medical training films involving medical and/or paramedical subjects.

★ 24722 ★ U.S. Department of Defense Army Medical Research and Materiel Command
Walter Reed Army Institute of Research Medicine Division
Washington, DC 20307-5100
Fax: (202)782-0703
Col. Charles E. McQueen, Dir.
Activities/Fields: Resolving military medical problems that fall within the general domain of the disciplines of internal medicine through study, laboratory experiments, and consultation. Divisional components include departments of Clinical Physiology, Gastroenterology, Hematology, Medical Research Fellowship, Nephrology, and Respiratory Research. **Pub:** *Proceedings.* • *Research Reports.*

★ 24723 ★ U.S. Department of Defense Army Medical Research and Materiel Command
Walter Reed Army Institute of Research (WRAIR)
Preventive Medicine Division
503 Robert Grant Rd.
Silver Spring, MD 20910
Phone: (301)319-9600 **Fax:** (301)319-9104
Col. Patrick W. Kelley, Dir.
Activities/Fields: Plans, conducts, and coordinates graduate education programs in the field of military preventive medicine; assists in the production of technical information concerned with this specialty; and designs and conducts epidemiologic studies. Division also provides epidemiologic consultation services. Components of this Division are departments of Advanced Preventive Medicine Studies, Epidemiology, and Field Studies, the Accession Medical Standards Analysis and Research Activity, and the Department of Defense Global Emerging Infections System.

★ 24724 ★ U.S. Department of Defense Army Medical Research and Materiel Command
Walter Reed Army Institute of Research Surgery Division
503 Robert Grant Ave., Rm. 1A34
Silver Spring, MD 20910-7500
Phone: (301)319-9761 **Fax:** (301)319-9839
Email: frederick.pearce@na.amedd.army.mil
Website: http://wrair-www.army.mil
Frederick Pearce, PhD, Chf.
Activities/Fields: Military medical problems of combat injury, shock, wounding, and resuscitation (singly or in combination) in order to establish optimal prophylactic and therapeutic care of severely injured patients. Division also develops adjuncts for the diagnosis and management of blast-induced injury to the lung and/or gastrointestinal tract; and develops and provides laboratory models for biomedical assessment of medical material systems. Branch components include Physiology of Combat Trauma, and Field Biomedical Engineering. **Frmly:** (2000) Surgery Division.

★ 24725 ★ U.S. Department of Education National Institute on Disability and Rehabilitation Research
Southeastern Michigan Spinal Cord Injury System (SEMSCIS)
Rehabilitation Institute of Michigan
261 Mack Blvd.
Detroit, MI 48201
Phone: (313)745-9770 **Fax:** (313)966-7502
Email: mdijkers@med.wayne.edu
Dr. Marcel Dijkers, Co-Project Dir.
Activities/Fields: Spinal cord injuries, including rehabilitation for patients with such injuries, reduction of such injuries, and new treatments.

★ 24726 ★ U.S. Department of Energy Department of Energy Program Offices—Environment, Safety and Health
Office of Biological and Environmental Research
((Medical Sciences Division)
Structural Biology Research Program)
19901 Germantown Rd., SC-73
Germantown, MD 20874-1290
Phone: (301)903-9009
Email: roland.hirsch@science.doe.gov
Website: http://www.sc.doe.gov/production/ober/msd_struct_bio.html
Roland F. Hirsch, PhD, Prog. Mgr.
Activities/Fields: Structural biology techniques aimed at determining three-dimensional structure of important proteins, nucleic acids, and other biological materials.

★ 24727 ★ U.S. Department of Energy Department of Energy Program Offices—Environment, Safety and Health
Office of Biological and Environmental Research
((Medical Sciences Division)
Boron Neutron Capture Therapy)
19901 Germantown Rd., SC-73
Germantown, MD 20874-1290
Phone: (301)903-9106
Email: peter.kirchner@science.doe.gov
Website: http://www.sc.doe.gov/production/ober/msd_bnct.html
Peter Kirchner, MD, Prog. Mgr.
Activities/Fields: Experimental approach to cancer treatment based on a dual step technique utilizing two linked treatment components. **Pub:** *Reports.*

★ 24728 ★ U.S. Department of Energy
Department of Energy Program Offices—Environment, Safety and Health
Office of Biological and Environmental Research
((Medical Sciences Division)
Laser Medicine Research Program)
19901 Germantown Rd., SC-73
Germantown, MD 20874-1290
Phone: (301)903-3268
Email: dean.cole@science.doe.gov
Website: http://www.sc.doe.gov/production/ober/msd_laser.html
Dean A. Cole, PhD, Prog. Mgr.
Activities/Fields: Laser applications for non-invasive medicine.

★ 24729 ★ U.S. Department of Energy
Department of Energy Program Offices—Environment, Safety and Health
Office of Biological and Environmental Research
((Medical Sciences Division)
Radiopharmaceutical Development Research Program)
19901 Germantown Rd., SC-73
Germantown, MD 20874-1290
Phone: (301)903-4071
Email: prem.srivastava@science.doe.gov
Website: http://www.sc.doe.gov/production/ober/msd_rad_pharm.html
Prem C. Srivastava, Prog. Mgr.
Activities/Fields: Radiochemistry and radiolabeling synthesis for attaching radioisotopes to organic structures, including positron emission tomography (PET) research.

★ 24730 ★ U.S. Department of Energy
Department of Energy Program Offices—Environment, Safety and Health
Office of Biological and Environmental Research
((Medical Sciences Division)
Advanced Imaging Instrumentation Research Program)
19901 Germantown Rd., SC-73
Germantown, MD 20874-1290
Phone: (301)903-3268
Email: dean.cole@science.doe.gov
Website: http://www.sc.doe.gov/production/ober/msd_med_image.html
Dean A. Cole, Prog. Mgr.
Activities/Fields: PET, single photon emission computing tomograph, magnetic resonance imaging, and magnetoencephalography; study of neurochemical status of the brain in patients with neurodegenerative diseases, substance abuse, and for improved confidence in management of disease such as cancer (diagnosis, design and planning treatment, and monitoring course of therapy); strives to make nuclear imaging more compatible to current and advancing future molecular medicine needs such as imaging gene expression and monitoring gene therapy.

★ 24731 ★ U.S. Department of Energy
Department of Energy Program Offices—Environment, Safety and Health
Office of Biological and Environmental Research
((Medical Sciences Division)
Molecular Nuclear Medicine)
19901 Germantown Rd., SC-73
Germantown, MD 20874-1290
Phone: (301)903-4071
Email: prem.srivastava@science.doe.gov
Website: http://www.sc.doe.gov/production/ober/msd_mol_med.html
Prem C. Srivastava, PhD, Prog. Mgr.
Activities/Fields: Biochemical dysfunctions and the mechanisms of dysfunctions associated with pathological states including development of new radiotracer/radiopharmaceutical tools and advanced medical imaging technologies for identification and detection of biomedical dysfunctions as early signs of disease (including cancer, brain diseases, and mental disorders), for molecular correction of biochemical defect and the treatment of disease and disorder.

★ 24732 ★ U.S. Department of Energy
Department of Energy Program Offices—Fossil Energy
Office of Biological and Environmental Research
(Medical Sciences Division)
19901 Germantown Rd., SC-73
Germantown, MD 20874-1290
Phone: (301)903-3213 **Fax:** (301)903-0567
Email: michael.viola@science.doe.gov
Website: http://www.sc.doe.gov/production/ober/msd_top.html
Michael Viola, MD, Dir.
Activities/Fields: Strives to develop beneficial applications of nuclear and other energy-related technologies for medical diagnosis and treatment of patient's problems.

★ 24733 ★ U.S. Department of Energy
Department of Energy Program Offices—Nuclear Energy, Science and Technology
Office of Science
((Office of High Energy and Nuclear Physics)
Division of High Energy Physics)
SC-22 Germantown Bldg.
1000 Independence Ave., SW
Germantown, MD 20874
Phone: (301)903-3624 **Fax:** (301)903-2597
Email: Marsha.Marsden@science.doe.gov
Website: http://doe-hep.hep.net/home.html
Marsha Marsden, Contact
Activities/Fields: Continuing research and development in the study of elementary particle physics, understanding both the experimental and theoretical consequences of this research.

★ 24734 ★ U.S. Department of Energy
Department of Energy Program Offices—Nuclear Energy, Science and Technology
Office of Science
((Office of High Energy and Nuclear Physics)
Division of Nuclear Physics)
19901 Germantown Rd., SC-23
Germantown, MD 20874-1290
Phone: (301)903-3613 **Fax:** (301)903-3833
Email: dennis.kovar@science.doe.gov
Website: http://www.sc.doe.gov/production/henp/np/index.html
Dennis Kovar, Dir.
Activities/Fields: Understanding the fundamental forces and particles of nature as manifested in nuclear matter.

★ 24735 ★ U.S. Department of Health and Human Services
Administration for Children and Families
National Center on Child Abuse and Neglect
330 C St., SW
Washington, DC 20447
Phone: (703)385-7565 **Free:** 800-FYI-3366
Fax: (703)385-3206
Email: nccanch@calib.com
Website: http://www.calib.com/nccanch
Mary Sullivan, Proj. Dir.
Activities/Fields: Conducts research; collects, analyzes, and disseminates information; provides assistance to states and communities in developing programs and activities related to the prevention, identification, and treatment of child abuse and neglect; and coordinates Federal efforts to combat child maltreatment.

★ 24736 ★ U.S. Department of Health and Human Services
Agency for Health Care Policy and Research
Center for Outcomes and Effectiveness Research
6010 Executive Blvd., Ste. 300
Rockville, MD 20852
Phone: (301)594-1485 **Fax:** (301)594-3211
Email: hhubbard@ahrq.gov
Website: http://www.ahrq.gov
Heddy Hubbard, RN,MPH, Actg. Dir.
Activities/Fields: Awards grants and contracts for patient outcomes research and studies on practice variations, outcomes research methodologies, clinical economics, and other medical effectiveness research topics. Supports studies on translating research for practice, therapeutics, and health disparities.

★ 24737 ★ U.S. Department of Health and Human Services
Agency for Toxic Substances and Disease Registry
1600 Clifton Rd., NE
Mail Stop E-28
Atlanta, GA 30333
Phone: (404)498-0004 **Fax:** (404)498-0086
Email: RY52@cdc.gov
Website: http://www.atsdr.cdc.gov
Dr. Henry Falk, Asst. Admin.
Activities/Fields: Epidemiologic studies on human health effects related to hazardous substance exposure, emphasizing substance-specific research on priority hazardous substances. Comprises Division of Health Studies, Division of Toxicology, Division of Health Assessment and Consultation, and Division of Health Education. **Pub:** *Biennial Report.* • *Health assessments.* • *Proceedings.* • *Research reports.* • *Toxicological profiles.*

★ 24738 ★ U.S. Department of Health and Human Services
Agency for Toxic Substances and Disease Registry
Division of Health Studies
1600 Clifton Rd., NE
Mail Stop E-31
Atlanta, GA 30333
Phone: (404)498-0105 **Fax:** (404)498-0077
G. David Williamson, Dir.
Activities/Fields: Epidemiology and other human health studies, evaluating the relationship between exposure to hazardous substances at waste sites and adverse health effects. Conducts health studies, surveillance programs, and registries. Subsidiary branches include Health Investigations Branch, Epidemiology and Surveillance Branch, and Exposure and Disease Registry Branch. Maintains National Exposure Registry and Emergency Event Surveillance System databases.

★ 24739 ★ U.S. Department of Health and Human Services
Agency for Toxic Substances and Disease Registry
Division of Toxicology
1600 Clifton Rd., NE
Mail Stop E-29
Atlanta, GA 30333
Phone: (404)498-0160 **Fax:** (404)498-0094
Email: cderosa@cdc.gov
Dr. Christopher DeRosa, Dir.
Activities/Fields: Priority hazardous substances. Sets priorities for research, initiates programs, and

identifies data needs for publication of *Toxicological Profiles.* Comprises Research Analysis Branch.

★ 24740 ★ U.S. Department of Health and Human Services
Centers for Disease Control and Prevention
1600 Clifton Rd., NE
Atlanta, GA 30333
Phone: (404)639-3311 **Fax:** (404)639-7111
Email: netinfo@cdc.gov
Website: http://www.cdc.gov
Dr. David W. Fleming, MD, Actg. Dir.
Activities/Fields: Responsible for protecting the public health of the nation by preventing disease, disability, and premature death and promoting healthy lifestyles for all Americans. Specifically, CDC research focuses on the prevention of infectious diseases, chronic diseases, injury or disease associated with environmental, home, and workplace hazards, and controllable risk factors such as poor nutrition, smoking, lack of exercise, high blood pressure, and lack of appropriate immunizations. **Pub:** *Chronic Disease Notes and Reports. • Health United States. • Morbidity and Mortality Weekly Report series. • NCHS Monthly Vital Statistics Report. • Vital and Health Statistics series.*

★ 24741 ★ U.S. Department of Health and Human Services
Centers for Disease Control and Prevention
Antinuclear Antibody Reference Laboratory
1600 Clifton Rd. NE, Rm. 17-3040
Mailstop A-25
Atlanta, GA 30333
Phone: (404)639-2727 **Fax:** (404)639-2108
Email: mgb1@cdc.gov
Dr. J. Steven McDougal, Chf.
Activities/Fields: Collaborating scientists from the Arthritis Foundation and CDC have prepared for distribution eleven antisera to nuclear components useful in the diagnosis and classification of certain autoimmune diseases. These reference antisera have been used in approximately 1900 laboratories and can be obtained by writing to the ANA Reference Laboratory at the above address. The eleven antisera currently available are: Homogeneous Pattern Antinuclear Antibody (ANA) and anti-native DNA; Speckled ANA (anti-SSB/La); Speckled ANA; Anti-U-1 RNP; Anti-Sm; Anti-Nucleolar; Anti-SSA/RO; Anti-centromere; Anti-Scl-70; Anti-Jo-1; Anti-PM-Scl.

★ 24742 ★ U.S. Department of Health and Human Services
Centers for Disease Control and Prevention
Epidemiology Program Office
Bldg. 1, Rm. 5009
1600 Clifton Rd., NE
Atlanta, GA 30333
Phone: (404)639-3661 **Fax:** (404)639-4088
Email: sbtl@cdc.gov
Website: http://www.cdc.gov/epo/index.htm
Stephen B. Thacker, Dir.
Activities/Fields: Public health surveillance, epidemiologic training and research, and consultation in statistical and epidemiologic methods. **Pub:** *MMWR Annual Summary. • MMWR Surveillance Summaries. • Morbidity and Mortality Weekly Report. • Recommendations and Reports.*

★ 24743 ★ U.S. Department of Health and Human Services
Centers for Disease Control and Prevention
Epidemiology Program Office
Division of Prevention Research and Analytic Methods
4770 Buford Hwy.
M.S K-73
Atlanta, GA 30341
Phone: (770)488-8188 **Fax:** (770)488-8461
Email: rdixon1@cdc.gov
Dr. Richard E. Dixon, Dir.
Activities/Fields: Methods for assessing the effectiveness of prevention strategies.

★ 24744 ★ U.S. Department of Health and Human Services
Centers for Disease Control and Prevention
National Center for Environmental Health
4770 Buford Hwy. NE (MS F-29)
Chamblee, GA 30341-3724
Phone: (770)488-7000 **Fax:** (770)488-7015
Email: rxj4@cdc.gov
Website: http://www.cdc.gov/nceh/default.htm
Richard J. Jackson, MD, Dir.
Activities/Fields: Administers national programs that promote a healthy environment and prevent premature death and avoidable illness and disability caused by non-infectious, non-occupational, environmental, and related factors. The Center is to be reorganized into divisions on Birth Defects and Pediatric Genetics, Childhood Development Disabilities and Health Environmental Hazards and Health Effects, and Laboratory Sciences.

★ 24745 ★ U.S. Department of Health and Human Services
Centers for Disease Control and Prevention
National Centers for Prevention Services
National Immunization Program
Mail Stop E-05
CDC NIP 1600 Clifton Rd, NE
Atlanta, GA 30333
Phone: (404)639-8200 **Fax:** (404)639-8626
Email: wa01@CDC.GOV
Website: http://www.nip.cdc.gov
Dr. Walter A. Orenstein, Dir.
Activities/Fields: Vaccine-preventable disease control.

★ 24746 ★ U.S. Department of Health and Human Services
Centers for Disease Control and Prevention
National Institute for Occupational Safety and Health
Division of Respiratory Disease Studies
1095 Willowdale Rd.
Morgantown, WV 26505
Phone: (304)285-5749 **Free:** 800-356-4676
Fax: (304)285-5861
Website: http://www.cdc.gov/niosh/im-drds.html
Gregory Wagner, MD, Dir.
Activities/Fields: Identification, evaluation, and prevention of occupational respiratory diseases, such as asthma, chronic obstructive pulmonary disease, and pneumoconiosis. Administers legislatively mandated medical services for coal miners; tests, evaluates, certifies, monitors, and conducts research on the quality of respiratory protective devices. **Pub:** *Reports.*

★ 24747 ★ U.S. Department of Health and Human Services
Centers for Disease Control and Prevention
National Institute for Occupational Safety and Health
Division of Safety Research
1095 Willowdale Rd.
Morgantown, WV 26505-2888
Phone: (304)285-5894 **Free:** 800-356-4676
Website: http://www.cdc.gov/niosh/im-dsr.html
Nancy Stout, EdD, Dir.
Activities/Fields: Occupational injury. Programs are organized around the public health approach to occupational injury prevention, including surveillance, analytic epidemiology, safety and human factors engineering, and health communication.

★ 24748 ★ U.S. Department of Health and Human Services
Centers for Disease Control and Prevention
National Institute for Occupational Safety and Health
Health Effects Laboratory Division
1095 Willowdale Rd.
Morgantown, WV 26505
Phone: (304)285-6121 **Free:** 800-356-4676
Website: http://www.cdc.gov/niosh/im-held.html
Albert E. Munson, PhD, Dir.
Activities/Fields: Workplace health and safety. Research involves causes, mechanisms, prevention and control of adverse health effects from workplace hazards, including ergonomics and toxins.

★ 24749 ★ U.S. Department of Health and Human Services
Centers for Disease Control and Prevention
National Institute for Occupational Safety and Health
National Occupational Research Agenda (Surveillance Research Methods)
Surveillance Branch
4676 Columbia Pkwy.
Cincinnati, OH 45226
Phone: (513)841-4303 **Free:** 800-356-4676
Fax: (513)841-4489
Email: jps4@cdc.gov
Website: http://www.cdc.gov/niosh/nrsurv.html
John P. Sestito, Team Ldr.
Activities/Fields: Surveillance systems, which describe where occupational injuries or illnesses are occurring, how frequent they are, whether they are increasing or decreasing, and whether prevention methods have been effective. **Pub:** *Papers, charts.*

★ 24750 ★ U.S. Department of Health and Human Services
Centers for Disease Control and Prevention
National Institute for Occupational Safety and Health
National Occupational Research Agenda (Traumatic Injuries)
Division of Safety Research
1095 Willowdale Rd.
Morgantown, WV 26505
Phone: (304)285-5894 **Free:** 800-356-4676
Fax: (304)285-6046
Email: nas5@cdc.gov
Website: http://www.cdc.gov/niosh/nrtram.html
Nancy Stout, EdD, Ch.
Activities/Fields: Reducing the incidence and toll of traumatic injuries at work through research and collaboration. **Pub:** *Reports.*

★ 24751 ★ U.S. Department of Health and Human Services
Centers for Disease Control and Prevention
National Institute for Occupational Safety and Health
National Occupational Research Agenda (Social and Economic Consequences of Workplace Illness and Injury)
1095 Willowdale Rd.
Morgantown, WV 26501
Phone: (304)285-6015 **Free:** 800-356-4676
Email: egb6@cdc.gov
Website: http://www.cdc.gov/niosh/nrsoce.html
Elyce Biddle, Contact
Activities/Fields: Social and economic consequences of workplace illness and injury.

★ 24752 ★ U.S. Department of Health and Human Services
Centers for Disease Control and Prevention
National Institute for Occupational Safety and Health
National Occupational Research Agenda (Special Populations at Risk)
4676 Columbia Pkwy.
Cincinnati, OH 45226
Phone: (513)458-7159 **Free:** 800-356-4676
Email: slb8@cdc.gov
Website: http://www.cdc.gov/niosh/nrspop.html
Sherry Baron, Team Ldr.
Activities/Fields: Special populations of workers, overlooked in the past, who may be at risk of injury and illness in the workplace. These populations are defined by biologic, social, and/or economic characteristics, including: age, gender, race, genetic susceptibility, disability, education, language, literacy, culture, lifestyle/lifework, low income, nationality, citizenship, and political vulnerability. **Pub:** *Reports.*

★ 24753 ★ U.S. Department of Health and Human Services
Centers for Disease Control and Prevention
National Institute for Occupational Safety and Health
National Occupational Research Agenda (Risk Assessment Methods)
Risk Evaluation Branch
4676 Columbia Pkwy., C15
Cincinnati, OH 45226
Phone: (513)533-8365 **Free:** 800-356-4676
Fax: (513)533-8224
Email: lts2@cdc.gov
Website: http://www.cdc.gov/niosh/nrram.html
Leslie Stayner, PhD, Team Ldr.
Activities/Fields: To promote the development of new methods that will improve ability to accurately predict the risks associated with occupational exposure, which will facilitate the development of policies to protect workers.

★ 24754 ★ U.S. Department of Health and Human Services
Centers for Disease Control and Prevention
National Institute for Occupational Safety and Health
National Occupational Research Agenda (Low Back Disorders)
MS R-12
4676 Columbia Pkwy.
Cincinnati, OH 45226
Phone: (513)841-4428 **Free:** 800-356-4676
Email: Twaters@cdc.gov
Website: http://www.cdc.gov/niosh/nrlowbck.html
Thomas R. Waters, Team Ldr.
Activities/Fields: Identify work activities and awkward postures that contribute to the causes of low back disorders.

★ 24755 ★ U.S. Department of Health and Human Services
Centers for Disease Control and Prevention
National Institute for Occupational Safety and Health
National Occupational Research Agenda (Organization of Work)
4676 Columbia Pkwy.
Cincinnati, OH 45226
Phone: (513)533-8383 **Free:** 800-356-4676
Email: sls4@cdc.gov
Website: http://www.cdc.gov/niosh/nrworg.html
Steven L. Sauter, Team Ldr.
Activities/Fields: Organization of work refers to the way work processes are structured and managed. In addition to job stress associated with aspects of work organization, studies are now identifying its contributions to other diverse health problems, including musculoskeletal disorders and cardiovascular diseases. Research areas include: surveillance, and etiologic studies of risk factors and intervention strategies to mitigate adverse work organization factors and outcomes.

★ 24756 ★ U.S. Department of Health and Human Services
Centers for Disease Control and Prevention
National Institute for Occupational Safety and Health
National Occupational Research Agenda (Musculoskeletal Disorders of the Upper Extremities)
MS R-12
4676 Columbia Pkwy.
Cincinnati, OH 45226
Phone: (513)841-4428 **Free:** 800-356-4676
Email: Twaters@cdc.gov
Website: http://www.cdc.gov/niosh/nrmusc.html
Thomas R. Waters, MD, Dir.
Activities/Fields: Work-related musculoskeletal disorders (MSD), such as low back pain, tendonitis, hand-arm vibration syndrome, and carpel tunnel syndrome.

★ 24757 ★ U.S. Department of Health and Human Services
Centers for Disease Control and Prevention
National Institute for Occupational Safety and Health
National Occupational Research Agenda (Infectious Diseases)
1095 Willowdale Rd.
Morgantown, WV 26505
Phone: (304)285-5943 **Free:** 800-356-4676
Email: dqw4@cdc.gov
Website: http://www.cdc.gov/niosh/nrinfc.html
David Weissman, MD, Team Ldr.
Activities/Fields: Research to determine the extent of occupational transmission of infectious diseases, to understand the barriers to the use of safe work practices and vaccines, and develop and evaluate new control methods.

★ 24758 ★ U.S. Department of Health and Human Services
Centers for Disease Control and Prevention
National Institute for Occupational Safety and Health
National Occupational Research Agenda (Intervention Effectiveness Research)
4686 Columbia Pkwy.
Cincinnati, OH 45226
Phone: (513)841-4493 **Free:** 800-356-4676
Email: RSinclair@cdc.gov
Website: http://www.cdc.gov/niosh/nriefr.html
Raymond Sinclair, Team Ldr.
Activities/Fields: Occupational disease and injury intervention, including safety and health training programs; health communications; changes in work environment or practices; control technologies (e.g., engineering techniques, recommending the use of protective equipment, and specific work practices); and regulatory and voluntary safety and health standards. **Pub:** *Evaluation Manual for Occupational Health & Safety Professionals.*

★ 24759 ★ U.S. Department of Health and Human Services
Centers for Disease Control and Prevention
National Institute for Occupational Safety and Health
National Occupational Research Agenda (Indoor Environment)
4676 Columbia Pkwy., R-16
Cincinnati, OH 45226
Phone: (513)841-4445 **Free:** 800-356-4676
Fax: (513)841-4486
Email: mfm0@cdc.gov
Website: http://www.cdc.gov/niosh/nrinev.html
Mark J. Mendell, PhD, Contact
Activities/Fields: Non-industrial workplace safety and health, including allergic and infectious diseases to non-specific symptoms such as headaches and eye irritation. **Pub:** *Articles.*

★ 24760 ★ U.S. Department of Health and Human Services
Centers for Disease Control and Prevention
National Institute for Occupational Safety and Health
National Occupational Research Agenda (Health Services Research)
Centers for Disease Control & Prevention
1600 Clifton Rd. NE, D40
Atlanta, GA 30333
Phone: (404)639-1534 **Free:** 800-356-4676
Fax: (404)639-2170
Email: sed2@cdc.gov
Website: http://www2.cdc.gov/NORA/noratopictemp.asp?rscharea=hsr
Scott Deitchman, MD, Dep. Dir.
Activities/Fields: Identify priority topics for occupational health services; identify priority topics to develop tools and methodology for occupational health services research; promote the study of occupational health to researchers in the field; and disseminate the results of occupational health services research in order to improve occupational health care. **Pub:** *Papers.*

★ 24761 ★ U.S. Department of Health and Human Services
Centers for Disease Control and Prevention
National Institute for Occupational Safety and Health
National Occupational Research Agenda (Hearing Loss)
Robert A. Taft Laboratories
4576 Columbia Pkwy., MS C-27
Cincinnati, OH 45226
Phone: (513)533-8482 **Free:** 800-356-4676
Fax: (513)533-8139
Email: jrf3@cdc.gov
Website: http://www.cdc.gov/niosh/nrhear.html
John R. Franks, PhD, Team Ldr.
Activities/Fields: Occupational hearing loss as a result of chronic exposure to ototraumatic (damaging to the ear or hearing process) agents, including noise, solvents, metals, asphyxiants (e.g. carbon monoxide), and heat. **Pub:** *Papers.*

★ 24762 ★ U.S. Department of Health and Human Services
Centers for Disease Control and Prevention
National Institute for Occupational Safety and Health
National Occupational Research Agenda (Exposure Assessment Methods Research)
4676 Columbia Pkwy.
Cincinnati, OH 45226
Phone: (513)533-8465 **Free:** 800-356-4676
Email: mlw2@cdc.gov
Website: http://www.cdc.gov/niosh/nrexpo.html
Mary Lynn Woebkenberg, Team Ldr.
Activities/Fields: Reduction of workplace exposures. Research includes defining exposure-response relationships in epidemiologic studies in order to better identify at-risk workers, develop cost-effective control and intervention strategies and improved baseline data for standard setting and risk management.

★ 24763 ★ U.S. Department of Health and Human Services
Centers for Disease Control and Prevention
National Institute for Occupational Safety and Health
National Occupational Research Agenda (Fertility and Pregnancy Abnormalities)
4676 Columbia Pkwy.
Cincinnati, OH 45226
Free: 800-356-4676
Email: ths1@cdc.gov
Website: http://www.cdc.gov/niosh/nrpreg.html
Teresa Schnorr, Contact
Activities/Fields: Physical and biological agents in the workplace that may affect fertility and pregnancy outcomes.

★ 24764 ★ U.S. Department of Health and Human Services
Centers for Disease Control and Prevention
National Institute for Occupational Safety and Health
National Occupational Research Agenda (Control Technology and Personal Protective Equipment)
Engineering Control Technology Branch
Division of Physical Sciences & Engineering
MS-R5
4676 Columbia Pkwy.
Cincinnati, OH 45226
Phone: (513)841-4221 **Free:** 800-356-4676
Fax: (513)841-4506
Email: ler3@cdc.gov
Website: http://www.cdc.gov/niosh/nrppe.html
Larry Reed, Team Ldr.
Activities/Fields: Reduction of worker exposures to occupational hazards by various methods, including design changes to equipment, modifications to training efforts, or the use of personal protective equipment.

★ 24765 ★ U.S. Department of Health and Human Services
Centers for Disease Control and Prevention
National Institute for Occupational Safety and Health
National Occupational Research Agenda (Occupational Asthma and Chronic Obstructive Pulmonary Disease)
NIOSH Field Studies Branch
H2800
1095 Willowdale Rd.
Morgantown, WV 26505
Phone: (304)285-5751 **Free:** 800-356-4676
Email: pkh0@cdc.gov
Paul Henneberger, PhD, Team Ldr.
Activities/Fields: Clarify the prevalence, risk factors, and exposure-disease relationships to occupationally-related airway diseases, including asthma and chronic obstructive disease (COPD); to refine techniques for monitoring worker health and the job environment; and to develop effective and practical means for preventing work-related airway diseases in at-risk workers. **Pub:** *Papers.*

★ 24766 ★ U.S. Department of Health and Human Services
Centers for Disease Control and Prevention
National Institute for Occupational Safety and Health
National Occupational Research Agenda (Cancer Research Methods)
NIOSH 4676
Columbia Pkwy. (C-14)
Cincinnati, OH 45226
Phone: (513)533-8481 **Free:** 800-356-4676
Fax: (513)533-8588
Email: pas4@cdc.gov
Website: http://www.cdc.gov/niosh/nrcanc.html
Paul A. Schulte, PhD, Team Ldr.
Activities/Fields: Prevention of occupational cancer by identifying exposures that have carcinogenic potential and eliminate or reduce their presence in the workplace.

★ 24767 ★ U.S. Department of Health and Human Services
Centers for Disease Control and Prevention
National Institute for Occupational Safety and Health
National Occupational Research Agenda (Allergic and Irritant Dermatitis)
PO Box 538707
Cincinnati, OH 45253
Phone: (513)841-4503 **Free:** 800-356-4676
Fax: (513)841-4483
Email: bdtl@cdc.gov
Website: http://www.cdc.gov/niosh/nrderm.html
Boris Lushniak, Med. Officer
Activities/Fields: Identify the prevalence, causes, exposure assessment methods, and early biologic markers of occupational skin diseases.

★ 24768 ★ U.S. Department of Health and Human Services
Centers for Disease Control and Prevention
National Institute for Occupational Safety and Health
National Occupational Research Agenda
Hubert H. Humphrey Bldg.
200 Independence Ave. SW, Rm. 715H
Washington, DC 20201
Phone: (202)401-6977 **Free:** 800-356-4676
Website: http://www.cdc.gov/niosh/nora
John Howard, Dir.
Activities/Fields: Occupational safety and health. **Pub:** *NORA News.*

★ 24769 ★ U.S. Department of Health and Human Services
Centers for Disease Control and Prevention—National Institute for Occupational Safety and Health
National Farm Medicine Center
Midwest Center for Agricultural Disease and Injury Research, Education, and Prevention
1000 N Oak Ave.
Marshfield, WI 54449-5790
Free: 800-662-6900 **Fax:** (715)389-3808
Email: nfmcsh@mfldclin.edu
Website: http://www.marshfieldclinic.org/nfmc/projects/default.htm
Dr. Anne Greenlee, Prin. Investigator
Activities/Fields: Investigating agricultural exposures, host susceptibility factors and risk of parkinson's disease; agromedicine training programs; safety education and prevention/intervention programs promoting sustained health of agricultural workers and families.

★ 24770 ★ U.S. Department of Health and Human Services
Food and Drug Administration
Rm. 1471
5600 Fishers Ln.
Rockville, MD 20857
Phone: (301)827-2410 **Fax:** (301)443-3100
Email: crawford@oc.fda.gov
Website: http://www.fda.gov
Lester Crawford, DVM, Dep. Commnr.
Activities/Fields: Public health of the nation as it may be impaired by foods, drugs, biological products, cosmetics, medical devices, ionizing and nonionizing radiation-emitting products and substances, poisons, pesticides, and food additives. FDA's functions are to ensure that: foods are safe, pure, and wholesome; drugs, medical devices, and biological products are safe and effective; cosmetics are harmless; that all of the above are honestly and informatively packaged; and that exposure to potentially injurious radiation is minimized. The principal components of FDA are: the Center for Biologics Evaluation and Research; Center for Devices and Radiological Health; Center for Drug Evaluation and Research; Center for Food Safety and Applied Nutrition; Center for Veterinary Medicine; the National Center for Toxicological Research; and the Office of Regulatory Affairs, which directs FDA's field operations. Research activities are also carried out in field laboratories and research centers located throughout the country–see entries that follow under FDA Regional Research Centers.

★ 24771 ★ U.S. Department of Health and Human Services
Food and Drug Administration
Center for Bilogics Evaluation and Research
Division of Bacterial Products
1401 Rockville Pike (HFM-422)
Bethesda, MD 20892
Phone: (301)496-1014 **Fax:** (301)402-2776
Dr. Richard Walker, MD, Dir.

Activities/Fields: Pathogenesis and prevention of medically important diseases due to bacteria and rickettsia. Emphasizes control of vaccines and immunotherapeutics. Conducts studies through the following laboratories: Mycobacteria, Pertussis, Enterics & Sexually Transmitted Diseases, Bacterial Polysaccharides, and Bacterial Toxins. **Pub:** *Annual Report.*

★ 24772 ★ U.S. Department of Health and Human Services
Food and Drug Administration
Center for Bilogics Evaluation and Research
Division of Cellular and Gene Therapies
1401 Rockville Pike, HFM-515
Rockville, MD 20852
Phone: (301)827-0680 **Fax:** (301)827-0449
Website: http://www.fda.gov/cber/research/dcgt.htm
Philip D. Noguchi, MD, Actg. Dir.
Activities/Fields: Cell and developmental biology, immunology, and tumor biology.

★ 24773 ★ U.S. Department of Health and Human Services
Food and Drug Administration
Center for Bilogics Evaluation and Research
Laboratory Cellular Immunology (Division of Cellular and Gene Therapies)
HFM 725 1401 Rockville Pike
Rockville, MD 20852-1448
Phone: (301)827-0452 **Fax:** (301)827-0449
Eda Bloom, PhD, Lab. Chf.
Activities/Fields: Regulation of lymphocyte activation and maturation at cellular and molecular levels, with emphasis on cytotoxic lymphocytes; roles of cytokines and cytokine-producing cells (lymphocytes and macrophages) in lymphocyte activation using models in vitro and invivo. **Pub:** *Proceedings.* • *Research Reports.*

★ 24774 ★ U.S. Department of Health and Human Services
Food and Drug Administration
Center for Bilogics Evaluation and Research
Laboratory of Hemostasis
1401 Rockville Pike, HFM 340
Rockville, MD 20852
Phone: (301)496-4833 **Fax:** (301)402-2780
Dr. Basil Goldstein, PhD, Actg. Chf.
Activities/Fields: Characterization of proteins involved in hemostasis and thrombosis. Biochemical research includes receptor and binding studies, and analysis of protein structure and function. Principal research efforts include studies on factor VIII and von Willebrand factor.

★ 24775 ★ U.S. Department of Health and Human Services
Food and Drug Administration
Center for Biologics Evaluation and Research
1401 Rockville Pike
Rockville, MD 20852
Phone: (301)827-0370 **Fax:** (301)827-0440
Website: http://www.fda.gov/cber
Kathryn C. Zoon, Dir.
Activities/Fields: Ensures the safety, efficacy, potency, and purity of biological products intended for use in the treatment, prevention, or cure of human diseases. Reviews the safety and effectiveness of vaccines, blood products, diagnostic products, and other biological and biotechnology-derived human products. Supports active applied research programs and provides regulatory review of biological products. Investigates viral and bacterial vaccines, immunology, developmental biology, parasitic diseases, cytokines, growth factors, and AIDS and related diseases.

★ 24776 ★ U.S. Department of Health and Human Services
Food and Drug Administration
Center for Biologics Evaluation and Research
Bone Marrow Growth Factors Staff
9000 Rockville Pike
Bldg. 37, Rm. 5C25
Bethesda, MD 20892
Phone: (301)496-6968 **Fax:** (301)480-3256
Dov H. Pluznik, PhD, Actg. Chf.
Activities/Fields: Cellular and molecular mechanisms involved in the production of hematopoietic growth factors and the differentiation of hematopoietic cells.

★ 24777 ★ U.S. Department of Health and Human Services
Food and Drug Administration
Center for Biologics Evaluation and Research
Division of Allergenic Products and Parasitology
1401 Rockville Pike
CBER HFM-410
Rockville, MD 20852
Phone: (301)496-2893 **Fax:** (301)496-4684
Email: tebull@gandalf.cber.nih.gov
Dr. Thomas Bull, Research Chemist
Activities/Fields: Biophysics, NMR, and molecular dynamics simulations. **Pub:** *Annual report.* **Frmly:** (1993) Division of Biochemistry and Biophysics.

★ 24778 ★ U.S. Department of Health and Human Services
Food and Drug Administration
Center for Biologics Evaluation and Research
Division of Cytokine Biology
1401 Rockville Pike
Rockville, MD 20852
Phone: (301)827-1735 **Fax:** (301)402-1659
Dr. David Finbloom, Dir.
Activities/Fields: Cytokine and growth factor products. Studies interferons, interleukins, colony stimulating factors; and growth factors. Emphasizes immunology, molecular biology, protein chemistry, and AIDS. Activities are carried out through the following Laboratories: Cell Biology, Chemical Biology, and Cytokine Research. **Pub:** *Annual Report.* • *Proceedings.* • *Reports.*

★ 24779 ★ U.S. Department of Health and Human Services
Food and Drug Administration
Center for Biologics Evaluation and Research
Division of Hematology (Laboratory of Plasma Derivatives)
1401 Rockville Pike, HFM 345
Rockville, MD 20852
Phone: (301)496-4396 **Fax:** (301)402-2780
Email: scott@cber.fda.gov
Dr. D. Scott, Chf.
Activities/Fields: Plasma volume expanders, immunoglobulins, and hepatitis B. Investigates thermally-induced albumin denaturation and thermal stabilization of albumin by saturated fatty acid anions; studies IgG dimer by electron microscopy and affinity chromatography; and conducts experiments to determine if the neutralization of hepatitis B virus infectivity could be achieved by formation of immune complexes with anti-HBs, which include antisera produced against a synthetic peptide of S region of the hepatitis B surface and antigen.

★ 24780 ★ U.S. Department of Health and Human Services
Food and Drug Administration
Center for Biologics Evaluation and Research
Division of Hematology
1401 Rockville Pike
Rockville, MD 20852
Phone: (301)496-4396 **Fax:** (301)402-2780
Email: goldingb@cber.fda.gov
Dr. Basil Golding, PhD, Actg. Dir.
Activities/Fields: Responsible for the safety, potency, purity, and efficacy of blood/plasma-derived/r-DNA biotechnology-derived therapeutic products. These include agents used in the management of clotting and bleeding disorders, immune deficiencies, hematologic malignancies, hypovolemia, anemia and related pathophysiologic states, and transplantation and autoimmune diseases. **Pub:** *Annual Report.*

★ 24781 ★ U.S. Department of Health and Human Services
Food and Drug Administration
Center for Biologics Evaluation and Research
Division of Monoclonal Antibodies
1401 Rockville Pike
HFM-555, NIH Bldg. 29B, Rm. 3NN-16
Rockville, MD 20852
Phone: (301)827-0850 **Fax:** (301)827-0852
Email: stein@cber.fda.gov
Website: http://www.fda.gov/cber
Kathryn E. Stein, PhD, Dir.
Activities/Fields: Monoclonal antibody structure and function; the regulation of antibody synthesis; the functions of radionuclide and toxin coupled monoclonal antibody therapeutics; and basic mechanisms involving the biology and physiology of cells involved in the immune system.

★ 24782 ★ U.S. Department of Health and Human Services
Food and Drug Administration
Center for Biologics Evaluation and Research
Laboratory of Biophysics
1401 Rockville Pike
Rockville, MD 20852-1448
Phone: (301)435-2035 **Fax:** (301)496-4684
Email: pastor@cber.fda.gov
Richard W. Pastor, PhD, Chf.
Activities/Fields: Development and application of high resolution NMR methods and light scattering for structural studies of biomacromolecules; development and application of computer modelling methods for studies of biomacromolecules; and characterization and development of adjuvants.

★ 24783 ★ U.S. Department of Health and Human Services
Food and Drug Administration
Center for Biologics Evaluation and Research
Laboratory of Cell Biology-Cytokine
1401 Rockville Pike
Rockville, MD 20852
Phone: (301)827-1735 **Fax:** (301)402-1659
David S. Finbloom, MD, Actg. Chf.
Activities/Fields: Characterization of new cytokines and growth factors, structure, functional relationship, and role in human growth. **Pub:** *Proceedings.* • *Research Reports.*

★ 24784 ★ U.S. Department of Health and Human Services
Food and Drug Administration
Center for Biologics Evaluation and Research
Laboratory of Cell Viral Regulations
FDA-CBER, HFM-541
Bldg. 29-A
Bethesda, MD 20892
Phone: (301)827-1806 **Fax:** (301)480-3256
Email: max@cber.fda.gov
Dr. Edward E. Max, Chf.
Activities/Fields: Regulation of immunoglobulin gene expression by cytokines and cell interactions focusing on the function of several immunoglobulin gene enhancers and the regulation of immunoglobulin isotype switching at the DNA level. Also focuses on the interaction of HIV with cells of the immune system centering on: the structural correlates of targets of neutralizing antibodies; and the activation of T cells by HIV through the T cell receptor and the surface molecules (other than CD4) that mediate viral entry into cells. **Frmly:** (2000) Laboratory of Cell Viral Regulation.

★ 24785 ★ U.S. Department of Health and Human Services
Food and Drug Administration
Center for Biologics Evaluation and Research
Laboratory of Cellular Hematology
1401 Rockville Pike, HFM-335
Rockville, MD 20852
Phone: (301)496-2577 **Fax:** (301)402-2780
Email: vostal@cber.fda.gov
Jaro Vostal, PhD, Acting Chief
Activities/Fields: Leukocytes, platelets, and signal transduction. Operates a hemoglobin and blood substitutes program. Principal area of research interest is blood cell physiology and platelet biochemistry, as related to transfusion. **Pub:** *Proceedings.* • *Reports.*

★ 24786 ★ U.S. Department of Health and Human Services
Food and Drug Administration
Center for Biologics Evaluation and Research
Laboratory of Chemical Biology
8800 Rockville Pike
Bethesda, MD 20892
Phone: (301)827-1777 **Fax:** (301)480-3256
Email: fraser@cber.fda.gov
Dr. Blair A. Fraser, Chf.
Activities/Fields: Biologically active peptides and proteins. Principal research efforts include isolation and structural analysis of novel neuropeptides, identification and isolation of precursor peptides, and identification of metabolic events responsible for post-translational protein processing. Conducts programs in regulation of membrane proteins and molecular pharmacology of signal transduction, developmental biology, and synthesis and use of modified oligodeoxyribonucleotides. Also develops methodologies and strategies for the microsequencing of proteins and the use of synthetic peptides.

★ 24787 ★ U.S. Department of Health and Human Services
Food and Drug Administration
Center for Biologics Evaluation and Research
Laboratory of Cytokine Research
29 Lincoln Dr.
Bethesda, MD 20892
Phone: (301)827-1720 **Fax:** (301)402-1659
David S. Finbloom, MD, Dir.
Activities/Fields: Structure and function of interferons and their receptors; identification and characterization of cytokines that modulate the function of monocytes and macrophages; mechanisms of interferon beta regulated gene expression; antitumor activities of cytokine or anticytokine receptor antibody toxin fusion proteins; and AIDS studies. **Pub:** *Proceedings.* • *Research Reports.*

★ 24788 ★ U.S. Department of Health and Human Services
Food and Drug Administration
Center for Biologics Evaluation and Research
Laboratory of Developement Biology
1401 Rockville Pike, HFM-730
Rockville, MD 20852-1448
Phone: (301)827-0450 **Fax:** (301)827-0449
Email: epstins@cber.fda.gov
Suzanne Epstein, MD, Chf.
Activities/Fields: Biology and developmental control of gene expression. Principal research efforts involve: identification of genetic elements that control the temporal and spatial expression of genes in *Drosophila*; elucidation of the role of homeobox genes in limb and organ development; and characterization of bone morphogenetic factors. **Pub:** *Proceedings.* • *Reports.* **Frmly:** Laboratory of Cellular and Molecular Biology.

★ 24789 ★ U.S. Department of Health and Human Services
Food and Drug Administration
Center for Biologics Evaluation and Research
Laboratory of DNA Virus Research
1401 Rockville Pike
Rockville, MD 20852
Phone: (301)827-0650 **Fax:** (301)496-1810
Dr. Andrew Lewis, Contact
Activities/Fields: Molecular biology of DNA viruses with emphasis on human herpesviruses and poxviruses. Focuses on gene expression, virus vectors, viral latency, viral replication, and immune responses. Conducts a program on the regulation of gene expression. **Pub:** *Proceedings.* • *Research Reports.*

★ 24790 ★ U.S. Department of Health and Human Services
Food and Drug Administration
Center for Biologics Evaluation and Research
Laboratory of Hepatitis Viruses
8800 Rockville Pike
Bethesda, MD 20892
Phone: (301)827-1880 **Fax:** (301)402-5585
Email: LABHR@HELIX.NIH.GOV
Dr. Stephen M. Feinstone, MD, Chf.
Activities/Fields: Molecular biology of the hepatitis C virus, emphasizing viral pathogenesis, replication, and antigenic structure. Supports a project on novel methods of producing hepatitis C vaccines. Operates a program focusing on non-A and non-B hepatitis, which includes hepatitis C virus and other yet to be identified hepatitis viruses.

★ 24791 ★ U.S. Department of Health and Human Services
Food and Drug Administration
Center for Biologics Evaluation and Research
Laboratory of Immuno-Chemistry
5510 Nicholson Ln.
Kensington, MD 20895
Phone: (301)594-6733
Walter Kuff, Contact
Activities/Fields: Chemical research involving the identification, structural elucidation, and quantitation of chemical constituents and impurities of vaccines and other biological products regulated by the Center. Laboratory is responsible for regulatory review of chemical aspects of biological products and for the testing of biological products to determine quantitatively the amounts of various preservatives, metals, stabilizers, adjuvants, chemical inactivators, nitrogen, and residual moisture present. Principal areas of research include inorganic and organic analysis; inductively coupled plasma emission and atomic absorption spectrometric aluminum analysis; residual moisture of freeze-dried biological products; and high-performance liquid chromatography of vaccine constituents. **Frmly:** Laboratory of Analytical Chemistry.

★ 24792 ★ U.S. Department of Health and Human Services
Food and Drug Administration
Center for Biologics Evaluation and Research
Laboratory of Immunobiochemistry
8800 Rockville Pike
Bethesda, MD 20892
Phone: (301)443-1544
Yuan L. Devries, PhD, Actg. Chf.
Activities/Fields: Characterization of allergenic extracts and the evaluation of the diagnostic and therapeutic safety and efficacy of allergenic extracts. Research program includes biochemical, biophysical, immunological, and molecular biology approaches to the characterization and human immune response to various allergens. Develops new methodologies, including using monoclonal antibodies and PCR techniques for the purification and characterization of allergens and HPLC or capillary electrophoresis. Evaluates the accuracy, precision, and sensitivity of allergen skin test procedures and defines potency of allergen extracts. **Frmly:** Laboratory of Allergy and Immunochemistry.

★ 24793 ★ U.S. Department of Health and Human Services
Food and Drug Administration
Center for Biologics Evaluation and Research
Laboratory of Immunoregulation
8800 Rockville Pike
Bethesda, MD 20892
Phone: (301)496-1870 **Fax:** (301)496-1810
Email: berkower@cber.fda.gov
Ira J. Berkower, MD,PhD, Chf.
Activities/Fields: Safety, efficacy, and potency of vaccines for human use including fundamental research into the immunogenicity of viral protein antigens. This includes antigen processing and presentation to antigen specific T cells; the mapping of a conserved neutralizing site that is shared across a broad spectrum of HIV-1 isolates, so antibodies to this site can neutralize diverse isolates; and novel vaccine constructs that assemble into particles for increased vaccine potency, while preserving the site in its native conformation.

★ 24794 ★ U.S. Department of Health and Human Services
Food and Drug Administration
Center for Biologics Evaluation and Research
Laboratory of Molecular and Developemental Immunology
29 Lincoln Dr.
NIH Bldg. 29-B
Bethesda, MD 20892-4555
Phone: (301)827-0717 **Fax:** (301)827-0852
Activities/Fields: Delineating the differences in the immune response to thymus-independent and thymus-dependent forms of polysaccharide antigens and the mechanism of signal transduction by thymus-independent antigens. Projects include: molecular analysis of monoclonal antibodies examining the roles of genetics and of the form of the antigen used for immunization. These studies have shown major differences in two sets of antibodies raised against bacterial levan in two different mouse strains in terms of fine specificity and immunoglobulin gene usage. Studies of two different forms of the meningococcal group C polysaccharide, the polysaccharide itself, and a polysaccharide-protein conjugate were used to examine the molecular consequences of altering the form of the vaccine on the subsequent antibody response. These

studies have demonstrated that the polysaccaharide-protein conjugate vaccine results in the development of antibodies with new specificities and of higher avidity than the polysaccharide, itself; employing a mutant strain of mice (*xid*) which is unresponsive to polysaccharide antigens to examine the role of a subpopulation of B lymphocytes, lacking in this strain, to examine the cellular requirements for mounting an immune response to polysaccharides; developing monoclonal antibodies to B lymphocytes; and examining signal transduction in B lymphocytes via polyclonal cross-linking of the Ig receptor. The last three studies will use subpopulations of B cells from normal mice as well as mice with the *xid* defect. Other studies involve the role of various adhesion molecular in the activitation/waive CD8T cells.

★ 24795 ★ U.S. Department of Health and Human Services
Food and Drug Administration
Center for Biologics Evaluation and Research
Laboratory of Mycobacteria
Bldg. 29, Rm. 502
29 Lincoln Dr.
Bethesda, MD 20892
Phone: (301)496-9559 **Fax:** (301)435-5675
Email: brennan@cber.fda.gov
Dr. Michael J. Brennan, PhD, Chf.
Activities/Fields: Development of novel vaccines for tuberculosis including research on DNA vaccines, immunopathogenesis of intracellular pathogens and bacterial adherene mechanisms. Areas of interest include molecular microbiology, immunology and bacterial pathogenesis. Regulatory duties include review of bacterial biologics including BCG vaccines and therapeutics, and skin test reagents.

★ 24796 ★ U.S. Department of Health and Human Services
Food and Drug Administration
Center for Biologics Evaluation and Research
Laboratory of Pertussis
8800 Rockville Pike
Bethesda, MD 20892
Phone: (301)402-3553 **Fax:** (301)402-2776
Drusilla Burns, PhD, Chf.
Activities/Fields: Regulation of bacterial vaccines (particularly pertussis vaccine). Initiates, directs, and participates in research on the immunochemistry of *Bordetella pertussis* and host parasite interactions in pertussis prerequisite to the development of improved pertussis vaccines and their control and clinical use. Activities involve biochemical,immunochemical, animal model, genetic, and serological studies. Current research programs focus on the mechanisms by which *Bordetella pertussis* attaches to and infects susceptible tissues and the cellular components responsible for local and systemic symptoms of whooping cough. Continuing research studies involve isolation and characterization of virulence factors and development of in vitro and animal laboratory models to study diseases and evaluate potential immunogens. **Pub:** *Proceedings.* • *Research Reports.*

★ 24797 ★ U.S. Department of Health and Human Services
Food and Drug Administration
Center for Biologics Evaluation and Research
Laboratory of Respiratory Viruses
8800 Rockville Pike
Bethesda, MD 20892
Phone: (301)827-1908 **Free:** 888-463-6332
Roland A. Levandowski, MD, Actg. Chf.
Activities/Fields: Human respiratory viral diseases, including influenza viruses, respiratory syncytial viruses, parainfluenza viruses, and rhinoviruses. Techniques employed are intended to permit understanding of the biology of the individual agents through genomic evaluation as well as the biology of the individual agents through in vivo and in vitro studies of cellular and humoral immune parameters.

★ 24798 ★ U.S. Department of Health and Human Services
Food and Drug Administration
Center for Biologics Evaluation and Research
Molecular Medical Genetics Staff
1401 Rockville Pike
Rockville, MD 20852
Phone: (301)827-0453 **Fax:** (301)827-0449
Email: gemarti@helix.nih.gov
Gerald Marti, Actg. Chf.
Activities/Fields: Molecular medical genetics.

★ 24799 ★ U.S. Department of Health and Human Services
Food and Drug Administration
Center for Biologics Evaluation and Research
Molecular Tumor Biology Staff
1401 Rockville Pike, HFM 710
Rockville, MD 20852
Phone: (301)827-0471 **Fax:** (301)827-0449
Email: puri@cber.fda.gov
Website: http://INTRANET.FDA.gov/CBER/
Raj Puri, MD,PhD, Chf.
Activities/Fields: Biology of receptors on human tumor cells; mechanisms of lentivirus infection and expression; MRNA editing. **Pub:** *Documents.* • *Points to Consider.*

★ 24800 ★ U.S. Department of Health and Human Services
Food and Drug Administration
Center for Biologics Evaluation and Research
Office of Therapeutics Research and Review
1401 Rockville Pike
HFM-500
Rockville, MD 20851
Phone: (301)827-5098 **Fax:** (301)827-5395
Email: siegel@cber.fda.gov
Website: http://www.fda.gov/cber/therapies.htm
J. Siegel, Dir.
Activities/Fields: Development, manufacture, testing, and activities of therapeutic biological products including those related to AIDS and those prepared by genetic engineering and synthetic procedures. This is done in order to develop and maintain a scientific base for establishing standards designed to ensure the continued safety, purity, potency, and effectiveness of biological therapeutics products.

★ 24801 ★ U.S. Department of Health and Human Services
Food and Drug Administration
Center for Biologics Evauluation and Research
Laboratory of Enteric and Sexually Transmitted Diseases
8800 Rockville Pike
Bethesda, MD 20892
Phone: (301)496-1893 **Fax:** (301)402-2776
Email: kopecko@cber.fda.gov
Website: http://www.fda.gov/cber/research/dbpa.htm
Dennis Kopecko, PhD, Chf.
Activities/Fields: Genetic and molecular bases of enteric bacterial disease pathogenesis and the host's immune response to infection. Biochemical, immunological, molecular genetic and cell biology methods (including recombinant DNA, in vitro cell cultures, electron and fluorescent microscopy, video/confocal imaging, and molecular immunological technologies) and animal model systems that are employed to analyze the determinants of bacterial virulence, gene expression control mechanisms, and their functional nature in pathogenesis. Current molecular events being analyzed in detail include the prokaryotic and eukaryotic mechanisms involved in: bacterial invasion of mucosal epithelial cells, bacterial intracellular survival, cellular and molecular bases of specific protective immunity to infection, and global regulatory mechanisms involved in controlling virulence gene expression. **Pub:** *Proceedings.* • *Research Reports.*

★ 24802 ★ U.S. Department of Health and Human Services
Food and Drug Administration
Center for Devices and Radiological Health
9200 Corporate Blvd., Rm. 100
Rockville, MD 20850
Phone: (301)443-4690 **Fax:** (301)594-1320
Website: http://www.fda.gov/cdrh/
David W. Feigal, Jr, Dir.
Activities/Fields: Develops and carries out a national program designed to control unnecessary exposures of humans to and assure the safe and efficacious use of ionizing and nonionizing radiation-emitting electronic products; and develops and carries out a national program to assure the safety, effectiveness, and proper labeling of medical devices for human use.

★ 24803 ★ U.S. Department of Health and Human Services
Food and Drug Administration
Center for Devices and Radiological Health
Biometric Sciences Division (Office of Surveillance and Biometrics)
Mail Code HFZ-540
5600 Fishers Ln.
Rockville, MD 20857
Phone: (301)443-7120 **Fax:** (301)443-0097
Activities/Fields: Statistical and epidemiologic review; medical devices evaluation, including risk assessment of post marketing long- and intermediate-term epidemiological effects; and review of pre-market approvals and post-market surveillance studies. Activities primarily involve epidemiological and experimental data collection, analysis, and interpretation; statistical methodology development; and statistical modeling of risk/benefit. Division comprises epidemiology, statistics, and post-market surveillance studies branches. **Pub:** *Proceedings.* • *Research Reports.*

★ 24804 ★ U.S. Department of Health and Human Services
Food and Drug Administration
Center for Devices and Radiological Health
Office of Device Evaluation
9200 Corporate Blvd.
Rockville, MD 20850
Phone: (301)594-2022 **Fax:** (301)594-2510
Website: http://www.fda.gov/cdrh
Bernanrd E. Statland, Dir.
Activities/Fields: Responsible for the evaluation of clinical and non-clinical data to establish the safety and effectiveness of medical devices and their marketability in the U.S.; and regulatory control of clinical trials involving medical devices. Principal areas of interest are health and physical sciences. **Pub:** *Research reports.*

★ 24805 ★ U.S. Department of Health and Human Services
Food and Drug Administration
Center for Devices and Radiological Health
Office of Science and Technology
9200 Corporate Blvd.
HFZ-100
Rockville, MD 20850
Phone: (301)827-4777 **Fax:** (301)827-4787
Email: dem@cdrh.fda.gov
Donald Marlowe, Dir.

Activities/Fields: Pysical, life, and engineering sciences. Specific activities involve: conducting research on the human health effects of radiation and medical devices and on existing and emerging health technologies; providing the Center and other units with laboratory support; and managing the research, development, and product testing engineering programs of the Center. Office comprises divisions for electronics and computer science, life sciences, mechanics and materials science, and physical sciences.

★ 24806 ★ U.S. Department of Health and Human Services
Food and Drug Administration
Center for Devices and Radiological Health
Office of Surveillance and Biometrics
(Division of Biostatistics)
Mail Code HFZ-542
1350 Piccard Dr.
Rockville, MD 20857
Phone: (301)594-0616 **Fax:** (301)443-8559
Email: gxc@cdrh.fda.gov
Dr. Gregory Campbell, PhD, Dir.
Activities/Fields: Statistical aspects of clinical trials submitted to the Center for Devices and Radiological Health (CDRH) as medical device applications. The division also performs statistical research and risk/benefit analyses on the safety, effectiveness, and use of medical devices and the risks of radiation. **Frmly:** Ionizing Radiation and Statistics Branch; Biometric Sciences Division, Statistics Branch.

★ 24807 ★ U.S. Department of Health and Human Services
Food and Drug Administration
Center for Drug Evaluation and Research
1451 Rockville Pike, Rm. 6027
Rockville, MD 20852
Phone: (301)594-5400 **Fax:** (301)594-6197
Website: http://www.fda.gov/cder/
Janet Woodcock, Dir.
Activities/Fields: Develops FDA policy with regard to the safety, effectiveness, and labeling of all drugs for human use; reviews and evaluates new drug applications and notices of claimed investigational exemption of new drugs; develops and implements standards for the safety and effectiveness of all over-the-counter drugs; monitors the quality of marketed drugs through product testing, surveillance, and compliance programs; develops guidelines on current Good Manufacturing Practices for use by the drug industry; develops and disseminates information and educational material on drugs to the medical community and the public; conducts research and develops scientific standards on the composition, quality, safety, and efficacy of human drugs; collects and evaluates information on the effects and use trends of marketed drugs; monitors prescription drug advertising and promotional labeling to assure their accuracy and integrity; analyzes data on accidental poisonings; and disseminates toxicity and treatment information on medicines. Principal Center components are the Office of Compliance, Office of +Drug Evaluation I, Office of +Drug Evaluation II, Office of +Drug Standards, Office of Epidemiology and Biostatistics, and Office of Research Resources.

★ 24808 ★ U.S. Department of Health and Human Services
Food and Drug Administration
Center for Drug Evaluation and Research
Division of Over-the-Counter Drug Products
(Office of Drug Evaluation)
9201 Corporate Blvd.
Rockville, MD 20850
Phone: (301)827-2241 **Fax:** (301)827-2316
Email: ganley@cder.fda.gov
Website: http://www.fda.gov/cder/otc/index.htm
Dr. Charles J. Ganley, MD, Dir.
Activities/Fields: Reviews over-the-counter (OTC) medications marketed in the United States.

★ 24809 ★ U.S. Department of Health and Human Services
Food and Drug Administration
Center for Drug Evaluation and Research
Office of Drug Standards
(Marketing Practices and Communications Branch)
Mail Code HFD-040
5600 Fishers Ln.
Rockville, MD 20857
Phone: (301)827-2828 **Fax:** (301)594-6759
Email: abramst@cder.fda.gov
Website: http://www.fda.gov/cder/ddmac/index.htm
Thomas Abrams, Dir.
Activities/Fields: Industry-wide marketing practices of the pharmaceutical industry and improvement of drug communications between FDA, health professionals, and the public. Specific research areas include prescription drugs, marketing practices, and health communications. **Frmly:** Drug Labeling Education and Research Branch.

★ 24810 ★ U.S. Department of Health and Human Services
Food and Drug Administration
Center for Drug Evaluation and Research
Office of Epidemiology and Biostatistics
(Surveillance and Data Processing Branch)
Mail Code HFD-737
5600 Fishers Ln.
Rockville, MD 20857
Phone: (301)443-6414
George Armstrong, Jr., Chf.
Activities/Fields: Receives, processes, and maintains data for the Adverse Drug and Biological Product Reaction Database, a compilation of data from adverse reaction reports submitted to the Food and Drug Administration primarily by drug manufacturers, physicians, pharmacists, other health professionals, and consumers. These data are used by the Epidemiology and Surveillance Division to generate alerts and to monitor and support special studies on adverse reactions to drugs and biological products. Also maintains the Drug Quality Reporting System, a drug product defect monitoring system. Receives, processes, and maintains data chiefly from pharmacists in hospital, nursing home, and retail practice. **Pub:** *DQRS Annual Review.* • *Drug Utilization Annual Review.*

★ 24811 ★ U.S. Department of Health and Human Services
Food and Drug Administration
Center for Drug Evaluation and Research
Office of Epidemiology and Biostatistics
Mail Code HFD-700
5600 Fishers Ln., Rm. 15B45
Rockville, MD 20857
Phone: (301)827-3209 **Fax:** (301)480-2825
Dr. Robert O'Neill, Chf.
Activities/Fields: Provides statistical and computational support for the Center for Drug Evaluation and Research. Areas of interest are statistics and drug safety, efficacy and quality.

★ 24812 ★ U.S. Department of Health and Human Services
Food and Drug Administration
Center for Drug Evaluation and Research
Office of Epidemiology and Biostatistics
(Statistical Evaluation and Research Branch)
Mail Code HFD-713
5600 Fishers Ln., Rm. 18B45
Rockville, MD 20857
Phone: (301)443-4594 **Fax:** (301)443-9279
Dr. Satya D. Dubey, Chf.
Activities/Fields: Clinical trials for assessing the efficacy and safety of pharmaceuticals; and conducts research in statistical methodologies involving applications of computers in improving review, evaluation, and research methods.

★ 24813 ★ U.S. Department of Health and Human Services
Food and Drug Administration
Center for Drug Evaluation and Research
Office of Generic Drugs
(Bioequivalence Division)
Metro Park North
7500 Standish Pl.
Rockville, MD 20855
Phone: (301)443-1544 **Fax:** (301)594-0181
Email: connerd@cder.fda.gov
Dale P. Conner, Dir.
Activities/Fields: Bioequivalence and dissolution testing data submitted by pharmaceutical firms in support of abbreviated new drug applications. Principal fields of research include biopharmaceutics, pharmacokinetics, and analytical methods. **Pub:** *Research Reports.* **Frmly:** Office of Drug Standards.

★ 24814 ★ U.S. Department of Health and Human Services
Food and Drug Administration
Center for Drug Evaluation and Research
Office of Testing and Research
(Division of Testing and Applied Analytical Development)
1114 Market St., Rm. 1002
Saint Louis, MO 63101
Phone: (314)539-2134 **Fax:** (314)539-2113
Email: layloff@ddastl.cder.fda.gov
Website: http://www.fda.gov/cder/dtaad/
Thomas P. Layloff, Jr., Dir.
Activities/Fields: Conducts method validation for new drug applications and analyzes drug substances for abbreviated new drug applications; serves as the FDA collaborating laboratory for the acceptance of reference standards for the United States Pharmacopeia; assists in monitoring the quality of marketed drugs through surveillance and compliance actions; conducts research to establish official laboratory techniques or methods to test drugs for compliance with standards of identity, strength, and purity; develops analytical methods, particularly automated methods adapted to large volumes of samples; and collects data to support bioavailability and bioequivalence reviews of drugs. Laboratory operations include long-range research activities related to analytical methods and analyses related to the FDA's surveillance programs and other aspects of drug monitoring. **Pub:** *Research Reports.* **Frmly:** Office of Research Resources; Drug Analysis Division.

★ 24815 ★ U.S. Department of Health and Human Services
Food and Drug Administration
Center for Food Safety and Applied Nutrition
5100 Paint Branch Pkwy.
College Park, MD 20740
Phone: (301)436-1600 **Fax:** (301)436-2668
Joseph Levitt, Dir.
Activities/Fields: Principal goals are to gather, analyze, and monitor published and unpublished information pertinent to the consumption, quality, and safety of foods and cosmetics; determine the nutritional needs of various population groups and develop strategies to improve the nutritional status of those at risk; isolate, purify, and identify potentially hazardous food and cosmetic constituents and adulterants, including biological, microbial, and chemical contaminants; develop, validate, and apply quantitative methods of analysis for potentially hazardous constituents, adulterants, and contaminants of foods and cosmetics, including environmental contaminants, animal drugs, and metabolites of microbial origin; develop, improve, and validate biological tests for various forms of human

toxicity, including chronic toxicity, fetal and neonatal toxicity, behavioral and immunotoxicity, and dermal and ocular toxicity; apply toxicity tests and epidemiological studies to determine the adverse effects (hazards) of food constituents and contaminants and of cosmetics ingredients, singly or in combination; improve the accuracy of methods used to assess potential risks to human health associated with the constituents and contaminants of foods and cosmetics; develop practical control technologies necessary to detect or prevent hazards resulting from the storage or processing of foods or cosmetics; and assess social, economic, and environmental determinants and impacts of Center actions. Research activities are primarily carried out in units of the Center's Office of Plant, Dairy Foods and Beverages, Office of Food Labeling, Office of Special Nutritionals, Office of Seafood, and Office of Special Research Skills.

★ 24816 ★ U.S. Department of Health and Human Services
Food and Drug Administration
Center for Food Safety and Applied Nutrition
Office of Plant and Diary Foods and Beverages
Rm. 4827, HFS-300
5100 Paint Branch Pkwy
College Park, MD 20740
Phone: (301)436-1700 **Fax:** (301)436-2632
Email: ttroxell@cfsan.fda.gov
Website: http://www.fda.gov/oc/orgcharts/orgchart.html
Dr. Terry C. Troxell, PhD, Dir.
Activities/Fields: Safety and quality of foods derived from plants, milk, eggs, and game foods, including studies on detection of inorganic and organic contaminants, pesticides and natural toxins; identification of virulence factors associated with foodborne pathogens; impact of foodborne pathogens on immune response; natural product chemistry of herbal products; and food processing and packaging; and risk assessment of harmful substances in foods. **Pub:** *Annual Pesticide Residue Monitoring Report.* • *Pesticide Analytical Manual.*

★ 24817 ★ U.S. Department of Health and Human Services
Food and Drug Administration
National Center for Toxicological Research
Biochemical Toxicology Division
HFT-110
3900 NCTR Dr.
Jefferson, AR 72079
Phone: (870)543-7202 **Fax:** (870)543-7136
Dr. Frederick A. Beland, Dir.
Activities/Fields: Biochemical mechanisms of toxicity and chemical carcinogenesis, including research on the metabolic activation of chemical toxicants; identification of cellular constituents modified by activated chemical toxicants; elucidation of biochemical and other mechanisms by which chemical carcinogenicity and mutagenicity are initiated and expressed; determination of critical detoxification pathways; studies on effects of cellular repair mechanisms on toxic response; and research on metabolism routes and rates.

★ 24818 ★ U.S. Department of Health and Human Services
Food and Drug Administration
National Center for Toxicological Research
Biometry Staff
NCTR Rd. 3900
Jefferson, AR 72079
Phone: (870)543-7008 **Fax:** (870)543-7662
Email: rkodell@nctr.sda.gov
Dr. Ralph Kodell, Dir.
Activities/Fields: Statistical design and analysis of toxicological experime nts. Principal area of research interest is biostatistics in toxicology, including survival analysis, time to tumor estimation and testing, and extrapolation of effects from high to low doses, and dose-response modeling for developmental defects. Focus is on quantitative risk estimation. **Pub:** *Research Reports.*

★ 24819 ★ U.S. Department of Health and Human Services
Food and Drug Administration
National Center for Toxicological Research
Chemistry Division
Bldg. 51, Mail Stop HFT-230
3900 NCTR Rd.
Jefferson, AR 72079
Phone: (870)543-7301 **Fax:** (870)543-7686
Email: rturesky@nctr.fda.gov
Website: http://www.fda.gov/nctr/science/divisions/chemistry.htm
Robert Turesky, PhD, Dir.

★ 24820 ★ U.S. Department of Health and Human Services
Food and Drug Administration
National Center for Toxicological Research
Genetic Toxicology Division
Bldg. 13
3900 NCTR Dr.
Jefferson, AR 72079
Phone: (870)543-7050 **Fax:** (870)543-7393
Email: mmmoore@nctr.fda.gov
Website: http://www.fda.gov/nctr/science/divisions/genreptox.htm
Martha Moore, PhD, Dir.
Activities/Fields: Directs an interdisciplinary toxicological research center emphasizing the use of genomic, proteomic and informatic tools to modify and develop standards that are applicable to The Food and Drug Administration's mission to protect the public health. **Frmly:** Genetic Toxicology Division.

★ 24821 ★ U.S. Department of Health and Human Services
Food and Drug Administration
National Center for Toxicological Research
Office of Research Support
3900 NCTR Rd.
Jefferson, AR 72079-9502
Phone: (870)543-7130 **Fax:** (870)543-7576
Website: http://www.fda.gov/oc/orgcharts.html
Rose Huber, Contact
Activities/Fields: Provides support to the NCTR by providing facility maintenance, animal husbandry, computer operations, and pathological services.

★ 24822 ★ U.S. Department of Health and Human Services
Food and Drug Administration
National Center for Toxicological Research
Pathology Associates
3900 NCTR Rd.
Jefferson, AR 72079
Phone: (870)543-7027 **Free:** 800-638-3321
Fax: (870)543-7030
Email: tbucci@nctr.foa.gov
John Latendresse, Prog. Dir.
Activities/Fields: Effects of a number of chemicals and their varying dosages for different time intervals of treated animals (including making inferences about the potential effect of the same chemicals upon the health of human beings); and studies on the toxicological effects of nerve agents (in cooperation with the Department of Defense), including standard teratology, delayed neuropathy, dominant-lethal, subchronic, and multigenerational protocols. Program also evaluates techniques required to recognize meaningful deviations from normal at earlier times or promise increased specificity in identifying these. Continuing cross-training of technical staff allows for comprehensive pathology services. **Frmly:** (2000) Pathology Associates.

★ 24823 ★ U.S. Department of Health and Human Services
Food and Drug Administration
Office of Orphan Products Development
5600 Fishers Ln.
HF-35, Rm. 6A-55
Rockville, MD 20857
Phone: (301)827-3666 **Fax:** (301)827-0017
Email: mhaffner@oc.fda.gov
Website: http://www.fda.gov/orphan/index.htm
Marlene E. Haffner, Dir.
Activities/Fields: Availability of orphan products. Orphan products are defined as drugs, biologics, medical devices, and foods for medical purposes which are indicated for a rare disease or condition (i.e., one affecting fewer than 200,000 people in the U.S.). Grants and contracts support clinical research intended to provide safety and efficacy data acceptable to the FDA which will either result in or substantially contribute to the approval of the products. **Pub:** *Request for Applications in the Federal Register*, annually.

★ 24824 ★ U.S. Department of Health and Human Services
Food and Drug Administration
Office of Planning and Evaluation
Evaluation and Analysis Staff
Mail Code HFP-10
5600 Fishers Ln., Rm. 1571
Rockville, MD 20857
Phone: (301)827-5252 **Fax:** (301)827-5260
Email: kmcevoy@oc.fda.gov
Website: http://www.fda.gov/ope/eval.html
John Uzzell, Dir.
Activities/Fields: In-house analytical consulting services to the FDA Commissioner and program managers. Activities involve evaluation, data collection, and analysis for all program policies and operations administered by the FDA, including pre-market review of drugs and medical devices.

★ 24825 ★ U.S. Department of Health and Human Services
Food and Drug Administration
Office of Women's Health
HF-8
Rm. 16-65
5600 Fishers Ln.
Rockville, MD 20857
Phone: (301)827-0350
Website: http://www.fda.gov/womens/
Activities/Fields: Funds research on women's health issues including breast and ovarian cancer, women and HIV, women and cardiovascular disease, osteoporosis, breast implant safety, the effects of estrogen, and on the safe and effective use of medications, therapeutic products, medical devices, food and cosmetics. Conducts intramural research on gender effects and regulatory science. Encourages industry to include women in their studies and promotes participation of women in clinical trials of FDA-regulated products. Encourages the analysis of clinical trial data for gender differences.

★ 24826 ★ U.S. Department of Health and Human Services
Health Care Financing Administration
Office of Research and Demonstrations
7500 Security Blvd., Rm. C3-20-11
Baltimore, MD 21244-1850
Phone: (410)786-6503 **Fax:** (410)786-6511
Email: ospinquiry@hcfa.gov
Website: http://cms.hhs.gov/about/agency/fak.asp
Thomas M. Kickham, PhD, Actg. Dir.

Activities/Fields: Develops and manages long-term strategic planning processes for the Health Care Financing Administration. Provides analytic support and information to Administration programs. Identifies and evaluates emerging trends in health care delivery and financing. Coordinates demonstration activities; participates in experimental health care delivery projects; develops research and educational materials. **Pub:** *Active Projects Report*, annually. • *Health Care Financing Review*, quarterly. **Frmly:** Office of Research and Demonstrations.

★ 24827 ★ U.S. Department of Health and Human Services
Health Resources and Services Administration
Bureau of Health Professions
Office of Policy and Research (Information Resource Management Branch)
5600 Fishers Ln., Rm. 8808
Park Lawn Bldg.
Rockville, MD 20857
Phone: (301)443-1355 **Fax:** (301)443-4414
Art Smith, Chf.

Activities/Fields: Provides health and health-related data available at the county level; compatible and consistent health-related data in a variety of forms in order to be of use to the broadest possible range of users; and flexible analytical capabilities for analysis of health and health-related data. **Frmly:** Information Systems Branch of the Office of Data Analysis and Management.

★ 24828 ★ U.S. Department of Health and Human Services
Health Resources and Services Administration
Gillis W. Long Hansen's Disease Center
1770 Physician Park Dr.
Baton Rouge, LA 70816
Phone: (225)756-3700 **Fax:** (225)756-3806
Website: http://bphc.hrsa.gov/nhdp/AMBULATORY_CARE_MAIN_PAGE.htm
Charles Stanley, Dir.

Activities/Fields: Care and rehabilitation of patients with Hansen's disease (leprosy) and for basic and applied research related to all aspects of the disease. In addition, Center provides a training facility for professionals and paraprofessionals involved with the diagnosis and treatment of Hansen's disease, both within the United States and abroad. Areas of research interest include studies of the causative organism of leprosy and its effect on the body as well as research in methods of clinical treatment and rehabilitation; mycobacterioses including tuberculosis. Accomplishments have included the infection of armadillos with the leprosy organism, the first experimental animal to be found naturally susceptible to the disseminated form of this disease, and earlier, the discovery of sulfone therapy, the first effective treatment for the disease. Tuberculosis studies include comprehensive evaluation of 50,000 candidate anti-TB drugs. **Pub:** *International Journal of Leprosy*, quarterly. • *The Star*, quarterly. **Frmly:** (2000) Gillis W. Long Hansen's Disease Center.

★ 24829 ★ U.S. Department of Health and Human Services
Indian Health Service
Office of Planning, Evaluation, and Legislation
Division of Program Statistics
Twinbrook Metro Plaza
12300 Twinbrook Pkwy., Ste. 450
Rockville, MD 20852
Phone: (301)443-1180 **Fax:** (301)443-1522
Email: epaisano@hqe.ihs.gov
Edna Paisano, Supv. Stat.

Activities/Fields: Main function is to satisfy the American Indian and Alaska Native health statistics information needs of its clients. The Division manages a number of information systems that provide data for measuring the health status of the American Indian and Alaska Native population and appraising IHS program activities. Division's primary duty is to serve IHS management, but it also has numerous dealings with other government agencies, government contractors, academia, researchers, the media, and the general public. Division is responsible for: vital events statistics, patient care statistics, and population statistics. In addition to providing statistical data, Division also provides statistical advice on analyzing the data. **Pub:** *Indian health status reports*, occasionally. • *Regional Differences in Indian Health*, annually. • *Trends in Indian Health*, annually.

★ 24830 ★ U.S. Department of Health and Human Services
National Cancer Institute
Cancer Information Products & Systems
6116 Executive Blvd. 300
Rockville, MD 20852
Phone: (301)496-9096 **Fax:** (301)480-8105
Email: gisele.sarosy@mail.nih.gov
Website: http://www.cancer.gov
Dr. Gisele Sarosy, PhD, Actg. Assoc. Dir.

Activities/Fields: Develops, maintains, and refines information on cancer treatment, screening, prevention, genetics, and supportive care for patients, health professionals, and the public, using editorial boards and scientific review processes. CIPS manages the production of this evidence-based information and its dissemination utilizing a variety of technologies (e.g., NCI Web sites such as CancerNet, facsimile, e-mail, etc.) and through partnerships with organizations that license NCI information. Also investigates new technologies and their applicability to gather, organize, and disseminate cancer information. ncer-related research and demonstration encompassing basic research, diagnosis, treatment, rehabilitation, and public and patient education. These centers also educate and train professionals in various clinical and research specialties. Research activities conducted at NCI's laboratories or supported through grants and contracts include many investigative approaches to cancer, including research in chemistry, biochemistry, biology, molecular biology, immunology, radiation physics, experimental chemotherapy, epidemiology, biometry, radiotherapy, and pharmacology. Major components of NCI include: Cancer Biology, Diagnosis and Centers Division; Cancer Etiology Division;

★ 24831 ★ U.S. Department of Health and Human Services
National Cancer Institute
Basic Sciences Division
Basic Research Laboratory
NCI-Frederick
Bldg. 469, Rm. 101
Frederick, MD 21702
Phone: (301)846-1318 **Fax:** (301)846-6164
Email: kcannon@mail.ncifcrf.gov
Karen Cannon, Sec.

Activities/Fields: Plans and conducts research on the cellular, molecular, genetic, biochemical and immunological mechanism affecting the progression, diagnosis and treatment of cancer; and collaborates with scientists from other research programs within the National Cancer Institute and the National Institutes of Health. **Pub:** *Proceedings*. • *Research Reports*. **Frmly:** (1996) Laboratory of Molecular Oncology.

★ 24832 ★ U.S. Department of Health and Human Services
National Cancer Institute
Chemistry of Carcinogenesis Laboratory
Bldg. 538, Rm. 115
PO Box B
Frederick, MD 21702-1201
Phone: (301)846-5852 **Fax:** (301)846-6146
Email: moschel@ncifcrf.gov
Website: http://web.ncifcrf.gov/research/ccl/default.asp
Dr. Robert Moschel, Ch.

Activities/Fields: Strives to improve the understanding of how certain chemicals initiate the process of carcinogenesis, and to use this understanding to help prevent or treat the disease.

★ 24833 ★ U.S. Department of Health and Human Services
National Cancer Institute
Division of Basic Sciences
Intramural Research Program
NIH Bldg. 31, Ste. 3A11
9000 Rockville Pike
Bethesda, MD 20892
Phone: (301)496-4345 **Fax:** (301)496-0775
Dr. J. Carl Barrett, Dir.

Activities/Fields: Program comprises branches for Immunology and laboratories for studies in biochemistry, cell biology, cellular oncology, genetics, immunobiology, mathematical biology, molecular biology, tumor immunology and biology.

★ 24834 ★ U.S. Department of Health and Human Services
National Cancer Institute
Division of Cancer Biology
Executive Pl. N, Ste. 5000
6130 Executive Blvd.
EPN Bldg., Ste. 500
Bethesda, MD 20892
Phone: (301)496-7028 **Fax:** (301)496-1037
Email: bs62d@nih.gov
Website: http://www3.cancer.gov/dcb/dcbhom.htm
Barbara Spalholz, PhD, Dir.

Activities/Fields: Extramural and basic and applied research on cancer cell biology and immunology, including the biological and health effects of exposures to ionizing and non-ionizing radiation, and the role of chemical, physical and biological agents, acting separately or together, in the development of cancer. Principal components include the Cancer Biology Branch, Cancer Immunology Branch, Cancer Genetics Branch Biological Carcinogenesis Branch, Chemical and Physical Carcinogenesis Branch, and Radiation Effects Branch. **Pub:** *Annual Report*.

★ 24835 ★ U.S. Department of Health and Human Services
National Cancer Institute
Division of Cancer Biology
Cancer Biology Branch
6130 Executive Blvd., Ste. 5000
Bethesda, MD 20892
Phone: (301)496-7028 **Fax:** (301)402-1037
Email: cf33a@nih.gov
Website: http://www3.cancer.gov/dcb/cbbhom.htm
Colette S. Freeman, PhD, Chf.

Activities/Fields: Facilitates and supports basic biological research aimed at defin ing elements of the phenotype of the malignant cell through interdisciplinary approaches. Areas of emphasis include both positive and negative regulation of cell growth and differentiation, mechanisms involved in the process of metastasis and of angiogenesis, the influence of the extracellular environment on the tumor cell, GENE EXPRESSION, PATHWAYS OF SIGNAL TRANSDUCTION, MODELS FOR CANCER BIOLOGY and the molecular biology of cancer cells.

★ 24836 ★ U.S. Department of Health and Human Services
National Cancer Institute
Division of Cancer Biology
Cancer Immunology Branch
Executive Plaza N, Rm. 501
6130 Executive Blvd.
Rockville, MD 20852
Phone: (301)496-7815 **Fax:** (301)480-2844
Email: am214t@nih.gov
Website: http://www.nci.nih.gov/dcb/cibhom.htm
Robert A. Mufson, PhD, Chf.

Activities/Fields: Molecular immunology and cellular immunology, with special emphasis on understanding the role of the immune system in the development, growth, and spread of tumors as it relates to the problems of cause, prevention, treatment, and diagnosis of malignant diseases.

★ 24837 ★ U.S. Department of Health and Human Services
National Cancer Institute
Division of Cancer Biology
Chemical and Physical Carcinogenesis Program
6130 Executive Blvd., Ste. 5000
MSC 7386
Bethesda, MD 20892-7055
Phone: (301)496-5471 **Fax:** (301)496-1040
Email: dl58s@nih.gov
Website: http://www.nci.nih.gov/DCB/DCBhom.htm
Dr. David Longfellow, Branch Chf.
Activities/Fields: Occurrence of cancer caused or promoted by chemical or physical agents, acting separately or together, or in combination with biological agents; and provides a broad spectrum of information, advice, and consultation to individual scientists and institutional science management officials relative to NIH and NCI funding and scientific review policies and procedures, preparation of grant applications, and choice of funding instruments. The Branch also: provides NCI management with recommendations as to funding needs, priorities, and strategies for the support of relevant research areas consistent with the current state of development of individual research activities and the promise of new initiatives; plans, develops, and manages research resources necessary for the conduct of the coordinated research program; and plans, organizes, and conducts meetings and workshops to further program objectives and maintains contact with the relevant scientific community to identify and evaluate new research trends relating to its program responsibilities. **Pub:** *National Cancer Institute's Annual Report.*

★ 24838 ★ U.S. Department of Health and Human Services
National Cancer Institute
Division of Cancer Biology
Radiation Effects Branch
6130 Executive Blvd.
Rockville, MD 20852-7391
Phone: (301)496-9326 **Fax:** (301)496-1224
Website: http://www.nih.gov
Bruce Wachholz, Chf.
Activities/Fields: Mechanisms of radiation-induced mutagenesis and carcinogenesis including supportive studies in radiation chemistry, radiation physics, molecular biology, cytogenetics and cell transformation; studies of cancer among selected populations exposed to radionuclides intentionally or accidentally released into the environment.

★ 24839 ★ U.S. Department of Health and Human Services
National Cancer Institute
Division of Cancer Control and Population Sciences
Extramural Epidemiology and Genetics Program
6130 Executive Blvd., Rm. 5114
MSC 7395
Bethesda, MD 20892-7395
Phone: (301)594-9499 **Fax:** (301)435-5477
Email: winnde@mail.nih.gov
Website: http://epi.grants.cancer.gov/index.html
Dr. Deborah Winn, PhD, Actg. Assoc. Dir.
Activities/Fields: Plans, develops, directs and manages a national extramural program of basic and applied research in biometry, epidemiology, and related multidisciplinary activities; establishes program priorities and evaluates program effectiveness; provides a broad spectrum of information, advice, and consultation to individual scientists and institutional sciences management officials concerning National Institutes of Health and National Cancer Institute (NCI) funding and scientific review policies and procedures, preparation of grant applications, and choice of funding instruments; provides (NCI) management with recommendations as to funding needs, priorities and strategies for the support of relevant research areas consistent with the current state of development of individual research activities and the promise of new initiatives; plans, develops, and manages research resources necessary for the conduct of the coordinated research program; and plans, organizes, and conducts meetings and workshops to further program objectives.

★ 24840 ★ U.S. Department of Health and Human Services
National Cancer Institute
Division of Cancer Epidemiology and Genetics
6120 Executive Blvd., Rm. 8070
Bethesda, MD 20892
Phone: (301)496-1611 **Fax:** (301)402-3256
Email: ncidcegnews@mail.nih.gov
Dr. Joseph F. Fraumeni, Jr., Contact
Activities/Fields: The Division of Cancer Epidemiology and Genetics (DCEG) is the primary focus within the National Cancer Institute for population-based research on environmental and genetic determinants of cancer. Intramural and collaborative interdisciplinary studies are conducted on the distribution, causes and natural history of cancer, and the means for its prevention. Research areas of special interest include genetic predisposition, lifestyle factors, environmental contaminants, occupational exposures, medications, radiation and infectious agents, as well as statistics and methods development.

★ 24841 ★ U.S. Department of Health and Human Services
National Cancer Institute
Division of Cancer Epidemiology and Genetics
Epidemiology and Biostatistics Program
EPS - 7018
Bethesda, MD 20892-7236
Phone: (301)496-4375 **Fax:** (301)402-4489
Dr. Peggy Tucker, Chf.
Activities/Fields: Activities of the Clinical Epidemiology Branch include: status and future prospects for research in specific areas of clinical observations of cancer patients and from clinical studies of families epistimology. and occupational groups and correlation of these results with laboratory findings; studies of the late effects of childhood cancer and the therapy of childhood cancer; operation of a clinic dealing with the genetics of human cancer to evaluate factors affecting risks of specific types of cancer such as neurofibromatosis; and preparation of analytical reviews to define current status and future prospects for research in specific areas of clinical epidemiology.

★ 24842 ★ U.S. Department of Health and Human Services
National Cancer Institute
Division of Cancer Prevention and Control
Cancer Control Research Program (Public Health Applications Branch)
6130 Executive Blvd., Rm. 241
Rockville, MD 20852
Phone: (301)496-8585 **Fax:** (301)496-8675
Mark Manley, Chf.
Activities/Fields: Responsible for the development, implementation, and evaluation of an extramural research program aimed at reducing risk factors for cancer and increasing early detection of cancer. **Pub:** *Monographs.* • *Professional journals.* **Frmly:** Health Promotion Science Branch.

★ 24843 ★ U.S. Department of Health and Human Services
National Cancer Institute
Division of Cancer Prevention and Control
Cancer Control Research Program
6130 Executive Blvd, Rm. 232
Rockville, MD 20852
Phone: (301)496-8594 **Fax:** (301)480-6637
Thomas J. Glynn, PhD, Chf.
Activities/Fields: Widespread use of proven health promotion and other cancer prevention and management techniques by health professionals, patients and their families, populations at elevated risk, and the general public; monitor basic and clinical research activities in order to identify new interventions that will reduce cancer rates in populations and to facilitate research on their application; provide training opportunities for research and/or application of cancer prevention and management interventions; establish program priorities, allocate resources, and integrate the projects of the various participating branches; and provide programmatic and consultative support to other divisional, institute, governmental, and private sector organizations that facilitate the application of proven cancer control interventions in populations. Program comprises branches for Cancer Control Applications, Health Promotion Science, and Special Population Studies. (A fourth unit, the Cancer Training Branch, no longer exists.).

★ 24844 ★ U.S. Department of Health and Human Services
National Cancer Institute
Division of Cancer Prevention and Control
Cancer Prevention Program (Chemoprevention Branch)
Executive Plaza N, Rm. 2118 M
6130 Executive Blvd.
M.S 7322
Bethesda, MD 20892
Phone: (301)496-8563 **Fax:** (301)402-0553
Dir. James Crowell, MD, Chf.
Activities/Fields: Chemoprevention involves the study and development of selected micronutrients or other small molecular weight substances for the purposes of reducing cancer incidence. Research has focused on identifying or demonstrating (in animal models, epidemiological studies, and human clinical trials) natural or synthetic agents that can lower cancer incidence. Activities include 68 ongoing clinical trials nationally and internationally with 200,000 subjects. Also develops drugs.

★ 24845 ★ U.S. Department of Health and Human Services
National Cancer Institute
Division of Cancer Prevention and Control
Cancer Prevention Program
9000 Rockville Pike
Bethesda, MD 20892
Phone: (301)496-8567 **Fax:** (301)402-0553
Dr. Winfred Malone, Actg. Assoc. Dir.
Activities/Fields: Cancer detection to determine which technique s for early detection of cancer can reduce morbidity and mortality from cancer; chemoprevention research to determine whether selected micronutrients or synthetic compounds can be shown in human trials to reduce cancer incidence; and diet and cancer research to determine whether changes in the diet can be shown to reduce cancer incidence in human trials. Principal components are the Prevention Program.

★ 24846 ★ U.S. Department of Health and Human Services
National Cancer Institute
Division of Cancer Prevention and Population Sciences
Cancer Surveillance Research Program
6116 Executive Blvd., MSC 8315
Bethesda, MD 20892-8315
Phone: (301)496-8506 **Fax:** (301)480-4077
Email: harshmat@mail.nih.gov
Website: http://surveillance.cancer.gov
Dr. Brenda K. Edwards, Assoc. Dir.
Activities/Fields: Impact of cancer and monitor the effects of cancer prevention and control activities in research, prevention, screening, treatment, and rehabilitation. Program also provides application research support for a broad range of activities in the Cancer Prevention and Control Division. Principal areas of interest are incidence, survival, and mortality of cancer in the United States as monitored through the Surveillance, Epidemiology, and End Results (SEER) Program; health behavior and practice patterns; economics of cancer; and cancer control resource allocations. Program comprises branches for Cancer Statistics and Statistical Applications and Research. **Pub:** *Annual Cancer Statistics Review.*

★ 24847 ★ U.S. Department of Health and Human Services
National Cancer Institute
Division of Cancer Treatment and Diagnosis
Developmental Therapeutics Program (Natural Products Branch)
NCI-Frederick
Fairview Center, Ste. 206
PO Box B 2-1201
Frederick, MD 21702-1201
Phone: (301)846-5387 **Fax:** (301)846-6178
Email: cragg@dtpax2.ncifcrf.gov
Website: http://dtp.nci.nih.gov/branches/npb/index.html
Dr. Gordon Cragg, Chf.
Activities/Fields: Acquisition of novel natural products for testing for anticancer anti-HIV activity via fermentation programs; and plant and marine organism collection and extraction projects.

★ 24848 ★ U.S. Department of Health and Human Services
National Cancer Institute (NCI)
Division of Cancer Treatment and Diagnosis (DCTD)
Developmental Therapeutics Program (DTP)
(Toxicology and Pharmacology Branch — T&PB)
Executive Plaza N, Ste. 8034
6130 Executive Blvd.
Bethesda, MD 20892-7451
Phone: (301)496-8777 **Fax:** (301)480-4836
Email: tomaszej@mail.nih.gov
Dr. Joseph E. Tomaszewski, Chf.
Activities/Fields: Provides the safety and toxicity information required for the scientific evaluation of new antitumor and anti-HIV drugs and vaccines by the Cancer Treatment Division's Drug Development Group or through the RAID Program for Phase I clinical trials. It is responsible for the acquisition of toxicology data on both new and established agents. The data accumulated are evaluated, and, for new drugs, provide the database for deriving the initial clinical dose and the toxicological base required for an Investigational New Drug Application to the Food and Drug Administration. The Branch also plans and guides developmental research for organ-specific toxicity assays such as bone marrow and heart, provides assistance for the development of new toxicology assays, tests new radiosensitizers and radioprotectors and assists the Pharmaceutical Resources Branch in the evaluation of experimental drug formulations.

★ 24849 ★ U.S. Department of Health and Human Services
National Cancer Institute
Division of Cancer Treatment and Diagnosis
Developmental Therapeutics Program (Grants and Contracts Operations Branch)
Executive Plaza N, Rm. 8153
9000 Rockville Pike
Bethesda, MD 20892-7456
Phone: (301)496-8783 **Fax:** (301)402-5200
Email: wolpertm@exchange.nih.gov
Website: http://dtp.nci.nih.gov
Dr. Mary Wolpert, Chf.
Activities/Fields: Preclinical anticancer drug discovery and development.

★ 24850 ★ U.S. Department of Health and Human Services
National Cancer Institute
Division of Cancer Treatment, Diagnosis, and Centers
NIH Bldg. 31, 3A44
31 Center Dr., MSC 2440
Bethesda, MD 20892-2440
Phone: (301)496-4291 **Fax:** (301)496-0826
Email: ef30d@nih.gov
Website: http://www3.cancer.gov/dctd/index.html
Dr. Ellen Feigal, Actg. Dir.
Activities/Fields: Cancer diagnostic and treatment activities with the objective of curing or controlling cancer in people; administers a total drug development program; and serves as the national focal point for information and data on cancer treatment studies. Division components are: Cancer Therapy Evaluation Program; Developmental Therapeutics Program; Radiation Research Program; Biomedical Imaging Program; Cancer Diagnosis Program; and Biometrics Research Branch.

★ 24851 ★ U.S. Department of Health and Human Services
National Cancer Institute
Division of Cancer Treatment, Diagnosis, and Centers
Biological Response Modifiers Program (Biological Resources Branch)
Frederick Cancer Research and Development Center
Bldg. 1052, Rm. 253
PO Box B
Frederick, MD 21701
Phone: (301)846-1098 **Fax:** (301)846-5429
Email: creekmor@nci.fcrf.gov
Website: http://web.ncifcrf.gov/research/brb
Dr. Stephen Creekmore, Chf.
Activities/Fields: Preclinical and clinical biological response modifiers re search in the biomedical community. The Branch monitors Phase I and early Phase II clinical studies that assess biological effects of biological response modifiers in cancer patients and correlate changes in the biological modifications with antitumor activity. In addition, Branch has established a preclinical screening program for the selection and preclinical assessment of the efficacy of biological response modifiers. A resource distribution system involving information acquisition and assessment as well as agent acquisition and testing has also been established.

★ 24852 ★ U.S. Department of Health and Human Services
National Cancer Institute
Division of Cancer Treatment, Diagnosis, and Centers
Cancer Centers Branch
6116 Executive Blvd., Ste. 700
MSC8345
Bethesda, MD 20892-8345
Phone: (301)496-8531 **Fax:** (301)402-0181
Email: lw187q@nih.gov
Website: http://www3.cancer.gov/cancercenters/
Linda K. Weiss, PhD, Chf.
Activities/Fields: Multidisciplinary cancer research efforts in the areas of basic, clinical and cancer prevention, control and population sciences. The Cancer Center Support Grant (CCSG) is intended to provide infrastructure for academic and research institutions for establishing and sustaining an interdisciplinary research focus on cancer. **Pub:** *Proceedings.*
• *Research Reports.*

★ 24853 ★ U.S. Department of Health and Human Services
National Cancer Institute
Division of Cancer Treatment, Diagnosis, and Centers
Clinical Oncology Program (Radiation Oncology Branch)
NIH Bldg. 10, Rm. B3B69
9000 Rockville Pike
Bethesda, MD 20892
Phone: (301)496-5457 **Fax:** (301)480-5439
Email: ccoleman@mail.nih.gov
Dr. C. Norm Coleman, Dir.
Activities/Fields: Clinical investigation of cancer treatment using X-ray technology; and laboratory investigation of radiobiology of mechanisms of action of various compounds and their effects on radiosensitization/radioprotection, and radioimmunotherapy. Emphasis is on radiation sensitizing compounds, radioprotecting compounds. Areas of investigation include primary breast cancer, small cell carcinoma of the lung, lymphoma, Hodgkin's disease, gliomas, mycosis fungoides, soft tissue sarcomas, and pediatric neoplasms, cancer and normal tissue. **Pub:** *Proceedings.*

★ 24854 ★ U.S. Department of Health and Human Services
National Cancer Institute
Division of Cancer Treatment, Diagnosis, and Centers
Clinical Oncology Program (NCI-Navy Medical Oncology Branch)
NCI-NNMC
8901 Wisconsin
Bethesda, MD 20889-5105
Phone: (301)496-0901 **Fax:** (301)496-0047
Dr. Barry Gause, Dir. of Fellowship Prog.
Activities/Fields: New modes of detection, staging, and treatment of human cancers by integrat ing clinical and laboratory research with an emphasis on understanding the fundamental biology of human tumor cells and applying these lessons to the clinic. By combining the most recent techniques of cellular and molecular biology with innovative clinical treatment studies, entering patients into other NCI protocols, and providing clinical care to Department of Defense patients for the Naval Hospital, the Branch represents a unique resource to both the National Cancer Institute and the Naval Hospital. The Branch is concerned with the primary care and clinical investigation of patients with a variety of solid tumors and hematologic malignancies. A major effort involves the staging and treatment of carcinomas of the breast, lung, and gastrointestinal tract. Performs chemotherapeutic protocols.

★ 24855 ★ U.S. Department of Health and Human Services
National Cancer Institute
Division of Cancer Treatment, Diagnosis, and Centers
Developmental Therapeutics Program (Information Technology Branch)
Executive Plaza N, Rm. 811
6130 Executive Blvd.
Rockville, MD 20852
Phone: (301)496-8747 **Fax:** (301)480-4808
Email: zaharevitz@dtpax2.ncifcrf.gov
Website: http://dtp.nci.nih.gov
Kenneth Paull, Chf.

Activities/Fields: All data associated with the Developmental Therapeutics Program. This includes data pertaining to the acquisition of chemicals and their structure and estimated properties as well as data derived from biological screening and from toxicology measurements. A developmental effort within the Branch is directed at improved methodologies of large file searching, new techniques for chemical structure manipulation, and studies of the relationships between chemical structure and physical and biological properties of molecules. **Pub:** *Proceedings.* • *Research Reports.*

★ 24856 ★ U.S. Department of Health and Human Services
National Cancer Institute
Division of Cancer Treatment, Diagnosis, and Centers
Developmental Therapeutics Program (Drug Synthesis and Chemistry Branch)
Executive Plaza N, Ste. 8028
6130 Executive Blvd.
Bethesda, MD 20892-7448
Phone: (301)496-8795 **Fax:** (301)480-4817
Dr. Ven Narayanan, Chf.
Activities/Fields: Acquiring and managing the flow of unique synthetic compounds for evaluation as potential anticancer agents.

★ 24857 ★ U.S. Department of Health and Human Services
National Cancer Institute
Division of Cancer Treatment, Diagnosis, and Centers
Developmental Therapeutics Program
Executive Plaza N, Rm. 8018
6130 Executive Blvd.
Rockville, MD 20852-7458
Phone: (301)496-8720 **Fax:** (301)402-0831
Email: eslb@nih.gov
Website: http://dtp.nci.nih.gov/
Dr. Edward A. Sausville, Assoc. Dir.
Activities/Fields: Preclinical discovery and development of anticancer and anti-HIV agents for the Division of Cancer Treatment and Diagnosis, focusing on chemotherapy. The Developmental Therapeutics Program includes nine branches: Biological Resources Branch; Biological Testing Branch; Drug Synthesis and Chemistry Branch; Grants and Contracts Operations Branch; Information Technology Branch; Natural Products Branch; Pharmaceutical Resources Branch; Pharmacology and Toxicology Branch; Screening Technologies Branch. Program is responsible for all preclinical phases of development, including acquisition and synthesis of materials, screening, production of diverse products, pharmaceutical development, toxicology, and pharmacology.

★ 24858 ★ U.S. Department of Health and Human Services
National Cancer Institute
Division of Cancer Treatment, Diagnosis, and Centers
Diagnostic Imaging Program
Executive Plaza N, Rm. 6000
6130 Executive Blvd.
Rockville, MD 20852
Phone: (301)496-9531 **Fax:** (301)480-5785
Email: sullivand@dtpepn.nci.nih.gov
Website: http://cancer.gov/bip
Dr. Daniel C. Sullivan, Assoc. Dir.
Activities/Fields: Responsible for both the stimulation of research in need-determined areas and the administration of grants, contracts, and cooperative agreements in support of development and evaluation of radiologic diagnostic imaging systems and related technology, including instrumentation and methodology to improve diagnosis of cancer and other diseases. This includes rapidly developing nonionizing modalities such as magnetic resonance imaging (MRI), diaphanography, and ultrasound as well as improvements in X-ray computed tomography (CT), digital radiography, positron emission tomography (PET), single photon emission computed tomography (SPECT), and other research in nuclear medicine and nuclide imaging such as the diagnostic applications of radio-labeled monoclonal antibodies.

★ 24859 ★ U.S. Department of Health and Human Services
National Cancer Institute
Division of Cancer Treatment, Diagnosis, and Centers
Radiation Research Program (Radiotherapy Development Branch)
Executive Plaza N, 6015-A
6130 Executive Blvd.
Bethesda, MD 20892-7440
Phone: (301)496-9360 **Fax:** (301)480-5785
Email: mahoneyf@mail.nih.gov
Dr. Francis J. Mahoney, PhD, Actg. Chf.
Activities/Fields: Cancer treatment. The scientific disciplines represented are radiation oncology, radi obiology, radiation chemistry, and radiation physics. Major areas of research in terms of funding are particle radiotherapy (photons, electrons, and particles), hyperthermia, radiation modifiers, radioimmunotherapy, radiobiology, expert systems, and radiation physics.

★ 24860 ★ U.S. Department of Health and Human Services
National Cancer Institute
Division of Cancer Treatment, Diagnosis, and Centers
Radiation Research Program
Executive Plaza N 6015-A
6130 Executive Blvd., MSC 7440
Bethesda, MD 20892-7440
Phone: (301)496-6111 **Fax:** (301)480-5785
Email: colemanc@mail.nih.gov
Dr. C. Norman Coleman, Assoc. Dir.
Activities/Fields: Diagnosis, staging, treatment, and post-treatmen t evaluation for the cancer patient for whom radiation and related forms of energy are used. It is an extramural radiation research program which establishes program priorities, allocates resources, maintains project integration, evaluates program effectiveness, and represents the program area in the management and scientific decision-making processes of the National Cancer Institute. This requires the coordination of research program activities with related programs elsewhere at NCI and NIH, with other federal agencies, and with national and international research organizations. The Program's branches are Diagnostic Imaging Research and Radiotherapy Development.

★ 24861 ★ U.S. Department of Health and Human Services
National Cancer Institute
Division of Clinical Sciences
NIH Bldg. 10, Rm. 12N214
10 Center Dr. MSC 1904
Bethesda, MD 20892-1904
Phone: (301)496-4251 **Fax:** (301)496-9962
Email: gc45e@nih.gov
Dr. Gregory A. Curt, Clin. Dir.
Activities/Fields: Intramural treatment-research arm of the e National Cancer Institute. It comprises branches for: Clinical Pharmacology, Medicine, NCI-Navy Medical Oncology, Pediatrics, Radiation Oncology, and Surgery.

★ 24862 ★ U.S. Department of Health and Human Services
National Cancer Institute
Division of Clinical Sciences
Cancer Prevention Studies Branch
Executive Plaza N, Rm. 211, MS 7326
6060 Executive Blvd.
Bethesda, MD 20892-7326
Phone: (301)496-8559 **Fax:** (301)435-8644
Email: pt1@nih.gov
Website: http://www-dcs.nci.nih.gov/branches/cpsb
Philip R. Taylor, MD, Chf.
Activities/Fields: Cancer control. It conducts intramural research in the areas of die t, nutrition, and cancer; genetics and cancer; cancer chemoprevention; and other cancer prevention strategies aimed at lowering human cancer risk. Current focus is on nutrition, primarily through development of prevention trials. Research includes studies in cancer epidemiology, clinical nutrition, and genetic epidemiology; and development of cancer prevention trials and epidemiologic methods.

★ 24863 ★ U.S. Department of Health and Human Services
National Cancer Institute
Division of Clinical Sciences
Cancer Therapy Evaluation Program
6130 Executive Blvd.
Suite 7018
Bethesda, MD 20892
Phone: (301)496-6138 **Fax:** (301)402-0084
Email: christianm@ctep.nci.nih.gov
Dr. Michele Christian, Assoc. Dir.
Activities/Fields: Responsible for the administration and coordination of the majority of the extramural clinical trials suppor ted by the Cancer Treatment Division. These programs include the activities of the clinical cooperative groups, the Phase I and Phase II drug development contractors, and the holders of investigator-initiated grants relating to cancer treatment. (Certain programs in developmental radiotherapy, such as high LET radiation, are administered in the Radiation Research Program; and the Phase I development of biologic response modifiers is handled by the Biological Response Modifiers Program.) Principal components of CTEP are: the Biometric Research Branch, Clinical Investigations Branch, Investigational Drug Branch, and the Regulatory Affairs Branch.

★ 24864 ★ U.S. Department of Health and Human Services
National Cancer Institute
Division of Clinical Sciences
Cancer Therapy Evaluation Program (Biometric Research Branch)
Executive Plaza N, Rm. 739
Bethesda, MD 20892
Phone: (301)496-4836 **Fax:** (301)402-0560
Website: http://ctep.info.nih.gov/BRB
Dr. Richard Simon, Chf.
Activities/Fields: Integral unit of Cancer Treatment and Diagnosis Division. It develops and evaluates clinical and biological data relating to cancer treatment.

★ 24865 ★ U.S. Department of Health and Human Services
National Cancer Institute
Division of Clinical Sciences
Dermatology Branch
37 Convent Dr.
Bldg. 10, Rm. 12N238
Bethesda, MD 20892
Phone: (301)496-2481 **Fax:** (301)496-5370
Email: skatz@boy-s.nih.gov
Website: http://www-dcs.nci.nih.gov/branches/dermatology/index.html
Stephen L. Katz, Chief
Activities/Fields: Etiology, diagnosis, and treatment of inflammatory and malignant diseases involving the skin and the host's response to these diseases.

★ 24866 ★ U.S. Department of Health and Human Services
National Cancer Institute
Division of Clinical Sciences
Hypoxia and Tumorigenesis Unit
Bldg. 37, Rm. 2C08
37 Convent Dr.
Bethesda, MD 20892-4255
Phone: (301)496-7279 **Fax:** (301)496-0497
Email: huange@mail.nih.gov
Website: http://www.nci.nih.gov/intra/LHC/hypoxia.htm
Eric Huang, Prin. Investigator
Activities/Fields: Mechanisms by which hypoxia contributes to tumorigenesis. Research focuses on hypoxia-inducible factor 1 (HIF1), and its role in tumor formation, progression, and metastasis.

★ 24867 ★ U.S. Department of Health and Human Services
National Cancer Institute
Division of Clinical Sciences
Intramural Research Program (Metabolism Branch)
NIH Bldg. 10, Rm. 4N115
10 Center Dr. MSC1374
Bethesda, MD 20892-1374
Phone: (301)496-6653 **Fax:** (301)496-9956
Email: tawald@helix.nih.gov
Dr. Thomas A. Waldmann, Chf.
Activities/Fields: Clinical and laboratory investigations focusing on performing molecular analyses of lymphocyte development and function, including purification of transactivating factors and the genes that encode them; functional genomics involving cDNA microarray analysis of human leukemia/lymphoma; developing antigen processing and the presentation to T lymphocytes with applications to vaccine design for AIDS and cancer; characterizing the multisubunit IL-2 and IL-15 receptors and developing their use as a target for immunotherapy using humanized monoclonal antibodies armed with toxins and alpha and beta emitting radionuclides; studying the arrangement of immunoglobulin and T-cell antigen receptor genes in normal and neoplastic cells; and evaluating biochemical events that accompany cell growth and the hormonal control of this growth as they relate to the study of malignancies.

★ 24868 ★ U.S. Department of Health and Human Services
National Cancer Institute
Division of Clinical Sciences
Laboratory of Human Carcinogenesis
37 Convent Dr.
Bldg. 37, Rm. 2COS
Bethesda, MD 20892-4255
Phone: (301)496-2048 **Fax:** (301)496-0497
Email: curtis_harris@nih.gov
Website: http://www.nci.nih.gov/intra/LHC/LHCPAGE.htm
Curtis C. Harris, MD, Ch.
Activities/Fields: Molecular mechanisms of human carcinogenesis; experimental approaches in biological systems for the extrapolation of carcinogenesis data and mechanisms from experimental animals to human situation; and host factors that determine differences in carcinogenesis susceptibility among individuals. **Pub:** *Bibliography*, annually.

★ 24869 ★ U.S. Department of Health and Human Services
National Cancer Institute
Division of Clinical Sciences
Medicine Branch
NIH Bldg. 10, Rm. 12N226
9000 Rockville Pike
Bethesda, MD 20892
Phone: (301)496-4916 **Fax:** (301)402-0172
Dr. Carmen Allegra, Actg. Ch.
Activities/Fields: Adult medical oncology unit with clinical programs emphasizing the broad area of internal medicine as related to cancer. Clinical emphasis is given to the diagnosis, staging, and treatment of Hodgkin's disease, malignant lymphomas, breast cancer, ovarian carcinoma, sarcomas, melanoma, AIDS/Kaposi's Sarcoma, chronic leukemias, and testicular carcinoma. The research program focuses on the general areas of drug resistance and cytogenetics of neoplastic and hemopoietic cells, tumor immunology, and the biochemical pharmacology of antineoplastic agents. A collaborative effort with the Clinical Pharmacology Branch and other groups concerned with pharmacokinetics is maintained. In addition, an active research program is in progress in the fields of hormone receptors and the molecular biology of hormone action.

★ 24870 ★ U.S. Department of Health and Human Services
National Cancer Institute
Division of Clinical Sciences
Surgery Branch
NIH Bldg. 10, Rm. 2B42
10 Center Drive
Bethesda, MD 20892
Phone: (301)496-4164 **Fax:** (301)402-1738
Email: sar@nih.gov
Dr. Steven Rosenberg, Chf.
Activities/Fields: Treatment of solid tumors and a broad program of laboratory research in c ancer. A wide variety of malignancies are studied, including melanomas, sarcomas, rectal cancer, breast carcinoma, pancreatic cancers, and head and neck cancers. The Branch investigates the use of adjuvant chemotherapy and immunotherapy and develops surgical techniques. Laboratory efforts of the Surgery Branch are closely related to its clinical activities and include programs in tumor immunology and surgical metabolism. Branch staff also serve as general surgeons to the entire National Institutes of Health and provide a variety of general surgical consultations not necessarily related to the field of cancer medicine.

★ 24871 ★ U.S. Department of Health and Human Services
National Cancer Institute
Division of Extramural Activities
6116 Executive Blvd., Ste. 8000
Mail Stop 8327
Bethesda, MD 20892
Phone: (301)496-5147 **Fax:** (301)402-0956
Email: mk74s@nih.gov
Website: http://www.nci.nih.gov
Marvin R. Kalt, PhD, Dir.
Activities/Fields: Administers and directs the National Cancer Institute's grant and contract review and processing activities; provides initial technical and scientific merit review of grants and contracts for the Institute; represents NCI on overall NIH extramural and collaborative program policy committees, coordinates such policy within NCI, and develops and recommends NCI policies and procedures as related to the review of grants and contracts; coordinates the Institute's review of research grant and training programs with the National Cancer Advisory Board; coordinates the implementation of committee management policies within NCI and provides the Institute's staff support for the National Cancer Advisory Board; coordinates program planning and evaluation in the extramural area; and provides scientific reports and analyses to the Institute's grant and contract programs. Principal components are the Research Programs Review Branch, Resources and Training Review Branch, Special Review and Logistics Branch, Program Coordination and Referral Branch, Applied Information Systems Branch, and the Research Analysis and Evaluation Branch, which analyzes and indexes the scientific content of all grants awarded by NCI as well as NCI contracts and extramural programs.

★ 24872 ★ U.S. Department of Health and Human Services
National Cancer Institute
Division of Extramural Activities
Special Review and Resources
6130 Executive Blvd. EPN Rm. 605
Bethesda, MD 20892
Phone: (301)496-7903 **Fax:** (301)402-0742
Wilna A. Woods, PhD, Ch.
Activities/Fields: Branch reviews the technical merit of all research and development, scientific resource, and scientific support contract proposals submitted to NCI in response to Requests for Proposals (RFPs).

★ 24873 ★ U.S. Department of Health and Human Services
National Cancer Institute
Frederick Cancer Research and Development Center
Bldg. 427, Rm. 1
PO Box B
Frederick, MD 21702-1201
Phone: (301)846-1113 **Fax:** (301)846-6628
Email: rd5lm@nih.gov
Website: http://web.ncifcrf.gov/
Dr. Ronald H. DeFelice, Chf.
Activities/Fields: Genetic and biochemical events related to the development and expression for the malignant phenotype; and develops strategies for therapeutic intervention in the malignant process based on these findings.

★ 24874 ★ U.S. Department of Health and Human Services
National Cancer Institute
International Cancer Information Center
6116 Executive Blvd.
Suite 300-A
Rockville, MD 20852
Phone: (301)496-9096 **Fax:** (301)480-8105
Email: gisele.sarosy@mail.nih.gov
Website: http://www.cancer.gov
Dr. Gisele Sarosy, MD, Actg. Assoc. Dir.
Activities/Fields: Purpose of ICRDB is to collect, analyze, and disseminate all data useful in prevention, diagnosis, treatment and supportive care of cancer and, as feasible, to disseminate results of cancer research undertaken in any country for the use of anyone conducting cancer research in any country. **Pub:** *Overviews.* • *Recent Reviews.*

★ 24875 ★ U.S. Department of Health and Human Services
National Cancer Institute
Laboratory of Biochemistry
NIH Bldg. 37, Rm. 6106C, MSC 4255
9000 Rockville Pike
Bethesda, MD 20892-4255
Phone: (301)496-5957
Email: ml4x@nih.gov
Dr. Michael Lichten, MD, Chf., Lab. of Biochem.
Activities/Fields: Relationship between structure and function in biological systems and on the regulation of cellular processes. The research involves prokaryotes and a range of eukaryote systems selected because of their potential for yielding important information on cellular structure, function, regulation, development, and differentiation. The study of regulation encompasses regulation of gene expression, regulation by interaction of macromolecules, and regulation of cells by hormones and ions. Work is carried out on both the molecular and cellular level. Techniques include those of biochemistry, physical chemistry, cell biology, and molecular genetics. **Pub:** *Proceedings.*

★ 24876 ★ U.S. Department of Health and Human Services
National Cancer Institute
Laboratory of Biological Chemistry
NIH Bldg. 37
9000 Rockville Pike
Bethesda, MD 20892
Phone: (301)496-4116 **Fax:** (301)496-5839
Dr. Richard Cysyk, Chf.
Activities/Fields: Cellular reactions that are critical to the control of tumor cell proliferation or differentiation. Recent advances in cell biology are evaluated for possible targets, and agents are designed to interact with these targets and are evaluated for biochemical and antitumor effectiveness. An important aspect of this mission is to develop appropriate in vivo systems to evaluate the chemotherapeutic effectiveness of agents shown to be active in simpler in vitro model systems. Accordingly, the Laboratory is involved in identifying endogenous factors present in vivo that modify drug action and influence differential toxicity with the aim of manipulating these factors to enhance antitumor activity.

★ 24877 ★ U.S. Department of Health and Human Services
National Cancer Institute
Laboratory of Cell Biology
NIH Bldg. 37, Rm. 1A09
Convent Dr., MSC 4254
Bethesda, MD 20892-4254
Phone: (301)496-1530 **Fax:** (301)402-0450
Email: mgottesman@nih.gov
Dr. Michael M. Gottesman, MD, Chf., Lab. of Cel Biology
Activities/Fields: Basic cell biology in relation to cancer immunology. Major emphasis is on characterization of tumor antigens biochemically and immunologically and the immune responses they evoke. Studies include antigens isolated from sarcomas, leukemias, and melanomas. As a corollary to this study, the biologic properties of alien histocompatibility antigens and variant antigens in neoplasms are also under study.

★ 24878 ★ U.S. Department of Health and Human Services
National Cancer Institute
Laboratory of Cellular Carcinogenesis and Tumor Promotion
National Cancer Institute Bldg. 37 Rm. 4068
37 Convent Dr. MSC 4255
Bethesda, MD 20892-4255
Phone: (301)496-2162 **Fax:** (301)496-8709
Email: yuspas@mail.nih.gov
Dr. Stuart Yuspa, Chf.
Activities/Fields: Molecular and biological changes that occur at the cellular and tissue level during the process of carcinogenesis. Objectives are to: define normal regulatory mechanisms for cellular growth and differentiation; determine the mechanism by which carcinogens alter normal regulation and the biological nature of these alterations; investigate the mechanism by which tumor promoters enhance the expression of carcinogen-induced alterations; identify cellular determinants for enhanced susceptibility or resistance to carcinogens and tumor promoters; and elucidate the mechanism by which certain pharmacologic agents inhibit carcinogenesis.

★ 24879 ★ U.S. Department of Health and Human Services
National Cancer Institute
Laboratory of Chemoprevention
NIH Bldg. 41, Rm. C629
4 Library Dr., MSC 5055
Bethesda, MD 20892
Phone: (301)496-6108 **Fax:** (301)496-8395
Email: Robertsa@dce41.nci.nih.gov
Website: http://rex.nci.nih.gov/RESEARCH/basic/lc/lcpage.htm
Dr. Anita Roberts, PhD, Chf.
Activities/Fields: Cell regulation by transfering growth factor-B; carcinogenesis. **Frmly:** (1998) Laboratory of Chemoprevention.

★ 24880 ★ U.S. Department of Health and Human Services
National Cancer Institute
Laboratory of Comparative Carcinogenesis
NCI At Frederick
Bldg. 538
Frederick, MD 21702-1201
Phone: (301)846-1241 **Fax:** (301)846-5946
Email: keefer@mail.ncifcrf.gov
Website: http://ccr.cancer.gov/Labs/Lab.asp?LabID=89
Dr. Larry Keefer, PhD, Chf.
Activities/Fields: Effects of chemical carcinogens in rodents and nonhuman primates in order to identify differences between species that are important for interspecies extrapolations of the effects of chemical agents, including extrapolations to man, and that afford experimental approaches to the elucidation of mechanisms in chemical carcinogenesis. Research is oriented toward identification of susceptibility and resistance to chemical carcinogenesis and toward identification, description, and investigation of mechanisms for interspecies differences and for cell and organ specificity in chemical carcinogenesis. The Laboratory investigates the roles of perinatal age period and pregnancy in modifying susceptibility to chemical carcinogens; studies mechanisms of action of the carcinogenic metals, cadmium, and nickel; and utilizes synthetic nitric oxide carrier compounds (NONOates) to investigate the biologic effects of this multifunctional bioregulatory compound.

★ 24881 ★ U.S. Department of Health and Human Services
National Cancer Institute
Laboratory of Experimental Carcinogenesis
NIH Bldg. 37, Rm. 3C28
37 Convent Dr.
Bethesda, MD 20892
Phone: (301)496-1935 **Fax:** (301)496-0734
Email: fran_williams@nih.gov
Website: http://neoplasia.nci.nih.gov
Dr. Snorri S. Thorgeirsson, Chf.
Activities/Fields: Elucidate mechanisms of malignant transformation in human and animal cells by chemical carcinogens; determine critical cellular and genetic factors involved in initiation, promotion, and progression of transformed cells; and apply the knowledge obtained from studying animal models toward effective prevention of cancer in man. Principal areas of research interest are the use of transgenic mouse models in cancer research, molecular and cellular aspects of hepatic stem cells; multidrug resistant gene family; chemical carcinogenesis and mutagenesis; molecular biology; and protein chemistry.

★ 24882 ★ U.S. Department of Health and Human Services
National Cancer Institute
Laboratory of Experimental Immunology
NCI-CCR
Bldg. 560, Rm. 3193 NCI
Frederick, MD 21702-1201
Phone: (301)846-1323 **Fax:** (301)846-1673
Email: ortaldo@ncifcrf.gov
Dr. John Ortaldo, Chf.
Activities/Fields: Cellular and humoral components of the immune response that may be involved in resistance to tumor growth; studies growth factors and other biological response modifiers (BRMs) that may be involved in the regulation of tumor growth; studies the mechanism of action of various biologicals at the cellular and molecular level; develops new biologicals and BRMs and investigates the effects of selected BRMs on the host and on tumor growth; and develops protocols for optimal biological response modification and evaluates the therapeutic efficacy of these substances in experimental animal tumor systems and cancer patients.

★ 24883 ★ U.S. Department of Health and Human Services
National Cancer Institute
Laboratory of Experimental Pathology
6116 Executive Blvd., 7064
Bethesda, MD 20892-8314
Phone: (301)496-2818 **Fax:** (301)402-1829
Email: saffiotti@nih.gov
Dr. Umberto Saffiotti, Chf.
Activities/Fields: Neoplastic transformation and its underlying mechanisms, with particular emphasis on epithelial target cells. It plans, develops, and implements research on the experimental pathology of carcinogenesis, and is especially concerned with the induction of neoplasia by chemical and physical factors in epithelial tissues. Activities include: development, characterization, and evaluation of experimental pathology models of human cancer, such as cancers of the respiratory tract, by in vivo and in vitro carcinogenesis methods; development and characterization of tissue culture systems for quantitative study of the effects of carcinogens alone or in combination; and research on mechanisms of carcinogenesis correlating different levels of biological organization, from human and animal whole organisms, organs, and tissue, to the cellular, subcellular, and molecular levels. **Pub:** *Proceedings.*

★ 24884 ★ U.S. Department of Health and Human Services
National Cancer Institute
Laboratory of Genetics
NIH Bldg. 37, Rm. 2B04
37 Convent Dr.
Bethesda, MD 20892-4256
Phone: (301)496-1734 **Fax:** (301)402-1031
Email: potter@helix.nih.gov
Dr. Michael Potter, Chf.
Activities/Fields: Role of genes that determine susceptibility and resistance to neoplastic development and special genes and their products that are associated with the neoplastic state (oncogenes, retroviral gene products, tumor associated antigens). Past activities have involved studies of the plasma cell tumor system in mice, and research continues on the organization of immunoglobulin genes and gene families and structure-function correlations with monoclonal antibodies. Areas of current research interest include: amino acid and DNA sequences, recombinant DNA technology, tissue culture, and hybridoma-monoclonal and antibody production.

★ 24885 ★ U.S. Department of Health and Human Services
National Cancer Institute
Laboratory of Human Carcinogenesis
NIH Bldg. 37, Rm. 2C05
37 Convent Dr.
Bethesda, MD 20892-4255
Phone: (301)496-2048 **Fax:** (301)496-0497
Curtis Harris, Chf.
Activities/Fields: Mechanisms of carcinogenesis in epithelial cells from humans and experimental animals; experimental approaches in biological systems for the extrapolation of carcinogenesis data and mechanisms from experimental animals to the human situation; and host factors that determine differences in carcinogenic susceptibility among individuals. Research is carried out in three areas: molecular and biochemical epidemiology; carcinogen macromolecular interaction; and in vitro carcinogenesis.

★ 24886 ★ U.S. Department of Health and Human Services
National Cancer Institute
Laboratory of Immunobiology
Frederick Cancer Research and Development Center
Ft. Detrick
Immunobiology Bldg. 560, Rm. 12-71
Frederick, MD 21702-1201
Phone: (301)846-1557 **Fax:** (301)846-6145
Email: bz5v@nih.gov
Dr. Berton Zbar, Chf.
Activities/Fields: Mechanisms of the effector arm of the immune system and cancer genetics. Its program comprises three interacting areas: the Office of the Chief, the Immunopathology Section, and the Cellular Immunity Section. Areas of research interest have included studies on cellular effectors of the immune system; the chemotaxis of leukocytes; the mechanisms of activation of macrophages to kill tumor cells; identification of genetic changes; human solid tumors; cloning of recessive oncogenes; and the suppression of malignant phenotype by gene replacement.

★ 24887 ★ U.S. Department of Health and Human Services
National Cancer Institute
Laboratory of Mathematical Biology
Frederick Cancer Research and Development Center
Bldg. 469, Rm. 151
Frederick, MD 21702-1201
Phone: (301)846-5532 **Fax:** (301)846-5598
Email: jmaizel@ncifcrf.gov
Website: http://www-lecb.ncifcrf.gov
Dr. Jacob V. Maizel, Chf.
Activities/Fields: Studies nucleic acid sequences, protein sequences, and macromolecular structure (including prediction of molecular structure) using methods of computation; kinetics of metabolic systems using computational and modeling methodology; applications of image analysis to micrographs and two-dimensional gels; theoretical immunology; and membrane biophysics and structure.

★ 24888 ★ U.S. Department of Health and Human Services
National Cancer Institute
Laboratory of Medicinal Chemistry
NIH Bldg. 376, Rm. 104
376 Boyles St.
Frederick, MD 21702
Phone: (301)846-5953 **Fax:** (301)846-6033
Victor E. Marquez, Chf.
Activities/Fields: Rational discovery of antitumor agents; implements basic research on the mechanisms of antitumor drug action and drug toxicity; incorporates knowledge of biochemical/molecular mechanisms into a drug synthesis program aimed at optimizing drug efficacy through enhancement of antitumor activity/selectivity and/or minimization of toxicity; and develops strategies for improving the clinical utility of new or existing anticancer drugs by overcoming tumor resistance and/or by protection of normal tissues against toxicity. Compounds with potential antitumor activity are synthesized and effects of such agents are assessed in experimental tumor systems in vitro and in vivo and on a variety of potential subcellular target sites (e.g., nucleic acids, nuclear proteins, microtubular protein, and enzyme systems). Analytical methodology for in vivo studies with new agents is developed, and, where warranted, biological studies with these agents are extended to the preclinical and Phase I stages. A wide range of methodologies is currently in use.

★ 24889 ★ U.S. Department of Health and Human Services
National Cancer Institute
Laboratory of Molecular Biology
NIH Bldg. 37, Rm. 5106
37 Convent Dr. MSC-4264
Bethesda, MD 20892-4264
Phone: (301)496-4797 **Fax:** (301)402-1344
Email: pasta@helix.nih.gov
Dr. Ira H. Pastan, Chf.
Activities/Fields: Immunotoxins for treatment of human cancer. To accomplish this, Pseudomonas exotoxin is coupled to monoclonal antibodies that react with specific human cancers. The activity of these conjugates is assessed in cell culture and animal models. Toxicity studies are conducted with monkeys, and the first promising immunotoxins are being prepared for clinical testing. The mechanisms by which immunotoxins enter and kill cells is studied by biochemical, genetic, and cell biological approaches in order to devise ways to improve the therapeutic efficiency of these agents. **Pub:** *Proceedings.*

★ 24890 ★ U.S. Department of Health and Human Services
National Cancer Institute
Laboratory of Molecular Carcinogenesis
NIH Bldg. 37, Rm. 3E24
9000 Rockville Pike
Bethesda, MD 20892
Phone: (301)496-6849 **Fax:** (301)496-8419
Harry V. Gelboin, PhD, Chf.
Activities/Fields: Cellular and biochemical events and mechanisms involved in carcinogenesis. Activities include: examination of the unusual properties of cells from patients who may be predisposed to cancer because of hereditary disease and investigation of various mechanisms of DNA repair using DNA transfection and sequencing to define the genomic changes observed; investigation of the genetics, multiplicity, and structure of the drug and carcinogen metabolizing enzyme systems; studies using monoclonal antibodies to gain an understanding of individual differences and their relationship to drug and carcinogen sensitivity; investigation of the mutation, recombination, and repair caused by carcinogen treatment using shuttle vectors that replicate in mammalian and bacterial cells; and studies of the relationship between the structure and function in chromatin (using biochemical and immunological methods), including evaluation of the regulatory properties of the non-histone proteins.

★ 24891 ★ U.S. Department of Health and Human Services
National Cancer Institute
Laboratory of Molecular Immunoregulation
Frederick Cancer Research and Development Center
Bldg. 560 Rm. 21-89A
Frederick, MD 21702-1201
Phone: (301)846-1551 **Fax:** (301)846-7042
Email: oppenhei@ncifcrf.gov
Website: http://rex.nci.nih.gov/RESEARCH/basic/lmi/lmipage.htm
Dr. Joost Oppenheim, Chf.
Activities/Fields: Biochemical and molecular effects of biological response modifiers on host resistance to cancer. It investigates at a molecular level the inter- and intracellular processes that regulate host defense mechanisms, including isolation of proteins, RNA, and DNA that regulate production and activities of lymphokines, cytokines, and their receptors. It utilizes in vitro and in vivo models to study the modulation by lymphokines/cytokines of cellular functions that participate in host defense. In addition, Laboratory devises new tests for diagnosis of cancer and for better definition of the immune status and more critical evaluation of biological response modifiers (BRMs). It evaluates the effects of BRMs on immunoregulatory pathways and host defense mechanisms; and generates BRMs that modify host defense mechanisms.

★ 24892 ★ U.S. Department of Health and Human Services
National Cancer Institute
Laboratory of Molecular Pharmacology
NIH Bldg. 37, Rm. 5968A
37 Convent Dr. MSC 4255
Bethesda, MD 20892-4255
Phone: (301)496-5944 **Fax:** (301)402-0752
Dr. Yves Pommier, Chf.
Activities/Fields: Mechanisms of action of anticancer agents are studied in culture and subcellular systems, with particular attention to effects involving DNA and nuclear proteins. Investigations focus on the relation between drug-induced macromolecular damage (and its repair) and cell survival. Drugs are also used as probes of the structure and function of DNA and chromatin. Experimental approaches include cell culture, DNA macromolecular damage measurements, DNA sequence analysis, and nuclear protein fractionation techniques. Major areas of current interest are the effects of anticancer drugs on topoisomerase enzymes and on cell cycle regulation. **Pub:** *Proceedings.* • *Research Reports.*

★ 24893 ★ U.S. Department of Health and Human Services
National Cancer Institute
Laboratory of Molecular Virology
NIH Bldg. 41, Rm. B602
41 Library Dr., MSC 5055
Bethesda, MD 20892
Phone: (301)496-9867 **Fax:** (301)496-4951
Email: hagerg@exchange.nih.gov
Website: http://rex.nci.nih.gov/RESEARCH/basic/lrbge/lrbge.htm
Dr. Gordon Hager, Ch.
Activities/Fields: Normal and abnormal regulation of gene expression. Studies employ methods from molecular biology, immunology, virology, and cell biology in an attempt to determine in specific cases what signals regulate gene expression. Current efforts involve both viral and eukaryotic genetic units. Research focuses on genes which are regulated at the level of transcription and which, in some cases, are responsive to induction by hormones or transacting proteins. Studies involve oncogenes and the mutations which are responsible for activation of these genes in neoplasia; and histocompatibility antigens and the roles of these genes in immune surveillance and tumor immunity. **Frmly:** (1996) Laboratory of Molecular Virology.

★ 24894 ★ U.S. Department of Health and Human Services
National Cancer Institute
Laboratory of Pathology
NIH Bldg. 10, Rm. 2A33
10 Center Dr. MSC 1500
Bethesda, MD 20892-1500
Phone: (301)496-3185 **Fax:** (301)402-0043
Dr. Lance Liotta, Chf.
Activities/Fields: Surgical pathology and autopsy services at the Clinical Center of the NIH. Offers diagnostic electron microscopy studies and cytopathologic services, including exfoliative and fine needle aspiration; provides all types of histological services and staining procedures for National Cancer Institute scientists; and conducts research programs in various areas of experimental cancer research. It also provides a fully accredited residency program in anatomic pathology. Component sections of the Laboratory are: Biochemical Pathology Section, Cytopathology Section, Gene Regulation Section, Hematopathology Section, Surgical +Pathology Section, Postmortem Section, Tumor Invasion and +Metastases Section, Ultrastructural Pathology Section, Molecular Pathology Section, Extracellular Matrix Pathology Section, Molecular Immune Activation Secion, and Women's Cancers Section. **Pub:** *Proceedings.* • *Research Reports.*

★ 24895 ★ U.S. Department of Health and Human Services
National Cancer Institute
Laboratory of Tumor Cell Biology
NIH Bldg. 37, Rm. 6A11
9000 Rockville Pike
Bethesda, MD 20892
Phone: (301)496-6007 **Fax:** (301)496-8394
Dr. Genoveffa Franchini, Chf.
Activities/Fields: Cellular proliferation, cell differentiation, and biochemical growth characteristics of normal and malignant mammalian cells both in vivo and in vitro, which will permit the optimal use of antitumor agents in the treatment of cancer and AIDS. Particular attention is given to human leukemias and lymphomas, acquired immunodeficiency syndrome (AIDS), Kaposi's sarcoma, antiviral agents, and vaccine development.

★ 24896 ★ U.S. Department of Health and Human Services
National Cancer Institute
Laboratory of Tumor Immunology and Biology
Laboratory of Tumor Immunology and Biology
NIH Bldg. 10, Rm. 8B07
10 Center Dr., MSC 1750
Bethesda, MD 20892
Phone: (301)496-4343 **Fax:** (301)496-2756
Email: js141c@nih.gov
Website: http://rex.nci.nih.gov/RESEARCH/basic/ltib/ltibpage.htm
Jeffrey Schlom, PhD, Chf.
Activities/Fields: Immunologic markers specific for or associated with various human neoplasms, with the ultimate aim of applying these toward the diagnosis, prognosis, and treatment of human cancer. Activities focus on: the generation and characterization of monoclonal antibodies to tumor-associated determinants, with particular emphasis on the study of human carcinomas; conjugation of monoclonal antibodies to isotopes or toxins to aid in the diagnosis, localization, and potential elimination of tumor cells; studies on the association between specific murine and human genetic elements and tumorigenesis using techniques of gene cloning and molecular hybridization; and development of immunoassays to aid in the characterization of human tumor cell populations and in the diagnosis or prognosis of certain human cancers.

★ 24897 ★ U.S. Department of Health and Human Services
National Cancer Institute
Laboratory of Viral Carcinogenesis
Frederick Cancer Research and Development Center
Bldg. 560, Rm. 21-105
Frederick, MD 21702-1201
Phone: (301)846-1296 **Fax:** (301)846-1686
Email: obrien@ncifcrf.gov
Dr. Stephen O'Brien, PhD, Chf.
Activities/Fields: Genetic and cellular mechanism of neoplastic transformation in man and mammalian model systems. Studies are conducted on the specific cellular genes that participate in transformation from several distinct approaches. Interests include studies on: endogenous mammalian retroviruses and their role in gene regulation and neoplasia; the expression of transforming viruses, their included oncogenes, and their ancestral cellular homologs during development and carcinogenesis using recombinant DNA technologies and systems; molecular processes of chemical carcinogenesis using gene cloning, cell transfection, and cell biology procedures; somatic cell genetic approaches to neoplastic transformation and the cytogenetic consequences of transformation; and activities of hormone-like growth factors and tumor promoters to determine their regulation of transformation sensitivity genes and transforming genes and of the progressive stages of transformation of cells in vitro and in vivo.

★ 24898 ★ U.S. Department of Health and Human Services
National Cancer Institute
Macromolecular Crystallogrophy Laboratory
Bldg. 536, Rm. 4
PO Box B
Frederick, MD 21702-1201
Phone: (301)846-5036 **Fax:** (301)846-6128
Email: wlodawer@ncifcrf.gov
Website: http://mcl1.ncifcrf.gov/
Dr. Alexander Wlodawer, Dir.
Activities/Fields: Macromolecular crystallography and its applications.

★ 24899 ★ U.S. Department of Health and Human Services
National Cancer Institute
Memorial Sloan-Kettering Cancer Center
Institute for Cancer Research
(Clinical Nutrition Research Unit)
1250 1st Ave.
New York, NY 10021
Phone: (212)639-2000 **Fax:** (212)639-5115
Dr. Richard S. Rivlin, Prog. Dir.
Activities/Fields: Nutrition and cancer prevention; bone and mineral metabolism; energy intake expenditure; immunology and infection; lipid metabolism; cellular growth; vitamins and trace elements; DNA repair and gene expression; hormonal regulation.

★ 24900 ★ U.S. Department of Health and Human Services
National Cancer Institute
Office of the Deputy Directory for Extramural Sciences
Comprehensive Minority Biomedical Section
6116 Exectutive Blvd., Ste. 7028
MSC 8350
Bethesda, MD 20892
Phone: (301)496-7344 **Fax:** (301)402-4551
Email: ss165i@nih.gov
Website: http://minorityopportunity.nci.nih.gov
Dr. Sanya A. Springfield, PhD, Chf.
Activities/Fields: Program reflects a broad-based approach to every aspect of the minority cancer problem, with particular focus on the cancer incidence mortality disparity between the black community and the general population. Emphasis is on increased funding for research by minority scientists, concerted enrollment of minority physicians and patients in clinical trials programs, cancer prevention and awareness heightening, and training and manpower development.

★ 24901 ★ U.S. Department of Health and Human Services
National Cancer Institute
Office of International Affairs
6130 Executive Blvd. Ste 100
Bethesda, MD 20892-7301
Phone: (301)496-4761 **Fax:** (301)496-3954
Email: nc6@cu.nih.gov
Website: http://www.nci.nih.gov/AboutNci/OIA
Dr. Federico Welsch, Assoc. Dir.
Activities/Fields: Promotes cooperative research through exchange programs with institutes in foreign countries; provides cancer research information worldwide, directly and through other institutions; and maintains liaison with international organizations and agencies involved in cancer research.

★ 24902 ★ U.S. Department of Health and Human Services
National Cancer Institute
Office of Technology Development
Executive Plaza South, Rm. 450
6120 Executive Blvd.
Rockville, MD 20852
Phone: (301)496-0477 **Fax:** (301)402-2117
Website: http://www-otd.nci.nih.gov/
Dr. Kathleen Sybert, Dir.
Activities/Fields: Responsible for administering cooperative research and development agreements with industry and universities; and providing patent management and licensing support.

★ 24903 ★ U.S. Department of Health and Human Services
National Center for Chronic Disease Prevention and Health Promotion
Mail Stop
4770 Buford Hwy., NE
Atlanta, GA 30341-3717
Phone: (770)488-5080 **Fax:** (770)488-5969
Email: ccdinfo@cdc.gov
Website: http://www.cdc.gov/nccdphp
Dr. James S. Marks, Dir.
Activities/Fields: Prevention of chronic diseases such as cardiovascular disease, diabetes, and cancer. Translates research findings into community programs and healthier lifestyles. Supports programs to improve nutrition, reproductive health, and exercise, and to discourage destructive behaviors, such as alcohol abuse and smoking. NCCDPHP's major organization units are: Office on Smoking and Health, the Division of Reproductive Health, the Division of Nutrition and Physical Activity, the Division of Adolescent and School Health, the Division of Diabetes Translation, the Division of Adult and Community Health, and the Division of Oral Health. **Frmly:** Center for Health Promotion and Education; (1991) Center for Chronic Disease Prevention and Health Promotion.

★ 24904 ★ U.S. Department of Health and Human Services
National Center for Chronic Disease Prevention and Health Promotion
Chronic Disease Control and Community Intervention Division
1600 Clifton Rd. NE
Atlanta, GA 30333
Phone: (770)488-5403 **Fax:** (770)488-5971
Email: dvm0@cdc.gov
David McQueen, Assoc. Dir.
Activities/Fields: Chronic diseases, including maternal and child health, breast and cervical cancer, diabetes, smoking, adolescents and school health, AIDS and women, and reproductive health. **Pub:** *Chronic Disease Notes and Reports.*

★ 24905 ★ U.S. Department of Health and Human Services
National Center for Environmental Health
Birth Defects and Developmental Disabilities Division
Health Studies Branch
4770 Buford Hwy, NE, F34
Chamblee, GA 30341-3724
Phone: (770)488-7366 **Fax:** (770)488-7361
Email: gpo1@cec.gov
Website: http://www.cdc.gov/ncbddd/default.htm
Dr. Colleen Boyle, Asst. Dir.
Activities/Fields: Surveillance research, intervention methods, and technical consultations leading to the design, conduct, analysis, and evaluation of epidemiologic studies of adverse reproductive outcomes (i.e., birth defects, developmental disabilities, genetic abnormalities, mental retardation, and spontaneous abortion). Activities include population-based surveillance, use of case-control methods, and randomized controlled trails. In addition, cooperative agreements with states have been developed in an effort to increase the Division's research capacity into prevention effectiveness. **Pub:** *Proceedings.* • *Research Reports.*

★ 24906 ★ U.S. Department of Health and Human Services
National Center for Environmental Health
Environmental Hazards and Health Effects Division
1600 Clifton Rd. M.S E-19
Atlanta, GA 30333
Phone: (404)498-1300 **Fax:** (404)498-1313
Email: mam7@cdc.gov
Dr. Michael McGeehin, Dir.
Activities/Fields: Environmental public health problems and their prevention. Specific areas of interest include toxic chemicals, natural environmental hazards, environmentally-induced disease, international environmental health, and indoor air pollution.

★ 24907 ★ U.S. Department of Health and Human Services
National Center for Environmental Health
Environmental Hazards and Health Effects Division
Health Studies Branch
1600 Clifton Rd. NE
MS-E23
Atlanta, GA 30333
Phone: (404)498-1340 **Fax:** (404)498-1355
Email: chr1@cdc.gov
Website: http://www.cdc.gov/nech/hsb
Carol Rubin, DVM, Chf.
Activities/Fields: Epidemiologic studies on environmental exposure and health effects. Also studies the epidemiology of natural disasters. This includes planning, implementing, and reporting epidemiologic research and providing technical assistance and assessment of risk from environmental hazards such as toxic chemicals, waste disposal, indoor air pollution, passive smoking, controlled substance analogs, and natural and man-made disasters.

★ 24908 ★ U.S. Department of Health and Human Services
National Center for Environmental Health
Environmental Health Laboratory Sciences Division
CDC
4770 Buford Hwy.
Chamblee, GA 30341-3724
Phone: (770)488-7950 **Fax:** (770)488-4839
Email: ejs1@cdc.gov
Website: http://www.cdc.gov/nceh/dls/default.htm
Dr. Eric J. Sampson, Dir.
Activities/Fields: Chronic disease and toxicant exposure. Laboratory methods development accounts for most of the activities related to problem definition in chronic disease. These activities include developing laboratory methods in cardiovascular disease, cancer, genetic markers of certain chronic diseases, and biomedical indices of nutritional status. To improve problem definition in toxicant exposure, Division is developing new and improving existing laboratory methods for detecting and measuring: body burdens of hazardous substances and their metabolites; and early stages of organ damage (using biochemical markers for organ-specific dysfunction). Services, including advice, assistance, and information, are available to state and local public health authorities, federal agencies, international organizations, academic, international, and private laboratories, and professional organizations in support of laboratory science in the fields of environmental health and non-infectious chronic diseases. The Division also collaborates with other CDC organizations as appropriate. Its consists of the Toxicology Branch, Clinical Biochemistry Branch, Nutritional Biochemistry Branch, Special Activities Branch, and Molecular +Biology Branch. **Pub:** *Proceedings.*

★ 24909 ★ U.S. Department of Health and Human Services
National Center for Health Statistics
6525 Belcrest Rd.
Hyattsville, MD 20782
Phone: (301)458-4500
Email: efs2@cdc.gov
Website: http://www.cdc.gov/nchs/
Edward Sondik, Dir.
Activities/Fields: National health statistics; conduct research in survey and statistical methodology; provide specialized training programs and technical assistance; and coordinate cooperative programs with state, national, and international organizations. Principal components include the Office of Analysis and Epidemiology, Office of Research and Methodology, and Office of Vital and Health Statistics Systems (Health Care Statistics Division, Health Examination Statistics Division, Health Interview Statistics Division, and Vital Statistics Division). Data Base NCHS maintains data systems that produce data in the following areas: extent of illness and disability in the population; distribution and normative standards for physiological and nutritional measurement; national vital statistics, including births, deaths, marriages, and divorces; hospital, nursing home, and ambulatory care utilization; health expenditures; family formation, growth, and dissolution; and other major health topics. **Pub:** *Advance Data.* • *Health U S*, annually. • *National Vital Statistics Report.* • *Vital and Health Statistics Series.* • *Vital Statistics of the U S*, annually.

★ 24910 ★ U.S. Department of Health and Human Services
National Center for Health Statistics
Office of Vital and Health Statistics Systems
Health Care Statistics Division
3311 Toledo Rd., Rm. 3409
Hyattsville, MD 20782
Phone: (301)458-4369 **Fax:** (301)458-4031
Email: ttm1@cdc.gov
Thomas McLemore, Dep. Dir.
Activities/Fields: Division's data collection and analysis program administers provider-based health care surveys, which monitor the nation's use of health care resources (including hospitals, nursing homes, and physicians). Specific areas of interest are health statistics, epidemiology, and health services research. Division comprised of branches for ambulatory care statistics, hospital care statistics, long-term care statistics, and technical services. **Pub:** *Vital and Health Statistics Report Series 13.*

★ 24911 ★ U.S. Department of Health and Human Services
National Center for Health Statistics
Office of Vital and Health Statistics Systems
Health Examination Statistics Division
6525 Belcrest Rd., Rm. 1000
Hyattsville, MD 20782
Phone: (301)458-4372 **Fax:** (301)436-5431
Clifford Johnson, Contact
Activities/Fields: Nutritional status for adults and children, growth and development of children, nominative or descriptive physiological data for children and adults, chronic disease in adults, and some environmental exposures. **Pub:** *Vital and Health Statistics Series II.*

★ 24912 ★ U.S. Department of Health and Human Services
National Center for Health Statistics
Office of Vital and Health Statistics Systems
Health Interview Statistics Division (Illness and Disability Statistics Branch)
6525 Belcrest Rd.
Hyattsville, MD 20782
Phone: (301)458-4004 **Fax:** (301)458-4035
Email: bzg5@cdc.gov
Website: http://www.cdc.gov/nchs/nhis
Dr. Jane F. Gentleman, PhD, Contact
Activities/Fields: Responsible for maintaining, analyzing, and preparing reports from National Health Interview Survey data. Areas of interest include estimates on illness and disability, use of health care services, and other health-related topics. **Pub:** *Series No. 10 National Health Interview Survey.* • *Summary Statistics*, annually.

★ 24913 ★ U.S. Department of Health and Human Services
National Center for Health Statistics
Office of Vital and Health Statistics Systems
Health Interview Statistics Division
6525 Belcrest Rd., Rm. 850
Hyattsville, MD 20782
Phone: (301)458-4001 **Fax:** (301)436-3484
Email: jgentleman@cdc.gov
Jane Gentleman, Dir.
Activities/Fields: Conducts the National Health Interview Survey (NHIS), a major data collection program of the National Center for Health Statistics. In accordance with the National Health Survey Act of 1956, NHIS provides continuing survey and special follow-up studies on major current health issues affecting the civilian noninstitutionalized population of the United States. NHIS data are obtained through personal interviews with household members conducted each week throughout the year in a probability sample of households; interviewing is performed by a staff employed by the Bureau of the Census. Specific activities involve collection and analysis of data concerning the incidence of acute illness and injuries, prevalence of chronic conditions and impairments, extent of disability, utilization of health care services, and other health-related topics. Data collected over a one-year period form the basis for the development of annual estimates of the health characteristics of the population and for the analysis of trends in those characteristics. Division comprises branches for Illness and Disability Statistics, Survey Planning and Development, Systems and Programming, and Utilization and Expenditures Statistics. **Pub:** *Advanced Data Reports.* • *Public use data files; peer-reviewed journal articles.* • *Vital and Health Statistics Series Reports.* **Frmly:** (2000) Health Interview Statistics Division.

★ 24914 ★ U.S. Department of Health and Human Services
National Center for Infectious Diseases
1600 Clifton Rd. NE, MSC-C12
Atlanta, GA 30333
Phone: (404)371-5329 **Fax:** (404)371-5449
Email: jem3@cdc.gov
Website: http://www.cdc.gov/ncidod/
Joseph E. McDade, Dep. Dir.
Activities/Fields: Coordinates a national program to improve the identification, investigation, diagnosis, prevention, and control of infectious diseases. Principal Center components include: Arctic Investigations Program; Bacterial and Mycotic Diseases Division; Hospital Infections Program; Division of AIDS, STD, DTB Lab Research; Division of Parisitic Diseases; Vector-Borne Infectious Diseases Division; and Division of Viral and Rickettsial Diseases; Division of Quarantine; and Scientific Resources Program.

★ 24915 ★ U.S. Department of Health and Human Services
National Center for Infectious Diseases
Arctic Investigations Program
4055 Tudor Centre Dr.
Anchorage, AK 99508
Phone: (907)729-3400 **Fax:** (907)729-3429
Email: jcb3@cdc.gov
Website: http://www.cdc.gov/ncidod/aip/aip.htm
Dr. Jay C. Butler, Dir.
Activities/Fields: Mission is to prevent infectious diseases and improve the quality of life of people living in the arctic and subarctic through: investigation of the causes of infectious diseases; evaluation of methods for disease prevention and control; dissemination of information; provision of epidemiologic, statistical, and laboratory consultation and technical assistance; and

assistance in training of personnel to perform studies of conditions that impact health. Activities focus on studies of conditions that occur at high incidence, are unique to, or may be of potential benefit to populations in (and outside of) the arctic and subarctic. Emphasis is on acute infectious diseases, but investigations are also conducted on select chronic diseases that are sequelae of infectious diseases and/or in which an infectious disease is suspected to play a role. Specific disease areas of interest include: Hepatitis B, Streptococcus pneumoniae, Haemophilus influenzae b, Helicobacter pylori, respiratory syncytial virus. **Pub:** *Proceedings.* • *Research Reports.*

★ 24916 ★ U.S. Department of Health and Human Services
National Center for Infectious Diseases
Division of AIDS, STD, and Tuberculosis Laboratory Research
Tuberculosis/Mycobacteriology Branch
1600 Clifton Rd. NE
Bldg. 17
MS F08
Atlanta, GA 30333
Phone: (404)639-1474 **Fax:** (404)639-1287
Email: tms1@cdc.gov
Dr. Thomas Shinnick, Ch.
Activities/Fields: Tuberculosis and other mycobacterial diseases, emphasizing etiologic agents of tuberculosis, leprosy, and other mycobacterioses; surveillance of the incidence of these diseases; and diagnostic procedures for rapid identification and drug resistance patterns. Principal research interest are moleucular biology, rapid diagnostic procedures, subtyping mechanisms, immunology, genetics, drug development, virulence factors, and taxonomy. **Pub:** *Proceedings.* **Frmly:** Division of Bacterial and Mycotic Diseases; Emerging Bacterial and Mycotic Diseases Branch; Tuberculosis and Other Mycobacteriosis Laboratory Section.

★ 24917 ★ U.S. Department of Health and Human Services
National Center for Infectious Diseases
Division of AIDS, STDS, Tuberculosis Laboratories
Immunology Branch
1600 Clifton Rd., NE, Bldg. 17 Rm. 3016 (MSA-25)
Atlanta, GA 30333
Phone: (404)639-3434 **Fax:** (404)639-2108
Email: jsm3@cdc.gov
Website: http://www.cdc.gov/ncidod/dastlr/immunology/default/htm
Dr. J. Steven McDougal, Chf.
Activities/Fields: Immunology and Acquired Immunodeficiency Syndrome (AIDS). **Frmly:** Division of Host Factors.

★ 24918 ★ U.S. Department of Health and Human Services
National Center for Infectious Diseases
Division of AIDS, STDS, and Tuberculosis Laboratories
Retrovirus Diseases Branch
1600 Clifton Rd. NE, G19
Atlanta, GA 30333
Phone: (404)639-1024 **Fax:** (404)639-1174
Email: TMF2@cdc.gov
Dr. Thomas M. Folks, PhD, Chf.
Activities/Fields: Retrovirus diseases and retroviral etiologies of chronic diseases. Develops HIV prevention tools, vaccines, microbicides; carries out global HIV and drug resistance surveillance. **Pub:** *Journal of Emerging Infectious Diseases,* monthly.

★ 24919 ★ U.S. Department of Health and Human Services
National Center for Infectious Diseases
Division of Bacterial and Mycotic Diseases
Childhood and Respirtory Diseases Branch
Mail Stop C23
1600 Clifton Rd., NE
Atlanta, GA 30333
Phone: (404)639-2215 **Fax:** (404)639-3970
Email: acs1@cdc.gov
Dr. Anne Schuchat, Chief
Activities/Fields: Laboratory and epidemiologic investigations of organisms except enteric and sexually transmitted diseases. Principal subjects of study are influenzae, type b; meningitidis; Group A streptococcus; Group B streptococcus; Brazilian purpuric fever, sipneumoniae, legionella infections, chlamydia and mycoplasma infections, and otitis media.

★ 24920 ★ U.S. Department of Health and Human Services
National Center for Infectious Diseases
Division of HIV / AIDS
1600 Clifton Rd., NE
Mail Stop E-49
Atlanta, GA 30333
Phone: (404)639-0900 **Fax:** (404)639-2007
Email: rxj1@cdc.gov
Website: http://www.cdc.gov/hiv/dhap.htm
Robert Janssen, Dir.
Activities/Fields: Epidemiologic and laboratory investigations, surveillance, and studies to determine risk factors, transmission patterns, prevalence/incidence of HIV/AIDS, and case reporting for acquired immunodeficiency syndrome. Program also develops and evaluates laboratory methods and procedures for the isolation and characterization of human immunodeficiency virus (HIV) and serodiagnosis and understanding of viral pathogenesis. Principal component units are: Office of the Director, Epidemiology Branch, Laboratory Investigations Branch, Statistics and Data Management Branch, HIV Seroepidemiology Branch, Field Services Branch, Technical Information Activity, International Activity, Surveillance Branch, Hematologic Diseases Branch, and Immunology Branch.

★ 24921 ★ U.S. Department of Health and Human Services
National Center for Infectious Diseases
Division of Parasitic Diseases
Entomology Branch
(Vector Biology and Toxicology Section)
4770 Buford Hwy., MS F22
Chamblee, GA 30341-3724
Phone: (770)488-4240 **Fax:** (770)488-4258
Email: bew5@cdc.gov
Website: http://www.cdc.gov/ncidod/dpd/aboutdpd/default.htmorg.structure
Robert A. Wirtz, Chf. Entomology Branch
Activities/Fields: Vector control strategies with a focus on malaria, Chagas disease, Leichmaniosis, and disseminates the results; conducts research on vector biology and the molecular and biochemical mechanisms for insecticide resistance; develops biochemical and bioassay field tests to assess vector insecticide susceptibility; develops and validates chemical tests for the detection of parasitic disease drugs and their metabolities in body fluids and tissues, and determines the pharmacologic response to such drugs; develops chemical procedures to detect new and existing pesticides in various formulations.

★ 24922 ★ U.S. Department of Health and Human Services
National Center for Infectious Diseases
Division of Parasitic Diseases
Epidemiology Branch
(Malaria Section)
4770 Buford Hwy., MS F22
Atlanta, GA 30341-3724
Phone: (770)488-7789 **Fax:** (770)488-4206
Email: ris1@cdc.gov
Rick Steketer, Chf.
Activities/Fields: Malaria in the U.S. and among U.S. citizens abroad; monitors the efficacy and safety of antimalarial drugs for chemoprophylaxis and chemotherapy; and provides clinical advice and epidemiologic assistance on the treatment, control, and prevention of malaria in the U.S. and abroad.

★ 24923 ★ U.S. Department of Health and Human Services
National Center for Infectious Diseases
Division of Parasitic Diseases
Epidemiology Branch
(Parasitic Diseases Section)
4770 Buford Hwy., MS F22
Atlanta, GA 30341-3724
Phone: (770)488-7760 **Fax:** (770)488-7794
Mark Eberhardt, Actg. Dir.
Activities/Fields: Surveillance and epidemiologic investigations of parasitic diseases, other than malaria, in the U.S. and abroad. Monitors the efficacy and safety of antiparasitic drugs. Monitors and investigates water source disease outbreaks. **Frmly:** (2000) Epidemiology Branch; Parasitic Diseases Section.

★ 24924 ★ U.S. Department of Health and Human Services
National Center for Infectious Diseases
Division of Parasitic Diseases
Epidemiology Branch
4770 Buford Hwy., MS F22
Atlanta, GA 30341-3724
Phone: (770)488-7760 **Fax:** (770)488-7761
James Maguire, Chf.
Activities/Fields: Parasitic diseases in the U.S. and abroad; monitors the efficacy and safety of antiparasitic drugs; provides clinical advice and epidemiologic assistance to state and local health departments, other federal agencies, and national and international health organizations, on the diagnosis, treatment, control, and prevention of parasitic diseases.

★ 24925 ★ U.S. Department of Health and Human Services
National Center for Infectious Diseases
Division of Vector-Borne Infectious Diseases
Dengue Branch
1324 Calle Canada
San Juan, PR 00920-3860
Phone: (787)706-2399 **Fax:** (787)706-2496
Email: ggc1@cdc.gov
Gary G. Clark, Chf.
Activities/Fields: Study of dengue, a viral disease spread by mosquitoes. Research includes investigation of vectors, reservoirs of disease, viruses that cause disease, and methods for surveillance prevention and control. **Pub:** *Dengue Surveillance Summary.* • *Research Reports.*

★ 24926 ★ U.S. Department of Health and Human Services
National Center for Infectious Diseases
Division of Viral and Rickettsial Diseases
1600 Clifton Rd. NE (MS A-30)
Atlanta, GA 30333
Phone: (404)639-3574 **Fax:** (404)639-3163
Website: http://www.cdc.gov/ncidod/dvrd/index.htm
James W. LeDuc, Actg. Dir.

Activities/Fields: Viral and rickettsial diseases of national and international importance. The Division addresses significant disease problems by the integrated application of modern virologic and epidemiologic methodologies–from molecular biologic methodologies (including nucleic acid and protein biochemistry) to immunologic and pathophysiologic methodologies to epidemiologic and statistical methodologies. Division comprises the Biometrics Activity, Infectious Disease Pathology Activity, Influenza Branch, Respiratory and Enteric Virus Branch, Special Pathogens Branch, Viral Exanthems and Herpesvirus Branch, and Viral and Rickettsial Zoonoses Branch. Branch. **Pub:** *Proceedings.* • *Research Reports.* **Frmly:** Viral Diseases Division.

★ 24927 ★ U.S. Department of Health and Human Services
National Center for Infectious Diseases Division of Viral and Rickettsial Diseases Hepatitis Branch
1600 Clifton Rd., NE, MS A33
MS G37
Atlanta, GA 30333
Phone: (404)371-5900 **Fax:** (404)371-5221
Email: hsm1@cdc.gov
Website: http://www.cdc.gov/ncidod/diseases/hepatitis/index.htm
Richard Conlon, MD, Actg. Dep. Dir.

Activities/Fields: Hepatitis A, B, C, D, and E. Works to implement hepatitis B and hepatitis A immunization programs nationally and internationally. **Pub:** *Hepatitis Surveillance Report*, annually.

★ 24928 ★ U.S. Department of Health and Human Services
National Center for Infectious Diseases Division of Viral and Rickettsial Diseases Influenza Branch
1600 Clifton Rd., NE
G-16
Atlanta, GA 30333
Phone: (404)639-3591 **Fax:** (404)639-2334
Email: NJC1@CDC.GOV
Website: http://www.cdc.gov/ncidol/diseases/flu/fluvirus.htm
Nancy Cox, Chf.

Activities/Fields: Focal point within CDC for studies pertaining to influenza viruses, their variation and occurrence in populations, and their control.

★ 24929 ★ U.S. Department of Health and Human Services
National Center for Infectious Diseases Division of Viral and Rickettsial Diseases Respiratory and Enteric Virus Branch
1600 Clifton Rd., NE
M.S A-34
Atlanta, GA 30333
Phone: (404)639-3596 **Fax:** (404)639-1307
Email: lja2@cdc.gov
Dr. Larry Anderson, Chf.

Activities/Fields: Respiratory viruses such as adenoviruses and respiratory syncytial virus, polio and other enteroviruses, and viruses causing gastroenteritis.

★ 24930 ★ U.S. Department of Health and Human Services
National Center for Infectious Diseases Division of Viral and Rickettsial Diseases Viral and Rickettsial Zoonoses Branch
Epidemiology Section
1600 Clifton Rd., NE
Atlanta, GA 30333
Phone: (404)639-1087 **Fax:** (404)639-4436
Email: jfc5@cdc.gov
Website: http://www.cdc.gov/ncidod/dvrd/branch/vrzb.htm
Dr. James Childs, Consult.

Activities/Fields: Rickettsial agents (such as those of Rocky Mountain spotted fever and Q fever).

★ 24931 ★ U.S. Department of Health and Human Services
National Center for Infectious Diseases Hospital Infections Program
1600 Clifton Rd. NE
Mail Stop E-69
Atlanta, GA 30333
Phone: (404)639-6400 **Fax:** (404)639-6459
Email: wrj1c@cdc.gov
Website: http://www.cdc.gov/ncidod/hip/hip.htm
Dr. William Jarvis, Chf.

Activities/Fields: Hospital-associated infections. The Program serves as the focal point within the National Center for Infectious Diseases for the issuance of recommendations and guidelines on prevention and control of hospital infections. The Program involves research on methods for preventing and controlling hospital infections and for rapid diagnosis of disease and identification of unusual sources of infection; and research to identify methods for antimicrobial susceptibility testing of groups of microorganisms and to determine the role of drug-resistant microorganisms in hospital infections. Program also provides epidemic aid and epidemiological consultation, upon request from state health departments, to institutions and public health organizations regarding the identification and control of nosocomial infections, provides basic diagnostic services in support of field investigations and cooperates with other components of CID for more definitive diagnosis of nosocomial infections and identification of etiologic agents, provides antimicrobial susceptibility consultation and services to other components of CID, provides intramural and extramural technical expertise and assistance in professional training activities; and serves as designated national and international reference centers for certain nosocomial infections. Components of the Hospital Infections Program are: Anti-Hospital Environmental Laboratory Branch, Nosocomial Pathogens Laboratory Branch, Investigation and Prevention Branch, and HIV Infectious Branch. **Pub:** *Guidelines for the Prevention and Control of Nosocomial Infections.* • *National Nosocomial Infections Surveillance System Reports.*

★ 24932 ★ U.S. Department of Health and Human Services
National Center for Infectious Diseases Scientific Resources Program
1600 Clifton Rd., NE
Atlanta, GA 30333
Phone: (404)639-3466 **Fax:** (404)639-3199
Email: bzm9@cdc.gov
Website: http://www.cdc.gov/ncidod/about.htm
Carolyn Black, Dir.

Activities/Fields: Procures, manages, and distributes the resources required by CDC investigators for research and service activities; conducts protocol reviews for research and diagnostic activities involving laboratory animals, and produces cell cultures, cell culture media, and microbiologic media, using modern methods and exhaustive quality assurance testing; maintains an active applied research program in cell biology, and conducts research leading to the development of new cell culture systems and cell lines; procures, prepares, and distributes sterile glassware and plasticware, and provides packing, shipping, and receiving services for etiologic agents, diagnostic specimens, and reagents from the CDC catalog; and provides services for maintaining and developing laboratory equipment; provides to the NCID research environments the instrumentation and expertise required to develop, refine, and apply modern technologies pertinent to the prevention and control of infectious, autoimmune, neoplastic, and hemotolgic diseases.

★ 24933 ★ U.S. Department of Health and Human Services
National Center for Injury Prevention and Control
4770 Buford Hwy. NE, MS K65
Atlanta, GA 30341-3724
Phone: (770)488-1506 **Fax:** (770)488-1667
Email: ohc@cdc.gov
Website: http://www.cdc.gov/ncipc
Sandra Bonzo, Dep. Dir.

Activities/Fields: Specific injury control research designed to: yield results directly applicable to identifying interventions to prevent injury occurrence or minimize disability; apply and evaluate the effect of known interventions on injury morbidity, mortality, disability, and costs; or elucidate the etiology and mechanisms of injuries. **Pub:** *Proceedings.* • *Research Reports.* **Frmly:** (1991) Injury Epidemiology and Control Division.

★ 24934 ★ U.S. Department of Health and Human Services
National Center for Prevention Services National Immunization Program Epidemiology and Surveillance Division
1600 Clifton Rd. NE, No. E-61
Atlanta, GA 30333
Phone: (404)639-8254 **Fax:** (404)639-8616
Email: mew2@cdc.gov
Dr. Melinda Wharton, Chf.

Activities/Fields: Incidence of diseases preventable by vaccination; and conducts studies on the safety and efficacy of new or existing vaccines. **Pub:** *Research Reports.*

★ 24935 ★ U.S. Department of Health and Human Services
National Center for Prevention Services Sexually Transmitted Disease / HIV Prevention Division (NCHSTP) Behavioral and Prevention Research Branch
Mail Stop E-44
1600 Clifton Rd., NE
Atlanta, GA 30333
Phone: (404)639-8376 **Fax:** (404)639-8622
Email: n2s4@odc.gov
Janet S. St. Lawrence, PhD, Chf.

Activities/Fields: Individual and group behavior patterns as they affect STD and HIV occurrence and transmission. Undertakes studies to evaluate new methods of prevention and intervention of HIV and STDs, and conducts surveys, studies, and methodological research on the sexual and drug-using behavior. Performs intervention research to prevent HIV/STD transmission. **Pub:** *MMWR.* • *Professional Journals.* **Frmly:** Epidemiology Research Branch; (2000) Sexually Transmitted Disease/HIV Prevention Division; Behavioral and Prevention Research Branch.

★ 24936 ★ U.S. Department of Health and Human Services
National Center for Research Resources Biological Models and Materials Resource Program Caenorhabditis Genetics Center
University of Minnesota
Department of GCD
6-160 Jackson Hall
321 Church St., SE
Minneapolis, MN 55455
Phone: (612)625-2265 **Fax:** (612)625-4648
Email: stier@biosci.cbs.umn.edu
Website: http://biosci.cbs.umb/cgc
Bob Herman, Dir.

Activities/Fields: Provides genetic stocks of Caenorhabditis elegans and other Caenorhabditis species for use by investigators initiating or continuing research on this nematode. The Center also acquires new strains described in current literature and evaluates methods for permanent storage of genetic stocks.

Current research includes: resolution of conflicting genetic data received from research laboratories, improving the resolution of the genetic map, and alignment of the genetic and physical maps. **Pub:** *Worm Breeders Gazette*. Newsletter.

★ 24937 ★ U.S. Department of Health and Human Services
National Center for Research Resources
Biomedical Engineering and Instrumentation Program
NIH Bldg. 13, Rm. 3N17
9000 Rockville Pike
Bethesda, MD 20892
Phone: (301)496-4741 **Fax:** (301)496-6608
Website: http://www.nih.gov/od/ors/dbeps/index.htm
Dr. Henry Eden, Dep. Dir.
Activities/Fields: Supports NIH intramural scientists in applications of engineering, mathematics, physics, and the physical sciences to the solution of problems in biology and medicine through collaborations involving measurement, imaging, mathematical modeling, or design of specialized equipment; and construction, modification, maintenance, repair, or lease of scientific equipment. **Frmly:** (2002) National Center for Research Resources; Biomedical Engineering and Instrumentation Program.

★ 24938 ★ U.S. Department of Health and Human Services
National Center for Research Resources
Biomedical Technology Program
1 Rockledge Centre, Rm. 6030
6705 Rockledge Rd., MSC 7965
Bethesda, MD 20892-7965
Phone: (301)435-0772 **Fax:** (301)480-3659
Dr. Michael Marron, Dir.
Activities/Fields: Physical sciences, mathematics, engineering, and computer sciences; biology; and medicine. Its purpose is to support and develop biomedically relevant technologies to be utilized by health scientists in solving biomedical and clinical research problems. Such technologies include mass spectrometers, high voltage electron microscopes, and nuclear magnetic and electron spin resonance spectrometers. BTP provides grants and contracts for establishing, maintaining, and developing these resources and for adapting technological capabilities developed in the commercial sector for use by the biomedical community. Support is currently provided in three main areas: computer resources; instruments and materials for studying biomolecular and cellular structure and function; and biomedical engineering and technology resources.

★ 24939 ★ U.S. Department of Health and Human Services
National Center for Research Resources
Comparative Medicine Program
Laboratory Animal Sciences Program
9000 Rockville Pike
Bldg 12A Rm 4007, MSC5662
Bethesda, MD 20892
Phone: (301)496-5795 **Fax:** (301)402-0006
Dr. Judith Vaitukaitis, Dir.
Activities/Fields: New animal models, to improve the care and health of animals used in research, and to train veterinarians in laboratory animal medicine. Focus is on the development of improved methods for diagnosing and controlling diseases among laboratory animals; and providing support to special breeding programs to ensure an adequate supply of animals that have been shown to be good models of human diseases or that serve as important research subjects.

★ 24940 ★ U.S. Department of Health and Human Services
National Eye Institute
Division of Biometry and Epidemiology
NIH Bldg. 31, Rm. 6A52
31 Center Dr. MSC 2510
Bethesda, MD 20892-2510
Phone: (301)496-1331 **Fax:** (301)496-2297
Website: http://www.nei.nih.gov
Fredrick Ferris, MD, Dir.
Activities/Fields: Plan, develop, and conduct human population studies concerned with the cause, prevention, and treatment of eye disease and vision disorders, with emphasis on the major causes of blindness. This includes studies of incidence and prevalencein defined populations, prospective and retrospective studies of risk factors, natural history studies, clinical trials, genetic studies, and studies to evaluate diagnostic procedures.

★ 24941 ★ U.S. Department of Health and Human Services
National Eye Institute
Division of Biometry and Epidemiology
Clinical Trials Branch
NIH Bldg. 31, Rm. 6A52
31 Center Dr. MSC 2510
Bethesda, MD 20892
Phone: (301)496-6583 **Fax:** (301)496-2297
Website: http://www.nei.nih.gov
Frederick L. Ferris, Chf.
Activities/Fields: Plan, develop, and conduct human population studies concerned with the cause, prevention, and treatment of eye disease and vision disorders, with emphasis on the major causes of blindness. This includes studies of incidence and prevalence on defined populations, prospective and retrospective studies of risk factors, natural history studies, clinical trials, genetic studies, and studies to evaluate diagnostic procedures.

★ 24942 ★ U.S. Department of Health and Human Services
National Eye Institute
Extramural Research
NIH EPS, Ste. 350
6120 Executive Blvd., MSC 7164
Bethesda, MD 20892-7164
Phone: (301)496-5301 **Fax:** (301)402-0528
Email: rh27v@nih.gov
Website: http://www.nei.nih.gov/
Dr. Ralph Helmsen, Res. Rsrcs. Off.
Activities/Fields: Improving the prevention, diagnosis, and treatment of visual disorders. This support includes the award of grants, cooperative agreements, fellowships, and contracts for research in retinal and choroidal diseases, corneal diseases, cataract, glaucoma, strabismus, amblyopia, visual processing, and low vision.

★ 24943 ★ U.S. Department of Health and Human Services
National Eye Institute
Extramural Research
Corneal Diseases Program
2020 Vision Place
Bethesda, MD 20892
Phone: (301)451-2020 **Fax:** (301)402-0528
Email: lam@nei.nih.gov/funding/nprp.htm
Website: http://www.nei.nih.gov
Richard S. Fischer, PhD, Contact
Activities/Fields: Ophthalmic research relating to corneal diseases and focusing on diseases of the cornea and the external ocular structures, including the conjunctiva and eyelids; corneal transplantation and wound healing; and contact lenses and surgical correction of refractive problems.

★ 24944 ★ U.S. Department of Health and Human Services
National Eye Institute
Extramural Research
Retinal Diseases Program
2020 Vision Place
Bethesda, MD 20892-7164
Phone: (301)451-2020 **Fax:** (301)402-0528
Email: pad@.nei.nih.gov
Website: http://www.nei.nih.gov/funding/nprp.htm
Peter A. Dudley, PhD, Contact
Activities/Fields: Structure and function of the retina and choroid in health and disease. NEI-fostered investigations include studies of the structure and metabolism of photoreceptor cells and their relationship to the underlying pigment epithelium; the retina's response to light and the initial processing of visual information transmitted to the visual centers of the brain; inflammation of the uveal tract (the iris, choroid, and ciliary body); and of the vitreous gel that fills the center of the eye. NEI also supports studies aimed at understanding causes of blindness such as developmental and hereditary retinal disorders; diabetic retinopathy and other vascular and circulatory abnormalities; myopia; ocular tumors; macular degeneration; retinal detachment; and inflammatory disorders, including uveitis. Also conducts clinical trials of the effects of treatment on retinal diseases.

★ 24945 ★ U.S. Department of Health and Human Services
National Eye Institute
Extramural Research
Strabismus, Amblyopia, Visual Processing, and Low Vision
NIH
Executive Plaza S, Ste. 350
6120 Executive Blvd., MSC 7164
Bethesda, MD 20892-7164
Phone: (301)451-2020 **Fax:** (301)402-0528
Email: oberdorfer@nei.nih.gov
Website: http://www.nei.nih.gov/
Michael D. Oberdorfer, PhD, Prog. Dir.
Activities/Fields: Contact person for extramural support for basic and clinical research on a broad range of studies concerned with the development and function of the neural pathways from the eye to the brain, the central processing of visual information, visual perception, optical properties of the eye, oculomotor function, functioning of the pupil, and control of the ocular muscles. A large number of congenital, developmental, and degenerative abnormalities affect the visual sensorimotor system, but two disorders are of primary concern–strabismus and amblyopia. These are frequent causes of visual impairment among children which may persist for life. Additional emphasis is placed on, and support provided for, research on optic neuropathies, eye movement disorders, the development of myopia, and the contact person for all research applications regarding low vision and blindness rehabilitation.

★ 24946 ★ U.S. Department of Health and Human Services
National Eye Institute
Intramural Research Program
NIH Bldg. 10, Rm. 31/6A20
31 Center Dr.
Bethesda, MD 20892-1858
Phone: (301)435-4543 **Fax:** (301)451-6764
Email: millers@nei.nih.gov
Dr. Sheldon Miller, Scientific Dir.
Activities/Fields: In-house research aimed at improving the prevention, diagnosis, and treatment of visual disorders. Major subject of research include retinal and choroidal diseases, corneal diseases, cataract, glaucoma, and sensory and motor disorders of vision. Program comprises a Clinical Branch and laboratories of Mechanisms of Ocular Diseases, Molecular and Developmental Biology, Ophthalmic Pathology, Retinal Cell and Molecular Biology, and Sensorimotor Research. **Pub:** *NEI's Annual Report.*

★ 24947 ★ U.S. Department of Health and Human Services
National Eye Institute
Intramural Research Program
Laboratory of Immunology
NIH Bldg. 10, Rm. 10/10 N 112
9000 Rockville Pike
Bethesda, MD 20892
Phone: (301)496-3123 **Fax:** (301)480-1122
Email: drbob@nei.nih.gov
Dr. Robert B. Nussenblatt, Lab. Chf.
Activities/Fields: Clinical research into the causes, preventions, diagnosis, and treatment of visual system disorders. It translates laboratory research results into clinical application, directs and administers the Institute's clinical care program, and assures functioning of the eye ward and clinic in the NIH Clinical Center. Principal Branch components are: the Cataract Section, Neuro-+Ophthalmology Section, Ocular +Immunology Section, Ophthalmic +Genetics and +Pediatric Ophthalmology Section, and Retinal and +Ocular Connective Tissue Diseases Section.

★ 24948 ★ U.S. Department of Health and Human Services
National Eye Institute
Laboratory on Mechanisms of Ocular Diseases
NIH Bldg. 6, Rm. 237/ 6 Center Dr. MSC 2735
9000 Rockville Pike
Bethesda, MD 20892-2735
Phone: (301)496-6669 **Fax:** (301)496-1759
Website: http://www.nei.nih.gov/intramural/lmod.htm
Dr. J. Samuel Zigler, Actg. Chf.
Activities/Fields: Mechanisms involved in cataract formation, pharmacologic and pathophysiologic aspects of aldose reductase in diabetic complications, molecular biology of a retinal dystrophy, and cataract caused by an enzyme deficiency. Laboratory also provides training opportunities in related diabetes and cataract research.

★ 24949 ★ U.S. Department of Health and Human Services
National Eye Institute
Laboratory of Molecular and Developmental Biology
NIH Bldg. 6, Rm. 201
6 Center Dr., MSC-2730
Bethesda, MD 20892
Phone: (301)496-9467 **Fax:** (301)402-0781
Email: joramp@nei.nih.gov
Dr. Joram Piatigorsky, Chf.
Activities/Fields: Cellular and molecular biology, with emphasis on molecular and developmental genetics. The research is designed to elucidate both normal and disease processes, and particular attention is given to hereditary diseases that can be studied at the gene level. Much (but not all) of the work uses eye tissue as models for general problems concerning cellular differentiation and gene expression. In addition, normal and pathogenic visual processes are related to the structure and function of genes; and phospholipid metabolism–particularly at the cell membrane–is investigated in order to advance knowledge of cellular differentiation and differential gene expression.

★ 24950 ★ U.S. Department of Health and Human Services
National Eye Institute
Laboratory of Retinal Cell and Molecular Biology
NIH Bldg. 6, Rm. 310
6 Center Dr. MSC 2740
Bethesda, MD 20892-2740
Phone: (301)496-3448 **Fax:** (301)402-1883
Email: bnwigg@helix.nih.gov
Website: http://www.nei.nih.gov/intramural/lrcmb.htm
Dr. Barbara N. Wiggert, Ch.
Activities/Fields: Biochemistry, molecular biology, and neurobiology of the retina.

★ 24951 ★ U.S. Department of Health and Human Services
National Heart, Lung, and Blood Institute
NIH Bldg. 31, Rm. 5A52
31 Center Dr., MSC 2486
Bethesda, MD 20892-2486
Phone: (301)496-5166 **Fax:** (301)402-0818
Email: lenfant@nhlbi.nih.gov
Website: http://www.nhlbi.nih.gov/
Claude Lenfant, Dir.
Activities/Fields: Responsible for a national program of research leading to the prevention and treatment of heart, lung, blood diseases, and sleep disorders. The scope of the Institute's effort encompasses all forms of heart and vascular disease (except the consequences of cerebrovascular disease), most forms of pulmonary disease (except cancers), sleep disorders, many blood diseases (including sickle cell disease), and the utilization of blood resources. Research scope is primarily basic and clinical but also includes applied research and clinical trials as well as demonstration and education research. The Institute also plans and directs research in the development, trial, and evaluation of drugs and devices relating to the prevention and treatment of these diseases and the rehabilitation of patients suffering from them; conducts studies into the clinical uses of blood and all aspects of the management of blood resources and supports training in basic and clinical research programs relating to heart, blood vessel, blood, and lung disease; conducts educational activities (including collection and dissemination of educational materials), with emphasis on prevention, for health professionals and the public and maintains relationships with various institutions, agencies, and organizations working in these areas; and awards pre- and postdoctoral fellowships and training grants to develop adequate numbers of research investigators. The NHLBI program also includes support for Specialized Centers of Research (SCORs), which are research units within institutions focusing on studies of a specific disease or group of diseases and the Women's Health Initiative, a multicenter observational study and clinical trail. Principal components of the Institute include divisions of: Blood Diseases and Resources, Epidemiology and Clinical Applications, Extramural Affairs, Heart and Vascular Diseases, Intramural Research, Lung Diseases, and the National Center on Sleep Disorders.

★ 24952 ★ U.S. Department of Health and Human Services
National Heart, Lung, and Blood Institute
Division of Epidemiology and Clinical Applications
2 Rockledge Centre
6701 Rockledge Dr. MSC 7938
Bethesda, MD 20892-7938
Phone: (301)435-0422 **Fax:** (301)480-1864
Email: savagep@nhlbi.nih.gov
Dr. Peter Savage, MD, Dir.
Activities/Fields: Epidemiological studies, clinical trials, basic and applied behavioral research, demonstration and education research, and projects for disease prevention and health promotion in heart, vascular, pulmonary, and blood diseases and blood resources. It maintains surveillance over developments in its program area and assesses the national need for research on the prevention, diagnosis, and treatment of these diseases by maintaining the necessary scientific management capability to foster and guide an effective attack upon them. Activities are carried out in the Clinical Applications and Prevention Program and Epidemiology and Biometry Program.

★ 24953 ★ U.S. Department of Health and Human Services
National Heart, Lung, and Blood Institute
Division of Epidemiology and Clinical Applications
Clinical Applications and Prevention Program
2 Rockledge Centre
6701 Rockledge Dr. MSC 7936
Bethesda, MD 20892-7936
Phone: (301)435-0414 **Fax:** (301)480-1773
Email: simonsd@nhlbi.nih.gov
Dr. Denise Simons-Morton, Actg. Dir.
Activities/Fields: Supports clinical trials, demonstration and educational research, basic and applied behavioral research, and projects for the prevention of cardiovascular, lung, and blood diseases as well as therapeutic measures. Principal areas of research are preventive medicine, nutrition, behavioral medicine, cardiology, and community demonstration and education projects. **Pub:** *Proceedings.* • *Research Reports.*

★ 24954 ★ U.S. Department of Health and Human Services
National Heart, Lung, and Blood Institute
Division of Extramural Affairs
6701 Rockledge Dr. MSC 7924, Ste. 7100
Bethesda, MD 20892-7924
Phone: (301)435-0260 **Fax:** (301)480-1124
Dr. Deborah Beebe, Dir.
Activities/Fields: Responsible for advising the Director of the Institute on research contract, grant, and research training program policies. It represents the Institute on overall NIH committees on extramural program policy, oversees compliance with such policy within NHLBI, and coordinates the Institute's research grant and research training and development programs with the National Heart, Lung, and Blood Advisory Council. Division also provides grant and contract management and processing services to the Institute's program divisions; and supplies initial scientific merit review of applications and proposals for project grants, program project and center grants, research training and development grants, and research contracts for the Institute.

★ 24955 ★ U.S. Department of Health and Human Services
National Heart, Lung, and Blood Institute
Division of Heart and Vascular Diseases
Two Rockledge Centre, Ste. 9044
6701 Rockledge Dr. MSC 7940
Bethesda, MD 20892-7940
Phone: (301)435-0466 **Fax:** (301)480-1336
Email: mockrins@nhlbi.nih.gov
Website: http://www.nhlbi.nih.gov/about/dhvd/index.htm
Dr. Stephen Mockrin, Dir.
Activities/Fields: Control of heart and vascular diseases. Major areas of investigat ion include arrythmias, congenital and infectious diseases, heart failure, ischemic heart disease, interventional cardiology, bioengineering, atherosclerosis, hypertension, vascular biology, vascular medicine, cardiovascular homeostasis and bionutrition, and molecular genetics and medicine. **Pub:** *Monographs.*

★ 24956 ★ U.S. Department of Health and Human Services
National Heart, Lung, and Blood Institute
Division of Heart and Vascular Diseases
Heart Research Program
(Arrhythmia Research Program)
2 Rockledge Ctr., Ste. 9192
6701 Rockledge Dr., MSC 7940
Bethesda, MD 20892-7940
Phone: (301)435-0507 **Fax:** (301)480-1454
Email: ps48j@nih.gov
Website: http://www.nhlbi.nih/gov/personal/laura/nhlbi/extlocal.html
Peter M. Spooner, PhD, Contact

Activities/Fields: Administers research grants and implements new research programs in the basic medical sciences as related to cardiology, physiology, anatomy, pharmacology, biochemistry, and bioengineering as they relate to cause and prevention of cardiac arrhythmias, sudden cardiac death, and cardiac ischemia. **Frmly:** (2000) Arrythmia Research Program.

★ 24957 ★ U.S. Department of Health and Human Services
National Heart, Lung, and Blood Institute
Division of Heart and Vascular Diseases
Heart Research Program
(Bioengineering Research Group)
2 Rockledge Center
6701 Rockledge Drive, Rm. 9166, MSC 7940
Bethesda, MD 20892-7940
Phone: (301)435-0555 **Fax:** (301)480-7940
Email: watsonj@nhlbi.nih.gov
Website: http://www.nhlbi.nih.gov
John T. Watson, PhD, Dir.
Activities/Fields: Mechanical circulatory support, biomaterials (blood-material interactions), and diagnostic and therapeutic devices, as well as technolgy transfer through Small Business Innovation Research Grants.

★ 24958 ★ U.S. Department of Health and Human Services
National Heart, Lung, and Blood Institute
Division of Heart and Vascular Diseases
Heart Research Program
Two Rockledge Centre
6701 Rockledge Dr., MSC 7940
Bethesda, MD 20892-7940
Phone: (301)435-0544 **Fax:** (301)480-1336
Email: fakundingj@nhlbi.nih.gov
Website: http://www.nhlbi.nih.gov/about/dhvd/index.htm
Dr. John Fakunding, PhD, Dir., Heart Research Prog.
Activities/Fields: Supports basic, applied, and clinical research in cardiac diseases, from embryonic life to adulthood. Targeted areas include heart arrhythmias and electrical abnormalities, cardiomyopathies, cardiac development, pediatric heart disease, heart failure and cardiogenic shock, exercise physiology, ischemic heart disease, inflammation and infectious disorders of the heart, heart transplantation, and myocardial preservation. Selected areas of focus are normal and abnormal cardiac development, diabetic cardiomyopathy, the pathogenesis of heart failure, electrical remodeling, single gene modifiers of cardiac disease, and interactive pediatric clinical research centers to promote the efficient evaluation of novel treatment methods and management strategies having potential benefit for children with structural congenital heart disease. Specialized Centers of Clinically Oriented Research support clinically relevant research studies on cardiac dysfunction and disease. The program comprises two Scientific Research Groups (SRG), the Heart Development, Function and Failure SRG, which supports broad areas of research in heart development, cardiac function and heart failure, and the Ischemia, Arrhythmia & Sudden Cardiac Death SRG, which includes basic, applied and clinical research studies dealing with the etiology and pathophysiology of ischemic heart disease and its consequences, as well as the control and treatment of cardiac electrical activity, rhythm and rate, especially as they relate to sudden cardiac death.

★ 24959 ★ U.S. Department of Health and Human Services
National Heart, Lung, and Blood Institute
Division of Heart and Vascular Diseases
Heart Research Training and Development Group
2 Rockledge Ctr., Ste. 9044
6701 Rockledge Dr., MSC 7940
Bethesda, MD 20892-7940
Phone: (301)435-0535 **Fax:** (301)480-1335
Email: mc63a@nih.gov
Beth Schucker, Trng. Ldr.
Activities/Fields: Administers training grants, fellowships, and career program awards to individuals and academic institutions for research training relating to cardiovascular disease.

★ 24960 ★ U.S. Department of Health and Human Services
National Heart, Lung, and Blood Institute
Division of Heart and Vascular Diseases
Specialized Centers of Research in Coronary and Peripheral Vascular Disease, Heart Failure, and Congenital Heart
2 Rockledge Ctr.
6701 Rockledge Dr.
Bethesda, MD 20892
Phone: (301)435-0466 **Fax:** (301)480-7971
Dr. Stephen Mockrin, Dir.
Activities/Fields: Supports cardiac and vascular disease research through grants.

★ 24961 ★ U.S. Department of Health and Human Services
National Heart, Lung, and Blood Institute
Division of Heart and Vascular Diseases
Vascular Research Program
Two Rockledge Center, Ste. 10198
6701 Rockledge Dr., MSC 7956
Bethesda, MD 20892-7956
Phone: (301)435-0545 **Fax:** (301)480-2849
Email: ss90g@nih.gov
Website: http://www.nhlbi.nih.gov/about/dhvd/index.htm
Sonia I. Skarlatos, PhD, Dir.
Activities/Fields: Arteriosclerosis, lipid metabolism, hypertension, vascular biology and medicine, and molecular genetics and medicine. This includes support for: research grants; Specialized Centers of Research (SCORs) in arteriosclerosis and hypertension; and nonhuman primate resources to facilitate study of disease states. Principal areas of research interest are: fundamental and metabolic research relating to the etiology, pathogenesis, and prevention of atherosclerosis; etiology, pathogenesis, and prevention of coronary artery and peripheral vascular arteriosclerosis; causes, development, complication, and prevention of cerebrovascular diseases that affect the vessels of the head and neck; the relationship of lipids and lipoproteins to coronary heart disease; and causes, mechanisms of development, treatment, and prevention of hypertension.

★ 24962 ★ U.S. Department of Health and Human Services
National Heart, Lung, and Blood Institute
Division of Intramural Research
Cardiology Branch
NIH Bldg. 10, Rm 7B-15
10 Center Dr. MSC 1650
Bethesda, MD 20892
Phone: (301)496-5817 **Fax:** (301)402-0888
Email: finkel@nih.gov
Dr. Toren Finkel, III, Chf.
Activities/Fields: Clinical and basic research efforts, including: studies into the genetic causes and pathophysiologic mechanisms responsible for hypertrophic cardiomyopathy; development of approaches to revascularize the ischemic heart, including the promotion of angiogenesis; studies into pathogenesis and treatment of coronary artery disease and of myocardial iscemia secondary to microvascular disease; elucidation of the mechanisms responsible for Syndrome X (chest pain in the presence of normal coronary arteries); elucidation of the molecular mechanisms responsible for restenosis; development of gene therapy for the treatment of restenosis and atherosclerosis; studies of vascular effects of estrogen and anti-estrogen therapies; and the development of techniques to detect stunned and hibernating myocardium and the elucidation of responsible mechanisms.

★ 24963 ★ U.S. Department of Health and Human Services
National Heart, Lung, and Blood Institute
Division of Intramural Research
Hematology Branch
NIH Bldg. 10, Rm. 7C103
10 Center Dr. MSC 1652
Bethesda, MD 20892-1652
Phone: (301)496-5093 **Fax:** (301)496-8396
Email: youngn@nhlbi.nih.gov
Dr. Neal S. Young, Chf.
Activities/Fields: Normal and abnormal hematopoiesis. Clinical research is conducted on patients with bone marrow failure syndromes, especially aplastic anemia, Fancon's anemia, and myelodysplasia; inherited anemias, including sickle cell anemia and thalassemia; and hematologic malignancies, including chronic myelogenous leukemia and multiple myeloma. The major areas of laboratory investigation are: immune suppression of hematopoiesis; viral interactions with bone marrow cells, especially of the human parvovirus; gene transduction into hematopoietic stem cells; and modulation of graft-versus-leukemia and graft-versus-host disease in allogeneic bone marrow transplantation. Techniques from cell biology, immunology, virology, and molecular biology are all employed in these efforts.

★ 24964 ★ U.S. Department of Health and Human Services
National Heart, Lung, and Blood Institute
Division of Intramural Research
Molecular Disease Branch
(Experimental Atherosclerosis Section)
NIH Bldg. 10, Rm. 5N113
10 Center Dr., MSC 1422
Bethesda, MD 20892-1422
Phone: (301)496-4826
Howard S. Kruth, MD, Chf.
Activities/Fields: Atherosclerosis.

★ 24965 ★ U.S. Department of Health and Human Services
National Heart, Lung, and Blood Institute
Division of Intramural Research
Molecular Disease Branch
NIH Bldg. 10, Rm. 7N115
10 Center Dr., MSC 1666
Bethesda, MD 20892-1666
Phone: (301)496-5095 **Fax:** (301)402-0190
Dr. H. Bryan Brewer, Chf.
Activities/Fields: Elucidation of the molecular mechanisms involved in lipid transport and metabolism in normal individuals and patients with disorders of lipid metabolism and atherosclerosis. Biochemical studies involve protein chemistry, immunology, tissue culture, molecular biology, and enzymology. Clinical research focuses on the effects of drugs and therapeutic diets on dyslipoproteinemia and on kinetic analysis of the metabolic defects in patients with these diseases.

★ 24966 ★ U.S. Department of Health and Human Services
National Heart, Lung, and Blood Institute
Division of Intramural Research
Pulmonary-Critical Care Medicine Branch
NIH Bldg. 10, Rm. 6D03
10 Center Dr. MSC-1590
Bethesda, MD 20892-1590
Phone: (301)496-1597 **Fax:** (301)496-2363
Joel Moss, Chf.
Activities/Fields: Structure and function of the lung in health and disease through cellular and biochemical methods. Both laboratory and clinical investigations are conducted and techniques of protein chemistry, molecular biology, tissue culture, and immunology are used. Emphasis is on the regulation of the inflammato-

ry and immune processes in the normal and diseased lung. Clinical research is directed toward correlating physiologic, biochemical, immunologic, and morphologic observations in patients with interstitial lung disease, destructive lung disease, hereditary disorders of connective tissue, hypersensitivity lung disease, and other lung disorders with an immunologic basis.

★ 24967 ★ U.S. Department of Health and Human Services
National Heart, Lung, and Blood Institute
Division of Lung Diseases
Two Rockledge Ctr., Ste. 10018
6701 Rockledge Dr. MSC 7952
Bethesda, MD 20892-7952
Phone: (301)435-0233 **Fax:** (301)480-3547
Email: kileyj@nhlbi.nih.gov
Website: http://www.nhlbi.nih.gov/about/dld/index.htm
Dr. James P. Kiley, PhD, Dir.
Activities/Fields: Focal point for planning and coordinating research and research training programs for all diseases of the respiratory system, including chronic obstructive pulmonary diseases; pediatric pulmonary diseases; occupational and immunologic lung diseases; pulmonary vascular diseases; acute lung injury; asthma; critical care; cystic fibrosis; lung cell biology; respiratory neurobiology and sleep; and pulmonary complications of AIDS. **Pub:** *and idiopathic pulmonary fibrosis. • Brochures on asthma, chronic obstructive pulmonary disease. • primary pulmonary hypertension. • sarcoidosis.*

★ 24968 ★ U.S. Department of Health and Human Services
National Heart, Lung, and Blood Institute
Division of Lung Diseases
Cell and Developmental Biology Branch (Lung Biology and Disease Program)
2 Rockledge Center, Ste. 10122
6701 Rockledge Dr., MSC 7952
Bethesda, MD 20892-7952
Phone: (301)435-0222 **Fax:** (301)480-3557
Email: gaild@nhlbi.nih.gov
Website: http://www.nhlbi.nih.gov/about/dld/index.htm
Dr. Dorothy Gail, PhD, Dir.
Activities/Fields: Pediatric pulmonary diseases, lung cell biology, acute lung injury, interstitial lung disease, pulmonary immunology, AIDS-related lung disease, and tuberculosis.

★ 24969 ★ U.S. Department of Health and Human Services
National Heart, Lung, and Blood Institute
Laboratory of Biochemical Genetics
NIH Bldg. 36, Rm. 1C-06
9000 Rockville Pike MSC 4036
Bethesda, MD 20892
Phone: (301)496-2401 **Fax:** (301)402-0270
Email: marshall@codon.nih.gov
Dr. Marshall Nirenberg, PhD, Chf.
Activities/Fields: Molecular Biology and Macromolecules. The Molecular Biology Section studies basic problems in molecular biology and biochemistry, particularly those that pertain to the development of the nervous system. Current research focuses on elucidating mechanisms that regulate gene expression using recombinant DNA techniques; and on cyclic nucleotides, ion channels, and cell recognition. The Macromolecules Section studies cellular control in *Escherichia coli.* Areas of interest include: the control of the synthesis and metabolism of cyclic AMP in bacterial cells; the regulation of expression of the gene for adenylate cyclase as well as the factors that regulate enzyme activity, using biological and recombinant DNA approaches; and analyses of structure, function, and repression mechanisms involving the *E. coli* cycle AMO receptor protein.

★ 24970 ★ U.S. Department of Health and Human Services
National Heart, Lung, and Blood Institute
Laboratory of Biophysical Chemistry
NIH Bldg. 50, Rm. 3403
50 South Dr.
Bethesda, MD 20892-1676
Phone: (301)496-2135 **Fax:** (301)402-3404
Email: ferrettj@nhlbi.nih.gov
Dr. James Ferretti, Chf.
Activities/Fields: Physical and chemical properties of molecules with a view to elucidating their biochemical functions. Specialties are nuclear magnetic resonance, mass spectrometry, computational chemistry, chromatography, and laboratory computer techniques. A special concern is the development of new techniques and their application to problems of current interest.

★ 24971 ★ U.S. Department of Health and Human Services
National Heart, Lung, and Blood Institute
Laboratory of Cardiac Energetics
NIH Bldg. 10, Rm. B1D 416
10 Center Dr. MSC 1061
Bethesda, MD 20892
Phone: (301)496-3658 **Fax:** (301)402-2389
Email: rsb@nih.gov
Dr. Robert Balaban, Chf.
Activities/Fields: Cardiology, nuclear magnetic resonance imaging/spectrography, cardiac energetics, and optical spectroscopy.

★ 24972 ★ U.S. Department of Health and Human Services
National Heart, Lung, and Blood Institute (NHLBI)
Laboratory of Cell Biology (LCB)
NIH Bldg. 50, Rm. 2517
9000 Rockville Pike
Bethesda, MD 20892
Phone: (301)496-1616 **Fax:** (301)402-1519
Email: edk@nih.gov
Edward Korn, PhD, Chf.
Activities/Fields: Structure/function studies of the regulation of non-muscle class II, and class I myosins by heavy and light chain phosphorylation in vitro and in vivo. The role of class II and class I myosins in vivo, particularly in the cellular slime mold Dictyostelium discoideum, for example, cytokinesis, differentiation and development, phagocytosis, motility and chemotaxis.

★ 24973 ★ U.S. Department of Health and Human Services
National Heart, Lung, and Blood Institute
Laboratory of Cell Signaling
NIH Bldg. 50, Rm. 3523
9000 Rockville Pike
Bethesda, MD 20892
Phone: (301)496-9646 **Fax:** (301)480-0357
Email: sgrhee@nih.gov
Dr. Sue Rhee, Chf.
Activities/Fields: Cell signaling in relation to the human heart, lung, and blood interaction.

★ 24974 ★ U.S. Department of Health and Human Services
National Heart, Lung, and Blood Institute
Laboratory of Kidney and Electrolyte Metabolism
NIH Bldg. 10, Rm. 6N260
10 Center Dr., MSC 1603
Bethesda, MD 20892
Phone: (301)496-3187 **Fax:** (301)402-1443
Dr. Mark Knepper, Chf.
Activities/Fields: Mechanism and regulation (hormonal and otherwise) of a variety of transport processes in systems, including the intact kidney, isolated perfused segments of renal tubules, and epithelial cell cultures. Emphasis is on electrophysiology, quantitative microscopy, nuclear magnetic resonance, and intermediary metabolism as related to transport. **Pub:** *Proceedings.*

★ 24975 ★ U.S. Department of Health and Human Services
National Heart, Lung, and Blood Institute
Laboratory of Molecular Cardiology
NIH Bldg. 10, Rm. 8N-202
10 Center Dr. MSC 1762
Bethesda, MD 20892
Phone: (301)496-1865 **Fax:** (301)402-1542
Email: adelster@nhlbi.nih.gov
Dr. Robert S. Adelstein, Chf.
Activities/Fields: Regulation function and expression of the contractile proteins in muscle and nonmuscle cells. The role of calcium, calmodulin, and phosphorylation in regulating actin-myosin interaction is of particular interest. Projects include studies of the mechanism by which phosphorylation alters contractile activity in smooth muscle and nonmuscle cells, regulation of contractile protein expression in cultured smooth muscle cells, and cloning the genes for selected contractile proteins. Current interest is the role these proteins and their genes play in cellular development, differentiation, and tumorigenicity.

★ 24976 ★ U.S. Department of Health and Human Services
National Heart, Lung, and Blood Institute
Molecular Hematology Branch
NIH Bldg. 10, Rm. 7D18
9000 Rockville Pike
Bethesda, MD 20892
Phone: (301)496-5844 **Fax:** (301)496-9985
Email: besafer@helix.nih.gov
Brian Safer, Actg. Chf.
Activities/Fields: Mechanism and regulation of mammalian gene expression to develop the understanding and technology necessary to carry out human gene therapy. The types of diseases being targeted are genetic cancer, viral, and cardiovascular. Major areas of research include gene cloning and adeno-associated virus (AAV) gene transfer, AAV vector development and isolation and characterization of genes, and expression of trans-acting factors involved in the regulation of gene expression, both at the transcriptional and translational level. **Pub:** *Proceedings. • Research Reports.*

★ 24977 ★ U.S. Department of Health and Human Services
National Heart, Lung, and Blood Institute
Sickle Cell Disease Scientific Research Group
2 Rockledge Centre
6701 Rockledge Dr. MSC 7950
Bethesda, MD 20892-7950
Phone: (301)435-0055 **Fax:** (301)480-0868
Email: evansg@nih.gov
Website: http://www.nhlbi.nih.gov
Greg Evans, PhD, Dir.
Activities/Fields: Provides a bridge for rapid translation and transfer of basic and clinical research on diseases to health care at the community level. The comprehensive sickle cell/red blood cell centers combine fundamental and clinical research, clinical trials, training and community service in an appproach designed to concentrate resources, facilities, and personnel in a focused approach to the problems posed by sickle cell disease. Specific research projects include: molecular, cellular, tissue, and organ studies, as well as clinical trials, training and education in sickle cell disease, Cooley's anemia, Fanconi anemia, and Diamond Blackfan anemia. **Frmly:** (2002) Sickle Cell Disease Scientific Research Group.

★ 24978 ★ U.S. Department of Health and Human Services
National Heart, Lung, and Blood Institute
Specialized Centers of Research on Arteriosclerosis
2 Rockledge Center, Ste. 10193
MSC 79516
6701 Rockledge Dr.
Bethesda, MD 20892-7956
Phone: (301)435-0550 **Fax:** (301)480-2858
Email: wassefm@nih.gov
Dr. Momtaz Wassef, Dir.
Activities/Fields: Hyperlipidemia and vascular diseases, including animal and tissue studies and other basic laboratory investigations. The research goal is to expidite development and application of new knowledge essential to improved diagnosis, treatment, and prevention of these disorders. **Frmly:** (2000) Specialized Centers of Research on Ateriosclerosis.

★ 24979 ★ U.S. Department of Health and Human Services
National Heart, Lung, and Blood Institute
Specialized Centers of Research on Ischemic Heart Disease
6701 Rockledge Dr., MSC 7940
Bethesda, MD 20892
Phone: (301)435-0544 **Fax:** (301)480-1336
Email: jf46f@nih.gov
Website: http://grants.nih.gov/grants/guide/RFA-files/RFA-HL-03-009.htm
Dr. John Fakunding, Contact
Activities/Fields: Myocardial infarction, angina pectoris, heart rhythum disturbances, heart failure. The research goal is to expedite development and application of new knowledge essential for improved diagnosis, treatment, and prevention of these disorders.

★ 24980 ★ U.S. Department of Health and Human Services
National Institute on Aging
Public Information Office
Bldg. 31., Rm. 5C27
31 Center Dr., MSC 2292
Bethesda, MD 20892-2292
Phone: (301)496-1752 **Free:** 800-222-2225
Fax: (301)496-2525
Email: hodesr@31.nia.nih.gov
Website: http://www.nia.nih.gov
Dr. Richard J. Hodes, Dir.
Activities/Fields: Biomedical, social, and behavioral aspects of aging. The Intramural Research Program is primarily conducted at the Gerontology Research Center in Baltimore, MD. In addition, the Institute's Neurosciences Laboratory operates basic and clinical research programs from the NIH Clinical Center in Bethesda, MD. The principal NIA extramural programs are the Behavioral and Social Research Program, the Biology of Aging Program, the Geriatrics Program, and the Neuroscience and Neuropsychology of Aging Program. Areas included in the program are: diagnostic assessment of the geriatric patient, dementia, incontinence, fall injuries, and musculoskeletal disorders producing functional disability in the geriatric population, among others.

★ 24981 ★ U.S. Department of Health and Human Services
National Institute on Aging
Behavioral and Social Research Program
Gateway Bldg., Rm 533
7201 Wisconsin Ave.
MSC 9205
Bethesda, MD 20892-9205
Phone: (301)496-3131 **Fax:** (301)402-0051
Email: BSRquery@EXMUR.NIA.NIH.GOV
Website: http://www.nia.nih.gov/research/extramural/behavior/
Dr. Richard M. Suzman, Assoc. Dir.
Activities/Fields: Social, psychological, cultural, demographic, and economic factors that affect both the process of growing old and the place of older people in society, as well as the ways in which behavioral and social processes interacting with biomedical processes influence particular aspects of health and functioning as people age. Its goals are to prolong the productive, healthy, middle years of life and to prevent or reverse such decrements of old age as memory loss, chronic ill health, sensory deficits, low self-esteem, and withdrawal from active participation in social and economic roles. The program focuses primarily on three broad categories: adult psychological development, with research supported that investigates social and behavioral influences upon cognitive functioning, personality, attitudes, and interpersonal relations over the adult life course, with emphasis on research relevant to maintaining and improving well being and independent functioning; social science research on aging, which is directed at understanding the social and environmental conditions influencing health, well being, and functioning of people in their middle and later years as well as the influence of social structures on aging and the interactions among psychosocial and biological processes on health and functioning; and demography and population epidemiology, involving research on the dynamics and consequences of population aging and aims to describe and understand the older population in terms of its social, demographic, economic, health, and functional characteristics and the impact of these changes on society as a whole.

★ 24982 ★ U.S. Department of Health and Human Services
National Institute on Aging
Biology of Aging Program
7201 Wisconsin Ave., Ste. 2C-231
Bethesda, MD 20892
Phone: (301)496-6402 **Fax:** (301)496-4996
Email: bapquery@nia.nih.gov
Website: http://www.nia.nih.gov/research/extramural/biology/
Dr. Richard L. Sprott, Assoc. Dir.
Activities/Fields: Basic mechanisms involved in aging processes and age-related disease. It funds research and training in ten main areas: biochemistry; genetics; endocrinology; immunology; nutrition and metabolism; molecular biology; pathobiology; cell biology, physiology; and biomarkers of aging. The Program also supports facilities that provide investigators with aging animals and cell cultures for use in aging research. **Frmly:** (1990) Biomedical Research and Clinical Medicine Program.

★ 24983 ★ U.S. Department of Health and Human Services
National Institute on Aging
Biology of Aging Program
Biology Branch
Gateway Bldg., Ste. 2C231
7201 Wisconsin Ave., MSC 9205
Bethesda, MD 20892-9205
Phone: (301)496-6402 **Fax:** (301)402-0010
Francis L. Bellino, Dep. Assoc. Dir.
Activities/Fields: Cellular aging research, which involves research using differentiated human cells in culture and the study of age-associated alterations in differentiated functions that are expressed by cells in vitro; fundamental molecular and genetics research and research training on the biology and mechanisms of aging at the cellular level and on vertebrate and invertebrate organisms, with particular interest in research that emphasizes the use of mammalian and human models; immunological research on the effects of aging on the various functions of the immune system; and research on age-related changes in endocrine function. **Frmly:** Molecular and Cell Biology Branch.

★ 24984 ★ U.S. Department of Health and Human Services
National Institute on Aging
Epidemiology, Demography, and Biometry Program
7201 Wisconsin Ave., Ste. 3C-309
Bethesda, MD 20892
Phone: (301)496-1178 **Fax:** (301)496-4006
Email: havlikr@gw.nia.nih.gov
Website: http://www.nia.nih.gov/research/intramural/edb
Richard J. Havlik, MD, Assoc. Dir.
Activities/Fields: Health and illness in older populations, including hip fractures and osteoporosis, dementia and other cognitive impairments, sleep disorders, predictive factors of mortality, bereavement behaviors, and events and conditions common among older persons prior to death. Gathers demographic information on the current and projected health, economic, social, and occupational status of older people.

★ 24985 ★ U.S. Department of Health and Human Services
National Institute on Aging
Geriatrics Program
7201 Wisconson Ave., St. 3E-327
Bethesda, MD 20892-9205
Phone: (301)496-1033 **Fax:** (301)402-1784
Dr. Evan Hadley, Chf.
Activities/Fields: Epidemiology, etiology, pathophysiology, diagnostic evaluation, and treatment of urinary incontinence in the elderly; studies on obesity, with particular interest in the effects of obesity on health and longevity, treatment of obesity, and contribution of overnutrition to aging of organ systems; research on infectious diseases in the elderly (cosponsored with the National Institute of Allergy and Infectious Diseases); studies on aspects of diabetes mellitus related to aging and the elderly and studies on the epidemiology of diabetes; and nutrition in relation to health of the aged and the aging process. Research also includes investigation of the function of the aging musculoskeletal system (including support for animal models or clinical studies in exercise physiology or orthopedic research); studies on enteral and parenteral nutritional support in elderly patients in acute and long-term care facilities (announced with five other institutes); research on the causes of age-related cardiovascular changes (and changes in risk factors for cardiovascular disease) and on the role of cardiovascular factors in age-related physiologic and pathologic changes; and studies on exercise physiology and aging.

★ 24986 ★ U.S. Department of Health and Human Services
National Institute on Aging
Intramural Research Program
Gerontology Research Center
5600 Nathan Shock Dr.
Baltimore, MD 21224
Phone: (410)558-8110 **Fax:** (410)558-8137
Email: longod@grc.nia.nih.gov
Dr. Dan L. Longo, Dir.
Activities/Fields: Process of aging in animals and man. Projects include the Baltimore Longitudinal Study of Aging, which involves the biennial observation of the same human subjects to determine changes and elucidate mechanisms underlying these changes. Program components include Behavioral Sciences Laboratory; Biological Chemistry Laboratory; Cardiovascular Science Laboratory; Cellular and Molecular Biology Laboratory; Clinical Physiology Laboratory; Longitudinal Studies Branch; Molecular Genetics Laboratory; Neurosciences Laboratory; and Personality and Cognition Laboratory.

★ 24987 ★ U.S. Department of Health and Human Services
National Institute on Aging
Intramural Research Program
Longitudinal Studies Section
(Laboratory of Clinical Investigation)
Gerontology Research Center
5600 Nathan Shock Dr.
Baltimore, MD 21224
Phone: (410)558-8364 **Fax:** (410)558-8321
Email: jf72d@nih.gov
Website: http://www.grc.nia.nih.gov
Jerome L. Fleg, MD, Interim Dir.
Activities/Fields: Longitudinal research on aging, particularly physiological and psychological aspects. **Pub:** *Proceedings.* • *Research reports.*

★ 24988 ★ U.S. Department of Health and Human Services
National Institute on Aging
Laboratory of Cardiovascular Science
Gerontology Research Center, Rm. 3B03
5600 Nathan Shock Dr.
Baltimore, MD 21224
Phone: (410)558-8202 **Fax:** (410)558-8150
Email: lakattae@grc.nia.nih.gov
Dr. Edward G. Lakatta, Chf.
Activities/Fields: Basic mechanisms that control myocardial and vascular function. Studies are extended to describe the influence of age and age-related chronic pathologic conditions in studies conducted in human and animal models. In humans, laboratory seeks to identify the adaptive changes in cardiovascular structure and function that occur with normative aging as well as those changes that predict or accompany the development of cardiovascular disease. Studies in animal models involve isolated cardiac and vascular cells and subcellular organelles. The biophysical mechanisms that govern excitation and contraction of myocardial cells are investigated with techniques that allow the simultaneous recording of contra c tility, cytosolic and membrane potential, or current in a single myocyte. Current research includes a program to study molecular mechanisms of vascular cell functions and pathology using molecular and tissue culture techniques. Also studies whether the blood vessels of adults and animals respond differently to injury by altered gene expression of growth factors and extracellular matrix proteins, and whether age alters endothelial cell growth and differentiation of in vivo systems. Also investigates the effects produced by cytokines, second messengers, aging, and cell cycle of in vitro models for angiogenesis.

★ 24989 ★ U.S. Department of Health and Human Services
National Institute on Aging
Laboratory of Cellular and Molecular Biology
Gerontology Research Center
Rm. 1-B-02, Stop 12
5600 Nathan Shock Dr.
Baltimore, MD 21224
Phone: (410)558-8443 **Fax:** (410)558-8335
Email: gorospem@grc.nia.nih.gov
Website: http://www.grc.nia.nih.gov/branches/lcmb/lcmb.htm
Myriam Gorospe, Actg. Ch.
Activities/Fields: Basic biological and biochemical mechanisms of aging. Activities include research into the mechanism of stress responses, hormone/neurotransmitter, signal transduction, neurodegeneration/protection, behavior, erythrocyte oxyradical production and aging, and NMR methodology and applications. Nutritional, pharmacological, exercise and other interventions into the aging process are also employed. Four groups make up the laboratory: Gene Expression and Aging Section; Molecular Dynamics Section; Molecular Physiology and Genetics Section; and NMR Unit. **Pub:** *Proceedings.*

★ 24990 ★ U.S. Department of Health and Human Services
National Institute on Aging
Laboratory of Clinical Physiology
Gerontology Research Center
5600 Nathan Shock Dr.
Baltimore, MD 21224
Phone: (410)558-8193 **Fax:** (410)558-8113
Dr. Reubin Andres, Chf.
Activities/Fields: Physiologic changes occurring over the entire adult lifespan. The Laboratory comprises sections on Applied Physiology, Clinical Immunology, Endocrinology, and Metabolism. The Applied +Physiology Section studies age changes in specific human systems, including renal, bone, and musculoskeletal. Investigations are concerned with interrelationships between age effects in different organ systems and in overall physiological changes in individuals, and efforts are made to differentiate between pathological disease changes and those secondary to pure age effects. In addition, Section develops and adapts computer techniques for kinetic modeling of physiological systems for the analysis of longitudinal data. In the Clinical +Immunology Section, studies are conducted on the decline in host immune responsiveness that is seen in aging. These studies involve the development of diagnostic procedures for the detection of relative immunodeficiencies in humans and the investigation of the mechanisms of these deficiencies in humans and experimental animals. The Endocrinology Section conducts studies on the molecular basis of age-related changes of hormone responses, especially those related to the biochemistry of the adenylate cyclase system and hormone receptors, aging and the endocrinology of the reproductive system, and neuroendocrinology. Clinical studies are conducted on subjects from the Baltimore Longitudinal Study of Human Aging; and studies on rodents are done on tissues from a variety of organs. The Metabolism Section emphasizes clinical research on such metabolic variables as: glucose-insulin homeostatic mechanisms and diabetes mellitus; obesity, patterns of fat distribution, and body composition; acute and sustained effects of physical activity; dietary and nutritional evaluation; and the interactive effects of these variables on rates of aging, disease developments, and longevity.

★ 24991 ★ U.S. Department of Health and Human Services
National Institute on Aging
Laboratory of Molecular Genetics
5600 Nathan Shock Dr.
Baltimore, MD 21224-6823
Phone: (410)558-8162 **Fax:** (410)558-8157
Email: vbohr@nih.gov
Dr. Vilhelm A. Bohr, Chf.
Activities/Fields: Fundamental nature of aging at the molecular level, including studies on changes in gene structure and function with aging. Researchers utilize the techniques of molecular genetics to examine age-related alterations in cellular function and the DNA repair processes.

★ 24992 ★ U.S. Department of Health and Human Services
National Institute on Aging (NIA)
Laboratory of Neurosciences
NIH Bldg. 10, Rm. 6N202
10 Center Dr., MSC 1582
Bethesda, MD 20892-1582
Phone: (301)496-1765 **Fax:** (301)402-0074
Email: sir@helix.nih.gov
Dr. Stanley Rapoport, Chf.
Activities/Fields: Function, structure, physiology, biochemistry, and pharmacology of the central and peripheral nervous system. Laboratory also examines changes that take place in these systems during development and aging in animal models and humans. The Laboratory comprises the Brain Aging and +Dementia Section, the Cerebral +Physiology and Metabolism Section, and the Neurochemistry and +Brain Transport Section. The Brain Aging and Dementia Section operates an eight-bed Patient Care Unit at the Clinical Center as well as an outpatient Dementia and Aging Clinic. Clinical methods involve positron emission tomography. Research activities focus primarily on aging of the central nervous system and on dementia and associated neurological diseases as these relate to the elderly. Subject groups include outpatient healthy men and women between 18 and 90 years of age, with syndrome and chronic hypertension. The Cerebral Physiology and Metabolism Section conducts fundamental research on animal models of human brain aging and disease using molecular biology, clinical in vivo brain imaging, neurochemistry involving phospholipid metabolism, electrophysiology, and cell culture techniques. The Neurochemistry and Brain Transport Section studies transport and regulation at the blood-brain and blood-nerve barriers, focusing on amino acids, toxic metals, and fatty acids. **Pub:** *Proceedings.*

★ 24993 ★ U.S. Department of Health and Human Services
National Institute on Aging
Laboratory of Personality and Cognition
Gerontology Research Center
5600 Nathan Shock Dr.
Baltimore, MD 21224
Phone: (410)558-8220 **Fax:** (410)558-8108
Email: lpcpsc@helix.nih.gov
Website: http://www.grc.nia.nih.gov/branches/lpc/lpc.htm
Dr. Paul T. Costa, Chf.
Activities/Fields: Individual differences in cognitive and personality processes and traits. Also investigated are the influence of age on these variables and their reciprocal influence on health, well-being, and adaptation. Studies employ longitudinal, experimental, and epidemiological methods in the analysis of psychological and psychosocial issues of aging, including health and health care needs, predictors of intellectual competence and decline, models of adult personality, and correlates of disease risk factors. Laboratory comprises sections on: Cognition and Personality, Stress, and Coping. The Cognition Section studies the psychological mechanisms underlying age-related changes in memory, learning, problem solving, and information processing. In addition, the roles of psychological and physiological characteristics in age differences and age changes in cognitive performance are analyzed. The Personality, +Stress, and Coping Section deals with the dimensions of personality and their influence on processes of adaptation in adult men and women. The objective is to determine methods and strategies for coping with the stresses of adult life and evaluate the effects of different coping mechanisms and personality dispositions on such outcomes as subjective well-being, social functioning, physical and psychiatric health and personality and psychological processes.

★ 24994 ★ U.S. Department of Health and Human Services
National Institute on Aging
Neuroscience and Neuropsychology of Aging Program
NIH Gateway Bldg., Ste. 350
7201 Wisconsin Ave. MSC9205
Bethesda, MD 20892-9205
Phone: (301)496-9350 **Fax:** (301)496-1494
Email: morrisom@nia.nih.gov
Marcelle Morrison-Bogorad, Assoc. Dir.
Activities/Fields: Normal and pathological aging of the nervous system and its behavioral consequences. Etiology or pathogenesis of Alzheimer's disease, improve diagnosis, and eventually provide a sound basis for effective therapy. Areas of particular interest are: differential diagnosis; clinical and basic studies of cerebral circulation, metabolism, neurochemistry, and neuroendocrinology; genetics; population studies; immunology-virology; and animal and other model systems. Other areas of interest include: research on role of infectious agents and immunolgoical processes that cause degeneration in the aging brain; identification of biological markers in the diagnosis of diseases, such

as Alzheimer's; epidemiological investigations of Alzheimer's disease and other dementing disorders of older age; research on diagnostic screening; development and validation of new measures for the diagnosis of Alzheimer's disease; studies designed to examine the nature and extent of age-related sensory and motor changes in older people, such as hearing and understanding of everyday speech, visual perception, taste, and smell as related to the effective functioning of older people in everyday contexts; neurobiological processes as they relate to the aging nervous system and behavior neuropsychological processes in aging animals and humans; sleep and circadian rhythms in aging and the treatment of disturbances; neural plasticity; and mechanisms underlying neural growth, survival, and death in the aging brain. **Frmly:** Physiology of Aging Branch.

★ 24995 ★ U.S. Department of Health and Human Services
National Institute on Aging
Office of Extramural Affairs
Gateway Bldg. 2C218
7201 Wisconsin Ave.
MSC 9205
Bethesda, MD 20892-9205
Phone: (301)496-9322 **Fax:** (301)402-2945
Email: mk46u@nih.gov
Website: http://www.nia.nih.gov
Dr. Miriam F. Kelty, Assoc. Dir.
Activities/Fields: Administers the funding programs through which NIA supports research and research training. Specific NIA funding mechanisms include: Research Project Grants; Research Program Project Grants; Research Career Development Awards; Clinical Investigator Awards; Academic Awards; National Research Service Awards; Physician Scientist Awards; Geriatric Leadership Academic Awards; Small Business Innovative Research Program; and Academic Research Enhancement Awards.

★ 24996 ★ U.S. Department of Health and Human Services
National Institute on Alcohol Abuse and Alcoholism
Willco Bldg., Ste. 400
6000 Executive Blvd.
Bethesda, MD 20892-7003
Phone: (301)443-3885 **Fax:** (301)443-7043
Email: rkington@mail.nih.gov
Website: http://www.niaaa.nih.gov
Raynard S. Kington, MD, Actg. Dir.
Activities/Fields: Prevention and treatment of alcohol-related problems and alcoholism. Seeks to develop new scientific knowledge that will reduce the incidence and prevalence of alcohol abuse and alcoholism and the associated morbidity and mortality. Conducts and supports research aimed at determining the causes of alcoholism, discovering how alcohol damages the organs of the body, and developing prevention and treatment strategies for application in the nation's health care system. Conducts policy studies with broad implications for alcohol prevention and treatment; and conducts epidemiological studies to assess the risks for and problems among various population groups.

★ 24997 ★ U.S. Department of Health and Human Services
National Institute on Alcohol Abuse and Alcoholism
Basic Research Division
Willco Bldg., Rm. 402
6000 Exec. Blvd.
Bethesda, MD 20892
Phone: (301)443-0799 **Fax:** (301)594-0673
Email: sz14w@nih.gov
Website: http://www.niaaa.nih.gov/extramural/resch-pro.htm
Samir Zakhari, Ch.
Activities/Fields: Multiple determinants and processes of alcoholism and other alcohol-related problems. Division administers the Institute's National +Alcohol Research Centers Program as well as its research scientists development and training programs. In addition, it collaborates with other national and international agencies, universities, and scientific organizations and provides technical assistance to universities, federal agencies, state and local governments, and community and voluntary organizations. Principal Division components are: Biomedical Research Branch and Neurosciences Research Branch. Research Branch and Neurosciences Research Branch.

★ 24998 ★ U.S. Department of Health and Human Services
National Institute on Alcohol Abuse and Alcoholism
Basic Research Division
Biomedical Research Branch
Willco Bldg., St. 402
6000 Executive Blvd., MSC 7003
Bethesda, MD 20892-7003
Phone: (301)443-4224 **Fax:** (301)594-0673
Email: szakhari@willco.miaaa.nih.gov
Dr. Samir Zakhari, PhD, Dir.
Activities/Fields: Supports and administers NIAAA extramural research grants and training programs on the effects of alcohol abuse and alcoholism as related to the central nervous system, the fetal alcohol syndrome, and neuroendocrine and pathological conditions. Research is aimed at reduction of morbidity and mortality associated with alcoholism and alcohol abuse and includes research in the areas of etiology, pathogenesis, identification, treatment, and prevention as well as in the development of basic research tools and methodologies. **Pub:** *Alcohol and Health Monograph Series.*

★ 24999 ★ U.S. Department of Health and Human Services
National Institute on Alcohol Abuse and Alcoholism
Basic Research Division
Neurosciences and Behavioral Research Branch
6000 Executive Blvd.
Bethesda, MD 20892-7003
Phone: (301)443-4223 **Fax:** (301)594-0673
Email: ewitt@willco.niaaa.nih.gov
Website: http://www.niaaa.nih.gov/extramural/resch-pro.htm
Ellen Witt, PhD, Contact
Activities/Fields: Effect of alcohol on the brain and behavior.

★ 25000 ★ U.S. Department of Health and Human Services
National Institute on Alcohol Abuse and Alcoholism
Biometry and Epidemiology Division
6000 Executive Blvd., MSC 7003
Bethesda, MD 20892-7003
Phone: (301)443-2193 **Fax:** (301)443-8614
Dr. Mary C. Dufor, MPH, Dir.
Activities/Fields: Incidence and prevalence of alcohol abuse and alcoholism (both nationally and in specific population groups); conducts national surveillance activities to collect and analyze alcohol-related program data through various information systems; and develops and maintains information systems to collect and analyze alcohol-related data. Division also collaborates with other organizations engaged in alcohol data collection activities, such as state-based information systems, in order to exchange pertinent data and to utilize existing data systems where appropriate.

★ 25001 ★ U.S. Department of Health and Human Services
National Institute on Alcohol Abuse and Alcoholism
Division of Clinical and Prevention Research
6000 Executive Blvd.
Willco Bldg., St. 505
Bethesda, MD 20892-7003
Phone: (301)443-1206 **Fax:** (301)443-8774
Email: rfuller@arswillco.niaaa.nih.gov
Website: http://www.niaaa.nih.gov/extramural/resch-pro.htm
Richard K. Fuller, MD, Dir.
Activities/Fields: Supports alcohol abuse and alcoholism treatment, prevention, and health services research through grants and cooperative agreements. Principal Division components are the Prevention Research Branch, the Treatment Research Branch, and the Health Services Research Program.

★ 25002 ★ U.S. Department of Health and Human Services
National Institute on Alcohol Abuse and Alcoholism
Intramural Clinical and Biological Research Division
JIH Bldg. 10, Rm. 3C103, MSC 1256
9000 Rockville Pike
Bethesda, MD 20892
Phone: (301)496-8996 **Fax:** (301)402-0445
Email: gkunos@mail.nih.gov
Dr. George Kunos, Dir.
Activities/Fields: Multiple determinants and processes of alcoholism and other alcohol-related problems and on prevention, diagnosis, treatment, and rehabilitation. It also provides in-house research scientist training in a variety of disciplines for work in alcohol-related research and collaborates with other agencies, universities, and scientific organizations. Division comprises laboratories of Clinical Studies; Metabolism; Membrane Biochemistry and Biophysics; Molecular and Cellular Neurobiology; and Neurogenetics.

★ 25003 ★ U.S. Department of Health and Human Services
National Institute on Alcohol Abuse and Alcoholism
Intramural Clinical and Biological Research Division
Clinical Studies Laboratory
NIH Bldg. 10, Rm. 3C114
9000 Rockville Pike
Bethesda, MD 20892
Phone: (301)496-5353 **Fax:** (301)402-0445
Paul Andreas, Contact
Activities/Fields: Neuroscience, clinical pharmacology, analytical biochemistry, internal medicine, and psychiatry, all as related to alcoholism.

★ 25004 ★ U.S. Department of Health and Human Services
National Institute on Alcohol Abuse and Alcoholism
Intramural Clinical and Biological Research Division
Laboratory of Molecular and Cellular Neurobiology
Park Bldg., Rm. 150
Bethesda, MD 20892-8115
Phone: (301)443-1234 **Fax:** (301)480-6882
Email: fweight@niaaa.nih.gov
Dr. Forrest Weight, Chf.
Activities/Fields: Alcohol and alcoholism, physiology, and pharmacology.

★ 25005 ★ U.S. Department of Health and Human Services
National Institute on Alcohol Abuse and Alcoholism
Prevention Research Center
Prevention Research Center (PIRE)
2150 Shattuck Ave., Ste. 900
Berkeley, CA 94704
Phone: (510)486-1111 **Fax:** (510)644-0594
Email: grube@prev.org
Website: http://www.pire.org
Dr. Joel Grube, Dir.
Activities/Fields: Prevention of alcohol-related problems. Research focuses on better understanding the social and physical environment that influences individual behavior and problems relating to alcohol abuse. Objectives are to: develop innovative research and approaches that contribute to informed decisions about cost-effective prevention programs and policies at the local, state, and national levels; contribute to broader theoretical frameworks in the prevention of alcohol-related problems, especially in the area of environmental factors; summarize new and existing knowledge about prevention theories, policies, and programs and disseminate information to professional, academic, and community audiences; and provide.

★ 25006 ★ U.S. Department of Health and Human Services
National Institute of Allergy and Infectious Diseases (NIAID)
Asthma and Allergic Diseases Cooperative Research Center
NIH, Bldg. 10, Rm. 11C205
10 Center Dr. MSC1881
Bethesda, MD 20892-1881
Phone: (301)496-2165 **Fax:** (301)480-8384
Email: dean_metcalfe@nih.gov
Dr. Dean Metcalfe, Chf.
Activities/Fields: Studies of the mast cell and its role in causing various allergic diseases, including asthma; and study of mast cell disorders including mastocytosis. **Frmly:** Asthma and Allergic Diseases Cooperative Research Center.

★ 25007 ★ U.S. Department of Health and Human Services
National Institute of Allergy and Infectious Diseases
Division of Acquired Immuniodeficiency Syndrome (AIDS)
Basic Science Program (Epidemiology Branch)
6700 B. Rockledge Dr., Rm. 4255
Bethesda, MD 20892
Phone: (301)402-0135 **Fax:** (301)402-4131
Email: cwilliams@niaid.nih.gov
Dr. Carolyn Williams, Contact
Activities/Fields: Coordinates population-based research that will advance the understanding of the biology and clinical course of HIV infection. Serves as a foundation for advancing treatment and prevention.

★ 25008 ★ U.S. Department of Health and Human Services
National Institute of Allergy and Infectious Diseases
Division of Acquired Immunodeficiency Syndrome (AIDS)
6007 Rockledge Dr.
Bldg. 6700 B, Rm. 4142
Bethesda, MD 20892
Phone: (301)496-0545 **Fax:** (301)402-1505
Email: et89f@nih.gov
Website: http://www.niaid.nih.gov/daids/default.htm
Dr. Edmond C. Tramont, MD, Dir.
Activities/Fields: Basic knowledge of the pathogenesis, natural history, and transmission of HIV. Promotes progress in the detection, treatment, and prevention of HIV.

★ 25009 ★ U.S. Department of Health and Human Services
National Institute of Allergy and Infectious Diseases
Division of Acquired Immunodeficiency Syndrome (AIDS)
Basic Science Program (Targeted Interventions Branch)
6700 B Rockledge Drive
Room 4254
Bethesda, MD 20892
Phone: (301)496-8197 **Fax:** (301)402-3211
Email: te35m@nih.gov
Dr. Sandra Bridges, Chf.
Activities/Fields: Discovery of effective vaccines and therapies for the prevention and treatment of HIV infection and disease.

★ 25010 ★ U.S. Department of Health and Human Services
National Institute of Allergy and Infectious Diseases
Division of Acquired Immunodeficiency Syndrome (AIDS)
Basic Science Program (Pathogenesis and Basic Research Branch)
Room 2140; Mail Stop 7610
6700B Rockledge Dr.
Bethesda, MD 20892-7610
Phone: (301)496-8666 **Fax:** (301)402-0369
Email: gm16s@nib.gov
Website: http://www.niaid.nih.gov
Gregory Milman, PhD, Dir.
Activities/Fields: Bioterrorism-related research, electronic research administration, small business opportunities, distance learning, and Internet training.

★ 25011 ★ U.S. Department of Health and Human Services
National Institute of Allergy and Infectious Diseases
Division of Acquired Immunodeficiency Syndrome (AIDS)
Basic Science Program
6700 B Rockledge Dr. MSC 7626
Bethesda, MD 20892-7626
Phone: (301)496-0637 **Fax:** (301)402-3211
Dr. Carl Dieffenbach, PhD, Assoc. Dir.
Activities/Fields: Pathogenesis, basic virology, immunobiology, pathobiology, the discovery of novel therapeutic approaches, and epidemiology.

★ 25012 ★ U.S. Department of Health and Human Services
National Institute of Allergy and Infectious Diseases
Division of Acquired Immunodeficiency Syndrome (AIDS)
Biostatistics Research Branch
6700-B Rockledge Dr., MSC 7609
Bethesda, MD 20892
Phone: (301)402-2306 **Fax:** (301)480-0912
Dennis Dixon, Chf.
Activities/Fields: Methodologic and biostatistical oversight and assistance.

★ 25013 ★ U.S. Department of Health and Human Services
National Institute of Allergy and Infectious Diseases
Division of Acquired Immunodeficiency Syndrome (AIDS)
Epidemiology Project Team
6700-B Rockledge Dr., Rm. 4131
Bethesda, MD 20892
Phone: (301)402-0135 **Fax:** (301)402-3211
Email: cwilliams@niaid.nih.gov
Dr. Carlie Williams, MD, Actg. Chf.
Activities/Fields: Epidemiology of HIV.

★ 25014 ★ U.S. Department of Health and Human Services
National Institute of Allergy and Infectious Diseases
Division of Acquired Immunodeficiency Syndrome (AIDS)
Office of Program Operations and Scientific Information
6007 Rockledge Dr., Rm. 4143
Bethesda, MD 20892
Phone: (301)496-0545 **Fax:** (301)402-1505
Email: tlasalvia@niaid.nih.gov
Website: http://www.niaid.nih.gov/daids/org/daidsorg.htm
Thomas Lasalvia, RN, Contact
Activities/Fields: Collects and maintains scientific data and composes reports for the Division of Acquired Immunodeficiency Syndrome.

★ 25015 ★ U.S. Department of Health and Human Services
National Institute of Allergy and Infectious Diseases
Division of Acquired Immunodeficiency Syndrome (AIDS)
Pediatric Project Team
6700-B Rockledge Dr. Rm. 5225
Bethesda, MD 20892
Phone: (301)402-2300 **Fax:** (301)402-3171
Email: jm74q@nih.gov
J. McNamara, MD, Chf.
Activities/Fields: HIV disease in relation to infants, children, and adolescents.

★ 25016 ★ U.S. Department of Health and Human Services
National Institute of Allergy and Infectious Diseases
Division of Acquired Immunodeficiency Syndrome (AIDS)
Pharmaceutical and Regulatory Affairs Branch
6700-B Rockledge Dr.
Bethesda, MD 20892
Phone: (301)496-8213 **Fax:** (301)402-1506
Email: am@niaid.nih.gov
Anna Martinez, PhD, Chf.
Activities/Fields: Assures that all clinical trials sponsored by DAIDS are conducted in accordance with FDA and Federal regulations.

★ 25017 ★ U.S. Department of Health and Human Services
National Institute of Allergy and Infectious Diseases
Division of Acquired Immunodeficiency Syndrome (AIDS)
Scientific Assessment and Resource Branch
6003 Executive Blvd.
Rockville, MD 20852
Phone: (301)402-0755 **Fax:** (301)480-5703
Activities/Fields: Conducts reviews to ensure that the Division's activities effectively address the stated scientific goals and priorities.

★ 25018 ★ U.S. Department of Health and Human Services
National Institute of Allergy and Infectious Diseases
Division of Acquired Immunodeficiency Syndrome (AIDS)
Therapeutics Research Program (Opportunistic Infections Research Branch)
6700-B Rockledge Dr., Rm. 5108
MSC 7624
Bethesda, MD 20892
Phone: (301)402-2304 **Fax:** (301)402-3171
Email: bl17u@nih.gov
Website: http://www.niaid.nih.gov/daids/org/daidstrp.htm
B. Laughon, PhD, Chf.
Activities/Fields: Improved therapies for the treatment and prophylaxis of OIs tuberculosis associated with HIV disease.

★ 25019 ★ U.S. Department of Health and Human Services
National Institute of Allergy and Infectious Diseases
Division of Acquired Immunodeficiency Syndrome (AIDS)
Therapeutics Research Program (Pediatric Medicine Branch)
Bldg. 31, Rm. 7A50
31 Center Dr.
Bethesda, MD 20892-2520
Phone: (301)402-2300 **Fax:** (301)402-0120
Dr. James G. McNamara, Chf.
Activities/Fields: Therapeutic strategies directed at: the clinical conditions associated with HIV infection in children and adolescents; and intervention to reduce the risk of transmission of HIV from infected mothers to the infant or fetus.

★ 25020 ★ U.S. Department of Health and Human Services
National Institute of Allergy and Infectious Diseases
Division of Acquired Immunodeficiency Syndrome (AIDS)
Therapeutics Research Program (HIV Research Branch)
6700-B Rockledge Dr., Rm. 5102
Bethesda, MD 20892
Phone: (301)496-0700 **Fax:** (301)480-4582
Email: cp22n@nih.gov
Carla Pettinelli, MD, Chf.
Activities/Fields: Preclinical and clinical research on: therapeutic strategies directed at the treatment of adult primary HIV infection; the augmentation of specific HIV immune responses and general host immunity in HIV-infected individuals; and the neurological complications of HIV infection.

★ 25021 ★ U.S. Department of Health and Human Services
National Institute of Allergy and Infectious Diseases
Division of Acquired Immunodeficiency Syndrome (AIDS)
Therapeutics Research Program (Clinical Site Management Branch)
6700-B Rockledge Dr., Rm. 5157
Bethesda, MD 20892
Phone: (301)402-0143 **Fax:** (301)480-4582
Email: mm154j@nih.gov
Margaret Matula, Actg. Chf.
Activities/Fields: Oversees the technical and administrative management of a program of research grants and contracts supporting clinical research sites carrying out DAIDS-supported clinical trials. These programs include: the Adult and Pediatric AIDS Clinical Trials Group (ACTG); the Terry Beirn Community Programs for Clinical Research on AIDS (CPCRA); the National Hemophilia Foundation (NHF); and the Acute Infection and Early Disease Research Program (AIEDRP).

★ 25022 ★ U.S. Department of Health and Human Services
National Institute of Allergy and Infectious Diseases
Division of Acquired Immunodeficiency Syndrome (AIDS)
Therapeutics Research Program (Coordinating Centers Branch)
6610 Rockledge Dr.
Bethesda, MD 20892-6603
Phone: (301)496-7728 **Fax:** (301)402-2508
D.M. Dixon, PhD, Chf.
Activities/Fields: Oversees the technical and administrative management of a program of research grants and contracts that provide coordinating support for the clinical trials organization supported by the TRP. This includes data management, biostatistical analysis, information processing, laboratory specimen tracking, coordinating, monitoring, and operations support. Oversight of the Division of AIDS Treatment Research Initiative (DATRI) is coordinated by this branch.

★ 25023 ★ U.S. Department of Health and Human Services
National Institute of Allergy and Infectious Diseases
Division of Acquired Immunodeficiency Syndrome (AIDS)
Therapeutics Research Program
6700-B Rockledge Dr., Rm. 5102
Bethesda, MD 20892
Phone: (301)496-8210 **Fax:** (301)480-4582
Email: fbl0C@nih.gov
Frederick Batzold, Actg. Dir.
Activities/Fields: Therapies against HIV disease, including associated opportunistic infections (OIs) and cancer in adults, infants, children, and adolescents.

★ 25024 ★ U.S. Department of Health and Human Services
National Institute of Allergy and Infectious Diseases
Division of Acquired Immunodeficiency Syndrome (AIDS)
Vaccine and Prevention Research Program (Preclinical Research Branch)
6700-B Rockledge Dr., Rm. 4102
Bethesda, MD 20892
Phone: (301)402-0121 **Fax:** (301)402-3684
Email: jbradac@niaid.nih.gov
Website: http://www.niaid.nih.gov/daids/vaccine
James Bradac, PhD, Chf.
Activities/Fields: Preclinical development and evaluation of safe and effective AIDS vaccines and adjuvants for the prevention of AIDS. **Frmly:** (2000) Preclinical Research Branch.

★ 25025 ★ U.S. Department of Health and Human Services
National Institute of Allergy and Infectious Diseases
Division of Acquired Immunodeficiency Syndrome (AIDS)
Vaccine and Prevention Research Program (Efficacy Trials Branch)
6700 B Rockledge Dr.
Bethesda, MD 20892
Phone: (301)496-6177 **Fax:** (301)402-3684
Margaret Johnson, Assoc. Dir.
Activities/Fields: Large-scale and domestic and international clinical trials of HIV vaccines and other biomedical and behavioral interventions.

★ 25026 ★ U.S. Department of Health and Human Services
National Institute of Allergy and Infectious Diseases
Division of Allergy, Immunology, and Transplantation
6700-B, Rm. 5142-MSC7640
Rockledge Dr.
Bethesda, MD 20892-7640
Phone: (301)496-1886 **Fax:** (301)402-2571
Email: dr17g@nih.gov
Website: http://www.niaid.nih.gov/research/dait.htm
Dr. Daniel Rotrosen, Ch.
Activities/Fields: Immune system as it functions in the maintenance of health and as it malfunctions in the production of disease. The Division provides leadership in the identification, design, and implementation of basic and clinical research initiatives encompassing a wide range of disorders including: autoimmune diseases such as childhood diabetes, rheumatoid arthritis and multiple sclerosis, allergic diseases such as asthma and occupational and environmental disorders and organ transplant rejection. **Frmly:** Immunology Allergic, and Immunologic Diseases Program, Allergy, Immunology, and Transplantation Program.

★ 25027 ★ U.S. Department of Health and Human Services
National Institute of Allergy and Infectious Diseases
Division of Allergy, Immunology, and Transplantation
Asthma, Allergy, and Inflamation Branch
6700-B Rockledge Dr.
Rm. 5142, MSC 7640
Bethesda, MD 20892-7640
Phone: (301)496-1886 **Fax:** (301)402-0175
Email: DR17G@NIH.GOV
Dr. Daniel Rotrosen, Chf.
Activities/Fields: Branch supports (through grants, cooperative agreements, career development awards, fellowships, and other mechanisms) basic and clinical research on the etiology, pathogenesis, diagnosis, prevention and treatment of allergic diseases and asthma; it also supports research on mucosal immunity, phagocyte biology and complement. Basic investigations include a study of the regulation of IgE antibody synthesis and IgE interactions with IgE receptors and other IgE binding molecules; studies of the epitopes of allergens and T cells that mediate allergic reations; assessment of the role of cytokines and adhesion molecules in regulating IgE synthesis and allergic inflammation in vitro and in vivo; and molecular and biochemical characterization of molecules expressed on, and in, mast cells, basophils and eosinophils. The diseases studies include asthma, allergic rhinitis, otitis, atopic dermatitis, and urticaria/angioedema. Also studies diseases induced by immune responses to specific antigens, notably IgE-mediated and T cell-mediated reactions to insect venoms, foods, industrial chemicals, contact sensitizers, airborne allergens, and drug hypersensitivity. The Asthma, Allergy and Inflammation Branch supports eight centers for the National Cooperative Inner City Asthma Study (NCICAS), which focuses on determining the mechanisms for the high morbidity and mortality from asthma of African American and Hispanic children ages 4-9 living in inner cities, and defining effective interventions to reduce that high morbidity and mortality. In addition, the Branch supports 15 (of 21) Asthma, Allergic and Immunologic Diseases Cooperative Research Centers, which integrate investigations of basic and clinical research related to human asthma, allergic diseases, and other immunologic diseases.

★ 25028 ★ U.S. Department of Health and Human Services
National Institute of Allergy and Infectious Diseases
Division of Allergy, Immunology, and Transplantation
Basic Immunology Branch
6700 B Rockledge Dr., Rm. 1128
MSC 7640
Bethesda, MD 20892
Phone: (301)496-7551 **Fax:** (301)480-2381
Email: hquill@hiaid.nih.gov
Dr. Helen Quill, Chf.
Activities/Fields: Biology and chemistry of the immune system and its products. Immunobiologic studies include: the origin, maturation, localization, and interactions of immunocyte (lymphocyte, plasmocyte, macrophage) populations and subpopulations; the cellular and biochemical mechanisms responsible for antigen processing, tolerance, and enhancement; research in the mechanisms responsible for induction and regulation of the immune response; and studies on lymphokines and other substances produced by immunocytes and other cells that regulate the immune system. Immunochemical studies include: the chemical structure and function of the immunoglobulin components of body fluids; the chemical structure, function, and biologic importance of naturally occurring antigens; the mechanisms of antigen-antibody reactions and the chemical basis of immunologic specificity; the regulation of immunoglobulin synthesis; the chemistry and function of immunopharmacologic agents; and chemical characterization of the molecular components and the function of accessory systems that participate in the immune response. **Frmly:** Immunobiology and Immunochemistry Branch.

★ 25029 ★ U.S. Department of Health and Human Services
National Institute of Allergy and Infectious Diseases
Division of Allergy, Immunology, and Transplantation
Clinical Immunology Branch
6700 B Rockledge Drive
Room 5135
Bethesda, MD 20892
Phone: (301)496-7104 **Fax:** (301)402-2571
Email: jwedgwood@niaid.nih.gov
Josiah Wedgwood, Chf.
Activities/Fields: Underlying cellular and molecular mechanisms responsible for the pathogenesis of immunologic diseases, as well as the application of basic knowledge to the etiology, prevention, and management of immunologic disorders, including autoimmune, immune complex, and immunodeficiency diseases and immunoregulatory dysfunctions. A special feature of this program is the support of Asthma, Allergic and Immunologic Disease Cooperative Research Centers (AAIDCRCs). An objective of AAIDCRCs is to accelerate the clinical application of new knowledge of the immune system. Programs are designed to integrate and coordinate research projects in clinical immunology that are being pursued in clinical specialties with those in basic research. AAIDCRC grants are awarded to an institution on behalf of a program director for support of a broadly based, multidisciplinary long-term research program that has a specific objective or basic theme. An AAIDCRC generally involves the organized efforts of groups of investigators who conduct research projects related to the overall program objective. The grant can provide support for the projects and for certain basic resources shared by individuals in a program where the sharing facilitates the total research effort. NIAID currently supports five CIRIDs (see following entries).

★ 25030 ★ U.S. Department of Health and Human Services
National Institute of Allergy and Infectious Diseases (NIAID)
Division of Allergy, Immunology, and Transplantation
Genetics and Transplantation Branch
6700B Rockledge Dr., Rm. 5142
Bethesda, MD 20892-7640
Phone: (301)496-1886 **Fax:** (301)402-2571
Email: dr17g@nih.gov
Website: http://www.niaid.nih.gov/organization/daitorg.htm
Dr. Daniel Rotrosen, Ch.
Activities/Fields: Genetic and immunologic mechanisms that are involved in responses to foreign substances such as infecting microorganisms and engrafted tissues. These mechanisms determine susceptibility or resistance to various diseases and the success or failure of organ or tissue grafts. The program supports investigations in animal species ranging from invertebrates to man, and the development of technologies and reagents. Research in genetics and transplantation is supported through the award of both grants and contracts. The research grant program supports studies on the molecular genetics of the immune system. The contract program in transplantation immunology supports the acquisition and distribution of reagents useful in research in immunogenetics and transplantation, evaluation of methodologies currently in use at the laboratory and the clinical level in those fields, development of new and more effective technologies for histocompatibility testing and immunologic manipulation, and collection and analysis of data to permit assessment of the efficacy of various transplant procedures.

★ 25031 ★ U.S. Department of Health and Human Services
National Institute of Allergy and Infectious Diseases
Division of Extramural Activities
6700 B Rockledge Drive
Bethesda, MD 20892
Phone: (301)496-7291 **Fax:** (301)402-0369
Dr. John McGowan, Dir.
Activities/Fields: Coordinates and provides administrative support for all NIAID program activities in the extramural area. The DEA staff work closely with scientific program staff, grantees, and potential grantees in providing management information, advice, and consultation as needed to fulfill the broad objectives of the NIAID research grants and contracts programs. DEA also directs and carries out the scientific and technical merit review of proposals and applications for research contracts, program projects, special research grants, and research training. Activities are organized in branches for contract management, grants management, program and project review, and research manpower development.

★ 25032 ★ U.S. Department of Health and Human Services
National Institute of Allergy and Infectious Diseases
Division of Extramural Activities
Contract Management Branch
6700-B Rockledge Dr., Rm. 2115
Bethesda, MD 20892
Phone: (301)496-0612 **Fax:** (301)402-0972
Email: bv4y@nih.gov
Website: http://www.niaid.nih.gov/contract/default.htm
Brenda J. Velez, Chf.
Activities/Fields: Contract management.

★ 25033 ★ U.S. Department of Health and Human Services
National Institute of Allergy and Infectious Diseases
Division of Extramural Activities
Grants Management Branch
National Inst. of Health
6700 B Rockledge Dr. Room 2116
Bethesda, MD 20892-7614
Phone: (301)402-6400 **Fax:** (301)480-3780
Email: mk35h@nih.gov
Mary Kirker, Chf.
Activities/Fields: Supports research activities through grant management.

★ 25034 ★ U.S. Department of Health and Human Services
National Institute of Allergy and Infectious Diseases
Division of Intramural Research
NIH Bldg. 10, Rm. 4A-31
10 Center Dr., MSC 1356
Bethesda, MD 20892-1356
Phone: (301)496-3006 **Fax:** (301)480-9324
Email: tk9c@nih.gov
Website: http://www.niaid.nih.gov/dir/default.htm
Dr. Thomas Kindt, Dir.
Activities/Fields: Causes of allergic, immunologic, and infectious diseases; research that has developed to the point of clinical application is pursued through clinical trials, performed at the Clinical Center of NIH or in collaboration with university centers. The NIAID Intramural Program has diverse components covering medical research relevant to the Institute's mission and includes laboratories for: Cellular and Molecular Immunology; Clinical Investigation; Host Defense; Immunogenetics; Immunology; Immunopathology; Immunoregulation; Infectious Diseases; Molecular Microbiology; Parasitic Diseases; Viral Diseases; Persistant Viral Diseases and Allergic Diseases. and Function Laboratory; and Persistant Viral Diseases. **Pub:** *Opportunities in the division of Intramural Research, NIAID, Annual Report.*

★ 25035 ★ U.S. Department of Health and Human Services
National Institute of Allergy and Infectious Diseases
Division of Microbiology and Infectious Diseases
Bacteriology and Mycology Branch
6610 B. Rockledge Dr., MSC-6603
Bethesda, MD 20892-6603
Phone: (301)496-7728 **Fax:** (301)402-2508
Email: dd24a@nih.gov
Dr. Dennis M. Dixon, Chf.
Activities/Fields: Diseases of man caused by bacteria and fungi, including: investigations on the biology and physiology of bacteria and fungi, their morphology, antigenic structure and composition, and toxins and endotoxins; and studies on pathogenesis, immunopathology, host defense mechanisms, diagnostic procedures, therapeutic measures, animal models, and the epidemiology of disease. Specific disease program areas include: medical mycology, turberculosis, and leprosy; hospital-associated infections; and streptococcal diseases and sequelae; and vector-borne bacterial diseases including Lyme disease. Other diseases and problem areas, such as Legionnaires' disease, listeriosis, mycoplasma infections, brucell osis, and anaerobic infections, are also investigated.

★ 25036 ★ U.S. Department of Health and Human Services
National Institute of Allergy and Infectious Diseases
Division of Microbiology and Infectious Diseases
Enteric Diseases Branch
6700 B Rockledge Drive
Room 3109
MSC 7630
Bethesda, MD 20892
Phone: (301)496-7051 **Fax:** (301)402-1456
Dr. Leslye Johnson, Chf.
Activities/Fields: Bacterial and viral enteric diseases, viral hepatitis, hepatitis antiviral drug development, hepatitis C, helicobacter pylori, and mucosal immunity.

★ 25037 ★ U.S. Department of Health and Human Services
National Institute of Allergy and Infectious Diseases
Division of Microbiology and Infectious Diseases
Parasitology and International Programs Branch
Solar Bldg., Rm. 3A10
Bethesda, MD 20892
Phone: (301)496-2544 **Fax:** (301)402-0659
Email: sj13y@nih.gov
Website: http://www.niaid.nih.gov/dmid/dmidover.htm
Dr. Stephanie James, Chf.
Activities/Fields: Host/parasite and vector relationships, with the ultimate goal of controlling parasitic diseases through such procedures as chemoprophylaxis, immunoprophylaxis, chemotherapy, and vector control. Research projects involve parasitology and medical entomology and use a broad spectrum of multidisciplinary approaches, including immunology, molecular biology, and biochemistry. Emphasis is directed toward studies on the infectious diseases of developing countries, through special programs on tropical disease research. As a means of stimulating research on schistosomiasis and filariasis, NIAID also supports two contracts to provide investigators with animals and vectors infected with various species of both these parasites.

★ 25038 ★ U.S. Department of Health and Human Services
National Institute of Allergy and Infectious Diseases
Division of Microbiology and Infectious Diseases
Respiratory Diseases Branch
6700B Rockledge Dr.
Room 3143
Bethesda, MD 20892
Phone: (301)496-1884 **Fax:** (301)480-4528
Email: pm23v@nih.gov
Website: http://www.niaid.nih.gov
Dr. Pamela McInnes, Deputy Director
Activities/Fields: Acute respiratory disease. Maintains programs in influenza, bacterial and viral respiratory disease, bacterial and viral vaccines, tuberculosis, pertussis, and pneumonia.

★ 25039 ★ U.S. Department of Health and Human Services
National Institute of Allergy and Infectious Diseases
Division of Mirobiology and Infectious Diseases
Virology Branch
6610 Rockledge Dr.
Bethesda, MD 20892
Phone: (301)496-7453 **Fax:** (301)480-1594
Email: cl28r@nih.gov
Dr. Catherine Laughlin, Chf.
Activities/Fields: SUPs grant and contract research on viral infections other than HIV and on prevention and treatment of these infections.

★ 25040 ★ U.S. Department of Health and Human Services
National Institute of Allergy and Infectious Diseases
Laboratory of Cellular and Molecular Immunology
NIH Bldg. 4, Rm. 111
9000 Rockville Pike
Bethesda, MD 20892-0420
Phone: (301)496-1257 **Fax:** (301)496-0877
Email: rs34r@nih.gov
Ronald H. Schwartz, Chf.
Activities/Fields: Cellular and molecular immunology.

★ 25041 ★ U.S. Department of Health and Human Services
National Institute of Allergy and Infectious Diseases
Laboratory of Clinical Investigation
NIH Bldg. 10, Rm. 11N228
10 Center Dr., MSC 1888
Bethesda, MD 20892-1888
Phone: (301)496-5807 **Fax:** (301)496-7383
Dr. Warren Strober, Chf.
Activities/Fields: Allergic, immunologic, and infectious diseases. Specific areas of research interest are: the molecular biology, pathogenesis, prevention and antiviral treatment of herpes virus infections in humans; the role of host defense mechanisms in prevention of infections; the pathogenesis, treatment, and prevention of cryptococcal and candida infections; the molecular basis of macrophage responses to infection; identification of genes that contribute to virulence in E. coli; mechanisms of regulation of immune reactivity in normal individuals and patients with immunologically mediated diseases; the biochemical response in lymphoid cells following antigenic stimulation in normal and immunologically impaired subjects; the immunologic abnormalities of asthma and other allergic diseases mechanisms of regulation of mucosal immune responses; the pathogenesis of inflammatory bowel diseases; the pathogenesis of immunodeficiency diseases; the biology of the mast cell; and the diagnosis and effective management of systemic mastocytosis.

★ 25042 ★ U.S. Department of Health and Human Services
National Institute of Allergy and Infectious Diseases
Laboratory of Immunogenetics
NIAID Twinbrook Facility
12441 Parklawn Dr., Rm. 200B
Rockville, MD 20852
Phone: (301)496-9589 **Fax:** (301)402-0259
Email: spierce@niaid.nih.gov
Website: http://www.niaid.nih.gov/dir/labs/lig.htm
Susan K. Pierce, PhD, Chf.
Activities/Fields: Multigene families that are involved in the control of immune function. Research emphasizes the structure and function of the genes and their products as well as mechanisms for gene regulation. Studies involve structural, serologic, and molecular genetic investigations. Techniques used include quantitative radioimmunoassays, protein structure determinations, recombinant DNA technologies (gene cloning and nucleotide sequencing) assays for DNA regulatory elements, and DNA-mediated gene transfer into mammalian cells; preparation and study of T- and B-cell hybridomas; and a variety of immunologic assays for cellular and humoral components of the immune response.

★ 25043 ★ U.S. Department of Health and Human Services
National Institute of Allergy and Infectious Diseases
Laboratory of Immunology
NIH Bldg. 10, Rm. 11N311
10 Center Dr. MSC 1892
Bethesda, MD 20892-1892
Phone: (301)496-5046 **Fax:** (301)496-0222
Website: http://www.nih.gov
William Paul, MD, Chf.
Activities/Fields: Various aspects of cellular, molecular, and developmental biology of lymphocytes; the regulation of immune responses; immunogenetics; and immunochemistry. Emphasis is on developing an understanding of how the various elements of the immune system function normally and of the role of immune mechanisms in the prevention and pathogenesis of diseases. Studies utilize a variety of techniques, including production and use of monoclonal antibodies, cloning and long-term growth of lymphocyte lines; molecular genetic analysis of cells of the immune system; and cell biological analysis of lymphocyte activation and differentiation. **Pub:** *Proceedings.*

★ 25044 ★ U.S. Department of Health and Human Services
National Institute of Allergy and Infectious Diseases
Laboratory of Immunopathology
NIH Bldg. 7, Rm. 304
7 Center Dr., MSC 0760
Bethesda, MD 20892-0760
Phone: (301)496-1150 **Fax:** (301)402-0077
Dr. Herbert C. Morse III, Chf.
Activities/Fields: Mechanisms by which retroviruses and adenoviruses induce disease. Activities involve: evaluation of the genetic organization of viruses in relation to their pathogenic properties; definition of the characteristics of normal target cell population and the effects of viruses on these cells; and identification of host characteristics that influence the outcome of virus infections. Methods involve molecular technology as well as in vivo analyses of viral pathogenicity in mice and hamsters, and immunologic studies of cells from normal, mutant, and virus-infected mice.

★ 25045 ★ U.S. Department of Health and Human Services
National Institute of Allergy and Infectious Diseases
Laboratory of Immunoregulation
NIH Bldg. 10, Rm. 11B13
9000 Rockville Pike
Bethesda, MD 20892
Phone: (301)496-1124 **Fax:** (301)402-0070
Dr. Anthony S. Fauci, Chf.
Activities/Fields: Mechanisms of activation and immunoregulation of human immune responses in normal individuals and in a variety of disease states characterized by abnormalities of immune function. Recent areas of research interest have included: acquired immunodeficiency syndrome (AIDS); immunoregulation of human lymphocyte function in normal and disease states; immunopathogenic features of immune-mediated diseases; clinical, immunopathogenic, and therapeutic studies in the spectrum of vasculitis; molecular biologic approach to the immune system; and immunopathogenesis of *Chlamydia trachomatis* infection. **Pub:** *Proceedings.*

★ 25046 ★ U.S. Department of Health and Human Services
National Institute of Allergy and Infectious Diseases
Laboratory of Infectious Diseases
NIH 50 Room 6134
9000 Rockville Pike
Bethesda, MD 20892

Phone: (301)496-2024 Fax: (301)496-8312
Dr. Robert M. Chanock, MD, Sr. Investigator
Activities/Fields: Defines the cause and epidemiology of medically important viral diseases and develops means for their control. Activities range from identification and antigenic characterization of viruses that cause acute disease of the respiratory and gastrointestinal tracts and liver to basic molecular studies of viral structure, function, and genome organization. Molecular biologic techniques are used to elucidate pathogenesis of disease as well as to develop purified subunit antigens and attenuated viral mutants for use in prevention of respiratory, gastrointestinal, and hepatic viral diseases.

★ 25047 ★ U.S. Department of Health and Human Services
National Institute of Allergy and Infectious Diseases
Laboratory of Microbial Structure and Function
Rocky Mountain Laboratories
903 S 4th St.
Hamilton, MT 59840
Phone: (406)363-3211 **Fax:** (406)363-9394
Email: jmusser@niaid.nih.gov
Website: http://www.niaid.nih.gov
Dr. James Musser, Chf.
Activities/Fields: Structural and functional elements of pathogenic bacterial surface components involved in pathogenesis and/or virulence of selected organisms or in genesis of host immunological responses to infections by these agents. Studies involve *Neissera gonorrhoeae, Borellia burgdorferi*, and others; both protein and nonprotein components of these gram-negative organism outer membrane are prime study candidates as mediators of interactions between bacterium and host and as likely vaccine components. Chemical characteristics, immunochemical properties, and genetic control of selected surface proponents are investigated to delineate their relationship to infectious disease phenomena of these bacteria. **Pub:** *Proceedings.* • *Research Reports.*

★ 25048 ★ U.S. Department of Health and Human Services
National Institute of Allergy and Infectious Diseases
Laboratory of Molecular Microbiology
NIH Bldg. 4, Rm. 315
4 Center Dr., MSC 0460
Bethesda, MD 20892-0460
Phone: (301)496-4012 **Fax:** (301)402-0226
Dr. Malcolm A. Martin, Chf.
Activities/Fields: Microorganisms and their capacity to produce disease in vertebrate hosts. Of prime importance in this effort is the biochemical characterization of viral genomes and the detailed analyses of gene products regulating expression or giving rise to mature structural proteins. A principal area of investigation has been the human immunodeficiency virus (HIV), with classical virological procedures used for the detection, quantitation, and biological characterization of HIV isolates of diverse origin. Biochemical and molecular biological techniques such as nucleic acid hybridization, gene cloning, DNA sequencing, in vitro mutagenesis, and transfection are used in combination with procedures such as immunoprecipitation or protein purification to study individual viral genes or potentially infectious proviral DNAs in order to assess structure/function relationships. Programs involving murine retroviruses concentrate on those portions of the viral genome that encode proteins that initiate and/or maintain the transformed state. The roles of host cellular determinants that augment or diminish disease/oncogenesis are also investigated.

★ 25049 ★ U.S. Department of Health and Human Services
National Institute of Allergy and Infectious Diseases (NIAID)
Laboratory of Molecular Structure
Twinbrook II
12441 Parklawn Dr., Rm. 205
Rockville, MD 20852
Phone: (301)496-8247 **Fax:** (301)480-2818
Email: jcoligan@niaid.nih.gov
John E. Coligan, PhD, Section Chf.
Activities/Fields: Molecular basis of the immune response. Also studies structural biology of immunologically relevant molecules. **Frmly:** Biological Resources Branch.

★ 25050 ★ U.S. Department of Health and Human Services
National Institute of Allergy and Infectious Diseases
Laboratory of Persistent Viral Diseases
Rocky Mountain Laboratories
903 S 4th St.
Hamilton, MT 59840
Phone: (406)363-9354 **Fax:** (406)363-9286
Email: bchesebro@nih.gov
Bruce Chesebro, MD, Chf.
Activities/Fields: Virus-host interaction, with the primary aim of elucidating mechanisms involved in establishment, maintenance, and elimination of persistent viral infections. Particular emphasis is placed on persistent viral infections involving cells of the hemopoietic and lymphoid systems and the central nervous system. The role of persistent infection in the development of autoimmune or immune complex disease is also studied. Models examined include human AIDS retrovirus and murine retroviruses, rabies virus, Aleutian disease virus of mink, and the agent of scrapie and other transmissible spongiform encephalopathies of humans and animals.

★ 25051 ★ U.S. Department of Health and Human Services
National Institute of Allergy and Infectious Diseases
Laboratory of Viral Diseases
NIH Bldg. 4, Rm. 229A
4 Center Dr., MSC0445
Bethesda, MD 20892-0445
Phone: (301)496-9869 **Fax:** (301)480-1147
Email: bmoss@nih.gov
Website: http://www.niaid.nih.gov/dir/labs/lvd.htm
Dr. Bernard Moss, Chf.
Activities/Fields: Genetic organization, expression, replication, assembly, and pathogenicity of viruses. Live recombinant viruses are genetically engineered for use as immunological tools and as vaccines against a variety of infectious agents. Current research topics include: regulation of gene expression in vitro and in vivo; mechanisms of DNA replication in vitro and in vivo; structure and function of RNA and DNA polymerases; genetic engineering of recombinant viruses as live vaccines; antiviral agents; determinants of virus virulence; host resistance genes; viral growth factors; and targets of humoral and cell-mediated immunity.

★ 25052 ★ U.S. Department of Health and Human Services
National Institute of Allergy and Infectious Diseases
Office of Administrative Management
Extramural Administrative Management Branch
6700 B. Rockledge Dr.
Bethesda, MD 20892
Phone: (301)496-7151 **Fax:** (301)402-0520
Marilyn Kunzweiler, Chf.
Activities/Fields: Extramural administrative management.

★ 25053 ★ U.S. Department of Health and Human Services
National Institute of Allergy and Infectious Diseases
Office of Communications
NIH Bldg. 31, Rm. 7A50
31 Center Dr., MSC2520
Bethesda, MD 20892-2520
Phone: (301)496-5717 **Fax:** (301)402-0120
Email: lf7j@nih.gov
Website: http://www.niaid.nih.gov/cgi-shl/contacts/contacts.cfm
Leslie Fink, Dir.
Activities/Fields: Supports the communication of research activities in the areas of AIDS, allergy, immunology, and infectious diseases.

★ 25054 ★ U.S. Department of Health and Human Services
National Institute of Allergy and Infectious Diseases
Office of Policy Analysis
NIH Bldg. 31, Rm. 7A52
9000 Rockville Pike
Bethesda, MD 20892
Phone: (301)496-6752 **Fax:** (301)402-0492
Email: lh28q@nih.gov
Website: http://www.niaid.nih.gov/cgi-shl/contacts/contacts.cfm
Lynn C. Hellinger, Actg. Dir.
Activities/Fields: Allergies and infectious diseases. **Pub:** *Profile*, annually.

★ 25055 ★ U.S. Department of Health and Human Services
National Institute of Allergy and Infectious Diseases
Rocky Mountain Laboratories
Administrative and Facilities Management Section
903 S 4th St.
RML/8207
Hamilton, MT 59840
Phone: (406)363-9324 **Fax:** (406)363-9218
Email: ps144e@nih.gov
Website: http://www.niaid.nih.gov/dir/labs.htm
Patricia A. Stewart, Chf.
Activities/Fields: Components include the Microbial Structure and Function Laboratory; Microscopy Branch; the Persistent Viral Diseases Laboratory; and Intracellular Parasites Laboratory. **Frmly:** Rocky Mountain Operations Branch.

★ 25056 ★ U.S. Department of Health and Human Services
National Institute of Arthritis and Musculoskeletal and Skin Diseases
NIH Bldg. 31, Rm. 4C32
31 Center Dr., MSC 2350
Bethesda, MD 20892
Phone: (301)496-4353 **Fax:** (301)480-6069
Website: http://www.niams.nih.gov
Dr. Stephen I. Katz, PhD, Dir.
Activities/Fields: Large number of diverse diseases, including rheumatoid arthritis, osteoarthritis, systemic lupus erythematosus, muscle diseases, osteoporosis, Paget's disease, back disorders, osteogenesis imperfecta, psoriasis, acne, ichthyosis, epidermolysis bullosa, and vitiligo. The Institute's Intramural Research Program conducts basic research studies in immunology, biophysics, biochemistry, molecular biology, structural biology, pathology and histochemistry, and pharmacology. Through its Arthritis and Rheumatism Branch, the Institute leads basic and clinical research and treatment programs in lupus erythematosus, rheumatoid arthritis, and other connective tissue diseases. The Institute's Extramural Activities Program is organized in five branches: Rheumatic Diseases Branch, Musculoskeletal Diseases Branch, Bone Biology and Bone Diseases Branch, Muscle Biology Branch, and Skin Diseases Branch. Other extramural

programs include the Centers Program. The Institute supports basic and clinical research through investigator-initiated research grants, research center grants, individual and institutional research training awards, career development awards, and contracts to public and private research institutions and organizations.

★ 25057 ★ U.S. Department of Health and Human Services
National Institute of Arthritis and Musculoskeletal and Skin Diseases
Extramural Activities Program
Centers Program
45 Center Dr., MSC 6500
Bethesda, MD 20892
Phone: (301)594-5052 **Fax:** (301)480-4543
Email: freemanb@exchange.nih.gov
Website: http://www.niams.nih.gov/rtac/funding/grants/centers_programs.htmP30
Julia B. Freeman, PhD, Dir.
Activities/Fields: Operates Multidisciplinary Clinical Research Centers (MCRC)s in Arthritis, Musculoskeletal and Skin Diseases. The goal of the Multidisciplinary Clinical Research Center (MCRC) program is to assess and improve outcomes for patients with arthritis and rheumatic diseases; musculoskeletal disorders including orthopedic and bone diseases; muscle diseases; and skin diseases. Maintains Specialized Centers of Research (SCORs) in rheumatoid arthritis, lupus, osteoarthritis, scleroderma, and osteoporosis. Sponsors Core Centers with programs in skin and rheumatic diseases and musculoskeletal disorders. **Frmly:** Multipurpose Arthritis Centers Program.

★ 25058 ★ U.S. Department of Health and Human Services
National Institute of Arthritis and Musculoskeletal and Skin Diseases
Extramural Activities Program
Muscle Biology Program
One Democracy Plz.
6701 Democracy Blvd., Ste. 800
Bethesda, MD 20892-4872
Phone: (301)594-5128 **Fax:** (301)480-4543
Email: lymnr@mail.nih.gov
Website: http://www.niams.nih.gov/rtac/index.htm
Richard W. Lymn, PhD, Dir.
Activities/Fields: Skeletal muscle development and function in normal and diseasd conditions, including studies on the structure and function of muscle, development and regeneration of muscle, normal and abnormal muscle metabolism, muscular dystrophy and other diseases and disorders of skeletal muscle.

★ 25059 ★ U.S. Department of Health and Human Services
National Institute of Arthritis and Musculoskeletal and Skin Diseases
Extramural Activities Program
Musculoskeletal Diseases Branch
Bldg. 31., Rm. 4-C-05
Bethesda, MD 20892
Phone: (301)495-4484 **Fax:** (301)480-2814
Email: niamsinfo@mail.nih.gov
Website: http://www.niams.nih.gov
Activities/Fields: Understanding of the structure, function, formation, metabolism, and biomechanics of bones, joints, and skeletal support structures. Research activity focuses on: osteoporosis and other metabolic diseases; joint replacement methods and materials; developmental disorders, including scoliosis, bone immunology, and transplantation; inherited connective tissue disorders; back disorders; and exercise pathophysiology.

★ 25060 ★ U.S. Department of Health and Human Services
National Institute of Arthritis and Musculoskeletal and Skin Diseases
Extramural Activities Program
Skin Diseases Branch
NIH
1 Democrary Plz.
6701 Democracy Blvd., No. 800
MSC 4872
Bethesda, MD 20892-4872
Phone: (301)594-5017 **Fax:** (301)480-4543
Email: moshella@ep.niams.nih.gov
Dr. Alan N. Moshell, MD, Dir. of Skin Disease & Branch Chf.
Activities/Fields: Structure, function, and physiology of skin as well as on the causes and improved treatment of a wide variety of skin diseases, including psoriasis, lupus, eczema, vitiligo, bullous skin diseases, acne, and ichthyosis.

★ 25061 ★ U.S. Department of Health and Human Services
National Institute of Arthritis and Musculoskeletal and Skin Diseases
Intramural Research Program
Arthritis and Rheumatism Branch
NIH Bldg. 10, Rm. 9N244
10 Center Dr., MSC 1820
Bethesda, MD 20892
Phone: (301)496-1474 **Fax:** (301)402-0012
Email: plotzp@mail.nih.gov
Website: http://www.irp.niams.nih.gov/NIAMS2/Labs-Branches_branch.jsp?branchId=14
Dr. Paul Plotz, Chf.
Activities/Fields: Arthritis, connective tissue diseases, and related areas, including immunology. Activities involve: disease-related studies on the etiology, pathology, and therapy of connective tissue disorders, with special emphasis on systemic lupus erythematosus, polymyositis, and rheumatoid arthritis (both human disease and animal models of these diseases are studied); and fundamental studies on immune regulation, with special emphasis on autoimmunity and mechanisms of immune responses at the cellular and molecular level. **Pub:** *Proceedings*.

★ 25062 ★ U.S. Department of Health and Human Services
National Institute of Arthritis and Musculoskeletal and Skin Diseases (NIAMS)
Intramural Research Program (IRP)
Laboratory of Physical Biology (LPB)
NIH Bldg. 50, Rm. 1140
900 Rockville Pike MSC 8024
Bethesda, MD 20892-8024
Phone: (301)496-5880 **Fax:** (301)402-0009
Email: wang@helix.nih.gov
Dr. Kuan Wang, PhD, Dir.
Activities/Fields: Mechanism of muscle contraction in intact cells and simplified preparations using time-resolved X-ray diffraction in conjunction with mechanochemical techniques. Electron microscopy is used with a wide variety of preparations, and digital image processing techniques are used to enhance resolution.

★ 25063 ★ U.S. Department of Health and Human Services
National Institute of Arthritis and Musculoskeletal and Skin Diseases
Intramural Research Program
Laboratory of Skin Biology
NIH Bldg. 50 Room 1523
9000 Rockville Pike
Bethesda, MD 20892-8023
Phone: (301)496-1578 **Fax:** (301)402-2886
Peter Steinert, Chf.
Activities/Fields: Structural, molecular, and cellular biology and genetics of skin proteins.

★ 25064 ★ U.S. Department of Health and Human Services
National Institute on Deafness and Other Communication Disorders
NIH Bldg. 31, Rm. 3C02
31 Center Dr.
Bethesda, MD 20892-2320
Phone: (301)402-0900 **Fax:** (301)402-1590
Dr. James F. Battey, Dir.
Activities/Fields: Biomedical and behavioral research and research training on normal processes and disorders of hearing, balance, smell, taste, voice, speech, and language, including hearing and deafness, hearing loss, hearing impairment, tinnitus, presbycusis, Waardenburg syndrome, Usher syndrome, dizziness, Meniere's disease, vestibular system, smell and taste disorders, voice disorders, spasmodic dysphonia, vocal cord paralysis, stuttering, speech disorders, language disorders, and aphasia.

★ 25065 ★ U.S. Department of Health and Human Services
National Institute on Deafness and Other Communication Disorders
Division Extramural Activities
31 Center Dr., MSC 2320
Bethesda, MD 20892
Phone: (301)496-8693 **Fax:** (301)402-6250
Website: http://www.nidcd.nih.gov/research/about/extramural.asp
Robert A. Dobie, MD, Dir.
Activities/Fields: Communication sciences and disorders. **Frmly:** (2000) Division of Extramural Activities.

★ 25066 ★ U.S. Department of Health and Human Services
National Institute on Deafness and Other Communication Disorders
Division of Human Communications
Executive Plaza S, Rm. 400C
6120 Executive Blvd.
MSC 7180
Bethesda, MD 20892-7180
Phone: (301)496-5061 **Fax:** (301)402-6251
Email: judih_cooper@nih.gov
Website: http://www.nidcd.nih.gov/about/org/der.htm
Judith Cooper, Chf.,Sci. Prog. Br.
Activities/Fields: Administers grants, contracts, and national research service awards for extramural research on hearing, balance, smell, taste, voice, speech, and language. Areas of research interest include diagnosis, treatment, and prevention of communication disorders, including the prevention and early diagnosis of hearing impairments that may result from exposure to noise or ototoxic drugs; the causes and treatment of tinnitus; the normal function of the central nervous system and the relationship of the taste and smell to the early detection of systemic disease; disorders such as stuttering, misarticulation, delayed language development, and voice disorders. **Frmly:** Communicative and Neurosensory Disorders Division.

★ 25067 ★ U.S. Department of Health and Human Services
National Institute on Deafness and Other Communication Disorders
Division of Intramural Research
50 South Dr., Rm. 4-4140
Bethesda, MD 20892
Phone: (301)496-6530 **Fax:** (301)402-2324
Email: wenthold@nidcd.nih.gov
Website: http://www.nidcd.nih.gov/intram/intram.htm
Dr. Robert J. Wenthold, PhD, Contact
Activities/Fields: Genetic and immune pathogenesis of head and neck neoplasms affecting human communication.

★ 25068 ★ U.S. Department of Health and Human Services
National Institute on Deafness and Other Communication Disorders
Division of Intramural Research
Audiology Unit
NIH Bldg. 10, Rm. 5C-306
9000 Rockville Pk.
Bethesda, MD 20892
Phone: (301)496-5368 **Fax:** (301)402-0409
Email: shotland@nidcd.nih.gov
Website: http://www.nih.gov/nidcd/
Lawrence L. Shotland, PhD, Chf.
Activities/Fields: Hearing and auditory function in various genetic, immunologic, or acquired conditions, including type 2 neurofibromatosis, Waardenburg syndrome, inherited metabolic degenerative disorders and non-syndromic hereditary hearing loss, and von-Hippel Lindau disease.

★ 25069 ★ U.S. Department of Health and Human Services
National Institute on Deafness and Other Communication Disorders
Division of Intramural Research
Voice and Speech Section
NIH Bldg. 10, Rm. 5D38
10 Center Dr., MSC 1416
Bethesda, MD 20892-1416
Phone: (301)496-9365 **Fax:** (301)480-0803
Christy L. Ludlow, PhD, Chf.
Activities/Fields: Speech and voice studies, including the neurophysiological and biomechanical bases of normal speech and voice production, pathophysiology of idiopathic speech and voice disorders such as spasmodic dysphonia and stuttering, and medical and surgical approaches to treatment of these disorders. Investigates sensorimotor regulation of the laryngeal musculature; motion and electromyographic analyses of laryngeal functioning during speech, respiration, and swallowing; magnetic and electrical stimulation of the central and peripheral laryngeal nervous system; and new treatment approaches including botulinum toxin, medication trials in patients with stuttering disorders, and phonosurgery for voice disorders. **Pub:** *Research Reports.*

★ 25070 ★ U.S. Department of Health and Human Services
National Institute of Dental Research
Division of Epidemiology and Oral Disease Prevention
45 Center Dr., MSC 6401, RM. 4A5-13D
5333 Westbard Ave., Rm. 528
Bethesda, MD 20892-6401
Phone: (301)594-7651 **Fax:** (301)480-8322
Dr. L. Jackson Brown, Dir.
Activities/Fields: Descriptive and analytical epidemiologic studies of the etiology, distribution, and trends in dental caries, periodontal diseases, and other oral diseases and disorders. Program's Disease Prevention and Health Promotion Branch manages activities involving health promotion research and application. Research is supported both through intramural projects and research and development contracts. **Pub:** *NIDR's Annual Report.* • *Symposia proceedings.*

★ 25071 ★ U.S. Department of Health and Human Services
National Institute of Dental Research
Division of Extramural Research
Natcher Bldg.
45 Center Dr., MSC-6402
Bethesda, MD 20892-2904
Phone: (301)480-8303 **Fax:** (301)480-8318
Email: george.hausch@nih.gov
Website: http://www.nidcr.nih.gov
H. George Hausch, Dir., Division of Extramural Acts.
Activities/Fields: Administers grant and contract funds for research and training research manpower. Support is provided for investigations ranging from basic laboratory studies on the causes of oral disorders to clinical trials of new therapies or means of disease prevention.

★ 25072 ★ U.S. Department of Health and Human Services
National Institute of Dental Research
Division of Extramural Research
Chronic Disabling Diseases Program
Natcher Bldg.
45 Center Dr., MSC 6402
Bethesda, MD 20892-6402
Phone: (301)594-4836 **Fax:** (301)480-8318
Website: http://www.nih.gov
Dr. Kenneth A. Gruber, Chief, Chronic Diseases Branch
Activities/Fields: Acquired chronic and disabling conditions of the craniofacial region, as well as this areas normal physiology. This includes, but is not limited to, osteoporosis and other bone diseases, autoimmune conditions, temporomandibular disorders, orofacial pain, normal physiology and pathological conditions of the salivary gland. **Frmly:** Craniofacial Anomalies Pain Control, and Behavioral Research Branch.

★ 25073 ★ U.S. Department of Health and Human Services
National Institute of Dental Research
Division of Extramural Research
Grants Management Section
45 Center Dr., Rm. 4AS-55
Bethesda, MD 20892
Phone: (301)594-4800 **Fax:** (301)480-3562
Email: md74u@nih.gov
Mary Daley, Chf.
Activities/Fields: Supports extramural research through grant and contract awards.

★ 25074 ★ U.S. Department of Health and Human Services
National Institute of Dental Research
Division of Extramural Research
Periodontal Disease Program
Bldg. 45, Ste. 4AN-18
Bethesda, MD 20892-6402
Phone: (301)594-2421 **Fax:** (301)480-8318
Email: dennis.mangan@nih.gov
Website: http://www.nidcr.nih.gov
Dr. Dennis Mangan, Chf., Infectious Disease Immunity Branch
Activities/Fields: Support of research on the microbiology and immunology of oral infectious diseases.

★ 25075 ★ U.S. Department of Health and Human Services
National Institute of Dental Research
Division of Extramural Research
Salivary Glands and Oral Biology Program
NIH 4S
45 Center Dr.
Bethesda, MD 20892
Phone: (301)594-5500 **Fax:** (301)480-8318
Gerassimos Roussos, Dir.
Activities/Fields: Development, structure, function, and diseases of the salivary glands in an attempt to determine the influence of salivary constituents on oral health.

★ 25076 ★ U.S. Department of Health and Human Services
National Institute of Dental Research
Division of Intramural Research
Bone Research Branch
NIH Bldg. 30, Rm. 228
30 Convent Dr., MSC 4320
Bethesda, MD 20892-4320
Phone: (301)496-4563 **Fax:** (301)402-0824
Email: probey@dir.nidcr.nih.gov
Website: http://wwwdir.nidcr.nih.gov/dirweb/csdb/csdb.asp
Pamela Gehron Robey, Chf.
Activities/Fields: Basic and clinical mineralized tissue research. **Pub:** *Research Reports.*

★ 25077 ★ U.S. Department of Health and Human Services
National Institute of Dental Research
Division of Intramural Research
Neurobiology and Anesthesiology Branch
NIH Bldg. 49, Rm. IA-04
10 Center Dr.
Bethesda, MD 20892
Phone: (301)496-6804 **Fax:** (301)402-0667
Email: rdionne@dir.nidcr.nih.gov
Raymond A. Dionne, PhD, Chf.
Activities/Fields: Oral-facial sensation, emphasizing mechanisms of pain and the development of new methods for controlling pain in humans. Branch sections utilize anatomical, physiological, behavioral, pharmacological, and psychophysical techniques to study neural function as it relates to the processing of sensory signals about the threat of tissue-damaging stimulation. **Frmly:** Neurobiology and Anesthesiology Branch.

★ 25078 ★ U.S. Department of Health and Human Services
National Institute of Dental Research
Laboratory of Developmental Biology
NIH Bldg. 30, Rm. 421
30 Convent Dr., MSC 4370
Bethesda, MD 20892-4370
Phone: (301)496-5974 **Fax:** (301)402-0897
Email: kenneth.yamada@nih.gov
Website: http://wwwdir.nidcr.nih.gov/dirweb/cdbrb/cdbrb.htm
Kenneth M. Yamada, Branch Chf.
Activities/Fields: Structure, function, and regulation of extracellular matrix molecules, their receptors, and other cell interaction systems. Research focuses on examining the functions and regulation of these systems in normal and abnormal development of craniofacial and other tissues; connective tissue remodeling; tumor metastasis and invasion; and other diseases and disorders involving extracellular molecules. Information on cell-matrix interaction mechanisms is applied to the development of biological and biochemical reagents for the understanding and therapy of oral and other diseases. **Frmly:** Developmental Biology and Anomalies Laboratory; (1997) Laboratory of Developmental Biology; (2000) National Institute of Dental Research; Craniofacial Developmental Biology and Regulation Branch.

★ 25079 ★ U.S. Department of Health and Human Services
National Institute of Dental Research
Laboratory of Microbial Ecology
NIH Bldg. 30, Rm. 316
9000 Rockville Pike
Bethesda, MD 20892
Phone: (301)496-2232 **Fax:** (301)402-0396
Activities/Fields: Microbial ecology.

★ 25080 ★ U.S. Department of Health and Human Services
National Institute of Diabetes and Digestive and Kidney Diseases
NIH Bldg. 31
31 Center Dr. MSC 2560
Bethesda, MD 20892-2560
Phone: (301)496-5877 **Fax:** (301)402-2125
Email: spiegela@extra.niddk.nih.gov
Website: http://www.niddk.nih.gov
Allen Spiegel, MD, Dir.
Activities/Fields: Serious diseases affecting public health. The Institute supports clinical research on the diseases of internal medicine and related subspecialty fields as well as in many basic science disciplines.

Institute activities include both intramural programs, which are carried out in the Institute's laboratory and clinical facilities on the NIH campus in Bethesda, MD and Phoenix, AZ; and extramural programs, which are supported by NIDDK and carried out at universities, private and public research facilities, and hospital-based clinical research centers. The Institute's Intramural Research Division encompasses the broad spectrum of metabolic diseases such as diabetes and other inborn errors of metabolism, endocrine disorders, mineral metabolism, digestive diseases, nutrition, urology and renal disease, and hematology. Basic research includes studies in biochemistry; nutrition; pathology; histochemistry; chemistry; physical, chemical, and molecular biology; pharmacology; and toxicology. NIDDK extramural research is organized in four divisions: Diabetes, Endocrinology, and Metabolic Diseases; Digestive Diseases and Nutrition; Kidney, Urologic, and Hematologic Diseases; and Extramural Activities. Mechanisms of NIDDK support for extramural programs include investigator-initiated grants, program project and center grants, and career development and training awards. The Institute also supports research and development projects and large-scale clinical trials through contracts.

★ 25081 ★ U.S. Department of Health and Human Services
National Institute of Diabetes and Digestive and Kidney Diseases
Clinical Nutrition Research Units Program
6707 Democracy Blvd.
MSC 5450
Bethesda, MD 20892-5450
Phone: (301)594-8883 **Fax:** (301)480-8300
Email: vh16h@nih.gov
Dr. Van S. Hubbard, Prog. Dir.

Activities/Fields: Integrated array of research, educational, and service activities focused on human nutrition in health and disease. Each unit serves as the focal point for an interdisciplinary approach to clinical nutrition research and for the stimulation of research in areas such as improved nutritional support of acutely and chronically ill persons, assessment of nutritional status, effects of disease states on nutrient needs, and effects of changes in nutritional status on disease. Funding for the CNRU program is provided through core center grants, which provide funds for: core resources such as cell culture, immunoassay, biostatistics, or other central research service facilities; pilot/feasibility projects, which support new investigators or investigators from other fields who wish to pursue new and innovative ideas to a point where they can compete for independent support; program enrichment funds to provide for small conferences or symposia and special consultants for the center; and a new investigator position. An existing base of high-quality nutrition-related research is a requirement for the establishment of a CNRU. Due to a restriction in the number of core center grants that can be made, investigator-initiated proposals are accepted only in response to a request for applications announced in the NIH Guide for Grants and Contracts.

★ 25082 ★ U.S. Department of Health and Human Services
National Institute of Diabetes and Digestive and Kidney Diseases
Division of Diabetes, Endocrinology, and Metabolic Diseases
NIH Bldg. 31, Rm. 9A16
31 Center Dr. MSC 2560
Bethesda, MD 20892-2560
Phone: (301)496-7349 **Fax:** (301)480-6792
Email: jf58s@nih.gov
Website: http://www.niddk.nih.gov
Judith Fradkin, MD, Dir.

Activities/Fields: Diabetes mellitus (both insulin dependent and noninsulin dependent diabetes); endocrinological diseases and disorders; and metabolic diseases, including research on the etiology, pathogenesis, and treatment of acquired or inborn errors of metabolism and cystic fibrosis. Support for basic and clinical biomedical research as well as epidemiologic and behavioral studies and clinical trials is provided through investigator-initiated research grants, new investigator awards, program project and center grants, and cooperative agreements. The Division also supports research fellowships, training grants, and a variety of career development awards as well as a limited number of resource and research and development contracts; and provides leadership in coordinating activities relating to diabetes and cystic fibrosis throughout the National Institutes of Health and various other federal agencies. Division's main branches are the Diabetes Programs Branch and the Endocrine and Metabolic Diseases Research Programs Branch.

★ 25083 ★ U.S. Department of Health and Human Services
National Institute of Diabetes and Digestive and Kidney Diseases
Division of Diabetes, Endocrinology, and Metabolic Diseases
Cystic Fibrosis Research Program
Natcher Bldg.
6707 Democracy Blvd.
Rm. 6103, MSC 5460
Bethesda, MD 20892-5460
Phone: (301)594-8810 **Fax:** (301)480-3503
Email: McKeonC@extra.niddk.nih.gov
Website: http://www.niddk.nih.gov/fund/program/a-elist.htmcystic
Dr. Catherine McKeon, Contact

Activities/Fields: Supports investigator-initiated research projects related to the etiology, pathogenesis, diagnosis, and treatment of cystic fibrosis (CF). In addition, the Program supports a cystic fibrosis research centers and small Business Innovation Research Grants.

★ 25084 ★ U.S. Department of Health and Human Services
National Institute of Diabetes and Digestive and Kidney Diseases
Division of Diabetes, Endocrinology, and Metabolic Diseases
Diabetes Center Program
6707 Democracy Blvd. MSC 5460
Room 697
Bethesda, MD 20892-5460
Phone: (301)594-8813 **Fax:** (301)480-3503
Email: eggermant@extra.niddk.nih.gov
Dr. Thomas Eggerman, Prog. Dir.

Activities/Fields: Administers two types of center awards: the Diabetes-+Endocrinology Research Centers (DERC) and the Diabetes Research and Training Centers (DRTC). The DERC is exclusively oriented toward biomedical research goals, while the DRTCs include training and translation components in addition to biomedical research. An existing base of high-quality diabetes-related research is a primary requirement for establishment of either type of center. Through shared resources (core facilities), both types of center grants provide a mechanism for integrating, coordinating, and fostering the interdisciplinary cooperation of a group of established investigators conducting programs of active high quality research in diabetes and related endocrine and metabolic disorders.

★ 25085 ★ U.S. Department of Health and Human Services
National Institute of Diabetes and Digestive and Kidney Diseases
Division of Diabetes, Endocrinology, and Metabolic Diseases
Diabetes Clinical Trials Program
6707 Democracy Blvd.
Bethesda, MD 20892
Phone: (301)594-8803 **Fax:** (301)402-6271
Email: garfields@extra.niddk.nih.gov
Website: http://www.niddk.nih.gov/patient/dpp/dpp.htm
Sanford Garfield, PhD, Sr.Adv. for Biometry and Behavioral Sci.

Activities/Fields: Supports a multicenter randomized clinical trial to determine whether interventions in high risk individuals can prevent the onset of type-2 diabetes. Participating in this study are 25 medical centers, a data coordinating center, and other supporting institutions that provide centralized technical and biochemical services. A group of expert consultants which is independent of the trial and external to the Institute continually reviews all operational aspects of the trial and provides policy advice to the Institute regarding the conduct of the study.

★ 25086 ★ U.S. Department of Health and Human Services
National Institute of Diabetes and Digestive and Kidney Diseases
Division of Diabetes, Endocrinology, and Metabolic Diseases
Endocrinology Research Section
45 Center Dr. MSC 6600
Bethesda, MD 20892-6600
Phone: (301)594-8819 **Fax:** (301)480-3503
Email: margolisr@extra.niddk.nih.gov
Dr. Ronald N. Margolis, Chf.

Activities/Fields: Supports (through research grants) investigator-initiated basic and clinical studies of normal and abnormal function of the pituitary, thyroid, parathyroid, adrenal, pineal, and thymus glands. Studies of the mode of action of hormones, their biosynthesis, secretion, and metabolism as well as their binding to protein carriers, subsequent release, and the kinetics of binding represent a major component of the Program. A substantial portion of the Program is devoted to structure/function studies of the hypothalamic releasing factors as they affect endocrine function as well as the physiology and pathophysiology of bone disease. In addition, studies of somatomedin and somatostatin and their effects on other hormones are supported, as is research on substances with hormone-like action such as prostaglandins and the brain peptides.

★ 25087 ★ U.S. Department of Health and Human Services
National Institute of Diabetes and Digestive and Kidney Diseases
Division of Diabetes, Endocrinology, and Metabolic Diseases
National Diabetes Data Group
45 Center Dr. MSC 5460
Bethesda, MD 20892-5460
Phone: (301)594-8801 **Fax:** (301)480-3503

Activities/Fields: Serves as the major federal focus for the collection, analysis, and dissemination of data on diabetes and its complications. Drawing upon the expertise of the research, medical, and lay communities, the Data Group initiates efforts to: define the data needed to address the scientific and public health issues in diabetes; foster and coordinate the collection of these data from multiple sources; promote the timely availability of reliable data to pertinent scientific, medical, and public organizations; modify data reporting systems to identify and categorize more appropriately the medical and socio-economic impact of diabetes; and promote the standardization of data collection and terminology in clinical and epidemiologic research. In addition, the NDDG staff works closely with members of the scientific community to stimulate development of new investigator-initiated research programs in diabetes epidemiology.

★ 25088 ★ U.S. Department of Health and Human Services
National Institute of Diabetes and Digestive and Kidney Diseases
Division of Diabetes, Endocrinology, and Metabolic Diseases
Research Career Development Program
45 Center Dr. MSC 6600
Bethesda, MD 20892-6600
Phone: (301)594-8819 **Fax:** (301)480-3503

Email: hydej@extra.niddk.nih.gov
Dr. Jim Hyde, Dir.

Activities/Fields: Administers a variety of research training and career development awards that span the full range of research programs falling within the Division. Prospective applicants are encouraged to contact the Research Career Development Program office regarding any questions about eligibility or provisions of the awards and to obtain current instructions for preparing applications. The available awards include National Research Service Awards, Physician Scientist Award, Clinical Investigator Award, and Research Career Development Award.

★ 25089 ★ U.S. Department of Health and Human Services
National Institute of Diabetes and Digestive and Kidney Diseases
Division of Diabetes, Endocrinology, and Metabolic Diseases
Special Program Branch
6707 Democracy Blvd., Rm. 609
Bethesda, MD 20892
Phone: (301)594-7692 **Fax:** (301)480-3503
Email: jh4862@nih.gov
Dr. James Hyde, PhD, Contact

Activities/Fields: Responsible for all of the Division-related research career development and training awards. These include individual and institutional National Research Service Awards (NRSA), Physician Scientist Awards (PSA), Clinical Investigator Awards (CIA), and Research Career Development Awards (RCDA). Branch components include the National Diabetes Data Group, Research Career Development Program; and the Special Programs Branch.

★ 25090 ★ U.S. Department of Health and Human Services
National Institute of Diabetes and Digestive and Kidney Diseases (NIDDK)
Division of Digestive Diseases and Nutrition (DDDN)
31 Center Dr., 9A27
Bethesda, MD 20892-2560
Phone: (301)496-1333 **Fax:** (301)480-7926
Email: hoofnaglej@extra.niddk.nih.gov
Dr. Jay H. Hoofnagle, Dir.

Activities/Fields: Fundamental and clinical studies of the normal functions of the digestive tract (esophagus, stomach, intestines) and changes associated with diseases of the liver, gallbladder, biliary tract, and exocrine pancreas; and basic nutrition, nutritional requirements, trace minerals, dietary fiber, obesity, and clinical nutrition. Principal Division components include the Digestive Diseases Branch, Nutritional Sciences Branch, and Special Programs Branch.

★ 25091 ★ U.S. Department of Health and Human Services
National Institute of Diabetes and Digestive and Kidney Diseases
Division of Digestive Diseases and Nutrition
Digestive Diseases Programs Branch (GI Transport and Absorption Program)
Two Democracy Plaza Room 663
6707 Democracy Blvd. MSC 5450
Bethesda, MD 20892-5450
Phone: (301)594-8884 **Fax:** (301)480-8300
Email: mm102i.@nih.gov
Dr. Michael Kenneth May, Prog. Dir.

Activities/Fields: Process of food digestion in the gastrointestinal tract (GIT). Other areas of research focus on the regulation of gene expression in the developing GIT; the structure and function of the gut mucosa; the cytoskeletal structure and contractility in brush border; the growth and differentiation of gastrointestinal cells in normal and disease states; intestinal transplantation, storage, and preservation; and gastrointestinal tissue injury, repair, and regeneration. Also supported are studies on gastrointestinal diseases such as maldigestion and malabsorption syndromes, celiac sprue, diarrhea, inflammatory bowel disease, gastric and duodenal ulcers, diseases of the salivary glands (excluding cystic fibrosis), and the effects of prostaglandins and other treatment modalities on the gastrointestinal tract and their possible role in the pathogenesis and treatment of digestive diseases.

★ 25092 ★ U.S. Department of Health and Human Services
National Institute of Diabetes and Digestive and Kidney Diseases
Division of Digestive Diseases and Nutrition
Digestive Diseases Programs Branch (Liver and Biliary Tract Diseases Program)
6700 Rockledge Dr., Rm. 5229
Bethesda, MD 20892
Phone: (301)435-3762 **Fax:** (301)402-3171
Email: tk13v@nih.gov
Thomas F. Kresina, PhD, Dir.

Activities/Fields: Office coordinates research to investigate opportunistic infections related to liver and enteric diseases, in particular, hepatitis C in the context of HIV infection, as well as, International Research related to HIV, liver disease, and substance abuse. Research focus also targets minority, and special populations with emphasis on specific issues related to HIV infection, and liver disease; safer behavior and health services; and impacr of HIV exposure in lives of the minority community. Both adults and children of all underrepresented racial, and ethnic populations are emphasized in this research focus. Biomedical research investigations support minority- related aspects of alcohol metabolism, organ damage to the liver and pancreas by alcohol and enhanced progression of AIDS-defining opportunistic infections, such as tuberculosis and hepatitis C by addiction to alcohol.

★ 25093 ★ U.S. Department of Health and Human Services
National Institute of Diabetes and Digestive and Kidney Diseases
Division of Digestive Diseases and Nutrition
Epidemiology and Clinical Trials Branch (Clinical Trials Program)
2 Democracy Plaza
6707 Democracy Blvd., MSC 5450
Bethesda, MD 20892-5450
Phone: (301)594-8879 **Fax:** (301)480-8300
Email: pr132q@nih.gov
Dr. Patricia R. Robuck, PhD, Dir.

Activities/Fields: Administers multi- and single center clinical trials in digestive and nutritional diseases and disorders. **Frmly:** Digestive Diseases Centers Branch.

★ 25094 ★ U.S. Department of Health and Human Services
National Institute of Diabetes and Digestive and Kidney Diseases
Division of Digestive Diseases and Nutrition
Nutritional Sciences Branch
6707 Democracy Blvd.
MSC 5450
Bethesda, MD 20892-5450
Phone: (301)594-8883 **Fax:** (301)480-8300
Email: van_hubbard@nih.gov
Dr. Van S. Hubbard, Ch. -Nutritional Sciences Branch

Activities/Fields: Basic, clinical, and behavioral research and training directed toward the improvement of human health. Priority areas of research are: human nutrition requirements, including environmental and host factors that may affect requirements, such as nutrient imbalance, drugs, disease, stress, and activity levels; physiological function of essential nutrients in health and disease, with emphasis on amino acids, calcium, magnesium, trace elements, and vitamins; and significance of proportion and amount of macronutrients (dietary proteins, fats, and carbohydrates) in metabolism. Studies are also conducted on the health significance of dietary fiber; prevention and control of obesity, including the relationship among genetic predisposition, induced metabolic change, and social, environmental, physiological, and behavioral factors; supportive nutrition of hospitalized patients; and assessment of nutritional status and dietary intake. Principal Branch components are the: Clinical Nutrition Research Units; Nutrient Metabolism Program; Obesity and Eating Disorders Program; and U.S.-Japan Malnutrition Panel. **Frmly:** Nutrition Program.

★ 25095 ★ U.S. Department of Health and Human Services
National Institute of Diabetes and Digestive and Kidney Diseases
Division of Digestive Diseases and Nutrition
Obesity and Eating Disorders Program
6707 Democracy Blvd.
Bethesda, MD 20892-5450
Phone: (301)594-8880 **Fax:** (301)480-8300
Email: sy29f@nih.gov
Dr. Susan Yanovski, Dir.

Activities/Fields: Biomedical and behavioral aspects of obesity, anorexia nervosa, bulimia, and other eating disorders. Goals are to establish a clear understanding of the etiology, prevention, and treatment of these multifaceted conditions. Studies focus on the physiological, metabolic, psychological, and genetic factors that affect food choices, food intake, eating behavior, appetite, and satiety; the effects of taste, smell, and gastric and humoral (including neurotransmitters) response in association with dietary intake and subsequent behavior; the physiologic and metabolic consequences of weight loss or weight gain; the effect of mild exercise on appetite and weight control; and individual variabilities in energy utilization and thermogenesis. The program also encourages investigations on the dietary determinants of the growth and control of adipocyte size and number; the responsiveness of the adipocyte to various metabolic and pharmacologic stimuli; the prevention of obesity and other eating disorders; improved methods of assessing body composition; examination of health risk factors associated with specific degrees of obesity or body composition; and determining the effect of exercise on body composition.

★ 25096 ★ U.S. Department of Health and Human Services
National Institute of Diabetes and Digestive and Kidney Diseases
Division of Digestive Diseases and Nutrition
Pancreas Program
Room 671, MSC 5450
6707 Democracy Blvd.
Bethesda, MD 20892
Phone: (301)594-8871 **Fax:** (301)480-8300
Website: http://www.niddk.nih.gov/fund/programs/m-rlist.htmpancreas
Dr. Jose Serrano, PhD, Dir.

Activities/Fields: Structure, function, and diseases (excluding cancer and cystic fibrosis) of the exocrine pancreas. Areas of research interest include: hormonal and neural regulation of electrolyte, fluid, and enzyme secretion; receptors for secretagogs; stimulus-secretion coupling mechanisms; gut-islet-acinar interrelations; organization and expression of pancreatic genes; protein synthesis and export; tissue injury, repair, and regeneration; physiology and pathology of trophic responses; neural innervention; transcapillary solute and fluid exchange; pancreatic tissue culture and storage, and preservation; imaging of the pancreas; pancreatic insufficiency; and acute and chronic pancreatitis and relevant experimental models.

★ 25097 ★ U.S. Department of Health and Human Services
National Institute of Diabetes and Digestive and Kidney Diseases
Division of Extramural Activities
6707 Democracy Dr., Rm. 715
MSC 5452
Bethesda, MD 20892-5452
Phone: (301)594-8834 **Fax:** (301)480-3505
Email: hammond2@extra.niddk.nih.gov
Website: http://www.niddk.nih.gov/funds/divisions/dea/deaintro.htm
Dr. Robert Hammond, Dir.

Activities/Fields: Serves as the service organization to the rest of the extramural division and is comprised of three branches: the review branch which reviews research grant applications; the grants management branch which prepares and issues grant awards; and the contracts and acquisition management branch which prepares and issues contracts.

★ 25098 ★ U.S. Department of Health and Human Services
National Institute of Diabetes and Digestive and Kidney Diseases
Division of Intramural Research
NIH Bldg. 10, Rm. 9M222
9000 Rockville Pike
Bethesda, MD 20892-1818
Phone: (301)496-4128 **Fax:** (301)496-9943
Email: marving@intra.niddk.nih.gov
Dr. Marvin C. Gershengorn, MD, Sci. Dir.

Activities/Fields: Metabolic diseases such as diabetes, other inborn errors of metabolism, endocrine disorders, mineral metabolism, digestive diseases, nutrition, urology and renal disease, and hematology. Basic research includes studies in biochemistry; nutrition; pathology; histochemistry; chemistry; physical, chemical, and molecular biology; pharmacology; and toxicology. Division comprises branches for: Clinical Endocrinology; Clinical Hematology; Diabetes; Digestive Diseases; Genetics and Biochemistry; Mathematical Research; Metabolic Diseases; Molecular, Cellular, and Nutritional Endocrinology; and Pediatric Metabolism; the Phoenix Epidemiology and Clinical Research Branch; and numerous laboratories.

★ 25099 ★ U.S. Department of Health and Human Services
National Institute of Diabetes and Digestive and Kidney Diseases
Division of Intramural Research
Digestive Diseases Branch
NIH Bldg. 10, Rm. 9C-103
10 Center Dr. MSC 1804
Bethesda, MD 20892-1804
Phone: (301)496-4201 **Fax:** (301)402-0600
Dr. Robert T. Jensen, Chf.

Activities/Fields: Diseases and disorders of the digestive tract, including the physiology, biochemistry, and etiology of diseases of the gastrointestinal tract and the liver, enzymes and metabolic pathways, disturbances in gastrointestinal tract function, and the effect of various treatments and therapies. Activities are carried out in sections for gastroenterology and liver diseases.

★ 25100 ★ U.S. Department of Health and Human Services
National Institute of Diabetes and Digestive and Kidney Diseases
Division of Intramural Research
Genetics and Biochemistry Branch
NIH Bldg. 5, Rm. 201
10 Center Dr. MSC 0538
Bethesda, MD 20892-0538
Phone: (301)496-2710 **Fax:** (301)496-9878
Dr. R. Daniel Camerini-Otero, Chf.

Activities/Fields: Clinical, biochemical, developmental, and molecular genetics. The range of current projects covers a wide field, from the very basic (e.g., mechanisms of genetic recombination and gene conversion in mammalian cells, DNA-mediated gene transfer, the regulation of gene expression, the molecular biology of early development in *Xenopus laevis*, biosynthesis and transport of lysosomal proteins, the molecular mechanisms of endocytosis, and the biochemical and molecular bases of human genetic disorders) to the more applied (i.e., development of new diagnostic tests and carrier detection for a number of human genetic diseases and the development of new techniques for gene purification and transfer).

★ 25101 ★ U.S. Department of Health and Human Services
National Institute of Diabetes and Digestive and Kidney Diseases
Division of Intramural Research
Mathematical Research Branch
BSA Bldg., Suite 350
9190 Rockville Pike
Bethesda, MD 20892-2690
Phone: (301)496-4325 **Fax:** (301)402-0535
Email: asherman@nih.gov
Website: http://www.niddk.nih.gov/intram/branchlb/mrb.htm
Dr. Arthur S. Sherman, Ch.

Activities/Fields: Mathematical and theoretical aspects of biological problems and the development of analytical and numerical methodology underlying such an approach. The research programs are designed to provide a formal basis and theoretical apparatus for the rational analysis and quantitative interpretation of biological phenomena. Research is organized around biological subject-matter areas rather than around subdisciplines of mathematics. Primary areas of research include neuroscience, physiology, cell biology, and endocrimology.

★ 25102 ★ U.S. Department of Health and Human Services
National Institute of Diabetes and Digestive and Kidney Diseases
Division of Intramural Research
Metabolic Diseases Branch
NIH Bldg. 10 /Rm. 9C-101
9000 Rockville Pike
Bethesda, MD 20892-1802
Phone: (301)496-5051 **Fax:** (301)496-0200
Dr. Stephen Marx, Actg. Chf.

Activities/Fields: Physiology and nature of metabolic diseases and disorders, with emphasis on the physiology, biochemistry, and mechanism of action of hormones controlling calcium metabolism. Investigations are directed at hormone-receptor interactions, regulation and characterization of adenylate cyclase, and cellular responses to hormones, particularly parathyroid hormone, calcitonin, and parathyroid related peptide. The clinical program involves studies of patients with disorders of mineral metabolism, including familial hyperparathyroid syndromes and patients with multiple endocrine neoplasia type I, hereditary resistance to parathyroid hormone or to calciferols. Patients with hyperparathyroidism are evaluated with arte riography, selective thyroid venous cath eterization, and radioimmunoassays for parathyroid hormone and cyclic AMP in plasma and/or urine. Excised parathyroid tissue is used for in vitro studies gene characterization and on control of hormone secretion.

★ 25103 ★ U.S. Department of Health and Human Services
National Institute of Diabetes and Digestive and Kidney Diseases
Division of Intramural Research
Molecular, Cellular, and Nutritional Endocrinology Branch
NIH Bldg. 10, Rm. 8D14
9000 Rockville Pike
Bethesda, MD 20892
Phone: (301)496-1540 **Fax:** (301)496-1649

Activities/Fields: Neuroendocrinology; experimental diabetes, metabolism, and nutrition; and growth and development. Research in neuroendocrinology includes basic and clinical investigations on the regulation of hypothalamic, pituitary, and placental polypeptide hormones. Studies in experimental diabetes, metabolism, and nutrition include investigation of the structure, function, and biosynthesis of integral membrane proteins involved in the hormonal regulation of carbohydrate and lipid metabolism; studies on the molecular and cellular basis of hormone action; and studies on the influence of altered metabolic and nutritional states on cellular function and its regulation by hormones. In the area of growth and development, Branch seeks to understand the mechanisms by which hormonal, nutritional, and cellular factors interact to regulate cell growth in different physiological states (e.g., fetal/embryonic development, post-natal growth, wound repair, neural cell growth, and maintenance), and how these controlled processes become deranged in pathological states involving excessive or inadequate cell growth (e.g., intrauterine growth retardation, dwarfism, neoplasia, atherosclerosis, diabetic retinopathy). The biosynthesis and action of polypeptide hormones/growth factors and their regulation is studied in appropriate model systems (e.g., cell cultures established from human subjects and animals) using state-of-the-art techniques of molecular and cell biology. Special emphasis is given to interactions between different cell types and their products, regulation of tissue responsiveness to growth factors, and alternative expression of growth factor genes resulting in novel peptides with biological functions not directly related to cell growth.

★ 25104 ★ U.S. Department of Health and Human Services
National Institute of Diabetes and Digestive and Kidney Diseases
Division of Kidney, Urologic, and Hematologic Diseases
NIH Bldg. 31, Rm. 9A-17
31 Center Dr.
MSC 2510
Bethesda, MD 20892-2510
Phone: (301)496-6325 **Fax:** (301)402-4874
Email: briggsj@hq.niddk.nih.gov
Website: http://www.niddk.nih.gov/fund/divisions/kuh/kuhintro.htm
Josephine P. Briggs, MD, Dir.

Activities/Fields: Kidney, urinary, and hematologic disorders, including epidemiologic studies and clinical trials. Offers investigator-initiated research grants and awards, program/project grants, center grants, and cooperative agreements. Also sponsors research fellowships, training grants, career development awards, and resource and research and development contracts. Scientific activities conducted through eleven major programs: Renal Physiology/Cell Biology Program, which focuses on the underlying mechanisms of kidney disease; Urology Program, which focuses on basic and clinical studies of normal and disease states of genitourinary system; Centers Program, which focuses on clinical studies in nephrology and urology; Manpower Program, which offers research training and career development awards; Chronic Renal Diseases Program, which supports basic and clinical research on chronic kidney diseases; End-Stage Renal Disease (ESRD) Program, which focuses on the mechanisms involved in ESRD; Clinical Trial Program, which focuses on clinical trials in urologicc and renal kidney diseases; Diabetic Nephropathy Program, which focuses on mechanisms of diabetic kidney disease and development of new therapies; Hematology Program, which focuses on normal and disease states of hematopoietic system; Epidemiology Program, which supports development of epidemiologic data related to major kidney, urologic, and hematologic diseases; HIV Program, which focuses on effects of HIV infection on renal, urinary, and hematopoietic function; and Small Business Innovation Research Program, which promotes commercialization of and small business involvement in federally funded research.

★ 25105 ★ U.S. Department of Health and Human Services
National Institute of Diabetes and Digestive and Kidney Diseases (NIDDK)
Division of Kidney, Urologic, and Hematologic Diseases (DKUHD)
Chronic Renal Diseases Program
6707 Democracy Blvd. 601
Bethesda, MD 20892-5458
Phone: (301)594-7717 **Fax:** (301)480-3510
Email: gladys_hirschman@nih.gov
Dr. Gladys H. Hirschman, MD, Prog. Dir.
Activities/Fields: Kidney diseases and develops treatments to prevent their onset and progression. Focuses on pathophysiology (including immunopathogenic mechanisms) of chronic renal diseases such as lupus nephritis, polycystic kidney disease, or interstitial nephritis, IgA nephropathy, and other glomerulopathies/glomerulonephritis; progressive renal disease; renial diseases of congenitial and genetic origins i.e., polycystic kidney disease; kidney disease in children and in minority populations; role of nutrition in renal disease; kidney disease caused by diabetes mellitus, including studies on pathogenic mechanisms, genetic morphologic and functional markers; and natural history of diabetic nephropathy, hypertensive renal disease and all of the above in the pediatric population.

★ 25106 ★ U.S. Department of Health and Human Services
National Institute of Diabetes and Digestive and Kidney Diseases
Division of Kidney, Urologic, and Hematologic Diseases
Hematology Program
6707 Democracy Blvd., Rm. 621
MSC 5458
Bethesda, MD 20892-5458
Phone: (301)594-7717 **Fax:** (301)480-3510
Email: badmand@extra.niddk.nih.gov
Website: http://www.niddk.nih.gov/fund/programs/f-list.htmbasic
David G. Badman, PhD, Prog. Dir.
Activities/Fields: Blood, including: hemoglobin structure and genetics; anemias of chronic diseases such as chronic renal failure; molecular and cellular role of erythropoietin; iron metabolism, transport, and storage; iron overload and deficiency; white blood cell metabolism and function; development of new iron chelating compounds for clinical use and testing the toxicity of these compounds; and hematologic aspects of AIDS, including bone marrow suppression; hematopoiesis, including stem cell biology; and gene therapy research.

★ 25107 ★ U.S. Department of Health and Human Services
National Institute of Diabetes and Digestive and Kidney Diseases
Division of Kidney, Urologic, and Hematologic Diseases
Renal Physiology / Cell Biology Program
Natcher Bldg. 5458
6707 Democracy Blvd.
Bethesda, MD 20892-5458
Phone: (301)594-7719 **Fax:** (301)480-3510
Dr. James Scherbenske, Contact
Activities/Fields: Underlying mechanisms of kidney disease. Studies in this program examine the normal structure and function of the kidney, including its biochemistry, metabolism, transport, and fluid-electrolyte dynamics. Research suppoorted is on the metabolic and physiologic transport processes that regulate solute and water excretion, as are studies on the adverse effects of drugs, nephrotoxins, and environmental toxins on the kidney. The program also has a primary interest in studies on analgesic abuse and heavy metal toxicities, as well as studies certain causes of acute renal failure such as hyppoxic injury.

★ 25108 ★ U.S. Department of Health and Human Services
National Institute of Diabetes and Digestive and Kidney Diseases
Division of Kidney, Urologic, and Hematologic Diseases
Urology and Women's Urological Health Program
Two Democracy Plaza Rm. 600
6707 Democracy Blvd. MSC 5458
Bethesda, MD 20892-5458
Phone: (301)594-7717 **Fax:** (301)480-3510
Email: nybergl@extra.niddk.nih.gov
Dr. Leroy M. Nyberg, Dir.
Activities/Fields: Normal and disease states of genitourinary system, including structure and function of the bladder, urethra, and prostate. Program interests include pyelonephritis, interstitial cystitis, urolithiasis, benign prostatic hyperplasia, prostatitis, impotence and sexual dysfunction, and urinary incontinence.

★ 25109 ★ U.S. Department of Health and Human Services
National Institute of Diabetes and Digestive and Kidney Diseases
Laboratory of Analytical Chemistry
NIH Bldg. 8, Rm. B2A-17
9000 Rockville Pike
Bethesda, MD 20892
Fax: (301)402-1967
Edwin Becker, Actg. Chf.
Activities/Fields: Provides consultation and technical assistance to Institute scientists in the area of instrumental and chemical analysis, particularly related to experimental design and interpretation of spectra.

★ 25110 ★ U.S. Department of Health and Human Services
National Institute of Diabetes and Digestive and Kidney Diseases
Laboratory of Bioorganic Chemistry
NIH Bldg. 8A, Rm. B1A02
8 Center Dr. MSC 0810
Bethesda, MD 20892-0810
Phone: (301)496-2619 **Fax:** (301)402-0008
Website: http://www.niddk.nih.gov/intram/branchlb/lbc.htm
Kenneth L. Kirk, Chf.
Activities/Fields: Mission is to elucidate the mechanism of interaction of pharmacologically active substances with biological systems. Research is designed to develop new chemical agents as tools for the study of membrane and cytosol functions of cells. New mechanisms of action or metabolism of such agents are also investigated for their potential use as therapeutics. Emphasis is on development and application of modern techniques of organic chemistry for the synthesis, separation, and spectral investigation of these chemical agents and their interactions with macromolecules. The goal is to provide insights into the normal and pathologic function of biological systems and to delineate the metabolic formation, fate, and action of physiologically active agents such as amino acids, biogenic amines, cyclic nucleotides, hormones, neurotransmitters, and steroids. Studies include pharmacologically active agents such as natural products, central stimulants, depressants, tranquilizers, anxiolytics, and other therapeutic agents, toxins, carcinogens, and mutagens.

★ 25111 ★ U.S. Department of Health and Human Services
National Institute of Diabetes and Digestive and Kidney Diseases
Laboratory of Cellular and Developmental Biology
Bldg. 50 Room 3134
9000 Rockville Pike MSC 8028
Bethesda, MD 20892-8028
Phone: (301)496-6125 **Fax:** (301)496-5239
Email: jurrien@helix.nih.gov
Dr. Jurrien Dean, MD, Chf.
Activities/Fields: Endocrinology, including research on hormonal regulation of enzymes involved in chylomicron uptake and metabolism in adipose and mammary tissues, the influence of hormones on cellular development and metabolism, and the disposition of fat and metabolites in the cell as viewed from ultrastructural studies; nutritional biochemistry, including studies on the structural and functional aspects of dihydrofolic reductase and other enzymes involved in folic acid metabolism and the intermediary metabolism of lipids, carbohydrates, and amino acids in the small intestine; membrane regulation, including studies on the mechanism of action of hormones on adenylate cyclase and other membrane regulatory processes; and developmental biochemistry, including studies on the structure and function of chromatin and the regulation of gene function during development.

★ 25112 ★ U.S. Department of Health and Human Services
National Institute of Diabetes and Digestive and Kidney Diseases
Laboratory of Chemical Biology
NIH Bldg. 10, Rm. 9N307
10 Center Dr. MSC-1822
Bethesda, MD 20892-1822
Phone: (301)496-5408 **Fax:** (301)402-0101
Email: aschecht@helix.nih.gov
Dr. Alan N. Schechter, Chf.
Activities/Fields: Chemical biology, including protein chemistry; and molecular genetics, including sickle cell anemia and thassemia. Research focuses on the control of gene expression, folding of proteins, and therapy of genetic diseases.

★ 25113 ★ U.S. Department of Health and Human Services
National Institute of Diabetes and Digestive and Kidney Diseases
Laboratory of Chemical Physics
NIH Bldg. 5
15 Center Dr. MSC-0520
Bethesda, MD 20892-0520
Phone: (301)496-1024 **Fax:** (301)435-2413
William A. Eaton, Chf.
Activities/Fields: Application of modern physical techniques to the study of a wide range of biological problems. Much of the research involves the use of a variety of spectroscopic methods (e.g., nuclear and electron magnetic resonance, laser-Raman and resonance Raman spectroscopy), electric-field-induced dichroism, ultraviolet and visible microspectrophotometry, and time-resolved absorption spectroscopy with nanosecond lasers.

★ 25114 ★ U.S. Department of Health and Human Services
National Institute of Diabetes and Digestive and Kidney Diseases
Laboratory of Molecular and Cellular Biology
NIH Bldg. 8, Rm. 2A19
9000 Rockville Pike
Bethesda, MD 20892
Phone: (301)496-1490 **Fax:** (301)402-0053
Email: ngn@helix.nih.gov
Dr. Nancy G. Nossal, Chf.
Activities/Fields: Molecular and cellular biology. Principal areas of research interest include: replication and gene regulation; development of adenoassociated virus vectors for genetic engineering and gene therapy; endocrine regulation of mammary gland development and tumors; growth factors; and glucocorticoid hormones.

★ 25115 ★ U.S. Department of Health and Human Services
National Institute of Environmental Health Sciences
MD B2-01
PO Box 12233
Research Triangle Park, NC 27709
Phone: (919)541-3201 **Fax:** (919)541-2260
Email: olden@niehs.nih.gov
Website: http://www.niehs.nih.gov
Dr. Kenneth Olden, Dir.
Activities/Fields: Conducts environmental health sciences research and supports research through its extramural and intramural programs. The Institute's Extramural Research and Training Division supports research within educational institutions, research institutes, and other public and private nonprofit organizations through individual grants, contracts, and Research Career Development Awards. Programs emphasize studies that provide information essential to an understanding of the way in which human health is adversely affected by environmental factors. Grant programs include support for Environmental Health Science Centers, Marine and Freshwater Biomedical Science Centers, Children's Environmental Health Centers, and research manpower development programs, as well as the Superfund Basic Research Program, a university-based program of basic research supported by NIEHS as part of the 1986 Superfund Amendments and Reauthorization Act. This Program combines basic research in the fields of ecology, engineering, and hydrogeology into a core program of biomedical research to provide a broader and more detailed body of scientific information to be used in decision-making related to the management of hazardous substances. In addition to the Basic Research Program, the Institute supports a model worker training program for workers involved in hazardous waste cleanup and emergency response. **Pub:** *Environmental Health Perspectives*, monthly. Journal.

★ 25116 ★ U.S. Department of Health and Human Services
National Institute of Environmental Health Sciences
Division of Extramural Research and Training
PO Box 12233
Research Triangle Park, NC 27709
Phone: (919)541-7723 **Fax:** (919)541-2843
Email: SASSAMAN@NIEHS.NIH.GOV
Website: http://www.niehs.nih.gov/dert/home.htm
Anne P. Sassaman, PhD, Dir.
Activities/Fields: Consequences of the exposure of humans and other biological systems to potentially toxic or harmful agents in the environment. Investigators at colleges, universities, and research foundations are supported through individual research grants, program project grants, and other support mechanisms. Research activities focus on the ways in which human health is adversely affected by chemical, physical, and other environmental factors. This involves: characterization of environmental health hazards; research on biological responses to environmental health hazards; applied toxicological research and testing; biometry and risk estimation; and resource and manpower development. (Research and training may span one, several, or all program areas.) The extramural program also includes support for Environmental Health Sciences Centers and for Marine and Freshwater Biomedical Science Centers. Environmental Health Sciences Centers serve as national focal points and resources for research and manpower development in health problems related to air, water, and food pollution; occupational and industrial neighborhood health and safety; heavy metal toxicity; agricultural chemical hazards; and the relationships of environment to cancer, birth defects, behavioral anomalies, respiratory and cardiovascular diseases, and diseases of other organs. Marine and +Freshwater +Biomedical Science Centers provide core support to foster multidisciplinary research on marine and freshwater organisms in the study of mechanisms of toxicity of environmental agents and as models for human diseases and disorders resulting from exposure to environmental toxicants.

★ 25117 ★ U.S. Department of Health and Human Services
National Institute of Environmental Health Sciences
Division of Intramural Research
PO Box 12233
Research Triangle Park, NC 27709
Phone: (919)541-3205 **Fax:** (919)541-4214
Email: lutzb@niehs.nih.gov
Dr. Lutz Birnbaumer, Actg. Sci. Dir.
Activities/Fields: Plans and conducts the Institute's basic laboratory and clinical research, which encompasses the environmental areas of medicine, biology, pharmacology, neurosciences and pulmonary pathobiology, chemistry, toxicology, genetics, and biophysics. Plans and conducts a program of toxicology and carcinogenesis studies to establish and characterize the toxicity of chemicals and other environmental agents, and to develop, validate, and evaluate such methods. Plans and conducts basic and applied research related to environmental health in the areas of risk assessment, statistics, biomathematics, and epidemiology. Ensures optimal utilization of available resources in the attainment of Institute objectives. Evaluates research efforts and establishes intramural priorities. Integrates ongoing and new research activities into the division structure. Collaborates with other NIH institutes, divisions and programs. Maintains an active association with peer groups in other federal agencies, academic and private institutions, and international organizations with similar environmental health research interests, and disseminates research results. Provides advice to the Institute Director and staff on matters of scientific interest. Comprises The Environmental Biology Program, The Environmental Diseases and Medicine Program, and The Environmental Toxicology Program.

★ 25118 ★ U.S. Department of Health and Human Services
National Institute of Environmental Health Sciences
Division of Intramural Research
Environmental Toxicology Program
PO Box 12233, MD A3-02
Research Triangle Park, NC 27709
Phone: (919)541-3802 **Fax:** (919)541-3647
Email: portier@niehs.nih.gov
Website: http://dir.niehs.nih.gov/diretp/
Dr. Christopher J. Portier, Dir.
Activities/Fields: Environmental toxicology.

★ 25119 ★ U.S. Department of Health and Human Services
National Institute of Environmental Health Sciences
Division of Intramural Research
Laboratory of Molecular Biophysics
PO Box 12233
Research Triangle Park, NC 27709
Phone: (919)541-3197 **Fax:** (919)541-5737
Email: pritchard@niehs.nih.gov
Dr. John B. Pritchard, Chf.
Activities/Fields: Spectroscopic methods to monitor the molecular interactions that occur between environmental agents and biological systems; develop, improve, and utilize analytical methodology for specified chemical agents; and conduct biochemical, physical, organic, and bio-organic studies of environmental agents and their conversion products, with emphasis on biomechanism elucidation.

★ 25120 ★ U.S. Department of Health and Human Services
National Institute of Environmental Health Sciences
Division of Intramural Researh
Laboratory of Pulmonary Pathobiology
Niehs Mail Drop A2-09
PO Box 12233
Research Triangle Park, NC 27709
Phone: (919)541-3540 **Fax:** (919)541-4133
Email: Nettesheim@Niehs.nih.gov
Dr. Paul Nettesheim, Chf.
Activities/Fields: Elucidate biochemical and molecular mechanisms of differentiation of airway epithelium; elucidate the role of growth factors in regulation of growth of normal and neoplastically transformed airway cells; explore pathogenetic mechanisms of inflammatory processes of the lung, particularly the cellular and biochemical basis of fibrogenesis; and elucidate the mechanisms of regulation of surfactant biosynthesis.

★ 25121 ★ U.S. Department of Health and Human Services
National Institute of Environmental Health Sciences
Environmental Toxicology Program
Toxicology Branch
Mail Drop A3-02
Research Triangle Park, NC 27709
Phone: (919)541-7992 **Fax:** (919)541-3647
Email: portier@niehs.nih.gov
Dr. Christopher Portier, Dir.
Activities/Fields: Activities are carried out in five work groups; the Chemical Dispositon Group studies the absorption, distribution,metabolism, and excretion of a range of chemicals to provide information useful in the design and interpretation of chemical toxicity and carcinogenicity activities; the Developmental and +Reproductive +Toxicology Group provides an in-house research program, consultation to program toxicologists on the design of special studies, and participation with National Institute for Occupational Safety and Health and National Center for Toxicological Research personnel in the organization, coordination, and long-range planning of the National Toxicology Program's reproductive and developmental toxicology program (in-house research activities include evaluating the reproductive toxicity of environmental and industrial chemicals, providing data on the toxic potential and mechanism of chemicals, and enhancing the development of new and more appropriate testing systems); the Immunologic +Toxicology Group selects, refines, and validates a panel of immunology and host resistance procedures to define immunotoxicity and correlating changes in immune function with alterations in host resistance; and the Inhalation +Toxicology Group conducts studies on compounds that enter the body primarily by inhalation; and works toward the technologic advancement of gas-vapor inhalation methodologies/facilities. (Further information on a fifth group, the Metal +Toxicology Group, was not available for this edition. In addition, the Biochemical +Toxicology Group that was previously listed in this Directory no longer exists.).

★ 25122 ★ U.S. Department of Health and Human Services
National Institute of General Medical Sciences
Biophysics and Physiological Sciences Program
45 Center Dr., MSC 6200
Bethesda, MD 20892-6200
Phone: (301)594-0828 **Fax:** (301)480-2004
Email: cassatj@nigms.nih.gov
Website: http://www.nigms.nih.gov
James Cassatt, Dir.
Activities/Fields: Works to further understanding of the structure and function of cells, cellular components, and the biological macromolecules that make up these components. Seeks to finds ways to prevent,

treat, and cure diseases that result from disturbed or abnormal cellular activity. Maintains a Biophysics Branch and a Cell Biology Branch. **Frmly:** (2000) Biophysics and Physiological Sciences Program.

★ 25123 ★ U.S. Department of Health and Human Services
National Institute of General Medical Sciences
Diagnostic Laboratory

1230 York Ave.
Box 2
New York, NY 10021
Phone: (212)327-8522 **Fax:** (212)327-8484
Email: keuterk@mail.rockfeller.edu
Kaci Keuter, Supv.

Activities/Fields: Provides diagnostic services and prospective and retrospective clinical studies in conjunction with disease screening and laboratory animal diagnostics at Rockefeller University. Research includes: transgenic animal technology; PCR; macrophage biology; and clinical case reviews. Provides a complete laboratory animal diagnostic program.

★ 25124 ★ U.S. Department of Health and Human Services
National Institute of General Medical Sciences
Division of Cell Biology and Biophysics
Biophysics Branch

45 Center Dr., MSC 6200
Bethesda, MD 20892-6200
Phone: (301)594-0828 **Fax:** (301)480-2004
Dr. Bert Shapiro, Dir.

Activities/Fields: Biophysics and bioengineering. Areas of emphasis in biophysical research include: the determination of the structures of proteins and nucleic acids; studies of the structural features that determine macromolecular conformation; the structural analysis of macromolecular interactions and of ligand-macro molecular interactions; the development of physical methodology for the analysis of molecular structure; and the development and use of theoretical methods to investigate biological systems. Bioengineering research interests include the development and refinement of instruments needed to conduct research in the areas described above. These instruments include: nuclear magnetic resonance spectroscopy, mass spectroscopy, and other forms of spectroscopy; x-ray and other scattering techniques; microscopy; and cell separation techniques. This area of research also includes the development of new bioanalytical methods and biomaterials.

★ 25125 ★ U.S. Department of Health and Human Services
National Institute of General Medical Sciences
Division of Cell Biology and Biophysics
Cell Biology Branch

45 Center Dr., MSC 6200
Bethesda, MD 20892-6200
Phone: (301)594-0828 **Fax:** (301)480-2004
James Cassatt, Div. Dir.

Activities/Fields: Molecular and biochemical activities of cells and subcellular components, as well as on the role of cellular dysfunction in disease. Emphasis is placed on research with applications to more than one cell type, model system, or disease state, as well as research that does not fall within the disease-oriented mission of another of the National Institutes of Health. Representative studies include those on: plasma and intracellular membranes, receptors, and signal transduction mechanisms; the structure and function of the cytoskeleton; cell motility; the regulation of protein and membrane synthesis and the activation of cell growth; subcellular organelles; cell division; and lipid biochemistry.

★ 25126 ★ U.S. Department of Health and Human Services
National Institute of General Medical Sciences
Division of Genetics and Developmental Biology

Bldg. 45, Rm. 2AS-25
45 Center Drive, MSC 6200
Bethesda, MD 20892-6200
Phone: (301)594-0943 **Fax:** (301)480-2228
Email: greenbej@nigms.nih.gov
Website: http://www.nih.gov/nigms
Judith H. Greenberg, PhD, Dir.

Activities/Fields: Genetics research and developmental biology to better understand the fundamental processes and mechanisms of inheritance. An objective of the program is the eventual prevention and improved treatment of genetic ills in man, including multifactoral diseases with a strong hereditary component, such as diabetes, atherosclerosis, hypertension, and schizophrenia. Research training support provided by the Division includes: institutional predoctoral programs, which sponsor research training in the broad field of genetic principles and mechanisms; individual postdoctoral awards, which support training for research that will lead to further understanding of genetics and development; and institutional postdoctoral programs (with emphasis on medical genetics), which provide advanced and special research training in genetics. Research is concerned with basic genetic and developmental studies. Research topics include the replication, repair, and recombination of DNA; regulation of gene expression; population genetics and evolution; cell cycle control; developmental genetics; chromosomal organization and mechanics; and neurogenetics.

★ 25127 ★ U.S. Department of Health and Human Services
National Institute of General Medical Sciences
Pharmacology and Biorelated Chemistry Program

45 Center Dr., MSC 6200
Bethesda, MD 20892-6200
Phone: (301)594-3827 **Fax:** (301)480-2802
Email: rogersm@nigms.nih.gov
Website: http://www.nigms.nih.gov
Dr. Michael E. Rogers, Dir.

Activities/Fields: Supports research and research training aimed at improving the molecular-level understanding of fundamental biological processes and discovering approaches to their control. Research supported by the Division takes a multi-faceted approach to problems in pharmacology, physiology, biochemistry, and biorelated chemistry that are either very basic in nature or that have implications for more than one disease area. The goals of supported research include an improved understanding of drug action and mechanisms of anesthesia; pharmacogenetics and mechanisms underlying individual responses to drugs; new methods and targets for drug discovery; advances in natural products synthesis; an enhanced understanding of biological catalysis; a greater knowledge of metabolic regulation and fundamental physiological processes; and the integration and application of basic physiological, pharmacological, and biochemical research to clinical issues in anesthesia, clinical pharmacology, and trauma and burn injury. The division also supports quantitative studies of complex systems involving areas within its scope.

★ 25128 ★ U.S. Department of Health and Human Services
National Institute of General Medical Sciences
Pharmacology Research Associate Program

Bldg. 45, Rm. 2AS-43
Bethesda, MD 20892-6200
Phone: (301)594-3583 **Fax:** (301)480-2802
Email: prat@nigms.nih.gov
Website: http://www.nigms.nih.gov/about_nigms/prat.html
Pamela A. Marino, PhD, CoDir.

Activities/Fields: Developing leaders in pharmacological research for key positions in academic, industrial, and government research laboratories. Each year 7 recently trained scientists are selected for a two-year period of postdoctoral research in laboratories of the National Institutes of Health. Fellows conduct research under the direction of one of more than 120 senior scientists and may take coursework in areas of their choice, such as applied mathematics, experimental statistics, medicinal chemistry, human biochemical genetics, and molecular biophysics. Since 1978, Program has specifically targeted several positions to clinical pharmacology (considered a shortage area). Applicants for such positions must have an M.D. degree, a minimum of one year of graduate medical training (internship or residency), and a demonstrated interest in a research career in clinical pharmacology.

★ 25129 ★ U.S. Department of Health and Human Services
National Institute of Mental Health

6001 Executive Blvd., Rm. 8235
Bethesda, MD 20892-9669
Phone: (301)443-3673 **Fax:** (301)443-2578
Email: rn3p@nih.gov
Website: http://www.nimh.nih.gov
Richard K. Nakamura, PhD, Actg. Dir.

Activities/Fields: Brain, mental illness, and mental health, particularly the causes, prevention, diagnosis, and treatment of mental illnesses. Principal components are: the Divisions of Neuroscience and Behavioral Science, Clinical and Treatment Research, Epidemiology and Services Research, Extramural Activities, and Intramural Research Programs; Offices of Prevention, Equal Employment Opportunity, Rural Mental Health Research, Legislative Analysis and Coordination, Scientific Information, Resource Management, and Science Policy and Program Planning; Office for Special Populations; and Office on AIDS. Operates the Neuropsychiatric Research Hospital on the St. Elizabeth's Hospital campus in Washington, D.C.

★ 25130 ★ U.S. Department of Health and Human Services
National Institute of Mental Health
Division of Clinical and Treatment Research

5600 Fishers Ln., Rm. 17C-20
Rockville, MD 20857
Phone: (301)443-3683 **Fax:** (301)443-7264
David Shore, MD, Actg. Dir.

Activities/Fields: Service delivery and health economics at the clinical, institutional, and systems levels; the understanding, treatment, and prevention of antisocial and violent behavior and their effects, including law and mental health interaction; and the prevention, control, and treatment of rape, other sexual assault, and their effects. The Division consists of: the Child and Family Support Branch, Services Research Branch, Statistical Research Branch, and Systems Development and Community Support Branch. **Frmly:** (1990) Biometry and Applied Sciences Division; Applied and Services Research Division.

★ 25131 ★ U.S. Department of Health and Human Services
National Institute of Mental Health
Division of Clinical and Treatment Research
Child and Adolescent Disorders Research Branch

6001 Executive Loop, Rm. 6200
MSC 9617
Bethesda, MD 20892-9617
Phone: (301)443-5944 **Fax:** (301)480-4415
Email: dkoretz@mail.nih.gov
Doreen Koretz, PhD, Chf.

Activities/Fields: Child and adolescent disorders, including attention deficit disorder, depression, conduct disorders, and autism. Also investigates suicide among children and adolescents. Focuses on classification, assessment, etiology, genetics, clinical course, outcome, and pharmacologic, somatic, and psychosocial treatment and rehabilitation of disorders affecting children and adolescents. **Frmly:** (1997) Division of Clinical and Treatment Research; Child and Adolescent Disorders Research Branch; (2000) Developmental Psychopathology Disorders Research Branch.

★ 25132 ★ U.S. Department of Health and Human Services
National Institute of Mental Health
Division of Clinical and Treatment Research
Mental Disorders of the Aging Research Branch
5600 Fishers Ln., Rm. 10-75
Rockville, MD 20857
Phone: (301)443-1185 **Fax:** (301)594-6784
Dr. Barry Lebowitz, Chf.

Activities/Fields: Mental health and illness implications of the aging process and old age. This includes studies on: causes, treatment, and prevention of Alzheimer's disease, senile dementia, and related disorders, with emphasis on differential diagnosis, test of memory-enhancing agents, and issues of coexisting illness and excess ability; causes, treatment, and prevention of depression in older persons (including investigations of the relationship of depression to dementing disorders, suicide, alcoholism, medical disease, and other behavioral disorders); causes, treatment, and prevention of behavioral disturbance and dysfunction, with special reference to agitation, assaultive/aggressive behavior, confusion, disorientation, and other behavioral problems; development and refinement of pharmacologic and psychosocial treatments, with special attention to efficacy, safety, side-effects, mechanisms of action, and drug/drug interaction; behavioral medicine and the interface of physical illness and mental disorders in later life; chronically mentally ill elderly, with special attention to treatment and management of schizophrenia and to psychosocial and behavioral approaches to quality of life; design and refinement of methods for treatment intervention, clinical trials, and service delivery models for the elderly; mental illness in nursing homes; effects of families, support systems, and self-help groups on the care of older persons with significant mental disorders; family stress and the care of Alzheimer's disease victims; and prevention of pathology among elderly at risk for mental illness. Support is provided through a wide range of mechanisms, including the Geriatric +Mental Health Academic Award; Scientist Development Awards; and National Research Service Awards, including individual fellowships and institutional awards at pre-doctoral or postdoctoral levels. In addition, the Clinical Research Centers on +Psychopathology of the +Elderly Program provides support to a limited number of centers situated in clinical treatment settings with demonstrable interest in the study of mental health and aging.

★ 25133 ★ U.S. Department of Health and Human Services
National Institute of Mental Health
Division of Extramural Activities
6001 Executive Blvd., Rm. 6154
MSC 9609
Bethesda, MD 20892-9609
Phone: (301)443-3367 **Fax:** (301)443-4720
Email: jsteinbe@nih.gov
Website: http://www.nimh.nih.gov/dea/index.htm
Jane Steinberg, PhD, Dir.

Activities/Fields: Provides leadership and advice in developing, implementing, and coordinating extramural programs and policies; represents the Institute on extramural program and policy issues within the Department and with outside organizations; provides scientific and technical review of applications for grants, cooperative agreements, and contracts; and oversees National Advisory Mental Health Council activities. The Division consists of the Office of the Director and the following branches: Clinical, Epidemiological, and Services Review Branch; Neuroscience and Behavioral Science Review Branch; Research Development and Special Projects Review Branch; and Extramural Policy Branch. Division does not provide direct grant support. Copies of all current grant announcements may be obtained from this office, but consultation with regard to the development of grant applications should be obtaned directly from the research support divisions of the National Institute of Mental Health.

★ 25134 ★ U.S. Department of Health and Human Services
National Institute of Mental Health
Division of State and Community Systems Development
Survey and Analysis Branch
5600 Fishers Ln.
Parklawn, Rm. 15C-04
Rockville, MD 20857
Phone: (301)443-3343 **Fax:** (301)443-7926
Email: rmanders@samhsa.gov
Website: http://www.mentalhealth.org
Ronald W. Manderscheid, Chf.

Activities/Fields: Statistics on the major characteristics of the nation's mental health service systems, their resources, staffing, utilization patterns, costs, and financing; develops methodology for statistical data collection and demography; and conducts ecological and demographic studies on the need and demand for mental health services. In addition, Branch provides consultation to state and local mental health agencies on statistical methodology, mental health information systems, and the use of data. **Pub:** *Information Systems Series.* • *Mental Health National Statistics Series.* • *Mental Health, United States*, biennially. **Frmly:** (1992) Statistical Research Branch.

★ 25135 ★ U.S. Department of Health and Human Services
National Institute of Mental Health
Epidemiology and Services Research Division
6001 Executive Blvd.
Bethesda, MD 20892-9629
Phone: (301)443-3648 **Fax:** (301)443-4045
Email: gnorquis@nih.gov
Website: http://www.nimh.nih.gov
Dr. Grayson Norquist, Dir.

Activities/Fields: Clinical epidemiology, classification, assessment, etiology, clinical course, outcome, treatment, and prevention of mental disorders and servcies research. **Frmly:** Clinical Research Division; Epidemiology and Services Research Division.

★ 25136 ★ U.S. Department of Health and Human Services
National Institute of Mental Health
Epidemiology and Services Research Division
Epidemiology and Psychopathology Research Branch
60001 Executive Blvd., Rm. 7219
MSC-9649
Bethesda, MD 20892-9649
Phone: (301)443-3774 **Fax:** (301)443-7895
Charles T. Kaelber, MD, Actg. Chf.

Activities/Fields: Assessing mental health/mental illness status of populations in terms of incidence and prevalence; describing the natural history of disorders and identifying illness syndromes in the community as well as in clinical patient populations; developing new epidemiologic, statistical, demographic, and other quantitatively oriented methodologies for assessing the mental illness/health of a population; conducting epidemiologic studies to identify etiologic factors of mental health/mental disorder in different groups in terms of inheritance, experience, behavior, biologic factors, and environment in community or patient populations; conducting case-control studies to test the efficacy of some positive action of intervention; and conducting clinical research in the classification, assessment, etiology, genetics, clinical course, outcome, and treatment of general psychopathology and other mental outcome and treatment of general psychopathology and other mental disorders. Support is provided through research grants, conference grants, small grants, specifically announced cooperative agreements, and institutional research training grants, as well as Research Scientist Development, Research Scientist, Clinical Scientist, and Physician Scientist Awards, and pre- and postdoctoral individual fellowships. Branch comprises the Development and Application of +Epidemiology Methods Section, Development and Testing of +Epidemiology Hypotheses Section, Experimental +Epidemiology and Evaluation Section, and General +Psychopathology Section.

★ 25137 ★ U.S. Department of Health and Human Services
National Institute of Mental Health
Epidemiology and Services Research Division
Prevention Research Branch
5600 Fishers Ln., Rm. 10C09
Rockville, MD 20857
Phone: (301)443-4283 **Fax:** (301)443-4045
Eve K. Moscicki, Chf.

Activities/Fields: Prevention of mental disorders and behavioral dysfunctions and the promotion of mental health, including preventing socio-emotional problems among infants and young children at risk; preventing conduct and other behavioral disorders in school-aged children; preventing anxiety and depressive disorders in children and adults; promoting mental health through the enhancement of protective factors, including coping mechanisms; preventing suicide and suicidality in preclinical populations; and preventing affective and anxiety disorders in HIV-infected individuals, people at high-risk for infection, their families, caretakers, and loved ones. **Pub:** *Proceedings.* • *Research Reports.*

★ 25138 ★ U.S. Department of Health and Human Services
National Institute of Mental Health
Epidemiology and Services Research Division
Violence and Traumatic Stress Research Branch
5600 Fishers Ln., Parklawn, 18C-14
Rockville, MD 20857
Phone: (301)443-3635 **Fax:** (301)443-4611
Doreen Koretz, PhD, Contact

Activities/Fields: Support research and research training concerned with the development and prevention of adult psychopathology and mental disorders. Included within the Branch are studies aimed at the major brain disorders (e.g., schizophrenia, bipolar disorder, major depression), antisocial and other personality disorders, and co-morbid physical and mental disorders, as well as cross cutting epidemiological studies and studies that examine traumatic stress and victimization as a risk factor for psychopathology. priority areas but are relevant to NIMH and Branch missions. The Branch does not support research that is not clearly relevant to mental health concerns or research that more appropriately falls within the mission of other federal programs. **Frmly:** Antisocial and Violent Behavior Branch.

★ 25139 ★ U.S. Department of Health and Human Services
National Institute of Mental Health
Intramural Research Programs Division
Bldg. 10, Rm. 4N222
MSC 2108
10 Central Dr.
Bethesda, MD 20892
Phone: (301)496-3501 **Fax:** (301)480-8348
Email: rd31o@nih.gov

Website: http://intramural.nimh.nih.gov
Robert Desimone, PhD, Dir.

Activities/Fields: Clinical and behavioral, biological, and special research dealing with the causes, diagnosis, treatment, and prevention of mental disorders and the biological and psychosocial factors that determine human behavior and development; provides a focus for national attention in the area of mental health research; and provides technical support through development and maintenance of electronic and mechanical instrumentation and equipment. **Pub:** *ADAMHA News*, biweekly. • *NIH Record*, biweekly.

★ 25140 ★ U.S. Department of Health and Human Services
National Institute of Mental Health
Intramural Research Programs Division
Experimental Therapeutic Branch
NIH Bldg. 10, Rm. 4F-229A
10 Center Dr., MSC 1380
Bethesda, MD 20892-1380
Phone: (301)496-4303 **Fax:** (301)480-5135
David Pickar, MD, Chf. of Expmt. Therapeutics

Activities/Fields: Basic and clinical neuroscience and attempts to integrate data on the biochemistry and pharmacology of the central nervous system with an understanding of the pathogenesis and treatment of major psychiatric diseases. Branch comprises the Clinical and Pharmacology Section, Clinical Studies Section, Molecular Neurogenetics Section, and Molecular Pharmacology Section. **Frmly:** Clinical Neuroscience Branch.

★ 25141 ★ U.S. Department of Health and Human Services
National Institute of Mental Health
Intramural Research Programs Division
Socio-Environmental Studies Laboratory
Federal Bldg., Rm. B1A-14
7550 Wisconsin Ave.
Bethesda, MD 20892-9005
Phone: (301)496-3383 **Fax:** (301)402-0621
Email: carmi.schooler@nih.gov
Carmi Schooler, PhD, Sect. Ch.

Activities/Fields: Social structure and personality, and cognition, including studies on basic cognitive and interpersonal processes in individuals throughout the life span.

★ 25142 ★ U.S. Department of Health and Human Services
National Institute of Mental Health
Intramural Research Programs Division (Basic Research)
Cell Biology Laboratory
NIH Bldg. 36, Rm. 2A-11
9000 Rockville Pike
Bethesda, MD 20892
Phone: (301)496-9444 **Fax:** (301)402-1748
Martin Zatz, Chf.

Activities/Fields: Light and electron microscope-level neuroanatomy, chronobiology, developmental neurobiology, biosynthesis of biologically active molecules, isolation of novel peptide hormones, and regulation of intracellular processes by chemical messenger. Laboratory has a section on biochemical pharmacology.

★ 25143 ★ U.S. Department of Health and Human Services
National Institute of Mental Health
Intramural Research Programs Division (Basic Research)
Cerebral Metabolism Laboratory
NIH Bldg. 36, Rm. 1A-05
9000 Rockville Pike
Bethesda, MD 20892
Phone: (301)496-1371 **Fax:** (301)480-1668
Website: http://intramural.nimh.nih.gov/research/lcm/
Louis Sokoloff, MD, Chf.

Activities/Fields: Neurochemistry and neurophysiology using biochemical methods for measuring local cerebral glucose utilization, local cerebral blood flow, and local cerebral protein synthesis in vivo. Laboratory comprises sections on clinical brain imaging and developmental neurochemistry.

★ 25144 ★ U.S. Department of Health and Human Services
National Institute of Mental Health
Intramural Research Programs Division (Basic Research)
General and Comparative Biochemistry Laboratory
NIH Bldg. 36, Rm. 3D28
36 Convent Dr., MSC 4094
Bethesda, MD 20892-4094
Phone: (301)496-3241 **Fax:** (301)402-4747
Giulio L. Cantoni, MD, Sci. Emeritus

Activities/Fields: Mechanisms and pathways of biological methylation, alkaloid biosynthesis, peptides, cellular differentiation, and gene expression in eukaryotes. Focus is on the enzymatic mechanisms in methyl transfer reactions, mechanism of drug addiction, muscle differentiation in cell culture, and genetic engineering. **Pub:** *Annual Report.*

★ 25145 ★ U.S. Department of Health and Human Services
National Institute of Mental Health
Intramural Research Programs Division (Basic Research)
Molecular Biology Laboratory
NIH Bldg. 36, Rm. 1B-08
9000 Rockville Pike
Bethesda, MD 20892
Phone: (301)496-6945 **Fax:** (301)402-0245
Email: davidn@helix.nih.gov
David Neville, MD, Chf.

Activities/Fields: Comprises sections on biophysical chemistry, molecular genetics, and regulatory proteins.

★ 25146 ★ U.S. Department of Health and Human Services
National Institute of Mental Health
Intramural Research Programs Division (Clinical Research)
Biological Psychiatry Branch
NIH Bldg. 10, Rm. 3S-239
10 Center Dr., MSC 1272
Bethesda, MD 20892-1272
Phone: (301)496-4805 **Fax:** (301)402-0052
Email: robert.post@nih.gov
Dr. Robert Post, Chf.

Activities/Fields: Clinical psychiatric problems, including manic-depressive and schizo-affective illness, recurrent depression, and panic-anxiety disorders. The Branch's goal is to develop programs to investigate psychologic, biochemical, and neuroanatomic contributions to the study of manic-depressive illness, anxiety disorders, and related symptoms. Focus is on psychobiology, involving studies in psychiatry, psychology, neurology, genetics, pharmacology, and biochemistry. Specific research interests are the biochemistry of neurotransmission and the action of mood stabilizers, brain imaging of affective illness, and the models of sensitization and kindling. Branch comprises Anxiety and +Affective Disorders Unit, Behavioral +Biology Unit, Psychobiology Section, Molecular +Neurobiology Section, and Behavioral Pharmacology Unit.

★ 25147 ★ U.S. Department of Health and Human Services
National Institute of Mental Health
Intramural Research Programs Division (Clinical Research)
Child Psychiatry Branch
NIH Bldg. 10, Rm. 3N-202
10 Center Dr., MSC 1600
Bethesda, MD 20892-1600
Phone: (301)496-6080 **Fax:** (301)402-0296
Email: rapoport@helix.nih.gov
Website: http://intramural.nimh.nih.gov/research/chp/index2.html
Judith L. Rapoport, MD, Chf.

Activities/Fields: Biological aspects of child psychiatry, including childhood schizophrenia, obsessive compulsive disorder, and hyperactivity. Areas of interest include pediatric psychopharmacology and brain imaging in child psychiatry. **Pub:** *Annual Report.*

★ 25148 ★ U.S. Department of Health and Human Services
National Institute of Mental Health
Intramural Research Programs Division (Clinical Research)
Clinical Neuroendocrinology Branch
NIH Bldg. 10, Rm. 2D-46
10 Center Dr.
Bethesda, MD 20892-1284
Phone: (301)496-6884 **Fax:** (301)402-1561
Philip W. Gold, MD, Chf.

Activities/Fields: Physiological organization of neuroendocrine systems and on the relevance of alterations in neuroendocrine function to the pathophysiology and etiology of major psychiatric disorders.

★ 25149 ★ U.S. Department of Health and Human Services
National Institute of Mental Health
Intramural Research Programs Division (Clinical Research)
Clinical Neurogenetics Branch
NIH Bldg. 10, Rm. 2D46
9000 Rockville Pike
Bethesda, MD 20892
Phone: (301)496-0373 **Fax:** (301)402-0859
Website: http://intramural.nimh.nih.gov/research/nsb/index.htm
Ellen Sidransky, MD, Sect. Ch.

Activities/Fields: Clinical and basic biologic and pharmacologic studies relating to the genetics of manic-depressive illness and schizophrenia. **Pub:** *Conference proceedings.*

★ 25150 ★ U.S. Department of Health and Human Services
National Institute of Mental Health
Intramural Research Programs Division (Clinical Research)
Clinical Psychobiology Branch
NIH Bldg. 10, Rm. 3S-231
10 Center Dr., MSC 1390
Bethesda, MD 20892-1390
Phone: (301)496-2141 **Fax:** (301)496-5439
Thomas A. Wehr, MD, Chf.

Activities/Fields: Clinical psychiatric and psychobiological research. Research interest includes sleep physiology and biological rythmns, seasonal affective disorder, (SAD) and light treatment. **Pub:** *Proceedings.*

★ 25151 ★ U.S. Department of Health and Human Services
National Institute of Mental Health
Intramural Research Programs Division (Clinical Research)
Laboratory of Clinical Science
NIH Bldg. 10, Rm. 3D41
10 Center Dr., MSC 1264
Bethesda, MD 20892-1264
Phone: (301)496-2757 **Fax:** (301)402-0188
Email: murphy.dl@helix.nih.gov
Dr. Dennis L. Murphy, MD, Chf.
Activities/Fields: Medical research related to mental health. Principal components include the Analytical +Biochemistry Section, Pharmacology Section, Geriatric +Psychiatry Section, Histopharmacology Section, and Clinical +Neuropharmacology Section. **Pub:** *Proceedings of national and international conferences.*

★ 25152 ★ U.S. Department of Health and Human Services
National Institute of Mental Health
Intramural Research Programs Division (Clinical Research)
Neurophsiology Laboratory
NIHAC Bldg. 110, Rm. 119
Poolesville, MD 20837
Phone: (301)443-4513 **Fax:** (301)402-0236
Charles Gerfen, Actg. Chf.
Activities/Fields: Neurophysiology.

★ 25153 ★ U.S. Department of Health and Human Services
National Institute of Mental Health
Intramural Research Programs Division (Clinical Research)
Neuropsychology Laboratory
NIH Bldg. 49, Rm. 1B80
49 Convent Dr., MSC 4415
Bethesda, MD 20892-4415
Phone: (301)496-5625 **Fax:** (301)402-0046
Email: bob@ln.nimh.nih.gov
Dr. Robert Desimore, Dir.
Activities/Fields: Relationships between neural structures and behavior in nonhuman primates using a multidisciplinary approach to study cognitive functions such as perception, attention, memory, and emotion in Old World monkeys.

★ 25154 ★ U.S. Department of Health and Human Services
National Institute of Mental Health
Intramural Research Programs Division (Clinical Research)
Psychology and Psychopathology Laboratory
5415 W Cedar Ln., Ste. 203B
Bethesda, MD 20892-2615
Phone: (301)496-2551 **Fax:** (301)594-5142
Email: alan.mirsky@nih.gov
Dr. Allan F. Mirsky, PhD, Section Chf.
Activities/Fields: Genetic and neurobehavioral factors in psychopathology, and on normal cognition, emphasizing the pathology of attention.

★ 25155 ★ U.S. Department of Health and Human Services
National Institute of Mental Health
Intramural Research Programs Division (Neuropsychiatric Research at Saint Elizabeth's Hospital)
Biochemical Genetics Laboratory
Bldg. 36, 3-D-20
9000 Rockville Pike
Bethesda, MD 20892
Phone: (301)435-3583 **Fax:** (301)480-9862
Email: merrilc@helix.nih.gov
Dr. Carl R. Merril, MD, Chf.
Activities/Fields: Affects of aging on the central nervous system. Primarily concerned with studies of protein variations in the brain, focusing on proteins and protein detection in normal and disease states. Exploring new approaches to increase the sensitivity of protein detection methods. Also, exploring the use of bacterial viruses, or bacteriophage, that display specific ligands or antibodies that can bind to proteins to provide a detection amplification system with a sensitivity to permit identification and characterization of proteins from single cells, or for the examination of trace proteins from tissues. Investigating the use of bacteriophage to treat infectious diseases caused by bacterial infections, as well as bacteriophage evolution, genomics, and molecular biology. The emergence of antibiotic-resistant bacterial strains requires the exploration of alternate antibacterial therapies, which led to study of the ability of bacterial viruses (bacteriophage, or phage) to rescue mice bacteremic from VRE. **Frmly:** Preclinical Pharmacology Laboratory.

★ 25156 ★ U.S. Department of Health and Human Services
National Institute of Mental Health
Intramural Research Programs Division (Neuropsychiatric Research at Saint Elizabeth's Hospital)
Clinical and Services Branch
Clinical Brain Disorders Branch
Bldg. 10 Center Dr., Rm. 4S-241
MSC1377
Bethesda, MD 20814-9692
Phone: (301)435-8966 **Fax:** (301)480-7795
Email: eganm@intra.nimh.nih.gov
Michael Egan, MD, Actg. Dir.
Activities/Fields: Schizophrenia, focusing on molecular genetic and epidemiological studies of the new physiological alternatives associated with schizophrenia using patients and their families.

★ 25157 ★ U.S. Department of Health and Human Services
National Institute of Mental Health
Mood and Anxiety Disorders Program (MAP)
10 Center Dr., Rm. 4N-222, MSC 1381
Bethesda, MD 20892-1381
Phone: (301)496-4183 **Free:** (866)627-6464
Fax: (301)480-8648
Email: nimhinfo@nih.gov
Website: http://intramural.nimh.gov/mood/
Dennis S. Charney, MD, Dir.
Activities/Fields: Mood and anxiety disorders, such as depression, bipolar disorder, anxiety disorders, posttraumatic stress disorder and obsessive compulsive disorder.

★ 25158 ★ U.S. Department of Health and Human Services
National Institute of Mental Health
Neuroscience and Behavioral Science Division
5600 Fishers Ln., Rm. 11-103
Rockville, MD 20857
Phone: (301)443-3563 **Fax:** (301)443-1731
Website: http://www.nimh.nih.gov
Stephen L. Foote, PhD, Actg. Dir.
Activities/Fields: Programs of research, research training, and resource development in basic and clinical neuroscience; reviews and assesses the performance of such programs; collaborates with other federal agencies and with outside organizations. The Division consists of the Behavioral and Integrative Neuroscience Research Branch, Molecular and Cellular Neuroscience Research Branch, Genetics Research Branch, Preclinical and Clinical Therapeutics Research Branch, the Reseearch Training and Research Development Program, and the Translational Research and Scientific Technology Program. **Pub:** *Conference proceedings.* **Frmly:** Basic Sciences Division; (1993) Basic Brain and Behavioral Sciences Division.

★ 25159 ★ U.S. Department of Health and Human Services
National Institute of Mental Health
Neuroscience and Behavioral Science Division
Behavioral, Cognitive, and Social Science Research Branch
6001 Exec. Blvd., Rm. 7215
Rockville, MD 20852
Phone: (301)443-3942 **Fax:** (301)443-9876
Email: moliveri@nih.gov
Dr. Mary Ellen Oliveri, Chf.
Activities/Fields: Programs of research, research training, and resource development in the behavioral sciences to increase understanding of psychological, psychosocial, emotional, and cognitive factors influencing behavior. **Frmly:** Behavioral Sciences Research Branch.

★ 25160 ★ U.S. Department of Health and Human Services
National Institute of Mental Health
Neuroscience and Behavioral Sciences Division
Molecular and Cellular Neuroscience Research Branch
Neuroscience Ctr. Bldg.
6001 Executive Blvd.
Rockville, MD 20857
Phone: (301)443-1504 **Fax:** (301)443-4822
Dr. Stephen Zalcman, Chf.
Activities/Fields: Behavior and brain function in order to develop knowledge of basic biological/molecular mechanisms underlying mental disorders and to understand the basic processes involved in the action of psychoactive drugs. Activities involve biobehavioral research, neurobiological research, and psychopharmacological research, which includes support for clinical and preclinical studies on the physiological sites and mechanisms of actions of psychoactive drugs. Branch comprises the Neuroimaging and Applied Neuroscience Research Branch.

★ 25161 ★ U.S. Department of Health and Human Services
National Institute of Mental Health
Office of Scientific Information
6001 Executive Blvd., Rm. 8184, MSC 9663
Bethesda, MD 20892-9663
Phone: (301)443-4513 **Free:** 800-421-4211
Fax: (301)443-4279
Website: http://www.nimh.nih.gov/
Clarissa Wittenberg, Dir.
Activities/Fields: Administers the Institute's public communication, scientific information dissemination, and media relations activities. Prepares materials for professionals and the general public based on current research developments. Is responsible for a national program to educate the public, primary care providers, and mental health specialists about mental disorders, including anxiety disorders and depressive illnesses. Office is comprised of two branches, the Public Affairs and Science Reports Branch and the Information Resources and Inquiries Branch.

★ 25162 ★ U.S. Department of Health and Human Services
National Institute of Neurological Disorders and Stroke
Bldg. 31, Rm. 8-A52
Bethesda, MD 20892-2540
Phone: (301)496-9746 **Fax:** (301)496-0296
Email: penna@ninds.nih.gov
Website: http://www.ninds.nih.gov
Audrey S. Penn, MD, Actg. Dir.
Activities/Fields: Causes, prevention, diagnosis, and treatment of neurological disorders and stroke. The

Institute conducts, fosters, and supports research and research training in neurological and muscle disorders through: intramural, collaborative, and field research in its own laboratories, branches, and clinics, and through contracts; research grants to scientific institutions and to individuals; individual and institutional research training awards to increase trained professional research manpower in neurological fields; and cooperation with various agencies in collecting and disseminating educational and informational material related to neurological disorders and stroke. The Institute is organized into: a division of extramural research, which plans and directs initiatives for grant and contract support for research, training, and career development; and a division of intramural research, which conducts basic and clinical research in neurological disorders and related disciplines.

★ 25163 ★ U.S. Department of Health and Human Services
National Institute of Neurological Disorders and Stroke
Division of Convulsive, Infectious, and Immune Disorders
Epilepsy Branch
NSC/2113
Bethesda, MD 20892
Phone: (301)496-1917 **Fax:** (301)496-2424
Website: http://www.ninds.nih.gov
Margaret Jacobs, Dir.

Activities/Fields: Epilepsy research. Goals are to promote research into the basic mechanisms, etiologies, prevention, diagnosis, and treatment of epilepsies. Branch implements its program through grant- and contract-supported research programs, with emphasis on: basic research (primarily grant-supported), identification of gap areas, and support of state-of-the-art monographs and international symposia; development of anticonvulsant drugs in conjunction with the Epilipsy Therapeutics Research Program (ETRP) conducted by the National Institute of Neurological Disorders and Stroke; and the development of clinical research centers in epilepsy. The ETRP Program comprises preclinical studies and clinical evaluations. Branch also supports comprehensive epilepsy programs for clinical and laboratory research in the diagnosis, treatment, prognosis, and prevention of epilepsy. These programs facilitate applied research and coordinate research and teaching with health care services. **Pub:** *Annual Report.*

★ 25164 ★ U.S. Department of Health and Human Services
National Institute of Neurological Disorders and Stroke
Division of Demyelinating, Atrophic, and Dementing Disorders
Federal Bldg., Rm. 810
7550 Wisconsin Ave.
Bethesda, MD 20892
Phone: (301)496-5679 **Fax:** (301)480-1080
Dr. Michael D. Walker, MD, Dir.

Activities/Fields: Understanding, diagnosis, treatment, and prevention of a broad scope of neurological disorders of adults and the aged. These diseases include Alzheimer's disease and other dementias, Parkinson's disease, Huntington's disease, and amyotrophic lateral sclerosis, as well as demyelinating disorders such as multiple sclerosis. In addition, research is funded on infectious diseases, including "slow" virus diseases, encephalitis, meningitis, and neurological aspects of AIDS. Biological research emphasizing neuroendocrinology and the neurological basis of pain is also supported. Research activities include studies of the physiology, biochemistry, pharmacology, anatomy, pathology, genetics, and epidemiology of these diseases and related conditions in humans and animal models.

★ 25165 ★ U.S. Department of Health and Human Services
National Institute of Neurological Disorders and Stroke
Division of Extramural Activities
6002 Executive Blvd., Rm. 3309
Bethesda, MD 20892
Phone: (301)402-9248 **Fax:** (301)402-4370
Email: atwellc@ninds.nih.gov
Website: http://www.ninds.nih.gov/about_ninds/organization.htmextramural
Contance W. Atwell, PhD, Dir.

Activities/Fields: Provides administrative support and coordination for the Institute's research grant, research training, and research contract activities. Division directs and carries out scientific and technical merit review of proposals for research contracts, program projects, clinical research centers, special research grants such as multi-institutional clinical trials, and career development and research training. Management services for research grant and contract activities are also provided. Division also coordinates training and career development of young investigators and research opportunities for minority scientists and minority institutions. Opportunities include institutional and individual training awards as well as support through new investigator research awards, research career development awards, and clinical investigator development awards. **Frmly:** (2000) Division of Extramural Activities.

★ 25166 ★ U.S. Department of Health and Human Services
National Institute of Neurological Disorders and Stroke (NINDS)
Division of Intramural Research (DIR)
Bldg. 36, Rm.5A-05
36 Convent Dr.
MSC 4150
Bethesda, MD 20892-4150
Phone: (301)435-2232 **Fax:** (301)480-5634
Email: landiss@ninds.nih.gov
Dr. Story Landis, PhD, Dir., Facilities Strategic Mgmt.

Activities/Fields: Neurological sciences and relevant disciplines, including drug therapies for debilitating neurological diseases such as Parkinsonism, new techniques to help scientists better understand how the brain and nervous system function, and major research advances in neurovirology, neurochemistry, and other fields. Current interests include central nervous system disorders, such as Creutzfeldt-Jakob disease, that appear to be slow infections caused by transmissible virus-like agents; Inherited disorders of lipid metabolism, such as Gaucher's disease, Niemann-Pick disease, Fabry's disease, Krabbe's disease, and Tay-Sachs disease. Studies with the PET scanner, which have shown a relationship between glucose uptake and brain tumor growth, allow scientists to obtain axial transverse or coronal images of the brain. Intramural research is organized in two program areas: Basic Neurosciences and Clinical Neurosciences. **Pub:** *Conference Proceedings.* • *Research Reports.*

★ 25167 ★ U.S. Department of Health and Human Services
National Institute of Neurological Disorders and Stroke
Division of Intramural Research (Basic Neurosciences Program)
Bldg. 36, Rm. 4-D04
9000 Rockville Pike
Bethesda, MD 20892
Phone: (301)496-6719 **Fax:** (301)402-1339
Email: gainerh@ninds.nih.gov
Website: http://intra.ninds.nih.gov
Dr. Harold Gainer, PhD, Lab. Chf.

Activities/Fields: Cell biology of neuropeptide and catecholamine cell-specific gene expression, biosynthesis and secretion.

★ 25168 ★ U.S. Department of Health and Human Services
National Institute of Neurological Disorders and Stroke
Division of Intramural Research (Basic Neurosciences Program)
Laboratory of Central Nervous System Studies
NIH Bldg. 36, Rm. 4A-05
36 Convent Dr., MSC4122
Bethesda, MD 20892
Phone: (301)496-4821 **Fax:** (301)496-9946
Dr. Clarence J. Gibbs, Jr., Chf.

Activities/Fields: Medical surveillance of disease patterns in many primitive and isolated populations; slow, latent, and temperate virus infections, particularly chronic degenerative neurologic diseases and their pathogenesis and mechanisms of virus persistence. Also studies configuration and change resulting in conversion of normal host precursors to infectious proteins in the transmissible amyloidoses of the brain. In addition, aging of the brain, Alzheimer's, Pick's, Parkinson's, and Huntington's diseases, multiple sclerosis, amyotrophic lateral sclerosis, chronic epilepsies, and other diseases are studied in microbiological, immunologic, genetic, and biochemical laboratories and clinics and in foci of high incidence throughout the world. Worldwide study of hemorrhagic fever with renal syndrome is conducted with isolation and molecular and virulence characterization of the hantavirus serotypes. HIV and HTLV I and II genetic variation, and involvement of the nervous system are studied worldwide.

★ 25169 ★ U.S. Department of Health and Human Services
National Institute of Neurological Disorders and Stroke
Division of Intramural Research (Basic Neurosciences Program)
Laboratory of Developmental Neurogenetics
NIH Bldg. 36, Rm. 5D06
36 Convent Dr.
Bethesda, MD 20892
Phone: (301)496-9106 **Fax:** (301)496-0899
Email: hudsonl@ninds.nih.gov
Dr. Lynn Hudson, Actg. Chf.

Activities/Fields: Molecular events that occur in the replication and expression of genetic materials in mammalian cells and their viruses. Genetic, biochemical, and recombinant DNA techniques are used to study gene replication and transcription. Post-transcriptional modification and translation of ribonucleic acids are also examined. The biological systems studied include: measles virus and vesicular stomatitis virus, two members of the negative strand RNA virus family, and glial cells of the central and peripheral nervous system, especially glial cell differentiation and development, with emphasis on the genes involved in myelin synthesis and maintenance. **Frmly:** Molecular Genetics Laboratory.

★ 25170 ★ U.S. Department of Health and Human Services
National Institute of Neurological Disorders and Stroke
Division of Intramural Research (Basic Neurosciences Program)
Laboratory of Molecular and Cellular Neurobiology
9000 Rockville Pike, Bldg. 49, Rm. 2A10
Bethesda, MD 20892
Phone: (301)496-6647 **Fax:** (301)496-8244
Email: quarlesr@ninds.nih.gov
Dr. Richard Quarles, Chf.

Activities/Fields: Molecular and cellular neurobiology, myelination, and cell surface receptors.

★ 25171 ★ U.S. Department of Health and Human Services
National Institute of Neurological Disorders and Stroke
Division of Intramural Research (Basic Neurosciences Program)
Laboratory of Neural Control
Bldg. 49, Rm. 3A50
49 Convent Drive, MSC 4455
Bethesda, MD 20892-4455
Phone: (301)496-4305 **Fax:** (301)402-4836
Email: reburke@helix.nih.gov
Website: http://intra.ninds.nih.gov/
Dr. Robert E. Burke, Chf.
Activities/Fields: Properties of mammalian nerve cells and the organization of neural circuits in the mammalian central nervous system, with particular reference to studies of the control of movement. Current experimental studies involve five main areas: the neurobiology of spinal cord motorneurons and motor units; the organization of interneuron circuits in the spinal cord; the development of motor systems in the embryonic avian and neonatal rodent spinal cord; and the generation of respiratory rhythms. Such studies utilize established as well as newly developed techniques for electrophysiologic recording from single neurons, but other methods, such as those of neuroanatomy and computer simulations, are also used as appropriate. The laboratory has facilities for the development of specialized experimental equipment and for computer-oriented data analysis and model building. **Pub:** *Conference Proceedings.* • *Monographs.*

★ 25172 ★ U.S. Department of Health and Human Services
National Institute of Neurological Disorders and Stroke
Division of Intramural Research (Basic Neurosciences Program)
Laboratory of Neurobiology
NIH Bldg. 36, Rm. 2A21
36 Convent Dr., MSC 4157
Bethesda, MD 20892
Phone: (301)496-1296 **Fax:** (301)480-1485
Email: reeset@ninds.nih.gov
Website: http://www.ninds.nih.gov/about_ninds/organization.htmintramural
Dr. Thomas S. Reese, Chf.
Activities/Fields: Structural research on the organization of the nervous system. Specific areas of interest are: synaptic transmission, neural membranes, the intracellular sequestration of ions, the blood-brain barrier, and axonal transport. Structural tools used include electron microscopy, X-ray spectroscopy, immunocytochemistry, cryotechniques, and computer processed imaging of light microscopy and electron microscopic images.

★ 25173 ★ U.S. Department of Health and Human Services
National Institute of Neurological Disorders and Stroke
Division of Intramural Research (Basic Neurosciences Program)
Laboratory of Neurochemistry
NIH Bldg. 36, Rm. 4D04
9000 Rockville Pike
Bethesda, MD 20892-4130
Phone: (301)496-1671 **Fax:** (301)496-1339
Email: gainerh@ninds.nih.gov
Dr. Harold Gainer, Chf.
Activities/Fields: Molecular events that underlie both the normal functioning of the developing and mature nervous system and the derangements that occur in neurological disease. Areas of study include: mechanisms of active ion transport, protein phosphorylaton, neuronal development and regeneration, gene expression of neuropeptides and their receptors, and neuronal cytoskeletal proteins.

★ 25174 ★ U.S. Department of Health and Human Services
National Institute of Neurological Disorders and Stroke
Division of Intramural Research (Basic Neurosciences Program)
Laboratory of Neurophysiology
NIH Bldg. 36, Rm. 4A21
9000 Rockville Pike
Bethesda, MD 20892
Phone: (301)496-2414 **Fax:** (301)402-1565
Email: barkerj@ninds.nih.gov
Website: http://intra.ninds.nih.gov/Lab.asp?Org_ID=91
Jeffery L. Barker, MD, Chf.
Activities/Fields: Physiological correlates and determinants of mammalian central nervous development, especially in the cortical, hippocampal and spinal cord regions. Methods are multidisciplinary, and include flow cytometry, imaging with physiological indicator dyes, electrophysiology, and immunocytochemistry. Flow cytometry in conjunction with surface phenotyping and indicator dyes has been used to provide a comprehensive account of physiologically relevant properties emerging during neuronal and glial lineage progressions. The absence of epitopes indicative of commitment or apoptosis has been used to sort uncommitted neutral stem cells, which can be expanded in vitro and induced to differentiate into neuronal or glial phenotypes. Similar physiological properties emerge among the progeny of these cells with the self-renewing and multi-potential characteristics of neural stem cells as arise in vivo. This novel strategy directly accesses physiological correlates and determinants of cell lineage progression. Two neurotransmitters (acetylcholine and GABA) play key roles during expansion and tissue histogenesis and form the primary focus of ongoing studies. **Pub:** *Annual Report.*

★ 25175 ★ U.S. Department of Health and Human Services
National Institute of Neurological Disorders and Stroke
Division of Intramural Research (Basic Neurosciences Program)
Neuroepidemiology Branch
NIH Campus
10 Center Dr.
Bldg. 10 Room 5-S-220
Bethesda, MD 20892-1447
Phone: (301)496-1714 **Fax:** (301)496-2358
Cecilia Blutstein, Off. Mgr.
Activities/Fields: Neuroepidemiology, the epidemiologic investigation of neurologic disorders, which requires a thorough knowledge of both clinical neurology and epidemiologic methods. The program focuses on research, education, and consultation in neuroepidemiology.

★ 25176 ★ U.S. Department of Health and Human Services
National Institute of Neurological Disorders and Stroke
Division of Intramural Research (Clinical Neurosciences Program)
NIH Bldg. 10, Rm. 5N234
10 Center Dr., MSC 1428
Bethesda, MD 20892-1428
Phone: (301)496-1561 **Fax:** (301)402-1007
Email: mcfarlandh@ninds.nih.gov
Website: http://neuroscience.nih.gov/study_areas.asp
Henry McFarland, MD, Dir.
Activities/Fields: Problems important in Clinical Neurology and Neurosurgery. The Office of the Clinical Director provides clinical neurological services to investigators within the Institute and other NIH institutes. Activities include clinical neurophysiological laboratory investigations, neurology consultations, and neuropathology. Principal branches include Biostatics, Developmental and Metabolic Neurology, Developmental and Metabolic Neurology, Epilepsy Research, Experimental Therapeutics, Medical Neurology, Neuroepidemiology, Neurogenetics, Neuroimmunology, Stroke, and Surgical Neurology, Clinical Neurocardiology, Cognitive Assistant Neurosciences, Neuromuscular Diseases.

★ 25177 ★ U.S. Department of Health and Human Services
National Institute of Neurological Disorders and Stroke
Division of Intramural Research (Clinical Neurosciences Program)
Clinical Neurosciences Branch
NIH Bldg. 10, Rm. 6N252
10 Center Dr., MSC 1620
Bethesda, MD 20892
Phone: (301)496-2103 **Fax:** (301)402-0180
Email: goldsteind@ninds.nih.gov
Dr. David S. Goldstein, Chf.
Activities/Fields: Neurosciences.

★ 25178 ★ U.S. Department of Health and Human Services
National Institute of Neurological Disorders and Stroke
Division of Intramural Research (Clinical Neurosciences Program)
Developmental and Metabolic Neurology Branch
NIH Bldg. 10, Rm. 3D04
10 Center Dr. MSC 1260
Bethesda, MD 20892-1260
Phone: (301)496-3285 **Fax:** (301)496-9480
Email: bradyr@ninds.nih.gov
Website: http://www.ninds.nih.gov/about_ninds/organization.htmintramurl
Dr. Roscoe O. Brady, Chf.
Activities/Fields: Genetic disorders of metabolism, demyelinating disorders, biochemistry of cell membranes, and signal transduction mechanisms in normal and neoplastic tissues. Principal areas of interest are biochemistry, genetics, neurochemistry, neuroimmunology, molecular genetics, and adult and pediatric neurology.

★ 25179 ★ U.S. Department of Health and Human Services
National Institute of Neurological Disorders and Stroke
Division of Intramural Research (Clinical Neurosciences Program)
Experimental Therapeutics Branch
NIH Bldg. 10, Rm. 5C103
10 Center Dr., MSC 1406
Bethesda, MD 20892-1406
Phone: (301)496-7993 **Fax:** (301)496-6609
Email: zawalich@ninds.nih.gov
Dr. Thomas N. Chase, Chf.
Activities/Fields: Improved pharmacotherapies for neurologic disease. The Branch operates a vertically integrated program of research, extending from basic molecular biology to clinical trials, focusing on neurodegenerative diseases such as Alzheimer's disease and Parkinson's disease. Current operating components are the Molecular Pharmacology Section which characterizes central transmitter receptors and information transduction processes; the Genetic Pharmacology Unit investigates pharmaceutical approaches to the selective regulation of gene expression; the Neurophysiology Pharmacology Section studies basal ganglia function in relation to transmitter system interactions; and Clinical Pharmacology Section works clinically and in animal models to elucidate pathophysiologic mechanisms and evaluate novel pharmacologic interventions. **Pub:** *Proceedings.* • *Research Reports.*

★ 25180 ★ U.S. Department of Health and Human Services
National Institute of Neurological Disorders and Stroke
Division of Intramural Research (Clinical Neurosciences Program)
Laboratory of Molecular Medicine and Neuroscience
NIH Bldg. 36, Rm. 5W21
36 Convent Dr.
Bethesda, MD 20892-4164
Phone: (301)496-1635 **Fax:** (301)594-5799
Email: majorg@ninds.nih.gov
Dr. Eugene Major, Chf.

Activities/Fields: Neurologic diseases at the clinical, biological, and molecular levels. Experimental emphasis is on the pathogenesis of diseases involving cellular dysfunctions caused by neurotropic viruses, toxic cytokines, or possible genetic alterations.

★ 25181 ★ U.S. Department of Health and Human Services
National Institute of Neurological Disorders and Stroke
Division of Intramural Research (Clinical Neurosciences Program)
Medical Neurology Branch
NIH Bldg. 10, Rm. 5N226
10 Center Dr., MSC 1428
Bethesda, MD 20892-1428
Phone: (301)496-9526 **Fax:** (301)480-2286
Email: hallettm@ninds.nih.gov
Website: http://www.ninds.nih.gov/Lab.asp?Org_ID=72
Mark Hallett, MD, Chf.

Activities/Fields: Basic and clinical aspects of a variety of neurologic disorders, including: pathophysiological mechanisms and treatment of movement disorders; pathophysiology of speech and language disorders; brain plasticity and rehabilitation.

★ 25182 ★ U.S. Department of Health and Human Services
National Institute of Neurological Disorders and Stroke
Division of Intramural Research (Clinical Neurosciences Program)
Neuroimmunology Branch
NIH Bldg. 10, Rm. 5B-16
10 Center Dr., MSC 1400
Bethesda, MD 20892-1400
Phone: (301)496-1801 **Fax:** (301)402-0373
Dr. Henry F. McFarland, Chf.

Activities/Fields: Activities of the Neuroimmunology Branch include basic and clinical investigations related to multiple sclerosis (MS) and other possible immunological-based diseases. Studies focus on examining basic or fundamental immunological questions, including a study of experimental animal models and the cellular immune response to potential antigens in the nervous system. Research studies also examine the role of human retroviruses, including HTLV-I and HTLV-II in diseases of the nervous system. Clinical studies focus on examining the natural history of MS using magnetic resonance imaging and assessing new innovative therapies in MS.

★ 25183 ★ U.S. Department of Health and Human Services
National Institute of Neurological Disorders and Stroke
Division of Intramural Research (Clinical Neurosciences Program)
Surgical Neurology Branch
NIH Bldg. 10, Rm. 5D37
10 Center Dr., MSC 1414
Bethesda, MD 20892-1414
Phone: (301)496-5728 **Fax:** (301)402-0380
Email: oldfield@box-o.nih.gov
Dr. Edward H. Oldfield, Chf.

Activities/Fields: Current areas of research, most of which integrate basic science, applied laboratory science, animal experimentation, and human studies include new therapeutic approaches (genetically-engineered immunotoxins, genetically-engineered viral vectors, new drug delivery techniques) for brain tumors and pituitary tumors, mechanisms of brain edema associated with brain tumors, mechanisms of tumor-associated angiogenesis, mechanisms of the beneficial recovery after cerebral implants or neurotrophic factors for Parkinson's disease, studies of certain types of cerebrovascular disease (vasospasm, regulation of cerebral blood flow, spinal arteriovenous malformations), von Hippel-Lindau syndrome, and functional neurosurgery (seizure surgery, development of implanted prosthesis for blindness).

★ 25184 ★ U.S. Department of Health and Human Services
National Institute of Neurological Disorders and Stroke
Division of Stroke, Trauma, and Neurodegenerative Disorders
7550 Wisconsin Ave.
Federal Bldg., 810
Bethesda, MD 20892
Phone: (301)496-2581 **Fax:** (301)480-1080
Dr. Michael Walker, Dir.

Activities/Fields: Stroke and central nervous system trauma, including support for basic, applied, and clinical research. This includes support for multidisciplinary cerebrovascular clinical research centers, a comprehensive stroke center program, spinal cord injury centers, a comprehensive CNS trauma center program, and head injury centers, as well as larger numbers of individual, investigator-initiated research grants. Program supports training of young investigators through formal institutional and individual training awards; support is also provided through new investigator research awards, research career development awards, and clinical teacher investigator development awards. In addition, Division administers grants to exploit the research opportunities presented by positron emission tomography (PET). Principal areas of research interest are: cerebrovascular disease (including stroke and its consequences); trauma to the brain, spinal cord, and peripheral nervous system; central nervous system regeneration; primary and metastatic tumors of the brain and/or spinal cord; headache; chronic pain; positron emission tomography; and manipulative therapy.

★ 25185 ★ U.S. Department of Health and Human Services
National Institute of Neurological Disorders and Stroke
Division of Stroke, Trauma, and Neurodegenerative Disorders
Neural Prosthesis Program
7550 Wisconsin Ave., Rm. 916
Bethesda, MD 20892
Phone: (301)496-5746 **Fax:** (301)402-1501
Email: fh2@cu.nih.gov
Dr. Frederick Terry Hambrecht, Hd.

Activities/Fields: Development of aids for the neurologically disabled based on direct interfaces with neural tissue. Principal areas of research interest are cochlear implants and cochlear nucleus implants for the deaf; visual prostheses for the blind; and motor prostheses for the paralyzed. Research is carried out under contract and through grants at universities and commercial research laboratories. **Pub:** *Proceedings.* • *Progress reports from contractors,* quarterly. • *Research Reports.*

★ 25186 ★ U.S. Department of Health and Human Services
National Institute of Neurological Disorders and Stroke
Small Business Innovation Research Program
Federal Bldg. 1016
Bethesda, MD 20892
Phone: (301)496-4188 **Fax:** (301)402-4370
Website: http://www.ninds.nih.gov
Sonny Kreitman, Dir.

Activities/Fields: Comprises awards for three phases of research: the objective of Phase I is to establish the technical merit and feasibility of proposed research efforts that may ultimately lead to commercial products or services; the objective of Phase II is to continue the research and development efforts initiated in Phase I that are likely to result in commercial products or services; and the objective of Phase III, where appropriate, is for the small business to pursue, with non-federal funds, the commercialization of the results of the research and development funded in Phases I and II. Recent areas of interest include: development of novel antiepileptic drugs; devices for automated seizure detection; research and development of magnetoencephalography (MEG); development of applications for evoked potentials; development of a portable EEG device; and development of instrumentation for monitoring autonomic nervous system (ANS) function.

★ 25187 ★ U.S. Department of Health and Human Services
National Institute of Nursing Research
NIH Bldg. 31, Rm. 5B-10
31 Center Dr.
Bethesda, MD 20892-2178
Phone: (301)496-0207 **Fax:** (301)480-8845
Email: info@ninr.nih.gov
Website: http://www.nih.gov/ninr
Dr. Patricia A. Grady, Dir.

Activities/Fields: Basic and clinical nursing research, training, and other programs in patient care research and information dissemination. The research programs of the Institute address actual and potential health problems. These programs focus on health promotion and disease prevention, understanding and mitigating the effects of acute and chronic illnesses and disabilities, and the delivery of nursing services. Nursing research examines the biological, biomedical, and behavioral processes in health care and its environment. Its purpose is to accomplish both short- and long-term improvements in nursing practice, patient health, and recovery from illness.

★ 25188 ★ U.S. Department of Health and Human Services
National Institute of Nursing Research
Division of Extramural Activities
Bldg. 31, Rm. 5B05
Bethesda, MD 20892-6300
Phone: (301)594-5963 **Fax:** (301)594-3405
Email: mleveck@exchange.nih.gov
Website: http://www.nih.gov/ninr/research/dea.html
Dr. Mary D. Leveck, Dep. Dir.

Activities/Fields: Human responses to illness and disability throughout the life span. Focus is on the biological, behavioral, and psychosocial factors that contribute to these conditions and on methods to improve responses or alleviate the effects of the illness or disease. Research topics of acute illness range from sleep-wake patterns of pre-term infants in the neonatal intensive care unit to the biobehavioral factors affecting recovery following a myocardial infarction. Research involving nursing care of patients with chronic illness addresses symptom management for conditions such as arthritis, diabetes, AIDS, and cancer. Additional research includes the assessment and management of pain, stress, cognitive impairment and urinary incontinence.

★ 25189 ★ U.S. Department of Health and Human Services
National Institute of Nursing Research
Intramural Research Division
Clinical Therapeutics Laboratory
Bldg. 10, Rm. 10C 103 (MSC1851)
9000 Rockville Pike
Bethesda, MD 20892-1851
Phone: (301)402-1833 **Fax:** (301)496-7184
Christine Grady, Chf.
Activities/Fields: Symptom management with emphasis on two primary groups: HIV-infected adults and the elderly.

★ 25190 ★ U.S. Department of Health and Human Services
National Institute of Nursing Research
Intramural Research Division
Laboratory for the Study of Human Responses to Health and Illness
Bldg. 9 Room 1-W-125
9 Central Drive
Bethesda, MD 20892-0967
Phone: (301)594-3752 **Fax:** (301)480-0726
Email: annette_wysocki@nih.gov
Dr. Annette B. Wysocki, PhD, Dir.
Activities/Fields: Research in wound healing.

★ 25191 ★ U.S. Department of Health and Human Services
National Institute for Occupational Safety and Health
Hubert H. Humphrey Bldg., Rm. 715 H
Centers for Disease Control & Prevention
200 Independence Ave. SW
Washington, DC 20201
Phone: (202)401-6997 **Free:** 800-356-4674
Fax: (202)260-4464
Email: pubstaff@cdc.gov
Website: http://www.cdc.gov/niosh/homepage.html
Linda Rosenstock, MDM, Dir.
Activities/Fields: Research to eliminate on-the-job hazards to health and safety. Institute is responsible for identifying occupational safety and health hazards, for determining methods to control them, and for recommending federal standards to limit the hazards. Institute is also responsible for administering the x-ray surveillance program for coal miners and for testing and certifying respirators and hazard measuring devices. In addition to research done in laboratories, NIOSH conducts health hazard evaluations in all types of workplaces (including mines), assists other agencies to investigate potentially hazardous situations, and supports research and training programs through extramural grants. To focus research efforts and resources, the Institute has identified ten leading work-related diseases and injuries and has developed a proposed prevention strategy for each. The Institute, in partnership with its stakholders, developed a national Occupational Research Agenda (NORA) with 21 research areas. The Institute is working with other groups, both local and national, to establish a comprehensive national surveillance system for occupational disease and injuries. NIOSH recommendations are transmitted to the Department of Labor, which is responsible for setting and enforcing occupational standards. NIOSH laboratory research is conducted at the Robert A. Taft Laboratory and the Alice Hamilton Laboratory for Occupational Safety and Health in Cincinnati, OH, and at the Appalachian Laboratory for Occupational Safety and Health in Morgantown, WV, the Pittsburgh Research Laboratory in Burceto, PA and the Spokane research Laboratory in Spokane, WA. Data Base NIOSH maintains the Registry of +Toxic Effects of +Chemical Substances (RTECS) and the NIOSHTIC database with 144,000 entries; both are available in a variety of formats. **Pub:** *Proceedings.* • *Research Reports.* • *Technical and research reports*, periodically.

★ 25192 ★ U.S. Department of Health and Human Services
National Institute for Occupational Safety and Health
Appalachian Laboratory for Occupational Safety and Health
1095 Willowdale Rd.
Morgantown, WV 26505-2888
Phone: (304)285-5704 **Fax:** (304)285-5717
Denzil Sloughter, Management Oper. Off.
Activities/Fields: Occupational safety and health, focusing on safe working environments, occupational-related respiratory diseases, cross-sectional prospective morbidity and mortality studies, and performance records of respirators and hazard measuring instruments. Maintains a national surveillance data system for the early detection and monitoring of occupational accidents and injuries, and NIOSHTIC database and microfiche collection.

★ 25193 ★ U.S. Department of Health and Human Services
National Institute for Occupational Safety and Health
Biomedical and Behavioral Science Division
Applied Biology Branch
Robert A. Taft Laboratories
4676 Columbia Pkwy.
Cincinnati, OH 45226-1998
Phone: (513)533-8433 **Fax:** (513)533-8494
Gayle DeBord, PhD, Chf.
Activities/Fields: Biological monitoring and immunochemistry/immunotoxicology studies, inhalation toxicology, animal husbandry, and pathology.

★ 25194 ★ U.S. Department of Health and Human Services
National Institute for Occupational Safety and Health
Biomedical and Behavioral Science Division
Applied Psychology and Ergonomics Branch
Robert A. Taft Laboratories
4676 Columbia Pkwy. M.S C-24
Cincinnati, OH 45226-1998
Phone: (513)533-8291 **Fax:** (513)533-8596
Email: sls4@cdc.gov
Steve Sauter, Chf.
Activities/Fields: Occupational stress and ergonomics.

★ 25195 ★ U.S. Department of Health and Human Services
National Institute for Occupational Safety and Health
Biomedical and Behavioral Science Division
Physical Agents Effects Branch
Robert A. Taft Laboratories, MS C-27
4676 Columbia Pkwy.
Cincinnati, OH 45226-1998
Phone: (513)533-8153 **Fax:** (513)533-8139
Email: wlotz@cdc.gov
Website: http://www.cdc.gov/niosh/homepage.html
W. Gregory Lotz, PhD, Sect. Chf.
Activities/Fields: Health effects of non-ionizing radiation and noise in the workplace.

★ 25196 ★ U.S. Department of Health and Human Services
National Institute for Occupational Safety and Health
Education and Information Division
Information Resources Branch
Robert A. Taft Laboratories
4676 Columbia Pkwy.
Cincinnati, OH 45226-1998
Phone: (513)533-8319 **Free:** 800-356-4674
Fax: (513)533-8347
Email: vep1@cdc.gov
Website: http://www.cdc.gov/niosh/im-eid.html
Vern Anderson, Chf.
Activities/Fields: Provides technical information support for NIOSH research programs. Its activities include collecting, organizing, and retrieving published and unpublished technical literature related to the field of occupational safety and health. **Pub:** *Audiovisual Catalog*, periodically. • *New Publication List*, periodically.

★ 25197 ★ U.S. Department of Health and Human Services
National Institute for Occupational Safety and Health
Physical Sciences and Engineering Division
Engineering Control Technology Branch
Robert A. Taft Laboratories
Mail Stop R-5
4676 Columbia Pkwy.
Cincinnati, OH 45226-1998
Phone: (513)841-4221 **Fax:** (513)841-4506
Larry Reed, Actg. Chf.
Activities/Fields: Planning and conducting worksite and laboratory research to identify and evaluate engineering control technology that will prevent worker exposure to toxic substances and harmful physical agents; promoting the transfer and widespread application of effective preventive engineering control measures for safeguarding worker health; providing engineering expertise in formulating effective and credible workplace standards; and providing technical consultation to other elements of the National Institute for Occupational Safety and Health and the Department of Labor in the application of new and improved techniques for hazard prevention and engineering controls. Branch comprises sections for chemical industry, minerals, materials processing, and general industry.

★ 25198 ★ U.S. Department of Health and Human Services
National Institute for Occupational Safety and Health
Physical Sciences and Engineering Division
Measurements Research Support Branch
Robert A. Taft Laboratories
4676 Columbia Pkwy.
Cincinnati, OH 45226-1998
Phone: (513)841-4241 **Fax:** (513)841-4500
Paul Schlect, Chf.
Activities/Fields: Sampling and analytical chemistry measurements for industrial hygiene field investigations and other National Institute for Occupational Safety and Health activities; and provides field industrial hygiene measurement support, including research, to develop new sampling and analysis techniques. Branch comprised of sections for measurement, development, and support. **Pub:** *Analytical Methods Studies.*

★ 25199 ★ U.S. Department of Health and Human Services
National Institute for Occupational Safety and Health
Physical Sciences and Engineering Division
Methods Research Branch
Robert A. Taft Laboratories
Mail Stop R-7
4676 Columbia Pkwy.
Cincinnati, OH 45226-1998
Phone: (513)841-4241 **Fax:** (513)841-4500
Email: erk1@cdc.gov
Website: http://www.cdc.gov/niosh/homepage.html
Dr. Eugene Kennedy, Chf.

Activities/Fields: Research that develops, improves and evaluates analytical methods for the evaluation of levels of toxic materials found in the work environment, and in industrial materials; providing expert consultation for the development of occupational health criteria and standards on methods for chemical analytical procedures; providing special consultation to the National Institute for Occupational Safety and Health and other government agencies; and providing validated NIOSH procedures for sampling and analytical methods. Branch comprises one section for special analyses for laboratory methods development. **Pub:** *NIOSH Manual of Analytical Methods*, biennially.

★ 25200 ★ U.S. Department of Health and Human Services
National Institute for Occupational Safety and Health
Physical Sciences and Engineering Division
Quality Assurance and Statistics Activity
Robert A. Taft Laboratories
4676 Columbia Pkwy. MS R-3
Cincinnati, OH 45226-1998
Phone: (513)841-4200 **Fax:** (513)841-4500
Email: pcs1@cdc.gov
Paul Schlecht, Actg. Chf.

Activities/Fields: Quality of NIOSH industrial hygiene laboratory services; conduct with the American Industrial Hygiene Association (AIHA) a proficiency testing program for industrial hygiene laboratories (the Proficiency Analytical Testing Program, covering a variety of metal and organic analyses, silica, and asbestos analyses); conduct with the U.S. Environmental Protection Agency and AIHA a proficiency testing program for environmental labs, including the Environmental Lead Proficiency Analytical Testing Program, which covers lead analyses in paint chips, soil, and dust wipes; and provide statistical support for NIOSH industrial hygiene chemistry and engineering control research. **Pub:** *NIOSH Manual of Analytical Methods.* **Frmly:** (1991) Monitoring and Control Research Branch; (2000) Physical Sciences and Engineering Division; Quality Assurance and Statistics Activity.

★ 25201 ★ U.S. Department of Health and Human Services
National Institute for Occupational Safety and Health
Surveillance, Hazard Evaluations, and Field Studies Division
Mail Stop R-12
Robert A. Taft Laboratories
4676 Columbia Pkwy.
Cincinnati, OH 45226-1998
Phone: (513)841-4428
Email: kjm3@cdc.gov
Website: http://www.cdc/gov/niosh/im-dshe.html
Kathy Masterson, Sec.

Activities/Fields: Epidemiologic field research and national surveillance in occupational health. Activities are carried out in four branches: Hazard Evaluations and Technical Assistance, Industrywide Studies, Surveillance and Health-related Energy Research. **Pub:** *Proceedings.* • *Research Reports.*

★ 25202 ★ U.S. Department of Health and Human Services
National Institute for Occupational Safety and Health
Surveillance, Hazard Evaluations, and Field Studies Division
Hazard Evaluations and Technical Assistance Branch
Robert A. Taft Laboratories
Mail Stop R-9
4676 Columbia Pkwy.
Cincinnati, OH 45226-4382
Phone: (513)841-4505 **Fax:** (513)841-4483
Email: dss2@nioshe1.em.cdc.gov
Website: http://www.cdc.gov/niosh/im-dshe.html
Mr. Dave Sundin, Dep. Dir.

Activities/Fields: General industry requests for assistance in evaluating potential health hazard situations, including requests from employers, employees, employee representatives, other federal agencies, and state and local agencies. Branch evaluates whether or not chemical, biological, or physical agents are hazardous as used or found in the workplace and makes recommendations for control procedures, improved work practices, and medical screening to reduce exposure levels and subsequent health effects. Branch comprises sections for industrial hygiene and medical studies.

★ 25203 ★ U.S. Department of Health and Human Services
National Institute for Occupational Safety and Health
Surveillance, Hazard Evaluations, and Field Studies Division
Industrywide Studies Branch
Robert A. Taft Laboratories
4676 Columbia Pkwy., Rm. 13
Cincinnati, OH 45226-1998
Phone: (513)841-4203 **Fax:** (513)841-4486
Email: dz7k@nih.gov
Teresa Schnorr, Chf.

Activities/Fields: Industrywide studies, through record studies and clinical/environmental studies, to: identify occupational causes of disease in the working population and their offspring; determine the incidence and prevalence of acute and chronic effects from work-related exposures to toxic and hazardous substances; and provide information needed to develop standards to control occupational health hazards. Branch comprises sections for industrial hygiene and epidemiology.

★ 25204 ★ U.S. Department of Health and Human Services
National Institute for Occupational Safety and Health
Surveillance, Hazard Evaluations, and Field Studies Division
Surveillance Branch
Robert A. Taft Laboratories
4676 Columbia Pkwy., ML-R19
Cincinnati, OH 45226-1998
Phone: (513)841-4208 **Fax:** (513)841-4483
Email: jps4@cdc.gov
Website: http://www.cdc.gov/niosh/im-dshe.html
John Sestito, Ch. Surveillance Branch

Activities/Fields: Surveillance system of the nation's work force and its environs and to make an early detection and continuous assessment of the magnitude and extent of job-related illnesses, exposures, and hazardous agents. Branch comprises sections for medical activity, hazards, and illness effects.

★ 25205 ★ U.S. Department of Health and Human Services
National Institutes of Health
1 Center Dr., MSC 0148
Bethesda, MD 20892-0148
Phone: (301)496-4000
Email: rk25n@nih.gov
Website: http://www.nih.gov
Dr. Ruth Kirschstein, Act. Dir.

Activities/Fields: Principal medical research arm of the federal government, with a mission to improve the health of the nation by increasing understanding of the processes underlying human health and by acquiring new knowledge to help prevent, detect, diagnose, and treat disease. NIH accomplishes this mission by: supporting research in universities, medical schools, hospitals, and research institutions in this country and abroad; conducting research in its own laboratories and clinics; supporting training for promising young researchers; helping to develop and maintain research resources; identifying research findings that can be applied to the care of patients and helping to transfer such advances to the health care system; promoting effective ways to communicate biomedical information to scientists, health practitioners, and the public; and developing and recommending policies related to the conduct and support of biomedical research. To carry out these functions, NIH is organized into 17 research Institutes (National Cancer Institute; National Eye Institute; National Heart, Lung and Blood Institute; National Institute on Aging; National Institute on Alcohol Abuse and Alcoholism; National Institute of Allergy and Infectious Diseases; National Institute of Arthritis and Musculoskeletal and Skin Diseases; National Institute of Child Health and Human Development; National Institute on Deafness and Other Communication Disorders; National Institute of Dental and Craniofacial Research; National Institute of Diabetes and Digestive and Kidney Diseases; National Institute on Drug Abuse; National Institute of Environmental Health Sciences; National Institute of General Medical Sciences; National Institute of Mental Health; National Institute of Neurological Disorders and Stroke; National Institute of Nursing Research); two divisions (Computer Research and Technology, and Research Grants); National Center for Nursing Research; the Warren Grant Magnuson Clinical Center; the John E. Fogarty International Center for Advanced Study in the Health Sciences; the National Center for Research Resources; and the National Library of Medicine.

★ 25206 ★ U.S. Department of Health and Human Services
National Institutes of Health
Baylor College of Medicine
Human Genome Sequencing Center
One Baylor Plaza
MSC-226
Houston, TX 77030
Phone: (713)798-6539 **Fax:** (713)798-5741
Email: hgsc-help@bcm.tmc.edu
Website: http://www.hgsc.bcm.tmc.edu/
Richard Gibbs, Dir.

Activities/Fields: Human Genome Project, Dictyostelium sequencing, Drosophila sequencing, Mouse sequencing, and cDNA sequencing.

★ 25207 ★ U.S. Department of Health and Human Services
National Institutes of Health
Fogarty International Center for Advanced Study in the Health Sciences
NIH Bldg. 31-B2C29
31 Center Dr., MSC 2220
Bethesda, MD 20892-2220
Phone: (301)496-2075 **Fax:** (301)594-1211
Email: ficinfo@nih.gov
Website: http://www.Fic.NIH.Gov
Irene Edwards, Info. Off.

Activities/Fields: Promotes international cooperation in biomedical and behavioral research through grants, fellowships, exchange awards, and int ernational agreements. **Pub:** *Directory of International Grants and Fellowships in the Health Sciences.*

★ 25208 ★ U.S. Department of Health and Human Services
National Institutes of Health
Fogarty International Center for Advanced Study in the Health Sciences
Division of International Training and Research
Bldg. 31, Rm. B2C39
31 Center Dr., MSC 2220
Bethesda, MD 20892
Phone: (301)496-1653 **Fax:** (301)402-0779
Email: kb16r@nih.gov
Website: http://www.nih.gov/fic/programs.html
Kenneth Bridbord, Dir.

Activities/Fields: Funds extramural research in order to enhance collaborative projects between U.S. principal investigators and non-U.S. principal investigators through research grants, fellowships, and training grants. Efforts are also made to foster scientific exchange between countries in all areas of biomedical and behavioral research.

★ 25209 ★ U.S. Department of Health and Human Services
National Institutes of Health
Frederick Cancer Research and Development Center
PO Box B
Frederick, MD 21702-1201
Phone: (301)846-1108 **Fax:** (301)846-1494
Email: c.reynolds@mcifcrf.gov
Dr. Craig Reynolds, Dir.
Activities/Fields: Cancer causes, biology, diagnosis, and treatment, and AIDS studies. The basic research program (operated by the biomedical research firm Advanced BioScience Laboratories, Inc.) and the NCI intramural research programs involve studies in macromolecular structure and function; mechanisms for inducing cancer using carcinogens; activation and expression of oncogenes; mechanisms, evolution, and control of transformation; in vitro and in vivo screening for cancer and AIDS therapeutic agents; regulation of host defense mechanisms; therapeutic use of immune effector mechanisms; phase I and II clinical trials of biological and chemotherapeutic agents; identification and regulation of AIDS virus genes and proteins; and genetics of cell differentiation and development. Support services are provided by the other four FCRDC contractors (see above). In addition, FCRDC provides research opportunities for researchers, pre- and postdoctoral fellows, professors on sabbatical from universities, clinicians, individuals sponsored by outside grants or fellowships, collaborative workers, student interns, and others in the scientific community to participate in research at the Center. **Pub:** *Research Reports.*

★ 25210 ★ U.S. Department of Health and Human Services
National Institutes of Health
National Cancer Institute
PO Box B
Frederick, MD 21702-1201
Phone: (301)846-1302 **Fax:** (301)846-1494
Email: reynoldsc@ncifcrf.gov
Website: http://web.ncifcrf.gov/
Craig W. Reynolds, Dir.
Activities/Fields: Causes of cancer, AIDS, and related diseases.

★ 25211 ★ U.S. Department of Health and Human Services
National Institutes of Health
National Cancer Institute
Analytical Chemistry Laboratory
PO Box B
Frederick, MD 21702-1201
Phone: (301)846-7286 **Fax:** (301)846-6037
Email: venstra@ncifcrf.gov
Website: http://web.ncifcrf.gov/rtp/labs/ACL/ACL.asp
Dr. Timothy D. Veenstra, Lab. Hd.
Activities/Fields: Techniques and methods for separating, analyzing, characterizing, and identifying compounds ranging from small molecules to complex biological samples such as proteins and polynucleotides.

★ 25212 ★ U.S. Department of Health and Human Services
National Institutes of Health
National Cancer Institute
Division of Basic Sciences
((Laboratory of Experimental Immunology) Leukocyte Cell Biology Section)
NCI-FCRDC
Bldg. 560, Rm. 31-93
Frederick, MD 21702-1201
Phone: (301)846-1323 **Fax:** (301)846-1673
Email: ORTALDO@NCIFCRF.GOV
Website: http://www3.cancer.gov/intra/lei/lcbs1.htm
John R. Ortaldo, PhD, Actg. Sect. Hd.
Activities/Fields: Differentiation and activation of human and murine leukocytes and the role of the cellular immune system in mediation antitumor immune responses.

★ 25213 ★ U.S. Department of Health and Human Services
National Institutes of Health
National Cancer Institute
Division of Basic Sciences
((Laboratory of Experimental Immunology) Cellular and Molecular Immunology Section)
NCI at Frederick
Bldg. 560, Rm. 31-23
Frederick, MD 21702-1201
Phone: (301)846-5700 **Fax:** (301)846-1673
Email: youngh@nciferf.gov
Website: http://www3.cancer.gov/intra/lei/cm1s1.htm
Howard A. Young, PhD, Sect. Hd.
Activities/Fields: Molecular regulation of gene expression.

★ 25214 ★ U.S. Department of Health and Human Services
National Institutes of Health
National Cancer Institute
Division of Basic Sciences
(Laboratory of Genomic Diversity — LGD)
Frederick Cancer Res. and Dev. Ctr.
Bldg. 560, Rm. 11-82
Frederick, MD 21702-1201
Phone: (301)846-1296 **Fax:** (301)846-1686
Email: obrien@.ncifcrf.gov
Website: http://home.ncifcrf.gov/ccr/lgd/
Stephen J. O'Brien, PhD, Chf.
Activities/Fields: Virus-host relationships in viral-induced cancers; the interaction of viral and cellular genes; host immune mechanisms related to the control of virus-induced cancers; and molecular processes in viral carcinogenesis.

★ 25215 ★ U.S. Department of Health and Human Services
National Institutes of Health
National Cancer Institute
Division of Basic Sciences
((Laboratory of Experimental Immunology) Experimental Therapeutics Section)
NCI-FCRDC
Bldg. 560, Rm. 31-93
Frederick, MD 21702-1201
Phone: (301)846-1258 **Fax:** (301)846-1673
Email: wiltroutr@mail.ncifcrf.gov
Robert H. Wiltrout, PhD, Sect. Hd.
Activities/Fields: Models that parallel the growth and dissemination observed clinically in human tumors; treatment of primary tumors and/or metastases; immunological and cell biological mechanisms by which biological response modifiers mediate antitumor/antimetastatic effects; regulation and mobilization of committed hematopoietic progenitor and pluripotent stem cells.

★ 25216 ★ U.S. Department of Health and Human Services
National Institutes of Health
National Cancer Institute
Division of Basic Sciences
(Laboratory of Leukocyte Biology)
Frederick Cancer Res. and Dev. Ctr.
Frederick, MD 21702-1201
Phone: (301)846-1504 **Fax:** (301)846-7034
Email: ruscettif@ncifcrf.gov
Website: http://rex.nci.nih.gov/RESEARCH/basic/llb/llbpage.htm
Francis W. Ruscetti, PhD, Chf.
Activities/Fields: Regulation of the biological response of hematopoietic and stem cells to humoral factors, the signal transduction pathways which control these stem cells, the cellular and viral aspects of pathogenesis caused by infection of these cells by human retroviruses and the application of these studies to the development of new therapies for cancer and AIDS.

★ 25217 ★ U.S. Department of Health and Human Services
National Institutes of Health
National Cancer Institute (NCI)
Division of Basic Sciences
(HIV Drug Resistance Program — DRP)
NCI-Frederick, Bldg 535, Room 109
PO Box B
Frederick, MD 21702-1201
Phone: (301)846-5943 **Fax:** (301)846-6013
Email: jcoffin@ncifcrf.gov
Website: http://www.ncifcrf.gov/hivdrp/index.html
John Coffin, PhD, Prog. Dir.
Activities/Fields: Effective antiviral therapy is the only hope for survival for the nearly one million Americans and 35 million individuals worldwide infected with HIV. Recognizing that evolution of resistant virus is the principal obstacle to such therapy, the HIV Drug Resistance Program is applying basic, translational, and clinical research to problems central to understanding the mechanism and evolution of antiviral drug resistance. Current research activities include: structural and biochemical analysis of reverse transcriptase variants; mechanism of genetic variation during virus replication; virion structure and assembly; virus-host interaction; development of model systems for the study of HIV in vivo; identification of novel replication inhibitors; clinical studies on the genetic structure and dynamics of HIV populations in vivo. Conducts in vitro drug resistance selection assays, genotypic and phenotypic analyses, and a range of other techniques, such as Polymerase Chain Reaction (PCR), site mutagenesis, viral load monitoring, and viral enzyme analysis for the HIV drug resistance program.

★ 25218 ★ U.S. Department of Health and Human Services
National Institutes of Health
National Cancer Institute
Division of Basic Sciences
(Laboratory of Molecular Cell Biology — LMCB)
Bethesda, MD 20892
Phone: (301)496-3029
Email: cw1m@nih.gov
Website: http://rex.nci.nih.gov/RESEARCH/basic/lmcb/lmcbpage.htm
Carl Wu, PhD, Chf.
Activities/Fields: The laboratory investigates basic cellular processes of homeostasis, growth, division, and differentiation, with an emphasis on the molecular biology of chromosomes and the cell nucleus.

★ 25219 ★ U.S. Department of Health and Human Services
National Institutes of Health
National Cancer Institute
Division of Basic Sciences
(Laboratory of Cell Regulation and Carcinogenesis)
NIH/NCI/LCRC, Bldg. 41, Rm. C629
41 Library Dr.
MSC 5055
Bethesda, MD 20892-5055
Phone: (301)496-6108 **Fax:** (301)496-8395
Email: robertsa@dce41.nci.nih.gov
Website: http://rex.nci.nih.gov/RESEARCH/basic/lc/lcpage.htm
Anita Roberts, PhD, Chf.
Activities/Fields: The laboratory focuses on mechanisms of carcinogenesis and on the role of the peptide growth factor, transforming growth factor-beta (TGF-beta), in homeostasis and pathophysiologic processes.

★ 25220 ★ U.S. Department of Health and Human Services
National Institutes of Health
National Cancer Institute
Division of Basic Sciences
(Laboratory of Metabolism)
Bldg. 37, Rm. 3E24
Bethesda, MD 20892
Phone: (301)496-9067 **Fax:** (301)496-8419
Email: fjgonz@helix.nih.gov
Website: http://home.ccr.cancer.gov/metabolism/lmpage.htm
Frank J. Gonzalez, PhD, Lab Chf.
Activities/Fields: Research for the National Cancer Institute on metabolism.

★ 25221 ★ U.S. Department of Health and Human Services
National Institutes of Health
National Cancer Institute
Division of Basic Sciences
(Laboratory of Immune Cell Biology — LICB)
NIH Bldg. 10, Rm. 1B40
Bethesda, MD 20892-1152
Phone: (301)496-4931 **Fax:** (301)102-4844
Email: jda@box-j.nih.gov
Website: http://www3.cancer.gov/intra/licb/licbpage.htm
Jonathan D. Ashwell, MD, Chf.
Activities/Fields: Biology of the immune system at the molecular and cellular levels, including the mechanisms and consequences of apoptosis (regulated cell death) and T cell receptor engagement.

★ 25222 ★ U.S. Department of Health and Human Services
National Institutes of Health
National Cancer Institute
Division of Basic Sciences
((Experimental Immunology Branch)
Dinah Singer Laboratory)
Bldg.10, Rm. 4B36, NIH
Bethesda, MD 20892-1360
Phone: (301)496-9097 **Fax:** (301)480-8499
Email: ds13j@nih.gov
Website: http://rex.nci.nih.gov/RESEARCH/basic/eib/singerd.htm
Dinah Singer, PhD, Chf., Molecular Regulation Sect.
Activities/Fields: Research interest is the molecular mechanisms regulating MHC gene expression.

★ 25223 ★ U.S. Department of Health and Human Services
National Institutes of Health
National Cancer Institute
Division of Basic Sciences
((Experimental Immunology Branch)
Andre Nussenzweig Laboratory)
Bldg.10, Rm. 4B36, NIH
Bethesda, MD 20892-1360
Phone: (301)402-1894 **Fax:** (301)496-0887
Email: an62h@nih.gov
Website: http://rex.nci.nih.gov/RESEARCH/basic/eib/nusenzwg.htm
Andre Nussenzweig, PhD, Investigator
Activities/Fields: Research interests include the function of DNA repair during lymphocyte development and aging.

★ 25224 ★ U.S. Department of Health and Human Services
National Institutes of Health
National Cancer Institute
Division of Basic Sciences
((Experimental Immunology Branch)
Alfred Singer Laboratory)
Bldg.10, Rm. 4B17, NIH
Bethesda, MD 20892-1360
Phone: (301)496-5461 **Fax:** (301)496-0887
Email: as38y@nih.gov
Website: http://rex.nci.nih.gov/RESEARCH/basic/eib/singera.htm
Alfred Singer, MD, Chf., Experimental Immunology Br.
Activities/Fields: Research interests include T cell development, T cell receptor structure and function and intrathymic signaling.

★ 25225 ★ U.S. Department of Health and Human Services
National Institutes of Health
National Cancer Institute
Division of Basic Sciences
((Experimental Immunology Branch)
Pierre Henkart Laboratory)
Bldg.10, Rm. 4B36, NIH
Bethesda, MD 20892-1360
Phone: (301)496-1554 **Fax:** (301)496-0887
Email: ph8j@nih.gov
Website: http://rex.nci.nih.gov/RESEARCH/basic/eib/henkart.htm
Pierre A. Henkart, PhD, Investigator
Activities/Fields: Research interests include molecular mechanisms of lymphocyte-mediated cytoxicity and molecular mechanisms of T lymphocyte apoptosis.

★ 25226 ★ U.S. Department of Health and Human Services
National Institutes of Health
National Cancer Institute
Division of Basic Sciences
((Experimental Immunology Branch)
Richard Hodes Laboratory)
Bldg.10, Rm. 4B17, NIH
Bethesda, MD 20892-1360
Phone: (301)496-3129 **Fax:** (301)496-0887
Email: rh32z@nih.gov
Website: http://rex.nci.nih.gov/RESEARCH/basic/eib/hodes.htm
Richard Hodes, MD, Chf., Immune Regulation Sect.
Activities/Fields: Research interests include cellular and molecular regulation of T cell and B cell activation.

★ 25227 ★ U.S. Department of Health and Human Services
National Institutes of Health
National Cancer Institute
Division of Basic Sciences
((Experimental Immunology Branch)
Michael Kuehn Laboratory)
Bldg.10, Rm. 4B17, NIH
10 Center Drive
Bethesda, MD 20892-1360
Phone: (301)496-9341 **Fax:** (301)496-0887
Email: mk16m@nih.gov
Website: http://rex.nci.nih.gov/RESEARCH/basic/eib/kuehn.htm
Michael Kuehn, PhD, Investigator
Activities/Fields: Research interest is genetic control of vertebrate embryonic development.

★ 25228 ★ U.S. Department of Health and Human Services
National Institutes of Health
National Cancer Institute
Division of Basic Sciences
((Experimental Immunology Branch)
Gene Shearer Laboratory)
Bldg.10, Rm. 4B17, NIH
Bethesda, MD 20892-1360
Phone: (301)402-3246 **Fax:** (301)496-0887
Email: gs22y@nih.gov
Website: http://rex.nci.nih.gov/RESEARCH/basic/eib/shearer.htm
Gene Shearer, PhD, Prin. Investg. /Sect. Chf.
Activities/Fields: Research areas include immune regulation and immune responses and AIDS immunology and tumor immunology.

★ 25229 ★ U.S. Department of Health and Human Services
National Institutes of Health
National Cancer Institute
Division of Basic Sciences
((Experimental Immunology Branch)
Paul Roche Laboratory)
Bldg.10, Rm. 4B36, NIH
9000 Rockville Pke.
Bethesda, MD 20892-1360
Phone: (301)496-7177 **Fax:** (301)496-0887
Email: pr17m@nih.gov
Website: http://rex.nci.nih.gov/RESEARCH/basic/eib/roche.htm
Paul A. Roche, PhD, Prin. Investg.
Activities/Fields: Research area is protein trafficking in lymphocytes.

★ 25230 ★ U.S. Department of Health and Human Services
National Institutes of Health
National Cancer Institute
Division of Basic Sciences
((Experimental Immunology Branch)
Stephen Shaw Laboratory)
Bldg.10, Rm. 4B36, NIH
Bethesda, MD 20892-1360
Phone: (301)435-6499 **Fax:** (301)496-0887
Email: sshaw@nih.gov
Website: http://rex.nci.nih.gov/RESEARCH/basic/eib/shaw.htm
Stephen Shaw, MD, Sec. Chf.
Activities/Fields: Research areas include genetics of the human histocompatability locus (HLA) and T cell differentiation, T cell adhesion, and their regulation.

★ 25231 ★ U.S. Department of Health and Human Services
National Institutes of Health
National Cancer Institute
Division of Basic Sciences
((Experimental Epidemiology Branch)
Flow Cytometry Laboratory)
Bldg.10, Rm. 4B17, NIH
Bethesda, MD 20892-1360
Phone: (301)496-2776 **Fax:** (301)496-0887
Email: ss71k@nih.gov
Website: http://rex.nci.nih.gov/RESEARCH/basic/eib/sharrow.htm
Susan Sharrow, Sr. Investg. & Fac. Mgr.
Activities/Fields: Research area is Flow Cytometry in Immunology.

★ 25232 ★ U.S. Department of Health and Human Services
National Institutes of Health
National Cancer Institute
Division of Basic Sciences
((Experimental Immunology Branch)
David Segal Laboratory)
Bldg.10, Rm. 4B36, NIH
9000 Rockville Pke.
Bethesda, MD 20892-1360
Phone: (301)496-4746 **Fax:** (301)496-0887
Email: dave_segal@nih.gov
Website: http://rex.nci.nih.gov/RESEARCH/basic/eib/segal.htm
David M. Segal, PhD, Prin. Investg. /Sect. Chf.
Activities/Fields: Research area is innate immunity.

★ 25233 ★ U.S. Department of Health and Human Services
National Institutes of Health
National Cancer Institute (NCI)
Division of Basic Sciences
((Laboratory of Biosystems and Cancer)
Structure and Function of Mammalian Centromere Section)
Bldg. 49, Rm. 4A56
Bethesda, MD 20892
Phone: (301)496-0541 **Fax:** (301)480-2772
Email: vl19x@nih.gov
Vladimir Larionov, PhD, Actg. Hd.
Activities/Fields: Centrometic regions of human chromosomes; determines minimal structural requirements for functional centromere and to generate portable human artificial chromosome (HAC) for gene delivery; isolation and characterization of human disease genes.

★ 25234 ★ U.S. Department of Health and Human Services
National Institutes of Health
National Cancer Institute
Division of Basic Sciences
(Laboratory of Biosystems and Cancer)
Bldg. 40, Rm. 2609
37 Convent Dr., MSC-4264
Bethesda, MD 20892
Phone: (301)594-8516
Email: barrett@mail.nih.gov
Website: http://rex.nci.nih.gov/RESEARCH/basic/LBCBarrettsLab.html
J. Carl Barrett, PhD, Ch.
Activities/Fields: Molecular and environmental causes of cancer; identification of new cancer genes; understanding mechanisms of action of specific genes in cell signaling cell proliferation, and cell death.

★ 25235 ★ U.S. Department of Health and Human Services
National Institutes of Health
National Cancer Institute (NCI)
Division of Basic Sciences
((Laboratory of Biosystems and Cancer)
Cancer and Aging Section)
Bldg. 40, Rm. 2609
Bethesda, MD 20892
Phone: (301)594-8516
Email: barrett@mail.nih.gov
Website: http://rex.nci.nih.gov/RESEARCH/basic/LBCCASBarrett.html
J. Carl Barrett, PhD, Ch.
Activities/Fields: Environmental causes of cancer as well as endogenous causes of cancer, including spontaneous mutations, aging, and hormones.

★ 25236 ★ U.S. Department of Health and Human Services
National Institutes of Health
National Cancer Institute
Division of Cancer Control and Population Sciences (DCCPS)
((Behavioral Research Program)
Tobacco Control Research Branch — TCRB)
Executive Pl. N, Rm. 4039B
6130 Executive Blvd.
Bethesda, MD 20892
Phone: (301)435-8638
Email: cb270r@nih.gov
Cathy Backinger, Br. Chf.
Activities/Fields: Tobacco use, with the aim of reversing the epidemic of tobacco-related cancers.

★ 25237 ★ U.S. Department of Health and Human Services
National Institutes of Health
National Cancer Institute
Division of Cancer Control and Population Sciences (DCCPS)
((Behavioral Research Program)
Helath Promotion Research Branch — HPRB)
6130 Executive Blvd., EPN 4080
Bethesda, MD 20892-7335
Phone: (301)451-9530 **Fax:** (301)480-2087
Website: http://www.healthpromotionresearch.cancer.gov
Linda Nebeling, Br. Chf.
Activities/Fields: Community-based behavioral intervention research to prevent cancer, including the areas of diet, physical activity, energy balance, sun and virus exposure.

★ 25238 ★ U.S. Department of Health and Human Services
National Institutes of Health
National Cancer Institute
Division of Cancer Control and Population Sciences (DCCPS)
((Behavioral Research Program)
Basic Biobehavioral Research Branch — BBRB)
6130 Executive Blvd./EPN 4074C
Bethesda, MD 20892
Phone: (301)496-8776 **Fax:** (301)435-7547
Email: ms496r@nih.gov
Website: http://dccps.nci.nih.gov/BBRB/default.html
Michael Stefanek, Br. Chf.
Activities/Fields: Preintervention research, including genetic testing for cancer, psychophysiological and genetic processes, genetic determinants of individual differences in the reinforcing effects of smoking, eating and/or physical activity and stress, immunity and cancer etiology and/or progression.

★ 25239 ★ U.S. Department of Health and Human Services
National Institutes of Health
National Cancer Institute
Division of Cancer Control and Population Sciences (DCCPS)
((Epidemiology and Genetics Research Program)
Clinical and Genetic Epidemiology Research Branch — CGERB)
6130 Executive Blvd., Rm. 5114, MSC 7395
Bethesda, MD 20892
Phone: (301)594-9499 **Fax:** (301)435-5477
Deborah M. Winn, Act. Chf.
Activities/Fields: Clinical and genetic epidemiology, ranging from elucidating determinants or progression and prognosis, pre-malignant conditions, clinical diagnostic strategies, clinical population genetics, clinical bioethics, genetic epidemiology, gene-gene and gene-modifier interactions, characterization of cancer susceptibility genes, and clinical and genetic networks and family registries.

★ 25240 ★ U.S. Department of Health and Human Services
National Institutes of Health
National Cancer Institute
Division of Cancer Control and Population Sciences (DCCPS)
((Epidemiology and Genetics Research Program)
Analytic Epidemiology Research Branch — AERB)
6130 Executive Blvd.
Rm. 5100
Bethesda, MD 20892
Phone: (301)435-4914 **Fax:** (301)402-4279
Email: sm33k@nih.gov
Sandra Melnick, Br. Chf.
Activities/Fields: Cancer etiology and modifying factors, in areas ranging from nutritional epidemiology, infectious disease epidemiology, hormonal studies, molecular epidemiology, metabolic/enzymatic pathways, physical and chemical agents, environmental epidemiology, to spatial studies.

★ 25241 ★ U.S. Department of Health and Human Services
National Institutes of Health
National Cancer Institute
Division of Cancer Control and Population Sciences (DCCPS)
((Applied Research Program)
Risk Factor Monitoring and Methods Branch)
6130 Executive Blvd.- MSC 7344
Bethesda, MD 20892-7344
Phone: (301)496-8500 **Fax:** (301)435-3710
Email: krebsms@mail.nih.gov
Website: http://riskfactor.cancer.gov
Sue Krebs-Smith, Branch. Chf.
Activities/Fields: The branch supports surveys designed to assess the prevalence of individual and societal risk factors in cancer prevention and research methods to improve their assessment.

★ 25242 ★ U.S. Department of Health and Human Services
National Institutes of Health
National Cancer Institute
Division of Cancer Control and Population Sciences (DCCPS)
((Surveillance Epidemiology and End Results Program — SRP)
Statistical Research and Applications Branch — SRAB)
Executive Plaza N, Ste. 504
6116 Executive Blvd., MSC 8317
Bethesda, MD 20892
Phone: (301)435-7739 **Fax:** (301)480-2046
Email: srab@nih.gov
Website: http://srab.cancer.gov
Eric Feuer, PhD, Br. Chf.
Activities/Fields: The branch plans, conducts, and supports statistical research, modeling, collaboration and consultation related to the cancer surveillance and the cancer control missions of the National Cancer Institute.

★ 25243 ★ U.S. Department of Health and Human Services
National Institutes of Health
National Cancer Institute
Division of Cancer Control and Population Sciences (DCCPS)
((Applied Research Program)
Health Services and Economics Branch)
6310 Executive Blvd.
Bethesda, MD 20892
Phone: (301)496-8500 **Fax:** (301)435-3710
Email: mbrown@mail.nih.gov
Website: http://healthservices.cancer.gov
Martin Brown, Branch Chf.
Activities/Fields: The study of cancer related health services for cancer sites which contribute most to cancer burden.

★ 25244 ★ U.S. Department of Health and Human Services
National Institutes of Health
National Cancer Institute
Division of Cancer Control and Population Sciences (DCCPS)
(Behavioral Research Program)
6130 Executive Blvd., MSC 7326
Bethesda, MD 20892-7326

Phone: (301)435-6816 **Fax:** (301)435-7547
Email: bc136e@.nih.gov
Website: http://dccps.nci.nih.gov/BRP
Robert T. Croyle, Assoc. Dir.

Activities/Fields: Behavioral research in areas such as tobacco use, screening, dietary behavior, health communication, and sun protection to increase cancer prevention.

★ 25245 ★ U.S. Department of Health and Human Services
National Institutes of Health
National Cancer Institute
Division of Cancer Control and Population Sciences (DCCPS)
((Applied Research Program)
Outcomes Research Branch — ORB)
6310 Executive Blvd.
Bethesda, MD 20892
Phone: (301)496-8500 **Fax:** (301)435-3710
Email: Joseph_Lipscomb@nih.gov
Website: http://outcomes.cancer.gov/
Joseph Liscomb, Branch Chf.

Activities/Fields: Cancer outcomes measurement and analysis.

★ 25246 ★ U.S. Department of Health and Human Services
National Institutes of Health
National Cancer Institute
Division of Cancer Control and Population Sciences (DCCPS)
(Epidemiology and Genetics Research Program — EGRP)
6130 Executive Blvd., Rm. 5114, MSC 8316
Bethesda, MD 20892
Phone: (301)496-8610 **Fax:** (301)435-9949
Email: winnde@mail.nih.gov
Website: http://epi.grants.cancer.gov
Deborah M. Winn, Ph.D, Act. Assoc. Dir.

Activities/Fields: The program plans, develops and manages a program of grant-supported, population-bases research on the etiology and prevention of cancer.

★ 25247 ★ U.S. Department of Health and Human Services
National Institutes of Health
National Cancer Institute
Division of Cancer Control and Population Sciences (DCCPS)
(Applied Research Program — ARP)
313 EPN
6130 Executive Blvd., MSC 7344
Bethesda, MD 20892
Phone: (301)594-6776 **Fax:** (301)594-6787
Email: stacey.vandor@nih.gov
Website: http://appliedresearch.cancer.gov
Stacy Vandor, Assc. Dir.

Activities/Fields: Patterns and trends in cancer related risk factors, health behaviors, economics, outcomes, and health services and influences of those factors, including databases for cancer related surveillance research.

★ 25248 ★ U.S. Department of Health and Human Services
National Institutes of Health
National Cancer Institute
Division of Cancer Control and Population Sciences (DCCPS)
(Surveillance, Epidemiology and End Results Program — SEER)
6116 Executive Blvd., Ste.504
Rockville, MD 20852
Phone: (301)496-8510 **Fax:** (301)496-9949
Email: bh43a@.nih.gov
Website: http://seer.cancer.gov
Benjamin F. Hankey, ScD, Br. Chf.

Activities/Fields: The program collects and publishes incidence and survival data from 11 population-based cancer registries and three supplemental registries covering approximately 14 percent of the U.S. population. **Pub:** *The Cancer Statistics Review 1973-1996.*

★ 25249 ★ U.S. Department of Health and Human Services
National Institutes of Health
National Cancer Institute
Division of Cancer Control and Population Sciences (DCCPS)
Office of the Director
6130 Executive Blvd.
Executive Plaza N, Rm. 6138
Rockville, MD 20852
Phone: (301)594-6776 **Fax:** (301)594-6787
Email: croyler@mail.nih.gov
Website: http://cancercontrol.cancer.gov
Dr. Robert T. Croyle, Act. Div. Dir.

Activities/Fields: Cancer genetic, epidemiologic, behavioral, social and surveillance research to reduce the risk, incidence and deaths from cancer.

★ 25250 ★ U.S. Department of Health and Human Services
National Institutes of Health
National Cancer Institute
Division of Cancer Epidemiology and Genetics
(Laboratory of Population Genetics)
Bldg. 41/D702
41 Library Dr.
Bethesda, MD 20892-5055
Phone: (301)435-8953 **Fax:** (301)435-8963
Email: kb52s@nih.gov
Dr. Kenneth H. Buetow, Chf.

Activities/Fields: The Laboratory investigates genetic determinants of cancer in human populations.

★ 25251 ★ U.S. Department of Health and Human Services
National Institutes of Health
National Cancer Institute
Division of Cancer Epidemiology and Genetics
(Human Genetics Program)
6120 Executive Blvd.
EPS Room 7016
Bethesda, MD 20892-7335
Phone: (301)496-4378 **Fax:** (301)402-4489
Email: fraumeni@nih.gov
Website: http://dceg.cancer.gov/hgp/index.html
Dr. Joseph F. Fraumeni, Jr., Actg. Dir.

Activities/Fields: The program plans, directs, manages and evaluates a diverse program of population-based research in genetic susceptibility to cancer, including clinical genetics, genetic epidemiology and population genetics.

★ 25252 ★ U.S. Department of Health and Human Services
National Institutes of Health
National Cancer Institute
Division of Cancer Epidemiology and Genetics
(Occupational Epidemiology Branch)
6120 Executive Blvd.
MSC 7240
EPS Rm. 8118
Bethesda, MD 20892-7335
Phone: (301)496-9093 **Fax:** (301)402-1819
Email: blaira@mail.nih.gov
Website: http://dceg.cancer.gov/ebp/oeb/index.html
Dr. Aaron Blair, Chf.

Activities/Fields: The Branch conducts studies to identify occupational groups at high risk of cancer.

★ 25253 ★ U.S. Department of Health and Human Services
National Institutes of Health
National Cancer Institute
Division of Cancer Epidemiology and Genetics
(Viral Epidemiology Branch)
6120 Executive Blvd.
MSC 7248
EPS Rm. 8012
Bethesda, MD 20892-7335
Phone: (301)496-8115 **Fax:** (301)402-0817
Email: goedertj@mail.nih.gov
Website: http://dceg.cancer.gov/ebp/veb/index.html
Dr. James J. Goedert, Chf.

Activities/Fields: The Branch conducts studies aimed at identifying the role of RNA and DNA viruses and other infectious agents in the etiology of human cancer.

★ 25254 ★ U.S. Department of Health and Human Services
National Institutes of Health
National Cancer Institute
Division of Cancer Epidemiology and Genetics
(Radiation Epidemiology Branch)
6120 Executive Blvd.
EPS Room 7048
Bethesda, MD 20892
Phone: (301)496-6600 **Fax:** (301)402-0207
Email: linetm@mail.nih.gov
Website: http://dceg.cancer.gov/ebp/reb/index.html
Dr. Martha Linet, Act. Chf.

Activities/Fields: The Branch conducts research to identify and quantify the risk of cancer in populations exposed to ionizing and non-ionizing radiation.

★ 25255 ★ U.S. Department of Health and Human Services
National Institutes of Health
National Cancer Institute
Division of Cancer Epidemiology and Genetics
(Nutritional Epidemiology Branch)
6120 Executive Blvd.
EPS Rm. 7040
Bethesda, MD 20892-7335
Phone: (301)594-2931 **Fax:** (301)496-6829
Email: schatzka@mail.nih.gov
Website: http://dceg.cancer.gov/ebp/neb/index.html
Dr. Arthur Schatzkin, Chf.

Activities/Fields: The Branch conducts population-base studies to assess etiologic hypotheses on the relationship of cancer risk to diet and nutrition; tests for associations between dietary factors, hormones, and risk at specific cancer; develops methods for nutritional epidemiology.

★ 25256 ★ U.S. Department of Health and Human Services
National Institutes of Health
National Cancer Institute
Division of Cancer Epidemiology and Genetics
(Environmental Epidemiology Branch)
6120 Executive Blvd.
MSC 7234
Bethesda, MD 20892-7335
Phone: (301)402-0916
Email: brintonl@mail.nih.gov
Website: http://dceg.cancer.gov/ebp/eeb/index.html
Dr. Louise A. Brinton, Chf.

Activities/Fields: The Branch conducts population-base studies to detect lifestyle, hormonal and other environmental and genetic determinants of cancer and coordinates studies to identify mechanisms of human carcinogenesis.

★ 25257 ★ U.S. Department of Health and Human Services
National Institutes of Health
National Cancer Institute
Division of Cancer Treatment and Diagnosis
((Cancer Diagnosis Program — CDP)
Resources Development Branch — RDB)
Executive Plaza N, Rm. 700
6130 Executive Blvd.
Bethesda, MD 20892
Fax: (301)496-7147
Email: ra32u@nih.gov
Website: http://www.cdp.ims.nci.nih.gov/rdb.html
Dr. Roger Aamodt, Branch Chf.
Activities/Fields: The Branch stimulates, develops and supports human tissue specimen resources to ensure availability of the tissue specimens needed to facilitate basic and translational cancer research.

★ 25258 ★ U.S. Department of Health and Human Services
National Institutes of Health
National Cancer Institute
Division of Cancer Treatment and Diagnosis
((Cancer Diagnosis Program — CDP)
Diagnostics Research Branch)
Executive Plaza N, Rm. 6035A
6130 Executive Blvd.
Bethesda, MD 20892
Phone: (301)496-1591 **Fax:** (301)402-7819
Email: TL82S@nih.gov
Website: http://www-cdp.ims.nci.nih.gov/drb.html
Tracy G. Lugo, PhD, Prog. Dir.
Activities/Fields: Supports research into new tools for cancer diagnosis, covering the entire process from the identification of potentially useful tumor cell characteristics to assuring that promising approaches to diagnosis and prognosis are moved from the laboratory to clinical practice in a timely way.

★ 25259 ★ U.S. Department of Health and Human Services
National Institutes of Health
National Cancer Institute
Division of Cancer Treatment and Diagnosis (DCTD)
((Cancer Diagnosis Program — CDP)
Technology Development Branch — TDB)
Executive Plaza N, Rm. 6035A
6130 Executive Blvd.
Rockville, MD 20852
Phone: (301)402-4185 **Fax:** (301)402-7819
Email: jj37d@nih.gov
Website: http://www-cdp.ims.nci.nih.gov/tdb.html
Dr. James Jacobson, Chf.
Activities/Fields: The Branch supports the development of novel technologies and devices that will result in better tools to aid in the clinical management of cancer patients.

★ 25260 ★ U.S. Department of Health and Human Services
National Institutes of Health
National Cancer Institute
Division of Cancer Treatment and Diagnosis
(Cancer Diagnosis Program — CDP)
9000 Rockville Pike
Bethesda, MD 20892
Phone: (301)496-8639
Email: liddellr@mail.nih.gov
Website: http://www.cancerdiagnosis.nci.nih.gov
Rebecca A. Liddell, PhD, Assoc. Dir.
Activities/Fields: Stimulates and supports research aimed at the development of better tools to aid in the clinical management of cancer patients.

★ 25261 ★ U.S. Department of Health and Human Services
National Institutes of Health
National Cancer Institute
Division of Clinical Sciences
(Urologic Oncology Branch)
10 Center Dr., MSC 1501
Bldg. 10, Rm. 2B47
Bethesda, MD 20892-1501
Phone: (301)496-6353 **Fax:** (301)402-0922
Email: linehanm@mail.nih.gov
Website: http://www-dcs.nci.nih.gov/branches/urology/
W. Marston Linehan, MD, Chf.
Activities/Fields: Cancer genes and molecular aspects of hereditary as well as sporadic forms of kidney, prostrate and bladder cancer.

★ 25262 ★ U.S. Department of Health and Human Services
National Institutes of Health
National Cancer Institute
Division of Clinical Sciences
(HIV and AIDS Malignancy Branch — HAMB)
Bldg. 10, Rm. 10S255
Bethesda, MD 20892-1868
Phone: (301)496-0328 **Fax:** (301)480-5955
Email: ry1n@nih.gov
Website: http://www-dcs.nci.nih.gov/branches/aidstrials/index.html
Robert Yarchoan, MD, Chf.
Activities/Fields: HIV infection and AIDS-related malignancies in children and adults.

★ 25263 ★ U.S. Department of Health and Human Services
National Institutes of Health
National Cancer Institute
Division of Clinical Sciences
(Laboratory of Pathology)
National Institutes of Health
Bldg. 10, Rm. 2A33
9000 Rockville Pike
Bethesda, MD 20892
Phone: (301)496-4345 **Fax:** (301)480-0853
Email: barrett@mail.nih.gov
Website: http://home.ccr.cancer.gov/lop/clinical
Dr. J. Carl Barrett, Dir.
Activities/Fields: Genetic mechanisms of human tumor progression, gene regulation, molecular immunology, invasion and metastasis, and cellular interaction with the extracellular matrix.

★ 25264 ★ U.S. Department of Health and Human Services
National Institutes of Health
National Cancer Institute
Division of Clinical Sciences
((HIV and AIDS Malignancy Branch — HAMB)
Pediatric HIV Working Group — PHWG)
Bldg. 10, Rm. 10s255
Bethesda, MD 20892
Phone: (301)402-1391 **Fax:** (301)480-1562
Email: yarchoan@helix.nih.gov
Robert Yarchoan, MD, Ch.
Activities/Fields: The group conducts clinical trials and provides family-centered care for HIV-infected children and families who participate in those trials.

★ 25265 ★ U.S. Department of Health and Human Services
National Institutes of Health
National Cancer Institute
Laboratory of Molecular Technology
PO Box B
Frederick, MD 21702-1201
Phone: (301)846-5676 **Fax:** (301)846-6100
Email: mtlseq@ncifcrf.gov
Website: http://web.ncifcrf.gov/rtp/lmt.asp
Dr. David J. Munroe, Hd.
Activities/Fields: Gene discovery and analysis capabilities, including advanced sequencing, genetics, genomics, and proteomics technologies.

★ 25266 ★ U.S. Department of Health and Human Services
National Institutes of Health
National Cancer Institute
Protein Chemistry Laboratory
PO Box B
Frederick, MD 21702-1000
Phone: (301)846-5154 **Fax:** (301)846-7269
Email: fisher@ncifcrf.gov
Website: http://web.ncifcrf.gov/rtp/PCL.asp
Dr. Robert J. Fisher, Hd.
Activities/Fields: N-terminal amino acid sequencing from PVDF-blotted proteins; GMP amino acid sequencing; protein digestion and separation resultant peptides by HPLC, MALDI-TOF mass spectrometry; and the study of macromolecular interactions using surface plasmon resonance spectroscopy (BIAcore analysis).

★ 25267 ★ U.S. Department of Health and Human Services
National Institutes of Health
National Center for Biotechnology Information
Bldg. 38A, 8-N-805
8600 Rockville Pike
Bethesda, MD 20894
Phone: (301)496-2475 **Fax:** (301)480-9241
Email: info@ncbi.nlm.nih.gov
Dr. David J. Lipman, MD, Dir.
Activities/Fields: Supports and develops biotechnology databases. Operates GenInfo Backbone Database.

★ 25268 ★ U.S. Department of Health and Human Services
National Institutes of Health
National Center for Complementary and Alternative Medicine (NCCAM)
NIH 31
9000 Rockville Pike
Bldg. 31, Rm. 2B11
Bethesda, MD 20892-2182
Phone: (301)435-5042 **Fax:** (301)594-6757
Email: nccam@nccam.nih.gov
Website: http://nccam.nih.gov/
Stephen E. Straus, MD, Dir.
Activities/Fields: Conducts and supports basic and applied research and training and disseminates information on complementary and alternative medicine to practitioners and the public.

★ 25269 ★ U.S. Department of Health and Human Services
National Institutes of Health
National Center for Research Resources
6705 Rockledge Dr., Ste. 5046
Bethesda, MD 20892-7965
Phone: (301)435-0888 **Fax:** (301)480-3558
Email: info@ncrr.nih.gov
Website: http://www.ncrr.nih.gov/
Dr. Judith Vaitukaitis, Dir.
Activities/Fields: Ensures that the essential tools, materials, and other research resources are readily available to the biomedical research community. Through grant programs, investigators across the nation have access to these technologies, instrumentation, specialized facilities, animal models and colonies (mammalian and nonmammalian), genetic stocks, and biomaterials such as cell lines, tissues, and organs. **Pub:** *Directories.* • *NCRR Reporter.* • *Reports.*

★ 25270 ★ U.S. Department of Health and Human Services
National Institutes of Health
National Eye Institute (NEI)
2020 Vision Pl.
Bethesda, MD 20892-3655
Phone: (301)496-5248 **Fax:** (301)402-1065
Email: 2020@nei.nih.gov
Website: http://www.nei.nih.gov/
Dr. Paul A. Sieving, PhD, Dir.
Activities/Fields: Improving prevention, diagnosis, and treatment of visual disorders. Specifically, the Institute: supports research and research training through grants, fellowships, and contracts to medical schools and research institutions; conducts laboratory and clinical research in its own facilities and fosters statistical and epidemiological studies of visual disorders in human populations; fosters research on rehabilitation of the visually handicapped; encourages the application of research findings to clinical practice; heightens public awareness of vision problems; and cooperates with voluntary organizations that engage in related activities. The NEI organization includes a Biometry and Epidemiology Program, Extramural and Collaborative Programs, and an Intramural Research Program. **Pub:** *Strategic Plan*, quinquenially. • *Eye diseases and disorders.*

★ 25271 ★ U.S. Department of Health and Human Services
National Institutes of Health
National Eye Institute
Intramural Research
(Ophthalmic Genetics and Visual Function Branch)
Bldg. 10, Rm. 10N226
10 Center Dr., MSC 1860
Bethesda, MD 20892-1860
Phone: (301)496-3577 **Fax:** (301)402-1214
Email: kaiserm@box-k.nih.gov
Website: http://www.nei.nih.gov/intramural/ogcsb.htmocg
Muriel I. Kaiser, Ch.
Activities/Fields: Gene expression and molecular interactions important to the eye to prevent, diagnose, and treat diseases of the eye and visual system, including corneal disease, cataract, retinal disease, and abnormalities of visual pathways.

★ 25272 ★ U.S. Department of Health and Human Services
National Institutes of Health
National Eye Institute
Intramural Research
(Section on Molecular Structure and Function)
Bldg. 10
10 Center Dr.
Bethesda, MD 20892
Phone: (301)402-3452
Email: graeme@helix.nih.gov
Website: http://www.nei.nih.gov/intramural/molstr.htm
Graeme J. Wistow, PhD, Hd.
Activities/Fields: Understanding important classes of proteins associated with the eye, using molecular biology, genomics, structural biology, and molecular evolution.

★ 25273 ★ U.S. Department of Health and Human Services
National Institutes of Health
National Eye Institute
Intramural Research
(Laboratory of Ocular Therapeutics)
Bldg. 6, Rm. 201
6 Center Dr., MSC 2730
Bethesda, MD 20892-2730
Phone: (301)496-4343 **Fax:** (301)402-0781
Email: kador@mge1.nei.nih.gov
Website: http://www.nei.nih.gov/intramural/lot.htm
Peter F. Kador, PhD, Ch.
Activities/Fields: Development, evaluation, and mechanism of action of new ophthalmic drugs to treat eye diseases, including aldose reductase inhibitors (ARI) and anticataract agents.

★ 25274 ★ U.S. Department of Health and Human Services
National Institutes of Health
National Eye Institute (NEI)
Intramural Research
((Laboratory of Mechanisms of Ocular Diseases)
Molecular Therapeutics)
Bldg. 6, Rm. 226
6 Center Dr., MSC 2735
Bethesda, MD 20892-2735
Phone: (301)496-2144
Email: carperd@nei.nih.gov
Website: http://www.nei.nih.gov/intramural/mt.htm
Deborah Carper, Hd.
Activities/Fields: Mechanisms responsible for cataract formation, including regulation of gene expression in oxidative stress models of cataract and in mechanisms responsible for gender-based differences in cataract development in aging populations.

★ 25275 ★ U.S. Department of Health and Human Services
National Institutes of Health
National Eye Institute
Intramural Research
((Laboratory of Mechanisms of Ocular Diseases)
Pathophysiology Group)
Bldg. 6, Rm. 316
6 Center Dr., MSC 2735
Bethesda, MD 20892-2735
Phone: (301)496-3161 **Fax:** (301)402-1570
Email: robisong@nei.nih.gov
Website: http://www.nei.nih.gov/intramural/patho.htm
W. Gerald Robison, Jr.,Ph, Hd.
Activities/Fields: Human tissues and experimental animals to elucidate underlying pathogenic mechanisms of ocular diseases, including retinopathy cataracts, and keratopathy, with emphasis on prevention of ocular complications of diabetes.

★ 25276 ★ U.S. Department of Health and Human Services
National Institutes of Health
National Eye Institute
Intramural Research
((Laboratory of Mechanisms of Ocular Diseases)
Lens and Cataract Biology Section)
Bldg. 6, Rm. 226
6 Center Dr., MSC 2735
Bethesda, MD 20892-2735
Phone: (301)496-6669 **Fax:** (301)402-1759
Email: ziglers@nei.nih.gov
Website: http://www.nei.nih.gov/intramural/lens.htm
J. Samuel Zigler, Jr.,Ph, Ch.
Activities/Fields: Structure, function, and evolution of lens crystallins and molecular mechanisms underlying cataract formation.

★ 25277 ★ U.S. Department of Health and Human Services
National Institutes of Health
National Eye Institute (NEI)
Intramural Research
((Laboratory of Mechanisms of Ocular Diseases)
Aging and Ocular Disease)
Bldg. 6, Rm. 226
6 Center Dr., MSC 2735
Bethesda, MD 20892-2735
Phone: (301)496-7471
Email: russelp@nei.nih.gov
Website: http://www.nei.nih.gov/intramural/aging.htm
Paul Russell, PhD, Hd.
Activities/Fields: Examination of changes in the eye, particularly the anterior segment, that occur with age and how some of these alterations may cause ocular disease. Research interests include cataract formation and primary open angle glaucoma.

★ 25278 ★ U.S. Department of Health and Human Services
National Institutes of Health
National Eye Institute
Intramural Research
(Division of Epidemiology and Clinical Research)
Bldg. 31, Rm. 6A52
31 Center Dr., MSC 2510
Bethesda, MD 20892-2510
Phone: (301)496-6583 **Fax:** (301)496-2297
Website: http://www.nei.nih.gov/intramural/biometry.htm
Frederick L. Ferris, III,MD, Dir.
Activities/Fields: Human population studies concerned with cause, prevention, and treatment of eye disease and vision disorders, with emphasis on major causes of blindness.

★ 25279 ★ U.S. Department of Health and Human Services
National Institutes of Health
National Heart, Lung, Blood Institute
Laboratory of Biochemistry
Bldg. 3, Rm. 222
3 Center Dr., MSC 0340
Bethesda, MD 20892
Phone: (301)592-8573 **Fax:** (301)592-8563
Email: bc50r@nih.gov
Website: http://www.nhlbi.nih.gov/labs/biochemistry/index.htm
Dr. Boon Chock, Ch.
Activities/Fields: Studies on the role of oxygen free radical mediated oxidation of enzymes in aging and various diseases (especially those involved in pulmonary dysfunction and arteriosclerosis); characterization of several bacterial selenoproteins, mechanism of biosynthesis of biosynthesis of selenophosphate and 2-selenouridine including EPR studies; regulation of protein ubiquitinating proteins, formation and utilization of free radicals, and cytosolic calcium oscillation; biochemical studies of the HIV-1 protease.

★ 25280 ★ U.S. Department of Health and Human Services
National Institutes of Health
National Heart, Lung, Blood Institute
Laboratory of Lymphocyte Biology
Bldg. 10, Rm. 5D49
10 Center Dr., MSC 1586
Bethesda, MD 20892
Phone: (301)402-6786 **Fax:** (301)480-1792
Email: biererb@nih.gov
Dr. Barbara Bierer, Dir.
Activities/Fields: Understanding of lymphocyte signal transduction and immune function.

★ 25281 ★ U.S. Department of Health and Human Services
National Institutes of Health
National Heart, Lung, Blood Institute
Laboratory of Molecular Biology
Bldg. 10, Rm. 7B14
10 Center Dr.
Bethesda, MD 20892
Phone: (301)541-8012 **Fax:** (301)402-0888
Email: finkelt@nhlbi.nih.gov
Website: http://www.nhlbi.nih.gov/labs/cardiology/molbio.htm
Dr. Toren Finkel, Ch.

Activities/Fields: Understanding the role of reactive oxygen species (ROS) as intracellular signaling molecules.

★ 25282 ★ U.S. Department of Health and Human Services
National Institutes of Health
National Heart, Lung, Blood Institute
Laboratory of Molecular Immunology
Bldg. 10, Rm. 7N244
10 Center. Dr.
Bethesda, MD 20892
Phone: (301)496-0098
Email: wl2w@nih.gov
Website: http://www.nhlbi.nih.gov/labs/molecularimmunology/index.htm
Dr. Warren Leonard, Ch.

Activities/Fields: T-cell activation process in normal and pathological states, including the elucidation of the interleukin-2 including the molecular regulation of the expression of its protein subunits.

★ 25283 ★ U.S. Department of Health and Human Services
National Institutes of Health
National Heart, Lung, Blood Institute
Vascular Biology Branch
Bldg. 10, Room 7B-15
10 Center Dr.
Bethesda, MD 20892-1650
Phone: (301)496-5817 **Fax:** (301)402-0888
Email: cannonr@nih.gov
Website: http://www.nhlbi.nih.gov/labs/cardiology/index.htm
Dr. Richard O. Cannon, III, Hd.

Activities/Fields: Pathophysiology of vascular diseases and novel therapeutics. Emphasis is on vessel wall biology and cell cycle regulation focusing on endothelial and smooth muscle cell biology.

★ 25284 ★ U.S. Department of Health and Human Services
National Institutes of Health
National Human Genome Research Institute (NHGRI)
31 Ctr. Dr., Rm. 4B09
Bethesda, MD 20892
Phone: (301)402-0911 **Fax:** (301)402-2218
Email: fc23a@nih.gov
Website: http://www.nhgri.nih.gov
Francis S. Collins, Dir.

Activities/Fields: The Institute's mission is to head the Human Genome Project for the National Institutes of Health.

★ 25285 ★ U.S. Department of Health and Human Services
National Institutes of Health
National Human Genome Research Institute (NHGRI)
Division of Extramural Research
(Ethical Legal and Social Implications Research Program — ELSI)
Bldg. 31, Rm. B2B07
31 Center Dr., MSC 2033
Bethesda, MD 20892-6050
Phone: (301)402-4997 **Fax:** (301)402-1950
Email: thmsone@mail.nih.gov
Website: http://www.nhgri.nih.gov/About_NHGRI/Der/Elsi/
Elizabeth Thomson, MS, Prog. Dir.

Activities/Fields: The program supports research that identifies and analyzes the ethical, legal, and social issues surrounding human genetics research.

★ 25286 ★ U.S. Department of Health and Human Services
National Institutes of Health
National Human Genome Research Institute (NHGRI)
Division of Extramural Research
(Model Organisms Program)
Bldg. 31, Rm. B2B07
31 Center Dr., MSC 2033
Bethesda, MD 20892-6050
Phone: (301)496-7531 **Fax:** (301)480-2770
Email: petersoj@odder.nhgri.nih.gov
Website: http://www.nhgri.nih.gov/About_NHGRI/Der/model.htm
Jane Peterson, PhD, Prog. Dir.

Activities/Fields: Mapping and sequencing of the genomes of model organisms, including E. coli, S. cerevisiae, C. elegans, D. melanogaster and the laboratory mouse.

★ 25287 ★ U.S. Department of Health and Human Services
National Institutes of Health
National Human Genome Research Institute (NHGRI)
Division of Extramural Research
(Genome Informatics Program)
Bldg. 31, Rm. B2B07
31 Ctr. Dr., MSC 2033
Bethesda, MD 20892
Phone: (301)435-5544 **Fax:** (301)480-2770
Email: brooksl@exchange.nih.gov
Website: http://www.nhgri.nih.gov/About_NHGRI/Der/ginform.htm
Lisa D. Brooks, PhD, Prog. Dir.

Activities/Fields: Fund grants on genomic data analysis, including sequence analysis, gene mapping, complex trait mapping and genetic variation; the development of database tools; and the development and maintenance of databases and genetic data.

★ 25288 ★ U.S. Department of Health and Human Services
National Institutes of Health
National Human Genome Research Institute (NHGRI)
Division of Extramural Research
(Genetic Variation Program)
Bldg. 31, Room B2B07
31 Center Dr., MSC 2033
National Institutes of Health
Bethesda, MD 20892-2033
Phone: (301)435-5544 **Fax:** (301)480-2770
Email: brooksl@exchange.nih.gov
Website: http://www.nhgri.nih.gov/About_NHGRI/Der/variat.htm
Lisa D. Brooks, PhD, Prog. Dir.

Activities/Fields: Funds research on the discovery Discovering and scoring of single nucleotide polymorphisms and other types of sequence variation, and the developmenting of high-resolution maps of genetic variation, and the developmenting of methods for the large-scale analysis of genetic variation, relating to phenotype and the analysis of complex traits.

★ 25289 ★ U.S. Department of Health and Human Services
National Institutes of Health
National Human Genome Research Institute (NHGRI)
Division of Extramural Research
(Sequencing Technology Program)
Bldg. 31, Rm. B2-B07
Bethesda, MD 20892-2033
Phone: (301)496-7531 **Fax:** (301)480-2770
Email: schlossj@exchange.nih.gov
Website: http://www.nhgri.nih.gov/About_NHGRI/Der/seqtech.htm
Jeffery Schloss, PhD, Prog. Dir.

Activities/Fields: Development of new methods, technologies, and instruments for rapid, low-cost determination of DNA sequence.

★ 25290 ★ U.S. Department of Health and Human Services
National Institutes of Health
National Human Genome Research Institute (NHGRI)
Division of Extramural Research
(Large Scale Sequencing Program)
Bldg. 31, Rm. B2B07
31 Center Dr., MSC 2033
Bethesda, MD 20892-2033
Phone: (301)496-7531 **Fax:** (301)480-2770
Email: jp22d@nih.gov
Jane Peterson, PhD, Prog. Dir.

Activities/Fields: Construction of physical maps and sequencing entire genomes, focusing on the human, mouse and Drosophila genomes.

★ 25291 ★ U.S. Department of Health and Human Services
National Institutes of Health
National Human Genome Research Institute (NHGRI)
Division of Extramural Research
(Functional Analysis of the Genome Program)
Bldg. 31, Rm. B2B07
31 Center Dr.
Bethesda, MD 20892
Phone: (301)496-7531 **Fax:** (301)480-2770
Email: feingole@exchange.nih.gov
Website: http://www.nhgri.nih.gov/About_NHGRI/Der/function.htm
Elise Feingold, PhD, Prog. Dir.

Activities/Fields: Development of improved techniques and strategies for efficient identification and functional analysis of genes, coding regions, and other functional elements of the genome on a high throughput, genome-wide basis.

★ 25292 ★ U.S. Department of Health and Human Services
National Institutes of Health
National Human Genome Research Institute (NHGRI)
Division of Intramural Research
(Cancer Genetics Branch)
49 Convent Dr., Bldg. 49, Rm. 4A22
Bethesda, MD 20892
Phone: (301)402-2023 **Fax:** (301)402-2040
Email: jtrent@nhgri.nih.gov
Website: http://www.nhgri.nih.gov/Intramural_research/Lab_cancer/
Jeffrey M. Trent, PhD, Chf.

Activities/Fields: The Branch's focus it to define the genetic changes that lead to the initiation and progression of cancer.

★ 25293 ★ U.S. Department of Health and Human Services
National Institutes of Health
National Human Genome Research Institute (NHGRI)
Division of Intramural Research
(Clinical Gene Therapy Branch)
10 Center Dr., Bldg. 10, Rm. 10C103
49 Convent Drive, MSC 4442
Bethesda, MD 20892
Phone: (301)435-2944 **Fax:** (301)496-7184
Email: fabio@nhgri.nih.gov
Website: http://www.nhgri.nih.gov/Intramural_research/Clinical_therapy/
Fabio Candotti, MD, Branch Hd.

Activities/Fields: Basic and applied science important to gene therapy and its application to the treatment of human diseases.

★ 25294 ★ U.S. Department of Health and Human Services
National Institutes of Health
National Human Genome Research Institute (NHGRI)
Division of Intramural Research
(Inherited Disease Research Branch)
49 Convent Dr., Bldg. 49, Rm. 4A72
Bethesda, MD 20892-4472
Phone: (301)402-2039 **Fax:** (301)402-2170
Email: rlnuss@nhgri.nih.gov
Website: http://www.nhgri.nih.gov/Intramural_research/IDRB/
Robert L. Nussbaum, MD, Chf.
Activities/Fields: The Branch's focus it to develop and apply tools in statistics, genetics and computer science to locate genes that contribute to multifactorial genetic disease.

★ 25295 ★ U.S. Department of Health and Human Services
National Institutes of Health
National Human Genome Research Institute (NHGRI)
Division of Intramural Research
(Genetic Disease Research Branch)
49 Convent Dr., Bldg. 49, Rm. 4A72
Bethesda, MD 20892
Phone: (301)402-2039 **Fax:** (301)402-2170
Email: rlnuss@nhgri.nih.gov
Website: http://www.nhgri.nih.gov/DIR/LGDR
Robert L. Nussbaum, MD, Chf.
Activities/Fields: The Branch's focus is to identify the genetic abnormalities responsible for human disease and elucidate the mechanisms by which they cause abnormalities in structure and function.

★ 25296 ★ U.S. Department of Health and Human Services
National Institutes of Health
National Human Genome Research Institute
Division of Intramural Research
(Medical Genetics Branch)
Triad Bldg., Ste. 3000
333 Cassell Dr.
Baltimore, MD 21224
Phone: (410)558-8201 **Fax:** (410)558-8087
Email: francomanocl@grc.nih.gov
Website: http://www.grc.nia.nih.gov/branches/lg/hgims/hgims.htm
Clair A. Francomano, MD, Chf.
Activities/Fields: The laboratory examines patients and families affected by inherited disorders to identify and characterize novel disorders of human development.

★ 25297 ★ U.S. Department of Health and Human Services
National Institutes of Health
National Human Genome Research Institute (NHGRI)
Division of Intramural Research
(Genetics and Molecular Biology Branch)
49 Convent Dr., Bldg. 49, Rm. 3A14
Bethesda, MD 20892-4442
Phone: (301)402-2194 **Fax:** (301)402-4929
Email: jp82a@nih.gov
Jennifer M. Puck, MD, Br. Chf.
Activities/Fields: The Branch uses molecular genes involved in the normal development and function of many tissues, including blood and epithelial cells, the immune system and the nervous system.

★ 25298 ★ U.S. Department of Health and Human Services
National Institutes of Health
National Human Genome Research Institute (NHGRI)
Division of Intramural Research
(Genome Technology Branch)
50 S Dr., Bldg. 50, Rm.5523
Bethesda, MD 20892
Phone: (301)402-0201 **Fax:** (301)402-4735
Email: egreen@nhgri.nih.gov
Website: http://www.nhgri.nih.gov/DIR/GTB/
Eric D. Green, MD, Chf.
Activities/Fields: The Branch's focus is contemporary technologies for performing genome analysis.

★ 25299 ★ U.S. Department of Health and Human Services
National Institutes of Health
National Human Genome Research Institute
Human Genome Project
Bldg. 31, Rm. 4B09
Bethesda, MD 20892
Phone: (301)402-0911 **Fax:** (301)402-2218
Email: francisc@exchange.nih.gov
Website: http://www.nhgri.nih.gov/index.html
Francis Collins, MD, Dir.
Activities/Fields: Constructs detailed genetic and physical maps of human genome to determine complete nucleotide sequence of human DNA in order to localize the estimated 50,000-100,000 genes within the human genome; performs analyses of genomes in several organisms.

★ 25300 ★ U.S. Department of Health and Human Services
National Institutes of Health
National Institute on Aging
Extramural Programs
(Geriatrics Program)
Bldg. 31, Rm. 5C27
31 Center Dr., MSC 2292
Bethesda, MD 20892
Phone: (301)496-6761
Email: gpquery@exmur.nia.nih.gov
Website: http://www.nia.nih.gov/research/extramural/geriatrics
Activities/Fields: Pathophysiology, diagnosis, treatment, and prevention of age-related diseases, degenerative conditions, and disabilities, especially physical frailty (deficits in strength, mobility, balance, and endurance); new diseases of old age; development of interventions and testing in controlled clinical trials.

★ 25301 ★ U.S. Department of Health and Human Services
National Institutes of Health
National Institute on Aging
Intramural Research Programs
(Laboratory of Molecular Gerontology)
Nathan W Shock Laboratories
Rm. 2-D-09, Stop 01
Baltimore, MD 21224
Phone: (410)558-8223 **Fax:** (410)558-8157
Email: bohrv@grc.nia.nih.gov
Website: http://www.grc.nia.nih.gov/branches/lmg/lmg.htm
Vilhelm A. Bohr, MD, Ch.
Activities/Fields: Molecular basis for aging and age-dependent diseases, notably cancer.

★ 25302 ★ U.S. Department of Health and Human Services
National Institutes of Health
National Institute on Aging
Intramural Research Programs
(Molecular Dynamics Section)
Gerontology Research Center
5600 Nathan Shock Dr.
Baltimore, MD 21224
Phone: (410)558-8168 **Fax:** (410)558-8173
Email: rifkindj@grc.nia.nih.gov
Website: http://www.grc.nia.nih.gov/branches/lcmb/mds/mds.htm
Joseph M. Rifkind, PhD, Ch.
Activities/Fields: Research on the interplay between structure dynamics and how these influence biological function.

★ 25303 ★ U.S. Department of Health and Human Services
National Institutes of Health
National Institute on Aging
Intramural Research Programs
(Laboratory of Immunology)
5600 Nathan Shock Dr.
Baltimore, MD 21224
Phone: (410)558-8159 **Fax:** (410)558-8284
Email: taubd@grc.nia.nih.gov
Website: http://www.grc.nia.nih.gov/branches/li/li.htm
Dennis D. Taub, PhD, Actg. Ch.
Activities/Fields: Dedicated to understanding the biological, biochemical, and molecular alterations in immune functions that occur within individuals during both normal and disease-associated aging processes.

★ 25304 ★ U.S. Department of Health and Human Services
National Institutes of Health
National Institute on Aging
Intramural Research Programs
(Cell Cycle Control Unit)
Gateway
7201 Wisconsin Ave., Ste. 3C309
Bethesda, MD 20892-9205
Email: gorospem@grc.nia.nih.gov
Website: http://www.grc.nia.nih.gov/branches/lbc/cccu.htm
Myriam Gorospe, PhD, Hd.
Activities/Fields: Cellular response to stress and gene expression; post-transcriptional control of cell cycle regulatory genes; functional analysis of the von Hippel-Lindau (VHL) tumor suppressor gene.

★ 25305 ★ U.S. Department of Health and Human Services
National Institutes of Health
National Institute on Aging
Intramural Research Programs
(Laboratory of Genetics)
Gerontology Research Center
5600 Nathan Shock Dr.
Baltimore, MD 21224
Phone: (410)558-8337
Email: schlessingerd@grc.nia.nih.gov
Website: http://www.grc.nia.nih.gov/branches/lg/lg.htm
David Schlessinger, PhD, Ch.
Activities/Fields: Studies of genetic determinants as an integrated part of human development.

★ 25306 ★ U.S. Department of Health and Human Services
National Institutes of Health
National Institute on Aging
Intramural Research Programs
(Cancer Molecular Genetics Unit)
Gerontology Research Center
5600 Nathan Shock Dr.
Baltimore, MD 21224-6825

Phone: (410)558-8506 **Fax:** (410)558-8386
Email: morinp@grc.nia.nih.gov
Website: http://www.grc.nia.nih.gov/branches/lbc/cmgu.htm
Patrice Jean-Luc Morin, PhD, Hd.
Activities/Fields: Ovarian cancer and the Wnt pathway in human cancer.

★ 25307 ★ U.S. Department of Health and Human Services
National Institutes of Health
National Institute on Aging
Intramural Research Programs
(Cardiac Function Unit)
Gerontology Research Center
5600 Nathan Shock Dr.
Baltimore, MD 21224
Phone: (410)558-8110
Email: lakattae@grc.nia.nih.gov
Website: http://www.grc.nia.nih.gov/branches/lcs/cardfunc/cardfunc.htm
Edward G. Lakatta, MD, Ch.
Activities/Fields: Cardiac dynamics and basic studies on isolated myocardial cells, including the influence of age on the intact cardiovascular system, especially the human myocardium; also studies the vascular structure, function, and mechanics of atherosclerosis, as well as gene therapy for age-related cardiovascular disease.

★ 25308 ★ U.S. Department of Health and Human Services
National Institutes of Health
National Institute on Aging
Intramural Research Programs
(Cell Stress and Aging Section Program)
Gerontology Research Center
5600 Nathan Shock Dr.
Baltimore, MD 21224
Phone: (410)558-8446
Email: holbroon@intra.nia.nih.gov
Website: http://www.grc.nia.nih.gov/branches/lbc/gea/gea.htm
Nikki Holbrook, PhD, Ch.
Activities/Fields: Cellular responses to stress and how they become altered with age.

★ 25309 ★ U.S. Department of Health and Human Services
National Institutes of Health
National Institute on Aging
Intramural Research Programs
(Laboratory of Epidemiology, Demography, and Biometry)
Gateway
7201 Wisconsin Ave., Ste. 3C309
Bethesda, MD 20892-9205
Phone: (301)496-1752
Website: http://www.nia.nih.gov/research/intramural/edb
Richard J. Havlik, MD, Assoc. Dir.
Activities/Fields: Chronic diseases and functional status and disability in the older population; physiologic risk factors for different dimensions of the dementing process, including cognitive decline and structural brain changes; geriatric epidemiology in areas of metabolism and nutritional risk factors, chronic inflammation, and comorbidity as they relate to functional outcomes, disease endpoints, and mortality in older persons; mathematical, statistical, and numerical aspects of aging and health.

★ 25310 ★ U.S. Department of Health and Human Services
National Institutes of Health
National Institute on Aging
Intramural Research Programs
(Behavioral Hypertension Section)
Gerontology Research Center
5600 Nathan Shock Dr.
Baltimore, MD 21224-6825
Email: andersond@grc.nia.nih.gov
Website: http://www.grc.nia.nih.gov/branches/lcs/bhs.htm
David E. Anderson, PhD, Ch.
Activities/Fields: Strives to clarify role of behavior in the etiology and pathogenesis of selected disorders of aging, to elucidate physiological and biochemical pathways by which behavioral factors influence disorders of aging, and to develop and apply behavioral interventions to prevent, ameliorate, or reverse disorders of aging.

★ 25311 ★ U.S. Department of Health and Human Services
National Institutes of Health
National Institute of Allergy and Infectious Diseases (NIAID)
NIH Bldg. 31, Rm. 7A03
31 Center Dr., MSC2520
Bethesda, MD 20892-2520
Phone: (301)496-2263 **Fax:** (301)402-0120
Email: afauci@niaid.nih.gov
Website: http://www.niaid.nih.gov
Dr. Anthony S. Fauci, MD, Dir.
Activities/Fields: Causes of allergic, immunologic, and infectious diseases and to the development of better means of preventing, diagnosing, and treating illnesses. Its mission involves studies on: genetic control, maturation, characteristics, and manipulation of the immune system; disorders of the immune system, including asthma and other allergies, immunodeficiency states, and autoimmunity; the role of the immune system in the pathogenesis of chronic diseases such as arthritis, the etiology, epidemiology, and pathogenesis of all types of infections (including those caused by viruses, mycoplasma, bacteria, fungi, and parasites) involving a variety of organ systems; the diagnosis, treatment, and prevention of all types of infections (including research on antimicrobial, antifungal, and antiviral therapy, and vaccines); and the role and mechanism of nucleic acid recombination in microbial agents. Fields of research include microbiology, parasitology, virology, bacteriology, genetics and transplantation biology, and mycology. The Institute is also concerned with enteric diseases and tropical diseases research. NIAID's program includes both inhouse (intramural) research and research conducted through grants, contracts, and interagency agreements (extramural). NIAID's extramural divisions are the Division of Acquired Immunodeficiency Syndrome (DAIDS), Division of Allergy, Immunology, and Transplantation (DAIT), and the Division of Microbiology and Infectious Diseases. NIAID's Division of Intramural Research (DIR) comprises 17 laboratories in Bethesda, MD, and the Rocky Mountain Laboratories in Hamilton, MT. Also supports a 52-bed inpatient service and outpatient research facility on the NIH campus.

★ 25312 ★ U.S. Department of Health and Human Services
National Institutes of Health
National Institute of Allergy and Infectious Diseases
Division of Intramural Research
(Laboratory of Intracellular Parasites)
Rocky Mountain Laboratories
903 S 4th St.
Hamilton, MT 59840
Phone: (406)363-9233 **Fax:** (406)363-9355
Email: harlan_caldwell@nih.gov
Website: http://www.niaid.nih.gov/dir/labs/licp.htm
Harlan D. Caldwell, PhD, Ch.
Activities/Fields: Immunologic and pathologic aspects of infections caused by intracellular prokaryotes, including chlamydia, mycobacteria, and chlamydia trachomatis.

★ 25313 ★ U.S. Department of Health and Human Services
National Institutes of Health
National Institute of Allergy and Infectious Diseases
Division of Intramural Research
(Laboratory of Host Defenses)
Bldg. 10, Rm. 11N113
10 Center Dr.
MSC 1886
Bethesda, MD 20892-1886
Phone: (301)496-1343 **Fax:** (301)402-4369
Email: jig@nih.gov
Website: http://www.niaid.nih.gov/dir/labs/lhd.htm
John I. Gallin, MD, Ch.
Activities/Fields: Mechanisms of host defense against bacterial and fungal infections, particularly the biochemistry, function and structure of phagocytic cells, including peripheral blood polymorphonuclear leukocytes (neutrophils), eosinophils, and monocytes, and fixed-tissue macrophages.

★ 25314 ★ U.S. Department of Health and Human Services
National Institutes of Health
National Institute of Child Health and Human Development
Division of Intramural Research
((Division of Epidemiology, Statistics and Prevention Research)
Biometry and Mathematical Statistics Branch)
Bldg. 6100, Rm. 7B05
9000 Rockville Pike
Bethesda, MD 20892-7510
Phone: (301)496-6813 **Fax:** (301)402-2084
Website: http://www.nichd.nih.gov/about/despr/bio.htm
Kai F. Yu, PhD, Ch.
Activities/Fields: Statistical theory and methodology relevant to problems under investigation in areas of maternal and child health.

★ 25315 ★ U.S. Department of Health and Human Services
National Institutes of Health
National Institute of Child Health and Human Development
Division of Intramural Research
(Division of Epidemiology, Statistics and Prevention Research)
6100 Bldg., Rm. 7B05
MSC 7510
Bethesda, MD 20892-7510
Phone: (301)496-5064 **Fax:** (301)402-2084
Email: mk90h@nih.gov
Website: http://www.nichd.nih.gov/about/despr/despr.htm
Mark A. Klebanoff, MD, Dir.
Activities/Fields: Epidemiologic, behavioral and biometric studies relating to reproductive, maternal, and child health, particularly reproductive processes, pregnancy, infant mortality and morbidity, child growth and development, clinical trials, vaccinology, and community-based interventions designed to promote healthful behaviors.

★ **25316** ★ **U.S. Department of Health and Human Services**
National Institutes of Health
National Institute of Child Health and Human Development
Division of Intramural Research
(Laboratory of Physical and Structural Biology)
12A/2041
Bethesda, MD 20892
Phone: (301)496-6561
Email: aparsegi@helix.nih.gov
Website: http://dir2.nichd.nih.gov/labs/lab.php3?16
V.A. Parsegian, Ch.
Activities/Fields: Aims to understand biological structures through the physical forces that animate them, in order to measure force vs. separation between molecules from all classes of bio-matter.

★ **25317** ★ **U.S. Department of Health and Human Services**
National Institutes of Health
National Institute of Child Health and Human Development
Division of Intramural Research
(Research Animal Management Branch)
Bldg. 6, Rm. 434
Bethesda, MD 20892
Phone: (301)496-9733
Email: barthoj@mail.nih.gov
Website: http://dir2.nichd.nih.gov/labs/lab.php3?19
John Bartholomew, Hd.
Activities/Fields: Animal disease control programs, including diagnosis, therapy, and prevention of disease from animals to humans (zoonoses).

★ **25318** ★ **U.S. Department of Health and Human Services**
National Institutes of Health
National Institute of Child Health and Human Development
Division of Intramural Research
(Laboratory of Mammalian Genes and Development)
Bldg.6B, Rm. 413
Bethesda, MD 20892
Phone: (301)496-1855
Email: hw@helix.nih.gov
Website: http://dir2.nichd.nih.gov/labs/lab.php3?13
Heinrich J. Westphal, Hd.
Activities/Fields: Advanced gene targeting and transgenic technologies to study genes that control specific stages of mouse development, particularly development of central and peripheral nervous systems, pituitary and thymus development and mechanisms of genomic imprinting.

★ **25319** ★ **U.S. Department of Health and Human Services**
National Institutes of Health
National Institute of Child Health and Human Development
Division of Intramural Research
(Laboratory of Gene Regulation and Development)
Bldg. 1st, Rm. 106
Bethesda, MD 20892-2425
Phone: (301)496-8391
Email: alanh@box-a.nih.gov
Website: http://dir2.nichd.nih.gov/labs/lab.php3?10
Alan Hinnebusch, Ch.
Activities/Fields: Regulation of gene expression in two model eukaryotic systems, the yeasts saccharomyces cerevisiae and Schizosaccharomyces pombe.

★ **25320** ★ **U.S. Department of Health and Human Services**
National Institutes of Health
National Institute of Child Health and Human Development
Division of Intramural Research
(Laboratory of Integrative and Medical Biophysics)
Bldg. 12A, Rm. 2001
Bethesda, MD 20892
Phone: (301)435-9233
Email: rjn@helix.nih.gov
Website: http://dir2.nichd.nih.gov/labs/lab.php3?11
Ralph Nossal, Ch.
Activities/Fields: Understanding basic biophysical mechanisms underlying cell and tissue function.

★ **25321** ★ **U.S. Department of Health and Human Services**
National Institutes of Health
National Institute of Child Health and Human Development
Division of Intramural Research
(Laboratory of Cellular and Molecular Neurophysiology)
Bldg. 36, Rm. 2B28
Bethesda, MD 20892
Phone: (301)496-9346
Email: mlm@helix.nih.gov
Website: http://dir2.nichd.nih.gov/labs/lab.php3?7
Dr. Mark Mayer, Ch.
Activities/Fields: Neurotransmitter receptors and ion channels and the cellular processes they control using patch clamp, imaging, molecular biological, biochemical, structural and neuroanatomical techniques applied to preparations, including transgenic mice, brain slices, cell cultures, in vitro expression systems including Xenopus oocytes and transiently transfected 293 cells, and proteins over-expressed in bacteria. **Pub:** *Papers.*

★ **25322** ★ **U.S. Department of Health and Human Services**
National Institutes of Health
National Institute of Child Health and Human Development
Division of Intramural Research
(Laboratory of Developmental Neurobiology)
Bldg. 49, Rm. 5A38
49 Convent Dr., MSC 4480
Bethesda, MD 20892-4480
Phone: (301)496-1463 **Fax:** (301)496-9939
Dr. Phillip G. Nelson, Ch.
Activities/Fields: Molecular and cellular mechanisms coupling electrical activity in neurons and muscle cells to development of the nervous system.

★ **25323** ★ **U.S. Department of Health and Human Services**
National Institutes of Health
National Institute of Child Health and Human Development
Division of Intramural Research
(Laboratories of the Scientific Director)
Bldg. 31, Rm. 2A50
31 Center Dr.
Bethesda, MD 20892
Phone: (301)496-2133
Website: http://dir2.nichd.nih.gov/labs/lab.php3?17
Igor Dawid, Ch.
Activities/Fields: Molecular events that influence fidelity of the genome, facilitating both evolution and species stability.

★ **25324** ★ **U.S. Department of Health and Human Services**
National Institutes of Health
National Institute of Child Health and Human Development
Division of Intramural Research
(Pediatric and Reproductive Endocrinology Branch)
Bldg. 10, Rm. 9D42
10 Center Dr., MSC 1583
Bethesda, MD 20892-1583
Phone: (301)496-5800 **Fax:** (301)402-0884
Email: chrousog@mail.nih.gov
Website: http://preb.nichd.nih.gov/
Dr. George Chrousos, Chf.
Activities/Fields: Pediatric and reproductive endocrinology and metabolism, especially physiology and pathophysiology of growth, development, metabolic, immune, and reproductive functions and study of major neurohormonal systems, hypothalamic-pituitary-adrenal (HPA) and -gonadal (HPG) axes and autonomic nervous system, that sub-serve these functions.

★ **25325** ★ **U.S. Department of Health and Human Services**
National Institutes of Health
National Institute of Child Health and Human Development
Division of Intramural Research
(Perinatology Research Branch)
Bldg. 31, Rm. 2A32
31 Center Dr., MSC 2425
Bethesda, MD 20892-2425
Phone: (301)993-2700
Email: romeror@mail.nih.gov
Website: http://dir2.nichd.nih.gov/labs/lab.php3?18
Roberto Romero, Hd.
Activities/Fields: Conditions responsible for perinatal morbidity and mortality, especially the study of human parturition (premature labor), intrauterine growth retardation, congenital anomalies, and pre-eclampsia.

★ **25326** ★ **U.S. Department of Health and Human Services**
National Institutes of Health
National Institute of Child Health and Human Development
Division of Intramural Research
(Heritable Disorders Branch)
Bldg. 31, Rm. 2A32, MSC 2425
31 Center Dr.
Bethesda, MD 20892
Phone: (301)496-6683
Email: marinij@mail.nih.gov
Website: http://dir2.nichd.nih.gov/labs/lab.php3?4
Joan C. Marini, Head
Activities/Fields: Etiology, diagnosis therapy of human genetic disorders, particularly clinically, inborn errors of metabolism and connective tissue disorders.

★ **25327** ★ **U.S. Department of Health and Human Services**
National Institutes of Health
National Institute of Dental and Craniofacial Research
31 Center Dr., MSC 2290
Bldg. 31, Rm. 2C39
Bethesda, MD 20892-2290
Phone: (301)496-3571 **Fax:** (301)402-2185
Email: lawrence.tabak@nih.gov
Website: http://www.nidcr.nih.gov
Lawrence A. Tabak, DDS,Ph, Dir.
Activities/Fields: Oral, dental, and craniofacial health, as well as prevention of those diseases and conditions; also develops new diagnostics and therapeutics.

★ 25328 ★ U.S. Department of Health and Human Services
National Institutes of Health
National Institute of Dental and Craniofacial Research
Division of Extramural Research (Neoplastic Diseases Branch)
Bldg. 45, Rm. 4AN-24A
45 Center Dr., MSC 6402
Bethesda, MD 20892-6402
Phone: (301)594-2419 **Fax:** (301)480-8318
Email: ann.sandberg@nih.gov
Ann L. Sandberg, PhD, Ch.
Activities/Fields: Basic, translational, clinical, and epidemiological research on cancers of the oral cavity, including etiology and early detection of oral cancers; progression of oral cancers; invasion and metastasis of oral cancer cells; therapy or oral cancers.

★ 25329 ★ U.S. Department of Health and Human Services
National Institutes of Health
National Institute of Dental and Craniofacial Research
Division of Extramural Research (Biomaterials, Biomimetics and Tissue Engineering Branch)
Bldg. 45, Rm. 4AN-18A
45 Center Dr.
Bethesda, MD 20892-6402
Phone: (301)594-2427 **Fax:** (301)480-8318
Email: eleni.kousvelari@nih.gov
Dr. Eleni Kousvelari, Dir.
Activities/Fields: Design, development and improvement of natural and novel synthetic biomaterials used in restoration, repair, and reconstruction of oral, dental and craniofacial tissues and organs.

★ 25330 ★ U.S. Department of Health and Human Services
National Institutes of Health
National Institute of Dental and Craniofacial Research
Division of Extramural Research (Craniofacial Anomalies and Injury Branch)
Bldg. 45, Rm. 4AN-24
45 Center Dr., MSC 6402
Bethesda, MD 20892-6402
Phone: (301)594-9898 **Fax:** (301)480-8318
Email: rochelle.small@nih.gov
Rochelle K. Small, PhD, Actg. Ch.
Activities/Fields: Understanding the development of head, face, and neck and to identify genetic and environmental contributions to craniofacial anomalies including biology of tooth and bone.

★ 25331 ★ U.S. Department of Health and Human Services
National Institutes of Health
National Institute of Dental and Craniofacial Research
Division of Extramural Research (Office of Clinical, Behavioral and Health Promotion Research)
Bldg. 45, Rm. 4AN-24B
45 Center Dr.
Bethesda, MD 20892-6402
Phone: (301)594-2089 **Fax:** (301)480-8318
Email: norman.braveman@nih.gov
Norman S. Braveman, PhD, Actg. Dir.
Activities/Fields: Development, evaluation and implementation of interventions to prevent or treat craniofacial, dental and oral diseases and disorders; assess behavioral and economic processes influencing health care delivery; researches alternative and complementary medicine; aims to improve end-of-life care.

★ 25332 ★ U.S. Department of Health and Human Services
National Institutes of Health
National Institute of Dental and Craniofacial Research
Division of Extramural Research (Clinical Trials Program)
Bldg. 45, Rm. 4AN-24B
45 Center Dr.
Bethesda, MD 20892-6402
Phone: (301)496-4261 **Fax:** (301)480-8318
Email: nidcrinfo@mail.nih.gov
Website: http://www.nidcr.nih.gov/research/CTP/clinical_trials.asp
Maryann Redford, PhD, Contact
Activities/Fields: Testing of interventions to prevent, inhibit, or reverse dental and craniofacial diseases and conditions; aims to promote and maintain oral health, using molecular biology, genetics, immunology and imaging.

★ 25333 ★ U.S. Department of Health and Human Services
National Institutes of Health
National Institute of Dental and Craniofacial Research
Division of Intramural Research (Matrix Metalloproteinase Section)
Bldg. 30, Rm. 132
30 Convent Dr., MSC 4326
Bethesda, MD 20892-4326
Phone: (301)496-1483 **Fax:** (301)402-1512
Email: henning.birkedal-hansen@nih.gov
Website: http://wwwdir.nidcr.nih.gov/dirweb/cores/mms/mms.asp
Dr. Henning Birkedal-Hansen, Actg. Ch.
Activities/Fields: Factors controlling synthesis, genetic regulation and function of matrix metalloproteinases in homeostasis and disease; defines role of metalloproteinases in cellular regulation and collagen degradation; characterizes biological function of matrix metalloproteinase inhibitors, TIMPs, and regulation of TIMP synthesis.

★ 25334 ★ U.S. Department of Health and Human Services
National Institutes of Health
National Institute of Dental and Craniofacial Research
Division of Intramural Research (Functional Genomics Unit)
Bldg. 30, Rm. 529
30 Convent Dr., MSC 4326
Bethesda, MD 20892-4326
Phone: (301)435-2887 **Fax:** (301)435-2888
Email: ashok.kulkarni@nih.gov
Website: http://wwwdir.nidcr.nih.gov/dirweb/cores/fgu/fgu.asp
Dr. Ashok Kulkarni, Dir.
Activities/Fields: Seeks to delineate precise in vivo functions of specific genes involved in molecular processes underlying disease conditions involving degenerative processes, metabolic defects and immune disorders.

★ 25335 ★ U.S. Department of Health and Human Services
National Institutes of Health
National Institute of Dental and Craniofacial Research
Division of Intramural Research (Immunopathology Section)
Bldg. 30, Rm. 325
30 Convent Dr., MSC 4352
Bethesda, MD 20892-4352
Phone: (301)496-9219 **Fax:** (301)402-1064
Email: larry.wahl@nih.gov
Website: http://wwwdir.nidcr.nih.gov/dirweb/cores/is/is.asp
Larry M. Wahl, PhD, Ch.
Activities/Fields: Factors and signal transduction pathways in the modulation of the immune response focusing on human moncytes.

★ 25336 ★ U.S. Department of Health and Human Services
National Institutes of Health
National Institute of Dental and Craniofacial Research
Division of Intramural Research (Cellular Neuroscience Section)
Bldg. 49, Rm. 1A11
30 Convent Dr., MSC 4410
Bethesda, MD 20892-4410
Phone: (301)402-4980 **Fax:** (301)402-0667
Email: maryann.ruda@nih.gov
Dr. M.A. Ruda, Ch.
Activities/Fields: Neuronal response to peripheral inflammation and hyperalgesia or nerve injury, representing neuronal plasticity at the level of the spinal cord and dorsal root ganglia, focused on the question of nociception.

★ 25337 ★ U.S. Department of Health and Human Services
National Institutes of Health
National Institute of Dental and Craniofacial Research
Division of Intramural Research (Molecular Therapeutics Unit)
Bldg. 30, Rm. 211
30 Convent Dr., MSC 4340
Bethesda, MD 20892-4340
Phone: (301)594-5270 **Fax:** (301)402-0823
Email: adrian.senderowicz@nih.gov
Website: http://wwwdir.nidcr.nih.gov/dirweb/opcb/mtu.htm
Dr. Adrian Senderowicz, Ch.
Activities/Fields: Mechanism-based therapeutic approaches for head and neck cancer, especially the study of antiproliferative mechanisms of novel small molecules, including the identification of pathways necessary for induction of apoptosis, differentiation, and cell cycle arrest.

★ 25338 ★ U.S. Department of Health and Human Services
National Institutes of Health
National Institute of Dental and Craniofacial Research
Division of Intramural Research (Oral Infection and Immunity Branch)
Bldg. 30, Rm. 332
30 Convent Dr., MSC 4352
Bethesda, MD 20892-4352
Phone: (301)496-9218 **Fax:** (301)402-1064
Email: sharon.wahl@nih.gov
Website: http://wwwdir.nidcr.nih.gov/dirweb/oiib/oiib.asp
Dr. Sharon M. Wahl, Dir.
Activities/Fields: Infectious pathogens, their unique attributes and virulence factors to provide insight into mechanisms of disarming them, especially the mucosal immune system.

★ 25339 ★ U.S. Department of Health and Human Services
National Institutes of Health
National Institute of Dental and Craniofacial Research
Division of Intramural Research (Proteases and Tissue Remodeling Unit)
Bldg. 30, Rm. 211
30 Convent Dr., MSC 4340
Bethesda, MD 20892-4340
Phone: (301)435-1840 **Fax:** (301)402-0823
Email: thomas.bugge@nih.gov
Website: http://wwwdir.nidcr.nih.gov/dirweb/opcb/ptru.asp
Dr. Thomas Bugge, Ch.

Activities/Fields: Understanding the function of matrix degrading proteolytic enzymes in physiological and pathological tissue remodeling processes, including cancer invasion and metastasis.

★ 25340 ★ U.S. Department of Health and Human Services National Institutes of Health National Institute of Dental and Craniofacial Research Division of Intramural Research (Molecular and Cellular Biochemistry Unit)

Bldg. 30, Rm. 211
30 Convent Dr., MSC 4340
Bethesda, MD 20892-4340
Phone: (301)496-4069 **Fax:** (301)402-0823
Email: mpark@yoda.nidcr.nih.gov
Website: http://wwwdir.nidcr.nih.gov/dirweb/opcb/mcbu.asp
Dr. Myung Hee Park, Dir.

Activities/Fields: Understanding normal control mechanisms underlying regulation of proliferation, differentiation and apoptosis of human oral keratinocytes and the multistep genotypic and phenotypic changes associated with oral carcinogenesis.

★ 25341 ★ U.S. Department of Health and Human Services National Institutes of Health National Institute of Dental and Craniofacial Research Division of Intramural Research (Peptide and Immunochemistry Unit)

Bldg. 30, Rm. B17B
30 Convent Dr., MSC 4340
Bethesda, MD 20892-4340
Phone: (301)496-4779 **Fax:** (301)402-0823
Email: frank.robey@nih.gov
Website: http://wwwdir.nidcr.nih.gov/dirweb/opcb/piu.asp
Dr. Frank Robey, Ch.

Activities/Fields: AIDS and cancer immunology, including immunosuppression in oral cancer.

★ 25342 ★ U.S. Department of Health and Human Services National Institutes of Health National Institute of Dental and Craniofacial Research Division of Intramural Research (Molecular Carcinogenesis Unit)

Bldg. 30, Rm. 211
30 Convent Dr., MSC 4340
Bethesda, MD 20892-4340
Phone: (301)496-6259 **Fax:** (301)402-0823
Email: silvio.gutkind@nih.gov
Website: http://wwwdir.nidcr.nih.gov/dirweb/opcb/mcs.asp
Dr. J. Silvio Gutkind, Ch.

Activities/Fields: Oral and pharyngeal cancer, including molecular mechanisms involved in squamous cell carcinogenesis.

★ 25343 ★ U.S. Department of Health and Human Services National Institutes of Health National Institute of Dental and Craniofacial Research Division of Intramural Research (Oral and Pharyngeal Cancer Branch)

Bldg. 30, Rm. 211
30 Convent Dr., MSC 4340
Bethesda, MD 20892-4340
Phone: (301)496-6259 **Fax:** (301)402-0823
Email: silvio.gutkind@nih.gov
Website: http://wwwdir.nidcr.nih.gov/dirweb/opcb/opcbhome.asp
J. Silvio Gutkind, PhD, Ch.

Activities/Fields: Normal and aberrant functions of tissues, cells, and molecules as they relate to oral disease states, with emphasis on etiology, diagnosis, treatment, and prevention of oral tumors.

★ 25344 ★ U.S. Department of Health and Human Services National Institutes of Health National Institute of Dental and Craniofacial Research Division of Intramural Research (Cell Growth Regulation Section)

Bldg. 30, Rm. Rm. 211
30 Convent Dr., MSC 4340
Bethesda, MD 20892-4340
Phone: (301)496-6259 **Fax:** (301)402-0823
Email: silvio.gutkind@nih.gov
Website: http://wwwdir.nidcr.nih.gov/dirweb/opcb/cgr.asp
Dr. J. Silvio Gutkind, Ch.

Activities/Fields: Oral and pharyngeal cancer, including molecular mechanisms controlling normal and aberrant cell growth.

★ 25345 ★ U.S. Department of Health and Human Services National Institutes of Health National Institute of Dental and Craniofacial Research Division of Intramural Research (Craniofacial Epidemiology and Genetics Branch)

Bldg. 30
30 Convent Dr., MSC 4326
Bethesda, MD 20892-4326
Phone: (301)496-1483 **Fax:** (301)402-1512
Email: henning.birkedal-hansen@nih.gov
Henning Birkedal-Hansen, DDS, Actg. Ch.

Activities/Fields: Seeks to improve and promote dental, oral and craniofacial health through epidemiology and health promotion.

★ 25346 ★ U.S. Department of Health and Human Services National Institutes of Health National Institute of Dental and Craniofacial Research Division of Intramural Research (Molecular and Genetic Epidemiology Section)

Bldg. 45, Rm. 4AS-43G
45 Center Dr., MSC 6401
Bethesda, MD 20892-6401
Phone: (301)594-4830 **Fax:** (301)480-8327
Email: sd31d@nih.gov
Dr. Scott R. Diehl, Contact

Activities/Fields: Basic causes of oral and craniofacial disorders, involving environmental risk factors such as smoking, drinking, and genetics. Research is focused on cleft lip and palate, Kartagener syndrome, early onset periodontitis, oral cancers, and nasopharyngeal carcinoma.

★ 25347 ★ U.S. Department of Health and Human Services National Institutes of Health National Institute of Dental and Craniofacial Research Division of Intramural Research

Bldg. 30, Rm. 132
30 Convent Dr., MSC 4326
Bethesda, MD 20892-4326
Phone: (301)496-1483 **Fax:** (301)402-1512
Email: henning.birkedal-hansen@nih.gov
Website: http://wwwdir.nidcr.nih.gov/dirweb/dirhome.asp
Henning Birkedal-Hansen, DDS, Dir.

Activities/Fields: Investigates biochemistry, structure, function and development of bone, teeth, salivary glands and connective tissues; studies role of bacteria and viruses in oral disease; genetic disorders and tumors of the oral cavity; cause and treatment of acute and chronic pain; development of new methods to diagnose oral diseases.

★ 25348 ★ U.S. Department of Health and Human Services National Institutes of Health National Institute of Diabetes and Digestive and Kidney Diseases Diabetic Nephropathy Program

2 Democracy Blvd., Rm. 639
Bethesda, MD 20892
Phone: (301)594-7713
Email: kimmelp@extra.niddk.nih.gov
Website: http://www.niddk.nih.gov/fund/program/A-Elist.htmdianep
Paul L. Kimmel, MD, Dir.

Activities/Fields: Pathophysiology and pathogenesis of diabetic nephropathy, natural history studies, and clinical trials through R01 mechanism, including molecular pathogenesis of extracellular matrix expansion and glomerulosclerosis, the role of the renin-angiotension system and growth factors, and the identification of treatments to prevent renal scarring.

★ 25349 ★ U.S. Department of Health and Human Services National Institutes of Health National Institute of Diabetes and Digestive and Kidney Diseases Division of Diabetes, Endocrinology, and Metabolic Diseases (Developmental Biology Research Program)

2 Democracy Plz., Rm. 6105
Bethesda, MD 20892
Phone: (301)594-8811
Email: satos@extra.niddk.nih.gov
Website: http://www.niddk.nih.gov/fund/program/A-Elist.htmdevelop
Sheryl Sato, PhD, Dir.

Activities/Fields: Understanding the signaling pathways and transcriptional programs underlying the formation of tissues and organs.

★ 25350 ★ U.S. Department of Health and Human Services National Institutes of Health National Institute of Diabetes and Digestive and Kidney Diseases Division of Diabetes, Endocrinology, and Metabolic Diseases (Endocrine Pancreas Program)

MSC-5460
6707 Democracy Blvd., Rm. 697
Bethesda, MD 20892-5460
Phone: (301)594-8802 **Fax:** (301)480-3503
Email: laughlinm@extra.niddk.nih.gov
Website: http://www.niddk.nih.gov/fund/program/A-Elist.htmendo
Maren Laughlin, PhD, Dir.

Activities/Fields: Endocrine cells (alpha, beta, delta, etc.) of the pancreas and the islets.

★ 25351 ★ U.S. Department of Health and Human Services National Institutes of Health National Institute of Diabetes and Digestive and Kidney Diseases Division of Diabetes, Endocrinology, and Metabolic Diseases (Cytoarchitecture and Matrix Research Program)

2 Democracy Plz., Rm. 6105
Bethesda, MD 20892
Phone: (301)594-8811
Email: satos@extra.niddk.nih.gov

Website: http://www.niddk.nih.gov/fund/program/A-Elist.htmAIDS
Sheryl Sato, PhD, Dir.
Activities/Fields: Properties and functions of intracellular and extracellular, filamentous suprastructures that are involved in hormone signaling and endocrine and metabolic disorders.

★ 25352 ★ U.S. Department of Health and Human Services
National Institutes of Health
National Institute of Diabetes and Digestive and Kidney Diseases
Division of Diabetes, Endocrinology, and Metabolic Diseases
(Bone and Mineral Research Program)
2 Democracy Plaza, Rm. 603
Bethesda, MD 20892
Phone: (301)451-9871 **Fax:** (301)480-3503
Email: mt270t@extra.niddk.nih.gov
Website: http://www.niddk.nih.gov/fund/program/A-Elist.htmb&m
Mehrdad Tondravi, PhD, Dir.
Activities/Fields: Basic and clinical research on the hormonal regulation of bone and mineral metabolism in health and disease.

★ 25353 ★ U.S. Department of Health and Human Services
National Institutes of Health
National Institute of Diabetes and Digestive and Kidney Diseases
Division of Diabetes, Endocrinology, and Metabolic Diseases
(Complications of Diabetes Program)
2 Democracy Plz., Rm. 699
Bethesda, MD 20892
Phone: (301)594-0021
Email: abrahamk@extra.niddk.nih.gov
Website: http://www.niddk.nih.gov/fund/program/A-Elist.htmcomplications
Kristin Abraham, PhD, Dir.
Activities/Fields: Classical diabetic complications and the effect of diabetes on any organ system.

★ 25354 ★ U.S. Department of Health and Human Services
National Institutes of Health
National Institute of Diabetes and Digestive and Kidney Diseases
Division of Diabetes, Endocrinology, and Metabolic Diseases
(Acquired Immunodeficiency Syndrome (AIDS) and Human Immunodeficiency Virus (HIV) Program)
2 Democracy Plz., Rm. 669
Bethesda, MD 20892
Phone: (301)594-8877
Email: hamiltonf@ep.niddk.nih.gov
Website: http://www.niddk.nih.gov/program/A-Elist.htmauto
Frank Hamilton, MD, Dir.
Activities/Fields: Characterization of intestinal injury, mechanisms of maldigestion, and intestinal mucosal functions, as well as hepatic and biliary dysfunction in patients with AIDS or in appropriate animal models.

★ 25355 ★ U.S. Department of Health and Human Services
National Institutes of Health
National Institute of Diabetes and Digestive and Kidney Diseases
Division of Diabetes, Endocrinology, and Metabolic Diseases
(Behavioral Research Program)
2 Democracy Plz.
Bethesda, MD 20892
Email: garfields@extra.niddk.nih.gov
Website: http://www.niddk.nih.gov/fund/program/A-Elist.htmbehavioral
Sanford Garfield, Sr. Adv.
Activities/Fields: Individual, family, and community-based strategies aimed at prevention of diabetes and its complications through lifestyle modifications, education, and other behavioral interventions, particularly on development of culturally sensitive, lifestyle interventions to prevent or treat diabetes in diverse high-risk populations including African-Americans, Hispanic Americans, and Native Americans.

★ 25356 ★ U.S. Department of Health and Human Services
National Institutes of Health
National Institute of Diabetes and Digestive and Kidney Diseases
Division of Diabetes, Endocrinology, and Metabolic Diseases
(Adipocyte Biology Research Program)
DEM 2/605
Bethesda, MD 20892
Phone: (301)594-7689 **Fax:** (301)435-6047
Email: naftc@extra.niddk.nih.gov
Website: http://www.niddk.nih.gov/fund/program/A-Elist.htmadipocyte
Carol Haft, PhD, Dir.
Activities/Fields: Development and physiology of the adipocyte cell, including studies on the properties of transcription factors that regulate adipocyte differentiation; consequences of insulin action on adipocyte physiology; and use of animal and tissue culture models to understand adipocyte biology.

★ 25357 ★ U.S. Department of Health and Human Services
National Institutes of Health
National Institute of Diabetes and Digestive and Kidney Diseases
Division of Diabetes, Endocrinology, and Metabolic Diseases
(Transcriptional Regulation of Metabolic Pathways Program)
2 Democracy Pl., Rm. 6105
Bethesda, MD 20892
Phone: (301)594-8811
Email: satos@extra.niddk.nih.gov
Website: http://www.niddk.nih.gov/fund/program/S-Zlist.htmTRMP
Sheryl Sato, PhD, Dir.
Activities/Fields: Understanding the significance of gene regulation to control of metabolism. Specific areas of support include (1) identifying and characterizing transcription factors and cis-acting regulatory elements in DNA using structural and functional approaches; (2) identifying mechanisms whereby signal transduction pathways elicit changes in gene expression; and (3) identifying the molecular response to environmental cues including hormonal stimulation, nutrients, development, and stress.

★ 25358 ★ U.S. Department of Health and Human Services
National Institutes of Health
National Institute of Diabetes and Digestive and Kidney Diseases
Division of Diabetes, Endocrinology, and Metabolic Diseases
(Type 2 Diabetes in the Pediatric Population Program)
2 Democracy Pl., Rm. 699
Bethesda, MD 20892
Phone: (301)594-0021
Email: linderb@extra.niddk.nih.gov
Website: http://www.niddk.nih.gov/fund/program/S-Zlist.htm
Barbara Linder, MD, Dir.
Activities/Fields: Pathophysiology, prevention, and treatment of Type 2 diabetes in children.

★ 25359 ★ U.S. Department of Health and Human Services
National Institutes of Health
National Institute of Diabetes and Digestive and Kidney Diseases
Division of Diabetes, Endocrinology, and Metabolic Diseases
(Thyroid Research Program)
2 Democracy Pl., Rm. 699
Bethesda, MD 20892
Phone: (301)594-0021
Email: linderb@extra.niddk.nih.gov
Website: http://www.niddk.nih.gov/fund/program/S-Zlist.htm
Barbara Linder, PhD, Dir.
Activities/Fields: Normal thyroid physiology and nonautoimmune thyroid disease including thyroid neoplasia. Specific areas of support include (1) physiologic regulation of the expression, processing, and secretion of thyroid hormones; (2) dysfunctional regulation of thyroid hormones that results in disease; (3) studies of the etiology, pathogenesis, diagnosis, and therapy of thyroid disorders; (4) studies on the deiodinase enzymes that convert inactive thyroid hormone to active thyroid hormone; and (5) studies on neural cells that are targets of regulation by and feedback to the thyroid.

★ 25360 ★ U.S. Department of Health and Human Services
National Institutes of Health
National Institute of Diabetes and Digestive and Kidney Diseases
Division of Diabetes, Endocrinology, and Metabolic Diseases
(Steroid Metabolism Program)
MSC 5460
2 Democracy Pl., Rm. 603
Bethesda, MD 20892-5460
Phone: (301)451-9871 **Fax:** (301)480-3503
Email: mt270t@nih.gov
Website: http://www.niddk.nih.gov/fund/program/S-Zlist.htm
Mehrdah Tondraui, PhD, Dir.
Activities/Fields: Biochemistry, molecular biology, genetics, metabolism, and biological function of steroids and similar molecules derived from cholesterol, including sex steroids and other hormones (glucocorticoids, mineralocorticoids), retinoids, cardiac glycosides, prostaglandins, eicosanoids, and bile acids. Specific areas of support include (1) structure and reaction mechanisms of enzymes and enzyme-substrate complexes in steroidogenesis and steroid interconversion pathways; (2) cholesterol activation for steroidogenesis, including cholesterol esterase and intramitochondrial translocation of cholesterol; (3) structure, function, and reaction mechanism of the p450 class of enzymes; (4) estrogens and androgens in development; and (5) structure and function of the mitochondrial cytochromes.

★ 25361 ★ U.S. Department of Health and Human Services
National Institutes of Health
National Institute of Diabetes and Digestive and Kidney Diseases
Division of Diabetes, Endocrinology, and Metabolic Diseases
(Therapeutic Approaches to Diabetes Mellitus Program)
MSC 5460
6707 Democracy Blvd., Rm. 6101
Bethesda, MD 20892-5460
Phone: (301)594-8802 **Fax:** (301)480-3503
Email: laughlinm@extra.niddk.nih.gov
Website: http://www.niddk.nih.gov/fund/program/S-Zlist.htm
Maren Laughlin, PhD, Dir.
Activities/Fields: Therapeutic approaches to achieving euglycemia. Specific areas of support include (1) studies on drug development; (2) transplantation of pancreas or pancreatic endocrine cells (islets or beta

cells); (3) glucose sensors (including their combination with insulin delivery systems to provide a closed-loop system); (4) cellular therapy, (including gene therapy approaches) that is being proposed to treat or prevent either type 1 or type 2 diabetes; (5) studies in cell culture to bioengineer or genetically manipulate cells to produce an insulin secreting cell or a glucose-responsive insulin secreting cell for the eventual treatment of diabetes; and (6) creation of animal models for therapeutic trials.

★ 25362 ★ U.S. Department of Health and Human Services
National Institutes of Health
National Institute of Diabetes and Digestive and Kidney Diseases
Division of Diabetes, Endocrinology, and Metabolic Diseases
(Reproductive Endocrinology Program)
2 Democracy Pl., Rm. 699
Bethesda, MD 20892
Phone: (301)594-0021
Email: linderb@extra.niddk.nih.gov
Website: http://www.niddk.nih.gov/program/M-Rlist.htmreproendo
Barbara Linder, MD, Dir.
Activities/Fields: Structure and function of gonadotropins including LH, FSH, and hCG and their receptors. Specific areas of support include (1) oligosaccharide modification and its effects on gonadotropin function; (2) metabolic responses of target tissue (e.g., prostate); (3) studies on the interaction of gonadotropins with their receptors; (4) physiological effects of the hormones (e.g., menopause, age at onset of menstruation); and (5) development and study of analogs of gonadotropins.

★ 25363 ★ U.S. Department of Health and Human Services
National Institutes of Health
National Institute of Diabetes and Digestive and Kidney Diseases
Division of Diabetes, Endocrinology, and Metabolic Diseases
(Protein Trafficing/Secretion/Processing Research Program)
2 Democracy Pl., Rm. 6101
Bethesda, MD 20892
Phone: (301)594-7689 **Fax:** (301)435-6047
Email: haftc@extra.niddk.nih.gov
Website: http://www.niddk.nih.gov/fund/program/M-Rlist.htm
Carol Haft, PhD, Dir.
Activities/Fields: Understanding the mechanisms accounting for the fate of proteins after initial translation. Specific areas of support include (1) protein folding; (2) post-translational modifications and the enzymes that catalyze them; (3) movement of proteins in vesicles from endoplasmic reticulum (ER) through the golgi and endosomes and their ultimate secretion; (4) mechanisms that account for vesicle formation (pinching-off) and vesicle fusion, which are paramount to understanding trafficking; (5) movement of proteins in the direction opposite of secretion, including endocytosis and retrograde transport; (6) proteins and small molecules that regulate protein trafficking; and (7) proteasomes, ubiquitin conjugation, and the N-end rule.

★ 25364 ★ U.S. Department of Health and Human Services
National Institutes of Health
National Institute of Diabetes and Digestive and Kidney Diseases
Division of Diabetes, Endocrinology, and Metabolic Diseases
(Regulation of Energy Balance and Body Composition Program)
MSC 5460
6707 Democracy Blvd., Rm. 693
Bethesda, MD 20892-5460
Phone: (301)594-8816 **Fax:** (301)480-3503
Email: smithp@.extra.niddk.nih.gov
Website: http://www.niddk.nih.gov/fund/program/M-Rlist.htm
Philip Smith, PhD, Dep. Dir
Activities/Fields: Regulation of body composition by the hypothalamus and circulating factors. Specific areas of support include (1) endocrinology of body composition including interactions between nutrition, exercise, and anabolic hormones; (2) neuropeptides and their receptors involved in regulatory pathways controlling feeding behavior, satiety, and energy expenditure; (3) interactions between hypothalamic-pituitary-adrenal axis and peripheral metabolic signals (e.g., insulin, leptin, glucocorticoids); (4) hormones and cytokines involved in wasting syndromes (cancer); (5) endocrine regulation of energy balance via uncoupling proteins; and (6) hypothalamic integration of peripheral endocrine and metabolic signals.

★ 25365 ★ U.S. Department of Health and Human Services
National Institutes of Health
National Institute of Diabetes and Digestive and Kidney Diseases
Division of Diabetes, Endocrinology, and Metabolic Diseases
(Protein Metabolism Program)
MSC 5460
6707 Democracy Blvd., Rm. 6101
Bethesda, MD 20892-5460
Phone: (301)594-8802 **Fax:** (301)480-3503
Email: laughlinm@.extra.niddk.nih.gov
Website: http://www.niddk.nih.gov/fund/program/M-Rlist.htm
Maren Laughlin, PhD, Dir.
Activities/Fields: Basic and clinical studies of protein, peptide, and amino acid metabolism, as well as studies of purified protein structure, kinetics, function, and enzyme reaction mechanism, including hormone regulation, effects of diet and exercise, and the pathology associated with metabolic diseases. Specific areas of support include (1) studies of flux or regulation of total protein synthesis and turnover in health and disease, including investigations of the specific enzymes of protein and amino acid metabolism; (2) amino acid and peptide membrane transport; (3) uptake, metabolism, and synthesis of specific amino acids; (4) regulation of urea production and nitrogen balance; (5) role of cofactors, vitamins, and minerals in metabolism and enzyme action; and (6) structure of specific classes of enzymes (redox, phosphate transfer, etc.) elucidated by x-ray, NMR, or electron microscopy.

★ 25366 ★ U.S. Department of Health and Human Services
National Institutes of Health
National Institute of Diabetes and Digestive and Kidney Diseases
Division of Diabetes, Endocrinology, and Metabolic Diseases
(Neuroendocrinology Program)
MSC 5460
2 Democracy Pl., Rm. 6105
Bethesda, MD 20892
Phone: (301)594-8811 **Fax:** (301)480-3503
Email: satos@extra.niddk.nih.gov
Website: http://www.niddk.nih.gov/program/M-Rlist.htmneuroendo
Sheryl Sato, PhD, Dir.
Activities/Fields: Neuropeptides of the hypothalamus. Specific areas of research support include (1) physiological response to stress through the hypothalamic-pituitary-adrenal axis; (2) neuropeptides and neuropeptide receptor signalling pathways; (3) gene regulation in the hypothalamus and pituitary gland; (4) diseases of the pituitary including neoplasia; (5) hypopituitary dwarfism; (6) identification and characterization of novel hypothalamic or pituitary hormones; (7) tissue specific and developmental expression of pituitary and hypothalamic genes; (8) pituitary hormone receptors and actions on target tissues (eg., GH IGF-1 axis); (9) neuropeptide receptors in diagnosis and treatment of disease; and (10) neuroendocrine-immune interactions.

★ 25367 ★ U.S. Department of Health and Human Services
National Institutes of Health
National Institute of Diabetes and Digestive and Kidney Diseases
Division of Diabetes, Endocrinology, and Metabolic Diseases
(Nuclear Hormone Superfamily Program)
MSC 5460
6707 Democracy Blvd., Rm. 6107
Bethesda, MD 20892-5460
Phone: (301)594-8819 **Fax:** (301)480-6047
Email: margolisr@extra.niddk.nih.gov
Website: http://www.niddk.nih.gov/fund/program/M-Rlist.htm
Ronald Margolis, PhD, Sr. Adv.
Activities/Fields: Basic and clinical research on members of the steroid hormone superfamily (also known as the nuclear receptor superfamily), including structure/function studies and the role in signal transduction and regulation of gene expression of the steroid hormones including glucocorticoids, mineralocorticoids, progesterone, estrogens, androgens (testosterone, DHEA) and the nuclear receptors including thyroid hormone, vitamin D, retinoids (RAR, RXR, vitamin A), PPARs, and orphan receptors (LXR, Nur77, COUP-TF, and others).

★ 25368 ★ U.S. Department of Health and Human Services
National Institutes of Health
National Institute of Diabetes and Digestive and Kidney Diseases
Division of Diabetes, Endocrinology, and Metabolic Diseases
(Lipid Metabolism Program)
MSC 5460
6707 Democracy Blvd., Rm. 6101
Bethesda, MD 20892-5460
Phone: (301)594-8802 **Fax:** (301)480-3503
Email: laughlinm@.extra.niddk.nih.gov
Website: http://www.niddk.nih.gov/fund/program/F-Llist.htm
Maren Laughlin, PhD, Dir.
Activities/Fields: Basic and clinical studies of the metabolism of fatty acid, triacylglycerols, cholesterol, and related molecules, which will lead to the development of effective treatments for diabetes, obesity, hypertriglyceridemia, hypercholesterolemia, burn injury, sepsis, and other metabolic diseases. Specific areas of support include (1) flux and regulation of oxidation, storage, and remodeling of dietary lipids in health and disease, and effects of diet and exercise; (2) regulation of lipid esterification, hormone-sensitive lipases, and phospholipid metabolism; (3) membrane transport and movement of lipids within the cell, or between organs (binding proteins, carnitine transferases); (4) lipid-protein interactions; (5) metabolism of bioactive lipids and their precursors; and (6) lipid peroxidation, especially associated with disease.

★ 25369 ★ U.S. Department of Health and Human Services
National Institutes of Health
National Institute of Diabetes and Digestive and Kidney Diseases
Division of Diabetes, Endocrinology, and Metabolic Diseases
(Minority Health Program)
6707 Democracy Blvd.
Bethesda, MD 20892
Phone: (301)496-4000
Email: agodoal@extra.niddk.nih.gov
Website: http://www.niddk.nih.gov/fund/program/M-Rlist.htmmhp
Lawrence Y. Agodoa, MD, Dir.

Activities/Fields: Disease that disproportionately affect minority populations, especially pathogenesis mechanisms, risk factors, and potential treatments for renal disease and hypertension, kidney disease of diabetes, and hemoglobinopathies such as sickle cell disease.

★ 25370 ★ U.S. Department of Health and Human Services
National Institutes of Health
National Institute of Diabetes and Digestive and Kidney Diseases
Division of Diabetes, Endocrinology, and Metabolic Diseases
(Intracellular Signal Transduction Research Program)
2 Democracy Pl., Rm. 607
Bethesda, MD 20892
Phone: (301)594-8817
Email: abrahamk@extra.niddk.nih.gov
Website: http://www.niddk.nih.gov/fund/program/F-Llist.htm
Kristin Abraham, PhD, Dir.
Activities/Fields: Understanding the structure and function of intracellular signal transducing molecules. Specific areas of support include (1) intracellular kinases, phosphatases, and anchoring proteins; (2) signaling mechanisms that have altered activity in response to protein phosphorylation, Ca2+ and cAMP; (3) approaches to solving the three-dimensional structure of signaling proteins including crystallography and NMR; (4) functional analysis of these proteins including comparison of wild-type and naturally occurring or synthetic, mutant proteins or expression of dominant-negative forms of the proteins; (5) microscopic techniques to localize these proteins within cells; (6) identification of substrates for these signaling proteins; and (7) analysis of crosstalk among distinct signal transduction pathways.

★ 25371 ★ U.S. Department of Health and Human Services
National Institutes of Health
National Institute of Diabetes and Digestive and Kidney Diseases
Division of Diabetes, Endocrinology, and Metabolic Diseases
(Insulin Receptor/Structure/Function/Action Program)
MSC 5460
2 Democracy Pl., Rm. 607
Bethesda, MD 20892-5460
Phone: (301)594-8817 **Fax:** (301)480-6047
Email: abrahamk@extra.niddk.nih.gov
Website: http://www.niddk.nih.gov/program/F-Llist.htminsulinRSFA
Kristin Abraham, PhD, Dir.
Activities/Fields: Structure, function, and action of the insulin receptor, including molecular analysis of ligand binding to receptor; activation of tyrosine kinase; subsequent insulin receptor function in signal transduction by serving as a platform for the attachment of downstream signaling molecules involved in insulin action; and the Insulin Receptor Signaling proteins ((IRS)-1,2,3,4) and other proteins containing Src Homology Domains (e.g., Sh(2)).

★ 25372 ★ U.S. Department of Health and Human Services
National Institutes of Health
National Institute of Diabetes and Digestive and Kidney Diseases
Division of Diabetes, Endocrinology, and Metabolic Diseases
(Insulin Resistance Program)
MSC 5460
6707 Democracy Blvd., Rm. 6101
Bethesda, MD 20892-5460
Phone: (301)594-8802 **Fax:** (301)480-3503
Email: laughinm@extra.niddk.nih.gov
Website: http://www.niddk.nih.gov/program/F-Llist.htminsulin
Maren Laughlin, PhD, Dir.
Activities/Fields: Role of insulin resistance in the pathogenesis of type 2 diabetes mellitus; relationship between insulin resistance and obesity; relationship between insulin resistance and physical activity; new methods to measure peripheral insulin resistance; molecular basis of decreased sensitivity to insulin; insulin receptor desensitization; uncoupling of receptor activation to downstream events; and animal models of insulin resistance.

★ 25373 ★ U.S. Department of Health and Human Services
National Institutes of Health
National Institute of Diabetes and Digestive and Kidney Diseases
Division of Diabetes, Endocrinology, and Metabolic Diseases
(Inborn Errors of Metabolism Program)
MS 5460
6707 Democracy Blvd., Rm. 6103
Bethesda, MD 20892-5460
Phone: (301)594-8810 **Fax:** (301)480-3503
Email: mckeonc@extra.niddk.nih.gov
Website: http://www.niddk.nih.gov/fund/program/F-Llist.htm
Catherine McKeon, PhD, Sr. Adv.
Activities/Fields: Pathophysiology and treatment of genetic metabolic diseases; including studies of etiology, pathogenesis, prevention, diagnosis, pathophysiology, and treatment of these diseases; characterization of the genes, gene defects, and regulatory alterations that underlie causes of these diseases; studies of the mutant enzyme and its effect on the structure and function of the protein; development of animal models for genetic disease; development of dietary, pharmacologic, and enzyme replacement therapies; and development of stem cell transplantation, both prenatally and postnatally, as a treatment for metabolic diseases.

★ 25374 ★ U.S. Department of Health and Human Services
National Institutes of Health
National Institute of Diabetes and Digestive and Kidney Diseases
Division of Diabetes, Endocrinology, and Metabolic Diseases
(Growth Factor/Receptor/Structure/Function Program)
MSC 5460
6707 Democracy Blvd., Rm. 693
Bethesda, MD 20892-5460
Phone: (301)594-8816 **Fax:** (301)480-3503
Email: smithp@extra.niddk.nih.gov
Website: http://www.niddk.nih.gov/fund/program/F-Llist.htm
Philip Smith, PhD, Dir.
Activities/Fields: Growth factors and cytokines and their receptors, binding proteins, and inhibitors. Specific areas of support include regulation of expression of growth factors and their receptors in endocrine cells and tissues; structure/function studies; role of growth factors in endocrine tumor progression; identification of genes that are downstream targets of growth factor receptor activation; modulation of growth factor action by binding proteins; autocrine and paracrine actions of growth factors and cytokines to regulate cell/tissue growth and function.

★ 25375 ★ U.S. Department of Health and Human Services
National Institutes of Health
National Institute of Diabetes and Digestive and Kidney Diseases
Division of Diabetes, Endocrinology, and Metabolic Diseases
(Hypoglycemia Program)
MSC 5460
2 Democracy Pl., Rm. 699
Bethesda, MD 20892
Phone: (301)594-0021 **Fax:** (301)480-3503
Email: linder@extra.niddk.nih.gov
Website: http://www.niddk.nih.gov/fund/program/A-Elist.htm
Barbara Linder, PhD, Dir.
Activities/Fields: Pathogenesis, prevention, treatment, and sequelae of hypoglycemia (low blood glucose) in both type 1 and type 2 diabetes.

★ 25376 ★ U.S. Department of Health and Human Services
National Institutes of Health
National Institute of Diabetes and Digestive and Kidney Diseases
Division of Diabetes, Endocrinology, and Metabolic Diseases
(Glucose Transport Program)
DEM 2605
6707 Democracy Blvd., Rm. 6101
Bethesda, MD 20892
Phone: (301)594-7689 **Fax:** (301)453-6047
Email: haftc@extra.niddk.nih.gov
Website: http://www.niddk.nih.gov/fund/program/F-Llist.htm
Carol Haft, PhD, Dir.
Activities/Fields: Glucose transport in health and disease, especially as relating to glucose homeostasis in diabetes and obesity.

★ 25377 ★ U.S. Department of Health and Human Services
National Institutes of Health
National Institute of Diabetes and Digestive and Kidney Diseases
Division of Diabetes, Endocrinology, and Metabolic Diseases
(Genetics of Diabetes Program)
6707 Democracy Blvd., Rm. 6103
Bethesda, MD 20892-5460
Phone: (301)594-8810 **Fax:** (301)480-3503
Email: mckeonc@extra.niddk.nih.gov
Website: http://www.niddk.nih.gov/fund/program/F-Llist.htm
Catherine McKeon, PhD, Sr. Adv.
Activities/Fields: Identification of genes that contribute to type 1 and 2 diabetes mellitus.

★ 25378 ★ U.S. Department of Health and Human Services
National Institutes of Health
National Institute of Diabetes and Digestive and Kidney Diseases
Division of Diabetes, Endocrinology, and Metabolic Diseases
(Glucose Metabolism Program)
MSC-5460
6707 Democracy Blvd., Rm. 6101
Bethesda, MD 20892-5460
Phone: (301)594-8802 **Fax:** (301)480-3503
Email: laughlinm@extra.niddk.nih.gov
Website: http://www.niddk.nih.gov/fund/program/F-Llist.htm
Maren Laughlin, PhD, Dir.
Activities/Fields: Glucose and glycogen metabolism; development of effective treatments for diabetes, glycogen storage disease, obesity, burn injury, sepsis and trauma, and other metabolic diseases.

★ 25379 ★ U.S. Department of Health and Human Services
National Institutes of Health
National Institute of Diabetes and Digestive and Kidney Diseases
Division of Diabetes, Endocrinology, and Metabolic Diseases
(Gene Therapy and Cystic Fibrosis Centers Program)
MSC-5460
6707 Democracy Blvd., Rm. 6103
Bethesda, MD 20892-5460
Phone: (301)594-8810 **Fax:** (301)480-3503
Email: mckeonc@extra.niddk.nih.gov
Website: http://www.niddk.nih.gov/fund/program/F-Llist.htm
Catherine McKeon, PhD, Sr. Adv.
Activities/Fields: Development of gene therapy techniques; fosters multidisciplinary collaboration in the development of clinical trials for the treatment of cystic fibrosis and other genetic metabolic diseases.

★ 25380 ★ U.S. Department of Health and Human Services
National Institutes of Health
National Institute of Diabetes and Digestive and Kidney Diseases
Division of Diabetes, Endocrinology, and Metabolic Diseases
(Genetics of Complications Program)
2 Democracy Pl., Rm. 699
Bethesda, MD 20892
Phone: (301)594-0021
Email: linderb@extra.niddk.nih.gov
Website: http://www.niddk.nih.gov/fund/program/A-Elist.htmepidT2
Barbara Linder, MD, Dir.
Activities/Fields: Discovery of genes that increase an individual's susceptibility to complications of diabetes. Basic mechanisms involved organs including kidneys, nervous system, eye, and vasculature.

★ 25381 ★ U.S. Department of Health and Human Services
National Institutes of Health
National Institute of Diabetes and Digestive and Kidney Diseases
Division of Diabetes, Endocrinology, and Metabolic Diseases
(Gene Therapy Program)
MSC-2560
Bldg. 31, Rm 9A04 Center Drive
Bethesda, MD 20892-5460
Phone: (301)594-8810 **Fax:** (301)480-3503
Email: mckeonc@extra.niddk.nih.gov
Website: http://www.niddk.nih.gov/fund/program/F-Llist.htm
Catherine McKeon, PhD, Sr. Adv.
Activities/Fields: Development of basic and applied gene therapy for genetic metabolic diseases, particularly pilot and feasibility studies to improve gene delivery systems; basic science of AAV, adenovirus, retrovirus, and lentivirus vectors; nonviral methods of gene transfer such as liposomes or DNA conjugates; studies targeting gene delivery to specific cell types; gene therapy of stem cells to treat genetic metabolic disease.

★ 25382 ★ U.S. Department of Health and Human Services
National Institutes of Health
National Institute of Diabetes and Digestive and Kidney Diseases
Division of Diabetes, Endocrinology, and Metabolic Diseases
(Epidemiology Type 2 Diabetes Research Program)
MSC-5460
6707 Democracy Blvd., Rm. 695
Bethesda, MD 20892-5460
Phone: (301)594-8801 **Fax:** (301)480-3503
Email: linderb@extra.niddk.nih.gov
Website: http://www.niddk.nih.gov/fund/program/A-Elist.htmepidT2
Barbara Linder, PhD, Dir.
Activities/Fields: Distribution and determinants of Type 2 diabetes, gestational diabetes, and complications of diabetes in populations, including community-based groups and large patient populations.

★ 25383 ★ U.S. Department of Health and Human Services
National Institutes of Health
National Institute of Diabetes and Digestive and Kidney Diseases
Division of Diabetes, Endocrinology, and Metabolic Diseases
(G-Protein Coupled Receptors Program)
MSC-5460
2 Democracy Plz., Rm. 607
Bethesda, MD 20892
Phone: (301)594-8817 **Fax:** (301)435-6047
Email: abrahamk@extra.niddk.nih.gov
Website: http://www.niddk.nih.gov/fund/program/F-Llist.htm
Kristin Abraham, PhD, Dir.
Activities/Fields: Studies on the G-protein coupled receptor superfamily, particularly cell surface, or seven transmembrane domain (7-TM), receptors coupled to GTP-binding ("G")-proteins for signal transduction; receptor structure; receptor down-regulation; role(s) of mutated receptors in disease; coupling of signaling through the receptor to other membrane-bound effectors or regulators such as adenylyl cyclase, ion channels, protein phosphatases or kinases, and other receptors.

★ 25384 ★ U.S. Department of Health and Human Services
National Institutes of Health
National Institute of Diabetes and Digestive and Kidney Diseases
Division of Diabetes, Endocrinology, and Metabolic Diseases
(Epidemiology Type 1 Diabetes Research Program)
Bldg. 31, Rm 9A04
MSC 2560
Bethesda, MD 20892-2560
Phone: (301)594-8801 **Fax:** (301)480-3503
Email: NIDDK_Inguiries@nih.gov
Website: http://www.niddk.nih.gov/fund/program/a-el-ist.htmepidt1
Allen Spiegel, PhD, Dir.
Activities/Fields: Distribution and determinants of Type 1 diabetes and its complications in populations, including community-based groups and large patient populations.

★ 25385 ★ U.S. Department of Health and Human Services
National Institutes of Health
National Institute of Diabetes and Digestive and Kidney Diseases
Division of Digestive Diseases and Nutrition
(Obesity/Nutrition Research Centers)
MSC 5461
2 Democracy Pl., Rm. 631
45 Center Dr.
Bethesda, MD 20892-5461
Phone: (301)594-8822 **Fax:** (301)480-3768
Email: hubbardv@extra.niddk.nih.gov
Website: http://www.niddk.nih.gov/fund/program/M-Rlist.htm
Van S. Hubbard, MD, Dir.
Activities/Fields: Biomedical research in obesity and nutrition; develop new knowledge concerning the development, treatment, and prevention of obesity and eating disorders; understand control and modulation of energy metabolism; understand and treat disorders associated with abnormalities of energy balance and weight management such as in anorexia nervosa, AIDS, and cancer.

★ 25386 ★ U.S. Department of Health and Human Services
National Institutes of Health
National Institute of Diabetes and Digestive and Kidney Diseases
Division of Digestive Diseases and Nutrition
(Nutrient Metabolism Program)
MSC 5450
6707 Democracy Blvd., Rm. 663
Bethesda, MD 20892-5450
Phone: (301)594-8884 **Fax:** (301)480-8300
Email: maym@extra.niddk.nih.gov
Website: http://www.niddk.nih.gov/fund/program/M-RLlist.htm
Michael Ken May, PhD, Dir.
Activities/Fields: Basic and clinical studies related to the requirement, bioavailability, and metabolism of nutrients and other dietary components at the organ, cellular, and subcellular levels in normal and diseased states. Areas of research include the understanding of physiologic function and mechanism of action/interaction of nutrients within the body; nutrient influence on gene regulation and expression; metabolism and function of nutrient antioxidants; effects of environment, heredity, stress, drug use, toxicants, and physical activity on problems of nutrient imbalance and nutrient requirements in health and disease; and specific metabolic considerations relating to alternative forms of nutrient delivery and use, such as total parenteral nutrition. Also supports research to improve methods of assessing nutritional status in health and disease.

★ 25387 ★ U.S. Department of Health and Human Services
National Institutes of Health
National Institute of Diabetes and Digestive and Kidney Diseases
Division of Digestive Diseases and Nutrition
(Gastrointestinal Neuroendocrinology Research Program)
MSC 5450
6707 Democracy Blvd., Rm. 663
Bethesda, MD 20892-5450
Phone: (301)594-8884 **Fax:** (301)480-8300
Email: maym@extra.niddk.nih.gov
Website: http://www.niddk.nih.gov/fund/program/F-Llist.htmGNP
Michael Ken May, PhD, Dir.
Activities/Fields: Basic and clinical studies on normal and abnormal function of both the enteric nervous system and the elements within the central nervous system that control the enteric nervous system, including histochemical and neurochemical analyses of the enteric nervous system, electrical properties of enteric ganglia, chemical neurotransmission, neural control of effector function, and extrinsic nervous input. Emphasis is on gastrointestinal hormones and peptides, including their structure, biological actions, structure-activity relationships, receptors, distribution, quantitation, metabolism, release, correlation with physiological events, deficiency, and the role of time variation in the data collected in the above studies. In addition, the program supports studies on disease conditions associated with excessive or inadequate secretion of neuropeptides.

★ 25388 ★ U.S. Department of Health and Human Services
National Institutes of Health
National Institute of Diabetes and Digestive and Kidney Diseases
Division of Digestive Diseases and Nutrition
(Gastrointestinal Transport and Absorption Program)
MSC 5450
6707 Democracy Blvd., Rm. 663
Bethesda, MD 20892-5450
Phone: (301)594-8884 **Fax:** (301)480-8300
Email: maym@extra.niddk.nih.gov
Website: http://www.niddk.nih.gov/fund/program/F-Llist.htmGTAP
Michael Ken May, PhD, Dir.
Activities/Fields: Process of food digestion, and absorption and transport in the gastrointestinal tract, including the synthesis and assembly of digestive enzymes; the transport of water, ions, sugars, amino acids, peptides, lipids, vitamins, and macromolecules; and the formation, structure, and function of chylomicrons. Other areas of research focus on the regulation of gene expression in the gastrointestinal tract; structure and function of the gut mucosa; cytoskeletal structure and contractility in brush borders; the growth and differentiation of gastrointestinal cells in normal and disease states; intestinal transplantation, storage, and preservation; and gastrointestinal tissue injury, repair, and regeneration. Also supported are studies on gastrointestinal diseases such as maldigestion and malabsorption syndromes.

★ 25389 ★ U.S. Department of Health and Human Services
National Institutes of Health
National Institute of Diabetes and Digestive and Kidney Diseases
Division of Digestive Diseases and Nutrition
(Epidemiology and Data Systems Program)
MSC 5450
6707 Democracy Blvd., Rm. 673
Bethesda, MD 20892-5450
Phone: (301)594-8878 **Fax:** (301)480-8300
Email: everhartj@extra.niddk.nih.gov
Website: http://www.niddk.nih.gov/fund/program/A-Elist.htmDDNE
James Everhart, MD, Ch.
Activities/Fields: Collection, analysis, and dissemination of data on digestive diseases and their complications.

★ 25390 ★ U.S. Department of Health and Human Services
National Institutes of Health
National Institute of Diabetes and Digestive and Kidney Diseases
Division of Digestive Diseases and Nutrition
(Clinical Nutrition Research Unit)
MSC 5461
6707 Democracy Blvd.
45 Center Dr.
Bethesda, MD 20892
Phone: (301)594-8822 **Fax:** (301)480-3768
Email: hubbardv@extra.niddk.nih.gov
Website: http://www.niddk.nih.gov/fund/program/A-Elist.htmCNRU
Van S. Hubbard, MD, Dir.
Activities/Fields: Research, educational, and service activities focused on human nutrition in health and disease; serves as focal point for an interdisciplinary approach to clinical nutrition research and for the stimulation of research in areas such as improved nutritional support of acutely and chronically ill persons, assessment of nutritional status, effects of disease states on nutrient needs, and effects of changes in nutritional status on disease.

★ 25391 ★ U.S. Department of Health and Human Services
National Institutes of Health
National Institute of Diabetes and Digestive and Kidney Diseases
Division of Digestive Diseases and Nutrition
(Clinical Trials in Digestive Diseases)
2 Democracy Pl., Rm. 659
Bethesda, MD 20892
Phone: (301)594-8879 **Fax:** (301)480-8300
Email: robuckp@extra.niddk.nih.gov
Website: http://www.niddk.nih.gov/fund/program/A-Elist.htmDDCT
Patrick R. Robuck, PhD, Dir.
Activities/Fields: Evaluation of experimental interventions in comparison with a standard treatment and/or placebo control in digestive diseases.

★ 25392 ★ U.S. Department of Health and Human Services
National Institutes of Health
National Institute of Diabetes and Digestive and Kidney Diseases
End-Stage Renal Disease Program
6707 Democracy Blvd.
Bethesda, MD 20892
Phone: (301)496-4000
Email: agodoal@extra.niddk.nih.gov
Website: http://www.niddk.nih.gov/fund/program/A-Elist.htmend
Lawrence Y. Agodoa, MD, Dir.
Activities/Fields: Strives to reduce morbidity and mortality from bone, blood, nervous system, metabolic, gastrointestinal, cardiovascular, and endocrine abnormalities in end-stage kidney failure; aims to improve the effectiveness of dialysis and transplantation. Special areas of interest include hemodialysis membrane reuse and alternative dialyzer sterilization methods; biocompatible membranes; high-flux hemodialysis; criteria for adequacy of dialysis.

★ 25393 ★ U.S. Department of Health and Human Services
National Institutes of Health
National Institute of Diabetes and Digestive and Kidney Diseases
Kidney, Urology, and Hematology Centers Program
MSC 5458
2 Democracu Blvd., Rm. 621
Bethesda, MD 20892-5458
Phone: (301)594-7717 **Fax:** (301)480-3510
Email: badmand@extra.niddk.nih.gov
Website: http://www.niddk.nih.gov/fund/program/F-Llist.htm
David Badman, PhD, Dir.
Activities/Fields: Strives to reduce adult and pediatric mortality and morbidity from kidney, urologic, and hematologic diseases.

★ 25394 ★ U.S. Department of Health and Human Services
National Institutes of Health
National Institute of Diabetes and Digestive and Kidney Diseases
Pediatric Nephrology Programs
630-2 Democracy Plz.
Bethesda, MD 20892-5458
Phone: (301)594-7717 **Fax:** (301)480-3510
Email: gladys_hirschman@nih.gov
Website: http://www.niddk.nih.gov/fund/program/M-Rlist.htmpednep
Gladys H. Hirschman, MD, Dir.
Activities/Fields: Aims to characterize the scope, nature, and impact of kidney diseases of children, including the causes, treatment, and prevention of these disorders.

★ 25395 ★ U.S. Department of Health and Human Services
National Institutes of Health
National Institute of Diabetes and Digestive and Kidney Diseases
Renal Diseases Epidemiology
Natcher Bldg.
45 Center Dr.
Bethesda, MD 20892
Email: jonesc@extra.niddk.nih.gov
Website: http://www.niddk.nih.gov/fund/program/M-Rlist.htmRDEP
Camille A. Jones, MD, Dir.
Activities/Fields: Descriptive and analytic research, including development and analysis of surveillance databases, cross-sectional surveys, prospective observational studies, and case-control studies (for evaluating rare diseases). Key areas include disease prevention; developing early markers of injury; defining risk factors for morbidity and mortality; increasing evaluation of kidney disease measurements and outcomes in ongoing observational studies.

★ 25396 ★ U.S. Department of Health and Human Services
National Institutes of Health
National Institute of Diabetes and Digestive and Kidney Diseases
Urologic Diseases Epidemiology Program
2 Democracy Pl., Rm. 615
Bethesda, MD 20892
Phone: (301)594-8305
Email: eggersp@extra.niddk.nih.gov
Website: http://www.niddk.nih.gov/fund/program/S-Zlist.htmUDEP
Paul Eggers, PhD, Dir.
Activities/Fields: Dedicated to preventing disease, developing early markers of injury, defining risk factors for morbidity and mortality, and increasing evaluation of urologic disease measurements and outcomes in ongoing observational studies. Dedicated to increasing availability of epidemiologic data through new databases and full utilization of existing federal, state, and private sources of data.

★ 25397 ★ U.S. Department of Health and Human Services
National Institutes of Health
National Institute of Diabetes and Digestive and Kidney Diseases
Urology Program
2 Democracy Blvd.
Bldg. 45, Rm. 6AS-136
Bethesda, MD 20892
Phone: (301)594-7717 **Fax:** (301)480-3510
Email: nybergl@ep.niddk.nih.gov
Website: http://www.niddk.nih.gov/fund/program/S-Zlist.htmuroprog
Dr. Leroy M. Nyberg, Jr.,MD, Dir.
Activities/Fields: Normal and abnormal development, structure, and function of the genitourinary tract and studies on the genitourinary effects of diabetes mellitus, spinal cord injury, and multiple sclerosis. Research includes etiology, diagnosis, pathophysiology, therapy, and prevention of major adult urological disease and disorders, including shock-wave and laser lithotripsy, urolithiasis inhibitors, bladder substitution procedures and devices, and prostate growth inhibitor and reduction therapies.

★ 25398 ★ U.S. Department of Health and Human Services
National Institutes of Health
National Institute of Environmental Health Sciences
Division of Extramural Research and Training
(Centers for Children's Environmental Health and Disease Prevention)
PO Box 12233
Research Triangle Park, NC 27709

Phone: (919)541-3254 Fax: (919)316-4606
Email: dearry@niehs.nih.gov
Website: http://www.niehs.nih.gov/translat/children/children.htm
Allen Dearry, PhD, Ch.
Activities/Fields: Applied intervention and prevention methods in connection with community-based prevention research; supports studies on the causes and mechanisms of children's disorders having an environmental etiology, identifies environmental exposures, intervenes to reduce hazardous exposures and their adverse health effects. Strives to decrease the prevalence, morbidity and mortality of environmentally related childhood diseases.

★ 25399 ★ U.S. Department of Health and Human Services
National Institutes of Health
National Institute of Environmental Health Sciences
Division of Extramural Research and Training
(Chemical Exposures and Molecular Biology Branch)
PO Box 12233
Research Triangle Park, NC 27709
Phone: (919)541-4943 **Fax:** (919)316-4606
Email: dearry@niehs.nih.gov
Website: http://www.niehs.nih.gov/dert/dertcemb/cembb.htm
Dr. Allen Dearry, Ch.
Activities/Fields: Environmental chemical exposures, environmental and molecular epidemiology.

★ 25400 ★ U.S. Department of Health and Human Services
National Institutes of Health
National Institute of Environmental Health Sciences
Division of Extramural Research and Training
(Program Analysis Branch)
PO Box 12233
Research Triangle Park, NC 27709
Phone: (919)541-7752 **Fax:** (919)541-4937
Email: vanhout1@niehs.nih.gov
Website: http://www.niehs.nih.gov/dert/dertpab/pab.htm
Dr. Bennett VanHouten, Ch.
Activities/Fields: Conducts long and short-term scientific analyses of grants portfolio; provides basis for priority setting, decision making, and strategic planning; develops methodologies to conduct impact analyses; identifies emerging emphasis areas for program development.

★ 25401 ★ U.S. Department of Health and Human Services
National Institutes of Health
National Institute of Environmental Health Sciences
Division of Extramural Research and Training
(Organs and Systems Toxicology Branch)
PO Box 12233
Research Triangle Park, NC 27709
Phone: (919)541-5327 **Fax:** (919)541-5064
Email: mcclure@niehs.nih.gov
Website: http://www.niehs.nih.gov/dert/dertostb/ostb.htm
Dr. Michael McClure, Dir.
Activities/Fields: Neurotoxicology, immunotoxicology, pulmonary/cardiovascular toxicology, and reproductive and developmental toxicology.

★ 25402 ★ U.S. Department of Health and Human Services
National Institutes of Health
National Institute of Environmental Health Sciences
Environmental Genome Project
PO Box 12233
111 Alexander Drive
Research Triangle Park, NC 27709
Phone: (919)541-4998 **Fax:** (919)316-4606
Email: velazqu1@niehs.nih.gov
Website: http://www.niehs.nih.gov/envgenom/home.htm
Jose M. Velazquez, PhD
Activities/Fields: Understanding the impact and interaction of environmental exposures on human health and disease.

★ 25403 ★ U.S. Department of Health and Human Services
National Institutes of Health
National Institute of Environmental Health Sciences
Environmental Genomic SNP Database Platform
PO Box 12233
Research Triangle Park, NC 27709
Phone: (919)541-2548 **Fax:** (919)541-5002
Email: selkirk@niehs.nih.gov
Dr. James Selkirk, Dir.
Activities/Fields: Identification of functionally important polymorphisms in environmental response genes that may determine differences in disease risks to environmental exposures.

★ 25404 ★ U.S. Department of Health and Human Services
National Institutes of Health
National Institute of Environmental Health Sciences
Epidemiology Branch
M/D A3-05
PO Box 12233
Research Triangle Park, NC 27709
Phone: (919)541-4660 **Fax:** (919)541-2511
Email: wilcox@niehs.nih.gov
Website: http://dir.niehs.nih.gov/direb/
Allen J. Wilcox, Ch.
Activities/Fields: Reproductive epidemiology and environmental and molecular epidemiology.

★ 25405 ★ U.S. Department of Health and Human Services
National Institutes of Health
National Institute of Environmental Health Sciences
Laboratory of Molecular Carcinogenesis
(Molecular and Genetic Epidemiology)
M/D A2-01
PO Box 12233
Research Triangle Park, NC 27709
Phone: (919)541-2511
Email: taylor@niehs.nih.gov
Website: http://dir.niehs.nih.gov/dirlmc/
Jack A. Taylor, PhD, Prin. Investigator
Activities/Fields: Interaction between genes and environmental exposures in human carcinogenesis, focus on understanding human genetic variation in susceptibility to DNA damage, and frequency and pattern of DNA mutation from environmental exposure.

★ 25406 ★ U.S. Department of Health and Human Services
National Institutes of Health
National Institute of Environmental Health Sciences
Laboratory of Molecular Carcinogenesis
(Eicosanoid Biochemistry Section)
M/D A2-01
PO Box 12233
Research Triangle Park, NC 27709
Phone: (919)541-3911
Email: eling@niehs.nih.gov
Website: http://dir.niehs.nih.gov/dirlmc/home.htm
Thomas Eling, PhD, Prin. Investigator
Activities/Fields: Enzymes (prostaglandin H synthase or Cox and lipoxygenases or Lox) which metabolize the cis-unsaturated fatty acids, arachidonic acid and linoleic acid to prostaglandins and other related metabolites.

★ 25407 ★ U.S. Department of Health and Human Services
National Institutes of Health
National Institute of Environmental Health Sciences
Laboratory of Molecular Carcinogenesis
(Regulatory Protein Section)
M/D2 - 04
PO Box 12233
Research Triangle Park, NC 27709
Phone: (919)541-1531 **Fax:** (919)541-4704
Email: merrick@niehs.nih.gov
Website: http://dir.niehs.nih.gov/dirlmc/
B. Alex Merrick, PhD, Prin. Investigator
Activities/Fields: Relates specific phosphorylation sites on p53 and p21-waf1 proteins with cell growth, DNA damage and apoptosis in normal and tumor cells.
Frmly: National Center for Toxicogenomics; Proteomics Group.

★ 25408 ★ U.S. Department of Health and Human Services
National Institutes of Health
National Institute of Environmental Health Sciences
Laboratory of Molecular Carcinogenesis
(Molecular Toxicology Group)
M/D A2-01
PO Box 12233
Research Triangle Park, NC 27709
Phone: (919)541-3241
Email: devereux@niehs.nih.gov
Website: http://dir.niehs.nih.gov/dirlmc/home.htm
Theodora Devereux, Prin. Investigator
Activities/Fields: Mechanisms of environmental carcinogenesis with emphasis on detection and identification of activated protooncogenes and inactivated tumor suppressor genes in human and rodent tumors.

★ 25409 ★ U.S. Department of Health and Human Services
National Institutes of Health
National Institute of Environmental Health Sciences
Laboratory of Molecular Carcinogenesis
(Hormones and Cancer Section)
M/D A2-01
PO Box 12233
Research Triangle Park, NC 27709
Phone: (919)541-7797
Email: diaugus2@niehs.nih.gov
Website: http://dir.niehs.nih.gov/dirlmc/home.htm
Dr. Richard DiAugustine, Prin. Investigator
Activities/Fields: Ovarian steroids and how they regulate growth and contribute to oncogenesis in target organs such as the uterus and mammary gland.

★ 25410 ★ U.S. Department of Health and Human Services
National Institutes of Health
National Institute of Environmental Health Sciences
Laboratory of Molecular Carcinogenesis (Gene Regulation Group)
M/D A2-01
PO Box 12233
Research Triangle Park, NC 27709
Phone: (919)541-7797
Email: afshari@niehs.nih.gov
Website: http://dir.niehs.nih.gov/dirlmc/home.htm
Cynthia A. Afshari, PhD, Prin. Investigator
Activities/Fields: Molecular events involved in the loss of negative growth controls and the evolution of cancer, including the discovery and cloning of novel tumor suppressor genes, function of thee genes from a cell biology and transduction approach.

★ 25411 ★ U.S. Department of Health and Human Services
National Institutes of Health
National Institute of Environmental Health Sciences
Laboratory of Molecular Carcinogenesis (Metastasis Section)
M/D A2-01
PO Box 12233
Research Triangle Park, NC 27709
Phone: (919)541-7797
Email: olden@niehs.nih.gov
Website: http://dir.niehs.nih.gov/dirlmc/
Ken Olden, PhD, Contact
Activities/Fields: Characteristics of metastatic tumor cells, such as the ability to adhere to and migrate on extracellular matrix molecules; activation of integrins in the adhesion of human breast carcinoma cells to basement membrane proteins (1,2).

★ 25412 ★ U.S. Department of Health and Human Services
National Institutes of Health
National Institute of Environmental Health Sciences
Laboratory of Molecular Carcinogenesis
M/D A2-01
PO Box 12233
Research Triangle Park, NC 27709
Phone: (919)541-7797
Email: barrent2@niehs.nih.gov
Website: http://dir.niehs.nih.gov/dirlmc/
Katie Barrentine, Sec.
Activities/Fields: Critical target genes in carcinogenesis to understand how chemicals act upon these genes to influence cancer development, including cancer prevention, diagnosis, and treatment.

★ 25413 ★ U.S. Department of Health and Human Services
National Institutes of Health
National Institute of Environmental Health Sciences
Laboratory of Molecular Carcinogenesis (Cell Adhesion and Migration)
M/D A2-01
PO Box 12233
Research Triangle Park, NC 27709
Phone: (919)541-7797
Email: akiyama@niehs.nih.gov
Website: http://dir.niehs.nih.gov/dirlmc/home.htm
Steven K. Akiyama, PhD, Prin. Investigator
Activities/Fields: Contributes to normal processes such as cellular differentiation, embryonic development, and would healing as well as to the progression of diseases and pathological conditions such as cancer, inflammatory responses, and developmental abnormalities that can arise from acute or chronic exposure to environmental toxicants.

★ 25414 ★ U.S. Department of Health and Human Services
National Institutes of Health
National Institute of Environmental Health Sciences
Laboratory of Signal Transduction (Ion Channel Physiology Group)
PO Box 12233
Research Triangle Park, NC 27709
Email: yakel@niehs.nih.gov
Website: http://dir.niehs.nih.gov/dirlst/groups/yakel.htm
Dr. Jerry Yakel, Hd.
Activities/Fields: 5-HT3 subtype of serotonin receptor; modulation of voltage-dependent calcium channels.

★ 25415 ★ U.S. Department of Health and Human Services
National Institutes of Health
National Institute of Environmental Health Sciences
Laboratory of Signal Transduction (Calcium Signaling Group)
PO Box 12233
Research Triangle Park, NC 27709
Phone: (919)541-1420 **Fax:** (919)541-1898
Email: putney@niehs.nih.gov
Website: http://dir.niehs.nih.gov/dirlst/groups/putney.htm
Dr. James W. Putney, Jr., Hd.
Activities/Fields: Cellular calcium regulation; neurotransmitter utilization of calcium.

★ 25416 ★ U.S. Department of Health and Human Services
National Institutes of Health
National Institute of Environmental Health Sciences
Laboratory of Signal Transduction (Inositol Signaling Group)
PO Box 12233
Research Triangle Park, NC 27709
Phone: (919)541-0793 **Fax:** (919)541-1898
Email: shears@niehs.nih.gov
Website: http://dir.niehs.nih.gov/dirlst/groups/shears.htm
Dr. Stephen B. Shears, Hd.
Activities/Fields: Inositol derivatives as regulators of cellular physiology.

★ 25417 ★ U.S. Department of Health and Human Services
National Institutes of Health
National Institute of Environmental Health Sciences
Laboratory of Signal Transduction (Cell Biology Group)
PO Box 12233
Research Triangle Park, NC 27709
Phone: (919)541-3873 **Fax:** (919)541-3385
Email: murphy1@niehs.nih.gov
Website: http://dir.niehs.nih.gov/dirlst/groups/murphy.htm
Dr. Elizabeth Murphy, Hd.
Activities/Fields: Stress induced alterations in signaling pathways and ionic homeostasis that induce protection and/or death.

★ 25418 ★ U.S. Department of Health and Human Services
National Institutes of Health
National Institute of Environmental Health Sciences
Laboratory of Signal Transduction (Receptor Tyrosine Kinsase Signaling and Regulation Group)
PO Box 12233
Research Triangle Park, NC 27709
Phone: (919)541-3619 **Fax:** (919)541-1898
Email: obryan@niehs.nih.gov
Website: http://dir.niehs.nih.gov/dirlst/groups/obryan.htm
Dr. John P. O'Bryan, Hd.
Activities/Fields: Integration of signal transduction cascades by adaptor proteins, particularly those which modulate the function of receptor tyrosine kinases.

★ 25419 ★ U.S. Department of Health and Human Services
National Institutes of Health
National Institute of Environmental Health Sciences
Laboratory of Signal Transduction (Molecular Endocrinology Group)
PO Box 12233
Research Triangle Park, NC 27709
Phone: (919)541-1564 **Fax:** (919)541-1367
Email: cidlowsk1@niehs.nih.gov
Website: http://dir.niehs.nih.gov/dirlst/groups/cidlowski.htm
Dr. John Cidlowski, Hd.
Activities/Fields: Mechanisms and control of apoptosis; glucocorticord receptors; orphan receptors.

★ 25420 ★ U.S. Department of Health and Human Services
National Institutes of Health
National Institute of Environmental Health Sciences
Laboratory of Signal Transduction (Membrane Biophysics Group)
PO Box 12233
Research Triangle Park, NC 27709
Phone: (919)541-0062 **Fax:** (919)541-1898
Email: armstro3@niehs.nih.gov
Website: http://dir.niehs.nih.gov/dirlst/groups/armstrong.htm
Dr. David L. Armstrong, Hd.
Activities/Fields: Patch clamp techniques; ion channel modulation at the molecular level.

★ 25421 ★ U.S. Department of Health and Human Services
National Institutes of Health
National Institute of Environmental Health Sciences
Laboratory of Signal Transduction (Studies in Polypeptide Hormone Action Group)
PO Box 12233
Research Triangle Park, NC 27709
Phone: (919)541-4899 **Fax:** (919)541-4571
Email: black009@niehs.nih.gov
Website: http://dir.niehs.nih.gov/dirlst/groups/blackshear.htm
Dr. Perry J. Blackshear, MD, Hd.
Activities/Fields: Signal transduction mechanisms and intracellular responses to surface acting agonists, with particular emphasis on the PKC pathway and on rapid transcriptional responses.

★ 25422 ★ U.S. Department of Health and Human Services
National Institutes of Health
National Institute of Environmental Health Sciences
Laboratory of Signal Transduction
PO Box 12233
Research Triangle Park, NC 27709
Phone: (919)541-1564 **Fax:** (919)541-1367
Email: cidlowski@niehs.nih.gov
Website: http://dir.niehs.nih.gov/dirlst/
Dr. John Cidlowski, Ch.
Activities/Fields: Mechanisms by which environmental agents can affect physiological processes and cause pathological outcomes by disrupting signal transduction pathways.

★ 25423 ★ U.S. Department of Health and Human Services
National Institutes of Health
National Institute of Environmental Health Sciences
Laboratory of Structural Biology (DNA Repair and Nucleic Acid Enzymology Group)
PO Box 12233
Research Triangle Park, NC 27709
Phone: (919)541-3267 **Fax:** (919)541-3592
Email: wilsons@niehs.nih.gov
Website: http://dir.niehs.nih.gov/dirlsb/naehome.htm
Dr. Samuel H. Wilson, Prin. Investigator
Activities/Fields: Physical, biochemical, cell and molecular biology studies of mammalian base excision repair enzymes and DNA polymerases, in particular studies gap-filling DNA synthesis and other gap repair reactions during Mammalian DNA repair.

★ 25424 ★ U.S. Department of Health and Human Services
National Institutes of Health
National Institute of Environmental Health Sciences
Laboratory of Structural Biology (Mass Spectrometry Group)
PO Box 12233
Research Triangle Park, NC 27709
Phone: (919)541-1966 **Fax:** (919)541-0022
Email: tomer@niehs.nih.gov
Website: http://dir.niehs.nih.gov/dirlsb/msshome.htm
Kenneth B. Tomer, PhD, Prin. Investigator
Activities/Fields: Mass spectrometry to identify unknown proteins and components of protein complexes and to study the macromolecular interactions within the complexes, including spermiation, protein-protein and protein-DNA interactions during mammalian base excision repair; investigates non-covalent complexes between CD4 and HIV gp120.

★ 25425 ★ U.S. Department of Health and Human Services
National Institutes of Health
National Institute of Environmental Health Sciences
Laboratory of Structural Biology (DNA Replication Fidelity Group)
PO Box 12233
Research Triangle Park, NC 27709
Phone: (919)541-2644 **Fax:** (919)541-7613
Email: kunkel@niehs.nih.gov
Website: http://dir.niehs.nih.gov/dirlsb/drfhome.htm
Thomas A. Kunkel, PhD, Prin. Investigator
Activities/Fields: Understanding the fidelity of normal DNA replication and repair processes that control spontaneous and induced mutation rates in organisms from viruses to humans, and understanding how these processes are perturbed by polymorphisms or mutations in critical genes or by DNA damage resulting from intracellular metabolism or exposure to the external environment.

★ 25426 ★ U.S. Department of Health and Human Services
National Institutes of Health
National Institute of Environmental Health Sciences
Laboratory of Structural Biology (Nuclear Magnetic Resonance Group)
PO Box 12233
Research Triangle Park, NC 27709
Phone: (919)541-4879 **Fax:** (919)541-5707
Email: london@niehs.nih.gov
Website: http://dir.niehs.nih.gov/dirlsb/nmrhome.htm
Robert E. London, PhD, Prin. Investigator
Activities/Fields: Structural characterizations of adducts which form between chemicals of environmental or pharmacological interest, and macromolecular targets or model systems; studies of intracellular ions and development of methods to determine ion levels in cells; intracellular magnesium and its measurement.

★ 25427 ★ U.S. Department of Health and Human Services
National Institutes of Health
National Institute of Environmental Health Sciences
Laboratory of Structural Biology (Macromolecular Structure Group)
PO Box 12233
Research Triangle Park, NC 27709
Phone: (919)541-1017 **Fax:** (919)316-4617
Email: hall4@niehs.nih.gov
Website: http://dir.niehs.nih.gov/dirlsb/hall_home.html
Traci Hall, Prin. Investigator
Activities/Fields: Structural biology, primarily x-ray crystallography, to study overlapping areas of embryonic development, cell signaling, and RNA-protein interactions.

★ 25428 ★ U.S. Department of Health and Human Services
National Institutes of Health
National Institute of Environmental Health Sciences
Laboratory of Structural Biology
M/D F3-02
PO Box 12233
Research Triangle Park, NC 27709
Phone: (919)541-3198 **Fax:** (919)541-7880
Email: london@niehs.nih.gov
Website: http://dir.niehs.nih.gov/dirlsb/
Robert E. London, Prin. Inv.
Activities/Fields: Provides insights into biological processes that impact human environmental health, including signal transduction processes, nucleic acid transactions, gene expression and protein translation and modification. Investigates relationship between atomic level structures of macromolecules and their biochemical properties, their abilities to interact with other macromolecules and with substrates, and their functions in vivo (requiring highly integrated approach wherein x-ray crystallography, nuclear magnetic resonance, mass spectroscopy and computational chemistry are combined with biochemical and genetic approaches).

★ 25429 ★ U.S. Department of Health and Human Services
National Institutes of Health
National Institute of Environmental Health Sciences
Laboratory of Structural Biology (Computational Chemistry/Molecular Modeling Group)
PO Box 12233
Research Triangle Park, NC 27709
Phone: (919)541-3198 **Fax:** (919)541-7880
Email: darden@niehs.nih.gov
Website: http://dir.niehs.nih.gov/dirlsb/cchome.htm
Tom Darden, PhD, Prin. Investigator
Activities/Fields: Understanding structural, mutational and sequence data generated using graphics, energy minimization, simulations, relative free energy, and homology-structure; provides current molecular modeling methodology. **Pub:** *Papers.*

★ 25430 ★ U.S. Department of Health and Human Services
National Institutes of Health
National Institute of Environmental Health Sciences
Microarray Center
111 Alexander Dr., Bldg. 101, Rm. D228
M/D F1-09
PO Box 12233
Research Triangle Park, NC 27709
Phone: (919)541-3710 **Fax:** (919)541-1460
Email: paules@niehs.nih.gov
Website: http://dir.niehs.nih.gov/microarray/
Dr. Rick Paules, Dir.
Activities/Fields: Identification of toxicants on the basis of tissue-specific patterns of gene expression (molecular signature); mechanisms of action of environmental agents through identification of gene expression networks; uses toxicant-induced gene expression as a biomarker to assess human exposure; effects of toxicants from one species to another; interactions of mixtures of chemicals; effects of low dose exposures versus high dose exposures; development of public database of expression profiles.

★ 25431 ★ U.S. Department of Health and Human Services
National Institutes of Health
National Institute of Environmental Health Sciences
National Center for Toxicogenomics
PO Box 12233, Mail Drop F1-05
111 TW Alexander Drive
Research Triangle Park, NC 27709
Phone: (919)541-4141 **Fax:** (919)541-1460
Email: tennant@niehs.nih.gov
Website: http://www.niehs.nih.gov/nct/home.htm
Dr. Raymond W. Tennant, Dir.
Activities/Fields: Genomics science to improve understanding of basic biological responses to environmental stressors/toxicants; aims to catalyze the application of toxicogenomics to improve human health.

★ 25432 ★ U.S. Department of Health and Human Services
National Institutes of Health
National Institute of General Medical Sciences
45 Center Dr., MSC 6200
Bethesda, MD 20892-6200
Phone: (301)594-2172 **Fax:** (301)402-0156
Email: cassmanm@nigms.nih.gov
Website: http://www.nigms.nih.gov/
Dr. Marvin Cassman, Dir.
Activities/Fields: Non-disease-targeted research and research training in the basic biomedical sciences; maintains no intramural (in-house) research. Program focuses on the areas of cell biology and biophysics; genetics and developmental biology; phamacology, physiology, and biological chemistry; and minority opportunities in research. The Institute fosters multidisciplinary approaches to research and employs the full range of support mechanisms–research project grants, program-project grants, research center grants, research career development awards, awards to new investigators, and institutional and individual fellowships.

★ 25433 ★ U.S. Department of Health and Human Services
National Institutes of Health
National Institute of Mental Health
Biological Psychiatry Branch
(Section on Molecular Neurobiology)
MSC 1381
Bldg. 10, Rm. 4n222
Bethesda, MD 20892-1381
Phone: (301)496-4183 **Fax:** (301)480-8348
Email: chuang@helix.nih.gov
Website: http://intramural.nimh.nih.gov/research/bpb/smn.htm
De-Maw Chuang, PhD, Ch.
Activities/Fields: Molecular mechanisms underlying programmed cell death (apoptosis) of neurons and its implication for central nervous system (CNS) development, as well as the pathogenesis of neuropsychiatric and neurodegenerative disorders.

★ 25434 ★ U.S. Department of Health and Human Services
National Institutes of Health
National Institute of Mental Health
Experimental Therapeutics Branch
(Section on Functional Imaging Methods)
MSC 1148
Bldg. 10, Rm. 1D80B
10 Center Dr.
Bethesda, MD 20892-1148
Phone: (301)402-1333 **Fax:** (301)402-1370
Email: nimhinfo@nih.gov
Website: http://fim.nimh.nih.gov/
Peter Bandettini, PhD, Ch.
Activities/Fields: Aims to increase the utility and interpretability of functional magnetic resonance imaging (fMRI), involving characterization of the neuronal, physiologic, and biophysical processes that contribute to blood oxygenation level dependent (BOLD) and perfusion-based contrast in fMRI; tailoring specific neuroscience questions to unique characteristics of fMRI processing and acquistion; development of pulse sequences, hardware, and processing techniques toward the direction of increased fMRI utility; exploration of measurement and quantification of previously unmeasured neuronal or physiological processes by MRI. **Pub:** *Papers.*

★ 25435 ★ U.S. Department of Health and Human Services
National Institutes of Health
National Institute of Mental Health
Experimental Therapeutics Branch
(Section on Clinical and Experimental Neurospychology)
MSC 1366
10 Center Dr., Rm. 4C104
9000 Rockville Pike
Bethesda, MD 20892
Phone: (301)496-2551 **Fax:** (301)594-5142
Email: nimhinfo@nih.gov
Website: http://lbc.nimh.nih.gov/research.html
Allan F. Mirsky, PhD, Ch.
Activities/Fields: Central nervous system (CNS) factors underlying normal and abnormal behavioral states, particularly on the interaction between environmental and genetic effects.

★ 25436 ★ U.S. Department of Health and Human Services
National Institutes of Health
National Institute of Mental Health
Experimental Therapeutics Branch
(Section on Cognitive Neuropsychology)
MSC 1366
10 Center Dr., Rm. 4C104
Bethesda, MD 20892-1366
Phone: (301)435-4931 **Fax:** (301)402-0921
Email: alex@codon.nih.gov
Website: http://lbc.nimh.nih.gov/research.htmlSection%20on%20Cognitive
Alex Martin, PhD, Ch.
Activities/Fields: Human cognitive systems through the study of how these systems break down in patients with brain injury or disease.

★ 25437 ★ U.S. Department of Health and Human Services
National Institutes of Health
National Institute of Mental Health
Experimental Therapeutics Branch
(Section on Neurocircuitry)
MSC 1366
10 Center Dr., Rm. 4C104
Bethesda, MD 20892-1366
Phone: (301)435-4932 **Fax:** (301)402-0921
Email: nimhinfo@nih.gov
Website: http://lbc.nimh.nih.gov/research.html
Leslie G. Ungerleider, PhD, Ch.
Activities/Fields: Understanding the role of the visual association cortex in perception and memory.

★ 25438 ★ U.S. Department of Health and Human Services
National Institutes of Health
National Institute of Mental Health
Experimental Therapeutics Branch
(Laboratory of Brain and Cognition)
MSC 1366
10 Center Dr., Rm. 4C104
Bethesda, MD 20892-1366
Phone: (301)435-4932 **Fax:** (301)402-0921
Email: nimhinfo@nih.gov
Website: http://lbc.nimh.nih.gov/
Leslie Ungerleider, Ch.
Activities/Fields: Basic and clinical research on normal and impaired attention, learning, memory and perception in humans, and on the underlying anatomical, genetic, neurophysiologic, and psychophysiologic mechanisms.

★ 25439 ★ U.S. Department of Health and Human Services
National Institutes of Health
National Institute of Mental Health
Experimental Therapeutics Branch
(Section on Fuctional Brain Imaging)
MSC 1366
10 Center Dr., Rm. 4C104
Bethesda, MD 20892-1366
Phone: (301)435-4925 **Fax:** (301)402-0921
Email: nimhinfo@nih.gov
Website: http://lbc.nimh.nih.gov/research.html
James V. Haxby, PhD, Ch.
Activities/Fields: Functional organization of intact human brain using functional brain imaging to measure local changes in cerebral blood flow associated with perceptual, cognitive, and mnemonic functions.

★ 25440 ★ U.S. Department of Health and Human Services
National Institutes of Health
National Institute of Mental Health
Experimental Therapeutics Branch
(Section on PET Radiopharmaceutical Sciences)
Bldg. 1, Rm. 3B310
1 Center Dr.
Bethesda, MD 20892-0135
Phone: (301)594-1089 **Fax:** (301)480-3610
Email: pikev@intra.nimh.nih.gov
Website: http://intramural.nimh.nih.gov/research/mib
Victor Pike, PhD, Ch.
Activities/Fields: Development and implementation of radioligands and radiotracers for selective PET (positron emission tomography) imaging of molecular targets in animal and human brain in order to understand causes of mental illness and of the mechanisms and efficacies of existing or proposed treatments.

★ 25441 ★ U.S. Department of Health and Human Services
National Institutes of Health
National Institute of Mental Health
Experimental Therapeutics Branch
(Section on PET Neuroimaging Sciences)
Bldg. 1, Rm. 3B310
1 Center Dr.
Bethesda, MD 20892-0135
Phone: (301)594-1089 **Fax:** (301)480-3610
Email: innisr@.intra.nimh.nih.gov
Website: http://intramural.nimh.nih.gov/research/mib/
Robert B. Innis, MD, Ch.
Activities/Fields: PET (positron emission tomography) tracers as molecular probes of physiology and pathophysiology in animals and humans; probes of intracellular signals transduction and gene expression as well as traditional receptor targets.

★ 25442 ★ U.S. Department of Health and Human Services
National Institutes of Health
National Institute of Mental Health
Experimental Therapeutics Branch
(Section on Neuroimaging)
Bldg. 1, Rm. 3B310
1 Center Dr.
Bethesda, MD 20892-0135
Phone: (301)594-1089 **Fax:** (301)480-3610
Email: drevetsw@intra.nimh.nih.gov
Website: http://intramural.nimh.nih.gov/research/mib/
Wayne Drevets, MD, Ch.
Activities/Fields: Functional and structural neuroimaging measures to investigate biological mechanisms of normal and pathological emotional states.

★ 25443 ★ U.S. Department of Health and Human Services
National Institutes of Health
National Institute of Mental Health
Experimental Therapeutics Branch
(Geriatric Psychiatry Branch)
MSC 1275
Bldg. 10, Rm. 3N226
Bethesda, MD 20892
Phone: (301)496-0948 **Fax:** (301)496-2847
Email: nimhinfo@nih.gov
Website: http://intramural.nimh.nih.gov/research/gpb/
P. Trey Sunderland, MD, Ch.
Activities/Fields: Alzheimer's disease (AD); tests for therapeutic synergy among available drugs, such as monoamine oxidase inhibitor selegline, cholinergic agent physostigmine, and serotonin uptake inhibitor fluoxetine.

★ 25444 ★ U.S. Department of Health and Human Services
National Institutes of Health
National Institute of Mental Health
Experimental Therapeutics Branch
(Molecular Imaging Branch)
Bldg. 1, Rm. 3B310
1 Center Dr.
Bethesda, MD 20892-0135
Phone: (301)594-1089 **Fax:** (301)480-3610
Email: innisr@intra.nimh.nih.gov
Website: http://intramural.nimh.nih.gov/research/mib/
Robert B. Innis, MD, Ch.
Activities/Fields: Neuroimaging techniques to explore molecular and chemical mechanisms associated with neural function in health and disease, investigates pathophysiological mechanisms associated with mental illnesses in order to enhance available treatments.

★ 25445 ★ U.S. Department of Health and Human Services
National Institutes of Health
National Institute of Mental Health
Experimental Therapeutics Branch
(Section on Neuroendocrine Immunology and Behavior)
Bldg. 10, Rm. 2D46
9000 Rockville Pike
Bethesda, MD 20892
Phone: (301)496-1891 **Fax:** (301)402-1561
Email: nimhinfo@nih.gov
Website: http://intramural.nimh.nih.gov/research/cne/
Esther M. Sternberg, MD, Contact
Activities/Fields: Bi-directional communication between the immune system and the central nervous system (CNS), whose genetic, infectious, toxic, or pharmacological dysregulation confers susceptibility to inflammatory and affective disorders; clinical studies in early inflammatory disease, depression, and fatigue states.

★ 25446 ★ U.S. Department of Health and Human Services
National Institutes of Health
National Institute of Mental Health
Experimental Therapeutics Branch
(Section on Neuropathology)
Bldg. 10, Rm. 4S235
9000 Rockville Pike
Bethesda, MD 20892
Phone: (301)402-7564 **Fax:** (301)402-0052
Email: nimhinfo@nih.gov
Website: http://intramural.nimh.nih.gov/research/cbdb/
Joel Kleinman, MD, Ch.
Activities/Fields: Postmortem studies of schizophrenia, suicide, alcohol, other drug addictions, movement disorders, and dementias.

★ 25447 ★ U.S. Department of Health and Human Services
National Institutes of Health
National Institute of Mental Health
Experimental Therapeutics Branch
(Clinical Neuroendocrinology Branch)
Bldg. 10, Rm. 2D46
9000 Rockville Pike
Bethesda, MD 20892
Phone: (301)496-1891 **Fax:** (301)402-1561
Email: nimhinfo@nih.gov
Website: http://intramural.nimh.nih.gov/research/cne/
Philip W. Gold, MD, Ch.
Activities/Fields: Committed to advancing knowledge to improve the diagnosis, treatment and overall health of patients suffering from depression.

★ 25448 ★ U.S. Department of Health and Human Services
National Institutes of Health
National Institute of Mental Health
Experimental Therapeutics Branch
(Section on Clinical Studies)
Bldg. 10, Rm. 4S235
9000 Rockville Pike
Bethesda, MD 20892
Phone: (301)402-7564 **Fax:** (301)402-0052
Email: nimhinfo@nih.gov
Website: http://intramural.nimh.nih.gov/research/cbdb/
Daniel R. Weinberger, MD, Ch.
Activities/Fields: Neuropsychiatric disorders, especially schizophrenia, Tourette's syndrome, and dementia.

★ 25449 ★ U.S. Department of Health and Human Services
National Institutes of Health
National Institute of Mental Health
Experimental Therapeutics Branch
(Unit on Reproduction Endocrine Studies)
MSC 1276
Bldg. 10, Rm. 3N238
Bethesda, MD 20892-1276
Phone: (301)496-9576 **Fax:** (301)496-2588
Email: nimhinfo@nih.gov
Website: http://intramural.nimh.nih.gov/research/beb/index2.htm
Peter Schmidt, MD, Ch.
Activities/Fields: Role of gonadal steroids in the regulation of neurophysiology and affective state in humans. Studies focus on the evaluation and treatment of mood disorders linked to the perimenopause and midlife, as well as, the psychotropic effects of gonadal steroids such as estradiol, testosterone, and dehydroepiandrosterone (DHEA).

★ 25450 ★ U.S. Department of Health and Human Services
National Institutes of Health
National Institute of Mental Health
Experimental Therapeutics Branch
(Behavioral Endocrinology Branch)
MSC 1276
Bldg. 10, Rm. 3N238
Bethesda, MD 20892-1276
Phone: (301)496-4588 **Fax:** (301)496-9576
Email: simpsonl@irp.nimh.gov
Website: http://intramural.nimh.nih.gov/research/beb/index2.htm
Linda Simpson-St.Clair, MD, contact
Activities/Fields: Impact of reproductive endocrine function on the brain, including mood, cerebral blood flow, immune function, cognition, circadian function, signal transduction effectors, and response to stressors.

★ 25451 ★ U.S. Department of Health and Human Services
National Institutes of Health
National Institute of Mental Health
Experimental Therapeutics Branch
(Section on Developmental Genetic Epidemiology)
MSC 1381
Bldg. 10, Rm. 4n222
Bethesda, MD 20892-1381
Phone: (301)496-4183 **Fax:** (301)480-8348
Email: nimhinfo@nih.gov
Website: http://intramural.nimh.nih.gov/research/etpb/
Kathleen R. Merikankangas, PhD, Ch.
Activities/Fields: Identification of risk factors for mood and anxiety disorders, their association with other psychiatric and medical disorders, including epidemiology, clinical psychology, developmental psychology, genetic epidemiology, psychiatry, and biostatistics.

★ 25452 ★ U.S. Department of Health and Human Services
National Institutes of Health
National Institute of Mental Health
Experimental Therapeutics Branch
(Section on Development and Affective Neuroscience)
MSC 1381
Bldg. 10, Rm. 4n222
Bethesda, MD 20892-1381
Phone: (301)496-4183 **Fax:** (301)480-8348
Email: nimhinfo@nih.gov
Website: http://intramural.nimh.nih.gov/research/etpb
Daniel S. Pine, MD, Ch.
Activities/Fields: Brain development, emotion regulation, and risk for mood and anxiety disorders in children and adolescents.

★ 25453 ★ U.S. Department of Health and Human Services
National Institutes of Health
National Institute of Mental Health
Experimental Therapeutics Branch
(Section on Behavioral Neuropharmacology)
MSC 1380
10 Center Dr., Rm. 4D11
Bethesda, MD 20892-1375
Phone: (301)496-7855 **Fax:** (301)480-1164
Email: jncrawle@codon.nih.gov
Website: http://intramural.nimh.nih.gov/research/etb/sbn/
Jacqueline N. Crawley, PhD, Ch.
Activities/Fields: Investigates behavior actions of brain neurotransmitters using rodent models of symptoms of neuropsychiatric diseases, including behavior neuopharmacology and behavioral genetics.

★ 25454 ★ U.S. Department of Health and Human Services
National Institutes of Health
National Institute of Mental Health
Experimental Therapeutics Branch
(Experimental Therapeutics and Pathophysiology Branch)
1 Center Drive
Bldg. 1, Rm. B3102
Bethesda, MD 20892
Phone: (301)494-1089 **Fax:** (301)480-3610
Email: nimhinfo@nih.gov
Website: http://intramural.nimh.nih.gov/research/etpb
Dennis S. Charney, MD, Ch.
Activities/Fields: Pathophysiology, etiology, and treatment of mood and anxiety disorders of children, adolescents, and adults; identification of neural circuits and neurochemicals.

★ 25455 ★ U.S. Department of Health and Human Services
National Institutes of Health
National Institute of Mental Health
Laboratory of Biochemical Genetics
Bldg. 10, Rm. 2D54
10 Center Dr.
Bethesda, MD 20892
Phone: (301)435-3583
Email: merrilc@helix.nih.gov
Website: http://intramural.nimh.nih.gov/research/lbg/index2.htm
Carl Merril, Ch.
Activities/Fields: Molecular variations in the central nervous system (CNS) in normal, aging and disease states, including proteome and the mitochondrial genome.

★ 25456 ★ U.S. Department of Health and Human Services
National Institutes of Health
National Institute of Mental Health
Laboratory of Cellular and Molecular Regulation
(Unit on Temporal Gene Expression)
9000 Rockville Pike
Bldg. 10, Room 3S231
Bethesda, MD 20892
Phone: (301)496-5590 **Fax:** (301)402-1748
Email: abri@codon.nih.gov
Website: http://intramural.nimh.nih.gov/lcmr/
Rubin Baler, PhD, Contact
Activities/Fields: Understanding the molecular underpinnings of transcriptional specificity in circadian transcriptional loops, focusing on the DNA determinants of circadian regulated genes and the identifica-

tion of circadian accessory proteins with role sin the fine tuning of key temporal parameters.

★ 25457 ★ U.S. Department of Health and Human Services
National Institutes of Health
National Institute of Mental Health
Laboratory of Cellular and Molecular Regulation
(Section on Molecular Neuroscience)
Bldg. 36, Rm. 2A-11
9000 Rockville Pike
Bethesda, MD 20892
Phone: (301)496-8287 **Fax:** (301)402-1748
Email: eiden@codon.nih.gov
Website: http://intramural.nimh.nih.gov/lcmr/smn/
Lee Eiden, PhD, Chf.
Activities/Fields: Molecular basis of cell-specific expression of neuropeptide, secretory protein and vesicular transporter genes responsible for chemically coded neurotransmission in the central and peripheral autonomic nervous systems.

★ 25458 ★ U.S. Department of Health and Human Services
National Institutes of Health
National Institute of Mental Health
Laboratory of Cellular and Molecular Regulation
(Section on Neural Gene Expression)
Bldg. 10, Rm. 2D06
9000 Rockville Pike
Bethesda, MD 20892
Phone: (301)496-8767
Email: scott@codon.nih.gov
Website: http://intramural.nimh.nih.gov/lcmr/snge/
Dr. W. Scott Young, III, Ch.
Activities/Fields: Regulation of genes in the central nervous system, particularly on those expressed within the paraventricular and supraoptic nuclei of the hypothalamus.

★ 25459 ★ U.S. Department of Health and Human Services
National Institutes of Health
National Institute of Mental Health
Laboratory of Cellular and Molecular Regulation
(Section on Functional Neuroanatomy)
Bldg. 36, Rm. 2D15
9000 Rockville Pike
Bethesda, MD 20892
Phone: (301)496-8287
Email: milesh@codon.nih.gov
Website: http://intramural.nimh.nih.gov/lcmr/sfn/
Miles A. Herkenham, PhD, Ch.
Activities/Fields: Investigates dynamic aspects of nervous system function in order to define and map regulatory events that occur in animals when they respond and adapt to immune challenges, repeated drug administration, or chronic stress.

★ 25460 ★ U.S. Department of Health and Human Services
National Institutes of Health
National Institute of Mental Health
Laboratory of Cellular and Molecular Regulation
(Section on Biochemical Pharmacology)
Bldg. 10, Rm. 3S231
9000 Rockville Pike
Bethesda, MD 20892
Phone: (301)496-5590 **Fax:** (301)402-1748
Email: zatz@codon.nih.gov
Website: http://intramural.nimh.nih.gov/research/lcmr
Martin Zatz, MD, Ch.
Activities/Fields: Cellular and biochemical mechanisms involved in the generation of circadian rhythms, their regulation by light, neurotransmitters, drugs, and their expression as behavioral and physiologic cycles. Relevant anatomic systems consist of pineal gland, supra chiasmatic nucleus of the hypothalamus, and the retina. Related research areas include regulation of photoreceptors, vitamin A, and phototransduction; receptors and second messenger systems; iorn transport and fluxes; enzyme induction, hormone synthesis, and release.

★ 25461 ★ U.S. Department of Health and Human Services
National Institutes of Health
National Institute of Mental Health
Laboratory of Cellular and Molecular Regulation
(Section on Molecular Virology)
Bldg. 10, Rm. 3A05
9000 Rockville Pike
Bethesda, MD 20892
Phone: (301)402-1641
Email: m_eiden@codon.nih.gov
Website: http://intramural.nimh.nih.gov/research/lcmr
Maribeth Eiden, PhD, Ch.
Activities/Fields: Use of retroviruses such as gibbon ape leukemia virus (GALV) to study the process of viral entry. Aims to identify new intracellular protein actors as well as development of efficient viral vectors.

★ 25462 ★ U.S. Department of Health and Human Services
National Institutes of Health
National Institute of Mental Health
Laboratory of Cellular and Molecular Regulation
Bldg. 10, Rm. 2A11
9000 Rockville Pike
Bethesda, MD 20892
Phone: (301)496-5590 **Fax:** (301)402-1748
Email: zatz@codon.nih.gov
Website: http://intramural.nimh.nih.gov/lcmr/index2.html
Martin Zats, MD, Ch.
Activities/Fields: Anatomical, cellular, physiological, pharmacological, biochemical and molecular bases of the expression and regulation of brain functions.

★ 25463 ★ U.S. Department of Health and Human Services
National Institutes of Health
National Institute of Mental Health
Laboratory of Cerebral Metabolism
(Unit on Neurobiology)
Bldg. 10, Rm. 3S231
9000 Rockville Pike
Bethesda, MD 20892
Phone: (301)496-1371
Email: nimhinfo@nih.gov
Website: http://intramural.nimh.nih.gov/research/lcm
Carolyn B. Smith, Ch.
Activities/Fields: Understanding of the biochemical events associated with development, plasticity, and involution of the nervous system.

★ 25464 ★ U.S. Department of Health and Human Services
National Institutes of Health
National Institute of Mental Health
Laboratory of Cerebral Metabolism
Bldg. 10, Rm. 3S231
9000 Rockville Pike
Bethesda, MD 20892
Phone: (301)496-1371 **Fax:** (301)480-1668
Email: nimhinfo@nih.gov
Website: http://intramural.nimh.nih.gov/research/lcm
Louis Sokoloff, MD, Ch.
Activities/Fields: Biochemical aspects of growth, development, maturation, and regulation of metabolism in the central nervous system (CNS).

★ 25465 ★ U.S. Department of Health and Human Services
National Institutes of Health
National Institute of Mental Health
Laboratory of Cerebral Metabolism
(Section on Developmental Neurochemistry)
Bldg. 10, Rm. 3S231
9000 Rockville Pike
Bethesda, MD 20892
Phone: (301)496-1371 **Fax:** (301)480-1668
Email: nimhinfo@nih.gov
Website: http://intramural.nimh.nih.gov/research/lcm
Louis Sokoloff, MD, Ch.
Activities/Fields: Development and application of methods that quantitatively measure the rates of physiological and biochemical processes in the individual structures of the nervous systems of conscious and behaving animals and humans, including cerebral blood flow, local cerebral glucose utilization, and local cerebral protein synthesis.

★ 25466 ★ U.S. Department of Health and Human Services
National Institutes of Health
National Institute of Mental Health
Laboratory of Clinical Sciences
(Section on Clinical Neuropharmacology)
Bldg. 10, Rm. 3D41
9000 Rockville Pike
Bethesda, MD 20892-1264
Phone: (301)496-3421 **Fax:** (301)402-0188
Email: theresad@codon.nih.gov
Website: http://intramural.nimh.nih.gov/research/lcs/index2.html
Dennis Murphy, MD, Ch.
Activities/Fields: Development of critical analysis of strategies and techniques for use in evaluating functional status of the brain, serotonergic neurotransmitter system, including genes and drugs and neuropeptide systems that affect it in normal behavior, including the dimensions of personality that may be relevant to psychopathology.

★ 25467 ★ U.S. Department of Health and Human Services
National Institutes of Health
National Institute of Mental Health
Laboratory of Genetics
(Unit on Cell Biology)
Bldg. 36, Rm. 3A31
9000 Rockville Pike
Bethesda, MD 20892
Phone: (301)496-5351
Email: nimhinfo@nih.gov
Website: http://intramural.nimh.nih.gov/research/log/
Ted Usdin, PhD, Ch.
Activities/Fields: Endogenous factors that modulate neuronal function, including pain perception and pituitary hormone secretion.

★ 25468 ★ U.S. Department of Health and Human Services
National Institutes of Health
National Institute of Mental Health
Laboratory of Genetics
(Gene Discovery Unit)
Bldg. 36, Rm. 3A31
9000 Rockville Pike
Bethesda, MD 20892
Phone: (301)496-5351
Email: nimhinfo@nih.gov
Website: http://intramural.nimh.nih.gov/research/log/
Tom Bonner, PhD, Ch.
Activities/Fields: Identification of candidate genes in restricted regions of the genome identified by linkage studies of complex genetic diseases, i.e. those that are not expected to show perfect cosegregation with any single locus.

★ 25469 ★ U.S. Department of Health and Human Services
National Institutes of Health
National Institute of Mental Health
Laboratory of Genetics
Bldg. 36, Rm. 3A31
9000 Rockville Pike
Bethesda, MD 20892
Phone: (301)496-5351
Email: nimhinfo@nih.gov
Website: http://intramural.nimh.nih.gov/research/log/
Michael Brownstein, PhD, Ch.
Activities/Fields: Complex genetic traits in humans and rodents, including whole genome genetic scans to the physiology of neuronal systems and protein structure activity relationships when appropriate.

★ 25470 ★ U.S. Department of Health and Human Services
National Institutes of Health
National Institute of Mental Health
Laboratory of Molecular Biology
(Unit on Lymphocyte Function)
Bldg. 36, Rm. 1B08
9000 Rockville Pike
Bethesda, MD 20892
Phone: (301)496-4864 **Fax:** (301)402-0245
Email: nimhinfo@nih.gov
Website: http://intramural.nimh.nih.gov/research/lmb/
Jon W. Marsh, PhD, Ch.
Activities/Fields: Immunological and central nervous system (CNS) dysfunction. Studies the cellular biochemical alterations generated by the expression of HIV accessory proteins, in particular, the HIV virulence factor NEF, the way this protein associated with an active serine kinase, Pak, and affects activation pathways critical to normal function of both the immunological and nervous systems, and the role these proteins play in pathogenesis.

★ 25471 ★ U.S. Department of Health and Human Services
National Institutes of Health
National Institute of Mental Health
Laboratory of Molecular Biology
(Section on Molecular Neurobiology)
Bldg. 36, Rm. 1B08
9000 Rockville Pike
Bethesda, MD 20892
Phone: (301)496-4864 **Fax:** (301)402-0245
Email: nimhinfo@nih.gov
Website: http://intramural.nimh.nih.gov/research/lmb/
Barry B. Kaplan, PhD, Ch.
Activities/Fields: Strives to define the function and origins of the mRNA population, and establish the existence of new inter- and/or intra-cellular macromolecular communication pathways in the nervous system.

★ 25472 ★ U.S. Department of Health and Human Services
National Institutes of Health
National Institute of Mental Health
Laboratory of Molecular Biology
(Section on Molecular Genetics)
Bldg. 36, Rm. 1B08
9000 Rockville Pike
Bethesda, MD 20892
Phone: (301)496-4864 **Fax:** (301)402-0245
Email: nimhinfo@nih.gov
Website: http://intramural.nimh.nih.gov/research/lmb/
Howard Nash, MD, Ch.
Activities/Fields: Identification of conserved genes that encode or control the physiological targets of an important class of pharmacological agents using molecular genetic and biochemical experiments.

★ 25473 ★ U.S. Department of Health and Human Services
National Institutes of Health
National Institute of Mental Health
Laboratory of Molecular Biology
(Section on Biophysical Chemistry)
Bldg. 36, Rm. 1B08
9000 Rockville Pike
Bethesda, MD 20892
Phone: (301)496-4864 **Fax:** (301)402-0245
Email: nimhinfo@nih.gov
Website: http://intramural.nimh.nih.gov/research/lmb/
David M. Neville, Jr., MD
Activities/Fields: Development of anti T-cell immunotoxins that deplete blood and lymph node T-cells by 2-3 logs in vivo; engineering these immunotoxins as both single fusion and coupled proteins for use in preclinical and clinical trials.

★ 25474 ★ U.S. Department of Health and Human Services
National Institutes of Health
National Institute of Mental Health
Laboratory of Molecular Biology
Bldg. 36, Rm. 1B08
9000 Rockville Pike
Bethesda, MD 20892
Phone: (301)496-4864 **Fax:** (301)402-0245
Email: nimhinfo@nih.gov
Website: http://intramural.nimh.nih.gov/research/lmb/
Howard Nash, MD, Ch.
Activities/Fields: Mechanistic aspects of diverse biological processes, including biochemistry coupled with genetics and cell and molecular biology.

★ 25475 ★ U.S. Department of Health and Human Services
National Institutes of Health
National Institute of Mental Health
Laboratory of Molecular Pathophysiology
Bldg. 49, Rm. B1EE16
49 Convent Dr., MSC 4405
Bethesda, MD 20892-4405
Phone: (301)496-9802 **Fax:** (301)480-0123
Email: manjih@intra.nimh.nih.gov
Website: http://intramural.nimh.nih.gov/research/lmp/
Husseini Manji, MD, Ch.
Activities/Fields: Investigation of disease- and treatment-induced changes in gene and protein expression profiles that regulate neuroplasticity and cellular resilience in mood disorders.

★ 25476 ★ U.S. Department of Health and Human Services
National Institutes of Health
National Institute of Mental Health
Laboratory of Neurochemistry
Bldg. 36, Rm. 3D32
9000 Rockville Pike
Bethesda, MD 20892
Phone: (301)496-3579 **Fax:** (301)480-9284
Email: nimhinfo@nih.gov
Website: http://intramural.nimh.nih.gov/research/lnc/
John Giovanelli, Contact
Activities/Fields: Regulation of synthesis of dopamine, norepinephrine, serotonin, and the endothelium-derived relaxing factor nitric oxide, including the characterization of phenylalanine, tyrosine, and tryptophan hydroxylases (the enzymes that catalyze the rate-limiting steps in the biosynthesis of these neurotransmitters).

★ 25477 ★ U.S. Department of Health and Human Services
National Institutes of Health
National Institute of Mental Health
Laboratory of Neurotoxicology
(Unit on Neuroimmunology)
10 Center Dr., Rm. 3D42
Bethesda, MD 20892-1262
Phone: (301)496-4022
Email: nimhinfo@nih.gov
Melvyn P. Heyes, PhD, Hd.
Activities/Fields: Clinical studies of patient groups with neurologic, genetic, or chronic inflammation disorders as well as patients with HIV.

★ 25478 ★ U.S. Department of Health and Human Services
National Institutes of Health
National Institute of Mental Health
Laboratory of Neurotoxicology
10 Center Dr., Rm. 3D42
Bethesda, MD 20892-1262
Phone: (301)496-4022 **Fax:** (301)451-5780
Email: nimhinfo@nih.gov
Website: http://intramural.nimh.nih.gov/research/lnt/index2.html
Dr. Sanford P. Markey, PhD, Ch.
Activities/Fields: Biochemical events that cause neuronal injury and degeneration produced by genetic disease, inflammation, trauma, and exposure to neurotoxic substances.

★ 25479 ★ U.S. Department of Health and Human Services
National Institutes of Health
National Institute of Mental Health
Laboratory of Neurotoxicology
(Section on Analytical Biochemistry)
10 Center Dr., Rm. 3D42
Bethesda, MD 20892-1262
Phone: (301)496-4022 **Fax:** (301)480-0198
Email: nimhinfo@nih.gov
Website: http://intramural.nimh.nih.gov/research/lnt/sab.html
Jeffrey A. Kowalak, PhD, Mgr.
Activities/Fields: Analytical methods for the characterization and quantification of bioactive components in physiological fluids and tissues.

★ 25480 ★ U.S. Department of Health and Human Services
National Institutes of Health
National Institute of Mental Health
Laboratory of System Neuroscience
(Section on Neuroanatomy)
Bldg. 36, Rm. 2D30
9000 Rockville Pike
Bethesda, MD 20892
Phone: (301)496-4341 **Fax:** (301)402-8960
Email: gerfen@helix.nih.gov
Charles R. Gerfen, PhD, Ch.
Activities/Fields: Understanding the role of basal ganglia in the frontal cortical function, using in situ hybridization histochemical techniques to quantify, at the cellular level, neurotransmitter receptor mediated changes in messenger RNAs encoding proteins or other substances that are utilized by striatal neurons, in connectionally identified subsets of neuron populations, particularly regulation of striatal neurons expressing D1 and D2 dopamine receptor subtypes.

★ 25481 ★ U.S. Department of Health and Human Services
National Institutes of Health
National Institute of Mental Health
Laboratory of System Neuroscience
(Unit of Neural Network Physiology)
Bldg. 36, Rm. 2D30
Bethesda, MD 20892
Phone: (301)402-2249 **Fax:** (301)402-8960
Email: dplenz@codon.nih.gov
Website: http://intramural.nimh.nih.gov/lsn/NeuralNetworkPhys/NNP_Homepage.htm
Dietmar Plenz, PhD, Ch.
Activities/Fields: Cortex-basal ganglia (Cx-BG) circuits, including reconstruction and analysis of Cx-BG systems in vitro using organotypic cultures from rats and mice.

★ 25482 ★ U.S. Department of Health and Human Services
National Institutes of Health
National Institute of Mental Health
Laboratory of System Neuroscience (Section on Neurophysiology)
MS Code 4401
Bldg. 36, Rm. 2D30
9000 Rockville Pike
Bethesda, MD 20892-4401
Phone: (301)402-5452 **Fax:** (301)402-5441
Email: arm@nih.gov
Website: http://nihac.info.nih.gov/
Andrew R. Mitz, PhD, Contact
Activities/Fields: Functional organization of the primate frontal cortex; monitors activity of single neurons in awake, behaving monkeys.

★ 25483 ★ U.S. Department of Health and Human Services
National Institutes of Health
National Institute of Mental Health
Laboratory of System Neuroscience
Bldg. 36, Rm. 2D30
9000 Rockville Pike
Bethesda, MD 20892
Phone: (301)496-4341 **Fax:** (301)402-8960
Email: gerfen@codon.nih.gov
Website: http://intramural.nimh.nih.gov/lsn/
Charles R. Gerfen, PhD, Ch.
Activities/Fields: Neurobiology of higher brain function, including physiologic organization of primate motor cortex other parts of the frontal lobe as well as mechanisms of regulating information flow into and within the cortex.

★ 25484 ★ U.S. Department of Health and Human Services
National Institutes of Health
National Institute of Mental Health
Molecular Neuropsychiatry Section
6001 Executive Blvd., Rm. 5213
MSC 2668
Bethesda, MD 20892-9561
Phone: (410)550-2953 **Fax:** (410)550-1477
Email: jcadet@intra.nida.nih.gov
Website: http://www.nida.nih.gov/DIR/molec-neuro.html
Jean Lud Cadet, MD, Ch.
Activities/Fields: Investigates biochemical, cellular and genetic abnormalities in neurobehavioral disorders; assesses effects of drugs at the cellular and molecular level; development of RNA isolation and gene cloning techniques to study disorders at the genomic level.

★ 25485 ★ U.S. Department of Health and Human Services
National Institutes of Health
National Institute of Mental Health
Pediatrics and Developmental Neuropsychiatry Branch
Bldg. 10, Rm. 4N208
9000 Rockville Pike
Bethesda, MD 20892
Phone: (301)496-5323 **Fax:** (301)402-8497
Email: swedos@irp.nimh.nih.gov
Website: http://intramural.nimh.nih.gov/research/pdn/
Susan Swedo, MD, Ch.
Activities/Fields: Identification of factors influencing the onset and expression of psychiatric symptomatology; development of treatment and prevention strategies for pediatric psychopathology.

★ 25486 ★ U.S. Department of Health and Human Services
National Institutes of Health
National Institute of Mental Health
Section on Biological Rhythms
Bldg. 10, Rm. 3S231
9000 Rockville Pike
Bethesda, MD 20892
Phone: (301)496-2141 **Fax:** (301)496-5439
Email: tawehr@box-t.nih.gov
Website: http://intramural.nimh.nih.gov/research/sbr/
Thomas A. Wehr, MD, Ch.
Activities/Fields: Human circadian and seasonal rhythms and their role in the pathogenesis of mood and sleep disorders; investigates how light regulates the timing of these rhythms and how it can be used for treatment.

★ 25487 ★ U.S. Department of Health and Human Services
National Institutes of Health
National Institute of Mental Health
Section on Developmental Neurobiology
Bldg. 31, Rm. 8A-52
9000 Rockville Pike
Bethesda, MD 20892
Phone: (301)443-4513
Email: nimhinfo@nih.gov
Website: http://intramural.nimh.nih.gov/research/sdn
Activities/Fields: Biochemical and molecular mechanisms involved in the development and function of chemical synapses; major focus in on trophic factors that promote differentiation and survival of nerve cells and the targets they innervate.

★ 25488 ★ U.S. Department of Health and Human Services
National Institutes of Health
National Institute of Mental Health
Section on Pharmacology
Bldg. 10, Rm. 2D57
9000 Rockville Pike
Bethesda, MD 20892
Phone: (301)496-0160 **Fax:** (301)402-0337
Email: saavedrj@irp.nimh.nih.org
Website: http://intramural.nimh.nih.gov/research/sop/
Dr. Juan M. Saavedra, MD, Contact
Activities/Fields: Effects of drugs and hormones on the central regulation of endocrine, autonomous and immune functions; biological rhythms; cerebral blood flow.

★ 25489 ★ U.S. Department of Health and Human Services
National Institutes of Health
National Institute of Mental Health
Section on Socio-Environmental Studies
Bldg. 10, Rm. 4N222
9000 Rockville Pike
Bethesda, MD 20892
Phone: (301)496-3383
Email: schoolec@irp.nimh.nih.gov
Website: http://intramural.nimh.nih.gov/research/ses
Carmi Schooler, PhD, Ch.
Activities/Fields: Determinants of normal and abnormal psychological functioning during the life span, including cognitive processing and self-direction or autonomy.

★ 25490 ★ U.S. Department of Health and Human Services
National Institutes of Health
National Institute of Neurological Disorders and Stroke
Division of Extramural Research (Neurogenetics Program)
NSC/2136
6001 Executive Blvd.
Bethesda, MD 20892
Phone: (301)496-5745 **Fax:** (301)402-1501
Email: rf45c@nih.gov
Website: http://www.ninds.nih.gov/about_ninds/clusters/neurogenetics.htm
Robert Finkelstein, PhD, Dir.
Activities/Fields: Identification of neurological disease genes; mechanisms by which genetic mutations cause neurological disease; aims to develop gene-based therapeutics for neurological disorders.

★ 25491 ★ U.S. Department of Health and Human Services
National Institutes of Health
National Institute of Neurological Disorders and Stroke
Division of Extramural Research (Channels, Synapses and Circuits Cluster)
NSC/2110
6001 Executive Blvd.
Bethesda, MD 20892-9523
Phone: (301)496-1917 **Fax:** (301)480-2424
Email: yl5o@nih.gov
Website: http://www.ninds.nih.gov/about_ninds/clusters/channels_synapses_and_circuits.htm
Yuan Liu, PhD, Dir.
Activities/Fields: Channels, synapses, and neural circuits that underlie normal brain functions and dysfunctions related to neurological disorders, such as epilepsy.

★ 25492 ★ U.S. Department of Health and Human Services
National Institutes of Health
National Institute of Neurological Disorders and Stroke
Division of Extramural Research (Clinical Trials Program)
NSC/2216
6001 Executive Blvd.
Bethesda, MD 20892-9531
Phone: (301)496-9520 **Fax:** (301)480-1080
Email: jm137f@nih.gov
Website: http://www.ninds.nih.gov/about_ninds/clusters/clinical_trials.htm
John Marler, MD, Assoc. Dir.
Activities/Fields: Neurological diseases, including stroke and managing the symptoms of stroke.

★ 25493 ★ U.S. Department of Health and Human Services
National Institutes of Health (NIH)
National Institute of Neurological Disorders and Stroke
Division of Extramural Research (Systems and Cognitive Neuroscience Cluster)
NSC/2109
6601 Executive Blvd.
Bethesda, MD 20892-9531
Phone: (301)496-9964 **Fax:** (301)402-2060
Email: ee48r@nih.gov
Website: http://ninds.nih.gov/about_ninds/clusters/systems_and_cognitive_neuroscience.htm
Emmeline Edwards, PhD, Dir.
Activities/Fields: Neurobiology of higher cognitive functions and complex behaviors; advances understanding of neuronal circuits underlying specific cognitive and motor functions.

★ 25494 ★ U.S. Department of Health and Human Services
National Institutes of Health
National Institute of Neurological Disorders and Stroke
Division of Extramural Research (Neural Environment Cluster Program)
NSC/2110
6001 Executive Blvd.
Bethesda, MD 20892-9521

Phone: (301)496-1431 **Fax:** (301)480-2424
Email: ap101d@nih.gov
Website: http://www.ninds.nih.gov/about_ninds/clusters/neural_environment.htm
Audrey Penn, PhD, Actng. Dir.
Activities/Fields: Strives to reduce the burden of neurological diseases by increasing knowledge of glial and cerebrovascular cell function in normal and pathological states, as well as immune cell function and infectious agents in diseased nervous systems.

★ 25495 ★ U.S. Department of Health and Human Services
National Institutes of Health
National Institute of Neurological Disorders and Stroke
Division of Extramural Research
(Neurodegeneration Cluster Program)
NSC/2223
6001 Executive Blvd.
Bethesda, MD 20892
Phone: (301)496-5680 **Fax:** (301)480-1080
Email: dm152o@nih.gov
Website: http://www.ninds.nih.gov/about_ninds/clusters/neurodegeneration.htm
Dr. Diane Murphy, PhD, Dir.
Activities/Fields: Understanding neuronal cell death, including Parkinson's disease, Alzheimer's disease, amyotrophic lateral sclerosis, Huntington's disease, Pick's disease, brain cell death.

★ 25496 ★ U.S. Department of Health and Human Services
National Institutes of Health (NIH)
National Institute of Neurological Disorders and Stroke
Division of Extramural Research
(Repair and Plasticity Program)
NSC/2206
6001 Executive Blvd.
Bethesda, MD 20892-9525
Phone: (301)496-1447 **Fax:** (301)480-1080
Email: ac207@nih.gov
Website: http://www.ninds.nih.gov/about_ninds/clusters/repair_and_plasticity.htm
Arlene Chiu, PhD, Dir.
Activities/Fields: Traumatic brain injury (TBI), including mechanisms of injury in the acute and chronic stages, clinical trail design for traumatic brain injury, and possible use of imaging technology to assess cognitive/behavioral changes after TBI.

★ 25497 ★ U.S. Department of Health and Human Services
National Institutes of Health (NIH)
National Institute of Neurological Disorders and Stroke
Division of Extramural Research
(Office of Minority Health and Research)
NSC/2150
6601 Executive Blvd.
Bethesda, MD 20892-9531
Phone: (301)496-3102 **Fax:** (301)594-5929
Email: gj62v@nih.gov
Website: http://www.ninds.nih.gov/about_ninds/clusters/special_programs_in_neuroscience.htm
Gayathri Jeyarasasingam, PhD, Dir.
Activities/Fields: Provides grants which support research groups aiming to reduce disease disparity of populations historically at increased risk for diseases and disorders of the brain, spinal cord, and peripheral nervous system.

★ 25498 ★ U.S. Department of Health and Human Services
National Institutes of Health
National Institute of Neurological Disorders and Stroke
Division of Intramural Research
(Behavioral Neuroscience Unit)
Bldg. 36, Rm. B205
36 Convent Dr., MSC 4124
Bethesda, MD 20892-4124
Phone: (301)496-3906 **Fax:** (301)402-2281
Email: schreurs@codon.nih.gov
Website: http://www.ninds.nih.gov/about_ninds/labs/archive/14.htm
Bernard G. Schreurs, PhD, Investigator
Activities/Fields: Behavior laws, or understanding what happens in the brain when learning occurs; aims to identify physiological basis of classical conditioning, an associative form of learning and memory.

★ 25499 ★ U.S. Department of Health and Human Services
National Institutes of Health
National Institute of Neurological Disorders and Stroke
Division of Intramural Research
(Clinical Stroke Research Unit)
Bldg. 36, Rm. 4A03
36 Convent Dr., MSC 4128
Bethesda, MD 20892-4128
Phone: (301)295-1755 **Fax:** (301)295-0863
Email: degrabat@ninds.nih.gov
Thomas J. DeGraba, MD, Investigator
Activities/Fields: Atherosclerosis, focused on the study of association of gene polymorphisms in the regulators of inflammation, T-lymphocyte profile, and altered gene expression in symptomatic versus asymptomatic patients.

★ 25500 ★ U.S. Department of Health and Human Services
National Institutes of Health
National Institute of Neurological Disorders and Stroke
Division of Intramural Research
(Analytical Cell Biology)
Bldg. 36, Rm. 2A21
36 Convent Dr., MSC 4062
Bethesda, MD 20892-4062
Phone: (301)435-2796 **Fax:** (301)480-1485
Email: sba@helix.nih.gov
Website: http://www.ninds.nih.gov/about_ninds/labs/38.htm
S. Brian Andrews, PhD, Sr. Investigator
Activities/Fields: Cell biology and physiology of neurons, especially the function of intracellular domains that regulate calcium (Ca) signaling following from synaptic activity; development of technologies for quantitative and molecular electron microscopy.

★ 25501 ★ U.S. Department of Health and Human Services
National Institutes of Health
National Institute of Neurological Disorders and Stroke
Division of Intramural Research
(Clinical Neurocardiology Section)
Bldg. 10, Rm. 6N252
10 Center Dr., MSC 1620
Bethesda, MD 20892-1620
Phone: (301)496-2103 **Fax:** (301)402-0180
Email: daveg@box-d.nih.gov
Website: http://www.ninds.nih.gov/about_ninds/labs/82.htm
David S. Goldstein, MD, Sr. Investigator
Activities/Fields: Clinical neurocardiology research about disorders of neuroendocrine regulation of the cardiovascular system, with emphasis on diseases where the symptomatic nervous system or catecholamines play important pathogenic roles, such as autonomic failures syndromes, pheochromocytoma, and neurogenetic conditions featuring abnormal catecholamine synthesis or metabolism.

★ 25502 ★ U.S. Department of Health and Human Services
National Institutes of Health
National Institute of Neurological Disorders and Stroke
Division of Intramural Research
(Cognitive Neuroscience Section)
Bldg. 10, Rm. 5C205
10 Center Dr., MSC 1440
Bethesda, MD 20892-1440
Phone: (301)496-0220 **Fax:** (301)480-2909
Email: grafmanj@ninds.nih.gov
Website: http://www.ninds.nih.gov/about_ninds/labs/83.htm
Jordan Grafman, PhD, Sr. Investigator
Activities/Fields: Studies the underlying cognitive architecture and number of circumscribed prefrontal cortex brain sectors subserving specific cognitive operations and/or knowledge; understanding types of information binding that occur in the human brain.

★ 25503 ★ U.S. Department of Health and Human Services
National Institutes of Health
National Institute of Neurological Disorders and Stroke
Division of Intramural Research
(Clinical Epilepsy Section)
Bldg. 10, Rm. 5N250
10 Center Dr., MSC 1408
Bethesda, MD 20892-1408
Phone: (301)496-1505 **Fax:** (301)402-2871
Email: theodorw@ninds.nih.gov
Website: http://www.ninds.nih.gov/about_ninds/labs/63.htm
William H. Theodore, MD, Sr. Investigator
Activities/Fields: Evaluation and treatment of uncontrolled epilepsy, emphasizing non-invasive approaches to localization of epileptic foci and cognitive mapping, using video-EEG monitoring, transcranial magnetic stimulation (TMS), positron emission tomography (PET), and magnetic resonance imaging (MRI), including functional MRI and MR spectroscopy.

★ 25504 ★ U.S. Department of Health and Human Services
National Institutes of Health
National Institute of Neurological Disorders and Stroke
Division of Intramural Research
(Brain Stimulation Unit)
Bldg. 10, Rm. 5N230
10 Center Dr., MSC 1430
Bethesda, MD 20892-1430
Phone: (301)496-0151 **Fax:** (301)402-1007
Email: wassermanne@ninds.nih.gov
Website: http://www.ninds.nih.gov/about_ninds/labs/104.htm
Eric Wassermann, MD, Chf.
Activities/Fields: Transcranial stimulation as a means of assessing and altering brain function in patients with neurological and psychiatric disorders, as well as, healthy individuals. Studies include measures of axonal excitability and synaptic influences on output cells of the motor cortex, and experimental treatments that alter these measures.

★ 25505 ★ U.S. Department of Health and Human Services
National Institutes of Health
National Institute of Neurological Disorders and Stroke
Division of Intramural Research (Cellular Immunology Section)
Bldg. 10, Rm. 5B16
10 Center Dr., MSC 1400
Bethesda, MD 20892-1400
Phone: (301)402-4488 **Fax:** (301)402-0373
Email: martinr@ninds.nih.gov
Website: http://www.ninds.nih.gov/about_ninds/labs/98.htm
Roland Martin, MD, Investigator
Activities/Fields: Understanding how the cellular immune system in multiple sclerosis (MS) patients reacts to autoantigens of the central nervous system. Research includes studies on molecular mechanisms of T-cell recognition.

★ 25506 ★ U.S. Department of Health and Human Services
National Institutes of Health (NIH)
National Institute of Neurological Disorders and Stroke
Division of Intramural Research (Advanced MRI Section)
Bldg. 10, Rm. B1D108
10 Center Dr., MSC 1065
Bethesda, MD 20892-1065
Phone: (301)402-1981 **Fax:** (301)402-3216
Email: jhd@helix.nih.gov
Website: http://www.ninds.nih.gov/about_ninds/labs/106.htm
Jeff H. Duyn, PhD, Investigator
Activities/Fields: Mechanisms behind MRI contrast, exploring avenues to manipulate contrast, and optimizing MRI data acquisition and analysis to achieve optimum sensitivity, resolution, reliability, and accuracy.

★ 25507 ★ U.S. Department of Health and Human Services
National Institutes of Health (NIH)
National Institute of Neurological Disorders and Stroke
Division of Intramural Research (Biochemistry Section)
Bldg. 10, Rm. 5D37
10 Center Dr., MSC 1414
Bethesda, MD 20892-1414
Phone: (301)496-6628 **Fax:** (301)402-0380
Email: youle@helix.nih.gov
Website: http://www.ninds.nih.gov/about_ninds/labs/81.htm
Richard J. Youle, PhD, Sr. Investigator
Activities/Fields: Immunotoxins, including protein toxins and chemeric toxins; understanding molecular basis of cell death.

★ 25508 ★ U.S. Department of Health and Human Services
National Institutes of Health (NIH)
National Library of Medicine
National Center for Biotechnology Information (Computational Biology Branch)
Bldg. 45, Rm. 6AN12J
45 Center Dr., MSC 6510
Bethesda, MD 20892-6510
Phone: (301)435-5981 **Fax:** (301)480-2288
Email: landsman@ncbi.nlm.nih.gov
Website: http://www.ncbi.nlm.nih.gov/CBBresearch/
David Landsman, PhD, Ch.
Activities/Fields: Theoretical, analytical and applied approaches to a broad range of fundamental problems in molecular biology. **Pub:** *Papers.* • *Reports.*

★ 25509 ★ U.S. Department of Health and Human Services
National Institutes of Health
Office of AIDS Research
Bldg. 2 Room 4E 14
Two Center Dr. MSC 0250
Bethesda, MD 20892
Phone: (301)496-0357 **Fax:** (301)496-2119
Dr. Jack Whitescarvre, Dir.
Activities/Fields: Advises the Director, NIH, and senior staff on the development of NIH-wide policy related to AIDS research, and coordinates NIH intramural and extramural AIDS research activities; Represents the Director, NIH, on all outside AIDS-related committees requiring NIH participation; Provides staff support to the NIH AIDS Advisory Committee; Recommends Intramural/Extramural AIDS research priorities to the Director, NIH; Develops an NIH annual plan and budget for AIDS research; Develops and maintains an information database on Intramural/Extramural AIDS activities and prepares special or recurring reports as needed; Develops information strategies to assure the public is informed of NIH AIDS research activities; Recommends solutions to ethical/legal issues arising from AIDS research; Facilitates cooperation in AIDS research between government, industry, and universities; and Fosters and develops plans for NIH involvement in international AIDS research activities.

★ 25510 ★ U.S. Department of Health and Human Services
National Institutes of Health
Office of Dietary Supplements
6100 Executive Blvd.,
Room 3B01, MSC 7517
Bethesda, MD 20892-7517
Phone: (301)435-2920 **Fax:** (301)480-1845
Email: ods@nih.gov
Website: http://ods.od.nih.gov/
Paul M. Coates, PhD, Dir.
Activities/Fields: Explore the role of dietary supplements to improve health care and promote scientific study of dietary supplements in maintaining health and preventing chronic disease. **Pub:** *Bibliography of Significant Advances in Dietary Supplements*, annually.

★ 25511 ★ U.S. Department of Health and Human Services
National Institutes of Health
Office of Extramural Research
NIH Bldg. 1, Rm. 144
1 Center Dr., Mail Stop 0152
Bethesda, MD 20892
Phone: (301)496-1096 **Fax:** (301)402-3469
Email: wendy_baldwin@nih.gov
Website: http://www.nih.gov/grants/oer.htm
Wendy Baldwin, PhD, Dep. Dir.
Activities/Fields: Adminsters the development and coordination of NIH policies and procedures for awarding funds in support of biomedical research, including policies for the conduct of biomedical and behavioral research involving human subjects or vertebrate animals; and provides policy guidance for the Research Grants Division.

★ 25512 ★ U.S. Department of Health and Human Services
National Institutes of Health
Office of Medical Applications of Research
Bldg. 31, Rm. 1B03
31 Center Dr., MSC-2082
Bethesda, MD 20892
Phone: (301)496-5641 **Free:** 888-644-2667
Fax: (301)402-0420
Email: bk76p@nih.gov
Website: http://consensus.nih.gov
Barnett S. Kramer, MD, MP, Dir.
Activities/Fields: Translation of results of biomedical research pertinent to health care into knowledge that can effectively be employed in the practice of medicine and public health. The Office facilitates and coordinates technical consensus development activities at the National Institutes of Health through the implementation of consensus conferences. These conferences bring together biomedical research scientists, practicing physicians, consumers, and others in an effort to reach general agreement on whether a given medical technology is safe and effective. OMAR works with NIH institutes to promote the effective dissemination of information derived from the consensus development process to the biomedical research and health care communities, the public, and other federal agencies. Principal area of research interest is health care technologies assessment, including drugs, devices, and medical and surgical procedures. **Pub:** *NIH Consensus and State-of-the-Science statements*, 5/year.

★ 25513 ★ U.S. Department of Health and Human Services
National Institutes of Health
Office of Recombinant DNA Activities
6000 Executive Blvd. Ste. 302
Bethesda, MD 20892-7010
Phone: (301)496-9838 **Fax:** (301)496-9839
Website: http://www.nih.gov/
Debra Knorr, Actg. Dir.
Activities/Fields: Administers the recombinant DNA research activities supported and monitored by the National Institutes of Health. (Recombinant DNA is prepared through laboratory transplantation or splicing of genes from one organism to another.) ORDA reviews all special requests submitted to NIH involving recombinant DNA technology and implements NIH policies and procedures for conducting this research. **Pub:** *NIH Guidelines for Research Involving Recombinant DNA Molecules.*

★ 25514 ★ U.S. Department of Health and Human Services
National Library of Medicine
Bldg. 38, 2S15
8600 Rockville Pike
Bethesda, MD 20894
Phone: (301)496-6308 **Fax:** (301)496-4450
Email: publicinfo@nlm.nih.gov
Website: http://www.nlm.nih.gov
Dr. Donald A.B. Lindberg, Dir.
Activities/Fields: World's largest research library in a single scientific and professional field. The Library collects materials in all major areas of the health sciences and, to a lesser degree, in chemistry, physics, botany, and zoology. The Library's extensive collections and information services may be used by health professionals and health-science students. In addition, NLM serves as a national resource for all U.S. health science libraries through its National Network of Libraries of Medicine. This network, which offers lending and other services, includes 4000 basic unit libraries (mostly at hospitals), 125 Resource Libraries (at medical schools), and eight Regional Medical Libraries (covering all geographic areas of the United States), and the NLM itself. **Pub:** *Index Medicus*, monthly.

★ 25515 ★ U.S. Department of Health and Human Services
National Library of Medicine
Extramural Programs Division
6705 Rockledge Dr., Ste. 301
Bethesda, MD 20894
Phone: (301)496-4621 **Fax:** (301)402-2952
Email: cornm@mail.nlm.nih.gov
Website: http://www.nlm.nih.gov/ep/extramural.html
Dr. Milton Corn, Dir.
Activities/Fields: Administers the National Library of Medicine's program of grants fo r support of fundamental and applied work in the organization, representation, utilization, and dissemination of health knowledge, with special interest in medical informatics and biotechnology information. Grants are generally awarded in three main categories: Research, Development, and Demonstration awards are investigator-initi-

ated projects that address problems of health information access, retrieval, and utilization. Projects may investigate fundamental research problems, may undertake development of theoretical findings into practical applications, or may demonstrate the value of new technologies in operating situations. First Independent Research Support and Transition (FIRST) Awards are small project awards to young investigators. Eligibility is limited to those who have received the doctorate within five years but have not yet served as principal investigator on a research grant or contract. Research Career Development Awards are available to young scientists with three or more years of postdoctoral experience. These awards enable the scientist to devote full time to research.

★ 25516 ★ U.S. Department of Health and Human Services
National Library of Medicine
Office of Computer and Communications Systems
Special Assistant for Research and Development
Bldg. 38A, Rm. 9F904
8600 Rockville Pike
Bethesda, MD 20894
Phone: (301)496-9300 **Fax:** (301)496-0673
Activities/Fields: Information processing, including information retrieval, ergonomics, natural language processing, artificial intelligence, and database management.

★ 25517 ★ U.S. Department of Health and Human Services
National Toxicology Program
PO Box 12233
Research Triangle Park, NC 27709
Phone: (919)541-3201 **Fax:** (919)541-2260
Email: hart@niehs.nih.gov
Website: http://ntp-server.niehs.nih.gov/
Dr. Kenneth Olden, Dir.
Activities/Fields: Reliable series of relatively inexpensive short-term tests and protocols useful for the public health regulation of toxic chemicals, including the development of test batteries to assess genetic, neurobehavioral, and immunological toxicities; expand the toxicological profiles of chemicals tested; increase the rate of testing of chemicals for such toxic effects as carcinogenicity, mutagenicity, and reproductive and developmental effects (NTP also examines the chemicals for neurobehavioral, immunological, and other toxic effects where appropriate) within funding limits; and disseminate results of NTP's testing and methods development programs to government research and regulatory agencies, industry, labor, environmental groups, the scientific community, and the public. Chemicals chosen for testing are those that involve widespread or intense human exposure, or those for which existing data on toxic effects are inadequate. Some chemicals are selected for testing because study of them may tell more about how structurally related chemicals are likely to affect human health. Other criteria include: amount produced, significant physical and chemical properties, interest by regulatory and research agencies, and possible public health significance. The NTP testing strategy is to identify the major toxic effects of each chemical studied (genetic mutations; damage to critical organs such as the lungs, liver, and nervous system; birth defects; or cancer). Chemicals are nominated for testing by a variety of sources, including representatives of the agencies on the NTP Executive Committee; government agencies not represented on the Committee; academic, industry, and labor groups; state and local governments; and individuals. Persons interested in proposing chemicals for testing should give the reasons for their nominations and, when known, include production and usage information, data on human exposures, results of toxicological studies, data on the chemical's reactions in the human body, information concerning the chemical's relationship to structurally similar chemicals about which there are data, and other pertinent information. **Pub:** *DOE and EPA Research Related to Toxicology.* • *NTP Annual Plan.* • *Report on Carcinogens*, annually. • *Review of Current DHHS.* • *Technical reports.*

★ 25518 ★ U.S. Department of Health and Human Services
Office of Assistant Secretary for Health
Office Of Research Integrity
Rockwall Bldg. 2
5515 Security Ln., Ste. 700
Rockville, MD 20852
Phone: (301)443-3400 **Fax:** (301)443-5351
Email: cpascal@osophs.dhhs.gov
Website: http://ori.dhhs.gov
Chris Pascal, Dir.
Activities/Fields: Responds to any allegations of scientific misconduct occurring in research supported by the Public Health Service.

★ 25519 ★ U.S. Department of Health and Human Services
Office of Assistant Secretary for Health
Office of Research Integrity
Research Investigations Division
Rockwall Bldg. 2
5515 Security Ln., Ste. 700
Rockville, MD 20852
Phone: (301)443-5330 **Fax:** (301)594-0043
Email: aprice@osophs.dhhs.gov
Website: http://ori.dhhs.gov/html/programs/rapidresponse.asp
Alan R. Price, Dir.
Activities/Fields: Responds to allegations of scientific misconduct occurring in research supported by the Public Health Service.

★ 25520 ★ U.S. Department of Health and Human Services
Office of Disease Prevention and Health Promotion
Humphrey Bldg.
200 Independence Ave. SW, Rm. 738G
Washington, DC 20201
Phone: (202)401-6295 **Fax:** (202)205-9478
Website: http://odphp.osophs.dhhs.gov/
Linda Meyers, Actg. Dir.
Activities/Fields: Develops and manages the National Health Goals and Objectives (known as Healthy People 2000) for the National Health Information Center. Coordinates policy and program for the Public Health Service.

★ 25521 ★ U.S. Department of Health and Human Services
Office of Family, Community and Long-Term Care Policy
Division of Disability, Aging and Long-Term Care Policy
200 Independence Ave. SW, Rm. 424E
Washington, DC 20201
Phone: (202)690-6443 **Fax:** (202)690-7733
Email: daltcp2@hhs.gov
Website: http://aspe.hhs.gov/daltcp/home.htm
Brenda Veazey, Staff Asst.
Activities/Fields: Financing, organization, and delivery of services to chronically impaired populations; informs the Department's policy development process. Recent work has centered on the needs of the impaired elderly, employment of working age adults with disabilities, and mentally disabled. Research areas include population characteristics, quality of care, home and community based services, disability issues, and data needs. **Pub:** *Reports.* • *Working papers.* **Frmly:** (2001) Office of Family, Community and Long-Term Care Policy; Division of Disability, Aging and Long-Term Care Policy.

★ 25522 ★ U.S. Department of Health and Human Services
Office of Research and Demonstrations
Beneficiary Studies Division
Research and Evaluation Group
C3-19-07
7500 Security Blvd.
Baltimore, MD 21244
Phone: (410)786-6692 **Fax:** (410)786-5515
Renee Mentnech, Dir.
Activities/Fields: Designs and conducts research and evaluations to study the impacts of CHFA and other health care programs, focusing particularly on beneficiary issues. Designs and conducts general studies related to beneficiaries. Evaluates demonstration projects, pilot projects and other innovations in HCFA programs. Designs demonstration projects. Develops data bases and evaluation methods/tools to evaluate the impact of HCFA programs on beneficiary issues. Provides technical research and evaluation related support to HCFA, HHS and others related to beneficiary issues. **Pub:** *Health Care Financing Annual Review.* **Frmly:** Office of Research and Demonstrations; Beneficiary Studies Division.

★ 25523 ★ U.S. Department of Health and Human Services
Office of Research and Demonstrations
Office of Demonstrations and Evaluations
Long-Term Care Experimentation Division (Division of Health Systems Research)
C3-20-17
7500 Security Blvd.
Baltimore, MD 21244
Phone: (410)786-6640 **Fax:** (410)786-6511
Brigid Goody, Dir.
Activities/Fields: Designs and conducts research and evaluations to study the impacts of HCFA and other health care programs; Designs and conducts general studies related to health care systems; Evaluates demonstration projects, pilot projects and other innovations in HCFA programs; Designs demonstration projects, particularly related to innovative delivery systems, models for long term care and dually-eligible beneficiaries; Develops databases and evaluation methods/tools to evaluate the impact of HCFA programs; Provides technical research and evaluation related support to HCFA, HHS, and others. **Frmly:** Office of Demonstrations and Evaluations; Long Term Care Experimentation Division.

★ 25524 ★ U.S. Department of Health and Human Services
Office of Research and Demonstrations
Office of Demonstrations and Evaluations
Research and Evaluation Group
C3-21-28
7500 Security Blvd.
Baltimore, MD 21244
Phone: (410)786-6500 **Fax:** (410)786-5515
Email: aesposito@cms.hha.gov
Al Esposito, Dir.
Activities/Fields: Research and Evaluation Group provides leadership and executive direction within CMS for a wide range of health care financing research and demonstration activities. Designs and conducts research and evaluation of the health care delivery system including CMS and other health care programs. Develops data bases and conducts analyses of the health care market. **Pub:** *Health Care Financing Review*, quarterly. • *Supplement*, annually.

★ 25525 ★ U.S. Department of Health and Human Services
Public Health Service
Agency for Health Care Policy and Research
Executive Office Center, Ste. 600
2101 E Jefferson St., Rm. 600
Rockville, MD 20852

Phone: (301)594-6662 **Free:** 800-358-9295
Fax: (301)594-2168
Email: info@ahrq.gov
Website: http://www.ahrq.gov
Dr. Carolyn M. Clancy, Actg. Dir.

Activities/Fields: Develops and disseminates research-based information to increase the scientific knowledge needed to enhance consumer and clinical decisionmaking, improve health care quality, and promote efficiency in the organization of public and private systems of health care delivery. Its programs evaluate the effectiveness of medical treatments and other health services and improve access to new scientific and technical information for health care practitioners, policymakers, administrators, insurers, researchers, educators, and consumers. AHRQ supports and conducts research and evaluation projects in eight areas: consumer choice; clinical improvement; health care cost, financing, and access; health information technology; outcomes and effectiveness of health care; health care organization and delivery; quality measurement and improvement; and technology assessment. **Frmly:** (2000) Agency for Health Care Policy and Research.

★ 25526 ★ U.S. Department of Health and Human Services
Public Health Service
Agency for Health Care Policy and Research
Center for General Health Services Extramural Research
6011 Executive Office Center, Rm. 200
Rockville, MD 20852-4993
Phone: (301)594-1349 **Fax:** (301)594-2155
Email: daniels@ahrq.gov
Dr. Daniel Scryer, Dir.

Activities/Fields: Delivery of health care service in rural areas and frontier areas; and the health of low-income groups, minority groups, and the elderly. Emphasizes the effectiveness, efficiency, and quality of health care services; the outcomes of health care services and procedures; clinical practice, including primary care and practice-oriented research; health care technologies, facilities, and equipment; health care costs, productivity, and market forces; health promotion and disease prevention; health statistics and epidemiology; and medical liability. **Pub:** *proceedings.* • *Research reports.*

★ 25527 ★ U.S. Department of Health and Human Services
Public Health Service
Agency for Health Care Policy and Research
Center for Organization and Delivery Studies
2101 E Jefferson St., Ste. 605
Rockville, MD 20852
Phone: (301)594-1410 **Fax:** (301)594-2314
Email: info@ahrq.gov
Website: http://www.ahcpr.gov/about/cods/
Irene Fraser, Dir.

Activities/Fields: Health care markets, health care delivery systems, and health care organizations. **Pub:** *Monographs.* • *Reports.*

★ 25528 ★ U.S. Department of Health and Human Services
Public Health Service
Office of Adolescent Pregnancy Programs
4350 East-West Hwy., ste. 200W
Bethesda, MD 20814
Phone: (301)594-4004 **Fax:** (301)594-5981
Email: opa@osophs.dhhs.gov
Website: http://opa.osophs.dhhs.gov/
Patrick J. Sheeran, DPA, Dir. of OAPP

Activities/Fields: Supports care demonstration projects to help pregnant teenagers and their children and families; and prevention demonstration projects to reach teenagers before they become sexually active. Programs include the award of research and evaluation grants and contracts for studies on the causes and consequences of adolescent sexual behavior, contraceptive use, and early childbearing; and evaluation of service delivery.

★ 25529 ★ U.S. Department of Health and Human Services
Research and Training Center on Rural Disabilities
Univ. of Montana
52 Corbin Hall
Missoula, MT 59812-7056
Phone: (406)243-5467 **Fax:** (406)243-2349
Email: ruraldoc@selway.umt.edu
Website: http://rtc.ruralinstitute.umt.edu
Dr. Tom Seekins, Dir.

Activities/Fields: Employment and vocational rehabilitation service needs of people with disabilities in rural areas; intervention development to improve employment outcomes; self-employment and economic development models; rural independent living; improvement of transportation, health care, housing, and accessibility; rural models for prevention of secondary disabilities; disability legislation and American Indian Tribes; and alternative models of delivery of rural rehabilitation services. **Pub:** *Newsletter.*

★ 25530 ★ U.S. Department of Health and Human Services
Social Security Administration
Office of Research and Statistics
Division of RSDI Research Statistics
Rm. 4-C 16, Operations Bldg.
6401 Security Blvd.
Baltimore, MD 21235
Phone: (410)965-0156 **Fax:** (410)966-3308
Barbara Lingg, Dir.

Activities/Fields: Preparation of statistical and analytical data pertaining to RSDI benefit provisions of Title II of the Social Security Act. **Pub:** *Annual statistical supplement.* **Frmly:** Division of RSD1 Research Statistics; (2001) Office of Research and Statistics; Division of RSDI Statistics and Evaluation Analysis.

★ 25531 ★ U.S. Department of Health and Human Services
Warren Grant Magnuson Clinical Center
NIH Bldg. 10
6100 Executive Blvd., Rm. 2C6-146
Bethesda, MD 20892
Phone: (301)496-2563 **Fax:** (301)402-2984
Email: jg21z@nih.gov
Website: http://www.cc.nih.gov
John I. Gallin, MD, Dir.

Activities/Fields: Designed to place patient care facilities close to research laboratories to promote the quick transfer of new findings of basic and clinical scientists to the treatment of patients. The Center provides high-quality patient care necessary for intramural clinical research conducted at the National Institutes of Health; performs research on methods and systems involved in patient care and study; disseminates information to professionals and to the public relevant to clinical investigation; develops and maintains training programs in the techniques and ethics of biomedical and clinical research; and interacts with scientists and physicians, nationally and internationally, on such mutual problems of clinical research as policy, education, ethics, and priorities. To be considered for admission to the Clinical Center, patients should be referred by their private physician and they can be admitted only if their medical condition meets the precise requirements of a specific research protocol. **Pub:** *Current Clinical Studies.* • *Medicine for the Public Booklets.* • *Patient Admission Procedures at NIH.*

★ 25532 ★ U.S. Department of Transportation
Coast Guard
Office of Health and Safety
Safety and Environmental Health Division
Coast Headquarters Bldg.
2100 2nd St. SW, G-WKS
Washington, DC 20593
Phone: (202)267-1883 **Fax:** (202)267-4355
Al Kotz, Chf.

Activities/Fields: Responsible for all internal mishap prevention, environmental health, and occupational health within the Coast Guard, including aircraft crashes, vessel collisions, fires, explosions, and chemical exposures.

★ 25533 ★ U.S. Department of Transportation
Federal Aviation Administration
Civil Aeromedical Institute (CAMI)
AAM-3
PO Box 25082
Oklahoma City, OK 73125-5060
Phone: (405)954-1000 **Fax:** (405)954-1010
Email: william_e_collins@mmacmail.jccbi.gov
Website: http://www.cami.jccbi.gov/
Dr. William E. Collins, Dir.

Activities/Fields: Civil aviation medicine directed toward preventing aircraft accidents and increasing survival rates associated with aircraft accidents. Studies are primarily in the fields of human factors, psychology, physiology, toxicology, cabin safety, restraint, ditching, and protective breathing equipment. Other areas of study include vision, human performance, and operator selection. Institute also conducts programs in aircraft accident investigation; medical certification (more than 640,000 airmen); statistical studies from the airman data bank; occupational health; and medical education of physicians, pilots, flight inspectors, accident investigators, and flight attendants. flight attendants. **Pub:** *Aeromedical safety brochures.* • *Federal Air Surgeon's Medical Bulletin.* • *Office of Aviation Medicine reports.*

★ 25534 ★ U.S. Department of Transportation
Federal Aviation Administration
Civil Aeromedical Institute
Aeromedical Research Division
(Protection and Survival Laboratory)
Mail Code AAM-630
6500 S MacArthur Blvd.
PO Box 25082
Oklahoma City, OK 73125
Phone: (405)954-5510 **Fax:** (405)954-4984
Email: van.gowdy@faa.gov
Website: http://www.cami.jccbi.gov/aam-600/630/600P&S-Lab.html
Van Gowdy, Mgr.

Activities/Fields: Problems concerning civil airmen and equipment in emergency conditions, such as function of seat/restraint/interior crash injury protection, emergency evacuation, flotation, and cabin safety. Principal areas of research interest are biomechanics of impact, human factors, and breathing equipment. Laboratory comprises the Biodynamics Research, and Cabin Safety Research units and Environmental Physiology. **Pub:** *Memorandums.* • *Research reports.*

★ 25535 ★ U.S. Department of Transportation
Federal Aviation Administration
Civil Aeromedical Institute
Aeromedical Research Division
(Toxicology and Accident Research Laboratory)
6500 S MacArthur Blvd.
PO Box 25082
Oklahoma City, OK 73125-5066
Phone: (405)954-4866 **Fax:** (405)954-3705

Email: dennis_canfield@mmacmail.jccbi.gov
Website: http://www.cami.jccbi.gov
Dennis Canfield, Mgr.

Activities/Fields: Human factor safety in civilian aviation. Studies are concerned with medical evidence available from aircraft accidents, including the genesis of the injuries experienced in those accidents; and effects of toxicants that may be present in post-crash fires or that may be otherwise introduced into the aviation environment. **Pub:** *Office of Aviation Medicine Technical Reports*. **Frmly:** (1991) Aviation Pathology and Toxicology Laboratory.

★ 25536 ★ U.S. Department of Transportation
Federal Aviation Administration
Civil Aeromedical Institute
Aeromedical Research Division
Mail Code AAM-600
PO Box 25082
Oklahoma City, OK 73125-5066
Phone: (405)954-4808 **Fax:** (405)954-0130
Email: james.e.whinnery@faa.gov
Website: http://www.cami.jccbi.gov
Dr. James E. Whinnery, PhD, M, Mgr.

Activities/Fields: Provides the Federal Aviation Administration (FAA) and the Federal Air Surgeon with the capability to: resolve operational, regulatory, and administrative problems related to medical certification of pilots; define and optimize workload and performance in aviation-related activities; and improve protection and survival in hostile and adverse aspects of general and commercial aviation. Division comprises the Toxicology and Accident Research Laboratory, Protection and Survival Laboratory, and Data Processing and Analysis Team. **Pub:** *Proceedings*. • *Research Reports*.

★ 25537 ★ U.S. Department of Transportation
Federal Aviation Administration
Civil Aeromedical Institute
Human Resources Research Division
Mail Code AAM-500
PO Box 25082
Oklahoma City, OK 73125
Phone: (405)954-4846 **Fax:** (405)954-4852
Email: david.schroeder@faa.gov
Dr. David J. Schroeder, Mgr.

Activities/Fields: Conducts an integrated program of applied field and laboratory performance research on organizational and human factors aspects of aviation work environments. Guidance for program development is obtained from the National Plan for Civil Aviation Human Factors, the FAA Strategic Plan, and senior agency management. Emphasis is placed on improving human performance through enhanced human machine/systems interfaces, equipment design, selection, training, opertating procedures, and business practices. **Pub:** *Office of Aerospace Medicine Technical Reports*.

★ 25538 ★ U.S. Department of Transportation
Federal Aviation Administration
Office of Aviation Medicine
Medical Specialities Division
800 Independence Ave. SW
Washington, DC 20593
Phone: (202)267-8035 **Fax:** (202)493-5006
Email: nicholas.lomangino@faa.gov
Dr. Nicholas Lomangino, Mgr.

Activities/Fields: Program office for medical standards, certification policy, and aeromedical research and development. Principal area of research interest is clinical medicine. **Pub:** *Guidelines*. • *Newsletters*. • *Research Reports*.

★ 25539 ★ U.S. Department of Veterans Affairs
GI Research Laboratory
4150 Clement St., 151-M2
San Francisco, CA 94121
Phone: (415)750-2095 **Fax:** (415)750-2196
Email: youngk@itsa.ucsf.edu
Dr. Young S. Kim, Dir.

Activities/Fields: Molecular biology and cell biology, including studies on DNA cloning and sequencing, PCR, vector construction, site-directed mutagenesis, eukaryotic gene transfection, and oncogene and tumor suppressor gene molecular biology.

★ 25540 ★ U.S. Department of Veterans Affairs
Hines Veterans Administration Hospital
Midwest Center for Health Services and Policy Research
151H
PO Box 5000
Hines, IL 60141
Phone: (708)202-2414 **Fax:** (708)202-2316
Email: weiss@research.hines.med.va.gov
Website: http://research.hines.med.va.gov
Kevin Weiss, MD, Dir.

Activities/Fields: Conduct relevant, high quality health services research; stimulate health services research and provide technical assistance in its development. Research objectives focus on accountability of the health care delivery system; examination of patient and health system outcomes including utilization, cost, mortality and morbidity, quality; evaluation of continuum of care for veterans with chronic conditions; assessing the effect of VA health care programs and policies on patient outcomes. **Pub:** *Newsbrief*, quarterly. Newsletter. • *Newsletter*, monthly.

★ 25541 ★ U.S. Department of Veterans Affairs
National Center for Post Traumatic Stress Disorder
Veterans Affairs Medical & Regional Office Center
215 N Main St.
White River Junction, VT 05009-0001
Phone: (802)296-5132 **Fax:** (802)296-5135
Email: ncptsd@ncptsd.org
Website: http://www.ncptsd.org
Matt Friedman, Dir.

Activities/Fields: Post Traumatic Stress Disorder, caused by the traumatic stress of war; dangerous peacekeeping operations; interpersonal violence, such as assault, rape, and child abuse; disaster; and severe accidental and violent trauma in the civilian arena. **Pub:** *PTSD Research Quarterly*, quarterly.

★ 25542 ★ U.S. Department of Veterans Affairs
National Center for Post-Traumatic Stress Disorder
Behavioral Science Division
VA Medical Center (116B-2)
150 S Huntington Ave.
Boston, MA 02130
Phone: (617)232-9500 **Fax:** (617)278-4501
Email: andrea.carney@med.va.gov
Website: http://www.ncptsd.org
Andrea Carney, Contact

Activities/Fields: Develops scientifically validated measures of post-traumatic stress disorder (PTSD), including psychological and psychophysiological procedures, identifies basic mechanisms of PTSD as related to neuroscience, psychological, and behavioral processes, and health-related aspects of stress and trauma.

★ 25543 ★ U.S. Department of Veterans Affairs
National Center for Post-Traumatic Stress Disorder
Clinical Neurosciences Division
VA Medical Center
Psychiatry Service 116A
950 Campbell Ave.
West Haven, CT 06516
Phone: (203)932-5711 **Fax:** (203)937-3481
Email: charney.dennis@west-haven.va.gov
Website: http://www.ncptsd.org/about/divisions/west_haven/index.html
Dennis Charney, MD, Dir.

Activities/Fields: Research on post-traumatic stress syndrome, including the effects of severe stress on brain function and new treatments for trauma victims.

★ 25544 ★ U.S. Department of Veterans Affairs
National Center for Post-Traumatic Stress Disorder
Education Division
VA Palo Alto Health Care System
3801 Miranda Ave.
Palo Alto, CA 94304
Phone: (650)493-5000 **Fax:** (650)617-2769
Email: gloria.galavez@med.va.gov
Website: http://www.ncptsd.org/about/divisions/education/index.html
Gloria Galavez, MSW, Contact

Activities/Fields: Research on post-traumatic stress disorder, including inpatient research protocols, sleep studies, and cross-cultural investigations.

★ 25545 ★ U.S. Department of Veterans Affairs
National Center for Post-Traumatic Stress Disorder
Executive Division
VA Medical Center (116D)
White River Junction, VT 05009
Phone: (802)296-5132 **Fax:** (802)296-5135
Email: ptsd@dartmouth.edu
Website: http://www.ncptsd.org
Matthew J. Friedman, PhD, Exec. Dir.

Activities/Fields: Directs the research operations of the Center and its divisions. **Pub:** *PTSD Research Quarterly*, quarterly. • *NCPTSD Clinical Quarterly*.

★ 25546 ★ U.S. Department of Veterans Affairs
National Center for Post-Traumatic Stress Disorder
Northeast Program Evaluation Center
VA Connecticut Health Care System (182)
950 Campbell Ave.
West Haven, CT 06516
Phone: (203)937-3851 **Fax:** (203)937-3433
Email: robert.rosenheck@yale.edu
Website: http://www.ncptsd.org/about/divisions/nepec/index.html
Linda Scelfo-Appio, Contact

Activities/Fields: Performs evaluation and monitoring of all VA hospital-based posttraumatic stress disorder programs throughout the nation.

★ 25547 ★ U.S. Department of Veterans Affairs
National Center for Post-Traumatic Stress Disorder
Pacific Islands Division
1132 Bishop St., Ste. 307
Honolulu, HI 96813
Phone: (808)566-1546 **Fax:** (808)566-1885
Email: renee.ishii@honolulu.va.gov
Website: http://www.ncptsd.org/about/divisions/pacific/index.html
Renee Ishii, Contact

Activities/Fields: Research on cross-cultural factors affecting the expression, assessment, and treatment of PTSD among ethnic minorities, particularly Pacific Islander and Asian Americans.

★ 25548 ★ U.S. Department of Veterans Affairs
National Center for Post-Traumatic Stress Disorder
Women's Health Sciences Division
VA Boston Health Care System
150 S Huntington St.
Boston, MA 02130
Phone: (617)232-9500 **Fax:** (617)278-4515
Email: sandra.tomasetti@med.va.gov
Website: http://www.ncptsd.org/about/divisions/womens/index.html
Sandra Tomasetti, Prog. Asst.
Activities/Fields: Research on the psychological impact of military service on women veterans, including the effect of post-traumatic stress disorder on women's health and medical problems.

★ 25549 ★ U.S. Department of Veterans Affairs
Rehabilitation Research and Development Center
VA Medical Center (153)
3801 Miranda Ave.
Palo Alto, CA 94304
Phone: (650)493-5000 **Fax:** (650)852-3474
Email: zajac@roses.stanford.edu
Website: http://www.palo-alto.med.va.gov/programs.htm
James Golf, Dir.
Activities/Fields: State-of-the-art technological aids and treatments for disabled veterans to improve their independence and quality of life, especially in their mobility. Specific research areas include orthopedic biomechanics, neuromuscular systems, human-machine integration, fracture healing and implant design, skeletal biology and physical activity, coordination of human movement, surgery simulation, neuromuscular diagnosis and repair, robotics, patient-handling, functional assessment, and technology transfer. **Pub:** *Conference proceedings.* • *Progress Report.*

★ 25550 ★ U.S. Department of Veterans Affairs
Rehabilitation Research and Development Center
Design Development
Laboratory of Neuromuscular Biomechanics
VA Medical Center
3801 Miranda Ave.
Palo Alto, CA 94304-1530
Phone: (650)493-5000 **Fax:** (650)493-4919
Christopher Jacobs, Dir.
Activities/Fields: Supports research on coordination of human lower extremity muscles during functional activities, such as standing, walking, and pedaling in able-bodied and disabled persons.

★ 25551 ★ U.S. Department of Veterans Affairs
Rehabilitation Research and Development Center
Design Development
Laboratory of Neuromuscular Electrophysiology
3801 Miranda Ave.
Palo Alto, CA 94304-1200
Phone: (650)493-5000 **Fax:** (650)493-4919
Christopher Jacobs, Dir.
Activities/Fields: Human neuromuscular electrophysiology data. Laboratory activities center around devices used to stimulate and record from both nerve and muscle tissue, and the associated computer peripheral devices to collect, analyze, and record this data.

★ 25552 ★ U.S. Department of Veterans Affairs
Rehabilitation Research and Development Service
Center for Anabolic Therapies in Spinal Cord Injury
VA Medical Center, Rm. 1E-02
130 W Kingsbridge Rd.
Bronx, NY 10468
Phone: (718)584-9000 **Fax:** (718)733-5291
Email: wabauman@earthlink.net
Website: http://www.vard.org/cent/bronx.htm
William A. Bauman, MD, Dir.
Activities/Fields: Use of anabolic steroids and other pharmaceuticals to treat secondary disabilities of spinal cord injury.

★ 25553 ★ U.S. Department of Veterans Affairs
Rehabilitation Research and Development Service
Center for Excellence in Functional Recovery in Chronic Spinal Cord Injury
Rehab R&D Center (128)
Miami VA Medical Center
1201 NW 16th St.
Miami, FL 33125
Phone: (305)324-3363 **Fax:** (305)324-3218
Email: m.sipski@miami.edu
Website: http://www.vard.org/cent/miami.htm
Marca L. Sipski, MD, Dir.
Activities/Fields: Spasticity, pain management, recovery of motor and sensory function, and other areas of critical importance to spinal cord injury patients seeking to regain their independence.

★ 25554 ★ U.S. Department of Veterans Affairs
Rehabilitation Research and Development Service
Center of Excellence on Geriatric Rehabilitation
1670 Clairmont Rd. (151R)
Decatur, GA 30033
Phone: (404)728-5064 **Fax:** (404)728-4837
Email: rschuch@emory.edu
Website: http://www.varrd.emory.edu/
Ronald A. Schuchard, PhD, Dir.
Activities/Fields: Improvement in the function, independence, and quality of life of veterans aging with disabilities and those acquiring disabilities as they age. The center focuses on vision rehabilitation research, environment and behavior research, physical performance and function research, and research that highlights the interaction among these areas. Research is directed towards understanding the mechanisms underlying impairments and disabilities, and applying this understanding to the design, testing, and evaluation of creative, rehabilitative interventions.

★ 25555 ★ U.S. Department of Veterans Affairs
Rehabilitation Research and Development Service
Center of Excellence on Healthy Aging with Disabilities
Houston VA Medical Center
2002 Holcombe Blvd.
Houston, TX 77030
Phone: (713)794-7254 **Fax:** (713)794-7623
Email: healthyaging@bcm.tmc.edu
Website: http://www.healthyagingva.org/
Trilok N. Monga, MD, Med. Dir.
Activities/Fields: Process of aging with disabilities in order to design, implement, and evaluate strategies that enhance the health, functioning, and well-being of veterans aging with disabilities, with an ultimate goal of establishing best rehabilitation practices for the benefit of veterans.

★ 25556 ★ U.S. Department of Veterans Affairs
Rehabilitation Research and Development Service
Center of Excellence for Innovative Visual Rehabilitation
Boston VA Medical Center
Mail Stop 151E
150 S Huntington Ave.
Boston, MA 02130
Phone: (617)264-6548 **Fax:** (617)264-6645
Email: joseph_rizzo@meei.harvard.edu
Website: http://www.bostonretinalimplant.org
Dr. Joseph F. Rizzo, III, Dir.
Activities/Fields: Development of a retinal prosthesis to restore vision in patients with retinitis pigmentosa and with age-related macular degeneration, the leading cause of blindness among veterans and the general population.

★ 25557 ★ U.S. Department of Veterans Affairs
Rehabilitation Research and Development Service
Center of Excellence for Limb Loss Prevention and Prosthetic Engineering
Seattle VAMC
1660 S Columbian Way, MS 151
Seattle, WA 98108
Phone: (206)764-2991 **Fax:** (206)764-2127
Email: bsangeor@u.washington.edu
Website: http://rehab.research.seattle.med.va.gov/
Bruce J. Sangeorzan, MD, Dir.
Activities/Fields: Prosthetics and amputation. Research focuses on preservation of the lower limb and its function, understanding deformities that lead to ulceration, the role of prophylactic correction of the deformity, and the role of protective footwear.

★ 25558 ★ U.S. Department of Veterans Affairs
Rehabilitation Research and Development Service
Center of Excellence on Restoration of Function in Spinal Cord Injury and Multiple Sclerosis
VA Connecticut Health Care System
950 Campbell Ave.
West Haven, CT 06516
Phone: (203)932-3802
Email: stephen.waxman@yale.edu
Website: http://www.vard.yale.edu/
Stephen G. Waxman, MD, Dir.
Activities/Fields: Understanding the molecular, cellular and physiological basis of abnormal impulse conduction, and applying this understanding to the development of strategies to restore function in people with spinal cord injury and multiple sclerosis. **Pub:** *Journal articles.*

★ 25559 ★ U.S. Department of Veterans Affairs
Rehabilitation Research and Development Service
Center for Restoring Function through Electrical Stimulation (FES)
11000 Cedar Ave., Ste. 230
Cleveland, OH 44106-3052
Phone: (216)231-3257 **Free:** 800-666-2353
Fax: (216)231-3258
Email: info@fes.org
Website: http://www.fesc.org
P. Hunter Peckham, PhD, Dir.
Activities/Fields: Restoration of function for persons with paralysis through functional electrical stimulation (FES) systems that improve health, productivity and quality of life. **Pub:** *Newsletter.*

★ 25560 ★ U.S. Department of Veterans Affairs
Research & Development Service
3710 SW Veterans Hospital Rd.
PO Box 1034
Portland, OR 97201
Phone: (503)273-5125 **Fax:** (503)273-5351
Email: michael.davey@med.va.gov
Dr. Michael P. Davey, Assoc. Ch., Res.
Activities/Fields: Genetics of alcoholism and substance abuse, osteoporosis in men, virology (CMV, HIV), immunology, diabetes, multiple sclerosis, hematology-oncology, spinal cord regeneration, tardive dyskinesia, Parkinson Disease, Hepatitis C, neurology health services research, hypertension, dermatology (malignant melanoma), etiology of rheumatoid arthritis, Alzheimer's disease, audiology, stroke, depression, schizophrenia, BI-polor disorders, and colon cancer. **Pub:** *R&D Newsletter*, quarterly. • *Research News*, quarterly. • *VA Regeneration Research Newsletter*, semiannually.

★ 25561 ★ U.S. Department of Veterans Affairs
Veterans Affairs Medical Center (West Los Angeles, CA)
Human Brain and Spinal Fluid Resource Center
Neurology Research (127A)
West Los Angeles Healthcare Center
11301 Wilshire Blvd.
Los Angeles, CA 90073
Phone: (310)268-3536 **Fax:** (310)268-4768
Email: rmnbbank@ucla.edu
Website: http://www.loni.ucla.edu/~nnrsb/nnrsb
Dr. Rashed M. Nagra, PhD, Dir.
Activities/Fields: Serves as a resource bank for cryopreserved human brain, spinal fluid, serum, and other tissue. Provides specimens to research community, particularly in the area of neurological and psychiatric diseases, including but not limited to Alzheimer's disease, Down's syndrome, Batten's disease, Huntington's disease multiple sclerosis, epilepsy, and Parkinson's disease. **Frmly:** National Neurological Research Specimen Bank.

★ 25562 ★ U.S. Department of Veterans Affairs
Veterans Health Administration
Office of Research and Development
U.S. Department of Veterans Affairs
810 Vermont Ave., NW
Washington, DC 20420
Phone: (202)273-8284 **Fax:** (202)273-6526
Email: david.thomas@mnil.va.gov
Website: http://www.va.gov/resdev/
John R. Feussner, MD, Chf. Res. Off.
Activities/Fields: Provides funding for intramural research performed by individual investigators at VA medical centers throughout the United States. These investigators are staff at the medical centers (physicians, basic scientists, nurses, dentists, psychologists, etc.) who apply for research funds from the Central Office of Research and Development through the medical centers' research and development committees. **Pub:** *Journal of Rehabilitation*, semimonthly.

★ 25563 ★ U.S. Department of Veterans Affairs
Veterans Health Administration
Office of Research and Development
Health Services Research and Development Service
(Service Directed Research Program)
810 Vermont Ave. NW
Washington, DC 20240
Phone: (202)273-5400 **Fax:** (202)273-6526
Activities/Fields: Addresses health care issues relating to the veteran population, the VA's system of health care networks, and the nation as a whole. Research projects are conducted in response to mandates and requests from a variety of constituencies, including Congress, federal agencies, the Secretary of Veterans Affairs and other VA administrators.

★ 25564 ★ U.S. Department of Veterans Affairs
Veterans Health Administration
Office of Research and Development
Health Services Research and Development Service
(Management Decision and Research Center)
VA Medical Center (152M)
150 S Huntington Ave.
Boston, MA 02130
Phone: (617)278-4433 **Fax:** (617)278-4438
Email: MDRC.Boston@med.va.gov
Website: http://www.hsrd.research.va.gov/about/centers/mdrc.cfc
Martin P. Charns, DBA, Dir.
Activities/Fields: Research associated with the organization and management of healthcare services. **Pub:** *Transition Watch.* • *Forum.* • *Management Brief.* • *Practice Matters.* • *Queri Quartly.*

★ 25565 ★ U.S. Department of Veterans Affairs
Veterans Health Administration
Office of Research and Development
Health Services Research and Development Service
(Investigator Initiated Research Program)
810 Vermont Ave. NW
Washington, DC 20240
Phone: (202)273-5400 **Fax:** (202)565-8440
Activities/Fields: Supports VA-funded health services research projects related to health care outcomes, access to care, cost and cost-effectiveness, assessment and assurance of quality, alternative organizational and delivery models, and development of new research methods and measurement tools.

★ 25566 ★ U.S. Department of Veterans Affairs
Veterans Health Administration
Office of Research and Development
Health Services Research and Development Service
(Center for the Study of Healthcare Provider Behavior)
Sepulveda Campus/VA Greater Los Angeles Healthcare System
16111 Plummer St. (152)
Sepulveda, CA 91343
Phone: (818)895-9449 **Fax:** (818)895-5838
Email: lisar@rand.org
Lisa V. Rubenstein, MD, Dir.
Activities/Fields: Research on provider behavior and practice patterns, health care quality and outcomes, quality improvement, clinical practice guideline implementation, and primary care/managed care evaluation.

★ 25567 ★ U.S. Department of Veterans Affairs
Veterans Health Administration
Office of Research and Development
Health Services Research and Development Service
(Center for Chronic Disease Outcomes Research)
VA Medical Center (152/2E)
1 Veterans Dr.
Minneapolis, MN 55417
Phone: (612)725-1979 **Fax:** (612)727-5699
Email: joanne.karvonen@med.va.gov
Website: http://www.hsrd.minneapolis.med.va.gov
Dr. Hanna B. Rubins, MPH, Dir.
Activities/Fields: Research on designing and testing health systems innovations to improve quality and outcomes of care, evaluating the effect of medical interventions on patient outcomes (efficiency trials and systematic reviews), defining the impact of patients' social and demographic characteristics on clinical decision making, and designing interventions to enhance patient participation in health care decisions.

★ 25568 ★ U.S. Department of Veterans Affairs
Veterans Health Administration
Office of Research and Development
Health Services Research and Development Service
(Northwest Center for Outcomes Research in Older Adults)
VA Puget Sound Health Care System
1660 S Columbia Way
Seattle, WA 98108
Phone: (206)764-2430 **Fax:** (206)764-2935
Email: sfihn@u.washington.edu
Website: http://www.hrsd.seattle.med.va.gov
Stephan D. Fihn, MD, Contact
Activities/Fields: Research on the care of the aging, veteran, ambulatory care, outcome research, and disease prevention/health promotion.

★ 25569 ★ U.S. Department of Veterans Affairs
Veterans Health Administration
Office of Research and Development
Health Services Research and Development Service
(Center for Mental Healthcare and Outcomes Research)
Central Arkansas Veteran's Health Care System
2200 Fort Roots Dr.
North Little Rock, AR 72114
Phone: (501)257-1710 **Fax:** (501)257-1707
Email: owenrichardr@uams.edu
Dr. Richard R. Owen, Dir.
Activities/Fields: Research on improving mental health care through the development, implementation, and dissemination of policy-relevant and clinically-relevant health services research, including cognitive impairment, cormobidity, depression, schizophrenia, and substance abuse.

★ 25570 ★ U.S. Department of Veterans Affairs
Veterans Health Administration
Office of Research and Development
Health Services Research and Development Service
(Center for Health Services Research in Primary Care)
VA Medical Center (152)
508 Fulton St.
Durham, NC 27705-3897
Phone: (919)286-6936 **Fax:** (919)416-5836
Email: Oddone.Eugene@durham.va.gov
Eugene Z. Oddone, MD, Dir.
Activities/Fields: Research on strategies that enhance the delivery, quality, and efficiency of primary care for veterans, including ambulatory care, women's health, geriatrics, and epidemiology of chronic diseases.

★ 25571 ★ U.S. Department of Veterans Affairs
Veterans Health Administration
Office of Research and Development
Medical Research Service
(Environmental Hazards Research Center)
VA Medical Center, 116B-4
150 S Huntington Ave.
Boston, MA 02130

Phone: (617)278-4517 **Fax:** (617)278-4448
Email: rwhite@bu.edu
Roberta F. White, PhD, Dir.

Activities/Fields: Research on behavioral toxicology.

★ 25572 ★ U.S. Department of Veterans Affairs
Veterans Health Administration
Office of Research and Development
Medical Research Service
(AIDS Research Center)
VA San Diego Health Care System
3350 La Jolla Village Dr.
San Diego, CA 92161
Phone: (858)552-7439 **Fax:** (858)552-7445
Email: drichman@ucsd.edu
Douglas Richman, MD, Dir.

Activities/Fields: Research on the molecular pathogenesis of HIV, as well as vaccines and chemotherapy.

★ 25573 ★ U.S. Department of Veterans Affairs
Veterans Health Administration
Office of Research and Development
Medical Research Service
(Alcoholism Research Center)
VA Connecticut Health Care System
950 Campbell Ave.
West Haven, CT 06516
Phone: (203)937-4790 **Fax:** (203)937-3468
John Harrison Krystal, MD, Dir.

Activities/Fields: Research on the neurobiology, genetics, and pharmacology of alcoholism.

★ 25574 ★ U.S. Department of Veterans Affairs
Veterans Health Administration
Office of Research and Development
Medical Research Service
(AIDS Research Center)
VA Medical Center
508 Fulton St.
Durham, NC 27705
Phone: (919)286-0411 **Fax:** (919)286-0441
Dr. John Hamilton, MD, Contact

Activities/Fields: Molecular and cellular characterization of HIV and related pathogens, including vaccine development, HIV gene regulation, virulence factors and common opportunistic infections in HIV-infected persons.

★ 25575 ★ U.S. Department of Veterans Affairs
Veterans Health Administration
Office of Research and Development
Medical Research Service
(Schizophrenia Research Center)
VA Connecticut Health Care System
950 Campbell Ave.
West Haven, CT 06516
Fax: (203)937-3878
Robert Innis, PhD, Dir.

Activities/Fields: Research on the clinical study of antipsychotic drugs in schizophrenia, including schizophrenia pathophysiology, abnormal chemical transmission in the brain, cellular neuroscience, neuroimaging, and clinical drug trials aimed at improving treatment for patients with schizophrenia.

★ 25576 ★ U.S. Department of Veterans Affairs
Veterans Health Administration
Office of Research and Development
Medical Research Service
(Schizophrenia Research Center)
Brockton VA Medical Center
940 Belmont St.
Brockton, MA 02301-5568
Phone: (508)583-4500 **Fax:** (508)586-0894
Email: robert.mccarley@med.va.gov
Dr. Robert McCarley, MD, Dir.

Activities/Fields: Research directed toward understanding the pathophysiology, clinical characteristics, and treatment of schizophrenia, including the role stress plays in the pathophysiology of schizophrenia, brain tissues studies to evaluate glutamatergic transmission in schizophrenics, the efficacy of dcycloserine on treating the symptoms of schizophrenia, and Magnetic Resonance Imaging (MRI) projects to evaluate activity in the brain.

★ 25577 ★ U.S. Department of Veterans Affairs
Veterans Health Administration
Office of Research and Development
Rehabilitation and Development Service
(Center for Mobility)
3801 Miranda Ave., MS-153
Rehabilitation Research & Development Center
Palo Alto, CA 94304
Phone: (650)493-5000 **Fax:** (650)493-4919
Email: cjacobs@roses.stanford.edu
Website: http://guide.stanford.edu
Christopher R. Jacobs, PhD, Dir.

Activities/Fields: The Clinical Emphasis of the Center is to improve mobility, either ambulation or manipulation, in individuals with Neurologic Impairments or Orthopaedic Impairments. We specifically target four conditions that cause significant loss of mobility to veterans and non-veterans alike: Stroke, Spinal Cord Injury, Arthritis, and Osteoporosis.

★ 25578 ★ U.S. Department of Veterans Affairs
Veterans Health Administration
Office of Research and Development
Rehabilitation and Development Service
(Center for Rehabilitative Auditory Research)
VA Medical Center
3710 SW U.S. Veterans Hosp. Rd.
R&D-NCPAR
Portland, OR 97207
Phone: (503)220-8262 **Fax:** (503)273-5021
Email: stephen.fausti@med.va.gov
Website: http://www.ncrar.org/home.htm
Stephen A. Fausti, PhD, ACCE & Dir.

Activities/Fields: Research on alleviating the communicative, social, and economic problems caused by auditory system impairment. **Pub:** *The Hearing Journal.* • *Journal of the International Neurophysical Society.* • *Journal Rehabilitation Research and Development (JRRD).* • *Journal of Speech and Hearing Research.* • *Newsletter*, quarterly. **Frmly:** (2000) Center for Rehabilitative Auditory Research.

★ 25579 ★ U.S. Department of Veterans Affairs
Veterans Health Administration
Office of Research and Development
Rehabilitation and Development Service
(Center for Functional Electric Stimulation)
11000 Cedar Ave., Ste. 230
Cleveland, OH 44106-3052
Phone: (216)231-3257 **Free:** 800-666-2353
Fax: (216)231-3258
Email: info@fesc.org
Website: http://www.fesc.org
P. Hunter Peckham, PhD, Dir.

Activities/Fields: Research on Functional Electrical Stimulation (FES), a technology that relies on controlled electric current to activate paralyzed muscles and plays a critical role in returning full or partial physical function to disabled persons.

★ 25580 ★ U.S. Department of Veterans Affairs
Veterans Health Administration
Office of Research and Development
Rehabilitation and Development Service
(Center for Healthy Aging with Disabilities)
VA Medical Center (39B)
2002 Holcombe Blvd.
Houston, TX 77030
Phone: (713)794-7254 **Fax:** (713)794-7623
Email: ams@bcm.tmc.edu
Arthur M. Sherwood, PhD, Dir.

Activities/Fields: The Center of Excellence on Healthy Aging with Disabilities (CHAD) has as its mission the understanding of the process of aging with disabilities in the design, implementation and evaluation of strategies to enhance health, functioning and well-being of veterans aging with disabilities.

Chapter 18
Medical & Allied Health Schools

This chapter includes 30 sections arranged alphabetically by occupational names. Educational programs in each section are arranged alphabetically by states, then by institution names within states. The last section of the chapter lists contacts for occupational categories not otherwise covered. For additional information, consult the "User's Guide" located at the front of this directory.

Alternative Health Care

Listed below are schools of alternative health. Individual specialties and techniques are listed for each school.

Alabama

★ 25581 ★ The PATH Foundation, Birmingham
1207 18th Ave. S
Birmingham, AL 35205
Phone: (205)322-7284
Cheryl W. Martin, Contact
Program(s): Hypnotherapy.

★ 25582 ★ Red Mountain Institute for the Healing Arts Inc.
1900 20th Ave. S, Ste. 220
Birmingham, AL 35209
Phone: (205)836-2024 **Fax:** (205)278-8802
Kitty Flewelling, Director
Program(s): Ayurvedic Medicine; Deep Tissue Massage; Massage Therapy; Neuromuscular Therapy; Swedish Massage.

Alaska

★ 25583 ★ Acupressure Institute of Alaska
119 Second St.
Juneau, AK 99801
Phone: (907)463-5560
Alexander Majewski, Director
Program(s): Acupressure; Aromatherapy; CranioSacroTherapy; Jin Shin Do; Qigong; Shiatsu.

★ 25584 ★ Gatekey School of Mind-Body Integration Studies
4041 B St., Flr. 300
Anchorage, AK 99503-5945
Phone: (907)561-7327 **Fax:** (907)561-6582
Carol Stiles, Contact
Program(s): Body-Mind Integration; Energy Work; Massage Therapy; Reiki.

Alberta

★ 25585 ★ Calgary College of Holistic Health and Clinics, Inc.
412 Silver Valley Rd. NW
Calgary, AB, Canada T3B 4B9
Phone: (403)288-4511 **Fax:** (403)288-0114
John Neumann, Contact
Program(s): Acupressure; Aromatherapy; Energy Work; Hypnotherapy; Massage Therapy; Reflexology; Shiatsu.

★ 25586 ★ Foothills College of Massage Therapy
7330 Fisher St., Ste. 400
Calgary, AB, Canada T2H 2H8
Phone: (403)255-4445 **Fax:** (403)255-4074
Beth Checkley, Contact
Program(s): Massage Therapy.

★ 25587 ★ Mount Royal College Centre for Complementary Haelth Education
2204 2nd St. SW
Calgary, AB, Canada T2S 1F5
Phone: (403)503-4886 **Fax:** (403)503-4899
Attiya Ghani, Contact
Program(s): Acupressure; Aromatherapy; Herbal Medicine; Massage Therapy; Reflexology; Sports Massage.

★ 25588 ★ School of Homeopathy-Devon, England
4 Oakvale Pl. SW
Calgary, AB, Canada T2V 1H4
Phone: (403)281-7976 **Fax:** (403)281-7976
Hana Stastny, Contact
Program(s): Anatomy and Physiology; Homeopathy; Pathology and Disease.

★ 25589 ★ Yoga Association of Alberta
Percy Page Center
11759 Groat Rd.
Edmonton, AB, Canada T5M 3K6
Phone: (403)427-8776 **Fax:** (403)427-0524
Margo Balog, Contact
Program(s): Yoga Teacher Training.

Arizona

★ 25590 ★ Arizona School of Integrative Studies
753 N Main St.
Cottonwood, AZ 86326
Phone: (520)639-3455 **Fax:** (520)639-3694
Jamie Rongo, Director
Program(s): Acupressure; Aromatherapy; CranioSacral Therapy; Energy Work; Homeopathy; Hydrotherapy; Massage Therapy; Polarity Therapy; Qigong; Reflexology; Shiatsu; Sports Massage; Structural Integration.

★ 25591 ★ Bonnie Prudden School of Physical Fitness and Myotherapy, LLC
4725 E Sunrise Dr., Ste. 346
Tucson, AZ 85718
Phone: (520)529-3979 **Free:** 800-221-4634
Fax: (520)529-6679
Email: info@bonnieprudden.com
Bonnie Prudden, Director
Program(s): Exercise Therapy; Myotherapy.

★ 25592 ★ Desert Institute of the Healing Arts
639 N 6th Ave.
Tucson, AZ 85705-8330
Phone: (520)882-0899 **Free:** 800-733-8098
Fax: (520)624-2996
Website: http://www.diha.com
Margaret Avery Moon, Director
Program(s): Aromatherapy; Hydrotherapy; Massage Therapy; Reflexology; Shiatsu; Sports Massage.

★ 25593 ★ Foundation for Holistic Health Therapy
80 Farmer Brothers Dr.
Sedona, AZ 86336
Phone: (520)204-1968 **Free:** 800-578-7312
Fax: (520)204-1968
Email: drbrown@cybertrails.com
Website: http://www.sedona-web.com/Lymphatic
William N. Brown, PhD, Director
Program(s): Energy Work; Lymphatic Massage.

★ 25594 ★ Institute for Natural Therapeutics
217 W University Dr.
Mesa, AZ 85201
Phone: (602)844-2255 **Fax:** (602)962-9907
Amy K. Hatch, Contact
Program(s): Aromatherapy; CranioSacral Therapy; Deep Tissue Massage; Massage Therapy; Reflexology; Reiki; Shiatsu.

★ 25595 ★ International Foundation of Bio-Magnetics
5447 E 5th st., Ste. 111
Tucson, AZ 85711
Phone: (520)751-7751 **Fax:** (520)751-7751
John Munno, Contact
Program(s): Bio-Magnetic Touch Healing; Energy Work.

★ 25596 ★ International Yoga Studies
13833 S 31st Pl.
Phoenix, AZ 85048
Phone: (602)759-1972 **Fax:** (602)704-9656
Sandra Summerfield Kozak, Director
Program(s): Ayurvedic Medicine; Yoga Teacher Training.

★ 25597 ★ Jin Shin Jyutsu, Inc.
8719 E San Alberto Dr.
Scottsdale, AZ 85258
Phone: (602)998-9331 **Fax:** (602)998-9335
David Burmeister, Director
Program(s): Jin Shin Jyutsu.

★ 25598 ★ Phoenix Institute of Herbal Medicine and Acupuncture
7501 E Oak, Ste. 114-115
Scottsdale, AZ 85252
Phone: (602)994-3648 **Fax:** (602)439-1511
Mary Beth Madden, Contact
Program(s): Acupuncture; Herbal Medicine; Traditional Chinese Medicine.

★ 25599 ★ Phoenix Therapeutic Massage College
609 N Scottsdale Rd.
Scottsdale, AZ 85257
Phone: (480)945-9461 **Fax:** (480)425-8247
Rose Taylor, Contact
Program(s): Massage Therapy; Swedish Massage.

★ 25600 ★ RainStar College
4130 N Goldwater Blvd.
Scottsdale, AZ 85251
Phone: (602)423-0375 **Fax:** (602)945-9824
Edvard R. Richards, Director
Program(s): Acupressure; Aromatherapy; Breathwork; Chinese Herbal Medicine; CranioSacral Therapy; Geriatric Massage; Herbal Medicine; Homeopathy; Hydrotherapy; Hypnotherapy; Iridology; Lymphatic Massage; Massage Therapy; Myofascial Release; On-Site Massage; Oriental Medicine; Pediatric Massage; Pregnancy Massage; Qigong; Reflexology; Reiki; Shiatsu; Spa Therapies; Sports Massage; Traditional Chinese Medicine; Trigger Point Therapy.

★ 25601 ★ Southwest College of Naturopathic Medicine and Health Sciences
2140 E Broadway Rd.
Tempe, AZ 85282
Phone: (602)858-9100 **Fax:** (602)858-9116
Website: http://www.scnm.edu
Melissa Winquist, Contact
Program(s): Acupuncture; Naturopathic Medicine.

★ 25602 ★ Southwest Institute of Healing Arts
1402 N Miller Rd., Ste. D-2
Scottsdale, AZ 85257
Phone: (602)994-9244 **Fax:** (602)994-3228
K.C. Miller, Director
Program(s): Acupressure; Acupuncture; Aromatherapy; Ayurvedic Medicine; Body-Mind Psychology; Childbirth Educator; CranioSacral Therapy; Doula; Energy Work; Equine Massage; Holistic Health; Herbal Medicine; Hypnotherapy; Massage Therapy; Oriental Medicine; Polarity Therapy; Qigong; Reflexology; Reiki; Shiatsu; Sports Massage; Traditional Chinese Medicine; Yoga Teacher Training.

★ 25603 ★ University of Arizona, College of Medicine
Program of Integrative Medicine
1249 N Mountain
Tucson, AZ 85724-5153
Phone: (520)626-7222 **Fax:** (520)626-6484
Website: http://www.ahsc.arizona.edu/integrative-medicine
Andrew Weil, MD, Contact
Program(s): Integrative Medicine.

★ 25604 ★ Wesland Institute
3367 N Country Club Rd.
Tucson, AZ 85716-1349
Phone: (520)881-1530 **Fax:** (520)881-1530
Richard Corvino, Director
Program(s): Hypnotherapy; Neuro-Linguistic Programming.

Arkansas

★ 25605 ★ American Academy of Healing Arts
School of Massage Therapy
1501 N University, Ste. 570
Little Rock, AR 72207
Phone: (501)666-9100 **Free:** 888-666-9101
Fax: (501)666-3133
Eileen Joyce, Contact
Program(s): CranioSacral Therapy; Deep Tissue Massage; Energy Work; Hydrotherapy; Massage Therapy; Polarity Therapy; Reflexology; Shiatsu.

★ 25606 ★ Body Wellness Therapeutic Massage Academy
11323 Arcade Dr.
Little Rock, AR 72212
Phone: (501)219-2639 **Fax:** (501)221-7626
Email: bodywellness@aristotle.net
Donna McGriff, Contact
Program(s): Acupressure; Aromatherapy; Ayurvedic Medicine; Deep Muscle Massage; Energy Work; Massage Therapy; Myofascial Release; Polarity Therapy; Reflexology; Reiki; Sports Massage; Swedish Massage.

★ 25607 ★ Center for Wellbeing
101 W Mountain
GCM Bldg., Ste. 107
Fayetteville, AR 72701
Phone: (501)442-2026 **Fax:** (501)442-2897
Email: cbeckerphd@aol.com
Chandana Becker, PhD, Director
Program(s): Polarity Therapy; Somatic Experiencing (Shock Trauma Renegotiaation Therapy).

★ 25608 ★ A Healing Touch, Inc.
Clinic and School of Massage Therapy
2201 Rogers Ave., Ste. F
Fort Smith, AR 72901
Phone: (501)783-7566
Wendy L. Morgan, Contact
Program(s): Acupressure; Aromatherapy; CranioSacral Therapy; Deep Tissue Massage; Energy Work; Herbal Medicine; Hypnotherapy; Massage Therapy; Shiatsu; Traditional Chinese Medicine.

★ 25609 ★ Hot Springs School of Therapy Technology
1415 N Moore Rd.
Hot Springs, AR 71913
Free: 800-844-0667
Ronald L. Wallace, Contact
Program(s): Acupressure; Aromatherapy; Herbal Medicine; Hydrotherapy; Massage Therapy; Reflexology; Shiatsu.

★ 25610 ★ Jean's School of Therapy Technology, Inc.
655 Park Ave.
Hot Springs, AR 71901
Phone: (501)623-9686 **Fax:** (501)623-0070
Jean R. Miller, Contact
Program(s): Acupressure; Deep Tissue Massage; Massage Therapy; Reflexology; Reiki; Shiatsu.

★ 25611 ★ White River School of Massage
48 Colt Square Dr.
Fayetteville, AR 72703
Phone: (501)521-2550 **Fax:** (501)521-2558
Ellen May, Director
Program(s): Aromatherapy; CranioSacral Therapy; Energy Work; Massage Therapy; Myofascial Release; Neuromuscular Therapy; Reflexology; Shiatsu; Sports Massage.

British Columbia

★ 25612 ★ Canadian College of Acupuncture and Oriental Medicine
855 Cormorant St.
Victoria, BC, Canada V8W 1R2
Phone: (250)384-2942 **Fax:** (250)360-2871
Diane St. Hilair, Contact
Program(s): Acupressure; Acupuncture; Herbal Medicine; Oriental Medicine; Traditional Chinese Medicine.

★ 25613 ★ Dominion Herbal College
7527 Kingsway
Burnaby, BC, Canada V3N 3C1
Phone: (604)521-5822 **Fax:** (604)526-1561
Bernice Birzneck, Contact
Program(s): Aromatherapy; Herbal Medicine.

★ 25614 ★ Meridian Institute
225 Canada Ave., Ste. 105
Duncan, BC, Canada V9L 1T6
Phone: (250)748-3588 **Fax:** (250)748-3578
Doris Gray, Contact
Program(s): Hypnotherapy.

★ 25615 ★ Vancouver Homeopathic Academy
PO Box 34095, Stn D
Vancouver, BC, Canada V6J 4M1
Phone: (604)708-9387 **Fax:** (604)708-1547
Kim Boutilier, Contact
Program(s): Homeopathy.

★ 25616 ★ West Coast College of Massage Therapy
555 W Hastings St., 6th Flr.
Vancouver, BC, Canada V6B 4N6
Phone: (604)689-3854 **Free:** 888-449-2242
Fax: (604)689-9804
Christine Mullie, Contact
Program(s): Acupuncture; Herbal Medicine; Humanistic Counseling; Hydrotherapy; Massage Therapy; Reflexology; Shiatsu.Nturopathic Medicine; Traditional Chinese Medicine.

California

★ 25617 ★ Academy of Chinese Culture & Health Sciences
1601 Clay St.
Oakland, CA 94612
Phone: (510)763-7787 **Fax:** (510)834-8646
Email: acchs@best.com
Program(s): Acupuncture; Herbal Medicine; Traditional Chinese Medicine.

★ 25618 ★ Academy for Guided Imagery
311 Miller Ave., Ste. G
PO Box 2070
Mill Valley, CA 94942
Free: 800-726-2070 **Fax:** (415)389-9342
Website: http://www.healthy.net/agi
Martin Rossman, MD, Director
Program(s): Guided Imagery.

★ 25619 ★ Academy of Health Professions
6784 El Cajon Blvd., Ste. G
San Diego, CA 92105
Phone: (619)464-3570 **Fax:** (619)461-5375
Karen Croft, Contact
Program(s): Aromatherapy; Deep Tissue Massage; Energy Work; Hawaiian Massage; Herbal Medicine; Holistic Health; Hypnotherapy; Massage Therapy; Nutrition; Passive Joint Movement; Pregnancy Massage; Reflexology; Reiki; Shiatsu; Sports Massage; Structural Alignment; Swedish Massage; Tui Na.

★ 25620 ★ Academy of Professional Careers
8376 Hercules St.
La Mesa, CA 91942
Phone: (619)461-5100 **Fax:** (619)461-1401
Juanita Cherry, Contact
Program(s): Energy Work; Holistic Health; Massage Therapy; Neuromuscular Therapy; Nutrition; Reflexology; Reiki; Shiatsu; Sports Massage.

★ 25621 ★ Acupressure Institute: Shiatsu, Massage & Asian Bodywork Trainings
1533 Shattuck Ave.
Berkeley, CA 94709
Phone: (510)845-1059 **Fax:** (510)845-1496
Email: colburn@acupressure.com
Website: http://www.acupressure.com
Pat Colburn, Contact
Program(s): Acupressure; Emotional Balancing; Energy Work; Massage Therapy; Oriental Medicine; Shiatsu; Sports Massage; Thai Massage; Traditional Chinese Medicine; Yoga Teacher Training.

★ 25622 ★ Advanced School of Massage Therapy
1414 E Thousand Oaks Blvd., Ste. 211, 213
Thousand Oaks, CA 91362
Phone: (805)495-1353 **Fax:** (805)379-1408
Jan Suckut, Contact
Program(s): CranioSacral Therapy; Energy Work; Facial Massage; Infant Massage; Massage Therapy; Pregnancy Massage; Reflexology; Sports Massage; Trigger Point Therapy.

★ 25623 ★ Alexander Educational Center
St. John Presbyterian Church
2727 College Ave., Rm. 207
Berkeley, CA 94705
Phone: (925)937-5746
Giora Pinkas, Director
Program(s): Alexander Technique.

★ 25624 ★ Alexander Training Institute of Los Angeles
1526 14th St., Ste. 110
Santa Monica, CA 90404
Phone: (310)395-9170
Lyn Charlsen, Director
Program(s): Alexander Technique.

★ 25625 ★ Alexander Training Institute of San Francisco
ACT
30 Grant Ave., 8th Fl.
San Francisco, CA 94108
Phone: (415)439-2465
Frank Ottiwell, Director
Program(s): Alexander Technique.

★ 25626 ★ Alive & Well! Institute of Conscious BodyWork
100 Shaw Dr.
San Anselmo, CA 94960
Phone: (415)258-0402 **Fax:** (415)258-0635
Email: alivewel@aol.com
Jocelyn Olivier, Director
Program(s): Acupressure; Aromatherapy; CranioSacral Therapy; Massage Therapy; Neuromuscular Reprogramming; Polarity Therapy; Qigong; Reflexology; Synergetic Studies.

★ 25627 ★ American Academy of Reflexology
606 E Magnolia Blvd., Ste. B
Burbank, CA 91501-2618
Phone: (818)841-7741 **Fax:** (818)841-2346
Bill Flocco, Contact
Program(s): Reflexology.

★ 25628 ★ American College of Traditional Chinese Medicine
455 Arkansas St.
San Francisco, CA 94107
Phone: (415)282-7600 **Fax:** (415)282-0856
Email: lhuang@actcm.org
Website: http://www.actcm.org
Lixin Huang, Contact
Program(s): Acupuncture; Herbal Medicine; Qigong; Traditional Chinese Medicine.

★ 25629 ★ American Institute of Hypnotherapy
16842 Von Karman Ave., Ste. 475
Irvine, CA 92606
Phone: (949)261-6400 **Free:** 800-872-9996
Fax: (949)251-4632
Guy Robert, Contact
Program(s): Hypnotherapy.

★ 25630 ★ American Institute of Massage Therapy, Inc., Costa Mesa
2156 Newport Blvd.
Costa Mesa, CA 92627
Phone: (949)642-0735 **Fax:** (949)642-1729
M.K. Hungerford, PhD, Contact
Program(s): Acupressure; Aromatherapy; CranioSacral Therapy; Massage Therapy; Neuromuscular Therapy; Reflexology; Reiki; Shiatsu; Sports Massage; Swedish Massage; Thai Massage.

★ 25631 ★ Ayurveda Institute of Massage and Spa Services
3140 Stone Station
Sebastopol, CA 95472
Phone: (707)523-9923 **Fax:** (707)824-4778
Dharmini Zelin, Contact
Program(s): Ayurvedic Medicine; Energy Work; Massage Therapy; Polarity Therapy; Reflexology; Spa Therapies.

★ 25632 ★ Belavi Institute for Facial Massage
1500 N Coast Hwy.
Laguna Beach, CA 92651
Phone: (714)443-1954 **Free:** 800-235-2844
Fax: (714)443-2292
Belle Tuckerman, Contact
Program(s): Facial Massage; Spa Therapies.

★ 25633 ★ Biofeedback Institute of Los Angeles
3710 S Robertson Blvd., Ste. 216
Culver City, CA 90232-2351
Phone: (310)841-4970 **Free:** 800-246-3526
Fax: (310)840-0923
Marjorie K. Toomin, PhD, Director
Program(s): Biofeedback; Neuromuscular Therapy.

★ 25634 ★ Biofeedback Training Institute - Stens Corp.
6451 Oakwood Dr.
Oakland, CA 94611
Free: 800-257-8367 **Fax:** (510)339-2222
Email: stensco@aol.com
Wendy Kesseler, Contact
Program(s): Biofeedback.

★ 25635 ★ Body Therapy Center
368 California Ave.
Palo Alto, CA 94306
Phone: (650)328-9400 **Fax:** (650)328-9478
Laura Skinner, Contact
Program(s): CranioSacral Therapy; Deep Tissue Massage; Esalen Massage; Massage Therapy; On-Site Massage; Reflexology; Reiki; Shiatsu; Sports Massage; Swedish Massage.

★ 25636 ★ Body Therapy Institute of Santa Barbara
835 N Milpas St.
Santa Barbara, CA 93103
Phone: (805)966-5802
Gael Ashwood, Contact
Program(s): Accupressure; CranioSacral Therapy; Deep Tissue Massage; Energy Work; Holistic Health; Massage Therapy; Polarity Therapy; Qigong; Reflexology; Reiki; Shiatsu.

★ 25637 ★ Breema Center
6076 Claremont Ave.
Oakland, CA 94618
Phone: (510)428-0937 **Fax:** (510)428-9235
Mary Cunio, Contact
Program(s): Breema Bodywork.

★ 25638 ★ British Institute of Homeopathy and Complementary Medicine
520 Washington Blvd., Ste. 423
Marina Del Rey, CA 90292
Phone: (310)557-2235 **Fax:** (310)577-0296
Email: bihus@thegrid.net
Dr. Trevor Cook, Contact
Program(s): Animal Therapy; Flower Essences; Herbal Medicine; Homeopathy.

★ 25639 ★ Calaveras College of Therapeutic Massage
96 Court St.
PO Box 274
San Andreas, CA 95249
Phone: (209)754-4876
Michelle Olkowski, Contact
Program(s): Acupressure; Aromatherapy; CranioSacral Therapy; Massage Therapy; Reflexology; Shiatsu; Swedish Massage.

★ 25640 ★ California College of Ayurveda
1117A E Main St.
Grass Valley, CA 95945
Phone: (530)274-9100 **Fax:** (530)274-7350
Marc Halpern, Contact
Program(s): Aromatherapy; Ayurvedic Medicine; Herbal Medicine.

★ 25641 ★ California College of Physical Arts, Inc.
18582 Beach Blvd., Ste. 11
Huntington Beach, CA 92648
Phone: (714)964-7744 **Fax:** (714)962-3934
Email: calcopa@gte.net
Website: http://www.fyi.com
Deborah S. Mulholland, Director
Program(s): Acupressure; Alexander Technique; Aromatherapy; Herbal Medicine; Holistic Health; Massage Therapy; Oriental Medicine; Reflexology; Reiki; Shiatsu; Sports Massage.

★ 25642 ★ California Graduate Institute
1145 Gayley Ave., Ste. 322
Los Angeles, CA 90024
Phone: (310)208-4240 **Fax:** (310)208-0684
Terry Oleson, PhD, Contact
Program(s): Biofeedback; Hypnotherapy.

★ 25643 ★ California Institute of Integral Sciences
1453 Mission St.
San Francisco, CA 94103
Phone: (415)575-6126 **Fax:** (415)575-1264

Email: iang@ciis.edu
Website: http://www.ciis.edu
Ian Grand, Director
Program(s): Somatic Education.

★ 25644 ★ California Institute of Massage and Spa Services
139 E Napa St.
730 Broadway
Sonoma, CA 95476
Phone: (707)939-9431
Kate Alves, Director
Program(s): Acupressure; Aromatherapy; CranioSacral Therapy; Energy Work; Massage Therapy; Polarity Therapy; Reflexology; Shiatsu; Spa Therapies; Swedish Massage.

★ 25645 ★ California Naturopathic College
1228 Camino Del Mar
Del Mar, CA 92014
Phone: (619)259-1222 **Fax:** (619)259-0730
Bettina Yelman, Contact
Program(s): Acupressure; Aromatherapy; Ayurvedic Medicine; CranioSacral Therapy; Energy Work; Herbal Medicine; Holistic Health; Homeopathy; Hypnotherapy; Massage Therapy; Naturopathic Medicine; Nutrition; Oriental Medicine; Polarity Therapy; Reflexology; Reiki; Shiatsu; Sports Massage.

★ 25646 ★ California School of Herbal Studies
9309 Hwy. 116
Forestville, CA 95436
Phone: (707)887-7457
James Green, Director
Program(s): Aromatherapy; Herbal Medicine.

★ 25647 ★ Calistoga Massage Therapy School
5959 Commerce Blvd., Ste. 13
Rohnert Park, CA 94928
Phone: (707)586-1953
Dr. Steven L. Ticen, Contact
Program(s): Massage Therapy.

★ 25648 ★ Caring Hands School of Massage
1484 E Main St.
Ventura, CA 93001
Phone: (805)643-3032
Program(s): Acupressure; LomiLomi Massage; Massage Therapy; Shiatsu.

★ 25649 ★ Center for the Alexander Technique
714 Nash Ave.
Menlo Park, CA 94025
Phone: (650)328-4736
Edward Avak, Director
Program(s): Alexander Technique.

★ 25650 ★ Center for Conscious Touch - Lupin Massage Institute
PO Box 1274
Los Gatos, CA 95031
Phone: (408)353-4231
Stuart Grace, Contact
Program(s): Acupressure; Anatomy and Phisiology; CranioSacral Therapy; Esalen Massage; Manual Lymph Drainage; Massage Therapy; Swedish Massage; Visceral Massage.

★ 25651 ★ Center for Hypnotherapy Certification
455 Newton Ave., Ste. 1
Oakland, CA 94606
Phone: (510)839-4800 **Free:** 800-398-0034
Fax: (510)836-0477
Marilyn Gordon, Director
Program(s): Hypnotherapy.

★ 25652 ★ Central California School of Body Therapy
1330 Southwood Dr., Ste. 7
San Luis Obispo, CA 93401
Phone: (805)783-2200 **Fax:** (805)783-2200
Email: siouxsun1@aol.com
Susan E. Stocks, Contact
Program(s): Acupressure; CranioSacral Therapy; Herbal Medicine; Homeopathy; Hypnotherapy; Massage Therapy; Shiatsu.

★ 25653 ★ Charles R. Drew University of Medicine and Sciences College of Allied Health Sciences Nurse-Midwifery Education Program
1621 E 120th St.
Los Angeles, CA 90059
Phone: (213)563-4951
H. Frances Hayes-Cushenberry, Director
Program(s): Midwifery.

★ 25654 ★ Chico Therapy: Wellness Center
1215 Mangrove Ave., Ste. B
Chico, CA 95926
Phone: (530)891-4301 **Fax:** (530)891-4359
Mike L. Metzger, Contact
Program(s): Acupressure; Aromatherapy; Ayurvedic Medicine; Deep Tissue Massage; Herbal Medicine; Infant Massage; Manual Lymph Drainage; Massage Therapy; Neuromuscular Therapy; Prenatal Massage; Reflexology; Shiatsu; Traditional Chinese Medicine.

★ 25655 ★ Chopra Center for Well Being
7630 Fay Ave.
La Jolla, CA 92037
Phone: (619)551-7788 **Fax:** (619)551-9570
David Simon, MD, Director
Program(s): Ayurvedic Medicine; Childbirth Education; Herbal Medicine; Meditation; Mind-Body Medicine.

★ 25656 ★ Circle of Friends
704 N Hwy. 101
Leucadia, CA 92024
Free: 800-434-9642 **Fax:** (619)753-5785
Email: rudra@unit.edu
Rudi M. Kadre, Director
Program(s): Yoga Teacher Training; Meditation.

★ 25657 ★ Cleveland Chiropractic College, Los Angeles
590 N Vermont Ave.
Los Angeles, CA 90004
Phone: (213)660-6166 **Free:** 800-466-2252
Fax: (213)660-5387
Carl S. Cleveland, Contact
Program(s): Chiropractic.

★ 25658 ★ College of Bio-Energetic Medicine
1955 Lucile, Ste. D
Stockton, CA 95209
Phone: (209)473-4993 **Fax:** (209)473-4997
Michael J. Eakin, Contact
Program(s): Acupressure; Aromatherapy; Deep Tissue Massage; Energy Work; Massage Therapy; Qigong; Reflexology; Reiki; Thai Massage; Traditional Chinese Medicine.

★ 25659 ★ Conscious Choice School of Massage and Integral Healing Arts
698 Azalea
Redding, CA 96002
Phone: (530)224-0957
Robert Newman, Contact
Program(s): Acupressure; Ayurvedic Medicine; CranioSacral Therapy; Deep Tissue Massage; Energy Work; Hypnotherapy; Massage Therapy; Polarity Therapy; Reflexology; Reiki.

★ 25660 ★ Curenter University
11543 Olympic Blvd.
Los Angeles, CA 90064
Phone: (310)914-4116 **Fax:** (310)479-3376
Marlan Goodwin, Contact
Program(s): Biofeedback; Holistic Health; Honeopathy; Iridology.

★ 25661 ★ Cypress Health Institute
PO Box 2941
Santa Cruz, CA 95063
Phone: (831)476-2115
Larry Bernstein, Contact
Program(s): Acupressure; CranioSacral Therapy; Deep Tissue Massage; Holistic Health; Hypnotherapy; Massage Therapy; Polarity Therapy; Reflexology; Sports Massage; Swedish Massage; Thai Massage.

★ 25662 ★ Dandelion Herbal Center
4803 Greenwood Hts. Dr.
Kneeland, CA 95549
Phone: (707)442-8157
Jane Bothwell, Director
Program(s): Herbal Medicine.

★ 25663 ★ Day Break Geriatric Massage Project
19091 N 5th St.
216 Pleasant Hill Ave. N
Sebastopol, CA 95472
Phone: (707)829-2798 **Fax:** (707)829-2799
Felicity Doyle, Contact
Program(s): Geriatric Massage.

★ 25664 ★ Desert Resorts School of Somatherapy
13100 Palm Dr.
Desert Hot Springs, CA 92240
Phone: (760)329-1175 **Fax:** (760)329-5925
Ramona Moody French, Director
Program(s): Acupressure; Aromatherapy; CranioSacral Therapy; Deep Tissue Massage; Holistic Health; Manual Lymph Drainage; Massage Therapy; Polarity Therapy; Reflexology; Shiatsu; Sports Massage; Swedish Massage.

★ 25665 ★ Desert Springs Therapy Center
Banning Massage School
66-705 E 6th St.
Desert Hot Springs, CA 92240
Phone: (760)329-5066 **Fax:** (760)251-6206
Email: dstc@gnn.com
Charles Thomas, Director
Program(s): Deep Tissue Massage; Hydrotherapy; Massage Therapy; Sports Massage.

★ 25666 ★ Diamond Light School of Massage and Healing Arts
45 San Clemente Dr.
Corte Madera, CA 94925
Phone: (415)454-6651
Vajra Matusow, Director
Program(s): Acupressure; Energy Work; Hypnotherapy; Massage Therapy; Reflexology; Reiki; Swedish Massage.

★ 25667 ★ Dongguk Royal University
440 Shatto Pl.
Los Angeles, CA 90020
Phone: (213)487-0110 **Free:** 800-303-1800
Fax: (213)487-0527
David Burciaga, Contact
Program(s): Acupressure; Acupuncture; Herbal Medicine; Oriental Medicine; Qigong; Traditional Chinese Medicine.

★ 25668 ★ Dry Creek Herb Farm and Learning Center
13935 Dry Creek Rd.
Auburn, CA 95602
Phone: (530)878-2441 **Fax:** (530)878-0613
Shatoiya de la Tour, Director
Program(s): Aromatherapy; Ayurvedic Medicine; Energy Work; Herbal Medicine; Qigong; Traditional Chinese Medicine.

★ 25669 ★ East West School of Herbology
PO Box 712
Santa Cruz, CA 95061
Free: 800-717-5010 **Fax:** (831)336-4548
Jill Agnello, Contact
Program(s): Herbal Medicine.

★ 25670 ★ Emperor's College of Traditional Oriental Medicine
1807 Wilshire Blvd.
Santa Monica, CA 90403
Phone: (310)453-8300 **Fax:** (310)829-3838
Email: dsl@emperors.edu
Website: http://www.emperors.edu
Leah McMahan, Contact
Program(s): Acupressure; Acupuncture; Herbal Medicine; Massage Therapy; Oriental Medicine; Qigong; Reflexology; Reiki; Traditional Chinese Medicine.

★ 25671 ★ Esalen Institute
Hwy. 1
Big Sur, CA 93920
Phone: (408)667-3000
Program(s): Esalen Massage.

★ 25672 ★ Evergreen Herb Garden and Learning Center
PO Box 1445
Placerville, CA 95667
Phone: (916)626-9288 **Fax:** (916)626-9288
Candis Cantin Packard, Contact
Program(s): Ayurvedic Medicine; Herbal Medicine; Polarity Therapy.

★ 25673 ★ Expanding Light at Ananda
14618 Tyler Foote Rd.
Nevada City, CA 95959
Free: 800-346-5350 **Fax:** (530)478-7519
Richard McCord, Contact
Program(s): Yoga Teacher Training.

★ 25674 ★ Feldenkrais Resources
830 Bancroft Way, Ste. 112
Berkeley, CA 94710
Phone: (510)540-7600 **Fax:** (510)540-7683
Email: feldenres@aol.com
Carol Kress, Contact
Program(s): Feldenkrais.

★ 25675 ★ Five Branches Institute of Traditional Chinese Medicine
200 7th Ave.
Santa Cruz, CA 95062
Phone: (831)476-9424 **Fax:** (831)476-8928
Email: tcm@fivebranches.edu
Website: http://www.fivebranches.edu
Meredith Bigley, Contact
Program(s): Acupuncture; Herbal Medicine; Traditional Chinese Medicine.

★ 25676 ★ Flower Essence Society
PO Box 459
Nevada City, CA 95959
Free: 800-736-9222 **Fax:** (530)265-0584
Email: mail@flowersociety.org
Website: http://www.flowersociety.org
Patricia Kaminski, Director
Program(s): Flower Essences.

★ 25677 ★ Foothills Massage School
PO Box 826
North San Juan, CA 95960
Phone: (530)292-3123 **Fax:** (530)292-3123
Saria Farr, Contact
Program(s): Acupressure; Aromatherapy; Deep Tissue Massage; Energy Work; Herbal Medicine; Massage Therapy; Polarity Therapy; Reflexology; Shiatsu; Yoga Teacher Training.

★ 25678 ★ Four Winds Seminars
187 Hillside Dr.
Fairfax, CA 94930
Phone: (415)457-2079 **Fax:** (415)457-2079
Email: mfairbanks@igc.apc.org
Melissa Fairbanks, Director
Program(s): Homeopathy.

★ 25679 ★ Friends Landing International Center for Conscious Living, Oakland
419 48th St.
Oakland, CA 94609
Whitewind Swan Fisher, Contact
Program(s): Hypnotherapy.

★ 25680 ★ Grof Transpersonal Training, Inc.
20 Sunnyside, Ste. A314
Mill Valley, CA 94941
Phone: (415)383-8779 **Fax:** (415)383-0965
Website: http://www.holotropic.com
Cary Sparks, Director
Program(s): Breathwork.

★ 25681 ★ Hahnemann College of Homeopathy
80 Nicholl Ave.
Richmond, CA 94801
Phone: (510)232-2079 **Fax:** (510)412-9044
Debra Callahan, Contact
Program(s): Homeopathy.

★ 25682 ★ Healing Arts Institute, Roseville
112 Douglas Blvd.
Roseville, CA 95678
Phone: (916)782-1275 **Free:** 800-718-6824
Fax: (916)783-4258
Joyce Meredith, Contact
Program(s): Acupressure; Alexander Technique; Aromatherapy; Deep Tissue Massage; Massage Therapy; Reflexology; Reiki; Shiatsu; Soft Tisuue Release; Sports Massage; Swedish Massage.

★ 25683 ★ Healing Hands School of Holistic Health
125 W Mission, Ste. 212
Escondido, CA 92025
Phone: (760)746-9364 **Free:** 800-355-6463
Paula Curtiss, Director
Program(s): Acupressure; Aromatherapy; CranioSacral Therapy; Deep Tissue Massage; Herbal Medicine; Homeopathy; Holistic Health; Hypnotherapy; Massage Therapy; Reflexology; Reiki; Shiatsu; Sports Massage.

★ 25684 ★ Heartwood Institute
220 Harmony Ln.
Garberville, CA 95542
Phone: (707)923-5000 **Fax:** (707)923-5010
Website: http://www.heartwoodinstitute.com
Chela Burger, Director
Program(s): Acupressure; CranioSacral Therapy; Deep Tissue Massage; Energy Work; Holistic Health; Hypnotherapy; Massage Therapy; Neuromuscular Therapy; Oriental Medicine; Polarity Therapy; Shiatsu; Sports Massage; Swedish Massage; Traditional Chinese Medicine.

★ 25685 ★ Hellerwork International LLC
406 Berry St.
Mount Shasta, CA 96067
Free: 800-392-3900 **Fax:** (916)926-6839
Website: http://www.hellerwork.com
Joseph Heller, Contact
Program(s): Hellerwork; Structural Integration.

★ 25686 ★ Hypnosis Clearing House
3702 Mount Diablo Blvd.
Lafayette, CA 94549
Phone: (510)283-3941 **Fax:** (510)283-9044
Email: hch@hypnotherapytraining.com
Website: http://www.hypnotherapytraining.com
Holly Holmes-Meredith, Director
Program(s): Hypnotherapy.

★ 25687 ★ Hypnosis Motivation Institute
18607 Ventura Blvd., Ste. 310
Tarzana, CA 91356
Phone: (818)758-2745
Candace Coleman, Contact
Program(s): Hypnotherapy.

★ 25688 ★ Hypnotherapy Training Institute
4730 Alta Vista Ave.
Santa Rosa, CA 95404
Phone: (707)579-9023 **Free:** 800-256-6448
Fax: (707)578-1033
Email: hypno@sonic.net
Website: http://www.hypnoschool.com
Randal Churchill, Director
Program(s): Hypnotherapy.

★ 25689 ★ Hypnotism Training Institute of Los Angeles
700 S Central Ave.
Glendale, CA 91204
Phone: (818)242-1159 **Fax:** (818)247-9379
Gil Boyne, Director
Program(s): Hypnotherapy.

★ 25690 ★ Inner Quest Awareness Center
13924 Taft St., Ste. 3
Garden Grove, CA 92843
Free: 800-769-1230 **Fax:** (714)539-2977
Jeanne A. Neher-Schurz, Contact
Program(s): Hypnotherapy; Reiki.

★ 25691 ★ Institute for Applied Iridology
PO Box 301
Laguna Beach, CA 92652
Free: 888-886-8985 **Fax:** 888-886-8985
Harri Wolf, Contact
Program(s): Iridology.

★ 25692 ★ **Institute of Chinese Herbology**
3871 Piedmont Ave., Ste. 363
Oakland, CA 94611
Phone: (510)428-2061 **Fax:** (510)428-2061
Kenneth Morris, Director
Program(s): Herbal Medicine; Traditional Chinese Medicine.

★ 25693 ★ **Institute of Classical Homeopathy**
Fort Mason Center
San Francisco, CA 94123
Phone: (707)963-7796 **Fax:** (707)963-6131
Stephanie Bero, Contact
Program(s): Homeopathy.

★ 25694 ★ **Institute of Orthopedic Massage**
406 Berkeley Park Blvd.
Kensington, CA 94706
Phone: (510)524-8256 **Fax:** (510)524-8242
Thomas Hendrickson, Director
Program(s): Massage Therapy; Orthopedic Massage.

★ 25695 ★ **Institute of Professional Practical Therapy**
1835 S La Cienega Blvd., Ste. 260
Los Angeles, CA 90035
Phone: (310)836-8811 **Fax:** (310)836-8857
Victor Dence, Contact
Program(s): Deep Tissue Massage; Massage Therapy.

★ 25696 ★ **Institute of Psycho-Structural Balancing**
3767 Overland Ave., Ste. 103
Los Angeles, CA 90034
Phone: (310)815-3675 **Fax:** (310)815-3670
Website: http://www.ipsb.com
Eileen Hamsa Henry, Director
Program(s): Acupressure; Aromatherapy; CranioSacral Therapy; Energy Work; Massage Therapy; Polarity Therapy; Qigong; Reflexology; Sports Massage; Tai Chi.

★ 25697 ★ **Institute for the Study of Somatic Education**
1158 Naples St.
San Francisco, CA 94112
Phone: (415)333-6644 **Fax:** (415)333-6644
Email: isse@aol.com
Paul Rubin, Director
Program(s): Feldenkrais; Somatic Education.

★ 25698 ★ **Internal Environment Institute**
11739 Washington Blvd.
Los Angeles, CA 90066
Phone: (310)572-6223 **Fax:** (310)572-6217
Conda J. Allred, Contact
Program(s): Colon Hydrotherapy.

★ 25699 ★ **International Association of Infant Massage**
1891 Goodyear Ave., Ste. 622
Ventura, CA 93003
Phone: (805)644-8524 **Free:** 800-248-5432
Fax: (805)644-7699
Susan Campbell, Contact
Program(s): Infant Massage.

★ 25700 ★ **International College of Homeopathy**
8306 Wilshire Blvd., Ste. 728
Beverly Hills, CA 90211
Phone: (310)645-0443 **Fax:** (310)645-1814
Email: registrar@qvius.edu
Cornella Franz, MD, Contact
Program(s): Energy Work; Homeopathy; Oriental Medicine.

★ 25701 ★ **International Professional School of Bodywork**
1366 Hornblend St.
San Diego, CA 92109
Phone: (619)272-4142 **Fax:** (619)272-4772
Email: beingipsb@aol.com
Website: http://www.webcom.com/ipsb
Barbara Clark, Director
Program(s): Acupressure; Alexander Technique; CranioSacral Therapy; Feldenkrais; Herbal Medicine; Massage Therapy; Qigong; Shiatsu; Sports Massage.

★ 25702 ★ **International Sivananda Yoga Vedanta Center**
14651 Ballantree Ln.
Grass Valley, CA 95949
Phone: (415)681-2731 **Free:** 800-469-9642
Fax: (415)681-5162
Email: swsita@ix.netcom.com
Website: http://www.sivananda.org
Swami Sitaramananda, Director
Program(s): Yoga Teacher Training.

★ 25703 ★ **Iyengar Yoga Institute**
2404 27th Ave.
San Francisco, CA 94116
Phone: (415)753-0909 **Fax:** (415)753-0913
Email: iyisf@sirius.com
Website: http://www.iyoga.com/iyisf
Janet MacLeod, Director
Program(s): Yoga Teacher Training.

★ 25704 ★ **Jin Shin Do Foundation for Bodymind Acupressure**
1084G San Miguel Canyon Rd.
Watsonville, CA 95076
Phone: (831)763-7702 **Fax:** (831)763-1151
Iona Teeguarden, Director
Program(s): Acupressure; Jin Shin Do.

★ 25705 ★ **John F. Kennedy University**
Graduate School for Holistic Studies
12 Altarinda Rd.
Orinda, CA 94563
Phone: (925)254-0105 **Fax:** (925)254-3322
Website: http://www.jfku.edu
K. Sue Duncan, Contact
Program(s): Holistic Health.

★ 25706 ★ **Just for Your Health College of Massage**
2075 Lincoln Ave., Ste. E
San Jose, CA 95125
Phone: (408)723-2131 **Fax:** (408)723-7389
Tina Garcia, Director
Program(s): Acupressure; Aromatherapy; Deep Tissue Massage; Energy Work; Homeopathy; Massage Therapy; Reflexology; Sports Massage; Tai Chi.

★ 25707 ★ **Kali Ray Tri Yoga Center**
PO Box 4287
Santa Cruz, CA 95063
Phone: (408)464-8100 **Fax:** (408)462-1945
Leela Vani, Contact
Program(s): Yoga Teacher Training.

★ 25708 ★ **Kate Jordan Seminars Bodywork for the Childbearing Year**
8950 Villa La Jolla Dr., Ste. 2162
La Jolla, CA 92037
Phone: (619)436-0418 **Free:** 888-287-6860
Fax: (619)457-3615
Email: pregmassge@aol.com
Kathy Sartain, Director
Program(s): Pregnancy Massage; Postpartum Massage.

★ 25709 ★ **Kyung San University USA School of Oriental Medicine**
8322 Garden Grove Blvd.
Garden Grove, CA 92844
Phone: (714)636-0337 **Fax:** (714)636-8459
Email: admin@kyungsan.edu
Eun Suk Lee, Contact
Program(s): Acupressure; Acupuncture; CranioSacral Therapy; Herbal Medicine; Oriental Medicine; Qigong; Reflexology; Shiatsu; Traditional Chinese Medicine.

★ 25710 ★ **Lake Tahoe Massage School**
1966 US Hwy 50
South Lake Tahoe, CA 96150
Phone: (530)544-1227
Jeannette Cunniff, Contact
Program(s): CranioSacral Therapy; Deep Tissue Massage; Massage Therapy; Medical Massage; Polarity Therapy; Reflexology; Reiki; Shiatsu; Sports Massage.

★ 25711 ★ **Life Chiropractic College West**
2005 Via Barrett
San Lorenzo, CA 94580
Free: 800-788-4476 **Fax:** (510)276-4893
Email: info@lifewest.edu
Website: http://www.lifewest.edu
Gerard W. Clum, Contact
Program(s): Chiropractic.

★ 25712 ★ **Linda Lack, Two-Snake Studios**
1637 S La Cienega Blvd.
Los Angeles, CA 90035
Phone: (310)273-4797 **Fax:** (310)932-1441
Linda Lack, Contact
Program(s): Movement Therapy; Yoga Teacher Training; Yoga Therapy.

★ 25713 ★ **Los Angeles College of Chiropractic**
16200 E Amber Valley Dr.
Whittier, CA 90609-1166
Phone: (562)947-8755 **Free:** 800-221-5222
Fax: (562)947-5724
Reed Phillips, PhD, Director
Program(s): Chiropractic.

★ 25714 ★ **Loving Hands Institute of Healing Arts**
639 11th St.
Fortuna, CA 95540-2346
Phone: (707)725-9627 **Fax:** (707)725-2471
Dr. Rosalind Skyhawk Ojala, Director
Program(s): Acupressure; Deep Tissue Massage; Esalen Massage; Holistic Health; Lymphatic Massage; Massage Therapy; Reflexology; Swedish Massage; Trigger Point Therapy.

★ 25715 ★ **Lu Ross Academy of Health & Beauty**
470 E Thompson Blvd.
Ventura, CA 93001
Phone: (805)643-5690
Chrys Huynh, Director
Program(s): Acupressure; Aromatherapy; CranioSacral Therapy; Energy Work; Herbal Medicine; Massage Therapy; Neuromuscular Therapy; Polarity Therapy; Qigong; Reflexology; Reiki; Shiatsu; Sports Massage.

★ 25716 ★ Massage School of Santa Monica
1453 Third St. Promenade, Ste. 340
Santa Monica, CA 90401
Phone: (310)393-7461 **Fax:** (310)453-2386
Bernadette Gessner, Director
Program(s): Acupressure; Aromatherapy; CranioSacral Therapy; Energy Work; Massage Therapy; Polarity Therapy; Qigong; Reflexology; Shiatsu; Sports Massage; Swedish Massage.

★ 25717 ★ Master Yoga Academy
7592 Fay Ave.
La Jolla, CA 92037
Phone: (619)454-6978 **Fax:** (619)454-5541
Rama Berch, Director
Program(s): Yoga Teacher Training.

★ 25718 ★ McKinnon Institute of Professional Massage and Bodywork
2940 Webster St.
Oakland, CA 94609-3407
Phone: (510)465-3488 **Fax:** (510)465-1533
Judith McKinnon, Director
Program(s): Acupressure; Anatomy and Physiology; CranioSacral Therapy; Deep Tissue Massage; Massage Therapy; On-Site Massage; Reflexology; Shiatsu; Sports Massage; Swedish Massage.

★ 25719 ★ Meiji College of Oriental Medicine
2550 Shattuck Ave.
Berkeley, CA 94704
Phone: (510)666-8248 **Fax:** (510)666-0111
Laura Pitre, Contact
Program(s): Acupuncture; Herbal Medicine; Oriental Medicine; Traditional Chinese Medicine.

★ 25720 ★ Mendocino School of Holistic Massage and Advanced Healing Arts
2680 Rd. B
Redwood Valley, CA 95470
Phone: (707)485-8197
Email: rammpack@pacific.net
Clark Ramm, Director
Program(s): Aromatherapy; Ayurvedic Medicine; Energy Work; Esalen Massage; Herbal Medicine; Holistic Health; Homeopathy; Hypnotherapy; Lymphatic Massage; Massage Therapy; Polarity Therapy; Rebirthing; Reflexology; Swedish Massage.

★ 25721 ★ Meridian Institute
99 Pacific St., Heritage Harbor Bldg. 375A
Monterey, CA 93940
Phone: (831)649-6684 **Fax:** (831)649-6688
Andy Seplow, Contact
Program(s): Acupuncture; Herbal Medicine; Massage Therapy; Traditional Chinese Medicine.

★ 25722 ★ Mesa Institute
150 N Felder
Orange, CA 92868
Phone: (714)937-4161 **Fax:** (714)937-6360
Chad Marta, Contact
Program(s): Acupressure; Aromatherapy; Ayurvedic Medicine; CranioSacral Therapy; Deep Tissue Massage; Energy Work; Holistic Health; Hypnotherapy; Massage Therapy; Polarity Therapy; Reflexology; Reiki; Shiatsu; Sports Massage.

★ 25723 ★ Michael Scholes School of Aromatic Studies
117 N Robertson Blvd.
Los Angeles, CA 90048
Phone: (310)276-1191 **Free:** 800-677-2368
Fax: (310)276-1156
Email: joanaroma@aol.com
Michael Scholes, Contact
Program(s): Aromatherapy; Energy Work.

★ 25724 ★ Midwifery Institute of California
3739 Balboa, Ste. 179
San Francisco, CA 94121
Shannon Ariton, Contact
Program(s): Midwifery.

★ 25725 ★ Montebello Career College
2465 W Whittier Blvd., Ste. 201
Montebello, CA 90640
Phone: (323)728-9636 **Fax:** (323)728-0952
Rosa Sanchez, Contact
Program(s): Massage Therapy.

★ 25726 ★ Monterey Institute of Touch
27820 Dorris Dr.
Carmel, CA 93923
Phone: (831)624-1006 **Fax:** (831)626-6916
Email: mit@redshift.com
Birgit Ball-Eisner, Contact
Program(s): Acupressure; Aromatherapy; CranioSacral Therapy; Massage Therapy; Polarity Therapy; Reflexology; Shiatsu; Sports Massage.

★ 25727 ★ Monterey Peninsula College
980 Fremont St.
Monterey, CA 93940
Phone: (831)646-4220 **Fax:** (831)645-1334
Dawn Sare, Contact
Program(s): Acupressure; Massage Therapy; Polarity Therapy; Refexology; Shiatsu; Sports Massage.

★ 25728 ★ Mount Madonna Center
445 Summit Rd.
Watsonville, CA 95076
Phone: (408)847-0406 **Fax:** (408)847-2683
Email: programs@mountmadonna.org
Website: http://www.mountmadonna.org
Gerald Friedberg, Director
Program(s): Ayurvedic Medicine; Yoga Teacher Training.

★ 25729 ★ Movement Studies Institute
1832 Second St.
Berkeley, CA 94710
Free: 800-342-3424 **Fax:** (510)548-4349
Email: info@movementstudies.com
Dr. Frank Wildman, Director
Program(s): Feldenkrais.

★ 25730 ★ Mueller College of Holistic Studies
4607 Park Blvd.
San Diego, CA 92116
Phone: (619)291-9811 **Fax:** (619)543-1113
Email: info@muellercollege.com
Website: http://www.muellercollege.com
Bill Mueller, Director
Program(s): Acupressure; Aromatherapy; Ayurvedic Medicine; CranioSacral Therapy; Herbal Medicine; Holistic Health; Massage Therapy; Oriental Madicine; Polarity Therapy; Qigong; Reflexology; Shiatsu; Traditional Chinese Medicine.

★ 25731 ★ National Holistic Institute
5900 Hollis St., Ste. J
Emeryville, CA 94608
Phone: (510)547-6442 **Free:** 800-315-3552
Fax: (510)547-6621
Email: nhi@nhimassage.com
Website: http://www.nhimassage.com
Nancy Seyfert, Director
Program(s): Holistic Health; Massage Therapy; Shiatsu; Sports Massage.

★ 25732 ★ National Institute of Massage
1150 E Palm Canyon Dr., Ste. 54
Palm Springs, CA 92264
Phone: (760)323-3535
Sharon Leeds, Contact
Program(s): Energy Work; Herbal Medicine; Massage Therapy; Polarity Therapy; Yoga Teacher Training.

★ 25733 ★ Natural Healing Institute of Naturopathy, Inc.
2146 Encinitas Blvd., Ste. 105
Encinitas, CA 92024
Phone: (760)943-8485 **Fax:** (760)943-9477
Patti Valentine, Contact
Program(s): Acupressure; Aromatherapy; Ayurvedic Medicine; Deep Tissue Massage; Energy Work; Herbal Medicine; Hypnotherapy; Massage Therapy; Naturopathic Medicine; Nutrition; Oriental Medicine; Reflexology; Shiatsu; Traditional Chinese Medicine.

★ 25734 ★ New Life Institute of Massage Therapy
1159 Hilltop Dr.
Redding, CA 96002
Phone: (530)222-1467 **Fax:** (530)222-3489
Shirley Latal, Contact
Program(s): CranioSacral Therapy; Massage Therapy; Myofascial Release; Reflexology.

★ 25735 ★ Oakendell School of Massage and Healing Arts
3585 Hawver Rd.
San Andreas, CA 95249
Phone: (209)754-0244 **Fax:** (209)754-1081
Steve Mertens, Contact
Program(s): Acupressure; Energy Work; Massage Therapy; Neuromuscular Therapy; Oriental Medicine; Qigong; Traditional Chinese Medicine.

★ 25736 ★ Pacific Academy of Homeopathy
1199 Sanchez St.
San Francisco, CA 94114
Phone: (415)458-8238 **Fax:** (415)695-8220
Richard Pitt, Contact
Program(s): Homeopathy.

★ 25737 ★ Pacific College
3160 Redhill Ave.
Costa Mesa, CA 92626
Phone: (714)662-4402 **Fax:** (714)662-1702
Betty Gross, Contact
Program(s): Acupressure; Aromatherapy; Massage Therapy; Reflexology; Shiatsu; Sports Massage.

★ 25738 ★ Pacific College of Alternative Therapies
19997 Stevens Creek Blvd., Ste. 2
Cupertino, CA 95014
Phone: (408)777-0102 **Fax:** (408)777-0188
Email: pcollege-atherapist@juno.com
Peter Hou, Director
Program(s): Acupressure; Massage Therapy; Qigong; Traditional Chinese Medicine; Tui Na.

★ 25739 ★ Pacific College of Oriental Medicine
7445 Mission Valley Rd., Ste. 105
San Diego, CA 92108
Phone: (619)574-6909 **Fax:** (619)574-6641
Email: jmiller@ormed.edu
Website: http://www.ormed.edu
Jack Miller, Contact
Program(s): Acupressure; Acupuncture; Energy Work; Herbal Medicine; Holistic Health; Massage Therapy; Oriental Medicine; Qigong; Reflexology; Shiatsu; Sports Massage; Traditional Chinese Medicine.

★ 25740 ★ Pacific Institute for the Alexander Technique
930 Alhambra Blvd., Ste. 270
Sacramento, CA 95816
Phone: (916)448-7424
Sherry Berjeron-Oliver, Contact
Program(s): Alexander Technique.

★ 25741 ★ Pacific Institute of Aromatherapy
PO Box 6723
San Rafael, CA 94903
Phone: (415)479-9121 **Fax:** (415)479-0119
Dr. Kurt Schnaubelt, Director
Program(s): Aromatherapy.

★ 25742 ★ Pacific School of Herbal Medicine
PO Box 2194
Berkeley, CA 94702
Phone: (510)685-4028
Adam Seller, Contact
Program(s): Aromatherapy; Ayurvedic Medicine; Herbal Medicine.

★ 25743 ★ Pacific School of Massage & Healing Arts
44800 Fish Rock Rd.
Gualala, CA 95445
Phone: (707)884-3138 **Fax:** (707)884-4106
Email: mitouer@mcn.org
Cheryl Mitouer, Director
Program(s): Massage Therapy; Transformational Bodywork.

★ 25744 ★ Palmer College of Chiropractic West
90 E Tasman Dr.
San Jose, CA 95134
Phone: (408)944-6000 **Free:** 800-442-4476
Fax: (408)944-6111
Peter A. Martin, Contact
Program(s): Chiropractic.

★ 25745 ★ Palo Alto School of Hypnotherapy
2443 Ash St., Ste. D
Palo Alto, CA 94306
Phone: (415)321-6419 **Free:** 800-774-9766
Fax: (650)941-2485
Josie Hadley, Contact
Program(s): Hypnotherapy; Qigong; Reiki.

★ 25746 ★ Polarity Therapy Center of Marin
PO Box 23
Tomales, CA 94971
Phone: (707)878-2278
Hanna Hammerli, Director
Program(s): Polarity Therapy.

★ 25747 ★ Polarity Wellness Center West
325 Shortt Rd.
Santa Rosa, CA 95405
Phone: (707)542-7966
Jan Milthaler, Director
Program(s): Polarity Therapy.

★ 25748 ★ Quantum-Veritas International University Systems
8306 Wilshire Blvd., Ste. 728
Beverly Hills, CA 90211
Phone: (310)645-0443 **Fax:** (310)645-1814
Cherie DeWonder, Contact
Program(s): Acupressure; Aromatherapy; Ayurvedic Medicine; CranioSacral Therapy; Deep Tissue Massage; Energy Work; Herbal Medicine; Kinesiology; Massage Therapy; Oriental Medicine; Polarity Therapy; Qigong; Reflexology; Shiatsu; Sports Massage; Traditional Chinese Medicine; Yoga Teacher Training.

★ 25749 ★ Reese Movement Institute, Inc.
2187 Newcastle
Cardiff, CA 92007
Phone: (760)436-9087 **Fax:** (760)436-9141
Email: rmiinc@aol.com
Mark Reese, Director
Program(s): Feldenkrais.

★ 25750 ★ Reflexology Institute
27636 Ynez Rd. L-7, Ste. 232
Temecula, CA 92591
Phone: (909)694-0225 **Fax:** (909)694-5910
Lynn Nelson, Contact
Program(s): Reflexology.

★ 25751 ★ Reiki Center of Los Angeles
16161 Ventura Blvd., Ste. 802
Encino, CA 91436
Phone: (818)881-5959 **Fax:** (818)881-1613
Joyce Morris, Contact
Program(s): Reiki.

★ 25752 ★ reSource
825 Bancroft Way
Berkeley, CA 94702
Phone: (510)433-7917 **Fax:** (510)841-3258
Gail Stewart, Director
Program(s): Deep Tissue Massage; Massage Therapy; Ortho-Bionomy; Trager.

★ 25753 ★ Rosa Institute of Aromatherapy
219 Carl St.
San Francisco, CA 94117-3804
Phone: (415)564-6785 **Fax:** (415)564-6799
Jeanne Rose, Contact
Program(s): Aromatherapy; Herbal Medicine.

★ 25754 ★ Rosen Method: The Berkeley Center
825 Bancroft Way
Berkeley, CA 94710
Phone: (510)845-6606 **Fax:** (510)845-8114
Abby Paige, Contact
Program(s): Rosen Method Bodywork.

★ 25755 ★ Samra University of Oriental Medicine
3000 S Robertson Blvd., 4th Flr.
Los Angeles, CA 90034
Phone: (310)202-6444 **Fax:** (310)202-6007
Email: admissions@samra.edu
Website: http://www.samra.edu
Kathryn P. White, PhD, Contact
Program(s): Acupressure; Acupuncture; Herbal Medicine; Oriental Medicine; Qigong; Traditional Chinese Medicine.

★ 25756 ★ San Francisco School of Massage
1327A Chestnut St.
San Francisco, CA 94123
Phone: (415)474-4600 **Fax:** (415)474-4601
Richard Bergess, Director
Program(s): Acupressure; Aromatherapy; Breema Bodywork; CranioSacral Therapy; Deep Tissue Massage; Esalen Massage; Lymphatic Massage; Massage Therapy; Reflexology; Reiki; Shiatsu; Sports Massage; Swedish Massage; Trigger Point Therapy.

★ 25757 ★ Santa Barbara College of Oriental Medicine
1919 State St., Ste. 204
Santa Barbara, CA 93101
Phone: (805)898-1180 **Fax:** (805)682-1864
Email: 76774.3507@compuserve.com
JoAnn Hickey, Contact
Program(s): Acupressure; Acupuncture; Chinese Herbal Medicine; Oriental Medicine; Qigong; Shiatsu; Traditional Chinese Medicine.

★ 25758 ★ Santa Barbara Yoga Center
32 E Micheltorena St.
Santa Barbara, CA 93101
Phone: (805)965-6045
Lais Da Silva, Contact
Program(s): Yoga Teacher Training.

★ 25759 ★ School of Healing Arts
1001 Garnet Ave., Ste. 200
San Diego, CA 92109
Phone: (619)581-9429 **Fax:** (619)490-2555
Seymour Koblin, Director
Program(s): Acupressure; Hypnotherapy; Holistic Health; Massage Therapy; Shiatsu.

★ 25760 ★ School of Homeopathy
2124 Kittredge St.
Berkeley, CA 94704
Phone: (510)649-0294 **Fax:** (510)649-1955
Email: mail@homeopathic.com
Website: http://www.homeopathic.com
Stuart Gracie, Contact
Program(s): Homeopathy.

★ 25761 ★ School of Intuitive Massage and Healing
503 Foxen Dr,
Santa Barbara, CA 93105
Phone: (805)687-2917 **Fax:** (805)563-0927
Anne Parks, Director
Program(s): Energy Work; Massage Therapy.

★ 25762 ★ School of Shiatsu and Massage
18424 Harbin Springs Rd.
PO Box 889
Middletown, CA 95461
Phone: (707)987-3801 **Fax:** (707)987-9638
Email: info@waba.edu
Website: http://www.waba.edu
Harold Dull, Director
Program(s): Acupressure; Massage Therapy; Shiatsu; Watsu Aquatic Bodywork.

★ 25763 ★ Sebastopol Massage Center
108 N Main, Ste. 5
Sebastopol, CA 95472
Phone: (707)823-3550
Patricia Oberg, Director
Program(s): Acupressure; CranioSacral Therapy; Energy Work; Esalen Massage; Massage Therapy; Ortho-Bionomy; Reflexology; Shiatsu; Swedish Massage.

★ 25764 ★ South Bay Massage College
3770 Highland Ave., Ste. 204
Manhattan Beach, CA 90266
Phone: (310)546-8774 **Fax:** (310)546-8775
Betsy Anderson, Contact
Program(s): Deep Tissue Massage; Massage Therapy; Refexology; Sports Massage.

★ 25765 ★ South Baylo University
1126 N Brookhurst St.
Anaheim, CA 92801
Phone: (714)533-1495 **Fax:** (714)533-6040

Email: ron@sbu.edu
Website: http://www.sbu.edu
Ronald Sokolsky, Director
Program(s): Acupuncture; Herbal Medicine; Qigong; Shiatsu; Traditional Chinese Medicine; Tui Na.

★ 25766 ★ Southern California School of Massage
12702 Magnolia Ave., Ste. 21
Riverside, CA 92503
Phone: (909)340-3336 **Fax:** (909)340-0154
Elizabeth Kelly, Contact
Program(s): Acupressure; Aromatherapy; Deep Tissue Massage; Energy Work; Holistic Health; Hypnotherapy; Massage Therapy; Polarity Therapy; Reflexology; Shiatsu; Sports Massage; Traditional Chinese Medicine.

★ 25767 ★ Taoist Institute
10630 Burbank Blvd.
North Hollywood, CA 91601
Phone: (818)760-4219
Carl Totton, Director
Program(s): Acupressure; Qigong; Tui Na.

★ 25768 ★ Therapeutic Learning Center
3636 N First St., Ste. 154
Fresno, CA 93727
Phone: (559)225-7772 **Fax:** (559)252-5313
Evangeline K. Hentrich, Contact
Program(s): Energy Work; Massage Therapy; Reflexology; Shiatsu; Swedish Massage.

★ 25769 ★ Touch for Health Kinesiology
11262 Washington Blvd.
Culver City, CA 90230
Phone: (310)313-5580 **Free:** 800-466-8342
Fax: (310)313-9319
Mark McCutcheon, Director
Program(s): Kinesiology; Touch for Health.

★ 25770 ★ Touch Therapy Institute
15720 Ventura Blvd., Ste. 101
Encino, CA 91436
Phone: (818)788-0824 **Fax:** (818)788-0875
Website: http://www.touchtherapyinstitute.com
Maria Grove, Director
Program(s): Acupressure; Alexander Technique; Anatomy and Physiology; Aromatherapy; Chair Massage; CPR/First Aid; CranioSacral Therapy; Energy Work; LomiLomi Massage; Lymphatic Massage; Massage Therapy; Myofascial Release; Pregnancy Massage; Qigong; Reflexology; Sports Massage; Swedish Massage; Therapeutic Touch; Trager.

★ 25771 ★ Touching for Health Center School of Professional Bodywork
628 Lincoln Ctr.
Stockton, CA 95207-2640
Phone: (209)474-9559 **Fax:** (209)474-9559
Roberta Baker, Director
Program(s): Acupressure; Aromatherapy; CranioSacral Therapy; Deep Tissue Massage; Manual Lymph Drainage; Massage Therapy; Myofascial Release; Polarity Therapy; Reflexology.

★ 25772 ★ TouchPro Institute of Chair Massage
584 Castro St., Ste. 555
San Francisco, CA 94114
Free: 800-999-5026 **Fax:** (415)621-1260
Douglas Hudson, Contact
Program(s): Chair Massage.

★ 25773 ★ Trager Institute
21 Locust Ave.
Mill Valley, CA 94941-2806
Phone: (415)388-2688 **Fax:** (415)388-2710
Email: admin@trager.com
Don Schwartz, PhD, Director
Program(s): Trager.

★ 25774 ★ Twin Lakes College of the Healing Arts
1210 Brommer St.
Santa Cruz, CA 95062
Phone: (831)476-2152
Becky Williams, Director
Program(s): Acupressure; Aromatherapy; Energy Work; Hypnotherapy; Massage Therapy; Polarity Therapy; Reflexology; Reiki; Shiatsu.

★ 25775 ★ United States Yoga Association
2159 Filbert St.
San Francisco, CA 94123
Phone: (415)931-9642 **Fax:** (415)921-6676
Sandy Wong, Contact
Program(s): Yoga Teacher Training.

★ 25776 ★ University of California, Los Angeles
Primary Care Division
Nurse-Midwifery Education Program
10833 LeConte Ave.
Los Angeles, CA 90099-4973
Phone: (310)794-4434 **Fax:** (310)206-3241
Email: mday@sonnet.ucla.edu
Mary Day, Contact
Program(s): Midwifery.

★ 25777 ★ University of California, San Diego
Division of Graduate Nursing Education
Nurse-Midwifery Program
9500 Gilman Dr.
La Jolla, CA 92093-0809
Phone: (619)543-5480 **Fax:** (619)543-7757
Lauren Hunter, Director
Program(s): Midwifery.

★ 25778 ★ University of Southern California
Nurse-Midwifery Education Program
1540 E Alcazar St.
CHP 222
Los Angeles, CA 90033
Phone: (323)442-2001 **Fax:** (323)442-2090
BJ Snell, Director
Program(s): Midwifery.

★ 25779 ★ Valley Hypnosis Center
3705 Sunnyside Dr.
Riverside, CA 92506
Phone: (909)781-0282
Sally Cernie, PhD, Contact
Program(s): Hypnotherapy; Pranic Healing; Reflexology; Reiki.

★ 25780 ★ Vitality Sciences Institute
70-A N El Camino Real
San Mateo, CA 94401-2866
Phone: (650)347-4565 **Fax:** (650)344-7783
Alicia Parnell, Contact
Program(s): Reposturing Dynamics.

★ 25781 ★ Vitality Training Center
243 N Hwy. 101, Ste. 5
Solana Beach, CA 92075
Phone: (619)259-9491 **Fax:** (619)259-2008
Annie Benefield, Director
Program(s): Acupressure; Aromatherapy; CranioSacral Therapy; Energy Work; Herbal Medicine; Holistic Health; Hypnotherapy; Massage Therapy; Neuromuscular Therapy; Reflexology; Reiki; Shiatsu; Sports Massage; Yoga Teacher Training.

★ 25782 ★ Wellness Holistic School of Massage
345 S E St.
Santa Rosa, CA 95404
Phone: (707)546-8115 **Free:** 800-939-6837
Virginia Romero, Director
Program(s): Energy Work; Esalen Massage; Kinesiology; Massage Therapy; Polarity Therapy; Reflexology; Swedish Massage; Touch for Health.

★ 25783 ★ West Pacific
434 N Lakeview Ave.
Anaheim, CA 92807
Phone: (714)998-8079 **Fax:** (714)998-8079
Joel Doti, Contact
Program(s): Deep Tissue Massage; Massage Therapy; Sports Massage.

★ 25784 ★ Western Institute of Neuromuscular Therapy
22981 Mill Creek Dr., Ste. A
Laguna Hills, CA 92653
Phone: (714)830-6151 **Fax:** (714)830-1729
Cynthia Ribeiro, Director
Program(s): Massage Therapy; Neuromuscular Therapy; Sports Massage.

★ 25785 ★ World School of Massage and Advanced Healing Arts
401 32nd Ave.
San Francisco, CA 94125
Phone: (415)221-2533 **Fax:** (415)221-0430
Patricia Cramer, Contact
Program(s): Aromatherapy; CranioSacral Therapy; Holistic Health; Massage Therapy; Reflexology; Vibrational Therapy.

★ 25786 ★ Wyrick Institute & Clinic
PO Box 99745
San Diego, CA 92169
Phone: (619)273-9764 **Fax:** (619)277-7358
Dana Wyrick, Director
Program(s): Manual Lymph Drainage.

★ 25787 ★ Yo San University of Traditional Chinese Medicine
1314 2nd St.
Santa Monica, CA 90401
Phone: (310)917-2202 **Fax:** (310)917-2203
Email: info@yosan.edu
Website: http://www.yosan.edu
Dr. Richard Hammerschlag, Director
Program(s): Acupuncture; Herbal Medicine; Lifestyle Counseling; Qigong; Traditional Chinese Medicine.

★ 25788 ★ Yoga Room
953-957 2nd St.
Encinitas, CA 92024
Phone: (619)753-1828 **Fax:** (619)753-4639
Peri Ness, Contact
Program(s): Yoga Teacher Training.

★ 25789 ★ Yoga Works, Inc.
1426 Montana Ave., 2nd Fl.
Santa Monica, CA 90403
Phone: (310)393-5150 **Fax:** (310)656-5892
Julie Jacobs, Contact
Program(s): Yoga Teacher Training.

★ 25790 ★ Zero Balancing Association
PO Box 1727
Capitola, CA 95010
Phone: (408)476-0665 **Fax:** (408)476-0665

Email: zbaoffice@aol.com
Fritz Smith, MD, Contact
Program(s): Zero Balancing.

Colorado

★ 25791 ★ Academy of Natural Therapy
123 Elm Ave.
Eaton, CO 80615
Phone: (970)454-2224 **Fax:** (303)454-3147
Email: mongan@ibm.net
Dorothy Mongan, Director
Program(s): Acupressure; Herbal Medicine; Massage Therapy; Reflexology; Shiatsu.

★ 25792 ★ Alexander Technique Institute, Colorado
2545 Vine Pl.
Boulder, CO 80304
Phone: (303)449-4143
Colin Egan, Director
Program(s): Alexander Technique.

★ 25793 ★ Ann Allen and Associates, Biofeedback and Stress Management
1660 S Albion St.
Denver, CO 80222
Phone: (303)757-0508 **Fax:** (303)758-9203
Ann Allen, Contact
Program(s): Biofeedback.

★ 25794 ★ Artemis Institute of Natural Therapies
875 Alpine Ave., Ste. 5
Boulder, CO 80304
Phone: (303)443-9289 **Fax:** (303)443-6361
Peter J. Holmes, Director
Program(s): Aromatherapy; Herbal Medicine.

★ 25795 ★ Association for Applied Psychophysiology and Biofeedback
10200 W 44th Ave., Ste. 304
Wheat Ridge, CO 80033
Phone: (303)422-8436 **Fax:** (303)422-8894
Francine Butler, Contact
Program(s): Biofeedback.

★ 25796 ★ BioSomatics
PO Box 206
Grand Junction, CO 81502
Phone: (970)245-8903 **Fax:** (970)241-5653
Carol Welch, Contact
Program(s): CranioSacral Therapy; Neuromuscular Therapy; Somatic Education.

★ 25797 ★ Boulder College of Massage Therapy
6255 Longbow
Boulder, CO 80301
Phone: (303)530-2100 **Free:** 800-442-5131
Fax: (303)530-2204
Christopher Quinn, Contact
Program(s): Chair Massage; Hydrotherapy; Infant Massage; Integrative Massage; Massage Therapy; Orthopedic Massage; Polarity Therapy; Prenatal Massage; Reflexology; Shiatsu; Sports Massage; Swedish Massage.

★ 25798 ★ Center of Advanced Therapeutics, Inc.
1221 S Clarkson St., Ste. 412
Denver, CO 80210
Phone: (303)765-2201
Mary Uhl, Contact
Program(s): CranioSacral Therapy; Deep Tissue Massage; Massage Therapy.

★ 25799 ★ Collinson School of Therapeutics & Massage
2596 Palmer Park Blvd.
Colorado Springs, CO 80909
Phone: (719)473-0145
Dr. Torry Collinson, Contact
Program(s): Acupressure; Aromatherapy; CranioSacral Therapy; Massage Therapy; Reflexology; Reiki; Shiatsu.

★ 25800 ★ Colorado Institute for Classical Homeopathy
2299 Pearl St., Ste. 401
Boulder, CO 80302
Phone: (303)440-3717
Barbara Seideneck, Director
Program(s): Homeopathy.

★ 25801 ★ Colorado Institute of Massage Therapy
2601 E St. Vrain
Colorado Springs, CO 80909
Phone: (719)634-7486 **Fax:** (719)447-9198
Website: http://www.coimt.com
Greg Smith, Contact
Program(s): Acupressure; Fitness Therapy; Massage Therapy; Neuromuscular Therapy; Reflexology; Sports Massage.

★ 25802 ★ Colorado School of Healing Arts
7655 W Mississippi, Ste. 100
Lakewood, CO 80226
Phone: (303)986-2320
Chris Smith, Director
Program(s): Aromatherapy; CranioSacral Therapy; Herbal Medicine; Massage Therapy; Neuromuscular Therapy; Reflexology; Sports Massage.

★ 25803 ★ Colorado School of Traditional Chinese Medicine
1441 York St., Ste. 202
Denver, CO 80210
Phone: (303)329-6355 **Fax:** (303)388-8165
Dr. George H. Kitchie, Contact
Program(s): Acupuncture; Chinese Herbal Medicine; Qigong; Traditional Chinese Medicine.

★ 25804 ★ Colorado Springs Academy of Therapeutic Massage
3612 Galley, Ste. A
Colorado Springs, CO 80909
Phone: (719)597-0017 **Fax:** (719)597-6647
Dr. Daniel A. Sollee, Director
Program(s): Deep Tissue Massage; Massage Therapy; Neuromuscular Therapy; Sports Massage; Swedish Massage; Trigger Point Therapy.

★ 25805 ★ Connecting Point School of Massage
104 Society Dr.
Telluride, CO 81435
Phone: (970)728-6424
Sefra Maples, Contact
Program(s): Acupressure; Aromatherapy; Deep Tissue Massage; Massage Therapy; Reflexology; Shiatsu; Spa Therapies.

★ 25806 ★ Cottonwood School of Massage Therapy
2620 S Parker Rd., Ste. 300
Aurora, CO 80014
Phone: (303)745-7725 **Fax:** (303)751-1861
Jackie Otey, Contact
Program(s): Aromatherapy; CranioSacral Therapy; Energy Work; Massage Therapy; Polarity Therapy; Reflexology; Reiki; Shiatsu; Sports Massage.

★ 25807 ★ Crestone Healing Arts Center
1689 Columbine Overlook
Crestone, CO 81131
Phone: (719)256-4036
Email: retuta@crestonehac.com
Dan Retuta, Director
Program(s): Acupressure; Anatomy and Physiology; CPR/First Aid; Herbal Medicine; Integrated Massage; Massage Therapy; On-Site Massage; Prenatal Massage; Qigong; Reflexology; Shiatsu; Swedish Massage.

★ 25808 ★ Day-Star Method of Yoga
2565 S Meade St.
Denver, CO 80219
Phone: (303)934-6309
Susan Flanders, Contact
Program(s): Yoga Teacher Training.

★ 25809 ★ Guild for Structural Integration
3107 28th St.
PO Box 1559
Boulder, CO 80301
Free: 800-447-0150 **Fax:** (303)447-0108
Email: gsi@rolfguild.org
Website: http://www.rolfguild.org
Susan Melchior, Director
Program(s): Structural Integration.

★ 25810 ★ Hahnemann Academy of North America
PO Box 3024
Pagosa Springs, CO 81147
Phone: (970)731-9681
Robin Murphy, Director
Program(s): Homeopathy.

★ 25811 ★ Institute of Taoist Education and Acupuncture, Inc.
1321 5th St.
Boulder, CO 80302
Phone: (303)440-3492 **Fax:** (303)440-3492
Sandra L. Lillie, Contact
Program(s): Acupuncture.

★ 25812 ★ Just for Health Enterprises, Inc.
480 S Holly St.
Denver, CO 80246
Phone: (303)341-4384 **Fax:** (303)360-9118
Rachel Lord, Contact
Program(s): Acupressure; Anatomy and Physiology; Deep Tissue Massage; Energy Work Herbal Medicine; Massage Therapy; Reflexology.

★ 25813 ★ Massage Therapy Institute of Colorado
1441 York St., Ste. 301
Denver, CO 80206
Phone: (303)329-6345 **Fax:** (303)388-8165
Mark Manton, Director
Program(s): Acupressure; Alexander Technique; Aromatherapy; Ayurvedic Medicine; CranioSacral Therapy; Energy Work; Feldenkrais; Herbal Medicine; Homeopathy; Hypnotherapy; Massage Therapy; Neuromuscular Therapy; Polarity Therapy; Qigong; Reflexology; Reiki; Shiatsu; Sports Massage.

★ 25814 ★ Modern Institute of Reflexology
7043 W Colfax
Denver, CO 80215
Phone: (303)237-1530 **Fax:** (303)237-1606
Zachary K. Brinkerhoff, Contact
Program(s): Reflexology.

★ 25815 ★ MountainHeart School of Bodywork and Transformational Therapy
719 5th, Unit A
Denver, CO 80224
Phone: (970)349-0473 **Free:** 800-673-0539
Fax: (970)349-0473
Christine McLaughlin, Contact
Program(s): Acupressure; Energy Work; Massage Therapy; Neuromuscular Therapy; Oriental Medicine; Reflexology.

★ 25816 ★ Polarity Center of Colorado
1721 Redwood Ave.
Boulder, CO 80304-1118
Phone: (303)443-9847 **Fax:** (303)415-1839
John Chitty, Director
Program(s): CranioSacral Therapy; Polarity Therapy.

★ 25817 ★ Qigong Research and Practice Center
PO Box 1727
Nederland, CO 80466
Phone: (303)258-0971 **Fax:** (303)258-0971
Rebecca D. Cohen, Contact
Program(s): Energy Work, Qigong; Tai Chi.

★ 25818 ★ Rocky Mountain Center for Botanical Studies
2639 Spruce St.
PO Box 19254
Boulder, CO 80302
Phone: (303)442-6861 **Fax:** (303)442-6294
Email: rmcbs@indra.com
Feather Jones, Director
Program(s): Aromatherapy; Ayurvedic Medicine; Herbal Medicine; Traditional Chinese Medicine.

★ 25819 ★ Rolf Institute of Structural Integration
205 Canyon Blvd.
Boulder, CO 80302
Phone: (303)449-5903 **Free:** 800-530-8875
Fax: (303)449-5978
Email: rolfinst@aol.com
Website: http://www.rolf.org
Holly Hamilton, Director
Program(s): Structural Integration.

★ 25820 ★ Ruseto College of Acupuncture and Chinese Medicine
2900 Valmont Rd., Ste. E-1
Boulder, CO 80301
Phone: (303)449-1686
Pao-Chin R. Huang, Director
Program(s): Acupuncture; Herbal Medicine; Massage Therapy; Polarity Therapy; Qigong; Reflexology; Shiatsu; Traditional Chinese Medicine; Tui Na.

★ 25821 ★ School of Natural Medicine
PO Box 7369
Boulder, CO 80306-7369
Phone: (303)443-4882 **Fax:** (303)443-8276
Email: snm@purehealth.com
Website: http://www.purehealth.com
Dr. Farida Sharan, Director
Program(s): Energy Work; Herbal Medicine; Iridology; Naturopathy.

★ 25822 ★ University of Colorado School of Nursing Nurse-Midwifery Option
Health Sciences Center
4200 E 9th Ave., Box C288-14
Denver, CO 80262
Phone: (303)315-8654 **Fax:** (303)315-5666
Email: laraine.guyette@uchsc.edu
Laraine Guyette, PhD, Director
Program(s): Midwifery.

Connecticut

★ 25823 ★ Connecticut Center for Massage Therapy, Inc.
25 Sylvan Rd. S
Westport, CT 06880
Phone: (203)221-7325 **Fax:** (203)221-0144
Email: info@ccmt.com
Website: http://www.ccmt.com
Susan Scoboria, Director
Program(s): Acupressure; Alexander Technique; Aromatherapy; CranioSacral Therapy; Energy Work; Feldenkrais; Massage Therapy; Neuromuscular Therapy; Polarity Therapy; Reflexology; Reiki; Shiatsu; Sports Massage.

★ 25824 ★ Connecticut Center for Massage Therapy, Inc.
75 Kitts Ln.
Newington, CT 06111
Phone: (860)667-1886 **Fax:** (860)667-2175
Email: info@ccmt.com
Website: http://www.ccmt.com
Wendy Dorsey, Director
Program(s): Acupressure; Energy Work; Massage Therapy; Meditation; Neuromuscular Therapy; Reflexology; Reiki; Shiatsu; Sports Massage.

★ 25825 ★ Connecticut Institute for Herbal Studies
87 Market Sq.
Newington, CT 06111
Phone: (860)666-5064 **Fax:** (860)666-5064
Email: laurachina@aol.com
Laura Mignosa, Director
Program(s): Herbal Medicine; Traditional Chinese Medicine.

★ 25826 ★ QiGong Institute
361 Post Rd. W
Westport, CT 06880
Email: akim.070972@aol.com
Dr. Richard M. Chin, Director
Program(s): Acupressure; CranioSacral Therapy; Energy Work; Herbal Medicine; Neuromuscular Therapy; Oriental Medicine; Polarity Therapy; Qigong; Reflexology; Shiatsu; Traditional Chinese Medicine.

★ 25827 ★ Rosen Center East, LLC
PO Box 5004
Westport, CT 06880
Phone: (203)319-1090 **Fax:** (203)319-0032
Sue Brenner, Director
Program(s): Rosen Method Bodywork.

★ 25828 ★ School of Homeopathy, Devon, England
82 E Pearl St.
New Haven, CT 06513
Phone: (203)624-8783 **Fax:** (203)624-8783
Betsy Levine, Contact
Program(s): Anatomy and Physiology; Homeopathy; Pathology and Disease.

★ 25829 ★ University of Bridgeport College of Chiropractic
75 Linden Ave.
Bridgeport, CT 06601
Phone: (203)576-4279 **Fax:** (203)576-4351
Website: http://www.bridgeport.edu/chiro/
Frank Zolli, Contact
Program(s): Chiropractic.

★ 25830 ★ University of Bridgeport, College of Naturopathic Medicine
60 Lafayette St.
Bridgeport, CT 06601
Phone: (203)576-4109 **Fax:** (203)576-4107
Miriam Madweb, Contact
Program(s): Acupuncture; Herbal Medicine; Homeopathy; Massage Therapy; Naturopathic Medicine; Nutrition.

★ 25831 ★ Yale University School of Nursing
100 Church St. S, Box 9740
New Haven, CT 06536-0740
Phone: (203)737-2344 **Fax:** (203)785-6455
Barbara Reif, Contact
Program(s): Midwifery.

Delaware

★ 25832 ★ Deep Muscle Therapy School
5317 Limestone Rd.
Wilmington, DE 19808
Phone: (302)239-1613 **Fax:** (302)239-5195
Velda Martin, Contact
Program(s): Deep Tissue Massage; Massage Therapy.

★ 25833 ★ Karen Carlson International Academy of Holistic Massage and Science
PO Box 3940
Greenville, DE 19807
Phone: (302)777-7307
Marilue Hartman, Contact
Program(s): Acupressure; Biofeedback; Energy Work; Feldenkrais; Herbal Medicine; Homeopathy; Massage Therapy; Reflexology.

District of Columbia

★ 25834 ★ Focus on Healing Reflexology Center
2808 Douglas St. NE
PO Box 26132
Washington, DC 20018
Phone: (301)779-8005 **Fax:** (301)779-8006
Njideka N. Olatunde, Director
Program(s): Reflexology.

★ 25835 ★ Georgetown University, School of Nursing
3700 Reservoir Rd. NW
Washington, DC 20007
Phone: (202)687-5041 **Fax:** (202)687-5553
Michele Havin, Contact
Program(s): Midwifery.

★ 25836 ★ Institute for Ethical and Clinical Hypnosis
2510 M St. NW
Washington, DC 20037
Phone: (202)331-1218 **Fax:** (202)659-9580
Masud Ansari, Contact
Program(s): Hypnotherapy.

★ 25837 ★ Potomac Massage Training Institute
4000 Albermarle St. NW 5th Fl.
Washington, DC 20016
Phone: (202)686-7046 **Fax:** (202)966-4579
Rose A. Gowdey, Director
Program(s): Alexander Technique; Aromatherapy; CranioSacral Therapy; Energy Work; Infant Massage; Massage Therapy; Myofascial Release; Neuromuscular Therapy; Polarity Therapy; Pregnancy Massage;

Qigong; Reflexology; Reiki; Shiatsu; Sports Massage; Traditional Chinese Medicine.

Florida

★ 25838 ★ Academy of Chinese Healing Arts, Inc.
505 S Orange Ave.
Sarasota, FL 34236
Phone: (941)955-4456 **Fax:** (941)330-1951
Email: acha@gte.net
Cynthia O'Donnell, Contact
Program(s): Acupressure; Acupuncture; Herbal Medicine; Homeopathy; Oriental Medicine; Qigong; Shiatsu; Traditional Chinese Medicine.

★ 25839 ★ Academy for Five Element Acupuncture
1170-A E Hallandale Beach Blvd.
Hallandale, FL 33009
Phone: (954)456-6336 **Fax:** (954)456-3944
Isaac Goren, Director
Program(s): Acupuncture; Herbal Medicine.

★ 25840 ★ Academy of Healing Arts, Massage and Facial Skin Care, Inc.
3141 S Military Trail
Lake Worth, FL 33463
Phone: (561)965-5550 **Fax:** (561)641-2603
Angela K. Artemik, Director
Program(s): Acupressure; Aromatherapy; Massage Therapy; Reflexology; Shiatsu.

★ 25841 ★ Academy of Lymphatic Studies
12651 W Sunrise Blvd.
Sunrise, FL 33323
Phone: (954)846-7855 **Free:** 800-863-5935
Fax: (954)845-9207
Joachim E. Zuther, Director
Program(s): Complete Decongestive Physiotherapy; Manual Lymph Drainage.

★ 25842 ★ Acupressure-Acupuncture Institute
10506 N Kendall Dr.
Miami, FL 33176
Phone: (305)595-9500 **Fax:** (305)595-2622
Email: aai@acupuncture.pair.com
Nancy Browne, Director
Program(s): Acupressure; Acupuncture; Herbal Medicine; Homeopathy; Massage Therapy; Oriental Medicine; Qigong; Reiki; Shiatsu; Traditional Chinese Medicine.

★ 25843 ★ Alpha Institute of South Florida, Inc.
904 Park Ave.
Lake Park, FL 33403
Phone: (561)845-1400 **Fax:** (561)845-1360
Douglas C. Espie, Director
Program(s): Aromatherapy; CranioSacral Therapy; Deep Tissue Massage; Energy Work; Hypnotherapy; Massage Therapy; Oriental Medicine; Polarity Therapy; Reflexology; Reiki; Shiatsu; Skin Care.

★ 25844 ★ Alpha School of Massage, Inc.
4642 San Juan Ave.
Jacksonville, FL 32210
Phone: (904)389-9117 **Fax:** (904)389-6496
Edward L. Driggers, Contact
Program(s): Acupressure; Aromatherapy; Energy Work; Herbal Medicine; Homeopathy; Massage Therapy; Neuromuscular Therapy; Reflexology; Reiki; Shiatsu; Sports Massage.

★ 25845 ★ American Institute of Massage Therapy, Inc., Fort Lauderdale
2101 N Federal Hwy.
Fort Lauderdale, FL 33301
Phone: (954)568-6200 **Fax:** (954)568-6100
Email: info@aimt.com
Website: http://www.aimt.com
Lexa Allin Sutherland, Director
Program(s): Aromatherapy; Colon Hydrotherapy; CranioSacral Therapy; Massage Therapy; Neuromuscular Therapy; Reflexology; Sports Massage.

★ 25846 ★ American Yoga Association
PO Box 19986
Sarasota, FL 34276
Phone: (941)927-4977 **Fax:** (941)921-9844
Patricia Rockwood, Director
Program(s): Yoga Teacher Training.

★ 25847 ★ Atlantic Institute of Aromatherapy
2514 W Kennedy Blvd.
Tampa, FL 33609
Phone: (813)265-2222 **Fax:** (813)265-2222
Sylla Sheppard-Hanger, Director
Program(s): Aromatherapy.

★ 25848 ★ Atlantic Institute of Oriental Medicine
1057 SE 17th St.
Fort Lauderdale, FL 33316
Phone: (954)463-3888 **Fax:** (954)463-3878
Edith Tonelli, Director
Program(s): Acupuncture; Herbal Medicine; Oriental Medicine; Traditional Chinese Medicine.

★ 25849 ★ Bhakti Academe School of Intuitive Massage and Healing
25400 US 19 N
Clearwater, FL 33763
Phone: (727)724-9727
Dale McNiff, Contact
Program(s): Bhakti Bodywork; Energy Work; Massage Therapy.

★ 25850 ★ Biofeedback Therapist Training Institute
1826 University Blvd. W
Jacksonville, FL 32217
Phone: (904)737-5821 **Fax:** (904)730-3821
Email: hartje@aol.com
Website: http://www.hartje.com
Jack C. Hartje, PhD, Director
Program(s): Biofeedback.

★ 25851 ★ Birth Buddies
5329 Buggy Whip Dr. N
Jacksonville, FL 32257
Phone: (904)268-5629 **Fax:** (904)363-6356
Susan Toffolon, Director
Program(s): Doula.

★ 25852 ★ Boca Raton Institute
5499 N Federal Hwy., Ste. A
Boca Raton, FL 33487
Phone: (561)241-8105 **Fax:** (561)241-9789
Constance M. Gregg, Director
Program(s): Acupressure; Aromatherapy; CranioSacral Therapy; Massage Therapy; Neuromuscular Therapy; Polarity Therapy; Reflexology; Shiatsu.

★ 25853 ★ Bonita Springs/Venice School of Massage Therapy
10915 Bonita Beach Rd., Ste. 2121
Bonita Springs, FL 34135
Phone: (941)495-0714 **Fax:** (941)498-7164
Fred Maehr, Director
Program(s): Aromatherapy; Colon Hydrotherapy; Herbal Medicine; Massage Therapy; Neuromuscular Therapy; Reflexology; Shiatsu; Spa Therapies.

★ 25854 ★ The Bramham Institute
1014 N Olive Ave.
West Palm Beach, FL 33401
Free: 800-575-0518 **Fax:** (561)832-6642
Sara Eavenson, Director
Program(s): Aromatherapy; Connective Tissue Massage; Hydrotherapy; Manual Lymph Drainage; Reflexology; Spa Therapies.

★ 25855 ★ Central Florida Hypnosis Institute
9737 Fairway Cir.
Leesburg, FL 34788
Phone: (352)315-0555 **Fax:** (352)315-0383
Earl J. Yawman, Director
Program(s): Hypnotherapy.

★ 25856 ★ Classical Acupuncture Institute
4237 Salisbury Rd., Ste. 108
Jacksonville, FL 32216
Phone: (904)296-0906
Debbie Rewis, Director
Program(s): Acupuncture.

★ 25857 ★ CORE Institute School of Massage Therapy and Structural Bodywork
223 W Carolina St.
Tallahassee, FL 32301
Phone: (850)222-8673 **Fax:** (850)561-6160
Email: core@nettally.com
Website: http://www.coreinstitute.com
George Kousealeos, Director
Program(s): Massage Therapy; Myofascial Release.

★ 25858 ★ Delphi Center for Midwifery Studies
3102 W Cypress St., Ste. B
Tampa, FL 33607-5108
Phone: (813)873-7135 **Fax:** (813)873-0274
Email: delphicntr@aol.com
Karin Kearns, Director
Program(s): Midwifery.

★ 25859 ★ Educating Hands of School Massage
120 SW 8th St.
Miami, FL 33130
Phone: (305)285-6991 **Fax:** (305)857-0298
Website: http://massagetherapynetwork.com/edhand1.html
Kathy Ozzard, Director
Program(s): Massage Therapy.

★ 25860 ★ Florida Academy of Massage
8695 College Pkwy., Ste. 110
Fort Myers, FL 33919
Phone: (941)489-2282 **Free:** 800-324-9543
Fax: (941)489-4065
Masud Ansari, Contact
Program(s): Massage Therapy.

★ 25861 ★ Florida College of Natural Health
8216 S Tamiami Trail
Sarasota, FL 34238
Phone: (941)966-7117 **Free:** 800-966-7117
Prudence Sterling, Director
Program(s): Acupressure; Acupuncture; Aromatherapy; Herbal Medicine; Homeopathy; Massage Therapy; Neuromuscular Therapy; Polarity Therapy; Reflexolo-

gy; Reiki; Shiatsu; Skin Care; Sports Massage; Traditional Chinese Medicine.

★ 25862 ★ Florida College of Natural Health
7925 NW 12th St., Ste. 201
Miami, FL 33126
Phone: (305)597-9599 **Free:** 800-599-9599
Fax: (305)597-9110
Lucy Bonilla, Director
Program(s): Acupressure; Acupuncture; Aromatherapy; CranioSacral Therapy; Massage Therapy; Myofascial Release; Neuromuscular Therapy; Polarity Therapy; Reflexology; Shiatsu; Sports Massage.

★ 25863 ★ Florida College of Natural Health
887 E Altamonte Dr.
Altamonte Springs, FL 32701
Phone: (407)261-0319 **Free:** 800-393-7337
Fax: (407)261-0342
Thea Depinto, Director
Program(s): Acupressure; Acupuncture; Aromatherapy; CranioSacral Therapy; Energy Work; Massage Therapy; Neuromuscular Therapy; Reflexology; Shiatsu; Skin Care; Sports Massage; Swedish Massage.

★ 25864 ★ Florida College of Natural Health, Pompano Beach
2001 W Sample Rd., Ste. 100
Pompano Beach, FL 33064
Phone: (954)975-6400 **Fax:** (954)975-9633
Kristi Mollis, Director
Program(s): Acupuncture; Massage Therapy; Skin Care.

★ 25865 ★ Florida Health Academy, Naples
261 Ninth St. S
Naples, FL 34102
Phone: (941)263-9391 **Fax:** (941)263-8680
Clara E. McElroy, Director
Program(s): Acupuncture; Aromatherapy; Herbal Medicine; Massage Therapy; Skin Care; Traditional Chinese Medicine.

★ 25866 ★ Florida Institute of Postural Integration
5837 Mariner Dr.
Tampa, FL 33609
Phone: (813)286-2273 **Fax:** (813)287-2870
Joy K. Johnson, Director
Program(s): Acupressure; Deep Tissue Massage.

★ 25867 ★ Florida Institute of Traditional Chinese Medicine
5335 66th St. N
Saint Petersburg, FL 33709
Phone: (813)546-6565 **Fax:** (813)547-0703
Dr. Su Liang Ku, Director
Program(s): Acupuncture; Herbal Medicine; Traditional Chinese Medicine; Tui Na.

★ 25868 ★ Florida School of Massage
6421 SW 13th St.
Gainesville, FL 32608
Phone: (352)378-7891 **Fax:** (352)376-7218
Email: info@massageonline.com
Website: http://www.massageonline.com
Paul Davenport, Director
Program(s): Anatomy and Physiology; CPR/First Aid; Colon Hydrotherapy; Connective Tissue Massage; Hydrotherapy; Massage Therapy; Neuromuscular Therapy; Polarity Therapy; Reflexology; Shiatsu; Sports Massage; Structural Integration; Swedish Massage.

★ 25869 ★ Florida School of Traditional Midwifery
6501 SW 13 St.
PO Box 5505
Gainesville, FL 32608
Phone: (352)338-0766 **Fax:** (352)338-2013
Jana Borino, Director
Program(s): Midwifery.

★ 25870 ★ Florida's Therapeutic Massage School
1300 E Gadsden St.
Pensacola, FL 32501
Phone: (850)433-8212
Geraldine Vaurigaud, Director
Program(s): Acupressure; Aromatherapy; Herbal Medicine; Hydrotherapy; Massage Therapy; Neuromuscular Therapy; Oriental Medicine; Polarity Therapy; Reflexology; Shiatsu; Sports Massage.

★ 25871 ★ HealthBuilders School of Therapeutic Massage Inc.
2180 State Rd. A1A
Saint Augustine, FL 32084
Phone: (904)471-8828 **Fax:** (904)471-8838
Karen Peters, Director
Program(s): Aromatherapy; Deep Tissue Massage; Energy Work; Massage Therapy; Polarity Therapy; Reflexology; Reiki.

★ 25872 ★ Holistic Health Services
1551 S 1st St., Ste. 701
Jacksonville Beach, FL 32250
Phone: (904)246-6064 **Fax:** (904)247-1266
Gail Greenfield, Director
Program(s): Reiki.

★ 25873 ★ Humanities Center Institute of Allied Health/School of Massage
4045 Park Blvd.
Pinellas Park, FL 33781
Phone: (727)541-5200 **Fax:** (727)545-0053
Sherry L. Fears, Director
Program(s): Massage Therapy; Neuromuscular Therapy.

★ 25874 ★ Integrated Health Care System
PO Box 67153
Saint Petersburg, FL 33736
Phone: (813)367-3063 **Fax:** (813)367-3170
Shirley Begley, Director
Program(s): Energy Work; Guided Imagery; Holistic Nursing; Hypnotherapy; Therapeutic Touch.

★ 25875 ★ International Institute of Reflexology
5650 1st Ave. N
PO Box 12642
Saint Petersburg, FL 33710
Phone: (727)343-4811 **Fax:** (727)381-2807
Dwight C. Byers, Contact
Program(s): Reflexology.

★ 25876 ★ Jacksonville School of Massage Therapy, Inc.
5305 San Juan Ave.
Jacksonville, FL 32210
Phone: (904)389-3878
Earl F. Kennedy, PhD, Director
Program(s): Acupressure; Aromatherapy; Ayurvedic Medicine; Biofeedback; Colon Hydrotherapy; Massage Therapy; Polarity Therapy; Reflexology; Reiki; Shiatsu; Traditional Chinese Medicine.

★ 25877 ★ National College of Oriental Medicine
7100 Lake Ellenor Dr.
Orlando, FL 32806
Phone: (407)888-8689 **Fax:** (407)888-8211
Email: info@acupunctureschool.com
Lloyd Buss, MD, Contact
Program(s): Acupuncture; Herbal Medicine; Oriental Medicine; Traditional Chinese Medicine.

★ 25878 ★ Omni Hypnosis Training Center
830 N Woodland Blvd.
Deland, FL 32720
Phone: (904)738-9188 **Fax:** (904)736-7598
Email: omni@omnihypnosis.com
Website: http://www.omnihypnosis.com
Gerald F. Kein, Director
Program(s): Hypnotherapy.

★ 25879 ★ Orlando Institute School of Massage Therapy, Inc.
3385 S Hwy. 17-92, Ste. 221
Casselberry, FL 32707
Phone: (407)331-1101 **Fax:** (407)331-8331
Stacee Diehl, Director
Program(s): Aromatherapy; Massage Therapy; Polarity Therapy; Reflexology; Shiatsu.

★ 25880 ★ Reiki Plus Institute
707 Barcelona Rd.
Key Largo, FL 33037
Phone: (305)451-9881
David G. Jarrell, Director
Program(s): Energy Work; Reiki.

★ 25881 ★ ReNew Life and Dotolo Institute School of Colon Hydrotherapy
1007 N MacDill
Tampa, FL 33607
Phone: (813)871-3200 **Fax:** (813)877-2640
Suzanne M. Gray, Contact
Program(s): Colon Hydrotherapy.

★ 25882 ★ Ridge Technical Center
7700 State Rd. 544
Winter Haven, FL 33881
Phone: (941)299-2512 **Fax:** (941)419-3060
Steve Strodman, Director
Program(s): Massage Therapy.

★ 25883 ★ Saint John Neuromuscular Pain Relief Institute
10710 Seminole Blvd., Ste. 1
Seminole, FL 33778
Phone: (727)397-5525 **Free:** 888-668-4325
Fax: (727)397-5808
Paul St. John, Director
Program(s): Neuromuscular Therapy.

★ 25884 ★ Sarasota School of Massage Therapy
1970 Main St., 3rd Fl.
Sarasota, FL 34236
Phone: (941)957-0577 **Fax:** (941)957-1049
Michael Rosen-Pyros, Director
Program(s): Aromatherapy; CranioSacral Therapy; Massage Therapy; Neuromuscular Therapy; Polarity Therapy; Reflexology.

★ 25885 ★ Seminar Network Intl., Inc. d/b/a SNI School of Massage and Allied Services
518 N Federal Hwy.
Lake Worth, FL 33460

Phone: (561)582-5349 **Free:** 800-882-0903
Fax: (561)582-0807
Nancy Putzan, Director
Program(s): Colon Hydrotherapy; Massage Therapy.

★ 25886 ★ Southeastern School of Neuromuscular and Massage Therapy, Inc.
9088 Golfside Dr.
Jacksonville, FL 32256
Phone: (904)448-9499 **Fax:** (904)448-9270
Kyle C. Wright, Contact
Program(s): Acupressure; CranioSacral Therapy; Feldenkrais; Herbal Medicine; Homeopathy; Massage Therapy; Neuromuscular Therapy; Polarity Therapy; Reflexology; Reiki; Shiatsu.

★ 25887 ★ University of Florida, Health Science Center
653 W 8th St., Bldg 1, 2nd Flr.
Jacksonville, FL 32209-6561
Phone: (904)549-3245
Alice H. Poe, Director
Program(s): Midwifery.

★ 25888 ★ University of Miami School of Nursing
5801 Red. Rd.
Coral Gables, FL 33124-3850
Phone: (305)284-6256
Virginia Crandall, Contact
Program(s): Midwifery.

★ 25889 ★ The Upledger Institute
11211 Prosperity Farms Rd., D-325
Palm Beach Gardens, FL 33410
Phone: (561)622-4334 **Free:** 800-233-5880
Fax: (561)622-4771
Email: upledger@upledger.com
Kevin Roberts, Director
Program(s): CranioSacral Therapy; Mechanical Link; Visceral Manipulation; Zero Blancing.

★ 25890 ★ Wood Hygienic Institute
2220 E Irlo Bronson Hwy.
Kissimmee, FL 34744
Phone: (407)933-0009
Program(s): Colon Hydrotherapy; Massage Therapy.

★ 25891 ★ Yoga Institute of Miami
9350 S Dadeland Blvd., Ste. 207
Miami, FL 33156
Phone: (305)670-0558 **Fax:** (305)661-9943
Bobbi Goldin, Director
Program(s): Yoga Teacher Training.

Georgia

★ 25892 ★ Academy of Somatic Healing Arts
1924 Cliff Valley Way
Atlanta, GA 30329
Phone: (404)315-0394 **Fax:** (404)633-1270
Jim Gabriel, Director
Program(s): Massage Therapy; Neuromuscular Therapy; Sports Massage.

★ 25893 ★ Alexander Technique of Atlanta
4246 Peachtree Rd., Ste. 6
Atlanta, GA 30319
Phone: (770)454-1177
Ron Dennis, Director
Program(s): Alexander Technique.

★ 25894 ★ Atlanta School of Massage
2300 Peachford Rd., Ste. 3200
Atlanta, GA 30338
Phone: (770)454-7167 **Free:** 888-276-6277
Fax: (770)454-7367
Program(s): Acupressure; Aromatherapy; Deep Tissue Massage; Integrative Massage; Massage Therapy; Polarity Therapy; Reflexology; Shiatsu; Spa Therapies.

★ 25895 ★ Capelli Learning Center
2581 Piedmont Rd., Ste. C-1000
Atlanta, GA 30324
Phone: (404)261-5261 **Fax:** (404)261-5069
Deb Elkin, Contact
Program(s): Deep Tissue Massage; Massage Therapy; Qigong; Reflexology; Thai Massage; Traditional Chinese Medicine.

★ 25896 ★ Emory University, Nell Hodgson Woodruff School of Nursing
Atlanta, GA 30322
Phone: (404)727-6961 **Fax:** (404)727-0536
L. Leush, Contact
Program(s): Midwifery.

★ 25897 ★ Georgia Institute of Therapeutic Massage, LLC
2160 Centra Ave.
PO Box 3657
Augusta, GA 30904
Phone: (706)738-7695 **Fax:** (706)738-6232
Vicki N. Platt, Director
Program(s): Acupressure; Massage Therapy; Neuromuscular Therapy; Polarity Therapy; Reflexology; Shiatsu; Sports Massage; Swedish Massage.

★ 25898 ★ Lake Lanier School of Massage
400 Brenau Ave.
Gainesville, GA 30501
Phone: (770)287-0377 **Fax:** (770)536-7350
Sandra Easterbrooks, Contact
Program(s): Massage Therapy.

★ 25899 ★ Life University, School of Chiropractic
1269 Barclay Cir.
Marietta, GA 30060
Phone: (770)426-2884 **Free:** 800-543-3345
Fax: (770)428-9886
Harry Harrison, Contact
Program(s): Chiropractic.

★ 25900 ★ New Life Institute Inc., School of Massage Excellence
4330 Georgetown Sq., Ste. 500
Atlanta, GA 30338
Phone: (770)457-2021 **Fax:** (770)457-5614
Sandy Jones, Contact
Program(s): Massage Therapy.

★ 25901 ★ Polarity Training Institute
566 Pharr Rd.
Atlanta, GA 30305
Phone: (770)704-5170
Will Leichnitz, Contact
Program(s): Polarity Therapy.

Hawaii

★ 25902 ★ Aisen Shiatsu School
1314 S King St., Ste. 601
Honolulu, HI 96814
Phone: (808)596-7354 **Fax:** (808)593-8282
Fumihiko Indei, Director
Program(s): Shiatsu.

★ 25903 ★ Aloha Kaui Massage Workshop
PO Box 622
Hanalei, HI 96714
Phone: (808)826-9990 **Fax:** (808)826-6180
Devaki Holman, Contact
Program(s): Massage Therapy.

★ 25904 ★ American Institute of Massage Therapy, Kailua
407 Uluniu St., Ste. 204A
Kailua, HI 96734
Phone: (808)266-2468 **Fax:** (808)266-2460
Elizabeth Reveley, Contact
Program(s): Acupressure; Aromatherapy; CranioSacral Therapy; Deep Tissue Massage; Energy Work; Healing Touch; Hypnotherapy; Massage Therapy; Reflexology.

★ 25905 ★ American Viniyoga Institute
PO Box 88
Makawao, HI 96768
Phone: (808)572-1414
Mary Lou Mellinger, Contact
Program(s): Yoga Teacher Training; Yoga Therapy.

★ 25906 ★ Big Island Academy of Massage, Inc.
211 Kinoole St.
Hilo, HI 96720
Phone: (808)935-1405
Paul Rambo, Contact
Program(s): Acupressure; Aromatherapy; Deep Tissue Massage; Energy Work; LomiLomi; Massage Therapy; Polarity Therapy; Reflexology; Reiki; Shiatsu; Sports Massage.

★ 25907 ★ Hawaii College of Health Sciences
1750 Kalakuna Ave., Ste. 2404
Honolulu, HI 96826
Phone: (808)941-8223 **Fax:** (808)944-8343
Evelyn James, Contact
Program(s): Acupressure; CranioSacral Therapy; Deep Tissue Massage; Herbal Medicine; Massage Therapy; Polarity Therapy; Reflexology; Shiatsu; Traditional Chinese Medicine.

★ 25908 ★ Hawaii College of Traditional Oriental Medicine
PO Box 457
Kula, HI 96790
Phone: (808)573-0899 **Fax:** (808)573-2450
Program(s): Acupressure; Acupuncture; Herbal Medicine; Oriental Medicine; Qigong; Shiatsu; Traditional Chinese Medicine.

★ 25909 ★ Hawaiian Islands School of Body Therapies
78-6739 Alii Dr.
PO Box 390188
Kailua Kona, HI 96740
Phone: (808)322-0048 **Fax:** (808)322-4971
Peter Wind, Director
Program(s): Aromatherapy; CranioSacral Therapy; Massage Therapy; Polarity Therapy; Reflexology; Restorative Treatment Therapy; Shiatsu.

★ 25910 ★ Honolulu School of Massage, Inc.
1136 12th Ave., Ste. 240
Honolulu, HI 96816
Phone: (808)733-0000 **Fax:** (808)733-0045
Email: hsminc@msn.com
Gayle E. Volger, Director

Program(s): Applied Kinesiology; CranioSacral Therapy; Deep Tissue Massage; Hydrotherapy; LomiLomi Massage; Massage Therapy; Neuromuscular Therapy; Reflexology; Shiatsu; Sports Massage.

★ 25911 ★ Institute of Clinical Acupuncture and Oriental Medicine
1270 Queen Emma St., Ste. 107
Honolulu, HI 96813
Phone: (808)521-2288 **Fax:** (808)521-2288
Catherine Low, Contact
Program(s): Acupuncture; Herbal Medicine; Oriental Medicine; Traditional Chinese Medicine.

★ 25912 ★ Maui Academy of the Healing Arts
1993 S Kihei Rd., Ste. 210
Kihei, HI 96753
Phone: (808)879-4266 **Fax:** (808)879-4484
Email: sancorp@maui.net
Website: http://www.maui.net/~sancorp/
John Sanderson, Director
Program(s): Acupressure; Esalen Massage; LomiLomi Massage; Lymphatic Massage; Massage Therapy; Reflexology; Shiatsu; Sports Massage; Swedish Massage; Thai Massage.

★ 25913 ★ Pacific Center for Awareness and Bodywork
7703 Koolau Rd.
PO Box 672
Kilauea, HI 96754
Phone: (808)828-6797 **Fax:** (808)828-6797
Website: http://www.oxford-intl.com/pacific
John Sanderson, Director
Program(s): Acupressure; Awareness Practices; Connective Bodywork; Hypnotherapy; Massage Therapy; Neuromuscular Therapy; Polarity Therapy; Reflexology; Structural Integration.

★ 25914 ★ Tai Hsuan Foundation: College of Acupuncture and Herbal Medicine
2600 S King St., Rm. 206
PO Box 11130
Honolulu, HI 96826
Free: 800-942-4788 **Fax:** (808)949-1005
Email: taihsuan@acupuncture-hi.com
Website: http://www.acupuncture-hi.com
Dr. Gayle Todoki, Contact
Program(s): Acupressure; Acupuncture; Herbal Medicine; Oriental Medicine; Qigong; Traditional Chinese Medicine.

★ 25915 ★ Traditional Chinese Medical College of Hawaii
PO Box 2288
Kamuela, HI 96743
Phone: (808)885-9226 **Fax:** (808)885-9226
Program(s): Acupuncture; Oriental Medicine; Traditional Chinese Medicine.

★ 25916 ★ University of Health Sciences
1778 Ala Moana Blvd., Ste. 1307
Honolulu, HI 96815
Phone: (808)951-8242 **Fax:** (808)951-8242
Lucy Han Lee, Contact
Program(s): Acupressure; Acupuncture; Herbal Medicine; Homeopathy; Iridology; Qigong; Reflexology; Shiatsu; Traditional Chinese Medicine.

Idaho

★ 25917 ★ Idaho Institute of Wholistic Studies
1412 W Washington
Boise, ID 83702
Phone: (208)345-2704 **Fax:** (208)367-9242
Barbera Bashan, Director
Program(s): Acupressure; Massage Therapy; Shiatsu; Sports Massage; Traditional Chinese Medicine.

★ 25918 ★ Idaho School of Massage Therapy
5353 Franklin Rd.
Boise, ID 83705
Phone: (208)343-1847
Cindy J. Langston, Contact
Program(s): Connective Tissue Massage; Deep Tissue Massage; Massage Therapy; Relexology; Shiatsu; Sports Massage; Swedish Massage.

★ 25919 ★ Moscow School of Massage
S 600 Main
Moscow, ID 83843
Phone: (208)882-7867
Lisa O'Leary, Director
Program(s): Deep Tissue Massage; Massage Therapy; Oriental Medicine; Qigong.

Illinois

★ 25920 ★ Best Institute of Hypnosis
832 16th Ave.
East Moline, IL 61244-2124
Phone: (309)755-2378 **Fax:** (309)755-1669
Kenn Geiger, Director
Program(s): Hypnotherapy.

★ 25921 ★ Center for Therapeutic Massage and Wellness
2704 Woodridge Rd.
Woodridge, IL 60517
Phone: (708)960-9053
Bea Stanton, Director
Program(s): CranioSacral Therapy; Energy Work; Massage Therapy; Qigong; Reflexology; Reiki; Sports Massage; Therapeutic Touch.

★ 25922 ★ Chicago National College of Naprapathy
3330 N Milwaukee Ave.
Chicago, IL 60641
Phone: (773)282-2686 **Fax:** (773)282-2688
Dr. Alexanne Osinski, Contact
Program(s): Naprapathy; Neuromuscular Therapy.

★ 25923 ★ Chicago School of Massage Therapy
2918 N Lincoln Ave.
Chicago, IL 60657
Phone: (773)477-9444 **Fax:** (773)477-7256
Jeff Marzano, Director
Program(s): Acupressure; Anatomy and Physiology; CranioSacral Therapy; Energy Work; Massage Therapy; Myofascial Release; Reflexology; Shiatsu; Sports Massage.

★ 25924 ★ Edens Institute of Alternative Therapy
212 N Park
Herrin, IL 62948
Phone: (618)942-8825
E. J. Engram, Director
Program(s): Massage Therapy.

★ 25925 ★ Integrative Yoag Therapy
1207 Lincoln Avee.
Galena, IL 61036
Phone: (815)777-6068 **Free:** 800-750-9642
Fax: (815)777-6629
Joseph LePage, Director
Program(s): Yoga Teacher Training.

★ 25926 ★ International Thai Therapist Association, Inc.
47 W Polk St., Ste. 100-329
Chicago, IL 60605
Phone: (773)792-4121 **Fax:** (773)326-6442
Email: itta@ix.netcom.com
Anthony B. James, PhD, Director
Program(s): Acupressure; Aromatherapy; Ayurvedic Medicine; CranioSacral Therapy; Energy Work; Herbal Medicine; Massage Therapy; Neuromuscular Therapy; Oriental Medicine; Qigong; Reflexology; Reiki; Shiatsu; Thai Massage; Traditional Chinese Medicine.

★ 25927 ★ Kurashova Institute, Inc.
PO Box 6246
Rock Island, IL 61201
Phone: (309)786-4888 **Fax:** (309)786-8687
Zhenya K. Wine, Director
Program(s): Massage Therapy; Neuromuscular Therapy; Russian Massage.

★ 25928 ★ Leidecker Institute
1901 N Roselle Rd., Ste. 800
Schaumburg, IL 60195
Phone: (847)844-1933
Lynsi Brule, Director
Program(s): Acupressure; Aromatherapy; Hypnotherapy; Reflexology; Reiki.

★ 25929 ★ LifePath School of Massage Therapy
7820 N University, Ste. 110
Peoria, IL 61614
Free: 888-254-3372 **Fax:** (309)693-7293
Email: rwasher@flink.com
Rhonda Washer, Director
Program(s): CranioSacral Therapy; Massage Therapy; Neuromuscular Therapy; Polarity Therapy; Reflexology; Shiatsu; Sports Massage; Swedish Massage.

★ 25930 ★ Midwest Center for the Study of Oriental Medicine
4334 N Hazel, Ste. 206
Chicago, IL 60613
Phone: (773)975-1295
William Dunbar, Director
Program(s): Acupressure; Acupuncture; Herbal Medicine; Oriental Medicine; Dtraditional Chinese Medicine.

★ 25931 ★ National College of Chiropractic
200 E Roosevelt Rd.
Lombard, IL 60148
Phone: (630)889-2000 **Free:** 800-826-6285
Fax: (630)889-6554
James F. Winterstein, Contact
Program(s): Acupuncture; Chiropractic.

★ 25932 ★ Northern Prairie School of Therapeutic Massage and Bodywork, Inc.
138 N Fair St.
Sycamore, IL 60178
Phone: (815)899-3382 **Fax:** (815)899-3381
Jeannette Vaupel, Director
Program(s): Acupressure; Aromatherapy; Ayurvedic Medicine; Biofeedback, CranioSacral Therapy; Energy Work; Herbal Medicine; Homeopathy; Hypnotherapy; Massage Therapy; Oriental Medicine; Polarity Therapy; Qigong; Reflexology, Reiki; Shiatsu; Traditional Chinese Medicine.

★ 25933 ★ Ohashiatsu Chicago
825 Chicago Ave.
Evanston, IL 60202
Phone: (847)864-1130 **Fax:** (847)733-9473
Matthew Sweigart, Director

Program(s): Acupressure; Shiatsu.

★ 25934 ★ Pamela Arwine
1701 Marguerite St.
Crystal Lake, IL 60014
Phone: (815)455-4502
Pamela Arwine, Director
Program(s): Hypnotherapy; Reiki.

★ 25935 ★ University of Illinois, Chicago School of Nursing
845 S Damen Ave.
Chicago, IL 60612
Phone: (312)996-7937
Janet Engstrom, Director
Program(s): Midwifery.

★ 25936 ★ Urbana Center for the Alexander Technique
508 W Washington St.
Urbana, IL 61801
Phone: (217)367-3172
Joan Murray, Director
Program(s): Alexander Technique.

★ 25937 ★ Wellness and Massage Training Institute
1051 Internationale Pkwy.
Woodridge, IL 60517
Phone: (630)325-3773
Email: info@wmti.com
Website: http://www.wmti.com
Raymond Miller, Director
Program(s): Aromatherapy; CranioSacral Therapy; Massage Therapy; Oriental Medicine; Ortho-Bionomy; Qigong; Reflexology; Shiatsu; Sports Massage; Traditional Chinese Medicine.

Indiana

★ 25938 ★ Academy of Reflexology and Health Therapy International
8397 E 10th St.
Indianapolis, IN 46219-5330
Phone: (317)897-5111 **Fax:** (317)897-5115
E. James O'Donnell, Director
Program(s): Acupressure; Alexander Technique; Energy Work; Feldenkrais; Homeopathy; Massage Therapy; Polarity Therapy; Reflexology; Sports Massage.

★ 25939 ★ Alexandria School of Scientific Therapeutics
809 S Harrison St.
PO Box 287
Alexandria, IN 46001
Phone: (765)724-9152 **Fax:** (765)724-9156
Herbert L. Hobbs, Contact
Program(s): Acupressure; Aromatherapy; Ayurvedic Medicine; Deep Muscle Massage; Energy Work; Feldenkrais; Herbal Medicine; Homeopathy; Massage Therapy; Neuromuscular Therapy; Oriental Medicine; Polarity Therapy; Reflexology; Sports Massage; Swedish Massage; Shiatsu.

★ 25940 ★ American Certified Massage School
109 ½ W Joliet St.
Crown Point, IN 46307
Phone: (219)661-9099 **Fax:** (219)661-8978
Gale Miller, Director
Program(s): Aromatherapy; Deep Tissue Massage; Massage Therapy; Reflexology; Sports Massage.

★ 25941 ★ Dancing Feet Yoga Center, Inc.
2501 Oriole Trl.
Long Beach, IN 46360
Phone: (219)872-9611 **Free:** 800-968-0694
Fax: (219)873-7612
Marsha Wenig, Director
Program(s): Yoga Teacher Training.

★ 25942 ★ Indiana University, Purdue University, Indianapolis Massage Therapy Program
620 N Union Dr., Rm. 102
Indianapolis, IN 46202
Phone: (317)274-2887 **Fax:** (317)274-2638
Janis Legendre, Contact
Program(s): Massage Therapy.

★ 25943 ★ Ivy Tech State College
3800 N Anthony Blvd.
Fort Wayne, IN 46805
Phone: (219)482-9171 **Fax:** (219)480-4149
Neal Davis, Director
Program(s): Massage Therapy.

★ 25944 ★ Midwest Training Institute of Hypnosis
2121 Engle Rd., Ste. 3A
Fort Wayne, IN 46809
Phone: (219)747-6774 **Fax:** (219)747-6774
Gisella Zukausky, Director
Program(s): Hypnotherapy.

Iowa

★ 25945 ★ Capri College, Davenport
425 E 59th St.
Davenport, IA 52807
Phone: (319)388-6642
Heather McClanahan, Director
Program(s): Acupressure; Aromatherapy; Massage Therapy; Neuromuscular Therapy; Polarity Therapy; Reflexology; Reiki; Shiatsu; Sports Massage.

★ 25946 ★ Capri College of Massage Therapy, Cedar Rapids
315 2nd Ave. SE
PO Box 74912
Cedar Rapids, IA 52401
Phone: (319)364-1541
Joni Westphall, Director
Program(s): Acupressure; Aromatherapy; Deep Tissue Massage; Massage Therapy; Reflexology.

★ 25947 ★ Carlson College of Massage Therapy
11809 County Rd., X 28
Anamosa, IA 52205
Phone: (319)462-3402 **Fax:** (319)462-5990
Ruth A. Carlson, Director
Program(s): Aromatherapy; Energy Work; Herbal Medicine; Massage Therapy; Polarity Therapy; Reflexology; Shiatsu; Sports Massage.

★ 25948 ★ Institute of Therapeutic Massage and Wellness
516 W 35th St.
Davenport, IA 52806
Phone: (319)445-1055 **Fax:** (319)285-5201
Bonita Howes, Director
Program(s): Acupressure; Aromatherapy; CranioSacral Therapy; Ennergy Work; Massage Therapy; Neuromuscular Therapy; Polarity Therapy; Reflexology; Reiki; Shiatsu; Sports Massage; Yoga Teacher Training.

★ 25949 ★ Maharishi University of Management
College of Maharishi Vedic Medicine
Fairfield, IA 52557
Phone: (515)472-1110 **Fax:** (515)472-1179
Email: admissions@mum.edu
Website: http://www.mum.edu
Robert Schneider, MD, Contact
Program(s): Ayurvedic Medicine; Herbal Medicine; Maharishi Vedic Medicine.

★ 25950 ★ Millenium College of Massage and Reflexology
934 S 17th St.
Fort Dodge, IA 50501
Phone: (515)955-2296 **Fax:** (515)955-7709
Angie Eldridge, Contact
Program(s): Acupressure; Aromatherapy; CranioSacral Therapy; Massage Therapy; Reflexology.

★ 25951 ★ MotherCare Doula Training
244 S Walnut
West Union, IA 52175
Phone: (319)422-8833 **Free:** 800-648-3662
Debbie Young, Director
Program(s): Doula.

★ 25952 ★ Palmer College of Chiropractic
1000 Brady St.
Davenport, IA 52803
Phone: (319)884-5000 **Fax:** (319)884-5897
Email: pcadmit@palmer.edu
David B. Anderson, Director
Program(s): Chiropractic.

Kansas

★ 25953 ★ BMSI Institute
8665 W 96th St., Ste. 300
Overland Park, KS 66212
Phone: (913)649-3322 **Fax:** (913)649-1010
Peggy Smith, Director
Program(s): Acupressure; Aromatherapy; CranioSacral Therapy; Energy Work; Massage Therapy; Polarity Therapy; Qigong; Reflexology; Reiki; Sports Massage; Traditional Chinese Medicine.

★ 25954 ★ Frontier School of Midwifery and Family Nursing
Hospital Hill
Hyden, KS 41749
Jeannette Woods, Director
Program(s): Midwifery.

★ 25955 ★ Johnson County Community College
9780 W 87th St.
Overland Park, KS 66212
Phone: (913)469-4422 **Fax:** (913)649-1050
Karen McDaniel, Director
Program(s): Aromatherapy; Cranial Sacral Therapy; Hydrotherapy; Massage Therapy; Reflexology.

★ 25956 ★ Kansas College of Chinese Medicine
9235 E Harry St., Bldg. 100, Ste. 1A
Wichita, KS 67207
Phone: (316)691-8822 **Fax:** (316)691-8868
Lawrence Scott, Director
Program(s): Acupressure; Acupuncture; Cranial Sacral Therapy; Deep Tissue Massage; Energy Work; Herbal Medicine; Massage Therapy; Oriental Medicine; Qigong; Shiatsu; Sports Massage; Traditional Chinese Medicine.

Kentucky

★ 25957 ★ Bluegrass Professional School of Massage Therapy
501 Darby Creek, Ste. 14
Lexington, KY 40509

Phone: (606)264-1450 **Fax:** (606)264-1450
Terri Sloan, Director
Program(s): Acupressure; Aromatherapy; Deep Tissue Massage; Massage Therapy; Reflexology; Sports Massage.

★ 25958 ★ Infinite Light Healing Studies Center, Inc.
3509 W Dogwood Cir.
LaGrange, KY 40031
Phone: (502)454-0430 **Fax:** (502)241-8732
Laurelle Gaia, Director
Program(s): Energy Work; Reiki.

★ 25959 ★ Louisville School of Massage
7410 New LaGrange Rd.
Louisville, KY 40222
Phone: (502)429-5765 **Fax:** (502)429-8581
Brent C. Williams, Director
Program(s): Massage Therapy.

★ 25960 ★ Sun Touch Massage School
914 W Broadway
Mayfield, KY 42066
Phone: (502)247-8923 **Fax:** (502)247-6110
Marilyn Gossett, Director
Program(s): Aromatherapy; Deep Tissue Massage; Massage Therapy; Polarity Therapy; Qigong; Reflexology; Swedish Massage.

Louisiana

★ 25961 ★ Blue Cliff School of Therapeutic Massage, Lafayette
103 Calco Blvd.
Lafayette, LA 70503
Phone: (318)269-0620 **Fax:** (318)269-0688
Claudette Hymel, Director
Program(s): CranioSacral Therapy; Massage Therapy; Neuromuscular Therapy; Shiatsu; Sports Massage.

★ 25962 ★ Blue Cliff School of Therapeutic Massage and Oriental Bodywork
1919 Veterans Blvd., Ste. 310
Kenner, LA 70062
Phone: (504)471-0294 **Fax:** (504)466-8514
Email: massage@ametro.net
J. Vernon Smith, PhD, Contact
Program(s): Acupressure; CranioSacral Therapy; Energy Work; Healing Touch; Massage Therapy; Neuromuscular Therapy; Oriental Medicine; Qigong; Reflexology; Shiatsu; Sports Massage; Traditional Chinese Medicine.

★ 25963 ★ Blue Cliff School of Therapeutic Massage, Shreveport
3823 Gilbret Dr., Ste. 103
Shreveport, LA 71104
Phone: (318)861-5959 **Fax:** (318)861-5957
Brenda Chadwick, Director
Program(s): Acupressure; CranioSacral Therapy; Deep Tissue Massage; Energy Work; Massage Therapy; Reflexology; Shiatsu.

★ 25964 ★ Career Training Specialists
Mid-City Plaza, 1611 Louisville Ave.
Monroe, LA 71201
Phone: (318)323-2889 **Fax:** (318)324-9883
Keith Hopkins, Director
Program(s): Aromatherapy; Deep Tissue Massage; Massage Therapy; Reflexology; Shiatsu.

★ 25965 ★ Central Louisiana School of Therapeutic Massage
2901 Hwy 28 E, Stes. C and D
Pineville, LA 71360
Phone: (318)449-1111 **Fax:** (318)445-5498
Andrea R. Martin, Director
Program(s): Acupressure; Deep Tissue Massage; Massage Therapy; Reflexology; Shiatsu.

★ 25966 ★ Louisiana Institute of Massage Therapy
1108 Lafitte St.
Lake Charles, LA 70601
Phone: (318)474-9435 **Fax:** (318)474-9432
Email: salvo.breaux@usaunwired.net
Susan Salvo, Director
Program(s): Hydrotherapy; Infant Massage; Massage Therapy; Pregnancy Massage; Reflexology; Sports Massage.

Maine

★ 25967 ★ Downeast School of Massage
99 Moose Meadow Ln.
PO Box 24
Waldoboro, ME 04572
Phone: (207)832-5531 **Fax:** (207)832-0504
Email: dsm@midcoast.com
Nancy Dail, Director
Program(s): Massage Therapy; Shiatsu; Sports Massage.

★ 25968 ★ Footloose, Inc., Professional Reflexology Training
Egypt Rd.
PO Box 112
Alna, ME 04535
Phone: (207)586-6751 **Fax:** (207)586-6702
Email: footloos@gwi.net
Janet E. Stetser, Director
Program(s): Hypnotherapy; Reflexology.

★ 25969 ★ New Hampshire Institute for Therapeutic Arts School for Massage Therapy
39 Main St.
Bridgton, ME 04009
Phone: (207)647-3794
Patrick Cowan, Director
Program(s): Acupressure; Lymphatic Massage; Massage Therapy; Neuromuscular Therapy; Polarity Therapy; Reflexology; Sports Massage; Swedish Massage.

★ 25970 ★ Polarity Realization Institute, Inc., Portland
222 St. John St., Ste. 300
Portland, ME 04101
Nancy Risley, Director
Program(s): Aromatherapy; CranioSacral Therapy; Deep Tissue Massage; Energy Work; Massage Therapy; Polarity Therapy; Reflexology; Yoga Teacher Training.

Manitoba

★ 25971 ★ Professional Institute of Massage Therapy, Winnipeg
570 Portage Ave.
Winnipeg, MB, Canada R3C 0G4
Phone: (204)775-1642 **Fax:** (204)775-1166
Sue Mamer, Contact
Program(s): Massage Therapy.

Maryland

★ 25972 ★ American Hypnosis Training Academy, Inc.
8750 Georgia Ave., Ste. 125E
Silver Spring, MD 20910
Phone: (301)565-0103 **Free:** 800-343-9915
Ron Klein, Director
Program(s): Hypnotherapy.

★ 25973 ★ Baltimore School of Massage
6401 Dogwood Rd.
Baltimore, MD 21207
Phone: (410)944-8855 **Fax:** (410)944-8859
Email: registrar@bhhc.com
Website: http://www.bsom.com
Cindi Pridgen, Contact
Program(s): Massage Therapy.

★ 25974 ★ Garrett Community College
687 Mosser Rd.
Mc Henry, MD 21541
Phone: (301)387-3084 **Fax:** (301)387-3096
Carol Newman, Director
Program(s): Deep Tissue Massage; Massage Therapy.

★ 25975 ★ Maryland Institute for Ericksonian Hypnosis and Psychotherapy
6118 Park Heights Ave.
Baltimore, MD 21215
Phone: (410)358-1381 **Fax:** (410)358-5815
Email: mehyp@aol.com
Hillel Zeitlin, Director
Program(s): Hypnotherapy.

★ 25976 ★ Maryland Institute of Traditional Chinese Medicine
4641 Montgomery Ave., Ste. 400
Bethesda, MD 20814
Phone: (301)718-7373 **Fax:** (301)718-0735
Website: http://www.mitcm.org
Hee Junj Sunj, Director
Program(s): Acupuncture; Herbal Medicine; Qigong; Traditional Chinese Medicine.

★ 25977 ★ Ohashiatsu Maryland
8659 Baltimore National Pike
Ellicott, MD 21043
Phone: (410)313-8501 **Fax:** (410)313-8500
Hazel Chung, Director
Program(s): Shiatsu.

★ 25978 ★ Polarity Center and Shamanic Studies
9 Philadelphia Ave.
Takoma Park, MD 20912
Rose Diana Khalsa, Director
Program(s): CranioSacral Therapy; Energy Work; Polarity Therapy; Qigong; Reflexology; Yoga.

★ 25979 ★ Traditional Acupuncture Institute
American City Bldg.
10227 Wincopin Circle, Ste. 100
Columbia, MD 21044-3422
Phone: (301)596-6006
Website: http://www.acupuncture.com/TCMSchools/TAI1.htm
Program(s): Acupuncture; Traditional Chinese Medicine.

★ 25980 ★ Unity Woods Yoga Center
4853 Cordell Ave., Ste. PH9
Bethesda, MD 20814

Phone: (301)656-8992 **Fax:** (301)656-7792
John Schumacher, Director
Program(s): Yoga Teacher Training.

★ 25981 ★ Yoga Center
8950 Rte. 108, Ste. 114
Columbia, MD 21045
Phone: (410)720-4340 **Fax:** (410)461-4799
Bob Glickstein, Director
Program(s): Yoga Teacher Training.

Massachusetts

★ 25982 ★ Alexander Technique School of New England
94 Lessey St.
Amherst, MA 01002
Phone: (413)253-2595
Email: mvine@netscape.com
Missy Vineyard, Director
Program(s): Alexander Technique.

★ 25983 ★ Alexander Technique Training Center
803 Boylston St.
Chestnut Hill, MA 02467
Phone: (617)734-6898
Email: kilroyr@tiac.net
Ruth Kilroy, Director
Program(s): Alexander Technique.

★ 25984 ★ American School for Energy Therapies
17 Spring St.
Watertown, MA 02472
Phone: (617)924-9150 **Free:** 800-875-6347
Fax: (617)924-2828
Douglas Jansenn, Director
Program(s): CranioSacral Therapy; Polarity Therapy.

★ 25985 ★ Association of Labor Assistants and Childbirth Educators
552 Massachusetts Ave.
Cambridge, MA 02139
Free: 888-222-5223 **Fax:** (617)441-3167
Jessica Porter, Director
Program(s): Childbirth Education; Doula.

★ 25986 ★ Bach International Education Program
100 Research Dr.
Wilmington, MA 01887
Phone: (978)988-3833 **Free:** 800-334-0843
Fax: (978)988-0233
Karen Zilinek, Director
Program(s): Flower Essences.

★ 25987 ★ Bancroft School of Massage Therapy
333 Shrewsbury St.
Worcester, MA 01604
Phone: (508)757-7923 **Fax:** (508)791-5930
Email: bsmttank@aol.com
Steven Tankanow, Director
Program(s): Massage Therapy.

★ 25988 ★ Baystate Medical Center Nurse-Midwifery Education Program
759 Chestnut St.
Springfield, MA 01199
Phone: (413)794-4448 **Fax:** (413)794-8770
Susan DeJoy, Director
Program(s): Midwifery.

★ 25989 ★ BKS Iyengar Yoga Center of Greater Boston
240A Elm St., Ste. 23
Somerville, MA 02144
Phone: (617)666-9551 **Fax:** (617)296-6194
Elizabeth Shields, Director
Program(s): Yoga Teacher Training.

★ 25990 ★ Blazing Star Herbal School
119 Pfersick Rd.
PO Box 6
Shelburne Falls, MA 01370
Phone: (413)625-6875 **Fax:** (413)625-6972
Gail Ulrich, Director
Program(s): Herbal Medicine; Plant Spirit.

★ 25991 ★ Boston University, School of Public Health
715 Albany St., Room A-207
Boston, MA 02118
Phone: (617)638-5012
Mary Barger, Director
Program(s): Midwifery.

★ 25992 ★ Center for Traditional Medicine
1770 Mass Ave., Ste. 624
Cambridge, MA 02140
Phone: (781)643-1918
Email: lekorn@wco.com
Website: http://www.halcyon.com/fwdp/medicine/tmp.html
Leslie Korn, PhD, Director
Program(s): CranioSacral Therapy; Energy Work; Herbal Medicine; Massage Therapy; Naturopathic Medicine; Polarity Therapy.

★ 25993 ★ Center for Universal and Holistic Studies, Worchester
3 Ruthaven Ave.
Worcester, MA 01606
Phone: (978)365-6104 **Fax:** (413)794-8770
Janice L. Lucht, Director
Program(s): Aromatherapy; Reflexology; Reiki.

★ 25994 ★ Central Mass School of Massage and Therapy
200 Main St.
Spencer, MA 01562
Phone: (508)885-0306 **Free:** 800-766-6572
Gregory St. Jacques, Director
Program(s): Acupressure; Aromatherapy, Deep Tissue Massage; Energy Work; Herbal Medicine; Massage Therapy; Meditation; Polarity Therapy; Reflexology; Reiki.

★ 25995 ★ Certificate Program in Holistic Nursing
PO Box 307
Shutesbury, MA 01072
Phone: (413)253-0443 **Fax:** (413)259-1034
Email: cphn@seedsandbridges.com
Website: http://www.seedsandbridges.com
Veda Andrus, Director
Program(s): Holistic Nursing.

★ 25996 ★ Dimon School for the Alexander Technique
15 Day St.
Cambridge, MA 02140
Phone: (617)876-3434
Ted Dimon, Director
Program(s): Alexander Technique.

★ 25997 ★ Dovestar Institute
120 Court St.
Plymouth, MA 02360
Phone: (508)830-0068 **Free:** 888-222-5603
Fax: (508)830-0288
Kamala Renner, Director
Program(s): Acupressure; Breathwork; Colon Hydrotherapy; Energy Work; Hypnotherapy; Kriya Massage; Massage Therapy; Qigong; Reflexology; Reiki; Shiatsu; Yoga Teacher Training.

★ 25998 ★ East/West Institute of Alternative Medicine
1972 Massachusetts Ave.
Cambridge, MA 02140
Phone: (617)876-4048 **Fax:** (617)497-4892
Erik Zutrau, Director
Program(s): Acupressure; Ayurvedic Medicine; Shiatsu; Traditional Chinese Medicine.

★ 25999 ★ Ellen Evert Hopman Introduction to Botanical Medicine and Self Care
PO Box 219
Amherst, MA 01004
Phone: (413)323-4494
Ellen Evert Hopman, Contact
Program(s): Aromatherapy; Herbal Medicine; Homeopathy.

★ 26000 ★ Greater New England Academy of Hypnosis, Inc.
PO Box 975
Andover, MA 01810
Phone: (978)474-4601 **Fax:** (978)474-4601
Alphonse M. Tatarunis, Director
Program(s): Hypnotherapy.

★ 26001 ★ Greenfield Community College
270 Main St.
PO Box 15
Greenfield, MA 01301
Phone: (413)775-1620 **Fax:** (413)774-2285
Laura Earl, Director
Program(s): Massage Therapy; Polarity Therapy; Reflexology; Shiatsu.

★ 26002 ★ International Ayurvedic Medicine Institute, Inc.
111 Elm St., Ste. 103-105
Worcester, MA 01609
Phone: (508)755-3744 **Fax:** (508)770-0618
Email: ayurveda@hotmail.com
Abbas Qutab, Director
Program(s): Ayurvedic Medicine.

★ 26003 ★ Kripalu Center for Yoga and Health
West St.
PO Box 793
Stockbridge, MA 01262
Free: 800-741-7353 **Fax:** (413)448-3384
Website: http://www.kripalu.org
John Willey, Director
Program(s): Holistic Health; Massage Therapy; Yoga Teacher Training.

★ 26004 ★ Massage Institute of New England
22 McGrath Hwy., Ste. 11
Somerville, MA 02143
Phone: (617)666-3700 **Fax:** (617)666-0109
Henry Corley, Director
Program(s): Energy Work; Massage Therapy; Neuromuscular Therapy; Sports Massage; Swedish Massage.

★ 26005 ★ Muscular Therapy Institute
122 Rindge Ave.
Cambridge, MA 02140

Phone: (617)576-1300 **Fax:** (617)864-8283
Website: http://www.mtti.com
Program(s): Massage Therapy.

★ 26006 ★ New England School of Acupuncture
30 Common St.
Watertown, MA 02472
Phone: (617)926-1788 **Fax:** (617)924-4167
Website: http://www.paris.maine.com/people/nesa
Daniel Seitz, Contact
Program(s): Acupuncture; Herbal Medicine; Oriental Medicine; Qigong; Traditional Chinese Medicine.

★ 26007 ★ New England School of Homeopathy
356 Middle St.
Amherst, MA 01002
Phone: (413)256-5949 **Fax:** (413)256-6223
Email: nesh@nesh.com
Dr. Amy Rothenberg, Contact
Program(s): Homeopathy.

★ 26008 ★ New England School of Whole Health Education
581 Boylston St., Ste. 506
Boston, MA 02216
Phone: (617)267-0516 **Fax:** (617)247-0896
Dr. Georgianna Donadio-McCormack, Director
Program(s): Holistic Health.

★ 26009 ★ New England School of Whole Health Education, Dover
60 Farm St.
Dover, MA 02030
Phone: (508)785-0309 **Fax:** (508)785-9743
Georgiana Donadio-McCormack, Director
Program(s): Holistic Health.

★ 26010 ★ Phoenix Rising Yoga Therapy
402 Park St.
PO Box 819
Housatonic, MA 01236
Phone: (413)274-3515 **Fax:** (413)274-6166
Email: moreinfo@pryt.com
Website: http://www.pryt.com
Becky McFarland, Contact
Program(s): Yoga Therapy.

★ 26011 ★ Polarity Realization Institute
126 High St.
Ipswich, MA 01938
Phone: (508)356-0980 **Fax:** (508)356-9818
Email: polaritytherapy@msn.com
Nancy Risley, Director
Program(s): Energy Work; Massage Therapy; Polarity Therapy.

★ 26012 ★ Polarity Realization Institute, Inc., Plymouth
59 Industrial Park Rd.
Plymouth, MA 02360
Phone: (978)356-0980 **Fax:** (978)356-9818
Nancy Risley, Director
Program(s): Aromatherapy, CranioSacral Therapy; Deep Tissue Massage; Energy Work; Massage Therapy; Polarity Therapy; Reflexology; Yoga Teacher Training.

★ 26013 ★ School for Body-Mind Centering
189 Pondview Dr.
Amherst, MA 01002-3230
Phone: (413)256-8615 **Fax:** (413)256-8239
Myra Avedon, Director
Program(s): Body-Mind Centering.

★ 26014 ★ Yoga Therapy Center
120A Westbourne Terrace
Brookline, MA 02446
Phone: (617)739-1146
Mukunda Stiles, Director
Program(s): Yoga Teacher Training.

Michigan

★ 26015 ★ Ann Arbor Institute of Massage Therapy
2835 Carpenter Rd.
Ann Arbor, MI 48108
Phone: (734)677-4430 **Fax:** (734)677-4520
Jocelyn Granger, Director
Program(s): Massage Therapy; Neuromuscular Therapy; Shiatsu; Sports Massage.

★ 26016 ★ Ann Arbor School of Massage and Bodywork
1530 Northwood
Ann Arbor, MI 48103-4667
Phone: (734)662-1572 **Fax:** (734)662-2246
Email: luisa@umich.edu
Barry Ryder, Director
Program(s): Massage Therapy.

★ 26017 ★ Blue Heron Academy of the Healing Arts and Sciences
2020 Raybrook SE, Ste. 203
Grand Rapids, MI 49546
Phone: (616)285-9999 **Fax:** (616)956-7777
Gregory T. Lawton, Director
Program(s): Acupressure; CranioSacral Therapy; Herbal Medicine; Homeopathy; Massage Therapy; Naturopathic Medicine; Neuromuscular Therapy; Oriental Medicine; Qigong; Sports Massage; Tai Chi; Traditional Chinese Medicine.

★ 26018 ★ Discovery Institute of Hypnotherapy
6451 Belding Ave.
Fenwick, MI 48834
Phone: (616)761-3453 **Fax:** (616)761-3710
Email: discovery@ud/ager.net
Charles Kinney, Director
Program(s): Hypnotherapy.

★ 26019 ★ Health Enrichment Center, Inc.
1820 N Lapeer Rd.
Lapeer, MI 48446
Phone: (810)667-9453 **Fax:** (810)667-4095
Email: hec@tir.com
Website: http://www.healthenrichment.com
Sandy Fritz, Director
Program(s): Acupressure; CranioSacral Therapy; Massage Therapy; Polarity Therapy; Reflexology; Shiatsu.

★ 26020 ★ Infinity International Institute of Hypnotherapy
4110 Edgeland, Ste. 800
Royal Oak, MI 48073-2285
Phone: (248)549-5594 **Fax:** (248)549-5421
Email: aspencer@infinityinst.com
Website: http://www.infinityinst.com
Anne H. Spencer, PhD, Director
Program(s): Hypnotherapy; Reiki; Therapeutic Touch.

★ 26021 ★ Institute of Natural Health Sciences
43000 Nine Mile Rd.
Novi, MI 48375
Phone: (248)473-8522 **Fax:** (248)473-8141
C. Lois Grice, Director
Program(s): Herbal Medicine; Homeopathy.

★ 26022 ★ Institute of Natural Therapies
PO Box 222
Hancock, MI 49930
Phone: (906)482-2222
Hal Rudnianin, Director
Program(s): Acupressure; CranioSacral Therapy; Massage Therapy; Qigong; Traditional Chinese Medicine.

★ 26023 ★ Institute of Transformational Hypnotherapy
PO Box 1293
East Lansing, MI 48826
Phone: (517)374-6156
Robert Ranger, Director
Program(s): Hypnotherapy.

★ 26024 ★ International Center for Reiki Training
21421 Hilltop, Ste. 28
Southfield, MI 48034
Free: 800-332-8112 **Fax:** (810)948-8112
Email: reikicen@aol.com
Website: http://www.reiki.org
William Lee Rand, Contact
Program(s): Reiki.

★ 26025 ★ Irene's Myomassology Institute, Inc.
18911 Ten Mile
Southfield, MI 48075
Phone: (248)569-4263 **Fax:** (248)569-4261
Kathleen Grogan, Contact
Program(s): Aromatherapy; CranioSacral Therapy; Herbal Medicine; Massage Therapy; Myomassology; Prenatal Massage; Polarity Therapy; Qigong; Reflexology; Shiatsu; Sports Massage; Thai Massage.

★ 26026 ★ Kalamazoo Center for the Healing Arts
3715 W Main, Ste. 3
Kalamazoo, MI 49006-2842
Phone: (616)373-0910 **Fax:** (616)373-0271
Email: kchands@aol.com
Jim Herweg, Director
Program(s): Acupressure; CranioSacral Therapy; Massage Therapy; Polarity Therapy; Reflexology.

★ 26027 ★ Michigan School of Myomassology
3270 Greenfield Rd.
Berkley, MI 48072
Phone: (248)542-7228 **Fax:** (248)542-5830
Karrie Sladewski, Director
Program(s): Accupressure; Aromatherapy; CranioSacral Therapy; Energy Work; Massage Therapy; Myomassology; Neuromuscular Therapy; Polarity Therapy; Reflexology; Reiki; Shiatsu; Sports Massage.

★ 26028 ★ Michigan School of Traditional Midwifery and Herbology
PO Box 162
Mikado, MI 48745
Phone: (517)736-6583
Casey Makela, Director
Program(s): Herbal Medicine; Midwifery.

★ 26029 ★ Naturopathic Institute of Therapies and Education
1410 S Mission
Mount Pleasant, MI 48858
Phone: (517)773-1714 **Fax:** (517)775-7319
Beth Flaugher, Director
Program(s): Aromatherapy; CranioSacral Therapy; Energy Work; Flower Essences; Herbal Medicine; Homeopathy; Iridology; Massage Therapy; Naturopathic Medicine; Neuromuscular Therapy; Nutrition;

Reflexology; Sports Massage; Traditional Chinese Medicine.

★ 26030 ★ Polarity Center of Dearborn
5824 Chase
Dearborn, MI 48126
Phone: (313)582-5034
John Bodary, Director
Program(s): CranioSacral Therapy; Polarity Therapy.

★ 26031 ★ Polarity Therapy Program
Lansing Community College
PO Box 40010
Lansing, MI 48901-7210
Phone: (517)887-1670
Sheila Cook, Director
Program(s): Polarity Therapy.

★ 26032 ★ University of Michigan School of Nursing
400 N Ingalls, Rm 3320
Ann Arbor, MI 48109-0482
Phone: (734)763-3710 **Fax:** (734)647-0351
Gloria Crothers, Director
Program(s): Midwifery.

★ 26033 ★ Wellspring Institute School of Therapeutic Bodywork
20312 Chalon St.
Saint Clair Shores, MI 48080
Phone: (810)772-8520
Sandra J. Todt, Director
Program(s): Acupressure; CranioSacral Therapy; Energy Work; Hypnotherapy; Massage Therapy; Polarity Therapy; Qigong; Reflexology; Shiatsu; Sports Massage; Therapeutic Touch.

★ 26034 ★ Yogic Sciences Research Foundation
1228 Daisy Ln.
East Lansing, MI 48823
Phone: (517)351-3056
Robert Eschbach, Director
Program(s): Yoga Teacher Training.

Minnesota

★ 26035 ★ Biofeedback Training and Treatment Center, Inc.
7300 France Ave. S, Ste. 200
Edina, MN 55435
Phone: (612)893-9400 **Fax:** (612)893-0615
Email: pills@aol.com
Lilli Ann Jeffrey-Smith, PhD, Director
Program(s): Biofeedback.

★ 26036 ★ BKS Iyengar Yoga Center
2736 Lyndale Ave. S
Minneapolis, MN 55408
Phone: (612)872-8708 **Fax:** (612)872-1893
Email: chirh001@tc.umn.edu
Lee Sverkerson, Director
Program(s): Yoga Teacher Training.

★ 26037 ★ Center for A Balanced Life, Inc.
1535 Livingston Ave., Ste. 105
West Saint Paul, MN 55118-3411
Phone: (612)455-0473
Sister M. Janine Rajkowski, Director
Program(s): Acupressure; Massage Therapy; Polarity Therapy; Reflexology.

★ 26038 ★ Hypnosis Research and Training Center
1960 Cliff Lake Rd., Stes. 112-200
Eagan, MN 55122
Phone: (612)707-1898 **Fax:** (612)707-1898
Kevin Hogan, Director
Program(s): Hypnotherapy; Neuro-Linguistic Programming.

★ 26039 ★ Lake Superior College
2101 Trinity Rd.
Duluth, MN 55811
Phone: (218)733-5921 **Free:** 800-432-2884
Dave Burson, Director
Program(s): Massage Therapy.

★ 26040 ★ Minneapolis School of Massage and Bodywork, Inc.
85 22nd Ave. NE
Minneapolis, MN 55418
Phone: (612)788-8907 **Fax:** (612)788-8907
Joan Crawford-Dietsch, Director
Program(s): Deep Tissue Massage; Massage Therapy; Sports Massage.

★ 26041 ★ Minnesota Center for Shiatsu Study
1313 5th St. SE, Ste. 336
Minneapolis, MN 55414
Phone: (612)379-3565 **Fax:** (612)379-3568
Email: shiatsumn@aol.com
Cari Johnson Pelava, Director
Program(s): Shiatsu; Traditional Chinese Medicine.

★ 26042 ★ Minnesota Institute of Acupuncture and Herbal Studies
1821 University Ave. W, Ste. 278-S
Saint Paul, MN 55104
Phone: (612)603-0994 **Fax:** (612)603-0995
Email: miahs@millcomm.com
Page Purdy, Contact
Program(s): Acupuncture; Herbal Medicine; Oriental Medicine; Traditional Chinese Medicine.

★ 26043 ★ Northern Lights School of Massage Therapy
1313 SE 5th St., Ste. 209
Minneapolis, MN 55414
Phone: (612)379-3822 **Fax:** (612)379-5971
Deni Dantis, Director
Program(s): Massage Therapy.

★ 26044 ★ Northwestern College of Chiropractic
2501 W 84th St.
Bloomington, MN 55431
Phone: (612)888-4777 **Fax:** (612)888-6713
John F. Allenburg, Contact
Program(s): Acupressure; Acupuncture; Chiropractic.

★ 26045 ★ Northwestern School of Homeopathy
10700 Old County Rd. 15, Ste. 350
Plymouth, MN 55441
Phone: (612)794-6445 **Fax:** (612)525-9518
Eric Sommermann, Contact
Program(s): Homeopathy.

★ 26046 ★ Sister Rosalind Gefre School of Professional Massage, Mankato
165 W Lind Ct.
Mankato, MN 56001
Phone: (507)344-0220
Program(s): Deep Tissue Massage; Massage Therapy; Reflexology.

★ 26047 ★ Sister Rosalind Gefre School of Professional Massage, Rochester
300 Elton Hills Dr. NW
Rochester, MN 55901
Phone: (507)286-8608 **Fax:** (507)282-2893
Rolf Bollingberg, Director
Program(s): Deep Tissue Massage; Massage Therapy; Reflexology.

★ 26048 ★ Sister Rosalind Gefre School of Professional Massage, Saint Paul
400 Selby Ave., Ste. G
Saint Paul, MN 55102
Phone: (651)228-0960 **Fax:** (651)698-7436
Audry Handland, Director
Program(s): Acupressure; Chair Massage; CranioSacral Therapy; Massage Therapy; Neuromuscular Therapy; On-Site Massage; Reflexology; Sports Massage.

★ 26049 ★ University of Minnesota Academic Health
308 Harvard St. SE 6-101
Minneapolis, MN 55455
Phone: (612)624-9459 **Fax:** (612)624-3174
Mary Jo Kreitzer, Director
Program(s): Midwifery.

Mississippi

★ 26050 ★ Blue Cliff School of Therapeutic Massage, Gulf Coast Campus
942 E Beach Blvd.
Gulfport, MS 39507
Phone: (228)896-9727 **Fax:** (228)896-8659
Richard Lee Berry, Director
Program(s): Acupressure; CraanioSacral Therapy; Healing Touch; Massage Therapy; Neuromuscular Therapy; Reflexology; Shiatsu; Sports Massage.

★ 26051 ★ Blue Cliff School of Therapeutic Massage, Jackson
5120 Galaxie Dr.
Jackson, MS 39206
Phone: (601)362-3624 **Fax:** (601)362-3694
Dee A. Meux, Director
Program(s): Aromatherapy; CranioSacral Therapy; Deep Tissue Massage; Energy Work; Massage Therapy; Neuromuscular Therapy; Reflexology; Reiki; Shiatsu.

Missouri

★ 26052 ★ Cleveland Chiropractic College. Kansas City
6401 Rockhill Rd.
Kansas City, MO 64131
Phone: (816)501-0100 **Fax:** (816)361-0272
Carl S. Cleveland, III, Contact
Program(s): Chiropractic.

★ 26053 ★ Inochi Institute, Inc.
70-D Grasso Plaza
Saint Louis, MO 63123
Phone: (314)544-9600 **Fax:** (314)631-0223
Thomas Duckworth, Director
Program(s): Acupressure; Acupuncture; Energy Work; Herbal Medicine; Homeopathy; Kototama Medicine; Massage Therapy; Naturopathic Medicine; Neuromuscular Therapy; Oriental Medicine; Shiatsu; Traditional Japanese Medicine.

★ 26054 ★ Logan College of Chiropractic
1851 Schoettler Rd.
PO Box 1065
Chesterfield, MO 63006-1065

Phone: (314)227-2100 **Free:** 800-533-9210
Fax: (314)207-2424
George A. Goodman, Contact
Program(s): Chiropractic.

★ 26055 ★ Massage Therapy Institute of Missouri (MTIM)
5 S 9th St., Ste. 202
Columbia, MO 65201
Phone: (573)875-7905 **Fax:** (573)443-7933
Email: eruvalca@digmo.org
Mirra Greenway, Director
Program(s): Deep Tissue Massage; Energy Work; Massage Therapy; Sports Massage; Swedish Massage.

★ 26056 ★ Massage Therapy Training Institute, LLC
9140 Ward Pkwy., Ste. 100
Kansas City, MO 64114
Phone: (816)523-9140
Terri Oglesby, Contact
Program(s): Aromatherapy; CranioSacral Therapy; Energy Work; Herbal Medicine; Massage Therapy; Myofascial Release; Neuromuscular Therapy; Polarity Therapy; Qigong; Reflexology; Shiatsu; Sports Massage; Therapeutic Touch; Trigger Point Therapy.

★ 26057 ★ Professional Massage Training Center
200 E Commercial
Springfield, MO 65803
Phone: (417)863-7682 **Fax:** (417)863-7652
Email: juliet@cland.net
Juliet Mee, Director
Program(s): Massage Therapy.

★ 26058 ★ Saint Charles School of Massage Therapy
2440 Executive Dr.
Saint Charles, MO 63301
Phone: (314)498-0777 **Fax:** (314)498-0708
Email: oasis@anet-stl.com
Website: http://www.britestar.net.oasis.com
Kathleen Crawford, Director
Program(s): Aromatherapy; CranioSacral Therapy; Massage Therapy; Polarity Therapy; Reflexology; Reiki; Shiatsu.

★ 26059 ★ University of Missouri, Columbia
Sinclair School of Nursing
Columbia, MO 65211
Phone: (573)882-0235 **Fax:** (573)884-4544
Nancy Johnson, Director
Program(s): Midwifery.

Montana

★ 26060 ★ Big Sky Somatic Institute
1802 11th Ave., Ste. A
Helena, MT 59601
Phone: (406)442-8998
Ron Floyd, Director
Program(s): Acupressure; Energy Work; Herbal Medicine; Massage Therapy; Neuromuscular Therapy; Qigong; Shiatsu; Thai Massage; Traditional Chinese Medicine.

★ 26061 ★ Rocky Mountain Herbal Institute
305 2nd Ave. S
PO Box 579
Hot Springs, MT 59845
Phone: (406)741-3811
Email: rmhi@rmhiherbal.org
Website: http://www.rmhiherbal.org
Roger W. Wicke, PhD, Director
Program(s): Herbal Medicine; Traditional Chinese Medicine.

★ 26062 ★ Starfire Massage School and Healing Center
9819 Waldo Rd.
Missoula, MT 59808
Phone: (406)721-7519 **Fax:** (406)721-7519
Mary Marron, Director
Program(s): Acupressure; Energy Work; Hydrotherapy; Massage Therapy; Reiki; Shamanic Healing; Shiatsu; Sound Healing.

Nebraska

★ 26063 ★ Gateway College of Massage Therapy
2607 Dakota Ave.
South Sioux City, NE 68776
Phone: (402)494-8390 **Fax:** (402)494-4561
Darrell J. Peck, PhD, Director
Program(s): Acupressure; CranioSacral Therapy; Massage Therapy; Neuromuscular Therapy; Reflexology; Sports Massage; Swedish Massage.

★ 26064 ★ Myotherapy Institute
6020 S 58th St.
Lincoln, NE 68516
Phone: (402)421-7410 **Fax:** (402)421-6736
Program(s): Hydrotherapy; Massage Therapy; Medical Massage; Spa Therapies.

★ 26065 ★ Omaha School of Massage Therapy
9748 Park Dr.
Omaha, NE 68127
Phone: (402)331-3694 **Fax:** (402)331-0280
Website: http://www.osmt.com
Ann Reuck, Director
Program(s): Acupressure; Aromatherapy; Energy Work; Massage Therapy; Reflexology; Sports Massage; Swedish Massage.

★ 26066 ★ Universal Center of Healing Arts
109 N 50th St.
Omaha, NE 68132
Phone: (402)556-4456 **Fax:** (402)561-0635
Patrick Davis, Director
Program(s): Acupressure; Aromatherapy; Ayurvedic Medicine; CranioSacral Therapy; Energy Work; Herbal Medicine; Massage Therapy; Neuromuscular Therapy; Oriental Medicine; Polarity Therapy; Qigong; Reflexology; Reiki; Shiatsu; Sports Massage; Tai Chi; Traditional Chinese Medicine; Yoga.

Nevada

★ 26067 ★ Aston-Patterning Training Center / A Continuing Education Service
PO Box 3568
Incline Village, NV 89450
Phone: (702)831-8228
Judith Aston, Director
Program(s): Aston-Patterning Bodywork and Movement.

★ 26068 ★ Dahan Institute of Massage Studies
3430 E Tropicana, Ste. 62
Las Vegas, NV 89121
Phone: (702)434-1338 **Fax:** (702)434-3449
Serge Dahan, Director
Program(s): Acupressure; Aromatherapy; Massage Therapy; Polarity Therapy; Reflexology; Shiatsu; Sports Massage.

★ 26069 ★ International BioMedical Research Institute
6490 S McCarran Blvd., C-24
Reno, NV 89509
Phone: (702)827-1444 **Fax:** (702)827-2424
Edna Edsig, Director
Program(s): Herbal Medicine; Homeopathy.

★ 26070 ★ Ralston School of Massage
Washoe Med. Ctr.
77 Pringle Way
Reno, NV 89520-0109
Phone: (702)982-5450 **Fax:** (702)982-5452
Email: 2relax@intercomm.com
Robert H. Oliver, Director
Program(s): Massage Therapy.

New Hampshire

★ 26071 ★ Dovestar Institute
50 Whitehall Rd.
Hooksett, NH 03106
Phone: (603)669-5104 **Free:** 888-222-5603
Fax: (603)625-1919
Kamala Renner, Director
Program(s): Acupressure; Colon Hydrotherapy; CranioSacral Therapy; Hypnotherapy; Kriya Massage; Qigong; Reflexology; Reiki; Shiatsu; Yoga Teacher Training.

★ 26072 ★ New England Academy of Therapeutic Sciences
402 Amherst St.
Nashua, NH 03063
Phone: (603)886-8433 **Fax:** (603)880-8654
Email: maureen@neats.com
Website: http://www.neats.com
Maureen J. Healy, Director
Program(s): Acupressure; Animal Therapy; CranioSacral Therapy; Equine Massage; Herbal Medicine; Homeopathy; Hypnotherapy; Massage Therapy; Neuromuscular Therapy; Polarity Therapy; Reflexology; Shiatsu; Swedish Massage; Traditional Chinese Medicine.

★ 26073 ★ New Hampshire Institute for Therapeutic Arts School of Massage Therapy, Hudson
153 Lowell Rd.
Hudson, NH 03051
Phone: (603)882-3022 **Fax:** (603)598-9101
Patrick Cowan, Contact
Program(s): Acupressure; Lymphatic Massage; Massage Therapy; Neuromuscular Therapy; Polarity Therapy; Reflexology; Sports Massage; Swedish Massage.

★ 26074 ★ North Eastern Institute of Whole Health, Inc.
22 Bridge St.
Manchester, NH 03101-1655
Phone: (603)623-5018 **Fax:** (603)641-5928
Dr. Douglas DuVerger, Director
Program(s): Acupressure; Anatomy and Physiology; Aromatherapy; Chair Massage; CPR/First Aid; CranioSacral Therapy; Esalen Therapy; Herbal Medicine; Hydrotherapy; Hypnotherapy; LomiLomi Massage; Lymphatic Massage; Massage Therapy; Neuromuscular Therapy; Oriental Medicine; Polarity Therapy; Pregnancy Massage; Qigong; Reflexology; Reiki; Shiatsu; Sports Massage; Traditional Chinese Medicine; Trigger Point Therapy.

New Jersey

★ 26075 ★ Academy of Massage Therapy
401 S Van Brunt St.
Englewood, NJ 07631
Phone: (201)568-3220 **Fax:** (201)568-5181
Joanna Sechuk, Director

Program(s): Aromatherapy; Massage Therapy; Medical Massage; Qigong; Reflexology; Reiki; Shiatsu; Sports Massage;Thai Massage.

★ 26076 ★ Academy of Natural Health Sciences
102 Green St.
Woodbridge, NJ 07095
Phone: (732)634-2155 **Fax:** (732)634-2155
Frank Auriemma, Director
Program(s): Acupressure; Aromatherapy; Ayurvedic Medicine; Energy Work; Herbal Medicine; Holistic Health; Homeopathy; Hypnotherapy; Massage Therapy; Neuromuscular Therapy; Nutrition; Polarity Therapy; Reflexology; Reiki; Shiatsu; Sports Massage.

★ 26077 ★ Academy of Professional Hypnosis
1358 Burnet Ave.
Union, NJ 07083
Phone: (908)964-4417 **Fax:** (908)810-0255
Dr. John Gatto, Contact
Program(s): Hypnotherapy.

★ 26078 ★ Body, Mind and Spirit Learning Alliance
917-2 N Main St.
Toms River, NJ 08753
Phone: (908)349-7153
Dianne O'Brien, Director
Program(s): Aromatherapy; CranioSacral Therapy; Massage Therapy; Reflexology; Reiki; Shiatsu; Swedish Massage.

★ 26079 ★ Center for TransPersonal BodyMind Studies
51 Upland Ave.
Metuchen, NJ 08840
Phone: (732)548-8579
Joanne Rossi, Director
Program(s): Aromatherapy; Energy Work; Massage Therapy; Polarity Therapy; Somatic Psychology.

★ 26080 ★ Center for Universal and Holistic Studies, Paramus
PO Box 1306
Paramus, NJ 07653
Phone: (973)686-9700
Elaine Gordon, Director
Program(s): Energy Work; Reflexology.

★ 26081 ★ Classic Center for Health and Healing
25 Orchard St., Ste. 101
Denville, NJ 07834-2160
Phone: (973)627-4833
Zoe Elva Putnam, Director
Program(s): Therapeutic Touch.

★ 26082 ★ Five Elements School of Classical Homeopathy
115 Rte. 46, Bldg. D-29
Mountain Lakes, NJ 07046
Phone: (201)402-8510 **Fax:** (201)402-9753
Jane Cicchetti, Director
Program(s): Homeopathy.

★ 26083 ★ Garden State Center for Holistic Health Care
1203 Airport Rd.
Rte. 70 W
Lakewood, NJ 08701
Phone: (732)364-0882 **Fax:** (732)364-7096
Gloria Coppola, Director
Program(s): Acupressure; Aromatherapy; CranioSacral Therapy; Energy Work; Massage Therapy; Neuromuscular Therapy; Reiki; Swedish Massage; Thai Massage.

★ 26084 ★ Healing Hands Institute for Massage Therapy
41 Bergenline Ave.
Westwood, NJ 07675
Phone: (201)722-0099 **Fax:** (201)722-0690
Email: hhi@aol.com
Eva Carey, Contact
Program(s): Acupressure; Aromatherapy; Massage Therapy; Medical Massage; Reflexology; Reiki; Shiatsu; Sports Massage; Swedish Massage; Traditional Chinese Medicine.

★ 26085 ★ Healing Hands School of Massage
515 Whitehorse Pike
Haddon Heights, NJ 08035
Phone: (609)546-7471 **Fax:** (609)546-7491
Kristina Shaw, Director
Program(s): Acupressure; CranioSacral Therapy; Deep Tissue Massage; Herbal Medicine; Hydrotherapy; Massage Therapy; Myofascial Release; Neuromuscular Therapy; Polarity Therapy; Reflexology; Reiki; Shiatsu; Swedish Massage; Traditional Chinese Medicine.

★ 26086 ★ Health Choices Center for the Healing Arts
170 Township Line Rd., Bldg. B
Belle Mead, NJ 08502
Phone: (908)359-3995 **Fax:** (908)359-3902
Renate M. Novak, Director
Program(s): Acupressure; Aromatherapy; Massage Therapy; Neuromuscular Therapy; Polarity Therapy; Qigong; Reflexology; Reiki; Shiatsu.

★ 26087 ★ Herbal Therapeutics School of Botanical Medicine
PO Box 553
Broadway, NJ 08808
Phone: (908)835-0822 **Fax:** (908)835-0824
David Winston, Director
Program(s): Herbal Medicine.

★ 26088 ★ Institute of Hypnotherapy
10 Darby Ct.
Manalapan, NJ 07726
Phone: (732)446-5995
Jaime Feldman, Director
Program(s): Hypnotherapy; Neuro-Linguistic Programming.

★ 26089 ★ Institute for Therapeutic Massage, Inc.
125 Wanaque Ave.
Pompton Lakes, NJ 07442
Phone: (201)839-6131 **Fax:** (201)839-9878
Lisa Helbig, Director
Program(s): Aromatherapy; Chair Massage; Energy Work; Geriatric Medicine; Massage Therapy; Pregnancy Massage; Reflexology; Reiki; Sports Massage.

★ 26090 ★ Massage Therapy Center for Healing and Learning
4 Deerfield Pl.
Flanders, NJ 07836
Phone: (973)927-3151
Jack Hicks, Director
Program(s): CranioSacral Therapy; Deep Tissue Massage; Massage Therapy; Reflexology; Reiki.

★ 26091 ★ Morris Institute of Natural Therapeutics
3108 Rte. 10 W
Denville, NJ 07834
Phone: (201)989-8939 **Fax:** (201)989-5554
Vincent R. Iuppo, Director
Program(s): Acupressure; Applied Kinesiology; Aromatherapy; Chair Massage; CranioSacral Therapy; Manual Lymph Drainage; Massage Therapy; Neuromuscular Therapy; Reflexology; Shiatsu; Sports Massage.

★ 26092 ★ Mother Love, Doula Training
584 Echo Glen Ave.
River Vale, NJ 07675
Phone: (201)358-2703 **Fax:** (201)664-4405
Debra Pascali-Bonaro, Director
Program(s): Doula.

★ 26093 ★ New Jersey Institute of Reflexology
155 Franklin Ave.
Long Branch, NJ 07740-6616
Free: 888-722-6547
Mary Alice Arre, Director
Program(s): Reflexology.

★ 26094 ★ New Jersey Massage Training Center
3699 Rt. 46E
Parsippany, NJ 07054
Phone: (973)263-2229 **Fax:** (973)402-1222
Larry Heisler, Director
Program(s): Acupressure; Massage Therapy; Neuromuscular Therapy; Qigong; Reflexology; Shiatsu; Sports Massage; Swedish Massage; Yoga Teacher Training.

★ 26095 ★ Ocean County Vo-Tech
1299 Old Freehold Rd.
Toms River, NJ 08753
Phone: (732)349-8444
Sharon Spaziani, Director
Program(s): Deep Tissue Massage; Massage Therapy.

★ 26096 ★ Our Lady of Lourdes Institute of Wholistic Studies
900 Haddon Ave., Ste. 118
Collingswood, NJ 08108
Phone: (609)869-3134 **Fax:** (609)869-3129
Erika MacWilliams, Contact
Program(s): Aromatherapy; Ayurvedic Medicine; Feldenkrais; Guided Imagery; Massage Therapy; Reflexology; Reiki; Shiatsu; Sports Massage; Therapeutic Touch; Traditional Chinese Medicine; Yoga Teacher Training.

★ 26097 ★ School of Asian Healing Arts
Executive Mews G-38
1930 E Marlton Park
Cherry Hill, NJ 08003
Phone: (609)424-7501 **Fax:** (609)424-7379
Ruth Dalphin, Director
Program(s): Acupressure; Qigong; Reflexology; Reiki; Shiatsu; Thai Massage; Traditional Chinese Medicine; Yoga Teacher Training.

★ 26098 ★ Seashore Healing Arts Center
505 New Rd., Stes. 5 and 7
Somers Point, NJ 08244
Phone: (609)601-9272
Edward Smith, Director
Program(s): Acupressure; Deep Tissue Massage; Energy Work; Massage Therapy; Meditation; Polarity Therapy; Qigong; Reflexology; Reiki; Yoga.

★ 26099 ★ Somerset School of Massage Therapy
7 Cedar Grove Ln.
Somerset, NJ 08873

Phone: (732)356-0787 **Fax:** (732)469-3494
Email: ssmt@massagecareer.com
Website: http://www.massagecareer.com
Deborah Scarpitto, Contact
Program(s): Massage Therapy; Neuromuscular Therapy; Reflexology; Shiatsu.

★ 26100 ★ Studio Yoga
2 Green Village Rd., Rm. 301
PO Box 99
Madison, NJ 07940
Phone: (973)966-5311 **Fax:** (973)966-1477
Theresa Rowland, Director
Program(s): Yoga Teacher Training.

★ 26101 ★ Swedish American Massage Institute (SAMI)
120 Maple Ave.
Red Bank, NJ 07701
Phone: (908)530-1188 **Fax:** (908)530-1919
Sharyn Ross, Director
Program(s): Aromatherapy; Massage Therapy; Neuromuscular Therapy; On-Site Massage; Reflexology; Sports Massage; Swedish Massage.

★ 26102 ★ Universal of Medicine and Dentistry of New Jersey
School of Health Related Professions
65 Bergen St.
Newark, NJ 07107-3001
Phone: (973)972-4298
Elaine Diegmann, Director
Program(s): Midwifery.

★ 26103 ★ Unlimited Potential
PO Box 64
Roseland, NJ 07068
Phone: (973)325-0900 **Fax:** (973)403-9789
Roxanne Louise, Director
Program(s): Hypnotherapy; Reiki.

New Mexico

★ 26104 ★ Academy Institute of Vedic Studies
1701 Santa Fe River Rd.
Santa Fe, NM 87501
Phone: (505)983-9385 **Fax:** (505)982-5807
Mira Foung, Director
Program(s): Ayurvedic Medicine.

★ 26105 ★ Ayurvedic Institute
11311 Menaul NE, Ste. A
PO Box 23445
Albuquerque, NM 87112
Phone: (505)291-9698 **Fax:** (505)294-7572
Website: http://www.ayurveda.com
Wynn Werner, Contact
Program(s): Anatomy and Physiology; Ayurvedic Medicine; Yoga.

★ 26106 ★ Body-Mind Centering
PO Box 4552
Taos, NM 87571
Phone: (505)758-1711 **Fax:** (505)751-0331
Ziji Beth Goren, Director
Program(s): Body-Mind Centering.

★ 26107 ★ Crystal Mountain Apprenticeship in the Healing Arts
118 Dartmouth SE
Albuquerque, NM 87106
Phone: (505)268-4411 **Free:** 800-967-5678
Fax: (505)268-4007
Rebecca Solomon, Director
Program(s): Anatomy and Physiology; Aromatherapy; CranioSacral Therapy; Energy Work; Esalen Massage; Herbal Medicine; Hydrotherapy; Kinesiology; LomiLomi Massage; Massage Therapy; Movement Education; Neuromuscular Therapy; Polarity Therapy; Reflexology; Shiatsu; Sports Massage; Traditional Chinese Medicine.

★ 26108 ★ Eastern New Mexico School of Massage Therapy
PO Box 2142
Clovis, NM 88101
Phone: (505)763-0551 **Fax:** (505)763-1405
Sue Pierce, Director
Program(s): CranioSacral Therapy; Energy Work; Herbal Medicine; Infant Massage; Manual Lymph Drainage; Massage Therapy; Polarity Therapy; Reflexology; Shiatsu.

★ 26109 ★ International Institute of Chinese Medicine
4884 La Junta del Alamo
PO Box 29988
Santa Fe, NM 87505
Phone: (505)473-5233 **Free:** 800-377-4561
Fax: (505)473-9279
Email: 102152.3463@compuserve.com
Website: http://www.thuntek.net/iicm
Dr. Michael Zeng, Contact
Program(s): Acupunture; Oriental Medicine; Qigong; Traditional Chinese Medicine; Tui Na.

★ 26110 ★ KRI
Rt. 2 Box 4 Shady Lane
Espanola, NM 87532
Phone: (505)753-0423 **Fax:** (505)753-5982
Nam K. Khalsa, Director
Program(s): Yoga Teacher Training.

★ 26111 ★ Maharishi College of Vedic Medicine
2721 Arizona, St. NE
Albuquerque, NM 87110
Phone: (505)830-0435 **Fax:** (505)830-0538
Email: desmithmd@aol.com
D. Edwards Smith, MD, Contact
Program(s): Ayurvedic Medicine; Maharishi Vedic Medicine.

★ 26112 ★ Medicine Wheel - A School of Holistic Therapies
1243 W Apache
Farmington, NM 87401
Free: 888-327-1914 **Fax:** (505)327-2234
Randy Barnes, Director
Program(s): Acupressure; Aromatherapy; CranioSacral Therapy; Herbal Medicine; Holistic Health; Massage Therapy; Neuromuscular Therapy; Polarity Therapy; Qigong; Traditional Chinese Medicine; Tui Na.

★ 26113 ★ Mesilla Valley School of Therapeutic Arts
741 N Alameda, Ste. 15
PO Box 1227
Las Cruces, NM 88005
Phone: (505)527-1239
Wanita Thompson, Director
Program(s): Massage Therapy.

★ 26114 ★ National College of Phytotherapy
3030 Isleta Blvd. SW
Albuquerque, NM 87105
Phone: (505)452-3468 **Fax:** (505)452-3468
Teresa Merriken, Contact
Program(s): Herbal Medicine.

★ 26115 ★ New Mexico Academy of Healing Arts
501 Franklin Ave.
PO Box 932
Santa Fe, NM 87501
Phone: (505)982-6271 **Free:** 888-808-5188
Fax: (505)988-2621
Website: http://www.nmaha.com
Lorin Parrish, Director
Program(s): Aromatherapy; CranioSacral Therapy; Feldenkrais; Massage Therapy; Polarity Therapy; Reflexology; Shiatsu; Sports Massage; Swedish Massage.

★ 26116 ★ New Mexico School of Natural Therapeutics
202 Morningside SE
Albuquerque, NM 87108
Phone: (505)268-6870 **Free:** 800-654-1675
Fax: (505)268-0818
Email: jpendry@swcp.com
Website: http://www.nmsnt.org
Robert Stevens, Director
Program(s): Deep Tissue Massage; Flower Essences; Herbal Medicine; Massage Therapy; Polarity Therapy; Pregnancy Massage; Reflexology; Shiatsu; Sports Massage; Swedish Massage.

★ 26117 ★ Rosen Method Center Southwest
PO Box 344
Santa Fe, NM 87504
Phone: (505)982-7149 **Fax:** (505)254-7048
Email: sw.touch@ix.netcom.com
Website: http://www.mcn.org/b/rosen
Sandra Wooten, Director
Program(s): Rosen Method Bodywork.

★ 26118 ★ Scherer Institute of Natural Healing
935 Alto St.
Santa Fe, NM 87501
Phone: (505)982-8398 **Fax:** (505)982-1825
Email: tsi@rt66.com
Website: http://www.newmexiconet.com/scher.htm
Lonnie Howard, Director
Program(s): Aromatherapy; CarnioSacral Therapy; Energy Work; Herbal Medicine; Massage Therapy; Polarity Therapy; Reflexology; Shiatsu; Sports Massage.

★ 26119 ★ Southwest Acupuncture College, Albuquerque
4308 Carlisle NE, Ste. 205
Albuquerque, NM 87107
Phone: (505)888-8898
Skya Gardner Abbate, Director
Program(s): Acupuncture; Herbal Medicine; Oriental Medicine; Qigong; Shiatsu; Traditional Chinese Medicine.

★ 26120 ★ Southwest Acupuncture College, Santa Fe
2960 Rodeo Park Dr. W
Santa Fe, NM 87505
Phone: (505)438-8884 **Fax:** (505)438-8883
Skya Gardner Abbate, Director
Program(s): Acupuncture; Herbal Medicine; Oriental Medicine; Qigong; Traditional Chinese Medicine.

★ 26121 ★ Taos School of Massage
1021 Salazar
Taos, NM 87571
Phone: (505)758-2725
Eric Ritchie, Director
Program(s): Acupressure; Applied Kinesiology; Ayurvedic Medicine; Body-Mind Clearing; Energy Work; Massage Therapy; Neuromuscular Therapy;

Qigong; Reflexology; Shiatsu; Sports Massage; Traditional Chinese Medicine.

★ 26122 ★ Universal Therapeutic Massage Institute, Inc.
3410 Aztec Rd. NE
Albuquerque, NM 87107
Free: 800-557-0020 **Fax:** (505)881-0749
Stacy Townsend, Contact
Program(s): CranioSacral Therapy; Massage Therapy; Myofascial Release; Neuromuscular Therapy; Polarity Therapy; Reflexology; Shiatsu; Sports Massaage; Traditional Chinese Medicine.

★ 26123 ★ University of New Mexico College of Nursing
Nursing/Pharmacy Bldg.
Albuquerque, NM 87131-1061
Phone: (505)272-1184
Barbara A. Overman, Director
Program(s): Midwifery.

★ 26124 ★ Wellness Institute
PO Box 2843
Taos, NM 87571
Phone: (505)776-1590 **Free:** 888-253-6331
Email: wellness@laplaza.taos.nm.us
Roger Gilchrist, Contact
Program(s): Polarity Therapy.

★ 26125 ★ Westbrook University
400 University Plaza
Aztec, NM 87410
Phone: (505)334-1115 **Free:** 800-447-6496
Fax: (505)334-7583
Email: admissions@cyberport.com
Website: http://www.westbrooku.edu
DeeAnne Greene, PhD, Contact
Program(s): Acupressure; Aromatherapy; Ayurvedic Medicine; Energy Work; Flower Essences; Herbal Medicine; Homeopathy; Midwifery; Naturopathic Medicine; Polarity Therapy; Reflexology.

★ 26126 ★ White Mountain School of Applied Healing
1204 Mechem, Ste. 10
Ruidoso, NM 88345
Phone: (505)258-3046
Pablo Falcon, Director
Program(s): Acupressure; Aromatherapy; Deep Tissue Massage; Energy Work; Manual Lymph Drainage; Massage Therapy; Reflexology; Reiki; Shiatsu.

New York

★ 26127 ★ Academy of Natural Healing
40 W 72nd St., Ste. 117
New York, NY 10023
Phone: (212)724-8782 **Fax:** (212)724-2535
Lewis Harrison, Director
Program(s): Acupressure; Aromatherapy; CranioSacral Therapy; Energy Work; Herbal Medicine; Homeopathy; Polarity Therapy; Qigong; Reflexology; Shiatsu.

★ 26128 ★ American Center for the Alexander Technique
129 W 67th St.
New York, NY 10023
Phone: (212)799-0468 **Fax:** (212)799-0468
Barbara Kent, Director
Program(s): Alexander Technique.

★ 26129 ★ American Taoist Healing Center
396 Broadway, Ste. 502
New York, NY 10013-3500
Phone: (212)274-0999 **Fax:** (212)274-9879
Louise Di Bello, Contact
Program(s): Acupressure; Acupuncture; Qigong; Traditional Chinese Medicine.

★ 26130 ★ Atlantic Academy of Classical Homeopathy
399 6th Ave., Ste. 3D
Brooklyn, NY 11215
Phone: (718)768-3811
Gerald Gewiss, Director
Program(s): Homeopathy.

★ 26131 ★ Ayurveda Holistic Center
82 A0 Bayville Ave.
Bayville, NY 11709
Phone: (516)628-8200
Email: mail@ayurvedahc.com
Website: http://www.ayurvedahc.com
Swami Sada Shiva Tirtha, Contact
Program(s): Ayurvedic Medicine.

★ 26132 ★ Barbara Brennan School of Healing
PO Box 2005
East Hampton, NY 11937
Phone: (516)329-0951 **Fax:** (516)324-9745
Website: http://www.barbarabrennan.com
Kay Conboy, Contact
Program(s): Brennan Healing Science; Energy Work.

★ 26133 ★ Biofeedback Training Associates
255 W 98th St.
New York, NY 10025
Phone: (212)222-5665 **Fax:** (212)222-5667
Email: ac@inx.net
Website: http://www.biof.com/biofeedback.html
Dr. Philip Brotman, Director
Program(s): Biofeedback; Hypnotherapy; Neurofeedback.

★ 26134 ★ Body Logic Institute
295 W 11th St., Ste. 1F
New York, NY 10014
Phone: (212)633-2143 **Free:** 800-877-8429
Fax: (212)633-6190
Yamuna Zake, Contact
Program(s): Body Logic; Body Rolling.

★ 26135 ★ Diana Kalfayan
150 W 80th St., Apt. 6C
New York, NY 10024
Phone: (212)877-9626
Diana Kalfayan, Director
Program(s): Esoteric Healing; Polarity Therapy.

★ 26136 ★ Finger Lakes School of Massage
1251 Trumansburg Rd.
Ithaca, NY 14850
Phone: (607)272-9024 **Fax:** (607)272-4271
Website: http://www.flsm.com
Cindy Black, Director
Program(s): Aromatherapy; Energy Work; Massage Therapy; Neuromuscular Therapy; Polarity Therapy; Reflexology; Shiatsu; Sports Massage; Thai Massage; Trager.

★ 26137 ★ Flynn's School of Herbology
60 E 4th St.
New York, NY 10003
Phone: (212)677-8140
Arcus Flynn, Contact
Program(s): Herbal Medicine.

★ 26138 ★ Hudson Valley School of Classical Homeopathy
321 McKinstry Rd.
Gardiner, NY 12525
Phone: (914)255-6141 **Fax:** (914)255-6241
David Kramer, Director
Program(s): Homeopathy.

★ 26139 ★ Hypnosis Institute
139 Fulton St., Ste. 304
New York, NY 10038
Phone: (212)227-8643 **Fax:** (212)791-9517
Email: hypno1@interport.net
Website: http://www.infaith.com
Barry Seedman, PhD, Director
Program(s): Hypnotherapy; Reiki.

★ 26140 ★ Institute for the Alexander Technique
853 Broadway, Ste. 1007
New York, NY 10003
Phone: (212)529-3211
Thomas Lemens, Contact
Program(s): Alexander Technique.

★ 26141 ★ Jivamukti Yoga Center
404 Lafayette St., 3rd Flr.
New York, NY 10003
Phone: (212)353-0214 **Fax:** (212)995-1313
Adrienne Burke, Director
Program(s): Yoga Teacher Training.

★ 26142 ★ Kundalini Yoga Center
401 Layfayette St.
New York, NY 10003
Phone: (212)475-0212
Email: ravi@ziplink.net
Website: http://www.ziplink.net/~ravi
Ravi Singh, Director
Program(s): Yoga Teacher Training.

★ 26143 ★ Kundalini Yoga East, Inc.
873 Broadway, Ste. 614
New York, NY 10003
Phone: (212)995-0521
Sat Jivan Kaur Khalsa, Director
Program(s): Energy Work; Yoga Teacher Training.

★ 26144 ★ Laura Norman Reflexology Training Center
41 Park Ave., Ste. 8A
New York, NY 10016
Phone: (212)532-4404 **Fax:** (212)532-4504
Laura Norman, Director
Program(s): Reflexology.

★ 26145 ★ Linden Tree Center for Holistic Health
8 Noxon Rd.
Poughkeepsie, NY 12603-2926
Phone: (914)471-8000
Gary Seigel, Director
Program(s): CranioSacral Therapy; Polarity Therapy.

★ 26146 ★ Long Island Reflexology Center
14 E Broadway
Port Jefferson, NY 11777
Phone: (516)474-3137 **Fax:** (516)287-3127
Geraldine Brill, Director
Program(s): Reflexology; Therapeutic Touch.

★ 26147 ★ Mathews School of the Alexander Technique
74 MacDougal St.
New York, NY 10012

Phone: (212)473-3247 **Fax:** (212)473-0341
Troup Mathews, Director
Program(s): Alexander Technique.

★ 26148 ★ Mercy College
555 Broadway
Dobbs Ferry, NY 10522
Phone: (914)674-7401 **Fax:** (914)674-7374
Douglas McDaniel, Director
Program(s): Acupuncture; Oriental Medicine.

★ 26149 ★ MotherMassage
108 E 16th St., Ste. 401
New York, NY 10003
Phone: (212)533-3188 **Fax:** (212)533-3148
Elaine Stillerman, Contact
Program(s): Prenatal Massage; Postpartum Massage.

★ 26150 ★ New Center College for Wholistic Health Education and Research
6801 Jericho Tpk., Ste. 300
Syosset, NY 11791
Phone: (516)364-0808 **Fax:** (516)364-0989
Steven Schenkman, Contact
Program(s): Acupuncture; Herbal Medicine; Holistic Nursing; Massage Therapy; Oriental Medicine; Traditional Chinese Medicine.

★ 26151 ★ New York Chiropractic College
2360 SR 89
Seneca Falls, NY 13148-0800
Phone: (315)568-3000 **Fax:** (315)568-3015
Email: enrolnow@nycc.edu
Website: http://www.nycc.edu
Kenneth W. Padgett, Contact
Program(s): Chiropractic.

★ 26152 ★ New York Institute of Massage
4701 Transit Rd.
Williamsville, NY 14221
Phone: (716)633-0355 **Free:** 800-884-6946
Fax: (716)633-0213
Sharon Boyd, Director
Program(s): Massage Therapy.

★ 26153 ★ New York Open Center
83 Spring St.
New York, NY 10012
Phone: (212)274-1829 **Fax:** (212)226-4056
Lisa Schimski, Director
Program(s): Polarity Therapy; Reflexology; Yoga Teacher Training.

★ 26154 ★ New York University Division of Nursing/School of Education
50 W 4th St.
425 Shimkin Hall
New York, NY 10012
Phone: (212)998-5895
Patricia Burkhardt, Director
Program(s): Midwifery.

★ 26155 ★ NLP Center of New York
24 E 12th St., Ste. 402
New York, NY 10003
Phone: (212)647-0860 **Fax:** (212)509-2326
Email: nlp@earthlink.net
Website: http://www.nlptraining.com
Steven Leeds, Director
Program(s): Hypnotherapy; Neuro-Linguistic Programming.

★ 26156 ★ Northeast School of Botanical Medicine
PO Box 6626
Ithaca, NY 14851
Phone: (607)564-1023
Program(s): Herbal Medicine.

★ 26157 ★ Ohashi Institute
12 W 27th St., 9th Fl.
New York, NY 10001
Free: 800-810-4190 **Fax:** (212)447-5819
Email: ohashiinst@aol.com
Website: http://www.ohashi.com
Program(s): Shiatsu.

★ 26158 ★ Omega Institute for Holistic Studies
260 Lake Dr.
Rhinebeck, NY 12572
Phone: (914)266-4444 **Fax:** (914)266-4828
Website: http://omega-inst.org
Laurie Zollo, Director
Program(s): Energy Work; Healing Touch; Massage Therapy; Mind-Body Medicine; Qigong; Reflexology; Yoga Teacher Training.

★ 26159 ★ Onondaga School of Therapeutic Massage
220 Walton St.
Syracuse, NY 13202
Phone: (315)424-1159 **Fax:** (315)424-0796
Jean Vatter, Director
Program(s): Massage Therapy.

★ 26160 ★ Pacific College of Oriental Medicine
915 Broadway, 3rd Fl.
New York, NY 10010
Phone: (212)982-3456 **Free:** 800-729-3468
Fax: (212)982-6514
Jennifer Park, Contact
Program(s): Acupuncture; Oriental Medicine; Traditional Chinese Medicine.

★ 26161 ★ R. J. Buckle Associates, LLC
PO Box 868
Hunter, NY 12442
Phone: (518)263-4402 **Fax:** (518)263-4031
Jane Buckle, Director
Program(s): Aromatherapy.

★ 26162 ★ Rainbow Reiki Center
1330 Main St.
Ruby, NY 12475
Phone: (914)336-4609
Joyce Kaessinger, Director
Program(s): Reiki.

★ 26163 ★ Reese Williams
270 Lafayette St., Ste. 805
New York, NY 10012
Phone: (212)343-9382
Reese Williams, Director
Program(s): CranioSacral Therapy; Polarity Therapy.

★ 26164 ★ Reflexhollogy - Science, Art and Heart
143-24 Poplar Ave.
Flushing, NY 11355
Phone: (718)961-2786
Holly Papa, Director
Program(s): Reflexology.

★ 26165 ★ Rubenfeld Synergy Center
115 Waverly Pl.
New York, NY 10011
Free: 800-747-6897 **Fax:** (212)254-1174
Email: rubenfeld@aol.com
Ilana Rubenfeld, Director
Program(s): Rubenfeld Synergy Method.

★ 26166 ★ School of Homeopathy
964 3rd Ave., 8th Flr.
New York, NY 10155-0003
Phone: (212)570-2576 **Fax:** (212)758-4079
Email: kathy@homeopathyschool.com
Website: http://www.homeopathyschool.com
Kathleen A. Lukas, Director
Program(s): Homeopathy.

★ 26167 ★ Sivananda Yoga Ranch
PO Box 195
Woodbourne, NY 12788
Phone: (914)436-6492 **Fax:** (914)434-1032
Email: yogaranch@sivanada.org
Website: http://www.sivananda.org/ranch.htm
Program(s): Yoga Teacher Training.

★ 26168 ★ State University of New York, Brooklyn Health Science Center
450 Clarkson Ave., Box 1227
Brooklyn, NY 11203-2908
Phone: (718)270-7740 **Fax:** (718)270-7634
Liliana Montano, Director
Program(s): Midwifery.

★ 26169 ★ State University of New York, Stony Brook School of Nursing
Health Sciences Center
Stony Brook, NY 11794-8240
Phone: (516)444-2879 **Fax:** (516)444-6049
Linda Sacino, Director
Program(s): Midwifery.

★ 26170 ★ Swedish Institute Inc.
226 W 26th St., 5th Fl.
New York, NY 10001
Phone: (212)924-5900 **Fax:** (212)924-7600
Program(s): Acupressure; Acupuncture; Massage Therapy; Oriental Medicine; Shiatsu.

★ 26171 ★ Teleosis School of Homeopathy
61 W 62nd St.
New York, NY 10023
Phone: (212)707-8481 **Fax:** (212)707-8481
Kim Kalina, Director
Program(s): Homeopathy.

★ 26172 ★ Traditional Reiki Network
Fire No. 602, Case Hill Rd.
Treadwell, NY 13846-0262
Phone: (607)829-3702 **Fax:** (914)254-4835
Ellen Sokolow, Director
Program(s): Reiki.

★ 26173 ★ Tri-State Institute of Traditional Chinese Acupuncture
80 8th Ave., Ste. 400
New York, NY 10024
Phone: (212)242-2255 **Fax:** (212)242-2920
Mark D. Seem, PhD, Contact
Program(s): Acupuncture; Herbal Medicine; Traditional Chinese Medicine.

★ 26174 ★ Wise Woman Center
416 Fishcreek
Saugerties, NY 12477
Phone: (914)246-8081 **Fax:** (914)246-8081
Susun S. Weed, Director

Program(s): Animal Therapy; Energy Work; Herbal Medicine.

★ 26175 ★ Woodstock Polarity Retreat Center
872 Buck Rd.
Stone Ridge, NY 12484
Phone: (914)687-4767 **Free:** 800-925-0159
Fax: (212)327-4049
Email: johnb310@aol.com
John Beaulieu, PhD, Director
Program(s): Polarity Therapy.

★ 26176 ★ Yoga and Polarity Center
32 Church St.
Malverne, NY 11565
Phone: (516)596-0397 **Fax:** (516)887-4747
Amy Bubser, Director
Program(s): Energy Work; Polarity Therapy; Reflexology; Yoga Teacher Training.

North Carolina

★ 26177 ★ Academy of Natural Therapies
5 Piney View Estates
PO Box 9223
Marshall, NC 28753
Phone: (828)683-1737 **Fax:** (828)363-0265
Angela Plum, PhD, Director
Program(s): Acupressure; Aroomatherapy; CranioSacral Therapy; Polarity Therapy.

★ 26178 ★ Asheville School of Massage
729 Haywood Rd.
Asheville, NC 28806
Phone: (828)236-9977 **Fax:** (828)254-5613
Tracy McMahon, Director
Program(s): Acupressure; Aromatherapy; CranioSacral Therapy; Deep Tissue Massage; Energy Work; Manual Lymph Drainage; Massage Therapy; Polarity Therapy; Reflexology; Shiatsu; Yoga Teacher Training.

★ 26179 ★ Body Therapy Institute
300 S Wind Rd.
Siler City, NC 27344
Phone: (919)663-3111 **Free:** 888-500-4500
Fax: (919)663-0369
Rick Rosen, Director
Program(s): Massage Therapy.

★ 26180 ★ Doula Training
1007 W Lady Diana Ct.
Apex, NC 27502
Phone: (919)362-5517 **Fax:** (919)387-6273
Ann Tumblin, Director
Program(s): Doula.

★ 26181 ★ East Carolina University School of Nursing
Greenville, NC 27858
Phone: (919)328-4298
Nancy Moss, Director
Program(s): Midwifery.

★ 26182 ★ G-Jo Institute
PO Box 1460.
Columbus, NC 28722
Phone: (828)863-4660
Barbara Gail Watson, Director
Program(s): Acupressure; Reflexology.

★ 26183 ★ Lighten Up Yoga Center
60 Biltmore Ave.
Asheville, NC 28801
Phone: (828)254-7756 **Fax:** (828)254-3797
Alice Dawson, Director
Program(s): Yoga Teacher Training.

★ 26184 ★ Listening Hands Polarity
605 Jones Ferry Rd., EE2
Carrboro, NC 27510
Phone: (919)942-1819
Gabriella Tal, Director
Program(s): Polarity Therapy.

★ 26185 ★ Natural Touch School of Massage Therapy, Greensboro
4007 W Wendover
Greensboro, NC 27407
Free: 877-799-0060
Wanda Adkins, Director
Program(s): Acupressure; CranioSacral Therapy; Energy Work; Massage Therapy; Myofascial Release; Polarity Therapy; Shiatsu.

★ 26186 ★ New Life Empowerment Center
129 S Long St.
Salisbury, NC 28144
Phone: (704)633-2700 **Fax:** (704)633-2046
Thomas Hartman, Director
Program(s): Acupressure; Aromatherapy; Energy Work; Hypnotherapy; Qigong; Reflexology; Reiki.

★ 26187 ★ North Carolina School of Natural Healing
20 Battery Park Ave., Rm. 570
Asheville, NC 28801
Phone: (704)252-7096
Craig Ellis, Director
Program(s): Acupressure; Aromatherapy; CranioSacral Therapy; Energy Work; Herbal Medicine; Massage Therapy; Meditation; Polarity Therapy; Reiki; Shiatsu.

★ 26188 ★ Professional Institute of Massage Therapy, Fargo
4553 9th Ave. SW, Ste. 2
Fargo, NC 58103
Phone: (704)281-5078
Michael Stafford, Director
Program(s): Massage Therapy.

★ 26189 ★ Southeastern School of Neuromuscular Massage Therapy of Charlotte, Inc.
4 Woodlawn Green, Ste. 200
Charlotte, NC 28217
Phone: (704)527-4979 **Fax:** (704)527-3104
Email: massage@ch.mindspring.com
Website: http://www.se-massage.com
Kimberly Williams, Contact
Program(s): Massage Therapy; Neuromuscular Therapy.

★ 26190 ★ Therapeutic Massage Training Institute
726 E Blvd.
Charlotte, NC 28203
Phone: (704)338-9660 **Fax:** (704)523-4389
Email: asktmti@aol.com
Lynda L. Clay, Director
Program(s): Massage Therapy.

★ 26191 ★ Tree of Life Polarity Center
PO Box 281
Saxapahaw, NC 27340
Phone: (336)376-8186
Janice Durand, Director
Program(s): Energy Work; Polarity Therapy.

★ 26192 ★ Wellness Training Center
231 Erwin Hills Rd.
Asheville, NC 28806
Phone: (828)683-3369
Robert Luka, Director
Program(s): Hypnotherapy.

★ 26193 ★ Whole You School of Massage and Bodywork
143 Woodview Dr.
Rutherfordton, NC 28139
Phone: (828)287-0955 **Fax:** (828)287-0067
Kenneth Shew, Director
Program(s): Acupressure; Aromatherapy; CranioSacral Therapy; Deep Tissue Massage; Massage Therapy; Neuromuscular Therapy; Reflexology; Reiki.

North Dakota

★ 26194 ★ Sister Rosalind Gefre School of Professional Massage, Fargo
McMerty Ctr., 619 7th St., Ste. L
Fargo, ND 58102
Phone: (701)297-5993
Program(s): Deep Tissue Massage; Massage Therapy; Reflexology.

Nova Scotia

★ 26195 ★ ICT Northumberland College
1660 Hollis St., Ste. 301
Halifax, NS, Canada B3J 1V7
Phone: (902)425-2869 **Fax:** (902)425-2858
Dawn Schmidt, Contact
Program(s): Massage Therapy.

Ohio

★ 26196 ★ Alexander Technique of Cincinnati
954 W Northbend Rd.
Cincinnati, OH 45224
Phone: (513)542-1010
Vivien Schapera, Director
Program(s): Alexander Technique.

★ 26197 ★ Bhumi's Yoga and Wellness Center
25068 Center Rideg Rd.
Cleveland, OH 44145
Phone: (440)899-9569 **Fax:** (440)899-9569
Email: healingbreath@mediaone.net
Harriet Russell, Director
Program(s): Acupressure; Energy Work; Meditation; Polarity Therapy; Reiki; Shiatsu; Yoga Teacher Training.

★ 26198 ★ Case Western Reserve University
Frances Payne Bolton School of Nursing
10900 Euclid Ave.
Cleveland, OH 44106-4904
Phone: (216)368-2532
Marcia Riegger, Director
Program(s): Midwifery.

★ 26199 ★ Central Ohio School of Massage
1120 Morse Rd., Ste. 250
Columbus, OH 43229
Phone: (614)841-1122 **Fax:** (614)841-0387
Email: admissions@cosm.org
Website: http://www.cosm.org
Program(s): Massage Therapy.

★ 26200 ★ Cleveland School of Massage/ Advanced Bodywork Institute
10683 Ravenna Rd.
Twinsburg, OH 44087
Phone: (330)405-1933
Jeff Kates, Director
Program(s): Aromatherapy; Deep Tissue Massage; Energy Work; Myofascial Release; Polarity Therapy; Reflexology; Swedish Massage.

★ 26201 ★ Columbus Academy of Medical Massage
3600 Main St.
Hilliard, OH 43026
Phone: (614)777-1161 **Fax:** (614)336-8478
Jennifer Hastings-Schunn, Contact
Program(s): Aromatherapy; Massage Therapy; Medical Massage; Myofascial Release; Trigger Point Therapy.

★ 26202 ★ Columbus Polarity Therapy Institute
170 W 5th Ave.
Columbus, OH 43201
Phone: (614)299-9438 **Fax:** (614)291-7252
Mary Jo Ruggieri, Director
Program(s): Acupressure; Aromatherapy; Ayurvedic Medicine; CranioSacral Therapy; Energy Work; Naturopathic Medicine; Polarity Therapy; Reflexology.

★ 26203 ★ Cuyahoga Community College
4250 Richmond Rd.
Highland Hills, OH 44122-6195
Phone: (216)987-2426 **Fax:** (216)987-2450
Sheila Batheja, Director
Program(s): Massage Therapy.

★ 26204 ★ Healing Heart Herbals
36254 McCumber Rd.
Rutland, OH 45775
Phone: (740)742-8901
Cindy Parker, Director
Program(s): Aromatherapy; Ayurvedic Medicine; Energy Work; Herbal Medicine; Homeopathy; Oriental Medicine; Polarity Therapy; Reflexology; Traditional Chinese Medicine.

★ 26205 ★ Integrated Touch Therapy, Inc, for Animals
7041 Zane Trail Rd.
Circleville, OH 43113
Phone: (740)474-6436 **Fax:** (740)474-2625
Patricia Whalen-Shaw, Director
Program(s): Acupressure; Animal Therapy; CranioSacral Therapy; Energy Work; Equine Massage; Herbal Medicine; Massage Therapy; Polarity Therapy.

★ 26206 ★ International Academy for Reflexology Studies
4759 Cornell Rd., Ste. D
Cincinnati, OH 45241
Phone: (513)489-9328 **Fax:** (513)489-9354
Marcia L. Aschendorf, Director
Program(s): Reflexology.

★ 26207 ★ Massage Away, Inc, School of Therapy
6685 Doubletree Ave.
Columbus, OH 43229
Phone: (614)825-6278 **Fax:** (614)825-6279
Gail Quinn, Director
Program(s): Massage Therapy.

★ 26208 ★ National Institute of Massotherapy
2110 Copley Rd.
Akron, OH 44320
Phone: (330)867-1996 **Fax:** (330)869-6422
Stephen Perkinson, Director
Program(s): Acupressure; CranioSacral Therapy; Massage Therapy; Neuromuscular Therapy; Polarity Therapy; Reflexology; Reiki; Shiatsu.

★ 26209 ★ National Institute of Massotherapy, Garfield Heights
12684 Rockside Rd.
Garfield Heights, OH 44125
Phone: (216)662-6955 **Fax:** (216)662-6980
Ewa Perkinson, Director
Program(s): Massage Therapy; Neuromuscular Therapy; Ortho-Bionomy; Polarity Therapy; Shiatsu.

★ 26210 ★ Northwest Academy of Massotherapy
1910 Indian Wood Circle, Ste. 301
Maumee, OH 43537
Phone: (419)893-6464
Eric Ritchie, Director
Program(s): Massage Therapy; Reflexology; Sports Massage.

★ 26211 ★ Ohio Academy of Holistic Health, Inc.
3033 Dayton-Xenia Rd.
Beavercreek, OH 45434
Phone: (937)427-0506 **Free:** 800-833-8122
Fax: (937)426-8883
Jedidiah Smith, Director
Program(s): Aromatherapy; Energy Work; Herbal Medicine; Hypnotherapy; Iridology; NeuroLinguistic Programming; Reflexology; Reiki; Touch for Health.

★ 26212 ★ Ohio College of Massotherapy
225 Heritage Woods Dr.
Akron, OH 44321
Phone: (330)665-1084 **Fax:** (330)665-5021
Ann K. Morrow, Contact
Program(s): Acupressure; Aromatherapy; CranioSacral Therapy; Massage Therapy; Myofascial Release; Neuromuscular Therapy; Reflexology; Sports Massage.

★ 26213 ★ Ohio State University College of Nursing
1585 Neil Ave.
Columbus, OH 43210-1289
Phone: (614)292-4041
Nancy K. Lowe, Director
Program(s): Midwifery.

★ 26214 ★ Reflexology Science Institute
1170 Old Henderson Rd., Ste. 206
Columbus, OH 43220
Phone: (614)457-5783 **Fax:** (614)442-0133
Eileen Motok, Director
Program(s): Acupressure; CranioSacral Therapy; Energy Work; Polarity Therapy; Reflexology; Reiki

★ 26215 ★ Retha J. Martin School of Hypnotherapy
5018 Mason Rd.
Berlin Heights, OH 44814
Phone: (419)433-2912
Retha J. Martin, Contact
Program(s): Energy Work; Hypnotherapy; Reiki.

★ 26216 ★ SHI, Integrative Medical Massage School
130 Cook Rd.
PO Box 474
Lebanon, OH 45036
Phone: (513)932-8712 **Fax:** (513)932-8180
Sharon L. Barnes, PhD, Director
Program(s): Alexander Technique; Biofeedback; CranioSacral Therapy; Energy Work; Feldenkrais; Massage Therapy; Medical Massage; Myofascial Release; Neuromuscular Therapy; Polarity Therapy; Somatic Education; Therapeutic Touch.

★ 26217 ★ University of Cincinnati, College of Nursing and Health
PO Box 210038
Cincinnati, OH 45221-0038
Phone: (513)558-5282
Mary Carol Akers, Director
Program(s): Midwifery.

★ 26218 ★ Youngstown College of Massotherapy
14 Highland Ave.
Struthers, OH 44471
Phone: (330)755-1406 **Fax:** (330)755-1605
Douglas M. Shodd, Sr., Contact
Program(s): Massage Therapy.

Oklahoma

★ 26219 ★ Massage Therapy Institute of Oklahoma
9433 E 51st St., Ste. H
Tulsa, OK 74145
Phone: (918)622-6644 **Fax:** (918)622-3401
Email: mtio@swbell.net
Xerlan Geiser, Director
Program(s): Acupressure; Aromatherapy; CranioSacral Therapy; Massage Therapy; Oriental Medicine; Reflexology; Shiatsu; Sports Massage.

★ 26220 ★ Oklahoma School of Natural Healing
1660 E 71st, Ste. 2-O
Tulsa, OK 74136-5191
Phone: (918)496-9401 **Fax:** (918)496-4461
Dr. Robert L. Groves, Director
Program(s): Acupressure; CranioSacral Therapy; Energy Work; Herbal Medicine; Homeopathy; Massage Therapy; Naturopathic Medicine; Neuromuscular Therapy; Ortho-Bionomy; Polarity Therapy; Qigong; Reflexology; Reiki; Shiatsu; Sports Massage; Traditional Chinese Medicine.

★ 26221 ★ Praxis College of Health Arts and Sciences
808 NW 88
Oklahoma City, OK 73114
Phone: (405)949-2244 **Fax:** (405)946-7040
Andre F. Fountain, Director
Program(s): Acupressure; Acupuncture; Aromatherapy; CranioSacral Therapy; Energy Work; Herbal Medicine; Hydrotherapy; Massage Therapy; Oriental Medicine; Polarity Therapy; Qigong; Reflexology; Shiatsu; Sports Massage; Traditional Chinese Medicine.

Ontario

★ 26222 ★ Artemisia Institute for Botanical and Preventive Health Care Education
PO Box 190
Jackson's Point, ON, Canada L0E 1L0
Phone: (905)722-1074
Christine E. DeVai, Contact
Program(s): Herbal Medicine.

★ 26223 ★ British Institute of Homeopathy
1445 St. Joseph Blvd.
Gloucester, ON, Canada K1C 7K9
Phone: (613)830-4759 **Free:** 800-579-4325
Fax: (613)830-9174
Patty Smith, Contact

Program(s): Animal Therapy; Herbal Medicine; Homeopathy; Midwifery; Naturopathic Medicine; Nutrition.

★ 26224 ★ Canadian College of Massage and Hydrotherapy, Newmarket
543 Timothy St.
Newmarket, ON, Canada L3Y 1R1
Phone: (905)853-5553 **Fax:** (905)853-5324
Kim Fountaine, Contact
Program(s): Acupuncture; Herbal Medicine; Humanistic Counseling; Hydrotherapy; Massage Therapy; Traditional Chinese Medicine.

★ 26225 ★ Canadian College of Massage and Hydrotherapy, North York
5160 Yonge St., Ste. 505
North York, ON, Canada M2N 6L7
Phone: (416)222-3586 **Fax:** (416)222-9424
Margaret Ward, Contact
Program(s): Acupuncture; Herbal Medicine; Humanistic Counseling; Hydrotherapy; Massage Therapy; Traditional Chinese Medicine.

★ 26226 ★ Canadian College of Naturopathic Medicine
2300 Yonge St., 18th Flr., Box 2431
Toronto, ON, Canada M4P 1E4
Phone: (416)486-8584 **Fax:** (416)484-6821
Catharine Shewell, Contact
Program(s): Acupuncture; Bodywork and Manipulation; Clinical Nutrition; Herbal Medicine; Homeopathy; Hydrotherapy; Naturopathic Medicine; Traditional Chinese Medicine.

★ 26227 ★ Canadian Memorial Chiropractic College
1900 Bayview Ave.
Toronto, ON, Canada M4G 3E6
Phone: (416)482-2340 **Fax:** (416)482-9745
Stefan Pallister, Contact
Program(s): Chiropractic.

★ 26228 ★ D'Arcy Lane Institute, D'AL School of Equine Massage Therapy
627 Maitland St.
London, ON, Canada N5Y 2V7
Phone: (519)673-4420 **Fax:** (519)673-0645
Marnie Byloo, Contact
Program(s): Animal Therapy; Equine Massage; Massage Therapy.

★ 26229 ★ Esther Myers Yoga Studio
390 Dupont St.
Toronto, ON, Canada M5R 1V9
Phone: (416)944-0838 **Fax:** (416)944-9151
Linda Cherney, Contact
Program(s): Yoga Teacher Training.

★ 26230 ★ Homeopathic College of Canada
280 Eglinton Ave. E
Toronto, ON, Canada M4P 1L4
Phone: (416)481-8816 **Fax:** (416)481-4444
Luba Plotkin, Contact
Program(s): Homeopathy.

★ 26231 ★ ICT Kikkawa College
1678 Bloor St. W
Toronto, ON, Canada M6P 1A9
Phone: (416)762-4857 **Fax:** (416)762-5733
Program(s): Massage Therapy.

★ 26232 ★ Institute of Traditional Chinese Medicine
368 Dupont St.
Toronto, ON, Canada M5R 1V9
Phone: (416)925-6752 **Fax:** (416)925-8920
David Lam, Contact
Program(s): Acupressure; Acupuncture; Herbal Medicine; Oriental Medicine; Qigong; Traditional Chinese Medicine.

★ 26233 ★ Michener Institute for Applied Health Sciences
222 St. Patrick St.
Toronto, ON, Canada M5T 1V4
Phone: (416)596-3177 **Fax:** (416)596-3180
Angi Gallupe, Contact
Program(s): Acupuncture; Traditional Chinese Medicine.

★ 26234 ★ Reaching Your Potential
11181 Yonge St., Room 141
Richmond Hill, ON, Canada L4S 1L2
Phone: (905)944-8867 **Fax:** (905)944-8869
Sher Smith, Contact
Program(s): CranioSacral Therapy; Polarity Therapy.

★ 26235 ★ Shiatsu Academy of Tokyo
320 Danforth Ave., Ste. 206
Toronto, ON, Canada M4K 1N8
Phone: (416)466-8780 **Fax:** (416)466-8719
Jan McClory, Contact
Program(s): Shiatsu.

★ 26236 ★ Shiatsu School of Canada, Inc
SSC Acupuncture Institute
547 College St.
Toronto, ON, Canada M6G 1A9
Phone: (416)323-1818 **Free:** 800-263-1703
Fax: (416)323-1681
Euza Ierullo, Contact
Program(s): Acupuncture; Shiatsu.

★ 26237 ★ Sutherland-Chan School and Teaching Clinic
330 Dupont St., 4th Flr.
Toronto, ON, Canada M6R 1K4
Phone: (416)924-1107 **Fax:** (416)924-9413
Marion Bishop, Contact
Program(s): Massage Therapy.

★ 26238 ★ Toronto School of Homeopathic Medicine
17 Yorkville Ave., Ste. 200
Toronto, ON, Canada M4W 1L1
Phone: (416)966-2350 **Free:** 800-572-6001
Fax: (416)966-1724
Shobhna Kapoor, Contact
Program(s): Homeopathy.

Oregon

★ 26239 ★ American Herbal Institute
3056 Lancaster Dr. NE
Salem, OR 97305
Phone: (503)364-7242
Constance Walker, Director
Program(s): Aromatherapy; Herbal Medicine; Hypnotherapy; Nutrition; Reflexology; Traditional Chinese Medicine.

★ 26240 ★ Ashland Massage Institute
PO Box 1233
Ashland, OR 97520
Phone: (541)482-5134
Beth Hoffman, Director
Program(s): Massage Therapy.

★ 26241 ★ Australasian College of Herbal Studies
530 1st St., Ste. A
PO Box 57
Lake Oswego, OR 97034
Phone: (503)635-6652 **Fax:** (503)636-0706
Email: achs@herbed.com
Website: http://www.herbed.com
Dorene Petersen, Contact
Program(s): Aromatherapy; Flower Essences; Herbal Medicine; Homeobotanical Therapy; Homeopathy; Iridology.

★ 26242 ★ Birthingway Midwifery Center
4620 N Maryland Ave.
Portland, OR 97217
Phone: (503)282-5729 **Fax:** (503)282-5729
Holly Scholles, Director
Program(s): Midwifery.

★ 26243 ★ Cascade Institute of Massage and Body Therapies
1250 Charnelton St.
Eugene, OR 97401
Phone: (541)687-8101 **Fax:** (541)687-0285
Wendy Doran, Contact
Program(s): Acupressure; Energy Work; Massage Therapy; Shiatsu; Swedish Massage.

★ 26244 ★ East-West College of the Healing Arts
4531 SE Belmont St.
Portland, OR 97215-1635
Phone: (503)231-1500 **Free:** 800-635-9141
Fax: (503)232-4087
Email: ewcha@aol.com
Richard Martin, Director
Program(s): Energy Work; Massage Therapy; Polarity Therapy; Shiatsu; Sports Massage.

★ 26245 ★ Friends Landing International Centers for Conscious Living
492 E 13th St., Ste. 101
Eugene, OR 97401
Phone: (541)484-6004 **Fax:** (541)741-1705
Whitewind Swan Fisher, Director
Program(s): Hypnotherapy.

★ 26246 ★ International Loving Touch Foundation, Inc.
PO Box 16374
Portland, OR 97292
Phone: (503)253-8482 **Fax:** (503)256-6753
Diana Moore, Director
Program(s): Infant Massage.

★ 26247 ★ National College of Naturopathic Medicine
049 SW Porter
Portland, OR 97201
Phone: (503)499-4343
Clyde Jensen, PhD, Contact
Program(s): Herbal Medicine; Homeopathy; Naturopathic Medicine; Oriental Medicine; Traditional Chinese Medicine.

★ 26248 ★ Northwest Acupressure Institute
966 Lorane Hwy.
Eugene, OR 97405
Phone: (503)345-2220
Kamala Quale, Director
Program(s): Acupressure; Jin Shin Do; Oriental Medicine; Qigong.

★ 26249 ★ Northwest Center for Herbal Studies
86437 Lorane Hwy.
Eugene, OR 97405
Phone: (541)484-6708
Email: herbs@ordata.com
Cherie Capps, Director
Program(s): Herbal Medicine.

★ 26250 ★ Oregon Coast School of Massage
1845 SW Hwy 101, Ste. 2
Lincoln City, OR 97367
Phone: (541)994-2728
Margaret Welch, Director
Program(s): Deep Tissue Massage; Energy Work; Massage Therapy; Shiatsu; Tai Chi.

★ 26251 ★ Oregon College of Oriental Medicine
10525 SE Cherry Blossom Dr.
Portland, OR 97216
Phone: (503)253-3443 **Fax:** (503)253-2701
Email: lpowell@teleport.com
Website: http://www.infinite.org/oregon.acupuncture
Linda Powell, Contact
Program(s): Acupressure; Acupuncture; Herbal Medicine; Oriental Medicine; Qigong; Shiatsu; Traditional Chinese Medicine.

★ 26252 ★ Oregon Health Sciences University
School of Nursing
3181 SW Sam Jackson Park Rd.
Portland, OR 97210
Phone: (503)494-3114 **Fax:** (503)494-3878
Carol Howe, Director
Program(s): Midwifery.

★ 26253 ★ Oregon School of Massage
9500 SW Barbur Blvd., Ste. 100
Portland, OR 97219
Phone: (503)244-3420 **Free:** 800-844-3420
Fax: (503)244-1815
Email: osmlbg@teleport.com
Ray Siderius, Director
Program(s): Acupressure; Alexander Technique; CranioSacral Therapy; Energy Work; Massage Therapy; Neuromuscular Therapy; Oriental Medicine; Polarity Therapy; Reflexology; Reiki; Shiatsu; Traditional Chinese Medicine.

★ 26254 ★ Oregon School of Massage, Salem
440 Ferry St. NE
Salem, OR 97302-3605
Phone: (503)585-8912 **Free:** 800-844-3420
Fax: (503)585-0988
Lisa Barck Garofalo, Director
Program(s): Alexander Technique; Anatomy and Physiology; Energy Work; Kinesiology; Massage Therapy; Polarity Therapy; Reflexology; Reiki; Shiatsu; Sports Massage; Traditional Chinese Medicine.

★ 26255 ★ Oregon School of Midwifery
342 E 12th Ave.
Eugene, OR 97401
Phone: (541)338-9778 **Fax:** (541)338-9783
Daphne Singingtree, Director
Program(s): Midwifery.

★ 26256 ★ Polarity Center of Salem
1940 Breyman NE
Salem, OR 97301
Phone: (503)581-6512
Ann Watters, Contact
Program(s): Polarity Therapy.

★ 26257 ★ Professional Course in Veterinary Homeopathy
1283 Lincoln St.
Eugene, OR 97401
Phone: (541)342-7665 **Fax:** (541)344-5356
Susan Pitcairn, Director
Program(s): Animal Therapy; Homeopathy.

★ 26258 ★ Sage Femme Midwifery School
PO Box 91
O Brien, OR 97534
Phone: (541)596-2543 **Free:** 800-247-8422
Fax: (541)596-2543
Patricia Downing, Director
Program(s): Childbirth Education; Doula; Herbal Medicine; Homeopathy; Midwifery.

★ 26259 ★ Western States Chiropractic College
2900 NE 132nd St.
Portland, OR 97230
Phone: (503)251-5734 **Fax:** (503)251-5723
William Dallas, Contact
Program(s): Chiropractic.

Pennsylvania

★ 26260 ★ Academy of Medical Arts and Business
2301 Academy Dr.
Harrisburg, PA 17112-1012
Phone: (717)545-4747 **Fax:** (717)901-9090
Gary Kay, Director
Program(s): Acupressure; Aromatherapy; CranioSacral Therapy; Deep Tissue Massage; Hypnotherapy; Massage Therapy; Prenatal Massage; Reflexology; Reiki; Shiatsu; Yoga Teacher Training.

★ 26261 ★ Academy for Myofascial Trigger Point Therapy
1312 E Carson St.
Pittsburgh, PA 15203
Phone: (412)481-2553 **Fax:** (412)481-3279
Joe Erdos, Director
Program(s): Trigger Point Therapy.

★ 26262 ★ Alternative Conjunction Clinic and School of Massage Therapy
716 State St.
Lemoyne, PA 17043
Phone: (717)737-6001 **Fax:** (717)737-6607
Melodie A. Adinolfi, Director
Program(s): Aromatherapy; Chair Massage; Esalen Massage; Massage Therapy; Neuromuscular Therapy; Russian Massage; Swedish Massage.

★ 26263 ★ Berks Technical Institute
2205 Ridgewood Dr.
Wyomissing, PA 19610
Phone: (610)372-1722 **Fax:** (610)376-4684
Tony Dooley, Director
Program(s): Massage Therapy; Swedish Massage.

★ 26264 ★ Career Training Academy (Monroeville)
Expo Mart
105 Mall Blvd., Ste. 300W
Monroeville, PA 15146
Phone: (412)372-3900 **Free:** 800-491-3470
Fax: (412)373-4262
Email: jreddy@careerta.com
Website: http://www.careerta.com
Maryagnes Luczak, Director
Program(s): Acupressure; Aromatherapy; Massage Therapy; Reflexology; Shiatsu; Sports Massage; Swedish Massage.

★ 26265 ★ Career Training Academy (New Kensington)
703 5th Ave.
New Kensington, PA 15068-6301
Phone: (724)337-1000 **Free:** 800-600-3470
Fax: (724)335-7140
John Reddy, Contact
Program(s): Acupressure; Aromatherapy; Massage Therapy; Reflexology; Shiatsu; Swedish Massage.

★ 26266 ★ Center for Human Integration
8400 Pine Rd.
Philadelphia, PA 19111
Phone: (215)742-3505 **Fax:** (215)742-3507
Kathy Schival, Director
Program(s): Acupressure; Aromatherapy; CranioSacral Therapy; Energy Work; Herbal Medicine; Hypnotherapy; Massage Therapy; Polarity Therapy; Reflexology; Reiki; Therapeutic Touch; Touch for Health; Zero Balancing.

★ 26267 ★ Central Pennsylvania School of Massage, Inc.
336 S Fraser St.
State College, PA 16801
Phone: (814)234-4900 **Fax:** (814)234-0440
Tom Broeren, Director
Program(s): Acupressure; Aromatherapy; Ayurvedic Medicine; Deep Tissue Massage; Energy Work; Geriatric Massage; Infant Massage; Massage Therapy; Oriental Medicine; Prenatal Massage; Qigong; Reflexology; Reiki; Shiatsu; Sports Massage; Traditional Chinese Medicine; Yoga Teacher Training.

★ 26268 ★ East-West School of Massage Therapy
504 Park Rd. N
Wyomissing, PA 19610
Phone: (610)375-7520 **Fax:** (610)375-7554
Elizabeth Brubaker, Director
Program(s): Acupressure; Aromatherapy; Energy Work; Massage Therapy; Polarity Therapy; Reflexology; Reiki; Shiatsu; Sports Massage.

★ 26269 ★ Endless Mountain School of Shiatsu
RR1, Box 1741
Factoryville, PA 18419
Phone: (570)942-4481 **Fax:** (570)942-6139
Samuel R. Kupetsky, Director
Program(s): Acupressure; Energy Work; Herbal Medicine; Oriental Medicine; Shiatsu; Traditional Chinese Medicine; Visualization.

★ 26270 ★ Esthetic Training Institute
702 Fountain Ave.
Lancaster, PA 17601
Free: 800-446-2260 **Fax:** (610)292-0299
Rose Ann Acuazzo-Linkens, Contact
Program(s): Aromatherapy; Massage Therapy; Reflexology; Reiki.

★ 26271 ★ Feldenkrais Professional Training Programs
59 Pebble Woods
Doylestown, PA 18901
Phone: (215)230-9208 **Fax:** (215)230-9086
David Zemach-Bersin, Director
Program(s): Feldenkrais.

★ 26272 ★ Health Options Institute
1410 Main St.
Northampton, PA 18067
Phone: (610)261-0880 **Fax:** (610)261-2964
Elizabeth Bieber, Director
Program(s): Acupressure; Aromatherapy; Deep Muscle Massage; Herbal Medicine; Massage Therapy; Neuromuscular Therapy; Reflexology; Reiki; Shiatsu.

★ 26273 ★ Himalayan Institute
RR 1, Box 400
Honesdale, PA 18431
Phone: (570)253-5551 **Free:** 800-822-4547
Fax: (570)253-9078
Program(s): Meditation; Yoga Teacher Training.

★ 26274 ★ Institute of Midwifery, Women, and Health
222 Hayward Hall, School House Lane and Henry Ave.
Philadelphia, PA 19144
Phone: (215)843-5775 **Fax:** (215)951-2526
Kate Siegrist, Director
Program(s): Midwifery.

★ 26275 ★ International School of Shiatsu
10 S Clinton St., Ste. 300
Doylestown, PA 18901
Phone: (215)340-9918 **Fax:** (215)340-9181
Megan Wilson, Director
Program(s): Acupressure; Shiatsu.

★ 26276 ★ Lancaster School of Massage
317 N Queen St.
Lancaster, PA 17603
Phone: (717)293-9698
Winona F. Bontrager, Director
Program(s): Connective Tissue Massage; CranioSacral Therapy; Massage Therapy; Neuromuscular Therapy; Polarity Therapy; Reflexology; Sports Massage; Swedish Massage.

★ 26277 ★ Lehigh Valley Healing Arts Academy
5412 Shimerville Rd.
Emmaus, PA 18049
Phone: (610)965-6165 **Fax:** (610)965-6165
Bonita A. Cassel-Beckwith, Director
Program(s): Acupressure; Alexander Technique; Aromatherapy; Ayurvedic Medicine; CranioSacral Therapy; Energy Work; Feldenkrais; Herbal Medicine; Homeopathy; Massage Therapy; Meditation; Polarity Therapy; Reflexology; Reiki; Shiatsu; Sports Massage; Therapeutic Touch; Traditional Chinese Medicine; Trager; Yoga.

★ 26278 ★ Massage Arts and Sciences Center of Philadelphia
1515 Locust St., 2nd Fl.
Philadelphia, PA 19102
Phone: (215)985-0674 **Fax:** (215)985-0175
Rosemarie Glaser, Director
Program(s): Massage Therapy; Reiki; Shiatsu; Sports Massage.

★ 26279 ★ Meridian Shiatsu Institute
998 Old Eagle School Rd., Ste. 1212
Wayne, PA 19087
Phone: (610)293-4030 **Fax:** (610)971-9860
Email: caroleepf@aol.com
Carolee Parker, Director
Program(s): Acupressure; Qigong; Reflexology; Reiki; Shiatsu; Traditional Chinese Medicine.

★ 26280 ★ Mount Nittany Institute of Natural Health
301 Shiloh Rd.
State College, PA 16801
Phone: (814)238-1121 **Fax:** (814)238-8145
Jennifer Welch, Director
Program(s): Acupressure; Anatomy and Physiology; Aromatherapy; Connective Tissue Massage; Energy Work; Herbal Medicine; Holistic Health; Massage Therapy; Neuromuscular Therapy; Polarity Therapy; Reflexology; Shiatsu; Sports Massage; Swedish Massage; Tai Chi; Yoga.

★ 26281 ★ Myofascial Release Seminars
222 W Lancaster Ave.
Paoli, PA 19301
Free: 800-327-2425 **Fax:** (610)644-1662
Email: fascia@erols.com
Website: http://www.vll.com/mfr/
Sandra Levengood, Director
Program(s): Myofascial Release.

★ 26282 ★ Northeastern School of Medical Massage, Inc.
2525 W Main, 2nd Flr.
Norristown, PA 19403
Phone: (610)631-5188
Constance J. Perry, Director
Program(s): Acupressure; Aromatherapy; Infant Massage; Massage Therapy; Medical Massage; Neuromuscular Therapy; Pregnancy Massage; Reflexology; Sports Massage; Swedish Massage.

★ 26283 ★ Pennsylvania Institute of Massage Therapy
93 SW End Blvd., Ste. 102
Quakertown, PA 18951-1150
Phone: (215)538-5339 **Fax:** (215)538-8896
Robert Tosh, Contact
Program(s): Animal Therapy; CPR/First Aid; Massage Therapy; Reflexology; Shiatsu; Tai Chi.

★ 26284 ★ Pennsylvania School of Muscle Therapy, Ltd.
994C Old Eagle School Rd., Ste. 1005
Wayne, PA 19087
Phone: (610)687-0888 **Fax:** (610)687-4726
Email: psmt@psmt.com
Website: http://www.psmt.com
MaryJo Myers, Contact
Program(s): Aromatherapy; Deep Muscle Massage; Massage Therapy; Qigong; Reflexology; Shiatsu; Sports Massage; Swedish Massage; Traditional Chinese Medicine.

★ 26285 ★ Pittsburgh School of Massage Therapy
10989 Frankstown Rd.
Pittsburgh, PA 15235
Free: 800-860-1114 **Fax:** (412)241-4933
Email: pghschmass@aol.com
Robert Jantsch, Director
Program(s): Acupressure; Alexander Technique; Aromatherapy; Energy Work; Massage Therapy; Neuromuscular Therapy; Reflexology; Shiatsu; Sports Massage; Swedish Massage.

★ 26286 ★ Professional School of Massage
131 E Maple Ave.
Langhorne, PA 19047
Phone: (215)750-0700
David Scott, Director
Program(s): Acupressure; Herbal Medicine; Massage Therapy; Polarity Therapy; Qigong; Reflexology; Reiki; Shiatsu.

★ 26287 ★ A Rose Therapeutics
352 E 6th Ave.
Conshohocken, PA 19428
Phone: (610)834-8140
Aura Rose, Director
Program(s): Acupressure; CranioSacral Therapy; Energy Work; Feldenkrais; Herbal Medicine; Hypnotherapy; Massage Therapy; Neuromuscular Therapy; Reflexology; Reiki; Shiatsu; Sports Massage; Swedish Massage; Yoga.

★ 26288 ★ School of Body Therapies
931 Langhorne-Yardley Rd.
Langhorne, PA 19047-1368
Phone: (215)752-7666 **Fax:** (215)752-1909
Lisa Barck Garofalo, Director
Program(s): Deep Muscle Massage; Massage Therapy; Thai Massage.

★ 26289 ★ Somatic Institute, Pittsburgh
8600 W Barkhurst Dr.
Pittsburgh, PA 15237
Phone: (412)366-5580 **Fax:** (412)367-1029
Kay Miller, Director
Program(s): Alexander Technique; Core Somatics; Feldenkrais; Somatic Education.

★ 26290 ★ Unergi School of Holistic Therapy
PO Box 335
Point Pleasant, PA 18950
Phone: (215)297-8006 **Fax:** (215)297-8199
Ute Arnold, Director
Program(s): Alexander Technique; Energy Work; Feldenkrais; Hypnotherapy; Unergi Integrated Therapy.

★ 26291 ★ University of Pennsylvania School of Nursing
420 Guardian Dr.
Philadelphia, PA 19104-6096
Phone: (215)898-4335
William McCool, Director
Program(s): Midwifery.

★ 26292 ★ Valley Forge Institute of Muscle Therapy
808 Valley Forge Rd.
Phoenixville, PA 19460
Phone: (610)935-3554
Thomas V. O'Ancona, Director
Program(s): Chair Massage; Neuromuscular Therapy; Polarity Therapy; Reflexology; Reiki; Sports Massage; Swedish Massage.

Puerto Rico

★ 26293 ★ University of Puerto Rico, Medical Sciences Campus
PO Box 365067
San Juan, PR 00936
Phone: (787)759-6546 **Fax:** (787)759-6719
Irene G. dela Torre, Director
Program(s): Midwifery.

Quebec

★ 26294 ★ Canadian Academy of Homeopathy
1173 Boul Mont Royal
Outremont, QC, Canada H2V 2H6
Phone: (514)279-6629 **Fax:** (514)279-0111
Francine Gauthier, Contact
Program(s): Homeopathy.

★ 26295 ★ Centre Psycho-Corporel, Inc.
675 Marguerite Bourgeoys
Quebec, QC, Canada G1S 3V8
Phone: (418)687-1165 **Fax:** (418)687-1166
Aline Dumas, Contact
Program(s): Acupressure; Kinesiology; Manual Lymph Drainage; Massage Therapy; Qigong; Reflexology; Shiatsu; Sports Massage; Swedish Massage.

★ 26296 ★ Health Training Group
3789 Hampton Ave.
Montreal, QC, Canada H4A 2K7
Phone: (514)485-6373
Howard Kiewe, Contact
Program(s): Polarity Therapy.

★ 26297 ★ Polarity Associates of Montreal
5535 Beaucort, Ste. 10
Montreal, QC, Canada H3W 2T7
Phone: (514)739-4673 **Fax:** (514)440-0251
Andrea Axt, Contact
Program(s): CranioSacral Therapy; Polarity Therapy.

★ 26298 ★ Psychovisual Therapy Training
7306 Sherbrooke W
Montreal, QC, Canada H4B 1R7
Phone: (514)489-6733 **Fax:** (514)485-3828
Bryan M. Knight, Contact
Program(s): Hypnotherapy; Psychovisual Therapy.

Rhode Island

★ 26299 ★ University of Rhode Island College of Nursing
2 Heathman Rd.
Kingston, RI 02881
Phone: (401)874-5328 **Fax:** (401)874-2061
Holly Kennedy, Director
Program(s): Midwifery.

Saskatchewan

★ 26300 ★ Professional Institute of Massage Therapy, Saskatoon
485 1st Ave. N
Saskatoon, SK, Canada S7K 1X5
Phone: (306)955-5833 **Fax:** (306)955-5864
Tracy Bazlak, Contact
Program(s): Massage Therapy.

South Carolina

★ 26301 ★ Charleston School of Massage, Inc.
778 Folly Rd., Ste. 3
Charleston, SC 29412
Phone: (843)762-7727 **Fax:** (843)762-1392
Mark Hendler, Director
Program(s): Acupressure; Aromatherapy; Ayurvedic Medicine; Deep Tissue Massage; Energy Work; Herbal Medicine; Massage Therapy; Reflexology; Reiki; Shiatsu; Spa Therapies.

★ 26302 ★ Dovestar Institute
4C Northridge Dr.
Hilton Head Island, SC 29928
Phone: (803)342-3361 **Free:** 888-222-5603
Fax: (803)342-3639
Kamala Renner, Director
Program(s): Acupressure; Breathwork; Colon Hydrotherapy; Energy Work; Kriya Massage; Hypnotherapy; Massage Therapy; Qigong; Reflexology; Reiki; Shiatsu; Yoga Teacher Training.

★ 26303 ★ Horry Georgetown Technical College
743 Hemlock Ave.
Myrtle Beach, SC 29577
Phone: (843)477-0808 **Fax:** (843)477-0775
Lisa Aglietti, Director
Program(s): Massage Therapy.

★ 26304 ★ Massage School of MTA, Inc.
1901 Laurens Rd., Ste. H
Greenville, SC 29607
Phone: (864)232-9001
Kenn Elrod, Director
Program(s): Acupressure; Aromatherapy; CranioSacral Therapy; Deep Tissue Massage; Energy Work; Massage Therapy; Polarity Therapy; Reflexology; Reiki; Shiatsu.

★ 26305 ★ Medical University of South Carolina
College of Nursing
99 Jonathon Lucas St.
Charleston, SC 29403
Phone: (843)792-2051
Deborah Williamsom, Director
Program(s): Midwifery.

★ 26306 ★ Sherman College of Straight Chiropractic
2020 Springfield Rd.
Boiling Springs, SC 29316
Phone: (864)578-8770 **Fax:** (864)599-7145
Susan S. Newlin, Director
Program(s): Chiropractic.

★ 26307 ★ Southeastern School of Neuromuscular and Massage Therapy, Inc.
7000 N Pine St., Ste. 2B Pinewood Mall
Spartanburg, SC 29303
Phone: (864)591-1134 **Fax:** (864)582-7805
Janice Schuelke, Director
Program(s): Aromatherapy; Massage Therapy; Myofascial Release; Neuromuscular Therapy; Swedish Massage.

South Dakota

★ 26308 ★ Carrie's Kadesh and School of Massage
112 E 3rd Ave.
Mitchell, SD 57301
Phone: (605)996-3916
Carrie Badker, Director
Program(s): Acupressure; Aromatherapy; Massage Therapy; Polarity Therapy; Reflexology; Sports Massage.

★ 26309 ★ Scientific Massage Institute
1523 ½ Deadwood Ave.
Rapid City, SD 57702
Phone: (605)341-5402 **Fax:** (605)342-0554
Sandy Feist, Director
Program(s): Acupressure; Chair Massage; Infant Massage; Massage Therapy; Reflexology.

★ 26310 ★ South Dakota School of Massage Therapy
902 W 22nd St.
Sioux Falls, SD 57105
Phone: (605)334-4422 **Fax:** (605)334-4422
Robin Jensen, Director
Program(s): Acupressure; Anatomy and Physiology; Aromatherapy; Deep Tissue Massage; Hydrotherapy; Kinesiology; Massage Therapy; Qigong; Rebirthing; Reflexology; Shiatsu; Sports Massage; Swedish Massage; Yoga.

★ 26311 ★ Stress Management Services, Inc.
Sioux Falls School of Massage Therapy
317 S Cleveland Ave.
Sioux Falls, SD 57103
Phone: (605)330-0175
Kristie R. Knudtson, Director
Program(s): Massage Therapy.

Tennessee

★ 26312 ★ American Academy of Medical Hypnoanalysts
5628 Murray Rd., Ste. 4
Memphis, TN 38119-3876
Free: 800-344-9766 **Fax:** (901)683-1224
David Leistikow, Director
Program(s): Hypnotherapy.

★ 26313 ★ Cumberland Institute for Wellness Education
500 Wilson Pike Circle, Ste. 121
PO Box 1527
Brentwood, TN 37027
Phone: (615)370-9794 **Fax:** (615)370-5869
Chad Porter, Director
Program(s): Acupressure; Aromatherapy; CranioSacral Therapy; Lymphatic Massage; Massage Therapy; Sports Massage.

★ 26314 ★ Institute of Therapeutic Massage and Movement
1161 Murfreesboro Rd., Ste. 405
Nashville, TN 37217
Phone: (615)360-8554
Angela Wood, Director
Program(s): Deep Tissue Massage; Massage Therapy.

★ 26315 ★ Massage Institute of Memphis
3445 Poplar, Ste. 4
Memphis, TN 38111
Phone: (901)324-4411 **Fax:** (901)324-4470
Karen E. Craig, Director
Program(s): Energy Work; Healing Touch; Massage Therapy; Reflexology; Sports Massage; Trigger Point Therapy.

★ 26316 ★ Middle Tennessee Institute of Therapeutic Massage
394 W Main St., Ste. A-15
Hendersonville, TN 37075
Phone: (615)826-9500 **Fax:** (615)826-9527
Shannon Dickson, Director
Program(s): Aromatherapy; CranioSacral Therapy; Massage Therapy; Neuromuscular Therapy; Polarity Therapy; Reflexology; Shiatsu; Sports Massage.

★ 26317 ★ Natural Health Institute
209 10th Ave. S, Ste. 212
Nashville, TN 37203
Phone: (615)242-6811 **Fax:** (615)242-6288
Angela Schlitt, Director
Program(s): Acupressure; Ayurvedic Medicine; Feldenkrais; Herbal Medicine; Hypnotherapy; Massage Therapy; Polarity Therapy; Reflexology; Reiki; Somatic Education.

★ 26318 ★ Tennessee Institute of Healing Arts
5779 Brainerd Rd.
Chattanooga, TN 37411
Phone: (423)892-9882 **Free:** 800-735-1910
Fax: (423)892-5006
Email: tiha@aol.com
Alan Jordan, Director
Program(s): Massage Therapy; Neuromuscular Therapy.

★ 26319 ★ Tennessee School of Massage
4726 Poplar, Ste. 4
Memphis, TN 38117
Phone: (901)767-8484
Email: relax@touchofhealth.com
Website: http://www.touchofhealth.com
Cissie Pryor, Director
Program(s): Acupressure; Aromatherapy; Hypnotherapy; Massage Therapy; Polarity Therapy; Reflexology; Shiatsu; Spa Therapies; Swedish Massage.

★ 26320 ★ Vanderbilt University School of Nursing
102 Godchaux Hall
Nashville, TN 37240-0008
Phone: (615)322-3800
Barbara Petersen, Director
Program(s): Midwifery.

Texas

★ 26321 ★ Academy of Oriental Medicine, Austin
2700 W Anderson Ln., Ste. 117
Austin, TX 78757
Phone: (512)454-1188 **Fax:** (512)454-7001
Email: info@aoma.edu
Website: http://www.aoma.edu
Stuart Watts, Director
Program(s): Acupressure; Acupuncture; Herbal Medicine; Jin Shin Do; Oriental Medicine; Qigong; Shiatsu; Tai Chi; Traditional Chinese Medicine, Tui Na.

★ 26322 ★ American College of Acupuncture and Oriental Medicine
9100 Park W Dr.
Houston, TX 77063
Phone: (713)780-9777 **Fax:** (713)781-5781
Email: 102657.1730@compuserve.com
Website: http://www.acaom.edu
Minmay Liang, Director
Program(s): Acupuncture; Herbal Medicine; Homeopathy; Oriental Medicine; Traditional Chinese Medicine.

★ 26323 ★ Anne King's Hypnosis TRaining
109 Smokey River N
Boerne, TX 78006
Phone: (830)537-5411 **Fax:** (830)537-5404
Anne King, Contact
Program(s): Hypnotherapy.

★ 26324 ★ Asten Center of Natural Therapeutics
797 N Grove Rd., Ste. 101
Richardson, TX 75081
Phone: (972)669-3245 **Fax:** (972)669-1191
Jill Townsend, Contact
Program(s): Massage Therapy; Polarity Therapy; Reflexology; Sports Massage; Swedish Massage; Trigger Point Therapy.

★ 26325 ★ Austin School of Massage Therapy
2600 W Stassney
Austin, TX 78745
Phone: (512)462-3005 **Free:** 800-276-2768
Fax: (512)462-3265
Bob Brock, Director
Program(s): Holistic Health; Massage Therapy; Neuromuscular Therapy; Polarity Therapy; Reflexology; Shiatsu.

★ 26326 ★ Baylor College of Medicine
6550 Fannin, Ste. 901
Houston, TX 77030
Phone: (713)798-7594 **Fax:** (713)798-3579
Betty Carter, Director
Program(s): Midwifery.

★ 26327 ★ Beijing School of Acupuncture and Oriental Medicine
4109 Cagle Dr., Ste. F
Fort Worth, TX 76107
Phone: (817)284-3037 **Fax:** (817)284-1047
Dr. Hadi Kareem, Contact
Program(s): Acupuncture; Oriental Medicine.

★ 26328 ★ El Paso Community College
100 W Rio Grande
El Paso, TX 79902
Phone: (915)831-4116 **Fax:** (915)831-4131
Marta de la Fuente, Director
Program(s): Massage Therapy; Reflexology.

★ 26329 ★ El Paso School of Massage
661 S Mesa Hills Dr., Ste. 100
El Paso, TX 79912
Phone: (915)833-2935 **Fax:** (915)833-3094
Hilda L. Chavez, Director
Program(s): Hydrotherapy; Massage Therapy; Neuromuscular Therapy; Swedish Massage.

★ 26330 ★ European Massage Therapy Institute
7220 Louis Pasteur, Ste. 140
San Antonio, TX 78229
Phone: (210)615-8207 **Fax:** (210)614-3732
Rosario Perez Garza, Director
Program(s): Aromatherapy; Manual Lymph Drainage; Massage Therapy; Postural Analysis; Reflexology.

★ 26331 ★ Fort Worth School of Massage
2929 Cleburne Rd.
Fort Worth, TX 76110
Phone: (817)923-9944 **Fax:** (817)923-9944
Joetta Payne, Director
Program(s): CranioSacral Therapy Massage Therapy; Reflexology; Reiki.

★ 26332 ★ Giving Tree Cottage
1808 S St.
Nacogdoches, TX 75964
Phone: (409)560-6299 **Fax:** (409)569-9400
Jo Harbison, Director
Program(s): Massage Therapy.

★ 26333 ★ Greater Beaumont School of Massage
229 Dowlen Rd., Ste. 15A
Beaumont, TX 77706
Phone: (409)866-8661 **Fax:** (409)866-4371
Jennifer Smith, Director
Program(s): Massage Therapy.

★ 26334 ★ Hands On Therapy School of Massage
1101 E 5th St.
Tyler, TX 75701
Phone: (903)535-7733 **Fax:** (903)535-7799
Jeannine Martin, Director
Program(s): Aromatherapy; Massage Therapy; Reflexology; Shiatsu; Swedish Massage; Deep Tissue Massage.

★ 26335 ★ Healing Arts Institute, Lubbock
5601 Aberdeen, Ste. G
Lubbock, TX 79414
Phone: (806)797-0034
Kay Nash, Director
Program(s): Aromatherapy; Deep Tissue Massage; Energy Work; Hydrotherapy; Massage Therapy; Polarity Therapy; Reflexology; Shiatsu.

★ 26336 ★ Heartsong Hypnotherapy Training Center
4314 W Lovers Ln.
PO Box 7972
Dallas, TX 75209
Phone: (214)358-3633 **Fax:** (214)352-1338
Bette Epstein, Director
Program(s): Aromatherapy; Biofeedback; Energy Work; Hypnotherapy; Reiki.

★ 26337 ★ Hypnosis Institute of Houston
13700 Veterans Memorial, Ste. 230
Houston, TX 77014
Phone: (281)587-1055 **Fax:** (281)379-3153
Gerald L. Schoonover, Director
Program(s): Hypnotherapy.

★ 26338 ★ Institute of Natural Healing Sciences, Inc.
4100 Felps Dr., Ste. E
Colleyville, TX 76034
Phone: (817)498-0716 **Free:** 800-448-4954
Fax: (817)281-1414
Email: hmmj@nkn.net
Website: http://www.body-mind-spirit.com
Hollis M. Morrow, Contact
Program(s): Acupressure; Chair Massage; CranioSacral Therapy; Massage Therapy; Polarity Therapy; Reflexology; Shiatsu; Sports Massage.

★ 26339 ★ Lauterstein-Conway Massage School
4701-B Burnet Rd.
Austin, TX 78756
Phone: (512)374-9222 **Free:** 800-474-0852
Fax: (512)374-9812
John Conway, Director
Program(s): Acupressure; CranioSacral Therapy; Energy Work; Massage Therapy; Reflexology; Shiatsu; Sports Massage; Swedish Massage; Zero Balancing.

★ 26340 ★ Massage Therapy Clinic and School
2045 Space Park Dr., Ste. 200
Houston, TX 77058
Phone: (281)333-0400 **Fax:** (281)333-9010
Charline L. Utley, Director
Program(s): Deep Tissue Massage; Energy Work; Massage Therapy; Polarity Therapy; Reflexology; Shiatsu; Swedish Massage.

★ 26341 ★ Maternidad La Luz, the Birth Place
1308 Magoffin
El Paso, TX 79901
Phone: (915)532-5895 **Fax:** (915)532-7127
Deborah Kalley, Director
Program(s): Midwifery.

★ 26342 ★ Midland College Health Sciences Continuing Education
3600 N Garfield
Midland, TX 79705
Phone: (915)685-6440
Norma Chavez, Director
Program(s): Massage Therapy.

★ 26343 ★ Mind Body Naturopathic and Holistic Health Institute
10911 W Ave.
San Antonio, TX 78213
Phone: (210)308-8888 **Fax:** (210)349-5679
Jeri C. Tiller, Contact
Program(s): Aromatherapy; Colon Hydrotherapy; Massage Therapy; Reflexology; Reiki; Yoga.

★ 26344 ★ MRC School of Massage
2990 Richmond, Ste. 142
Houston, TX 77098
Phone: (713)522-1423 **Fax:** (713)522-1446
Robert I. Garza, Director
Program(s): Massage Therapy; Swedish Massage.

★ 26345 ★ Neuromuscular Concepts School of Massage
8607 Wurzbach Rd., Bldg. Q, Ste. 101
San Antonio, TX 78240

Phone: (210)558-3148 **Fax:** (210)558-3114
Paul Frizzell, Director
Program(s): Acupressure; Aromatherapy; Ayurvedic Medicine; CranioSacral Therapy; Energy Work; Feldenkrais; Herbal Medicine; Homeopathy; Massage Therapy; Neuromuscular Therapy; Oriental Medicine; Polarity Therapy; Qigong; Reflexology; Reiki; Shiatsu; Sports Massage; Traditional Chinese Medicine; Yoga Teacher Training.

★ 26346 ★ Parker College of Chiropractic
2500 Walnut Hill Ln.
Dallas, TX 75229
Phone: (214)438-6932 **Free:** 800-438-6932
Fax: (214)357-3620
Website: http://www.parkercc.edu
Reba Sexton, Contact
Program(s): Chiropractic.

★ 26347 ★ Parkland School of Nurse-Midwifery
5201 Harry Hines Blvd., MS 6107A
Dallas, TX 75235
Phone: (214)590-2580
Mary C. Brucker, Director
Program(s): Midwifery.

★ 26348 ★ PATH Foundation
1006 Burning Tree
Kingwood, TX 77339
Phone: (281)358-3700 **Fax:** (281)359-5700
Ed R. Martin, PhD, Director
Program(s): Hypnotherapy.

★ 26349 ★ Relax Station School of Massage Therapy
1409 Kingwood Dr.
Kingwood, TX 77339
Phone: (281)358-0600 **Fax:** (281)358-4089
Allen Boxman, Director
Program(s): Acupressure; Aromatherapy; CranioSacral Therapy; Massage Therapy; Neuromuscular Therapy; Sports Massage.

★ 26350 ★ Saint Phillip's College
1801 Martin Luther King Blvd.
San Antonio, TX 78203
Phone: (210)531-4770 **Fax:** (210)531-4774
Barbara Witte-Howell, Director
Program(s): Massage Therapy.

★ 26351 ★ School of Natural Therapy
4309 N 10th, Stes. A, B, C
McAllen, TX 78504
Phone: (956)630-0928 **Fax:** (956)630-6103
Lorena Granados, Director
Program(s): Deep Tissue Massage; Massage Therapy; Reflexology.

★ 26352 ★ South Texas Educational Center for Classical Homeopathy
13526 George Rd., Ste. 101
San Antonio, TX 78230-3002
Phone: (210)493-0561 **Fax:** (210)492-8013
Sandra J. Perko, Director
Program(s): Clinical Nutrition; Herbal Medicine; Homeopathy.

★ 26353 ★ Sterling Health Center
15070 Beltwood Pkwy.
Dallas, TX 75244
Phone: (972)991-9293 **Fax:** (972)991-3292
Dianna Lee, Director
Program(s): Anatomy and Physiology; Aromatherapy; Chair Massage; Deep Tissue Massage; Manual Lymph Drainage; Massage Therapy; Myofascial Release; Pregnancy Massage; Reflexology; Shiatsu; Sports Massage; Trigger Point Therapy.

★ 26354 ★ Texas Chiropractic College
5912 Spencer Hwy.
Pasadena, TX 77505-1699
Phone: (281)487-1170 **Free:** 800-468-6839
Fax: (281)991-4871
Email: gabbygreen@ol.com
S.M. Elliott, Contact
Program(s): Chiropractic.

★ 26355 ★ Texas College of Oriental Medicine, Inc.
3917 Booth Calloway Rd.
Richland Hills, TX 76118
Phone: (817)595-2339 **Fax:** (817)284-1047
Hadi Kareem, Director
Program(s): Acupressure; Herbal Medicine; Oriental Medicine; Traditional Chinese Medicine.

★ 26356 ★ Texas Healing Arts Institute, LLC, and School of Massage
2704 Rio Grande, Ste. 11
Austin, TX 78705
Phone: (512)236-8424 **Fax:** (512)236-1040
Jo Bunny, Director
Program(s): CranioSacral Therapy; Deep Tissue Massage; Hydrotherapy; Massage Therapy; Myofascial Release; Reflexology; Shiatsu.

★ 26357 ★ Texas Institute of Traditional Chinese Medicine
4005 Manchaca Rd., Ste. 102
Austin, TX 78704
Phone: (512)444-8082 **Free:** 800-252-5088
Fax: (512)444-6345
Email: texastcm@texastcm.edu
Website: http://www.texastcm.edu
Kermit Heimann, Director
Program(s): Acupuncture; Herbal Medicine; Oriental Medicine; Qigong; Traditional Chinese Medicine.

★ 26358 ★ Therapeutic Body Concepts
6162 Wurzbach Rd.
San Antonio, TX 78238
Phone: (210)684-6563 **Fax:** (210)680-2782
Leon Gosset, Contact
Program(s): Massage Therapy.

★ 26359 ★ University of North Texas
PO Box 311337
Denton, TX 76203-1337
Phone: (940)565-2910 **Fax:** (940)565-2905
Michael Attekruse, Director
Program(s): Biofeedback; Mental Health Counseling.

★ 26360 ★ University of Texas, El Paso/ Texas Tech University
4800 Alberta Ave.
El Paso, TX 79905
Phone: (915)545-6490
Carolyn Simmons, Director
Program(s): Midwifery.

★ 26361 ★ University of Texas, Galveston School of Nursing
1100 Mechanic
Galveston, TX 77555-1029
Phone: (409)772-8347 **Fax:** (409)772-3770
JoAnn Mahoney, Director
Program(s): Midwifery.

★ 26362 ★ Wellness Skills, Inc., Dallas
6102 E Mockingbird Ln., Ste. 401
Dallas, TX 75214-2620
Phone: (214)828-4000 **Fax:** (214)828-0065
Richard Nottingham, Director
Program(s): Aromatherapy; Massage Therapy; Polarity Therapy; Relexology; Shiatsu; Trigger Point Therapy.

★ 26363 ★ Wellness Skills, Inc., Fort Worth
6301 Airport Fwy., Ste. 200
Fort Worth, TX 76117-5360
Phone: (817)838-3800 **Fax:** (817)838-2933
Kelli Eager, Director
Program(s): Aromatherapy; Massage Therapy; Polarity Therapy; Reflexology; Shiatsu; Sports Massage; Trigger Point Therapy.

★ 26364 ★ Winters School Inc.
4625 SW Fwy., Ste. 142
Houston, TX 77027
Phone: (713)626-2200 **Fax:** (713)626-2230
Cari Denson West, Director
Program(s): Deep Tissue Massage; Massage Therapy; Polarity Therapy; Reflexology; Shiatsu.

★ 26365 ★ Yoga Institute and Bookshop
3830 Villanova St.
Houston, TX 77002-3640
Free: 800-524-6674
Lex Gillan, Director
Program(s): Yoga Teacher Training.

Utah

★ 26366 ★ Myotherapy College of Utah
1174 E 2700 S, Ste. 19
Salt Lake City, UT 84106
Phone: (801)484-7624 **Fax:** (801)484-1928
Sheriden Black, Director
Program(s): Aromatherapy; CranioSacral Therapy; Deep Tissue Massage; Energy Work; Homeopathy; Massage Therapy; Polarity Therapy; Reflexology; Reiki; Shiatsu.

★ 26367 ★ Ogden Institute of Massage Therapy
3500 Harrison Blvd.
Ogden, UT 84403
Phone: (801)627-8227 **Fax:** (801)627-2228
Craig S. Anderson, Director
Program(s): CranioSacral Therapy; Deep Tissue Massage; Massage Therapy; Shiatsu.

★ 26368 ★ School of Natural Healing
25 W 200 S
PO Box 412
Springville, UT 84663
Free: 800-372-8255 **Fax:** (801)489-8341
Email: snh@qi3.com
Website: http://www.homestar.net/school
David W. Christopher, Director
Program(s): Herbal Medicine.

★ 26369 ★ Sensory Development Institute
1871 W Canyon View Dr.
Saint George, UT 84770
Phone: (435)652-9003 **Fax:** (435)652-8949
Pam Shelline, Director
Program(s): Aromatherapy; Energy Work; Massage Therapy; Oriental Medicine; Reflexology; Shiatsu; Spa Therapies.

★ 26370 ★ University of Utah College of Nursing
10 S 2000 E Front
Salt Lake City, UT 84112-5880
Phone: (801)581-8274 **Fax:** (801)581-4642
Marilyn Stewart, Director
Program(s): Midwifery.

★ 26371 ★ Utah College of Massage Therapy
25 S 300 E
Salt Lake City, UT 84111
Free: 800-617-3302 **Fax:** (801)521-3339
Email: info@ucmt.com
Website: http://www.ucmt.com
Norman Cohn, Director
Program(s): Acupressure; CranioSacral Therapy; Deep Tissue Massage; Feldenkrais; Injury Massage; Infant Massage; Massage Therapy; Qigong; Reflexology; Shiatsu; Russian Massage; Touch for Health; Trigger Point Therapy.

★ 26372 ★ Utah College of Massage Therapy, Utah Valley Campus
135 S State St., Ste. 12
Lindon, UT 84042
Phone: (801)796-0300 **Fax:** (801)796-0309
Karyn Grant, Director
Program(s): Acupressure; CranioSacral Therapy; Energy Work; Feldenkrais; Massage Therapy; Neuromuscular Therapy; Reflexology; Shiatsu; Sports Massage.

★ 26373 ★ Utah College of Midwifery
230 W 170 N
Orem, UT 84057
Phone: (801)764-9068 **Free:** 888-489-1238
Suzanne Smith, Director
Program(s): Childbirth Educator; Doula; Midwifery.

Vermont

★ 26374 ★ Partner Earth Education Center
PO Box 298
Pawlet, VT 05761-0298
Phone: (802)325-2121 **Fax:** (802)325-2121
Pam Montgomery, Director
Program(s): Herbal Medicine; Plant Spirit Medicine.

★ 26375 ★ Sage Mountain Retreat Center and Botanical Sanctuary
PO Box 420
East Barre, VT 05649
Phone: (802)479-9825 **Fax:** (802)476-3722
Rosemary Gladstar, Director
Program(s): Herbal Medicine.

★ 26376 ★ Universal Institute of Healing Arts
RFD 3
Box 5285
Montpelier, VT 05602
Phone: (802)229-4844
Bob Onne, Director
Program(s): Acupressure; Deep Tissue Massage; Reflexology; Shiatsu.

★ 26377 ★ Vermont Institute of Massage Therapy
10 Cottage Grove Ave.
South Burlington, VT 05403
Phone: (802)862-1111 **Fax:** (802)660-3733
Kathleen Wright, Director
Program(s): Acupressure; Energy Work; Massage Therapy; Reflexology.

★ 26378 ★ Vermont School of Professional Massage
14 Merchant St.
Barre, VT 05641
Phone: (802)479-2340
Faeterri Silver, Director
Program(s): Massage Therapy.

Virginia

★ 26379 ★ Alexander Technique Center of Washington DC
PO Box 449
McLean, VA 22101
Phone: (703)821-4277
Marian Goldberg, Director
Program(s): Alexander Technique.

★ 26380 ★ Applied Kinesthetic Studies School of Massage
692 Pine St.
Herndon, VA 20170
Phone: (703)464-0333 **Fax:** (703)464-5999
Katharine Hunter, Director
Program(s): Swedish Massage.

★ 26381 ★ Blue Ridge School of Massage and Yoga
201 S Main St.
Blacksburg, VA 24060
Phone: (540)552-2177
Colleen A. Kelly, Director
Program(s): Acupressure; Alexander Technique; Deep Tissue Massage; Energy Work; Massage Therapy; Meditation; Polarity Therapy; Qigong; Reflexology; Reiki; Shiatsu; Traditional Chinese Medicine; Yoga.

★ 26382 ★ Cayce/Reilly School of Massotherapy
215 67th St.
Virginia Beach, VA 23451
Phone: (757)437-7202 **Fax:** (757)428-0398
Email: are@are-cayce.com
Website: http://www.are-cayce.com
Dwight Zieman, Contact
Program(s): Acupressure; Alexander Technique; Aromatherapy; CranioSacral Therapy; Hypnotherapy; Massage Therapy; Neuromuscular Therapy; Reflexology; Reiki; Sports Massage.

★ 26383 ★ Eastern Institute of Hypnotherapy
PO Box 249
Goshen, VA 24439-0249
Phone: (540)997-0325 **Free:** 800-296-6463
Fax: (540)997-0324
Email: hyptrainer@aol.com
Allen S. Chips, Director
Program(s): Hypnotherapy; Neuro-Linguistic Programming.

★ 26384 ★ Eastern Institute of Reiki Therapy
Transpersonal Reiki Institute
956 Knob Rd.
PO Box 249
Goshen, VA 24439-0249
Phone: (540)997-0325 **Free:** 800-296-6463
Fax: (540)997-0324
Email: hyptrainer@aol.com
Dee Chips, Director
Program(s): Reiki.

★ 26385 ★ Equissage, Inc.
15715 Southern Cross Ln.
Round Hill, VA 20141
Free: 800-843-0224 **Fax:** (540)338-5569
Nelson R. Schreiber, Director
Program(s): Animal Therapy; Deep Tissue Massage; Equine Massage.

★ 26386 ★ Fuller School of Massage Therapy
3500 Virginia Beach Blvd.
Virginia Beach, VA 23452
Phone: (757)340-7132 **Fax:** (757)486-2192
Nancy Bender, Director
Program(s): Aromatherapy; CranioSacral Therapy; Herbal Medicine; Homeopathy; Massage Therapy; Polarity Therapy; Prenatal Massage; Qigong; Reflexology; Reiki; Shiatsu; Sports Massage.

★ 26387 ★ Institute for Integrated Therapies
3708 N Rosser St., Ste. 201
Alexandria, VA 22311
Phone: (703)931-8340 **Fax:** (703)931-8567
Margaret L. D'Urso, Director
Program(s): CranioSacral Therapy; Massage Therapy; Reflexology; Vibrational Therapy.

★ 26388 ★ National Center for Instruction of Homeopathy and Homeotherapeutics
National Center for Homeopathy Annual Summer School
801 N Fairfax St., Ste. 306
Alexandria, VA 22314
Phone: (703)548-7790 **Fax:** (703)548-7792
Email: nchinfo@igc.apc.org
Website: http://www.healthy.net
Stephen Messer, Contact
Program(s): Animal Therapy; Homeopathy.

★ 26389 ★ Natural Touch School of Massage Therapy
291 Park Ave.
Danville, VA 24541
Phone: (804)799-0060
Wanda Adkins, Director
Program(s): Acupressure; CranioSacral Therapy; Energy Work; Massage Therapy; Myofascial Release; Polarity Therapy; Shiatsu.

★ 26390 ★ Natural Touch School of Massage Therapy
1202 Main St.
Lynchburg, VA 24504
Phone: (804)845-3003
Wanda Adkins, Director
Program(s): Acupressure; CranioSacral Therapy; Energy Work; Massage Therapy; Myofascial Release; Polarity Therapy; Shiatsu.

★ 26391 ★ Piedmont School of Professional Massage
12712 Directors Loop
Woodbridge, VA 22192
Phone: (703)497-4437
Alan Coyne, Director
Program(s): Massage Therapy.

★ 26392 ★ Richmond Academy of Massage
2004 Bremo Rd., Ste. 102
Richmond, VA 23226
Phone: (804)282-5003 **Fax:** (804)288-7356
D.C. Ashburn, Director
Program(s): Massage Therapy.

★ 26393 ★ Satchidananda Ashram - Yogaville
Rt. 1, Box 1720
Buckingham, VA 23921

Phone: (804)969-3121 **Free:** 800-858-9642
Fax: (804)969-1303
Program(s): Yoga Teacher Training.

★ 26394 ★ Shenandoah University
1775 N Sector Ct.
Winchester, VA 22601
Phone: (540)678-4382 **Fax:** (540)665-5519
Juliana Fehr, Director
Program(s): Midwifery.

★ 26395 ★ Virginia Academy of Massage Therapy
5314 George Washington Memorial Hwy.
Yorktown, VA 23692
Phone: (757)872-0934 **Fax:** (757)898-0620
Barbara Marker, Director
Program(s): Acupressure; CranioSacral Therapy; Deep Tissue Massage; Energy Work; Hypnotherapy; Massage Therapy; Reflexology; Traditional Chinese Medicine.

★ 26396 ★ Virginia School for Alexander Technique
1021 Sheridan Ave.
Charlottesville, VA 22901
Phone: (804)977-7186
Daria T. Okugawa, Director
Program(s): Alexander Technique.

★ 26397 ★ Virginia School of Massage
2008 Morton Dr.
Charlottesville, VA 22903
Phone: (804)293-4031 **Fax:** (804)293-4190
Email: registrar@vasom.com
Sue Ellis Dyar, Contact
Program(s): Massage Therapy.

★ 26398 ★ Virginia School of Massage, Blacksburg
106B Southpark Dr.
Blacksburg, VA 24060
Phone: (804)293-4031 **Fax:** (804)293-4190
Lori Nicolaysen, Director
Program(s): Massage Therapy.

★ 26399 ★ Virginia School of Massage, Winchester
2820 Valley Ave.
Winchester, VA 22601
Phone: (804)293-4031 **Fax:** (804)293-4190
Lori Nicolaysen, Director
Program(s): Massage Therapy.

Washington

★ 26400 ★ Ashmead College, Everett
2721 Wetmore Ave.
Everett, WA 98201
Phone: (425)339-2678 **Fax:** (425)258-2620
Website: http://www.ashmeadcollege.com
Cheryl France, Director
Program(s): Anatomy and Physiology; Aromatherapy; CPR/First Aid; Geriatric Massage; Hydrotherapy; Kinesiology; Massage Therapy; Pregnancy Massage; Spa Therapies; Sports Massage.

★ 26401 ★ Ashmead College, Seattle
7120 Woodlawn Ave. NE
Seattle, WA 98115
Phone: (206)527-0807 **Fax:** (206)527-1957
Website: http://www.ashmeadcollege.com
Marsha Aldinger, Director
Program(s): Anatomy and Physiology; Aromatherapy; First Aid/CPR; Geriatric Massage; Hydrotherapy; Kinesiology; Massage Therapy; Pregnancy Massage; Spa Therapies; Sports Massage.

★ 26402 ★ Ashmead College, Tacoma Campus
5005 Pacific Hwy. E, Ste. 20
Fife, WA 98424
Phone: (253)926-1435
Website: http://www.ashmeadcollege.com
Julie Currier, Director
Program(s): Anatomy and Physiology; Aromatherapy; CPR/First Aid; Geriatric Massage; Hydrotherapy; Kinesiology; Massage Therapy; Pregnancy Massage; Spa Therapies; Sports Massage.

★ 26403 ★ Ayur-vedic Medicine, Yoga Therapy, UltraNutrition School
819 NE 65th St.
Seattle, WA 98115
Phone: (206)729-9999 **Fax:** (206)729-0164
Program(s): Aromatherapy; Ayurvedic Medicine; Herbal Medicine; Naturopathic Medicine; Yoga Therapy.

★ 26404 ★ Bastyr University
14500 Juanita Dr. NE
Kenmore, WA 98028-4966
Phone: (425)823-1300 **Fax:** (425)823-6222
Sandra Lane, Director
Program(s): Acupuncture; Ayurvedic Medicine; Herbal Medicine; Homeopathy; Midwifery; Naturopathic Medicine; Nutrition; Qigong; Shiatsu; Traditional Chinese Medicine.

★ 26405 ★ Bellevue Massage School
16301 NE 8th St., Ste. 106
Bellevue, WA 98008
Phone: (425)641-3409 **Fax:** (425)641-3409
Elise Hockett, Director
Program(s): Deep Tissue Massage; Energy Work; Massage Therapy; Reflexology; Touch for Health.

★ 26406 ★ BodyMind Academy
1247 120th Ave. NE
Bellevue, WA 98005
Phone: (425)635-0145 **Fax:** (425)635-3588
Thomas J. Johnston, Director
Program(s): Breathwork; Hypnotherapy; Massage Therapy; Shiatsu.

★ 26407 ★ BodyMind Energetics Institute
15832 34th Ave. NE
Seattle, WA 98155
Phone: (206)361-4700
Reed Svadesh Johnson, Director
Program(s): Orgodynamics; Qigong; Shiatsu; Trager.

★ 26408 ★ Brenneke School of Massage
160 Roy St.
Seattle, WA 98109
Phone: (206)282-1233 **Fax:** (206)282-9183
Heida Brenneke, Director
Program(s): CranioSacral Therapy; Massage Therapy; Polarity Therapy; Relexology; Reiki; Shiatsu; Sports Massage.

★ 26409 ★ Brian Utting School of Massage
900 Thomas St.
Seattle, WA 98109
Phone: (206)292-8055 **Free:** 800-842-8731
Fax: (206)292-0113
Brian Utting, Director
Program(s): Connective Tissue Massage; Deep Tissue Massage; Hydrotherapy; Injury Treatment and Evaluation; Massage Therapy; Neuromuscular Therapy; Sports Massage.

★ 26410 ★ Cedar Mountain Center for Massage, Inc.
5601 NE St. John's Rd.
Vancouver, WA 98661
Phone: (360)696-2210 **Fax:** (360)696-0130
Sandra V. Hattan, Director
Program(s): Aromatherapy; Massage Therapy; Polarity Therapy; Reflexology; Shiatsu; Sports Massage.

★ 26411 ★ Heartspring Transformation Trainings
5404 Meridian Ave. N
Seattle, WA 98103
Phone: (206)547-4064
Email: byheart@wolfenet.com
Pamela Grace, Director
Program(s): Hypnotherapy; Reiki.

★ 26412 ★ Inland Massage Institute
111 E Magnesium Rd., Ste. F
Spokane, WA 99208
Phone: (509)465-3033 **Fax:** (509)326-1236
Sheryl L. Storro, Contact
Program(s): Massage Therapy; Swedish Massage.

★ 26413 ★ Institute of Dynamic Aromatherapy
2000 2nd Ave., Ste. 206
Seattle, WA 98121
Phone: (206)374-8773 **Free:** 800-260-7401
Fax: (206)374-9020
Jade Shutes, Director
Program(s): Aromatherapy; Herbal Medicine; Reflexology.

★ 26414 ★ Institute for Therapeutic Learning
9322 21st Ave. NW
Seattle, WA 98117
Phone: (206)783-1838
Email: jelias@sprynet.com
Website: http://www.home.sprynet.com/sprynet/jelias
Jack Elias, Director
Program(s): Energy Work; Hypnotherapy.

★ 26415 ★ North American Institute of Neuro-Therapy
117 E Louisa. Ste. 188
Seattle, WA 98102
Phone: (206)322-0633
Marilyn Michael, Director
Program(s): Neuro-Therapy.

★ 26416 ★ Northwest Institute of Acupuncture and Oriental Medicine
701 N 34th St., Ste 300
Seattle, WA 98103
Phone: (206)633-2419 **Fax:** (206)633-5578
Email: niaom@halcyon.com
Website: http://www.halcyon.com/niaom
Frederick O. Lanphear, PhD, Contact
Program(s): Acupuncture; Oriental Medicine; Traditional Chinese Medicine.

★ 26417 ★ Peninsula College
1502 E Lauridsen Blvd.
Port Angeles, WA 98362
Phone: (360)417-6569
Dona Smasal, Director
Program(s): Aromatherapy; Deep Muscle Massage; Energy Work; Massage Therapy; Oriental Medicine; Shiatsu.

★ 26418 ★ Seattle Institute of Oriental Medicine
916 NE 65th St., Ste. B
Seattle, WA 98115

Phone: (206)517-4541 Fax: (206)526-1932
Email: info@siom.com
Website: http://www.siom.com
Dan Bensky, Director
Program(s): Acupuncture; Oriental Medicine; Traditional Chinese Medicine.

★ 26419 ★ Seattle Midwifery School
2524 16th Ave. S, Room 300
Seattle, WA 98109
Phone: (206)322-8834
Melissa Hicks, Director
Program(s): Childbirth Education; Doula; Midwifery.

★ 26420 ★ Soma Institute
730 Klink
Buckley, WA 98321
Phone: (360)829-1025 **Fax:** (360)829-2805
Karen L. Bolesky, Director
Program(s): Soma Neuromuscular Integration.

★ 26421 ★ Spectrum Center School of Massage
12506 18th St. NE, Ste. 1
Lake Stevens, WA 98258
Phone: (425)334-5409
Barbara Collins, Director
Program(s): CranioSacral Therapy; Massage Therapy; Polarity Therapy; Sports Massage.

★ 26422 ★ Tacoma Community College Alliance Hypnotherapy Professional Hypnosis Training
30640 Pacific Hwy. S, Ste. E
Federal Way, WA 98003
Phone: (206)927-8888 **Fax:** (206)566-5020
Roy Hunter, Contact
Program(s): Hypnotherapy.

★ 26423 ★ Tri City School of Massage
26 E 3rd Ave.
Kennewick, WA 99336
Phone: (509)586-6434
Patty J. Kruschke, Director
Program(s): Massage Therapy.

★ 26424 ★ University of Washington School of Nursing
PO Box 357262
Seattle, WA 98195-7262
Phone: (206)543-8241
Aileen MacClaren, Director
Program(s): Midwifery.

★ 26425 ★ Wellness Institute
3716 274th Ave. SE
Issaquah, WA 98029
Phone: (425)391-9716 **Fax:** (425)391-9737
David Hartman, Director
Program(s): Breathwork; Energy Work; Hypnotherapy.

★ 26426 ★ Yoga Centers
2255 140th Ave. NE, Stes. E and F
Bellevue, WA 98005
Phone: (425)746-7476 **Fax:** (425)746-3961
Mona Renner, Director
Program(s): Aromatherapy; Energy Work; Yoga Teacher Training.

West Virginia

★ 26427 ★ Mountain State School of Massage
3407 River Lane Dr.
PO Box 4487
Malden, WV 25306
Phone: (304)926-8822 **Fax:** (304)926-8837
Robert Rogers, Director
Program(s): Anatomy and Physiology; Chair Massage; Connective Tissue Massage; Hydrotherapy; Kinesiology; Massage Therapy; Neuromuscular Therapy; Polarity Therapy; Reflexology; Shiatsu; Sports Massage; Swedish Massage.

Wisconsin

★ 26428 ★ Blue Sky Educational Foundation, Professional School of Massage and Therapeutic Bodywork
220 Oak St.
Grafton, WI 53024
Phone: (414)376-1011 **Fax:** (414)376-7707
Vicki Chossek, Director
Program(s): Massage Therapy.

★ 26429 ★ Capri College Massage Therapy Program
6414 Odana Rd.
Madison, WI 53719
Phone: (608)274-5390 **Fax:** (608)274-1215
Program(s): Acupressure; Aromatherapy; Massage Therapy; Reflexology; Reiki; Shiatsu; Swedish Massage.

★ 26430 ★ Fox Valley School of Massage
2003 N Meade St.
Appleton, WI 54914
Phone: (920)722-3271 **Fax:** (920)882-9412
Tom Finch, Director
Program(s): Aromatherapy; Massage Therapy; Neuromuscular Therapy; Polarity Therapy; Qigong; Reiki.

★ 26431 ★ Institute for Wholistic Education
33719 116th St.
Twin Lakes, WI 53181
Phone: (414)877-9396 **Fax:** (414)889-8591
Santosh Krinsky, Contact
Program(s): Ayurvedic Medicine.

★ 26432 ★ Lakeside School of Massage Therapy
1726 N 1st St., Ste. 100
Milwaukee, WI 53212
Phone: (414)372-4345 **Fax:** (414)372-5350
Email: lakeschool@aol.com
Claude Gagnon, Director
Program(s): Acupressure; Massage Therapy; Reflexology; Shiatsu.

★ 26433 ★ Marquette University College of Nursing
PO Box 1881
Milwaukee, WI 53201-1881
Phone: (414)288-3842
Leona Vandevusse, Director
Program(s): Midwifery.

★ 26434 ★ Midwest Center for the Study of Oriental Medicine
6226 Bankers Rd., Ste. 8
Racine, WI 53403
Phone: (414)554-2010 **Fax:** (414)554-7475
Email: dunbardoc@aol.com
Dr. William Dunbar, Contact
Program(s): Acupressure; Acupuncture; Herbal Medicine; Oriental Medicine; Traditional Chinese Medicine.

★ 26435 ★ Milwaukee School of Massage
830 E Chambers St.
Milwaukee, WI 53212
Phone: (414)347-1151
Wanda M. Beals, Director
Program(s): Acupressure; Ayurvedic Medicine; CranioSacral Therapy; Energy Work; Feldenkrais; Massage Therapy; Myofascial Release; Oriental Medicine; Reiki; Swedish Massage.

★ 26436 ★ Saint Croix Center for the Healing Arts, Ltd.
411 County Hwy UU
Hudson, WI 54016
Phone: (715)381-1402 **Fax:** (715)381-1502
June Motzer-Trollen, Director
Program(s): Acupressure; Aromatherapy; Massage Therapy; Reflexology; Sports Massage.

★ 26437 ★ SpiriTouch Institute, Inc.
6225 University
Madison, WI 53705
Phone: (608)236-9042 **Fax:** (608)236-9570
Lori Hellenbrand, Director
Program(s): Energy Work; Massage Therapy; Reiki.

★ 26438 ★ Wisconsin Institute of Chinese Herbology
6921 Mariner Dr.
Racine, WI 53406
Phone: (414)886-5858 **Fax:** (414)886-5858
Email: herbalstudies@aol.com
Arthur D. Shattuck, Director
Program(s): Animal Therapy; Herbal Medicine; Oriental Medicine; Traditional Chinese Medicine.

★ 26439 ★ Wisconsin Institute of Natural Wellness
6921 Mariner Dr.
Racine, WI 53406
Phone: (414)886-3344 **Fax:** (414)632-9533
Arthur D. Shattuck, Director
Program(s): Acupressure; Massage Therapy; Reflexology; Reiki; Shiatsu; Tai Chi; Traditional Chinese Medicine.

Blood Bank Technology

Facilities listed below offer Specialist in Blood Bank (SBB) education programs accredited by the American Association of Blood Banks (8101 Glenbrook Rd., Bethesda, MD 20814-2749, (301)907-6977, http://www.aabb.org) in collaboration with the Commission on Accreditation of Allied Health Education Programs (35 E Wacker Dr., Ste. 1970, Chicago, IL 60601-2208, (312)553-9355, http://www.caahep.org/).

District of Columbia

★ 26440 ★ Walter Reed Army Medical Center
Department of Pathology and ALS
U.S. Army Blood Bank Fellowship Program
Specialist in Blood Bank Technology Program
6900 Georgia Ave. NW
Washington, DC 20307-5001
Phone: (202)782-6210 **Fax:** (202)782-4502
Email: william.turcan@na.amedd.army.mil

Website: http://www.wramc.army.mil
William Turcan, Director
Maj. D. Joe Chaffin, MD, Contact

Florida

★ 26441 ★ Florida Blood Services Transfusion Medicine Academic Center Specialist in Blood Bank Technology Program
10100 Ninth St. N
Saint Petersburg, FL 33713
Phone: (727)568-5433 **Fax:** (727)568-1177
Email: mdoty@fbsblood.org
Website: http://www.fbsblood.org/academic.asp
Marjorie Doty, Director
German Felix LeParc, MD, Contact

Illinois

★ 26442 ★ University of Illinois, Chicago College of Applied Health Sciences Specialist in Blood Bank Technology Program
1919 W Taylor St.
M/C 530
Chicago, IL 60612-7249
Phone: (312)996-6721 **Fax:** (312)996-8342
Email: veronica@uic.edu
Website: http://www.sbhis.uic.edu/
Veronica N. Lewis, Director
Sanobar Kahn, MD, CNT

Louisiana

★ 26443 ★ Medical Center of Louisiana Charity Hospital Specialist in Blood Bank Technology Program
1532 Tulane Ave.
New Orleans, LA 70112-2860
Phone: (504)903-2466 **Fax:** (504)903-2635
Email: kkirkl@lsumc.edu
Karen C. Kirkley, Contact
Yuan S Kao, MD, CNT

Maryland

★ 26444 ★ Johns Hopkins Hospital Specialist in Blood Bank Technology Program
Carnegie Bldg., Rm. 656
600 N Wolfe St.
Baltimore, MD 21287-6667
Phone: (410)955-6580 **Fax:** (410)955-0618
Email: cberite1@jhmi.edu
Christine M. Beritela, Director
Paul Ness, MD, CNT

★ 26445 ★ U.S. Department of Health and Human Services National Institutes of Health (NIH) Clinical Center Blood Bank Specialist in Blood Bank Technology Program
NIH/CC/DTM Bldg. 10, Rm. 1C711
10 Center Dr., MSC 1184
Bethesda, MD 20892-1184
Phone: (301)496-8335 **Fax:** (301)402-9990
Email: kbyrne@mail.cc.nih.gov
Website: http://www.nih.gov
Karen Byrne, Contact
David F. Stroncek, MD, Contact

Ohio

★ 26446 ★ Ohio State University Medical Center Blood Bank American Red Cross Blood Services, Central Ohio Region Specialist in Blood Bank Technology Program
995 E Broad St.
Columbus, OH 43205
Phone: (614)253-2740 **Fax:** (614)253-2487
Email: kosankej@usa.redcross.org
Joanne Kosanke, Director
Mary Wissel, MD, CNT

★ 26447 ★ University of Cincinnati Medical Center Hoxworth Blood Center Specialist in Blood Bank Technology Program
3130 Highland Ave.
PO Box 670055
Cincinnati, OH 45267-0055
Phone: (513)558-1259 **Fax:** (513)558-1279
Email: catherine.beiting@uc.edu
Website: http://www2.hoxworth.org/hoxworth/ed-uopp.htm
Catherine Beiting, Contact
Thomas Zuck, MD, CNT

Texas

★ 26448 ★ Gulf Coast School of Blood Bank Technology Specialist in Blood Bank Technology Program
1400 La Concha Ln.
Houston, TX 77054-1802
Phone: (713)791-6201 **Fax:** (713)791-6610
Email: cwong@giveblood.org
Website: http://www.giveblood.org
Clare Wong, Director
Arthur Bracey, MD, Contact

★ 26449 ★ University of Texas Health Science Center at San Antonio Department of Clinical Laboratory Sciences Specialist in Blood Bank Technology Program
7703 Floyd Curl Dr.
San Antonio, TX 78229-3900
Phone: (210)567-8869 **Fax:** (210)567-8875
Email: smithla@uthscsa.edu
Website: http://www.uthscsa.edu
Linda A. Smith, PhD, Director
Chantal Harrison, MD, CNT

★ 26450 ★ University of Texas Medical Branch, Galveston Specialist in Blood Bank Technology Program
301 University Blvd.
Galveston, TX 77555-0717
Phone: (409)772-4866 **Fax:** (409)772-5683
Email: jvincent@utmb.edu
Website: http://www.utmb.edu/sbb
Janet Vincent, DIR
Alexander Indrikovs, MD, Contact

★ 26451 ★ University of Texas Southwestern Medical Center Specialist in Blood Bank Technology Program
5323 Harry Hines Blvd.
Dallas, TX 75390-8878
Phone: (214)648-1785 **Fax:** (214)648-1029
Email: barbara.fryer@utsouthwestern.edu
Website: http://www.swmed.edu/education/allied/
Barbara Laird-Fryer, Contact
Harold Kaplan, MD, Contact

Wisconsin

★ 26452 ★ Blood Center of Southeastern Wisconsin Specialist in Blood Bank Technology Program
638 N 18th St.
Milwaukee, WI 53233
Phone: (414)937-6403 **Fax:** (414)937-6202
Email: lrlemense@bcsew.edu
Website: http://www.bloodctrwise.org
Lynne R. LeMense, Contact
Janice G. McFarland, MD, CNT

Chiropractic

Listed below are programs and institutions accredited by The Council on Chiropractic Education, 8049 N 85th Way, Scottsdale, AZ 85258, (480)443-8877, http://ace-usa.org. Information on chiropractic as a career is available from the American Chiropractic Association, 1701 Clarendon Blvd., Arlington, VA 22209, (800)986-4636, http://www.amerchiro.org.

California

★ 26453 ★ Cleveland Chiropractic College, Los Angeles
590 N Vermont Ave.
Los Angeles, CA 90004
Phone: (323)660-6166 **Free:** 800-466-2252
Fax: (323)906-2090
Email: givradm@cleveland.edu
Website: http://www.clevelandchiropractic.edu

★ 26454 ★ Life Chiropractic College, West
25001 Industrial Blvd.
Hayward, CA 94545
Phone: (510)780-4500 **Free:** 800-788-4476
Fax: (510)780-4515
Email: gclum@LifeWest.edu
Website: http://www.lifewest.edu
Gerard W. Clum, President

★ 26455 ★ Palmer College of Chiropractic, West
90 E Tasman Dr.
San Jose, CA 95134
Phone: (408)944-6005 **Free:** 800-442-4476
Fax: (408)944-6111
Email: riekeman_g@palmer.edu
Website: http://www.palmer.edu
Guy Riekeman, President

★ 26456 ★ Southern California University of Health Sciences Los Angeles College of Chiropractic
16200 E Amber Valley Dr.
PO Box 1166
Whittier, CA 90609-1166
Phone: (562)902-3330 **Free:** 800-221-5222
Fax: (562)947-7863
Email: reedphillips@scuhs.edu
Website: http://www.scuhs.edu
Reed B. Phillips, PhD, President

Connecticut

★ 26457 ★ University of Bridgeport College of Chiropractic
75 Linden Ave.
Bridgeport, CT 06601
Phone: (203)576-4278 **Free:** 888-822-4476
Fax: (203)576-4483
Email: frank.zolli@snet.net
Website: http://www.bridgeport.edu/chiro
Frank A. Zolli, Contact

Georgia

★ 26458 ★ Life University College of Chiropractic
1269 Barclay Circle
Marietta, GA 30060
Phone: (770)424-0554 **Free:** 800-543-3202
Fax: (770)429-4819
Email: drsid@life.edu
Website: http://www.life.edu
Sid E. Williams, President

Illinois

★ 26459 ★ National University of Health Sciences
College of Professional Studies
Doctor of Chiropractic Degree Program
200 E Roosevelt Rd.
Lombard, IL 60148-4583
Phone: (630)889-6604 **Free:** 800-826-6285
Fax: (630)889-6600
Email: jwinterstein@nuhs.edu
Website: http://www.nuhs.edu
James F. Winterstein, President

Iowa

★ 26460 ★ Palmer College of Chiropractic
1000 Brady St.
Davenport, IA 52803
Phone: (563)884-5621 **Free:** 800-722-2586
Fax: (563)884-5409
Email: riekeman_g@palmer.edu
Website: http://www.palmer.edu

Minnesota

★ 26461 ★ Northwestern Health Sciences University
Northwestern College of Chiropractic
2501 W 84th St.
Bloomington, MN 55431
Phone: (952)885-5410 **Free:** 800-888-4777
Fax: (952)886-7583
Email: njohnson@nwhealth.edu
Website: http://www.nwhealth.edu
Alfred D. Traina, President

Missouri

★ 26462 ★ Cleveland Chiropractic College, Kansas City
6401 Rockhill Rd.
Kansas City, MO 64131
Phone: (816)501-0100 **Free:** 800-467-2252
Fax: (816)361-0272
Email: drcsciii@cleveland.edu
Website: http://www.clevelandchiropractic.edu
Carl S. Cleveland, III, President

★ 26463 ★ Logan College of Chiropractic
1851 Schoettler Rd.
PO Box 1065
Chesterfield, MO 63006-1065
Phone: (636)227-2100 **Free:** 800-782-3344
Fax: (636)207-2420
Email: goodman@logan.edu
Website: http://www.logan.edu
George A. Goodman, President

New York

★ 26464 ★ New York Chiropractic College
2360 State Rd. 89
PO Box 800
Seneca Falls, NY 13148-0800
Phone: (315)568-3100 **Free:** 800-234-6922
Fax: (315)568-3012
Email: fnicchi@nycc.edu
Website: http://www.nycc.edu
Frank Nicchi, President

Ontario

★ 26465 ★ Canadian Memorial Chiropractic College
1900 Bayview Ave.
Toronto, ON, Canada M4G 3E6
Phone: (416)482-2340 **Fax:** (416)482-9745
Website: http://www.cmcc.ca
Jean A. Moss, President

Oregon

★ 26466 ★ Western States Chiropractic College
2900 NE 132nd Ave.
Portland, OR 97230
Phone: (503)251-5712 **Free:** 800-641-5641
Fax: (503)251-2817
Email: whdallas@wschiro.edu
Website: http://www.wschiro.edu
William H. Dallas, President

Quebec

★ 26467 ★ University of Quebec, Trois Rivieres
Chiropractic Program
CP 500
Trois Rivieres, QC, Canada G9A 5H7
Phone: (819)376-5186 **Fax:** (819)376-5204
Email: andre_m_gonthier@uqtr.uquebec.ca
Dr. Andre-Marie Gonthier, Director

South Carolina

★ 26468 ★ Sherman College of Straight Chiropractic
2020 Springfield Rd.
PO Box 1452
Spartanburg, SC 29304
Phone: (864)578-8770 **Free:** 800-849-8771
Fax: (864)599-7145
Email: jhardee@sherman.edu
Website: http://www.sherman.edu
Jerry L. Hardee, President

Texas

★ 26469 ★ Parker College of Chiropractic
2500 Walnut Hill Ln., Ste. 100E
Dallas, TX 75229-5668
Phone: (214)902-3470 **Free:** 800-438-6932
Fax: (214)352-6603
Email: president@parkercc.edu
Website: http://www.parkercc.edu
Fabrizio Mancini, President

★ 26470 ★ Texas Chiropractic College
5912 Spencer Hwy.
Pasadena, TX 77505-1699
Phone: (281)487-1170 **Free:** 800-468-6839
Fax: (281)487-0329
Email: smelliott@txchiro.edu
Website: http://www.txchiro.edu
Shelby M. Elliott, President

Dentistry

The following dental schools are accredited by the Commission on Dental Accreditation of the American Dental Association (ADA). For information on all dental programs, including advanced dental education, dental hygiene, dental assistant, and dental laboratory technician, contact the ADA at 211 E Chicago Ave., Chicago, IL 60611, (312)440-2500, http://www.ada.org/.

Alabama

★ 26471 ★ University of Alabama, Birmingham
School of Dentistry
1919 7th Ave. S
Birmingham, AL 35294
Phone: (205)934-4720 **Fax:** (205)934-9283
Website: http://www.dental.uab.edu
Dr. Mary Lynne Capilouto, Director

California

★ 26472 ★ Loma Linda University
School of Dentistry
Loma Linda, CA 92350
Phone: (909)558-1200 **Free:** 800-422-4558
Fax: (714)824-4211
Website: http://www.llu.edu/llu/dentistry
Dr. Charles J. Goodacre, Director

★ 26473 ★ University of California, Los Angeles
School of Dentistry
Center for the Health Sciences
10833 Leconte Ave., Rm. 53-038
Los Angeles, CA 90095-1668
Phone: (310)825-7354 **Fax:** (310)206-5539
Website: http://www.dent.ucla.edu
Dr. No-Hee Park, Director

★ 26474 ★ University of California, San Francisco
School of Dentistry
513 Parnassus Ave., S-630
San Francisco, CA 94143
Phone: (415)476-1323 **Fax:** (415)476-4226
Website: http://www.ucsf.edu
Dr. Charles Bertolami, Director

★ 26475 ★ University of the Pacific
School of Dentistry
2155 Webster St.
San Francisco, CA 94115
Phone: (415)929-6400 **Fax:** (415)929-6654
Website: http://www.dental.uop.edu
Dr. Arthur A. Dugoni, Director

★ 26476 ★ University of Southern California
School of Dentistry
University Park, MC-0641, Rm. 203
Los Angeles, CA 90089-0641
Phone: (213)740-2800 **Fax:** (213)740-3607
Website: http://www.usc.edu/hsc/dental
Dr. Harold Slavkin, Director

Colorado

★ 26477 ★ University of Colorado Medical Center
School of Dentistry
4200 E 9th Ave.
Box C-284
Denver, CO 80262
Phone: (303)315-8752 **Fax:** (303)315-8773
Website: http://www.uchsc.edu/sd/sd
Dr. Howard M. Landesman, Director

Connecticut

★ 26478 ★ University of Connecticut
School of Dental Medicine
263 Farmington Ave.
Farmington, CT 06032-5332
Phone: (203)679-2808 **Fax:** (203)679-1330
Website: http://sdm.uchc.edu
Dr. Peter J. Robinson, Director

District of Columbia

★ 26479 ★ Howard University
College of Dentistry
600 W St. NW
Washington, DC 20059
Phone: (202)806-0440 **Fax:** (202)806-0354
Website: http://www.howard.edu
Dr. Charles Sanders, Director

Florida

★ 26480 ★ Nova Southeastern University
College of Dental Medicine
3200 S University Dr.
Fort Lauderdale, FL 33328
Phone: (954)262-7319 **Fax:** (954)262-1782
Website: http://www.nova.edu/cwis/centers/hpd/dental
Dr. Robert Uchin, Director

★ 26481 ★ University of Florida
College of Dentistry
PO Box 100405
Gainesville, FL 32610-0405
Phone: (352)392-2911 **Fax:** (352)392-3070
Website: http://www.dental.ufl.edu
Dr. Frank A. Catalanotto, Director

Georgia

★ 26482 ★ Medical College of Georgia
School of Dentistry
1459 Laney Walker Blvd.
Augusta, GA 30912-0200
Phone: (706)721-3587 **Fax:** (706)721-6276
Website: http://www.mcg.edu/SOD
Dr. Brad J. Potter, Director

Illinois

★ 26483 ★ Southern Illinois University
School of Dental Medicine
Bldg. 273/2300
2800 College Ave.
Alton, IL 62002
Phone: (618)474-7170 **Fax:** (618)474-7150
Website: http://www.siue.edu/DMSCH
Dr. Patrick Ferrillo, Jr., Director

★ 26484 ★ University of Illinois, Chicago
College of Dentistry
801 S Paulina St.
Chicago, IL 60612
Phone: (312)996-7520 **Fax:** (312)996-1022
Website: http://dentistry.uic.edu
Dr. Bruce S. Graham, Director

Indiana

★ 26485 ★ Indiana University
School of Dentistry
1121 W Michigan St.
Indianapolis, IN 46202
Phone: (317)274-7957 **Fax:** (317)274-2419
Website: http://www.iusd.iupui.edu
Dr. Lawrence Goldblatt, Director

Iowa

★ 26486 ★ University of Iowa
College of Dentistry
Dental Bldg.
Iowa City, IA 52242
Phone: (319)335-9650 **Fax:** (319)335-7155
Website: http://www.uiowa.edu/homepage/academics
Dr. David Johnsen, Director

Kentucky

★ 26487 ★ University of Kentucky
College of Dentistry
Medical Center
800 Rose St.
Lexington, KY 40536-0084
Phone: (606)233-5850 **Fax:** (606)258-1042
Website: www.mc.uky.edu/Dentistry
Dr. Leon A. Assael, Director

★ 26488 ★ University of Louisville
School of Dentistry
Health Sciences Center
Louisville, KY 40202
Phone: (502)588-5293 **Fax:** (502)588-7163
Website: http://www.dental.louisville.edu/dental
Dr. John N. Williams, Director

Louisiana

★ 26489 ★ Louisiana State University
School of Dentistry
1100 Florida Ave., Bldg. 101
New Orleans, LA 70119
Phone: (504)619-8700
Website: http://www.lsusd.lsumc.edu
Dr. Eric J. Hovland, Contact

Maryland

★ 26490 ★ University of Maryland
Baltimore College of Dental Surgery
666 W Baltimore St., Rm. 4-A-11
Baltimore, MD 21201
Phone: (410)706-7461 **Fax:** (410)706-0406
Website: http://www.dental.umaryland.edu
Dr. Richard Ranney, Director

Massachusetts

★ 26491 ★ Boston University
Henry M. Goldman School of Dental Medicine
100 E Newton St.
Boston, MA 02118
Phone: (617)638-4700 **Fax:** (617)638-4490
Website: http://dentalschool.bu.edu
Dr. Spencer N. Frankl, Director

★ 26492 ★ Harvard University
School of Dental Medicine
188 Longwood Ave.
Boston, MA 02115
Phone: (617)432-1405 **Fax:** (617)432-4266
Website: http://www.hsdm.med.harvard.edu
Dr. R. Bruce Donoff, Director

★ 26493 ★ Tufts University
School of Dental Medicine
1 Kneeland St.
Boston, MA 02111
Phone: (617)636-7000 **Fax:** (617)636-0309
Website: http://www.tufts.edu/dental
Dr. Lonnie H. Norris, Director

Michigan

★ 26494 ★ University of Detroit Mercy
School of Dentistry
8200 W Outer Dr.
PO Box 98
Detroit, MI 48219-0900
Phone: (313)446-1800 **Free:** 800-635-5020
Fax: (313)446-1839
Dr. H. Robert Steiman, Director

★ 26495 ★ University of Michigan
School of Dentistry
1234 Dental Bldg.
Ann Arbor, MI 48109-1078
Phone: (734)763-6933 **Fax:** (313)747-4024
Website: http://www.dent.umich.edu
Dr. William E. Kotowicz, Director

Minnesota

★ 26496 ★ University of Minnesota
School of Dentistry
515 SE Delaware St.
Minneapolis, MN 55455
Phone: (612)625-9982 **Fax:** (612)626-2654
Website: http://www.umn.edu/dental
Dr. Peter Polverini, Director

Mississippi

★ 26497 ★ University of Mississippi
School of Dentistry
Medical Center
2500 N State St.
Jackson, MS 39216-4505
Phone: (601)984-6028
Website: http://www.dentistry.umc.edu
Dr. Willie J. Hill, Director

Missouri

★ 26498 ★ University of Missouri, Kansas City
School of Dentistry
650 E 25th St.
Kansas City, MO 64108
Phone: (816)235-2100 **Fax:** (816)235-2157
Website: http://www.umkc.edu/dentistry
Dr. Michael J. Reed, Director

Nebraska

★ 26499 ★ Creighton University
School of Dentistry
2500 California St.
Omaha, NE 68178
Phone: (402)280-5060 **Fax:** (402)280-5094
Website: http://cudental.creighton.edu
Dr. Wayne W. Barkmeier, Director

★ 26500 ★ University of Nebraska Medical Center
College of Dentistry
Medical Center
40th and Holdrege Sts.
Lincoln, NE 68583-0740
Phone: (402)472-1363 **Free:** 800-626-8431
Fax: (402)472-6681
Website: http://www.unmc.edu/dentistry
Dr. John Reinhardt, Director

New Jersey

★ 26501 ★ University of Medicine and Dentistry of New Jersey
Dental School
110 Bergen St.
Newark, NJ 07103-2425
Website: http://www.umdnj.edu
Dr. Cecile Feldman, Director

New York

★ 26502 ★ Columbia University
School of Dental and Oral Surgery
630 W 168th St.
New York, NY 10032
Phone: (212)305-2500 **Fax:** (212)305-7134
Website: http://cpmcnet.columbia.edu/dept/dental
Dr. Ira B. Lamster, Director

★ 26503 ★ New York University
College of Dentistry
345 E 24th St.
New York, NY 10010
Phone: (212)998-9800 **Fax:** (212)995-4080
Website: http://www.nyu.edu/Dental
Dr. Michael C. Alfano, Director

★ 26504 ★ State University of New York, Buffalo
School of Dental Medicine
325 Squire Hall
Buffalo, NY 14214
Phone: (716)829-2836 **Fax:** (716)829-2387
Website: http://www.sdm.buffalo.edu
Dr. Richard N. Buchanan, Director

★ 26505 ★ State University of New York, Stony Brook
School of Dental Medicine
Rockland Hall
Stony Brook, NY 11794-8700
Phone: (516)632-8950 **Fax:** (516)632-9105
Website: http://www.informatics.sunysb.edu/dental
Dr. Barry R. Rifkin, Director

North Carolina

★ 26506 ★ University of North Carolina, Chapel Hill
School of Dentistry
104 Brauer Hall, 211-H
Chapel Hill, NC 27599-7450
Phone: (919)966-1161 **Fax:** (919)966-4049
Website: http://www.dent.unc.edu
Dr. John W. Stamm, Director

Ohio

★ 26507 ★ Case Western Reserve University
School of Dentistry
2123 Abington Rd.
Cleveland, OH 44106
Phone: (216)368-3200 **Fax:** (216)368-3204
Website: http://www.cwru.edu/dental/casewebsite
Dr. Jerold Goldberg, Director

★ 26508 ★ Ohio State University
College of Dentistry
305 W 12th Ave.
Columbus, OH 43210
Phone: (614)292-9755 **Fax:** (614)292-7619
Website: www.dent.ohio-state.edu
Dr. Jan E. Kronmiller, Director

Oklahoma

★ 26509 ★ University of Oklahoma
College of Dentistry
PO Box 26901
Oklahoma City, OK 73190
Phone: (405)271-5444 **Fax:** (405)271-3423
Email: dentistry@ouhsc.edu
Website: http://dentistry.ouhsc.edu
Dr. Stephen K. Young, Director

Oregon

★ 26510 ★ Oregon Health Sciences University
School of Dentistry, Sam Jackson Pk.
611 SW Campus Dr.
Portland, OR 97201
Phone: (503)494-8801 **Fax:** (503)494-8801
Website: http://www.ohsu.edu/sod-A
Dr. Sharon P. Turner, Director

Pennsylvania

★ 26511 ★ Temple University
School of Dentistry
3223 N Broad St.
Philadelphia, PA 19140
Phone: (215)221-2803 **Fax:** (215)221-2802
Website: http://www.temple.edu
Dr. Martin F. Tansy, Director

★ 26512 ★ University of Pennsylvania
School of Dental Medicine
4001 W Spruce St.
Philadelphia, PA 19104
Phone: (215)898-8961 **Fax:** (215)898-5243
Website: http://www.dental.upenn.edu
Dr. Raymond Fonseca, Director

★ 26513 ★ University of Pittsburgh
School of Dental Medicine
3501 Terrace St.
Pittsburgh, PA 15261
Phone: (412)648-8900 **Fax:** (412)648-8219
Website: http://www.dental.pitt.edu
Dr. Thomas Braun, Director

Puerto Rico

★ 26514 ★ University of Puerto Rico
School of Dentistry
Medical Sciences Campus
PO Box 365067
San Juan, PR 00936-5067
Phone: (787)758-2525 **Fax:** (787)751-0990
Dr. Fernadndo Haddock, Director

South Carolina

★ 26515 ★ Medical University of South Carolina
College of Dental Medicine
171 Ashley Ave.
Charleston, SC 29425
Phone: (803)792-3811 **Fax:** (803)792-0390
Website: http://www2.musc.edu/dentistry/dental.html
Dr. Richard De Champlain, Director

Tennessee

★ 26516 ★ Meharry Medical College
School of Dentistry
1005 Dr. D.B. Todd Blvd.
Nashville, TN 37208
Phone: (615)327-6207 **Fax:** (615)327-6213
Dr. William B. Butler, Director

★ 26517 ★ University of Tennessee, Memphis
College of Dentistry
875 Union Ave.
Memphis, TN 38163
Phone: (901)448-6204 **Free:** 800-788-0040
Fax: (901)448-7104
Website: http://www.utmem.edu/dentistry
Dr. William F. Slagle, Director

Texas

★ 26518 ★ Texas A&M University
Baylor College of Dentistry
3302 Gaston Ave.
Dallas, TX 75246
Phone: (214)828-8100 **Fax:** (214)828-8496
Website: http://www.tambcd.edu
Dr. James Cole, Director

★ 26519 ★ University of Texas Health Science Center, Houston
Dental Branch
6516 John Freeman Ave.
Houston, TX 77030
Phone: (713)792-4021 **Fax:** (713)792-4189
Website: http://www.db.uth.tmc.edu
Dr. Ronald Johnson, Director

★ 26520 ★ University of Texas Health Science Center, San Antonio
Dental School
7703 Floyd Curl Dr.
San Antonio, TX 78284-7914
Phone: (512)567-3160 **Fax:** (512)567-6721
Website: http://www.dental.uthscsa.edu
Dr. Kenneth L. Kalkwarf, Director

Virginia

★ 26521 ★ Virginia Commonwealth University
School of Dentistry
PO Box 980566
Richmond, VA 23298-0566
Phone: (804)828-9196 **Fax:** (804)371-6072
Website: http://www.dentistry.vcu.edu
Dr. Ronald J. Hunt, Jr., Director

Washington

★ 26522 ★ University of Washington
School of Dentistry
Health Sciences Bldg., Room D-322
PO Box 356365
Seattle, WA 98195
Phone: (206)543-5840 **Fax:** (206)616-2612
Website: http://www.dental.washington.edu
Dr. James C. Steiner, Director

West Virginia

★ 26523 ★ West Virginia University
School of Dentistry
The Medical Ctr.
PO Box 9400
Morgantown, WV 26506-9400
Phone: (304)293-3511 **Fax:** (304)293-2859
Dr. James J. Koelbl, Director

Wisconsin

★ 26524 ★ **Marquette University School of Dentistry**
PO Box 1881
Milwaukee, WI 53201
Phone: (414)288-3532 **Fax:** (414)288-6505
Website: http://www.dental.mu.edu
Dr. William K. Lobb, Director

Dietetics

Listed below are coordinated dietetic programs accredited by the Commission on Accreditation/ Approval for Dietetics Education of the American Dietetic Association. These programs offer academic preparation and clinical experience at the bachelor and master's levels. The Association also accredits post-baccalaureate dietetic internships and pre-professional practice programs and approves didactic programs in dietetics, as well as dietetic technician programs. For more information, contact the American Dietetic Association, 120 S Riverside Plaza, Ste. 2000, Chicago, IL 60606-6995, (312)899-0040, http://www.eatright.org/.

X123Q8

★ 26525 ★ **Syracuse University Department of Nutrition and Hospitality Management Coordinated Program in Dietetics**
034 Slocum Hall
Syracuse, 13244-1250
Phone: (315)443-9326 **Fax:** (315)443-2735
Email: ksbrueni@syr.edu
Website: http://hshp.syr.edu/nutrition.html
Kay Stearns Bruening, PhD, Contact

Alabama

★ 26526 ★ **Alabama A & M University Department of Family and Consumer Sciences Nutrition and Hospitality Management**
PO Box 639
Normal, AL 35762-0639
Phone: (256)858-4103 **Fax:** (256)851-5433
Email: awarren@aamu.edu
Ann P. Warren, Contact

★ 26527 ★ **Auburn University Nutrition and Food Science Dietetics-Didactic Program**
328 Spidle Hall
Auburn, AL 36849-5605
Phone: (334)844-4261 **Fax:** (334)844-3268
Email: rfellers@auburn.edu
Website: http://www.humsci.auburn.edu/
Robin B. Fellers, PhD, Director

★ 26528 ★ **Jacksonville State University Family and Consumer Sciences Dietetics-Didactic Program**
125 E Mason Hall
Jacksonville, AL 36265
Phone: (256)782-5053 **Fax:** (256)782-5916
Email: dgoodwin@jsucc_jsu.edu
Debra K. Goodwin, Contact

★ 26529 ★ **Oakwood College Family and Consumer Science Dietetics-Preprofessional Practice Program**
7000 Adventist Blvd.
Huntsville, AL 35896
Phone: (256)726-7228 **Fax:** (256)726-7233
Email: msovyanhadi@oakwood.edu
Website: http://www.oakwood.edu/fcs/dip2002.html
Marta L. Sovyanhadi, PhD, Contact

★ 26530 ★ **Oakwood College Family and Consumer Sciences Dietetics-Didactic Program**
7000 Adventist Blvd.
Huntsville, AL 35896
Phone: (256)726-7230 **Fax:** (256)726-7233
Email: dsmith@oakwood.edu
Website: http://www.oakwood.edu/fcs/
Donna A. Smith, Contact

★ 26531 ★ **Samford University Family and Consumer Sciences Dietetics-Didactic Program**
800 Lakeshore Dr.
Birmingham, AL 35229-2239
Phone: (205)726-2930 **Fax:** (205)726-2068
Email: pchart@samford.edu
Website: http://www.samford.edu/
Patricia H. Terry, PhD, Director

★ 26532 ★ **Tuskegee University Food and Nutrition Sciences**
204 Campbell Hall
Tuskegee University, AL 36088
Phone: (334)727-8326 **Fax:** (334)727-8493
Email: ghebwp@tusk.edu
Beatrice W. Phillips, EdD, Contact

★ 26533 ★ **University of Alabama Department of Human Nutrition and Hospitality Management**
PO Box 870158
206 Doster Hall
Tuscaloosa, AL 35487-0158
Phone: (205)348-8130 **Fax:** (205)348-3789
Email: dmorriso@ches.ua.edu
Website: http://www.ches.ua.edu
Debra W. Morrison, Director

★ 26534 ★ **University of Alabama Department of Human Nutrition and Hospitality Management Dietetics-Didactic Program**
PO Box 870158
Tuscaloosa, AL 35487-0158
Phone: (205)348-4710 **Fax:** (205)348-3789
Email: shancock@ches.ua.edu
Website: http://www.ches.ua.edu
Shelley R. Hancock, Director
Debra W. Morrison, Contact

★ 26535 ★ **University of Montevallo Family and Consumer Sciences Dietetics-Didactic Program**
Station 6385
Bloch Hall
Montevallo, AL 35115-6000
Phone: (205)665-6385 **Fax:** (205)665-6387
Email: andrews@um.montevallo.edu
Website: http://www.montevallo.edu/
Frances E. Andrews, PhD, Contact

Alaska

★ 26536 ★ **University of Alaska, Anchorage Culinary Arts and Hospitality**
3211 Providence Dr.
108 Cuddy Center
Anchorage, AK 99508
Phone: (907)786-1362 **Fax:** (907)786-1402
Email: afnlo@uaa.alaska.edu
Website: http://www.eatrightalaska.org/ap4.html
Nancy Overpeck, EdD, Director

Arizona

★ 26537 ★ **Arizona State University East Department of Nutrition Dietetic Internship Program**
7001 E Williams Field Rd., Bldg. 20
Mesa, AZ 85212
Phone: (480)727-1748 **Fax:** (480)727-1064
Email: tina.shepard@asu.edu
Website: http://www.east.asu.edu/ecollege/nutrition
Christina W. Shepard, Contact

★ 26538 ★ **Arizona State University East Department of Nutrition Dietetics-Didactic Program**
7001 E Williams Field Rd.
Mesa, AZ 85212
Phone: (480)727-1731 **Fax:** (480)727-1064
Email: linda.vaughan@asu.edu
Linda A. Vaughan, PhD, Contact

★ 26539 ★ **Carondelet St. Mary's Hospital Department of Nutrition Services Dietetic Internship Program**
1601 W St. Mary's Rd.
Tucson, AZ 85745
Phone: (520)872-6109 **Fax:** (520)740-6108
Email: kyee@carondelet.org
Website: http://www.azdpac.org/prgramin-fo.cfm?PID=100020
Kelli Jo Yee, Contact

★ 26540 ★ **Central Arizona College Dietetic Technician Program**
8470 N Overfield Rd.
Coolidge, AZ 85228-9030
Phone: (520)426-4497 **Fax:** (520)426-4476
Email: glenna_mccollum@centralaz.edu
Website: http://www.centralaz.edu
Glenna R. McCollum, Contact

★ 26541 ★ **Chandler-Gilbert Community College Dietetic Technician Consortium Nutrition Faculty**
2626 E Pecos Rd.
Chandler, AZ 85225-2499
Phone: (480)732-7142 **Fax:** (480)857-5122
Email: susan.gaumont@cgcmail.maricopa.edu
Susan A. Gaumont, Contact

★ 26542 ★ **Maricopa County Department of Public Health Office of Nutrition Services Dietetic Internship Program**
1414 W Broadway, Ste. 237
Tempe, AZ 85282
Phone: (480)966-3090 **Fax:** (480)966-3233
Email: shirleystrembel@mail.maricopa.gov
Website: http://www.eatrightarizona.org
Shirley K. Strembel, Contact

★ 26543 ★ **Paradise Valley Community College Dietetic Technology Consortium Nutrition Faculty and Program Director Dietetic Technician Program**
18401 North 32nd St.
Phoenix, AZ 85032-1210
Phone: (602)787-7295 **Fax:** (602)787-7285
Email: lori.anonsen@pvmail.maricopa.edu
Website: http://www.cgc.maricopa.edu/pecos/aca-demics/
Lori J. Anonsen, Contact

★ 26544 ★ Paradise Valley Unified School District
Dietetics-Preprofessional Practice Program
20621 N 32nd St.
Phoenix, AZ 85050
Phone: (602)493-6330 **Fax:** (602)493-6334
Email: kglindmeier@pvusd.k12.az.us
Website: http://www.pvusd.k12.az.us
Kathleen M. Glindmeier, Contact

★ 26545 ★ University of Arizona
Department of Nutritional Sciences
Dietetics-Didactic Program
309 Shantz Bldg.
PO Box 210038
Tucson, AZ 85721-0038
Phone: (520)621-1619 **Fax:** (520)621-9446
Email: whhowell@ag.arizona.edu
Website: http://ag.arizona.edu/NSC/nschome.htm
Wanda Howell, PhD, Contact

★ 26546 ★ University of Arizona
Medical Center Support Services
Dietetic Internship Program
1501 N Campbell Ave.
PO Box 245088
Tucson, AZ 85724-5088
Phone: (520)694-6622 **Fax:** (520)694-6276
Email: sbristol@umcaz.edu
Website: http://www.azdpac.org
Susan E. Bristol, Contact

★ 26547 ★ Yavapai County Health Department
Dietetic Internship Program
930 Division St.
Prescott, AZ 86301
Phone: (928)771-3138 **Fax:** (928)771-3369
Email: judy.lee-morris@co.Yavapai.az.us
Website: http://www.co.Yavapai.az.us
Judy S. Lee-Norris, Contact

Arkansas

★ 26548 ★ Black River Technical College
Dietetic Technician Program
PO Box 468
Pocahontas, AR 72455
Phone: (870)248-4000 **Fax:** (870)248-4100
Email: angelac@blackrivertech.org
Website: http://www.blackrivertech.org
Angela C. Caldwell, Contact

★ 26549 ★ Harding University
Department of Family and Consumer Sciences
Dietetics-Didactic Program
PO Box 12233
900 E Center Ave.
Searcy, AR 72149-0001
Phone: (501)279-4472 **Fax:** (501)279-4098
Email: lritchie@harding.edu
Lisa Ritchie, EdD, Contact

★ 26550 ★ Henderson State University
Department of Family and Consumer Sciences
Dietetics-Didactic Program
PO Box 7504
Arkadelphia, AR 71999-0001
Phone: (870)230-5542 **Fax:** (870)230-5172
Email: lockwol@hsu.edu
Website: http://www.hsu.edu/dept/fcs/index.html
Laura P. Lockwood, Contact

★ 26551 ★ Ouachita Baptist University
Dietetics-Didactic Program
PO Box 3769
410 Ouachita
Arkadelphia, AR 71998-0001
Phone: (870)245-5542 **Fax:** (870)245-5500
Email: freemans@obu.edu
Website: http://www.obu.edu/biology/program_in_dietetics.htm
Stacy L. Freeman, Director

★ 26552 ★ University of Arkansas
School of Human Environmental Sciences
Dietetics-Didactic Program
118 HOEC
Fayetteville, AR 72701
Phone: (479)575-6815 **Fax:** (479)575-7171
Email: mfitch@comp.uark.edu
Website: http://www.uark.edu/depts/hesweb/index.html
Marjorie E. Fitch-Hilgenberg, PhD, Contact

★ 26553 ★ University of Arkansas for Medical Sciences
Central Arkansas Veterans Healthcare System
Dietetic Internship Program
4301 W Markham St., Slot 627
Little Rock, AR 72205-7199
Phone: (501)686-5714 **Fax:** (501)686-5716
Email: carrollpollya@uams.edu
Website: http://www.uams.edu/chrp/diet.htm
Polly A. Carroll, Contact

★ 26554 ★ University of Arkansas, Pine Bluff
Department of Human Sciences
Dietetics-Didactic Program
Mail Slot 4971
1200 N University Dr.
Pine Bluff, AR 71601
Phone: (870)575-8817 **Fax:** (870)543-8823
Email: neal_e@vx4500.uapb.edu
Lucille Meadows, Contact

★ 26555 ★ University of Central Arkansas
Family and Consumer Sciences
Dietetic Internship Program
McAlister Hall 100
Conway, AR 72035
Phone: (501)450-5954 **Fax:** (501)450-5958
Email: lizc@mail.uca.edu
Website: http://uca.edu/chas/diet.html
Elizabeth L. Coffman, Contact

★ 26556 ★ University of Central Arkansas
Family and Consumer Sciences
Dietetics-Didactic Program
McAlister Hall, Rm. 100
Conway, AR 72035
Phone: (501)450-5950 **Fax:** (501)450-5958
Email: maryh@mail.uca.edu
Website: http://www.uca.edu/divisions/academic/chas/facs/dietetic.htm
Mary H. Harlan, EdD, Contact

California

★ 26557 ★ California Polytechnic State University
Food Science & Nutrition Department
Dietetics-Didactic Program
San Luis Obispo, CA 93407
Phone: (805)756-7383 **Fax:** (805)756-1146
Email: lmnichol@calpoly.edu
Website: http://www.calpoly.edu/~fsn/
Lisa M. Nicholson, PhD, Director

★ 26558 ★ California State Polytechnic University
Human Nutrition and Food Science
Dietetic-Didactic Program
3801 W Temple Ave.
Pomona, CA 91768-2557
Phone: (909)869-4877 **Fax:** (909)869-5078
Email: msmeskin@cusupomona.edu
Website: http://www.csupomona.edu
Mark S. Meskin, PhD, Contact

★ 26559 ★ California State Polytechnic University
Human Nutrition and Food Science Department
3801 W Temple Ave.
Pomona, CA 91768-2557
Phone: (909)869-2163 **Fax:** (909)869-5078
Email: kcaldwellfreeman@csupomona.edu
Website: http://www.csupomona.edu/~kcaldwellfreeman/
Kara Caldwell-Freeman, PhD, Director

★ 26560 ★ California State University, Chico
Nutrition and Food Sciences
Department of Biological Sciences
Dietetic Internship Program
Chico, CA 95929-0002
Phone: (530)898-6805 **Fax:** (530)898-5586
Email: bkirks@csuchico.edu
Website: http://www.csuchico.edu/bio/nfsc
Barbara A. Kirks, EdD, Contact

★ 26561 ★ California State University, Chico
Program in Nutrition and Food Science
Dietetics-Didactic Program
Tehama Hall, 124
Chico, CA 95929-0002
Phone: (530)898-6805 **Fax:** (530)898-4363
Email: fjohnson@csuchico.edu
Website: http://www.csuchico.edu/nfsc
Faye C. Johnson, EdD, Contact

★ 26562 ★ California State University, Fresno
Department of Food Science and Nutrition
5300 N Campus Dr., M/S FF17
Fresno, CA 93740-8019
Phone: (559)278-8009 **Fax:** (559)278-7623
Email: mollie_smith@csufresno.edu
Website: http://www.cast.scufresno.edu/fsn
Mollie M. Smith, Contact

★ 26563 ★ California State University, Fresno
Department of Food Science and Nutrition
Dietetics-Didactic Program
5300 N Campus Dr.
M/S FF17
Fresno, CA 93740-8019
Phone: (559)278-2164 **Fax:** (559)278-7623
Email: sandraw@csufresno.edu
Website: http://cast.csufresno.edu/fsn/
Sandra S. Witte, PhD, Director

★ 26564 ★ California State University, Long Beach
Department of Family and Consumer Sciences
Dietetics-Didactic Program
1250 Bellflower Blvd.
Long Beach, CA 90840-0501
Phone: (562)985-4545 **Fax:** (562)985-4414
Email: jjlee@csulb.edu

Website: http://www.csulb.edu/colleges/chhs/dpd
Jacqueline D. Lee, PhD, Director

★ 26565 ★ California State University, Long Beach
Family and Consumer Sciences
Dietetic Internship Program
1250 N Bellflower Blvd.
Long Beach, CA 90840-0501
Phone: (562)985-4494 **Fax:** (562)985-4414
Email: gcfrank@csulb.edu
Website: http://www.csulb.edu/~gcfrank
Gail C. Frank, PhD, Director

★ 26566 ★ California State University, Los Angeles
Deparment of Health and Nutritional Sciences
Coordinated Program in Dietetics
5151 State University Dr.
Los Angeles, CA 90032-8172
Phone: (323)343-5439 **Fax:** (323)343-6482
Email: lcalder@calstatela.edu
Website: http://www.calstatela.edu/dept/hnut sci/dept pro.htm
Laura L. Calderon, DrPH, Director

★ 26567 ★ California State University, Los Angeles
Department of Kinesiology and Nutritional Sciences
Dietetics-Didactic Program
5151 State University Dr.
Los Angeles, CA 90032-8162
Phone: (323)343-4666 **Fax:** (323)343-6482
Email: jgota@calstatela.edu
Website: http://www.calstatela.edu/dept/hnut_sci/dept_pro.htm
Joyce Y. Gota, Director
Laura Calderon, DrPH, Contact

★ 26568 ★ California State University, Northridge
Department of Family and Consumer Sciences
Dietetics-Didactic Program
18111 Nordhoff St.
Northridge, CA 91330-8308
Phone: (818)677-3051 **Fax:** (818)677-4778
Email: nbenmaor@msn.com
Nilda S. Benmaor, Contact

★ 26569 ★ California State University, Northridge
Family Environmental Sciences
Dietetic Internship Program
18111 Nordhoff St.
Northridge, CA 91330-8308
Phone: (818)677-3051 **Fax:** (818)677-4778
Email: TeriDeWolfeMS_RD@aol.com
Website: http://www.csundi.com
Teri DeWolfe, Contact

★ 26570 ★ California State University, Sacramento
Department of Family and Consumer Sciences
Dietetic Internship Program
6000 J St.
Sacramento, CA 95819-6053
Phone: (916)278-6732 **Fax:** (916)278-7520
Email: wcunningham@csus.edu
Website: http://www.csus.edu/indiv/c/cunninghamw/
Wendy M. Mueller-Cunningham, PhD, Director

★ 26571 ★ California State University, Sacramento
Department of Family and Consumer Sciences
Dietetics-Didactic Program
6000 J St.
Sacramento, CA 95819-6053
Phone: (916)278-7320 **Fax:** (916)278-7520
Email: dhyson@csus.edu
Website: http://www.csus.edu/facs
Dianne A. Hyson, PhD, Director

★ 26572 ★ California State University, San Bernardino
Department of Health Science and Human Ecology
Dietetics-Didactic Program
5500 University Pkwy.
San Bernardino, CA 92407-2318
Phone: (909)880-5340 **Fax:** (909)880-7037
Email: dchen@csusb.edu
Website: http://health.csusb.edu/dchen/
Dorothy C. Chen-Maynard, PhD, Director

★ 26573 ★ Central Valley WIC
Dietetic Internship Program
1560 E Manning Ave.
Reedley, CA 93654-2346
Phone: (559)646-6611 **Fax:** (559)646-6615
Email: beth@cvwdi.org
Website: http://www.cvwdi.org
Beth M. Arrindell, Director

★ 26574 ★ Chaffey College
Food Service Management
Dietetic Technician Program
5885 Haven Ave.
Rancho Cucamonga, CA 91737-3002
Phone: (909)941-2711 **Fax:** (909)466-2831
Email: dsuzannej@excite.com
D. Suzanne Johnson, Contact

★ 26575 ★ Children's Hospital of Los Angeles
Center for Child Development and Developmental Disabilities/UAP
Dietetic Internship Program
Mailstop 53
PO Box 54700
Los Angeles, CA 90054-0700
Phone: (323)669-2300 **Fax:** (323)671-3842
Email: aharris@chla.usc.edu
Anne B. Harris, Contact

★ 26576 ★ Clinica Sierra Vista
Dietetic Internship Program
1430 Truxtun Ave., Ste. 120
Bakersfield, CA 93301-3834
Phone: (661)587-5781 **Fax:** (661)587-5794
Email: wallacel@clinicasieravista.org
Laurie J. Wallace, Director

★ 26577 ★ Cosumnes Rivre College
Nutrition Department
Dietetic Technician Program
8401 Center Pkwy.
Sacramento, CA 95823-5799
Phone: (916)691-7514 **Fax:** (916)691-7146
Email: wassmed@crc.losrios.cc.ca.us
Website: http://www.crc.losrios.cc.ca
Dana W. Wassmer, Contact

★ 26578 ★ Glendale Memorial Hospital and Health Center
Food and Nutrition Services
Dietetic Internship Program
1420 S Central Ave.
Glendale, CA 91204-2594
Phone: (818)502-2248 **Fax:** (818)507-4665
Email: ncarvalh@chw.edu
Website: http://www.glendalememorial.com/dietary/index.html
Nicole K. Carvalho, Contact

★ 26579 ★ Loma Linda University
School of Allied Health Professions
Department of Nutrition and Dietetics
Coordinated Program in Dietetics
Loma Linda, CA 92354
Phone: (909)558-4593 **Fax:** (909)558-4291
Email: bert-connell@sahp.llu.edu
Website: http://www.llu.edu/llu/nutrition
Bertrum C. Connell, PhD, Contact

★ 26580 ★ Loma Linda University
School of Allied Health Professions
Department of Nutrition and Dietetics
Dietetic Technician Program
Loma Linda, CA 92350
Phone: (909)558-4593 **Fax:** (909)558-4291
Email: ghodgkin@sahp.llu.edu
Website: http://www.llu.edu/llu/nutrition
Georgia E. Hodgkin, EdD, Contact

★ 26581 ★ Loma Linda University
School of Public Health
Department of Nutrition
Coordinated Program in Dietetics
Nichol Hall, Rm. 1102
Loma Linda, CA 92350
Phone: (909)558-4598 **Fax:** (909)558-4095
Email: ehaddad@sph.llu.edu
Website: http://www.llu.edu/llu/nutrition/
Ella H. Haddad, DrPH, Director

★ 26582 ★ Long Beach City College
Liberal Arts Campus
Family and Consumer Studies Division
Dietetic Technician Program
4901 E Carson St.
Long Beach, CA 90808-1706
Phone: (562)938-4550 **Fax:** (562)938-4118
Email: lhuy@lbcc.edu
Linda A. Huy, EdD, Contact

★ 26583 ★ Los Angeles City College
Family and Consumer Studies
Dietetic Technician Program
855 N Vermont Ave.
Los Angeles, CA 90029-3590
Phone: (323)953-4000 **Fax:** (714)777-3862
Email: janiceyung@aol.com
Website: http://www.lacc.cc.ca.us
Janice M. Young, Contact

★ 26584 ★ Los Angeles County/USC Healthcare Network
Dietetic Internship Program
1200 N State St., Rm. 1506
Los Angeles, CA 90033-4525
Phone: (323)226-6901 **Fax:** (323)222-3422
Email: emalacusc@juno.com
Website: http://lacuscdi.org
Elizabeth H. Ma, Contact

★ 26585 ★ Merritt College
Dietetic Technician Program
12500 Campus Dr.
Oakland, CA 94619-3107
Phone: (510)436-2521 **Fax:** (510)434-3873
Email: shouston@peralta.cc.ca.us
Website: http://www.merritt.edu
Susan M. Houston, Contact

★ 26586 ★ Napa State Hospital
Dietetic Internship Program
2100 Napa-Vallejo Hwy.
Napa, CA 94558-6293
Phone: (707)253-5428 **Fax:** (707)254-2422
Email: wpao@dmhnsh.state.ca.us
Website: http://www.dmh.ca.gov/job/napa/napa.asp
Wen F. Pao, Contact

★ 26587 ★ Northeast Valley Health Corp.
WIC Program
Dietetic Internship Program
1172 N Maclay Ave.
San Fernando, CA 91340-1328
Phone: (818)898-1388 **Fax:** (818)898-3424
Email: annetteb-wic@nevhc.org
Annette A. Besnilian, Director

★ 26588 ★ Olive View/UCLA Medical Center
Department of Food and Nutrition Services
Dietetic Internship Program
14445 Olive View Dr., Rm. 1C112
Sylmar, CA 91342-1438
Phone: (818)364-4220 **Fax:** (818)364-3998
Email: robmmck@cs.com
Robin M. McKelvey, Director

★ 26589 ★ Orange Coast College
Dietetic Technician Program
2701 Fairview Rd.
Costa Mesa, CA 92628-5005
Phone: (714)432-5835 **Fax:** (714)432-5609
Email: ehuang@mail.occ.cccd.edu
Eleanor B. Huang, Contact

★ 26590 ★ Patton State Hospital
Dietetic Internship Program
3102 E Highland Ave.
Patton, CA 92369
Phone: (909)425-7575 **Fax:** (909)425-7069
Email: asimoran@dmhspsh.state.ca.us
Anneke G. Simorangkir, Contact

★ 26591 ★ Pepperdine University
RAC108C, Nutritional Sciences
Dietetics-Didactic Program
24255 Pacific Coast Hwy.
Malibu, CA 90263-4325
Phone: (310)506-4325 **Fax:** (310)506-4785
Email: susan.helm@pepperdine.edu
Website: http://www.pepperdine.edu/
Susan E. Helm, PhD, Contact

★ 26592 ★ Porterville Development Center
Dietetic Internship Program
PO Box 2000
Porterville, CA 93258-2000
Phone: (559)782-2753 **Fax:** (559)782-2756
Email: chahesy@pdc.dds.ca.gov
Christine N. Hahesy, Director

★ 26593 ★ Public Health Foundation Enterprises
WIC Program
Dietetic Internship Program
12781 Schabarum Ave.
Irwindale, CA 91706-6802
Phone: (626)856-6618 **Fax:** (626)813-9390
Email: robin@phfewic.org
Website: http://www.phfewic.org
Robin B. Evans, Contact

★ 26594 ★ San Bernardino Valley College
Dietetic Technician Program
North Hall - FCS Office
701 S Mount Vernon
San Bernardino, CA 92410-2798
Phone: (909)384-8542 **Fax:** (909)384-9725
Email: jmartin@sbccd.cc.ca.us
Denise D. Whisler, DrPH, Contact

★ 26595 ★ San Diego State University
Department of Exercise and Nutritional Sciences
Dietetics-Didactic Program
5500 Campanile Dr.
San Diego, CA 92182-7251
Phone: (619)594-3045 **Fax:** (619)594-6553
Email: spindler@mail.sdsu.edu
Website: http://www.sdsu.edu
Audrey A. Spindler, PhD, Director

★ 26596 ★ San Diego State University
Exercise and Nutritional Sciences
Dietetic Internship Program
5500 Campanile Dr.
San Diego, CA 92182-7251
Phone: (619)594-1341 **Fax:** (619)594-6553
Email: didirector-sdsu@cox.net
Website: http://rohan.sdsu.edu/dept/extstd/dietetic.html
Michelle R. Snyder, Director

★ 26597 ★ San Diego WIC
Dietetic Internship Program
8057 Vickers St.
San Diego, CA 92111-1917
Phone: (858)505-3065 **Fax:** (858)569-7906
Email: eanderson@projects.sdsu.edu
Website: http://www.wic-sdsu.org
Ellen L. Anderson, Director

★ 26598 ★ San Francisco State University
Consumer and Family Studies/Dietetics
Dietetic Internship Program
1600 Holloway Ave.
San Francisco, CA 94132-1722
Phone: (415)338-1219 **Fax:** (415)338-0947
Email: ajrigby@sfsu.edu
Website: http://www.sfsu.edu/~sda/
Alison J. Rigby, PhD, Director

★ 26599 ★ San Francisco State University
Consumer and Family Studies/Dietetics
Dietetics-Didactic Program
1600 Holloway Ave.
San Francisco, CA 94132-1722
Phone: (415)338-1219 **Fax:** (415)338-0947
Email: vijay@sfsu.edu
Website: http://www.sfsu.edu/
Vijay Ganji, PhD, Director

★ 26600 ★ San Jose State University
Department of Nutrition and Food Science
Dietetic Internship Program
1 Washington Sq.
San Jose, CA 95192-0058
Phone: (408)924-3104 **Fax:** (408)924-3114
Email: ksucher@email.sjsu.edu
Kathryn P. Sucher, ScD, Director

★ 26601 ★ San Jose State University
Department of Nutrition and Food Science
Dietetics-Didactic Program
San Jose, CA 95192-0058
Phone: (408)924-3109 **Fax:** (408)924-3114
Email: nancyclu@email.sjsu.edu
Nancy C. Lu, PhD, Director

★ 26602 ★ Univeristy of California, San Francisco Medical Center
Nutrition Services
Dietetic Internship Program
Medical Center, Box 0212, Rm. M-294
San Francisco, CA 94143-0212
Phone: (415)353-1355 **Fax:** (415)353-8705
Email: patricia.booth@ucsfmedctr.org
Patricia A. Booth, Director

★ 26603 ★ University of California, Berkeley
Department of Nutritional Sciences and Toxicology
Dietetics-Didactic Program
119 Morgan Hall
Berkeley, CA 94720-3104
Phone: (510)642-4090 **Fax:** (510)642-0535
Email: hudson@nature.berkeley.edu
Website: http://nutrition.berkeley.edu
Nancy R. Hudson, Contact

★ 26604 ★ University of California, Berkeley
School of Public Health
Dietetic Internship Program
140 Warren Hall
Berkeley, CA 94720-7360
Phone: (510)643-0969 **Fax:** (510)642-9891
Email: kmcburne@uclink.berkeley.edu
Website: http://sph.Berkeley.edu:7047/call?inf970954944.dtl
Kathleen A. McBurney, PhD, Contact

★ 26605 ★ University of California, Davis
Department of Nutrition
Dietetics-Didactic Program
1 Shields Ave.
Davis, CA 95616-8669
Phone: (530)752-0160 **Fax:** (530)752-8966
Email: fmsteinberg@ucdavis.edu
Website: http://nutrition.ucdavis.edu
Francene M. Steinberg, PhD, Director

★ 26606 ★ University of California, Davis
UC Davis Health System
Food and Nutrition Services
Dietetic Internship Program
2315 Stockton Blvd.
Sacramento, CA 95817-2201
Phone: (916)734-1302
Email: angelita.fan@udmc.ucdavis.edu
Angelita K. Fan, Contact

★ 26607 ★ VA San Diego Healthcare System
Dietetic Internship Program
Dietetics and Clinical Nutrition Services 120
3350 La Jolla Village Dr.
San Diego, CA 92161-0002
Phone: (858)552-8585 **Fax:** (858)552-4340
Email: teresa.bush-zurn@med.va.gov
Teresa Bush-Zurn, Director

★ 26608 ★ Veterans Affairs Greater Los Angeles Healthcare System
Dietetic Internship Program
Nutrition and Food Department 120
11301 Wilshire Blvd.
Los Angeles, CA 90073
Phone: (310)268-3120 **Fax:** (310)268-4787
Email: carrie.johnsen@med.va.gov

Website: http://www.va.gov/nfs/DieteticInternships.htm
Carrie C. Johnsen, Contact

Colorado

★ 26609 ★ Colorado State University
Department of Food Science and Human Nutrition
Dietetics-Didactic Program or Dietetic Internship Program
Gifford Bldg., Rm. 205
Fort Collins, CO 80523-1571
Phone: (970)491-7462 **Fax:** (970)491-7252
Email: harris@cahs.colostate.edu
Website: http://www.cahs.colostate.edu/fshn/
Mary Harris, PhD, Director

★ 26610 ★ Front Range Community College
Dietetic Technician Program
3645 West 112th Ave.
23
Westminster, CO 80031-2199
Phone: (303)404-5260 **Fax:** (303)404-2178
Email: louann.dixon@wc.frcc.cccoes.edu
Lou Ann H. Dixon, Contact

★ 26611 ★ Penrose-St. Francis Health Services
Nutrition Services
Dietetic Internship Program
PO Box 7021
Colorado Springs, CO 80933-7021
Phone: (719)776-5863 **Fax:** (719)776-2500
Email: suzannelogan@centura.org
Suzanne M. Logan, Director

★ 26612 ★ Tri-County Health Department
Nutrition Services
Dietetic Internship Program
4857 S Broadway
Englewood, CO 80110-6894
Phone: (303)761-1340 **Fax:** (303)761-1528
Email: Bennett@tchd.org
Anne E. Bennett, Director

★ 26613 ★ University of Northern Colorado
Community Health and Nutrition
Dietetic Internship Program
CHN, Box 93
501 20th St.
Greeley, CO 80639
Phone: (970)351-1769 **Fax:** (970)351-1489
Email: Alana.cline@unco.edu
Website: http://www.unco.edu/dietetic
Alana D. Cline, Director

★ 26614 ★ University of Northern Colorado
Department of Community Health and Nutrition
Dietetics-Didactic Program
Gunter 2320
Greeley, CO 80639
Phone: (970)351-1706 **Fax:** (970)351-1489
Email: jamie.erskine@unco.edu
Website: http://www.hhs.unco.edu/Diet.htm
Jamie M. Erskine, PhD, Director

Connecticut

★ 26615 ★ Briarwood College
Dietetic Technician Program
2279 Mount Vernon Rd.
Southington, CT 06489-1007
Phone: (860)628-4751 **Fax:** (860)628-6444
Email: leibovitzp@briarwood.edu
Paula K. Leibovitz, Contact

★ 26616 ★ Danbury Hospital
Preprofessional Practice Program in Dietetics
24 Hospital Ave.
Danbury, CT 06810-6099
Phone: (203)797-7942 **Fax:** (203)797-7619
Email: Janice.cannon@danhosp.org
Janice D. Cannon, Director

★ 26617 ★ Gateway Community College
Dietetic Technician Program
88 Bassett Rd.
North Haven, CT 06473
Phone: (203)285-2389 **Fax:** (203)285-2400
Email: mdoran@gwcc.commnet.edu
Website: http://www.gwctc.commnet.edu
Marcia Swan Doran, Contact

★ 26618 ★ Saint Joseph College
Department of Nutrition and Family Studies
Coordinated Program in Dietetics
1678 Asylum Ave.
West Hartford, CT 06117-2700
Phone: (860)231-5534 **Fax:** (860)231-8396
Email: mgaughan@sjc.edu
Margaret E. Gaughan, PhD, Director

★ 26619 ★ Saint Joseph College
Department of Nutrition and Family Studies
Dietetics-Didactic Program
1678 Asylum Ave.
West Hartford, CT 06117-2700
Phone: (860)231-5769 **Fax:** (860)231-8396
Email: saffenito@sjc.edu
Website: http://www.sjc.edu
Sandra M. Affenito, PhD, Director
Margaret E. Gaughan, PhD, Contact

★ 26620 ★ Saint Joseph College
Nutrition and Family Studies
Dietetic Internship Program
1678 Asylum Ave.
West Hartford, CT 06117-2700
Phone: (860)232-5254 **Fax:** (860)231-8396
Email: dcorcora@sjc.edu
Donna W. Corcoran, Director

★ 26621 ★ University of Connecticut
Department of Nutritional Sciences
Dietetics-Didactic Program
U-4017
3624 Horsebarn Rd. Extension
Storrs, CT 06269
Phone: (860)486-0119 **Fax:** (860)486-3674
Email: eshanley@canrl.uconn.edu
Website: http://www.canr.uconn.edu/nusci/
Ellen Rosa Shanley, Director

★ 26622 ★ University of Connecticut
School of Allied Health
Coordinated Program in Dietetics
358 Mansfield Rd., Unit 2101
Storrs, CT 06269-2101
Phone: (860)486-0016 **Fax:** (860)486-5375
Email: robin.abourizk@uconn.edu
Website: http://www.alliedhealth.uconn.edu
Robin H. Abourizk, Contact

★ 26623 ★ University of Connecticut
School of Allied Health
Coordinated Program in Dietetics or Dietetic Internship Program
358 Mansfield Rd., U-101
Storrs, CT 06269-2101
Phone: (860)486-0016 **Fax:** (860)486-5375
Email: robin.abourizk@uconn.edu
Website: http://www.alliedhealth.conn.edu
Robin H. Abourizk, Director

★ 26624 ★ University of New Haven
Department of Biology and Environmental Science
Dietetics-Didactic Program
300 Orange Ave.
West Haven, CT 06516-1916
Phone: (203)932-7410 **Fax:** (203)932-7083
Email: gchavent@newhaven.edu
Website: http://www.newhaven.edu
Georgia A. Chavent, Director

★ 26625 ★ Yale-New Haven Hospital
Food & Nutrition
Dietetic Internship Program
20 York St., GBB
New Haven, CT 06504
Phone: (203)688-5074 **Fax:** (203)688-2412
Email: ford@gwpo.ynhh.org
Website: http://www.ynhh.org/general/training.htmldiet
Deborah F. Flanel, Director

Delaware

★ 26626 ★ Delaware State University
Department of Family and Consumer Sciences
Dietetics-Didactic Program
1200 N Dupont Highway
Dover, DE 19901-2277
Phone: (302)857-6440 **Fax:** (302)857-6441
Email: mclausel@dsc.edu
Website: http://www.dsc.edu
Maggie R. Clausell, PhD, Director

★ 26627 ★ University of Delaware
Department of Nutrition and Dietetics
Dietetics-Didactic Program
234A Alison Hall
Newark, DE 19716-3301
Phone: (302)831-2798 **Fax:** (302)831-4186
Email: connie.vickery@udel.edu
Website: http://napa.ntdt.udel.edu
Constance E. Vickery, PhD, Director

★ 26628 ★ University of Delaware
Nutrition and Dietetics
Dietetic Internship Program
315 Alison Hall
Newark, DE 19716
Phone: (302)831-1677 **Fax:** (302)831-4186
Email: hamilton@udel.edu
Charlene M. Hamilton, PhD, Director

District of Columbia

★ 26629 ★ Howard University
Department of Nutritional Sciences
Division of Allied Helath Sciences
Coordinated Program in Dietetics
Sixth and Bryant Sts. NW
Washington, DC 20059
Phone: (202)806-5648 **Fax:** (202)806-9233
Email: tbaker@fac.howard.edu
Thelma B. Baker, PhD, Director

★ 26630 ★ University of the District of Columbia
Department of Biological and Environmental Sciences
Dietetics-Didactic Program
4200 Connecticut Ave. NW
Bldg. 44, Rm. 200-02
Washington, DC 20008-1173
Phone: (202)274-5516 **Fax:** (202)274-5845
Email: pganganna@udc.edu
Prema Ganganna, PhD, Director

★ 26631 ★ Walter Reed Army Medical Center
Nutrition Care Directorate
Dietetic Internship Program
6900 Georgia Ave. NW
Washington, DC 20307-5001
Phone: (202)782-0387 **Fax:** (202)782-9289
Email: Melanie.craig@na.amedd.army.mil
Website: http://www.amsc.amedd.army.mil/frames-et.htm
Melanie J. Craig, Director

Florida

★ 26632 ★ Florida Community College at Jacksonville-North Campus
Dietetic Technician Program
4501 Capper Rd.
Jacksonville, FL 32218-4436
Phone: (904)766-6743 **Fax:** (904)766-6654
Email: mwolson@fccj.org
Website: http://www.fccj.org
Margaret R. Wolson, Contact

★ 26633 ★ Florida International University
Department of Dietetics and Nutrition
Coordinated Program in Dietetics
11200 SW 8th St.
Miami, FL 33199
Phone: (305)348-1611 **Fax:** (305)348-1996
Email: monsejj@fiu.edu
Website: http://w3.fiu.edu/dietetics
Jorge J. Monserrate, Director

★ 26634 ★ Florida International University
Department of Dietetics and Nutrition
Dietetic Internship Program
University Park
Health Bldg. Rm 206
Miami, FL 33199
Phone: (305)348-2878 **Fax:** (305)348-1996
Amy D. Jaffe, Director

★ 26635 ★ Florida International University
Department of Dietetics and Nutrition
Dietetics-Didactic Program
11200 SW 8th St.
Miami, FL 33199
Phone: (305)348-2878 **Fax:** (305)348-1996
Email: brownjj@fiu.edu
Website: http://w3.fiu.edu/dietetics/
Jordana J. Brown, Director
Zisca R. Dixon, PhD, Director

★ 26636 ★ Florida State University
College of Human Sciences
Department of Nutrition, Food, and Exercise Sciences
436 Sandels Bldg.
Tallahassee, FL 32306-1493
Phone: (850)644-4794 **Fax:** (850)645-5000
Email: jdorsey@mailer.fsu.edu
Website: http://www.chs.fsu.edu/nfes/
Jodee L. Dorsey, PhD, Director

★ 26637 ★ Florida State University
Department of Nutrition, Food and Exercise Sciences
Dietetic Internship Program
400 Sandels Bldg.
Tallahassee, FL 32306-1493
Phone: (850)644-1828 **Fax:** (850)644-5000
Email: lcook@mailer.fsu.edu
Website: http://www.fsu.edu~human
Laura R. Cook, PhD, Director

★ 26638 ★ James A. Haley Veterans Hospital
Department of Nutrition and Food Service
Dietetic Internship Program
13000 N Bruce B. Downs Blvd.
Tampa, FL 33612-4745
Phone: (813)972-2000 **Fax:** (813)978-5838
Email: anne.brezina@med.va.gov
Anne E. Brezina, Director

★ 26639 ★ Miami-Dade Community College
Dietetic Technician Program
Mitchell Wolfson Campus
300 Northeast 2nd Ave.
Suite 3704
Miami, FL 33132-2297
Phone: (305)237-3162 **Fax:** (305)237-3802
Email: smyers@mdcc.edu
Website: http://www.mdcc.edu/wolfson/departments/natsciences
Susan J. Myers, Contact

★ 26640 ★ Palm Beach Community College
Dietetic Technician Program
4200 Congress Ave.
Mail Station 32
Lake Worth, FL 33461-4796
Phone: (561)868-3352 **Fax:** (561)868-3753
Email: froehlit@pbcc.edu
Website: http://www.pbcc.edu/acad/programs/dietetic/index.htm
Trish Froehlich, Contact

★ 26641 ★ Pasco County Health Department
Nutrition Division
Dietetic Internship Program
10841 Little Rd.
New Port Richey, FL 34654-2533
Phone: (727)869-3900 **Fax:** (727)863-9734
Email: clara_lawhead@doh.state.fl.us
Website: http://www9.myflorida.com/chdpasco/DI_Web/dihome.htm
Clara R. Lawhead, Director

★ 26642 ★ St. Luke's Hospital/Mayo Clinic Jacksonville
Dietetic Internship Program
4500 San Pablo Rd.
Jacksonville, FL 32224
Phone: (904)953-2753 **Fax:** (904)953-2954
Email: robinson.nell@mayo.edu
Nell E. Robinson, Director

★ 26643 ★ Sarasota District Schools
Food and Nutrition Services
Dietetic Internship Program
101 Old Venice Rd.
Osprey, FL 34229-9023
Phone: (941)486-2199 **Fax:** (941)486-2021
Email: dietetic_internship@sarasota.k12.fl.us
Website: http://www.Sarasota.k12.fl.us/fns
Beverly L. Girard, Director

★ 26644 ★ Sarasota Memorial Hospital
Food and Nutrition Services
Dietetic Internship Program
1700 S Tamiami Trail
Sarasota, FL 34239-3555
Phone: (941)917-6041 **Fax:** (941)917-6196
Email: joan-disley@smh.com
Website: http://www.smh.com/newdeptpage
Joan E. Disley, Director

★ 26645 ★ University of Florida
Food Science and Human Nutrition Department
Dietetic Internship Program
359 FSB
PO Box 110370
Gainesville, FL 32611
Phone: (352)392-1991 **Fax:** (352)392-9467
Email: gpk@mail.ifas.ufl.edu
Gail Abbott Kauwell, PhD, Director

★ 26646 ★ University of Florida
Food Science and Human Nutrition Department
Dietetics-Didactic Program
PO Box 110370
Gainesville, FL 32611-0370
Phone: (352)392-1512 **Fax:** (352)392-9467
Email: psmcmahon@mail.ifas.ufl.edu
Website: http://fshn.ifas.ufl.edu/
Pamela J. McMahon, PhD, Director

★ 26647 ★ University of North Florida
College of Health
Dietetics-Didactic Program
4567 St. Johns Bluff Rd. S
Jacksonville, FL 32224-2645
Phone: (904)620-2840 **Fax:** (904)620-2848
Email: jrodrigu@unf.edu
Website: http://www.unf.edu/
Judith C. Rodriguez, PhD, Director

★ 26648 ★ University of North Florida
Department of Health Science
Dietetic Internship Program
4567 St. Johns Bluff Rd. S
Jacksonville, FL 32224-2645
Phone: (904)620-2840 **Fax:** (904)620-2848
Email: cchristi@unf.edu
Website: http://www.unf.edu/coh/mshnutri.htm
Catherine W. Christie, PhD, Director

Georgia

★ 26649 ★ Emory Hospitals
Food and Nutrition Services
Dietetic Internship Program
1364 Clifton Rd. NE
Room FG06
Atlanta, GA 30322
Phone: (404)712-4178 **Fax:** (404)712-7452
Email: dietetic_internship@emory.org
Website: http://medshare.emory.org/EHC/FNSWeb.nsf
Maureen C. McAndrews, Director

★ 26650 ★ Fort Valley State University
Department of Family and Consumer Sciences
Dietetics-Didactic Program
1005 State University Dr.
PO Box 4622 FVSU
Fort Valley, GA 31030
Phone: (912)825-6234 **Fax:** (912)825-6078
Email: hunts@mail.fvsu.edu
Sharon K. Hunt, Director

★ **26651** ★ **Georgia Department of Human Resources**
Division of Public Health
Family Health Branch, Nutrition Section
Dietetic Internship Program
2 Peachtree St. NW, Ste. 11-254
Atlanta, GA 30303-3142
Phone: (404)657-2884 **Fax:** (404)657-2886
Email: frcook@dhr.state.ga.us
Website: http://www.ph.dhr.state.ga.us/programs
Frances H. Cook, Director

★ **26652** ★ **Georgia Southern University**
Department of Family and Consumer Sciences
Dietetics-Didactic Program
Box 8034
Statesboro, GA 30460
Phone: (912)681-5345 **Fax:** (912)681-0276
Email: fbrown2@gsaix2.cc.gasou.edu
Elfrieda F. Brown, Director

★ **26653** ★ **Georgia State University**
Department of Nutrition and Dietetics
Dietetic Internship Program
University Plaza
Atlanta, GA 30303-3083
Phone: (404)651-1082 **Fax:** (404)651-1235
Email: bhopkins@gsu.edu
Barbara L. Hopkins, Director

★ **26654** ★ **Georgia State University**
Department of Nutrition and Dietetics
Dietetics-Didactic Program
33 Gilmir St. SE, U-2
Atlanta, GA 30303-3082
Phone: (404)651-1108 **Fax:** (404)651-1235
Email: dbaxter@gsu.edu
Website: http://www.gsu.edu/nutrition
Delia H. Baxter, PhD, Director

★ **26655** ★ **Life University**
Department of Nutrition
Dietetics-Didactic Program
1269 Barclay Circle
Marietta, GA 30060-2903
Phone: (770)426-2736 **Fax:** (770)426-2698
Email: tbrigman@life.edu
Tracey B. Brigman, Director

★ **26656** ★ **Life University**
Nutrition Department
Dietetic Internship Program
1269 Barclay Circle SE
Marietta, GA 30060-2903
Phone: (770)426-2736 **Fax:** (770)426-2697
Email: jalehd@life.edu
Jaleh Dehpahlavan, Director

★ **26657** ★ **Life University**
Nutrition Department
Dietetic Technician Program
1269 Barclay Circle, SE
110 Annex B
Marietta, GA 30060-2903
Phone: (770)426-2736 **Fax:** (770)426-2697
Email: jalehd@life.edu
Jaleh Dehpahlavan, Contact

★ **26658** ★ **Southern Regional Medical Center**
Dietetic Internship Program
11 Upper Riverdale Rd. SW
Riverdale, GA 30274-2600
Phone: (770)991-8030 **Fax:** (770)991-8690
Email: crocker_stephanie@promina.org
Website: http://www.southernregional.org
Stephanie L. Crocker, Director

★ **26659** ★ **University of Georgia**
Department of Foods and Nutrition
College of Family and Consumer Sciences
Dietetics-Didactic Program
Dawson Hall
Athens, GA 30602
Phone: (706)542-7983 **Fax:** (706)542-5059
Email: jfischer@fcs.uga.edu
Joan G. Fischer, PhD, Director

★ **26660** ★ **University of Georgia**
Department of Foods and Nutrition
Dietetic Internship Program
Dawson Hall
Athens, GA 30602
Phone: (706)542-4908 **Fax:** (706)542-5059
Email: bgrossma@fcs.uga.edu
Website: http://www.fcs.uga.edu
Barbara M. Grossman, PhD, Director

★ **26661** ★ **University Health Care System**
Dietetic Internship Program
1350 Walton Way
Augusta, GA 30901-2629
Phone: (706)774-8897 **Fax:** (706)774-8671
Email: jlee@uh.org
Website: http://www.universityhealth.org
Jeanne B. Lee, Director

Hawaii

★ **26662** ★ **University of Hawaii, Manoa**
Department of Human Nutrition, Food, and Animal Science
Dietetics-Didactic Program
1955 East West Rd., Rm. 3141
Honolulu, HI 96822-2218
Phone: (808)956-3847 **Fax:** (808)956-4024
Email: shovic@hawaii.edu
Website: http://www.hawaii.edu/dietetics
Anne C. Shovic, PhD, Director

Idaho

★ **26663** ★ **Idaho State University**
Department of Health and Nutrition Sciences
Dietetic Internship Program
Campus Box 8109
Pocatello, ID 83209-8109
Phone: (208)282-2352 **Fax:** (208)282-4903
Email: dundmary@isu.edu
Mary L. Dundas, PhD, Director

★ **26664** ★ **Idaho State University**
Department of Health and Nutrition Sciences
Dietetics-Didactic Program
Campus Box 8109
1291 E Terry/MLK Way
Pocatello, ID 83209-8109
Phone: (208)282-2961 **Fax:** (208)282-4903
Email: mcknlaur@isu.edu
Laura E. G. McKnight, Contact

★ **26665** ★ **University of Idaho**
School of Family and Consumer Sciences
College of Agriculture
Coordinated Program in Dietetics
Moscow, ID 83844-3183
Phone: (208)885-6026 **Fax:** (208)885-5751
Email: kgabel@uidaho.edu
Website: http://www.uidaho.edu/fcs
Kathleen A. Gabel, PhD, Director

Illinois

★ **26666** ★ **Benedictine University**
Department of Nutrition
Dietetic Internship Program
5700 College Rd.
Lisle, IL 60532-0900
Phone: (630)829-6548 **Fax:** (630)829-6547
Email: jmoreschi@ben.edu
Website: http://www.ben.edu
Julie Moreschi, Director

★ **26667** ★ **Benedictine University**
Department of Nutrition
Dietetics-Didactic Program
5700 College Rd.
Lisle, IL 60532-0900
Phone: (630)829-6521 **Fax:** (630)829-6547
Email: jdavis@ben.edu
Website: http://www.ben.edu/nutrition/index.html
Julie J. Davis, Director

★ **26668** ★ **Bradley University**
Family and Consumer Sciences Department
Dietetics-Didactic Program
1501 W Bradley Ave.
Peoria, IL 61625-0115
Phone: (309)677-2436 **Fax:** (309)677-3813
Email: jad@bradley.edu
Website: http://www.bradley.edu/
Jeannette Davidson, PhD, Director

★ **26669** ★ **Dominican University**
Department of Nutrition Sciences
Dietetics-Didactic Program
7900 W Division St.
River Forest, IL 60305-1066
Phone: (708)524-6906 **Fax:** (708)366-5360
Email: judybeto@email.dom.edu
Website: http://www.dom.edu
Judith A. Beto, PhD, Director

★ **26670** ★ **Eastern Illinois University**
School of Family and Consumer Sciences
Dietetics-Didactic Program or Dietetic Internship Program
600 Lincoln Ave.
Klehm Hall 1433
Charleston, IL 61920-3099
Phone: (217)581-6680 **Fax:** (217)581-6090
Email: mdburns@eiu.edu
Website: http://www.eiu.edu/~famsci/
Melanie T. Burns, PhD, Director

★ **26671** ★ **Edward Hines Jr. VA Hospital**
Dietetic Internship Program
Nutrition and Food Service (120D)
PO Box 5000
Hines, IL 60141
Phone: (708)202-2343 **Fax:** (708)202-2252
Email: foley.sharon@hines.va.gov
Website: http://www.hinesvainternship.com
Sharon Foley, Director

★ **26672** ★ **Illinois State University**
Department of Family and Consumer Sciences
Dietetic Internship Program
Campus Box 5060
Normal, IL 61790-5060
Phone: (309)438-7031 **Fax:** (309)438-5659
Email: mawilso@ilstu.edu
Website: http://www.cast.ilstu.edu/isudi
Mardell A. Wilson, EdD, Director

★ 26673 ★ Illinois State University
Department of Family and Consumer Sciences
Dietetics-Didactic Program
Campus Box 5060
Normal, IL 61790-5060
Phone: (309)438-8850 **Fax:** (309)438-5659
Email: rcullen@ilstu.edu
Website: http://www.cast.ilstu.edu/fcs/food/index.shtml
Robert W. Cullen, PhD, Director

★ 26674 ★ Ingalls Memorial Hospital
Dietetic Internship Program
1 Ingalls Dr.
Harvey, IL 60426
Phone: (708)915-5723 **Fax:** (708)915-3110
Email: mvaughn@ingalls.org
Website: http://www.ingalls.org
Mary Keith Vaughn, Director

★ 26675 ★ Loyola University, Chicago
Department of Food and Nutrition
Dietetic Internship Program
6525 N Sheridan Rd.
Chicago, IL 60626-5311
Phone: (773)508-8298 **Fax:** (773)508-8296
Email: jkouba@luc.edu
Website: http://www.luc.edu/depts/nutrition/internsh.htm
Joanne Kouba, Director

★ 26676 ★ Loyola University, Chicago
Food and Nutrition Programs
Dietetics-Didactic Program
6525 N Sheridan Rd.
Chicago, IL 60626-5311
Phone: (773)508-8299 **Fax:** (773)508-8296
Email: tcarlyl@wpo.it.luc.edu
Website: http://www.luc.edu/depts/nutrition
Tracey L. Carlyle, Director

★ 26677 ★ Malcolm X College
City Colleges of Chicago
Dietetic Technician Program
1900 W Van Buren
Chicago, IL 60612-3145
Phone: (312)850-7383 **Fax:** (312)850-7453
Email: pkushida@ccc.edu
Perla M. Kushida, Edd, Contact

★ 26678 ★ Northern Illinois University
School of Family, Consumer, and Nutrition Sciences
Dietetic Internship Program
DeKalb, IL 60115-2854
Phone: (815)753-6386 **Fax:** (815)753-1321
Email: lrobins@niu.edu
Website: http://www.fcns.niu.edu/ndha
Lucy C. Robinson, Director

★ 26679 ★ Northern Illinois University
School of Family, Consumer, and Nutrition Sciences
Dietetics-Didactic Program
DeKalb, IL 60115-2854
Phone: (815)753-6352 **Fax:** (815)753-1321
Email: jmlukaszuk@niu.edu
Website: http://www.niu.edu
Judith M. Lukaszuk, PhD, Director

★ 26680 ★ Olivet Nazarene University
Department of Family and Consumer Sciences
Dietetics-Didactic Program
1 University Dr.
Bourbonnais, IL 60914
Phone: (815)928-5571 **Fax:** (815)935-4990
Email: canstrom@olivet.edu
Website: http://web.olivet.edu/facs/
Cantherine N. Anstrom, Director

★ 26681 ★ OSF St. Francis Medical Center
Dietetic Internship Program
530 NE Glen Oak Ave.
Peoria, IL 61637-0001
Phone: (309)655-3707 **Fax:** (309)655-4022
Email: mei-ling.lin@osfhealthcare.org
Website: http://www.osaintfrancis.org/SchoolsDieteticIntern/
Mei-Ling C. Lin, Director

★ 26682 ★ Rush Presbyterian-St. Luke's Medical Center
Dietetic Internship Program
1653 W Congress Pkwy.
Chicago, IL 60612-3864
Phone: (312)942-3349 **Fax:** (312)942-5203
Email: annalynn_skipper@rush.edu
Website: http://www.rushu.rush.edu/nutrition
Annalynn Skipper, Director

★ 26683 ★ St. John's Hospital
School of Dietetics/Food and Nutrition Services
Dietetic Internship Program
800 E Carpenter St.
Springfield, IL 62769
Phone: (217)544-6464 **Fax:** (217)757-6871
Email: slopinsk@st-johns.org
Website: http://www.st-johns.org
Sara A. Lopinski, Director

★ 26684 ★ Southern Illinois University, Carbondale
Animal Science, Food and Nutrition
Dietetics-Didactic Program
Mail Code 4417
875 S Normal Ave
Carbondale, IL 62901-4317
Phone: (618)453-7512 **Fax:** (618)453-7517
Email: saraland@siu.edu
Website: http://www.siu.edu/departments/coagr/animal/dietetic/
Sara Long, PhD, Director

★ 26685 ★ Southern Illinois University, Carbondale
Food and Nutrition
Dietetic Internship Program
Mail Code 4317
Carbondale, IL 62901-4317
Phone: (618)453-5192 **Fax:** (618)453-7517
Email: jans01@siu.edu
Website: http://www.siu.edu/departments/coagr/animal/dietetic/grad
Janet A. Sundberg, Director

★ 26686 ★ University of Illinois, Chicago
Department of Human Nutrition and Dietetics
Coordinated Program in Dietetics
1919 W Taylor St.
M/C 517
Chicago, IL 60612-7256
Phone: (312)996-8055 **Fax:** (312)413-0319
Email: braunsch@uic.edu
Carol L. Braunschweig, PhD, Director

★ 26687 ★ University of Illinois, Chicago
Department of Human Nutrition (M/C 517)
Dietetics-Didactic Program
1919 W Taylor St.
Chicago, IL 60612-7256
Phone: (773)508-8299 **Fax:** (773)508-8296
Email: braunsch@uic.edu
Website: http://www.uic.edu
Carol L. Braunschweig, PhD, Director

★ 26688 ★ University of Illinois, Urbana-Champaign
Department of Food Science and Human Nutrition
Dietetic Internship Program
443 Bevier Hall
905 S Goodwin Ave.
Urbana, IL 61801
Phone: (217)333-2987 **Fax:** (217)265-0925
Email: tappende@uiuc.edu
Website: http://www.aces.uiuc.edu/~dietetic/Default.htm
Kelly A. Tappenden, PhD, Director

★ 26689 ★ University of Illinois, Urbana, Champaign
Department of Food Science and Human Nutrition
Dietetics-Didactic Program
345 Bevier Hall
905 S Goodwin Ave.
Urbana, IL 61801-3852
Phone: (217)244-2884 **Fax:** (217)265-0925
Email: plawecki@uiuc.edu
Website: http://www.fshn.uiuc.edu/Dietetics/index.html
Karen L. Plawecki, Director

★ 26690 ★ Western Illinois University
Department of Family and Consumer Sciences
Dietetics-Didactic Program
Macomb, IL 61455
Phone: (309)298-1581 **Fax:** (309)298-2688
Email: KR-Greathouse@wiu.edu
Website: http://www.wiu.edu/users/mifcs
Karen R. Greathouse, PhD, Director

★ 26691 ★ William Rainey Harper College
Dietetic Technician Program
1200 W Algonquin Rd.
Palatine, IL 60067-7398
Phone: (847)925-6537 **Fax:** (847)925-6047
Email: jallendo@harper.cc.il.us
Website: http://www.harpercollege.edu
Jane F. Allendorph, Contact

Indiana

★ 26692 ★ Ball Memorial Hospital
Department of Dietetics
Dietetic Internship Program
2401 W University Ave.
Muncie, IN 47303-3499
Phone: (765)747-3273 **Fax:** (765)741-2994
Email: kshields@chs.cami3.com
Website: http://www.cardinalhealthsystem.org
Karen S. Shields, Director

★ 26693 ★ Ball State University
Department of Family and Consumer Sciences
Dietetic Technician Program
150 Applied Technology
Muncie, IN 47306-0250
Phone: (765)285-2255 **Fax:** (765)285-2314
Email: ccarr@bsu.edu
Corine M. Carr, EdD, Contact

★ 26694 ★ Ball State University
Department of Family and Consumer Sciences
Dietetics-Didactic Program
Muncie, IN 47306-0250

Phone: (765)285-5931 **Fax:** (765)285-2314
Email: jlowe2@bsu.edu
Website: http://www.bsu.edu/cast/fcs
Judith B. Lowe, Director

★ 26695 ★ Ball State University
Family and Consumer Sciences
Dietetic Internship Program
150 Applied Technology Bldg.
Muncie, IN 47306
Phone: (765)285-5940 **Fax:** (765)285-2314
Email: mskurtz@bsu.edu
Marla S. Kurtz, Director

★ 26696 ★ Indiana State University
Department of Family and Consumer Sciences
Coordinated Program in Dietetics
Terre Haute, IN 47809
Phone: (812)237-3925 **Fax:** (812)237-3304
Email: hereed@ruby.indstate.edu
Carol A. Reed, Contact

★ 26697 ★ Indiana State University
Department of Family and Consumer Sciences
Coordinated Program in Dietetics
Terre Haute, IN 47809
Phone: (812)237-3295 **Fax:** (812)237-3304
Email: hereed@ruby.indstate.edu
Carol A. Reed, Director

★ 26698 ★ Indiana University, Bloomington
Department of Applied Health Science
Dietetics-Didactic Program
HPER 116
1025 E Seventh St.
Bloomington, IN 47405-7109
Phone: (812)855-1531 **Fax:** (812)855-3936
Email: vgetty@indiana.edu
Victoria M. Getty, MEd, Director

★ 26699 ★ Indiana University School of Medicine
School of Allied Health
Nutrition/Dietetics Program
Dietetic Internship Program
Ball Residence BR114
Indianapolis, IN 46202-5180
Phone: (317)278-0933 **Fax:** (317)278-3940
Email: jopalka@iupui.edu
Jacquelynn O'Palka, PhD, Director

★ 26700 ★ Marian College
Department of Food and Nutrition Sciences
Food and Nutrition Sciences Program
Coordinated Program in Dietetics
3200 Cold Spring Rd.
Indianapolis, IN 46222-1997
Phone: (317)955-6340 **Fax:** (317)955-6448
Email: cstrain@marian.edu
Website: http://www.marian.edu
Catherine H. Strain, Contact

★ 26701 ★ Marian College
Department of Nursing and Nutritional Sciences
Food amd Nutrition Sciences Program
Dietetics-Didactic Program or Coordinated Program in Dietetics
3200 Cold Springs Rd.
Indianapolis, IN 46222-1997
Phone: (317)955-6340 **Fax:** (317)955-6448
Email: cstrain@marian.edu
Website: http://www.marian.edu/
Catherine H. Strain, Director

★ 26702 ★ Purdue University
Department of Foods and Nutrition
Coordinated Program in Dietetics
700 W State St.
West Lafayette, IN 47907-2059
Phone: (765)496-6569 **Fax:** (765)494-0674
Email: bousheyc@cfs.purdue.edu
Website: http://www.cfs.purdue.edu/fn/
Carol J. Boushey, Director

★ 26703 ★ Purdue University
Department of Foods and Nutrition
Dietetics-Didactic Program
1264 Stone Hall
West Lafayette, IN 47907-1264
Phone: (765)494-8238 **Fax:** (765)494-0674
Email: woodo@cfs.purdue.edu
Website: http://www.cfs.purdue.edu/fdsnutr
Olivia B. Wood, Director
Carol J. Boushey, PhD, Contact

★ 26704 ★ Purdue University, Calumet
Department of Behavioral Sciences
Preprofessional Practice Program in Dietetics
2200 169th St.
Hammond, IN 46323-2094
Phone: (219)989-2940 **Fax:** (219)989-2008
Email: fields@calumet.purdue.edu
Rita A. Fields, Director

Iowa

★ 26705 ★ Iowa State University
Department of Food Science and Human Nutrition
Dietetic Internship Program
220 Mackay Hall
Ames, IA 50011
Phone: (515)294-7316 **Fax:** (515)294-6193
Email: janderso@iastate.edu
Website: http://www.dietetics.iastate.edu
Jean A. Anderson, Director

★ 26706 ★ Iowa State University
Department of Food Science and Human Nutrition
Dietetics-Didactic Program
220 MacKay Hall
Ames, IA 50011-1120
Phone: (515)294-2321 **Fax:** (515)294-5390
Email: moakland@iastate.edu
Website: http://www.dietetics.iastate.edu
Mary Jane Oakland, PhD, Director

★ 26707 ★ University of Iowa Hospitals and Clinics
Dietetic Internship Program
200 Hawkins Dr.
W146GH
Iowa City, IA 52242-1051
Phone: (319)356-1240 **Fax:** (319)356-8674
Email: laurie-kroymann@uiowa.edu
Website: http://www.uihc.uiowa.edu/fns/internship
Laurie L. Kroymann, Director

★ 26708 ★ University of Northern Iowa
Department of Design, Family and Consumer Sciences
Dietetics-Didactic Program
219 Latham Hall
1227 W 27th St.
Cedar Falls, IA 50614-0332
Phone: (319)273-2418 **Fax:** (319)273-7096
Email: Tammie.collum@uni.edu
Website: http://csbsnt.csbs.uni.edu/dept/dfcs/index.html
Tammie Collum, Director

Kansas

★ 26709 ★ Kansas State University
Department of Hotel, Restaurant, Institution Management, and Dietetics
Coordinated Program in Dietetics
Justin Hall, Rm. 104
Manhattan, KS 66506-1404
Phone: (785)532-2216 **Fax:** (785)532-5522
Email: canter@ksu.edu
Website: http://www.humec.ksu.edu/humec/hrimd/programs/dietetics/
Deborah D. Canter, PhD, Director

★ 26710 ★ Kansas State University
Department of Hotel, Restaurant, Institution Management and Dietetics
Department of Food and Nutrition
Dietetics-Didactic Program
Manhattan, KS 66506-1404
Phone: (785)532-2208 **Fax:** (785)532-5522
Email: barrett@humec.ksu.edu
Website: http://www.ksu.edu/humec/hrimd/hr_diet.htm
Elizabeth B. Barrett, PhD, Contact

★ 26711 ★ University of Kansas Medical Center
Department of Dietetics and Nutrition
Dietetic Internship Program
3901 Rainbow Blvd.
Kansas City, KS 66160-7250
Phone: (913)588-7683 **Fax:** (913)588-8946
Email: rbarkley@kumc.edu
Rachel S. Barkley, Director

Kentucky

★ 26712 ★ Berea College
Department of Child and Family Studies
Dietetics-Didactic Program
CPO 2192
Berea, KY 40404
Phone: (859)985-3743 **Fax:** (859)985-3917
Email: janice_blythe@berea.edu
Website: http://www.berea.edu/CFS/CFS.home.htmlfaculty
Janice B. Blythe, PhD, Director

★ 26713 ★ Eastern Kentucky University
Department of Family and Consumer Sciences
Dietetics-Didactic Program or Dietetic Internship Program
102 Burrier Bldg.
Richmond, KY 40475
Phone: (859)622-3445 **Fax:** (859)622-1163
Email: sara.sutton@eku.edu
Website: http://www.fcs.eku.edu
Sara W. Sutton, Director

★ 26714 ★ Morehead State University
College of Science and Technology
Dietetics-Didactic Program or Dietetic Internship Program
Reed Hall 246
UPO 721
Morehead, KY 40351-1689
Phone: (606)783-2023 **Fax:** (606)783-5007
Email: m.sampley@morehead-st.edu
Marilyn T. Sampley, PhD, Director

★ 26715 ★ Murray State University
Department of Wellness and Therapeutic Sciences
Division of Nutrition, Dietetics and Food Management
Dietetics-Didactic Program or Dietetic Internship Program
Applied Sciences Bldg.
200 N Oakley
Murray, KY 42071-3345
Phone: (270)762-3387 **Fax:** (270)762-6950
Email: kathy.timmons@murraystate.edu
Website: http://www.mursurky.edu/gacd/CIT/FCS/
Kathryn L. Timmons, Director

★ 26716 ★ Spalding University
Dietetic Internship Program
851 S Fourth St.
Louisville, KY 40203-2115
Phone: (502)585-9911 **Fax:** (502)588-7175
Email: krapp@spalding.edu
Website: http://www.spalding.edu
Kathy R. Rapp, Director

★ 26717 ★ University of Kentucky
Department of Nutrition and Food Sciences
Dietetics-Didactic Program
204 Funkhouser Bldg.
Lexington, KY 40506-0050
Phone: (859)257-1661 **Fax:** (859)257-1275
Email: mecook0@uky.edu
Website: http://www.uky.edu/HES
Margaret E. Cook-Newell, Director
Hazel W. Forsythe, PhD, Contact

★ 26718 ★ University of Kentucky
Human Environmental Sciences
Nutrition and Food Science Department
204 Funkhouser Bldg.
Lexington, KY 40506-0054
Phone: (606)257-3800 **Fax:** (606)257-3707
Email: vabl@pop.uky.edu
Website: http://www.uky.edu
Hazel W. Forsythe, PhD, Director

★ 26719 ★ University of Kentucky Hospital
Nutrition Services
Dietetic Internship Program
800 Rose St.
H507 UKCMC
Lexington, KY 40536-0293
Phone: (606)323-5154 **Fax:** (606)257-4588
Email: bsvivi0@uky.edu
Beverly S. Vivian, Director

★ 26720 ★ Western Kentucky University
Department of Consumer and Family Sciences
Dietetics-Didactic Program
Academic Complex 302F
1 Big Red Way
Bowling Green, KY 42101-3576
Phone: (270)745-4352 **Fax:** (270)745-3999
Email: Danita.Kelley@wku.edu
Website: http://www.wku.edu/dietetics
Danita M. Saxon Kelley, PhD, Director

Louisiana

★ 26721 ★ Delgado Community College
Dietetic Technician Program
615 City Park Ave.
New Orleans, LA 70119
Phone: (504)483-4330 **Fax:** (504)483-4324
Email: dmpace@dcc.edu
Website: http://www/dcc/edi
Donna M. Pace, Contact

★ 26722 ★ Louisiana State University
School of Human Ecology
Dietetic Internship Program
Tower Drive
Baton Rouge, LA 70803-4301
Phone: (225)578-1729 **Fax:** (225)578-2697
Email: chanmugam@aol.com
Website: http://sun.huec.lsu.edu/hnf.html
Prithiva S. Chanmugam, PhD, Director

★ 26723 ★ Louisiana State University
School of Human Ecology
Dietetics-Didactic Program
Baton Rouge, LA 70803-4300
Phone: (225)578-1631 **Fax:** (225)578-2697
Email: ceoneil@lsu.edu
Website: http://sun.huec.lsu.edu
Carol E. O'Neill, PhD, Director

★ 26724 ★ Louisiana Tech University
School of Human Ecology
Dietetic Internship Program
PO Box 3167 T.S
Ruston, LA 71272
Phone: (318)257-3043 **Fax:** (318)257-4014
Email: Erickson@ans.latech.edu
Website: http://www.ans.latech.edu/humaneco-intern.html
Dawn M. Erickson, Director

★ 26725 ★ Louisiana Tech University
School of Human Ecology
Dietetics-Didactic Program
PO Box 3167
Ruston, LA 71272
Phone: (318)257-2607 **Fax:** (318)257-4014
Email: molaison@hec.latech.edu
Website: http://www.ans.latech.edu/humaneco-index.html
Elaine F. Molaison, PhD, Director

★ 26726 ★ McNeese State University
Dietectics-Didactic Program
PO Box 92820
Lake Charles, LA 70609
Phone: (337)475-5970 **Fax:** (337)475-5681
Email: bfonteno@mail.mcneese.edu
Website: http://www.faculty.mcneese.edu/bfonteno
Beth Fontenot, Director

★ 26727 ★ McNeese State University
Dietetic Internship Program
PO Box 92820 MSU
Lake Charles, LA 70609-2820
Phone: (337)475-5684 **Fax:** (337)475-5681
Email: dholl205@aol.com
Debra S. Hollingsworth, PhD, Director

★ 26728 ★ Nicholls State University
Department of Family, Consumer, and Agricultural Sciences
Dietetics-Didactic Program
Box 2014
Thibodaux, LA 70310
Phone: (985)448-4690 **Fax:** (985)449-7073
Email: facs-cgl@nicholls.edu
Colette G. Leistner, PhD, Director

★ 26729 ★ North Oaks Health System
Nutritional Services
Dietetic Internship Program
PO Box 2668
Hammond, LA 70404-2668
Phone: (985)230-6548 **Fax:** (985)230-6563
Email: pelegrinv@northoaks.org
Website: http://www.northoaks.org
Virginia M. Pelegrin, Director

★ 26730 ★ Southern University and A&M College
College of Agricultural, Family and Consumer Science
Human Nutrition and Food Program
Dietetics-Didactic Program or Dietetic Internship Program
PO Box 11342
Baton Rouge, LA 70813-1342
Phone: (225)771-4660 **Fax:** (225)771-3107
Email: bmcgee@subr.edu
Bernestine B. McGee, PhD, Director

★ 26731 ★ Touro Infirmary
Dietetic Internship Program
1401 Foucher St.
New Orleans, LA 70115-3515
Phone: (504)897-8034 **Fax:** (504)897-8093
Email: fitzpatrickp@touro.com
Patricia A. Fitzpatrick, Director

★ 26732 ★ Tulane University
School of Public Health
Community Health Sciences
Dietetic Internship Program
1440 Canal St.,Ste. 2317
New Orleans, LA 70112-2699
Phone: (504)584-2672 **Fax:** (504)584-3540
Email: jzighel@mailhost.tcs.tulane.edu
Jodi E. Zighelboim, Director

★ 26733 ★ University of Louisiana, Lafayette
College of Applied Life Sciences
School of Human Resources
Dietetics-Didactic Program or Dietetic Internship Program
McKinley St.
PO Box 40399
Lafayette, LA 70504-0399
Phone: (337)482-6577 **Fax:** (337)482-5395
Email: boa5197@louisiana.edu
Website: http://www.sustainablelouisiana/humr.org
Bernice O. Adeleye, PhD, Director

Maine

★ 26734 ★ Southern Maine Technical College
Dietetic Technician Program
Fort Rd.
South Portland, ME 04106
Phone: (207)767-9606 **Fax:** (207)767-2731
Email: igabrielson@smtc.edu
Website: http://www.smtc.net/
Linda W. Gabrielson, Contact

★ 26735 ★ University of Maine
Department of Food Science and Human Nutrition
Dietetics-Didactic Program
5735 Hitchner Hall
Orono, ME 04469-5735
Phone: (207)581-3130 **Fax:** (207)581-1636
Email: sullivan@umenfa.maine.edu
Website: http://www.fsn.umaine.edu
Susan S. Sullivan, DSc, Director

★ 26736 ★ University of Maine, Orono
Department of Food Science and Human Nutrition
Dietetic Internship Program
5735 Hitchner Hall, Rm. 113
Orono, ME 04469-5749
Phone: (207)581-3134 **Fax:** (207)581-1636
Email: aawhite@umenfa.maine.edu
Website: http://www.ume.maine.edu/~nfa/fsn/
Adrienne A. White, PhD, Director

★ 26737 ★ Washington County Technical College
Department of Food/Hospitality and Dietetics Studies
Dietetic Technician Program
RR 1 Box 22
Calais, ME 04619
Phone: (207)454-1091 **Fax:** (207)454-1006
Email: dharris@wctc.org
Website: http://www.wctc.org
Denise E. Harris, Contact

Maryland

★ 26738 ★ Baltimore City Community College
Department of Allied Health and Human Services
Dietetic Technician Program
2901 Liberty Heights Ave.
Baltimore, MD 21215-7893
Phone: (410)462-7724 **Fax:** (410)462-7734
Email: jcampbell@bccc.state.md.us
Jolene R. Campbell, MEd, Contact

★ 26739 ★ Johns Hopkins Bayview Medical Center
Clinical Nutrition Department
Dietetic Internship Program
4940 Eastern Ave.
Baltimore, MD 21224-2735
Phone: (410)550-1319 **Fax:** (410)550-0650
Email: ckoch@jhmi.edu
Website: http://www.jhbmc.jhu.edu/nutria/index.html
Cheryl R. Koch, Director

★ 26740 ★ Morgan State University
Department of Family and Consumer Sciences
Dietetics-Didactic Program
1700 E Cold Spring Ln.
Jenkins Bldg., 403-A
Baltimore, MD 21251
Phone: (443)885-3905 **Fax:** (443)319-3787
Email: iforand@morgan.edu
Website: http://www.morgan.edu
Ivis T. Forrester-Anderson, PhD, Director

★ 26741 ★ National Institutes of Health Clinical Center, Nutrition Department
Dietetic Internship Program
Bldg. 10, Rm. B1S-234
10 Center Dr., MSC 1078
Bethesda, MD 20892-1078
Phone: (301)496-6349 **Fax:** (301)496-0622
Email: mleser@nih.gov
Website: http://www.cc.nih.gov/nutr/
Maureen G. Leser, Director

★ 26742 ★ Sodexho Health Care Services, Mid Atlantic
Dietetic Internship Program
10500 Little Patuxent Pkwy., Ste. 620
Columbia, MD 21044
Phone: (410)715-1201 **Fax:** (410)715-1694
Email: jdebelius@sodexhousa.com
Website: http://www.sodexhousa.com/car_dietetic.html
Janet L. Debelius, Director

★ 26743 ★ University of Maryland, College Park
Department of Nutrition and Food Science
Dietetic Internship Program
0112 Skinner Bldg.
College Park, MD 20742
Phone: (301)405-4525 **Fax:** (301)574-3842
Email: pml64@umail.umd.edu
Website: http://www.agnr.umd.edu/users/nfsc/internship
Phyllis E. Fatzinger-McShane, Director

★ 26744 ★ University of Maryland, College Park
Department of Nutrition and Food Sciences
Dietetics-Didactic Program
College Park, MD 20742-7521
Phone: (301)405-4532 **Fax:** (301)314-9327
Email: nb81@umail.umd.edu
Website: http://www.agnr.umd.edu/users/nfsc
Nancy J. Brenowitz, Director

★ 26745 ★ University of Maryland, Eastern Shore
Department of Human Ecology
Dietetic Internship Program
Princess Anne, MD 21853-1299
Phone: (410)651-6066 **Fax:** (410)651-6207
Email: bwblakely@umes.edu
Website: http://www.umes.edu/ecology/ap4.htm
Bettie W. Blakely, PhD, Director

★ 26746 ★ University of Maryland, Eastern Shore
Department of Human Ecology
Dietetics-Didactic Program or Dietetics-Preprofessional Practice Program
Princess Anne, MD 21853-1299
Phone: (410)651-6066 **Fax:** (410)651-6207
Email: bwblakely@mail.umes.edu
Website: http://www.umes.edu/ecology/undergraduate.htm
Bettie W. Blakely, PhD, Director

★ 26747 ★ University of Maryland Medical System
Food and Nutrition Services
Dietetic Internship Program
22 S Greene St.
Baltimore, MD 21201-1595
Phone: (410)328-2561 **Fax:** (410)328-1007
Email: lwohlberg@umm.edu
Laura K. Wohlberg, Director

Massachusetts

★ 26748 ★ Beth Israel Deaconess Medical Center
Nutrition Services
Dietetic Internship Program
330 Brookline Ave.
Boston, MA 02215-5491
Phone: (617)667-2580 **Fax:** (617)632-7180
Email: psamour@caregroup.harvard.edu
Website: http://www.bidmc.Harvard.edu/dietetic
Patricia Queen Samour, Director

★ 26749 ★ Boston University Sargent College
Graduate Nutrition Division
Dietetic Internship Program
635 Commonwealth Ave.
Boston, MA 02215-1605
Phone: (617)353-7470 **Fax:** (617)353-7567
Email: salge@bu.edu
Website: http://www.bu.edu/sargent/hs
Joan Salge Blake, Director

★ 26750 ★ Boston University/Sargent College
Department of Health Sciences
Dietetics-Didactic Program
635 Commonwealth Ave.
Boston, MA 02215-1605
Phone: (617)353-7488 **Fax:** (617)353-7567
Email: rdurschl@bu.edu
Website: http://www.bu.edu/sargent/programs
Roberta P. Durschlag, PhD, Director

★ 26751 ★ Brigham and Women's Hospital
Dietetic Internship Program
75 Francis St.
Boston, MA 02115-6195
Phone: (617)732-5577 **Fax:** (617)278-6929
Email: amccarley@partners.org
Website: http://www.brighamandwomens.org/
Alice M. McCarley, Director

★ 26752 ★ Framingham State College
Department of Family and Consumer Sciences
Dietetics-Didactic Program or Coordinated Program in Dietetics
100 State St.
Framingham, MA 01701-9101
Phone: (508)626-4757 **Fax:** (508)626-4003
Email: maberne@frc.mass.edu
Website: http://www.framingham.edu
Marilyn M. Abernethy, DrPH, Director
Suzanne H. Neubauer, Contact

★ 26753 ★ Frances Stern Nutrition Center
New England Medical Center
Tufts University
Dietetic Internship Program
750 Washington St., Box 783
Boston, MA 02111-1533
Phone: (617)636-5273 **Fax:** (617)636-8325
Email: jdwyer1@tufts-nemc.org
Website: http://www.tufts.edu/nutrition/program/dietetic_internship/
Johanna T. Dwyer, DSc, Director

★ 26754 ★ Laboure College
Dietetic Technician Program
2120 Dorchester Ave.
Boston, MA 02124-5698
Phone: (617)296-8300 **Fax:** (617)296-7947
Email: anne_manion@laboure.edu
Website: http://www.labourecollege.org
Anne S. Manion, Contact

★ 26755 ★ Massachusetts General Hospital
Department of Nutrition and Food Services
Dietetic Internship Program
Boston, MA 02114
Phone: (617)726-2589 **Fax:** (617)726-7649
Email: kcreedon@partners.org
Website: http://www.massgeneral.org/visitor/nutrition_dietetics.htm
Kathleen E. Creedon, Director

★ 26756 ★ Mount Auburn Hospital
Dietetic Internship Program
330 Mount Auburn St.
Cambridge, MA 02138
Phone: (617)499-5159 **Fax:** (617)499-5673
Email: mta.nutr.dmb@mahhosp.org
Website: http://www.mtauburn.caregroup.org/mededu/mededu.asp
Donna M. Belcher, Director

★ 26757 ★ North Shore Community College
Division of Health Professions
Department of Nutritional Sciences and Diet Technology
Dietetic Technician Program
1 Ferncroft Rd.
Danvers, MA 01923-4093
Phone: (978)762-4000 **Fax:** (978)762-4002
Email: blucas@northshore.edu
Bernadette S. Lucas, Contact

★ 26758 ★ Simmons College
Department of Nutrition
Dietetic Internship Program
300 The Fenway
Boston, MA 02115
Phone: (617)521-2718 **Fax:** (617)521-3137
Email: herbold@simmons.edu
Website: http://www.simmons.edu
Nancie H. Herbold, EdD, Director

★ 26759 ★ Simmons College
Department of Nutrition
Dietetics-Didactic Program
300 The Fenway
Boston, MA 02115-5898
Phone: (617)521-2708 **Fax:** (617)521-3137
Email: metallin@simmons.edu
Website: http://www.simmons.edu/
Elizabeth S. Metallinos-Katsaras, PhD, Director

★ 26760 ★ Sodexho Health Care Services
Distance Education
Dietetic Internship Program
45 Hayden Ave.
Lexington, MA 02420
Free: 800-926-7429 **Fax:** (603)487-5293
Email: DistLearningIntern@sodexhoUSA.com
Website: http://www.dieteticintern.com
Barbara J. Woodland, EdD, Director

★ 26761 ★ Sodexho Health Care Services
Southcoast Hospitals Group
Dietetic Internship Program
101 Page St.
New Bedford, MA 02740-3464
Phone: (508)961-5161 **Fax:** (508)961-5166
Email: nutrition@southcoast.org
Website: http://www.southcoast.org/jobs/interns-dietary.html
Elizabeth F. Winthrop, Director

★ 26762 ★ University of Massachusetts, Amherst
Department of Nutrition
Dietetic Internship Program
358 N Pleasant St.
Amherst, MA 01003-9296
Phone: (413)545-2484 **Fax:** (413)577-3838
Email: aszlosek@contined.umass.edu
Website: http://www.umasss.edu/dieteticinternship/
Alice E. Szlosek, Director

★ 26763 ★ University of Massachusetts, Amherst
Department of Nutrition
Dietetics-Didactic Program
213 Chenoweth Laboratory
100 Holdsworth Way
Amherst, MA 01003-9282
Phone: (413)577-0671 **Fax:** (413)545-1074
Email: aszlosek@contined.umass.edu
Website: http://www.umass.edu/sphhs/nutrition
Alice E. Szlosek, Director

Michigan

★ 26764 ★ Andrews University
Department of Nutrition
Dietetics-Didactic Program or Dietetics-Preprofessional Practice Program
Berrien Springs, MI 49104-0210
Phone: (616)471-3370 **Fax:** (616)471-3485
Email: wcraig@andrews.edu
Website: http://www.andrews.edu/NUFS
Winston J. Craig, Director

★ 26765 ★ Central Michigan University
Human Environmental Studies
Dietetic Internship Program
Wightman Hall 205
Mount Pleasant, MI 48859-3652
Phone: (989)879-4357 **Fax:** (989)879-4378
Email: jaylaf@cmich.edu
Website: http://nutrition.ehs.cmich.edu/CMUDI.htm
Ann F. Jay, Director

★ 26766 ★ Central Michigan University
Human Environmental Studies
Dietetics-Didactic Program or Dietetic Internship Program
Wightman Hall 205
Mount Pleasant, MI 48859
Phone: (989)774-2004 **Fax:** (989)774-2435
Email: jack.logomarsino@cmich.edu
Website: http://www.nutrition.ehs.cmich.edu
John V. Logomarsino, PhD, Director

★ 26767 ★ Detroit Health Department
Nutrition Division
Dietetic Internship Program
1151 Taylor
Detroit, MI 48202-1732
Phone: (313)876-4090 **Fax:** (313)876-4645
Email: aryai@health.ci.Detroit.mi.us
Indira D. Arya, Director

★ 26768 ★ Eastern Michigan University
Department of Human, Environmental, and Consumer Resources
Coordinated Program in Dietetics
206 Roosevelt Hall
Ypsilanti, MI 48197
Phone: (734)487-7862 **Fax:** (734)487-7087
Email: judi.brooks@emich.edu
Website: http://www.emich.edu
Judith T. Brooks, PhD, Director

★ 26769 ★ Harper University Hospital
Department of Nutrition and Food Services
Dietetic Internship Program
3990 John R St.
Detroit, MI 48201-2018
Phone: (313)745-2037 **Fax:** (313)993-8509
Email: mlearnman2@dmc.org
Website: http://www.dmc.org/harper/diet/
Diane L. Trippett, Director

★ 26770 ★ Henry Ford Hospital
Department of Food and Nutrition Services
Dietetic Internship Program
2799 W Grand Blvd.
Detroit, MI 48202-2689
Phone: (313)916-3473 **Fax:** (313)916-0761
Email: lhufnagl@hfhs.org
Lynne A. Hufnagle, Director

★ 26771 ★ Hurley Medical Center
Nutrition Service Department
Dietetic Internship Program
One Hurley Plaza
Flint, MI 48503-5993
Phone: (810)257-6674 **Fax:** (810)424-4780
Email: jcardanl@hurleymc.com
Jennifer J. Gardner-Cardani, Director

★ 26772 ★ Madonna University
Department of Biological and Health Sciences
Dietetics-Didactic Program
36600 Schoolcraft Rd.
Livonia, MI 48150-1173
Phone: (734)432-5534 **Fax:** (734)432-5393
Email: kschmitz@madonna.edu
Website: http://www.madonna.edu
Karen J. Schmitz, PhD, Director

★ 26773 ★ Marygrove College
Department of Human Nutrition and Foods
8425 W McNichols Rd.
Detroit, MI 48221
Phone: (313)927-1322 **Fax:** (313)927-1345
Email: mnettles@marygrove.edu
Website: http://www.msu.edu/unit/fshn
Ethel M. Nettles, PhD, Director

★ 26774 ★ Michigan State University
Department of Food Science and Human Nutrition
Dietetic Internship Program
2100 Anthony Hall
East Lansing, MI 48824-1225
Phone: (517)355-7713 **Fax:** (517)353-1676
Email: rogersg3@msu.edu
Website: http://www.msu.edu/unit/fshn/grad/intern.html
Gail J. Rogers, Director

★ 26775 ★ Michigan State University
Department of Food Science and Human Nutrition
Dietetics-Didactic Program
210 Trout FSHN Bldg.
East Lansing, MI 48824-1224
Phone: (517)355-8474 **Fax:** (517)353-8963
Email: chenowel@msu.edu
Website: http://www.msu.edu/unit/fshn
Wanda L. Chenoweth, PhD, Director

★ 26776 ★ Northern Michigan University
Department of Health, Physical Education and Recreation
Dietetics-Didactic Program
Marquette, MI 49855
Phone: (906)227-2366 **Fax:** (906)227-2181
Email: mmowafy@nmu.edu
Mohey A. Mowafy, PhD, Director

★ 26777 ★ Oakland County Health Division
Health Education, Nutrition, and Substance Abuse Services
Dietetic Internship Program
27725 Greenfield Rd.
Southfield, MI 48076-3625
Phone: (248)424-7133 **Fax:** (248)424-7144
Email: eatonl@co.Oakland.mi.us
Linda H. Eaton, Director

★ 26778 ★ University of Michigan Hospitals and Health Centers
Dietetic Internship Program
UH2C227/0056
1500 E Medical Center Dr.
Ann Arbor, MI 48109-0056
Phone: (734)936-5197 **Fax:** (734)936-5195
Email: joyceks@umich.edu
Joyce Kerestes-Smith, Director

★ 26779 ★ University of Michigan School of Public Health
Human Nutrition Program
Dietetics-Didactic Program
1420 Washington Heights
M6150
Ann Arbor, MI 48109-2029
Phone: (734)764-0214 **Fax:** (734)764-5233
Email: hanmark@umich.edu
Theresa L. Han-Markey, Director

★ 26780 ★ University of Michigan School of Public Health
Preprofessional Practice Program in Dietetics
1420 Washington Heights, M6150
Ann Arbor, MI 48109-2029
Phone: (734)764-3277 **Fax:** (734)647-5865
Email: apfdir@med.umich.edu
Andrea J. Lasichak, Director

★ 26781 ★ Wayne State University
Department of Nutrition and Food Sciences
Coordinated Program in Dietetics
3009 Science Hall
Detroit, MI 48202
Phone: (313)577-2500 **Fax:** (313)577-8616
Email: treinha@lifesci.wayne.edu
Website: http://www.science.wayne.edu/~nfs/dietetics.htm
Tonia G. Reinhard, Director

★ 26782 ★ Western Michigan University
Department of Family and Consumer Sciences
Dietetics-Didactic Program
3024 Kohrman Hall
Kalamazoo, MI 49008
Phone: (616)387-3729 **Fax:** (616)387-3353
Email: rojhani@wmich.edu
Website: http://www.wmich.edu
Arezoo Rojhani, PhD, Director

★ 26783 ★ Western Michigan University
Family and Consumer Sciences
Dietetic Internship Program
3025 Kohrman Hall
Kalamazoo, MI 49008-5067
Phone: (616)387-3710 **Fax:** (616)387-3353
Email: mpeterso@wmich.edu
Website: http://unix.cc.wmich.edu/~mpeterso
Maija Peterson, PhD, Director

Minnesota

★ 26784 ★ College of Saint Catherine
Family, Consumer and Nutritional Sciences
Dietetics-Didactic Program
2004 Randolph Ave.
Saint Paul, MN 55105-1750
Phone: (651)690-6204 **Fax:** (651)690-6958
Email: peode@stkate.edu
Patricia J. Ode, Director

★ 26785 ★ Concordia College
Department of Family and Nutrition Sciences
Dietetics-Didactic Program
Moorhead, MN 56562
Phone: (218)299-3748 **Fax:** (218)299-4308
Email: blarson@gloria.cord.edu
Website: http://www.cord.edu
Betty J. Larson, EdD, Director

★ 26786 ★ Concordia College
Dietetic Internship and Dining Services
901 S 8th St.
Moorhead, MN 56562
Phone: (218)299-3706 **Fax:** (218)299-4409
Email: dcadwell@cord.edu
Website: http://www.cord.edu/dept/auxservices/ccdi-web.htm
Debra Lee-Cadwell, Director

★ 26787 ★ Minneapolis Veterans Affairs Medical Center
Nutrition and Food Service
Dietetic Internship Program
One Veterans Dr.
Minneapolis, MN 55417
Phone: (612)725-2004 **Fax:** (612)727-5997
Email: heidi.hoover@med.va.gov
Website: http://www.va.gov/nfs
Heidi H. Hoover, Director

★ 26788 ★ Minnesota State University, Mankato
Family Consumer Science Department
Dietetics-Didactic Program
102 Wiecking Center
Mankato, MN 56001
Phone: (507)389-6016 **Fax:** (507)389-2411
Email: sally.weerts@mnsu.edu
Website: http://www.mankato.msus.edu/
Sally Weerts, PhD, Director

★ 26789 ★ Regions Hospital
Dietetic Internship Program
640 Jackson St.
Saint Paul, MN 55101-2502
Phone: (651)254-2712 **Fax:** (651)254-9927
Email: betty.l.orchard@healthpartners.com
Elizabeth L. Orchard, Director

★ 26790 ★ Saint John's University
College of Saint Benedict
Nutrition Department, ASC 151
Coordinated Program in Dietetics
37 S College Ave.
Saint Joseph, MN 56374-2099
Phone: (320)363-5976 **Fax:** (320)363-5582
Email: djones@csbsju.edu
Website: http://www.CSBSJU.edu/nutrition/
Diane Veale Jones, Director

★ 26791 ★ St. Mary's Hospital/Mayo Medical Center
Dietetic Internship Program
1216 Second St. SW
Rochester, MN 55902-1906
Phone: (507)255-5617 **Fax:** (507)255-7379
Email: grant.jeanne@mayo.edu
Website: http://www.mayo.edu
Jeanne E. Grant, Director

★ 26792 ★ University of Minnesota
Coordinated Program in Dietetics
268 Food Science and Nutrition
1334 Eckles Ave.
Saint Paul, MN 55108-6099
Phone: (612)624-9278 **Fax:** (612)625-5272
Email: cearthma@umn.edu
Website: http://www.fsci.umn.edu/
Carrie P. Earthman, PhD, Director

★ 26793 ★ University of Minnesota
Department of Food Science and Nutrition
Dietetics-Didactic Program
225 Food Science and Nutrition
1334 Eckles Ave.
Saint Paul, MN 55108-6099
Phone: (612)624-3255 **Fax:** (612)264-5272
Email: lmarquar@umn.edu
Website: http://www.fscn.che.umn.edu
Leonard F. Marquart, PhD, Director

★ 26794 ★ University of Minnesota
Dietetic Internship Program
225 Food Science and Nutrition
Saint Paul, MN 55108-6099
Phone: (612)625-5285 **Fax:** (612)624-5272
Email: cmpeters@umn.edu
Website: http://fscn.che.umn.edu/digs/
Carolyn M. Peterson, Director

★ 26795 ★ University of Minnesota, Crookston
Center for Health and Human Services
Dietetic Technician Program
2900 University Ave.
Crookston, MN 56716-5001
Phone: (218)281-8202 **Fax:** (218)281-8050
Email: sstewwart@mail.crk.umn.edu
Website: http://www.crk.umn.edu
Sharon S. Stewart, PhD, Contact

Mississippi

★ 26796 ★ Alcorn State University
Department of Family and Consumer Sciences
Dietetics-Didactic Program
1000 ASU Dr., Ste. 839
Alcorn State, MS 39096-7500
Phone: (601)877-6258 **Fax:** (601)877-3960
Email: mrasco@lorman.alcorn.edu
Mattie R. Russo, Director

★ 26797 ★ Alcorn State University
Department of Family and Consumer Sciences
Dietetics-Didactic Program
1000 ASU Dr., Ste. 839
Lorman, MS 39096-7500
Phone: (601)877-6258 **Fax:** (601)877-3960
Email: mrasco@lorman.alcorn.edu
Mattie R. Rasco, Director

★ 26798 ★ Delta State University
Division of Family and Consumer Sciences
Coordinated Program in Dietetics
PO Box 3273
Cleveland, MS 38733
Phone: (662)846-4317 **Fax:** (662)846-4314
Email: awelch@dsu.deltast.edu
Anne S. Welch, PhD, Director

★ 26799 ★ Mississippi State University
School of Human Sciences
Dietetics-Didactic Program
PO Box 9745
Mississippi State, MS 39762-9745
Phone: (662)325-2950 **Fax:** (662)325-8188
Email: cabailey1978@humansci.msstate.edu
Website: http://www.msstate.edu/school/humansciences
Carolyn A. Bailey, Director

★ 26800 ★ Mississippi State University Schoolof Human Sciences
Dietetic Internship Program
PO Box 9745
128 Lloyd Ricks
Mississippi State, MS 39762-9745
Phone: (662)325-0919 **Fax:** (662)325-8188
Email: shbyrd@humansci.misstate.edu
Website: http://www.misstate.edu/school/humansciences/
Sylvia H. Byrd, PhD, Director

★ 26801 ★ St. Dominic-Jackson Memorial Hospital
Nutrition and Food Service Department
Dietetic Internship Program
969 Lakeland Dr.
Jackson, MS 39216-4699
Phone: (601)200-6935 **Fax:** (601)200-0799
Email: dietitian@stdom.com
Website: http://www.stdom.com
Jana J. Long, Director

★ 26802 ★ University of Mississippi
Department of Family and Consumer Sciences
Dietetics-Didactic Program
110 Meek Hall
PO Box 1848
University, MS 38677-1848
Phone: (662)915-7371 **Fax:** (662)915-7039
Email: smithd@olemiss.edu
Erskine R. Smith, PhD, Director

★ 26803 ★ University of Southern Mississippi
School of Family and Consumer Sciences
Dietetic Internship Program
PO Box 5035
Hattiesburg, MS 39406-5053
Phone: (601)924-9769 **Fax:** (601)924-1119
Email: rabroome@netdoor.com
Website: http://www.hhs.usm.edu/fcs/nfs_di.html
Ruth Ann Broome, Director

★ 26804 ★ University of Southern Mississippi
School of Family and Consumer Sciences
Dietetics-Didactic Program
P.O.Box 5035
Hattiesburg, MS 39406
Phone: (601)266-4679 **Fax:** (601)266-4680
Email: mary.nettles@usm.edu
Website: http://www.usm.edu/
Mary F. Nettles, PhD, Director

Missouri

★ 26805 ★ ARAMARK Healthcare Support Services-Kansas City
Saint Joseph Health Center
Dietetic Internship Program
1000 Carondelet Dr.
Kansas City, MO 64114-4802
Phone: (816)943-2146 **Fax:** (816)943-4719
Email: linhart-kathy@aramark.com
Website: http://www.aramark.com
Kathy Linhart, Director

★ 26806 ★ Central Missouri State University
Department of Health and Human Performance
Dietetics-Didactic Program
Hudson 008
Warrensburg, MO 64093
Phone: (660)543-4361 **Fax:** (660)543-8295
Email: dassenko@cmsul.cmsu.edu
Website: http://www.cmsu.edu/dietetics/
Sandra A. Dassenko, PhD, Director

★ 26807 ★ College of the Ozarks
Dietetics Education
Dietetics-Didactic Program
PO Box 17
Point Lookout, MO 65726-0017
Phone: (417)334-6411 **Fax:** (417)335-2618
Email: bhuddleston@cofo.edu
Elizabeth A. Huddleston, Director

★ 26808 ★ DVA Medical Center
Jefferson Barracks Divsion
Dietetic Internship Program
1 Jefferson Barracks Dr. (120/JB)
Saint Louis, MO 63125
Phone: (314)894-6631 **Fax:** (314)845-5023
Email: amy.knobloc-hahn@med.va.gov
Website: http://www.va.gov/nfs/StLouisVA
Amy L. Knoblock-Hahn, Director

★ 26809 ★ Fontbonne College
Department of Human Environmental Sciences
Dietetics-Didactic Program
6800 Wydown Blvd.
Saint Louis, MO 63105-3098
Phone: (314)889-1415 **Fax:** (314)719-8015
Email: chouston@fontbonne.edu
Cheryl A. Houston, PhD, Director

★ 26810 ★ Jewish Hospital-College of Nursing/Allied Health
Dietetic Internship Program
306 S Kingshighway
Mailstop 90-30-625
Saint Louis, MO 63110
Phone: (314)454-5307 **Fax:** (314)454-5239
Email: mpf3837@bjc.org
Website: http://www.jhconah.edu
Mary P. Fuhrman, Director

★ 26811 ★ Missouri Department of Health and Senior Services
Nutritional Health and Services
Bureau of Nutrition Policy and Education
Dietetic Internship Program
920 Wildwood
Jefferson City, MO 65102-0570
Phone: (573)751-6183 **Fax:** (573)522-3244
Email: wilkir@dhss.state.mo.us
Website: http://www.dhss.state.mos.us/MissouriNutrition
Rosalind M. Wilkins, Director

★ 26812 ★ Northwest Missouri State University
College of Education and Human Services
Department of Human Environmental Sciences
Dietetics-Didactic Program
Administration Bldg., Rm. 309
Maryville, MO 64468-6001
Phone: (660)562-1167 **Fax:** (660)562-1900
Email: jciak@mail.nwmissouri.edu
Website: http://www.nwmissouri.edu
Jenell D. Ciak, PhD, Director

★ 26813 ★ St. Louis community College at Florissant Valley
Department of Family and Consumer Sciences
Dietetic Technician Program
3400 Pershall Rd.
Saint Louis, MO 63135-1499
Phone: (314)595-4378 **Fax:** (314)595-2047
Email: jflorin@sticc.cc.mo.us
Website: http://www.sticc.cc.mo.us
Jeanne R. Pranger Florini, Contact

★ 26814 ★ Saint Louis University
Edward and Margaret Doisy School of Allied Health Professions
Department of Nutrition and Dietetics
Dietetic Internship Program
Rm. 3076
Saint Louis, MO 63104-1111
Phone: (314)577-8523 **Fax:** (314)577-8520
Email: mattfeld@slu.edu
Website: http://www.slu.edu/colleges/AH
Mildred K. Mattfeldt-Berman, PhD, Director

★ 26815 ★ Saint Louis University
School of Allied Health Professions
Dietetics-Didactic Program
Dietetics-Didactic Program or Dietetic Internship Program
Department of Nutrition and Dietetics, Rm. 3076
Saint Louis, MO 63104-1111
Phone: (314)577-8523 **Fax:** (314)577-8520
Email: shortje@slu.edu
Website: http://www.slu.edu/colleges/AH/ND
Joy Short, Director

★ 26816 ★ Southeast Missouri State University
Department of Human Environmental Studies
Dietetic Internship Program
1 University Plaza
Cape Girardeau, MO 63701-4799
Phone: (573)651-2733 **Fax:** (573)651-2949
Email: abmarietta@semo.edu
Website: http://www5.semo.edu/dietetic_internship/
Ann B. Marietta, PhD, Director

★ 26817 ★ Southwest Missouri State University
Department of Biomedical Sciences
Dietetics-Didactic Program
Springfield, MO 65804
Phone: (417)836-5603 **Fax:** (417)836-5588
Email: hcr678f@smsu.edu
Website: http://www.smsu.edu/
Helen C. Reid, PhD, Director

★ 26818 ★ University of Missouri, Columbia
Coordinated Program in Dietetics
103 Rothwell
Columbia, MO 65211
Phone: (573)882-4136 **Fax:** (573)884-4885
Email: umchesdietetics@missouri.edu
Website: http://www.missouri.edu/~nutsci/
Catherine A. Peterson, PhD, Director

Montana

★ 26819 ★ Montana State University
Department of Health and Human Development
Dietetics-Didactic Program
201 Romney
Bozeman, MT 59717
Phone: (406)994-6075 **Fax:** (406)994-2013

Email: betties@montana.edu
Website: http://www.montana.edu/nutrition
Bettie C. Stanislao, PhD, Director

Nebraska

★ 26820 ★ Southeast Community College
Dietetic Technician Program
800 O St.
Lincoln, NE 68520-1227
Phone: (402)437-2465 **Fax:** (402)437-2404
Email: jtaylor@southeast.edu
Bernardine J. Taylor, Contact

★ 26821 ★ University of Nebraska, Kearney
Department of Family and Consumer Sciences
Dietetics-Didactic Program
Otto Olsen Bldg., Rm. 205C
00-905 W 25th St.
Kearney, NE 68849-2130
Phone: (308)865-8229 **Fax:** (308)865-8040
Email: daviss@unk.edu
Website: http://www.unk.edu/
Sharon L. Davis, Director

★ 26822 ★ University of Nebraska, Lincoln
Department of Nutritional Science and Dietetics
Dietetic Internship Program
202 Ruth Leverton Hall
Lincoln, NE 68583-0806
Phone: (402)472-7966 **Fax:** (402)472-1587
Email: wkoszewskil@unl.edu
Website: http://nsd.unl.edu/nsd/intern/diintern.htm
Wanda M. Koszewski, PhD, Director

★ 26823 ★ University of Nebraska, Lincoln
Department of Nutritional Science and Dietetics
Dietetics-Didactic Program
202 Ruth Leverton Hall
Lincoln, NE 68583-0806
Phone: (402)472-2925 **Fax:** (402)472-1587
Email: lyoung3@unl.edu
Website: http://www.unl.edu
Linda O. Young, Director

★ 26824 ★ University of Nebraska Medical Center
Dietetic Internship Program
981200 Nebraska Medical Center
Omaha, NE 68198-1200
Phone: (402)559-7365 **Fax:** (402)559-6010
Email: gwoscyna@unmc.edu
Glenda R. Woscyna, Director

Nevada

★ 26825 ★ Truckee Meadows Community College
Dietetic Technician Program
7000 Dandini Blvd.
RDMT 334J
Reno, NV 89512-3999
Phone: (775)673-8218 **Fax:** (775)674-7983
Email: jgrover@tmcc.edu
Website: http://www.tmcc.edu
Janice L. Grover, Contact

★ 26826 ★ University of Nevada, Las Vegas
Department of Nutrition Sciences
Dietetics-Didactic Program
Box 453026
4505 S Maryland Pkwy.
Las Vegas, NV 89154-3026
Phone: (702)895-1169 **Fax:** (702)895-2616
Email: smeacham@ccmail.nevada.edu
Susan L. Meacham, PhD, Contact

★ 26827 ★ University of Nevada, Reno
Department of Nutrition
Dietetic Internship Program
Mail Stop 142
Reno, NV 89557
Phone: (775)784-6442 **Fax:** (775)784-6449
Email: dswilson@equinox.unr.edu
Website: http://www.unr.edu/hcs/nutrition
David S. Wilson, PhD, Director

★ 26828 ★ University of Nevada, Reno
Department of Nutrition
Dietetics-Didactic Program
Mail Stop 142
Reno, NV 89557
Phone: (775)784-6442 **Fax:** (775)784-6449
Email: dswilson@equinox.unr.edu
Website: http://www.unr.edu/hcs/nutrition
David S. Wilson, PhD, Director

New Hampshire

★ 26829 ★ Keene State College
Health Sciences/Nutrition
Dietetics-Didactic Program
Joslin House
MS 2903
229 Main St.
Keene, NH 03435-2903
Phone: (603)358-2423 **Fax:** (603)358-2892
Email: rdunn@keene.edu
Website: http://www.keene.edu/programs/hlsc/
Rebecca L. Dunn, Contact

★ 26830 ★ Keene State College
Home Economics/Human Services
Dietetic Internship Program
229 Main St., M2903
Keene, NH 03431
Phone: (603)358-2915 **Fax:** (603)358-2892
Email: lprosper@keene.edu
Website: http://www.keene.edu/academics/dietetics
Pamela J. Smith, EdD, Director

★ 26831 ★ University of New Hampshire
Department of Animal and Nutritional Sciences
Human Nutrition Center
Dietetics-Didactic Program
Colovos Rd.
Durham, NH 03824
Phone: (603)862-1723 **Fax:** (603)862-0308
Email: chjs@cisunix.unh.edu
Website: http://arethusa.unh.edu/colsa/ansci/ans.htm
Colette Janson-Sand, PhD, Director

★ 26832 ★ University of New Hampshire
Nutrition Assessment and Counseling Service
Human Nutrition Center
Dietetic Internship Program
Colovos Rd.
Durham, NH 03824
Phone: (603)862-2811 **Fax:** (603)862-0308
Email: cfg@christa.unh.edu
Website: http://www.dieteticinternship.unh.edu
Caroline F. Giles, Director

★ 26833 ★ University of New Hampshire Thompson School of Applied Science
Dietetic Technician Program
6A Putnam Hall
Durham, NH 03824
Phone: (603)862-1050 **Fax:** (603)862-2915
Email: njohnson@cisunix.unh.edu
Website: http://www.unh.edu
Nancy M. Johnson, MEd, Contact

New Jersey

★ 26834 ★ Camden County College
Math, Science, Health Careers, and Dietetic Technology
Dietetic Technician Program
PO Box 200
College Dr.
Blackwood, NJ 08012-0200
Phone: (856)227-7200 **Fax:** (856)374-4862
Email: mfisher@mail.camdencc.edu
Website: http://www.camdencc.edu
Michele C. Fisher, PhD, Contact

★ 26835 ★ College of Saint Elizabeth
Department of Foods and Nutrition
Dietetic Internship Program
Henderson Hall
2 Convent Rd.
Morristown, NJ 07960-6989
Phone: (973)290-4125 **Fax:** (973)290-4138
Email: diet@cse.edu
Website: http://www.cse.edu
Monica W. Luby, Director

★ 26836 ★ College of Saint Elizabeth
Department of Foods and Nutrition
Dietetics-Didactic Program
2 Convent Rd.
Morristown, NJ 07960-6989
Phone: (973)290-4127 **Fax:** (973)290-4138
Email: jburge@cse.edu
Website: http://www.cse.edu
Jean C. Burge, PhD, Director

★ 26837 ★ Middlesex County College
Dietetic Technician Program
PO Box 3050
Edison, NJ 08818-3050
Phone: (732)906-2538 **Fax:** (732)906-7745
Email: mary-pat_maciolek@middlesexcc.edu
Website: http://www.middlesexcc.edu
Mary-Pat Maciolek, Contact

★ 26838 ★ Montclair State University
Department of Home Ecology
Preprofessional Practice Program in Dietetics
Upper Montclair, NJ 07043
Phone: (973)655-4375 **Fax:** (973)655-4399
Email: sokolikc@mail.Montclair.edu
Carol A. Sokolik, Director

★ 26839 ★ Montclair State University
Department of Human Ecology
Dietetics-Didactic Program
111 Finley
Upper Montclair, NJ 07043
Phone: (973)655-4416 **Fax:** (973)655-7467
Email: lioud@mail.montclair.edu
Website: http://www.montclair.edu/pages/HECO/Food-Dietetics.html
Doreen Liou, EdD, Director

★ 26840 ★ New Jersey Department of Health and Senior Services
Family Health Services-WIC
Dietetic Internship Program
50 E State St.
PO Box 364
Trenton, NJ 08625-0364
Phone: (609)292-9560 **Fax:** (609)292-3580
Email: mlynch@doh.state.nj.us
Marilyn A. Lynch, Director

★ 26841 ★ Rutgers, the State University of New Jersey
Department of Nutritional Sciences
Dietetics-Didactic Program
2298 Davison Hall
26 Nichol Ave.
New Brunswick, NJ 08901-2882
Phone: (732)932-9570 **Fax:** (732)932-6522
Email: bltangel@rci.rutgers.edu
Website: http://aesop.rutgers.edu/~nutrition
Barbara L. Tangel, Director

★ 26842 ★ University of Medicine and Dentistry of New Jersey
School of Health Related Professions
Coordinated Program in Dietetics
1776 Raritan Rd.
Scotch Plains, NJ 07076
Phone: (908)889-2435 **Fax:** (908)889-2487
Email: oconnoja@umdnj.edu
Website: http://shrp.umdnj.edu/catalog/Primary_Care/
Joyce A. O'Connor, PhD, Director

★ 26843 ★ University of Medicine and Dentistry of New Jersey
School of Health Related Professions
Dietetic Internship Program
1776 Raritan Rd.
Scotch Plains, NJ 07076
Phone: (908)889-2488 **Fax:** (908)889-2487
Email: langevdd@umdnj.edu
Website: http://shrp.umdnj.edu/programs/dietetic/index.htm
Denise D. Langevin, Director

New Mexico

★ 26844 ★ New Mexico State University
Department of Family and Consumer Sciences
Dietetics-Didactic Program
Box 30003/MSC 3470
Las Cruces, NM 88003-8003
Phone: (505)646-1178 **Fax:** (505)646-1889
Email: abock@nmsuvm1.nmsu.edu
Website: http://www.nmsu.edu/~famcom
Margaret A. Bock, PhD, Director

★ 26845 ★ University of New Mexico
Division of Individual, Family, and Community Education
Dietetic Internship Program
216 Education Office Bldg.
Albuquerque, NM 87131-1231
Phone: (505)277-0937 **Fax:** (505)277-4362
Email: ggarza@unm.edu
Mary V. Garza, PhD, Director

★ 26846 ★ University of New Mexico
Division of Individual, Family, and Community Education
Dietetics-Didactic Program
108 Education Office Bldg
College Of Education
Albuquerque, NM 87131-1231
Phone: (505)277-3160 **Fax:** (505)277-4362
Email: kheller@unm.edu
Karen E. Heller, PhD, Director

New York

★ 26847 ★ ARAMARK Healthcare Support Services
Mary Immaculate Hosptial
Metropolitan New York Dietetic Internship Program
152-11 89th Ave.
Jamaica, NY 11432
Free: 800-378-5348 **Fax:** (718)738-5228
Email: charny-allison@ARAMARK.com
Allison Charny, Director

★ 26848 ★ Brooklyn College
Department of Health and Nutrition Sciences
Dietetic Internship Program
2900 Bedford Ave.
Brooklyn, NY 11210-2889
Phone: (718)951-5909 **Fax:** (718)951-4670
Email: diprog@brooklyn.cuny.edu
Website: http://academic.Brooklyn.cuny.edu/hns
Roseanne Schnoll, PhD, Director

★ 26849 ★ Brooklyn College
Department of Health and Nutrition Sciences
Dietetics-Didactic Program
Dietetics-Didactic Program or Preprofessional Practice Program in Dietetics
2900 Bedford Ave.
Brooklyn, NY 11210-2889
Phone: (718)951-5541 **Fax:** (718)951-4670
Email: ahlawson@brooklyn.cuny.edu
Website: http://academic.brooklyn.cuny.edu/hns
Annie S. Hauck-Lawson, PhD, Director

★ 26850 ★ City University of New York
Herbert H. Lehman College
Department of Health Sciences
Dietetic Internship Program
250 Bedford Park Blvd. W
Bronx, NY 10468-1589
Phone: (718)960-8796 **Fax:** (718)960-8908
Email: aboersma@lehman.cuny.edu
Website: http://www.lehman.cuny.edu/
Anne Boersma, PhD, Director

★ 26851 ★ City University of New York
Herbert H. Lehman College
Department of Health Services, Dietetics, Food, and Nutrition
Dietetics-Didactic Program
Bedford Park Blvd. W
Bronx, NY 10468-1589
Phone: (718)960-8775 **Fax:** (718)960-8908
Website: http://www.lehman.cuny.edu
Alice Tobias, EdD, Director

★ 26852 ★ City University of New York
Hunter College
School of Health Sciences
Dietetic Internship Program
425 E 25th St., Box 896
New York, NY 10010-2590
Phone: (212)481-5165 **Fax:** (212)481-5260
Email: allimarshall1234@aol.com
Website: http://www.hunter.cuny.edu/schoolhp/phn/dietetic_internship
Allison R. Marshall, Director

★ 26853 ★ City University of New York
Hunter College
School of Health Sciences
Dietetics-Didactic Program
Brookdale Health Science Center
425 E 25th St.
New York, NY 10010-2590
Phone: (212)481-5118 **Fax:** (212)481-5260
Email: knavder@hunter.cuny.edu
Khursheed P. Navder, PhD, Director

★ 26854 ★ City University of New York
LaGuardia Community College
Dietetic Technician Program
E300
Long Island City, NY 11101-3071
Phone: (718)482-5758 **Fax:** (718)609-2052
Email: oppolitoro@lagcc.cuny.edu
Website: http://www.lagcc.cuny.edu
Rosann T. Ippolito, Contact

★ 26855 ★ City University of New York
Queens College
Department of Family, Nutrition, and Exercise Sciences
Dietetic Internship Program
65-30 Kissena Blvd.
Flushing, NY 11367-1597
Phone: (718)997-4155 **Fax:** (718)997-4163
Email: susan_braverman@qc.edu
Website: http://www.qc.edu/FNES/dietintern.html
Susan P. Braverman, Director

★ 26856 ★ City University of New York
Queens College
Department of Family, Nutrition, and Exercise Sciences
Dietetics-Didactic Program
65-30 Kissena Blvd.
Flushing, NY 11367-1597
Phone: (718)997-4152 **Fax:** (718)997-4163
Email: pminer@qcl.qc.edu
Website: http://www.qc.edu/
Patricia K. Miner, Director

★ 26857 ★ Columbia University Teachers College
Health and Behavior Studies
Dietetic Internship Program
525 W 120th St., Box 137
New York, NY 10027-6625
Phone: (212)678-3950 **Fax:** (212)678-4048
Email: cc2005@columbia.edu
Website: http://www.tc.Columbia.edu/~academic/nutri
Christina Costa, Director

★ 26858 ★ Cornell University
Division of Nutritional Sciences
Dietetic Internship Program
373 Martha Van Rensselaer Hall
Ithaca, NY 14853
Phone: (607)255-2613 **Fax:** (607)255-0178
Email: set6@cornell.edu
Website: http://www.nutrition.cornell.edu/grad/diet.html
Susan E. Travis, Director

★ 26859 ★ Cornell University
Division of Nutritional Sciences
Dietetics-Didactic Program or Dietetic Internship Program
373 Martha Van Renssalaer Hall
Ithaca, NY 14853-4401
Phone: (607)255-2613 **Fax:** (607)255-0178
Email: set6@cornell.edu
Website: http://www.nutrition.cornell.edu/diet.html
Susan E. Travis, Director

★ 26860 ★ Cornell University - Ithaca
Division of Nutritional Sciences
373 Martha Van Rensselaer Hall
Ithaca, NY 14853-4401
Phone: (607)255-2613 **Fax:** (607)255-0178
Email: set6@cornell.edu
Website: http://www.nutrition.cornell.edu/diet.html
Susan E. Travis, Contact

★ 26861 ★ Dutchess Community College
Dietetic Technician Program
53 Pendell Rd.
Poughkeepsie, NY 12601-1512
Phone: (845)431-8323 **Fax:** (845)431-8329
Email: hirning@sunydutchess.edu
Website: http://www.sunydutchess.edu
Felicia Hirning, Contact

★ 26862 ★ D'Youville College
Coordinated Program in Dietetics
320 Porter Ave.
Buffalo, NY 14201-1084
Phone: (716)881-7752 **Fax:** (716)881-7790
Email: baumgartc@dyc.edu
Website: http://www.dyc.edu
Charlotte W. Baumgart, PhD, Director

★ 26863 ★ Erie Community College North Campus
Dietetic Technician Program
6205 Main St.
Williamsville, NY 14221-7095
Phone: (716)851-1598 **Fax:** (716)851-1429
Email: garfoot@ecc.edu
Website: http://www.ecc.edu
Margaret E. Garfoot, Contact

★ 26864 ★ Long Island University C.W. Post Campus
Department of Nutrition
Dietetic Internship Program
720 Northern Blvd.
Brookville, NY 11548
Phone: (516)299-3224 **Fax:** (516)299-3106
Email: asarcona@liu.edu
Website: http://www.liu.edu/nutrit
Alessandra R. Sarcona, Director

★ 26865 ★ Long Island University, C W Post Campus
Department of Nutrition
Dietetics-Didactic Program
720 Northern Blvd.
Brookville, NY 11548
Phone: (516)299-3046 **Fax:** (516)299-3106
Email: bshorter@liu.edu
Website: http://www.liu.edu/nutrit
Barbara J. Shorter, EdD, Director

★ 26866 ★ Marymount College, Fordham University
Department of Human Ecology
Dietetics-Didactic Program
100 Marymount Ave.
Tarrytown, NY 10591
Phone: (914)332-6559 **Fax:** (914)631-8586
Email: gezo@mmc.marymt.edu
Website: http://www.marymt.edu
Evelyn Gezo, Director

★ 26867 ★ New York Institute of Technology
Clinical Nutrition Department
Dietetics-Didactic Program
NYCOM II, Room 342
35 W Fourth St., 10th Fl.
Old Westbury, NY 11568-8000
Phone: (516)686-3803 **Fax:** (516)686-3795
Email: settinge@nyit.edu
Website: http://www.nyit.edu/
Susan E. Ettinger, PhD, Director

★ 26868 ★ New York Institute of Technology
Dietetic Internship Program
NYCOM II, Rm. 334
Old Westbury, NY 11568-8000
Phone: (516)686-3803 **Fax:** (516)686-3795
Email: settinge@nyit.edu
Susan E. Ettinger, PhD, Director

★ 26869 ★ New York-Presbyterian Hospital
Dietetic Internship Program
525 E 68th St., AN-833
New York, NY 10021-4873
Phone: (212)746-0836 **Fax:** (212)746-8287
Email: erosenth@nyp.org
Website: http://www.nyp.org/nutrition
Elaine M. Rosenthal, Director

★ 26870 ★ New York University
Department of Nutrition and Food Studies
Dietetic Internship Program
35 W 4th St., 10th Fl.
New York, NY 10011
Phone: (212)998-5580 **Fax:** (212)995-4194
Email: lisa.sasson@nyu.edu
Website: http://www.nyu.edu/education/nutrition
Lisa M. Sasson, Director

★ 26871 ★ New York University
Department of Nutrition and Food Studies
Dietetics-Didactic Program
35 W Fourth St.
10th Flr., Rm 1077
New York, NY 10012-1172
Phone: (212)998-5580 **Fax:** (212)995-4194
Email: judith.gilbride@nyu.edu
Website: http://www.nyu.edu/education/nutrition
Judith A. Gilbride, PhD, Director

★ 26872 ★ North Shore-Long Island Jewish Health System
Dietetic Internship Program
300 Community Dr.
Manhasset, NY 11030
Phone: (516)562-4113 **Fax:** (516)562-1298
Lisa Carmody, Director

★ 26873 ★ Rochester Institute of Technology
Hospitality and Service Management
Coordinated Program in Dietetics
14 Lomb Memorial Dr.
Rochester, NY 14623-5604
Phone: (585)475-2357 **Fax:** (585)475-5099
Email: eakism@rit.isc.edu
Website: http://www.rit.edu
Elizabeth A. Kmiecinski, Director

★ 26874 ★ Rochester Institute of Technology
Hospitality and Service Management
Dietetics-Didactic Program
14 Lomb Memorial Dr.
Rochester, NY 14623-5604
Phone: (585)475-2352 **Fax:** (585)475-5099
Email: bxcism@rit.edu
Website: http://www.rit.edu
Barbara Cerio, Director
Elizabeth A. Kmiecinski, Contact

★ 26875 ★ The Sage Colleges
Dietetic Internship Program
45 Ferry St.
Troy, NY 12180-4115
Phone: (518)244-2044 **Fax:** (518)244-4586
Email: severp@sage.edu
Website: http://www.sage.edu
Patricia S. Wager, Director

★ 26876 ★ The Sage Colleges
Division of Health and Rehabilitation Sciences
Dietetics-Didactic Program
Ackerman Hall
45 Ferry St.
Troy, NY 12180-4115
Phone: (518)244-2043 **Fax:** (518)244-4586
Email: estesc@Sage.edu
Website: http://www.sage.edu/divisions/hrs/nutrition.html
Carmela T. Estes, Director

★ 26877 ★ Sodexho Health Care Services
New York Metropolitan
Dietetic Internship Program
90 Merrick Ave., Ste. 210
East Meadow, NY 11554
Phone: (516)794-9150 **Fax:** (516)794-9154
Email: bonnie.giller@sodexhousa.com
Website: http://www.sodexho-usa.com/car_dietetic.html
Bonnie R. Giller, Director

★ 26878 ★ State University of New York Agriculture and Technical College
Dietetic Technician Program
Bailey Annex
Morrisville, NY 13408
Phone: (315)684-6213 **Fax:** (315)684-6592
Email: smithml@morrisville.edu
Marie L. Smith, MEd, Contact

★ 26879 ★ State University of New York Rockland Community College
Dietetic Technician Program
145 College Rd.
Suffern, NY 10901-3699
Phone: (845)574-4130 **Fax:** (845)574-4498
Email: ghowell@sunyrockland.edu
Website: http://www.sunyrockland.edu
Georgette Howell, Contact

★ 26880 ★ State University of New York, Buffalo
Dietetic Internship Program
15 Farber Hall
3435 Main St.
Buffalo, NY 14214
Phone: (716)829-3680 **Fax:** (716)829-3700
Email: platek@buffalo.edu
Website: http://www.wings.buffalo.edu/ptens/pos-nu-internship.html
Mary E. Platek, Director

★ 26881 ★ State University of New York, Buffalo
Dietetics and Nutrition Department
Coordinated Program in Dietetics
Caudell Hall 207
Buffalo, NY 14222-1095
Phone: (716)878-5634 **Fax:** (716)878-5834
Email: hayesdm@buffalostate.edu
Donna M. Hayes, Director

★ 26882 ★ State University of New York, Buffalo
Dietetics and Nutrition Program
Dietetics-Didactic Program
1300 Elmwood Ave.
Buffalo, NY 14222-1095
Phone: (716)878-4333 **Fax:** (716)878-5834
Email: raot@buffalostate.edu
Website: http://www.buffalostate.eud
Tejaswini Rao, PhD, Director
Donna M. Hayes, Contact

★ 26883 ★ State University of New York, Oneonta
Department of Human Ecology
Dietetic Internship Program
39 Denison Hall
Oneonta, NY 13820
Phone: (607)436-2705 **Fax:** (607)436-3084
Email: haessicj@oneonta.edu
Website: http://www.ONEONTA.EDU/dieteticinternship
Carolyn J. Haessig, PhD, Director

★ 26884 ★ State University of New York, Oneonta
Department of Human Ecology
Dietetics-Didactic Program
28 Denison Hall
Oneonta, NY 13820-4015
Phone: (607)436-2112 **Fax:** (607)436-2051
Email: dowdelma@oneonta.edu
Website: http://www.oneonta.edu/academics/huec/diet_food.html
Mary Ann Dowdell, PhD, Contact

★ 26885 ★ State University of New York, Plattsburgh
Food and Nutrition Program
Dietetics-Didactic Program
101 Broad St.
Plattsburgh, NY 12901-2681
Phone: (518)564-4222 **Fax:** (518)564-3100
Email: jean.coates@plattsburgh.edu
Jean A. Ostasz-Coates, PhD, Director

★ 26886 ★ State University of New York, Stony Brook
Department of Family Medicine
Dietetic Internship Program
Health Sciences Center, Level 4
Stony Brook, NY 11794-8461
Phone: (516)444-8246 **Fax:** (516)444-7552
Email: jconnoll@notes.cc.sunysb.edu
Website: http://www.famed.sunysb.edu
Josephine Connolly-Schoonen, Director

★ 26887 ★ Sufflok County Community College
Eastern Campus
Dietetic Technician Program
121 Speonk-Riverhead Rd.
Riverhead, NY 11901-3499
Phone: (631)548-2590 **Fax:** (631)548-2617
Email: newmanj@sunysuffolk.edu
Website: http://www.sunysuffolk.edu
Jodi N. Levine, Contact

★ 26888 ★ Syracuse University
Department of Nutrition and Hospitality Management
Dietetic Internship Program
034 Slocum Hall
Syracuse, NY 13244-1250
Phone: (315)443-2386 **Fax:** (315)443-2735
Email: dzconnol@syr.edu
Website: http://hshp.syr.edu/nutrition_grad.html
Debra Connolly, Director

★ 26889 ★ Syracuse University
Department of Nutrition and Hospitality Management
Dietetics-Didactic Program
034 Slocum Hall
Syracuse, NY 13244-1250
Phone: (315)443-2386 **Fax:** (315)443-2735
Email: thoracek@mailbox.syr.edu
Tanya M. Horacek, PhD, Director
Kay Stearns Bruening, PhD, Contact

★ 26890 ★ VA Medical Center
Nutrition and Food Program (120)
Dietetic Internship Program
130 W Kingsbridge Rd.
Bronx, NY 10468-3904
Phone: (718)584-9000 **Fax:** (718)741-4238
Email: susan.spector@med.va.gov
Website: http://www.va.gov/visns/visn03/diethome.asp
Susan B. Spector, Director

★ 26891 ★ Westchester Community College
Foods Service Administration Department
Dietetic Technician Program
Student Center Bldg.
111
75 Grasslands Rd.
Valhalla, NY 10595-1698
Phone: (914)785-6182 **Fax:** (914)785-7989
Email: theresa.cousins@sunywcc.edu
Website: http://www.wcc.co.westchester.ny.us
Theresa A. Cousins, Contact

★ 26892 ★ Westchester Medical Center
Food Services Divsion
Dietetic Internship Program
Grasslands Rd.
Valhalla, NY 10595-1689
Phone: (914)493-8978 **Fax:** (914)493-1376
Email: delucac@wcmc.com
Joan C. O'Brien, Director

North Carolina

★ 26893 ★ Appalachian State University
Department of Family and Consumer Sciences
Dietetic Internship Program
PO Box 32056
Boone, NC 28608-2056
Phone: (828)262-2631 **Fax:** (828)265-8620
Email: bogardussl@appstate.edu
Susan L. Bogardus, PhD, Director

★ 26894 ★ Appalachian State University
Department of Family and Consumer Sciences
Dietetics-Didactic Program
Boone, NC 28608-2630
Phone: (828)262-2630 **Fax:** (828)265-8620
Email: mcanultyl@appstate.edu
Website: http://www.appstate.edu/
Lisa McAnulty, PhD, Director

★ 26895 ★ East Carolina University
School of Human Environmental Sciences
Department of Nutrition and Hospitality Management
Dietetics-Didactic Program or Dietetic Internship Program
Greenville, NC 27858-4353
Phone: (252)328-6917 **Fax:** (252)328-4276
Email: escottstumps@mail.ecu.edu
Website: http://www.ecu.edu/hes/nuhm/NUHMhome.htm
Sylvia Escott-Stump, Director

★ 26896 ★ Lenoir Community College
Dietetic Technician Program
PO Box 600
Lincolnton, NC 28093-0600
Phone: (704)748-1065 **Fax:** (704)748-1074
Email: gunnell.juanita@gaston.cc.nc.us
Juanita O. Gunnell, Contact

★ 26897 ★ Meredith College
Department of Human Environmental Sciences
Dietetic Internship Program
3800 Hillsborough St.
Raleigh, NC 27607-5298
Phone: (919)760-8419 **Fax:** (919)760-2819
Email: barishd@meredith.edu
Website: http://www.Meredith.edu/hes/foods_dietetic.htm
Debrah Barish, Director

★ 26898 ★ Meredith College
Department of Human Environmental Sciences
Dietetics-Didactic Program
3800 Hillsborough St.
Raleigh, NC 27607-5298
Phone: (919)760-8079 **Fax:** (919)760-2819
Email: fishers@meredith.edu
Susan G. Fisher, PhD, Director

★ 26899 ★ North Carolina A & T State University
Department of Human Environment and Family Sciences
Dietetics-Didactic Program
102 Benbow Hall
1601 E Market St.
Greensboro, NC 27411-1064
Phone: (336)334-7850 **Fax:** (336)334-7265
Email: lizette@ncat.edu
Lizette Sanchez-Lugo, PhD, Director

★ 26900 ★ North Carolina Central University
Department of Human Sciences
Dietetics-Didactic Program or Dietetic Internship Program
PO Box 19615
Durham, NC 27707-0099
Phone: (919)530-7439 **Fax:** (919)530-7983
Email: eokeiyi@wpo.nccu.edu
Esther C. Okeiyi, PhD, Director

★ 26901 ★ University of North Carolina, Chapel Hill
Department of Nutrition
Dietetics-Didactic Program or Coordinated Program in Dietetics
McGavran-Greenburg Hall
CB 7400
Chapel Hill, NC 27599-7461
Phone: (919)966-7214 **Fax:** (919)966-7216
Email: carolyn_barrett@unc.edu
Website: http://www.sph.unc.edu/nutr
Carolyn H. Barrett, Director

★ 26902 ★ University of North Carolina, Greensboro
Department of Nutrition and Foodservice Systems
Dietetic Internship Program
318 Stone Bldg.
PO Box 26170
Greensboro, NC 27412
Phone: (336)256-0326 **Fax:** (336)334-4129
Email: martha_taylor@uncg.edu
Website: http://www.uncg.edu/nfs
Martha L. Taylor, PhD, Director

★ 26903 ★ University of North Carolina, Greensboro
Nutrition and Foodservice Systems
Dietetics-Didactic Program
PO Box 26170
Greensboro, NC 27402-6170
Phone: (336)334-5313 **Fax:** (336)334-4129
Email: cheryl_lovelady@uncg.edu
Website: http://www.uncg.edu/nfs
Cheryl A. Lovelady, PhD, Director

★ 26904 ★ Western Carolina University
Department of Health Sciences
Dietetics-Didactic Program
Cullowhee, NC 28723
Phone: (828)227-7113 **Fax:** (828)227-7446
Email: hosig@email.wcu.edu
Website: http://www.wcu.edu/aps/healths/HS_UG-ND.htm
Kathryn W. Hosig, PhD, Director

★ 26905 ★ Western Carolina University
Department of Health Sciences
Nutrition/Dietetics
Dietetic Internship Program
Cullowhee, NC 28723
Phone: (828)227-7114 **Fax:** (828)227-7446
Email: plsmith1@mindspring.com
Website: http://www.wcu.edu/aps/healths/HS_UG-ND_DI.htm
Nancy L. Williams, Director

North Dakota

★ 26906 ★ North Dakota State University
Department of Health, Nutrition and Exercise Sciences
Dietetics-Didactic Program
351 EML Hall
Box 5057
Fargo, ND 58105-5057
Phone: (701)231-7480 **Fax:** (701)231-7174
Email: lynwrrw.qinrwea@ndsu.nodak.edu
Website: http://www.ndsu.nodak.edu/
Lynette S. Winters, Contact

★ 26907 ★ North Dakota State University
Department of Health, Nutrition, and Exercise Sciences
Coordinated Program in Dietetics
EML Hall 351
Fargo, ND 58105-5057
Phone: (701)231-7480 **Fax:** (701)231-7174
Email: lynette.winters@ndsu.nodak.edu
Website: http://www.ndsu.nodak.edu/
Lynette S. Winters, Director

★ 26908 ★ North Dakota State University
Department of Health, Nutrition, and Exercise Sciences
Dietetics-Didactic Program
351 EML Hall, Box 5057
Fargo, ND 58105-5057
Phone: (701)231-7480 **Fax:** (701)231-7174
Email: lynette.winters@ndsu.nodak.edu
Website: http://www.ndsu.nodak.edu
Lynette S. Winters, Director

★ 26909 ★ University of North Dakota
Department of Nutrition and Dietetics
Coordinated Program in Dietetics
PO Box 8237
Grand Forks, ND 58202-8237
Phone: (701)777-3752 **Fax:** (701)777-3268
Email: judy_hall@mail.und.nodak.edu
Website: http://www.und.edu/dept/nursing/nutrition.html
Judith H. Hall, Director

Ohio

★ 26910 ★ Bluffton College
Family and Consumer Sciences
Dietetics-Didactic Program
280 W College Ave.
Box 1346
Bluffton, OH 45817-1196
Phone: (419)358-3229 **Fax:** (419)358-3323
Email: myersd@bluffton.edu
Website: http://www.bluffton.edu/fcs
Deborah I. Myers, Director

★ 26911 ★ Bowling Green State University
Department of Family and Consumer Sciences
Dietetics-Didactic Program
206 Johnston Hall
Bowling Green, OH 43403-0254
Phone: (419)372-8941 **Fax:** (419)372-7854
Email: chaar@bgnet.bgsu.edu
Website: http://www.bgsu.edu/colleges/edhd/FCS
Christine M. Haar, Director

★ 26912 ★ Bowling Green State University
School of Family and Consumer Sciences
Dietetic Internship Program
Bowling Green, OH 43403-0254
Phone: (419)372-8941 **Fax:** (419)372-7854
Email: chaar@bgnet.bgsu.edu
Website: http://www.bgsu.edu/colleges/edhd/FCS/di
Christine M. Haar, Director

★ 26913 ★ Case Western Reserve University
Department of Nutrition
Dietetics-Didactic Program
10900 Euclid Ave
Cleveland, OH 44106-4906
Phone: (216)368-2442 **Fax:** (216)368-6644
Email: mmc3@po.cwru.edu
Website: http://www.cwru.edu/med/nutrition/home.html
Margaret M. Cicirella, Director

★ 26914 ★ Case Western Reserve University
School of Medicine
Department of Nutrition
Dietetic Internship Program
10900 Euclid Ave.
Cleveland, OH 44106-1712
Phone: (216)368-6626 **Fax:** (216)368-6644
Email: imp@po.cwru.edu
Isabel M. Parraga, PhD, Director

★ 26915 ★ Christ Hospital
Food and Nutrition Services
Dietetic Internship Program
2139 Auburn Ave.
Cincinnati, OH 45219-2906
Phone: (513)585-2283 **Fax:** (513)585-3033
Email: dvoraksv@healthall.com
Website: http://www.health-alliance.com/Christ_dietetic_internship.html
Susan V. Dvorak, Director

★ 26916 ★ Cincinnati Children's Division of Developmental Disabilities
Children's Hospital Medical Center
University Center of Excellence on Disabilities
Dietetic Internship Program
3333Burnet Ave., PAV Bldg. 3713
Cincinnati, OH 45229-3039
Phone: (513)636-4614 **Fax:** (513)636-7361
Email: ekvalls@chmcc.org
Shirley M. Ekvall, PhD, Director

★ 26917 ★ Cincinnati State Technical and Community College
Health Technologies Division
Dietetic Technician Program
3520 Central Pkwy.
Cincinnati, OH 45223-2690
Phone: (513)569-1479 **Fax:** (513)569-1659
Email: charalee.allen@cincinnatistate.edu
Website: http://www.cinstate.cc.oh.us
Charalee Allen, MEd, Contact

★ 26918 ★ Cleveland Clinic Foundation
Dietetic Internship Program
Nutrition Therapy M17
9500 Euclid Ave.
Cleveland, OH 44195
Phone: (216)444-6487 **Fax:** (216)444-9415
Email: kents@ccf.org
Website: http://www.clevelandclinic.org/education/diet
Sue Kent, Director

★ 26919 ★ Columbus State Community College
Hospitality Management Department
Dietetic Technician Program
550 E Spring St.
PO Box 1609
Columbus, OH 43216-1609
Phone: (614)287-2580 **Fax:** (614)287-5973
Email: lconway@cscc.edu
Website: http://www.cscc.edu
Louise G. Conway, Contact

★ 26920 ★ Cuyahoga Community College
Dietetic Technician Program
2900 Community College Ave.
Cleveland, OH 44115-3196
Phone: (216)987-4497 **Fax:** (216)987-4386
Email: barbara.mikuszewski@tri-c.edu
Website: http://www.tri-c.edu
Barbara S. Mikuszewski, Contact

★ 26921 ★ Good Samaritan Hospital
Nutrition Department
Dietetic Internship Program
375 Dixmyth Ave.
Cincinnati, OH 45220-2489
Phone: (513)872-1983 **Fax:** (513)872-4986
Email: jackene_Laverty@trihealth.com
Jackene M. Laverty, Director

★ 26922 ★ Hocking Technical College
Dietetic Technician Program
3301 Hocking Pkwy.
Nelsonville, OH 45764-9704
Phone: (614)753-3591 **Fax:** (740)753-5105
Email: murray_d@hocking.edu
Website: http://www.hocking.edu
Deborah H. Murray, Contact

★ 26923 ★ Kent State University
School of Family and Consumer Studies
Nutrition and Dietetics
Dietetic Internship Program
100 Nixson Hall
Kent, OH 44242
Phone: (330)672-2064 **Fax:** (330)672-2194
Email: nburzmin@mvh.org
Website: http://www.kent.edu/f&cs/
Nancy H. Burzminski, Director

★ 26924 ★ Kent State University
School of Family and Consumer Studies
Nutrition and Dietetics
Dietetics-Didactic Program
Nixson Hall
Kent, OH 44242
Phone: (330)672-2197 **Fax:** (330)672-2194
Email: klowry@kent.edu
Website: http://www.kent.edu/f&cs
Karen R. Gordon, PhD, Director

★ 26925 ★ Louis Stokes Cleveland VA Medical Center
Dietetic Internship Program
10701 East Blvd.
Cleveland, OH 44106-1702
Phone: (216)791-3800 **Fax:** (216)421-3014
Email: anne.raguso@med.va.gov
Website: http://www.cwru.edu/med/nutrition/clevanc.html
Anne O. Raguso, PhD, Director

★ 26926 ★ MetroHealth Medical Center
Clinical Nutrition
Dietetic Internship Program
2500 MetroHealth Dr.
Cleveland, OH 44109-1998
Phone: (216)778-2718 **Fax:** (216)778-8363
Email: lbonacuse@metrohealth.org
Website: http://www.metrohealth.org/nutrition/dietetic.asp
Lisa M. Bonacuse, Director

★ 26927 ★ Miami University
Department of Physical Education, Health and Sports Studies
Dietetics-Didactic Program
100A Phillips Hall
Oxford, OH 45056
Phone: (513)529-5036 **Fax:** (513)529-5006
Email: rudgesj@muohio.edu
Susan J. Rudge, PhD, Director

★ 26928 ★ Miami Valley Hospital
Dietetic Internship Program
1 Wyoming St.
Dayton, OH 45409
Phone: (937)208-2448 **Fax:** (937)341-8193
Email: rmlee@mvh.org
Website: http://www.miamivalleyhospital.com
Rebecca H. Lee, Director

★ 26929 ★ Mount Carmel College of Nursing
Dietetic Internship Program
127 S Davis Ave.
Columbus, OH 43222-1504
Phone: (614)234-5439 **Fax:** (614)234-2875
Email: kblancha@mchs.com
Website: http://www.mccn.edu
Kathleen M. Blanchard, Director

★ 26930 ★ Ohio State University
College of Human Ecology
Department of Human Nutrition
Dietetic Internship Program
325 Campbell Hall
Columbus, OH 43210-1295
Phone: (614)292-8189 **Fax:** (614)292-8880
Email: Mitchell.15@osu.edu
Website: http://hec.osu.edu/hnfm/dietetics/internship.htm
Mary C. Mitchell, PhD, Director

★ 26931 ★ Ohio State University
Department of Human Nutrition
Dietetics-Didactic Program
1787 Neil Ave.
Columbus, OH 43210-1220
Phone: (614)292-0715 **Fax:** (614)292-8880
Email: smith.23@osu.edu
Website: http://www.hec.ohio-state.edu/hn/index.htm
Anne M. Smith, PhD, Director

★ 26932 ★ Ohio State University
School of Allied Medical Professions
Coordinated Program in Dietetics
1583 Perry St.
Columbus, OH 43210-1234
Phone: (614)292-0635 **Fax:** (614)292-0210
Email: schiller.l@osu.edu
Website: http://www.amp.ohio-state.edu
M. Rosita Schiller, PhD, Director

★ 26933 ★ The Ohio State University
School of Allied Medical Professions
Medical Dietetics Division
Dietetic Internship Program
1583 Perry St.
Columbus, OH 43210-1234
Phone: (614)292-0635 **Fax:** (614)292-0210
Email: schiller.1@osu.edu
Website: http://www.amp.ohio-state.edu
M. Rosita Schiller, PhD, Director

★ 26934 ★ Ohio University
School of Human and Consumer Sciences
Dietetics-Didactic Program
Grover Center W324
Athens, OH 45701-2979
Phone: (740)593-2875 **Fax:** (740)593-0289
Email: holben@ohio.edu
Website: http://www.ohiou.edu/humanandconsumer/school.html
David H. Holben, PhD, Director

★ 26935 ★ Owens Community College
Dietetic Technician Program
PO Box 10,000
Oregon Rd.
Toledo, OH 43699-1947
Phone: (419)661-7214 **Fax:** (419)661-7251
Email: tmadaras@owens.edu
Website: http://www.owens.edu
Tekla M. Madaras, MEd, Contact

★ 26936 ★ Sinclair Community College
Dietetic Technician Program
444 West 3rd St.
Dayton, OH 45402-1460
Phone: (937)512-2756 **Fax:** (937)512-3092
Email: betty.dykes@sinclair.edu
Website: http://www.sinclair.edu
Beatriz U. Dykes, PhD, Contact

★ 26937 ★ University of Akron
School of Family and Consumer Sciences
Coordinated Program in Dietetics
215 Schrank Hall S
Akron, OH 44325-6103
Phone: (330)972-6043 **Fax:** (330)972-4934
Email: slhudak@uakron.edu
Website: http://www.uakron.edu/faa/schools/homeec.html
Sandra L. Hudak, Director

★ 26938 ★ University of Akron
School of Family and Consumer Sciences
Dietetics-Didactic Program
215 Schrank Hall S
Akron, OH 44325-6103
Phone: (330)972-6046 **Fax:** (330)972-4934
Email: sue@uakron.edu
Website: http://www.uakron.edu/faa/schools/homeec.html
Sue A. Rasor-Greenslag, Director
Eston B. Brown, Contact

★ 26939 ★ University of Cincinnati
College of Allied Health Sciences
Dietetics-Didactic Program
363C Hastings and William French Bldg.
Cincinnati, OH 45267-0394
Phone: (513)558-7504 **Fax:** (513)558-7500
Email: couchsc@email.uc.edu
Website: http://www.cahs.uc.edu/departments/dietetics.cfm
Sarah Collins Couch, Director

★ 26940 ★ University of Dayton
Health and Sports Science
Food and Health Program
Dietetics-Didactic Program
300 College Park Ave.
Dayton, OH 45469-1210
Phone: (937)229-4203 **Fax:** (937)229-4244
Email: patricia.dolan@notes.udayton.edu
Website: http://homepages.udayton.edu/~dolanp
Patricia Dolan, Director

★ 26941 ★ University Hospitals of Cleveland
Department of Nutrition Services
Dietetic Internship Program
11100 Euclid Ave.
Lakeside 5021 Mailstop
Cleveland, OH 44106-5000
Phone: (216)844-1310 **Fax:** (216)844-8188
Email: Sharon.schwartz@uhhs.com
Website: http://www.cwru.edu/med/nutrition/uhocle.html
Sharon K. Schwartz, Director

★ 26942 ★ Youngstown State University
Coordinated Program in Dietetics
1 University Plaza
Youngstown, OH 44555-0001
Phone: (330)941-3344 **Fax:** (330)941-1824
Email: jhassell@cc.ysu.edu
Website: http://www.ysu.edu
Jean H. Hassell, Director

★ 26943 ★ Youngstown State University
Department of Human Ecology
Dietetic Technician Program
1 University Plaza
Youngstown, OH 44555-3344
Phone: (330)941-1823 **Fax:** (330)941-1824
Email: smleson@ysu.edu
Website: http://www.ysu.edu
Suzanne M. Leson, Contact

★ 26944 ★ Youngstown State University
Department of Human Ecology
Dietetics-Didactic Program
1 University Plaza
Youngstown, OH 44555-0001
Phone: (330)941-3345 **Fax:** (330)941-1824
Email: mrshayes@cc.ysu.edu
Website: http://www.ysu.edu
Mohammad R. Shayesteh, PhD, Director
Jean H. Hassel, Contact

Oklahoma

★ 26945 ★ Langston University
Department of Human Ecology
Dietetics-Didactic Program
308/304 Jones Hall
Langston, OK 73050
Phone: (405)466-3337 **Fax:** (405)466-3364
Email: aknight@lunet.edu
Ada Pearl Knight, PhD, Director

★ 26946 ★ Northeastern State University
College of Business and Industry
Dietetics-Didactic Program
600 N Grand
210A PA Bldg.
Tahlequah, OK 74464-2399
Phone: (918)456-5511 **Fax:** (918)458-2337
Email: millerak@nsuok.edu
Website: http://arapaho.nsuok.edu/~fcs
Alexandria R. Miller, PhD, Director

★ 26947 ★ Oklahoma State University
Department of Nutritional Sciences
Dietetic Internship Program
HES 425
Stillwater, OK 74078-6141
Phone: (405)744-8294 **Fax:** (405)744-7113
Email: gobucks@okstate.edu
Website: http://www.okstate.edu/hes/nsci/
Lea L. Ebro, PhD, Director

★ 26948 ★ Oklahoma State University
Department of Nutritional Sciences
Dietetics-Didactic Program
HES 425
Stillwater, OK 74078-6141
Phone: (405)744-5041 **Fax:** (405)744-1357
Email: nutsci@okstate.edu
Website: http://www.okstate.edu/hes/nsci
Kathryn S. Keim, PhD, Director

★ 26949 ★ Oklahoma State University
Hospitality Services Technology
Dietetic Technician Program
1801 E Fourth St.
Okmulgee, OK 74447-3901
Phone: (918)293-5004 **Fax:** (918)293-4618
Email: downer@osu-okmulgee.eud
Website: http://www.osu-okmulgee.edu/hosp
Nelda G. Downer, Contact

★ 26950 ★ University of Central Oklahoma
College of Education
Department of Human Environmental Sciences
Dietetics-Didactic Program
Edmond, OK 73034
Phone: (405)974-5805 **Fax:** (405)974-3850
Email: mwaters@ucok.edu
Website: http://204.154.115.1/
Marilyn S. Waters, PhD, Director

★ 26951 ★ University of Central Oklahoma
Human Environmental Sciences
Dietetic Internship Program
100 N University Dr.
Edmond, OK 73034
Phone: (405)974-5369 **Fax:** (405)974-3850
Email: kmeyers@ucok.edu
Website: http://www.educ.edu
Karen D. Meyers, Director

★ 26952 ★ University of Oklahoma Health Sciences Center
Department of Nutritional Sciences
Coordinated Program in Dietetics
801 NE 13th
Oklahoma City, OK 73190
Phone: (405)271-2113 **Fax:** (405)271-1560
Email: Karen-funderburg@ouhsc.edu
Website: http://moon.ouhsc.edu/mguild
Karen M. Funderburg, Director

★ 26953 ★ University of Oklahoma Health Sciences Center, College of Allied Health
Nutritional Sciences Department
Dietetics-Didactic Program
PO Box 26901
Oklahoma City, OK 73190
Phone: (405)271-2113 **Fax:** (405)271-1560
Email: Stephen-glore@ouhsc.edu
Website: http://www.ah.ouhsc.edu/main/Programs/prog1.asp?prog_1d=5
Stephen R. Glore, PhD, Director

★ 26954 ★ University of Oklahoma Health Sciences Center
College of Allied Health
Department of Nutritional Sciences
Dietetic Internship Program
Box 26901, CHB
Oklahoma City, OK 73190
Phone: (405)271-2113 **Fax:** (405)271-1560
Email: Kathy-onley@ouhsc.edu
Website: http://www.ah.ouhsc.edu/main/
Kathy Onley, PhD, Director

Oregon

★ 26955 ★ Mid-Willamette Valley Dietetic Internship
Capital Manor Retirement Community
1955 Dallas Rd. NW, Ste. 1200
Salem, OR 97304
Phone: (503)362-4101 **Fax:** (503)371-9021
Email: ndunton@capitalmanor.com
Nancy J. Dunton, PhD, Director

★ 26956 ★ Oregon Health Sciences University
Dietetic Internship Program
EJH-10
3181 SW Sam Jackson Park Rd.
Portland, OR 97201-3098
Phone: (503)494-7596 **Fax:** (503)494-7076
Email: hagand@ohsu.edu
Website: http://www.ohsu.edu/som-dietetic/
Dorothy W. Hagan, PhD, Director

★ 26957 ★ Oregon State University
Nutrition and Food Management
Dietetics-Didactic Program
212 Milam Hall
Corvallis, OR 97331-5103
Phone: (541)737-0960 **Fax:** (541)737-6914
Email: cluskeym@orst.edu
Website: http://www.orst.edu
Mary M. Cluskey, PhD, Director

Pennsylvania

★ 26958 ★ ARAMARK Corp.
Mid-Atlantic Dietetic Internship
Philadelphia Area
41 Pebble Ridge Rd.
Warrington, PA 18976
Free: 800-666-4272 **Fax:** (215)918-1607
Email: Richards-pat@ARAMARK.com
Patricia M. Richards, Director

★ 26959 ★ Cedar Crest College
Allen Center for Nutrition
Dietetics-Didactic Program
100 College Dr.
Allentown, PA 18104-6196
Phone: (610)606-4666 **Fax:** (610)606-4624
Email: jeziegle@cedarcrest.edu
Website: http://www2.cedarcrest.edu
Jane E. Ziegler, Director

★ 26960 ★ Community College of Allegheny County
Allegheny Campus
Dietetic Technician Program
808 Ridge Ave.
Pittsburgh, PA 15212-6097
Phone: (412)237-2640 **Fax:** (412)237-4521
Email: evargo@ccac.edu
Website: http://www.ccac.edu
Elizabeth C. Vargo, Contact

★ 26961 ★ Community College of Philadelphia
Dietetic Technician Program
1700 Spring Garden St.
Philadelphia, PA 19130-3991
Phone: (215)751-8948 **Fax:** (215)751-8937
Email: dkoteski@ccp.cc.pa.us
Website: http://faculty.ccp.cc.pa.us/dept/diet
Dorothy R. Koteski, Contact

★ 26962 ★ Crozer-Chester Medical Center
Medical Nutrition Therapy
Dietetic Internship Program
One Medical Center Blvd.
Upland, PA 19013-3902
Phone: (610)447-2304 **Fax:** (610)447-2325
Email: Kathleen.yerger@crozer.org
Website: http://www.crozer.org
Kathleen G. Yerger, Director

★ 26963 ★ Drexel University
Department of Bioscience and Biotechnology
Dietetics-Didactic Program
3141 Chestnut St.
Philadelphia, PA 19104-2875
Phone: (215)895-2413 **Fax:** (215)895-1273
Email: egford@drexel.edu
Website: http://www.bioscience.drexel.edu/
Eileen G. Ford, Director

★ 26964 ★ Edinboro University of Pennsylvania
Department of Biology and Health Services
Coordinated Program in Dietetics
Edinboro, PA 16444
Phone: (814)732-2458 **Fax:** (814)732-2422
Email: lanz@edinboro.edu
Sally J. Lanz, Director

★ 26965 ★ Family Health Council, Inc.
Dietetic Internship Program
960 Penn Ave., Ste. 600
Pittsburgh, PA 15222-1417
Phone: (412)288-2130 **Fax:** (412)288-9036
Email: pwebb@fhcinc.org
Website: http://www.fhcinc.org
Karen A. Virostek, Director

★ 26966 ★ Gannon University
College of Sciences, Engineering and Health Sciences
Coordinated Program in Dietetics
109 University Square
Erie, PA 16541-0001
Phone: (814)871-5452 **Fax:** (814)871-5662

Email: mughal@gannon.edu
Website: http:www.gannon.edu
Dawna T. Mughal, PhD, Director

★ 26967 ★ Geisinger Medical Center
Clinical Nutrition 01-15
Dietetic Internship Program
100 N Academy Ave.
Danville, PA 17822-0115
Phone: (570)271-6468 **Fax:** (570)271-7805
Email: kkieselhorst@geisinger.edu
Website: http://www.geisinger.org
Kessey J. Kieselhorst, Director

★ 26968 ★ Immaculata College
Department of Fashion, Foods, and Nutrition
Dietetics-Didactic Program
PO Box 722
Immaculata, PA 19345-0722
Phone: (610)647-4400 **Fax:** (610)251-1668
Email: sjohnston@immaculata.edu
Website: http://www.immaculate.edu/HTM/ACADEMIC/departments.html
Susan W. Johnston, Director

★ 26969 ★ Immaculata College
Department of Nutrition Education
Dietetic Internship Program
Box 500-Graduate Division
Immaculata, PA 19345-0500
Phone: (610)647-4400 **Fax:** (610)953-8550
Email: sjohnston@immaculata.edu
Website: http://www.immaculata.edu
Susan W. Johnston, Director

★ 26970 ★ Indiana University of Pennsylvania
Department of Food and Nutrition
Dietetic Internship Program
10 Ackerman Hall
911 South Drive
Indiana, PA 15705-1087
Phone: (724)357-4440 **Fax:** (724)357-7582
Email: stdavis@iup.edu
Website: http://www.hhs.iup.edu/fn/
Stephanie A. Taylor-Davis, PhD, Director

★ 26971 ★ Indiana University of Pennsylvania
Department of Food and Nutrition
Dietetics-Didactic Program
10 Ackerman Hall
911 South Dr.
Indiana, PA 15705-1087
Phone: (724)357-4440 **Fax:** (724)357-7582
Email: rjohnson@iup.edu
Website: http://www.hhs.iup.edu/fn/
Rita M. Johnson, PhD, Director

★ 26972 ★ La Salle University
School of Nursing
Coordinated Program in Dietetics
1900 W Olney Ave.
Philadelphia, PA 19141-1199
Phone: (215)951-1258 **Fax:** (215)951-1896
Email: henstenb@lasalle.edu
Website: http://www.lasalle.edu/academ/nutrition
Jule Anne D. Henstenburg, Contact

★ 26973 ★ La Salle University
School of Nursing
Dietetics-Didactic Program
1900 W Olney Ave.
Philadelphia, PA 19141-1108
Phone: (215)951-1258 **Fax:** (215)951-1772
Email: henstenb@lasalle.edu
Website: http://www.lasalle.edu/academ/nursing/nutrition/home.htm
Jule Anne D. Henstenburg, Director

★ 26974 ★ Mansfield University
Department of Health Sciences
Dietetics-Didactic Program
203C Elliott Hall
Mansfield, PA 16933
Phone: (570)662-4628 **Fax:** (570)662-4137
Email: kwright@mnsfld.edu
Website: http://www.mnsfld.edu/~health/index.htm
Kathy J. Wright, PhD, Director

★ 26975 ★ Marywood University
Department of Nutrition and Dietetics
Coordinated Program in Dietetics
2300 Adams Ave.
Scranton, PA 18509-1598
Phone: (570)348-6277 **Fax:** (570)348-6029
Email: nutrition@ac.marywood.edu
Website: http://www.marywood.edu/departments/nutr_diet/home.html
Marianne E. Borja, EdD, Director

★ 26976 ★ Marywood University
Department of Nutrition and Dietetics
Dietetic Internship Program
2300 Adams Ave.
Scranton, PA 18509-1514
Phone: (570)348-6211 **Fax:** (570)340-6029
Email: harrisonl@ac.marywood.edu
Website: http://www.marywood.edu
Lee M. Harrison, PhD, Director

★ 26977 ★ Marywood University
Department of Nutrition and Dietetics
Dietetics-Didactic Program
2300 Adams Ave.
Scranton, PA 18509-1514
Phone: (570)348-6211 **Fax:** (570)348-6029
Email: winters@es.marywood.edu
Website: http://www.marywood.edu/departments/nutr_diet/home.html
Barbara L. Winters, PhD, Director
Marianne E. Borja, EdD, Contact

★ 26978 ★ Marywood University
Department of Nutrition and Dietetics
Distance Education Dietetic Internship
2300 Adams Ave.
Scranton, PA 18509-1514
Phone: (570)348-6211 **Fax:** (570)345-6029
Email: dunnetouhey@es.marywood.edu
Website: http://www.marywood.edu/departments/nutr_diet/home.html
Maureen Dunne-Touhey, Contact

★ 26979 ★ Mercyhurst College
Department of Human Ecology
Coordinated Program in Dietetics
501 E 38th St.
Erie, PA 16546
Phone: (814)824-2462 **Fax:** (814)824-3053
Email: cglispy@mercyhurst.edu
Website: http://www.mercyhurst.edu/
Charlene J. Glispy, Director

★ 26980 ★ Messiah College
Department of Natural Sciences
Dietetics-Didactic Program
One College Ave
PO Box 3030
Grantham, PA 17027
Phone: (717)766-2511 **Fax:** (717)691-6046
Email: mmihok@messiah.edu
Mary Ann Mihok, PhD, Director

★ 26981 ★ Pennsylvania State University
College of Health and Human Development
Nutrition Department
Dietetics-Didactic Program
University Park, PA 16802-6500
Phone: (814)865-9150 **Fax:** (814)863-6103
Email: myk2@psu.edu
Website: http://nutrition.hhdev.psu.edu
Marie Y. Kamp, Director

★ 26982 ★ Pennsylvania State University
College of Health and Human Development
School of Hotel, Restaurant, and Recreation Management
Dietetic Technician Program
University Park, PA 16802-1307
Phone: (814)863-2676 **Fax:** (814)863-4257
Email: dpde@psu.edu
Website: http://www.worldcampus.psu.edu
Ellen W. Barbrow, MEd, Contact

★ 26983 ★ Pennsylvania State University
Department of Nutritional Sciences
Dietetic Internship Program
121-A Henderson Bldg. South
University Park, PA 16802
Phone: (814)865-9150 **Fax:** (814)863-6103
Email: myk2@psu.edu
Website: http://nutrition.psu.edu/internship
Marie Y. Kamp, Director

★ 26984 ★ Seton Hill University
Division of Natural and Health Sciences
Coordinated Program in Nutrition/Dietetics
Greensburg, PA 15601
Phone: (724)830-1045 **Fax:** (724)830-1571
Email: sandrick@setonhill.edu
Website: http://www.setonhill.edu
Janice G. Sandrick, PhD, Director

★ 26985 ★ Sodexho Health Care Services
NJ/Philadelphia Metro Dietetic Internship
Route 532 and General Sullivan Rd.
PO Box 602-0601
Washington Crossing, PA 18977
Phone: (215)493-4025 **Fax:** (215)612-5302
Email: gwolset@fhcs.org
Website: http://www.sodexho-usa.com/car_dietetic.html
Gayanne R. Wolset, Director

★ 26986 ★ Sodexho Health Care Services Allentown
Dietetic Internship Program
6081 Hamilton Blvd.
Allentown, PA 18106-0501
Phone: (610)366-5237 **Fax:** (610)366-5454
Email: areyes@woodco.com
Website: http://www.woodco.com
Alison B. Reyes, Director

★ 26987 ★ University of Pittsburgh
School of Health and Rehabilitation Sciences
Dietetics-Didactic Program or Coordinated Program in Dietetics
4048 Forbes Tower
Pittsburgh, PA 15260-1802
Phone: (412)383-6534 **Fax:** (412)383-6636
Email: kcrawfor@pitt.edu
Website: http://www.shrs.pitt.edu/cdn
Kim Crawford, Director

★ 26988 ★ University of Pittsburgh Medical Center
Presbyterian Shadyside
Dietetic Internship Program
5230 Centre Ave.
Pittsburgh, PA 15232-1304
Phone: (412)623-2114 **Fax:** (412)623-2429
Email: scottsmithjl@msx.upmc.edu
Joyce Scott-Smith, Director

★ 26989 ★ West Chester University
Sturzebecker Health Sciences Center
Department of Health
Dietetics-Didactic Program
H302 Department of Health
West Chester, PA 19383
Phone: (610)436-2655 **Fax:** (610)436-2860
Email: jharris@wcupa.edu
Website: http://www.wcupa.edu/
Jeffrey E. Harris, DrPH, Director

★ 26990 ★ Westmoreland County Community College
Dietetic Technician Program
Commissioners Hall
400 Armbrust Rd.
Youngwood, PA 15697
Phone: (724)925-4235 **Fax:** (724)925-4293
Email: shiplec@astro.westmoreland.cc.pa.us
Website: http://www.westmoreland.cc.pa.us/
Cheryl B. Shipley, Contact

Puerto Rico

★ 26991 ★ Puerto Rico Department of Health
Dietetic Internship Program
PO Box 70184
San Juan, PR 00936
Phone: (787)274-6831 **Fax:** (787)274-8345
Email: aerivera@salud.gov.pr
Ana E. Rivera, Director

★ 26992 ★ University of Puerto Rico
College of Health Related Professions
Dietetic Internship Program
Medical Sciences Campus
PO Box 365067
San Juan, PR 00936-5067
Phone: (787)758-2525 **Fax:** (787)756-8529
Email: ritalucca@cprs.tcm.upr.edu
Rita L. De Delgado, Director

★ 26993 ★ University of Puerto Rico
Rio Piedras Campus
School of Family Ecology and Nutrition
Dietetics-Didactic Program
Box 23347, UPR Station
San Juan, PR 00931-3347
Phone: (787)764-0000 **Fax:** (787)772-1422
Email: ihernan1@rrpac.upr.clu.edu
Iris Z. Hernandez, Director

★ 26994 ★ VA Medical Center San Juan
Dietetic Internship Program
10 Calle Casia
San Juan, PR 00921-3201
Phone: (787)641-2962 **Fax:** (787)641-8366
Email: awilda.Ortiz@med.va.gov
Awilda Ortiz, Director

Rhode Island

★ 26995 ★ Johnson and Wales University
College of Culinary Arts
Dietetics-Didactic Program
1 Washington Ave.
Providence, RI 02905
Phone: (401)598-1881 **Fax:** (401)598-1161
Email: suzanne.vieira@jwu.edu
Website: http://www.jwu.edu
Suzanne P. Vieira, Director

★ 26996 ★ University of Rhode Island
Department of Nutrition and Food Sciences
Dietetic Internship Program
106 Ranger Hall
Kingston, RI 02881
Phone: (401)874-4028 **Fax:** (401)874-5974
Email: gwg@uri.edu
Website: http://www.uri.edu/cels/fsn
Geoffrey W. Greene, PhD, Director

★ 26997 ★ University of Rhode Island
Department of Nutrition and Food Sciences
Dietetics-Didactic Program
110 Ranger Hall
Kingston, RI 02881-0804
Phone: (401)874-5869 **Fax:** (401)874-5974
Email: cathy@uri.edu
Website: http://www.uri.edu/cels/fsn
Catherine English, PhD, Director

South Carolina

★ 26998 ★ Clemson University
Department of FHSN
Dietetic Internship Program
224 Poole Agricultural Center
Box 340371
Clemson, SC 29634-0001
Phone: (864)656-7614
Email: rhln@clemson.edu
Website: http://www.Clemson.edu/foodscience
Rita H. Haliena, Director

★ 26999 ★ Clemson University
Department of Food Science and Human Nutrition
Dietetics-Didactic Program
223 Poole, Agricultural Center
Box 340371
Clemson, SC 29634-0371
Phone: (864)656-5690 **Fax:** (864)656-0331
Email: bkunkel@clemson.edu
Website: http://www.clemson.edu/foodscience
Mary E. Kunkel, PhD, Director

★ 27000 ★ Medical University of South Carolina
Dietetic Internship Program
Digestive Disease Center
96 Jonathan Lucas St.
Charleston, SC 29425
Phone: (843)792-1454 **Fax:** (843)792-4183
Email: tranen@musc.edu
Website: http://www.musc.edu/dieteticinternship
Stephanie S. Tranen, Director

★ 27001 ★ South Carolina Department of Health and Environmental Control
Dietetic Internship Program
Mills Complex, Box 101106
Columbia, SC 29211-0106
Phone: (803)898-0819 **Fax:** (803)898-0557
Email: spannsh@dhec.state.sc.us
Website: http://www.scdhec.net/hs/proservices/pro-services.htm
Sandra H. Spann, Director

★ 27002 ★ South Carolina State University
Department of Family and Consumer Sciences
Dietetics-Didactic Program
Staley Hall
PO Box 7084
Orangeburg, SC 29117-0001
Phone: (803)536-8620 **Fax:** (803)533-3628
Email: zs_bowensj@scsu.edu
Juanita Bowens-Seabrook, PhD, Director

★ 27003 ★ Winthrop University
Department of Human Nutrition
Dietetic Internship Program
302 Life Sciences Bldg.
Rock Hill, SC 29733
Phone: (803)323-4521 **Fax:** (803)323-2254
Email: thomasjh@winthrop.edu
Website: http://www.Winthrop.edu/nutrition/missionstatement.htm
Judy H. Thomas, Director

★ 27004 ★ Winthrop University
Department of Human Nutrition
Dietetics-Didactic Program
Rock Hill, SC 29733
Phone: (803)323-4520 **Fax:** (803)323-2254
Email: wolmanp@winthrop.edu
Website: http://www.winthrop.edu/nutrition
Patricia G. Wolman, EdD, Director

South Dakota

★ 27005 ★ Mount Marty College
Department of Nutrition and Food Science
Dietetics-Didactic Program or Coordinated Program in Dietetics
1105 W Eighth St.
Yankton, SD 57078-3724
Phone: (605)668-1520 **Fax:** (605)668-1607
Email: tholzbauer@mtmc.edu
Website: http://www.mtmc.edu
Sister Thecla M. Holzbauer, Director

★ 27006 ★ South Dakota State University
College of Family and Consumer Sciences
Department Nutrition, Food Science, and Hospitality
Dietetics-Didactic Program
PO Box 2275A
Brookings, SD 57007-0497
Phone: (605)688-5683 **Fax:** (605)688-5603
Email: kendra_kattelmann@sdstate.edu
Website: http://www.sdstate.edu
Kendra K. Kattelmann, PhD, Director

★ 27007 ★ University of South Dakota
School of Medicine
Preprofessional Practice Program in Dietetics
1400 W 22nd St.
Sioux Falls, SD 57105
Phone: (605)357-1581 **Fax:** (605)357-1438
Email: mmpeters@usd.edu
Website: http://www.usd.edu/cd/dieteticinternship
Mary M. Peterson, Director

Tennessee

★ 27008 ★ Carson-Newman College
Division of Family and Consumer Sciences
Dietetics-Didactic Program
Box 71881
Jefferson City, TN 37760-7001
Phone: (865)471-3295 **Fax:** (865)471-3502
Email: kcoffey@cn.edu
Website: http://www.cn.edu/
Kitty R. Coffey, PhD, Director

★ 27009 ★ East Tennessee State University
College of Applied Science and Technology
Department of Applied Human Sciences
Dietetic Internship Program
PO Box 70671
Johnson City, TN 37614-1709
Phone: (423)439-7537 **Fax:** (423)439-7539
Email: lowee@etsu.edu
Website: http://www.etsu.edu/scitech/ahsc/clnu.htm
Elizabeth C. Lowe, Director

★ 27010 ★ East Tennessee State University
Department of Applied Human Sciences
Dietetics-Didactic Program
PO Box 70671
Johnson City, TN 37614-0671
Phone: (423)439-7532 **Fax:** (423)439-7539
Email: verheggr@etsu.edu
Website: http://www.etsu.edu/
Ruth D. Verhegge, Director

★ 27011 ★ Lipscomb University
Department of Family and Consumer Sciences
Dietetic Internship Program
3901 Granny White Pike
Nashville, TN 37204-3951
Phone: (615)279-6106 **Fax:** (615)269-1808
Email: Autumn.Marshall@lipscomb.edu
Website: http://www.lipscomb.edu
Autumn C. Marshall, PhD, Director

★ 27012 ★ Lipscomb University
Department of Family and Consumer Sciences
Dietetics-Didactic Program
3901 Granny White Pike
Nashville, TN 37204-3951
Phone: (615)279-5767 **Fax:** (615)269-1808
Email: nancy.hunt@lipscomb.edu
Website: http://www.lipscomb.edu
Nancy H. Hunt, Director

★ 27013 ★ Middle Tennessee State University
Department of Human Sciences
Dietetics-Didactic Program
PO Box 86
Murfreesboro, TN 37132
Phone: (615)904-8076 **Fax:** (615)898-5130
Email: dewalker@mtsu.edu
Website: http://www.mtsu.edu
Dellmar Walker, PhD, Director

★ 27014 ★ National Health Care Corp.
Dietetic Internship Program
PO Box 1398
Murfreesboro, TN 37133-1398
Phone: (615)890-2020 **Fax:** (615)890-0123
Email: pope@nhccare.com
Website: http://www.nhccare.com/di.htm
Patty T. Poe, Director

★ 27015 ★ Southwest Tennessee Community College
Dietetic Technician Program
PO Box 780
Memphis, TN 38101-0780
Phone: (901)333-5673 **Fax:** (901)333-5057
Email: tharris@southwest.edu
Website: http://www.southwest.tn.edu
Thelma J. Harris, Contact

★ 27016 ★ Tennessee State University
Department of Family and Consumer Sciences
Dietetics-Didactic Program
PO Box 9598
3500 John A. Merritt Blvd.
Nashville, TN 37209-1561
Phone: (615)963-5619 **Fax:** (615)963-5033
Email: sgodwin@tnstate.edu
Website: http://www.tnstate.edu/sacs
Sandria L. Godwin, PhD, Director

★ 27017 ★ Tennessee Technological University
School of Human Ecology
Dietetics-Didactic Program
Box 5035
Cookeville, TN 38505
Phone: (931)372-3376 **Fax:** (931)372-3150
Email: ccunningham@tntech.edu
Website: http://iweb.tntech.edu/abrunt
Cathy Hix Cunningham, PhD, Director

★ 27018 ★ University of Memphis
Consumer Science and Education
Dietetic Internship Program
Manning Hall
Memphis, TN 38152
Phone: (901)678-3108 **Fax:** (901)678-5324
Email: lhclemens@memphis.edu
Website: http://csed.Memphis.edu/ClinicalNutrition.asp
Linda H. Clemens, EdD, Director

★ 27019 ★ University of Memphis
Department of Consumer Science and Education
Dietetic Internship Program
Manning Hall
Memphis, TN 38152
Phone: (901)678-3108 **Fax:** (901)678-5324
Email: lhclemns@memphis.edu
Website: http://csed.Memphis.edu/ClinicalNutrition.asp
Linda H. Clemens, EdD, Director

★ 27020 ★ University of Memphis
Department of Consumer Science and Education
Dietetics-Didactic Program
Memphis, TN 38152
Phone: (901)678-3110 **Fax:** (901)678-5324
Email: rroach@memphis.edu
Website: http://www.coe.memphis.edu
Robin R. Roach, EdD, Director

★ 27021 ★ University of Tennessee, Chattanooga
Department of Human Ecology
Dietetics-Didactic Program
615 McCallie Ave.
Chattanooga, TN 37403
Phone: (423)425-5379 **Fax:** (423)425-4479
Email: holly-dieken@utc.edu
Website: http://www.utc.edu/~hecodept/academic.html
Holly A. Dieken, PhD, Director

★ 27022 ★ University of Tennessee, Knoxville
College of Human Ecology
Department of Nutrition
Dietetics-Didactic Program
229 Jessie Harris Bldg.
1215 W Cumberland Ave.
Knoxville, TN 37996-1920
Phone: (865)974-6264 **Fax:** (865)974-3491
Email: phansen@utk.edu
Melissa B. Hansen-Petrik, PhD, Director

★ 27023 ★ University of Tennessee, Knoxville
Department of Nutrition
College of Human Ecology
Dietetic Internship Program
1215 Cumberland Ave., Rm. 229
Knoxville, TN 37996-1920
Phone: (865)974-6256 **Fax:** (865)974-3491
Email: kbalnick@utk.edu
Website: http://nutrition.he.utk.edu/
Karen B. Wetherall, Director

★ 27024 ★ The University of Tennessee, Martin
Department of Family and Consumer Sciences
Dietetics-Didactic Program
340 Gooch Hall
Martin, TN 38238-5045
Phone: (731)587-7101 **Fax:** (731)587-7106
Email: gawipi@utm.edu
Website: http://www.utm.edu/departments/agr/humenvir/diet.htm
Georgina M. Awipi, PhD, Contact

★ 27025 ★ University of Tennessee, Martin
Department of Human Environmental Sciences
Dietetic Internship Program
340 Gooch Hall
Martin, TN 38238-5045
Phone: (901)587-7107 **Fax:** (901)587-7106
Email: loril@utm.edu
Website: http://www.utm.edu/departments/agr/humenvir/ap4grad.htm
Lori H. Littleton, Director

★ 27026 ★ Vanderbilt University Medical Center
Dietetic Internship Program
B-802TVC
1301 22nd Ave. S
Nashville, TN 37232-5510
Phone: (615)322-0062 **Fax:** (615)343-8810
Email: cynthia.broadhurst@mcmail.vanderbilt.edu
Website: http://mc.Vanderbilt.edu/alliedhealth
Cynthia B. Broadhurst, Director

★ 27027 ★ Vanderbilt University Medical Center
Dietetic Internship Program
B-802TVC
1301 22nd Ave. S
Nashville, TN 37232-5510
Phone: (615)322-0062 **Fax:** (615)343-8810
Email: Cynthia.Broadhurst@vanderbilt.edu
Website: http://www.mc.Vanderbilt.edu/alliedhealth/
Cynthia B. Broadhurst, Director

Texas

★ 27028 ★ Abilene Christian University
Department of Family and Consumer Sciences
Dietetics-Didactic Program
ACU Box 28155
Abilene, TX 79699
Phone: (915)674-2089 **Fax:** (915)674-2086
Email: joness@acu.edu
Website: http://www.acu.edu/academics/fcs
Sheila A. Jones, Director

★ 27029 ★ Baylor University
Department of Family and Consumer Sciences
Dietetics-Didactic Program
BU Box 97346
Waco, TX 76798-7346
Phone: (254)710-6258 **Fax:** (254)710-3629
Email: LuAnn_Soliah@baylor.edu
LuAnn Soliah, PhD, Director

★ 27030 ★ Baylor University Medical Center
Dietetic Internship Program
3500 Gaston Ave.
Dallas, TX 75246-2045
Phone: (214)820-4019 **Fax:** (214)820-2263
Email: ja.grim@bhcs.com
Website: http://www.baylorhealth.com/dietetic_internship
Julie A. Grim, Director

★ 27031 ★ El Paso Community College
Dietetic Technician Program
100 W Rio Grande Ave.
El Paso, TX 79902
Phone: (915)831-4470 **Fax:** (915)831-4114
Email: marshac@epcc.edu
Website: http://www.epcc.edu
Marsha K. Cummings, MEd, Contact

★ 27032 ★ Houston VA Medical Center
Nutrition and Food Service (120)
Dietetic Internship Program
2002 Holcombe Blvd.
Houston, TX 77030-4298
Phone: (713)791-1414 **Fax:** (713)794-7448
Email: caroline.nelson@med.va.gov
Website: http://www.va.gov/nfs/HoustonVAMC
Caroline J. Nelson, Director

★ 27033 ★ Lamar University
Department of Family and Consumer Sciences
Dietetics-Didactic Program
PO Box 10035
Beaumont, TX 77710-0035
Phone: (409)880-8663 **Fax:** (409)880-8666
Email: ruizcs@hal.lamar.edu
Website: http://www.lamar.edu
Connie S. Ruiz, PhD, Director

★ 27034 ★ Lamar University
Department of Family and Consumer Sciences
Preprofessional Practice Program in Dietetics
PO Box 10035
Beaumont, TX 77710-0035
Phone: (409)880-8663 **Fax:** (409)880-8666
Email: pembertoar@hal.lamar.edu
Website: http://www.lamar.edu
Amy Pemberton-Shows, PhD, Director

★ 27035 ★ Prairie View A&M University
Department of Agriculture, Nutrition, and Human Ecology
Dietetics-Didactic Program
PO Box 4329
Prairie View, TX 77446-4329
Phone: (936)857-4417 **Fax:** (936)857-4441
Email: sharon_mcwhinney@pvamu.edu
Website: http://www.pvamu.edu
Sharon L. McWhinney, PhD, Director

★ 27036 ★ Prairie View A&M University
Dietetic Internship Program
PO Box 4329
Prairie View, TX 77446
Phone: (936)857-4417 **Fax:** (936)857-2200
Email: Sharon_mcwhinney@pvamu.edu
Website: http://www.pvamu.edu
Sharon L. McWhinney, PhD, Director

★ 27037 ★ Presbyterian Hospital of Dallas
Dietetic Internship Program
8200 Walnut Hill Lane
Dallas, TX 75231-4402
Phone: (214)345-7558 **Fax:** (214)345-8473
Email: lyndamanson@texashealth.org
Website: http://www.phscare.org/phd/dietetics
Lynda M. Manson, PhD, Director

★ 27038 ★ St. Philip's College
Dietetic Technician Program
1801 Martin Luther King
San Antonio, TX 78203-2098
Phone: (210)531-3315 **Fax:** (210)531-3351
Email: mkunz@accd.edu
Website: http://www.accd.edu/spc/tourism
Mary A. Kunz, Contact

★ 27039 ★ Sam Houston State University
Department of Family and Consumer Sciences
Dietetic Internship Program
PO Box 2177
1700 Sam Houston Ave.
Huntsville, TX 77341-2177
Phone: (936)294-1242 **Fax:** (936)294-4204
Email: hec_azk@shsu.edu
Website: http://www.shsu.edu/~hec_www/
Zaheer A. Kirmani, PhD, Director

★ 27040 ★ Sam Houston State University
Family and Consumer Sciences
Dietetics-Didactic Program
SHSU Box 2177
Huntsville, TX 77341-2177
Fax: (936)294-4204
Email: hec_zak@shsu.edu
Website: http://www.shsu.edu/~hec_www/
Zaheer A. Kirmani, PhD, Director

★ 27041 ★ San Jacinto College Central
Dietetic Technology
Dietetic Technician Program
8060 Spencer Hwy.
PO Box 2007
Pasadena, TX 77505
Phone: (281)476-1501 **Fax:** (281)478-2790
Email: edsmith@sjcd.cc.tx.us
Website: http://www.sjcd.cc.tx.us
Robert E. Smith, EdD, Contact

★ 27042 ★ Southwest Texas State University
Department of Family and Consumer Sciences
Dietetic Internship Program
601 University Dr.
San Marcos, TX 78666-4616
Phone: (512)245-2155 **Fax:** (512)245-3829
Email: bf04@swt.edu
Website: http://www.fcs.swt.edu/fcs_dept/dietint.htm
B.J. Friedman, PhD, Director

★ 27043 ★ Southwest Texas State University
Family and Consumer Sciences
Dietetics-Didactic Program
601 University Dr.
San Marcos, TX 78666-4616
Phone: (512)245-2482 **Fax:** (512)245-3829
Email: sh07@swt.edu
Website: http://www.fcs.swt.edu/fcs_dept/NF.html
Sylvia L. Crixell, PhD, Director

★ 27044 ★ Stephen F. Austin State University
Department of Human Sciences
Dietetics-Didactic Program
SFA Station
P.O.Box 13014
Nacogdoches, TX 75962-3014
Phone: (936)468-4502 **Fax:** (936)468-2140
Email: sweems@sfasu.edu
Website: http://www.sfasu.edu/sweems
Mary Suzy K. Weems, PhD, Director

★ 27045 ★ Stephen F. Austin State University
Department of Human Sciences
Preprofessional Practice Program in Dietetics
PO Box 13014-SFA Station
Nacogdoches, TX 75962-3014
Phone: (409)468-4502 **Fax:** (409)468-2140
Email: bmarques@sfasu.edu
Website: http://www.sfasu.edu/di
Brenda G. Marques, PhD, Director

★ 27046 ★ Tarleton State University
Department of Human Sciences
Dietetics-Didactic Program
Box T-0380
Stephenville, TX 76402
Phone: (254)968-9196 **Fax:** (254)968-9728
Email: ltalley@tarleton.edu
Website: http://www.tarleton.edu/~hs
Linda J. Talley, PhD, Director

★ 27047 ★ Tarrant County College
Business and Technology Division
Dietetic Technician Program
2100 Southeast Pkwy.
Arlington, TX 76018
Phone: (817)515-3621 **Fax:** (817)515-3581
Email: shrriss@tcjc.cc.tx.us
Website: http://www.tccd.net
Sheryl O. Harris, Contact

★ 27048 ★ Texas A&M University
Department of Animal Science
Human Nutrition Section
Dietetic Internship Program
212D Kleberg Center
College Station, TX 77843-2471
Phone: (979)458-4642 **Fax:** (979)862-2378
Email: mb-george@tamu.edu
Website: http://dieteticinternship.tamu.edu
Mary Beth George, Director

★ 27049 ★ Texas A&M University
Human Nutrition Section
Dietetics-Didactic Program
2471 TAMU
College Station, TX 77843-2471
Phone: (979)845-2142 **Fax:** (979)862-2378
Email: karen-beathard@ansc.tamu.edu
Website: http://nutr.tamu.edu
Karen A. Beathard, Director

★ 27050 ★ Texas A&M University, Kingsville
Department of Human Sciences
Dietetic Internship Program
MSC 168
700 University Blvd.
Kingsville, TX 78363-8202
Phone: (361)593-2206 **Fax:** (361)593-2230
Email: kagg000@tamuk.edu
Website: http://www.tamuk.edu/aghs/hsci/brochure.html
Gloria I. Fernandez-Van Zante, Director

★ 27051 ★ Texas A&M University, Kingsville
Department of Human Sciences
Dietetics-Didactic Program
MSC 168
700 University Blvd.
Kingsville, TX 78363
Phone: (361)593-2206 **Fax:** (361)593-2230
Email: deyhim@hotmail.com
Website: http://www.tamuk.edu/aghs/hsci
Farzad Deyhim, Director

★ 27052 ★ Texas Christian University
Department of Nutrition Sciences
Coordinated Program in Dietetics
TCU Box 298600
Anne Richardson Bass Bldg.
Room 106
Fort Worth, TX 76129
Phone: (817)257-7309 **Fax:** (817)257-5849
Email: a.vanbeber@tcu.edu
Website: http://www.tcu.edu
Anne D. VanBeber, PhD, Director
Marla D. Murphy, PhD, Contact

★ 27053 ★ Texas Christian University
Department of Nutritional Sciences
Dietetics-Didactic Program
Box 298600
Fort Worth, TX 76129
Phone: (817)257-7309 **Fax:** (817)257-5849
Email: m.gorman@tcu.edu
Website: http://www.tcu.edu
Mary Anne Sullivan Gorman, PhD, Director

★ 27054 ★ Texas Department of Health
Bureau of Nutrition Services
Dietetic Internship Program
1100 W 49th St.
Austin, TX 78756
Phone: (512)458-7111 **Fax:** (512)458-7446
Email: sherry.clark@tdh.state.tx.us
Website: http://www.tdh.state.tx.us/wichd/nut/intern-intro.htm
Sherry Clark, Director

★ 27055 ★ Texas Southern University
Department of Human Services and Consumer Sciences
Dietetics-Didactic Program
3100 Cleburne Ave.
Houston, TX 77004-4575
Phone: (713)313-7637 **Fax:** (713)313-7228
Email: morgan_amW@tsu.edu
Website: http://www.tsu.edu
Annie M. Morgan, Director

★ 27056 ★ Texas Tech University
Department of Education, Nutrition, Restaurant-Hotel Management
Dietetics-Didactic Program
PO Box 41162
Lubbock, TX 79409-1162
Phone: (806)742-3068 **Fax:** (806)742-3042
Email: c.roman-shriver@ttu.edu
Website: http://www.hs.ttu.edu
Carmen R. Roman-Shriver, PhD, Director

★ 27057 ★ Texas Tech University
Department of Education, Nutrition, Restaurant, and Hotel Management
Dietetic Internship Program
PO Box 41162
Lubbock, TX 79409-1162
Phone: (806)742-3068 **Fax:** (806)742-3042
Email: c.roman-shriver@hs.ttu.edu
Website: http://www.hs.ttu.edu/intern
Carmen R. Roman-Shriver, PhD, Director

★ 27058 ★ Texas Woman's University
Department of Nutrition and Food Sciences
Dietetic Internship Program
1130 M.D. Anderson Blvd.
Houston, TX 77030-2897
Phone: (713)794-2371 **Fax:** (713)794-2374
Email: nfs_houston@twu.edu
Website: http://www.twu.edu/hs/nfs/hintern.htm
Rose M. Bush, Director

★ 27059 ★ Texas Woman's University
Department of Nutrition and Food Sciences
Dietetics-Didactic Program
304 Administration Dr.,
Clock Tower
Denton, TX 76201
Phone: (940)898-2650 **Fax:** (940)898-2634
Email: f_imrhan@twu.edu
Website: http://www.twu.edu/hs/nfs/nfs
Victoria L. Imrhan, PhD, Director

★ 27060 ★ Texas Woman's University
Nutrition and Food Sciences
Dietetic Internship Program
PO Box 425888
Denton, TX 76204-5888
Phone: (940)898-2657 **Fax:** (940)898-2634
Email: mrew@twu.edu
Website: http://www.twu.edu/hs/nfs/intern.htm
Martha L. Rew, Director

★ 27061 ★ U.S. Military Dietetic Internship Consortium
Brooke Army Medical Center
Nutrition Care Division
Dietetic Internship Program
Bldg. 3600, 3851 Roger Brooke Dr.
Fort Sam Houston, TX 78234-6200
Phone: (210)916-4332 **Fax:** (210)916-4152
Email: danny.jaghab@amedd.army.mil
Website: http://www.amsc.amedd.army.mil/frameset.htm
Danny Jaghab, Director

★ 27062 ★ U.S. Military Dietetic Internship Consortium
Wilford Hall Medical Center
U.S. Air Force
Dietetic Internship Program
959 MDTS/MTN
2200 Bergquist Dr., Ste. 1
San Antonio, TX 78236-5300
Phone: (210)292-6289 **Fax:** (210)292-7826
Email: donna.smith@lackland.af.mil
Donna C. Smith, Contact

★ 27063 ★ University of Houston
Department of Human Development and Consumer Sciences
Dietetics-Didactic Program
4800 Calhoun Rd.
Houston, TX 77204-6861
Phone: (713)743-4117 **Fax:** (713)743-4033
Email: kmatalon@uh.edu
Website: http://www.tech.uh.edu/hdcs/hnf.htm
Kimberlee Michals-Matalon, PhD, Director

★ 27064 ★ University of Houston
Human Development and Consumer Sciences
Dietetic Internship Program
4800 Calhoun
Houston, TX 77204-6020
Phone: (713)743-4112 **Fax:** (713)743-4033
Email: dietintern@uh.edu
Website: http://www.coe.uh.edu/HHP/internship
Sharon K. Bode, PhD, Director

★ 27065 ★ University of the Incarnate Word
Dietetic Internship Program
4301 Broadway, Box 311
San Antonio, TX 78209
Phone: (210)829-3152 **Fax:** (210)829-3153
Email: josephb@universe.uiwtx.edu
Website: http://www.uiw.edu
Joseph C. Bonilla, PhD, Director

★ 27066 ★ University of the Incarnate Word
Dietetic Internship Program
4301 Broadway,
San Antonio, TX 78209-6318
Phone: (210)829-3167 **Fax:** (210)829-3153
Email: josephb@universe.uiwtx.edu
Website: http://www.uiw.edu
Joseph C. Bonilla, PhD, Director

★ 27067 ★ University of the Incarnate Word
Dietetics-Didactic Program
4301 Broadway
San Antonio, TX 78209-6318
Phone: (210)829-3167 **Fax:** (210)829-3153
Email: josephb@universe.uiwtx.edu
Website: http://www.uiw.edu
Joseph C. Bonilla, PhD, Director

★ 27068 ★ University of Texas Southwestern Medical Center at Dallas
Department of Clinical Nutrition
Coordinated Program in Dietetics
5323 Harry Hines Blvd.
Dallas, TX 75390-8877
Phone: (214)648-1520 **Fax:** (214)648-1514
Email: clindiet@utsouthwestern.edu
Website: http://www.utsouthwestern.edu/clinnut
Bernadette B. Latson, Director

★ 27069 ★ University of Texas, Austin
Department of Human Ecology
Coordinated Program in Dietetics
GEA117 (A2700)
Austin, TX 78712-1097
Phone: (512)471-0637 **Fax:** (512)471-5630
Email: ksworth@mail.utexas.edu
Website: http://www.utexas.edu/depts/he/CoordinatedProgram.htm
Katherine Y. Southworth, Director

★ 27070 ★ University of Texas, Austin
Department of Human Ecology
Dietetics-Didactic Program
GEA 117
Austin, TX 78712
Phone: (512)471-7639 **Fax:** (512)471-5630
Email: mljt@mail.utexas.edu
Website: http://www.utexas.edu/depts/he/
Jane F. Tillman, Director

★ 27071 ★ University of Texas Health Science Center, Houston
School of Public Health
Dietetic Internship Program
1200 Herman Pressler St.
Human Nutrition Center, W 908RAS
Houston, TX 77030
Phone: (713)500-9347 **Fax:** (713)500-9329
Email: jmartin@sph.uth.tmc.edu
Website: http://www.sph.uth.tmc.edu/
Jeanne B. Martin, PhD, Director

★ 27072 ★ University of Texas, Pan American
College of Health Sciences and Human Services
Coordinated Program in Dietetics
1201 W University Dr.
Edinburg, TX 78539-2999
Phone: (956)318-5264 **Fax:** (956)318-5265
Email: ebriones@panam.edu
Website: http://www.panam.edu
Esperanza R. Briones, PhD, Director

Utah

★ 27073 ★ Brigham Young University
Department of Nutrition, Dietectics, and Food Science
Dietetics-Didactic Program or Dietetic Internship Program
S219 ESC
PO Box 24620
Provo, UT 84602-4620
Phone: (801)422-6676 **Fax:** (801)422-8714
Email: nora_nyland@byu.edu
Website: http://bioag.byu.edu
Nora K. Nyland, PhD, Director

★ 27074 ★ University of Utah/College of Health
Division of Foods and Nutrition
Coordinated Program in Dietetics
Dietetic Internship Program
250 S 1850 E, No. 239
Salt Lake City, UT 84112
Phone: (801)585-3218 **Fax:** (801)585-3218
Email: joseph.carlson@hsc.utah.edu
Website: http://www.health.utah.edu/fdnu
Joseph J. Carlson, PhD, Director

★ 27075 ★ Utah State University
Department of Nutrition and Food Sciences
Dietetics-Didactic Program or Coordinated Program in Dietetics
Logan, UT 84322-8700
Phone: (435)797-2105 **Fax:** (435)797-2379
Email: noreens@cc.usu.edu
Website: http://www.usu.edu/~dietetic
Noreen B. Schvaneveldt, Director

★ 27076 ★ Utah State University, Salt Lake
Dietetic Internship Program
5250 S Commerce Dr, Ste. 300
Murray, UT 84107
Phone: (801)269-9422 **Fax:** (801)266-7907
Email: annmil@ext.usu.edu
Website: http://extension.usu.edu/conted/intern
Ann Martin Mildenhall, Director

Vermont

★ 27077 ★ University of Vermont
Department of Nutrition and Food Sciences
Dietetics-Didactic Program
Terrill Hall
Burlington, VT 05405
Phone: (802)656-0539 **Fax:** (802)656-0407
Email: jross@zoo.uvm.edu
Website: http://nutrition.uvm.edu/
Jane K. Ross, PhD, Director

Virginia

★ 27078 ★ James Madison University
Department of Health Sciences
Dietetic Internship Program
MSC 4301
800 S Main St.
Harrisonburg, VA 22807
Phone: (540)568-7084 **Fax:** (540)568-3336
Email: gloeckjw@jmu.edu
Website: http://www.jmu.edu/healthsci/
Janet W. Gloeckner, PhD, Director

★ 27079 ★ James Madison University
Department of Health Sciences
Dietetics-Didactic Program
MSC 4301
HHS 3140
Harrisonburg, VA 22807
Phone: (540)568-6362 **Fax:** (540)568-3336
Email: brevarpb@jmu.edu
Website: http://www.jmu.edu/
Patricia B. Brevard, PhD, Director

★ 27080 ★ Norfolk State University
Food Science and Nutrition Program
Dietetics-Didactic Program
700 Park Ave.
James B. Bowser Bldg., Rm. 202
Norfolk, VA 23504
Phone: (757)823-9532 **Fax:** (757)823-2909
Email: latubbs@nsu.edu
Website: http://www.sci.nsu.edu
Lori A. Tubbs, Director

★ 27081 ★ Northern Virginia Community College
Business Division/Hospitality Management
Dietetic Technician Program
8333 Little River Turnpike
Annandale, VA 22003-3796
Phone: (703)323-3458 **Fax:** (703)323-3509
Email: jsass@nvcc.edu
Website: http://www.nvcc.edu
Janet M. Sass, Contact

★ 27082 ★ Radford University
Food and Nutrition Program
Dietetics-Didactic Program
PO Box 6962
Radford, VA 24142-5826
Phone: (540)831-7680 **Fax:** (540)831-7736
Email: m-miller@radford.edu
Website: http://www.radford.edu/~fdsn-web
Mary J. Miller, Director

★ 27083 ★ Radford University
Foods and Nutrition Program
Dietetic Internship Program
PO Box 6962
Radford, VA 24142-6962
Phone: (540)831-7679 **Fax:** (540)831-7736
Email: sfclark@radford.edu
Website: http://www.Radford.edu/~mntintern
Susan F. Clark, PhD, Director

★ 27084 ★ Tidewater Community College
Dietetic Technician Program
1700 College Crescent
Virginia Beach, VA 23456-1918
Phone: (757)822-7336 **Fax:** (757)427-1338
Email: cmedlin@tcc.edu
Christine L. Medlin, PhD, Contact

★ 27085 ★ University of Virginia Health System
Department of Nutrition Services
Dietetic Internship Program
Box 800673
Charlottesville, VA 22908
Phone: (434)924-2286 **Fax:** (434)982-3957
Email: ara6t@virginia.edu
Website: http://hsc.Virginia.edu/nutrition/dietetics/home.htm
Ana Abad-Sinden, Director

★ 27086 ★ Virginia Commonwealth University Health System
Dietetic Internship Program
PO Box 980294
Richmond, VA 23298-0294
Phone: (804)828-9108 **Fax:** (804)628-0921
Email: aerobbin@hsc.vcu.edu
Website: http://views.vcu.edu/dietetic
Ann E. Robbins, Director

★ 27087 ★ Virginia Department of Health
Division of WIC and Community Nutrition Services
Dietetic Internship Program
1500 E Main St., Rm. 132
Richmond, VA 23219
Phone: (804)786-5420 **Fax:** (804)371-6162
Email: lfoster@vdh.state.va.us
Linda H. Foster, Director

★ 27088 ★ Virginia Polytechnic Institute and State University
College of Human Resources and Education
Department of Human Nutrition, Foods and Exercise
Dietetics-Didactic Program or Dietetic Internship Program
Blacksburg, VA 24061-0430
Phone: (540)231-5104 **Fax:** (540)231-3916
Email: snrichar@vt.edu
Website: http://www.chre.vt.edu/HNFE/
Sharon M. Nickols-Richardson, PhD, Director

★ 27089 ★ Virginia Polytechnic Institute and State University
Dietetic Internship Program
338 Wallace Hall
Blacksburg, VA 24061-0430
Phone: (540)231-5540 **Fax:** (540)231-3916
Email: Rdinternship@vt.edu
Website: http://www.hnfe.vt.edu/internship/default.html
Carol B. Papillon, Director

★ 27090 ★ Virginia State University
Department of Agriculture and Human Ecology
Dietetics-Didactic Program or Dietetic Internship Program
Box 9211
Petersburg, VA 23806
Phone: (804)524-5502 **Fax:** (804)524-5048

Email: bmalinau@vsu.edu
Website: http://www.vsu.edu
Brenda M. Malinauskas, PhD, Director

Washington

★ 27091 ★ Bastyr University
Department of Food Science and Human Nutrition
Dietetics-Didactic Program
14500 Juanita Dr. NE
Kenmore, WA 98028-4966
Phone: (425)602-3099 **Fax:** (425)823-6222
Email: bkindbla@bastyr.edu
Website: http://www.bastyr.edu
Beverly D. Kinblade, Director

★ 27092 ★ Bastyr University
Nutrition Program
Dietetic Internship Program
14500 Juanita Dr. NE
Kenmore, WA 98028-4966
Phone: (425)602-3124 **Fax:** (425)823-6222
Email: smyer@bastyr.edu
Suzzanne N. Myer, Director

★ 27093 ★ Central Washington University
Department of Family and Consumer Sciences
Dietetic Internship Program
400 E 8th Ave.
Ellensburg, WA 98926-7565
Phone: (509)963-3360 **Fax:** (509)963-2787
Email: buergeln@cwu.edu
Website: http://www.cwu.edu/~fandcs/page6.html
Nancy S. Buergel, Director

★ 27094 ★ Central Washington University
Department of Family and Consumer Sciences
Dietetics-Didactic Program
400 E Eighth Ave.
Ellensburg, WA 98926-7565
Phone: (509)963-2366 **Fax:** (509)963-2787
Email: bergmane@cwu.edu
Website: http://www.cwu.edu
Ethan A. Bergman, PhD, Director

★ 27095 ★ Sea Mar Community Health Center
Dietetic Internship Program
8915 14th Ave. S
Seattle, WA 98108-4807
Phone: (206)762-0876 **Fax:** (206)763-1856
Website: http://www.seamar.org
Debra A. Boutin, Director

★ 27096 ★ Seattle Pacific University
Department of Family and Consumer Sciences
Dietetics-Didactic Program
3307 Third Ave. W
Seattle, WA 98119-1997
Phone: (206)281-2708 **Fax:** (206)281-2035
Email: ehackman@spu.edu
Website: http://www.spu.edu
Evette M. Hackman, PhD, Director

★ 27097 ★ Shoreline Community College
Nutrition and Dietetic Technology
Dietetic Technician Program
16101 Greenwood Ave. North
Rm 5334
Seattle, WA 98133-5696
Phone: (206)546-5891 **Fax:** (206)546-5869
Email: aleahy@ctc.edu
Website: http://shoreline.ctc.edu/
Alison P. Leahy, Contact

★ 27098 ★ Spokane Community College
Dietetic Technician Program
North 1810 Greene St.
MS 2090
Spokane, WA 99217-5399
Phone: (509)533-7314 **Fax:** (509)533-8621
Email: eclason@scc.spokane.edu
Website: http://www.scc.spokane.cc.wa.us/hes/alliedh/ntt/htm
Erin L. Clason, Contact

★ 27099 ★ University of Washington
Department of Nutritional Sciences
Dietetics-Didactic Program
305 Raitt Hall
PO Box 353410
Seattle, WA 98195-3410
Phone: (206)616-7382 **Fax:** (206)685-1696
Email: bbruemme@u.Washington.edu
Website: http://depts.Washington.edu/nutr/
Barbara A. Bruemmer, PhD, Director

★ 27100 ★ University of Washington
Nutritional Science Program
Dietetic Internship Program
PO Box 353410
305 Raitt Hall
Seattle, WA 98195
Phone: (206)543-2501 **Fax:** (206)685-1698
Email: jleader@u.washington.edu
Website: http://depts.washington.edu/nutr/
Janet K. Leader, Director

★ 27101 ★ Washington State University
Department of Food Science and Human Nutrition
Dietetics-Didactic Program
FSHN 120
PO Box 646376
Pullman, WA 99164-6376
Phone: (509)335-1395 **Fax:** (509)335-4815
Email: medlefsen@wsu.edu
Website: http://av.fshn.wsu.edu
Miriam S. Edlefsen, PhD, Director

★ 27102 ★ Washington State University
Department of Food Sciences and Human Nutrition
Coordinated Program in Dietetics
106 FSHN Bldg.
PO Box 646376
Pullman, WA 99164-6376
Phone: (509)335-4763 **Fax:** (509)335-4815
Email: susan.scheunemann@nw.amedd.army.mil
Website: http://av.fshn.wsu.edu
Susan J. Scheunemann, Director

★ 27103 ★ Washington State University, Spokane
Dietetic Internship Program
310 N Riverpoint Blvd.
Box M
Spokane, WA 99202-1675
Phone: (509)358-7562 **Fax:** (509)358-7627
Email: beary@wsu.edu
Website: http://www.dietetic-internship.Spokane.wsu.edu
Janet K. Beary, PhD, Director

West Virginia

★ 27104 ★ West Virginia University
College of Agriculture, Forestry, and Consumer Sciences
Dietetics-Didactic Program or Dietetic Internship Program
PO Box 6124
702-G Allen Hall
Morgantown, WV 26506-6124
Phone: (304)293-3402 **Fax:** (304)293-2750
Email: bforbes3@wvu.edu
Website: http://www.caf.wvu.edu/
Betty J. Forbes, Director

★ 27105 ★ West Virginia University Hospitals, Inc.
Department of Nutrition and Environmental Services
Dietetic Internship Program
Medical Center Dr.
PO Box 8016
Morgantown, WV 26506-8016
Phone: (304)598-4105 **Fax:** (304)598-4119
Email: johnstonj@rcbhsc.wvu.edu
Website: http://www.hsc.wvu.edu/di
Jill L. Johnston, Director

Wisconsin

★ 27106 ★ Madison Area Technical College
Dietetic Technician Program
3550 Anderson St.
Madison, WI 53704-2599
Phone: (608)246-6319 **Fax:** (608)246-6880
Email: bhundt@madison.tec.wi.us
Website: http://madison.tec.wi.us
Barbara A. Hundt, EdS, Contact

★ 27107 ★ Milwaukee Area Technical College
West Campus
Dietetic Technician Program
1200 South 71st St.
West Allis, WI 53214-3110
Phone: (414)456-5364 **Fax:** (414)456-5425
Email: dueling@matc.edu
Website: http://www.matc.edu
Jean L. Dueling, Contact

★ 27108 ★ Mount Mary College
Department of Dietetics
Coordinated Program in Dietetics
2900 N Menomonee River Pkwy.
Milwaukee, WI 53222-4545
Phone: (414)256-1216 **Fax:** (414)256-1224
Email: fischej@mtmary.edu
Website: http://www.mtmary.edu/dept_dietetics.htm
Janet A. Fischer, Director

★ 27109 ★ Mount Mary College
Graduate Program in Dietetics
Dietetic Internship Program
2900 N Menomonee River Pkwy.
Milwaukee, WI 53222-4597
Phone: (414)256-1216 **Fax:** (414)256-1224
Email: starkl@mtmary.edu
Website: http://www.mtmary.edu/dietetics.htm
Lisa K. Stark, Director

★ 27110 ★ University of Wisconsin, Green Bay
Department of Human Biology
Dietetic Internship Program or Dietetics-Didactic Program
2420 Nicolet Dr.
ES 301
Green Bay, WI 54311-7001
Phone: (920)465-2332 **Fax:** (920)465-2769
Email: laceyk@uwgb.edu
Website: http://www.uwgb.edu/humbio/
Karen P. Lacey, Director

★ 27111 ★ University of Wisconsin Hospitals and Clinics
Food and Nutrition Services
Dietetic Internship Program
Food and Nutrition Services F4/120
600 Highland Ave.
Madison, WI 53792-1510
Phone: (608)263-8237 **Fax:** (608)262-1636
Email: me.morgan@uwmsg.hosp.wisc.edu
Marjorie U. Morgan, Director

★ 27112 ★ University of Wisconsin, Madison
Department of Nutritional Sciences
Coordinated Program in Dietetics
1415 Linden Dr.
Madison, WI 53706-1571
Phone: (608)262-5847 **Fax:** (608)262-5860
Email: karls@nutrisci.wisc.edu
Lynette M. Karls, Director

★ 27113 ★ University of Wisconsin, Madison
Department of Nutritional Sciences
Dietetics-Didactic Program
1415 Linden Dr.
Madison, WI 53706-1571
Phone: (608)262-2727 **Fax:** (608)262-5860
Email: ney@nutrisci.wisc.edu
Website: http://nutrisci.wisc.edu
Denise M. Ney, PhD, Director
Lynette M. Karls, Contact

★ 27114 ★ University of Wisconsin, Stevens Point
School of Health Promotion and Human Development
Dietetics-Didactic Program
Stevens Point, WI 54481
Phone: (715)346-4087 **Fax:** (715)346-3751
Email: jchithar@uwsp.edu
Website: http://www.uwsp.edu/hphd/academics/
Jayne S. Chitharanjan, Director

★ 27115 ★ University of Wisconsin, Stout
College of Human Development
Food and Nutrition Department
Dietetics-Didactic Program
Menomonie, WI 54751-0790
Phone: (715)232-2216 **Fax:** (715)232-2317
Email: seabornc@uwstout.edu
Website: http://www.uwstout.edu/programs/bsd/
Carol D. Seaborn, PhD, Director

★ 27116 ★ University of Wisconsin, Stout
Department of Food and Nutrition
Dietetic Internship Program
220 Home Economics Bldg.
415 10th Ave.
Menomonie, WI 54751
Phone: (715)232-1994 **Fax:** (715)232-2317
Email: hansonmeli@uwstout.edu
Website: http://www.uwstout.edu/programs/msfns/intern/
Melinda A. Hanson, Director

★ 27117 ★ Viterbo College
Nutrition and Dietetics Department
Coordinated Program in Dietetics or Dietetic Internship Program
815 S Ninth St.
La Crosse, WI 54601-4797
Phone: (608)796-3660 **Fax:** (608)796-3668
Email: lclewis@viterbo.edu
Website: http://www.viterbo.edu/academic/ug/sls/majors/Dietetics/
Lorraine C. Lewis, Director

Wyoming

★ 27118 ★ University of Wyoming
Department of Family and Consumer Sciences
Dietetics-Didactic Program
PO Box 3354
Laramie, WY 82071-3354
Phone: (307)766-4145 **Fax:** (307)766-5686
Email: schantz@uwyo.edu
Website: http://www.uwyo.edu/family
Rhoda M. Schantz, PhD, Director

Environmental Health

The following institutions offer undergraduate and graduate environmental health programs accredited by the National Environmental Health Association, 720 S Colorado Blvd., South Tower, Ste. 970, Denver, CO 80246-1925, (303)756-9090, http://www.neha.org/.

California

★ 27119 ★ California State University, Fresno
Health Science Department
Box 38
Fresno, CA 93740-0038
Phone: (559)278-4747 **Fax:** (559)278-4179
Email: sdonohue@csufresno.edu
Website: http://www.csufresno.edu/schoolofhealth/school.html
Sandra Donohue, Contact

★ 27120 ★ California State University, Northridge
College of Health and Human Development
Department of Environmental and Occupational Health
1811 Nordhoff St.
Northridge, CA 91330-8285
Phone: (818)677-4719 **Fax:** (818)677-2045
Email: peter.bellin@csun1.csun.edu
Website: http://www.csun.edu/~vchsc00b/Program.html
Peter Bellin, PhD, Contact

Colorado

★ 27121 ★ Colorado State University
Department of Environmental Health
Fort Collins, CO 80523-1676
Phone: (970)491-6074 **Fax:** (970)491-2940
Email: ehinfo@colostate.edu
Website: http://www.bernardino.colostate.edu/enhealth
John S. Reif, Contact

Georgia

★ 27122 ★ University of Georgia
College of Agricultural and Environmental Sciences
Environmental Health Science
206 Environmental Health Bldg.
Athens, GA 30602-2102
Phone: (706)542-2454 **Fax:** (706)542-7472
Email: jwfisher@arches.uga.edu
Website: http://www.uga.edu/~ehs
Jeff Fisher, PhD, Contact

Idaho

★ 27123 ★ Boise State University
College of Health Sciences
Environmental Health Program
1910 University Dr.
M/S 1835
Boise, ID 83725
Phone: (208)426-3795 **Fax:** (208)426-2199
Email: gshook@boisestate.edu
Website: http://hs.boisestate.edu/envhlth
Gary Shook, MD, Contact

Illinois

★ 27124 ★ Illinois State University
Environmental Health Program
Department of Health Sciences
Campus Box 5220
Normal, IL 61790-5220
Phone: (309)438-7121 **Fax:** (309)438-2450
Email: tbierma@ilstu.edu
Website: http://www.cast.ilstu.edu/hsc/EnHealth/Eh-home.htm
Thomas J. Bierma, Contact

★ 27125 ★ University of Illinois, Springfield
Department of Environmental Studies
PO Box 19243
Springfield, IL 62794-9243
Email: lafollette.sharron@uis.edu
Sharron LaFollette, PhD, Contact

Indiana

★ 27126 ★ Indiana State University
Environmental Health Program
School of Health and Human Performance
Health and Human Performance Bldg., Rm. B-83
Terre Haute, IN 47809
Phone: (812)237-3079 **Fax:** (812)237-4338
Email: hselieze@scifac.indstate.edu
Website: http://web.indstate.edu/hlthsfty/eh/eh.htm
Eliezer Bermudez, PhD, Contact

Kentucky

★ 27127 ★ Eastern Kentucky University
Department of Environmental Health Sciences
521 Lancaster Ave.
Richmond, KY 40475-3102
Phone: (606)622-1939
Email: carolyn.harvey@eku.edu
Website: http://www.environmentalhealth.eku.edu
Carolyn H. Harvey, PhD, Contact

Maryland

★ 27128 ★ Salisbury State University
Environmental Health Program
Salisbury, MD 21801
Phone: (410)543-6499 **Fax:** (410)548-3318
Email: eavenso@ssu.edu
Website: http://www.ssu.edu/schools/Henson/Dept.html
Elicia A. Venso, PhD, Contact

Missouri

★ 27129 ★ Missouri Southern University
Environmental Health Program
3950 E Newman Rd.
Joplin, MO 64801-1595
Phone: (417)625-9765 **Fax:** (417)625-3169
Email: fletcher-m@mail.mssc.edu

Website: http://www.mssc.edu/biology/home.htm
Michael Fletcher, Contact

New Jersey

★ 27130 ★ Richard Stockton College of New Jersey
Public Health Program
Environmental Health Track
PO Box 195
Pomona, NJ 08240-0195
Phone: (609)652-4395 **Fax:** (609)652-4858
Email: Bruce.DeLussa@Stockton.Edu
Website: http://loki.stockton.edu/~calamide/phealth.htm
Bruce DeLussa, Contact

New Mexico

★ 27131 ★ New Mexico State University
Department of Health Sciences
Environmental Health Program
Las Cruces, NM 88005
Phone: (505)646-8194 **Fax:** (505)646-4343
Email: sarnold@nmsu.edu
Stephen D. Arnold, PhD, Contact

North Carolina

★ 27132 ★ East Carolina University
Department of Environmental Health Sciences, Safety, and Technology
School of Industry and Technology
Bldg. 310
Greenville, NC 27858-4353
Phone: (252)328-4249 **Fax:** (919)328-0380
Email: spraud@mail.ecu.edu
Website: http://www.ecu.edu/ehlt
Daniel D. Sprau, PhD, Contact

Ohio

★ 27133 ★ Bowling Green University
College of Health and Human Services
Environmental Health Program
214 Health Center
Bowling Green, OH 43403-0280
Phone: (419)372-7774 **Fax:** (419)372-2897
Email: Silverma@bgnet.bgsu.edu
Website: http://www.bgsu.edu/departments/envh/envh-hp.htm
Gary Silverman, Contact

★ 27134 ★ Ohio University
Environmental Health Science Program
School of Health Sciences
416 The Tower
Athens, OH 45701-2979
Phone: (740)593-1223 **Fax:** (740)593-0555
Email: morrone@ohiou.edu
Website: http://cscwww.cats.ohiou.edu/healthsciences/envrhlth.htm
Michele Morrone, PhD, Contact

★ 27135 ★ Wright State University
Institute for Environmental Quality
3640 Colonel Glenn Hwy.
Dayton, OH 45435
Phone: (937)775-2201 **Fax:** (937)775-4997
Email: allen.burton@wright.edu
Website: http://www.wright.edu/academics/ieq
G. Allen Burton, Jr., P, Contact

Oregon

★ 27136 ★ Oregon State University
College of Health and Human Performance
Department of Public Health
Environmental Health and Safety Program
310 Waldo Hall
Corvallis, OR 97331-6406
Phone: (541)737-3833 **Fax:** (541)737-4001
Email: cathy.neuman@orst.edu
Website: http://www.orst.edu/dept/HHP/PH/ph_undergrad.html
Catherine Neumann, PhD, Contact

Pennsylvania

★ 27137 ★ Indiana University of Pennsylvania
Department of Biology
Environmental Health Program
315 Weyandt Hall
Indiana, PA 15705
Phone: (724)357-4898 **Fax:** (724)357-5700
Email: tsimmons@grove.iup.edu
Tom Simmons, PhD, Contact

Tennessee

★ 27138 ★ East Tennessee State University
Environmental Health Department
PO Box 70682
Johnson City, TN 37614-0682
Phone: (423)439-7633 **Fax:** (423)439-5238
Email: philsche@etsu.edu
Website: http://www.etsu-TN.edu/cpah/environ.htm
Phil Scheuerman, PhD, Contact

Washington

★ 27139 ★ University of Washington
School of Public Health and Community Medicine
Environmental Health Department
PO Box 357234
Seattle, WA 98195-7234
Phone: (206)543-4207 **Fax:** (206)616-2651
Email: ctreser@u.washington.edu
Website: http://depts.washington.edu/envhlth
Charles D. Treser, Contact

Wisconsin

★ 27140 ★ University of Wisconsin, Eau Claire
Environmental and Public Health
Division of Allied Health Professions
Environmental and Public Health Program
School of Arts and Sciences
Eau Claire, WI 54702-4004
Phone: (715)836-2628 **Fax:** (715)836-3379
Email: nelsonr@uwec.edu
Website: http://www.uwec.edu/academic/ah/enph
Robert Nelson, PhD, Contact

Health Information Administration

The following baccalaureate, post-baccalaureate, and master's degree programs in health information (medical record) administration have been accredited by the Commission on Accreditation of Allied Health Education Programs (35 E Wacker Dr., Ste. 1970, Chicago, IL 60601-2208, (312)553-9355, http://www.caahep.org/) in collaboration with the Council on Accreditation of the American Health Information Management Association, 233 N Michigan Ave., Ste. 2150, Chicago, IL 60601-5519, (312)233-1100, http://www.ahima.org/. Contact either of these organizations for a listing of accredited academic programs for health information (medical record) technicians.

Alabama

★ 27141 ★ Alabama State University
Health Information Administrator Program
PO Box 271
915 S Jackson St.
Montgomery, AL 36101-0271
Phone: (334)229-5058 **Fax:** (334)229-4964
Email: sholt@asunet.alasu.edu
Sandria K. Holt, Director

★ 27142 ★ University of Alabama, Birmingham
Health Information Management Program
1675 University Blvd.
411 Webb Bldg.
Birmingham, AL 35294-3361
Phone: (205)934-1678 **Fax:** (205)975-5980
Email: sgrostic@uab.edu
Website: http://www.uab.edu
Sara S. Grostick, Director
Remarks: The school also offers a master's degree in Health Information Management. Contact Helmuth Orthner at 205934-3529 for more information.

Arkansas

★ 27143 ★ Arkansas Tech University
Health Information Administrator Program
105 Wilson Hall
Russellville, AR 72801
Phone: (501)968-0441 **Fax:** (501)964-0504
Email: melinda.wilkins@mail.atu.edu
Website: http://pls.atu.edu/biosci/him/him.htm
Melinda Wilkins, Director

California

★ 27144 ★ Loma Linda University
Health Information Administrator Program
1905 Nichol Hall
Loma Linda, CA 92350
Phone: (909)824-4976 **Fax:** (909)824-4291
Email: mdavidian@sahp.llu.edu
Website: http://www.llu.edu/llu/sahp/
Marilyn R. Davidian, Director
Remarks: The school also offers a master's degree in Health Information Management.

Colorado

★ 27145 ★ Regis University
Health Information Management Program
3333 Regis Blvd.
Mail Stop G-10
Denver, CO 80221-1099
Phone: (303)458-4157 **Fax:** (303)964-5533
Email: scarlon@regis.edu
Website: http://www.regis.edu/shcp/hsam.htm
Sheila A. Carlon, PhD, Director
Remarks: The school also offers a master's degree in Health Services Administration.

Florida

★ 27146 ★ Florida A&M University
Health Information Administrator Program
Ware-Rhaney Bldg., Rm. 223D
Tallahassee, FL 32307
Phone: (904)599-3822 **Fax:** (904)561-2457

Website: http://www.famu.edu/ahs/him.html
Barbara W. Mosley, PhD, Director

★ 27147 ★ Florida International University
Health Information Administrator Program
North Campus
3000 NE 151st St.
ACI 200
North Miami, FL 33181
Phone: (305)919-5631 **Fax:** (305)919-4864
Email: mcdons@fiu.edu
Website: http://www.fiu.edu/~cohealth/
Sandra McDonald, Director

★ 27148 ★ University of Central Florida
Health Information Management Program
PO Box 162200
Orlando, FL 32816-2200
Phone: (407)823-2369 **Fax:** (407)823-6138
Email: tfalen@mail.ucf.edu
Website: http://www.cohpa.ucf.edu/health.pro/
Thomas J. Falen, Director

Georgia

★ 27149 ★ Macon State College
Health Information Administrator Program
100 College Station Dr.
Macon, GA 31206-5144
Phone: (912)471-2788 **Fax:** (912)417-2787
Email: nsayles@mail.maconstate.edu
Nanette Sayles, Director

★ 27150 ★ Medical College of Georgia
School of Allied Health Sciences
Health Information Management Program
AL-122
Augusta, GA 30912-0400
Phone: (706)721-3436 **Fax:** (706)721-6067
Email: cacampbe@mail.mcg.edu
Website: http://www.mcg.edu/sah/him
Carol Campbell, Director

Illinois

★ 27151 ★ Chicago State University
Health Information Administrator Program
9501 S King Dr.
BHS 610
Chicago, IL 60628-1598
Phone: (773)995-2593 **Fax:** (773)995-4484
Email: l_thomas@email.com
Website: http://www.csu.edu/CollegeOfHealthSciences/HealthInformationAdministration/
Leona M. Thomas, Director

★ 27152 ★ Illinois State University
Health Information Management Program
103 Moulton Hall
5220 Health Sciences
Normal, IL 61761
Phone: (309)438-8329 **Fax:** (309)438-2450
Email: fwaterst@ilstu.edu
Website: http://www.cast.ilstu.edu/hsc/courses/under/hsc-u.htm
Francis L. Waterstraat, Director

★ 27153 ★ University of Illinois, Chicago
Health Information Management Program
1919 W Taylor, Rm. 811
M/C520
Chicago, IL 60612
Phone: (312)996-1444 **Fax:** (312)413-0205
Email: patena@uic.edu
Website: http://www.sbhis.uic.edu/GradBk98-99/him_main.htm
Karen Patena, Director
Remarks: The school also offers a master's degree in Public Health Informatics. Contact Aimee Wiebel at 312966-3818 or e-mail PHI@uic.edu for more information.

Indiana

★ 27154 ★ Indiana University School of Informatics
Health Information Administrator Program
719 Indiana Ave., Ste. 316
Indianapolis, IN 46202-5119
Phone: (317)274-1572 **Fax:** (317)278-7669
Email: dforgey@iupui.edu
Danita Forgey, Contact

Kansas

★ 27155 ★ University of Kansas Medical Center
Department of Health Information Management
Health Information Administrator Program
3901 Rainbow Blvd.
Mail Stop 2008
Kansas City, KS 66160-7607
Phone: (913)588-2423 **Fax:** (913)588-2428
Email: kkoob@kumc.edu
Website: http://www.kumc.edu/SAH/HIM/
Karl J. Koob, Director

Kentucky

★ 27156 ★ Eastern Kentucky University
Health Information Management Program
Dizney 117
Richmond, KY 40475-3135
Phone: (606)622-1915 **Fax:** (606)622-1140
Email: hrshinds@acs.eku.edu
Website: http://www.healthinfo.eku.edu
Frances A. Hindsman, Director

Louisiana

★ 27157 ★ Louisiana Tech University
Health Information Management Program
PO Box 3171
Ruston, LA 71272
Phone: (318)257-2854 **Fax:** (318)257-4896
Email: kennedy@him.latech.edu
Website: http://www.ans.latech.edu/him-index.html
Angela Kennedy, Director

★ 27158 ★ University of Louisiana, Lafayette
Health Information Management Program
PO Box 41007
Lafayette, LA 70504
Phone: (337)482-6629 **Fax:** (337)482-5902
Email: venable@louisiana.edu
Website: http://www.usl.edu/departments/HealthInfoMgmt/
Carol A. Venable, Director

Massachusetts

★ 27159 ★ Northeastern University
Health Information Administrator Program
266 Ryder Hall
360 Huntington Ave.
Boston, MA 02115
Phone: (617)373-2525 **Fax:** (617)373-2325
Email: ancollin@lynx.neu.edu
Website: http://www.neu.edu/uc/
Annalee Collins, Director

Michigan

★ 27160 ★ Ferris State University
College of Allied Health Sciences
Health Information Management Program
200 Ferris Dr.
VFS 402
Big Rapids, MI 49307-2740
Phone: (616)592-2313 **Fax:** (616)592-3788
Email: ellen_j_haneline@ferris.edu
Website: http://www.ferris.edu/htmls/colleges/alliedhe/hinfoman.htm
Ellen J. Haneline, Director

Minnesota

★ 27161 ★ College of St. Catherine
Health Information Administrator Program
601 25th Ave. S
Minneapolis, MN 55454
Phone: (651)690-7756 **Fax:** (651)690-7849
Email: jdvalerius@stkate.edu
Joanne Valerius, Contact

★ 27162 ★ College of Saint Scholastica
Health Information Management Program
1200 Kenwood Ave.
Duluth, MN 55811-0000
Phone: (218)723-6011 **Fax:** (218)733-2239
Email: klatour@css.edu
Website: http://www.css.edu/him
Kathleen M. LaTour, Director
Remarks: The school also offers a master's degree in Health Information Management. Contact Shirley Eichenwald at 888876-1030 for more information.

Mississippi

★ 27163 ★ University of Mississippi Medical Center
Health Information Management Program
2500 N State St.
Jackson, MS 39216
Phone: (601)984-6305 **Fax:** (601)984-6344
Email: byates@shrp.umsmed.edu
Website: http://shrp3.unsmed.edu/him/index.html
Rebecca J. Yates, Director

Missouri

★ 27164 ★ Saint Louis University Health Sciences Center
School of Allied Health Professions
Health Information Administrator Program
3437 Caroline St., Rm. 3087
Saint Louis, MO 63104
Phone: (314)577-8516 **Fax:** (314)268-5135
Email: smithjk@lan.slu.edu
Website: http://www.slu.edu/colleges/AH/Departments/him.html
K. Jody Smith, Director

★ 27165 ★ Stephens College
School of Graduate and Continuing Education
Health Information Administrator Program
Campus Box 2083
1200 E Broadway
Columbia, MO 65215
Free: 800-388-7579 **Fax:** (573)876-7237
Email: sce@stephens.edu
Website: http://www.stephens.edu/www/PR/GradConEd/GCE_HIM.html
Barbara Nicholson, Director

Nebraska

★ 27166 ★ College of Saint Mary
Health Information Administrator Program
1901 S 72nd St.
Omaha, NE 68124
Phone: (402)399-2405 **Free:** 800-926-5534
Fax: (402)399-2657
Email: ejacobs@csm.edu
Website: http://www.csm.edu
Ellen B. Jacobs, Director

New York

★ 27167 ★ Long Island University
Health Information Administrator Program
CW Post Campus, Rm. 257
720 Northern Blvd.
Greenvale, NY 11548
Phone: (718)470-7448 **Fax:** (718)347-8961
Email: healprof@cwpost.liu.edu
Website: http://www.cwpost.liunet.edu/cwis/cwp/hscience/healinfo/healinfo.html
Joann Johansmeyer, Director

★ 27168 ★ State University of New York Institute of Technology, Utica/Rome
Health Information Administrator Program
PO Box 3050
Utica, NY 13504-3050
Phone: (315)792-7391 **Fax:** (315)792-7138
Email: fdlsl@sunyit.edu
Website: http://www.sunyit.edu/pubm/academic/undrgrad/hlthinfo/degrees.htm
Donna L. Silsbee, Director

North Carolina

★ 27169 ★ East Carolina University
School of Allied Health Sciences
Health Information Administrator Program
Belk Bldg.
Greenville, NC 27858
Phone: (252)328-2202 **Fax:** (252)328-4470
Email: laymane@mail.ecu.edu
Website: http://www.news.ecu.edu/experts/healthinfo_manage.html
Elizabeth Layman, PhD, Director

★ 27170 ★ Western Carolina University
Health Information Administrator Program
121 Moore Hall
Cullowhee, NC 28723
Phone: (704)227-7113 **Fax:** (704)227-7446
Email: floreani@wpoff.wcu.edu
Website: http://www.wcu.edu/aps/healths/himhome.html
Walter R. Floreani, Director

Ohio

★ 27171 ★ Ohio State University
Health Information Administrator Program
1583 Perry St.
Columbus, OH 43210-1234
Phone: (614)292-0567 **Fax:** (614)292-0210
Email: brodnik.2@osu.edu
Website: http://www.amp.ohio-state.edu/!sampweb/hi-1.htm
Melanie Brodnik, PhD, Director
Remarks: The school also offers a master's degree in Health Information Management.

Oklahoma

★ 27172 ★ East Central University
Department of Health Information Management
Health Information Administrator Program
Ada, OK 74820
Phone: (580)332-8000 **Fax:** (580)332-4616
Email: sdixon@mailclerk.ecok.edu
Website: http://www.ecok.edu/acaddept/him/
Sandra A. Dixon, Director

★ 27173 ★ Southwestern Oklahoma State University
Health Information Administrator Program
100 Campus Dr.
Weatherford, OK 73096
Phone: (580)774-3287 **Fax:** (580)774-3795
Email: pricham@swosu.edu
Website: http://164.58.39.105/academic/arts_sci.htm
Marion Prichard, Director

Pennsylvania

★ 27174 ★ Duquesne University
Department of Health Management Systems
Health Information Administrator Program
600 Forbes Ave.
Pittsburgh, PA 15282
Phone: (412)396-5424 **Fax:** (412)396-4467
Email: begler@duq.edu
Website: http://www.duq.edu/index.html
Kathleen Begler, Director
Remarks: The school also offers a master's degree in Health Information Management. Contact Joan Kiel at 412396-4772 for more information.

★ 27175 ★ Gwynedd-Mercy College
Health Information Administrator Program
PO Box 901
1325 Sumneytown Pike
Gwynedd Valley, PA 19437
Phone: (215)646-7300 **Fax:** (215)641-5559
Email: hornung.j@gmc.edu
Website: http://www.gmc.edu/academic/schools/alliedhealth/himgmt.htm
Jennifer Hornung, Director

★ 27176 ★ Temple University
Health Information Administrator Program
3307 N Broad St.
Philadelphia, PA 19140
Phone: (215)707-4823 **Fax:** (215)707-5852
Email: lharman@vm.temple.edu
Website: http://www.temple.edu/HIM/
Laurinda Harman, PhD, Director

★ 27177 ★ University of Pittsburgh
Health Information Administrator Program
6051 Forbes Tower
Pittsburgh, PA 15260
Phone: (412)647-1190 **Fax:** (412)647-1199
Email: madelhak@pitt.edu
Website: http://www.him.upmc.edu
Mervat Abdelhak, PhD, Director
Remarks: The school also offers a master's degree in Health Information Systems.

Puerto Rico

★ 27178 ★ University of Puerto Rico
Health Information Administrator Program
Medical Science Campus
GPO Box 5067
San Juan, PR 00936-5067
Phone: (787)764-3609 **Fax:** (787)759-3645
Email: anaorabona@cprs.rcm.upr.edu
Website: http://cprsweb.rcm.upr.edu/HealthInfoAdministration.htm
Anna Orabona-Ocasio, Director
Remarks: The school also offers a master's degree in Health Informatics.

South Carolina

★ 27179 ★ Medical University of South Carolina
Master's of Health Science
171 Ashley Ave.
Charleston, SC 29425
Phone: (843)792-4492
Email: wagerka@musc.edu
Karen Wager, PhD, Director

South Dakota

★ 27180 ★ Dakota State University
Health Information Administrator Program
C.B. Kennedy Center 151
Madison, SD 57042-1799
Phone: (605)256-5170 **Fax:** (605)256-5316
Email: bennettd@columbia.dsu.edu
Website: http://www.dsu.edu
Dorine Bennett, Director

Tennessee

★ 27181 ★ Tennessee State University
Health Information Administrator Program
3500 John A. Merritt Blvd.
Nashville, TN 37209-1561
Phone: (615)963-7441 **Fax:** (615)963-7498
Email: kunnu@harpo.tnstate.edu
Website: http://www.tnstate.edu/alhp/
Elizabeth Kunnu, Director

★ 27182 ★ University of Tennessee Health Science Center
Health Information Administrator Program
822 Beale St., Rm. 300
Memphis, TN 38163
Phone: (901)448-6486 **Fax:** (901)448-7545
Email: mmccain@utmem.edu
Website: http://www.utmen.edu/him/homepage.htm
Mary C. McCain, Director

Texas

★ 27183 ★ Southwest Texas State University
Health Information Management Program
601 University Dr.
San Marcos, TX 78666-4616
Phone: (512)245-8242 **Fax:** (512)245-8258
Email: sb02@swt.edu
Website: http://www.health.swt.edu/catalog/himmajor.html
Sue E. Biedermann, Director

★ 27184 ★ Texas Southern University
College of Pharmacy and Health Sciences
Health Information Administrator Program
3100 Cleburne St.
Houston, TX 77004
Phone: (713)313-7265 **Fax:** (713)313-1094
Email: fannyhawkins@hotmail.com
Website: http://www.tsu.edu/pharmacy/index.htm
Fanny Hawkins, Director

Utah

★ 27185 ★ Weber State University
Health Information Administrator Program
3911 University Circle
Ogden, UT 84408-3911
Phone: (801)626-7298 **Fax:** (801)626-7683
Email: celliott@weber.edu
Website: http://weber.edu/has/Default.html
Chris Elliott, Director

Washington

★ 27186 ★ University of Washington
Health Information Management Program
1107 NE 45th, Ste. 400
Seattle, WA 98105
Phone: (206)543-8810 **Fax:** (206)685-4719
Email: gcmurphy@u.washington.edu
Website: http://www.edoutreach.washington.edu/extinfo/certprog/hia/default.htm
Gretchen Murphy, Director

Health Services Administration

The following health services administration programs are accredited by the Accrediting Commission on Education for Health Services Administration. For further information on these programs, and for listings of undergraduate programs, contact the Association of University Programs in Health Administration, 730 11th St. NW, 4th Floor, Washington, DC 20001-4510, (202) 638-1448, http://www.aupha.org/.

Alabama

★ 27187 ★ University of Alabama, Birmingham
Department of Health Services Administration
Master of Science in Health Administration Program
506 Webb Bldg.
1530 3rd Ave. S
Birmingham, AL 35294-3361
Phone: (205)934-1735 **Fax:** (205)975-6608
Email: msha@uab.edu
Website: http://www.hsa.uab.edu
Stephen J. O'Conner, PhD, Director
Fnded: 1965.

Alberta

★ 27188 ★ University of Alberta
Department of Public Health Sciences
Graduate Program in Health Services Administration
13-103 Clinical Sciences Bldg.
University of Alberta
Edmonton, AB, Canada T6G 2G3
Phone: (780)492-8608 **Fax:** (780)492-0364
Email: kent.rondeau@alberta.ca
Website: http://www.med.ualberta.ca/PHS/
Kent V. Rondeau, PhD, Director

Arizona

★ 27189 ★ Arizona State University
College of Business
School of Health Administration and Policy
Graduate Program in Health Services Administration
Box 874506
Tempe, AZ 85287-4506
Phone: (602)965-7778 **Fax:** (602)965-6654
Email: asuhap@asu.edu
Website: http://www.cob.asu.edu/hap/index.html
Eugene S. Schneller, Director

★ 27190 ★ Arizona State University
School of Health Administration and Policy
Graduate Program in Health Services and Policy
College of Business
Box 874506
Tempe, AZ 85287-4506
Email: asuhap@atsasu.edu
Website: http://www.cob.asu.edu/hap/index/html

Arkansas

★ 27191 ★ University of Arkansas, Little Rock
College of Professional Professional Studies
Graduate Program in Health Services Administration
2801 S University Ave.
Little Rock, AR 72204-1099
Phone: (501)569-3293 **Fax:** (501)569-8365
Email: jbwayne@ualr.edu
Website: http://www.ualr.edu/~hsadmin/index.htm
John B. Wayne, PhD, Director

California

★ 27192 ★ San Diego State University
Graduate School of Public Health
Division of Health Services Administration
San Diego, CA 92182-4162
Phone: (619)594-4443 **Fax:** (619)594-6112
Email: swilliam@mail.sdsu.edu
Website: http://www.sdsu.edu
Stephen J. Williams, Director

★ 27193 ★ University of California, Berkeley
Haas School of Business
Graduate Program in Health Services Management
Haas School of Business, mail code 1900
Berkeley, CA 94720
Phone: (510)643-1399 **Fax:** (510)642-4700
Email: raube@haas.berkeley.edu
Website: http://www.haas.berkeley.edu/advantage/health.htm
Kristiana Raube, PhD, Exec Director

★ 27194 ★ University of California, Los Angeles
School of Public Health
Department of Health Services
Health Policy and Management Program
PO Box 951772
10833 Le Conte Ave.
Los Angeles, CA 90095-1772
Phone: (310)825-7863 **Fax:** (310)825-3317
Email: almer@ph.ucla.edu
Website: http://www.ph.ucla.edu/hs
Diana W. Hilberman, Dr.PH, Director
Fnded: 1960.

★ 27195 ★ University of Southern California
School of Policy, Planning and Development
Health Services Administration Program
Los Angeles, CA 90089-0626
Phone: (213)740-4280 **Fax:** (213)740-1801
Email: myrtle@usc.edu
Website: http://www.usc.edu/dept/sppd
LaVonna Lewis, PhD, Director

Colorado

★ 27196 ★ University of Colorado, Denver
Graduate School of Business Administration
Programs in Health Services Administration
Campus Box 165
PO Box 173364
Denver, CO 80217-3364
Phone: (303)556-5845 **Fax:** (303)556-5899
Email: elbiggs@aol.com
Website: http://www.business.cudenver.edu
Errol L. Biggs, PhD, Director

★ 27197 ★ University of Colorado, Denver
Network for Healthcare Management
Executive Master of Business Administration in Health Administration
PO Box 480006
Denver, CO 80248-0006
Phone: (303)623-1888 **Fax:** (303)623-6228
Email: peter_taffe@cao.cudenver.edu
Website: http://www.execed.colorado.edu
Errol L. Biggs, PhD, Director

Connecticut

★ 27198 ★ University of Connecticut
School of Business
Center for Health Systems Management
368 Fairfield Rd., U-41
Storrs, CT 06269-2041
Phone: (860)486-4122 **Fax:** (860)486-4230
Email: jkramer@sba.uconn.edu
Website: http://www.sba.uconn.edu/HealthSystems/
Jeffrey A. Kramer, PhD, Director

★ 27199 ★ Yale University
School of Medicine
Department of Epidemiology and Public Health
Division of Health Policy and Administration
60 College St.
PO Box 208034
New Haven, CT 06520-8034
Phone: (203)785-2854 **Fax:** (203)785-6287
Website: http://www.yale.edu/yaleinfo/gradprof.html
Mark Schlesinger, PhD, Director
Fnded: 1947.

District of Columbia

★ 27200 ★ The George Washington University
Department of Health Services Management and Policy
2175 K St. NW, Ste. 700
Washington, DC 20037
Phone: (202)467-2288 **Fax:** (202)416-0075
Website: http://www.gwumc.edu/sphhs/heaser.htm
Brian Biles, MD, Director

Fnded: 1959.

Florida

★ 27201 ★ Florida International University
Program in Health Services Administration
N Miami Campus
3000 NE 151st St.
North Miami, FL 33181-3600
Phone: (305)919-5890 **Fax:** (305)919-5848
Email: spm@fiu.edu
Website: http://www.fiu.edu/~cupa/hsa-grad.html
Gloria J. Deckard, PhD, Director

★ 27202 ★ University of Central Florida
College of Health and Public Affairs
Health Services Administration Program
13-103 Clinical Sciences Bldg.
University of Alberta
Orlando, FL 32816
Phone: (407)823-6318 **Fax:** (407)823-6318
Email: hsainfo@mail.ucf.edu
Website: http://www.cohpa.ucf.edu/health.pro/hsa/graduate/
Myron Fottler, PhD, Exec Director

★ 27203 ★ University of Florida
Colleges of Health Professions
Graduate Program in Health Administration
PO Box 100195
Gainesville, FL 32610-0195
Phone: (352)392-7590 **Fax:** (352)392-7109
Email: hsa-info@hp.ufl.edu
Website: http://www.hp.ufl/hsa
Niccie L. McKay, PhD, Director

★ 27204 ★ University of Miami
Academic Programs in Health Administration and Policy
PO Box 248505
Coral Gables, FL 33124-6524
Phone: (305)284-5926 **Fax:** (305)284-5905
Email: mfrench@miami.edu
Website: http://www.bus.miami.edu/gbp/ealth/index.html
Michael T. French, PhD, Director

★ 27205 ★ University of South Florida
College of Public Health
Department of Health Policy and Management
13201 Bruce B. Downs Blvd.
MDC 56
Tampa, FL 33612-3805
Free: 888-873-2674 **Fax:** (813)974-6741
Email: advisor@hsc.usf.edu
Website: http://www.hsc.usf.edu/PUBHEALTH/hpm
Barbara Langland Orban, PhD, Director
Fnded: 1988.

Georgia

★ 27206 ★ Georgia State University
Graduate Program in Health Administration
Institute of Health Administration
University Plaza
Atlanta, GA 30303
Phone: (404)651-2637 **Fax:** (404)651-1230
Email: asumner@gsu.edu
Website: http://www.gsu.edu/~wwwiha/
Andrew T. Sumner, Director
Fnded: 1965.

Illinois

★ 27207 ★ Governors State University
College of Health Professions
Health Administration Program
University Park, IL 60466
Phone: (708)534-4032 **Fax:** (708)534-8041
Email: c-crawford@atsgovst.edu
Website: http://www.govst.edu
Catherine M. Crawford, PhD, Director

★ 27208 ★ Northwestern University
Kellogg Graduate School of Management
Program in Health Industry Management
Nathaniel Leverone Hall
2001 Sheridan Rd.
Evanston, IL 60208
Phone: (847)491-5540 **Fax:** (847)491-2683
Email: myrogers@nwu.edu
Website: http://www.kellogg.nwu.edu
Joel I. Shalowitz, MD, Director

★ 27209 ★ Rush University
Health Systems Management
Rush-Presbyterian /St. Luke's Medical Center
1653 W Congress Pkwy.
Chicago, IL 60612-3833
Phone: (312)942-5402 **Fax:** (312)942-4957
Email: rushhsm@rushu.rush.edu
Website: http://www.rushu.rush.edu/hsm
Denise M. Oleske, PhD, Director

★ 27210 ★ University of Chicago
Graduate Program in Health Administration and Policy
969 E 60th St.
Box 6011
Chicago, IL 60637
Phone: (773)702-1324 **Fax:** (773)702-7222
Email: lawlor@atschas.uchicago.edu
Website: http://www.uchicago.edu
Edward F. Lawlor, PhD, Director
Fnded: 1934.

Indiana

★ 27211 ★ Indiana University
School of Public and Environmental Affairs
Graduate Program in Health Administration
1110 W Michigan St.
Rm. LO 227
Indianapolis, IN 46202-5152
Phone: (317)278-4898 **Free:** 877-292-9321
Fax: (317)274-4444
Email: MHASPEA@iupui.edu
Website: http://www.mha.iupui.edu/
Stephen L. Walston, PhD, Director

Iowa

★ 27212 ★ Des Moines University
Health Care Administration Program
3200 Grand Ave.
Des Moines, IA 50312
Phone: (515)271-1364 **Free:** 800-240-2767
Fax: (515)271-1614
Email: HM.Admit@dmu.edu
Website: http://www.dmu.edu/cohs/dhm/hca/index.htm
Mary Pat Wohlford-Wessels, Director

★ 27213 ★ University of Iowa
College of Medicine and Graduate College
A Division of Health Management and Policy
2700 Steindler Bldg.
Iowa City, IA 52242
Phone: (319)335-9814 **Fax:** (319)335-9772
Email: student-affairs-administrator@mail.pmeh.uiowa.edu
Website: http://www.pmeh.uiowa.edu/hmp/MHAdegree.html
Douglas S. Wakefield, PhD, Director

Kansas

★ 27214 ★ University of Kansas
School of Medicine
Department of Health Policy and Management
Student Services Office
Edwards Campus
12600 Quivira Rd.
Overland Park, KS 66213
Phone: (913)897-8585 **Fax:** (913)897-8681
Email: ks_hsa@kumc.edu
Website: http://www.kumc.edu/som/hpm
Cynthia Carter Haddock, PhD, Director

Kentucky

★ 27215 ★ University of Kentucky
Martin School of Public Policy & Administration
Master of Health Administration Program
419 Patterson Office Tower
Lexington, KY 40506-0027
Phone: (859)252-5594 **Fax:** (859)323-1937
Email: rcr@pop.uky.edu
Website: http://www.uky.edu/RGS/Martin School
Robert C. Rodgers, PhD, Director
Alt. Contact: For Program information: 413 Patterson Office Tower, Lexington, KY 40506-0027; email: (Sarah Lee) solee@pop.uky.edu.

Louisiana

★ 27216 ★ Tulane University
School of Public Health and Tropical Medicine
Tulane University Health Sciences Center
Department of Health Systems Management
1440 Canal St., Ste. 1900
New Orleans, LA 70112
Phone: (504)988-7700 **Fax:** (504)988-7701
Email: hsm@hsm.tulane.edu
Website: http://www.tulane.hsm.edu
Judith W. Overall, Director

Maryland

★ 27217 ★ The Johns Hopkins University
School of Hygiene and Public Health
Department of Health Policy and Management
Masters of Health Science in Health Finance and Management
624 N Broadway, Rm. 406
Baltimore, MD 21205-1995
Phone: (410)955-5317 **Fax:** (410)955-6959
Email: dshiloh@jhsph.edu
Website: http://www.jhsph.edu/Departments/HPM/mhs/htm
William J. Ward, Jr., Director
Fnded: 1972.

Massachusetts

★ 27218 ★ Boston University
School of Management
Health Care Management Program
595 Commonwealth Ave., Rm. 106
Boston, MA 02215
Phone: (617)353-2730 **Fax:** (617)353-9498
Email: smghcmp@bu.edu
Website: http://management.bu.edu
Alan B. Cohen, ScD, Director

★ 27219 ★ Clark University
Graduate School of Management
Health Administration Program
Carlson Hall
950 Main St.
Worcester, MA 01610-1477
Phone: (508)793-7670 **Fax:** (508)793-8822
Email: eottensmeyer@atsclark.edu
Website: http://www.mba.clark.edu
Edward Ottensmeyer, PhD, Director

★ 27220 ★ Simmons College
Graduate Program in Health Care Administration
300 The Fenway
S309
Boston, MA 02115
Phone: (617)521-2377 **Fax:** (617)521-3406
Email: gshsadm@simmons.edu
Website: http://www.simmons.edu/programs/gshs/gphca.html
Linda Roemer, PhD, Director

Michigan

★ 27221 ★ University of Michigan
School of Public Health
Department of Health Management and Policy
University of Michigan
School of Public Health
Ann Arbor, MI 48109-2029
Phone: (734)763-9900 **Fax:** (734)764-4338
Email: sph.hmp.inquiries@umich.edu
Website: http://www.sph.umich.edu
William G. Weissert, PhD, Director

Minnesota

★ 27222 ★ University of Minnesota
Program in Healthcare Administration
Carlson School of Management, Rm. 3-140
321 19th Ave. S
Minneapolis, MN 55455-9940
Phone: (612)624-8818 **Free:** 877-MHA-UOFM
Fax: (612)624-8804
Email: mha@carlsonschool.umn.edu
Website: http://www.carlsonschool.umn.edu/mha
James W. Begun, PhD, Director
Fnded: 1946.

Missouri

★ 27223 ★ Saint Louis University
School of Public Health
Department of Health Administration
3663 Lindell Blvd.
Saint Louis, MO 63108
Phone: (314)977-8112 **Free:** 800-782-6769
Fax: (314)977-8150
Email: laxm@slu.edu
Website: http://www.slu.edu/colleges/sph/
Claudia R. Campbell, PhD, Director
Fnded: 1947.

★ 27224 ★ University of Missouri, Columbia
Health Services Management
324 Clark Hall
Columbia, MO 65211
Phone: (573)882-1849 **Free:** 800-877-4764
Fax: (573)882-6158
Email: mha@health.missouri.edu
Website: http://www.hmi.missouri.edu
Gordon D. Brown, PhD, Director

★ 27225 ★ Washington University
School of Medicine
Health Administration Program
4547 Clayton Ave.
Saint Louis, MO 63110-1501
Phone: (314)362-4277 **Fax:** (314)362-3265
Email: marilyn@medicine.wustl.edu
Website: http://www.medicine.wustl.edu/~hap
Stuart B. Boxerman, Director
Fnded: 1946.

Nebraska

★ 27226 ★ Creighton University
Master of Health Services Administration
2500 California Plaza
Omaha, NE 68178
Phone: (402)280-3268 **Fax:** (402)280-3332
Email: mclean@creighton.edu
Website: http://hsa.creighton.edu
Robert A. McLean, Director

New Hampshire

★ 27227 ★ University of New Hampshire
School of Health and Human Services
Department of Health Management and Policy
Master of Health Administration Program
Hewitt Hall
4 Library Way
Durham, NH 03824
Phone: (603)862-2733 **Fax:** (603)862-3461
Email: mha.info@unh.edu
Website: http://www.unh.edu.hmp/
James B. Lewis, Director

New Jersey

★ 27228 ★ Seton Hall University
Graduate Department of Public and Health Administration
Seton Hall University
South Orange, NJ 07079
Phone: (973)761-9510 **Fax:** (973)275-2463
Email: wishnaom@shu.edu
Website: http://www.setonworldwide.com
Naomi Wish, PhD, Contact

New York

★ 27229 ★ City University of New York
Baruch College
Mount Sinai School of Medicine
Graduate Program in Health Care Administration
17 Lexington Ave., Box F1215
New York, NY 10010
Phone: (212)802-6706 **Fax:** (212)802-6705
Email: Ted_Joyce@Baruch.cuny.edu
Website: http://www.baruch.cuny.edu
Ted Joyce, PhD, Director

★ 27230 ★ Cornell University
College of Human Ecology
Department of Policy Analysis and Management
Sloan Program in Health Services Administration
N231 Martha Van Rensselaer Hall
Ithaca, NY 14853-4401
Phone: (607)255-2594 **Fax:** (607)255-4071
Email: dsk@cornell.edu
Website: http://www.human.cornell.edu/pam/sloan
Donald S. Kenkel, PhD, Director

★ 27231 ★ New York University
Robert F. Wagner Graduate School of Public Service
Program in Health Policy and Management
40 W 4th St.
Tisch Hall, Rm. 600
New York, NY 10012-1118
Phone: (212)998-7440 **Fax:** (212)995-4162
Email: wagner.admissions@nyu.edu
Website: http://www.nyu.edu/wagner
Anthony Kovner, PhD, Director

★ 27232 ★ Union College
Graduate Management Institute
Program in Health Systems Administration
807 Union Ave.
Lamont House Graduate Center
Schenectady, NY 12308
Phone: (518)388-6238 **Fax:** (518)388-6754
Email: mba@union.edu
Website: http://www.mba.union.edu
Martin A. Strosberg, PhD, Director

North Carolina

★ 27233 ★ Duke University
The Fuqua School of Businesss
Health Sector Management Program
PO Box 90120
Durham, NC 27708-0120
Phone: (919)660-7989 **Fax:** (919)660-7843
Email: hsm@fuqua.duke.edu
Website: http://www.fuqua.duke.edu/programs/hsm
Kevin A. Schulman, MD, Director

★ 27234 ★ University of North Carolina, Chapel Hill
School of Public Health
Department of Health Policy and Administration
CB 7400, McGavran-Greenburg Hall
Chapel Hill, NC 27599-7400
Phone: (919)966-7350 **Fax:** (919)966-6961
Email: kkilpatr@sph.unc.edu
Website: http://www.sph.unc.edu/hpaa/
Kerry E. Kilpatrick, PhD, Director

★ 27235 ★ University of North Carolina, Charlotte
Health Administration
9201 University City Boulevard
Macy 103
Charlotte, NC 28223
Phone: (704)687-4522 **Fax:** (704)687-4347
Email: WFPilkin@email.uncc.edu
Website: http://www.uncc.edu/gradmiss/hltad-mas.htm
William F. Pilkington, Director

Nova Scotia

★ 27236 ★ Dalhousie University
Faculty of Health Professions
School of Health Services Administration
5599 Fenwick St.
Halifax, NS, Canada B3H 1R2
Phone: (902)494-7097 **Fax:** (902)494-6849
Email: health.services.administration@dal.ca
Website: http://www.dal.ca/shsa
Thomas A. Rathwell, PhD, Director

Ohio

★ 27237 ★ Cleveland State University
College of Business Administration
Graduate Study in Health Care Administration
College of Business Administration Bldg. 434
Cleveland, OH 44112
Phone: (216)687-4711 **Fax:** (216)687-9354
Email: b.marshall@csuohio.edu
Website: http://www.csuohio.edu/hca/
Brenda Stevenson Marshall, PhD, Director

★ 27238 ★ Ohio State University
Graduate Program in Health Services Management and Policy
1583 Perry St., Rm. 246
Columbus, OH 43210-1234
Phone: (614)292-9708 **Fax:** (614)292-3572
Email: hsmp@sosu.edu
Website: http://www.med.ohio-state.edu/hsmp/
Stephen F. Loebs, PhD, Director

★ 27239 ★ Xavier University
Graduate Program in Health Services Administration
3800 Victory Pkwy.
Cincinnati, OH 45207-7331
Phone: (513)745-3392 **Fax:** (513)745-4301
Email: schicki@admin.xu.edu
Website: http://www.xu.edu/dpets/mhsa
Ida Critelli Schick, PhD, Director
Fnded: 1958.

Oklahoma

★ 27240 ★ University of Oklahoma
Health Sciences Center
College of Public Health
Department of Health Administration and Policy
PO Box 26901
Oklahoma City, OK 73190
Phone: (405)271-2114 **Fax:** (405)271-1868
Email: edward-brandt@ouhsc.edu
Website: http://w3.uokhsc.edu/hap
Edward N. Brandt, Jr,PhD, Director

Ontario

★ 27241 ★ University of Ottawa
Master's Program in Health Administration
136 Jean-Jacques Lussier Private
Vanier Bldg.
Faculty of Administration
Ottawa, ON, Canada K1N 6N5
Phone: (613)562-5884 **Fax:** (613)562-5912
Email: mha@admin.uottowa.ca
Website: http://www.admin.uottowa.ca.mha
Douglas E. Angus, Director

★ 27242 ★ University of Toronto
Health Administration Program
2nd Fl., McMurrich Bldg.
12 Queen's Park Crescent W
Toronto, ON, Canada M5S 1A8
Phone: (416)946-3023 **Fax:** (416)978-7350
Email: tina.smith@utoronto.ca
Website: http://www.utoronto.ca/hltadmin/
Tina Smith, Director

Oregon

★ 27243 ★ Oregon State University
Department of Public Health
Health Care Administration Program
Waldo Hall 256
Corvallis, OR 97331-6406
Phone: (541)737-2686 **Fax:** (541)737-4001
Email: leonard.friedman@atsorst.edu
Website: http://www.osu.orst.edu
Leonard H. Friedman, PhD, Director

Pennsylvania

★ 27244 ★ King's College
McGowan School of Business
Master of Science Health Care Administration
133 N River St.
Wilkes Barre, PA 18711
Phone: (570)208-6083 **Fax:** (570)208-5989
Email: bjhealey@kings.edu
Website: http://www.kings.edu/hca
Bernard J. Healey, PhD, Director

★ 27245 ★ Penn State Great Valley
The Pennsylvania State University
Great Valley School of Graduate Professional Studies
Health Care Master of Business Administration Program
30 E Swedesford Rd.
Malvern, PA 19355
Phone: (610)648-3269 **Fax:** (610)889-1334
Email: jld13@psu.edu
Website: http://www.gv.psu.edu
Janice L. Dreachslin, Director

★ 27246 ★ Pennsylvania State University
Department of Health Policy and Administration
Concurrent Master Business Administration/Master Health Administration Program
116 Henderson Bldg.
University Park, PA 16802
Phone: (814)863-2859 **Fax:** (814)865-2905
Email: bgf2@psu.edu
Website: http://www.hhdev.psu.edu/hpa/hpa.htm
S. Diane Brannon, PhD, Director

★ 27247 ★ Temple University
School of Business and Management
Department of Risk, Insurance, and Healthcare Management
Graduate Program in Health Management
Ritter Annex (004-00)
Philadelphia, PA 19122
Phone: (215)204-8468 **Fax:** (215)204-3851
Email: zinn@vm.temple.edu
Website: http://www.sbm.temple.edu
Jacqueline Zinn, PhD, Director

★ 27248 ★ University of Pennsylvania
The Wharton School
Graduate Program in Health Care Management
Colonial Penn Center
3641 Locust Walk
Philadelphia, PA 19104-6218
Phone: (215)898-6861 **Fax:** (215)573-2157
Email: pauly@wharton.upenn.edu
Website: http://www.wharton.upenn.edu
Mark V. Pauly, PhD, Director

★ 27249 ★ University of Pittsburgh
Health Administration Program
A-646 Crabtree Hall
130 DeSoto St.
Pittsburgh, PA 15261
Phone: (412)624-3123 **Fax:** (412)624-3146
Email: lave@pitt.edu
Website: http://www.edc.gsph.pitt.edu/hsa/
Judith R. Lave, PhD, Director

★ 27250 ★ University of Scranton
Panuska College of Professional Studies
Graduate Program in Health Administration
417 McGurrin Hall
Scranton, PA 18510-4597
Phone: (570)941-4242 **Fax:** (570)941-5882
Email: oldenp1@uofs.edu
Website: http://www.academic.uofs.edu/department/HAHR/mha_program.htm
Peter C. Olden, PhD, Director

★ 27251 ★ Widener University
Graduate Program in Health and Medical Services Administration
One University Place
Chester, PA 19013
Phone: (610)499-4384 **Fax:** (610)499-4615
Email: health.administration@widener.edu
Website: http://www.sba.widener.edu/hmsahome/html
Caryl E. Carpenter, PhD, Director

Puerto Rico

★ 27252 ★ University of Puerto Rico
Graduate School of Public Health
Master in Health Services Administration
Medical Sciences Campus Bldg.
GPO Box 5067
San Juan, PR 00936-5067
Phone: (787)758-2525 **Fax:** (787)758-2783
Email: roramirez@rcm.upr.edu
Website: http://www.rcm.upr.edu
Roberto Ramirez, PhD, Director

South Carolina

★ 27253 ★ Medical University of South Carolina
Department of Health Administration and Policy
Master of Health Administration Program
19 Hagwood Ave., Ste. 408
PO Box 250807
Charleston, SC 29425
Phone: (843)792-2118 **Fax:** (843)792-3327
Email: dhapinfo@musc.edu
Website: http://www.musc.edu/hap/
Andrea W. White, PhD, Director

★ 27254 ★ University of South Carolina
School of Public Health
Graduate Program in Health Services Administration
Department of Health Administration
Columbia, SC 29208

Phone: (803)777-6096 **Fax:** (803)777-1836
Email: dcdodson@sph.sc.edu
Website: http://www.hadm.sc.edu
Don C. Dodson, PhD, Director

Tennessee

★ 27255 ★ Meharry Medical College
Health Services Administration Program
1005 D.B. Todd Blvd.
Box 53-A
Nashville, TN 37208-9989
Phone: (615)327-6069 **Fax:** (615)327-6717
Email: elbrown@mail.mmc.edu
Website: http://www.mmc.edu
Herman M. Ellis, MD, Director

★ 27256 ★ University of Memphis
McCord Hall, Rm. 119
Memphis, TN 38152
Phone: (901)678-1465 **Fax:** (901)678-2981
Email: peftzgrl@memphis.edu
Website: http://www.people.memphis.edu/~gahealthadmin
Paul E. Fitzgerald, Jr,PhD, Director

Texas

★ 27257 ★ Houston Baptist University
Center For Health Studies
Graduate Programs in Health Administration
7502 Fondren Rd.
Houston, TX 77074-3298
Phone: (281)649-3419 **Fax:** (281)649-3340
Email: hgriffin@hbu.edu
Website: http://www.hbu.edu/Pages/acad/H3Fmsha.html
Harold Ray Griffin, PhD, Director

★ 27258 ★ Midwestern State University
College of Health and Human Services
Health and Public Administration
3410 Taft Blvd.
Wichita Falls, TX 76308
Phone: (940)397-4752 **Fax:** (940)397-4845
Email: russell.porter@nexus.mwsu.edu
Website: http://www.mwsu.edu/~hsa/hsaintro.html
Russel D. Porter, PhD, Director

★ 27259 ★ Southwest Texas State University
Graduate Program in Health Care Administration
601 University Dr.
San Marcos, TX 78666-4616
Phone: (512)245-3556 **Fax:** (512)245-8712
Email: ws06@swt.edu
Website: http://www.health.swt.edu
Wayne B. Sorensen, PhD, Director
Fnded: 1973.

★ 27260 ★ Texas Tech University
College of Business Administration
The MBA & MD/MBA Program in Health Organization Management
Lubbock, TX 79409-2101
Phone: (806)742-1236 **Fax:** (806)742-2308
Email: hom@ba.ttu.edu
Website: http://www.ba.ttu.edu
Timothy W. Nix, PhD, Director

★ 27261 ★ Texas Woman's University, Houston
Program in Health Care Administration
1130 MD Anderson Blvd.
Houston, TX 77030
Phone: (713)794-2061 **Fax:** (713)794-2350
Email: kmoseley@twu.edu
Website: http://www.twu.edu/houston/
S. Kelley Moseley, PhD, Director

★ 27262 ★ Trinity University
On-Campus Graduate Program in Health Care Administration
715 Stadium Dr., No. 58
Chapman Graduate Center-N400
San Antonio, TX 78212-7200
Phone: (210)999-8107 **Fax:** (210)999-8108
Email: hca@trinity.edu
Website: http://www.trinity.edu/departments/health-care
Stephen L. Tucker, Contact
Fnded: 1965.

★ 27263 ★ U.S. Army/Baylor University
Center for Healthcare Education and Studies
Academy of Health Sciences
Graduate Program in Health Care Administration
3151 Scott Rd. (MCCS-HRA)
Fort Sam Houston, TX 78234-6135
Phone: (210)221-6345 **Fax:** (210)221-6051
Email: charles.wainright@cen.amedd.army.mil
Website: http://www.cs.amedd.army.mil/baylorhca
LTC Charles F. Wainright, III, PhD, Director

★ 27264 ★ University of Houston, Clear Lake
School of Business and Public Administration
Healthcare Administration Program
2700 Bay Area Blvd.
Mail Code 73
Houston, TX 77058-1098
Phone: (281)283-3130 **Fax:** (281)283-3136
Email: hadm@cl.uh.edu
Website: http://www.cl.uh.edu/bpa/hadm
Phillip J. Decker, Director

★ 27265 ★ University of Mary Hardin-Baylor
Graduate Program in Health Services Management
900 College St.
UMHB Station Box 8405
Belton, TX 76513-2599
Phone: (254)295-4558 **Free:** 800-727-UNMB
Fax: (254)295-5300
Email: mhsm@umhb.edu
Website: http://www.umhb.edu/programs/Graduate/MHSM.htm
Dr. Mary Anne Franklin, Contact

Virginia

★ 27266 ★ Virginia Commonwealth University
Medical College of Virginia
School of Allied Health Professions
Department of Health Administration
Box 980203
Richmond, VA 23298-0203
Phone: (804)828-0719 **Fax:** (804)828-1894
Email: shavasy@hsc.vcu.edu
Website: http://www.had.vcu.edu
Jan Clement, PhD, Director

Washington

★ 27267 ★ University of Washington, Seattle
Graduate Program in Health Services Administration
Box 357660
Seattle, WA 98195-7660
Phone: (206)543-8778 **Fax:** (206)543-3964
Email: alinew@u.washington.edu
Website: http://depts.washington.edu/mhap
Dr. William E. Welton, PhD, Director

★ 27268 ★ Washington State University
Graduate Program in Health Policy and Administration
668 N Riverpoint Blvd., Box B
Spokane, WA 99202-1162
Phone: (509)358-7980 **Fax:** (509)358-7900
Email: venzon@wsu.edu
Website: http://www.hpa.spokane.wsu.edu
Winsor C. Schmidt, Contact

Wisconsin

★ 27269 ★ University of Wisconsin, Madison
Administrative Medicine Program
734 WARF Bldg.
610 N Walnut St.
Madison, WI 53705-2397
Phone: (608)263-4889 **Fax:** (608)262-6404
Email: hwilde@facstaff.wisc.edu
Website: http://www.medsch.wisc.edu/adminmed/
David Kindig, MD,PhD, Director
Mark Covaleski, PhD, Director

Medical Illustration

Schools listed below offer degree programs that are accredited by the Association of Medical Illustrators (5475 Mark Daubling Blvd., Ste. 108, Colorado Springs, CO 80918, (719)598-8622, http://www.ami.org) in conjunction with the Commission on Accreditation of Allied Health Education Programs (35 E Wacker Dr., Ste. 1970, Chicago, IL 60601-2208, (312)553-9355, http://www.caahep.org/).

Georgia

★ 27270 ★ Medical College of Georgia
School of Graduate Studies
Graduate Program in Medical Illustration
1120 15th St.
Augusta, GA 30912-0300
Phone: (706)721-3266 **Fax:** (706)721-7855
Email: medart@mcg.edu
Website: http://www.mcg.edu/medart/

Illinois

★ 27271 ★ University of Illinois, Chicago
College of Associated Health Professions
Department of Biomedical Visualization
Graduate Program in Medical Illustration
1919 W Taylor St., Rm. 213
M/C 527
Chicago, IL 60612
Phone: (312)996-7337 **Fax:** (312)996-8342
Email: aakatz@uic.edu
Website: http://www.uic.edu/ahs/sbhis/bvis/index.htm

Maryland

★ 27272 ★ Johns Hopkins School of Medicine
Department of Art as Applied to Medicine
Graduate Program in Medical Illustration
1830 E Monument St., Ste. 7000
Baltimore, MD 21205-2100
Phone: (410)955-3213 **Fax:** (410)955-1085
Email: glees@medart.jhu.edu
Website: http://www.med.jhu.edu/medart/

Michigan

★ 27273 ★ University of Michigan
School of Art and Design
M.F.A. Program in Medical and Biological Illustration
2000 Bonisteel Blvd., Rm. 1075
Ann Arbor, MI 48109-2069
Phone: (734)763-5247 **Fax:** (734)936-0469
Email: brdsmith@umich.edu
Website: http://www.rackham.umich.edu/programs/biohealth.sci/medill.html

Ontario

★ 27274 ★ University of Toronto
Department of Surgery
Division of Biomedical Communications
Graduate Program in Medical Illustration
One King's College Circle
Medical Sciences Bldg., Rm. 2356
Toronto, ON, Canada M5S 1A8
Phone: (416)978-2659 **Fax:** (416)978-6891
Email: l.wilson.pauwels@utoronto.ca
Website: http://www.bmc.med.utoronto.ca/bmc/

Texas

★ 27275 ★ University of Texas Southwestern Medical Center, Dallas
Department of Biomedical Communications
Biomedical Communication Graduate Program
5323 Hines Blvd.
Dallas, TX 75235-8881
Phone: (214)648-4699 **Fax:** (214)648-5353
Email: lewis.calver@utsouthwestern.edu
Website: http://www.swmed.edu/medillus/

Medicine

The following are accredited U.S. medical schools. Professional associations to contact for further information on medical education include the Association of American Medical Colleges (2450 N St. NW, Washington, DC 20037-1126, (202)828-0400, http://www.aamc.org/) and the American Medical Association (515 N State St., Chicago, IL 60610, (312)464-5000, http://www.ama-assn.org/).

Alabama

★ 27276 ★ University of Alabama, Birmingham
School of Medicine
1813 6th Ave., S
Birmingham, AL 35294-3293
Phone: (205)934-4011 **Fax:** (205)934-0333
Website: http://www.uab.edu/uasom
William B. Deal, MD, Director
Fnded: 1945.

★ 27277 ★ University of South Alabama College of Medicine
307 University Blvd.
Mobile, AL 36688
Phone: (334)460-7174 **Fax:** (334)460-6073
Website: http://www.southalabama.edu
Robert A. Kreisberg, MD, Director
Fnded: 1973.

Alberta

★ 27278 ★ University of Alberta
Faculty of Medicine and Dentistry
2J2 Walter Mackenzie Health Sciences Center
8440 112th St.
Edmonton, AB, Canada T6G 2R7
Phone: (780)492-6350 **Fax:** (780)492-7303
Website: http://www.med.ualberta.ca
D. L. J. Tyrrell, MD,PhD, Director
Fnded: 1913.

★ 27279 ★ University of Calgary
Faculty of Medicine
3330 Hospital Dr., NW
Calgary, AB, Canada T2N 4N1
Phone: (403)220-6848 **Fax:** (403)283-4740
Email: staylors@ucalgary.ca
Website: http://www.med.ucalgary.ca/
D. G. Gall, MD, Director
Fnded: 1970.

Arizona

★ 27280 ★ University of Arizona
College of Medicine
PO Box 245018
Tucson, AZ 85724-5018
Phone: (520)626-6214 **Fax:** (520)626-4884
Website: http://www.ahsc.arizona.edu/
Raymond L. Woolsey, MD,PhD, Director
Fnded: 1967.

Arkansas

★ 27281 ★ University of Arkansas
College of Medicine
4301 W Markham St.
Little Rock, AR 72205
Phone: (501)686-5000 **Fax:** (501)686-8160
Website: http://www.uams.edu/com/
John P. Shock, MD, Director
Fnded: 1879.

British Columbia

★ 27282 ★ University of British Columbia
Faculty of Medicine
317-2194 Health Sciences Mall
Vancouver, BC, Canada V6T 1Z3
Phone: (604)822-2421 **Fax:** (604)822-6061
Website: http://www.med.ubc.ca
John A. Cairns, MD, Director
Fnded: 1950.

California

★ 27283 ★ Loma Linda University
School of Medicine
Loma Linda, CA 92350
Phone: (909)558-4462 **Fax:** (909)558-0292
Email: cbender@som.llu.edu
Website: http://www.llu.edu/llu/medicine/
Brian S. Bull, MD, Director
Fnded: 1961. **Frmly:** (1909) College of Medical Evangelists.

★ 27284 ★ Stanford University
School of Medicine
300 Pasteur Dr.
Stanford, CA 94305-5519
Phone: (650)725-3900 **Fax:** (650)725-7368
Website: http://www.med.stanford.edu
Philip A. Pizzo, MD, Director
Fnded: 1908.

★ 27285 ★ University of California, Davis
School of Medicine
Davis, CA 95616
Phone: (916)752-0331 **Fax:** (916)752-3512
Website: http://www.med.ucdavis.edu/
Dr. Joseph Silva, Jr., Director
Fnded: 1968.

★ 27286 ★ University of California, Irvine
College of Medicine
Irvine, CA 92697-3950
Phone: (949)824-6119 **Fax:** (949)824-2676
Website: http://www.ucihs.uci.edu
Thomas C. Cesario, MD, Director
Fnded: 1965. **Frmly:** (1898) California College of Medicine.

★ 27287 ★ University of California, Los Angeles
UCLA School of Medicine
10833 Le Conte Ave.
Los Angeles, CA 90024
Phone: (310)825-9111 **Fax:** (310)206-5046
Website: http://www.medsch.ucla.edu
Gerald S. Levey, MD, Director
Fnded: 1951.

★ 27288 ★ University of California, San Diego
School of Medicine
Office of Admissions, 0621
La Jolla, CA 92093
Phone: (858)534-3713 **Fax:** (858)534-6573
Website: http://medicine.ucsd.edu
Edward W. Holmes, MD, Director
Fnded: 1968.

★ 27289 ★ University of California, San Francisco
School of Medicine
513 Parnassus Ave., Rm. S-224
San Francisco, CA 94143-0410
Phone: (415)476-9000 **Fax:** (415)476-0689
Website: http://www.som.ucsf.edu
Haile T. Debas, MD, Director
Fnded: 1873. **Alt. Contact:** Admissions, c-200, Box 0408, San Francisco, CA 92350; (415)476-4044. **Frmly:** (1864) Toland Medical College.

★ 27290 ★ University of Southern California
Keck School of Medicine
1975 Zonal Ave.
Los Angeles, CA 90033
Phone: (323)442-1900 **Fax:** (323)442-2722
Website: http://www.usc.edu/schools/medicine
Stephen J. Ryan, MD, Director
Fnded: 1885.

Colorado

★ 27291 ★ University of Colorado, Denver
School of Medicine
4200 E 9th Ave.
Box C290
Denver, CO 80262
Phone: (303)372-0000 **Fax:** (303)315-8494

Email: som@uchsc.edu
Website: http://www.uchsc.edu/sm/sm
Richard D. Krugman, MD, Director
Fnded: 1883.

Connecticut

★ 27292 ★ University of Connecticut School of Medicine
263 Farmington Ave.
Farmington, CT 06030
Phone: (860)679-2000 **Fax:** (860)679-1371
Website: http://www.uchc.edu
Peter J. Deckers, MD, Director
Fnded: 1968.

★ 27293 ★ Yale University School of Medicine
PO Box 208055
333 Cedar St.
New Haven, CT 06520-8055
Phone: (203)785-4672 **Fax:** (203)785-7437
Website: http://info.med.yale.edu/
David A. Kessler, MD, Director
Fnded: 1813.

District of Columbia

★ 27294 ★ George Washington University School of Medicine and Health Sciences
2300 Eye St. NW
Washington, DC 20037
Phone: (202)994-1000 **Fax:** (202)994-0926
Website: http://www.gwu.edu/~gwumc
Dr. John F. Williams, Jr., Director
Fnded: 1974. **Frmly:** (1821) Medical Department of the Columbian College.

★ 27295 ★ Georgetown University School of Medicine
3900 Reservoir Rd. NW
Washington, DC 20007
Phone: (202)687-1612 **Fax:** (202)687-2792
Website: http://www.dml.georgetown.edu/schmed/
S. Ray Mitchell, MD, Director
Fnded: 1851.

★ 27296 ★ Howard University College of Medicine
520 W St. NW
Washington, DC 20059
Phone: (202)806-6270 **Fax:** (202)806-7934
Website: http://www.med.howard.edu
Floyd J. Malveaux, MD,PhD, Director
Fnded: 1867.

Florida

★ 27297 ★ University of Florida College of Medicine
Box 100014, JHMHC
Gainesville, FL 32610-0014
Phone: (352)392-2761 **Fax:** (352)392-9395
Website: http://www.med.ufl.edu
Kenneth I. Burns, MD,PhD, Director
Fnded: 1956.

★ 27298 ★ University of Miami School of Medicine
PO Box 016099 (R699)
1600 NW 10th Ave.
Miami, FL 33101
Phone: (305)243-6545 **Fax:** (305)243-4888
Email: jclarkson@miami.edu
Website: http://www.miami.edu
John G. Clarkson, MD, Director
Fnded: 1952.

★ 27299 ★ University of South Florida College of Medicine
12901 Bruce B. Downs Blvd., MDC 2
Tampa, FL 33612-4742
Phone: (813)974-2196 **Fax:** (813)974-3886
Website: http://www.med.usf.edu/med.html
Dr. Robert M. Daugherty, Jr., Director
Fnded: 1971.

Georgia

★ 27300 ★ Emory University School of Medicine
Woodruff Health Sciences Center Administration Bldg.
1440 Clifton Rd., NE
Atlanta, GA 30322-4510
Phone: (404)727-5640 **Fax:** (404)727-0473
Website: http://www.emory.edu/WHSC/MED/med.html
Thomas J. Lawley, MD, Director
Fnded: 1854.

★ 27301 ★ Medical College of Georgia School of Medicine
1120 15th St.
Augusta, GA 30912
Phone: (706)721-0211 **Fax:** (706)721-7035
Website: http://www.mcg.edu/SOM/index.html
Betty B. Ray, MD, Director
Fnded: 1833. **Frmly:** (1828) Medical Academy of Georgia.

★ 27302 ★ Mercer University School of Medicine
1550 College St.
Macon, GA 31207
Phone: (912)301-2600 **Fax:** (912)301-2547
Website: http://www.mercer.edu
Ann C. Jobe, MD, Director
Fnded: 1972.

★ 27303 ★ Morehouse School of Medicine
720 Westview Dr. SW
Atlanta, GA 30310
Phone: (404)752-1500 **Fax:** (404)752-1594
Website: http://www.msm.edu/
Louis W. Sullivan, MD, Director
Fnded: 1978.

Hawaii

★ 27304 ★ University of Hawaii, Manoa John A. Burns School of Medicine
1960 East-West Rd.
Honolulu, HI 96822
Phone: (808)956-8287 **Fax:** (808)956-5506
Website: http://www.hawaiimed.hawaii.edu
Edwin C. Cadman, MD, Director
Fnded: 1965.

Illinois

★ 27305 ★ Finch University of Health Sciences/Chicago Medical School
3333 Green Bay Rd.
North Chicago, IL 60064
Phone: (847)578-3301 **Fax:** (847)578-3343
Email: barsanoc@finchcms.edu
Website: http://www.finchcms.edu
Charles P. Barsano, MD,PhD, Director
Fnded: 1912.

★ 27306 ★ Loyola University, Chicago Stritch School of Medicine
2160 S First Ave.
Maywood, IL 60153
Phone: (708)216-9000 **Fax:** (708)216-4305
Website: http://www.meddean.luc.edu/
Stephen Slogoff, MD, Director
Fnded: 1915.

★ 27307 ★ Northwestern University Medical School
303 E Chicago Ave.
Chicago, IL 60611-3008
Phone: (312)503-8649 **Fax:** (312)503-7757
Website: http://www.nums.nwu.edu
Lewis Landsberg, MD, Director
Fnded: 1859.

★ 27308 ★ Rush University Rush Medical College
1653 W Congress Pkwy
Chicago, IL 60612
Phone: (312)942-6913 **Fax:** (312)942-2828
Email: medcol@rush.edu
Website: http://www.rush.edu
Larry J. Goodman, MD, Director
Fnded: 1837.

★ 27309 ★ Southern Illinois University School of Medicine
801 N Rutledge
PO Box 19230
Springfield, IL 62794-9230
Phone: (217)782-3318 **Fax:** (217)524-0786
Email: cgetto@siumed.edu
Website: http://www.siumed.edu
Carl J. Getto, MD, Director
Fnded: 1969.

★ 27310 ★ University of Chicago Division of the Biological Sciences Pritzker School of Medicine
5841 S Maryland Ave.
Chicago, IL 60637
Phone: (773)702-9000 **Fax:** (773)702-1897
Website: http://www.uchicago.edu
Bruce Weir, MD, Director
Fnded: 1968. **Frmly:** (1927) The School of Medicine of the University of Chicago.

★ 27311 ★ University of Illinois, Chicago College of Medicine
1853 W Polk St. (M/C 784)
Chicago, IL 60612
Phone: (312)996-3500 **Fax:** (312)996-9006
Website: http://www.uic.edu/depts/mcam/
Gerald S. Moss, MD, Director
Fnded: 1900. **Frmly:** (1881) College of Physicians and Surgeons of Chicago.

Indiana

★ 27312 ★ Indiana University School of Medicine
Indiana University Medical Center
1120 South Dr.
Indianapolis, IN 46202-5114
Phone: (317)274-8157 **Fax:** (317)274-8439
Website: http://www.medicine.iu.edu
D. Craig Brater, MD, Director
Fnded: 1903.

Iowa

★ 27313 ★ University of Iowa College of Medicine
200 Medicine Admin. Bldg.
100 Medicine Admin. Bldg.
Iowa City, IA 52242-1101
Phone: (319)335-8050 **Fax:** (319)335-8049
Website: http://www.medadmin.uiowa.edu
Robert P. Kelch, MD, Director
Fnded: 1850.

Kansas

★ 27314 ★ University of Kansas School of Medicine
3901 Rainbow Blvd.
Kansas City, KS 66160-7300
Phone: (913)588-5200 **Fax:** (913)588-5259
Website: http://www.kumc.edu/som
Deborah E. Powell, MD, Director
Fnded: 1906.

Kentucky

★ 27315 ★ University of Kentucky College of Medicine
A. B. Chandler Medical Center
800 Rose St. (MN-150)
Lexington, KY 40536-0298
Phone: (859)323-5000 **Fax:** (859)323-2039
Website: http://www.mc.uky.edu/medicine
Emery A. Wilson, MD, Director
Fnded: 1960.

★ 27316 ★ University of Louisville School of Medicine
Health Sciences Center
Abell Administration Center
323 E Chestnut St.
Louisville, KY 40202
Phone: (502)852-5184 **Fax:** (502)852-6849
Website: http://www.louisville.edu/medschool/
Joel A. Kaplan, MD, Director
Fnded: 1833.

Louisiana

★ 27317 ★ Louisiana State University School of Medicine in New Orleans
1542 Tulane Ave.
New Orleans, LA 70112-2822
Phone: (504)568-4007 **Fax:** (504)568-4008
Website: http://www.lsumc.edu
Robert L. Marier, MD, Director
Fnded: 1931.

★ 27318 ★ Louisiana State University School of Medicine in Shreveport
Office of Student Admissions
PO Box 33932
Shreveport, LA 71130-3932
Phone: (318)675-5000 **Fax:** (318)675-5244
Website: http://lib-sh.lsumc.edu
John C. McDonald, MD, Director
Fnded: 1965.

★ 27319 ★ Tulane University School of Medicine
1430 Tulane Ave.
New Orleans, LA 70112
Phone: (504)588-5462 **Fax:** (504)584-2945
Email: medsch@tmcpop.tmc.tulane.edu
Website: http://www.mcl.tulane.edu/tumc
Ian L. Taylor, MD, Director
Fnded: 1834.

Manitoba

★ 27320 ★ University of Manitoba Faculty of Medicine
753 McDermot Ave.
Winnipeg, MB, Canada R3E 0W3
Phone: (204)789-3557 **Fax:** (204)789-3928
B. K. Hennen, MD, Director
Fnded: 1883.

Maryland

★ 27321 ★ Johns Hopkins University School of Medicine
720 Rutland Ave.
Baltimore, MD 21205
Phone: (410)955-5000 **Fax:** (410)955-0889
Website: http://www.hopkins.med.jhu.edu
Dr. Edward D. Miller, Jr., Director
Fnded: 1893.

★ 27322 ★ Uniformed Services University of the Health Sciences F. Edward Hebert School of Medicine
4301 Jones Bridge Rd.
Bethesda, MD 20814-4799
Phone: (301)295-3016 **Fax:** (301)295-3542
Website: http://www.usuhs.mil
Val G. Hemming, MD, Director
Fnded: 1972.

★ 27323 ★ University of Maryland School of Medicine
655 W Baltimore St.
Baltimore, MD 21201
Phone: (410)706-3100 **Fax:** (410)706-0235
Email: deanmed@som.umaryland.edu
Website: http://medschool.umaryland.edu
Donald E. Wilson, MD, Director
Fnded: 1807.

Massachusetts

★ 27324 ★ Boston University School of Medicine
715 Albany St.
Boston, MA 02118
Phone: (617)638-8000 **Fax:** (617)638-5258
Website: http://www.bumc.bu.edu
Aram V. Chobanian, MD, Director
Fnded: 1873.

★ 27325 ★ Harvard Medical School
25 Shattuck St.
Boston, MA 02115
Phone: (617)432-1000 **Fax:** (617)432-3907
Website: http://www.med.harvard.edu
Joseph B. Martin, MD,PhD, Director
Fnded: 1782.

★ 27326 ★ Tufts University School of Medicine
136 Harrison Ave.
Boston, MA 02111
Phone: (617)636-7000 **Fax:** (617)636-0375
Email: jharrington@infonet.tufts.edu
Website: http://www.tufts.edu/med
John T. Harrington, MD, Director
Fnded: 1893.

★ 27327 ★ University of Massachusetts Medical School
55 Lake Ave. N
Worcester, MA 01655
Phone: (508)856-8100 **Fax:** (508)856-8181
Email: aaron.lazare@umassmed.edu
Website: http://www.umassmed.edu
Aaron Lazare, MD, Director
Fnded: 1962.

Michigan

★ 27328 ★ Michigan State University College of Human Medicine
A-110 East Fee Hall
East Lansing, MI 48824
Phone: (517)353-1730 **Fax:** (517)355-0342
Website: http://www.chm.msu.edu
Glenn C. Davis, MD, Director
Fnded: 1964.

★ 27329 ★ University of Michigan Medical School
1301 Catherine Rd.
Medical Science Bldg. I
Ann Arbor, MI 48109-0624
Phone: (734)763-9600 **Fax:** (734)763-4936
Website: http://www.med.umich.edu/medschool
Allen S. Lichter, MD, Director
Fnded: 1850.

★ 27330 ★ Wayne State University School of Medicine
540 E Canfield
Detroit, MI 48201
Phone: (313)577-1460 **Fax:** (313)577-8777
Website: http://www.med.wayne.edu
John D. Crissman, MD, Director
Fnded: 1956. **Frmly:** (1868) Detroit Medical College.

Minnesota

★ 27331 ★ Mayo Medical School
200 First St. SW
Rochester, MN 55905
Phone: (507)284-3671 **Fax:** (507)284-2634
Website: http://www.mayo.edu/mms
Anthony J. Windebank, MD, Director
Fnded: 1972.

★ 27332 ★ University of Minnesota, Duluth School of Medicine
10 University Dr.
Duluth, MN 55812
Phone: (218)726-7571 **Fax:** (218)726-7383
Email: med@d.umn.edu
Website: http://www.d.umn.edu/medweb/
Richard J. Ziegler, PhD, Director
Fnded: 1972.

★ 27333 ★ University of Minnesota, Minneapolis Medical School
Mayo Mail Code 293
420 Delaware St. SE
Minneapolis, MN 55455
Phone: (612)624-1188
Website: http://www.med.umn.edu
Alfred F. Michael, MD, Director
Fnded: 1888.

Mississippi

★ 27334 ★ University of Mississippi School of Medicine
2500 N State St.
Jackson, MS 39216-4505
Phone: (601)984-1000 **Fax:** (601)984-1011
Website: http://umc.edu
A. Wallace Conerly, MD, Director
Fnded: 1903.

Missouri

★ 27335 ★ Saint Louis University School of Medicine
1402 S Grand Blvd.
Saint Louis, MO 63104
Phone: (314)577-8000 **Fax:** (314)577-8645
Website: http://www.slu.edu/colleges/med/
Patricia L. Monteleone, MD, Director
Fnded: 1903. **Frmly:** Marion Sims-Beaumont College of Medicine.

★ 27336 ★ University of Missouri, Columbia School of Medicine
MA202 Medical Sciences Bldg.
1 Hospital Dr.
Columbia, MO 65212
Phone: (573)882-2923 **Fax:** (573)884-4808
Website: http://www.muhealth.org
Daniel H. Winship, MD, Director
Fnded: 1841.

★ 27337 ★ University of Missouri, Kansas City School of Medicine
2411 Holmes St.
Kansas City, MO 64108-2792
Phone: (816)235-1808 **Fax:** (816)235-5277
Website: http://www.med.umkc.edu
Betty M. Dress, MD, Director
Fnded: 1971.

★ 27338 ★ Washington University School of Medicine
660 S Euclid Ave., Box. 8106
Saint Louis, MO 63110
Phone: (314)362-5000 **Fax:** (314)367-6666
Website: http://medinfo.wustl.edu
William A. Peck, MD, Director
Fnded: 1891.

Nebraska

★ 27339 ★ Creighton University School of Medicine
2500 California Plaza
Omaha, NE 68178
Phone: (402)280-2900 **Fax:** (402)280-4027
Website: http://medicine.creighton.edu
M. Roy Wilson, MD, Director
Fnded: 1892.

★ 27340 ★ University of Nebraska College of Medicine
986545 Nebraska Medical Ctr
Omaha, NE 68198-6545
Phone: (402)559-4000 **Fax:** (402)559-4148
Website: http://www.unmc.edu
James O. Armitage, MD, Director
Fnded: 1902. **Frmly:** (1881) Omaha Medical College.

Nevada

★ 27341 ★ University of Nevada School of Medicine
2040 W Charleston Blvd.
Ste. 400
Reno, NV 89557-0046
Phone: (775)784-6001 **Fax:** (702)671-2277
Website: http://www.unr.edu/med/
Robert H. Miller, MD, Director
Fnded: 1969.

New Hampshire

★ 27342 ★ Dartmouth Medical School
7020 Remsen, Rm. 306
Hanover, NH 03755-3833
Phone: (603)650-1481 **Fax:** (603)650-1202
Website: http://www.dartmouth.edu/dms
John C. Baldwin, MD, Director
Fnded: 1797.

New Jersey

★ 27343 ★ University of Medicine and Dentistry of New Jersey New Jersey Medical School
185 S Orange Ave.
Newark, NJ 07103-2714
Phone: (973)972-4300 **Fax:** (973)972-7104
Website: http://njms.umdnj.edu/
Russell T. Joffe, MD, Director
Fnded: 1965. **Frmly:** (1954) Seton Hall College of Medicine and Dentistry.

★ 27344 ★ University of Medicine and Dentistry of New Jersey Robert Wood Johnson Medical School
125 Paterson St., Ste. 1400
New Brunswick, NJ 08901
Phone: (732)235-5600 **Fax:** (732)235-6315
Harold L. Paz, MD, Director
Fnded: 1970.

New Mexico

★ 27345 ★ University of New Mexico School of Medicine
Albuquerque, NM 87131
Phone: (505)272-2321 **Fax:** (505)272-6581
Website: http://medlab1.unm.edu
Paul B. Roth, MD, Director
Fnded: 1961.

New York

★ 27346 ★ Albany Medical College
47 New Scotland Ave.
Albany, NY 12208
Phone: (518)262-5582 **Fax:** (518)262-6515
Website: http://www.amc.edu
Vincent P. Verdile, MD, Director
Fnded: 1839.

★ 27347 ★ Columbia University College of Physicians and Surgeons
630 W 168th St.
New York, NY 10032
Phone: (212)305-3592 **Fax:** (212)305-3545
Website: http://www.columbia.edu
Gerald D. Fischbach, MD, Director
Fnded: 1814.

★ 27348 ★ Cornell University Joan and Sanford I. Weill Medical College Graduate School of Medical Sciences
New York, NY 10021
Phone: (212)746-5454 **Fax:** (212)746-8424
Email: dean@mail.med.cornell.edu
Website: http://www.med.cornell.edu
Dr. Antonio M. Gotto, Jr., Director
Fnded: 1898.

★ 27349 ★ New York Medical College
Administration Bldg.
Valhalla, NY 10595
Phone: (914)594-4000 **Fax:** (914)594-4145
Website: http://www.nymc.edu
Francis L. Belloni, PhD, Director
Fnded: 1860.

★ 27350 ★ New York University Mount Sinai School of Medicine
1 Gustave L. Levy Pl.
New York, NY 10029-6574
Phone: (212)241-6500 **Fax:** (212)410-6111
Website: http://www.mssm.edu
Nathan Kase, MD, Director
Fnded: 1963.

★ 27351 ★ New York University School of Medicine
550 1st Ave.
New York, NY 10016
Phone: (212)263-7300 **Fax:** (212)545-8846
Website: http://www.med.nyu.edu
Robert M. Glickman, MD, Director
Fnded: 1841.

★ 27352 ★ State University of New York Downstate Medical Center College of Medicine
450 Clarkson Ave., Box 97
Brooklyn, NY 11203-2098
Phone: (718)270-1000 **Fax:** (718)270-4074
Email: efeigelson@netmail.hscbklyn.edu
Website: http://www.downstate.edu
Eugene B. Feigelson, MD, Director
Fnded: 1860.

★ 27353 ★ State University of New York Upstate Medical Center College of Medicine
750 E Adams St.
Syracuse, NY 13210-2399
Phone: (315)464-9720 **Fax:** (315)464-9721
Website: http://www.upstate.edu
Michael F. Roizen, MD, Director
Fnded: 1834.

★ 27354 ★ State University of New York, Buffalo School of Medicine and Biomedical Sciences
3435 Main St.
Buffalo, NY 14214
Phone: (716)829-2771 **Fax:** (716)829-3395
Website: http://www.smbs.buffalo.edu
John R. Wright, MD, Director
Fnded: 1846.

★ 27355 ★ State University of New York, Stony Brook Health Sciences Center School of Medicine
HSC Level 4-170
Level 4, Rm. 170
Stony Brook, NY 11794-8430
Phone: (631)444-2080 **Fax:** (631)444-6266
Website: http://www.uhmc.sunysb.edu/hsc/
Norman H. Edelman, MD, Director
Fnded: 1971.

★ 27356 ★ University of Rochester School of Medicine and Dentistry
601 Elmwood Ave.
Rochester, NY 14642
Phone: (716)275-7181 **Fax:** (716)256-1131
Website: http://www.rochester.edu
Edward M. Hundert, MD, Director
Fnded: 1920.

★ 27357 ★ Yeshiva University
Albert Einstein College of Medicine
1300 Morris Park Ave.
Bronx, NY 10461
Phone: (718)430-2000 **Fax:** (718)430-8822
Website: http://www.aecom.yu.edu
Dominick P. Purpura, MD, Director
Fnded: 1955.

Newfoundland and Labrador

★ 27358 ★ Memorial University of Newfoundland
Faculty of Medicine
Health Sciences Centre
Prince Philip Dr.
Saint John's, NL, Canada A1B 3V6
Phone: (709)777-6602 **Fax:** (709)777-6746
Website: http://www.med.mun.ca/med
M. I. Bowmer, MD, Director
Fnded: 1967.

North Carolina

★ 27359 ★ Duke University
School of Medicine
PO Box 2927
Durham, NC 27710
Phone: (919)684-2455 **Fax:** (919)684-0208
Website: http://www.mc.duke.edu/depts/som
R. Sanders Williams, MD, Director
Fnded: 1390.

★ 27360 ★ East Carolina University
Brody School of Medicine
Greenville, NC 27858-4354
Phone: (252)816-2201 **Fax:** (252)816-3192
Website: http://www.med.ecu.edu
Peter J. Kragel, MD, Director
Fnded: 1972.

★ 27361 ★ University of North Carolina, Chapel Hill
School of Medicine
Chapel Hill, NC 27599
Phone: (919)966-4161 **Fax:** (919)966-8623
Website: http://www.med.unc.edu
Jeffrey L. Houpt, MD, Director
Fnded: 1879.

★ 27362 ★ Wake Forest University
School of Medicine
Medical Center Blvd.
Winston-Salem, NC 27157
Phone: (336)716-2011 **Fax:** (336)716-5139
Website: http://isnet.is.wfu.edu
James N. Thompson, MD, Director
Fnded: 1902.

North Dakota

★ 27363 ★ University of North Dakota
School of Medicine and Health Sciences
501 N Columbia Rd.
Box 9037
Grand Forks, ND 58202-9037
Phone: (701)777-2514 **Fax:** (701)777-3527
Website: http://www.med.und.nodak.edu
H. David Wilson, MD, Director
Fnded: 1905.

Nova Scotia

★ 27364 ★ Dalhousie University
Faculty of Medicine
Clinical Research Ctr
5849 University Ave
Halifax, NS, Canada B3H 4H7
Phone: (902)494-6592 **Fax:** (902)494-7119
Website: http://www.medicine.dal.ca
N. MacDonald, MD, Director
Fnded: 1868.

Ohio

★ 27365 ★ Case Western Reserve University
School of Medicine
10900 Euclid Ave.
Cleveland, OH 44106-4915
Phone: (216)368-2000 **Fax:** (216)368-3013
Website: http://mediswww.cwru.edu
Nathan A. Berger, MD, Director
Fnded: 1843. **Frmly:** Cleveland Medical College.

★ 27366 ★ Medical College of Ohio
PO Box 10008
Toledo, OH 43699-0008
Phone: (419)383-4172 **Fax:** (419)383-6100
Website: http://www.mco.edu/smed
Amira F. Gohara, MD, Director
Fnded: 1967. **Frmly:** (1964) Toledo State College of Medicine.

★ 27367 ★ Northeastern Ohio Universities
College of Medicine
4209 State Rte. 44
PO Box 95
Rootstown, OH 44272-0095
Phone: (330)325-2511 **Fax:** (330)325-5919
Website: http://www.neoucom.edu
Robert S. Blacklow, MD, Director
Fnded: 1973.

★ 27368 ★ Ohio State University
College of Medicine and Public Health
200A Meiling Hall
370 W 9th Ave.
Columbus, OH 43210
Phone: (614)292-2220 **Fax:** (614)292-1301
Website: http://www.med.ohio-state.edu
Fred Sanfilippo, MD, Director
Fnded: 1914.

★ 27369 ★ University of Cincinnati
College of Medicine
PO Box 670555
Cincinnati, OH 45267-0555
Phone: (513)558-7391 **Fax:** (513)558-1165
Website: http://www.med.uc.edu
John J. Hutton, MD, Director
Fnded: 1819.

★ 27370 ★ Wright State University
School of Medicine
PO Box 927
Dayton, OH 45401-0927
Phone: (937)775-3010 **Fax:** (937)775-2211
Email: howard.part@wright.edu
Website: http://www.med.wright.edu
Howard M. Part, MD, Director
Fnded: 1973.

Oklahoma

★ 27371 ★ University of Oklahoma
College of Medicine
PO Box 26901
Oklahoma City, OK 73190
Phone: (405)271-2265 **Fax:** (405)271-3032
Website: http://medicine.ouhsc.edu
Jerry B. Vannatta, MD, Director
Fnded: 1900.

Ontario

★ 27372 ★ McMaster University
Faculty of Health Sciences
1200 Main St. W
Hamilton, ON, Canada L8S 4J9
Phone: (905)525-9140 **Fax:** (905)546-0800
J. G. Kelton, MD, Director
Fnded: 1967.

★ 27373 ★ Queen's University
Faculty of Health Sciences
Kingston, ON, Canada K7L 3N6
Phone: (613)533-2542 **Fax:** (613)553-6884
Website: http://meds.queensu.ca
David M. C. Walker, MD, Director
Fnded: 1854.

★ 27374 ★ University of Ottawa
Faculty of Medicine
451 Smyth Rd.
Ottawa, ON, Canada K1H 8M5
Phone: (613)562-5400 **Fax:** (613)562-5457
Peter Walker, MD, Director
Fnded: 1945.

★ 27375 ★ University of Toronto
Faculty of Medicine
1 King's College Cr.
Toronto, ON, Canada M5S 1A8
Phone: (416)978-6585 **Fax:** (416)978-1774
Email: medicine.web@utoronto.ca
Website: http://utl2.library.utoronto.ca/www/medicine
C. D. Naylor, MD, Contact
Fnded: 1843.

★ 27376 ★ University of Western Ontario
Faculty of Medicine and Dentistry
Richmond St., N
London, ON, Canada N6A 5C1
Phone: (519)661-3744 **Fax:** (519)661-3797
C. P. Herbert, MD, Director
Fnded: 1882.

Oregon

★ 27377 ★ Oregon Health Sciences University
School of Medicine
3181 SW Sam Jackson Park Rd.
Portland, OR 97201-3098
Phone: (503)494-8311 **Fax:** (503)494-3400
Website: http://www.ohsu.edu/som
Dr. Joseph E. Robertson, Jr., Director
Fnded: 1887.

Pennsylvania

★ 27378 ★ MCP Hahnemann School of Medicine
Medical Program
2900 Queen Lane
Philadelphia, PA 19129
Phone: (215)991-8560 **Fax:** (215)843-0214
Website: http://www.mcphu.edu
Warren E. Ross, MD, Director

Fnded: 1998.

★ 27379 ★ Pennsylvania State University College of Medicine
500 University Dr.
PO Box 850
Hershey, PA 17033
Phone: (717)531-8521 **Fax:** (717)531-5351
Email: dkirch@psu.edu
Website: http://www.hmc.psu.edu
Darrell G. Kirch, MD, Director
Fnded: 1963.

★ 27380 ★ Temple University School of Medicine
3420 N Broad St.
Philadelphia, PA 19140
Phone: (215)707-7000 **Fax:** (215)707-8431
Email: tusmdean@vm.temple.edu
Website: http://www.temple.edu/medschool/
Leon S. Malmud, MD, Director
Fnded: 1901.

★ 27381 ★ Thomas Jefferson University Jefferson Medical College
1025 Walnut St.
Philadelphia, PA 19107-5083
Phone: (215)955-6000 **Fax:** (215)503-2654
Email: dean.jmc@mail.tju.edu
Website: http://www.tju.edu
Thomas J. Nasca, MD, Director
Fnded: 1824.

★ 27382 ★ University of Pennsylvania School of Medicine
36th and Hamilton Walk
Philadelphia, PA 19104-6055
Phone: (215)898-8034 **Fax:** (215)573-2030
Website: http://www.med.upenn.edu
Arthur H. Rubenstein, MBBCh, Director
Fnded: 1765.

★ 27383 ★ University of Pittsburgh School of Medicine
Alan Magee Scaife Hall of the Health Professions
Pittsburgh, PA 15261
Phone: (412)648-9891 **Fax:** (412)648-1236
Website: http://www.omed.pitt.edu
Arthur S. Levine, MD, Director
Fnded: 1908. **Frmly:** (1886) Western Pennsylvania Medical College.

Puerto Rico

★ 27384 ★ Ponce School of Medicine
PO Box 7004
Ponce, PR 00732
Phone: (787)840-2575 **Fax:** (787)840-9756
Email: psm004@caribe.net
Website: http://www.psm.edu
Manuel Martinez-Maldonado, MD, Director
Fnded: 1977. **Alt. Contact:** Fax: (787)841-1040.

★ 27385 ★ Universidad Central del Caribe School of Medicine
PO Box 60-327
Bayamon, PR 00960-6032
Phone: (787)798-3001 **Fax:** (787)798-4990
Website: http://www.ucaribe.edu
Helen Rosa, MD, Director
Fnded: 1976.

★ 27386 ★ University of Puerto Rico School of Medicine
Medical Sciences Campus
PO Box 365067
San Juan, PR 00936-5067
Phone: (787)758-2525 **Fax:** (787)756-8475
Email: fjoglar@rcm.upr.edu
Website: http://www.rcm.upr.edu
Francisco M. Joglar, MD, Director
Fnded: 1950.

Quebec

★ 27387 ★ Laval University Faculty of Medicine
Quebec City, QC, Canada G1K 7P4
Phone: (418)656-2331 **Fax:** (418)656-5062
Marc Desmeules, MD, Director
Fnded: 1852.

★ 27388 ★ McGill University Faculty of Medicine
3655 Promenade Sir-William-Osler
Montreal, QC, Canada H3G 1Y6
Phone: (514)398-3515 **Fax:** (514)398-3595
Email: recepmed@med.mcgill.ca
Website: http://www.med.mcgill.ca
Abraham Fuks, MD, Director
Fnded: 1829.

★ 27389 ★ University of Montreal Faculty of Medicine
2900 Blvd. Edouard-Montpetit
PO Box 6128, Succ. Centre-ville
Montreal, QC, Canada H3C 3J7
Phone: (514)343-6267 **Fax:** (514)343-2068
Email: vinaypa@alize.ere.umontreal.ca
Patrick Vinay, MD,PhD, Director
Fnded: 1843.

★ 27390 ★ University of Sherbrooke Faculty of Medicine
3001 12th Ave. N
Sherbrooke, QC, Canada J1H 5N4
Phone: (819)564-5200 **Fax:** (819)564-5420
Website: http://www.crc.cuse.usherb.ca/facmed
Michel Baron, MD, Director
Fnded: 1961.

Rhode Island

★ 27391 ★ Brown University School of Medicine
97 Waterman St.
Providence, RI 02912
Phone: (401)863-3971 **Fax:** (401)863-3431
Website: http://biomedics.biomed.brown.edu
Donald J. Marsh, MD, Director
Fnded: 1973.

South Carolina

★ 27392 ★ Medical University of South Carolina College of Medicine
171 Ashley Ave.
Charleston, SC 29425
Phone: (843)792-2300 **Fax:** (843)792-2967
Website: http://www2.musc.edu
J. G. Reves, MD, Director
Fnded: 1824.

★ 27393 ★ University of South Carolina School of Medicine
Columbia, SC 29208
Phone: (803)733-3200 **Fax:** (803)733-3335
Email: faulkner@med.sc.edu
Website: http://www.med.sc.edu
Larry R. Faulkner, MD, Director
Fnded: 1973.

South Dakota

★ 27394 ★ University of South Dakota School of Medicine
1400 W 22nd
Sioux Falls, SD 57105-1570
Phone: (605)357-1300 **Fax:** (605)357-1311
Website: http://www.usd.edu/med/som
Robert C. Talley, MD, Director
Fnded: 1907.

Tennessee

★ 27395 ★ East Tennessee State University James H. Quillen College of Medicine
PO Box 70694
Johnson City, TN 37614
Phone: (423)439-1000 **Fax:** (423)439-8090
Email: medcom@etsu.edu
Website: http://www.qcom.etsu.edu
Ronald D. Franks, MD, Director
Fnded: 1974.

★ 27396 ★ Meharry Medical College School of Medicine
1005 Dr. D.B. Todd Jr. Blvd.
Nashville, TN 37208
Phone: (615)327-6204 **Fax:** (615)327-6568
Email: meharrysom@ccvax.mmc.edu
Website: http://www.mmc.edu
A. Cherrie Epps, PhD, Director
Fnded: 1876.

★ 27397 ★ University of Tennessee Health Science Center College of Medicine
62 S Dunlap, Rm. 420
Memphis, TN 38163
Phone: (901)448-5529 **Fax:** (901)448-7683
Website: http://www.utmem.edu
Henry G. Herrod, MD, Director
Fnded: 1851.

★ 27398 ★ Vanderbilt University School of Medicine
21st Ave. S at Garland Ave.
Nashville, TN 37232
Phone: (615)322-5000 **Fax:** (615)343-7286
Email: steven.gabbe@mcmail.vanderbilt.edu
Website: http://www.mc.vanderbilt.edu/medschool/
Steven G. Gabbe, MD, Director
Fnded: 1875.

Texas

★ 27399 ★ Baylor College of Medicine
1 Baylor Plaza
Houston, TX 77030
Phone: (713)798-4951 **Fax:** (713)798-8811
Website: http://www.bcm.tmc.edu
Bobby R. Alford, MD, Director
Fnded: 1969.

★ 27400 ★ Texas A&M University Health Science Center College of Medicine
147 Joe H. Reynolds Medical Bldg.
College Station, TX 77843-1114
Phone: (979)845-7743 **Fax:** (979)847-8663
Website: http://tamushsc.tamu.edu
Nancy W. Dickey, MD, Director
Fnded: 1971.

★ 27401 ★ Texas Tech University Health Sciences Center
School of Medicine
3601 4th St.
Lubbock, TX 79430
Phone: (806)743-1000 **Fax:** (806)743-3021
Website: http://www.ttuhsc.edu
Joel Kupersmith, MD, Director
Fnded: 1969.

★ 27402 ★ University of Texas
Houston Medical School
6431 Fannin
Houston, TX 77030
Phone: (713)500-5160 **Fax:** (713)500-0602
Website: http://www.med.uth.tmc.edu/
L. Maximilian Buja, MD, Director
Fnded: 1969.

★ 27403 ★ University of Texas
University of Texas Medical School, Galveston
301 University Blvd.
Galveston, TX 77555-0133
Phone: (409)772-1011 **Fax:** (409)772-9598
Email: smlemon@utmb.edu
Website: http://www.utmb.edu
Stanley M. Lemon, MD, Director
Fnded: 1881.

★ 27404 ★ University of Texas, San Antonio
Medical School
7703 Floyd Curl Dr.
San Antonio, TX 78284-7790
Phone: (210)567-4420 **Fax:** (210)567-6962
Website: http://www.uthscsa.edu/som/som_main.htm
Steven A. Wartman, MD, Director
Fnded: 1959.

★ 27405 ★ University of Texas Southwestern Medical Center, Dallas
5323 Harry Hines Blvd.
Dallas, TX 75390
Phone: (214)648-3111 **Fax:** (214)648-8955
Website: http://www.swmed.edu
Robert J. Alpern, MD, Director
Fnded: 1972. **Frmly:** (1943) Southwestern Medical College.

Utah

★ 27406 ★ University of Utah
School of Medicine
50 N Medical Dr.
Salt Lake City, UT 84132
Phone: (801)581-7201 **Fax:** (801)585-3300
Website: http://www.med.utah.edu/som
A. Lorris Betz, MD,PhD, Director
Fnded: 1905.

Vermont

★ 27407 ★ University of Vermont
College of Medicine
Burlington, VT 05405
Phone: (802)656-2150 **Fax:** (802)656-8577
Website: http://salus.uvm.edu
Joseph B. Warshaw, MD, Director
Fnded: 1803.

Virginia

★ 27408 ★ Medical College of Hampton Roads
Eastern Virginia Medical School
PO Box 1980
Norfolk, VA 23501
Phone: (757)446-5600 **Fax:** (757)446-8444
Website: http://www.evms.edu
Evan R. Farmer, MD, Director
Fnded: 1964.

★ 27409 ★ University of Virginia
School of Medicine
Health System
PO Box 800793, McKim Hall
Charlottesville, VA 22908-0793
Phone: (804)924-0211 **Fax:** (804)982-0874
Website: http://www.med.virginia.edu
Robert M. Carey, MD, Director
Fnded: 1825.

★ 27410 ★ Virginia Commonwealth University
School of Medicine
PO Box 980565
Richmond, VA 23298
Phone: (804)828-9000 **Fax:** (804)371-7628
Website: http://www.medschool.vcu.edu
Dr. Heber H. Newsome, Jr., Director
Fnded: 1838.

Washington

★ 27411 ★ University of Washington
School of Medicine
Box 356340
Seattle, WA 98195
Phone: (206)543-1515 **Fax:** (206)543-3639
Website: http://www.washington.edu/medical.som
Paul G. Ramsey, MD, Director
Fnded: 1945.

West Virginia

★ 27412 ★ Marshall University
Joan C. Edwards School of Medicine
1600 Medical Center Dr., Ste. 3400
Huntington, WV 25701-3655
Phone: (304)691-1700 **Fax:** (304)691-1726
Website: http://musom.marshall.edu/
Dr. Charles H. McKown, Jr., Director
Fnded: 1972.

★ 27413 ★ West Virginia University
School of Medicine
Robert C. Byrd Health Sciences Center
Box 9000
Morgantown, WV 26506-9000
Phone: (304)293-0111 **Fax:** (304)293-4973
Email: cwhyte@hsc.wvu.edu
Website: http://www.hsc.wvu.edu
Robert M. D'Alessandri, MD, Director
Fnded: 1902.

Wisconsin

★ 27414 ★ Medical College of Wisconsin
8701 Watertown Plank Rd.
Milwaukee, WI 53226
Phone: (414)456-8296 **Fax:** (414)456-6560
Website: http://www.mcw.edu
Michael J. Dunn, MD, Director
Fnded: 1913.

★ 27415 ★ University of Wisconsin
Medical School
1300 University Ave.
Madison, WI 53706
Phone: (608)263-4900 **Fax:** (608)262-2327
Website: http://www.biostat.wisc.edu
Philip M. Farrell, MD,PhD, Director
Fnded: 1979.

Mortuary Science

The following colleges and programs in funeral service education and mortuary science are accredited by the American Board of Funeral Service Education, 38 Florida Ave., Portland, ME 04103, (207) 878-6530, http://www.abfse.org/.

Alabama

★ 27416 ★ Bishop State Community College
Funeral Service Education Program
1365 Dr. Martin Luther King Jr. Ave.
Mobile, AL 36603-5362
Phone: (251)405-4400 **Fax:** (251)405-4427
Email: wthompson@bscc.cc.al.us
Website: http://www.bscc.cc.al.us/
William Thompson, Director

★ 27417 ★ Jefferson State Community College
Funeral Service Education Program
2601 Carson Rd.
Birmingham, AL 35215
Phone: (205)856-7844 **Fax:** (205)856-7803
Email: wcounce@jeffstateonline.com
Website: http://www.jeffstateonline.com
Dr. William Counce, Director

Arizona

★ 27418 ★ Mesa Community College
Mortuary Science Program
Williams Education Ctr.
7440 E Tahoe Ave.
Mesa, AZ 85212-0908
Phone: (480)988-8501 **Fax:** (480)988-8520
Email: tom.taggart@mcmail.maricopa.edu
Website: http://www.mc.maricopa.edu/academic/mort_sci
Dr. Thomas R. Taggart, Director

Arkansas

★ 27419 ★ Arkansas State University Mountain Home
Funeral Service Program
1600 S College St.
Mountain Home, AR 72653
Phone: (870)508-6100 **Fax:** (870)508-6283
Email: rschofield@brook.asumh.edu
Website: http://www.asumh.edu/funeral.htm
Ron Schofield, Director

★ 27420 ★ University of Arkansas Community College at Hope
Funeral Service Program
PO Box 140
Hope, AR 71802-0140
Phone: (870)722-8206 **Fax:** (870)777-5957
Email: kdavis@mail.uacch.cc.ar.us
Website: http://uacch.cc.ar.us
Karen Davis, Director

California

★ 27421 ★ American River College
Funeral Service Education
4700 College Oak Dr.
Sacramento, CA 95841
Phone: (916)484-8902 **Fax:** (916)484-8817
Website: http://www.arc.losrios.edu

★ 27422 ★ Cypress College
Mortuary Science Department
9200 Valley View St.
Cypress, CA 90630
Phone: (714)484-7278 **Fax:** (714)484-7417
Email: mortsci@express.cc.ca.us
Website: http://www.cypress.college.org
Douglas Metz, Director

Colorado

★ 27423 ★ Arapahoe Community College
Mortuary Science Program
PO Box 9002
Littleton, CO 80160-9002
Phone: (303)797-5954
Email: martha.gaidies@arapahoe.edu
Website: http://www.arapahoe.edu/Programs/Mortuary/
Martha L. Gaidies, Chairman of the Board

Connecticut

★ 27424 ★ Briarwood College
Mortuary Science Program
2279 Mt. Vernon Rd.
Southington, CT 06489
Phone: (860)628-4751 **Free:** 800-952-2444
Fax: (860)628-6444
Email: laskowskib@briarwood.edu
Website: http://www.briarwood.edu
Bernard Laskowski, Director

District of Columbia

★ 27425 ★ University of the District of Columbia
Van Ness Campus
Mortuary Science Department
4200 Connecticut Ave. NW
MB4407
Washington, DC 20008
Phone: (202)274-5858
Courtney Terry, Director

Florida

★ 27426 ★ Miami-Dade Community College
W.L. Philbrick School of Funeral Sciences
11380 NW 27th Ave.
Miami, FL 33167
Phone: (305)237-1245 **Fax:** (305)237-8195
Email: rcovert@mdcc.edu
Website: http://www.mdcc.edu
Ralph Covert, Director

★ 27427 ★ Saint Petersburg College
Funeral Services Program
PO Box 13489
Saint Petersburg, FL 33733-3489
Phone: (727)341-3781 **Fax:** (727)341-3770
Email: davisk@spcollege.edu
Website: http://www.spcollege.edu
Kevin Davis, Director

Georgia

★ 27428 ★ Gupton-Jones College of Funeral Service
5141 Snapfinger Woods Dr.
Decatur, GA 30035-4022
Phone: (770)593-2257 **Free:** 800-848-5352
Fax: (770)593-1891
Email: gjcfs@mindspring.com
Website: http://www.gupton-jones.edu/
Patty S. Hutcheson, President

★ 27429 ★ Ogeechee Technical College
Department of Funeral Service Education
1 Joe Kennedy Blvd.
Statesboro, GA 30458
Phone: (912)681-5500 **Free:** 800-646-1316
Fax: (912)486-7604
Email: jbarnes@ogeechee.org
Website: http://www.ogeechee.org
Jarvis Barnes, Director

Illinois

★ 27430 ★ Carl Sandburg College
Mortuary Science Program
2400 Tom L. Wilson Blvd.
PO Box 1407
Galesburg, IL 61401-9576
Phone: (309)341-0831 **Fax:** (309)341-1040
Email: tkrause@csc.cc.il.us
Website: http://www.csc.cc.il.us
Tim Krause, Contact

★ 27431 ★ Malcolm X College
Department of Mortuary Science
1900 W Van Buren St.
Chicago, IL 60612
Fax: (312)850-7453
Email: alwilliams@ccc.edu
Website: http://www.ccc.edu/malcolmx
Alta L. Williams, Director

★ 27432 ★ Southern Illinois University
Mortuary Science and Funeral Service
ASA-MC6615
Carbondale, IL 62901-6615
Phone: (618)453-7214 **Fax:** (618)453-7020
Email: cgriffit@siu.edu
Website: http://www.siu.edu/~hcp/msfs/mshome.html
Cydney Griffith, Director

★ 27433 ★ Worsham College of Mortuary Science
495 Northgate Pkwy.
Wheeling, IL 60090-2646
Phone: (847)808-8444 **Fax:** (847)808-8493
Email: soulfillet@aol.com
Website: http://www.worshamcollege.com
Stephanie J. Kann, Director

Indiana

★ 27434 ★ Mid-America College of Funeral Service
3111 Hamburg Pike
Jeffersonville, IN 47130
Phone: (812)288-8878 **Free:** 800-221-6158
Fax: (812)288-5942
Email: macfs@mindspring.com
Website: http://www.mid-america.edu
John R. Braboy, President

★ 27435 ★ Vincennes University
Funeral Service Education Program
1002 N 1st St.
Vincennes, IN 47591
Phone: (812)888-5469 **Fax:** (812)888-4550
Email: jalsobro@indian.vinu.edu
Website: http://www.vinu.edu
John Alsobrooks, Chairman of the Board

Kansas

★ 27436 ★ Kansas City Kansas Community College
Mortuary Science Department
7250 State Ave.
Kansas City, KS 66112
Phone: (913)288-7607 **Fax:** (913)288-7677
Email: wwright@toto.net
Website: http://www.kckcc.edu
Wiley Wright, Contact

Louisiana

★ 27437 ★ Delgado Community College
City Park Campus
Department of Funeral Service Education
615 City Park Ave.
New Orleans, LA 70119-4399
Phone: (504)483-4014 **Fax:** (504)483-4609
Email: mgibson@dcc.edu
Website: http://www.dcc.edu
Malcolm L. Gibson, Contact

Maryland

★ 27438 ★ Community College of Baltimore County
Catonsville Campus
Mortuary Science Program
800 S Rolling Rd.
Baltimore, MD 21228
Phone: (410)455-4162 **Fax:** (410)719-6547
Email: jdoe151@aol.com
Website: http://www.ccbc.cc.md.us
William C. Gonce, Chairman of the Board

Massachusetts

★ 27439 ★ Funeral Institute of the North East
Mortuary College
77 University Ave.
Westwood, MA 02090
Phone: (781)461-9080 **Fax:** (781)461-8787
Email: lynlou@tiac.net
Website: http://www.fine-ne.com
Louis Misantone, President

★ 27440 ★ Mount Ida College
New England Institute of Funeral Service Education
777 Dedham St.
Newton Centre, MA 02459
Phone: (617)928-4714 **Fax:** (617)928-4713
Email: jstaylor@mountida.edu
Website: http://www.mountida.edu
Jacquelyn Taylor, Director

Michigan

★ 27441 ★ Wayne State University
Department of Mortuary Science
5439 Woodward Ave.
Detroit, MI 48202
Phone: (313)577-2050 **Fax:** (313)577-4456
Email: ab8123@wayne.edu
Website: http://mortuarysciencewayne.org
Michael Wilk, Director

Minnesota

★ 27442 ★ University of Minnesota Program of Mortuary Science
MMC 740
420 Delaware St. SE
Minneapolis, MN 55455
Phone: (612)624-6464 **Fax:** (612)626-4163
Email: mortsci@umn.edu
Website: http://www.med.umn.edu/mortsci
Michael LuBrant, Director

Mississippi

★ 27443 ★ East Mississippi Community College
Funeral Service Technology
PO Box 158
Scooba, MS 39358
Phone: (662)476-5100 **Fax:** (662)476-5086
Email: odickerson@emcc.cc.ms.us
Website: http://www.emcc.cc.ms.us
Don Webb, Director

★ 27444 ★ Holmes Community College
Funeral Services Technology
412 W Ridgeland Ave.
Ridgeland, MS 39157
Phone: (601)605-3323 **Fax:** (601)605-3410
Email: bdepriest@holmes.cc.ms.us
Website: http://www.holmes.cc.ms.us/fst/index.html
Bill W. DePriest, Director

★ 27445 ★ Mississippi Gulf Coast Community College
Funeral Service Technology
PO Box 548
Perkinston, MS 39573
Phone: (601)528-8909 **Fax:** (601)528-8422
Email: michael.normansr@mgccc.cc.ms.us
Website: http://www.mgccc.cc.ms.us
Michael Norman, Contact

★ 27446 ★ Northwest Mississippi Community College
Funeral Service Technology Program
Desoto Center
5197 WE Ross Pkwy.
Southaven, MS 38671
Phone: (662)280-6137 **Fax:** (662)280-6161
Email: landerson@northwest.ms.edu
Website: http://www.northwest.ms.edu
Larry Anderson, Director

Missouri

★ 27447 ★ Saint Louis Community College at Forest Park
Department of Funeral Service Education
5600 Oakland Ave.
Saint Louis, MO 63110
Phone: (314)644-9327 **Fax:** (314)644-9752
Email: skoosmann@stlcc.edu
Website: http://www.stlcc.edu
Steven B. Koosmann, Director

New Jersey

★ 27448 ★ Mercer County Community College
Funeral Service Curriculum
1200 Old Trenton Rd.
PO Box B
Trenton, NJ 08690
Phone: (609)586-4800 **Fax:** (609)586-5602
Email: smithr@mccc.edu
Website: http://www.mccc.edu
Robert C. Smith III, Director

New York

★ 27449 ★ American Academy McAllister Institute of Funeral Service, Inc.
450 W 56th St.
New York, NY 10019
Phone: (212)757-1190 **Fax:** (212)765-5923
Email: info@a-a-m-i.org
Website: http://www.a-a-m-i.org
Meg Dunn, President

★ 27450 ★ Hudson Valley Community College
Mortuary Science Department
80 Vandenburgh Ave.
Troy, NY 12180
Phone: (518)629-7113 **Fax:** (518)629-8025
Email: reinhela@hvcc.edu
Website: http://www.hvcc.edu
D. Elaine Reinhard, Chairman of the Board

★ 27451 ★ Nassau Community College
Mortuary Science Department
357 East Rd.
Garden City, NY 11530-6793
Phone: (516)572-7277 **Fax:** (516)572-0626
Email: lieblaj@sunynassau.edu
Website: http://www.sunynassau.edu
John M. Lieblang, Chairman of the Board

★ 27452 ★ Simmons Institute of Funeral Service
1828 South Ave.
Syracuse, NY 13207
Phone: (315)475-5142 **Fax:** (315)475-3817
Email: mcwightman20@aol.com
Website: http://www.simmonsinstitute.com
Maurice C. Wightman, President

★ 27453 ★ State University of New York College of Technology at Canton
Mortuary Science Program
Canton, NY 13617
Phone: (315)386-7110 **Fax:** (315)386-7959
Email: walch@canton.edu
Website: http://www.canton.edu
Barry Walch, Contact

North Carolina

★ 27454 ★ Fayetteville Technical Community College
Funeral Service Education Department
PO Box 35236
Fayetteville, NC 28303
Phone: (910)678-8301 **Fax:** (910)484-6600
Email: landonm@faytechcc.edu
Website: http://www.faytechcc.edu
Michael Landon, Chairman of the Board

Ohio

★ 27455 ★ Cincinnati College of Mortuary Science
645 W North Bend Rd.
Cincinnati, OH 45224-1462
Phone: (513)761-2020 **Free:** 888-377-8433
Fax: (513)761-3333
Email: generalinfo@ccms.edu
Website: http://www.ccms.edu
Dan Flory, President

Oklahoma

★ 27456 ★ University of Central Oklahoma
Department of Funeral Service Education
Edmond, OK 73034-5209
Phone: (405)974-5192 **Fax:** (405)974-3848
Email: cburkey@ucok.edu
Website: http://www.ucok.edu/funeral
Chris Burkey, Chairman of the Board

Oregon

★ 27457 ★ Mount Hood Community College
Department of Funeral Service Education
26000 SE Stark St.
Gresham, OR 97030
Phone: (503)491-6941 **Fax:** (503)491-6050
Email: malcomw@mhcc.edu
Website: http://www.mhcc.edu
William Malcolm, Director

Pennsylvania

★ 27458 ★ Northampton Community College
Department of Funeral Service Education
3835 Green Pond Rd.
Bethlehem, PA 18017
Phone: (610)861-5388 **Fax:** (610)861-4581
Email: jlunsford@northampton.edu
Website: http://www.northampton.edu
John Lunsford, Director

★ 27459 ★ Pittsburgh Institute of Mortuary Science
5808 Baum Blvd.
Pittsburgh, PA 15206
Phone: (412)362-8500 **Fax:** (412)362-1684
Email: pims5808@aol.com
Website: http://www.p-i-m-s.com
Eugene C. Ogrodnik, President

South Carolina

★ 27460 ★ Piedmont Technical College
Funeral Service Program
PO Drawer 1467
Emerald Rd.
Greenwood, SC 29648-1467
Phone: (864)941-8690 **Fax:** (864)941-8711
Email: vessels.g@ptc.edu
Website: http://www.ptc.edu
Gloria Walker Vessels, Contact

Tennessee

★ 27461 ★ John A. Gupton College
1616 Church St.
Nashville, TN 37203
Phone: (615)327-3927 **Fax:** (615)321-4518
Email: spann@guptoncollege.com
Website: http://www.guptoncollege.com
B. Steven Spann, President

Texas

★ 27462 ★ Amarillo College
Mortuary Science Program
PO Box 447
Amarillo, TX 79178-0001
Phone: (806)856-3631 **Fax:** (806)854-6096
Email: altieri-jc@actx.edu
Website: http://www.actx.edu
Jason Altieri, Director

★ 27463 ★ Commonwealth Institute of Funeral Service
415 Barren Springs
Houston, TX 77090
Phone: (281)873-0262 **Fax:** (281)873-5232
Email: tvanbeck@pdg.net
Website: http://www.commonwealthinst.org/
Todd W. Van Beck, President

★ 27464 ★ Dallas Institute of Funeral Service
3909 S Buckner Blvd.
Dallas, TX 75227
Phone: (214)388-5466 **Free:** 800-235-5444
Fax: (214)388-0316
Email: difs@dallasinstitute.edu
Website: http://www.dallasinstitute.edu
James Shoemake, President

★ 27465 ★ San Antonio College
Mortuary Science Program
1300 San Pedro Ave.
NTC 124
San Antonio, TX 78212-4299
Phone: (210)733-2905 **Fax:** (210)733-2907
Email: fsolis@accdvm.accd.edu
Website: http://www.accd.edu/sac/mortuary/home.html
Francisco E. Solis, Contact

Virginia

★ 27466 ★ John Tyler Community College
Funeral Service Program
Chester, VA 23831
Phone: (804)706-5113 **Fax:** (804)796-4362
Rick Sikon, Director

Wisconsin

★ 27467 ★ Milwaukee Area Technical College
West Campus
Funeral Service Department
1200 S 71st St.
West Allis, WI 53214
Phone: (414)456-5320 **Fax:** (414)456-5360
Email: pludeman@matc.edu
Website: http://matc.edu
John Pludeman, Contact

Nurse Anesthesia

Listed below are nurse anesthesia educational programs accredited by the Council on Accreditation of Nurse Anesthesia Educational Programs, 222 S Prospect Ave., Park Ridge, IL 60068, (847)692-7050, http://www.aana.com/coa/.

Alabama

★ 27468 ★ University of Alabama, Birmingham
Nurse Anesthesia Program
Webb Bldg., Rm. 637
1530 3rd Ave. S
Birmingham, AL 35294
Phone: (205)934-3209 **Fax:** (205)934-3212
Email: williams@uab.edu
Website: http://www.uab.edu/dcdc/na/home.htm
Joe R. Williams, Director

California

★ 27469 ★ California State University, Fullerton
Department of Nursing
Kaiser Permanente School of Anesthesia
100 S Los Robles, Ste. 550
Pasadena, CA 91188
Phone: (626)564-3000 **Fax:** (626)564-3099
Email: john.j.nagelhout@kp.org
Website: http://www.kpsan.org
John J. Nagelhout, Director

★ 27470 ★ Samuel Merritt College
Program of Nurse Anesthesia
435 Hawthorne Ave.
Oakland, CA 94609
Phone: (510)869-8926 **Fax:** (510)869-6677
Email: sfoster@samuelmerritt.edu
Website: http://www.samuelmerritt.edu
Scott D. Foster, Director

★ 27471 ★ University of Southern California
Program of Nurse Anesthesia
1540 Alcazar St., CHP 222
Los Angeles, CA 90089
Phone: (323)442-2012 **Fax:** (323)442-2090
Email: mgold@hsc.usc.edu
Website: http://www.usc.edu/hsc
Michele E. Gold, Director

Connecticut

★ 27472 ★ Central Connecticut State University
New Britain School of Nurse Anesthesia
100 Grand St.
New Britain, CT 06050
Phone: (860)224-5612 **Fax:** (860)826-4992
Email: joancrna@aol.com
Website: http://www.biology.ccsu.edu/gradprograms.html
Joan H. Dobbins, Director

★ 27473 ★ Hospital of St. Raphael
School of Nurse Anesthesia
1423 Chapel St.
New Haven, CT 06511
Phone: (203)789-3351 **Fax:** (203)789-3352
Email: hsrsna@snet.net
Website: http://www.vaness.com/hsr/hsr.htm
Judy Thompson, Director

★ 27474 ★ Southern Connecticut State University/Bridgeport Hospital
Nurse Anesthesia Program
267 Grant St.
Bridgeport, CT 06610
Phone: (203)384-3280 **Fax:** (203)384-3855
Email: napbpthosp@aol.com
Website: http://www.bpthospnap.org
Diane M. Mericnyak, Director

District of Columbia

★ 27475 ★ Georgetown University
School of Nursing
Nurse Anesthesia Program
Box 571107
3700 Reservoir Rd. NW
Washington, DC 20057
Phone: (202)687-4612 **Fax:** (202)687-5553
Email: jasinskd@georgetown.edu
Website: http://www.georgetown.edu
Donna M. Jasinski, Director

Florida

★ 27476 ★ Barry University
Master of Science Program in Anesthesiology
11300 NE 2nd Ave.
Miami Shores, FL 33161
Phone: (305)899-3230 **Free:** 800-756-6000
Fax: (305)899-3366
Email: mrodriguez@mail.barry.edu
Website: http://www2.barry.edu/vpaa-snhs/anesthe.htm
Dolores M. Gibbs, Director

★ 27477 ★ Bay Medical Center
Gooding Institute of Nurse Anesthesia
615 N Bonita Ave.
Panama City, FL 32401
Phone: (850)747-6918 **Free:** 800-422-2418
Fax: (850)747-6115
Email: gooding@baymedical.org
Website: http://www.baymedical.org
David R. Ely, Director

★ 27478 ★ Florida Gulf Coast University
Norman R. Wolford School of Nurse Anesthesia
PO Box 413012
Naples, FL 34101
Phone: (941)436-5370 **Fax:** (941)436-5639
Email: nrw@fgcu.edu
Website: http://www.fgcu.edu
Susan Campbell, Director

★ 27479 ★ Florida International University
School of Nursing
Anesthesiology Nursing Program
3000 NE 151 St.
North Miami, FL 33181
Phone: (305)919-5350 **Fax:** (305)919-5209
Email: mcdonoug@fiu.edu
Website: http://w3.fiu.edu/nursing/anesthesiology
John P. McDonough, Director

Georgia

★ 27480 ★ Medical College of Georgia
Nursing Anesthesia Program
1120 15th St., EB-229
Augusta, GA 30912
Phone: (706)721-9558 **Fax:** (706)721-8206
Email: emonti@mail.mcg.edu
Website: http://www.mcg.edu
Elizabeth J. Monti, Director

Illinois

★ 27481 ★ Bradley University/Decatur Memorial Hospital
Nurse Anesthesia Program
2300 N Edward St.
Decatur, IL 62526
Phone: (217)876-2578 **Fax:** (217)876-2587
Email: susang@dmhhs.org
Website: http://www.dmhhs.com
Sue M. Kiefer-Griffin, Director

★ 27482 ★ Evanston Northwestern Healthcare/DePaul University
School of Anesthesia
2650 Ridge Ave.
Evanston, IL 60201
Phone: (847)570-1959 **Fax:** (847)733-5392
Email: broche@enh.org
Website: http://www.advocatehealth.com/rhmcsa
Bernadette T. Roche, Director

★ 27483 ★ Rush University
College of Nursing
Nurse Anesthesia Program
600 S Paulina St., No. 1072B
Chicago, IL 60612
Phone: (312)942-7100 **Fax:** (312)942-3043
Email: mfaut-callahan@rushu.rush.edu
Website: http://www.rushu.rush.edu/nursing
Margaret Faut-Callahan, Director

★ 27484 ★ Southern Illinois University, Edwardsville
School of Nursing
Anesthesia Nursing Specialization
Campus Box 1066
Edwardsville, IL 62026-1066
Phone: (618)650-3906 **Free:** 800-234-4844
Fax: (618)650-3854
Email: wellis@siue.edu
Website: http://www.siue.edu
Wayne E. Ellis, Director

Iowa

★ 27485 ★ University of Iowa
College of Nursing
Anesthesia Nursing Program
Rm. 6613 JCP, UIHC
200 Hawkins Dr.
Iowa City, IA 52242
Phone: (319)384-7354 **Free:** 800-553-4692
Fax: (319)384-7286
Email: e-s-thompson@uiowa.edu
Website: http://www.anesth.uiowa.edu/srna
Edward S. Thompson, Director

Kansas

★ 27486 ★ Newman University
Nurse Anesthesia Program
3100 McCormick Ave., Ste. 214 ECK
Wichita, KS 67213
Phone: (316)942-4291 **Fax:** (316)942-4483
Email: chipasa@newmanu.edu
Website: http://www.newmanu.edu/gradnan.html
Anthony Chipas, Director

★ 27487 ★ University of Kansas Medical Center
Program of Nurse Anesthesia Education
3901 Rainbow Blvd.
Kansas City, KS 66160
Phone: (913)588-6612 **Fax:** (913)588-3334
Email: nanesthe@kumc.edu
Website: http://www2.kumc.edu/sah/nurseanesthesia
Carol G. Elliott, Chairman of the Board

Kentucky

★ 27488 ★ Trover Foundation/Murray State University
Program of Anesthesia
435 N Kentucky Ave., Ste. A
Madisonville, KY 42431
Phone: (270)824-3460 **Fax:** (270)824-3469
Email: anesprog@trover.org
Website: http://www.crnaky.com
W. Gray McCall, Director

Louisiana

★ 27489 ★ Louisiana State University Health Sciences Center
School of Nursing
Nurse Anesthesia Program
1900 Gravier St.
Box G-4
New Orleans, LA 70112
Phone: (504)568-7505 **Fax:** (504)568-4136
Email: kwren@lsuhsc.edu
Website: http://nursing.lsuhsc.edu/sonweb/mn/crna_program/default.htm
Kathleen R. Wren, Director

Maine

★ 27490 ★ University of New England
School of Nurse Anesthesia
716 Stevens Ave.
Portland, ME 04103
Phone: (207)797-7261 **Fax:** (207)797-7225
Email: ldeisering@une.edu
Website: http://www.une.edu
Leon F. Deisering, Director

Maryland

★ 27491 ★ Uniformed Services University of the Health Sciences
Graduate School of Nursing
Nurse Anesthesia Program
1335 East-West Hwy., Ste. 9-700
Silver Spring, MD 20910
Phone: (301)295-0979 **Fax:** (301)295-1722
Email: paustin@usuhs.mil
Website: http://www.usuhs.mil
Lt. Col. Paul Austin, Director

★ 27492 ★ U.S. Navy
Nurse Corps Anesthesia Program
NSHS-Code ON1
8901 Wisconsin Ave.
Bethesda, MD 20889
Phone: (301)295-6091 **Fax:** (301)295-0827
Email: lheindel@nsh10.med.navy.mil
Website: http://www-nshs.med.navy.mil/nncapwww/nrsanes.htm
Louis Heindel, Director

Massachusetts

★ 27493 ★ Northeastern University/New England Medical Center
Nurse Anesthesia Program
207 Robinson Hall
Boston, MA 02115
Phone: (617)373-7962 **Fax:** (617)373-8672
Email: st.alves@neu.edu
Website: http://www.neu.edu
Steve L. Alves, Director

Michigan

★ 27494 ★ Henry Ford Hospital/ University of Detroit Mercy
Graduate Program of Nurse Anesthesiology
Clara Ford Pavilion, Rm. 303
2799 W Grand Blvd.
Detroit, MI 48202
Phone: (313)916-2934 **Fax:** (313)916-2606
Email: schanes@hfhs.org
Website: http://ids.udmercy.edu/naprogram
Patrick J. Quinn, Director

★ 27495 ★ Oakland University
Beaumont Graduate Program of Nurse Anesthesia
(Beaumont Royal Oak and Troy)
3601 W 13 Mile Rd.
Royal Oak, MI 48073
Phone: (248)551-8075 **Fax:** (248)551-8285
Email: kzaglaniczny@beaumont.edu
Website: http://www.beaumont.edu/crna
Karen L. Zaglaniczny, Director

★ 27496 ★ University of Detroit Mercy
Graduate Program of Nurse Anesthesiology
St. Joseph Mercy Oakland
44405 Woodward Ave.
Pontiac, MI 48341
Phone: (248)858-6593 **Fax:** (248)859-6599
Email: doschm@trinity-health.org
Website: http://www.udmercy.edu/naprogram
Michael P. Dosch, Director

★ 27497 ★ University of Michigan, Flint
Hurley Medical Center
Master of Science in Anesthesia Program
Hurley Medical Center
1 Hurley Plaza
Flint, MI 48503
Phone: (810)257-9264 **Fax:** (810)760-0839
Email: dmcfarl1@hurleymc.com
Website: http://www.hurleymc.com/education/anesthes/index.htm
Francis Gerbasi, Director

★ 27498 ★ Wayne State University
College of Pharmacy and Allied Health Professions
Nurse Anesthesia Program
4201 St. Antoine, Rm. 2V-4
Detroit, MI 48201
Phone: (313)745-3610 **Fax:** (313)993-7729
Email: pworth@dmc.org
Website: http://wizard.pharm.wayne.edu/anesth
Prudentia Worth, Chairman of the Board

Minnesota

★ 27499 ★ Mayo School of Health Sciences
Master of Nurse Anesthesia Program
1108 Siebens Bldg.
200 1st St. SW
Rochester, MN 55905
Phone: (507)284-8331 **Free:** 800-626-9041
Fax: (507)284-0656
Email: marienau.mary@mayo.edu
Website: http://www.mayo.edu/hrs/hrs_nam.htm
Mary E. Shirk Marienau, Director

★ 27500 ★ Minneapolis School of Anesthesia
6715 Minnetonka Blvd.
Saint Louis Park, MN 55426
Phone: (952)925-5222 **Fax:** (952)925-6004
Email: gombkoto.msa@worldnet.att.net
Website: http://www.nurseanesthesia.org
Rebecca L. Gombkoto, Director

★ 27501 ★ Minneapolis VA School of Anesthesia
1 Veterans Dr., 112A
Minneapolis, MN 55417
Phone: (612)725-2000 **Fax:** (612)970-5887
Email: fager003@umn.edu
Kathleen A. Fagerlund, Director

★ 27502 ★ Saint Mary's University of Minnesota/Abbott Northwestern Hospital
Graduate Program in Nurse Anesthesia
2500 Park Ave.
Minneapolis, MN 55404
Phone: (612)728-5133 **Fax:** (612)728-5167
Email: mmoody@smumn.edu
Website: http://www.smumn.edu
Merri L. Moody, Director

Missouri

★ 27503 ★ Southwest Missouri School of Anesthesia
1235 E Cherokee
Springfield, MO 65804
Phone: (417)885-6890 **Fax:** (417)885-6895
Email: as14293@sprg.smhs.com
Website: http://www.smsu.edu/faculty/jmg230f/ronis/naopen.html
William O. Kirk, Director

★ 27504 ★ Truman Medical Center
School of Nurse Anesthesia
2301 Holmes St.
Kansas City, MO 64108
Phone: (816)556-3216 **Fax:** (816)556-3963
Email: tmcanes@tmcmed.org
Website: http://www.trumanmed.org/crna
Mark Lipari, Director

★ 27505 ★ Webster University
MS in Nurse Anesthesia
470 E Lockwood Ave.
Saint Louis, MO 63119
Phone: (314)968-5916 **Fax:** (314)968-7194
Email: clarkga@webster.edu
Website: http://www.webster.edu
Gary D. Clark, Director

Nebraska

★ 27506 ★ Bryan LGH Medical Center/ University of Kansas
School of Nurse Anesthesia
1600 S 48 St.
Lincoln, NE 68506
Phone: (402)481-3135 **Free:** 800-742-7844
Fax: (402)481-8404
Email: jcuddeford@bryanlgh.org
Website: http://www.bryanlgh.org
James D. Cuddeford, Director

New Jersey

★ 27507 ★ University of Medicine and Dentistry of New Jersey
Our Lady of Lourdes Medical Center
Nurse Anesthesia Program
1600 Haddon Ave.
Camden, NJ 08103
Phone: (856)757-3897 **Fax:** (856)968-2568
Email: roddend@lourdesnet.org
F. David Rodden, Director

New York

★ 27508 ★ Albany Medical College
Nurse Anesthesiology Program
43 New Scotland Ave., MC-131
Albany, NY 12208
Phone: (518)262-4303 **Fax:** (518)262-5170
Email: amcnap@mail.amc.edu
Website: http://www.amc.edu/gradstu
Kathleen M. O'Donnell, Director

★ 27509 ★ Columbia University
School of Nursing
Program in Nurse Anesthesia
630 W 168th St.
New York, NY 10032
Phone: (212)305-4196 **Fax:** (212)305-6937
Email: tjl2@columbia.edu
Website: http://www.columbia.edu
Timothy J. Lehey, Director

★ 27510 ★ State University of New York, Brooklyn (SUNY-HSCB)
Health Science Center
Nurse Anesthesia with Harlem Hospital Center
Nurse Anesthesia with Kings County Hospital Center
450 Clarkson Ave.
Box 22
Brooklyn, NY 11203
Phone: (212)939-3575 **Fax:** (212)939-3574
Email: varirao@netmail.hscbklyn.edu
Website: http://www.downstate.edu
Visitacion T. Arirao, Director

★ 27511 ★ State University of New York, Buffalo
School of Nursing
Nurse Anesthesia Program
1116 Kimball Tower
3435 Main St.
Buffalo, NY 14214
Phone: (716)829-2410 **Fax:** (716)829-2021
Email: tobst@buffalo.edu
Website: http://nursing.buffalo.edu
Thomas E. Obst, Director

North Carolina

★ 27512 ★ Carolinas HealthCare System/ University of North Carolina, Charlotte
Nurse Anesthesia Program
PO Box 32861
Charlotte, NC 28232
Phone: (704)355-2375 **Fax:** (704)355-7263
Email: ymobley@carolinas.org
Website: http://www.carolinas.org/education
Jacqueline M. Hall, Director

★ 27513 ★ Duke University
Nurse Anesthesia Program
Box 3322 DUMC
Durham, NC 27710
Phone: (919)684-3786 **Free:** 877-415-3853
Fax: (919)681-8899
Email: mary.karlet@duke.edu
Website: http://www.nursing.duke.edu
Mary Karlet, Director

★ 27514 ★ University of North Carolina, Greensboro
Raleigh School of Nurse Anesthesia
23 Sunnybrook Rd., Ste. 163
Raleigh, NC 27610
Phone: (919)250-9740 **Fax:** (919)250-0348
Email: rsna@earthlink.net
Website: http://home.earthlink.net/~rsna
Nancy Bruton-Maree, Director

★ 27515 ★ Wake Forest University Baptist Medical Center
The University of North Carolina, Greensboro
Nurse Anesthesia Program
Medical Center Blvd.
Winston Salem, NC 27157
Phone: (336)716-1411 **Fax:** (336)716-1412
Email: vcbeane@wfubmc.edu
Website: http://www.wfubmc.edu
Sandra M. Ouellette, Director

North Dakota

★ 27516 ★ University of North Dakota
College of Nursing
Nurse Anesthesiology Program
PO Box 9025
Grand Forks, ND 58202
Phone: (701)777-4509 **Fax:** (701)777-4096
Email: rick_brown@mail.und.nodak.edu
Website: http://www.und.nodak.edu/dept/nursing/anesmstr.html
Rick Brown, Director

Ohio

★ 27517 ★ Case Western Reserve University
Cleveland Clinic Foundation
Frances Payne Bolton School of Nursing
School of Nurse Anesthesia
9500 Euclid Ave., E-31
Cleveland, OH 44195
Phone: (216)444-6547 **Free:** 800-223-2273
Fax: (216)444-9247
Email: blakelp@ccf.org
Website: http://fpb.cwru.edu/Program%20Areas/Right/NAMSN.htm
Paul R. Blakeley, Director

★ 27518 ★ Case Western Reserve University
Frances Payne Bolton School of Nursing
Program in Nurse Anesthesia
10900 Euclid Ave.
Cleveland, OH 44106
Phone: (216)368-0221 **Free:** 800-825-2540
Fax: (216)368-3542
Email: jrk@po.cwru.edu
Website: http://fpb.cwru.edu
Jack R. Kless, Director

★ 27519 ★ St. Elizabeth Health Center
School for Nurse Anesthetists, Inc.
1044 Belmont Ave.
Youngstown, OH 44501
Phone: (330)480-3444 **Fax:** (330)480-5202
Email: brodgers@belpark.net
Website: http://www.belpark.net/crnaschool
Beverly A. Rodgers, Director

★ 27520 ★ University of Akron
College of Nursing
Graduate Anesthesia Program
209 Carroll St.
Akron, OH 44325
Phone: (330)972-5406 **Fax:** (330)972-6632
Email: barton@uakron.edu
Website: http://www.uakron.edu/nursing/academic/anesthesia.htm
Charles R. Barton, Director

★ 27521 ★ University of Cincinnati
College of Nursing
Masters Program in Nurse Anesthesia
PO Box 210038
Cincinnati, OH 45221
Phone: (513)558-5500 **Fax:** (513)558-7523
Email: wanda.wilson@uc.edu
Website: http://www.nursing@uc.edu
Wanda O. Wilson, Director

Pennsylvania

★ 27522 ★ Allegheny Valley Hospital/ LaRoche College
School of Nurse Anesthesia
1301 Carlisle St.
Natrona Heights, PA 15065
Phone: (724)226-7013 **Fax:** (724)226-7199
Email: dadcrna@hotmail.com
Website: http://nursing.auhs.edu/john_pages/napo.htm
Deborah A. Davison, Director

★ 27523 ★ Hamot Medical Center
School of Anesthesia
Gannon University
201 State St.
Erie, PA 16550
Phone: (814)877-2938 **Free:** 800-937-9133
Fax: (814)877-6070
Email: steve.anderson@hamot.org
Website: http://www.hamot.org
K. Stephen Anderson, Director

★ 27524 ★ Lankenau Hospital
School of Anesthesia
100 Lancaster Ave.
Wynnewood, PA 19096
Phone: (610)645-2145 **Fax:** (610)645-3411
Email: wildgustb@mlhs.org

Website: http://www.nursing.villanova.edu/msn/gradstdy/anesth.htm
Bette M. Wildgust, Director

★ 27525 ★ MCP Hahnemann University
Nurse Anesthesia Program
245 N 15th St., MS 501
Philadelphia, PA 19102-1192
Phone: (215)762-4309 **Fax:** (215)762-1259
Email: booth@drexel.edu
Website: http://nursing.mcphu.edu/sonbasics/napo.htm
Michael J. Booth, Director

★ 27526 ★ Montgomery Hospital
Frank J. Tornetta School of Anesthesia
1301 Powell St.
PO Box 992
Norristown, PA 19404
Phone: (610)270-2139 **Fax:** (610)270-2318
Email: philacrna@aol.com
Michael T. Kost, Director

★ 27527 ★ Nazareth Hospital
School of Nurse Anesthesiology
2601 Holme Ave.
Philadelphia, PA 19152
Phone: (215)335-6217 **Fax:** (215)335-6668
Email: jwoods@che-east.org
Joan E. Woods, Director

★ 27528 ★ Pennsylvania Hospital
School of Nurse Anesthesia
800 Spruce St.
Philadelphia, PA 19107
Phone: (215)829-3320 **Fax:** (215)829-8757
Email: phsa@pahosp.com
Website: http://www.med.upenn.edu/pahosp/pahpe/nurse_anesth/index.html
Kathleen Kinslow, Director

★ 27529 ★ St. Francis Medical Center/LaRoche College
School of Anesthesia
400 45th St.
Pittsburgh, PA 15201
Phone: (412)622-4369 **Fax:** (412)688-3883
Email: loefflera@sfhs.edu
Website: http://www.sfhs.edu/library/schools/anesth
Arlene S. Loeffler, Director

★ 27530 ★ University of Pittsburgh
School of Nursing
Nurse Anesthesia Program
336 Victoria Bldg.
3500 Victoria St.
Pittsburgh, PA 15261
Phone: (412)624-4860 **Fax:** (412)383-7227
Email: napcrna@pitt.edu
Website: http://www.pitt.edu/~napcrna
John M. O'Donnell, Director

★ 27531 ★ Westmoreland-Latrobe Hospitals/LaRoche College
School of Anesthesia
532 W Pittsburgh St.
Greensburg, PA 15601
Phone: (724)832-4144 **Fax:** (724)832-4164
Email: bighoward@aol.com
Website: http://www.laroche.edu/TOC/academic/academic.html
Howard F. Armour, Director

★ 27532 ★ Wyoming Valley Health Care System
University of Scranton
School of Nurse Anesthesia
575 N River St.
Wilkes Barre, PA 18764
Phone: (570)552-7290 **Fax:** (570)552-7299
Email: eevanina@wvhcs.org
Website: http://www.scranton.edu/graduateschool
Eileen Evanina, Director

Puerto Rico

★ 27533 ★ Inter American University of Puerto Rico
Master of Science in Anesthesia
PO Box 4050
Arecibo, PR 00614
Phone: (787)878-5475 **Fax:** (787)881-3831
Email: imolina@arecibo.inter.edu
Website: http://www.arecibo.inter.edu
Ivan J. Molina, Director

★ 27534 ★ University of Puerto Rico
School of Nursing
Nurse Anesthesia Program
Medial Sciences Campus
PO Box 365067
San Juan, PR 00936
Phone: (787)758-2525 **Fax:** (787)281-0721
Email: mplaza@rcm.upr.edu
Website: http://www.rcm.upr.edu/pagenursing3.html
Crucita Mattei, Director

Rhode Island

★ 27535 ★ Memorial Hospital of Rhode Island
School of Nurse Anesthesia
111 Brewster St.
Pawtucket, RI 02860
Phone: (401)729-2485 **Fax:** (401)729-3476
Email: foster@ids.net
Website: http://www.mhri.org/anesth
Mark A. Foster, Director

★ 27536 ★ Saint Joseph Hospital
School of Anesthesia for Nurses
200 High Service Ave.
North Providence, RI 02904
Phone: (401)456-3639 **Fax:** (401)752-8140
Email: saintjoes@aol.com
Website: http://www.saintjosephri.com
Lucille S. Buono, Director

South Carolina

★ 27537 ★ Medical University of South Carolina
Anesthesia for Nurses Program
165 Cannon St., Ste. 402
PO Box 250855
Charleston, SC 29425
Phone: (843)792-3785 **Fax:** (843)792-1984
Email: truverl@musc.edu
Website: http://www.musc.edu/afn
Lawrence H. Truver, Director

★ 27538 ★ USC/PRMH
Graduate Program in Nurse Anesthesia
15 Medical Park, Ste. 221
Columbia, SC 29203
Phone: (803)434-6344 **Fax:** (803)434-4099
Email: kwilliam@richmed.medpark.sc.edu
Website: http://www.med.sc.edu:88/mnuran.htm
Kristi H. Williams, Director

South Dakota

★ 27539 ★ Mount Marty College
Graduate Program in Nurse Anesthesiology
3932 S Western Ave.
Sioux Falls, SD 57105
Phone: (605)322-8090 **Free:** 877-727-8672
Fax: (605)322-8095
Email: msna@mtmc.edu
Website: http://www.mtmc.edu/~ans
Larry L. Dahlen, Director

Tennessee

★ 27540 ★ Erlanger Health System/University of Tennessee, Chattanooga
School of Nursing
Nurse Anesthesia Concentration
615 McCallie Ave.
Chattanooga, TN 37403
Phone: (423)755-4750 **Fax:** (423)755-4668
Email: zacharra@erlanger.org
Website: http://www.utc.edu/~utcnurse/index.htm
Dana H. Wertenberger, Director

★ 27541 ★ Middle Tennessee School of Anesthesia
Nurse Anesthesia Program
PO Box 6414
Madison, TN 37116
Phone: (615)868-6503 **Fax:** (615)868-9885
Email: dean@mtsa.edu
Website: http://www.mtsa.edu
Mary E. DeVasher, Director

★ 27542 ★ University of Tennessee
College of Nursing
Nurse Anesthesia Concentration
1924 Alcoa Hwy.
Box U-109
Knoxville, TN 37920
Phone: (865)544-9222 **Fax:** (865)544-6852
Email: jpreston@mc.utmck.edu
Website: http://nightingale.con.utk.edu
John C. Preston, Director

★ 27543 ★ University of Tennessee
Health Sciences Center
College of Nursing
Nurse Anesthesia Option
877 Madison Ave.
Memphis, TN 38163
Phone: (901)448-6102 **Fax:** (901)448-4121
Email: lhill@utmem.edu
Website: http://www.utmem.edu/nursing
Linda Hill, Director

Texas

★ 27544 ★ Baylor College of Medicine
Graduate Program in Nurse Anesthesia
6550 Fannin St., Ste. 1003
Houston, TX 77030
Phone: (713)873-2860 **Fax:** (713)873-2867
Email: jrwalker@bcm.tmc.edu
Website: http://www.bcm.tmc.edu/gpna
James R. Walker, Director

★ 27545 ★ Texas Wesleyan University
Graduate Program of Nurse Anesthesia
1201 Wesleyan St.
Fort Worth, TX 76105
Phone: (817)531-4406 **Fax:** (817)531-6508
Email: ksanders@txwes.edu
Website: http://www.txwesleyan.edu
Kay K. Sanders, Chairman of the Board

★ 27546 ★ U.S. Army
Graduate Program in Anesthesia Nursing
MCCS-HNE, Anesthesia Branch
2250 Stanley Rd., Ste. 214
San Antonio, TX 78234
Phone: (210)221-6905 **Fax:** (210)221-8114
Email: norma.garrett@amedd.army.mil
Website: http://www.dns.amedd.army.mil/crna
Normalynn Garrett, Director

★ 27547 ★ University of Texas
Houston Health Science Center
School of Nursing
Nurse Anesthesia Division
1100 Holcombe Blvd., Ste. 6, 150
Houston, TX 77030
Phone: (713)500-2159 **Fax:** (713)500-2171
Email: rlester@son1.nur.uth.tmc.edu
Website: http://son1.nur.uth.tmc.edu
Rodney C. Lester, Director

Virginia

★ 27548 ★ Old Dominion University
School of Nursing
Nurse Anesthesia Program
Technology Bldg., Rm. 363
4608 Hampton Blvd.
Norfolk, VA 23529
Phone: (757)683-5068 **Free:** 800-572-2762
Fax: (757)683-5124
Email: joswaks@odu.edu
Website: http://web.odu.edu
Jill S. Detty Oswaks, Director

★ 27549 ★ Virginia Commonwealth University
Department of Nurse Anesthesia
PO Box 980226
Richmond, VA 23298
Phone: (804)828-9808 **Fax:** (804)828-0581
Email: mdfallac@hsc.vcu.edu
Website: http://views.vcu.edu/sahp/rngas
Michael D. Fallacaro, Chairman of the Board

Washington

★ 27550 ★ Gonzaga University
Sacred Heart Medical Center
Master of Anesthesiology Education Program
101 W 8th Ave.
PO Box 2555
Spokane, WA 99220
Phone: (509)474-4971 **Fax:** (509)474-3113
Email: meyersmr@shmc.org
Website: http://www.gonzaga.edu/academic/Education/Masters/aci/aeindex.html
Margaret R. Meyers, Director

West Virginia

★ 27551 ★ Charleston Area Medical Center
School of Nurse Anesthesia
3110 MacCorkle Ave. SE, Rm. 2041
Charleston, WV 25304
Phone: (304)388-9950 **Fax:** (304)388-9955
Email: nancy.tierney@camcare.com
Website: http://www.anesthesiaschool.org
Nancy L. Tierney, Director

Wisconsin

★ 27552 ★ Franciscan Skemp Healthcare
School of Anesthesia
700 West Ave.
La Crosse, WI 54601
Phone: (608)785-0940 **Fax:** (608)791-9799
Email: jochman.barbara@mayo.edu
Website: http://perth.uwlax.edu/biology/graduate/crna.htm
Barbara J. Jochman, Director

Nurse-Midwifery

The following are certificate and graduate nurse-midwifery programs accredited by the Division of Accreditation of the American College of Nurse-Midwives, 818 Connecticut Ave. NW, Ste. 900, Washington, DC 20006, (202)728-9860, http://www.acnm.org/.

California

★ 27553 ★ Charles R. Drew University of Medicine and Science
College of Allied Health Sciences
Nurse-Midwifery Certificate Education Program
1621 E 120th St.
Mail Point 22
Los Angeles, CA 90059
Phone: (323)563-4951
Email: frcushen@cdrewu.edu
Website: http://www.cdrewu.edu
H. Frances Hayes-Cushenberry, JD, Director

★ 27554 ★ San Diego State University/University of California, San Diego
USCD Division of Graduate Nursing Education
Nurse-Midwifery Graduate Program
9500 Gilman Dr.
Department 0809
La Jolla, CA 92093-0809
Phone: (619)543-5480
Lauren Hunter, Director

★ 27555 ★ University of California, Los Angeles
UCLA School of Nursing
Nurse-Midwifery Graduate Program
Factor Bldg., Rm. 5934-A
Box 956819
Los Angeles, CA 90095-6919
Phone: (310)794-4434
Email: shuser@sonnet.ucla.edu
Website: http://www.nursing.ucla.edu/son
Susan Huser, Director

★ 27556 ★ University of California, San Francisco
San Francisco General Hospital
Interdepartmental Nurse-Midwifery Graduate Education Program
San Francisco General Hospital, Ward 6D, Rm. 21
1001 Potrero Ave.
San Francisco, CA 94110
Phone: (415)206-5106
Email: linda@ob.ucsf.edu
Website: http://nurseweb.ucsf.edu/www/speclist.htm
Linda Ennis, Director

★ 27557 ★ University of Southern California
Nurse-Midwifery Graduate Program
1540 Alcazar St., CHP 222
Los Angeles, CA 90033
Phone: (323)442-2001
Email: bjsnell@hsc.usc.edu
Website: http://uscnurse.usc.edu
B.J. Snell, PhD, Director

Colorado

★ 27558 ★ University of Colorado
Health Sciences Center
School of Nursing
Nurse-Midwifery Graduate Program
4200 E 9th Ave.
Box C288-14
Denver, CO 80262
Phone: (303)724-1183
Email: marie.hastings-tolsma@uchsc.edu
Website: http://freenet.uchsc.edu/son
Marie Hastings-Tolsma, PhD, Director

Connecticut

★ 27559 ★ Yale University
School of Nursing
Nurse-Midwifery Graduate Program
100 Church St. S
PO Box 9740
New Haven, CT 06536-0740
Phone: (203)785-2389 **Fax:** (203)785-6455
Email: lynette.ament@yale.edu
Website: http://info.med.yale.edu/nursing
Lynette Ament, PhD, Director

District of Columbia

★ 27560 ★ Georgetown University
School of Nursing and Health Studies
Graduate Program in Nurse-Midwifery
3700 Reservoir Rd. NW
PO Box 571107
Washington, DC 20007
Phone: (202)687-4772 **Fax:** (202)687-5553
Email: midwife@gunet.georgetown.edu
Website: http://www.dml.georgetown.edu/schnurs/midwife1.html
Ann Silvonek, Director

Florida

★ 27561 ★ University of Florida
UFHSC-J College of Nursing
Nurse-Midwifery Graduate Program
653 W 8th St., Bldg. 1, 2nd Fl.
Jacksonville, FL 32209-6561
Phone: (904)244-5174
Email: poeah@nursing.ufl.edu
Website: http://con.ufl.edu
Alice H. Poe, Director

★ 27562 ★ University of Miami
School of Nursing
Nurse-Midwifery Graduate Program
5801 Red Rd.
PO Box 248153
Coral Gables, FL 33124-3850
Phone: (305)284-6256
Email: jgottlieb@miami.edu
Website: http://www.miami.edu/nur/net20/graduate/midwife.htm
Jeanne Gottlieb, Director

Georgia

★ 27563 ★ Emory University
Neil Hodgson Woodruff School of Nursing
Nurse-Midwifery Graduate Program
Atlanta, GA 30322
Phone: (404)727-6961 **Fax:** (404)727-0536
Email: makelle@nurse.emory.edu
Website: http://www.nurse.emory.edu
Maureen Kelley, PhD, Director

Illinois

★ 27564 ★ University of Illinois, Chicago College of Nursing M/C 802
Nurse-Midwifery Graduate Program
845 S Damen Ave.
Chicago, IL 60612
Phone: (312)996-1867 **Fax:** (312)996-8871
Email: engstrom@uic.edu
Website: http://www.nurs.uic.edu
Janet Engstrom, PhD, Director

Kansas

★ 27565 ★ University of Kansas
Nurse-Midwifery Graduate Program
3901 Rainbow Blvd.
Kansas City, KS 66160-7502
Phone: (913)588-1683 **Fax:** (913)588-8299
Email: gbreedlove@kumc.edu
Website: http://www2.kumc.edu/midwife
Ginger Breedlove, PhD, Director

Kentucky

★ 27566 ★ Frontier School of Midwifery and Family Nursing
Community-Based Nurse-Midwifery Certificate Education Program (CNEP)
195 School St.
PO Box 528
Hyden, KY 41749
Phone: (606)672-2312 **Fax:** (606)672-3776
Email: CNEP@midwives.org
Website: http://www.midwives.org
Susan Ulrich, PhD, Director

Maryland

★ 27567 ★ University of Maryland
School of Nursing
Nurse-Midwifery Graduate Program
655 W Lombard St., Ste. 575
Baltimore, MD 21201
Phone: (410)706-8625
Email: stom@son.umaryland.edu
Website: http://nursing.umaryland.edu
Sally Tom, Director

Massachusetts

★ 27568 ★ Baystate Medical Center
Midwifery Certificate Education Program
689 Chestnut St.
Springfield, MA 01199
Phone: (413)794-4448 **Fax:** (413)794-8770
Email: barbara.graves@bhs.org
Website: http://www.baystatehealth.com/baystatemidwifery
Barbara W. Graves, Director

★ 27569 ★ Boston University
School of Public Health
Department of Maternal and Child Health
Nurse-Midwifery Graduate Education Program T-5W
715 Albany St.
Boston, MA 02118
Phone: (617)638-5012
Email: mbarger@bu.edu
Website: http://www.bumc.bu.edu/shp/mc
Mary Barger, Director

Michigan

★ 27570 ★ University of Michigan
School of Nursing
Nurse-Midwifery Graduate Program
400 N Ingalls, Rm. 3320
Ann Arbor, MI 48109-0482
Phone: (313)763-3710 **Fax:** (313)647-0351
Email: dswalker@umich.edu
Website: http://www-personal.umich.edu/~dswalker/umhome.html
Deborah Walker, DNSc, Director

Minnesota

★ 27571 ★ University of Minnesota
School of Nursing
Nurse-Midwifery Graduate Program
6-101 Weaver-Densford Hall
308 Harvard St. SE
Minneapolis, MN 55455
Phone: (612)624-6494
Email: avery003@tc.umn.edu
Website: http://www.nursing.umn.edu/MS/MSmidwifery.html
Melissa Avery, PhD, Director

Missouri

★ 27572 ★ University of Missouri, Columbia
Sinclair School of Nursing
Nurse-Midwifery Graduate Program
Columbia, MO 65211
Phone: (573)882-0235
Email: chelinik@health.missouri.edu
Website: http://www.muhealth.org/~son/docs/midwifery.html
Katherine Chelini, Director

New Jersey

★ 27573 ★ University of Medicine and Dentistry of New Jersey
School of Health Related Professions
Nurse-Midwifery Certificate Program
65 Bergen St.
Newark, NJ 07107-3001
Phone: (973)972-4298
Email: diegmaek@umdnj.edu
Website: http://www.umdnj.edu/shrpweb/programs/midwife
Elaine Diegmann, N.D., Director

New Mexico

★ 27574 ★ University of New Mexico
College of Nursing
Nurse-Midwifery Graduate Program
Nursing/Pharmacy Bldg.
Albuquerque, NM 87131-1061
Phone: (505)272-1184 **Fax:** (505)272-8901
Email: midwyfe@unm.edu
Website: http://hsc.unm.edu/consg/msn_midw.html
Julie Gorwoda, Director

New York

★ 27575 ★ Columbia University
School of Nursing
Graduate Program in Midwifery
630 W 168th St.
Box 49
New York, NY 10032
Phone: (212)305-5236 **Fax:** (212)305-3680
Email: jed19@columbia.edu
Website: http://cpmcnet.columbia.edu/dept/nursing
Jennifer Dohrn, Director

★ 27576 ★ New York University
Nurse-Midwifery Graduate Education Program
246 Greene St.
New York, NY 10003-6677
Phone: (212)998-5895
Email: patricia.burkhardt@nyu.edu
Website: http://www.nyu.edu/education/nursing
Patricia Burkhardt, DrPH, Director

★ 27577 ★ State University of New York, Brooklyn
Health Science Center
College of Health Related Professions
Nurse-Midwifery Graduate Education Program
450 Clarkson Ave.
Box 1227
Brooklyn, NY 11203
Phone: (718)270-7740 **Fax:** (718)270-7634
Email: lhsia@downstate.edu
Website: http://www.hscbklyn.edu/CHRP/Midwif
Lily Hsia, Director

★ 27578 ★ State University of New York, Stony Brook
School of Nursing
Nurse-Midwifery Graduate Program
Health Sciences Center
Stony Brook, NY 11794-8240
Phone: (516)444-2867
Email: peter.johnson@stonybrook.edu
Website: http://www.pathwaystomidwifery.org
Peter Johnson, PhD, Director

North Carolina

★ 27579 ★ East Carolina University
School of Nursing
Nurse-Midwifery Graduate Program
Greenville, NC 27858-1818
Phone: (252)328-4303 **Fax:** (252)328-2332
Email: mossn@mail.ecu.edu
Website: http://www.ecu.edu/nursing
Nancy Moss, PhD, Director

Ohio

★ 27580 ★ Case Western Reserve University
Frances Payne Bolton School of Nursing
Nurse-Midwifery Graduate Program
10900 Euclid Ave.
Cleveland, OH 44106-1712
Phone: (216)368-2532
Email: ggm@po.cwru.edu
Website: http://cwru4.nurs.cwru.edu
Gretchen Mettler, Director

★ 27581 ★ Ohio State University
College of Nursing
Nurse-Midwifery Graduate Program
1585 Neil Ave.
Columbus, OH 43210-1289
Phone: (614)292-4041 **Fax:** (614)494-3878
Email: nursing@osu.edu
Website: http://www.con.ohio-state.edu
Nancy K. Lowe, PhD, Director

★ 27582 ★ University of Cincinnati
College of Nursing and Health
Nurse-Midwifery Graduate Program
PO Box 210038
Cincinnati, OH 45221-0038
Phone: (513)558-5282
Email: mary.akers@uc.edu
Website: http://www.uc.edu/www/nursing
Mary Carol Akers, Director

Oregon

★ 27583 ★ Oregon Health Sciences University
School of Nursing
Nurse-Midwifery Graduate Program
3181 SW Sam Jackson Park Rd.
Portland, OR 97201
Phone: (503)494-3822
Email: howec@ohsu.edu
Website: http://www.ohsu.edu/son-primcare/indexnmwh.html
Carol Howe, DNSc, Director

Pennsylvania

★ 27584 ★ Institute of Midwifery, Women and Health
Midwifery Certificate Program
Hayward Hall, Rm. 222
Schoolhouse Lane and Henry Ave.
Philadelphia, PA 19144
Phone: (215)951-2525 **Fax:** (215)951-2526
Email: instituteofmidwifery@philau.edu
Website: http://www.instituteofmidwifery.org
Jerrilyn Hobdy, Director

★ 27585 ★ University of Pennsylvania
School of Nursing
Graduate Program in Nurse-Midwifery
Nursing Education Bldg.
420 Guardian Dr.
Philadelphia, PA 19104-6096
Phone: (215)898-4335
Email: mccoolwf@nursing.upenn.edu
Website: http://www.nursing.upenn.edu/midwifery
William F. McCool, PhD, Director

Puerto Rico

★ 27586 ★ University of Puerto Rico
Graduate School of Public Health
Nurse-Midwifery Graduate Program
Medical Sciences Campus
PO Box 5067
San Juan, PR 00936-5067
Phone: (787)281-7355
Website: http://www.upr.edu/upri
Irene dela Torre, Director

Rhode Island

★ 27587 ★ University of Rhode Island
College of Nursing
Graduate Program in Nurse-Midwifery
White Hall
Kingston, RI 02881-0814
Phone: (401)874-5327
Email: jmercer@uri.edu
Website: http://www.uri.edu/nursing/programs/msmidwife.html
Judith Mercer, Director

South Carolina

★ 27588 ★ Medical University of South Carolina
College of Nursing
Nurse-Midwifery Graduate Program
99 Jonathan Lucas St.
Charleston, SC 29403
Phone: (843)792-4642 **Fax:** (843)792-1741
Email: hickeym@musc.edu
Website: http://www.musc.edu
Marcella Hickey, Director

Tennessee

★ 27589 ★ Vanderbilt University
School of Nursing
Nurse-Midwifery Graduate Program
102 Godchaux Hall
21st Ave. S
Nashville, TN 37240-0008
Phone: (615)322-3800
Email: vusn_admissions@mcmail.vanderbilt.edu
Website: http://www.mc.vanderbilt.edu/nursing
Barbara Petersen, EdD, Director

Texas

★ 27590 ★ Baylor College of Medicine
Nurse-Midwifery Graduate Program
6550 Fannin, Ste. 954
Houston, TX 77030
Phone: (713)793-8895 **Fax:** (713)793-8647
Email: sbarry@bcm.tmc.edu
Website: http://www.bcm.tmc.edu/midwifery
Susan E. Barry, Director

★ 27591 ★ University of Texas Southwestern Medical Center at Dallas
Parkland School of Nurse-Midwifery
Nurse-Midwifery Certificate Program
5201 Harry Hines Blvd.
MS 6107A
Dallas, TX 75235
Phone: (214)590-2580 **Fax:** (214)590-0436
Email: mbruck@parknet.pmh.org
Website: http://www.swmed.edu/home_pages/parkland/midwifery/midwifehome.html
Mary C. Brucker, Director

★ 27592 ★ University of Texas, El Paso/ Texas Tech University
Department of OB/GYN
Nurse-Midwifery Graduate Program
Texas Tech University Health Sciences Center
4800 Alberta Ave.
El Paso, TX 79905
Phone: (915)545-6490
Email: midwifery@ttmcelp.ttuhsc.edu
Website: http://www.nurse.utep.edu/nursing/degree.programs/midwife.htm
Carlene Nelson, PhD, Director

★ 27593 ★ University of Texas Medical Branch, Galveston
School of Nursing
Collaborative Nurse-Midwifery Graduate Education Program
1100 Mechanic
Galveston, TX 77555-1029
Phone: (409)772-8347
Email: bcamune@utmb.edu
Website: http://www.utmb.edu
Barbara Camune, Director

Utah

★ 27594 ★ University of Utah
College of Nursing
Nurse-Midwifery Graduate Program
10 South 2000 East Front
Salt Lake City, UT 84112-5880
Phone: (801)581-8274
Email: jane.dyer@nurse.utah.edu
Website: http://medstat.med.utah.edu/nmw
Jane Dyer, Director

Virginia

★ 27595 ★ Shenandoah University
Division of Nursing
Nurse-Midwifery Graduate Program
1775 N Sector Ct.
Winchester, VA 22601
Phone: (540)678-4382
Email: jfehr@su.edu
Website: http://www.su.edu/nursing/mas_mid.html
Juliana Fehr, PhD, Director

Washington

★ 27596 ★ University of Washington
School of Nursing
Nurse-Midwifery Graduate Program
Box 357262
Seattle, WA 98195-7262
Phone: (206)543-8241
Email: midwife@u.washington.edu
Website: http://www.son.washington.edu/departments/fcn/midwifery
Aileen Macharen, PhD, Director

Wisconsin

★ 27597 ★ Marquette University
College of Nursing
Graduate Program in Nurse-Midwifery
PO Box 1881
Milwaukee, WI 53201-1881
Phone: (414)288-3842
Email: leona.vandevusse@marquette.edu
Website: http://www.mu.edu
Leona VandeVusse, PhD, Director

Nursing

The institutions listed below offer programs in nursing. For more information, contact the National League for Nursing, 61 Broadway, New York, NY 10006, (800)669-1656, http://www.nln.org/.

Alabama

★ 27598 ★ Auburn University, Montgomery
School of Nursing
PO Box 244023
Montgomery, AL 36124-4023
Phone: (334)244-3863 **Fax:** (334)244-3243
Email: lstutheit@mickey.aum.edu
Website: http://www.aum.edu
Lorinda B. Stutheit, Contact
Fnded: 1967. **Degrees Offered:** BSN.

★ 27599 ★ Jacksonville State University
College of Nursing and Health Sciences
Graduate Studies
700 Pelham Rd. N
Jacksonville, AL 36265-1602
Phone: (256)782-5276 **Fax:** (256)782-5406
Email: bhembree@jsucc.jsu.edu
Website: http://www.jsu.edu/depart/nursing
Dr. Beth Hembree, Contact
Fnded: 1883. **Degrees Offered:** BSN, MSN.

★ 27600 ★ Samford University
Ida V. Moffett School of Nursing
800 Lakeshore Dr.
Birmingham, AL 35229
Phone: (205)726-2626 **Fax:** (205)726-2219
Email: gsmcdani@samford.edu
Website: http://www.samford.edu
Dr. Gretchen McDaniel, Contact

Fnded: 1841. **Degrees Offered:** BSN, MSN, MSN/MBA.

★ 27601 ★ Spring Hill College
Division of Nursing
4000 Dauphin St.
Mobile, AL 36608
Phone: (334)380-4492 **Fax:** (334)380-4495
Email: charrison@shc.edu
Website: http://faculty.shc.edu/nursing
Dr. Carol Harrison, Contact
Fnded: 1830. **Degrees Offered:** BSN.

★ 27602 ★ Troy State University
School of Nursing
400 Pell Ave.
Troy, AL 36082
Phone: (334)670-3428 **Fax:** (334)670-3744
Email: shalley@trojan.troyst.edu
Website: http://www.troyst.edu
Susan Halley, Contact
Fnded: 1887. **Degrees Offered:** BSN, MSN.

★ 27603 ★ Tuskegee University
Program in Nursing
Basil O'Connor Hall, Rm. 209
Tuskegee, AL 36083
Phone: (334)727-8382 **Fax:** (334)727-5461
Email: dholeman@acd.tusk.edu
Website: http://www.tusk.edu
Dr. Doris S. Holeman, Contact
Fnded: 1881. **Degrees Offered:** BSN.

★ 27604 ★ University of Alabama
Capstone College of Nursing
Nursing Student Recruitment
PO Box 870358
Tuscaloosa, AL 35487-0358
Phone: (205)348-6640 **Fax:** (205)348-5559
Email: pmcculla@bama.ua.edu
Website: http://nursing.ua.edu
Pat McCullar, Contact
Fnded: 1831. **Degrees Offered:** BSN, MSN, MSN/MA, MSN/MBA.

★ 27605 ★ University of Alabama, Birmingham
School of Nursing
1530 3rd Ave. S, NB 108
Birmingham, AL 35294-1210
Phone: (205)934-6787 **Fax:** (205)975-6142
Email: galfob@son.uab.edu
Website: http://www.uab.edu/son/
Dr. Elizabeth S. Galford, Contact
Fnded: 1969. **Degrees Offered:** BSN, MSN, MSN/MPH, PhD.

★ 27606 ★ University of Alabama, Huntsville
College of Nursing
Nursing Student Affairs
College of Nursing
Huntsville, AL 35899
Phone: (256)824-6742 **Fax:** (256)824-6026
Email: wilsonol@uah.edu
Website: http://www.uah.edu/nursing
Lavan Wilson, Contact
Fnded: 1950. **Degrees Offered:** BSN, MSN.

★ 27607 ★ University of Mobile
School of Nursing
PO Box 13220
Mobile, AL 36663-0220
Phone: (251)442-2227 **Fax:** (251)442-2520
Email: elizabethflanagan@free.umobile.edu
Website: http://www.umobile.edu/
Dr. Elizabeth Flanagan, Contact
Fnded: 1961. **Degrees Offered:** BSN, MSN.

★ 27608 ★ University of North Alabama
College of Nursing and Allied Health
Florence, AL 35632
Phone: (256)765-4311 **Fax:** (256)765-4935
Website: http://www.una.edu/
Fnded: 1830. **Degrees Offered:** BSN.

★ 27609 ★ University of South Alabama
College of Nursing
USA Springhill CON 1004
Mobile, AL 36688-0002
Phone: (251)434-3410 **Fax:** (251)434-3413
Email: rrhodes@usouthal.edu
Website: http://usaonline.southalabama.edu
Dr. Rosemary S. Rhodes, Contact
Fnded: 1963. **Degrees Offered:** BSN, MSN.

Alberta

★ 27610 ★ Athabasca University
Centre for Nursing and Health Sciences
One University Dr.
Athabasca, AB, Canada T9S 3A3
Free: 800-788-9041 **Fax:** (780)675-6468
Email: marge@athabascau.ca
Website: http://www.athabascau.ca/cnhs/
Dr. Margaret Edwards, Contact
Fnded: 1970. **Degrees Offered:** BN, MHS.

★ 27611 ★ University of Alberta
Faculty of Nursing
Edmonton, AB, Canada T6G 2G3
Phone: (780)492-6251 **Fax:** (780)492-6029
Email: elaine.carswell@ualberta.ca
Website: http://www.us-nursing.ualberta.ca/
Elaine Carswell, Contact
Fnded: 1906. **Degrees Offered:** BSCN, MN, PhD.

★ 27612 ★ University of Calgary
Faculty of Nursing
2500 University Dr. NW
Calgary, AB, Canada T2N 1N4
Phone: (403)220-7288 **Fax:** (403)284-4803
Email: pjolly@ucalgary.ca
Website: http://www.ucalgary.ca/nu
Pat Jolly, Contact
Fnded: 1945. **Degrees Offered:** BN, MN, PhD.

★ 27613 ★ University of Lethbridge
School of Health Sciences
4401 University Dr.
Lethbridge, AB, Canada T1K 3M4
Phone: (403)329-2649 **Fax:** (403)329-2668
Email: tom.samuel@uleth.ca
Website: http://home.uleth.ca/hlsc/
Tom Samuel, Contact
Fnded: 1967. **Degrees Offered:** BN, M SC.

Arizona

★ 27614 ★ Arizona State University
College of Nursing
Office of Student Services
Box 872602
Tempe, AZ 85287-2602
Phone: (480)965-2987 **Fax:** (480)965-8468
Email: maurine.lee@asu.edu
Website: http://nursing.asu.edu
Maurine Lee, Contact
Fnded: 1885. **Degrees Offered:** BSN, MS, MS/MHA

★ 27615 ★ Grand Canyon University
Samaritan College of Nursing
3300 W Camelback Rd.
Phoenix, AZ 85017
Phone: (602)589-2431 **Fax:** (602)589-2098
Email: crussell@grand-canyon.edu
Website: http://www.grand-canyon.edu
Dr. Cynthia Russell, Contact
Fnded: 1949. **Degrees Offered:** BSN.

★ 27616 ★ Northern Arizona University
Department of Nursing
Box 15035
Flagstaff, AZ 86011
Phone: (928)523-6717 **Fax:** (928)523-7171
Website: http://www.nau.edu/hp/dept/nurse
Fnded: 1899. **Degrees Offered:** BSN, MS.

★ 27617 ★ University of Arizona
College of Nursing
1305 N Martin St.
PO Box 210203
Tucson, AZ 85721-0203
Phone: (520)626-3808 **Fax:** (520)626-6424
Email: abeaudrie@nursing.arizona.edu
Website: http://www.nursing.arizona.edu
Alan Beaudrie, Contact
Fnded: 1885. **Degrees Offered:** BSN, MS, PhD.

★ 27618 ★ University of Phoenix, Phoenix Campus
Health Care Sciences and Nursing
4635 E Elwood St.
Phoenix, AZ 85040-1958
Phone: (480)804-7600
Website: http://www.phoenix.edu/
Fnded: 1976. **Degrees Offered:** BSN, MSN, MSN/MBA.

★ 27619 ★ University of Phoenix, Southern Arizona Campus
College of Health Care Sciences and Nursing
5099 E Grant Rd.
Tucson, AZ 85712
Phone: (520)881-6512
Website: http://www.phoenix.edu/
Degrees Offered: BSN, MSN, MSN/MBA.

Arkansas

★ 27620 ★ Arkansas State University
Department of Nursing
PO Box 910
State University, AR 72467-0069
Phone: (870)972-3074 **Fax:** (870)972-2954
Email: pskorga@astate.edu
Website: http://www.conhp.astate.edu/Nursing/
Dr. Phyllis Skorga, Contact
Fnded: 1909. **Degrees Offered:** BSN, MSN

★ 27621 ★ Arkansas Tech University
Program in Nursing
224 G Dean Hall
Russellville, AR 72801
Phone: (479)968-0383 **Fax:** (479)968-0219
Email: rebecca.burris@mail.atu.edu
Website: http://www.atu.edu
Dr. Rebecca Francis Burris, Contact
Fnded: 1909. **Degrees Offered:** BSN.

★ 27622 ★ Harding University
College of Nursing
PO Box 12265
Searcy, AR 72149-0001
Phone: (501)279-4682 **Fax:** (501)305-8902
Email: dkemper@harding.edu
Website: http://www.harding.edu
Deborah G. Kemper, Contact
Fnded: 1924. **Degrees Offered:** BSN, MSN.

★ 27623 ★ Henderson State University
Department of Nursing
Box 7803
1100 Henderson St.
Arkadelphia, AR 71999-0001
Phone: (870)230-5015 **Fax:** (870)230-5390
Website: http://www.hsu.edu
Fnded: 1890. **Degrees Offered:** BSN.

★ 27624 ★ University of Arkansas, Fayetteville
Eleanor Mann School of Nursing
217 Ozark Hall
Fayetteville, AR 72701
Phone: (501)575-3907 **Fax:** (501)575-3218
Email: neighbo@uark.edu
Website: http://www.uark.edu/coehp
Dr. Marianne Neighbors, Contact
Fnded: 1871. **Degrees Offered:** BSN.

★ 27625 ★ University of Arkansas, Monticello
Division of Nursing
PO Box 3606
Monticello, AR 71656
Phone: (870)460-1069 **Fax:** (870)460-1969
Email: eustace@uamont.edu
Website: http://uamont.edu
Dr. Larry W. Eustace, Contact
Fnded: 1909. **Degrees Offered:** BSN.

★ 27626 ★ University of Arkansas, Pine Bluff
Department of Nursing
1200 University Dr.
Mail Slot 4973
Pine Bluff, AR 71601
Phone: (870)575-8220 **Fax:** (870)575-8229
Email: henderson_i@uapb.edu
Website: http://www.uapb.com
Dr. Irene T. Henderson, Contact
Fnded: 1873. **Degrees Offered:** BSN.

★ 27627 ★ University of Central Arkansas
Department of Nursing
201 S Donaghey Ave.
Conway, AR 72035
Phone: (501)450-3119 **Fax:** (501)450-5503
Email: annm@mail.uca.edu
Website: http://www.uca.edu/divisions/academic/nursing/
Ann Mattison, Contact
Fnded: 1907. **Degrees Offered:** BSN, MSN.

British Columbia

★ 27628 ★ British Columbia Institute of Technology
School of Health Sciences
3700 Willingdon Ave.
Burnaby, BC, Canada V5G 3H2
Phone: (604)434-1610 **Fax:** (604)432-1816
Website: http://www.health.bcit.ca/nursing/
Fnded: 1964. **Degrees Offered:** BSN.

★ 27629 ★ Kwantlen University College
Faculty of Community and Health Sciences
12666 72nd Ave.
Surrey, BC, Canada V3W 2M8
Phone: (604)599-2234
Email: heather.mcmann@kwantlen.ca
Website: http://www.kwantlen.bc.ca/
Heather McMann, Contact
Degrees Offered: BSN.

★ 27630 ★ Malaspina University-College
Department of Nursing
900 5th St.
Nanaimo, BC, Canada V9R 5S5
Phone: (250)740-6410
Website: http://www.mala.bc.ca/www/discover/health/index.htm
Fnded: 1969. **Degrees Offered:** BSCN.

★ 27631 ★ Okanagan University College
Nursing Department
3333 College Way
Kelowna, BC, Canada V1V 1V7
Phone: (250)762-5445 **Fax:** (250)470-6085
Email: dcallaghan@ouc.bc.ca
Website: http://www.ouc.bc.ca/
Doris Callaghan, Contact
Degrees Offered: BSN.

★ 27632 ★ Trinity Western University
Department of Nursing
7600 Glover Rd.
Langley, BC, Canada V2Y 1Y1
Phone: (604)888-7511 **Fax:** (604)513-2018
Email: pesut@twu.ca
Website: http://www.twu.ca/
Barbara Pesut, Contact
Fnded: 1962. **Degrees Offered:** BSCN.

★ 27633 ★ University of British Columbia
School of Nursing
T201-2211 Wesbrook Mall
Vancouver, BC, Canada V6T 2B5
Phone: (604)822-7498 **Fax:** (604)822-7466
Email: hilton@nursing.ubc.ca
Website: http://www.nursing.ubc.ca
Ann Hilton, Contact
Fnded: 1915. **Degrees Offered:** BSN, MSN, PhD.

★ 27634 ★ University College of the Cariboo
School of Nursing
PO Box 3010
900 College Dr.
Kamloops, BC, Canada V2C 5N3
Phone: (250)828-5435 **Fax:** (250)828-5450
Website: http://www.cariboo.bc.ca/nursing/index.html
Fnded: 1970. **Degrees Offered:** BSN.

★ 27635 ★ University of Northern British Columbia
Nursing Programme
3333 University Way
Prince George, BC, Canada V2N 4Z9
Phone: (250)960-5645 **Fax:** (250)960-5744
Email: fayled@unbc.ca
Website: http://www.unbc.ca/
Deanna Fayle, Contact
Degrees Offered: BSN.

★ 27636 ★ University of Victoria
School of Nursing
PO Box 1700
Victoria, BC, Canada V8W 2Y2
Phone: (250)721-7961 **Fax:** (250)721-6231
Email: jgillie@uvic.ca
Website: http://web.uvic.ca/nurs/
Joan Gillie, Contact
Fnded: 1963. **Degrees Offered:** BSN, MN, PhD.

California

★ 27637 ★ Azusa Pacific University
School of Nursing
901 E Alosta Ave.
Azusa, CA 91702
Phone: (626)815-5386 **Fax:** (626)815-5414
Website: http://www.apu.edu/nursing/grad/
Fnded: 1899. **Degrees Offered:** BSN, MSN.

★ 27638 ★ Biola University
Department of Nursing
13800 Biola Ave.
La Mirada, CA 90639
Phone: (562)903-4850 **Fax:** (562)903-4803
Email: cindy.westcott@biola.edu
Website: http://www.biola.edu/
Cynthia L. Westcott, Contact
Fnded: 1908. **Degrees Offered:** BS

★ 27639 ★ California State University, Bakersfield
Program in Nursing
9001 Stockdale Hwy.
Bakersfield, CA 93311-1099
Phone: (661)664-2093 **Fax:** (661)665-6347
Email: cmeares@csub.edu
Website: http://www.csubak.edu
Dr. Candace Meares, Contact
Fnded: 1970. **Degrees Offered:** BSN, MSN.

★ 27640 ★ California State University, Chico
School of Nursing
Chico, CA 95929-0200
Phone: (530)898-6207 **Fax:** (530)898-4363
Email: syoung@facultypo.csuchico.edu
Website: http://www.csuchico.edu/nurs/nurs.html
Shelley Young, Contact
Fnded: 1887. **Degrees Offered:** BSN, MSN.

★ 27641 ★ California State University, Dominguez Hills
Program in Nursing
Student Services Center
James Welch Hall, 3rd Fl.
Carson, CA 90747
Free: 800-344-5484 **Fax:** (310)516-3542
Email: sohadvising@soh.csudh.edu
Website: http://www.csudh.edu/soh/don/index.htm
Fnded: 1960. **Degrees Offered:** BSN, MSN.

★ 27642 ★ California State University, Fresno
Department of Nursing
2345 E San Ramon Ave.
Fresno, CA 93740-8031
Phone: (559)278-2041 **Fax:** (559)278-6360
Email: michael_russler@csufresno.edu
Website: http://www.csufresno.edu
Mike Russler, Contact
Fnded: 1911. **Degrees Offered:** BSN, MSN.

★ 27643 ★ California State University, Fullerton
Department of Nursing
EC-199
PO Box 6868
Fullerton, CA 92834-6868
Phone: (714)278-3336 **Fax:** (714)278-3338
Email: nursing@fullerton.edu
Website: http://my.fullerton.edu/nursing/
Fnded: 1957. **Degrees Offered:** BSN, MSN.

★ 27644 ★ California State University, Hayward
Department of Nursing and Health Sciences
25800 Carlos Bee Blvd.
Hayward, CA 94542
Phone: (510)885-3481 **Fax:** (510)885-2156
Email: lcondit@csuhayward.edu
Website: http://www.csuhayward.edu
Lynn Condit, Contact

Fnded: 1957. **Degrees Offered:** BSN.

★ 27645 ★ California State University, Long Beach
Department of Nursing
1250 Bellflower Blvd.
Long Beach, CA 90840-0119
Phone: (562)985-4473 **Fax:** (562)985-2382
Email: akliachk@csulb.edu
Website: http://www.csulb.edu/~nursing/
Alison Kliachko-Trafas, Contact
Fnded: 1949. **Degrees Offered:** BSN, MSN, MSN/MPH.

★ 27646 ★ California State University, Los Angeles
Department of Nursing
5151 State University Dr.
Los Angeles, CA 90032
Phone: (323)343-4700 **Fax:** (323)343-6454
Email: jpapen@calstatela.edu
Website: http://www.calstatela.edu/dept/nursing
Dr. Judith Papenhausen, Contact
Fnded: 1947. **Degrees Offered:** BS, MS.

★ 27647 ★ California State University, Northridge
Nursing Program
18111 Nordhoff St.
Northridge, CA 91330-8285
Phone: (818)677-2423 **Fax:** (818)677-2045
Email: ellen.mcfadden@csun.edu
Website: http://www.csun.edu
Dr. Ellen McFadden, Contact
Fnded: 1958. **Degrees Offered:** BSN.

★ 27648 ★ California State University, Sacramento
Division of Nursing
6000 J St.
Sacramento, CA 95819-6096
Phone: (916)278-7298 **Fax:** (916)278-6311
Email: jarviska@csus.edu
Website: http://www.csus.edu/
Kathleen Jarvis, Contact
Fnded: 1947. **Degrees Offered:** BS, MS.

★ 27649 ★ California State University, San Bernardino
Department of Nursing
5500 University Pkwy.
San Bernardino, CA 92407
Phone: (909)880-5380 **Fax:** (909)880-7089
Email: slloyd@csusb.edu
Website: http://nursing.csusb.edu
Dr. Susan Lloyd, Contact
Fnded: 1965. **Degrees Offered:** BSN, MSN.

★ 27650 ★ California State University, Stanislaus
Department of Nursing
801 W Monte Vista Ave.
Turlock, CA 95382
Phone: (209)667-3141 **Fax:** (209)667-3690
Email: iworthington@csustan.edu
Website: http://www.csustan.edu/Nursing/index.htm
Ilene M. Worthington, Contact
Fnded: 1957. **Degrees Offered:** BSN.

★ 27651 ★ Dominican University of California
Division of Health Sciences
Nursing Program
50 Acacia Ave.
San Rafael, CA 94901-2298
Phone: (415)458-3754 **Fax:** (415)485-3214
Email: lcrivello@dominican.edu
Website: http://www.dominican.edu/
Lorrie Crivello, Contact
Fnded: 1890. **Degrees Offered:** BSN, MSN.

★ 27652 ★ Holy Names College
Department of Nursing
3500 Mountain Blvd.
Oakland, CA 94619-1699
Phone: (510)436-1351
Email: adulted@hnc.edu
Website: http://www.hnc.edu/site/academic/programs/adult_undergradprog/nurs.html
Fnded: 1868. **Degrees Offered:** BSN, MSN.

★ 27653 ★ Humboldt State University
Department of Nursing
1 Harpst St.
Arcata, CA 95521
Phone: (707)826-3215 **Fax:** (707)826-5141
Email: nurs@humboldt.edu
Website: http://www.humboldt.edu/~nurs
Dr. Betty J. Jensen, Contact
Fnded: 1913. **Degrees Offered:** BSN.

★ 27654 ★ Loma Linda University
School of Nursing
Loma Linda, CA 92350
Phone: (909)558-8061 **Fax:** (909)558-4134
Email: jbates@sn.llu.edu
Website: http://www.llu.edu/llu/nursing/
Joyce Bates, Contact
Fnded: 1905. **Degrees Offered:** BS, MS, MS/MA, MS/MPH, PhD.

★ 27655 ★ Mount Saint Mary's College
Department of Nursing
12001 Chalon Rd.
Los Angeles, CA 90049-1599
Free: 800-999-9893
Email: admissions@msmc.la.edu
Website: http://www.msmc.la.edu/nursing/
Fnded: 1925. **Degrees Offered:** BSN, MSN.

★ 27656 ★ National University
Department of Nursing
11255 N Torrey Pines Rd.
La Jolla, CA 92037
Free: 800-628-8648 **Fax:** (858)642-8715
Email: rvainer@nu.edu
Website: http://www.nu.edu/nursing-handbook
Renata Vainer, Contact
Fnded: 1971. **Degrees Offered:** BSN.

★ 27657 ★ Pacific Union College
Department of Nursing
One Angwin Ave.
Angwin, CA 94508
Phone: (707)965-7262 **Fax:** (707)965-6499
Email: jlpearce@puc.edu
Website: http://www.puc.edu
Dr. Julia L. Pearce, Contact
Fnded: 1882. **Degrees Offered:** BSN.

★ 27658 ★ Point Loma Nazarene University
Department of Nursing
3900 Lomaland Dr.
San Diego, CA 92106-2899
Phone: (619)849-2236 **Fax:** (619)849-2672
Email: dcrummy@ptloma.edu
Website: http://www.ptloma.edu/nursing
Dottie E. Crummy, Contact
Fnded: 1902. **Degrees Offered:** BSN, MSN.

★ 27659 ★ Saint Mary's College of California
Samuel Merritt-Saint Mary's Intercollegiate Nursing Consortium
Moraga, CA
Email: admission@samuelmerritt.edu
Website: http://www.stmarys-ca.edu/
Fnded: 1863. **Degrees Offered:** BSN, MSN.

★ 27660 ★ Samuel Merritt College
Samuel Merritt-Saint Mary's Intercollegiate Nursing Consortium
370 Hawthorne Ave.
Oakland, CA 94609
Phone: (510)869-6576 **Free:** 800-607-6377
Fax: (510)869-6525
Email: admission@samuelmerritt.edu
Website: http://www.samuelmerritt.edu
Fnded: 1909. **Degrees Offered:** BSN, MSN.

★ 27661 ★ San Diego State University
School of Nursing
5500 Campanile Dr.
San Diego, CA 92182-4158
Phone: (619)594-2540 **Fax:** (619)594-2765
Email: rreed@mail.sdsu.edu
Website: http://www-rohan.sdsu.edu/chhs/nursing/index.html
Dr. Richard C. Reed, Contact
Fnded: 1897. **Degrees Offered:** BSN, MSN.

★ 27662 ★ San Francisco State University
School of Nursing
1600 Holloway Ave.
371 Burk Hall
San Francisco, CA 94132-4161
Phone: (415)338-1802 **Fax:** (415)338-0555
Email: anichols@sfsu.edu
Website: http://www.sfsu.edu/
Dr. Amy Nichols, Contact
Fnded: 1899. **Degrees Offered:** BSN, MSN.

★ 27663 ★ San Jose State University
School of Nursing
1 Washington Sq.
San Jose, CA 95192
Phone: (408)924-3144 **Fax:** (408)924-3135
Email: connollydr@son.sjsu.edu
Website: http://www.sjsu.edu
Dr. Phyllis Connolly, Contact
Fnded: 1857. **Degrees Offered:** BS, MS.

★ 27664 ★ Sonoma State University
Department of Nursing
1801 E Cotati Ave.
Rohnert Park, CA 94928
Phone: (707)664-2465 **Fax:** (707)664-2653
Email: becky.cohen@sonoma.edu
Website: http://www.sonoma.edu/nursing
Becky Schroeder Cohen, Contact
Fnded: 1960. **Degrees Offered:** BSN, MSN

★ 27665 ★ University of California, Los Angeles
School of Nursing
Box 951702
Los Angeles, CA 90095-1702
Phone: (310)825-7181 **Fax:** (310)206-7433
Email: sonsaff@ucla.edu
Website: http://www.nursing.ucla.edu/son
Kathy Scrivner, Contact
Fnded: 1919. **Degrees Offered:** BS, MSN, MSN/MBA, PhD.

★ 27666 ★ **University of California, San Francisco**
School of Nursing
2 Kirkham St., Rm. N319X
San Francisco, CA 94143-0602
Phone: (415)476-1435 **Fax:** (415)476-9707
Email: jeff.kilmer@nursing.ucsf.edu
Website: http://nurseweb.ucsf.edu
Jeff Kilmer, Contact
Fnded: 1864. **Degrees Offered:** MS, PhD.

★ 27667 ★ **University of Phoenix, Northern California Campus**
College of Health Care Sciences and Nursing
Pleasanton, CA
Phone: 877—4-STUDENT
Website: http://www.phoenix.edu/
Degrees Offered: BSN, MSN, MSN/MBA.

★ 27668 ★ **University of Phoenix, Sacramento Campus**
College of Health Care Sciences and Nursing
Sacramento, CA
Free: 800-266-2107
Website: http://www.phoenix.edu/
Degrees Offered: BSN, MSN, MSN/MBA.

★ 27669 ★ **University of Phoenix, San Diego Campus**
College of Health Care Sciences and Nursing
San Diego, CA
Free: 888-867-4636
Website: http://www.phoenix.edu/sandiego/
Degrees Offered: BSN, MSN, MSN/MBA.

★ 27670 ★ **University of Phoenix, Southern California Campus**
College of Health Care Sciences and Nursing
10540 Talbert Ave.
West Tower, Ste. 120
Fountain Valley, CA 92708
Free: 800-697-8223
Website: http://www.phoenix.edu/
Degrees Offered: BSN, MSN, MSN/MBA.

★ 27671 ★ **University of San Diego**
Hahn School of Nursing and Health Sciences
Student Services
5998 Alcala Pk.
San Diego, CA 92110-2492
Phone: (619)260-4548 **Fax:** (619)260-6814
Email: cmm@sandiego.edu
Website: http://www.sandiego.edu/nursing
Cathleen Mumper, Contact
Fnded: 1949. **Degrees Offered:** BSN, MSN, MSN/MBA, PhD.

★ 27672 ★ **University of San Francisco**
School of Nursing
2130 Fulton St.
Cowell Hall 110
San Francisco, CA 94117-1080
Phone: (415)422-2961 **Fax:** (415)422-6877
Email: reedr@usfca.edu
Website: http://www.usfca.edu/
Robert J. Reed, Contact
Fnded: 1855. **Degrees Offered:** BSN, MSN, MSN/MS.

★ 27673 ★ **University of Southern California**
Department of Nursing
1540 Alcazar St.
CHP 22
Los Angeles, CA 90089
Phone: (323)442-2012
Email: mgold@usc.edu
Website: http://uscnurse.usc.edu/
Dr. Michele Gold, Contact
Fnded: 1880. **Degrees Offered:** MSN.

★ 27674 ★ **Western University of Health Sciences**
College of Graduate Nursing
309 E 2nd St.
College Plaza
Pomona, CA 91766
Phone: (909)469-5523 **Fax:** (909)469-5521
Website: http://www.westernu.edu/cogn.html
Fnded: 1975. **Degrees Offered:** MSN.

Colorado

★ 27675 ★ **Mesa State College**
Department of Nursing and Radiologic Sciences
1100 North Ave.
Grand Junction, CO 81501
Phone: (970)248-1774 **Fax:** (970)248-1133
Website: http://www.mesastate.edu/
Judy Goodhart, Contact
Fnded: 1925. **Degrees Offered:** BSN.

★ 27676 ★ **Metropolitan State College of Denver**
Department of Health Professions
Campus Box 33
PO Box 173362
Denver, CO 80217-3362
Phone: (303)556-8415 **Fax:** (303)556-3439
Email: hillsro@mscd.edu
Website: http://www.mscd.edu/~nursing/
Roberta Hills, Contact
Fnded: 1963. **Degrees Offered:** BS.

★ 27677 ★ **Regis University**
Department of Nursing
3333 Regis Blvd., G-9
Denver, CO 80221-1099
Phone: (303)458-4938 **Fax:** (303)964-5533
Email: acampbel@regis.edu
Website: http://www.regis.edu
Allison Campbell, Contact
Fnded: 1877. **Degrees Offered:** BSN, MS.

★ 27678 ★ **University of Colorado Health Sciences Center**
School of Nursing
4200 E 9th Ave., Box C288-6
Denver, CO 80262
Phone: (303)315-5592 **Fax:** (303)315-5648
Email: chris.muller@uchsc.edu
Website: http://www.uchsc.edu/nursing
Christine Muller, Contact
Fnded: 1883. **Degrees Offered:** BS, MS, MSN/MBA, PhD.

★ 27679 ★ **University of Colorado, Colorado Springs**
Beth-El College of Nursing and Health Sciences
1420 Austin Bluffs Pkwy.
PO Box 7150
Colorado Springs, CO 80933-7150
Phone: (719)262-4411 **Fax:** (719)262-4416
Email: klasala@uccs.edu
Website: http://www.uccs.edu
Dr. Kathy LaSala, Contact
Fnded: 1965. **Degrees Offered:** BSN, MSN.

★ 27680 ★ **University of Northern Colorado**
School of Nursing
Box 125
Greeley, CO 80639
Phone: (303)351-2663 **Fax:** (303)351-1707
Email: judy.richter@unco.edu
Website: http://www.unco.edu/HHS/son/son.htm
Dr. Judy Richter, Contact
Fnded: 1890. **Degrees Offered:** BS, MS.

★ 27681 ★ **University of Phoenix, Colorado Campus**
College of Health Care Sciences and Nursing
10004 Park Meadow Dr.
Lone Tree, CO 80124-9909
Phone: (303)600-1307
Website: http://www.phoenix.edu/
Degrees Offered: BSN, MSN, MSN/MBA.

★ 27682 ★ **University of Phoenix—Southern Colorado Campus**
College of Health Care Sciences and Nursing
Colorado Springs, CO
Phone: (719)599-5282
Website: http://www.phoenix.edu/
Degrees Offered: BSN, MSN, MSN/MBA.

★ 27683 ★ **University of Southern Colorado**
Department of Nursing
2220 Bonforte Blvd.
Pueblo, CO 81001
Phone: (719)549-2100 **Fax:** (719)549-2732
Email: steen@uscolo.edu
Website: http://www.uscolo.edu
Dr. Melva J. Steen, Contact
Fnded: 1933. **Degrees Offered:** BSN.

Connecticut

★ 27684 ★ **Central Connecticut State University**
Department of Health and Human Service Professions
1615 Stanley St.
New Britain, CT 06050-4010
Phone: (860)832-2154 **Fax:** (860)832-2188
Email: williamsmj@ccsu.edu
Website: http://www.ccsu.edu
Dr. Mary Jane Williams, Contact
Fnded: 1849. **Degrees Offered:** BSN.

★ 27685 ★ **Fairfield University**
School of Nursing
1073 N Benson Rd.
Fairfield, CT 06824
Phone: (203)254-4000 **Fax:** (203)254-4126
Website: http://www.fairfield.edu/academic/nursing/
Fnded: 1942. **Degrees Offered:** BS, MSN.

★ 27686 ★ **Quinnipiac College**
Department of Nursing
275 Mount Carmel Ave.
Hamden, CT 06518
Phone: (203)582-8672 **Fax:** (203)582-3443
Email: graduate@quinnipiac.edu
Website: http://www.quinnipiac.edu
Scott Farber, Contact
Fnded: 1929. **Degrees Offered:** BS, MSN.

★ 27687 ★ Sacred Heart University
Program in Nursing
5151 Park Ave.
Fairfield, CT 06432
Phone: (203)371-7715 **Fax:** (203)365-7662
Email: halucha@sacredheart.edu
Website: http://nursing.sacredheart.edu/
Alma C. Haluch, Contact
Fnded: 1963. **Degrees Offered:** BS, MSN, MSN/MBA.

★ 27688 ★ Saint Joseph College
Department of Nursing
1678 Asylum Ave.
West Hartford, CT 06117-2700
Phone: (860)231-5316 **Fax:** (860)231-8396
Email: ndrew@sjc.edu
Website: http://www.sjc.edu
Dr. Nancy Drew, Contact
Fnded: 1932. **Degrees Offered:** BS, MS.

★ 27689 ★ Southern Connecticut State University
Department of Nursing
501 Crescent St.
New Haven, CT 06515
Phone: (203)392-6482 **Fax:** (203)392-6493
Email: killion@scsu.ctstateu.edu
Website: http://www.southernct.edu/departments/nursing
Dr. Susan Killion, Contact
Fnded: 1893. **Degrees Offered:** BSN, MSN.

★ 27690 ★ University of Connecticut
School of Nursing
Office of Academic Advising Services
231 Glenbrook Rd.
Unit 2026
Storrs, CT 06269-2026
Phone: (860)486-1968 **Fax:** (860)486-0906
Email: nuradm11@uconnvm.uconn.edu
Website: http://www.nursing.uconn.edu
Fnded: 1881. **Degrees Offered:** BS, MS, MSN/MBA, MSN/MPH, PhD.

★ 27691 ★ University of Hartford
College of Education, Nursing and Health Professions
200 Bloomfield Ave.
West Hartford, CT 06117-1599
Phone: (860)768-5116 **Fax:** (860)768-5346
Email: mhall@hartford.edu
Website: http://www.hartford.edu/enhp
Marlene J. Hall, Contact
Fnded: 1877. **Degrees Offered:** BSN, MSN, MSN/MSOB.

★ 27692 ★ Western Connecticut State University
Department of Nursing
181 White St.
Danbury, CT 06810
Phone: (203)837-8557 **Fax:** (203)837-8550
Email: piscopob@wcsu.edu
Website: http://www.wcsu.edu
Dr. Barbara Piscopo, Contact
Fnded: 1903. **Degrees Offered:** BSN, MSN.

★ 27693 ★ Yale University
School of Nursing
100 Church St. S
PO Box 9740
New Haven, CT 06536-0740
Phone: (203)737-2557 **Fax:** (203)737-5409
Email: sharon.sanderson@yale.edu
Website: http://nursing.yale.edu
Sharon Sanderson, Contact
Fnded: 1701. **Degrees Offered:** DN SC, MSN, MSN/MBA, MSN/MPH.

Delaware

★ 27694 ★ Delaware State University
Department of Nursing
1200 N DuPont Hwy.
Dover, DE 19901-2277
Phone: (302)857-6750 **Fax:** (302)857-6753
Email: mwatkins@dsc.edu
Website: http://www.dsc.edu/
Dr. Mary P. Watkins, Contact
Fnded: 1891. **Degrees Offered:** BSN.

★ 27695 ★ University of Delaware
Department of Nursing
391 McDowell Hall
Newark, DE 19716
Phone: (302)831-1255 **Fax:** (302)831-2382
Email: ud-gradnursing@udel.edu
Website: http://www.udel.edu/nursing/udnursing.html
Elizabeth Bonavita, Contact
Fnded: 1743. **Degrees Offered:** BSN, MSN.

★ 27696 ★ Wesley College
Department of Nursing
120 N State St.
Dulany Hall
Dover, DE 19901
Phone: (302)736-2512 **Fax:** (302)736-2550
Email: gambarlu@wesley.edu
Website: http://www.wesley.edu
Dr. Lucille Gambardella, Contact
Fnded: 1873. **Degrees Offered:** BSN, MSN.

★ 27697 ★ Wilmington College
Division of Nursing
320 DuPont Hwy.
New Castle, DE 19720
Phone: (302)328-9401 **Fax:** (302)328-1147
Email: kchri@wilmcoll.edu
Website: http://www.wilmcoll.edu/
Kim Christensen, Contact
Fnded: 1967. **Degrees Offered:** BSN, MSN, MSN/MBA, MSN/MS.

District of Columbia

★ 27698 ★ Catholic University of America
School of Nursing
124 Gowan Hall
Washington, DC 20064
Phone: (202)319-6457
Email: queenr@cua.edu
Website: http://nursing.cua.edu
Rose Queen, Contact
Fnded: 1887. **Degrees Offered:** BSN, DN SC, MA/MSM, MSN.

★ 27699 ★ Georgetown University
School of Nursing and Health Studies
3700 Reservoir Rd. NW
Washington, DC 20007
Phone: (202)687-8439 **Fax:** (202)687-5553
Email: ADL6@georgetown.edu
Website: http://snhs.georgetown.edu
David Lewis, Contact
Fnded: 1789. **Degrees Offered:** BSN, MS.

★ 27700 ★ Howard University
Division of Nursing
501 Bryant St. NW
Washington, DC 20059
Phone: (202)806-7460 **Fax:** (202)806-5978
Email: rjohnson@howard.edu
Website: http://www.howard.edu
Dr. Ruth Johnson, Contact
Fnded: 1867. **Degrees Offered:** BSN, MSN.

★ 27701 ★ University of the District of Columbia
Nursing Education Program
4200 Connecticut Ave. NW
Washington, DC 20008
Phone: (202)274-5899 **Fax:** (202)274-5952
Website: http://www.udc.edu
Fnded: 1976. **Degrees Offered:** BS.

Florida

★ 27702 ★ Barry University
School of Nursing
11300 NE 2nd Ave.
Miami Shores, FL 33161-6695
Phone: (305)899-3800 **Fax:** (305)899-3831
Email: jdyer@mail.barry.edu
Website: http://www.barry.edu
Dr. Janyce Dyer, Contact
Fnded: 1940. **Degrees Offered:** BSN, MSN, MSN/MBA, PhD.

★ 27703 ★ Bethune-Cookman College
Division of Nursing
640 Dr. Mary McLeod Bethune Blvd.
Daytona Beach, FL 32114
Phone: (904)323-2031 **Fax:** (904)257-5338
Email: dixona@cookman.edu
Website: http://www.cookman.edu/Nursing
Dr. Alma Dixon, Contact
Fnded: 1904. **Degrees Offered:** BSN.

★ 27704 ★ Florida Agricultural and Mechanical University
School of Nursing
PO Box 136
Tallahassee, FL 32307
Phone: (850)599-3017 **Fax:** (850)599-3849
Email: mlewis@famu.edu
Website: http://www.famu.edu/acad/colleges/son
Dr. Margaret Lewis, Contact
Fnded: 1887. **Degrees Offered:** BSN, MSN, PhD.

★ 27705 ★ Florida Atlantic University
College of Nursing
777 Glades Rd.
Boca Raton, FL 33431-0991
Phone: (561)297-3384 **Fax:** (561)297-0088
Email: ldunphy@fau.edu
Website: http://www.fau.edu/nursing
Dr. Lynne M. Dunphy, Contact
Fnded: 1961. **Degrees Offered:** BSN, DNS, MSN.

★ 27706 ★ Florida Gulf Coast University
School of Nursing
10501 Florida Gulf Coast University Blvd. S
Fort Myers Beach, FL 33931
Phone: (941)590-7512 **Fax:** (941)590-7474
Email: kmiles@fgcu.edu
Website: http://www.fgcu.edu
Dr. Karen Miles, Contact
Fnded: 1991. **Degrees Offered:** BSN, MSN.

★ 27707 ★ Florida Hospital College of Health Sciences
Department of Nursing
800 Lake Estelle Dr.
Orlando, FL 32803
Phone: (407)303-9798 **Fax:** (407)303-9408
Email: fhcinfo@fhchs.edu
Website: http://204.4.13.166/edu/fhcweb
Degrees Offered: BS.

★ 27708 ★ Florida International University
School of Nursing
3000 NE 151st St., ACII-230
North Miami, FL 33181
Phone: (305)919-5915 **Fax:** (305)919-5395
Email: jeany@fiu.edu
Website: http://www.fiu.edu
Paula Delpech, Contact
Fnded: 1965. **Degrees Offered:** BSN, MSN.

★ 27709 ★ Florida Southern College
Department of Nursing
111 Lake Hollingsworth Dr.
Lakeland, FL 33801
Phone: (863)680-4315 **Fax:** (863)680-4120
Email: smarks@flsouthern.edu
Website: http://www.flsouthern.edu/nursing/
Sheila F. Marks, Contact
Fnded: 1885. **Degrees Offered:** BSN.

★ 27710 ★ Florida State University
School of Nursing
461C Vivian M. Duxbury Hall
Tallahassee, FL 32306-4310
Phone: (850)644-5638 **Fax:** (850)644-7660
Email: epage@nursing.fsu.edu
Website: http://www.fsu.edu
Eddie Page, Contact
Fnded: 1851. **Degrees Offered:** BSN, MSN, NSN/MS.

★ 27711 ★ Jacksonville University
School of Nursing
2800 University Blvd. N
Jacksonville, FL 32211
Phone: (904)256-5363 **Fax:** (904)256-7287
Email: jmcdani@ju.edu
Website: http://www.ju.edu
Dr. Goodlett McDaniel, Contact
Fnded: 1934. **Degrees Offered:** BSN, MSN, MSN/MBA.

★ 27712 ★ University of Central Florida
School of Nursing
PO Box 162210
Orlando, FL 32816-2210
Phone: (407)823-2744 **Fax:** (407)823-5675
Email: kijek@mail.ucf.edu
Website: http://www.cohpa.ucf.edu/nursing
Dr. Jean Kijek, Contact
Fnded: 1963. **Degrees Offered:** BSN, MSN.

★ 27713 ★ University of Florida
College of Nursing
PO Box 100197
Gainesville, FL 32610-0197
Phone: (352)273-6331 **Fax:** (352)392-8100
Email: couramm@nursing.ufl.edu
Website: http://con.ufl.edu/
Dr. Myrna M. Courage, Contact
Fnded: 1853. **Degrees Offered:** BSN, MSN, MSN/MBA, MSN/MPH, MSN/PhD.

★ 27714 ★ University of Miami
School of Nursing
5801 Red Rd.
Coral Gables, FL 33143-2343
Phone: (305)284-3666 **Fax:** (305)284-4827
Website: http://www.miami.edu/UMH
Fnded: 1925. **Degrees Offered:** BSN, MSN, PhD.

★ 27715 ★ University of North Florida
School of Nursing
College of Health Advising Office
Rm. 3025A, Bldg. 39
Jacksonville, FL 32224-2673
Phone: (904)620-2684 **Fax:** (904)620-2848
Website: http://www.unf.edu/coh/cohnursi.htm
Dr. Li Loriz, Contact
Fnded: 1965. **Degrees Offered:** BSN, MSN.

★ 27716 ★ University of Phoenix, Fort Lauderdale Campus
College of Health Care Sciences and Nursing
Fort Lauderdale, FL
Phone: (954)382-5303
Website: http://www.phoenix.edu/
Degrees Offered: BSN, MSN, MSN/MBA.

★ 27717 ★ University of Phoenix—Jacksonville Campus
College of Health Care and Nursing
4500 Salisbury Rd., Ste. 200
Jacksonville, FL 32216
Phone: (904)636-6645
Website: http://www.phoenix.edu/
Degrees Offered: BSN, MSN, MSN/MBA.

★ 27718 ★ University of Phoenix, Orlando Campus
College of Health Care Sciences and Nursing
Maitland, FL 32751
Phone: (407)667-0555
Website: http://www.phoenix.edu/
Degrees Offered: BSN, MSN, MSN/MBA.

★ 27719 ★ University of Phoenix, Tampa Campus
College of Health Care Sciences and Nursing
Tampa, FL
Phone: (813)626-7911
Website: http://www.phoenix.edu/
Degrees Offered: BSN, MSN, MSN/MBA.

★ 27720 ★ University of South Florida
College of Nursing
12901 Bruce B. Downs Blvd.
MDC Box 22
Tampa, FL 33612-4766
Phone: (813)974-9305 **Fax:** (813)974-5418
Email: pmartini@hsc.usf.edu
Website: http://hsc.usf.edu/nrusing/51
Dr. Patricia Martini Clark, Contact
Fnded: 1956. **Degrees Offered:** BS, MS, MSN/MPH, PhD.

★ 27721 ★ University of Tampa
Department of Nursing
401 W Kennedy Blvd.
Tampa, FL 33606-1490
Phone: (813)258-3333 **Fax:** (813)258-7214
Email: nross@alpha.utampa.edu
Website: http://www.utampa.edu/academics/libera-larts/departments/nursingbsn.html
Dr. Nancy Ross, Contact
Fnded: 1931. **Degrees Offered:** BSN, MSN.

★ 27722 ★ University of West Florida
Department of Nursing
Office of Admissions
11000 University Pkwy.
Pensacola, FL 32514
Phone: (850)474-2884 **Fax:** (850)474-3360
Email: admissions@uwf.edu
Website: http://www.uwf.edu
Fnded: 1963. **Degrees Offered:** BSN.

Georgia

★ 27723 ★ Albany State University
College of Health Professions
504 College Dr.
Albany, GA 31705
Phone: (229)430-4727 **Fax:** (229)430-3937
Email: lgrimsl@asurams.edu
Website: http://asuweb.asurams.edu
Linda P. Grimsley, Contact
Fnded: 1903. **Degrees Offered:** BSN, MSN.

★ 27724 ★ Armstrong Atlantic State University
Program in Nursing
11935 Abercorn St.
Savannah, GA 31419-1997
Phone: (912)927-5311 **Fax:** (912)920-6579
Email: sterncam@mail.armstrong.edu
Website: http://www.armstrong.edu
Dr. Camille Stern, Contact
Fnded: 1935. **Degrees Offered:** BSN, MN/MHSA, MSN.

★ 27725 ★ Brenau University
School of Health and Science
1 Centennial Circle
Gainesville, GA 30501
Phone: (770)534-6162
Email: lminish@lib.brenau.edu
Website: http://www.brenau.edu
Dr. Lynn Minish, Contact
Fnded: 1878. **Degrees Offered:** BSN, MSN.

★ 27726 ★ Clayton College & State University
Department of Nursing
5900 N Lee St.
Morrow, GA 30260
Phone: (770)961-3484 **Fax:** (770)961-3639
Email: lydiamcallister@mail.clayton.edu
Website: http://healthsci.clayton.edu
Dr. Lydia E. McAllister, Contact
Fnded: 1969. **Degrees Offered:** BSN.

★ 27727 ★ Columbus State University
Nursing Program
4225 University Ave.
Columbus, GA 31907-2079
Phone: (706)565-3649 **Fax:** (706)569-3101
Email: goyne_june@colstate.edu
Website: http://nursing.colstate.edu
Dr. June Goyne, Contact
Fnded: 1958. **Degrees Offered:** BSN.

★ 27728 ★ Emory University
Nell Hodgson Woodruff School of Nursing
1520 Clifton Rd. NE
Atlanta, GA 30322
Phone: (404)727-7980 **Fax:** (404)727-8509
Email: admit@nurse.emory.edu
Website: http://www.nursing.emory.edu
Dr. Nancy Halloran, Contact
Fnded: 1836. **Degrees Offered:** BSN, MN/MPH, MSN, PhD.

★ 27729 ★ Georgia Baptist College of Nursing of Mercer University
Department of Nursing
3001 Mercer University Dr.
Atlanta, GA 30341
Phone: (678)547-6774 **Fax:** (678)547-6777
Email: streit_la@mercer.edu
Website: http://nursing.mercer.edu
Dr. Linda Streit, Contact
Fnded: 1988. **Degrees Offered:** BSN, MSN.

★ 27730 ★ Georgia College and State University
School of Health Sciences
CBX 64
231 W Hancock St.
Milledgeville, GA 31061
Phone: (478)445-1795 **Fax:** (478)445-1913
Email: kfrith@gcsu.edu
Website: http://www.gcsu.edu/acad_affairs/school_healthsci
Dr. Karen Frith, Contact
Fnded: 1889. **Degrees Offered:** BSN, MSN, MSN/MBA.

★ 27731 ★ Georgia Southern University
School of Nursing
PO Box 8158
Statesboro, GA 30460-8158
Phone: (912)681-5056 **Fax:** (912)681-0536
Email: dhodnicki@gsvms2.cc.gasou.edu
Website: http://www.gasou.edu
Dr. Donna Hodnicki, Contact
Fnded: 1906. **Degrees Offered:** BSN, MSN.

★ 27732 ★ Georgia Southwestern State University
School of Nursing
800 Wheatley St.
Americus, GA 31709
Phone: (229)931-2275 **Fax:** (229)931-2274
Email: nkh@canes.gsw.edu
Website: http://www.gsw.edu
Nancy K. Hunt, Contact
Fnded: 1906. **Degrees Offered:** BSN.

★ 27733 ★ Georgia State University
School of Nursing
Office of Academic Assistance
33 Gilmer St., A0965
Atlanta, GA 30302
Phone: (404)651-3064 **Fax:** (404)651-4871
Email: bbsmith@gsu.edu
Website: http://chhs.gsu.edu/nursing
Barbara Smith, Contact
Fnded: 1913. **Degrees Offered:** BS, MS, PhD.

★ 27734 ★ Kennesaw State University
School of Nursing
1000 Chastain Rd.
Kennesaw, GA 30144
Phone: (770)423-6061 **Fax:** (770)423-6627
Email: gdorman@ksumail.kennesaw.edu
Website: http://www.kennesaw.edu/nursing
Dr. Regina Dorman, Contact
Fnded: 1963. **Degrees Offered:** BSN, MSN.

★ 27735 ★ La Grange College
Department of Nursing
601 Broad St.
LaGrange, GA 30240-2999
Phone: (706)880-8220 **Fax:** (706)880-8029
Email: msauter@lagrange.edu
Website: http://www.lagrange.edu
Dr. Maranah A. Sauter, Contact
Fnded: 1831. **Degrees Offered:** BSN.

★ 27736 ★ Medical College of Georgia
School of Nursing
AA-170-Kelly Bldg.
Augusta, GA 30912
Phone: (706)721-2725 **Fax:** (706)721-0186
Email: gradadm@mail.mcg.edu
Website: http://www.mcg.edu/son
Fnded: 1828. **Degrees Offered:** BSN, MSN, PhD.

★ 27737 ★ North Georgia College and State University
Department of Nursing
Rte. 60
Dahlonega, GA 30597
Phone: (706)864-1930 **Fax:** (706)864-1845
Email: tbarnett@ngcsu.edu
Website: http://www.ngcsu.edu
Toni Barnett, Contact
Fnded: 1873. **Degrees Offered:** BSN, MSN.

★ 27738 ★ State University of West Georgia
Department of Nursing
1601 Maple St.
Carrollton, GA 30118
Phone: (770)836-6552 **Fax:** (770)836-4409
Email: ltaylor@westga.edu
Website: http://www.westga.edu/~nurs/
Dr. Laurie Taylor, Contact
Fnded: 1933. **Degrees Offered:** BSN, MSN.

★ 27739 ★ Thomas University
Division of Nursing
1501 Millpond Rd.
Thomasville, GA 31792-7490
Free: 800-538-9784 **Fax:** (229)226-1653
Email: dsmith@thomasu.edu
Website: http://www.thomasu.edu/nursing.htm
Dr. Diane Smith, Contact
Fnded: 1950. **Degrees Offered:** BSN.

★ 27740 ★ Valdosta State University
College of Nursing
1300 N Patterson St.
Valdosta, GA 31698-0130
Phone: (229)333-5959 **Fax:** (229)333-7300
Email: mreichen@valdosta.edu
Website: http://www.valdosta.edu/nursing/
Dr. MaryAnn Reichenbach, Contact
Fnded: 1906. **Degrees Offered:** BSN, MSN.

Guam

★ 27741 ★ University of Guam
College of Nursing and Health Sciences
Office of Admissions and Records
UOG Station
Mangilao, GU 96923
Phone: (671)735-2210 **Fax:** (671)734-4245
Email: admitme@uog9.uog.edu
Website: http://uog.edu
Dr. Deborah Leon Guerrero, Contact
Fnded: 1952. **Degrees Offered:** BSN.

Hawaii

★ 27742 ★ Hawaii Pacific University
School of Nursing
45-045 Kamehameha Hwy.
Kaneohe, HI 96744-5297
Phone: (808)236-3552 **Fax:** (808)236-5818
Email: plangeot@hpu.edu
Website: http://www.hpu.edu
Patricia Lange-Otsuka, Contact
Fnded: 1965. **Degrees Offered:** BSN, MSN, MSN/MBA.

★ 27743 ★ University of Hawaii, Hilo
Department of Nursing
200 W Kawili St.
UCB 236
Hilo, HI 96720
Phone: (808)974-7761 **Fax:** (808)974-7665
Email: cmukai@hawaii.edu
Website: http://www.uhh.hawaii.edu
Dr. Cecilia Mukai, Contact
Fnded: 1970. **Degrees Offered:** BSN.

★ 27744 ★ University of Hawaii, Manoa
School of Nursing and Dental Hygiene
2528 McCarthy Mall
Honolulu, HI 96822
Phone: (808)956-5326 **Fax:** (808)956-5296
Email: jinouye@hawaii.edu
Website: http://www.nursing.hawaii.edu
Dr. Jillian Inouye, Contact
Fnded: 1907. **Degrees Offered:** BS, MS, PhD.

★ 27745 ★ University of Phoenix, Hawaii Campus
College of Health Care Sciences and Nursing
Honolulu, HI 96801
Phone: (866)236-7655
Website: http://www.phoenix.edu/
Degrees Offered: BSN, MSN, MSN/MBA.

Idaho

★ 27746 ★ Boise State University
Department of Nursing
1910 University Dr.
Boise, ID 83725-0399
Phone: (208)426-3783 **Fax:** (208)426-1370
Email: ptaylor@boisestate.edu
Website: http://nursing.boisestate.edu
Pat Taylor, Contact
Fnded: 1932. **Degrees Offered:** BSN.

★ 27747 ★ Idaho State University
Department of Nursing
Campus Box 8101
Pocatello, ID 83209-8101
Phone: (208)282-2443 **Fax:** (208)282-4476
Email: ashtcaro@isu.edu
Website: http://www.isu.edu/departments/nursing
Dr. Carol Ashton, Contact
Fnded: 1901. **Degrees Offered:** BSN, MS.

★ 27748 ★ Lewis-Clark State College
Division of Nursing
500 8th Ave.
Lewiston, ID 83501
Phone: (208)792-2250 **Fax:** (208)792-2062
Email: dblum@lcsc.edu
Website: http://www.lcsc.edu/Nurdiv/
Dianne Blum, Contact
Fnded: 1893. **Degrees Offered:** BSN.

Illinois

★ 27749 ★ Aurora University
School of Nursing
347 S Gladstone Ave.
Aurora, IL 60506-4892
Phone: (630)844-5130 **Fax:** (630)844-7822
Email: mlocklin@aurora.edu
Website: http://www.aurora.edu
Dr. Maryanne Locklin, Contact
Fnded: 1893. **Degrees Offered:** BSN.

★ 27750 ★ Benedictine University
Department of Nursing
5700 College Rd.
Lisle, IL 60532
Phone: (630)829-6567 **Fax:** (630)829-6551
Email: smoore@ben.edu
Website: http://www.ben.edu/
Dr. Shirley A. Moore, Contact
Fnded: 1887. **Degrees Offered:** BSN.

★ 27751 ★ Blessing-Rieman College of Nursing
Broadway at 11th St.
Quincy, IL 62305-7005

Phone: (217)228-5520 **Fax:** (217)223-4661
Email: brcnadmissions@blessinghospital.com
Website: http://www.brcn.edu/
Kelli Collins, Contact
Heather Tourney, Contact
Degrees Offered: BSN.

★ 27752 ★ Bradley University
Department of Nursing
Student Records Coordinator
Peoria, IL 61625
Phone: (309)677-2530 **Fax:** (309)677-2527
Email: mmiller@bradley.edu
Website: http://www.bradley.edu/academics/ehs/nur/nur_index.html
Marilyn Miller, Contact
Fnded: 1897. **Degrees Offered:** BSN, MSN.

★ 27753 ★ Chicago State University
College of Nursing and Allied Health Professions
9501 S Martin Luther King Dr.
Chicago, IL 60628
Phone: (773)995-3992 **Fax:** (773)821-2438
Website: http://www.csu.edu
Dr. Linda B. Hureston, Contact
Fnded: 1867. **Degrees Offered:** BSN.

★ 27754 ★ Concordia University
Concordia University and West Suburban College of Nursing
3 Erie Ct.
Oak Park, IL 60302
Phone: (708)763-6538 **Fax:** (708)763-1531
Degrees Offered: BSN.

★ 27755 ★ DePaul University
Department of Nursing
990 W Fullerton Ave.
Chicago, IL 60614
Phone: (773)325-7280 **Fax:** (773)325-7282
Email: cwerdric@depaul.edu
Website: http://www.depaul.edu/~nursing
Christine Werdrick, Contact
Fnded: 1898. **Degrees Offered:** BS, MS.

★ 27756 ★ Elmhurst College
Deicke Center for Nursing Education
Elmhurst, IL 60126
Phone: (630)617-3344 **Fax:** (630)617-3237
Email: lindan@elmhurst.edu
Website: http://www.elmhurst.edu/
Dr. Linda Niedringhaus, Contact
Fnded: 1871. **Degrees Offered:** BSN.

★ 27757 ★ Governors State University
Division of Nursing, Communication Disorders, Occupational Therapy and Physical Therapy
University Park, IL 60466
Phone: (708)235-2133 **Fax:** (708)235-2197
Email: j-krawcz@govst.edu
Website: http://www.govst.edu/
Dr. June Krawczak, Contact
Fnded: 1969. **Degrees Offered:** BS, MS.

★ 27758 ★ Illinois State University
Mennonite College of Nursing
5810 Edwards Hall
Normal, IL 61790-5810
Phone: (309)438-2358 **Fax:** (309)438-2280
Email: ddwilso2@ilstu.edu
Website: http://www.mcn.ilstu.edu/
Dr. Denise Wilson, Contact
Fnded: 1857. **Degrees Offered:** BSN, MSN.

★ 27759 ★ Illinois Wesleyan University
School of Nursing
PO Box 2900
Bloomington, IL 61701-2900
Phone: (309)556-3051 **Fax:** (309)556-3043
Email: dhartweg@titan.iwu.edu
Website: http://titan.iwu.edu/~nursing
Dr. Donna L. Hartweg, Contact
Fnded: 1850. **Degrees Offered:** BSN.

★ 27760 ★ Lakeview College of Nursing
903 N Logan Ave.
Danville, IL 61832
Phone: (217)443-5238 **Fax:** (217)442-2279
Email: kholden@lakeviewcol.edu
Website: http://www.lakeviewcol.edu
Kelly Holden, Contact
Fnded: 1987. **Degrees Offered:** BSN.

★ 27761 ★ Lewis University
Program in Nursing
One University Pkwy.
Romeoville, IL 60446-2298
Phone: (815)836-5355 **Fax:** (815)838-8306
Email: stephelo@lewisu.edu
Website: http://www.lewisu.edu/academics/nursing/index.htm
Lois Stephens, Contact
Fnded: 1932. **Degrees Offered:** BSN, MSN, MSN/MBA.

★ 27762 ★ Loyola University, Chicago
Marcella Niehoff School of Nursing
6525 N Sheridan Rd.
Chicago, IL 60626
Phone: (773)508-3249 **Fax:** (773)508-3241
Email: lgroves@luc.edu
Website: http://www.luc.edu/schools/nursing
Lauren Groves, Contact
Fnded: 1870. **Degrees Offered:** BSN, MSN, MSN/MBA, PhD.

★ 27763 ★ MacMurray College
Department of Nursing
447 E College Ave.
Jacksonville, IL 62650
Phone: (217)479-7083 **Fax:** (217)479-7078
Email: macbsn@mac.edu
Website: http://www.mac.edu/academ/nurs.htm
Devonna L. Dugan, Contact
Fnded: 1846. **Degrees Offered:** BSN.

★ 27764 ★ McKendree College
Department of Nursing
701 College Rd.
Lebanon, IL 62254
Free: 800-232-7228 **Fax:** (618)537-6259
Email: pchamber@mckendree.edu
Website: http://www.mckendree.edu/
Pamela Chambers, Contact
Fnded: 1828. **Degrees Offered:** BSN.

★ 27765 ★ Millikin University
School of Nursing
1184 W Main St.
Decatur, IL 62522
Phone: (217)424-6348 **Fax:** (217)424-3993
Email: ncreason@mail.millikin.edu
Website: http://www.millikin.edu
Dr. Nancy Creason, Contact
Fnded: 1901. **Degrees Offered:** BSN.

★ 27766 ★ North Park University
School of Nursing
3225 W Foster Ave.
Chicago, IL 60625
Phone: (773)244-5508 **Fax:** (773)279-7994
Email: tjames@northpark.edu
Website: http://www.northpark.edu
Trevor James, Contact
Fnded: 1891. **Degrees Offered:** BS, MS, MS/MA, MS/MBA.

★ 27767 ★ Northern Illinois University
School of Nursing
1240 Normal Rd.
DeKalb, IL 60115-2864
Phone: (815)753-6557 **Fax:** (815)753-0814
Email: selder@niu.edu
Website: http://www.nursing.niu.edu
Stacie Elder, Contact
Fnded: 1895. **Degrees Offered:** BS, MS, MSN/MPH.

★ 27768 ★ Olivet Nazarene University
Division of Nursing
One University Ave.
Bourbonnais, IL 60914
Phone: (815)939-5186 **Fax:** (815)935-4991
Email: linda.westerberg@apollogrp.edu
Website: http://www.olivet.edu/academics/divisions/nursing
Linda Westerberg, Contact
Fnded: 1907. **Degrees Offered:** BS, MSN.

★ 27769 ★ Rockford College
Department of Nursing
5050 E State St.
Rockford, IL 61108-2393
Phone: (815)226-4050 **Fax:** (815)226-2822
Email: paul_hartzog@rockford.edu
Website: http://www.rockford.edu
Paul Hartzog, Contact
Fnded: 1847. **Degrees Offered:** BSN.

★ 27770 ★ Rush University
College of Nursing
Armour Academic Center
600 S Paulina St., Rm. 440, AAC
Chicago, IL 60612
Phone: (312)942-7100 **Fax:** (312)942-2219
Email: ruadmissions@rushu.rush.edu
Website: http://www.rushu.rush.edu/nursing
Hicela Castruita-Woods, Contact
Fnded: 1969. **Degrees Offered:** BSN, DN SC, MSN, MSN/MBA.

★ 27771 ★ Saint Anthony College of Nursing
5658 E State St.
Rockford, IL 61108-2468
Phone: (815)227-2141 **Fax:** (815)395-2275
Email: cheryldelgado@sacn.edu
Website: http://www.sacn.edu
Cheryl Delgado, Contact
Fnded: 1915. **Degrees Offered:** BSN.

★ 27772 ★ Saint Francis Medical Center
College of Nursing
511 NE Greenleaf St.
Peoria, IL 61603
Phone: (309)655-2230 **Fax:** (309)655-3648
Email: jan.f.boundy@osfhealthcare.org
Website: http://www.sfmccon.edu
Janice F. Boundy, Contact
Fnded: 1986. **Degrees Offered:** BSN, MSN.

★ 27773 ★ Saint John's College
Department of Nursing
421 N 9th St.
Springfield, IL 62702
Phone: (217)525-5628 **Fax:** (217)757-6870
Email: bbeasley@st-johns.org
Website: http://www.st-johns.org
Beth Beasley, Contact
Fnded: 1886. **Degrees Offered:** BSN.

★ 27774 ★ Saint Xavier University
School of Nursing
3700 W 103rd St.
Chicago, IL 60655
Phone: (773)298-3708 Fax: (773)298-3704
Email: filipski@sxu.edu
Website: http://www.sxu.edu/academ/nursing
Dr. Ann Filipski, Contact
Fnded: 1847. Degrees Offered: BS, MS, MS/MBA.

★ 27775 ★ Southern Illinois University, Edwardsville
School of Nursing
Alumni Hall, Rm. 2107
Edwardsville, IL 62026-1066
Phone: (618)650-3930 Fax: (618)650-3854
Email: angewhi@siue.edu
Website: http://www.siue.edu/NURSING
Angela White, Contact
Fnded: 1957. Degrees Offered: BS, MS.

★ 27776 ★ Trinity Christian College
Department of Nursing
6601 W College Dr.
Palos Heights, IL 60463
Free: 800-748-0085 Fax: (708)385-5665
Email: admissions@trnty.edu
Website: http://www.trnty/depts/nursing/
Fnded: 1959. Degrees Offered: BSN.

★ 27777 ★ University of Illinois, Chicago
College of Nursing
845 S Damen Ave.
Chicago, IL 60612-7350
Phone: (312)996-2184 Fax: (312)996-8066
Email: kdiana@uic.edu
Website: http://www.nurs.uic.edu
Kate DiAna, Contact
Fnded: 1946. Degrees Offered: BSN, MS, MS/MBA, MS/MPH, PhD.

★ 27778 ★ University of Saint Francis
Saint Joseph College of Nursing and Allied Health
500 Wilcox St.
Joliet, IL 60435
Free: 800-735-7500 Fax: (815)740-3431
Email: cjakielski@stfrancis.edu
Website: http://www.stfrancis.edu
Caryn Jakielski, Contact
Fnded: 1920. Degrees Offered: BSN, MSN.

Indiana

★ 27779 ★ Anderson University
Department of Nursing
1100 E 5th St.
Anderson, IN 46012
Phone: (765)641-4390 Fax: (765)641-3851
Website: http://www.anderson.edu/academics/nurs/
Fnded: 1917. Degrees Offered: BSN

★ 27780 ★ Ball State University
School of Nursing
Muncie, IN 47306-0265
Phone: (765)285-5764 Fax: (765)285-2169
Email: mryan@bsu.edu
Website: http://www.bsu.edu
Dr. Marilyn Ryan, RN, Contact
Fnded: 1918. Degrees Offered: BS, MS.

★ 27781 ★ Bethel College
Department of Nursing
1001 W McKinley St.
Mishawaka, IN 46545
Phone: (574)257-2594 Fax: (574)257-3326
Email: davidhr@bethel-in.edu
Website: http://www.bethelcollege.edu
Dr. Ruth E. Davidhizar, Contact
Fnded: 1947. Degrees Offered: BSN.

★ 27782 ★ Goshen College
Department of Nursing
1700 S Main St.
Goshen, IN 46526
Phone: (219)535-7535 Fax: (219)535-7609
Email: admissions@goshen.edu
Website: http://www.goshen.edu
Fnded: 1894. Degrees Offered: BSN.

★ 27783 ★ Indiana State University
School of Nursing
749 Chestnut St.
Terre Haute, IN 47809
Phone: (812)237-2317 Fax: (812)237-4300
Email: nufoster@isugw.indstate.edu
Website: http://web.indstate.edu
Lynn C. Foster, Contact
Fnded: 1865. Degrees Offered: BS, MS.

★ 27784 ★ Indiana University, Bloomington
Department of Nursing-Bloomington Division
Sycamore Hall, Rm. 401
Bloomington, IN 47405
Phone: (812)855-2592 Fax: (812)855-6986
Email: lwrasse@indiana.edu
Website: http://www.indiana.edu
Lisa Wrasse, Contact
Fnded: 1820. Degrees Offered: BSN.

★ 27785 ★ Indiana University, East
Division of Nursing
2325 Chester Blvd.
Richmond, IN 47374-1289
Phone: (765)973-8242 Fax: (765)973-8220
Email: krclark@indiana.edu
Website: http://www.indiana.edu/nursing
Karen R. Clark, Contact
Fnded: 1971. Degrees Offered: BSN.

★ 27786 ★ Indiana University, Kokomo
Indiana University School of Nursing
2300 S Washington St.
PO Box 9003
Kokomo, IN 46904-9003
Phone: (765)455-9384 Fax: (765)455-9421
Email: mstarke@iuk.edu
Website: http://www.iuk.indiana.edu
Morris Starkey, Contact
Fnded: 1945. Degrees Offered: BSN.

★ 27787 ★ Indiana University, Northwest
School of Nursing and Health Professions
3400 Broadway
Gary, IN 46408
Phone: (219)980-6549 Fax: (219)980-6578
Email: lgraves@iun.edu
Website: http://www.iun.indiana.edu/nursing
Laura J. Graves, Contact
Fnded: 1959. Degrees Offered: BSN.

★ 27788 ★ Indiana University—Purdue University, Fort Wayne
Department of Nursing
2101 E Coliseum Blvd.
Fort Wayne, IN 46805-1499
Phone: (260)481-6284 Fax: (260)481-5767
Email: lemirej@ipfw.edu
Website: http://www.ipfw.edu/nursing
Dr. Judith Lemire, Contact
Fnded: 1917. Degrees Offered: BS, MS.

★ 27789 ★ Indiana University—Purdue University, Indianapolis
School of Nursing
1111 Middle Dr., NU 136
Indianapolis, IN 46202
Phone: (317)274-3115 Fax: (317)274-2996
Email: warnerjr@iupui.edu
Website: http://www.nursing.iupui.edu
Dr. Joanne R. Warner, Contact
Fnded: 1969. Degrees Offered: BSN, MSN, MSN/MPH, PhD.

★ 27790 ★ Indiana University, South Bend
Division of Nursing and Health Professions
1700 Mishawaka Ave.
PO Box 7111
South Bend, IN 46634-7111
Phone: (219)237-4571 Fax: (219)237-4461
Email: nursing@iusb.edu
Website: http://www.iusb.edu/~health/
Fnded: 1922. Degrees Offered: BSN.

★ 27791 ★ Indiana University, Southeast
Division of Nursing
4201 Grant Line Rd., LF-102
New Albany, IN 47150
Phone: (812)941-2560 Fax: (812)941-2687
Website: http://www.ius.indiana.edu/Nursing
Fnded: 1941. Degrees Offered: BSN.

★ 27792 ★ Indiana Wesleyan University
Division of Nursing Education
4201 S Washington St.
Marion, IN 46953
Phone: (765)677-2357 Fax: (765)677-2380
Email: barb.schulz@indwes.edu
Website: http://www.indwes.edu/academics/Nursing
Barbara Schulz, Contact
Fnded: 1920. Degrees Offered: BS, MS.

★ 27793 ★ Marian College
Department of Nursing and Nutritional Science
3200 Cold Spring Rd.
Indianapolis, IN 46222-1997
Phone: (317)955-6157 Fax: (317)955-6135
Email: bhart@marian.edu
Website: http://www.marian.edu/academ/departments/nursing
Barbara Hart, RN, Contact
Fnded: 1851. Degrees Offered: BSN.

★ 27794 ★ Purdue University
School of Nursing
Schleman Hall of Student Services
West Lafayette, IN 47907
Phone: (765)494-1776 Fax: (765)494-0544
Email: admissions@purdue.edu
Website: http://www.nursing.purdue.edu
Dr. Douglas Christiansen, Contact
Fnded: 1869. Degrees Offered: BS.

★ 27795 ★ Purdue University, Calumet
School of Nursing
2200 169th St.
Hammond, IN 46323-2094
Phone: (219)989-2815 Fax: (219)989-2848
Email: walkerj@calumet.purdue.edu
Website: http://www.calumet.purdue.edu
Dr. Jane Walker, Contact
Fnded: 1951. Degrees Offered: BS, MS.

★ 27796 ★ Saint Mary's College
Department of Nursing
124 LeMans
Notre Dame, IN 46556
Phone: (574)284-4587 **Fax:** (574)284-4716
Email: mpnolan@saintmarys.edu
Website: http://www.saintmarys.edu
Mary Pat Nolan, Contact
Fnded: 1844. **Degrees Offered:** BS.

★ 27797 ★ University of Evansville
Department of Nursing
1800 Lincoln Ave.
Evansville, IN 47722
Phone: (812)479-2584 **Fax:** (812)479-2717
Email: ja2@evansville.edu
Website: http://www.evansville.edu
Jane P. Allen, Contact
Fnded: 1854. **Degrees Offered:** BSN.

★ 27798 ★ University of Indianapolis
School of Nursing
1400 E Hanna Ave.
Indianapolis, IN 46227-3697
Phone: (317)788-3471 **Fax:** (317)788-3542
Email: siccardi@uindy.edu
Website: http://www.uindy.edu
Anita Siccardi, Contact
Fnded: 1902. **Degrees Offered:** BSN, MSN, MSN/MBA.

★ 27799 ★ University of Saint Francis
Department of Nursing
2701 Spring St.
Fort Wayne, IN 46808-3994
Phone: (260)434-7687 **Fax:** (260)434-7404
Email: nsweeney@sf.edu
Website: http://www.sf.edu
Dr. Nancy Sweeney, Contact
Fnded: 1890. **Degrees Offered:** BSN, MSN.

★ 27800 ★ University of Southern Indiana
School of Nursing and Health Professions
8600 University Blvd.
Evansville, IN 47712
Phone: (812)465-1173 **Fax:** (812)465-7092
Email: awhite@usi.edu
Website: http://www.usi.edu
Dr. Ann H. White, Contact
Fnded: 1965. **Degrees Offered:** BSN, MSN.

★ 27801 ★ Valparaiso University
College of Nursing
836 LaPorte Ave.
Valparaiso, IN 46383-6493
Phone: (219)464-5289 **Fax:** (219)464-5425
Email: janet.brown@valpo.edu
Website: http://www.valpo.edu/nursing
Dr. Janet M. Brown, Contact
Fnded: 1859. **Degrees Offered:** BSN, MSN.

Iowa

★ 27802 ★ Allen College
Program in Nursing
1825 Logan Ave.
Waterloo, IA 50703
Phone: (319)226-2002 **Fax:** (319)226-2020
Website: http://www.allencollege.edu
Barb Seible, Contact
Fnded: 1989. **Degrees Offered:** BSN, MSN.

★ 27803 ★ Briar Cliff University
Department of Nursing
3303 Rebecca St.
PO Box 2100
Sioux City, IA 51104
Phone: (712)279-5458 **Fax:** (712)279-5497
Email: daumer@briarcliff.edu
Website: http://www.briarcliff.edu
Dr. Ruth Daumer, Contact
Fnded: 1930. **Degrees Offered:** BSN.

★ 27804 ★ Clarke College
Department of Nursing and Health
1550 Clark Dr.
Dubuque, IA 52001
Phone: (563)588-6361 **Fax:** (563)588-8684
Email: kay.frommelt@clarke.edu
Website: http://www.clarke.edu
Dr. Katherine Helen Frommelt, Contact
Fnded: 1843. **Degrees Offered:** BS, MSN.

★ 27805 ★ Coe College
Department of Nursing
1220 1st Ave. NE
Cedar Rapids, IA 52402
Phone: (319)369-8120 **Fax:** (319)369-8121
Email: johrt@coe.edu
Website: http://www.coe.edu/
H. Jule Ohrt, Contact
Fnded: 1851. **Degrees Offered:** BSN.

★ 27806 ★ Grand View College
Division of Nursing
1200 Grandview Ave.
Des Moines, IA 50316
Phone: (515)263-2800 **Fax:** (515)263-6077
Website: http://www.gvc.edu
Fnded: 1896. **Degrees Offered:** BSN.

★ 27807 ★ Iowa Wesleyan College
Division of Nursing
601 N Main St.
Mount Pleasant, IA 52641
Free: 800-582-2383 **Fax:** (319)385-6296
Email: cowens@iwc.edu
Website: http://www.iwc.edu
Cary Owens, Contact
Fnded: 1842. **Degrees Offered:** BSN.

★ 27808 ★ Luther College
Department of Nursing
700 College Dr.
Decorah, IA 52101
Phone: (563)387-1057 **Fax:** (563)387-2149
Email: greenru@luther.edu
Website: http://www.luther.edu
Ruth Green, Contact
Fnded: 1861. **Degrees Offered:** BA.

★ 27809 ★ Mercy College of Health Sciences
Division of Nursing
928 6th Ave.
Des Moines, IA 50309
Phone: (515)643-3180 **Fax:** (515)643-6698
Email: information@mchs.edu
Website: http://www.mchs.edu/nursing/nursing_main.htm
Fnded: 1995. **Degrees Offered:** BSN.

★ 27810 ★ Morningside College
Department of Nursing Education
1501 Morningside Ave.
Sioux City, IA 51106
Phone: (712)274-5154 **Fax:** (712)274-5101
Email: kovarna@morningside.edu
Website: http://www.morningside.edu/
Mary Kovarna, Contact
Fnded: 1894. **Degrees Offered:** BSN.

★ 27811 ★ Mount Mercy College
Department of Nursing
1330 Elmhurst Dr. NE
Cedar Rapids, IA 52402
Free: 800-248-4504 **Fax:** (319)368-6479
Email: mtarbox@mmc.mtmercy.edu
Website: http://www.mtmercy.edu
Dr. Mary P. Tarbox, Contact
Fnded: 1928. **Degrees Offered:** BSN.

★ 27812 ★ University of Iowa
College of Nursing
444 Nursing Bldg.
Iowa City, IA 52242
Phone: (319)334-4667 **Fax:** (319)335-9990
Email: tracy-middleton@uiowa.edu
Website: http://www.nursing.uiowa.edu
Tracy Middleton, Contact
Fnded: 1847. **Degrees Offered:** BSN, MSN, MSN/MBA, PhD.

Kansas

★ 27813 ★ Baker University
School of Nursing
1500 SW 10th St.
Topeka, KS 66604-1353
Phone: (785)354-5851 **Fax:** (785)354-5832
Email: peggy.geier@bakeru.edu
Website: http://www.bakeru.edu
Peggy Geier, Contact
Fnded: 1858. **Degrees Offered:** BSN.

★ 27814 ★ Bethel College
Department of Nursing
300 E 27th St.
North Newton, KS 67117
Phone: (316)283-2500 **Fax:** (316)284-5286
Email: moore@bethelks.edu
Website: http://www.bethelks.edu
Dr. Carol Moore, Contact
Fnded: 1887. **Degrees Offered:** BSN.

★ 27815 ★ Emporia State University
Newman Division of Nursing
1127 Chestnut St.
Emporia, KS 66801-2523
Phone: (620)343-6800 **Fax:** (620)341-7871
Email: calhounj@emporia.edu
Website: http://www.emporia.edu/ndn
Dr. Judith E. Calhoun, Contact
Fnded: 1863. **Degrees Offered:** BSN.

★ 27816 ★ Fort Hays State University
Department of Nursing
600 Park St.
Stroup Hall 122D
Hays, KS 67601-4099
Phone: (785)628-4511 **Fax:** (785)628-4080
Email: lconnell@fhsu.edu
Website: http://www.fhsu.edu/nursing/
Dr. Liane Connelly, Contact
Fnded: 1902. **Degrees Offered:** BSN, MSN.

★ 27817 ★ Kansas Wesleyan University
Department of Nursing Education
Peters Hall of Science
100 E Claflin Ave.
Salina, KS 67401-6196
Phone: (785)827-5541 **Fax:** (785)827-0927
Email: pkissell@kwu.edu
Website: http://www.kwu.edu/nursing
Dr. Patricia D. Kissell, Contact
Fnded: 1886. **Degrees Offered:** BSN.

★ 27818 ★ MidAmerica Nazarene University
Division of Nursing
2030 E College Way
Olathe, KS 66062
Phone: (913)782-3750 **Fax:** (913)791-3408
Email: psmith@mnu.edu
Website: http://www.mnu.edu
Dr. Palma Lenn Smith, Contact
Fnded: 1966. **Degrees Offered:** BSN.

★ 27819 ★ Newman University
Division of Nursing
3100 McCormick Ave.
Wichita, KS 67213
Phone: (316)942-4291 **Fax:** (316)942-4483
Email: chipasa@newmanu.edu
Website: http://www.newmanu.edu
Dr. Anthony Chipas, Contact
Fnded: 1933. **Degrees Offered:** BSN, M SC N.

★ 27820 ★ Pittsburg State University
Department of Nursing
1701 S Broadway
Pittsburg, KS 66762
Phone: (316)235-4435 **Fax:** (316)235-4449
Email: sbowling@pittstate.edu
Website: http://www.pittstate.edu/nurs
Dr. Sharon Bowling, Contact
Fnded: 1903. **Degrees Offered:** BSN, MSN

★ 27821 ★ Southwestern College
Nursing Program
100 College St.
Winfield, KS 67156
Phone: (620)229-6236 **Fax:** (620)229-6344
Email: scadmit@sckans.edu
Website: http://www.sckans.edu
Todd Moore, Contact
Fnded: 1885. **Degrees Offered:** BSN.

★ 27822 ★ Tabor College
Department of Nursing
400 S Jefferson
Hillsboro, KS 67063
Phone: (620)947-3121
Email: bsn@tabor.edu
Website: http://www.tabor.edu/tcw/nursing.htm
Fnded: 1908. **Degrees Offered:** BSN.

★ 27823 ★ University of Kansas
School of Nursing
3901 Rainbow Blvd.
Kansas City, KS 66160-7501
Phone: (913)588-1619 **Fax:** (913)588-1615
Email: soninfo@kumc.edu
Website: http://www.kumc.edu/instruction/nursing/degrees.htm
Dr. Rita Clifford, Contact
Fnded: 1866. **Degrees Offered:** BSN, MS, MS/MHSA, MS/MPH, PhD.

★ 27824 ★ Washburn University of Topeka
School of Nursing
1700 SW College Ave.
Topeka, KS 66621
Phone: (785)231-1032 **Fax:** (785)231-1032
Email: mary.allen@washburn.edu
Website: http://www.washburn.edu/sonu/index.html
Mary V. Allen, Contact
Fnded: 1865. **Degrees Offered:** BSN.

★ 27825 ★ Wichita State University
School of Nursing
1845 Fairmount St.
Wichita, KS 67260-0041
Phone: (316)978-3610 **Fax:** (316)978-3094
Email: alicia.huckstadt@wichita.edu
Website: http://www.chp.wichita.edu/nurs
Dr. Alicia Huckstadt, Contact
Fnded: 1895. **Degrees Offered:** BSN, MSN, MSN/MBA.

Kentucky

★ 27826 ★ Bellarmine University
Donna and Allan Lansing School of Nursing and Health Sciences
Miles Hall
2001 Newburg Rd.
Louisville, KY 40205-0671
Phone: (502)452-8149 **Fax:** (502)452-8058
Email: scronin@bellarmine.edu
Website: http://www.bellarmine.edu
Dr. Sherill N. Cronin, Contact
Fnded: 1950. **Degrees Offered:** BSN, MSN, MSN/MBA.

★ 27827 ★ Berea College
Department of Nursing
CPO 1794
Berea, KY 40404
Phone: (859)985-3384 **Fax:** (859)985-3917
Email: pam_farley@berea.edu
Website: http://www.berea.edu
Dr. Pam Farley, Contact
Fnded: 1855. **Degrees Offered:** BS.

★ 27828 ★ Eastern Kentucky University
Department of Baccalaureate and Graduate Nursing
223 Rowlett Bldg.
Richmond, KY 40475
Phone: (859)622-1827 **Fax:** (859)622-1972
Website: http://www.bsn-gn.edku.edu
Fnded: 1906. **Degrees Offered:** BSN, MSN.

★ 27829 ★ Midway College
Program in Nursing (Baccalaureate)
512 E Stephens St.
Midway, KY 40347
Phone: (859)846-5725
Email: bkitchen@midway.edu
Website: http://www.midway.edu
Barbara Kitchen, Contact
Fnded: 1847. **Degrees Offered:** BSN.

★ 27830 ★ Morehead State University
Department of Nursing and Allied Health Sciences
UPO 715
Morehead, KY 40351
Phone: (606)783-5173 **Fax:** (606)783-9104
Email: j.gross@moreheadstate.edu
Website: http://www.moreheadstate.edu/colleges/science/nahs
Dr. Janet J. Gross, Contact
Fnded: 1922. **Degrees Offered:** BSN.

★ 27831 ★ Murray State University
Department of Nursing
PO Box 9
120 Mason Hall
Murray, KY 42071-0009
Phone: (502)762-6671 **Fax:** (270)762-6662
Email: nancey.france@murraystate.edu
Website: http://www.mursuky.edu/qacd/cos/nur/nursing.htm
Dr. Nancey E. M. France, Contact
Fnded: 1922. **Degrees Offered:** BSN, MSN.

★ 27832 ★ Northern Kentucky University
Department of Nursing
Highland Heights, KY 41099
Phone: (859)572-5178 **Fax:** (859)572-6098
Email: robinson@nku.edu
Website: http://www.nku.edu
Dr. Denise Robinson, Contact
Fnded: 1968. **Degrees Offered:** BSN, MSN.

★ 27833 ★ Spalding University
School of Nursing and Health Sciences
851 S 4th St.
Louisville, KY 40203-2188
Phone: (502)585-7125 **Fax:** (502)588-7175
Email: ccrabtree@spalding.edu
Website: http://www.spalding.edu
Dr. Cynthia R. Crabtree, Contact
Fnded: 1814. **Degrees Offered:** BSN, MSN.

★ 27834 ★ Thomas More College
Program in Nursing
Crestview Hills, KY 41017
Phone: (859)344-3508 **Fax:** (859)344-3345
Website: http://www.thomasmore.edu
Fnded: 1921. **Degrees Offered:** BSN.

★ 27835 ★ University of Kentucky
College of Nursing
Rm. 309 CON/HSLC
Lexington, KY 40536-0232
Phone: (859)323-5108 **Fax:** (859)323-1057
Email: conss@uky.edu
Website: http://www.mc.uky.edu/nursing
Fnded: 1865. **Degrees Offered:** BSN, MSN, PhD.

★ 27836 ★ University of Louisville
School of Nursing
555 S Floyd St.
Louisville, KY 40292
Phone: (502)852-5366 **Fax:** (502)852-8783
Email: camccu01@louisville.edu
Website: http://www.louisville.edu/nursing
Dr. Cynthia McCurren, Contact
Fnded: 1798. **Degrees Offered:** BSN, MSN.

★ 27837 ★ Western Kentucky University
Department of Nursing
One Big Red Way
Academic Complex 108G
Bowling Green, KY 42101-3576
Phone: (270)745-3490 **Fax:** (502)745-3392
Email: beverly.siegrist@wku.edu
Website: http://www.wku.edu
Dr. Beverly C. Siegrist, Contact
Fnded: 1906. **Degrees Offered:** BSN, MSN.

Louisiana

★ 27838 ★ Dillard University
Division of Nursing
2601 Gentilly Blvd.
New Orleans, LA 70122
Phone: (504)286-4717 **Fax:** (504)286-4861
Website: http://www.dillard.edu/academic/nursing
Fnded: 1869. **Degrees Offered:** BSN.

★ 27839 ★ Grambling State University
School of Nursing
PO Box 1192
Grambling, LA 71245
Phone: (318)274-2897 **Fax:** (318)274-3491
Email: hensleyr@alpha0.gram.edu
Rhonda Hensley, Contact
Fnded: 1901. **Degrees Offered:** BSN, MSN.

★ 27840 ★ Louisiana College
Department of Nursing
PO Box 556
Pineville, LA 71359-0556
Phone: (318)487-7127 **Fax:** (318)487-7488
Website: http://www.lacollege.edu

Fnded: 1906. **Degrees Offered:** BSN.

★ 27841 ★ Louisiana State University Health Sciences Center
School of Nursing
1900 Gravier St.
New Orleans, LA 70112
Phone: (504)568-4133 **Fax:** (504)568-5853
Website: http://nursing.lsuhsc.edu
Fnded: 1931. **Degrees Offered:** BSN, DNS, MN.

★ 27842 ★ Loyola University, New Orleans
Program in Nursing
6363 Saint Charles Ave.
Campus Box 14
New Orleans, LA 70118
Phone: (504)865-3142 **Fax:** (504)865-3254
Email: bwilson@loyno.edu
Website: http://www.loyno.edu/~nursing
Dr. Billie Ann Wilson, Contact
Fnded: 1912. **Degrees Offered:** BSN, MSN.

★ 27843 ★ McNeese State University
College of Nursing
PO Box 90415
Lake Charles, LA 70609-0415
Phone: (337)475-5753 **Fax:** (337)475-5702
Email: rbrewer@acc.mcneese.edu
Website: http://www.mcneese.edu
Dr. Ruth Brewer, Contact
Fnded: 1939. **Degrees Offered:** BSN, MSN.

★ 27844 ★ Nicholls State University
Department of Nursing
PO Box 2143
Thibodaux, LA 70310
Phone: (504)448-4696 **Fax:** (504)448-4932
Email: nurs-tjs@mail.nich.edu
Website: http://www.nicholls.edu/nursing/
Dr. Thomas Smith, Contact
Fnded: 1948. **Degrees Offered:** BSN.

★ 27845 ★ Northwestern State University of Louisiana
College of Nursing
1800 Line Ave.
Shreveport, LA 71101
Phone: (318)677-3100 **Fax:** (318)677-3127
Email: porterfieldd@nsula.edu
Website: http://www.nsula.edu
Dr. Deborah Porterfield, Contact
Fnded: 1884. **Degrees Offered:** BSN, MSN.

★ 27846 ★ Our Lady of Holy Cross College
Division of Nursing
4123 Woodland Dr.
New Orleans, LA 70131
Phone: (504)394-7744 **Fax:** (504)391-2421
Email: smcneely@olhcc.edu
Website: http://www.olhcc.edu
Stanton McNeely, Contact
Fnded: 1916. **Degrees Offered:** BSN.

★ 27847 ★ Our Lady of the Lake College
Division of Nursing
7434 Perkins Rd.
Baton Rouge, LA 70808
Phone: (225)768-1700
Email: admission@ololcollege.edu
Website: http://www.ololcollege.edu
Fnded: 1990. **Degrees Offered:** BSN.

★ 27848 ★ Southeastern Louisiana University
College of Nursing and Health Sciences
SLU 835
Hammond, LA 70402
Phone: (985)549-5045
Email: cprestholdt@selu.edu
Website: http://www.selu.edu/Academics/Nursing
Dr. Cynthia Prestholdt, Contact
Fnded: 1925. **Degrees Offered:** BS, MSN.

★ 27849 ★ Southern University and Agricultural and Mechanical College
School of Nursing
PO Box 11784
Baton Rouge, LA 70813
Phone: (225)771-2663 **Fax:** (225)771-3547
Email: ladonnastrauss@suson.subr.edu
Website: http://www.subr.edu/suson
Ladonna Strauss, Contact
Fnded: 1880. **Degrees Offered:** BSN, MSN, PhD.

★ 27850 ★ University of Louisiana, Lafayette
College of Nursing
PO Box 43810
Lafayette, LA 70504-3810
Phone: (337)482-5617 **Fax:** (337)482-5053
Email: carolyn@louisiana.edu
Website: http://www.louisiana.edu
Dr. Carolyn Delahoussaye, Contact
Fnded: 1898. **Degrees Offered:** BSN, MSN.

★ 27851 ★ University of Louisiana, Monroe
College of Nursing
700 University Ave.
Monroe, LA 71209-0460
Phone: (318)342-1460 **Fax:** (318)342-1567
Email: corder@ulm.edu
Website: http://www.ulm.edu
Dr. Jan B. Corder, Contact
Fnded: 1931. **Degrees Offered:** BS.

★ 27852 ★ University of Phoenix, Louisiana Campus
College of Health Care Sciences and Nursing
2431 S Acadian Thruway, Ste. 110
Baton Rouge, LA 70808
Phone: (225)927-4443
Website: http://www.phoenix.edu/
Degrees Offered: BSN, MSN, MSN/MBA.

Maine

★ 27853 ★ Husson College
School of Nursing
One College Cir.
Bangor, ME 04401-2999
Phone: (207)941-7080 **Fax:** (207)941-7883
Email: caseg@husson.edu
Website: http://www.husson.edu
George L. Case, Contact
Fnded: 1898. **Degrees Offered:** BSN, MSN.

★ 27854 ★ Saint Joseph's College of Maine
Department of Nursing
278 Whites Bridge Rd.
Standish, ME 04084-5263
Phone: (207)893-7957 **Fax:** (207)892-7423
Email: lconover@sjcme.edu
Website: http://www.sjcme.edu
Dr. Linda Conover, Contact
Fnded: 1912. **Degrees Offered:** BSN, MSN.

★ 27855 ★ University of Maine
School of Nursing
218 Dunn Hall
Orono, ME 04469
Phone: (207)581-2605 **Fax:** (207)581-2585
Email: cwood@maine.edu
Website: http://www.ume.maine.edu/~graduate/
Dr. Carol Wood, Contact
Fnded: 1865. **Degrees Offered:** BSN, MSN.

★ 27856 ★ University of Maine, Fort Kent
Department of Nursing
23 University Dr.
Fort Kent, ME 04743-1292
Phone: (207)834-7586 **Fax:** (207)834-7577
Email: radsma@maine.edu
Website: http://www.umfk.maine.edu/academics/programs/nursing/
Jenny Radsma, Contact
Fnded: 1878. **Degrees Offered:** BSN.

★ 27857 ★ University of New England
Department of Nursing
11 Hills Beach Rd.
Biddeford, ME 04005
Phone: (207)283-0171 **Fax:** (207)282-6379
Email: cspirito@mailbox.une.edu
Website: http://www.uned.edu/chp/nursing/
Dr. Carl Spirito, Contact
Fnded: 1831. **Degrees Offered:** BSN, MSN.

★ 27858 ★ University of Southern Maine
College of Nursing and Health Professions
PO Box 9300
Portland, ME 04104-9300
Phone: (207)780-4808 **Fax:** (207)780-4997
Email: mrodgers@usm.maine.edu
Website: http://www.usm.maine.edu/conhp
Dr. Marianne Rodgers, Contact
Fnded: 1878. **Degrees Offered:** BS, MS, MS/MBA.

Manitoba

★ 27859 ★ Brandon University
School of Health Studies
270 18th St.
Brandon, MB, Canada R7A 6A9
Phone: (204)727-7403 **Fax:** (204)728-7292
Email: demas@brandonu.ca
Website: http://www.brandonu.ca/
Cathy Demas, Contact
Fnded: 1899. **Degrees Offered:** BSC PN.

★ 27860 ★ University of Manitoba
Faculty of Nursing
Helen Glass Centre for Nursing
Winnipeg, MB, Canada R3T 2N2
Phone: (204)474-9317 **Fax:** (204)474-7682
Email: karen_chalmers@umanitoba.ca
Website: http://www.umanitoba.ca/faculties/nursing/
Dr. Karen Chalmers, Contact
Fnded: 1877. **Degrees Offered:** BN, MN.

Maryland

★ 27861 ★ Bowie State University
Program in Nursing
14000 Jericho Park Rd.
Bowie, MD 20715
Phone: (301)860-4000 **Fax:** (301)860-3222
Website: http://www.bowiestate.edu/dptnurs/
Fnded: 1865. **Degrees Offered:** BSN, MSN.

★ 27862 ★ College of Notre Dame of Maryland
Department of Nursing
4701 N Charles St.
Baltimore, MD 21210-2476
Phone: (410)532-5500
Email: wec@ndm.edu
Website: http://206.205.71.30/academics/departments/nd_aca_nursing.cfm
Fnded: 1873. **Degrees Offered:** BS.

★ 27863 ★ Columbia Union College
Nursing Department
7600 Flower Ave.
Takoma Park, MD 20912
Phone: (301)891-4144 **Fax:** (301)891-4191
Email: jessex@cuc.edu
Website: http://www.cuc.edu
Joy Essex, Contact
Fnded: 1904. **Degrees Offered:** BS.

★ 27864 ★ Coppin State College
Helene Fuld School of Nursing
2500 W North Ave.
Baltimore, MD 21216-3698
Phone: (410)951-3988 **Fax:** (410)462-3032
Email: dboyd@coppin.edu
Website: http://www.coppin.edu
Darryl A. Boyd, Contact
Fnded: 1900. **Degrees Offered:** BSN, MSN.

★ 27865 ★ Johns Hopkins University
School of Nursing
525 N Wolfe St.
Baltimore, MD 21205-2110
Phone: (410)955-7548 **Fax:** (410)614-7086
Email: orourke@son.jhmi.edu
Website: http://www.son.jhmi.edu
Mary O'Rourke, Contact
Fnded: 1876. **Degrees Offered:** BS, MSN, MSN/MBA, MSN/MPH, MSN/PhD.

★ 27866 ★ Salisbury University
Program in Nursing
1101 Camden Ave.
Salisbury, MD 21801
Phone: (410)543-6420 **Fax:** (410)548-3313
Email: kkbadros@salisbury.edu
Website: http://www.ssu.edu/Schools/Henson/NursingDept.html
Dr. Karen K. Badros, Contact
Fnded: 1925. **Degrees Offered:** BS, MS.

★ 27867 ★ Towson University
Department of Nursing
8000 York Rd.
Towson, MD 21252-0001
Phone: (410)704-4209 **Fax:** (410)704-4325
Email: jjordan@towson.edu
Website: http://www.towson.edu
Dr. Joan C. Jordan, Contact
Fnded: 1866. **Degrees Offered:** BS, MS.

★ 27868 ★ University of Maryland
School of Nursing
655 W Lombard St., Rm. 102
Baltimore, MD 21201-1579
Phone: (410)706-0501 **Fax:** (410)706-7238
Email: cornblat@son.umaryland.edu
Website: http://www.umaryland.edu
Robin Becker-Cornblatt, Contact
Fnded: 1807. **Degrees Offered:** BSN, MS, MS/MBA, PhD.

★ 27869 ★ Villa Julie College
Nursing Division
1525 Greenspring Valley Rd.
Stevenson, MD 21153-0641
Phone: (410)486-7000 **Fax:** (410)486-3552
Email: nursing@mail.vjc.edu
Website: http://www4.vjc.edu/Nursing
Fnded: 1952. **Degrees Offered:** BS.

Massachusetts

★ 27870 ★ American International College
Division of Nursing
1000 State St.
Springfield, MA 01109
Phone: (413)205-3800 **Fax:** (413)205-3943
Email: pmiller@acad.aic.edu
Website: http://www.aic.edu
Dr. Peter J. Miller, Contact
Fnded: 1885. **Degrees Offered:** BSN

★ 27871 ★ Anna Maria College
Department of Nursing
50 Sunset Ln.
Paxton, MA 01612-1198
Phone: (508)829-3316 **Fax:** (508)849-3343
Email: asilveri@annamaria.edu
Website: http://www.annamaria.edu
Dr. Audrey Marie Silveri, Director
Fnded: 1946. **Degrees Offered:** BSN

★ 27872 ★ Atlantic Union College
Department of Nursing
BS Coordinator
338 Main St.
South Lancaster, MA 01561
Phone: (978)368-2402 **Fax:** (978)368-2015
Email: mrittenhouse@atlanticuc.edu
Website: http://www.atlanticuc.edu
Marguerite Rittenhouse, Contact
Fnded: 1882. **Degrees Offered:** BS.

★ 27873 ★ Boston College
School of Nursing
140 Commonwealth Ave.
Chestnut Hill, MA 02467-3812
Phone: (617)552-4059 **Fax:** (617)552-0745
Email: parentkr@bc.edu
Website: http://www.bc.edu/nursing
Kristin Parent, Contact
Fnded: 1863. **Degrees Offered:** BS, MS, MS/MA, MS/MBA, PhD.

★ 27874 ★ Curry College
Division of Nursing and Health Sciences
1071 Blue Hill Ave.
Milton, MA 02186
Free: 800-669-0686 **Fax:** (617)333-2114
Email: bweckwor@curry.edu
Website: http://www.curry.edu
Bruce Weckworth, Contact
Fnded: 1879. **Degrees Offered:** BS.

★ 27875 ★ Emmanuel College
Department of Nursing
400 The Fenway
Boston, MA 02115
Phone: (617)735-9935 **Fax:** (617)735-9797
Email: riley@emmanuel.edu
Website: http://www.emmanuel.edu
Dr. Joan M. Riley, Contact
Fnded: 1919. **Degrees Offered:** BSN.

★ 27876 ★ Endicott College
Program in Nursing
376 Hale St.
Beverly, MA 01915
Phone: (978)921-1000 **Fax:** (978)232-2500
Email: admissio@endicott.edu
Website: http://www.endicott.edu
Thomas J. Redman, Contact
Fnded: 1939. **Degrees Offered:** BS.

★ 27877 ★ Fitchburg State College
Department of Nursing
160 Pearl St.
Fitchburg, MA 01420-2697
Phone: (978)665-3365 **Fax:** (978)665-3658
Email: bcammuso@fsc.edu
Website: http://www.fsc.edu
Dr. Barbara Cammuso, Contact
Fnded: 1894. **Degrees Offered:** BSN, M SC.

★ 27878 ★ Framingham State College
Department of Nursing
100 State St.
Framingham, MA 01701
Phone: (508)626-4715 **Fax:** (508)626-4746
Email: sconrad@frc.mass.edu
Website: http://www.frc.mass.edu/sconrad
Dr. Susan L. Conrad, Contact
Fnded: 1839. **Degrees Offered:** BS.

★ 27879 ★ MGH Institute of Health Professions
Program in Nursing
Charlestown Navy Yard
36 First Ave.
Boston, MA 02129
Phone: (617)726-3140 **Fax:** (617)726-8010
Email: admissions@mghihp.edu
Website: http://www.mghihp.edu
Fnded: 1977. **Degrees Offered:** MSN.

★ 27880 ★ Northeastern University
School of Nursing
203 Mugar Hall
360 Huntington Ave.
Boston, MA 02115
Phone: (617)373-3829 **Fax:** (617)373-4701
Email: w.purnell@neu.edu
Website: http://www.bouve.neu.edu/nursing.html
Bill Purnell, Contact
Fnded: 1898. **Degrees Offered:** BSN, MS, MSN/MBA.

★ 27881 ★ Regis College
Division of Nursing
235 Wellesley St.
Weston, MA 02493
Phone: (781)768-7188 **Fax:** (781)768-7071
Email: lisa.krug@regiscollege.edu
Website: http://www.regiscollege.edu
Lisa Krug, Contact
Fnded: 1927. **Degrees Offered:** BSN, MSN.

★ 27882 ★ Salem State College
Nursing Department
352 Lafayette St.
Salem, MA 01970
Phone: (978)542-6310 **Fax:** (978)542-7215
Email: susan.anderson@salemstate.edu
Website: http://www.salemstate.edu
Dr. Susan Anderson, Contact
Fnded: 1854. **Degrees Offered:** BSN, MSN, MSN/MBA.

★ 27883 ★ Simmons College
Department of Nursing
300 The Fenway
Boston, MA 02115
Phone: (617)521-2139 **Fax:** (617)521-3045
Email: judy.beal@simmons.edu
Website: http://www.simmons.edu/gshs/nursing/
Dr. Judith Beal, Contact
Fnded: 1899. **Degrees Offered:** BSN, MSN.

★ 27884 ★ University of Massachusetts, Amherst
School of Nursing
229 Arnold House
715 N Pleasant St.
Amherst, MA 01003-9304
Phone: (413)545-1302 **Fax:** (413)577-2550
Email: kcarlson@nursing.umass.edu
Website: http://www.umass.edu/nursing
Karen Ayotte, Contact
Fnded: 1863. **Degrees Offered:** BS, MS, MS/MPH, PhD.

★ 27885 ★ University of Massachusetts, Boston
College of Nursing and Health Sciences
100 Morrissey Blvd.
Boston, MA 02125
Phone: (617)287-6000 **Fax:** (617)265-7173
Email: enrollment.information@umb.edu
Website: http://www.nursing.umb.edu/
Jon Hutton, Contact
Fnded: 1964. **Degrees Offered:** BS, MS, PhD.

★ 27886 ★ University of Massachusetts, Dartmouth
College of Nursing
285 Old Westport Rd.
North Dartmouth, MA 02747-2300
Phone: (508)999-8159 **Fax:** (508)999-9127
Email: ndluhy@umassd.edu
Website: http://www.umassd.edu
Dr. Nancy Dluhy, Contact
Fnded: 1895. **Degrees Offered:** BSN, MS.

★ 27887 ★ University of Massachusetts, Lowell
Department of Nursing
3 Solomont Way, Ste. 2
Lowell, MA 01854-5126
Phone: (978)934-4467 **Fax:** (978)934-3006
Email: may_futrell@uml.edu
Website: http://www.uml.edu
Dr. May Futrell, Contact
Fnded: 1894. **Degrees Offered:** BS, MS, PhD.

★ 27888 ★ University of Massachusetts, Worcester
Graduate School of Nursing
55 Lake Ave. N
Worcester, MA 01655-0115
Phone: (508)856-5801 **Fax:** (508)856-5851
Email: elizabeth.flodin@umassmed.edu
Website: http://www.umassmed.edu/gsn/
Elizabeth Flodin, Contact
Fnded: 1962. **Degrees Offered:** MS, PhD.

★ 27889 ★ Worcester State College
Department of Nursing
486 Chandler St.
Worcester, MA 01602
Phone: (508)929-8685 **Fax:** (508)929-8186
Email: asamar@worcester.edu
Website: http://www.worcester.edu
Dr. Annmarie Samar, Contact
Fnded: 1874. **Degrees Offered:** BS, MS.

Michigan

★ 27890 ★ Andrews University
Department of Nursing
Berrien Springs, MI 49104
Phone: (616)471-3192 **Fax:** (616)471-3454
Email: francesj@andrews.edu
Website: http://www.andrews.edu
Dr. Frances Johnson, Contact
Fnded: 1874. **Degrees Offered:** BS, MS.

★ 27891 ★ Eastern Michigan University
Department of Nursing
301 Marshall Bldg.
Ypsilanti, MI 48197
Phone: (734)487-2310 **Fax:** (734)487-6946
Website: http://www.emich.edu/nursing
Dr. Susan Pfoutz, Contact
Fnded: 1849. **Degrees Offered:** BSN, MSN.

★ 27892 ★ Ferris State University
Department of Nursing and Dental Hygiene
200 Ferris Dr., Rm. 400A
Big Rapids, MI 49307
Phone: (231)591-2267 **Fax:** (231)591-2325
Email: coonj@ferris.edu
Website: http://www.ferris.edu
Dr. Julie A. Coon, Contact
Fnded: 1884. **Degrees Offered:** BSN.

★ 27893 ★ Grand Valley State University
Russell B. Kirkhof School of Nursing
DeVos Center, Rm. 338C
Allendale, MI 49401-9403
Phone: (616)331-7163 **Fax:** (616)895-2510
Email: bondl@gvsu.edu
Website: http://www4.gvsu.edu/kson/
Dr. Linda Bond, Contact
Fnded: 1960. **Degrees Offered:** BSN, MSN, MSN/MBA.

★ 27894 ★ Lake Superior State University
Department of Nursing
650 W Easterday Ave.
Sault Sainte Marie, MI 49783
Phone: (906)635-2446 **Fax:** (906)635-2266
Email: danleitner@lssu.edu
Website: http://www.lssu.edu
Donna Anleitner, Contact
Fnded: 1946. **Degrees Offered:** BSN.

★ 27895 ★ Madonna University
College of Nursing and Health
36600 Schoolcraft Rd.
Livonia, MI 48150-1173
Phone: (734)432-5461 **Fax:** (734)432-5463
Email: noconnor@maddona.edu
Website: http://www.munet.edu
Dr. Nancy O'Connor, Contact
Fnded: 1947. **Degrees Offered:** BSN, MSN, MSN/MBA.

★ 27896 ★ Michigan State University
College of Nursing
A-230 Life Sciences Bldg.
East Lansing, MI 48824
Phone: (517)353-4827 **Fax:** (517)353-9553
Email: nuro7@msu.edu
Website: http://nursing.msu.edu/
Renee B. Canady, Contact
Fnded: 1855. **Degrees Offered:** BSN, MSN, PhD.

★ 27897 ★ Northern Michigan University
College of Nursing and Allied Health Science
2310 New Science Facility
Marquette, MI 49855
Phone: (906)227-2487 **Fax:** (906)227-1658
Email: mwallace@nmu.edu
Website: http://www.nmu.edu/departments/nursing.html
Mary A. Wallace, Contact
Fnded: 1899. **Degrees Offered:** BSN, MSN.

★ 27898 ★ Oakland University
School of Nursing
452 O'Dowd Hall
Rochester, MI 48309-4401
Phone: (248)370-4082 **Fax:** (248)370-2996
Email: mullin@oakland.edu
Website: http://www2.oakland.edu/nursing
Sarah Mullin, Contact
Fnded: 1957. **Degrees Offered:** BSN, MSN.

★ 27899 ★ Saginaw Valley State University
Crystal M. Lange College of Nursing and Health Sciences
7400 Bay Rd.
University Center, MI 48710-0001
Phone: (989)964-4130
Email: blecke@svsu.edu
Website: http://www.svsu.edu/acadprog/nhs/
Dr. Janalou Blecke, Contact
Fnded: 1963. **Degrees Offered:** BSN, MSN.

★ 27900 ★ University of Detroit Mercy
McAuley School of Nursing
PO Box 19900
Detroit, MI 48219-0900
Phone: (313)993-6423 **Fax:** (313)993-6175
Email: baiardjm@udmercy.edu
Website: http://www.udmercy.edu
Janet Baiardi, Contact
Fnded: 1877. **Degrees Offered:** BSN, MSN.

★ 27901 ★ University of Michigan
School of Nursing
400 N Ingalls Bldg., Rm. 1154
Ann Arbor, MI 48109-0482
Phone: (734)764-7188 **Fax:** (734)647-1419
Email: loveland@umich.edu
Website: http://www.nursing.umich.edu
Dr. Carol J. Loveland-Cherry, Contact
Fnded: 1817. **Degrees Offered:** BSN, MS, MS/MHSA, PhD.

★ 27902 ★ University of Michigan, Flint
Department of Nursing
2180 William S White Bldg.
303 E Kearsley
Flint, MI 48502-1950
Phone: (810)762-3420 **Fax:** (810)766-6851
Email: nursing@list.flint.umich.edu
Website: http://www.flint.umich.edu
Margaret A. Hathaway, Contact
Fnded: 1956. **Degrees Offered:** BSN, MSN.

★ 27903 ★ University of Phoenix, Metro Detroit Campus
College of Health Care Sciences and Nursing
5480 Corporate Dr.
Ste. 240
Troy, MI 48098-9729
Free: 800-834-2438
Website: http://www.phoenix.edu/
Degrees Offered: BSN, MSN, MSN/MBA.

★ 27904 ★ University of Phoenix, West Michigan Campus
College of Health Care Sciences and Nursing
Grand Rapids, MI
Free: 888-345-9699
Website: http://www.phoenix.edu/
Degrees Offered: BSN, MSN, MSN/MBA.

★ 27905 ★ Wayne State University
College of Nursing
10 Cohn Bldg.
5557 Cass Ave.
Detroit, MI 48202
Phone: (313)577-4082 **Fax:** (313)577-6949
Email: jharden@wayne.edu
Website: http://www.nursing.wayne.edu
Janet Harden, Contact
Fnded: 1868. **Degrees Offered:** BSN, MSN, PhD.

★ 27906 ★ Western Michigan University
College of Health and Human Services
1903 W Michigan Ave.
Kalamazoo, MI 49008
Phone: (616)387-8150 **Fax:** (616)387-8170
Email: marsha.mahan@wmich.edu
Website: http://www.wmich.edu
Marsha Ann Mahan, Contact
Fnded: 1903. **Degrees Offered:** BS.

Minnesota

★ 27907 ★ Augsburg College
Program in Nursing
2211 Riverside Ave. S
Minneapolis, MN 55454
Phone: (612)330-1204 **Fax:** (612)330-1649
Email: watson@augsburg.edu
Website: http://www.augsburg.edu
Luann Watson, Contact
Fnded: 1869. **Degrees Offered:** BS, MA.

★ 27908 ★ Bemidji State University
Department of Nursing
Deputy Hall 105, Box 15
1500 Birchmont Dr. NE
Bemidji, MN 56601
Phone: (218)755-3892 **Fax:** (218)755-4402
Email: rscheela@bemidjistate.edu
Website: http://www.bemidji.msus.edu
Dr. Rochelle A. Scheela, Contact
Fnded: 1919. **Degrees Offered:** BS.

★ 27909 ★ Bethel College
Department of Nursing
3900 Bethel Dr.
Saint Paul, MN 55112
Phone: (651)638-6298 **Fax:** (651)635-1965
Email: m-schaffer@bethel.edu
Website: http://www.bethel.edu/cgcs/
Dr. Marjorie Schaffer, Contact
Fnded: 1871. **Degrees Offered:** BSN, MA.

★ 27910 ★ College of Saint Benedict
Department of Nursing
37 College Ave. S
Saint Joseph, MN 56374
Phone: (320)363-5404 **Fax:** (320)363-6099
Email: ktwohy@csbsju.edu
Website: http://www.csbsju.edu/nursing/
Dr. Kathleen M. Twohy, Contact
Fnded: 1887. **Degrees Offered:** BS.

★ 27911 ★ College of Saint Catherine
Department of Nursing
2004 Randolph Ave.
F-22
Saint Paul, MN 55105
Phone: (651)690-6575 **Fax:** (651)690-6941
Email: rebrink@stkate.edu
Website: http://www.stkate.edu
Dr. Ruth Brink, Contact
Fnded: 1905. **Degrees Offered:** BS, MA.

★ 27912 ★ College of Saint Scholastica
Department of Nursing
1200 Kenwood Ave.
Duluth, MN 55811
Phone: (218)723-6452 **Fax:** (218)723-6472
Email: cmaynard@css.edu
Website: http://www.css.edu
Dr. Carleen Maynard, Contact
Fnded: 1912. **Degrees Offered:** BA, MA.

★ 27913 ★ Concordia College
Tri-College University Nursing Consortium
901 S 8th St.
Moorhead, MN 56562
Phone: (218)299-4102 **Fax:** (218)299-4308
Email: cpeterso@cord.edu
Website: http://www.cord.edu/dept/nursing/index.htm
Connie Peterson, Contact
Fnded: 1891. **Degrees Offered:** BA.

★ 27914 ★ Gustavus Adolphus College
Minnesota Intercollegiate Nursing Consortium
Saint Peter, MN 56082
Website: http://www.gustavus.edu/
Remarks: For more information see listing under Minnesota Intercollegiate Nursing Consortium.

★ 27915 ★ Metropolitan State University
School of Nursing
700 E 7th St.
Saint Paul, MN 55106-5000
Phone: (651)793-1378 **Fax:** (651)793-1382
Email: lynda.zimmerman@metrostate.edu
Website: http://www.metrostate.edu
Lynda Zimmerman, Contact
Fnded: 1971. **Degrees Offered:** BSN, MSN.

★ 27916 ★ Minnesota Intercollegiate Nursing Consortium
1520 St. Olaf Ave.
Northfield, MN 55057-1098
Phone: (507)646-3265 **Fax:** (507)646-3733
Email: glazebro@stolaf.edu
Dr. Rita S. Glazebrook, Contact
Degrees Offered: BA.

★ 27917 ★ Minnesota State University, Mankato
School of Nursing
360 Wissink Hall, MSU 27
Mankato, MN 56001
Phone: (507)389-1317 **Fax:** (507)389-6516
Email: sonja.meiers@mnsu.edu
Website: http://www.mankato.msus.edu/
Dr. Sonja J. Meiers, Contact
Fnded: 1868. **Degrees Offered:** BS, MSN.

★ 27918 ★ Minnesota State University, Moorhead
Tri-College University Nursing Consortium
1104 S 7th Ave.
Moorhead, MN 56563
Phone: (218)236-4699 **Fax:** (218)299-5990
Email: giedt@mnstate.edu
Website: http://www.moorhead.msus.edu/
Dr. Jane Giedt, Contact
Fnded: 1885. **Degrees Offered:** BSN, MS.

★ 27919 ★ Saint Olaf College
Minnesota Intercollegiate Nursing Consortium
Northfield, MN 55057
Website: http://www.stolaf.edu/
Remarks: For more information see listing under Minnesota Intercollegiate Nursing Consortium.

★ 27920 ★ University of Minnesota, Twin Cities Campus
School of Nursing
5-160 Weaver-Densford Hall
308 Harvard St. SE
Minneapolis, MN 55455-0213
Phone: (612)625-5965 **Fax:** (612)624-3174
Email: rosan003@umn.edu
Website: http://www.nursing.umn.edu
Jennifer Rosand, Contact
Fnded: 1851. **Degrees Offered:** BSN, MS, MS/MPH, PhD.

★ 27921 ★ Winona State University
College of Nursing
859 SE 30th Ave.
Rochester, MN 55904
Phone: (507)285-7489 **Fax:** (507)292-5127
Email: wmcbreen@winona.msus.edu
Website: http://www.winona.edu/nursing/
Dr. William McBreen, Contact
Fnded: 1858. **Degrees Offered:** BSN, MS.

Mississippi

★ 27922 ★ Alcorn State University
School of Nursing
15 Campus Dr.
Natchez, MS 39120
Phone: (601)442-3901 **Fax:** (601)446-5942
Email: stiner@lorman.alcorn.edu
Website: http://www.alcorn.edu/academic/academ/nurses.htm
Dr. Evelyn Stiner, Contact
Fnded: 1871. **Degrees Offered:** BSN, MSN.

★ 27923 ★ Delta State University
School of Nursing
PO Box 3343
Cleveland, MS 38733
Phone: (662)846-4255 **Fax:** (662)846-4267
Email: dlamar@dsu.deltast.edu
Website: http://www.deltastate.edu
Dr. Dana Lamar, Contact
Fnded: 1924. **Degrees Offered:** BSN, MSN.

★ 27924 ★ Mississippi College
School of Nursing
Box 4037
200 S Capitol St.
Clinton, MS 39058
Phone: (601)925-3278 **Fax:** (601)925-3379
Email: padgett@mc.edu
Website: http://mc.edu
Dr. Mary Jean Padgett, Contact
Fnded: 1826. **Degrees Offered:** BSN.

★ 27925 ★ Mississippi University for Women
Division of Nursing
PO Box W-910
15th St. N
Columbus, MS 39701
Phone: (662)329-7323 **Fax:** (662)329-7372
Email: mcurtis@muw.edu
Website: http://www.muw.edu/nursing
Dr. Mary Pat Curtis, Contact
Fnded: 1884. **Degrees Offered:** BSN, MSN.

★ 27926 ★ University of Mississippi Medical Center
School of Nursing
2500 N State St.
Jackson, MS 39216-4505
Phone: (601)984-6256 **Fax:** (601)815-5957
Email: oallen@son.umsmed.edu
Website: http://son.umc.edu/
Dr. Ola Allen, Contact

Fnded: 1955. **Degrees Offered:** BSN, MSN, PhD.

★ 27927 ★ University of Southern Mississippi
College of Nursing
Box 5095
Hattiesburg, MS 39406-5095
Phone: (601)266-5788 **Fax:** (601)266-5927
Email: helen.rassier@usm.edu
Website: http://www.nursing.usm.edu
Helen C. Rassier, Contact
Fnded: 1910. **Degrees Offered:** BSN, MSN, PhD.

★ 27928 ★ William Carey College
School of Nursing
498 Tuscan Ave.
Hattiesburg, MS 39401
Phone: (601)318-6147 **Fax:** (601)318-6446
Email: mware@wmcarey.edu
Website: http://www.wmcarey.edu
Dr. Mary A. Ware, Contact
Fnded: 1906. **Degrees Offered:** BSN.

Missouri

★ 27929 ★ Avila University
Department of Nursing
Office of Admissions
11901 Wornall Rd.
Kansas City, MO 64145
Phone: (816)501-2400 **Fax:** (816)501-2453
Email: admissions@mail.avila.edu
Website: http://www.avila.edu/catalog/degrees/nursing_.htm
Fnded: 1916. **Degrees Offered:** BSN.

★ 27930 ★ Central Missouri State University
Department of Nursing
Graduate Studies, WDE 1800
Warrensburg, MO 64093
Phone: (660)543-4621
Email: perrin@cmsu1.cmsu.edu
Website: http://www.cmsu.edu/nursing/dept.html
Dr. Novella Perrin, Contact
Fnded: 1871. **Degrees Offered:** BS, MSN.

★ 27931 ★ Culver-Stockton College
Blessing-Rieman College of Nursing
Canton, MO 63435
Website: http://www.culver.edu/
Remarks: For more information see description under Blessing-Rieman College of Nursing, Quincy, Illinois.

★ 27932 ★ Deaconess College of Nursing
6150 Oakland Ave.
Saint Louis, MO 63139
Free: 800-942-4310 **Fax:** (314)768-3044
Email: lisa.mancini@tenethealth.com
Website: http://www.deaconess.edu
Lisa Mancini, Contact
Fnded: 1889. **Degrees Offered:** BSN.

★ 27933 ★ Graceland University
School of Nursing
1401 W Truman Rd.
Independence, MO 64050-3434
Phone: (816)833-0524 **Fax:** (816)833-2990
Email: karenf@graceland.edu
Website: http://outreach.graceland.edu
Karen Fernengel, Contact
Fnded: 1895. **Degrees Offered:** BSN, MSN

★ 27934 ★ Jewish Hospital College of Nursing and Allied Health
Division of Nursing
306 S Kingshighway Blvd.
Saint Louis, MO 63116
Phone: (314)454-8416 **Fax:** (314)454-5239
Email: sjb@bjcmail.carenet.org
Dr. Elizabeth A. Buck, Contact
Fnded: 1902. **Degrees Offered:** BSN, MSN.

★ 27935 ★ Maryville University, Saint Louis
School of Health Professions
Nursing Program
13550 Conway Rd.
Saint Louis, MO 63141
Phone: (314)529-9435
Email: sstopke@maryville.edu
Website: http://www.maryville.edu
Sherry Stopke, Contact
Fnded: 1872. **Degrees Offered:** BSN, MSN.

★ 27936 ★ Missouri Southern State College
Department of Nursing
3950 E Newman Rd.
Kuhn Hall
Joplin, MO 64801-1595
Phone: (417)625-9322 **Fax:** (417)625-3186
Email: box-b@mail.mssc.edu
Website: http://www.mssc.edu
Dr. Barbara J. Box, Contact
Fnded: 1937. **Degrees Offered:** BSN.

★ 27937 ★ Missouri Western State College
Department of Nursing
4525 Downs Dr.
Saint Joseph, MO 64507
Phone: (816)271-4415 **Fax:** (816)271-5849
Email: nursing@mwsc.edu
Website: http://www.mwsc.edu/nursing
Fnded: 1915. **Degrees Offered:** BSN.

★ 27938 ★ Research College of Nursing
College of Nursing
2316 E Meyer Blvd.
Kansas City, MO 64132-1199
Phone: (816)276-4733 **Fax:** (816)276-3526
Email: lamendenhall@healthmidwest.org
Leslie Mendenhall, Contact
Fnded: 1980. **Degrees Offered:** BSN, MSN.

★ 27939 ★ Saint Louis University
School of Nursing
3525 Caroline Mall
Saint Louis, MO 63104
Phone: (314)577-8931 **Fax:** (314)577-8949
Email: edele@slu.edu
Website: http://www.slu.edu/colleges/NR
Dr. Margie Edel, Contact
Fnded: 1818. **Degrees Offered:** BSN, MSN, MSN/MPH, PhD.

★ 27940 ★ Saint Luke's College
Nursing College
4426 Wornall Rd.
Kansas City, MO 64111
Phone: (816)932-2073 **Fax:** (816)932-3831
Email: mjthomas@saint-lukes.org
Website: http://www.saint-lukes.org/meded/slc.htm
Marsha Thomas, Contact
Fnded: 1903. **Degrees Offered:** BSN.

★ 27941 ★ Southeast Missouri State University
Department of Nursing
One University Plaza
Mail Stop 8300
Cape Girardeau, MO 63701-4799
Phone: (573)651-2871 **Fax:** (573)651-2142
Email: ejackson@semo.edu
Website: http://www2.semo.edu/nursing
Dr. Elaine Jackson, Contact
Fnded: 1873. **Degrees Offered:** BSN, MSN.

★ 27942 ★ Southwest Missouri State University
Department of Nursing
901 S National
Springfield, MO 65804
Phone: (417)836-5310 **Fax:** (417)836-5484
Email: kathrynhope@smsu.edu
Website: http://www.smsu.edu/nursing
Dr. Kathryn L. Hope, Contact
Fnded: 1905. **Degrees Offered:** BSN, MSN.

★ 27943 ★ Truman State University
Program in Nursing
Barnett Hall 223
100 E Normal St.
Kirksville, MO 63501
Phone: (660)785-4557 **Fax:** (660)785-7424
Email: spowelso@truman.edu
Website: http://nursing.truman.edu
Dr. Stephanie A. Powelson, Contact
Fnded: 1867. **Degrees Offered:** BSN.

★ 27944 ★ University of Missouri, Columbia
Sinclair School of Nursing
S235 Sinclair School of Nursing
Columbia, MO 65211
Phone: (573)882-0277 **Fax:** (573)884-4544
Email: johnsonn@missouri.edu
Website: http://www.muhealth.org/
Nancy Lee Johnson, Contact
Fnded: 1839. **Degrees Offered:** BSN, MS, PhD.

★ 27945 ★ University of Missouri, Kansas City
School of Nursing
2220 Holmes St.
Kansas City, MO 64108
Phone: (816)235-1740 **Fax:** (816)235-1701
Email: jellisonj@umkc.edu
Website: http://www.umkc.edu
Judy A. Jellison, Contact
Fnded: 1929. **Degrees Offered:** BSN, MSN, PhD.

★ 27946 ★ University of Missouri, Saint Louis
College of Nursing
8001 Natural Bridge Rd.
Saint Louis, MO 63121-4499
Phone: (314)516-7087 **Fax:** (314)516-7519
Email: canda@umsl.edu
Website: http://www.umsl.edu/divisions/nursing/
Kathern Canda, Contact
Fnded: 1963. **Degrees Offered:** BSN, MSN, PhD.

★ 27947 ★ Webster University
Department of Nursing
470 E Lockwood Ave.
Saint Louis, MO 63119
Phone: (314)968-7483 **Fax:** (314)963-6101
Email: headysa@websteruniv.edu
Website: http://www.webster.edu/depts/artsci/nursing/nursing.html
Dr. Susan Heady, Contact
Fnded: 1915. **Degrees Offered:** BSN, MSN.

★ 27948 ★ William Jewell College
Department of Nursing
500 College Hill, Box 2002
Liberty, MO 64068
Phone: (816)781-7700 **Fax:** (816)415-5024
Email: godfreyn@william.jewell.edu
Website: http://jewell.edu
Dr. Nelda S. Godfrey, Contact
Fnded: 1849. **Degrees Offered:** BS.

Montana

★ 27949 ★ Carroll College
Department of Nursing
Helena, MT 59625
Phone: (406)447-5482 **Fax:** (406)447-4533
Email: mbrown@carroll.edu
Website: http://www.carroll.edu
Mike Brown, Contact
Fnded: 1909. **Degrees Offered:** BA.

★ 27950 ★ Montana State University, Bozeman
College of Nursing
Sherrick Hall
PO Box 173560
Bozeman, MT 59717-3560
Phone: (406)994-3784 **Fax:** (406)994-6020
Email: gmcneely@montana.edu
Website: http://www.montana.edu/nursing
Dr. A. Gretchen McNeely, Contact
Fnded: 1893. **Degrees Offered:** BSN, MN.

★ 27951 ★ Montana State University, Northern
College of Nursing
2100 16th Ave. S
PO Box 6010
Great Falls, MT 59406
Free: 800-446-2698 **Fax:** (406)771-4426
Email: rmunson@msun.edu
Website: http://www.msun.edu/academics/nursing
Renae Munson, Contact
Fnded: 1929. **Degrees Offered:** BSN.

Nebraska

★ 27952 ★ Clarkson College
Department of Nursing
101 S 42nd St.
Omaha, NE 68131-2739
Free: 800-647-5500 **Fax:** (402)552-6057
Website: http://www.clarksoncollege.edu
Fnded: 1888. **Degrees Offered:** BSN, MSN.

★ 27953 ★ College of Saint Mary
School of Health Care Professions
1901 S 72nd St.
Omaha, NE 68124
Phone: (402)399-2636 **Fax:** (402)399-2654
Email: phawkins@csm.edu
Website: http://www.csm.edu
Dr. Peggy L. Hawkins, Contact
Fnded: 1923. **Degrees Offered:** BSN.

★ 27954 ★ Creighton University
School of Nursing
2500 California Plaza
Omaha, NE 68178
Phone: (402)280-2041 **Fax:** (402)280-2045
Email: bbevans@creighton.edu
Website: http://nursing.creighton.edu/
Dr. Brenda Bergman-Evans, Contact
Fnded: 1878. **Degrees Offered:** BSN, MS

★ 27955 ★ Midland Lutheran College
Department of Nursing
900 N Clarkson
Fremont, NE 68025
Phone: (402)721-5480 **Fax:** (402)721-0250
Email: watson@mlc.edu
Website: http://www.mlc.edu
Doug Watson, Contact
Fnded: 1883. **Degrees Offered:** BSN.

★ 27956 ★ Nebraska Methodist College
Department of Nursing
8501 W Dodge Rd.
Omaha, NE 68114-3426
Phone: (402)354-2270 **Fax:** (402)354-8875
Website: http://www.methodistcollege.edu
Marilyn Valerio, Contact
Fnded: 1891. **Degrees Offered:** BSN, MSN.

★ 27957 ★ Nebraska Wesleyan University
Department of Nursing
5000 Saint Paul Ave.
Lincoln, NE 68504
Phone: (402)465-2334 **Fax:** (402)465-2179
Email: pjm@nebrwesleyan.edu
Website: http://www.nebrwesleyan.edu
Dr. Patricia Jean Morin, Contact
Fnded: 1887. **Degrees Offered:** BSN, MSN.

★ 27958 ★ Union College
Division of Health Sciences
3800 S 48th St.
Lincoln, NE 68506
Phone: (402)486-2524 **Fax:** (402)486-2559
Email: kaminear@ucollege.edu
Website: http://www.ucollege.edu
Karen W. Minear, Contact
Fnded: 1891. **Degrees Offered:** BSN.

★ 27959 ★ University of Nebraska Medical Center
College of Nursing
985330 Nebraska Medical Center
Omaha, NE 68198-5330
Phone: (402)559-7457 **Fax:** (402)559-4303
Email: mwilson@unmc.edu
Website: http://www.unmc.edu/nursing/
Dr. Margaret Wilson, Contact
Fnded: 1869. **Degrees Offered:** BSN, MSN, PhD.

Nevada

★ 27960 ★ University of Nevada, Las Vegas
Department of Nursing
4505 Maryland Pkwy.
Las Vegas, NV 89154-3018
Phone: (702)895-3360 **Fax:** (702)895-4807
Email: cbowles@ccmail.nevada.edu
Website: http://www.unlv.edu
Dr. Cheryl Bowles, Contact
Fnded: 1957. **Degrees Offered:** BSN, MSN.

★ 27961 ★ University of Nevada, Reno
Orvis School of Nursing
Mail Stop 134
Reno, NV 89557
Phone: (775)784-6841 **Fax:** (775)784-4262
Email: jaynem@unr.edu
Website: http://www.unr.edu
Jayne Moore, Contact
Fnded: 1874. **Degrees Offered:** BSN, MS, MSN/MPH.

New Brunswick

★ 27962 ★ Universite de Moncton
School of Nursing
Pavillon Leopold Taillon
Moncton, NB, Canada E1A 3E9
Phone: (506)858-4443 **Fax:** (506)858-4544
Email: bordely@umoncton.ca
Website: http://www.umoncton.ca/
Yoland Bordeleau, Contact
Fnded: 1963. **Degrees Offered:** BSCN, M SC N.

★ 27963 ★ University of New Brunswick, Fredericton
Faculty of Nursing
PO Box 4400
Fredericton, NB, Canada E3B 5A3
Phone: (506)451-6844 **Fax:** (506)447-3374
Email: anderson@unb.ca
Website: http://www.unbf.ca/nursing/
Fnded: 1785. **Degrees Offered:** BN, MN.

New Hampshire

★ 27964 ★ Colby-Sawyer College
Department of Nursing
541 Main St.
New London, NH 03257-4648
Phone: (603)526-3646 **Fax:** (603)526-3452
Email: kthies@colby-sawyer.edu
Website: http://www.colby-sawyer.edu/academic/nursing
Dr. Kathleen M. Thies, Contact
Fnded: 1837. **Degrees Offered:** BS.

★ 27965 ★ Rivier College
Department of Nursing and Health Sciences
420 Main St.
Nashua, NH 03060-5086
Phone: (603)897-8478 **Fax:** (603)897-8884
Email: ipattison@rivier.edu
Website: http://www.rivier.edu
Dr. Ivor Pattison, Contact
Fnded: 1933. **Degrees Offered:** BS, MS, MS/MBA.

★ 27966 ★ Saint Anselm College
Department of Nursing
100 Saint Anselm Dr.
Manchester, NH 03102-1310
Phone: (603)641-7500 **Fax:** (603)641-7550
Email: ngriffin@anselm.edu
Website: http://www.anselm.edu
Nancy Davis Griffin, Contact
Fnded: 1889. **Degrees Offered:** BS.

★ 27967 ★ University of New Hampshire
Department of Nursing
Hewitt Hall
4 Library Way
Durham, NH 03824-3563
Phone: (603)862-2260 **Fax:** (603)862-4771
Email: geh@christa.unh.edu
Website: http://www.unh.edu/nursing
Gene Harkless, Contact
Fnded: 1866. **Degrees Offered:** BS, MS.

New Jersey

★ 27968 ★ Bloomfield College
Division of Nursing
One Park Pl.
1 Park Pl.
Bloomfield, NJ 07003
Phone: (973)748-9000 **Fax:** (973)748-0916
Email: lourdes_delgado@bloomfield.edu
Website: http://www.bloomfield.edu
Lourdes Delgado, Contact

Fnded: 1868. **Degrees Offered:** BSN.

★ 27969 ★ College of New Jersey
School of Nursing
PO Box 7718
2000 Pennington Rd.
Ewing, NJ 08628-0718
Phone: (609)771-2591 **Fax:** (609)637-5159
Email: lindberg@tcnj.edu
Website: http://www.tcnj.edu/~nursing
Dr. Claire Lindberg, Contact
Fnded: 1855. **Degrees Offered:** BSN, MSN.

★ 27970 ★ College of Saint Elizabeth
Department of Nursing
2 Convent Rd.
Morristown, NJ 07960-6989
Phone: (973)290-4056 **Fax:** (973)290-4177
Email: jlehmann@cse.edu
Website: http://www.cse.edu/sgcs_continuingstudies.htm
Sr. Janet Lehmann, Contact
Fnded: 1899. **Degrees Offered:** BSN.

★ 27971 ★ Fairleigh Dickinson University, Metropolitan Campus
Henry P. Becton School of Nursing and Allied Health
Dickinson Hall-444A
1000 River Rd.
Teaneck, NJ 07666
Phone: (201)692-2888 **Fax:** (201)692-2388
Email: swarren@mailbox.fdu.edu
Website: http://www.fdu.edu
Dr. Susan Warren, Contact
Fnded: 1942. **Degrees Offered:** BSN, MSN.

★ 27972 ★ Felician College
Department of Professional Nursing-BSN
262 S Main St.
Lodi, NJ 07644
Phone: (201)559-6055
Website: http://www.felician.edu
Elizabeth Griffin, Contact
Fnded: 1942. **Degrees Offered:** BSN, MSN.

★ 27973 ★ Kean University
Department of Nursing
1000 Morris Ave.
Townsend 112
Union, NJ 07083-0411
Phone: (908)737-3386 **Fax:** (908)737-3393
Email: dpacquia@kean.edu
Website: http://www.kean.edu/
Dr. Dula Pacquiao, Contact
Fnded: 1855. **Degrees Offered:** BSN, MSN, MSN/MPA.

★ 27974 ★ Monmouth University
Marjorie K. Unterberg School of Nursing
West Long Branch, NJ 07764
Phone: (732)571-3443 **Fax:** (732)263-5131
Email: sstark@monmouth.edu
Website: http://www.monmouth.edu
Dr. Sharon Stark, Contact
Fnded: 1933. **Degrees Offered:** BSN, MSN.

★ 27975 ★ New Jersey City University
Department of Nursing
2039 Kennedy Blvd., P449
Jersey City, NJ 07305
Phone: (201)200-3157 **Fax:** (201)200-3222
Email: gboseman@njcu.edu
Website: http://www.njcu.edu/dept/ProfStudies/nursing2/rnbsn.htm
Dr. Gloria Boseman, Contact
Fnded: 1927. **Degrees Offered:** BSN, MS.

★ 27976 ★ Richard Stockton College of New Jersey
Program in Nursing
Office of Enrollment Management
PO Box 195
Pomona, NJ 08240
Phone: (609)652-4837
Email: admissions@stockton.edu
Website: http://www.stockton.edu
Fnded: 1969. **Degrees Offered:** BSN, MSN.

★ 27977 ★ Rutgers, the State University of New Jersey
Camden College of Arts and Sciences
Department of Nursing
Armitage Hall
311 N 5th St.
Camden, NJ 08102
Phone: (856)225-6526 **Fax:** (856)225-6541
Email: otoolem@crab.rutgers.edu
Website: http://www.rutgers.edu
Marie O'Toole, Contact
Fnded: 1927. **Degrees Offered:** BS, MS.

★ 27978 ★ Rutgers, the State University of New Jersey
College of Nursing
180 University Ave.
Newark, NJ 07102-1803
Phone: (973)353-5293 **Fax:** (973)353-1277
Email: dolinsky@nightingale.rutgers.edu
Website: http://www.rutgers.edu
Dr. Elaine Dolinsky, Contact
Fnded: 1956. **Degrees Offered:** BS, MS, MS/MPH, PhD.

★ 27979 ★ Saint Peter's College
Nursing Program
Hudson Terrace
Englewood Cliffs, NJ 07632
Phone: (201)568-5208 **Fax:** (201)569-1254
Email: yam_m@spcvxa.spc.edu
Website: http://www.spc.edu
Dr. Marylou Yam, Contact
Fnded: 1872. **Degrees Offered:** BSN, MSN.

★ 27980 ★ Seton Hall University
College of Nursing
400 S Orange Ave.
South Orange, NJ 07079-2693
Phone: (973)761-9285 **Fax:** (973)761-9607
Email: bugelmar@shu.edu
Website: http://www.shu.edu
Mary Jo Bugel, Contact
Fnded: 1856. **Degrees Offered:** BSN, MSN, MSN/MA, MSN/MBA.

★ 27981 ★ Thomas Edison State College
Program in Nursing
101 W State St.
Trenton, NJ 08608-1176
Email: info@tesc.edu
Website: http://www.tesc.edu
Fnded: 1983. **Degrees Offered:** BSN.

★ 27982 ★ University of Medicine and Dentistry of New Jersey
School of Nursing
65 Bergen St., Rm. 1126
University Heights
Newark, NJ 07107-3001
Phone: (973)972-5336 **Fax:** (973)972-7453
Email: shieldjo@umdnj.edu
Website: http://sn.umdnj.edu/school/
Joan Zadrozny Shields, Contact
Fnded: 1954. **Degrees Offered:** BSN, MSN, PhD.

★ 27983 ★ William Paterson University of New Jersey
Department of Nursing
300 Pompton Rd., W240
Wayne, NJ 07470
Phone: (973)720-3495 **Fax:** (973)720-3517
Email: barefordc@wpunj.edu
Website: http://www.wpunj.edu
Dr. Connie Gleim Bareford, Contact
Fnded: 1855. **Degrees Offered:** BSN, MSN.

New Mexico

★ 27984 ★ Eastern New Mexico University
Department of Allied Health—Nursing
Station No. 12
Portales, NM 88130
Phone: (505)562-2403 **Fax:** (505)562-2293
Email: ellen.bral@enmu.edu
Website: http://www.enmu.edu
Dr. Ellen E. Bral, Contact
Fnded: 1934. **Degrees Offered:** BSN.

★ 27985 ★ New Mexico State University
Department of Nursing
Department 3185
PO Box 30001
Las Cruces, NM 88003-8001
Phone: (505)646-3812 **Fax:** (505)646-2527
Email: mpase@nmsu.edu
Website: http://www.nmsu.edu/~nursing
Marilyn Pase, Contact
Fnded: 1888. **Degrees Offered:** BSN, MSN.

★ 27986 ★ University of New Mexico
College of Nursing
2502 Marble NE
NRPH Bldg.
Albuquerque, NM 87131-5688
Phone: (505)272-4223 **Fax:** (505)272-3970
Email: erowe@salud.unm.edu
Website: http://hsc.unm.edu/consg/
Elizabeth Rowe, Contact
Fnded: 1889. **Degrees Offered:** BSN, MSN, MSN/MALAS, MSN/MPA, MSN/MPH.

★ 27987 ★ University of Phoenix, New Mexico Campus
College of Health Care Sciences and Nursing
Albuquerque, NM
Phone: (505)821-4800
Website: http://www.phoenix.edu/
Degrees Offered: BSN, MSN, MSN/MBA.

New York

★ 27988 ★ Adelphi University
School of Nursing
One South Ave.
Levermore Hall
Garden City, NY 11530
Phone: (516)877-3052 **Fax:** (516)877-3039
Email: posillic@adelphi.edu
Website: http://www.adelphi.edu
Joseph Posillico, Contact
Fnded: 1896. **Degrees Offered:** BS, MS, MS/MBA.

★ 27989 ★ City University of New York
College of Staten Island
Department of Nursing
2800 Victory Blvd.
Staten Island, NY 10314
Phone: (718)982-3845 **Fax:** (718)982-3813
Email: lunney@postbox.csi.cuny.edu
Website: http://www.csi.cuny.edu/nursing
Dr. Margaret Lunney, Contact

Fnded: 1955. Degrees Offered: BS, MS.

★ 27990 ★ City University of New York Herbert H. Lehman College
Department of Nursing
250 Bedford Park Blvd. W
Bronx, NY 10468
Phone: (718)960-8374 **Fax:** (718)960-8488
Website: http://www.lehman.cuny.edu
Fnded: 1931. **Degrees Offered:** BS, MS.

★ 27991 ★ City University of New York Hunter College
Hunter-Bellevue School of Nursing
425 E 25th St.
New York, NY 10010
Phone: (212)481-4465 **Fax:** (212)481-4427
Email: vmalinsk@hunter.cuny.edu
Website: http://www.hunter.cuny.edu/schoolhp/nursing
Dr. Violet M. Malinski, Contact
Fnded: 1870. **Degrees Offered:** BS, MS, MS/MPH.

★ 27992 ★ City University of New York Medgar Evers College
Department of Nursing
BSN Program Coordinator
C-302B
Brooklyn, NY 11225
Phone: (718)270-6230 **Fax:** (718)270-6496
Email: emccarroll@mec.cuny.edu
Website: http://www.mec.cuny.edu/academic_affairs/science_tech_school/nursing/nurse_home.htm
Dr. Ellen McCarroll, Contact
Fnded: 1969. **Degrees Offered:** BS.

★ 27993 ★ City University of New York York College
Program in Nursing
94-20 Guy R. Brewer Blvd.
Jamaica, NY 11451
Phone: (718)262-2165
Website: http://www.york.cuny.edu/~healthsci/nuprogram.html
Fnded: 1967. **Degrees Offered:** BS.

★ 27994 ★ College of Mount Saint Vincent
Division of Nursing
6301 Riverdale Ave.
Riverdale, NY 10471-1093
Phone: (718)405-3354 **Fax:** (718)405-3286
Website: http://www.mountsaintvincent.edu/academics/majors_and_programs/nursing2/nursing.htm
Fnded: 1911. **Degrees Offered:** BS, MSN.

★ 27995 ★ College of New Rochelle
School of Nursing
29 Castle Pl.
New Rochelle, NY 10805-2308
Phone: (914)654-5454 **Fax:** (914)654-5994
Email: ddemarest@cnr.edu
Website: http://cnr.edu
Dr. Donna J. Demarest, Contact
Fnded: 1904. **Degrees Offered:** BSN, MS.

★ 27996 ★ Columbia University
School of Nursing
630 W 168th St.
Box 6
New York, NY 10032
Phone: (212)305-5756 **Fax:** (212)305-3680
Email: nursing@columbia.edu
Website: http://www.nursing.hs.columbia.edu
Amy Duschenchuk, Contact
Fnded: 1754. **Degrees Offered:** BS, DN SC, MN/MPH, MS, MSN/MBA.

★ 27997 ★ Daemen College
Department of Nursing
4380 Main St.
Amherst, NY 14226
Phone: (716)839-8408 **Fax:** (716)839-8516
Email: dwydysh@daemen.edu
Website: http://www.daemen.edu
Deborah Wydysh, Contact
Fnded: 1947. **Degrees Offered:** BS, MS.

★ 27998 ★ Dominican College
Division of Nursing
Orangeburg, NY 10962-1210
Phone: (845)359-7800 **Fax:** (845)398-4999
Website: http://www.dc.edu
Fnded: 1952. **Degrees Offered:** BSN, MS.

★ 27999 ★ D'Youville College
Department of Nursing
320 Porter Ave.
Buffalo, NY 14201
Phone: (716)881-7744 **Fax:** (716)515-0679
Email: fisherl@dyc.edu
Website: http://www.dyc.edu
Linda Fisher, Contact
Fnded: 1908. **Degrees Offered:** BSN, MS.

★ 28000 ★ Elmira College
Program in Nursing Education
One Park Pl.
Elmira, NY 14901
Phone: (607)735-1724 **Fax:** (607)735-1718
Email: bneal@elmira.edu
Website: http://www.elmira.edu
William S. Neal, Contact
Fnded: 1855. **Degrees Offered:** BS.

★ 28001 ★ Excelsior College
School of Nursing
7 Columbia Cir.
Albany, NY 12203
Phone: (518)464-8500 **Fax:** (518)464-8777
Email: msn@regents.edu
Website: http://www.regents.edu
Deborah L. Sopczyk, Contact
Fnded: 1970. **Degrees Offered:** BSN, MS.

★ 28002 ★ Hartwick College
Department of Nursing
One Hartwick College Dr.
Miller Science Ctr.
Oneonta, NY 13820
Phone: (607)431-4780 **Fax:** (607)431-4850
Email: dettenriedes@hartwick.edu
Website: http://www.hartwick.edu
Sharon D. Dettenrieder, Contact
Fnded: 1797. **Degrees Offered:** BS.

★ 28003 ★ Keuka College
Division of Nursing
PO Box 98
Keuka Park, NY 14478-0098
Phone: (315)536-5273 **Fax:** (315)531-5660
Email: lrrossi@mail.keuka.edu
Website: http://www.keuka.edu/asap/nursing.htm
Dr. Linda R. Rossi, Contact
Fnded: 1890. **Degrees Offered:** BS.

★ 28004 ★ Long Island University C.W. Post Campus
Program in Nursing
Rm. 270
720 Northern Blvd.
Brookville, NY 11548-1300
Phone: (516)299-2320 **Fax:** (516)299-2352
Email: lknapp@hornet.liunet.edu
Website: http://www.cwpost.liunet.edu/cwis/cwp/post.html
Dr. Lori Knapp, Contact
Fnded: 1954. **Degrees Offered:** BS, MS.

★ 28005 ★ Long Island University, Brooklyn Campus
School of Nursing
One University Plaza
Brooklyn, NY 11201
Phone: (718)488-1059 **Fax:** (718)780-4019
Email: susanne.flower@liu.edu
Website: http://www.liunet.edu
Susanne Flower, Contact
Fnded: 1926. **Degrees Offered:** BS, MS.

★ 28006 ★ Mercy College
Program in Nursing
555 Broadway
Hudson Hall
Dobbs Ferry, NY 10522
Phone: (914)674-9331 **Fax:** (914)674-9457
Email: mford@mercy.edu
Website: http://www.mercynet.edu
Miriam Ford, Contact
Fnded: 1951. **Degrees Offered:** BS, MS.

★ 28007 ★ Molloy College
Department of Nursing
1000 Hempstead Ave.
PO Box 5002
Rockville Centre, NY 11571-5002
Phone: (516)256-2218 **Fax:** (516)678-9718
Email: fpemberton@molloy.edu
Website: http://www.molloy.edu/
Dr. Freida Pemberton, Contact
Fnded: 1955. **Degrees Offered:** BS, MS.

★ 28008 ★ Mount Saint Mary College
Division of Nursing
330 Powell Ave.
Newburgh, NY 12550
Phone: (845)569-3138 **Fax:** (845)562-6762
Email: deboer@msmc.edu
Website: http://www.msmc.edu/webdex/divnurs/index.htm
Sr. Leona DeBoer, Contact
Fnded: 1960. **Degrees Offered:** BSN, MS.

★ 28009 ★ Nazareth College of Rochester
Department of Nursing
4245 East Ave.
Rochester, NY 14618-3790
Phone: (585)389-2711 **Fax:** (585)389-2714
Email: pahanson@naz.edu
Website: http://www.naz.edu
Dr. Patricia A. Hanson, Contact
Fnded: 1924. **Degrees Offered:** BS, MS.

★ 28010 ★ New York University
Division of Nursing
246 Greene St.
New York, NY 10003
Phone: (212)992-9418 **Fax:** (212)995-4302
Email: nursing.programs@nyu.edu
Website: http://www.nyu.edu/education/nursing
Vida Samuel-Wheeler, Contact
Fnded: 1831. **Degrees Offered:** BS, MA, MS/MA, PhD.

★ 28011 ★ Pace University
Lienhard School of Nursing
861 Bedford Rd.
Pleasantville, NY 10570
Phone: (914)773-3553 **Fax:** (914)773-3345
Email: kkeith@pace.edu

Website: http://www.pace.edu
Dr. Karen Keith, Contact
Fnded: 1906. **Degrees Offered:** BS, MS.

★ 28012 ★ Pace University, Pleasantville/ Briarcliff Campus
Lienhard School of Nursing
861 Bedford Rd.
Pleasantville, NY 10570
Phone: (914)773-3553 **Fax:** (914)773-3345
Email: kkeith@pace.edu
Website: http://www.pace.edu
Dr. Karen Keith, Contact
Degrees Offered: BS, MS.

★ 28013 ★ Roberts Wesleyan College
Division of Nursing
2301 Westside Dr.
Rochester, NY 14624
Phone: (585)594-6400 **Fax:** (585)549-6371
Email: admissions@roberts.edu
Website: http://www.roberts.edu
Linda Kurtz, Contact
Fnded: 1866. **Degrees Offered:** BS.

★ 28014 ★ Sage Colleges
Division of Nursing
Troy, NY 12180-4115
Phone: (518)244-2384 **Fax:** (518)244-2009
Email: nursing@sage.edu
Website: http://www.sage.edu/departments/nur
Dr. Joan Dacher, Contact
Degrees Offered: BS, MS, MSN/MBA.

★ 28015 ★ Saint John Fisher College
Nursing Program
3690 East Ave.
Rochester, NY 14618
Phone: (585)385-8471 **Fax:** (585)385-8466
Email: mccloskey@sjfc.edu
Website: http://www.sjfc.edu
Dr. Cynthia McCloskey, Contact
Fnded: 1948. **Degrees Offered:** BS, MS.

★ 28016 ★ Saint Joseph's College, New York
Department of Nursing
245 Clinton Ave.
Brooklyn, NY 11205-3688
Phone: (718)399-0185 **Fax:** (718)638-8839
Email: bsands@sjcny.edu
Website: http://www.sjcny.edu
Dr. Barbara L. Sands, Contact
Fnded: 1916. **Degrees Offered:** BSN.

★ 28017 ★ State University of New York Brockport College
Department of Nursing
350 New Campus Dr.
Brockport, NY 14420-2988
Phone: (585)395-5320 **Fax:** (585)395-5312
Email: lsnell@brockport.edu
Website: http://www.brockport.edu
Dr. Linda Snell, Contact
Fnded: 1867. **Degrees Offered:** BSN, MS.

★ 28018 ★ State University of New York Institute of Technology, Utica/Rome
School of Nursing
PO Box 3050
Utica, NY 13504-3050
Phone: (315)792-7295 **Fax:** (315)792-7555
Email: snlr@sunyit.edu
Website: http://www.sunyit.edu
Nancy Rickard, Contact
Fnded: 1966. **Degrees Offered:** BS, MS.

★ 28019 ★ State University of New York Upstate Medical Center
College of Nursing
750 E Adams St.
Syracuse, NY 13210
Phone: (315)464-4276 **Fax:** (315)464-5168
Email: gavanc@upstate.edu
Website: http://nursepro.hscsyr.edu
Dr. Carol Gavan, Contact
Fnded: 1950. **Degrees Offered:** BS, MS.

★ 28020 ★ State University of New York, Binghamton
School of Nursing
PO Box 6000
Binghamton, NY 13902-6000
Phone: (607)777-4964 **Fax:** (607)777-4440
Email: jferrari@binghamton.edu
Website: http://dson.binghamton.edu
Joyce Ferrario, Contact
Fnded: 1946. **Degrees Offered:** BS, MS, PhD.

★ 28021 ★ State University of New York, Brooklyn
Health Science Center
College of Nursing
450 Clarkson Ave.
Box 22
Brooklyn, NY 11203-2098
Phone: (718)270-7605 **Fax:** (718)270-7636
Email: laila.sedhom@downstate.edu
Website: http://www.downstate.edu
Dr. Laila N. Sedhom, Contact
Fnded: 1858. **Degrees Offered:** BS, MS, MS/MPH.

★ 28022 ★ State University of New York, Buffalo
School of Nursing
1023 Kimball Tower
3435 Main St., Bldg. No. 37
Buffalo, NY 14214-3079
Phone: (716)829-2537 **Fax:** (716)829-2021
Email: nurse-studentaffairs@buffalo.edu
Website: http://wings.buffalo.edu/nursing
Dr. Elaine R. Cusker, Contact
Fnded: 1846. **Degrees Offered:** BS, DNS, MS.

★ 28023 ★ State University of New York, New Paltz
Department of Nursing
WSB 01B
New Paltz, NY 12561
Phone: (845)257-2949 **Fax:** (845)257-2926
Email: holmbers@newpaltz.edu
Website: http://www.newpaltz.edu
Dr. Sharon Holmberg, Contact
Fnded: 1828. **Degrees Offered:** BSN, MSN.

★ 28024 ★ State University of New York, Plattsburgh
Department of Nursing
101 Broad St.
Hawkins Hall 209B
Plattsburgh, NY 12901
Phone: (518)564-4225 **Fax:** (518)564-3100
Email: beebegc@plattsburgh.edu
Website: http://www.plattsburgh.edu/nursing
Dr. Gretchen Crawford Beebe, Contact
Fnded: 1889. **Degrees Offered:** BS.

★ 28025 ★ State University of New York, Stony Brook
School of Nursing
Health Sciences Center
Stony Brook, NY 11794-8240
Phone: (631)444-3200 **Fax:** (631)444-6628
Website: http://www.uhmc.sunysb.edu/nursing
Fnded: 1957. **Degrees Offered:** BS, MS.

★ 28026 ★ University of Rochester
School of Nursing
Box SON
601 Elmwood Ave.
Rochester, NY 14642
Phone: (585)275-2375 **Fax:** (585)756-8299
Email: son_admissions@urmc.rochester.edu
Website: http://www.urmc.rochester.edu/son
Elaine M. Andolina, Contact
Fnded: 1850. **Degrees Offered:** BS, MS, MSN/PhD.

★ 28027 ★ Utica College
Department of Nursing
1600 Burrstone Rd.
Utica, NY 13502
Phone: (315)792-3006 **Fax:** (315)792-3003
Email: pquinn@utica.edu
Website: http://www.utica.edu
Patrick A. Quinn, Contact
Fnded: 1946. **Degrees Offered:** BS.

★ 28028 ★ Wagner College
Department of Nursing
One Campus Rd.
Campus Hall, 3rd Fl.
Staten Island, NY 10301
Phone: (718)390-3444 **Fax:** (718)420-4009
Email: kahern@wagner.edu
Website: http://www.wagner.edu
Dr. Kathleen Ahern, Contact
Fnded: 1883. **Degrees Offered:** BS, MS.

Newfoundland and Labrador

★ 28029 ★ Memorial University of Newfoundland
School of Nursing
Health Science Centre
Prince Philip Pkwy.
Saint John's, NL, Canada A1B 3V6
Phone: (709)777-6679 **Fax:** (709)777-7037
Email: agaudine@mun.ca
Website: http://www.mun.ca/nurs
Dr. Alice Gaudine, Contact
Fnded: 1925. **Degrees Offered:** BN, MN.

North Carolina

★ 28030 ★ Barton College
School of Nursing
PO Box 5000
Wilson, NC 27893-7000
Phone: (252)399-6400 **Fax:** (252)399-6416
Email: ppruden@barton.edu
Website: http://www.barton.edu/nursing
Dr. Pet S. Pruden, Contact
Fnded: 1902. **Degrees Offered:** BSN.

★ 28031 ★ Cabarrus College of Health Sciences
Louise Harkey School of Nursing
431 Copperfield Blvd. NE
Concord, NC 28025-2405
Phone: (704)783-1756 **Fax:** (704)783-2077
Email: esmall@northeastmedical.org
Dr. Ernestine Small, Contact
Fnded: 1942. **Degrees Offered:** BSN.

★ 28032 ★ Duke University
School of Nursing
Box 3322
Durham, NC 27710
Phone: 877-415-3853 **Fax:** (919)681-8899
Email: admissions@son3.mc.duke.edu
Website: http://www.nursing.duke.edu
Jennifer Avery, Contact
Fnded: 1838. **Degrees Offered:** BSN, MSN, MSN/MBA, MSN/MCM.

★ 28033 ★ East Carolina University
School of Nursing
Rivers Bldg., Rm. 130
Greenville, NC 27858-4353
Phone: (252)328-4302 **Fax:** (252)328-4300
Email: bernhardtj@mail.ecu.edu
Website: http://www.ecu.edu
Dr. Judy Bernhardt, Contact
Fnded: 1907. **Degrees Offered:** BSN, MSN, PhD.

★ 28034 ★ Gardner-Webb University
School of Nursing
PO Box 7268
Boiling Springs, NC 28017
Phone: (704)406-4358 **Fax:** (704)406-3919
Email: rbeck-little@gardner-webb.edu
Website: http://www.gardner-webb.edu
Dr. Susie Beck-Little, Contact
Fnded: 1905. **Degrees Offered:** BSN, MSN, MSN/MBA.

★ 28035 ★ Lenoir-Rhyne College
Department of Nursing
PO Box 7292
Hickory, NC 28603
Phone: (828)328-7282 **Fax:** (828)328-7284
Email: reecel@lrc.edu
Website: http://www.lrc.edu
Dr. Linda W. Reece, Contact
Fnded: 1891. **Degrees Offered:** BS.

★ 28036 ★ North Carolina Agricultural and Technical State University
School of Nursing
1601 E Market St.
Greensboro, NC 27411
Phone: (336)334-7752 **Fax:** (336)334-7637
Email: daviss@ncat.edu
Website: http://www.ncat.edu/~nursing/index.html
Sophia Davis, Contact
Fnded: 1891. **Degrees Offered:** BSN.

★ 28037 ★ North Carolina Central University
Department of Nursing
PO Box 19798
Durham, NC 27707
Phone: (919)530-6381 **Fax:** (919)530-5343
Email: bpdennis@wpo.nccu.edu
Website: http://ariel.acc.nccu.edu/artsci/nursing/
Dr. Betty Pierce Dennis, Contact
Fnded: 1910. **Degrees Offered:** BSN.

★ 28038 ★ Queens University of Charlotte
Division of Nursing
1900 Selwyn Ave.
Charlotte, NC 28274
Phone: (704)337-2363 **Fax:** (704)337-2477
Email: martink@queens.edu
Website: http://www.queens.edu
Dr. Karen J. Martin, Contact
Fnded: 1857. **Degrees Offered:** BSN, MSN, MSN/MBA.

★ 28039 ★ Southeastern North Carolina Nursing Consortium
PO Box 1510
Pembroke, NC 28372
Phone: (910)521-6522 **Fax:** (910)521-6178
Email: tonya.locklear@uncp.edu
Tonya Locklear, Contact
Degrees Offered: BSN.

★ 28040 ★ University of North Carolina, Chapel Hill
School of Nursing
Campus Box 7460
Chapel Hill, NC 27599-7460
Phone: (919)966-4260 **Fax:** (919)966-3540
Email: kathy_moore@unc.edu
Website: http://www.unc.edu/depts/nursing
Katherine Moore, Contact
Fnded: 1789. **Degrees Offered:** BSN, MSN, MSN/MS, PhD.

★ 28041 ★ University of North Carolina, Charlotte
School of Nursing
9201 University City Blvd.
Charlotte, NC 28223-0001
Phone: (704)687-4684 **Fax:** (704)687-3180
Email: mksloss@email.uncc.edu
Website: http://www.uncc.edu
Martha Sloss, Contact
Fnded: 1946. **Degrees Offered:** BSN, MSN, MSN/MHA.

★ 28042 ★ University of North Carolina, Greensboro
School of Nursing
PO Box 26172
Greensboro, NC 27402-6172
Phone: (336)334-5561 **Fax:** (336)334-3628
Email: eileen_kohlenberg@uncg.edu
Website: http://www.uncg.edu/nur/
Eileen Kohlenberg, Contact
Fnded: 1891. **Degrees Offered:** BSN, MSN, MSN/MBA.

★ 28043 ★ University of North Carolina, Wilmington
School of Nursing
601 S College Rd.
Wilmington, NC 28403-5995
Phone: (910)962-3208 **Fax:** (910)962-3723
Email: nursing@uncwil.edu
Website: http://www.uncwil.edu/inside
Nancy L. McLemore, Contact
Fnded: 1947. **Degrees Offered:** BS, MSN.

★ 28044 ★ Western Carolina University
Department of Nursing
Cullowhee, NC 28723
Phone: (828)227-6157 **Fax:** (828)232-2408
Email: sswain@email.wcu.edu
Website: http://www.wcu.edu
Sharon Swain, Contact
Fnded: 1889. **Degrees Offered:** BSN, MSN.

★ 28045 ★ Winston-Salem State University
Department of Nursing
601 Martin Luther King Jr. Dr.
Winston-Salem, NC 27110
Phone: (336)750-2660 **Fax:** (336)750-2568
Email: mcgadneyj@wssu.edu
Website: http://www.wssu.edu
Dr. Joanette McGadney, Contact
Fnded: 1892. **Degrees Offered:** BSN, MSN.

North Dakota

★ 28046 ★ Dickinson State University
Department of Nursing
291 Campus Dr.
Dickinson, ND 58601-4896
Phone: (701)483-2480 **Fax:** (701)483-2524
Website: http://www.dsu.nodak.edu/Catalog/nursing.htm
Mary Anne Marsh, Contact
Fnded: 1918. **Degrees Offered:** BSN.

★ 28047 ★ Jamestown College
Department of Nursing
Admissions Department
6081 College Ln.
Jamestown, ND 58405
Phone: (701)252-3467 **Fax:** (701)253-4318
Website: http://www.jc.edu
Fnded: 1883. **Degrees Offered:** BSN.

★ 28048 ★ Medcenter One College of Nursing
512 N 7th St.
Bismarck, ND 58501
Phone: (701)323-6271 **Fax:** (701)323-6967
Email: msmith@mohs.org
Website: http://medcenterone.com/nursing/nursing.htm
Mary Smith, Contact
Fnded: 1988. **Degrees Offered:** BSN.

★ 28049 ★ Minot State University
Department of Nursing
500 University Ave. W
Minot, ND 58707-0002
Phone: (701)858-3101 **Fax:** (701)858-4309
Email: petterse@misu.nodak.edu
Website: http://www.misu.nodak.edu/nursing/home.htm
Linda Pettersen, Contact
Fnded: 1913. **Degrees Offered:** BSN.

★ 28050 ★ North Dakota State University
Tri-College University Nursing Consortium
136 Sudro Hall
PO Box 5055
Fargo, ND 58105-5055
Phone: (218)236-4699 **Fax:** (218)299-5990
Email: giedt@mnstate.edu
Website: http://www.ndsu.nodak.edu/instruct/nysveen/nursing
Dr. Jane Giedt, Contact
Fnded: 1890. **Degrees Offered:** BSN, MS.

★ 28051 ★ University of Mary
Division of Nursing
7500 University Dr.
Bismarck, ND 58504
Phone: (701)255-7500 **Fax:** (701)255-7687
Website: http://www.umary.edu/AcadInfo/NurDiv
Fnded: 1959. **Degrees Offered:** BSN, MSN.

★ 28052 ★ University of North Dakota
College of Nursing
PO Box 9025
Grand Forks, ND 58202-9025
Phone: (701)777-4552 **Fax:** (701)777-4096
Email: ginny_guido@mail.und.nodak.edu
Website: http://www.und.nodak.edu/dept/nursing
Dr. Ginny W. Guido, Contact
Fnded: 1883. **Degrees Offered:** BSN, MS, PhD.

Nova Scotia

★ 28053 ★ Dalhousie University
School of Nursing
5869 University Ave.
Halifax, NS, Canada B3H 3J5
Phone: (902)494-2391 **Fax:** (902)494-3487
Email: joan.evans@dal.ca
Website: http://www.dal.ca/nursing
Dr. Joan Evans, Contact
Fnded: 1818. **Degrees Offered:** BSCN, MN, MN/MHSA.

★ 28054 ★ Saint Francis Xavier University
Department of Nursing
PO Box 5000
Antigonish, NS, Canada B2G 2W5
Phone: (902)867-5386 **Fax:** (902)867-2329
Email: lpushor@stfx.ca
Website: http://www.stfx.ca
Laurie Pushor, Contact
Fnded: 1853. **Degrees Offered:** BSCN.

Ohio

★ 28055 ★ Ashland University
Department of Nursing
401 College Ave.
Ashland, OH 44805
Phone: (419)289-5242 **Fax:** (419)258-5989
Email: dstitzle@ashland.edu
Website: http://www.ashland.edu
Dr. Dorothy A. Stitzlein, Contact
Fnded: 1878. **Degrees Offered:** BSN.

★ 28056 ★ Capital University
School of Nursing
2199 E Main St.
Columbus, OH 43209-2394
Phone: (614)236-6331 **Fax:** (614)236-6157
Email: gglasgow@capital.edu
Website: http://www.capital.edu/nursing/nurshome.shtml
Dr. Gretchen Glasgow, Contact
Fnded: 1830. **Degrees Offered:** BSN, MSN, MSN/JD, MSN/MBA.

★ 28057 ★ Case Western Reserve University
Frances Payne Bolton School of Nursing
10900 Euclid Ave.
Cleveland, OH 44106-4904
Phone: (216)368-5977 **Fax:** (216)368-0124
Email: jes16@po.cwru.edu
Website: http://fpb.cwru.edu
Janet Ziol, Contact
Fnded: 1826. **Degrees Offered:** BSN, MSN, MSN/MA, MSN/MBA, MSN/MPH, MSN/PhD.

★ 28058 ★ Cedarville University
Department of Nursing
251 N Main St.
Cedarville, OH 45314-0601
Free: 800-233-2784 **Fax:** (937)766-7575
Email: admissions@cedarville.edu
Website: http://www.cedarville.edu
Roscoe Smith, Contact
Fnded: 1887. **Degrees Offered:** BSN.

★ 28059 ★ Cleveland State University
Department of Nursing
2121 Euclid Ave., RT 915
Cleveland, OH 44115
Phone: (216)687-3558 **Fax:** (216)687-3556
Email: s.radzyminski@csuohio.edu
Website: http://www.csuohio.edu
Dr. Sharon Radzyminski, Contact
Fnded: 1964. **Degrees Offered:** BSN, MSN.

★ 28060 ★ College of Mount Saint Joseph
Department of Nursing
5701 Delhi Rd.
Cincinnati, OH 45233-1670
Phone: (513)244-4511 **Fax:** (513)451-2547
Email: darla_vale@mail.msj.edu
Website: http://www.msj.edu
Dr. Darla Vale, Contact
Fnded: 1920. **Degrees Offered:** BSN.

★ 28061 ★ Franciscan University of Steubenville
Department of Nursing
Steubenville, OH 43952
Phone: (740)284-7245 **Fax:** (740)283-6449
Email: jdavis@franciscan.edu
Website: http://www.franuniv.edu
Dr. Joan Davis, Contact
Fnded: 1946. **Degrees Offered:** BSN, MSN.

★ 28062 ★ Kent State University
College of Nursing
PO Box 5190
Kent, OH 44242
Phone: (330)672-7930 **Fax:** (330)672-2433
Email: cstopper@kent.edu
Website: http://www.kent.edu/nursing
Connie Stopper, Contact
Fnded: 1910. **Degrees Offered:** BSN, MSN, PhD.

★ 28063 ★ Lourdes College
Nursing Department
6832 Convent Blvd.
Sylvania, OH 43560
Phone: (419)824-3793 **Fax:** (419)824-3985
Email: sbernhei@lourdes.edu
Website: http://www.lourdes.edu
Susan Bernheisel, Contact
Fnded: 1958. **Degrees Offered:** BSN.

★ 28064 ★ Malone College
School of Nursing
515 25th St. NW
Canton, OH 44709
Phone: (330)471-8366 **Fax:** (330)471-8478
Email: lreinhart2@malone.edu
Website: http://www.malone.edu
Dr. Loretta M. Reinhart, Contact
Fnded: 1892. **Degrees Offered:** BSN, MSN.

★ 28065 ★ Medical College of Ohio
School of Nursing
3015 Arlington Ave.
Toledo, OH 43614-5803
Phone: (419)383-5892 **Fax:** (419)383-5894
Email: jrobinson@mco.edu
Website: http://www.mco.edu/snur/index.html
Dr. Janet H. Robinson, Contact
Fnded: 1964. **Degrees Offered:** BSN, MSN.

★ 28066 ★ Miami University
Department of Nursing
1601 Peck Blvd.
Hamilton, OH 45011
Phone: (513)785-3280 **Fax:** (513)785-3284
Email: millsem@muohio.edu
Website: http://www.ham.muohio.edu/nursing/
Dr. Eugenia M. Mills, Contact
Fnded: 1809. **Degrees Offered:** BSN.

★ 28067 ★ Mount Carmel College of Nursing
Baccalaureate Nursing Program
127 S Davis Ave.
Columbus, OH 43222-1504
Phone: (614)234-5144 **Fax:** (614)234-2875
Email: mmenefield@mchs.com
Website: http://www.mccn.edu/index.html
Merchel Menefield, Contact
Degrees Offered: BSN.

★ 28068 ★ Ohio State University
College of Nursing
1585 Neil Ave.
Columbus, OH 43210-1289
Phone: (614)292-4945 **Fax:** (614)292-9399
Email: cody.12@osu.edu
Website: http://www.con.ohio-state.edu
Sandy Cody, Contact
Fnded: 1870. **Degrees Offered:** BSN, MS, PhD.

★ 28069 ★ Ohio University
School of Nursing
Grover Center E365
Athens, OH 45701
Phone: (740)593-4494 **Fax:** (740)593-0286
Email: nursing@ohio.edu
Website: http://www.ohio.edu/nursing/
Emily Harman, Contact
Fnded: 1804. **Degrees Offered:** BSN.

★ 28070 ★ Otterbein College
Program in Nursing
Science Bldg.
Campus Mail: NURS
Westerville, OH 43081
Phone: (614)823-1614
Email: sbuxton@otterbein.edu
Website: http://www.otterbein.edu/dept/NURS
Fnded: 1847. **Degrees Offered:** BSN, MSN.

★ 28071 ★ Shawnee State University
Department of Nursing
940 2nd St.
Portsmouth, OH 45662
Phone: (740)351-3378 **Fax:** (740)351-3354
Email: cboyd@shawnee.edu
Website: http://www.shawnee.edu
Dr. Cheryl A. Boyd, Contact
Fnded: 1986. **Degrees Offered:** BSN.

★ 28072 ★ University of Akron
College of Nursing
209 Carroll St.
Akron, OH 44325-3701
Phone: (330)972-7555 **Fax:** (330)972-5737
Email: kr1@uakron.edu
Website: http://odin.chemistry.uakron.edu/nursing
Dr. Kathy Ross-Alaolmolki, Contact
Fnded: 1870. **Degrees Offered:** BSN, MSN, PhD.

★ 28073 ★ University of Cincinnati
College of Nursing
PO Box 210038
Cincinnati, OH 45221-0038
Phone: (513)558-5072 **Fax:** (513)558-7523
Email: loren.carter@uc.edu
Website: http://www.nursing.uc.edu
Loren Carter, Contact
Fnded: 1819. **Degrees Offered:** BSN, MSN, MSN/MBA, PhD.

★ 28074 ★ Ursuline College
The Breen School of Nursing
2550 Lander Rd.
Pepper Pike, OH 44124
Phone: (440)449-3425 **Fax:** (440)449-4267
Email: cwaggoner@ursuline.edu
Website: http://www.ursuline.edu
Dr. Carol Waggoner, Contact
Fnded: 1871. **Degrees Offered:** BSN, MSN.

★ 28075 ★ Walsh University
Department of Nursing
2020 Easton St. NW
North Canton, OH 44720
Phone: (330)490-7250 **Fax:** (330)490-7206
Email: jcampbell@walsh.edu
Website: http://www.walsh.edu/
Dr. Janis M. Campbell, Contact
Fnded: 1958. **Degrees Offered:** BSN.

★ 28076 ★ Wright State University
College of Nursing and Health
3640 Colonel Glenn Hwy.
Dayton, OH 45435
Phone: (937)775-3132 **Fax:** (937)775-4571
Email: theresa.haghnazarian@wright.edu
Website: http://www.nursing.wright.edu
Theresa A. Haghnazarian, Contact
Fnded: 1964. **Degrees Offered:** BSN, MS, MS/MBA.

★ 28077 ★ Xavier University
Department of Nursing
3800 Victory Pkwy.
Cincinnati, OH 45207-7351
Phone: (513)745-4392 **Fax:** (513)745-1087
Email: gomez@admin.xavier.edu
Website: http://www.xu.edu
Marilyn Volk Gomez, Contact
Fnded: 1831. **Degrees Offered:** BSN, MSN, MSN/MBA.

★ 28078 ★ Youngstown State University
Department of Nursing
One University Plaza
Youngstown, OH 44555
Phone: (330)941-1796 **Fax:** (330)941-2309
Email: spshipton@ysu.edu
Website: http://www.ysu.edu
Dr. Sharon Shipton, Contact
Fnded: 1908. **Degrees Offered:** BSN, MSN.

Oklahoma

★ 28079 ★ Bacone College
Department of Nursing
Admissions Officer
2299 Old Bacone Rd.
Muskogee, OK 74403
Free: 888-682-5514
Email: info@bacone.edu
Fnded: 1880. **Degrees Offered:** BSN.

★ 28080 ★ East Central University
Department of Nursing
1100 E 14th St.
Ada, OK 74820
Phone: (580)310-5434 **Fax:** (580)310-5785
Email: jcatalan@mailclerk.ecok.edu
Website: http://www.ecok.edu
Dr. Joseph T. Catalano, Contact
Fnded: 1909. **Degrees Offered:** BS.

★ 28081 ★ Langston University
School of Nursing and Health Professions
302 University Women Bldg.
Langston, OK 73050
Phone: (405)466-3411 **Fax:** (405)466-2195
Email: fjhinds@lunet.edu
Website: http://www.lunet.ed/nurs5.html
Farretta Hinds, Contact
Fnded: 1897. **Degrees Offered:** BSN.

★ 28082 ★ Northeastern State University
Department of Nursing
PO Box 549
Muskogee, OK 74402-0549
Phone: (918)781-5410 **Fax:** (918)781-5411
Email: vannostr@nsuok.edu
Website: http://www.nsuok.edu
Dr. Joyce A. Van Nostrand, Contact
Fnded: 1846. **Degrees Offered:** BSN.

★ 28083 ★ Northwestern Oklahoma State University
Division of Nursing
709 Oklahoma Blvd.
Alva, OK 73717-2799
Phone: (580)327-8489 **Fax:** (580)327-8434
Email: flbuechner@nwosu.edu
Website: http://www.nwosu.edu/nursing
Dr. Frankie L. Buechner, Contact
Fnded: 1897. **Degrees Offered:** BSN.

★ 28084 ★ Oklahoma Baptist University
School of Nursing
500 W University
Shawnee, OK 74804
Phone: (405)878-2081 **Fax:** (405)878-2083
Email: lana_bolhouse@mail.okbu.edu
Website: http://www.okbu.edu
Dr. Lana Bolhouse, Contact
Fnded: 1910. **Degrees Offered:** BSN.

★ 28085 ★ Oklahoma City University
Kramer School of Nursing
2501 N Blackwelder
Oklahoma City, OK 73106
Phone: (405)521-5901 **Fax:** (405)521-5914
Email: gkirkham@okcu.edu
Website: http://www.okcu.edu
Glenda Kirkham, Contact
Fnded: 1904. **Degrees Offered:** BSN.

★ 28086 ★ Oklahoma Panhandle State University
Bachelor of Science in Nursing Program
PO Box 430
323 W Eagle Blvd.
Goodwell, OK 73939
Phone: (580)349-1528 **Fax:** (580)349-2302
Email: renej@opsu.edu
Website: http://www.opsu.edu
Rene Johnson, Contact
Fnded: 1909. **Degrees Offered:** BSN.

★ 28087 ★ Oklahoma Wesleyan College
Division of Nursing
2201 Silver Lake Rd.
Bartlesville, OK 74006
Phone: (918)335-6254 **Fax:** (918)335-6204
Email: pgiles@okwu.edu
Website: http://nursing.okwu.edu
Pamela Ann Giles, Contact
Fnded: 1909. **Degrees Offered:** BSN.

★ 28088 ★ Oral Roberts University
Anna Vaughn School of Nursing
Tulsa, OK 74171
Phone: (918)495-6198 **Fax:** (918)495-6020
Email: kjezek@oru.edu
Website: http://www.oru.edu
Dr. Kenda Jezek, Contact
Fnded: 1963. **Degrees Offered:** BSN.

★ 28089 ★ Southern Nazarene University
School of Nursing
6729 NW 39th Expressway
Bethany, OK 73008
Phone: (405)491-6365 **Fax:** (405)717-6264
Email: aferguso@snu.edu
Website: http://www.snu.edu
Dr. Ann Ferguson, Contact
Fnded: 1899. **Degrees Offered:** BS.

★ 28090 ★ Southwestern Oklahoma State University
Division of Nursing
100 Campus Dr.
Weatherford, OK 73096-3098
Phone: (580)774-3261 **Fax:** (580)774-7075
Email: killgoc@swosu.edu
Website: http://www.swosu.edu/academic/nurse
Charlene Killgore, Contact
Fnded: 1901. **Degrees Offered:** BSN.

★ 28091 ★ University of Central Oklahoma
Department of Nursing
100 N University Dr.
Edmond, OK 73034-5209
Phone: (405)974-5000
Email: vaddison@ucok.edu
Website: http://nursing.ucok.edu
Vicki Hodges, Contact
Fnded: 1890. **Degrees Offered:** BSN.

★ 28092 ★ University of Oklahoma Health Sciences Center
College of Nursing
PO Box 26901
1100 N Stonewall Ave.
Oklahoma City, OK 73190
Phone: (405)271-2125 **Fax:** (405)271-7341
Website: http://www.nursing.ouhsc.edu/
Fnded: 1890. **Degrees Offered:** BSN, MS.

★ 28093 ★ University of Phoenix—Oklahoma City Campus
College of Nursing and Health Care Sciences
Oklahoma City, OK
Phone: (405)842-8007
Website: http://www.phoenix.edu/
Degrees Offered: BSN, MSN, MSN/MBA.

★ 28094 ★ University of Phoenix—Tulsa Campus
College of Nursing and Health Care Sciences
Tulsa, OK
Phone: (918)622-4877
Website: http://www.phoenix.edu/
Degrees Offered: BSN, MSN, MSN/MBA.

★ 28095 ★ University of Tulsa
School of Nursing
600 S College Ave.
Tulsa, OK 74104-3189
Phone: (918)631-3116 **Fax:** (918)631-2068
Email: susan-gaston@utulsa.edu
Website: http://www.cba.utulsa.edu/nsg
Dr. Susan Gaston, Contact
Fnded: 1894. **Degrees Offered:** BSN.

Ontario

★ 28096 ★ Lakehead University
School of Nursing
955 Oliver Rd.
Thunder Bay, ON, Canada P7B 5E1
Phone: (807)343-8643 **Fax:** (807)343-8246
Email: dpallen@sky.lakeheadu.ca
Website: http://www.lakeheadu.ca
Darlene Steven, Contact
Fnded: 1965. **Degrees Offered:** BSN.

★ 28097 ★ Laurentian University
School of Nursing
935 Ramsey Lake Rd.
Sudbury, ON, Canada P3E 2C6
Phone: (705)675-1151 **Fax:** (705)675-4861
Email: erukholm@nickel.laurentian.ca
Website: http://www.laurentian.ca/
Dr. Ellen Rukholm, Contact
Fnded: 1960. **Degrees Offered:** BSCN.

★ 28098 ★ McMaster University
School of Nursing
1200 Main St. W
Rm. 3N10
Hamilton, ON, Canada L8N 3Z5
Phone: (905)525-9140 **Fax:** (905)546-1129
Website: http://www.fhs.mcmaster.ca/nursing
Fnded: 1887. **Degrees Offered:** BSCN, M SC, PhD.

★ 28099 ★ Queen's University, Kingston
School of Nursing
Cataraqui Bldg.
90 Barrie St.
Kingston, ON, Canada K7L 3N6
Phone: (613)533-6000 **Fax:** (613)533-6770
Email: kisilevb@post.queensu.ca
Website: http://meds-ss10.meds.queensu.ca/nursing/
Dr. Barbara Kisilevsky, Contact
Fnded: 1841. **Degrees Offered:** BNSC, M SC.

★ 28100 ★ Ryerson University
Program in Nursing
350 Victoria St.
Toronto, ON, Canada M5B 2K3
Phone: (416)979-5000 **Fax:** (416)979-5332
Email: rperras@ryerson.ca
Website: http://www.ryerson.ca/nursing
Richard Perras, Contact
Fnded: 1948. **Degrees Offered:** BSCN.

★ 28101 ★ University of Ottawa
School of Nursing
451 Smyth Rd.
Ottawa, ON, Canada K1H 8M5
Phone: (613)562-5800
Email: jellis@uottawa.ca
Website: http://www.health.uottawa.ca/sn/
Jacqueline Ellis, Contact
Fnded: 1848. **Degrees Offered:** BSCN, M SC N.

★ 28102 ★ University of Toronto
Faculty of Nursing
Office of Student Affairs
50 Saint George St.
Toronto, ON, Canada M5S 3H4
Phone: (416)978-2863 **Fax:** (416)978-8222
Email: inquiry.nursing@utoronto.ca
Website: http://www.nursing.utoronto.ca
Fnded: 1827. **Degrees Offered:** BSCN, MN, MN/MBA, PhD.

★ 28103 ★ University of Western Ontario
School of Nursing
London, ON, Canada N6A 5C1
Phone: (519)661-3409 **Fax:** (519)850-2514
Email: nursweb@uwo.ca
Website: http://www.uwo.ca/
Lori Johnson, Contact
Fnded: 1878. **Degrees Offered:** BSCN, M SC N, PhD.

★ 28104 ★ University of Windsor
School of Nursing
401 Sunset Ave.
Windsor, ON, Canada N9B 3P4
Phone: (519)253-3000 **Fax:** (519)973-7084
Email: bear@uwindsor.ca
Website: http://www.uwindsor.ca/nursing
Dr. Kaye Fawdry, Contact
Fnded: 1857. **Degrees Offered:** BSCN, M SC.

★ 28105 ★ York University
School of Nursing
Atkinson Faculty of Liberal and Professional Studies
Atkinson Rm. 418
4700 Keele St.
Toronto, ON, Canada M3J 1P3
Phone: (416)736-5271 **Fax:** (416)736-5714
Email: kathem@yorku.ca
Website: http://www.yorku.ca/
Dr. Kathleen Macdonald, Contact
Fnded: 1959. **Degrees Offered:** BSCN.

Oregon

★ 28106 ★ Linfield College
School of Nursing, Portland Campus
2255 NW Northrup St.
Portland, OR 97210
Phone: (503)413-8481 **Fax:** (503)413-6283
Email: bwoodwar@linfield.edu
Website: http://www.linfield.edu/portland
Beth A. Woodward, Contact
Fnded: 1849. **Degrees Offered:** BSN.

★ 28107 ★ Oregon Health and Science University
School of Nursing
3455 SW U.S. Veterans Hospital Rd.
SN-4N
Portland, OR 97239-2491
Phone: (503)494-7725 **Fax:** (503)494-4350
Website: http://www.ohsu.edu/son
Fnded: 1974. **Degrees Offered:** BS, MS, MSN/MPH, PhD.

★ 28108 ★ University of Portland
School of Nursing
5000 N Willamette Blvd.
Portland, OR 97203-5798
Phone: (503)943-7211 **Fax:** (503)943-7729
Email: nursing@up.edu
Website: http://www.up.edu
Dr. Terry R. Misener, Contact
Fnded: 1901. **Degrees Offered:** BSN, MS.

★ 28109 ★ Walla Walla College
School of Nursing
10345 SE Market St.
Portland, OR 97216
Phone: (503)251-6115 **Fax:** (503)261-6249
Email: thurnja@wwc.edu
Website: http://www.wwc.edu/academics/department/nursing
Jan Thurnhofer, Contact
Fnded: 1892. **Degrees Offered:** BS.

Pennsylvania

★ 28110 ★ Alvernia College
Department of Nursing
400 Saint Bernardine St.
NRC 110
Reading, PA 19607
Phone: (610)796-8306 **Fax:** (610)796-8464
Email: karen.thacker@alvernia.edu
Website: http://www.alvernia.edu
Karen S. Thacker, Contact
Fnded: 1958. **Degrees Offered:** BSN.

★ 28111 ★ Bloomsburg University of Pennsylvania
Department of Nursing
MCHS 3121
Bloomsburg, PA 17815
Phone: (570)389-4602 **Fax:** (570)389-5008
Email: haymaker@husky.bloomu.edu
Website: http://www.bloomu.edu/nursing
Dr. Sharon Haymaker, Contact
Fnded: 1839. **Degrees Offered:** BSN, MSN, MSN/MBA.

★ 28112 ★ California University of Pennsylvania
Department of Nursing
250 University Ave.
Box 60
California, PA 15419-1394
Phone: (724)938-5739 **Fax:** (724)938-1612
Email: marcinek@cup.edu
Website: http://www.cup.edu
Dr. Margaret Marcinek, Contact
Fnded: 1852. **Degrees Offered:** BSC PN.

★ 28113 ★ Carlow College
Division of Nursing
3333 5th Ave.
Pittsburgh, PA 15213
Phone: (412)578-6092 **Fax:** (412)578-6321
Email: lwaigand@carlow.edu
Website: http://www.carlow.edu/academic/nursing.html
Lee Waigand, Contact
Fnded: 1929. **Degrees Offered:** BSN, MSN.

★ 28114 ★ Cedar Crest College
Department of Nursing
100 College Dr.
Allentown, PA 18104-6196
Phone: (610)606-4606 **Fax:** (610)606-4615
Email: lrmurray@cedarcrest.edu
Website: http://www.cedarcrest.edu
Dr. Laurie R. Murray, Contact
Fnded: 1867. **Degrees Offered:** BS.

★ 28115 ★ Clarion University of Pennsylvania
School of Nursing
Strain Behavioral Science Bldg.
Slippery Rock, PA 16057-1326
Phone: (724)738-2323 **Fax:** (724)738-2881
Email: joyce.white@sru.edu
Website: http://www.clarion.edu/academic/nursing/index.htm
Dr. Joyce White, Contact
Fnded: 1867. **Degrees Offered:** BSN, MSN.

★ 28116 ★ College Misericordia
Department of Nursing
301 Lake St.
Dallas, PA 18612
Phone: (717)674-6451 **Fax:** (570)674-8902
Email: lbrown@misericordia.edu
Website: http://www.miseri.edu
Larree Brown, Contact
Fnded: 1924. **Degrees Offered:** BSN, MSN.

★ 28117 ★ DeSales University
Department of Nursing and Health
2755 Station Ave.
Center Valley, PA 18034
Phone: (610)282-1100 **Fax:** (610)282-2254
Email: carol.mest@desales.edu
Website: http://www.desales.edu
Dr. Carol G. Mest, Contact
Fnded: 1964. **Degrees Offered:** BSN, MSN, MSN/MBA.

★ 28118 ★ Drexel University
College of Nursing and Health Professions
1505 Race St.
Mail Stop 501
Philadelphia, PA 19102-1192
Phone: (215)762-1336 **Fax:** (215)762-7778
Email: joyce.segal@drexel.edu
Website: http://www.drexel.edu
Joyce Segal, Contact
Fnded: 1891. **Degrees Offered:** BSN, MSN.

★ 28119 ★ Duquesne University School of Nursing
630A College Hall
600 Forbes Ave.
Pittsburgh, PA 15282-1760
Phone: (412)396-6540 **Fax:** (412)396-6346
Email: lockhart@duq.edu
Website: http://www.nursing.duq.edu
Dr. Joanne Lockhart, Contact
Fnded: 1878. **Degrees Offered:** BSN, MSN, MSN/MBA, PhD.

★ 28120 ★ East Stroudsburg University of Pennsylvania Department of Nursing
200 Prospect St.
East Stroudsburg, PA 18301-2999
Phone: (570)422-3563 **Fax:** (570)422-3848
Website: http://www.esu.edu
Dr. Cecile Champagne, Contact
Fnded: 1893. **Degrees Offered:** BS.

★ 28121 ★ Eastern University Program in Nursing
1300 Eagle Rd.
Saint Davids, PA 19087
Phone: (610)341-5896 **Fax:** (610)225-5016
Email: mlacey@eastern.edu
Website: http://www.eastern.edu
Dr. Margaret Lacey, Contact
Fnded: 1952. **Degrees Offered:** BSN.

★ 28122 ★ Edinboro University of Pennsylvania Department of Nursing
125 Centennial Hall
Edinboro, PA 16444
Phone: (814)732-1127 **Fax:** (814)732-2536
Email: nosel@edinboro.edu
Website: http://www.edinboro.edu/cwis/nursing/nursing.html
Patricia Louise Nosel, Contact
Fnded: 1857. **Degrees Offered:** BS, MSN.

★ 28123 ★ Gannon University Villa Maria School of Nursing
109 University Sq.
Erie, PA 16541-0001
Phone: (814)871-5363 **Fax:** (814)871-5662
Email: shoemake001@gannon.edu
Website: http://www.gannon.edu
Ruth Ellen Shoemaker, Contact
Fnded: 1925. **Degrees Offered:** BSN, MSN.

★ 28124 ★ Gwynedd-Mercy College School of Nursing
PO Box 901
Gwynedd Valley, PA 19437-0901
Phone: (215)646-7300 **Fax:** (215)641-5517
Website: http://www.gmc.edu
Dr. Barbara A. Jones, Contact
Fnded: 1948. **Degrees Offered:** BSN, MSN.

★ 28125 ★ Holy Family College School of Nursing and Allied Health Professions
Grant and Frankford Aves.
Philadelphia, PA 19114-2094
Phone: (215)637-7700 **Fax:** (215)637-1478
Email: schiavo@hfc.edu
Website: http://www.hfc.edu
Dr. Antoinette Schiavo, Contact
Fnded: 1954. **Degrees Offered:** BSN, MSN.

★ 28126 ★ Immaculata University Department of Nursing
1145 King Rd.
Immaculata, PA 19345
Phone: (610)647-4400 **Fax:** (610)251-1668
Email: jcranmer@immaculata.edu
Website: http://www.immaculata.edu/nursing/
Dr. Janice Cranmer, Contact
Fnded: 1920. **Degrees Offered:** BSN.

★ 28127 ★ Indiana University of Pennsylvania Department of Nursing and Allied Health
Rm. 129 Stright Hall
Indiana, PA 15705-1087
Phone: (724)357-2222 **Fax:** (724)357-7518
Email: avlinzey@iup.edu
Website: http://www.iup.edu
Dr. Alicia Linzey, Contact
Fnded: 1875. **Degrees Offered:** BSN, MSN.

★ 28128 ★ Kutztown University of Pennsylvania Department of Nursing
219 Beekey Bldg.
Kutztown, PA 19530
Phone: (610)683-4328 **Fax:** (610)683-4708
Email: kjohnsto@kutztown.edu
Website: http://www.kutztown.edu
Dr. Kimberly Anne Johnston, Contact
Fnded: 1866. **Degrees Offered:** BSN.

★ 28129 ★ La Roche College Department of Nursing and Nursing Management
9000 Babcock Blvd.
Pittsburgh, PA 15237
Phone: (412)536-1262 **Fax:** (412)536-1283
Email: bowersr1@laroche.edu
Website: http://www.laroche.edu
Renee A. Bowers, Contact
Fnded: 1963. **Degrees Offered:** BSN, MSN.

★ 28130 ★ La Salle University School of Nursing
1900 W Olney Ave.
Philadelphia, PA 19141-1199
Phone: (215)951-1413 **Fax:** (215)951-1896
Email: vito@lasalle.edu
Website: http://www.lasalle.edu/academ/nursing
Dr. Kathleen O. Vito, Contact
Fnded: 1863. **Degrees Offered:** BSN, MSN, MSN/MBA.

★ 28131 ★ Mansfield University of Pennsylvania Robert Packer Department of Health Sciences
Admissions Office
Alumni Hall
Mansfield, PA 16933
Phone: (570)662-4243 **Fax:** (570)662-4121
Email: admissns@mnsfld.edu
Website: http://www.mansfield.edu
Fnded: 1857. **Degrees Offered:** BSN.

★ 28132 ★ Marywood University Department of Nursing
2300 Adams Ave.
Scranton, PA 18509
Phone: (570)348-6211 **Fax:** (570)961-4761
Email: golden@ac.marywood.edu
Website: http://www.marywood.edu/uscat/nurs.htm
Dr. Mary Alice Elizabeth Golden, Contact
Fnded: 1915. **Degrees Offered:** BSN, MSN.

★ 28133 ★ Messiah College Department of Nursing
One College Ave.
Grantham, PA 17027
Phone: (717)691-6000 **Fax:** (717)796-5374
Email: strausba@messiah.edu
Website: http://www.messiah.edu
William Strausbaugh, Contact
Fnded: 1909. **Degrees Offered:** BSN.

★ 28134 ★ Millersville University of Pennsylvania Department of Nursing
PO Box 1002
Millersville, PA 17551-0302
Phone: (717)871-5276 **Fax:** (717)872-3985
Email: barbara.haus@millersville.edu
Website: http://www.millersv.edu
Dr. Barbara Haus, Contact
Fnded: 1855. **Degrees Offered:** BSN, MSN.

★ 28135 ★ Mount Aloysius College Department of Nursing
7373 Admiral Peary Hwy.
Cresson, PA 16630
Phone: (814)886-6427 **Fax:** (814)886-6374
Email: cnickerson@mtaloy.edu
Website: http://www.mtaloy.edu
Dr. Carolyn Nickerson, Contact
Fnded: 1939. **Degrees Offered:** BSN.

★ 28136 ★ Neumann College Program in Nursing and Health Sciences Program in Nursing
One Neumann Dr.
Aston, PA 19014-1298
Free: 800-963-8626 **Fax:** (610)459-1370
Email: nursediv@neumann.edu
Website: http://www.neumann.edu
Dr. Gregg E. Newschwander, Contact
Fnded: 1965. **Degrees Offered:** BS, MS.

★ 28137 ★ Pennsylvania State University, University Park Campus School of Nursing
203 Health and Human Development E
University Park, PA 16802
Phone: (814)863-2211 **Fax:** (814)865-3779
Email: amk20@psu.edu
Website: http://www.hhdev.psu.edu/nurs/nurs.htm
Dr. Ann Kolanowski, Contact
Fnded: 1855. **Degrees Offered:** BS, MS, PhD.

★ 28138 ★ Saint Francis University Department of Nursing
Box 600
Loretto, PA 15940-0600
Phone: (814)472-3027 **Fax:** (814)472-3849
Email: jsamii@francis.edu
Website: http://www.sfcpa.edu
Dr. Jean M. Samii, Contact
Fnded: 1847. **Degrees Offered:** BSN.

★ 28139 ★ Slippery Rock University of Pennsylvania Department of Nursing
115A Behavioral Sciences Bldg.
Slippery Rock, PA 16057
Phone: (724)738-2323 **Fax:** (724)738-2881
Email: joyce.white@sru.edu
Website: http://www.sru.edu/depts/chhs/Nursing/nursing.htm
Dr. Joyce White, Contact
Fnded: 1889. **Degrees Offered:** BSN, MSN.

★ 28140 ★ Temple University Department of Nursing
3307 N Broad St.
Philadelphia, PA 19140
Phone: (215)707-4617 **Fax:** (215)707-1599
Email: margaret.shepard@temple.edu
Website: http://www.temple.edu/nursing
Dr. Margaret Shepard, Contact

Fnded: 1884. **Degrees Offered:** BSN, MSN.

★ 28141 ★ Thomas Jefferson University
Department of Nursing
130 S 9th St., Ste. 1200
Philadelphia, PA 19107
Phone: (215)503-6057 **Fax:** (215)932-1468
Email: mary.bowen@mail.tju.edu
Website: http://www.tju.edu
Dr. Mary E. Bowen, Contact
Fnded: 1824. **Degrees Offered:** BSN, MSN.

★ 28142 ★ University of Pennsylvania
School of Nursing
420 Guardian Dr.
Philadelphia, PA 19104-6096
Phone: (215)898-3301 **Fax:** (215)573-8439
Email: szentesy@nursing.upenn.edu
Website: http://www.nursing.upenn.edu
Kari Szentesy, Contact
Fnded: 1740. **Degrees Offered:** BSN, MSN, MSN/MBA, MSN/MPH, MSN/PhD.

★ 28143 ★ University of Pittsburgh
School of Nursing
239 Victoria Bldg.
3500 Victoria St.
Pittsburgh, PA 15261
Phone: (412)624-4586 **Fax:** (412)624-2409
Email: gartley@pitt.edu
Website: http://www.nursing.pitt.edu
Rosanna Gartley, Contact
Degrees Offered: BSN, MSN, PhD.

★ 28144 ★ University of Pittsburgh, Bradford
Department of Nursing
Admissions Department
300 Campus Dr.
Bradford, PA 16701
Free: 800-872-1787
Website: http://www.pitt.edu
Fnded: 1963. **Degrees Offered:** BSN.

★ 28145 ★ University of Scranton
Department of Nursing
McGurrin Hall
Scranton, PA 18510
Phone: (570)941-4060 **Fax:** (570)941-7093
Email: hansonm2@scranton.edu
Website: http://www.uofs.edu
Dr. Mary Jane Hanson, Contact
Fnded: 1888. **Degrees Offered:** BS, MS.

★ 28146 ★ Villanova University
College of Nursing
Villanova, PA 19085-1690
Phone: (610)519-4934 **Fax:** (610)519-7997
Email: claire.manfredi@villanova.edu
Website: http://www.nursing.villanova.edu/
Dr. Claire Manfredi, Contact
Fnded: 1842. **Degrees Offered:** BSN, MSN.

★ 28147 ★ Waynesburg College
Department of Nursing
1001 Corporate Dr.
Canonsburg, PA 15317
Phone: (724)743-4420 **Fax:** (724)743-4425
Email: hitt@waynesburg.edu
Website: http://www.waynesburg.edu
Dr. Stacie Hitt, Contact
Fnded: 1849. **Degrees Offered:** BSN, MSN, MSN/MBA.

★ 28148 ★ West Chester University of Pennsylvania
Department of Nursing
100 S Church St.
West Chester, PA 19383
Phone: (610)436-2258
Email: jhickman@wcupa.edu
Website: http://health-sciences.wcupa.edu/nursing
Dr. Janet S. Hickman, Contact
Fnded: 1871. **Degrees Offered:** BSN, MSN.

★ 28149 ★ Widener University
School of Nursing
One University Pl.
Chester, PA 19013
Phone: (610)499-4208 **Fax:** (610)499-4216
Email: mary.b.walker@widener.edu
Website: http://www.widener.edu
Dr. Mary Walker, Contact
Fnded: 1821. **Degrees Offered:** BSN, DN SC, MSN.

★ 28150 ★ Wilkes University
Department of Nursing
109 S Franklin St.
Wilkes Barre, PA 18766
Phone: (570)408-4076 **Fax:** (570)408-7807
Email: telban@wilkes.edu
Website: http://www.wilkes.edu
Dr. Sharon Telban, Contact
Fnded: 1933. **Degrees Offered:** BS, MS.

★ 28151 ★ York College of Pennsylvania
Department of Nursing
York, PA 17405
Phone: (717)815-1212 **Fax:** (717)849-1651
Website: http://www.ycp.edu
Dr. Lynn Warner, Contact
Fnded: 1787. **Degrees Offered:** BS, MS.

Prince Edward Island

★ 28152 ★ University of Prince Edward Island
School of Nursing
550 University Ave.
Charlottetown, PE, Canada C1A 4P3
Phone: (902)566-0733 **Fax:** (902)566-0777
Email: mlaustin@upei.ca
Website: http://upei.ca/
Mary-Lou Austin, Contact
Fnded: 1834. **Degrees Offered:** BSCN.

Puerto Rico

★ 28153 ★ Inter American University of Puerto Rico, Metropolitan Campus
Carmen Torres de Tiburcio School of Nursing
PO Box 191293
San Juan, PR 00919-1293
Phone: (787)763-3066 **Fax:** (787)250-1242
Email: geortiz@inter.edu
Website: http://www.metro.inter.edu/progacad/enfe/nursing/index.html
Dr. Gloria E. Ortiz, Contact
Fnded: 1960. **Degrees Offered:** BSN.

★ 28154 ★ Pontifical Catholic University of Puerto Rico
Department of Nursing
Ave. Las Americas, Station 6
Ponce, PR 00732
Phone: (787)841-2000
Website: http://www.pucpr.edu/catalogo/espanol/ciencias/dep_enf.htm
Alma Albizu, Contact
Fnded: 1948. **Degrees Offered:** BSN.

★ 28155 ★ Universidad Adventista de las Antillas
Department of Nursing
PO Box 118
Mayaguez, PR 00681-0118
Phone: (787)834-9595 **Fax:** (787)834-9597
Email: ycancel@uaa.edu
Website: http://www.uaa.edu
Maria L. Cruz, Contact
Fnded: 1957. **Degrees Offered:** BSN.

★ 28156 ★ Universidad Metropolitana
Department of Nursing
PO Box 21150
San Juan, PR 00928-1150
Phone: (787)766-1717 **Fax:** (787)769-7663
Email: um_mpedroza@suagm.edu
Website: http://umet_mie.suagm.edu/
Mayra Pedroza, Contact
Fnded: 1980. **Degrees Offered:** BSN.

★ 28157 ★ University of Puerto Rico, Arecibo
Department of Nursing
Arecibo, PR
Phone: (787)878-2830 **Fax:** (787)880-4972
Website: http://upra.edu/asuntosacademicos/enfermia/menu_enfe.htm
Fnded: 1967. **Degrees Offered:** BSN.

★ 28158 ★ University of Puerto Rico, Humacao
Department of Nursing
Humacao, PR 00792
Phone: (787)850-0000 **Fax:** (787)850-9411
Website: http://cuhwww.upr.clu.edu/~enfe/
Fnded: 1962. **Degrees Offered:** BS.

★ 28159 ★ University of Puerto Rico, Mayaguez Campus
Department of Nursing
PO Box 9015
Mayaguez, PR 00681
Phone: (787)263-3482 **Fax:** (787)832-3875
Email: z_torres@rumac.uprm.edu
Website: http://www.uprm.edu
Zaida Lina Torres, Contact
Fnded: 1911. **Degrees Offered:** BSN.

★ 28160 ★ University of Puerto Rico, Medical Sciences Campus
School of Nursing
MSN Department
PO Box 365067
San Juan, PR 00936-5067
Phone: (787)758-2525 **Fax:** (787)281-0721
Website: http://www.rcm.upr.clu.edu/
Gladys Velez, Contact
Fnded: 1950. **Degrees Offered:** BSN, MSN.

★ 28161 ★ University of the Sacred Heart
Program in Nursing
Box 12383
Loiza Station
Santurce, PR 00914-0383
Phone: (787)728-1515 **Fax:** (787)728-1250
Email: pcruz@sagrado.edu
Website: http://www.sagrado.edu/
Pura Julia Cruz, Contact
Fnded: 1935. **Degrees Offered:** BSN, MSN.

Quebec

★ 28162 ★ McGill University
School of Nursing
Wilson Hall
3506 University St.
Montreal, QC, Canada H3A 2A7
Phone: (514)398-4151 **Fax:** (514)398-8455
Email: anna.santandrea@mcgill.ca
Website: http://www.nursing.mcgill.ca
Anna M. Santandrea, Contact
Fnded: 1821. **Degrees Offered:** BSCN, M SC, PhD.

★ 28163 ★ Universite Laval
Faculty of Nursing
Pavillion Paul-Comtois
Bureau 4106
Sainte-Foy, QC, Canada G1K 7P4
Phone: (418)656-3356 **Fax:** (418)656-7304
Email: fsi@fsi.ulaval.ca
Website: http://www.fsi.ulaval.ca
Fnded: 1852. **Degrees Offered:** BSCN, MSN, PhD.

★ 28164 ★ Universite de Montreal
Faculty of Nursing
CP 6128
Succursale Centre-Ville
Montreal, QC, Canada H3C 3J7
Phone: (514)343-6111 **Fax:** (514)343-2306
Email: louise.gagnon@umontreal.ca
Website: http://www.scinf.umontreal.ca
Louise Gagnon, PhD, Contact
Fnded: 1920. **Degrees Offered:** BSCN, M SC, PhD.

★ 28165 ★ Universite du Quebec en Abitibi-Temiscamingue
Departement des sciences sociales et de la sante
445 Boulevard de l'Universite
Rouyn-Noranda, QC, Canada J9X 5E4
Phone: (819)762-0971 **Fax:** (819)797-4727
Email: lyne.fecteau@uqat.ca
Website: http://www.uqat.uquebec.ca/gestac/prg/7855.asp
Lyne Fecteau, Contact
Fnded: 1983. **Degrees Offered:** BN.

★ 28166 ★ Universite du Quebec a Chicoutimi
Program in Nursing
555 Blvd. de L'Universite
Chicoutimi, QC, Canada G7H 2B1
Phone: (418)545-5011 **Fax:** (418)545-5012
Email: francoise_courville@uqac.ca
Website: http://www.uqac.uquebec.ca/
Francoise Courville, Contact
Fnded: 1969. **Degrees Offered:** BA, MSN.

★ 28167 ★ Universite du Quebec en Outaouais
Departement des Sciences Infirmieres
C-3333
Hull, QC, Canada J8X 3X7
Phone: (819)595-3900 **Fax:** (819)595-2384
Email: chantal_stpierre@uqah.uquebec.ca
Website: http://www.uquebec.ca/
Chantal Saint-Pierre, Contact
Fnded: 1981. **Degrees Offered:** BSCN, M SC N.

★ 28168 ★ Universite du Quebec a Rimouski
Program in Nursing
300 Allee des Ursulines
Rimouski, QC, Canada G5H 3K6
Phone: (418)723-1986 **Fax:** (418)724-1849
Email: guy_belanger@uqar.qc.ca
Website: http://www.uquebec.ca/mscinf/
Guy Belanger, Contact
Fnded: 1973. **Degrees Offered:** BSCN, M SC N.

★ 28169 ★ Universite du Quebec a Trois-Rivieres
Program in Nursing
Casier Postal 500
Trois Rivieres, QC, Canada G9A 5H7
Phone: (819)376-5011
Email: lisette_richard@uqtr.ca
Website: http://www.uqtr.uquebec.ca/
Lisette Richard, Contact
Fnded: 1969. **Degrees Offered:** BS, MSN.

★ 28170 ★ Universite de Sherbrooke
Department of Nursing
Sherbrooke, QC, Canada J1H 5N4
Phone: (819)564-5358 **Fax:** (819)820-6816
Email: dstcyr@courrier.usherb.ca
Website: http://scinf.med.usherb.ca
Dr. Denise St. Cyr-Tribble, Contact
Fnded: 1954. **Degrees Offered:** BSCN, M SC, PhD.

Rhode Island

★ 28171 ★ Rhode Island College
Department of Nursing
600 Mount Pleasant Ave.
Providence, RI 02908-1991
Phone: (401)456-8014 **Fax:** (401)456-8206
Email: jwilliams@ric.edu
Website: http://www.ric.edu
Dr. Jane Williams, Contact
Fnded: 1854. **Degrees Offered:** BS.

★ 28172 ★ Salve Regina University
Department of Nursing
100 Ochre Point Ave.
Newport, RI 02840-4192
Free: 888-467-2583 **Fax:** (401)848-2823
Email: sruadmis@salve.edu
Website: http://www.salve.edu/dept_nursing/index.html
Laura E. McPhie Oliveira, Contact
Fnded: 1934. **Degrees Offered:** BS.

★ 28173 ★ University of Rhode Island
College of Nursing
White Hall
Kingston, RI 02881
Phone: (401)874-2766 **Fax:** (401)874-2061
Email: dsb@uri.edu
Website: http://www.uri.edu/nursing
Dr. Donna Schwartz-Barcott, Contact
Fnded: 1892. **Degrees Offered:** BS, MS, PhD.

Saskatchewan

★ 28174 ★ University of Saskatchewan
College of Nursing
107 Wiggins Rd.
Saskatoon, SK, Canada S7N 5E5
Phone: (306)966-6229 **Fax:** (306)966-6703
Email: gail.laing@sask.usask.ca
Website: http://www.usask.ca/nursing/
Dr. Gail Laing, Contact
Fnded: 1907. **Degrees Offered:** BSN, MN.

South Carolina

★ 28175 ★ Charleston Southern University
Wingo School of Nursing
PO Box 118087
9200 University Blvd.
Charleston, SC 29423-8087
Phone: (843)863-7075 **Fax:** (843)863-7540
Email: mlarisey@csuniv.edu
Website: http://www.csuniv.edu
Dr. Marian M. Larisey, Contact
Fnded: 1964. **Degrees Offered:** BSN.

★ 28176 ★ Clemson University
School of Nursing
Advising Center
309 Edwards Hall
Clemson, SC 29634-0744
Phone: (864)656-5495 **Fax:** (864)656-1688
Email: mary2@clemson.edu
Website: http://www.clemson.edu/
Beth Hearn, Contact
Fnded: 1889. **Degrees Offered:** BS, MS.

★ 28177 ★ Lander University
School of Nursing
Stanley Ave.
Greenwood, SC 29649
Phone: (864)388-8307 **Fax:** (864)388-8125
Email: tnelson@lander.edu
Website: http://www.lander.edu
Thomas Nelson, Contact
Fnded: 1872. **Degrees Offered:** BSN.

★ 28178 ★ Medical University of South Carolina
College of Nursing
99 Jonathan Lucas St.
PO Box 250160
Charleston, SC 29425
Phone: (843)792-8515 **Fax:** (843)792-9258
Email: pagecf@musc.edu
Website: http://www.musc.edu/Nursing
Carolyn Page, Contact
Fnded: 1824. **Degrees Offered:** BSN, MSN, PhD.

★ 28179 ★ University of South Carolina
College of Nursing
1601 Greene St.
Williams Brice Bldg.
Columbia, SC 29208
Phone: (803)777-3754 **Fax:** (803)777-0616
Email: cyjackso@nrwpo.nurs.sc.edu
Website: http://www.sc.edu/nursing
Cheryl Nelson-Jackson, Contact
Fnded: 1801. **Degrees Offered:** BSN, MSN, MSN/MPH, PhD.

★ 28180 ★ University of South Carolina, Aiken
School of Nursing
471 University Pkwy.
Aiken, SC 29801
Phone: (803)648-6851 **Fax:** (803)641-3362
Email: trudyg@aiken.sc.edu
Website: http://www.usca.edu/nursing/
Dr. Trudy Groves, Contact
Fnded: 1961. **Degrees Offered:** BSN.

★ 28181 ★ University of South Carolina, Spartanburg
Mary Black School of Nursing
800 University Way
Spartanburg, SC 29303
Free: 888-551-3858 **Fax:** (864)503-5411
Website: http://www.uscs.edu/academics/mbsn/
Fnded: 1967. **Degrees Offered:** BSN.

South Dakota

★ 28182 ★ Augustana College
Department of Nursing
2001 S Summit Ave.
Sioux Falls, SD 57197
Phone: (605)274-4729 **Fax:** (605)274-4723
Email: margot_nelson@augie.edu

Website: http://www.augie.edu
Dr. Margot Nelson, Contact
Fnded: 1860. **Degrees Offered:** BA, MA.

★ 28183 ★ Mount Marty College
Nursing Program
1105 W 8th St.
Yankton, SD 57078-3724
Phone: (605)668-1594 **Fax:** (605)668-1607
Email: jstephens@mtmc.edu
Website: http://www.mtmc.edu
Dr. Janice E. Stephens, Contact
Fnded: 1936. **Degrees Offered:** BSN.

★ 28184 ★ Presentation College
Department of Nursing
1500 N Main St.
Aberdeen, SD 57401
Phone: (605)229-8472 **Fax:** (605)229-8489
Email: janicesw@presentation.edu
Website: http://www.presentation.edu
Dr. Janice Williams, Contact
Fnded: 1951. **Degrees Offered:** BSN.

★ 28185 ★ South Dakota State University
College of Nursing
Rotunda Lane, NFA 217
Box 2275
Brookings, SD 57007-0098
Phone: (605)688-4114 **Fax:** (605)688-5827
Email: penny_powers@sdstate.edu
Website: http://www.sdstate.org/Academics/CollegeOfNursing/
Dr. Penny Powers, Contact
Fnded: 1881. **Degrees Offered:** BS, MS.

Tennessee

★ 28186 ★ Austin Peay State University
College of Human Services and Nursing
PO Box 4658
Clarksville, TN 37044
Phone: (931)221-7710 **Fax:** (931)221-7595
Website: http://www.apsu.edu/nursing01
Fnded: 1927. **Degrees Offered:** BSN.

★ 28187 ★ Baptist College of Health Sciences
Nursing Division
1003 Monroe
Memphis, TN 38104
Phone: (901)575-2247
Email: admissions@bchs.edu
Fnded: 1994. **Degrees Offered:** BSN.

★ 28188 ★ Belmont University
School of Nursing
1900 Belmont Blvd.
Nashville, TN 37212-3757
Phone: (615)460-6107 **Fax:** (615)460-6125
Email: hendonc@mail.belmont.edu
Website: http://www.belmont.edu/nursing
Cathy Hendon, Contact
Fnded: 1951. **Degrees Offered:** BSN, MSN.

★ 28189 ★ Carson-Newman College
Department of Nursing
1646 Russell Ave.
C-NC Box 71883
Jefferson City, TN 37760
Phone: (865)471-3426 **Fax:** (865)471-4574
Email: chuff@cn.edu
Website: http://www.cn.edu
Dr. Cynthia Huff, Contact
Fnded: 1851. **Degrees Offered:** BSN, MSN.

★ 28190 ★ Cumberland University
Division of Nursing
One Cumberland Sq.
Lebanon, TN 37087-3554
Phone: (615)444-2562 **Fax:** (615)443-8427
Email: nursing@cumberland.edu
Website: http://www.cumberland.edu/academics/nursing/index.html
Dr. Leanne Busby, Contact
Fnded: 1842. **Degrees Offered:** BSN.

★ 28191 ★ East Tennessee State University
College of Nursing
PO Box 70617
Johnson City, TN 37614-0617
Phone: (423)439-4578 **Fax:** (423)439-4522
Email: admitnur@etsu.edu
Website: http://www.etsu.edu/etsu.com
Rebecca Brewster, Contact
Fnded: 1911. **Degrees Offered:** BSN, DSN, MSN.

★ 28192 ★ King College
School of Nursing
1350 King College Rd.
Bristol, TN 37620
Phone: (423)652-4748 **Fax:** (423)968-4456
Dr. Johanne A. Quinn, Contact
Fnded: 1867. **Degrees Offered:** BSN.

★ 28193 ★ Lincoln Memorial University
Department of Nursing
Cumberland Gap Pkwy.
Harrogate, TN 37752
Phone: (423)869-6326 **Fax:** (423)869-6244
Email: ebarr@lmunet.edu
Website: http://www.lmunet.edu
Dr. Elisa Barr, Contact
Fnded: 1897. **Degrees Offered:** BSN.

★ 28194 ★ Middle Tennessee State University
School of Nursing
1301 E Main St.
PO Box 81
Murfreesboro, TN 37132-0001
Phone: (615)898-2437 **Fax:** (615)898-5441
Email: pgholder@mtsu.edu
Website: http://www.mtsu.edu/~nursing/
Dr. Pamela G. Holder, Contact
Fnded: 1911. **Degrees Offered:** BSN.

★ 28195 ★ Southern Adventist University
School of Nursing
PO Box 370
Collegedale, TN 37315
Phone: (423)238-2941 **Fax:** (423)238-3004
Email: lmarlowe@southern.edu
Website: http://www.southern.edu/
Linda Marlowe, Contact
Fnded: 1892. **Degrees Offered:** BS, MSN, MSN/MBA.

★ 28196 ★ Tennessee State University
School of Nursing
3500 John A. Merritt Blvd.
Box 9590
Nashville, TN 37209-1561
Phone: (615)963-5261 **Fax:** (615)963-7614
Email: bbrown@tnstate.edu
Website: http://www.tnstate.edu
Dr. Barbara E. Brown, Contact
Fnded: 1912. **Degrees Offered:** BSN, MSN.

★ 28197 ★ Tennessee Technological University
School of Nursing
PO Box 5001
Cookeville, TN 38505-0001
Phone: (931)372-3203 **Fax:** (931)372-6244
Email: nursing@tntech.edu
Website: http://www.tntech.edu/www/acad/nursing/
Margaret Chaffin, Contact
Fnded: 1915. **Degrees Offered:** BSN.

★ 28198 ★ Tennessee Wesleyan College
Fort Sanders Nursing Department
9821 Cogdill Rd., Ste. 2
Knoxville, TN 37932
Phone: (865)777-5100 **Fax:** (865)777-5114
Website: http://www.twcnet.edu/academics/nursing
Fnded: 1857. **Degrees Offered:** BSN.

★ 28199 ★ Union University
School of Nursing
1050 Union University Dr.
Jackson, TN 38305
Phone: (731)661-5235 **Fax:** (731)661-5504
Email: jwebb@uu.edu
Jill Webb, Contact
Fnded: 1823. **Degrees Offered:** BSN, MSN.

★ 28200 ★ University of Memphis
Loewenberg School of Nursing
105 Newport Hall
Memphis, TN 38152
Phone: (901)678-2003 **Fax:** (901)678-4906
Email: shall@memphis.edu
Website: http://www.nursing.memphis.edu
Sheila Hall, Contact
Fnded: 1912. **Degrees Offered:** BSN.

★ 28201 ★ University of Tennessee
College of Nursing
1200 Volunteer Blvd.
Knoxville, TN 37996-4180
Phone: (865)974-4151 **Fax:** (865)974-3569
Email: smcguire@utk.edu
Website: http://www.nightingale.com.utk.edu
Dr. Sandra L. McGuire, Contact
Fnded: 1794. **Degrees Offered:** BSN, MSN, PhD.

★ 28202 ★ University of Tennessee, Chattanooga
School of Nursing
615 McCallie Ave.
Chattanooga, TN 37403-2598
Phone: (423)755-4750 **Fax:** (423)755-4668
Email: kay-lindgren@utc.edu
Website: http://www.utc.edu/~utcnurse/index.htm
Dr. Katherine Russell Lindgren, Contact
Fnded: 1886. **Degrees Offered:** BSN, MSN.

★ 28203 ★ University of Tennessee Health Science Center
College of Nursing
877 Madison Ave., Ste. 637
Memphis, TN 38163
Phone: (901)448-6139 **Fax:** (901)448-4121
Email: cgraff@utmem.edu
Website: http://www.utmem.edu/nursing
Dr. Carolyn Graff, Contact
Fnded: 1911. **Degrees Offered:** DN SC, MSN.

★ 28204 ★ University of Tennessee, Martin
Department of Nursing
Gooch Hall 136J
Martin, TN 38238
Phone: (731)587-7138 **Fax:** (731)587-7939
Email: brendac@utm.edu

Website: http://www.utm.edu
Brenda W. Campbell, Contact
Fnded: 1900. **Degrees Offered:** BSN.

★ 28205 ★ Vanderbilt University
School of Nursing
229C Godchaux Hall
Nashville, TN 37240
Phone: (615)322-3800 **Fax:** (615)343-0333
Email: karen.stevens@vanderbilt.edu
Website: http://www.mc.vanderbilt.edu/nursing/
Karen Stevens, Contact
Fnded: 1873. **Degrees Offered:** MSN, MSN/MBA, PhD.

Texas

★ 28206 ★ Abilene Intercollegiate School of Nursing
2149 Hickory St.
Abilene, TX 79601
Phone: (915)672-2441 **Fax:** (915)672-5026
Email: aisnadv@abilene.com
Jo Garcia, Contact
Degrees Offered: BSN, MSN.

★ 28207 ★ Angelo State University
Department of Nursing
PO Box 10902
San Angelo, TX 76909
Phone: (915)942-2224 **Fax:** (915)942-2236
Email: leslie.mayrand@angelo.edu
Website: http://www.angelo.edu/dept/nur/
Dr. Leslie Mayrand, Contact
Fnded: 1928. **Degrees Offered:** BSN, MSN.

★ 28208 ★ Baylor University
Louise Herrington School of Nursing
3700 Worth St.
Dallas, TX 75246
Phone: (214)820-3361 **Fax:** (214)820-4770
Email: pauline_johnson@baylor.edu
Website: http://www.baylor.edu
Dr. Pauline Johnson, Contact
Fnded: 1845. **Degrees Offered:** BSN, MSN.

★ 28209 ★ East Texas Baptist University
Department of Nursing
1209 N Grove St.
Marshall, TX 75670
Phone: (903)935-7963 **Fax:** (903)938-9225
Email: charvey@etbu.edu
Website: http://www.etbu.edu
Dr. Carolyn Harvey, Contact
Fnded: 1912. **Degrees Offered:** BSN.

★ 28210 ★ Houston Baptist University
College of Nursing
7502 Fondren St.
Houston, TX 77074
Phone: (281)649-3300 **Fax:** (281)649-3340
Email: bbinder@hbu.edu
Website: http://www.hbu.edu/
Dr. Brenda Binder, Contact
Fnded: 1960. **Degrees Offered:** BSN, MSN.

★ 28211 ★ Lamar University
Department of Nursing
PO Box 10081
Beaumont, TX 77710
Phone: (409)880-7720 **Fax:** (409)880-8698
Email: carrollal@hal.lamar.edu
Website: http://www.lamar.edu
Dr. Anita Carroll, Contact
Fnded: 1923. **Degrees Offered:** BSN, MSN.

★ 28212 ★ Lubbock Christian University
Department of Nursing
5601 W 19th St.
Lubbock, TX 79407
Email: nursing@lcu.edu
Fnded: 1957. **Degrees Offered:** BSN.

★ 28213 ★ Midwestern State University
Nursing Program
3410 Taft Blvd.
Wichita Falls, TX 76308
Phone: (940)397-4599 **Fax:** (940)397-4513
Email: deborah.garrison@mwsu.edu
Website: http://www.mwsu.edu/
Dr. Deborah Garrison, Contact
Fnded: 1922. **Degrees Offered:** BSN, MSN.

★ 28214 ★ Prairie View A&M University
College of Nursing
1801 Main St., Ste. 1002
Houston, TX 77002
Phone: (713)797-7003 **Fax:** (713)797-7012
Email: chloe_gaines@pvamu.edu
Website: http://www.pvamu.edu/PVnursing/
Dr. Chloe Gaines, Contact
Fnded: 1878. **Degrees Offered:** BSN, MSN.

★ 28215 ★ Southwestern Adventist University
Department of Nursing
Keene, TX 76059
Phone: (817)645-3921 **Fax:** (817)556-4713
Email: moorep@swau.edu
Website: http://www.swau.edu/
Dr. Penny Moore, Contact
Fnded: 1894. **Degrees Offered:** BS.

★ 28216 ★ Stephen F. Austin State University
Division of Nursing
SFA Box 6156
Nacogdoches, TX 75962
Phone: (936)468-3604 **Fax:** (936)468-1696
Website: http://www.sfasu.edu/
Dr. Glenda C. Walker, Contact
Fnded: 1923. **Degrees Offered:** BSN.

★ 28217 ★ Tarleton State University
Department of Nursing
Box T-0500
Stephenville, TX 76402
Phone: (254)968-9139 **Fax:** (254)968-9716
Email: skinner@tarleton.edu
Website: http://www.tarleton.edu/~nursing
Fnded: 1899. **Degrees Offered:** BSN.

★ 28218 ★ Texas A&M International University
Canseco School of Nursing
5201 University Blvd.
Laredo, TX 78041-1900
Phone: (956)326-2450 **Fax:** (956)326-2449
Email: sbaker@tamiu.edu
Website: http://www.tamiu.edu/
Dr. Susan Scoville Baker, Contact
Fnded: 1969. **Degrees Offered:** BSN.

★ 28219 ★ Texas A&M University, Corpus Christi
School of Nursing and Health Sciences
6300 Ocean Dr.
FC167
Corpus Christi, TX 78412
Phone: (361)825-2798 **Fax:** (361)825-2484
Email: kolson@falcon.tamucc.edu
Website: http://www.sci.tamucc.edu/nursing/
Dr. Karen Olson, Contact
Fnded: 1947. **Degrees Offered:** BSN, MSN.

★ 28220 ★ Texas Christian University
Harris School of Nursing
TCU Box 298620
2800 W Bowie
Fort Worth, TX 76129
Phone: (817)257-7650 **Fax:** (817)257-7944
Email: k.baldwin@tcu.edu
Website: http://www.tcu.edu/
Kathleen Baldwin, Contact
Fnded: 1873. **Degrees Offered:** BSN.

★ 28221 ★ Texas Tech University Health Sciences Center
School of Nursing
3601 4th St.
Lubbock, TX 79430
Phone: (806)743-3055
Email: barbara.johnston@ttuhsc.edu
Website: http://www.ttunursing.com
Barbara Johnston, Contact
Fnded: 1969. **Degrees Offered:** BSN, MSN, MSN/MBA.

★ 28222 ★ Texas Woman's University
College of Nursing
1810 Inwood Rd.
Dallas, TX 75235-7299
Phone: (214)689-6551 **Fax:** (214)689-6539
Email: cmobley@twu.edu
Website: http://www.twu.edu/nursing/
Dr. Caryl Mobley, Contact
Fnded: 1901. **Degrees Offered:** BS, MS, MSN/MHA, PhD.

★ 28223 ★ University of the Incarnate Word
Program in Nursing
4301 Broadway
San Antonio, TX 78209
Phone: (210)829-3988 **Fax:** (210)829-3174
Email: strickla@universe.uiwtx.edu
Website: http://www.uiw.edu/
Dr. Sandra Strickland, Contact
Fnded: 1881. **Degrees Offered:** BSN, MSN, MSN/MBA.

★ 28224 ★ University of Mary Hardin-Baylor
School of Nursing
900 College St.
UMHB Box 8015
Belton, TX 76513-2599
Phone: (254)295-4662 **Fax:** (254)295-4141
Website: http://www.umhb.edu/
Dr. Grace Labaj, Contact
Fnded: 1845. **Degrees Offered:** BSN.

★ 28225 ★ University of Texas, Arlington
School of Nursing
UTA Box 19407
411 S Nedderman Dr.
Arlington, TX 76019-0407
Phone: (817)272-7086 **Fax:** (817)272-5006
Email: grove@uta.edu
Website: http://www.uta.edu/nursing
Dr. Susan K. Grove, Contact
Fnded: 1895. **Degrees Offered:** BSN, MS/MPH, MSN, MSN/MBA, MSN/MHA, MSN/MPH.

★ 28226 ★ University of Texas, Austin
School of Nursing
Student Affairs Office, Graduate Admissions
1700 Red River St.
Austin, TX 78701-1499
Phone: (512)471-7927 **Fax:** (512)232-4777
Email: nugrad@uts.cc.utexas.edu

Website: http://www.utexas.edu/nursing
Fnded: 1883. **Degrees Offered:** BSN, MSN, MSN/MBA, PhD.

★ 28227 ★ University of Texas, Brownsville
Department of Nursing
Brownsville, TX 78520
Phone: (956)574-6690 **Fax:** (956)544-8881
Email: eherriage@utb.edu
Website: http://www.utb.edu/
Dr. Ella Herriage, Contact
Fnded: 1973. **Degrees Offered:** BSN, MS.

★ 28228 ★ University of Texas, El Paso
School of Nursing
1101 N Campbell St.
El Paso, TX 79902
Phone: (915)747-7246 **Fax:** (915)747-7207
Email: dstuppy@utep.edu
Website: http://chs.utep.edu/nursing
Dr. Dorothy Stuppy, Contact
Fnded: 1913. **Degrees Offered:** BSN, DSN, MSN.

★ 28229 ★ University of Texas Health Science Center, Houston
School of Nursing
School of Nursing Admissions
1100 Holcombe Blvd.
Houston, TX 77030
Free: 800-232-8876 **Fax:** (713)500-2007
Email: www@son1.nur.uth.tmc.edu
Website: http://sonser4.nur.uth.tmc.edu
Fnded: 1972. **Degrees Offered:** BSN, DSN, MSN, MSN/MPH.

★ 28230 ★ University of Texas Health Science Center, San Antonio
School of Nursing
7703 Floyd Curl Dr.
Mail Code 7945
San Antonio, TX 78229-3900
Phone: (210)567-5815
Email: robinsonb@uthscsa.edu
Website: http://nursing.uthscsa.edu
Dr. Beverly Robinson, Contact
Fnded: 1976. **Degrees Offered:** BSN, MSN, MSN/MPH, PhD.

★ 28231 ★ University of Texas Medical Branch
School of Nursing
301 University Blvd.
Galveston, TX 77555-1029
Phone: (409)772-8310 **Fax:** (409)772-3770
Email: cbray@utmb.edu
Website: http://www.son.utmb.edu
Christelle Bray, Contact
Fnded: 1891. **Degrees Offered:** BSN, MSN, PhD.

★ 28232 ★ University of Texas, Pan American
Department of Nursing
1201 W University Dr.
Edinburg, TX 78539
Phone: (956)316-7082 **Fax:** (956)381-2875
Email: btucker@panam.edu
Website: http://www.panam.edu
Dr. Barbara Tucker, Contact
Fnded: 1927. **Degrees Offered:** BSN, MSN.

★ 28233 ★ University of Texas, Tyler
Program in Nursing
3900 University Blvd.
Tyler, TX 75799
Phone: (903)566-7220 **Fax:** (903)565-5533
Email: syarbrough@mail.uttyl.edu
Website: http://www.uttyler.edu/nursing
Dr. Susan Yarbrough, Contact
Fnded: 1971. **Degrees Offered:** BSN, MSN, MSN/MBA.

★ 28234 ★ West Texas A&M University
Division of Nursing
WTAMU Box 60969
Canyon, TX 79016-0001
Phone: (806)651-2661 **Fax:** (806)651-2632
Email: lrobinson@mail.wtamu.edu
Website: http://www.wtamu.edu/nursing
Lynda Robinson, Contact
Fnded: 1909. **Degrees Offered:** BSN, MSN.

Utah

★ 28235 ★ Brigham Young University
College of Nursing
500F SWKT
PO Box 25426
Provo, UT 84602-5426
Phone: (801)422-4142 **Fax:** (801)422-0536
Email: denise_gibbons@byu.edu
Website: http://www.nurse.byu.edu/
Denise Gibbons Davis, Contact
Fnded: 1875. **Degrees Offered:** BS, MS.

★ 28236 ★ University of Phoenix, Utah Campus
College of Nursing and Health Care Sciences
5251 Green St.
Salt Lake City, UT 84123-4617
Phone: (801)263-1444
Email: scott.jones@phoenix.edu
Website: http://www.universities.com/Schools/U/University_Of_Phoenix_Utah_Campus.asp
Scott Jones, Contact
Degrees Offered: BSN, MSN, MSN/MBA.

★ 28237 ★ University of Utah
College of Nursing
10 S 2000 East
Salt Lake City, UT 84112-5880
Phone: (801)581-3414 **Fax:** (801)581-4642
Email: joyce.rathbun@nurs.utah.edu
Website: http://www.utah.edu/
Joyce Rathbun, Contact
Fnded: 1850. **Degrees Offered:** BS, MS, PhD.

★ 28238 ★ Weber State University
Program in Nursing
3903 University Circle
Ogden, UT 84408-3903
Phone: (801)626-6128 **Fax:** (801)626-6397
Email: rholt@weber.edu
Website: http://www.weber.edu/
Rob Holt, Contact
Fnded: 1889. **Degrees Offered:** BSN.

★ 28239 ★ Westminster College
Saint Mark's-Westminster School of Nursing and Health Sciences
1840 S 1300 East
Salt Lake City, UT 84105
Phone: (801)832-2150 **Fax:** (801)832-3110
Email: kemrich@westminstercollege.edu
Website: http://www.westminstercollege.edu
Kathleen Emrich, EdD, Contact
Fnded: 1875. **Degrees Offered:** BS, MS.

Vermont

★ 28240 ★ Norwich University
Division of Nursing
Office of Admissions
158 Harmon Dr.
Northfield, VT 05663
Phone: (802)485-2008 **Fax:** (802)485-2032
Email: nuadm@norwich.edu
Website: http://www.norwich.edu
Rose Myers, Contact
Fnded: 1819. **Degrees Offered:** BSN.

★ 28241 ★ Southern Vermont College
Department of Nursing
982 Mansion Dr.
Bennington, VT 05201
Phone: (802)447-4656 **Fax:** (802)447-4652
Website: http://www.svc.edu/academics/divisions/nursing.html
Holly Madison, Contact
Fnded: 1926. **Degrees Offered:** BSN.

★ 28242 ★ University of Vermont
School of Nursing
Rowell Bldg., Rm. 216
Burlington, VT 05405-0068
Phone: (802)656-2018 **Fax:** (802)656-8306
Email: gail.havens@uvm.edu
Website: http://www.uvm.edu/
Dr. Gail Havens, Contact
Fnded: 1791. **Degrees Offered:** BS, MS.

Virgin Islands

★ 28243 ★ University of the Virgin Islands
Division of Nursing
2 John Brewer's Bay
St. Thomas, VI 00802-9990
Phone: (340)693-1291 **Fax:** (340)693-1285
Email: gcallwo@uvi.edu
Website: http://manta.uvi.edu/
Dr. Gloria B. Callwood, Contact
Fnded: 1962. **Degrees Offered:** BS.

Virginia

★ 28244 ★ Community Hospital of Roanoke Valley
College of Health Sciences
Nursing Education Program
PO Box 13186
Roanoke, VA 24013
Phone: (540)985-8311 **Fax:** (540)985-9773
Email: becky@chs.edu
Website: http://www.chs.edu
Dr. Rebecca Culver Clark, Contact
Fnded: 1982. **Degrees Offered:** BSN.

★ 28245 ★ Eastern Mennonite University
Department of Nursing
1200 Park Rd.
Harrisonburg, VA 22802
Free: 800-368-2665 **Fax:** (540)432-4444
Email: millerlw@emu.edu
Website: http://www.emu.edu/
Lawrence W. Miller, Contact
Fnded: 1917. **Degrees Offered:** BSN.

★ 28246 ★ George Mason University
College of Nursing and Health Science
Mail Stop 3C4
4400 University Dr.
Fairfax, VA 22030-4444
Phone: (703)993-1904 **Fax:** (703)993-6303
Email: clangley@gmu.edu

Website: http://cnhs.gmu.edu/
Dr. Chris Langley, Contact
Fnded: 1957. Degrees Offered: BSN, MSN, MSN/MBA, PhD.

★ 28247 ★ Hampton University Department of Nursing
Freeman Hall
Hampton, VA 23668
Phone: (757)727-5251 Fax: (757)727-5423
Email: nursing@hamptonu.edu
Website: http://www.hamptonu.edu/nursing/Index.htm
Mrs. Johnnie Bunch, Contact
Fnded: 1868. Degrees Offered: BS, MS, PhD.

★ 28248 ★ James Madison University Department of Nursing
701 Carrier Dr.
Health and Human Services Bldg., MSC 4305
Harrisonburg, VA 22807
Phone: (540)568-6314 Fax: (540)568-7896
Email: hedricts@jmu.edu
Website: http://www.nursing.jmu.edu
Tonia Simmons Hedrick, Contact
Fnded: 1908. Degrees Offered: BSN.

★ 28249 ★ Liberty University Department of Nursing
1971 University Blvd.
Lynchburg, VA 24502
Phone: (434)582-2519
Email: hspear@liberty.edu
Website: http://www.liberty.edu
Dr. Hila Spear, Contact
Fnded: 1971. Degrees Offered: BSN, MSN.

★ 28250 ★ Lynchburg College School of Health Sciences and Human Performance
McMillan Nursing Bldg.
1501 Lakeside Dr.
Lynchburg, VA 24501-3199
Phone: (804)544-8324 Fax: (804)544-8323
Email: whitman_n@mail.lynchburg.edu
Website: http://www.lynchburg.edu/schools/NRSG.htm
Dr. Nancy I. Whitman, Contact
Fnded: 1903. Degrees Offered: BS.

★ 28251 ★ Marymount University School of Health Professions
2807 N Glebe Rd.
Arlington, VA 22207-4299
Phone: (703)284-5906
Email: francesca.reed@marymount.edu
Website: http://marymount.edu
Francesca Reed, Contact
Fnded: 1950. Degrees Offered: BSN, MSN.

★ 28252 ★ Norfolk State University Department of Nursing
700 Park Ave., Rm. 420 Robinson
Norfolk, VA 23504-8026
Phone: (757)823-9013 Fax: (757)823-8241
Email: wfwhite-parson@nsu.edu
Website: http://www.nsu.edu/schools/sciencetech/nursing/
Dr. Willar White-Parson, Contact
Fnded: 1935. Degrees Offered: BSN.

★ 28253 ★ Old Dominion University Department of Nursing
Norfolk, VA 23529-0500
Phone: (757)683-4298 Fax: (757)683-5253
Email: lgarzon@odu.edu
Website: http://www.odu.edu/nursson
Dr. Laurel Garzon, Contact
Fnded: 1930. Degrees Offered: BSN, MSN.

★ 28254 ★ Radford University School of Nursing
Box 6964
RU Station
Waldron Hall
Radford, VA 24142
Phone: (540)831-7700 Fax: (540)831-7716
Email: nurse-web@radford.edu
Website: http://www.radford.edu/nurs-web
Dr. Karolyn Givens, Contact
Fnded: 1910. Degrees Offered: BSN, MSN.

★ 28255 ★ Shenandoah University Division of Nursing
1775 N Sector Ct.
Winchester, VA 22601
Phone: (540)665-5508 Fax: (540)665-5519
Email: mmorrow@su.edu
Website: http://www.su.edu
Dr. Martha Morrow, Contact
Fnded: 1875. Degrees Offered: BSN, MSN.

★ 28256 ★ University of Virginia College at Wise Department of Nursing
One College Ave.
Smiddy Hall, Rm. 243
Wise, VA 24293-4400
Phone: (540)328-0275 Fax: (540)328-0247
Website: http://www.wise.virginia.edu/nursing
Fnded: 1954. Degrees Offered: BSN.

★ 28257 ★ University of Virginia School of Nursing
PO Box 800782
McLeod Hall
Charlottesville, VA 22908
Free: 888-283-8703 Fax: (434)982-0528
Email: nur-osa@virginia.edu
Website: http://www.nursing.virginia.edu
Clay D. Hysell, Contact
Fnded: 1819. Degrees Offered: BSN, MSN, MSN/HSM, MSN/MA, MSN/MBA, MSN/PhD.

★ 28258 ★ Virginia Commonwealth University School of Nursing
PO Box 567
1220 E Broad St.
Richmond, VA 23298-0567
Phone: (804)828-5171 Fax: (804)828-7743
Email: slipp@hsc.vcu.edu
Website: http://views.vcu.edu/son/son.html
Susan L. Lipp, Contact
Fnded: 1838. Degrees Offered: BS, MS, PhD.

Washington

★ 28259 ★ Gonzaga University Intercollegiate College of Nursing/ Washington State University
Spokane, WA 99258-0038
Website: http://www.gu.gonzaga.edu/
Remarks: For more information on this program, see listing under Intercollegiate College of Nursing/Washington State University.

★ 28260 ★ Intercollegiate College of Nursing/Washington State University
2917 W Fort George Wright Dr.
Spokane, WA 99224-5291
Phone: (509)324-7334 Fax: (509)324-7336
Email: mruby@wsu.edu
Margaret Ruby, Contact
Degrees Offered: BSN, MN.

★ 28261 ★ Northwest College Mark and Huldah Buntain School of Nursing
5520 108th Ave. NE
Kirkland, WA 98033
Free: 800-669-3781
Website: http://www.nwcollege.edu/
Carl Christiansen, Contact
Fnded: 1934. Degrees Offered: BS.

★ 28262 ★ Pacific Lutheran University School of Nursing
Tacoma, WA 98447-0029
Phone: (253)536-8264 Fax: (253)535-7590
Email: mizeeb@plu.edu
Website: http://www.plu.edu/~nurs/
Emily Mize, Contact
Fnded: 1890. Degrees Offered: BSN, MSN.

★ 28263 ★ Seattle Pacific University School of Health Sciences
Marston Hall, No. 320
3307 3rd Ave. W
Seattle, WA 98119-1997
Phone: (206)281-2649 Fax: (206)281-2649
Email: ehitchens@spu.edu
Website: http://www.spu.edu/dept/bsc/
Dr. Emily Hitchens, Contact
Fnded: 1891. Degrees Offered: BSN, MN/MBA, MSN.

★ 28264 ★ Seattle University School of Nursing
900 Broadway
Seattle, WA 98122-4340
Phone: (206)296-5666 Fax: (206)296-5544
Email: kathryna@seattleu.edu
Website: http://www.seattleu.edu/nurs
Dr. Kathryn Anderson, Contact
Fnded: 1891. Degrees Offered: BSN, MSN.

★ 28265 ★ University of Washington School of Nursing
Health Sciences Bldg.
Box 357260
Seattle, WA 98195
Phone: (206)543-8736 Fax: (206)685-1613
Email: egg@u.washington.edu
Website: http://www.son.washington.edu
Carolyn Chow, Contact
Fnded: 1861. Degrees Offered: BSN, MN, MN/MPH, MSN/MHA, PhD.

West Virginia

★ 28266 ★ Alderson-Broaddus College Department of Nursing
Box 2003
Philippi, WV 26416
Phone: (304)457-1700 Fax: (304)457-6308
Email: boni@ab.edu
Website: http://www.ab.edu
Dr. M. Sharon Boni, Contact
Fnded: 1871. Degrees Offered: BSN.

★ 28267 ★ Bluefield State College Program in Nursing
219 Rock St.
Bluefield, WV 24701
Phone: (304)327-4139 Fax: (304)327-4219
Email: bpritchett@bluefield.wvnet.edu
Website: http://www.bluefieldstate.edu
Beth Pritchett, Contact
Fnded: 1895. Degrees Offered: BSN.

★ 28268 ★ Fairmont State College School of Health Careers
1201 Locust Ave.
Fairmont, WV 26554
Phone: (304)367-4761 **Fax:** (304)367-4268
Email: mmeighen@mail.fscwv.edu
Website: http://www.fscwv.edu/
Dr. Mary G. Meighen, Contact
Fnded: 1865. **Degrees Offered:** BSN.

★ 28269 ★ Marshall University College of Nursing and Health Professions
One John Marshall Dr.
Huntington, WV 25755-9500
Phone: (304)696-2618 **Fax:** (304)696-6739
Email: conhp@marshall.edu
Website: http://www.marshall.edu/conhp
Dr. Linda Scott, Contact
Fnded: 1837. **Degrees Offered:** BSN, MSN.

★ 28270 ★ Mountain State University Program in Nursing
Box 9003
Beckley, WV 25802-9003
Phone: (304)929-1425 **Fax:** 800-766-6067
Email: jsharp@mountainstate.edu
Website: http://www.cwv.edu/
Dr. Jessica Sharp, Contact
Fnded: 1933. **Degrees Offered:** BSN, MSN.

★ 28271 ★ Shepherd College Department of Nursing Education
Shepherdstown, WV 25443
Phone: (304)876-5341 **Fax:** (304)876-5169
Email: kgaberso@shepherd.edu
Website: http://www.shepherd.edu
Dr. Kathleen Gaberson, Contact
Fnded: 1871. **Degrees Offered:** BSN.

★ 28272 ★ University of Charleston Department of Nursing
2300 MacCorkle Ave. SE
Charleston, WV 25304
Phone: (304)357-4750 **Fax:** (304)357-4781
Email: admissions@uchaswv.edu
Website: http://www.ucwv.edu/dhs/bsn
Kim Scranage, Contact
Fnded: 1888. **Degrees Offered:** BSN.

★ 28273 ★ West Liberty State College Department of Health Sciences
West Liberty, WV 26074
Phone: (304)336-8108 **Fax:** (304)336-5104
Website: http://www.wlsc.edu/nursing/index.htm
Fnded: 1837. **Degrees Offered:** BSN.

★ 28274 ★ West Virginia University School of Nursing
6417 RCB Health Science Center S
PO Box 9640
Morgantown, WV 26506-9600
Phone: (304)293-4298 **Fax:** (304)293-2784
Email: mjsmith@wvu.edu
Website: http://www.hsc.wvu.edu/son/
Mary Jane Smith, Contact
Fnded: 1867. **Degrees Offered:** BSN, DSN, MSN.

★ 28275 ★ West Virginia Wesleyan College Department of Nursing
59 College Ave.
Buckhannon, WV 26201-2995
Phone: (304)473-8224 **Fax:** (304)473-8435
Email: aurelio_s@wvwc.edu
Website: http://www.wvwc.edu/
Shauna Lively Aurelio, Contact
Fnded: 1890. **Degrees Offered:** BSN.

★ 28276 ★ Wheeling Jesuit University Department of Nursing
316 Washington Ave.
Wheeling, WV 26003-6233
Phone: (304)243-2344 **Fax:** (304)243-2608
Website: http://www.wju.edu/academics/nursing
Fnded: 1954. **Degrees Offered:** BSN, MSN.

Wisconsin

★ 28277 ★ Alverno College Division of Nursing
3400 S 43rd St.
PO Box 343922
Milwaukee, WI 53234-3922
Phone: (414)382-6284 **Fax:** (414)382-6279
Email: judeen.schulte@alverno.edu
Website: http://www.alverno.edu
Dr. Judeen A. Schulte, Contact
Fnded: 1887. **Degrees Offered:** BSN

★ 28278 ★ Bellin College of Nursing Nursing Program
725 S Webster Ave.
Green Bay, WI 54301
Phone: (920)433-5803 **Fax:** (920)433-7416
Email: pcroghan@bcon.edu
Website: http://www.bcon.edu
Dr. Penny Croghan, Contact
Fnded: 1909. **Degrees Offered:** BSN.

★ 28279 ★ Cardinal Stritch University College of Nursing
6801 N Yates Rd.
Milwaukee, WI 53217-3985
Phone: (414)410-4042 **Fax:** (414)410-4239
Email: gradadm@stritch.edu
Website: http://www.stritch.edu/nursing/main.html
Fnded: 1937. **Degrees Offered:** BSN, MSN.

★ 28280 ★ Columbia College of Nursing/ Mount Mary College Nursing Program
Nursing Recruiter
2900 N Menomonee River Pkwy.
Milwaukee, WI 53222
Phone: (414)256-1219 **Fax:** (414)256-0180
Email: bondr@mtmary.edu
Website: http://www.mtmary.edu/nursing.html
Ronda Bond, Contact
Fnded: 2002. **Degrees Offered:** BSN.

★ 28281 ★ Concordia University Wisconsin Division of Nursing
12800 N Lake Shore Dr.
Mequon, WI 53097
Phone: (262)243-4452 **Fax:** (262)243-4506
Email: ruth.gresley@cuw.edu
Website: http://cuw.edu
Dr. Ruth Gresley, Contact
Fnded: 1881. **Degrees Offered:** BSN, MSN.

★ 28282 ★ Edgewood College Program in Nursing
1000 Edgewood College Dr.
Madison, WI 53711
Phone: (608)663-2292 **Fax:** (608)663-2863
Email: mkellypowell@edgewood.edu
Website: http://www.edgewood.edu/
Dr. Mary L. Kelly-Powell, Contact
Fnded: 1927. **Degrees Offered:** BS, MS.

★ 28283 ★ Marian College of Fond du Lac Nursing Studies Division
45 S National Ave.
Fond du Lac, WI 54935-4699
Phone: (920)923-8094 **Fax:** (920)923-8755
Email: admissions@mariancollege.edu
Website: http://www.mariancollege.edu
Fnded: 1936. **Degrees Offered:** BSN, MSN.

★ 28284 ★ Marquette University College of Nursing
PO Box 1881
Clark Hall
Milwaukee, WI 53201-1881
Phone: (414)288-3810 **Fax:** (414)288-1597
Email: maureen.o'brien@marquette.edu
Website: http://www.marquette.edu/nursing
Dr. Maureen O'Brien, Contact
Fnded: 1881. **Degrees Offered:** BSN, MSN, MSN/MBA, PhD.

★ 28285 ★ Milwaukee School of Engineering School of Nursing
1025 N Broadway St.
Milwaukee, WI 53202-3109
Phone: (414)277-4516 **Fax:** (414)277-4540
Email: brown@msoe.edu
Website: http://www.msoe.edu/nursing
Dr. Mary Louise Brown, Contact
Fnded: 1903. **Degrees Offered:** BSN.

★ 28286 ★ University of Wisconsin, Eau Claire School of Nursing
Eau Claire, WI 54702-4004
Phone: (715)836-5287 **Fax:** (715)836-5925
Email: wendtle@uwec.edu
Website: http://www.uwec.edu/Academic/Nurs/
Dr. Linda Elaine Wendt, Contact
Fnded: 1916. **Degrees Offered:** BSN, MSN.

★ 28287 ★ University of Wisconsin, Green Bay Professional Program in Nursing
2420 Nicolet Dr.
Green Bay, WI 54311-7001
Phone: (920)465-2826 **Fax:** (920)465-2854
Email: wuellind@uwgb.edu
Website: http://www.uwgb.edu/nursing/index.htm
Dawn M. Wuelling, Contact
Fnded: 1968. **Degrees Offered:** BSN.

★ 28288 ★ University of Wisconsin, Milwaukee School of Nursing
Student Affairs
PO Box 413
Milwaukee, WI 53201
Phone: (414)229-5473 **Fax:** (414)229-5554
Email: schulgal@uwm.edu
Website: http://www.nursing.uwm.edu
Lisa Schulga, Contact
Fnded: 1956. **Degrees Offered:** BSN, MS, PhD.

★ 28289 ★ University of Wisconsin, Oshkosh College of Nursing
800 Algoma Blvd.
Oshkosh, WI 54901-8660
Phone: (920)424-2106 **Fax:** (920)424-0123
Email: smithr@uwosh.edu
Website: http://www.uwosh.edu/colleges/con
Dr. Rosemary Smith, Contact
Fnded: 1871. **Degrees Offered:** BSN, MSN.

★ 28290 ★ Viterbo University
School of Nursing
815 S 9th St.
La Crosse, WI 54601
Phone: (608)796-3010 **Fax:** (608)796-3050
Email: adm.buzz@viterbo.edu
Website: http://www.viterbo.edu
Dr. Roland Nelson, Contact
Fnded: 1890. **Degrees Offered:** BSN, MSN.

Wyoming

★ 28291 ★ University of Wyoming
School of Nursing
PO Box 3065
Laramie, WY 82071-3065
Phone: (307)766-4291 **Fax:** (307)766-4294
Email: nurs.inq@uwyo.edu
Website: http://marshal.uwyo.edu/nursing/home/welcome.htm
Claire Hitchcock, Contact
Fnded: 1886. **Degrees Offered:** BSN, MS.

Occupational Therapy

The following programs (baccalaureate and graduate) for the occupational therapist are accredited by the Accreditation Council for Occupational Therapy Education of the American Occupational Therapy Association. For career information, and for a listing of approved entry level programs (associate and certificate) for occupational therapy assistants, contact the American Occupational Therapy Association at 4720 Montgomery Lane, Bethesda, MD 20824, (301)652-2682, http://www.aota.org/.

Alabama

★ 28292 ★ Alabama State University
College of Health Sciences
Occupational Therapy Program
915 S Jackson St.
Montgomery, AL 36101-0271
Phone: (334)229-4615 **Fax:** (334)229-4964
Email: dtoole@asunet.alasu.edu
Website: http://www.alasu.edu
Donna R. Toole, EdD, Director

★ 28293 ★ Tuskegee University
Department of Allied Health
Occupational Therapy Program
Basil O'Connor Hall
Tuskegee University, AL 36088-1696
Phone: (334)727-8696 **Fax:** (334)727-8259
Email: grayg@tusk.edu
Website: http://svmc107.tusk.edu/tu/nah/occuthera-py.html
Gwendolyn Gray, Director

★ 28294 ★ University of Alabama, Birmingham
School of Health Related Professions
Occupational Therapy Program
102 Bishop Bldg.
1530 3rd Ave. S
Birmingham, AL 35294-2030
Phone: (205)934-3568 **Fax:** (205)975-7787
Email: cpeyton@uab.edu
Website: http://www.uab.edu
Claudia Peyton, Director

★ 28295 ★ University of South Alabama
Springhill Academic Campus
Occupational Therapy Program
1504 Springhill Ave., Rm. 5108
Mobile, AL 36604
Phone: (334)434-3939 **Fax:** (334)434-3934
Email: mscaffa@jaguar1.usouthal.edu
Website: http://www.southal.edu
Marjorie E. Scaffa, PhD, Director

Arizona

★ 28296 ★ Kirksville College
Arizona School of Health Sciences
Occupational Therapy Program
5850 E Still Cir.
Mesa, AZ 85206
Phone: (480)219-6000
Email: melvinj@az.swc.kcom.edu
Website: http://www.ashs.edu
Judith A. Melvin, PhD, Director

★ 28297 ★ Midwestern University, Glendale
Occupational Therapy Program
19555 N 59th Ave.
Glendale, AZ 85308
Phone: (623)572-3630 **Free:** 888-247-9277
Fax: (623)572-3635
Email: cmerch@arizona.midwestern.edu
Website: http://www.midwestern.edu
Christine Merchant, Director

Arkansas

★ 28298 ★ University of Central Arkansas
Occupational Therapy Program
201 Donaghey Ave., HSC Ste. 300
Box 5001
Conway, AR 72035-0001
Phone: (501)450-3192 **Fax:** (501)450-3622
Email: LindaS@mail.uca.edu
Website: http://www.uca.edu/divisions/academic/chas/ot.html
Linda D. Shalik, PhD, Director

California

★ 28299 ★ California State University, Dominguez Hills
Occupational Therapy Program
1000 E Victoria St., LCH B-102
Carson, CA 90747
Phone: (310)243-2726 **Fax:** (310)516-3317
Email: mnoriega@soh.csudh.edu
Website: http://www.csudh.edu
Marilyn Masunaka-Noriega, Director

★ 28300 ★ Dominican University of California
Occupational Therapy Program
50 Acacia Ave.
San Rafael, CA 94901-2298
Phone: (415)458-3731 **Fax:** (415)458-3774
Email: rramsey@dominican.edu
Website: http://www.dominican.edu
Ruth Ramsey, Director

★ 28301 ★ Loma Linda University
School of Allied Health Professions
Occupational Therapy Program
SAHP-Nichol Hall, Rm. A902
Loma Linda, CA 92350-0001
Phone: (909)558-4628 **Fax:** (909)558-0239
Email: liane-hewitt@sahp.llu.edu
Website: http://www.llu.edu
Liane Hewitt, Director

★ 28302 ★ Samuel Merritt College
Occupational Therapy Program
370 Hawthorne Ave.
Oakland, CA 94609-3108
Phone: (510)869-8925 **Fax:** (510)869-6282
Email: gmccorma@samuelmerritt.edu
Website: http://www.samuelmerritt.edu
Guy L. McCormack, PhD, Director

★ 28303 ★ San Jose State University
College of Applied Sciences and Arts
Occupational Therapy Program
1 Washington Sq.
San Jose, CA 95192-0059
Phone: (408)924-3070 **Fax:** (408)924-3088
Email: guburton@email.sjsu.edu
Website: http://www.sjsu.edu
Gordon V. Burton, PhD, Director

★ 28304 ★ University of Southern California
Department of Occupational Science and Occupational Therapy
Occupational Therapy Program
1540 Alcazar, CHP 133
Los Angeles, CA 90089-9003
Phone: (323)442-2850 **Fax:** (323)442-1540
Email: otdept@usc.edu
Website: http://www.usc.edu/OT
Florence A. Clark, PhD, Director

Colorado

★ 28305 ★ Colorado State University
Occupational Therapy Program
228 Occupational Therapy Bldg.
Fort Collins, CO 80523
Phone: (970)491-6253 **Fax:** (970)491-6290
Email: hanzlik@cahs.colostate.edu
Website: http://www.cahs.colostate.edu/ot
Jodie Redditi-Hanzlik, PhD, Director

Connecticut

★ 28306 ★ Quinnipiac University
School of Health Sciences
Occupational Therapy Program
275 Mt. Carmel Ave.
Hamden, CT 06518-0569
Phone: (203)582-8204 **Fax:** (203)281-8706
Email: hartmann@quinnipiac.edu
Website: http://www.quinnipiac.edu
Kimberly D. Hartmann, Director

★ 28307 ★ University of Hartford
College of Education, Nursing and Health Professions
Occupational Therapy Program
Dana Hall, Rm. 232
200 Bloomfield Ave.
West Hartford, CT 06117-1599
Phone: (860)768-4377 **Fax:** (860)768-5244
Email: bsmith@mail.hartford.edu
Website: http://uhavax.hartford.edu/~healthpro
Betsey C. Smith, Director

District of Columbia

★ 28308 ★ Howard University
Division of Allied Health Sciences
Occupational Therapy Program
6th and Bryant Sts. NW
Washington, DC 20059-0001
Phone: (202)806-7614 **Fax:** (202)462-5248
Email: sjackson@fac.howard.edu
Website: http://www.howard.edu
Shirley Jackson, Director

Florida

★ 28309 ★ Barry University
Occupational Therapy Program
11300 NE 2nd Ave.
Miami Shores, FL 33161-6695
Phone: (305)899-3213 **Fax:** (305)899-2958
Email: mmitchell@mail.barry.edu
Website: http://www.barry.edu/snhs/Msprograms/OccupationalTherapy
Douglas Mitchell, Director

★ 28310 ★ Florida Agricultural and Mechanical (A&M) University
Occupational Therapy Program
223 Ware-Rhaney Bldg.
Tallahassee, FL 32307
Phone: (850)561-2185 **Fax:** (850)561-2457
Website: http://www.famu.edu
Jacquelyn Anderson Bolden, PhD, Director

★ 28311 ★ Florida Gulf Coast University
Occupational Therapy Program
10501 FGCU Blvd. S
Fort Myers, FL 33965-6565
Phone: (941)590-7550 **Fax:** (941)590-7474
Email: lcampani@fgcu.edu
Website: http://www.fgcu.edu
Loredana Campanile, Director

★ 28312 ★ Florida International University
Occupational Therapy Program
University Park Campus, CH-101
Miami, FL 33199
Phone: (305)348-2263 **Fax:** (305)348-1240
Email: shaffner@fiu.edu
Website: http://w3.fiu.edu/ot
Pamela Shaffner, Director

★ 28313 ★ Nova Southeastern University College of Allied Health Health Professions Division
Occupational Therapy Program
3200 S University Dr.
Fort Lauderdale, FL 33328
Phone: (954)262-1110 **Fax:** (954)262-2290
Email: reba@hpd.acast.nova.edu
Website: http://www.nova.edu/cwis/centers/hpd/ot/index.html
Carol Niman Reed, EdD, Director

★ 28314 ★ University of Florida
Occupational Therapy Program
PO Box 100164, HSC
Gainesville, FL 32610-0164
Phone: (352)392-2617 **Fax:** (352)846-1042
Email: walker.hrp@mail.health.efl.edu
Website: http://www.hp.ufl.edu/ot
William C. Mann, PhD, Director

★ 28315 ★ University of St. Augustine for Health Sciences
Institute of Occupational Therapy
1 University Blvd.
Saint Augustine, FL 32086
Phone: (904)826-0084 **Free:** 800-241-1027
Fax: (904)827-0069
Email: ksclayto@usa.edu
Website: http://www.usa.edu
Karen S. Clayton, PhD, Director

Georgia

★ 28316 ★ Brenau University
Occupational Therapy Program
1 Centennial Cir.
Gainesville, GA 30501
Phone: (770)534-6139 **Fax:** (770)534-6186
Email: bschell@lib.brenau.edu
Website: http://www.brenau.edu/OT
Barbara A. Schell, PhD, Director

★ 28317 ★ Medical College of Georgia School of Allied Health Sciences
Occupational Therapy Program
EF 102
1120 15th St.
Augusta, GA 30912-0700
Phone: (706)721-2725 **Fax:** (706)721-9718
Email: kbradley@mail.mcg.edu
Website: http://www.mcg.edu/sah/ot/index.html
Kathy P. Bradley, EdD, Director

★ 28318 ★ Medical College of Georgia/ Columbus State University
Occupational Therapy Program
Illges Hall, Rm. 107
4225 University Ave.
Columbus, GA 31907
Phone: (706)568-2242 **Fax:** (706)568-2073
Email: jjedlick@mail.mcg.edu
Website: http://www.mcg.edu/sah/ot/index.html
Kathy Bradley, EdD, Director

Idaho

★ 28319 ★ Idaho State University
Occupational Therapy Program
Campus Box 8045
Pocatello, ID 83209-8045
Phone: (208)282-4095
Website: http://www.isu.edu/departments/dpot

Illinois

★ 28320 ★ Chicago State University College of Health Sciences
Occupational Therapy Program
9501 S King Dr.
Chicago, IL 60628-1598
Phone: (773)995-2366 **Fax:** (773)995-2839
Email: bahgkks@csu.edu
Website: http://www.csu.edu
Kuzhilethu K. Kshepakaran, Director

★ 28321 ★ Governors State University College of Health Professions
Occupational Therapy Program
University Park, IL 60466-0975
Phone: (708)534-7293 **Fax:** (708)534-1647
Email: b-cada@govst.edu
Website: http://www.govst.edu
Elizabeth Cada, Director

★ 28322 ★ Midwestern University College of Health Sciences
Occupational Therapy Program
555 31st St.
Downers Grove, IL 60515
Phone: (630)515-6188 **Fax:** (630)515-7224
Email: tlaster@midwestern.edu
Website: http://www.midwestern.edu
Thomas Evans Laster, Director

★ 28323 ★ Rush University Rush-Presbyterian-St. Luke's Medical Center
Occupational Therapy Program
600 S Paulina, Ste. 1009-B
Chicago, IL 60612-3833
Phone: (312)942-5099 **Fax:** (312)942-6989
Email: jbachelder@rushu.rush.edu
Website: http://www.rushu.rush.edu
Judy Bachelder, PhD, Director

★ 28324 ★ University of Illinois, Chicago College of Health and Human Development Sciences
Occupational Therapy Program
1919 W Taylor St., M/C 811
Chicago, IL 60612
Phone: (312)996-6901 **Fax:** (312)413-0256
Email: Kielhfnr@uic.edu
Website: http://www.uic.edu/ahp/OT
Gary Kielhofner, DrPH, Director

Indiana

★ 28325 ★ Indiana University School of Allied Health Sciences
Occupational Therapy Program
Coleman Hall 316
1140 W Michigan St.
Indianapolis, IN 46202-5119
Phone: (317)274-8006 **Fax:** (317)274-2150
Email: chamant@iupui.edu
Website: http://www.iupui.edu/it/iusahs
Celestine Hamant, Director

★ 28326 ★ University of Indianapolis School of Occupational Therapy
1400 E Hanna Ave.
Indianapolis, IN 46227-3697
Phone: (317)788-3432 **Fax:** (317)788-3542
Email: moyers@uindy.edu
Website: http://www.ot.uindy.edu
Penelope A. Moyers, EdD, Director

★ 28327 ★ University of Southern Indiana
Occupational Therapy Program
8600 University Blvd.
Evansville, IN 47712-3534
Phone: (812)465-1179 **Fax:** (812)465-7092
Email: otinfo@usi.edu
Website: http://health.usi.edu/acadprog/ot/index.htm
Aimee J. Luebben, EdD, Director

Iowa

★ 28328 ★ Saint Ambrose University
Occupational Therapy Program
518 W Locust
Davenport, IA 52803-2898
Phone: (563)333-6277 **Fax:** (563)333-6410
Email: pwenthe@saunix.sau.edu
Website: http://www.sau.edu
Phyllis Wenthe, Director

Kansas

★ 28329 ★ Newman University
Occupational Therapy Program
3100 McCormick Ave.
Wichita, KS 67213-2097
Phone: (316)942-4291 **Fax:** (316)942-4483
Email: sowersj@newmanu.edu
Website: http://www.newmanu.edu/ot
Jeanne Sowers, Director

★ 28330 ★ University of Kansas Medical Center
School of Allied Health
Occupational Therapy Program
3033 Robinson
3901 Rainbow Blvd.
Kansas City, KS 66160-7602
Phone: (913)588-7174 **Fax:** (913)588-4568
Email: wdunn@kumc.edu
Website: http://www.kumc.edu/SAH/OTEd/index.html
Winnie Dunn, PhD, Director

Kentucky

★ 28331 ★ Eastern Kentucky University
Occupational Therapy Program
Dizney 103
Richmond, KY 40475-3135
Phone: (859)622-3300 **Fax:** (859)622-1605
Email: otsbenne@acs.eku.edu
Website: http://www.health.eku.edu
Onda Bennett, PhD, Director

★ 28332 ★ Spalding University
Occupational Therapy Program
851 S 4th St.
Louisville, KY 40203-2188
Phone: (502)585-7125 **Fax:** (502)588-7175
Email: rstrickland@spalding.edu
Website: http://www.spalding.edu
L. Randy Strickland, EdD, Director

Louisiana

★ 28333 ★ Louisiana State University Health Sciences Center, New Orleans
School of Allied Health Professions
Occupational Therapy Program
1900 Gravier St.
New Orleans, LA 70112-2223
Phone: (504)568-4302 **Fax:** (504)568-4306
Email: taylor@lsuhsc.edu
Website: http://www.lsumc.edu
Eve Taylor, PhD, Director

★ 28334 ★ Louisiana State University Health Sciences Center, Shreveport
School of Allied Health Professions
Occupational Therapy Program
1501 Kings Hwy.
PO Box 33932
Shreveport, LA 71130-3932
Phone: (318)675-6827 **Fax:** (318)675-6937
Email: kseidn@lsumc.edu
Website: http://www.lsumc.edu
Kristin Seidner, Director

★ 28335 ★ University of Louisiana, Monroe
College of Allied Health and Rehabilitation Professions
Occupational Therapy Program
Monroe, LA 71209-0430
Phone: (318)342-1610 **Fax:** (318)342-5584
Email: aldavis@alpha.ulm.edu
Website: http://www.ulm.edu/ot/OT.html
Kathryn H. Davis, Director

Maine

★ 28336 ★ University of New England
College of Arts and Sciences
Occupational Therapy Program
Biddeford, ME 04005-9599
Phone: (207)283-0171 **Fax:** (207)282-6379
Email: nmacrae@mailbox.une.edu
Website: http://www.une.edu
Nancy MacRae, Director

★ 28337 ★ University of Southern Maine
Lewiston-Auburn College
Occupational Therapy Program
51 Westminster St.
Lewiston, ME 04240-3534
Phone: (207)753-6523 **Fax:** (207)753-6555
Email: rblack@usm.maine.edu
Website: http://www.usm.maine.edu/~lac/ot
Roxie M. Black, Director

Maryland

★ 28338 ★ Towson University
Department of Occupational Therapy and Occupational Science
Occupational Therapy Program
8000 York Rd.
Towson, MD 21252-0001
Phone: (410)704-4170
Email: mreitz@towson.edu
Website: http://www.towson.edu/OT
S. Maggie Reitz, PhD, Director

Massachusetts

★ 28339 ★ American International College
Occupational Therapy Program
1000 State St.
Box 46
Springfield, MA 01109-3189
Phone: (413)205-3321
Email: dowroyer@acad.aic.edu
Website: http://www.aic.edu
Cathy A. Dow-Royer, Director

★ 28340 ★ Bay Path College
Occupational Therapy Program
588 Longmeadow St.
Longmeadow, MA 01106
Phone: (413)565-1331 **Fax:** (413)565-1102
Email: ksladyk@baypath.edu
Website: http://www.baypath.edu
Karen Sladyk, PhD, Director

★ 28341 ★ Boston University
Sargent College of Health and Rehabilitation Sciences
Occupational Therapy Program
635 Commonwealth Ave.
Boston, MA 02215
Phone: (617)353-2000 **Fax:** (617)353-2926
Email: wjcoster@bu.edu
Website: http://www.bu.edu/sargent/ot
Wendy Coster, PhD, Director

★ 28342 ★ Springfield College
Occupational Therapy Program
263 Alden St.
Springfield, MA 01109-3797
Phone: (413)748-3762 **Fax:** (413)748-3796
Email: kpost@spfldcol.edu
Website: http://www.spfldcol.edu/ot
Katherine M. Post, Director

★ 28343 ★ Tufts University
Boston School of Occupational Therapy
Occupational Therapy Program
26 Winthrop St.
Medford, MA 02155-7084
Phone: (617)627-3720 **Fax:** (617)627-3722
Email: sschwartz@emerald.tufts.edu
Website: http://www.tufts.edu
Sharan Schwartzberg, EdD, Director

★ 28344 ★ Worcester State College
Occupational Therapy Program
486 Chandler St.
Worcester, MA 01602-2597
Phone: (508)929-8624 **Fax:** (508)929-8178
Email: djoss@worcester.edu
Website: http://www.worc.mass.edu
Mark S. Rosenfeld, PhD, Director

Michigan

★ 28345 ★ Baker College of Flint
Occupational Therapy Program
G-1050 W Bristol Rd.
Flint, MI 48507-5508
Phone: (810)766-4100 **Fax:** (810)766-4049
Email: hagen_d@flint.baker.edu
Website: http://www.baker.edu
Darrell Hagen, Director

★ 28346 ★ Eastern Michigan University
Department of Associated Health Professions
Occupational Therapy Program
322 Everett Marshall Hall
Ypsilanti, MI 48197-2239
Phone: (734)487-4094 **Fax:** (734)487-4095
Website: http://www.emich.edu
Betsy Francis, PhD, Director

★ 28347 ★ Grand Valley State University
Occupational Therapy Program
322 Henry Hall
1 Campus Dr.
Allendale, MI 49401-9403
Phone: (616)895-3356 **Fax:** (616)895-3350
Email: grapczyc@gvsu.edu
Website: http://www4.gvsu.edu/otp
Cynthia Grapczynski, EdD, Director

★ 28348 ★ Saginaw Valley State University
Occupational Therapy Program
Ryder Center W, Rm. 105
7400 Bay Rd.
University Center, MI 48710-0001
Phone: (989)791-7356 **Fax:** (989)790-0545
Website: http://www.svsu.edu
Alfred G. Bracciano, EdD, Director

★ 28349 ★ Wayne State University
Eugene Applebaum College of Pharmacy and Health Sciences
Occupational Therapy Program
Detroit, MI 48202-3489
Phone: (313)577-1435 **Fax:** (313)577-5822
Website: http://wizard.pharm.wayne.edu/OT
Nancy J. Powell, PhD, Director

★ 28350 ★ Western Michigan University
Occupational Therapy Program
EWB Bldg.
1903 W Michigan Ave.
Kalamazoo, MI 49008-5051
Phone: (616)387-7260 **Fax:** (616)387-7262
Email: petersonc@wmich.edu
Website: http://www.wmich.edu
Cindee Peterson, PhD, Director

Minnesota

★ 28351 ★ College of Saint Catherine
Occupational Therapy Program
2004 Randolph Ave.
Mail No. 4092
Saint Paul, MN 55105-1794
Phone: (651)690-6606 **Fax:** (651)690-8804
Email: jdbhaugen@stkate.edu
Website: http://www.stkate.edu/ot
Julie D. Bass Haugen, PhD, Director

★ 28352 ★ College of Saint Scholastica
Occupational Therapy Program
1200 Kenwood Ave.
Duluth, MN 55811
Phone: (218)723-6099 **Fax:** (218)723-6472
Email: rberkela@css.edu

Website: http://www.css.edu
Ron Berkeland, Director

★ 28353 ★ University of Minnesota
Occupational Therapy Program
MMC 388
420 Delaware St. SE
Minneapolis, MN 55455-0392
Phone: (612)626-5887 **Fax:** (612)625-7192
Email: otprog@tc.umn.edu
Website: http://www.ot.umn.edu
Judith Reisman, PhD, Director

Mississippi

★ 28354 ★ University of Mississippi Medical Center
School of Related Health Professions
Occupational Therapy Program
2500 N State St.
Jackson, MS 39216-4505
Phone: (601)984-6350 **Fax:** (601)984-6344
Email: bgroat@shrp.umsmed.edu
Website: http://shrp.umc.edu
Bette A. Groat, Director

Missouri

★ 28355 ★ Maryville University
Occupational Therapy Program
13550 Conway Rd.
Saint Louis, MO 63141
Phone: (314)529-9515 **Fax:** (314)529-9085
Email: lhunt@maryville.edu
Website: http://www.maryville.edu/sohp/programs/ot.htm
Linda Hunt, Director

★ 28356 ★ Rockhurst University
College of Arts and Sciences
Occupational Therapy Program
1100 Rockhurst Rd.
Kansas City, MO 64110-2561
Phone: (816)501-4635 **Fax:** (816)501-4643
Email: jane.rues@rockhurst.edu
Website: http://www.rockhurst.edu/ot
Jane P. Rues, EdD, Director

★ 28357 ★ Saint Louis University (SLU)
Edward and Margaret Doisey School of Allied Health Professions
Occupational Therapy Program
3437 Caroline St.
Saint Louis, MO 63104
Phone: (314)577-8514 **Fax:** (314)268-5414
Email: behrsk@slu.edu
Website: http://www.slu.edu/colleges/AH/OT
Shirley K. Behr, PhD, Director

★ 28358 ★ University of Missouri, Columbia
School of Health Related Professions
Occupational Therapy Program
407 Lewis Hall
Columbia, MO 65211
Phone: (573)882-3988 **Fax:** (573)884-2610
Email: baldwin@healthmissouri.edu
Website: http://www.missouri.edu
Diana J. Baldwin, Director

★ 28359 ★ Washington University
School of Medicine
Occupational Therapy Program
4444 Forest Park Ave.
Campus Box 8505
Saint Louis, MO 63108
Phone: (314)286-1600 **Fax:** (314)286-1601
Email: cbaum@ot-link.wustl.edu
Website: http://www.ot.wustl.edu
M. Carolyn Baum, PhD, Director

Nebraska

★ 28360 ★ College of Saint Mary
Occupational Therapy Program
1901 S 72nd St.
Omaha, NE 68124-2377
Phone: (402)399-2400 **Free:** 800-926-5534
Fax: (402)399-2647
Email: pgromak@csm.edu
Website: http://www.csm.edu
Patricia A. Gromak, Director

★ 28361 ★ Creighton University
School of Pharmacy and Allied Health
Occupational Therapy Program
2500 California Plaza
Omaha, NE 68178-0259
Phone: (402)280-5957 **Free:** 800-325-2830
Fax: (402)280-5692
Email: rpadilla@creighton.edu
Website: http://ot.creighton.edu
Rene Padilla, Director

New Hampshire

★ 28362 ★ University of New Hampshire
School of Health and Human Services
Occupational Therapy Program
Hewitt Hall
4 Library Way
Durham, NH 03824-3563
Phone: (603)862-2167 **Fax:** (603)862-0778
Email: acseidel@christa.unh.edu
Website: http://www.unh.edu
Alice Seidel, EdD, Director

New Jersey

★ 28363 ★ Kean University
School of Natural Applied and Health Sciences
Occupational Therapy Program
Townsend T209
PO Box 411
Union, NJ 07083-9982
Phone: (908)527-2590 **Fax:** (908)527-3222
Email: ot@turbo.kean.edu
Website: http://www.kean.edu/~ot
Karen Stern, EdD, Director

★ 28364 ★ Richard Stockton College of New Jersey
Professional Studies Division
Occupational Therapy Program
Jim Leeds Rd.
PO Box 195
Pomona, NJ 08240-0195
Phone: (609)652-4687
Website: http://www.stockton.edu

★ 28365 ★ Seton Hall University
Occupational Therapy Program
McQuaid Hall
400 S Orange Ave.
South Orange, NJ 07079-2689
Phone: (973)761-7145
Email: breinees@shu.edu
Website: http://gradmeded.shu.edu/graduateprograms/msot.html
Estelle B. Breines, PhD, Director

New Mexico

★ 28366 ★ University of New Mexico
School of Medicine
Occupational Therapy Program
Health Science and Services Bldg., Rm. 215
Albuquerque, NM 87131-5641
Phone: (505)272-1753 **Fax:** (505)272-8079
Email: tkcrowe@salud.unm.edu
Website: http://hsc.unm.edu/ot
Terry K. Crowe, PhD, Director

New York

★ 28367 ★ City University of New York (CUNY)
York College
Occupational Therapy Program
94-20 Guy R. Brewer Blvd.
Jamaica, NY 11451-9902
Phone: (718)262-2720 **Fax:** (718)262-2767
Email: kaplan@york.cuny.edu
Website: http://www.york.cuny.edu/~healthsci/index.html
Lillian Kaplan, Director

★ 28368 ★ Columbia University
Occupational Therapy Program
Neurological Institute, 8th Fl.
710 W 168th St.
New York, NY 10032
Phone: (212)305-3781 **Fax:** (212)305-4569
Email: jf6@columbia.edu
Website: http://columbiaOT.org
Janet Falk-Kessler, EdD, Director

★ 28369 ★ Dominican College
Occupational Therapy Program
470 Western Hwy.
Orangeburg, NY 10962-1299
Phone: (845)359-7800 **Fax:** (845)359-2313
Website: http://www.dc.edu
Sandra F. Countee, PhD, Director

★ 28370 ★ D'Youville College
Occupational Therapy Program
320 Porter Ave.
Buffalo, NY 14201-1084
Phone: (716)881-7600 **Fax:** (716)881-8137
Email: gingherm@dyc.edu
Website: http://www.dyc.edu
Merlene C. Gingher, EdD, Director

★ 28371 ★ Ithaca College
Occupational Therapy Program
200 Smiddy Hall
Ithaca, NY 14850
Phone: (607)274-1975 **Fax:** (607)274-3055
Email: catheyg@ithaca.edu
Website: http://www.ithaca.edu/hshp/ot
Catherine Y. Gordon, EdD, Director

★ 28372 ★ Keuka College
Occupational Therapy Program
Keuka Park, NY 14478-0098
Phone: (315)279-5255
Email: ptalty@mail.keuka.edu
Website: http://www.keuka.edu
Peter M. Talty, Director

★ 28373 ★ Long Island University, Brooklyn
Occupational Therapy Program
1 University Plaza
Brooklyn, NY 11201
Phone: (718)488-1011
Website: http://www.liu.edu

★ 28374 ★ Mercy College
Occupational Therapy Program
555 Broadway
Dobbs Ferry, NY 10522-1189
Phone: (914)674-9331 **Fax:** (914)674-9457
Email: otprogram@mercy.edu
Website: http://grad.mercy.edu/occupationaltherapy
Joan Toglia, Director

★ 28375 ★ New York Institute of Technology
Occupational Therapy Program
PO Box 8000
Old Westbury, NY 11568-8000
Phone: (516)686-3738 **Fax:** (516)686-3795
Email: hplotnick@iris.nyit.edu
Website: http://www.nyit.edu
Hermine Plotnick, Director

★ 28376 ★ New York University
School of Education
Occupational Therapy Program
35 W 4th St., 11th Fl.
New York, NY 10012-1172
Phone: (212)998-5825 **Fax:** (212)995-4044
Email: labovitz@is2.nyu.edu
Website: http://www.nyu.edu/education/ot
Jim Hinojosa, PhD, Director

★ 28377 ★ Sage Colleges
Occupational Therapy Program
45 Ferry St.
Troy, NY 12180-4115
Phone: (518)244-2217 **Free:** 800-999-3772
Fax: (518)244-4524
Email: frankm@sage.edu
Website: http://www.sage.edu
Martha M. Frank, Director

★ 28378 ★ State University of New York, Brooklyn (SUNY)
Health Science Center
College of Health Related Professions
Occupational Therapy Program
450 Clarkson Ave., Box 81
Brooklyn, NY 11203-2098
Phone: (718)270-7730 **Fax:** (718)270-7464
Email: jsabari@netmail.hscbklyn.edu
Website: http://www.downstate.edu/chrp.ot
Joyce Sabari, PhD, Director

★ 28379 ★ State University of New York, Buffalo
Occupational Therapy Program
515 Stockton Kimball Tower
3435 Main St.
Buffalo, NY 14214-3079
Phone: (716)829-3141 **Fax:** (716)829-3217
Email: nochajsk@buffalo.edu
Website: http://wings.buffalo.edu/academic/department/hrp/ot
Susan M. Nochajski, PhD, Director

★ 28380 ★ State University of New York, Stony Brook
School of Health Technology and Management
Division of Rehabilitation Sciences
Occupational Therapy Program
L2-031
Stony Brook, NY 11794-8201
Phone: (631)444-8160 **Fax:** (631)444-7621
Email: dcosta@epo.hsc.sunysb.edu
Website: http://www.sunysb.edu
Donna M. Costa, Director

★ 28381 ★ Syracuse University
Utica College
Division of Health and Human Studies
Occupational Therapy Program
1600 Burrstone Rd.
Utica, NY 13502-4892
Phone: (315)792-3006 **Fax:** (315)792-3248
Email: pcarey@utica.ucsu.edu
Website: http://www.utica.edu
Paula D. Carey, Director

★ 28382 ★ Touro College, Bay Shore
Occupational Therapy Program
1700 Union Blvd.
Bay Shore, NY 11706
Phone: (631)665-1600 **Fax:** (631)665-6084
Email: tonyh@touro.edu
Website: http://www.touro.edu/shs
Anthony Hollander, PhD, Director

★ 28383 ★ Touro College, Manhattan
School of Health Sciences
Occupational Therapy Program
27-33 W 23rd St.
New York, NY 10010-4202
Phone: (212)463-0400
Email: tonyh@touro.edu
Website: http://www.touro.edu/shs
Anthony C. Hollander, PhD, Director

North Carolina

★ 28384 ★ East Carolina University
School of Allied Health Sciences
Occupational Therapy Program
Greenville, NC 27858-4353
Phone: (252)328-4441 **Fax:** (252)328-4470
Email: dickersona@mail.ecu.edu
Website: http://www.ecu.edu/ot
Anne Dickerson, PhD, Director

★ 28385 ★ Lenoir-Rhyne College
Occupational Therapy Program
Box 7547
Hickory, NC 28603
Phone: (828)328-7300 **Fax:** (828)328-7364
Email: sssahler@lrc.edu
Website: http://www.lrc.edu/departments/ot/oth_department.html
Susan Stallings-Sahler, PhD, Director

★ 28386 ★ University of North Carolina, Chapel Hill
Division of Occupational Science
Occupational Therapy Program
Medical School, Wing E
Campus Box 7120
Chapel Hill, NC 27599-7120
Phone: (919)966-2451 **Fax:** (919)966-9007
Website: http://www.alliedhealth.unc.edu/ocsci
Cathy Nielson, Director

★ 28387 ★ Winston-Salem State University
Occupational Therapy Program
601 Martin Luther King, Jr. Dr.
Campus Box 19368
Winston-Salem, NC 27110
Phone: (336)750-3170 **Fax:** (336)750-3173
Email: baldwinlc@wssu.edu
Website: http://www.wssu.edu
Lynda C. Baldwin, Director

North Dakota

★ 28388 ★ University of Mary
Occupational Therapy Program
7500 University Dr.
Bismarck, ND 58504-9652
Phone: (701)255-7500 **Free:** 800-408-6279
Fax: (701)255-7687
Email: ikensl@umary.edu
Website: http://www.umary.edu
Stacie L. Iken, Director

★ 28389 ★ University of North Dakota
Occupational Therapy Program
Box 7126, University Station
Grand Forks, ND 58202-7126
Phone: (701)777-2209 **Fax:** (701)777-2212
Email: smcintyr@mail.med.und.nodak.edu
Website: http://www.med.und.nodak.edu/depts/ot/home.htm
Sue McIntyre, Director

Ohio

★ 28390 ★ Cleveland State University
Occupational Therapy Program
Health Sciences 103
1983 E 24th St.
Cleveland, OH 44115-2440
Phone: (216)687-3567 **Fax:** (216)687-9316
Email: j.bazyk@csuohio.edu
Website: http://www.csuohio.edu/healthsci/hs.htm
John J. Bazyk, Director

★ 28391 ★ Medical College of Ohio, Toledo
School of Allied Health
Occupational Therapy Program
3015 Arlington Ave.
Toledo, OH 43614-5803
Phone: (419)383-4160 **Fax:** (419)383-5880
Email: jthomas@mco.edu
Website: http://www.mco.edu
Julie J. Thomas, PhD, Director

★ 28392 ★ Ohio State University
School of Allied Medical Professions
Occupational Therapy Program
1583 Perry St., 406 SAMP
Columbus, OH 43210-1234
Phone: (614)292-1706 **Fax:** (614)292-0210
Website: http://www.amp.ohio-state.edu
H. Kay Grant, PhD, Director

★ 28393 ★ Shawnee State University
Occupational Therapy Program
940 2nd St.
Portsmouth, OH 45662-4303
Phone: (740)351-3209
Email: swheeler@shawnee.edu
Website: http://www.shawnee.edu
Steve D. Wheeler, Director

★ 28394 ★ University of Findlay
Occupational Therapy Program
1000 N Main St.
Findlay, OH 45840-3695
Phone: (419)424-5314 **Free:** 800-472-9502
Fax: (419)424-6977
Email: owens@mail.findlay.edu
Website: http://www.findlay.edu
Peggy Owens, Director

★ 28395 ★ Xavier University
Occupational Therapy Program
3800 Victory Pkwy.
Cincinnati, OH 45207-7341
Phone: (513)745-3150 **Fax:** (513)745-3261
Email: jpecin@aol.com

Website: http://www.xu.edu
Joanne Phillips Estes, Director

Oklahoma

★ 28396 ★ University of Oklahoma Schusterman Health Sciences Center
Occupational Therapy Program
4502 E 41st St.
Tulsa, OK 74135
Phone: (918)838-4660
Website: http://w3.uokhsc.edu/rehab

★ 28397 ★ University of Oklahoma Health Sciences Center, Oklahoma City
College of Allied Health
Occupational Therapy Program
801 NE 13th St.
Oklahoma City, OK 73190-1090
Phone: (405)271-2411 **Fax:** (405)271-2432
Email: toby-hamilton@uokhsc.edu
Website: http://w3.uokhsc.edu/rehab
Toby B. Hamilton, Director

Oregon

★ 28398 ★ Pacific University
School of Occupational Therapy
2043 College Way
Forest Grove, OR 97116-1797
Phone: (503)359-2789 **Free:** 800-933-9308
Fax: (503)359-2980
Email: mcewenm@pacificu.edu
Website: http://www.ot.pacificu.edu
Molly McEwen, Director

Pennsylvania

★ 28399 ★ Alvernia College
Occupational Therapy Program
400 St. Bernardine St.
Reading, PA 19607-1799
Phone: (610)796-8339 **Fax:** (610)796-8422
Email: pennyne@alvernia.edu
Website: http://www.alvernia.edu
Neil Penny, Director

★ 28400 ★ Chatham College
Occupational Therapy Program
Woodland Rd.
Pittsburgh, PA 15233
Phone: (412)365-1290 **Fax:** (412)365-1213
Email: henry@chatham.edu
Website: http://www.chatham.edu
Eileen Henry, EdD, Director

★ 28401 ★ College Misericordia
Division of Health Sciences
Occupational Therapy Program
301 Lake St.
Dallas, PA 18612-1098
Phone: (866)262-6363
Email: jciprian@miseri.edu
Website: http://www.misericordia.edu
Joseph A. Cipriani Jr., EdD, Director

★ 28402 ★ Duquesne University
John G. Rangos, Sr. School of Health Sciences
Occupational Therapy Program
Health Sciences Bldg., Rm. 234
Pittsburgh, PA 15282-0020
Phone: (412)396-5945 **Fax:** (412)396-4343
Email: crist@duq.edu
Website: http://www.healthsciences.duq.edu/ot/oth-ome.html
Patricia Crist, PhD, Director

★ 28403 ★ Elizabethtown College
Occupational Therapy Program
1 Alpha Dr.
Elizabethtown, PA 17022-2298
Phone: (717)361-1174 **Fax:** (717)361-1176
Email: gillardm@etown.edu
Website: http://www.etown.edu
Marian Gillard, PhD, Director

★ 28404 ★ Gannon University
Occupational Therapy Program
109 University Sq.
Erie, PA 16541-0001
Phone: (814)871-7663 **Fax:** (814)871-5662
Email: dijoseph@gannon.edu
Website: http://www.gannon.edu
Linda M. DiJoseph, Director

★ 28405 ★ Mount Aloysius College
Occupational Therapy Program
7373 Admiral Peary Hwy.
Cresson, PA 16630
Phone: (814)886-6522 **Fax:** (814)886-4906
Email: tclark@mtaloy.edu
Website: http://www.mtaloy.edu
Threese A. Clark, Director

★ 28406 ★ Pennsylvania State University, Mont Alto
Occupational Therapy Program
1 Campus Dr.
Mont Alto, PA 17237-9703
Phone: (717)749-6130 **Fax:** (717)749-6166
Email: jvd102@psu.edu
Website: http://www.ma.psu.edu/ot.htm
Janet DeLany, D Ed, Director

★ 28407 ★ Philadelphia University
Occupational Therapy Program
School House Ln. and Henry Ave.
Philadelphia, PA 19144-5497
Phone: (215)951-2943
Email: admissions@philacol.edu
Website: http://www.philau.edu

★ 28408 ★ Saint Francis University
Occupational Therapy Program
PO Box 600
Loretto, PA 15940-0600
Phone: (814)472-3899
Website: http://www.saintfrancisuniversity.edu

★ 28409 ★ Temple University
College of Allied Health Professions
Occupational Therapy Program
3307 N Broad St.
Philadelphia, PA 19140
Phone: (215)707-4813 **Fax:** (215)707-7656
Email: mkinneal@astro.temple.edu
Website: http://www.temple.edu/OT
Moya Kinnealey, PhD, Director

★ 28410 ★ Thomas Jefferson University
College of Health Professions
Occupational Therapy Program
Edison Bldg., Rm. 810
130 S 9th St.
Philadelphia, PA 19107-5233
Phone: (215)503-8010 **Fax:** (215)503-3499
Email: janice.burke@mail.tju.edu
Website: http://jeffline.tju.edu/cwis/chp/index2.html
Janice P. Burke, PhD, Director

★ 28411 ★ University of Pittsburgh
School of Health and Rehabilitation Sciences
Occupational Therapy Program
5012 Forbes Tower
Pittsburgh, PA 15260
Phone: (412)383-6620
Email: jcr@pitt.edu
Website: http://www.shrs.pitt.edu/ot/index.html
Joan Rogers, PhD, Director

★ 28412 ★ University of the Sciences in Philadelphia
Occupational Therapy Program
600 S 43rd St.
Box 24
Philadelphia, PA 19104-4495
Phone: (215)596-8810 **Fax:** (215)596-8690
Email: r.ideish@usip.edu
Website: http://www.usip.edu
Paula Kramer, PhD, Director

★ 28413 ★ University of Scranton
Occupational Therapy Program
Scranton, PA 18510-4501
Phone: (570)941-7540 **Fax:** (570)941-4380
Email: kasarjl@uofs.edu
Website: http://www.scranton.edu
Jack Kasar, PhD, Director

Puerto Rico

★ 28414 ★ University of Puerto Rico
Occupational Therapy Program
Medical Sciences Campus - CHRP
PO Box 365067
San Juan, PR 00936-5067
Phone: (787)758-2525 **Fax:** (787)282-8174
Website: http://www.upr.clu.edu/englishv2/home.htm
Migdalia Morales, Director

South Carolina

★ 28415 ★ Medical University of South Carolina
College of Health Professions
Occupational Therapy Program
171 Ashley Ave., Rm. 123-CHP
Charleston, SC 29425-2701
Phone: (843)792-2961
Email: trickeyb@musc.edu
Website: http://www.musc.edu/chp-rehab/ot/oth-ome.htm
Becki A. Trickey, PhD, Director

South Dakota

★ 28416 ★ University of South Dakota
Occupational Therapy Program
414 E Clark St.
Vermillion, SD 57069-2390
Phone: (605)677-5600 **Fax:** (605)677-6581
Website: http://www.usd.edu/usdot
Barbara Brockevelt, Director

Tennessee

★ 28417 ★ Belmont University
School of Occupational Therapy
1900 Belmont Blvd.
Nashville, TN 37212-3757
Phone: (615)460-6700 **Fax:** (615)460-6475
Email: mcphees@mail.belmont.edu
Website: http://www.belmont.edu/ot
Scott D. McPhee, DrPH, Director

★ 28418 ★ Milligan College
Occupational Therapy Program
PO Box 130
Milligan College, TN 37682
Phone: (423)975-8010 **Fax:** (423)975-8019
Email: dwpoff@milligan.edu
Website: http://www.milligan.edu
Daniel W. Poff, PhD, Director

★ 28419 ★ Tennessee State University
School of Allied Health Professions
Occupational Therapy Program
3500 John A. Merritt Blvd.
Nashville, TN 37209-1561
Phone: (615)963-5891 **Fax:** (615)963-5926
Email: snyderl@harpo.tnstate.edu
Website: http://duke.tnstate.edu/ot
Larry Snyder, Director

★ 28420 ★ University of Tennessee, Chattanooga
Occupational Therapy Program
1 Provident W Bldg.
Chattanooga, TN 37402
Phone: (423)785-2357
Website: http://www.utc.edu/~chhs.rehab.htm

★ 28421 ★ University of Tennessee, Memphis
Health Science Center
Occupational Therapy Program
822 Beale St., Rm. 350
Memphis, TN 38163
Phone: (901)448-8393 **Fax:** (901)448-7545
Email: anolen@utmem.edu
Website: http://www.utmem.edu/occ_therapy/home.html
Ann H. Nolen, PsyD, Director

Texas

★ 28422 ★ Texas Tech University Health Sciences Center, Amarillo
School of Allied Health Professions
Occupational Therapy Program
1300 Wallace Blvd.
Amarillo, TX 79106
Phone: (806)743-3220
Website: http://www.ttuhsc.edu

★ 28423 ★ Texas Tech University Health Sciences Center, Lubbock
School of Allied Health
Occupational Therapy Program
STOP 6220, Rm. 2C212
3601 4th St.
Lubbock, TX 79430
Phone: (806)743-3220 **Fax:** (806)743-2515
Email: alhsb@ttuhsc.edu
Website: http://www.ttuhsc.edu
Susan C. Burwash, Director

★ 28424 ★ Texas Tech University Health Sciences Center, Odessa
School of Allied Health
Occupational Therapy Program
800 W 4th St.
Odessa, TX 79763
Phone: (906)743-3220
Website: http://www.ttuhsc.edu

★ 28425 ★ Texas Woman's University, Dallas
Occupational Therapy Program
Dallas, TX
Phone: (940)898-2801
Email: ot@twu.edu
Website: http://www.twu.edu/ot

★ 28426 ★ Texas Woman's University, Denton
School of Occupational Therapy
Box 425648, TWU Station
Denton, TX 76204-5648
Phone: (940)898-2801 **Fax:** (940)898-2806
Email: ot@twu.edu
Website: http://www.twu.edu/ot
Janette Schkade, PhD, Director

★ 28427 ★ Texas Woman's University, Houston
Occupational Therapy Program
Houston, TX
Phone: (940)898-2801
Email: ot@twu.edu
Website: http://www.twu.edu/ot

★ 28428 ★ University of Texas, El Paso
College of Health Professions
Occupational Therapy Program
1101 N Campbell St.
El Paso, TX 79902
Phone: (915)747-7270
Website: http://www.utep.edu

★ 28429 ★ University of Texas Health Science Center, San Antonio
Occupational Therapy Program
7703 Floyd Curl Dr.
Mail Code 6245
San Antonio, TX 78229-3900
Phone: (210)567-8880 **Fax:** (210)567-8893
Email: haradon@uthscsa.edu
Website: http://www.uthscsa.edu
Gale L. Haradon, PhD, Director

★ 28430 ★ University of Texas Medical Branch, Galveston
School of Allied Health Sciences
Occupational Therapy Program
301 University Blvd.
Galveston, TX 77555-1028
Phone: (409)772-3060 **Fax:** (409)747-1615
Email: laprimea@utmb.edu
Website: http://www.sahs.utmb.edu/programs/ot
Loree Primeau, PhD, Director

★ 28431 ★ University of Texas, Pan-American
Occupational Therapy Program
1201 W University Dr.
Edinburg, TX 78539-2999
Phone: (956)381-2475 **Fax:** (956)381-2476
Email: jebowen@panam.edu
Website: http://www.panam.edu
Judith E. Bowen, Director

Utah

★ 28432 ★ University of Utah
Occupational Therapy Program
520 Wakara Way
Salt Lake City, UT 84108-1290
Phone: (801)585-9135
Website: http://www.health.utah.edu/occh

Virginia

★ 28433 ★ College of Health Sciences
Community Hospital of Roanoke Valley
Occupational Therapy Program
920 S Jefferson St.
Roanoke, VA 24016
Phone: (540)985-8594 **Fax:** (540)985-9773
Website: http://www.chs.edu
David A. Hayes, Director

★ 28434 ★ James Madison University
College of Integrated Science and Technology
Department of Health Sciences
Occupational Therapy Program
MSC 4301
Harrisonburg, VA 22807
Phone: (540)568-2399
Website: http://www.jmu.edu

★ 28435 ★ Shenandoah University
Occupational Therapy Program
333 W Cork St., 5th Fl.
Winchester, VA 22601
Phone: (540)665-5559 **Fax:** (540)665-5564
Email: gstone@su.edu
Website: http://www.su.edu
Gretchen V.M. Stone, PhD, Director

★ 28436 ★ Virginia Commonwealth University
Occupational Therapy Program
PO Box 980008
Richmond, VA 23298-0008
Phone: (804)828-2219 **Fax:** (804)828-0782
Email: sjlane@vcu.edu
Website: http://views.vcu.edu/sahp/occu
Shelly J. Lane, PhD, Director

Washington

★ 28437 ★ Eastern Washington University
Occupational Therapy Program
Riverpoint Higher Education Park, Health Sciences Bldg.
310 N Riverpoint Blvd., Box R
Spokane, WA 99202-1675
Phone: (509)368-6560
Website: http://www.csmt.ewu.edu/csmt/ot/ot-dept.htm

★ 28438 ★ University of Puget Sound
School of Occupational Therapy
1500 N Warner
Tacoma, WA 98416-0510
Phone: (253)879-3281 **Fax:** (253)879-2933
Email: tomlin@ups.edu
Website: http://www.ups.edu/ot
George Tomlin, PhD, Director

★ 28439 ★ University of Washington
Department of Rehabilitation Medicine
Occupational Therapy Program
Box 356490
Seattle, WA 98195
Phone: (206)598-5410 **Fax:** (206)685-3244
Email: ot@u.washington.edu
Website: http://depts.washington.edu/rehab/education/ot.shtml
Elizabeth M. Kanny, PhD, Director

West Virginia

★ 28440 ★ West Virginia University
Occupational Therapy Program
Robert C. Byrd Health Sciences Center
PO Box 9139 - HSN
Morgantown, WV 26506-9139
Phone: (304)293-8828 **Fax:** (304)293-7105
Email: rmccombi@wvu.edu
Website: http://www.hsc.wvu.edu/som/ot
Randy McCombie, PhD, Director

Wisconsin

★ 28441 ★ Concordia University, Wisconsin
Occupational Therapy Program
12800 N Lake Shore Dr.
Mequon, WI 53092-2402
Phone: (414)243-4429 **Fax:** (414)243-4506
Email: peggy.denton@cuw.edu
Website: http://www.cuw.edu/occupationaltherapy
Peggy L. Denton, PhD, Director

★ 28442 ★ Mount Mary College
Occupational Therapy Program
2900 N Menomonee River Pkwy.
Milwaukee, WI 53222-4597
Phone: (414)256-1246 **Fax:** (414)256-1224
Email: olsonj@mtmary.edu
Website: http://www.mtmary.edu
Jane Olson, PhD, Director

★ 28443 ★ University of Wisconsin, LaCrosse
Occupational Therapy Program
4043 Health Science Center
1725 State St.
La Crosse, WI 54601
Phone: (608)785-6620 **Fax:** (608)785-6647
Email: marti_pm@mail.uwlax.edu
Website: http://perth.uwlax.edu/ot
Peggy M. Martin, Director

★ 28444 ★ University of Wisconsin, Madison
Occupational Therapy Program
1300 University Ave., 2110 MSC
Madison, WI 53706-1532
Phone: (608)262-2936
Email: hohlstein@education.wisc.edu
Website: http://www.soemadison.wisc.edu/kinesiology/ugrad/ot.htm
Rita Hohlstein, Director

★ 28445 ★ University of Wisconsin, Milwaukee
School of Allied Health Professions
Occupational Therapy Program
PO Box 413
Milwaukee, WI 53201-0413
Phone: (414)229-4713 **Fax:** (414)229-3930
Email: smithro@uwm.edu
Website: http://www.uwm.edu/SAHP
Roger O. Smith, PhD, Director

Wyoming

★ 28446 ★ University of North Dakota
Casper College
Occupational Therapy Program
125 College Dr.
Casper, WY 82601
Phone: (307)268-2867 **Fax:** (307)268-3099
Email: mwonser@acad.cc.whecn.edu
Website: http://www.cc.whecn.edu
Marla Wonser, Director

Optometry

Schools and colleges listed below are accredited by the Council on Optometric Education of the American Optometric Association (AOA), 243 N Lindbergh Blvd., St. Louis, MO 63141, (314)991-4100, http://www.aoanet.org. For general information about the profession, contact the AOA or the Association of Schools and Colleges of Optometry, 6110 Executive Blvd., Ste. 510, Rockville, MD 20852, (301)231-5944, http://www.opted.org/.

Alabama

★ 28447 ★ University of Alabama, Birmingham
School of Optometry
HPB 124
1530 3rd Ave. S
Birmingham, AL 35294-0010
Phone: (205)934-6150
Email: admissions@icare.opt.uab.edu
Website: http://www.icare..opt.uab.edu

California

★ 28448 ★ Southern California College of Optometry
2575 Yorba Linda Blvd.
Fullerton, CA 92831
Phone: (714)449-7444
Email: leswalls@scco.edu
Website: http://www.scco.edu/second.html

★ 28449 ★ University of California, Berkeley
School of Optometry
360 Minor Hall
Berkeley, CA 94720-2020
Phone: (510)642-9537
Email: ubcso@spectacle.berkeley.edu
Website: http://spectacle.berkeley.edu

Florida

★ 28450 ★ Nova Southeastern University
Health Professions Division
College of Optometry
3200 S University Dr.
Fort Lauderdale, FL 33328
Phone: (954)723-1125
Email: astella@hpd.nov.edu
Website: http://www.nova.edu/cwis/centers/hpd/optometry

Illinois

★ 28451 ★ Illinois College of Optometry
3241 S Michigan Ave.
Chicago, IL 60616
Phone: (312)225-1700
Email: admissions@eyecare.ico.edu
Website: http://www.ico.edu/ico2/flindex.html

Indiana

★ 28452 ★ Indiana University
School of Optometry
800 E Atwater Ave.
Bloomington, IN 47405
Phone: (812)855-1917
Email: iuopt@indiana.edu
Website: http://www.opt.indiana.edu

Massachusetts

★ 28453 ★ New England College of Optometry
424 Beacon St.
Boston, MA 02115
Phone: (617)266-2030
Email: admissio@ne-optometry.edu
Website: http://www.ne-optometry.edu

Michigan

★ 28454 ★ Ferris State University
Michigan College of Optometry
1310 Cramer Cir.
Big Rapids, MI 49307
Phone: (231)591-3700
Email: olsonc@ferris.edu
Website: http://www.ferris.edu/mco

Missouri

★ 28455 ★ University of Missouri, Saint Louis
School of Optometry
8001 Natural Bridge Rd.
Saint Louis, MO 63121
Phone: (314)516-6263
Email: sdavis@umsl.edu
Website: http://www.umsl.edu/~optometry.html

New York

★ 28456 ★ State University of New York
State College of Optometry
33 W 42nd St.
New York, NY 10036
Phone: (212)780-5100
Email: admissions@sunyopt.edu
Website: http://www.sunyopt.edu

Ohio

★ 28457 ★ Ohio State University
College of Optometry
320 W 10th Ave.
PO Box 182342
Columbus, OH 43218-2342
Phone: (614)292-2647
Email: optometry@osu.edu
Website: http://www.optometry.ohio-state.edu

Oklahoma

★ 28458 ★ Northeastern State University
College of Optometry
600 N Grand Ave.
Tahlequah, OK 74464
Phone: (918)456-5511
Email: stratton@cherokee.nsuok.edu
Website: http://arapaho.nsuok.edu/~optometry

Ontario

★ 28459 ★ University of Waterloo
School of Optometry
Waterloo, ON, Canada N2L 3G1
Phone: (519)888-4567
Graham Strong, OD,PhD, Director

Oregon

★ 28460 ★ Pacific University
College of Optometry
2043 College Way
Forest Grove, OR 97116
Phone: (503)359-2900 **Free:** 800-933-9308
Fax: (503)359-2900
Email: admissions@pacificu.edu
Website: http://www.opt.pacificu.edu/opt/index.shtml

Pennsylvania

★ 28461 ★ Pennsylvania College of Optometry
8360 Old York Rd.
Elkins Park, PA 19027
Phone: (215)780-1301 **Free:** 800-824-6262

Email: admissions@pco.edu
Website: http://www.pco.edu

Puerto Rico

★ 28462 ★ Inter American University of Puerto Rico
School of Optometry
PO Box 191049
San Juan, PR 00919-1049
Phone: (787)765-1915
Email: jcolon@inter.edu
Website: http://www.optonet.inter.edu

Quebec

★ 28463 ★ University of Montreal
School of Optometry
3744 Jean-Brillant, Ste. 260-7
Montreal, QC, Canada H3T 1P1
Phone: (514)343-6325
Pierre Simonet, PhD, Director

Tennessee

★ 28464 ★ Southern College of Optometry
1245 Madison Ave.
Memphis, TN 38104
Phone: (901)722-3225 **Free:** 800-238-0180
Email: jhauser@sco.edu
Website: http://www.sco.edu

Texas

★ 28465 ★ University of Houston
College of Optometry
4800 Calhoun Rd.
Houston, TX 77204-6052
Phone: (713)743-2040
Website: http://www.opt.uh.edu

Osteopathic Medicine

The following schools of osteopathic medicine are accredited by the American Osteopathic Association, Bureau of Professional Education. Professional associations to contact for general information on osteopathic medical education are the American Osteopathic Association (142 E Ontario St., Chicago, IL 60611, (800)621-1773, http://www.aoa-net.org/) and the American Association of Colleges of Osteopathic Medicine (5550 Friendship Blvd., Ste. 310, Chevy Chase, MD 20815-7231, (301)968-4100, http://www.aacom.org/).

Arizona

★ 28466 ★ Arizona College of Osteopathic Medicine (AZCOM)
19555 N 59th Ave.
Glendale, AZ 85308
Phone: (623)572-3215 **Free:** 888-247-9277
Website: http://www.midwestern.edu/Pages/AZCOM.html

California

★ 28467 ★ Touro University College of Osteopathic Medicine (TUCOM)
Mare Island, Quarters C
832 Walnut Ave.
Vallejo, CA 94592
Phone: (707)562-5100
Website: http://www.tucom.edu

★ 28468 ★ Western University of Health Sciences
College of Osteopathic Medicine of the Pacific (COMP)
309 E 2nd St. and College Plaza
Pomona, CA 91766-1889
Phone: (909)623-6116
Website: http://www.westernu.edu/comp.html

Florida

★ 28469 ★ Nova Southeastern University
College of Osteopathic Medicine (NSU-COM)
3200 S University Dr.
Fort Lauderdale, FL 33328
Phone: (954)262-1407 **Free:** 800-356-0026
Fax: (954)262-2250
Website: http://medicine.nova.edu

Illinois

★ 28470 ★ Midwestern University
Chicago College of Osteopathic Medicine (CCOM)
555 31st St.
Downers Grove, IL 60515
Phone: (630)515-6171 **Free:** 800-458-6253
Website: http://www.midwestern.edu/Pages/CCOM.html

Iowa

★ 28471 ★ Des Moines University
College of Osteopathic Medicine and Surgery
3200 Grand Ave.
Des Moines, IA 50312
Phone: (515)271-1450
Website: http://www.uomhs.edu

Kentucky

★ 28472 ★ Pikeville College
School of Osteopathic Medicine (PCSOM)
147 Sycamore St.
Pikeville, KY 41501
Phone: (606)218-5250
Website: http://pcsom.pc.edu

Maine

★ 28473 ★ University of New England
College of Osteopathic Medicine (UNE/COM)
11 Hills Beach Rd.
Biddeford, ME 04005
Free: 800-477-4863
Website: http://www.une.edu/com/main.html

Michigan

★ 28474 ★ Michigan State University
College of Osteopathic Medicine (MSU/COM)
E Fee Hall, A-309
East Lansing, MI 48824
Phone: (517)353-7740
Website: http://www.com.msu.edu

Missouri

★ 28475 ★ Kirksville College of Osteopathic Medicine (KCOM)
800 W Jefferson St.
Kirksville, MO 63501
Phone: (660)626-2237
Website: http://www.kcom.edu

★ 28476 ★ University of Health Sciences
College of Osteopathic Medicine (UHS-COM)
1750 Independence Ave.
Kansas City, MO 64106
Free: 800-234-4847
Website: http://www.uhs.edu

New Jersey

★ 28477 ★ University of Medicine and Dentistry of New Jersey
School of Osteopathic Medicine (UMDNJ-SOM)
Academic Center
1 Medical Center Dr.
Stratford, NJ 08084
Phone: (856)566-6000
Website: http://som.umdnj.edu

New York

★ 28478 ★ New York Institute of Technology
New York College of Osteopathic Medicine (NYCOM)
PO Box 8000
Old Westbury, NY 11568
Phone: (516)626-6947
Website: http://www.nyit.edu

Ohio

★ 28479 ★ Ohio University
College of Osteopathic Medicine (OUCOM)
Grosvenor and Irvine Halls
Athens, OH 45701
Free: 800-345-1560
Website: http://www.tcom.ohiou.edu/oucom

Oklahoma

★ 28480 ★ Oklahoma State University
College of Osteopathic Medicine (OSUCOM)
1111 W 17th St.
Tulsa, OK 74107
Free: 800-677-1972
Website: http://osu.com.okstate.edu/osucom.html

Pennsylvania

★ 28481 ★ Lake Erie College of Osteopathic Medicine (LECOM)
1858 W Grandview Blvd.
Erie, PA 16509
Phone: (814)866-6641
Website: http://www.lecom.edu

★ 28482 ★ Philadelphia College of Osteopathic Medicine (PCOM)
4170 City Ave.
Philadelphia, PA 19131
Phone: (215)871-6701 **Free:** 800-999-6998
Website: http://www.pcom.edu

Texas

★ 28483 ★ University of North Texas, Fort Worth (UNT)
Health Science Center (HSCFW)
Texas College of Osteopathic Medicine (TCOM)
3500 Camp Bowie Blvd.
Fort Worth, TX 76107-2970
Phone: (817)735-2205
Website: http://www.hsc.unt.edu/education/tcom

West Virginia

★ 28484 ★ West Virginia School of Osteopathic Medicine (WVSOM)
400 N Lee St.
Lewisburg, WV 24901
Phone: (304)647-6373
Website: http://www.wvsom.edu

Perfusion

The following perfusion training programs are accredited by the Commission on Accreditation of Allied Health Education Programs, 35 E Wacker Dr., Ste. 1970, Chicago, IL 60601-2208, (312)553-9355, http://www.caahep.org/. For information on careers in this field, contact the American Society of Extra-Corporeal Technology, 503 Carlisle Dr., Ste. 125, Herndon, VA 20170, (703)435-8556, http://www.amsect.org/.

Arizona

★ 28485 ★ University of Arizona Health Sciences Center
Cardiothoracic Surgery Services
Circulatory Sciences Graduate Program
1501 N Campbell Ave., Rm. 4402
Tucson, AZ 85724
Phone: (520)626-6339 **Fax:** (520)626-4042
Email: dflarson@u.arizona.edu
Website: http://www.pharmacology.arizona.edu/pharm_tox
Douglas Larson, PhD, Contact

Connecticut

★ 28486 ★ Quinnipiac College
Cardiovascular Perfusion Program
275 Mt. Carmel Ave.
Hamden, CT 06518
Phone: (203)582-3427 **Fax:** (203)582-8706
Email: michael.smith@quinnipiac.edu
Website: http://www.quinnipiac.edu
Michael Smith, PhD, Contact

District of Columbia

★ 28487 ★ Walter Reed Army Medical Center
Cardiothoracic Physician Assistant/ Perfusion Training Program
6825 16th St. NW, Bldg. 2, Rm. 4655
Washington, DC 20307-5001
Phone: (202)782-4865 **Fax:** (202)782-8253
Email: jogletree@erols.com
James M. Ogletree, Contact

Florida

★ 28488 ★ Barry University
Cardiovascular Perfusion Program
11300 NE Second Ave.
Miami Shores, FL 33161-6695
Phone: (305)899-3214 **Fax:** (305)899-3845
Email: jfreed@mail.barry.edu
Website: http://www.barry.edu/snhs/bsprograms/cardioperfusion/default.htm
Jason Freed, Contact

Illinois

★ 28489 ★ Rush University
College of Health Sciences
Department of Perfusion Technology
600 S Paulina
Chicago, IL 60612
Phone: (312)942-2305 **Fax:** (312)942-4048
Email: robin_g_sutton@rush.edu
Website: http://www.rush.edu/perfusion
Robin Sutton, Contact

Iowa

★ 28490 ★ University of Iowa Hospitals and Clinics
Perfusion Technology Program
Perfusion Technology Education Program
200 Hawkins Dr., 1601 JCP
Iowa City, IA 52242-1086
Phone: (319)356-8496 **Fax:** (319)353-7174
Email: scott-niles@uiowa.edu
Website: http://www.surgery.uiowa.edu:80/surgery/ptep/
Scott Niles, Contact

Maryland

★ 28491 ★ Johns Hopkins Hospital
School of Perfusion Science
600 N Wolfe St./814 Blalock
Baltimore, MD 21287-4814
Phone: (410)955-5168 **Fax:** (410)955-4163
Email: rmogh@jhmi.edu
Website: http://www.med.jhu.edu/perfusion
Roshi Etemad-Moghadam, Contact

Massachusetts

★ 28492 ★ Northeastern University
Bouve College of Health Sciences
Perfusion Technology Program
360 Huntington Ave.
Boston, MA 02115
Phone: (617)373-4183 **Fax:** (617)373-2968
Email: e.pepin@neu.edu
Website: http://www.bouve.neu.edu/department/cps/perfusion.html
Eric Pepin, EdD, Contact

Nebraska

★ 28493 ★ University of Nebraska Medical Center
Division of Clinical Perfusion Education
985155 Nebraska Medical Center
Omaha, NE 68198-5155
Phone: (402)559-7227 **Fax:** (402)559-6455
Email: cskarda@unmc.edu
Website: http://www.unmc.edu/cpe
Reba A. Benschoter, PhD, Director

New Jersey

★ 28494 ★ Cooper Health System
University of Medicine and Dentistry of New Jersey
School of Cardiovascular Perfusion
One Cooper Plaza
310 Sarah Cooper Bldg.
Camden, NJ 08103
Phone: (856)342-3277 **Fax:** (856)968-8529
Email: fowler-sally@cooperhealth.edu
Website: http://www.cooperhealth.org/programs/allied/allied_cardiovascular_perfusion.htm
Sally Fowler, Contact

New York

★ 28495 ★ Northshore University Hospital
Long Island University—CW Post Campus
School of Cardiovascular Perfusion
Manhasset, NY 11030
Phone: (516)562-1399 **Fax:** (516)562-1521
Email: ehiscvp@aol.com
Website: http://www.cwpost.liunet.edu/cwis/cwp/hscience/medbio/cardio.html
Richard Chann, Contact

★ 28496 ★ State University of New York Upstate Medical Center
Department of Cardiovascular Perfusion
750 E Adams St.
Syracuse, NY 13210
Phone: (315)464-6933 **Fax:** (315)464-6914
Email: searlesb@upstate.edu
Website: http://perfusion.upstate.edu
Bruce Searles, Contact

Ohio

★ 28497 ★ Christ Hospital
School of Perfusion Science
2139 Auburn Ave.
Cincinnati, OH 45219
Phone: (513)585-1106 **Fax:** (513)585-3241
Email: warmutcr@healthall.com
Website: http://www.health-alliance.com/hospitals/christ/christ_schools_perfusion.html
Craig Warmuth, Contact

★ 28498 ★ Cleveland Clinic Foundation
School of Perfusion
G-33
9500 Euclid Ave.
Cleveland, OH 44195-5001
Phone: (216)444-3895 **Fax:** (216)445-2725
Email: moyersc@cesmtp.ccf.org
Website: http://www.clevelandclinic.org/heartcenter/pub/professionals/education/special/perfusion.htm
Carolyn Moyers, Contact

★ 28499 ★ Ohio State University
1583 Perry St.
Columbus, OH 43210
Phone: (614)292-7261 **Fax:** (614)292-0210
Email: beckley.1@osu.edu
Website: http://circ-tech.amp.ohio-state.edu
Philip Beckley, PhD, Contact

Pennsylvania

★ 28500 ★ MCP Hahneman University
Drexel University
Program in Cardiovascular Perfusion Technology
Broad and Vine Sts.
Mail Stop 508
Philadelphia, PA 19102-1192
Phone: (215)762-7895 **Fax:** (215)246-5347

Email: stroud@mcphu.edu
Website: http://www.mcphu.edu/shp/shpprogs/cardioperf.html
Robert Stroud, Contact
Frmly: Allegheny University of the Health Sciences

★ 28501 ★ University of Pittsburgh Medical Center
School of Cardiovascular Perfusion
5230 Center Ave.
Pittsburgh, PA 15232
Phone: (412)623-2482 **Fax:** (412)623-1091
Email: rushrd@shy.edu
Website: http://www.carlow.edu/academic/bioperfusion.html
Robert Rush, Contact

South Carolina

★ 28502 ★ Medical University of South Carolina
College of Health Professions
Extracorporeal Technology Educational Program
101 Doughty St., 2nd Fl., Rm. 206
Charleston, SC 29401
Phone: (843)792-2298 **Fax:** (843)792-4417
Email: sistinoj@musc.edu
Website: http://www.musc.edu/chp-clin/ect/ect.htm
Joe Sistino, Contact

Tennessee

★ 28503 ★ Vanderbilt University Medical Center
Programs in Allied Health
Program in Cardiovascular Perfusion Technology
The Vanderbilt Clinic, Ste. 2986 TVC
Nashville, TN 37232-5734
Phone: (615)343-9195 **Fax:** (615)322-0742
Email: james.ramsey@vanderbilt.edu
Website: http://www.mc.vanderbilt.edu/cvpt
James J. Ramsey, Contact

Texas

★ 28504 ★ Texas Heart Institute
PO Box 20345
MC-1-224
Houston, TX 77225
Phone: (713)791-4026 **Fax:** (713)791-8677
Email: rmcinnis@heart.thi.tmc.edu
Website: http://www.tmc.edu/thi/perfuse.html
Raymond McInnis, Contact

Wisconsin

★ 28505 ★ Milwaukee School of Engineering
Perfusion Technology
1025 N Broadway
Milwaukee, WI 53202-3109
Phone: (414)277-7209 **Fax:** (414)277-7465
Email: altenber@msoe.edu
Website: http://www.msoe.edu/grad/msp/
Charles Altenbern, Contact

Pharmacology

Listed below are schools of medicine, schools of osteopathic medicine, schools of pharmacy, and schools of veterinary medicine that offer programs in pharmacology. To obtain general information on these programs, including specialties offered, contact the American Society for Pharmacology and Experimental Therapeutics, 9650 Rockville Pike, Bethesda, MD 20814-3995, (301)634-7060, http://www.aspet.org.

Alabama

★ 28506 ★ Auburn University
College of Veterinary Medicine
Department of Anatomy, Physiology, and Pharmacology
Graduate Program in Pharmacology
Hargis Hall
Auburn, AL 36849
Phone: (334)844-4425 **Fax:** (334)884-5388
Email: gradadm@mail.auburn.edu
Website: http://www.vetmed.auburn.edu/anatphys/

★ 28507 ★ Auburn University
School of Pharmacy
Department of Pharmacal Sciences
Graduate Study in Pharmaceutical Sciences
Office of Academic and Student Affairs
209 Pharmacy Bldg.
Auburn, AL 36849-5501
Phone: (334)844-8358 **Fax:** (334)844-8353
Email: raviswr@mail.auburn.edu

★ 28508 ★ University of Alabama, Birmingham
Graduate School
Department of Pharmacology
1400 University Blvd., Ste. 511
Birmingham, AL 35294-1150
Phone: (205)934-8227 **Fax:** (205)934-8413
Email: inquire@gradschool.huc.uab.edu
Website: http://main.uab.edu/show.asp?durki=26060

★ 28509 ★ University of South Alabama
College of Medicine
Pharmacology and Toxicology Department
251 CSAB
Mobile, AL 36688-0002
Phone: (334)460-6153
Email: jayling@jaguar1.usouthal.edu
Website: http://www.southalabama.edu/pharmacology/index.html

Arizona

★ 28510 ★ University of Arizona
Cancer Biology Interdisciplinary Graduate Program
Arizona Cancer Center, Room 4999
1515 N Campbell Ave.
Tucson, AZ 85724-5024
Phone: (520)626-7479 **Fax:** (520)626-4979
Email: acione@azcc.arizona.edu

★ 28511 ★ University of Arizona
College of Pharmacy
Pharmaceutical Sciences Graduate Program
PO Box 210207
Tucson, AZ 85721
Phone: (520)626-4351
Email: phscgradprog@pharmacy.arizona.edu

★ 28512 ★ University of Arizona
Pharmacology and Toxicology Department
AHSC 5103, Box 24-5050
Tucson, AZ 85724-5050
Phone: (520)626-7281 **Fax:** (520)626-2204
Email: gradprog@email.arizona.edu

Arkansas

★ 28513 ★ University of Arkansas for Medical Sciences
Department of Pharmacology and Toxicology
Biomedical Research Ctr.
4301 W Markham St., Slot 611
Little Rock, AR 72205
Phone: (501)686-8895 **Fax:** (501)686-5521
Email: mayeuxphilipr@uams.edu
Website: http://www.uams.edu/pharmtox/pharmtox.htm

California

★ 28514 ★ Alliant International University
California School of Professional Psychology
Clinical Psychopharmacology Program
1005 Atlantic Ave.
Alameda, CA 94501
Phone: (510)523-2300 **Fax:** (415)931-8322
Email: stulkin@alliant.edu
Website: http://www.alliant.edu/

★ 28515 ★ Loma Linda University
Graduate School of Medicine
Department of Physiology and Pharmacology
Graduate School Admissions
Office of the Dean
Loma Linda, CA 92354-9965
Phone: (909)558-1800 **Free:** 800-422-4558
Fax: (909)558-4859
Email: gradschool@univ.llu.edu
Website: http://www.llu.edu/llu/medicine/bulletin/phys.htm

★ 28516 ★ Stanford University
School of Medicine
Department of Molecular Pharmacology
Graduate Admissions Office
Room 137, Old Union
Stanford, CA 94305
Phone: (650)723-4291
Website: http://www.stanford.edu/dept/molepharm/

★ 28517 ★ University of California, Davis
Pharmacology and Toxicology Graduate Group
4117 Meyer Hall
1 Shields Ave.
Davis, CA 95616-8588
Phone: (530)752-4516 **Fax:** (530)752-3394
Email: cdwinter@ucdavis.edu
Website: http://etx.ucdavis.edu/ptx

★ 28518 ★ University of California, Irvine
College of Medicine
Department of Pharmacology
360 Med Surge II
Irvine, CA 92697-4625
Phone: (949)824-7651 **Fax:** (949)824-2095
Email: pharm@uci.edu
Website: http://www.ucihs.uci.edu/pharmaco/

★ 28519 ★ University of California, Los Angeles
School of Medicine
Department of Molecular and Medical Pharmacology
10833 Le Conte Ave.
Los Angeles, CA 90095-1735
Phone: (310)794-7726
Email: gradinfo@pharm.medsch.ucla.edu
Website: http://www.nuc.ucla.edu/

★ 28520 ★ University of California, San Francisco
Department of Pharmaceutical Sciences and Pharmacogenomics
513 Parnassus, Room S840
San Francisco, CA 94143-0446
Phone: (415)476-1947 **Fax:** (415)502-4322
Email: pspg@itsa.ucsf.edu
Website: http://www.pharmchem.ucsf.edu/grad-page.html

★ 28521 ★ University of the Pacific
School of Pharmacy
Department of Pharmaceutical Sciences
3601 Pacific Ave.
Stockton, CA 95211
Phone: (209)946-2261 **Fax:** (209)946-2858
Email: gradschool@uop.edu
Website: http://www.uop.edu/uop.nsf/

★ 28522 ★ University of Southern California
School of Medicine
Programs in Biomedical and Biological Sciences
Office of Academic and Scientific Affairs
1975 Zonal Ave.
KAM-110
Los Angeles, CA 90033
Phone: (323)442-1609 **Fax:** (323)442-1610
Email: acadsci@hsc.usc.edu
Website: http://www.usc.edu/medicine/pibbs

★ 28523 ★ University of Southern California
School of Pharmacy
Department of Molecular Pharmacology and Toxicology
Stouffer Pharmaceutical Sciences Center 207
1985 Zonal Ave.
Los Angeles, CA 90033
Phone: (213)342-1474
Email: admitusc@usc.edu
Website: http://www.usc.edu/hsc/pharmacy/

Colorado

★ 28524 ★ University of Colorado Health Sciences Center
Department of Pharmacology
Campus Box C-236
4200 E 9th St.
Denver, CO 80262
Phone: (303)315-8120 **Fax:** (303)315-7097
Email: grad.pharm@uchsc.edu
Website: http://prosche.uchsc.edu/pharm/

Connecticut

★ 28525 ★ University of Connecticut
School of Pharmacy
Department of Pharmaceutical Science
372 Fairfield Rd., U-92
PO Box U-92
Storrs, CT 06269-2092
Phone: (860)486-2493
Email: Phrmacy8@uconnvm.uconn.edu
Website: http://pharmacy.uconn.edu/

★ 28526 ★ University of Connecticut Health Center
Graduate School
Department of Cellular and Molecular Pharmacology
263 Farmington Ave., MC-3906
Farmington, CT 06030
Phone: (860)679-4306 **Fax:** (860)679-1899
Email: robertson@nso2.uchc.edu
Website: http://grad.uchc.edu

★ 28527 ★ Yale University
Graduate School of Arts and Sciences
Department of Pharmacology
PO Box 208084
New Haven, CT 06520-8084
Phone: (203)785-3735
Email: bbs@yale.edu
Website: http://info.med.yale.edu/bbs/

District of Columbia

★ 28528 ★ George Washington University
Columbian School of Arts and Sciences
Department of Biomedical Sciences
Phillips Hall, Rm. 107
801 22nd St. NW
Washington, DC 20052
Phone: (202)994-6211 **Fax:** (202)994-6213
Email: askcsas@gwu.edu
Website: http://www.gwu.edu/~gwibs/

★ 28529 ★ Georgetown University Graduate School
School of Medicine
PhD Program
3900 Reservoir Rd. NW
NW 103 Medical-Dental Bldg.
Graduate Biomedical Education
Office of the Dean of Research and Graduate Education
Washington, DC 20007
Phone: (202)687-1379 **Fax:** (202)687-2585
Email: johnsonw@georgetown.edu

★ 28530 ★ Georgetown University Medical Center
School of Medicine
Pharmacological Sciences Training Program
3900 Reservoir Rd. NW
Medical Dental Bldg. SE-404
Washington, DC 20007
Phone: (202)687-6939 **Fax:** (202)687-4872
Email: bwolfe01@georgetown.edu
Website: http://www.dml.georgetown.edu/depts/pharmacology/

★ 28531 ★ Howard University
Graduate School of Arts and Sciences
Department of Pharmacology
Office of Admissions
Fourth and College Sts. NW
Washington, DC 20059
Phone: (202)806-5805 **Fax:** (202)462-4053
Email: hugsadmission@howard.edu
Website: http://www.hucmlrc.howard.edu/Pharmacology/default.htm

Florida

★ 28532 ★ Florida A&M University
Division of Graduate Studies, Research, and Continuing Education
Pharmacology and Toxicology Program
Graduate Admission Office
G-9 Foote-Hilyer Administration Bldg.
Tallahassee, FL 32307
Phone: (850)599-3796 **Fax:** (850)599-3952
Email: admissions@famu.edu
Website: http://www.famu2.famu.edu/acad/colleges/copps/

★ 28533 ★ University of Florida
College of Medicine
Department of Physiology and Pharmacology
PO Box 100215
Gainesville, FL 32610-0215
Phone: (352)392-0740
Email: OHP@phys.med.ufl.edu
Website: http://rgp.ufl.edu/education/

★ 28534 ★ University of Miami
School of Medicine
Department of Biochemistry and Molecular Biology
PO Box 016129
Miami, FL 33101
Phone: (305)243-6265 **Fax:** (305)243-5665
Email: r.werner@miami.edu

★ 28535 ★ University of South Florida
College of Medicine
Department of Pharmacology and Therapeutics
MDC Box 9
12901 Bruce B. Downs Blvd.
Tampa, FL 33612-4799
Phone: (813)974-9922 **Fax:** (813)974-3081
Website: http://www.med.usf.edu/PHD/

Georgia

★ 28536 ★ Emory University
Graduate Division of Biological and Biomedical Sciences
Program in Molecular and Systems Pharmacology
1462 Clifton Rd., Ste. 314
Atlanta, GA 30322
Phone: (404)727-2545 **Fax:** (404)727-3322
Website: http://www.biomed.emory.edu/program_msp.html

★ 28537 ★ Morehouse School of Medicine
Office of Graduate Education in the Biomedical Sciences
Doctoral Program in Biomedical Sciences
720 Westview Dr.
Atlanta, GA 30310-1495
Phone: (404)752-1755 **Fax:** (404)752-1164
Email: paulsen@msm.edu

★ 28538 ★ University of Georgia
College of Pharmacy
Department of Pharmaceutical and Biomedical Science
Athens, GA 30602
Phone: (706)542-5403 **Fax:** (706)542-5358
Email: jwilson@rx.uga.edu
Website: http://www.gradsch.uga.edu/

★ 28539 ★ University of Georgia
College of Pharmacy
Non-traditional Pharm.D. Program
Athens, GA 30602
Phone: (706)542-1911 **Fax:** (706)542-5269
Email: ntpharmd@rx.uga.edu

★ 28540 ★ University of Georgia
Department of Pharmacology
Department of Pharmaceutical and Biomedical Science
Athens, GA 30602
Phone: (706)542-5339 **Fax:** (706)542-5358
Email: tcapomac@rx.uga.edu

Hawaii

★ 28541 ★ University of Hawaii, Manoa
Department of Pharmacology
Graduate Division Admissions Office
2540 Maile Way
Honolulu, HI 96822
Phone: (808)956-8544
Email: admissions@admin.grad.hawaii.edu

Idaho

★ 28542 ★ Idaho State University
College of Pharmacy
Department of Pharmaceutical Sciences
Campus Box 8334
Pocatello, ID 83209
Phone: (208)282-2682 **Fax:** (208)282-4482
Email: btaylor@otc.isu.edu
Website: http://rx.isu.edu/

Illinois

★ 28543 ★ Finch University of Health Sciences
School of Graduate and Postdoctoral Studies
Department of Cellular and Molecular Biology
Office of Graduate Admissions
3333 Green Bay Rd.
North Chicago, IL 60064
Phone: (847)578-3271
Email: pastor@finchcms.edu

★ 28544 ★ Illinois State University
Department of Biological Sciences
Campus Box 4120
Normal, IL 61790-4120
Phone: (309)438-3664 **Fax:** (309)438-3722
Email: cawinch@ilstu.edu
Website: http://www.bio.ilstu.edu/

★ 28545 ★ Loyola University/Chicago Medical Center
Biomedical Sciences Department
Pharmacology and Experimental Therapeutics
2160 S 1st Ave.
Bldg. 102, Rm. 3621
Maywood, IL 60153
Phone: (708)216-6594 **Fax:** (708)216-6596
Email: kmartinez@lumc.edu
Website: http://www.meddean.luc.edu/lumen/DeptWebs/PHARM/Index.htm

★ 28546 ★ Northwestern University
Medical School
Integrated Graduate Program in the Life Sciences
303 E Chicago Ave.
Ward 12-373/W150
Chicago, IL 60611-3008
Free: 800-255-4166 **Fax:** (312)908-5253
Email: igp@northwestern.edu
Website: http://www.nums.northwestern.edu/igp/

★ 28547 ★ Rush University
The Graduate College
Department of Pharmacology
2242 W Harrison St.
Chicago, IL 60612
Phone: (312)942-6247 **Fax:** (312)942-8112
Email: ruinfo@rushu.rush.edu
Website: http://www.rushu.rush.edu/pharm/dept/

★ 28548 ★ Southern Illinois University
Graduate School
Department of Pharmacology
Carbondale, IL 62901-4716
Phone: (618)536-7791
Email: gradschl@siu.edu

★ 28549 ★ Southern Illinois University
School of Medicine
Department of Pharmacology
PO Box 19629
Springfield, IL 62794-9629
Phone: (217)545-2875 **Fax:** (217)545-0145
Email: dsmith@siumed.edu
Website: http://www.siumed.edu/pharm/home.html

★ 28550 ★ University of Chicago
Division of the Biological Sciences
Department of Neurobiology, Pharmacology, and Physiology
947 E 58th St.
MC0926
Chicago, IL 60637-5416
Phone: (773)702-6371 **Fax:** (773)702-1216

★ 28551 ★ University of Illinois, Chicago
College of Medicine
Department of Molecular and Cellular Pharmacology
835 S Wolcott
M/C 868
Chicago, IL 60612-7243
Phone: (312)996-7635 **Fax:** (312)413-0185
Email: pharmacology-gs@uic.edu
Website: http://www.uic.edu/depts/mcph/

Indiana

★ 28552 ★ Butler University
College of Pharmacy
Pharmacology Program
Indianapolis, IN 46208
Phone: (317)940-9969 **Free:** 800-368-6852
Fax: (317)940-6172
Email: admission@butler.edu

★ 28553 ★ Indiana University
Graduate School, IUPI Campus
Department of Pharmacology
Union Bldg., Room 518
620 Union Dr.
Indianapolis, IN 46202-5167
Phone: (317)274-4023
Website: http://www.iupui.edu/~iuphtx/home1.html

★ 28554 ★ Indiana University
School of Medicine
Medical Sciences Graduate Program
104 Jordan Hall
Bloomington, IN 47405
Phone: (812)855-9066 **Fax:** (812)855-4436
Email: slhall@indiana.edu
Website: http://www.indiana.edu/~medsci/

★ 28555 ★ Purdue University
School of Pharmacy and Pharmaceutical Sciences
Department of Medicinal Chemistry and Molecular Pharmacology
1333 Pharmacy Bldg.
West Lafayette, IN 47907-1330
Phone: (765)494-5968 **Fax:** (765)494-7880
Email: gradprog@pharmacy.purdue.edu
Website: http://www.pharmacy.purdue.edu/~mcmp/

★ 28556 ★ Purdue University
School of Veterinary Medicine
Department of Basic Medical Sciences
School of Veterinary Medicine
Department of Basic Medical Sciences
West Lafayette, IN 47907-1246
Phone: (317)494-8632 **Fax:** (317)494-0781
Email: gradinfo@purdue.edu

Iowa

★ 28557 ★ University of Iowa
College of Medicine
Department of Biomedical Sciences
1189 Medical Laboratories
Iowa City, IA 52242-1181
Phone: (319)335-8305 **Fax:** (319)335-7656
Email: biosciences@uiowa.edu

★ 28558 ★ University of Iowa
College of Medicine
Department of Pharmacology
BSB 2-532
Iowa City, IA 52242-1109
Phone: (319)335-7965 **Fax:** (319)335-8930
Email: pharmacology@uiowa.edu

Kansas

★ 28559 ★ University of Kansas
Graduate Study in Pharmacology and Toxicology
Department of Pharmacology and Toxicology
300 Strong Hall
Lawrence, KS 66045-1729
Phone: (785)864-4141 **Fax:** (785)864-4555
Email: graduate@raven.cc.ukans.edu
Website: http://www.pharm.ukans.edu/pharmtox/index.html

★ 28560 ★ University of Kansas Medical Center
Interdisciplinary Graduate Program in Biomedical Sciences
2nd Flr BRF Bldg
2035 Lied
3901 Rainbow Blvd.
Kansas City, KS 66160-7836
Phone: (913)588-7140 **Free:** 800-408-2039
Email: igpbs@kumc.edu
Website: http://www.kumc.edu/research/medicine/pharmacology/dhp.html

Kentucky

★ 28561 ★ University of Kentucky
College of Medicine
Department of Biomedical Pharmacology
Graduate Program in Cell and Molecular Biology
800 Rose St.
A.B. Chandler Medical Center, MS 305
Lexington, KY 40536-0084
Phone: (859)323-6085 **Fax:** (859)323-1981
Email: dturner@pop.uky.edu
Website: http://www.mc.uky.edu/pharmacology/default.asp

★ 28562 ★ University of Kentucky
College of Pharmacy
Department of Pharmaceutical Sciences
511 Pharmacy Bldg.
Lexington, KY 40536-0082
Phone: (859)257-1998 **Fax:** (859)323-6886
Email: nlhump2@uky.edu
Website: http://www.mc.uky.edu/pharmacology/default.asp

★ **28563** ★ **University of Louisville**
Graduate School
Department of Pharmacology and Toxicology
Office of Research and Graduate Programs
Louisville, KY 40292
Phone: (502)852-6495
Email: gradadm@louisville.edu
Website: http://www.louisville.edu/medschool/pharmacology/

★ **28564** ★ **University of Louisville**
Office of Research and Graduate Programs
Department of Pharmacology and Toxicology
Louisville, KY 40292
Phone: (502)852-8367
Website: http://www.louisville.edu/medschool/pharmacology/

Louisiana

★ **28565** ★ **Louisiana State University Health Sciences Center**
Department of Pharmacology and Experimental Therapeutics
1901 Perdido St.
New Orleans, LA 70112
Phone: (504)568-4740 **Fax:** (504)568-2361
Email: emize@lsuhsc.edu
Website: http://www.medschool.lsuhsc.edu/phar/

★ **28566** ★ **Louisiana State University**
School of Medicine
Department of Pharmacology and Therapeutics
PO Box 33932
Shreveport, LA 71130-3932
Phone: (318)675-7867 **Fax:** (318)675-7857
Email: tdugas@lsumc.edu
Website: http://gradsch.shreveport.lsumc.edu/Pharm/Pharm.html

★ **28567** ★ **Tulane University**
Graduate School of Arts and Sciences
Department of Pharmacology
Gibson Hall, Room 324
New Orleans, LA 70118
Phone: (504)865-5100
Email: graduate.school@tulane.edu
Website: http://www.tmc.tulane.edu/departments/pharmacology/

★ **28568** ★ **Tulane University**
School of Medicine
Department of Pharmacology
Office of Graduate Studies
1430 Tulane Ave. (SL 00)
New Orleans, LA 70112-9962
Phone: (504)588-5187 **Fax:** (504)588-3721
Email: medsch@tmcpop.tmc.tulane.edu
Website: http://www1.omi.tulane.edu/departments/pharmacology/pharm.html

Maryland

★ **28569** ★ **Johns Hopkins University**
Arts and Sciences Advanced Academic Programs
Biotechnology Program
3003 N Charles St.
Ste. 150
Baltimore, MD 21218
Free: 800-847-3330 **Fax:** (410)516-6017
Email: advanced@jhu.edu

★ **28570** ★ **Johns Hopkins University**
School of Medicine
Department of Pharmacology and Molecular Sciences
Graduate Program in Pharmacology and Molecular Sciences
725 N Wolfe St.
Baltimore, MD 21205
Phone: (410)955-7117
Email: mguercio@bs.jhmi.edu
Website: http://www.med.jhu.edu/pharmacology/

★ **28571** ★ **Uniformed Services University of the Health Sciences**
Graduate Education Office
Pharmacology Department
4301 Jones Bridge Rd., USUHS
Bethesda, MD 20814-4799
Phone: (301)295-9474 **Free:** 800-772-1747
Fax: (301)295-6772
Website: http://www.usuhs.mil/geo/gradpgm_index.html

★ **28572** ★ **University of Maryland**
School of Medicine
Department of Pharmacology and Experimental Therapeutics
Graduate Program Coordinator
20 N Pine St.
Baltimore, MD 21201
Phone: (410)706-7131 **Fax:** (410)706-3473
Email: gradinfo@umaryland.edu
Website: http://som1.umaryland.edu/~smPharm/pharm.html

Massachusetts

★ **28573** ★ **Boston University**
School of Medicine
Division of Graduate Medical Sciences
Department of Pharmacology
80 E Concord St.
Boston, MA 02118
Phone: (617)638-5120 **Fax:** (617)638-4842
Email: wilcox@bu.edu

★ **28574** ★ **Massachusetts College of Pharmacy and Allied Health Sciences**
Department of Pharmaceutical Sciences
Coordinator of Graduate Admissions
179 Longwood Ave.
Boston, MA 02115
Phone: (617)732-2850 **Fax:** (617)732-2801
Email: admissions@mcp.edu
Website: http://www.mcp.edu/ps/pharms.htm

★ **28575** ★ **Northeastern University**
Bouve College of Pharmacy and Health Sciences, Counseling, Psychology, Rehabilitation and Special Needs
Pharmacology Program
203 Mugar Life Sciences Bldg.
360 Huntington Ave.
Boston, MA 02115
Phone: (617)373-2708 **Fax:** (617)373-3216
Email: w.purnell@nunet.neu.edu
Website: http://www.bouve.neu.edu/department/phar/pharmsci/bms.html

★ **28576** ★ **Tufts University**
Sackler School of Graduate Biomedical Sciences
Department of Pharmacology and Experimental Therapeutics
136 Harrison Ave.
Boston, MA 02111
Phone: (617)636-7000 **Fax:** (617)636-0309
Email: sschool@infonet.tufts.edu
Website: http://www.tufts.edu/sackler/pharmacology/

★ **28577** ★ **University of Massachusetts Medical Center at Worcester**
Department of Biochemistry and Molecular Pharmacology
55 Lake Ave. N
Worcester, MA 01655-0122
Phone: (508)856-2405 **Fax:** (508)856-5080
Email: gsbs@umassmed.edu
Website: http://www.umassmed.edu/pharmacology/

Michigan

★ **28578** ★ **Michigan State University**
College of Human Medicine
Department of Pharmacology and Toxicology
B440 Life Sciences Bldg.
East Lansing, MI 48824
Phone: (517)353-7146
Email: hummeld@pilot.msu.edu
Website: http://www.phmtox.msu.edu/

★ **28579** ★ **University of Michigan**
Medical School
Department of Pharmacology
1301 MSRB III
Ann Arbor, MI 48109-0632
Phone: (734)764-8166 **Fax:** (734)763-4450
Email: effergie@umich.edu
Website: http://www.med.umich.edu/pharm/homepage.html

★ **28580** ★ **Wayne State University**
School of Medicine
Department of Pharmacology
6374 Scott Hall
Detroit, MI 48202
Phone: (313)577-6737 **Fax:** (313)577-6739
Email: s.r.terlecky@wayne.edu
Website: http://www.med.wayne.edu/pharm/home.htm

Minnesota

★ **28581** ★ **Mayo Graduate School**
Molecular Pharmacology and Experimental Therapeutics
200 First St. SW
Rochester, MN 55905
Phone: (507)538-1160 **Fax:** (507)284-0999
Email: phd.training@mayo.edu
Website: http://www.mayo.edu/research/mpet/

★ **28582** ★ **University of Minnesota**
Medical School
Department of Pharmacology
6-120 Jackson Hall
321 Church St. SE
Minneapolis, MN 55455
Phone: (612)625-9997 **Fax:** (612)625-8408
Email: campb034@umn.edu
Website: http://www.pharmacology.med.umn.edu/

★ **28583** ★ **University of Minnesota**
School of Law
Drug Research and Development
429 Law Center, 229-19th Ave S
Minneapolis, MN 55455
Phone: (612)625-0055 **Fax:** (612)625-2011
Email: biosciences@uiowa.edu

Mississippi

★ 28584 ★ University of Mississippi School of Medicine
Graduate Programs in the Basic Medical Sciences
Department of Pharmacology and Toxicology
Division of Student Services and Records
2500 N State St.
Jackson, MS 39216-4505
Phone: (601)984-1100
Website: http://pharmacology.umc.edu/

★ 28585 ★ University of Mississippi School of Pharmacognosy
Faser Hall
University, MS 38677
Phone: (662)915-7026 **Fax:** (662)915-7026
Email: chufford@olemiss.edu
Website: http://www.olemiss.edu/depts/pharmacology

★ 28586 ★ University of Mississippi School of Pharmacy
Department of Pharmacology
303A Faser
University, MS 38677
Phone: (662)915-7330 **Fax:** (662)915-5118
Email: phcol1@olemiss.edu
Website: http://www.olemiss.edu/depts/pharmacology

Missouri

★ 28587 ★ Saint Louis University
Department of Pharmacological and Physiological Science
3663 Lindell Blvd.
Saint Louis, MO 63108-3342
Phone: (314)977-2240 **Fax:** (314)977-3943
Email: grequest@slu.edu

★ 28588 ★ Saint Louis University
Department of Pharmacological and Physiological Science
School of Medicine
1402 S Grand Blvd. (M228)
Saint Louis, MO 63104
Phone: (314)577-8418 **Fax:** (314)268-5396
Email: grequest@slu.edu
Website: http://www.slu.edu/departments/pharm_phys/

★ 28589 ★ University of Missouri, Columbia
School of Medicine
Department of Pharmacology
M-517B Medical Sciences Bldg.
Columbia, MO 65212
Phone: (573)882-7188 **Fax:** (573)884-4558
Email: gradschl@missouri.edu
Website: http://www.muhealth.org/~pharmacology/gradprog.html

★ 28590 ★ University of Missouri, Kansas City
Department of Pharmaceutical Science
5100 Rockhill Rd.
Kansas City, MO 64110-2499
Phone: (816)235-1111 **Fax:** (816)235-1717
Email: admit@umkc.edu
Website: http://www.umkc.edu/pharm/PHARMSCI.HTML

Montana

★ 28591 ★ University of Montana
School of Pharmacy and Allied Health Sciences
Department of Pharmaceutical Sciences
SB 271
Missoula, MT 59812-1075
Phone: (406)243-4765 **Fax:** (406)243-5228
Email: pharmsci@selway.umt.edu

Nebraska

★ 28592 ★ Creighton University
Graduate School
Department of Pharmacology
2500 California Plaza
Omaha, NE 68178
Phone: (402)280-2870
Email: gradsch@creighton.edu
Website: http://spahp.creighton.edu/

★ 28593 ★ University of Nebraska Medical Center
Biomedical Research Training Program
Department of Pharmacology
Office of the Dean for Graduate Studies and Research
986810 Nebraska Medical Center
Omaha, NE 68198-6810
Phone: (402)559-6531 **Free:** 800-626-8431
Fax: (402)559-7845
Email: dbulling@unmc.edu
Website: http://www.unmc.edu/Pharmacology/

★ 28594 ★ University of Nebraska Medical Center
Eppley Institute for Research in Cancer and Allied Diseases
Cancer Research Training Program
986805 Nebraska Medical Center
Omaha, NE 68198-6805
Phone: (402)559-4401 **Fax:** (402)559-4651
Email: dbulling@unmc.edu
Website: http://www.unmc.edu/Eppley/crtp.htm

Nevada

★ 28595 ★ University of Nevada, Reno
School of Medicine
Department of Cell and Molecular Pharmacology and Physiology
Graduate School, Rm. 326
Reno, NV 89557-0035
Phone: (775)784-6869 **Fax:** (775)784-6064
Email: gradadmissions@unr.edu

★ 28596 ★ University of Nevada, Reno
School of Medicine
Department of Cellular and Molecular Pharmacology and Physiology
Department of Physiology and Cell Biology, Rm. 352
Reno, NV 89557-0046
Phone: (702)784-6908
Email: burt@physio.unr.edu

New Hampshire

★ 28597 ★ Dartmouth College
Medical School
Department of Pharmacology and Toxicology
Office of Admissions
7650 Remsen, Rm. 522
Hanover, NH 03755-3833
Phone: (603)650-1667
Email: pharmacology.and.toxicology@dartmouth.edu
Website: http://www.dartmouth.edu/dms/pharmtox/

New Jersey

★ 28598 ★ Rutgers, the State University of New Jersey
Division of Life Sciences
Doctorate Programs in Molecular Biosciences
Nelson Biological Laboratory, Rm. A102
Piscataway, NJ 08854
Phone: (732)445-3430 **Fax:** (732)445-6370
Email: ambrose@biology.rutgers.edu
Website: http://lifesci.rutgers.edu/~molbiosci/

★ 28599 ★ Rutgers, the State University of New Jersey
Graduate School
Department of Cellular and Molecular Pharmacology
Office of Graduate and Professional Admissions
Van Nest Hall
PO Box 5053
New Brunswick, NJ 08903-5053
Phone: (732)932-1766 **Fax:** (732)932-8231
Email: mcnamame@umdnj.edu
Website: http://pharmacy.rutgers.edu/graduate-programs.htm

★ 28600 ★ University of Medicine and Dentistry of New Jersey
Department of Pharmacology and Physiology
185 S Orange Ave.
Newark, NJ 07103
Phone: (973)972-4444 **Fax:** (973)972-7950
Email: njms-dpp@umdnj.edu

★ 28601 ★ University of Medicine and Dentistry of New Jersey
Graduate School of Biomedical Sciences, Piscataway
Department of Cellular and Molecular Pharmacology
675 Hoes Lane
Piscataway, NJ 08854-5635
Phone: (732)235-5016
Email: gsbspisc@umdnj.edu
Website: http://www2.umdnj.edu/~pharm/gradphrm.htm

New Mexico

★ 28602 ★ University of New Mexico
School of Medicine
Biomedical Sciences Graduate Program
Box 520
Albuquerque, NM 87131-5196
Phone: (505)272-1887 **Fax:** (505)272-8738
Email: bsgp@salud.unm.edu
Website: http://hsc.unm.edu/som/bsgs/info.html

New York

★ 28603 ★ Albany Medical College
Department of Vascular Biology
Graduate Studies Program Office
47 New Scotland Ave., MC-16
Albany, NY 12208-3479
Phone: (518)262-5253 **Fax:** (518)262-5183
Email: graduate-studies@mail.amc.edu
Website: http://www.amc.edu/Academic/GradStudies/gradstudies.htm

★ 28604 ★ Albany Medical College
Neuropharmacology and Neuroscience Program
47 New Scotland Ave., MC-16
Albany, NY 12208
Phone: (518)262-5253 **Fax:** (518)262-5183
Email: graduate-studies@mail.amc.edu
Website: http://www.amc.edu/Academic/GradStudies/gradstudies.htm

★ 28605 ★ Columbia University
College of Physicians and Surgeons
Department of Pharmacology
630 W 168th St.
New York, NY 10032
Phone: (212)305-8058 **Fax:** (212)305-1031
Email: GSASatPandS@columbia.edu
Website: http://cpmcnet.columbia.edu/dept/gsas

★ 28606 ★ Cornell University
Graduate School
Department of Pharmacology
1300 York Ave., Rm. E409
New York, NY 10021
Phone: (212)746-6565
Email: jat2008@med.cornell.edu
Website: http://web.vet.cornell.edu/public/research/graded/index.html

★ 28607 ★ Long Island University, Brooklyn
Arnold and Marie Schwartz College of Pharmacy and Health Sciences
Division of Pharmacology, Toxicology, and Medicinal Chemistry
1 University Plaza
Brooklyn, NY 11201
Phone: (718)488-1062 **Fax:** (718)797-2399
Email: attend@liu.edu

★ 28608 ★ Mount Sinai School of Medicine
Graduate Program in the Biomedical Sciences
PO Box 1022
1 Gustave L. Levy Pl.
New York, NY 10029-6574
Phone: (212)241-6546 **Fax:** (212)241-0651
Email: grads@smtplink.mssm.edu
Website: http://www.mssm.edu/gradschool/

★ 28609 ★ New York Medical College
Graduate School of Basic Medical Sciences
Department of Pharmacology
Director of Admissions
95 Grasslands Rd.
Valhalla, NY 10595
Phone: (914)594-4110 **Fax:** (914)594-4944

★ 28610 ★ New York University
Graduate School of Arts and Science
Basic Medical Sciences
Graduate Enrollment Services
One Half 5th Ave.
New York, NY 10003
Phone: (212)998-8050 **Fax:** (212)995-4557
Email: gsas.admissions@nyu.edu

★ 28611 ★ New York University
Sackler Institute of Graduate Biomedical Sciences
Program in Molecular Pharmacology and Signal Transduction
550 1st Ave.
New York, NY 10016
Phone: (212)263-5648 **Fax:** (212)263-7600
Email: sackler-info@nyumed.med.nyu.edu
Website: http://www.med.nyu.edu/Sackler/HomePage.html

★ 28612 ★ St. John's University
College of Pharmacy and Allied Health Professions
Department of Medicinal Chemistry
8000 Utopia Pkwy.
Jamaica, NY 11439
Phone: (718)990-6132
Email: admissions@stjohns.edu

★ 28613 ★ State University of New York Upstate Medical Center
College of Graduate Studies
Department of Pharmacology
SUNY Health Science Center
750 E Adams St.
Syracuse, NY 13210
Phone: (315)464-4538 **Fax:** (315)464-4544
Email: gradstud@hscsyr.edu

★ 28614 ★ State University of New York, Buffalo
Department of Chemistry, College of Arts and Sciences
Department of Medicinal Chemistry
457 Cooke Hall
Buffalo, NY 14260
Phone: (716)645-6369 **Fax:** (716)645-2393
Email: podolic@acsu.buffalo.edu

★ 28615 ★ State University of New York, Buffalo
School of Medicine and Biomedical Sciences
Department of Pharmacology and Toxicology, Department of Pathology Interdisciplinary Graduate Program in Biomedical Sciences
128 Biomedical Education Bldg.
3435 Main St.
Buffalo, NY 14214-3000
Phone: (716)829-3398 **Fax:** (716)829-2437
Email: ehayden@buffalo.edu

★ 28616 ★ State University of New York, Buffalo
School of Pharmacy and Pharmaceutical Sciences
Department of Pharmaceutics
545 Hochstetter Hall
Buffalo, NY 14260-1200
Phone: (716)645-2842 **Fax:** (716)645-3850
Email: ljanos@buffalo.edu

★ 28617 ★ State University of New York, Stony Brook
Department of Pharmacological Sciences
Molecular and Cellular Pharmacology
BST 8-196 Z=8651
Stony Brook, NY 11794-8651
Phone: (631)444-3057 **Fax:** (631)444-3218
Email: grad@pharm.sunysb.edu
Website: http://www.pharm.sunysb.edu/

★ 28618 ★ University of Buffalo
Roswell Park Cancer Institute
Department of Molecular Pharmacology and Cancer Therapeutics
420 Research Studies Center
Buffalo, NY 14263
Phone: (716)845-8225 **Fax:** (716)845-8857
Email: gradapp@roswellpark.org
Website: http://www.roswellpark.org/gradeducation/

★ 28619 ★ University of Buffalo
Roswell Park Cancer Institute
Interdisciplinary Program in Cancer Research
Elm and Carlton Sts.
Buffalo, NY 14263-0001
Free: 800-685-6825 **Fax:** (716)845-8178
Email: gradapp@roswellpark.org

★ 28620 ★ University of Rochester
School of Medicine and Dentistry
Department of Pharmacology and Physiology, Graduate Program in Biomedical Sciences
Cellular and Molecular Basis of Medicine
601 Elmwood Ave.
PO Box 711
Rochester, NY 14642
Phone: (585)275-0447 **Fax:** (585)273-2652
Email: cmm@urmc.rochester.edu
Website: http://www.urmc.rochester.edu/phph/

★ 28621 ★ Weill Graduate School of Medical Sciences of Cornell University
Department of Pharmacology
445 E 69th St.
New York, NY 10021-4896
Phone: (212)746-6565 **Fax:** (212)746-8906
Email: gsms@med.cornell.edu

★ 28622 ★ Weill Medical School of Cornell University
Department of Pharmacology
1300 York Ave., Rm. E409
New York, NY 10021
Phone: (212)746-6250 **Fax:** (212)746-8835
Email: jat2008@med.cornell.edu

★ 28623 ★ Yeshiva University
Albert Einstein College of Medicine
Department of Molecular Pharmacology
Bronx, NY 10461-1602
Phone: (718)430-2505
Email: rubin@aecom.yu.edu

★ 28624 ★ Yeshiva University
Albert Einstein College of Medicine
Department of Molecular Pharmacology
1300 Morris Park Ave.
Bronx, NY 10461
Phone: (718)430-2345 **Fax:** (718)430-8655
Email: phd@aecom.yu.edu

North Carolina

★ 28625 ★ Duke University Medical Center
Department of Pharmacology and Cancer Biology
Pharmacology and Cancer Biology Graduate Program
Box 3813
Durham, NC 27710
Phone: (919)613-8650
Website: http://pharmacology.mc.duke.edu/

★ 28626 ★ East Carolina University
School of Medicine
Department of Pharmacology
Greenville, NC 27858-4353
Phone: (252)816-2758
Email: tschetterp@mail.ecu.edu
Website: http://www.research2.ecu.edu/grad/

★ 28627 ★ University of North Carolina, Chapel Hill
Department of Pharmacology
CB 7365
Chapel Hill, NC 27599-7365
Phone: (919)966-1153 **Fax:** (919)966-5640
Email: phcograd@med.unc.edu
Website: http://www.med.unc.edu/pharm/

★ 28628 ★ Wake Forest University
Bowman Gray School of Medicine
Department of Pharmacology
Dean of the Graduate School
Medical Center Blvd.
Winston-Salem, NC 27199-0603
Phone: (336)716-4303 **Free:** 800-438-4723
Fax: (336)716-4204
Email: bggrad@wfubmc.edu
Website: http://isnet.is.wfu.edu/physpharm/homepage.html

North Dakota

★ 28629 ★ University of North Dakota
Graduate School
Department of Pharmacology and Toxicology
501 N Columbia Rd.
Grand Forks, ND 58202-9037
Phone: (701)777-3975 **Fax:** (701)777-4490
Email: pharmphys@medicine.nodak.edu
Website: http://www.med.und.nodak.edu

Ohio

★ 28630 ★ Case Western Reserve University
School of Medicine
Biomedical Sciences Training Program
10900 Euclid Ave. (WG46)
Cleveland, OH 44106-4934
Phone: (216)368-3347 **Fax:** (216)368-0795
Email: bstp@po.cwru.edu
Website: http://www.cwru.edu/med/bstp/info.html

★ 28631 ★ Case Western Reserve University
School of Medicine
Department of Pharmacology
Office of Graduate Admissions
10900 Euclid Ave.
Cleveland, OH 44106-7027
Phone: (216)368-2000 **Fax:** (216)368-3395
Email: rak5@po.cwru.edu
Website: http://www.cwru.edu/med/bstp/info.html

★ 28632 ★ Kent State University
School of Biomedical Sciences
110 Cunningham Hall
Kent, OH 44242-0001
Phone: (330)672-2263 **Fax:** (330)672-9391

★ 28633 ★ Medical College of Ohio
Department of Pharmacology
3035 Arlington Ave.
Toledo, OH 43614
Phone: (419)383-4182 **Fax:** (419)383-2871
Email: mheck@mco.edu

★ 28634 ★ Medical College of Ohio
Graduate School
Department of Molecular and Cellular Biology
Department of Molecular Basis of Disease
3000 Arlington Ave.
Toledo, OH 43614
Phone: (419)383-4918 **Fax:** (419)383-3089
Email: rruch@mco.edu

★ 28635 ★ Northeastern Ohio Universities
Basics Medical Sciences
PO Box 95
Rootstown, OH 44272-0095
Phone: (216)325-2511 **Fax:** (330)325-8372

★ 28636 ★ Ohio State University
College of Pharmacy
500 W 12th St.
Columbus, OH 43210-1291
Phone: (614)292-2266 **Fax:** (614)292-2588
Email: gadmbrks@dendrite.pharmacy.ohio-state.edu
Website: http://www.pharmacy.ohio-state.edu/

★ 28637 ★ Ohio State University
Integrated Biomedical Science Graduate Program
Meiling Hall, Room 268
370 W 9th Ave.
Columbus, OH 43210
Phone: (614)292-0857 **Fax:** (614)247-7175
Email: yates.1@osu.edu
Website: http://www.ibgp.org/

★ 28638 ★ University of Cincinnati
College of Medicine
Department of Pharmacology and Cell Biophysics
231 Bethesda Ave.
PO Box 670555
Cincinnati, OH 45267-0575
Phone: (513)558-2366 **Fax:** (513)558-1169
Email: nancy.thyberg@uc.edu
Website: http://www.med.us.edu/pharmacology/

★ 28639 ★ University of Cincinnati
College of Pharmacy
Pharmacology and Toxicology Program
3223 Eden Ave.
PO Box 670004
Cincinnati, OH 45267-0004
Phone: (513)558-3784 **Fax:** (513)558-4372
Email: marcia.sedam@uc.edu

★ 28640 ★ Wright State University
School of Medicine
Department of Pharmacology and Toxicology
Dayton, OH 45435
Phone: (937)775-2159 **Fax:** (937)775-7221
Email: robert.grubbs@wright.edu
Website: http://www.med.wright.edu/som/academic/pharm/pharm.html

Oklahoma

★ 28641 ★ University of Oklahoma Health Sciences Center
Graduate College
Department of Cell Biology
PO Box 26901
Oklahoma City, OK 73190
Phone: (405)271-2406 **Fax:** (405)271-3548
Email: brenda-callahan@ouhsc.edu

Pennsylvania

★ 28642 ★ Drexel University
College of Medicine, Biomedical Graduate Studies
Department of Pharmacology and Physiology
2900 Queen Ln.
Ste. 239
Philadelphia, PA 19129
Phone: (215)991-8570 **Free:** (866)624-6633
Fax: (215)843-5810
Email: Tracey.M.Bracale@drexel.edu

★ 28643 ★ Drexel University College of Medicine
Biomedical Graduate Program
2900 Queen Ln.
Ste. 239
Philadelphia, PA 19129
Phone: (215)762-2383 **Free:** (866)624-6633
Fax: (215)843-5810
Email: biograd@drexel.edu

★ 28644 ★ Duquesne University
Graduate School of Pharmaceutical Sciences
Pharmacy Department
449 Mellon Hall of Science
Pittsburgh, PA 15282
Phone: (412)396-5662 **Fax:** (412)396-5593
Email: gsps-adm@duq.edu

★ 28645 ★ Pennsylvania State University
College of Medicine
Cell and Molecular Biology Graduate Program
H133, PO Box 850
500 University Dr.
Hershey, PA 17033
Phone: (717)531-1045 **Fax:** (717)531-0102
Email: cmb-grad-hmc@psu.edu

★ 28646 ★ Pennsylvania State University
College of Medicine
Department of Pharmacology
Department of Pharmacology H-078
500 University Dr.
Hershey, PA 17033
Phone: (717)531-8285 **Fax:** (717)531-5013
Email: pharm-grad-hmc@psu.edu
Website: http://www.hmc.psu.edu/pharmacology_program/index.html

★ 28647 ★ Pennsylvania State University
College of Medicine
Neuroscience Graduate Program
H-109, P. O. Box 850
500 University Dr.
Hershey, PA 17033
Phone: (717)531-8650 **Fax:** (717)531-5184
Email: grad-hmc@psu.edu

★ 28648 ★ Pennsylvania State University
Milton Hershey Medical Center
College of Medicine
Graduate Programs in Biomedical Sciences
H-170, Office of Graduate Education
500 University Dr.
Hershey, PA 17033
Phone: (717)531-8892 **Fax:** (717)531-4139
Email: grad-hmc@psu.edu

★ 28649 ★ Temple University
School of Medicine
Department of Pharmacology
3400 N Broad St.
Philadelphia, PA 19140-9630
Phone: (215)204-1380
Email: tu_grad@blue.temple.edu
Website: http://www.temple.edu/pharmacology/

★ 28650 ★ Thomas Jefferson University
College of Graduate Studies
Department of Pharmacology
1020 Locust St., M-46
Philadelphia, PA 19107-6799
Phone: (215)503-4400 **Fax:** (215)503-3433
Email: cgs-info@mail.tju.edu

★ 28651 ★ Thomas Jefferson University
College of Graduate Studies
Molecular Pharmacology and Structural Biology
1020 Locust St., M-46
Philadelphia, PA 19107-6799
Phone: (215)503-4400 **Fax:** (215)503-3433
Email: cgs-info@mail.tju.edu

★ 28652 ★ University of Pennsylvania
School of Medicine
Biomedical Graduate Studies
240 John Morgan Bldg.
Philadelphia, PA 19104-6064
Phone: (215)898-1030
Email: bgs@mail.med.upenn.edu

★ 28653 ★ University of Pennsylvania
School of Medicine
Department of Pharmacological Sciences
Philadelphia, PA 19104
Phone: (215)898-8025
Email: leroy@pharm.med.upenn.edu

★ 28654 ★ University of Pittsburgh
School of Medicine
Department of Molecular Pharmacology
INTBP, 524 Scaife Hall
3550 Terrace St.
Pittsburgh, PA 15261
Phone: (412)648-8957 **Fax:** (412)648-1077
Email: gradstudies@medschool.pitt.edu

★ 28655 ★ University of the Sciences in Philadelphia
Graduate School
Department of Chemistry and Pharmacognosy
600 S 43rd St.
Philadelphia, PA 19104
Phone: (215)596-8937 **Fax:** (215)895-1185
Email: Graduate@usip.edu

★ 28656 ★ University of the Sciences in Philadelphia
Graduate School
Department of Pharmacology and Toxicology
600 S 43rd St.
Philadelphia, PA 19104
Phone: (215)596-8937 **Fax:** (215)895-1185
Email: Graduate@usip.edu
Website: http://www.usip.edu/graduate/pharmacology_toxicology.htm

Puerto Rico

★ 28657 ★ University of Puerto Rico
School of Medicine
Department of Pharmacology and Toxicology
UPR, Medical Sciences Campus
GPO 5067
San Juan, PR 00936
Phone: (787)724-1006 **Fax:** (787)282-0568
Email: scorey@neurobio.upr.clu.edu

Rhode Island

★ 28658 ★ Brown University
Division of Biology and Medicine
Graduate Program in Molecular Pharmacology and Physiology
Box G-B3
Providence, RI 02912
Phone: (401)863-2574
Email: Cheryl_Pariseau@brown.edu

★ 28659 ★ University of Rhode Island
College of Pharmacy
Department of Pharmacology
117 Fogarty Hall
Kingston, RI 02881-0809
Phone: (401)874-5842
Email: urigrad@uriacc.uri.edu

South Carolina

★ 28660 ★ Medical University of South Carolina
College of Graduate Studies
Department of Cell and Molecular Pharmacology
41 Bee St.
PO Box 250203
Charleston, SC 29425
Phone: (843)792-8710 **Fax:** (843)792-6615
Email: oes-web@musc.edu

★ 28661 ★ Medical University of South Carolina
College of Graduate Studies
Marine Biomedicine and Environmental Sciences
41 Bee St.
PO Box 250203
Charleston, SC 29425
Phone: (843)792-8710 **Fax:** (843)792-6615
Email: oes-web@musc.edu

★ 28662 ★ Medical University of South Carolina
Marine Biomedicine and Environmental Sciences
Graduate Programs in Molecular, Cell Biology, and Pathophysiology
221 Ft. Johnson Rd.
Charleston, SC 29412
Phone: (843)762-5530 **Fax:** (843)762-5535
Email: morrisp@musc.edu

South Dakota

★ 28663 ★ University of South Dakota
School of Medicine
Basic Biomedical Sciences
414 E Clark St.
Vermillion, SD 57069-2390
Phone: (605)677-5254 **Fax:** (605)677-6381
Email: biomed@usd.edu

★ 28664 ★ University of South Dakota
School of Medicine
Department of Pharmacology
414 E Clark St.
Vermillion, SD 57069-2390
Phone: (605)677-5254 **Fax:** (605)677-6381
Email: biomed@usd.edu

Tennessee

★ 28665 ★ East Tennessee State University
James H. Quillen College of Medicine
Graduate Department of Biomedical Science
PO Box 70407
Johnson City, TN 37614
Phone: (423)439-5652 **Fax:** (423)439-4020
Email: biomed@etsu.edu
Website: http://www.etsu.edu/gradstud/index.htm

★ 28666 ★ University of Tennessee, Memphis
College of Graduate Health Sciences
Department of Pharmacology
894 Union Ave.
Memphis, TN 38163
Phone: (901)448-4465 **Fax:** (901)448-7126
Email: schneide@Physio1.utmem.edu
Website: http://www.utmem.edu/grad/PROGRAMS/program_pharmacol.html

★ 28667 ★ Vanderbilt University
The Graduate School
Department of Pharmacology
411 Kirkland Hall
Nashville, TN 37240
Phone: (615)343-2727 **Free:** 800-810-8993
Fax: (615)322-3827
Email: vugs@nwfs1.gs.vanderbilt.edu

★ 28668 ★ Vanderbilt University
Interdisciplinary Graduate Program
Department of Pharmacology
340 Light Hall
Nashville, TN 37232-0301
Phone: (615)343-2573 **Free:** 800-810-8993
Fax: (615)343-0749
Email: michelle.grundy@vanderbilt.edu

Texas

★ 28669 ★ Baylor College of Medicine
Department of Pharmacology
One Baylor Plaza
Houston, TX 77030
Phone: (713)798-7902 **Fax:** (713)798-3145
Email: pchan@bcm.tmc.edu

★ 28670 ★ Baylor College of Medicine
Graduate School of Biomedical Sciences
Interdepartmental Program in Cell and Molecular Biology
One Baylor Plaza
Houston, TX 77030
Phone: (713)798-6557 **Fax:** (713)798-6325
Email: cmbprog@bcm.tmc.edu

★ 28671 ★ Texas Tech University Health Sciences Center
Graduate School of Biomedical Sciences
Department of Pharmacology
3601 4th St.
Lubbock, TX 79430
Phone: (806)743-2556 **Free:** 800-528-5391
Fax: (806)743-2656
Email: acagsbs@ttuhsc.edu

Website: http://www2.ttuhsc.edu/pages/grad/default.htm

★ 28672 ★ University of Houston
College of Pharmacy
Department of Pharmacological and Pharmaceutical Sciences
141 Science & Research Bldg. 2
Houston, TX 77204-5000
Phone: (713)743-1222 **Fax:** (713)743-1229
Email: vigreen@uh.edu

★ 28673 ★ University of North Texas Health Science Center
Graduate School of Biomedical Sciences
Biomedical Sciences
3500 Camp Bowie Blvd.
Fort Worth, TX 76107
Phone: (817)735-2000 **Free:** 800-511-GRAD
Fax: (817)735-0243
Website: http://www.hsc.unt.edu/education/gsbs/

★ 28674 ★ University of Texas, Austin
College of Pharmacy
Department of Pharmacology
Division of Pharmacology/Toxicology
College of Pharmacy
Austin, TX 78712-1074
Phone: (512)471-1737
Email: adgrd@utxdp.dp.utexas.edu

★ 28675 ★ University of Texas, Austin
College of Pharmacy
Department of Pharmacology and Toxicology
Division of Pharmacology/Toxicology
College of Pharmacy
Austin, TX 78712-1074
Phone: (512)471-5158 **Fax:** (512)471-5002
Email: KehrerJim@mail.utexas.edu

★ 28676 ★ University of Texas Health Science Center, San Antonio
Graduate School of Biomedical Sciences
Department of Pharmacology
7703 Floyd Curl Dr.
Mail Code 7764
San Antonio, TX 78229-3900
Phone: (210)567-4220 **Fax:** (210)567-4303
Email: pharmgrad@uthscsa.edu
Website: http://pharmacology.uthscsa.edu/

★ 28677 ★ University of Texas, Houston
Graduate School of Biomedical Sciences
Department of Cell and Regulatory Biology
PO Box 20334
Houston, TX 77225
Phone: (713)500-9850 **Fax:** (713)500-9877
Email: Victoria.P.Knutson@uth.tmc.edu

★ 28678 ★ University of Texas Medical Branch, Galveston
Graduate School of Biomedical Sciences
Department of Pharmacology and Toxicology
5106 Administration Bldg.
301 University Blvd.
Galveston, TX 77555-0132
Phone: (409)772-2665 **Fax:** (409)747-0772
Email: grad.school@utmb.edu

★ 28679 ★ University of Texas Southwestern Medical Center, Dallas
Graduate School of Biomedical Sciences
Division of Cell and Molecular Biology
Division of Pharmacological Sciences
5323 Harry Hines Blvd.
Dallas, TX 75390-9004
Phone: (214)648-8099 **Fax:** (214)648-2978
Email: dcmbinfo@utsouthwestern.edu
Website: http://swnt240.swmed.edu/gradschool/webpages/dcmbhpg.htm

Utah

★ 28680 ★ University of Utah
College of Pharmacy
Department of Pharmacology and Toxicology
30 S 2000 E, Rm. 201
Salt Lake City, UT 84112
Phone: (801)581-6447 **Fax:** (801)581-4049
Email: gradapplicants@deans.pharm.utah.edu

Vermont

★ 28681 ★ University of Vermont
Graduate Studies in Pharmacology and Physiology
Department of Pharmacology
Given Medical Bldg.
Burlington, VT 05405
Phone: (802)656-2500 **Fax:** (802)656-4523
Email: jhayes@zoo.uvm.edu

Virginia

★ 28682 ★ University of Virginia
Graduate School of Arts and Sciences
Department of Pharmacology
437 Cabell Hall
Charlottesville, VA 22903
Phone: (434)924-7184 **Fax:** (804)924-6737
Email: pharmgrad@virginia.edu

★ 28683 ★ University of Virginia
UVa Health System, Department of Pharmacology
Cellular and Molecular Pharmacology
800735 UVa Health System
1300 Jefferson Park Ave.
Charlottesville, VA 22908
Phone: (434)924-1919

★ 28684 ★ Virginia Commonwealth University
School of Medicine
Department of Pharmacology and Toxicology
PO Box 980613
Richmond, VA 23298
Phone: (804)828-8400 **Fax:** (804)828-1532
Email: ssawyer@hsc.vcu.edu
Website: http://www.vcu.edu/gradweb/programs/pfmed.htmphar

Washington

★ 28685 ★ University of Washington
School of Medicine
Department of Pharmacology
PO Box 357280
Seattle, WA 98195-7280
Phone: (206)685-9252 **Fax:** (206)685-3822
Email: uwgrad@u.washington.edu

★ 28686 ★ Washington State University
Department of Pharmaceutical Sciences
Program in Pharmacology and Toxicology
PO Box 646534
Pullman, WA 99164-6534
Phone: (509)335-7598 **Fax:** (509)335-5902
Email: pharmtox@wsu.edu

West Virginia

★ 28687 ★ Marshall University
School of Medicine
Department of Biomedical Sciences
Office of Research and Graduate Education
1542 Spring Valley Dr.
Huntington, WV 25704
Phone: (304)696-7326 **Fax:** (304)696-7171
Email: gruettem@marshall.edu
Website: http://meb.marshall.edu/graduate/course.htm

★ 28688 ★ West Virginia University
School of Medicine
Department of Pharmacology and Toxicology
PO Box 9024
Morgantown, WV 26506-9024
Phone: (304)293-7116 **Fax:** (304)293-7038
Email: cnoel@hsc.wvu.edu

Wisconsin

★ 28689 ★ Medical College of Wisconsin
Graduate School of Biomedical Sciences
Department of Pharmacology and Toxicology
8701 Watertown Plank Rd.
PO Box 26509
Milwaukee, WI 53226-0509
Phone: (414)456-8218 **Fax:** (414)456-6554
Email: gradschool@mcw.edu

★ 28690 ★ University of Wisconsin, Madison
Medical School
Department of Pharmacology
Molecular and Cellular Pharmacology
3750 Medical Sciences Center
1300 University Ave.
Madison, WI 53706
Phone: (608)262-9826 **Fax:** (608)262-1257
Email: lsquire@facstaff.wisc.edu

Pharmacy

The following colleges and schools of pharmacy offer programs accredited by the American Council on Pharmaceutical Education, 20 N Clark St., Ste. 2500, Chicago, IL 60602-5109, (312)664-3575, http://www.acpe-accredit.org. For additional information on the colleges or pharmacy as a career, contact the American Association of Colleges of Pharmacy, 1426 Prince St., Alexandria, VA 22314, (703)739-2330, http://www.aacp.org/.

Alabama

★ 28691 ★ Auburn University
Harrison School of Pharmacy
217 Walker Bldg.
Auburn University, AL 36849-5501
Phone: (334)844-8348 **Fax:** (334)844-8353
Email: evansrl@auburn.edu
Website: http://pharmacy.auburn.edu
R. Lee Evans, Jr., Director

★ 28692 ★ Samford University
McWhorter School of Pharmacy
800 Lakeshore Dr.
Birmingham, AL 35229
Phone: (205)726-2820 **Fax:** (205)726-2759
Email: jodean@samford.edu
Website: http://www.samford.edu/schools/pharmacy.html
Joseph O. Dean, Jr., Director

Arizona

★ 28693 ★ Midwestern University, Glendale
College of Pharmacy
19555 N 59th Ave.
Glendale, AZ 85308
Phone: (623)572-3500 **Fax:** (623)572-3510
Email: dslark@arizona.midwestern.edu
Website: http://www.midwestern.edu/Pages/CPG.html
David J. Slatkin, PhD, Director

★ 28694 ★ University of Arizona
College of Pharmacy
1703 E Mabel St.
PO Box 210207
Tucson, AZ 85721
Phone: (520)626-1427 **Fax:** (520)626-4063
Email: bootman@pharmacy.arizona.edu
Website: http://www.pharmacy.arizona.edu
J. Lyle Bootman, PhD, Director

Arkansas

★ 28695 ★ University of Arkansas for Medical Sciences
College of Pharmacy
4301 W Markham St., Slot 522
Little Rock, AR 72205
Phone: (501)686-5557 **Fax:** (501)686-8315
Email: MilneLarryD@uams.edu
Website: http://www.uams.edu/cop
L. D. Milne, PhD, Director

California

★ 28696 ★ University of California, San Francisco
School of Pharmacy
521 Parnassus Ave., Rm. C-156
Box 0622
San Francisco, CA 94143-0622
Phone: (415)476-1225 **Fax:** (415)476-6632
Email: makx@itsa.ucsf.edu
Website: http://www.sop.ucsf.edu
Mary Anne Koda-Kimble, Director

★ 28697 ★ University of the Pacific
Thomas J. Long School of Pharmacy and Health Sciences
3601 Pacific Ave.
Stockton, CA 95211
Phone: (209)946-2561 **Fax:** (209)946-2410
Email: poppenhe@uop.edu
Website: http://www.uop.edu/pharmacy/index.html
Phillip R. Oppenheimer, Director

★ 28698 ★ University of Southern California
School of Pharmacy
1985 Zonal Ave.
Los Angeles, CA 90089-9121
Phone: (323)442-1369 **Fax:** (323)442-1681
Email: knipe@hsc.usc.edu
Website: http://pharmacy.usc.edu
Dr. Timothy M. Chan, Director

★ 28699 ★ Western University of Health Sciences
College of Pharmacy
309 E 2nd St.
Pomona, CA 91766-1854
Phone: (909)469-5500 **Fax:** (909)469-5539
Email: mdray@westernu.edu
Website: http://www.westernu.edu
Max Ray, PhD, Director

Colorado

★ 28700 ★ University of Colorado Health Sciences Center
School of Pharmacy
4200 E 9th Ave., C-238
Denver, CO 80262
Phone: (303)315-5055 **Fax:** (303)315-6281
Email: louis.diamond@uchsc.edu
Website: http://www.uchsc.edu/sp/sp
Louis Diamond, PhD, Director

Connecticut

★ 28701 ★ University of Connecticut
School of Pharmacy
372 Fairfield Rd., Unit 2092
Storrs, CT 06269-2092
Phone: (860)486-2129 **Fax:** (860)486-1553
Email: michael.gerald@uconn.edu
Website: http://pharmacy.uconn.edu
Michael C. Gerald, PhD, Director

District of Columbia

★ 28702 ★ Howard University
College of Pharmacy
2300 4th St. NW
Washington, DC 20059
Phone: (202)806-5431 **Fax:** (202)234-1375
Email: plecca@howard.edu
Website: http://www.howard.edu
Pedro J. Lecca, PhD, Director

Florida

★ 28703 ★ Florida Agricultural and Mechanical (A&M) University
College of Pharmacy and Pharmaceutical Sciences
201 Dyson Pharmacy Bldg.
Tallahassee, FL 32307
Phone: (850)559-3301 **Fax:** (850)559-3347
Email: henry.lewisiii@famu.edu
Website: http://www.famu.edu/copps
Henry Lewis, III, Director

★ 28704 ★ Nova Southeastern University
College of Pharmacy
3200 S University Dr.
Fort Lauderdale, FL 33328
Phone: (954)262-1300 **Fax:** (954)262-2278
Email: hardigan@nova.edu
Website: http://www.nova.edu/cwis/centers/hdp/pharmacy
William D. Hardigan, PhD, Director

★ 28705 ★ Palm Beach Atlantic College
School of Pharmacy
901 S Flagler Dr.
PO Box 24708
West Palm Beach, FL 33416-4708
Phone: (561)803-2700 **Fax:** (561)803-2703
Email: swigarts@pbac.edu
Website: http://www.pbac.edu
Scott Swigart, Director

★ 28706 ★ University of Florida
College of Pharmacy
J. Hillis Miller Health Center
1600 SE Archer Rd., Rm. 454
Box 100484
Gainesville, FL 32610
Phone: (352)392-9714 **Fax:** (352)392-3480
Website: http://www.cop.ufl.edu
William H. Riffee, PhD, Director

Georgia

★ 28707 ★ Mercer University
Southern School of Pharmacy
3001 Mercer University Dr.
Atlanta, GA 30341-4415
Phone: (678)547-6304 **Fax:** (678)547-6315
Email: matthews_h@mercer.edu
Website: http://www.mercer.edu/dean_phm.htm
H. W. Matthews, PhD, Director

★ 28708 ★ University of Georgia
College of Pharmacy
Athens, GA 30602-2351
Phone: (706)542-1914 **Fax:** (706)542-5269
Email: soie@mail.rx.uga.edu
Website: http://www.rx.uga.edu
Svein Oie, PhD, Director

Idaho

★ 28709 ★ Idaho State University
College of Pharmacy
Box 8288
Pocatello, ID 83209
Phone: (208)282-2175 **Fax:** (208)282-4482
Email: jsteiner@pharmacy.isu.edu
Website: http://rx.isu.edu
Joseph F. Steiner, Director

Illinois

★ 28710 ★ Midwestern University
Chicago College of Pharmacy
555 31st St.
Downers Grove, IL 60515
Phone: (630)971-6417 **Fax:** (630)971-6097
Email: mleexx@midwestern.edu
Website: http://www.midwestern.edu/Pages/CCP.html
Mary Lee, Director

★ 28711 ★ University of Illinois, Chicago
College of Pharmacy
833 S Wood St.
M/C 874
Chicago, IL 60612
Phone: (312)996-7240 **Fax:** (312)996-3272
Email: sagraves@uic.edu
Website: http://www.uic.edu/pharmacy
Rosalie Sagraves, Director

Indiana

★ 28712 ★ Butler University
College of Pharmacy and Health Sciences
4600 Sunset Ave.
Indianapolis, IN 46208
Phone: (317)940-9735 **Fax:** (317)940-6172
Email: pchase@butler.edu
Website: http://www.butler.edu/www/cophs
Patricia Chase, PhD, Director

★ 28713 ★ Purdue University
School of Pharmacy and Pharmacal Sciences
1330 Heine Pharmacy Bldg.
West Lafayette, IN 47907
Phone: (765)494-1368 **Fax:** (765)494-7880
Email: chipr@pharmacy.purdue.edu
Website: http://www.pharmacy.purdue.edu/index.html
Charles O. Rutledge, PhD, Director

Iowa

★ 28714 ★ Drake University
College of Pharmacy and Health Sciences
25th and University Aves.
Des Moines, IA 50311
Phone: (515)271-1814 **Fax:** (515)271-4171
Email: stephen.hoag@drake.edu
Website: http://www.pharmacy.drake.edu
Stephen G. Hoag, PhD, Director

★ 28715 ★ University of Iowa
College of Pharmacy
Iowa City, IA 52242
Phone: (319)335-8794 **Fax:** (319)335-5594
Email: jordan-cohen@uiowa.edu
Website: http://www.uiowa.edu/~pharmacy
Jordan Cohen, PhD, Director

Kansas

★ 28716 ★ University of Kansas
School of Pharmacy
Malott Hall, Rm. 2056
1251 Wescoe Hall Dr.
Lawrence, KS 66045-2500
Phone: (785)864-3591 **Fax:** (785)864-5265
Email: jfincham@ku.edu
Website: http://www.pharm.ukans.edu/dean/index.htm
Jack E. Fincham, PhD, Director

Kentucky

★ 28717 ★ University of Kentucky
College of Pharmacy
907 Rose St., Ste. 327
Lexington, KY 40536-0082
Phone: (859)323-7601 **Fax:** (859)257-2128
Email: krobe2@pop.uky.edu
Website: http://www.uky.edu/Pharmacy
Kenneth B. Roberts, PhD, Director

Louisiana

★ 28718 ★ University of Louisiana, Monroe
College of Pharmacy
700 University Ave.
Monroe, LA 71209-0400
Phone: (318)342-1600 **Fax:** (318)342-1606
Email: pybourn@ulm.edu
Website: http://www.ulm.edu
William M. Bourn, PhD, Director

★ 28719 ★ Xavier University of Louisiana
College of Pharmacy
1 Drexel Dr.
New Orleans, LA 70125
Phone: (504)483-7424 **Fax:** (504)485-7930
Email: wharris@xula.edu
Website: http://www.xula.edu
Wayne T. Harris, PhD, Director

Maryland

★ 28720 ★ University of Maryland
School of Pharmacy
20 N Pine St., Rm. 730
Baltimore, MD 21201-1180
Phone: (410)706-7651 **Fax:** (410)706-4012
Email: dknapp@rx.umaryland.edu
Website: http://www.pharmacy.umaryland.edu
David A. Knapp, PhD, Director

Massachusetts

★ 28721 ★ Massachusetts College of Pharmacy and Health Sciences, Boston
179 Longwood Ave.
Boston, MA 02115
Phone: (617)732-2108 **Fax:** (617)732-2244
Email: abelmonte@mcp.edu
Website: http://www.mcp.edu
Albert A. Belmonte, PhD, Director

★ 28722 ★ Massachusetts College of Pharmacy and Health Sciences, Worcester
School of Pharmacy
19 Foster St.
Worcester, MA 01608
Phone: (508)890-8855 **Fax:** (508)890-8515
Email: dpisano@mcp.edu
Website: http://www.mcp.edu
Douglas Pisano, PhD, Director

★ 28723 ★ Northeastern University
School of Pharmacy
206 Mugar Hall
Boston, MA 02115
Phone: (617)373-8917 **Fax:** (617)373-7655
Email: d.robinson@neu.edu
Website: http://www.neu.edu/bouve/pharma.html
Daniel C. Robinson, Director

Michigan

★ 28724 ★ Ferris State University
College of Pharmacy
220 Ferris Dr.
Big Rapids, MI 49307
Phone: (231)591-2254 **Fax:** (231)591-3829
Email: Ian_Mathison@ferris.edu
Website: http://www.pharmacy.ferris.edu
Ian W. Mathison, PhD, Director

★ 28725 ★ University of Michigan
College of Pharmacy
428 Church St.
Ann Arbor, MI 48109-1065
Phone: (734)764-7312 **Fax:** (734)763-2022
Email: gkenyon@umich.edu
Website: http://www.umich.edu/~pharmacy
George L. Kenyon, PhD, Director

★ 28726 ★ Wayne State University
Eugene Applebaum College of Pharmacy and Health Sciences
105 Shapero Hall
Detroit, MI 48202
Phone: (313)577-1574 **Fax:** (313)577-0457
Email: bschmoll@wizard.pharm.wayne.edu
Website: http://wizard.pharm.wayne.edu/welcome.html
Beverly J. Schmoll, PhD, Director

Minnesota

★ 28727 ★ University of Minnesota
College of Pharmacy
308 Harvard St. SE
5-130 Weaver-Densford Hall
Minneapolis, MN 55455-0343
Phone: (612)624-1900 **Fax:** (612)624-2974
Email: speed001@tc.umn.edu
Website: http://www.pharmacy.umn.edu
Marilyn K. Speedie, PhD, Director

Mississippi

★ 28728 ★ University of Mississippi
School of Pharmacy
PO Box 1848
University, MS 38677
Phone: (662)915-7265 **Fax:** (662)915-5118
Email: wells@olemiss.edu
Website: http://www.olemiss.edu/depts/pharm_school
Barbara G. Wells, Director

Missouri

★ 28729 ★ Saint Louis College of Pharmacy
4588 Parkview Pl.
Saint Louis, MO 63110
Phone: (314)367-8700 **Fax:** (314)367-2784
Email: kkirk@stlcop.edu
Website: http://www.stlcop.edu
Kenneth W. Kirk, PhD, Director

★ 28730 ★ University of Missouri, Kansas City
School of Pharmacy
5005 Rockhill Rd.
Kansas City, MO 64110-2499
Phone: (816)235-1609 **Fax:** (816)235-5190
Email: rpiepho@cctr.umkc.edu
Website: http://www.umkc.edu/pharmacy
Robert W. Piepho, PhD, Director

Montana

★ 28731 ★ University of Montana
School of Pharmacy and Allied Health Sciences
340 Skaggs Bldg.
Missoula, MT 59812-1512
Phone: (406)243-4621 **Fax:** (406)243-4209
Email: forbesds@selway.umt.edu
Website: http://www.umt.edu/pharmacy
David S. Forbes, PhD, Director

Nebraska

★ 28732 ★ Creighton University
School of Pharmacy and Allied Health Professions
2500 California Plaza
Omaha, NE 68178
Phone: (402)280-2950 **Fax:** (402)280-5738
Email: stohs@creighton.edu
Website: http://www.spahp.creighton.edu
Sidney J. Stohs, PhD, Director

★ 28733 ★ University of Nebraska Medical Center
College of Pharmacy
986000 Nebraska Medical Center
Omaha, NE 68198-6000
Phone: (402)559-4333 **Fax:** (402)559-5060
Email: cueda@unmc.edu
Website: http://www.unmc.edu/Pharmacy/college.html
Clarence T. Ueda, PhD, Director

New Jersey

★ 28734 ★ Rutgers, the State University of New Jersey
Ernest Mario School of Pharmacy
William Levine Hall
160 Frelinghuysen Rd.
Piscataway, NJ 08854-8020
Phone: (732)445-2675 **Fax:** (732)445-5767
Email: jlcolaiz@rci.rutgers.edu
Website: http://www.pharmacy.rutgers.edu
John L. Colaizzi, PhD, Director

New Mexico

★ 28735 ★ University of New Mexico
College of Pharmacy
2502 Marble NE
Albuquerque, NM 87131-5691
Phone: (505)272-3241 **Fax:** (505)272-6749
Email: wmhadley@unm.edu
Website: http://www.hsc.unm.edu/Pharmacy.html
William Hadley, PhD, Director

New York

★ 28736 ★ Albany College of Pharmacy
106 New Scotland Ave.
Albany, NY 12208
Phone: (518)445-7200 **Fax:** (518)445-7294
Email: andritzm@acp.edu
Website: http://www.acp.edu
Mary H. Andritz, Director

★ 28737 ★ Long Island University
Arnold and Marie Schwartz College of Pharmacy and Health Sciences
75 DeKalb Ave. at University Plaza
Brooklyn, NY 11201
Phone: (718)488-1004 **Fax:** (718)488-0628
Email: sgross@liu.edu
Website: http://www.liunet.edu
Stephen M. Gross, PhD, Director

★ 28738 ★ Saint John's University
College of Pharmacy and Allied Health Professions
8000 Utopia Pkwy.
Jamaica, NY 11439
Phone: (718)990-6411 **Fax:** (718)990-1871
Email: mangionr@stjohns.edu
Website: http://www.stjohns.edu
Robert A. Mangione, EdD, Director

★ 28739 ★ University of Buffalo/State University of New York
School of Pharmacy and Pharmaceutical Sciences
126 Cooke Hall
Amherst, NY 14260-1200
Phone: (716)645-2823 **Fax:** (716)645-3688
Email: wka@buffalo.edu
Website: http://www.pharmacy.buffalo.edu
Wayne K. Anderson, PhD, Director

North Carolina

★ 28740 ★ Campbell University
School of Pharmacy
Buies Creek, NC 27506
Phone: (910)893-1200 **Fax:** (910)893-1943
Email: maddox@mailcenter.edu
Website: http://www.campbell.edu/pharmacy
Ronald W. Maddox, PhD, Director

★ 28741 ★ University of North Carolina, Chapel Hill
School of Pharmacy
Beard Hall
Campus Box 7360
Chapel Hill, NC 27599
Phone: (919)966-1121 **Fax:** (919)966-6919
Email: bill_campbell@unc.edu
Website: http://www.pharmacy.unc.edu
William H. Campbell, PhD, Director

North Dakota

★ 28742 ★ North Dakota State University
College of Pharmacy
123 Sudro Hall
Fargo, ND 58105-5055
Phone: (701)231-7609 **Fax:** (701)231-7606
Email: charles.peterson@ndsu.nodak.edu
Website: http://www.ndsu.nodak.edu/pharmacy
Charles D. Peterson, PhD, Director

Ohio

★ 28743 ★ Ohio Northern University
College of Pharmacy
Ada, OH 45810
Phone: (419)772-2277 **Fax:** (419)772-2720
Email: b-bryant@onu.edu
Website: http://www.onu.edu/Pharmacy
Bobby Bryant, Director

★ 28744 ★ Ohio State University
College of Pharmacy
500 W 12th Ave.
Columbus, OH 43210
Phone: (614)292-5711 **Fax:** (614)292-3113
Email: cassady.l@osu.edu
Website: http://www.pharmacy.ohio-state.edu
John M. Cassady, PhD, Director

★ 28745 ★ University of Cincinnati
College of Pharmacy
PO Box 670004
Cincinnati, OH 45267-0004
Phone: (513)558-3326 **Fax:** (513)558-4372
Email: Daniel.Acosta@uc.edu
Website: http://www.pharmacy.uc.edu
Daniel Acosta, Jr., P, Director

★ 28746 ★ University of Toledo
College of Pharmacy
2801 W Bancroft St.
Toledo, OH 43606-3390
Phone: (419)530-1931 **Fax:** (419)530-1907
Email: johnnie.early@utoledo.edu
Website: http://www.utoledo.edu/pharmacy
Johnnie L. Early, II, Ph, Director

Oklahoma

★ 28747 ★ Southwestern Oklahoma State University
School of Pharmacy
100 Campus Dr.
Weatherford, OK 73096
Phone: (580)774-3105 **Fax:** (580)774-7020
Email: bergmad@swosu.edu
Website: http://www.swosu.edu/depts/pharmacy/index.html
H. David Bergman, PhD, Director

★ 28748 ★ University of Oklahoma
College of Pharmacy
1110 N Stonewall Ave.
PO Box 26901
Oklahoma City, OK 73190
Phone: (405)271-6485 **Fax:** (405)271-3830
Email: carl-buckner@ouhsc.edu
Website: http://www.oupharmacy.com
Carl K. Buckner, PhD, Director

Oregon

★ 28749 ★ Oregon State University
College of Pharmacy
203 Pharmacy Bldg.
Corvallis, OR 97331-3507
Phone: (541)737-3424 **Fax:** (541)737-3999
Email: Wayne.Kradjan@orst.edu
Website: http://pharmacy.orst.edu
Wayne A. Kradjan, Director

Pennsylvania

★ 28750 ★ Duquesne University
Mylan School of Pharmacy
306 Bayer Learning Ctr.
Pittsburgh, PA 15282-1504
Phone: (412)396-6377 **Fax:** (412)396-1810
Email: vanderveen@duq.edu
Website: http://www.duq.edu/pharmacy/pharmacy.htm
R. Pete Vanderveen, PhD, Director

★ 28751 ★ Lake Erie College of Osteopathic Medicine
School of Pharmacy
1858 W Grandview Blvd.
Erie, PA 16509
Phone: (814)866-6641 **Fax:** (814)866-8123
Email: dswaffar@lecom.edu
Website: http://www.lecom.edu/pharmacy
Diane Swaffar, PhD, Director

★ 28752 ★ Temple University
School of Pharmacy
3307 N Broad St.
Philadelphia, PA 19140
Phone: (215)707-4990 **Fax:** (215)707-3678
Email: peter.doukas@temple.edu
Website: http://www.temple.edu/pharmacy
Peter H. Doukas, PhD, Director

★ 28753 ★ University of Pittsburgh
School of Pharmacy
1104 Salk Hall
3501 Terrace St.
Pittsburgh, PA 15261
Phone: (412)624-3270 **Fax:** (412)648-1086
Email: rjuhl@pitt.edu
Website: http://www.pharmacy.pitt.edu
Randy P. Juhl, PhD, Director

★ 28754 ★ University of the Sciences in Philadelphia
Philadelphia College of Pharmacy
600 S 43rd St.
Philadelphia, PA 19104-4495
Phone: (215)596-8870 **Fax:** (215)596-8977
Email: gdowns@usip.edu
Website: http://www.usip.edu
George E. Downs, PhD, Director

★ 28755 ★ Wilkes University
Nesbitt School of Pharmacy
Wilkes Barre, PA 18766
Phone: (570)408-4280 **Fax:** (570)408-7828
Email: grahamb@wilkes.edu
Website: http://www.pharmacy.wilkes.edu
Bernard W. Graham, PhD, Director

Puerto Rico

★ 28756 ★ University of Puerto Rico Medical Sciences Campus
School of Pharmacy
PO Box 365067
San Juan, PR 00936-5067
Phone: (787)758-2525 **Fax:** (787)751-5680
Email: ioquendo@rcm.upr.edu
Website: http://www.upr.clu.edu
Ilia Oquendo, PhD, Director

Rhode Island

★ 28757 ★ University of Rhode Island
College of Pharmacy
41 Lower College Rd.
Kingston, RI 02881
Phone: (401)874-2761 **Fax:** (401)874-2181
Email: del@uri.edu
Website: http://www.uri.edu/pharm
Donald E. Letendre, Director

South Carolina

★ 28758 ★ Medical University of South Carolina
College of Pharmacy
280 Calhoun St.
PO Box 250141
Charleston, SC 29425
Phone: (843)792-8450 **Fax:** (843)792-9081
Email: cormierj@musc.edu
Website: http://www.musc.edu/pharmacy
John Cormier, Director

★ 28759 ★ University of South Carolina
College of Pharmacy
Columbia, SC 29208
Phone: (803)777-4151 **Fax:** (803)777-4945
Email: sadikf@cop.sc.edu
Website: http://www.pharm.sc.edu
Farid Sadik, PhD, Director

South Dakota

★ 28760 ★ South Dakota State University
College of Pharmacy
Box 2202-C
Brookings, SD 57007-0099
Phone: (605)688-6197 **Fax:** (605)688-6232
Email: danny-lattin@sdstate.edu
Website: http://www3.sdstate.edu/Academics/CollegeOfPharmacy
Danny L. Lattin, PhD, Director

Tennessee

★ 28761 ★ University of Tennessee, Memphis
College of Pharmacy
847 Monroe Ave., Ste. 226
Memphis, TN 38163
Phone: (901)448-6036 **Fax:** (901)448-7053
Email: dgourley@utmem.edu
Website: http://www.pharmacy.utmem.edu
Dick R. Gourley, PhD, Director

Texas

★ 28762 ★ Texas Southern University
College of Pharmacy and Health Sciences
3100 Cleburne Ave.
Houston, TX 77004
Phone: (713)313-7164 **Fax:** (713)313-1091
Email: hayes_be@tsu.edu
Website: http://www.tsu.edu
Dick Gourley, Director

★ 28763 ★ Texas Tech University Health Sciences Center
School of Pharmacy
1300 S Coulter
Amarillo, TX 79106
Phone: (806)354-5463 **Fax:** (806)356-4613
Email: arthur@cortex.ama.ttuhsc.edu
Website: http://www.pharmacy.ama.ttuhsc.edu
Arthur A. Nelson, Jr., P, Director

★ 28764 ★ University of Houston
College of Pharmacy
141 Sciences and Research 2 Bldg.
Houston, TX 77204-5000
Phone: (713)743-1300 **Fax:** (713)743-5678
Email: mlokhandwala@uh.edu
Website: http://www.pharmacy.uh.edu
Mustafa F. Lokhandwala, PhD, Director

★ 28765 ★ University of Texas, Austin
College of Pharmacy
Austin, TX 78712-1074
Phone: (512)471-1737 **Fax:** (512)471-8783
Email: sleslie@mail.utexas.ed
Website: http://www.utexas.edu/pharmacy
Steven W. Leslie, PhD, Director

Utah

★ 28766 ★ University of Utah
College of Pharmacy
30 South 2000 East, Rm. 201
Salt Lake City, UT 84112-5820
Phone: (801)581-6731 **Fax:** (801)581-3716
Email: jmauger@deans.pharm.utah.edu
Website: http://www.pharmacy.utah.edu
John W. Mauger, PhD, Director

Virginia

★ 28767 ★ Hampton University
School of Pharmacy
Hampton, VA 23668
Phone: (757)727-5071 **Fax:** (757)727-5840
Email: arcelia.johnson-fannin@hamptonu.edu
Website: http://www.hamptonu.edu
Arcelia Johnson-Fannin, Director

★ 28768 ★ Shenandoah University
Bernard J. Dunn School of Pharmacy
1460 University Dr.
Winchester, VA 22601
Phone: (540)665-1282 **Fax:** (540)665-1283
Email: amckay@su.edu
Website: http://www.su.edu/pharmacy
Alan B. McKay, PhD, Director

★ 28769 ★ Virginia Commonwealth University
Medical College of Virginia
School of Pharmacy
410 N 12th St.
MCV Box 980581
Richmond, VA 23298-0581
Phone: (804)828-3006 **Fax:** (804)827-0002
Email: vayanchi@vcu.edu
Website: http://www.pharmacy.vcu.edu
Victor A. Yanchick, PhD, Director

Washington

★ 28770 ★ University of Washington
School of Pharmacy
H364 Health Sciences
Box 357631
Seattle, WA 98195-7631
Phone: (206)543-2030 **Fax:** (206)685-9297
Email: sidnels@u.washington.edu
Website: http://www.depts.washington.edu/pha
Sidney D. Nelson, Jr., P, Director

★ 28771 ★ Washington State University
College of Pharmacy
PO Box 646510
Pullman, WA 99164-6510
Phone: (509)335-4750 **Fax:** (509)335-2530
Email: fassett@mail.wsu.edu
Website: http://www.pharmacy.wsu.edu
William E. Fassett, PhD, Director

West Virginia

★ 28772 ★ West Virginia University
School of Pharmacy
1136 Health Sciences Center N
PO Box 9500
Morgantown, WV 26506-9500
Phone: (304)293-5101 **Fax:** (304)293-5483
Email: gspratto@hsc.wvu.edu
Website: http://www.hsc.wvu.edu/sop/index.html
George R. Spratto, PhD, Director

Wisconsin

★ 28773 ★ University of Wisconsin, Madison
School of Pharmacy
777 Highland Ave.
Madison, WI 53705-2222
Phone: (608)262-1414 **Fax:** (608)262-3397
Email: mhw@pharmacy.wisc.edu
Website: http://www.wisc.edu/pharmacy
Melvin H. Weinswig, PhD, Director

Wyoming

★ 28774 ★ University of Wyoming
School of Pharmacy
Box 3375
Laramie, WY 82071-3375
Phone: (307)766-6120 **Fax:** (307)766-2953
Email: uwpharmacy@uwyo.edu
Website: http://www.uwyo.edu/pharmacy
Paul L. Ranelli, PhD, Director

Physical Therapy

The following programs for physical therapists are accredited by the American Physical Therapy Association (APTA), 1111 N Fairfax St., Alexandria, VA 22314, (800)999-APTA, http://www.apta.org/. The APTA also accredits and maintains a listing of educational programs for physical therapy assistants.

Alabama

★ 28775 ★ University of Alabama, Birmingham
School of Health Related Professions
Physical Therapist Program
Bishop Bldg., Rm. 102
1530 3rd Ave. S
Birmingham, AL 35294-2030
Phone: (205)934-3566 **Fax:** (205)975-7787
Email: sshaw@uab.edu
Website: http://main.uab.edu/show.asp?durki=3415
Sharon Shaw, DrPH, Director

★ 28776 ★ **University of South Alabama**
Department of Physical Therapy
Physical Therapist Program
1504 Springhill Ave., Rm. 1214
Mobile, AL 36604
Phone: (251)434-3575 **Fax:** (251)434-3822
Website: http://www.usouthal.edu/usa/allhealth/pt.htm
Dennis W. Fell, MD, Director

Arizona

★ 28777 ★ **Arizona School for Health Sciences**
Kirksville College of Osteopathic Medicine
Physical Therapy Program
5850 E Still Cir.
Mesa, AZ 85206
Phone: (480)219-6000 **Fax:** (480)219-6100
Email: sbrown@ashs.edu
Website: http://www.ashs.edu/discpl_pt.htm
Suzanne Robben Brown, Director

★ 28778 ★ **Northern Arizona University**
Department of Physical Therapy
Physical Therapist Program
PO Box 15105
Flagstaff, AZ 86011
Phone: (928)523-4092 **Fax:** (928)523-9289
Email: carl.derosa@nau.edu
Website: http://www.nau.edu
Carl DeRosa, PhD, Director

Arkansas

★ 28779 ★ **Arkansas State University**
College of Nursing and Health Professions
Physical Therapy Program
PO Box 910
State University, AR 72467-0910
Phone: (870)972-3591 **Fax:** (870)972-3652
Email: jguffey@astate.edu
Website: http://pt.astate.edu
J. Stephen Guffey, EdD, Director

★ 28780 ★ **University of Central Arkansas**
Department of Physical Therapy
Physical Therapist Program
201 Donaghey, PTC 300
Conway, AR 72035-0001
Phone: (501)450-3611 **Fax:** (501)450-5822
Email: venitaL@mail.uca.edu
Website: http://www.uca.edu/divisions/academic/pt
Venita Lovelace-Chandler, PhD, Director

California

★ 28781 ★ **Azusa Pacific University**
Physical Therapist Program
901 E Alosta Ave.
Azusa, CA 91702-7000
Phone: (626)815-5020 **Fax:** (626)815-5017
Email: mlaymon@apu.edu
Website: http://www.apu.edu/clas/grad/pt
Michael Laymon, Director

★ 28782 ★ **California State University, Fresno**
Physical Therapist Program
2345 E San Ramon Ave., MS-MH 29
Fresno, CA 93740-8031
Phone: (559)278-2625 **Fax:** (559)278-3635
Email: janetd@csufresno.edu
Website: http://www.csufresno.edu/physicaltherapy
Janet K. Duttarer, PhD, Director

★ 28783 ★ **California State University, Long Beach**
College of Health and Human Services
Physical Therapist Program
1250 Bellflower Blvd.
Long Beach, CA 90840
Phone: (562)985-4072 **Fax:** (562)985-4069
Email: rjmorris@csulb.edu
Website: http://www.csulb.edu
Ray J. Morris, Director

★ 28784 ★ **California State University, Northridge**
Department of Health Sciences
Physical Therapist Program
Northridge, CA 91330-8285
Phone: (818)677-4081 **Fax:** (818)677-3101
Email: george.wolfe@csun.edu
Website: http://www.csun.edu
George A. Wolfe, PhD, Director

★ 28785 ★ **California State University, Sacramento**
College of Health and Human Services
Physical Therapist Program
6000 J St.
Sacramento, CA 95819-6020
Phone: (916)278-6426 **Fax:** (916)278-5053
Email: mcgintys@csus.edu
Website: http://www.hhs.csus.edu
Susan M. McGinty, EdD, Director

★ 28786 ★ **Chapman University**
Department of Physical Therapy
Physical Therapist Program
1 University Dr.
Orange, CA 92866
Phone: (714)744-7620 **Fax:** (714)744-7621
Email: gabard@chapman.edu
Website: http://www.chapman.edu/wilkinson/pt
Donald L. Gabard, PhD, Director

★ 28787 ★ **Loma Linda University**
School of Allied Health Professions
Department of Physical Therapy
Physical Therapist Program
Loma Linda, CA 92350
Phone: (909)824-4632 **Fax:** (909)824-4291
Email: lchinnock@sahp.llu.edu
Website: http://www.llu.edu
Larry Chinnock, EdD, Director

★ 28788 ★ **Mount Saint Mary's College**
Department of Physical Therapy
Physical Therapist Program
12001 Chalon Rd.
Los Angeles, CA 90049-1599
Phone: (310)954-4171 **Fax:** (310)954-4179
Email: cmoore@msmc.la.edu
Website: http://www.msmc.la.edu/Academics/Majors-Programs/Master%20Physical%20Therapy/PT.htm
Cynthia L. Moore, Director

★ 28789 ★ **Samuel Merritt College**
Physical Therapist Program
370 Hawthorne Ave.
Oakland, CA 94609
Phone: (510)869-6241 **Fax:** (510)869-6282
Email: mjewell@samuelmerritt.edu
Website: http://www.samuelmerritt.edu
Martha J. Jewell, PhD, Director

★ 28790 ★ **University of California, San Francisco/San Francisco State University**
Department of Physical Therapy and Rehabilitation Science
Physical Therapist Program
1320 7th Ave.
Box 0736
San Francisco, CA 94143-0736
Phone: (415)338-2001 **Fax:** (415)338-0907
Email: gppt@sfsu.edu
Website: http://www.ucsf.edu
Nancy Byl, PhD, Director

★ 28791 ★ **University of the Pacific**
School of Pharmacy and Health Sciences
Department of Physical Therapy
Physical Therapist Program
Stockton, CA 95211
Phone: (209)946-2886 **Fax:** (209)946-2367
Email: dumphred@uop.edu
Website: http://www.uop.edu
Darcy Umphred, PhD, Director

★ 28792 ★ **University of Southern California**
Department of Biokinesiology & Physical Therapy
Physical Therapist Program
1540 E Alcazar St., CHP 155
Los Angeles, CA 90089-9006
Phone: (323)442-2890 **Fax:** (323)442-1515
Email: jamesgor@usc.edu
Website: http://www.usc.edu
James Gordon, EdD, Director

★ 28793 ★ **Western University of Health Sciences**
Department of Physical Therapy Education
Physical Therapist Program
309 E 2nd St.
Pomona, CA 91766-1854
Phone: (909)469-5294 **Fax:** (909)469-5692
Email: dredmanbentley@westernu.edu
Website: http://www.westernu.edu/cahp.html
Donna Redman-Bentley, PhD, Director

Colorado

★ 28794 ★ **Regis University**
Department of Physical Therapy
Physical Therapist Program
3333 Regis Blvd.
Mail Code G-4
Denver, CO 80221-1099
Phone: (303)458-4066 **Fax:** (303)964-5474
Email: btschoep@regis.edu
Website: http://www.regis.edu
Barbara A. Tschoepe, PhD, Director

★ 28795 ★ **University of Colorado Health Science Center**
Physical Therapist Program
4200 E 9th Ave.
Box C244
Denver, CO 80262
Phone: (303)372-9144 **Fax:** (303)372-9016
Email: carolyn.heriza@uchsc.edu
Website: http://www.uchsc.edu/gs/pt
Carolyn B. Heriza, EdD, Director

Connecticut

★ 28796 ★ Quinnipiac University
School of Health Sciences
Physical Therapist Program
Mt. Carmel Ave.
Hamden, CT 06518
Phone: (203)582-5251 **Fax:** (203)582-8706
Email: tantorski@quinnipiac.edu
Website: http://www.quinnipiac.edu
Edward P. Tantorski, Director

★ 28797 ★ Sacred Heart University
Physical Therapist Program
5151 Park Ave.
Fairfield, CT 06432-1000
Phone: (203)365-7656 **Fax:** (203)365-4723
Email: emerym@sacredheart.edu
Website: http://www.sacredheart.edu
Michael J. Emery, EdD, Director

★ 28798 ★ University of Connecticut
School of Allied Health Professions
Department of Physical Therapy
Physical Therapist Program
358 Mansfield Rd., U-101
Storrs, CT 06269-2101
Phone: (860)486-2834 **Fax:** (860)486-1588
Email: hasson@uconnvm.uconn.edu
Website: http://www.alliedhealth.uconn.edu
Scott Hasson, EdD, Director

★ 28799 ★ University of Hartford
Department of Physical Therapy
Physical Therapist Program
200 Bloomfield Ave.
West Hartford, CT 06117-1599
Phone: (860)768-5303 **Fax:** (860)768-5244
Email: certo@hartford.edu
Website: http://www.hartford.edu
Catherine M. E. Certo, ScD, Director

Delaware

★ 28800 ★ University of Delaware
Department of Physical Therapy
Physical Therapist Program
303 McKinly Laboratory
Newark, DE 19716
Phone: (302)831-8910 **Fax:** (302)831-4234
Email: sbinder@udel.edu
Website: http://www.udel.edu/PT/index.html
Stuart A. Binder-MacLeod, PhD, Director

District of Columbia

★ 28801 ★ The George Washington University
School of Medicine and Health Sciences
Program in Physical Therapy
2100 M St. NW, Ste. 203
Washington, DC 20037
Phone: (202)496-8370 **Fax:** (202)496-6288
Email: hspglr@gwumc.edu
Website: http://www.gwumc.edu/healthsci
Gloria L. Rogers, Director

★ 28802 ★ Howard University
College of Pharmacy, Nursing, and Allied Health Sciences
Physical Therapist Program
6th and Bryant Sts. NW
Washington, DC 20059
Phone: (202)806-7613 **Fax:** (202)806-2820
Email: ktavakol@howard.edu
Website: http://www.howard.edu
Kamran Tavakol, PhD, Director

Florida

★ 28803 ★ Florida Agricultural and Mechanical (A&M) University
School of Allied Health Sciences
Physical Therapist Program
Ware-Rhaney Bldg., Rm. 223
Tallahassee, FL 32307-3500
Phone: (850)599-3820 **Fax:** (850)561-2457
Email: dowery@lycos.com
Website: http://www.famu.edu
Evelyn S. Dowery, EdD, Director

★ 28804 ★ Florida Gulf Coast University
Department of Physical Therapy
10501 FGCU Blvd. S
Fort Myers, FL 33965-6565
Phone: (941)590-1000 **Fax:** (941)590-1010
Email: ekwill@fgcu.edu
Website: http://www.fgcu.edu/chp/pt
Ellen Kroog Williamson, Chairman of the Board

★ 28805 ★ Florida International University
College of Health Sciences
Department of Physical Therapy
Physical Therapist Program
Miami, FL 33199
Phone: (305)348-3831 **Fax:** (305)348-1240
Email: elbauml@fiu.edu
Website: http://w3.fiu.edu/pt
Leonard Elbaum, EdD, Director

★ 28806 ★ Nova Southeastern University
College of Allied Health
Health Profession Division
Physical Therapist Program
3200 S University Dr.
Fort Lauderdale, FL 33328
Phone: (954)262-1662 **Fax:** (954)262-1783
Email: hill@nova.edu
Website: http://www.nova.edu/pt
Cheryl J. Hill, Director

★ 28807 ★ University of Central Florida
Physical Therapist Program
4000 Central Florida Blvd.
HPAI, Ste. 256
Orlando, FL 32816-2205
Phone: (407)823-3462 **Fax:** (407)823-3464
Email: kparry@mail.ucf.edu
Website: http://www.cohpa.ucf.edu/health.pro
Katherine K. Parry, PhD, Director

★ 28808 ★ University of Florida
College of Health Professions
Department of Physical Therapy
Physical Therapist Program
Box 100154 HSC
Gainesville, FL 32610-0154
Phone: (352)265-0085 **Fax:** (352)265-0731
Email: rgarrigu@hp.ufl.edu
Website: http://www.ufl.edu
Robert Garrigues, PhD, Director

★ 28809 ★ University of Miami
School of Medicine
Physical Therapist Program
5915 Ponce de Leon Blvd., 5th Fl.
Coral Gables, FL 33146
Phone: (305)284-4535 **Fax:** (305)284-6128
Email: shayes@miami.edu
Website: http://www.miami.edu
Sherrill H. Hayes, PhD, Director

★ 28810 ★ University of North Florida
College of Health
Physical Therapist Program
4567 St. John's Bluff Rd. S
Jacksonville, FL 32224
Phone: (904)620-2841 **Fax:** (904)620-2848
Email: mnonnema@unf.edu
Website: http://www.unf.edu
Margaret Nonnemacher, PhD, Director

★ 28811 ★ University of Saint Augustine for Health Sciences
Institute of Physical Therapy
Physical Therapist Program
1 University Blvd.
Saint Augustine, FL 32086
Phone: (904)826-0084 **Fax:** (904)826-0085
Email: gcgornia@usa.edu
Website: http://www.usa.edu
Gerard C. Gorniak, PhD, Director

★ 28812 ★ University of South Florida
School of Physical Therapy
12901 Bruce B Downs Blvd., MDC 77
Tampa, FL 33612
Phone: (813)974-8870 **Fax:** (813)974-8915
Email: mclenden@hsc.usf.edu
Website: http://www.hsc.usf.edu/COM/physicaltherapy
Martha Clendenin, PhD, Director

Georgia

★ 28813 ★ Armstrong Atlantic State University
Physical Therapist Program
11935 Abercorn St.
Savannah, GA 31419-1997
Phone: (912)921-2327 **Fax:** (912)921-5838
Email: lakedavi@mail.armstrong.edu
Website: http://www.pt.armstrong.edu
David A. Lake, PhD, Director

★ 28814 ★ Emory University
Division of Physical Therapy
Physical Therapist Program
1441 Clifton Rd. NE, Ste. 423
Atlanta, GA 30322
Phone: (404)712-5660 **Fax:** (404)712-4130
Email: pcatlin@emory.edu
Website: http://www.cc.emory.edu/MED/AH/PT
Pamela A. Catlin, EdD, Director

★ 28815 ★ Georgia State University
Department of Physical Therapy
Physical Therapist Program
University Plaza
Atlanta, GA 30303
Phone: (404)651-3091 **Fax:** (404)651-1584
Email: mpearl@gsu.edu
Website: http://www.gsu.edu
Marcia Pearl, PhD, Director

★ 28816 ★ Medical College of Georgia
School of Allied Health Sciences
Department of Physical Therapy
Physical Therapist Program
Augusta, GA 30912-0800
Phone: (706)721-2141 **Fax:** (706)721-3209
Email: dkeskula@mail.mcg.edu
Website: http://www.mcg.edu
Douglas R. Keskula, PhD, Director

★ 28817 ★ North Georgia College and State University
Physical Therapist Program
Barnes Hall, Rm. A-8
Dahlonega, GA 30597

Phone: (706)864-1422 **Fax:** (706)864-1493
Email: rlaird@ngcsu.edu
Website: http://www.ngc.peachnet.edu/academic/sciences/pt/pthome.htm
Robert J. Laird, PhD, Director

Idaho

★ 28818 ★ Idaho State University
Kasiska College of Health Professions
Department of Physical and Occupational Therapy
Physical Therapist Program
Box 8045
Pocatello, ID 83209
Phone: (208)282-4095 **Fax:** (208)282-4962
Email: physther@isu.edu
Website: http://www.isu.edu/departments/dpot
Alexander G. Urfer, PhD, Director

Illinois

★ 28819 ★ Bradley University
Department of Physical Therapy
Physical Therapist Program
1501 W Bradley Ave.
Peoria, IL 61625
Phone: (309)677-3489 **Fax:** (309)677-4053
Email: jun@bumail.bradley.edu
Website: http://www.bradley.edu/academics/ehs/pt/pt_index.html
Mary Jo Mays, PhD, Director

★ 28820 ★ Governors State University
College of Health Professions
Physical Therapist Program
University Park, IL 60466
Phone: (708)534-7290 **Fax:** (708)534-1647
Email: r-carter@govst.edu
Website: http://www.govst.edu/mpt
Russell E. Carter, EdD, Director

★ 28821 ★ The Herman M. Finch University of Health Sciences /Chicago Medical School
School of Related Health Sciences
Physical Therapist Program
3333 Green Bay Rd.
North Chicago, IL 60064
Phone: (847)578-3307 **Fax:** (847)578-8816
Email: schuitd@finchcms.edu
Website: http://www.finchcms.edu
Dale Schuit, PhD, Director

★ 28822 ★ Midwestern University
College of Health Sciences
Physical Therapist Program
555 31st St.
Downers Grove, IL 60515
Phone: (630)515-6462 **Free:** 800-458-6253
Fax: (630)515-7224
Email: dcechx@midwestern.edu
Website: http://www.midwestern.edu/Pages/PTP.html
Donna Cech, Director

★ 28823 ★ Northern Illinois University
School of Allied Health Professions
Physical Therapist Program
DeKalb, IL 60115
Phone: (815)753-1383 **Fax:** (815)753-0720
Email: mblascha@niu.edu
Website: http://www.niu.edu
M. J. Blaschak, PhD, Director

★ 28824 ★ Northwestern University Medical School
Department of Physical Therapy and Human Movement Sciences
Physical Therapist Program
645 N Michigan Ave., Ste. 1100
Chicago, IL 60611-2814
Phone: (312)908-8160 **Fax:** (312)908-0741
Email: k-hayes@northwestern.edu
Website: http://www.nupt.nwu.edu
Karen W. Hayes, PhD, Director

★ 28825 ★ University of Illinois, Chicago
College of Applied Health Sciences
Physical Therapist Program
1919 W Taylor St., M/C 898
Chicago, IL 60612
Phone: (312)996-7764 **Fax:** (312)996-3807
Email: astorto@uic.edu
Website: http://www.uic.edu/ahp/pt
Suzann K. Campbell, PhD, Director

Indiana

★ 28826 ★ Indiana University
School of Allied Health Sciences
Physical Therapist Program
Coleman Hall 120
1140 W Michigan St.
Indianapolis, IN 46202-5119
Phone: (317)278-1875 **Fax:** (317)278-1876
Email: wsquille@iupui.edu
Website: http://www.indiana.edu/
William S. Quillen, PhD, Director

★ 28827 ★ University of Evansville
Department of Physical Therapy
Physical Therapist Program
1800 Lincoln Ave.
Evansville, IN 47722
Phone: (812)479-2345 **Free:** 800-423-8633
Fax: (812)479-2717
Email: mk43@evansville.edu
Website: http://www.evansville.edu
Mary P. Kessler, Director

★ 28828 ★ University of Indianapolis
Krannert School of Physical Therapy
Physical Therapist Program
1400 E Hanna Ave.
Indianapolis, IN 46227-3697
Phone: (317)788-3500 **Fax:** (317)788-3542
Email: cgraham@uindy.edu
Website: http://www.uindy.edu
Cecilia Graham, PhD, Director

Iowa

★ 28829 ★ Clarke College
Department of Physical Therapy
Physical Therapist Program
1550 Clarke Dr.
Dubuque, IA 52001-3198
Phone: (319)588-6382 **Fax:** (319)588-6789
Email: jbrasseu@clarke.edu
Website: http://www.clarke.edu
Jeannette Brasseur, PhD, Director

★ 28830 ★ Des Moines University, Osteopathic Medical Center
College of Health Sciences
Physical Therapist Program
3200 Grand Ave.
Des Moines, IA 50312
Phone: (515)271-1634 **Free:** 800-240-2767
Fax: (515)271-1714
Email: Susan.Cigelman@dmu.edu
Website: http://www.dmu.edu/pt/index.htm
M. Susan Cigelman, EdD, Director

★ 28831 ★ Saint Ambrose University
College of Human Services
Department of Physical Therapy
Physical Therapist Program
518 W Locust
Davenport, IA 52803
Phone: (563)333-6403 **Fax:** (563)333-6410
Email: pt@sau.edu
Website: http://web.sau.edu/mpt
Sandra L. Cassady, PhD, Director

★ 28832 ★ University of Iowa
College of Medicine
Physical Therapist Program
2600 Steindler Bldg.
Iowa City, IA 52242-1008
Phone: (319)335-9791 **Fax:** (319)335-9707
Email: david-nielsen@uiowa.edu
Website: http://www.uiowa.edu
David H. Nielsen, PhD, Director

Kansas

★ 28833 ★ University of Kansas Medical Center
Department of Physical Therapy Education
Physical Therapist Program
3056 Robinson Hall
3901 Rainbow Blvd.
Kansas City, KS 66160-7601
Phone: (913)588-6799 **Fax:** (913)588-4568
Email: Enwemeka@kumc.edu
Website: http://www.kumc.edu/SAH/pted/
Chukuka Enwemeka, PhD, Director

★ 28834 ★ Wichita State University
College of Health Professions
Physical Therapist Program
1845 Fairmont
Wichita, KS 67260-0043
Phone: (316)978-3604 **Fax:** (316)978-3025
Email: wilson@chp.twsu.edu
Website: http://chp.wichita.edu/pt
Camilla M. Wilson, PhD, Director

Kentucky

★ 28835 ★ Bellarmine University
Lansing School of Nursing and Health Sciences
Physical Therapist Program
Miles Hall, Rm. 105
2001 Newburg Rd.
Louisville, KY 40205
Phone: (502)852-7816 **Fax:** (502)852-4597
Email: mwiegand@bellarmine.edu
Mark Wiegand, PhD, Director

★ 28836 ★ University of Kentucky
Physical Therapist Program
213 CAHP Bldg.
121 Washington Ave.
Lexington, KY 40506-0003
Phone: (859)323-1100 **Fax:** (859)257-1816
Email: trmalo1@pop.uky.edu
Website: http://www.uky.edu/
Terry R. Malone, EdD, Director

Louisiana

★ 28837 ★ Louisiana State University Health Sciences Center, New Orleans
School of Allied Health Professions
Physical Therapist Program
1900 Gravier St.
LSU Health Sciences Center
New Orleans, LA 70112
Phone: (504)568-4288 **Fax:** (504)568-6552

Website: http://www.lsumc.edu
Elizabeth Weiss, PhD, Director

★ 28838 ★ Louisiana State University Health Sciences Center, Shreveport
School of Allied Health Professions
Physical Therapist Program
1501 Kings Hwy.
PO Box 33932
Shreveport, LA 71130-3932
Phone: (318)675-6820 **Fax:** (318)675-6937
Email: sdunn2@lsumc.edu
Website: http://www.lsumc.edu
Sharon Dunn, Director

Maine

★ 28839 ★ Husson College
Physical Therapist Program
1 College Circle
Bangor, ME 04401
Phone: (207)941-7101 **Fax:** (207)941-7883
Email: sidaway@husson.edu
Website: http://www.husson.edu/pt
Ben Sidaway, PhD, Director

★ 28840 ★ University of New England
Department of Physical Therapy
Physical Therapist Program
11 Hills Beach Rd.
Biddeford, ME 04005
Phone: (207)283-0171 **Fax:** (207)294-5926
Email: msheldon@une.edu
Website: http://www.une.edu
Mike Sheldon, Director

Maryland

★ 28841 ★ University of Maryland, Baltimore
School of Medicine
Physical Therapist Program
100 Penn St., Rm. 115
Baltimore, MD 21201
Phone: (410)706-7720 **Fax:** (410)706-6387
Email: mrodgers@umaryland.edu
Website: http://pt.umaryland.edu
Mary M. Rodgers, PhD, Director

★ 28842 ★ University of Maryland, Eastern Shore
Department of Physical Therapy
Physical Therapist Program
Kiah Hall, 1st Fl.
Princess Anne, MD 21853-1299
Phone: (410)651-6360 **Fax:** (410)651-6259
Email: rlblakely@mail.umes.edu
Website: http://www.umes.edu/pt
Raymond L. Blakely, PhD, Director

Massachusetts

★ 28843 ★ American International College
Physical Therapist Program
1000 State St.
Springfield, MA 01109-9983
Phone: (413)205-3412 **Fax:** (413)788-9961
Email: eswanson@acad.aic.edu
Website: http://www.aic.edu/web/ptherapy/index.htm
Edward Swanson, Director

★ 28844 ★ Boston University
Sargent College of Health and Rehabilitation Sciences
Department of Physical Therapy
Physical Therapist Program
635 Commonwealth Ave.
Boston, MA 02215
Phone: (617)353-2720 **Fax:** (617)353-9463
Email: fetters@bu.edu
Website: http://www.bu.edu/sargent
Linda Fetters, PhD, Director

★ 28845 ★ MGH Institute of Health Professions
Physical Therapist Program
Charleston Navy Yard
36 1st Ave.
Boston, MA 02129
Phone: (617)724-4841 **Fax:** (617)724-4854
Email: Lportney@mghihp.edu
Website: http://www.mghihp.edu
Leslie G. Portney, PhD, Director

★ 28846 ★ Northeastern University
Physical Therapist Program
Mugar Life Science Bldg., Rm. 117-A
360 Huntington Ave.
Boston, MA 02115
Phone: (617)373-3160 **Fax:** (617)373-3161
Email: mharris@neu.edu
Website: http://www.northeastern.edu/
Meredith H. Harris, EdD, Director

★ 28847 ★ Simmons College
Graduate School for Health Studies
Program in Physical Therapy
300 The Fenway
Boston, MA 02115
Phone: (617)521-2635 **Fax:** (617)521-3137
Email: djette@simmons.edu
Website: http://www.simmons.edu/gshs
Diane Jette, Director

★ 28848 ★ Springfield College
Department of Physical Therapy
Physical Therapist Program
263 Alden St.
Springfield, MA 01109
Phone: (413)748-3590 **Fax:** (413)748-3371
Email: ltsoumas@spfldcol.edu
Website: http://www.spfldcol.edu/pt
Linda J. Tsoumas, Director

★ 28849 ★ University of Massachusetts, Lowell
Physical Therapist Program
Weed Hall
3 Solomon Way, Ste. 5
Lowell, MA 01854-5095
Phone: (978)934-4517 **Fax:** (978)934-3006
Email: sally_healey@uml.edu
Website: http://www.uml.edu/
Joseph A. Dorsey, EdD, Director

Michigan

★ 28850 ★ Andrews University
Department of Physical Therapy
Physical Therapist Program
Berrien Springs, MI 49104-0420
Phone: (616)471-6551 **Free:** 800-827-2878
Fax: (616)471-2866
Email: perryw@andrews.edu
Website: http://www.andrews.edu/PHTH
Wayne L. Perry, PhD, Director

★ 28851 ★ Central Michigan University
Physical Therapist Program
134 Pearce Hall
Mount Pleasant, MI 48859
Phone: (517)774-2347 **Fax:** (517)774-2908
Email: herman.l.triezenberg@cmich.edu
Website: http://www.cmich.edu/~physther/
Herm Triezenberg, PhD, Director

★ 28852 ★ Grand Valley State University
Physical Therapist Program
328 Henry Hall
Allendale, MI 49401
Phone: (616)895-3356 **Fax:** (616)895-3350
Email: peckj@gvsu.edu
Website: http://www.gvsu.edu/pt
John Peck, PhD, Director

★ 28853 ★ Oakland University
School of Health Sciences
Physical Therapist Program
Rochester, MI 48309-4482
Phone: (248)370-4041 **Fax:** (248)370-4287
Email: marcoux@oakland.edu
Website: http://www.acs.oakland.edu
Beth C. Marcoux, PhD, Director

★ 28854 ★ University of Michigan, Flint
School of Health Professions and Studies
Physical Therapist Program
Flint, MI 48502-1950
Phone: (810)762-3373 **Fax:** (810)766-6668
Email: pkc@umflint.edu
Website: http://www.flint.umich.edu/Departments/PT
Paulette Cebulski, PhD, Director

★ 28855 ★ Wayne State University
Physical Therapist Program
439 Shapero Hall
Detroit, MI 48202
Phone: (313)577-1432 **Fax:** (313)577-8586
Email: aa4944@wayne.edu
Website: http://www.wayne.edu
Louis R. Amundsen, PhD, Director

Minnesota

★ 28856 ★ College of Saint Catherine, Minneapolis
Physical Therapist Program
601 25th Ave. S
Minneapolis, MN 55454
Phone: (651)690-7822 **Fax:** (651)690-7876
Email: dosellheim@stkate.edu
Website: http://www.stkate.edu/
Debra Sellheim, PhD, Director

★ 28857 ★ College of Saint Scholastica
Department of Physical Therapy
Graduate Physical Therapist Program
1200 Kenwood Ave.
Duluth, MN 55811
Phone: (218)723-6786 **Fax:** (218)723-6472
Email: dwise@css.edu
Website: http://www.css.edu
Denise Wise, PhD, Director

★ 28858 ★ Mayo Foundation
Mayo School of Sciences
Physical Therapist Program
200 1st St. SW
Rochester, MN 55905
Phone: (507)284-2054 **Fax:** (507)284-0656
Email: cummings.john@mayo.edu
Website: http://www.mayo.edu
John P. Cummings, PhD, Director

★ 28859 ★ University of Minnesota
Physical Therapist Program
Box 388 UMHC
Minneapolis, MN 55455
Phone: (612)624-0427 **Fax:** (612)625-7192
Email: carey007@maroon.tc.umn.edu
Website: http://www.physther.med.umn.edu/
James R. Carey, PhD, Director

Mississippi

★ 28860 ★ University of Mississippi Medical Center
School of Health Related Professions
Physical Therapist Program
2500 N State St.
Jackson, MS 39216-4505
Phone: (601)984-6330 **Fax:** (601)815-1715
Email: ngreenwald@shrp.umsmed.edu
Website: http://shrp.umc.edu/programs/pt.html
Neva F. Greenwald, Director

Missouri

★ 28861 ★ Maryville University, Saint Louis
Department of Physical Therapy
Physical Therapist Program
13550 Conway Rd.
Saint Louis, MO 63141
Phone: (314)529-9523 **Fax:** (314)529-9495
Email: chuckpt@maryville.edu
Website: http://www.maryville.edu
Charles Gulas, Director

★ 28862 ★ Rockhurst University
Physical Therapist Program
1100 Rockhurst Rd.
Kansas City, MO 64110
Phone: (816)501-4059 **Fax:** (816)501-4643
Email: spake@vax1.rockhurst.edu
Website: http://www.rockhurst.edu
Ellen Spake, Director

★ 28863 ★ Saint Louis University
Department of Physical Therapy
Physical Therapist Program
3437 Caroline St., Rm. 1026
Saint Louis, MO 63104
Phone: (314)577-8505 **Fax:** (314)577-8513
Email: ruebling@slu.edu
Website: http://www.slu.edu/colleges/AH/PTH
Irma S. Ruebling, Director

★ 28864 ★ Southwest Baptist University
Department of Physical Therapy
Physical Therapist Program
1600 University Ave.
Bolivar, MO 65613-2496
Phone: (417)328-1672 **Fax:** (417)328-1658
Email: dhash@sbuniv.edu
Website: http://falcon.sbuniv.edu/pt/index.html
Dorothy Hash, DPT, Director

★ 28865 ★ University of Missouri, Columbia
School of Health Professions
Physical Therapist Program
106 Lewis Hall
Columbia, MO 65211
Phone: (573)882-7103 **Fax:** (573)884-8369
Email: denbighb@ext.missouri.edu
Website: http://www.missouri.edu
Marilyn K. Sanford, PhD, Director

★ 28866 ★ Washington University
Department of Physical Therapy
Physical Therapist Program
4444 Forest Park Blvd., Ste. 1101
Saint Louis, MO 63108
Phone: (314)286-1400 **Fax:** (314)286-1410
Email: deusingers@msnotes.wustl.edu
Website: http://medicine.wustl.edu/~ptprog/
Susan S. Deusinger, PhD, Director

Montana

★ 28867 ★ University of Montana, Missoula
Department of Physical Therapy
Physical Therapist Program
Skaggs Bldg. 135
Missoula, MT 59812
Phone: (406)243-4753 **Fax:** (406)243-2795
Email: williams@selway.umt.edu
Website: http://www.umt.edu/pt
Ann K. Williams, PhD, Director

Nebraska

★ 28868 ★ Creighton University
School of Pharmacy and Allied Health Professions
Physical Therapist Program
2500 California Plaza
Omaha, NE 68178
Phone: (402)280-5675 **Fax:** (402)280-5692
Email: rsandstr@creighton.edu
Website: http://spahp.creighton.edu
Robert Sandstrom, PhD, Director

★ 28869 ★ University of Nebraska Medical Center
Division of Physical Therapy Education
Physical Therapist Program
984420 Nebraska Medical Ctr.
Omaha, NE 68198-4420
Phone: (402)559-4259 **Fax:** (402)559-8626
Email: phageman@unmc.edu
Website: http://www.unmc.edu/PhysicalTherapy/ptedu.htm
Patricia A. Hageman, PhD, Director

Nevada

★ 28870 ★ University of Nevada, Las Vegas
Physical Therapist Program
4505 Maryland Pkwy.
Box 453029
Las Vegas, NV 89154-3029
Phone: (702)895-3003 **Fax:** (702)895-4883
Email: hwallmann@ccmail.nevada.edu
Website: http://www.unlv.edu/Colleges/Health_Sciences/Physical_Therapy/index.html
Harvey Wallmann, Chairman of the Board

New Hampshire

★ 28871 ★ Notre Dame College
Physical Therapist Program
2321 Elm St.
Manchester, NH 03104-2299
Phone: (603)647-5500 **Fax:** (603)222-7520
Email: Ehaskvitz@notredame.edu
Esther Haskvitz, PhD, Director

New Jersey

★ 28872 ★ Richard Stockton College of New Jersey
Physical Therapist Program
Jim Leeds Rd.
Pomona, NJ 08240
Phone: (609)652-4261 **Fax:** (609)652-4858
Email: bkathrins@stockton.edu
Website: http://loki.stockton.edu/index.html
Bess Kathrins, Director

★ 28873 ★ Rutgers, the State University of New Jersey/University of Medicine and Dentistry of New Jersey
Camden Campus
Physical Therapist Program
Primary Care Center, Ste. 228
40 E Laurel Rd.
Stratford, NJ 08084-1353
Phone: (856)566-6456 **Fax:** (856)566-6458
Email: mnardone@umdnj.edu
Website: http://camden-www.rutgers.edu/
Marie Koval Nardone, Director

★ 28874 ★ University of Medicine and Dentistry of New Jersey
School of Health Related Professions
Physical Therapist Program
65 Bergen St.
Newark, NJ 07107-3001
Phone: (973)972-5454 **Fax:** (973)972-3717
Email: merians@umdnj.edu
Website: http://www.umdnj.edu/~shrpweb
Alma S. Merians, PhD, Director

New Mexico

★ 28875 ★ University of New Mexico
Physical Therapist Program
Health Sciences and Services Bldg., Rm. 204
Albuquerque, NM 87131-5661
Phone: (505)272-5755 **Fax:** (505)272-8079
Email: randrews@salud.unm.edu
Website: http://www.unm.edu/
Ronald Andrews, PhD, Director

New York

★ 28876 ★ City University of New York College of Staten Island
Physical Therapist Program
2800 Victory Blvd.
Staten Island, NY 10314
Phone: (718)982-3153 **Fax:** (718)982-2984
Email: rothmanj@postbox.csi.cuny.edu
Website: http://www.library.csi.cuny.edu/dept/pt/main.htm
Jeffrey Rothman, EdD, Director

★ 28877 ★ City University of New York Hunter College
School of Health Sciences
Physical Therapist Program
425 E 25th St.
New York, NY 10010
Phone: (212)481-4469 **Fax:** (212)481-8618
Email: gkrasilo@hunter.cuny.edu
Website: http://www.hunter.cuny.edu/health/pt
Gary Krasilovsky, PhD, Director

★ 28878 ★ Clarkson University
Department of Physical Therapy
PO Box 5880
Potsdam, NY 13699-5880
Phone: (315)268-3786 **Fax:** (315)268-1539
Email: feitelsb@clarkson.edu
Website: http://www.clarkson.edu
Samuel B. Feitelberg, Director

★ 28879 ★ **Columbia University**
Physical Therapist Program
710 W 168th St., 8th Fl.
New York, NY 10032
Phone: (212)305-3781 **Fax:** (212)305-4569
Email: kh111@columbia.edu
Website: http://cpmcnet.columbia.edu/dept/pt
Kenneth J. Harwood, PhD, Director

★ 28880 ★ **Daemen College**
Physical Therapist Program
4380 Main St.
Amherst, NY 14226-3592
Phone: (716)839-8345 **Fax:** (716)839-8537
Email: mbrogan@daemen.edu
Website: http://www.daemen.edu/departments/pt/default.html
Michael S. Brogan, Director

★ 28881 ★ **D'Youville College**
Physical Therapist Program
1 D'Youville Sq.
320 Porter Ave.
Buffalo, NY 14201-1084
Phone: (716)881-7702 **Fax:** (716)881-8137
Email: riversl@dyc.edu
Website: http://www.koolnet.org
Lynn Rivers, Director

★ 28882 ★ **Ithaca College**
Department of Physical Therapy
Physical Therapist Program
332 Smiddy Hall
Ithaca, NY 14850-7183
Phone: (607)274-3342 **Fax:** (607)274-1137
Email: rbrown@ithaca.edu
Website: http://www.ithaca.edu/hshp/pt/pt2/icpt2/html
Renee Brown, PhD, Director

★ 28883 ★ **Long Island University, Brooklyn**
Zeckendorf Health Sciences Center
Division of Physical Therapy
1 University Plaza
Brooklyn, NY 11201-5372
Phone: (718)488-1063 **Fax:** (718)780-4002
Email: wsusman@liu.edu
Website: http://www.brooklyn.liunet.edu/cwis/bklyn/health/bsphythe.html
William M. Susman, PhD, Director

★ 28884 ★ **Mercy College**
Physical Therapist Program
Graduate Center
555 Broadway
Dobbs Ferry, NY 10522
Phone: (914)674-9331 **Free:** 800-637-2969
Fax: (914)674-9457
Email: cfendersn@mercy.edu
Website: http://www.mercynet.edu/programs/index.htmlgrad
Claudia B. Fenderson, EdD, Director

★ 28885 ★ **Nazareth College of Rochester**
Physical Therapy Department
4245 East Ave.
Rochester, NY 14618-3790
Phone: (716)389-2900 **Fax:** (716)389-2908
Email: jwbloss@naz.edu
Website: http://www.naz.edu/dept/physical_therapy/index.html
Jill W. Bloss, Director

★ 28886 ★ **New York Institute of Technology**
Department of Physical Therapy
Wheatley Rd.
Box 8000
Old Westbury, NY 11568-8000
Phone: (516)686-7696 **Fax:** (516)686-7699
Email: pdouris@nyit.edu
Website: http://iris.nyit.edu/~physther
Peter C. Douris, EdD, Director

★ 28887 ★ **New York Medical College**
Graduate School of Health Sciences
Physical Therapist Program
Learning Center, Rm. 302
Valhalla, NY 10595
Phone: (914)594-4517 **Fax:** (914)594-4292
Email: michael_majsak@nymc.edu
Website: http://www.nymc.edu/admit/gshs/phys_therapy.htm
Michael J. Majsak, EdD, Director

★ 28888 ★ **New York University**
Physical Therapist Program
380 2nd Ave., 4th Fl.
New York, NY 10010-4086
Phone: (212)998-9400 **Fax:** (212)995-4190
Email: wk1@is2.nyu.edu
Website: http://www.nyu.edu/education/pt
Wen Ling, PhD, Director

★ 28889 ★ **The Sage Colleges**
Division of Health and Rehabilitation Sciences
Physical Therapist Program
Troy, NY 12180
Phone: (518)244-2266 **Fax:** (518)244-4524
Email: sellem@sage.edu
Website: http://www.sage.edu/html/RSC/prrsc.html
Marjane Selleck, Director

★ 28890 ★ **State University of New York Upstate Medical Center**
College of Health Professions
Physical Therapist Program
750 E Adams St.
Syracuse, NY 13210
Phone: (315)464-0881 **Fax:** (315)464-6887
Email: grametp@upstate.edu
Website: http://www.ec.hscsyr.edu/CHRP/pt/physical_therapy.html
Pamela Gramet, PhD, Director

★ 28891 ★ **State University of New York, Brooklyn (SUNY)**
Health Science Center
Physical Therapist Program
450 Clarkson Ave., Box 16
Brooklyn, NY 11203-2098
Phone: (718)270-7720 **Fax:** (718)270-7439
Email: jkatz@downstate.edu
Website: http://www.hscbklyn.edu/CHRP/pt.html
Joanne S. Katz, PhD, Director

★ 28892 ★ **State University of New York, Buffalo**
Department of Physical Therapy, Exercise and Nutrition Sciences
Physical Therapist Program
405 Kimball Tower
3435 Main St.
Buffalo, NY 14214-3079
Phone: (716)829-2941 **Fax:** (716)829-2428
Email: sbennett@buffalo.edu
Website: http://wings.buffalo.edu
Susan E. Bennett, EdD, Director

★ 28893 ★ **State University of New York, Stony Brook**
School of Health Technology and Management
Physical Therapist Program
Health Sciences Center
Stony Brook, NY 11794-8201
Phone: (631)444-3250 **Fax:** (631)444-7621
Email: rjohnson@epo.hsc.sunysb.edu
Website: http://www.sunysb.edu/
Richard W. Johnson, Director

★ 28894 ★ **Syracuse University**
Utica College
Health and Human Studies Division
Physical Therapist Program
1600 Burrstone Rd.
Utica, NY 13502-4892
Phone: (315)792-3059 **Fax:** (315)792-3248
Email: dscalise-smith@utica.ucsu.edu
Website: http://www.ucsu.edu/academic/majors/ptmajor.html
Dale Scalise-Smith, PhD, Director

★ 28895 ★ **Touro College**
School of Health Sciences
Physical Therapist Program
1700 Union Blvd.
Bay Shore, NY 11706
Phone: (631)665-1600 **Fax:** (631)665-4986
Email: josephw@touro.edu
Website: http://www.touro.edu/HEALTH/pt.htm
Kevin Wong, Director

North Carolina

★ 28896 ★ **Duke University Medical Center**
Physical Therapist Program
PO Box 3965
Durham, NC 27710
Phone: (919)684-2445 **Fax:** (919)684-6708
Email: richa052@mc.duke.edu
Jan K. Richardson, PhD, Director

★ 28897 ★ **East Carolina University**
Department of Physical Therapy
Physical Therapist Program
Greenville, NC 27858-4353
Phone: (252)328-4450 **Fax:** (252)328-0707
Email: albrightb@ecu.edu
Website: http://www.ecu.edu/pt/
Bruce C. Albright, PhD, Director

★ 28898 ★ **Elon University**
Department of Physical Therapy Education
Physical Therapist Program
Campus Box 2085
Elon, NC 27244-2010
Phone: (336)278-6400 **Free:** 800-334-8448
Fax: (336)278-6414
Email: rogers@elon.edu
Elizabeth Rogers, EdD, Director

★ 28899 ★ **University of North Carolina, Chapel Hill**
Division of Physical Therapy
Physical Therapist Program
Medical School Wing E
CB 7135
Chapel Hill, NC 27599-7135
Phone: (919)966-4708 **Fax:** (919)966-3678
Email: dsekerak@med.unc.edu
Website: http://www.med.unc.edu/mahp/physical/
Darlene K. Sekerak, PhD, Director

★ 28900 ★ Western Carolina University
Physical Therapist Program
312 Moore Bldg.
Cullowhee, NC 28723-9646
Phone: (828)227-7070 **Fax:** (828)227-7071
Email: klunnen@email.wcu.edu
Website: http://www.wcu.edu/aps/pt/
Karen Y. Lennen, EdD, Director

★ 28901 ★ Winston-Salem State University
Physical Therapist Program
601 Martin Luther King Jr. Dr.
Winston-Salem, NC 27110
Fax: (336)750-2192
Email: greengj@wssu.edu
Gloria J. Green, Director

North Dakota

★ 28902 ★ University of Mary
Division of Human Performance Sciences
Physical Therapist Program
7500 University Dr.
Bismarck, ND 58504-9652
Phone: (701)255-7500 **Free:** 800-408-6279
Fax: (701)255-7687
Email: mparker@umary.edu
Website: http://www.umary.edu/pt.htm
Michael G. Parker, PhD, Director

★ 28903 ★ University of North Dakota
School of Medicine and Health Sciences
Physical Therapist Program
501 N Columbia Rd.
PO Box 9037
Grand Forks, ND 58202-9037
Phone: (701)777-2831 **Fax:** (701)777-4199
Email: tommohr@medicine.nodak.edu
Website: http://www.med.und.nodak.edu/depts/pt/home.htm
Thomas M. Mohr, PhD, Director

Ohio

★ 28904 ★ Andrews University, Dayton
Department of Physical Therapy
Physical Therapist Program
2912 Springboro W, Ste. 301
Dayton, OH 45439
Phone: (937)298-2878 **Fax:** (937)298-9500
Email: daryls@andrews.edu
Website: http://www.andrews.edu/PHTH/
Daryl Stuart, EdD, Director

★ 28905 ★ Cleveland State University
Department of Health Sciences
Physical Therapist Program
Health Sciences Bldg., No. 109
2121 Euclid Ave.
Cleveland, OH 44115
Phone: (216)687-3567 **Fax:** (216)687-9316
Email: m.wagner@csuohio.edu
Website: http://www.csuohio.edu
Marilyn B . Wagner, PhD, Director

★ 28906 ★ College of Mount St. Joseph
Physical Therapist Program
5701 Delhi Rd.
Cincinnati, OH 45233-1672
Phone: (513)244-4890 **Fax:** (513)451-2547
Email: terri_glenn@mail.msj.edu
Terri M. Glenn, PhD, Director

★ 28907 ★ Medical College of Ohio
Physical Therapist Program
4418 Collier Bldg.
3015 Arlington Ave.
Toledo, OH 43614
Phone: (419)383-3518 **Fax:** (419)383-5880
Email: chornbeck@mco.edu
Website: http://www.mco.edu/
Catherine L. Hornbeck, Director

★ 28908 ★ Ohio State University
Physical Therapist Program
306 Allied Medical Professions
1583 Perry St.
Columbus, OH 43210
Phone: (614)292-5921 **Fax:** (614)292-0210
Email: nichols.3@osu.edu
Website: http://www.amp.ohio-state.edu/
Deborah S. Nichols, PhD, Director

★ 28909 ★ Ohio University
School of Physical Therapy
Physical Therapist Program
Grover Center, W290
Athens, OH 45701
Phone: (740)593-1225 **Fax:** (740)593-0292
Email: overbya@ohio.edu
Website: http://www.ohiou.edu/
Averell S. Overby, DrPH, Director

★ 28910 ★ University of Cincinnati
College of Allied Health Sciences
Physical Therapy Program
French East
PO Box 670394
Cincinnati, OH 45267-0394
Phone: (513)558-7477 **Fax:** (513)558-7474
Email: mulligea@uc.edu
Website: http://www.uc.edu/cahs/
Lizanne Mulligan, PhD, Director

★ 28911 ★ University of Findlay
Physical Therapist Program
1000 N Main St.
Findlay, OH 45840
Phone: (419)424-4863 **Fax:** (419)424-6977
Email: dutton@lucy.findlay.edu
Website: http://www.findlay.edu/academic/science/health/index.html
Lisa L. Dutton, Director

★ 28912 ★ Walsh University
Division of Physical Therapy
2020 Easton St. NW
North Canton, OH 44720-3396
Phone: (330)490-7286 **Fax:** (330)490-7371
Email: sbemis@alex.walsh.edu
Susan A. Bemis, EdD, Director

★ 28913 ★ Youngstown State University
Physical Therapist Program
B080 Cushwa Hall
Youngstown, OH 44555-2558
Phone: (330)742-2558 **Fax:** (330)742-1898
Email: mmcclell@cc.ysu.edu
Website: http://www.ysu.edu/colleges/hhs/hhsindex.htm
Marleen McClelland, PhD, Director

Oklahoma

★ 28914 ★ University of Oklahoma Health Sciences Center
Physical Therapist Program
PO Box 26901
Oklahoma City, OK 73190
Phone: (405)271-2131 **Fax:** (405)271-2432
Website: http://w3.ouhsc.edu/ahealth/rehab.htm
Martha J. Ferretti, Director

Ontario

★ 28915 ★ University of Toronto
Physical Therapist Program
256 McCaul St.
Toronto, ON, Canada M5T 1W5
Phone: (416)978-2769 **Fax:** (416)978-4363
Email: m.verrier@utoronto.ca
Molly Verrier, Director

Oregon

★ 28916 ★ Pacific University
School of Physical Therapy
Physical Therapist Program
2043 College Way
Forest Grove, OR 97116
Phone: (503)352-2846 **Fax:** (503)352-2995
Email: banaitid@pacificu.edu
Website: http://nellie.pacificu.edu/PT/index.html
Daiva A. Banaitis, PhD, Director

Pennsylvania

★ 28917 ★ Arcadia University
Department of Physical Therapy
Physical Therapist Program
450 S Easton Rd.
Glenside, PA 19038-3295
Phone: (215)572-2950 **Fax:** (215)572-2157
Email: craik@arcadia.edu
Rebecca L. Craik, PhD, Director

★ 28918 ★ Chatham College
Physical Therapist Program
Woodland Rd.
Pittsburgh, PA 15232-2826
Phone: (412)365-1409 **Fax:** (412)365-1213
Email: rpatterson@chatham.edu
Website: http://www.chatham.edu/academic/pt/physther1.htm
Ray M. Patterson, EdD, Director

★ 28919 ★ College Misericordia
Physical Therapist Program
301 Lake St.
Dallas, PA 18612-1098
Phone: (570)674-6465 **Fax:** (570)674-3052
Email: cwilkins@miseri.edu
Website: http://www.miseri.edu/academic/Undergrad/healthweb/PTWeb/DeptHome.htm
Catherine Perry Wilkinson, EdD, Director

★ 28920 ★ Duquesne University
School of Health Sciences
Physical Therapist Program
109 Health Sciences Bldg.
Pittsburgh, PA 15282
Phone: (412)396-5541 **Fax:** (412)396-4399
Email: morgan@duq2.cc.duq.edu
Website: http://www.duq.edu/
Robert C. Morgan, PhD, Director

★ 28921 ★ Gannon University
College of Sciences, Engineering and Health Sciences
Physical Therapist Program
109 University Sq.
Erie, PA 16541-0001
Phone: (814)871-5639 **Fax:** (814)871-5662
Email: meacci001@gannon.edu
Website: http://www.gannon.edu/
Charles Meacci, EdD, Director

★ 28922 ★ MCP Hahnemann University Programs in Rehabilitation Sciences
Physical Therapist Program
Mail Stop 502
245 N 15th St.
Philadelphia, PA 19102-1192
Phone: (215)762-4973 **Fax:** (215)762-3886
Email: jane.k.oeffner@drexel.edu
Website: http://www.auhs.edu/shp/depts/pt
Jane K. Oeffner, Director

★ 28923 ★ Neumann College
Division of Nursing and Health Sciences
Physical Therapy Program
1 Neumann Dr.
Aston, PA 19014-1298
Phone: (610)558-5534 **Fax:** (610)361-5290
Email: postr@neumann.edu
Website: http://www.neumann.edu
Robert E. Post, PhD, Director

★ 28924 ★ Saint Francis University
Physical Therapist Program
PO Box 600
Loretto, PA 15940-0600
Phone: (814)472-3123 **Fax:** (814)472-3140
Email: episarski@francis.edu
Edward M. Pisarski, EdD, Director

★ 28925 ★ Slippery Rock University of Pennsylvania
Graduate School of Physical Therapy
Physical Therapist Program
Physical Therapy Bldg.
North Rd.
Slippery Rock, PA 16057
Phone: (724)738-2080 **Fax:** (724)738-2113
Email: barbara.billek@sru.edu
Website: http://www.sru.edu/
Barbara Billek-Sawhney, EdD, Director

★ 28926 ★ Temple University
College of Allied Health Professions
Physical Therapist Program
3307 N Broad St.
Philadelphia, PA 19140
Phone: (215)707-4816 **Fax:** (215)707-7500
Email: lhack001@astro.ocis.temple.edu
Website: http://astro.ocis.temple.edu/
Laurita M. Hack, PhD, Director

★ 28927 ★ Thomas Jefferson University
College of Health Professions
Physical Therapist Program
130 S 9th St., Ste. 830 Edison
Philadelphia, PA 19107-5233
Phone: (215)503-8025 **Fax:** (215)503-3499
Email: marcus.besser@mail.tju.edu
Website: http://www.tju.edu
Marcus P. Besser, PhD, Director

★ 28928 ★ University of Pittsburgh
School of Health and Rehabilitation Sciences
Physical Therapist Program
6035 Forbes Tower
Pittsburgh, PA 15260
Phone: (412)647-1252 **Fax:** (412)647-1222
Email: delitto@pitt.edu
Website: http://www.pitt.edu/
Anthony Delitto, PhD, Director

★ 28929 ★ University of the Sciences in Philadelphia
Physical Therapist Program
600 S 43rd St.
Philadelphia, PA 19104
Phone: (215)596-8849 **Fax:** (215)895-3121
Email: a.iglars@usip.edu
Website: http://www.pcps.edu
Annette Iglarsh, PhD, Director

★ 28930 ★ University of Scranton
Physical Therapist Program
800 Linden St.
Scranton, PA 18510-4586
Phone: (570)941-7499 **Fax:** (570)941-7940
Email: kosmahle1@scranton.edu
Website: http://academic.uofs.edu/department/pt/default.htm
Edmund M. Kosmahl, EdD, Director

★ 28931 ★ Widener University
School of Human Service Professions
Physical Therapist Program
1 University Pl.
Chester, PA 19013
Phone: (610)499-1277 **Fax:** (610)499-1231
Email: robin.l.dole@widener.edu
Website: http://www.widener.edu/widener1.html
Robin L. Dole, EdD, Director

Rhode Island

★ 28932 ★ University of Rhode Island
Physical Therapist Program
Independence Square II
25 W Independence Way
Kingston, RI 02881-0180
Phone: (401)874-5001 **Fax:** (401)874-5630
Email: rowinski@uri.edu
Website: http://www.uri.edu/hss/pt/index.html
Mark J. Rowinski, PhD, Director

South Carolina

★ 28933 ★ Medical University of South Carolina
Department of Rehabilitation Sciences
Physical Therapist Program
171 Ashley Ave.
Charleston, SC 29425-2730
Phone: (843)792-2961 **Fax:** (843)792-0710
Email: morrisetted@musc.edu
Website: http://www.musc.edu/chp-rehab/
David Morrisette, PhD, Director

South Dakota

★ 28934 ★ University of South Dakota
Department of Physical Therapy
Physical Therapist Program
414 E Clark St.
Vermillion, SD 57069
Phone: (605)677-5915 **Fax:** (605)677-6529
Website: http://www.usd.edu/med/som/somdept/pt/
Lana R. Svien, Director

Tennessee

★ 28935 ★ Belmont University
Physical Therapist Program
1900 Belmont Blvd.
Nashville, TN 37212-3757
Phone: (615)460-6727 **Fax:** (615)460-6729
Email: greathoused@mail.belmont.edu
David G. Greathouse, PhD, Director

★ 28936 ★ East Tennessee State University
Physical Therapist Program
Box 70624
Johnson City, TN 37614-1709
Phone: (423)439-8793 **Fax:** (423)439-8077
Email: williada@etsu.edu
Website: http://www.etsu.edu/cpah/physther/pt/index.htm
Duane A. Williams, Director

★ 28937 ★ University of Tennessee, Chattanooga
School of Rehabilitation Professions
Physical Therapist Program
302 Health and Human Services Bldg.
615 McCallie Ave.
Chattanooga, TN 37403-2598
Phone: (423)755-4747 **Fax:** (423)785-2215
Email: randy-walker@utc.edu
Website: http://www.utc.edu/
J. Randy Walker, PhD, Director

★ 28938 ★ University of Tennessee Health Science Center
Physical Therapist Program
822 Beale St., Ste. 337
Memphis, TN 38163
Phone: (901)448-5888 **Fax:** (901)448-7545
Email: bconnolly@utmem.edu
Website: http://www.utmen.edu/physther/intro.html
Barbara H. Connolly, EdD, Director

Texas

★ 28939 ★ Hardin-Simmons University
Physical Therapist Program
2200 Hickory
PO Box 16065
Abilene, TX 79698-6065
Phone: (915)670-5860 **Free:** 888-820-0218
Fax: (915)670-5868
Email: joconnel@hsutx.edu
Website: http://www.hsutx.edu/grad/pt.htm
Janelle O'Connell, PhD, Director

★ 28940 ★ Southwest Texas State University
Health Science Center
Physical Therapist Program
601 University Dr.
San Marcos, TX 78666-4616
Phone: (512)245-8351 **Fax:** (512)245-8736
Email: bs04@swt.edu
Website: http://www.swt.edu
Barbara Sanders, PhD, Director

★ 28941 ★ Texas Tech University Health Sciences Center, Lubbock
Physical Therapist Program
3601 4th St.
Lubbock, TX 79430
Phone: (806)743-3220 **Fax:** (806)743-1262
Email: alhap@ttuhsc.edu
Website: http://www.ttuhsc.edu/pages/alhpt/alhpt_homepage.html
Andrew Priest, EdD, Director

★ 28942 ★ Texas Woman's University
School of Physical Therapy
Physical Therapist Program
PO Box 425766, TWU Station
Denton, TX 76204-5766
Phone: (940)898-2460 **Fax:** (940)898-2486
Email: crozier@twu.edu
Website: http://www.twu.edu/pt/
Carolyn Rozier, PhD, Director

★ 28943 ★ U.S. Army/Baylor University Academy of Health Sciences
MCCS-HMT Physical Therapy Branch
Physical Therapist Program
3151 Scott Rd.
Fort Sam Houston, TX 78234-6138
Phone: (210)221-8410 **Fax:** (210)221-7585
Email: timothy.flynn@cen.amedd.army.mil

Website: http://www.cs.amedd.army.mil/baylorpt/65b.htm
Lt. Col. Timothy W. Flynn, PhD, Director

★ 28944 ★ University of Texas, El Paso
Physical Therapist Program
1101 N Campbell
El Paso, TX 79902-0581
Phone: (915)747-8207 **Fax:** (915)747-8211
Email: ryberg@miners.utep.edu
Website: http://www.nurse.utep.edu/pt/index.htm
J. Alan Ryberg, PhD, Director

★ 28945 ★ University of Texas Health Science Center, San Antonio
Physical Therapist Program
7703 Floyd Curl Dr.
San Antonio, TX 78229-3900
Phone: (210)567-8862 **Fax:** (210)567-8774
Email: dedomenico@uthscsa.edu
Website: http://www.uthscsa.edu/sah_main.html
Giovanni de Domenico, PhD, Director

★ 28946 ★ University of Texas Medical Branch, Galveston
School of Allied Health Sciences
Physical Therapist Program
301 University Blvd.
Galveston, TX 77555-1028
Phone: (409)772-3068 **Fax:** (409)747-1613
Email: mhinman@utmb.edu
Website: http://www.utmb.edu
Martha Hinman, EdD, Director

★ 28947 ★ University of Texas Southwestern Medical Center, Dallas
Southwestern Allied Health Sciences School
Physical Therapist Program
5323 Harry Hines Blvd.
Dallas, TX 75390-8876
Phone: (214)648-1551 **Fax:** (214)648-1511
Email: pwinch@mednet.swmed.edu
Website: http://www.swmed.edu/
Patricia Winchester, PhD, Director

Utah

★ 28948 ★ University of Utah
Division of Physical Therapy
Physical Therapist Program
520 Wakara Way, Ste. 302
Salt Lake City, UT 84108
Phone: (801)581-8681 **Fax:** (801)585-5629
Email: scott.ward@hsc.utah.edu
Website: http://www.utah.edu/
R. Scott Ward, PhD, Director

Vermont

★ 28949 ★ University of Vermont
School of Allied Health Sciences
Physical Therapist Program
305 Rowell Bldg.
Burlington, VT 05405-0068
Phone: (802)656-3252 **Fax:** (802)656-6586
Email: jheld@zoo.uvm.edu
Website: http://www.uvm.edu/
Jean M. Held, EdD, Director

Virginia

★ 28950 ★ Marymount University
Physical Therapist Program
2807 N Glebe Rd.
Arlington, VA 22207-4299
Phone: (703)284-5980 **Fax:** (703)284-5981
Email: diana.venskus@marymount.edu
Diana Gilroy Venskus, Director

★ 28951 ★ Old Dominion University
School of Community Health Professions and Physical Therapy
Physical Therapist Program
Health Science Bldg.
Norfolk, VA 23529-0288
Phone: (757)683-4519 **Fax:** (757)683-4410
Email: gmaihafe@odu.edu
Website: http://www.odu.edu
George Maihafer, PhD, Director

★ 28952 ★ Shenandoah University
School of Health Professions
Physical Therapist Program
333 W Cork St.
Winchester, VA 22601
Phone: (540)665-5520 **Free:** 800-432-2266
Fax: (540)665-5530
Email: stepper@su.edu
Website: http://www.su.edu/pt/
Steven H. Tepper, PhD, Director

★ 28953 ★ Virginia Commonwealth University
Medical College of Virginia
Physical Therapist Program
Box 980224
Richmond, VA 23298-0224
Phone: (804)828-0234 **Fax:** (804)828-8111
Email: tmayhew@hsc.vcu.edu
Website: http://views.vcu.edu/pt/
Thomas Mayhew, PhD, Director

Washington

★ 28954 ★ Eastern Washington University
Department of Physical Therapy
310 N Riverpoint Blvd.
Box T
Spokane, WA 99202-1675
Phone: (509)368-6601 **Fax:** (509)368-6623
Email: deldin@mail.ewu.edu
Website: http://www.ewu.edu
Donna El-Din, PhD, Chairman of the Board

★ 28955 ★ University of Puget Sound
Physical Therapist Program
1500 N Warner
Tacoma, WA 98416
Phone: (253)879-3281 **Fax:** (253)879-2933
Email: hummel@ups.edu
Website: http://www.ups.edu
Kathie Hummel-Berry, PhD, Director

★ 28956 ★ University of Washington
Department of Rehabilitation Medicine
Physical Therapist Program
1959 NE Pacific St.
Seattle, WA 98195-6490
Phone: (206)598-5333 **Fax:** (206)685-3244
Email: mguthrie@u.washington.edu
Website: http://weber.u.washington.edu/~rehab
Mark R. Guthrie, PhD, Director

West Virginia

★ 28957 ★ West Virginia University
School of Medicine
Physical Therapist Program
PO Box 9226
Morgantown, WV 26506-9226
Phone: (304)293-3610 **Fax:** (304)293-7105
Email: mmandich@hsc.wvu.edu
Website: http://www.hsc.wvu.edu/som/pther
MaryBeth Mandich, PhD, Director

★ 28958 ★ Wheeling Jesuit University
Physical Therapist Program
316 Washington Ave.
Wheeling, WV 26003
Phone: (304)243-2432 **Free:** (866)243-2068
Fax: (304)243-2042
Email: lezook@wju.edu
Letha Zook, EdD, Director

Wisconsin

★ 28959 ★ Carroll College
Physical Therapist Program
100 N East Ave.
Waukesha, WI 53186
Phone: (262)524-1294 **Fax:** (262)524-7690
Email: jhopp@carroll1.cc.edu
Website: http://www.cc.edu/pt
Jane F. Hopp, PhD, Director

★ 28960 ★ Concordia University, Wisconsin
Physical Therapist Program
12800 N Lake Shore Dr.
Mequon, WI 53092-7699
Phone: (262)243-4433 **Fax:** (414)243-4506
Email: terry.steffen@cuw.edu
Website: http://www.cuw.edu
Teresa M. Steffen, PhD, Director

★ 28961 ★ Marquette University
Physical Therapist Program
PO Box 1881
Milwaukee, WI 53201-1881
Phone: (414)288-7194 **Fax:** (414)288-5987
Email: lawrence.pan@marquette.edu
Website: http://www.marquette.edu/chs
Lawrence G. Pan, PhD, Director

★ 28962 ★ University of Wisconsin, La Crosse
Department of Physical Therapy
Physical Therapist Program
4071 Health Science Ctr.
1725 State St.
La Crosse, WI 54601
Phone: (608)785-8470 **Fax:** (608)785-8460
Email: straker.gwyn@uwlax.edu
Website: http://www.uwlax.edu/SAH/PT/PhysicalTherapy.html
Gwyneth Straker, Director

★ 28963 ★ University of Wisconsin, Madison
Physical Therapist Program
5175 Medical Sciences Ctr.
1300 University Ave.
Madison, WI 53706-1532
Phone: (608)263-7131 **Fax:** (608)263-6434
Email: steinkam@surgery.wisc.edu
Website: http://www.medsch.wisc.edu/pt
Lisa Steinkamp, Director

Physician Assistant

The physician assistant educational programs listed in this section are accredited by the Commission on Accreditation of Allied Health Education Programs, 35 E Wacker Dr., Ste. 1970, Chicago, IL 60601-2208, (312)553-9355, http://www.caahep.org/. For information on the profession, contact the Association of Physician Assistant Programs, 950 N Washington St., Alexandria,

VA 22314, (703)548-5538, or the American Academy of Physician Assistants, 950 N Washington St., Alexandria, VA 22314 (703)836-2272, http://www.aapa.org/.

Alabama

★ 28964 ★ University of Alabama, Birmingham
School of Health Related Professions
Surgical Physician Assistant Program
RMSB 481
1530 3rd Ave. S
Birmingham, AL 35294
Phone: (205)934-4407
Email: bsspa@shrp.uab.edu

★ 28965 ★ University of South Alabama
College of Allied Health Professions
Department of Physician Assistant Studies
1504 Springhill Ave., Ste. 4410
Mobile, AL 36604-3273
Phone: (334)434-3641 **Fax:** (334)434-3646
Email: pastudies@usamail.usouthal.edu

Arizona

★ 28966 ★ Arizona School of Health Sciences
Physician Assistant Program
5850 E Still Cir.
Mesa, AZ 85206
Email: paprogram@ashs.edu

★ 28967 ★ Midwestern University
Physician Assistant Program
Office of Admissions
19555 N 59th Ave.
Glendale, AZ 85308
Phone: (623)572-3215

California

★ 28968 ★ Charles R. Drew University of Medicine and Science
College of Health Sciences
Physician Assistant Program
1731 E 120th St.
Los Angeles, CA 90059
Phone: (323)563-5879
Email: caspauld@cdrewu.edu
Website: http://www.cdrewu.edu

★ 28969 ★ Loma Linda University
School of Allied Health Professions
Physician Assistant Program
Nichol Hall, Rm. 2033
Loma Linda, CA 92350
Phone: (909)558-7295
Email: bstocker@sahp.llu.edu

★ 28970 ★ Riverside Community College
Riverside County Regional Medical Center
Primary Care Physician Assistant Program
16130 Lasselle St.
Moreno Valley, CA 92551
Phone: (909)571-6166

★ 28971 ★ Samuel Merritt College
Physician Assistant Program
450 30th St., Ste. 4708
Oakland, CA 94609
Phone: (510)869-6576
Email: admission@samuelmerritt.edu

★ 28972 ★ Stanford University
School of Medicine
Primary Care Associate Program
703 Welch Rd., Ste. F-1
Palo Alto, CA 94304
Phone: (650)725-6959
Email: pcap-information@lists.stanford.edu

★ 28973 ★ Touro University at Mare Island College of Health Sciences
Physician Assistant Program
Office of Admissions
1310 Johnson Ln.
Vallejo, CA 94592
Free: 888-887-7336
Email: sdavis@touro.edu

★ 28974 ★ University of California, Davis Medical Center
Department of Family and Community Medicine
Physician Assistant Program/Family Nurse Practitioner Program
2516 Stockton Blvd., Ste. 254
Sacramento, CA 95817-2297
Phone: (916)734-3551
Email: patty.frank@ucdmc.ucdavis.edu
Website: http://www-med.ucdavis.edu/adm_edu/fnp_pa_program/index.htm

★ 28975 ★ University of Southern California
Keck School of Medicine
Physician Assistant Program
Unit 7, Bldg. A-6, Rm. 6429
1000 S Fremont Ave.
Alhambra, CA 91803
Phone: (626)457-4240
Email: woehrle@usc.edu

★ 28976 ★ Western University of Health Sciences
Primary Care Physician Assistant Program
College Plaza
Pomona, CA 91766-1854
Phone: (909)469-5378
Email: admissions@westernu.edu

Colorado

★ 28977 ★ Red Rocks Community College
Physician Assistant Program
13300 W 6th Ave.
Denver, CO 80228
Phone: (303)914-6386
Email: arlene.duran@rrcc.edu

★ 28978 ★ University of Colorado Health Science Center
Child Health Associate/Physician Assistant Program
PO Box 6508
Mail Stop F543
Aurora, CO 80045
Phone: (303)315-7963
Email: chapa-info@uchsc.edu
Website: http://www.uchsc.edu/sm/chapa

Connecticut

★ 28979 ★ Quinnipiac University
Office of Graduate Admissions
Physician Assistant Program
275 Mt. Carmel Ave.
Hamden, CT 06518
Phone: (203)582-8672
Email: graduate@quinnipiac.edu
Website: http://www.quinnipiac.edu/grad_adm/physicn.html

★ 28980 ★ Yale University
School of Medicine
Physician Associate Program
47 College St., Ste. 220
New Haven, CT 06510
Phone: (203)785-4252
Email: janet.liscio@yale.edu
Website: http://info.med.yale.edu/phyassoc/

District of Columbia

★ 28981 ★ George Washington University
Physician Assistant Program
900 23rd St. NW, Ste. 6148
Washington, DC 20037
Phone: (202)994-7644
Email: npamag@gwumc.edu
Website: http://www.gwu.edu/~gwu_pa

★ 28982 ★ Howard University
College of Pharmacy, Nursing, and Allied Health Sciences
Physician Assistant Program
Sixth and Bryant Sts. NW, Annex I
Washington, DC 20059
Phone: (202)806-7536
Email: mbarnard@howard.edu
Website: http://www.howard.edu/CollegeAlliedHealth/paprog.html

Florida

★ 28983 ★ Barry University
School of Graduate Medical Sciences
Physician Assistant Program
11300 NE 2nd Ave.
Miami Shores, FL 33161
Phone: (305)899-3964
Email: mweiner@mail.barry.edu
Website: http://www2.barry.edu/vpaa-gms/pa/paprog.htm

★ 28984 ★ Miami-Dade Community College
Medical Center Campus
Physician Assistant Program
950 NW 20th St.
Miami, FL 33127-4693
Phone: (305)237-4420
Email: taylow@mdcc.edu
Website: http://www.mdcc.edu/medical/

★ 28985 ★ Nova Southeastern University
Physician Assistant Program
3200 S University Dr.
Fort Lauderdale, FL 33328
Phone: (954)262-1250
Email: marquard@nova.edu
Website: http://www.nova.edu/cwis/centers/hpd/pap

★ 28986 ★ University of Florida
Physician Assistant Program
PO Box 100176
Gainesville, FL 32610-0176
Phone: (352)265-7955
Email: ops@medicine.ufl.edu

Georgia

★ 28987 ★ Emory University School of Medicine Physician Assistant Program
1462 Clifton Rd. NE, Ste. 280
Atlanta, GA 30322
Phone: (404)727-7825
Email: emory-pa-admit@learnlink.emory.edu

★ 28988 ★ Medical College of Georgia Physician Assistant Program
AE 1032
Augusta, GA 30912
Phone: (706)721-3246
Email: underadm@mail.mcg.edu
Website: http://www.mcg.edu/SAH/PhyAsst/index.html

★ 28989 ★ South University Physician Assistant Program
709 Mall Blvd.
Savannah, GA 31406
Phone: (912)201-8023
Email: paprogram@southuniversity.edu
Website: http://www.southcollege.edu

Idaho

★ 28990 ★ Idaho State University Physician Assistant Program
Campus Box 8253
Pocatello, ID 83209-8253
Phone: (208)282-4705
Email: kingnore@isu.edu

Illinois

★ 28991 ★ Finch University of Health Sciences/Chicago Medical School Physician Assistant Program
3333 Green Bay Rd., Bldg. 51
North Chicago, IL 60064-3095
Phone: (847)578-3312
Email: stewarts@finchcms.edu
Website: http://www.finchcms.edu

★ 28992 ★ Malcolm X College /Cook County Hospital Physician Assistant Program
1900 W Van Buren St., Ste. 3241
Chicago, IL 60612
Phone: (312)850-7255
Website: http://www.ccc.edu/malcolmx/malcolmx1/CD_physassist.htm

★ 28993 ★ Midwestern University Physician Assistant Program
555 W 31st St.
Downers Grove, IL 60515
Free: 800-458-6253
Email: admissil@midwestern.edu
Website: http://www.midwestern.edu

★ 28994 ★ Southern Illinois University, Carbondale Physician Assistant Program
Lindegren Hall, Rm. 129
MC 6516
Carbondale, IL 62901-6516
Phone: (618)453-5527
Website: http://www.siu.edu/~hcp/pa.html

Indiana

★ 28995 ★ Butler University/Clarian Health College of Pharmacy and Health Sciences Physician Assistant Program
4600 Sunset Ave.
Indianapolis, IN 46208
Phone: (317)940-9969
Email: dpearson@butler.edu
Website: http://www.butler.edu/www/cophs

★ 28996 ★ University of Saint Francis Physician Assistant Program
2701 Spring St.
Fort Wayne, IN 46808
Email: jroth@sf.edu
Website: http://www.sf.edu

Iowa

★ 28997 ★ Des Moines University Osteopathic Medical Center Physician Assistant Program
3200 Grand Ave.
Des Moines, IA 50312
Phone: (515)271-1603
Email: pam.chambers@dmu.edu
Website: http://www.dmu.edu/cohs/pa/index.htm

★ 28998 ★ University of Iowa College of Medicine Physician Assistant Program
5167 Westlawn
Iowa City, IA 52242
Phone: (319)335-8922
Email: paprogram@uiowa.edu
Website: http://www.medicine.uiowa.edu/pa/pa.htm

Kansas

★ 28999 ★ Wichita State University College of Health Professions Physician Assistant Program
Campus Box 43
Wichita, KS 67260-0043
Phone: (316)978-3011
Email: jennifer.biddle@wichita.edu

Kentucky

★ 29000 ★ University of Kentucky College of Health Sciences Physician Assistant Program
900 S Limestone St., Ste. 205
Lexington, KY 40536
Phone: (859)323-1100
Email: hadleyr@uky.edu

Louisiana

★ 29001 ★ Louisiana State University Health Sciences Center School of Allied Health Professions Physician Assistant Program
1501 Kings Hwy.
PO Box 33932
Shreveport, LA 71130-3932
Phone: (318)675-7317
Email: kwilli6@lsuhsc.edu
Website: http://www.lsuhsc.edu/

Maine

★ 29002 ★ University of New England Physician Assistant Program
11 Hills Beach Rd.
Biddeford, ME 04005
Phone: (207)797-7261
Email: dfarrell@mailbox.une.edu
Website: http://www.une.edu

Maryland

★ 29003 ★ Anne Arundel Community College School of Health Professions, Wellness, and Physical Education Physician Assistant Program
101 College Pkwy.
Arnold, MD 21012
Phone: (410)777-7310
Email: laramos@aacc.edu

★ 29004 ★ Towson University/Community College of Baltimore, Essex Physician Assistant Program
7201 Rossville Blvd.
Baltimore, MD 21237
Phone: (410)780-6579
Email: sshaw@ccbc.cc.md.us

★ 29005 ★ University of Maryland, Eastern Shore Physician Assistant Program
Modular 934-5
Princess Anne, MD 21853
Phone: (410)651-7584
Email: pa@mail.umes.edu

Massachusetts

★ 29006 ★ Massachusetts College of Pharmacy and Health Sciences Physician Assistant Studies Program
179 Longwood Ave., WB01
Boston, MA 02115
Phone: (617)732-2140
Email: gbottomley@mcp.edu

★ 29007 ★ Northeastern University Physician Assistant Program
202 Robinson Hall
Boston, MA 02115
Phone: (617)373-3195
Email: paprogram@neu.edu
Website: http://www.dac.neu.edu/pap/physasst.html

★ 29008 ★ Springfield College/Baystate Health System Physician Assistant Program
263 Alden St.
Springfield, MA 01109
Free: 800-343-1257
Website: http://www.springfieldcollege.edu/home-page.nsf

Michigan

★ 29009 ★ Central Michigan University Physician Assistant Program
101 Foust Hall
Mount Pleasant, MI 48859
Phone: (989)774-2478
Email: chpadmit@cmich.edu
Website: http://www.cmich.edu/pa-pro.html

★ 29010 ★ Grand Valley State University Medical Education and Research Center Physician Assistant Program
1000 Monroe NW
Grand Rapids, MI 49503
Phone: (616)233-6500
Email: pas@gvsu.edu
Website: http://www4.gvsu.edu/pas/index.htm

★ 29011 ★ University of Detroit Mercy Physician Assistant Program
8200 W Outer Dr.
PO Box 130
Detroit, MI 48219-0900
Phone: (313)993-6177
Email: chpgrad@udmercy.edu
Website: http://www.udmercy.edu

★ 29012 ★ Wayne State University College of Pharmacy and Allied Health Professions Department of Physician Assistant Studies
Detroit, MI 48202
Phone: (313)577-1368
Email: ab4754@wayne.edu
Website: http://wizard.pharm.wayne.edu/pastudies/pa.htm

★ 29013 ★ Western Michigan University Physician Assistant Program
1903 W Michigan Ave.
Kalamazoo, MI 49008-5138
Phone: (616)387-5314
Website: http://www.wmich.edu/paprog/

Minnesota

★ 29014 ★ Augsburg College Physician Assistant Program
2211 Riverside Ave.
Campus Box 149
Minneapolis, MN 55454
Phone: (612)330-1039
Email: paprog@augsburg.edu
Website: http://www.augsburg.edu/pap/index.html

Missouri

★ 29015 ★ Saint Louis University School of Allied Health Professions Physician Assistant Program
3437 Caroline St.
Saint Louis, MO 63104
Phone: (314)577-8521
Email: mayj@slu.edu
Website: http://www.slu.edu/colleges/AH/PA

★ 29016 ★ Southwest Missouri State University Department of Physician Assistant Studies
901 S National Ave.
Springfield, MO 65804
Phone: (417)836-6151
Email: physicianasststudies@smsu.edu

Montana

★ 29017 ★ Rocky Mountain College Physician Assistant Program
1511 Poly Dr.
Billings, MT 59102-1797
Phone: (406)657-1190
Email: pa@rocky.edu
Website: http://www.rocky.edu

Nebraska

★ 29018 ★ Union College Physician Assistant Program
3800 S 4th St.
Lincoln, NE 68506
Phone: (402)486-2527
Email: paprog@ucollege.edu
Website: http://www.college.edu/pa/home.htm

★ 29019 ★ University of Nebraska Medical Center Physician Assistant Program
984300 NE Medical Ctr.
Omaha, NE 68198-4300
Phone: (402)559-5266
Email: dklandon@unmc.edu
Website: http://www.unmc.edu/AlliedHealth/pa

New Hampshire

★ 29020 ★ Massachusetts College of Pharmacy and Health Sciences, Manchester Physician Assistant Program
Office of Graduate Admissions and Continuing Education
1260 Elm St.
Manchester, NH 03101
Free: 800-225-5506
Email: admissions.manchester@mcp.edu

New Jersey

★ 29021 ★ Seton Hall University Physician Assistant Program
400 South Orange Ave.
South Orange, NJ 07079-2689
Phone: (973)275-2596
Email: gradmeded@shu.edu
Website: http://www.shu.edu/academic/arts_sci/Undergraduate/biology/pa.html

★ 29022 ★ University of Medicine and Dentistry of New Jersey Physician Assistant Program
65 Bergen St.
Newark, NJ 07107-3001
Phone: (973)972-5954

★ 29023 ★ University of Medicine and Dentistry of New Jersey /Rutgers, the State University of New Jersey Robert Wood Johnson Medical School Physician Assistant Program
675 Hoes Ln.
Piscataway, NJ 08854-5635
Phone: (732)235-4444
Website: http://www2.umdnj.edu/paweb

New Mexico

★ 29024 ★ University of New Mexico School of Medicine Department of Family & Community Medicine Physician Assistant Program
2400 Tucker NE
Albuquerque, NM 87131-5241
Phone: (505)272-9678
Email: paprogram@salud.unm.edu
Website: http://hsc.unm.edu/fcm/

★ 29025 ★ University of St. Francis Physician Assistant Program
4401 Silver Ave. SE, Ste. B
Albuquerque, NM 87108
Phone: (505)266-5565 **Free:** 888-446-4657
Email: pa@stfrancis.edu

New York

★ 29026 ★ Bronx Lebanon Hospital Center Physician Assistant Program
1650 Selwyn Ave., Ste. 11D
Bronx, NY 10457
Phone: (718)960-1255

★ 29027 ★ Brooklyn Hospital Center/ Long Island University Physician Assistant Program
121 DeKalb Ave.
Brooklyn, NY 11201
Phone: (718)260-2780 **Fax:** (718)260-2780
Email: tbhcpap@aol.com
Website: http://www.brooklyn.liunet.edu/cwis/bklyn/health/bsphyass.html

★ 29028 ★ City University of New York Harlem Hospital Center Sophie Davis School of Biomedical Education Physician Assistant Program
506 Lennox Ave.
WP 619
New York, NY 10037
Phone: (212)939-2525
Email: paprogram@ccny.cuny.edu
Website: http://www.ccny.cuny.edu

★ 29029 ★ Daemen College Physician Assistant Department
4380 Main St.
Amherst, NY 14226-3592
Free: 800-462-7652
Email: admissions@daemen.edu
Website: http://www.daemen.edu/departments/pa

★ 29030 ★ D'Youville College Physician Assistant Program
320 Porter Ave.
Buffalo, NY 14201
Phone: (716)881-7713
Website: http://www.dyc.edu/academics/

★ 29031 ★ Hofstra University Physician Assistant Studies Program
113 Monroe Lecture Hall
127 Hofstra University
Hempstead, NY 11549
Phone: (516)463-4074
Email: paprogram@hofstra.edu

★ 29032 ★ Hudson Valley Community College Albany Medical College Physician Assistant Program
47 New Scotland Ave.
Mail Code 4
Albany, NY 12208
Phone: (518)262-5251
Email: daisr@mail.amc.edu
Website: http://www.hvcc.edu/academ/schools/health/pas/pas.html

★ 29033 ★ Le Moyne College Physician Assistant Program
Department of Biology
1419 Salt Springs Rd.
Syracuse, NY 13214-1399
Phone: (315)445-4745
Email: simonpa@mail.lemoyne.edu

Website: http://www.lemoyne.edu/academic_affairs/programs/pa/PApage.htm
Patricia Simone, Contact

★ 29034 ★ Mercy College
Graduate Program in Physician Assistant Studies
555 Broadway
Dobbs Ferry, NY 10522
Phone: (914)674-7635
Email: paprogram@mercynet.edu

★ 29035 ★ New York Institute of Technology
Physician Assistant Program
PO Box 8000
Old Westbury, NY 11568-8000
Phone: (516)686-3881
Email: sbarese@nyit.edu

★ 29036 ★ Pace University, Lenox Hill Hospital
Physician Assistant Program
1 Pace Plaza, Rm. Y-31
New York, NY 10038
Phone: (212)346-1357
Email: paprogram@pace.edu

★ 29037 ★ Rochester Institute of Technology
Physician Assistant Program
85 Lomb Memorial Dr.
Rochester, NY 14623-5603
Phone: (716)475-2978
Email: hbmscl@rit.edu
Website: http://www.rit.edu/~930www/Proj/UGrad/UGradCat/colleges/cos/phyassist.html

★ 29038 ★ St. Vincent Catholic Medical Centers of New York
Brooklyn and Queens Region
Physician Assistant Program
175-05 Horace Harding Expy.
Fresh Meadows, NY 11365
Phone: (718)357-0500
Email: tsimone@cmcny.com

★ 29039 ★ St. Vincent Catholic Medical Centers of New York
Physician Assistant Program
75 Vanderbilt Ave.
Staten Island, NY 10304-3850
Phone: (718)354-5570

★ 29040 ★ State University of New York, Brooklyn
Health Science Center
Physician Assistant Program
450 Clarkson Ave.
Box 1222
Brooklyn, NY 11203
Phone: (718)270-2324
Email: admissions@downstate.edu
Website: http://www.hscbklyn.edu/CHRP/pa.html

★ 29041 ★ State University of New York, Stony Brook
School of Health Technology and Management
Physician Assistant Program
Health Sciences Center, L2-424
Stony Brook, NY 11794-8202
Phone: (631)444-3190
Email: paprogram@sunysb.edu
Website: http://www.uhmc.sunysb.edu/shtm/pa/pa_welcome.html

★ 29042 ★ Touro College
School of Health Sciences
Physician Assistant Program
1700 Union Blvd.
Bay Shore, NY 11706
Phone: (631)665-1600
Website: http://www.touro.edu

★ 29043 ★ Touro College, Manhattan Campus
School of Health Sciences
Physician Assistant Program
27-33 W 23rd St.
New York, NY 10010
Phone: (212)463-0400
Email: ngraff@touro.edu

★ 29044 ★ Wagner College /Staten Island University Hospital
Physician Assistant Program
74 Melville St.
Staten Island, NY 10309-4035
Phone: (718)226-2928
Email: nlowy@siuh.edu
Website: http://www.siuh.edu/pa/pa.html

★ 29045 ★ Weill Cornell Medical College
Physician Assistant Program
1300 York Ave.
Box 195
New York, NY 10021
Phone: (212)746-5133
Email: lfw2001@med.cornell.edu
Website: http://www.med.cornell.edu/dept/index.html

North Carolina

★ 29046 ★ Duke University Medical Center
Physician Assistant Program
DUMC 3848
Durham, NC 27710
Phone: (919)681-3161
Email: paadmission@mc.duke.edu
Website: http://dmi-www.mc.duke.edu/cfm/pap

★ 29047 ★ East Carolina University
School of Allied Health Sciences
Physician Assistant Program
West Research Campus
1157 VOA Site "C" Rd.
Greenville, NC 27834
Phone: (252)744-1100
Email: trubeg@mail.edu.edu
Website: http://www.ecu.edu/pa

★ 29048 ★ Methodist College
Physician Assistant Program
5107B College Centre Dr.
Fayetteville, NC 28311
Phone: (910)630-7495
Email: paprog@methodist.edu
Website: http://www.apcnet.com/methodist/methodist.html

★ 29049 ★ Wake Forest University
School of Medicine
Physician Assistant Program
Medical Center Blvd.
Winston Salem, NC 27157-1006
Phone: (336)716-4356
Email: kscales@wfubmc.edu
Website: http://mero.lib.wfubmc.edu/paprogram/

North Dakota

★ 29050 ★ University of North Dakota
School of Medicine and Health Sciences
Department of Community Medicine
Physician Assistant Program
PO Box 9037
Grand Forks, ND 58202-9037
Phone: (701)777-2344
Email: painfo@medicine.nodak.edu
Website: http://www.med.und.nodak.edu/depts/Commed/Home.html
Rhonda McDaniel, Contact

Ohio

★ 29051 ★ Cuyahoga Community College
Physician Assistant Program
11000 Pleasant Valley Rd.
Parma, OH 44130
Phone: (216)987-5363
Email: lisa.jozwiak@tri-c.edu

★ 29052 ★ Cuyahoga Community College
Surgical Physician Assistant Program
11000 Pleasant Valley Rd.
Parma, OH 44130
Phone: (216)987-5363
Email: lisa.jozwiak@tri-c.edu

★ 29053 ★ Kettering College of Medical Arts
Physician Assistant Program
3737 Southern Blvd.
Kettering, OH 45429
Phone: (937)296-7238
Email: sue.wulff@kmcnetwork.org
Website: http://www.kcma.edu/

★ 29054 ★ Marietta College
Physician Assistant Program
215 5th St.
Marietta, OH 45750
Phone: (740)376-4458
Email: paprog@marietta.edu

★ 29055 ★ Medical College of Ohio
School of Allied Health
Physician Assistant Program
3015 Arlington Ave.
Toledo, OH 43614-5803
Phone: (419)383-5408
Email: tlangenderfe@mco.edu
Website: http://www.mco.edu

★ 29056 ★ University of Findlay
Physician Assistant Program
1000 N Main St.
Findlay, OH 45840-3695
Phone: (419)424-4529
Email: davis@mail.findlay.edu

Oklahoma

★ 29057 ★ University of Oklahoma Health Sciences Center
Physician Associate Program
Health Sciences Center
PO Box 26901
Oklahoma City, OK 73190
Phone: (405)271-2058
Website: http://www.medicine.ouhsc.edu/education/pafset.html

Oregon

★ 29058 ★ Oregon Health Sciences University
Physician Assistant Program
3181 SW Sam Jackson Park Rd.
Mailcode GH219
Portland, OR 97201-3098
Phone: (503)494-1484
Email: paprgm@ohsu.edu
Website: http://www.ohsu.edu/ah-pa

★ 29059 ★ Pacific University
School of Physician Assistant Studies
Physician Assistant Program
2043 College Way
Forest Grove, OR 97116
Phone: (503)352-2898
Email: pa@pacificu.edu
Website: http://www.pacificu.edu/academics/pa.html

Pennsylvania

★ 29060 ★ Arcadia University
Physician Assistant Program
Brubaker Hall, Health Science Center
450 S Easton Rd.
Glenside, PA 19038
Phone: (215)572-2082
Email: benchouk@arcadia.edu

★ 29061 ★ Chatham College
Physician Assistant Program
Woodland Rd.
Pittsburgh, PA 15232
Phone: (412)365-1412
Email: admissions@chatham.edu
Website: http://www.chatham.edu/academic/PA/pac1.html

★ 29062 ★ DeSales University
Physician Assistant Program
2755 Station Ave.
Center Valley, PA 18034-9568
Phone: (610)282-1100
Email: paprog@desales.edu

★ 29063 ★ Drexel University
College of Nursing and Health Professions
Physician Assistant Program
1505 Race St., 8th Fl.
MS 504
Philadelphia, PA 19102-1192
Phone: (215)762-7135
Email: enroll@mcphu.edu

★ 29064 ★ Duquesne University
John G. Rangos Sr. School of Health Sciences
Physician Assistant Program
323 Health Sciences Bldg.
Pittsburgh, PA 15282
Free: 800-456-0590
Email: calhoun@duq.edu
Website: http://www.duq.edu/healthsciences/pa/pa-home.html

★ 29065 ★ Gannon University
Physician Assistant Program
109 University Sq.
Erie, PA 16541-0001
Phone: (814)871-7474
Email: cfal@gannon.edu
Website: http://www.gannon.edu/programs/under/phyasst.html

★ 29066 ★ King's College
Physician Assistant Program
133 N River St.
Wilkes Barre, PA 18711
Phone: (570)208-5853
Email: sesedon@kings.edu
Website: http://www.kings.edu/home/majors/pa_program.htm

★ 29067 ★ Lock Haven University of Pennsylvania
Physician Assistant Program
Lock Haven, PA 17745
Phone: (570)893-2541
Email: weisenha@lhup.edu
Website: http://www.lhup.edu/academic/acad_affairs/academ_grad_phyas.html

★ 29068 ★ Marywood University
Physician Assistant Program
2300 Adams Ave.
Scranton, PA 18509
Phone: (570)348-6298
Email: ugadm@ac.marywood.edu
Website: http://www.marywood.edu/ug_cat/departments/phys_asst.stm

★ 29069 ★ Pennsylvania College of Technology
Physician Assistant Program
1 College Ave., DIF 123
Williamsport, PA 17701-5799
Phone: (570)327-4779
Email: pholmes@pct.edu
Website: http://www.pct.edu

★ 29070 ★ Philadelphia College of Osteopathic Medicine
Department of Physician Assistant Studies
Evans Hall
4170 City Ave., Ste. 005
Philadelphia, PA 19131
Phone: (215)871-6772
Email: kennethha@pcom.edu
Website: http://www.pcom.edu/academicprograms/pa/index.html

★ 29071 ★ Philadelphia University
Physician Assistant Program
School House Ln. and Henry Ave.
Philadelphia, PA 19144
Phone: (215)951-2908
Email: mccombs@philau.edu
Website: http://www.philau.edu

★ 29072 ★ Saint Francis University
Department of Physician Assistant Sciences
PO Box 600
Loretto, PA 15940-0600
Phone: (814)472-3020
Email: admissions@francis.edu
Website: http://www.sfcpa.edu

★ 29073 ★ Seton Hill University
Physician Assistant Program
Seton Hill Dr.
Greensburg, PA 15601
Free: 800-826-6234
Email: admit@setonhill.edu
Website: http://maura.setonhill.edu/~msct/fmsc15.htm

South Carolina

★ 29074 ★ Medical University of South Carolina
College of Health Professions
Physician Assistant Program
PO Box 250856
Charleston, SC 29425
Phone: (843)792-0376
Email: jonesmo@musc.edu
Website: http://www.musc.edu/pa_program

South Dakota

★ 29075 ★ University of South Dakota
School of Medicine
Physician Assistant Studies Program
414 E Clark St.
Vermillion, SD 57069-2390
Phone: (605)677-5128
Email: usdpa@usd.edu
Website: http://www.usd.edu/med/som/somdept/pa

Tennessee

★ 29076 ★ Bethel College
Physician Assistant Program
325 Cherry Ave.
PO Box 329
Mc Kenzie, TN 38201
Phone: (731)352-4247
Email: taylore@bethel-college.edu

★ 29077 ★ Trevecca Nazarene University
Physician Assistant Program
333 Murfreesboro Rd.
Nashville, TN 37210-2877
Phone: (615)248-1225
Email: admissions_pa@trevecca.edu
Website: http://www.trevecca.edu/academics/nas/gradphysasst/

Texas

★ 29078 ★ Academy of Health Sciences
Interservice Physician Assistant Program
3151 Scott Rd., Ste. 1202
Attn: MCCS HMP
Fort Sam Houston, TX 78234-6138
Phone: (210)221-8004

★ 29079 ★ Baylor College of Medicine
Physician Assistant Program
1 Baylor Plaza, Rm. 633E
Houston, TX 77030
Phone: (713)798-4619
Email: melodym@bcm.tmc.edu
Website: http://www.bcm.tmc.edu

★ 29080 ★ Texas Tech University Health Sciences Center
School of Allied Health
Department of Diagnostic and Primary Care
Physician Assistant Program
3600 N Garfield
Midland, TX 79705
Phone: (915)620-9905
Email: jrunyan@midland.cc.tx.us

★ 29081 ★ University of North Texas Health Science Center
Physician Assistant Studies
3500 Camp Bowie Blvd.
Fort Worth, TX 76107-2699
Phone: (817)735-2301
Email: paadmissions@hsc.unt.edu

Website: http://www.hsc.unt.edu/departments/fammed/assist.htm

★ 29082 ★ University of Texas Southwestern Medical Center
Physician Assistant Program
6011 Harry Hines Blvd.
Dallas, TX 75390-9090
Phone: (214)648-1701
Email: isela.perez@utsouthwestern.edu
Website: http://www.swmed.edu/home_pages/allied/hcpa.htm

★ 29083 ★ University of Texas Health Science Center, San Antonio
Department of Physician Assistant Studies
Physician Assistant Program
7703 Floyd Curl Dr.
Mail Code 6249
San Antonio, TX 78229-3900
Phone: (210)567-8811
Email: pastudies@uthscsa.edu

★ 29084 ★ University of Texas Medical Branch
School of Allied Health Sciences
Physician Assistant Program
301 University Blvd.
Galveston, TX 77555
Phone: (409)772-3046
Email: rrahr@utmb.edu
Website: http://www.sahs.utmb.edu/sahs/physician_assistant_studies

★ 29085 ★ University of Texas, Pan-American
Physician Assistant Program
1201 W University Dr.
Edinburg, TX 78539
Phone: (956)381-2292

Utah

★ 29086 ★ University of Utah
Physician Assistant Program
375 Chipeta Way
Salt Lake City, UT 84108
Phone: (801)581-7766
Email: drobinson@upap.utah.edu
Website: http://www.utah.edu/upap/

Virginia

★ 29087 ★ College of Health Sciences
Physician Assistant Program
920 S Jefferson St.
Roanoke, VA 24016
Phone: (540)985-4016
Email: pa@mail.chs.edu
Website: http://www.chs.edu

★ 29088 ★ Eastern Virginia Medical School
Physician Assistant Program
700 W Olney Rd.
PO Box 1980
Norfolk, VA 23507
Phone: (757)446-7158
Email: paprog@evms.edu
Website: http://www.evms.edu/hlthprof/mpa.html

★ 29089 ★ James Madison University
Department of Health Sciences
Physician Assistant Program
MSC 4301
Harrisonburg, VA 22807
Phone: (540)568-2395
Email: paprogram@jmu.edu

★ 29090 ★ Shenandoah University
Division of Physician Assistant Studies
1460 University Dr.
Winchester, VA 22601
Phone: (540)542-6208
Email: pa@su.edu

Washington

★ 29091 ★ University of Washington MEDEX Northwest
Physician Assistant Program
4311 11th Ave. NE, Ste. 200
Seattle, WA 98105
Phone: (206)616-4001
Email: medex@u.washington.edu
Website: http://www.washington.edu/medical/som/depts/medes

West Virginia

★ 29092 ★ Alderson-Broaddus College
Physician Assistant Department
PO Box 2036
Philippi, WV 26416
Phone: (304)457-6283
Email: holt_m@ab.edu
Website: http://blue.ab.edu/

★ 29093 ★ Mountain State University
Physician Assistant Program
609 S Kanawha St.
PO Box 9003
Beckley, WV 25802
Phone: (304)253-7351
Website: http://www.cwv.edu/nhs/pa/index.html

Wisconsin

★ 29094 ★ Marquette University
College of Health Sciences
Department of Physician Assistant Studies
1700 Bldg.
PO Box 1881
Milwaukee, WI 53201-1881
Phone: (414)288-5688
Website: http://www.marquette.edu/chs/phas/

★ 29095 ★ University of Wisconsin
Gunderson Lutheran Medical Foundation/ Mayo School of Health-Related Sciences
Physician Assistant Program
4031 Health Science Center
1725 State St.
La Crosse, WI 54601-3767
Phone: (608)785-6620
Email: paprogram@uwlax.edu
Website: http://www.uwlax.edu/SAH/PhysicianAssistant/

★ 29096 ★ University of Wisconsin, Madison
Physician Assistant Program
Medical Sciences Center, Rm. 1050
1300 University Ave.
Madison, WI 53706
Phone: (608)263-5620
Website: http://www.medsch.wisc.edu/pa/

Podiatry

The following colleges of podiatric medicine are accredited by the Council on Podiatric Medical Education. For further information, contact the Council, or the American Podiatric Medical Association, at 9312 Old Georgetown Rd., Bethesda, MD 20814-1698, (301)571-9200, http://www.apma.org.

California

★ 29097 ★ California College of Podiatric Medicine
100 Corporate Pl., Ste. C
Vallejo, CA 94590
Phone: (707)558-1333 **Free:** 800-443-2276
Website: http://www.ccpm.edu
Clyde Taylor, President
Jeffrey C. Page, Director

Florida

★ 29098 ★ Barry University School of Graduate Medical Sciences
College of Podiatric Medicine
11300 NE 2nd Ave.
Miami Shores, FL 33161
Phone: (305)899-3249
Website: http://www2.barry.edu/vpaa-gms/podiatry.html
Jeanne O'Laughlin, PhD, Director
Chester A. Evans, Director

Illinois

★ 29099 ★ Finch University
Dr. William M. Scholl College of Podiatric Medicine
1001 N Dearborn St.
Chicago, IL 60610
Phone: (312)280-2880
Website: http://www.scholl.edu
Terence B. Albright, DPM, Director

Iowa

★ 29100 ★ Des Moines University
College of Podiatric Medicine
3200 Grand Ave.
Des Moines, IA 50312
Phone: (515)271-1464
Website: http://www.uomhs.edu/cpms/index.html
Robert T. Yoho, DPM, Director

New York

★ 29101 ★ New York College of Podiatric Medicine
1800 Park Ave.
New York, NY 10035
Phone: (212)410-8000
Website: http://www.nycpm.edu
Louis L. Levine, Director
Michael J. Trepal, DPM, Director

Ohio

★ 29102 ★ Ohio College of Podiatric Medicine
10515 Carnegie Ave.
Cleveland, OH 44106
Phone: (216)231-3300
Website: http://www.ocpm.edu
Thomas V. Melillo, DPM, Director
Vincent J. Hetherington, DPM, Director

Pennsylvania

★ 29103 ★ Temple University School of Podiatric Medicine
8th at Race St.
Philadelphia, PA 19107
Phone: (215)625-5400
Website: http://www.pcpm.edu
John A. Mattiacci, Director

Psychoanalysis

The psychoanalytic training institutes listed below are accredited by the National Association for the Advancement of Psychoanalysis, 80 8th Ave., Ste. 1501, New York, NY 10011, (212)741-0515, http://www.naap.org.

Colorado

★ 29104 ★ Colorado Center for Modern Psychoanalytic Studies
2240 Linden Ave.
Boulder, CO 80304-1617
Phone: (303)447-1159 **Fax:** (303)473-1963
Email: lbloom2240@aol.com
Miriam K. Bloom, PhD, Director

New Jersey

★ 29105 ★ New Jersey Center for Modern Psychoanalysis
14-25 Plaza Rd. Ste. 215
Fair Lawn, NJ 07410
Phone: (201)794-1222 **Fax:** (201)796-3432
Stanley Hayden, PhD, Director

★ 29106 ★ Psychoanalytic Center of Northern New Jersey
769 Northfield Ave., No LL2
West Orange, NJ 07052
Phone: (973)736-7600 **Fax:** (973)736-6519
Email: SPEUD@aol.com
Vicki Semel, PsyD, Director

★ 29107 ★ Psychoanalytic Training Institute of New Jersey
800 Catalpa Ave.
Teaneck, NJ 07666
Phone: (201)836-1065 **Fax:** (201)836-3902
Email: njinstitut@aol.com
Neil Wilson, PhD, Director

New York

★ 29108 ★ Blanton-Peale Graduate Institute
3 West 29 St.
New York, NY 10001
Phone: (212)725-7850 **Fax:** (212)689-3212
Dr. Holly Harrison Johnson, Director

★ 29109 ★ C.G. Jung Institute of New York
28 E 39th St.
New York, NY 10016-2587
Phone: (212)986-5458 **Fax:** (212)867-0920
Email: cgjungnyc@worldnet.att.net
Website: http://www.cgjungpage.com
Soren Ekstrom, PhD, President

★ 29110 ★ Institute for Expressive Analysis
240 East 93 St., Ste. 12
New York, NY 10024
Phone: (212)362-2167 **Fax:** (212)595-6053
Email: SMRSTN@aol.com
Website: http://iea-ny.org/
Joel M. Gavriele-Gold, PhD, Director

★ 29111 ★ International University for Graduate Studies
239 Central Park West, Ste. 1AS
New York, NY 10019
Free: 888-660-0686 **Fax:** 888-660-0686
Email: CarolynWest@compuserve.com
Norma Ross, Director

★ 29112 ★ Mid-Manhattan Institute for Psychoanalysis
239 Central Park West, Ste. 1AS
New York, NY 10024
Phone: (212)799-8558 **Fax:** (212)799-8135
Email: mmi@mmi.edu
Deborah Bershatsky, PhD, Director

★ 29113 ★ National Psychological Association for Psychoanalysis Training Institute
150 W 13th St.
New York, NY 10011
Phone: (212)924-7440 **Fax:** (212)989-7543
Email: info@npap.org
Website: http://www.npap.org
Gary Ahlskog, PhD, President

★ 29114 ★ New York Center for Jungian Studies
41 Park Ave., Ste. 1D
New York, NY 10016
Phone: (212)689-8238 **Fax:** (212)889-7634
Email: aryeh@hvi.com
Aryeh Maidenbaum, PhD, Director

★ 29115 ★ Psychoanalytic Psychotherapy Study Center
80 Fifth Ave., Ste. 903
New York, NY 10011
Phone: (212)254-4422 **Fax:** (212)675-4386
Email: ppsc@worldnet.att.net
Website: http://www.nonprofitpages.com/ppsc/
Judy Levitz, PhD, Director

★ 29116 ★ Training and Research Institute for Self Psychology
15 W 96 St.Ste. 2
New York, NY 10025
Phone: (212)663-3508
Email: TrispNYC@msn.com
Website: http://www.selfpsychology.org/trisp/
R.B. Ulman, PhD, Director

★ 29117 ★ Washington Square Institute
41 E 11th St.
New York, NY 10003
Phone: (212)477-2600 **Fax:** (212)477-2600
Email: info@WSI.org
Website: http://www.wsi.org/
Gerd H. Fenchel, PhD, Director

★ 29118 ★ Westchester Institute for Training in Psychoanalysis and Psychotherapy
105 S Bedford Rd., Ste. 302
PO Box 89
Mount Kisco, NY 10549
Phone: (914)666-0163 **Fax:** (914)666-0390
Donald E. Kalsched, PhD, Director

Pennsylvania

★ 29119 ★ Institute for Psychoanalytic Psychotherapies
26 Summit Grove Ave., Ste. 217
Bryn Mawr, PA 19010
Phone: (215)635-5368 **Fax:** (215)635-5601
Email: HHCOVITZ@aol.com
Howard H. Covitz, PhD, Director

★ 29120 ★ Philadelphia School of Psychoanalysis
313 S 16 St.
Philadelphia, PA 19102
Phone: (215)732-8244 **Fax:** (215)732-8454
Email: psp@libertynet.org
Website: http://www.libertynet.org/psp/
Stephen Day Ellis, PhD, Contact

Public Health

The following graduate schools of public health are members of the Association of Schools of Public Health (1101 15th St. NW, Ste. 910, Washington, DC 20005, (202)296-1099, http://www.asph.org/) and are accredited by the Council on Education for Public Health, 800 Eye St., NW, Ste. 202, Washington, DC 20001-3710, (202)789-1050, http://www.ceph.org/.

Alabama

★ 29121 ★ University of Alabama, Birmingham School of Public Health
1665 University Blvd.
120 Ryals Bldg.
Birmingham, AL 35294-0022
Phone: (205)934-4993
Website: http://www.uab.edu/PublicHealth/

California

★ 29122 ★ Loma Linda University School of Public Health
Loma Linda, CA 92350
Phone: (909)824-4694 **Free:** 800-422-4558
Fax: (909)824-4087
Website: http://www.llu.edu/llu/grad/grad.html

★ 29123 ★ San Diego State University College of Health & Human Services Graduate School of Public Health
5500 Campanile Dr.
San Diego, CA 92182-4162
Phone: (619)594-6317 **Fax:** (619)594-6112
Website: http://www-rohan.edu/dept/gsphsdsu/web/gsph.html

★ 29124 ★ University of California, Berkeley School of Public Health
19 Earl Warren Hall
Berkeley, CA 94720
Phone: (510)643-0881
Website: http://ist_socrates.berkeley.edu/~sph/

★ 29125 ★ University of California, Los Angeles School of Public Health
Center for Health Sciences, Rm. 16-071
Box 951722
Los Angeles, CA 90095
Phone: (310)825-5516 **Fax:** (310)825-8440
Website: http://www.ph.ucla.edu

Connecticut

★ 29126 ★ University of Connecticut Health Center
Graduate Program in Public Health
236 Farmington Ave.
Farmington, CT 06030-1910
Phone: (860)679-3351 **Fax:** (860)679-2374
Email: mph@nso.uchc.edu
Website: http://grad.uchc.edu/

★ 29127 ★ Yale University
School of Medicine
Department of Epidemiology and Public Health
60 College St., Rm. 208
New Haven, CT 06520-8034
Phone: (203)785-2844 **Fax:** (203)785-7296
Website: http://info.med.yale.edu/eph/

District of Columbia

★ 29128 ★ George Washington University
School of Public Health and Health Services
2300 Eye St. NW, Rm. 719
Washington, DC 20037
Phone: (202)994-0248
Website: http://www.gwumc.edu/sphhs

Florida

★ 29129 ★ University of South Florida
College of Public Health
13201 Bruce B. Downs Blvd.
MDC-56
Tampa, FL 33612-3805
Phone: (813)974-3623 **Fax:** (813)974-4718
Website: http://com1.med.usf.edu/pubhealth/coph1.html

Georgia

★ 29130 ★ Emory University
Rollins School of Public Health
1518 Clifton Rd. NE
Atlanta, GA 30322
Phone: (404)727-3956 **Fax:** (404)727-3996
Website: http://www.sph.emory.edu

Hawaii

★ 29131 ★ University of Hawaii
School of Public Health
1960 East-West Rd.
Honolulu, HI 96822
Phone: (808)956-8267 **Fax:** (808)956-4585
Website: http://www2.hawaii.edu/~sphdean

Illinois

★ 29132 ★ University of Illinois, Chicago
School of Public Health
2121 W Taylor St.
Chicago, IL 60612
Phone: (312)996-6625 **Fax:** (312)996-1374
Website: http://www.uic.edu/sph/

Indiana

★ 29133 ★ Indiana University
Committee for the School of Public Health
Robert Long Hospital, LO-211
1110 W Michigan St.
Indianapolis, IN 46202-5102
Phone: (317)278-0377
Email: skeough@indiana.edu
Website: http://www.indiana.edu/~aphs/phed.html
Dr. Mohammad R. Torabi, Contact

Iowa

★ 29134 ★ University of Iowa
Department of Preventive Medicine and Environmental Health
Public Health Program
2800 Steindler Bldg.
Iowa City, IA 52242-1008
Phone: (319)335-8992 **Free:** 800-553-IOWA
Fax: (319)335-9200
Email: program-director@mail.public-health.uiowa.edu
Website: http://www.public-health.uiowa.edu/

Louisiana

★ 29135 ★ Tulane University
School of Public Health and Tropical Medicine
1430 Tulane Ave.
New Orleans, LA 70112
Phone: (504)588-5387 **Fax:** (504)588-5718
Website: http://www.sph.tulane.edu

Maryland

★ 29136 ★ Johns Hopkins University
School of Hygiene and Public Health
615 N Wolfe St.
Baltimore, MD 21205-2179
Phone: (410)955-3543 **Fax:** (410)955-0121
Website: http://www.jhsph.edu

Massachusetts

★ 29137 ★ Boston University
School of Public Health
80 E Concord St., A-403
Boston, MA 02118-2394
Phone: (617)638-4640 **Fax:** (617)638-5299
Website: http://www-busph.bu.edu

★ 29138 ★ Harvard University
School of Public Health
677 Huntington Ave., Rm. G-4
Boston, MA 02115
Phone: (617)432-1031 **Fax:** (617)277-5320
Website: http://www.hsph.harvard.edu/

★ 29139 ★ University of Massachusetts
School of Public Health
101 Arnold House
Amherst, MA 01003-0037
Phone: (413)545-1303 **Fax:** (413)545-1264
Website: http://www.umass.edu/soph/

Michigan

★ 29140 ★ University of Michigan
School of Public Health
109 S Observatory St.
Ann Arbor, MI 48109-2029
Phone: (734)764-5425 **Fax:** (734)763-5455
Website: http://www.sph.umich.edu/

Minnesota

★ 29141 ★ University of Minnesota
School of Public Health
420 Delaware St. SE
Box 197 Mayo
Minneapolis, MN 55455
Phone: (612)626-3500 **Free:** 800-774-8636
Fax: (612)626-6931
Website: http://www.sph.umn.edu/

Missouri

★ 29142 ★ Saint Louis University
School of Public Health
3663 Lindell Ave.
Saint Louis, MO 63108-3342
Phone: (314)977-8144 **Fax:** (314)977-8150
Website: http://www.slu.edu/colleges/sph/slusph/Default.htm

New Jersey

★ 29143 ★ University of Medicine and Dentistry of New Jersey / Rutgers, the State University of New Jersey / New Jersey Institute of Technology
Public Health Program
675 Hoes Ln.
Piscataway, NJ 08854-5635
Phone: (732)235-4549 **Fax:** (732)235-4569
Email: rmcintyr@umdnj.edu
Website: http://www2.umdnj.edu/ethicweb/
Russell L. McIntyre, Contact

New York

★ 29144 ★ Columbia University
School of Public Health
600 W 168th St.
New York, NY 10032
Phone: (212)305-3927 **Fax:** (212)305-1460
Website: http://cpmcnet.columbia.edu/dept/sph/

★ 29145 ★ State University of New York, Albany
School of Public Health
1 University Pl.
Rensselaer, NY 12144-3456
Phone: (518)402-0300 **Fax:** (518)485-5565
Website: http://www.albany.edu/sph/

North Carolina

★ 29146 ★ University of North Carolina, Chapel Hill
School of Public Health
Campus Box 7400
Chapel Hill, NC 27599-7400
Phone: (919)966-7676 **Fax:** (919)966-7678
Website: http://www.sph.unc.edu

Ohio

★ 29147 ★ Ohio State University
School of Public Health
320 W 10th Ave.
M120 Starling-Loving Hall
Columbus, OH 43210-1240
Phone: (614)293-3907
Website: http://medicine.osu.edu/

Oklahoma

★ 29148 ★ University of Oklahoma
College of Public Health
Health Sciences Center, CHB 139
PO Box 26901
Oklahoma City, OK 73190
Phone: (405)271-2308 **Fax:** (405)271-3039
Website: http://www.ouhsc.edu

Pennsylvania

★ 29149 ★ MCP Hahnemann University School of Public Health
Broad & Vine Sts.
Bellet Bldg., 11th Fl.
Mail Stop 660
Philadelphia, PA 19102-1192
Phone: (215)762-8288 **Fax:** (215)246-5347
Email: enroll@mcphu.edu
Website: http://www.drexel.edu/pubhealth
Frmly: Allegheny University of the Health Sciences

★ 29150 ★ University of Pittsburgh Graduate School of Public Health
114 Parran Hall
Pittsburgh, PA 15261
Phone: (412)624-3002 **Fax:** (412)624-3309
Website: http://www.pitt.edu/~gsphhome/

Puerto Rico

★ 29151 ★ University of Puerto Rico School of Public Health
Health Sciences Center
GPO Box 365067
San Juan, PR 00936-5067
Phone: (787)764-5975
Website: http://wwwrcm.upr.clu.edu

South Carolina

★ 29152 ★ University of South Carolina School of Public Health
Health Sciences Bldg.
Columbia, SC 29208
Phone: (803)777-5031 **Fax:** (803)777-4783
Website: http://www.sph.sc.edu

Tennessee

★ 29153 ★ University of Tennessee, Memphis School of Public Health
66 N Pauline St., Ste. 633
Memphis, TN 38163
Phone: (901)448-5826
Website: http://www.utmem.edu/

Texas

★ 29154 ★ Texas A&M University School of Rural Public Health
Health Science Center
260 Centeq Bldg.
TAMU 1266
College Station, TX 77843-1266
Phone: (409)845-2387
Website: http://hsc.tamu.edu/SRPH/

★ 29155 ★ University of North Texas Department of Public Health and Preventive Medicine
Health Science Center
3500 Camp Bowie Blvd.
Fort Worth, TX 76107-2699
Phone: (817)735-2204 **Free:** 800-535-TCOM
Fax: (817)735-2225
Email: studaffr@hsc.unt.edu
Website: http://www.hsc.unt.edu/

★ 29156 ★ University of Texas Health Sciences Center at Houston School of Public Health
PO Box 20186
Houston, TX 77225
Phone: (713)500-9100 **Fax:** (713)791-1369
Website: http://www.sph.uth.tmc.edu

Washington

★ 29157 ★ University of Washington School of Public Health and Community Medicine
Box 357230
Seattle, WA 98195-7230
Phone: (206)543-1144 **Fax:** (206)543-3813
Website: http://weber.u.washington.edu/~sphcm/sphcm.html

Rehabilitation

The institutions listed below offer programs in rehabilitation education. All are members of the National Council on Rehabilitation Education, c/o California State University—Fresno, Rehabilitation Counseling Program, 5005 N Maple Ave., MS 3, Fresno, CA 93740-8025, (559)278-0325, http://www.rehabeducators.org.

Alabama

★ 29158 ★ Auburn University Department of Rehabilitation and Special Education Rehabilitation Counseling Program
1228 Haley Center
Auburn University, AL 36849
Phone: (334)844-5943 **Fax:** (334)844-2080
Email: mcdanrs@mail.auburn.edu
Website: http://www.auburn.edu/academic/education/rse/
Randall S. McDaniel, Contact

★ 29159 ★ Troy State University Department of Human Services Rehabilitation Program
104 McCartha Hall
Troy, AL 36082
Phone: (334)670-3366 **Fax:** (334)670-3473
Email: rmillard@troyst.net
Richard P. Millard, RhD, Contact

★ 29160 ★ University of Alabama Rehabilitation Counseling Program
Box 870231
Tuscaloosa, AL 35487-0231
Phone: (205)348-1190 **Fax:** (205)348-7584
Email: jsatcher@bamaed.ua.edu
Website: http://www.bamaed.ua.edu/Counsed.htm
Jamie Satcher, PhD, Contact

Alberta

★ 29161 ★ University of Calgary Community Rehabilitation and Disability Studies Community Rehabilitation Program
2500 University Dr. NW
Calgary, AB, Canada T2N 1N4
Phone: (403)220-3543 **Fax:** (403)220-6494
Email: marlett@ucalgary.ca
Nancy Marlett, PhD, Director

Arizona

★ 29162 ★ Northern Arizona University American Indian Rehabilitation Research and Training Center Arizona University Center on Disabilities
PO Box 5630
Northern Arizona University, AZ
Phone: (928)523-4791 **Fax:** (928)523-9127
Email: priscilla.sanderson@nau.edu
Priscilla Sanderson, PhD, Director

★ 29163 ★ University of Arizona College of Education Department of Special Education, Rehabilitation and School Psychology Rehabilitation Counseling Program
Rm. 412
PO Box 210069
Tucson, AZ 85721-0069
Phone: (520)621-7822 **Fax:** (520)621-3821
Email: sales@u.arizona.edu
Website: http://www.ed.arizona.edu/departs/SER/ser-info.htm
Amos Sales, EdD, Contact

Arkansas

★ 29164 ★ Arkansas State University Department of Psychology and Counseling Rehabilitation Counseling Program MRC Program
PO Box 1560
State University, AR 72467
Phone: (870)972-3064 **Fax:** (870)972-3962
Email: tturner@astate.edu
Website: http://147.97.11.245/cep/mrc/index.html
Tyra Turner, RhD, Contact

★ 29165 ★ Arkansas Tech University Rehabilitation Science
348 Witherspoon Hall
Russellville, AR 72801
Phone: (479)968-0283 **Fax:** (479)964-0544
Email: lyman.harris@mail.atu.edu
Lyman Harris, Director

★ 29166 ★ University of Arkansas, Fayetteville Department of Rehabilitation Education and Research Rehabilitation Counseling Program
346 N West Ave.
WAAX 319
West Ave. Annex
Fayetteville, AR 72701
Phone: (501)575-3658 **Fax:** (501)575-3253
Email: btwilli@uark.edu
Website: http://comp.uark.edu/~rehab/grad.html
Brent Williams, PhD, Contact

★ 29167 ★ University of Arkansas, Little Rock Department of Counseling, Adult, and Rehabilitation Education
2801 S University Ave.
Little Rock, AR 72204
Phone: (501)569-3169 **Fax:** (501)569-3428
Email: lrdickerson@ualr.edu
Larry R. Dickerson, Contact

California

★ 29168 ★ California State University, Fresno School of Education and Human Development Rehabilitation Counseling Program
5005 N Maple Ave., ED 3
Fresno, CA 93740-8025
Phone: (559)278-0325 **Fax:** (559)278-0016
Email: charlesa@csufresno.edu
Website: http://caracas.soehd.csufresno.edu/
Charles Arokiasamy, RhD, Contact

★ 29169 ★ California State University, Los Angeles
Division of Administration and Counseling
Rehabilitation Counseling Program
5151 State University Dr.
Los Angeles, CA 90032
Phone: (323)343-4250 **Fax:** (323)343-4252
Email: mbrodwi@calstatela.edu
Website: http://www.calstatela.edu/dept/edac/index.htm
Martin Brodwin, Contact

★ 29170 ★ California State University, Sacramento
School of Education
Department of Special Education, Rehabilitation and School Psychology
Vocational Rehabilitation and Counseling Programs
6000 J St.
Sacramento, CA 95819-6079
Phone: (916)278-6622 **Fax:** (916)278-3498
Email: kochr@educserver.educ.csus.edu
Website: http://edweb.csus.edu/eds/default.html
Richard A. Koch, EdD, Contact

★ 29171 ★ San Diego State University
Department of Administration, Rehabilitation and Post-secondary Education
Rehabilitation Counseling Program
Interwork Institute
3590 Camino del Rio North
San Diego, CA 92108
Phone: (619)594-6406 **Fax:** (619)594-0991
Email: fmcfarla@mail.sdsu.edu
Website: http://www.interwork.sdsu.edu/~dwright/EdLdr/
Fred McFarlane, PhD, Contact

★ 29172 ★ San Francisco State University
Department of Counseling
Rehabilitation Counseling Program
1600 Holloway Ave.
San Francisco, CA 94132
Phone: (415)338-2005 **Fax:** (415)338-0594
Email: ali1212@sfsu.edu
Website: http://www.sfsu.edu/~counsel/html/program/RC.htm
Anita Leal-Idrogo, PhD, Contact

Colorado

★ 29173 ★ University of Northern Colorado
Department of Human Services
Rehabilitation Counseling Program
Gunter Hall, Rm. 1250
Greeley, CO 80639
Phone: (970)351-2403 **Fax:** (970)351-1255
Email: juliet.fried@unco.edu
Website: http://www.hhs.unco.edu/Rehab.htm
Juliet H. Fried, EdD, Contact

District of Columbia

★ 29174 ★ George Washington University
Rehabilitation Counseling Program
2011 Eye St. NW
Ste. 300
Washington, DC 20052
Phone: (202)973-1550 **Fax:** (202)775-0053
Email: dondew@gwu.edu
Website: http://www.gwu.edu/~chaos/
Donald W. Dew, CNT, Director

Florida

★ 29175 ★ Florida State University
Department of Rehabilitation and Counseling Services
College of Education
215 Stone Bldg.
Tallahassee, FL 32301
Phone: (850)644-3854 **Fax:** (850)644-4335
Email: debener@garnet.acns.fsu.edu
Website: http://www.fsu.edu/~coe/departments/hss.html
Deborah Ebener, PhD, Contact

★ 29176 ★ University of Florida
Department of Rehabilitation Counseling
Rehabilitation Counseling Program and Rehabilitative Services
PO Box 100175
Gainesville, FL 32610-0175
Phone: (352)265-0745 **Fax:** (352)265-0744
Email: hsawter@hp.ufl.edu
Horace W. Sawyer, Contact

★ 29177 ★ University of North Florida
Department of Health Science
Rehabilitation Counseling Program
4567 St. Johns Bluff Rd. S
Jacksonville, FL 32224-2645
Phone: (904)620-2840 **Fax:** (904)620-2848
Email: jpatters@unf.edu
Website: http://www.unf.edu or http://www.unf.edu/coh/cohrehab.htm
Jeanne Patterson, EdD, Contact

★ 29178 ★ University of South Florida
College of Arts and Sciences
Department of Rehabilitation and Mental Health Counseling
4202 E Fowler Ave., BEH 315
Tampa, FL 33620-8100
Phone: (813)974-2855 **Fax:** (813)974-8080
Email: dixon@chuma1.cas.usf.edu
Website: http://www.cas.usf.edu/rehab_counseling/index.html
Charlotte G. Dixon, Contact

Georgia

★ 29179 ★ Fort Valley State University
Counseling Psychology, Rehabilitation Counseling, and Case Management
1005 State University Dr.
Fort Valley, GA 31030-4313
Phone: (478)825-6237 **Fax:** (478)827-3097
Email: edwardsd@fvsu.edu
Dothell W. Edwards, Jr., Contact

★ 29180 ★ Georgia State University
Department of Counseling and Psychological Services
Rehabilitation Counseling Program
College of Education, 9th Fl.
Atlanta, GA 30303-3083
Phone: (404)651-2550 **Fax:** (404)651-1160
Email: rweed@gsu.edu
Website: http://www.gsu.edu/~wwwcps/
Roger O. Weed, PhD, Contact

★ 29181 ★ Thomas University
Division of Human Services
Rehabilitation Studies Program
1501 Millpond Rd.
Thomasville, GA 31792-7499
Phone: (229)226-1621 **Fax:** (912)226-1653
Email: schandler@thomasu.edu
Shirley K. Chandler, PhD, Director

Hawaii

★ 29182 ★ University of Hawaii, Manoa
Department of Counselor Education
Rehabilitation Counseling Program
1776 University Ave.
WA2-221
Honolulu, HI 96822
Phone: (808)956-7904 **Fax:** (808)956-3814
Email: dwwong@hawaii.edu
Website: http://www.hawaii.edu/97catalog/education/counseling.html
Daniel Wong, PhD, Contact

Idaho

★ 29183 ★ University of Idaho
Division of Adult, Counselor, and Technology Education
Rehabilitation/Community Counseling Program
College of Education
Moscow, ID 83843-3083
Phone: (208)885-6556 **Fax:** (208)885-6869
Email: jfischer@uidaho.edu
Website: http://www.uidaho.edu/ed/acte/
Jerry Fischer, RhD, Contact

Illinois

★ 29184 ★ Illinois Institute of Technology
Institute of Psychology
Rehabilitation Counseling Program
3101 S Dearborn St.
Chicago, IL 60616
Phone: (312)567-3515 **Fax:** (312)567-3493
Email: lam@iit.edu
Website: http://www.iit.edu/colleges/psych/
Chow Lam, PhD, Director

★ 29185 ★ Northern Illinois University
Department of Communicative Disorders
Rehabilitation Counseling Program
DeKalb, IL 60115-2899
Phone: (815)753-1484 **Fax:** (815)753-9123
Email: glong@niu.edu
Website: http://www.chhs.niu.edu/comd/
Gregory Long, PhD, Contact

★ 29186 ★ Southern Illinois University, Carbondale
Rehabilitation Institute
Rehabilitation Counseling and Rehabilitation Services Programs
Rehn Hall 317
Carbondale, IL 62901-4609
Phone: (618)536-7704 **Fax:** (618)453-8271
Email: bordieri@siu.edu
Website: http://www.siu.edu/~rehabrct/
James Bordieri, PhD, Director

★ 29187 ★ University of Illinois
Department of Community Health
Rehabilitation Counseling Program
120 Huff Hall
MC-588
Champaign, IL 61820
Phone: (217)333-2307 **Fax:** (217)333-2766
Email: alston@uiuc.edu
Website: http://www.als.uiuc.edu/chlth/chlth-home.html
Reginald Alston, PhD, Contact

Iowa

★ 29188 ★ Drake University
School of Education
Rehabilitation Counseling Program
3206 University Ave.
Des Moines, IA 50311
Phone: (515)271-3061 **Fax:** (515)271-4848
Email: bs6991r@acad.drake.edu
Website: http://www.educ.drake.edu/nri/default.html
Robert Stensrud, EdD, Contact

★ 29189 ★ University of Iowa
Graduate Programs in Rehabilitation
N362 Lindquist Center N
Iowa City, IA 52242-1529
Phone: (319)335-5275 **Fax:** (319)335-5291
Email: vilia-tarvydas@uiowa.edu
Website: http://www.coe164.education.uiowa.edu:8180/crsd
Vilia Tarvydas, PhD, Contact

Kansas

★ 29190 ★ Emporia State University
Department of Counselor Education and Rehabilitation Programs
1200 Commercial
Campus Box 4036
Emporia, KS 66801
Phone: (620)341-5220 **Fax:** (620)341-6200
Email: kuehnmar@emporia.edu
Website: http://www.emporia.edu/counre/index.htm
Marvin D. Kuehn, EdD, Contact

Kentucky

★ 29191 ★ University of Kentucky
Special Education and Rehabilitation Counseling Program
224 Taylor Education Bldg.
Lexington, KY 40506
Phone: (859)257-3834 **Fax:** (859)257-3835
Email: crystal@uky.edu
Website: http://www.uky.edu/Education/EDP/cpoption.html
Ralph Crystal, PhD, Contact

Louisiana

★ 29192 ★ Louisiana State University Health Sciences Center
School of Allied Health Professions
Department of Rehabilitation Counseling
Rehabilitation Counseling Program
1900 Gravier St.
Rm. 8C1, Box G6-2
New Orleans, LA 70112-2262
Phone: (504)568-4315 **Fax:** (504)568-4324
Email: dstroh@lsuhsc.edu
Website: http://AlliedHealth.lsuhsc.edu
Douglas Strohmer, PhD, Contact

★ 29193 ★ Louisiana Tech University
Professional Development and Research Institute on Blindness
Box 3158
Ruston, LA 71272
Phone: (318)257-4554 **Fax:** (318)257-2259
Email: rgardner@latech.edu
Ronald J. Gardner, Director

★ 29194 ★ Southern University
Rehabilitation Counseling and Services
Department of Psychology
229 Blanks Hall
Baton Rouge, LA 70813
Phone: (225)771-2819 **Fax:** (225)771-2293
Email: kundusubr@aol.com
Website: http://www.subr.edu/academic/science/
Madan M. Kundu, PhD, Contact

Maine

★ 29195 ★ University of Maine, Farmington
Department of Special Education and Rehabilitation Services
University of Maine at Farmington
Farmington, ME 04938
Phone: (207)778-7260 **Fax:** (207)778-7157
Email: pullo@maine.edu
Robert E. Pullo, PhD, Contact

★ 29196 ★ University of Southern Maine
Rehabilitation Counseling Program
400 Bailey Hall
Gorham, ME 04038
Phone: (207)780-5316 **Fax:** (207)780-5043
Email: smurphy@usm.maine.edu
Website: http://www.usm.maine.edu/~coe/hrd/ce.htm
Stephen Murphy, PhD, Contact

Maryland

★ 29197 ★ Coppin State College
Department of Applied Psychology and Rehabilitation Counseling
Rehabilitation Counseling Program
2500 West North Ave.
Baltimore, MD 21216-3698
Phone: (410)383-5791 **Fax:** (410)383-5791
Email: jspry@coe.coppin.umd.edu
Website: http://www.coppin.edu/academic/academic.html
Janet Denise Spry, PhD, Contact

★ 29198 ★ University of Maryland
Counseling and Personnel Services Department
Rehabilitation Counseling Program
College of Education
Benjamin Bldg., Rm. 3214
College Park, MD 20742
Phone: (301)405-2858 **Fax:** (301)405-9995
Email: ef24@umail.umd.edu
Website: http://www.inform.umd.edu/EDUC/Depts/EDCP/Rehab/index.html
Ellen Fabian, PhD, Contact

★ 29199 ★ University of Maryland Eastern Shore
Department of Rehabilitation Services
Rehabilitation Services and Counseling Programs
934-5 Backbone Rd.
Princess Anne, MD 21853-1299
Phone: (410)651-6262 **Fax:** (410)651-6736
Email: jmfobbs@mail.umes.edu
Joan Fobbs, PhD, Contact

Massachusetts

★ 29200 ★ Assumption College
Institute for Social and Rehabilitation Services
500 Salisbury St.
Worcester, MA 01609
Phone: (508)767-7370 **Fax:** (508)798-2872
Email: sabelli@assumption.edu
Website: http://www.assumption.edu:80/dept/SocRehab/socmain.html
Susan Sabelli, RhD, Contact

★ 29201 ★ Boston University
Sargent College of Health and Rehabilitation Sciences
Rehabilitation Counseling Program
Department of Rehabilitation Sciences
635 Commonwealth Ave.
Boston, MA 02215
Phone: (617)353-2725 **Fax:** (617)353-8914
Email: ado@bu.edu
Website: http://www.bu.edu/sargent
Arthur E. Dell Orto, PhD, Exec Director

★ 29202 ★ Springfield College
Rehabilitation and Disability Studies Department
263 Alden St.
Springfield, MA 01109
Phone: (413)748-3318 **Fax:** (413)748-3787
Email: truscioj@spfldcol.edu
Website: http://www.springfieldcollege.edu/homepage.nsf
Thomas Ruscio, Contact

★ 29203 ★ University of Massachusetts, Boston
Counseling and School Psychology
100 Morrissey Blvd.
Boston, MA 02125
Phone: (617)287-7602 **Fax:** (617)287-7664
Email: Nanzhang.Hampton@umb.edu
Nan Zhang Hampton, PhD, Contact

Michigan

★ 29204 ★ Michigan State University
Office of Rehabilitation and Disability Studies
Counseling, Educational Psychology and Special Education
Rehabilitation Counseling Program
College of Education
237 Erickson Hall
East Lansing, MI 48824-1034
Phone: (517)355-1838 **Fax:** (517)353-6393
Email: leahym@msu.edu
Website: http://ed-web3.educ.msu.edu/ord/default.htm
Michael Leahy, PhD, Director

★ 29205 ★ Wayne State University
Rehabilitation Counseling and Community Inclusion
Rehabilitation Counseling Program
5425 Gullen Mall
311 Education
Detroit, MI 48202
Phone: (313)577-1743 **Fax:** (313)577-5235
Email: a_coven@wayne.edu
Website: http://www.coe.wayne.edu/org/TBF/tbf.html
Arnold B. Coven, EdD, Contact

★ 29206 ★ Western Michigan University
Departments of Counselor Education and Counseling Psychology and Blind Rehabilitation
Rehabilitation Counseling Program
3404 Sangren Hall
Kalamazoo, MI 49008-5111
Phone: (616)387-3455 **Fax:** (616)387-3567
Email: william.wiener@wmich.edu
Website: http://www.wmich.edu/hhs/blrh/html/rtc.htm
William R. Wiener, PhD, Contact

Minnesota

★ 29207 ★ Minnesota State University, Mankato
Department of Speech, Hearing and Rehabilitation Services
Rehabilitation Counseling Program
College of Allied Health and Nursing
103 Armstrong Hall
Mankato, MN 56001
Phone: (507)389-1414 **Fax:** (507)389-2821
Email: gerald.schneck@mnsu.edu
Website: http://www.mnsu.edu/dept/rehbcnsig/
Gerald Schneck, PhD, Contact

★ 29208 ★ Saint Cloud State University
Department of counselor education and Educational Psychology
Rehabilitation Counseling Program
720 Fourth Ave. S
Saint Cloud, MN 56301
Phone: (320)255-3131 **Fax:** (320)255-4082
Email: jhotz@stcloudstate.edu
Website: http://condor.stcloudstate.edu/~bulletin/apsy/brochure1.html
John C. Hotz, RhD, Contact

Mississippi

★ 29209 ★ Jackson State University
Rehabilitation Counseling Program
PO Box 17501
Jackson, MS 39217
Phone: (601)979-2380 **Fax:** (601)979-4190
Email: fgiles@ccaix.jsums.edu
Website: http://ccaix.jsums.edu/~www/soe/html/sped-rehab.html
Frank L. Giles, PhD, Contact

★ 29210 ★ Mississippi State University
Department of Counseling, Educational Psychology, and Special Education
Rehabilitation Counseling Program
Mail Stop 9727
Mississippi State, MS 39762
Phone: (662)325-3426 **Fax:** (662)325-3263
Email: ghendren@colled.msstate.edu
Website: http://www.educ.msstate.edu/CEdEPy/cedepy.html
Glen Hendren, PhD, Contact

Missouri

★ 29211 ★ Maryville University, Saint Louis
Department of Rehabilitation Counseling
Rehabilitation Counseling Program
13550 Conway Rd.
Saint Louis, MO 63141-7299
Phone: (314)529-9625 **Fax:** (314)529-9139
Email: lcarlucc@maryville.edu
Lance W. Carluccio, PhD, Director

★ 29212 ★ University of Missouri, Columbia
Department of Educational and Counseling Psychology
Rehabilitation Counseling Program
6 Hill Hall
Columbia, MO 65211
Phone: (573)882-7731 **Fax:** (573)884-5989
Email: robertsc@missouri.edu
Website: http://tiger.coe.missouri.edu/~ecp/
C. David Roberts, PhD, Director

New Jersey

★ 29213 ★ University of Medicine and Dentistry of New Jersey
Department of Psychiatric Rehabilitation
School of Health-Related Professions
1776 Raritan Rd.
Rm. 517
Scotch Plains, NJ 07076
Phone: (908)889-2430 **Fax:** (908)889-2432
Kenneth J. Gill, PhD, Contact

New Mexico

★ 29214 ★ Western New Mexico University
Department of Occupational Therapy and Rehabilitation
PO Box 680
Silver City, NM 88062
Phone: (505)574-5170 **Fax:** (505)574-5150
Email: casselg@silver.wnmu.edu
Gwen Cassel, Contact

New York

★ 29215 ★ City University of New York Hunter College
Department of Educational Foundations and Counseling Programs
Rehabilitation Counseling Program
695 Park Ave.
New York, NY 10021
Phone: (212)772-4755 **Fax:** (212)650-3198
Website: http://discovery.hunter.cuny.edu/~bettye/couns.html
John O'Neill, PhD, Contact

★ 29216 ★ Cornell University
Program on Employment and Disability
School of Industrial and Labor Relations
331 Ives Hall
Ithaca, NY 14853-3901
Phone: (607)255-7727 **Fax:** (607)255-2763
Email: smb23@cornell.edu
Susanne M. Bruyere, PhD, Director

★ 29217 ★ Hofstra University
Department of Counseling, Research, Special Education and Rehabilitation
Rehabilitation Counseling Program
Rehabilitation Administration Program
124 Hofstra University
111 Mason Hall
Hempstead, NY 11549
Phone: (516)463-5782 **Fax:** (516)463-6415
Email: edajsl@hofstra.edu
Website: http://www.hofstra.edu/Communities/?uri=/Graduate&bounce=/Graduate/
Joseph Lechowicz, PhD, Director

★ 29218 ★ New York University
Rehabilitation Counseling
Department of Applied Psychology
239 Greene St.
Ste. 400
New York, NY 10003
Phone: (212)998-5293 **Fax:** (212)995-4358
Email: david.peterson@nyu.edu
Website: http://www.nyu.edu/education/health/rehab/index.html
David B. Peterson, PhD, Director

★ 29219 ★ St. John's University
Rehabilitational Counseling Program
Division of Human Services and Counseling
School of Education
8000 Utopia Pkwy.
Jamaica, NY 11439
Phone: (718)990-6455 **Fax:** (718)990-7468
Email: gsampson@si.rr.com
Gene Sampson, PhD, Contact

★ 29220 ★ State University of New York, Albany
Department of Education and Counseling Psychology
1400 Washington Ave.
(Education 220)
Albany, NY 12222
Phone: (518)442-5050 **Fax:** (518)442-4953
Email: sgrand@nycap.rr.com
Website: http://www.albany.edu/counseling_psych/
Sheldon Grand, PhD, Contact

★ 29221 ★ State University of New York, Buffalo
Department of Counseling and Educational Psychology
Rehabilitation Counseling Program
409 Christopher Baldy Hall
Buffalo, NY 14260-1000
Phone: (716)645-2484 **Fax:** (716)645-6661
Email: tjanikow@buffalo.edu
Website: http://www.gse.buffalo.edu/DC/CEP/RC.html
Timothy P. Janikowski, PhD, Director

★ 29222 ★ Syracuse University
Rehabilitation Counseling Program
259 Huntington Hall
Syracuse, NY 13244-2340
Phone: (315)443-9624 **Fax:** (315)443-5732
Email: DdGilbri@syr.edu
Website: http://soeweb.syr.edu/chs/index.htm
Dennis Gilbride, PhD, Contact

North Carolina

★ 29223 ★ East Carolina University
School of Allied Health Sciences
Department of Rehabilitation Studies
Rehabilitation Counseling Program
Greenville, NC 27858-4353
Phone: (252)328-4455 **Fax:** (252)328-4470
Email: thomass@mail.ecu.edu
Website: http://www.ecu.edu/rehb/rc.htm
Stephen W. Thomas, EdD, Contact

★ 29224 ★ University of North Carolina, Chapel Hill
Division of Rehabilitation Psychology and Counseling
Rehabilitation Psychology and Counseling Program
224 Medical School Wing E, CB 7205
Chapel Hill, NC 27599-7205
Phone: (919)966-3351 **Fax:** (919)966-9125
Email: eburker@css.unc.edu
Website: http://www.alliedhealth.unc.edu/rps/
Eileen Burker, PhD, Contact

Ohio

★ 29225 ★ Bowling Green State University
Department of Special Education
Rehabilitation Counseling Program
Bowling Green, OH 43403-0255
Phone: (419)372-7293 **Fax:** (419)372-8265

Email: jstewar@bgnet.bgsu.edu
Website: http://www.bgsu.edu/colleges/edhd/EIS/DIS/
Jay R. Stewart, PhD, Director

★ 29226 ★ Kent State University
Educational Foundations and Special Services
Rehabilitation Counseling Program
405 White Hall
Kent, OH 44242
Phone: (330)672-2294 **Fax:** (330)672-2512
Email: prumrill@kent.edu
Website: http://www.educ.kent.edu/CoE/EFSS/Programs/RCE/rce.html
Phillip Rumrill, PhD, Contact

★ 29227 ★ Ohio State University
Rehabilitation Services
Rehabilitation Counseling Program
356 Arps Hall
1945 N High St.
Columbus, OH 43210-1120
Phone: (614)292-8183 **Fax:** (614)292-4255
Email: klein.3@osu.edu
Website: http://www.coe.ohio-state.edu/paes/Default.htm
Michael Klein, PhD, Contact

★ 29228 ★ Ohio University
Department of Counseling and Higher Education
Rehabilitation Counseling Program
201 McCracken Hall
Athens, OH 45701-2979
Phone: (740)593-4440 **Fax:** (740)593-0799
Email: olsheski@ohiou.edu
Website: http://www.ohiou.edu/che/index.html
Jerry Olsheski, PhD, Contact

★ 29229 ★ Wright State University
Rehabilitation Counseling Programs
Department of Human Services
MO52 Creative Arts Center
3640 Colonel Glenn Hwy.
Dayton, OH 45435-0001
Phone: (937)775-2075 **Fax:** (937)775-2042
Email: stephen.fortson@wright.edu
Website: http://www.ed.wright.edu/departments/hs/programs.html
Stephen Fortson, PhD, Contact

Oklahoma

★ 29230 ★ East Central University
Department of Human Resources
Rehabilitation Counseling Program
Box Z-2
Ada, OK 74820
Phone: (580)332-8000 **Fax:** (580)436-3329
Email: rbmgrtnr@mailclerk.ecok.edu
Website: http://www.ecok.edu/acaddept/humres/rehbmast.html
Richard Baumgartner, EdD, Contact

★ 29231 ★ Langston University, Oklahoma City
Rehabilitation Counseling Program
4205 N Lincoln Blvd.
Oklahoma City, OK 73105
Phone: (405)962-1671 **Fax:** (405)962-1621
Email: clmoore@lunet.edu
Corey Moore, RhD, Director

★ 29232 ★ Oklahoma State University
National Clearinghouse of Rehabilitation Training Materials
5202 N Richmond Hill Dr.
Stillwater, OK 74078-4080
Phone: (405)744-2000 **Free:** 800-223-5219
Fax: (405)744-2001
Email: seefelj@okstate.edu
Website: http://www.nchrtm.okstate.edu
Judy Seefeldt, Director

★ 29233 ★ University of Oklahoma
National Center for Disability Education and Training
106 W Constitution, Bldg. 158
Norman, OK 73072-7820
Phone: (405)325-4913 **Fax:** (405)325-1632
Charles E. Young, Director

Oregon

★ 29234 ★ Portland State University
School of Education
Rehabilitation Counseling Program
PO Box 751
Portland, OR 97207
Phone: (503)725-4619 **Fax:** (503)725-5599
Email: livnehh@pdx.edu
Website: http://www.ed.pdx.edu/spedcoun/rehab/
Hanoch Livneh, PhD, Contact

★ 29235 ★ Western Oregon University
Division of Special Education
Rehabilitation Counselor Education Program
Education Bldg., Rm. 220
Monmouth, OR 97361
Phone: (503)838-8444 **Fax:** (503)838-8228
Email: kellerl@wou.edu
Website: http://www.wou.edu/education/sped/rc.html
Linda Keller, PhD, Contact

Pennsylvania

★ 29236 ★ East Stroudsburg University
Department of Special Education/ Rehabilitation
Rehabilitative Services
200 Prospect St.
East Stroudsburg, PA 18301-2999
Phone: (570)422-3558 **Fax:** (570)422-3777
Email: dsteere@po-box.esu.edu
Daniel Steere, PhD, Contact

★ 29237 ★ Pennsylvania State University
Department of Counselor Education, Counseling Psychology and Rehabilitation Services
Rehabilitation Counseling Program
327 Cedar Bldg.
University Park, PA 16802-3110
Phone: (814)865-6643 **Fax:** (814)863-7750
Email: exm31@psu.edu
Website: http://www.ed.psu.edu/cned/rehab/
Elias Mpofu, PhD, Contact

★ 29238 ★ University of Scranton
Department of Counseling and Human Services
Rehabilitation Counseling Programs
Scranton, PA 18510-4523
Phone: (570)941-4236 **Fax:** (570)941-5882
Email: bruchl1@scranton.edu
Website: http://academic.uofs.edu/department/chs/grad.html
Lori A. Bruch, EdD, Contact

Puerto Rico

★ 29239 ★ University of Puerto Rico
Rio Piedras Campus
Rehabilitation Counseling School
PO Box 23345
San Juan, PR 00931-3345
Phone: (787)764-0000 **Fax:** (787)763-4199
Hilda E. Gonzalez de Perez, Contact

South Carolina

★ 29240 ★ South Carolina State University
Department of Human Services
Rehabilitation Counseling Program
300 College St.
PO Box 7356
Orangeburg, SC 29117-0001
Phone: (803)536-8600 **Fax:** (803)533-3636
Email: dstaten@scsu.edu
Website: http://www.scsu.edu/academic/S_Applie/Rehib_Co/index.htm
David Staten, PhD, Contact

★ 29241 ★ University of South Carolina
School of Medicine
Rehabilitation Counseling Program
3555 Harden St. Extension, Ste. B-20
Columbia, SC 29208
Phone: (803)434-4296 **Fax:** (803)434-4231
Email: lleech@medpark.sc.edu
Website: http://www.med.sc.edu/REHAB/PROGRAM/HOMEPG.htm
Linda L. Leech, PhD, Director

Tennessee

★ 29242 ★ University of Memphis
Department of Counseling, Educational Psychology and Research
Rehabilitation Counseling Program
Ball Education Bldg., Rm. 100
Memphis, TN 38152
Phone: (901)678-2841 **Fax:** (901)678-4778
Email: cdonnell@memphis.edu
Website: http://www.people.memphis.edu/~coe_cepr/rehab.htm
Chandra Donnell, PhD, Contact

★ 29243 ★ University of Tennessee, Knoxville
Department of Educational Psychology and Counseling
Rehabilitation Counseling Program
A207 Claxton Complex
Knoxville, TN 37996-3452
Phone: (865)974-8145 **Fax:** (865)974-0135
Email: askinner@utk.edu
Website: http://www.coe.utk.edu/units/rdhs.html
Amy Skinner, PhD, Contact

Texas

★ 29244 ★ Stephen F. Austin State University
Department of Counseling and Special Education Programs
Rehabilitation Counseling Program
PO Box 13019, SFA Sta.
Nacogdoches, TX 75962
Phone: (936)468-2906 **Fax:** (936)468-1342
Email: rchoate@sfasu.edu
Website: http://www.education.sfasu.edu/csped/rehabcn.htm
Robert Choate, EdD, Director

★ 29245 ★ University of North Texas
Department of Rehabilitation, Social Work and Addictions
Rehabilitation Counseling Program
PO Box 311456
Denton, TX 76203-1456
Phone: (940)565-2488 **Fax:** (940)565-3960
Email: pleung@scs.cmm.unt.edu
Website: http://www.scs.unt.edu/depts/rswa/msrhab.htm
Paul Leung, PhD, Contact

★ 29246 ★ University of Texas Southwestern Medical Center at Dallas
Department of Rehabilitation Counseling
Rehabilitative Counseling Program
5323 Harry Hines Blvd.
Dallas, TX 75390
Phone: (214)648-1740 **Fax:** (214)648-1771
Email: dpool@mednet.swmed.edu
Website: http://www.swmed.edu/home_pages/publish/ahs_catalog/rehab.html
Donald A. Pool, PhD, Contact

★ 29247 ★ University of Texas, Austin
Department of Special Education and Rehabilitation Counselor Education
Rehabilitation Counseling Program
University Station D5300
Austin, TX 78712
Phone: (512)232-5687 **Fax:** (512)232-5686
Email: r.parker@mail.utexas.edu
Website: http://www.edb.utexas.edu/coe/depts/sped/Rehab/homepage.html
Randall M. Parker, PhD, Contact

★ 29248 ★ University of Texas, Pan American
College of Health Sciences and Human Services
Rehabilitative Services Program
1201 W University Dr.
Edinburg, TX 78539-2999
Phone: (956)316-7036 **Fax:** (956)318-5237
Email: bjreed@panam.edu
Bruce Reed, PhD, Contact

Utah

★ 29249 ★ Utah State University
Department of Special Education and Rehabilitation
Rehabilitation Counseling Program
2865 Old Main Hill
Logan, UT 84322-2865
Phone: (435)797-3243 **Fax:** (435)797-3572
Email: jsmart@cc.usu.edu
Website: http://www.rce.usu.edu/
Julie F. Smart, PhD, Contact

Virginia

★ 29250 ★ Virginia Commonwealth University
Medical College of Virginia
Department of Rehabilitation Counseling
1121 E Clay St.
PO Box 980330
Richmond, VA 23298-0330
Phone: (804)828-1132 **Fax:** (804)828-1321
Email: mntucker@vcu.edu
Website: http://views.vcu.edu/sahp/rehab/
Christine Reid, PhD, Contact

Washington

★ 29251 ★ Western Washington University
Center for Continuing Education in Rehabilitation
Rehabilitation Counseling Program
6912 220th St. SW, Ste. 105
Mountlake Terrace, WA 98043
Phone: (425)774-4446 **Free:** 888-377-0100
Fax: (425)774-9303
Email: geri.hansen@wwu.edu
Geraldine Hansen, EdD, Director

West Virginia

★ 29252 ★ West Virginia University
Department of Counseling, Rehabilitation Counseling and Counseling Psychology
Rehabilitation Counseling Program
PO Box 6122
502 Allen Hall
Morgantown, WV 26506-6122
Phone: (304)293-3807 **Fax:** (304)293-4082
Email: mglenn@wvu.edu
Website: http://www.wvu.edu/~hre/
Margaret Glenn, EdD, Contact

Wisconsin

★ 29253 ★ University of Wisconsin, Madison
Department of Rehabilitation Psychology and Special Education
Rehabilitation Counseling Program
432 N Murray St.
Madison, WI 53706-1496
Phone: (608)263-5860 **Fax:** (608)262-8108
Email: rlynch@education.wisc.edu
Website: http://www.soemadison.wisc.edu/rpse/
Ruth Torkelson Lynch, PhD, Contact

★ 29254 ★ University of Wisconsin, Milwaukee
Department of Educational Psychology
Rehabilitation Counseling Program
709 Enderis Hall
PO Box 413
Milwaukee, WI 53201-0413
Phone: (414)229-4767 **Fax:** (414)229-4939
Email: pichette@uwn.edu
Website: http://www.uwm.edu/Dept/EdPsych/msinf.html
Gene Pichette, PhD, Contact

★ 29255 ★ University of Wisconsin, Stout
Department of Rehabilitation and Counseling
Rehabilitation Counseling Program
221 10th Ave., Rm. 250 VR
Menomonie, WI 54751
Phone: (715)232-2499 **Fax:** (715)232-2356
Email: stewarts@uwstout.edu
Website: http://www.uwstout.edu/programs/bsvr/
Shirley Stewart, PhD, Contact

Respiratory Therapy

Listed below are respiratory therapist educational programs accredited by the Commission on Accreditation of Allied Health Education Programs (35 E Wacker Dr., Ste. 1970, Chicago, IL 60601-2208, (312)553-9355, http://www.caahep.org/) in collaboration with the Committee on Accreditation for Respiratory Care (CoARC). Information on accredited respiratory therapy technician programs may be obtained by contacting CoARC at 1248 Harwood Rd., Bedford, TX 76021-4244, (817)283-2835, http://www.coarc.com/.

Alabama

★ 29256 ★ George C. Wallace State Community College
Advanced Respiratory Therapist Program
Rte. 6
Box 62
Dothan, AL 36303
Phone: (334)983-3521
Email: dodom@wallace.edu
Website: http://www.wallace.edu/wccpages/index.html
Henry D. Odom, Contact

★ 29257 ★ Shelton State Community College
Advanced Respiratory Therapist Program
3401 Martin Luther King Jr. Blvd.
Tuscaloosa, AL 35401
Phone: (205)391-2641
Email: bspruell@sheltonstate.edu
Website: http://207.157.109.131/
Bruce E. Spruell, Contact

★ 29258 ★ University of Alabama, Birmingham
Respiratory Therapy Program
1705 University Blvd.
RMSB 486
Birmingham, AL 35294-1212
Phone: (205)934-3783
Email: grangerw@uab.edu
Website: http://main.uab.edu/show.asp?durki=3418
Wesley M. Granger, PhD, Contact

★ 29259 ★ University of South Alabama
Advanced Respiratory Therapist Program
Department of Cardiorespiratory Care
1504 Springhill Ave., Rm. 2545
Mobile, AL 36604-3273
Phone: (251)434-3405
Email: wwojciec@jaguar1.usouthal.edu
Website: http://www.southalabama.edu/usa/allhealth/crc.htm
William V. Wojciechowski, Contact

★ 29260 ★ Wallace State College
Advanced Respiratory Therapist Program
PO Box 2000
Hanceville, AL 35077-2000
Phone: (256)352-8310
Email: p_taylor@bellsouth.net
Website: http://www.wallacestatehanceville.edu/
Paul D. Taylor, Contact

Arizona

★ 29261 ★ Apollo College Tri-City
Advanced Respiratory Therapist Program
630 W Southern Ave.
Mesa, AZ 85210
Phone: (480)831-6585
Email: vspear@apollocollege.com
Website: http://www.apollocollege.com/
Valerie S. Spear, Contact

★ 29262 ★ Apollo College, Phoenix Campus
Advanced Respiratory Therapist Program
8503 N 27th Ave.
Phoenix, AZ 85051
Phone: (602)864-1571

Email: andersonaz2000@yahoo.com
Website: http://www.apollocollege.com/rt.htm
Pamela M. Nelson-Artibey, Contact

★ 29263 ★ Gateway Community College
Advanced Respiratory Therapist Program
108 N 40th St.
Phoenix, AZ 85034-1795
Phone: (602)392-5000
Email: toni.rodriguez@gwmail.maricopa.edu
Website: http://www.gwc.maricopa.edu/aop/resp.html
Toni L. Rodriguez, EdD, Contact

★ 29264 ★ Long Technical College
Advanced Respiratory Therapist Program
13450 N Black Canyon Hwy.
Phoenix, AZ 85029
Phone: (602)548-1955
Email: randerson@longtechnicalcollege.com
Ronda D. Anderson, Contact

★ 29265 ★ Pima Community College
Advanced Respiratory Therapist Program
2202 W Anklam Rd.
Tucson, AZ 85709-0080
Phone: (520)206-3107
Email: rpatze@pimacc.pima.edu
Website: http://www.pimacc.pima.edu/~curonline/cat-curr/RTH-P.HTM
Richard A. Patze, Contact

★ 29266 ★ Pima Medical Institute—Mesa
Advanced Respiratory Therapist Program
957 S Dobson Rd.
Mesa, AZ 85202
Phone: (480)345-7777
Email: pmifaculty@aol.com
Website: http://pimamedical.com/
Cynthia Smathers, Contact

★ 29267 ★ Pima Medical Institute-Tucson
Advanced Respiratory Therapist Program
3350 E Grant
Tucson, AZ 85716-2800
Phone: (520)326-1600
Email: leanna@qwest.net
Website: http://pimamedical.com/
Leanna Konechne, Contact

Arkansas

★ 29268 ★ Arkansas Valley Technical Institute
Respiratory Care Program
1311 S I St.
Fort Smith, AR 72901-4915
Phone: (501)441-5256
Email: frpayne@medscape.com
F. Ross Payne, Contact

★ 29269 ★ Black River Technical College
Advanced Respiratory Therapist Program
PO Box 468
Hwy. 304 E
Pocahontas, AR 72455
Phone: (870)248-4000
Email: briang@blackrivertech.org
Brian Garrett, Contact

★ 29270 ★ NorthWest Arkansas Community College
Advanced Respiratory Therapist Program
One College Dr.
Bentonville, AR 72712-5091
Phone: (501)619-4250
Email: aclark@nwacc.net
Alan Clark, Contact

★ 29271 ★ Pulaski Technical College
Advanced Respiratory Therapist Program
3000 W Scenic Dr.
North Little Rock, AR 72118
Phone: (501)812-2223
Email: jdavis@mail.ptc.tec.ar.us
Jim C. Davis, Contact

★ 29272 ★ University of Arkansas Community College at Hope
Advanced Respiratory Therapist Program
PO Box 140
2500 S Main St.
Hope, AR 71802-0140
Phone: (870)777-5722
Email: klejeune@uacch.cc.ar.us
J. Kenneth Le Jeune, Contact

★ 29273 ★ University of Arkansas for Medical Sciences
Advanced Respiratory Therapist Program
AHEC-Southwest
300 E Sixth St.
Texarkana, AR 71854
Phone: (870)779-6033
Email: evansdennisp@uams.edu
D. Patrick Evans, Contact

★ 29274 ★ University of Arkansas for Medical Sciences
College of Health Related Professions
Advanced Respiratory Therapist Program
4301 W Markham, Slot 704 (14B/NLR)
Little Rock, AR 72205
Phone: (501)257-2343
Email: booneernal@uams.edu
Website: http://www.uams.edu/ahec/ahec12.htm
Erna Boone, Contact

California

★ 29275 ★ American River College
Advanced Respiratory Therapist Program
4700 College Oak Dr.
Sacramento, CA 95841
Phone: (916)484-8876
Email: warmanj@arc.losrios.cc.ca.us
Website: http://www.arc.losrios.cc.ca.us/scihlth/resp-care.html
James L. Warman, PhD, Contact

★ 29276 ★ Bryman College
Advanced Respiratory Therapist Program
1245 S Winchester Blvd.
San Jose, CA 95128
Phone: (408)246-0859
Email: vfadal@cci.edu
Victor T. Fadal, Contact

★ 29277 ★ Butte Glenn Community College
Advanced Respiratory Therapist Program
3536 Butte Campus Dr.
Oroville, CA 95965-8399
Phone: (530)895-2423
Email: solomonda@butte.cc.ca.us
Website: http://www.butte.cc.ca.us/catalog_htmls/RT.html
Daniel J. Solomon, Contact

★ 29278 ★ California College for Health Sciences
Advanced Respiratory Therapist Program
2423 Hoover Ave.
National City, CA 91950
Free: 800-221-7374
Email: jwelsh@cchs.edu
Website: http://www.cchs.edu/bachelors/respcare/
Jeffrey Welsh, PhD, Contact

★ 29279 ★ California Paramedical and Technical College—Riverside
Advanced Respiratory Therapist Program
4550 La Sierra Ave.
Riverside, CA 92505-2907
Phone: (909)687-9006
Email: wwalls@cptc-riverside.com
Website: http://www.pe.net/~compcptc/Respth.htm
Wayne A. Walls, Contact

★ 29280 ★ ConCorde Career Institute
Advanced Respiratory Therapist Program
12412 Victory Blvd.
North Hollywood, CA 91606
Phone: (818)753-6860
Email: mhaberwood@concordecareercolleges.com
Marlyn H. Haberwood, Contact

★ 29281 ★ Crafton Hills College
Advanced Respiratory Therapist Program
11711 Sand Canyon Rd.
Yucaipa, CA 92399-1799
Phone: (909)389-3284
Email: kbryson@crafton.sbccd.cc.ca.us
Website: http://www.sbccd.cc.ca.us/chc/index.htm
Kenneth R. Bryson, Contact

★ 29282 ★ East Los Angeles College/ Santa Monica College
Advanced Respiratory Therapist Program
1301 Avienda Cesar Chavez
Monterey Park, CA 91754-6099
Phone: (323)265-8612
Email: mcarr89774@aol.com
Website: http://www.elac.cc.ca.us/respiratorycat.htm
Michael R. Carr, Contact

★ 29283 ★ El Camino Community College
Advanced Respiratory Therapist Program
16007 Crenshaw Blvd.
Torrance, CA 90506
Phone: (310)660-3248
Email: sinopoli@elcamino.cc.ca.us
Website: http://www.elcamino.cc.ca.us/respiratory-care/default.htm
Louis M. Sinopoli, EdD, Contact

★ 29284 ★ Foothill College
Advanced Respiratory Therapist Program
12345 El Monte Rd.
Los Altos Hills, CA 94022
Phone: (650)949-7292
Email: treanor@fhda.edu
Website: http://www.foothill.fhda.edu/bio/programs/respther/
Shirley Treanor Barker, EdD, Contact

★ 29285 ★ Fresno City College
Advanced Respiratory Therapist Program
1101 E University Ave.
Fresno, CA 93741
Phone: (559)244-2631
Email: steven.boyd@do1.scccd.cc.ca.us
Website: http://www.fcc.cc.ca.us/healthsci/hsdivision.htmlrcp
Steven L. Boyd, Contact

★ 29286 ★ Grossmont College
Advanced Respiratory Therapist Program
8800 Grossmont College Dr.
El Cajon, CA 92020
Phone: (619)644-7448
Email: lorenda.seibold-phalan@gcccd.net
Website: http://grossmont.gcccd.cc.ca.us/healthprofessions/RTWebPage/Default.htm
Lorenda J. Seibold-Phalan, Contact

★ 29287 ★ Hacienda La Puente Adult Education
Willow Adult Center
Respiratory Therapy Program
14101 E Nelson Ave., Rm. 26
La Puente, CA 91746
Phone: (626)855-3138
Email: kmbooth@hlpusd.k12.ca.us
Kevin Booth, Contact

★ 29288 ★ Loma Linda University
Advanced Respiratory Therapist Program
Department of Cardiopulmonary Science
Nichol Hall, Rm. 1926
Loma Linda, CA 92350
Phone: (909)558-4932
Email: david-stanton@sahp.llu.edu
Website: http://www.llu.edu/llu/sahp/resp.htmlanchor401949
David Stanton, Contact

★ 29289 ★ Los Angeles Valley College
Advanced Respiratory Therapist Program
5800 Fulton Ave.
Van Nuys, CA 91401-4096
Phone: (818)947-2845
Email: sinshefa@lavc.edu
Website: http://www.lavc.cc.ca.us/catalog/rt.html
Frank Sinsheimer, EdD, Contact

★ 29290 ★ Modesto Junior College
Advanced Respiratory Therapist Program
435 College Ave.
Modesto, CA 95350
Phone: (209)575-6388
Email: lylet@yosemite.cc.ca.us
Website: http://virtual.yosemite.cc.ca.us/catalog/programs/respcarepgm.htm
Terry P. Lyle, Contact

★ 29291 ★ Mount San Antonio College
Advanced Respiratory Therapist Program
1100 N Grand Ave.
Walnut, CA 91789
Phone: (909)594-5611
Email: zin@earthlink.net
Website: http://www.mtsac.edu/instruction/dept686.html
Terrance M. Krider, Contact

★ 29292 ★ Napa Valley College
Advanced Respiratory Therapist Program
2277 Napa Vallejo Hwy.
Napa, CA 94558
Phone: (707)253-3147
Email: rchudnofsky@campus.nvc.cc.ca.us
Website: http://www.nvc.cc.ca.us/html/repiratory_therapy.html
Robert S. Chudnofsky, Contact

★ 29293 ★ Ohlone College
Advanced Respiratory Therapist Program
43600 Mission Blvd.
PO BOX 3909
Fremont, CA 94539-0390
Phone: (510)659-6029
Email: cmcnamee-cole@ohlone.cc.ca.us
Website: http://www.ohlone.cc.ca.us/instr/resp_ther/
Carol McNamee-Cole, Contact

★ 29294 ★ Orange Coast College
Advanced Respiratory Therapist Program
2701 Fairview Rd.
PO Box 5005
Costa Mesa, CA 92628-5005
Phone: (714)432-5541
Email: dadelman@mail.occ.cccd.edu
Website: http://www.occ.cccd.edu/departments/alh/respcinfo.html
Daniel S. Adelmann, Contact

★ 29295 ★ San Joaquin Valley College
Advanced Respiratory Therapist Program
8400 W Mineral King
Visalia, CA 93291-9283
Phone: (559)651-2500
Email: barryw@sjvc.com
Website: http://www.sjvc.com/
Barry Westling, Contact

★ 29296 ★ San Joaquin Valley College
Advanced Respiratory Therapist Program
201 New Stine Rd.
Bakersfield, CA 93309
Phone: (661)834-0126
Email: jeffreyc@sjvc.com
Website: http://www.sjvc.com/
Jeffrey E. Cox, Contact

★ 29297 ★ Simi Valley Adult School and Career Institute
Advanced Respiratory Therapist Program
3192 Los Angeles Ave.
Simi Valley, CA 93065
Phone: (805)579-6262
Email: ckingston@simi.tec.ca.us
Christine R. Kingston, Contact

★ 29298 ★ Skyline College
Advanced Respiratory Therapist Program
3300 College Dr.
San Bruno, CA 94066
Phone: (650)738-4382
Email: williamsonm@smccd.net
Website: http://www.smcccd.cc.ca.us/smcccd/skyline/smt/rpth.htmlanchor242942
Michael Williamson, Contact

★ 29299 ★ Victor Valley College
Advanced Respiratory Therapist Program
18422 Bear Valley Rd.
Victorville, CA 92392-5849
Phone: (760)245-4271
Email: lboutcher@vvc.cc.ca.us
Website: http://www.vvcconline.com/allhealth/index_rt.htm
Larry Boutcher, PhD, Contact

Colorado

★ 29300 ★ Front Range Community College
Advanced Respiratory Therapist Program
3645 W 112th Ave.
Campus Box 41
Westminster, CO 80030-2199
Phone: (303)404-5222
Email: jim.hannaford@wc.frcc.cccoes.edu
Website: http://frcc.cc.co.us/about/pubs/cat/programs/respiratory_care.html
James E. Hannaford, Contact

★ 29301 ★ Pima Medical Institute—Denver
Advanced Respiratory Therapist Program
1701 W 72nd Ave.
Denver, CO 80221
Phone: (303)426-1800
Email: clydewentworth@msn.com
Website: http://pimamedical.com/
C. Allen Wentworth, Contact

★ 29302 ★ Pueblo Community College
Advanced Respiratory Therapist Program
900 W Orman Ave.
Pueblo, CO 81004
Phone: (719)549-3266
Email: delia.lechtenberg@pcc.cccoes.edu
Website: http://www.pcc.cccoes.edu/resp_care/welcome.htm
Delia Lechtenberg, Contact

★ 29303 ★ T. H. Pickens Technical Center
Advanced Respiratory Therapist Program
500 Airport Blvd.
Aurora, CO 80011
Phone: (303)344-4910
Email: leigho@pickens.aps.k12.co.us
Website: http://www.pickenstech.org/Programs/programs.respiratory.care.tech.html
Leigh E. Otto, Contact

Connecticut

★ 29304 ★ Manchester Community College
Advanced Respiratory Therapist Program
Great Path, MS 17
PO Box 1046
Manchester, CT 06045-1046
Phone: (860)512-2714
Email: kmilikowski@mcc.commnet.edu
Website: http://www.mcc.commnet.edu/programs/healthcareers/RespCare/home.html
Karen A. Milikowski, Contact

★ 29305 ★ Naugatuck Valley Community College
Advanced Respiratory Therapist Program
750 Chase Pkwy.
Waterbury, CT 06708
Phone: (203)596-8662
Email: sbaer@nvcc.commnet.edu
Sharon A. Baer, Contact

★ 29306 ★ Norwalk Hospital/Norwalk Community Technical College
Advanced Respiratory Therapist Program
Maple St.
Norwalk, CT 06856-5050
Phone: (203)852-2479
Email: edward.reardon@norwalkhealth.org
Website: http://www.nctc.commnet.edu/pages/degree/programs/resp-p.htm
Edward A. Reardon, Contact

★ 29307 ★ Quinnipiac College
Advanced Respiratory Therapist Program
275 Mt. Carmel Ave.
Hamden, CT 06518
Phone: (203)582-8682
Email: ronald.beckett@quinnipiac.edu
Website: http://www.quinnipiac.edu/academics/department.asp?School=HS&Dept=115
Ronald G. Beckett, PhD, Contact

★ 29308 ★ University of Hartford
Advanced Respiratory Therapist Program
200 Bloomfield Ave.
West Hartford, CT 06117-1599
Phone: (860)768-4823
Email: pkennedy@mail.hartford.edu
Website: http://uhavax.hartford.edu/~healthpro/rt.html
Peter W. Kennedy, PhD, Contact

Delaware

★ 29309 ★ Delaware Technical and Community College—Owens Campus
Advanced Respiratory Therapist Program
PO Box 610, Rt. 18
Georgetown, DE 19947
Phone: (302)856-5400
Email: jlittle@outland.dtcc.edu
Website: http://www.dtcc.edu/
James G. Little, Contact

★ 29310 ★ Delaware Technical and Community College—Wilmington
Advanced Respiratory Therapist Program
Riverside Medical Arts Complex
700 W Lea Blvd., Ste 101
Wilmington, DE 19802
Phone: (302)765-4598
Email: rlang@christiancare.org
Website: http://www.dtcc.edu/
Robert M. Lang, Contact

District of Columbia

★ 29311 ★ University of the District of Columbia
Advanced Respiratory Therapist Program
4200 Connecticut Ave. NW
Washington, DC 20008
Phone: (202)274-5925
Email: slockwood@udc.edu
Website: http://udc2.org
Susan D. Lockwood, Contact

Florida

★ 29312 ★ ATI Health Education Centers, Campus No. 150
Advanced Respiratory Therapist Program
1395 NW 167 St., 2nd Fl.
Miami, FL 33169
Phone: (305)628-1000
Email: mgrassi@atienterprises.com
Website: http://www.aticareertraining.com/
Michele A. Grassi, Contact

★ 29313 ★ Broward Community College
Advanced Respiratory Therapist Program
1000 Coconut Creek Blvd.
Coconut Creek, FL 33066
Phone: (954)969-2082
Email: jprince@broward.cc.fl.us
Website: http://fs.broward.cc.fl.us/~jprince/index.htm
John Prince, Contact

★ 29314 ★ D.G. Erwin Technical Center
Advanced Respiratory Therapist Program
2010 E Hillsborough Ave.
Tampa, FL 33610
Phone: (813)231-1800
Email: leroux_1@firn.edu
L. Kelli LeRoux, Contact

★ 29315 ★ Daytona Beach Community College
Advanced Respiratory Therapist Program
1200 W International Speedway Blvd.
PO Box 2811
Daytona Beach, FL 32114-2811
Phone: (386)255-8131
Email: mccumbm@dbcc.edu
Website: http://www.dbcc.cc.fl.us/
Michael R. McCumber, EdD, Contact

★ 29316 ★ Edison Community College
Advanced Respiratory Therapist Program
8099 College Pkwy. SW
PO Box 60210
Fort Myers, FL 33906-6210
Phone: (941)489-9430
Email: jelsberr@edison.edu
Website: http://www.edison.edu/departments/health-science/respiratory.htm
Jeffrey B. Elsberry, PhD, Contact

★ 29317 ★ Florida A&M University (LB)
School of Allied Health Science
Advanced Respiratory Therapist Program
223 Ware-Rhaney Bldg.
Tallahassee, FL 32307-3500
Phone: (850)561-2027
Email: alphonso.baldwin@worldnet.att.net
Website: http://www.famu2.famu.edu/acad/colleges/ahs/rt.html
Alphonso Baldwin, PhD, Contact

★ 29318 ★ Florida Community College—Jacksonville
Advanced Respiratory Therapist Program
4501 Capper Rd.
Jacksonville, FL 32218
Phone: (904)766-6516
Email: jwoods@fccj.edu
Website: http://www.fccj.cc.fl.us/catalog/pos/as/RespiratoryCare-22440.html
James R. Woods, Contact

★ 29319 ★ Gulf Coast Community College
Advanced Respiratory Therapist Program
5230 W Hwy. 98
Panama City, FL 32401-1058
Phone: (850)872-3827
Email: bkillion@gulfcoast.edu
Bradley E. Killion, Contact

★ 29320 ★ Hillsborough Community College
Advanced Respiratory Therapist Program
4001 Tampa Bay Blvd.
Tampa, FL 33614
Phone: (813)253-7318
Email: marjiewilk@hcc.cc.fl.us
Marjorie J. Wilkins, Contact

★ 29321 ★ Indian River Community College (LB)
Advanced Respiratory Therapist Program
3209 Virginia Ave.
Fort Pierce, FL 34981-5599
Phone: (561)462-4358
Email: grosenfe@ircc.cc.fl.us
Website: http://www.ircc.cc.fl.us/index.htm
Georgette Rosenfeld, Contact

★ 29322 ★ Manatee Community College
Advanced Respiratory Therapist Program
PO Box 1849
Bradenton, FL 34206-1849
Phone: (941)752-5518
Email: hainesl@mccfl.edu
Website: http://www.mcc.cc.fl.us/Courses/as-frame.htm
J. Lynn Haines, Contact

★ 29323 ★ Miami-Dade Community College (LB)
Advanced Respiratory Therapist Program
950 NW 20th St.
Miami, FL 33127-4693
Phone: (305)237-4423
Email: rabreu@mdcc.edu
Website: http://www.mdcc.edu/medical/
Rolando Abreu, Contact

★ 29324 ★ Palm Beach Community College, Eissey Campus
Advanced Respiratory Therapist Program
Lewis Center 107
3160 PGA Blvd.
Palm Beach Gardens, FL 33410
Phone: (561)207-5068
Email: rogersj@pbcc.edu
Website: http://www.pbcc.cc.fl.us/
Jacqueline Rogers, Contact

★ 29325 ★ Pinellas Technical Education Centers
Advanced Respiratory Therapist Program
901 34th St. S
Saint Petersburg, FL 33711-2298
Phone: (727)893-2500
Email: cmartinetto@ptec.pinellas.k12.fl.us
Marsha E. Karkheck, Contact

★ 29326 ★ Saint Petersburg College
Advanced Respiratory Therapist Program
Health Education Center/Respiratory Care Program
7200 66th St. N
Pinellas Park, FL 33781
Phone: (727)341-3627
Email: mikless@spcollege.edu
Website: http://www.spjc.cc.fl.us/webcentral/acad/respcare.htm
Stephen P. Mikles, Contact

★ 29327 ★ Santa Fe Community College
Advanced Respiratory Therapist Program
3000 NW 83rd St.
Gainesville, FL 32606-6200
Phone: (352)395-5683
Email: paul.stephan@santafe.cc.fl.us
Website: http://inst.santafe.cc.fl.us/~health/respcare/
Paul J. Stephan, Contact

★ 29328 ★ Seminole Community College (LB)
Advanced Respiratory Therapist Program
100 Weldon Blvd.
Sanford, FL 32773-6199
Phone: (407)328-2293
Email: shideles@scc-fl.com
Website: http://www.seminole.cc.fl.us/Respiratory/
R. Steven Shideler, Contact

★ 29329 ★ Tallahassee Community College
Advanced Respiratory Therapist Program
444 Appleyard Dr.
Tallahassee, FL 32304-2895
Phone: (850)922-8103
Email: streetmd@tcc.cc.fl.us
Website: http://www.tallahassee.cc.fl.us/generalinfo/asrespiratory.htmBridge
Dewey E. Streetman, Contact

★ 29330 ★ University of Central Florida
Cardiopulmonary Sciences Program
Health and Public Affairs
Advanced Respiratory Therapist Program
Orlando, FL 32816-2205
Phone: (407)823-2214
Email: worrell@pegasus.cc.ucf.edu
Website: http://www.ucf.edu/catalog/9798/Degree_Programs/cardiopulmonary_sciences.html
L. Timothy Worrell, Contact

★ 29331 ★ Valencia Community College
Advanced Respiratory Therapist Program
PO Box 3028
Orlando, FL 32802-3028
Phone: (407)299-5000
Email: lcapraun@gwmail.valencia.cc.fl.us
Website: http://faculty.valencia.cc.fl.us/rescare/
Lynn W. Capraun, Contact

Georgia

★ 29332 ★ Armstrong Atlantic State University (LB)
Advanced Respiratory Therapist Program
11935 Abercorn St.
Savannah, GA 31419
Phone: (912)921-7446
Email: bowersro@mail.armstrong.edu
Website: http://www.rt.armstrong.edu/rcp.html
Ross L. Bowers, Contact

★ 29333 ★ Athens Area Technical Institute (LB)
Advanced Respiratory Therapist Program
800 Hwy. 29 N
Athens, GA 30601-1800
Phone: (706)355-5104
Email: ott@aati.edu
Website: http://admin1.athens.tec.ga.us/rtweb.html
Bruce A. Ott, EdD, Contact

★ 29334 ★ Augusta Technical College
Advanced Respiratory Therapist Program
3200 Augusta Tech Dr.
Augusta, GA 30906
Phone: (706)771-4194
Email: rwaller@augusta.tec.ga.us
Website: http://www.augusta.tec.ga.us/academic/A_rtt.htm
Rita Waller, Contact
Frmly: Augusta Technical Institute.

★ 29335 ★ Coosa Valley Technical Institute (LB)
Advanced Respiratory Therapist Program
One Maurice Culberson Dr.
Rome, GA 30161
Phone: (706)295-6910
Email: lpapp@cvtcollege.org
Leann I. Papp, Contact

★ 29336 ★ Darton College
Division of Allied Health
Advanced Respiratory Therapist Program
2400 Gillionville Rd.
Albany, GA 31707-3098
Phone: (229)430-6896
Email: thomasb@darton.edu
Website: http://www.dartnet.peachnet.edu/Programs/AlliedHealth/respcare.htm
William F. Thomas, Jr., Contact

★ 29337 ★ Georgia State University (LB)
Advanced Respiratory Therapist Program
Cardiopulmonary Care Sciences
C2 Kell Hall, University Plaza
Atlanta, GA 30303-3083
Phone: (404)651-1490
Email: resjlr@langate.gsu.edu
Website: http://www.gsu.edu/~wwwchs/dept/card/index.htm
Joseph L. Rau, PhD, Contact

★ 29338 ★ Griffin Technical College
Advanced Respiratory Therapist Program
501 Varsity Rd.
Griffin, GA 30223
Phone: (770)233-6169
Email: keatons@griftec.org
Shana D. Keaton, Contact

★ 29339 ★ Gwinnett Technical Institute
Advanced Respiratory Therapist Program
5150 Sugarloaf Pkwy.
PO Box 1505
Lawrenceville, GA 30046-1505
Phone: (770)962-7580
Email: bdelorme@gwinnett.tec.ga.us
Website: http://www.gwinnett-tech.org/programs/respiratory_therapist_aatd.html
Robert P. DeLorme, Contact

★ 29340 ★ Heart of Georgia Technical College
Advanced Respiratory Therapist Program
560 Pinehill Rd.
Dublin, GA 31021
Phone: (478)274-7881
Email: natalies@heartga.tec.ga.us
Natalie A. Smith, Contact

★ 29341 ★ Macon State College
Advanced Respiratory Therapist Program
100 College Station Dr.
Macon, GA 31206-5144
Phone: (912)471-2789
Email: cmatson@mail.maconstate.edu
Website: http://www.maconstate.edu/
Charles R. Matson, Contact

★ 29342 ★ Medical College of Georgia (LB)
Advanced Respiratory Therapist Program
Department of Respiratory Therapy
HM-143
Augusta, GA 30912-0850
Phone: (706)721-3554
Email: ataft@mail.mcg.edu
Website: http://www.mcg.edu/SAH/respther/index.html
Shelley C. Mishoe, PhD, Contact

★ 29343 ★ National Institute of Technology
Advanced Respiratory Therapist Program
1706 NE Expressway
Atlanta, GA 30329
Phone: (404)327-8787
Terri L. McQuiddy, Contact

★ 29344 ★ Southwest Georgia Technical College
Advanced Respiratory Therapist Program
15689 U.S. Hwy. 19 N
Thomasville, GA 31792
Phone: (229)225-4078
Email: tmiller@swgtc.net
Website: http://www.thomas.tec.ga.us/
Tammy A. Miller, Contact

Hawaii

★ 29345 ★ Kapiolani Community College
Advanced Respiratory Therapist Program
Health Sciences Department
4303 Diamond Head Rd.
Honolulu, HI 96816
Phone: (808)734-9243
Email: wehrman@hawaii.edu
Website: http://www.kcc.hawaii.edu/academics/catalog/programs/health/index.htm
Stephen F. Wehrman, Contact

Idaho

★ 29346 ★ Boise State University (LB)
Advanced Respiratory Therapist Program
1910 University Dr.
Boise, ID 83725-1320
Phone: (208)426-3670
Email: ccolby@boisestate.edu
Website: http://selland.boisestate.edu/academic_divisions/heal_serv/resp_ther.htm
Conrad Colby, PhD, Contact

Illinois

★ 29347 ★ Central Illinois College/Saint Francis Medical Center (LB)
Advanced Respiratory Therapist Program
201 SW Adams
Peoria, IL 61635-0001
Phone: (309)999-4663
Email: kcrawfordjones@icc.cc.il.us
Website: http://www.icc.cc.il.us/haps/HCprgms4.htmtherapist
Carole K. Crawford-Jones, Contact

★ 29348 ★ College of DuPage
Advanced Respiratory Therapist Program
425 Fawell Blvd.
Glen Ellyn, IL 60137-6599
Phone: (630)942-2518
Email: bretlk@cdnet.cod.edu
Website: http://www.cod.edu/Academic/AcadProg/Occ_Voc/RespCare.htm
Kenneth M. Bretl, Contact

★ 29349 ★ Kankakee Community College
Advanced Respiratory Therapist Program
PO Box 888
River Rd.
Kankakee, IL 60901-0888
Phone: (815)933-0276
Email: nfrey@kcc.cc.il.us
Website: http://www.kcc.cc.il.us/
Nichola Frey, Contact

★ 29350 ★ Kaskaskia College
Advanced Respiratory Therapist Program
27210 College Rd.
Centralia, IL 62801
Phone: (618)543-3352
Email: burban@kc.cc.il.us
Sharon Beth Urban, Contact

★ 29351 ★ Lincoln Land Community College
Advanced Respiratory Therapist Program
5250 Shepherd Rd.
PO Box 19256
Springfield, IL 62794-9256
Phone: (217)786-2814
Email: randy.prather@llcc.cc.il.us
Website: http://www.llcc.cc.il.us/ahp/rcp.htm
Randel A. Prather, Contact

★ 29352 ★ Malcolm X College
Advanced Respiratory Therapist Program
1900 W Van Buren St.
Chicago, IL 60612
Phone: (312)850-7382
George West, Contact

★ 29353 ★ Moraine Valley Community College
Department of Health Sciences
Advanced Respiratory Therapist Program
10900 S 88th Ave.
Palos Hills, IL 60465
Phone: (708)974-5380
Email: lehner@moraine.cc.il.us

Website: http://www.moraine.cc.il.us/aca_info/health.html
Raymond F. Lehner, Contact

★ 29354 ★ National-Louis University
Advanced Respiratory Therapist Program
2840 Sheridan Rd.
Evanston, IL 60201-1796
Phone: (847)256-5150
Email: sthompson@nl.edu
Website: http://www.nl.edu/nlu_cas/divisions/hhs/undergraduate/allied_health/index.html
Stephen L. Thompson, PhD, Contact

★ 29355 ★ Parkland College
Advanced Respiratory Therapist Program
2400 W Bradley Ave.
Champaign, IL 61821-1899
Phone: (217)351-2296
Email: tdesjardins@parkland.cc.il.us
Website: http://www.parkland.cc.il.us/hp/rc/rtweb.html
Terry Des Jardins, Contact

★ 29356 ★ Rock Valley College
Advanced Respiratory Therapist Program
3301 N Mulford Rd.
Rockford, IL 61114-5699
Phone: (815)921-3220
Email: j.sills@rvc.cc.il.us
Website: http://www.rvc.cc.il.us/classes/helthser/pages/health.htmrespiratory
James R. Sills, Contact

★ 29357 ★ St. Augustine College
Advanced Respiratory Therapist Program
1345 W Argyle St.
Chicago, IL 60640-3593
Phone: (773)878-8756
Email: cortizcolombia@aol.com
Shirley Thomason, Contact

★ 29358 ★ St. John's Hospital
Elgin Community College
Advanced Respiratory Therapist Program
800 E Carpenter
Springfield, IL 62769-0001
Phone: (217)544-6464
Email: jszoke@st-johns.org
Jan M. Szoke, Contact

★ 29359 ★ Southern Illinois University, Carbondale
College of Applied Science and Arts
Advanced Respiratory Therapist Program
1365 Douglas Dr.
Carbondale, IL 62901-6615
Phone: (618)453-7221
Email: stanman@saluki-mail.siu.edu
Website: http://www.siu.edu/~hcp/
Stanley M. Pearson, II, Contact

★ 29360 ★ Southwestern Illinois College
Respiratory Care Technology Program
211 S Third St.
PO Box 694
Belleville, IL 62222-0694
Phone: (618)234-2121
Email: mmcmilli@sebh.org
Margaret J. McMillin, Contact

★ 29361 ★ Triton College
Advanced Respiratory Therapist Program
2000 Fifth Ave.
River Grove, IL 60171
Phone: (708)456-0300
Email: kanderso@triton.cc.il.us
Website: http://www.triton.cc.il.us/faculty/kanderson/
Kristine Anderson, Contact

★ 29362 ★ Waubonsee Community College (LB)
Advanced Respiratory Therapist Program
Rte. 47 at Waubonsee Dr.
Sugar Grove, IL 60554-9799
Phone: (630)466-7900
Email: csolarski@mail.wcc.cc.il.us
Carleton A. Solarski, Contact

Indiana

★ 29363 ★ Indiana University Northwest (LB)
Advanced Respiratory Therapist Program
3400 Broadway
Gary, IN 46408
Phone: (219)980-6548
Email: spearson@iun.edu
Website: http://www.iun.edu/~ahealth/resp.htm
Susan T. Pearson, Contact

★ 29364 ★ Indiana University School of Medicine
Advanced Respiratory Therapist Program
1140 W Michigan St.
Coleman Hall, Rm. 224
Indianapolis, IN 46202-5119
Phone: (317)278-7381
Email: dcullen@iupui.edu
Website: http://www.iupui.edu/it/iusahs/bulletin/97-99/prog/resp/
Deborah L. Cullen, EdD, Contact

★ 29365 ★ Ivy Tech State College
Advanced Respiratory Therapist Program
Halstead Professional Arts Bldg.
3714 Franklin St.
Michigan City, IN 46360
Phone: (219)879-9137
Email: slayhew@ivytech.edu
Susan J. Layhew, Contact

★ 29366 ★ Ivy Tech State College—Central Indiana (LB)
Advanced Respiratory Therapist Program
One W 26th St.
Indianapolis, IN 46206
Phone: (317)921-4410
Email: mstowe@ivy.tec.in.us
Marcus D. Stowe, Contact

★ 29367 ★ Ivy Tech State college—Fort Wayne (LB)
Advanced Respiratory Therapist Program
3800 N Anthony Blvd.
Fort Wayne, IN 46805
Phone: (260)480-4270
Email: jbrink@ivytech.edu
Website: http://www.ivy.tec.in.us/FortWayne/
Jennifer K. Brink, Contact
Frmly: Indiana Vocational Technical College.

★ 29368 ★ Ivy Tech State College—Lafayette
Advanced Respiratory Therapist Program
3101 S Creasy Ln.
Lafayette, IN 47903-6299
Phone: (765)772-9100
Email: pjames@ivy.tec.in.us
Website: http://www.laf.ivy.tec.in.us/degree_programs/health/respiratory.html
Peggy S. James, Contact
Frmly: Indiana Vocational Technical College.

★ 29369 ★ University of Southern Indiana (LB)
Advanced Respiratory Therapist Program
8600 University Blvd.
Evansville, IN 47712-3534
Phone: (812)464-1702
Email: rhooper@usi.edu
Robert Hooper, Contact

Iowa

★ 29370 ★ Des Moines Area Community College (LB)
Advanced Respiratory Therapist Program
2006 S Ankeny Blvd.
Ankeny, IA 50021-3993
Phone: (515)964-6298
Email: kegeorge@dmacc.edu
Website: http://www.dmacc.cc.ia.us/
Kerry E. George, Contact

★ 29371 ★ Hawkeye Community College
Advanced Respiratory Therapist Program
1501 E Orange Rd.
PO Box 8015
Waterloo, IA 50704-8015
Phone: (319)296-2320
Email: ldahl@hawkeye.ia.cc.us
Lawrence A. Dahl, EdD, Contact

★ 29372 ★ Kirkwood Community College
Advanced Respiratory Therapist Program
6301 Kirkwood Blvd. SW
PO Box 2068
Cedar Rapids, IA 52406-9973
Phone: (319)398-4987
Email: kbronkh@kirkwood.cc.ia.us
Website: http://www.kirkwood.cc.ia.us/healthscience/rt.html
H. Kenneth Bronkhorst, Contact

★ 29373 ★ Northeast Iowa Community College
Advanced Respiratory Therapist Program
10250 Sundown Rd.
Peosta, IA 52068-9988
Free: 800-728-7367
Email: rauscha@nicc.edu
Website: http://www.nicc.cc.ia.us/peo_tech.html35
Amy M. Rausch, Contact

★ 29374 ★ Southeastern Community College
Advanced Respiratory Therapist Program
1015 S Gear Ave.
West Burlington, IA 52655
Phone: (319)752-2731
Email: ldvorak@secc.cc.is.us
Lori A. Dvorak, Contact

Kansas

★ 29375 ★ Bethany Medical Center / Kansas City Kansas Community College
Advanced Respiratory Therapist Program
7250 State Ave.
Kansas City, KS 66112-9978
Phone: (913)288-7245
Email: mparrett@toto.net
Website: http://www.kckcc.cc.ks.us/rtp/index.htm
C. Michael Parrett, Contact

★ 29376 ★ Johnson County Community College
Advanced Respiratory Therapist Program
12345 College Blvd.
Overland Park, KS 66210-1299

Phone: (913)469-8500
Email: ccraig@jccc.net
Website: http://www.jccc.net/acad/resp/
Clarissa M. Craig, Contact

★ 29377 ★ Labette Community College
Advanced Respiratory Therapist Program
200 S 14th St.
Parsons, KS 67357
Phone: (620)820-1160
Email: conniec@labette.edu
Website: http://www.labette.cc.ks.us/dept/resp-care.htm
Connie S. Crooks, Contact

★ 29378 ★ Newman University
Allied Health Division
Respiratory Care Program
3100 McCormick Ave.
Wichita, KS 67213-2097
Phone: (316)942-4291
Email: trumppm@newmanu.edu
Website: http://www.ksnewman.edu/depts.htmRESPIRATORY CARE
Margaret L. Trumpp, Contact

★ 29379 ★ Seward County Community College
Advanced Respiratory Therapist Program
1801 N Kansas
PO Box 1137
Liberal, KS 67905-1137
Phone: (316)626-3026
Email: eanderso@sccc.cc.ks.us
Website: http://www.sccc.cc.ks.us/RT.html
Edward B. Anderson, Contact

★ 29380 ★ University of Kansas Medical Center (LB)
Advanced Respiratory Therapist Program
Respiratory Care Education
3901 Rainbow Blvd.
Kansas City, KS 66160-7606
Phone: (913)588-4634
Email: bludwig@kumc.edu
Website: http://www.kumc.edu/SAH/resp_care/
Barbara A. Ludwig, Contact

★ 29381 ★ Washburn University
Allied Health Department
Advanced Respiratory Therapist Program
1700 SW College
Topeka, KS 66621
Phone: (785)231-1010
Email: zzmunz@washburn.edu
Website: http://www.washburn.edu/sas/ah/rt/index.html
Patricia M. Munzer, Contact

Kentucky

★ 29382 ★ Bellarmine University (LB)
Cardiopulmonary Science Program
2001 Newburg Rd.
Louisville, KY 40205
Phone: (502)452-8415
Email: jwalker@bellarmine.edu
Jerome F. Walker, EdD, Contact

★ 29383 ★ Bowling Green Technical College
Advanced Respiratory Therapist Program
1845 Loop Dr.
Bowling Green, KY 42101
Phone: (270)746-7461
Email: brian.harlan@kctcs.net
Brian Harlan, Contact

★ 29384 ★ Jefferson Community College
Advanced Respiratory Therapist Program
109 E Broadway
Louisville, KY 40202
Phone: (502)213-2197
Email: joan.kruse@kctcs.net
Website: http://www.jcc.uky.edu/dt/Campus_Information/Academic_Programs/Career_Prog/Respiratory_Care/default.htm
Joan L. Kruse, Contact

★ 29385 ★ Laurel Technical College—Rockcastle Campus
Advanced Respiratory Therapist Program
955 W Main
PO Box 275
Mount Vernon, KY 40456
Phone: (606)256-4346
Email: carl.baker@kctcs.net
Carl Baker, Jr., Contact

★ 29386 ★ Lexington Community College (LB)
Advanced Respiratory Therapist Program
Cooper Dr.
330F Oswald Bldg.
Lexington, KY 40506-0235
Phone: (606)257-4872
Email: jkmatc1@pop.uky.edu
Website: http://www.uky.edu/LCC/RCP/
James K. Matchuny, Contact

★ 29387 ★ Madison Consortium for Respiratory Care Education
Advanced Respiratory Therapist Program
750 N Laffoon St.
Madisonville, KY 42431
Phone: (270)824-7552
Email: david.pennaman@kctcs.edu
David F. Pennaman, Contact

★ 29388 ★ Mayo Technical College/Prestonburg Community College
Advanced Respiratory Therapist Program
513 Third St.
Paintsville, KY 41240
Phone: (606)789-5321
Email: melissa.steele@kctcs.net
Melissa B. Steele, Contact

★ 29389 ★ Northern Kentucky University (LB)
Respiratory Care Program
Nunn Dr.
Albright Health Center, Rm. 225C
Highland Heights, KY 41099-2104
Phone: (859)572-5557
Email: langenderfer@nku.edu
Website: http://www.nku.edu/~ahhssw/respiratorycare.htmlx
Robert Langenderfer, Contact

★ 29390 ★ Rowan Technical College
Advanced Respiratory Therapist Program
609 Viking Dr.
Morehead, KY 40351
Phone: (606)783-1538
Email: marlene.vice@kctcs.net
Marlene K. Vice, Contact

★ 29391 ★ St. Catharine College
Advanced Respiratory Therapist Program
2735 Bardstown Rd.
Saint Catharine, KY 40061
Phone: (502)348-0388
Kathleen Sheeley, Contact

★ 29392 ★ Southeast Community College
Advanced Respiratory Therapist Program
3300 S Hwy. 25E
Pineville, KY 40977
Phone: (606)337-3106
Email: mike.good@kctcs.edu
Website: http://www.uky.edu/CommunityColleges/Sou/respiratory.html
Michael S. Good, Contact

★ 29393 ★ West Kentucky Technical College
Advanced Respiratory Therapist Program
5200 Alben Barkley Dr.
PO Box 7408
Paducah, KY 42002-7408
Phone: (270)554-6244
Email: ruth.thompson@kctcs.edu
Website: http://www.wkytech.com/respir.html
Ruth P. Thompson, Contact

Louisiana

★ 29394 ★ Bossier Parish Community College
Advanced Respiratory Therapist Program
2719 Airline Dr. N
Bossier City, LA 71111-5601
Phone: (318)675-6814
Email: dmeren@lsumc.edu
Website: http://www.bpcc.cc.la.us/asrt.htmlTOP
Diana T. Merendino, Contact

★ 29395 ★ Delgado Community College
Advanced Respiratory Therapist Program
615 City Park Ave.
New Orleans, LA 70119
Phone: (504)483-4007
Email: dolsen@dcc.edu
Website: http://www.dcc.edu/ahealth/respcare.htm
Diane M. Olsen-Rawls, Contact

★ 29396 ★ Louisiana State University Health Sciences Center
Department of Cardiopulmonary Science
Advanced Respiratory Therapist Program
1900 Gravier St.
New Orleans, LA 70112-2262
Phone: (504)568-4235
Email: jcairo@lsuhsc.edu
Website: http://www.lsuhsc.edu/Schools/AlliedHealth/CardiopulmonaryScience/cps1.htm
J. M. Cairo, PhD, Contact

★ 29397 ★ Louisiana State University, Eunice
Advanced Respiratory Therapist Program
PO Box 1129
2048 Johnson Hwy.
Eunice, LA 70535
Phone: (337)457-7311
Email: kreynold@lsue.edu
Kathleen B. Reynolds, Contact

★ 29398 ★ Louisiana Technical College—West Jefferson Campus
Advanced Respiratory Therapist Program
475 Manhattan Blvd.
Harvey, LA 70058-4441
Phone: (504)361-6388
Email: tsmootwj@yahoo.com
Toy B. Smoot, Contact

★ 29399 ★ Nicholls State University (LB)
Department of Allied Health Sciences
Advanced Respiratory Therapist Program
235 Civic Center Blvd.
Houma, LA 70360
Phone: (985)876-8852

Email: ahsc-ejc@nicholls.edu
Website: http://server.nich.edu/acad/bulletin/bltnalhe.htmlresp
Errol J. Champagne, Contact

★ 29400 ★ Our Lady of Holy Cross College
Ochsner School of Allied Health Sciences
Advanced Respiratory Therapist Program
1514 Jefferson Hwy.
New Orleans, LA 70121-2484
Phone: (504)842-3736
Email: mlabiche@ochsner.org
Website: http://www.ochsner.org/gmeweb/ahs.htm
Mary LaBiche, Contact

★ 29401 ★ Our Lady of the Lake College
Louisiana State University Health Sciences Center Consortium
Advanced Respiratory Therapist Program
5345 Brittany Dr.
Baton Rouge, LA 70808-4345
Phone: (225)768-1786
Email: jbush@ololcollege.edu
Jackie Bush, Contact

★ 29402 ★ Southern University, Shreveport
Advanced Respiratory Therapist Program
3050 Martin Luther King Jr. Dr.
Shreveport, LA 71107
Phone: (318)674-3452
Email: jwarren@susla.edu
Website: http://www.susbo.edu/science.htm
Jo A. Warren, Contact

Maine

★ 29403 ★ Kennebec Valley Technical College
Advanced Respiratory Therapist Program
92 Western Ave.
Fairfield, ME 04937-1367
Phone: (207)453-5161
Email: kblarsso@kvtc.net
Website: http://www.kvtc.mtcs.tec.me.us/rt.htm
Barbara A. Larsson, Contact

★ 29404 ★ Southern Maine Technical College
Advanced Respiratory Therapist Program
2 Fort Rd.
South Portland, ME 04106
Phone: (207)767-9592
Email: wchop@smtc.net
Website: http://www.smtc.net/programs/respiratory.htm
Walter C. Chop, Contact

Maryland

★ 29405 ★ Allegany College of Maryland
Advanced Respiratory Therapist Program
12401 Willowbrook Rd. SE
Cumberland, MD 21502-2596
Phone: (301)784-5522
Email: brocks@ac.cc.md.us
Website: http://www.ac.cc.md.us/Department/respther.htm
William R. Rocks, Contact
Frmly: Allegany Community College.

★ 29406 ★ Baltimore City Community College
Respiratory Care Program
2901 Liberty Heights Ave.
Baltimore, MD 21215-7893
Phone: (410)462-7717
Email: jross@bccc.state.md.us
Joe N. Ross, Contact

★ 29407 ★ Columbia Union College (LB)
Advanced Respiratory Therapist Program
7600 Flower Ave.
Takoma Park, MD 20912
Phone: (301)891-4181
Website: http://www.cuc.edu/academics/resp_care.html
Alvin R. Tucker, Contact

★ 29408 ★ Community College of Baltimore County—Essex Campus
Respiratory Care Therapist Program
7201 Rossville Blvd.
Baltimore, MD 21237-3899
Phone: (443)777-7000
Email: barbsc@helix.org
Website: http://www.ccbc.cc.md.us/campuses/essex/academics/career/aas/e_rc.htm
Barbara M. Schenk, Contact

★ 29409 ★ Frederick Community College (LB)
Advanced Respiratory Therapist Program
7932 Opossumtown Pike
Frederick, MD 21702
Phone: (301)846-2528
Email: mpaugh@fcc.cc.md.us
Website: http://www.fcc.cc.md.us/academic_programs/allied_health_wellness.cfmrtp
Mark L. Paugh, PhD, Contact

★ 29410 ★ Prince George's Community College (LB)
Allied Health Department
Advanced Respiratory Therapist Program
301 Largo Rd.
Largo, MD 20774-2199
Phone: (301)322-0740
Email: smithla1@pg.cc.md.us
Website: http://pgweb.pg.cc.md.us/
Linda A. Smith, Contact

★ 29411 ★ Salisbury University (LB)
Advanced Respiratory Therapist Program
1101 Camden Ave.
Salisbury, MD 21801
Phone: (410)543-6409
Email: srschneider@salisbury.edu
Website: http://www.ssu.edu/Schools/Henson.html
Sidney R. Schneider, PhD, Contact

Massachusetts

★ 29412 ★ Berkshire Community College
Advanced Respiratory Therapist Program
1350 West St.
Pittsfield, MA 01201
Phone: (413)499-4660
Email: tcarey@cc.berkshire.org
Website: http://cc.berkshire.org/perl-cgi/showPage.cgi?deptDatarsp
Thomas P. Carey, Jr., Contact

★ 29413 ★ Massachusetts Bay Community College
Advanced Respiratory Therapist Program
50 Oakland St.
Wellesley Hills, MA 02481
Phone: (781)239-2273
Email: stanleys@mbcc.mass.edu
Website: http://www.mbcc.mass.edu/mbcc/Programs/PROGRAMS.HTMLRespiratory AS
Scott A. Stanley, Contact

★ 29414 ★ Massasoit Community College (LB)
Advanced Respiratory Therapist Program
One Massasoit Blvd.
Brockton, MA 02302
Phone: (508)588-9100
Email: mdesilva@massasoit.mass.edu
Website: http://www.massasoit.mass.edu/resp.htm
Martha T. DeSilva, Contact

★ 29415 ★ North Shore Community College (LB)
Advanced Respiratory Therapist Program
One Ferncroft Rd.
Danvers, MA 01923-0840
Phone: (978)762-4166
Email: gtwomey@nscc.mass.edu
Website: http://www.nscc.cc.ma.us/
Geraldine Twomey, Contact

★ 29416 ★ Northeastern University (LB)
Respiratory Therapy Program
100 Dockser Hall
360 Huntington Ave.
Boston, MA 02115-5000
Phone: (617)373-3667
Email: t.barnes@neu.edu
Website: http://www.dac.neu.edu/cps/RTPROG.HTM
Thomas A. Barnes, EdD, Contact

★ 29417 ★ Northern Essex Community College
Advanced Respiratory Therapist Program
45 Franklin St.
Lawrence, MA 01841-4911
Phone: (978)738-7514
Email: crowse@necc.mass.edu
Website: http://www.necc.mass.edu/acaprds5.htmRESPIRATORY
Christopher Rowse, Contact

★ 29418 ★ Quinsigamond Community College
Advanced Respiratory Therapist Program
670 W Boylston St.
Worcester, MA 01606-2092
Phone: (508)854-4398
Email: lyndan@qcc.mass.edu
Website: http://www.qcc.mass.edu/
Lynda A. Nesbitt, Contact

★ 29419 ★ Springfield Technical Community College
Advanced Respiratory Therapist Program
One Armory Sq.
Springfield, MA 01105-9000
Phone: (413)755-4829
Email: robinson@stcc.mass.edu
Website: http://www.stcc.mass.edu/academics/Descriptions/Respiratory.asp
Lee J. Robinson, Contact

Michigan

★ 29420 ★ Delta College
Advanced Respiratory Therapist Program
1961 Delta Rd.
University Center, MI 48710
Phone: (517)686-9489
Email: ebgregory@alpha.delta.edu
Website: http://www.delta.edu/classes/catalog/RT.html
Earl B. Gregory, Contact

★ 29421 ★ Ferris State University (LB)
College of Allied Health Sciences
Advanced Respiratory Therapist Program
200 Ferris Dr., VFS 210A
Big Rapids, MI 49307-2740

Phone: (231)591-2261
Email: easterj@ferris.edu
Website: http://www.ferris.edu/htmls/colleges/allied-he/respirat.htm
Julian F. Easter, Contact

★ 29422 ★ Henry Ford Community College
Advanced Respiratory Therapist Program
5101 Evergreen
Dearborn, MI 48128-1495
Phone: (313)317-6580
Email: dszyman@hfcc.net
Website: http://www.henryford.cc.mi.us/
Debra A. Szymanski, Contact

★ 29423 ★ Kalamazoo Valley Community College
Respiratory Care Program
6767 W O Ave.
PO Box 4070
Kalamazoo, MI 49003-4070
Phone: (616)372-5288
Email: amoss@kvcc.edu
Website: http://puma.kvcc.edu/respirat/
Albert W. Moss, Contact

★ 29424 ★ Macomb Community College/ Detroit Macomb Hospital Corp.
Advanced Respiratory Therapist Program
Health and Human Services
44575 Garfield Rd.
Clinton Township, MI 48038-1139
Phone: (586)286-2150
Email: alsteadm@macomb.edu
Website: http://www.macomb.cc.mi.us/Courses98LibArts/RSP.htm
Mary E. Alstead, Contact

★ 29425 ★ Marygrove College
Advanced Respiratory Therapist Program
8425 W McNichols
Detroit, MI 48221-2599
Phone: (313)927-1421
Email: kmiller@marygrove.edu
Website: http://www.marygrove.edu/respirat%20care.htm
Kathy A. Miller, Contact

★ 29426 ★ Monroe County Community College
Advanced Respiratory Therapist Program
1555 S Raisinville Rd.
Monroe, MI 48161-9746
Phone: (734)384-4268
Email: bboggs@mail.monroe.cc.mi.us
Website: http://www.monroe.cc.mi.us/academicdept/health.htm
Bonnie E. Boggs, Contact

★ 29427 ★ Mott Community College
Division of Health Sciences
Advanced Respiratory Therapist Program
1401 E Court St.
Flint, MI 48503-2809
Phone: (810)232-6563
Email: dpanzlau@mcc.edu
Website: http://www.programs.mcc.edu/respiratory_therapy/
David L. Panzlau, Contact

★ 29428 ★ Muskegon Community College
Advanced Respiratory Therapist Program
221 S Quarterline Rd.
Muskegon, MI 49442
Phone: (231)777-0370
Email: knued@muskegon.cc.mi.us
Website: http://www.muskegon.cc.mi.us/courses/schedule/resp.htm
Daniel B. Knue, Contact

★ 29429 ★ Oakland Community College—Southfield Campus
Advanced Respiratory Therapist Program
22322 Rutland Dr.
Southfield, MI 48075-4793
Phone: (248)233-2921
Email: sjwork@occ.cc.mi.us
Sue J. Work, Contact

★ 29430 ★ Wayne County Community College District
Advanced Respiratory Therapist Program
801 W Fort St.
Detroit, MI 48226
Phone: (313)496-2798
Email: debrahak@aol.com
Debraha K. Watson, PhD, Contact

Minnesota

★ 29431 ★ College of Saint Catherine
Advanced Respiratory Therapist Program
601 25th Ave. S
Minneapolis, MN 55454
Phone: (651)690-7819
Email: jeboatright@stkate.edu
Website: http://www.stkate.edu/Admission/
John E. Boatright, Contact

★ 29432 ★ Lake Superior College
Advanced Respiratory Therapist Program
2101 Trinity Rd.
Duluth, MN 55811
Phone: (218)733-7600
Email: c.annable@lsc.mnscu.edu
Website: http://www.lsc.cc.mn.us/programs/rcpmain.htm
Cynthia Annable, Contact

★ 29433 ★ Northwest Technical College—East Grand Forks
Advanced Respiratory Therapist Program
2202 Central Ave. NE
East Grand Forks, MN 56721
Phone: (218)773-3441
Email: tony.sorum@ntcmn.edu
Website: http://www.ntc-online.com/ntc/cat/resp_ats.htm
Tony D. Sorum, Contact

★ 29434 ★ Rochester Community and Technical College /Mayo Foundation (LB)
Respiratory Care Program
851 30th Ave. SE
Rochester, MN 55904-4999
Phone: (507)284-0174
Email: ward.jeffrey@mayo.edu
Website: http://www.mayo.edu/hrs/hrs_rt.htm
Jeffrey J. Ward, Contact

★ 29435 ★ Saint Paul Technical College
Advanced Respiratory Therapist Program
235 Marshall Ave.
Saint Paul, MN 55102
Phone: (651)846-1501
Email: grant.jones@sptc.mnscu.edu
Website: http://www.sptc.tec.mn.us/programs/health/respitory.asp
D. Grant Jones, Contact

Mississippi

★ 29436 ★ Coahoma Community College
Advanced Respiratory Therapist Program
3240 Friars Point Rd.
Clarksdale, MS 38614
Phone: (662)624-3462
Email: anthony.brooks@nwmrmc.hma-corp.com
Anthony E. Brooks, Contact

★ 29437 ★ Copiah-Lincoln Community College
Vocational-Technical Division
Advanced Respiratory Therapist Program
30 Campus Dr.
Natchez, MS 39120
Phone: (601)446-1161
Email: walt.wilson@colin.edu
Website: http://www.colin.cc.ms.us/Natchez/Default.htm
Walton B. Wilson, Contact

★ 29438 ★ Hinds Community College (LB)
Advanced Respiratory Therapist Program
Nursing/Allied Health Center
1750 Chadwick Dr.
Jackson, MS 39204-3402
Phone: (601)371-3517
Email: dsylvester@hinds.cc.ms.us
Website: http://www.hinds.cc.ms.us/
Diane H. Sylvester, Contact

★ 29439 ★ Itawamba Community College
Advanced Respiratory Therapist Program
602 Hill St.
Fulton, MS 38843
Phone: (662)862-8348
Email: hjplunkett@icc.cc.ms.us
Website: http://www.icc.cc.ms.us/
James H. Plunkett, Contact

★ 29440 ★ Meridian Community College
Advanced Respiratory Therapist Program
910 Hwy. 19 N
Meridian, MS 39307
Phone: (601)484-8752
Steve W. Arinder, Contact

★ 29441 ★ Mississippi Gulf Coast Community College
Advanced Respiratory Therapist Program
2300 Hwy. 90
PO Box 100
Gautier, MS 39553
Phone: (228)497-7711
Email: donald.hayes@mgccc.cc.ms.us
Website: http://www.mgc.cc.ms.us/
Donald W. Hayes, Contact

★ 29442 ★ Northeast Mississippi Community College
Advanced Respiratory Therapist Program
101 Cunningham Blvd.
Booneville, MS 38829-1726
Phone: (662)720-7387
Email: bprince@necc.cc.ms.us
Website: http://www.necc.cc.ms.us/
Beverly D. Prince, Contact

★ 29443 ★ Northwest Mississippi Community College (LB)
Advanced Respiratory Therapist Program
5197 WE Ross Pkwy.
Southaven, MS 38671
Phone: (662)280-6151
Email: r_clark@nwcc.cc.ms.us
Website: http://www.necc.cc.ms.us
Regina K. Clark, Contact

★ 29444 ★ Pearl River Community College (LB)
Vocational Technical Center/Forrest County Center
Advanced Respiratory Therapist Program
5448 U.S. Hwy. 49 S
5448 US Hwy. 49 S
Hattiesburg, MS 39401
Phone: (601)554-9089
Email: slking@prcc.cc.ms.us
Website: http://www.prcc.cc.ms.us/cat-tecp.htmRESPIRATORY CARE TECHNOLOGY
S. Lee King, Contact

Missouri

★ 29445 ★ Cape Girardeau Career & Technology Center
Advanced Respiratory Therapist Program
1080 S Silver Springs Rd.
Cape Girardeau, MO 63703
Phone: (573)334-0826
Email: pfauk@cape.k12.mo.us
Kenneth F. Pfau, Contact

★ 29446 ★ ConCorde Career Institute, Inc.
Advanced Respiratory Therapist Program
3239 Broadway
Kansas City, MO 64111
Phone: (816)531-5223
Email: lbass@concordecareercolleges.com
Website: http://www.concordecareercolleges.com/
Lana C. Bass, Contact

★ 29447 ★ Hannibal LaGrange College
Hannibal Career and Technical Center
Advanced Respiratory Therapist Program
4550 McMasters Ave.
Hannibal, MO 63401-2285
Phone: (573)221-4430
Email: dbach@hannibal.k12.mo.us
David D. Bach, Contact

★ 29448 ★ Missouri Southern State College (LB)
Advanced Respiratory Therapist Program
MSSC Allied Health Bldg.
3950 E Newman Rd.
Joplin, MO 64801-1595
Phone: (417)659-4405
Email: pippin-g@mail.mssc.edu
Website: http://www.mssc.edu/catalog99-01/technology/rt/index.htm
Glenda A. Pippin, Contact

★ 29449 ★ Ozarks Technical Community College
Advanced Respiratory Therapist Program
PO Box 5958
Springfield, MO 65801
Phone: (417)895-7127
Email: bishops@otc.edu
Website: http://www.otc.cc.mo.us/degrees/alldhlth/rt/index.htm
Stephen I. Bishop, PhD, Contact

★ 29450 ★ Rolla Technical Center
Advanced Respiratory Therapist Program
500 Forum Dr.
Rolla, MO 65401-4678
Phone: (573)458-0160
Email: doldfather@rolla.k12.mo.us
Diane R. Oldfather, Contact

★ 29451 ★ St. Louis Community College—Forest Park (LB)
Advanced Respiratory Therapist Program
5600 Oakland Ave.
Saint Louis, MO 63110-1316
Phone: (314)644-9079
Email: jbrennan@stlcc.cc.mo.us
Website: http://www.stlcc.cc.mo.us/fp/respira/
James R. Brennan, Contact

★ 29452 ★ Sanford-Brown College
Respiratory Therapy Program
1203 Smizer Mill Rd.
Fenton, MO 63026
Phone: (636)349-4900
Email: monica.skaggs@wix.net
Monica Skaggs, Contact

★ 29453 ★ South Central Career Center
Advanced Respiratory Therapist Program
1009 Jackson St.
West Plains, MO 65775
Phone: (417)256-8883
Email: cschuttler@wphs.k12.mo.us
Mary Catherine Schuttler, Contact

★ 29454 ★ University of Missouri—Columbia (LB)
Respiratory Therapy Program
SHP/Cardiopulmonary and Diagnostic Sciences Department
605 Lewis Hall
Columbia, MO 65211-4230
Phone: (573)882-8422
Email: hoganr@health.missouri.edu
Website: http://www.muhealth.org/~shrp/rtwww/docs/rt.html
Rosemary G. Hogan, Contact

Montana

★ 29455 ★ Montana State University College of Technology—Great Falls
Advanced Respiratory Therapist Program
2100 16th Ave. S
PO Box 6010
Great Falls, MT 59406-6010
Phone: (406)771-4360
Email: lbates@msugf.edu
Website: http://msucotgf.montana.edu/~msucotgf/programs/respirat.html
Leonard Bates, Contact

★ 29456 ★ The University of Montana—Missoula
Advanced Respiratory Therapist Program
32 Campus Dr.
Missoula, MT 59812
Phone: (406)243-7821
Email: bwafstet@selway.umt.edu
Robert W. Wafstet, Contact

Nebraska

★ 29457 ★ Alegent/IMC Midland Lutheran College
Advanced Respiratory Therapist Program
6901 N 72nd St.
Omaha, NE 68122-1799
Phone: (402)572-2314
Email: tklopfen@alegent.org
Website: http://www.mlc.edu/acadmenu.html
Steven L. Carper, Contact

★ 29458 ★ Metropolitan Community College
Respiratory Care Program
PO Box 3777
Omaha, NE 68103-0777
Phone: (402)738-4653
Email: jmoss@metropo.mccneb.edu
Website: http://www.mccneb.edu/pr/catalog2.htmRCT
Jerald A. Moss, Contact

★ 29459 ★ Nebraska Methodist College of Nursing and Allied Health (LB)
Advanced Respiratory Therapist Program
8501 W Dodge Rd.
Omaha, NE 68114-3426
Phone: (402)354-4913
Email: chamil1@methodistcollege.edu
Website: http://www.methodistcollege.edu/
Christine A. Hamilton, Contact

★ 29460 ★ Southeast Community College—Lincoln
Advanced Respiratory Therapist Program
8800 O St.
Lincoln, NE 68520-1299
Phone: (402)437-2781
Email: cpasco@scc.cc.ne.us
Website: http://www.college.sccm.cc.ne.us/2b6.htmRespiratory Care Program
Charlotte L. Pasco, Contact

Nevada

★ 29461 ★ Community College of Southern Nevada
Advanced Respiratory Therapist Program
6375 W Charleston Blvd.
Las Vegas, NV 89146-1124
Phone: (702)651-5665
Email: randy_insley@ccsn.nevada.edu
Carlton R. Insley, III, Contact

New Hampshire

★ 29462 ★ New Hampshire Community Technical College
Advanced Respiratory Therapist Program
One College Dr.
Claremont, NH 03743-0907
Phone: (603)542-7744
Email: j_marcle@tec.nh.us
Website: http://www.claremont.tec.nh.us/
John F. Marcley, Contact

New Jersey

★ 29463 ★ Bergen Community College
Advanced Respiratory Therapist Program
400 Paramus Rd.
Paramus, NJ 07652
Phone: (201)447-7944
Email: rmuller@bergen.edu
Website: http://www.bergen.cc.nj.us/
Robert A. Muller, Contact

★ 29464 ★ Brookdale Community College
Advanced Respiratory Therapist Program
Respiratory Therapy/Health Science
765 Newman Springs Rd.
Lincroft, NJ 07738-1597
Phone: (732)224-2606
Email: pfusaro@brookdale.cc.nj.us
Website: http://www2.brookdale.cc.nj.us/brookdale/storiescc/dsaasrtt.htm
Patricia A. Fusaro, Contact

★ 29465 ★ Gloucester County College
Advanced Respiratory Therapist Program
1400 Tanyard Rd.
Sewell, NJ 08080
Phone: (856)415-2192
Email: aleder@gccnj.edu
Anna P. Leder, Contact

★ 29466 ★ Northwest New Jersey Consortium for Respiratory Care Education
Advanced Respiratory Therapist Program
Saint Clare's Health Services
400 W Blackwell St.
Dover, NJ 07801-2525
Phone: (973)537-3906
Email: dadams@saintclares.org
Dianne A. Adams, Contact

★ 29467 ★ Passaic County Community College
Advanced Respiratory Therapist Program
One College Blvd.
Paterson, NJ 07505-1179
Phone: (973)684-5280
Email: smccleaster@pccc.cc.nj.us
Website: http://www.pccc.cc.nj.us/courses/therapy.html
Sandra McCleaster, Contact

★ 29468 ★ Union County College
Advanced Respiratory Therapist Program
1033 Springfield Ave.
Cranford, NJ 07016
Phone: (908)412-3574
Email: handrews@hawk.ucc.edu
Website: http://www.ucc.edu
Harlan Andrews, Contact

★ 29469 ★ University of Medicine and Dentistry of New Jersey
Primary Care Center
Advanced Respiratory Therapist Program
40 E Laurel Rd.
Stratford, NJ 08084-1353
Phone: (856)566-2893
Email: gross@umdnj.edu
Website: http://www.umdnj.edu/shrpweb/catalog/Cardiopulmonary_Sciences/rsj-program.htm
G. Woodard Gross, Contact

★ 29470 ★ University of Medicine and Dentistry of New Jersey
School of Health Related Professions
Advanced Respiratory Therapist Program
65 Bergen St.
Newark, NJ 07107-3001
Phone: (973)972-7228
Email: wclark@umdnj.edu
Website: http://www.umdnj.edu/shrpweb/catalog/Cardiopulmonary_Sciences/index-rnj.htm
William F. Clark, PhD, Contact

New Mexico

★ 29471 ★ Albuquerque Technical Vocational Institute
Advanced Respiratory Therapist Program
Health Occupations Department
525 Buena Vista SE
Albuquerque, NM 87106-4096
Phone: (505)224-4111
Email: rgentile@tvi.cc.nm.us
Website: http://www.tvi.cc.nm.us/health/resp.html
Richard J. Gentile, Jr., Contact

★ 29472 ★ Dona Ana Branch Community College
Advanced Respiratory Therapist Program
3400 S Espina
Las Cruces, NM 88003-8001
Phone: (505)527-7634
Email: thayth@nmsu.edu
Website: http://dabcc-www.nmsu.edu/Catalog/respiratory.html
Thomas Hayth, Contact

★ 29473 ★ Eastern New Mexico University—Roswell
Advanced Respiratory Therapist Program
PO Box 6000
Roswell, NM 88202-6000
Phone: (505)624-7217
Email: gina.buldra@roswell.enmu.edu
Gina Buldra, Contact

New York

★ 29474 ★ City University of New York Manhattan Community College
Department of Allied Health Sciences
Advanced Respiratory Therapist Program
199 Chambers St.
New York, NY 10007
Phone: (212)220-8336
Email: eflannery@bmcc.cuny.edu
Website: http://www.bmcc.cuny.edu/acaprogs/respprog.htm
Everett W. Flannery, Contact

★ 29475 ★ Erie Community College
Advanced Respiratory Therapist Program
6205 Main St.
Williamsville, NY 14221-7095
Phone: (716)851-1531
Email: bierl@ecc.edu
Website: http://nstaff.sunyerie.edu/home/crcn/ah.htm
James J. Bierl, Contact

★ 29476 ★ Genesee Community College
Advanced Respiratory Therapist Program
One College Rd.
Batavia, NY 14020-9704
Phone: (716)343-0055
Email: rmjacobs@genesee.suny.edu
Website: http://www.sunygenesee.cc.ny.us/dept/health.htm
Ronald M. Jacobs, Contact

★ 29477 ★ Hudson Valley Community College
Respiratory Care Program
80 Vandenburg Ave.
Troy, NY 12180
Phone: (518)629-7454
Email: hylanpat@hvcc.edu
Website: http://www.hvcc.edu/academ/schools/health/res/
Patricia G. Hyland, Contact

★ 29478 ★ Long Island University, Brooklyn Campus (LB)
Advanced Respiratory Therapist Program
Division of Respiratory Care
One University Plaza
Brooklyn, NY 11201-5372
Phone: (718)488-1492
Email: tjohnson@liu.edu
Website: http://www.brooklyn.liunet.edu/cwis/bklyn/health/bsrescar.html
Thomas J. Johnson, Contact

★ 29479 ★ Mohawk Valley Community College
Advanced Respiratory Therapist Program
1101 Sherman Dr.
Utica, NY 13501-5394
Phone: (315)792-5664
Email: lphillips@mvcc.edu
Website: http://www.mvcc.edu/catalog/health/resp1.htm
Lorie Phillips, Contact

★ 29480 ★ Molloy College (LB)
Advanced Respiratory Therapist Program
1000 Hempstead Ave.
Rockville Centre, NY 11571-5002
Phone: (516)677-5000
Email: rtralongo@molloy.edu
Website: http://www.molloy.edu/academic/allied.htm
Robert J. Tralongo, Contact

★ 29481 ★ Nassau Community College
Advanced Respiratory Therapist Program
One Education Dr.
Garden City, NY 11530-6793
Phone: (516)572-7560
Email: hostetw@ncc.edu
Website: http://www.sunynassau.edu/catalog/acaddep/acadep.htm
Warren Hostetter, Contact

★ 29482 ★ New York University (LB)
Center for Allied Health
Advanced Respiratory Therapist Program
11 W 42nd St., Rm. 518
New York, NY 10036-8083
Phone: (212)790-1630
Email: cqs3166@is4.nyu.edu
Website: http://www.scps.nyu.edu/dyncon/heac/cour_alli_resp.html
Carole Smith, Contact

★ 29483 ★ Onondaga Community College
Advanced Respiratory Therapist Program
4941 Onondaga Rd.
Syracuse, NY 13215-2099
Phone: (315)498-2471
Email: clevelad@sunyocc.edu
Website: http://www.sunyocc.edu/
Daniel V. Cleveland, Contact

★ 29484 ★ State University of New York Upstate Medical Center
Advanced Respiratory Therapist Program
750 E Adams St.
Syracuse, NY 13210
Phone: (315)464-5580
Email: morfeij@upstate.edu
Website: http://www.ec.hscsyr.edu/CHRP/resp/Respiratory_Care.html
Joseph J. Morfei, Contact

★ 29485 ★ State University of New York, Stony Brook
School of Health Technology and Management
Respiratory Care Program
Stony Brook, NY 11794-8203
Phone: (631)444-3184
Email: james.ganetis@sunysb.edu
Website: http://www.uhmc.sunysb.edu/shtm/rc/rc_homepage.html
James A. Ganetis, Contact

★ 29486 ★ Westchester Community College (LB)
Advanced Respiratory Therapist Program
75 Grasslands Rd.
Health Science 19
Valhalla, NY 10595-1698

Phone: (914)785-6883
Email: jose.quinones@sunywcc.edu
Website: http://www.sunywcc.edu/
Jose Quinones, Contact

North Carolina

★ 29487 ★ Carteret Community College
Advanced Respiratory Therapist Program
3505 Arendell St.
Morehead City, NC 28557-2989
Phone: (252)222-6281
Email: lap@carteret.cc.nc.us
Website: http://gofish.carteret.cc.nc.us/
Laurie A. Pratt, Contact

★ 29488 ★ Catawba Valley Community College
Advanced Respiratory Therapist Program
2550 Hwy. 70 SE
Hickory, NC 28602
Phone: (828)327-7000
Email: cbitsche@cvcc.cc.nc.us
Website: http://www.cvcc.cc.nc.us/programs/health/RCPAGE.HTM
Catherine A. Bitsche, Contact

★ 29489 ★ Central Piedmont Community College
Advanced Respiratory Therapist Program
PO Box 35009
Charlotte, NC 28235
Phone: (704)330-6274
Email: tom_morris@cpcc.edu
Website: http://www.cpcc.cc.nc.us/Health_Sciences/Respiratory_Care/
Thomas R. Morris, Contact

★ 29490 ★ Durham Technical Community College
Advanced Respiratory Therapist Program
Department of Respiratory Care
1637 Lawson St.
Durham, NC 27713
Phone: (919)686-3643
Email: millerr@gwmail.dtcc.cc.nc.us
Website: http://209.86.110.158/career/progstud/rctech/rctech.htm
Richard D. Miller, PhD, Contact

★ 29491 ★ Edgecombe Community College
Advanced Respiratory Therapist Program
225 Tarboro St.
Rocky Mount, NC 27801-5430
Phone: (252)446-0436
Email: webbrd@edgecombe.cc.nc.us
Website: http://www.edgecombe.cc.nc.us/RESPCARE.HTM
Ralph D. Webb, Contact

★ 29492 ★ Fayetteville Technical Community College
Advanced Respiratory Therapist Program
PO Box 35236
Fayetteville, NC 28303-0236
Phone: (910)678-8316
Email: baldwinr@ftccmail.faytech.cc.nc.us
Website: http://atlas.faytech.cc.nc.us/edprog/curr/a45720.html
Ruth A. Baldwin, Contact

★ 29493 ★ Forsyth Technical Community College
Advanced Respiratory Therapist Program
2100 Silas Creek Pkwy.
Winston-Salem, NC 27103-5197
Phone: (336)723-0371
Email: psheppard@forsyth.cc.nc.us
Website: http://www.forsyth.tec.nc.us/
Perry W. Sheppard, Contact

★ 29494 ★ Pitt Community College (LB)
Advanced Respiratory Therapist Program
PO Drawer 7007
Hwy. 11 S
Greenville, NC 27835-7007
Phone: (252)321-4619
Email: cstrickl@pcc.pitt.cc.nc.us
Website: http://www.pitt.cc.nc.us/
M. Carolyn Strickland, Contact

★ 29495 ★ Robeson Community College
Advanced Respiratory Therapist Program
PO Box 1420
5160 Fayetteville Rd.
Lumberton, NC 28358
Phone: (910)738-7101
Email: kheustes@robeson.cc.nc.us
Website: http://www.robeson.cc.nc.us/health.htmRespiratory
Kelli Heustess, Contact

★ 29496 ★ Rockingham Community College
Advanced Respiratory Therapist Program
PO Box 38
Wentworth, NC 27375-0038
Phone: (336)342-4261
Email: hardingt@rcc.cc.ns.us
Thomas W. Harding, Contact

★ 29497 ★ Sandhills Community College
Advanced Respiratory Therapist Program
3395 Airport Rd.
Pinehurst, NC 28374
Phone: (910)695-3836
Email: croftb@email.sandhills.cc.nc.us
Website: http://www.sandhills.cc.nc.us/rct/rct-index.html
William L. Croft, Contact

★ 29498 ★ Southwestern Community College (LB)
Advanced Respiratory Therapist Program
447 College Dr.
Sylva, NC 28779
Phone: (828)586-4091
Email: shatfield@southwest.cc.nc.us
Website: http://www.southwest.cc.nc.us/Acadprog/rsp.htm
Sharon Hatfield, Contact

★ 29499 ★ Stanly Community College
Advanced Respiratory Therapist Program
141 College Dr.
Albemarle, NC 28001
Phone: (704)991-0267
Email: crumptp@stanly.cc.nc.us
Website: http://www.stanly.cc.nc.us/STUSER/CRSCAT/course_schedule/respcare.htm
Tammy P. Crump, PhD, Contact

North Dakota

★ 29500 ★ North Dakota State University / MeritCare Hospital Consortium (LB)
Respiratory Care Program
MeritCare Hospital
PO Box MC
Fargo, ND 58122-0118
Phone: (701)234-6147
Email: garybrown@meritcare.com
Website: http://www.ndsu.nodak.edu/instruct/poolson/rt/
Gary Brown, Contact

★ 29501 ★ University of Mary / Saint Alexius Medical Center
School of Respiratory Care
Advanced Respiratory Therapist Program
900 E Broadway
Bismarck, ND 58502
Phone: (701)530-7757
Email: wbeachey@primecare.org
Website: http://www.umary.edu/course/co_respcare.htm
Will D. Beachey, Contact

Ohio

★ 29502 ★ Bowling Green State University/Firelands College
Advanced Respiratory Therapist Program
One University Dr.
Huron, OH 44839
Phone: (419)433-5560
Email: rroark@bgnet.bgsu.edu
Website: http://www.firelands.bgsu.edu/as/rt/
Roddy C. Roark, Contact

★ 29503 ★ Cincinnati State Technical and Community College
Advanced Respiratory Therapist Program
3520 Central Pkwy.
Cincinnati, OH 45223-9984
Phone: (513)569-1690
Email: debra.lierl@cincinnatistate.edu
Website: http://www.cinstate.cc.oh.us/htd-rc.htm
Debra Lierl, Contact

★ 29504 ★ Collins Career Center
Advanced Respiratory Therapist Program
11627 State Rte. 243
Chesapeake, OH 45619-7962
Phone: (740)867-6641
Email: katerry@collins-cc.k12.oh.us
Website: http://www.collins-cc.k12.oh.us/
Keith Terry, Contact

★ 29505 ★ Columbus State Community College (LB)
Advanced Respiratory Therapist Program
550 E Spring St.
Columbus, OH 43215-1609
Phone: (614)287-2513
Email: dwallace@cscc.edu
David U. Wallace, Contact

★ 29506 ★ Cuyahoga Community College (LB)
Advanced Respiratory Therapist Program
11000 Pleasant Valley Rd.
Respiratory Therapy, A208
Parma, OH 44130-5199
Phone: (216)987-5267
Email: david.lucas@tri-c.edu
Website: http://www.tri-c.cc.oh.us/HEALTH/RCWEB/Frmset1.htm
David A. Lucas, Contact

★ 29507 ★ James A. Rhodes State College (LB)
Advanced Respiratory Therapist Program
Cook Hall
4240 Campus Dr.
Lima, OH 45804-3597
Phone: (419)995-8366
Email: woodfield.r@rhodesstate.edu
Website: http://www.ltc.tec.oh.us/academic/health/resp_care.htm
Richard N. Woodfield, Jr., Contact
Frmly: Lima Technical College.

★ 29508 ★ Jefferson Community College
Advanced Respiratory Therapist Program
4000 Sunset Blvd.
Steubenville, OH 43952
Phone: (740)264-5591
Email: lake536@clover.net
Website: http://ns3.jeffersoncc.org/jcc/programinfo.asp?programid=40
Cynthia Carducci, Contact

★ 29509 ★ Kettering College of Medical Arts (LB)
Advanced Respiratory Therapist Program
3737 Southern Blvd.
Kettering, OH 45429-1299
Phone: (937)298-3399
Email: nancy.colletti@kmcnetwork.org
Website: http://www.kcma.edu/
Nancy E. Colletti, Contact

★ 29510 ★ Lakeland Community College
Advanced Respiratory Therapist Program
7700 Clocktower Dr.
Kirtland, OH 44094-5198
Phone: (440)953-7343
Email: ckenny@lakeland.cc.oh.us
Website: http://www.lakeland.cc.oh.us/ACADEMIC/SH/resp/index.htm
Catherine J. Kenny, Contact

★ 29511 ★ North Central State College (LB)
Advanced Respiratory Therapist Program
2441 Kenwood Cir.
PO Box 698
Mansfield, OH 44901-0698
Phone: (419)755-4891
Email: rslabod@ncstate.tec.oh.us
Website: http://www.nctc.tec.oh.us/pages/respther.html
Robert A. Slabodnick, Contact

★ 29512 ★ Ohio State University (LB)
Advanced Respiratory Therapist Program
Respiratory Therapy Division
1583 Perry St.
Columbus, OH 43210-1234
Phone: (614)292-8445
Email: douce.2@osu.edu
Website: http://www.amp.ohio-state.edu/!SAMPWEB/rt-1.htm
F. Herbert Douce, Contact

★ 29513 ★ Shawnee State University (LB)
Advanced Respiratory Therapist Program
940 Second St.
Portsmouth, OH 45662
Phone: (740)351-3235
Email: dthomas@shawnee.edu
Website: http://www.shawnee.edu/prospective/academics/aca%20deptment/health/parts/mids/respiratory.htm
Donald L. Thomas, Contact

★ 29514 ★ Sinclair Community College (LB)
Advanced Respiratory Therapist Program
444 W Third St.
Dayton, OH 45402
Phone: (937)512-2849
Email: cynthia.beckett@sinclair.edu
Website: http://www.sinclair.edu/departments/ret/
Cynthia A. Beckett, PhD, Contact

★ 29515 ★ Stark State College of Technology
Advanced Respiratory Therapist Program
6200 Frank Ave. NW
Canton, OH 44720-7299
Phone: (330)966-5458
Email: pcastillo@starkstate.edu
Website: http://www.stark.cc.oh.us/academic/health/respiratory_care.htm
Peter R. Castillo, Contact
Frmly: Stark Technical College.

★ 29516 ★ University of Akron
Advanced Respiratory Therapist Program
302 Buchtel Ave.
Akron, OH 44325-3702
Phone: (330)972-7906
Email: laverne@uakron.edu
Website: http://www.commtech.uakron.edu/commtech/a_health/respcare.htm
LaVerne C. Yousey, Contact

★ 29517 ★ University of Toledo (LB)
Advanced Respiratory Therapist Program
2801 W Bancroft St.
Toledo, OH 43606-3390
Phone: (419)530-5308
Email: margaret.traband@utoledo.edu
Website: http://www.hhs.utoledo.edu/
Margaret F. Traband, Contact

★ 29518 ★ Washington State Community College
Advanced Respiratory Therapist Program
710 Colegate Dr.
Marietta, OH 45750
Phone: (740)374-8716
Email: rkinker@wscc.edu
J. Robert Kinker, Jr., PhD, Contact

★ 29519 ★ Youngstown State University
Advanced Respiratory Therapist Program
One University Plaza
Youngstown, OH 44555
Phone: (330)742-1764
Email: lnharris@cc.ysu.edu
Website: http://www.ysu.edu/colleges/hhs/healthp/index.htm
Louis N. Harris, EdD, Contact

Oklahoma

★ 29520 ★ Francis Tuttle Area Vo-Tech Oklahoma City Community College
Advanced Respiratory Therapist Program
12777 N Rockwell Ave.
Oklahoma City, OK 73142-2789
Phone: (405)717-4269
Email: lheyland@francistuttle.com
Website: http://www.francistuttle.com/index.htm
Lezli Heyland, Contact
Frmly: Francis Tuttle Technology Center.

★ 29521 ★ Great Plains Technology Center (LB)
Advanced Respiratory Therapist Program
4500 W Lee Blvd.
Lawton, OK 73505
Phone: (580)250-5572
Email: jpowers@gptech.org
Jack A. Powers, Contact

★ 29522 ★ Pioneer Technical Center
Advanced Respiratory Therapist Program
2101 N Ash
Ponca City, OK 74601
Phone: (580)762-8336
Email: miket@pioneertech.org
Michael L. Taylor, Contact

★ 29523 ★ Rose State College
Advanced Respiratory Therapist Program
6420 SE 15th St.
Midwest City, OK 73110-2799
Phone: (405)733-7571
Email: nlorance@rose.edu
Website: http://www.rose.cc.ok.us/hsdiv/programs/resther.htm
Nancy J. Lorance, Contact

★ 29524 ★ Tulsa Community College
Advanced Respiratory Therapist Program
Allied Health Division, Metro Campus
909 S Boston Ave.
Rm. MP458
Tulsa, OK 74119-2095
Phone: (918)595-7016
Email: gpersing@tulsa.cc.ok.us
Website: http://www.tulsa.cc.ok.us/respirat.html
Gary E. Persing, Contact

Oregon

★ 29525 ★ Lane Community College
Advanced Respiratory Therapist Program
4000 E 30th Ave.
Eugene, OR 97405-0640
Phone: (541)463-5624
Email: hechtr@lanecc.edu
Website: http://lanecc.edu/fahealth/rc1.htm
Roger H. Hecht, Contact

★ 29526 ★ Mount Hood Community College
Allied Health Division
Advanced Respiratory Therapist Program
26000 SE Stark St.
Gresham, OR 97030
Phone: (503)491-7172
Email: hicksg@mhcc.cc.or.us
Website: http://www.mhcc.cc.or.us/catalog/programs/respir.htm
George Hicks, Contact

★ 29527 ★ Rogue Community College
Advanced Respiratory Therapist Program
202 S Riverside Ave.
Medford, OR 97501
Phone: (541)245-7500
Email: jhulse@rogue.cc.or.us
Website: http://www2.rogue.cc/alliedhealth/Respiratory/home.htm
James L. Hulse, Contact

Pennsylvania

★ 29528 ★ Community College of Allegheny County
Advanced Respiratory Therapist Program
808 Ridge Ave.
Allied Health Department
Milton Hall, Rm. 606
Pittsburgh, PA 15212
Phone: (412)237-2607
Email: troop@ccac.edu
Website: http://www.acd.ccac.edu/allied-health/programs/resphome.htm
Thomas A. Roop, Contact

★ 29529 ★ Community College of Philadelphia
Advanced Respiratory Therapist Program
1700 Spring Garden St.
Philadelphia, PA 19130-3991
Phone: (215)751-4823
Email: falsis@ccp.cc.pa.us

Website: http://inet.ccp.cc.pa.us/vpacaff/PROG&CRS/CREDIT/DIVBS&T/resp/
Frank M. Alsis, EdD, Contact

★ 29530 ★ Delaware County Community College
Crozer-Chester Medical Center
Advanced Respiratory Therapist Program
One Medical Center Blvd.
Upland, PA 19013
Phone: (610)447-2440
Email: paul.swietlik@crozer.org
Paul A. Swietlik, Contact

★ 29531 ★ Gannon University
Advanced Respiratory Therapist Program
109 University Sq.
Erie, PA 16541-0001
Phone: (814)871-5637
Email: cornfield@gannon.edu
Website: http://WWW.GANNON.EDU/RESOURCE/DEPT/respcare/index.html
Charles Cornfield, Contact

★ 29532 ★ Gwynedd Mercy College (LB)
Advanced Respiratory Therapist Program
PO Box 901
Gwynedd Valley, PA 19437
Phone: (215)641-5536
Email: galvin.w@gmc.edu
Website: http://www.gmc.edu/academic/schools/alliedhealth/resp_care.htm
William F. Galvin, Contact

★ 29533 ★ Harrisburg Area Community College
Advanced Respiratory Therapist Program
One HACC Dr.
Harrisburg, PA 17110
Phone: (717)780-2315
Email: baleidic@hacc.edu
Website: http://www.hacc.edu/
Bradley A. Leidich, Contact

★ 29534 ★ Indiana University of Pennsylvania (LB)
Western Pennsylvania Hospital
Advanced Respiratory Therapist Program
4800 Friendship Ave.
Pittsburgh, PA 15224
Phone: (412)578-7003
Email: bmalley@wpahs.org
Website: http://www.iup.edu/schedu/catalog/hhumsvc/resp.htmlx
William J. Malley, Contact

★ 29535 ★ Luzerne County Community College
Advanced Respiratory Therapist Program
1333 S Prospect St.
Nanticoke, PA 18634
Phone: (570)740-0467
Christopher Tino, Contact

★ 29536 ★ Mansfield University
Health Sciences Department
Advanced Respiratory Therapist Program
Guthrie Sq.
Sayre, PA 18840
Phone: (570)882-4513
Email: lvosburg@inet.guthrie.org
Website: http://www.mnsfld.edu/
Larry B. Vosburgh, Contact

★ 29537 ★ Millersville University
Advanced Respiratory Therapist Program
PO Box 1002
Roddy Science Ctr.
Millersville, PA 17551-0302
Phone: (717)290-5511
Email: jhughes@marauder.millersv.edu
Website: http://muweb.millersv.edu/~rtp/
John M. Hughes, Contact

★ 29538 ★ Reading Area Community College
Advanced Respiratory Therapist Program
10 S Second St.
Reading, PA 19603-1706
Phone: (610)372-4721
Email: rlamme@email.racc.cc.pa.us
Website: http://www.racc.cc.pa.us/health.html
Robert D. Lamme, Contact

★ 29539 ★ University of Pittsburgh, Johnstown
Advanced Respiratory Therapist Program
227 Krebs Hall
Johnstown, PA 15904
Phone: (814)269-2958
Email: bcolbert@pitt.edu
Website: http://www.pitt.edu/~upjweb/admissions/programs/allied_health_programs.html
Bruce J. Colbert, Contact

★ 29540 ★ West Chester University / Bryn Mawr Hospital (LB)
Advanced Respiratory Therapist Program
130 S Bryn Mawr Ave.
Bryn Mawr, PA 19010-3160
Phone: (610)526-3347
Email: kellarb@mlhs.org
Website: http://www.wcupa.edu/_academics/sch_shs.hea/UNDERGRA.HTM
Brian Kellar, Contact

★ 29541 ★ Western School of Health and Business Careers
Advanced Respiratory Therapist Program
421 Seventh Ave.
Pittsburgh, PA 15219-1907
Phone: (412)281-7083
Email: kmclark12@hotmail.com
Website: http://www.westernschool.com/programs/respiratory.html
Kimberly M. Clark, Contact

★ 29542 ★ York College of Pennsylvania/ York Hospital
Advanced Respiratory Therapist Program
School of Respiratory Care
1001 S George St.
York, PA 17405-7198
Phone: (717)851-2464
Email: msimmons@wellspan.org
Website: http://goose.ycp.edu/department/biology/index.html
Mark Simmons, Contact

Puerto Rico

★ 29543 ★ Sistema Universitario Ana G. Mendez
Advanced Respiratory Therapist Program
PO Box 21150
San Juan, PR 00928-1150
Phone: (787)766-1717
Email: um_ltorres@suagm.edu
Leyda Luz Torres-Lopez, Contact
Frmly: Universidad Metropolitana.

★ 29544 ★ Universidad Adventista de las Antillas
Advanced Respiratory Therapist Program
PO Box 118
Mayaguez, PR 00681-0118
Phone: (787)834-9595
Email: darypr@hotmail.com
Website: http://www.uaa.edu/
Damaria Cruz, Contact

Rhode Island

★ 29545 ★ Community College of Rhode Island
CardioRespiratory Care Program
1762 Louisquisset Pike
Lincoln, RI 02865-4585
Phone: (401)333-7024
Email: jjacobs@ccri.cc.ri.us
Website: http://www.ccri.cc.ri.us/FRAMES/box24FR.htm
Joanne Jacobs, Contact

South Carolina

★ 29546 ★ Florence-Darlington Technical College
Advanced Respiratory Therapist Program
PO Box 100548
Florence, SC 29501-0548
Phone: (843)661-8148
Email: evansj@flo.tec.sc.us
Website: http://www.flo.tec.sc.us/
John A. Evans, Contact

★ 29547 ★ Greenville Technical College (LB)
Advanced Respiratory Therapist Program
PO Box 5616
Station B
Greenville, SC 29606-5616
Phone: (864)250-8037
Email: woodyjaw@gvltec.edu
Website: http://www.greenvilletech.com/resptherac.htm
James A. Woody, Contact

★ 29548 ★ Midlands Technical College (LB)
Advanced Respiratory Therapist Program
PO Box 2408
Columbia, SC 29202
Phone: (803)822-3433
Email: ackermanl@midlandstech.com
Website: http://www.mid.tec.sc.us/edu/home.html
Linda Ackerman, Contact

★ 29549 ★ Orangeburg-Calhoun Technical College (LB)
Advanced Respiratory Therapist Program
3250 St. Matthews Rd.
Orangeburg, SC 29118
Phone: (803)535-1344
Email: stinchcomba@octech.edu
Audrey T. Stinchcomb, Contact

★ 29550 ★ Piedmont Technical College
Advanced Respiratory Therapist Program
PO Drawer 1467
Greenwood, SC 29646
Phone: (864)941-8533
Email: allen_a@piedmont.tec.sc.us
Website: http://www.piedmont.tec.sc.us/academic/respcare.htm
Ann M. Allen, Contact

★ 29551 ★ Spartanburg Technical College
Advanced Respiratory Therapist Program
PO Box 4386
Spartanburg, SC 29305-4386
Phone: (864)591-3938
Email: andersonr@stcsc.edu
Website: http://199.5.204.101/hs_rc_ad.htm
Randall W. Anderson, Contact

★ 29552 ★ Tri-County Technical College
Advanced Respiratory Therapist Program
PO Box 587
Pendleton, SC 29670
Phone: (864)646-1354
Thomas D. Baxter, Contact

★ 29553 ★ Trident Technical College
Advanced Respiratory Therapist Program
PO Box 118067
7000 Rivers Ave.
Charleston, SC 29423-8067
Phone: (843)574-6101
Email: ann.moore@tridenttech.edu
Website: http://www.trident.tec.sc.us/alliedhealth/respiratory.html
Ann R. Moore, Contact

South Dakota

★ 29554 ★ Dakota State University
Respiratory Care Program
Science Center
820 N Washington Ave.
Madison, SD 57042-1799
Phone: (605)322-8613
Email: bruce.feistner@dsu.edu
Website: http://www.departments.dsu.edu/sciences/m_respcare.htm
Bruce A. Feistner, Contact

Tennessee

★ 29555 ★ Baptist College of Health Sciences
Advanced Respiratory Therapist Program
1003 Monroe Ave.
Memphis, TN 38104
Phone: (901)572-2650
Email: andrew.mazzoli@bchs.edu
Andrew J. Mazzoli, PhD, Contact

★ 29556 ★ Chattanooga State Technical Community College
Advanced Respiratory Therapist Program
4501 Amnicola Hwy.
Chattanooga, TN 37406
Phone: (423)697-4450
Email: mickey.rountree@chattanoogastate.edu
Website: http://www.cstcc.cc.tn.us/www/academics/alliedhealth/index.htm
McIver Rountree, Jr., Contact

★ 29557 ★ Columbia State Community College
Advanced Respiratory Therapist Program
PO Box 1315
Columbia, TN 38402-1315
Phone: (931)540-2663
Email: rdavid@coscc.coscc.cc.tn.us
Website: http://www.coscc.cc.tn.us/academic/83-139.htmrct
R. David Johnson, Contact

★ 29558 ★ ConCorde Career College
Advanced Respiratory Therapist Program
5100 Poplar Ave., Ste. 132
Memphis, TN 38137
Phone: (901)761-9494
Email: mcamp@concordecareercolleges.com
Michael Camp, Contact

★ 29559 ★ East Tennessee State University (LB)
Advanced Respiratory Therapist Program
1000 W East St.
Elizabethton, TN 37643
Phone: (423)547-4900
Email: mack@access.etsu.edu
Website: http://www.etsu.edu/cpah/hrelated/hrelrttr.htm
Delmar Mack, EdD, Contact

★ 29560 ★ Jackson State Community College
Advanced Respiratory Therapist Program
2046 N Parkway St.
Jackson, TN 38301-3797
Phone: (731)424-3520
Email: cgarner@jscc.edu
Website: http://www.jscc.cc.tn.us/users/allied/
Cathy K. Garner, Contact

★ 29561 ★ Roane State Community College
Advanced Respiratory Therapist Program
276 Patton Ln.
Harriman, TN 37748-5011
Phone: (865)354-3000
Email: hill_la@rscc.cc.tn.us
Website: http://www.rscc.cc.tn.us/academic/health-sci/RespTherapy/
Lesha A. Hill, Contact

★ 29562 ★ Tennessee State University
Advanced Respiratory Therapist Program
3500 John A. Merritt Blvd.
Nashville, TN 37209-1561
Phone: (615)963-7420
Email: tjohn@tnstate.edu
Website: http://www.tnstate.edu/alhp/
Thomas John, PhD, Contact

★ 29563 ★ Tennessee Technology Center at Memphis
Advanced Respiratory Therapist Program
550 Alabama Ave.
Memphis, TN 38105-3604
Phone: (901)543-6186
Email: bfaulkner56@hotmail.com
Brenda S. Faulkner, Contact

★ 29564 ★ Volunteer State Community College
Advanced Respiratory Therapist Program
1480 Nashville Pike
Gallatin, TN 37066-3188
Phone: 888-335-8722
Email: cory.martin@vscc.cc.tn.us
Website: http://www.vscc.cc.tn.us/academic/health/resp.html
Cory E. Martin, Contact

★ 29565 ★ Walters State Community College
Advanced Respiratory Therapist Program
500 S Davy Crockett Pkwy.
Morristown, TN 37813-6899
Phone: (423)798-7941
Email: robert.mcgee@ws.edu
Robert G. McGee, Jr., Contact

Texas

★ 29566 ★ Alvin Community College (LB)
Advanced Respiratory Therapist Program
3110 Mustang Rd.
Alvin, TX 77511-4898
Phone: (281)756-3658
Email: dflatland@alvin.cc.tx.us
Website: http://www.alvin.cc.tx.us/DEPT/resp/resp.htm
Diane Flatland, Contact

★ 29567 ★ Amarillo College (LB)
Advanced Respiratory Therapist Program
PO Box 447
Amarillo, TX 79178
Phone: (806)354-6058
Email: young-wa@actx.edu
Website: http://www.actx.edu/~respiratory_care/
William A. Young, Contact

★ 29568 ★ Angelina College
Advanced Respiratory Therapist Program
USPS 803-000
PO Box 1768
Lufkin, TX 75902-1768
Phone: (936)633-5419
Email: mparks@angelina.cc.tx.us
Website: http://eagle.angelina.cc.tx.us/respiratory/index.htm
William M. Parks, Contact

★ 29569 ★ ATI Career Training Center (LB)
Advanced Respiratory Therapist Program
10003 Technology Blvd. W
Dallas, TX 75220
Phone: (214)902-8191
Email: jsaunders@atienterprises.com
James R. Saunders, Contact

★ 29570 ★ Collin County Community College
Advanced Respiratory Therapist Program
2200 W University Dr.
McKinney, TX 75070
Phone: (972)548-6870
Email: dgibson@ccccd.edu
Website: http://www.ccccd.edu/divisions/hpc/RESPTHER.HTM
David R. Gibson, Contact

★ 29571 ★ Del Mar College
Advanced Respiratory Therapist Program
101 Baldwin
Corpus Christi, TX 78404
Phone: (361)698-1108
Email: jwatson@delmar.edu
Website: http://www.delmar.edu/rt/rtweb.htm
Jeffrey T. Watson, Contact

★ 29572 ★ El Centro College
Advanced Respiratory Therapist Program
Main and Lamar Sts.
Dallas, TX 75202-3604
Phone: (214)860-2279
Email: glp5547@dcccd.edu
Website: http://www.ecc.dcccd.edu/health-ls/respiratory/RCP.HTM
Gary L. Peschka, Contact

★ 29573 ★ El Paso Community College
Advanced Respiratory Therapist Program
PO Box 20500
El Paso, TX 79998
Phone: (915)831-2000
Email: paulan@epcc.edu
Website: http://www.epcc.edu/
Paul Andrade, Contact

★ 29574 ★ Houston Community College System
Advanced Respiratory Therapist Program
Respiratory Therapist Program
Coleman Health Science Bldg.
1900 Galen
Houston, TX 77030
Phone: (713)718-7379
Email: reynolds_t@hccs.cc.tx.us
Website: http://www.hccs.cc.tx.us/SEcollege/RespCareTechnician.html
Thomas W. Reynolds, Contact

★ 29575 ★ Howard College—San Angelo Campus (LB)
Advanced Respiratory Therapist Program
3197 Executive Dr.
San Angelo, TX 76904
Phone: (915)481-8300
Email: cvoyce@hc.cc.tx.us
Cynthia K. Voyce, Contact

★ 29576 ★ Kingwood College-NHMCCD
Advanced Respiratory Therapist Program
20000 Kingwood Dr.
Kingwood, TX 77339
Phone: (281)312-1608
Email: kmccowen@nhmccd.edu
Website: http://kcweb.nhmccd.edu/programs/shas/respcare/respcare.htm
Kenny P. McCowen, Contact

★ 29577 ★ Lamar University Institute of Technology (LB)
Respiratory Care Program
PO Box 10061
Beaumont, TX 77710
Phone: (409)880-8852
Email: bronsonpa@lit-mail.lamar.edu
Website: http://www.theinstitute.lamar.edu/programs/respiratorycare.htm
Paul A. Bronson, Contact

★ 29578 ★ McLennan Community College
Advanced Respiratory Therapist Program
1400 College Dr.
Waco, TX 76708
Phone: (254)299-8369
Email: dgg@mccadm.cc.tx.us
Douglas G. Gibson, Contact

★ 29579 ★ Midland College (LB)
Advanced Respiratory Therapist Program
3600 N Garfield
Midland, TX 79705
Phone: (915)685-4600
Email: rweidmann@midland.edu
Website: http://www.midland.cc.tx.us/courses/p-r.htmlresp care
Robert Weidmann, Contact

★ 29580 ★ Midwestern State University (LB)
Advanced Respiratory Therapist Program
3410 Taft Blvd.
Wichita Falls, TX 76308-2099
Phone: (940)397-4653
Email: ann.medford@mwsu.edu
Website: http://www.mwsu.edu/htmldocs/departments/resphom.html
Annette O. Medford, Contact

★ 29581 ★ Odessa College
Advanced Respiratory Therapist Program
201 W University
Odessa, TX 79764
Phone: (915)335-6456
Email: jsullivan@odessa.edu
Website: http://coyote.odessa.edu/
Jacquelyn R. Sullivan, Contact

★ 29582 ★ St. Philip's College (LB)
Advanced Respiratory Therapist Program
1801 Martin Luther King Blvd.
San Antonio, TX 78203-2098
Phone: (210)531-3473
Email: bfisher@accd.edu
Bruce W. Fisher, Contact

★ 29583 ★ San Jacinto College
Advanced Respiratory Therapist Program
8060 Spencer Hwy.
Pasadena, TX 77501-2007
Phone: (281)476-1501
Email: lvandi@central.sjcd.cc.tx.us
Website: http://www.sjcd.cc.tx.us/central/resc/index.htm
Larry P. Vandiver, Contact

★ 29584 ★ South Plains College-Lubbock Campus
Respiratory Care Program
Reese Ctr.
528 Gilbert Dr.
Lubbock, TX 79416
Phone: (806)885-3048
Email: vstalcup@southplainscollege.edu
Website: http://www.spc.cc.tx.us/
Valorie A. Stalcup, Contact

★ 29585 ★ Southwest Texas State University
Advanced Respiratory Therapist Program
601 University Dr.
San Marcos, TX 78666-4616
Phone: (512)245-8243
Email: ch03@swt.edu
Website: http://www.health.swt.edu/
Cade J. Harkins, III, Contact

★ 29586 ★ Southwest Texas State University
Hospital Management Consortium
Respiratory Care School Consortium
Advanced Respiratory Therapist Program
1242 N 19th
Abilene, TX 79601
Phone: (915)670-2380
Email: jlawrenc@hendrickhealth.org
Jeff Lawrence, Contact

★ 29587 ★ Tarrant County College, Northeast Campus
Respiratory Care Program
828 Harwood Rd.
Hurst, TX 76054-3299
Phone: (817)515-6574
Email: john.hiser@tccd.net
Website: http://www.tcjc.cc.tx.us/campus_ne/resp/
John D. Hiser, Contact

★ 29588 ★ Temple College (LB)
Advanced Respiratory Therapist Program
2600 S First St.
Temple, TX 76504-7453
Phone: (254)778-4811
Email: bill.cornel@templejc.edu
Website: http://www.templejc.edu/
William M. Cornelius, III, Contact

★ 29589 ★ Texas Southern University
Advanced Respiratory Therapist Program
3100 Cleburne
Houston, TX 77004
Phone: (713)313-7265
Email: hampton_jm@tsu.edu
Website: http://www.tsu.edu/pharmacy/index.htm
Jean M. Hampton, PhD, Contact

★ 29590 ★ Tyler Junior College (LB)
Advanced Respiratory Therapist Program
PO Box 9020
Tyler, TX 75711-9020
Phone: (903)510-2472
Email: pbru@tjc.edu
Website: http://www.tyler.cc.tx.us/
Phyllis W. Brunner, Contact

★ 29591 ★ United States Air Force School of Healthcare Sciences
Cardiopulmonary Program
381 TRS/XWBH 917 Missile Rd.
Sheppard AFB, TX 76311-2246
Phone: (940)676-3812
Email: steven.smith3@sheppard.af.mil
MSgt. Steven M. Smith, Contact

★ 29592 ★ U.S. Army Medical Department Center and School (AMEDD)
Advanced Respiratory Therapist Program
McIdoe Rd., Bldg. 1151
Fort Sam Houston, TX 78234-6100
Phone: (210)295-4411
Email: jon.o'hora@cen.amedd.army.mil
Jon P. O'Hora, Contact

★ 29593 ★ University of Texas Health Science Center at San Antonio
Advanced Respiratory Therapist Program
Department of Respiratory Care
7703 Floyd Curl Dr., Mail Code 6248
San Antonio, TX 78229-3900
Phone: (210)567-8850
Email: shelledy@uthscsa.edu
Website: http://www.uthscsa.edu/sah/rc.html
David C. Shelledy, PhD, Contact

★ 29594 ★ University of Texas, Brownsville
Texas Southmost College
Advanced Respiratory Therapist Program
80 Ft. Brown
Brownsville, TX 78520-4993
Phone: (956)554-5017
Email: jmccabe@utb1.utb.edu
Website: http://unix.utb.edu/~kgarcia/rthp.htm
John L. McCabe, PhD, Contact

★ 29595 ★ University of Texas Medical Branch, Galveston
School of Allied Health Sciences
Advanced Respiratory Therapist Program
301 University Blvd.
Galveston, TX 77555-1028
Phone: (409)772-5693
Email: jnilsest@utmb.edu
Website: http://www.rc.utmb.edu/
Jon O. Nilsestuen, PhD, Contact

★ 29596 ★ Victoria College (LB)
Advanced Respiratory Therapist Program
2200 E Red River
Victoria, TX 77901
Phone: (361)572-6491
Email: ckallus@victoriacollege.edu
Website: http://www.vc.cc.tx.us/programs/rescare.html
Chris E. Kallus, Contact

★ 29597 ★ Weatherford College
Advanced Respiratory Therapist Program
225 College Park Dr.
Weatherford, TX 76086

Phone: (817)598-6451
Email: sbutler@wc.edu
Sheila Butler, Contact

Utah

★ 29598 ★ Weber State University (LB)
Respiratory Therapy Program
3904 University Cir.
Ogden, UT 84408-3904
Phone: (801)626-7071
Email: gbills@weber.edu
Website: http://weber.edu/resptherapy/
Georgine W. Bills, Contact

Vermont

★ 29599 ★ Champlain College
Advanced Respiratory Therapist Program
163 S Willard St.
Burlington, VT 05402-0670
Phone: (802)865-6491
Email: baconf@champlain.edu
Website: http://www.champlain.edu/CLnD/respiratory.htm
Faye T. Bacon, Contact

Virginia

★ 29600 ★ Central Virginia Community College
Advanced Respiratory Therapist Program
3506 Wards Rd.
Lynchburg, VA 24502
Phone: (434)832-7685
Email: crawleym@cv.cc.va.us
Martha N. Crawley, Contact

★ 29601 ★ Community Hospital of Roanoke Valley
College of Health Sciences
Advanced Respiratory Therapist Program
PO Box 13186
Roanoke, VA 24031-3186
Phone: (540)985-8483
Email: paul@health.chs.edu
Website: http://www.chs.edu/respiratory_care_education.html
Paul M. Lemons, Contact

★ 29602 ★ J. Sargeant Reynolds Community College
Advanced Respiratory Therapist Program
PO Box 85622
Richmond, VA 23285-5622
Phone: (804)786-3009
Email: dodonohue@jsr.vccs.edu
Website: http://www.jsr.cc.va.us/Catalog/programs/RespiratoryTherapyAAS.htm
Donald K. O'Donohue, Contact

★ 29603 ★ Mountain Empire Community College
Advanced Respiratory Therapist Program
PO Drawer 700
Big Stone Gap, VA 24219
Phone: (540)523-2400
Email: mcook@me.cc.va.us
Website: http://www.me.cc.va.us/dept/nurse/respiratory/RESPCARE.HTML
Michael W. Cook, Contact

★ 29604 ★ Northern Virginia Community College (LB)
Advanced Respiratory Therapist Program
8333 Little River Trnpk.
Annandale, VA 22003-3796
Phone: (703)323-3280
Email: lstone@nv.cc.va.us
Website: http://www.nv.cc.va.us/annandale/health/rth/rthhome.htm
Linda L. Stone, Contact

★ 29605 ★ Shenandoah University
Advanced Respiratory Therapist Program
1460 University Dr.
Winchester, VA 22601
Phone: (540)665-5516
Email: woneill@su.edu
Website: http://www.su.edu/respcare/index.htm
William A. O'Neill, Contact

★ 29606 ★ Southwest Virginia Community College (LB)
Advanced Respiratory Therapist Program
PO Box SVCC
Richlands, VA 24641-1510
Phone: (540)964-7306
Email: joe_dipietro@sw.cc.va.us
Website: http://www.sw.cc.va.us/M&NS/HLTECH.html
Joseph S. DiPietro, PhD, Contact

★ 29607 ★ Tidewater Community College (LB)
Advanced Respiratory Therapist Program
1700 College Crescent
Virginia Beach, VA 23456
Phone: (757)822-7263
Email: tccrosg@tc.cc.va.us
Website: http://www.tc.cc.va.us/vabeach/hstdiv/rth/
Gary Cross, Contact

Washington

★ 29608 ★ Highline Community College
Advanced Respiratory Therapist Program
2400 S 240th St.
PO Box 98000
Des Moines, WA 98198-9800
Phone: (206)878-3710
Email: bbonner@highline.edu
Website: http://www.highline.ctc.edu/highlinehome/home.htm
Robert A. Bonner, Contact

★ 29609 ★ Seattle Central Community College
Advanced Respiratory Therapist Program
1701 Broadway/2BE3210
Seattle, WA 98122-3803
Phone: (206)587-4056
Email: rmccallum@sccd.ctc.edu
Website: http://seattlecentral.org/learn/respiratory/120_resp.html
Robert I.C. McCallum, Contact

★ 29610 ★ Spokane Community College
Advanced Respiratory Therapist Program
N 1810 Greene St.
MS 2090
Spokane, WA 99217-5399
Phone: (509)533-7307
Email: darkell@scc.spokane.cc.wa.us
Website: http://www.scc.spokane.cc.wa.us/hes/alliedh/respcare.htm
Diana K. Arkell, Contact

★ 29611 ★ Tacoma Community College
Advanced Respiratory Therapist Program
6501 S 19th St.
Allied Health Bldg.
Tacoma, WA 98466-6100
Phone: (253)566-5231
Email: jcoad@tcc.ctc.edu
Website: http://www.tacoma.ctc.edu/home/bleffler/index.htm
Jan Coad, Contact

West Virginia

★ 29612 ★ Carver Career Center (LB)
Advanced Respiratory Therapist Program
4799 Midland Dr.
Charleston, WV 25306
Phone: (304)348-1965
Email: kdcrrt@yahoo.com
Website: http://www.wvonline.com/carver/health/advresp.htm
Kym Chaffin, Contact
Frmly: Carver Career and Technical Education Center.

★ 29613 ★ Mountain State University (LB)
Advanced Respiratory Therapist Program
PO Box 9003
Beckley, WV 25802-9003
Phone: (304)253-7351
Email: smills@mountainstate.edu
Website: http://www.cwv.edu/nhs/resp/index.html
Sandra Mills, Contact
Frmly: College of West Virginia.

★ 29614 ★ University of Charleston (LB)
Advanced Respiratory Therapist Program
2300 MacCorkle Ave. SE
Charleston, WV 25304
Phone: (304)357-4837
Email: aparkman@ucwv.edu
Website: http://www.uchaswv.edu/dhs/respcare/
Anna W. Parkman, PhD, Contact

★ 29615 ★ West Virginia Northern Community College
Advanced Respiratory Therapist Program
1704 Market St.
Wheeling, WV 26003-3551
Phone: (304)233-5900
Email: rlucki@northern.wvnet.edu
Website: http://techctr1.northern.wvnet.edu/catalog/respiratory.htm
Ralph C. Lucki, Contact

★ 29616 ★ Wheeling Jesuit University
Advanced Respiratory Therapist Program
316 Washington Ave.
Wheeling, WV 26003-6295
Phone: (304)243-2372
Email: amaran@wju.edu
Website: http://www.wju.edu/academics/departments/rt/
Allen H. Marangoni, Contact

Wisconsin

★ 29617 ★ Madison Area Technical College
Advanced Respiratory Therapist Program
3550 Anderson St.
Madison, WI 53704-2599
Phone: (608)246-6686
Email: ghojem@matcmadison.edu
Website: http://www.madison.tec.wi.us/catalog/PROG_CRS/PD/PD105151.ssi
Glenn N. Hojem, Contact

★ 29618 ★ Mid-State Technical College
Advanced Respiratory Therapist Program
2600 W Fifth St.
Marshfield, WI 54449-3299
Phone: (715)389-7033
Email: sosborne@mstc.edu

Website: http://www.midstate.tec.wi.us/respcare.htm
Scott S. Osborne, Contact

★ 29619 ★ Milwaukee Area Technical College
Advanced Respiratory Therapist Program
700 W State St.
Milwaukee, WI 53233-1443
Phone: (414)297-7130
Email: hoffmanm@matc.edu
Website: http://www.milwaukee.tec.wi.us/utility/clas/prog/alli/resp.htm
Mark J. Hoffman, Contact

★ 29620 ★ Northeast Wisconsin Technical College (LB)
Advanced Respiratory Therapist Program
2740 W Mason St.
PO Box 19042
Green Bay, WI 54307-9042
Phone: (920)498-5533
Email: kschlitz@nwtc.edu
Website: http://www.nwtc.tec.wi.us/DegreesDiplomas/healthcom.htm
Katherine A. Schlitz, Contact

★ 29621 ★ Western Wisconsin Technical College
Advanced Respiratory Therapist Program
304 N Sixth St.
La Crosse, WI 54601
Phone: (608)785-9244
Email: milischr@wwtc.edu
Website: http://www.western.tec.wi.us/
Robert A. Milisch, Contact

Social Work

The following institutions offer accredited programs in social work. For information on these programs, contact the Council on Social Work Education, 1725 Duke St., Ste. 500, Alexandria, VA 22314, (703)683-8080, http://www.cswe.org/.

Alabama

★ 29622 ★ Alabama A & M University
Graduate Social Work Department
Graduate Program in Social Work
PO Box 302
Normal, AL 35762
Phone: (256)851-5478 **Fax:** (256)851-5484
Email: swycoff@aamu.edu
Website: http://www.aamu.edu
Shelley Ann Wyckoff, Chairman of the Board

★ 29623 ★ University of Alabama
School of Social Work
Graduate Program in Social Work
Box 870314
Tuscaloosa, AL 35487-0314
Phone: (205)348-7027 **Fax:** (205)348-9419
Email: dean@sw.ua.edu
Website: http://www.ua.edu/academic/colleges/socwork
James P. Adams, Jr., Director

Alaska

★ 29624 ★ University of Alaska, Anchorage
School of Social Work
College of Health, Education, and Social Welfare
Graduate Program in Social Work
3211 Providence Dr.
Anchorage, AK 99508-8230
Phone: (907)786-6907 **Fax:** (907)786-6912
Email: afeas1@uaa.alaska.edu
Website: http://www.uaa.alaska.edu/socwork
Elizabeth A. Sirles, Director

Arizona

★ 29625 ★ Arizona State University
School of Social Work
Graduate Program in Social Work
Box 871802
Tempe, AZ 85287-1802
Phone: (480)965-2795 **Fax:** (480)965-2799
Email: kegerdes@asu.edu
Website: http://ssw.asu.edu/
Leslie Leighninger, Director

Arkansas

★ 29626 ★ University of Arkansas, Little Rock
School of Social Work
Graduate Program in Social Work
2801 S University
Little Rock, AR 72204
Phone: (501)569-3240 **Fax:** (501)569-3184
Email: hmturney@ualr.edu
Website: http://www.ualr.edu/~swdept/
Howard M. Turney, Director

California

★ 29627 ★ California State University, Fresno
Department of Social Work Education
Graduate Program in Social Work
5310 Campus Dr., PH 102
Fresno, CA 93740-8019
Phone: (559)278-3992 **Fax:** (559)278-7191
Email: jane_middleton@csufresno.edu
Website: http://www.csufresno.edu/
E. Jane Middleton, Director

★ 29628 ★ California State University, Long Beach
Department of Social Work
Graduate Program in Social Work
1250 Bellflower Blvd.
Long Beach, CA 90840-0902
Phone: (562)985-7774 **Fax:** (562)985-5514
Email: joliver@csulb.edu
Website: http://www.csulb.edu/~socialwk/
John Oliver, Director

★ 29629 ★ California State University, Los Angeles
Department of Social Work
Graduate Program in Social Work
5151 State University Dr.
Los Angeles, CA 90008
Phone: (323)343-4680 **Fax:** (213)343-5009
Email: fanders@cslanet.calstatela.edu
Website: http://www.calstatela.edu
E. Frederick Anderson, Director

★ 29630 ★ California State University, Sacramento
Division of Social Work
Graduate Program in Social Work
6000 J St.
Sacramento, CA 95819-6090
Phone: (916)278-6943 **Fax:** (916)278-7167
Website: http://www.hhs.csus.edu/SWRK
Robin Carter, Director

★ 29631 ★ California State University, San Bernardino
Department of Social Work
Graduate Program in Social Work
5500 University Pkwy.
San Bernardino, CA 92407-2397
Phone: (909)880-5501 **Fax:** (909)880-7029
Email: tmorris@csusb.edu
Website: http://socialwork.csusb.edu
Teresa Morris, Director

★ 29632 ★ California State University, Stanislaus
Social Work Department
Graduate Program in Social Work
801 W Monte Vista Ave.
Turlock, CA 95382
Phone: (209)667-3091 **Fax:** (209)667-3869
Email: edunbar@stan.csustan.edu
Website: http://www.csustan.edu/Social_Work/index.htm
Ellen R. Dunbar, Director

★ 29633 ★ Loma Linda University
Department of Social Work
Graduate Program in Social Work
Griggs Hall
Loma Linda, CA 92350
Phone: (909)558-8548 **Fax:** (909)558-0450
Email: bbuckles@univ.llu.edu
Website: http://www.llu.edu/llu/
Beverly J. Buckles, Chairman of the Board

★ 29634 ★ San Diego State University
School of Social Work
Graduate Program in Social Work
5500 Campanile Dr.
San Diego, CA 92182-4119
Phone: (619)594-6865 **Fax:** (619)594-5991
Email: aharbert@mail.sdsu.edu
Website: http://www-rohan.sdsu.edu/dept/chhs/sw/sw.html
Anita S. Harbert, Director

★ 29635 ★ San Francisco State University
School of Social Work
Graduate Program in Social Work
1600 Holloway Ave.
San Francisco, CA 94132
Phone: (415)338-1003 **Fax:** (415)338-0591
Website: http://www.sfsu.edu/~socwork
Eileen F. Levy, Director

★ 29636 ★ San Jose State University
College of Social Work
Graduate Program in Social Work
1 Washington Sq., Ste. 215
San Jose, CA 95192-0124
Phone: (408)924-5800 **Fax:** (408)924-5892
Website: http://www.sjsu.edu/depts/SocialWork
Sylvia R. Andrew, Director

★ 29637 ★ University of California, Berkeley
School of Social Welfare
Graduate Program in Social Work
120 Haviland Hall
Berkeley, CA 94720-7400
Phone: (510)642-4341 **Fax:** (510)643-6126
Email: lmidanik@uclink4.berkeley.edu
Website: http://socialwelfare.berkeley.edu
James Midgley, Director

★ 29638 ★ University of California, Los Angeles
School of Public Policy and Social Research
Department of Social Welfare
Graduate Program in Social Work
3250 Public Policy Bldg.
PO Box 951656
Los Angeles, CA 90095-1656
Phone: (310)825-2892 **Fax:** (310)206-7564
Email: swinfor@sppsr.ucla.edu
Website: http://www.sppsr.ucla.edu/sw
A. E. Benjamin, Chairman of the Board

★ 29639 ★ University of Southern California
School of Social Work
Graduate Program in Social Work
699 W 34th St.
Montgomery Ross Fisher Bldg., Rm. 214
Los Angeles, CA 90089-0411
Phone: (213)740-2711 **Fax:** (213)740-3301
Email: mflynn@usc.edu
Website: http://www.usc.edu/dept/socialwork/
Marilyn S. Flynn, Director

Colorado

★ 29640 ★ Colorado State University
School of Social Work
Graduate Program in Social Work
127 Education Bldg.
Fort Collins, CO 80523-1586
Phone: (970)491-6612 **Fax:** (970)491-7280
Email: granger@.cahs.colostate.edu
Website: http://www.cahs.colostate.edu/sw
Ben P. Granger, Director

★ 29641 ★ University of Denver
Graduate School of Social Work
2148 S High St.
Denver, CO 80208-2886
Phone: (303)871-2203 **Fax:** (303)871-2845
Email: caalter@du.edu
Website: http://www.du.edu
Catherine F. Alter, Director

Connecticut

★ 29642 ★ Southern Connecticut State University
Department of Social Work
Graduate Social Work Program
101 Farnham Ave.
New Haven, CT 06515
Phone: (203)392-6580 **Fax:** (203)392-6580
Website: http://www.southernct.edu
Todd William Rofuth, Director

★ 29643 ★ University of Connecticut
School of Social Work
Graduate Program in Social Work
1798 Asylum Ave.
West Hartford, CT 06117
Phone: (860)570-9141 **Fax:** (860)570-9264
Email: kay.davidson@uconn.edu
Website: http://www.socialwork.uconn.edu/
Kay Davidson, Director

Delaware

★ 29644 ★ Delaware State University
Department of Social Work
Graduate Program in Social Work
1200 N DuPont Hwy.
Dover, DE 19901
Phone: (302)857-6770 **Fax:** (302)857-6794
Email: jaustin@dsc.edu
Website: http://www.dsc.edu/
John N. Austin, Chairman of the Board

District of Columbia

★ 29645 ★ Catholic University of America
National Catholic School of Social Service
Graduate Program in Social Work
Shahan Hall
Cardinal Station
Washington, DC 20064
Phone: (202)319-5454 **Fax:** (202)319-5093
Website: http://ncsss.cua.edu
Ann Patrick Conrad, Director

★ 29646 ★ Gallaudet University
Department of Social Work
Graduate Program in Social Work
800 Florida Ave. NE
Washington, DC 20002-3695
Phone: (202)651-5160 **Fax:** (202)651-5817
Email: janet.pray@gallaudet.edu
Website: http://depts.gallaudet.edu/social.work
Barbara J. White, Chairman of the Board

★ 29647 ★ Howard University
School of Social Work
Graduate Program in Social Work
601 Howard Pl. NW
Washington, DC 20059
Phone: (202)806-7300 **Fax:** (202)387-4309
Email: renglish@howard.edu
Website: http://www.socialwork.howard.edu/
Richard A. English, Director

Florida

★ 29648 ★ Barry University
School of Social Work
Graduate Program in Social Work
11300 NE 2nd Ave.
Miami Shores, FL 33161
Phone: (305)899-3900 **Fax:** (305)899-3934
Website: http://www2.barry.edu/vpaa-ssw.default.htm
Stephen M. Holloway, Director

★ 29649 ★ Florida International University
School of Social Work
Graduate Program in Social Work
11200 SW 8th St.
ECS 460
Miami, FL 33199
Phone: (305)348-5880 **Fax:** (305)348-5313
Email: thomlisr@.fiu.edu
Website: http://www.fiu.edu/~cupa/social-work.html
Ray Thomlison, Director

★ 29650 ★ Florida State University
School of Social Work
Graduate Program in Social Work
UCC 2505
Tallahassee, FL 32306-2570
Phone: (850)644-4751 **Fax:** (850)644-9750
Website: http://ssw.fsu.edu/
C. Aaron McNeece, Director

★ 29651 ★ University of Central Florida
School of Social Work
Graduate Program in Social Work
PO Box 163358
Orlando, FL 32828
Phone: (407)823-2114 **Fax:** (407)823-5697
Email: mvanhook@pegasus.cc.ucf.edu
Website: http://www.cohpa.ucf.edu/social/
Mary P. Van Hook, Director

★ 29652 ★ University of South Florida
School of Social Work
Graduate Program in Social Work
4202 E Fowler Ave.
MGY 132
Tampa, FL 33620-8100
Phone: (813)974-2063 **Fax:** (813)974-4675
Email: amuso@chuma1.cas.usf.edu
Website: http://www.cas.usf.edu/social_work/index.html
Jean F. Amuso, Director

Georgia

★ 29653 ★ Clark Atlanta University
School of Social Work
Graduate Program in Social Work
James P. Brawley Dr. at Fair St. SW
Atlanta, GA 30314-4391
Phone: (404)880-8548 **Fax:** (404)880-6434
Website: http://www.cau.edu
Dorcas Davis Bowles, Director

★ 29654 ★ Georgia State University
College of Health and Human Sciences
School of Social Work
Graduate Program in Social Work
University Plaza
Atlanta, GA 30303-3083
Phone: (404)651-3526 **Fax:** (404)651-1863
Website: http://chhs.gsu.edu/socialwork
James L. Wolk, Director

★ 29655 ★ Savannah State University
College of Liberal Arts and Social Sciences
Master's Department of Social Work
PO Box 20553
Savannah, GA 31404
Phone: (912)356-2410 **Fax:** (912)356-2458
Email: bswmsw@tigerpaw.savstate.edu
Website: http://www.savstate.edu
James Maury, Chairman of the Board

★ 29656 ★ University of Georgia
School of Social Work
Graduate Program in Social Work
Tucker Hall
Athens, GA 30602-7016
Phone: (706)542-5424 **Fax:** (706)542-3282
Email: byegidis@arches.uga.edu
Website: http://www.ssw.uga.edu/
Bonnie Yegidis, Director

★ 29657 ★ Valdosta State University
Division of Social Work
Graduate Program in Social Work
1500 Patterson St.
Valdosta, GA 31698
Phone: (912)249-4864 **Fax:** (912)245-4341
Email: marchiba@valdosta.edu
Website: http://www.valdosta.peachnet.edu/sowk
Martha M. Giddings, Director

Hawaii

★ 29658 ★ University of Hawaii, Manoa
School of Social Work
Graduate Program in Social Work
1800 East-West Rd.
Honolulu, HI 96822
Phone: (808)956-6300 **Fax:** (808)956-5964
Email: jmatsuok@hawaii.edu
Website: http://www2.hawaii.edu/sswork/welcome.html
Jon K. Matsuoka, Director

Idaho

★ 29659 ★ Boise State University
School of Social Work
Graduate Program in Social Work
1910 University Dr.
Boise, ID 83725
Phone: (208)426-1568 **Fax:** (208)426-4291
Email: mwilson@boisestate.edu
Website: http://www.idbsu.edu/socwork/
Martha Wilson, Director

Illinois

★ 29660 ★ Aurora University
George Williams College
School of Social Work
Graduate Program in Social Work
347 S Gladstone Ave.
Aurora, IL 60506-4892
Phone: (630)844-5419 **Fax:** (630)844-4923
Website: http://www.aurora.edu/
Sandra S. Alcorn, Director

★ 29661 ★ Loyola University, Chicago
School of Social Work
Graduate Program in Social Work
820 N Michigan Ave.
Chicago, IL 60611
Phone: (312)915-7005 **Fax:** (312)915-7645
Email: jwalsh3@luc.edu
Website: http://www.luc.edu/schools/socialwork/
Joseph A. Walsh, Director

★ 29662 ★ Southern Illinois University, Carbondale
School of Social Work
Graduate Program in Social Work
Quigley Hall, Room 4
Mail Code 4329
Carbondale, IL 62901-4329
Phone: (618)453-2243 **Fax:** (618)453-4291
Email: mnemet@siu.edu
Website: http://www.siu.edu/~socwork
Mizanur R. Miah, Director

★ 29663 ★ University of Chicago
School of Social Service Administration
Graduate Program in Social Work
969 E 60th St.
Chicago, IL 60637
Phone: (773)702-1250 **Fax:** (773)834-1582
Email: e-lawlor@uchicago.edu
Website: http://www.ssa.uchicago.edu/
Edward F. Lawlor, Director

★ 29664 ★ University of Illinois, Chicago
Jane Addams College of Social Work
Graduate Program in Social Work
1040 W Harrison St.
Mail Code 309
Chicago, IL 60607-7134
Phone: (312)996-3219 **Fax:** (312)996-1802
Website: http://www.uic.edu/jaddams/college/
Creasie Finney Hairston, Director

★ 29665 ★ University of Illinois, Urbana, Champaign
School of Social Work
Graduate Program in Social Work
1207 W Oregon St.
Urbana, IL 61801
Phone: (217)333-2261 **Fax:** (217)244-5220
Email: social@uiuc.edu
Website: http://www.social.uiuc.edu/
John Poertner, Director

Indiana

★ 29666 ★ Indiana University
School of Social Work
Graduate Program in Social Work
902 W New York St., ES 4138
Indianapolis, IN 46202-5156
Phone: (317)274-6705 **Fax:** (317)274-8630
Email: rbrock@iupui.edu
Website: http://iussw.iupui.edu/
Michael A. Patchner, Director

★ 29667 ★ University of Southern Indiana
Social Work Department
Graduate Program in Social Work
8600 University Blvd.
Evansville, IN 47712
Phone: (812)464-1843 **Fax:** (812)464-1116
Website: http://www.usi.edu/EDU/SOC_WORK/SOCIAL.HTM
David Charles Cousert, Chairman of the Board

Iowa

★ 29668 ★ Saint Ambrose University
School of Social Work
518 W Locust St.
Davenport, IA 52803
Phone: (563)333-6379 **Fax:** (563)333-6097
Email: ksiska@sau.edu
Website: http://www.sau.edu/msw
Brenda L. DuBois, Director

★ 29669 ★ University of Iowa
School of Social Work
Graduate Program in Social Work
308 North Hall
Iowa City, IA 52242-1223
Phone: (319)335-1250 **Fax:** (319)335-1711
Email: salome-raheim@uiowa.edu
Website: http://www.uiowa.edu/~socialwk/
Salome Raheim, Director

Kansas

★ 29670 ★ University of Kansas
School of Social Welfare
Graduate Program in Social Work
1545 Lilac Ln.
Lawrence, KS 66044-3184
Phone: (785)864-4720 **Fax:** (785)864-5277
Email: annw@ukans.edu
Website: http://www.socwel.ukans.edu/
Ann Weick, Director

★ 29671 ★ Washburn University
Department of Social Work
Graduate Program in Social Work
1700 College Ave.
Topeka, KS 66621
Phone: (785)231-1010 **Fax:** (785)231-1027
Email: zzdpsw@washburn.edu
Website: http://www.washburn.edu/sas/social-work/index.html
Mark Kaufman, Director

Kentucky

★ 29672 ★ Spalding University
School of Social Work
Graduate Program in Social Work
851 S 4th St.
Louisville, KY 40203-2115
Phone: (502)585-9911 **Fax:** (502)992-2413
Website: http://www.spalding.edu/university/professionalstudies/socialwork/index.ht
Helen Deines, Director

★ 29673 ★ University of Kentucky
College of Social Work
Graduate Program in Social Work
619 Patterson Office Tower
Lexington, KY 40506-0027
Phone: (859)257-6654 **Fax:** (859)323-1030
Email: khoffma@pop.uky.edu
Website: http://www.uky.edu/SocialWork/welcome.html
Kay S. Hoffman, Director

★ 29674 ★ University of Louisville
Raymond A. Kent School of Social Work
Graduate School of Social Work
Oppenheimer Hall
Louisville, KY 40292
Phone: (502)852-3944 **Fax:** (502)852-0422
Email: terry.singer@louisville.edu
Website: http://www.louisville.edu/kent/
Terry L. Singer, Director

Louisiana

★ 29675 ★ Grambling State University
School of Social Work
Graduate Program in Social Work
PO Box 907
Grambling, LA 71245
Phone: (318)274-3305 **Fax:** (318)274-3254
Website: http://www.gram.edu/sosw/sosw.htm
Valiyaveetil Thomas Samuel, Director

★ 29676 ★ Louisiana State University
School of Social Work
Graduate Program in Social Work
Huey P. Long Field House
Baton Rouge, LA 70803
Phone: (225)578-1351 **Fax:** (225)578-1357
Email: socialwork@lsu.edu
Website: http://www.socialwork.lsu.edu
Steven R. Rose, Director

★ 29677 ★ Southern University, New Orleans
School of Social Work
Graduate Program in Social Work
6400 Press Dr.
New Orleans, LA 70126
Phone: (504)286-5376 **Fax:** (504)286-5387
Website: http://www.suno.edu/
Millie M. Charles, Director

★ 29678 ★ Tulane University
School of Social Work
Graduate Program in Social Work
6823 St. Charles Ave.
New Orleans, LA 70118-5672
Phone: (504)865-5314 **Fax:** (504)862-8727
Email: sengland@mailhost.tcs.tulane.edu
Website: http://www.tulane.edu/~tssw/
Ronald Marks, Director

Maine

★ 29679 ★ University of Maine
School of Social Work
Graduate Program in Social Work
5770 Social Work Bldg.
Orono, ME 04469
Phone: (207)581-2389 **Fax:** (207)581-2396
Email: gail.werrbach@umit.maine.edu
Website: http://www.ume.maine.edu/~soclwork
Gail Werrbach, Director

★ 29680 ★ University of New England
School of Social Work
Graduate Program in Social Work
11 Hills Beach Rd.
Biddeford, ME 04005
Phone: (207)797-7261 **Fax:** (207)541-3100
Email: jthompson@mailbox.une.edu
Website: http://www.une.edu/chp/socialwork/index.html
Joanne J. Thompson, Director

Maryland

★ 29681 ★ University of Maryland, Baltimore
School of Social Work
Graduate Program in Social Work
Louis L. Kaplan Hall
525 W Redwood St.
Baltimore, MD 21201-1777
Phone: (410)706-7794 **Fax:** (410)706-0273
Email: jharris@ssw.umaryland.edu
Website: http://ssw.umaryland.edu/
Jesse J. Harris, Director

Massachusetts

★ 29682 ★ Boston College
Graduate School of Social Work
McGuinn Hall
140 Commonwealth Ave.
Chestnut Hill, MA 02467-3807
Phone: (617)552-4020 **Fax:** (617)552-2374
Website: http://www.bc.edu/gssw
Alberto A. Godenzi, Director

★ 29683 ★ Boston University
School of Social Work
Graduate Program in Social Work
264 Bay State Rd.
Boston, MA 02215
Phone: (617)353-3750 **Fax:** (617)353-5612
Email: wpeebles@bu.edu
Website: http://www.bu.edu/ssw/
Wilma Peebles-Wilkins, Director

★ 29684 ★ Salem State College
School of Social Work
Graduate Program in Social Work
352 Lafayette St.
Salem, MA 01970
Phone: (978)542-6650 **Fax:** (978)542-6936
Email: donald.riley@salem.mass.edu
Website: http://www.salemstate.edu/socialwork
Donald P. Riley, Director

★ 29685 ★ Simmons College
Graduate School of Social Work
51 Commonwealth Ave.
Boston, MA 02116
Phone: (617)521-3900 **Fax:** (617)521-3956
Email: jregan@simmons.edu
Website: http://www.simmons.edu/programs/ssw/
Joseph M. Regan, Director

★ 29686 ★ Smith College
School for Social Work
Graduate Program in Social Work
Lilly Hall
Northampton, MA 01063
Phone: (413)585-7952 **Fax:** (413)585-7994
Website: http://www.smith.edu/ssw/
Carolyn Jacobs, Director

★ 29687 ★ Springfield College
School of Social Work
Graduate Program in Social Work
263 Alden St.
Springfield, MA 01109-3797
Phone: (413)748-3065 **Fax:** (413)748-3069
Email: francine_vecchiolla@spfldcol.edu
Website: http://www.spfldcol.edu/
Francine J. Vecchiolla, Director

Michigan

★ 29688 ★ Andrews University
Social Work Department
Graduate Program in Social Work
Nethery Hall
Berrien Springs, MI 49104
Phone: (616)471-6135 **Fax:** (616)471-3686
Email: spittman@andrews.edu
Website: http://www.andrews.edu
Sharon Pittman, Director

★ 29689 ★ Eastern Michigan University
Graduate Program in Social Work
317 Marshall Bldg.
Ypsilanti, MI 48197
Phone: (734)487-4169 **Fax:** (734)487-6832
Email: wanda.bracy@emich.edu
Website: http://www.emich.edu/public/swk/swkhome.htm
John Gunther, Director

★ 29690 ★ Grand Valley State University
School of Social Work
Graduate Program in Social Work
De Vos Center, 3rd Fl.
401 W Fulton
Grand Rapids, MI 49504
Phone: (616)771-6550 **Fax:** (616)771-6570
Email: mulderr@gvsu.edu
Website: http://www4.gvsu.edu/ssw
Rodney Mulder, Director

★ 29691 ★ Michigan State University
School of Social Work
Graduate Program in Social Work
254 Baker Hall
East Lansing, MI 48824
Phone: (517)353-8632 **Fax:** (517)353-3038
Email: social.work@ssc.msu.edu
Website: http://www.ssc.msu.edu/~sw/
Gary Anderson, Director

★ 29692 ★ University of Michigan
School of Social Work
Graduate Program in Social Work
1080 S University
Ann Arbor, MI 48109-1106
Phone: (734)764-5340 **Fax:** (734)764-9954
Email: pameares@umich.edu
Website: http://www.ssw.umich.edu/
Paula Allen-Meares, Director

★ 29693 ★ Wayne State University
School of Social Work
Graduate Program in Social Work
201 Thompson Home
4756 Cass Ave.
Detroit, MI 48202
Phone: (313)577-4400 **Fax:** (313)577-8770
Email: aa8773@wayne.edu
Website: http://www.socialwork.wayne.edu
Phyllis Ivory Vroom, Director

★ 29694 ★ Western Michigan University
School of Social Work
Graduate Program in Social Work
1903 Western Ave.
Kalamazoo, MI 49008-5034
Phone: (616)387-3170 **Fax:** (616)387-3183
Email: mabrey@wmich.edu
Website: http://www.wmich.edu/hhs/sw
Earlie M. Washington, Director

Minnesota

★ 29695 ★ Augsburg College
Department of Social Work
Graduate Program in Social Work
2211 Riverside Ave.
Minneapolis, MN 55454
Phone: (612)330-1189 **Fax:** (612)330-1493
Email: bosch@augsberg.edu
Website: http://www.augsburg.edu
Anthony A. Bibus, Chairman of the Board

★ 29696 ★ College of Saint Catherine/ University of Saint Thomas
School of Social Work
Graduate Program in Social Work
2115 Summit Ave.
Mail LOR 406
Saint Paul, MN 55105
Phone: (651)962-5800 **Fax:** (651)962-5819
Email: bwshank@stthomas.edu
Website: http://department.stthomas.edu/grad/index.cfm
Barbara W. Shank, Director

★ 29697 ★ University of Minnesota, Duluth
Department of Social Work
Graduate Program in Social Work
220 Bohannon Hall
Duluth, MN 55812-2496
Phone: (218)726-7245 **Fax:** (218)726-7185
Email: sw@d.umn.edu
Website: http://www.d.umn.edu/sw/
Michael Raschick, Director

★ 29698 ★ University of Minnesota, Twin Cities
School of Social Work
Graduate Program in Social Work
1404 Gortner Ave.
Saint Paul, MN 55108
Phone: (612)625-1220 **Fax:** (612)624-3744
Email: jguam@che1.che.umn.edu
Website: http://ssw.che.umn.edu/
Jean K. Quam, Director

Mississippi

★ 29699 ★ Jackson State University
Graduate Program in Social Work
3825 Ridgewood Rd., Ste. 9
Jackson, MS 39211
Phone: (601)432-6819 **Fax:** (601)432-6827
Email: mswprog@ccaix.jsums.edu
Website: http://www.jsums.edu/
Gwendolyn Spencer Prater, Director

★ 29700 ★ University of Southern Mississippi
School of Social Work
Graduate Program in Social Work
PO Box 5114
Hattiesburg, MS 39406

Phone: (601)266-4163 Fax: (601)266-4165
Website: http://www-dept.usm.edu/~socwork/
Michael Forster, Director

Missouri

★ 29701 ★ Saint Louis University
School of Social Service
Graduate Program in Social Work
3550 Lindell Blvd.
Saint Louis, MO 63103
Phone: (314)977-2730 **Fax:** (314)977-2731
Email: tebbsc@slu.edu
Website: http://www.slu.edu/colleges/socsvc/
Susan C. Tebb, Director

★ 29702 ★ Southwest Missouri State University
School of Social Work
Graduate Program in Social Work
Professional Bldg., Ste. 200
901 S National Ave.
Springfield, MO 65804
Phone: (417)836-6953 **Fax:** (417)836-7688
Email: JOG495@mail.smsu.edu
Website: http://www.smsu.edu/swk/
Mary Ann Jennings, Director

★ 29703 ★ University of Missouri, Columbia
School of Social Work
Graduate Program in Social Work
729 Clark Hall
Columbia, MO 65211-4470
Phone: (573)882-4447 **Fax:** (573)882-8926
Email: cowgerc@missouri.edu
Website: http://web.missouri.edu/~sswmain
Charles Cowger, Director

★ 29704 ★ Washington University
George Warren Brown School of Social Work
Graduate Program in Social Work
1 Brookings Dr.
Campus Box 1196
Saint Louis, MO 63130-4899
Phone: (314)935-6693 **Fax:** (314)935-8511
Email: mswadmis@gwbssw.wustl.edu
Website: http://gwbweb.wustl.edu/
Shanti K. Khinduka, Director

Nebraska

★ 29705 ★ University of Nebraska, Omaha
School of Social Work
Graduate Program in Social Work
60th and Dodge Sts.
Annex 40
Omaha, NE 68182-0293
Phone: (402)554-2793 **Fax:** (402)554-3788
Website: http://cid.unomaha.edu/~wwwpa/sw/swhome.html
Sunny Andrews, Director

Nevada

★ 29706 ★ University of Nevada, Las Vegas
School of Social Work
Graduate Program in Social Work
4505 Maryland Pkwy.
Box 455032
Las Vegas, NV 89154-5032
Phone: (702)895-4338 **Fax:** (702)895-4079
Email: elangston@ccmail.nevada.edu
Website: http://www.nscee.edu/unlv/Colleges/Urban
Esther Jones Langston, Director

★ 29707 ★ University of Nevada, Reno
School of Social Work
Graduate Program in Social Work
Business Bldg., Rm. 523
Mail Stop 090
Reno, NV 89557-0068
Phone: (775)784-6542 **Fax:** (775)784-4573
Email: pierce@unr.edu
Website: http://www.unr.edu/hcs/ssw/index.html
Dean Pierce, Director

New Hampshire

★ 29708 ★ University of New Hampshire
Department of Social Work
Graduate Program in Social Work
Pettee Hall
50 College Rd.
Durham, NH 03824-3596
Phone: (603)862-1799 **Fax:** (603)862-4374
Email: rej@christa.unh.edu
Website: http://www.unh.edu/social-work/index.html
Robert E. Jolley, Chairman of the Board

New Jersey

★ 29709 ★ Kean University
Department of Social Work
Master of Social Work Program
1000 Morris Ave.
Hutchinson Hall, Rm. 305
Union, NJ 07083-7131
Phone: (908)527-2634 **Fax:** (908)289-5633
Website: http://www.kean.edu/
Patricia G. Pearson, Chairman of the Board

★ 29710 ★ Monmouth University
Social Work Department
Graduate Program in Social Work
Norwood and Cedar Ave.
West Long Branch, NJ 07764-1898
Phone: (732)571-3543 **Fax:** (732)263-5217
Website: http://www.monmouth.edu/socialwork
Mark E. Rodgers, Director

★ 29711 ★ Rutgers, the State University of New Jersey
School of Social Work
Graduate Program in Social Work
536 George St.
New Brunswick, NJ 08901-1167
Phone: (732)932-7253 **Fax:** (732)932-8915
Website: http://www.rutgers.edu
Mary Edna Davidson, Director

New Mexico

★ 29712 ★ New Mexico Highlands University
School of Social Work
Master of Social Work Program
Las Vegas, NM 87701
Phone: (505)454-3563 **Fax:** (505)454-3454
Email: a_garcia@nmhu.edu
Website: http://www.nmhu.edu/academics/schsocwork
Alfredo A. Garcia, Director

★ 29713 ★ New Mexico State University
School of Social Work
Graduate Program in Social Work
PO Box 30001, MSC 3SW
Las Cruces, NM 88003-8001
Phone: (505)646-2143 **Fax:** (505)646-4116
Email: socwork@nmsu.edu
Website: http://www.nmsu.edu/~socwork
Stephen C. Anderson, Director

New York

★ 29714 ★ Adelphi University
School of Social Work
Graduate Program in Social Work
South Ave.
Garden City, NY 11530
Phone: (516)877-4355 **Fax:** (516)877-4436
Email: levin@adlibv.adelphi.edu
Website: http://www.adelphi.edu/socialwork/
Brooke E. Spiro, Director

★ 29715 ★ City University of New York Hunter College
School of Social Work
Master of Social Work Program
129 E 79th St.
New York, NY 10021
Phone: (212)452-7085 **Fax:** (212)452-7150
Email: bleashore@shiva.hunter.cuny.edu
Website: http://www.hunter.cuny.edu/socwork/
Bogart R. Leashore, Director

★ 29716 ★ Columbia University
School of Social Work
Master of Social Work Program
622 W 113th St.
New York, NY 10025
Phone: (212)854-5189 **Fax:** (212)854-4585
Email: rafl@columbia.edu
Website: http://www.columbia.edu/cu/ssw/
Sheila B. Kamerman, Director

★ 29717 ★ Fordham University
Graduate School of Social Service
Master of Social Work Program
Lincoln Center Campus
113 W 60th St., Rm. 726
New York, NY 10023-7479
Phone: (212)636-6600 **Fax:** (212)636-7876
Email: quaranta@mary.fordham.edu
Website: http://www.fordham.edu/gss/index.html
Peter B. Vaughan, Director

★ 29718 ★ New York University
Shirley M. Ehrenkranz School of Social Work
Graduate Program in Social Work
1 Washington Sq. N
New York, NY 10003
Phone: (212)998-5959 **Fax:** (212)995-4172
Email: essw.admissions@nyu.edu
Website: http://www.nyu.edu/socialwork/
Suzanne E. England, Director

★ 29719 ★ Roberts Wesleyan College
Master of Social Work Program
2301 Westside Dr.
Rochester, NY 14624-1997
Phone: (716)594-6410 **Fax:** (716)594-6480
Email: descoteauxw@roberts.edu
Website: http://www.rwc.edu/academic/social_w_s/index.htm
William R. Descoteaux, Director

★ 29720 ★ State University of New York, Albany
School of Social Welfare
Graduate Program in Social Work
135 Western Ave.
Albany, NY 12222
Phone: (518)442-5320 **Fax:** (518)442-5380
Email: kbl@csc.albany.edu
Website: http://www.albany.edu/ssw/index.html
Katharine Briar-Lawson, Director

★ 29721 ★ State University of New York, Buffalo
School of Social Work
Graduate Program in Social Work
685 Baldy Hall
PO Box 601050
Buffalo, NY 14260-1050
Phone: (716)645-3381 **Fax:** (716)645-3883
Email: shulman@acsu.buffalo.edu
Website: http://www.socialwork.buffalo.edu/
Lawrence Shulman, Director

★ 29722 ★ State University of New York, Stony Brook
School of Social Welfare
Graduate Program in Social Work
Health Sciences Center, Level 2, Rm. 093
Stony Brook, NY 11794-8231
Phone: (631)444-2139 **Fax:** (631)444-8908
Email: francesb@ssw.hsc.sunysb.edu
Website: http://www.uhmc.sunysb.edu/socwelf/
Frances L. Brisbane, Director

★ 29723 ★ Syracuse University
School of Social Work
Graduate Program in Social Work
Sims Hall
Syracuse, NY 13244-1230
Phone: (315)443-5550 **Fax:** (315)443-5576
Email: wlpoll@social.syr.edu
Website: http://www.social.syr.edu/
Bruce W. Lagay, Director

★ 29724 ★ Yeshiva University
Wurzweiler School of Social Work
Graduate Program in Social Work
Belfer Hall
2495 Amsterdam Ave.
New York, NY 10033
Phone: (212)960-0820 **Fax:** (212)960-0822
Email: srgelman@ymail.yu.edu
Website: http://www.yu.edu/wurzweiler
Sheldon R. Gelman, Director

North Carolina

★ 29725 ★ East Carolina University
School of Social Work and Criminal Justice Studies
Graduate Program in Social Work
Ragsdale Bldg., Rm. 134
Greenville, NC 27858-4353
Phone: (252)328-4208 **Fax:** (252)328-4196
Email: griffinl@mail.ecu.edu
Website: http://www.ecu.edu/
W. David Harrison, Director

★ 29726 ★ University of North Carolina, Chapel Hill
School of Social Work
Graduate Program in Social Work
Tate-Turner-Kuralt Bldg.
301 Pittsboro St.
CB 3550
Chapel Hill, NC 27599-3550
Phone: (919)962-1225 **Fax:** (919)962-0890
Email: stromgot@email.unc.edu
Website: http://ssw.unc.edu
Jack Richman, Director

★ 29727 ★ University of North Carolina, Greensboro/North Carolina A & T State University
Joint Master of Social Work Program
PO Box 26170
Greensboro, NC 27402-6170
Phone: (336)334-4100 **Fax:** (336)334-5210
Email: jcrife@uncg.edu
Website: http://www.uncg.edu/swk/joint_msw.htm
John C. Rife, Director

North Dakota

★ 29728 ★ University of North Dakota
Department of Social Work
Graduate Program in Social Work
Gillette Hall
Box 7135
Grand Forks, ND 58202-7135
Phone: (701)777-2669 **Fax:** (701)777-4257
Email: mike_jacobsen@mail.und.nodak.edu
Website: http://www.und.nodak.edu
Ralph Woehle, Director

Ohio

★ 29729 ★ Case Western Reserve University
Mandel School of Applied Social Sciences
Master in Social Work Program
10900 Euclid Ave.
Cleveland, OH 44106-7164
Phone: (216)368-2270 **Fax:** (216)368-2850
Email: msassdean@po.cwru.edu
Website: http://msass.cwru.edu
Darlyne Bailey, Director

★ 29730 ★ Ohio State University
College of Social Work
Graduate Program in Social Work
300 Stillman Hall
1947 College Rd.
Columbus, OH 43210-1162
Phone: (614)292-2972 **Fax:** (614)292-6940
Email: tripodi.5@osu.edu
Website: http://www.csw.ohio-state.edu/
Tony Tripodi, Director

★ 29731 ★ University of Akron/Cleveland State University
School of Social Work
Joint Master of Social Work Program
Polsky Bldg., Room 411
Akron, OH 44325-8001
Phone: (330)972-5275 **Fax:** (330)972-5739
Email: vfitch@uakron.edu
Virginia Fitch, Director

★ 29732 ★ University of Cincinnati
School of Social Work
Graduate Program in Social Work
PO Box 210108
Cincinnati, OH 45221-0108
Phone: (513)556-4615 **Fax:** (513)556-2077
Email: philip.jackson@uc.edu
Website: http://www.uc.edu/socialwork/
Philip Jackson, Director

Oklahoma

★ 29733 ★ University of Oklahoma
School of Social Work
Graduate Program in Social Work
1005 Jenkins Ave.
Norman, OK 73019
Phone: (405)325-2821 **Fax:** (405)325-7072
Website: http://www.ou.edu/socialwork/
Roosevelt Wright, Jr., Director

Oregon

★ 29734 ★ Portland State University
Graduate School of Social Work
PO Box 751
Portland, OR 97207-0751
Phone: (503)725-4712 **Fax:** (503)725-5545
Email: wardj@rri.pdx.edu
Website: http://www.ssw.pdx.edu/
James H. Ward, Director

Pennsylvania

★ 29735 ★ Bryn Mawr College
Graduate School of Social Work and Social Research
300 Airdale Rd.
Bryn Mawr, PA 19010-1697
Phone: (610)520-2600 **Fax:** (610)520-2655
Email: rmayden@brnymawr.edu
Website: http://www.brynmawr.edu/gsswsr
Ruth W. Mayden, Director

★ 29736 ★ Marywood University
School of Social Work
Graduate Program in Social Work
2300 Adams Ave.
Scranton, PA 18509-1598
Phone: (570)348-6282 **Fax:** (570)961-4742
Email: whitaker@ac.marywood.edu
Website: http://www.marywood.edu/goals.htm
William H. Whitaker, Director

★ 29737 ★ Temple University
School of Social Administration
Graduate Program in Social Work
Ritter Hall Annex, Rm. 555
1301 Cecil B. Moore Ave.
Philadelphia, PA 19122
Phone: (215)204-8623 **Fax:** (215)204-9606
Email: leonard@vm.temple.edu
Website: http://www.temple.edu/socialwork/
Curtis A. Leonard, Director

★ 29738 ★ University of Pennsylvania
School of Social Work
Graduate Program in Social Work
3701 Locust Walk
Philadelphia, PA 19104-6214
Phone: (215)898-5511 **Fax:** (215)573-2099
Email: iram@ssw.upenn.edu
Website: http://www.ssw.upenn.edu/
Roberta R. Iversen, Director

★ 29739 ★ University of Pittsburgh
School of Social Work
Graduate Program in Social Work
2117 Cathedral of Learning
Pittsburgh, PA 15260
Phone: (412)624-6304 **Fax:** (412)624-6323
Email: deesw@vms.cis.pitt.edu
Website: http://www.pitt.edu/~pittssw/
Sandra Wexler, Director

★ 29740 ★ West Chester University
Department of Graduate Social Work
Reynolds Hall
West Chester, PA 19383
Phone: (610)436-2664 **Fax:** (610)738-0375
Website: http://www.wcupa.edu
Ann A. Abbott, Chairman of the Board

★ 29741 ★ Widener University
Center for Social Work Education
Graduate Program in Social Work
1 University Place
Chester, PA 19013
Phone: (610)499-1153 **Fax:** (610)499-4617
Email: paula.t.silver@.widener.edu
Website: http://muse.widener.edu/socialwork/
Paula T. Silver, Director

Puerto Rico

★ 29742 ★ Universidad Interamericana de Puerto Rico, Recinto Metropolitano
Graduate Social Work Program
PO Box 191293
San Juan, PR 00919-1293
Phone: (787)250-1912 **Fax:** (787)250-6843
Rosalie Rosa Soderal, Director

★ 29743 ★ University of Puerto Rico, Rio Piedra Campus
Beatriz Lassalle Graduate School of Social Work
PO Box 23345
San Juan, PR 00931-3345
Phone: (787)763-3725 **Fax:** (787)763-3725
Website: http://www.upr.edu/
Norma Rodriguez-Roldan, Director

Rhode Island

★ 29744 ★ Rhode Island College
School of Social Work
Graduate Program in Social Work
600 Mt. Pleasant Dr.
Providence, RI 02908
Phone: (401)456-8042 **Fax:** (401)456-8620
Website: http://www.ric.edu/socwk/
George D. Metrey, Director

South Carolina

★ 29745 ★ University of South Carolina
College of Social Work
Graduate Program in Social Work
Columbia, SC 29208
Phone: (803)777-5291 **Fax:** (803)777-3498
Email: frank.raymond@sc.edu
Website: http://www.sc.edu/cosw/
Frank B. Raymond, III, Director

Tennessee

★ 29746 ★ University of Tennessee
College of Social Work
Graduate Program in Social Work
109 Henson Hall
Knoxville, TN 37996-3333
Phone: (865)974-3176 **Fax:** (865)974-4803
Email: jfiene@utk.edu
Website: http://www.csw.utk.edu/
Karen M. Sowers, Director

Texas

★ 29747 ★ Baylor University
School of Social Work
Graduate Program in Social Work
PO Box 97320
Waco, TX 76798-7320
Phone: (254)710-6400 **Fax:** (254)710-6455
Website: http://www.baylor.edu
Diana R. Garland, Chairman of the Board

★ 29748 ★ Our Lady of the Lake University
Worden School of Social Service
Graduate Program in Social Work
411 SW 24th St.
San Antonio, TX 78207-4689
Phone: (210)434-3969 **Fax:** (210)431-4028
Email: zimmc@lake.ollusa.edu
Website: http://www.ollusa.edu/academic/worden/worden.htm
James Allen, Director

★ 29749 ★ Southwest Texas State University
School of Social Work
Graduate Program in Social Work
601 University Dr.
San Marcos, TX 78666-4616
Phone: (512)245-8833 **Fax:** (512)245-8097
Email: kb01@swt.edu
Dorinda N. Noble, Director

★ 29750 ★ Stephen F. Austin State University
School of Social Work
Master of Social Work Program
SFA Station
PO Box 6104
Nacogdoches, TX 75962-6104
Phone: (936)468-4020 **Fax:** (936)468-7201
Website: http://www.sfasu.edu/aas/socwk
Michael R. Daley, Director

★ 29751 ★ University of Houston
Graduate School of Social Work
237 Social Work Bldg.
Houston, TX 77204-4013
Phone: (713)743-8085 **Fax:** (713)743-3267
Email: lcolby@uh.edu
Website: http://www.sw.uh.edu/
Ira C. Colby, Director

★ 29752 ★ University of Texas, Arlington
School of Social Work
Graduate Program in Social Work
Box 19129
Arlington, TX 76019
Phone: (817)272-3181 **Fax:** (817)272-5229
Email: granvold@uta.edu
Website: http://www.uta.edu/ssw/utassw.html
Santos H. Hernandez, Director

★ 29753 ★ University of Texas, Austin
School of Social Work
Graduate Program in Social Work
1925 San Jacinto Blvd.
Austin, TX 78712
Phone: (512)471-1937 **Fax:** (512)471-7268
Email: bwwhite@mail.utexas.edu
Website: http://utexas.edu/depts/sswork/
Barbara W. White, Director

Utah

★ 29754 ★ Brigham Young University
School of Social Work
Master of Social Work Program
217 Knight Mangum Bldg.
PO Box 24476
Provo, UT 84602-4476
Phone: (801)378-3282 **Fax:** (801)378-4049
Email: socialwork@byu.edu
Website: http://fhss.byu.edu/socwork/
Elaine Walton, Director

★ 29755 ★ University of Utah
Graduate School of Social Work
395 S 1500 E, Rm. 111
Salt Lake City, UT 84112-0260
Phone: (801)581-6192 **Fax:** (801)585-3219
Email: jmather@ocwk.utah.edu
Website: http://www.socwk.utah.edu
Jannah Hurn Mather, Director

Vermont

★ 29756 ★ University of Vermont
Department of Social Work
Graduate Program in Social Work
288 Waterman Bldg.
Burlington, VT 05405
Phone: (802)656-8800 **Fax:** (802)656-8565
Email: dmpratt@zoo.uvm.edu
Website: http://www.uvm.edu/~socwork/index.html
Gale Burford, Director

Virginia

★ 29757 ★ Norfolk State University
Ethelyn R. Strong School of Social Work
Graduate Program in Social Work
700 Park Ave.
Norfolk, VA 23504
Phone: (757)823-8668 **Fax:** (757)823-2556
Website: http://www.nsu.edu/schools/swork/index.htm
Marvin D. Feit, Director

★ 29758 ★ Radford University
School of Social Work
Graduate Program in Social Work
Box 6958
Radford, VA 24142
Phone: (540)831-7689 **Fax:** (540)831-7670
Email: mrigby@runet.edu
Website: http://www.runet.edu/~sowk-web/
Marilyn A. Rigby, Director

★ 29759 ★ Virginia Commonwealth University
School of Social Work
Graduate Program in Social Work
1001 W Franklin St.
PO Box 842027
Richmond, VA 23284-2027
Phone: (804)828-1030 **Fax:** (804)828-7541
Email: fbaskind@vcu.edu
Website: http://www.vcu.edu/slwweb/index.htm
Frank R. Baskind, Director

Washington

★ 29760 ★ Eastern Washington University
Inland Empire School of Social Work and Human Services
Graduate Program in Social Work
526 5th St.
Cheney, WA 99004-2431
Phone: (509)359-6482 **Fax:** (509)359-6475
Email: socialwork@ewu.edu
Website: http://sswhs.ewu.edu/socialwork.html
Michael L. Frumkin, Director

★ 29761 ★ University of Washington
School of Social Work
Graduate Program in Social Work
4101 15th Ave. NE
Seattle, WA 98105-6299
Phone: (206)685-1662 **Fax:** (206)543-1228
Email: hooy@u.washington.edu
Website: http://depts.u.washington.edu/sswweb
Dorothy Van Soest, Director

★ 29762 ★ Walla Walla College
Graduate School of Social Work
204 S College Ave.
College Place, WA 99324-1198
Phone: (509)527-2590 **Fax:** (509)527-2434
Website: http://www.wwc.edu
Wilma Hepker, Director

West Virginia

★ 29763 ★ West Virginia University
School of Applied Social Sciences
Division of Social Work
Graduate Program in Social Work
PO Box 6830
Morgantown, WV 26506-6830
Phone: (304)293-3501 **Fax:** (304)293-5936
Email: blocke2@wvu.edu
Website: http://www.wvu.edu/~socialwk/
Virginia Stadler Majewski, Director

Wisconsin

★ 29764 ★ University of Wisconsin, Madison
School of Social Work
Graduate Program in Social Work
1350 University Ave.
Madison, WI 53706-1510
Phone: (608)263-3561 **Fax:** (608)263-3836
Email: socwork@macc.wisc.edu
Website: http://www.wisc.edu
Daniel R. Meyer, Director

★ 29765 ★ University of Wisconsin, Milwaukee
School of Social Welfare
Graduate Program in Social Work
PO Box 786
Milwaukee, WI 53201
Phone: (414)229-4400 **Fax:** (414)229-5311
Email: jmj2@cds.wm.edu
Website: http://www.uwm.edu/Dept/SSW/
James A. Blackburn, Director

Wyoming

★ 29766 ★ University of Wyoming
Division of Social Work
Graduate Program in Social Work
Box 3632
Laramie, WY 82071
Phone: (307)766-6112 **Fax:** (307)766-6839
Email: debval@uwyo.edu
Website: http://uwacadweb.uwyo.edu/SocialWork/sowk.html
Deborah Valentine, Director

Veterinary Medicine

Colleges of veterinary medicine listed in this section are accredited by the American Veterinary Medical Association, 1931 N Meacham Rd., Ste. 100, Schaumburg, IL 60173, (847)925-8070, http://www.avma.org/.

Alabama

★ 29767 ★ Auburn University
College of Veterinary Medicine
Auburn University, AL 36849
Phone: (334)844-3691
Website: http://www.vetmed.auburn.edu

★ 29768 ★ Tuskegee University
School of Veterinary Medicine
Tuskegee University, AL 36088
Phone: (334)727-8173
Website: http://svmc107.tusk.edu

California

★ 29769 ★ University of California, Davis
School of Veterinary Medicine
Davis, CA 95616-8734
Phone: (530)752-1360
Website: http://www.vetmed.ucdavis.edu

★ 29770 ★ Western University of Health Sciences
College of Veterinary Medicine
309 E 2nd St., College Plaza
Pomona, CA 91766
Phone: (909)469-5628
Website: http://www.westernu.edu/cvm.html

Colorado

★ 29771 ★ Colorado State University
College of Veterinary Medicine and Biomedical Sciences
Fort Collins, CO 80523
Phone: (970)491-7051
Website: http://www.cvmbs.colostate.edu

Florida

★ 29772 ★ University of Florida
College of Veterinary Medicine
Gainesville, FL 32610-0125
Phone: (352)392-4700
Website: http://www.vetmed.ufl.edu

Georgia

★ 29773 ★ University of Georgia
College of Veterinary Medicine
Athens, GA 30602
Phone: (706)542-3461
Website: http://www.vet.uga.edu

Illinois

★ 29774 ★ University of Illinois
College of Veterinary Medicine
2001 S Lincoln
Urbana, IL 61801
Phone: (217)333-2760
Website: http://www.cvm.uiuc.edu

Indiana

★ 29775 ★ Purdue University
School of Veterinary Medicine
1240 Lynn Hall
West Lafayette, IN 47907-1240
Phone: (765)494-7607
Website: http://www.vet.purdue.edu

Iowa

★ 29776 ★ Iowa State University
College of Veterinary Medicine
Ames, IA 50011
Phone: (515)294-1242
Website: http://www.vetmed.iastate.edu

Kansas

★ 29777 ★ Kansas State University
College of Veterinary Medicine
Manhattan, KS 66506
Phone: (785)532-6011
Website: http://www.vet.ksu.edu

Louisiana

★ 29778 ★ Louisiana State University
School of Veterinary Medicine
Baton Rouge, LA 70803
Phone: (225)346-3100
Website: http://www.vetmed.lsu.edu

Massachusetts

★ 29779 ★ Tufts University
School of Veterinary Medicine
200 Westboro Rd.
North Grafton, MA 01536
Phone: (508)839-5302
Website: http://www.tufts.edu/vet

Michigan

★ 29780 ★ Michigan State University
College of Veterinary Medicine
East Lansing, MI 48824-1314
Phone: (517)355-6509
Website: http://www.cvm.msu.edu

Minnesota

★ 29781 ★ University of Minnesota
College of Veterinary Medicine
Saint Paul, MN 55108
Phone: (612)624-9227
Website: http://www.cvm.umn.edu

Mississippi

★ 29782 ★ Mississippi State University
College of Veterinary Medicine
Mississippi State, MS 39762
Phone: (662)325-3432
Website: http://www.cvm.msstate.edu

Missouri

★ 29783 ★ University of Missouri
College of Veterinary Medicine
Columbia, MO 65211
Phone: (573)882-3877
Website: http://www.cvm.missouri.edu

New York

★ 29784 ★ Cornell University
College of Veterinary Medicine
Ithaca, NY 14853-6401
Phone: (607)253-3700
Website: http://www.vet.cornell.edu

North Carolina

★ 29785 ★ North Carolina State University
College of Veterinary Medicine
4700 Hillsborough St.
Raleigh, NC 27606
Phone: (919)513-6200
Website: http://www.cvm.ncsu.edu

Ohio

★ 29786 ★ Ohio State University
College of Veterinary Medicine
Columbus, OH 43210
Phone: (614)292-1171
Website: http://www.vet.ohio-state.edu

Oklahoma

★ 29787 ★ Oklahoma State University College of Veterinary Medicine
Stillwater, OK 74078
Phone: (405)744-6648
Website: http://www.cvm.okstate.edu

Ontario

★ 29788 ★ University of Guelph Ontario Veterinary College
Guelph, ON, Canada N1G 2W1
Fax: (519)837-3230

Oregon

★ 29789 ★ Oregon State University College of Veterinary Medicine
Corvallis, OR 97331-4801
Phone: (541)737-2141
Website: http://www.vet.orst.edu

Pennsylvania

★ 29790 ★ University of Pennsylvania School of Veterinary Medicine
3800 Spruce St.
Philadelphia, PA 19104-6044
Phone: (215)898-5434
Website: http://www.vet.upenn.edu

Prince Edward Island

★ 29791 ★ University of Prince Edward Island Atlantic Veterinary College
Charlottetown, PE, Canada C1A 4P3
Phone: (902)566-0800 **Fax:** (902)566-0958

Quebec

★ 29792 ★ University of Montreal Faculty of Veterinary Medicine
Saint Hyancinthe, QC, Canada J2S 7C6
Phone: (514)345-8521 **Fax:** (514)778-8114

Saskatchewan

★ 29793 ★ University of Saskatchewan Western College of Veterinary Medicine
52 Campus Dr.
Saskatoon, SK, Canada S7N 5B4
Fax: (306)966-8747

Tennessee

★ 29794 ★ University of Tennessee College of Veterinary Medicine
Knoxville, TN 37901
Phone: (865)974-7262
Website: http://www.vet.utk.edu

Texas

★ 29795 ★ Texas A&M University College of Veterinary Medicine
College Station, TX 77843-4461
Phone: (409)845-5051
Website: http://www.cvm.tamu.edu

Virginia

★ 29796 ★ University of Maryland/ Virginia Tech Virginia-Maryland Regional College of Veterinary Medicine
Blacksburg, VA 24061-0442
Phone: (540)231-4621
Website: http://www.vetmed.vt.edu

Washington

★ 29797 ★ Washington State University College of Veterinary Medicine
Pullman, WA 99164-7010
Phone: (509)335-9515
Website: http://www.vetmed.wsu.edu

Wisconsin

★ 29798 ★ University of Wisconsin, Madison School of Veterinary Medicine
Madison, WI 53706
Phone: (608)263-6716
Website: http://www.vetmed.wisc.edu

Other Allied Health Educational Programs

This section lists professional organizations to contact for information on occupational fields not covered in preceding sections. Educational programs in many of these areas are accredited by the Commission on Accreditation of Allied Health Education Programs, 35 E Wacker Dr., Ste. 1970, Chicago, IL 60601, (312)553-9355, http://www.caahep.org/.

Anesthesiologist's Assistant

★ 29799 ★ American Academy of Anesthesiologist Assistants
PO Box 13978
Tallahassee, FL 32317
Phone: (850)656-8848 **Fax:** (850)656-3038
Email: info@anesthetist.org
Website: http://www.shoestringnet.com/AAAA/

Athletic Training

★ 29800 ★ National Athletic Trainers Association
2952 Stemmons Fwy., Ste. 200
Dallas, TX 75247
Phone: (214)637-6282 **Free:** 800-TRY-NATA
Fax: (214)637-2206
Email: ebd@nata.org
Website: http://www.nata.org/
Eve Becker-Doyle, Exec Director

Cardiovascular Technology

★ 29801 ★ Alliance of Cardiovascular Professionals
Thalia Landing Offices, Bldg. 2
4356 Bonney Rd., No. 103
Virginia Beach, VA 23452-1200
Phone: (757)497-1225 **Fax:** (757)497-0010
Email: peggymcelgunn@comcast.net
Website: http://www.acp-online.org/
Peggy McElgunn, Contact

★ 29802 ★ American Society of Echocardiography
1500 Sunday Dr., Ste. 102
Raleigh, NC 27607
Phone: (919)861-5574 **Fax:** (919)787-4916
Email: smilton@asecho.org
Website: http://asecho.org/index.shtml
Shawnette Milton, Contact

★ 29803 ★ Society for Vascular Ultrasound
4601 Presidents Dr., Ste. 260
Lanham, MD 20706-4365
Phone: (301)459-7550 **Fax:** (301)459-5651
Email: svuinfo@svunet.org
Website: http://www.svunet.org/
Frmly: Society of Vascular Technology.

Cytotechnology

★ 29804 ★ American Society of Cytopathology
400 W Ninth St., Ste. 201
Wilmington, DE 19801
Phone: (302)429-8802 **Fax:** (302)429-8807
Email: asc@cytopathology.org
Website: http://www.cytopathology.org/

Electroneurodiagnostic Technology

★ 29805 ★ American Society of Electroneurodiagnostic Technologists
426 W 42nd St.
Kansas City, MO 64111
Phone: (816)931-1120 **Fax:** (816)931-1145
Email: info@aset.org
Website: http://www.aset.org/

Emergency Medical Services

★ 29806 ★ National Association of Emergency Medical Technicians
PO Box 1400
Clinton, MS 39060
Phone: (601)924-7744 **Free:** 800-34-NAEMT
Fax: (601)924-7325
Email: info@naemt.org
Website: http://www.naemt.org/public/default.htm

Medical Assisting

★ 29807 ★ American Association of Medical Assistants
20 N Wacker Dr., Ste. 1575
Chicago, IL 60606-2903
Phone: (312)899-1500 **Free:** 800-228-2262
Website: http://www.aama-ntl.org/

Ophthalmic Medical Technology

★ 29808 ★ Joint Commission on Allied Health Personnel in Ophthalmology (JCAHPO)
2025 Woodlane Dr.
Saint Paul, MN 55125-2995
Phone: (651)731-2944 **Free:** 800-284-3937
Fax: (651)731-0410
Email: jcahpo@jcahpo.org
Website: http://www.jcahpo.org/

Orthotics & Prosthetics

★ 29809 ★ National Commission on Orthotic and Prosthetic Education
330 John Carlyle St., Ste. 200
Alexandria, VA 22314
Phone: (703)836-7114

Email: info@ncope.org
Website: http://www.ncope.org/

Sonography

★ 29810 ★ Society of Diagnostic Medical Sonography
2745 Dallas Pkwy., Ste. 350
Plano, TX 75093-8730
Phone: (214)473-8057 **Free:** 800-229-9506
Fax: (214)473-8563
Email: info@sdms.org
Website: http://www.sdms.org/

Surgical Technology

★ 29811 ★ Association of Surgical Technologists
7108-C, S Alton Way, Ste. 100
Englewood, CO 80112-2106
Phone: (303)694-9130 **Fax:** (303)694-9169
Email: pprice@ast.org
Website: http://www.ast.org/
Paul Price, Contact

Alphabetical Name and Keyword Index

This is an alphabetical listing of all resources included in this directory as well as former or alternate names of the resources. Index references are to entry numbers rather than page numbers. Entry numbers appear in lightface type if the reference is to a former or alternate name; otherwise, entry numbers appear in boldface type. Consult the "User's Guide" at the beginning of this directory for more detailed information about the index.

A

Index

Index

B

C

Index

Index

Index

D

Index

F

Index

G

Index

H

Index

Index

J

K

L

M

Index

Index

Index

P

Index

Index

Q

R

S

Index

Index

Index

V

X

Y

Z